The 2007 PDR® Library - for all of your drug information needs.

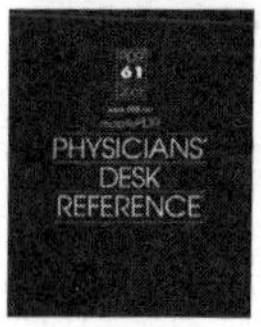

2007 Physicians' Desk Reference®

Physicians have turned to the PDR® for the latest word on prescription drugs for over 60 years. Today, PDR® is still considered the standard prescription drug reference and can be found in virtually every physician's office, hospital and pharmacy in the United States. You can search the more than 4,000 drugs by using one of many indices and look at more than 2,100 full-color photos of drugs cross-referenced to the label information.

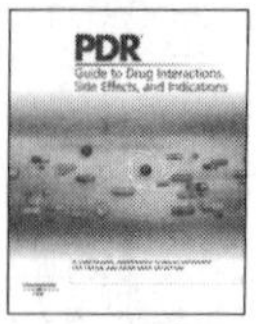

2007 PDR® Guide to Drug Interactions, Side Effects, and Indications

Now you can manage the risks inherent in today's complex drug environment. Cross-referenced to the 2007 PDR® and designed to be highly accessible for busy healthcare professionals, this title covers all the bases by ensuring safe drug management. It's an all-in-one resource that contains eight critical checkpoints including Drug Interactions, Side Effects, and Indications.

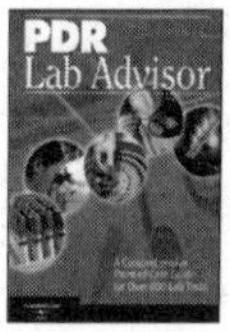

PDR® Lab Advisor

Comprehensive point-of-care reference guide for over 600 lab tests. Designed to be used at the point of care, the PDR® Lab Advisor enables the busy health-care professional to quickly look up the most relevant tests to order to confirm a diagnosis and then assist the patient in interpreting and, if necessary, act on the results. This authoritative guide facilitates clinical decision-making, saves time, and reduces the number of marginal, costly tests ordered.

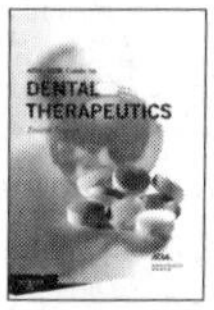

ADA®/PDR® Guide to Dental Therapeutics

The definitive guide to making the best medication decisions for dental practices. Updated, comprehensive, highly relevant, and now produced by the American Dental Association® in partnership with PDR®, the new ADA®/PDR® Guide to Dental Therapeutics, Fourth Edition is the most authoritative guide to dental therapeutics currently available and is essential for today's busy dental practice.

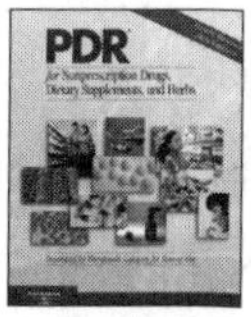

2007 PDR® for Nonprescription Drugs, Dietary Supplements, and Herbs

Now more than ever, you need to stay current on the OTC drugs, dietary supplements, and herbal remedies your patients are taking. This title includes complete descriptions of the most commonly used OTC medications, all organized by therapeutic categories for fast access. You'll also find full-color images of nearly 300 products.

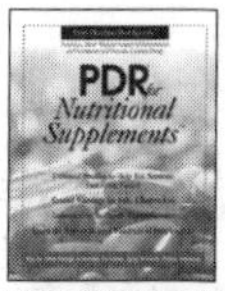

PDR® for Nutritional Supplements - 1st Edition

The definitive information source for more than 300 nutritional supplements. This unique, comprehensive, unbiased source of solid, evidence-based information about nutritional supplements provides practitioners with more than 700 pages of the most reliable information available.

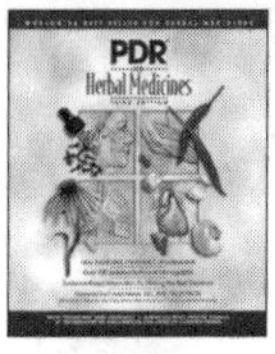

PDR® for Herbal Medicines - 3rd Edition

The third edition goes far beyond the original source, adding a new section on Nutritional Supplements and new information aimed at greatly enhancing patient management by medical practitioners. All monographs have been updated to include recent scientific findings on efficacy, safety and potential interactions; clinical trials (including abstracts); case reports; and meta-analysis results. This new information has resulted in greatly expanded Effects, Contraindications, Precautions and Adverse Reactions, and Dosage sections of each monograph.

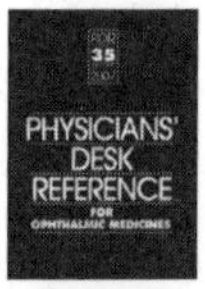

2007 PDR® for Ophthalmic Medicines

The definitive reference for the eye-care professional offers more than 200 pages of detailed information on drugs and equipment used in the fields of ophthalmology and optometry. With five full indices and information on specialized instruments, lenses and much more, this guide is the most comprehensive of its kind.

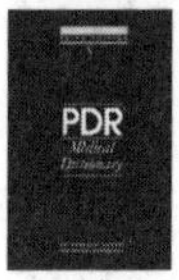

PDR® Medical Dictionary - 3rd Edition

With today's rapidly changing medical technology, it is more challenging than ever for medical professionals to stay up-to-date. The ***PDR® Medical Dictionary, Third Edition*** has been thoroughly updated to make this dictionary the most reliable resource. This new edition includes over 107,000 terms and definitions—more than 5,000 new to this edition!

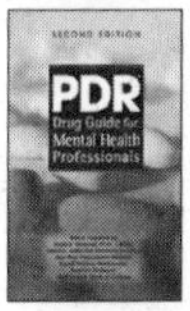

PDR® Drug Guide for Mental Health Professionals - 2nd Edition

The ***PDR® Drug Guide for Mental Health Professionals*** was created to help you understand the beneficial effects—and the dangerous side effects—of today's potent psychotherapeutic medications. Over 75 common psychotropic drugs are profiled by brand name. All this vital information is presented in a easy-to-read format, written in nontechnical language, and drawn from the FDA-approved PDR database.

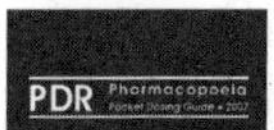

2007 PDR® Pharmacopoeia Pocket Dosing Guide - 7th Edition

This pocket dosing guide brings important dispensing information to the practitioner's fingertips. Organized in tabular format, this pocket-sized, 300-page quick reference is easy to navigate and gives important FDA-approved dosing information, black box warning summaries and much more, whenever it is needed. At the point of care, rely on ***PDR® Pharmacopoeia*** for quick dosing information.

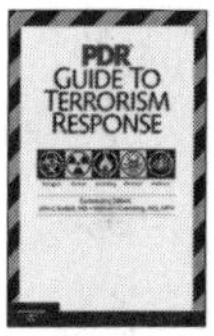

PDR® Guide to Terrorism Response

Treating mass casualties of a terrorism attack is too important to rely on anything less than the most authoritative advice. That's why **PDR®**, the most trusted name in healthcare, teamed up with world-class medical experts to produce a one-of-kind guide for physicians and other healthcare personnel who need answers stat on treating victims of every major CDC-designated biological and chemical weapon, as well as suicide bombings, incendiary attacks, nuclear/radiation explosions, and more.

Complete Your 2007 PDR® Library NOW! Enclose payment and save shipping costs.

Quantity	Description	Price	S & H	Total only for Bill Me
_____ copies	2007 Physicians' Desk Reference®	$94.95 each	$9.95 each	$_______
_____ copies	2007 PDR® Guide to Drug Interactions, Side Effects, and Indications	$73.95 each	$9.95 each	$_______
_____ copies	The PDR® Lab Advisor ***NEW!***	$44.95 each	$6.95 each	$_______
_____ copies	ADA®/PDR® Guide to Dental Therapeutics (4th Edition) ***NEW!***	$69.95 each	$9.95 each	$_______
_____ copies	2007 PDR® for Nonprescription Drugs, Dietary Supplements, and Herbs	$59.95 each	$9.95 each	$_______
_____ copies	PDR® for Nutritional Supplements	$49.95 each	$9.95 each	$_______
_____ copies	PDR® for Herbal Medicines (3rd Edition)	$59.95 each	$9.95 each	$_______
_____ copies	2007 PDR® for Ophthalmic Medicines	$69.95 each	$9.95 each	$_______
_____ copies	PDR® Medical Dictionary (3rd Edition)	$49.95 each	$9.95 each	$_______
_____ copies	PDR® Drug Guide for Mental Health Professionals (2nd Edition)	$39.95 each	$6.95 each	$_______
_____ copies	2007 PDR® Pharmacopoeia Pocket Dosing Guide	$9.95 each	$1.95 each	$_______
_____ copies	PDR® Guide to Terrorism Response ***NEW!***	$59.95 each	$9.95 each	$_______

Valid for 2007 editions only, prices and shipping & handling higher outside U.S.

Sales Tax (FL, KY, & NJ) $_______

TOTAL AMOUNT $_______

SAVE TIME AND MONEY EVERY YEAR AS A STANDING ORDER SUBSCRIBER

☐ Check here to enter your standing order for future editions of publications ordered. They will be shipped to you automatically, after advance notice. As a standing order subscriber, you are **guaranteed** our lowest price offer, earliest delivery and FREE shipping and handling.

FREE Shipping & Handling if Paying NOW!

Mail this order form to:
PDR®
Thomson Healthcare
PO Box 6911
Florence, KY 41022-9700
e-mail: PDR.customerservice@thomson.com

For Faster Service—
FAX YOUR ORDER 1-800-735-0419
or CALL TOLL-FREE 1-800-678-5689
Do not mail a confirmation order in addition to this fax.

PLEASE INDICATE METHOD OF PAYMENT:

Payment Enclosed (Shipping & Handling FREE)

☐ Check payable to PDR
☐ VISA ☐ MasterCard
☐ Discover ☐ American Express

Account No. ____________

Exp. Date ____________

D0753447

Address ____________

City ____________

State/Zip ____________

Email (*Requested for shipping confirmation*) ____________

☐ **Bill me later** (Add Shipping & Handling only if paying later)

KEY C90080001

KEYED TO PDR®
61
EDITION
2007

PDR®

Guide to Drug Interactions, Side Effects, and Indications

Executive Vice President, PDR: Kevin D. Sanborn; **Senior Vice President, PDR Sales:** Roseanne McCauley; **Vice President, Marketing:** William T. Hicks; **Vice President, Regulatory Affairs:** Mukesh Mehta, RPh; **Vice President, PDR Services:** Brian Holland; **Senior Director, Pharmaceutical Solutions Sales:** Anthony Sorce; **National Solutions Managers:** Frank Karkowsky, Elaine Musco, Marion Reid, RPh; **Senior Solutions Managers:** Debra Goldman, Warner Stuart, Suzanne E. Yarrow, RN; **Solutions Managers:** Joseph Gross, Marjorie A. Jaxel, Lois Smith, Krista Turpin; **Sales Coordinators:** Dawn McPartland, Janet Wallendal; **Director of Trade Sales:** Bill Gaffney; **Senior Manager, Direct Marketing:** Amy Cheong; **Senior Director of Product Management, Electronic Solutions:** Valerie E. Berger; **Director of Product Management, Monographs:** Jeffrey D. Schaefer; **Senior Marketing Manager:** Kim Marich; **Senior Director, Client Services:** Stephanie Struble; **Director of Operations:** Robert Klein; **Director of Finance:** Mark S. Ritchin; **Director, Editorial Services:** Bette LaGow; **Manager, Professional Services:** Michael DeLuca, PharmD, MBA; **Drug Information Specialists:** Majid Kerolous, PharmD; Nermin Shenouda, PharmD; Greg Tallis, RPh; **Project Editor:** Lori Murray; **Manager, Client Services:** Travis Northern; **Customer Service Supervisor:** Todd Taccetta; **Manager, Production Purchasing:** Thomas Westburgh; **PDR Production Manager:** Steven Maher; **Sr. Index Editor:** Noel Deloughery; **Index Editor:** Allison O'Hare; **Senior Production Coordinators:** Gianna Caradonna, Yasmin Hernández; **Production Coordinator:** Nick W. Clark; **Traffic Assistant:** Kim Condon; **Production Design Supervisor:** Adeline Rich; **Senior Electronic Publishing Designer:** Livio Udina; **Electronic Publishing Designers:** Deana DiVizio, Carrie Faeth, Monika Popowitz; **Production Associate:** Joan K. Akerlind; **Digital Imaging Manager:** Christopher Husted; **Digital Imaging Coordinator:** Michael Labruyere

THOMSON PDR™

Officers of Thomson Healthcare, Inc.: *President and Chief Executive Officer:* Bob Cullen; *Chief Financial Officer:* Paul Hilger; *Chief Medical Officer:* Rich Klasco, MD, FACEP; *Executive Vice President, Medstat:* Carol Diephuis; *Executive Vice President, Micromedex:* Jeff Reihl; *Executive Vice President, PDR:* Kevin D. Sanborn; *Senior Vice President, Technology:* Michael Karaman; *Vice President, Finance:* Joseph Scarfone; *Vice President, Human Resources:* Pamela M. Bilash; *Vice President, Planning and Business Development:* Ray Zoeller; *Vice President, Product Strategy:* Anita Brown; *Vice President, Strategic Initiatives:* Timothy Murray

ISBN: 1-56363-581-X

FOREWORD

Welcome to one of the most useful drug references in current clinical practice, the 2007 edition of the *PDR® Guide to Drug Interactions, Side Effects, and Indications*. Cross-referenced with key facts from the *2007 Physicians' Desk Reference®*, this unique handbook can help you to provide safe drug management. From its Indications Index, which permits you to instantly identify the full range of pharmaceutical alternatives for any given illness, to its Contraindications Index, which just as swiftly singles out alternatives to avoid, this *PDR* guide is designed to make safe, effective prescribing as fast, easy, and accurate as possible. Whether the challenge is identification of an unknown tablet or capsule, detecting the source of an adverse reaction, or avoiding a negative interaction, the *PDR® Guide to Drug Interactions, Side Effects, and Indications* provides the tools you need to quickly find the answer. Here's a brief overview of the many features offered in the 2007 edition:

Interactions Index. In this section you'll find an entry for each product described in *PDR* and its companion volumes. Listed are generic compounds and dietary items that may interact with the product, as well as the specific brands containing each generic ingredient. A brief description of the interaction also appears. (Because product labeling varies in the scope of its interaction reporting, be sure to check the listing for each product in the patient's regimen.)

Food Interactions Cross-Reference. If you suspect an interaction with a specific dietary item, turn to this section. There you will find potential drug/food and drug/alcohol interactions cross-referenced alphabetically by the name or type of food. Each entry includes a list of implicated drugs and a brief description of each interaction.

Side Effects Index. When a multidrug regimen masks the source of a side effect, this section provides the solution. It contains an alphabetical list of the more than 3,600 distinct reactions cited throughout *PDR* and its companion volumes. Each entry includes an alphabetical list of the brands that have been associated with the problem. To help target the most likely offenders, incidence data are included whenever found in the official labeling.

Indications Index. If you need to locate an alternative to a problem medication—or simply want to review the full range of options for a particular diagnosis—turn to this part of the book. Here each indication cited in *PDR* and its companions is listed alphabetically, with a cross-reference to all brands approved for that purpose. For easy comparison, the listings include the generic name and manufacturer of each product. (Only FDA-approved indications are referenced.)

Contraindications Index. When therapy is complicated by other medical conditions, this convenient index will enable you to eliminate quickly any contraindicated drugs from consideration. Here each contraindication cited in *PDR* is listed alphabetically, together with the drugs to avoid when the problem occurs.

International Drug Name Index. This section enables you to determine quickly a U.S. equivalent when you're confronted with a medication from another country. The index describes the product's country of origin, the closest domestic generic equivalent, all associated *PDR* brand-name entries and their *PDR* page number. Included are more than 33,000 entries covering products from more than 25 nations. Prescribing a U.S. substitute has never been easier!

Generic Availability Guide. If you've ever had trouble remembering whether there's a generic alternative for a particular brand, you're sure to appreciate this handy guide. It alerts you to the existence of alternatives, form by form, and strength by strength. Included are all prescription drugs described in *PDR* and *PDR® for Ophthalmic Medicines.*

Imprint Identification Guide. This comprehensive table permits you to establish quickly the identity of virtually any unknown tablet or capsule. Organized alphabetically by imprint, it supplies the brand or generic name of the drug, its strength and manufacturer, and, to confirm its identity, the color, form, and shape.

Based on the FDA-approved labeling in the 2007 editions of *Physicians' Desk Reference, PDR for Ophthalmic Medicines,* and *PDR for Nonprescription Drugs, Dietary Supplements, and Herbs*—and augmented with a wealth of authoritative data from such *PDR* affiliates as *Red Book®* and Micromedex, Inc.—the entries in the *PDR® Guide to Drug Interactions, Side Effects, and Indications* cover some 3,000 domestic drug products. Please note, however, that because the entries in the Indications, Contraindications, Interactions, and Side Effects indices are derived directly from the FDA-sanctioned prescribing information published by *PDR*, only products described in *Physicians' Desk Reference* and its main companion volumes are cited in these sections.

Please note, also, that the publisher cannot guarantee that all entries are totally accurate or complete, nor is the publisher responsible for misuse of a product due to typographical error. Remember that important qualifications of the information listed in these indices may reside in the underlying text. Use this Guide as a convenient cross-reference, but consult the *PDR* text, as well as the medical literature, when more detailed information is needed.

New Evidence-Based Application for Your PDA

We are pleased to announce the launch of **Thomson Clinical Xpert**™, a powerful medical reference for Palm® OS and Pocket PC handhelds developed by PDR. Designed specifically for use at the point of care, this decision-support tool puts drug, disease, and laboratory information instantly into the hands of physicians and other clinical professionals via their PDA.

Much more than a quick drug lookup, Thomson Clinical Xpert provides medical references and point-of-care tools you need in your daily workflow, including:

- **Drug labeling:** Search more than 4,000 trade names
- **Interaction checker:** Check up to 32 medications at one time
- **Toxicology information:** Screen 200 of the most common poisonings and drug overdoses
- **Medical calculators:** Convenient calculators: dosing, metric conversions, and more
- **News and alerts:** Get FDA announcements, clinical updates, and upcoming drug launches
- **Laboratory test information:** Identify and interpret details of more than 500 laboratory tests
- **Disease database:** Find current evidence-based treatment recommendations
- **Alternative medicine database:** Consult information on more than 300 popular herbs and dietary supplements

Thomson Clinical Xpert is available **free** to registered members of PDR.net, your medical professional web portal for drug information and much more. Go to *www.PDR.net* to put this clinical-decision support tool to work for you now.

Web-Based Clinical Resources

PDR.net, a web portal designed specifically for healthcare professionals, provides a wealth of clinical information, including full drug and disease monographs, specialty-specific resource centers, patient education, clinical news, and conference information. PDR.net gives prescribers online access to authoritative, evidence-based information they need to support or confirm diagnosis and treatment decisions, including:

- Daily feeds of specialty news, conference coverage, and monthly summaries
- FDA-approved and other manufacturer-provided product labeling for more than 4,000 brand-name drugs
- Multi-drug interaction checker and other tools
- Extensive disease diagnosis and treatment information
- Customizable patient education
- Professional resources

PDR.net is also home to our **Clinical Resource Centers**, giving you the latest medical news and disease information all in one easy place. Log on to *www.PDR.net* to visit one of these clinical specialties:

- Allergy and Immunology
- Cardiovascular
- Dermatology
- Diabetes and Endocrinology
- Nephrology
- Neurology
- Pediatrics
- Psychiatry
- Pulmonology
- Rheumatology
- Urology
- Women's Health
- And more

Online access is **free** for U.S.-based MDs, DOs, dentists, NPs, and PAs in full-time patient practice, as well as for medical students, residents, and other select prescribing allied health professionals. Register today at *www.PDR.net*.

Other Clinical Information Products from PDR

For complicated cases and special patient problems, there is no substitute for the in-depth data contained in *Physicians' Desk Reference*. But for those times when you need quick access to critical prescribing information, you'll want to consult the **PDR® Monthly Prescribing Guide**™, the essential drug reference designed specifically for use at the point of care. Distilled from the pages of *PDR*, this digest-sized reference presents the key facts on more than 1,500 drug formulations, including therapeutic class, indications and contraindications, warnings and precautions, pregnancy rating, drug interactions and side effects, and adult and pediatric dosages. Most entries also give the PDR page number to turn to for further information. In addition, a full-color insert of pill images allows you to correctly identify each product. Issued monthly, the guide is regularly updated with detailed descriptions of new drugs to receive FDA approval, as well as FDA-approved revisions to existing product information. You'll also find bulletins about major new developments in the pharmaceutical industry, an overview of important new agents nearing approval, and recent clinical findings on common nutritional supplements. To learn more about this useful publication and to inquire about subscription rates, call 800-232-7379.

For those times when all you need is quick confirmation of a particular dosage, you will want to have a copy of the 2007 **PDR® Pharmacopoeia Pocket Dosing Guide**. Only slightly larger than an index card and a half inch thick, it fits easily into any pocket, and provides you with FDA-approved dosing recommendations for more than 1,500 drugs. Unlike other condensed drug references, the information is drawn almost exclusively from the FDA-approved drug labeling published in *Physicians' Desk Reference*. And its tabular presentation makes lookups a breeze. The *2007 PDR Pharmacopoeia Pocket Dosing Guide* is a tool you really can't afford to be without.

To help you counsel patients who use over-the-counter supplements, the **PDR® for Nutritional Supplements** offers the latest available scientific consensus on hundreds of popular products, including amino acids, fatty acids, probiotics, phytoestrogens, phytosterols, over-the-counter hormones, and much more. Focused on the scientific evidence for each supplement's claims, this unique reference offers you today's most detailed, informed, and objective overview of a burgeoning new area in the field of self-treatment.

For counseling patients who favor herbal remedies, the newly updated **PDR® for Herbal Medicines Third Edition** provides you with the latest science-based assessment of more than 700 botanicals. Indexed by scientific and common names (as well as Western, Asian, and homeopathic indications), this volume also includes a Side Effects Index, a Drug/Herb Interactions Guide, an Herb Identification Guide with nearly 400 color photos, and a Safety Guide that lists herbs to be avoided during pregnancy and herbs to be used only under professional supervision. Although botanical products are not officially regulated or monitored in the United States, *PDR for Herbal Medicines* provides you with authoritative information—the findings of the German Regulatory Authority's expert committee on herbal medicines, Commission E.

PDR and its major companion volumes are also found in the **PDR® Electronic Library** on CD-ROM. This Windows-compatible disc provides users with a complete database of *PDR* prescribing information, electronically searchable for instant retrieval. A standard subscription includes *PDR's* sophisticated search software and an extensive file of chemical structures, illustrations, and full-color product photographs. Optional enhancements include the complete contents of *The Merck Manual Seventeenth Edition, Stedman's Medical Dictionary*, and *Stedman's Spellchecker*. For anyone who wants to run a fast double check on a proposed prescription, there's also the *PDR® Drug Interactions and Side Effects System* — sophisticated software capable of automatically screening a 20-drug regimen for conflicts, then proposing alternatives for any problematic medication. This unique decision-making tool comes free with the *PDR Electronic Library*.

For more information on these or any other members of the growing family of *PDR* products, please call, toll-free, 800-232-7379 or fax 201-722-2680.

CONTENTS

Section 1
Interactions Index 1

Section 2
Food Interactions Cross-Reference 1517

Section 3
Side Effects Index 1529

Section 4
Indications Index 1811

Section 5
Contraindications Index 1875

Section 6
International Drug Name Index 1891

Section 7
Generic Availability Guide 2025

Section 8
Imprint Identification Guide 2037

Poison Control Centers 2147
A national directory arranged alphabetically by state and city.

Key to Controlled Substances Categories 2153
Gives the definition of each category and the prescribing limitations that apply.

Key to FDA Use-in-Pregnancy Ratings 2153
Provides a description of each risk/benefit rating.

SECTION 1

INTERACTIONS INDEX

Cataloged in this section are all interactions found during a review of the labeling published in *PDR®, PDR For Nonprescription Drugs and Dietary Supplements and Herbs™,* and *PDR For Ophthalmic Medicines™*. The list is arranged alphabetically by brand or, when applicable, generic name.

Whenever appropriate, each brand-name heading is followed by a summary of the major pharmaceutical categories with which the product is said to interact. Beneath this summary is an alphabetical list of the compounds in these categories, each followed by a brief notation regarding the results of concurrent administration with the brand in question. After each notation is an alphabetical list of the brands of the compound found in *PDR®* and its companion volumes. Page numbers refer to the 2007 editions of

PDR®, PDR for Ophthalmic Medicines™ and the *PDR for Nonprescription Drugs and Dietary Supplements and Herbs™,* which is published later each year. A key to the symbols denoting the companion volumes appears in the bottom margin of every other page.

Following the list of interactive drugs is a similar list of foods. Note that interactions with alcohol are listed here as well.

This index lists only interactions cited in official prescribing information as published by *PDR®*. Because product labeling varies in the scope of its interaction reporting, the most prudent course is to check each product in the patient's regimen. Note also that cross-sensitivity reactions and effects on laboratory results are not included in the listings.

ABELCET INJECTION
(Amphotericin B Lipid Complex) 1141
May interact with aminoglycosides, antineoplastics, corticosteroids, curariform skeletal muscle relaxants, cardiac glycosides, imidazoles, and certain other agents. Compounds in these categories include:

ACTH (Concurrent use may potentiate hypokalemia which could predispose the patient to cardiac dysfunction).
> No products indexed under this heading.

Altretamine (Concurrent use may enhance the potential for renal toxicity, bronchospasm and hypotension).
> No products indexed under this heading.

Amikacin Sulfate (Concurrent use may enhance the potential for drug-induced renal toxicity).
> No products indexed under this heading.

Anastrozole (Concurrent use may enhance the potential for renal toxicity, bronchospasm and hypotension). Products include:
> Arimidex Tablets 673

Asparaginase (Concurrent use may enhance the potential for renal toxicity, bronchospasm and hypotension). Products include:
> Elspar for Injection 2463
> Elspar for Injection 1960

Atracurium Besylate (Amphotericin B-induced hypokalemia may enhance the curariform effect of skeletal relaxants).
> No products indexed under this heading.

Betamethasone Acetate (Concurrent use may potentiate hypokalemia which could predispose the patient to cardiac dysfunction).
> No products indexed under this heading.

Betamethasone Sodium Phosphate (Concurrent use may potentiate hypokalemia which could predispose the patient to cardiac dysfunction).
> No products indexed under this heading.

Bicalutamide (Concurrent use may enhance the potential for renal toxicity, bronchospasm and hypotension).
> No products indexed under this heading.

Bleomycin Sulfate (Concurrent use may enhance the potential for renal toxicity, bronchospasm and hypotension).
> No products indexed under this heading.

Busulfan (Concurrent use may enhance the potential for renal toxicity, bronchospasm and hypotension). Products include:
> I.V. Busulfex 2493
> Myleran Tablets 1525

Carboplatin (Concurrent use may enhance the potential for renal toxicity, bronchospasm and hypotension).
> No products indexed under this heading.

Carmustine (BCNU) (Concurrent use may enhance the potential for renal toxicity, bronchospasm and hypotension).
> No products indexed under this heading.

Chlorambucil (Concurrent use may enhance the potential for renal toxicity, bronchospasm and hypotension). Products include:
> Leukeran Tablets 1504

Cisatracurium Besylate (Amphotericin B-induced hypokalemia may enhance the curariform effect of skeletal relaxants). Products include:
> Nimbex Injection 498

Cisplatin (Concurrent use may enhance the potential for renal toxicity, bronchospasm and hypotension).
> No products indexed under this heading.

Clotrimazole (Antagonism between amphotericin B and imidazole derivatives, which inhibit ergosterol synthesis, has been reported; clinical significance of this finding has not been determined). Products include:
> Desenex Athlete's Foot Cream ▣◫635
> Lotrimin 3039
> Lotrisone 3040

Cortisone Acetate (Concurrent use may potentiate hypokalemia which could predispose the patient to cardiac dysfunction).
> No products indexed under this heading.

Cyclophosphamide (Concurrent use may potentiate for renal toxicity, bronchospasm and hypotension).
> No products indexed under this heading.

Cyclosporine (Concurrent initiation of cyclosporine and Abelcet within several days of bone marrow ablation may be associated with increased nephrotoxicity). Products include:
> Gengraf Capsules 459
> Neoral Oral Solution 2259
> Neoral Soft Gelatin Capsules 2259
> Restasis Ophthalmic Emulsion 575
> Sandimmune 2275

Dacarbazine (Concurrent use may enhance the potential for renal toxicity, bronchospasm and hypotension).
> No products indexed under this heading.

Daunorubicin Citrate (Concurrent use may enhance the potential for renal toxicity, bronchospasm and hypotension).
> No products indexed under this heading.

Daunorubicin Hydrochloride (Concurrent use may enhance the potential for renal toxicity, bronchospasm and hypotension).
> No products indexed under this heading.

IMPORTANT NOTE: Always consult each drug listing in the patient's regimen for possible interactions.

Denileukin Diftitox (Concurrent use may enhance the potential for renal toxicity, bronchospasm and hypotension). Products include:
- Ontak Vials 1745

Deslanoside (Concurrent use may induce hypokalemia and may potentiate digitalis toxicity).
- No products indexed under this heading.

Dexamethasone (Concurrent use may potentiate hypokalemia which could predispose the patient to cardiac dysfunction). Products include:
- Ciprodex Otic Suspension 559
- Decadron Tablets 1951
- TobraDex Ophthalmic Ointment 562
- TobraDex Ophthalmic Suspension ... 563

Dexamethasone Acetate (Concurrent use may potentiate hypokalemia which could predispose the patient to cardiac dysfunction).
- No products indexed under this heading.

Dexamethasone Sodium Phosphate (Concurrent use may potentiate hypokalemia which could predispose the patient to cardiac dysfunction).
- No products indexed under this heading.

Digitalis Glycoside Preparations (Concurrent use may induce hypokalemia and may potentiate digitalis toxicity).
- No products indexed under this heading.

Digitoxin (Concurrent use may induce hypokalemia and may potentiate digitalis toxicity).
- No products indexed under this heading.

Digoxin (Concurrent use may induce hypokalemia and may potentiate digitalis toxicity). Products include:
- Lanoxicaps Capsules 1490
- Lanoxin Injection 1494
- Lanoxin Injection Pediatric 1497
- Lanoxin Tablets 1500

Docetaxel (Concurrent use may enhance the potential for renal toxicity, bronchospasm and hypotension). Products include:
- Taxotere Injection Concentrate 2932

Doxacurium Chloride (Amphotericin B-induced hypokalemia may enhance the curariform effect of skeletal relaxants).
- No products indexed under this heading.

Doxorubicin Hydrochloride (Concurrent use may enhance the potential for renal toxicity, bronchospasm and hypotension).
- No products indexed under this heading.

Epirubicin Hydrochloride (Concurrent use may enhance the potential for renal toxicity, bronchospasm and hypotension).
- No products indexed under this heading.

Estramustine Phosphate Sodium (Concurrent use may enhance the potential for renal toxicity, bronchospasm and hypotension). Products include:
- Emcyt Capsules 2634

Etoposide (Concurrent use may enhance the potential for renal toxicity, bronchospasm and hypotension).
- No products indexed under this heading.

Exemestane (Concurrent use may enhance the potential for renal toxicity, bronchospasm and hypotension). Products include:
- Aromasin Tablets 2600

Floxuridine (Concurrent use may enhance the potential for renal toxicity, bronchospasm and hypotension).
- No products indexed under this heading.

Fluconazole (Antagonism between amphotericin B and imidazole derivatives, which inhibit ergosterol synthesis, has been reported; clinical significance of this finding has not been determined).
- No products indexed under this heading.

Flucytosine (Concurrent use may increase the toxicity of flucytosine by possibly increasing its cellular uptake and/or impairing its renal excretion).
- No products indexed under this heading.

Fludrocortisone Acetate (Concurrent use may potentiate hypokalemia which could predispose the patient to cardiac dysfunction).
- No products indexed under this heading.

Fluorouracil (Concurrent use may enhance the potential for renal toxicity, bronchospasm and hypotension). Products include:
- Carac Cream, 0.5% 2879
- Efudex 3363

Flutamide (Concurrent use may enhance the potential for renal toxicity, bronchospasm and hypotension). Products include:
- Eulexin Capsules 3009

Gemcitabine Hydrochloride (Concurrent use may enhance the potential for renal toxicity, bronchospasm and hypotension). Products include:
- Gemzar for Injection 1771

Gentamicin Sulfate (Concurrent use may enhance the potential for drug-induced renal toxicity). Products include:
- Garamycin Injectable 3014
- Pred-G Ophthalmic Ointment ...... ⊙237
- Pred-G Ophthalmic Suspension ...... ⊙236

Hydrocortisone (Concurrent use may potentiate hypokalemia which could predispose the patient to cardiac dysfunction). Products include:
- Colocort Rectal Suspension, USP (Retention) 100 mg/60 mL 2476
- Hydrocortone Tablets 1989
- Preparation H Hydrocortisone Cream ...... ▣646

Hydrocortisone Acetate (Concurrent use may potentiate hypokalemia which could predispose the patient to cardiac dysfunction). Products include:
- Analpram-HC 1159
- Pramosone 1161
- ProctoFoam-HC 3099

Hydrocortisone Sodium Phosphate (Concurrent use may potentiate hypokalemia which could predispose the patient to cardiac dysfunction).
- No products indexed under this heading.

Hydrocortisone Sodium Succinate (Concurrent use may potentiate hypokalemia which could predispose the patient to cardiac dysfunction).
- No products indexed under this heading.

Hydroxyurea (Concurrent use may enhance the potential for renal toxicity, bronchospasm and hypotension).
- No products indexed under this heading.

Idarubicin Hydrochloride (Concurrent use may enhance the potential for renal toxicity, bronchospasm and hypotension).
- No products indexed under this heading.

Ifosfamide (Concurrent use may enhance the potential for renal toxicity, bronchospasm and hypotension).
- No products indexed under this heading.

Interferon alfa-2a, Recombinant (Concurrent use may enhance the potential for renal toxicity, bronchospasm and hypotension).
- No products indexed under this heading.

Interferon alfa-2b, Recombinant (Concurrent use may enhance the potential for renal toxicity, bronchospasm and hypotension). Products include:
- Intron A for Injection 3024
- Rebetron Combination Therapy 3063

Irinotecan Hydrochloride (Concurrent use may enhance the potential for renal toxicity, bronchospasm and hypotension). Products include:
- Camptosar Injection 2604

Kanamycin Sulfate (Concurrent use may enhance the potential for drug-induced renal toxicity).
- No products indexed under this heading.

Ketoconazole (Antagonism between amphotericin B and imidazole derivatives, which inhibit ergosterol synthesis, has been reported; clinical significance of this finding has not been determined). Products include:
- Nizoral A-D Shampoo, 1% 1868

Leukocyte Transfusions (Concurrent use has resulted in acute pulmonary toxicity; concurrent use should be avoided).
- No products indexed under this heading.

Levamisole Hydrochloride (Concurrent use may enhance the potential for renal toxicity, bronchospasm and hypotension).
- No products indexed under this heading.

Lomustine (CCNU) (Concurrent use may enhance the potential for renal toxicity, bronchospasm and hypotension).
- No products indexed under this heading.

Mechlorethamine Hydrochloride (Concurrent use may enhance the potential for renal toxicity, bronchospasm and hypotension). Products include:
- Mustargen for Injection 2468

Megestrol Acetate (Concurrent use may enhance the potential for renal toxicity, bronchospasm and hypotension). Products include:
- Megace ES Oral Suspension 2481

Melphalan (Concurrent use may enhance the potential for renal toxicity, bronchospasm and hypotension). Products include:
- Alkeran Tablets 956

Mercaptopurine (Concurrent use may enhance the potential for renal toxicity, bronchospasm and hypotension).
- No products indexed under this heading.

Methotrexate Sodium (Concurrent use may enhance the potential for renal toxicity, bronchospasm and hypotension).
- No products indexed under this heading.

Methylprednisolone Acetate (Concurrent use may potentiate hypokalemia which could predispose the patient to cardiac dysfunction). Products include:
- Depo-Medrol Injectable Suspension 2617
- Depo-Medrol Single-Dose Vial 2619

Methylprednisolone Sodium Succinate (Concurrent use may potentiate hypokalemia which could predispose the patient to cardiac dysfunction).
- No products indexed under this heading.

Metocurine Iodide (Amphotericin B-induced hypokalemia may enhance the curariform effect of skeletal relaxants).
- No products indexed under this heading.

Miconazole (Antagonism between amphotericin B and imidazole derivatives, which inhibit ergosterol synthesis, has been reported; clinical significance of this finding has not been determined).
- No products indexed under this heading.

Miconazole Nitrate (Antagonism between amphotericin B and imidazole derivatives, which inhibit ergosterol synthesis, has been reported; clinical significance of this finding has not been determined). Products include:
- Desenex ...... ▣635
- Desenex Jock Itch Spray Powder ...... ▣635

Mitomycin (Mitomycin-C) (Concurrent use may enhance the potential for renal toxicity, bronchospasm and hypotension).
- No products indexed under this heading.

Mitotane (Concurrent use may enhance the potential for renal toxicity, bronchospasm and hypotension).
- No products indexed under this heading.

Mitoxantrone Hydrochloride (Concurrent use may enhance the potential for renal toxicity, bronchospasm and hypotension).
- No products indexed under this heading.

Mivacurium Chloride (Amphotericin B-induced hypokalemia may enhance the curariform effect of skeletal relaxants). Products include:
- Mivacron Injection 493

Oxaliplatin (Concurrent use may enhance the potential for renal toxicity, bronchospasm and hypotension). Products include:
- Eloxatin for Injection 2892

Paclitaxel (Concurrent use may enhance the potential for renal toxicity, bronchospasm and hypotension).
- No products indexed under this heading.

Pancuronium Bromide (Amphotericin B-induced hypokalemia may enhance the curariform effect of skeletal relaxants).
No products indexed under this heading.

Pentamidine Isethionate (Concurrent use may enhance the potential for drug-induced renal toxicity).
No products indexed under this heading.

Pipecuronium Bromide (Amphotericin B-induced hypokalemia may enhance the curariform effect of skeletal relaxants).
No products indexed under this heading.

Prednisolone Acetate (Concurrent use may potentiate hypokalemia which could predispose the patient to cardiac dysfunction). Products include:
Blephamide Ophthalmic Ointment 568
Blephamide Ophthalmic Suspension 569
Poly-Pred Ophthalmic Suspension .... ⊙233
Pred Forte Ophthalmic Suspension .... ⊙235
Pred Mild Ophthalmic Suspension .... ⊙238
Pred-G Ophthalmic Ointment .... ⊙237
Pred-G Ophthalmic Suspension .... ⊙236

Prednisolone Sodium Phosphate (Concurrent use may potentiate hypokalemia which could predispose the patient to cardiac dysfunction).
No products indexed under this heading.

Prednisolone Tebutate (Concurrent use may potentiate hypokalemia which could predispose the patient to cardiac dysfunction).
No products indexed under this heading.

Prednisone (Concurrent use may potentiate hypokalemia which could predispose the patient to cardiac dysfunction).
No products indexed under this heading.

Procarbazine Hydrochloride (Concurrent use may enhance the potential for renal toxicity, bronchospasm and hypotension). Products include:
Matulane Capsules 3191

Rapacuronium Bromide (Amphotericin B-induced hypokalemia may enhance the curariform effect of skeletal relaxants).
No products indexed under this heading.

Rocuronium Bromide (Amphotericin B-induced hypokalemia may enhance the curariform effect of skeletal relaxants). Products include:
Zemuron Injection 2346

Streptomycin Sulfate (Concurrent use may enhance the potential for drug-induced renal toxicity).
No products indexed under this heading.

Streptozocin (Concurrent use may enhance the potential for renal toxicity, bronchospasm and hypotension).
No products indexed under this heading.

Tamoxifen Citrate (Concurrent use may enhance the potential for renal toxicity, bronchospasm and hypotension). Products include:
Soltamox Oral Solution 3527

Teniposide (Concurrent use may enhance the potential for renal toxicity, bronchospasm and hypotension).
No products indexed under this heading.

Thioguanine (Concurrent use may enhance the potential for renal toxicity, bronchospasm and hypotension). Products include:
Tabloid Tablets 1575

Thiotepa (Concurrent use may enhance the potential for renal toxicity, bronchospasm and hypotension).
No products indexed under this heading.

Tobramycin (Concurrent use may enhance the potential for drug-induced renal toxicity). Products include:
TOBI Solution for Inhalation 2298
TobraDex Ophthalmic Ointment 562
TobraDex Ophthalmic Suspension 563
Zylet Ophthalmic Suspension .... ⊙259

Tobramycin Sulfate (Concurrent use may enhance the potential for drug-induced renal toxicity).
No products indexed under this heading.

Topotecan Hydrochloride (Concurrent use may enhance the potential for renal toxicity, bronchospasm and hypotension). Products include:
Hycamtin for Injection 1458

Toremifene Citrate (Concurrent use may enhance the potential for renal toxicity, bronchospasm and hypotension).
No products indexed under this heading.

Triamcinolone (Concurrent use may potentiate hypokalemia which could predispose the patient to cardiac dysfunction).
No products indexed under this heading.

Triamcinolone Acetonide (Concurrent use may potentiate hypokalemia which could predispose the patient to cardiac dysfunction). Products include:
Azmacort Inhalation Aerosol 1726
Nasacort AQ Nasal Spray 2922

Triamcinolone Diacetate (Concurrent use may potentiate hypokalemia which could predispose the patient to cardiac dysfunction).
No products indexed under this heading.

Triamcinolone Hexacetonide (Concurrent use may potentiate hypokalemia which could predispose the patient to cardiac dysfunction).
No products indexed under this heading.

Tubocurarine Chloride (Amphotericin B-induced hypokalemia may enhance the curariform effect of skeletal muscle relaxants).
No products indexed under this heading.

Valrubicin (Concurrent use may enhance the potential for renal toxicity, bronchospasm and hypotension).
No products indexed under this heading.

Vecuronium Bromide (Amphotericin B-induced hypokalemia may enhance the curariform effect of skeletal relaxants).
No products indexed under this heading.

Vincristine Sulfate (Concurrent use may enhance the potential for renal toxicity, bronchospasm and hypotension).
No products indexed under this heading.

Vinorelbine Tartrate (Concurrent use may enhance the potential for renal toxicity, bronchospasm and hypotension).
No products indexed under this heading.

Zidovudine (Potential for increased myelotoxicity and nephrotoxicity). Products include:
Combivir Tablets 1411
Retrovir 1560
Retrovir IV Infusion 1564
Trizivir Tablets 1589

ABILIFY ORAL SOLUTION
(Aripiprazole) 882
See Abilify Tablets

ABILIFY ORAL SOLUTION
(Aripiprazole) 2450
See Abilify Tablets

ABILIFY DISCMELT ORALLY DISINTEGRATING TABLETS
(Aripiprazole) 882
See Abilify Tablets

ABILIFY DISCMELT ORALLY DISINTEGRATING TABLETS
(Aripiprazole) 2450
See Abilify Tablets

ABILIFY TABLETS
(Aripiprazole) 882
May interact with cytochrome p450 2d6 inhibitors (selected), cytochrome p450 3a4 inducers (selected), cytochrome p450 3a4 inhibitors (selected), and certain other agents. Compounds in these categories include:

Acetazolamide (Inhibitors of CYP3A4 or CYP2D6 can inhibit aripiprazole elimination and cause increased blood levels).
No products indexed under this heading.

Allium sativum (Agents that induce CYP3A4 could cause an increase in aripiprazole clearance and lower blood levels).
No products indexed under this heading.

Amiodarone Hydrochloride (Inhibitors of CYP3A4 or CYP2D6 can inhibit aripiprazole elimination and cause increased blood levels).
No products indexed under this heading.

Amitriptyline Hydrochloride (Inhibitors of CYP3A4 or CYP2D6 can inhibit aripiprazole elimination and cause increased blood levels).
No products indexed under this heading.

Amoxapine (Inhibitors of CYP3A4 or CYP2D6 can inhibit aripiprazole elimination and cause increased blood levels).
No products indexed under this heading.

Amprenavir (Inhibitors of CYP3A4 or CYP2D6 can inhibit aripiprazole elimination and cause increased blood levels). Products include:
Agenerase Capsules 1327
Agenerase Oral Solution 1332

Anastrozole (Inhibitors of CYP3A4 or CYP2D6 can inhibit aripiprazole elimination and cause increased blood levels). Products include:
Arimidex Tablets 673

Aprepitant (Inhibitors of CYP3A4 or CYP2D6 can inhibit aripiprazole elimination and cause increased blood levels). Products include:
Emend Capsules 1963

Betamethasone Acetate (Agents that induce CYP3A4 could cause an increase in aripiprazole clearance and lower blood levels).
No products indexed under this heading.

Betamethasone Sodium Phosphate (Agents that induce CYP3A4 could cause an increase in aripiprazole clearance and lower blood levels).
No products indexed under this heading.

Bupropion Hydrochloride (Inhibitors of CYP3A4 or CYP2D6 can inhibit aripiprazole elimination and cause increased blood levels). Products include:
Wellbutrin Tablets 1603
Wellbutrin SR Sustained-Release Tablets 1607
Wellbutrin XL Extended-Release Tablets 1613
Zyban Sustained-Release Tablets 1644

Carbamazepine (Agents that induce CYP3A4 could cause an increase in aripiprazole clearance and lower blood levels). Products include:
Carbatrol Capsules 3171
Equetro Extended-Release Capsules 3180
Tegretol/Tegretol-XR 2295

Celecoxib (Inhibitors of CYP3A4 or CYP2D6 can inhibit aripiprazole elimination and cause increased blood levels). Products include:
Celebrex Capsules 3134

Chloroquine Hydrochloride (Inhibitors of CYP3A4 or CYP2D6 can inhibit aripiprazole elimination and cause increased blood levels).
No products indexed under this heading.

Chloroquine Phosphate (Inhibitors of CYP3A4 or CYP2D6 can inhibit aripiprazole elimination and cause increased blood levels).
No products indexed under this heading.

Chlorpheniramine (Inhibitors of CYP3A4 or CYP2D6 can inhibit aripiprazole elimination and cause increased blood levels).
No products indexed under this heading.

Chlorpheniramine Maleate (Inhibitors of CYP3A4 or CYP2D6 can inhibit aripiprazole elimination and cause increased blood levels). Products include:
Advil Allergy Sinus Caplets .... ■□770
Advil Multi-Symptom Cold Caplets .... ■□770
BC Allergy Sinus Cold Powder .... ■□677
Comtrex Maximum Strength Cold & Cough Day/Night Caplets - Night Formulation .... ■□726
Comtrex Maximum Strength Day/Night Severe Cold & Sinus Caplets - Night Formulation .... ■□725
Contac Cold and Flu Maximum Strength Caplets .... ■□728
Contac Cold and Flu Day and Night Caplets (Night Formulation Only) .... ■□727
Children's Dimetapp Long Acting Cough Plus Cold Syrup .... ■□731
Robitussin Cough & Cold Long-Acting Liquid .... ■□735
Robitussin Cough & Allergy Syrup .... ■□736
Robitussin Cough & Cold Nighttime Liquid .... ■□736

Chlorpheniramine Polistirex
(Inhibitors of CYP3A4 or CYP2D6
can inhibit aripiprazole elimination
and cause increased blood levels).
Products include:

Chlorpheniramine Tannate
(Inhibitors of CYP3A4 or CYP2D6
can inhibit aripiprazole elimination
and cause increased blood levels).
 No products indexed under this
 heading.

Cimetidine (Inhibitors of CYP3A4 or
CYP2D6 can inhibit aripiprazole elimination and cause increased blood
levels). Products include:

Cimetidine Hydrochloride (Inhibitors of CYP3A4 or CYP2D6 can
inhibit aripiprazole elimination and
cause increased blood levels).
 No products indexed under this
 heading.

Ciprofloxacin (Inhibitors of CYP3A4
or CYP2D6 can inhibit aripiprazole
elimination and cause increased
blood levels). Products include:

Ciprofloxacin Hydrochloride
(Agents that induce CYP3A4 could
cause an increase in aripiprazole
clearance and lower blood levels).
Products include:

Cisplatin (Agents that induce
CYP3A4 could cause an increase in
aripiprazole clearance and lower
blood levels).
 No products indexed under this
 heading.

Citalopram Hydrobromide (Inhibitors of CYP3A4 or CYP2D6 can

inhibit aripiprazole elimination and
cause increased blood levels).
Products include:

Clarithromycin (Inhibitors of
CYP3A4 or CYP2D6 can inhibit aripiprazole elimination and cause
increased blood levels). Products
include:

Clomipramine Hydrochloride
(Inhibitors of CYP3A4 or CYP2D6
can inhibit aripiprazole elimination
and cause increased blood levels).
 No products indexed under this
 heading.

Clotrimazole (Inhibitors of CYP3A4
or CYP2D6 can inhibit aripiprazole
elimination and cause increased
blood levels). Products include:

Cocaine Hydrochloride (Inhibitors
of CYP3A4 or CYP2D6 can inhibit
aripiprazole elimination and cause
increased blood levels).
 No products indexed under this
 heading.

Cortisone Acetate (Agents that
induce CYP3A4 could cause an
increase in aripiprazole clearance
and lower blood levels).
 No products indexed under this
 heading.

Cyclosporine (Inhibitors of CYP3A4
or CYP2D6 can inhibit aripiprazole
elimination and cause increased
blood levels). Products include:

Dalfopristin (Inhibitors of CYP3A4
or CYP2D6 can inhibit aripiprazole
elimination and cause increased
blood levels).
 No products indexed under this
 heading.

Danazol (Inhibitors of CYP3A4 or
CYP2D6 can inhibit aripiprazole elimination and cause increased blood
levels).
 No products indexed under this
 heading.

Delavirdine Mesylate (Inhibitors of
CYP3A4 or CYP2D6 can inhibit aripiprazole elimination and cause
increased blood levels). Products
include:

Desipramine Hydrochloride
(Inhibitors of CYP3A4 or CYP2D6
can inhibit aripiprazole elimination
and cause increased blood levels).
 No products indexed under this
 heading.

Dexamethasone (Agents that
induce CYP3A4 could cause an
increase in aripiprazole clearance
and lower blood levels). Products
include:

Dexamethasone Acetate (Agents
that induce CYP3A4 could cause an
increase in aripiprazole clearance
and lower blood levels).
 No products indexed under this
 heading.

**Dexamethasone Sodium Phos-
phate** (Agents that induce CYP3A4
could cause an increase in aripiprazole clearance and lower blood
levels).
 No products indexed under this
 heading.

Diltiazem Hydrochloride (Inhibitors of CYP3A4 or CYP2D6 can
inhibit aripiprazole elimination and
cause increased blood levels).
Products include:

Diltiazem Maleate (Inhibitors of
CYP3A4 or CYP2D6 can inhibit aripiprazole elimination and cause
increased blood levels).
 No products indexed under this
 heading.

Diphenhydramine (Inhibitors of
CYP3A4 or CYP2D6 can inhibit aripiprazole elimination and cause
increased blood levels). Products
include:

Diphenhydramine Hydrochloride
(Inhibitors of CYP3A4 or CYP2D6
can inhibit aripiprazole elimination
and cause increased blood levels).
Products include:

Doxepin Hydrochloride (Inhibitors
of CYP3A4 or CYP2D6 can inhibit
aripiprazole elimination and cause
increased blood levels).
 No products indexed under this
 heading.

Doxorubicin Hydrochloride
(Agents that induce CYP3A4 could
cause an increase in aripiprazole
clearance and lower blood levels).
 No products indexed under this
 heading.

Efavirenz (Inhibitors of CYP3A4 or
CYP2D6 can inhibit aripiprazole elimination and cause increased blood
levels). Products include:

Erythromycin (Inhibitors of
CYP3A4 or CYP2D6 can inhibit aripiprazole elimination and cause
increased blood levels). Products
include:

Erythromycin Estolate (Inhibitors
of CYP3A4 or CYP2D6 can inhibit
aripiprazole elimination and cause
increased blood levels).
 No products indexed under this
 heading.

Erythromycin Ethylsuccinate
(Inhibitors of CYP3A4 or CYP2D6
can inhibit aripiprazole elimination
and cause increased blood levels).
Products include:

Erythromycin Gluceptate (Inhibitors of CYP3A4 or CYP2D6 can
inhibit aripiprazole elimination and
cause increased blood levels).
 No products indexed under this
 heading.

Erythromycin Lactobionate
(Inhibitors of CYP3A4 or CYP2D6
can inhibit aripiprazole elimination
and cause increased blood levels).
 No products indexed under this
 heading.

Erythromycin Stearate (Inhibitors
of CYP3A4 or CYP2D6 can inhibit
aripiprazole elimination and cause
increased blood levels). Products
include:

Escitalopram Oxalate (Inhibitors
of CYP3A4 or CYP2D6 can inhibit
aripiprazole elimination and cause
increased blood levels). Products
include:

Esomeprazole Magnesium
(Inhibitors of CYP3A4 or CYP2D6
can inhibit aripiprazole elimination
and cause increased blood levels).
Products include:

Ethosuximide (Agents that induce
CYP3A4 could cause an increase in
aripiprazole clearance and lower
blood levels).
 No products indexed under this
 heading.

Felbamate (Agents that induce
CYP3A4 could cause an increase in
aripiprazole clearance and lower
blood levels).
 No products indexed under this
 heading.

Fluconazole (Inhibitors of CYP3A4
or CYP2D6 can inhibit aripiprazole
elimination and cause increased
blood levels).
 No products indexed under this
 heading.

Fludrocortisone Acetate (Agents
that induce CYP3A4 could cause an
increase in aripiprazole clearance
and lower blood levels).
 No products indexed under this
 heading.

Fluoxetine (Inhibitors of CYP3A4 or
CYP2D6 can inhibit aripiprazole elimination and cause increased blood
levels).
 No products indexed under this
 heading.

Fluoxetine Hydrochloride (Inhibitors of CYP3A4 or CYP2D6 can
inhibit aripiprazole elimination and
cause increased blood levels).
Products include:

Fluphenazine Decanoate (Inhibitors of CYP3A4 or CYP2D6 can inhibit aripiprazole elimination and cause increased blood levels).
No products indexed under this heading.

Fluphenazine Enanthate (Inhibitors of CYP3A4 or CYP2D6 can inhibit aripiprazole elimination and cause increased blood levels).
No products indexed under this heading.

Fluphenazine Hydrochloride (Inhibitors of CYP3A4 or CYP2D6 can inhibit aripiprazole elimination and cause increased blood levels).
No products indexed under this heading.

Fluvoxamine Maleate (Inhibitors of CYP3A4 or CYP2D6 can inhibit aripiprazole elimination and cause increased blood levels).
No products indexed under this heading.

Fosamprenavir Calcium (Inhibitors of CYP3A4 or CYP2D6 can inhibit aripiprazole elimination and cause increased blood levels). Products include:
Lexiva1505

Fosphenytoin Sodium (Agents that induce CYP3A4 could cause an increase in aripiprazole clearance and lower blood levels).
No products indexed under this heading.

Garlic Extract (Agents that induce CYP3A4 could cause an increase in aripiprazole clearance and lower blood levels).
No products indexed under this heading.

Garlic Oil (Agents that induce CYP3A4 could cause an increase in aripiprazole clearance and lower blood levels).
No products indexed under this heading.

Halofantrine Hydrochloride (Inhibitors of CYP3A4 or CYP2D6 can inhibit aripiprazole elimination and cause increased blood levels).
No products indexed under this heading.

Haloperidol (Inhibitors of CYP3A4 or CYP2D6 can inhibit aripiprazole elimination and cause increased blood levels).
No products indexed under this heading.

Haloperidol Decanoate (Inhibitors of CYP3A4 or CYP2D6 can inhibit aripiprazole elimination and cause increased blood levels).
No products indexed under this heading.

Hydrocortisone (Agents that induce CYP3A4 could cause an increase in aripiprazole clearance and lower blood levels). Products include:
Colocort Rectal Suspension, USP (Retention) 100 mg/60 mL2476
Hydrocortone Tablets1989
Preparation H Hydrocortisone Cream ..646

Hydrocortisone Acetate (Agents that induce CYP3A4 could cause an increase in aripiprazole clearance and lower blood levels). Products include:
Analpram-HC1159
Pramosone1161
ProctoFoam-HC3099

Hydrocortisone Butyrate (Agents that induce CYP3A4 could cause an

increase in aripiprazole clearance and lower blood levels). Products include:
Locoid Lipocream Cream1160

Hydrocortisone Cypionate (Agents that induce CYP3A4 could cause an increase in aripiprazole clearance and lower blood levels).
No products indexed under this heading.

Hydrocortisone Hemisuccinate (Agents that induce CYP3A4 could cause an increase in aripiprazole clearance and lower blood levels).
No products indexed under this heading.

Hydrocortisone Probutate (Agents that induce CYP3A4 could cause an increase in aripiprazole clearance and lower blood levels).
No products indexed under this heading.

Hydrocortisone Sodium Phosphate (Agents that induce CYP3A4 could cause an increase in aripiprazole clearance and lower blood levels).
No products indexed under this heading.

Hydrocortisone Sodium Succinate (Agents that induce CYP3A4 could cause an increase in aripiprazole clearance and lower blood levels).
No products indexed under this heading.

Hydrocortisone Valerate (Agents that induce CYP3A4 could cause an increase in aripiprazole clearance and lower blood levels).
No products indexed under this heading.

Hydroxychloroquine Sulfate (Inhibitors of CYP3A4 or CYP2D6 can inhibit aripiprazole elimination and cause increased blood levels).
No products indexed under this heading.

Hypericum (Agents that induce CYP3A4 could cause an increase in aripiprazole clearance and lower blood levels). Products include:
Satiete Tablets832

Hypericum Perforatum (Agents that induce CYP3A4 could cause an increase in aripiprazole clearance and lower blood levels).
No products indexed under this heading.

Imatinib Mesylate (Inhibitors of CYP3A4 or CYP2D6 can inhibit aripiprazole elimination and cause increased blood levels). Products include:
Gleevec Tablets2227

Imipramine Hydrochloride (Inhibitors of CYP3A4 or CYP2D6 can inhibit aripiprazole elimination and cause increased blood levels).
No products indexed under this heading.

Imipramine Pamoate (Inhibitors of CYP3A4 or CYP2D6 can inhibit aripiprazole elimination and cause increased blood levels).
No products indexed under this heading.

Indinavir Sulfate (Inhibitors of CYP3A4 or CYP2D6 can inhibit aripiprazole elimination and cause increased blood levels). Products include:
Crixivan Capsules1940

Isoniazid (Inhibitors of CYP3A4 or CYP2D6 can inhibit aripiprazole elimination and cause increased blood levels).
No products indexed under this heading.

Itraconazole (Inhibitors of CYP3A4 or CYP2D6 can inhibit aripiprazole elimination and cause increased blood levels).
No products indexed under this heading.

Ketoconazole (Inhibitors of CYP3A4 or CYP2D6 can inhibit aripiprazole elimination and cause increased blood levels). Products include:
Nizoral A-D Shampoo, 1%1868

Lopinavir (Inhibitors of CYP3A4 or CYP2D6 can inhibit aripiprazole elimination and cause increased blood levels). Products include:
Kaletra ...476

Loratadine (Inhibitors of CYP3A4 or CYP2D6 can inhibit aripiprazole elimination and cause increased blood levels). Products include:
Alavert Allergy & Sinus D-12 Hour Tablets ..771
Alavert ...771
Children's Claritin Allergy Oral Solution771
Claritin Non-Drowsy 24 Hour Tablets ..772
Claritin Reditabs 24 Hour Non-Drowsy Tablets772
Claritin-D Non-Drowsy 12 Hour Tablets ..772
Claritin-D Non-Drowsy 24 Hour Tablets ..772

Maprotiline Hydrochloride (Inhibitors of CYP3A4 or CYP2D6 can inhibit aripiprazole elimination and cause increased blood levels).
No products indexed under this heading.

Mephenytoin (Agents that induce CYP3A4 could cause an increase in aripiprazole clearance and lower blood levels).
No products indexed under this heading.

Methadone Hydrochloride (Inhibitors of CYP3A4 or CYP2D6 can inhibit aripiprazole elimination and cause increased blood levels).
No products indexed under this heading.

Methsuximide (Agents that induce CYP3A4 could cause an increase in aripiprazole clearance and lower blood levels).
No products indexed under this heading.

Methylprednisolone (Agents that induce CYP3A4 could cause an increase in aripiprazole clearance and lower blood levels).
No products indexed under this heading.

Methylprednisolone Acetate (Agents that induce CYP3A4 could cause an increase in aripiprazole clearance and lower blood levels). Products include:
Depo-Medrol Injectable Suspension2617
Depo-Medrol Single-Dose Vial2619

Methylprednisolone Sodium Succinate (Agents that induce CYP3A4 could cause an increase in aripiprazole clearance and lower blood levels).
No products indexed under this heading.

Metronidazole (Inhibitors of CYP3A4 or CYP2D6 can inhibit arip-

iprazole elimination and cause increased blood levels). Products include:
Metrogel 1%1211
MetroGel-Vaginal Gel1855
Vandazol Vaginal Gel3338

Metronidazole Benzoate (Inhibitors of CYP3A4 or CYP2D6 can inhibit aripiprazole elimination and cause increased blood levels).
No products indexed under this heading.

Metronidazole Hydrochloride (Inhibitors of CYP3A4 or CYP2D6 can inhibit aripiprazole elimination and cause increased blood levels).
No products indexed under this heading.

Mibefradil Dihydrochloride (Inhibitors of CYP3A4 or CYP2D6 can inhibit aripiprazole elimination and cause increased blood levels).
No products indexed under this heading.

Miconazole (Inhibitors of CYP3A4 or CYP2D6 can inhibit aripiprazole elimination and cause increased blood levels).
No products indexed under this heading.

Miconazole Nitrate (Inhibitors of CYP3A4 or CYP2D6 can inhibit aripiprazole elimination and cause increased blood levels). Products include:
Desenex ..635
Desenex Jock Itch Spray Powder ...635

Moclobemide (Inhibitors of CYP3A4 or CYP2D6 can inhibit aripiprazole elimination and cause increased blood levels).
No products indexed under this heading.

Modafinil (Agents that induce CYP3A4 could cause an increase in aripiprazole clearance and lower blood levels). Products include:
Provigil Tablets988

Nefazodone Hydrochloride (Inhibitors of CYP3A4 or CYP2D6 can inhibit aripiprazole elimination and cause increased blood levels).
No products indexed under this heading.

Nelfinavir Mesylate (Inhibitors of CYP3A4 or CYP2D6 can inhibit aripiprazole elimination and cause increased blood levels). Products include:
Viracept ..2577

Nevirapine (Inhibitors of CYP3A4 or CYP2D6 can inhibit aripiprazole elimination and cause increased blood levels). Products include:
Viramune Oral Suspension873
Viramune Tablets873

Niacinamide (Inhibitors of CYP3A4 or CYP2D6 can inhibit aripiprazole elimination and cause increased blood levels).
No products indexed under this heading.

Nicotinamide (Inhibitors of CYP3A4 or CYP2D6 can inhibit aripiprazole elimination and cause increased blood levels). Products include:
Nicomide Tablets1088

Nifedipine (Inhibitors of CYP3A4 or CYP2D6 can inhibit aripiprazole elimination and cause increased blood levels). Products include:
Adalat CC Tablets2964

Norfloxacin (Inhibitors of CYP3A4 or CYP2D6 can inhibit aripiprazole elimination and cause increased blood levels). Products include:

IMPORTANT NOTE: Always consult each drug listing in the patient's regimen for possible interactions.

Noroxin Tablets 2032

Nortriptyline Hydrochloride (Inhibitors of CYP3A4 or CYP2D6 can inhibit aripiprazole elimination and cause increased blood levels).
No products indexed under this heading.

Omeprazole (Inhibitors of CYP3A4 or CYP2D6 can inhibit aripiprazole elimination and cause increased blood levels). Products include:
Zegerid Capsules 2958
Zegerid Powder for Oral Solution 2958

Oxcarbazepine (Agents that induce CYP3A4 could cause an increase in aripiprazole clearance and lower blood levels). Products include:
Trileptal Tablets 2300
Trileptal Oral Suspension 2300

Paroxetine Hydrochloride (Inhibitors of CYP3A4 or CYP2D6 can inhibit aripiprazole elimination and cause increased blood levels). Products include:
Paxil CR Controlled-Release Tablets 1538
Paxil 1530

Perphenazine (Inhibitors of CYP3A4 or CYP2D6 can inhibit aripiprazole elimination and cause increased blood levels).
No products indexed under this heading.

Phenobarbital (Agents that induce CYP3A4 could cause an increase in aripiprazole clearance and lower blood levels). Products include:
Donnatal Extentabs 2493

Phenobarbital Sodium (Agents that induce CYP3A4 could cause an increase in aripiprazole clearance and lower blood levels).
No products indexed under this heading.

Phenytoin (Agents that induce CYP3A4 could cause an increase in aripiprazole clearance and lower blood levels).
No products indexed under this heading.

Phenytoin Sodium (Agents that induce CYP3A4 could cause an increase in aripiprazole clearance and lower blood levels). Products include:
Phenytek Capsules 2160

Prednisolone Acetate (Agents that induce CYP3A4 could cause an increase in aripiprazole clearance and lower blood levels). Products include:
Blephamide Ophthalmic Ointment 568
Blephamide Ophthalmic Suspension.................................. 569
Poly-Pred Ophthalmic Suspension .... ⊙233
Pred Forte Ophthalmic Suspension .... ⊙235
Pred Mild Ophthalmic Suspension .... ⊙238
Pred-G Ophthalmic Ointment .... ⊙237
Pred-G Ophthalmic Suspension ...... ⊙236

Prednisolone Sodium Phosphate (Agents that induce CYP3A4 could cause an increase in aripiprazole clearance and lower blood levels).
No products indexed under this heading.

Prednisolone Tebutate (Agents that induce CYP3A4 could cause an increase in aripiprazole clearance and lower blood levels).
No products indexed under this heading.

Prednisone (Agents that induce CYP3A4 could cause an increase in aripiprazole clearance and lower blood levels).
No products indexed under this heading.

Primidone (Agents that induce CYP3A4 could cause an increase in aripiprazole clearance and lower blood levels).
No products indexed under this heading.

Propafenone Hydrochloride (Inhibitors of CYP3A4 or CYP2D6 can inhibit aripiprazole elimination and cause increased blood levels). Products include:
Rythmol SR Capsules 2727

Propoxyphene Hydrochloride (Inhibitors of CYP3A4 or CYP2D6 can inhibit aripiprazole elimination and cause increased blood levels).
No products indexed under this heading.

Propoxyphene Napsylate (Inhibitors of CYP3A4 or CYP2D6 can inhibit aripiprazole elimination and cause increased blood levels).
No products indexed under this heading.

Protriptyline Hydrochloride (Inhibitors of CYP3A4 or CYP2D6 can inhibit aripiprazole elimination and cause increased blood levels).
No products indexed under this heading.

Quinacrine Hydrochloride (Inhibitors of CYP3A4 or CYP2D6 can inhibit aripiprazole elimination and cause increased blood levels).
No products indexed under this heading.

Quinidine (Inhibitors of CYP3A4 or CYP2D6 can inhibit aripiprazole elimination and cause increased blood levels).
No products indexed under this heading.

Quinidine Gluconate (Inhibitors of CYP3A4 or CYP2D6 can inhibit aripiprazole elimination and cause increased blood levels).
No products indexed under this heading.

Quinidine Hydrochloride (Inhibitors of CYP3A4 or CYP2D6 can inhibit aripiprazole elimination and cause increased blood levels).
No products indexed under this heading.

Quinidine Polygalacturonate (Inhibitors of CYP3A4 or CYP2D6 can inhibit aripiprazole elimination and cause increased blood levels).
No products indexed under this heading.

Quinidine Sulfate (Inhibitors of CYP3A4 or CYP2D6 can inhibit aripiprazole elimination and cause increased blood levels).
No products indexed under this heading.

Quinine (Inhibitors of CYP3A4 or CYP2D6 can inhibit aripiprazole elimination and cause increased blood levels).
No products indexed under this heading.

Quinine Sulfate (Inhibitors of CYP3A4 or CYP2D6 can inhibit aripiprazole elimination and cause increased blood levels).
No products indexed under this heading.

Quinupristin (Inhibitors of CYP3A4 or CYP2D6 can inhibit aripiprazole elimination and cause increased blood levels).
No products indexed under this heading.

Ranitidine Bismuth Citrate (Inhibitors of CYP3A4 or CYP2D6 can inhibit aripiprazole elimination and cause increased blood levels).
No products indexed under this heading.

Ranitidine Hydrochloride (Inhibitors of CYP3A4 or CYP2D6 can inhibit aripiprazole elimination and cause increased blood levels). Products include:
Zantac 1624
Zantac Injection 1619
Zantac Injection Pharmacy Bulk Package 1622

Rifabutin (Agents that induce CYP3A4 could cause an increase in aripiprazole clearance and lower blood levels).
No products indexed under this heading.

Rifampicin (Agents that induce CYP3A4 could cause an increase in aripiprazole clearance and lower blood levels).
No products indexed under this heading.

Rifampin (Agents that induce CYP3A4 could cause an increase in aripiprazole clearance and lower blood levels).
No products indexed under this heading.

Rifapentine (Agents that induce CYP3A4 could cause an increase in aripiprazole clearance and lower blood levels).
No products indexed under this heading.

Ritonavir (Inhibitors of CYP3A4 or CYP2D6 can inhibit aripiprazole elimination and cause increased blood levels). Products include:
Kaletra 476
Norvir 503

Saquinavir (Inhibitors of CYP3A4 or CYP2D6 can inhibit aripiprazole elimination and cause increased blood levels).
No products indexed under this heading.

Saquinavir Mesylate (Inhibitors of CYP3A4 or CYP2D6 can inhibit aripiprazole elimination and cause increased blood levels). Products include:
Invirase 2772

Sertraline Hydrochloride (Inhibitors of CYP3A4 or CYP2D6 can inhibit aripiprazole elimination and cause increased blood levels). Products include:
Zoloft 2586

Sulfinpyrazone (Agents that induce CYP3A4 could cause an increase in aripiprazole clearance and lower blood levels).
No products indexed under this heading.

Telithromycin (Inhibitors of CYP3A4 or CYP2D6 can inhibit aripiprazole elimination and cause increased blood levels). Products include:
Ketek Tablets 2903

Terbinafine Hydrochloride (Inhibitors of CYP3A4 or CYP2D6 can inhibit aripiprazole elimination and cause increased blood levels). Products include:
Lamisil Tablets 2232
Lamisil AT Creams (Athlete's Foot & Jock Itch)................................. ▣636

Theophylline (Agents that induce CYP3A4 could cause an increase in aripiprazole clearance and lower blood levels).
No products indexed under this heading.

Thioridazine Hydrochloride (Inhibitors of CYP3A4 or CYP2D6 can inhibit aripiprazole elimination and cause increased blood levels). Products include:
Thioridazine Hydrochloride Tablets 2163

Triamcinolone (Agents that induce CYP3A4 could cause an increase in aripiprazole clearance and lower blood levels).
No products indexed under this heading.

Triamcinolone Acetonide (Agents that induce CYP3A4 could cause an increase in aripiprazole clearance and lower blood levels). Products include:
Azmacort Inhalation Aerosol 1726
Nasacort AQ Nasal Spray 2922

Triamcinolone Diacetate (Agents that induce CYP3A4 could cause an increase in aripiprazole clearance and lower blood levels).
No products indexed under this heading.

Triamcinolone Hexacetonide (Agents that induce CYP3A4 could cause an increase in aripiprazole clearance and lower blood levels).
No products indexed under this heading.

Trimipramine Maleate (Inhibitors of CYP3A4 or CYP2D6 can inhibit aripiprazole elimination and cause increased blood levels).
No products indexed under this heading.

Troglitazone (Agents that induce CYP3A4 could cause an increase in aripiprazole clearance and lower blood levels).
No products indexed under this heading.

Troleandomycin (Inhibitors of CYP3A4 or CYP2D6 can inhibit aripiprazole elimination and cause increased blood levels).
No products indexed under this heading.

Valproate Sodium (Inhibitors of CYP3A4 or CYP2D6 can inhibit aripiprazole elimination and cause increased blood levels). Products include:
Depacon Injection 412

Verapamil Hydrochloride (Inhibitors of CYP3A4 or CYP2D6 can inhibit aripiprazole elimination and cause increased blood levels). Products include:
Covera-HS Tablets 3139
Tarka Tablets 524
Verelan PM Extended-Release Capsules, Controlled-Onset 3106

Voriconazole (Inhibitors of CYP3A4 or CYP2D6 can inhibit aripiprazole elimination and cause increased blood levels). Products include:
VFEND I.V. 2564
VFEND Oral Suspension 2564
VFEND Tablets 2564

Zafirlukast (Inhibitors of CYP3A4 or CYP2D6 can inhibit aripiprazole elimination and cause increased blood levels). Products include:
Accolate Tablets 671

Zileuton (Inhibitors of CYP3A4 or CYP2D6 can inhibit aripiprazole elimination and cause increased blood levels). Products include:
Zyflo Tablets 1023

Food Interactions

Grapefruit (Inhibitors of CYP3A4 or CYP2D6 can inhibit aripiprazole elimination and cause increased blood levels).

Grapefruit Juice (Inhibitors of CYP3A4 or CYP2D6 can inhibit aripiprazole elimination and cause increased blood levels).

ABILIFY TABLETS

(Aripiprazole) 2450
May interact with antihypertensives, central nervous system depressants, central nervous system stimulants, cytochrome p450 2d6 inhibitors (selected), cytochrome p450 3a4 inducers (selected), cytochrome p450 3a4 inhibitors (selected), quinidine, and certain other agents. Compounds in these categories include:

Acebutolol Hydrochloride (Due to its alpha-1-adrenergic receptor antagonism, aripiprazole has the potential to enhance the effect of certain antihypertensive agents).
No products indexed under this heading.

Acetazolamide (Inhibitors of CYP3A4 can inhibit aripiprazole elimination and cause increased blood levels).
No products indexed under this heading.

Alfentanil Hydrochloride (Given the primary CNS effects of aripiprazole, caution should be used when co-administered with other centrally acting drugs).
No products indexed under this heading.

Allium sativum (Agents that induce CYP3A4 could cause an increase in aripiprazole clearance and lower blood levels).
No products indexed under this heading.

Alprazolam (Given the primary CNS effects of aripiprazole, caution should be used when co-administered with other centrally acting drugs). Products include:
Niravam Orally Disintegrating Tablets 3092

Amiodarone Hydrochloride (Inhibitors of CYP3A4 can inhibit aripiprazole elimination and cause increased blood levels).
No products indexed under this heading.

Amitriptyline Hydrochloride (Inhibitors of CYP2D6 can inhibit aripiprazole elimination and cause increased blood levels).
No products indexed under this heading.

Amlodipine Besylate (Due to its alpha-1-adrenergic receptor antagonism, aripiprazole has the potential to enhance the effect of certain antihypertensive agents). Products include:
Caduet Tablets 2508
Lotrel Capsules 2249
Norvasc Tablets 2545

Amoxapine (Inhibitors of CYP2D6 can inhibit aripiprazole elimination and cause increased blood levels).
No products indexed under this heading.

Amphetamine Resins (Given the primary CNS effects of aripiprazole, caution should be used when co-administered with other centrally acting drugs).
No products indexed under this heading.

Amprenavir (Inhibitors of CYP3A4 can inhibit aripiprazole elimination and cause increased blood levels). Products include:
Agenerase Capsules 1327
Agenerase Oral Solution 1332

Anastrozole (Inhibitors of CYP3A4 can inhibit aripiprazole elimination and cause increased blood levels). Products include:
Arimidex Tablets 673

Aprepitant (Agents that induce CYP3A4 could cause an increase in aripiprazole clearance and lower blood levels). Products include:
Emend Capsules 1963

Aprobarbital (Given the primary CNS effects of aripiprazole, caution should be used when co-administered with other centrally acting drugs).
No products indexed under this heading.

Atenolol (Due to its alpha-1-adrenergic receptor antagonism, aripiprazole has the potential to enhance the effect of certain antihypertensive agents).
No products indexed under this heading.

Benazepril Hydrochloride (Due to its alpha-1-adrenergic receptor antagonism, aripiprazole has the potential to enhance the effect of certain antihypertensive agents). Products include:
Lotensin Tablets 2243
Lotensin HCT Tablets 2246
Lotrel Capsules 2249

Bendroflumethiazide (Due to its alpha-1-adrenergic receptor antagonism, aripiprazole has the potential to enhance the effect of certain antihypertensive agents).
No products indexed under this heading.

Betamethasone Acetate (Agents that induce CYP3A4 could cause an increase in aripiprazole clearance and lower blood levels).
No products indexed under this heading.

Betamethasone Sodium Phosphate (Agents that induce CYP3A4 could cause an increase in aripiprazole clearance and lower blood levels).
No products indexed under this heading.

Betaxolol Hydrochloride (Due to its alpha-1-adrenergic receptor antagonism, aripiprazole has the potential to enhance the effect of certain antihypertensive agents). Products include:
Betoptic S Ophthalmic Suspension 558

Bisoprolol Fumarate (Due to its alpha-1-adrenergic receptor antagonism, aripiprazole has the potential to enhance the effect of certain antihypertensive agents).
No products indexed under this heading.

Buprenorphine Hydrochloride (Given the primary CNS effects of aripiprazole, caution should be used when co-administered with other centrally acting drugs). Products include:
Buprenex Injectable 2716
Suboxone Tablets 2717
Subutex Tablets 2717

Bupropion Hydrochloride (Inhibitors of CYP2D6 can inhibit aripiprazole elimination and cause increased blood levels). Products include:
Wellbutrin Tablets 1603
Wellbutrin SR Sustained-Release Tablets 1607
Wellbutrin XL Extended-Release Tablets 1613
Zyban Sustained-Release Tablets 1644

Buspirone Hydrochloride (Given the primary CNS effects of aripiprazole, caution should be used when co-administered with other centrally acting drugs).
No products indexed under this heading.

Butabarbital (Given the primary CNS effects of aripiprazole, caution should be used when co-administered with other centrally acting drugs).
No products indexed under this heading.

Butalbital (Given the primary CNS effects of aripiprazole, caution should be used when co-administered with other centrally acting drugs).
No products indexed under this heading.

Candesartan Cilexetil (Due to its alpha-1-adrenergic receptor antagonism, aripiprazole has the potential to enhance the effect of certain antihypertensive agents). Products include:
Atacand Tablets 649
Atacand HCT 651

Captopril (Due to its alpha-1-adrenergic receptor antagonism, aripiprazole has the potential to enhance the effect of certain antihypertensive agents). Products include:
Captopril Tablets 2149

Carbamazepine (Co-administration of carbamazepine, a potent CYP3A4 inducer, with aripiprazole resulted in an approximate 70% decrease in Cmax and AUC values of both aripiprazole and its active metabolite, dehydro-aripiprazole. When carbamazepine is added to aripiprazole therapy, aripiprazole dose should be doubled. When carbamazepine is withdrawn from combination therapy, aripiprazole dose should then be reduced). Products include:
Carbatrol Capsules 3171
Equetro Extended-Release Capsules 3180
Tegretol/Tegretol-XR 2295

Carteolol Hydrochloride (Due to its alpha-1-adrenergic receptor antagonism, aripiprazole has the potential to enhance the effect of certain antihypertensive agents). Products include:
Carteolol Hydrochloride Ophthalmic Solution USP, 1% .... ⊙ 249

Celecoxib (Inhibitors of CYP2D6 can inhibit aripiprazole elimination and cause increased blood levels). Products include:
Celebrex Capsules 3134

Chlordiazepoxide (Given the primary CNS effects of aripiprazole, caution should be used when co-administered with other centrally acting drugs).
No products indexed under this heading.

Chlordiazepoxide Hydrochloride (Given the primary CNS effects of aripiprazole, caution should be used when co-administered with other centrally acting drugs). Products include:
Librium Capsules 3347

Chloroquine Hydrochloride (Inhibitors of CYP2D6 can inhibit aripiprazole elimination and cause increased blood levels).
No products indexed under this heading.

Chloroquine Phosphate (Inhibitors of CYP2D6 can inhibit aripiprazole elimination and cause increased blood levels).
No products indexed under this heading.

Chlorothiazide (Due to its alpha-1-adrenergic receptor antagonism, aripiprazole has the potential to enhance the effect of certain antihypertensive agents). Products include:
Diuril Oral Suspension 1954

Chlorothiazide Sodium (Due to its alpha-1-adrenergic receptor antagonism, aripiprazole has the potential to enhance the effect of certain antihypertensive agents). Products include:
Diuril Sodium Intravenous 2467

Chlorpheniramine (Inhibitors of CYP2D6 can inhibit aripiprazole elimination and cause increased blood levels).
No products indexed under this heading.

Chlorpheniramine Maleate (Inhibitors of CYP2D6 can inhibit aripiprazole elimination and cause increased blood levels). Products include:
Advil Allergy Sinus Caplets .... ▣ 770
Advil Multi-Symptom Cold Caplets .... ▣ 770
BC Allergy Sinus Cold Powder .... ▣ 677
Comtrex Maximum Strength Cold & Cough Day/Night Caplets - Night Formulation .... ▣ 726
Comtrex Maximum Strength Day/Night Severe Cold & Sinus Caplets - Night Formulation .... ▣ 725
Contac Cold and Flu Maximum Strength Caplets .... ▣ 728
Contac Cold and Flu Day and Night Caplets (Night Formulation Only) .... ▣ 727
Children's Dimetapp Long Acting Cough Plus Cold Syrup .... ▣ 731
Robitussin Cough & Cold Long-Acting Liquid .... ▣ 735
Robitussin Cough & Allergy Syrup .. ▣ 736
Robitussin Cough & Cold Nighttime Liquid .... ▣ 736
Robitussin Cough, Cold & Flu Nighttime Liquid .... ▣ 738
Robitussin Pediatric Cough & Cold Long-Acting Liquid .... ▣ 735
Robitussin Pediatric Cough & Cold Nighttime Liquid .... ▣ 736
Triaminic Cold & Allergy Liquid .... ▣ 746
Triaminic Cough & Runny Nose Softchews .... ▣ 748
Children's Tylenol Plus Flu Oral Suspension .... ▣ 749
Tylenol Allergy Multi-Symptom Caplets with Cool Burst and Gelcaps 1872
Children's Tylenol Plus Cold Suspension Liquid 1879
Children's Tylenol Plus Cough & Runny Nose Suspension Liquid 1879
Children's Tylenol Plus Flu Suspension Liquid 1881
Children's Tylenol Plus Multi-Symptom Cold Suspension Liquid 1879
Tylenol Cold Head Congestion Nighttime Caplets with Cool Burst 1873

Tylenol Cold Multi-Symptom Nighttime Caplets with Cool Burst 1874
Tylenol Sinus Congestion & Pain Nighttime Caplets with Cool Burst 1876
Vicks 44M Cough, Cold & Flu Relief Liquid 2680
Pediatric Vicks 44m Cough & Cold Relief Liquid 2676
Children's Vicks NyQuil Cold/Cough Relief .... ■ 756
Children's Vicks NyQuil Cold/Cough Relief Liquid 2680
Zicam Maximum Strength Flu Daytime .... ■ 768

Chlorpheniramine Polistirex (Inhibitors of CYP2D6 can inhibit aripiprazole elimination and cause increased blood levels). Products include:
Tussionex Pennkinetic Extended-Release Suspension 3327

Chlorpheniramine Tannate (Inhibitors of CYP2D6 can inhibit aripiprazole elimination and cause increased blood levels).
No products indexed under this heading.

Chlorpromazine (Given the primary CNS effects of aripiprazole, caution should be used when co-administered with other centrally acting drugs).
No products indexed under this heading.

Chlorpromazine Hydrochloride (Given the primary CNS effects of aripiprazole, caution should be used when co-administered with other centrally acting drugs).
No products indexed under this heading.

Chlorprothixene (Given the primary CNS effects of aripiprazole, caution should be used when co-administered with other centrally acting drugs).
No products indexed under this heading.

Chlorprothixene Hydrochloride (Given the primary CNS effects of aripiprazole, caution should be used when co-administered with other centrally acting drugs).
No products indexed under this heading.

Chlorprothixene Lactate (Given the primary CNS effects of aripiprazole, caution should be used when co-administered with other centrally acting drugs).
No products indexed under this heading.

Chlorthalidone (Due to its alpha-1-adrenergic receptor antagonism, aripiprazole has the potential to enhance the effect of certain antihypertensive agents). Products include:
Clorpres Tablets 2153

Cimetidine (Inhibitors of CYP3A4 can inhibit aripiprazole elimination and cause increased blood levels). Products include:
Tagamet HB 200 Tablets .... ■ 664

Cimetidine Hydrochloride (Inhibitors of CYP3A4 can inhibit aripiprazole elimination and cause increased blood levels).
No products indexed under this heading.

Ciprofloxacin (Inhibitors of CYP3A4 can inhibit aripiprazole elimination and cause increased blood levels). Products include:
Cipro Oral Suspension 2977
Cipro I.V. 2984
Cipro XR Tablets 2990
Ciprodex Otic Suspension 559

Ciprofloxacin Hydrochloride (Agents that induce CYP3A4 could cause an increase in aripiprazole clearance and lower blood levels). Products include:
Ciloxan Ophthalmic Ointment 559
Ciloxan Ophthalmic Solution .... ⊙ 206
Cipro Tablets 2977
Proquin XR Tablets 1153

Cisplatin (Agents that induce CYP3A4 could cause an increase in aripiprazole clearance and lower blood levels).
No products indexed under this heading.

Citalopram Hydrobromide (Inhibitors of CYP2D6 can inhibit aripiprazole elimination and cause increased blood levels). Products include:
Celexa 1176

Clarithromycin (Inhibitors of CYP3A4 can inhibit aripiprazole elimination and cause increased blood levels). Products include:
Biaxin/Biaxin XL 402
PREVPAC 3284

Clomipramine Hydrochloride (Inhibitors of CYP2D6 can inhibit aripiprazole elimination and cause increased blood levels).
No products indexed under this heading.

Clonidine (Due to its alpha-1-adrenergic receptor antagonism, aripiprazole has the potential to enhance the effect of certain antihypertensive agents). Products include:
Catapres-TTS 844

Clonidine Hydrochloride (Due to its alpha-1-adrenergic receptor antagonism, aripiprazole has the potential to enhance the effect of certain antihypertensive agents). Products include:
Catapres Tablets 843
Clorpres Tablets 2153

Clorazepate Dipotassium (Given the primary CNS effects of aripiprazole, caution should be used when co-administered with other centrally acting drugs). Products include:
Tranxene 2474

Clotrimazole (Inhibitors of CYP3A4 can inhibit aripiprazole elimination and cause increased blood levels). Products include:
Desenex Athlete's Foot Cream .... ■ 635
Lotrimin 3039
Lotrisone 3040

Clozapine (Given the primary CNS effects of aripiprazole, caution should be used when co-administered with other centrally acting drugs). Products include:
Clozaril Tablets 2184
FazaClo Orally Disintegrating Tablets 551

Cocaine Hydrochloride (Inhibitors of CYP2D6 can inhibit aripiprazole elimination and cause increased blood levels).
No products indexed under this heading.

Codeine Phosphate (Given the primary CNS effects of aripiprazole, caution should be used when co-administered with other centrally acting drugs). Products include:
Tylenol with Codeine Tablets 2391

Cortisone Acetate (Agents that induce CYP3A4 could cause an increase in aripiprazole clearance and lower blood levels).
No products indexed under this heading.

Cyclosporine (Inhibitors of CYP3A4 can inhibit aripiprazole elimination and cause increased blood levels). Products include:
Gengraf Capsules 459
Neoral Oral Solution 2259
Neoral Soft Gelatin Capsules 2259
Restasis Ophthalmic Emulsion 575
Sandimmune 2275

Dalfopristin (Inhibitors of CYP3A4 can inhibit aripiprazole elimination and cause increased blood levels).
No products indexed under this heading.

Danazol (Inhibitors of CYP3A4 can inhibit aripiprazole elimination and cause increased blood levels).
No products indexed under this heading.

Delavirdine Mesylate (Inhibitors of CYP3A4 can inhibit aripiprazole elimination and cause increased blood levels). Products include:
Rescriptor Tablets 2551

Deserpidine (Due to its alpha-1-adrenergic receptor antagonism, aripiprazole has the potential to enhance the effect of certain antihypertensive agents).
No products indexed under this heading.

Desflurane (Given the primary CNS effects of aripiprazole, caution should be used when co-administered with other centrally acting drugs).
No products indexed under this heading.

Desipramine Hydrochloride (Inhibitors of CYP2D6 can inhibit aripiprazole elimination and cause increased blood levels).
No products indexed under this heading.

Dexamethasone (Agents that induce CYP3A4 could cause an increase in aripiprazole clearance and lower blood levels). Products include:
Ciprodex Otic Suspension 559
Decadron Tablets 1951
TobraDex Ophthalmic Ointment 562
TobraDex Ophthalmic Suspension 563

Dexamethasone Acetate (Agents that induce CYP3A4 could cause an increase in aripiprazole clearance and lower blood levels).
No products indexed under this heading.

Dexamethasone Sodium Phosphate (Agents that induce CYP3A4 could cause an increase in aripiprazole clearance and lower blood levels).
No products indexed under this heading.

Dextroamphetamine Sulfate (Given the primary CNS effects of aripiprazole, caution should be used when co-administered with other centrally acting drugs). Products include:
Adderall Tablets 3164
Adderall XR Capsules 3166
Dexedrine 1420
DextroStat Tablets 3179

Dezocine (Given the primary CNS effects of aripiprazole, caution should be used when co-administered with other centrally acting drugs).
No products indexed under this heading.

Diazepam (Given the primary CNS effects of aripiprazole, caution should be used when co-administered with other centrally acting drugs). Products include:
Diastat Rectal Delivery System 3343
Valium Tablets 2819

Diazoxide (Due to its alpha-1-adrenergic receptor antagonism, aripiprazole has the potential to enhance the effect of certain antihypertensive agents). Products include:
Hyperstat I.V. 3017

Diltiazem Hydrochloride (Due to its alpha-1-adrenergic receptor antagonism, aripiprazole has the potential to enhance the effect of certain antihypertensive agents). Products include:
Cardizem LA Extended Release Tablets 1728
Tiazac Capsules 1201

Diltiazem Maleate (Inhibitors of CYP3A4 can inhibit aripiprazole elimination and cause increased blood levels).
No products indexed under this heading.

Diphenhydramine (Inhibitors of CYP2D6 can inhibit aripiprazole elimination and cause increased blood levels). Products include:
Tylenol Sore Throat Nighttime Liquid with Cool Burst 1877

Diphenhydramine Hydrochloride (Inhibitors of CYP2D6 can inhibit aripiprazole elimination and cause increased blood levels). Products include:
Nytol QuickCaps Caplets .... ■ 615
Nytol QuickGels Softgels Maximum Strength .... ■ 616
Simply Sleep Caplets 1868
Sominex Original Formula Tablets .... ■ 616
TheraFlu Warming Relief Nighttime Severe Cold .... ■ 743
TheraFlu Thin Strips Multi Symptom .... ■ 744
Triaminic Nighttime Cold & Cough Liquid .... ■ 746
Triaminic Thin Strips Cough & Runny Nose .... ■ 749
Extra Strength Tylenol PM Caplets, Vanilla Caplets, Geltabs, Gelcaps and Liquid 1875
Tylenol Sore Throat Nighttime Liquid with Cool Burst .... ■ 790
Tylenol Allergy Multi-Symptom Nighttime Caplets with Cool Burst 1872
Tylenol Severe Allergy Caplets 1872
Children's Tylenol Plus Cold & Allergy Suspension Liquid 1878

Doxazosin Mesylate (Due to its alpha-1-adrenergic receptor antagonism, aripiprazole has the potential to enhance the effect of certain antihypertensive agents). Products include:
Cardura XL Tablets 2515

Doxepin Hydrochloride (Inhibitors of CYP2D6 can inhibit aripiprazole elimination and cause increased blood levels).
No products indexed under this heading.

Doxorubicin Hydrochloride (Agents that induce CYP3A4 could cause an increase in aripiprazole clearance and lower blood levels).
No products indexed under this heading.

Droperidol (Given the primary CNS effects of aripiprazole, caution should be used when co-administered with other centrally acting drugs).
No products indexed under this heading.

Efavirenz (Agents that induce CYP3A4 could cause an increase in aripiprazole clearance and lower blood levels). Products include:
Atripla Tablets 945
Sustiva Capsules 930
Sustiva Tablets 930

Enalapril Maleate (Due to its alpha-1-adrenergic receptor antagonism, aripiprazole has the potential to enhance the effect of certain antihypertensive agents). Products include:
Vasotec I.V. Injection 2103

Enalaprilat (Due to its alpha-1-adrenergic receptor antagonism, aripiprazole has the potential to enhance the effect of certain antihypertensive agents).
No products indexed under this heading.

Enflurane (Given the primary CNS effects of aripiprazole, caution should be used when co-administered with other centrally acting drugs).
No products indexed under this heading.

Eprosartan Mesylate (Due to its alpha-1-adrenergic receptor antagonism, aripiprazole has the potential to enhance the effect of certain antihypertensive agents). Products include:
Teveten Tablets 1735
Teveten HCT Tablets 1737

Erythromycin (Inhibitors of CYP3A4 can inhibit aripiprazole elimination and cause increased blood levels). Products include:
Ery-Tab Tablets 449
Erythromycin Base Filmtab Tablets 455
Erythromycin Delayed-Release Capsules, USP 457
PCE Dispertab Tablets 515

Erythromycin Estolate (Inhibitors of CYP3A4 can inhibit aripiprazole elimination and cause increased blood levels).
No products indexed under this heading.

Erythromycin Ethylsuccinate (Inhibitors of CYP3A4 can inhibit aripiprazole elimination and cause increased blood levels). Products include:
E.E.S. 451
EryPed 447

Erythromycin Gluceptate (Inhibitors of CYP3A4 can inhibit aripiprazole elimination and cause increased blood levels).
No products indexed under this heading.

Erythromycin Lactobionate (Inhibitors of CYP3A4 can inhibit aripiprazole elimination and cause increased blood levels).
No products indexed under this heading.

Erythromycin Stearate (Inhibitors of CYP3A4 can inhibit aripiprazole elimination and cause increased blood levels). Products include:
Erythrocin Stearate Filmtab Tablets 453

Escitalopram Oxalate (Inhibitors of CYP2D6 can inhibit aripiprazole elimination and cause increased blood levels). Products include:
Lexapro Oral Solution 1190
Lexapro Tablets 1190

Esmolol Hydrochloride (Due to its alpha-1-adrenergic receptor antagonism, aripiprazole has the potential to enhance the effect of certain antihypertensive agents).
No products indexed under this heading.

Esomeprazole Magnesium (Inhibitors of CYP3A4 can inhibit aripiprazole elimination and cause increased blood levels). Products include:
Nexium Delayed-Release Capsules 655

Estazolam (Given the primary CNS effects of aripiprazole, caution should be used when co-administered with other centrally acting drugs). Products include:
ProSom Tablets 517

Ethanol (Given the primary CNS effects of aripiprazole, caution should be used when co-administered with other centrally acting drugs).
No products indexed under this heading.

Ethchlorvynol (Given the primary CNS effects of aripiprazole, caution should be used when co-administered with other centrally acting drugs).
No products indexed under this heading.

Ethinamate (Given the primary CNS effects of aripiprazole, caution should be used when co-administered with other centrally acting drugs).
No products indexed under this heading.

Ethosuximide (Agents that induce CYP3A4 could cause an increase in aripiprazole clearance and lower blood levels).
No products indexed under this heading.

Ethyl Alcohol (Given the primary CNS effects of aripiprazole, caution should be used when co-administered with other centrally acting drugs).
No products indexed under this heading.

Felbamate (Agents that induce CYP3A4 could cause an increase in aripiprazole clearance and lower blood levels).
No products indexed under this heading.

Felodipine (Due to its alpha-1-adrenergic receptor antagonism, aripiprazole has the potential to enhance the effect of certain antihypertensive agents).
No products indexed under this heading.

Fentanyl (Given the primary CNS effects of aripiprazole, caution should be used when co-administered with other centrally acting drugs). Products include:
Duragesic Transdermal System 2373
Ionsys Transdermal System 2379

Fentanyl Citrate (Given the primary CNS effects of aripiprazole, caution should be used when co-administered with other centrally acting drugs). Products include:
Actiq 979

Fluconazole (Inhibitors of CYP3A4 can inhibit aripiprazole elimination and cause increased blood levels).
No products indexed under this heading.

Fludrocortisone Acetate (Agents that induce CYP3A4 could cause an increase in aripiprazole clearance and lower blood levels).
No products indexed under this heading.

Fluoxetine (Co-administration with quinidine, a potent inhibitor of CYP2D6, increased the AUC of aripiprazole by 112% but decreased the AUC of its active metabolite, dehydro-aripiprazole, by 35%. Aripiprazole dose should be reduced to one-half of its normal dose when concomitant administration of quinidine with aripiprazole occurs. Other significant inhibitors of CYP2D6, such as fluoxetine, would be expected to have similar effects and should be accompanied by similar dose reductions. When the CYP2D6 inhibitor iswithdrawn from the combination therapy, aripiprazole dose should then be increased).
No products indexed under this heading.

Fluoxetine Hydrochloride (Co-administration with quinidine, a potent inhibitor of CYP2D6, increased the AUC of aripiprazole by 112% but decreased the AUC of its active metabolite, dehydro-aripiprazole, by 35%. Aripiprazole dose should be reduced to one-half of its normal dose when concomitant administration of quinidine with aripiprazole occurs. Other significant inhibitors of CYP2D6, such as fluoxetine, would be expected to have similar effects and should be accompanied by similar dose reductions. When the CYP2D6 inhibitor iswithdrawn from the combination therapy, aripiprazole dose should then be increased). Products include:
Prozac Pulvules and Liquid 1801
Symbyax Capsules 1819

Fluphenazine Decanoate (Inhibitors of CYP2D6 can inhibit aripiprazole elimination and cause increased blood levels).
No products indexed under this heading.

Fluphenazine Enanthate (Inhibitors of CYP2D6 can inhibit aripiprazole elimination and cause increased blood levels).
No products indexed under this heading.

Fluphenazine Hydrochloride (Inhibitors of CYP2D6 can inhibit aripiprazole elimination and cause increased blood levels).
No products indexed under this heading.

Flurazepam Hydrochloride (Given the primary CNS effects of aripiprazole, caution should be used when co-administered with other centrally acting drugs). Products include:
Dalmane Capsules 3342

Fluvoxamine Maleate (Inhibitors of CYP3A4 can inhibit aripiprazole elimination and cause increased blood levels).
No products indexed under this heading.

Fosamprenavir Calcium (Inhibitors of CYP3A4 can inhibit aripiprazole elimination and cause increased blood levels). Products include:
Lexiva Tablets 1505

Fosinopril Sodium (Due to its alpha-1-adrenergic receptor antagonism, aripiprazole has the potential to enhance the effect of certain antihypertensive agents).
No products indexed under this heading.

Fosphenytoin Sodium (Agents that induce CYP3A4 could cause an increase in aripiprazole clearance and lower blood levels).
No products indexed under this heading.

Furosemide (Due to its alpha-1-adrenergic receptor antagonism, aripiprazole has the potential to enhance the effect of certain antihypertensive agents). Products include:
Furosemide Tablets 2154

Garlic Extract (Agents that induce CYP3A4 could cause an increase in aripiprazole clearance and lower blood levels).
No products indexed under this heading.

Garlic Oil (Agents that induce CYP3A4 could cause an increase in aripiprazole clearance and lower blood levels).
No products indexed under this heading.

Glutethimide (Given the primary CNS effects of aripiprazole, caution should be used when co-administered with other centrally acting drugs).
No products indexed under this heading.

Guanabenz Acetate (Due to its alpha-1-adrenergic receptor antagonism, aripiprazole has the potential to enhance the effect of certain antihypertensive agents).
No products indexed under this heading.

Guanethidine Monosulfate (Due to its alpha-1-adrenergic receptor antagonism, aripiprazole has the potential to enhance the effect of certain antihypertensive agents).
No products indexed under this heading.

Halofantrine Hydrochloride (Inhibitors of CYP2D6 can inhibit aripiprazole elimination and cause increased blood levels).
No products indexed under this heading.

Haloperidol (Inhibitors of CYP2D6 can inhibit aripiprazole elimination and cause increased blood levels).
No products indexed under this heading.

Haloperidol Decanoate (Inhibitors of CYP2D6 can inhibit aripiprazole elimination and cause increased blood levels).
No products indexed under this heading.

Hydralazine Hydrochloride (Due to its alpha-1-adrenergic receptor antagonism, aripiprazole has the potential to enhance the effect of certain antihypertensive agents). Products include:

BiDil Tablets 2171

Hydrochlorothiazide (Due to its alpha-1-adrenergic receptor antagonism, aripiprazole has the potential to enhance the effect of certain antihypertensive agents). Products include:

- Aldoril Tablets 1910
- Atacand HCT 651
- Avalide Tablets 888
- Avalide Tablets 2874
- Benicar HCT Tablets 1044
- Diovan HCT Tablets 2196
- Dyazide Capsules 1423
- Hyzaar 50-12.5 Tablets 1990
- Hyzaar 100-12.5 Tablets 1990
- Hyzaar 100-25 Tablets 1990
- Lopressor HCT 50/25 Tablets 2241
- Lopressor HCT 100/25 Tablets 2241
- Lopressor HCT 100/50 Tablets 2241
- Lotensin HCT Tablets 2246
- Micardis HCT Tablets 856
- Moduretic Tablets 2028
- Prinzide Tablets 2056
- Teveten HCT Tablets 1737
- Timolide Tablets 2086
- Uniretic Tablets 3100

Hydrocodone Bitartrate (Given the primary CNS effects of aripiprazole, caution should be used when co-administered with other centrally acting drugs). Products include:

- Hycodan 1116
- Hycotuss Expectorant Syrup 1117
- Vicodin Tablets 535
- Vicodin ES Tablets 536
- Vicodin HP Tablets 538
- Vicoprofen Tablets 539
- Zydone Tablets 1139

Hydrocodone Polistirex (Given the primary CNS effects of aripiprazole, caution should be used when co-administered with other centrally acting drugs). Products include:

- Tussionex Pennkinetic Extended-Release Suspension 3327

Hydrocortisone (Agents that induce CYP3A4 could cause an increase in aripiprazole clearance and lower blood levels). Products include:

- Colocort Rectal Suspension, USP (Retention) 100 mg/60 mL 2476
- Hydrocortone Tablets 1989
- Preparation H Hydrocortisone Cream .... ■ 646

Hydrocortisone Acetate (Agents that induce CYP3A4 could cause an increase in aripiprazole clearance and lower blood levels). Products include:

- Analpram-HC 1159
- Pramosone 1161
- ProctoFoam-HC 3099

Hydrocortisone Butyrate (Agents that induce CYP3A4 could cause an increase in aripiprazole clearance and lower blood levels). Products include:

- Locoid Lipocream Cream 1160

Hydrocortisone Cypionate (Agents that induce CYP3A4 could cause an increase in aripiprazole clearance and lower blood levels).

No products indexed under this heading.

Hydrocortisone Hemisuccinate (Agents that induce CYP3A4 could cause an increase in aripiprazole clearance and lower blood levels).

No products indexed under this heading.

Hydrocortisone Probutate (Agents that induce CYP3A4 could cause an increase in aripiprazole clearance and lower blood levels).

No products indexed under this heading.

Hydrocortisone Sodium Phosphate (Agents that induce CYP3A4 could cause an increase in aripiprazole clearance and lower blood levels).

No products indexed under this heading.

Hydrocortisone Sodium Succinate (Agents that induce CYP3A4 could cause an increase in aripiprazole clearance and lower blood levels).

No products indexed under this heading.

Hydrocortisone Valerate (Agents that induce CYP3A4 could cause an increase in aripiprazole clearance and lower blood levels).

No products indexed under this heading.

Hydroflumethiazide (Due to its alpha-1-adrenergic receptor antagonism, aripiprazole has the potential to enhance the effect of certain antihypertensive agents).

No products indexed under this heading.

Hydromorphone Hydrochloride (Given the primary CNS effects of aripiprazole, caution should be used when co-administered with other centrally acting drugs). Products include:

- Dilaudid 440
- Dilaudid Non-Sterile Powder 440
- Dilaudid Oral Liquid 445
- Dilaudid Rectal Suppositories 440
- Dilaudid Tablets 440
- Dilaudid Tablets - 8 mg 445
- Dilaudid-HP 442

Hydroxychloroquine Sulfate (Inhibitors of CYP2D6 can inhibit aripiprazole elimination and cause increased blood levels).

No products indexed under this heading.

Hydroxyzine Hydrochloride (Given the primary CNS effects of aripiprazole, caution should be used when co-administered with other centrally acting drugs).

No products indexed under this heading.

Hypericum (Agents that induce CYP3A4 could cause an increase in aripiprazole clearance and lower blood levels). Products include:

- Satiete Tablets .... ■ 832

Hypericum Perforatum (Agents that induce CYP3A4 could cause an increase in aripiprazole clearance and lower blood levels).

No products indexed under this heading.

Imatinib Mesylate (Inhibitors of CYP2D6 can inhibit aripiprazole elimination and cause increased blood levels). Products include:

- Gleevec Tablets 2227

Imipramine Hydrochloride (Inhibitors of CYP2D6 can inhibit aripiprazole elimination and cause increased blood levels).

No products indexed under this heading.

Imipramine Pamoate (Inhibitors of CYP2D6 can inhibit aripiprazole elimination and cause increased blood levels).

No products indexed under this heading.

Indapamide (Due to its alpha-1-adrenergic receptor antagonism, aripiprazole has the potential to enhance the effect of certain antihypertensive agents). Products include:

- Indapamide Tablets 2156

Indinavir Sulfate (Inhibitors of CYP3A4 can inhibit aripiprazole elimination and cause increased blood levels). Products include:

- Crixivan Capsules 1940

Irbesartan (Due to its alpha-1-adrenergic receptor antagonism, aripiprazole has the potential to enhance the effect of certain antihypertensive agents). Products include:

- Avalide Tablets 888
- Avalide Tablets 2874
- Avapro Tablets 891
- Avapro Tablets 2871

Isoflurane (Given the primary CNS effects of aripiprazole, caution should be used when co-administered with other centrally acting drugs).

No products indexed under this heading.

Isoniazid (Inhibitors of CYP3A4 can inhibit aripiprazole elimination and cause increased blood levels).

No products indexed under this heading.

Isradipine (Due to its alpha-1-adrenergic receptor antagonism, aripiprazole has the potential to enhance the effect of certain antihypertensive agents). Products include:

- DynaCirc CR Tablets 2721

Itraconazole (Co-administration with ketoconazole increased the AUC of aripiprazole and its active metabolite by 63% and 77%, respectively. When concomitant administration of ketoconazole with aripiprazole occurs, aripiprazole dose should be reduced to one-half of its normal dose. Other strong inhibitors of CYP3A4 (itraconazole) would be expected to have similar effects and need similar dose reductions. When the CYP3A4 inhibitor is withdrawn from the combination therapy, aripiprazole dose should then be increased).

No products indexed under this heading.

Ketamine Hydrochloride (Given the primary CNS effects of aripiprazole, caution should be used when co-administered with other centrally acting drugs).

No products indexed under this heading.

Ketoconazole (Co-administration with ketoconazole increased the AUC of aripiprazole and its active metabolite by 63% and 77%, respectively. When concomitant administration of ketoconazole with aripiprazole occurs, aripiprazole dose should be reduced to one-half of its normal dose. When the CYP3A4 inhibitor is withdrawn from the combination therapy, aripiprazole dose should then be increased). Products include:

- Nizoral A-D Shampoo, 1% 1868

Labetalol Hydrochloride (Due to its alpha-1-adrenergic receptor antagonism, aripiprazole has the potential to enhance the effect of certain antihypertensive agents).

No products indexed under this heading.

Levomethadyl Acetate Hydrochloride (Given the primary CNS effects of aripiprazole, caution should be used when co-administered with other centrally acting drugs).

No products indexed under this heading.

Levorphanol Tartrate (Given the primary CNS effects of aripiprazole, caution should be used when co-administered with other centrally acting drugs).

No products indexed under this heading.

Lisinopril (Due to its alpha-1-adrenergic receptor antagonism, aripiprazole has the potential to enhance the effect of certain antihypertensive agents). Products include:

- Prinivil Tablets 2052
- Prinzide Tablets 2056

Lopinavir (Inhibitors of CYP3A4 can inhibit aripiprazole elimination and cause increased blood levels). Products include:

- Kaletra 476

Loratadine (Inhibitors of CYP3A4 can inhibit aripiprazole elimination and cause increased blood levels). Products include:

- Alavert Allergy & Sinus D-12 Hour Tablets .... ■ 771
- Alavert .... ■ 771
- Children's Claritin Allergy Oral Solution .... ■ 771
- Claritin Non-Drowsy 24 Hour Tablets .... ■ 772
- Claritin Reditabs 24 Hour Non-Drowsy Tablets .... ■ 772
- Claritin-D Non-Drowsy 12 Hour Tablets .... ■ 772
- Claritin-D Non-Drowsy 24 Hour Tablets .... ■ 772

Lorazepam (Given the primary CNS effects of aripiprazole, caution should be used when co-administered with other centrally acting drugs).

No products indexed under this heading.

Losartan Potassium (Due to its alpha-1-adrenergic receptor antagonism, aripiprazole has the potential to enhance the effect of certain antihypertensive agents). Products include:

- Cozaar Tablets 1935
- Hyzaar 50-12.5 Tablets 1990
- Hyzaar 100-12.5 Tablets 1990
- Hyzaar 100-25 Tablets 1990

Loxapine Hydrochloride (Given the primary CNS effects of aripiprazole, caution should be used when co-administered with other centrally acting drugs).

No products indexed under this heading.

Loxapine Succinate (Given the primary CNS effects of aripiprazole, caution should be used when co-administered with other centrally acting drugs).

No products indexed under this heading.

Maprotiline Hydrochloride (Inhibitors of CYP2D6 can inhibit aripiprazole elimination and cause increased blood levels).

No products indexed under this heading.

Mecamylamine Hydrochloride (Due to its alpha-1-adrenergic receptor antagonism, aripiprazole has the potential to enhance the effect of certain antihypertensive agents).

No products indexed under this heading.

Meperidine Hydrochloride (Given the primary CNS effects of aripiprazole, caution should be used when co-administered with other centrally acting drugs).
No products indexed under this heading.

Mephenytoin (Agents that induce CYP3A4 could cause an increase in aripiprazole clearance and lower blood levels).
No products indexed under this heading.

Mephobarbital (Given the primary CNS effects of aripiprazole, caution should be used when co-administered with other centrally acting drugs).
No products indexed under this heading.

Meprobamate (Given the primary CNS effects of aripiprazole, caution should be used when co-administered with other centrally acting drugs).
No products indexed under this heading.

Mesoridazine Besylate (Given the primary CNS effects of aripiprazole, caution should be used when co-administered with other centrally acting drugs).
No products indexed under this heading.

Methadone Hydrochloride (Inhibitors of CYP2D6 can inhibit aripiprazole elimination and cause increased blood levels).
No products indexed under this heading.

Methamphetamine Hydrochloride (Given the primary CNS effects of aripiprazole, caution should be used when co-administered with other centrally acting drugs). Products include:
Desoxyn Tablets, USP 2462

Methohexital Sodium (Given the primary CNS effects of aripiprazole, caution should be used when co-administered with other centrally acting drugs).
No products indexed under this heading.

Methotrimeprazine (Given the primary CNS effects of aripiprazole, caution should be used when co-administered with other centrally acting drugs).
No products indexed under this heading.

Methoxyflurane (Given the primary CNS effects of aripiprazole, caution should be used when co-administered with other centrally acting drugs).
No products indexed under this heading.

Methsuximide (Agents that induce CYP3A4 could cause an increase in aripiprazole clearance and lower blood levels).
No products indexed under this heading.

Methyclothiazide (Due to its alpha-1-adrenergic receptor antagonism, aripiprazole has the potential to enhance the effect of certain antihypertensive agents).
No products indexed under this heading.

Methyldopa (Due to its alpha-1-adrenergic receptor antagonism, aripiprazole has the potential to enhance the effect of certain antihypertensive agents). Products include:
Aldoril Tablets 1910

Methyldopate Hydrochloride (Due to its alpha-1-adrenergic receptor antagonism, aripiprazole has the potential to enhance the effect of certain antihypertensive agents).
No products indexed under this heading.

Methylphenidate (Given the primary CNS effects of aripiprazole, caution should be used when co-administered with other centrally acting drugs). Products include:
Daytrana Transdermal Patch 3174

Methylphenidate Hydrochloride (Given the primary CNS effects of aripiprazole, caution should be used when co-administered with other centrally acting drugs). Products include:
Concerta Extended-Release Tablets 1881
Metadate CD Capsules 3323
Ritalin Hydrochloride Tablets 2269
Ritalin LA Capsules 2271
Ritalin-SR Tablets 2269

Methylprednisolone (Agents that induce CYP3A4 could cause an increase in aripiprazole clearance and lower blood levels).
No products indexed under this heading.

Methylprednisolone Acetate (Agents that induce CYP3A4 could cause an increase in aripiprazole clearance and lower blood levels). Products include:
Depo-Medrol Injectable Suspension 2617
Depo-Medrol Single-Dose Vial 2619

Methylprednisolone Sodium Succinate (Agents that induce CYP3A4 could cause an increase in aripiprazole clearance and lower blood levels).
No products indexed under this heading.

Metolazone (Due to its alpha-1-adrenergic receptor antagonism, aripiprazole has the potential to enhance the effect of certain antihypertensive agents).
No products indexed under this heading.

Metoprolol Succinate (Due to its alpha-1-adrenergic receptor antagonism, aripiprazole has the potential to enhance the effect of certain antihypertensive agents). Products include:
Toprol-XL Tablets 668

Metoprolol Tartrate (Due to its alpha-1-adrenergic receptor antagonism, aripiprazole has the potential to enhance the effect of certain antihypertensive agents). Products include:
Lopressor Injection 2238
Lopressor Tablets 2238
Lopressor HCT 50/25 Tablets 2241
Lopressor HCT 100/25 Tablets 2241
Lopressor HCT 100/50 Tablets 2241

Metronidazole (Inhibitors of CYP3A4 can inhibit aripiprazole elimination and cause increased blood levels). Products include:
Metrogel 1% 1211
MetroGel-Vaginal Gel 1855
Vandazole Vaginal Gel 3338

Metronidazole Benzoate (Inhibitors of CYP3A4 can inhibit aripiprazole elimination and cause increased blood levels).
No products indexed under this heading.

Metronidazole Hydrochloride (Inhibitors of CYP3A4 can inhibit aripiprazole elimination and cause increased blood levels).
No products indexed under this heading.

Metyrosine (Due to its alpha-1-adrenergic receptor antagonism, aripiprazole has the potential to enhance the effect of certain antihypertensive agents). Products include:
Demser Capsules 1953

Mibefradil Dihydrochloride (Due to its alpha-1-adrenergic receptor antagonism, aripiprazole has the potential to enhance the effect of certain antihypertensive agents).
No products indexed under this heading.

Miconazole (Inhibitors of CYP3A4 can inhibit aripiprazole elimination and cause increased blood levels).
No products indexed under this heading.

Miconazole Nitrate (Inhibitors of CYP3A4 can inhibit aripiprazole elimination and cause increased blood levels). Products include:
Desenex 635
Desenex Jock Itch Spray Powder 635

Midazolam Hydrochloride (Given the primary CNS effects of aripiprazole, caution should be used when co-administered with other centrally acting drugs).
No products indexed under this heading.

Minoxidil (Due to its alpha-1-adrenergic receptor antagonism, aripiprazole has the potential to enhance the effect of certain antihypertensive agents). Products include:
Men's Rogaine Extra Strength Hair Regrowth Treatment Topical Solution, Ocean Rush Scent and Original Unscented 633
Men's Rogaine Foam Hair Regrowth Treatment 633
Women's Rogaine Hair Regrowth Treatment Topical Solution, Spring Bloom Scent and Original Unscented 634

Moclobemide (Inhibitors of CYP2D6 can inhibit aripiprazole elimination and cause increased blood levels).
No products indexed under this heading.

Modafinil (Agents that induce CYP3A4 could cause an increase in aripiprazole clearance and lower blood levels). Products include:
Provigil Tablets 988

Moexipril Hydrochloride (Due to its alpha-1-adrenergic receptor antagonism, aripiprazole has the potential to enhance the effect of certain antihypertensive agents). Products include:
Uniretic Tablets 3100
Univasc Tablets 3104

Molindone Hydrochloride (Given the primary CNS effects of aripiprazole, caution should be used when co-administered with other centrally acting drugs). Products include:
Moban Tablets 1119

Morphine Sulfate (Given the primary CNS effects of aripiprazole, caution should be used when co-administered with other centrally acting drugs). Products include:
Avinza Capsules 1741
Kadian Capsules 577
MS Contin Tablets 2701

Nadolol (Due to its alpha-1-adrenergic receptor antagonism, aripiprazole has the potential to enhance the effect of certain antihypertensive agents). Products include:
Nadolol Tablets 2159

Nefazodone Hydrochloride (Inhibitors of CYP3A4 can inhibit aripiprazole elimination and cause increased blood levels).
No products indexed under this heading.

Nelfinavir Mesylate (Inhibitors of CYP3A4 can inhibit aripiprazole elimination and cause increased blood levels). Products include:
Viracept 2577

Nevirapine (Agents that induce CYP3A4 could cause an increase in aripiprazole clearance and lower blood levels). Products include:
Viramune Oral Suspension 873
Viramune Tablets 873

Niacinamide (Inhibitors of CYP3A4 can inhibit aripiprazole elimination and cause increased blood levels).
No products indexed under this heading.

Nicardipine Hydrochloride (Due to its alpha-1-adrenergic receptor antagonism, aripiprazole has the potential to enhance the effect of certain antihypertensive agents). Products include:
Cardene I.V. 2497

Nicotinamide (Inhibitors of CYP3A4 can inhibit aripiprazole elimination and cause increased blood levels). Products include:
Nicomide Tablets 1088

Nifedipine (Due to its alpha-1-adrenergic receptor antagonism, aripiprazole has the potential to enhance the effect of certain antihypertensive agents). Products include:
Adalat CC Tablets 2964

Nisoldipine (Due to its alpha-1-adrenergic receptor antagonism, aripiprazole has the potential to enhance the effect of certain antihypertensive agents). Products include:
Sular Tablets 3122

Nitroglycerin (Due to its alpha-1-adrenergic receptor antagonism, aripiprazole has the potential to enhance the effect of certain antihypertensive agents). Products include:
Nitro-Dur Transdermal Infusion System 3046
Nitrolingual Pumpspray 3120

Norfloxacin (Inhibitors of CYP3A4 can inhibit aripiprazole elimination and cause increased blood levels). Products include:
Noroxin Tablets 2032

Nortriptyline Hydrochloride (Inhibitors of CYP2D6 can inhibit aripiprazole elimination and cause increased blood levels).
No products indexed under this heading.

Olanzapine (Given the primary CNS effects of aripiprazole, caution should be used when co-administered with other centrally acting drugs). Products include:
Symbyax Capsules 1819
Zyprexa Tablets 1830
Zyprexa IntraMuscular 1830
Zyprexa ZYDIS Orally Disintegrating Tablets 1830

Omeprazole (Inhibitors of CYP3A4 can inhibit aripiprazole elimination and cause increased blood levels). Products include:
- Zegerid Capsules 2958
- Zegerid Powder for Oral Solution 2958

Oxazepam (Given the primary CNS effects of aripiprazole, caution should be used when co-administered with other centrally acting drugs).
No products indexed under this heading.

Oxcarbazepine (Agents that induce CYP3A4 could cause an increase in aripiprazole clearance and lower blood levels). Products include:
- Trileptal Tablets 2300
- Trileptal Oral Suspension 2300

Oxycodone Hydrochloride (Given the primary CNS effects of aripiprazole, caution should be used when co-administered with other centrally acting drugs). Products include:
- OxyContin Tablets 2703
- OxyFast Oral Concentrate Solution 2708
- OxyIR Capsules 2708
- Percocet Tablets 1131
- Percodan Tablets 1132

Paroxetine Hydrochloride (Co-administration with quinidine, a potent inhibitor of CYP2D6, increased the AUC of aripiprazole by 112% but decreased the AUC of its active metabolite, dehydro-aripiprazole, by 35%. Aripiprazole dose should be reduced to one-half of its normal dose when concomitant administration of quinidine with aripiprazole occurs. Other significant inhibitors of CYP2D6, such as paroxetine, would be expected to have similar effects and should be accompanied by similar dose reductions. When the CYP2D6 inhibitor iswithdrawn from the combination therapy, aripiprazole dose should then be increased). Products include:
- Paxil CR Controlled-Release Tablets 1538
- Paxil 1530

Paroxetine Mesylate (Co-administration with quinidine, a potent inhibitor of CYP2D6, increased the AUC of aripiprazole by 112% but decreased the AUC of its active metabolite, dehydro-aripiprazole, by 35%. Aripiprazole dose should be reduced to one-half of its normal dose when concomitant administration of quinidine with aripiprazole occurs. Other significant inhibitors of CYP2D6, such as paroxetine, would be expected to have similar effects and should be accompanied by similar dose reductions. When the CYP2D6 inhibitor iswithdrawn from the combination therapy, aripiprazole dose should then be increased). Products include:
- Pexeva Tablets 1694

Pemoline (Given the primary CNS effects of aripiprazole, caution should be used when co-administered with other centrally acting drugs).
No products indexed under this heading.

Penbutolol Sulfate (Due to its alpha-1-adrenergic receptor antagonism, aripiprazole has the potential to enhance the effect of certain antihypertensive agents).
No products indexed under this heading.

Pentobarbital Sodium (Given the primary CNS effects of aripiprazole, caution should be used when co-administered with other centrally acting drugs). Products include:
- Nembutal Sodium Solution, USP 2470

Perindopril Erbumine (Due to its alpha-1-adrenergic receptor antagonism, aripiprazole has the potential to enhance the effect of certain antihypertensive agents). Products include:
- Aceon Tablets (2 mg, 4 mg, 8 mg) 3194

Perphenazine (Inhibitors of CYP2D6 can inhibit aripiprazole elimination and cause increased blood levels).
No products indexed under this heading.

Phenobarbital (Agents that induce CYP3A4 could cause an increase in aripiprazole clearance and lower blood levels). Products include:
- Donnatal Extentabs 2493

Phenobarbital Sodium (Agents that induce CYP3A4 could cause an increase in aripiprazole clearance and lower blood levels).
No products indexed under this heading.

Phenoxybenzamine Hydrochloride (Due to its alpha-1-adrenergic receptor antagonism, aripiprazole has the potential to enhance the effect of certain antihypertensive agents). Products include:
- Dibenzyline Capsules 3399

Phentolamine Mesylate (Due to its alpha-1-adrenergic receptor antagonism, aripiprazole has the potential to enhance the effect of certain antihypertensive agents).
No products indexed under this heading.

Phenytoin (Agents that induce CYP3A4 could cause an increase in aripiprazole clearance and lower blood levels).
No products indexed under this heading.

Phenytoin Sodium (Agents that induce CYP3A4 could cause an increase in aripiprazole clearance and lower blood levels). Products include:
- Phenytek Capsules 2160

Pindolol (Due to its alpha-1-adrenergic receptor antagonism, aripiprazole has the potential to enhance the effect of certain antihypertensive agents).
No products indexed under this heading.

Polythiazide (Due to its alpha-1-adrenergic receptor antagonism, aripiprazole has the potential to enhance the effect of certain antihypertensive agents).
No products indexed under this heading.

Prazepam (Given the primary CNS effects of aripiprazole, caution should be used when co-administered with other centrally acting drugs).
No products indexed under this heading.

Prazosin Hydrochloride (Due to its alpha-1-adrenergic receptor antagonism, aripiprazole has the potential to enhance the effect of certain antihypertensive agents).
No products indexed under this heading.

Prednisolone Acetate (Agents that induce CYP3A4 could cause an increase in aripiprazole clearance and lower blood levels). Products include:
- Blephamide Ophthalmic Ointment 568
- Blephamide Ophthalmic Suspension 569
- Poly-Pred Ophthalmic Suspension .... ⊙233
- Pred Forte Ophthalmic Suspension .... ⊙235
- Pred Mild Ophthalmic Suspension .... ⊙238
- Pred-G Ophthalmic Ointment .... ⊙237
- Pred-G Ophthalmic Suspension ...... ⊙236

Prednisolone Sodium Phosphate (Agents that induce CYP3A4 could cause an increase in aripiprazole clearance and lower blood levels).
No products indexed under this heading.

Prednisolone Tebutate (Agents that induce CYP3A4 could cause an increase in aripiprazole clearance and lower blood levels).
No products indexed under this heading.

Prednisone (Agents that induce CYP3A4 could cause an increase in aripiprazole clearance and lower blood levels).
No products indexed under this heading.

Primidone (Agents that induce CYP3A4 could cause an increase in aripiprazole clearance and lower blood levels).
No products indexed under this heading.

Prochlorperazine (Given the primary CNS effects of aripiprazole, caution should be used when co-administered with other centrally acting drugs).
No products indexed under this heading.

Promethazine Hydrochloride (Given the primary CNS effects of aripiprazole, caution should be used when co-administered with other centrally acting drugs). Products include:
- Phenergan Tablets and Suppositories 3440

Propafenone Hydrochloride (Inhibitors of CYP2D6 can inhibit aripiprazole elimination and cause increased blood levels). Products include:
- Rythmol SR Capsules 2727

Propofol (Given the primary CNS effects of aripiprazole, caution should be used when co-administered with other centrally acting drugs).
No products indexed under this heading.

Propoxyphene Hydrochloride (Inhibitors of CYP3A4 can inhibit aripiprazole elimination and cause increased blood levels).
No products indexed under this heading.

Propoxyphene Napsylate (Inhibitors of CYP3A4 can inhibit aripiprazole elimination and cause increased blood levels).
No products indexed under this heading.

Propranolol Hydrochloride (Due to its alpha-1-adrenergic receptor antagonism, aripiprazole has the potential to enhance the effect of certain antihypertensive agents). Products include:
- Inderal LA Long-Acting Capsules 3429
- InnoPran XL Capsules 2723

Protriptyline Hydrochloride (Inhibitors of CYP2D6 can inhibit aripiprazole elimination and cause increased blood levels).
No products indexed under this heading.

Quazepam (Given the primary CNS effects of aripiprazole, caution should be used when co-administered with other centrally acting drugs).
No products indexed under this heading.

Quetiapine Fumarate (Given the primary CNS effects of aripiprazole, caution should be used when co-administered with other centrally acting drugs). Products include:
- Seroquel Tablets 690

Quinacrine Hydrochloride (Inhibitors of CYP2D6 can inhibit aripiprazole elimination and cause increased blood levels).
No products indexed under this heading.

Quinapril Hydrochloride (Due to its alpha-1-adrenergic receptor antagonism, aripiprazole has the potential to enhance the effect of certain antihypertensive agents).
No products indexed under this heading.

Quinidine (Co-administration with quinidine, a potent inhibitor of CYP2D6, increased the AUC of aripiprazole by 112% but decreased the AUC of its active metabolite, dehydro-aripiprazole, by 35%. Aripiprazole dose should be reduced to one-half of its normal dose when concomitant administration of quinidine with aripiprazole occurs. When the CYP2D6 inhibitor is withdrawn from the combination therapy, aripiprazole dose should then be increased).
No products indexed under this heading.

Quinidine Gluconate (Co-administration with quinidine, a potent inhibitor of CYP2D6, increased the AUC of aripiprazole by 112% but decreased the AUC of its active metabolite, dehydro-aripiprazole, by 35%. Aripiprazole dose should be reduced to one-half of its normal dose when concomitant administration of quinidine with aripiprazole occurs. When the CYP2D6 inhibitor is withdrawn from the combination therapy, aripiprazole dose should then be increased).
No products indexed under this heading.

Quinidine Hydrochloride (Co-administration with quinidine, a potent inhibitor of CYP2D6, increased the AUC of aripiprazole by 112% but decreased the AUC of its active metabolite, dehydro-aripiprazole, by 35%. Aripiprazole dose should be reduced to one-half of its normal dose when concomitant administration of quinidine with aripiprazole occurs. When the CYP2D6 inhibitor is withdrawn from the combination therapy, aripiprazole dose should then be increased).
No products indexed under this heading.

Quinidine Polygalacturonate (Co-administration with quinidine, a potent inhibitor of CYP2D6, increased the AUC of aripiprazole by 112% but decreased the AUC of its active metabolite, dehydro-aripiprazole, by 35%. Aripiprazole

dose should be reduced to one-half of its normal dose when concomitant administration of quinidine with aripiprazole occurs. When the CYP2D6 inhibitor is withdrawn from the combination therapy, aripiprazole dose should then be increased).
No products indexed under this heading.

Quinidine Sulfate (Co-administration with quinidine, a potent inhibitor of CYP2D6, increased the AUC of aripiprazole by 112% but decreased the AUC of its active metabolite, dehydro-aripiprazole, by 35%. Aripiprazole dose should be reduced to one-half of its normal dose when concomitant administration of quinidine with aripiprazole occurs. When the CYP2D6 inhibitor is withdrawn from the combination therapy, aripiprazole dose should then be increased).
No products indexed under this heading.

Quinine (Inhibitors of CYP3A4 can inhibit aripiprazole elimination and cause increased blood levels).
No products indexed under this heading.

Quinine Sulfate (Inhibitors of CYP3A4 can inhibit aripiprazole elimination and cause increased blood levels).
No products indexed under this heading.

Quinupristin (Inhibitors of CYP3A4 can inhibit aripiprazole elimination and cause increased blood levels).
No products indexed under this heading.

Ramipril (Due to its alpha-1-adrenergic receptor antagonism, aripiprazole has the potential to enhance the effect of certain antihypertensive agents). Products include:
Altace Capsules 1702

Ranitidine Bismuth Citrate (Inhibitors of CYP3A4 can inhibit aripiprazole elimination and cause increased blood levels).
No products indexed under this heading.

Ranitidine Hydrochloride (Inhibitors of CYP3A4 can inhibit aripiprazole elimination and cause increased blood levels). Products include:
Zantac 1624
Zantac Injection 1619
Zantac Injection Pharmacy Bulk Package 1622

Rauwolfia Serpentina (Due to its alpha-1-adrenergic receptor antagonism, aripiprazole has the potential to enhance the effect of certain antihypertensive agents).
No products indexed under this heading.

Remifentanil Hydrochloride (Given the primary CNS effects of aripiprazole, caution should be used when co-administered with other centrally acting drugs).
No products indexed under this heading.

Rescinnamine (Due to its alpha-1-adrenergic receptor antagonism, aripiprazole has the potential to enhance the effect of certain antihypertensive agents).
No products indexed under this heading.

Reserpine (Due to its alpha-1-adrenergic receptor antagonism, aripiprazole has the potential to enhance the effect of certain antihypertensive agents).
No products indexed under this heading.

Rifabutin (Agents that induce CYP3A4 could cause an increase in aripiprazole clearance and lower blood levels).
No products indexed under this heading.

Rifampicin (Agents that induce CYP3A4 could cause an increase in aripiprazole clearance and lower blood levels).
No products indexed under this heading.

Rifampin (Agents that induce CYP3A4 could cause an increase in aripiprazole clearance and lower blood levels).
No products indexed under this heading.

Rifapentine (Agents that induce CYP3A4 could cause an increase in aripiprazole clearance and lower blood levels).
No products indexed under this heading.

Risperidone (Given the primary CNS effects of aripiprazole, caution should be used when co-administered with other centrally acting drugs). Products include:
Risperdal 1676
Risperdal Consta Long-Acting Injection 1682
Risperdal M-Tab Orally Disintegrating Tablets 1676

Ritonavir (Inhibitors of CYP3A4 can inhibit aripiprazole elimination and cause increased blood levels). Products include:
Kaletra 476
Norvir 503

Saquinavir (Inhibitors of CYP3A4 can inhibit aripiprazole elimination and cause increased blood levels).
No products indexed under this heading.

Saquinavir Mesylate (Inhibitors of CYP3A4 can inhibit aripiprazole elimination and cause increased blood levels). Products include:
Invirase 2772

Secobarbital Sodium (Given the primary CNS effects of aripiprazole, caution should be used when co-administered with other centrally acting drugs).
No products indexed under this heading.

Sertraline Hydrochloride (Inhibitors of CYP3A4 can inhibit aripiprazole elimination and cause increased blood levels). Products include:
Zoloft 2586

Sevoflurane (Given the primary CNS effects of aripiprazole, caution should be used when co-administered with other centrally acting drugs). Products include:
Ultane Liquid for Inhalation 531

Sodium Nitroprusside (Due to its alpha-1-adrenergic receptor antagonism, aripiprazole has the potential to enhance the effect of certain antihypertensive agents).
No products indexed under this heading.

Sodium Oxybate (Given the primary CNS effects of aripiprazole, caution should be used when co-administered with other centrally acting drugs). Products include:
Xyrem Oral Solution 1688

Sotalol Hydrochloride (Due to its alpha-1-adrenergic receptor antagonism, aripiprazole has the potential to enhance the effect of certain antihypertensive agents).
No products indexed under this heading.

Spirapril Hydrochloride (Due to its alpha-1-adrenergic receptor antagonism, aripiprazole has the potential to enhance the effect of certain antihypertensive agents).
No products indexed under this heading.

Sufentanil Citrate (Given the primary CNS effects of aripiprazole, caution should be used when co-administered with other centrally acting drugs).
No products indexed under this heading.

Sulfinpyrazone (Agents that induce CYP3A4 could cause an increase in aripiprazole clearance and lower blood levels).
No products indexed under this heading.

Telithromycin (Inhibitors of CYP3A4 can inhibit aripiprazole elimination and cause increased blood levels). Products include:
Ketek Tablets 2903

Telmisartan (Due to its alpha-1-adrenergic receptor antagonism, aripiprazole has the potential to enhance the effect of certain antihypertensive agents). Products include:
Micardis Tablets 854
Micardis HCT Tablets 856

Temazepam (Given the primary CNS effects of aripiprazole, caution should be used when co-administered with other centrally acting drugs). Products include:
Restoril Capsules 1860

Terazosin Hydrochloride (Due to its alpha-1-adrenergic receptor antagonism, aripiprazole has the potential to enhance the effect of certain antihypertensive agents). Products include:
Hytrin Capsules 471

Terbinafine Hydrochloride (Inhibitors of CYP2D6 can inhibit aripiprazole elimination and cause increased blood levels). Products include:
Lamisil Tablets 2232
Lamisil AT Creams (Athlete's Foot & Jock Itch) 636

Theophylline (Agents that induce CYP3A4 could cause an increase in aripiprazole clearance and lower blood levels).
No products indexed under this heading.

Thiamylal Sodium (Given the primary CNS effects of aripiprazole, caution should be used when co-administered with other centrally acting drugs).
No products indexed under this heading.

Thioridazine Hydrochloride (Inhibitors of CYP2D6 can inhibit aripiprazole elimination and cause increased blood levels). Products include:
Thioridazine Hydrochloride Tablets 2163

Thiothixene (Given the primary CNS effects of aripiprazole, caution should be used when co-administered with other centrally acting drugs). Products include:
Thiothixene Capsules 2165

Timolol Maleate (Due to its alpha-1-adrenergic receptor antagonism, aripiprazole has the potential to enhance the effect of certain antihypertensive agents). Products include:
Blocadren Tablets 1916
Cosopt Sterile Ophthalmic Solution 1931
Timolide Tablets 2086
Timoptic Sterile Ophthalmic Solution 2088
Timoptic in Ocudose 2091
Timoptic-XE Sterile Ophthalmic Gel Forming Solution 2092

Torsemide (Due to its alpha-1-adrenergic receptor antagonism, aripiprazole has the potential to enhance the effect of certain antihypertensive agents). Products include:
Demadex Injection 2759
Demadex Tablets 2759

Trandolapril (Due to its alpha-1-adrenergic receptor antagonism, aripiprazole has the potential to enhance the effect of certain antihypertensive agents). Products include:
Mavik Tablets 486
Tarka Tablets 524

Triamcinolone (Agents that induce CYP3A4 could cause an increase in aripiprazole clearance and lower blood levels).
No products indexed under this heading.

Triamcinolone Acetonide (Agents that induce CYP3A4 could cause an increase in aripiprazole clearance and lower blood levels). Products include:
Azmacort Inhalation Aerosol 1726
Nasacort AQ Nasal Spray 2922

Triamcinolone Diacetate (Agents that induce CYP3A4 could cause an increase in aripiprazole clearance and lower blood levels).
No products indexed under this heading.

Triamcinolone Hexacetonide (Agents that induce CYP3A4 could cause an increase in aripiprazole clearance and lower blood levels).
No products indexed under this heading.

Triazolam (Given the primary CNS effects of aripiprazole, caution should be used when co-administered with other centrally acting drugs).
No products indexed under this heading.

Trifluoperazine Hydrochloride (Given the primary CNS effects of aripiprazole, caution should be used when co-administered with other centrally acting drugs).
No products indexed under this heading.

Trimethaphan Camsylate (Due to its alpha-1-adrenergic receptor antagonism, aripiprazole has the potential to enhance the effect of certain antihypertensive agents).
No products indexed under this heading.

Trimipramine Maleate (Inhibitors of CYP2D6 can inhibit aripiprazole elimination and cause increased blood levels).
No products indexed under this heading.

Troglitazone (Agents that induce CYP3A4 could cause an increase in aripiprazole clearance and lower blood levels).
No products indexed under this heading.

Troleandomycin (Inhibitors of CYP3A4 can inhibit aripiprazole elimination and cause increased blood levels).
No products indexed under this heading.

Valproate Sodium (Inhibitors of CYP3A4 can inhibit aripiprazole elimination and cause increased blood levels). Products include:
Depacon Injection 412

Valsartan (Due to its alpha-1-adrenergic receptor antagonism, aripiprazole has the potential to enhance the effect of certain antihypertensive agents). Products include:
Diovan Tablets 2193
Diovan HCT Tablets 2196

Verapamil Hydrochloride (Due to its alpha-1-adrenergic receptor antagonism, aripiprazole has the potential to enhance the effect of certain antihypertensive agents). Products include:
Covera-HS Tablets 3139
Tarka Tablets 524
Verelan PM Extended-Release Capsules, Controlled-Onset 3106

Voriconazole (Inhibitors of CYP3A4 can inhibit aripiprazole elimination and cause increased blood levels). Products include:
VFEND I.V. 2564
VFEND Oral Suspension 2564
VFEND Tablets 2564

Zafirlukast (Inhibitors of CYP3A4 can inhibit aripiprazole elimination and cause increased blood levels). Products include:
Accolate Tablets 671

Zaleplon (Given the primary CNS effects of aripiprazole, caution should be used when co-administered with other centrally acting drugs). Products include:
Sonata Capsules 1717

Zileuton (Inhibitors of CYP3A4 can inhibit aripiprazole elimination and cause increased blood levels). Products include:
Zyflo Tablets 1023

Ziprasidone Hydrochloride (Given the primary CNS effects of aripiprazole, caution should be used when co-administered with other centrally acting drugs). Products include:
Geodon Capsules 2529

Zolpidem Tartrate (Given the primary CNS effects of aripiprazole, caution should be used when co-administered with other centrally acting drugs). Products include:
Ambien Tablets 2851
Ambien CR Tablets 2855

Food Interactions

Alcohol (Given the primary CNS effects of aripiprazole, caution should be use when co-administered with alcohol; patients should be advised to avoid alcohol while taking aripiprazole).

Grapefruit (Inhibitors of CYP3A4 can inhibit aripiprazole elimination and cause increased blood levels).

Grapefruit Juice (Inhibitors of CYP3A4 can inhibit aripiprazole elimination and cause increased blood levels).

ABREVA CREAM

(Docosanol) .... ▣710
None cited in PDR database.

ACCOLATE TABLETS

(Zafirlukast) 671
May interact with dihydropyridine calcium channel blockers, erythromycin, phenytoin, xanthines, and certain other agents. Compounds in these categories include:

Aminophylline (Rare cases of patients experiencing increased theophylline levels with or without clinical signs or symptoms of theophylline toxicity after addition of zafirlukast to an existing theophylline regimen have been reported; co-administration with liquid theophylline products has resulted in a decrease in the mean plasma levels of zafirlukast by approximately 30%).
No products indexed under this heading.

Amlodipine Besylate (Zafirlukast is a known inhibitor of CYP3A4 in vitro; co-administration with other drugs known to be metabolized by this isoenzyme, such as dihydropyridine calcium channel blockers, should be undertaken with reasonable clinical monitoring; no formal interaction studies have been conducted). Products include:
Caduet Tablets 2508
Lotrel Capsules 2249
Norvasc Tablets 2545

Aspirin (Co-administration has resulted in mean increased plasma levels of zafirlukast by approximately 45%). Products include:
Aggrenox Capsules 822
Bayer Aspirin 744
BC Allergy Sinus Cold Powder .... ▣677
BC Headache Powder .... ▣677
Arthritis Strength BC Powder .... ▣677
BC Sinus Cold Powder .... ▣677
Excedrin Extra Strength Caplets/Tablets/Geltabs .... ▣684
Excedrin Migraine Caplets/Tablets/Geltabs .... ▣609
Goody's Body Pain Formula Powder .... ▣684
Goody's Extra Strength Headache Powders .... ▣611
Goody's Extra Strength Pain Relief Tablets .... ▣685
Percodan Tablets 1132
St. Joseph 81 mg Aspirin Chewable and Enteric Coated Tablets 1869

Astemizole (Zafirlukast is a known inhibitor of CYP3A4 in vitro; co-administration with other drugs known to be metabolized by this isoenzyme, such as astemizole, should be undertaken with reasonable clinical monitoring; no formal interaction studies have been conducted).
No products indexed under this heading.

Carbamazepine (Zafirlukast is a known inhibitor of the cytochrome P4502C9 isoenzyme; co-administration with other drugs known to be metabolized by this isoenzyme, such as carbamazepine, should be undertaken with caution; no formal interaction studies have been conducted). Products include:
Carbatrol Capsules 3171
Equetro Extended-Release Capsules 3180
Tegretol/Tegretol-XR 2295

Cisapride (Zafirlukast is a known inhibitor of CYP3A4 in vitro; co-administration with other drugs known to be metabolized by this isoenzyme, such as cisapride, should be undertaken with reasonable clinical monitoring; no formal interaction studies have been conducted).
No products indexed under this heading.

Cyclosporine (Zafirlukast is a known inhibitor of CYP3A4 in vitro; co-administration with other drugs known to be metabolized by this isoenzyme, such as cyclosporine, should be undertaken with reasonable clinical monitoring; no formal interaction studies have been conducted). Products include:
Gengraf Capsules 459
Neoral Oral Solution 2259
Neoral Soft Gelatin Capsules 2259
Restasis Ophthalmic Emulsion 575
Sandimmune 2275

Dyphylline (Rare cases of patients experiencing increased theophylline levels with or without clinical signs or symptoms of theophylline toxicity after addition of zafirlukast to an existing theophylline regimen have been reported; co-administration with liquid theophylline products has resulted in a decrease in the mean plasma levels of zafirlukast by approximately 30%).
No products indexed under this heading.

Erythromycin (Co-administration results in a decrease in the mean plasma levels of zafirlukast by approximately 40% due to decrease in zafirlukast bioavailability). Products include:
Ery-Tab Tablets 449
Erythromycin Base Filmtab Tablets 455
Erythromycin Delayed-Release Capsules, USP 457
PCE Dispertab Tablets 515

Erythromycin Estolate (Co-administration results in a decrease in the mean plasma levels of zafirlukast by approximately 40% due to decrease in zafirlukast bioavailability).
No products indexed under this heading.

Erythromycin Ethylsuccinate (Co-administration results in a decrease in the mean plasma levels of zafirlukast by approximately 40% due to decrease in zafirlukast bioavailability). Products include:
E.E.S. 451
EryPed 447

Erythromycin Gluceptate (Co-administration results in a decrease in the mean plasma levels of zafirlukast by approximately 40% due to decrease in zafirlukast bioavailability).
No products indexed under this heading.

Erythromycin Lactobionate (Co-administration results in a decrease in the mean plasma levels of zafirlukast by approximately 40% due to decrease in zafirlukast bioavailability).
No products indexed under this heading.

Erythromycin Stearate (Co-administration results in a decrease in the mean plasma levels of zafirlukast by approximately 40% due to decrease in zafirlukast bioavailability). Products include:
Erythrocin Stearate Filmtab Tablets 453

Felodipine (Zafirlukast is a known inhibitor of CYP3A4 in vitro; co-administration with other drugs known to be metabolized by this isoenzyme, such as dihydropyridine calcium channel blockers, should be undertaken with reasonable clinical monitoring; no formal interaction studies have been conducted).
No products indexed under this heading.

Fosphenytoin Sodium (Zafirlukast is a known inhibitor of the cytochrome P4502C9 isoenzyme; co-administration with other drugs known to be metabolized by this isoenzyme, such as phenytoin, should be undertaken with caution; no formal interaction studies have been conducted).
No products indexed under this heading.

Isradipine (Zafirlukast is a known inhibitor of CYP3A4 in vitro; co-administration with other drugs known to be metabolized by this isoenzyme, such as dihydropyridine calcium channel blockers, should be undertaken with reasonable clinical monitoring; no formal interaction studies have been conducted). Products include:
DynaCirc CR Tablets 2721

Nicardipine Hydrochloride (Zafirlukast is a known inhibitor of CYP3A4 in vitro; co-administration with other drugs known to be metabolized by this isoenzyme, such as dihydropyridine calcium channel blockers, should be undertaken with reasonable clinical monitoring; no formal interaction studies have been conducted). Products include:
Cardene I.V. 2497

Nifedipine (Zafirlukast is a known inhibitor of CYP3A4 in vitro; co-administration with other drugs known to be metabolized by this isoenzyme, such as dihydropyridine calcium channel blockers, should be undertaken with reasonable clinical monitoring; no formal interaction studies have been conducted). Products include:
Adalat CC Tablets 2964

Nimodipine (Zafirlukast is a known inhibitor of CYP3A4 in vitro; co-administration with other drugs known to be metabolized by this isoenzyme, such as dihydropyridine calcium channel blockers, should be undertaken with reasonable clinical monitoring; no formal interaction studies have been conducted). Products include:
Nimotop Capsules 749

Phenytoin (Zafirlukast is a known inhibitor of the cytochrome P4502C9 isoenzyme; co-administration with other drugs known to be metabolized by this isoenzyme, such as phenytoin, should be undertaken with caution; no formal interaction studies have been conducted).
No products indexed under this heading.

Phenytoin Sodium (Zafirlukast is a known inhibitor of the cytochrome P4502C9 isoenzyme; co-administration with other drugs known to be metabolized by this isoenzyme, such as phenytoin, should be undertaken with caution; no formal interaction studies have been conducted). Products include:
Phenytek Capsules 2160

Terfenadine (Co-administration results in a decrease in the mean Cmax (66%) and AUC (54%) of zafirlukast; no effect of zafirlukast on terfenadine plasma concentrations or ECG parameters).
No products indexed under this heading.

Theophylline (Rare cases of patients experiencing increased theophylline levels with or without clinical signs or symptoms of theophylline toxicity after addition of zafirlukast to an existing theophylline regimen have been reported; co-administration with liquid theophylline products has resulted in a decrease in the mean plasma levels of zafirlukast by approximately 30%).
No products indexed under this heading.

Theophylline Anhydrous (Rare cases of patients experiencing increased theophylline levels with or without clinical signs or symptoms of theophylline toxicity after addition of zafirlukast to an existing theophylline regimen have been reported; co-administration with liquid theophylline products has resulted in a decrease in the mean plasma levels of zafirlukast by approximately 30%). Products include:
Uniphyl Tablets 2710

Theophylline Calcium Salicylate (Rare cases of patients experiencing increased theophylline levels with or without clinical signs or symptoms of theophylline toxicity after addition of zafirlukast to an existing theophylline regimen have been reported; co-administration with liquid theophylline products has resulted in a decrease in the mean plasma levels of zafirlukast by approximately 30%).
No products indexed under this heading.

Theophylline Dihydroxypropyl (Glyceryl) (Rare cases of patients experiencing increased theophylline levels with or without clinical signs or symptoms of theophylline toxicity after addition of zafirlukast to an existing theophylline regimen have been reported; co-administration with liquid theophylline products has resulted in a decrease in the mean plasma levels of zafirlukast by approximately 30%).
No products indexed under this heading.

Theophylline Ethylenediamine (Rare cases of patients experiencing increased theophylline levels with or without clinical signs or symptoms of theophylline toxicity after addition of zafirlukast to an existing theophylline regimen have been reported; co-administration with liquid theophylline products has resulted in a decrease in the mean plasma levels of zafirlukast by approximately 30%).
No products indexed under this heading.

Theophylline Sodium Glycinate (Rare cases of patients experiencing increased theophylline levels with or without clinical signs or symptoms of theophylline toxicity after addition of zafirlukast to an existing theophylline regimen have been reported; co-administration with liquid theophylline products has resulted in a decrease in the mean plasma levels of zafirlukast by approximately 30%).
No products indexed under this heading.

Tolbutamide (Zafirlukast is a known inhibitor of the cytochrome P4502C9 isoenzyme; co-administration with other drugs known to be metabolized by this isoenzyme, such as tolbutamide, should be undertaken with caution; no formal interaction studies have been conducted).
No products indexed under this heading.

Warfarin Sodium (Co-administration results in a significant increase in the mean AUC and half-life of S-warfarin producing a clinically significant increase in prothrombin time). Products include:
Coumadin for Injection 898
Coumadin Tablets 898

Food Interactions

Food, unspecified (Co-administration with food reduces mean bioavailability by approximately 40%; patients should be instructed to take Accolate at least 1 hour before or 2 hours after meals).

ACCUNEB INHALATION SOLUTION

(Albuterol Sulfate) 1055
May interact with beta blockers, monoamine oxidase inhibitors, potassium-depleting diuretics, sympathomimetics, tricyclic antidepressants, and certain other agents. Compounds in these categories include:

Acebutolol Hydrochloride (Co-administration with beta blockers inhibits the effects of each other).
No products indexed under this heading.

Albuterol (Co-administration with other sympathomimetic agents increases the risk of adverse cardiovascular effects). Products include:
Proventil Inhalation Aerosol 3053

Amitriptyline Hydrochloride (Co-administration with tricyclic antidepressants can potentiate the action of albuterol on the cardiovascular system).
No products indexed under this heading.

Amoxapine (Co-administration with tricyclic antidepressants can potentiate the action of albuterol on the cardiovascular system).
No products indexed under this heading.

Atenolol (Co-administration with beta blockers inhibits the effects of each other).
No products indexed under this heading.

Bendroflumethiazide (Co-administration with non-potassium sparing diuretics can result in acute worsening of ECG changes and/or hypokalemia, especially when recommended dose of the beta agonist is exceeded; clinical significance of this interaction is unknown).
No products indexed under this heading.

Betaxolol Hydrochloride (Co-administration with beta blockers inhibits the effects of each other). Products include:
Betoptic S Ophthalmic Suspension 558

Bisoprolol Fumarate (Co-administration with beta blockers inhibits the effects of each other).
No products indexed under this heading.

Bumetanide (Co-administration with non-potassium sparing diuretics can result in acute worsening of ECG changes and/or hypokalemia, especially when recommended dose of the beta agonist is exceeded; clinical significance of this interaction is unknown). Products include:
Bumex Tablets 2746

Carteolol Hydrochloride (Co-administration with beta blockers inhibits the effects of each other). Products include:
Carteolol Hydrochloride Ophthalmic Solution USP, 1%...... ⊙249

Chlorothiazide (Co-administration with non-potassium sparing diuretics can result in acute worsening of ECG changes and/or hypokalemia, especially when recommended dose of the beta agonist is exceeded; clinical significance of this interaction is unknown). Products include:
Diuril Oral Suspension 1954

Chlorothiazide Sodium (Co-administration with non-potassium sparing diuretics can result in acute worsening of ECG changes and/or hypokalemia, especially when recommended dose of the beta agonist is exceeded; clinical significance of this interaction is unknown). Products include:
Diuril Sodium Intravenous 2467

Clomipramine Hydrochloride (Co-administration with tricyclic antidepressants can potentiate the action of albuterol on the cardiovascular system).
No products indexed under this heading.

Desipramine Hydrochloride (Co-administration with tricyclic antidepressants can potentiate the action of albuterol on the cardiovascular system).
No products indexed under this heading.

Digoxin (Mean decreases of 16% to 22% in serum digoxin levels were demonstrated after single dose IV and oral albuterol, respectively; the clinical significance of this interaction is unknown). Products include:
Lanoxicaps Capsules 1490
Lanoxin Injection 1494
Lanoxin Injection Pediatric 1497
Lanoxin Tablets 1500

Dobutamine Hydrochloride (Co-administration with other sympathomimetic agents increases the risk of adverse cardiovascular effects).
No products indexed under this heading.

Dopamine Hydrochloride (Co-administration with other sympathomimetic agents increases the risk of adverse cardiovascular effects).
No products indexed under this heading.

Doxepin Hydrochloride (Co-administration with tricyclic antidepressants can potentiate the action of albuterol on the cardiovascular system).
No products indexed under this heading.

Ephedrine Hydrochloride (Co-administration with other sympathomimetic agents increases the risk of adverse cardiovascular effects).
No products indexed under this heading.

Ephedrine Sulfate (Co-administration with other sympathomimetic agents increases the risk of adverse cardiovascular effects).
No products indexed under this heading.

Ephedrine Tannate (Co-administration with other sympathomimetic agents increases the risk of adverse cardiovascular effects).
No products indexed under this heading.

Epinephrine (Co-administration with other sympathomimetic agents increases the risk of adverse cardiovascular effects). Products include:
EpiPen 1061
Primatene Mist .... ▣719
Twinject 0.15 3379
Twinject 0.3 3378

Epinephrine Bitartrate (Co-administration with other sympathomimetic agents increases the risk of adverse cardiovascular effects).
No products indexed under this heading.

Epinephrine Hydrochloride (Co-administration with other sympathomimetic agents increases the risk of adverse cardiovascular effects).
No products indexed under this heading.

Esmolol Hydrochloride (Co-administration with beta blockers inhibits the effects of each other).
No products indexed under this heading.

Ethacrynic Acid (Co-administration with non-potassium sparing diuretics can result in acute worsening of ECG changes and/or hypokalemia, especially when recommended dose of the beta agonist is exceeded; clinical significance of this interaction is unknown). Products include:
Edecrin Tablets 1959

Furosemide (Co-administration with non-potassium sparing diuretics can result in acute worsening of ECG changes and/or hypokalemia, especially when recommended dose of the beta agonist is exceeded; clinical significance of this interaction is unknown). Products include:
Furosemide Tablets 2154

Hydrochlorothiazide (Co-administration with non-potassium sparing diuretics can result in acute worsening of ECG changes and/or hypokalemia, especially when recommended dose of the beta agonist is exceeded; clinical significance of this interaction is unknown). Products include:
Aldoril Tablets 1910
Atacand HCT 651
Avalide Tablets 888
Avalide Tablets 2874
Benicar HCT Tablets 1044
Diovan HCT Tablets 2196
Dyazide Capsules 1423
Hyzaar 50-12.5 Tablets 1990
Hyzaar 100-12.5 Tablets 1990
Hyzaar 100-25 Tablets 1990
Lopressor HCT 50/25 Tablets 2241
Lopressor HCT 100/25 Tablets 2241
Lopressor HCT 100/50 Tablets 2241
Lotensin HCT Tablets 2246
Micardis HCT Tablets 856
Moduretic Tablets 2028
Prinzide Tablets 2056
Teveten HCT Tablets 1737
Timolide Tablets 2086
Uniretic Tablets 3100

Hydroflumethiazide (Co-administration with non-potassium sparing diuretics can result in acute worsening of ECG changes and/or hypokalemia, especially when recommended dose of the beta agonist is exceeded; clinical significance of this interaction is unknown).
No products indexed under this heading.

Imipramine Hydrochloride (Co-administration with tricyclic antidepressants can potentiate the action of albuterol on the cardiovascular system).
No products indexed under this heading.

Imipramine Pamoate (Co-administration with tricyclic antidepressants can potentiate the action of albuterol on the cardiovascular system).
No products indexed under this heading.

Isocarboxazid (Co-administration with MAO inhibitors can potentiate the action of albuterol on the cardiovascular system).
No products indexed under this heading.

Isoproterenol Hydrochloride (Co-administration with other sympathomimetic agents increases the risk of adverse cardiovascular effects).
No products indexed under this heading.

Isoproterenol Sulfate (Co-administration with other sympathomimetic agents increases the risk of adverse cardiovascular effects).
No products indexed under this heading.

Labetalol Hydrochloride (Co-administration with beta blockers inhibits the effects of each other).
No products indexed under this heading.

Levalbuterol Hydrochloride (Co-administration with other sympathomimetic agents increases the risk of adverse cardiovascular effects). Products include:
- Xopenex Inhalation Solution 3146
- Xopenex Inhalation Solution Concentrate 3150

Levobunolol Hydrochloride (Co-administration with beta blockers inhibits the effects of each other). Products include:
- Betagan Ophthalmic Solution, USP .... ⊙220

Maprotiline Hydrochloride (Co-administration with tricyclic antidepressants can potentiate the action of albuterol on the cardiovascular system).
No products indexed under this heading.

Metaproterenol Sulfate (Co-administration with other sympathomimetic agents increases the risk of adverse cardiovascular effects). Products include:
- Alupent Inhalation Aerosol 826

Metaraminol Bitartrate (Co-administration with other sympathomimetic agents increases the risk of adverse cardiovascular effects).
No products indexed under this heading.

Methoxamine Hydrochloride (Co-administration with other sympathomimetic agents increases the risk of adverse cardiovascular effects).
No products indexed under this heading.

Methyclothiazide (Co-administration with non-potassium sparing diuretics can result in acute worsening of ECG changes and/or hypokalemia, especially when recommended dose of the beta agonist is exceeded; clinical significance of this interaction is unknown).
No products indexed under this heading.

Metipranolol Hydrochloride (Co-administration with beta blockers inhibits the effects of each other).
No products indexed under this heading.

Metoprolol Succinate (Co-administration with beta blockers inhibits the effects of each other). Products include:
- Toprol-XL Tablets 668

Metoprolol Tartrate (Co-administration with beta blockers inhibits the effects of each other). Products include:
- Lopressor Injection 2238
- Lopressor Tablets 2238
- Lopressor HCT 50/25 Tablets 2241
- Lopressor HCT 100/25 Tablets 2241
- Lopressor HCT 100/50 Tablets 2241

Moclobemide (Co-administration with MAO inhibitors can potentiate the action of albuterol on the cardiovascular system).
No products indexed under this heading.

Nadolol (Co-administration with beta blockers inhibits the effects of each other). Products include:
- Nadolol Tablets 2159

Norepinephrine Bitartrate (Co-administration with other sympathomimetic agents increases the risk of adverse cardiovascular effects).
No products indexed under this heading.

Nortriptyline Hydrochloride (Co-administration with tricyclic antidepressants can potentiate the action of albuterol on the cardiovascular system).
No products indexed under this heading.

Pargyline Hydrochloride (Co-administration with MAO inhibitors can potentiate the action of albuterol on the cardiovascular system).
No products indexed under this heading.

Penbutolol Sulfate (Co-administration with beta blockers inhibits the effects of each other).
No products indexed under this heading.

Phenelzine Sulfate (Co-administration with MAO inhibitors can potentiate the action of albuterol on the cardiovascular system).
No products indexed under this heading.

Phenylephrine Bitartrate (Co-administration with other sympathomimetic agents increases the risk of adverse cardiovascular effects).
No products indexed under this heading.

Phenylephrine Hydrochloride (Co-administration with other sympathomimetic agents increases the risk of adverse cardiovascular effects). Products include:
- Comtrex Maximum Strength Non-Drowsy Cold & Cough Caplets .... ▣725
- Comtrex Maximum Strength Day/Night Severe Cold & Sinus Caplets - Day Formulation .... ▣725
- Comtrex Maximum Strength Day/Night Severe Cold & Sinus Caplets - Night Formulation .... ▣725
- Contac Cold and Flu Maximum Strength Caplets .... ▣728
- Contac Cold and Flu Day and Night Caplets (Day Formulation Only) .... ▣727
- Contac Cold and Flu Day and Night Caplets (Night Formulation Only) .... ▣727
- Contac Cold and Flu Non-Drowsy Caplets .... ▣728
- Contac-D Cold Non-Drowsy Tablets .... ▣729
- Children's Dimetapp Cold & Allergy Elixir .... ▣730
- Children's Dimetapp Cold & Allergy Chewable Tablets .... ▣730
- Children's Dimetapp DM Cold & Cough Elixir .... ▣731
- Toddler's Dimetapp Cold and Cough Drops .... ▣732
- Excedrin Sinus Headache Caplets/Tablets .... ▣610
- 4-Way Fast Acting Nasal Spray .... ▣775
- 4-Way Menthol Nasal Spray .... ▣775
- Preparation H Maximum Strength Cream .... ▣666
- Preparation H Cooling Gel .... ▣666
- Preparation H .... ▣666
- Refenesen PE Caplets .... ▣721
- Robitussin Cough & Allergy Syrup .... ▣736
- Robitussin Cough & Cold Nighttime Liquid .... ▣736
- Robitussin Cough, Cold & Flu Nighttime Liquid .... ▣738
- Robitussin Head & Chest Congestion PE Syrup .... ▣739
- Robitussin Pediatric Cough & Cold Nighttime Liquid .... ▣736
- TheraFlu Cold & Cough Hot Liquid .... ▣740
- TheraFlu Cold & Sore Throat Hot Liquid .... ▣741
- TheraFlu Flu & Sore Throat Hot Liquid .... ▣742
- TheraFlu Daytime Severe Cold Hot Liquid .... ▣742
- TheraFlu Nighttime Severe Cold Hot Liquid .... ▣740
- TheraFlu Warming Relief Daytime Severe Cold .... ▣743
- TheraFlu Warming Relief Nighttime Severe Cold .... ▣743
- Triaminic Chest & Nasal Congestion Liquid .... ▣746
- Triaminic Cold & Allergy Liquid .... ▣746
- Triaminic Daytime Cold & Cough Liquid .... ▣745
- Triaminic Nighttime Cold & Cough Liquid .... ▣746
- Triaminic Thin Strips Cold .... ▣748
- Triaminic Thin Strips Cold & Cough .... ▣778
- Triaminic Infant Thin Strips Decongestant .... ▣747
- Triaminic Infant Thin Strips Decongestant Plus Cough .... ▣747
- Children's Tylenol Plus Flu Oral Suspension .... ▣749
- Tylenol Cold Head Congestion Daytime Caplets with Cool Burst and Gelcaps .... ▣750
- Tylenol Cold Multi-Symptom Daytime Liquid .... ▣752
- Tylenol Cold Multi-Symptom Severe Daytime Liquid .... ▣752
- Concentrated Tylenol Infants' Drops Plus Cold & Cough .... ▣754
- Tylenol Allergy Multi-Symptom Caplets with Cool Burst and Gelcaps 1872
- Tylenol Allergy Multi-Symptom Nighttime Caplets with Cool Burst 1872
- Children's Tylenol Plus Cold Suspension Liquid 1879
- Children's Tylenol Plus Cold & Allergy Suspension Liquid 1878
- Children's Tylenol Plus Flu Suspension Liquid 1881
- Children's Tylenol Plus Multi-Symptom Cold Suspension Liquid 1879
- Tylenol Cold Head Congestion Daytime Caplets with Cool Burst 1873
- Tylenol Cold Head Congestion Nighttime Caplets with Cool Burst 1873
- Tylenol Cold Head Congestion Severe Caplets with Cool Burst 1873
- Tylenol Cold Multi-Symptom Daytime Caplets with Cool Burst and Gelcaps 1874
- Tylenol Cold Multi-Symptom Daytime Liquid with Citrus Burst 1874
- Tylenol Cold Multi-Symptom Nighttime Caplets with Cool Burst 1874
- Tylenol Cold Multi-Symptom Nighttime Liquid with Cool Burst 1874
- Tylenol Cold Multi-Symptom Severe Caplets with Cool Burst 1874
- Tylenol Cold Multi-Symptom Severe Daytime Liquid with Citrus Burst 1874
- Tylenol Sinus Congestion & Pain Daytime Caplets with Cool Burst and Gelcaps 1876
- Tylenol Sinus Congestion & Pain Nighttime Caplets with Cool Burst 1876
- Tylenol Sinus Congestion & Pain Severe Caplets with Cool Burst 1876
- Vicks 44D Cough & Head Congestion Relief Liquid .... ▣760
- Vicks DayQuil LiquiCaps/Liquid Multi-Symptom Cold/Flu Relief .... ▣761
- Zicam Cough Plus D Cough Spray .... ▣767

Phenylephrine Tannate (Co-administration with other sympathomimetic agents increases the risk of adverse cardiovascular effects).
No products indexed under this heading.

Phenylpropanolamine Hydrochloride (Co-administration with other sympathomimetic agents increases the risk of adverse cardiovascular effects).
No products indexed under this heading.

Pindolol (Co-administration with beta blockers inhibits the effects of each other).
No products indexed under this heading.

Pirbuterol Acetate (Co-administration with other sympathomimetic agents increases the risk of adverse cardiovascular effects). Products include:
- Maxair Autohaler 1852

Polythiazide (Co-administration with non-potassium sparing diuretics can result in acute worsening of ECG changes and/or hypokalemia, especially when recommended dose of the beta agonist is exceeded; clinical significance of this interaction is unknown).
No products indexed under this heading.

Procarbazine Hydrochloride (Co-administration with MAO inhibitors can potentiate the action of albuterol on the cardiovascular system). Products include:
- Matulane Capsules 3191

Propranolol Hydrochloride (Co-administration with beta blockers inhibits the effects of each other). Products include:
- Inderal LA Long-Acting Capsules 3429
- InnoPran XL Capsules 2723

Protriptyline Hydrochloride (Co-administration with tricyclic antidepressants can potentiate the action of albuterol on the cardiovascular system).
No products indexed under this heading.

Pseudoephedrine Hydrochloride (Co-administration with other sympathomimetic agents increases the risk of adverse cardiovascular effects). Products include:
- Advil Allergy Sinus Caplets .... ▣770
- Advil Cold & Sinus .... ▣723
- Advil Multi-Symptom Cold Caplets .... ▣770
- Aleve Cold & Sinus Caplets 744
- Allegra-D 12 Hour Extended-Release Tablets 2846

Allegra-D 24 Hour Extended-Release Tablets 2849
BC Cold Powder 677
Comtrex Maximum Strength Cold & Cough Day/Night Caplets - Day Formulation 726
Comtrex Maximum Strength Cold & Cough Day/Night Caplets - Night Formulation 726
Children's Motrin Cold Oral Suspension 1867
Mucinex D Extended-Release Bi-Layer Tablets 776
Robitussin Cough & Cold CF Liquid 735
Robitussin Cough & Cold Pediatric Drops 735
Tylenol Sinus Congestion & Pain Nighttime Caplets with Cool Burst 778
Tylenol Cold Severe Congestion Non-Drowsy Caplets with Cool Burst 1874
Tylenol Sinus Severe Congestion Caplets with Cool Burst 1876
Vicks 44D Cough & Head Congestion Relief Liquid 2679
Vicks 44M Cough, Cold & Flu Relief Liquid 2680
Vicks DayQuil Multi-Symptom Cold/Flu Relief LiquiCaps 2678
Vicks DayQuil Multi-Symptom Cold/Flu Relief Liquid 2678
Vicks NyQuil Multi-Symptom Cold/Flu Relief Liquid 2681
Vicks NyQuil Multi-Symptom Cold/Flu Relief LiquiCaps 2681
Children's Vicks NyQuil Cold/Cough Relief Liquid 2680
Zyrtec-D 12 Hour Extended Release Tablets 2597

Pseudoephedrine Sulfate (Co-administration with other sympathomimetic agents increases the risk of adverse cardiovascular effects). Products include:
Alavert Allergy & Sinus D-12 Hour Tablets 771
Clarinex-D 24-Hour Extended-Release Tablets 2998
Claritin-D Non-Drowsy 12 Hour Tablets 772
Claritin-D Non-Drowsy 24 Hour Tablets 772

Salmeterol Xinafoate (Co-administration with other sympathomimetic agents increases the risk of adverse cardiovascular effects). Products include:
Advair Diskus 100/50 1308
Advair Diskus 250/50 1308
Advair Diskus 500/50 1308
Advair HFA Inhalation Aerosol 1318
Serevent Diskus 1568

Selegiline Hydrochloride (Co-administration with MAO inhibitors can potentiate the action of albuterol on the cardiovascular system). Products include:
Eldepryl Capsules 3208
Zelapar Tablets 3372

Sotalol Hydrochloride (Co-administration with beta blockers inhibits the effects of each other).
No products indexed under this heading.

Terbutaline Sulfate (Co-administration with other sympathomimetic agents increases the risk of adverse cardiovascular effects).
No products indexed under this heading.

Timolol Hemihydrate (Co-administration with beta blockers inhibits the effects of each other). Products include:
Betimol Ophthalmic Solution 3382
Betimol Ophthalmic Solution .... ⊙ 295

Timolol Maleate (Co-administration with beta blockers inhibits the effects of each other). Products include:
Blocadren Tablets 1916
Cosopt Sterile Ophthalmic Solution 1931
Timolide Tablets 2086
Timoptic Sterile Ophthalmic Solution 2088
Timoptic in Ocudose 2091
Timoptic-XE Sterile Ophthalmic Gel Forming Solution 2092

Torsemide (Co-administration with non-potassium sparing diuretics can result in acute worsening of ECG changes and/or hypokalemia, especially when recommended dose of the beta agonist is exceeded; clinical significance of this interaction is unknown). Products include:
Demadex Injection 2759
Demadex Tablets 2759

Tranylcypromine Sulfate (Co-administration with MAO inhibitors can potentiate the action of albuterol on the cardiovascular system). Products include:
Parnate Tablets 1527

Trimipramine Maleate (Co-administration with tricyclic antidepressants can potentiate the action of albuterol on the cardiovascular system).
No products indexed under this heading.

ACCUTANE CAPSULES

(Isotretinoin) 2731
May interact with corticosteroids, phenytoin, tetracyclines, and certain other agents. Compounds in these categories include:

Betamethasone Acetate (Systemic corticosteroids are known to cause osteoporosis; caution is advised if used concurrently because of potential interactive effect on bone loss between systemic corticosteroids and Accutane).
No products indexed under this heading.

Betamethasone Sodium Phosphate (Systemic corticosteroids are known to cause osteoporosis; caution is advised if used concurrently because of potential interactive effect on bone loss between systemic corticosteroids and Accutane).
No products indexed under this heading.

Cortisone Acetate (Systemic corticosteroids are known to cause osteoporosis; caution is advised if used concurrently because of potential interactive effect on bone loss between systemic corticosteroids and Accutane).
No products indexed under this heading.

Demeclocycline Hydrochloride (Concomitant treatment with Accutane and tetracyclines should be avoided because Accutane is associated with a number of cases of pseudotumor cerebri, some of which involved concomitant use of tetracyclines).
No products indexed under this heading.

Dexamethasone (Systemic corticosteroids are known to cause osteoporosis; caution is advised if used concurrently because of potential interactive effect on bone loss between systemic corticosteroids and Accutane). Products include:
Ciprodex Otic Suspension 559
Decadron Tablets 1951
TobraDex Ophthalmic Ointment 562
TobraDex Ophthalmic Suspension 563

Dexamethasone Acetate (Systemic corticosteroids are known to cause osteoporosis; caution is advised if used concurrently because of potential interactive effect on bone loss between systemic corticosteroids and Accutane).
No products indexed under this heading.

Dexamethasone Sodium Phosphate (Systemic corticosteroids are known to cause osteoporosis; caution is advised if used concurrently because of potential interactive effect on bone loss between systemic corticosteroids and Accutane).
No products indexed under this heading.

Doxycycline Calcium (Concomitant treatment with Accutane and tetracyclines should be avoided because Accutane is associated with a number of cases of pseudotumor cerebri, some of which involved concomitant use of tetracyclines).
No products indexed under this heading.

Doxycycline Hyclate (Concomitant treatment with Accutane and tetracyclines should be avoided because Accutane is associated with a number of cases of pseudotumor cerebri, some of which involved concomitant use of tetracyclines).
No products indexed under this heading.

Doxycycline Monohydrate (Concomitant treatment with Accutane and tetracyclines should be avoided because Accutane is associated with a number of cases of pseudotumor cerebri, some of which involved concomitant use of tetracyclines). Products include:
Oracea Capsules 1000

Fludrocortisone Acetate (Systemic corticosteroids are known to cause osteoporosis; caution is advised if used concurrently because of potential interactive effect on bone loss between systemic corticosteroids and Accutane).
No products indexed under this heading.

Fosphenytoin Sodium (Phenytoin is known to cause osteomalacia; caution is advised if used concurrently because of potential interactive effect on bone loss between phenytoin and Accutane).
No products indexed under this heading.

Hydrocortisone (Systemic corticosteroids are known to cause osteoporosis; caution is advised if used concurrently because of potential interactive effect on bone loss between systemic corticosteroids and Accutane). Products include:
Colocort Rectal Suspension, USP (Retention) 100 mg/60 mL 2476
Hydrocortone Tablets 1989
Preparation H Hydrocortisone Cream 646

Hydrocortisone Acetate (Systemic corticosteroids are known to cause osteoporosis; caution is advised if used concurrently because of potential interactive effect on bone loss between systemic corticosteroids and Accutane). Products include:
Analpram-HC 1159
Pramosone 1161
ProctoFoam-HC 3099

Hydrocortisone Sodium Phosphate (Systemic corticosteroids are known to cause osteoporosis; caution is advised if used concurrently because of potential interactive effect on bone loss between systemic corticosteroids and Accutane).
No products indexed under this heading.

Hydrocortisone Sodium Succinate (Systemic corticosteroids are known to cause osteoporosis; caution is advised if used concurrently because of potential interactive effect on bone loss between systemic corticosteroids and Accutane).
No products indexed under this heading.

Hypericum (Avoid St. John's Wort due to a possible interaction based on reports of breakthrough bleeding being reported on oral contraceptives shortly after starting St. John's Wort. Pregnancies have been reported by users of combined hormonal contraceptives who also used some form of St. John's Wort). Products include:
Satiete Tablets 832

Methacycline Hydrochloride (Concomitant treatment with Accutane and tetracyclines should be avoided because Accutane is associated with a number of cases of pseudotumor cerebri, some of which involved concomitant use of tetracyclines).
No products indexed under this heading.

Methylprednisolone Acetate (Systemic corticosteroids are known to cause osteoporosis; caution is advised if used concurrently because of potential interactive effect on bone loss between systemic corticosteroids and Accutane). Products include:
Depo-Medrol Injectable Suspension 2617
Depo-Medrol Single-Dose Vial 2619

Methylprednisolone Sodium Succinate (Systemic corticosteroids are known to cause osteoporosis; caution is advised if used concurrently because of potential interactive effect on bone loss between systemic corticosteroids and Accutane).
No products indexed under this heading.

Minocycline Hydrochloride (Concomitant treatment with Accutane and tetracyclines should be avoided because Accutane is associated with a number of cases of pseudotumor cerebri, some of which involved concomitant use of tetracyclines). Products include:
Solodyn Extended Release Tablets 1890

Norethindrone (Microdosed progesterone preparations (minipills) may be an inadequate method of contraception during Accutane therapy). Products include:
Ortho Micronor Tablets 2426

Oxytetracycline Hydrochloride (Concomitant treatment with Accutane and tetracyclines should be avoided because Accutane is associated with a number of cases of pseudotumor cerebri, some of which involved concomitant use of tetracyclines).
No products indexed under this heading.

Phenytoin (Phenytoin is known to cause osteomalacia; caution is advised if used concurrently because of potential interactive effect on bone loss between phenytoin and Accutane).
No products indexed under this heading.

Phenytoin Sodium (Phenytoin is known to cause osteomalacia; caution is advised if used concurrently because of potential interactive effect on bone loss between phenytoin and Accutane). Products include:
Phenytek Capsules 2160

Prednisolone Acetate (Systemic corticosteroids are known to cause osteoporosis; caution is advised if used concurrently because of potential interactive effect on bone loss between systemic corticosteroids and Accutane). Products include:
Blephamide Ophthalmic Ointment 568
Blephamide Ophthalmic Suspension.................................. 569
Poly-Pred Ophthalmic Suspension .... ⊙ 233
Pred Forte Ophthalmic Suspension .... ⊙ 235
Pred Mild Ophthalmic Suspension .... ⊙ 238
Pred-G Ophthalmic Ointment .... ⊙ 237
Pred-G Ophthalmic Suspension ...... ⊙ 236

Prednisolone Sodium Phosphate (Systemic corticosteroids are known to cause osteoporosis; caution is advised if used concurrently because of potential interactive effect on bone loss between systemic corticosteroids and Accutane).
No products indexed under this heading.

Prednisolone Tebutate (Systemic corticosteroids are known to cause osteoporosis; caution is advised if used concurrently because of potential interactive effect on bone loss between systemic corticosteroids and Accutane).
No products indexed under this heading.

Prednisone (Systemic corticosteroids are known to cause osteoporosis; caution is advised if used concurrently because of potential interactive effect on bone loss between systemic corticosteroids and Accutane).
No products indexed under this heading.

Tetracycline Hydrochloride (Concomitant treatment with Accutane and tetracyclines should be avoided because Accutane is associated with a number of cases of pseudotumor cerebri, some of which involved concomitant use of tetracyclines).
No products indexed under this heading.

Triamcinolone (Systemic corticosteroids are known to cause osteoporosis; caution is advised if used concurrently because of potential interactive effect on bone loss between systemic corticosteroids and Accutane).
No products indexed under this heading.

Triamcinolone Acetonide (Systemic corticosteroids are known to cause osteoporosis; caution is advised if used concurrently because of potential interactive effect on bone loss between systemic corticosteroids and Accutane). Products include:
Azmacort Inhalation Aerosol 1726
Nasacort AQ Nasal Spray 2922

Triamcinolone Diacetate (Systemic corticosteroids are known to cause osteoporosis; caution is advised if used concurrently because of potential interactive effect on bone loss between systemic corticosteroids and Accutane).
No products indexed under this heading.

Triamcinolone Hexacetonide (Systemic corticosteroids are known to cause osteoporosis; caution is advised if used concurrently because of potential interactive effect on bone loss between systemic corticosteroids and Accutane).
No products indexed under this heading.

Vitamin A (Additive Vitamin A toxicity). Products include:
Visutein Capsules 3329

ACCUZYME DEBRIDING OINTMENT

(Papain, Urea) 1662
None cited in PDR database.

ACCUZYME SE SPRAY EMULSION

(Papain, Urea) 1662
May interact with:

Heavy metal salts, unspecified (Papain may be inactivated by the salts of heavy metals).
No products indexed under this heading.

Hydrogen Peroxide (May inactivate papain).
No products indexed under this heading.

ACEON TABLETS (2 MG, 4 MG, 8 MG)

(Perindopril Erbumine) 3194
May interact with diuretics, lithium preparations, potassium preparations, potassium sparing diuretics, and certain other agents. Compounds in these categories include:

Amiloride Hydrochloride (Co-administration of perindopril with potassium-sparing diuretics may increase the risk of hyperkalemia). Products include:
Midamor Tablets 2026
Moduretic Tablets 2028

Bendroflumethiazide (Patients on diuretics, and especially those started recently, may occasionally experience an excessive reduction in blood pressure after initiation of perindopril therapy; co-administration has resulted in reduced bioavailability of perindopril).
No products indexed under this heading.

Bumetanide (Patients on diuretics, and especially those started recently, may occasionally experience an excessive reduction in blood pressure after initiation of perindopril therapy; co-administration has resulted in reduced bioavailability of perindopril). Products include:
Bumex Tablets 2746

Chlorothiazide (Patients on diuretics, and especially those started recently, may occasionally experience an excessive reduction in blood pressure after initiation of perindopril therapy; co-administration has resulted in reduced bioavailability of perindopril). Products include:
Diuril Oral Suspension 1954

Chlorothiazide Sodium (Patients on diuretics, and especially those started recently, may occasionally experience an excessive reduction in blood pressure after initiation of perindopril therapy; co-administration has resulted in reduced bioavailability of perindopril). Products include:
Diuril Sodium Intravenous 2467

Chlorthalidone (Patients on diuretics, and especially those started recently, may occasionally experience an excessive reduction in blood pressure after initiation of perindopril therapy; co-administration has resulted in reduced bioavailability of perindopril). Products include:
Clorpres Tablets 2153

Cyclosporine (Co-administration of perindopril with other drugs capable of increasing serum potassium, such as cyclosporine, may increase the risk of hyperkalemia). Products include:
Gengraf Capsules 459
Neoral Oral Solution 2259
Neoral Soft Gelatin Capsules 2259
Restasis Ophthalmic Emulsion 575
Sandimmune 2275

Ethacrynic Acid (Patients on diuretics, and especially those started recently, may occasionally experience an excessive reduction in blood pressure after initiation of perindopril therapy; co-administration has resulted in reduced bioavailability of perindopril). Products include:
Edecrin Tablets 1959

Furosemide (Patients on diuretics, and especially those started recently, may occasionally experience an excessive reduction in blood pressure after initiation of perindopril therapy; co-administration has resulted in reduced bioavailability of perindopril). Products include:
Furosemide Tablets 2154

Gentamicin Sulfate (Animal data has suggested the possibility of an interaction between gentamicin and perindopril; co-administration should proceed with caution). Products include:
Garamycin Injectable 3014
Pred-G Ophthalmic Ointment .... ⊙ 237
Pred-G Ophthalmic Suspension ...... ⊙ 236

Heparin Sodium (Co-administration of perindopril with other drugs capable of increasing serum potassium, such as heparin, may increase the risk of hyperkalemia).
No products indexed under this heading.

Hydrochlorothiazide (Patients on diuretics, and especially those started recently, may occasionally experience an excessive reduction in blood pressure after initiation of perindopril therapy; co-administration has resulted in reduced bioavailability of perindopril). Products include:
Aldoril Tablets 1910
Atacand HCT 651
Avalide Tablets 888
Avalide Tablets 2874
Benicar HCT Tablets 1044
Diovan HCT Tablets 2196
Dyazide Capsules 1423
Hyzaar 50-12.5 Tablets 1990
Hyzaar 100-12.5 Tablets 1990
Hyzaar 100-25 Tablets 1990
Lopressor HCT 50/25 Tablets 2241
Lopressor HCT 100/25 Tablets 2241
Lopressor HCT 100/50 Tablets 2241
Lotensin HCT Tablets 2246
Micardis HCT Tablets 856
Moduretic Tablets 2028
Prinzide Tablets 2056
Teveten HCT Tablets 1737
Timolide Tablets 2086
Uniretic Tablets 3100

Hydroflumethiazide (Patients on diuretics, and especially those started recently, may occasionally experience an excessive reduction in blood pressure after initiation of perindopril therapy; co-administration has resulted in reduced bioavailability of perindopril).
No products indexed under this heading.

Indapamide (Patients on diuretics, and especially those started recently, may occasionally experience an excessive reduction in blood pressure after initiation of perindopril therapy; co-administration has resulted in reduced bioavailability of perindopril). Products include:
Indapamide Tablets 2156

Indomethacin (Co-administration of perindopril with other drugs capable of increasing serum potassium, such as indomethacin, may increase the risk of hyperkalemia). Products include:
Indocin 1995

Lithium (Co-administration of ACE inhibitors and lithium has resulted in increased serum lithium levels and symptoms of lithium toxicity).
No products indexed under this heading.

Lithium Carbonate (Co-administration of ACE inhibitors and lithium has resulted in increased serum lithium levels and symptoms of lithium toxicity). Products include:
Lithobid Tablets 1692

Lithium Citrate (Co-administration of ACE inhibitors and lithium has resulted in increased serum lithium levels and symptoms of lithium toxicity).
No products indexed under this heading.

Methyclothiazide (Patients on diuretics, and especially those started recently, may occasionally experience an excessive reduction in blood pressure after initiation of perindopril therapy; co-administration has resulted in reduced bioavailability of perindopril).
No products indexed under this heading.

Metolazone (Patients on diuretics, and especially those started recently, may occasionally experience an excessive reduction in blood pressure after initiation of perindopril therapy; co-administration has resulted in reduced bioavailability of perindopril).
No products indexed under this heading.

Polythiazide (Patients on diuretics, and especially those started recently, may occasionally experience an excessive reduction in blood pressure after initiation of perindopril therapy; co-administration has resulted in reduced bioavailability of perindopril).
No products indexed under this heading.

Potassium Acid Phosphate (Co-administration of perindopril with potassium supplements may increase the risk of hyperkalemia). Products include:
K-Phos Original (Sodium Free) Tablets 760

Potassium Bicarbonate (Co-administration of perindopril with potassium supplements may increase the risk of hyperkalemia).
No products indexed under this heading.

Potassium Chloride (Co-administration of perindopril with potassium supplements may increase the risk of hyperkalemia). Products include:
- Colyte with Flavor Packs for Oral Solution 3088
- HalfLytely and Bisacodyl Tablets Bowel Prep Kit with Flavors Packs 881
- K-Dur Extended-Relase Tablets 3033
- K-Lor Oral Solution 474
- K-Tab Tablets 475
- MoviPrep Oral Solution 2839
- TriLyte with Flavor Packs for Oral Solution 3100

Potassium Citrate (Co-administration of perindopril with potassium supplements may increase the risk of hyperkalemia). Products include:
- Urocit-K Tablets 2144

Potassium Gluconate (Co-administration of perindopril with potassium supplements may increase the risk of hyperkalemia).
No products indexed under this heading.

Potassium Phosphate (Co-administration of perindopril with potassium supplements may increase the risk of hyperkalemia). Products include:
- K-Phos Neutral Tablets 760

Spironolactone (Co-administration of perindopril with potassium-sparing diuretics may increase the risk of hyperkalemia).
No products indexed under this heading.

Torsemide (Patients on diuretics, and especially those started recently, may occasionally experience an excessive reduction in blood pressure after initiation of perindopril therapy; co-administration has resulted in reduced bioavailability of perindopril). Products include:
- Demadex Injection 2759
- Demadex Tablets 2759

Triamterene (Co-administration of perindopril with potassium-sparing diuretics may increase the risk of hyperkalemia). Products include:
- Dyazide Capsules 1423
- Dyrenium Capsules 3400

Food Interactions

Food, unspecified (The presence of food in the GI tract does not affect the rate or extent of absorption of perindopril but reduces bioavailability of perindoprilat by about 35%; in clinical trials, perindopril was generally administered in a non-fasting state).

ACETADOTE INJECTION

(Acetylcysteine) 1031
None cited in PDR database.

ACIPHEX TABLETS

(Rabeprazole Sodium) 1090
May interact with iron containing oral preparations and certain other agents. Compounds in these categories include:

Bacampicillin Hydrochloride (Rabeprazole produces sustained inhibition of gastric acid secretion; rabeprazole may interfere with the absorption of certain drugs, such as bacampicillin, where gastric pH is an important determinant of the bioavailability).
No products indexed under this heading.

Digoxin (Co-administration has resulted in an increase in the AUC and Cmax for digoxin of 19% and 29%, respectively). Products include:
- Lanoxicaps Capsules 1490
- Lanoxin Injection 1494
- Lanoxin Injection Pediatric 1497
- Lanoxin Tablets 1500

Ferrous Fumarate (Rabeprazole produces sustained inhibition of gastric acid secretion; rabeprazole may interfere with the absorption of certain drugs, such as iron salts, where gastric pH is an important determinant of the bioavailability).
No products indexed under this heading.

Ferrous Gluconate (Rabeprazole produces sustained inhibition of gastric acid secretion; rabeprazole may interfere with the absorption of certain drugs, such as iron salts, where gastric pH is an important determinant of the bioavailability).
No products indexed under this heading.

Ferrous Sulfate (Rabeprazole produces sustained inhibition of gastric acid secretion; rabeprazole may interfere with the absorption of certain drugs, such as iron salts, where gastric pH is an important determinant of the bioavailability). Products include:
- Slow Fe Iron Tablets 818
- Slow Fe with Folic Acid Tablets 819

Iron (Rabeprazole produces sustained inhibition of gastric acid secretion; rabeprazole may interfere with the absorption of certain drugs, such as iron salts, where gastric pH is an important determinant of the bioavailability).
No products indexed under this heading.

Ketoconazole (Co-administration has resulted in an approximately 30% decrease in the bioavailability of ketoconazole and an increase in the AUC). Products include:
- Nizoral A-D Shampoo, 1% 1868

Polysaccharide Iron Complex (Rabeprazole produces sustained inhibition of gastric acid secretion; rabeprazole may interfere with the absorption of certain drugs, such as iron salts, where gastric pH is an important determinant of the bioavailability). Products include:
- Nu-Iron 150 Capsules 2127

Warfarin Sodium (Co-administration has resulted in increased INR and prothrombin time, which may lead to abnormal bleeding and even death). Products include:
- Coumadin for Injection 898
- Coumadin Tablets 898

ACLOVATE CREAM

(Alclometasone Dipropionate) 2660
None cited in PDR database.

ACLOVATE OINTMENT

(Alclometasone Dipropionate) 2660
None cited in PDR database.

ACTIMMUNE

(Interferon Gamma-1B) 1671
May interact with:

Bone Marrow Depressants, unspecified (Caution should be exercised when administering with other potentially myelosuppressive agents).
No products indexed under this heading.

ACTIQ

(Fentanyl Citrate) 979
May interact with antihistamines, central nervous system depressants, erythromycin, general anesthetics, hypnotics and sedatives, monoamine oxidase inhibitors, narcotic analgesics, phenothiazines, tranquilizers, and certain other agents. Compounds in these categories include:

Acrivastine (Co-administration may result in increased depressant effects).
No products indexed under this heading.

Alfentanil Hydrochloride (Co-administration may result in increased depressant effects; hypoventilation, hypotension, and profound sedation may occur).
No products indexed under this heading.

Alprazolam (Co-administration may result in increased depressant effects; hypoventilation, hypotension, and profound sedation may occur). Products include:
- Niravam Orally Disintegrating Tablets 3092

Aprobarbital (Co-administration may result in increased depressant effects; hypoventilation, hypotension, and profound sedation may occur).
No products indexed under this heading.

Astemizole (Co-administration may result in increased depressant effects).
No products indexed under this heading.

Azatadine Maleate (Co-administration may result in increased depressant effects).
No products indexed under this heading.

Bromodiphenhydramine Hydrochloride (Co-administration may result in increased depressant effects).
No products indexed under this heading.

Brompheniramine Maleate (Co-administration may result in increased depressant effects). Products include:
- Children's Dimetapp Cold & Allergy Elixir 730
- Children's Dimetapp Cold & Allergy Chewable Tablets 730
- Children's Dimetapp DM Cold & Cough Elixir 731

Buprenorphine Hydrochloride (Co-administration may result in increased depressant effects; hypoventilation, hypotension, and profound sedation may occur). Products include:
- Buprenex Injectable 2716
- Suboxone Tablets 2717
- Subutex Tablets 2717

Buspirone Hydrochloride (Co-administration may result in increased depressant effects; hypoventilation, hypotension, and profound sedation may occur).
No products indexed under this heading.

Butabarbital (Co-administration may result in increased depressant effects; hypoventilation, hypotension, and profound sedation may occur).
No products indexed under this heading.

Butalbital (Co-administration may result in increased depressant effects; hypoventilation, hypotension, and profound sedation may occur).
No products indexed under this heading.

Cetirizine Hydrochloride (Co-administration may result in increased depressant effects). Products include:
- Zyrtec Chewable Tablets 2594
- Zyrtec 2594
- Zyrtec-D 12 Hour Extended Release Tablets 2597

Chlordiazepoxide (Co-administration may result in increased depressant effects; hypoventilation, hypotension, and profound sedation may occur).
No products indexed under this heading.

Chlordiazepoxide Hydrochloride (Co-administration may result in increased depressant effects; hypoventilation, hypotension, and profound sedation may occur). Products include:
- Librium Capsules 3347

Chlorpheniramine Maleate (Co-administration may result in increased depressant effects). Products include:
- Advil Allergy Sinus Caplets 770
- Advil Multi-Symptom Cold Caplets 770
- BC Allergy Sinus Cold Powder 677
- Comtrex Maximum Strength Cold & Cough Day/Night Caplets - Night Formulation 726
- Comtrex Maximum Strength Day/Night Severe Cold & Sinus Caplets - Night Formulation 725
- Contac Cold and Flu Maximum Strength Caplets 728
- Contac Cold and Flu Day and Night Caplets (Night Formulation Only) 727
- Children's Dimetapp Long Acting Cough Plus Cold Syrup 731
- Robitussin Cough & Cold Long-Acting Liquid 735
- Robitussin Cough & Allergy Syrup 736
- Robitussin Cough & Cold Nighttime Liquid 736
- Robitussin Cough, Cold & Flu Nighttime Liquid 738
- Robitussin Pediatric Cough & Cold Long-Acting Liquid 735
- Robitussin Pediatric Cough & Cold Nighttime Liquid 736
- Triaminic Cold & Allergy Liquid 746
- Triaminic Cough & Runny Nose Softchews 748
- Children's Tylenol Plus Flu Oral Suspension 749
- Tylenol Allergy Multi-Symptom Caplets with Cool Burst and Gelcaps 1872
- Children's Tylenol Plus Cold Suspension Liquid 1879
- Children's Tylenol Plus Cough & Runny Nose Suspension Liquid 1879
- Children's Tylenol Plus Flu Suspension Liquid 1881

IMPORTANT NOTE: Always consult each drug listing in the patient's regimen for possible interactions.

Children's Tylenol Plus Multi-Symptom Cold Suspension Liquid 1879
Tylenol Cold Head Congestion Nighttime Caplets with Cool Burst 1873
Tylenol Cold Multi-Symptom Nighttime Caplets with Cool Burst 1874
Tylenol Sinus Congestion & Pain Nighttime Caplets with Cool Burst 1876
Vicks 44M Cough, Cold & Flu Relief Liquid 2680
Pediatric Vicks 44m Cough & Cold Relief Liquid 2676
Children's Vicks NyQuil Cold/Cough Relief .... ▣ 756
Children's Vicks NyQuil Cold/Cough Relief Liquid 2680
Zicam Maximum Strength Flu Daytime .... ▣ 768

Chlorpheniramine Polistirex (Co-administration may result in increased depressant effects). Products include:
Tussionex Pennkinetic Extended-Release Suspension 3327

Chlorpheniramine Tannate (Co-administration may result in increased depressant effects).
No products indexed under this heading.

Chlorpromazine (Co-administration may result in increased depressant effects; hypoventilation, hypotension, and profound sedation may occur).
No products indexed under this heading.

Chlorpromazine Hydrochloride (Co-administration may result in increased depressant effects; hypoventilation, hypotension, and profound sedation may occur).
No products indexed under this heading.

Chlorprothixene (Co-administration may result in increased depressant effects; hypoventilation, hypotension, and profound sedation may occur).
No products indexed under this heading.

Chlorprothixene Hydrochloride (Co-administration may result in increased depressant effects; hypoventilation, hypotension, and profound sedation may occur).
No products indexed under this heading.

Chlorprothixene Lactate (Co-administration may result in increased depressant effects; hypoventilation, hypotension, and profound sedation may occur).
No products indexed under this heading.

Clemastine Fumarate (Co-administration may result in increased depressant effects).
No products indexed under this heading.

Clorazepate Dipotassium (Co-administration may result in increased depressant effects; hypoventilation, hypotension, and profound sedation may occur). Products include:
Tranxene 2474

Clozapine (Co-administration may result in increased depressant effects; hypoventilation, hypotension, and profound sedation may occur). Products include:
Clozaril Tablets 2184
FazaClo Orally Disintegrating Tablets 551

Codeine Phosphate (Co-administration may result in increased depressant effects; hypoventilation, hypotension, and profound sedation may occur). Products include:
Tylenol with Codeine Tablets 2391

Cyproheptadine Hydrochloride (Co-administration may result in increased depressant effects).
No products indexed under this heading.

Desflurane (Co-administration may result in increased depressant effects; hypoventilation, hypotension, and profound sedation may occur).
No products indexed under this heading.

Dexchlorpheniramine Maleate (Co-administration may result in increased depressant effects).
No products indexed under this heading.

Dezocine (Co-administration may result in increased depressant effects; hypoventilation, hypotension, and profound sedation may occur).
No products indexed under this heading.

Diazepam (Co-administration may result in increased depressant effects; hypoventilation, hypotension, and profound sedation may occur). Products include:
Diastat Rectal Delivery System 3343
Valium Tablets 2819

Diphenhydramine Citrate (Co-administration may result in increased depressant effects). Products include:
Advil PM Caplets .... ▣ 615
Excedrin PM Caplets/Tablets/Geltabs .... ▣ 610
Goody's PM Powder for Pain with Sleeplessness .... ▣ 612

Diphenhydramine Hydrochloride (Co-administration may result in increased depressant effects). Products include:
Nytol QuickCaps Caplets .... ▣ 615
Nytol QuickGels Softgels Maximum Strength .... ▣ 616
Simply Sleep Caplets 1868
Sominex Original Formula Tablets .... ▣ 616
TheraFlu Warming Relief Nighttime Severe Cold .... ▣ 743
TheraFlu Thin Strips Multi Symptom .... ▣ 744
Triaminic Nighttime Cold & Cough Liquid .... ▣ 746
Triaminic Thin Strips Cough & Runny Nose .... ▣ 749
Extra Strength Tylenol PM Caplets, Vanilla Caplets, Geltabs, Gelcaps and Liquid 1875
Tylenol Sore Throat Nighttime Liquid with Cool Burst .... ▣ 790
Tylenol Allergy Multi-Symptom Nighttime Caplets with Cool Burst 1872
Tylenol Severe Allergy Caplets 1872
Children's Tylenol Plus Cold & Allergy Suspension Liquid 1878

Diphenylpyraline Hydrochloride (Co-administration may result in increased depressant effects).
No products indexed under this heading.

Droperidol (Co-administration may result in increased depressant effects; hypoventilation, hypotension, and profound sedation may occur).
No products indexed under this heading.

Enflurane (Co-administration may result in increased depressant effects; hypoventilation, hypotension, and profound sedation may occur).
No products indexed under this heading.

Erythromycin (Co-administration with potent inhibitors of CYP450 3A4 isoform, such as erythromycin, may increase the bioavailability of swallowed fentanyl by decreasing intestinal and hepatic first pass metabolism and may decrease the systemic clearance resulting in increased or prolonged opioid effects). Products include:
Ery-Tab Tablets 449
Erythromycin Base Filmtab Tablets 455
Erythromycin Delayed-Release Capsules, USP 457
PCE Dispertab Tablets 515

Erythromycin Estolate (Co-administration with potent inhibitors of CYP450 3A4 isoform, such as erythromycin, may increase the bioavailability of swallowed fentanyl by decreasing intestinal and hepatic first pass metabolism and may decrease the systemic clearance resulting in increased or prolonged opioid effects).
No products indexed under this heading.

Erythromycin Ethylsuccinate (Co-administration with potent inhibitors of CYP450 3A4 isoform, such as erythromycin, may increase the bioavailability of swallowed fentanyl by decreasing intestinal and hepatic first pass metabolism and may decrease the systemic clearance resulting in increased or prolonged opioid effects). Products include:
E.E.S. 451
EryPed 447

Erythromycin Gluceptate (Co-administration with potent inhibitors of CYP450 3A4 isoform, such as erythromycin, may incréase the bioavailability of swallowed fentanyl by decreasing intestinal and hepatic first pass metabolism and may decrease the systemic clearance resulting in increased or prolonged opioid effects).
No products indexed under this heading.

Erythromycin Lactobionate (Co-administration with potent inhibitors of CYP450 3A4 isoform, such as erythromycin, may increase the bioavailability of swallowed fentanyl by decreasing intestinal and hepatic first pass metabolism and may decrease the systemic clearance resulting in increased or prolonged opioid effects).
No products indexed under this heading.

Erythromycin Stearate (Co-administration with potent inhibitors of CYP450 3A4 isoform, such as erythromycin, may increase the bioavailability of swallowed fentanyl by decreasing intestinal and hepatic first pass metabolism and may decrease the systemic clearance resulting in increased or prolonged opioid effects). Products include:
Erythrocin Stearate Filmtab Tablets 453

Estazolam (Co-administration may result in increased depressant effects; hypoventilation, hypotension, and profound sedation may occur). Products include:
ProSom Tablets 517

Ethanol (Co-administration may result in increased depressant effects; hypoventilation, hypotension, and profound sedation may occur).
No products indexed under this heading.

Ethchlorvynol (Co-administration may result in increased depressant effects; hypoventilation, hypotension, and profound sedation may occur).
No products indexed under this heading.

Ethinamate (Co-administration may result in increased depressant effects; hypoventilation, hypotension, and profound sedation may occur).
No products indexed under this heading.

Ethyl Alcohol (Co-administration may result in increased depressant effects; hypoventilation, hypotension, and profound sedation may occur).
No products indexed under this heading.

Fentanyl (Co-administration may result in increased depressant effects; hypoventilation, hypotension, and profound sedation may occur). Products include:
Duragesic Transdermal System 2373
Ionsys Transdermal System 2379

Fexofenadine Hydrochloride (Co-administration may result in increased depressant effects). Products include:
Allegra 2844
Allegra-D 12 Hour Extended-Release Tablets 2846
Allegra-D 24 Hour Extended-Release Tablets 2849

Fluphenazine Decanoate (Co-administration may result in increased depressant effects; hypoventilation, hypotension, and profound sedation may occur).
No products indexed under this heading.

Fluphenazine Enanthate (Co-administration may result in increased depressant effects; hypoventilation, hypotension, and profound sedation may occur).
No products indexed under this heading.

Fluphenazine Hydrochloride (Co-administration may result in increased depressant effects; hypoventilation, hypotension, and profound sedation may occur).
No products indexed under this heading.

Flurazepam Hydrochloride (Co-administration may result in increased depressant effects; hypoventilation, hypotension, and profound sedation may occur). Products include:
Dalmane Capsules 3342

Glutethimide (Co-administration may result in increased depressant effects; hypoventilation, hypotension, and profound sedation may occur).
No products indexed under this heading.

Haloperidol (Co-administration may result in increased depressant effects; hypoventilation, hypotension, and profound sedation may occur).
No products indexed under this heading.

Haloperidol Decanoate (Co-administration may result in increased depressant effects; hypoventilation, hypotension, and profound sedation may occur).
No products indexed under this heading.

Hydrocodone Bitartrate (Co-administration may result in increased depressant effects; hypoventilation, hypotension, and profound sedation may occur). Products include:
- Hycodan 1116
- Hycotuss Expectorant Syrup 1117
- Vicodin Tablets 535
- Vicodin ES Tablets 536
- Vicodin HP Tablets 538
- Vicoprofen Tablets 539
- Zydone Tablets 1139

Hydrocodone Polistirex (Co-administration may result in increased depressant effects; hypoventilation, hypotension, and profound sedation may occur). Products include:
- Tussionex Pennkinetic Extended-Release Suspension 3327

Hydromorphone Hydrochloride (Co-administration may result in increased depressant effects; hypoventilation, hypotension, and profound sedation may occur). Products include:
- Dilaudid 440
- Dilaudid Non-Sterile Powder 440
- Dilaudid Oral Liquid 445
- Dilaudid Rectal Suppositories 440
- Dilaudid Tablets 440
- Dilaudid Tablets - 8 mg 445
- Dilaudid-HP 442

Hydroxyzine Hydrochloride (Co-administration may result in increased depressant effects; hypoventilation, hypotension, and profound sedation may occur).
No products indexed under this heading.

Isocarboxazid (Concurrent and/or sequential use with MAO inhibitors is not recommended; potential for severe and unpredictable potentiation of MAO inhibitors has been reported with opioid analgesics).
No products indexed under this heading.

Isoflurane (Co-administration may result in increased depressant effects; hypoventilation, hypotension, and profound sedation may occur).
No products indexed under this heading.

Itraconazole (Co-administration with potent inhibitors of CYP450 3A4 isoform, such as azole antifungal itraconazole, may increase the bioavailability of swallowed fentanyl by decreasing intestinal and hepatic first pass metabolism and may decrease the systemic clearance resulting in increased or prolonged opioid effects).
No products indexed under this heading.

Ketamine Hydrochloride (Co-administration may result in increased depressant effects; hypoventilation, hypotension, and profound sedation may occur).
No products indexed under this heading.

Ketoconazole (Co-administration with potent inhibitors of CYP450 3A4 isoform, such as azole antifungal ketoconazole, may increase the bioavailability of swallowed fentanyl by decreasing intestinal and hepatic first pass metabolism and may decrease the systemic clearance resulting in increased or prolonged opioid effects). Products include:
- Nizoral A-D Shampoo, 1% 1868

Levomethadyl Acetate Hydrochloride (Co-administration may result in increased depressant effects; hypoventilation, hypotension, and profound sedation may occur).
No products indexed under this heading.

Levorphanol Tartrate (Co-administration may result in increased depressant effects; hypoventilation, hypotension, and profound sedation may occur).
No products indexed under this heading.

Loratadine (Co-administration may result in increased depressant effects). Products include:
- Alavert Allergy & Sinus D-12 Hour Tablets 771
- Alavert 771
- Children's Claritin Allergy Oral Solution 771
- Claritin Non-Drowsy 24 Hour Tablets 772
- Claritin Reditabs 24 Hour Non-Drowsy Tablets 772
- Claritin-D Non-Drowsy 12 Hour Tablets 772
- Claritin-D Non-Drowsy 24 Hour Tablets 772

Lorazepam (Co-administration may result in increased depressant effects; hypoventilation, hypotension, and profound sedation may occur).
No products indexed under this heading.

Loxapine Hydrochloride (Co-administration may result in increased depressant effects; hypoventilation, hypotension, and profound sedation may occur).
No products indexed under this heading.

Loxapine Succinate (Co-administration may result in increased depressant effects; hypoventilation, hypotension, and profound sedation may occur).
No products indexed under this heading.

Meperidine Hydrochloride (Co-administration may result in increased depressant effects; hypoventilation, hypotension, and profound sedation may occur).
No products indexed under this heading.

Mephobarbital (Co-administration may result in increased depressant effects; hypoventilation, hypotension, and profound sedation may occur).
No products indexed under this heading.

Meprobamate (Co-administration may result in increased depressant effects; hypoventilation, hypotension, and profound sedation may occur).
No products indexed under this heading.

Mesoridazine Besylate (Co-administration may result in increased depressant effects; hypoventilation, hypotension, and profound sedation may occur).
No products indexed under this heading.

Methadone Hydrochloride (Co-administration may result in increased depressant effects; hypoventilation, hypotension, and profound sedation may occur).
No products indexed under this heading.

Methdilazine Hydrochloride (Co-administration may result in increased depressant effects).
No products indexed under this heading.

Methohexital Sodium (Co-administration may result in increased depressant effects; hypoventilation, hypotension, and profound sedation may occur).
No products indexed under this heading.

Methotrimeprazine (Co-administration may result in increased depressant effects; hypoventilation, hypotension, and profound sedation may occur).
No products indexed under this heading.

Methoxyflurane (Co-administration may result in increased depressant effects; hypoventilation, hypotension, and profound sedation may occur).
No products indexed under this heading.

Midazolam Hydrochloride (Co-administration may result in increased depressant effects; hypoventilation, hypotension, and profound sedation may occur).
No products indexed under this heading.

Moclobemide (Concurrent and/or sequential use with MAO inhibitors is not recommended; potential for severe and unpredictable potentiation of MAO inhibitors has been reported with opioid analgesics).
No products indexed under this heading.

Molindone Hydrochloride (Co-administration may result in increased depressant effects; hypoventilation, hypotension, and profound sedation may occur). Products include:
- Moban Tablets 1119

Morphine Sulfate (Co-administration may result in increased depressant effects; hypoventilation, hypotension, and profound sedation may occur). Products include:
- Avinza Capsules 1741
- Kadian Capsules 577
- MS Contin Tablets 2701

Olanzapine (Co-administration may result in increased depressant effects; hypoventilation, hypotension, and profound sedation may occur). Products include:
- Symbyax Capsules 1819
- Zyprexa Tablets 1830
- Zyprexa IntraMuscular 1830
- Zyprexa ZYDIS Orally Disintegrating Tablets 1830

Oxazepam (Co-administration may result in increased depressant effects; hypoventilation, hypotension, and profound sedation may occur).
No products indexed under this heading.

Oxycodone Hydrochloride (Co-administration may result in increased depressant effects; hypoventilation, hypotension, and profound sedation may occur). Products include:
- OxyContin Tablets 2703
- OxyFast Oral Concentrate Solution 2708
- OxyIR Capsules 2708
- Percocet Tablets 1131
- Percodan Tablets 1132

Pargyline Hydrochloride (Concurrent and/or sequential use with MAO inhibitors is not recommended; potential for severe and unpredictable potentiation of MAO inhibitors has been reported with opioid analgesics).
No products indexed under this heading.

Pentobarbital Sodium (Co-administration may result in increased depressant effects; hypoventilation, hypotension, and profound sedation may occur). Products include:
- Nembutal Sodium Solution, USP 2470

Perphenazine (Co-administration may result in increased depressant effects; hypoventilation, hypotension, and profound sedation may occur).
No products indexed under this heading.

Phenelzine Sulfate (Concurrent and/or sequential use with MAO inhibitors is not recommended; potential for severe and unpredictable potentiation of MAO inhibitors has been reported with opioid analgesics).
No products indexed under this heading.

Phenobarbital (Co-administration may result in increased depressant effects; hypoventilation, hypotension, and profound sedation may occur). Products include:
- Donnatal Extentabs 2493

Prazepam (Co-administration may result in increased depressant effects; hypoventilation, hypotension, and profound sedation may occur).
No products indexed under this heading.

Procarbazine Hydrochloride (Concurrent and/or sequential use with MAO inhibitors is not recommended; potential for severe and unpredictable potentiation of MAO inhibitors has been reported with opioid analgesics). Products include:
- Matulane Capsules 3191

Prochlorperazine (Co-administration may result in increased depressant effects; hypoventilation, hypotension, and profound sedation may occur).
No products indexed under this heading.

Promethazine Hydrochloride (Co-administration may result in increased depressant effects). Products include:
- Phenergan Tablets and Suppositories 3440

Propofol (Co-administration may result in increased depressant effects; hypoventilation, hypotension, and profound sedation may occur).
No products indexed under this heading.

Propoxyphene Hydrochloride (Co-administration may result in increased depressant effects; hypoventilation, hypotension, and profound sedation may occur).
No products indexed under this heading.

Propoxyphene Napsylate (Co-administration may result in increased depressant effects; hypoventilation, hypotension, and profound sedation may occur).
No products indexed under this heading.

Pyrilamine Maleate (Co-administration may result in increased depressant effects).
No products indexed under this heading.

Pyrilamine Tannate (Co-administration may result in increased depressant effects).
No products indexed under this heading.

Quazepam (Co-administration may result in increased depressant effects; hypoventilation, hypotension, and profound sedation may occur).
No products indexed under this heading.

Quetiapine Fumarate (Co-administration may result in increased depressant effects; hypoventilation, hypotension, and profound sedation may occur). Products include:
Seroquel Tablets 690

Ramelteon (Co-administration may result in increased depressant effects; hypoventilation, hypotension, and profound sedation may occur). Products include:
Rozerem Tablets 3231

Remifentanil Hydrochloride (Co-administration may result in increased depressant effects; hypoventilation, hypotension, and profound sedation may occur).
No products indexed under this heading.

Risperidone (Co-administration may result in increased depressant effects; hypoventilation, hypotension, and profound sedation may occur). Products include:
Risperdal 1676
Risperdal Consta Long-Acting Injection 1682
Risperdal M-Tab Orally Disintegrating Tablets 1676

Ritonavir (Co-administration with potent inhibitors of CYP450 3A4 isoform, such as protease inhibitor ritonavir, may increase the bioavailability of swallowed fentanyl by decreasing intestinal and hepatic first pass metabolism and may decrease the systemic clearance resulting in increased or prolonged opioid effects). Products include:
Kaletra 476
Norvir 503

Secobarbital Sodium (Co-administration may result in increased depressant effects; hypoventilation, hypotension, and profound sedation may occur).
No products indexed under this heading.

Selegiline Hydrochloride (Concurrent and/or sequential use with MAO inhibitors is not recommended; potential for severe and unpredictable potentiation of MAO inhibitors has been reported with opioid analgesics). Products include:
Eldepryl Capsules 3208
Zelapar Tablets 3372

Sevoflurane (Co-administration may result in increased depressant effects; hypoventilation, hypotension, and profound sedation may occur). Products include:
Ultane Liquid for Inhalation 531

Sodium Oxybate (Co-administration may result in increased depressant effects; hypoventilation, hypotension, and profound sedation may occur). Products include:
Xyrem Oral Solution 1688

Sufentanil Citrate (Co-administration may result in increased depressant effects; hypoventilation, hypotension, and profound sedation may occur).
No products indexed under this heading.

Temazepam (Co-administration may result in increased depressant effects; hypoventilation, hypotension, and profound sedation may occur). Products include:
Restoril Capsules 1860

Terfenadine (Co-administration may result in increased depressant effects).
No products indexed under this heading.

Thiamylal Sodium (Co-administration may result in increased depressant effects; hypoventilation, hypotension, and profound sedation may occur).
No products indexed under this heading.

Thioridazine Hydrochloride (Co-administration may result in increased depressant effects; hypoventilation, hypotension, and profound sedation may occur). Products include:
Thioridazine Hydrochloride Tablets 2163

Thiothixene (Co-administration may result in increased depressant effects; hypoventilation, hypotension, and profound sedation may occur). Products include:
Thiothixene Capsules 2165

Tranylcypromine Sulfate (Concurrent and/or sequential use with MAO inhibitors is not recommended; potential for severe and unpredictable potentiation of MAO inhibitors has been reported with opioid analgesics). Products include:
Parnate Tablets 1527

Triazolam (Co-administration may result in increased depressant effects; hypoventilation, hypotension, and profound sedation may occur).
No products indexed under this heading.

Trifluoperazine Hydrochloride (Co-administration may result in increased depressant effects; hypoventilation, hypotension, and profound sedation may occur).
No products indexed under this heading.

Trimeprazine Tartrate (Co-administration may result in increased depressant effects).
No products indexed under this heading.

Tripelennamine Hydrochloride (Co-administration may result in increased depressant effects).
No products indexed under this heading.

Triprolidine Hydrochloride (Co-administration may result in increased depressant effects).
No products indexed under this heading.

Zaleplon (Co-administration may result in increased depressant effects; hypoventilation, hypotension, and profound sedation may occur). Products include:
Sonata Capsules 1717

Ziprasidone Hydrochloride (Co-administration may result in increased depressant effects; hypoventilation, hypotension, and profound sedation may occur). Products include:
Geodon Capsules 2529

Zolpidem Tartrate (Co-administration may result in increased depressant effects; hypoventilation, hypotension, and profound sedation may occur). Products include:
Ambien Tablets 2851
Ambien CR Tablets 2855

Food Interactions

Alcohol (Concurrent use with alcoholic beverages may result in increased depressant effects; hypoventilation, hypotension, and profound sedation may occur).

ACTIVASE I.V.

(Alteplase) 1223
May interact with ACE inhibitors, vitamin K antagonists, and certain other agents. Compounds in these categories include:

Abciximab (Drugs that alter platelet function, such as abciximab, may increase the risk of bleeding if administered prior to or after alteplase therapy). Products include:
ReoPro Vials 1809

Aspirin (Drugs that alter platelet function, such as aspirin, may increase the risk of bleeding if administered prior to or after alteplase therapy). Products include:
Aggrenox Capsules 822
Bayer Aspirin 744
BC Allergy Sinus Cold Powder .... ◙ 677
BC Headache Powder .... ◙ 677
Arthritis Strength BC Powder .... ◙ 677
BC Sinus Cold Powder .... ◙ 677
Excedrin Extra Strength Caplets/Tablets/Geltabs .... ◙ 684
Excedrin Migraine Caplets/Tablets/Geltabs .... ◙ 609
Goody's Body Pain Formula Powder .... ◙ 684
Goody's Extra Strength Headache Powders .... ◙ 611
Goody's Extra Strength Pain Relief Tablets .... ◙ 685
Percodan Tablets 1132
St. Joseph 81 mg Aspirin Chewable and Enteric Coated Tablets 1869

Benazepril Hydrochloride (Post-marketing reports of orolingual angioedema associated with alteplase have primarily been in acute ischemic stroke patients receiving concomitant ACE inhibitors). Products include:
Lotensin Tablets 2243
Lotensin HCT Tablets 2246
Lotrel Capsules 2249

Captopril (Post-marketing reports of orolingual angioedema associated with alteplase have primarily been in acute ischemic stroke patients receiving concomitant ACE inhibitors). Products include:
Captopril Tablets 2149

Clopidogrel Bisulfate (Drugs that alter platelet function, such as clopidogrel, may increase the risk of bleeding if administered prior to or after alteplase therapy). Products include:
Plavix Tablets 917
Plavix Tablets 2926

Dicumarol (Co-administration increases the risk of bleeding).
No products indexed under this heading.

Dipyridamole (Drugs that alter platelet function, such as dipyridamole, may increase the risk of bleeding if administered prior to or after alteplase therapy). Products include:
Aggrenox Capsules 822
Persantine Tablets 868

Enalapril Maleate (Post-marketing reports of orolingual angioedema associated with alteplase have primarily been in acute ischemic stroke patients receiving concomitant ACE inhibitors). Products include:
Vasotec I.V. Injection 2103

Enalaprilat (Post-marketing reports of orolingual angioedema associated with alteplase have primarily been in acute ischemic stroke patients receiving concomitant ACE inhibitors).
No products indexed under this heading.

Eptifibatide (Drugs that alter platelet function, such as eptifibatide, may increase the risk of bleeding if administered prior to or after alteplase therapy). Products include:
Integrilin Injection 3020

Fosinopril Sodium (Post-marketing reports of orolingual angioedema associated with alteplase have primarily been in acute ischemic stroke patients receiving concomitant ACE inhibitors).
No products indexed under this heading.

Heparin Sodium (Co-administration increases the risk of bleeding).
No products indexed under this heading.

Lisinopril (Post-marketing reports of orolingual angioedema associated with alteplase have primarily been in acute ischemic stroke patients receiving concomitant ACE inhibitors). Products include:
Prinivil Tablets 2052
Prinzide Tablets 2056

Moexipril Hydrochloride (Post-marketing reports of orolingual angioedema associated with alteplase have primarily been in acute ischemic stroke patients receiving concomitant ACE inhibitors). Products include:
Uniretic Tablets 3100
Univasc Tablets 3104

Perindopril Erbumine (Post-marketing reports of orolingual angioedema associated with alteplase have primarily been in acute ischemic stroke patients receiving concomitant ACE inhibitors). Products include:
Aceon Tablets (2 mg, 4 mg, 8 mg) 3194

Quinapril Hydrochloride (Post-marketing reports of orolingual angioedema associated with alteplase have primarily been in acute ischemic stroke patients receiving concomitant ACE inhibitors).
No products indexed under this heading.

Ramipril (Post-marketing reports of orolingual angioedema associated with alteplase have primarily been in acute ischemic stroke patients receiving concomitant ACE inhibitors). Products include:
Altace Capsules 1702

Spirapril Hydrochloride (Post-marketing reports of orolingual angioedema associated with alteplase have primarily been in acute ischemic stroke patients receiving concomitant ACE inhibitors).
No products indexed under this heading.

Ticlopidine Hydrochloride (Drugs that alter platelet function, such as ticlopidine, may increase the risk of bleeding if administered prior to or after alteplase therapy). Products include:
Ticlid Tablets 2810

Tirofiban Hydrochloride (Drugs that alter platelet function, such as tirofiban, may increase the risk of bleeding if administered prior to or after alteplase therapy). Products include:
Aggrastat 1907

Trandolapril (Post-marketing reports of orolingual angioedema associated with alteplase have primarily been in acute ischemic stroke patients receiving concomitant ACE inhibitors). Products include:
Mavik Tablets 486
Tarka Tablets 524

Warfarin Sodium (Co-administration increases the risk of bleeding). Products include:
Coumadin for Injection 898
Coumadin Tablets 898

ACTIVE CALCIUM TABLETS

(Calcium Citrate, Vitamin D) 3339
None cited in PDR database.

ACTONEL TABLETS

(Risedronate Sodium) 2683
May interact with antacids containing aluminum, calcium and magnesium, calcium preparations, and certain other agents. Compounds in these categories include:

Aluminum Carbonate (Antacids may interfere with the absorption of risedronate sodium; antacids should be taken at a different time of the day).
No products indexed under this heading.

Aluminum Hydroxide (Antacids may interfere with the absorption of risedronate sodium; antacids should be taken at a different time of the day). Products include:
Gaviscon Regular Strength Liquid .. ■658
Gaviscon Regular Strength Tablets .... ■658
Gaviscon Extra Strength Liquid ...... ■658
Gaviscon Extra Strength Tablets .... ■658
Maalox Regular Strength Antacid/Antigas Liquid 2175
Maalox Max Maximum Strength Antacid/Anti-Gas Liquid 2176

Aspirin (The incidence of gastrointestinal adverse events is, in general, higher with co-administration; caution should be used). Products include:
Aggrenox Capsules 822
Bayer Aspirin 744
BC Allergy Sinus Cold Powder .... ■677
BC Headache Powder .... ■677
Arthritis Strength BC Powder .... ■677
BC Sinus Cold Powder .... ■677
Excedrin Extra Strength Caplets/Tablets/Geltabs .... ■684
Excedrin Migraine Caplets/Tablets/Geltabs .... ■609
Goody's Body Pain Formula Powder .... ■684
Goody's Extra Strength Headache Powders .... ■611
Goody's Extra Strength Pain Relief Tablets .... ■685
Percodan Tablets 1132
St. Joseph 81 mg Aspirin Chewable and Enteric Coated Tablets 1869

Calcium Carbonate (Calcium-containing preparations may interfere with the absorption of risedronate sodium; calcium preparations should be taken at a different time of the day). Products include:
Actonel with Calcium Tablets 2688
Calcet Tablets 2138
Caltrate 600 PLUS .... ■809
Caltrate 600 + D Tablets .... ■809
D-Cal Chewable Caplets .... ■812
Gas-X with Maalox .... ■656
Maalox Regular Strength Antacid Chewable Tablets 2177
Maalox Max Maximum Strength Antacid/Antigas Chewable Tablets 2176
Maalox Max Maximum Strength Chewable Tablets .... ■660
Os-Cal Chewable Tablets .... ■818
Pepcid Complete Chewable Tablets 1701
Children's Pepto 2674
PremCal Light, Regular, and Extra Strength Tablets .... ■818
Tums .... ■664

Calcium Chloride (Calcium-containing preparations may interfere with the absorption of risedronate sodium; calcium preparations should be taken at a different time of the day).
No products indexed under this heading.

Calcium Citrate (Calcium-containing preparations may interfere with the absorption of risedronate sodium; calcium preparations should be taken at a different time of the day). Products include:
Active Calcium Tablets 3339
Citracal Caplets .... ■703
Citracal Lemon Cream Creamy Bites 2139
Citracal Prenatal + DHA Tablets and Capsules 2139

Calcium Glubionate (Calcium-containing preparations may interfere with the absorption of risedronate sodium; calcium preparations should be taken at a different time of the day).
No products indexed under this heading.

Magaldrate (Antacids may interfere with the absorption of risedronate sodium; antacids should be taken at a different time of the day).
No products indexed under this heading.

Magnesium Hydroxide (Antacids may interfere with the absorption of risedronate sodium; antacids should be taken at a different time of the day). Products include:
Maalox Regular Strength Antacid/Antigas Liquid 2175
Maalox Max Maximum Strength Antacid/Anti-Gas Liquid 2176
Pepcid Complete Chewable Tablets 1701

Magnesium Oxide (Antacids may interfere with the absorption of risedronate sodium; antacids should be taken at a different time of the day). Products include:
Beelith Tablets 759
PremCal Light, Regular, and Extra Strength Tablets .... ■818

Food Interactions

Food, unspecified (Mean oral bioavailability is decreased when risedronate is administered with food; risedronate sodium is effective when administered at least 30 minutes before breakfast).

ACTONEL WITH CALCIUM TABLETS

(Calcium Carbonate, Risedronate Sodium) 2688
May interact with antacids, antacids containing aluminum, calcium and magnesium, bisphosphonates, calcium preparations, cations, fluoroquinolone antibiotics, glucocorticoids, iron containing oral preparations, tetracyclines, thiazides, and certain other agents. Compounds in these categories include:

Alatrofloxacin Mesylate (Concomitant administration of a fluoroquinolone and calcium carbonate may decrease the absorption of the flouroquinolone).
No products indexed under this heading.

Alendronate Sodium (Co-administration with calcium may lead to a decrease in biphosphonate absorption). Products include:
Fosamax 1969
Fosamax Plus D Tablets 1977

Aluminum Carbonate (Antacids may interfere with the absorption of risedronate sodium; antacids should be taken at a different time of the day).
No products indexed under this heading.

Aluminum-containing Compounds, unspecified (Co-administration of risedronate sodium and calcium, antacids, or oral medications containing divalent cations will interfere with the absorption of risedronate sodium).
No products indexed under this heading.

Aluminum Hydroxide (Antacids may interfere with the absorption of risedronate sodium; antacids should be taken at a different time of the day). Products include:
Gaviscon Regular Strength Liquid .. ■658
Gaviscon Regular Strength Tablets .... ■658
Gaviscon Extra Strength Liquid ...... ■658
Gaviscon Extra Strength Tablets .... ■658
Maalox Regular Strength Antacid/Antigas Liquid 2175
Maalox Max Maximum Strength Antacid/Anti-Gas Liquid 2176

Aspirin (The incidence of gastrointestinal adverse events is, in general, higher with co-administration; caution should be used). Products include:
Aggrenox Capsules 822
Bayer Aspirin 744
BC Allergy Sinus Cold Powder .... ■677
BC Headache Powder .... ■677
Arthritis Strength BC Powder .... ■677
BC Sinus Cold Powder .... ■677
Excedrin Extra Strength Caplets/Tablets/Geltabs .... ■684
Excedrin Migraine Caplets/Tablets/Geltabs .... ■609
Goody's Body Pain Formula Powder .... ■684
Goody's Extra Strength Headache Powders .... ■611
Goody's Extra Strength Pain Relief Tablets .... ■685
Percodan Tablets 1132
St. Joseph 81 mg Aspirin Chewable and Enteric Coated Tablets 1869

Bendroflumethiazide (Reduced urinary excretion of calcium has been reported during concomitant use of calcium carbonate and thiazide diuretics).
No products indexed under this heading.

Betamethasone Acetate (Calcium absorption is reduced when calcium carbonate is taken concomitantly with systemic glucocorticoids).
No products indexed under this heading.

Betamethasone Sodium Phosphate (Calcium absorption is reduced when calcium carbonate is taken concomitantly with systemic glucocorticoids).
No products indexed under this heading.

Calcitriol (Absorption of calcium may be increased when calcium carbonate is given concomitantly with vitamin D analogues). Products include:
Calcijex Injection 411
Rocaltrol Capsules 2798
Rocaltrol Oral Solution 2798

Calcium (Co-administration of risedronate sodium and calcium, antacids, or oral medications containing divalent cations will interfere with the absorption of risedronate sodium). Products include:
Os-Cal 250 + D Tablets .... ■817
Os-Cal 500 Tablets .... ■817
Os-Cal 500 + D Tablets .... ■817

Calcium Chloride (Co-administration of risedronate sodium and calcium, antacids, or oral medications containing divalent cations will interfere with the absorption of risedronate sodium).
No products indexed under this heading.

Calcium Citrate (Co-administration of risedronate sodium and calcium, antacids, or oral medications containing divalent cations will interfere with the absorption of risedronate sodium). Products include:
Active Calcium Tablets 3339
Citracal Caplets .... ■703
Citracal Lemon Cream Creamy Bites 2139
Citracal Prenatal + DHA Tablets and Capsules 2139

Calcium Glubionate (Co-administration of risedronate sodium and calcium, antacids, or oral medications containing divalent cations will interfere with the absorption of risedronate sodium).
No products indexed under this heading.

Chlorothiazide (Reduced urinary excretion of calcium has been reported during concomitant use of calcium carbonate and thiazide diuretics). Products include:
Diuril Oral Suspension 1954

Chlorothiazide Sodium (Reduced urinary excretion of calcium has been reported during concomitant use of calcium carbonate and thiazide diuretics). Products include:
Diuril Sodium Intravenous 2467

Ciprofloxacin (Concomitant administration of a fluoroquinolone and calcium carbonate may decrease the absorption of the flouroquinolone). Products include:
Cipro Oral Suspension 2977
Cipro I.V. 2984
Cipro XR Tablets 2990
Ciprodex Otic Suspension 559

Ciprofloxacin Hydrochloride (Concomitant administration of a fluoroquinolone and calcium carbonate may decrease the absorption of the flouroquinolone). Products include:
- Ciloxan Ophthalmic Ointment 559
- Ciloxan Ophthalmic Solution .... ⊙206
- Cipro Tablets 2977
- Proquin XR Tablets 1153

Cortisone Acetate (Calcium absorption is reduced when calcium carbonate is taken concomitantly with systemic glucocorticoids).
No products indexed under this heading.

Demeclocycline Hydrochloride (Concomitant administration of a tetracycline and a calcium carbonate may decrease the absorption of the tetracycline).
No products indexed under this heading.

Dexamethasone (Calcium absorption is reduced when calcium carbonate is taken concomitantly with systemic glucocorticoids). Products include:
- Ciprodex Otic Suspension 559
- Decadron Tablets 1951
- TobraDex Ophthalmic Ointment 562
- TobraDex Ophthalmic Suspension 563

Dexamethasone Acetate (Calcium absorption is reduced when calcium carbonate is taken concomitantly with systemic glucocorticoids).
No products indexed under this heading.

Dexamethasone Sodium Phosphate (Calcium absorption is reduced when calcium carbonate is taken concomitantly with systemic glucocorticoids).
No products indexed under this heading.

Doxercalciferol (Absorption of calcium may be increased when calcium carbonate is given concomitantly with vitamin D analogues). Products include:
- Hectorol Capsules 1275
- Hectorol Injection 1278

Doxycycline Calcium (Concomitant administration of a tetracycline and a calcium carbonate may decrease the absorption of the tetracycline).
No products indexed under this heading.

Doxycycline Hyclate (Concomitant administration of a tetracycline and a calcium carbonate may decrease the absorption of the tetracycline).
No products indexed under this heading.

Doxycycline Monohydrate (Concomitant administration of a tetracycline and a calcium carbonate may decrease the absorption of the tetracycline). Products include:
- Oracea Capsules 1000

Enoxacin (Concomitant administration of a fluoroquinolone and calcium carbonate may decrease the absorption of the flouroquinolone).
No products indexed under this heading.

Etidronate Disodium (Co-administration with calcium may lead to a decrease in biphosphonate absorption). Products include:
- Didronel Tablets 2697

Ferrous Fumarate (Calcium may interfere with the absorption of iron. Patients being treated for iron-deficiency should take iron and calcium at different times of the day).
No products indexed under this heading.

Ferrous Gluconate (Calcium may interfere with the absorption of iron. Patients being treated for iron-deficiency should take iron and calcium at different times of the day).
No products indexed under this heading.

Ferrous Sulfate (Calcium may interfere with the absorption of iron. Patients being treated for iron-deficiency should take iron and calcium at different times of the day). Products include:
- Slow Fe Iron Tablets .... ■818
- Slow Fe with Folic Acid Tablets .... ■819

Fludrocortisone Acetate (Calcium absorption is reduced when calcium carbonate is taken concomitantly with systemic glucocorticoids).
No products indexed under this heading.

Grepafloxacin Hydrochloride (Concomitant administration of a fluoroquinolone and calcium carbonate may decrease the absorption of the flouroquinolone).
No products indexed under this heading.

Hydrochlorothiazide (Reduced urinary excretion of calcium has been reported during concomitant use of calcium carbonate and thiazide diuretics). Products include:
- Aldoril Tablets 1910
- Atacand HCT 651
- Avalide Tablets 888
- Avalide Tablets 2874
- Benicar HCT Tablets 1044
- Diovan HCT Tablets 2196
- Dyazide Capsules 1423
- Hyzaar 50-12.5 Tablets 1990
- Hyzaar 100-12.5 Tablets 1990
- Hyzaar 100-25 Tablets 1990
- Lopressor HCT 50/25 Tablets 2241
- Lopressor HCT 100/25 Tablets 2241
- Lopressor HCT 100/50 Tablets 2241
- Lotensin HCT Tablets 2246
- Micardis HCT Tablets 856
- Moduretic Tablets 2028
- Prinzide Tablets 2056
- Teveten HCT Tablets 1737
- Timolide Tablets 2086
- Uniretic Tablets 3100

Hydrocortisone (Calcium absorption is reduced when calcium carbonate is taken concomitantly with systemic glucocorticoids). Products include:
- Colocort Rectal Suspension, USP (Retention) 100 mg/60 mL 2476
- Hydrocortone Tablets 1989
- Preparation H Hydrocortisone Cream .... ■646

Hydrocortisone Acetate (Calcium absorption is reduced when calcium carbonate is taken concomitantly with systemic glucocorticoids). Products include:
- Analpram-HC 1159
- Pramosone 1161
- ProctoFoam-HC 3099

Hydrocortisone Sodium Phosphate (Calcium absorption is reduced when calcium carbonate is taken concomitantly with systemic glucocorticoids).
No products indexed under this heading.

Hydrocortisone Sodium Succinate (Calcium absorption is reduced when calcium carbonate is taken concomitantly with systemic glucocorticoids).
No products indexed under this heading.

Hydroflumethiazide (Reduced urinary excretion of calcium has been reported during concomitant use of calcium carbonate and thiazide diuretics).
No products indexed under this heading.

Iron (Calcium may interfere with the absorption of iron. Patients being treated for iron-deficiency should take iron and calcium at different times of the day).
No products indexed under this heading.

Levothyroxine Sodium (Concomitant intake of levothyroxine and calcium carbonate was found to reduce levothyroxine absorption and increase serum thyrotropin levels). Products include:
- Levothroid Tablets 1186
- Levoxyl Tablets 1712
- Synthroid Tablets 520
- Westhroid Tablets 3403

Lomefloxacin Hydrochloride (Concomitant administration of a fluoroquinolone and calcium carbonate may decrease the absorption of the flouroquinolone).
No products indexed under this heading.

Magaldrate (Antacids may interfere with the absorption of risedronate sodium; antacids should be taken at a different time of the day).
No products indexed under this heading.

Magnesium (Co-administration of risedronate sodium and calcium, antacids, or oral medications containing divalent cations will interfere with the absorption of risedronate sodium).
No products indexed under this heading.

Magnesium Hydroxide (Antacids may interfere with the absorption of risedronate sodium; antacids should be taken at a different time of the day). Products include:
- Maalox Regular Strength Antacid/Antigas Liquid 2175
- Maalox Max Maximum Strength Antacid/Anti-Gas Liquid 2176
- Pepcid Complete Chewable Tablets 1701

Magnesium Oxide (Antacids may interfere with the absorption of risedronate sodium; antacids should be taken at a different time of the day). Products include:
- Beelith Tablets 759
- PremCal Light, Regular, and Extra Strength Tablets .... ■818

Methacycline Hydrochloride (Concomitant administration of a tetracycline and a calcium carbonate may decrease the absorption of the tetracycline).
No products indexed under this heading.

Methyclothiazide (Reduced urinary excretion of calcium has been reported during concomitant use of calcium carbonate and thiazide diuretics).
No products indexed under this heading.

Methylprednisolone Acetate (Calcium absorption is reduced when calcium carbonate is taken concomitantly with systemic glucocorticoids). Products include:
- Depo-Medrol Injectable Suspension 2617
- Depo-Medrol Single-Dose Vial 2619

Methylprednisolone Sodium Succinate (Calcium absorption is reduced when calcium carbonate is taken concomitantly with systemic glucocorticoids).
No products indexed under this heading.

Minocycline Hydrochloride (Concomitant administration of a tetracycline and a calcium carbonate may decrease the absorption of the tetracycline). Products include:
- Solodyn Extended Release Tablets 1890

Moxifloxacin Hydrochloride (Concomitant administration of a fluoroquinolone and calcium carbonate may decrease the absorption of the flouroquinolone). Products include:
- Avelox 2970
- Vigamox Ophthalmic Solution 564

Norfloxacin (Concomitant administration of a fluoroquinolone and calcium carbonate may decrease the absorption of the flouroquinolone). Products include:
- Noroxin Tablets 2032

Ofloxacin (Concomitant administration of a fluoroquinolone and calcium carbonate may decrease the absorption of the flouroquinolone). Products include:
- Floxin Otic Solution 1049

Oxytetracycline Hydrochloride (Concomitant administration of a tetracycline and a calcium carbonate may decrease the absorption of the tetracycline).
No products indexed under this heading.

Paricalcitol (Absorption of calcium may be increased when calcium carbonate is given concomitantly with vitamin D analogues). Products include:
- Zemplar Capsules 541
- Zemplar Injection 543

Polysaccharide Iron Complex (Calcium may interfere with the absorption of iron. Patients being treated for iron-deficiency should take iron and calcium at different times of the day). Products include:
- Nu-Iron 150 Capsules 2127

Polythiazide (Reduced urinary excretion of calcium has been reported during concomitant use of calcium carbonate and thiazide diuretics).
No products indexed under this heading.

Prednisolone Acetate (Calcium absorption is reduced when calcium carbonate is taken concomitantly with systemic glucocorticoids). Products include:
- Blephamide Ophthalmic Ointment 568
- Blephamide Ophthalmic Suspension 569
- Poly-Pred Ophthalmic Suspension .... ⊙233
- Pred Forte Ophthalmic Suspension .... ⊙235
- Pred Mild Ophthalmic Suspension .... ⊙238
- Pred-G Ophthalmic Ointment .... ⊙237
- Pred-G Ophthalmic Suspension .... ⊙236

Prednisolone Sodium Phosphate (Calcium absorption is reduced when calcium carbonate is taken concomitantly with systemic glucocorticoids).
No products indexed under this heading.

Prednisolone Tebutate (Calcium absorption is reduced when calcium carbonate is taken concomitantly with systemic glucocorticoids).
No products indexed under this heading.

Prednisone (Calcium absorption is reduced when calcium carbonate is taken concomitantly with systemic glucocorticoids).
No products indexed under this heading.

Sodium Bicarbonate (Co-administration of risedronate sodium and calcium, antacids, or oral medications containing divalent cations will interfere with the absorption of risedronate sodium). Products include:
Colyte with Flavor Packs for Oral Solution 3088
HalfLytely and Bisacodyl Tablets Bowel Prep Kit with Flavors Packs 881
TriLyte with Flavor Packs for Oral Solution 3100

Tetracycline Hydrochloride (Concomitant administration of a tetracycline and a calcium carbonate may decrease the absorption of the tetracycline).
No products indexed under this heading.

Tiludronate Disodium (Co-administration with calcium may lead to a decrease in biphosphonate absorption).
No products indexed under this heading.

Triamcinolone (Calcium absorption is reduced when calcium carbonate is taken concomitantly with systemic glucocorticoids).
No products indexed under this heading.

Triamcinolone Acetonide (Calcium absorption is reduced when calcium carbonate is taken concomitantly with systemic glucocorticoids). Products include:
Azmacort Inhalation Aerosol 1726
Nasacort AQ Nasal Spray 2922

Triamcinolone Diacetate (Calcium absorption is reduced when calcium carbonate is taken concomitantly with systemic glucocorticoids).
No products indexed under this heading.

Triamcinolone Hexacetonide (Calcium absorption is reduced when calcium carbonate is taken concomitantly with systemic glucocorticoids).
No products indexed under this heading.

Trovafloxacin Mesylate (Concomitant administration of a fluoroquinolone and calcium carbonate may decrease the absorption of the flouroquinolone).
No products indexed under this heading.

Vitamin D (Absorption of calcium may be increased when calcium carbonate is given concomitantly with vitamin D analogues). Products include:
Active Calcium Tablets 3339
Caltrate 600 PLUS 809
Caltrate 600 + D Tablets 809
D-Cal Chewable Caplets 812
Os-Cal 250 + D Tablets 817
Os-Cal 500 + D Tablets 817

Zinc (Co-administration of risedronate sodium and calcium, antacids, or oral medications containing divalent cations will interfere with the absorption of risedronate sodium). Products include:
Visutein Capsules 3329

Food Interactions

Food, unspecified (Mean oral bioavailability is decreased when risedronate is administered with food; risedronate sodium is effective when administered at least 30 minutes before breakfast).

ACTOPLUS MET TABLETS

(Metformin Hydrochloride, Pioglitazone Hydrochloride) 3214
May interact with cationic drugs that are eliminated by renal tubular, calcium channel blockers, corticosteroids, cytochrome p450 3a4 substrates (selected), diuretics, estrogens, oral hypoglycemic agents, insulin, oral contraceptives, phenothiazines, phenytoin, sympathomimetics, thiazides, thyroid preparations, and certain other agents. Compounds in these categories include:

Acarbose (Pioglitazone, like other thiazolidinediones, can cause fluid retention when used alone or in combination with other antihyperglycemic agents, including insulin). Products include:
Precose Tablets 751

Albuterol (Certain drugs, including sympathomimetics, tend to produce hyperglycemia and may lead to loss of glycemic control. When such drugs are administered to a patient receiving Actoplus Met, the patient should be closely observed to maintain adequate glycemic control). Products include:
Proventil Inhalation Aerosol 3053

Albuterol Sulfate (Certain drugs, including sympathomimetics, tend to produce hyperglycemia and may lead to loss of glycemic control. When such drugs are administered to a patient receiving Actoplus Met, the patient should be closely observed to maintain adequate glycemic control). Products include:
AccuNeb Inhalation Solution 1055
Combivent Inhalation Aerosol 847
DuoNeb Inhalation Solution 1058
ProAir HFA Inhalation Aerosol 3300
Proventil Inhalation Solution 0.083% 3055
Proventil HFA Inhalation Aerosol 3056
Ventolin HFA Inhalation Aerosol 1600
VoSpire ER Tablets 1052

Alfentanil Hydrochloride (Studies have suggested that pioglitazone may be a weak inducer of CYP450 isoform 3A4 substrate).
No products indexed under this heading.

Alprazolam (Studies have suggested that pioglitazone may be a weak inducer of CYP450 isoform 3A4 substrate). Products include:
Niravam Orally Disintegrating Tablets 3092

Amiloride Hydrochloride (Cationic drugs that are eliminated by renal tubular secretion theoretically have the potential for interaction with metformin by competing for common renal tubular transport systems. Although such interactions remain theoretical, careful patient monitoring and dose adjustment of Actoplus Met and/or the interfering drug is recommended in patients who are taking cationic medications that are excreted via the proximal renal tubular secretory system). Products include:
Midamor Tablets 2026
Moduretic Tablets 2028

Amitriptyline Hydrochloride (Studies have suggested that pioglitazone may be a weak inducer of CYP450 isoform 3A4 substrate).
No products indexed under this heading.

Amlodipine Besylate (Certain drugs, including calcium channel blockers, tend to produce hyperglycemia and may lead to loss of glycemic control. When such drugs are administered to a patient receiving Actoplus Met, the patient should be closely observed to maintain adequate glycemic control). Products include:
Caduet Tablets 2508
Lotrel Capsules 2249
Norvasc Tablets 2545

Aprepitant (Studies have suggested that pioglitazone may be a weak inducer of CYP450 isoform 3A4 substrate). Products include:
Emend Capsules 1963

Astemizole (Studies have suggested that pioglitazone may be a weak inducer of CYP450 isoform 3A4 substrate).
No products indexed under this heading.

Atorvastatin Calcium (Studies have suggested that pioglitazone may be a weak inducer of CYP450 isoform 3A4 substrate). Products include:
Caduet Tablets 2508
Lipitor Tablets 2483

Belladonna Ergotamine (Studies have suggested that pioglitazone may be a weak inducer of CYP450 isoform 3A4 substrate).
No products indexed under this heading.

Bendroflumethiazide (Certain drugs, including thiazide diuretics, tend to produce hyperglycemia and may lead to loss of glycemic control. When such drugs are administered to a patient receiving Actoplus Met, the patient should be closely observed to maintain adequate glycemic control).
No products indexed under this heading.

Bepridil Hydrochloride (Certain drugs, including calcium channel blockers, tend to produce hyperglycemia and may lead to loss of glycemic control. When such drugs are administered to a patient receiving Actoplus Met, the patient should be closely observed to maintain adequate glycemic control).
No products indexed under this heading.

Betamethasone Acetate (Certain drugs, including corticosteroids, tend to produce hyperglycemia and may lead to loss of glycemic control. When such drugs are administered to a patient receiving Actoplus Met, the patient should be closely observed to maintain adequate glycemic control).
No products indexed under this heading.

Betamethasone Sodium Phosphate (Certain drugs, including corticosteroids, tend to produce hyperglycemia and may lead to loss of glycemic control. When such drugs are administered to a patient receiving Actoplus Met, the patient should be closely observed to maintain adequate glycemic control).
No products indexed under this heading.

Bumetanide (Certain drugs, including diuretics, tend to produce hyperglycemia and may lead to loss of glycemic control. When such drugs are administered to a patient receiving Actoplus Met, the patient should be closely observed to maintain adequate glycemic control). Products include:
Bumex Tablets 2746

Buspirone Hydrochloride (Studies have suggested that pioglitazone may be a weak inducer of CYP450 isoform 3A4 substrate).
No products indexed under this heading.

Busulfan (Studies have suggested that pioglitazone may be a weak inducer of CYP450 isoform 3A4 substrate). Products include:
I.V. Busulfex 2493
Myleran Tablets 1525

Carbamazepine (Studies have suggested that pioglitazone may be a weak inducer of CYP450 isoform 3A4 substrate). Products include:
Carbatrol Capsules 3171
Equetro Extended-Release Capsules 3180
Tegretol/Tegretol-XR 2295

Cerivastatin Sodium (Studies have suggested that pioglitazone may be a weak inducer of CYP450 isoform 3A4 substrate).
No products indexed under this heading.

Chlorothiazide (Certain drugs, including thiazide diuretics, tend to produce hyperglycemia and may lead to loss of glycemic control. When such drugs are administered to a patient receiving Actoplus Met, the patient should be closely observed to maintain adequate glycemic control). Products include:
Diuril Oral Suspension 1954

Chlorothiazide Sodium (Certain drugs, including thiazide diuretics, tend to produce hyperglycemia and may lead to loss of glycemic control. When such drugs are administered to a patient receiving Actoplus Met, the patient should be closely observed to maintain adequate glycemic control). Products include:
Diuril Sodium Intravenous 2467

Chlorotrianisene (Certain drugs, including estrogens, tend to produce hyperglycemia and may lead to loss of glycemic control. When such drugs are administered to a patient receiving Actoplus Met, the patient should be closely observed to maintain adequate glycemic control).
No products indexed under this heading.

Chlorpheniramine (Studies have suggested that pioglitazone may be a weak inducer of CYP450 isoform 3A4 substrate).
No products indexed under this heading.

Chlorpheniramine Maleate (Studies have suggested that pioglitazone may be a weak inducer of CYP450 isoform 3A4 substrate). Products include:

Advil Allergy Sinus Caplets .... ▣770
Advil Multi-Symptom Cold Caplets .... ▣770
BC Allergy Sinus Cold Powder .... ▣677
Comtrex Maximum Strength Cold & Cough Day/Night Caplets - Night Formulation .... ▣726
Comtrex Maximum Strength Day/Night Severe Cold & Sinus Caplets - Night Formulation .... ▣725
Contac Cold and Flu Maximum Strength Caplets .... ▣728
Contac Cold and Flu Day and Night Caplets (Night Formulation Only) .... ▣727
Children's Dimetapp Long Acting Cough Plus Cold Syrup .... ▣731
Robitussin Cough & Cold Long-Acting Liquid .... ▣735
Robitussin Cough & Allergy Syrup .. ▣736
Robitussin Cough & Cold Nighttime Liquid .... ▣736
Robitussin Cough, Cold & Flu Nighttime Liquid .... ▣738
Robitussin Pediatric Cough & Cold Long-Acting Liquid .... ▣735
Robitussin Pediatric Cough & Cold Nighttime Liquid .... ▣736
Triaminic Cold & Allergy Liquid .... ▣746
Triaminic Cough & Runny Nose Softchews .... ▣748
Children's Tylenol Plus Flu Oral Suspension .... ▣749
Tylenol Allergy Multi-Symptom Caplets with Cool Burst and Gelcaps 1872
Children's Tylenol Plus Cold Suspension Liquid 1879
Children's Tylenol Plus Cough & Runny Nose Suspension Liquid 1879
Children's Tylenol Plus Flu Suspension Liquid 1881
Children's Tylenol Plus Multi-Symptom Cold Suspension Liquid 1879
Tylenol Cold Head Congestion Nighttime Caplets with Cool Burst 1873
Tylenol Cold Multi-Symptom Nighttime Caplets with Cool Burst 1874
Tylenol Sinus Congestion & Pain Nighttime Caplets with Cool Burst 1876
Vicks 44M Cough, Cold & Flu Relief Liquid 2680
Pediatric Vicks 44m Cough & Cold Relief Liquid 2676
Children's Vicks NyQuil Cold/Cough Relief .... ▣756
Children's Vicks NyQuil Cold/Cough Relief Liquid 2680
Zicam Maximum Strength Flu Daytime .... ▣768

Chlorpheniramine Polistirex (Studies have suggested that pioglitazone may be a weak inducer of CYP450 isoform 3A4 substrate). Products include:

Tussionex Pennkinetic Extended-Release Suspension 3327

Chlorpheniramine Tannate (Studies have suggested that pioglitazone may be a weak inducer of CYP450 isoform 3A4 substrate).

No products indexed under this heading.

Chlorpromazine (Certain drugs, including phenothiazines, tend to produce hyperglycemia and may lead to loss of glycemic control. When such drugs are administered to a patient receiving Actoplus Met, the patient should be closely observed to maintain adequate glycemic control).

No products indexed under this heading.

Chlorpromazine Hydrochloride (Certain drugs, including phenothiazines, tend to produce hyperglycemia and may lead to loss of glycemic control. When such drugs are administered to a patient receiving Actoplus Met, the patient should be closely observed to maintain adequate glycemic control).

No products indexed under this heading.

Chlorpropamide (Pioglitazone, like other thiazolidinediones, can cause fluid retention when used alone or in combination with other antihyperglycemic agents, including insulin).

No products indexed under this heading.

Chlorthalidone (Certain drugs, including diuretics, tend to produce hyperglycemia and may lead to loss of glycemic control. When such drugs are administered to a patient receiving Actoplus Met, the patient should be closely observed to maintain adequate glycemic control). Products include:

Clorpres Tablets 2153

Cimetidine (Cationic drugs that are eliminated by renal tubular secretion and theoretically have the potential for interaction with metformin by competing for common renal tubular transport systems. Although such interactions remain theoretical (except for cimetidine), careful patient monitoring and dose adjustment of Actolus Met and/or the interfering drug is recommended in patients who are taking cationic medications that are excreted via the proximal renal tubular secretory system). Products include:

Tagamet HB 200 Tablets .... ▣664

Cimetidine Hydrochloride (Cationic drugs that are eliminated by renal tubular secretion and theoretically have the potential for interaction with metformin by competing for common renal tubular transport systems. Although such interactions remain theoretical (except for cimetidine), careful patient monitoring and dose adjustment of Actolus Met and/or the interfering drug is recommended in patients who are taking cationic medications that are excreted via the proximal renal tubular secretory system).

No products indexed under this heading.

Cisapride (Studies have suggested that pioglitazone may be a weak inducer of CYP450 isoform 3A4 substrate).

No products indexed under this heading.

Clarithromycin (Studies have suggested that pioglitazone may be a weak inducer of CYP450 isoform 3A4 substrate). Products include:

Biaxin/Biaxin XL 402
PREVPAC 3284

Cortisone Acetate (Certain drugs, including corticosteroids, tend to produce hyperglycemia and may lead to loss of glycemic control. When such drugs are administered to a patient receiving Actoplus Met, the patient should be closely observed to maintain adequate glycemic control).

No products indexed under this heading.

Cyclosporine (Studies have suggested that pioglitazone may be a weak inducer of CYP450 isoform 3A4 substrate). Products include:

Gengraf Capsules 459
Neoral Oral Solution 2259
Neoral Soft Gelatin Capsules 2259
Restasis Ophthalmic Emulsion 575
Sandimmune 2275

Desogestrel (Certain drugs, including oral contraceptives, tend to produce hyperglycemia and may lead to loss of glycemic control. When such drugs are administered to a patient receiving Actoplus Met, the patient should be closely observed to maintain adequate glycemic control). Products include:

Mircette Tablets 1066

Dexamethasone (Certain drugs, including corticosteroids, tend to produce hyperglycemia and may lead to loss of glycemic control. When such drugs are administered to a patient receiving Actoplus Met, the patient should be closely observed to maintain adequate glycemic control). Products include:

Ciprodex Otic Suspension 559
Decadron Tablets 1951
TobraDex Ophthalmic Ointment 562
TobraDex Ophthalmic Suspension ... 563

Dexamethasone Acetate (Certain drugs, including corticosteroids, tend to produce hyperglycemia and may lead to loss of glycemic control. When such drugs are administered to a patient receiving Actoplus Met, the patient should be closely observed to maintain adequate glycemic control).

No products indexed under this heading.

Dexamethasone Sodium Phosphate (Certain drugs, including corticosteroids, tend to produce hyperglycemia and may lead to loss of glycemic control. When such drugs are administered to a patient receiving Actoplus Met, the patient should be closely observed to maintain adequate glycemic control).

No products indexed under this heading.

Diazepam (Studies have suggested that pioglitazone may be a weak inducer of CYP450 isoform 3A4 substrate). Products include:

Diastat Rectal Delivery System 3343
Valium Tablets 2819

Dienestrol (Certain drugs, including estrogens, tend to produce hyperglycemia and may lead to loss of glycemic control. When such drugs are administered to a patient receiving Actoplus Met, the patient should be closely observed to maintain adequate glycemic control).

No products indexed under this heading.

Diethylstilbestrol (Certain drugs, including estrogens, tend to produce hyperglycemia and may lead to loss of glycemic control. When such drugs are administered to a patient receiving Actoplus Met, the patient should be closely observed to maintain adequate glycemic control).

No products indexed under this heading.

Digoxin (Cationic drugs that are eliminated by renal tubular secretion theoretically have the potential for interaction with metformin by competing for common renal tubular transport systems. Although such interactions remain theoretical, careful patient monitoring and dose adjustment of Actoplus Met and/or the interfering drug is recommended in patients who are taking cationic medications that are excreted via the proximal renal tubular secretory system). Products include:

Lanoxicaps Capsules 1490
Lanoxin Injection 1494
Lanoxin Injection Pediatric 1497
Lanoxin Tablets 1500

Dihydroergotamine Mesylate (Studies have suggested that pioglitazone may be a weak inducer of CYP450 isoform 3A4 substrate). Products include:

Migranal Nasal Spray 3348

Diltiazem Hydrochloride (Certain drugs, including calcium channel blockers, tend to produce hyperglycemia and may lead to loss of glycemic control. When such drugs are administered to a patient receiving Actoplus Met, the patient should be closely observed to maintain adequate glycemic control). Products include:

Cardizem LA Extended Release Tablets 1728
Tiazac Capsules 1201

Diltiazem Maleate (Studies have suggested that pioglitazone may be a weak inducer of CYP450 isoform 3A4 substrate).

No products indexed under this heading.

Disopyramide (Studies have suggested that pioglitazone may be a weak inducer of CYP450 isoform 3A4 substrate).

No products indexed under this heading.

Disopyramide Phosphate (Studies have suggested that pioglitazone may be a weak inducer of CYP450 isoform 3A4 substrate).

No products indexed under this heading.

Disulfiram (Studies have suggested that pioglitazone may be a weak inducer of CYP450 isoform 3A4 substrate).

No products indexed under this heading.

Dobutamine Hydrochloride (Certain drugs, including sympathomimetics, tend to produce hyperglycemia and may lead to loss of glycemic control. When such drugs are administered to a patient receiving Actoplus Met, the patient should be closely observed to maintain adequate glycemic control).

No products indexed under this heading.

Dopamine Hydrochloride (Certain drugs, including sympathomimetics, tend to produce hyperglycemia and may lead to loss of glycemic control. When such drugs are administered to a patient receiving Actoplus Met, the patient should be closely observed to maintain adequate glycemic control).

No products indexed under this heading.

Doxorubicin Hydrochloride (Studies have suggested that pioglitazone may be a weak inducer of CYP450 isoform 3A4 substrate).

No products indexed under this heading.

Dronabinol (Studies have suggested that pioglitazone may be a weak inducer of CYP450 isoform 3A4 substrate). Products include:

Marinol Capsules 3333

Ephedrine Hydrochloride (Certain drugs, including sympathomimetics, tend to produce hyperglycemia and may lead to loss of glycemic control. When such drugs are administered to a patient receiving Actoplus Met, the patient should be closely observed to maintain adequate glycemic control).
No products indexed under this heading.

Ephedrine Sulfate (Certain drugs, including sympathomimetics, tend to produce hyperglycemia and may lead to loss of glycemic control. When such drugs are administered to a patient receiving Actoplus Met, the patient should be closely observed to maintain adequate glycemic control).
No products indexed under this heading.

Ephedrine Tannate (Certain drugs, including sympathomimetics, tend to produce hyperglycemia and may lead to loss of glycemic control. When such drugs are administered to a patient receiving Actoplus Met, the patient should be closely observed to maintain adequate glycemic control).
No products indexed under this heading.

Epinephrine (Certain drugs, including sympathomimetics, tend to produce hyperglycemia and may lead to loss of glycemic control. When such drugs are administered to a patient receiving Actoplus Met, the patient should be closely observed to maintain adequate glycemic control). Products include:
EpiPen **1061**
Primatene Mist **719**
Twinject 0.15 .... **3379**
Twinject 0.3 .... **3378**

Epinephrine Bitartrate (Certain drugs, including sympathomimetics, tend to produce hyperglycemia and may lead to loss of glycemic control. When such drugs are administered to a patient receiving Actoplus Met, the patient should be closely observed to maintain adequate glycemic control).
No products indexed under this heading.

Epinephrine Hydrochloride (Certain drugs, including sympathomimetics, tend to produce hyperglycemia and may lead to loss of glycemic control. When such drugs are administered to a patient receiving Actoplus Met, the patient should be closely observed to maintain adequate glycemic control).
No products indexed under this heading.

Ergotamine Tartrate (Studies have suggested that pioglitazone may be a weak inducer of CYP450 isoform 3A4 substrate).
No products indexed under this heading.

Erythromycin (Studies have suggested that pioglitazone may be a weak inducer of CYP450 isoform 3A4 substrate). Products include:
Ery-Tab Tablets **449**
Erythromycin Base Filmtab Tablets **455**
Erythromycin Delayed-Release Capsules, USP **457**
PCE Dispertab Tablets **515**

Erythromycin Estolate (Studies have suggested that pioglitazone may be a weak inducer of CYP450 isoform 3A4 substrate).
No products indexed under this heading.

Erythromycin Ethylsuccinate (Studies have suggested that pioglitazone may be a weak inducer of CYP450 isoform 3A4 substrate). Products include:
E.E.S. **451**
EryPed **447**

Erythromycin Gluceptate (Studies have suggested that pioglitazone may be a weak inducer of CYP450 isoform 3A4 substrate).
No products indexed under this heading.

Erythromycin Lactobionate (Studies have suggested that pioglitazone may be a weak inducer of CYP450 isoform 3A4 substrate).
No products indexed under this heading.

Erythromycin Stearate (Studies have suggested that pioglitazone may be a weak inducer of CYP450 isoform 3A4 substrate). Products include:
Erythrocin Stearate Filmtab Tablets **453**

Estradiol (Certain drugs, including estrogens, tend to produce hyperglycemia and may lead to loss of glycemic control. When such drugs are administered to a patient receiving Actoplus Met, the patient should be closely observed to maintain adequate glycemic control). Products include:
Angeliq Tablets **762**
Climara Transdermal System **771**
Climara Pro Transdermal System **776**
Estrasorb Topical Emulsion **1147**
Estring Vaginal Ring **2635**
Menostar Transdermal System **782**
Vagifem Tablets **2334**

Estradiol Benzoate (Studies have suggested that pioglitazone may be a weak inducer of CYP450 isoform 3A4 substrate).
No products indexed under this heading.

Estradiol Cypionate (Studies have suggested that pioglitazone may be a weak inducer of CYP450 isoform 3A4 substrate).
No products indexed under this heading.

Estradiol Valerate (Studies have suggested that pioglitazone may be a weak inducer of CYP450 isoform 3A4 substrate).
No products indexed under this heading.

Estrogens, Conjugated (Certain drugs, including estrogens, tend to produce hyperglycemia and may lead to loss of glycemic control. When such drugs are administered to a patient receiving Actoplus Met, the patient should be closely observed to maintain adequate glycemic control). Products include:
Premarin Intravenous **3442**
Premarin Tablets **3446**
Premarin Vaginal Cream **3452**
Premphase Tablets **3456**
Prempro Tablets **3456**

Estrogens, Esterified (Certain drugs, including estrogens, tend to produce hyperglycemia and may lead to loss of glycemic control. When such drugs are administered to a patient receiving Actoplus Met, the patient should be closely observed to maintain adequate glycemic control). Products include:
Estratest Tablets **3199**
Estratest H.S. Tablets **3199**

Estropipate (Certain drugs, including estrogens, tend to produce hyperglycemia and may lead to loss of glycemic control. When such drugs are administered to a patient receiving Actoplus Met, the patient should be closely observed to maintain adequate glycemic control).
No products indexed under this heading.

Ethacrynic Acid (Certain drugs, including diuretics, tend to produce hyperglycemia and may lead to loss of glycemic control. When such drugs are administered to a patient receiving Actoplus Met, the patient should be closely observed to maintain adequate glycemic control). Products include:
Edecrin Tablets **1959**

Ethinyl Estradiol (Certain drugs, including oral contraceptives, tend to produce hyperglycemia and may lead to loss of glycemic control. When such drugs are administered to a patient receiving Actoplus Met, the patient should be closely observed to maintain adequate glycemic control). Products include:
Mircette Tablets **1066**
NuvaRing **2340**
Ortho-Cyclen/Ortho Tri-Cyclen **2429**
Ortho Evra Transdermal System **2417**
Ortho Tri-Cyclen Lo Tablets **2436**
Seasonique Tablets **1077**
Yasmin 28 Tablets **796**
Yaz Tablets **803**

Ethosuximide (Studies have suggested that pioglitazone may be a weak inducer of CYP450 isoform 3A4 substrate).
No products indexed under this heading.

Ethyl Alcohol (Alcohol is known to potentiate the effect of metformin on lactate metabolism. Patients, therefore, should be warned against excessive alcohol intake, acute or chronic, while receiving Actoplus Met).
No products indexed under this heading.

Ethynodiol Diacetate (Certain drugs, including oral contraceptives, tend to produce hyperglycemia and may lead to loss of glycemic control. When such drugs are administered to a patient receiving Actoplus Met, the patient should be closely observed to maintain adequate glycemic control).
No products indexed under this heading.

Etoposide (Studies have suggested that pioglitazone may be a weak inducer of CYP450 isoform 3A4 substrate).
No products indexed under this heading.

Etoposide Phosphate (Studies have suggested that pioglitazone may be a weak inducer of CYP450 isoform 3A4 substrate).
No products indexed under this heading.

Felodipine (Certain drugs, including calcium channel blockers, tend to produce hyperglycemia and may lead to loss of glycemic control. When such drugs are administered to a patient receiving Actoplus Met, the patient should be closely observed to maintain adequate glycemic control).
No products indexed under this heading.

Fentanyl (Studies have suggested that pioglitazone may be a weak inducer of CYP450 isoform 3A4 substrate). Products include:
Duragesic Transdermal System **2373**
Ionsys Transdermal System **2379**

Fentanyl Citrate (Studies have suggested that pioglitazone may be a weak inducer of CYP450 isoform 3A4 substrate). Products include:
Actiq **979**

Fludrocortisone Acetate (Certain drugs, including corticosteroids, tend to produce hyperglycemia and may lead to loss of glycemic control. When such drugs are administered to a patient receiving Actoplus Met, the patient should be closely observed to maintain adequate glycemic control).
No products indexed under this heading.

Fluphenazine Decanoate (Certain drugs, including phenothiazines, tend to produce hyperglycemia and may lead to loss of glycemic control. When such drugs are administered to a patient receiving Actoplus Met, the patient should be closely observed to maintain adequate glycemic control).
No products indexed under this heading.

Fluphenazine Enanthate (Certain drugs, including phenothiazines, tend to produce hyperglycemia and may lead to loss of glycemic control. When such drugs are administered to a patient receiving Actoplus Met, the patient should be closely observed to maintain adequate glycemic control).
No products indexed under this heading.

Fluphenazine Hydrochloride (Certain drugs, including phenothiazines, tend to produce hyperglycemia and may lead to loss of glycemic control. When such drugs are administered to a patient receiving Actoplus Met, the patient should be closely observed to maintain adequate glycemic control).
No products indexed under this heading.

Fosphenytoin Sodium (Certain drugs, including phenytoin, tend to produce hyperglycemia and may lead to loss of glycemic control. When such drugs are administered to a patient receiving Actoplus Met, the patient should be closely observed to maintain adequate glycemic control).
No products indexed under this heading.

Furosemide (A single-dose, metformin-furosemide drug interaction study in healthy subjects demonstrated that pharmacokinetic parameters of both compounds were affected by co-administration. Furosemide increased the metformin plasma and blood Cmax by 22% and blood AUC by 15%, without any significant change in metformin renal clearance. When administered with metformin, the Cmax and AUC of furosemide were 31% and 12% smaller, respectively, than when administered alone and the terminal half-life was decreased by 31%,without any significant change in furosemide renal clearance. No information is available about the interaction of metformin and furosemide when co-administerd chronically). Products include:

Furosemide Tablets 2154

Glimepiride (Pioglitazone, like other thiazolidinediones, can cause fluid retention when used alone or in combination with other antihyperglycemic agents, including insulin). Products include:

Avandaryl Tablets 1379
Duetact Tablets 3226

Glipizide (Pioglitazone, like other thiazolidinediones, can cause fluid retention when used alone or in combination with other antihyperglycemic agents, including insulin).

No products indexed under this heading.

Glyburide (Pioglitazone, like other thiazolidinediones, can cause fluid retention when used alone or in combination with other antihyperglycemic agents, including insulin).

No products indexed under this heading.

Haloperidol (Studies have suggested that pioglitazone may be a weak inducer of CYP450 isoform 3A4 substrate).

No products indexed under this heading.

Haloperidol Decanoate (Studies have suggested that pioglitazone may be a weak inducer of CYP450 isoform 3A4 substrate).

No products indexed under this heading.

Haloperidol Lactate (Studies have suggested that pioglitazone may be a weak inducer of CYP450 isoform 3A4 substrate).

No products indexed under this heading.

Hydrochlorothiazide (Certain drugs, including thiazide diuretics, tend to produce hyperglycemia and may lead to loss of glycemic control. When such drugs are administered to a patient receiving Actoplus Met, the patient should be closely observed to maintain adequate glycemic control). Products include:

Aldoril Tablets 1910
Atacand HCT 651
Avalide Tablets 888
Avalide Tablets 2874
Benicar HCT Tablets 1044
Diovan HCT Tablets 2196
Dyazide Capsules 1423
Hyzaar 50-12.5 Tablets 1990
Hyzaar 100-12.5 Tablets 1990
Hyzaar 100-25 Tablets 1990
Lopressor HCT 50/25 Tablets 2241
Lopressor HCT 100/25 Tablets 2241
Lopressor HCT 100/50 Tablets 2241
Lotensin HCT Tablets 2246
Micardis HCT Tablets 856
Moduretic Tablets 2028
Prinzide Tablets 2056
Teveten HCT Tablets 1737
Timolide Tablets 2086
Uniretic Tablets 3100

Hydrocortisone (Certain drugs, including corticosteroids, tend to produce hyperglycemia and may lead to loss of glycemic control. When such drugs are administered to a patient receiving Actoplus Met,

the patient should be closely observed to maintain adequate glycemic control). Products include:

Colocort Rectal Suspension, USP (Retention) 100 mg/60 mL........... 2476
Hydrocortone Tablets 1989
Preparation H Hydrocortisone Cream .. ▣646

Hydrocortisone Acetate (Certain drugs, including corticosteroids, tend to produce hyperglycemia and may lead to loss of glycemic control. When such drugs are administered to a patient receiving Actoplus Met, the patient should be closely observed to maintain adequate glycemic control). Products include:

Analpram-HC 1159
Pramosone 1161
ProctoFoam-HC 3099

Hydrocortisone Sodium Phosphate (Certain drugs, including corticosteroids, tend to produce hyperglycemia and may lead to loss of glycemic control. When such drugs are administered to a patient receiving Actoplus Met, the patient should be closely observed to maintain adequate glycemic control).

No products indexed under this heading.

Hydrocortisone Sodium Succinate (Certain drugs, including corticosteroids, tend to produce hyperglycemia and may lead to loss of glycemic control. When such drugs are administered to a patient receiving Actoplus Met, the patient should be closely observed to maintain adequate glycemic control).

No products indexed under this heading.

Hydroflumethiazide (Certain drugs, including thiazide diuretics, tend to produce hyperglycemia and may lead to loss of glycemic control. When such drugs are administered to a patient receiving Actoplus Met, the patient should be closely observed to maintain adequate glycemic control).

No products indexed under this heading.

Indapamide (Certain drugs, including diuretics, tend to produce hyperglycemia and may lead to loss of glycemic control. When such drugs are administered to a patient receiving Actoplus Met, the patient should be closely observed to maintain adequate glycemic control). Products include:

Indapamide Tablets 2156

Indinavir Sulfate (Studies have suggested that pioglitazone may be a weak inducer of CYP450 isoform 3A4 substrate). Products include:

Crixivan Capsules 1940

Insulin, Human, Zinc Suspension (Pioglitazone, like other thiazolidinediones, can cause fluid retention when used alone or in combination with other antihyperglycemic agents, including insulin). Products include:

Humulin L, 100 Units 1794
Humulin U, 100 Units 1800

Insulin, Human NPH (Pioglitazone, like other thiazolidinediones, can cause fluid retention when used alone or in combination with other antihyperglycemic agents, including insulin). Products include:

Humulin N, 100 Units 1795
Humulin N Pen 1797

Insulin, Human Regular (Pioglitazone, like other thiazolidinediones, can cause fluid retention when used

alone or in combination with other antihyperglycemic agents, including insulin). Products include:

Humulin R, 100 Units 1798

Insulin, Human Regular and Human NPH Mixture (Pioglitazone, like other thiazolidinediones, can cause fluid retention when used alone or in combination with other antihyperglycemic agents, including insulin). Products include:

Humulin 50/50, 100 Units 1791
Humulin 70/30 Pen 1793

Insulin, NPH (Pioglitazone, like other thiazolidinediones, can cause fluid retention when used alone or in combination with other antihyperglycemic agents, including insulin).

No products indexed under this heading.

Insulin, Regular (Pioglitazone, like other thiazolidinediones, can cause fluid retention when used alone or in combination with other antihyperglycemic agents, including insulin).

No products indexed under this heading.

Insulin, Zinc Crystals (Pioglitazone, like other thiazolidinediones, can cause fluid retention when used alone or in combination with other antihyperglycemic agents, including insulin).

No products indexed under this heading.

Insulin, Zinc Suspension (Pioglitazone, like other thiazolidinediones, can cause fluid retention when used alone or in combination with other antihyperglycemic agents, including insulin).

No products indexed under this heading.

Insulin Aspart, Human Regular (Pioglitazone, like other thiazolidinediones, can cause fluid retention when used alone or in combination with other antihyperglycemic agents, including insulin). Products include:

NovoLog Injection 2326

Insulin glargine (Pioglitazone, like other thiazolidinediones, can cause fluid retention when used alone or in combination with other antihyperglycemic agents, including insulin). Products include:

Lantus Injection 2909

Insulin Lispro, Human (Pioglitazone, like other thiazolidinediones, can cause fluid retention when used alone or in combination with other antihyperglycemic agents, including insulin). Products include:

Humalog-Pen 1781
Humalog Mix 50/50-Pen 1783
Humalog Mix 75/25-Pen 1785

Insulin Lispro Protamine, Human (Pioglitazone, like other thiazolidinediones, can cause fluid retention when used alone or in combination with other antihyperglycemic agents, including insulin). Products include:

Humalog Mix 50/50-Pen 1783
Humalog Mix 75/25-Pen 1785

Isoniazid (Certain drugs, including isoniazid, tend to produce hyperglycemia and may lead to loss of glycemic control. When such drugs are administered to a patient receiving Actoplus Met, the patient should be closely observed to maintain adequate glycemic control).

No products indexed under this heading.

Isoproterenol Hydrochloride (Certain drugs, including sympathomimetics, tend to produce hyperglycemia and may lead to loss of glycemic control. When such drugs are administered to a patient receiving Actoplus Met, the patient should be closely observed to maintain adequate glycemic control).

No products indexed under this heading.

Isoproterenol Sulfate (Certain drugs, including sympathomimetics, tend to produce hyperglycemia and may lead to loss of glycemic control. When such drugs are administered to a patient receiving Actoplus Met, the patient should be closely observed to maintain adequate glycemic control).

No products indexed under this heading.

Isradipine (Certain drugs, including calcium channel blockers, tend to produce hyperglycemia and may lead to loss of glycemic control. When such drugs are administered to a patient receiving Actoplus Met, the patient should be closely observed to maintain adequate glycemic control). Products include:

DynaCirc CR Tablets 2721

Itraconazole (Studies have suggested that pioglitazone may be a weak inducer of CYP450 isoform 3A4 substrate).

No products indexed under this heading.

Ketoconazole (Studies have suggested that pioglitazone may be a weak inducer of CYP450 isoform 3A4 substrate). Products include:

Nizoral A-D Shampoo, 1% 1868

Levalbuterol Hydrochloride (Certain drugs, including sympathomimetics, tend to produce hyperglycemia and may lead to loss of glycemic control. When such drugs are administered to a patient receiving Actoplus Met, the patient should be closely observed to maintain adequate glycemic control). Products include:

Xopenex Inhalation Solution 3146
Xopenex Inhalation Solution Concentrate 3150

Levonorgestrel (Certain drugs, including oral contraceptives, tend to produce hyperglycemia and may lead to loss of glycemic control. When such drugs are administered to a patient receiving Actoplus Met, the patient should be closely observed to maintain adequate glycemic control). Products include:

Climara Pro Transdermal System 776
Mirena Intrauterine System 787
Plan B Tablets 1076
Seasonique Tablets 1077

Levothyroxine Sodium (Certain drugs, including thyroid products, tend to produce hyperglycemia and may lead to loss of glycemic control. When such drugs are administered to a patient receiving Actoplus Met, the patient should be closely observed to maintain adequate glycemic control). Products include:

Levothroid Tablets 1186
Levoxyl Tablets 1712
Synthroid Tablets 520
Westhroid Tablets 3403

Lidocaine (Studies have suggested that pioglitazone may be a weak inducer of CYP450 isoform 3A4 substrate). Products include:

Lidoderm Patch 1118
Synera Topical Patch 1137

Lidocaine Hydrochloride (Studies have suggested that pioglitazone may be a weak inducer of CYP450 isoform 3A4 substrate).
No products indexed under this heading.

Liothyronine Sodium (Certain drugs, including thyroid products, tend to produce hyperglycemia and may lead to loss of glycemic control. When such drugs are administered to a patient receiving Actoplus Met, the patient should be closely observed to maintain adequate glycemic control). Products include:
Cytomel Tablets 1710
Westhroid Tablets 3403

Liotrix (Certain drugs, including thyroid products, tend to produce hyperglycemia and may lead to loss of glycemic control. When such drugs are administered to a patient receiving Actoplus Met, the patient should be closely observed to maintain adequate glycemic control). Products include:
Thyrolar Tablets 1199

Lovastatin (Studies have suggested that pioglitazone may be a weak inducer of CYP450 isoform 3A4 substrate). Products include:
Advicor Tablets 1722
Altoprev Extended-Release Tablets 3109
Mevacor Tablets 2021

Mesoridazine Besylate (Certain drugs, including phenothiazines, tend to produce hyperglycemia and may lead to loss of glycemic control. When such drugs are administered to a patient receiving Actoplus Met, the patient should be closely observed to maintain adequate glycemic control).
No products indexed under this heading.

Mestranol (Certain drugs, including oral contraceptives, tend to produce hyperglycemia and may lead to loss of glycemic control. When such drugs are administered to a patient receiving Actoplus Met, the patient should be closely observed to maintain adequate glycemic control).
No products indexed under this heading.

Metaproterenol Sulfate (Certain drugs, including sympathomimetics, tend to produce hyperglycemia and may lead to loss of glycemic control. When such drugs are administered to a patient receiving Actoplus Met, the patient should be closely observed to maintain adequate glycemic control). Products include:
Alupent Inhalation Aerosol 826

Metaraminol Bitartrate (Certain drugs, including sympathomimetics, tend to produce hyperglycemia and may lead to loss of glycemic control. When such drugs are administered to a patient receiving Actoplus Met, the patient should be closely observed to maintain adequate glycemic control).
No products indexed under this heading.

Methadone Hydrochloride (Studies have suggested that pioglitazone may be a weak inducer of CYP450 isoform 3A4 substrate).
No products indexed under this heading.

Methotrimeprazine (Certain drugs, including phenothiazines, tend to produce hyperglycemia and may lead to loss of glycemic control. When such drugs are administered to a patient receiving Actoplus Met, the patient should be closely observed to maintain adequate glycemic control).
No products indexed under this heading.

Methoxamine Hydrochloride (Certain drugs, including sympathomimetics, tend to produce hyperglycemia and may lead to loss of glycemic control. When such drugs are administered to a patient receiving Actoplus Met, the patient should be closely observed to maintain adequate glycemic control).
No products indexed under this heading.

Methyclothiazide (Certain drugs, including thiazide diuretics, tend to produce hyperglycemia and may lead to loss of glycemic control. When such drugs are administered to a patient receiving Actoplus Met, the patient should be closely observed to maintain adequate glycemic control).
No products indexed under this heading.

Methylprednisolone Acetate (Certain drugs, including corticosteroids, tend to produce hyperglycemia and may lead to loss of glycemic control. When such drugs are administered to a patient receiving Actoplus Met, the patient should be closely observed to maintain adequate glycemic control). Products include:
Depo-Medrol Injectable Suspension 2617
Depo-Medrol Single-Dose Vial 2619

Methylprednisolone Sodium Succinate (Certain drugs, including corticosteroids, tend to produce hyperglycemia and may lead to loss of glycemic control. When such drugs are administered to a patient receiving Actoplus Met, the patient should be closely observed to maintain adequate glycemic control).
No products indexed under this heading.

Metolazone (Certain drugs, including diuretics, tend to produce hyperglycemia and may lead to loss of glycemic control. When such drugs are administered to a patient receiving Actoplus Met, the patient should be closely observed to maintain adequate glycemic control).
No products indexed under this heading.

Mibefradil Dihydrochloride (Certain drugs, including calcium channel blockers, tend to produce hyperglycemia and may lead to loss of glycemic control. When such drugs are administered to a patient receiving Actoplus Met, the patient should be closely observed to maintain adequate glycemic control).
No products indexed under this heading.

Midazolam Hydrochloride (Studies have suggested that pioglitazone may be a weak inducer of CYP450 isoform 3A4 substrate).
No products indexed under this heading.

Miglitol (Pioglitazone, like other thiazolidinediones, can cause fluid retention when used alone or in combination with other antihyperglycemic agents, including insulin).
No products indexed under this heading.

Morphine Sulfate (Cationic drugs that are eliminated by renal tubular secretion theoretically have the potential for interaction with metformin by competing for common renal tubular transport systems. Although such interactions remain theoretical, careful patient monitoring and dose adjustment of Actoplus Met and/or the interfering drug is recommended in patients who are taking cationic medications that are excreted via the proximal renal tubular secretory system). Products include:
Avinza Capsules 1741
Kadian Capsules 577
MS Contin Tablets 2701

Nefazodone Hydrochloride (Studies have suggested that pioglitazone may be a weak inducer of CYP450 isoform 3A4 substrate).
No products indexed under this heading.

Nelfinavir Mesylate (Studies have suggested that pioglitazone may be a weak inducer of CYP450 isoform 3A4 substrate). Products include:
Viracept 2577

Nicardipine Hydrochloride (Certain drugs, including calcium channel blockers, tend to produce hyperglycemia and may lead to loss of glycemic control. When such drugs are administered to a patient receiving Actoplus Met, the patient should be closely observed to maintain adequate glycemic control). Products include:
Cardene I.V. 2497

Nicotinic Acid (Certain drugs, including nicotinic acid, tend to produce hyperglycemia and may lead to loss of glycemic control. When such drugs are administered to a patient receiving Actoplus Met, the patient should be closely observed to maintain adequate glycemic control).
No products indexed under this heading.

Nifedipine (A single-dose, metformin-nifedipine drug interaction study in normal healthy volunteers demonstrated that co-administration of nifedipine increased plasma metformin Cmax and AUC by 20% and 9%, respectively, and increased the amount excreted in the urine.Tmax and half-life were unaffected. Nifedipine appears to enhance the absorption of metformin. Metformin had minimal effects on nifedipine). Products include:
Adalat CC Tablets 2964

Nimodipine (Certain drugs, including calcium channel blockers, tend to produce hyperglycemia and may lead to loss of glycemic control. When such drugs are administered to a patient receiving Actoplus Met, the patient should be closely observed to maintain adequate glycemic control). Products include:
Nimotop Capsules 749

Nisoldipine (Certain drugs, including calcium channel blockers, tend to produce hyperglycemia and may lead to loss of glycemic control. When such drugs are administered to a patient receiving Actoplus Met, the patient should be closely observed to maintain adequate glycemic control). Products include:
Sular Tablets 3122

Nitrendipine (Studies have suggested that pioglitazone may be a weak inducer of CYP450 isoform 3A4 substrate).
No products indexed under this heading.

Norepinephrine Bitartrate (Certain drugs, including sympathomimetics, tend to produce hyperglycemia and may lead to loss of glycemic control. When such drugs are administered to a patient receiving Actoplus Met, the patient should be closely observed to maintain adequate glycemic control).
No products indexed under this heading.

Norethindrone (Certain drugs, including oral contraceptives, tend to produce hyperglycemia and may lead to loss of glycemic control. When such drugs are administered to a patient receiving Actoplus Met, the patient should be closely observed to maintain adequate glycemic control). Products include:
Ortho Micronor Tablets 2426

Norethindrone Acetate (Studies have suggested that pioglitazone may be a weak inducer of CYP450 isoform 3A4 substrate).
No products indexed under this heading.

Norethynodrel (Certain drugs, including oral contraceptives, tend to produce hyperglycemia and may lead to loss of glycemic control. When such drugs are administered to a patient receiving Actoplus Met, the patient should be closely observed to maintain adequate glycemic control).
No products indexed under this heading.

Norgestimate (Certain drugs, including oral contraceptives, tend to produce hyperglycemia and may lead to loss of glycemic control. When such drugs are administered to a patient receiving Actoplus Met, the patient should be closely observed to maintain adequate glycemic control). Products include:
Ortho-Cyclen/Ortho Tri-Cyclen 2429
Ortho Tri-Cyclen Lo Tablets 2436

Norgestrel (Certain drugs, including oral contraceptives, tend to produce hyperglycemia and may lead to loss of glycemic control. When such drugs are administered to a patient receiving Actoplus Met, the patient should be closely observed to maintain adequate glycemic control).
No products indexed under this heading.

Ondansetron (Studies have suggested that pioglitazone may be a weak inducer of CYP450 isoform 3A4 substrate). Products include:
Zofran ODT Orally Disintegrating Tablets 1639

Ondansetron Hydrochloride (Studies have suggested that pioglitazone may be a weak inducer of CYP450 isoform 3A4 substrate). Products include:
Zofran Injection 1634
Zofran 1639

Paclitaxel (Studies have suggested that pioglitazone may be a weak inducer of CYP450 isoform 3A4 substrate).

No products indexed under this heading.

Perphenazine (Certain drugs, including phenothiazines, tend to produce hyperglycemia and may lead to loss of glycemic control. When such drugs are administered to a patient receiving Actoplus Met, the patient should be closely observed to maintain adequate glycemic control).

No products indexed under this heading.

Phenylephrine Bitartrate (Certain drugs, including sympathomimetics, tend to produce hyperglycemia and may lead to loss of glycemic control. When such drugs are administered to a patient receiving Actoplus Met, the patient should be closely observed to maintain adequate glycemic control).

No products indexed under this heading.

Phenylephrine Hydrochloride (Certain drugs, including sympathomimetics, tend to produce hyperglycemia and may lead to loss of glycemic control. When such drugs are administered to a patient receiving Actoplus Met, the patient should be closely observed to maintain adequate glycemic control). Products include:

- Comtrex Maximum Strength Non-Drowsy Cold & Cough Caplets .... ▣ 725
- Comtrex Maximum Strength Day/Night Severe Cold & Sinus Caplets - Day Formulation .... ▣ 725
- Comtrex Maximum Strength Day/Night Severe Cold & Sinus Caplets - Night Formulation .... ▣ 725
- Contac Cold and Flu Maximum Strength Caplets .... ▣ 728
- Contac Cold and Flu Day and Night Caplets (Day Formulation Only) .... ▣ 727
- Contac Cold and Flu Day and Night Caplets (Night Formulation Only) .... ▣ 727
- Contac Cold and Flu Non-Drowsy Caplets .... ▣ 728
- Contac-D Cold Non-Drowsy Tablets .... ▣ 729
- Children's Dimetapp Cold & Allergy Elixir .... ▣ 730
- Children's Dimetapp Cold & Allergy Chewable Tablets .... ▣ 730
- Children's Dimetapp DM Cold & Cough Elixir .... ▣ 731
- Toddler's Dimetapp Cold and Cough Drops .... ▣ 732
- Excedrin Sinus Headache Caplets/Tablets .... ▣ 610
- 4-Way Fast Acting Nasal Spray .... ▣ 775
- 4-Way Menthol Nasal Spray .... ▣ 775
- Preparation H Maximum Strength Cream .... ▣ 666
- Preparation H Cooling Gel .... ▣ 666
- Preparation H .... ▣ 666
- Refenesen PE Caplets .... ▣ 721
- Robitussin Cough & Allergy Syrup .... ▣ 736
- Robitussin Cough & Cold Nighttime Liquid .... ▣ 736
- Robitussin Cough, Cold & Flu Nighttime Liquid .... ▣ 738
- Robitussin Head & Chest Congestion PE Syrup .... ▣ 739
- Robitussin Pediatric Cough & Cold Nighttime Liquid .... ▣ 736
- TheraFlu Cold & Cough Hot Liquid .... ▣ 740
- TheraFlu Cold & Sore Throat Hot Liquid .... ▣ 741
- TheraFlu Flu & Sore Throat Hot Liquid .... ▣ 742
- TheraFlu Daytime Severe Cold Hot Liquid .... ▣ 742
- TheraFlu Nighttime Severe Cold Hot Liquid .... ▣ 740
- TheraFlu Warming Relief Daytime Severe Cold .... ▣ 743
- TheraFlu Warming Relief Nighttime Severe Cold .... ▣ 743
- Triaminic Chest & Nasal Congestion Liquid .... ▣ 746
- Triaminic Cold & Allergy Liquid .... ▣ 746
- Triaminic Daytime Cold & Cough Liquid .... ▣ 745
- Triaminic Nighttime Cold & Cough Liquid .... ▣ 746
- Triaminic Thin Strips Cold .... ▣ 748
- Triaminic Thin Strips Cold & Cough .... ▣ 778
- Triaminic Infant Thin Strips Decongestant .... ▣ 747
- Triaminic Infant Thin Strips Decongestant Plus Cough .... ▣ 747
- Children's Tylenol Plus Flu Oral Suspension .... ▣ 749
- Tylenol Cold Head Congestion Daytime Caplets with Cool Burst and Gelcaps .... ▣ 750
- Tylenol Cold Multi-Symptom Daytime Liquid .... ▣ 752
- Tylenol Cold Multi-Symptom Severe Daytime Liquid .... ▣ 752
- Concentrated Tylenol Infants' Drops Plus Cold & Cough .... ▣ 754
- Tylenol Allergy Multi-Symptom Caplets with Cool Burst and Gelcaps 1872
- Tylenol Allergy Multi-Symptom Nighttime Caplets with Cool Burst 1872
- Children's Tylenol Plus Cold Suspension Liquid 1879
- Children's Tylenol Plus Cold & Allergy Suspension Liquid 1878
- Children's Tylenol Plus Flu Suspension Liquid 1881
- Children's Tylenol Plus Multi-Symptom Cold Suspension Liquid 1879
- Tylenol Cold Head Congestion Daytime Caplets with Cool Burst 1873
- Tylenol Cold Head Congestion Nighttime Caplets with Cool Burst 1873
- Tylenol Cold Head Congestion Severe Caplets with Cool Burst 1873
- Tylenol Cold Multi-Symptom Daytime Caplets with Cool Burst and Gelcaps 1874
- Tylenol Cold Multi-Symptom Daytime Liquid with Citrus Burst 1874
- Tylenol Cold Multi-Symptom Nighttime Caplets with Cool Burst 1874
- Tylenol Cold Multi-Symptom Nighttime Liquid with Cool Burst 1874
- Tylenol Cold Multi-Symptom Severe Caplets with Cool Burst 1874
- Tylenol Cold Multi-Symptom Severe Daytime Liquid with Citrus Burst 1874
- Tylenol Sinus Congestion & Pain Daytime Caplets with Cool Burst and Gelcaps 1876
- Tylenol Sinus Congestion & Pain Nighttime Caplets with Cool Burst 1876
- Tylenol Sinus Congestion & Pain Severe Caplets with Cool Burst 1876
- Vicks 44D Cough & Head Congestion Relief Liquid .... ▣ 760
- Vicks DayQuil LiquiCaps/Liquid Multi-Symptom Cold/Flu Relief .... ▣ 761
- Zicam Cough Plus D Cough Spray .... ▣ 767

Phenylephrine Tannate (Certain drugs, including sympathomimetics, tend to produce hyperglycemia and may lead to loss of glycemic control. When such drugs are administered to a patient receiving Actoplus Met, the patient should be closely observed to maintain adequate glycemic control).

No products indexed under this heading.

Phenylpropanolamine Hydrochloride (Certain drugs, including sympathomimetics, tend to produce hyperglycemia and may lead to loss of glycemic control. When such drugs are administered to a patient receiving Actoplus Met, the patient should be closely observed to maintain adequate glycemic control).

No products indexed under this heading.

Phenytoin (Certain drugs, including phenytoin, tend to produce hyperglycemia and may lead to loss of glycemic control. When such drugs are administered to a patient receiving Actoplus Met, the patient should be closely observed to maintain adequate glycemic control).

No products indexed under this heading.

Phenytoin Sodium (Certain drugs, including phenytoin, tend to produce hyperglycemia and may lead to loss of glycemic control. When such drugs are administered to a patient receiving Actoplus Met, the patient should be closely observed to maintain adequate glycemic control). Products include:

- Phenytek Capsules 2160

Pimozide (Studies have suggested that pioglitazone may be a weak inducer of CYP450 isoform 3A4 substrate).

No products indexed under this heading.

Pirbuterol Acetate (Certain drugs, including sympathomimetics, tend to produce hyperglycemia and may lead to loss of glycemic control. When such drugs are administered to a patient receiving Actoplus Met, the patient should be closely observed to maintain adequate glycemic control). Products include:

- Maxair Autohaler 1852

Polyestradiol Phosphate (Certain drugs, including estrogens, tend to produce hyperglycemia and may lead to loss of glycemic control. When such drugs are administered to a patient receiving Actoplus Met, the patient should be closely observed to maintain adequate glycemic control).

No products indexed under this heading.

Polythiazide (Certain drugs, including thiazide diuretics, tend to produce hyperglycemia and may lead to loss of glycemic control. When such drugs are administered to a patient receiving Actoplus Met, the patient should be closely observed to maintain adequate glycemic control).

No products indexed under this heading.

Prednisolone Acetate (Certain drugs, including corticosteroids, tend to produce hyperglycemia and may lead to loss of glycemic control. When such drugs are administered to a patient receiving Actoplus Met, the patient should be closely observed to maintain adequate glycemic control). Products include:

- Blephamide Ophthalmic Ointment 568
- Blephamide Ophthalmic Suspension 569
- Poly-Pred Ophthalmic Suspension .... ⊙ 233
- Pred Forte Ophthalmic Suspension .... ⊙ 235
- Pred Mild Ophthalmic Suspension .... ⊙ 238
- Pred-G Ophthalmic Ointment .... ⊙ 237
- Pred-G Ophthalmic Suspension .... ⊙ 236

Prednisolone Sodium Phosphate (Certain drugs, including corticosteroids, tend to produce hyperglycemia and may lead to loss of glycemic control. When such drugs are administered to a patient receiving Actoplus Met, the patient should be closely observed to maintain adequate glycemic control).

No products indexed under this heading.

Prednisolone Tebutate (Certain drugs, including corticosteroids, tend to produce hyperglycemia and may lead to loss of glycemic control. When such drugs are administered to a patient receiving Actoplus Met, the patient should be closely observed to maintain adequate glycemic control).

No products indexed under this heading.

Prednisone (Certain drugs, including corticosteroids, tend to produce hyperglycemia and may lead to loss of glycemic control. When such drugs are administered to a patient receiving Actoplus Met, the patient should be closely observed to maintain adequate glycemic control).

No products indexed under this heading.

Procainamide Hydrochloride (Cationic drugs that are eliminated by renal tubular secretion theoretically have the potential for interaction with metformin by competing for common renal tubular transport systems. Although such interactions remain theoretical, careful patient monitoring and dose adjustment of Actoplus Met and/or the interfering drug is recommended in patients who are taking cationic medications that are excreted via the proximal renal tubular secretory system).

No products indexed under this heading.

Prochlorperazine (Certain drugs, including phenothiazines, tend to produce hyperglycemia and may lead to loss of glycemic control. When such drugs are administered to a patient receiving Actoplus Met, the patient should be closely observed to maintain adequate glycemic control).

No products indexed under this heading.

Promethazine Hydrochloride (Certain drugs, including phenothiazines, tend to produce hyperglycemia and may lead to loss of glycemic control. When such drugs are administered to a patient receiving Actoplus Met, the patient should be closely observed to maintain adequate glycemic control). Products include:

- Phenergan Tablets and Suppositories 3440

Pseudoephedrine Hydrochloride (Certain drugs, including sympathomimetics, tend to produce hyperglycemia and may lead to loss of glycemic control. When such drugs are administered to a patient receiving Actoplus Met, the patient should be closely observed to maintain adequate glycemic control). Products include:

- Advil Allergy Sinus Caplets .... ▣ 770
- Advil Cold & Sinus .... ▣ 723
- Advil Multi-Symptom Cold Caplets .... ▣ 770
- Aleve Cold & Sinus Caplets 744
- Allegra-D 12 Hour Extended-Release Tablets 2846

Allegra-D 24 Hour Extended-Release Tablets 2849
BC Cold Powder .... ■ 677
Comtrex Maximum Strength Cold & Cough Day/Night Caplets - Day Formulation........................ ■ 726
Comtrex Maximum Strength Cold & Cough Day/Night Caplets - Night Formulation...................... ■ 726
Children's Motrin Cold Oral Suspension 1867
Mucinex D Extended-Release Bi-Layer Tablets .... ■ 776
Robitussin Cough & Cold CF Liquid .... ■ 735
Robitussin Cough & Cold Pediatric Drops.......................... ■ 735
Tylenol Sinus Congestion & Pain Nighttime Caplets with Cool Burst .... ■ 778
Tylenol Cold Severe Congestion Non-Drowsy Caplets with Cool Burst 1874
Tylenol Sinus Severe Congestion Caplets with Cool Burst 1876
Vicks 44D Cough & Head Congestion Relief Liquid 2679
Vicks 44M Cough, Cold & Flu Relief Liquid 2680
Vicks DayQuil Multi-Symptom Cold/Flu Relief LiquiCaps 2678
Vicks DayQuil Multi-Symptom Cold/Flu Relief Liquid 2678
Vicks NyQuil Multi-Symptom Cold/Flu Relief Liquid 2681
Vicks NyQuil Multi-Symptom Cold/Flu Relief LiquiCaps 2681
Children's Vicks NyQuil Cold/Cough Relief Liquid 2680
Zyrtec-D 12 Hour Extended Release Tablets 2597

Pseudoephedrine Sulfate (Certain drugs, including sympathomimetics, tend to produce hyperglycemia and may lead to loss of glycemic control. When such drugs are administered to a patient receiving Actoplus Met, the patient should be closely observed to maintain adequate glycemic control). Products include:

Alavert Allergy & Sinus D-12 Hour Tablets .... ■ 771
Clarinex-D 24-Hour Extended-Release Tablets 2998
Claritin-D Non-Drowsy 12 Hour Tablets .... ■ 772
Claritin-D Non-Drowsy 24 Hour Tablets .... ■ 772

Quinestrol (Certain drugs, including estrogens, tend to produce hyperglycemia and may lead to loss of glycemic control. When such drugs are administered to a patient receiving Actoplus Met, the patient should be closely observed to maintain adequate glycemic control).

No products indexed under this heading.

Quinidine Gluconate (Cationic drugs that are eliminated by renal tubular secretion theoretically have the potential for interaction with metformin by competing for common renal tubular transport systems. Although such interactions remain theoretical, careful patient monitoring and dose adjustment of Actoplus Met and/or the interfering drug is recommended in patients who are taking cationic medications that are excreted via the proximal renal tubular secretory system).

No products indexed under this heading.

Quinidine Polygalacturonate (Cationic drugs that are eliminated by renal tubular secretion theoretically have the potential for interaction with metformin by competing for common renal tubular transport systems. Although such interactions remain theoretical, careful patient monitoring and dose adjustment of Actoplus Met and/or the interfering drug is recommended in patients who are taking cationic medications that are excreted via the proximal renal tubular secretory system).

No products indexed under this heading.

Quinidine Sulfate (Cationic drugs that are eliminated by renal tubular secretion theoretically have the potential for interaction with metformin by competing for common renal tubular transport systems. Although such interactions remain theoretical, careful patient monitoring and dose adjustment of Actoplus Met and/or the interfering drug is recommended in patients who are taking cationic medications that are excreted via the proximal renal tubular secretory system).

No products indexed under this heading.

Quinine Sulfate (Cationic drugs that are eliminated by renal tubular secretion theoretically have the potential for interaction with metformin by competing for common renal tubular transport systems. Although such interactions remain theoretical, careful patient monitoring and dose adjustment of Actoplus Met and/or the interfering drug is recommended in patients who are taking cationic medications that are excreted via the proximal renal tubular secretory system).

No products indexed under this heading.

Ranitidine Hydrochloride (Cationic drugs that are eliminated by renal tubular secretion theoretically have the potential for interaction with metformin by competing for common renal tubular transport systems. Although such interactions remain theoretical, careful patient monitoring and dose adjustment of Actoplus Met and/or the interfering drug is recommended in patients who are taking cationic medications that are excreted via the proximal renal tubular secretory system). Products include:

Zantac 1624
Zantac Injection 1619
Zantac Injection Pharmacy Bulk Package 1622

Repaglinide (Pioglitazone, like other thiazolidinediones, can cause fluid retention when used alone or in combination with other antihyperglycemic agents, including insulin).

No products indexed under this heading.

Rifabutin (Studies have suggested that pioglitazone may be a weak inducer of CYP450 isoform 3A4 substrate).

No products indexed under this heading.

Ritonavir (Studies have suggested that pioglitazone may be a weak inducer of CYP450 isoform 3A4 substrate). Products include:

Kaletra 476
Norvir 503

Rosiglitazone Maleate (Pioglitazone, like other thiazolidinediones, can cause fluid retention when used alone or in combination with other antihyperglycemic agents, including insulin). Products include:

Avandamet Tablets 1373
Avandaryl Tablets 1379
Avandia Tablets 1384

Salmeterol Xinafoate (Certain drugs, including sympathomimetics, tend to produce hyperglycemia and may lead to loss of glycemic control. When such drugs are administered to a patient receiving Actoplus Met, the patient should be closely observed to maintain adequate glycemic control). Products include:

Advair Diskus 100/50 1308
Advair Diskus 250/50 1308
Advair Diskus 500/50 1308
Advair HFA Inhalation Aerosol 1318
Serevent Diskus 1568

Saquinavir (Studies have suggested that pioglitazone may be a weak inducer of CYP450 isoform 3A4 substrate).

No products indexed under this heading.

Saquinavir Mesylate (Studies have suggested that pioglitazone may be a weak inducer of CYP450 isoform 3A4 substrate). Products include:

Invirase 2772

Sertraline Hydrochloride (Studies have suggested that pioglitazone may be a weak inducer of CYP450 isoform 3A4 substrate). Products include:

Zoloft 2586

Sildenafil Citrate (Studies have suggested that pioglitazone may be a weak inducer of CYP450 isoform 3A4 substrate). Products include:

Revatio Tablets 2557
Viagra Tablets 2573

Simvastatin (Studies have suggested that pioglitazone may be a weak inducer of CYP450 isoform 3A4 substrate). Products include:

Vytorin 10/10 Tablets 2114
Vytorin 10/10 Tablets 3077
Vytorin 10/20 Tablets 2114
Vytorin 10/20 Tablets 3077
Vytorin 10/40 Tablets 2114
Vytorin 10/40 Tablets 3077
Vytorin 10/80 Tablets 2114
Vytorin 10/80 Tablets 3077
Zocor Tablets 2105

Sirolimus (Studies have suggested that pioglitazone may be a weak inducer of CYP450 isoform 3A4 substrate). Products include:

Rapamune Oral Solution and Tablets 3475

Spironolactone (Certain drugs, including diuretics, tend to produce hyperglycemia and may lead to loss of glycemic control. When such drugs are administered to a patient receiving Actoplus Met, the patient should be closely observed to maintain adequate glycemic control).

No products indexed under this heading.

Tacrolimus (Studies have suggested that pioglitazone may be a weak inducer of CYP450 isoform 3A4 substrate). Products include:

Prograf Capsules and Injection 632
Protopic Ointment 638

Tamoxifen Citrate (Studies have suggested that pioglitazone may be a weak inducer of CYP450 isoform 3A4 substrate). Products include:

Soltamox Oral Solution 3527

Terbutaline Sulfate (Certain drugs, including sympathomimetics, tend to produce hyperglycemia and may lead to loss of glycemic control. When such drugs are administered to a patient receiving Actoplus Met, the patient should be closely observed to maintain adequate glycemic control).

No products indexed under this heading.

Thioridazine Hydrochloride (Certain drugs, including phenothiazines, tend to produce hyperglycemia and may lead to loss of glycemic control. When such drugs are administered to a patient receiving Actoplus Met, the patient should be closely observed to maintain adequate glycemic control). Products include:

Thioridazine Hydrochloride Tablets 2163

Thyroglobulin (Certain drugs, including thyroid products, tend to produce hyperglycemia and may lead to loss of glycemic control. When such drugs are administered to a patient receiving Actoplus Met, the patient should be closely observed to maintain adequate glycemic control).

No products indexed under this heading.

Thyroid (Certain drugs, including thyroid products, tend to produce hyperglycemia and may lead to loss of glycemic control. When such drugs are administered to a patient receiving Actoplus Met, the patient should be closely observed to maintain adequate glycemic control).

No products indexed under this heading.

Thyroxine (Certain drugs, including thyroid products, tend to produce hyperglycemia and may lead to loss of glycemic control. When such drugs are administered to a patient receiving Actoplus Met, the patient should be closely observed to maintain adequate glycemic control).

No products indexed under this heading.

Thyroxine Sodium (Certain drugs, including thyroid products, tend to produce hyperglycemia and may lead to loss of glycemic control. When such drugs are administered to a patient receiving Actoplus Met, the patient should be closely observed to maintain adequate glycemic control).

No products indexed under this heading.

Tiagabine Hydrochloride (Studies have suggested that pioglitazone may be a weak inducer of CYP450 isoform 3A4 substrate). Products include:

Gabitril Tablets 984

Tolazamide (Pioglitazone, like other thiazolidinediones, can cause fluid retention when used alone or in combination with other antihyperglycemic agents, including insulin).

No products indexed under this heading.

Tolbutamide (Pioglitazone, like other thiazolidinediones, can cause fluid retention when used alone or in combination with other antihyperglycemic agents, including insulin).

No products indexed under this heading.

Tolterodine Tartrate (Studies have suggested that pioglitazone may be a weak inducer of CYP450 isoform 3A4 substrate). Products include:
Detrol Tablets 2628
Detrol LA Capsules 2631

Torsemide (Certain drugs, including diuretics, tend to produce hyperglycemia and may lead to loss of glycemic control. When such drugs are administered to a patient receiving Actoplus Met, the patient should be closely observed to maintain adequate glycemic control). Products include:
Demadex Injection 2759
Demadex Tablets 2759

Trazodone Hydrochloride (Studies have suggested that pioglitazone may be a weak inducer of CYP450 isoform 3A4 substrate).
No products indexed under this heading.

Triamcinolone (Certain drugs, including corticosteroids, tend to produce hyperglycemia and may lead to loss of glycemic control. When such drugs are administered to a patient receiving Actoplus Met, the patient should be closely observed to maintain adequate glycemic control).
No products indexed under this heading.

Triamcinolone Acetonide (Certain drugs, including corticosteroids, tend to produce hyperglycemia and may lead to loss of glycemic control. When such drugs are administered to a patient receiving Actoplus Met, the patient should be closely observed to maintain adequate glycemic control). Products include:
Azmacort Inhalation Aerosol 1726
Nasacort AQ Nasal Spray 2922

Triamcinolone Diacetate (Certain drugs, including corticosteroids, tend to produce hyperglycemia and may lead to loss of glycemic control. When such drugs are administered to a patient receiving Actoplus Met, the patient should be closely observed to maintain adequate glycemic control).
No products indexed under this heading.

Triamcinolone Hexacetonide (Certain drugs, including corticosteroids, tend to produce hyperglycemia and may lead to loss of glycemic control. When such drugs are administered to a patient receiving Actoplus Met, the patient should be closely observed to maintain adequate glycemic control).
No products indexed under this heading.

Triamterene (Cationic drugs that are eliminated by renal tubular secretion theoretically have the potential for interaction with metformin by competing for common renal tubular transport systems. Although such interactions remain theoretical, careful patient monitoring and dose adjustment of Actoplus Met and/or the interfering drug is recommended in patients who are taking cationic medications that are excreted via the proximal renal tubular secretory system). Products include:
Dyazide Capsules 1423
Dyrenium Capsules 3400

Triazolam (Studies have suggested that pioglitazone may be a weak inducer of CYP450 isoform 3A4 substrate).
No products indexed under this heading.

Trifluoperazine Hydrochloride (Certain drugs, including phenothiazines, tend to produce hyperglycemia and may lead to loss of glycemic control. When such drugs are administered to a patient receiving Actoplus Met, the patient should be closely observed to maintain adequate glycemic control).
No products indexed under this heading.

Trimethoprim (Cationic drugs that are eliminated by renal tubular secretion theoretically have the potential for interaction with metformin by competing for common renal tubular transport systems. Although such interactions remain theoretical, careful patient monitoring and dose adjustment of Actoplus Met and/or the interfering drug is recommended in patients who are taking cationic medications that are excreted via the proximal renal tubular secretory system).
No products indexed under this heading.

Trimethoprim Sulfate (Cationic drugs that are eliminated by renal tubular secretion theoretically have the potential for interaction with metformin by competing for common renal tubular transport systems. Although such interactions remain theoretical, careful patient monitoring and dose adjustment of Actoplus Met and/or the interfering drug is recommended in patients who are taking cationic medications that are excreted via the proximal renal tubular secretory system). Products include:
Polytrim Ophthalmic Solution 574

Troglitazone (Pioglitazone, like other thiazolidinediones, can cause fluid retention when used alone or in combination with other antihyperglycemic agents, including insulin).
No products indexed under this heading.

Vancomycin Hydrochloride (Cationic drugs that are eliminated by renal tubular secretion theoretically have the potential for interaction with metformin by competing for common renal tubular transport systems. Although such interactions remain theoretical, careful patient monitoring and dose adjustment of Actoplus Met and/or the interfering drug is recommended in patients who are taking cationic medications that are excreted via the proximal renal tubular secretory system). Products include:
Vancocin HCl Capsules, USP 3380

Verapamil Hydrochloride (Certain drugs, including calcium channel blockers, tend to produce hyperglycemia and may lead to loss of glycemic control. When such drugs are administered to a patient receiving Actoplus Met, the patient should be closely observed to maintain adequate glycemic control). Products include:
Covera-HS Tablets 3139
Tarka Tablets 524
Verelan PM Extended-Release Capsules, Controlled-Onset 3106

Vinblastine Sulfate (Studies have suggested that pioglitazone may be a weak inducer of CYP450 isoform 3A4 substrate).
No products indexed under this heading.

Vincristine Sulfate (Studies have suggested that pioglitazone may be a weak inducer of CYP450 isoform 3A4 substrate).
No products indexed under this heading.

Warfarin Sodium (Studies have suggested that pioglitazone may be a weak inducer of CYP450 isoform 3A4 substrate). Products include:
Coumadin for Injection 898
Coumadin Tablets 898

Food Interactions

Alcohol (Alcohol is known to potentiate the effect of metformin on lactate metabolism. Patients, therefore, should be warned against excessive alcohol intake, acute or chronic, while receiving Actoplus Met).

ACTOS TABLETS

(Pioglitazone Hydrochloride) 3219
May interact with oral contraceptives and certain other agents. Compounds in these categories include:

Atorvastatin Calcium (Atorvastatin appears to induce the metabolism of pioglitazone; pioglitazone appears to induce the metabolism of atorvastatin). Products include:
Caduet Tablets 2508
Lipitor Tablets 2483

Desogestrel (Co-administration of pioglitazone hydrochloride (45mg once daily) and an oral contraceptive (1mg norethindrone plus 0.035mg ethinyl estradiol once daily) for 21 days, resulted in an 11% decrease in ethinyl estradiol AUC (0-24h) and an 11% to 14% decrease in Cmax. There were no significant changes in norethindrone AUC (0-24h) and Cmax). Products include:
Mircette Tablets 1066

Ethinyl Estradiol (Co-administration of pioglitazone hydrochloride (45mg once daily) and an oral contraceptive (1mg norethindrone plus 0.035mg ethinyl estradiol once daily) for 21 days, resulted in an 11% decrease in ethinyl estradiol AUC (0-24h) and an 11% to 14% decrease in Cmax. There were no significant changes in norethindrone AUC (0-24h) and Cmax). Products include:
Mircette Tablets 1066
NuvaRing 2340
Ortho-Cyclen/Ortho Tri-Cyclen 2429
Ortho Evra Transdermal System 2417
Ortho Tri-Cyclen Lo Tablets 2436
Seasonique Tablets 1077
Yasmin 28 Tablets 796
Yaz Tablets 803

Ethynodiol Diacetate (Co-administration of pioglitazone hydrochloride (45mg once daily) and an oral contraceptive (1mg norethindrone plus 0.035mg ethinyl estradiol once daily) for 21 days, resulted in an 11% decrease in ethinyl estradiol AUC (0-24h) and an 11% to 14% decrease in Cmax. There were no significant changes in norethindrone AUC (0-24h) and Cmax).
No products indexed under this heading.

Ketoconazole (In vitro, ketoconazole appears to significantly inhibit metabolism of pioglitazone). Products include:
Nizoral A-D Shampoo, 1% 1868

Levonorgestrel (Co-administration of pioglitazone hydrochloride (45mg once daily) and an oral contraceptive (1mg norethindrone plus 0.035mg ethinyl estradiol once daily) for 21 days, resulted in an 11% decrease in ethinyl estradiol AUC (0-24h) and an 11% to 14% decrease in Cmax. There were no significant changes in norethindrone AUC (0-24h) and Cmax). Products include:
Climara Pro Transdermal System 776
Mirena Intrauterine System 787
Plan B Tablets 1076
Seasonique Tablets 1077

Mestranol (Co-administration of pioglitazone hydrochloride (45mg once daily) and an oral contraceptive (1mg norethindrone plus 0.035mg ethinyl estradiol once daily) for 21 days, resulted in an 11% decrease in ethinyl estradiol AUC (0-24h) and an 11% to 14% decrease in Cmax. There were no significant changes in norethindrone AUC (0-24h) and Cmax).
No products indexed under this heading.

Midazolam Hydrochloride (Pioglitazone appears to induce the metabolism of midazolam with a 26% reduction of midazolam Cmax and AUC).
No products indexed under this heading.

Nifedipine (Co-administration of pioglitazone and nifedipine ER has resulted in increased metabolism of nifedipine; in view of the high variability of nifedipine pharmacokinetics, the clinical significance of the finding is unknown). Products include:
Adalat CC Tablets 2964

Norethindrone (Co-administration of pioglitazone hydrochloride (45mg once daily) and an oral contraceptive (1mg norethindrone plus 0.035mg ethinyl estradiol once daily) for 21 days, resulted in an 11% decrease in ethinyl estradiol AUC (0-24h) and an 11% to 14% decrease in Cmax. There were no significant changes in norethindrone AUC (0-24h) and Cmax). Products include:
Ortho Micronor Tablets 2426

Norethynodrel (Co-administration of pioglitazone hydrochloride (45mg once daily) and an oral contraceptive (1mg norethindrone plus 0.035mg ethinyl estradiol once daily) for 21 days, resulted in an 11% decrease in ethinyl estradiol AUC (0-24h) and an 11% to 14% decrease in Cmax. There were no significant changes in norethindrone AUC (0-24h) and Cmax).
No products indexed under this heading.

Norgestimate (Co-administration of pioglitazone hydrochloride (45mg once daily) and an oral contraceptive (1mg norethindrone plus 0.035mg ethinyl estradiol once daily) for 21 days, resulted in an 11% decrease in ethinyl estradiol AUC (0-24h) and an 11% to 14% decrease in Cmax, There were no significant changes in norethindrone AUC (0-24h) and Cmax). Products include:
Ortho-Cyclen/Ortho Tri-Cyclen 2429
Ortho Tri-Cyclen Lo Tablets 2436

Norgestrel (Co-administration of pioglitazone hydrochloride (45mg once daily) and an oral contraceptive (1mg norethindrone plus 0.035mg ethinyl estradiol once daily) for 21 days, resulted in an 11% decrease in ethinyl estradiol AUC (0-24h) and an 11% to 14% decrease in Cmax. There were no significant changes in norethindrone AUC (0-24h) and Cmax).
No products indexed under this heading.

ACULAR OPHTHALMIC SOLUTION

(Ketorolac Tromethamine) 565
May interact with:

Warfarin Sodium (Potential for increased bleeding time; concurrent use with other agents which prolong bleeding time requires caution). Products include:
Coumadin for Injection 898
Coumadin Tablets 898

ACULAR LS OPHTHALMIC SOLUTION

(Ketorolac Tromethamine) 566
None cited in PDR database.

ADACEL VACCINE

(Diphtheria & Tetanus Toxoids and Acellular Pertussis Vaccine Adsorbed) 2945
May interact with alkylating agents, antimetabolites, corticosteroids, cytotoxic drugs, and immunosuppressive agents. Compounds in these categories include:

Azathioprine (Concurrent immunosuppressive therapy may reduce the immune response to vaccine).
No products indexed under this heading.

Basiliximab (Concurrent immunosuppressive therapy may reduce the immune response to vaccine). Products include:
Simulect for Injection 2284

Betamethasone Acetate (Concurrent immunosuppressive therapy with greater than physiologic doses of corticosteroids may reduce the immune response to vaccine).
No products indexed under this heading.

Betamethasone Sodium Phosphate (Concurrent immunosuppressive therapy with greater than physiologic doses of corticosteroids may reduce the immune response to vaccine).
No products indexed under this heading.

Bleomycin Sulfate (Cytotoxic drugs may reduce the immune response to vaccine).
No products indexed under this heading.

Busulfan (Alkylating drugs may reduce the immune response to vaccine). Products include:
I.V. Busulfex 2493
Myleran Tablets 1525

Capecitabine (Immunosuppressive therapies may reduce the immune response to vaccines). Products include:
Xeloda Tablets 2822

Carmustine (BCNU) (Alkylating drugs may reduce the immune response to vaccine).
No products indexed under this heading.

Chlorambucil (Alkylating drugs may reduce the immune response to vaccine). Products include:
Leukeran Tablets 1504

Cladribine (Immunosuppressive therapies may reduce the immune response to vaccines). Products include:
Leustatin Injection 2357

Cortisone Acetate (Concurrent immunosuppressive therapy with greater than physiologic doses of corticosteroids may reduce the immune response to vaccine).
No products indexed under this heading.

Cyclophosphamide (Alkylating drugs may reduce the immune response to vaccine).
No products indexed under this heading.

Cyclosporine (Concurrent immunosuppressive therapy may reduce the immune response to vaccine). Products include:
Gengraf Capsules 459
Neoral Oral Solution 2259
Neoral Soft Gelatin Capsules 2259
Restasis Ophthalmic Emulsion 575
Sandimmune 2275

Cytarabine (Immunosuppressive therapies may reduce the immune response to vaccines).
No products indexed under this heading.

Dacarbazine (Alkylating drugs may reduce the immune response to vaccine).
No products indexed under this heading.

Daunorubicin Hydrochloride (Cytotoxic drugs may reduce the immune response to vaccine).
No products indexed under this heading.

Dexamethasone (Concurrent immunosuppressive therapy with greater than physiologic doses of corticosteroids may reduce the immune response to vaccine). Products include:
Ciprodex Otic Suspension 559
Decadron Tablets 1951
TobraDex Ophthalmic Ointment 562
TobraDex Ophthalmic Suspension ... 563

Dexamethasone Acetate (Concurrent immunosuppressive therapy with greater than physiologic doses of corticosteroids may reduce the immune response to vaccine).
No products indexed under this heading.

Dexamethasone Sodium Phosphate (Concurrent immunosuppressive therapy with greater than physiologic doses of corticosteroids may reduce the immune response to vaccine).
No products indexed under this heading.

Doxorubicin Hydrochloride (Cytotoxic drugs may reduce the immune response to vaccine).
No products indexed under this heading.

Epirubicin Hydrochloride (Cytotoxic drugs may reduce the immune response to vaccine).
No products indexed under this heading.

Floxuridine (Immunosuppressive therapies may reduce the immune response to vaccines).
No products indexed under this heading.

Fludarabine Phosphate (Immunosuppressive therapies may reduce the immune response to vaccines).
No products indexed under this heading.

Fludrocortisone Acetate (Concurrent immunosuppressive therapy with greater than physiologic doses of corticosteroids may reduce the immune response to vaccine).
No products indexed under this heading.

Fluorouracil (Immunosuppressive therapies may reduce the immune response to vaccines). Products include:
Carac Cream, 0.5% 2879
Efudex 3363

Gemcitabine Hydrochloride (Immunosuppressive therapies may reduce the immune response to vaccines). Products include:
Gemzar for Injection 1771

Hydrocortisone (Concurrent immunosuppressive therapy with greater than physiologic doses of corticosteroids may reduce the immune response to vaccine). Products include:
Colocort Rectal Suspension, USP (Retention) 100 mg/60 mL 2476
Hydrocortone Tablets 1989
Preparation H Hydrocortisone Cream .... ⊡ 646

Hydrocortisone Acetate (Concurrent immunosuppressive therapy with greater than physiologic doses of corticosteroids may reduce the immune response to vaccine). Products include:
Analpram-HC 1159
Pramosone 1161
ProctoFoam-HC 3099

Hydrocortisone Sodium Phosphate (Concurrent immunosuppressive therapy with greater than physiologic doses of corticosteroids may reduce the immune response to vaccine).
No products indexed under this heading.

Hydrocortisone Sodium Succinate (Concurrent immunosuppressive therapy with greater than physiologic doses of corticosteroids may reduce the immune response to vaccine).
No products indexed under this heading.

Hydroxyurea (Cytotoxic drugs may reduce the immune response to vaccine).
No products indexed under this heading.

Lomustine (CCNU) (Alkylating drugs may reduce the immune response to vaccine).
No products indexed under this heading.

Mechlorethamine Hydrochloride (Alkylating drugs may reduce the immune response to vaccine). Products include:
Mustargen for Injection 2468

Melphalan (Alkylating drugs may reduce the immune response to vaccine). Products include:
Alkeran Tablets 956

Mercaptopurine (Immunosuppressive therapies may reduce the immune response to vaccines).
No products indexed under this heading.

Methotrexate (Immunosuppressive therapies may reduce the immune response to vaccines).
No products indexed under this heading.

Methotrexate Sodium (Cytotoxic drugs may reduce the immune response to vaccine).
No products indexed under this heading.

Methylprednisolone Acetate (Concurrent immunosuppressive therapy with greater than physiologic doses of corticosteroids may reduce the immune response to vaccine). Products include:
Depo-Medrol Injectable Suspension 2617
Depo-Medrol Single-Dose Vial 2619

Methylprednisolone Sodium Succinate (Concurrent immunosuppressive therapy with greater than physiologic doses of corticosteroids may reduce the immune response to vaccine).
No products indexed under this heading.

Mitotane (Cytotoxic drugs may reduce the immune response to vaccine).
No products indexed under this heading.

Mitoxantrone Hydrochloride (Cytotoxic drugs may reduce the immune response to vaccine).
No products indexed under this heading.

Muromonab-CD3 (Concurrent immunosuppressive therapy may reduce the immune response to vaccine). Products include:
Orthoclone OKT3 Sterile Solution 2360

Mycophenolate Mofetil (Concurrent immunosuppressive therapy may reduce the immune response to vaccine). Products include:
CellCept Capsules 2747
CellCept Oral Suspension 2747
CellCept Tablets 2747

Pentostatin (Immunosuppressive therapies may reduce the immune response to vaccines). Products include:
Nipent for Injection 1863

Prednisolone Acetate (Concurrent immunosuppressive therapy with greater than physiologic doses of corticosteroids may reduce the immune response to vaccine). Products include:
Blephamide Ophthalmic Ointment 568
Blephamide Ophthalmic Suspension................................. 569
Poly-Pred Ophthalmic Suspension .... ⊙ 233
Pred Forte Ophthalmic Suspension .... ⊙ 235
Pred Mild Ophthalmic Suspension .... ⊙ 238
Pred-G Ophthalmic Ointment .... ⊙ 237
Pred-G Ophthalmic Suspension .... ⊙ 236

Prednisolone Sodium Phosphate (Concurrent immunosuppressive therapy with greater than physiologic doses of corticosteroids may reduce the immune response to vaccine).
No products indexed under this heading.

Prednisolone Tebutate (Concurrent immunosuppressive therapy with greater than physiologic doses of corticosteroids may reduce the immune response to vaccine).
No products indexed under this heading.

Prednisone (Concurrent immunosuppressive therapy with greater than physiologic doses of corticosteroids may reduce the immune response to vaccine).
No products indexed under this heading.

Procarbazine Hydrochloride (Cytotoxic drugs may reduce the immune response to vaccine). Products include:
Matulane Capsules 3191

Sirolimus (Concurrent immunosuppressive therapy may reduce the immune response to vaccine). Products include:
Rapamune Oral Solution and Tablets 3475

Tacrolimus (Concurrent immunosuppressive therapy may reduce the immune response to vaccine). Products include:
Prograf Capsules and Injection 632
Protopic Ointment 638

Tamoxifen Citrate (Cytotoxic drugs may reduce the immune response to vaccine). Products include:
Soltamox Oral Solution 3527

Thioguanine (Immunosuppressive therapies may reduce the immune response to vaccines). Products include:
Tabloid Tablets 1575

Thiotepa (Alkylating drugs may reduce the immune response to vaccine).
No products indexed under this heading.

Triamcinolone (Concurrent immunosuppressive therapy with greater than physiologic doses of corticosteroids may reduce the immune response to vaccine).
No products indexed under this heading.

Triamcinolone Acetonide (Concurrent immunosuppressive therapy with greater than physiologic doses of corticosteroids may reduce the immune response to vaccine). Products include:
Azmacort Inhalation Aerosol 1726
Nasacort AQ Nasal Spray 2922

Triamcinolone Diacetate (Concurrent immunosuppressive therapy with greater than physiologic doses of corticosteroids may reduce the immune response to vaccine).
No products indexed under this heading.

Triamcinolone Hexacetonide (Concurrent immunosuppressive therapy with greater than physiologic doses of corticosteroids may reduce the immune response to vaccine).
No products indexed under this heading.

Vincristine Sulfate (Cytotoxic drugs may reduce the immune response to vaccine).
No products indexed under this heading.

ADALAT CC TABLETS

(Nifedipine) 2964

May interact with antihypertensives, beta blockers, oral anticoagulants, cytochrome p450 3a4 inducers (selected), cytochrome p450 3a4 inhibitors (selected), cytochrome p450 3a substrates (selected), erythromycin, cardiac glycosides, narcotic analgesics, phenytoin, and certain other agents. Compounds in these categories include:

Acarbose (Nifedipine tends to produce hyperglycemia and may lead to loss of glucose control. Blood glucose levels should be monitored when used in combination with nifedipine). Products include:
Precose Tablets 751

Acebutolol Hydrochloride (Combination of nifedipine and beta-blockers may increase the likelihood of congestive heart failure, severe hypotension, or exacerbation of angina).
No products indexed under this heading.

Acetazolamide (Nifedipine is mainly eliminated by metabolism and is a substrate of CYP3A4. Inhibitors of CYP3A4 can impact the exposure to nifedipine and consequently its desirable and undesirable effects).
No products indexed under this heading.

Alfentanil Hydrochloride (Potential for severe hypotension and/or increased fluid volume requirements cannot be ruled out when nifedipine is co-administered with a beta-blocker and a narcotic analgesic).
No products indexed under this heading.

Allium sativum (Nifedipine is mainly eliminated by metabolism and is a substrate of CYP3A4. Inducers of CYP3A4 can impact the exposure to nifedipine and consequently its desirable and undesirable effects).
No products indexed under this heading.

Alprazolam (Data indicates that nifedipine can inhibit the metabolism of drugs that are substrates of CYP3A, thereby increasing the exposure to other drugs). Products include:
Niravam Orally Disintegrating Tablets 3092

Aminophylline (Data indicates that nifedipine can inhibit the metabolism of drugs that are substrates of CYP3A, thereby increasing the exposure to other drugs).
No products indexed under this heading.

Amiodarone Hydrochloride (Nifedipine is mainly eliminated by metabolism and is a substrate of CYP3A4. Inhibitors of CYP3A4 can impact the exposure to nifedipine and consequently its desirable and undesirable effects).
No products indexed under this heading.

Amitriptyline Hydrochloride (Data indicates that nifedipine can inhibit the metabolism of drugs that are substrates of CYP3A, thereby increasing the exposure to other drugs).
No products indexed under this heading.

Amlodipine Besylate (Data indicates that nifedipine can inhibit the metabolism of drugs that are substrates of CYP3A, thereby increasing the exposure to other drugs). Products include:
Caduet Tablets 2508
Lotrel Capsules 2249
Norvasc Tablets 2545

Amprenavir (Co-administration of nifedipine with CYP3A4 inhibitors, such as amprenavir, may cause an increase in nifedipine plasma concentrations; a reduction in nifedipine dosage may be considered). Products include:
Agenerase Capsules 1327
Agenerase Oral Solution 1332

Anastrozole (Nifedipine is mainly eliminated by metabolism and is a substrate of CYP3A4. Inhibitors of CYP3A4 can impact the exposure to nifedipine and consequently its desirable and undesirable effects). Products include:
Arimidex Tablets 673

Anisindione (There have been rare reports of increased prothrombin time in patients taking coumarin anticoagulants to whom nifedipine was administered). Products include:
Miradon Tablets 3042

Aprepitant (Nifedipine is mainly eliminated by metabolism and is a substrate of CYP3A4. Inhibitors of CYP3A4 can impact the exposure to nifedipine and consequently its desirable and undesirable effects). Products include:
Emend Capsules 1963

Astemizole (Data indicates that nifedipine can inhibit the metabolism of drugs that are substrates of CYP3A, thereby increasing the exposure to other drugs).
No products indexed under this heading.

Atanazavir (Co-administration of nifedipine with CYP3A4 inhibitors, such as atanazavir, may cause an increase in nifedipine plasma concentrations; a reduction in nifedipine dosage may be considered).
No products indexed under this heading.

Atenolol (Combination of nifedipine and beta-blockers may increase the likelihood of congestive heart failure, severe hypotension, or exacerbation of angina).
No products indexed under this heading.

Atorvastatin Calcium (Data indicates that nifedipine can inhibit the metabolism of drugs that are substrates of CYP3A, thereby increasing the exposure to other drugs). Products include:
Caduet Tablets 2508
Lipitor Tablets 2483

Benazepril Hydrochloride (Co-administration with nifedipine can cause a hypotensive effect and attenuate the tachycardic effect of nifedipine). Products include:
Lotensin Tablets 2243
Lotensin HCT Tablets 2246
Lotrel Capsules 2249

Bendroflumethiazide (Nifedipine is a vasodilator, and co-administration of other drugs affecting blood pressure may result in pharmacodynamic interactions).
No products indexed under this heading.

Betamethasone Acetate (Nifedipine is mainly eliminated by metabolism and is a substrate of CYP3A4. Inducers of CYP3A4 can impact the exposure to nifedipine and consequently its desirable and undesirable effects).
No products indexed under this heading.

Betamethasone Sodium Phosphate (Nifedipine is mainly eliminated by metabolism and is a substrate of CYP3A4. Inducers of CYP3A4 can impact the exposure to nifedipine and consequently its desirable and undesirable effects).
No products indexed under this heading.

Betaxolol Hydrochloride (Combination of nifedipine and beta-blockers may increase the likelihood of congestive heart failure, severe hypotension, or exacerbation of angina). Products include:
Betoptic S Ophthalmic Suspension.................................. 558

Bisoprolol Fumarate (Combination of nifedipine and beta-blockers may increase the likelihood of congestive heart failure, severe hypotension, or exacerbation of angina).
No products indexed under this heading.

Buprenorphine Hydrochloride (Potential for severe hypotension and/or increased fluid volume requirements cannot be ruled out when nifedipine is co-administered with a beta-blocker and a narcotic analgesic). Products include:
Buprenex Injectable 2716
Suboxone Tablets 2717
Subutex Tablets 2717

Buspirone Hydrochloride (Data indicates that nifedipine can inhibit the metabolism of drugs that are substrates of CYP3A, thereby increasing the exposure to other drugs).
No products indexed under this heading.

Busulfan (Data indicates that nifedipine can inhibit the metabolism of drugs that are substrates of CYP3A, thereby increasing the exposure to other drugs). Products include:
I.V. Busulfex 2493
Myleran Tablets 1525

Candesartan Cilexetil (Nifedipine is a vasodilator, and co-administration of other drugs affecting blood pressure may result in pharmacodynamic interactions). Products include:
Atacand Tablets 649
Atacand HCT 651

Captopril (Nifedipine is a vasodilator, and co-administration of other drugs affecting blood pressure may result in pharmacodynamic interactions). Products include:
Captopril Tablets 2149

Carbamazepine (Carbamazepine has been shown to reduce plasma concentrations of other calcium channel blockers due to enzyme induction; a similar interaction with nifedipine leading to a decrease in nifedipine plasma concentrations and a decrease in efficacy cannot be excluded; a dosage adjustment of nifedipine may be needed). Products include:
Carbatrol Capsules 3171
Equetro Extended-Release Capsules 3180
Tegretol/Tegretol-XR 2295

Carteolol Hydrochloride (Combination of nifedipine and beta-blockers may increase the likelihood of congestive heart failure, severe hypotension, or exacerbation of angina). Products include:
Carteolol Hydrochloride Ophthalmic Solution USP, 1% ....⊙ 249

Cerivastatin Sodium (Data indicates that nifedipine can inhibit the metabolism of drugs that are substrates of CYP3A, thereby increasing the exposure to other drugs).
No products indexed under this heading.

Chlorothiazide (Nifedipine is a vasodilator, and co-administration of other drugs affecting blood pressure may result in pharmacodynamic interactions). Products include:
Diuril Oral Suspension 1954

Chlorothiazide Sodium (Nifedipine is a vasodilator, and co-administration of other drugs affect-

ing blood pressure may result in pharmacodynamic interactions). Products include:
- Diuril Sodium Intravenous 2467

Chlorpheniramine (Data indicates that nifedipine can inhibit the metabolism of drugs that are substrates of CYP3A, thereby increasing the exposure to other drugs).
No products indexed under this heading.

Chlorpheniramine Maleate (Data indicates that nifedipine can inhibit the metabolism of drugs that are substrates of CYP3A, thereby increasing the exposure to other drugs). Products include:
- Advil Allergy Sinus Caplets 770
- Advil Multi-Symptom Cold Caplets 770
- BC Allergy Sinus Cold Powder 677
- Comtrex Maximum Strength Cold & Cough Day/Night Caplets - Night Formulation 726
- Comtrex Maximum Strength Day/Night Severe Cold & Sinus Caplets - Night Formulation 725
- Contac Cold and Flu Maximum Strength Caplets 728
- Contac Cold and Flu Day and Night Caplets (Night Formulation Only) 727
- Children's Dimetapp Long Acting Cough Plus Cold Syrup 731
- Robitussin Cough & Cold Long-Acting Liquid 735
- Robitussin Cough & Allergy Syrup .. 736
- Robitussin Cough & Cold Nighttime Liquid 736
- Robitussin Cough, Cold & Flu Nighttime Liquid 738
- Robitussin Pediatric Cough & Cold Long-Acting Liquid 735
- Robitussin Pediatric Cough & Cold Nighttime Liquid 736
- Triaminic Cold & Allergy Liquid 746
- Triaminic Cough & Runny Nose Softchews 748
- Children's Tylenol Plus Flu Oral Suspension 749
- Tylenol Allergy Multi-Symptom Caplets with Cool Burst and Gelcaps 1872
- Children's Tylenol Plus Cold Suspension Liquid 1879
- Children's Tylenol Plus Cough & Runny Nose Suspension Liquid 1879
- Children's Tylenol Plus Flu Suspension Liquid 1881
- Children's Tylenol Plus Multi-Symptom Cold Suspension Liquid 1879
- Tylenol Cold Head Congestion Nighttime Caplets with Cool Burst 1873
- Tylenol Cold Multi-Symptom Nighttime Caplets with Cool Burst 1874
- Tylenol Sinus Congestion & Pain Nighttime Caplets with Cool Burst 1876
- Vicks 44M Cough, Cold & Flu Relief Liquid 2680
- Pediatric Vicks 44m Cough & Cold Relief Liquid 2676
- Children's Vicks NyQuil Cold/Cough Relief 756
- Children's Vicks NyQuil Cold/Cough Relief Liquid 2680
- Zicam Maximum Strength Flu Daytime 768

Chlorpheniramine Polistirex (Data indicates that nifedipine can inhibit the metabolism of drugs that are substrates of CYP3A, thereby increasing the exposure to other drugs). Products include:
- Tussionex Pennkinetic Extended-Release Suspension 3327

Chlorpheniramine Tannate (Data indicates that nifedipine can inhibit the metabolism of drugs that are substrates of CYP3A, thereby increasing the exposure to other drugs).
No products indexed under this heading.

Chlorthalidone (Nifedipine is a vasodilator, and co-administration of other drugs affecting blood pressure may result in pharmacodynamic interactions). Products include:
- Clorpres Tablets 2153

Cimetidine (Both the peak plasma level of nifedipine and AUC may increase in the presence of cimetidine. Cautious titration of nifedipine is advised; relevant changes in blood pressure was experienced; a reduction in nifedipine dosage may be considered). Products include:
- Tagamet HB 200 Tablets 664

Cimetidine Hydrochloride (Both the peak plasma level of nifedipine and AUC may increase in the presence of cimetidine. Cautious titration of nifedipine is advised; relevant changes in blood pressure was experienced; a reduction in nifedipine dosage may be considered).
No products indexed under this heading.

Ciprofloxacin (Nifedipine is mainly eliminated by metabolism and is a substrate of CYP3A4. Inhibitors of CYP3A4 can impact the exposure to nifedipine and consequently its desirable and undesirable effects). Products include:
- Cipro Oral Suspension 2977
- Cipro I.V. 2984
- Cipro XR Tablets 2990
- Ciprodex Otic Suspension 559

Ciprofloxacin Hydrochloride (Nifedipine is mainly eliminated by metabolism and is a substrate of CYP3A4. Inducers of CYP3A4 can impact the exposure to nifedipine and consequently its desirable and undesirable effects). Products include:
- Ciloxan Ophthalmic Ointment 559
- Ciloxan Ophthalmic Solution .... ⊙206
- Cipro Tablets 2977
- Proquin XR Tablets 1153

Cisapride (Concomitant administration may lead to increased plasma concentrations of nifedipine).
No products indexed under this heading.

Cisplatin (Nifedipine is mainly eliminated by metabolism and is a substrate of CYP3A4. Inducers of CYP3A4 can impact the exposure to nifedipine and consequently its desirable and undesirable effects).
No products indexed under this heading.

Clarithromycin (Nifedipine is mainly eliminated by metabolism and is a substrate of CYP3A4. Inhibitors of CYP3A4 can impact the exposure to nifedipine and consequently its desirable and undesirable effects). Products include:
- Biaxin/Biaxin XL 402
- PREVPAC 3284

Clonidine (Nifedipine is a vasodilator, and co-administration of other drugs affecting blood pressure may result in pharmacodynamic interactions). Products include:
- Catapres-TTS 844

Clonidine Hydrochloride (Nifedipine is a vasodilator, and co-administration of other drugs affecting blood pressure may result in pharmacodynamic interactions). Products include:
- Catapres Tablets 843
- Clorpres Tablets 2153

Clotrimazole (Nifedipine is mainly eliminated by metabolism and is a substrate of CYP3A4. Inhibitors of CYP3A4 can impact the exposure to nifedipine and consequently its desirable and undesirable effects). Products include:
- Desenex Athlete's Foot Cream 635
- Lotrimin 3039
- Lotrisone 3040

Codeine Phosphate (Potential for severe hypotension and/or increased fluid volume requirements cannot be ruled out when nifedipine is co-administered with a beta-blocker and a narcotic analgesic). Products include:
- Tylenol with Codeine Tablets 2391

Cortisone Acetate (Nifedipine is mainly eliminated by metabolism and is a substrate of CYP3A4. Inducers of CYP3A4 can impact the exposure to nifedipine and consequently its desirable and undesirable effects).
No products indexed under this heading.

Cyclosporine (Nifedipine is mainly eliminated by metabolism and is a substrate of CYP3A4. Inhibitors of CYP3A4 can impact the exposure to nifedipine and consequently its desirable and undesirable effects). Products include:
- Gengraf Capsules 459
- Neoral Oral Solution 2259
- Neoral Soft Gelatin Capsules 2259
- Restasis Ophthalmic Emulsion 575
- Sandimmune 2275

Dalfopristin (Concomitant administration may lead to increased plasma concentrations of nifedipine; a reduction in nifedipine dosage may be considered).
No products indexed under this heading.

Danazol (Nifedipine is mainly eliminated by metabolism and is a substrate of CYP3A4. Inhibitors of CYP3A4 can impact the exposure to nifedipine and consequently its desirable and undesirable effects).
No products indexed under this heading.

Delavirdine Mesylate (Nifedipine is mainly eliminated by metabolism and is a substrate of CYP3A4. Inhibitors of CYP3A4 can impact the exposure to nifedipine and consequently its desirable and undesirable effects). Products include:
- Rescriptor Tablets 2551

Delavirine (Co-administration of nifedipine with CYP3A4 inhibitors, such as delavirine, may cause an increase in nifedipine plasma concentrations; a reduction in nifedipine dosage may be considered).
No products indexed under this heading.

Deserpidine (Nifedipine is a vasodilator, and co-administration of other drugs affecting blood pressure may result in pharmacodynamic interactions).
No products indexed under this heading.

Deslanoside (Potential of elevated digoxin levels).
No products indexed under this heading.

Desogestrel (Data indicates that nifedipine can inhibit the metabolism of drugs that are substrates of CYP3A, thereby increasing the exposure to other drugs). Products include:
- Mircette Tablets 1066

Dexamethasone (Nifedipine is mainly eliminated by metabolism and is a substrate of CYP3A4. Inducers of CYP3A4 can impact the exposure to nifedipine and consequently its desirable and undesirable effects). Products include:
- Ciprodex Otic Suspension 559
- Decadron Tablets 1951
- TobraDex Ophthalmic Ointment 562
- TobraDex Ophthalmic Suspension ... 563

Dexamethasone Acetate (Nifedipine is mainly eliminated by metabolism and is a substrate of CYP3A4. Inducers of CYP3A4 can impact the exposure to nifedipine and consequently its desirable and undesirable effects).
No products indexed under this heading.

Dexamethasone Phosphate (Data indicates that nifedipine can inhibit the metabolism of drugs that are substrates of CYP3A, thereby increasing the exposure to other drugs).
No products indexed under this heading.

Dexamethasone Sodium (Data indicates that nifedipine can inhibit the metabolism of drugs that are substrates of CYP3A, thereby increasing the exposure to other drugs).
No products indexed under this heading.

Dexamethasone Sodium Phosphate (Nifedipine is mainly eliminated by metabolism and is a substrate of CYP3A4. Inducers of CYP3A4 can impact the exposure to nifedipine and consequently its desirable and undesirable effects).
No products indexed under this heading.

Dezocine (Potential for severe hypotension and/or increased fluid volume requirements cannot be ruled out when nifedipine is co-administered with a beta-blocker and a narcotic analgesic).
No products indexed under this heading.

Diazepam (Data indicates that nifedipine can inhibit the metabolism of drugs that are substrates of CYP3A, thereby increasing the exposure to other drugs). Products include:
- Diastat Rectal Delivery System 3343
- Valium Tablets 2819

Diazoxide (Nifedipine is a vasodilator, and co-administration of other drugs affecting blood pressure may result in pharmacodynamic interactions). Products include:
- Hyperstat I.V. 3017

Dicumarol (There have been rare reports of increased prothrombin time in patients taking coumarin anticoagulants to whom nifedipine was administered).
No products indexed under this heading.

Digitalis Glycoside Preparations (Potential of elevated digoxin levels).
No products indexed under this heading.

Digitoxin (Potential of elevated digoxin levels).
No products indexed under this heading.

Digoxin (Potential of elevated digoxin levels). Products include:
Lanoxicaps Capsules 1490
Lanoxin Injection 1494
Lanoxin Injection Pediatric 1497
Lanoxin Tablets 1500

Dihydroergotamine Mesylate (Data indicates that nifedipine can inhibit the metabolism of drugs that are substrates of CYP3A, thereby increasing the exposure to other drugs). Products include:
Migranal Nasal Spray 3348

Diltiazem Hydrochloride (Co-administration can increase nifedipine Cmax and AUC by 2.0 and 2.2 respectively; use with caution and consider dose reducation of nifedipine). Products include:
Cardizem LA Extended Release Tablets 1728
Tiazac Capsules 1201

Diltiazem Maleate (Nifedipine is mainly eliminated by metabolism and is a substrate of CYP3A4. Inhibitors of CYP3A4 can impact the exposure to nifedipine and consequently its desirable and undesirable effects).
No products indexed under this heading.

Disopyramide Phosphate (Data indicates that nifedipine can inhibit the metabolism of drugs that are substrates of CYP3A, thereby increasing the exposure to other drugs).
No products indexed under this heading.

Doxazosin Mesylate (Co-administration of nifedipine with CYP3A4 inhibitors, such as doxazosin, may cause an increase in nifedipine plasma concentrations; a reduction in nifedipine dosage may be considered). Products include:
Cardura XL Tablets 2515

Doxorubicin Hydrochloride (Nifedipine is mainly eliminated by metabolism and is a substrate of CYP3A4. Inducers of CYP3A4 can impact the exposure to nifedipine and consequently its desirable and undesirable effects).
No products indexed under this heading.

Dronabinol (Data indicates that nifedipine can inhibit the metabolism of drugs that are substrates of CYP3A, thereby increasing the exposure to other drugs). Products include:
Marinol Capsules 3333

Dyphylline (Data indicates that nifedipine can inhibit the metabolism of drugs that are substrates of CYP3A, thereby increasing the exposure to other drugs).
No products indexed under this heading.

Efavirenz (Nifedipine is mainly eliminated by metabolism and is a substrate of CYP3A4. Inhibitors of CYP3A4 can impact the exposure to nifedipine and consequently its desirable and undesirable effects).
Products include:
Atripla Tablets 945
Sustiva Capsules 930
Sustiva Tablets 930

Enalapril Maleate (Nifedipine is a vasodilator, and co-administration of other drugs affecting blood pressure may result in pharmacodynamic interactions). Products include:
Vasotec I.V. Injection 2103

Enalaprilat (Nifedipine is a vasodilator, and co-administration of other drugs affecting blood pressure may result in pharmacodynamic interactions).
No products indexed under this heading.

Eprosartan Mesylate (Nifedipine is a vasodilator, and co-administration of other drugs affecting blood pressure may result in pharmacodynamic interactions). Products include:
Teveten Tablets 1735
Teveten HCT Tablets 1737

Ergotamine Tartrate (Data indicates that nifedipine can inhibit the metabolism of drugs that are substrates of CYP3A, thereby increasing the exposure to other drugs).
No products indexed under this heading.

Erythromycin (Co-administration of nifedipine with CYP3A4 inhibitors, such as erythromycin, may cause an increase in nifedipine plasma concentrations; a reduction in nifedipine dosage may be considered).
Products include:
Ery-Tab Tablets 449
Erythromycin Base Filmtab Tablets 455
Erythromycin Delayed-Release Capsules, USP 457
PCE Dispertab Tablets 515

Erythromycin Estolate (Co-administration of nifedipine with CYP3A4 inhibitors, such as erythromycin, may cause an increase in nifedipine plasma concentrations; a reduction in nifedipine dosage may be considered).
No products indexed under this heading.

Erythromycin Ethylsuccinate (Co-administration of nifedipine with CYP3A4 inhibitors, such as erythromycin, may cause an increase in nifedipine plasma concentrations; a reduction in nifedipine dosage may be considered). Products include:
E.E.S. 451
EryPed 447

Erythromycin Gluceptate (Co-administration of nifedipine with CYP3A4 inhibitors, such as erythromycin, may cause an increase in nifedipine plasma concentrations; a reduction in nifedipine dosage may be considered).
No products indexed under this heading.

Erythromycin Lactobionate (Co-administration of nifedipine with CYP3A4 inhibitors, such as erythromycin, may cause an increase in nifedipine plasma concentrations; a reduction in nifedipine dosage may be considered).
No products indexed under this heading.

Erythromycin Stearate (Co-administration of nifedipine with CYP3A4 inhibitors, such as erythromycin, may cause an increase in nifedipine plasma concentrations; a reduction in nifedipine dosage may be considered). Products include:
Erythrocin Stearate Filmtab Tablets 453

Esmolol Hydrochloride (Combination of nifedipine and beta-blockers may increase the likelihood of congestive heart failure, severe hypotension, or exacerbation of angina).
No products indexed under this heading.

Esomeprazole Magnesium (Nifedipine is mainly eliminated by metabolism and is a substrate of CYP3A4. Inhibitors of CYP3A4 can impact the exposure to nifedipine and consequently its desirable and undesirable effects). Products include:
Nexium Delayed-Release Capsules 655

Estrogen (Data indicates that nifedipine can inhibit the metabolism of drugs that are substrates of CYP3A, thereby increasing the exposure to other drugs).
No products indexed under this heading.

Estrogens, Conjugated (Data indicates that nifedipine can inhibit the metabolism of drugs that are substrates of CYP3A, thereby increasing the exposure to other drugs).
Products include:
Premarin Intravenous 3442
Premarin Tablets 3446
Premarin Vaginal Cream 3452
Premphase Tablets 3456
Prempro Tablets 3456

Estrogens, Conjugated, Synthetic A (Data indicates that nifedipine can inhibit the metabolism of drugs that are substrates of CYP3A, thereby increasing the exposure to other drugs).
No products indexed under this heading.

Estrogens, Esterified (Data indicates that nifedipine can inhibit the metabolism of drugs that are substrates of CYP3A, thereby increasing the exposure to other drugs).
Products include:
Estratest Tablets 3199
Estratest H.S. Tablets 3199

Ethinyl Estradiol (Data indicates that nifedipine can inhibit the metabolism of drugs that are substrates of CYP3A, thereby increasing the exposure to other drugs). Products include:
Mircette Tablets 1066
NuvaRing 2340
Ortho-Cyclen/Ortho Tri-Cyclen 2429
Ortho Evra Transdermal System 2417
Ortho Tri-Cyclen Lo Tablets 2436
Seasonique Tablets 1077
Yasmin 28 Tablets 796
Yaz Tablets 803

Ethosuximide (Nifedipine is mainly eliminated by metabolism and is a substrate of CYP3A4. Inducers of CYP3A4 can impact the exposure to nifedipine and consequently its desirable and undesirable effects).
No products indexed under this heading.

Ethynodiol Diacetate (Data indicates that nifedipine can inhibit the metabolism of drugs that are substrates of CYP3A, thereby increasing the exposure to other drugs).
No products indexed under this heading.

Etoposide (Data indicates that nifedipine can inhibit the metabolism of drugs that are substrates of CYP3A, thereby increasing the exposure to other drugs).
No products indexed under this heading.

Etoposide Phosphate (Data indicates that nifedipine can inhibit the metabolism of drugs that are substrates of CYP3A, thereby increasing the exposure to other drugs).
No products indexed under this heading.

Felbamate (Nifedipine is mainly eliminated by metabolism and is a substrate of CYP3A4. Inducers of CYP3A4 can impact the exposure to nifedipine and consequently its desirable and undesirable effects).
No products indexed under this heading.

Felodipine (Data indicates that nifedipine can inhibit the metabolism of drugs that are substrates of CYP3A, thereby increasing the exposure to other drugs).
No products indexed under this heading.

Fentanyl (Severe hypotension and/or increased fluid volume requirements have been reported when nifedipine was co-administered with a beta-blocker and high-dose fentanyl anesthesia. If permitted, sufficient time (at least 36 hours) should be allowed for nifedipine to be washed out of the body prior to surgery).
Products include:
Duragesic Transdermal System 2373
Ionsys Transdermal System 2379

Fentanyl Citrate (Severe hypotension and/or increased fluid volume requirements have been reported when nifedipine was co-administered with a beta-blocker and high-dose fentanyl anesthesia. If permitted, sufficient time (at least 36 hours) should be allowed for nifedipine to be washed out of the body prior to surgery). Products include:
Actiq 979

Fluconazole (Co-administration of nifedipine with CYP3A4 inhibitors, such as fluconazole, may cause an increase in nifedipine plasma concentrations; a reduction in nifedipine dosage may be considered).
No products indexed under this heading.

Fludrocortisone Acetate (Nifedipine is mainly eliminated by metabolism and is a substrate of CYP3A4. Inducers of CYP3A4 can impact the exposure to nifedipine and consequently its desirable and undesirable effects).
No products indexed under this heading.

Fluoxetine (Co-administration of nifedipine with CYP3A4 inhibitors, such as fluoxetine, may cause an increase in nifedipine plasma concentrations; a reduction in nifedipine dosage may be considered).
No products indexed under this heading.

Fluoxetine Hydrochloride (Co-administration of nifedipine with CYP3A4 inhibitors, such as fluoxetine, may cause an increase in nifedipine plasma concentrations; a reduction in nifedipine dosage may be considered). Products include:
Prozac Pulvules and Liquid 1801
Symbyax Capsules 1819

Fluvoxamine Maleate (Nifedipine is mainly eliminated by metabolism and is a substrate of CYP3A4. Inhibitors of CYP3A4 can impact the exposure to nifedipine and consequently its desirable and undesirable effects).
No products indexed under this heading.

Fosamprenavir Calcium (Nifedipine is mainly eliminated by metabolism and is a substrate of CYP3A4. Inhibitors of CYP3A4 can impact the

exposure to nifedipine and consequently its desirable and undesirable effects). Products include:

Fosinopril Sodium (Nifedipine is a vasodilator, and co-administration of other drugs affecting blood pressure may result in pharmacodynamic interactions).

No products indexed under this heading.

Fosphenytoin Sodium (Co-administration of nifedipine and phenytoin, an inducer of CYP3A4, lowered AUC and Cmax of nifedipine by approximately 70%).

No products indexed under this heading.

Furosemide (Nifedipine is a vasodilator, and co-administration of other drugs affecting blood pressure may result in pharmacodynamic interactions). Products include:

Garlic Extract (Nifedipine is mainly eliminated by metabolism and is a substrate of CYP3A4. Inducers of CYP3A4 can impact the exposure to nifedipine and consequently its desirable and undesirable effects).

No products indexed under this heading.

Garlic Oil (Nifedipine is mainly eliminated by metabolism and is a substrate of CYP3A4. Inducers of CYP3A4 can impact the exposure to nifedipine and consequently its desirable and undesirable effects).

No products indexed under this heading.

Glyburide (Data indicates that nifedipine can inhibit the metabolism of drugs that are substrates of CYP3A, thereby increasing the exposure to other drugs).

No products indexed under this heading.

Guanabenz Acetate (Nifedipine is a vasodilator, and co-administration of other drugs affecting blood pressure may result in pharmacodynamic interactions).

No products indexed under this heading.

Guanethidine Monosulfate (Nifedipine is a vasodilator, and co-administration of other drugs affecting blood pressure may result in pharmacodynamic interactions).

No products indexed under this heading.

Haloperidol (Data indicates that nifedipine can inhibit the metabolism of drugs that are substrates of CYP3A, thereby increasing the exposure to other drugs).

No products indexed under this heading.

Haloperidol Decanoate (Data indicates that nifedipine can inhibit the metabolism of drugs that are substrates of CYP3A, thereby increasing the exposure to other drugs).

No products indexed under this heading.

Hydralazine Hydrochloride (Nifedipine is a vasodilator, and co-administration of other drugs affecting blood pressure may result in pharmacodynamic interactions). Products include:

Hydrochlorothiazide (Nifedipine is a vasodilator, and co-administration of other drugs affecting blood pressure may result in pharmacodynamic interactions). Products include:

Hydrocodone Bitartrate (Potential for severe hypotension and/or increased fluid volume requirements cannot be ruled out when nifedipine is co-administered with a beta-blocker and a narcotic analgesic). Products include:

Hydrocodone Polistirex (Potential for severe hypotension and/or increased fluid volume requirements cannot be ruled out when nifedipine is co-administered with a beta-blocker and a narcotic analgesic). Products include:

Hydrocortisone (Nifedipine is mainly eliminated by metabolism and is a substrate of CYP3A4. Inducers of CYP3A4 can impact the exposure to nifedipine and consequently its desirable and undesirable effects). Products include:

Hydrocortisone Acetate (Nifedipine is mainly eliminated by metabolism and is a substrate of CYP3A4. Inducers of CYP3A4 can impact the exposure to nifedipine and consequently its desirable and undesirable effects). Products include:

Hydrocortisone Butyrate (Nifedipine is mainly eliminated by metabolism and is a substrate of CYP3A4. Inducers of CYP3A4 can impact the exposure to nifedipine and consequently its desirable and undesirable effects). Products include:

Hydrocortisone Cypionate (Nifedipine is mainly eliminated by metabolism and is a substrate of CYP3A4. Inducers of CYP3A4 can impact the exposure to nifedipine and consequently its desirable and undesirable effects).

No products indexed under this heading.

Hydrocortisone Hemisuccinate (Nifedipine is mainly eliminated by metabolism and is a substrate of CYP3A4. Inducers of CYP3A4 can impact the exposure to nifedipine and consequently its desirable and undesirable effects).

No products indexed under this heading.

Hydrocortisone Probutate (Nifedipine is mainly eliminated by metabolism and is a substrate of CYP3A4. Inducers of CYP3A4 can impact the exposure to nifedipine and consequently its desirable and undesirable effects).

No products indexed under this heading.

Hydrocortisone Sodium Phosphate (Nifedipine is mainly eliminated by metabolism and is a substrate of CYP3A4. Inducers of CYP3A4 can impact the exposure to nifedipine and consequently its desirable and undesirable effects).

No products indexed under this heading.

Hydrocortisone Sodium Succinate (Nifedipine is mainly eliminated by metabolism and is a substrate of CYP3A4. Inducers of CYP3A4 can impact the exposure to nifedipine and consequently its desirable and undesirable effects).

No products indexed under this heading.

Hydrocortisone Valerate (Nifedipine is mainly eliminated by metabolism and is a substrate of CYP3A4. Inducers of CYP3A4 can impact the exposure to nifedipine and consequently its desirable and undesirable effects).

No products indexed under this heading.

Hydroflumethiazide (Nifedipine is a vasodilator, and co-administration of other drugs affecting blood pressure may result in pharmacodynamic interactions).

No products indexed under this heading.

Hydromorphone Hydrochloride (Potential for severe hypotension and/or increased fluid volume requirements cannot be ruled out when nifedipine is co-administered with a beta-blocker and a narcotic analgesic). Products include:

Hypericum (Co-administration of nifedipine with CYP3A4 inducers, such as St. John's Wort, may cause a decrease in nifedipine plasma concentrations; a dosage adjustment may be needed). Products include:

Hypericum Perforatum (Nifedipine is mainly eliminated by metabolism and is a substrate of CYP3A4. Inducers of CYP3A4 can impact the exposure to nifedipine and consequently its desirable and undesirable effects).

No products indexed under this heading.

Imipramine Hydrochloride (Data indicates that nifedipine can inhibit the metabolism of drugs that are substrates of CYP3A, thereby increasing the exposure to other drugs).

No products indexed under this heading.

Imipramine Pamoate (Data indicates that nifedipine can inhibit the metabolism of drugs that are substrates of CYP3A, thereby increasing the exposure to other drugs).

No products indexed under this heading.

Indapamide (Nifedipine is a vasodilator, and co-administration of other drugs affecting blood pressure may result in pharmacodynamic interactions). Products include:

Indinavir Sulfate (Co-administration of nifedipine with CYP3A4 inhibitors, such as indinavir, may cause an increase in nifedipine plasma concentrations; a reduction in nifedipine dosage may be considered). Products include:

Irbesartan (Nifedipine is a vasodilator, and co-administration of other drugs affecting blood pressure may result in pharmacodynamic interactions). Products include:

Isoniazid (Nifedipine is mainly eliminated by metabolism and is a substrate of CYP3A4. Inhibitors of CYP3A4 can impact the exposure to nifedipine and consequently its desirable and undesirable effects).

No products indexed under this heading.

Isradipine (Data indicates that nifedipine can inhibit the metabolism of drugs that are substrates of CYP3A, thereby increasing the exposure to other drugs). Products include:

Itraconazole (Co-administration of nifedipine with CYP3A4 inhibitors, such as itraconazole, may cause an increase in nifedipine plasma concentrations; a reduction in nifedipine dosage may be considered).

No products indexed under this heading.

Ketoconazole (Co-administration of nifedipine with CYP3A4 inhibitors, such as ketoconazol, may cause an increase in nifedipine plasma concentrations; a reduction in nifedipine dosage may be considered). Products include:

Labetalol Hydrochloride (Combination of nifedipine and beta-blockers may increase the likelihood of congestive heart failure, severe hypotension, or exacerbation of angina).

No products indexed under this heading.

Levobunolol Hydrochloride (Combination of nifedipine and beta-blockers may increase the likelihood of congestive heart failure, severe hypotension, or exacerbation of angina). Products include:

Levonorgestrel (Data indicates that nifedipine can inhibit the metabolism of drugs that are substrates of

CYP3A, thereby increasing the exposure to other drugs). Products include:

- Climara Pro Transdermal System 776
- Mirena Intrauterine System 787
- Plan B Tablets 1076
- Seasonique Tablets 1077

Levorphanol Tartrate (Potential for severe hypotension and/or increased fluid volume requirements cannot be ruled out when nifedipine is co-administered with a beta-blocker and a narcotic analgesic).
No products indexed under this heading.

Lidocaine (Data indicates that nifedipine can inhibit the metabolism of drugs that are substrates of CYP3A, thereby increasing the exposure to other drugs). Products include:

- Lidoderm Patch 1118
- Synera Topical Patch 1137

Lidocaine Hydrochloride (Data indicates that nifedipine can inhibit the metabolism of drugs that are substrates of CYP3A, thereby increasing the exposure to other drugs).
No products indexed under this heading.

Lisinopril (Nifedipine is a vasodilator, and co-administration of other drugs affecting blood pressure may result in pharmacodynamic interactions). Products include:

- Prinivil Tablets 2052
- Prinzide Tablets 2056

Lopinavir (Nifedipine is mainly eliminated by metabolism and is a substrate of CYP3A4. Inhibitors of CYP3A4 can impact the exposure to nifedipine and consequently its desirable and undesirable effects). Products include:

- Kaletra 476

Loratadine (Nifedipine is mainly eliminated by metabolism and is a substrate of CYP3A4. Inhibitors of CYP3A4 can impact the exposure to nifedipine and consequently its desirable and undesirable effects). Products include:

- Alavert Allergy & Sinus D-12 Hour Tablets .... ▣ 771
- Alavert .... ▣ 771
- Children's Claritin Allergy Oral Solution .... ▣ 771
- Claritin Non-Drowsy 24 Hour Tablets .... ▣ 772
- Claritin Reditabs 24 Hour Non-Drowsy Tablets .... ▣ 772
- Claritin-D Non-Drowsy 12 Hour Tablets .... ▣ 772
- Claritin-D Non-Drowsy 24 Hour Tablets .... ▣ 772

Losartan Potassium (Nifedipine is a vasodilator, and co-administration of other drugs affecting blood pressure may result in pharmacodynamic interactions). Products include:

- Cozaar Tablets 1935
- Hyzaar 50-12.5 Tablets 1990
- Hyzaar 100-12.5 Tablets 1990
- Hyzaar 100-25 Tablets 1990

Lovastatin (Data indicates that nifedipine can inhibit the metabolism of drugs that are substrates of CYP3A, thereby increasing the exposure to other drugs). Products include:

- Advicor Tablets 1722
- Altoprev Extended-Release Tablets 3109
- Mevacor Tablets 2021

Mecamylamine Hydrochloride (Nifedipine is a vasodilator, and co-administration of other drugs affecting blood pressure may result in pharmacodynamic interactions).
No products indexed under this heading.

Meperidine Hydrochloride (Potential for severe hypotension and/or increased fluid volume requirements cannot be ruled out when nifedipine is co-administered with a beta-blocker and a narcotic analgesic).
No products indexed under this heading.

Mephenytoin (Nifedipine is mainly eliminated by metabolism and is a substrate of CYP3A4. Inducers of CYP3A4 can impact the exposure to nifedipine and consequently its desirable and undesirable effects).
No products indexed under this heading.

Mestranol (Data indicates that nifedipine can inhibit the metabolism of drugs that are substrates of CYP3A, thereby increasing the exposure to other drugs).
No products indexed under this heading.

Metformin Hydrochloride (Co-administration with nifedipine can increase Cmax of metformin hydrochloride, AUC of metformin hydrochloride and amount of metformin hydrochloride excreted in urine). Products include:

- ActoPlus Met Tablets 3214
- Avandamet Tablets 1373
- Fortamet Extended-Release Tablets 3115

Methadone Hydrochloride (Potential for severe hypotension and/or increased fluid volume requirements cannot be ruled out when nifedipine is co-administered with a beta-blocker and a narcotic analgesic).
No products indexed under this heading.

Methsuximide (Nifedipine is mainly eliminated by metabolism and is a substrate of CYP3A4. Inducers of CYP3A4 can impact the exposure to nifedipine and consequently its desirable and undesirable effects).
No products indexed under this heading.

Methyclothiazide (Nifedipine is a vasodilator, and co-administration of other drugs affecting blood pressure may result in pharmacodynamic interactions).
No products indexed under this heading.

Methyldopa (Nifedipine is a vasodilator, and co-administration of other drugs affecting blood pressure may result in pharmacodynamic interactions). Products include:

- Aldoril Tablets 1910

Methyldopate Hydrochloride (Nifedipine is a vasodilator, and co-administration of other drugs affecting blood pressure may result in pharmacodynamic interactions).
No products indexed under this heading.

Methylprednisolone (Nifedipine is mainly eliminated by metabolism and is a substrate of CYP3A4. Inducers of CYP3A4 can impact the exposure to nifedipine and consequently its desirable and undesirable effects).
No products indexed under this heading.

Methylprednisolone Acetate (Nifedipine is mainly eliminated by metabolism and is a substrate of CYP3A4. Inducers of CYP3A4 can impact the exposure to nifedipine and consequently its desirable and undesirable effects). Products include:

- Depo-Medrol Injectable Suspension 2617
- Depo-Medrol Single-Dose Vial 2619

Methylprednisolone Sodium Succinate (Nifedipine is mainly eliminated by metabolism and is a substrate of CYP3A4. Inducers of CYP3A4 can impact the exposure to nifedipine and consequently its desirable and undesirable effects).
No products indexed under this heading.

Metipranolol Hydrochloride (Combination of nifedipine and beta-blockers may increase the likelihood of congestive heart failure, severe hypotension, or exacerbation of angina).
No products indexed under this heading.

Metolazone (Nifedipine is a vasodilator, and co-administration of other drugs affecting blood pressure may result in pharmacodynamic interactions).
No products indexed under this heading.

Metoprolol Succinate (Combination of nifedipine and beta-blockers may increase the likelihood of congestive heart failure, severe hypotension, or exacerbation of angina). Products include:

- Toprol-XL Tablets 668

Metoprolol Tartrate (Combination of nifedipine and beta-blockers may increase the likelihood of congestive heart failure, severe hypotension, or exacerbation of angina). Products include:

- Lopressor Injection 2238
- Lopressor Tablets 2238
- Lopressor HCT 50/25 Tablets 2241
- Lopressor HCT 100/25 Tablets 2241
- Lopressor HCT 100/50 Tablets 2241

Metronidazole (Nifedipine is mainly eliminated by metabolism and is a substrate of CYP3A4. Inhibitors of CYP3A4 can impact the exposure to nifedipine and consequently its desirable and undesirable effects). Products include:

- Metrogel 1% 1211
- MetroGel-Vaginal Gel 1855
- Vandazole Vaginal Gel 3338

Metronidazole Benzoate (Nifedipine is mainly eliminated by metabolism and is a substrate of CYP3A4. Inhibitors of CYP3A4 can impact the exposure to nifedipine and consequently its desirable and undesirable effects).
No products indexed under this heading.

Metronidazole Hydrochloride (Nifedipine is mainly eliminated by metabolism and is a substrate of CYP3A4. Inhibitors of CYP3A4 can impact the exposure to nifedipine and consequently its desirable and undesirable effects).
No products indexed under this heading.

Metyrosine (Nifedipine is a vasodilator, and co-administration of other drugs affecting blood pressure may result in pharmacodynamic interactions). Products include:

- Demser Capsules 1953

Mibefradil Dihydrochloride (Nifedipine is a vasodilator, and co-administration of other drugs affecting blood pressure may result in pharmacodynamic interactions).
No products indexed under this heading.

Miconazole (Nifedipine is mainly eliminated by metabolism and is a substrate of CYP3A4. Inhibitors of CYP3A4 can impact the exposure to nifedipine and consequently its desirable and undesirable effects).
No products indexed under this heading.

Miconazole Nitrate (Nifedipine is mainly eliminated by metabolism and is a substrate of CYP3A4. Inhibitors of CYP3A4 can impact the exposure to nifedipine and consequently its desirable and undesirable effects). Products include:

- Desenex .... ▣ 635
- Desenex Jock Itch Spray Powder ... ▣ 635

Midazolam Hydrochloride (Data indicates that nifedipine can inhibit the metabolism of drugs that are substrates of CYP3A, thereby increasing the exposure to other drugs).
No products indexed under this heading.

Minoxidil (Nifedipine is a vasodilator, and co-administration of other drugs affecting blood pressure may result in pharmacodynamic interactions). Products include:

- Men's Rogaine Extra Strength Hair Regrowth Treatment Topical Solution, Ocean Rush Scent and Original Unscented ..... ▣ 633
- Men's Rogaine Foam Hair Regrowth Treatment .... ▣ 633
- Women's Rogaine Hair Regrowth Treatment Topical Solution, Spring Bloom Scent and Original Unscented .... ▣ 634

Modafinil (Nifedipine is mainly eliminated by metabolism and is a substrate of CYP3A4. Inducers of CYP3A4 can impact the exposure to nifedipine and consequently its desirable and undesirable effects). Products include:

- Provigil Tablets 988

Moexipril Hydrochloride (Nifedipine is a vasodilator, and co-administration of other drugs affecting blood pressure may result in pharmacodynamic interactions). Products include:

- Uniretic Tablets 3100
- Univasc Tablets 3104

Morphine Sulfate (Potential for severe hypotension and/or increased fluid volume requirements cannot be ruled out when nifedipine is co-administered with a beta-blocker and a narcotic analgesic). Products include:

- Avinza Capsules 1741
- Kadian Capsules 577
- MS Contin Tablets 2701

Nadolol (Combination of nifedipine and beta-blockers may increase the likelihood of congestive heart failure, severe hypotension, or exacerbation of angina). Products include:

- Nadolol Tablets 2159

Nefazodone Hydrochloride (Co-administration of nifedipine with CYP3A4 inhibitors, such as nefazodone, may cause an increase in nifedipine plasma concentrations; a reduction in nifedipine dosage may be considered).
No products indexed under this heading.

Nelfinavir Mesylate (Co-administration of nifedipine with CYP3A4 inhibitors, such as nelfinavir, may cause an increase in nifedipine plasma concentrations; a reduction in nifedipine dosage may be considered). Products include:

Viracept 2577

Nevirapine (Nifedipine is mainly eliminated by metabolism and is a substrate of CYP3A4. Inhibitors of CYP3A4 can impact the exposure to nifedipine and consequently its desirable and undesirable effects). Products include:

Viramune Oral Suspension 873
Viramune Tablets 873

Niacinamide (Nifedipine is mainly eliminated by metabolism and is a substrate of CYP3A4. Inhibitors of CYP3A4 can impact the exposure to nifedipine and consequently its desirable and undesirable effects).

No products indexed under this heading.

Nicardipine (Data indicates that nifedipine can inhibit the metabolism of drugs that are substrates of CYP3A, thereby increasing the exposure to other drugs).

No products indexed under this heading.

Nicardipine Hydrochloride (Data indicates that nifedipine can inhibit the metabolism of drugs that are substrates of CYP3A, thereby increasing the exposure to other drugs). Products include:

Cardene I.V. 2497

Nicotinamide (Nifedipine is mainly eliminated by metabolism and is a substrate of CYP3A4. Inhibitors of CYP3A4 can impact the exposure to nifedipine and consequently its desirable and undesirable effects). Products include:

Nicomide Tablets 1088

Nimodipine (Data indicates that nifedipine can inhibit the metabolism of drugs that are substrates of CYP3A, thereby increasing the exposure to other drugs). Products include:

Nimotop Capsules 749

Nisoldipine (Data indicates that nifedipine can inhibit the metabolism of drugs that are substrates of CYP3A, thereby increasing the exposure to other drugs). Products include:

Sular Tablets 3122

Nitroglycerin (Nifedipine is a vasodilator, and co-administration of other drugs affecting blood pressure may result in pharmacodynamic interactions). Products include:

Nitro-Dur Transdermal Infusion System 3046
Nitrolingual Pumpspray 3120

Norethindrone (Data indicates that nifedipine can inhibit the metabolism of drugs that are substrates of CYP3A, thereby increasing the exposure to other drugs). Products include:

Ortho Micronor Tablets 2426

Norfloxacin (Nifedipine is mainly eliminated by metabolism and is a substrate of CYP3A4. Inhibitors of CYP3A4 can impact the exposure to nifedipine and consequently its desirable and undesirable effects). Products include:

Noroxin Tablets 2032

Norgestrel (Data indicates that nifedipine can inhibit the metabolism of drugs that are substrates of CYP3A, thereby increasing the exposure to other drugs).

No products indexed under this heading.

Omeprazole (Nifedipine is mainly eliminated by metabolism and is a substrate of CYP3A4. Inhibitors of CYP3A4 can impact the exposure to nifedipine and consequently its desirable and undesirable effects). Products include:

Zegerid Capsules 2958
Zegerid Powder for Oral Solution 2958

Ondansetron Hydrochloride (Data indicates that nifedipine can inhibit the metabolism of drugs that are substrates of CYP3A, thereby increasing the exposure to other drugs). Products include:

Zofran Injection 1634
Zofran 1639

Oxcarbazepine (Nifedipine is mainly eliminated by metabolism and is a substrate of CYP3A4. Inducers of CYP3A4 can impact the exposure to nifedipine and consequently its desirable and undesirable effects). Products include:

Trileptal Tablets 2300
Trileptal Oral Suspension 2300

Oxycodone Hydrochloride (Potential for severe hypotension and/or increased fluid volume requirements cannot be ruled out when nifedipine is co-administered with a beta-blocker and a narcotic analgesic). Products include:

OxyContin Tablets 2703
OxyFast Oral Concentrate Solution 2708
OxyIR Capsules 2708
Percocet Tablets 1131
Percodan Tablets 1132

Paclitaxel (Data indicates that nifedipine can inhibit the metabolism of drugs that are substrates of CYP3A, thereby increasing the exposure to other drugs).

No products indexed under this heading.

Paroxetine Hydrochloride (Nifedipine is mainly eliminated by metabolism and is a substrate of CYP3A4. Inhibitors of CYP3A4 can impact the exposure to nifedipine and consequently its desirable and undesirable effects). Products include:

Paxil CR Controlled-Release Tablets 1538
Paxil 1530

Penbutolol Sulfate (Combination of nifedipine and beta-blockers may increase the likelihood of congestive heart failure, severe hypotension, or exacerbation of angina).

No products indexed under this heading.

Perindopril Erbumine (Nifedipine is a vasodilator, and co-administration of other drugs affecting blood pressure may result in pharmacodynamic interactions). Products include:

Aceon Tablets (2 mg, 4 mg, 8 mg) 3194

Phenobarbital (Phenobarbital has been shown to reduce plasma concentrations of other calcium channel blockers due to enzyme induction; a similar interaction with nifedipine leading to a decrease in nifedipine plasma concentrations and a decrease in efficacy cannot be excluded; a dosage adjustment of nifedipine may be needed). Products include:

Donnatal Extentabs 2493

Phenobarbital Sodium (Phenobarbital has been shown to reduce plasma concentrations of other calcium channel blockers due to enzyme induction; a similar interaction with nifedipine leading to a decrease in nifedipine plasma concentrations and a decrease in efficacy cannot be excluded, a dosage adjustment of nifedipine may be needed).

No products indexed under this heading.

Phenoxybenzamine Hydrochloride (Nifedipine is a vasodilator, and co-administration of other drugs affecting blood pressure may result in pharmacodynamic interactions). Products include:

Dibenzyline Capsules 3399

Phentolamine Mesylate (Nifedipine is a vasodilator, and co-administration of other drugs affecting blood pressure may result in pharmacodynamic interactions).

No products indexed under this heading.

Phenytoin (Co-administration of nifedipine and phenytoin, an inducer of CYP3A4, lowered AUC and Cmax of nifedipine by approximately 70%; a dosage adjustment of nifedipine may be needed).

No products indexed under this heading.

Phenytoin Sodium (Co-administration of nifedipine and phenytoin, an inducer of CYP3A4, lowered AUC and Cmax of nifedipine by approximately 70%; a dosage adjustment of nifedipine may be needed). Products include:

Phenytek Capsules 2160

Pimozide (Data indicates that nifedipine can inhibit the metabolism of drugs that are substrates of CYP3A, thereby increasing the exposure to other drugs).

No products indexed under this heading.

Pindolol (Combination of nifedipine and beta-blockers may increase the likelihood of congestive heart failure, severe hypotension, or exacerbation of angina).

No products indexed under this heading.

Polythiazide (Nifedipine is a vasodilator, and co-administration of other drugs affecting blood pressure may result in pharmacodynamic interactions).

No products indexed under this heading.

Prazosin Hydrochloride (Nifedipine is a vasodilator, and co-administration of other drugs affecting blood pressure may result in pharmacodynamic interactions).

No products indexed under this heading.

Prednisolone Acetate (Nifedipine is mainly eliminated by metabolism and is a substrate of CYP3A4. Inducers of CYP3A4 can impact the exposure to nifedipine and consequently its desirable and undesirable effects). Products include:

Blephamide Ophthalmic Ointment 568
Blephamide Ophthalmic Suspension 569
Poly-Pred Ophthalmic Suspension .... ⊙233
Pred Forte Ophthalmic Suspension .... ⊙235
Pred Mild Ophthalmic Suspension .... ⊙238
Pred-G Ophthalmic Ointment .... ⊙237
Pred-G Ophthalmic Suspension .... ⊙236

Prednisolone Sodium Phosphate (Nifedipine is mainly eliminated by metabolism and is a substrate of CYP3A4. Inducers of CYP3A4 can impact the exposure to nifedipine and consequently its desirable and undesirable effects).

No products indexed under this heading.

Prednisolone Tebutate (Nifedipine is mainly eliminated by metabolism and is a substrate of CYP3A4. Inducers of CYP3A4 can impact the exposure to nifedipine and consequently its desirable and undesirable effects).

No products indexed under this heading.

Prednisone (Nifedipine is mainly eliminated by metabolism and is a substrate of CYP3A4. Inducers of CYP3A4 can impact the exposure to nifedipine and consequently its desirable and undesirable effects).

No products indexed under this heading.

Primidone (Nifedipine is mainly eliminated by metabolism and is a substrate of CYP3A4. Inducers of CYP3A4 can impact the exposure to nifedipine and consequently its desirable and undesirable effects).

No products indexed under this heading.

Propoxyphene Hydrochloride (Potential for severe hypotension and/or increased fluid volume requirements cannot be ruled out when nifedipine is co-administered with a beta-blocker and a narcotic analgesic).

No products indexed under this heading.

Propoxyphene Napsylate (Potential for severe hypotension and/or increased fluid volume requirements cannot be ruled out when nifedipine is co-administered with a beta-blocker and a narcotic analgesic).

No products indexed under this heading.

Propranolol Hydrochloride (Combination of nifedipine and beta-blockers may increase the likelihood of congestive heart failure, severe hypotension, or exacerbation of angina). Products include:

Inderal LA Long-Acting Capsules 3429
InnoPran XL Capsules 2723

Quinapril Hydrochloride (Nifedipine is a vasodilator, and co-administration of other drugs affecting blood pressure may result in pharmacodynamic interactions).

No products indexed under this heading.

Quinidine (Nifedipine is mainly eliminated by metabolism and is a substrate of CYP3A4. Inhibitors of CYP3A4 can impact the exposure to nifedipine and consequently its desirable and undesirable effects).

No products indexed under this heading.

Quinidine Gluconate (Co-administration with nifedipine can increase nifedipine Cmax and AUC by 2.30 and 1.37 respectively. Heart rate will increase by 17.9 beats/minute).

No products indexed under this heading.

Quinidine Hydrochloride (Nifedipine is mainly eliminated by metabolism and is a substrate of CYP3A4. Inhibitors of CYP3A4 can impact the exposure to nifedipine and consequently its desirable and undesirable effects).
　　No products indexed under this heading.

Quinidine Polygalacturonate (Co-administration with nifedipine can increase nifedipine Cmax and AUC by 2.30 and 1.37 respectively. Heart rate will increase by 17.9 beats/minute).
　　No products indexed under this heading.

Quinidine Sulfate (Co-administration with nifedipine can increase nifedipine Cmax and AUC by 2.30 and 1.37 respectively. Heart rate will increase by 17.9 beats/minute).
　　No products indexed under this heading.

Quinine (Nifedipine is mainly eliminated by metabolism and is a substrate of CYP3A4. Inhibitors of CYP3A4 can impact the exposure to nifedipine and consequently its desirable and undesirable effects).
　　No products indexed under this heading.

Quinine Sulfate (Nifedipine is mainly eliminated by metabolism and is a substrate of CYP3A4. Inhibitors of CYP3A4 can impact the exposure to nifedipine and consequently its desirable and undesirable effects).
　　No products indexed under this heading.

Quinupristin (Concomitant administration may lead to increased plasma concentrations of nifedipine; a reduction in nifedipine dosage may be considered).
　　No products indexed under this heading.

Ramipril (Nifedipine is a vasodilator, and co-administration of other drugs affecting blood pressure may result in pharmacodynamic interactions). Products include:
　　Altace Capsules 1702

Ranitidine Bismuth Citrate (Nifedipine is mainly eliminated by metabolism and is a substrate of CYP3A4. Inhibitors of CYP3A4 can impact the exposure to nifedipine and consequently its desirable and undesirable effects).
　　No products indexed under this heading.

Ranitidine Hydrochloride (Produces smaller, non-significant increases in peak nifedipine plasma levels and AUC). Products include:
　　Zantac ... 1624
　　Zantac Injection 1619
　　Zantac Injection Pharmacy Bulk
　　　Package 1622

Rauwolfia Serpentina (Nifedipine is a vasodilator, and co-administration of other drugs affecting blood pressure may result in pharmacodynamic interactions).
　　No products indexed under this heading.

Remifentanil Hydrochloride (Potential for severe hypotension and/or increased fluid volume requirements cannot be ruled out when nifedipine is co-administered with a beta-blocker and a narcotic analgesic).
　　No products indexed under this heading.

Rescinnamine (Nifedipine is a vasodilator, and co-administration of other drugs affecting blood pressure may result in pharmacodynamic interactions).
　　No products indexed under this heading.

Reserpine (Nifedipine is a vasodilator, and co-administration of other drugs affecting blood pressure may result in pharmacodynamic interactions).
　　No products indexed under this heading.

Rifabutin (Nifedipine is mainly eliminated by metabolism and is a substrate of CYP3A4. Inducers of CYP3A4 can impact the exposure to nifedipine and consequently its desirable and undesirable effects).
　　No products indexed under this heading.

Rifampicin (Rifampicin strongly induces CYP3A4, and upon co-administration with rifampicin, the bioavailability of nifedipine is distinctly reduced and its efficacy weakened. Rifampicin should be avoided in patients receiving nifedipine).
　　No products indexed under this heading.

Rifampin (Co-administration with nifedipine can decrease the exposure of oral nifedipine; a dosage adjustment of nifedipine may be needed).
　　No products indexed under this heading.

Rifapentine (Co-administration with a CYP3A4 inducer, such as rifapentine, will decrease the exposure to nifedipine; a dosage adjustment of nifedipine may be needed).
　　No products indexed under this heading.

Ritonavir (Co-administration of nifedipine with CYP3A4 inhibitors, such as ritonavir, may cause an increase in nifedipine plasma concentrations; a reduction in nifedipine dosage may be considered). Products include:
　　Kaletra ... 476
　　Norvir .. 503

Saquinavir (Co-administration of nifedipine with CYP3A4 inhibitors, such as saquinavir, may cause an increase in nifedipine plasma concentrations; a reduction in nifedipine dosage may be considered).
　　No products indexed under this heading.

Saquinavir Mesylate (Co-administration of nifedipine with CYP3A4 inhibitors, such as saquinavir, may cause an increase in nifedipine plasma concentrations; a reduction in nifedipine dosage may be considered). Products include:
　　Invirase .. 2772

Sertraline Hydrochloride (Nifedipine is mainly eliminated by metabolism and is a substrate of CYP3A4. Inhibitors of CYP3A4 can impact the exposure to nifedipine and consequently its desirable and undesirable effects). Products include:
　　Zoloft .. 2586

Sildenafil Citrate (Data indicates that nifedipine can inhibit the metabolism of drugs that are substrates of CYP3A, thereby increasing the exposure to other drugs). Products include:
　　Revatio Tablets 2557
　　Viagra Tablets 2573

Simvastatin (Data indicates that nifedipine can inhibit the metabolism

of drugs that are substrates of CYP3A, thereby increasing the exposure to other drugs). Products include:
　　Vytorin 10/10 Tablets 2114
　　Vytorin 10/10 Tablets 3077
　　Vytorin 10/20 Tablets 2114
　　Vytorin 10/20 Tablets 3077
　　Vytorin 10/40 Tablets 2114
　　Vytorin 10/40 Tablets 3077
　　Vytorin 10/80 Tablets 2114
　　Vytorin 10/80 Tablets 3077
　　Zocor Tablets 2105

Sirolimus (Data indicates that nifedipine can inhibit the metabolism of drugs that are substrates of CYP3A, thereby increasing the exposure to other drugs). Products include:
　　Rapamune Oral Solution and
　　　Tablets .. 3475

Sodium Nitroprusside (Nifedipine is a vasodilator, and co-administration of other drugs affecting blood pressure may result in pharmacodynamic interactions).
　　No products indexed under this heading.

Sotalol Hydrochloride (Combination of nifedipine and beta-blockers may increase the likelihood of congestive heart failure, severe hypotension, or exacerbation of angina).
　　No products indexed under this heading.

Spirapril Hydrochloride (Nifedipine is a vasodilator, and co-administration of other drugs affecting blood pressure may result in pharmacodynamic interactions).
　　No products indexed under this heading.

Sufentanil Citrate (Potential for severe hypotension and/or increased fluid volume requirements cannot be ruled out when nifedipine is co-administered with a beta-blocker and a narcotic analgesic).
　　No products indexed under this heading.

Sulfinpyrazone (Nifedipine is mainly eliminated by metabolism and is a substrate of CYP3A4. Inducers of CYP3A4 can impact the exposure to nifedipine and consequently its desirable and undesirable effects).
　　No products indexed under this heading.

Tacrolimus (If co-administered with nifedipine, tacrolimus plasma concentrations should be monitored and a reduction in tacrolimus dosage may be considered). Products include:
　　Prograf Capsules and Injection 632
　　Protopic Ointment 638

Tamoxifen Citrate (Data indicates that nifedipine can inhibit the metabolism of drugs that are substrates of CYP3A, thereby increasing the exposure to other drugs). Products include:
　　Soltamox Oral Solution 3527

Telithromycin (Nifedipine is mainly eliminated by metabolism and is a substrate of CYP3A4. Inhibitors of CYP3A4 can impact the exposure to nifedipine and undesirable effects). Products include:
　　Ketek Tablets 2903

Telmisartan (Nifedipine is a vasodilator, and co-administration of other drugs affecting blood pressure may result in pharmacodynamic interactions). Products include:
　　Micardis Tablets 854
　　Micardis HCT Tablets 856

Terazosin Hydrochloride (Nifedipine is a vasodilator, and co-administration of other drugs affecting blood pressure may result in pharmacodynamic interactions). Products include:
　　Hytrin Capsules 471

Terfenadine (Data indicates that nifedipine can inhibit the metabolism of drugs that are substrates of CYP3A, thereby increasing the exposure to other drugs).
　　No products indexed under this heading.

Testosterone (Data indicates that nifedipine can inhibit the metabolism of drugs that are substrates of CYP3A, thereby increasing the exposure to other drugs). Products include:
　　AndroGel 3329
　　Striant Mucoadhesive 1007
　　Testim 1% Gel 695

Testosterone Cypionate (Data indicates that nifedipine can inhibit the metabolism of drugs that are substrates of CYP3A, thereby increasing the exposure to other drugs).
　　No products indexed under this heading.

Testosterone Enanthate (Data indicates that nifedipine can inhibit the metabolism of drugs that are substrates of CYP3A, thereby increasing the exposure to other drugs).
　　No products indexed under this heading.

Testosterone Propionate (Data indicates that nifedipine can inhibit the metabolism of drugs that are substrates of CYP3A, thereby increasing the exposure to other drugs).
　　No products indexed under this heading.

Theophylline (Nifedipine is mainly eliminated by metabolism and is a substrate of CYP3A4. Inducers of CYP3A4 can impact the exposure to nifedipine and consequently its desirable and undesirable effects).
　　No products indexed under this heading.

Theophylline Anhydrous (Data indicates that nifedipine can inhibit the metabolism of drugs that are substrates of CYP3A, thereby increasing the exposure to other drugs). Products include:
　　Uniphyl Tablets 2710

Theophylline Calcium Salicylate (Data indicates that nifedipine can inhibit the metabolism of drugs that are substrates of CYP3A, thereby increasing the exposure to other drugs).
　　No products indexed under this heading.

Theophylline Sodium Glycinate (Data indicates that nifedipine can inhibit the metabolism of drugs that are substrates of CYP3A, thereby increasing the exposure to other drugs).
　　No products indexed under this heading.

Tiagabine Hydrochloride (Data indicates that nifedipine can inhibit the metabolism of drugs that are substrates of CYP3A, thereby increasing the exposure to other drugs). Products include:
　　Gabitril Tablets 984

Timolol Hemihydrate (Combination of nifedipine and beta-blockers

may increase the likelihood of congestive heart failure, severe hypotension, or exacerbation of angina). Products include:
Betimol Ophthalmic Solution 3382
Betimol Ophthalmic Solution .... ⊙295

Timolol Maleate (Combination of nifedipine and beta-blockers may increase the likelihood of congestive heart failure, severe hypotension, or exacerbation of angina). Products include:
Blocadren Tablets 1916
Cosopt Sterile Ophthalmic Solution....................................... 1931
Timolide Tablets 2086
Timoptic Sterile Ophthalmic Solution....................................... 2088
Timoptic in Ocudose 2091
Timoptic-XE Sterile Ophthalmic Gel Forming Solution 2092

Tolterodine Tartrate (Data indicates that nifedipine can inhibit the metabolism of drugs that are substrates of CYP3A, thereby increasing the exposure to other drugs). Products include:
Detrol Tablets 2628
Detrol LA Capsules 2631

Torsemide (Nifedipine is a vasodilator, and co-administration of other drugs affecting blood pressure may result in pharmacodynamic interactions). Products include:
Demadex Injection 2759
Demadex Tablets 2759

Trandolapril (Nifedipine is a vasodilator, and co-administration of other drugs affecting blood pressure may result in pharmacodynamic interactions). Products include:
Mavik Tablets 486
Tarka Tablets 524

Trazodone Hydrochloride (Data indicates that nifedipine can inhibit the metabolism of drugs that are substrates of CYP3A, thereby increasing the exposure to other drugs).
No products indexed under this heading.

Triamcinolone (Nifedipine is mainly eliminated by metabolism and is a substrate of CYP3A4. Inducers of CYP3A4 can impact the exposure to nifedipine and consequently its desirable and undesirable effects).
No products indexed under this heading.

Triamcinolone Acetonide (Nifedipine is mainly eliminated by metabolism and is a substrate of CYP3A4. Inducers of CYP3A4 can impact the exposure to nifedipine and consequently its desirable and undesirable effects). Products include:
Azmacort Inhalation Aerosol 1726
Nasacort AQ Nasal Spray 2922

Triamcinolone Diacetate (Nifedipine is mainly eliminated by metabolism and is a substrate of CYP3A4. Inducers of CYP3A4 can impact the exposure to nifedipine and consequently its desirable and undesirable effects).
No products indexed under this heading.

Triamcinolone Hexacetonide (Nifedipine is mainly eliminated by metabolism and is a substrate of CYP3A4. Inducers of CYP3A4 can impact the exposure to nifedipine and consequently its desirable and undesirable effects).
No products indexed under this heading.

Triazolam (Data indicates that nifedipine can inhibit the metabolism of drugs that are substrates of CYP3A, thereby increasing the exposure to other drugs).
No products indexed under this heading.

Trimethaphan Camsylate (Nifedipine is a vasodilator, and co-administration of other drugs affecting blood pressure may result in pharmacodynamic interactions).
No products indexed under this heading.

Troglitazone (Nifedipine is mainly eliminated by metabolism and is a substrate of CYP3A4. Inhibitors of CYP3A4 can impact the exposure to nifedipine and consequently its desirable and undesirable effects).
No products indexed under this heading.

Troleandomycin (Nifedipine is mainly eliminated by metabolism and is a substrate of CYP3A4. Inhibitors of CYP3A4 can impact the exposure to nifedipine and consequently its desirable and undesirable effects).
No products indexed under this heading.

Valproate Sodium (Nifedipine is mainly eliminated by metabolism and is a substrate of CYP3A4. Inhibitors of CYP3A4 can impact the exposure to nifedipine and consequently its desirable and undesirable effects). Products include:
Depacon Injection 412

Valproic Acid (Valproic acid has been shown to elevate plasma concentrations of other calcium channel blockers due to enzyme inhibition; a similar interaction with nifedipine leading to an increase in nifedipine plasma concentrations and an increase in efficacy cannot be excluded). Products include:
Depakene 417

Valsartan (Nifedipine is a vasodilator, and co-administration of other drugs affecting blood pressure may result in pharmacodynamic interactions). Products include:
Diovan Tablets 2193
Diovan HCT Tablets 2196

Venlafaxine Hydrochloride (Data indicates that nifedipine can inhibit the metabolism of drugs that are substrates of CYP3A, thereby increasing the exposure to other drugs). Products include:
Effexor Tablets 3411
Effexor XR Capsules 3417

Verapamil Hydrochloride (Co-administration of nifedipine with CYP3A4 inhibitors, such as verapamil hydrochloride, may cause an increase in nifedipine plasma concentration; a reduction in nifedipine dosage may be considered). Products include:
Covera-HS Tablets 3139
Tarka Tablets 524
Verelan PM Extended-Release Capsules, Controlled-Onset........... 3106

Vinblastine Sulfate (Data indicates that nifedipine can inhibit the metabolism of drugs that are substrates of CYP3A, thereby increasing the exposure to other drugs).
No products indexed under this heading.

Vincristine Sulfate (Data indicates that nifedipine can inhibit the metabolism of drugs that are substrates of CYP3A, thereby increasing the exposure to other drugs).
No products indexed under this heading.

Voriconazole (Nifedipine is mainly eliminated by metabolism and is a substrate of CYP3A4. Inhibitors of CYP3A4 can impact the exposure to nifedipine and consequently its desirable and undesirable effects). Products include:
VFEND I.V. 2564
VFEND Oral Suspension 2564
VFEND Tablets 2564

Warfarin Sodium (There have been rare reports of increased prothrombin time in patients taking coumarin anticoagulants to whom nifedipine was administered). Products include:
Coumadin for Injection 898
Coumadin Tablets 898

Zafirlukast (Nifedipine is mainly eliminated by metabolism and is a substrate of CYP3A4. Inhibitors of CYP3A4 can impact the exposure to nifedipine and consequently its desirable and undesirable effects). Products include:
Accolate Tablets 671

Zileuton (Nifedipine is mainly eliminated by metabolism and is a substrate of CYP3A4. Inhibitors of CYP3A4 can impact the exposure to nifedipine and consequently its desirable and undesirable effects). Products include:
Zyflo Tablets 1023

Food Interactions

Diet, high-lipid (High-fat meal increases peak plasma nifedipine concentrations by 60%, a prolongation in the time to peak concentration, but no significant change in the AUC; administer on an empty stomach).

Grapefruit (Nifedipine is mainly eliminated by metabolism and is a substrate of CYP3A4. Inhibitors of CYP3A4 can impact the exposure to nifedipine and consequently its desirable and undesirable effects).

Grapefruit Juice (Co-administration of nifedipine with grapefruit juice results in up to a 2-fold increase in AUC and Cmax, due to inhibition of CYP3A4-related first-pass metabolism. This effect of grapefruit juice may last for at least 3 days; co-administration should beavoided).

ADDERALL TABLETS

(Amphetamine Aspartate, Amphetamine Sulfate, Dextroamphetamine Saccharate, Dextroamphetamine Sulfate).............. 3164
See Adderall XR Capsules

ADDERALL XR CAPSULES

(Amphetamine Aspartate, Amphetamine Sulfate, Dextroamphetamine Saccharate, Dextroamphetamine Sulfate).............. 3166
May interact with antacids, antihistamines, antihypertensives, beta blockers, monoamine oxidase inhibitors, methenamine, phenytoin, thiazides, tricyclic antidepressants, urinary alkalinizing agents, veratrum alkaloids, and certain other agents. Compounds in these categories include:

Acebutolol Hydrochloride (Adrenergic blockers are inhibited by amphetamines; amphetamines may antagonize the hypotensive effects of antihypertensives).
No products indexed under this heading.

Acetazolamide (Co-administration with urinary alkalinizing agents, such as acetazolamide, increase the concentration of the non-ionized species of the amphetamine molecule, thereby decreasing urinary excretion resulting in increased blood levels and potentiate the actions of amphetamines).
No products indexed under this heading.

Acetazolamide Sodium (Co-administration with urinary alkalinizing agents, such as acetazolamide, increase the concentration of the non-ionized species of the amphetamine molecule, thereby decreasing urinary excretion resulting in increased blood levels and potentiate the actions of amphetamines).
No products indexed under this heading.

Acrivastine (Amphetamines may counteract the sedative effect of antihistamines).
No products indexed under this heading.

Aluminum Carbonate (Co-administration with gastrointestinal alkalinizing agents, such as antacids, may increase the absorption of amphetamines; concurrent use should be avoided).
No products indexed under this heading.

Aluminum Hydroxide (Co-administration with gastrointestinal alkalinizing agents, such as antacids, may increase the absorption of amphetamines; concurrent use should be avoided). Products include:
Gaviscon Regular Strength Liquid .. ▣658
Gaviscon Regular Strength Tablets.. ▣658
Gaviscon Extra Strength Liquid ...... ▣658
Gaviscon Extra Strength Tablets .... ▣658
Maalox Regular Strength Antacid/Antigas Liquid................. 2175
Maalox Max Maximum Strength Antacid/Anti-Gas Liquid................ 2176

Amitriptyline Hydrochloride (Enhanced activity of tricyclic antidepressants or sympathomimetics; possible increases in d-amphetamine resulting in potentiation of cardiovascular effects).
No products indexed under this heading.

Amlodipine Besylate (Amphetamines may antagonize the hypotensive effects of antihypertensives). Products include:
Caduet Tablets 2508
Lotrel Capsules 2249
Norvasc Tablets 2545

Ammonium Chloride (Co-administration with urinary acidifying agents increases the concentration of the ionized species of the amphetamine molecule, thereby increasing urinary excretion resulting in reduced blood levels and efficacy of amphetamines).
No products indexed under this heading.

Amoxapine (Enhanced activity of tricyclic antidepressants or sympathomimetics; possible increases in d-amphetamine resulting in potentiation of cardiovascular effects).
No products indexed under this heading.

Astemizole (Amphetamines may counteract the sedative effect of antihistamines).
No products indexed under this heading.

Atenolol (Adrenergic blockers are inhibited by amphetamines; amphetamines may antagonize the hypotensive effects of antihypertensives).
No products indexed under this heading.

Azatadine Maleate (Amphetamines may counteract the sedative effect of antihistamines).
No products indexed under this heading.

Benazepril Hydrochloride (Amphetamines may antagonize the hypotensive effects of antihypertensives). Products include:
Lotensin Tablets 2243
Lotensin HCT Tablets 2246
Lotrel Capsules 2249

Bendroflumethiazide (Co-administration with urinary alkalinizing agents, such as certain thiazides, increase the concentration of the non-ionized species of the amphetamine molecule, thereby decreasing urinary excretion resulting in increased blood levels and potentiation ofactions of amphetamines; amphetamines may antagonize the hypotensive effects of antihypertensives).
No products indexed under this heading.

Betaxolol Hydrochloride (Adrenergic blockers are inhibited by amphetamines; amphetamines may antagonize the hypotensive effects of antihypertensives). Products include:
Betoptic S Ophthalmic Suspension 558

Bisoprolol Fumarate (Adrenergic blockers are inhibited by amphetamines; amphetamines may antagonize the hypotensive effects of antihypertensives).
No products indexed under this heading.

Bromodiphenhydramine Hydrochloride (Amphetamines may counteract the sedative effect of antihistamines).
No products indexed under this heading.

Brompheniramine Maleate (Amphetamines may counteract the sedative effect of antihistamines). Products include:
Children's Dimetapp Cold & Allergy Elixir .... ■ 730
Children's Dimetapp Cold & Allergy Chewable Tablets .... ■ 730
Children's Dimetapp DM Cold & Cough Elixir .... ■ 731

Candesartan Cilexetil (Amphetamines may antagonize the hypotensive effects of antihypertensives). Products include:
Atacand Tablets 649
Atacand HCT 651

Captopril (Amphetamines may antagonize the hypotensive effects of antihypertensives). Products include:
Captopril Tablets 2149

Carteolol Hydrochloride (Adrenergic blockers are inhibited by amphetamines; amphetamines may antagonize the hypotensive effects of antihypertensives). Products include:
Carteolol Hydrochloride Ophthalmic Solution USP, 1% .... ⊙ 249

Cetirizine Hydrochloride (Amphetamines may counteract the sedative effect of antihistamines). Products include:
Zyrtec Chewable Tablets 2594
Zyrtec 2594
Zyrtec-D 12 Hour Extended Release Tablets 2597

Chlorothiazide (Co-administration with urinary alkalinizing agents, such as certain thiazides, increase the concentration of the non-ionized species of the amphetamine molecule, thereby decreasing urinary excretion resulting in increased blood levels and potentiation ofactions of amphetamines; amphetamines may antagonize the hypotensive effects of antihypertensives). Products include:
Diuril Oral Suspension 1954

Chlorothiazide Sodium (Co-administration with urinary alkalinizing agents, such as certain thiazides, increase the concentration of the non-ionized species of the amphetamine molecule, thereby decreasing urinary excretion resulting in increased blood levels and potentiation ofactions of amphetamines; amphetamines may antagonize the hypotensive effects of antihypertensives). Products include:
Diuril Sodium Intravenous 2467

Chlorpheniramine Maleate (Amphetamines may counteract the sedative effect of antihistamines). Products include:
Advil Allergy Sinus Caplets .... ■ 770
Advil Multi-Symptom Cold Caplets .... ■ 770
BC Allergy Sinus Cold Powder .... ■ 677
Comtrex Maximum Strength Cold & Cough Day/Night Caplets - Night Formulation .... ■ 726
Comtrex Maximum Strength Day/Night Severe Cold & Sinus Caplets - Night Formulation .... ■ 725
Contac Cold and Flu Maximum Strength Caplets .... ■ 728
Contac Cold and Flu Day and Night Caplets (Night Formulation Only) .... ■ 727
Children's Dimetapp Long Acting Cough Plus Cold Syrup .... ■ 731
Robitussin Cough & Cold Long-Acting Liquid .... ■ 735
Robitussin Cough & Allergy Syrup .. ■ 736
Robitussin Cough & Cold Nighttime Liquid .... ■ 736
Robitussin Cough, Cold & Flu Nighttime Liquid .... ■ 738
Robitussin Pediatric Cough & Cold Long-Acting Liquid .... ■ 735
Robitussin Pediatric Cough & Cold Nighttime Liquid .... ■ 736
Triaminic Cold & Allergy Liquid .... ■ 746
Triaminic Cough & Runny Nose Softchews .... ■ 748
Children's Tylenol Plus Flu Oral Suspension .... ■ 749
Tylenol Allergy Multi-Symptom Caplets with Cool Burst and Gelcaps 1872
Children's Tylenol Plus Cold Suspension Liquid 1879
Children's Tylenol Plus Cough & Runny Nose Suspension Liquid 1879
Children's Tylenol Plus Flu Suspension Liquid 1881
Children's Tylenol Plus Multi-Symptom Cold Suspension Liquid 1879
Tylenol Cold Head Congestion Nighttime Caplets with Cool Burst 1873
Tylenol Cold Multi-Symptom Nighttime Caplets with Cool Burst 1874
Tylenol Sinus Congestion & Pain Nighttime Caplets with Cool Burst 1876
Vicks 44M Cough, Cold & Flu Relief Liquid 2680
Pediatric Vicks 44m Cough & Cold Relief Liquid 2676
Children's Vicks NyQuil Cold/Cough Relief .... ■ 756
Children's Vicks NyQuil Cold/Cough Relief Liquid 2680
Zicam Maximum Strength Flu Daytime .... ■ 768

Chlorpheniramine Polistirex (Amphetamines may counteract the sedative effect of antihistamines). Products include:
Tussionex Pennkinetic Extended-Release Suspension 3327

Chlorpheniramine Tannate (Amphetamines may counteract the sedative effect of antihistamines).
No products indexed under this heading.

Chlorpromazine (Blocks the dopamine and norepinephrine receptors, thus inhibiting the central stimulant effects of amphetamines).
No products indexed under this heading.

Chlorpromazine Hydrochloride (Blocks the dopamine and norepinephrine receptors, thus inhibiting the central stimulant effects of amphetamines).
No products indexed under this heading.

Chlorthalidone (Amphetamines may antagonize the hypotensive effects of antihypertensives). Products include:
Clorpres Tablets 2153

Clemastine Fumarate (Amphetamines may counteract the sedative effect of antihistamines).
No products indexed under this heading.

Clomipramine Hydrochloride (Enhanced activity of tricyclic antidepressants or sympathomimetics; possible increases in d-amphetamine resulting in potentiation of cardiovascular effects).
No products indexed under this heading.

Clonidine (Amphetamines may antagonize the hypotensive effects of antihypertensives). Products include:
Catapres-TTS 844

Clonidine Hydrochloride (Amphetamines may antagonize the hypotensive effects of antihypertensives). Products include:
Catapres Tablets 843
Clorpres Tablets 2153

Cryptenamine Preparations (Amphetamines inhibit the hypotensive effect of veratrum alkaloids).
No products indexed under this heading.

Cyproheptadine Hydrochloride (Amphetamines may counteract the sedative effect of antihistamines).
No products indexed under this heading.

Deserpidine (Amphetamines may antagonize the hypotensive effects of antihypertensives).
No products indexed under this heading.

Desipramine Hydrochloride (Enhanced activity of tricyclic antidepressants or sympathomimetics; possible increases in d-amphetamine resulting in potentiation of cardiovascular effects).
No products indexed under this heading.

Dexchlorpheniramine Maleate (Amphetamines may counteract the sedative effect of antihistamines).
No products indexed under this heading.

Diazoxide (Amphetamines may antagonize the hypotensive effects of antihypertensives). Products include:
Hyperstat I.V. 3017

Diltiazem Hydrochloride (Amphetamines may antagonize the hypotensive effects of antihypertensives). Products include:
Cardizem LA Extended Release Tablets 1728
Tiazac Capsules 1201

Diphenhydramine Citrate (Amphetamines may counteract the sedative effect of antihistamines). Products include:
Advil PM Caplets .... ■ 615
Excedrin PM Caplets/Tablets/Geltabs .... ■ 610
Goody's PM Powder for Pain with Sleeplessness .... ■ 612

Diphenhydramine Hydrochloride (Amphetamines may counteract the sedative effect of antihistamines). Products include:
Nytol QuickCaps Caplets .... ■ 615
Nytol QuickGels Softgels Maximum Strength .... ■ 616
Simply Sleep Caplets 1868
Sominex Original Formula Tablets .. ■ 616
TheraFlu Warming Relief Nighttime Severe Cold .... ■ 743
TheraFlu Thin Strips Multi Symptom .... ■ 744
Triaminic Nighttime Cold & Cough Liquid .... ■ 746
Triaminic Thin Strips Cough & Runny Nose .... ■ 749
Extra Strength Tylenol PM Caplets, Vanilla Caplets, Geltabs, Gelcaps and Liquid 1875
Tylenol Sore Throat Nighttime Liquid with Cool Burst .... ■ 790
Tylenol Allergy Multi-Symptom Nighttime Caplets with Cool Burst 1872
Tylenol Severe Allergy Caplets 1872
Children's Tylenol Plus Cold & Allergy Suspension Liquid 1878

Diphenylpyraline Hydrochloride (Amphetamines may counteract the sedative effect of antihistamines).
No products indexed under this heading.

Doxazosin Mesylate (Amphetamines may antagonize the hypotensive effects of antihypertensives). Products include:
Cardura XL Tablets 2515

Doxepin Hydrochloride (Enhanced activity of tricyclic antidepressants or sympathomimetics; possible increases in d-amphetamine resulting in potentiation of cardiovascular effects).
No products indexed under this heading.

Enalapril Maleate (Amphetamines may antagonize the hypotensive effects of antihypertensives). Products include:
Vasotec I.V. Injection 2103

Enalaprilat (Amphetamines may antagonize the hypotensive effects of antihypertensives).
No products indexed under this heading.

Eprosartan Mesylate (Amphetamines may antagonize the hypotensive effects of antihypertensives). Products include:
Teveten Tablets 1735
Teveten HCT Tablets 1737

Esmolol Hydrochloride (Adrenergic blockers are inhibited by amphetamines; amphetamines may antagonize the hypotensive effects of antihypertensives).
No products indexed under this heading.

Ethosuximide (Amphetamines may delay intestinal absorption of ethosuximide).
No products indexed under this heading.

Felodipine (Amphetamines may antagonize the hypotensive effects of antihypertensives).
No products indexed under this heading.

Fexofenadine Hydrochloride (Amphetamines may counteract the sedative effect of antihistamines). Products include:
Allegra 2844
Allegra-D 12 Hour Extended-Release Tablets 2846
Allegra-D 24 Hour Extended-Release Tablets 2849

Fosinopril Sodium (Amphetamines may antagonize the hypotensive effects of antihypertensives).
No products indexed under this heading.

Fosphenytoin Sodium (Amphetamines may delay intestinal absorption of phenytoin; co-administration may produce a synergistic anticonvulsant action).
No products indexed under this heading.

Furazolidone (Concurrent use with metabolite of furazolidone may result in hypertensive crises; may slow the metabolism of amphetamines with resultant increase in their effect on release of norepinephrine and other monoamines from adrenergic nerve ending; this can cause headaches and other signs of hypertensice crises).
No products indexed under this heading.

Furosemide (Amphetamines may antagonize the hypotensive effects of antihypertensives). Products include:
Furosemide Tablets 2154

Glutamic Acid Hydrochloride (Co-administration with gastrointestinal acidifying agents, such as glutamic acid, lowers absorption of amphetamines resulting in reduced blood levels and efficacy of amphetamines).
No products indexed under this heading.

Guanabenz Acetate (Amphetamines may antagonize the hypotensive effects of antihypertensives).
No products indexed under this heading.

Guanethidine Monosulfate (Co-administration with gastrointestinal acidifying agents, such as guanethidine, lowers absorption of amphetamines resulting in reduced blood levels and efficacy of amphetamines; amphetamines may antagonize the hypotensive effects of antihypertensives).
No products indexed under this heading.

Haloperidol (Blocks the dopamine receptors, thus inhibiting the central stimulant effects of amphetamines).
No products indexed under this heading.

Haloperidol Decanoate (Blocks the dopamine receptors, thus inhibiting the central stimulant effects of amphetamines).
No products indexed under this heading.

Hydralazine Hydrochloride (Amphetamines may antagonize the hypotensive effects of antihypertensives). Products include:
BiDil Tablets 2171

Hydrochlorothiazide (Co-administration with urinary alkalinizing agents, such as certain thiazides, increase the concentration of the non-ionized species of the amphetamine molecule, thereby decreasing urinary excretion resulting in increased blood levels and potentiation ofactions of amphetamines; amphetamines may antagonize the hypotensive effects of antihypertensives). Products include:
Aldoril Tablets 1910
Atacand HCT 651
Avalide Tablets 888
Avalide Tablets 2874
Benicar HCT Tablets 1044
Diovan HCT Tablets 2196
Dyazide Capsules 1423
Hyzaar 50-12.5 Tablets 1990
Hyzaar 100-12.5 Tablets 1990
Hyzaar 100-25 Tablets 1990
Lopressor HCT 50/25 Tablets 2241
Lopressor HCT 100/25 Tablets 2241
Lopressor HCT 100/50 Tablets 2241
Lotensin HCT Tablets 2246
Micardis HCT Tablets 856
Moduretic Tablets 2028
Prinzide Tablets 2056
Teveten HCT Tablets 1737
Timolide Tablets 2086
Uniretic Tablets 3100

Hydroflumethiazide (Co-administration with urinary alkalinizing agents, such as certain thiazides, increase the concentration of the non-ionized species of the amphetamine molecule, thereby decreasing urinary excretion resulting in increased blood levels and potentiation ofactions of amphetamines; amphetamines may antagonize the hypotensive effects of antihypertensives).
No products indexed under this heading.

Imipramine Hydrochloride (Enhanced activity of tricyclic antidepressants or sympathomimetics; possible increases in d-amphetamine resulting in potentiation of cardiovascular effects).
No products indexed under this heading.

Imipramine Pamoate (Enhanced activity of tricyclic antidepressants or sympathomimetics; possible increases in d-amphetamine resulting in potentiation of cardiovascular effects).
No products indexed under this heading.

Indapamide (Amphetamines may antagonize the hypotensive effects of antihypertensives). Products include:
Indapamide Tablets 2156

Irbesartan (Amphetamines may antagonize the hypotensive effects of antihypertensives). Products include:
Avalide Tablets 888
Avalide Tablets 2874
Avapro Tablets 891
Avapro Tablets 2871

Isocarboxazid (Concurrent and/or sequential use may result in hypertensive crises; MAOI may slow the metabolism of amphetamines with resultant increase in their effect on release of norepinephrine and other monoamines from adrenergic nerve ending; this can cause headaches and other signs of hypertensive crises; concurrent and/or sequential use is contraindicated).
No products indexed under this heading.

Isradipine (Amphetamines may antagonize the hypotensive effects of antihypertensives). Products include:
DynaCirc CR Tablets 2721

Labetalol Hydrochloride (Adrenergic blockers are inhibited by amphetamines; amphetamines may antagonize the hypotensive effects of antihypertensives).
No products indexed under this heading.

Levobunolol Hydrochloride (Adrenergic blockers are inhibited by amphetamines; amphetamines may antagonize the hypotensive effects of antihypertensives). Products include:
Betagan Ophthalmic Solution, USP .... ⊙ 220

Lisinopril (Amphetamines may antagonize the hypotensive effects of antihypertensives). Products include:
Prinivil Tablets 2052
Prinzide Tablets 2056

Lithium Carbonate (Anorectic and stimulatory effects of amphetamines may be inhibited by lithium carbonate). Products include:
Lithobid Tablets 1692

Loratadine (Amphetamines may counteract the sedative effect of antihistamines). Products include:
Alavert Allergy & Sinus D-12 Hour Tablets 771
Alavert 771
Children's Claritin Allergy Oral Solution 771
Claritin Non-Drowsy 24 Hour Tablets 772
Claritin Reditabs 24 Hour Non-Drowsy Tablets 772
Claritin-D Non-Drowsy 12 Hour Tablets 772
Claritin-D Non-Drowsy 24 Hour Tablets 772

Losartan Potassium (Amphetamines may antagonize the hypotensive effects of antihypertensives). Products include:
Cozaar Tablets 1935
Hyzaar 50-12.5 Tablets 1990
Hyzaar 100-12.5 Tablets 1990
Hyzaar 100-25 Tablets 1990

Magaldrate (Co-administration with gastrointestinal alkalinizing agents, such as antacids, may increase the absorption of amphetamines; concurrent use should be avoided).
No products indexed under this heading.

Magnesium Hydroxide (Co-administration with gastrointestinal alkalinizing agents, such as antacids, may increase the absorption of amphetamines; concurrent use should be avoided). Products include:
Maalox Regular Strength Antacid/Antigas Liquid 2175
Maalox Max Maximum Strength Antacid/Anti-Gas Liquid 2176
Pepcid Complete Chewable Tablets 1701

Magnesium Oxide (Co-administration with gastrointestinal alkalinizing agents, such as antacids, may increase the absorption of amphetamines; concurrent use should be avoided). Products include:
Beelith Tablets 759
PremCal Light, Regular, and Extra Strength Tablets 818

Maprotiline Hydrochloride (Enhanced activity of tricyclic antidepressants or sympathomimetics; possible increases in d-amphetamine resulting in potentiation of cardiovascular effects).
No products indexed under this heading.

Mecamylamine Hydrochloride (Amphetamines may antagonize the hypotensive effects of antihypertensives).
No products indexed under this heading.

Meperidine Hydrochloride (Amphetamines potentiate the analgesic effect of meperidine).
No products indexed under this heading.

Methdilazine Hydrochloride (Amphetamines may counteract the sedative effect of antihistamines).
No products indexed under this heading.

Methenamine (Urinary excretion of amphetamines is increased, and efficacy is reduced by acidifying agents used in methenamine therapy). Products include:
Prosed/DS Tablets 1157

Methenamine Hippurate (Urinary excretion of amphetamines is increased, and efficacy is reduced by acidifying agents used in methenamine therapy).
No products indexed under this heading.

Methenamine Mandelate (Urinary excretion of amphetamines is increased, and efficacy is reduced by acidifying agents used in methenamine therapy). Products include:
Uroqid-Acid No. 2 Tablets 760

Methyclothiazide (Co-administration with urinary alkalinizing agents, such as certain thiazides, increase the concentration of the non-ionized species of the amphetamine molecule, thereby decreasing urinary excretion resulting in increased blood levels and potentiation ofactions of amphetamines; amphetamines may antagonize the hypotensive effects of antihypertensives).
No products indexed under this heading.

Methyldopa (Amphetamines may antagonize the hypotensive effects of antihypertensives). Products include:
Aldoril Tablets 1910

Methyldopate Hydrochloride (Amphetamines may antagonize the hypotensive effects of antihypertensives).
No products indexed under this heading.

Metipranolol Hydrochloride (Adrenergic blockers are inhibited by amphetamines; amphetamines may antagonize the hypotensive effects of antihypertensives).
No products indexed under this heading.

Metolazone (Amphetamines may antagonize the hypotensive effects of antihypertensives).
No products indexed under this heading.

Metoprolol Succinate (Adrenergic blockers are inhibited by amphetamines; amphetamines may antagonize the hypotensive effects of antihypertensives). Products include:
Toprol-XL Tablets 668

Metoprolol Tartrate (Adrenergic blockers are inhibited by amphetamines; amphetamines may antagonize the hypotensive effects of antihypertensives). Products include:
Lopressor Injection 2238
Lopressor Tablets 2238
Lopressor HCT 50/25 Tablets 2241
Lopressor HCT 100/25 Tablets 2241
Lopressor HCT 100/50 Tablets 2241

Metyrosine (Amphetamines may antagonize the hypotensive effects of antihypertensives). Products include:
Demser Capsules 1953

Mibefradil Dihydrochloride (Amphetamines may antagonize the hypotensive effects of antihypertensives).
No products indexed under this heading.

Minoxidil (Amphetamines may antagonize the hypotensive effects of antihypertensives). Products include:
Men's Rogaine Extra Strength Hair Regrowth Treatment Topical Solution, Ocean Rush Scent and Original Unscented .... ▣633
Men's Rogaine Foam Hair Regrowth Treatment .... ▣633
Women's Rogaine Hair Regrowth Treatment Topical Solution, Spring Bloom Scent and Original Unscented .... ▣634

Moclobemide (Concurrent and/or sequential use may result in hypertensive crises; MAOI may slow the metabolism of amphetamines with resultant increase in their effect on release of norepinephrine and other monoamines from adrenergic nerve ending; this can cause headaches and other signs of hypertensive crises; concurrent and/or sequential use is contraindicated).
No products indexed under this heading.

Moexipril Hydrochloride (Amphetamines may antagonize the hypotensive effects of antihypertensives). Products include:
Uniretic Tablets 3100
Univasc Tablets 3104

Nadolol (Adrenergic blockers are inhibited by amphetamines; amphetamines may antagonize the hypotensive effects of antihypertensives). Products include:
Nadolol Tablets 2159

Nicardipine Hydrochloride (Amphetamines may antagonize the hypotensive effects of antihypertensives). Products include:
Cardene I.V. 2497

Nifedipine (Amphetamines may antagonize the hypotensive effects of antihypertensives). Products include:
Adalat CC Tablets 2964

Nisoldipine (Amphetamines may antagonize the hypotensive effects of antihypertensives). Products include:
Sular Tablets 3122

Nitroglycerin (Amphetamines may antagonize the hypotensive effects of antihypertensives). Products include:
Nitro-Dur Transdermal Infusion System 3046
Nitrolingual Pumpspray 3120

Norepinephrine Bitartrate (Amphetamines enhance the adrenergic effect of norepinephrine).
No products indexed under this heading.

Nortriptyline Hydrochloride (Enhanced activity of tricyclic antidepressants or sympathomimetics; possible increases in d-amphetamine resulting in potentiation of cardiovascular effects).
No products indexed under this heading.

Pargyline Hydrochloride (Concurrent and/or sequential use may result in hypertensive crises; MAOI may slow the metabolism of amphetamines with resultant increase in their effect on release of norepinephrine and other monoamines from adrenergic nerve ending; this can cause headaches and other signs of hypertensive crises; concurrent and/or sequential use is contraindicated).
No products indexed under this heading.

Penbutolol Sulfate (Adrenergic blockers are inhibited by amphetamines; amphetamines may antagonize the hypotensive effects of antihypertensives).
No products indexed under this heading.

Perindopril Erbumine (Amphetamines may antagonize the hypotensive effects of antihypertensives). Products include:
Aceon Tablets (2 mg, 4 mg, 8 mg) 3194

Phenelzine Sulfate (Concurrent and/or sequential use may result in hypertensive crises; MAOI may slow the metabolism of amphetamines with resultant increase in their effect on release of norepinephrine and other monoamines from adrenergic nerve ending; this can cause headaches and other signs of hypertensive crises; concurrent and/or sequential use is contraindicated).
No products indexed under this heading.

Phenobarbital (Amphetamines may delay intestinal absorption of phenobarbital; co-administration may produce a synergistic anticonvulsant action). Products include:
Donnatal Extentabs 2493

Phenoxybenzamine Hydrochloride (Amphetamines may antagonize the hypotensive effects of antihypertensives). Products include:
Dibenzyline Capsules 3399

Phentolamine Mesylate (Amphetamines may antagonize the hypotensive effects of antihypertensives).
No products indexed under this heading.

Phenytoin (Amphetamines may delay intestinal absorption of phenytoin; co-administration may produce a synergistic anticonvulsant action).
No products indexed under this heading.

Phenytoin Sodium (Amphetamines may delay intestinal absorption of phenytoin; co-administration may produce a synergistic anticonvulsant action). Products include:
Phenytek Capsules 2160

Pindolol (Adrenergic blockers are inhibited by amphetamines; amphetamines may antagonize the hypotensive effects of antihypertensives).
No products indexed under this heading.

Polythiazide (Co-administration with urinary alkalinizing agents, such as certain thiazides, increase the concentration of the non-ionized species of the amphetamine molecule, thereby decreasing urinary excretion resulting in increased blood levels and potentiation ofactions of amphetamines; amphetamines may antagonize the hypotensive effects of antihypertensives).
No products indexed under this heading.

Potassium Citrate (Co-administration with urinary acidifying agents increases the concentration of the ionized species of the amphetamine molecule, thereby increasing urinary excretion resulting in reduced blood levels and efficacy of amphetamines). Products include:
Urocit-K Tablets 2144

Prazosin Hydrochloride (Amphetamines may antagonize the hypotensive effects of antihypertensives).
No products indexed under this heading.

Procarbazine Hydrochloride (Concurrent and/or sequential use may result in hypertensive crises; MAOI may slow the metabolism of amphetamines with resultant increase in their effect on release of norepinephrine and other monoamines from adrenergic nerve ending; this can cause headaches and other signs of hypertensive crises; concurrent and/or sequential use is contraindicated). Products include:
Matulane Capsules 3191

Promethazine Hydrochloride (Amphetamines may counteract the sedative effect of antihistamines). Products include:
Phenergan Tablets and Suppositories 3440

Propoxyphene Hydrochloride (In cases of propoxyphene overdosage, amphetamine CNS stimulation is potentiated and fatal convulsions can occur).
No products indexed under this heading.

Propoxyphene Napsylate (In cases of propoxyphene overdosage, amphetamine CNS stimulation is potentiated and fatal convulsions can occur).
No products indexed under this heading.

Propranolol Hydrochloride (Adrenergic blockers are inhibited by amphetamines; amphetamines may antagonize the hypotensive effects of antihypertensives). Products include:
Inderal LA Long-Acting Capsules 3429
InnoPran XL Capsules 2723

Protriptyline Hydrochloride (Enhanced activity of tricyclic antidepressants or sympathomimetics; possible increases in d-amphetamine resulting in potentiation of cardiovascular effects).
No products indexed under this heading.

Pyrilamine Maleate (Amphetamines may counteract the sedative effect of antihistamines).
No products indexed under this heading.

Pyrilamine Tannate (Amphetamines may counteract the sedative effect of antihistamines).
No products indexed under this heading.

Quinapril Hydrochloride (Amphetamines may antagonize the hypotensive effects of antihypertensives).
No products indexed under this heading.

Ramipril (Amphetamines may antagonize the hypotensive effects of antihypertensives). Products include:
Altace Capsules 1702

Rauwolfia Serpentina (Amphetamines may antagonize the hypotensive effects of antihypertensives).
No products indexed under this heading.

Rescinnamine (Amphetamines may antagonize the hypotensive effects of antihypertensives).
No products indexed under this heading.

Reserpine (Co-administration with gastrointestinal acidifying agents, such as reserpine, lowers absorption of amphetamines resulting in reduced blood levels and efficacy of amphetamines; amphetamines may antagonize the hypotensive effects of antihypertensives).
No products indexed under this heading.

Selegiline Hydrochloride (Concurrent and/or sequential use may result in hypertensive crises; MAOI may slow the metabolism of amphetamines with resultant increase in their effect on release of norepinephrine and other monoamines from adrenergic nerve ending; this can cause headaches and other signs of hypertensive crises; concurrent and/or sequential use is contraindicated). Products include:
Eldepryl Capsules 3208
Zelapar Tablets 3372

Sodium Bicarbonate (Co-administration with gastrointestinal alkalinizing agents, such as systemic disodium bicarbonate, increases the absorption of amphetamines). Products include:
Colyte with Flavor Packs for Oral Solution 3088
HalfLytely and Bisacodyl Tablets Bowel Prep Kit with Flavors Packs 881
TriLyte with Flavor Packs for Oral Solution 3100

Sodium Citrate (Co-administration with urinary acidifying agents increases the concentration of the ionized species of the amphetamine molecule, thereby increasing urinary excretion resulting in reduced blood levels and efficacy of amphetamines).
No products indexed under this heading.

Sodium Nitroprusside (Amphetamines may antagonize the hypotensive effects of antihypertensives).
No products indexed under this heading.

Sotalol Hydrochloride (Adrenergic blockers are inhibited by amphetamines; amphetamines may antagonize the hypotensive effects of antihypertensives).
No products indexed under this heading.

Spirapril Hydrochloride (Amphetamines may antagonize the hypotensive effects of antihypertensives).
No products indexed under this heading.

Telmisartan (Amphetamines may antagonize the hypotensive effects of antihypertensives). Products include:
Micardis Tablets 854
Micardis HCT Tablets 856

Terazosin Hydrochloride (Amphetamines may antagonize the hypotensive effects of antihypertensives). Products include:
Hytrin Capsules 471

Terfenadine (Amphetamines may counteract the sedative effect of antihistamines).
No products indexed under this heading.

Timolol Hemihydrate (Adrenergic blockers are inhibited by amphetamines; amphetamines may antagonize the hypotensive effects of antihypertensives). Products include:
Betimol Ophthalmic Solution 3382
Betimol Ophthalmic Solution .... ⊙ 295

Timolol Maleate (Adrenergic blockers are inhibited by amphetamines; amphetamines may antagonize the hypotensive effects of antihypertensives). Products include:
Blocadren Tablets 1916
Cosopt Sterile Ophthalmic Solution 1931
Timolide Tablets 2086
Timoptic Sterile Ophthalmic Solution 2088
Timoptic in Ocudose 2091
Timoptic-XE Sterile Ophthalmic Gel Forming Solution 2092

Torsemide (Amphetamines may antagonize the hypotensive effects of antihypertensives). Products include:
Demadex Injection 2759
Demadex Tablets 2759

Trandolapril (Amphetamines may antagonize the hypotensive effects of antihypertensives). Products include:
Mavik Tablets 486
Tarka Tablets 524

Tranylcypromine Sulfate (Concurrent and/or sequential use may result in hypertensive crises; MAOI may slow the metabolism of amphetamines with resultant increase in their effect on release of norepinephrine and other monoamines from adrenergic nerve ending; this can cause headaches and other signs of hypertensive crises; concurrent and/or sequential use is contraindicated). Products include:
Parnate Tablets 1527

Trimeprazine Tartrate (Amphetamines may counteract the sedative effect of antihistamines).
No products indexed under this heading.

Trimethaphan Camsylate (Amphetamines may antagonize the hypotensive effects of antihypertensives).
No products indexed under this heading.

Trimipramine Maleate (Enhanced activity of tricyclic antidepressants or sympathomimetics; possible increases in d-amphetamine resulting in potentiation of cardiovascular effects).
No products indexed under this heading.

Tripelennamine Hydrochloride (Amphetamines may counteract the sedative effect of antihistamines).
No products indexed under this heading.

Triprolidine Hydrochloride (Amphetamines may counteract the sedative effect of antihistamines).
No products indexed under this heading.

Valsartan (Amphetamines may antagonize the hypotensive effects of antihypertensives). Products include:
Diovan Tablets 2193
Diovan HCT Tablets 2196

Verapamil Hydrochloride (Amphetamines may antagonize the hypotensive effects of antihypertensives). Products include:
Covera-HS Tablets 3139
Tarka Tablets 524
Verelan PM Extended-Release Capsules, Controlled-Onset 3106

Vitamin C (Co-administration with gastrointestinal acidifying agents, such as vitamin C, lowers absorption of amphetamines resulting in reduced blood levels and efficacy of amphetamines). Products include:
Bausch & Lomb Ocuvite Adult Eye Vitamin and Mineral Supplement Soft Gels .... ▣ 706
Bausch & Lomb Ocuvite Adult 50+ Eye Vitamin and Mineral Supplement Soft Gels .... ▣ 706
Ocuvite Adult Vitamin and Mineral Supplement .... ⊙ 253
Ocuvite Adult 50+ Vitamin and Mineral Supplement .... ⊙ 253
Peridin-C Vitamin C Supplement .... ▣ 818

Food Interactions

Food, unspecified (Concurrent use with food prolongs T_{max} by 2.5 hours, however, food does not affect the extent of absorption).

ADENOCARD INJECTION

(Adenosine) 617
May interact with cardiac glycosides, xanthines, and certain other agents. Compounds in these categories include:

Aminophylline (The effects of adenosine are antagonized by co-administration with methylxanthines, such as theophylline; larger doses of adenosine may be required or adenosine may not be effective).
No products indexed under this heading.

Caffeine (The effects of adenosine are antagonized by co-administration with methylxanthines, such as caffeine; larger doses of adenosine may be required or adenosine may not be effective). Products include:
BC Headache Powder .... ▣ 677
Arthritis Strength BC Powder .... ▣ 677
Excedrin Extra Strength Caplets/Tablets/Geltabs .... ▣ 684
Excedrin Migraine Caplets/Tablets/Geltabs .... ▣ 609
Excedrin Tension Headache Caplets/Tablets/Geltabs .... ▣ 611
Goody's Extra Strength Headache Powders .... ▣ 611
Goody's Extra Strength Pain Relief Tablets .... ▣ 685
Vivarin .... ▣ 602
Winrgy Dietary Supplement .... ▣ 823

Carbamazepine (Adenosine decreases the conduction through AV node, higher degrees of heart block may be produced in the presence of carbamazepine). Products include:
Carbatrol Capsules 3171
Equetro Extended-Release Capsules 3180
Tegretol/Tegretol-XR 2295

Deslanoside (The use of adenosine in patients receiving digitalis may be rarely associated with ventricular fibrillation).
No products indexed under this heading.

Digitalis Glycoside Preparations (The use of adenosine in patients receiving digitalis may be rarely associated with ventricular fibrillation).
No products indexed under this heading.

Digitoxin (The use of adenosine in patients receiving digitalis may be rarely associated with ventricular fibrillation).
No products indexed under this heading.

Digoxin (The use of adenosine in patients receiving digitalis may be rarely associated with ventricular fibrillation). Products include:
Lanoxicaps Capsules 1490
Lanoxin Injection 1494
Lanoxin Injection Pediatric 1497
Lanoxin Tablets 1500

Dipyridamole (Adenosine effects are potentiated by dipyridamole; smaller doses of adenosine may be effective with concurrent use). Products include:
Aggrenox Capsules 822
Persantine Tablets 868

Dyphylline (The effects of adenosine are antagonized by co-administration with methylxanthines, such as theophylline; larger doses of adenosine may be required or adenosine may not be effective).
No products indexed under this heading.

Theophylline (The effects of adenosine are antagonized by co-administration with methylxanthines, such as theophylline; larger doses of adenosine may be required or adenosine may not be effective).
No products indexed under this heading.

Theophylline Anhydrous (The effects of adenosine are antagonized by co-administration with methylxanthines, such as theophylline; larger doses of adenosine may be required or adenosine may not be effective). Products include:
Uniphyl Tablets 2710

Theophylline Calcium Salicylate (The effects of adenosine are antagonized by co-administration with methylxanthines, such as theophylline; larger doses of adenosine may be required or adenosine may not be effective).
No products indexed under this heading.

Theophylline Dihydroxypropyl (Glyceryl) (The effects of adenosine are antagonized by co-administration with methylxanthines, such as theophylline; larger doses of adenosine may be required or adenosine may not be effective).
No products indexed under this heading.

Theophylline Ethylenediamine (The effects of adenosine are antagonized by co-administration with methylxanthines, such as theophylline; larger doses of adenosine may be required or adenosine may not be effective).
No products indexed under this heading.

Theophylline Sodium Glycinate (The effects of adenosine are antagonized by co-administration with methylxanthines, such as theophylline; larger doses of adenosine may be required or adenosine may not be effective).
No products indexed under this heading.

Verapamil Hydrochloride (Digoxin and verapamil use may be rarely associated with ventricular fibrillation when combined with adenosine; potential for additive or synergistic depressant effects on the SA and AV nodes). Products include:
Covera-HS Tablets 3139
Tarka Tablets 524
Verelan PM Extended-Release Capsules, Controlled-Onset 3106

ADENOSCAN

(Adenosine) 619
May interact with adenosine receptor antagonists, beta blockers, calcium channel blockers, cardiac glycosides, and nucleoside transport inhibitors. Compounds in these categories include:

Acebutolol Hydrochloride (Potential for additive or synergistic depressant effects on the SA or AV nodes; adenosine should be used with caution in the presence of these agents; no adverse interactions have been reported when co-administered).
No products indexed under this heading.

Aminophylline (The vasoactive effects of adenosine are inhibited by adenosine receptor antagonists such as methylxanthines).
No products indexed under this heading.

Amlodipine Besylate (Potential for additive or synergistic depressant effects on the SA or AV nodes; adenosine should be used with caution in the presence of these agents; no adverse interactions have been reported when co-administered). Products include:
Caduet Tablets 2508
Lotrel Capsules 2249
Norvasc Tablets 2545

Atenolol (Potential for additive or synergistic depressant effects on the SA or AV nodes; adenosine should be used with caution in the presence of these agents; no adverse interactions have been reported when co-administered).
No products indexed under this heading.

Bepridil Hydrochloride (Potential for additive or synergistic depressant effects on the SA or AV nodes; adenosine should be used with caution in the presence of these agents; no adverse interactions have been reported when co-administered).
No products indexed under this heading.

Betaxolol Hydrochloride (Potential for additive or synergistic depressant effects on the SA or AV nodes; adenosine should be used with caution in the presence of these agents;

no adverse interactions have been reported when co-administered). Products include:
- Betoptic S Ophthalmic Suspension 558

Bisoprolol Fumarate (Potential for additive or synergistic depressant effects on the SA or AV nodes; adenosine should be used with caution in the presence of these agents; no adverse interactions have been reported when co-administered).
No products indexed under this heading.

Caffeine (The vasoactive effects of adenosine are inhibited by adenosine receptor antagonists such as methylxanthines). Products include:
- BC Headache Powder .... ▣677
- Arthritis Strength BC Powder .... ▣677
- Excedrin Extra Strength Caplets/Tablets/Geltabs .... ▣684
- Excedrin Migraine Caplets/Tablets/Geltabs .... ▣609
- Excedrin Tension Headache Caplets/Tablets/Geltabs .... ▣611
- Goody's Extra Strength Headache Powders .... ▣611
- Goody's Extra Strength Pain Relief Tablets .... ▣685
- Vivarin .... ▣602
- Winrgy Dietary Supplement .... ▣823

Carteolol Hydrochloride (Potential for additive or synergistic depressant effects on the SA or AV nodes; adenosine should be used with caution in the presence of these agents; no adverse interactions have been reported when co-administered). Products include:
- Carteolol Hydrochloride Ophthalmic Solution USP, 1% .... ⊙249

Deslanoside (Potential for additive or synergistic depressant effects on the SA or AV nodes; adenosine should be used with caution in the presence of these agents; no adverse interactions have been reported when co-administered).
No products indexed under this heading.

Digitalis Glycoside Preparations (Potential for additive or synergistic depressant effects on the SA or AV nodes; adenosine should be used with caution in the presence of these agents; no adverse interactions have been reported when co-administered).
No products indexed under this heading.

Digitoxin (Potential for additive or synergistic depressant effects on the SA or AV nodes; adenosine should be used with caution in the presence of these agents; no adverse interactions have been reported when co-administered).
No products indexed under this heading.

Digoxin (Potential for additive or synergistic depressant effects on the SA or AV nodes; adenosine should be used with caution in the presence of these agents; no adverse interactions have been reported when co-administered). Products include:
- Lanoxicaps Capsules 1490
- Lanoxin Injection 1494
- Lanoxin Injection Pediatric 1497
- Lanoxin Tablets 1500

Diltiazem Hydrochloride (Potential for additive or synergistic depressant effects on the SA or AV nodes; adenosine should be used with caution in the presence of these agents; no adverse interactions have been reported when co-administered). Products include:
- Cardizem LA Extended Release Tablets 1728
- Tiazac Capsules 1201

Dipyridamole (Vasoactive effects of adenosine are potentiated by nucleoside transport inhibitors). Products include:
- Aggrenox Capsules 822
- Persantine Tablets 868

Dyphylline (The vasoactive effects of adenosine are inhibited by adenosine receptor antagonists such as methylxanthines).
No products indexed under this heading.

Esmolol Hydrochloride (Potential for additive or synergistic depressant effects on the SA or AV nodes; adenosine should be used with caution in the presence of these agents; no adverse interactions have been reported when co-administered).
No products indexed under this heading.

Felodipine (Potential for additive or synergistic depressant effects on the SA or AV nodes; adenosine should be used with caution in the presence of these agents; no adverse interactions have been reported when co-administered).
No products indexed under this heading.

Isradipine (Potential for additive or synergistic depressant effects on the SA or AV nodes; adenosine should be used with caution in the presence of these agents; no adverse interactions have been reported when co-administered). Products include:
- DynaCirc CR Tablets 2721

Labetalol Hydrochloride (Potential for additive or synergistic depressant effects on the SA or AV nodes; adenosine should be used with caution in the presence of these agents; no adverse interactions have been reported when co-administered).
No products indexed under this heading.

Levobunolol Hydrochloride (Potential for additive or synergistic depressant effects on the SA or AV nodes; adenosine should be used with caution in the presence of these agents; no adverse interactions have been reported when co-administered). Products include:
- Betagan Ophthalmic Solution, USP .... ⊙220

Metipranolol Hydrochloride (Potential for additive or synergistic depressant effects on the SA or AV nodes; adenosine should be used with caution in the presence of these agents; no adverse interactions have been reported when co-administered).
No products indexed under this heading.

Metoprolol Succinate (Potential for additive or synergistic depressant effects on the SA or AV nodes; adenosine should be used with caution in the presence of these agents; no adverse interactions have been reported when co-administered). Products include:
- Toprol-XL Tablets 668

Metoprolol Tartrate (Potential for additive or synergistic depressant effects on the SA or AV nodes; adenosine should be used with caution in the presence of these agents; no adverse interactions have been reported when co-administered). Products include:
- Lopressor Injection 2238
- Lopressor Tablets 2238
- Lopressor HCT 50/25 Tablets 2241
- Lopressor HCT 100/25 Tablets 2241
- Lopressor HCT 100/50 Tablets 2241

Mibefradil Dihydrochloride (Potential for additive or synergistic depressant effects on the SA or AV nodes; adenosine should be used with caution in the presence of these agents; no adverse interactions have been reported when co-administered).
No products indexed under this heading.

Nadolol (Potential for additive or synergistic depressant effects on the SA or AV nodes; adenosine should be used with caution in the presence of these agents; no adverse interactions have been reported when co-administered). Products include:
- Nadolol Tablets 2159

Nicardipine Hydrochloride (Potential for additive or synergistic depressant effects on the SA or AV nodes; adenosine should be used with caution in the presence of these agents; no adverse interactions have been reported when co-administered). Products include:
- Cardene I.V. 2497

Nifedipine (Potential for additive or synergistic depressant effects on the SA or AV nodes; adenosine should be used with caution in the presence of these agents; no adverse interactions have been reported when co-administered). Products include:
- Adalat CC Tablets 2964

Nimodipine (Potential for additive or synergistic depressant effects on the SA or AV nodes; adenosine should be used with caution in the presence of these agents; no adverse interactions have been reported when co-administered). Products include:
- Nimotop Capsules 749

Nisoldipine (Potential for additive or synergistic depressant effects on the SA or AV nodes; adenosine should be used with caution in the presence of these agents; no adverse interactions have been reported when co-administered). Products include:
- Sular Tablets 3122

Penbutolol Sulfate (Potential for additive or synergistic depressant effects on the SA or AV nodes; adenosine should be used with caution in the presence of these agents; no adverse interactions have been reported when co-administered).
No products indexed under this heading.

Pindolol (Potential for additive or synergistic depressant effects on the SA or AV nodes; adenosine should be used with caution in the presence of these agents; no adverse interactions have been reported when co-administered).
No products indexed under this heading.

Propranolol Hydrochloride (Potential for additive or synergistic depressant effects on the SA or AV nodes; adenosine should be used with caution in the presence of these agents; no adverse interactions have been reported when co-administered). Products include:
- Inderal LA Long-Acting Capsules 3429
- InnoPran XL Capsules 2723

Sotalol Hydrochloride (Potential for additive or synergistic depressant effects on the SA or AV nodes; adenosine should be used with caution in the presence of these agents; no adverse interactions have been reported when co-administered).
No products indexed under this heading.

Theophylline (The vasoactive effects of adenosine are inhibited by adenosine receptor antagonists such as methylxanthines).
No products indexed under this heading.

Theophylline Calcium Salicylate (The vasoactive effects of adenosine are inhibited by adenosine receptor antagonists such as methylxanthines).
No products indexed under this heading.

Theophylline Sodium Glycinate (The vasoactive effects of adenosine are inhibited by adenosine receptor antagonists such as methylxanthines).
No products indexed under this heading.

Timolol Hemihydrate (Potential for additive or synergistic depressant effects on the SA or AV nodes; adenosine should be used with caution in the presence of these agents; no adverse interactions have been reported when co-administered). Products include:
- Betimol Ophthalmic Solution 3382
- Betimol Ophthalmic Solution .... ⊙295

Timolol Maleate (Potential for additive or synergistic depressant effects on the SA or AV nodes; adenosine should be used with caution in the presence of these agents; no adverse interactions have been reported when co-administered). Products include:
- Blocadren Tablets 1916
- Cosopt Sterile Ophthalmic Solution 1931
- Timolide Tablets 2086
- Timoptic Sterile Ophthalmic Solution 2088
- Timoptic in Ocudose 2091
- Timoptic-XE Sterile Ophthalmic Gel Forming Solution 2092

Verapamil Hydrochloride (Potential for additive or synergistic depressant effects on the SA or AV nodes; adenosine should be used with caution in the presence of these agents; no adverse interactions have been reported when co-administered). Products include:
- Covera-HS Tablets 3139
- Tarka Tablets 524
- Verelan PM Extended-Release Capsules, Controlled-Onset 3106

ADIPEX-P CAPSULES

(Phentermine Hydrochloride) 1215

See Adipex-P Tablets

ADIPEX-P TABLETS

(Phentermine Hydrochloride) 1215

May interact with insulin, monoamine oxidase inhibitors, selective serotonin reuptake inhibitors, and certain other agents. Compounds in these categories include:

Citalopram Hydrobromide (The safety and efficacy of combination therapy with phentermine and any other drug products for weight loss, including selective serotonin reuptake inhibitors, have not been established; co-administration of these products for weight loss is not recommended). Products include:

Celexa 1176

Dexfenfluramine Hydrochloride (Co-administration has resulted in primary pulmonary hypertension, a rare, frequently fatal disease of the lungs and serious regurgitant cardiac valvular disease).

No products indexed under this heading.

Escitalopram Oxalate (The safety and efficacy of combination therapy with phentermine and any other drug products for weight loss, including selective serotonin reuptake inhibitors, have not been established; co-administration of these products for weight loss is not recommended). Products include:

Lexapro Oral Solution 1190
Lexapro Tablets 1190

Fenfluramine Hydrochloride (Co-administration has resulted in primary pulmonary hypertension, a rare, frequently fatal disease of the lungs and serious regurgitant cardiac valvular disease).

No products indexed under this heading.

Fluoxetine Hydrochloride (The safety and efficacy of combination therapy with phentermine and any other drug products for weight loss, including selective serotonin reuptake inhibitors, have not been established; co-administration of these products for weight loss is not recommended). Products include:

Prozac Pulvules and Liquid 1801
Symbyax Capsules 1819

Fluvoxamine Maleate (The safety and efficacy of combination therapy with phentermine and any other drug products for weight loss, including selective serotonin reuptake inhibitors, have not been established; co-administration of these products for weight loss is not recommended).

No products indexed under this heading.

Guanethidine Monosulfate (Decreased hypotensive effect of guanethidine).

No products indexed under this heading.

Insulin, Human, Zinc Suspension (Insulin requirement may be altered). Products include:

Humulin L, 100 Units 1794
Humulin U, 100 Units 1800

Insulin, Human NPH (Insulin requirement may be altered). Products include:

Humulin N, 100 Units 1795
Humulin N Pen 1797

Insulin, Human Regular (Insulin requirement may be altered). Products include:

Humulin R, 100 Units 1798

Insulin, Human Regular and Human NPH Mixture (Insulin requirement may be altered). Products include:

Humulin 50/50, 100 Units 1791
Humulin 70/30 Pen 1793

Insulin, NPH (Insulin requirement may be altered).

No products indexed under this heading.

Insulin, Regular (Insulin requirement may be altered).

No products indexed under this heading.

Insulin, Zinc Crystals (Insulin requirement may be altered).

No products indexed under this heading.

Insulin, Zinc Suspension (Insulin requirement may be altered).

No products indexed under this heading.

Insulin Aspart, Human Regular (Insulin requirement may be altered). Products include:

NovoLog Injection 2326

Insulin glargine (Insulin requirement may be altered). Products include:

Lantus Injection 2909

Insulin Lispro, Human (Insulin requirement may be altered). Products include:

Humalog-Pen 1781
Humalog Mix 50/50-Pen 1783
Humalog Mix 75/25-Pen 1785

Insulin Lispro Protamine, Human (Insulin requirement may be altered). Products include:

Humalog Mix 50/50-Pen 1783
Humalog Mix 75/25-Pen 1785

Isocarboxazid (Concurrent and/or sequential administration with MAO inhibitors may result in hypertensive crises; co-administration is contraindicated).

No products indexed under this heading.

Moclobemide (Concurrent and/or sequential administration with MAO inhibitors may result in hypertensive crises; co-administration is contraindicated).

No products indexed under this heading.

Pargyline Hydrochloride (Concurrent and/or sequential administration with MAO inhibitors may result in hypertensive crises; co-administration is contraindicated).

No products indexed under this heading.

Paroxetine Hydrochloride (The safety and efficacy of combination therapy with phentermine and any other drug products for weight loss, including selective serotonin reuptake inhibitors, have not been established; co-administration of these products for weight loss is not recommended). Products include:

Paxil CR Controlled-Release Tablets 1538
Paxil 1530

Phenelzine Sulfate (Concurrent and/or sequential administration with MAO inhibitors may result in hypertensive crises; co-administration is contraindicated).

No products indexed under this heading.

Procarbazine Hydrochloride (Concurrent and/or sequential administration with MAO inhibitors may result in hypertensive crises; co-administration is contraindicated). Products include:

Matulane Capsules 3191

Selegiline Hydrochloride (Concurrent and/or sequential administration with MAO inhibitors may result in hypertensive crises; co-administration is contraindicated). Products include:

Eldepryl Capsules 3208
Zelapar Tablets 3372

Sertraline Hydrochloride (The safety and efficacy of combination therapy with phentermine and any other drug products for weight loss, including selective serotonin reuptake inhibitors, have not been established; co-administration of these products for weight loss is not recommended). Products include:

Zoloft 2586

Tranylcypromine Sulfate (Concurrent and/or sequential administration with MAO inhibitors may result in hypertensive crises; co-administration is contraindicated). Products include:

Parnate Tablets 1527

Food Interactions

Alcohol (May result in adverse drug interaction).

ADVAIR DISKUS 100/50

(Fluticasone Propionate, Salmeterol Xinafoate) 1308

May interact with beta blockers, monoamine oxidase inhibitors, potassium-depleting diuretics, tricyclic antidepressants, and certain other agents. Compounds in these categories include:

Acebutolol Hydrochloride (Co-administration with beta-blockers not only blocks the pulmonary effect of beta-agonists, such as salmeterol, but may produce severe bronchospasm in patients with asthma).

No products indexed under this heading.

Amitriptyline Hydrochloride (Concurrent and/or sequential administration with tricyclic antidepressants may potentiate the action of salmeterol on the vascular system).

No products indexed under this heading.

Amoxapine (Concurrent and/or sequential administration with tricyclic antidepressants may potentiate the action of salmeterol on the vascular system).

No products indexed under this heading.

Atenolol (Co-administration with beta-blockers not only blocks the pulmonary effect of beta-agonists, such as salmeterol, but may produce severe bronchospasm in patients with asthma).

No products indexed under this heading.

Bendroflumethiazide (The ECG changes and/or hypokalemia that may result from the administration of non-potassium sparing diuretics can be acutely worsened by beta-agonists, especially when the recommended dose of beta-agonist is exceeded).

No products indexed under this heading.

Betaxolol Hydrochloride (Co-administration with beta-blockers not only blocks the pulmonary effect of beta-agonists, such as salmeterol, but may produce severe bronchospasm in patients with asthma). Products include:

Betoptic S Ophthalmic Suspension 558

Bisoprolol Fumarate (Co-administration with beta-blockers not only blocks the pulmonary effect of beta-agonists, such as salmeterol, but may produce severe bronchospasm in patients with asthma).

No products indexed under this heading.

Bumetanide (The ECG changes and/or hypokalemia that may result from the administration of non-potassium sparing diuretics can be acutely worsened by beta-agonists, especially when the recommended dose of beta-agonist is exceeded). Products include:

Bumex Tablets 2746

Carteolol Hydrochloride (Co-administration with beta-blockers not only blocks the pulmonary effect of beta-agonists, such as salmeterol, but may produce severe bronchospasm in patients with asthma). Products include:

Carteolol Hydrochloride Ophthalmic Solution USP, 1% .... ⊙ 249

Chlorothiazide (The ECG changes and/or hypokalemia that may result from the administration of non-potassium sparing diuretics can be acutely worsened by beta-agonists, especially when the recommended dose of beta-agonist is exceeded). Products include:

Diuril Oral Suspension 1954

Chlorothiazide Sodium (The ECG changes and/or hypokalemia that may result from the administration of non-potassium sparing diuretics can be acutely worsened by beta-agonists, especially when the recommended dose of beta-agonist is exceeded). Products include:

Diuril Sodium Intravenous 2467

Clomipramine Hydrochloride (Concurrent and/or sequential administration with tricyclic antidepressants may potentiate the action of salmeterol on the vascular system).

No products indexed under this heading.

Desipramine Hydrochloride (Concurrent and/or sequential administration with tricyclic antidepressants may potentiate the action of salmeterol on the vascular system).

No products indexed under this heading.

Doxepin Hydrochloride (Concurrent and/or sequential administration with tricyclic antidepressants may potentiate the action of salmeterol on the vascular system).

No products indexed under this heading.

Esmolol Hydrochloride (Co-administration with beta-blockers not only blocks the pulmonary effect of beta-agonists, such as salmeterol, but may produce severe bronchospasm in patients with asthma).

No products indexed under this heading.

Ethacrynic Acid (The ECG changes and/or hypokalemia that may result from the administration of non-potassium sparing diuretics can be acutely worsened by beta-agonists, especially when the recommended dose of beta-agonist is exceeded). Products include:

Edecrin Tablets 1959

Furosemide (The ECG changes and/or hypokalemia that may result from the administration of non-potassium sparing diuretics can be acutely worsened by beta-agonists, especially when the recommended dose of beta-agonist is exceeded). Products include:

Furosemide Tablets 2154

Hydrochlorothiazide (The ECG changes and/or hypokalemia that may result from the administration of non-potassium sparing diuretics can be acutely worsened by beta-agonists, especially when the recommended dose of beta-agonist is exceeded). Products include:

Hydroflumethiazide (The ECG changes and/or hypokalemia that may result from the administration of non-potassium sparing diuretics can be acutely worsened by beta-agonists, especially when the recommended dose of beta-agonist is exceeded).

No products indexed under this heading.

Imipramine Hydrochloride (Concurrent and/or sequential administration with tricyclic antidepressants may potentiate the action of salmeterol on the vascular system).

No products indexed under this heading.

Imipramine Pamoate (Concurrent and/or sequential administration with tricyclic antidepressants may potentiate the action of salmeterol on the vascular system).

No products indexed under this heading.

Isocarboxazid (Concurrent and/or sequential administration with MAO inhibitors may potentiate the action of salmeterol on the vascular system).

No products indexed under this heading.

Ketoconazole (Co-administration of a single dose of fluticasone with multiple doses of ketoconazole, a potent CYP3A4 inhibitor, to steady state has resulted in increased fluticasone exposure, a reduction in plasma cortisol AUC and no effect on urinary excretion of cortisol). Products include:

Labetalol Hydrochloride (Co-administration with beta-blockers not only blocks the pulmonary effect of beta-agonists, such as salmeterol, but may produce severe bronchospasm in patients with asthma).

No products indexed under this heading.

Levobunolol Hydrochloride (Co-administration with beta-blockers not only blocks the pulmonary effect of beta-agonists, such as salmeterol, but may produce severe bronchospasm in patients with asthma). Products include:

Maprotiline Hydrochloride (Concurrent and/or sequential administration may potentiate the action of salmeterol on the vascular system).

No products indexed under this heading.

Methyclothiazide (The ECG changes and/or hypokalemia that may result from the administration of non-potassium sparing diuretics can be acutely worsened by beta-agonists, especially when the recommended dose of beta-agonist is exceeded).

No products indexed under this heading.

Metipranolol Hydrochloride (Co-administration with beta-blockers not only blocks the pulmonary effect of beta-agonists, such as salmeterol, but may produce severe bronchospasm in patients with asthma).

No products indexed under this heading.

Metoprolol Succinate (Co-administration with beta-blockers not only blocks the pulmonary effect of beta-agonists, such as salmeterol, but may produce severe bronchospasm in patients with asthma). Products include:

Metoprolol Tartrate (Co-administration with beta-blockers not only blocks the pulmonary effect of beta-agonists, such as salmeterol, but may produce severe bronchospasm in patients with asthma). Products include:

Moclobemide (Concurrent and/or sequential administration with MAO inhibitors may potentiate the action of salmeterol on the vascular system).

No products indexed under this heading.

Nadolol (Co-administration with beta-blockers not only blocks the pulmonary effect of beta-agonists, such as salmeterol, but may produce severe bronchospasm in patients with asthma). Products include:

Nortriptyline Hydrochloride (Concurrent and/or sequential administration with tricyclic antidepressants may potentiate the action of salmeterol on the vascular system).

No products indexed under this heading.

Pargyline Hydrochloride (Concurrent and/or sequential administration with MAO inhibitors may potentiate the action of salmeterol on the vascular system).

No products indexed under this heading.

Penbutolol Sulfate (Co-administration with beta-blockers not only blocks the pulmonary effect of beta-agonists, such as salmeterol, but may produce severe bronchospasm in patients with asthma).

No products indexed under this heading.

Phenelzine Sulfate (Concurrent and/or sequential administration with MAO inhibitors may potentiate the action of salmeterol on the vascular system).

No products indexed under this heading.

Pindolol (Co-administration with beta-blockers not only blocks the pulmonary effect of beta-agonists, such as salmeterol, but may produce severe bronchospasm in patients with asthma).

No products indexed under this heading.

Polythiazide (The ECG changes and/or hypokalemia that may result from the administration of non-potassium sparing diuretics can be acutely worsened by beta-agonists, especially when the recommended dose of beta-agonist is exceeded).

No products indexed under this heading.

Procarbazine Hydrochloride (Concurrent and/or sequential administration with MAO inhibitors may potentiate the action of salmeterol on the vascular system). Products include:

Propranolol Hydrochloride (Co-administration with beta-blockers not only blocks the pulmonary effect of beta-agonists, such as salmeterol, but may produce severe bronchospasm in patients with asthma). Products include:

Protriptyline Hydrochloride (Concurrent and/or sequential administration with tricyclic antidepressants may potentiate the action of salmeterol on the vascular system).

No products indexed under this heading.

Ritonavir (Ritonavir, a potent CYP3A4 inhibitor, can significantly increase plasma fluticasone exposure, resulting in reduced serum cortisol concentrations. Cushing syndrome and adrenal suppression have been reported; therefore, co-administration is not recommended unless the potential benefit outweighs the risks). Products include:

Selegiline Hydrochloride (Concurrent and/or sequential administration with MAO inhibitors may potentiate the action of salmeterol on the vascular system). Products include:

Sotalol Hydrochloride (Co-administration with beta-blockers not only blocks the pulmonary effect of beta-agonists, such as salmeterol, but may produce severe bronchospasm in patients with asthma).

No products indexed under this heading.

Timolol Hemihydrate (Co-administration with beta-blockers not only blocks the pulmonary effect of beta-agonists, such as salmeterol, but may produce severe bronchospasm in patients with asthma). Products include:

Timolol Maleate (Co-administration with beta-blockers not only blocks the pulmonary effect of beta-agonists, such as salmeterol, but

may produce severe bronchospasm in patients with asthma). Products include:

Torsemide (The ECG changes and/or hypokalemia that may result from the administration of non-potassium sparing diuretics can be acutely worsened by beta-agonists, especially when the recommended dose of beta-agonist is exceeded). Products include:

Tranylcypromine Sulfate (Concurrent and/or sequential administration with MAO inhibitors may potentiate the action of salmeterol on the vascular system). Products include:

Trimipramine Maleate (Concurrent and/or sequential administration with tricyclic antidepressants may potentiate the action of salmeterol on the vascular system).

No products indexed under this heading.

ADVAIR DISKUS 250/50
(Fluticasone Propionate,
Salmeterol Xinafoate) 1308
See Advair Diskus 100/50

ADVAIR DISKUS 500/50
(Fluticasone Propionate,
Salmeterol Xinafoate) 1308
See Advair Diskus 100/50

ADVAIR HFA INHALATION AEROSOL
(Fluticasone Propionate,
Salmeterol Xinafoate) 1318
See Advair Diskus 100/50

ADVATE INJECTION
(Antihemophilic Factor
(Recombinant)) 712
None cited in PDR database.

ADVICOR TABLETS
(Lovastatin, Niacin) 1722
May interact with azole antifungals, beta blockers, calcium channel blockers, oral anticoagulants, erythromycin, fibrates, nitrates and nitrites, protease inhibitors, and certain other agents. Compounds in these categories include:

Acebutolol Hydrochloride (Co-administration of niacin with vasoactive drugs, such as adrenergic blocking agents, may result in postural hypotension, particularly in patients with unstable angina or acute phase of myocardial infarction).

No products indexed under this heading.

Amlodipine Besylate (Co-administration of niacin with vasoactive drugs, such as calcium channel blockers, may result in postural hypotension, particularly in patients with unstable angina or acute phase of myocardial infarction). Products include:

Amprenavir (Co-administration results in serious skeletal muscle disorders, such as rhabdomyolysis and myopathy). Products include:

Agenerase Capsules ... 1327
Agenerase Oral Solution ... 1332

Amyl Nitrite (Co-administration of niacin with vasoactive drugs, such as nitrates, may result in postural hypotension, particularly in patients with unstable angina or acute phase of myocardial infarction).

No products indexed under this heading.

Anisindione (Co-administration has resulted in increased bleeding and/or prothrombin time). Products include:

Miradon Tablets ... 3042

Aspirin (May decrease the metabolic clearance of niacin; the clinical relevance of this finding is unclear). Products include:

Aggrenox Capsules ... 822
Bayer Aspirin ... 744
BC Allergy Sinus Cold Powder ... 677
BC Headache Powder ... 677
Arthritis Strength BC Powder ... 677
BC Sinus Cold Powder ... 677
Excedrin Extra Strength Caplets/Tablets/Geltabs ... 684
Excedrin Migraine Caplets/Tablets/Geltabs ... 609
Goody's Body Pain Formula Powder ... 684
Goody's Extra Strength Headache Powders ... 611
Goody's Extra Strength Pain Relief Tablets ... 685
Percodan Tablets ... 1132
St. Joseph 81 mg Aspirin Chewable and Enteric Coated Tablets ... 1869

Atenolol (Co-administration of niacin with vasoactive drugs, such as adrenergic blocking agents, may result in postural hypotension, particularly in patients with unstable angina or acute phase of myocardial infarction).

No products indexed under this heading.

Bepridil Hydrochloride (Co-administration of niacin with vasoactive drugs, such as calcium channel blockers, may result in postural hypotension, particularly in patients with unstable angina or acute phase of myocardial infarction).

No products indexed under this heading.

Betaxolol Hydrochloride (Co-administration of niacin with vasoactive drugs, such as adrenergic blocking agents, may result in postural hypotension, particularly in patients with unstable angina or acute phase of myocardial infarction). Products include:

Betoptic S Ophthalmic Suspension ... 558

Bisoprolol Fumarate (Co-administration of niacin with vasoactive drugs, such as adrenergic blocking agents, may result in postural hypotension, particularly in patients with unstable angina or acute phase of myocardial infarction).

No products indexed under this heading.

Carteolol Hydrochloride (Co-administration of niacin with vasoactive drugs, such as adrenergic blocking agents, may result in postural hypotension, particularly in patients with unstable angina or acute phase of myocardial infarction). Products include:

Carteolol Hydrochloride Ophthalmic Solution USP, 1% ... ⊙249

Cholestyramine (In-vitro study resulted in approximately 10% to 30% of available niacin bound to cholestyramine; 4 to 6 hours should elapse between ingestion of bile acid-binding resins and the administration of Advicor).

No products indexed under this heading.

Clarithromycin (Co-administration results in serious skeletal muscle disorders, such as rhabdomyolysis and myopathy). Products include:

Biaxin/Biaxin XL ... 402
PREVPAC ... 3284

Clofibrate (The incidence and severity of myopathy are increased by co-administration of Advicor with drugs that cause myopathy when given alone, such as fibrates; combined use should be avoided).

No products indexed under this heading.

Clotrimazole (Co-administration results in serious skeletal muscle disorders, such as rhabdomyolysis and myopathy). Products include:

Desenex Athlete's Foot Cream ... 635
Lotrimin ... 3039
Lotrisone ... 3040

Colestipol Hydrochloride (In-vitro study resulted in approximately 90% of available niacin bound to colestipol; 4 to 6 hours should elapse between ingestion of bile acid-binding resins and the administration of Advicor).

No products indexed under this heading.

Cyclosporine (Co-administration results in serious skeletal muscle disorders, such as rhabdomyolysis and myopathy). Products include:

Gengraf Capsules ... 459
Neoral Oral Solution ... 2259
Neoral Soft Gelatin Capsules ... 2259
Restasis Ophthalmic Emulsion ... 575
Sandimmune ... 2275

Danazol (Co-administration results in serious skeletal muscle disorders, such as rhabdomyolysis and myopathy).

No products indexed under this heading.

Dicumarol (Co-administration has resulted in increased bleeding and/or prothrombin time).

No products indexed under this heading.

Diltiazem Hydrochloride (Co-administration of niacin with vasoactive drugs, such as calcium channel blockers, may result in postural hypotension, particularly in patients with unstable angina or acute phase of myocardial infarction). Products include:

Cardizem LA Extended Release Tablets ... 1728
Tiazac Capsules ... 1201

Erythrityl Tetranitrate (Co-administration of niacin with vasoactive drugs, such as nitrates, may result in postural hypotension, particularly in patients with unstable angina or acute phase of myocardial infarction).

No products indexed under this heading.

Erythromycin (Co-administration results in serious skeletal muscle disorders, such as rhabdomyolysis and myopathy). Products include:

Ery-Tab Tablets ... 449
Erythromycin Base Filmtab Tablets ... 455
Erythromycin Delayed-Release Capsules, USP ... 457
PCE Dispertab Tablets ... 515

Erythromycin Estolate (Co-administration results in serious skeletal muscle disorders, such as rhabdomyolysis and myopathy).

No products indexed under this heading.

Erythromycin Ethylsuccinate (Co-administration results in serious skeletal muscle disorders, such as rhabdomyolysis and myopathy). Products include:

E.E.S. ... 451
EryPed ... 447

Erythromycin Gluceptate (Co-administration results in serious skeletal muscle disorders, such as rhabdomyolysis and myopathy).

No products indexed under this heading.

Erythromycin Lactobionate (Co-administration results in serious skeletal muscle disorders, such as rhabdomyolysis and myopathy).

No products indexed under this heading.

Erythromycin Stearate (Co-administration results in serious skeletal muscle disorders, such as rhabdomyolysis and myopathy). Products include:

Erythrocin Stearate Filmtab Tablets ... 453

Esmolol Hydrochloride (Co-administration of niacin with vasoactive drugs, such as adrenergic blocking agents, may result in postural hypotension, particularly in patients with unstable angina or acute phase of myocardial infarction).

No products indexed under this heading.

Felodipine (Co-administration of niacin with vasoactive drugs, such as calcium channel blockers, may result in postural hypotension, particularly in patients with unstable angina or acute phase of myocardial infarction).

No products indexed under this heading.

Fenofibrate (The incidence and severity of myopathy are increased by co-administration of Advicor with drugs that cause myopathy when given alone, such as fibrates; combined use should be avoided). Products include:

Lofibra Tablets ... 1219
Lofibra Capsules ... 1216
Tricor Tablets ... 527
Triglide Tablets ... 3123

Fluconazole (Co-administration results in serious skeletal muscle disorders, such as rhabdomyolysis and myopathy).

No products indexed under this heading.

Gemfibrozil (The incidence and severity of myopathy are increased by co-administration of Advicor with drugs that cause myopathy when given alone, such as fibrates; combined use should be avoided).

No products indexed under this heading.

Indinavir Sulfate (Co-administration results in serious skeletal muscle disorders, such as rhabdomyolysis and myopathy). Products include:

Crixivan Capsules ... 1940

Isosorbide Dinitrate (Co-administration of niacin with vasoactive drugs, such as nitrates, may result in postural hypotension, particularly in patients with unstable angina or acute phase of myocardial infarction). Products include:

BiDil Tablets ... 2171

Isosorbide Mononitrate (Co-administration of niacin with vasoactive drugs, such as nitrates, may result in postural hypotension, particularly in patients with unstable angina or acute phase of myocardial infarction). Products include:

Imdur Tablets ... 3018

Isradipine (Co-administration of niacin with vasoactive drugs, such as calcium channel blockers, may result in postural hypotension, particularly in patients with unstable angina or acute phase of myocardial infarction). Products include:

DynaCirc CR Tablets ... 2721

Itraconazole (Co-administration results in serious skeletal muscle disorders, such as rhabdomyolysis and myopathy).

No products indexed under this heading.

Ketoconazole (Co-administration results in serious skeletal muscle disorders, such as rhabdomyolysis and myopathy). Products include:

Nizoral A-D Shampoo, 1% ... 1868

Labetalol Hydrochloride (Co-administration of niacin with vasoactive drugs, such as adrenergic blocking agents, may result in postural hypotension, particularly in patients with unstable angina or acute phase of myocardial infarction).

No products indexed under this heading.

Levobunolol Hydrochloride (Co-administration of niacin with vasoactive drugs, such as adrenergic blocking agents, may result in postural hypotension, particularly in patients with unstable angina or acute phase of myocardial infarction). Products include:

Betagan Ophthalmic Solution, USP ... ⊙220

Lopinavir (Co-administration results in serious skeletal muscle disorders, such as rhabdomyolysis and myopathy). Products include:

Kaletra ... 476

Metipranolol Hydrochloride (Co-administration of niacin with vasoactive drugs, such as adrenergic blocking agents, may result in postural hypotension, particularly in patients with unstable angina or acute phase of myocardial infarction).

No products indexed under this heading.

Metoprolol Succinate (Co-administration of niacin with vasoactive drugs, such as adrenergic blocking agents, may result in postural hypotension, particularly in patients with unstable angina or acute phase of myocardial infarction). Products include:

Toprol-XL Tablets ... 668

Metoprolol Tartrate (Co-administration of niacin with vasoactive drugs, such as adrenergic blocking agents, may result in postural hypotension, particularly in patients with unstable angina or acute phase of myocardial infarction). Products include:

Lopressor Injection ... 2238
Lopressor Tablets ... 2238

IMPORTANT NOTE: Always consult each drug listing in the patient's regimen for possible interactions.

Lopressor HCT 50/25 Tablets 2241
Lopressor HCT 100/25 Tablets 2241
Lopressor HCT 100/50 Tablets 2241

Mibefradil Dihydrochloride (Co-administration of niacin with vasoactive drugs, such as calcium channel blockers, may result in postural hypotension, particularly in patients with unstable angina or acute phase of myocardial infarction).
No products indexed under this heading.

Miconazole (Co-administration results in serious skeletal muscle disorders, such as rhabdomyolysis and myopathy).
No products indexed under this heading.

Nadolol (Co-administration of niacin with vasoactive drugs, such as adrenergic blocking agents, may result in postural hypotension, particularly in patients with unstable angina or acute phase of myocardial infarction). Products include:
Nadolol Tablets 2159

Nefazodone Hydrochloride (Co-administration results in serious skeletal muscle disorders, such as rhabdomyolysis and myopathy).
No products indexed under this heading.

Nelfinavir Mesylate (Co-administration results in serious skeletal muscle disorders, such as rhabdomyolysis and myopathy). Products include:
Viracept 2577

Nicardipine Hydrochloride (Co-administration of niacin with vasoactive drugs, such as calcium channel blockers, may result in postural hypotension, particularly in patients with unstable angina or acute phase of myocardial infarction). Products include:
Cardene I.V. 2497

Nicotinamide (May potentiate the adverse effects of Advicor). Products include:
Nicomide Tablets 1088

Nifedipine (Co-administration of niacin with vasoactive drugs, such as calcium channel blockers, may result in postural hypotension, particularly in patients with unstable angina or acute phase of myocardial infarction). Products include:
Adalat CC Tablets 2964

Nimodipine (Co-administration of niacin with vasoactive drugs, such as calcium channel blockers, may result in postural hypotension, particularly in patients with unstable angina or acute phase of myocardial infarction). Products include:
Nimotop Capsules 749

Nisoldipine (Co-administration of niacin with vasoactive drugs, such as calcium channel blockers, may result in postural hypotension, particularly in patients with unstable angina or acute phase of myocardial infarction). Products include:
Sular Tablets 3122

Nitroglycerin (Co-administration of niacin with vasoactive drugs, such as nitrates, may result in postural hypotension, particularly in patients with unstable angina or acute phase of myocardial infarction). Products include:
Nitro-Dur Transdermal Infusion System... 3046
Nitrolingual Pumpspray 3120

Oxiconazole Nitrate (Co-administration results in serious skeletal muscle disorders, such as rhabdomyolysis and myopathy). Products include:
Oxistat 2667

Penbutolol Sulfate (Co-administration of niacin with vasoactive drugs, such as adrenergic blocking agents, may result in postural hypotension, particularly in patients with unstable angina or acute phase of myocardial infarction).
No products indexed under this heading.

Pentaerythritol Tetranitrate (Co-administration of niacin with vasoactive drugs, such as nitrates, may result in postural hypotension, particularly in patients with unstable angina or acute phase of myocardial infarction).
No products indexed under this heading.

Pindolol (Co-administration of niacin with vasoactive drugs, such as adrenergic blocking agents, may result in postural hypotension, particularly in patients with unstable angina or acute phase of myocardial infarction).
No products indexed under this heading.

Propranolol Hydrochloride (Co-administration of niacin with vasoactive drugs, such as adrenergic blocking agents, may result in postural hypotension, particularly in patients with unstable angina or acute phase of myocardial infarction). Products include:
Inderal LA Long-Acting Capsules 3429
InnoPran XL Capsules 2723

Ritonavir (Co-administration results in serious skeletal muscle disorders, such as rhabdomyolysis and myopathy). Products include:
Kaletra 476
Norvir 503

Saquinavir (Co-administration results in serious skeletal muscle disorders, such as rhabdomyolysis and myopathy).
No products indexed under this heading.

Saquinavir Mesylate (Co-administration results in serious skeletal muscle disorders, such as rhabdomyolysis and myopathy). Products include:
Invirase 2772

Sotalol Hydrochloride (Co-administration of niacin with vasoactive drugs, such as adrenergic blocking agents, may result in postural hypotension, particularly in patients with unstable angina or acute phase of myocardial infarction).
No products indexed under this heading.

Telithromycin (Co-administration results in serious skeletal muscle disorders, such as rhabdomyolysis and myopathy). Products include:
Ketek Tablets 2903

Terconazole (Co-administration results in serious skeletal muscle disorders, such as rhabdomyolysis and myopathy).
No products indexed under this heading.

Timolol Hemihydrate (Co-administration of niacin with vasoactive drugs, such as adrenergic blocking agents, may result in postural hypotension, particularly in patients with unstable angina or acute phase of myocardial infarction). Products include:
Betimol Ophthalmic Solution 3382
Betimol Ophthalmic Solution .... ⊙295

Timolol Maleate (Co-administration of niacin with vasoactive drugs, such as adrenergic blocking agents, may result in postural hypotension, particularly in patients with unstable angina or acute phase of myocardial infarction). Products include:
Blocadren Tablets 1916
Cosopt Sterile Ophthalmic Solution.. 1931
Timolide Tablets 2086
Timoptic Sterile Ophthalmic Solution.. 2088
Timoptic in Ocudose 2091
Timoptic-XE Sterile Ophthalmic Gel Forming Solution 2092

Verapamil Hydrochloride (Co-administration of niacin with vasoactive drugs, such as calcium channel blockers, may result in postural hypotension, particularly in patients with unstable angina or acute phase of myocardial infarction). Products include:
Covera-HS Tablets 3139
Tarka Tablets 524
Verelan PM Extended-Release Capsules, Controlled-Onset........... 3106

Warfarin Sodium (Co-administration has resulted in increased bleeding and/or prothrombin time). Products include:
Coumadin for Injection 898
Coumadin Tablets 898

Food Interactions

Alcohol (Concomitant alcohol may increase the flushing and its use should be avoided around the time of Advicor administration).

Drinks, hot, unspecified (Concomitant hot drinks may increase the flushing and its use should be avoided around the time of Advicor administration).

Grapefruit Juice (Inhibits CYP3A4 and can increase the plasma concentration of lovastatin; concurrent use should be avoided).

ADVIL ALLERGY SINUS CAPLETS

(Chlorpheniramine Maleate, Ibuprofen, Pseudoephedrine Hydrochloride)................................ ▣770

May interact with anticoagulants, corticosteroids, parenterally administered corticosteroids, hypnotics and sedatives, monoamine oxidase inhibitors, non-steroidal anti-inflammatory agents, potassium-depleting corticosteroids, sex steroids, topical nonsteroidal anti-inflammatory agents, tranquilizers, and certain other agents. Compounds in these categories include:

Alprazolam (Concurrent use with sedatives or tranquilizers may increase drowsiness). Products include:
Niravam Orally Disintegrating Tablets... 3092

Anisindione (Concurrent use of anticoagulants may increase the risk of stomach bleeding). Products include:
Miradon Tablets 3042

Ardeparin Sodium (Concurrent use of anticoagulants may increase the risk of stomach bleeding).
No products indexed under this heading.

Betamethasone Acetate (Concurrent use of steroid drugs may increase the risk of stomach bleeding).
No products indexed under this heading.

Betamethasone Sodium Phosphate (Concurrent use of steroid drugs may increase the risk of stomach bleeding).
No products indexed under this heading.

Buspirone Hydrochloride (Concurrent use with sedatives or tranquilizers may increase drowsiness).
No products indexed under this heading.

Celecoxib (Concurrent use of other non-steroidal anti-inflammatory agents may increase the risk of stomach bleeding). Products include:
Celebrex Capsules 3134

Chlordiazepoxide (Concurrent use with sedatives or tranquilizers may increase drowsiness).
No products indexed under this heading.

Chlordiazepoxide Hydrochloride (Concurrent use with sedatives or tranquilizers may increase drowsiness). Products include:
Librium Capsules 3347

Chlorpromazine (Concurrent use with sedatives or tranquilizers may increase drowsiness).
No products indexed under this heading.

Chlorpromazine Hydrochloride (Concurrent use with sedatives or tranquilizers may increase drowsiness).
No products indexed under this heading.

Chlorprothixene (Concurrent use with sedatives or tranquilizers may increase drowsiness).
No products indexed under this heading.

Chlorprothixene Hydrochloride (Concurrent use with sedatives or tranquilizers may increase drowsiness).
No products indexed under this heading.

Clorazepate Dipotassium (Concurrent use with sedatives or tranquilizers may increase drowsiness). Products include:
Tranxene 2474

Cortisone Acetate (Concurrent use of steroid drugs may increase the risk of stomach bleeding).
No products indexed under this heading.

Dalteparin Sodium (Concurrent use of anticoagulants may increase the risk of stomach bleeding). Products include:
Fragmin Injection 1097

Danaparoid Sodium (Concurrent use of anticoagulants may increase the risk of stomach bleeding).
No products indexed under this heading.

Desogestrel (Concurrent use of steroid drugs may increase the risk of stomach bleeding). Products include:
Mircette Tablets 1066

Dexamethasone (Concurrent use of steroid drugs may increase the risk of stomach bleeding). Products include:
Ciprodex Otic Suspension 559
Decadron Tablets 1951
TobraDex Ophthalmic Ointment 562
TobraDex Ophthalmic Suspension ... 563

Dexamethasone Acetate (Concurrent use of steroid drugs may increase the risk of stomach bleeding).
No products indexed under this heading.

Dexamethasone Sodium Phosphate (Concurrent use of steroid drugs may increase the risk of stomach bleeding).
No products indexed under this heading.

Diazepam (Concurrent use with sedatives or tranquilizers may increase drowsiness). Products include:
Diastat Rectal Delivery System 3343
Valium Tablets 2819

Diclofenac Potassium (Concurrent use of other non-steroidal anti-inflammatory agents may increase the risk of stomach bleeding).
No products indexed under this heading.

Diclofenac Sodium (Concurrent use of other non-steroidal anti-inflammatory agents may increase the risk of stomach bleeding). Products include:
Arthrotec Tablets 3129
Voltaren Ophthalmic Solution 2309
Voltaren Tablets 2307
Voltaren-XR Tablets 2310

Dicumarol (Concurrent use of anticoagulants may increase the risk of stomach bleeding).
No products indexed under this heading.

Droperidol (Concurrent use with sedatives or tranquilizers may increase drowsiness).
No products indexed under this heading.

Enoxaparin Sodium (Concurrent use of anticoagulants may increase the risk of stomach bleeding). Products include:
Lovenox Injection 2915

Estazolam (Concurrent use with sedatives or tranquilizers may increase drowsiness). Products include:
ProSom Tablets 517

Estradiol (Concurrent use of steroid drugs may increase the risk of stomach bleeding). Products include:
Angeliq Tablets 762
Climara Transdermal System 771
Climara Pro Transdermal System 776
Estrasorb Topical Emulsion 1147
Estring Vaginal Ring 2635
Menostar Transdermal System 782
Vagifem Tablets 2334

Estrogens, Conjugated (Concurrent use of steroid drugs may increase the risk of stomach bleeding). Products include:
Premarin Intravenous 3442
Premarin Tablets 3446
Premarin Vaginal Cream 3452
Premphase Tablets 3456
Prempro Tablets 3456

Ethchlorvynol (Concurrent use with sedatives or tranquilizers may increase drowsiness).
No products indexed under this heading.

Ethinamate (Concurrent use with sedatives or tranquilizers may increase drowsiness).
No products indexed under this heading.

Ethinyl Estradiol (Concurrent use of steroid drugs may increase the risk of stomach bleeding). Products include:
Mircette Tablets 1066
NuvaRing 2340
Ortho-Cyclen/Ortho Tri-Cyclen 2429
Ortho Evra Transdermal System 2417
Ortho Tri-Cyclen Lo Tablets 2436
Seasonique Tablets 1077
Yasmin 28 Tablets 796
Yaz Tablets 803

Ethynodiol Diacetate (Concurrent use of steroid drugs may increase the risk of stomach bleeding).
No products indexed under this heading.

Etodolac (Concurrent use of other non-steroidal anti-inflammatory agents may increase the risk of stomach bleeding).
No products indexed under this heading.

Fenoprofen Calcium (Concurrent use of other non-steroidal anti-inflammatory agents may increase the risk of stomach bleeding). Products include:
Nalfon Capsules 2502

Fludrocortisone Acetate (Concurrent use of steroid drugs may increase the risk of stomach bleeding).
No products indexed under this heading.

Fluoxymesterone (Concurrent use of steroid drugs may increase the risk of stomach bleeding). Products include:
Androxy Tablets 3335

Fluphenazine Decanoate (Concurrent use with sedatives or tranquilizers may increase drowsiness).
No products indexed under this heading.

Fluphenazine Enanthate (Concurrent use with sedatives or tranquilizers may increase drowsiness).
No products indexed under this heading.

Fluphenazine Hydrochloride (Concurrent use with sedatives or tranquilizers may increase drowsiness).
No products indexed under this heading.

Flurazepam Hydrochloride (Concurrent use with sedatives or tranquilizers may increase drowsiness). Products include:
Dalmane Capsules 3342

Flurbiprofen (Concurrent use of other non-steroidal anti-inflammatory agents may increase the risk of stomach bleeding).
No products indexed under this heading.

Flurbiprofen Sodium (Concurrent use of other non-steroidal anti-inflammatory agents may increase the risk of stomach bleeding). Products include:
Ocufen Ophthalmic Solution .... ⊙232

Fondaparinux Sodium (Concurrent use of anticoagulants may increase the risk of stomach bleeding). Products include:
Arixtra Injection 1351

Glutethimide (Concurrent use with sedatives or tranquilizers may increase drowsiness).
No products indexed under this heading.

Haloperidol (Concurrent use with sedatives or tranquilizers may increase drowsiness).
No products indexed under this heading.

Haloperidol Decanoate (Concurrent use with sedatives or tranquilizers may increase drowsiness).
No products indexed under this heading.

Heparin Calcium (Concurrent use of anticoagulants may increase the risk of stomach bleeding).
No products indexed under this heading.

Heparin Sodium (Concurrent use of anticoagulants may increase the risk of stomach bleeding).
No products indexed under this heading.

Hydrocortisone (Concurrent use of steroid drugs may increase the risk of stomach bleeding). Products include:
Colocort Rectal Suspension, USP (Retention) 100 mg/60 mL 2476
Hydrocortone Tablets 1989
Preparation H Hydrocortisone Cream .... ▣646

Hydrocortisone Acetate (Concurrent use of steroid drugs may increase the risk of stomach bleeding). Products include:
Analpram-HC 1159
Pramosone 1161
ProctoFoam-HC 3099

Hydrocortisone Sodium Phosphate (Concurrent use of steroid drugs may increase the risk of stomach bleeding).
No products indexed under this heading.

Hydrocortisone Sodium Succinate (Concurrent use of steroid drugs may increase the risk of stomach bleeding).
No products indexed under this heading.

Hydroxyzine Hydrochloride (Concurrent use with sedatives or tranquilizers may increase drowsiness).
No products indexed under this heading.

Indomethacin (Concurrent use of other non-steroidal anti-inflammatory agents may increase the risk of stomach bleeding). Products include:
Indocin 1995

Indomethacin Sodium Trihydrate (Concurrent use of other non-steroidal anti-inflammatory agents may increase the risk of stomach bleeding). Products include:
Indocin I.V. 2465

Isocarboxazid (Do not use while taking, or for up to two weeks after stopping, MAO inhibitors).
No products indexed under this heading.

Ketoprofen (Concurrent use of other non-steroidal anti-inflammatory agents may increase the risk of stomach bleeding).
No products indexed under this heading.

Ketorolac Tromethamine (Concurrent use of other non-steroidal anti-inflammatory agents may increase the risk of stomach bleeding). Products include:
Acular Ophthalmic Solution 565
Acular LS Ophthalmic Solution 566

Levonorgestrel (Concurrent use of steroid drugs may increase the risk of stomach bleeding). Products include:
Climara Pro Transdermal System 776
Mirena Intrauterine System 787
Plan B Tablets 1076
Seasonique Tablets 1077

Lorazepam (Concurrent use with sedatives or tranquilizers may increase drowsiness).
No products indexed under this heading.

Low Molecular Weight Heparins (Concurrent use of anticoagulants may increase the risk of stomach bleeding).
No products indexed under this heading.

Loxapine Hydrochloride (Concurrent use with sedatives or tranquilizers may increase drowsiness).
No products indexed under this heading.

Loxapine Succinate (Concurrent use with sedatives or tranquilizers may increase drowsiness).
No products indexed under this heading.

Meclofenamate Sodium (Concurrent use of other non-steroidal anti-inflammatory agents may increase the risk of stomach bleeding).
No products indexed under this heading.

Mefenamic Acid (Concurrent use of other non-steroidal anti-inflammatory agents may increase the risk of stomach bleeding).
No products indexed under this heading.

Meloxicam (Concurrent use of other non-steroidal anti-inflammatory agents may increase the risk of stomach bleeding). Products include:
Mobic Oral Suspension 863
Mobic Tablets 863

Meprobamate (Concurrent use with sedatives or tranquilizers may increase drowsiness).
No products indexed under this heading.

Mesoridazine Besylate (Concurrent use with sedatives or tranquilizers may increase drowsiness).
No products indexed under this heading.

Mestranol (Concurrent use of steroid drugs may increase the risk of stomach bleeding).
No products indexed under this heading.

Methylprednisolone Acetate (Concurrent use of steroid drugs may increase the risk of stomach bleeding). Products include:
Depo-Medrol Injectable Suspension 2617
Depo-Medrol Single-Dose Vial 2619

Methylprednisolone Sodium Succinate (Concurrent use of steroid drugs may increase the risk of stomach bleeding).
No products indexed under this heading.

Methyltestosterone (Concurrent use of steroid drugs may increase the risk of stomach bleeding). Products include:
Estratest Tablets 3199
Estratest H.S. Tablets 3199

Midazolam Hydrochloride (Concurrent use with sedatives or tranquilizers may increase drowsiness).
No products indexed under this heading.

Moclobemide (Do not use while taking, or for up to two weeks after stopping, MAO inhibitors).
No products indexed under this heading.

Molindone Hydrochloride (Concurrent use with sedatives or tranquilizers may increase drowsiness). Products include:
- Moban Tablets 1119

Nabumetone (Concurrent use of other non-steroidal anti-inflammatory agents may increase the risk of stomach bleeding).
- No products indexed under this heading.

Naproxen (Concurrent use of other non-steroidal anti-inflammatory agents may increase the risk of stomach bleeding). Products include:
- EC-Naprosyn Delayed-Release Tablets 2761
- Naprosyn Suspension 2761
- Naprosyn Tablets 2761
- Prevacid NapraPAC 3280

Naproxen Sodium (Concurrent use of other non-steroidal anti-inflammatory agents may increase the risk of stomach bleeding). Products include:
- Aleve Caplets 742
- Aleve Gelcaps 743
- Aleve Tablets 743
- Aleve Cold & Sinus Caplets 744
- Anaprox Tablets 2761
- Anaprox DS Tablets 2761

Norethindrone (Concurrent use of steroid drugs may increase the risk of stomach bleeding). Products include:
- Ortho Micronor Tablets 2426

Norethindrone Acetate (Concurrent use of steroid drugs may increase the risk of stomach bleeding).
- No products indexed under this heading.

Norgestimate (Concurrent use of steroid drugs may increase the risk of stomach bleeding). Products include:
- Ortho-Cyclen/Ortho Tri-Cyclen 2429
- Ortho Tri-Cyclen Lo Tablets 2436

Oxaprozin (Concurrent use of other non-steroidal anti-inflammatory agents may increase the risk of stomach bleeding).
- No products indexed under this heading.

Oxazepam (Concurrent use with sedatives or tranquilizers may increase drowsiness).
- No products indexed under this heading.

Pargyline Hydrochloride (Do not use while taking, or for up to two weeks after stopping, MAO inhibitors).
- No products indexed under this heading.

Perphenazine (Concurrent use with sedatives or tranquilizers may increase drowsiness).
- No products indexed under this heading.

Phenelzine Sulfate (Do not use while taking, or for up to two weeks after stopping, MAO inhibitors).
- No products indexed under this heading.

Phenylbutazone (Concurrent use of other non-steroidal anti-inflammatory agents may increase the risk of stomach bleeding).
- No products indexed under this heading.

Piroxicam (Concurrent use of other non-steroidal anti-inflammatory agents may increase the risk of stomach bleeding).
- No products indexed under this heading.

Prazepam (Concurrent use with sedatives or tranquilizers may increase drowsiness).
- No products indexed under this heading.

Prednisolone Acetate (Concurrent use of steroid drugs may increase the risk of stomach bleeding). Products include:
- Blephamide Ophthalmic Ointment 568
- Blephamide Ophthalmic Suspension 569
- Poly-Pred Ophthalmic Suspension .... ⊙233
- Pred Forte Ophthalmic Suspension .... ⊙235
- Pred Mild Ophthalmic Suspension .... ⊙238
- Pred-G Ophthalmic Ointment .... ⊙237
- Pred-G Ophthalmic Suspension .... ⊙236

Prednisolone Sodium Phosphate (Concurrent use of steroid drugs may increase the risk of stomach bleeding).
- No products indexed under this heading.

Prednisolone Tebutate (Concurrent use of steroid drugs may increase the risk of stomach bleeding).
- No products indexed under this heading.

Prednisone (Concurrent use of steroid drugs may increase the risk of stomach bleeding).
- No products indexed under this heading.

Procarbazine Hydrochloride (Do not use while taking, or for up to two weeks after stopping, MAO inhibitors). Products include:
- Matulane Capsules 3191

Prochlorperazine (Concurrent use with sedatives or tranquilizers may increase drowsiness).
- No products indexed under this heading.

Promethazine Hydrochloride (Concurrent use with sedatives or tranquilizers may increase drowsiness). Products include:
- Phenergan Tablets and Suppositories 3440

Propofol (Concurrent use with sedatives or tranquilizers may increase drowsiness).
- No products indexed under this heading.

Quazepam (Concurrent use with sedatives or tranquilizers may increase drowsiness).
- No products indexed under this heading.

Ramelteon (Concurrent use with sedatives or tranquilizers may increase drowsiness). Products include:
- Rozerem Tablets 3231

Rofecoxib (Concurrent use of other non-steroidal anti-inflammatory agents may increase the risk of stomach bleeding).
- No products indexed under this heading.

Secobarbital Sodium (Concurrent use with sedatives or tranquilizers may increase drowsiness).
- No products indexed under this heading.

Selegiline Hydrochloride (Do not use while taking, or for up to two weeks after stopping, MAO inhibitors). Products include:
- Eldepryl Capsules 3208
- Zelapar Tablets 3372

Sulindac (Concurrent use of other non-steroidal anti-inflammatory agents may increase the risk of stomach bleeding). Products include:
- Clinoril Tablets 1924

Suprofen (Concurrent use of other non-steroidal anti-inflammatory agents may increase the risk of stomach bleeding).
- No products indexed under this heading.

Temazepam (Concurrent use with sedatives or tranquilizers may increase drowsiness). Products include:
- Restoril Capsules 1860

Testosterone (Concurrent use of steroid drugs may increase the risk of stomach bleeding). Products include:
- AndroGel 3329
- Striant Mucoadhesive 1007
- Testim 1% Gel 695

Thioridazine Hydrochloride (Concurrent use with sedatives or tranquilizers may increase drowsiness). Products include:
- Thioridazine Hydrochloride Tablets 2163

Thiothixene (Concurrent use with sedatives or tranquilizers may increase drowsiness). Products include:
- Thiothixene Capsules 2165

Tinzaparin Sodium (Concurrent use of anticoagulants may increase the risk of stomach bleeding).
- No products indexed under this heading.

Tolmetin Sodium (Concurrent use of other non-steroidal anti-inflammatory agents may increase the risk of stomach bleeding).
- No products indexed under this heading.

Tranylcypromine Sulfate (Do not use while taking, or for up to two weeks after stopping, MAO inhibitors). Products include:
- Parnate Tablets 1527

Triamcinolone (Concurrent use of steroid drugs may increase the risk of stomach bleeding).
- No products indexed under this heading.

Triamcinolone Acetonide (Concurrent use of steroid drugs may increase the risk of stomach bleeding). Products include:
- Azmacort Inhalation Aerosol 1726
- Nasacort AQ Nasal Spray 2922

Triamcinolone Diacetate (Concurrent use of steroid drugs may increase the risk of stomach bleeding).
- No products indexed under this heading.

Triamcinolone Hexacetonide (Concurrent use of steroid drugs may increase the risk of stomach bleeding).
- No products indexed under this heading.

Triazolam (Concurrent use with sedatives or tranquilizers may increase drowsiness).
- No products indexed under this heading.

Trifluoperazine Hydrochloride (Concurrent use with sedatives or tranquilizers may increase drowsiness).
- No products indexed under this heading.

Valdecoxib (Concurrent use of other non-steroidal anti-inflammatory agents may increase the risk of stomach bleeding).
- No products indexed under this heading.

Warfarin Sodium (Concurrent use of anticoagulants may increase the risk of stomach bleeding). Products include:
- Coumadin for Injection 898
- Coumadin Tablets 898

Zaleplon (Concurrent use with sedatives or tranquilizers may increase drowsiness). Products include:
- Sonata Capsules 1717

Zolpidem Tartrate (Concurrent use with sedatives or tranquilizers may increase drowsiness). Products include:
- Ambien Tablets 2851
- Ambien CR Tablets 2855

Food Interactions

Alcohol (Consuming 3 or more alcoholic beverages while using this product may increase the risk of stomach bleeding).

ADVIL CAPLETS

(Ibuprofen) .... ▣674

May interact with anticoagulants, corticosteroids, parenterally administered corticosteroids, non-steroidal anti-inflammatory agents, potassium-depleting corticosteroids, sex steroids, topical nonsteroidal anti-inflammatory agents, and certain other agents. Compounds in these categories include:

Anisindione (Concurrent use of anticoagulants may increase the risk of stomach bleeding). Products include:
- Miradon Tablets 3042

Ardeparin Sodium (Concurrent use of anticoagulants may increase the risk of stomach bleeding).
- No products indexed under this heading.

Betamethasone Acetate (Concurrent use of steroid drugs may increase the risk of stomach bleeding).
- No products indexed under this heading.

Betamethasone Sodium Phosphate (Concurrent use of steroid drugs may increase the risk of stomach bleeding).
- No products indexed under this heading.

Celecoxib (Concurrent use of other non-steroidal anti-inflammatory agents may increase the risk of stomach bleeding). Products include:
- Celebrex Capsules 3134

Cortisone Acetate (Concurrent use of steroid drugs may increase the risk of stomach bleeding).
- No products indexed under this heading.

Dalteparin Sodium (Concurrent use of anticoagulants may increase the risk of stomach bleeding). Products include:
- Fragmin Injection 1097

Danaparoid Sodium (Concurrent use of anticoagulants may increase the risk of stomach bleeding).
- No products indexed under this heading.

Desogestrel (Concurrent use of steroid drugs may increase the risk of stomach bleeding). Products include:

agents may increase the risk of stomach bleeding). Products include:
Clinoril Tablets 1924

Suprofen (Concurrent use of other non-steroidal anti-inflammatory agents may increase the risk of stomach bleeding).
No products indexed under this heading.

Testosterone (Concurrent use of steroid drugs may increase the risk of stomach bleeding). Products include:
AndroGel 3329
Striant Mucoadhesive 1007
Testim 1% Gel 695

Tinzaparin Sodium (Concurrent use of anticoagulants may increase the risk of stomach bleeding).
No products indexed under this heading.

Tolmetin Sodium (Concurrent use of other non-steroidal anti-inflammatory agents may increase the risk of stomach bleeding).
No products indexed under this heading.

Triamcinolone (Concurrent use of steroid drugs may increase the risk of stomach bleeding).
No products indexed under this heading.

Triamcinolone Acetonide (Concurrent use of steroid drugs may increase the risk of stomach bleeding). Products include:
Azmacort Inhalation Aerosol 1726
Nasacort AQ Nasal Spray 2922

Triamcinolone Diacetate (Concurrent use of steroid drugs may increase the risk of stomach bleeding).
No products indexed under this heading.

Triamcinolone Hexacetonide (Concurrent use of steroid drugs may increase the risk of stomach bleeding).
No products indexed under this heading.

Valdecoxib (Concurrent use of other non-steroidal anti-inflammatory agents may increase the risk of stomach bleeding).
No products indexed under this heading.

Warfarin Sodium (Concurrent use of anticoagulants may increase the risk of stomach bleeding). Products include:
Coumadin for Injection 898
Coumadin Tablets 898

Food Interactions

Alcohol (Consuming 3 or more alcoholic beverages while using this product may increase the risk of stomach bleeding).

CHILDREN'S ADVIL ORAL SUSPENSION

(Ibuprofen) .... ▣603

May interact with anticoagulants, corticosteroids, parenterally administered corticosteroids, non-steroidal anti-inflammatory agents, potassium-depleting corticosteroids, sex steroids, and topical nonsteroidal anti-inflammatory agents. Compounds in these categories include:

Anisindione (Concurrent use of anticoagulants may increase the risk of stomach bleeding). Products include:
Miradon Tablets 3042

Ardeparin Sodium (Concurrent use of anticaogulants may increase the risk of stomach bleeding).
No products indexed under this heading.

Betamethasone Acetate (Concurrent use of steroid drugs may increase the risk of stomach bleeding).
No products indexed under this heading.

Betamethasone Sodium Phosphate (Concurrent use of steroid drugs may increase the risk of stomach bleeding).
No products indexed under this heading.

Celecoxib (Concurrent use of other non-steroidal anti-inflammatory agents may increase the risk of stomach bleeding). Products include:
Celebrex Capsules 3134

Cortisone Acetate (Concurrent use of steroid drugs may increase the risk of stomach bleeding).
No products indexed under this heading.

Dalteparin Sodium (Concurrent use of anticaogulants may increase the risk of stomach bleeding). Products include:
Fragmin Injection 1097

Danaparoid Sodium (Concurrent use of anticaogulants may increase the risk of stomach bleeding).
No products indexed under this heading.

Desogestrel (Concurrent use of steroid drugs may increase the risk of stomach bleeding). Products include:
Mircette Tablets 1066

Dexamethasone (Concurrent use of steroid drugs may increase the risk of stomach bleeding). Products include:
Ciprodex Otic Suspension 559
Decadron Tablets 1951
TobraDex Ophthalmic Ointment 562
TobraDex Ophthalmic Suspension ... 563

Dexamethasone Acetate (Concurrent use of steroid drugs may increase the risk of stomach bleeding).
No products indexed under this heading.

Dexamethasone Sodium Phosphate (Concurrent use of steroid drugs may increase the risk of stomach bleeding).
No products indexed under this heading.

Diclofenac Potassium (Concurrent use of other non-steroidal anti-inflammatory agents may increase the risk of stomach bleeding).
No products indexed under this heading.

Diclofenac Sodium (Concurrent use of other non-steroidal anti-inflammatory agents may increase the risk of stomach bleeding). Products include:
Arthrotec Tablets 3129
Voltaren Ophthalmic Solution 2309
Voltaren Tablets 2307
Voltaren-XR Tablets 2310

Dicumarol (Concurrent use of anticaogulants may increase the risk of stomach bleeding).
No products indexed under this heading.

Enoxaparin Sodium (Concurrent use of anticaogulants may increase the risk of stomach bleeding). Products include:
Lovenox Injection 2915

Estradiol (Concurrent use of steroid drugs may increase the risk of stomach bleeding). Products include:
Angeliq Tablets 762
Climara Transdermal System 771
Climara Pro Transdermal System 776
Estrasorb Topical Emulsion 1147
Estring Vaginal Ring 2635
Menostar Transdermal System 782
Vagifem Tablets 2334

Estrogens, Conjugated (Concurrent use of steroid drugs may increase the risk of stomach bleeding). Products include:
Premarin Intravenous 3442
Premarin Tablets 3446
Premarin Vaginal Cream 3452
Premphase Tablets 3456
Prempro Tablets 3456

Ethinyl Estradiol (Concurrent use of steroid drugs may increase the risk of stomach bleeding). Products include:
Mircette Tablets 1066
NuvaRing 2340
Ortho-Cyclen/Ortho Tri-Cyclen 2429
Ortho Evra Transdermal System 2417
Ortho Tri-Cyclen Lo Tablets 2436
Seasonique Tablets 1077
Yasmin 28 Tablets 796
Yaz Tablets 803

Ethynodiol Diacetate (Concurrent use of steroid drugs may increase the risk of stomach bleeding).
No products indexed under this heading.

Etodolac (Concurrent use of other non-steroidal anti-inflammatory agents may increase the risk of stomach bleeding).
No products indexed under this heading.

Fenoprofen Calcium (Concurrent use of other non-steroidal anti-inflammatory agents may increase the risk of stomach bleeding). Products include:
Nalfon Capsules 2502

Fludrocortisone Acetate (Concurrent use of steroid drugs may increase the risk of stomach bleeding).
No products indexed under this heading.

Fluoxymesterone (Concurrent use of steroid drugs may increase the risk of stomach bleeding). Products include:
Androxy Tablets 3335

Flurbiprofen (Concurrent use of other non-steroidal anti-inflammatory agents may increase the risk of stomach bleeding).
No products indexed under this heading.

Fondaparinux Sodium (Concurrent use of anticaogulants may increase the risk of stomach bleeding). Products include:
Arixtra Injection 1351

Heparin Calcium (Concurrent use of anticaogulants may increase the risk of stomach bleeding).
No products indexed under this heading.

Heparin Sodium (Concurrent use of anticaogulants may increase the risk of stomach bleeding).
No products indexed under this heading.

Hydrocortisone (Concurrent use of steroid drugs may increase the risk of stomach bleeding). Products include:
Colocort Rectal Suspension, USP (Retention) 100 mg/60 mL.......... 2476
Hydrocortone Tablets 1989
Preparation H Hydrocortisone Cream .... ▣646

Hydrocortisone Acetate (Concurrent use of steroid drugs may increase the risk of stomach bleeding). Products include:
Analpram-HC 1159
Pramosone 1161
ProctoFoam-HC 3099

Hydrocortisone Sodium Phosphate (Concurrent use of steroid drugs may increase the risk of stomach bleeding).
No products indexed under this heading.

Hydrocortisone Sodium Succinate (Concurrent use of steroid drugs may increase the risk of stomach bleeding).
No products indexed under this heading.

Indomethacin (Concurrent use of other non-steroidal anti-inflammatory agents may increase the risk of stomach bleeding). Products include:
Indocin 1995

Indomethacin Sodium Trihydrate (Concurrent use of other non-steroidal anti-inflammatory agents may increase the risk of stomach bleeding). Products include:
Indocin I.V. 2465

Ketoprofen (Concurrent use of other non-steroidal anti-inflammatory agents may increase the risk of stomach bleeding).
No products indexed under this heading.

Ketorolac Tromethamine (Concurrent use of other non-steroidal anti-inflammatory agents may increase the risk of stomach bleeding). Products include:
Acular Ophthalmic Solution 565
Acular LS Ophthalmic Solution 566

Levonorgestrel (Concurrent use of steroid drugs may increase the risk of stomach bleeding). Products include:
Climara Pro Transdermal System 776
Mirena Intrauterine System 787
Plan B Tablets 1076
Seasonique Tablets 1077

Low Molecular Weight Heparins (Concurrent use of anticaogulants may increase the risk of stomach bleeding).
No products indexed under this heading.

Meclofenamate Sodium (Concurrent use of other non-steroidal anti-inflammatory agents may increase the risk of stomach bleeding).
No products indexed under this heading.

Mefenamic Acid (Concurrent use of other non-steroidal anti-inflammatory agents may increase the risk of stomach bleeding).
No products indexed under this heading.

Meloxicam (Concurrent use of other non-steroidal anti-inflammatory agents may increase the risk of stomach bleeding). Products include:
Mobic Oral Suspension 863
Mobic Tablets 863

Mestranol (Concurrent use of steroid drugs may increase the risk of stomach bleeding).
No products indexed under this heading.

Methylprednisolone Acetate (Concurrent use of steroid drugs may increase the risk of stomach bleeding). Products include:
Depo-Medrol Injectable Suspension 2617
Depo-Medrol Single-Dose Vial 2619

Methylprednisolone Sodium Succinate (Concurrent use of steroid drugs may increase the risk of stomach bleeding).
No products indexed under this heading.

Methyltestosterone (Concurrent use of steroid drugs may increase the risk of stomach bleeding). Products include:
Estratest Tablets 3199
Estratest H.S. Tablets 3199

Nabumetone (Concurrent use of other non-steroidal anti-inflammatory agents may increase the risk of stomach bleeding).
No products indexed under this heading.

Naproxen (Concurrent use of other non-steroidal anti-inflammatory agents may increase the risk of stomach bleeding). Products include:
EC-Naprosyn Delayed-Release Tablets 2761
Naprosyn Suspension 2761
Naprosyn Tablets 2761
Prevacid NapraPAC 3280

Naproxen Sodium (Concurrent use of other non-steroidal anti-inflammatory agents may increase the risk of stomach bleeding). Products include:
Aleve Caplets 742
Aleve Gelcaps 743
Aleve Tablets 743
Aleve Cold & Sinus Caplets 744
Anaprox Tablets 2761
Anaprox DS Tablets 2761

Norethindrone (Concurrent use of steroid drugs may increase the risk of stomach bleeding). Products include:
Ortho Micronor Tablets 2426

Norethindrone Acetate (Concurrent use of steroid drugs may increase the risk of stomach bleeding).
No products indexed under this heading.

Norgestimate (Concurrent use of steroid drugs may increase the risk of stomach bleeding). Products include:
Ortho-Cyclen/Ortho Tri-Cyclen 2429
Ortho Tri-Cyclen Lo Tablets 2436

Oxaprozin (Concurrent use of other non-steroidal anti-inflammatory agents may increase the risk of stomach bleeding).
No products indexed under this heading.

Phenylbutazone (Concurrent use of other non-steroidal anti-inflammatory agents may increase the risk of stomach bleeding).
No products indexed under this heading.

Piroxicam (Concurrent use of other non-steroidal anti-inflammatory agents may increase the risk of stomach bleeding).
No products indexed under this heading.

Prednisolone Acetate (Concurrent use of steroid drugs may increase the risk of stomach bleeding). Products include:
Blephamide Ophthalmic Ointment 568
Blephamide Ophthalmic Suspension 569
Poly-Pred Ophthalmic Suspension .... ⊙233
Pred Forte Ophthalmic Suspension .... ⊙235
Pred Mild Ophthalmic Suspension .... ⊙238
Pred-G Ophthalmic Ointment .... ⊙237
Pred-G Ophthalmic Suspension .... ⊙236

Prednisolone Sodium Phosphate (Concurrent use of steroid drugs may increase the risk of stomach bleeding).
No products indexed under this heading.

Prednisolone Tebutate (Concurrent use of steroid drugs may increase the risk of stomach bleeding).
No products indexed under this heading.

Prednisone (Concurrent use of steroid drugs may increase the risk of stomach bleeding).
No products indexed under this heading.

Rofecoxib (Concurrent use of other non-steroidal anti-inflammatory agents may increase the risk of stomach bleeding).
No products indexed under this heading.

Sulindac (Concurrent use of other non-steroidal anti-inflammatory agents may increase the risk of stomach bleeding). Products include:
Clinoril Tablets 1924

Testosterone (Concurrent use of steroid drugs may increase the risk of stomach bleeding). Products include:
AndroGel 3329
Striant Mucoadhesive 1007
Testim 1% Gel 695

Tinzaparin Sodium (Concurrent use of anticaogulants may increase the risk of stomach bleeding).
No products indexed under this heading.

Tolmetin Sodium (Concurrent use of other non-steroidal anti-inflammatory agents may increase the risk of stomach bleeding).
No products indexed under this heading.

Triamcinolone (Concurrent use of steroid drugs may increase the risk of stomach bleeding).
No products indexed under this heading.

Triamcinolone Acetonide (Concurrent use of steroid drugs may increase the risk of stomach bleeding). Products include:
Azmacort Inhalation Aerosol 1726
Nasacort AQ Nasal Spray 2922

Triamcinolone Diacetate (Concurrent use of steroid drugs may increase the risk of stomach bleeding).
No products indexed under this heading.

Triamcinolone Hexacetonide (Concurrent use of steroid drugs may increase the risk of stomach bleeding).
No products indexed under this heading.

Valdecoxib (Concurrent use of other non-steroidal anti-inflammatory agents may increase the risk of stomach bleeding).
No products indexed under this heading.

Warfarin Sodium (Concurrent use of anticaogulants may increase the risk of stomach bleeding). Products include:
Coumadin for Injection 898
Coumadin Tablets 898

CHILDREN'S ADVIL CHEWABLE TABLETS

(Ibuprofen) 603
May interact with anticoagulants, corticosteroids, parenterally administered corticosteroids, non-steroidal anti-inflammatory agents, potassium-depleting corticosteroids, sex steroids, and topical nonsteroidal anti-inflammatory agents. Compounds in these categories include:

Anisindione (Concurrent use of anticaogulants may increase the risk of stomach bleeding). Products include:
Miradon Tablets 3042

Ardeparin Sodium (Concurrent use of anticaogulants may increase the risk of stomach bleeding).
No products indexed under this heading.

Betamethasone Acetate (Concurrent use of steroid drugs may increase the risk of stomach bleeding).
No products indexed under this heading.

Betamethasone Sodium Phosphate (Concurrent use of steroid drugs may increase the risk of stomach bleeding).
No products indexed under this heading.

Celecoxib (Concurrent use of other non-steroidal anti-inflammatory agents may increase the risk of stomach bleeding). Products include:
Celebrex Capsules 3134

Cortisone Acetate (Concurrent use of steroid drugs may increase the risk of stomach bleeding).
No products indexed under this heading.

Dalteparin Sodium (Concurrent use of anticaogulants may increase the risk of stomach bleeding). Products include:
Fragmin Injection 1097

Danaparoid Sodium (Concurrent use of anticaogulants may increase the risk of stomach bleeding).
No products indexed under this heading.

Desogestrel (Concurrent use of steroid drugs may increase the risk of stomach bleeding). Products include:
Mircette Tablets 1066

Dexamethasone (Concurrent use of steroid drugs may increase the risk of stomach bleeding). Products include:
Ciprodex Otic Suspension 559
Decadron Tablets 1951
TobraDex Ophthalmic Ointment 562
TobraDex Ophthalmic Suspension 563

Dexamethasone Acetate (Concurrent use of steroid drugs may increase the risk of stomach bleeding).
No products indexed under this heading.

Dexamethasone Sodium Phosphate (Concurrent use of steroid drugs may increase the risk of stomach bleeding).
No products indexed under this heading.

Diclofenac Potassium (Concurrent use of other non-steroidal anti-inflammatory agents may increase the risk of stomach bleeding).
No products indexed under this heading.

Diclofenac Sodium (Concurrent use of other non-steroidal anti-inflammatory agents may increase the risk of stomach bleeding). Products include:
Arthrotec Tablets 3129
Voltaren Ophthalmic Solution 2309
Voltaren Tablets 2307
Voltaren-XR Tablets 2310

Dicumarol (Concurrent use of anticoagulants may increase the risk of stomach bleeding).
No products indexed under this heading.

Enoxaparin Sodium (Concurrent use of anticoagulants may increase the risk of stomach bleeding). Products include:
Lovenox Injection 2915

Estradiol (Concurrent use of steroid drugs may increase the risk of stomach bleeding). Products include:
Angeliq Tablets 762
Climara Transdermal System 771
Climara Pro Transdermal System 776
Estrasorb Topical Emulsion 1147
Estring Vaginal Ring 2635
Menostar Transdermal System 782
Vagifem Tablets 2334

Estrogens, Conjugated (Concurrent use of steroid drugs may increase the risk of stomach bleeding). Products include:
Premarin Intravenous 3442
Premarin Tablets 3446
Premarin Vaginal Cream 3452
Premphase Tablets 3456
Prempro Tablets 3456

Ethinyl Estradiol (Concurrent use of steroid drugs may increase the risk of stomach bleeding). Products include:
Mircette Tablets 1066
NuvaRing 2340
Ortho-Cyclen/Ortho Tri-Cyclen 2429
Ortho Evra Transdermal System 2417
Ortho Tri-Cyclen Lo Tablets 2436
Seasonique Tablets 1077
Yasmin 28 Tablets 796
Yaz Tablets 803

Ethynodiol Diacetate (Concurrent use of steroid drugs may increase the risk of stomach bleeding).
No products indexed under this heading.

Etodolac (Concurrent use of other non-steroidal anti-inflammatory agents may increase the risk of stomach bleeding).
No products indexed under this heading.

Fenoprofen Calcium (Concurrent use of other non-steroidal anti-inflammatory agents may increase the risk of stomach bleeding). Products include:
Nalfon Capsules 2502

Fludrocortisone Acetate (Concurrent use of steroid drugs may increase the risk of stomach bleeding).
No products indexed under this heading.

Fluoxymesterone (Concurrent use of steroid drugs may increase the risk of stomach bleeding). Products include:
- Androxy Tablets 3335

Flurbiprofen (Concurrent use of other non-steroidal anti-inflammatory agents may increase the risk of stomach bleeding).
- No products indexed under this heading.

Flurbiprofen Sodium (Concurrent use of other non-steroidal anti-inflammatory agents may increase the risk of stomach bleeding). Products include:
- Ocufen Ophthalmic Solution .... ⊙232

Fondaparinux Sodium (Concurrent use of anticoagulants may increase the risk of stomach bleeding). Products include:
- Arixtra Injection 1351

Heparin Calcium (Concurrent use of anticoagulants may increase the risk of stomach bleeding).
- No products indexed under this heading.

Heparin Sodium (Concurrent use of anticoagulants may increase the risk of stomach bleeding).
- No products indexed under this heading.

Hydrocortisone (Concurrent use of steroid drugs may increase the risk of stomach bleeding). Products include:
- Colocort Rectal Suspension, USP (Retention) 100 mg/60 mL 2476
- Hydrocortone Tablets 1989
- Preparation H Hydrocortisone Cream .... ▣646

Hydrocortisone Acetate (Concurrent use of steroid drugs may increase the risk of stomach bleeding). Products include:
- Analpram-HC 1159
- Pramosone 1161
- ProctoFoam-HC 3099

Hydrocortisone Sodium Phosphate (Concurrent use of steroid drugs may increase the risk of stomach bleeding).
- No products indexed under this heading.

Hydrocortisone Sodium Succinate (Concurrent use of steroid drugs may increase the risk of stomach bleeding).
- No products indexed under this heading.

Indomethacin (Concurrent use of other non-steroidal anti-inflammatory agents may increase the risk of stomach bleeding). Products include:
- Indocin 1995

Indomethacin Sodium Trihydrate (Concurrent use of other non-steroidal anti-inflammatory agents may increase the risk of stomach bleeding). Products include:
- Indocin I.V. 2465

Ketoprofen (Concurrent use of other non-steroidal anti-inflammatory agents may increase the risk of stomach bleeding).
- No products indexed under this heading.

Ketorolac Tromethamine (Concurrent use of other non-steroidal anti-inflammatory agents may increase the risk of stomach bleeding). Products include:
- Acular Ophthalmic Solution 565
- Acular LS Ophthalmic Solution 566

Levonorgestrel (Concurrent use of steroid drugs may increase the risk of stomach bleeding). Products include:
- Climara Pro Transdermal System 776
- Mirena Intrauterine System 787
- Plan B Tablets 1076
- Seasonique Tablets 1077

Low Molecular Weight Heparins (Concurrent use of anticoagulants may increase the risk of stomach bleeding).
- No products indexed under this heading.

Meclofenamate Sodium (Concurrent use of other non-steroidal anti-inflammatory agents may increase the risk of stomach bleeding).
- No products indexed under this heading.

Mefenamic Acid (Concurrent use of other non-steroidal anti-inflammatory agents may increase the risk of stomach bleeding).
- No products indexed under this heading.

Meloxicam (Concurrent use of other non-steroidal anti-inflammatory agents may increase the risk of stomach bleeding). Products include:
- Mobic Oral Suspension 863
- Mobic Tablets 863

Mestranol (Concurrent use of steroid drugs may increase the risk of stomach bleeding).
- No products indexed under this heading.

Methylprednisolone Acetate (Concurrent use of steroid drugs may increase the risk of stomach bleeding). Products include:
- Depo-Medrol Injectable Suspension 2617
- Depo-Medrol Single-Dose Vial 2619

Methylprednisolone Sodium Succinate (Concurrent use of steroid drugs may increase the risk of stomach bleeding).
- No products indexed under this heading.

Methyltestosterone (Concurrent use of steroid drugs may increase the risk of stomach bleeding). Products include:
- Estratest Tablets 3199
- Estratest H.S. Tablets 3199

Nabumetone (Concurrent use of other non-steroidal anti-inflammatory agents may increase the risk of stomach bleeding).
- No products indexed under this heading.

Naproxen (Concurrent use of other non-steroidal anti-inflammatory agents may increase the risk of stomach bleeding). Products include:
- EC-Naprosyn Delayed-Release Tablets 2761
- Naprosyn Suspension 2761
- Naprosyn Tablets 2761
- Prevacid NapraPAC 3280

Naproxen Sodium (Concurrent use of other non-steroidal anti-inflammatory agents may increase the risk of stomach bleeding). Products include:
- Aleve Caplets 742
- Aleve Gelcaps 743
- Aleve Tablets 743
- Aleve Cold & Sinus Caplets 744
- Anaprox Tablets 2761
- Anaprox DS Tablets 2761

Norethindrone (Concurrent use of steroid drugs may increase the risk of stomach bleeding). Products include:
- Ortho Micronor Tablets 2426

Norethindrone Acetate (Concurrent use of steroid drugs may increase the risk of stomach bleeding).
- No products indexed under this heading.

Norgestimate (Concurrent use of steroid drugs may increase the risk of stomach bleeding). Products include:
- Ortho-Cyclen/Ortho Tri-Cyclen 2429
- Ortho Tri-Cyclen Lo Tablets 2436

Oxaprozin (Concurrent use of other non-steroidal anti-inflammatory agents may increase the risk of stomach bleeding).
- No products indexed under this heading.

Phenylbutazone (Concurrent use of other non-steroidal anti-inflammatory agents may increase the risk of stomach bleeding).
- No products indexed under this heading.

Piroxicam (Concurrent use of other non-steroidal anti-inflammatory agents may increase the risk of stomach bleeding).
- No products indexed under this heading.

Prednisolone Acetate (Concurrent use of steroid drugs may increase the risk of stomach bleeding). Products include:
- Blephamide Ophthalmic Ointment 568
- Blephamide Ophthalmic Suspension 569
- Poly-Pred Ophthalmic Suspension .... ⊙233
- Pred Forte Ophthalmic Suspension .... ⊙235
- Pred Mild Ophthalmic Suspension .... ⊙238
- Pred-G Ophthalmic Ointment .... ⊙237
- Pred-G Ophthalmic Suspension .... ⊙236

Prednisolone Sodium Phosphate (Concurrent use of steroid drugs may increase the risk of stomach bleeding).
- No products indexed under this heading.

Prednisolone Tebutate (Concurrent use of steroid drugs may increase the risk of stomach bleeding).
- No products indexed under this heading.

Prednisone (Concurrent use of steroid drugs may increase the risk of stomach bleeding).
- No products indexed under this heading.

Rofecoxib (Concurrent use of other non-steroidal anti-inflammatory agents may increase the risk of stomach bleeding).
- No products indexed under this heading.

Sulindac (Concurrent use of other non-steroidal anti-inflammatory agents may increase the risk of stomach bleeding). Products include:
- Clinoril Tablets 1924

Suprofen (Concurrent use of other non-steroidal anti-inflammatory agents may increase the risk of stomach bleeding).
- No products indexed under this heading.

Testosterone (Concurrent use of steroid drugs may increase the risk of stomach bleeding). Products include:
- AndroGel 3329
- Striant Mucoadhesive 1007
- Testim 1% Gel 695

Tinzaparin Sodium (Concurrent use of anticoagulants may increase the risk of stomach bleeding).
- No products indexed under this heading.

Tolmetin Sodium (Concurrent use of other non-steroidal anti-inflammatory agents may increase the risk of stomach bleeding).
- No products indexed under this heading.

Triamcinolone (Concurrent use of steroid drugs may increase the risk of stomach bleeding).
- No products indexed under this heading.

Triamcinolone Acetonide (Concurrent use of steroid drugs may increase the risk of stomach bleeding). Products include:
- Azmacort Inhalation Aerosol 1726
- Nasacort AQ Nasal Spray 2922

Triamcinolone Diacetate (Concurrent use of steroid drugs may increase the risk of stomach bleeding).
- No products indexed under this heading.

Triamcinolone Hexacetonide (Concurrent use of steroid drugs may increase the risk of stomach bleeding).
- No products indexed under this heading.

Valdecoxib (Concurrent use of other non-steroidal anti-inflammatory agents may increase the risk of stomach bleeding).
- No products indexed under this heading.

Warfarin Sodium (Concurrent use of anticoagulants may increase the risk of stomach bleeding). Products include:
- Coumadin for Injection 898
- Coumadin Tablets 898

ADVIL COLD & SINUS CAPLETS

(Ibuprofen, Pseudoephedrine Hydrochloride) .... ▣723

May interact with anticoagulants, corticosteroids, parenterally administered corticosteroids, non-steroidal anti-inflammatory agents, potassium-depleting corticosteroids, sex steroids, topical nonsteroidal anti-inflammatory agents, and certain other agents. Compounds in these categories include:

Anisindione (Concurrent use of anticoagulants may increase the risk of stomach bleeding). Products include:
- Miradon Tablets 3042

Ardeparin Sodium (Concurrent use of anticoagulants may increase the risk of stomach bleeding).
- No products indexed under this heading.

Betamethasone Acetate (Concurrent use of steroid drugs may increase the risk of stomach bleeding).
- No products indexed under this heading.

IMPORTANT NOTE: Always consult each drug listing in the patient's regimen for possible interactions.

Pred-G Ophthalmic Ointment .... ⊙237
Pred-G Ophthalmic Suspension ...... ⊙236

Prednisolone Sodium Phosphate (Concurrent use of steroid drugs may increase the risk of stomach bleeding).
No products indexed under this heading.

Prednisolone Tebutate (Concurrent use of steroid drugs may increase the risk of stomach bleeding).
No products indexed under this heading.

Prednisone (Concurrent use of steroid drugs may increase the risk of stomach bleeding).
No products indexed under this heading.

Rofecoxib (Concurrent use of other non-steroidal anti-inflammatory agents may increase the risk of stomach bleeding).
No products indexed under this heading.

Sulindac (Concurrent use of other non-steroidal anti-inflammatory agents may increase the risk of stomach bleeding). Products include:
Clinoril Tablets 1924

Suprofen (Concurrent use of other non-steroidal anti-inflammatory agents may increase the risk of stomach bleeding).
No products indexed under this heading.

Testosterone (Concurrent use of steroid drugs may increase the risk of stomach bleeding). Products include:
AndroGel 3329
Striant Mucoadhesive 1007
Testim 1% Gel 695

Tinzaparin Sodium (Concurrent use of anticoagulants may increase the risk of stomach bleeding).
No products indexed under this heading.

Tolmetin Sodium (Concurrent use of other non-steroidal anti-inflammatory agents may increase the risk of stomach bleeding).
No products indexed under this heading.

Triamcinolone (Concurrent use of steroid drugs may increase the risk of stomach bleeding).
No products indexed under this heading.

Triamcinolone Acetonide (Concurrent use of steroid drugs may increase the risk of stomach bleeding). Products include:
Azmacort Inhalation Aerosol 1726
Nasacort AQ Nasal Spray 2922

Triamcinolone Diacetate (Concurrent use of steroid drugs may increase the risk of stomach bleeding).
No products indexed under this heading.

Triamcinolone Hexacetonide (Concurrent use of steroid drugs may increase the risk of stomach bleeding).
No products indexed under this heading.

Valdecoxib (Concurrent use of other non-steroidal anti-inflammatory agents may increase the risk of stomach bleeding).
No products indexed under this heading.

Warfarin Sodium (Concurrent use of anticoagulants may increase the risk of stomach bleeding). Products include:
Coumadin for Injection 898
Coumadin Tablets 898

ADVIL COLD & SINUS LIQUI-GELS

(Ibuprofen, Pseudoephedrine Hydrochloride)................................ ▣723
See Advil Cold & Sinus Caplets

ADVIL GEL CAPLETS

(Ibuprofen) .... ▣674
See Advil Caplets

INFANTS' ADVIL CONCENTRATED DROPS

(Ibuprofen) .... ▣604
May interact with anticoagulants, corticosteroids, parenterally administered corticosteroids, non-steroidal anti-inflammatory agents, potassium-depleting corticosteroids, sex steroids, and topical nonsteroidal anti-inflammatory agents. Compounds in these categories include:

Anisindione (Concurrent use of anticoagulants may increase the risk of stomach bleeding). Products include:
Miradon Tablets 3042

Ardeparin Sodium (Concurrent use of anticoagulants may increase the risk of stomach bleeding).
No products indexed under this heading.

Betamethasone Acetate (Concurrent use of steroid drugs may increase the risk of stomach bleeding).
No products indexed under this heading.

Betamethasone Sodium Phosphate (Concurrent use of steroid drugs may increase the risk of stomach bleeding).
No products indexed under this heading.

Celecoxib (Concurrent use of other non-steroidal anti-inflammatory agents may increase the stomach bleeding). Products include:
Celebrex Capsules 3134

Cortisone Acetate (Concurrent use of steroid drugs may increase the risk of stomach bleeding).
No products indexed under this heading.

Dalteparin Sodium (Concurrent use of anticoagulants may increase the risk of stomach bleeding). Products include:
Fragmin Injection 1097

Danaparoid Sodium (Concurrent use of anticoagulants may increase the risk of stomach bleeding).
No products indexed under this heading.

Desogestrel (Concurrent use of steroid drugs may increase the risk of stomach bleeding). Products include:
Mircette Tablets 1066

Dexamethasone (Concurrent use of steroid drugs may increase the risk of stomach bleeding). Products include:
Ciprodex Otic Suspension 559
Decadron Tablets 1951
TobraDex Ophthalmic Ointment 562
TobraDex Ophthalmic Suspension ... 563

Dexamethasone Acetate (Concurrent use of steroid drugs may increase the risk of stomach bleeding).
No products indexed under this heading.

Dexamethasone Sodium Phosphate (Concurrent use of steroid drugs may increase the risk of stomach bleeding).
No products indexed under this heading.

Diclofenac Potassium (Concurrent use of other non-steroidal anti-inflammatory agents may increase the stomach bleeding).
No products indexed under this heading.

Diclofenac Sodium (Concurrent use of other non-steroidal anti-inflammatory agents may increase the stomach bleeding). Products include:
Arthrotec Tablets 3129
Voltaren Ophthalmic Solution 2309
Voltaren Tablets 2307
Voltaren-XR Tablets 2310

Dicumarol (Concurrent use of anticoagulants may increase the risk of stomach bleeding).
No products indexed under this heading.

Enoxaparin Sodium (Concurrent use of anticoagulants may increase the risk of stomach bleeding). Products include:
Lovenox Injection 2915

Estradiol (Concurrent use of steroid drugs may increase the risk of stomach bleeding). Products include:
Angeliq Tablets 762
Climara Transdermal System 771
Climara Pro Transdermal System 776
Estrasorb Topical Emulsion 1147
Estring Vaginal Ring 2635
Menostar Transdermal System 782
Vagifem Tablets 2334

Estrogens, Conjugated (Concurrent use of steroid drugs may increase the risk of stomach bleeding). Products include:
Premarin Intravenous 3442
Premarin Tablets 3446
Premarin Vaginal Cream 3452
Premphase Tablets 3456
Prempro Tablets 3456

Ethinyl Estradiol (Concurrent use of steroid drugs may increase the risk of stomach bleeding). Products include:
Mircette Tablets 1066
NuvaRing 2340
Ortho-Cyclen/Ortho Tri-Cyclen 2429
Ortho Evra Transdermal System 2417
Ortho Tri-Cyclen Lo Tablets 2436
Seasonique Tablets 1077
Yasmin 28 Tablets 796
Yaz Tablets 803

Ethynodiol Diacetate (Concurrent use of steroid drugs may increase the risk of stomach bleeding).
No products indexed under this heading.

Etodolac (Concurrent use of other non-steroidal anti-inflammatory agents may increase the stomach bleeding).
No products indexed under this heading.

Fenoprofen Calcium (Concurrent use of other non-steroidal anti-inflammatory agents may increase the stomach bleeding). Products include:
Nalfon Capsules 2502

Fludrocortisone Acetate (Concurrent use of steroid drugs may increase the risk of stomach bleeding).
No products indexed under this heading.

Fluoxymesterone (Concurrent use of steroid drugs may increase the risk of stomach bleeding). Products include:
Androxy Tablets 3335

Flurbiprofen (Concurrent use of other non-steroidal anti-inflammatory agents may increase the stomach bleeding).
No products indexed under this heading.

Fondaparinux Sodium (Concurrent use of anticoagulants may increase the risk of stomach bleeding). Products include:
Arixtra Injection 1351

Heparin Calcium (Concurrent use of anticoagulants may increase the risk of stomach bleeding).
No products indexed under this heading.

Heparin Sodium (Concurrent use of anticoagulants may increase the risk of stomach bleeding).
No products indexed under this heading.

Hydrocortisone (Concurrent use of steroid drugs may increase the risk of stomach bleeding). Products include:
Colocort Rectal Suspension, USP (Retention) 100 mg/60 mL 2476
Hydrocortone Tablets 1989
Preparation H Hydrocortisone Cream .... ▣646

Hydrocortisone Acetate (Concurrent use of steroid drugs may increase the risk of stomach bleeding). Products include:
Analpram-HC 1159
Pramosone 1161
ProctoFoam-HC 3099

Hydrocortisone Sodium Phosphate (Concurrent use of steroid drugs may increase the risk of stomach bleeding).
No products indexed under this heading.

Hydrocortisone Sodium Succinate (Concurrent use of steroid drugs may increase the risk of stomach bleeding).
No products indexed under this heading.

Indomethacin (Concurrent use of other non-steroidal anti-inflammatory agents may increase the stomach bleeding). Products include:
Indocin 1995

Indomethacin Sodium Trihydrate (Concurrent use of other non-steroidal anti-inflammatory agents may increase the stomach bleeding). Products include:
Indocin I.V. 2465

Ketoprofen (Concurrent use of other non-steroidal anti-inflammatory agents may increase the stomach bleeding).
No products indexed under this heading.

Ketorolac Tromethamine (Concurrent use of other non-steroidal anti-inflammatory agents may increase the stomach bleeding). Products include:
Acular Ophthalmic Solution 565
Acular LS Ophthalmic Solution 566

Levonorgestrel (Concurrent use of steroid drugs may increase the risk of stomach bleeding). Products include:
Climara Pro Transdermal System 776
Mirena Intrauterine System 787
Plan B Tablets 1076
Seasonique Tablets 1077

Low Molecular Weight Heparins (Concurrent use of anticoagulants may increase the risk of stomach bleeding).
No products indexed under this heading.

Meclofenamate Sodium (Concurrent use of other non-steroidal anti-inflammatory agents may increase the stomach bleeding).
No products indexed under this heading.

Mefenamic Acid (Concurrent use of other non-steroidal anti-inflammatory agents may increase the stomach bleeding).
No products indexed under this heading.

Meloxicam (Concurrent use of other non-steroidal anti-inflammatory agents may increase the stomach bleeding). Products include:
Mobic Oral Suspension 863
Mobic Tablets 863

Mestranol (Concurrent use of steroid drugs may increase the risk of stomach bleeding).
No products indexed under this heading.

Methylprednisolone Acetate (Concurrent use of steroid drugs may increase the risk of stomach bleeding). Products include:
Depo-Medrol Injectable Suspension 2617
Depo-Medrol Single-Dose Vial 2619

Methylprednisolone Sodium Succinate (Concurrent use of steroid drugs may increase the risk of stomach bleeding).
No products indexed under this heading.

Methyltestosterone (Concurrent use of steroid drugs may increase the risk of stomach bleeding). Products include:
Estratest Tablets 3199
Estratest H.S. Tablets 3199

Nabumetone (Concurrent use of other non-steroidal anti-inflammatory agents may increase the stomach bleeding).
No products indexed under this heading.

Naproxen (Concurrent use of other non-steroidal anti-inflammatory agents may increase the stomach bleeding). Products include:
EC-Naprosyn Delayed-Release Tablets 2761
Naprosyn Suspension 2761
Naprosyn Tablets 2761
Prevacid NapraPAC 3280

Naproxen Sodium (Concurrent use of other non-steroidal anti-inflammatory agents may increase the stomach bleeding). Products include:
Aleve Caplets 742
Aleve Gelcaps 743
Aleve Tablets 743
Aleve Cold & Sinus Caplets 744
Anaprox Tablets 2761
Anaprox DS Tablets 2761

Norethindrone (Concurrent use of steroid drugs may increase the risk of stomach bleeding). Products include:
Ortho Micronor Tablets 2426

Norethindrone Acetate (Concurrent use of steroid drugs may increase the risk of stomach bleeding).
No products indexed under this heading.

Norgestimate (Concurrent use of steroid drugs may increase the risk of stomach bleeding). Products include:
Ortho-Cyclen/Ortho Tri-Cyclen 2429
Ortho Tri-Cyclen Lo Tablets 2436

Oxaprozin (Concurrent use of other non-steroidal anti-inflammatory agents may increase the stomach bleeding).
No products indexed under this heading.

Phenylbutazone (Concurrent use of other non-steroidal anti-inflammatory agents may increase the stomach bleeding).
No products indexed under this heading.

Piroxicam (Concurrent use of other non-steroidal anti-inflammatory agents may increase the stomach bleeding).
No products indexed under this heading.

Prednisolone Acetate (Concurrent use of steroid drugs may increase the risk of stomach bleeding). Products include:
Blephamide Ophthalmic Ointment 568
Blephamide Ophthalmic Suspension 569
Poly-Pred Ophthalmic Suspension .... ⊙233
Pred Forte Ophthalmic Suspension .... ⊙235
Pred Mild Ophthalmic Suspension .... ⊙238
Pred-G Ophthalmic Ointment .... ⊙237
Pred-G Ophthalmic Suspension ...... ⊙236

Prednisolone Sodium Phosphate (Concurrent use of steroid drugs may increase the risk of stomach bleeding).
No products indexed under this heading.

Prednisolone Tebutate (Concurrent use of steroid drugs may increase the risk of stomach bleeding).
No products indexed under this heading.

Prednisone (Concurrent use of steroid drugs may increase the risk of stomach bleeding).
No products indexed under this heading.

Rofecoxib (Concurrent use of other non-steroidal anti-inflammatory agents may increase the stomach bleeding).
No products indexed under this heading.

Sulindac (Concurrent use of other non-steroidal anti-inflammatory agents may increase the stomach bleeding). Products include:
Clinoril Tablets 1924

Testosterone (Concurrent use of steroid drugs may increase the risk of stomach bleeding). Products include:
AndroGel 3329
Striant Mucoadhesive 1007
Testim 1% Gel 695

Tinzaparin Sodium (Concurrent use of anticoagulants may increase the risk of stomach bleeding).
No products indexed under this heading.

Tolmetin Sodium (Concurrent use of other non-steroidal anti-inflammatory agents may increase the stomach bleeding).
No products indexed under this heading.

Triamcinolone (Concurrent use of steroid drugs may increase the risk of stomach bleeding).
No products indexed under this heading.

Triamcinolone Acetonide (Concurrent use of steroid drugs may increase the risk of stomach bleeding). Products include:
Azmacort Inhalation Aerosol 1726
Nasacort AQ Nasal Spray 2922

Triamcinolone Diacetate (Concurrent use of steroid drugs may increase the risk of stomach bleeding).
No products indexed under this heading.

Triamcinolone Hexacetonide (Concurrent use of steroid drugs may increase the risk of stomach bleeding).
No products indexed under this heading.

Valdecoxib (Concurrent use of other non-steroidal anti-inflammatory agents may increase the stomach bleeding).
No products indexed under this heading.

Warfarin Sodium (Concurrent use of anticoagulants may increase the risk of stomach bleeding). Products include:
Coumadin for Injection 898
Coumadin Tablets 898

INFANTS' ADVIL CONCENTRATED DROPS - WHITE GRAPE (DYE-FREE)

(Ibuprofen) 604
See Infants' Advil Concentrated Drops

JUNIOR STRENGTH ADVIL SWALLOW TABLETS

(Ibuprofen) 605
May interact with anticoagulants, corticosteroids, parenterally administered corticosteroids, non-steroidal anti-inflammatory agents, potassium-depleting corticosteroids, sex steroids, and topical nonsteroidal anti-inflammatory agents. Compounds in these categories include:

Anisindione (Concurrent use of anticoagulants may increase the risk of stomach bleeding). Products include:
Miradon Tablets 3042

Ardeparin Sodium (Concurrent use of anticoagulants may increase the risk of stomach bleeding).
No products indexed under this heading.

Betamethasone Acetate (Concurrent use of steroid drugs may increase the risk of stomach bleeding).
No products indexed under this heading.

Betamethasone Sodium Phosphate (Concurrent use of steroid drugs may increase the risk of stomach bleeding).
No products indexed under this heading.

Celecoxib (Concurrent use of other non-steroidal anti-inflammatory agents may increase the risk of stomach bleeding). Products include:
Celebrex Capsules 3134

Cortisone Acetate (Concurrent use of steroid drugs may increase the risk of stomach bleeding).
No products indexed under this heading.

Dalteparin Sodium (Concurrent use of anticoagulants may increase the risk of stomach bleeding). Products include:
Fragmin Injection 1097

Danaparoid Sodium (Concurrent use of anticoagulants may increase the risk of stomach bleeding).
No products indexed under this heading.

Desogestrel (Concurrent use of steroid drugs may increase the risk of stomach bleeding). Products include:
Mircette Tablets 1066

Dexamethasone (Concurrent use of steroid drugs may increase the risk of stomach bleeding). Products include:
Ciprodex Otic Suspension 559
Decadron Tablets 1951
TobraDex Ophthalmic Ointment 562
TobraDex Ophthalmic Suspension ... 563

Dexamethasone Acetate (Concurrent use of steroid drugs may increase the risk of stomach bleeding).
No products indexed under this heading.

Dexamethasone Sodium Phosphate (Concurrent use of steroid drugs may increase the risk of stomach bleeding).
No products indexed under this heading.

Diclofenac Potassium (Concurrent use of other non-steroidal anti-inflammatory agents may increase the risk of stomach bleeding).
No products indexed under this heading.

Diclofenac Sodium (Concurrent use of other non-steroidal anti-inflammatory agents may increase the risk of stomach bleeding). Products include:
Arthrotec Tablets 3129
Voltaren Ophthalmic Solution 2309
Voltaren Tablets 2307
Voltaren-XR Tablets 2310

Dicumarol (Concurrent use of anticoagulants may increase the risk of stomach bleeding).
No products indexed under this heading.

Enoxaparin Sodium (Concurrent use of anticoagulants may increase the risk of stomach bleeding). Products include:
Lovenox Injection 2915

Estradiol (Concurrent use of steroid drugs may increase the risk of stomach bleeding). Products include:
Angeliq Tablets 762
Climara Transdermal System 771
Climara Pro Transdermal System 776
Estrasorb Topical Emulsion 1147
Estring Vaginal Ring 2635
Menostar Transdermal System 782
Vagifem Tablets 2334

Estrogens, Conjugated (Concurrent use of steroid drugs may increase the risk of stomach bleeding). Products include:
Premarin Intravenous 3442
Premarin Tablets 3446
Premarin Vaginal Cream 3452
Premphase Tablets 3456
Prempro Tablets 3456

Ethinyl Estradiol (Concurrent use of steroid drugs may increase the risk of stomach bleeding). Products include:
- Mircette Tablets 1066
- NuvaRing 2340
- Ortho-Cyclen/Ortho Tri-Cyclen 2429
- Ortho Evra Transdermal System 2417
- Ortho Tri-Cyclen Lo Tablets 2436
- Seasonique Tablets 1077
- Yasmin 28 Tablets 796
- Yaz Tablets 803

Ethynodiol Diacetate (Concurrent use of steroid drugs may increase the risk of stomach bleeding).
- No products indexed under this heading.

Etodolac (Concurrent use of other non-steroidal anti-inflammatory agents may increase the risk of stomach bleeding).
- No products indexed under this heading.

Fenoprofen Calcium (Concurrent use of other non-steroidal anti-inflammatory agents may increase the risk of stomach bleeding). Products include:
- Nalfon Capsules 2502

Fludrocortisone Acetate (Concurrent use of steroid drugs may increase the risk of stomach bleeding).
- No products indexed under this heading.

Fluoxymesterone (Concurrent use of steroid drugs may increase the risk of stomach bleeding). Products include:
- Androxy Tablets 3335

Flurbiprofen (Concurrent use of other non-steroidal anti-inflammatory agents may increase the risk of stomach bleeding).
- No products indexed under this heading.

Flurbiprofen Sodium (Concurrent use of other non-steroidal anti-inflammatory agents may increase the risk of stomach bleeding). Products include:
- Ocufen Ophthalmic Solution .... ⊙232

Fondaparinux Sodium (Concurrent use of anticoagulants may increase the risk of stomach bleeding). Products include:
- Arixtra Injection 1351

Heparin Calcium (Concurrent use of anticoagulants may increase the risk of stomach bleeding).
- No products indexed under this heading.

Heparin Sodium (Concurrent use of anticoagulants may increase the risk of stomach bleeding).
- No products indexed under this heading.

Hydrocortisone (Concurrent use of steroid drugs may increase the risk of stomach bleeding). Products include:
- Colocort Rectal Suspension, USP (Retention) 100 mg/60 mL 2476
- Hydrocortone Tablets 1989
- Preparation H Hydrocortisone Cream .... ■646

Hydrocortisone Acetate (Concurrent use of steroid drugs may increase the risk of stomach bleeding). Products include:
- Analpram-HC 1159
- Pramosone 1161
- ProctoFoam-HC 3099

Hydrocortisone Sodium Phosphate (Concurrent use of steroid drugs may increase the risk of stomach bleeding).
- No products indexed under this heading.

Hydrocortisone Sodium Succinate (Concurrent use of steroid drugs may increase the risk of stomach bleeding).
- No products indexed under this heading.

Indomethacin (Concurrent use of other non-steroidal anti-inflammatory agents may increase the risk of stomach bleeding). Products include:
- Indocin 1995

Indomethacin Sodium Trihydrate (Concurrent use of other non-steroidal anti-inflammatory agents may increase the risk of stomach bleeding). Products include:
- Indocin I.V. 2465

Ketoprofen (Concurrent use of other non-steroidal anti-inflammatory agents may increase the risk of stomach bleeding).
- No products indexed under this heading.

Ketorolac Tromethamine (Concurrent use of other non-steroidal anti-inflammatory agents may increase the risk of stomach bleeding). Products include:
- Acular Ophthalmic Solution 565
- Acular LS Ophthalmic Solution 566

Levonorgestrel (Concurrent use of steroid drugs may increase the risk of stomach bleeding). Products include:
- Climara Pro Transdermal System 776
- Mirena Intrauterine System 787
- Plan B Tablets 1076
- Seasonique Tablets 1077

Low Molecular Weight Heparins (Concurrent use of anticoagulants may increase the risk of stomach bleeding).
- No products indexed under this heading.

Meclofenamate Sodium (Concurrent use of other non-steroidal anti-inflammatory agents may increase the risk of stomach bleeding).
- No products indexed under this heading.

Mefenamic Acid (Concurrent use of other non-steroidal anti-inflammatory agents may increase the risk of stomach bleeding).
- No products indexed under this heading.

Meloxicam (Concurrent use of other non-steroidal anti-inflammatory agents may increase the risk of stomach bleeding). Products include:
- Mobic Oral Suspension 863
- Mobic Tablets 863

Mestranol (Concurrent use of steroid drugs may increase the risk of stomach bleeding).
- No products indexed under this heading.

Methylprednisolone Acetate (Concurrent use of steroid drugs may increase the risk of stomach bleeding). Products include:
- Depo-Medrol Injectable Suspension 2617
- Depo-Medrol Single-Dose Vial 2619

Methylprednisolone Sodium Succinate (Concurrent use of steroid drugs may increase the risk of stomach bleeding).
- No products indexed under this heading.

Methyltestosterone (Concurrent use of steroid drugs may increase the risk of stomach bleeding). Products include:
- Estratest Tablets 3199
- Estratest H.S. Tablets 3199

Nabumetone (Concurrent use of other non-steroidal anti-inflammatory agents may increase the risk of stomach bleeding).
- No products indexed under this heading.

Naproxen (Concurrent use of other non-steroidal anti-inflammatory agents may increase the risk of stomach bleeding). Products include:
- EC-Naprosyn Delayed-Release Tablets 2761
- Naprosyn Suspension 2761
- Naprosyn Tablets 2761
- Prevacid NapraPAC 3280

Naproxen Sodium (Concurrent use of other non-steroidal anti-inflammatory agents may increase the risk of stomach bleeding). Products include:
- Aleve Caplets 742
- Aleve Gelcaps 743
- Aleve Tablets 743
- Aleve Cold & Sinus Caplets 744
- Anaprox Tablets 2761
- Anaprox DS Tablets 2761

Norethindrone (Concurrent use of steroid drugs may increase the risk of stomach bleeding). Products include:
- Ortho Micronor Tablets 2426

Norethindrone Acetate (Concurrent use of steroid drugs may increase the risk of stomach bleeding).
- No products indexed under this heading.

Norgestimate (Concurrent use of steroid drugs may increase the risk of stomach bleeding). Products include:
- Ortho-Cyclen/Ortho Tri-Cyclen 2429
- Ortho Tri-Cyclen Lo Tablets 2436

Oxaprozin (Concurrent use of other non-steroidal anti-inflammatory agents may increase the risk of stomach bleeding).
- No products indexed under this heading.

Phenylbutazone (Concurrent use of other non-steroidal anti-inflammatory agents may increase the risk of stomach bleeding).
- No products indexed under this heading.

Piroxicam (Concurrent use of other non-steroidal anti-inflammatory agents may increase the risk of stomach bleeding).
- No products indexed under this heading.

Prednisolone Acetate (Concurrent use of steroid drugs may increase the risk of stomach bleeding). Products include:
- Blephamide Ophthalmic Ointment 568
- Blephamide Ophthalmic Suspension 569
- Poly-Pred Ophthalmic Suspension .... ⊙233
- Pred Forte Ophthalmic Suspension .... ⊙235
- Pred Mild Ophthalmic Suspension .... ⊙238
- Pred-G Ophthalmic Ointment .... ⊙237
- Pred-G Ophthalmic Suspension .... ⊙236

Prednisolone Sodium Phosphate (Concurrent use of steroid drugs may increase the risk of stomach bleeding).
- No products indexed under this heading.

Prednisolone Tebutate (Concurrent use of steroid drugs may increase the risk of stomach bleeding).
- No products indexed under this heading.

Prednisone (Concurrent use of steroid drugs may increase the risk of stomach bleeding).
- No products indexed under this heading.

Rofecoxib (Concurrent use of other non-steroidal anti-inflammatory agents may increase the risk of stomach bleeding).
- No products indexed under this heading.

Sulindac (Concurrent use of other non-steroidal anti-inflammatory agents may increase the risk of stomach bleeding). Products include:
- Clinoril Tablets 1924

Suprofen (Concurrent use of other non-steroidal anti-inflammatory agents may increase the risk of stomach bleeding).
- No products indexed under this heading.

Testosterone (Concurrent use of steroid drugs may increase the risk of stomach bleeding). Products include:
- AndroGel 3329
- Striant Mucoadhesive 1007
- Testim 1% Gel 695

Tinzaparin Sodium (Concurrent use of anticoagulants may increase the risk of stomach bleeding).
- No products indexed under this heading.

Tolmetin Sodium (Concurrent use of other non-steroidal anti-inflammatory agents may increase the risk of stomach bleeding).
- No products indexed under this heading.

Triamcinolone (Concurrent use of steroid drugs may increase the risk of stomach bleeding).
- No products indexed under this heading.

Triamcinolone Acetonide (Concurrent use of steroid drugs may increase the risk of stomach bleeding). Products include:
- Azmacort Inhalation Aerosol 1726
- Nasacort AQ Nasal Spray 2922

Triamcinolone Diacetate (Concurrent use of steroid drugs may increase the risk of stomach bleeding).
- No products indexed under this heading.

Triamcinolone Hexacetonide (Concurrent use of steroid drugs may increase the risk of stomach bleeding).
- No products indexed under this heading.

Valdecoxib (Concurrent use of other non-steroidal anti-inflammatory agents may increase the risk of stomach bleeding).
- No products indexed under this heading.

Warfarin Sodium (Concurrent use of anticoagulants may increase the risk of stomach bleeding). Products include:
- Coumadin for Injection 898
- Coumadin Tablets 898

ADVIL LIQUI-GELS
(Ibuprofen) .... ▣674
See Advil Caplets

ADVIL MIGRAINE LIQUIGELS
(Ibuprofen) .... ▣608
May interact with anticoagulants, corticosteroids, parenterally administered corticosteroids, oral anticoagulants, non-steroidal anti-inflammatory agents, potassium-depleting corticosteroids, sex steroids, topical nonsteroidal anti-inflammatory agents, and certain other agents. Compounds in these categories include:

Anisindione (Concurrent use of an anticoagulant may increase the risk of stomach bleeding). Products include:
- Miradon Tablets 3042

Ardeparin Sodium (Concurrent use of an anticoagulant may increase the risk of stomach bleeding).
- No products indexed under this heading.

Betamethasone Acetate (Concurrent use of a steroid drug may increase the risk of stomach bleeding).
- No products indexed under this heading.

Betamethasone Sodium Phosphate (Concurrent use of a steroid drug may increase the risk of stomach bleeding).
- No products indexed under this heading.

Celecoxib (Concurrent use of non-steroidal anti- inflammatory drug may increase the risk of stomach bleeding). Products include:
- Celebrex Capsules 3134

Cortisone Acetate (Concurrent use of a steroid drug may increase the risk of stomach bleeding).
- No products indexed under this heading.

Dalteparin Sodium (Concurrent use of an anticoagulant may increase the risk of stomach bleeding). Products include:
- Fragmin Injection 1097

Danaparoid Sodium (Concurrent use of an anticoagulant may increase the risk of stomach bleeding).
- No products indexed under this heading.

Desogestrel (Concurrent use of a steroid drug may increase the risk of stomach bleeding). Products include:
- Mircette Tablets 1066

Dexamethasone (Concurrent use of a steroid drug may increase the risk of stomach bleeding). Products include:
- Ciprodex Otic Suspension 559
- Decadron Tablets 1951
- TobraDex Ophthalmic Ointment 562
- TobraDex Ophthalmic Suspension ... 563

Dexamethasone Acetate (Concurrent use of a steroid drug may increase the risk of stomach bleeding).
- No products indexed under this heading.

Dexamethasone Sodium Phosphate (Concurrent use of a steroid drug may increase the risk of stomach bleeding).
- No products indexed under this heading.

Diclofenac Potassium (Concurrent use of non-steroidal anti- inflammatory drug may increase the risk of stomach bleeding.).
- No products indexed under this heading.

Diclofenac Sodium (Concurrent use of non- steroidal anti-inflammatory drug may increase the risk of stomach bleeding). Products include:
- Arthrotec Tablets 3129
- Voltaren Ophthalmic Solution 2309
- Voltaren Tablets 2307
- Voltaren-XR Tablets 2310

Dicumarol (Concurrent use of an anticoagulant may increase the risk of stomach bleeding).
- No products indexed under this heading.

Enoxaparin Sodium (Concurrent use of an anticoagulant may increase the risk of stomach bleeding). Products include:
- Lovenox Injection 2915

Estradiol (Concurrent use of a steroid drug may increase the risk of stomach bleeding). Products include:
- Angeliq Tablets 762
- Climara Transdermal System 771
- Climara Pro Transdermal System 776
- Estrasorb Topical Emulsion 1147
- Estring Vaginal Ring 2635
- Menostar Transdermal System 782
- Vagifem Tablets 2334

Estrogens, Conjugated (Concurrent use of a steroid drug may increase the risk of stomach bleeding). Products include:
- Premarin Intravenous 3442
- Premarin Tablets 3446
- Premarin Vaginal Cream 3452
- Premphase Tablets 3456
- Prempro Tablets 3456

Ethinyl Estradiol (Concurrent use of a steroid drug may increase the risk of stomach bleeding). Products include:
- Mircette Tablets 1066
- NuvaRing 2340
- Ortho-Cyclen/Ortho Tri-Cyclen 2429
- Ortho Evra Transdermal System 2417
- Ortho Tri-Cyclen Lo Tablets 2436
- Seasonique Tablets 1077
- Yasmin 28 Tablets 796
- Yaz Tablets 803

Ethynodiol Diacetate (Concurrent use of a steroid drug may increase the risk of stomach bleeding).
- No products indexed under this heading.

Etodolac (Concurrent use of non-steroidal anti- inflammatory drug may increase the risk of stomach bleeding.).
- No products indexed under this heading.

Fenoprofen Calcium (Concurrent use of non-steroidal anti- inflammatory drug may increase the risk of stomach bleeding). Products include:
- Nalfon Capsules 2502

Fludrocortisone Acetate (Concurrent use of a steroid drug may increase the risk of stomach bleeding).
- No products indexed under this heading.

Fluoxymesterone (Concurrent use of a steroid drug may increase the risk of stomach bleeding). Products include:
- Androxy Tablets 3335

Flurbiprofen (Concurrent use of non-steroidal anti- inflammatory drug may increase the risk of stomach bleeding.).
- No products indexed under this heading.

Flurbiprofen Sodium (Concurrent use of non- steroidal anti-inflammatory drug may increase the risk of stomach bleeding). Products include:
- Ocufen Ophthalmic Solution .... ⊙232

Fondaparinux Sodium (Concurrent use of an anticoagulant may increase the risk of stomach bleeding). Products include:
- Arixtra Injection 1351

Heparin Calcium (Concurrent use of an anticoagulant may increase the risk of stomach bleeding).
- No products indexed under this heading.

Heparin Sodium (Concurrent use of an anticoagulant may increase the risk of stomach bleeding).
- No products indexed under this heading.

Hydrocortisone (Concurrent use of a steroid drug may increase the risk of stomach bleeding). Products include:
- Colocort Rectal Suspension, USP (Retention) 100 mg/60 mL........... 2476
- Hydrocortone Tablets 1989
- Preparation H Hydrocortisone Cream .... ▣646

Hydrocortisone Acetate (Concurrent use of a steroid drug may increase the risk of stomach bleeding). Products include:
- Analpram-HC 1159
- Pramosone 1161
- ProctoFoam-HC 3099

Hydrocortisone Sodium Phosphate (Concurrent use of a steroid drug may increase the risk of stomach bleeding).
- No products indexed under this heading.

Hydrocortisone Sodium Succinate (Concurrent use of a steroid drug may increase the risk of stomach bleeding).
- No products indexed under this heading.

Indomethacin (Concurrent use of non-steroidal anti- inflammatory drug may increase the risk of stomach bleeding). Products include:
- Indocin 1995

Indomethacin Sodium Trihydrate (Concurrent use of non-steroidal anti- inflammatory drug may increase the risk of stomach bleeding). Products include:
- Indocin I.V. 2465

Ketoprofen (Concurrent use of non-steroidal anti- inflammatory drug may increase the risk of stomach bleeding.).
- No products indexed under this heading.

Ketorolac Tromethamine (Concurrent use of non-steroidal anti-inflammatory drug may increase the risk of stomach bleeding). Products include:
- Acular Ophthalmic Solution 565
- Acular LS Ophthalmic Solution 566

Levonorgestrel (Concurrent use of a steroid drug may increase the risk of stomach bleeding). Products include:
- Climara Pro Transdermal System 776
- Mirena Intrauterine System 787
- Plan B Tablets 1076
- Seasonique Tablets 1077

Low Molecular Weight Heparins (Concurrent use of an anticoagulant may increase the risk of stomach bleeding).
- No products indexed under this heading.

Meclofenamate Sodium (Concurrent use of non-steroidal anti- inflammatory drug may increase the risk of stomach bleeding.).
- No products indexed under this heading.

Mefenamic Acid (Concurrent use of non-steroidal anti- inflammatory drug may increase the risk of stomach bleeding.).
- No products indexed under this heading.

Meloxicam (Concurrent use of non-steroidal anti- inflammatory drug may increase the risk of stomach bleeding). Products include:
- Mobic Oral Suspension 863
- Mobic Tablets 863

Mestranol (Concurrent use of a steroid drug may increase the risk of stomach bleeding).
- No products indexed under this heading.

Methylprednisolone Acetate (Concurrent use of a steroid drug may increase the risk of stomach bleeding). Products include:
- Depo-Medrol Injectable Suspension 2617
- Depo-Medrol Single-Dose Vial 2619

Methylprednisolone Sodium Succinate (Concurrent use of a steroid drug may increase the risk of stomach bleeding).
- No products indexed under this heading.

Methyltestosterone (Concurrent use of a steroid drug may increase the risk of stomach bleeding). Products include:
- Estratest Tablets 3199
- Estratest H.S. Tablets 3199

Nabumetone (Concurrent use of non-steroidal anti- inflammatory drug may increase the risk of stomach bleeding.).
- No products indexed under this heading.

Naproxen (Concurrent use of non-steroidal anti- inflammatory drug may increase the risk of stomach bleeding). Products include:
- EC-Naprosyn Delayed-Release Tablets 2761
- Naprosyn Suspension 2761
- Naprosyn Tablets 2761
- Prevacid NapraPAC 3280

Naproxen Sodium (Concurrent use of non-steroidal anti- inflammatory drug may increase the risk of stomach bleeding). Products include:
- Aleve Caplets 742
- Aleve Gelcaps 743
- Aleve Tablets 743
- Aleve Cold & Sinus Caplets 744
- Anaprox Tablets 2761
- Anaprox DS Tablets 2761

Norethindrone (Concurrent use of a steroid drug may increase the risk of stomach bleeding). Products include:
- Ortho Micronor Tablets 2426

Norethindrone Acetate (Concurrent use of a steroid drug may increase the risk of stomach bleeding).
No products indexed under this heading.

Norgestimate (Concurrent use of a steroid drug may increase the risk of stomach bleeding). Products include:
Ortho-Cyclen/Ortho Tri-Cyclen 2429
Ortho Tri-Cyclen Lo Tablets 2436

Oxaprozin (Concurrent use of non-steroidal anti- inflammatory drug may increase the risk of stomach bleeding.).
No products indexed under this heading.

Phenylbutazone (Concurrent use of non-steroidal anti- inflammatory drug may increase the risk of stomach bleeding.).
No products indexed under this heading.

Piroxicam (Concurrent use of non-steroidal anti- inflammatory drug may increase the risk of stomach bleeding.).
No products indexed under this heading.

Prednisolone Acetate (Concurrent use of a steroid drug may increase the risk of stomach bleeding). Products include:
Blephamide Ophthalmic Ointment 568
Blephamide Ophthalmic Suspension................................. 569
Poly-Pred Ophthalmic Suspension .... ⊙233
Pred Forte Ophthalmic Suspension .... ⊙235
Pred Mild Ophthalmic Suspension .... ⊙238
Pred-G Ophthalmic Ointment .... ⊙237
Pred-G Ophthalmic Suspension ...... ⊙236

Prednisolone Sodium Phosphate (Concurrent use of a steroid drug may increase the risk of stomach bleeding).
No products indexed under this heading.

Prednisolone Tebutate (Concurrent use of a steroid drug may increase the risk of stomach bleeding).
No products indexed under this heading.

Prednisone (Concurrent use of a steroid drug may increase the risk of stomach bleeding).
No products indexed under this heading.

Rofecoxib (Concurrent use of non-steroidal anti- inflammatory drug may increase the risk of stomach bleeding.).
No products indexed under this heading.

Sulindac (Concurrent use of non-steroidal anti- inflammatory drug may increase the risk of stomach bleeding). Products include:
Clinoril Tablets 1924

Suprofen (Concurrent use of non-steroidal anti-inflammatory drug may increase the risk of stomach bleeding).
No products indexed under this heading.

Testosterone (Concurrent use of a steroid drug may increase the risk of stomach bleeding). Products include:
AndroGel 3329
Striant Mucoadhesive 1007
Testim 1% Gel 695

Tinzaparin Sodium (Concurrent use of an anticoagulant may increase the risk of stomach bleeding).
No products indexed under this heading.

Tolmetin Sodium (Concurrent use of non-steroidal anti- inflammatory drug may increase the risk of stomach bleeding.).
No products indexed under this heading.

Triamcinolone (Concurrent use of a steroid drug may increase the risk of stomach bleeding).
No products indexed under this heading.

Triamcinolone Acetonide (Concurrent use of a steroid drug may increase the risk of stomach bleeding). Products include:
Azmacort Inhalation Aerosol 1726
Nasacort AQ Nasal Spray 2922

Triamcinolone Diacetate (Concurrent use of a steroid drug may increase the risk of stomach bleeding).
No products indexed under this heading.

Triamcinolone Hexacetonide (Concurrent use of a steroid drug may increase the risk of stomach bleeding).
No products indexed under this heading.

Valdecoxib (Concurrent use of non-steroidal anti- inflammatory drug may increase the risk of stomach bleeding.).
No products indexed under this heading.

Warfarin Sodium (Concurrent use of an anticoagulant may increase the risk of stomach bleeding). Products include:
Coumadin for Injection 898
Coumadin Tablets 898

Food Interactions

Alcohol (Consumption of 3 or more alcoholic beverage the risk of stomach bleeding).

ADVIL MULTI-SYMPTOM COLD CAPLETS

(Chlorpheniramine Maleate, Ibuprofen, Pseudoephedrine Hydrochloride)................................. ■770
See Advil Allergy Sinus Caplets

ADVIL PM CAPLETS

(Diphenhydramine Citrate, Ibuprofen).. ■615
May interact with anticoagulants and certain other agents. Compounds in these categories include:

Anisindione (Increases the chance of stomach bleeding). Products include:
Miradon Tablets 3042

Ardeparin Sodium (Increases the chance of stomach bleeding).
No products indexed under this heading.

Dalteparin Sodium (Increases the chance of stomach bleeding). Products include:
Fragmin Injection 1097

Danaparoid Sodium (Increases the chance of stomach bleeding).
No products indexed under this heading.

Dicumarol (Increases the chance of stomach bleeding).
No products indexed under this heading.

Enoxaparin Sodium (Increases the chance of stomach bleeding). Products include:
Lovenox Injection 2915

Fondaparinux Sodium (Increases the chance of stomach bleeding). Products include:
Arixtra Injection 1351

Heparin Calcium (Increases the chance of stomach bleeding).
No products indexed under this heading.

Heparin Sodium (Increases the chance of stomach bleeding).
No products indexed under this heading.

Low Molecular Weight Heparins (Increases the chance of stomach bleeding).
No products indexed under this heading.

Tinzaparin Sodium (Increases the chance of stomach bleeding).
No products indexed under this heading.

Warfarin Sodium (Increases the chance of stomach bleeding). Products include:
Coumadin for Injection 898
Coumadin Tablets 898

Food Interactions

Alcohol (Having 3 or more alcoholic beverages will increase the chances of stomach bleeding).

ADVIL TABLETS

(Ibuprofen) .... ■674
See Advil Caplets

AEROBID INHALER SYSTEM

(Flunisolide) 1171
None cited in PDR database.

AEROBID-M INHALER SYSTEM

(Flunisolide) 1171
None cited in PDR database.

AEROCHAMBER PLUS AND AEROCHAMBER PLUS WITH MASK

(Spacer, Inhalation) 1173
None cited in PDR database.

AGENERASE CAPSULES

(Amprenavir) 1327
See Agenerase Oral Solution

AGENERASE ORAL SOLUTION

(Amprenavir) 1332
May interact with antacids containing aluminum, calcium and magnesium, calcium channel blockers, dexamethasone, ergot-containing drugs, oral hypoglycemic agents, insulin, oral contraceptives, phenytoin, protease inhibitors, quinidine, and certain other agents. Compounds in these categories include:

Acarbose (New onset diabetes mellitus, exacerbation of pre-existing diabetes mellitus, and hyperglycemia have been reported in HIV-infected patients receiving protease inhibitors; some patients may require dose adjustments). Products include:
Precose Tablets 751

Alprazolam (Increased benzodiazepine plasma concentrations; clinical significance is unknown; however, a decrease in benzodiazepine dose may be needed). Products include:
Niravam Orally Disintegrating Tablets 3092

Aluminum Carbonate (Antacids decrease amprenavir plasma concentrations; Agenerase should be taken at least one hour before or after antacids).
No products indexed under this heading.

Aluminum Hydroxide (Antacids decrease amprenavir plasma concentrations; Agenerase should be taken at least one hour before or after antacids). Products include:
Gaviscon Regular Strength Liquid .. ■658
Gaviscon Regular Strength Tablets.. ■658
Gaviscon Extra Strength Liquid ...... ■658
Gaviscon Extra Strength Tablets .... ■658
Maalox Regular Strength Antacid/Antigas Liquid.................. 2175
Maalox Max Maximum Strength Antacid/Anti-Gas Liquid................ 2176

Amiodarone Hydrochloride (Increases antiarrhythmics plasma concentrations).
No products indexed under this heading.

Amitriptyline Hydrochloride (Increase in tricyclic antidepressant plasma concentrations).
No products indexed under this heading.

Amlodipine Besylate (Increased calcium channel blockers plasma concentrations). Products include:
Caduet Tablets 2508
Lotrel Capsules 2249
Norvasc Tablets 2545

Amoxapine (Co-administration could result in serious and/or life-threatening drug interactions).
No products indexed under this heading.

Atorvastatin Calcium (Increased atorvastatin plasma concentrations). Products include:
Caduet Tablets 2508
Lipitor Tablets 2483

Bepridil Hydrochloride (Increases bepridil plasma concentrations; increased bepridil exposure may be associated with life-threatening reactions, such as cardiac arrhythmias).
No products indexed under this heading.

Carbamazepine (Decreases amprenavir plasma concentrations potentially reducing effectiveness of amprenavir). Products include:
Carbatrol Capsules 3171
Equetro Extended-Release Capsules.. 3180
Tegretol/Tegretol-XR 2295

Chlorpropamide (New onset diabetes mellitus, exacerbation of pre-existing diabetes mellitus, and hyperglycemia have been reported in HIV-infected patients receiving protease inhibitors; some patients may require dose adjustments).
No products indexed under this heading.

Cisapride (Co-administration of amprenavir is contraindicated with drugs that are highly dependant of CYP3A4 for clearance and for which elevated plasma concentrations are associated with serious and/or life-threatening events).
No products indexed under this heading.

Clarithromycin (Co-administration has resulted in 15% increase in Cmax, 18% increase in AUC, and 39% increase in Cmin of amprenavir;

10% decrease in clarithromycin Cmax was reported). Products include:

Clomipramine Hydrochloride (Co-administration could result in serious and/or life-threatening drug interactions).

No products indexed under this heading.

Clorazepate Dipotassium (Increased benzodiazepine plasma concentrations; clinical significance is unknown; however, a decrease in benzodiazepine dose may be needed). Products include:

Clozapine (May result in increased plasma concentrations of clozapine). Products include:

Cyclosporine (Increased immuno-suppressant plasma concentrations). Products include:

Dapsone (Co-administration with dapsone may result in increased plasma concentrations of dapsone). Products include:

Delavirdine Mesylate (Co-administration may lead to loss of virologic response and possible resistance to delavirdine. Co-administration has resulted in a 40% increase in Cmax, 130% increase in AUC, and 125% increase in Cmin of amprenavir. A 47% decrease in delavirdine Cmax, 61% decrease in delavirdine AUC, and 88% decrease in delavirdine Cmin). Products include:

Desogestrel (May lead to loss of virologic response and possible resistance to amprenavir; alternative methods of non-hormonal contraception are recommended). Products include:

Dexamethasone (Decreases amprenavir plasma concentrations potentially reducing effectiveness of amprenavir). Products include:

Dexamethasone Acetate (Decreases amprenavir plasma concentrations potentially reducing effectiveness of amprenavir).

No products indexed under this heading.

Dexamethasone Sodium Phosphate (Decreases amprenavir plasma concentrations potentially reducing effectiveness of amprenavir).

No products indexed under this heading.

Diazepam (Increased benzodiazepine plasma concentrations; clinical significance is unknown; however, a decrease in benzodiazepine dose may be needed). Products include:

Didanosine (Didanosine secondary to the antacid content has not been specifically studied; however, based upon data with other protease inhibitors, it is advisable that antacids not be taken at the same time as amprenavir because of potential interference with absorption; it is recommended that their administration be separated by at least an hour).

No products indexed under this heading.

Dihydroergotamine Mesylate (Co-administration of amprenavir is contraindicated with drugs that are highly dependant of CYP3A4, such as ergot derivatives, for clearance and for which elevated plasma concentrations are associated with serious and/or life-threatening events, such as acute ergot toxicity characterized by peripheral vasospasm and ischemia of the extremities and other tissues). Products include:

Diltiazem Hydrochloride (Increased calcium channel blockers plasma concentrations). Products include:

Disulfiram (Agenerase Oral Solution contains a large amount of propylene glycol and because of the potential risk of toxicity from the large amount of this excipient; co-administration with disulfiram is contraindicated).

No products indexed under this heading.

Ergonovine Maleate (Co-administration of amprenavir is contraindicated with drugs that are highly dependant of CYP3A4, such as ergot derivatives, for clearance and for which elevated plasma concentrations are associated with serious and/or life-threatening events, such as acute ergot toxicity characterized by peripheral vasospasm and ischemia of the extremities and other tissues).

No products indexed under this heading.

Ergotamine Tartrate (Co-administration of amprenavir is contraindicated with drugs that are highly dependant of CYP3A4, such as ergot derivatives, for clearance and for which elevated plasma concentrations are associated with serious and/or life-threatening events, such as acute ergot toxicity characterized by peripheral vasospasm and ischemia of the extremities and other tissues).

No products indexed under this heading.

Ethinyl Estradiol (Co-administration has resulted in a 22% decrease in AUC and 20% decrease in Cmin of amprenavir. Ethinyl estradiol Cmin also increased 32%). Products include:

Ethynodiol Diacetate (May lead to loss of virologic response and possible resistance to amprenavir; alternative methods of non-hormonal contraception are recommended).

No products indexed under this heading.

Felodipine (Increased calcium channel blockers plasma concentrations).

No products indexed under this heading.

Flecainide Acetate (If amprenavir is co-administered with ritonavir capsules, concurrent use of flecainide is contraindicated). Products include:

Flurazepam Hydrochloride (Increased benzodiazepine plasma concentrations; clinical significance is unknown; however, a decrease in benzodiazepine dose may be needed). Products include:

Fluticasone Propionate (Concurrent use will result in significantly decreased serum cortisol concentrations). Products include:

Fosphenytoin Sodium (Decreases amprenavir plasma concentrations potentially reducing effectiveness of amprenavir).

No products indexed under this heading.

Glimepiride (New onset diabetes mellitus, exacerbation of pre-existing diabetes mellitus, and hyperglycemia have been reported in HIV-infected patients receiving protease inhibitors; some patients may require dose adjustments). Products include:

Glipizide (New onset diabetes mellitus, exacerbation of pre-existing diabetes mellitus, and hyperglycemia have been reported in HIV-infected patients receiving protease inhibitors; some patients may require dose adjustments).

No products indexed under this heading.

Glyburide (New onset diabetes mellitus, exacerbation of pre-existing diabetes mellitus, and hyperglycemia have been reported in HIV-infected patients receiving protease inhibitors; some patients may require dose adjustments).

No products indexed under this heading.

Hypericum (Co-administration of amprenavir and St. John's Wort or products containing St. John's Wort is expected to substantially decrease protease inhibitor concentrations and may result in suboptimal levels of amprenavir and lead to loss of virologic response and possible resistance to amprenavir; concurrent use is not recommended). Products include:

Imipramine Hydrochloride (Increase in tricyclic antidepressant plasma concentrations).

No products indexed under this heading.

Imipramine Pamoate (Increase in tricyclic antidepressant plasma concentrations).

No products indexed under this heading.

Indinavir Sulfate (Increases amprenavir plasma concentrations). Products include:

Insulin, Human, Zinc Suspension (New onset diabetes mellitus, exacerbation of pre-existing diabetes mellitus, and hyperglycemia have been reported in HIV-infected patients receiving protease inhibitors; some patients may require dose adjustments). Products include:

Insulin, Human NPH (New onset diabetes mellitus, exacerbation of pre-existing diabetes mellitus, and hyperglycemia have been reported in HIV-infected patients receiving protease inhibitors; some patients may require dose adjustments). Products include:

Insulin, Human Regular (New onset diabetes mellitus, exacerbation of pre-existing diabetes mellitus, and hyperglycemia have been reported in HIV-infected patients receiving protease inhibitors; some patients may require dose adjustments). Products include:

Insulin, Human Regular and Human NPH Mixture (New onset diabetes mellitus, exacerbation of pre-existing diabetes mellitus, and hyperglycemia have been reported in HIV-infected patients receiving protease inhibitors; some patients may require dose adjustments). Products include:

Insulin, NPH (New onset diabetes mellitus, exacerbation of pre-existing diabetes mellitus, and hyperglycemia have been reported in HIV-infected patients receiving protease inhibitors; some patients may require dose adjustments).

No products indexed under this heading.

Insulin, Regular (New onset diabetes mellitus, exacerbation of pre-existing diabetes mellitus, and hyperglycemia have been reported in HIV-infected patients receiving protease inhibitors; some patients may require dose adjustments).

No products indexed under this heading.

Insulin, Zinc Crystals (New onset diabetes mellitus, exacerbation of pre-existing diabetes mellitus, and hyperglycemia have been reported in HIV-infected patients receiving protease inhibitors; some patients may require dose adjustments).

No products indexed under this heading.

IMPORTANT NOTE: Always consult each drug listing in the patient's regimen for possible interactions.

Insulin, Zinc Suspension (New onset diabetes mellitus, exacerbation of pre-existing diabetes mellitus, and hyperglycemia have been reported in HIV-infected patients receiving protease inhibitors; some patients may require dose adjustments).
No products indexed under this heading.

Insulin Aspart, Human Regular (New onset diabetes mellitus, exacerbation of pre-existing diabetes mellitus, and hyperglycemia have been reported in HIV-infected patients receiving protease inhibitors; some patients may require dose adjustments). Products include:
NovoLog Injection 2326

Insulin glargine (New onset diabetes mellitus, exacerbation of pre-existing diabetes mellitus, and hyperglycemia have been reported in HIV-infected patients receiving protease inhibitors; some patients may require dose adjustments). Products include:
Lantus Injection 2909

Insulin Lispro, Human (New onset diabetes mellitus, exacerbation of pre-existing diabetes mellitus, and hyperglycemia have been reported in HIV-infected patients receiving protease inhibitors; some patients may require dose adjustments). Products include:
Humalog-Pen 1781
Humalog Mix 50/50-Pen 1783
Humalog Mix 75/25-Pen 1785

Insulin Lispro Protamine, Human (New onset diabetes mellitus, exacerbation of pre-existing diabetes mellitus, and hyperglycemia have been reported in HIV-infected patients receiving protease inhibitors; some patients may require dose adjustments). Products include:
Humalog Mix 50/50-Pen 1783
Humalog Mix 75/25-Pen 1785

Isradipine (Increased calcium channel blockers plasma concentrations). Products include:
DynaCirc CR Tablets 2721

Itraconazole (Increased itraconazole plasma concentrations; dose reduction of itraconazole may be needed for patients receiving more than 400 mg itraconazole per day).
No products indexed under this heading.

Ketoconazole (Increased ketoconazole plasma concentrations; dose reduction of ketoconazole may be needed for patients receiving more than 400 mg ketoconazole per day). Products include:
Nizoral A-D Shampoo, 1% 1868

Levonorgestrel (May lead to loss of virologic response and possible resistance to amprenavir; alternative methods of non-hormonal contraception are recommended). Products include:
Climara Pro Transdermal System 776
Mirena Intrauterine System 787
Plan B Tablets 1076
Seasonique Tablets 1077

Lidocaine Hydrochloride (Increases antiarrhythmics plasma concentrations).
No products indexed under this heading.

Lopinavir (Increases amprenavir plasma concentrations). Products include:
Kaletra 476

Loratadine (May result in increased plasma concentrations of loratadine). Products include:
Alavert Allergy & Sinus D-12 Hour Tablets .... ▣771
Alavert .... ▣771
Children's Claritin Allergy Oral Solution .... ▣771
Claritin Non-Drowsy 24 Hour Tablets .... ▣772
Claritin Reditabs 24 Hour Non-Drowsy Tablets .... ▣772
Claritin-D Non-Drowsy 12 Hour Tablets .... ▣772
Claritin-D Non-Drowsy 24 Hour Tablets .... ▣772

Lovastatin (Co-administration increases the serum concentrations of lovastatin resulting in increased activity as well as toxicity, such as myopathy and rhabdomyolysis; concurrent use is not recommended). Products include:
Advicor Tablets 1722
Altoprev Extended-Release Tablets 3109
Mevacor Tablets 2021

Magaldrate (Antacids decrease amprenavir plasma concentrations; Agenerase should be taken at least one hour before or after antacids).
No products indexed under this heading.

Magnesium Hydroxide (Antacids decrease amprenavir plasma concentrations; Agenerase should be taken at least one hour before or after antacids). Products include:
Maalox Regular Strength Antacid/Antigas Liquid 2175
Maalox Max Maximum Strength Antacid/Anti-Gas Liquid 2176
Pepcid Complete Chewable Tablets 1701

Magnesium Oxide (Antacids decrease amprenavir plasma concentrations; Agenerase should be taken at least one hour before or after antacids). Products include:
Beelith Tablets 759
PremCal Light, Regular, and Extra Strength Tablets .... ▣818

Mestranol (May lead to loss of virologic response and possible resistance to amprenavir; alternative methods of non-hormonal contraception are recommended).
No products indexed under this heading.

Metformin Hydrochloride (New onset diabetes mellitus, exacerbation of pre-existing diabetes mellitus, and hyperglycemia have been reported in HIV-infected patients receiving protease inhibitors; some patients may require dose adjustments). Products include:
ActoPlus Met Tablets 3214
Avandamet Tablets 1373
Fortamet Extended-Release Tablets 3115

Methadone Hydrochloride (Co-administration of amprenavir and methadone can decrease plasma levels of methadone. Co-administration of amprenavir and methadone as compared to a non-matched historical control group resulted in a 30%, 27% and 25% decrease in serum amprenavir AUC, Cmax and Cmin, respectively. Alternative antiretroviral therapy should be considered).
No products indexed under this heading.

Methylergonovine Maleate (Co-administration of amprenavir is contraindicated with drugs that are highly dependant of CYP3A4, such as ergot derivatives, for clearance and for which elevated plasma concentrations are associated with serious and/or life-threatening events, such as acute ergot toxicity characterized by peripheral vasospasm and ischemia of the extremities and other tissues).
No products indexed under this heading.

Methysergide Maleate (Co-administration of amprenavir is contraindicated with drugs that are highly dependant of CYP3A4, such as ergot derivatives, for clearance and for which elevated plasma concentrations are associated with serious and/or life-threatening events, such as acute ergot toxicity characterized by peripheral vasospasm and ischemia of the extremities and other tissues).
No products indexed under this heading.

Metronidazole (Agenerase Oral Solution contains a large amount of propylene glycol and because of the potential risk of toxicity from the large amount of this excipient; co-administration with metronidazole is contraindicated). Products include:
Metrogel 1% 1211
MetroGel-Vaginal Gel 1855
Vandazole Vaginal Gel 3338

Metronidazole Hydrochloride (Agenerase Oral Solution contains a large amount of propylene glycol and because of the potential risk of toxicity from the large amount of this excipient; co-administration with metronidazole is contraindicated).
No products indexed under this heading.

Mibefradil Dihydrochloride (Increased calcium channel blockers plasma concentrations).
No products indexed under this heading.

Midazolam Hydrochloride (Co-administration of amprenavir is contraindicated with drugs that are highly dependant of CYP3A4 for clearance and for which elevated plasma concentrations are associated with serious and/or life-threatening events, such as prolonged or increased sedation or respiratory depression).
No products indexed under this heading.

Miglitol (New onset diabetes mellitus, exacerbation of pre-existing diabetes mellitus, and hyperglycemia have been reported in HIV-infected patients receiving protease inhibitors; some patients may require dose adjustments).
No products indexed under this heading.

Nelfinavir Mesylate (Increases amprenavir plasma concentrations). Products include:
Viracept 2577

Nicardipine Hydrochloride (Increased calcium channel blockers plasma concentrations). Products include:
Cardene I.V. 2497

Nifedipine (Increased calcium channel blockers plasma concentrations). Products include:
Adalat CC Tablets 2964

Nimodipine (Increased calcium channel blockers plasma concentrations). Products include:
Nimotop Capsules 749

Nisoldipine (Increased calcium channel blockers plasma concentrations). Products include:
Sular Tablets 3122

Norethindrone (Co-administration has resulted in a 22% decrease in AUC and 20% decrease in Cmin of amprenavir. Norethindrone AUC and Cmin increased 18% and 45%, respectively). Products include:
Ortho Micronor Tablets 2426

Norethynodrel (May lead to loss of virologic response and possible resistance to amprenavir; alternative methods of non-hormonal contraception are recommended).
No products indexed under this heading.

Norgestimate (May lead to loss of virologic response and possible resistance to amprenavir; alternative methods of non-hormonal contraception are recommended). Products include:
Ortho-Cyclen/Ortho Tri-Cyclen 2429
Ortho Tri-Cyclen Lo Tablets 2436

Norgestrel (May lead to loss of virologic response and possible resistance to amprenavir; alternative methods of non-hormonal contraception are recommended).
No products indexed under this heading.

Phenobarbital (Decreases amprenavir plasma concentrations potentially reducing effectiveness of amprenavir). Products include:
Donnatal Extentabs 2493

Phenytoin (Decreases amprenavir plasma concentrations potentially reducing effectiveness of amprenavir).
No products indexed under this heading.

Phenytoin Sodium (Decreases amprenavir plasma concentrations potentially reducing effectiveness of amprenavir). Products include:
Phenytek Capsules 2160

Pimozide (Co-administration of amprenavir is contraindicated with drugs that are highly dependant of CYP3A4 for clearance and for which elevated plasma concentrations are associated with serious and/or life-threatening events, such as cardiac arrhythmias).
No products indexed under this heading.

Pioglitazone Hydrochloride (New onset diabetes mellitus, exacerbation of pre-existing diabetes mellitus, and hyperglycemia have been reported in HIV-infected patients receiving protease inhibitors; some patients may require dose adjustments). Products include:
ActoPlus Met Tablets 3214
Actos Tablets 3219
Duetact Tablets 3226

Pravastatin Sodium (Co-administration increases the serum concentrations of pravastatin resulting in increased activity as well as toxicity, such as myopathy and rhabdomyolysis; caution should be exercised if used concurrently).
No products indexed under this heading.

Propafenone Hydrochloride (If amprenavir is co-administered with ritonavir capsules; concurrent use of propafenone is contraindicated). Products include:

Rythmol SR Capsules 2727

Protriptyline Hydrochloride (Co-administration could result in serious and/or life-threatening drug interactions).

No products indexed under this heading.

Quinidine (Increases quinidine plasma concentrations; caution is warranted and therapeutic monitoring is recommended).

No products indexed under this heading.

Quinidine Gluconate (Increases quinidine plasma concentrations; caution is warranted and therapeutic monitoring is recommended).

No products indexed under this heading.

Quinidine Hydrochloride (Increases quinidine plasma concentrations; caution is warranted and therapeutic monitoring is recommended).

No products indexed under this heading.

Quinidine Polygalacturonate (Increases quinidine plasma concentrations; caution is warranted and therapeutic monitoring is recommended).

No products indexed under this heading.

Quinidine Sulfate (Increases quinidine plasma concentrations; caution is warranted and therapeutic monitoring is recommended).

No products indexed under this heading.

Rapamycin (Increased immunosuppressant plasma concentrations).

No products indexed under this heading.

Repaglinide (New onset diabetes mellitus, exacerbation of pre-existing diabetes mellitus, and hyperglycemia have been reported in HIV-infected patients receiving protease inhibitors; some patients may require dose adjustments).

No products indexed under this heading.

Rifabutin (Increased rifabutin and rifabutin metabolite plasma concentrations; dosage reduction of rifabutin to at least half the recommended dose is required when used concurrently).

No products indexed under this heading.

Rifampin (Co-administration may lead to loss of virologic response and possible resistance to amprenavir or the class of protease inhibitors).

No products indexed under this heading.

Ritonavir (Concurrent use of Agenerase Oral Solution and Norvir Oral Solution is not recommended because the large amount of propylene glycol in Agenerase Oral Solution and ethanol in Norvir Oral Solution may compete for the same metabolic pathway for elimination; concurrent use has been associated with elevation of ALT and AST as well as cholesterol and triglycerides). Products include:

Kaletra 476
Norvir 503

Rosiglitazone Maleate (New onset diabetes mellitus, exacerbation of pre-existing diabetes mellitus, and hyperglycemia have been reported in HIV-infected patients receiving protease inhibitors; some patients may require dose adjustments). Products include:

Avandamet Tablets 1373
Avandaryl Tablets 1379
Avandia Tablets 1384

Saquinavir (Decreases amprenavir plasma concentrations).

No products indexed under this heading.

Saquinavir Mesylate (Decreases amprenavir plasma concentrations). Products include:

Invirase 2772

Sildenafil Citrate (Increase in sildenafil plasma concentrations; use with caution at reduced doses of 25 mg every 48 hours with increased monitoring for adverse events). Products include:

Revatio Tablets 2557
Viagra Tablets 2573

Simvastatin (Co-administration increases the serum concentrations of simvastatin resulting in increased activity as well as toxicity, such as myopathy and rhabdomyolysis; concurrent use is not recommended). Products include:

Vytorin 10/10 Tablets 2114
Vytorin 10/10 Tablets 3077
Vytorin 10/20 Tablets 2114
Vytorin 10/20 Tablets 3077
Vytorin 10/40 Tablets 2114
Vytorin 10/40 Tablets 3077
Vytorin 10/80 Tablets 2114
Vytorin 10/80 Tablets 3077
Zocor Tablets 2105

Tacrolimus (Increased immunosuppressant plasma concentrations). Products include:

Prograf Capsules and Injection 632
Protopic Ointment 638

Tolazamide (New onset diabetes mellitus, exacerbation of pre-existing diabetes mellitus, and hyperglycemia have been reported in HIV-infected patients receiving protease inhibitors; some patients may require dose adjustments).

No products indexed under this heading.

Tolbutamide (New onset diabetes mellitus, exacerbation of pre-existing diabetes mellitus, and hyperglycemia have been reported in HIV-infected patients receiving protease inhibitors; some patients may require dose adjustments).

No products indexed under this heading.

Trazodone Hydrochloride (Concomitant use may increase plasma concentrations of trazodone).

No products indexed under this heading.

Triazolam (Co-administration of amprenavir is contraindicated with drugs that are highly dependant of CYP3A4 for clearance and for which elevated plasma concentrations are associated with serious and/or life-threatening events, such as prolonged or increased sedation or respiratory depression).

No products indexed under this heading.

Trimipramine Maleate (Co-administration could result in serious and/or life-threatening drug interactions).

No products indexed under this heading.

Troglitazone (New onset diabetes mellitus, exacerbation of pre-existing diabetes mellitus, and hyperglycemia have been reported in HIV-infected patients receiving protease inhibitors; some patients may require dose adjustments).

No products indexed under this heading.

Verapamil Hydrochloride (Increased calcium channel blockers plasma concentrations). Products include:

Covera-HS Tablets 3139
Tarka Tablets 524
Verelan PM Extended-Release Capsules, Controlled-Onset...... 3106

Vitamin E (Amprenavir formulations contain large amounts of vitamin E; high vitamin E doses may exacerbate the blood coagulation defect of vitamin K deficiency caused by anticoagulant therapy; concurrent use with additional vitamin E should be avoided). Products include:

Bausch & Lomb Ocuvite Adult Eye Vitamin and Mineral Supplement Soft Gels...... 706
Bausch & Lomb Ocuvite Adult 50+ Eye Vitamin and Mineral Supplement Soft Gels...... 706
MarineOmega Softgel Capsules 2672
Ocuvite Adult Vitamin and Mineral Supplement...... 253
Ocuvite Adult 50+ Vitamin and Mineral Supplement...... 253

Warfarin Sodium (Concentrations of warfarin may be affected with concurrent use; monitor INR). Products include:

Coumadin for Injection 898
Coumadin Tablets 898

Zidovudine (Co-administration has resulted in 13% increase in AUC of amprenavir; 40% increase in Cmax and 31% increase in AUC for zidovudine have been reported). Products include:

Combivir Tablets 1411
Retrovir 1560
Retrovir IV Infusion 1564
Trizivir Tablets 1589

Food Interactions

Alcohol (Concurrent use of Agenerase Oral Solution with alcoholic beverages is not recommended).

Food, unspecified (High-fat meals may decrease the absorption of Agenerase and should be avoided; Agenerase may be taken with meals of normal fat content).

AGGRASTAT INJECTION

(Tirofiban Hydrochloride) 1907

May interact with glycoprotein (GP) IIb/IIIa inhibitors and certain other agents. Compounds in these categories include:

Abciximab (Concomitant use with another parenteral GP IIb/IIIa inhibitor is contraindicated). Products include:

ReoPro Vials 1809

Aspirin (The use of tirofiban in combination with aspirin has been associated with an increase in bleeding compared to aspirin alone). Products include:

Aggrenox Capsules 822
Bayer Aspirin 744
BC Allergy Sinus Cold Powder 677
BC Headache Powder 677
Arthritis Strength BC Powder 677
BC Sinus Cold Powder 677
Excedrin Extra Strength Caplets/Tablets/Geltabs...... 684
Excedrin Migraine Caplets/Tablets/Geltabs...... 609
Goody's Body Pain Formula Powder...... 684
Goody's Extra Strength Headache Powders...... 611
Goody's Extra Strength Pain Relief Tablets...... 685
Percodan Tablets 1132
St. Joseph 81 mg Aspirin Chewable and Enteric Coated Tablets...... 1869

Eptifibatide (Concomitant use with another parenteral GP IIb/IIIa inhibitor is contraindicated). Products include:

Integrilin Injection 3020

Heparin Sodium (The use of tirofiban in combination with heparin has been associated with an increase in bleeding compared to heparin alone).

No products indexed under this heading.

Levothyroxine Sodium (Co-administration has resulted in a higher rate of clearance of tirofiban; the clinical significance of this is unknown). Products include:

Levothroid Tablets 1186
Levoxyl Tablets 1712
Synthroid Tablets 520
Westhroid Tablets 3403

Omeprazole (Co-administration has resulted in a higher rate of clearance of tirofiban; the clinical significance of this is unknown). Products include:

Zegerid Capsules 2958
Zegerid Powder for Oral Solution 2958

AGGRASTAT INJECTION PREMIXED

(Tirofiban Hydrochloride) 1907

See Aggrastat Injection

AGGRENOX CAPSULES

(Aspirin, Dipyridamole) 822

May interact with ACE inhibitors, anticholinesterase drugs, beta blockers, anticoagulants, diuretics, oral hypoglycemic agents, non-steroidal anti-inflammatory agents, phenytoin, valproate, and certain other agents. Compounds in these categories include:

Acarbose (Moderate doses of aspirin may increase the effectiveness of renal hypoglycemic drugs, leading to hypoglycemia). Products include:

Precose Tablets 751

Acebutolol Hydrochloride (The hypertensive effects of beta-blockers may be diminished by the concomitant administration of aspirin due to inhibition of renal prostaglandins, leading to decreased renal blood flow and salt and fluid retention).

No products indexed under this heading.

Acetazolamide (Co-administration can lead to high serum concentrations of acetazolamide (and toxicity) due to competition at the renal tube for secretion).

No products indexed under this heading.

Acetazolamide Sodium (Co-administration can lead to high serum concentrations of acetazolamide (and toxicity) due to competition at the renal tube for secretion).

No products indexed under this heading.

Adenosine (Dipyridamole has been reported to increase the plasma levels and cardiovascular effects of adenosine). Products include:

Adenocard Injection 617

Adenoscan 619

Amiloride Hydrochloride (The effectiveness of diuretics in patients with underlying renal or cardiovascular disease may be diminished by co-administration of aspirin due to inhibition of renal prostaglandins, leading to decreased renal blood flow and salt and fluid retention). Products include:
- Midamor Tablets 2026
- Moduretic Tablets 2028

Anisindione (Patients on anticoagulation therapy are at risk for bleeding). Products include:
- Miradon Tablets 3042

Ardeparin Sodium (Patients on anticoagulation therapy are at risk for bleeding).
No products indexed under this heading.

Atenolol (The hypertensive effects of beta-blockers may be diminished by the concomitant administration of aspirin due to inhibition of renal prostaglandins, leading to decreased renal blood flow and salt and fluid retention).
No products indexed under this heading.

Benazepril Hydrochloride (Co-administration can result in diminished hypotensive and hyponatremic effects of ACE inhibitors due to the effect of aspirin on the renin-angiotensin conversion pathway). Products include:
- Lotensin Tablets 2243
- Lotensin HCT Tablets 2246
- Lotrel Capsules 2249

Bendroflumethiazide (The effectiveness of diuretics in patients with underlying renal or cardiovascular disease may be diminished by co-administration of aspirin due to inhibition of renal prostaglandins, leading to decreased renal blood flow and salt and fluid retention).
No products indexed under this heading.

Betaxolol Hydrochloride (The hypertensive effects of beta-blockers may be diminished by the concomitant administration of aspirin due to inhibition of renal prostaglandins, leading to decreased renal blood flow and salt and fluid retention). Products include:
- Betoptic S Ophthalmic Suspension 558

Bisoprolol Fumarate (The hypertensive effects of beta-blockers may be diminished by the concomitant administration of aspirin due to inhibition of renal prostaglandins, leading to decreased renal blood flow and salt and fluid retention).
No products indexed under this heading.

Bumetanide (The effectiveness of diuretics in patients with underlying renal or cardiovascular disease may be diminished by co-administration of aspirin due to inhibition of renal prostaglandins, leading to decreased renal blood flow and salt and fluid retention). Products include:
- Bumex Tablets 2746

Captopril (Co-administration can result in diminished hypotensive and hyponatremic effects of ACE inhibitors due to the effect of aspirin on the renin-angiotensin conversion pathway). Products include:
- Captopril Tablets 2149

Carteolol Hydrochloride (The hypertensive effects of beta-blockers may be diminished by the concomitant administration of aspirin due to inhibition of renal prostaglandins, leading to decreased renal blood flow and salt and fluid retention). Products include:
- Carteolol Hydrochloride Ophthalmic Solution USP, 1%....... ⊙ 249

Celecoxib (Co-administration of non-steroidal anti-inflammatory drugs with aspirin may increase bleeding or lead to decreased renal function). Products include:
- Celebrex Capsules 3134

Chlorothiazide (The effectiveness of diuretics in patients with underlying renal or cardiovascular disease may be diminished by co-administration of aspirin due to inhibition of renal prostaglandins, leading to decreased renal blood flow and salt and fluid retention). Products include:
- Diuril Oral Suspension 1954

Chlorothiazide Sodium (The effectiveness of diuretics in patients with underlying renal or cardiovascular disease may be diminished by co-administration of aspirin due to inhibition of renal prostaglandins, leading to decreased renal blood flow and salt and fluid retention). Products include:
- Diuril Sodium Intravenous 2467

Chlorpropamide (Moderate doses of aspirin may increase the effectiveness of renal hypoglycemic drugs, leading to hypoglycemia).
No products indexed under this heading.

Chlorthalidone (The effectiveness of diuretics in patients with underlying renal or cardiovascular disease may be diminished by co-administration of aspirin due to inhibition of renal prostaglandins, leading to decreased renal blood flow and salt and fluid retention). Products include:
- Clorpres Tablets 2153

Dalteparin Sodium (Patients on anticoagulation therapy are at risk for bleeding). Products include:
- Fragmin Injection 1097

Danaparoid Sodium (Patients on anticoagulation therapy are at risk for bleeding).
No products indexed under this heading.

Diclofenac Potassium (Co-administration of non-steroidal anti-inflammatory drugs with aspirin may increase bleeding or lead to decreased renal function).
No products indexed under this heading.

Diclofenac Sodium (Co-administration of non-steroidal anti-inflammatory drugs with aspirin may increase bleeding or lead to decreased renal function). Products include:
- Arthrotec Tablets 3129
- Voltaren Ophthalmic Solution 2309
- Voltaren Tablets 2307
- Voltaren-XR Tablets 2310

Dicumarol (Patients on anticoagulation therapy are at risk for bleeding).
No products indexed under this heading.

Divalproex Sodium (Salicylic acid can displace protein-bound valproic acid leading to an increase in serum valproic acid levels). Products include:
- Depakote Sprinkle Capsules 422
- Depakote Tablets 427
- Depakote ER Tablets 434

Donepezil Hydrochloride (Dipyridamole may counteract the anticholinesterase effect of cholinesterase inhibitors, thereby potentially aggravating myasthenia gravis). Products include:
- Aricept Tablets 1094
- Aricept ODT Tablets 1094

Enalapril Maleate (Co-administration can result in diminished hypotensive and hyponatremic effects of ACE inhibitors due to the effect of aspirin on the renin-angiotensin conversion pathway). Products include:
- Vasotec I.V. Injection 2103

Enalaprilat (Co-administration can result in diminished hypotensive and hyponatremic effects of ACE inhibitors due to the effect of aspirin on the renin-angiotensin conversion pathway).
No products indexed under this heading.

Enoxaparin Sodium (Patients on anticoagulation therapy are at risk for bleeding). Products include:
- Lovenox Injection 2915

Esmolol Hydrochloride (The hypertensive effects of beta-blockers may be diminished by the concomitant administration of aspirin due to inhibition of renal prostaglandins, leading to decreased renal blood flow and salt and fluid retention).
No products indexed under this heading.

Ethacrynic Acid (The effectiveness of diuretics in patients with underlying renal or cardiovascular disease may be diminished by co-administration of aspirin due to inhibition of renal prostaglandins, leading to decreased renal blood flow and salt and fluid retention). Products include:
- Edecrin Tablets 1959

Etodolac (Co-administration of non-steroidal anti-inflammatory drugs with aspirin may increase bleeding or lead to decreased renal function).
No products indexed under this heading.

Fenoprofen Calcium (Co-administration of non-steroidal anti-inflammatory drugs with aspirin may increase bleeding or lead to decreased renal function). Products include:
- Nalfon Capsules 2502

Flurbiprofen (Co-administration of non-steroidal anti-inflammatory drugs with aspirin may increase bleeding or lead to decreased renal function).
No products indexed under this heading.

Fondaparinux Sodium (Patients on anticoagulation therapy are at risk for bleeding). Products include:
- Arixtra Injection 1351

Fosinopril Sodium (Co-administration can result in diminished hypotensive and hyponatremic effects of ACE inhibitors due to the effect of aspirin on the renin-angiotensin conversion pathway).
No products indexed under this heading.

Fosphenytoin Sodium (Salicylic acid can displace protein-bound phenytoin leading to a decrease in the total concentration of phenytoin).
No products indexed under this heading.

Furosemide (The effectiveness of diuretics in patients with underlying renal or cardiovascular disease may be diminished by co-administration of aspirin due to inhibition of renal prostaglandins, leading to decreased renal blood flow and salt and fluid retention). Products include:
- Furosemide Tablets 2154

Galantamine Hydrobromide (Dipyridamole may counteract the anticholinesterase effect of cholinesterase inhibitors, thereby potentially aggravating myasthenia gravis). Products include:
- Razadyne 2399
- Razadyne ER Extended-Release Capsules 2399

Glimepiride (Moderate doses of aspirin may increase the effectiveness of renal hypoglycemic drugs, leading to hypoglycemia). Products include:
- Avandaryl Tablets 1379
- Duetact Tablets 3226

Glipizide (Moderate doses of aspirin may increase the effectiveness of renal hypoglycemic drugs, leading to hypoglycemia).
No products indexed under this heading.

Glyburide (Moderate doses of aspirin may increase the effectiveness of renal hypoglycemic drugs, leading to hypoglycemia).
No products indexed under this heading.

Heparin Calcium (Patients on anticoagulation therapy are at risk for bleeding).
No products indexed under this heading.

Heparin Sodium (Aspirin can increase the anticoagulant activity of heparin, increasing bleeding risk).
No products indexed under this heading.

Hydrochlorothiazide (The effectiveness of diuretics in patients with underlying renal or cardiovascular disease may be diminished by co-administration of aspirin due to inhibition of renal prostaglandins, leading to decreased renal blood flow and salt and fluid retention). Products include:
- Aldoril Tablets 1910
- Atacand HCT 651
- Avalide Tablets 888
- Avalide Tablets 2874
- Benicar HCT Tablets 1044
- Diovan HCT Tablets 2196
- Dyazide Capsules 1423
- Hyzaar 50-12.5 Tablets 1990
- Hyzaar 100-12.5 Tablets 1990
- Hyzaar 100-25 Tablets 1990
- Lopressor HCT 50/25 Tablets 2241
- Lopressor HCT 100/25 Tablets 2241
- Lopressor HCT 100/50 Tablets 2241
- Lotensin HCT Tablets 2246
- Micardis HCT Tablets 856
- Moduretic Tablets 2028
- Prinzide Tablets 2056
- Teveten HCT Tablets 1737
- Timolide Tablets 2086
- Uniretic Tablets 3100

Hydroflumethiazide (The effectiveness of diuretics in patients with underlying renal or cardiovascular disease may be diminished by co-administration of aspirin due to inhibition of renal prostaglandins, leading to decreased renal blood flow and salt and fluid retention).
No products indexed under this heading.

Ibuprofen (Co-administration of non-steroidal anti-inflammatory drugs with aspirin may increase bleeding or lead to decreased renal function). Products include:
- Advil Allergy Sinus Caplets .... ▣ 770
- Advil .... ▣ 674
- Children's Advil Oral Suspension .... ▣ 603
- Children's Advil Chewable Tablets .... ▣ 603
- Advil Cold & Sinus .... ▣ 723
- Infants' Advil Concentrated Drops .... ▣ 604
- Infants' Advil Concentrated Drops - White Grape (Dye-Free) .... ▣ 604
- Junior Strength Advil Swallow Tablets .... ▣ 605
- Advil Migraine Liquigels .... ▣ 608
- Advil Multi-Symptom Cold Caplets .... ▣ 770
- Advil PM Caplets .... ▣ 615
- Motrin IB Tablets and Caplets 1866
- Children's Motrin Oral Suspension 1867
- Children's Motrin Non-Staining Dye-Free Oral Suspension 1867
- Children's Motrin Cold Oral Suspension 1867
- Infants' Motrin Concentrated Drops 1867
- Infants' Motrin Non-Staining Dye-Free Concentrated Drops 1867
- Junior Strength Motrin Caplets and Chewable Tablets 1867
- Vicoprofen Tablets 539

Indapamide (The effectiveness of diuretics in patients with underlying renal or cardiovascular disease may be diminished by co-administration of aspirin due to inhibition of renal prostaglandins, leading to decreased renal blood flow and salt and fluid retention). Products include:
- Indapamide Tablets 2156

Indomethacin (Co-administration of non-steroidal anti-inflammatory drugs with aspirin may increase bleeding or lead to decreased renal function). Products include:
- Indocin 1995

Indomethacin Sodium Trihydrate (Co-administration of non-steroidal anti-inflammatory drugs with aspirin may increase bleeding or lead to decreased renal function). Products include:
- Indocin I.V. 2465

Ketoprofen (Co-administration of non-steroidal anti-inflammatory drugs with aspirin may increase bleeding or lead to decreased renal function).
No products indexed under this heading.

Ketorolac Tromethamine (Co-administration of non-steroidal anti-inflammatory drugs with aspirin may increase bleeding or lead to decreased renal function). Products include:
- Acular Ophthalmic Solution 565
- Acular LS Ophthalmic Solution 566

Labetalol Hydrochloride (The hypertensive effects of beta-blockers may be diminished by the concomitant administration of aspirin due to inhibition of renal prostaglandins, leading to decreased renal blood flow and salt and fluid retention).
No products indexed under this heading.

Levobunolol Hydrochloride (The hypertensive effects of beta-blockers may be diminished by the concomitant administration of aspirin due to inhibition of renal prostaglandins, leading to decreased renal blood flow and salt and fluid retention). Products include:
- Betagan Ophthalmic Solution, USP .... ⊙ 220

Lisinopril (Co-administration can result in diminished hypotensive and hyponatremic effects of ACE inhibitors due to the effect of aspirin on the renin-angiotensin conversion pathway). Products include:
- Prinivil Tablets 2052
- Prinzide Tablets 2056

Low Molecular Weight Heparins (Patients on anticoagulation therapy are at risk for bleeding).
No products indexed under this heading.

Meclofenamate Sodium (Co-administration of non-steroidal anti-inflammatory drugs with aspirin may increase bleeding or lead to decreased renal function).
No products indexed under this heading.

Mefenamic Acid (Co-administration of non-steroidal anti-inflammatory drugs with aspirin may increase bleeding or lead to decreased renal function).
No products indexed under this heading.

Meloxicam (Co-administration of non-steroidal anti-inflammatory drugs with aspirin may increase bleeding or lead to decreased renal function). Products include:
- Mobic Oral Suspension 863
- Mobic Tablets 863

Metformin Hydrochloride (Moderate doses of aspirin may increase the effectiveness of renal hypoglycemic drugs, leading to hypoglycemia). Products include:
- ActoPlus Met Tablets 3214
- Avandamet Tablets 1373
- Fortamet Extended-Release Tablets 3115

Methotrexate Sodium (Salicylic acid can inhibit renal clearance of methotrexate, leading to bone marrow toxicity, especially in the elderly or renal impaired).
No products indexed under this heading.

Methyclothiazide (The effectiveness of diuretics in patients with underlying renal or cardiovascular disease may be diminished by co-administration of aspirin due to inhibition of renal prostaglandins, leading to decreased renal blood flow and salt and fluid retention).
No products indexed under this heading.

Metipranolol Hydrochloride (The hypertensive effects of beta-blockers may be diminished by the concomitant administration of aspirin due to inhibition of renal prostaglandins, leading to decreased renal blood flow and salt and fluid retention).
No products indexed under this heading.

Metolazone (The effectiveness of diuretics in patients with underlying renal or cardiovascular disease may be diminished by co-administration of aspirin due to inhibition of renal prostaglandins, leading to decreased renal blood flow and salt and fluid retention).
No products indexed under this heading.

Metoprolol Succinate (The hypertensive effects of beta-blockers may be diminished by the concomitant administration of aspirin due to inhibition of renal prostaglandins, leading to decreased renal blood flow and salt and fluid retention). Products include:
- Toprol-XL Tablets 668

Metoprolol Tartrate (The hypertensive effects of beta-blockers may be diminished by the concomitant administration of aspirin due to inhibition of renal prostaglandins, leading to decreased renal blood flow and salt and fluid retention). Products include:
- Lopressor Injection 2238
- Lopressor Tablets 2238
- Lopressor HCT 50/25 Tablets 2241
- Lopressor HCT 100/25 Tablets 2241
- Lopressor HCT 100/50 Tablets 2241

Miglitol (Moderate doses of aspirin may increase the effectiveness of renal hypoglycemic drugs, leading to hypoglycemia).
No products indexed under this heading.

Moexipril Hydrochloride (Co-administration can result in diminished hypotensive and hyponatremic effects of ACE inhibitors due to the effect of aspirin on the renin-angiotensin conversion pathway). Products include:
- Uniretic Tablets 3100
- Univasc Tablets 3104

Nabumetone (Co-administration of non-steroidal anti-inflammatory drugs with aspirin may increase bleeding or lead to decreased renal function).
No products indexed under this heading.

Nadolol (The hypertensive effects of beta-blockers may be diminished by the concomitant administration of aspirin due to inhibition of renal prostaglandins, leading to decreased renal blood flow and salt and fluid retention). Products include:
- Nadolol Tablets 2159

Naproxen (Co-administration of non-steroidal anti-inflammatory drugs with aspirin may increase bleeding or lead to decreased renal function). Products include:
- EC-Naprosyn Delayed-Release Tablets 2761
- Naprosyn Suspension 2761
- Naprosyn Tablets 2761
- Prevacid NapraPAC 3280

Naproxen Sodium (Co-administration of non-steroidal anti-inflammatory drugs with aspirin may increase bleeding or lead to decreased renal function). Products include:
- Aleve Caplets 742
- Aleve Gelcaps 743
- Aleve Tablets 743
- Aleve Cold & Sinus Caplets 744
- Anaprox Tablets 2761
- Anaprox DS Tablets 2761

Neostigmine Bromide (Dipyridamole may counteract the anticholinesterase effect of cholinesterase inhibitors, thereby potentially aggravating myasthenia gravis).
No products indexed under this heading.

Neostigmine Methylsulfate (Dipyridamole may counteract the anticholinesterase effect of cholinesterase inhibitors, thereby potentially aggravating myasthenia gravis).
No products indexed under this heading.

Oxaprozin (Co-administration of non-steroidal anti-inflammatory drugs with aspirin may increase bleeding or lead to decreased renal function).
No products indexed under this heading.

Penbutolol Sulfate (The hypertensive effects of beta-blockers may be diminished by the concomitant administration of aspirin due to inhibition of renal prostaglandins, leading to decreased renal blood flow and salt and fluid retention).
No products indexed under this heading.

Perindopril Erbumine (Co-administration can result in diminished hypotensive and hyponatremic effects of ACE inhibitors due to the effect of aspirin on the renin-angiotensin conversion pathway). Products include:
- Aceon Tablets (2 mg, 4 mg, 8 mg) 3194

Phenylbutazone (Co-administration of non-steroidal anti-inflammatory drugs with aspirin may increase bleeding or lead to decreased renal function).
No products indexed under this heading.

Phenytoin (Salicylic acid can displace protein-bound phenytoin leading to a decrease in the total concentration of phenytoin).
No products indexed under this heading.

Phenytoin Sodium (Salicylic acid can displace protein-bound phenytoin leading to a decrease in the total concentration of phenytoin). Products include:
- Phenytek Capsules 2160

Pindolol (The hypertensive effects of beta-blockers may be diminished by the concomitant administration of aspirin due to inhibition of renal prostaglandins, leading to decreased renal blood flow and salt and fluid retention).
No products indexed under this heading.

Pioglitazone Hydrochloride (Moderate doses of aspirin may increase the effectiveness of renal hypoglycemic drugs, leading to hypoglycemia). Products include:
- ActoPlus Met Tablets 3214
- Actos Tablets 3219
- Duetact Tablets 3226

Piroxicam (Co-administration of non-steroidal anti-inflammatory drugs with aspirin may increase bleeding or lead to decreased renal function).
No products indexed under this heading.

Polythiazide (The effectiveness of diuretics in patients with underlying renal or cardiovascular disease may be diminished by co-administration of aspirin due to inhibition of renal prostaglandins, leading to decreased renal blood flow and salt and fluid retention).
No products indexed under this heading.

Probenecid (Salicylates antagonize the uricosuric action of uricosuric agents, such as probenecid).
No products indexed under this heading.

Propranolol Hydrochloride (The hypertensive effects of beta-blockers may be diminished by the concomitant administration of aspirin due to inhibition of renal prostaglandins, leading to decreased renal blood flow and salt and fluid retention). Products include:
Inderal LA Long-Acting Capsules 3429
InnoPran XL Capsules 2723

Pyridostigmine Bromide (Dipyridamole may counteract the anticholinesterase effect of cholinesterase inhibitors, thereby potentially aggravating myasthenia gravis).
No products indexed under this heading.

Quinapril Hydrochloride (Co-administration can result in diminished hypotensive and hyponatremic effects of ACE inhibitors due to the effect of aspirin on the renin-angiotensin conversion pathway).
No products indexed under this heading.

Ramipril (Co-administration can result in diminished hypotensive and hyponatremic effects of ACE inhibitors due to the effect of aspirin on the renin-angiotensin conversion pathway). Products include:
Altace Capsules 1702

Repaglinide (Moderate doses of aspirin may increase the effectiveness of renal hypoglycemic drugs, leading to hypoglycemia).
No products indexed under this heading.

Rivastigmine Tartrate (Dipyridamole may counteract the anticholinesterase effect of cholinesterase inhibitors, thereby potentially aggravating myasthenia gravis). Products include:
Exelon Capsules 2206
Exelon Oral Solution 2206

Rofecoxib (Co-administration of non-steroidal anti-inflammatory drugs with aspirin may increase bleeding or lead to decreased renal function).
No products indexed under this heading.

Rosiglitazone Maleate (Moderate doses of aspirin may increase the effectiveness of renal hypoglycemic drugs, leading to hypoglycemia). Products include:
Avandamet Tablets 1373
Avandaryl Tablets 1379
Avandia Tablets 1384

Sotalol Hydrochloride (The hypertensive effects of beta-blockers may be diminished by the concomitant administration of aspirin due to inhibition of renal prostaglandins, leading to decreased renal blood flow and salt and fluid retention).
No products indexed under this heading.

Spirapril Hydrochloride (Co-administration can result in diminished hypotensive and hyponatremic effects of ACE inhibitors due to the effect of aspirin on the renin-angiotensin conversion pathway).
No products indexed under this heading.

Spironolactone (The effectiveness of diuretics in patients with underlying renal or cardiovascular disease may be diminished by co-administration of aspirin due to inhibition of renal prostaglandins, leading to decreased renal blood flow and salt and fluid retention).
No products indexed under this heading.

Sulfinpyrazone (Salicylates antagonize the uricosuric action of uricosuric agents, such as sulfinpyrazone).
No products indexed under this heading.

Sulindac (Co-administration of non-steroidal anti-inflammatory drugs with aspirin may increase bleeding or lead to decreased renal function). Products include:
Clinoril Tablets 1924

Tacrine Hydrochloride (Dipyridamole may counteract the anticholinesterase effect of cholinesterase inhibitors, thereby potentially aggravating myasthenia gravis).
No products indexed under this heading.

Timolol Hemihydrate (The hypertensive effects of beta-blockers may be diminished by the concomitant administration of aspirin due to inhibition of renal prostaglandins, leading to decreased renal blood flow and salt and fluid retention). Products include:
Betimol Ophthalmic Solution 3382
Betimol Ophthalmic Solution .... ⊙295

Timolol Maleate (The hypertensive effects of beta-blockers may be diminished by the concomitant administration of aspirin due to inhibition of renal prostaglandins, leading to decreased renal blood flow and salt and fluid retention). Products include:
Blocadren Tablets 1916
Cosopt Sterile Ophthalmic Solution....................................... 1931
Timolide Tablets 2086
Timoptic Sterile Ophthalmic Solution....................................... 2088
Timoptic in Ocudose 2091
Timoptic-XE Sterile Ophthalmic Gel Forming Solution.................... 2092

Tinzaparin Sodium (Patients on anticoagulation therapy are at risk for bleeding).
No products indexed under this heading.

Tolazamide (Moderate doses of aspirin may increase the effectiveness of renal hypoglycemic drugs, leading to hypoglycemia).
No products indexed under this heading.

Tolbutamide (Moderate doses of aspirin may increase the effectiveness of renal hypoglycemic drugs, leading to hypoglycemia).
No products indexed under this heading.

Tolmetin Sodium (Co-administration of non-steroidal anti-inflammatory drugs with aspirin may increase bleeding or lead to decreased renal function).
No products indexed under this heading.

Torsemide (The effectiveness of diuretics in patients with underlying renal or cardiovascular disease may be diminished by co-administration of aspirin due to inhibition of renal prostaglandins, leading to decreased renal blood flow and salt and fluid retention). Products include:
Demadex Injection 2759
Demadex Tablets 2759

Trandolapril (Co-administration can result in diminished hypotensive and hyponatremic effects of ACE inhibitors due to the effect of aspirin on the renin-angiotensin conversion pathway). Products include:
Mavik Tablets 486
Tarka Tablets 524

Triamterene (The effectiveness of diuretics in patients with underlying renal or cardiovascular disease may be diminished by co-administration of aspirin due to inhibition of renal prostaglandins, leading to decreased renal blood flow and salt and fluid retention). Products include:
Dyazide Capsules 1423
Dyrenium Capsules 3400

Troglitazone (Moderate doses of aspirin may increase the effectiveness of renal hypoglycemic drugs, leading to hypoglycemia).
No products indexed under this heading.

Valdecoxib (Co-administration of non-steroidal anti-inflammatory drugs with aspirin may increase bleeding or lead to decreased renal function).
No products indexed under this heading.

Valproate Sodium (Salicylic acid can displace protein-bound valproic acid leading to an increase in serum valproic acid levels). Products include:
Depacon Injection 412

Valproic Acid (Salicylic acid can displace protein-bound valproic acid leading to an increase in serum valproic acid levels). Products include:
Depakene 417

Warfarin Sodium (Aspirin can displace warfarin from protein binding sites, leading to a prolongation of both the prothrombin time and the bleeding time). Products include:
Coumadin for Injection 898
Coumadin Tablets 898

Food Interactions

Alcohol (Patients who consume three or more alcoholic drinks every day should be counseled about the bleeding risks involved with chronic, heavy alcohol use while taking aspirin).

AGRYLIN CAPSULES

(Anagrelide Hydrochloride) 3169

May interact with aspirin-acetylsalicylic acid, cytochrome p450 1a2 inhibitors (selected), cytochrome p450 1a2 substrates (selected), and certain other agents. Compounds in these categories include:

Acetaminophen (Anagrelide demonstrates some limited inhibitory activity towards CYP1A2 which may present a theoretical potential for interaction with other co-administered medicinal products sharing that clearance mechanism). Products include:
Comtrex Maximum Strength Cold & Cough Day/Night Caplets - Day Formulation......................... ▣726
Comtrex Maximum Strength Cold & Cough Day/Night Caplets - Night Formulation .... ▣726
Comtrex Maximum Strength Non-Drowsy Cold & Cough Caplets...................................... ▣725
Comtrex Maximum Strength Day/Night Severe Cold & Sinus Caplets - Day Formulation .... ▣725
Comtrex Maximum Strength Day/Night Severe Cold & Sinus Caplets - Night Formulation .... ▣725
Contac Cold and Flu Maximum Strength Caplets......................... ▣728
Contac Cold and Flu Day and Night Caplets (Day Formulation Only).. ▣727
Contac Cold and Flu Day and Night Caplets (Night Formulation Only)............................ ▣727
Contac Cold and Flu Non-Drowsy Caplets.. ▣728
Excedrin Extra Strength Caplets/Tablets/Geltabs............ ▣684
Excedrin Migraine Caplets/Tablets/Geltabs............ ▣609
Excedrin PM Caplets/Tablets/Geltabs............ ▣610
Excedrin Sinus Headache Caplets/Tablets .... ▣610
Excedrin Tension Headache Caplets/Tablets/Geltabs............ ▣611
Goody's Body Pain Formula Powder.. ▣684
Goody's Extra Strength Headache Powders..................... ▣611
Goody's Extra Strength Pain Relief Tablets .... ▣685
Goody's PM Powder for Pain with Sleeplessness .... ▣612
Percocet Tablets 1131
Robitussin Cough, Cold & Flu Nighttime Liquid......................... ▣738
TheraFlu Cold & Sore Throat Hot Liquid .... ▣741
TheraFlu Flu & Chest Congestion Hot Liquid .... ▣741
TheraFlu Flu & Sore Throat Hot Liquid .... ▣742
TheraFlu Daytime Severe Cold Hot Liquid .... ▣742
TheraFlu Nighttime Severe Cold Hot Liquid .... ▣740
TheraFlu Warming Relief Daytime Severe Cold............................... ▣743
TheraFlu Warming Relief Nighttime Severe Cold................ ▣743
Triaminic Cough & Sore Throat Liquid .... ▣747
Regular Strength Tylenol Tablets 1870
Children's Tylenol with Flavor Creator.. ▣679
Children's Tylenol Plus Flu Oral Suspension................................ ▣749
Tylenol Cold Head Congestion Daytime Caplets with Cool Burst and Gelcaps .... ▣750
Tylenol Cold Multi-Symptom Daytime Liquid............................ ▣752
Tylenol Cold Multi-Symptom Severe Daytime Liquid .... ▣752
Tylenol 8 Hour Extended Release Caplets.. 1870
Tylenol 1870
Extra Strength Tylenol PM Caplets, Vanilla Caplets, Geltabs, Gelcaps and Liquid.......... 1875
Extra Strength Tylenol Rapid Release Gels.............................. 1870
Concentrated Tylenol Infants' Drops Plus Cold & Cough............ ▣754
Tylenol with Codeine Tablets 2391
Tylenol Allergy Multi-Symptom Caplets with Cool Burst and Gelcaps.. 1872
Tylenol Allergy Multi-Symptom Nighttime Caplets with Cool Burst.. 1872
Tylenol Severe Allergy Caplets 1872
Tylenol Arthritis Pain Extended Release Caplets and Geltabs 1870
Tylenol Chest Congestion Caplets with Cool Burst............................ 1872
Tylenol Chest Congestion Liquid with Cool Burst............................ 1872
Children's Tylenol Suspension Liquid and Meltaways................... 1878

Children's Tylenol Plus Cold Suspension Liquid 1879
Children's Tylenol Plus Cold & Allergy Suspension Liquid 1878
Children's Tylenol Plus Cough & Runny Nose Suspension Liquid 1879
Children's Tylenol Plus Cough & Sore Throat Suspension Liquid 1879
Children's Tylenol Suspension with Flavor Creator 1878
Children's Tylenol Plus Flu Suspension Liquid 1881
Children's Tylenol Plus Multi-Symptom Cold Suspension Liquid 1879
Tylenol Cold Severe Congestion Non-Drowsy Caplets with Cool Burst 1874
Tylenol Cold Head Congestion Daytime Caplets with Cool Burst 1873
Tylenol Cold Head Congestion Nighttime Caplets with Cool Burst 1873
Tylenol Cold Head Congestion Severe Caplets with Cool Burst 1873
Tylenol Cold Multi-Symptom Daytime Caplets with Cool Burst and Gelcaps 1874
Tylenol Cold Multi-Symptom Daytime Liquid with Citrus Burst 1874
Tylenol Cold Multi-Symptom Nighttime Caplets with Cool Burst 1874
Tylenol Cold Multi-Symptom Nighttime Liquid with Cool Burst 1874
Tylenol Cold Multi-Symptom Severe Caplets with Cool Burst 1874
Tylenol Cold Multi-Symptom Severe Daytime Liquid with Citrus Burst 1874
Tylenol Cough & Sore Throat Daytime Liquid with Cool Burst 1877
Tylenol Cough & Sore Throat Nighttime Liquid with Cool Burst 1877
Concentrated Tylenol Infants' Drops 1878
Concentrated Tylenol Infants' Drops Plus Cold 1879
Concentrated Tylenol Infants' Drops Plus Cold and Cough 1879
Jr. Tylenol Meltaways 1878
Tylenol Sinus Severe Congestion Caplets with Cool Burst 1876
Tylenol Sinus Congestion & Pain Daytime Caplets with Cool Burst and Gelcaps 1876
Tylenol Sinus Congestion & Pain Nighttime Caplets with Cool Burst 1876
Tylenol Sinus Congestion & Pain Severe Caplets with Cool Burst 1876
Tylenol Sore Throat Daytime Liquid with Cool Burst 1877
Tylenol Sore Throat Nighttime Liquid with Cool Burst 1877
Women's Tylenol Menstrual Relief Caplets 1877
Vicks 44M Cough, Cold & Flu Relief Liquid 2680
Vicks DayQuil LiquiCaps/Liquid Multi-Symptom Cold/Flu Relief 761
Vicks DayQuil Multi-Symptom Cold/Flu Relief LiquiCaps 2678
Vicks DayQuil Multi-Symptom Cold/Flu Relief Liquid 2678
Vicks NyQuil Multi-Symptom Cold/Flu Relief Liquid 2681
Vicks NyQuil Multi-Symptom Cold/Flu Relief LiquiCaps 2681
Vicks NyQuil LiquiCaps/Liquid Multi-Symptom Cold/Flu Relief 763
Vicodin Tablets 535
Vicodin ES Tablets 536
Vicodin HP Tablets 538
Zicam Maximum Strength Flu Daytime 768
Zicam Maximum Strength Flu Nighttime 768
Zydone Tablets 1139

Alatrofloxacin Mesylate (Anagrelide is metabolized at least in part by CYP1A2. Therefore, CYP1A2 inhibitors could theoretically adversely influence the clearance of anagrelide).
No products indexed under this heading.

Amiodarone Hydrochloride (Anagrelide is metabolized at least in part by CYP1A2. Therefore, CYP1A2 inhibitors could theoretically adversely influence the clearance of anagrelide).
No products indexed under this heading.

Amitriptyline Hydrochloride (Anagrelide demonstrates some limited inhibitory activity towards CYP1A2 which may present a theoretical potential for interaction with other co-administered medicinal products sharing that clearance mechanism).
No products indexed under this heading.

Amoxapine (Anagrelide demonstrates some limited inhibitory activity towards CYP1A2 which may present a theoretical potential for interaction with other co-administered medicinal products sharing that clearance mechanism).
No products indexed under this heading.

Amrinone Lactate (Anagrelide is an inhibitor of AMP PDE III. The effects of medicinal products with similar properties, such as amrinone, may be exacerbated by anagrelide).
No products indexed under this heading.

Anastrozole (Anagrelide is metabolized at least in part by CYP1A2. Therefore, CYP1A2 inhibitors could theoretically adversely influence the clearance of anagrelide). Products include:
Arimidex Tablets 673

Aspirin (Anagrelide may slightly enhance the inhibition of platelet aggregation by aspirin). Products include:
Aggrenox Capsules 822
Bayer Aspirin 744
BC Allergy Sinus Cold Powder 677
BC Headache Powder 677
Arthritis Strength BC Powder 677
BC Sinus Cold Powder 677
Excedrin Extra Strength Caplets/Tablets/Geltabs 684
Excedrin Migraine Caplets/Tablets/Geltabs 609
Goody's Body Pain Formula Powder 684
Goody's Extra Strength Headache Powders 611
Goody's Extra Strength Pain Relief Tablets 685
Percodan Tablets 1132
St. Joseph 81 mg Aspirin Chewable and Enteric Coated Tablets 1869

Aspirin, Enteric Coated (Anagrelide may slightly enhance the inhibition of platelet aggregation by aspirin).
No products indexed under this heading.

Aspirin Buffered (Anagrelide may slightly enhance the inhibition of platelet aggregation by aspirin). Products include:
Bufferin Extra Strength Tablets 678
Bufferin Regular Strength Tablets 678

Caffeine (Anagrelide demonstrates some limited inhibitory activity towards CYP1A2 which may present a theoretical potential for interaction with other co-administered medicinal products sharing that clearance mechanism). Products include:
BC Headache Powder 677
Arthritis Strength BC Powder 677
Excedrin Extra Strength Caplets/Tablets/Geltabs 684
Excedrin Migraine Caplets/Tablets/Geltabs 609
Excedrin Tension Headache Caplets/Tablets/Geltabs 611
Goody's Extra Strength Headache Powders 611
Goody's Extra Strength Pain Relief Tablets 685
Vivarin 602
Winrgy Dietary Supplement 823

Caffeine Anhydrous (Anagrelide demonstrates some limited inhibitory activity towards CYP1A2 which may present a theoretical potential for interaction with other co-administered medicinal products sharing that clearance mechanism).
No products indexed under this heading.

Chlordiazepoxide (Anagrelide demonstrates some limited inhibitory activity towards CYP1A2 which may present a theoretical potential for interaction with other co-administered medicinal products sharing that clearance mechanism).
No products indexed under this heading.

Chlordiazepoxide Hydrochloride (Anagrelide demonstrates some limited inhibitory activity towards CYP1A2 which may present a theoretical potential for interaction with other co-administered medicinal products sharing that clearance mechanism). Products include:
Librium Capsules 3347

Cilostazol (Anagrelide is an inhibitor of AMP PDE III. The effects of medicinal products with similar properties, such as cilostazol, may be exacerbated by anagrelide). Products include:
Pletal Tablets 2455

Cimetidine (Anagrelide is metabolized at least in part by CYP1A2. Therefore, CYP1A2 inhibitors could theoretically adversely influence the clearance of anagrelide). Products include:
Tagamet HB 200 Tablets 664

Cimetidine Hydrochloride (Anagrelide is metabolized at least in part by CYP1A2. Therefore, CYP1A2 inhibitors could theoretically adversely influence the clearance of anagrelide).
No products indexed under this heading.

Ciprofloxacin (Anagrelide is metabolized at least in part by CYP1A2. Therefore, CYP1A2 inhibitors could theoretically adversely influence the clearance of anagrelide). Products include:
Cipro Oral Suspension 2977
Cipro I.V. 2984
Cipro XR Tablets 2990
Ciprodex Otic Suspension 559

Ciprofloxacin Hydrochloride (Anagrelide is metabolized at least in part by CYP1A2. Therefore, CYP1A2 inhibitors could theoretically adversely influence the clearance of anagrelide). Products include:
Ciloxan Ophthalmic Ointment 559
Ciloxan Ophthalmic Solution .... ⊙ 206
Cipro Tablets 2977
Proquin XR Tablets 1153

Clarithromycin (Anagrelide is metabolized at least in part by CYP1A2. Therefore, CYP1A2 inhibitors could theoretically adversely influence the clearance of anagrelide). Products include:
Biaxin/Biaxin XL 402
PREVPAC 3284

Clomipramine Hydrochloride (Anagrelide demonstrates some limited inhibitory activity towards CYP1A2 which may present a theoretical potential for interaction with other co-administered medicinal products sharing that clearance mechanism).
No products indexed under this heading.

Clopidogrel Bisulfate (Anagrelide demonstrates some limited inhibitory activity towards CYP1A2 which may present a theoretical potential for interaction with other co-administered medicinal products sharing that clearance mechanism). Products include:
Plavix Tablets 917
Plavix Tablets 2926

Clozapine (Anagrelide demonstrates some limited inhibitory activity towards CYP1A2 which may present a theoretical potential for interaction with other co-administered medicinal products sharing that clearance mechanism). Products include:
Clozaril Tablets 2184
FazaClo Orally Disintegrating Tablets 551

Cyclobenzaprine (Anagrelide demonstrates some limited inhibitory activity towards CYP1A2 which may present a theoretical potential for interaction with other co-administered medicinal products sharing that clearance mechanism).
No products indexed under this heading.

Cyclobenzaprine Hydrochloride (Anagrelide demonstrates some limited inhibitory activity towards CYP1A2 which may present a theoretical potential for interaction with other co-administered medicinal products sharing that clearance mechanism).
No products indexed under this heading.

Desipramine Hydrochloride (Anagrelide demonstrates some limited inhibitory activity towards CYP1A2 which may present a theoretical potential for interaction with other co-administered medicinal products sharing that clearance mechanism).
No products indexed under this heading.

Desogestrel (Anagrelide is metabolized at least in part by CYP1A2. Therefore, CYP1A2 inhibitors could theoretically adversely influence the clearance of anagrelide). Products include:
Mircette Tablets 1066

Diazepam (Anagrelide demonstrates some limited inhibitory activity towards CYP1A2 which may present a theoretical potential for interaction with other co-administered medicinal products sharing that clearance mechanism). Products include:
Diastat Rectal Delivery System 3343
Valium Tablets 2819

Diltiazem Hydrochloride (Anagrelide demonstrates some limited inhibitory activity towards CYP1A2 which may present a theoretical potential for interaction with other co-administered medicinal products sharing that clearance mechanism). Products include:
Cardizem LA Extended Release Tablets 1728

other co-administered medicinal products sharing that clearance mechanism). Products include:
Uniphyl Tablets 2710

Ticlopidine Hydrochloride (Anagrelide is metabolized at least in part by CYP1A2. Therefore, CYP1A2 inhibitors could theoretically adversely influence the clearance of anagrelide). Products include:
Ticlid Tablets 2810

Trimethaphan Camsylate (Anagrelide demonstrates some limited inhibitory activity towards CYP1A2 which may present a theoretical potential for interaction with other co-administered medicinal products sharing that clearance mechanism).
No products indexed under this heading.

Trimipramine Maleate (Anagrelide demonstrates some limited inhibitory activity towards CYP1A2 which may present a theoretical potential for interaction with other co-administered medicinal products sharing that clearance mechanism).
No products indexed under this heading.

Troleandomycin (Anagrelide is metabolized at least in part by CYP1A2. Therefore, CYP1A2 inhibitors could theoretically adversely influence the clearance of anagrelide).
No products indexed under this heading.

Trovafloxacin Mesylate (Anagrelide is metabolized at least in part by CYP1A2. Therefore, CYP1A2 inhibitors could theoretically adversely influence the clearance of anagrelide).
No products indexed under this heading.

Verapamil Hydrochloride (Anagrelide demonstrates some limited inhibitory activity towards CYP1A2 which may present a theoretical potential for interaction with other co-administered medicinal products sharing that clearance mechanism). Products include:
Covera-HS Tablets 3139
Tarka Tablets 524
Verelan PM Extended-Release Capsules, Controlled-Onset........... 3106

Warfarin Sodium (Anagrelide demonstrates some limited inhibitory activity towards CYP1A2 which may present a theoretical potential for interaction with other co-administered medicinal products sharing that clearance mechanism). Products include:
Coumadin for Injection 898
Coumadin Tablets 898

Zileuton (Anagrelide is metabolized at least in part by CYP1A2. Therefore, CYP1A2 inhibitors could theoretically adversely influence the clearance of anagrelide). Products include:
Zyflo Tablets 1023

Zolmitriptan (Anagrelide demonstrates some limited inhibitory activity towards CYP1A2 which may present a theoretical potential for interaction with other co-administered medicinal products sharing that clearance mechanism). Products include:
Zomig Tablets 3519
Zomig Nasal Spray 3523
Zomig-ZMT Tablets 3519

Food Interactions

Grapefruit Juice (Anagrelide is metabolized at least in part by CYP1A2. Therefore, CYP1A2 inhibitors could theoretically adversely influence the clearance of anagrelide).

ALAMAST OPHTHALMIC SOLUTION

(Pemirolast Potassium) 3381
None cited in PDR database.

ALAVERT ALLERGY & SINUS D-12 HOUR TABLETS

(Loratadine, Pseudoephedrine Sulfate) .... ■□771
May interact with monoamine oxidase inhibitors. Compounds in these categories include:

Isocarboxazid (Do not use while taking, or for two weeks after stopping, MAO inhibitors).
No products indexed under this heading.

Moclobemide (Do not use while taking, or for two weeks after stopping, MAO inhibitors).
No products indexed under this heading.

Pargyline Hydrochloride (Do not use while taking, or for two weeks after stopping, MAO inhibitors).
No products indexed under this heading.

Phenelzine Sulfate (Do not use while taking, or for two weeks after stopping, MAO inhibitors).
No products indexed under this heading.

Procarbazine Hydrochloride (Do not use while taking, or for two weeks after stopping, MAO inhibitors). Products include:
Matulane Capsules 3191

Selegiline Hydrochloride (Do not use while taking, or for two weeks after stopping, MAO inhibitors). Products include:
Eldepryl Capsules 3208
Zelapar Tablets 3372

Tranylcypromine Sulfate (Do not use while taking, or for two weeks after stopping, MAO inhibitors). Products include:
Parnate Tablets 1527

ALAVERT ORALLY DISINTEGRATING TABLETS

(Loratadine) .... ■□771
None cited in PDR database.

ALAVERT SWALLOW TABLETS

(Loratadine) .... ■□771
None cited in PDR database.

ALBALON OPHTHALMIC SOLUTION

(Naphazoline Hydrochloride) .... ⊙218
May interact with monoamine oxidase inhibitors, tricyclic antidepressants, and certain other agents. Compounds in these categories include:

Amitriptyline Hydrochloride (May potentiate the pressor effect of naphazoline).
No products indexed under this heading.

Amoxapine (May potentiate the pressor effect of naphazoline).
No products indexed under this heading.

Clomipramine Hydrochloride (May potentiate the pressor effect of naphazoline).
No products indexed under this heading.

Desipramine Hydrochloride (May potentiate the pressor effect of naphazoline).
No products indexed under this heading.

Doxepin Hydrochloride (May potentiate the pressor effect of naphazoline).
No products indexed under this heading.

Imipramine Hydrochloride (May potentiate the pressor effect of naphazoline).
No products indexed under this heading.

Imipramine Pamoate (May potentiate the pressor effect of naphazoline).
No products indexed under this heading.

Isocarboxazid (Severe hypertensive crisis).
No products indexed under this heading.

Maprotiline Hydrochloride (May potentiate the pressor effect of naphazoline).
No products indexed under this heading.

Moclobemide (Severe hypertensive crisis).
No products indexed under this heading.

Nortriptyline Hydrochloride (May potentiate the pressor effect of naphazoline).
No products indexed under this heading.

Pargyline Hydrochloride (Severe hypertensive crisis).
No products indexed under this heading.

Phenelzine Sulfate (Severe hypertensive crisis).
No products indexed under this heading.

Procarbazine Hydrochloride (Severe hypertensive crisis). Products include:
Matulane Capsules 3191

Protriptyline Hydrochloride (May potentiate the pressor effect of naphazoline).
No products indexed under this heading.

Selegiline Hydrochloride (Severe hypertensive crisis). Products include:
Eldepryl Capsules 3208
Zelapar Tablets 3372

Tranylcypromine Sulfate (Severe hypertensive crisis). Products include:
Parnate Tablets 1527

Trimipramine Maleate (May potentiate the pressor effect of naphazoline).
No products indexed under this heading.

ALBENZA TABLETS

(Albendazole) 1338
May interact with:

Cimetidine (Co-administration has resulted in increased albendazole sulfoxide concentrations in bile and cystic fluid in hydatid cyst). Products include:
Tagamet HB 200 Tablets .... ■□664

Cimetidine Hydrochloride (Co-administration has resulted in increased albendazole sulfoxide concentrations in bile and cystic fluid in hydatid cyst).
No products indexed under this heading.

Dexamethasone (Co-administration has resulted in higher steady-state trough concentrations of albendazole sulfoxide). Products include:
Ciprodex Otic Suspension 559
Decadron Tablets 1951
TobraDex Ophthalmic Ointment 562
TobraDex Ophthalmic Suspension ... 563

Dexamethasone Acetate (Co-administration has resulted in higher steady-state trough concentrations of albendazole sulfoxide).
No products indexed under this heading.

Dexamethasone Sodium Phosphate (Co-administration has resulted in higher steady-state trough concentrations of albendazole sulfoxide).
No products indexed under this heading.

Praziquantel (Co-administration has resulted in increased mean maximum plasma concentration and area under the curve of albendazole sulfoxide). Products include:
Biltricide Tablets 2976

Food Interactions

Diet, high-lipid (Oral bioavailability appears to be enhanced when albendazole is co-administered with a fatty meal).

ALBUTEIN 5%, ALBUMIN (HUMAN)

(Albumin (human)) 1652
None cited in PDR database.

ALBUTEIN 25% , ALBUMIN (HUMAN)

(Albumin (human)) 1653
None cited in PDR database.

ALDARA CREAM, 5%

(Imiquimod) 1846
None cited in PDR database.

ALDORIL TABLETS

(Hydrochlorothiazide, Methyldopa) 1910
May interact with antihypertensives, barbiturates, corticosteroids, general anesthetics, cardiac glycosides, oral hypoglycemic agents, insulin, lithium preparations, monoamine oxidase inhibitors, narcotic analgesics, non-steroidal anti-inflammatory agents, and certain other agents. Compounds in these categories include:

Acarbose (Dosage adjustment of the antidiabetic drug may be required). Products include:
Precose Tablets 751

Acebutolol Hydrochloride (Potentiation of antihypertensive effect).
No products indexed under this heading.

ACTH (Hypokalemia may result).
No products indexed under this heading.

Alfentanil Hydrochloride (Aggravates orthostatic hypotension).
No products indexed under this heading.

Amlodipine Besylate (Potentiation of antihypertensive effect). Products include:

Caduet Tablets 2508
Lotrel Capsules 2249
Norvasc Tablets 2545

Aprobarbital (Aggravates orthostatic hypotension).
No products indexed under this heading.

Atenolol (Potentiation of antihypertensive effect).
No products indexed under this heading.

Benazepril Hydrochloride (Potentiation of antihypertensive effect). Products include:
Lotensin Tablets 2243
Lotensin HCT Tablets 2246
Lotrel Capsules 2249

Bendroflumethiazide (Potentiation of antihypertensive effect).
No products indexed under this heading.

Betamethasone Acetate (Hypokalemia may result).
No products indexed under this heading.

Betamethasone Sodium Phosphate (Hypokalemia may result).
No products indexed under this heading.

Betaxolol Hydrochloride (Potentiation of antihypertensive effect). Products include:
Betoptic S Ophthalmic Suspension 558

Bisoprolol Fumarate (Potentiation of antihypertensive effect).
No products indexed under this heading.

Buprenorphine Hydrochloride (Aggravates orthostatic hypotension). Products include:
Buprenex Injectable 2716
Suboxone Tablets 2717
Subutex Tablets 2717

Butabarbital (Aggravates orthostatic hypotension).
No products indexed under this heading.

Butalbital (Aggravates orthostatic hypotension).
No products indexed under this heading.

Candesartan Cilexetil (Potentiation of antihypertensive effect). Products include:
Atacand Tablets 649
Atacand HCT 651

Captopril (Potentiation of antihypertensive effect). Products include:
Captopril Tablets 2149

Carteolol Hydrochloride (Potentiation of antihypertensive effect). Products include:
Carteolol Hydrochloride Ophthalmic Solution USP, 1% .... ⊙ 249

Celecoxib (May result in reduced diuretic effect). Products include:
Celebrex Capsules 3134

Chlorothiazide (Potentiation of antihypertensive effect). Products include:
Diuril Oral Suspension 1954

Chlorothiazide Sodium (Potentiation of antihypertensive effect). Products include:
Diuril Sodium Intravenous 2467

Chlorpropamide (Dosage adjustment of the antidiabetic drug may be required).
No products indexed under this heading.

Chlorthalidone (Potentiation of antihypertensive effect). Products include:
Clorpres Tablets 2153

Cholestyramine (Binds the hydrochlorothiazide and reduces its absorption from gastrointestinal tract by up to 85%).
No products indexed under this heading.

Clonidine (Potentiation of antihypertensive effect). Products include:
Catapres-TTS 844

Clonidine Hydrochloride (Potentiation of antihypertensive effect). Products include:
Catapres Tablets 843
Clorpres Tablets 2153

Codeine Phosphate (Aggravates orthostatic hypotension). Products include:
Tylenol with Codeine Tablets 2391

Colestipol Hydrochloride (Binds the hydrochlorothiazide and reduces its absorption from gastrointestinal tract by up to 43%).
No products indexed under this heading.

Cortisone Acetate (Hypokalemia may result).
No products indexed under this heading.

Deserpidine (Potentiation of antihypertensive effect).
No products indexed under this heading.

Deslanoside (Hypokalemia may exaggerate cardiac toxicity of digitalis).
No products indexed under this heading.

Dexamethasone (Hypokalemia may result). Products include:
Ciprodex Otic Suspension 559
Decadron Tablets 1951
TobraDex Ophthalmic Ointment 562
TobraDex Ophthalmic Suspension 563

Dexamethasone Acetate (Hypokalemia may result).
No products indexed under this heading.

Dexamethasone Sodium Phosphate (Hypokalemia may result).
No products indexed under this heading.

Dezocine (Aggravates orthostatic hypotension).
No products indexed under this heading.

Diazoxide (Potentiation of antihypertensive effect). Products include:
Hyperstat I.V. 3017

Diclofenac Potassium (May result in reduced diuretic effect).
No products indexed under this heading.

Diclofenac Sodium (May result in reduced diuretic effect). Products include:
Arthrotec Tablets 3129
Voltaren Ophthalmic Solution 2309
Voltaren Tablets 2307
Voltaren-XR Tablets 2310

Digitalis Glycoside Preparations (Hypokalemia may exaggerate cardiac toxicity of digitalis).
No products indexed under this heading.

Digitoxin (Hypokalemia may exaggerate cardiac toxicity of digitalis).
No products indexed under this heading.

Digoxin (Hypokalemia may exaggerate cardiac toxicity of digitalis). Products include:
Lanoxicaps Capsules 1490
Lanoxin Injection 1494
Lanoxin Injection Pediatric 1497
Lanoxin Tablets 1500

Diltiazem Hydrochloride (Potentiation of antihypertensive effect). Products include:
Cardizem LA Extended Release Tablets 1728
Tiazac Capsules 1201

Doxazosin Mesylate (Potentiation of antihypertensive effect). Products include:
Cardura XL Tablets 2515

Enalapril Maleate (Potentiation of antihypertensive effect). Products include:
Vasotec I.V. Injection 2103

Enalaprilat (Potentiation of antihypertensive effect).
No products indexed under this heading.

Enflurane (May require reduced dose of anesthetics).
No products indexed under this heading.

Eprosartan Mesylate (Potentiation of antihypertensive effect). Products include:
Teveten Tablets 1735
Teveten HCT Tablets 1737

Esmolol Hydrochloride (Potentiation of antihypertensive effect).
No products indexed under this heading.

Etodolac (May result in reduced diuretic effect).
No products indexed under this heading.

Felodipine (Potentiation of antihypertensive effect).
No products indexed under this heading.

Fenoprofen Calcium (May result in reduced diuretic effect). Products include:
Nalfon Capsules 2502

Fentanyl (Aggravates orthostatic hypotension). Products include:
Duragesic Transdermal System 2373
Ionsys Transdermal System 2379

Fentanyl Citrate (Aggravates orthostatic hypotension). Products include:
Actiq 979

Ferrous Gluconate (Co-administration results in a decrease in the bioavailability of methyldopa; this may adversely affect blood pressure control in patients treated with methlydopa; concurrent use is not recommended).
No products indexed under this heading.

Ferrous Sulfate (Co-administration results in a decrease in the bioavailability of methyldopa; this may adversely affect blood pressure control in patients treated with methlydopa; concurrent use is not recommended). Products include:
Slow Fe Iron Tablets .... ▣ 818
Slow Fe with Folic Acid Tablets .... ▣ 819

Fludrocortisone Acetate (Hypokalemia may result).
No products indexed under this heading.

Flurbiprofen (May result in reduced diuretic effect).
No products indexed under this heading.

Fosinopril Sodium (Potentiation of antihypertensive effect).
No products indexed under this heading.

Furosemide (Potentiation of antihypertensive effect). Products include:
Furosemide Tablets 2154

Glimepiride (Dosage adjustment of the antidiabetic drug may be required). Products include:
Avandaryl Tablets 1379
Duetact Tablets 3226

Glipizide (Dosage adjustment of the antidiabetic drug may be required).
No products indexed under this heading.

Glyburide (Dosage adjustment of the antidiabetic drug may be required).
No products indexed under this heading.

Guanabenz Acetate (Potentiation of antihypertensive effect).
No products indexed under this heading.

Guanethidine Monosulfate (Potentiation of antihypertensive effect).
No products indexed under this heading.

Hydralazine Hydrochloride (Potentiation of antihypertensive effect). Products include:
BiDil Tablets 2171

Hydrocodone Bitartrate (Aggravates orthostatic hypotension). Products include:
Hycodan 1116
Hycotuss Expectorant Syrup 1117
Vicodin Tablets 535
Vicodin ES Tablets 536
Vicodin HP Tablets 538
Vicoprofen Tablets 539
Zydone Tablets 1139

Hydrocodone Polistirex (Aggravates orthostatic hypotension). Products include:
Tussionex Pennkinetic Extended-Release Suspension 3327

Hydrocortisone (Hypokalemia may result). Products include:
Colocort Rectal Suspension, USP (Retention) 100 mg/60 mL 2476
Hydrocortone Tablets 1989
Preparation H Hydrocortisone Cream .... ▣ 646

Hydrocortisone Acetate (Hypokalemia may result). Products include:
Analpram-HC 1159
Pramosone 1161
ProctoFoam-HC 3099

Hydrocortisone Sodium Phosphate (Hypokalemia may result).
No products indexed under this heading.

Hydrocortisone Sodium Succinate (Hypokalemia may result).
No products indexed under this heading.

Hydroflumethiazide (Potentiation of antihypertensive effect).
No products indexed under this heading.

Hydromorphone Hydrochloride (Aggravates orthostatic hypotension). Products include:
Dilaudid 440
Dilaudid Non-Sterile Powder 440
Dilaudid Oral Liquid 445
Dilaudid Rectal Suppositories 440
Dilaudid Tablets 440
Dilaudid Tablets - 8 mg 445
Dilaudid-HP 442

Ibuprofen (May result in reduced diuretic effect). Products include:
Advil Allergy Sinus Caplets .... ▣ 770
Advil .... ▣ 674
Children's Advil Oral Suspension .... ▣ 603
Children's Advil Chewable Tablets .... ▣ 603
Advil Cold & Sinus .... ▣ 723
Infants' Advil Concentrated Drops .... ▣ 604
Infants' Advil Concentrated Drops - White Grape (Dye-Free) .... ▣ 604
Junior Strength Advil Swallow Tablets .... ▣ 605

IMPORTANT NOTE: Always consult each drug listing in the patient's regimen for possible interactions.

Advil Migraine Liquigels ▣ 608
Advil Multi-Symptom Cold Caplets ▣ 770
Advil PM Caplets ▣ 615
Motrin IB Tablets and Caplets 1866
Children's Motrin Oral Suspension ... 1867
Children's Motrin Non-Staining Dye-Free Oral Suspension 1867
Children's Motrin Cold Oral Suspension 1867
Infants' Motrin Concentrated Drops 1867
Infants' Motrin Non-Staining Dye-Free Concentrated Drops 1867
Junior Strength Motrin Caplets and Chewable Tablets 1867
Vicoprofen Tablets 539

Indapamide (Potentiation of antihypertensive effect). Products include:
Indapamide Tablets 2156

Indomethacin (May result in reduced diuretic effect). Products include:
Indocin 1995

Indomethacin Sodium Trihydrate (May result in reduced diuretic effect). Products include:
Indocin I.V. 2465

Insulin, Human, Zinc Suspension (Insulin requirement may be altered). Products include:
Humulin L, 100 Units 1794
Humulin U, 100 Units 1800

Insulin, Human NPH (Insulin requirement may be altered). Products include:
Humulin N, 100 Units 1795
Humulin N Pen 1797

Insulin, Human Regular (Insulin requirement may be altered). Products include:
Humulin R, 100 Units 1798

Insulin, Human Regular and Human NPH Mixture (Insulin requirement may be altered). Products include:
Humulin 50/50, 100 Units 1791
Humulin 70/30 Pen 1793

Insulin, NPH (Insulin requirement may be altered).
No products indexed under this heading.

Insulin, Regular (Insulin requirement may be altered).
No products indexed under this heading.

Insulin, Zinc Crystals (Insulin requirement may be altered).
No products indexed under this heading.

Insulin, Zinc Suspension (Insulin requirement may be altered).
No products indexed under this heading.

Insulin Aspart, Human Regular (Insulin requirement may be altered). Products include:
NovoLog Injection 2326

Insulin glargine (Insulin requirement may be altered). Products include:
Lantus Injection 2909

Insulin Lispro, Human (Insulin requirement may be altered). Products include:
Humalog-Pen 1781
Humalog Mix 50/50-Pen 1783
Humalog Mix 75/25-Pen 1785

Insulin Lispro Protamine, Human (Insulin requirement may be altered). Products include:
Humalog Mix 50/50-Pen 1783
Humalog Mix 75/25-Pen 1785

Irbesartan (Potentiation of antihypertensive effect). Products include:
Avalide Tablets 888
Avalide Tablets 2874
Avapro Tablets 891
Avapro Tablets 2871

Isocarboxazid (Concurrent use is contraindicated).
No products indexed under this heading.

Isoflurane (May require reduced dose of anesthetics).
No products indexed under this heading.

Isradipine (Potentiation of antihypertensive effect). Products include:
DynaCirc CR Tablets 2721

Ketamine Hydrochloride (May require reduced dose of anesthetics).
No products indexed under this heading.

Ketoprofen (May result in reduced diuretic effect).
No products indexed under this heading.

Ketorolac Tromethamine (May result in reduced diuretic effect). Products include:
Acular Ophthalmic Solution 565
Acular LS Ophthalmic Solution 566

Labetalol Hydrochloride (Potentiation of antihypertensive effect).
No products indexed under this heading.

Levorphanol Tartrate (Aggravates orthostatic hypotension).
No products indexed under this heading.

Lisinopril (Potentiation of antihypertensive effect). Products include:
Prinivil Tablets 2052
Prinzide Tablets 2056

Lithium (High risk of lithium toxicity).
No products indexed under this heading.

Lithium Carbonate (High risk of lithium toxicity). Products include:
Lithobid Tablets 1692

Lithium Citrate (High risk of lithium toxicity).
No products indexed under this heading.

Losartan Potassium (Potentiation of antihypertensive effect). Products include:
Cozaar Tablets 1935
Hyzaar 50-12.5 Tablets 1990
Hyzaar 100-12.5 Tablets 1990
Hyzaar 100-25 Tablets 1990

Mecamylamine Hydrochloride (Potentiation of antihypertensive effect).
No products indexed under this heading.

Meclofenamate Sodium (May result in reduced diuretic effect).
No products indexed under this heading.

Mefenamic Acid (May result in reduced diuretic effect).
No products indexed under this heading.

Meloxicam (May result in reduced diuretic effect). Products include:
Mobic Oral Suspension 863
Mobic Tablets 863

Meperidine Hydrochloride (Aggravates orthostatic hypotension).
No products indexed under this heading.

Mephobarbital (Aggravates orthostatic hypotension).
No products indexed under this heading.

Metformin Hydrochloride (Dosage adjustment of the antidiabetic drug may be required). Products include:
ActoPlus Met Tablets 3214
Avandamet Tablets 1373
Fortamet Extended-Release Tablets 3115

Methadone Hydrochloride (Aggravates orthostatic hypotension).
No products indexed under this heading.

Methohexital Sodium (May require reduced dose of anesthetics).
No products indexed under this heading.

Methoxyflurane (May require reduced dose of anesthetics).
No products indexed under this heading.

Methyclothiazide (Potentiation of antihypertensive effect).
No products indexed under this heading.

Methyldopate Hydrochloride (Potentiation of antihypertensive effect).
No products indexed under this heading.

Methylprednisolone Acetate (Hypokalemia may result). Products include:
Depo-Medrol Injectable Suspension 2617
Depo-Medrol Single-Dose Vial 2619

Methylprednisolone Sodium Succinate (Hypokalemia may result).
No products indexed under this heading.

Metolazone (Potentiation of antihypertensive effect).
No products indexed under this heading.

Metoprolol Succinate (Potentiation of antihypertensive effect). Products include:
Toprol-XL Tablets 668

Metoprolol Tartrate (Potentiation of antihypertensive effect). Products include:
Lopressor Injection 2238
Lopressor Tablets 2238
Lopressor HCT 50/25 Tablets 2241
Lopressor HCT 100/25 Tablets 2241
Lopressor HCT 100/50 Tablets 2241

Metyrosine (Potentiation of antihypertensive effect). Products include:
Demser Capsules 1953

Mibefradil Dihydrochloride (Potentiation of antihypertensive effect).
No products indexed under this heading.

Miglitol (Dosage adjustment of the antidiabetic drug may be required).
No products indexed under this heading.

Minoxidil (Potentiation of antihypertensive effect). Products include:
Men's Rogaine Extra Strength Hair Regrowth Treatment Topical Solution, Ocean Rush Scent and Original Unscented ▣ 633
Men's Rogaine Foam Hair Regrowth Treatment ▣ 633
Women's Rogaine Hair Regrowth Treatment Topical Solution, Spring Bloom Scent and Original Unscented ▣ 634

Moclobemide (Concurrent use is contraindicated).
No products indexed under this heading.

Moexipril Hydrochloride (Potentiation of antihypertensive effect). Products include:
Uniretic Tablets 3100
Univasc Tablets 3104

Morphine Sulfate (Aggravates orthostatic hypotension). Products include:
Avinza Capsules 1741
Kadian Capsules 577
MS Contin Tablets 2701

Nabumetone (May result in reduced diuretic effect).
No products indexed under this heading.

Nadolol (Potentiation of antihypertensive effect). Products include:
Nadolol Tablets 2159

Naproxen (May result in reduced diuretic effect). Products include:
EC-Naprosyn Delayed-Release Tablets 2761
Naprosyn Suspension 2761
Naprosyn Tablets 2761
Prevacid NapraPAC 3280

Naproxen Sodium (May result in reduced diuretic effect). Products include:
Aleve Caplets 742
Aleve Gelcaps 743
Aleve Tablets 743
Aleve Cold & Sinus Caplets 744
Anaprox Tablets 2761
Anaprox DS Tablets 2761

Nicardipine Hydrochloride (Potentiation of antihypertensive effect). Products include:
Cardene I.V. 2497

Nifedipine (Potentiation of antihypertensive effect). Products include:
Adalat CC Tablets 2964

Nisoldipine (Potentiation of antihypertensive effect). Products include:
Sular Tablets 3122

Nitroglycerin (Potentiation of antihypertensive effect). Products include:
Nitro-Dur Transdermal Infusion System 3046
Nitrolingual Pumpspray 3120

Norepinephrine Bitartrate (Decreased arterial responsiveness to norepinephrine).
No products indexed under this heading.

Oxaprozin (May result in reduced diuretic effect).
No products indexed under this heading.

Oxycodone Hydrochloride (Aggravates orthostatic hypotension). Products include:
OxyContin Tablets 2703
OxyFast Oral Concentrate Solution 2708
OxyIR Capsules 2708
Percocet Tablets 1131
Percodan Tablets 1132

Pargyline Hydrochloride (Concurrent use is contraindicated).
No products indexed under this heading.

Penbutolol Sulfate (Potentiation of antihypertensive effect).
No products indexed under this heading.

Pentobarbital Sodium (Aggravates orthostatic hypotension). Products include:
Nembutal Sodium Solution, USP 2470

Perindopril Erbumine (Potentiation of antihypertensive effect). Products include:
Aceon Tablets (2 mg, 4 mg, 8 mg) 3194

Phenelzine Sulfate (Concurrent use is contraindicated).
No products indexed under this heading.

Phenobarbital (Aggravates orthostatic hypotension). Products include:
Donnatal Extentabs 2493

Phenoxybenzamine Hydrochloride (Potentiation of antihypertensive effect). Products include:
Dibenzyline Capsules 3399

Phentolamine Mesylate (Potentiation of antihypertensive effect).
No products indexed under this heading.

Phenylbutazone (May result in reduced diuretic effect).
No products indexed under this heading.

Pindolol (Potentiation of antihypertensive effect).
No products indexed under this heading.

Pioglitazone Hydrochloride (Dosage adjustment of the antidiabetic drug may be required). Products include:
ActoPlus Met Tablets 3214
Actos Tablets 3219
Duetact Tablets 3226

Piroxicam (May result in reduced diuretic effect).
No products indexed under this heading.

Polythiazide (Potentiation of antihypertensive effect).
No products indexed under this heading.

Prazosin Hydrochloride (Potentiation of antihypertensive effect).
No products indexed under this heading.

Prednisolone Acetate (Hypokalemia may result). Products include:
Blephamide Ophthalmic Ointment 568
Blephamide Ophthalmic Suspension................................. 569
Poly-Pred Ophthalmic Suspension .... ⊙ 233
Pred Forte Ophthalmic Suspension .... ⊙ 235
Pred Mild Ophthalmic Suspension .... ⊙ 238
Pred-G Ophthalmic Ointment .... ⊙ 237
Pred-G Ophthalmic Suspension ...... ⊙ 236

Prednisolone Sodium Phosphate (Hypokalemia may result).
No products indexed under this heading.

Prednisolone Tebutate (Hypokalemia may result).
No products indexed under this heading.

Prednisone (Hypokalemia may result).
No products indexed under this heading.

Procarbazine Hydrochloride (Concurrent use is contraindicated). Products include:
Matulane Capsules 3191

Propofol (May require reduced dose of anesthetics).
No products indexed under this heading.

Propoxyphene Hydrochloride (Aggravates orthostatic hypotension).
No products indexed under this heading.

Propoxyphene Napsylate (Aggravates orthostatic hypotension).
No products indexed under this heading.

Propranolol Hydrochloride (Potentiation of antihypertensive effect). Products include:
Inderal LA Long-Acting Capsules 3429
InnoPran XL Capsules 2723

Quinapril Hydrochloride (Potentiation of antihypertensive effect).
No products indexed under this heading.

Ramipril (Potentiation of antihypertensive effect). Products include:
Altace Capsules 1702

Rauwolfia Serpentina (Potentiation of antihypertensive effect).
No products indexed under this heading.

Remifentanil Hydrochloride (Aggravates orthostatic hypotension).
No products indexed under this heading.

Repaglinide (Dosage adjustment of the antidiabetic drug may be required).
No products indexed under this heading.

Rescinnamine (Potentiation of antihypertensive effect).
No products indexed under this heading.

Reserpine (Potentiation of antihypertensive effect).
No products indexed under this heading.

Rofecoxib (May result in reduced diuretic effect).
No products indexed under this heading.

Rosiglitazone Maleate (Dosage adjustment of the antidiabetic drug may be required). Products include:
Avandamet Tablets 1373
Avandaryl Tablets 1379
Avandia Tablets 1384

Secobarbital Sodium (Aggravates orthostatic hypotension).
No products indexed under this heading.

Selegiline Hydrochloride (Concurrent use is contraindicated). Products include:
Eldepryl Capsules 3208
Zelapar Tablets 3372

Sevoflurane (May require reduced dose of anesthetics). Products include:
Ultane Liquid for Inhalation 531

Sodium Nitroprusside (Potentiation of antihypertensive effect).
No products indexed under this heading.

Sotalol Hydrochloride (Potentiation of antihypertensive effect).
No products indexed under this heading.

Spirapril Hydrochloride (Potentiation of antihypertensive effect).
No products indexed under this heading.

Sufentanil Citrate (Aggravates orthostatic hypotension).
No products indexed under this heading.

Sulindac (May result in reduced diuretic effect). Products include:
Clinoril Tablets 1924

Telmisartan (Potentiation of antihypertensive effect). Products include:
Micardis Tablets 854
Micardis HCT Tablets 856

Terazosin Hydrochloride (Potentiation of antihypertensive effect). Products include:
Hytrin Capsules 471

Thiamylal Sodium (Aggravates orthostatic hypotension).
No products indexed under this heading.

Timolol Maleate (Potentiation of antihypertensive effect). Products include:
Blocadren Tablets 1916
Cosopt Sterile Ophthalmic Solution.. 1931
Timolide Tablets 2086
Timoptic Sterile Ophthalmic Solution.. 2088
Timoptic in Ocudose 2091
Timoptic-XE Sterile Ophthalmic Gel Forming Solution.................. 2092

Tolazamide (Dosage adjustment of the antidiabetic drug may be required).
No products indexed under this heading.

Tolbutamide (Dosage adjustment of the antidiabetic drug may be required).
No products indexed under this heading.

Tolmetin Sodium (May result in reduced diuretic effect).
No products indexed under this heading.

Torsemide (Potentiation of antihypertensive effect). Products include:
Demadex Injection 2759
Demadex Tablets 2759

Trandolapril (Potentiation of antihypertensive effect). Products include:
Mavik Tablets 486
Tarka Tablets 524

Tranylcypromine Sulfate (Concurrent use is contraindicated). Products include:
Parnate Tablets 1527

Triamcinolone (Hypokalemia may result).
No products indexed under this heading.

Triamcinolone Acetonide (Hypokalemia may result). Products include:
Azmacort Inhalation Aerosol 1726
Nasacort AQ Nasal Spray 2922

Triamcinolone Diacetate (Hypokalemia may result).
No products indexed under this heading.

Triamcinolone Hexacetonide (Hypokalemia may result).
No products indexed under this heading.

Trimethaphan Camsylate (Potentiation of antihypertensive effect).
No products indexed under this heading.

Troglitazone (Dosage adjustment of the antidiabetic drug may be required).
No products indexed under this heading.

Tubocurarine Chloride (Increased responsiveness to tubocurarine).
No products indexed under this heading.

Valdecoxib (May result in reduced diuretic effect).
No products indexed under this heading.

Valsartan (Potentiation of antihypertensive effect). Products include:
Diovan Tablets 2193
Diovan HCT Tablets 2196

Verapamil Hydrochloride (Potentiation of antihypertensive effect). Products include:
Covera-HS Tablets 3139
Tarka Tablets 524
Verelan PM Extended-Release Capsules, Controlled-Onset........... 3106

Food Interactions

Alcohol (Aggravates orthostatic hypotension).

ALDURAZYME FOR INTRAVENOUS INFUSION

(Laronidase) 1268
None cited in PDR database.

ALEVE CAPLETS

(Naproxen Sodium) 742
May interact with corticosteroids, oral anticoagulants, non-steroidal anti-inflammatory agents, and certain other agents. Compounds in these categories include:

Anisindione (Taking with anticoagulant drugs may increase chances of stomach bleeding). Products include:
Miradon Tablets 3042

Betamethasone Acetate (Taking with steroid drugs may increase chances of stomach bleeding).
No products indexed under this heading.

Betamethasone Sodium Phosphate (Taking with steroid drugs may increase chances of stomach bleeding).
No products indexed under this heading.

Celecoxib (Taking with other NSAIDs may increase chances of stomach bleeding). Products include:
Celebrex Capsules 3134

Cortisone Acetate (Taking with steroid drugs may increase chances of stomach bleeding).
No products indexed under this heading.

Dexamethasone (Taking with steroid drugs may increase chances of stomach bleeding). Products include:
Ciprodex Otic Suspension 559
Decadron Tablets 1951
TobraDex Ophthalmic Ointment 562
TobraDex Ophthalmic Suspension ... 563

Dexamethasone Acetate (Taking with steroid drugs may increase chances of stomach bleeding).
No products indexed under this heading.

Dexamethasone Sodium Phosphate (Taking with steroid drugs may increase chances of stomach bleeding).
No products indexed under this heading.

Diclofenac Potassium (Taking with other NSAIDs may increase chances of stomach bleeding).
No products indexed under this heading.

Diclofenac Sodium (Taking with other NSAIDs may increase chances of stomach bleeding). Products include:
Arthrotec Tablets 3129
Voltaren Ophthalmic Solution 2309
Voltaren Tablets 2307
Voltaren-XR Tablets 2310

Dicumarol (Taking with anticoagulant drugs may increase chances of stomach bleeding).
No products indexed under this heading.

Etodolac (Taking with other NSAIDs may increase chances of stomach bleeding).
No products indexed under this heading.

Fenoprofen Calcium (Taking with other NSAIDs may increase chances of stomach bleeding). Products include:
- Nalfon Capsules 2502

Fludrocortisone Acetate (Taking with steroid drugs may increase chances of stomach bleeding).
- No products indexed under this heading.

Flurbiprofen (Taking with other NSAIDs may increase chances of stomach bleeding).
- No products indexed under this heading.

Hydrocortisone (Taking with steroid drugs may increase chances of stomach bleeding). Products include:
- Colocort Rectal Suspension, USP (Retention) 100 mg/60 mL 2476
- Hydrocortone Tablets 1989
- Preparation H Hydrocortisone Cream .... ▣646

Hydrocortisone Acetate (Taking with steroid drugs may increase chances of stomach bleeding). Products include:
- Analpram-HC 1159
- Pramosone 1161
- ProctoFoam-HC 3099

Hydrocortisone Sodium Phosphate (Taking with steroid drugs may increase chances of stomach bleeding).
- No products indexed under this heading.

Hydrocortisone Sodium Succinate (Taking with steroid drugs may increase chances of stomach bleeding).
- No products indexed under this heading.

Ibuprofen (Taking with other NSAIDs may increase chances of stomach bleeding). Products include:
- Advil Allergy Sinus Caplets .... ▣770
- Advil .... ▣674
- Children's Advil Oral Suspension .... ▣603
- Children's Advil Chewable Tablets .... ▣603
- Advil Cold & Sinus .... ▣723
- Infants' Advil Concentrated Drops .... ▣604
- Infants' Advil Concentrated Drops - White Grape (Dye-Free) .... ▣604
- Junior Strength Advil Swallow Tablets .... ▣605
- Advil Migraine Liquigels .... ▣608
- Advil Multi-Symptom Cold Caplets .... ▣770
- Advil PM Caplets .... ▣615
- Motrin IB Tablets and Caplets 1866
- Children's Motrin Oral Suspension 1867
- Children's Motrin Non-Staining Dye-Free Oral Suspension 1867
- Children's Motrin Cold Oral Suspension 1867
- Infants' Motrin Concentrated Drops 1867
- Infants' Motrin Non-Staining Dye-Free Concentrated Drops 1867
- Junior Strength Motrin Caplets and Chewable Tablets 1867
- Vicoprofen Tablets 539

Indomethacin (Taking with other NSAIDs may increase chances of stomach bleeding). Products include:
- Indocin 1995

Indomethacin Sodium Trihydrate (Taking with other NSAIDs may increase chances of stomach bleeding). Products include:
- Indocin I.V. 2465

Ketoprofen (Taking with other NSAIDs may increase chances of stomach bleeding).
- No products indexed under this heading.

Ketorolac Tromethamine (Taking with other NSAIDs may increase chances of stomach bleeding). Products include:
- Acular Ophthalmic Solution 565
- Acular LS Ophthalmic Solution 566

Meclofenamate Sodium (Taking with other NSAIDs may increase chances of stomach bleeding).
- No products indexed under this heading.

Mefenamic Acid (Taking with other NSAIDs may increase chances of stomach bleeding).
- No products indexed under this heading.

Meloxicam (Taking with other NSAIDs may increase chances of stomach bleeding). Products include:
- Mobic Oral Suspension 863
- Mobic Tablets 863

Methylprednisolone Acetate (Taking with steroid drugs may increase chances of stomach bleeding). Products include:
- Depo-Medrol Injectable Suspension 2617
- Depo-Medrol Single-Dose Vial 2619

Methylprednisolone Sodium Succinate (Taking with steroid drugs may increase chances of stomach bleeding).
- No products indexed under this heading.

Nabumetone (Taking with other NSAIDs may increase chances of stomach bleeding).
- No products indexed under this heading.

Naproxen (Taking with other NSAIDs may increase chances of stomach bleeding). Products include:
- EC-Naprosyn Delayed-Release Tablets 2761
- Naprosyn Suspension 2761
- Naprosyn Tablets 2761
- Prevacid NapraPAC 3280

Oxaprozin (Taking with other NSAIDs may increase chances of stomach bleeding).
- No products indexed under this heading.

Phenylbutazone (Taking with other NSAIDs may increase chances of stomach bleeding).
- No products indexed under this heading.

Piroxicam (Taking with other NSAIDs may increase chances of stomach bleeding).
- No products indexed under this heading.

Prednisolone Acetate (Taking with steroid drugs may increase chances of stomach bleeding). Products include:
- Blephamide Ophthalmic Ointment 568
- Blephamide Ophthalmic Suspension 569
- Poly-Pred Ophthalmic Suspension .... ⊙233
- Pred Forte Ophthalmic Suspension .... ⊙235
- Pred Mild Ophthalmic Suspension .... ⊙238
- Pred-G Ophthalmic Ointment .... ⊙237
- Pred-G Ophthalmic Suspension .... ⊙236

Prednisolone Sodium Phosphate (Taking with steroid drugs may increase chances of stomach bleeding).
- No products indexed under this heading.

Prednisolone Tebutate (Taking with steroid drugs may increase chances of stomach bleeding).
- No products indexed under this heading.

Prednisone (Taking with steroid drugs may increase chances of stomach bleeding).
- No products indexed under this heading.

Rofecoxib (Taking with other NSAIDs may increase chances of stomach bleeding).
- No products indexed under this heading.

Sulindac (Taking with other NSAIDs may increase chances of stomach bleeding). Products include:
- Clinoril Tablets 1924

Tolmetin Sodium (Taking with other NSAIDs may increase chances of stomach bleeding).
- No products indexed under this heading.

Triamcinolone (Taking with steroid drugs may increase chances of stomach bleeding).
- No products indexed under this heading.

Triamcinolone Acetonide (Taking with steroid drugs may increase chances of stomach bleeding). Products include:
- Azmacort Inhalation Aerosol 1726
- Nasacort AQ Nasal Spray 2922

Triamcinolone Diacetate (Taking with steroid drugs may increase chances of stomach bleeding).
- No products indexed under this heading.

Triamcinolone Hexacetonide (Taking with steroid drugs may increase chances of stomach bleeding).
- No products indexed under this heading.

Valdecoxib (Taking with other NSAIDs may increase chances of stomach bleeding).
- No products indexed under this heading.

Warfarin Sodium (Taking with anticoagulant drugs may increase chances of stomach bleeding). Products include:
- Coumadin for Injection 898
- Coumadin Tablets 898

Food Interactions

Alcohol (Taking with alcohol may increase chances of stomach bleeding).

ALEVE GELCAPS

(Naproxen Sodium) 743

May interact with corticosteroids, oral anticoagulants, non-steroidal anti-inflammatory agents, and certain other agents. Compounds in these categories include:

Anisindione (Taking anticoagulant drugs may increase chances of stomach bleeding). Products include:
- Miradon Tablets 3042

Betamethasone Acetate (Taking with steroid drugs may increase chances of stamch bleeding).
- No products indexed under this heading.

Betamethasone Sodium Phosphate (Taking with steroid drugs may increase chances of stamch bleeding).
- No products indexed under this heading.

Celecoxib (Taking with other NSAIDs may increase chances of stomach bleeding). Products include:
- Celebrex Capsules 3134

Cortisone Acetate (Taking with steroid drugs may increase chances of stamch bleeding).
- No products indexed under this heading.

Dexamethasone (Taking with steroid drugs may increase chances of stamch bleeding). Products include:
- Ciprodex Otic Suspension 559
- Decadron Tablets 1951
- TobraDex Ophthalmic Ointment 562
- TobraDex Ophthalmic Suspension 563

Dexamethasone Acetate (Taking with steroid drugs may increase chances of stamch bleeding).
- No products indexed under this heading.

Dexamethasone Sodium Phosphate (Taking with steroid drugs may increase chances of stamch bleeding).
- No products indexed under this heading.

Diclofenac Potassium (Taking with other NSAIDs may increase chances of stomach bleeding).
- No products indexed under this heading.

Diclofenac Sodium (Taking with other NSAIDs may increase chances of stomach bleeding). Products include:
- Arthrotec Tablets 3129
- Voltaren Ophthalmic Solution 2309
- Voltaren Tablets 2307
- Voltaren-XR Tablets 2310

Dicumarol (Taking anticoagulant drugs may increase chances of stomach bleeding).
- No products indexed under this heading.

Etodolac (Taking with other NSAIDs may increase chances of stomach bleeding).
- No products indexed under this heading.

Fenoprofen Calcium (Taking with other NSAIDs may increase chances of stomach bleeding). Products include:
- Nalfon Capsules 2502

Fludrocortisone Acetate (Taking with steroid drugs may increase chances of stamch bleeding).
- No products indexed under this heading.

Flurbiprofen (Taking with other NSAIDs may increase chances of stomach bleeding).
- No products indexed under this heading.

Hydrocortisone (Taking with steroid drugs may increase chances of stamch bleeding). Products include:
- Colocort Rectal Suspension, USP (Retention) 100 mg/60 mL 2476
- Hydrocortone Tablets 1989
- Preparation H Hydrocortisone Cream .... ▣646

Hydrocortisone Acetate (Taking with steroid drugs may increase chances of stamch bleeding). Products include:
- Analpram-HC 1159
- Pramosone 1161
- ProctoFoam-HC 3099

Food Interactions

ALEVE COLD & SINUS CAPLETS

May interact with corticosteroids, oral anticoagulants, monoamine oxidase inhibitors, non-steroidal anti-inflammatory agents, and certain other agents. Compounds in these categories include:

Advil Multi-Symptom Cold
Caplets 🔲770
Advil PM Caplets 🔲615
Motrin IB Tablets and Caplets 1866
Children's Motrin Oral Suspension ... 1867
Children's Motrin Non-Staining
Dye-Free Oral Suspension............. 1867
Children's Motrin Cold Oral
Suspension 1867
Infants' Motrin Concentrated
Drops.. 1867
Infants' Motrin Non-Staining
Dye-Free Concentrated Drops....... 1867
Junior Strength Motrin Caplets
and Chewable Tablets.................. 1867
Vicoprofen Tablets 539

Indomethacin (Taking with other
NSAIDs may increase chances of
stomach bleeding). Products
include:
Indocin .. 1995

**Indomethacin Sodium Trihy-
drate** (Taking with other NSAIDs
may increase chances of stomach
bleeding). Products include:
Indocin I.V. 2465

Isocarboxazid (Do not take concurrently with MAO inhibitors or for 2
weeks after stopping MAO
inhibitors).
No products indexed under this
heading.

Ketoprofen (Taking with other
NSAIDs may increase chances of
stomach bleeding).
No products indexed under this
heading.

Ketorolac Tromethamine (Taking
with other NSAIDs may increase
chances of stomach bleeding).
Products include:
Acular Ophthalmic Solution 565
Acular LS Ophthalmic Solution 566

Meclofenamate Sodium (Taking
with other NSAIDs may increase
chances of stomach bleeding).
No products indexed under this
heading.

Mefenamic Acid (Taking with other
NSAIDs may increase chances of
stomach bleeding).
No products indexed under this
heading.

Meloxicam (Taking with other
NSAIDs may increase chances of
stomach bleeding). Products
include:
Mobic Oral Suspension 863
Mobic Tablets 863

Methylprednisolone Acetate (Tak-
ing with steroid drugs may increase
chances of stomach bleeding).
Products include:
Depo-Medrol Injectable
Suspension 2617
Depo-Medrol Single-Dose Vial 2619

**Methylprednisolone Sodium
Succinate** (Taking with steroid
drugs may increase chances of
stomach bleeding).
No products indexed under this
heading.

Moclobemide (Do not take concurrently with MAO inhibitors or for 2
weeks after stopping MAO
inhibitors).
No products indexed under this
heading.

Nabumetone (Taking with other
NSAIDs may increase chances of
stomach bleeding).
No products indexed under this
heading.

Naproxen (Taking with other
NSAIDs may increase chances of
stomach bleeding). Products
include:

EC-Naprosyn Delayed-Release
Tablets 2761
Naprosyn Suspension 2761
Naprosyn Tablets 2761
Prevacid NapraPAC 3280

Oxaprozin (Taking with other
NSAIDs may increase chances of
stomach bleeding).
No products indexed under this
heading.

Pargyline Hydrochloride (Do not
take concurrently with MAO inhibitors
or for 2 weeks after stopping MAO
inhibitors).
No products indexed under this
heading.

Phenelzine Sulfate (Do not take
concurrently with MAO inhibitors or
for 2 weeks after stopping MAO
inhibitors).
No products indexed under this
heading.

Phenylbutazone (Taking with other
NSAIDs may increase chances of
stomach bleeding).
No products indexed under this
heading.

Piroxicam (Taking with other
NSAIDs may increase chances of
stomach bleeding).
No products indexed under this
heading.

Prednisolone Acetate (Taking with
steroid drugs may increase chances
of stomach bleeding). Products
include:
Blephamide Ophthalmic Ointment 568
Blephamide Ophthalmic
Suspension................................. 569
Poly-Pred Ophthalmic
Suspension ⊙233
Pred Forte Ophthalmic
Suspension ⊙235
Pred Mild Ophthalmic
Suspension ⊙238
Pred-G Ophthalmic Ointment ⊙237
Pred-G Ophthalmic Suspension ⊙236

Prednisolone Sodium Phosphate
(Taking with steroid drugs may
increase chances of stomach
bleeding).
No products indexed under this
heading.

Prednisolone Tebutate (Taking
with steroid drugs may increase
chances of stomach bleeding).
No products indexed under this
heading.

Prednisone (Taking with steroid
drugs may increase chances of
stomach bleeding).
No products indexed under this
heading.

Procarbazine Hydrochloride (Do
not take concurrently with MAO
inhibitors or for 2 weeks after stopping MAO inhibitors). Products
include:
Matulane Capsules 3191

Rofecoxib (Taking with other
NSAIDs may increase chances of
stomach bleeding).
No products indexed under this
heading.

Selegiline Hydrochloride (Do not
take concurrently with MAO inhibitors
or for 2 weeks after stopping MAO
inhibitors). Products include:
Eldepryl Capsules 3208
Zelapar Tablets 3372

Sulindac (Taking with other NSAIDs
may increase chances of stomach
bleeding). Products include:
Clinoril Tablets 1924

Tolmetin Sodium (Taking with other NSAIDs may increase chances of
stomach bleeding).
No products indexed under this
heading.

Tranylcypromine Sulfate (Do not
take concurrently with MAO inhibitors
or for 2 weeks after stopping MAO
inhibitors). Products include:
Parnate Tablets 1527

Triamcinolone (Taking with steroid
drugs may increase chances of
stomach bleeding).
No products indexed under this
heading.

Triamcinolone Acetonide (Taking
with steroid drugs may increase
chances of stomach bleeding).
Products include:
Azmacort Inhalation Aerosol 1726
Nasacort AQ Nasal Spray 2922

Triamcinolone Diacetate (Taking
with steroid drugs may increase
chances of stomach bleeding).
No products indexed under this
heading.

Triamcinolone Hexacetonide
(Taking with steroid drugs may
increase chances of stomach
bleeding).
No products indexed under this
heading.

Valdecoxib (Taking with other
NSAIDs may increase chances of
stomach bleeding).
No products indexed under this
heading.

Warfarin Sodium (Taking with anti-
coagulant drugs may increase
chances of stomach bleeding).
Products include:
Coumadin for Injection 898
Coumadin Tablets 898

Food Interactions

Alcohol (Taking with alcohol may
increase chances of stomach bleeding).

ALEVE TABLETS

(Naproxen Sodium) 743
May interact with corticosteroids,
oral anticoagulants, non-steroidal anti-inflammatory agents, and certain
other agents. Compounds in these
categories include:

Anisindione (Taking with anticoagulant drugs may increase chances of
stomach bleeding). Products
include:
Miradon Tablets 3042

Betamethasone Acetate (Taking
with steroid drugs may increase
chances of stomach bleeding).
No products indexed under this
heading.

**Betamethasone Sodium Phos-
phate** (Taking with steroid drugs
may increase chances of stomach
bleeding).
No products indexed under this
heading.

Celecoxib (Taking with other
NSAIDs may increase chances of
stomach bleeding). Products
include:
Celebrex Capsules 3134

Cortisone Acetate (Taking with
steroid drugs may increase chances
of stomach bleeding).
No products indexed under this
heading.

Dexamethasone (Taking with steroid drugs may increase chances of
stomach bleeding). Products
include:
Ciprodex Otic Suspension 559

Decadron Tablets 1951
TobraDex Ophthalmic Ointment 562
TobraDex Ophthalmic Suspension ... 563

Dexamethasone Acetate (Taking
with steroid drugs may increase
chances of stomach bleeding).
No products indexed under this
heading.

**Dexamethasone Sodium Phos-
phate** (Taking with steroid drugs
may increase chances of stomach
bleeding).
No products indexed under this
heading.

Diclofenac Potassium (Taking with
other NSAIDs may increase chances
of stomach bleeding).
No products indexed under this
heading.

Diclofenac Sodium (Taking with
other NSAIDs may increase chances
of stomach bleeding). Products
include:
Arthrotec Tablets 3129
Voltaren Ophthalmic Solution 2309
Voltaren Tablets 2307
Voltaren-XR Tablets 2310

Dicumarol (Taking with anticoagulant drugs may increase chances of
stomach bleeding).
No products indexed under this
heading.

Etodolac (Taking with other NSAIDs
may increase chances of stomach
bleeding).
No products indexed under this
heading.

Fenoprofen Calcium (Taking with
other NSAIDs may increase chances
of stomach bleeding). Products
include:
Nalfon Capsules 2502

Fludrocortisone Acetate (Taking
with steroid drugs may increase
chances of stomach bleeding).
No products indexed under this
heading.

Flurbiprofen (Taking with other
NSAIDs may increase chances of
stomach bleeding).
No products indexed under this
heading.

Hydrocortisone (Taking with ste-
roid drugs may increase chances of
stomach bleeding). Products
include:
Colocort Rectal Suspension, USP
(Retention) 100 mg/60 mL.......... 2476
Hydrocortone Tablets 1989
Preparation H Hydrocortisone
Cream 🔲646

Hydrocortisone Acetate (Taking
with steroid drugs may increase
chances of stomach bleeding).
Products include:
Analpram-HC 1159
Pramosone 1161
ProctoFoam-HC 3099

**Hydrocortisone Sodium Phos-
phate** (Taking with steroid drugs
may increase chances of stomach
bleeding).
No products indexed under this
heading.

**Hydrocortisone Sodium Succin-
ate** (Taking with steroid drugs may
increase chances of stomach
bleeding).
No products indexed under this
heading.

Ibuprofen (Taking with other
NSAIDs may increase chances of
stomach bleeding). Products
include:
Advil Allergy Sinus Caplets 🔲770
Advil .. 🔲674

(🔲 Described in PDR For Nonprescription Drugs) (⊙ Described in PDR For Ophthalmic Medicines™)

Children's Advil Oral Suspension .... ■603
Children's Advil Chewable Tablets .. ■603
Advil Cold & Sinus .... ■723
Infants' Advil Concentrated Drops .. ■604
Infants' Advil Concentrated Drops - White Grape (Dye-Free)............. ■604
Junior Strength Advil Swallow Tablets....................................... ■605
Advil Migraine Liquigels .... ■608
Advil Multi-Symptom Cold Caplets....................................... ■770
Advil PM Caplets .... ■615
Motrin IB Tablets and Caplets 1866
Children's Motrin Oral Suspension ... 1867
Children's Motrin Non-Staining Dye-Free Oral Suspension............ 1867
Children's Motrin Cold Oral Suspension 1867
Infants' Motrin Concentrated Drops.. 1867
Infants' Motrin Non-Staining Dye-Free Concentrated Drops....... 1867
Junior Strength Motrin Caplets and Chewable Tablets.................. 1867
Vicoprofen Tablets 539

Indomethacin (Taking with other NSAIDs may increase chances of stomach bleeding). Products include:
Indocin 1995

Indomethacin Sodium Trihydrate (Taking with other NSAIDs may increase chances of stomach bleeding). Products include:
Indocin I.V. 2465

Ketoprofen (Taking with other NSAIDs may increase chances of stomach bleeding).
No products indexed under this heading.

Ketorolac Tromethamine (Taking with other NSAIDs may increase chances of stomach bleeding). Products include:
Acular Ophthalmic Solution 565
Acular LS Ophthalmic Solution 566

Meclofenamate Sodium (Taking with other NSAIDs may increase chances of stomach bleeding).
No products indexed under this heading.

Mefenamic Acid (Taking with other NSAIDs may increase chances of stomach bleeding).
No products indexed under this heading.

Meloxicam (Taking with other NSAIDs may increase chances of stomach bleeding). Products include:
Mobic Oral Suspension 863
Mobic Tablets 863

Methylprednisolone Acetate (Taking with steroid drugs may increase chances of stomach bleeding). Products include:
Depo-Medrol Injectable Suspension 2617
Depo-Medrol Single-Dose Vial 2619

Methylprednisolone Sodium Succinate (Taking with steroid drugs may increase chances of stomach bleeding).
No products indexed under this heading.

Nabumetone (Taking with other NSAIDs may increase chances of stomach bleeding).
No products indexed under this heading.

Naproxen (Taking with other NSAIDs may increase chances of stomach bleeding). Products include:
EC-Naprosyn Delayed-Release Tablets 2761
Naprosyn Suspension 2761
Naprosyn Tablets 2761
Prevacid NapraPAC 3280

Oxaprozin (Taking with other NSAIDs may increase chances of stomach bleeding).
No products indexed under this heading.

Phenylbutazone (Taking with other NSAIDs may increase chances of stomach bleeding).
No products indexed under this heading.

Piroxicam (Taking with other NSAIDs may increase chances of stomach bleeding).
No products indexed under this heading.

Prednisolone Acetate (Taking with steroid drugs may increase chances of stomach bleeding). Products include:
Blephamide Ophthalmic Ointment 568
Blephamide Ophthalmic Suspension.................................. 569
Poly-Pred Ophthalmic Suspension .... ⊙233
Pred Forte Ophthalmic Suspension .... ⊙235
Pred Mild Ophthalmic Suspension .... ⊙238
Pred-G Ophthalmic Ointment .... ⊙237
Pred-G Ophthalmic Suspension ...... ⊙236

Prednisolone Sodium Phosphate (Taking with steroid drugs may increase chances of stomach bleeding).
No products indexed under this heading.

Prednisolone Tebutate (Taking with steroid drugs may increase chances of stomach bleeding).
No products indexed under this heading.

Prednisone (Taking with steroid drugs may increase chances of stomach bleeding).
No products indexed under this heading.

Rofecoxib (Taking with other NSAIDs may increase chances of stomach bleeding).
No products indexed under this heading.

Sulindac (Taking with other NSAIDs may increase chances of stomach bleeding). Products include:
Clinoril Tablets 1924

Tolmetin Sodium (Taking with other NSAIDs may increase chances of stomach bleeding).
No products indexed under this heading.

Triamcinolone (Taking with steroid drugs may increase chances of stomach bleeding).
No products indexed under this heading.

Triamcinolone Acetonide (Taking with steroid drugs may increase chances of stomach bleeding). Products include:
Azmacort Inhalation Aerosol 1726
Nasacort AQ Nasal Spray 2922

Triamcinolone Diacetate (Taking with steroid drugs may increase chances of stomach bleeding).
No products indexed under this heading.

Triamcinolone Hexacetonide (Taking with steroid drugs may increase chances of stomach bleeding).
No products indexed under this heading.

Valdecoxib (Taking with other NSAIDs may increase chances of stomach bleeding).
No products indexed under this heading.

Warfarin Sodium (Taking with anticoagulant drugs may increase chances of stomach bleeding). Products include:
Coumadin for Injection 898
Coumadin Tablets 898

Food Interactions

Alcohol (Taking with alcohol may increase chances of stomach bleeding).

ALEVE COLD & SINUS CAPLETS

(Naproxen Sodium, Pseudoephedrine Hydrochloride)....... ■724

May interact with corticosteroids, oral anticoagulants, monoamine oxidase inhibitors, non-steroidal anti-inflammatory agents, and certain other agents. Compounds in these categories include:

Anisindione (Taking with anticoagulant drugs may increase chances of stomach bleeding). Products include:
Miradon Tablets 3042

Betamethasone Acetate (Taking with steroid drugs may increase chances of stomach bleeding).
No products indexed under this heading.

Betamethasone Sodium Phosphate (Taking with steroid drugs may increase chances of stomach bleeding).
No products indexed under this heading.

Celecoxib (Taking with other NSAIDs may increase chances of stomach bleeding). Products include:
Celebrex Capsules 3134

Cortisone Acetate (Taking with steroid drugs may increase chances of stomach bleeding).
No products indexed under this heading.

Dexamethasone (Taking with steroid drugs may increase chances of stomach bleeding). Products include:
Ciprodex Otic Suspension 559
Decadron Tablets 1951
TobraDex Ophthalmic Ointment 562
TobraDex Ophthalmic Suspension ... 563

Dexamethasone Acetate (Taking with steroid drugs may increase chances of stomach bleeding).
No products indexed under this heading.

Dexamethasone Sodium Phosphate (Taking with steroid drugs may increase chances of stomach bleeding).
No products indexed under this heading.

Diclofenac Potassium (Taking with other NSAIDs may increase chances of stomach bleeding).
No products indexed under this heading.

Diclofenac Sodium (Taking with other NSAIDs may increase chances of stomach bleeding). Products include:
Arthrotec Tablets 3129
Voltaren Ophthalmic Solution 2309
Voltaren Tablets 2307
Voltaren-XR Tablets 2310

Dicumarol (Taking with anticoagulant drugs may increase chances of stomach bleeding).
No products indexed under this heading.

Etodolac (Taking with other NSAIDs may increase chances of stomach bleeding).
No products indexed under this heading.

Fenoprofen Calcium (Taking with other NSAIDs may increase chances of stomach bleeding). Products include:
Nalfon Capsules 2502

Fludrocortisone Acetate (Taking with steroid drugs may increase chances of stomach bleeding).
No products indexed under this heading.

Flurbiprofen (Taking with other NSAIDs may increase chances of stomach bleeding).
No products indexed under this heading.

Hydrocortisone (Taking with steroid drugs may increase chances of stomach bleeding). Products include:
Colocort Rectal Suspension, USP (Retention) 100 mg/60 mL........... 2476
Hydrocortone Tablets 1989
Preparation H Hydrocortisone Cream .... ■646

Hydrocortisone Acetate (Taking with steroid drugs may increase chances of stomach bleeding). Products include:
Analpram-HC 1159
Pramosone 1161
ProctoFoam-HC 3099

Hydrocortisone Sodium Phosphate (Taking with steroid drugs may increase chances of stomach bleeding).
No products indexed under this heading.

Hydrocortisone Sodium Succinate (Taking with steroid drugs may increase chances of stomach bleeding).
No products indexed under this heading.

Ibuprofen (Taking with other NSAIDs may increase chances of stomach bleeding). Products include:
Advil Allergy Sinus Caplets .... ■770
Advil .... ■674
Children's Advil Oral Suspension .... ■603
Children's Advil Chewable Tablets .. ■603
Advil Cold & Sinus .... ■723
Infants' Advil Concentrated Drops .. ■604
Infants' Advil Concentrated Drops - White Grape (Dye-Free)............. ■604
Junior Strength Advil Swallow Tablets....................................... ■605
Advil Migraine Liquigels .... ■608
Advil Multi-Symptom Cold Caplets....................................... ■770
Advil PM Caplets .... ■615
Motrin IB Tablets and Caplets 1866
Children's Motrin Oral Suspension ... 1867
Children's Motrin Non-Staining Dye-Free Oral Suspension............ 1867
Children's Motrin Cold Oral Suspension 1867
Infants' Motrin Concentrated Drops.. 1867
Infants' Motrin Non-Staining Dye-Free Concentrated Drops....... 1867
Junior Strength Motrin Caplets and Chewable Tablets.................. 1867
Vicoprofen Tablets 539

Indomethacin (Taking with other NSAIDs may increase chances of stomach bleeding). Products include:
Indocin 1995

Indomethacin Sodium Trihydrate (Taking with other NSAIDs may increase chances of stomach bleeding). Products include:
Indocin I.V. 2465

Isocarboxazid (Do not take concurrently with MAO inhibitors or for 2 weeks after stopping MAO inhibitors).
No products indexed under this heading.

Ketoprofen (Taking with other NSAIDs may increase chances of stomach bleeding).
No products indexed under this heading.

Ketorolac Tromethamine (Taking with other NSAIDs may increase chances of stomach bleeding). Products include:
Acular Ophthalmic Solution 565
Acular LS Ophthalmic Solution 566

Meclofenamate Sodium (Taking with other NSAIDs may increase chances of stomach bleeding).
No products indexed under this heading.

Mefenamic Acid (Taking with other NSAIDs may increase chances of stomach bleeding).
No products indexed under this heading.

Meloxicam (Taking with other NSAIDs may increase chances of stomach bleeding). Products include:
Mobic Oral Suspension 863
Mobic Tablets 863

Methylprednisolone Acetate (Taking with steroid drugs may increase chances of stomach bleeding). Products include:
Depo-Medrol Injectable Suspension 2617
Depo-Medrol Single-Dose Vial 2619

Methylprednisolone Sodium Succinate (Taking with steroid drugs may increase chances of stomach bleeding).
No products indexed under this heading.

Moclobemide (Do not take concurrently with MAO inhibitors or for 2 weeks after stopping MAO inhibitors).
No products indexed under this heading.

Nabumetone (Taking with other NSAIDs may increase chances of stomach bleeding).
No products indexed under this heading.

Naproxen (Taking with other NSAIDs may increase chances of stomach bleeding). Products include:
EC-Naprosyn Delayed-Release Tablets 2761
Naprosyn Suspension 2761
Naprosyn Tablets 2761
Prevacid NapraPAC 3280

Oxaprozin (Taking with other NSAIDs may increase chances of stomach bleeding).
No products indexed under this heading.

Pargyline Hydrochloride (Do not take concurrently with MAO inhibitors or for 2 weeks after stopping MAO inhibitors).
No products indexed under this heading.

Phenelzine Sulfate (Do not take concurrently with MAO inhibitors or for 2 weeks after stopping MAO inhibitors).
No products indexed under this heading.

Phenylbutazone (Taking with other NSAIDs may increase chances of stomach bleeding).
No products indexed under this heading.

Piroxicam (Taking with other NSAIDs may increase chances of stomach bleeding).
No products indexed under this heading.

Prednisolone Acetate (Taking with steroid drugs may increase chances of stomach bleeding). Products include:
Blephamide Ophthalmic Ointment 568
Blephamide Ophthalmic Suspension 569
Poly-Pred Ophthalmic Suspension .... ⊙233
Pred Forte Ophthalmic Suspension .... ⊙235
Pred Mild Ophthalmic Suspension .... ⊙238
Pred-G Ophthalmic Ointment .... ⊙237
Pred-G Ophthalmic Suspension .... ⊙236

Prednisolone Sodium Phosphate (Taking with steroid drugs may increase chances of stomach bleeding).
No products indexed under this heading.

Prednisolone Tebutate (Taking with steroid drugs may increase chances of stomach bleeding).
No products indexed under this heading.

Prednisone (Taking with steroid drugs may increase chances of stomach bleeding).
No products indexed under this heading.

Procarbazine Hydrochloride (Do not take concurrently with MAO inhibitors or for 2 weeks after stopping MAO inhibitors). Products include:
Matulane Capsules 3191

Rofecoxib (Taking with other NSAIDs may increase chances of stomach bleeding).
No products indexed under this heading.

Selegiline Hydrochloride (Do not take concurrently with MAO inhibitors or for 2 weeks after stopping MAO inhibitors). Products include:
Eldepryl Capsules 3208
Zelapar Tablets 3372

Sulindac (Taking with other NSAIDs may increase chances of stomach bleeding). Products include:
Clinoril Tablets 1924

Tolmetin Sodium (Taking with other NSAIDs may increase chances of stomach bleeding).
No products indexed under this heading.

Tranylcypromine Sulfate (Do not take concurrently with MAO inhibitors or for 2 weeks after stopping MAO inhibitors). Products include:
Parnate Tablets 1527

Triamcinolone (Taking with steroid drugs may increase chances of stomach bleeding).
No products indexed under this heading.

Triamcinolone Acetonide (Taking with steroid drugs may increase chances of stomach bleeding). Products include:
Azmacort Inhalation Aerosol 1726
Nasacort AQ Nasal Spray 2922

Triamcinolone Diacetate (Taking with steroid drugs may increase chances of stomach bleeding).
No products indexed under this heading.

Triamcinolone Hexacetonide (Taking with steroid drugs may increase chances of stomach bleeding).
No products indexed under this heading.

Valdecoxib (Taking with other NSAIDs may increase chances of stomach bleeding).
No products indexed under this heading.

Warfarin Sodium (Taking with anticoagulant drugs may increase chances of stomach bleeding). Products include:
Coumadin for Injection 898
Coumadin Tablets 898

Food Interactions

Alcohol (Taking with alcohol may increase chances of stomach bleeding).

ALFERON N INJECTION

(Interferon alfa-N3 (Human Leukocyte Derived)) 1665
None cited in PDR database.

ALIMTA FOR INJECTION

(Pemetrexed) 1750
May interact with nephrotoxic agents, non-steroidal anti-inflammatory agents, and certain other agents. Compounds in these categories include:

Abacavir Sulfate (Concomitant administration of nephrotoxic drugs could result in delayed clearance of pemetrexed). Products include:
Epzicom Tablets 1436
Trizivir Tablets 1589
Ziagen 1626

Acyclovir (Concomitant administration of nephrotoxic drugs could result in delayed clearance of pemetrexed). Products include:
Zovirax 1643
Zovirax Cream 820
Zovirax Ointment 821

Acyclovir Sodium (Concomitant administration of nephrotoxic drugs could result in delayed clearance of pemetrexed).
No products indexed under this heading.

Alatrofloxacin Mesylate (Concomitant administration of nephrotoxic drugs could result in delayed clearance of pemetrexed).
No products indexed under this heading.

Aldesleukin (Concomitant administration of nephrotoxic drugs could result in delayed clearance of pemetrexed). Products include:
Proleukin for Injection 2266

Amikacin Sulfate (Concomitant administration of nephrotoxic drugs could result in delayed clearance of pemetrexed).
No products indexed under this heading.

Amoxicillin (Concomitant administration of nephrotoxic drugs could result in delayed clearance of pemetrexed). Products include:
Amoxil Capsules 1343
Amoxil Chewable Tablets 1343
Amoxil Pediatric Drops for Oral Suspension 1343
Amoxil Powder for Oral Suspension 1343
Amoxil Tablets 1343
Augmentin 1360
Augmentin Tablets 1363
Augmentin XR Extended-Release Tablets 1369
Augmentin ES-600 Powder for Oral Suspension 1366
PREVPAC 3284

Amoxicillin Trihydrate (Concomitant administration of nephrotoxic drugs could result in delayed clearance of pemetrexed).
No products indexed under this heading.

Amphotericin B (Concomitant administration of nephrotoxic drugs could result in delayed clearance of pemetrexed).
No products indexed under this heading.

Amphotericin B, liposomal (Concomitant administration of nephrotoxic drugs could result in delayed clearance of pemetrexed). Products include:
AmBisome for Injection 620

Amphotericin B Cholesteryl Sulfate (Concomitant administration of nephrotoxic drugs could result in delayed clearance of pemetrexed).
No products indexed under this heading.

Amphotericin B Lipid Complex (Concomitant administration of nephrotoxic drugs could result in delayed clearance of pemetrexed). Products include:
Abelcet Injection 1141

Ampicillin (Concomitant administration of nephrotoxic drugs could result in delayed clearance of pemetrexed).
No products indexed under this heading.

Ampicillin Sodium (Concomitant administration of nephrotoxic drugs could result in delayed clearance of pemetrexed).
No products indexed under this heading.

Ampicillin Trihydrate (Concomitant administration of nephrotoxic drugs could result in delayed clearance of pemetrexed).
No products indexed under this heading.

Amprenavir (Concomitant administration of nephrotoxic drugs could result in delayed clearance of pemetrexed). Products include:
Agenerase Capsules 1327
Agenerase Oral Solution 1332

Aspirin (Concomitant administration of nephrotoxic drugs could result in delayed clearance of pemetrexed). Products include:
Aggrenox Capsules 822
Bayer Aspirin 744
BC Allergy Sinus Cold Powder .... ▣677
BC Headache Powder .... ▣677
Arthritis Strength BC Powder .... ▣677
BC Sinus Cold Powder .... ▣677
Excedrin Extra Strength Caplets/Tablets/Geltabs .... ▣684
Excedrin Migraine Caplets/Tablets/Geltabs .... ▣609
Goody's Body Pain Formula Powder .... ▣684
Goody's Extra Strength Headache Powders .... ▣611
Goody's Extra Strength Pain Relief Tablets .... ▣685
Percodan Tablets 1132
St. Joseph 81 mg Aspirin Chewable and Enteric Coated Tablets 1869

Atazanavir (Concomitant administration of nephrotoxic drugs could result in delayed clearance of pemetrexed).
No products indexed under this heading.

Atorvastatin Calcium (Concomitant administration of nephrotoxic drugs could result in delayed clearance of pemetrexed). Products include:
Caduet Tablets 2508
Lipitor Tablets 2483

Azithromycin Dihydrate (Concomitant administration of nephrotoxic drugs could result in delayed clearance of pemetrexed).
No products indexed under this heading.

Azlocillin Sodium (Concomitant administration of nephrotoxic drugs could result in delayed clearance of pemetrexed).
No products indexed under this heading.

Aztreonam (Concomitant administration of nephrotoxic drugs could result in delayed clearance of pemetrexed).
No products indexed under this heading.

Bacampicillin Hydrochloride (Concomitant administration of nephrotoxic drugs could result in delayed clearance of pemetrexed).
No products indexed under this heading.

Balsalazide Disodium (Concomitant administration of nephrotoxic drugs could result in delayed clearance of pemetrexed). Products include:
Colazal Capsules 2838

Benazepril Hydrochloride (Concomitant administration of nephrotoxic drugs could result in delayed clearance of pemetrexed). Products include:
Lotensin Tablets 2243
Lotensin HCT Tablets 2246
Lotrel Capsules 2249

Bendroflumethiazide (Concomitant administration of nephrotoxic drugs could result in delayed clearance of pemetrexed).
No products indexed under this heading.

Caffeine (Concomitant administration of nephrotoxic drugs could result in delayed clearance of pemetrexed). Products include:
BC Headache Powder 677
Arthritis Strength BC Powder 677
Excedrin Extra Strength Caplets/Tablets/Geltabs 684
Excedrin Migraine Caplets/Tablets/Geltabs 609
Excedrin Tension Headache Caplets/Tablets/Geltabs 611
Goody's Extra Strength Headache Powders 611
Goody's Extra Strength Pain Relief Tablets 685
Vivarin 602
Winrgy Dietary Supplement 823

Captopril (Concomitant administration of nephrotoxic drugs could result in delayed clearance of pemetrexed). Products include:
Captopril Tablets 2149

Carbenicillin Disodium (Concomitant administration of nephrotoxic drugs could result in delayed clearance of pemetrexed).
No products indexed under this heading.

Carbenicillin Indanyl Sodium (Concomitant administration of nephrotoxic drugs could result in delayed clearance of pemetrexed).
No products indexed under this heading.

Carboplatin (Concomitant administration of nephrotoxic drugs could result in delayed clearance of pemetrexed).
No products indexed under this heading.

Carmustine (BCNU) (Concomitant administration of nephrotoxic drugs could result in delayed clearance of pemetrexed).
No products indexed under this heading.

Cefaclor (Concomitant administration of nephrotoxic drugs could result in delayed clearance of pemetrexed).
No products indexed under this heading.

Cefadroxil (Concomitant administration of nephrotoxic drugs could result in delayed clearance of pemetrexed).
No products indexed under this heading.

Cefamandole Nafate (Concomitant administration of nephrotoxic drugs could result in delayed clearance of pemetrexed).
No products indexed under this heading.

Cefazolin Sodium (Concomitant administration of nephrotoxic drugs could result in delayed clearance of pemetrexed).
No products indexed under this heading.

Cefdinir (Concomitant administration of nephrotoxic drugs could result in delayed clearance of pemetrexed). Products include:
Omnicef Capsules 511
Omnicef for Oral Suspension 511

Cefepime Hydrochloride (Concomitant administration of nephrotoxic drugs could result in delayed clearance of pemetrexed). Products include:
Maxipime for Injection 1105

Cefixime (Concomitant administration of nephrotoxic drugs could result in delayed clearance of pemetrexed). Products include:
Suprax 1843

Cefmetazole Sodium (Concomitant administration of nephrotoxic drugs could result in delayed clearance of pemetrexed).
No products indexed under this heading.

Cefonicid Sodium (Concomitant administration of nephrotoxic drugs could result in delayed clearance of pemetrexed).
No products indexed under this heading.

Cefoperazone Sodium (Concomitant administration of nephrotoxic drugs could result in delayed clearance of pemetrexed).
No products indexed under this heading.

Ceforanide (Concomitant administration of nephrotoxic drugs could result in delayed clearance of pemetrexed).
No products indexed under this heading.

Cefotaxime Sodium (Concomitant administration of nephrotoxic drugs could result in delayed clearance of pemetrexed).
No products indexed under this heading.

Cefotetan (Concomitant administration of nephrotoxic drugs could result in delayed clearance of pemetrexed).
No products indexed under this heading.

Cefoxitin Sodium (Concomitant administration of nephrotoxic drugs could result in delayed clearance of pemetrexed). Products include:
Mefoxin for Injection 2012
Mefoxin Premixed Intravenous Solution 2016

Cefpodoxime Proxetil (Concomitant administration of nephrotoxic drugs could result in delayed clearance of pemetrexed). Products include:
Vantin Tablets and Oral Suspension 2645

Cefprozil (Concomitant administration of nephrotoxic drugs could result in delayed clearance of pemetrexed).
No products indexed under this heading.

Ceftazidime (Concomitant administration of nephrotoxic drugs could result in delayed clearance of pemetrexed). Products include:
Fortaz 1453

Ceftizoxime Sodium (Concomitant administration of nephrotoxic drugs could result in delayed clearance of pemetrexed).
No products indexed under this heading.

Ceftriaxone Sodium (Concomitant administration of nephrotoxic drugs could result in delayed clearance of pemetrexed). Products include:
Rocephin Injectable Vials, ADD-Vantage, Galaxy, Bulk 2800

Cefuroxime Axetil (Concomitant administration of nephrotoxic drugs could result in delayed clearance of pemetrexed). Products include:
Ceftin 1407

Cefuroxime Sodium (Concomitant administration of nephrotoxic drugs could result in delayed clearance of pemetrexed).
No products indexed under this heading.

Celecoxib (Patients with mild to moderate renal insufficiency should avoid NSAIDs with short elimination half-lives two days before, the day of, and two days following administration of pemetrexed. All patients should avoid NSAIDs with longer half-lives at least five days before, the day of, and two days following pemetrexed administration. If concomitant administration of an NSAID is necessary, patients should be monitored closely for toxicity, especially myelosuppression, renal and gastrointestinal toxicity). Products include:
Celebrex Capsules 3134

Cephalexin (Concomitant administration of nephrotoxic drugs could result in delayed clearance of pemetrexed). Products include:
Keflex Capsules 549

Cephalothin Sodium (Concomitant administration of nephrotoxic drugs could result in delayed clearance of pemetrexed).
No products indexed under this heading.

Cephapirin Sodium (Concomitant administration of nephrotoxic drugs could result in delayed clearance of pemetrexed).
No products indexed under this heading.

Cephradine (Concomitant administration of nephrotoxic drugs could result in delayed clearance of pemetrexed).
No products indexed under this heading.

Cerivastatin Sodium (Concomitant administration of nephrotoxic drugs could result in delayed clearance of pemetrexed).
No products indexed under this heading.

Chlorothiazide (Concomitant administration of nephrotoxic drugs could result in delayed clearance of pemetrexed). Products include:
Diuril Oral Suspension 1954

Chlorothiazide Sodium (Concomitant administration of nephrotoxic drugs could result in delayed clearance of pemetrexed). Products include:
Diuril Sodium Intravenous 2467

Chlorpropamide (Concomitant administration of nephrotoxic drugs could result in delayed clearance of pemetrexed).
No products indexed under this heading.

Cidofovir (Concomitant administration of nephrotoxic drugs could result in delayed clearance of pemetrexed).
No products indexed under this heading.

Cilastatin Sodium (Concomitant administration of nephrotoxic drugs could result in delayed clearance of pemetrexed). Products include:
Primaxin I.M. 2045
Primaxin I.V. 2048

Cimetidine (Concomitant administration of nephrotoxic drugs could result in delayed clearance of pemetrexed). Products include:
Tagamet HB 200 Tablets 664

Cimetidine Hydrochloride (Concomitant administration of nephrotoxic drugs could result in delayed clearance of pemetrexed).
No products indexed under this heading.

Cisplatin (Concomitant administration of nephrotoxic drugs could result in delayed clearance of pemetrexed).
No products indexed under this heading.

Cladribine (Concomitant administration of nephrotoxic drugs could result in delayed clearance of pemetrexed). Products include:
Leustatin Injection 2357

Clozapine (Concomitant administration of nephrotoxic drugs could result in delayed clearance of pemetrexed). Products include:
Clozaril Tablets 2184
FazaClo Orally Disintegrating Tablets 551

Colistimethate Sodium (Concomitant administration of nephrotoxic drugs could result in delayed clearance of pemetrexed).
No products indexed under this heading.

Colistin Sulfate (Concomitant administration of nephrotoxic drugs could result in delayed clearance of pemetrexed).
No products indexed under this heading.

Cyclophosphamide (Concomitant administration of nephrotoxic drugs could result in delayed clearance of pemetrexed).
No products indexed under this heading.

Cyclosporine (Concomitant administration of nephrotoxic drugs could result in delayed clearance of pemetrexed). Products include:
- Gengraf Capsules 459
- Neoral Oral Solution 2259
- Neoral Soft Gelatin Capsules 2259
- Restasis Ophthalmic Emulsion 575
- Sandimmune 2275

Cytarabine (Concomitant administration of nephrotoxic drugs could result in delayed clearance of pemetrexed).
No products indexed under this heading.

Cytarabine Liposome (Concomitant administration of nephrotoxic drugs could result in delayed clearance of pemetrexed). Products include:
- DepoCyt Injection 1143

Delavirdine Mesylate (Concomitant administration of nephrotoxic drugs could result in delayed clearance of pemetrexed). Products include:
- Rescriptor Tablets 2551

Diatrizoate Meglumine (Concomitant administration of nephrotoxic drugs could result in delayed clearance of pemetrexed).
No products indexed under this heading.

Diatrizoate Sodium (Concomitant administration of nephrotoxic drugs could result in delayed clearance of pemetrexed).
No products indexed under this heading.

Diclofenac Potassium (Patients with mild to moderate renal insufficiency should avoid NSAIDs with short elimination half-lives two days before, the day of, and two days following administration of pemetrexed. All patients should avoid NSAIDs with longer half-lives at least five days before, the day of, and two days following pemetrexed administration. If concomitant administration of an NSAID is necessary, patients should be monitored closely for toxicity, especially myelosuppression, renal and gastrointestinal toxicity).
No products indexed under this heading.

Diclofenac Sodium (Patients with mild to moderate renal insufficiency should avoid NSAIDs with short elimination half-lives two days before, the day of, and two days following administration of pemetrexed. All patients should avoid NSAIDs with longer half-lives at least five days before, the day of, and two days following pemetrexed administration. If concomitant administration of an NSAID is necessary, patients should be monitored closely for toxicity, especially myelosuppression, renal and gastrointestinal toxicity). Products include:
- Arthrotec Tablets 3129
- Voltaren Ophthalmic Solution 2309
- Voltaren Tablets 2307
- Voltaren-XR Tablets 2310

Dicloxacillin Sodium (Concomitant administration of nephrotoxic drugs could result in delayed clearance of pemetrexed).
No products indexed under this heading.

Didanosine (Concomitant administration of nephrotoxic drugs could result in delayed clearance of pemetrexed).
No products indexed under this heading.

Efavirenz (Concomitant administration of nephrotoxic drugs could result in delayed clearance of pemetrexed). Products include:
- Atripla Tablets 945
- Sustiva Capsules 930
- Sustiva Tablets 930

Emtricitabine (Concomitant administration of nephrotoxic drugs could result in delayed clearance of pemetrexed). Products include:
- Atripla Tablets 945
- Emtriva Capsules 1287
- Emtriva Oral Solution 1287
- Truvada Tablets 1296

Enalapril Maleate (Concomitant administration of nephrotoxic drugs could result in delayed clearance of pemetrexed). Products include:
- Vasotec I.V. Injection 2103

Enalaprilat (Concomitant administration of nephrotoxic drugs could result in delayed clearance of pemetrexed).
No products indexed under this heading.

Enfuvirtide (Concomitant administration of nephrotoxic drugs could result in delayed clearance of pemetrexed). Products include:
- Fuzeon Injection 2767

Ethiodized Oil (Concomitant administration of nephrotoxic drugs could result in delayed clearance of pemetrexed).
No products indexed under this heading.

Etodolac (Patients with mild to moderate renal insufficiency should avoid NSAIDs with short elimination half-lives two days before, the day of, and two days following administration of pemetrexed. All patients should avoid NSAIDs with longer half-lives at least five days before, the day of, and two days following pemetrexed administration. If concomitant administration of an NSAID is necessary, patients should be monitored closely for toxicity, especially myelosuppression, renal and gastrointestinal toxicity).
No products indexed under this heading.

Fenoprofen Calcium (Patients with mild to moderate renal insufficiency should avoid NSAIDs with short elimination half-lives two days before, the day of, and two days following administration of pemetrexed. All patients should avoid NSAIDs with longer half-lives at least five days before, the day of, and two days following pemetrexed administration. If concomitant administration of an NSAID is necessary, patients should be monitored closely for toxicity, especially myelosuppression, renal and gastrointestinal toxicity). Products include:
- Nalfon Capsules 2502

Filgrastim (Concomitant administration of nephrotoxic drugs could result in delayed clearance of pemetrexed). Products include:
- Neupogen for Injection 603

Fluorouracil (Concomitant administration of nephrotoxic drugs could result in delayed clearance of pemetrexed). Products include:
- Carac Cream, 0.5% 2879
- Efudex 3363

Flurbiprofen (Patients with mild to moderate renal insufficiency should avoid NSAIDs with short elimination half-lives two days before, the day of, and two days following administration of pemetrexed. All patients should avoid NSAIDs with longer half-lives at least five days before, the day of, and two days following pemetrexed administration. If concomitant administration of an NSAID is necessary, patients should be monitored closely for toxicity, especially myelosuppression, renal and gastrointestinal toxicity).
No products indexed under this heading.

Fluvastatin Sodium (Concomitant administration of nephrotoxic drugs could result in delayed clearance of pemetrexed). Products include:
- Lescol Capsules 2233
- Lescol XL Tablets 2233

Foscarnet Sodium (Concomitant administration of nephrotoxic drugs could result in delayed clearance of pemetrexed).
No products indexed under this heading.

Fosinopril Sodium (Concomitant administration of nephrotoxic drugs could result in delayed clearance of pemetrexed).
No products indexed under this heading.

Furosemide (Concomitant administration of nephrotoxic drugs could result in delayed clearance of pemetrexed). Products include:
- Furosemide Tablets 2154

Gadopentetate Dimeglumine (Concomitant administration of nephrotoxic drugs could result in delayed clearance of pemetrexed).
No products indexed under this heading.

Gentamicin (Concomitant administration of nephrotoxic drugs could result in delayed clearance of pemetrexed).
No products indexed under this heading.

Gentamicin Sulfate (Concomitant administration of nephrotoxic drugs could result in delayed clearance of pemetrexed). Products include:
- Garamycin Injectable 3014
- Pred-G Ophthalmic Ointment .... ⊙237
- Pred-G Ophthalmic Suspension .... ⊙236

Glipizide (Concomitant administration of nephrotoxic drugs could result in delayed clearance of pemetrexed).
No products indexed under this heading.

Globulin, Immune (Human) (Concomitant administration of nephrotoxic drugs could result in delayed clearance of pemetrexed). Products include:
- Flebogamma 5%, Immune Globulin Intravenous (Human) 1658
- GamaSTAN 3234

Glyburide (Concomitant administration of nephrotoxic drugs could result in delayed clearance of pemetrexed).
No products indexed under this heading.

Gold Therapy (Concomitant administration of nephrotoxic drugs could result in delayed clearance of pemetrexed).
No products indexed under this heading.

HMG-CoA Reductase Inhibitors (Concomitant administration of nephrotoxic drugs could result in delayed clearance of pemetrexed).
No products indexed under this heading.

Hydrochlorothiazide (Concomitant administration of nephrotoxic drugs could result in delayed clearance of pemetrexed). Products include:
- Aldoril Tablets 1910
- Atacand HCT 651
- Avalide Tablets 888
- Avalide Tablets 2874
- Benicar HCT Tablets 1044
- Diovan HCT Tablets 2196
- Dyazide Capsules 1423
- Hyzaar 50-12.5 Tablets 1990
- Hyzaar 100-12.5 Tablets 1990
- Hyzaar 100-25 Tablets 1990
- Lopressor HCT 50/25 Tablets 2241
- Lopressor HCT 100/25 Tablets 2241
- Lopressor HCT 100/50 Tablets 2241
- Lotensin HCT Tablets 2246
- Micardis HCT Tablets 856
- Moduretic Tablets 2028
- Prinzide Tablets 2056
- Teveten HCT Tablets 1737
- Timolide Tablets 2086
- Uniretic Tablets 3100

Hydroflumethiazide (Concomitant administration of nephrotoxic drugs could result in delayed clearance of pemetrexed).
No products indexed under this heading.

Ibuprofen (Caution should be used when administering ibuprofen concurrently with pemetrexed to patients with mild to moderate renal insufficiency (CrCl 45-79 mL/min)). Products include:
- Advil Allergy Sinus Caplets .... ▣770
- Advil .... ▣674
- Children's Advil Oral Suspension .... ▣603
- Children's Advil Chewable Tablets .... ▣603
- Advil Cold & Sinus .... ▣723
- Infants' Advil Concentrated Drops .... ▣604
- Infants' Advil Concentrated Drops - White Grape (Dye-Free) .... ▣604
- Junior Strength Advil Swallow Tablets .... ▣605
- Advil Migraine Liquigels .... ▣608
- Advil Multi-Symptom Cold Caplets .... ▣770
- Advil PM Caplets .... ▣615
- Motrin IB Tablets and Caplets 1866
- Children's Motrin Oral Suspension 1867
- Children's Motrin Non-Staining Dye-Free Oral Suspension 1867
- Children's Motrin Cold Oral Suspension 1867
- Infants' Motrin Concentrated Drops 1867
- Infants' Motrin Non-Staining Dye-Free Concentrated Drops 1867
- Junior Strength Motrin Caplets and Chewable Tablets 1867
- Vicoprofen Tablets 539

Idarubicin Hydrochloride (Concomitant administration of nephrotoxic drugs could result in delayed clearance of pemetrexed).
No products indexed under this heading.

Ifosfamide (Concomitant administration of nephrotoxic drugs could result in delayed clearance of pemetrexed).
No products indexed under this heading.

Imipenem (Concomitant administration of nephrotoxic drugs could result in delayed clearance of pemetrexed). Products include:
Primaxin I.M. 2045
Primaxin I.V. 2048

Immune Globulin Intravenous (Human) (Concomitant administration of nephrotoxic drugs could result in delayed clearance of pemetrexed). Products include:
Carimune NF 3499
Gammagard Liquid 721
Gammagard S/D 724
Gamunex Immune Globulin I.V., 10% 3235

Indinavir Sulfate (Concomitant administration of nephrotoxic drugs could result in delayed clearance of pemetrexed). Products include:
Crixivan Capsules 1940

Indomethacin (Patients with mild to moderate renal insufficiency should avoid NSAIDs with short elimination half-lives two days before, the day of, and two days following administration of pemetrexed. All patients should avoid NSAIDs with longer half-lives at least five days before, the day of, and two days following pemetrexed administration. If concomitant administration of an NSAID is necessary, patients should be monitored closely for toxicity, especially myelosuppression, renal and gastrointestinal toxicity). Products include:
Indocin 1995

Indomethacin Sodium Trihydrate (Patients with mild to moderate renal insufficiency should avoid NSAIDs with short elimination half-lives two days before, the day of, and two days following administration of pemetrexed. All patients should avoid NSAIDs with longer half-lives at least five days before, the day of, and two days following pemetrexed administration. If concomitant administration of an NSAID is necessary, patients should be monitored closely for toxicity, especially myelosuppression, renal and gastrointestinal toxicity). Products include:
Indocin I.V. 2465

Interferon Beta-1b (Concomitant administration of nephrotoxic drugs could result in delayed clearance of pemetrexed). Products include:
Betaseron for SC Injection 767

Interleuken-2 (Concomitant administration of nephrotoxic drugs could result in delayed clearance of pemetrexed).
No products indexed under this heading.

Iodamide Meglumine (Concomitant administration of nephrotoxic drugs could result in delayed clearance of pemetrexed).
No products indexed under this heading.

Iohexol (Concomitant administration of nephrotoxic drugs could result in delayed clearance of pemetrexed).
No products indexed under this heading.

Iopamidol (Concomitant administration of nephrotoxic drugs could result in delayed clearance of pemetrexed).
No products indexed under this heading.

Iopanoic Acid (Concomitant administration of nephrotoxic drugs could result in delayed clearance of pemetrexed).
No products indexed under this heading.

Iothalamate Meglumine (Concomitant administration of nephrotoxic drugs could result in delayed clearance of pemetrexed).
No products indexed under this heading.

Ioxaglate Meglumine (Concomitant administration of nephrotoxic drugs could result in delayed clearance of pemetrexed).
No products indexed under this heading.

Ioxaglate Sodium (Concomitant administration of nephrotoxic drugs could result in delayed clearance of pemetrexed).
No products indexed under this heading.

Kanamycin Sulfate (Concomitant administration of nephrotoxic drugs could result in delayed clearance of pemetrexed).
No products indexed under this heading.

Ketoprofen (Patients with mild to moderate renal insufficiency should avoid NSAIDs with short elimination half-lives two days before, the day of, and two days following administration of pemetrexed. All patients should avoid NSAIDs with longer half-lives at least five days before, the day of, and two days following pemetrexed administration. If concomitant administration of an NSAID is necessary, patients should be monitored closely for toxicity, especially myelosuppression, renal and gastrointestinal toxicity).
No products indexed under this heading.

Ketorolac Tromethamine (Patients with mild to moderate renal insufficiency should avoid NSAIDs with short elimination half-lives two days before, the day of, and two days following administration of pemetrexed. All patients should avoid NSAIDs with longer half-lives at least five days before, the day of, and two days following pemetrexed administration. If concomitant administration of an NSAID is necessary, patients should be monitored closely for toxicity, especially myelosuppression, renal and gastrointestinal toxicity). Products include:
Acular Ophthalmic Solution 565
Acular LS Ophthalmic Solution 566

Lamium album (Concomitant administration of nephrotoxic drugs could result in delayed clearance of pemetrexed).
No products indexed under this heading.

Lisinopril (Concomitant administration of nephrotoxic drugs could result in delayed clearance of pemetrexed). Products include:
Prinivil Tablets 2052
Prinzide Tablets 2056

Lithium (Concomitant administration of nephrotoxic drugs could result in delayed clearance of pemetrexed).
No products indexed under this heading.

Lithium Carbonate (Concomitant administration of nephrotoxic drugs could result in delayed clearance of pemetrexed). Products include:
Lithobid Tablets 1692

Lithium Citrate (Concomitant administration of nephrotoxic drugs could result in delayed clearance of pemetrexed).
No products indexed under this heading.

Lopinavir (Concomitant administration of nephrotoxic drugs could result in delayed clearance of pemetrexed). Products include:
Kaletra 476

Loracarbef (Concomitant administration of nephrotoxic drugs could result in delayed clearance of pemetrexed).
No products indexed under this heading.

Lovastatin (Concomitant administration of nephrotoxic drugs could result in delayed clearance of pemetrexed). Products include:
Advicor Tablets 1722
Altoprev Extended-Release Tablets 3109
Mevacor Tablets 2021

Meclofenamate Sodium (Patients with mild to moderate renal insufficiency should avoid NSAIDs with short elimination half-lives two days before, the day of, and two days following administration of pemetrexed. All patients should avoid NSAIDs with longer half-lives at least five days before, the day of, and two days following pemetrexed administration. If concomitant administration of an NSAID is necessary, patients should be monitored closely for toxicity, especially myelosuppression, renal and gastrointestinal toxicity).
No products indexed under this heading.

Mefenamic Acid (Patients with mild to moderate renal insufficiency should avoid NSAIDs with short elimination half-lives two days before, the day of, and two days following administration of pemetrexed. All patients should avoid NSAIDs with longer half-lives at least five days before, the day of, and two days following pemetrexed administration. If concomitant administration of an NSAID is necessary, patients should be monitored closely for toxicity, especially myelosuppression, renal and gastrointestinal toxicity).
No products indexed under this heading.

Meloxicam (Patients with mild to moderate renal insufficiency should avoid NSAIDs with short elimination half-lives two days before, the day of, and two days following administration of pemetrexed. All patients should avoid NSAIDs with longer half-lives at least five days before, the day of, and two days following pemetrexed administration. If concomitant administration of an NSAID is necessary, patients should be monitored closely for toxicity, especially myelosuppression, renal and gastrointestinal toxicity). Products include:
Mobic Oral Suspension 863
Mobic Tablets 863

Melphalan Hydrochloride (Concomitant administration of nephrotoxic drugs could result in delayed clearance of pemetrexed). Products include:
Alkeran for Injection 955

Mesalamine (Concomitant administration of nephrotoxic drugs could result in delayed clearance of pemetrexed). Products include:
Asacol Delayed-Release Tablets 2692
Canasa Rectal Suppositories 699
Pentasa Capsules 3185

Methimazole (Concomitant administration of nephrotoxic drugs could result in delayed clearance of pemetrexed).
No products indexed under this heading.

Methotrexate (Concomitant administration of nephrotoxic drugs could result in delayed clearance of pemetrexed).
No products indexed under this heading.

Methotrexate Sodium (Concomitant administration of nephrotoxic drugs could result in delayed clearance of pemetrexed).
No products indexed under this heading.

Methyclothiazide (Concomitant administration of nephrotoxic drugs could result in delayed clearance of pemetrexed).
No products indexed under this heading.

Mezlocillin Sodium (Concomitant administration of nephrotoxic drugs could result in delayed clearance of pemetrexed).
No products indexed under this heading.

Minocycline Hydrochloride (Concomitant administration of nephrotoxic drugs could result in delayed clearance of pemetrexed). Products include:
Solodyn Extended Release Tablets 1890

Mitomycin (Mitomycin-C) (Concomitant administration of nephrotoxic drugs could result in delayed clearance of pemetrexed).
No products indexed under this heading.

Moexipril Hydrochloride (Concomitant administration of nephrotoxic drugs could result in delayed clearance of pemetrexed). Products include:
Uniretic Tablets 3100
Univasc Tablets 3104

Muromonab-CD3 (Concomitant administration of nephrotoxic drugs could result in delayed clearance of pemetrexed). Products include:
Orthoclone OKT3 Sterile Solution 2360

Nabumetone (Patients with mild to moderate renal insufficiency should avoid NSAIDs with short elimination half-lives two days before, the day of, and two days following administration of pemetrexed. All patients should avoid NSAIDs with longer half-lives at least five days before, the day of, and two days following pemetrexed administration. If concomitant administration of an NSAID is necessary, patients should be monitored closely for toxicity, especially myelosuppression, renal and gastrointestinal toxicity).
No products indexed under this heading.

Nafcillin Sodium (Concomitant administration of nephrotoxic drugs could result in delayed clearance of pemetrexed).

 No products indexed under this heading.

Naproxen (Patients with mild to moderate renal insufficiency should avoid NSAIDs with short elimination half-lives two days before, the day of, and two days following administration of pemetrexed. All patients should avoid NSAIDs with longer half-lives at least five days before, the day of, and two days following pemetrexed administration. If concomitant administration of an NSAID is necessary, patients should be monitored closely for toxicity, especially myelosuppression, renal and gastrointestinal toxicity). Products include:

Naproxen Sodium (Patients with mild to moderate renal insufficiency should avoid NSAIDs with short elimination half-lives two days before, the day of, and two days following administration of pemetrexed. All patients should avoid NSAIDs with longer half-lives at least five days before, the day of, and two days following pemetrexed administration. If concomitant administration of an NSAID is necessary, patients should be monitored closely for toxicity, especially myelosuppression, renal and gastrointestinal toxicity). Products include:

Nelfinavir Mesylate (Concomitant administration of nephrotoxic drugs could result in delayed clearance of pemetrexed). Products include:

Neomycin (Concomitant administration of nephrotoxic drugs could result in delayed clearance of pemetrexed). Products include:

Neomycin, oral (Concomitant administration of nephrotoxic drugs could result in delayed clearance of pemetrexed).

 No products indexed under this heading.

Neomycin Sulfate (Concomitant administration of nephrotoxic drugs could result in delayed clearance of pemetrexed). Products include:

Nevirapine (Concomitant administration of nephrotoxic drugs could result in delayed clearance of pemetrexed). Products include:

Norfloxacin (Concomitant administration of nephrotoxic drugs could result in delayed clearance of pemetrexed). Products include:

Olsalazine Sodium (Concomitant administration of nephrotoxic drugs could result in delayed clearance of pemetrexed).

 No products indexed under this heading.

Omeprazole (Concomitant administration of nephrotoxic drugs could result in delayed clearance of pemetrexed). Products include:

Oxaprozin (Patients with mild to moderate renal insufficiency should avoid NSAIDs with short elimination half-lives two days before, the day of, and two days following administration of pemetrexed. All patients should avoid NSAIDs with longer half-lives at least five days before, the day of, and two days following pemetrexed administration. If concomitant administration of an NSAID is necessary, patients should be monitored closely for toxicity, especially myelosuppression, renal and gastrointestinal toxicity).

 No products indexed under this heading.

Pamidronate Disodium (Concomitant administration of nephrotoxic drugs could result in delayed clearance of pemetrexed). Products include:

Paroxetine Hydrochloride (Concomitant administration of nephrotoxic drugs could result in delayed clearance of pemetrexed). Products include:

Penicillamine (Concomitant administration of nephrotoxic drugs could result in delayed clearance of pemetrexed). Products include:

Penicillin G Benzathine (Concomitant administration of nephrotoxic drugs could result in delayed clearance of pemetrexed). Products include:

Penicillin G Potassium (Concomitant administration of nephrotoxic drugs could result in delayed clearance of pemetrexed).

 No products indexed under this heading.

Penicillin G Procaine (Concomitant administration of nephrotoxic drugs could result in delayed clearance of pemetrexed). Products include:

Penicillin G Sodium (Concomitant administration of nephrotoxic drugs could result in delayed clearance of pemetrexed).

 No products indexed under this heading.

Penicillin V Potassium (Concomitant administration of nephrotoxic drugs could result in delayed clearance of pemetrexed).

 No products indexed under this heading.

Pentamidine Isethionate (Concomitant administration of nephrotoxic drugs could result in delayed clearance of pemetrexed).

 No products indexed under this heading.

Perindopril Erbumine (Concomitant administration of nephrotoxic

drugs could result in delayed clearance of pemetrexed). Products include:

Phenylbutazone (Patients with mild to moderate renal insufficiency should avoid NSAIDs with short elimination half-lives two days before, the day of, and two days following administration of pemetrexed. All patients should avoid NSAIDs with longer half-lives at least five days before, the day of, and two days following pemetrexed administration. If concomitant administration of an NSAID is necessary, patients should be monitored closely for toxicity, especially myelosuppression, renal and gastrointestinal toxicity).

 No products indexed under this heading.

Piroxicam (Patients with mild to moderate renal insufficiency should avoid NSAIDs with short elimination half-lives two days before, the day of, and two days following administration of pemetrexed. All patients should avoid NSAIDs with longer half-lives at least five days before, the day of, and two days following pemetrexed administration. If concomitant administration of an NSAID is necessary, patients should be monitored closely for toxicity, especially myelosuppression, renal and gastrointestinal toxicity).

 No products indexed under this heading.

Plicamycin (Concomitant administration of nephrotoxic drugs could result in delayed clearance of pemetrexed).

 No products indexed under this heading.

Polymyxin (Concomitant administration of nephrotoxic drugs could result in delayed clearance of pemetrexed).

 No products indexed under this heading.

Polymyxin B Sulfate (Concomitant administration of nephrotoxic drugs could result in delayed clearance of pemetrexed). Products include:

Polythiazide (Concomitant administration of nephrotoxic drugs could result in delayed clearance of pemetrexed).

 No products indexed under this heading.

Pravastatin Sodium (Concomitant administration of nephrotoxic drugs could result in delayed clearance of pemetrexed).

 No products indexed under this heading.

Probenecid (Concomitant administration of substances that are also tubularly secreted (e.g., probenecid) could potentially result in delayed clearance of pemetrexed).

 No products indexed under this heading.

Quinapril Hydrochloride (Concomitant administration of nephrotoxic drugs could result in delayed clearance of pemetrexed).

 No products indexed under this heading.

Rabeprazole Sodium (Concomitant administration of nephrotoxic drugs could result in delayed clearance of pemetrexed). Products include:

Ramipril (Concomitant administration of nephrotoxic drugs could result in delayed clearance of pemetrexed). Products include:

Rifampin (Concomitant administration of nephrotoxic drugs could result in delayed clearance of pemetrexed).

 No products indexed under this heading.

Riluzole (Concomitant administration of nephrotoxic drugs could result in delayed clearance of pemetrexed). Products include:

Ritonavir (Concomitant administration of nephrotoxic drugs could result in delayed clearance of pemetrexed). Products include:

Rofecoxib (Patients with mild to moderate renal insufficiency should avoid NSAIDs with short elimination half-lives two days before, the day of, and two days following administration of pemetrexed. All patients should avoid NSAIDs with longer half-lives at least five days before, the day of, and two days following pemetrexed administration. If concomitant administration of an NSAID is necessary, patients should be monitored closely for toxicity, especially myelosuppression, renal and gastrointestinal toxicity).

 No products indexed under this heading.

Saquinavir (Concomitant administration of nephrotoxic drugs could result in delayed clearance of pemetrexed).

 No products indexed under this heading.

Sibutramine Hydrochloride Monohydrate (Concomitant administration of nephrotoxic drugs could result in delayed clearance of pemetrexed). Products include:

Simvastatin (Concomitant administration of nephrotoxic drugs could result in delayed clearance of pemetrexed). Products include:

Spirapril Hydrochloride (Concomitant administration of nephrotoxic drugs could result in delayed clearance of pemetrexed).

 No products indexed under this heading.

Stavudine (Concomitant administration of nephrotoxic drugs could result in delayed clearance of pemetrexed).
No products indexed under this heading.

Streptomycin Sulfate (Concomitant administration of nephrotoxic drugs could result in delayed clearance of pemetrexed).
No products indexed under this heading.

Streptozocin (Concomitant administration of nephrotoxic drugs could result in delayed clearance of pemetrexed).
No products indexed under this heading.

Sulfacytine (Concomitant administration of nephrotoxic drugs could result in delayed clearance of pemetrexed).
No products indexed under this heading.

Sulfamethizole (Concomitant administration of nephrotoxic drugs could result in delayed clearance of pemetrexed).
No products indexed under this heading.

Sulfamethoxazole (Concomitant administration of nephrotoxic drugs could result in delayed clearance of pemetrexed).
No products indexed under this heading.

Sulfasalazine (Concomitant administration of nephrotoxic drugs could result in delayed clearance of pemetrexed).
No products indexed under this heading.

Sulfinpyrazone (Concomitant administration of nephrotoxic drugs could result in delayed clearance of pemetrexed).
No products indexed under this heading.

Sulfisoxazole Acetyl (Concomitant administration of nephrotoxic drugs could result in delayed clearance of pemetrexed).
No products indexed under this heading.

Sulfisoxazole Diolamine (Concomitant administration of nephrotoxic drugs could result in delayed clearance of pemetrexed).
No products indexed under this heading.

Sulindac (Patients with mild to moderate renal insufficiency should avoid NSAIDs with short elimination half-lives two days before, the day of, and two days following administration of pemetrexed. All patients should avoid NSAIDs with longer half-lives at least five days before, the day of, and two days following pemetrexed administration. If concomitant administration of an NSAID is necessary, patients should be monitored closely for toxicity, especially myelosuppression, renal and gastrointestinal toxicity). Products include:
Clinoril Tablets 1924

Tacrolimus (Concomitant administration of nephrotoxic drugs could result in delayed clearance of pemetrexed). Products include:
Prograf Capsules and Injection 632
Protopic Ointment 638

Tenofovir Disoproxil Fumarate (Concomitant administration of nephrotoxic drugs could result in delayed clearance of pemetrexed). Products include:
Atripla Tablets 945
Truvada Tablets 1296
Viread Tablets 1301

Thioguanine (Concomitant administration of nephrotoxic drugs could result in delayed clearance of pemetrexed). Products include:
Tabloid Tablets 1575

Ticarcillin Disodium (Concomitant administration of nephrotoxic drugs could result in delayed clearance of pemetrexed). Products include:
Timentin ADD-Vantage 1580
Timentin Injection Galaxy Container 1583
Timentin IV Infusion 1577
Timentin Pharmacy Bulk Package 1586

Tobramycin (Concomitant administration of nephrotoxic drugs could result in delayed clearance of pemetrexed). Products include:
TOBI Solution for Inhalation 2298
TobraDex Ophthalmic Ointment 562
TobraDex Ophthalmic Suspension ... 563
Zylet Ophthalmic Suspension .... ⊙259

Tobramycin Sulfate (Concomitant administration of nephrotoxic drugs could result in delayed clearance of pemetrexed).
No products indexed under this heading.

Tolazamide (Concomitant administration of nephrotoxic drugs could result in delayed clearance of pemetrexed).
No products indexed under this heading.

Tolbutamide (Concomitant administration of nephrotoxic drugs could result in delayed clearance of pemetrexed).
No products indexed under this heading.

Tolmetin Sodium (Patients with mild to moderate renal insufficiency should avoid NSAIDs with short elimination half-lives two days before, the day of, and two days following administration of pemetrexed. All patients should avoid NSAIDs with longer half-lives at least five days before, the day of, and two days following pemetrexed administration. If concomitant administration of an NSAID is necessary, patients should be monitored closely for toxicity, especially myelosuppression, renal and gastrointestinal toxicity).
No products indexed under this heading.

Trandolapril (Concomitant administration of nephrotoxic drugs could result in delayed clearance of pemetrexed). Products include:
Mavik Tablets 486
Tarka Tablets 524

Triamterene (Concomitant administration of nephrotoxic drugs could result in delayed clearance of pemetrexed). Products include:
Dyazide Capsules 1423
Dyrenium Capsules 3400

Trimethadione (Concomitant administration of nephrotoxic drugs could result in delayed clearance of pemetrexed).
No products indexed under this heading.

Trovafloxacin Mesylate (Concomitant administration of nephrotoxic drugs could result in delayed clearance of pemetrexed).
No products indexed under this heading.

Tyropanoate Sodium (Concomitant administration of nephrotoxic drugs could result in delayed clearance of pemetrexed).
No products indexed under this heading.

Valacyclovir Hydrochloride (Concomitant administration of nephrotoxic drugs could result in delayed clearance of pemetrexed). Products include:
Valtrex Caplets 1597

Valdecoxib (Patients with mild to moderate renal insufficiency should avoid NSAIDs with short elimination half-lives two days before, the day of, and two days following administration of pemetrexed. All patients should avoid NSAIDs with longer half-lives at least five days before, the day of, and two days following pemetrexed administration. If concomitant administration of an NSAID is necessary, patients should be monitored closely for toxicity, especially myelosuppression, renal and gastrointestinal toxicity).
No products indexed under this heading.

Vancomycin Hydrochloride (Concomitant administration of nephrotoxic drugs could result in delayed clearance of pemetrexed). Products include:
Vancocin HCl Capsules, USP 3380

Voriconazole (Concomitant administration of nephrotoxic drugs could result in delayed clearance of pemetrexed). Products include:
VFEND I.V. 2564
VFEND Oral Suspension 2564
VFEND Tablets 2564

Zalcitabine (Concomitant administration of nephrotoxic drugs could result in delayed clearance of pemetrexed).
No products indexed under this heading.

Zidovudine (Concomitant administration of nephrotoxic drugs could result in delayed clearance of pemetrexed). Products include:
Combivir Tablets 1411
Retrovir 1560
Retrovir IV Infusion 1564
Trizivir Tablets 1589

Zoledronic acid (Concomitant administration of nephrotoxic drugs could result in delayed clearance of pemetrexed). Products include:
Zometa for Intravenous Infusion 2315

ALINIA FOR ORAL SUSPENSION

(Nitazoxanide) 2835
May interact with highly protein bound drugs (selected). Compounds in these categories include:

Amiodarone Hydrochloride (Metabolite is highly bound to plasma protein. Use caution when administering nitazoxanide concurrently with other highly plasma protein-bound drugs with narrow therapeutic indices).
No products indexed under this heading.

Amitriptyline Hydrochloride (Metabolite is highly bound to plasma protein. Use caution when administering nitazoxanide concurrently with other highly plasma protein-bound drugs with narrow therapeutic indices).
No products indexed under this heading.

Atovaquone (Metabolite is highly bound to plasma protein. Use caution when administering nitazoxanide concurrently with other highly plasma protein-bound drugs with narrow therapeutic indices). Products include:
Malarone Pediatric Tablets 1517
Malarone Tablets 1517
Mepron Suspension 1521

Cefonicid Sodium (Metabolite is highly bound to plasma protein. Use caution when administering nitazoxanide concurrently with other highly plasma protein-bound drugs with narrow therapeutic indices).
No products indexed under this heading.

Celecoxib (Metabolite is highly bound to plasma protein. Use caution when administering nitazoxanide concurrently with other highly plasma protein-bound drugs with narrow therapeutic indices). Products include:
Celebrex Capsules 3134

Chlordiazepoxide (Metabolite is highly bound to plasma protein. Use caution when administering nitazoxanide concurrently with other highly plasma protein-bound drugs with narrow therapeutic indices).
No products indexed under this heading.

Chlordiazepoxide Hydrochloride (Metabolite is highly bound to plasma protein. Use caution when administering nitazoxanide concurrently with other highly plasma protein-bound drugs with narrow therapeutic indices). Products include:
Librium Capsules 3347

Chlorpromazine (Metabolite is highly bound to plasma protein. Use caution when administering nitazoxanide concurrently with other highly plasma protein-bound drugs with narrow therapeutic indices).
No products indexed under this heading.

Chlorpromazine Hydrochloride (Metabolite is highly bound to plasma protein. Use caution when administering nitazoxanide concurrently with other highly plasma protein-bound drugs with narrow therapeutic indices).
No products indexed under this heading.

Clomipramine Hydrochloride (Metabolite is highly bound to plasma protein. Use caution when administering nitazoxanide concurrently with other highly plasma protein-bound drugs with narrow therapeutic indices).
No products indexed under this heading.

Clozapine (Metabolite is highly bound to plasma protein. Use caution when administering nitazoxanide concurrently with other highly plasma protein-bound drugs with narrow therapeutic indices). Products include:
Clozaril Tablets 2184
FazaClo Orally Disintegrating Tablets 551

Cyclosporine (Metabolite is highly bound to plasma protein. Use caution when administering nitazoxanide concurrently with other highly plasma protein-bound drugs with narrow therapeutic indices). Products include:
Gengraf Capsules 459
Neoral Oral Solution 2259
Neoral Soft Gelatin Capsules 2259
Restasis Ophthalmic Emulsion 575

Sandimmune 2275

Diazepam (Metabolite is highly bound to plasma protein. Use caution when administering nitazoxanide concurrently with other highly plasma protein-bound drugs with narrow therapeutic indices). Products include:

Diastat Rectal Delivery System 3343
Valium Tablets 2819

Diclofenac Potassium (Metabolite is highly bound to plasma protein. Use caution when administering nitazoxanide concurrently with other highly plasma protein-bound drugs with narrow therapeutic indices).

No products indexed under this heading.

Diclofenac Sodium (Metabolite is highly bound to plasma protein. Use caution when administering nitazoxanide concurrently with other highly plasma protein-bound drugs with narrow therapeutic indices). Products include:

Arthrotec Tablets 3129
Voltaren Ophthalmic Solution 2309
Voltaren Tablets 2307
Voltaren-XR Tablets 2310

Dipyridamole (Metabolite is highly bound to plasma protein. Use caution when administering nitazoxanide concurrently with other highly plasma protein-bound drugs with narrow therapeutic indices). Products include:

Aggrenox Capsules 822
Persantine Tablets 868

Fenoprofen Calcium (Metabolite is highly bound to plasma protein. Use caution when administering nitazoxanide concurrently with other highly plasma protein-bound drugs with narrow therapeutic indices). Products include:

Nalfon Capsules 2502

Flurazepam Hydrochloride (Metabolite is highly bound to plasma protein. Use caution when administering nitazoxanide concurrently with other highly plasma protein-bound drugs with narrow therapeutic indices). Products include:

Dalmane Capsules 3342

Flurbiprofen (Metabolite is highly bound to plasma protein. Use caution when administering nitazoxanide concurrently with other highly plasma protein-bound drugs with narrow therapeutic indices).

No products indexed under this heading.

Glipizide (Metabolite is highly bound to plasma protein. Use caution when administering nitazoxanide concurrently with other highly plasma protein-bound drugs with narrow therapeutic indices).

No products indexed under this heading.

Ibuprofen (Metabolite is highly bound to plasma protein. Use caution when administering nitazoxanide concurrently with other highly plasma protein-bound drugs with narrow therapeutic indices). Products include:

Advil Allergy Sinus Caplets .... ◘770
Advil .... ◘674
Children's Advil Oral Suspension .... ◘603
Children's Advil Chewable Tablets .. ◘603
Advil Cold & Sinus .... ◘723
Infants' Advil Concentrated Drops .. ◘604
Infants' Advil Concentrated Drops - White Grape (Dye-Free)............. ◘604
Junior Strength Advil Swallow Tablets.. ◘605
Advil Migraine Liquigels .... ◘608
Advil Multi-Symptom Cold Caplets.. ◘770
Advil PM Caplets .... ◘615
Motrin IB Tablets and Caplets 1866
Children's Motrin Oral Suspension ... 1867
Children's Motrin Non-Staining Dye-Free Oral Suspension............ 1867
Children's Motrin Cold Oral Suspension 1867
Infants' Motrin Concentrated Drops.. 1867
Infants' Motrin Non-Staining Dye-Free Concentrated Drops....... 1867
Junior Strength Motrin Caplets and Chewable Tablets.................. 1867
Vicoprofen Tablets 539

Imipramine Hydrochloride (Metabolite is highly bound to plasma protein. Use caution when administering nitazoxanide concurrently with other highly plasma protein-bound drugs with narrow therapeutic indices).

No products indexed under this heading.

Imipramine Pamoate (Metabolite is highly bound to plasma protein. Use caution when administering nitazoxanide concurrently with other highly plasma protein-bound drugs with narrow therapeutic indices).

No products indexed under this heading.

Indomethacin (Metabolite is highly bound to plasma protein. Use caution when administering nitazoxanide concurrently with other highly plasma protein-bound drugs with narrow therapeutic indices). Products include:

Indocin 1995

Indomethacin Sodium Trihydrate (Metabolite is highly bound to plasma protein. Use caution when administering nitazoxanide concurrently with other highly plasma protein-bound drugs with narrow therapeutic indices). Products include:

Indocin I.V. 2465

Ketoprofen (Metabolite is highly bound to plasma protein. Use caution when administering nitazoxanide concurrently with other highly plasma protein-bound drugs with narrow therapeutic indices).

No products indexed under this heading.

Ketorolac Tromethamine (Metabolite is highly bound to plasma protein. Use caution when administering nitazoxanide concurrently with other highly plasma protein-bound drugs with narrow therapeutic indices). Products include:

Acular Ophthalmic Solution 565
Acular LS Ophthalmic Solution 566

Meclofenamate Sodium (Metabolite is highly bound to plasma protein. Use caution when administering nitazoxanide concurrently with other highly plasma protein-bound drugs with narrow therapeutic indices).

No products indexed under this heading.

Mefenamic Acid (Metabolite is highly bound to plasma protein. Use caution when administering nitazoxanide concurrently with other highly plasma protein-bound drugs with narrow therapeutic indices).

No products indexed under this heading.

Midazolam Hydrochloride (Metabolite is highly bound to plasma protein. Use caution when administering nitazoxanide concurrently with other highly plasma protein-bound drugs with narrow therapeutic indices).

No products indexed under this heading.

Naproxen (Metabolite is highly bound to plasma protein. Use caution when administering nitazoxanide concurrently with other highly plasma protein-bound drugs with narrow therapeutic indices). Products include:

EC-Naprosyn Delayed-Release Tablets 2761
Naprosyn Suspension 2761
Naprosyn Tablets 2761
Prevacid NapraPAC 3280

Naproxen Sodium (Metabolite is highly bound to plasma protein. Use caution when administering nitazoxanide concurrently with other highly plasma protein-bound drugs with narrow therapeutic indices). Products include:

Aleve Caplets 742
Aleve Gelcaps 743
Aleve Tablets 743
Aleve Cold & Sinus Caplets 744
Anaprox Tablets 2761
Anaprox DS Tablets 2761

Nortriptyline Hydrochloride (Metabolite is highly bound to plasma protein. Use caution when administering nitazoxanide concurrently with other highly plasma protein-bound drugs with narrow therapeutic indices).

No products indexed under this heading.

Oxaprozin (Metabolite is highly bound to plasma protein. Use caution when administering nitazoxanide concurrently with other highly plasma protein-bound drugs with narrow therapeutic indices).

No products indexed under this heading.

Oxazepam (Metabolite is highly bound to plasma protein. Use caution when administering nitazoxanide concurrently with other highly plasma protein-bound drugs with narrow therapeutic indices).

No products indexed under this heading.

Phenylbutazone (Metabolite is highly bound to plasma protein. Use caution when administering nitazoxanide concurrently with other highly plasma protein-bound drugs with narrow therapeutic indices).

No products indexed under this heading.

Piroxicam (Metabolite is highly bound to plasma protein. Use caution when administering nitazoxanide concurrently with other highly plasma protein-bound drugs with narrow therapeutic indices).

No products indexed under this heading.

Propranolol Hydrochloride (Metabolite is highly bound to plasma protein. Use caution when administering nitazoxanide concurrently with other highly plasma protein-bound drugs with narrow therapeutic indices). Products include:

Inderal LA Long-Acting Capsules 3429
InnoPran XL Capsules 2723

Sulindac (Metabolite is highly bound to plasma protein. Use caution when administering nitazoxanide concurrently with other highly plasma protein-bound drugs with narrow therapeutic indices). Products include:

Clinoril Tablets 1924

Temazepam (Metabolite is highly bound to plasma protein. Use caution when administering nitazoxanide concurrently with other highly plasma protein-bound drugs with narrow therapeutic indices). Products include:

Restoril Capsules 1860

Tolbutamide (Metabolite is highly bound to plasma protein. Use caution when administering nitazoxanide concurrently with other highly plasma protein-bound drugs with narrow therapeutic indices).

No products indexed under this heading.

Tolmetin Sodium (Metabolite is highly bound to plasma protein. Use caution when administering nitazoxanide concurrently with other highly plasma protein-bound drugs with narrow therapeutic indices).

No products indexed under this heading.

Trimipramine Maleate (Metabolite is highly bound to plasma protein. Use caution when administering nitazoxanide concurrently with other highly plasma protein-bound drugs with narrow therapeutic indices).

No products indexed under this heading.

Warfarin Sodium (Metabolite is highly bound to plasma protein. Use caution when administering nitazoxanide concurrently with other highly plasma protein-bound drugs with narrow therapeutic indices). Products include:

Coumadin for Injection 898
Coumadin Tablets 898

ALINIA TABLETS

(Nitazoxanide) 2835
See Alinia for Oral Suspension

ALKERAN FOR INJECTION

(Melphalan Hydrochloride) 955
May interact with:

Carmustine (BCNU) (Reduced threshold for BCNU lung toxicity).

No products indexed under this heading.

Cisplatin (Affects melphalan kinetics by inducing renal dysfunction and subsequently altering melphalan clearance).

No products indexed under this heading.

Cyclosporine (Potential for severe renal failure). Products include:

Gengraf Capsules 459
Neoral Oral Solution 2259
Neoral Soft Gelatin Capsules 2259
Restasis Ophthalmic Emulsion 575
Sandimmune 2275

Nalidixic Acid (Increased incidence of severe hemorrhagic necrotic enterocolitis).

No products indexed under this heading.

ALKERAN TABLETS

(Melphalan) 956
None cited in PDR database.

ALLEGRA CAPSULES

(Fexofenadine Hydrochloride) 2844
May interact with erythromycin and certain other agents. Compounds in these categories include:

Aluminum Hydroxide (Administration of fexofenadine within 15 minutes of an aluminum and magnesium containing antacid decreased fexofenadine AUC by 41% and Cmax by 43%; Allegra should not be taken closely in time with aluminum and magnesium containing antacids). Products include:

Gaviscon Regular Strength Liquid .. 658
Gaviscon Regular Strength Tablets 658
Gaviscon Extra Strength Liquid 658
Gaviscon Extra Strength Tablets 658
Maalox Regular Strength Antacid/Antigas Liquid 2175
Maalox Max Maximum Strength Antacid/Anti-Gas Liquid 2176

Erythromycin (Co-administration with erythromycin enhances fexofenadine gastrointestinal absorption thereby increasing plasma levels of fexofenadine; in vivo animal studies suggest that erythromycin may also decrease biliary excretion). Products include:

Ery-Tab Tablets 449
Erythromycin Base Filmtab Tablets 455
Erythromycin Delayed-Release Capsules, USP 457
PCE Dispertab Tablets 515

Erythromycin Estolate (Co-administration with erythromycin enhances fexofenadine gastrointestinal absorption thereby increasing plasma levels of fexofenadine; in vivo animal studies suggest that erythromycin may also decrease biliary excretion).

No products indexed under this heading.

Erythromycin Ethylsuccinate (Co-administration with erythromycin enhances fexofenadine gastrointestinal absorption thereby increasing plasma levels of fexofenadine; in vivo animal studies suggest that erythromycin may also decrease biliary excretion). Products include:

E.E.S. 451
EryPed 447

Erythromycin Gluceptate (Co-administration with erythromycin enhances fexofenadine gastrointestinal absorption thereby increasing plasma levels of fexofenadine; in vivo animal studies suggest that erythromycin may also decrease biliary excretion).

No products indexed under this heading.

Erythromycin Lactobionate (Co-administration with erythromycin enhances fexofenadine gastrointestinal absorption thereby increasing plasma levels of fexofenadine; in vivo animal studies suggest that erythromycin may also decrease biliary excretion).

No products indexed under this heading.

Erythromycin Stearate (Co-administration with erythromycin enhances fexofenadine gastrointestinal absorption thereby increasing plasma levels of fexofenadine; in vivo animal studies suggest that erythromycin may also decrease biliary excretion). Products include:

Erythrocin Stearate Filmtab Tablets 453

Ketoconazole (Co-administration with ketoconazole enhances fexofenadine gastrointestinal absorption thereby increasing plasma levels of fexofenadine; in vivo animal studies suggest that ketoconazole may also decrease fexofenadine gastrointestinal secretion). Products include:

Nizoral A-D Shampoo, 1% 1868

Magnesium Hydroxide (Administration of fexofenadine within 15 minutes of an aluminum and magnesium containing antacid decreased fexofenadine AUC by 41% and Cmax by 43%; Allegra should not be taken closely in time with aluminum and magnesium containing antacids). Products include:

Maalox Regular Strength Antacid/Antigas Liquid 2175
Maalox Max Maximum Strength Antacid/Anti-Gas Liquid 2176
Pepcid Complete Chewable Tablets 1701

Food Interactions

Fruit juices, unspecified (Grapefruit, orange and apple may reduce the bioavailability and exposure of fexofenadine; it is recommended that fexofenadine should be taken with water).

ALLEGRA TABLETS

(Fexofenadine Hydrochloride) 2844
See Allegra Capsules

ALLEGRA-D 12 HOUR EXTENDED-RELEASE TABLETS

(Fexofenadine Hydrochloride, Pseudoephedrine Hydrochloride) 2846

May interact with antacids, erythromycin, cardiac glycosides, monoamine oxidase inhibitors, sympathomimetics, and certain other agents. Compounds in these categories include:

Albuterol (Combined effects of pseudoephedrine with other sympathomimetics on cardiovascular system may be harmful to the patient). Products include:

Proventil Inhalation Aerosol 3053

Albuterol Sulfate (Combined effects of pseudoephedrine with other sympathomimetics on cardiovascular system may be harmful to the patient). Products include:

AccuNeb Inhalation Solution 1055
Combivent Inhalation Aerosol 847
DuoNeb Inhalation Solution 1058
ProAir HFA Inhalation Aerosol 3300
Proventil Inhalation Solution 0.083% 3055
Proventil HFA Inhalation Aerosol 3056
Ventolin HFA Inhalation Aerosol 1600
VoSpire ER Tablets 1052

Aluminum Carbonate (Co-administration with fexofenadine HCL may decrease fexofenadine AUC by 41% and Cmax by 43%).

No products indexed under this heading.

Aluminum Hydroxide (Co-administration with fexofenadine HCL may decrease fexofenadine AUC by 41% and Cmax by 43%). Products include:

Gaviscon Regular Strength Liquid .. 658
Gaviscon Regular Strength Tablets 658
Gaviscon Extra Strength Liquid 658
Gaviscon Extra Strength Tablets 658
Maalox Regular Strength Antacid/Antigas Liquid 2175
Maalox Max Maximum Strength Antacid/Anti-Gas Liquid 2176

Apple Juice (Co-administration with grapefruit, orange or apple juice will reduce the bioavailability and exposure or fexofenadine).

No products indexed under this heading.

Deslanoside (Increased ectopic pacemaker activity can occur when pseudoephedrine is used concomitantly with digitalis).

No products indexed under this heading.

Digitalis Glycoside Preparations (Increased ectopic pacemaker activity can occur when pseudoephedrine is used concomitantly with digitalis).

No products indexed under this heading.

Digitoxin (Increased ectopic pacemaker activity can occur when pseudoephedrine is used concomitantly with digitalis).

No products indexed under this heading.

Digoxin (Increased ectopic pacemaker activity can occur when pseudoephedrine is used concomitantly with digitalis). Products include:

Lanoxicaps Capsules 1490
Lanoxin Injection 1494
Lanoxin Injection Pediatric 1497
Lanoxin Tablets 1500

Dobutamine Hydrochloride (Combined effects of pseudoephedrine with other sympathomimetics on cardiovascular system may be harmful to the patient).

No products indexed under this heading.

Dopamine Hydrochloride (Combined effects of pseudoephedrine with other sympathomimetics on cardiovascular system may be harmful to the patient).

No products indexed under this heading.

Ephedrine Hydrochloride (Combined effects of pseudoephedrine with other sympathomimetics on cardiovascular system may be harmful to the patient).

No products indexed under this heading.

Ephedrine Sulfate (Combined effects of pseudoephedrine with other sympathomimetics on cardiovascular system may be harmful to the patient).

No products indexed under this heading.

Ephedrine Tannate (Combined effects of pseudoephedrine with other sympathomimetics on cardiovascular system may be harmful to the patient).

No products indexed under this heading.

Epinephrine (Combined effects of pseudoephedrine with other sympathomimetics on cardiovascular system may be harmful to the patient). Products include:

EpiPen 1061
Primatene Mist 719
Twinject 0.15 3379
Twinject 0.3 3378

Epinephrine Bitartrate (Combined effects of pseudoephedrine with other sympathomimetics on cardiovascular system may be harmful to the patient).

No products indexed under this heading.

Epinephrine Hydrochloride (Combined effects of pseudoephedrine with other sympathomimetics on cardiovascular system may be harmful to the patient).

No products indexed under this heading.

Erythromycin (Co-administration with erythromycin enhances fexofenadine gastrointestinal absorption thereby increasing plasma levels of fexofenadine; in vivo animal studies suggest that erythromycin may also decrease biliary excretion). Products include:

Ery-Tab Tablets 449
Erythromycin Base Filmtab Tablets 455
Erythromycin Delayed-Release Capsules, USP 457
PCE Dispertab Tablets 515

Erythromycin Estolate (Co-administration with erythromycin enhances fexofenadine gastrointestinal absorption thereby increasing plasma levels of fexofenadine; in vivo animal studies suggest that erythromycin may also decrease biliary excretion).

No products indexed under this heading.

Erythromycin Ethylsuccinate (Co-administration with erythromycin enhances fexofenadine gastrointestinal absorption thereby increasing plasma levels of fexofenadine; in vivo animal studies suggest that erythromycin may also decrease biliary excretion). Products include:

E.E.S. 451
EryPed 447

Erythromycin Gluceptate (Co-administration with erythromycin enhances fexofenadine gastrointestinal absorption thereby increasing plasma levels of fexofenadine; in vivo animal studies suggest that erythromycin may also decrease biliary excretion).

No products indexed under this heading.

Erythromycin Lactobionate (Co-administration with erythromycin enhances fexofenadine gastrointestinal absorption thereby increasing plasma levels of fexofenadine; in vivo animal studies suggest that erythromycin may also decrease biliary excretion).

No products indexed under this heading.

Erythromycin Stearate (Co-administration with erythromycin enhances fexofenadine gastrointestinal absorption thereby increasing plasma levels of fexofenadine; in vivo animal studies suggest that erythromycin may also decrease biliary excretion). Products include:

Erythrocin Stearate Filmtab Tablets 453

Isocarboxazid (Concurrent and/or sequential use with MAO inhibitors is contraindicated).

No products indexed under this heading.

Isoproterenol Hydrochloride (Combined effects of pseudoephedrine with other sympathomimetics on cardiovascular system may be harmful to the patient).

No products indexed under this heading.

Isoproterenol Sulfate (Combined effects of pseudoephedrine with other sympathomimetics on cardiovascular system may be harmful to the patient).

No products indexed under this heading.

Ketoconazole (Co-administration with ketoconazole enhances fexofenadine gastrointestinal absorption thereby increasing plasma levels of fexofenadine; in vivo animal studies suggest that ketoconazole may also decrease fexofenadine gastrointestinal secretion). Products include:

Nizoral A-D Shampoo, 1% 1868

Levalbuterol Hydrochloride (Combined effects of pseudoephedrine with other sympathomimetics on cardiovascular system may be harmful to the patient). Products include:
Xopenex Inhalation Solution 3146
Xopenex Inhalation Solution Concentrate 3150

Magaldrate (Co-administration with fexofenadine HCL may decrease fexofenadine AUC by 41% and Cmax by 43%).
No products indexed under this heading.

Magnesium Hydroxide (Co-administration with fexofenadine HCL may decrease fexofenadine AUC by 41% and Cmax by 43%). Products include:
Maalox Regular Strength Antacid/Antigas Liquid................ 2175
Maalox Max Maximum Strength Antacid/Anti-Gas Liquid............... 2176
Pepcid Complete Chewable Tablets 1701

Magnesium Oxide (Co-administration with fexofenadine HCL may decrease fexofenadine AUC by 41% and Cmax by 43%). Products include:
Beelith Tablets 759
PremCal Light, Regular, and Extra Strength Tablets................ ▣ 818

Mecamylamine Hydrochloride (Reduced antihypertensive effects).
No products indexed under this heading.

Metaproterenol Sulfate (Combined effects of pseudoephedrine with other sympathomimetics on cardiovascular system may be harmful to the patient). Products include:
Alupent Inhalation Aerosol 826

Metaraminol Bitartrate (Combined effects of pseudoephedrine with other sympathomimetics on cardiovascular system may be harmful to the patient).
No products indexed under this heading.

Methoxamine Hydrochloride (Combined effects of pseudoephedrine with other sympathomimetics on cardiovascular system may be harmful to the patient).
No products indexed under this heading.

Methyldopa (Reduced antihypertensive effects). Products include:
Aldoril Tablets 1910

Methyldopate Hydrochloride (Reduced antihypertensive effects).
No products indexed under this heading.

Moclobemide (Concurrent and/or sequential use with MAO inhibitors is contraindicated).
No products indexed under this heading.

Norepinephrine Bitartrate (Combined effects of pseudoephedrine with other sympathomimetics on cardiovascular system may be harmful to the patient).
No products indexed under this heading.

Pargyline Hydrochloride (Concurrent and/or sequential use with MAO inhibitors is contraindicated).
No products indexed under this heading.

Phenelzine Sulfate (Concurrent and/or sequential use with MAO inhibitors is contraindicated).
No products indexed under this heading.

Phenylephrine Bitartrate (Combined effects of pseudoephedrine with other sympathomimetics on cardiovascular system may be harmful to the patient).
No products indexed under this heading.

Phenylephrine Hydrochloride (Combined effects of pseudoephedrine with other sympathomimetics on cardiovascular system may be harmful to the patient). Products include:
Comtrex Maximum Strength Non-Drowsy Cold & Cough Caplets...................................... ▣ 725
Comtrex Maximum Strength Day/Night Severe Cold & Sinus Caplets - Day Formulation .... ▣ 725
Comtrex Maximum Strength Day/Night Severe Cold & Sinus Caplets - Night Formulation .... ▣ 725
Contac Cold and Flu Maximum Strength Caplets........................ ▣ 728
Contac Cold and Flu Day and Night Caplets (Day Formulation Only)... ▣ 727
Contac Cold and Flu Day and Night Caplets (Night Formulation Only)...................... ▣ 727
Contac Cold and Flu Non-Drowsy Caplets...................................... ▣ 728
Contac-D Cold Non-Drowsy Tablets.. ▣ 729
Children's Dimetapp Cold & Allergy Elixir............................... ▣ 730
Children's Dimetapp Cold & Allergy Chewable Tablets............ ▣ 730
Children's Dimetapp DM Cold & Cough Elixir .... ▣ 731
Toddler's Dimetapp Cold and Cough Drops .... ▣ 732
Excedrin Sinus Headache Caplets/Tablets .... ▣ 610
4-Way Fast Acting Nasal Spray ...... ▣ 775
4-Way Menthol Nasal Spray .... ▣ 775
Preparation H Maximum Strength Cream .... ▣ 666
Preparation H Cooling Gel .... ▣ 666
Preparation H .... ▣ 666
Refenesen PE Caplets .... ▣ 721
Robitussin Cough & Allergy Syrup .. ▣ 736
Robitussin Cough & Cold Nighttime Liquid............................ ▣ 736
Robitussin Cough, Cold & Flu Nighttime Liquid.......................... ▣ 738
Robitussin Head & Chest Congestion PE Syrup................. ▣ 739
Robitussin Pediatric Cough & Cold Nighttime Liquid.................. ▣ 736
TheraFlu Cold & Cough Hot Liquid .... ▣ 740
TheraFlu Cold & Sore Throat Hot Liquid .... ▣ 741
TheraFlu Flu & Sore Throat Hot Liquid .... ▣ 742
TheraFlu Daytime Severe Cold Hot Liquid................................. ▣ 742
TheraFlu Nighttime Severe Cold Hot Liquid .... ▣ 740
TheraFlu Warming Relief Daytime Severe Cold.............................. ▣ 743
TheraFlu Warming Relief Nighttime Severe Cold .... ▣ 743
Triaminic Chest & Nasal Congestion Liquid....................... ▣ 746
Triaminic Cold & Allergy Liquid .... ▣ 746
Triaminic Daytime Cold & Cough Liquid .... ▣ 745
Triaminic Nighttime Cold & Cough Liquid............................... ▣ 746
Triaminic Thin Strips Cold .... ▣ 748
Triaminic Thin Strips Cold & Cough.. ▣ 778
Triaminic Infant Thin Strips Decongestant.............................. ▣ 747
Triaminic Infant Thin Strips Decongestant Plus Cough........... ▣ 747
Children's Tylenol Plus Flu Oral Suspension............................... ▣ 749
Tylenol Cold Head Congestion Daytime Caplets with Cool Burst and Gelcaps .... ▣ 750
Tylenol Cold Multi-Symptom Daytime Liquid............................... ▣ 752
Tylenol Cold Multi-Symptom Severe Daytime Liquid .... ▣ 752
Concentrated Tylenol Infants' Drops Plus Cold & Cough........... ▣ 754
Tylenol Allergy Multi-Symptom Caplets with Cool Burst and Gelcaps.. 1872
Tylenol Allergy Multi-Symptom Nighttime Caplets with Cool Burst... 1872
Children's Tylenol Plus Cold Suspension Liquid 1879
Children's Tylenol Plus Cold & Allergy Suspension Liquid............ 1878
Children's Tylenol Plus Flu Suspension Liquid 1881
Children's Tylenol Plus Multi-Symptom Cold Suspension Liquid 1879
Tylenol Cold Head Congestion Daytime Caplets with Cool Burst... 1873
Tylenol Cold Head Congestion Nighttime Caplets with Cool Burst... 1873
Tylenol Cold Head Congestion Severe Caplets with Cool Burst..... 1873
Tylenol Cold Multi-Symptom Daytime Caplets with Cool Burst and Gelcaps 1874
Tylenol Cold Multi-Symptom Daytime Liquid with Citrus Burst... 1874
Tylenol Cold Multi-Symptom Nighttime Caplets with Cool Burst... 1874
Tylenol Cold Multi-Symptom Nighttime Liquid with Cool Burst... 1874
Tylenol Cold Multi-Symptom Severe Caplets with Cool Burst..... 1874
Tylenol Cold Multi-Symptom Severe Daytime Liquid with Citrus Burst 1874
Tylenol Sinus Congestion & Pain Daytime Caplets with Cool Burst and Gelcaps 1876
Tylenol Sinus Congestion & Pain Nighttime Caplets with Cool Burst... 1876
Tylenol Sinus Congestion & Pain Severe Caplets with Cool Burst..... 1876
Vicks 44D Cough & Head Congestion Relief Liquid............. ▣ 760
Vicks DayQuil LiquiCaps/Liquid Multi-Symptom Cold/Flu Relief..... ▣ 761
Zicam Cough Plus D Cough Spray.. ▣ 767

Phenylephrine Tannate (Combined effects of pseudoephedrine with other sympathomimetics on cardiovascular system may be harmful to the patient).
No products indexed under this heading.

Phenylpropanolamine Hydrochloride (Combined effects of pseudoephedrine with other sympathomimetics on cardiovascular system may be harmful to the patient).
No products indexed under this heading.

Pirbuterol Acetate (Combined effects of pseudoephedrine with other sympathomimetics on cardiovascular system may be harmful to the patient). Products include:
Maxair Autohaler 1852

Procarbazine Hydrochloride (Concurrent and/or sequential use with MAO inhibitors is contraindicated). Products include:
Matulane Capsules 3191

Pseudoephedrine Sulfate (Combined effects of pseudoephedrine with other sympathomimetics on cardiovascular system may be harmful to the patient). Products include:
Alavert Allergy & Sinus D-12 Hour Tablets.. ▣ 771
Clarinex-D 24-Hour Extended-Release Tablets............ 2998
Claritin-D Non-Drowsy 12 Hour Tablets.. ▣ 772
Claritin-D Non-Drowsy 24 Hour Tablets.. ▣ 772

Reserpine (Reduced antihypertensive effects).
No products indexed under this heading.

Salmeterol Xinafoate (Combined effects of pseudoephedrine with other sympathomimetics on cardiovascular system may be harmful to the patient). Products include:
Advair Diskus 100/50 1308
Advair Diskus 250/50 1308
Advair Diskus 500/50 1308
Advair HFA Inhalation Aerosol 1318
Serevent Diskus 1568

Selegiline Hydrochloride (Concurrent and/or sequential use with MAO inhibitors is contraindicated). Products include:
Eldepryl Capsules 3208
Zelapar Tablets 3372

Sodium Bicarbonate (Co-administration with fexofenadine HCL may decrease fexofenadine AUC by 41% and Cmax by 43%). Products include:
Colyte with Flavor Packs for Oral Solution.. 3088
HalfLytely and Bisacodyl Tablets Bowel Prep Kit with Flavors Packs.. 881
TriLyte with Flavor Packs for Oral Solution.. 3100

Terbutaline Sulfate (Combined effects of pseudoephedrine with other sympathomimetics on cardiovascular system may be harmful to the patient).
No products indexed under this heading.

Tranylcypromine Sulfate (Concurrent and/or sequential use with MAO inhibitors is contraindicated). Products include:
Parnate Tablets 1527

Food Interactions

Diet, high-lipid (Co-administration with a high-fat meal decreased fexofenadine plasma concentrations Cmax and AUC, and Tmax was delayed by 50%; the rate of extent of pseudoephedrine absorption was not affected by food; administration of Allegra-D with food should be avoided).

Grapefruit Juice (Co-administration with grapefruit, orange or apple juice will reduce the bioavailability and exposure or fexofenadine).

Orange Juice (Co-administration with grapefruit, orange or apple juice will reduce the bioavailability and exposure or fexofenadine).

ALLEGRA-D 24 HOUR EXTENDED-RELEASE TABLETS

(Fexofenadine Hydrochloride, Pseudoephedrine Hydrochloride)........ 2849
See Allegra-D 12 Hour Extended-Release Tablets

ALOPRIM FOR INJECTION

(Allopurinol Sodium) **2167**
May interact with cytotoxic drugs, thiazides, and certain other agents. Compounds in these categories include:

Amoxicillin Trihydrate (Co-administration of amoxicillin with allopurinol increases the frequency of rash).
No products indexed under this heading.

Ampicillin (Co-administration of ampicillin with allopurinol increases the frequency of rash).
No products indexed under this heading.

Ampicillin Sodium (Co-administration of ampicillin with allopurinol increases the frequency of rash).
No products indexed under this heading.

Azathioprine (Allopurinol inhibits the enzymatic oxidation of azathioprine to 6-thiouric acid; this interaction has been observed with oral allopurinol, usually with longer term therapy, reduction in oral dose of allopurinol has been suggested).
No products indexed under this heading.

Bendroflumethiazide (Co-administration of allopurinol and thiazide diuretics contribute to increased allopurinol toxicity).
No products indexed under this heading.

Bleomycin Sulfate (Co-administration of allopurinol with cytotoxic agents including cyclophosphamide in patients with neoplastic disease, except leukemia, enhances the bone marrow suppression).
No products indexed under this heading.

Chlorothiazide (Co-administration of allopurinol and thiazide diuretics contribute to increased allopurinol toxicity). Products include:
Diuril Oral Suspension **1954**

Chlorothiazide Sodium (Co-administration of allopurinol and thiazide diuretics contribute to increased allopurinol toxicity).
Products include:
Diuril Sodium Intravenous **2467**

Chlorpropamide (The half-life of chlorpropamide in the plasma may be prolonged by allopurinol, since allopurinol and chlorpropamide may compete for excretion in the renal tubule; the risk of hypoglycemia secondary to this interaction may be increased if used concurrently).
No products indexed under this heading.

Cyclophosphamide (Co-administration of allopurinol with cyclophosphamide in patients with neoplastic disease, except leukemia, enhances the bone marrow suppression).
No products indexed under this heading.

Cyclosporine (Co-administration may result in increased cyclosporine levels). Products include:
Gengraf Capsules **459**
Neoral Oral Solution **2259**
Neoral Soft Gelatin Capsules **2259**
Restasis Ophthalmic Emulsion **575**
Sandimmune **2275**

Daunorubicin Hydrochloride (Co-administration of allopurinol with cytotoxic agents including cyclophosphamide in patients with neoplastic disease, except leukemia, enhances the bone marrow suppression).
No products indexed under this heading.

Dicumarol (Allopurinol prolongs the half-life of dicumarol).
No products indexed under this heading.

Doxorubicin Hydrochloride (Co-administration of allopurinol with cytotoxic agents including cyclophosphamide in patients with neoplastic disease, except leukemia, enhances the bone marrow suppression).
No products indexed under this heading.

Epirubicin Hydrochloride (Co-administration of allopurinol with cytotoxic agents including cyclophosphamide in patients with neoplastic disease, except leukemia, enhances the bone marrow suppression).
No products indexed under this heading.

Fluorouracil (Co-administration of allopurinol with cytotoxic agents including cyclophosphamide in patients with neoplastic disease, except leukemia, enhances the bone marrow suppression). Products include:
Carac Cream, 0.5% **2879**
Efudex **3363**

Hydrochlorothiazide (Co-administration of allopurinol and thiazide diuretics contribute to increased allopurinol toxicity).
Products include:
Aldoril Tablets **1910**
Atacand HCT **651**
Avalide Tablets **888**
Avalide Tablets **2874**
Benicar HCT Tablets **1044**
Diovan HCT Tablets **2196**
Dyazide Capsules **1423**
Hyzaar 50-12.5 Tablets **1990**
Hyzaar 100-12.5 Tablets **1990**
Hyzaar 100-25 Tablets **1990**
Lopressor HCT 50/25 Tablets **2241**
Lopressor HCT 100/25 Tablets **2241**
Lopressor HCT 100/50 Tablets **2241**
Lotensin HCT Tablets **2246**
Micardis HCT Tablets **856**
Moduretic Tablets **2028**
Prinzide Tablets **2056**
Teveten HCT Tablets **1737**
Timolide Tablets **2086**
Uniretic Tablets **3100**

Hydroflumethiazide (Co-administration of allopurinol and thiazide diuretics contribute to increased allopurinol toxicity).
No products indexed under this heading.

Hydroxyurea (Co-administration of allopurinol with cytotoxic agents including cyclophosphamide in patients with neoplastic disease, except leukemia, enhances the bone marrow suppression).
No products indexed under this heading.

Mercaptopurine (Allopurinol inhibits the enzymatic oxidation of mercaptopurine to 6-thiouric acid; this interaction has been observed with oral allopurinol, usually with longer term therapy, reduction in oral dose of allopurinol has been suggested).
No products indexed under this heading.

Methotrexate Sodium (Co-administration of allopurinol with cytotoxic agents including cyclophosphamide in patients with neoplastic disease, except leukemia, enhances the bone marrow suppression).
No products indexed under this heading.

Methyclothiazide (Co-administration of allopurinol and thiazide diuretics contribute to increased allopurinol toxicity).
No products indexed under this heading.

Mitotane (Co-administration of allopurinol with cytotoxic agents including cyclophosphamide in patients with neoplastic disease, except leukemia, enhances the bone marrow suppression).
No products indexed under this heading.

Mitoxantrone Hydrochloride (Co-administration of allopurinol with cytotoxic agents including cyclophosphamide in patients with neoplastic disease, except leukemia, enhances the bone marrow suppression).
No products indexed under this heading.

Polythiazide (Co-administration of allopurinol and thiazide diuretics contribute to increased allopurinol toxicity).
No products indexed under this heading.

Probenecid (Co-administration of uricosuric agents decreases the inhibition of xanthine by oxypurinol and increases the urinary excretion of uric acid).
No products indexed under this heading.

Procarbazine Hydrochloride (Co-administration of allopurinol with cytotoxic agents including cyclophosphamide in patients with neoplastic disease, except leukemia, enhances the bone marrow suppression). Products include:
Matulane Capsules **3191**

Sulfinpyrazone (Co-administration of uricosuric agents decreases the inhibition of xanthine by oxypurinol and increases the urinary excretion of uric acid).
No products indexed under this heading.

Tamoxifen Citrate (Co-administration of allopurinol with cytotoxic agents including cyclophosphamide in patients with neoplastic disease, except leukemia, enhances the bone marrow suppression). Products include:
Soltamox Oral Solution **3527**

Vincristine Sulfate (Co-administration of allopurinol with cytotoxic agents including cyclophosphamide in patients with neoplastic disease, except leukemia, enhances the bone marrow suppression).
No products indexed under this heading.

ALOXI INJECTION

(Palonosetron Hydrochloride) **2127**
None cited in PDR database.

ALPHAGAN P OPHTHALMIC SOLUTION

(Brimonidine Tartrate) **567**
May interact with anesthetics, antihypertensives, barbiturates, beta blockers, central nervous system depressants, cardiac glycosides, hypnotics and sedatives, monoamine oxidase inhibitors, narcotic analgesics, tricyclic antidepressants, and certain other agents. Compounds in these categories include:

Acebutolol Hydrochloride (Concurrent use of brimonidine, an alpha adrenergic agonist, with beta blockers (ophthalmic and systemic) may reduce pulse and blood pressure, however, in clinical trials brimonidine did not have any significant effects on pulse and blood pressure).
No products indexed under this heading.

Alfentanil Hydrochloride (Possible additive or potentiating effect with CNS depressants).
No products indexed under this heading.

Alprazolam (Possible additive or potentiating effect with CNS depressants). Products include:
Niravam Orally Disintegrating Tablets **3092**

Amitriptyline Hydrochloride (Tricyclic antidepressants have been reported to blunt the hypotensive effect of systemic clonidine, an alpha adrenergic agonist; it is not known whether the concurrent use of these agents with brimonidine can lead to interference in IOP-lowering effect; caution is advised).
No products indexed under this heading.

Amlodipine Besylate (Concurrent use of brimonidine, an alpha adrenergic agonist, with antihypertensives may reduce pulse and blood pressure, however, in clinical trials brimonidine did not have any significant effects on pulse and blood pressure). Products include:
Caduet Tablets **2508**
Lotrel Capsules **2249**
Norvasc Tablets **2545**

Amoxapine (Tricyclic antidepressants have been reported to blunt the hypotensive effect of systemic clonidine, an alpha adrenergic agonist; it is not known whether the concurrent use of these agents with brimonidine can lead to interference in IOP-lowering effect; caution is advised).
No products indexed under this heading.

Aprobarbital (Possible additive or potentiating effect with CNS depressants).
No products indexed under this heading.

Atenolol (Concurrent use of brimonidine, an alpha adrenergic agonist, with beta blockers (ophthalmic and systemic) may reduce pulse and blood pressure, however, in clinical trials brimonidine did not have any significant effects on pulse and blood pressure).
No products indexed under this heading.

Benazepril Hydrochloride (Concurrent use of brimonidine, an alpha adrenergic agonist, with antihypertensives may reduce pulse and blood pressure, however, in clinical trials brimonidine did not have any significant effects on pulse and blood pressure). Products include:

Bendroflumethiazide (Concurrent use of brimonidine, an alpha adrenergic agonist, with antihypertensives may reduce pulse and blood pressure, however, in clinical trials brimonidine did not have any significant effects on pulse and blood pressure).

No products indexed under this heading.

Betaxolol Hydrochloride (Concurrent use of brimonidine, an alpha adrenergic agonist, with beta blockers (ophthalmic and systemic) may reduce pulse and blood pressure, however, in clinical trials brimonidine did not have any significant effects on pulse and blood pressure). Products include:

Bisoprolol Fumarate (Concurrent use of brimonidine, an alpha adrenergic agonist, with beta blockers (ophthalmic and systemic) may reduce pulse and blood pressure, however, in clinical trials brimonidine did not have any significant effects on pulse and blood pressure).

No products indexed under this heading.

Buprenorphine Hydrochloride (Possible additive or potentiating effect with CNS depressants). Products include:

Buspirone Hydrochloride (Possible additive or potentiating effect with CNS depressants).

No products indexed under this heading.

Butabarbital (Possible additive or potentiating effect with CNS depressants).

No products indexed under this heading.

Butalbital (Possible additive or potentiating effect with CNS depressants).

No products indexed under this heading.

Candesartan Cilexetil (Concurrent use of brimonidine, an alpha adrenergic agonist, with antihypertensives may reduce pulse and blood pressure, however, in clinical trials brimonidine did not have any significant effects on pulse and blood pressure). Products include:

Captopril (Concurrent use of brimonidine, an alpha adrenergic agonist, with antihypertensives may reduce pulse and blood pressure, however, in clinical trials brimonidine did not have any significant effects on pulse and blood pressure). Products include:

Carteolol Hydrochloride (Concurrent use of brimonidine, an alpha adrenergic agonist, with beta blockers (ophthalmic and systemic) may

reduce pulse and blood pressure, however, in clinical trials brimonidine did not have any significant effects on pulse and blood pressure). Products include:

Chlordiazepoxide (Possible additive or potentiating effect with CNS depressants).

No products indexed under this heading.

Chlordiazepoxide Hydrochloride (Possible additive or potentiating effect with CNS depressants). Products include:

Chlorothiazide (Concurrent use of brimonidine, an alpha adrenergic agonist, with antihypertensives may reduce pulse and blood pressure, however, in clinical trials brimonidine did not have any significant effects on pulse and blood pressure). Products include:

Chlorothiazide Sodium (Concurrent use of brimonidine, an alpha adrenergic agonist, with antihypertensives may reduce pulse and blood pressure, however, in clinical trials brimonidine did not have any significant effects on pulse and blood pressure). Products include:

Chlorpromazine (Possible additive or potentiating effect with CNS depressants).

No products indexed under this heading.

Chlorpromazine Hydrochloride (Possible additive or potentiating effect with CNS depressants).

No products indexed under this heading.

Chlorprothixene (Possible additive or potentiating effect with CNS depressants).

No products indexed under this heading.

Chlorprothixene Hydrochloride (Possible additive or potentiating effect with CNS depressants).

No products indexed under this heading.

Chlorprothixene Lactate (Possible additive or potentiating effect with CNS depressants).

No products indexed under this heading.

Chlorthalidone (Concurrent use of brimonidine, an alpha adrenergic agonist, with antihypertensives may reduce pulse and blood pressure, however, in clinical trials brimonidine did not have any significant effects on pulse and blood pressure). Products include:

Clomipramine Hydrochloride (Tricyclic antidepressants have been reported to blunt the hypotensive effect of systemic clonidine, an alpha adrenergic agonist; it is not known whether the concurrent use of these agents with brimonidine can lead to interference in IOP-lowering effect; caution is advised).

No products indexed under this heading.

Clonidine (Concurrent use of brimonidine, an alpha adrenergic agonist, with antihypertensives may reduce pulse and blood pressure, however, in clinical trials brimonidine

did not have any significant effects on pulse and blood pressure). Products include:

Clonidine Hydrochloride (Concurrent use of brimonidine, an alpha adrenergic agonist, with antihypertensives may reduce pulse and blood pressure, however, in clinical trials brimonidine did not have any significant effects on pulse and blood pressure). Products include:

Clorazepate Dipotassium (Possible additive or potentiating effect with CNS depressants). Products include:

Clozapine (Possible additive or potentiating effect with CNS depressants). Products include:

Codeine Phosphate (Possible additive or potentiating effect with CNS depressants). Products include:

Deserpidine (Concurrent use of brimonidine, an alpha adrenergic agonist, with antihypertensives may reduce pulse and blood pressure, however, in clinical trials brimonidine did not have any significant effects on pulse and blood pressure).

No products indexed under this heading.

Desflurane (Possible additive or potentiating effect with CNS depressants).

No products indexed under this heading.

Desipramine Hydrochloride (Tricyclic antidepressants have been reported to blunt the hypotensive effect of systemic clonidine, an alpha adrenergic agonist; it is not known whether the concurrent use of these agents with brimonidine can lead to interference in IOP-lowering effect; caution is advised).

No products indexed under this heading.

Deslanoside (Concurrent use of brimonidine, an alpha adrenergic agonist, with cardiac glycosides may reduce pulse and blood pressure, however, in clinical trials brimonidine did not have any significant effects on pulse and blood pressure).

No products indexed under this heading.

Dezocine (Possible additive or potentiating effect with CNS depressants).

No products indexed under this heading.

Diazepam (Possible additive or potentiating effect with CNS depressants). Products include:

Diazoxide (Concurrent use of brimonidine, an alpha adrenergic agonist, with antihypertensives may reduce pulse and blood pressure, however, in clinical trials brimonidine did not have any significant effects on pulse and blood pressure). Products include:

Digitalis Glycoside Preparations (Concurrent use of brimonidine, an alpha adrenergic agonist, with cardiac glycosides may reduce pulse and blood pressure, however, in clinical trials brimonidine did not have any significant effects on pulse and blood pressure).

No products indexed under this heading.

Digitoxin (Concurrent use of brimonidine, an alpha adrenergic agonist, with cardiac glycosides may reduce pulse and blood pressure, however, in clinical trials brimonidine did not have any significant effects on pulse and blood pressure).

No products indexed under this heading.

Digoxin (Concurrent use of brimonidine, an alpha adrenergic agonist, with cardiac glycosides may reduce pulse and blood pressure, however, in clinical trials brimonidine did not have any significant effects on pulse and blood pressure). Products include:

Diltiazem Hydrochloride (Concurrent use of brimonidine, an alpha adrenergic agonist, with antihypertensives may reduce pulse and blood pressure, however, in clinical trials brimonidine did not have any significant effects on pulse and blood pressure). Products include:

Doxazosin Mesylate (Concurrent use of brimonidine, an alpha adrenergic agonist, with antihypertensives may reduce pulse and blood pressure, however, in clinical trials brimonidine did not have any significant effects on pulse and blood pressure). Products include:

Doxepin Hydrochloride (Tricyclic antidepressants have been reported to blunt the hypotensive effect of systemic clonidine, an alpha adrenergic agonist; it is not known whether the concurrent use of these agents with brimonidine can lead to interference in IOP-lowering effect; caution is advised).

No products indexed under this heading.

Droperidol (Possible additive or potentiating effect with CNS depressants).

No products indexed under this heading.

Enalapril Maleate (Concurrent use of brimonidine, an alpha adrenergic agonist, with antihypertensives may reduce pulse and blood pressure, however, in clinical trials brimonidine did not have any significant effects on pulse and blood pressure). Products include:

Enalaprilat (Concurrent use of brimonidine, an alpha adrenergic agonist, with antihypertensives may reduce pulse and blood pressure, however, in clinical trials brimonidine did not have any significant effects on pulse and blood pressure).

No products indexed under this heading.

Enflurane (Possible additive or potentiating effect with CNS depressants).

No products indexed under this heading.

Eprosartan Mesylate (Concurrent use of brimonidine, an alpha adrenergic agonist, with antihypertensives may reduce pulse and blood pressure, however, in clinical trials brimonidine did not have any significant effects on pulse and blood pressure). Products include:

Teveten Tablets 1735
Teveten HCT Tablets 1737

Esmolol Hydrochloride (Concurrent use of brimonidine, an alpha adrenergic agonist, with beta blockers (ophthalmic and systemic) may reduce pulse and blood pressure, however, in clinical trials brimonidine did not have any significant effects on pulse and blood pressure).

No products indexed under this heading.

Estazolam (Possible additive or potentiating effect with CNS depressants). Products include:

ProSom Tablets 517

Ethanol (Possible additive or potentiating effect with CNS depressants).

No products indexed under this heading.

Ethchlorvynol (Possible additive or potentiating effect with CNS depressants).

No products indexed under this heading.

Ethinamate (Possible additive or potentiating effect with CNS depressants).

No products indexed under this heading.

Ethyl Alcohol (Possible additive or potentiating effect with CNS depressants).

No products indexed under this heading.

Felodipine (Concurrent use of brimonidine, an alpha adrenergic agonist, with antihypertensives may reduce pulse and blood pressure, however, in clinical trials brimonidine did not have any significant effects on pulse and blood pressure).

No products indexed under this heading.

Fentanyl (Possible additive or potentiating effect with CNS depressants). Products include:

Duragesic Transdermal System 2373
Ionsys Transdermal System 2379

Fentanyl Citrate (Possible additive or potentiating effect with CNS depressants). Products include:

Actiq ... 979

Fluphenazine Decanoate (Possible additive or potentiating effect with CNS depressants).

No products indexed under this heading.

Fluphenazine Enanthate (Possible additive or potentiating effect with CNS depressants).

No products indexed under this heading.

Fluphenazine Hydrochloride (Possible additive or potentiating effect with CNS depressants).

No products indexed under this heading.

Flurazepam Hydrochloride (Possible additive or potentiating effect with CNS depressants). Products include:

Dalmane Capsules 3342

Fosinopril Sodium (Concurrent use of brimonidine, an alpha adrenergic agonist, with antihypertensives may reduce pulse and blood pressure, however, in clinical trials brimonidine did not have any significant effects on pulse and blood pressure).

No products indexed under this heading.

Furosemide (Concurrent use of brimonidine, an alpha adrenergic agonist, with antihypertensives may reduce pulse and blood pressure, however, in clinical trials brimonidine did not have any significant effects on pulse and blood pressure). Products include:

Furosemide Tablets 2154

Glutethimide (Possible additive or potentiating effect with CNS depressants).

No products indexed under this heading.

Guanabenz Acetate (Concurrent use of brimonidine, an alpha adrenergic agonist, with antihypertensives may reduce pulse and blood pressure, however, in clinical trials brimonidine did not have any significant effects on pulse and blood pressure).

No products indexed under this heading.

Guanethidine Monosulfate (Concurrent use of brimonidine, an alpha adrenergic agonist, with antihypertensives may reduce pulse and blood pressure, however, in clinical trials brimonidine did not have any significant effects on pulse and blood pressure).

No products indexed under this heading.

Haloperidol (Possible additive or potentiating effect with CNS depressants).

No products indexed under this heading.

Haloperidol Decanoate (Possible additive or potentiating effect with CNS depressants).

No products indexed under this heading.

Halothane (Possible additive or potentiating effect with CNS depressants).

No products indexed under this heading.

Hydralazine Hydrochloride (Concurrent use of brimonidine, an alpha adrenergic agonist, with antihypertensives may reduce pulse and blood pressure, however, in clinical trials brimonidine did not have any significant effects on pulse and blood pressure). Products include:

BiDil Tablets 2171

Hydrochlorothiazide (Concurrent use of brimonidine, an alpha adrenergic agonist, with antihypertensives may reduce pulse and blood pressure, however, in clinical trials brimonidine did not have any significant effects on pulse and blood pressure). Products include:

Aldoril Tablets 1910
Atacand HCT 651
Avalide Tablets 888
Avalide Tablets 2874
Benicar HCT Tablets 1044
Diovan HCT Tablets 2196
Dyazide Capsules 1423
Hyzaar 50-12.5 Tablets 1990
Hyzaar 100-12.5 Tablets 1990
Hyzaar 100-25 Tablets 1990
Lopressor HCT 50/25 Tablets 2241

Lopressor HCT 100/25 Tablets 2241
Lopressor HCT 100/50 Tablets 2241
Lotensin HCT Tablets 2246
Micardis HCT Tablets 856
Moduretic Tablets 2028
Prinzide Tablets 2056
Teveten HCT Tablets 1737
Timolide Tablets 2086
Uniretic Tablets 3100

Hydrocodone Bitartrate (Possible additive or potentiating effect with CNS depressants). Products include:

Hycodan .. 1116
Hycotuss Expectorant Syrup 1117
Vicodin Tablets 535
Vicodin ES Tablets 536
Vicodin HP Tablets 538
Vicoprofen Tablets 539
Zydone Tablets 1139

Hydrocodone Polistirex (Possible additive or potentiating effect with CNS depressants). Products include:

Tussionex Pennkinetic
Extended-Release Suspension 3327

Hydroflumethiazide (Concurrent use of brimonidine, an alpha adrenergic agonist, with antihypertensives may reduce pulse and blood pressure, however, in clinical trials brimonidine did not have any significant effects on pulse and blood pressure).

No products indexed under this heading.

Hydromorphone Hydrochloride (Possible additive or potentiating effect with CNS depressants). Products include:

Dilaudid .. 440
Dilaudid Non-Sterile Powder 440
Dilaudid Oral Liquid 445
Dilaudid Rectal Suppositories 440
Dilaudid Tablets 440
Dilaudid Tablets - 8 mg 445
Dilaudid-HP 442

Hydroxyzine Hydrochloride (Possible additive or potentiating effect with CNS depressants).

No products indexed under this heading.

Imipramine Hydrochloride (Tricyclic antidepressants have been reported to blunt the hypotensive effect of systemic clonidine, an alpha adrenergic agonist; it is not known whether the concurrent use of these agents with brimonidine can lead to interference in IOP-lowering effect; caution is advised).

No products indexed under this heading.

Imipramine Pamoate (Tricyclic antidepressants have been reported to blunt the hypotensive effect of systemic clonidine, an alpha adrenergic agonist; it is not known whether the concurrent use of these agents with brimonidine can lead to interference in IOP-lowering effect; caution is advised).

No products indexed under this heading.

Indapamide (Concurrent use of brimonidine, an alpha adrenergic agonist, with antihypertensives may reduce pulse and blood pressure, however, in clinical trials brimonidine did not have any significant effects on pulse and blood pressure). Products include:

Indapamide Tablets 2156

Irbesartan (Concurrent use of brimonidine, an alpha adrenergic agonist, with antihypertensives may reduce pulse and blood pressure, however, in clinical trials brimonidine

did not have any significant effects on pulse and blood pressure). Products include:

Avalide Tablets 888
Avalide Tablets 2874
Avapro Tablets 891
Avapro Tablets 2871

Isocarboxazid (Concurrent use of brimonidine, an alpha adrenergic agonist, and MAO inhibitor is contraindicated).

No products indexed under this heading.

Isoflurane (Possible additive or potentiating effect with CNS depressants).

No products indexed under this heading.

Isradipine (Concurrent use of brimonidine, an alpha adrenergic agonist, with antihypertensives may reduce pulse and blood pressure, however, in clinical trials brimonidine did not have any significant effects on pulse and blood pressure). Products include:

DynaCirc CR Tablets 2721

Ketamine Hydrochloride (Possible additive or potentiating effect with CNS depressants).

No products indexed under this heading.

Labetalol Hydrochloride (Concurrent use of brimonidine, an alpha adrenergic agonist, with beta blockers (ophthalmic and systemic) may reduce pulse and blood pressure, however, in clinical trials brimonidine did not have any significant effects on pulse and blood pressure).

No products indexed under this heading.

Levobunolol Hydrochloride (Concurrent use of brimonidine, an alpha adrenergic agonist, with beta blockers (ophthalmic and systemic) may reduce pulse and blood pressure, however, in clinical trials brimonidine did not have any significant effects on pulse and blood pressure). Products include:

Betagan Ophthalmic Solution,
USP .. ⊙220

Levomethadyl Acetate Hydrochloride (Possible additive or potentiating effect with CNS depressants).

No products indexed under this heading.

Levorphanol Tartrate (Possible additive or potentiating effect with CNS depressants).

No products indexed under this heading.

Lisinopril (Concurrent use of brimonidine, an alpha adrenergic agonist, with antihypertensives may reduce pulse and blood pressure, however, in clinical trials brimonidine did not have any significant effects on pulse and blood pressure). Products include:

Prinivil Tablets 2052
Prinzide Tablets 2056

Lorazepam (Possible additive or potentiating effect with CNS depressants).

No products indexed under this heading.

Losartan Potassium (Concurrent use of brimonidine, an alpha adrenergic agonist, with antihypertensives may reduce pulse and blood pressure, however, in clinical trials brimonidine did not have any significant effects on pulse and blood pressure). Products include:

IMPORTANT NOTE: Always consult each drug listing in the patient's regimen for possible interactions.

Loxapine Hydrochloride (Possible additive or potentiating effect with CNS depressants).

No products indexed under this heading.

Loxapine Succinate (Possible additive or potentiating effect with CNS depressants).

No products indexed under this heading.

Maprotiline Hydrochloride (Tricyclic antidepressants have been reported to blunt the hypotensive effect of systemic clonidine, an alpha adrenergic agonist; it is not known whether the concurrent use of these agents with brimonidine can lead to interference in IOP-lowering effect; caution is advised).

No products indexed under this heading.

Mecamylamine Hydrochloride (Concurrent use of brimonidine, an alpha adrenergic agonist, with antihypertensives may reduce pulse and blood pressure, however, in clinical trials brimonidine did not have any significant effects on pulse and blood pressure).

No products indexed under this heading.

Meperidine Hydrochloride (Possible additive or potentiating effect with CNS depressants).

No products indexed under this heading.

Mephobarbital (Possible additive or potentiating effect with CNS depressants).

No products indexed under this heading.

Meprobamate (Possible additive or potentiating effect with CNS depressants).

No products indexed under this heading.

Mesoridazine Besylate (Possible additive or potentiating effect with CNS depressants).

No products indexed under this heading.

Methadone Hydrochloride (Possible additive or potentiating effect with CNS depressants).

No products indexed under this heading.

Methohexital Sodium (Possible additive or potentiating effect with CNS depressants).

No products indexed under this heading.

Methotrimeprazine (Possible additive or potentiating effect with CNS depressants).

No products indexed under this heading.

Methoxyflurane (Possible additive or potentiating effect with CNS depressants).

No products indexed under this heading.

Methyclothiazide (Concurrent use of brimonidine, an alpha adrenergic agonist, with antihypertensives may reduce pulse and blood pressure, however, in clinical trials brimonidine did not have any significant effects on pulse and blood pressure).

No products indexed under this heading.

Methyldopa (Concurrent use of brimonidine, an alpha adrenergic

agonist, with antihypertensives may reduce pulse and blood pressure, however, in clinical trials brimonidine did not have any significant effects on pulse and blood pressure).
Products include:

Methyldopate Hydrochloride (Concurrent use of brimonidine, an alpha adrenergic agonist, with antihypertensives may reduce pulse and blood pressure, however, in clinical trials brimonidine did not have any significant effects on pulse and blood pressure).

No products indexed under this heading.

Metipranolol Hydrochloride (Concurrent use of brimonidine, an alpha adrenergic agonist, with beta blockers (ophthalmic and systemic) may reduce pulse and blood pressure, however, in clinical trials brimonidine did not have any significant effects on pulse and blood pressure).

No products indexed under this heading.

Metolazone (Concurrent use of brimonidine, an alpha adrenergic agonist, with antihypertensives may reduce pulse and blood pressure, however, in clinical trials brimonidine did not have any significant effects on pulse and blood pressure).

No products indexed under this heading.

Metoprolol Succinate (Concurrent use of brimonidine, an alpha adrenergic agonist, with beta blockers (ophthalmic and systemic) may reduce pulse and blood pressure, however, in clinical trials brimonidine did not have any significant effects on pulse and blood pressure). Products include:

Metoprolol Tartrate (Concurrent use of brimonidine, an alpha adrenergic agonist, with beta blockers (ophthalmic and systemic) may reduce pulse and blood pressure, however, in clinical trials brimonidine did not have any significant effects on pulse and blood pressure). Products include:

Metyrosine (Concurrent use of brimonidine, an alpha adrenergic agonist, with antihypertensives may reduce pulse and blood pressure, however, in clinical trials brimonidine did not have any significant effects on pulse and blood pressure).
Products include:

Mibefradil Dihydrochloride (Concurrent use of brimonidine, an alpha adrenergic agonist, with antihypertensives may reduce pulse and blood pressure, however, in clinical trials brimonidine did not have any significant effects on pulse and blood pressure).

No products indexed under this heading.

Midazolam Hydrochloride (Possible additive or potentiating effect with CNS depressants).

No products indexed under this heading.

Minoxidil (Concurrent use of brimonidine, an alpha adrenergic agonist, with antihypertensives may reduce pulse and blood pressure,

however, in clinical trials brimonidine did not have any significant effects on pulse and blood pressure).
Products include:
Men's Rogaine Extra Strength Hair Regrowth Treatment Topical Solution, Ocean Rush Scent and Original Unscented □□ 633
Men's Rogaine Foam Hair Regrowth Treatment □□ 633
Women's Rogaine Hair Regrowth Treatment Topical Solution, Spring Bloom Scent and Original Unscented □□ 634

Moclobemide (Concurrent use of brimonidine, an alpha adrenergic agonist, and MAO inhibitor is contraindicated).

No products indexed under this heading.

Moexipril Hydrochloride (Concurrent use of brimonidine, an alpha adrenergic agonist, with antihypertensives may reduce pulse and blood pressure, however, in clinical trials brimonidine did not have any significant effects on pulse and blood pressure). Products include:

Molindone Hydrochloride (Possible additive or potentiating effect with CNS depressants). Products include:

Morphine Sulfate (Possible additive or potentiating effect with CNS depressants). Products include:

Nadolol (Concurrent use of brimonidine, an alpha adrenergic agonist, with beta blockers (ophthalmic and systemic) may reduce pulse and blood pressure, however, in clinical trials brimonidine did not have any significant effects on pulse and blood pressure). Products include:

Nicardipine Hydrochloride (Concurrent use of brimonidine, an alpha adrenergic agonist, with antihypertensives may reduce pulse and blood pressure, however, in clinical trials brimonidine did not have any significant effects on pulse and blood pressure). Products include:

Nifedipine (Concurrent use of brimonidine, an alpha adrenergic agonist, with antihypertensives may reduce pulse and blood pressure, however, in clinical trials brimonidine did not have any significant effects on pulse and blood pressure).
Products include:

Nisoldipine (Concurrent use of brimonidine, an alpha adrenergic agonist, with antihypertensives may reduce pulse and blood pressure, however, in clinical trials brimonidine did not have any significant effects on pulse and blood pressure).
Products include:

Nitroglycerin (Concurrent use of brimonidine, an alpha adrenergic agonist, with antihypertensives may reduce pulse and blood pressure, however, in clinical trials brimonidine did not have any significant effects on pulse and blood pressure).
Products include:

Nortriptyline Hydrochloride (Tricyclic antidepressants have been reported to blunt the hypotensive effect of systemic clonidine, an alpha adrenergic agonist; it is not known whether the concurrent use of these agents with brimonidine can lead to interference in IOP-lowering effect; caution is advised).

No products indexed under this heading.

Olanzapine (Possible additive or potentiating effect with CNS depressants). Products include:

Oxazepam (Possible additive or potentiating effect with CNS depressants).

No products indexed under this heading.

Oxycodone Hydrochloride (Possible additive or potentiating effect with CNS depressants). Products include:

Pargyline Hydrochloride (Concurrent use of brimonidine, an alpha adrenergic agonist, and MAO inhibitor is contraindicated).

No products indexed under this heading.

Penbutolol Sulfate (Concurrent use of brimonidine, an alpha adrenergic agonist, with beta blockers (ophthalmic and systemic) may reduce pulse and blood pressure, however, in clinical trials brimonidine did not have any significant effects on pulse and blood pressure).

No products indexed under this heading.

Pentobarbital Sodium (Possible additive or potentiating effect with CNS depressants). Products include:

Perindopril Erbumine (Concurrent use of brimonidine, an alpha adrenergic agonist, with antihypertensives may reduce pulse and blood pressure, however, in clinical trials brimonidine did not have any significant effects on pulse and blood pressure). Products include:

Perphenazine (Possible additive or potentiating effect with CNS depressants).

No products indexed under this heading.

Phenelzine Sulfate (Concurrent use of brimonidine, an alpha adrenergic agonist, and MAO inhibitor is contraindicated).

No products indexed under this heading.

Phenobarbital (Possible additive or potentiating effect with CNS depressants). Products include:

Phenoxybenzamine Hydrochloride (Concurrent use of brimonidine, an alpha adrenergic agonist, with antihypertensives may reduce pulse and blood pressure, however, in clinical trials brimonidine did not have any significant effects on pulse and blood pressure). Products include:

Dibenzyline Capsules 3399

Phentolamine Mesylate (Concurrent use of brimonidine, an alpha adrenergic agonist, with antihypertensives may reduce pulse and blood pressure, however, in clinical trials brimonidine did not have any significant effects on pulse and blood pressure).
No products indexed under this heading.

Pindolol (Concurrent use of brimonidine, an alpha adrenergic agonist, with beta blockers (ophthalmic and systemic) may reduce pulse and blood pressure, however, in clinical trials brimonidine did not have any significant effects on pulse and blood pressure).
No products indexed under this heading.

Polythiazide (Concurrent use of brimonidine, an alpha adrenergic agonist, with antihypertensives may reduce pulse and blood pressure, however, in clinical trials brimonidine did not have any significant effects on pulse and blood pressure).
No products indexed under this heading.

Prazepam (Possible additive or potentiating effect with CNS depressants).
No products indexed under this heading.

Prazosin Hydrochloride (Concurrent use of brimonidine, an alpha adrenergic agonist, with antihypertensives may reduce pulse and blood pressure, however, in clinical trials brimonidine did not have any significant effects on pulse and blood pressure).
No products indexed under this heading.

Procarbazine Hydrochloride (Concurrent use of brimonidine, an alpha adrenergic agonist, and MAO inhibitor is contraindicated). Products include:
Matulane Capsules 3191

Prochlorperazine (Possible additive or potentiating effect with CNS depressants).
No products indexed under this heading.

Promethazine Hydrochloride (Possible additive or potentiating effect with CNS depressants). Products include:
Phenergan Tablets and Suppositories 3440

Propofol (Possible additive or potentiating effect with CNS depressants).
No products indexed under this heading.

Propoxyphene Hydrochloride (Possible additive or potentiating effect with CNS depressants).
No products indexed under this heading.

Propoxyphene Napsylate (Possible additive or potentiating effect with CNS depressants).
No products indexed under this heading.

Propranolol Hydrochloride (Concurrent use of brimonidine, an alpha adrenergic agonist, with beta blockers (ophthalmic and systemic) may reduce pulse and blood pressure, however, in clinical trials brimonidine did not have any significant effects on pulse and blood pressure). Products include:
Inderal LA Long-Acting Capsules 3429
InnoPran XL Capsules 2723

Protriptyline Hydrochloride (Tricyclic antidepressants have been reported to blunt the hypotensive effect of systemic clonidine, an alpha adrenergic agonist; it is not known whether the concurrent use of these agents with brimonidine can lead to interference in IOP-lowering effect; caution is advised).
No products indexed under this heading.

Quazepam (Possible additive or potentiating effect with CNS depressants).
No products indexed under this heading.

Quetiapine Fumarate (Possible additive or potentiating effect with CNS depressants). Products include:
Seroquel Tablets 690

Quinapril Hydrochloride (Concurrent use of brimonidine, an alpha adrenergic agonist, with antihypertensives may reduce pulse and blood pressure, however, in clinical trials brimonidine did not have any significant effects on pulse and blood pressure).
No products indexed under this heading.

Ramelteon (Possible additive or potentiating effect with CNS depressants). Products include:
Rozerem Tablets 3231

Ramipril (Concurrent use of brimonidine, an alpha adrenergic agonist, with antihypertensives may reduce pulse and blood pressure, however, in clinical trials brimonidine did not have any significant effects on pulse and blood pressure). Products include:
Altace Capsules 1702

Rauwolfia Serpentina (Concurrent use of brimonidine, an alpha adrenergic agonist, with antihypertensives may reduce pulse and blood pressure, however, in clinical trials brimonidine did not have any significant effects on pulse and blood pressure).
No products indexed under this heading.

Remifentanil Hydrochloride (Possible additive or potentiating effect with CNS depressants).
No products indexed under this heading.

Rescinnamine (Concurrent use of brimonidine, an alpha adrenergic agonist, with antihypertensives may reduce pulse and blood pressure, however, in clinical trials brimonidine did not have any significant effects on pulse and blood pressure).
No products indexed under this heading.

Reserpine (Concurrent use of brimonidine, an alpha adrenergic agonist, with antihypertensives may reduce pulse and blood pressure, however, in clinical trials brimonidine did not have any significant effects on pulse and blood pressure).
No products indexed under this heading.

Risperidone (Possible additive or potentiating effect with CNS depressants). Products include:
Risperdal 1676
Risperdal Consta Long-Acting Injection 1682
Risperdal M-Tab Orally Disintegrating Tablets 1676

Secobarbital Sodium (Possible additive or potentiating effect with CNS depressants).
No products indexed under this heading.

Selegiline Hydrochloride (Concurrent use of brimonidine, an alpha adrenergic agonist, and MAO inhibitor is contraindicated). Products include:
Eldepryl Capsules 3208
Zelapar Tablets 3372

Sevoflurane (Possible additive or potentiating effect with CNS depressants). Products include:
Ultane Liquid for Inhalation 531

Sodium Nitroprusside (Concurrent use of brimonidine, an alpha adrenergic agonist, with antihypertensives may reduce pulse and blood pressure, however, in clinical trials brimonidine did not have any significant effects on pulse and blood pressure).
No products indexed under this heading.

Sodium Oxybate (Possible additive or potentiating effect with CNS depressants). Products include:
Xyrem Oral Solution 1688

Sotalol Hydrochloride (Concurrent use of brimonidine, an alpha adrenergic agonist, with beta blockers (ophthalmic and systemic) may reduce pulse and blood pressure, however, in clinical trials brimonidine did not have any significant effects on pulse and blood pressure).
No products indexed under this heading.

Spirapril Hydrochloride (Concurrent use of brimonidine, an alpha adrenergic agonist, with antihypertensives may reduce pulse and blood pressure, however, in clinical trials brimonidine did not have any significant effects on pulse and blood pressure).
No products indexed under this heading.

Sufentanil Citrate (Possible additive or potentiating effect with CNS depressants).
No products indexed under this heading.

Telmisartan (Concurrent use of brimonidine, an alpha adrenergic agonist, with antihypertensives may reduce pulse and blood pressure, however, in clinical trials brimonidine did not have any significant effects on pulse and blood pressure). Products include:
Micardis Tablets 854
Micardis HCT Tablets 856

Temazepam (Possible additive or potentiating effect with CNS depressants). Products include:
Restoril Capsules 1860

Terazosin Hydrochloride (Concurrent use of brimonidine, an alpha adrenergic agonist, with antihypertensives may reduce pulse and blood pressure, however, in clinical trials brimonidine did not have any significant effects on pulse and blood pressure). Products include:
Hytrin Capsules 471

Thiamylal Sodium (Possible additive or potentiating effect with CNS depressants).
No products indexed under this heading.

Thioridazine Hydrochloride (Possible additive or potentiating effect with CNS depressants). Products include:
Thioridazine Hydrochloride Tablets 2163

Thiothixene (Possible additive or potentiating effect with CNS depressants). Products include:
Thiothixene Capsules 2165

Timolol Hemihydrate (Concurrent use of brimonidine, an alpha adrenergic agonist, with beta blockers (ophthalmic and systemic) may reduce pulse and blood pressure, however, in clinical trials brimonidine did not have any significant effects on pulse and blood pressure). Products include:
Betimol Ophthalmic Solution 3382
Betimol Ophthalmic Solution .... ⊙295

Timolol Maleate (Concurrent use of brimonidine, an alpha adrenergic agonist, with beta blockers (ophthalmic and systemic) may reduce pulse and blood pressure, however, in clinical trials brimonidine did not have any significant effects on pulse and blood pressure). Products include:
Blocadren Tablets 1916
Cosopt Sterile Ophthalmic Solution 1931
Timolide Tablets 2086
Timoptic Sterile Ophthalmic Solution 2088
Timoptic in Ocudose 2091
Timoptic-XE Sterile Ophthalmic Gel Forming Solution 2092

Torsemide (Concurrent use of brimonidine, an alpha adrenergic agonist, with antihypertensives may reduce pulse and blood pressure, however, in clinical trials brimonidine did not have any significant effects on pulse and blood pressure). Products include:
Demadex Injection 2759
Demadex Tablets 2759

Trandolapril (Concurrent use of brimonidine, an alpha adrenergic agonist, with antihypertensives may reduce pulse and blood pressure, however, in clinical trials brimonidine did not have any significant effects on pulse and blood pressure). Products include:
Mavik Tablets 486
Tarka Tablets 524

Tranylcypromine Sulfate (Concurrent use of brimonidine, an alpha adrenergic agonist, and MAO inhibitor is contraindicated). Products include:
Parnate Tablets 1527

Triazolam (Possible additive or potentiating effect with CNS depressants).
No products indexed under this heading.

Trifluoperazine Hydrochloride (Possible additive or potentiating effect with CNS depressants).
No products indexed under this heading.

Trimethaphan Camsylate (Concurrent use of brimonidine, an alpha adrenergic agonist, with antihypertensives may reduce pulse and blood pressure, however, in clinical trials brimonidine did not have any significant effects on pulse and blood pressure).
No products indexed under this heading.

Trimipramine Maleate (Tricyclic antidepressants have been reported to blunt the hypotensive effect of systemic clonidine, an alpha adrenergic agonist; it is not known whether the concurrent use of these agents with brimonidine can lead to interference in IOP-lowering effect; caution is advised).
No products indexed under this heading.

Valsartan (Concurrent use of brimonidine, an alpha adrenergic agonist, with antihypertensives may reduce pulse and blood pressure, however, in clinical trials brimonidine did not have any significant effects on pulse and blood pressure). Products include:
Diovan Tablets 2193
Diovan HCT Tablets 2196

Verapamil Hydrochloride (Concurrent use of brimonidine, an alpha adrenergic agonist, with antihypertensives may reduce pulse and blood pressure, however, in clinical trials brimonidine did not have any significant effects on pulse and blood pressure). Products include:
Covera-HS Tablets 3139
Tarka Tablets 524
Verelan PM Extended-Release Capsules, Controlled-Onset 3106

Zaleplon (Possible additive or potentiating effect with CNS depressants). Products include:
Sonata Capsules 1717

Ziprasidone Hydrochloride (Possible additive or potentiating effect with CNS depressants). Products include:
Geodon Capsules 2529

Zolpidem Tartrate (Possible additive or potentiating effect with CNS depressants). Products include:
Ambien Tablets 2851
Ambien CR Tablets 2855

Food Interactions

Alcohol (Possible additive or potentiating effect with CNS depressants).

ALPHANATE, ANTIHEMOPHILIC FACTOR (HUMAN)

(Antihemophilic Factor (Human), Factor VIII (AHF, AHG)) 1654
None cited in PDR database.

ALPHANINE SD, COAGULATION FACTOR IX (HUMAN)

(Factor IX (Human)) 1656
None cited in PDR database.

ALREX OPHTHALMIC SUSPENSION 0.2%

(Loteprednol Etabonate) ..... ⊙246
None cited in PDR database.

ALTACE CAPSULES

(Ramipril) 1702
May interact with diuretics, oral hypoglycemic agents, insulin, lithium preparations, non-steroidal anti-inflammatory agents, potassium preparations, potassium sparing diuretics, and certain other agents. Compounds in these categories include:

Acarbose (There have been rare reports of hypoglycemia reported during ramipril therapy when given to patients concomitantly taking oral hypoglycemic agents or insulin). Products include:
Precose Tablets 751

Amiloride Hydrochloride (May result in excessive reduction of blood pressure after initiation of therapy; increased risk of hyperkalemia). Products include:
Midamor Tablets 2026
Moduretic Tablets 2028

Bendroflumethiazide (May result in excessive reduction of blood pressure after initiation of therapy).
No products indexed under this heading.

Bumetanide (May result in excessive reduction of blood pressure after initiation of therapy). Products include:
Bumex Tablets 2746

Celecoxib (Co-administration of ACE inhibitors with NSAIDs have been associated with worsening of renal failure and hyperkalemia). Products include:
Celebrex Capsules 3134

Chlorothiazide (May result in excessive reduction of blood pressure after initiation of therapy). Products include:
Diuril Oral Suspension 1954

Chlorothiazide Sodium (May result in excessive reduction of blood pressure after initiation of therapy). Products include:
Diuril Sodium Intravenous 2467

Chlorpropamide (There have been rare reports of hypoglycemia reported during ramipril therapy when given to patients concomitantly taking oral hypoglycemic agents or insulin).
No products indexed under this heading.

Chlorthalidone (May result in excessive reduction of blood pressure after initiation of therapy). Products include:
Clorpres Tablets 2153

Diclofenac Potassium (Co-administration of ACE inhibitors with NSAIDs have been associated with worsening of renal failure and hyperkalemia).
No products indexed under this heading.

Diclofenac Sodium (Co-administration of ACE inhibitors with NSAIDs have been associated with worsening of renal failure and hyperkalemia). Products include:
Arthrotec Tablets 3129
Voltaren Ophthalmic Solution 2309
Voltaren Tablets 2307
Voltaren-XR Tablets 2310

Ethacrynic Acid (May result in excessive reduction of blood pressure after initiation of therapy). Products include:
Edecrin Tablets 1959

Etodolac (Co-administration of ACE inhibitors with NSAIDs have been associated with worsening of renal failure and hyperkalemia).
No products indexed under this heading.

Fenoprofen Calcium (Co-administration of ACE inhibitors with NSAIDs have been associated with worsening of renal failure and hyperkalemia). Products include:
Nalfon Capsules 2502

Flurbiprofen (Co-administration of ACE inhibitors with NSAIDs have been associated with worsening of renal failure and hyperkalemia).
No products indexed under this heading.

Furosemide (May result in excessive reduction of blood pressure after initiation of therapy). Products include:
Furosemide Tablets 2154

Glimepiride (There have been rare reports of hypoglycemia reported during ramipril therapy when given to patients concomitantly taking oral hypoglycemic agents or insulin). Products include:
Avandaryl Tablets 1379
Duetact Tablets 3226

Glipizide (There have been rare reports of hypoglycemia reported during ramipril therapy when given to patients concomitantly taking oral hypoglycemic agents or insulin).
No products indexed under this heading.

Glyburide (There have been rare reports of hypoglycemia reported during ramipril therapy when given to patients concomitantly taking oral hypoglycemic agents or insulin).
No products indexed under this heading.

Hydrochlorothiazide (May result in excessive reduction of blood pressure after initiation of therapy). Products include:
Aldoril Tablets 1910
Atacand HCT 651
Avalide Tablets 888
Avalide Tablets 2874
Benicar HCT Tablets 1044
Diovan HCT Tablets 2196
Dyazide Capsules 1423
Hyzaar 50-12.5 Tablets 1990
Hyzaar 100-12.5 Tablets 1990
Hyzaar 100-25 Tablets 1990
Lopressor HCT 50/25 Tablets 2241
Lopressor HCT 100/25 Tablets 2241
Lopressor HCT 100/50 Tablets 2241
Lotensin HCT Tablets 2246
Micardis HCT Tablets 856
Moduretic Tablets 2028
Prinzide Tablets 2056
Teveten HCT Tablets 1737
Timolide Tablets 2086
Uniretic Tablets 3100

Hydroflumethiazide (May result in excessive reduction of blood pressure after initiation of therapy).
No products indexed under this heading.

Ibuprofen (Co-administration of ACE inhibitors with NSAIDs have been associated with worsening of renal failure and hyperkalemia). Products include:
Advil Allergy Sinus Caplets ..... ▣770
Advil ..... ▣674
Children's Advil Oral Suspension ..... ▣603
Children's Advil Chewable Tablets ..... ▣603
Advil Cold & Sinus ..... ▣723
Infants' Advil Concentrated Drops ..... ▣604
Infants' Advil Concentrated Drops - White Grape (Dye-Free) ..... ▣604
Junior Strength Advil Swallow Tablets ..... ▣605
Advil Migraine Liquigels ..... ▣608
Advil Multi-Symptom Cold Caplets ..... ▣770
Advil PM Caplets ..... ▣615
Motrin IB Tablets and Caplets 1866
Children's Motrin Oral Suspension 1867
Children's Motrin Non-Staining Dye-Free Oral Suspension 1867
Children's Motrin Cold Oral Suspension 1867
Infants' Motrin Concentrated Drops 1867
Infants' Motrin Non-Staining Dye-Free Concentrated Drops 1867
Junior Strength Motrin Caplets and Chewable Tablets 1867
Vicoprofen Tablets 539

Indapamide (May result in excessive reduction of blood pressure after initiation of therapy). Products include:
Indapamide Tablets 2156

Indomethacin (Co-administration of ACE inhibitors with NSAIDs have been associated with worsening of renal failure and hyperkalemia). Products include:
Indocin 1995

Indomethacin Sodium Trihydrate (Co-administration of ACE inhibitors with NSAIDs have been associated with worsening of renal failure and hyperkalemia). Products include:
Indocin I.V. 2465

Insulin, Human, Zinc Suspension (There have been rare reports of hypoglycemia reported during ramipril therapy when given to patients concomitantly taking oral hypoglycemic agents or insulin). Products include:
Humulin L, 100 Units 1794
Humulin U, 100 Units 1800

Insulin, Human NPH (There have been rare reports of hypoglycemia reported during ramipril therapy when given to patients concomitantly taking oral hypoglycemic agents or insulin). Products include:
Humulin N, 100 Units 1795
Humulin N Pen 1797

Insulin, Human Regular (There have been rare reports of hypoglycemia reported during ramipril therapy when given to patients concomitantly taking oral hypoglycemic agents or insulin). Products include:
Humulin R, 100 Units 1798

Insulin, Human Regular and Human NPH Mixture (There have been rare reports of hypoglycemia reported during ramipril therapy when given to patients concomitantly taking oral hypoglycemic agents or insulin). Products include:
Humulin 50/50, 100 Units 1791
Humulin 70/30 Pen 1793

Insulin, NPH (There have been rare reports of hypoglycemia reported during ramipril therapy when given to patients concomitantly taking oral hypoglycemic agents or insulin).
No products indexed under this heading.

Insulin, Regular (There have been rare reports of hypoglycemia reported during ramipril therapy when given to patients concomitantly taking oral hypoglycemic agents or insulin).
No products indexed under this heading.

Insulin, Zinc Crystals (There have been rare reports of hypoglycemia reported during ramipril therapy when given to patients concomitantly taking oral hypoglycemic agents or insulin).
No products indexed under this heading.

Insulin, Zinc Suspension (There have been rare reports of hypoglycemia reported during ramipril therapy when given to patients concomitantly taking oral hypoglycemic agents or insulin).
No products indexed under this heading.

Insulin Aspart, Human Regular (There have been rare reports of hypoglycemia reported during ramipril therapy when given to patients

concomitantly taking oral hypoglycemic agents or insulin). Products include:
NovoLog Injection 2326

Insulin glargine (There have been rare reports of hypoglycemia reported during ramipril therapy when given to patients concomitantly taking oral hypoglycemic agents or insulin). Products include:
Lantus Injection 2909

Insulin Lispro, Human (There have been rare reports of hypoglycemia reported during ramipril therapy when given to patients concomitantly taking oral hypoglycemic agents or insulin). Products include:
Humalog-Pen 1781
Humalog Mix 50/50-Pen 1783
Humalog Mix 75/25-Pen 1785

Insulin Lispro Protamine, Human (There have been rare reports of hypoglycemia reported during ramipril therapy when given to patients concomitantly taking oral hypoglycemic agents or insulin). Products include:
Humalog Mix 50/50-Pen 1783
Humalog Mix 75/25-Pen 1785

Ketoprofen (Co-administration of ACE inhibitors with NSAIDs have been associated with worsening of renal failure and hyperkalemia).
No products indexed under this heading.

Ketorolac Tromethamine (Co-administration of ACE inhibitors with NSAIDs have been associated with worsening of renal failure and hyperkalemia). Products include:
Acular Ophthalmic Solution 565
Acular LS Ophthalmic Solution 566

Lithium (Increased serum lithium levels and symptoms of lithium toxicity).
No products indexed under this heading.

Lithium Carbonate (Increased serum lithium levels and symptoms of lithium toxicity). Products include:
Lithobid Tablets 1692

Lithium Citrate (Increased serum lithium levels and symptoms of lithium toxicity).
No products indexed under this heading.

Meclofenamate Sodium (Co-administration of ACE inhibitors with NSAIDs have been associated with worsening of renal failure and hyperkalemia).
No products indexed under this heading.

Mefenamic Acid (Co-administration of ACE inhibitors with NSAIDs have been associated with worsening of renal failure and hyperkalemia).
No products indexed under this heading.

Meloxicam (Co-administration of ACE inhibitors with NSAIDs have been associated with worsening of renal failure and hyperkalemia). Products include:
Mobic Oral Suspension 863
Mobic Tablets 863

Metformin Hydrochloride (There have been rare reports of hypoglycemia reported during ramipril therapy when given to patients concomitantly taking oral hypoglycemic agents or insulin). Products include:
ActoPlus Met Tablets 3214
Avandamet Tablets 1373
Fortamet Extended-Release Tablets 3115

Methyclothiazide (May result in excessive reduction of blood pressure after initiation of therapy).
No products indexed under this heading.

Metolazone (May result in excessive reduction of blood pressure after initiation of therapy).
No products indexed under this heading.

Miglitol (There have been rare reports of hypoglycemia reported during ramipril therapy when given to patients concomitantly taking oral hypoglycemic agents or insulin).
No products indexed under this heading.

Nabumetone (Co-administration of ACE inhibitors with NSAIDs have been associated with worsening of renal failure and hyperkalemia).
No products indexed under this heading.

Naproxen (Co-administration of ACE inhibitors with NSAIDs have been associated with worsening of renal failure and hyperkalemia). Products include:
EC-Naprosyn Delayed-Release Tablets 2761
Naprosyn Suspension 2761
Naprosyn Tablets 2761
Prevacid NapraPAC 3280

Naproxen Sodium (Co-administration of ACE inhibitors with NSAIDs have been associated with worsening of renal failure and hyperkalemia). Products include:
Aleve Caplets 742
Aleve Gelcaps 743
Aleve Tablets 743
Aleve Cold & Sinus Caplets 744
Anaprox Tablets 2761
Anaprox DS Tablets 2761

Oxaprozin (Co-administration of ACE inhibitors with NSAIDs have been associated with worsening of renal failure and hyperkalemia).
No products indexed under this heading.

Phenylbutazone (Co-administration of ACE inhibitors with NSAIDs have been associated with worsening of renal failure and hyperkalemia).
No products indexed under this heading.

Pioglitazone Hydrochloride (There have been rare reports of hypoglycemia reported during ramipril therapy when given to patients concomitantly taking oral hypoglycemic agents or insulin). Products include:
ActoPlus Met Tablets 3214
Actos Tablets 3219
Duetact Tablets 3226

Piroxicam (Co-administration of ACE inhibitors with NSAIDs have been associated with worsening of renal failure and hyperkalemia).
No products indexed under this heading.

Polythiazide (May result in excessive reduction of blood pressure after initiation of therapy).
No products indexed under this heading.

Potassium Acid Phosphate (Increased risk of hyperkalemia). Products include:
K-Phos Original (Sodium Free) Tablets 760

Potassium Bicarbonate (Increased risk of hyperkalemia).
No products indexed under this heading.

Potassium Chloride (Increased risk of hyperkalemia). Products include:
Colyte with Flavor Packs for Oral Solution 3088
HalfLytely and Bisacodyl Tablets Bowel Prep Kit with Flavors Packs 881
K-Dur Extended-Release Tablets 3033
K-Lor Oral Solution 474
K-Tab Tablets 475
MoviPrep Oral Solution 2839
TriLyte with Flavor Packs for Oral Solution 3100

Potassium Citrate (Increased risk of hyperkalemia). Products include:
Urocit-K Tablets 2144

Potassium Gluconate (Increased risk of hyperkalemia).
No products indexed under this heading.

Potassium Phosphate (Increased risk of hyperkalemia). Products include:
K-Phos Neutral Tablets 760

Repaglinide (There have been rare reports of hypoglycemia reported during ramipril therapy when given to patients concomitantly taking oral hypoglycemic agents or insulin).
No products indexed under this heading.

Rofecoxib (Co-administration of ACE inhibitors with NSAIDs have been associated with worsening of renal failure and hyperkalemia).
No products indexed under this heading.

Rosiglitazone Maleate (There have been reports of hypoglycemia reported during ramipril therapy when given to patients concomitantly taking oral hypoglycemic agents or insulin). Products include:
Avandamet Tablets 1373
Avandaryl Tablets 1379
Avandia Tablets 1384

Spironolactone (May result in excessive reduction of blood pressure after initiation of therapy; increased risk of hyperkalemia).
No products indexed under this heading.

Sulindac (Co-administration of ACE inhibitors with NSAIDs have been associated with worsening of renal failure and hyperkalemia). Products include:
Clinoril Tablets 1924

Tolazamide (There have been rare reports of hypoglycemia reported during ramipril therapy when given to patients concomitantly taking oral hypoglycemic agents or insulin).
No products indexed under this heading.

Tolbutamide (There have been rare reports of hypoglycemia reported during ramipril therapy when given to patients concomitantly taking oral hypoglycemic agents or insulin).
No products indexed under this heading.

Tolmetin Sodium (Co-administration of ACE inhibitors with NSAIDs have been associated with worsening of renal failure and hyperkalemia).
No products indexed under this heading.

Torsemide (May result in excessive reduction of blood pressure after initiation of therapy). Products include:
Demadex Injection 2759
Demadex Tablets 2759

Triamterene (May result in excessive reduction of blood pressure after initiation of therapy; increased risk of hyperkalemia). Products include:
Dyazide Capsules 1423
Dyrenium Capsules 3400

Troglitazone (There have been rare reports of hypoglycemia reported during ramipril therapy when given to patients concomitantly taking oral hypoglycemic agents or insulin).
No products indexed under this heading.

Valdecoxib (Co-administration of ACE inhibitors with NSAIDs have been associated with worsening of renal failure and hyperkalemia).
No products indexed under this heading.

Food Interactions

Food, unspecified (The rate of absorption is reduced, not the extent of absorption).

Salt Substitutes, Potassium-Containing (Increases risk of hyperkalemia).

ALTOPREV EXTENDED-RELEASE TABLETS

(Lovastatin) 3109
May interact with oral anticoagulants, erythromycin, fibrates, protease inhibitors, and certain other agents. Compounds in these categories include:

Amiodarone Hydrochloride (Co-administration with potent CYP3A4 inhibitors, such as cyclosporine, increases the risk of myopathy/rhabdomyolysis; the dose of lovastatin should not exceed 40 mg/day).
No products indexed under this heading.

Amprenavir (Co-administration with potent CYP3A4 inhibitors, such as HIV protease inhibitors, increases the risk of myopathy/rhabdomyolysis; concurrent use should be avoided). Products include:
Agenerase Capsules 1327
Agenerase Oral Solution 1332

Anisindione (Co-administration has resulted in increased bleeding and/or prothrombin time in a few patients). Products include:
Miradon Tablets 3042

Cimetidine (May blunt adrenal and/or gonadal steroid production. Co-administration with drugs that may decrease the levels or activity of endogenous steroid hormones, like cimetidine, should be done with caution). Products include:
Tagamet HB 200 Tablets 664

Cimetidine Hydrochloride (May blunt adrenal and/or gonadal steroid production. Co-administration with drugs that may decrease the levels or activity of endogenous steroid hormones, like cimetidine, should be done with caution).
No products indexed under this heading.

Clarithromycin (Co-administration with potent CYP3A4 inhibitors, such as cyclosporine, increases the risk of myopathy/rhabdomyolysis; the dose of lovastatin should not exceed 20 mg/day). Products include:
Biaxin/Biaxin XL 402
PREVPAC 3284

Clofibrate (Co-administration with other lipid lowering drugs that can cause myopathy when given alone, such as fibrates, increases the risk of myopathy/rhabdomyolysis; concurrent use should be avoided unless the benefit outweights the risk. The dose of lovastatin should not exceed 20 mg/day if given concurrently).
 No products indexed under this heading.

Cyclosporine (Co-administration with potent CYP3A4 inhibitors, such as cyclosporine, increases the risk of myopathy/rhabdomyolysis; the dose of lovastatin should not exceed 20 mg/day). Products include:

Dicumarol (Co-administration has resulted in increased bleeding and/or prothrombin time in a few patients).
 No products indexed under this heading.

Erythromycin (Co-administration with potent CYP3A4 inhibitors, such as erythromycin, increases the risk of myopathy/rhabdomyolysis; concurrent use should be avoided. Products include:

Erythromycin Estolate (Co-administration with potent CYP3A4 inhibitors, such as erythromycin, increases the risk of myopathy/rhabdomyolysis; concurrent use should be avoided).
 No products indexed under this heading.

Erythromycin Ethylsuccinate (Co-administration with potent CYP3A4 inhibitors, such as erythromycin, increases the risk of myopathy/rhabdomyolysis; concurrent use should be avoided). Products include:

Erythromycin Gluceptate (Co-administration with potent CYP3A4 inhibitors, such as erythromycin, increases the risk of myopathy/rhabdomyolysis; concurrent use should be avoided).
 No products indexed under this heading.

Erythromycin Lactobionate (Co-administration with potent CYP3A4 inhibitors, such as erythromycin, increases the risk of myopathy/rhabdomyolysis; concurrent use should be avoided).
 No products indexed under this heading.

Erythromycin Stearate (Co-administration with potent CYP3A4 inhibitors, such as erythromycin, increases the risk of myopathy/rhabdomyolysis; concurrent use should be avoided). Products include:

Fenofibrate (Co-administration with other lipid lowering drugs that can cause myopathy when given alone, such as fibrates, increases the risk of myopathy/rhabdomyolysis; con-

current use should be avoided unless the benefit outweights the risk. The dose of lovastatin should not exceed 20 mg/day if given currently). Products include:

Gemfibrozil (Co-administration with other lipid lowering drugs that can cause myopathy when given alone, such as fibrates, increases the risk of myopathy/rhabdomyolysis; concurrent use should be avoided unless the benefit outweights the risk. The dose of lovastatin should not exceed 20 mg/day if given concurrently).
 No products indexed under this heading.

Indinavir Sulfate (Co-administration with potent CYP3A4 inhibitors, such as HIV protease inhibitors, increases the risk of myopathy/rhabdomyolysis; concurrent use should be avoided). Products include:

Itraconazole (Co-administration with potent CYP3A4 inhibitors, such as itraconazole, increases the risk of myopathy/rhabdomyolysis; concurrent use should be avoided).
 No products indexed under this heading.

Ketoconazole (Co-administration with potent CYP3A4 inhibitors, such as ketoconazole, increases the risk of myopathy/rhabdomyolysis; concurrent use should be avoided). Products include:

Lopinavir (Co-administration with potent CYP3A4 inhibitors, such as HIV protease inhibitors, increases the risk of myopathy/rhabdomyolysis; concurrent use should be avoided). Products include:

Nefazodone Hydrochloride (Co-administration with the potent CYP3A4 inhibitors, such as nefazodone, increases the risk of myopathy/rhabdomyolysis; concurrent use should be avoided).
 No products indexed under this heading.

Nelfinavir Mesylate (Co-administration with potent CYP3A4 inhibitors, such as HIV protease inhibitors, increases the risk of myopathy/rhabdomyolysis; concurrent use should be avoided). Products include:

Niacin (Co-administration with niacin (greater than or equal to 1 g/day) increases the risk of myopathy/rhabdomyolysis; concurrent use should be avoided unless the benefit outweighs the risk. The dose of lovastatin should not exceed 20 mg/day if given concurrently). Products include:

Ritonavir (Co-administration with potent CYP3A4 inhibitors, such as HIV protease inhibitors, increases the risk of myopathy/rhabdomyolysis; concurrent use should be avoided). Products include:

Saquinavir (Co-administration with potent CYP3A4 inhibitors, such as HIV protease inhibitors, increases the risk of myopathy/rhabdomyolysis; concurrent use should be avoided).
 No products indexed under this heading.

Saquinavir Mesylate (Co-administration with potent CYP3A4 inhibitors, such as HIV protease inhibitors, increases the risk of myopathy/rhabdomyolysis; concurrent use should be avoided). Products include:

Spironolactone (May blunt adrenal and/or gonadal steroid production. Co-administration with drugs that may decrease the levels or activity of endogenous steroid hormones, like spironolactone, should be done with caution).
 No products indexed under this heading.

Verapamil Hydrochloride (Co-administration with potent CYP3A4 inhibitors, such as verapamil, increases the risk of myopathy/rhabdomyolysis; the dose of lovastatin should not exceed 40 mg/day). Products include:

Warfarin Sodium (Co-administration has resulted in increased bleeding and/or prothrombin time in a few patients). Products include:

Food Interactions

Food, unspecified (Decreases the bio-availability of Altoprev).

Grapefruit Juice (Co-administration with potent CYP3A4 inhibitors, such as large quantities of grapefruit juice (greater than 1 quart daily), increases the risk of myopathy/rhabdomyolysis; concurrent use should be avoided).

ALUPENT INHALATION AEROSOL

May interact with monoamine oxidase inhibitors, sympathomimetic aerosol bronchodilators, and tricyclic antidepressants. Compounds in these categories include:

Albuterol (Possible potentiation of adrenergic effects with beta adrenergic aerosol bronchodilators). Products include:

Amitriptyline Hydrochloride (The action of beta adrenergic agonists on the vascular system may be potentiated).
 No products indexed under this heading.

Amoxapine (The action of beta adrenergic agonists on the vascular system may be potentiated).
 No products indexed under this heading.

Bitolterol Mesylate (Possible potentiation of adrenergic effects with beta adrenergic aerosol bronchodilators).
 No products indexed under this heading.

Clomipramine Hydrochloride (The action of beta adrenergic agonists on the vascular system may be potentiated).
 No products indexed under this heading.

Desipramine Hydrochloride (The action of beta adrenergic agonists on the vascular system may be potentiated).
 No products indexed under this heading.

Doxepin Hydrochloride (The action of beta adrenergic agonists on the vascular system may be potentiated).
 No products indexed under this heading.

Imipramine Hydrochloride (The action of beta adrenergic agonists on the vascular system may be potentiated).
 No products indexed under this heading.

Imipramine Pamoate (The action of beta adrenergic agonists on the vascular system may be potentiated).
 No products indexed under this heading.

Isocarboxazid (The action of beta adrenergic agonists on the vascular system may be potentiated).
 No products indexed under this heading.

Isoetharine (Possible potentiation of adrenergic effects with beta adrenergic aerosol bronchodilators).
 No products indexed under this heading.

Isoproterenol Hydrochloride (Possible potentiation of adrenergic effects with beta adrenergic aerosol bronchodilators).
 No products indexed under this heading.

Levalbuterol Hydrochloride (Possible potentiation of adrenergic effects with beta adrenergic aerosol bronchodilators). Products include:

Maprotiline Hydrochloride (The action of beta adrenergic agonists on the vascular system may be potentiated).
 No products indexed under this heading.

Moclobemide (The action of beta adrenergic agonists on the vascular system may be potentiated).
 No products indexed under this heading.

Nortriptyline Hydrochloride (The action of beta adrenergic agonists on the vascular system may be potentiated).
 No products indexed under this heading.

Pargyline Hydrochloride (The action of beta adrenergic agonists on the vascular system may be potentiated).
 No products indexed under this heading.

Phenelzine Sulfate (The action of beta adrenergic agonists on the vascular system may be potentiated).
 No products indexed under this heading.

Pirbuterol Acetate (Possible potentiation of adrenergic effects with beta adrenergic aerosol bronchodilators). Products include:

Maxair Autohaler 1852

Procarbazine Hydrochloride (The action of beta adrenergic agonists on the vascular system may be potentiated). Products include:
Matulane Capsules 3191

Protriptyline Hydrochloride (The action of beta adrenergic agonists on the vascular system may be potentiated).
No products indexed under this heading.

Salmeterol Xinafoate (Possible potentiation of adrenergic effects with beta adrenergic aerosol bronchodilators). Products include:
Advair Diskus 100/50 1308
Advair Diskus 250/50 1308
Advair Diskus 500/50 1308
Advair HFA Inhalation Aerosol 1318
Serevent Diskus 1568

Selegiline Hydrochloride (The action of beta adrenergic agonists on the vascular system may be potentiated). Products include:
Eldepryl Capsules 3208
Zelapar Tablets 3372

Terbutaline Sulfate (Possible potentiation of adrenergic effects with beta adrenergic aerosol bronchodilators).
No products indexed under this heading.

Tranylcypromine Sulfate (The action of beta adrenergic agonists on the vascular system may be potentiated). Products include:
Parnate Tablets 1527

Trimipramine Maleate (The action of beta adrenergic agonists on the vascular system may be potentiated).
No products indexed under this heading.

AMBIEN TABLETS

(Zolpidem Tartrate) 2851

May interact with central nervous system depressants and certain other agents. Compounds in these categories include:

Alfentanil Hydrochloride (Potential for enhanced CNS depressant effects of zolpidem).
No products indexed under this heading.

Alprazolam (Potential for enhanced CNS depressant effects of zolpidem). Products include:
Niravam Orally Disintegrating Tablets 3092

Aprobarbital (Potential for enhanced CNS depressant effects of zolpidem).
No products indexed under this heading.

Buprenorphine Hydrochloride (Potential for enhanced CNS depressant effects of zolpidem). Products include:
Buprenex Injectable 2716
Suboxone Tablets 2717
Subutex Tablets 2717

Buspirone Hydrochloride (Potential for enhanced CNS depressant effects of zolpidem).
No products indexed under this heading.

Butabarbital (Potential for enhanced CNS depressant effects of zolpidem).
No products indexed under this heading.

Butalbital (Potential for enhanced CNS depressant effects of zolpidem).
No products indexed under this heading.

Chlordiazepoxide (Potential for enhanced CNS depressant effects of zolpidem).
No products indexed under this heading.

Chlordiazepoxide Hydrochloride (Potential for enhanced CNS depressant effects of zolpidem). Products include:
Librium Capsules 3347

Chlorpromazine (Additive effect of decreased alertness and psychomotor performance; potential for enhanced CNS depressant effects of zolpidem).
No products indexed under this heading.

Chlorpromazine Hydrochloride (Additive effect of decreased alertness and psychomotor performance; potential for enhanced CNS depressant effects of zolpidem).
No products indexed under this heading.

Chlorprothixene (Potential for enhanced CNS depressant effects of zolpidem).
No products indexed under this heading.

Chlorprothixene Hydrochloride (Potential for enhanced CNS depressant effects of zolpidem).
No products indexed under this heading.

Chlorprothixene Lactate (Potential for enhanced CNS depressant effects of zolpidem).
No products indexed under this heading.

Clorazepate Dipotassium (Potential for enhanced CNS depressant effects of zolpidem). Products include:
Tranxene 2474

Clozapine (Potential for enhanced CNS depressant effects of zolpidem). Products include:
Clozaril Tablets 2184
FazaClo Orally Disintegrating Tablets 551

Codeine Phosphate (Potential for enhanced CNS depressant effects of zolpidem). Products include:
Tylenol with Codeine Tablets 2391

Desflurane (Potential for enhanced CNS depressant effects of zolpidem).
No products indexed under this heading.

Dezocine (Potential for enhanced CNS depressant effects of zolpidem).
No products indexed under this heading.

Diazepam (Potential for enhanced CNS depressant effects of zolpidem). Products include:
Diastat Rectal Delivery System 3343
Valium Tablets 2819

Droperidol (Potential for enhanced CNS depressant effects of zolpidem).
No products indexed under this heading.

Enflurane (Potential for enhanced CNS depressant effects of zolpidem).
No products indexed under this heading.

Estazolam (Potential for enhanced CNS depressant effects of zolpidem). Products include:
ProSom Tablets 517

Ethanol (Potential for enhanced CNS depressant effects of zolpidem).
No products indexed under this heading.

Ethchlorvynol (Potential for enhanced CNS depressant effects of zolpidem).
No products indexed under this heading.

Ethinamate (Potential for enhanced CNS depressant effects of zolpidem).
No products indexed under this heading.

Ethyl Alcohol (Potential for enhanced CNS depressant effects of zolpidem).
No products indexed under this heading.

Fentanyl (Potential for enhanced CNS depressant effects of zolpidem). Products include:
Duragesic Transdermal System 2373
Ionsys Transdermal System 2379

Fentanyl Citrate (Potential for enhanced CNS depressant effects of zolpidem). Products include:
Actiq 979

Flumazenil (Zolpidem's sedative/hypnotic effect was reversed by flumazenil; however, no significant alterations in zolpidem pharmacokinetics was found). Products include:
Romazicon Injection 2804

Fluoxetine Hydrochloride (Co-administration during multiple doses of both drugs at steady-state concentrations has resulted in a 17% increase in the zolpidem half-life; there was no evidence of an additive effect in psychomotor performance). Products include:
Prozac Pulvules and Liquid 1801
Symbyax Capsules 1819

Fluphenazine Decanoate (Potential for enhanced CNS depressant effects of zolpidem).
No products indexed under this heading.

Fluphenazine Enanthate (Potential for enhanced CNS depressant effects of zolpidem).
No products indexed under this heading.

Fluphenazine Hydrochloride (Potential for enhanced CNS depressant effects of zolpidem).
No products indexed under this heading.

Flurazepam Hydrochloride (Potential for enhanced CNS depressant effects of zolpidem). Products include:
Dalmane Capsules 3342

Glutethimide (Potential for enhanced CNS depressant effects of zolpidem).
No products indexed under this heading.

Haloperidol (Co-administration in a single study revealed no effect on the pharmacokinetics or pharmacodynamics of zolpidem; however, there is a potential for enhanced CNS depressant effect of zolpidem).
No products indexed under this heading.

Haloperidol Decanoate (Co-administration in a single study revealed no effect on the pharmacokinetics or pharmacodynamics of zolpidem; however, there is a potential for enhanced CNS depressant effect of zolpidem).
No products indexed under this heading.

Hydrocodone Bitartrate (Potential for enhanced CNS depressant effects of zolpidem). Products include:
Hycodan 1116
Hycotuss Expectorant Syrup 1117
Vicodin Tablets 535
Vicodin ES Tablets 536
Vicodin HP Tablets 538
Vicoprofen Tablets 539
Zydone Tablets 1139

Hydrocodone Polistirex (Potential for enhanced CNS depressant effects of zolpidem). Products include:
Tussionex Pennkinetic Extended-Release Suspension 3327

Hydromorphone Hydrochloride (Potential for enhanced CNS depressant effects of zolpidem). Products include:
Dilaudid 440
Dilaudid Non-Sterile Powder 440
Dilaudid Oral Liquid 445
Dilaudid Rectal Suppositories 440
Dilaudid Tablets 440
Dilaudid Tablets - 8 mg 445
Dilaudid-HP 442

Hydroxyzine Hydrochloride (Potential for enhanced CNS depressant effects of zolpidem).
No products indexed under this heading.

Imipramine Hydrochloride (Co-administration produces 20% decrease in peak levels of imipramine with an additive effect of decreased alertness).
No products indexed under this heading.

Imipramine Pamoate (Co-administration produces 20% decrease in peak levels of imipramine with an additive effect of decreased alertness).
No products indexed under this heading.

Isoflurane (Potential for enhanced CNS depressant effects of zolpidem).
No products indexed under this heading.

Itraconazole (Co-administration has resulted in a 34% increse in AUCO-infinity of zolpidem; there were no significant pharmacodynamic effects of zolpidem on subjective drowsiness, postural sway, or pychomotor performance).
No products indexed under this heading.

Ketamine Hydrochloride (Potential for enhanced CNS depressant effects of zolpidem).
No products indexed under this heading.

Levomethadyl Acetate Hydrochloride (Potential for enhanced CNS depressant effects of zolpidem).
No products indexed under this heading.

Levorphanol Tartrate (Potential for enhanced CNS depressant effects of zolpidem).
No products indexed under this heading.

Lorazepam (Potential for enhanced CNS depressant effects of zolpidem).
No products indexed under this heading.

Loxapine Hydrochloride (Potential for enhanced CNS depressant effects of zolpidem).
No products indexed under this heading.

Loxapine Succinate (Potential for enhanced CNS depressant effects of zolpidem).
No products indexed under this heading.

Meperidine Hydrochloride (Potential for enhanced CNS depressant effects of zolpidem).
No products indexed under this heading.

Mephobarbital (Potential for enhanced CNS depressant effects of zolpidem).
No products indexed under this heading.

Meprobamate (Potential for enhanced CNS depressant effects of zolpidem).
No products indexed under this heading.

Mesoridazine Besylate (Potential for enhanced CNS depressant effects of zolpidem).
No products indexed under this heading.

Methadone Hydrochloride (Potential for enhanced CNS depressant effects of zolpidem).
No products indexed under this heading.

Methohexital Sodium (Potential for enhanced CNS depressant effects of zolpidem).
No products indexed under this heading.

Methotrimeprazine (Potential for enhanced CNS depressant effects of zolpidem).
No products indexed under this heading.

Methoxyflurane (Potential for enhanced CNS depressant effects of zolpidem).
No products indexed under this heading.

Midazolam Hydrochloride (Potential for enhanced CNS depressant effects of zolpidem).
No products indexed under this heading.

Molindone Hydrochloride (Potential for enhanced CNS depressant effects of zolpidem). Products include:
Moban Tablets 1119

Morphine Sulfate (Potential for enhanced CNS depressant effects of zolpidem). Products include:
Avinza Capsules 1741
Kadian Capsules 577
MS Contin Tablets 2701

Olanzapine (Potential for enhanced CNS depressant effects of zolpidem). Products include:
Symbyax Capsules 1819
Zyprexa Tablets 1830
Zyprexa IntraMuscular 1830
Zyprexa ZYDIS Orally Disintegrating Tablets 1830

Oxazepam (Potential for enhanced CNS depressant effects of zolpidem).
No products indexed under this heading.

Oxycodone Hydrochloride (Potential for enhanced CNS depressant effects of zolpidem). Products include:
OxyContin Tablets 2703
OxyFast Oral Concentrate Solution 2708
OxyIR Capsules 2708
Percocet Tablets 1131
Percodan Tablets 1132

Pentobarbital Sodium (Potential for enhanced CNS depressant effects of zolpidem). Products include:
Nembutal Sodium Solution, USP 2470

Perphenazine (Potential for enhanced CNS depressant effects of zolpidem).
No products indexed under this heading.

Phenobarbital (Potential for enhanced CNS depressant effects of zolpidem). Products include:
Donnatal Extentabs 2493

Prazepam (Potential for enhanced CNS depressant effects of zolpidem).
No products indexed under this heading.

Prochlorperazine (Potential for enhanced CNS depressant effects of zolpidem).
No products indexed under this heading.

Promethazine Hydrochloride (Potential for enhanced CNS depressant effects of zolpidem). Products include:
Phenergan Tablets and Suppositories 3440

Propofol (Potential for enhanced CNS depressant effects of zolpidem).
No products indexed under this heading.

Propoxyphene Hydrochloride (Potential for enhanced CNS depressant effects of zolpidem).
No products indexed under this heading.

Propoxyphene Napsylate (Potential for enhanced CNS depressant effects of zolpidem).
No products indexed under this heading.

Quazepam (Potential for enhanced CNS depressant effects of zolpidem).
No products indexed under this heading.

Quetiapine Fumarate (Potential for enhanced CNS depressant effects of zolpidem). Products include:
Seroquel Tablets 690

Remifentanil Hydrochloride (Potential for enhanced CNS depressant effects of zolpidem).
No products indexed under this heading.

Rifampin (Co-administration has resulted in significant reductions of the AUC, Cmax, and T½ of zolpidem together with significant reductions in the pharmacodynamic effects of zolpidem).
No products indexed under this heading.

Risperidone (Potential for enhanced CNS depressant effects of zolpidem). Products include:
Risperdal 1676
Risperdal Consta Long-Acting Injection 1682
Risperdal M-Tab Orally Disintegrating Tablets 1676

Secobarbital Sodium (Potential for enhanced CNS depressant effects of zolpidem).
No products indexed under this heading.

Sertraline Hydrochloride (Co-administration following consecutive nightly doses has resulted in significantly higher (43%) Cmax and significantly lower Tmax (53%) of zolpidem). Products include:
Zoloft 2586

Sevoflurane (Potential for enhanced CNS depressant effects of zolpidem). Products include:
Ultane Liquid for Inhalation 531

Sufentanil Citrate (Potential for enhanced CNS depressant effects of zolpidem).
No products indexed under this heading.

Temazepam (Potential for enhanced CNS depressant effects of zolpidem). Products include:
Restoril Capsules 1860

Thiamylal Sodium (Potential for enhanced CNS depressant effects of zolpidem).
No products indexed under this heading.

Thioridazine Hydrochloride (Potential for enhanced CNS depressant effects of zolpidem). Products include:
Thioridazine Hydrochloride Tablets 2163

Thiothixene (Potential for enhanced CNS depressant effects of zolpidem). Products include:
Thiothixene Capsules 2165

Triazolam (Potential for enhanced CNS depressant effects of zolpidem).
No products indexed under this heading.

Trifluoperazine Hydrochloride (Potential for enhanced CNS depressant effects of zolpidem).
No products indexed under this heading.

Zaleplon (Potential for enhanced CNS depressant effects of zolpidem). Products include:
Sonata Capsules 1717

Ziprasidone Hydrochloride (Potential for enhanced CNS depressant effects of zolpidem). Products include:
Geodon Capsules 2529

Food Interactions

Alcohol (Co-administration produces additive effects on psychomotor performance).

Meal, unspecified (Mean AUC and Cmax decreased by 15% and 25% respectively, while Tmax was prolonged by 60%; for faster sleep onset, Ambien should not be administered with or immediately after meal).

AMBIEN CR TABLETS

(Zolpidem Tartrate) 2855
May interact with:

Chlorpromazine (Chlorpromazine in combination with zolpidem tartrate produced no pharmacokinetic interaction, but there was an additive effect of decreased alertness and psychomotor performance).
No products indexed under this heading.

Chlorpromazine Hydrochloride (Chlorpromazine in combination with zolpidem tartrate produced no pharmacokinetic interaction, but there was an additive effect of decreased alertness and psychomotor performance).
No products indexed under this heading.

Flumazenil (The sedative/hypnotic effect of zolpidem was reversed by flumazenil; however, no significant alterations in zolpidem pharmacokinetics were found). Products include:
Romazicon Injection 2804

Fluoxetine (When multiple doses of zolpidem tartrate and fluoxetine at steady-state concentrations were evaluated, the only significant change was a 17% increase in the zolpidem half-life. There was no evidence of an additive effect in psychomotor performance).
No products indexed under this heading.

Fluoxetine Hydrochloride (When multiple doses of zolpidem tartrate and fluoxetine at steady-state concentrations were evaluated, the only significant change was a 17% increase in the zolpidem half-life. There was no evidence of an additive effect in psychomotor performance). Products include:
Prozac Pulvules and Liquid 1801
Symbyax Capsules 1819

Haloperidol (Haloperidol and zolpidem tartrate revealed no effect of haloperidol on the pharmacokinetics or pharmacodynamics of zolpidem; however, there is potential for an additive effect of decreased alertness and psychomotor performance).
No products indexed under this heading.

Haloperidol Decanoate (Haloperidol and zolpidem tartrate revealed no effect of haloperidol on the pharmacokinetics or pharmacodynamics of zolpidem; however, there is potential for an additive effect of decreased alertness and psychomotor performance).
No products indexed under this heading.

Haloperidol Lactate (Haloperidol and zolpidem tartrate revealed no effect of haloperidol on the pharmacokinetics or pharmacodynamics of zolpidem; however, there is potential for an additive effect of decreased alertness and psychomotor performance).
No products indexed under this heading.

Imipramine Hydrochloride (Imipramine in combination with zolpidem tartrate produced no pharmacokinetic interaction other than a 20% decrease in peak levels of imipramine; however, there is potential for an additive effect of decreased alertness and psychomotor performance).
No products indexed under this heading.

Imipramine Pamoate (Imipramine in combination with zolpidem tartrate produced no pharmacokinetic interaction other than a 20% decrease in peak levels of imipramine; however, there is potential for an additive effect of decreased alertness and psychomotor performance).
No products indexed under this heading.

Itraconazole (Co-administration resulted in a 34% increase in AUC of zolpidem. There were no significant pharmacodynamic effects of zolpidem on subjective drowsiness, postural sway, or psychomotor performance).
No products indexed under this heading.

Rifampin (Co-administration with rifampin showed significant reductions of the AUC (-73%), Cmax (-58%), and T1/2 (-36%) of zolpidem together with significant reductions in the pharmacodynamic effects of zolpidem).
No products indexed under this heading.

Sertraline Hydrochloride (Co-administration following five consecutive nightly doses has resulted in significantly higher (43%) Cmax and significantly lower Tmax (53%) of zolpidem). Products include:
Zoloft 2586

Food Interactions

Alcohol (An additive effect on psychomotor performance between alcohol and zolpidem tartrate was demonstrated).

AMBISOME FOR INJECTION

(Amphotericin B, liposomal) 620
May interact with aminoglycosides, antineoplastics, corticosteroids, curariform skeletal muscle relaxants, cardiac glycosides, imidazoles, and certain other agents. Compounds in these categories include:

ACTH (Concurrent use of ACTH and amphotericin B may potentiate hypokalemia which could predispose the patient to cardiac dysfunction).
No products indexed under this heading.

Altretamine (Concurrent use of antineoplastic agents and amphotericin B may enhance the potential for renal toxicity, bronchospasm, and hypotension).
No products indexed under this heading.

Amikacin Sulfate (Concurrent use of amphotericin B and other nephrotoxic agents, such as aminoglycosides, may enhance the potential for drug-induced renal toxicity).
No products indexed under this heading.

Anastrozole (Concurrent use of antineoplastic agents and amphotericin B may enhance the potential for renal toxicity, bronchospasm, and hypotension). Products include:
Arimidex Tablets 673

Asparaginase (Concurrent use of antineoplastic agents and amphotericin B may enhance the potential for renal toxicity, bronchospasm, and hypotension). Products include:
Elspar for Injection 2463
Elspar for Injection 1960

Atracurium Besylate (Amphotericin B-induced hypokalemia may enhance the curariform effect of skeletal relaxants).
No products indexed under this heading.

Betamethasone Acetate (Concurrent use of corticosteroids and amphotericin B may potentiate hypokalemia which could predispose the patient to cardiac dysfunction).
No products indexed under this heading.

Betamethasone Sodium Phosphate (Concurrent use of corticosteroids and amphotericin B may potentiate hypokalemia which could predispose the patient to cardiac dysfunction).
No products indexed under this heading.

Bicalutamide (Concurrent use of antineoplastic agents and amphotericin B may enhance the potential for renal toxicity, bronchospasm, and hypotension).
No products indexed under this heading.

Bleomycin Sulfate (Concurrent use of antineoplastic agents and amphotericin B may enhance the potential for renal toxicity, bronchospasm, and hypotension).
No products indexed under this heading.

Busulfan (Concurrent use of antineoplastic agents and amphotericin B may enhance the potential for renal toxicity, bronchospasm, and hypotension). Products include:
I.V. Busulfex 2493
Myleran Tablets 1525

Carboplatin (Concurrent use of antineoplastic agents and amphotericin B may enhance the potential for renal toxicity, bronchospasm, and hypotension).
No products indexed under this heading.

Carmustine (BCNU) (Concurrent use of antineoplastic agents and amphotericin B may enhance the potential for renal toxicity, bronchospasm, and hypotension).
No products indexed under this heading.

Chlorambucil (Concurrent use of antineoplastic agents and amphotericin B may enhance the potential for renal toxicity, bronchospasm, and hypotension). Products include:
Leukeran Tablets 1504

Cisatracurium Besylate (Amphotericin B-induced hypokalemia may enhance the curariform effect of skeletal relaxants). Products include:
Nimbex Injection 498

Cisplatin (Concurrent use of antineoplastic agents and amphotericin B may enhance the potential for renal toxicity, bronchospasm, and hypotension).
No products indexed under this heading.

Clotrimazole (Imidazoles may induce fungal resistance to amphotericin B; combination therapy should be administered with caution, especially in immunocompromised patients). Products include:
Desenex Athlete's Foot Cream 635
Lotrimin 3039
Lotrisone 3040

Cortisone Acetate (Concurrent use of corticosteroids and amphotericin B may potentiate hypokalemia which could predispose the patient to cardiac dysfunction).
No products indexed under this heading.

Cyclophosphamide (Concurrent use of antineoplastic agents and amphotericin B may enhance the potential for renal toxicity, bronchospasm, and hypotension).
No products indexed under this heading.

Cyclosporine (Concurrent use of amphotericin B and other nephrotoxic agents, such as cyclosporine, may enhance the potential for drug-induced renal toxicity). Products include:
Gengraf Capsules 459
Neoral Oral Solution 2259
Neoral Soft Gelatin Capsules 2259
Restasis Ophthalmic Emulsion 575
Sandimmune 2275

Dacarbazine (Concurrent use of antineoplastic agents and amphotericin B may enhance the potential for renal toxicity, bronchospasm, and hypotension).
No products indexed under this heading.

Daunorubicin Citrate (Concurrent use of antineoplastic agents and amphotericin B may enhance the potential for renal toxicity, bronchospasm, and hypotension).
No products indexed under this heading.

Daunorubicin Hydrochloride (Concurrent use of antineoplastic agents and amphotericin B may enhance the potential for renal toxicity, bronchospasm, and hypotension).
No products indexed under this heading.

Denileukin Diftitox (Concurrent use of antineoplastic agents and amphotericin B may enhance the potential for renal toxicity, bronchospasm, and hypotension). Products include:
Ontak Vials 1745

Deslanoside (Concurrent use of digitalis and amphotericin B may induce hypokalemia and may potentiate digitalis toxicity).
No products indexed under this heading.

Dexamethasone (Concurrent use of corticosteroids and amphotericin B may potentiate hypokalemia which could predispose the patient to cardiac dysfunction). Products include:
Ciprodex Otic Suspension 559
Decadron Tablets 1951
TobraDex Ophthalmic Ointment 562
TobraDex Ophthalmic Suspension ... 563

Dexamethasone Acetate (Concurrent use of corticosteroids and amphotericin B may potentiate hypokalemia which could predispose the patient to cardiac dysfunction).
No products indexed under this heading.

Dexamethasone Sodium Phosphate (Concurrent use of corticosteroids and amphotericin B may potentiate hypokalemia which could predispose the patient to cardiac dysfunction).
No products indexed under this heading.

Digitalis Glycoside Preparations (Concurrent use of digitalis and amphotericin B may induce hypokalemia and may potentiate digitalis toxicity).
No products indexed under this heading.

Digitoxin (Concurrent use of digitalis and amphotericin B may induce hypokalemia and may potentiate digitalis toxicity).
No products indexed under this heading.

Digoxin (Concurrent use of digitalis and amphotericin B may induce hypokalemia and may potentiate digitalis toxicity). Products include:
Lanoxicaps Capsules 1490
Lanoxin Injection 1494
Lanoxin Injection Pediatric 1497
Lanoxin Tablets 1500

Docetaxel (Concurrent use of antineoplastic agents and amphotericin B may enhance the potential for renal toxicity, bronchospasm, and hypotension). Products include:
Taxotere Injection Concentrate 2932

Doxacurium Chloride (Amphotericin B-induced hypokalemia may enhance the curariform effect of skeletal relaxants).
No products indexed under this heading.

Doxorubicin Hydrochloride (Concurrent use of antineoplastic agents and amphotericin B may enhance the potential for renal toxicity, bronchospasm, and hypotension).
No products indexed under this heading.

Epirubicin Hydrochloride (Concurrent use of antineoplastic agents and amphotericin B may enhance the potential for renal toxicity, bronchospasm, and hypotension).
No products indexed under this heading.

Estramustine Phosphate Sodium (Concurrent use of antineoplastic agents and amphotericin B may enhance the potential for renal toxicity, bronchospasm, and hypotension). Products include:
Emcyt Capsules 2634

Etoposide (Concurrent use of antineoplastic agents and amphotericin B may enhance the potential for renal toxicity, bronchospasm, and hypotension).
No products indexed under this heading.

Exemestane (Concurrent use of antineoplastic agents and amphotericin B may enhance the potential for renal toxicity, bronchospasm, and hypotension). Products include:
Aromasin Tablets 2600

Floxuridine (Concurrent use of antineoplastic agents and amphotericin B may enhance the potential for renal toxicity, bronchospasm, and hypotension).
No products indexed under this heading.

Fluconazole (Imidazoles may induce fungal resistance to amphotericin B; combination therapy should be administered with caution, especially in immunocompromised patients).
No products indexed under this heading.

Flucytosine (Concurrent use may increase the toxicity of flucytosine by possibly increasing its cellular uptake and/or impairing its renal excretion).
No products indexed under this heading.

Fludrocortisone Acetate (Concurrent use of corticosteroids and amphotericin B may potentiate hypokalemia which could predispose the patient to cardiac dysfunction).
No products indexed under this heading.

Fluorouracil (Concurrent use of antineoplastic agents and amphotericin B may enhance the potential for renal toxicity, bronchospasm, and hypotension). Products include:
Carac Cream, 0.5% 2879
Efudex 3363

Flutamide (Concurrent use of antineoplastic agents and amphotericin B may enhance the potential for renal toxicity, bronchospasm, and hypotension). Products include:

Eulexin Capsules 3009

Gemcitabine Hydrochloride (Concurrent use of antineoplastic agents and amphotericin B may enhance the potential for renal toxicity, bronchospasm, and hypotension). Products include:

Gemzar for Injection 1771

Gentamicin Sulfate (Concurrent use of amphotericin B and other nephrotoxic agents, such as aminoglycosides, may enhance the potential for drug-induced renal toxicity). Products include:

Garamycin Injectable 3014
Pred-G Ophthalmic Ointment .... ⊙237
Pred-G Ophthalmic Suspension ...... ⊙236

Hydrocortisone (Concurrent use of corticosteroids and amphotericin B may potentiate hypokalemia which could predispose the patient to cardiac dysfunction). Products include:

Colocort Rectal Suspension, USP (Retention) 100 mg/60 mL........... 2476
Hydrocortone Tablets 1989
Preparation H Hydrocortisone Cream .... ▣646

Hydrocortisone Acetate (Concurrent use of corticosteroids and amphotericin B may potentiate hypokalemia which could predispose the patient to cardiac dysfunction). Products include:

Analpram-HC 1159
Pramosone 1161
ProctoFoam-HC 3099

Hydrocortisone Sodium Phosphate (Concurrent use of corticosteroids and amphotericin B may potentiate hypokalemia which could predispose the patient to cardiac dysfunction).

No products indexed under this heading.

Hydrocortisone Sodium Succinate (Concurrent use of corticosteroids and amphotericin B may potentiate hypokalemia which could predispose the patient to cardiac dysfunction).

No products indexed under this heading.

Hydroxyurea (Concurrent use of antineoplastic agents and amphotericin B may enhance the potential for renal toxicity, bronchospasm, and hypotension).

No products indexed under this heading.

Idarubicin Hydrochloride (Concurrent use of antineoplastic agents and amphotericin B may enhance the potential for renal toxicity, bronchospasm, and hypotension).

No products indexed under this heading.

Ifosfamide (Concurrent use of antineoplastic agents and amphotericin B may enhance the potential for renal toxicity, bronchospasm, and hypotension).

No products indexed under this heading.

Interferon alfa-2a, Recombinant (Concurrent use of antineoplastic agents and amphotericin B may enhance the potential for renal toxicity, bronchospasm, and hypotension).

No products indexed under this heading.

Interferon alfa-2b, Recombinant (Concurrent use of antineoplastic agents and amphotericin B may enhance the potential for renal toxicity, bronchospasm, and hypotension). Products include:

Intron A for Injection 3024
Rebetron Combination Therapy 3063

Irinotecan Hydrochloride (Concurrent use of antineoplastic agents and amphotericin B may enhance the potential for renal toxicity, bronchospasm, and hypotension). Products include:

Camptosar Injection 2604

Kanamycin Sulfate (Concurrent use of amphotericin B and other nephrotoxic agents, such as aminoglycosides, may enhance the potential for drug-induced renal toxicity).

No products indexed under this heading.

Ketoconazole (Imidazoles may induce fungal resistance to amphotericin B; combination therapy should be administered with caution, especially in immunocompromised patients). Products include:

Nizoral A-D Shampoo, 1% 1868

Levamisole Hydrochloride (Concurrent use of antineoplastic agents and amphotericin B may enhance the potential for renal toxicity, bronchospasm, and hypotension).

No products indexed under this heading.

Lomustine (CCNU) (Concurrent use of antineoplastic agents and amphotericin B may enhance the potential for renal toxicity, bronchospasm, and hypotension).

No products indexed under this heading.

Mechlorethamine Hydrochloride (Concurrent use of antineoplastic agents and amphotericin B may enhance the potential for renal toxicity, bronchospasm, and hypotension). Products include:

Mustargen for Injection 2468

Megestrol Acetate (Concurrent use of antineoplastic agents and amphotericin B may enhance the potential for renal toxicity, bronchospasm, and hypotension). Products include:

Megace ES Oral Suspension 2481

Melphalan (Concurrent use of antineoplastic agents and amphotericin B may enhance the potential for renal toxicity, bronchospasm, and hypotension). Products include:

Alkeran Tablets 956

Mercaptopurine (Concurrent use of antineoplastic agents and amphotericin B may enhance the potential for renal toxicity, bronchospasm, and hypotension).

No products indexed under this heading.

Methotrexate Sodium (Concurrent use of antineoplastic agents and amphotericin B may enhance the potential for renal toxicity, bronchospasm, and hypotension).

No products indexed under this heading.

Methylprednisolone Acetate (Concurrent use of corticosteroids and amphotericin B may potentiate hypokalemia which could predispose the patient to cardiac dysfunction). Products include:

Depo-Medrol Injectable Suspension 2617
Depo-Medrol Single-Dose Vial 2619

Methylprednisolone Sodium Succinate (Concurrent use of corticosteroids and amphotericin B may potentiate hypokalemia which could predispose the patient to cardiac dysfunction).

No products indexed under this heading.

Metocurine Iodide (Amphotericin B-induced hypokalemia may enhance the curariform effect of skeletal relaxants).

No products indexed under this heading.

Miconazole (Imidazoles may induce fungal resistance to amphotericin B; combination therapy should be administered with caution, especially in immunocompromised patients).

No products indexed under this heading.

Miconazole Nitrate (Imidazoles may induce fungal resistance to amphotericin B; combination therapy should be administered with caution, especially in immunocompromised patients). Products include:

Desenex .... ▣635
Desenex Jock Itch Spray Powder .... ▣635

Mitomycin (Mitomycin-C) (Concurrent use of antineoplastic agents and amphotericin B may enhance the potential for renal toxicity, bronchospasm, and hypotension).

No products indexed under this heading.

Mitotane (Concurrent use of antineoplastic agents and amphotericin B may enhance the potential for renal toxicity, bronchospasm, and hypotension).

No products indexed under this heading.

Mitoxantrone Hydrochloride (Concurrent use of antineoplastic agents and amphotericin B may enhance the potential for renal toxicity, bronchospasm, and hypotension).

No products indexed under this heading.

Mivacurium Chloride (Amphotericin B-induced hypokalemia may enhance the curariform effect of skeletal relaxants). Products include:

Mivacron Injection 493

Oxaliplatin (Concurrent use of antineoplastic agents and amphotericin B may enhance the potential for renal toxicity, bronchospasm, and hypotension). Products include:

Eloxatin for Injection 2892

Paclitaxel (Concurrent use of antineoplastic agents and amphotericin B may enhance the potential for renal toxicity, bronchospasm, and hypotension).

No products indexed under this heading.

Pancuronium Bromide (Amphotericin B-induced hypokalemia may enhance the curariform effect of skeletal relaxants).

No products indexed under this heading.

Pentamidine Isethionate (Concurrent use of amphotericin B and other nephrotoxic agents, such as pentamidine, may enhance the potential for drug-induced renal toxicity).

No products indexed under this heading.

Pipecuronium Bromide (Amphotericin B-induced hypokalemia may enhance the curariform effect of skeletal relaxants).

No products indexed under this heading.

Prednisolone Acetate (Concurrent use of corticosteroids and amphotericin B may potentiate hypokalemia which could predispose the patient to cardiac dysfunction). Products include:

Blephamide Ophthalmic Ointment 568
Blephamide Ophthalmic Suspension 569
Poly-Pred Ophthalmic Suspension .... ⊙233
Pred Forte Ophthalmic Suspension .... ⊙235
Pred Mild Ophthalmic Suspension .... ⊙238
Pred-G Ophthalmic Ointment .... ⊙237
Pred-G Ophthalmic Suspension ...... ⊙236

Prednisolone Sodium Phosphate (Concurrent use of corticosteroids and amphotericin B may potentiate hypokalemia which could predispose the patient to cardiac dysfunction).

No products indexed under this heading.

Prednisolone Tebutate (Concurrent use of corticosteroids and amphotericin B may potentiate hypokalemia which could predispose the patient to cardiac dysfunction).

No products indexed under this heading.

Prednisone (Concurrent use of corticosteroids and amphotericin B may potentiate hypokalemia which could predispose the patient to cardiac dysfunction).

No products indexed under this heading.

Procarbazine Hydrochloride (Concurrent use of antineoplastic agents and amphotericin B may enhance the potential for renal toxicity, bronchospasm, and hypotension). Products include:

Matulane Capsules 3191

Rapacuronium Bromide (Amphotericin B-induced hypokalemia may enhance the curariform effect of skeletal relaxants).

No products indexed under this heading.

Rocuronium Bromide (Amphotericin B-induced hypokalemia may enhance the curariform effect of skeletal relaxants). Products include:

Zemuron Injection 2346

Streptomycin Sulfate (Concurrent use of amphotericin B and other nephrotoxic agents, such as aminoglycosides, may enhance the potential for drug-induced renal toxicity).

No products indexed under this heading.

Streptozocin (Concurrent use of antineoplastic agents and amphotericin B may enhance the potential for renal toxicity, bronchospasm, and hypotension).

No products indexed under this heading.

Tamoxifen Citrate (Concurrent use of antineoplastic agents and amphotericin B may enhance the potential for renal toxicity, bronchospasm, and hypotension). Products include:

Soltamox Oral Solution 3527

Teniposide (Concurrent use of antineoplastic agents and amphotericin B may enhance the potential for renal toxicity, bronchospasm, and hypotension).

No products indexed under this heading.

Thioguanine (Concurrent use of antineoplastic agents and amphoteri-

(▣ Described in PDR For Nonprescription Drugs) (⊙ Described in PDR For Ophthalmic Medicines™)

cin B may enhance the potential for renal toxicity, bronchospasm, and hypotension). Products include:
Tabloid Tablets 1575

Thiotepa (Concurrent use of antineoplastic agents and amphotericin B may enhance the potential for renal toxicity, bronchospasm, and hypotension).
No products indexed under this heading.

Tobramycin (Concurrent use of amphotericin B and other nephrotoxic agents, such as aminoglycosides, may enhance the potential for drug-induced renal toxicity). Products include:
TOBI Solution for Inhalation 2298
TobraDex Ophthalmic Ointment 562
TobraDex Ophthalmic Suspension ... 563
Zylet Ophthalmic Suspension .... ⊙259

Tobramycin Sulfate (Concurrent use of amphotericin B and other nephrotoxic agents, such as aminoglycosides, may enhance the potential for drug-induced renal toxicity).
No products indexed under this heading.

Topotecan Hydrochloride (Concurrent use of antineoplastic agents and amphotericin B may enhance the potential for renal toxicity, bronchospasm, and hypotension). Products include:
Hycamtin for Injection 1458

Toremifene Citrate (Concurrent use of antineoplastic agents and amphotericin B may enhance the potential for renal toxicity, bronchospasm, and hypotension).
No products indexed under this heading.

Triamcinolone (Concurrent use of corticosteroids and amphotericin B may potentiate hypokalemia which could predispose the patient to cardiac dysfunction).
No products indexed under this heading.

Triamcinolone Acetonide (Concurrent use of corticosteroids and amphotericin B may potentiate hypokalemia which could predispose the patient to cardiac dysfunction). Products include:
Azmacort Inhalation Aerosol 1726
Nasacort AQ Nasal Spray 2922

Triamcinolone Diacetate (Concurrent use of corticosteroids and amphotericin B may potentiate hypokalemia which could predispose the patient to cardiac dysfunction).
No products indexed under this heading.

Triamcinolone Hexacetonide (Concurrent use of corticosteroids and amphotericin B may potentiate hypokalemia which could predispose the patient to cardiac dysfunction).
No products indexed under this heading.

Tubocurarine Chloride (Amphotericin B-induced hypokalemia may enhance the curariform effect of skeletal relaxants).
No products indexed under this heading.

Valrubicin (Concurrent use of antineoplastic agents and amphotericin B may enhance the potential for renal toxicity, bronchospasm, and hypotension).
No products indexed under this heading.

Vecuronium Bromide (Amphotericin B-induced hypokalemia may enhance the curariform effect of skeletal relaxants).
No products indexed under this heading.

Vincristine Sulfate (Concurrent use of antineoplastic agents and amphotericin B may enhance the potential for renal toxicity, bronchospasm, and hypotension).
No products indexed under this heading.

Vinorelbine Tartrate (Concurrent use of antineoplastic agents and amphotericin B may enhance the potential for renal toxicity, bronchospasm, and hypotension).
No products indexed under this heading.

AMBROTOSE AO CAPSULES
(Herbals with Vitamins) .... ■826
None cited in PDR database.

AMBROTOSE CAPSULES
(Herbals, Multiple) .... ■826
None cited in PDR database.

AMBROTOSE POWDER
(Glucosamine Hydrochloride, Herbals, Multiple).............................. ■826
None cited in PDR database.

AMBROTOSE WITH LECITHIN CAPSULES
(Herbals, Multiple, Lecithin) .... ■826
None cited in PDR database.

AMERGE TABLETS
(Naratriptan Hydrochloride) 1339
May interact with 5HT1-receptor agonists, ergot-containing drugs, oral contraceptives, and selective serotonin reuptake inhibitors. Compounds in these categories include:

Citalopram Hydrobromide (Cases of life-threatening serotonin syndrome, including mental status changes, autonomic instability, neuromuscular aberrations, and/or GI symptoms, have been reported during combination use of selective serotonin reuptake inhibitors and triptans. If concomitant treatment with naratriptan and an SSRI is clinically warranted, careful observation of the patient is advised, particularly during treatment initiation and dose increases). Products include:
Celexa 1176

Desogestrel (Co-administration with oral contraceptives has resulted in reduced clearance by 32% and volume of distribution by 22%, producing slightly higher concentrations of naratriptan). Products include:
Mircette Tablets 1066

Dihydroergotamine Mesylate (Ergot-containing drugs have been reported to cause prolonged vasospastic reactions; because there is a theoretical basis that these effects may be additive, use of ergot-type agents and naratriptan within 24 hours is contraindicated). Products include:
Migranal Nasal Spray 3348

3-Diphenylacrylate (Co-administration with other 5-HT_1 agonists within 24 hours of each other is contraindicated because of the vasospastic effects may be additive).
No products indexed under this heading.

Duloxetine Hydrochloride (Cases of life-threatening serotonin syndrome, including mental status changes, autonomic instability, neuromuscular aberrations, and/or GI symptoms, have been reported during combination use of serotonin and norepinephrine reuptake inhibitors and triptans. If concomitant treatment with naratriptan and an SNRI is clinically warranted, careful observation of the patient is advised, particularly during treatment initiation and dose increases). Products include:
Cymbalta Delayed-Release Capsules 1757

Ergonovine Maleate (Ergot-containing drugs have been reported to cause prolonged vasospastic reactions; because there is a theoretical basis that these effects may be additive, use of ergot-type agents and naratriptan within 24 hours is contraindicated).
No products indexed under this heading.

Ergotamine Tartrate (Ergot-containing drugs have been reported to cause prolonged vasospastic reactions; because there is a theoretical basis that these effects may be additive, use of ergot-type agents and naratriptan within 24 hours is contraindicated).
No products indexed under this heading.

Escitalopram Oxalate (Cases of life-threatening serotonin syndrome, including mental status changes, autonomic instability, neuromuscular aberrations, and/or GI symptoms, have been reported during combination use of selective serotonin reuptake inhibitors and triptans. If concomitant treatment with naratriptan and an SSRI is clinically warranted, careful observation of the patient is advised, particularly during treatment initiation and dose increases). Products include:
Lexapro Oral Solution 1190
Lexapro Tablets 1190

Ethinyl Estradiol (Co-administration with oral contraceptives has resulted in reduced clearance by 32% and volume of distribution by 22%, producing slightly higher concentrations of naratriptan). Products include:
Mircette Tablets 1066
NuvaRing 2340
Ortho-Cyclen/Ortho Tri-Cyclen 2429
Ortho Evra Transdermal System 2417
Ortho Tri-Cyclen Lo Tablets 2436
Seasonique Tablets 1077
Yasmin 28 Tablets 796
Yaz Tablets 803

Ethynodiol Diacetate (Co-administration with oral contraceptives has resulted in reduced clearance by 32% and volume of distribution by 22%, producing slightly higher concentrations of naratriptan).
No products indexed under this heading.

Fluoxetine Hydrochloride (Cases of life-threatening serotonin syndrome, including mental status changes, autonomic instability, neuromuscular aberrations, and/or GI symptoms, have been reported during combination use of selective serotonin reuptake inhibitors and triptans. If concomitant treatment with naratriptan and an SSRI is clinically warranted, careful observation of the patient is advised, particularly during treatment initiation and dose increases). Products include:
Prozac Pulvules and Liquid 1801
Symbyax Capsules 1819

Fluvoxamine Maleate (Cases of life-threatening serotonin syndrome, including mental status changes, autonomic instability, neuromuscular aberrations, and/or GI symptoms, have been reported during combination use of selective serotonin reuptake inhibitors and triptans. If concomitant treatment with naratriptan and an SSRI is clinically warranted, careful observation of the patient is advised, particularly during treatment initiation and dose increases).
No products indexed under this heading.

Levonorgestrel (Co-administration with oral contraceptives has resulted in reduced clearance by 32% and volume of distribution by 22%, producing slightly higher concentrations of naratriptan). Products include:
Climara Pro Transdermal System 776
Mirena Intrauterine System 787
Plan B Tablets 1076
Seasonique Tablets 1077

Mestranol (Co-administration with oral contraceptives has resulted in reduced clearance by 32% and volume of distribution by 22%, producing slightly higher concentrations of naratriptan).
No products indexed under this heading.

Methylergonovine Maleate (Ergot-containing drugs have been reported to cause prolonged vasospastic reactions; because there is a theoretical basis that these effects may be additive, use of ergot-type agents and naratriptan within 24 hours is contraindicated).
No products indexed under this heading.

Methysergide Maleate (Ergot-containing drugs have been reported to cause prolonged vasospastic reactions; because there is a theoretical basis that these effects may be additive, use of ergot-type agents and naratriptan within 24 hours is contraindicated).
No products indexed under this heading.

Nefazodone Hydrochloride (Cases of life-threatening serotonin syndrome, including mental status changes, autonomic instability, neuromuscular aberrations, and/or GI symptoms, have been reported during combination use of serotonin and norepinephrine reuptake inhibitors and triptans. If concomitant treatment with naratriptan and an SNRI is clinically warranted, careful observation of the patient is advised, particularly during treatment initiation and dose increases).
No products indexed under this heading.

Norethindrone (Co-administration with oral contraceptives has resulted in reduced clearance by 32% and volume of distribution by 22%, producing slightly higher concentrations of naratriptan). Products include:
Ortho Micronor Tablets 2426

Norethynodrel (Co-administration with oral contraceptives has resulted in reduced clearance by 32% and volume of distribution by 22%, producing slightly higher concentrations of naratriptan).
No products indexed under this heading.

Norgestimate (Co-administration with oral contraceptives has resulted in reduced clearance by 32% and volume of distribution by 22%, producing slightly higher concentrations of naratriptan). Products include:
Ortho-Cyclen/Ortho Tri-Cyclen 2429
Ortho Tri-Cyclen Lo Tablets 2436

Norgestrel (Co-administration with oral contraceptives has resulted in reduced clearance by 32% and volume of distribution by 22%, producing slightly higher concentrations of naratriptan).
No products indexed under this heading.

Paroxetine Hydrochloride (Cases of life-threatening serotonin syndrome, including mental status changes, autonomic instability, neuromuscular aberrations, and/or GI symptoms, have been reported during combination use of selective serotonin reuptake inhibitors and triptans. If concomitant treatment with naratriptan and an SSRI is clinically warranted, careful observation of the patient is advised, particularly during treatment initiation and dose increases). Products include:
Paxil CR Controlled-Release Tablets 1538
Paxil 1530

Rizatriptan Benzoate (Co-administration with other 5-HT$_1$ agonists within 24 hours of each other is contraindicated because of the vasospastic effects may be additive). Products include:
Maxalt Tablets 2008
Maxalt-MLT Orally Disintegrating Tablets 2008

Sertraline Hydrochloride (Cases of life-threatening serotonin syndrome, including mental status changes, autonomic instability, neuromuscular aberrations, and/or GI symptoms, have been reported during combination use of selective serotonin reuptake inhibitors and triptans. If concomitant treatment with naratriptan and an SSRI is clinically warranted, careful observation of the patient is advised, particularly during treatment initiation and dose increases). Products include:
Zoloft 2586

Sumatriptan (Co-administration with other 5-HT$_1$ agonists within 24 hours of each other is contraindicated because of the vasospastic effects may be additive). Products include:
Imitrex Nasal Spray 1467

Sumatriptan Succinate (Co-administration with other 5-HT$_1$ agonists within 24 hours of each other is contraindicated because of the vasospastic effects may be additive). Products include:
Imitrex Injection 1463
Imitrex Tablets 1471

Venlafaxine Hydrochloride (Cases of life-threatening serotonin syndrome, including mental status changes, autonomic instability, neuromuscular aberrations, and/or GI symptoms, have been reported during combination use of serotonin and norepinephrine reuptake inhibitors and triptans. If concomitant treatment with naratriptan and an SNRI is clinically warranted, careful observation of the patient is advised, particularly during treatment initiation and dose increases). Products include:
Effexor Tablets 3411
Effexor XR Capsules 3417

Zolmitriptan (Co-administration with other 5-HT$_1$ agonists within 24 hours of each other is contraindicated because of the vasospastic effects may be additive). Products include:
Zomig Tablets 3519
Zomig Nasal Spray 3523
Zomig-ZMT Tablets 3519

AMEVIVE

(Alefacept) 626
None cited in PDR database.

AMINOHIPPURATE SODIUM PAH INJECTION

(Aminohippurate Sodium) 1913
May interact with sulfonamides and certain other agents. Compounds in these categories include:

Bendroflumethiazide (Co-administration with sulfonamides interfere with chemical color development essential to the analytical procedures).
No products indexed under this heading.

Chlorothiazide (Co-administration with sulfonamides interfere with chemical color development essential to the analytical procedures). Products include:
Diuril Oral Suspension 1954

Chlorothiazide Sodium (Co-administration with sulfonamides interfere with chemical color development essential to the analytical procedures). Products include:
Diuril Sodium Intravenous 2467

Chlorpropamide (Co-administration with sulfonamides interfere with chemical color development essential to the analytical procedures).
No products indexed under this heading.

Glipizide (Co-administration with sulfonamides interfere with chemical color development essential to the analytical procedures).
No products indexed under this heading.

Glyburide (Co-administration with sulfonamides interfere with chemical color development essential to the analytical procedures).
No products indexed under this heading.

Hydrochlorothiazide (Co-administration with sulfonamides interfere with chemical color development essential to the analytical procedures). Products include:
Aldoril Tablets 1910
Atacand HCT 651
Avalide Tablets 888
Avalide Tablets 2874
Benicar HCT Tablets 1044
Diovan HCT Tablets 2196
Dyazide Capsules 1423
Hyzaar 50-12.5 Tablets 1990
Hyzaar 100-12.5 Tablets 1990
Hyzaar 100-25 Tablets 1990
Lopressor HCT 50/25 Tablets 2241
Lopressor HCT 100/25 Tablets 2241
Lopressor HCT 100/50 Tablets 2241
Lotensin HCT Tablets 2246
Micardis HCT Tablets 856
Moduretic Tablets 2028
Prinzide Tablets 2056
Teveten HCT Tablets 1737
Timolide Tablets 2086
Uniretic Tablets 3100

Hydroflumethiazide (Co-administration with sulfonamides interfere with chemical color development essential to the analytical procedures).
No products indexed under this heading.

Methyclothiazide (Co-administration with sulfonamides interfere with chemical color development essential to the analytical procedures).
No products indexed under this heading.

Polythiazide (Co-administration with sulfonamides interfere with chemical color development essential to the analytical procedures).
No products indexed under this heading.

Probenecid (Tubular secretion of PAH depressed).
No products indexed under this heading.

Procaine Hydrochloride (Renal clearance measurements impaired).
No products indexed under this heading.

Sulfacytine (Co-administration with sulfonamides interfere with chemical color development essential to the analytical procedures).
No products indexed under this heading.

Sulfamethizole (Co-administration with sulfonamides interfere with chemical color development essential to the analytical procedures).
No products indexed under this heading.

Sulfamethoxazole (Co-administration with sulfonamides interfere with chemical color development essential to the analytical procedures).
No products indexed under this heading.

Sulfasalazine (Co-administration with sulfonamides interfere with chemical color development essential to the analytical procedures).
No products indexed under this heading.

Sulfinpyrazone (Co-administration with sulfonamides interfere with chemical color development essential to the analytical procedures).
No products indexed under this heading.

Sulfisoxazole Acetyl (Co-administration with sulfonamides interfere with chemical color development essential to the analytical procedures).
No products indexed under this heading.

Sulfisoxazole Diolamine (Co-administration with sulfonamides interfere with chemical color development essential to the analytical procedures).
No products indexed under this heading.

Tolazamide (Co-administration with sulfonamides interfere with chemical color development essential to the analytical procedures).
No products indexed under this heading.

Tolbutamide (Co-administration with sulfonamides interfere with chemical color development essential to the analytical procedures).
No products indexed under this heading.

AMITIZA CAPSULES

(Lubiprostone) 3224
None cited in PDR database.

AMOXIL CAPSULES

(Amoxicillin) 1343
See Amoxil Tablets

AMOXIL CHEWABLE TABLETS

(Amoxicillin) 1343
See Amoxil Tablets

AMOXIL PEDIATRIC DROPS FOR ORAL SUSPENSION

(Amoxicillin) 1343
May interact with:

See (Amoxil Tablets).
No products indexed under this heading.

AMOXIL POWDER FOR ORAL SUSPENSION

(Amoxicillin) 1343
See Amoxil Tablets

AMOXIL TABLETS

(Amoxicillin) 1343
May interact with macrolide antibiotics, tetracyclines, and certain other agents. Compounds in these categories include:

Azithromycin Dihydrate (May interfere with bactericidal effects of penicillin. This has been demonstrated in vitro; however, the clinical significance of the interaction is not well documented).
No products indexed under this heading.

Chloramphenicol Sodium Succinate (May interfere with bactericidal effects of penicillin. This has been demonstrated in vitro; however, the clinical significance of the interaction is not well documented).
No products indexed under this heading.

Clarithromycin (May interfere with bactericidal effects of penicillin. This has been demonstrated in vitro; however, the clinical significance of the interaction is not well documented). Products include:
Biaxin/Biaxin XL 402
PREVPAC 3284

Demeclocycline Hydrochloride (May interfere with bactericidal effects of penicillin. This has been demonstrated in vitro; however, the clinical significance of the interaction is not well documented).
No products indexed under this heading.

Dirithromycin (May interfere with bactericidal effects of penicillin. This has been demonstrated in vitro; however, the clinical significance of the interaction is not well documented).
No products indexed under this heading.

Doxycycline Calcium (May interfere with bactericidal effects of penicillin. This has been demonstrated in vitro; however, the clinical significance of the interaction is not well documented).
No products indexed under this heading.

Doxycycline Hyclate (May interfere with bactericidal effects of penicillin. This has been demonstrated in vitro; however, the clinical significance of the interaction is not well documented).
No products indexed under this heading.

Doxycycline Monohydrate (May interfere with bactericidal effects of penicillin. This has been demonstrated in vitro; however, the clinical significance of the interaction is not well documented). Products include:
Oracea Capsules **1000**

Erythromycin (May interfere with bactericidal effects of penicillin. This has been demonstrated in vitro; however, the clinical significance of the interaction is not well documented). Products include:
Ery-Tab Tablets **449**
Erythromycin Base Filmtab Tablets **455**
Erythromycin Delayed-Release Capsules, USP **457**
PCE Dispertab Tablets **515**

Erythromycin Estolate (May interfere with bactericidal effects of penicillin. This has been demonstrated in vitro; however, the clinical significance of the interaction is not well documented).
No products indexed under this heading.

Erythromycin Ethylsuccinate (May interfere with bactericidal effects of penicillin. This has been demonstrated in vitro; however, the clinical significance of the interaction is not well documented). Products include:
E.E.S. **451**
EryPed **447**

Erythromycin Gluceptate (May interfere with bactericidal effects of penicillin. This has been demonstrated in vitro; however, the clinical significance of the interaction is not well documented).
No products indexed under this heading.

Erythromycin Stearate (May interfere with bactericidal effects of penicillin. This has been demonstrated in vitro; however, the clinical significance of the interaction is not well documented). Products include:
Erythrocin Stearate Filmtab Tablets **453**

Methacycline Hydrochloride (May interfere with bactericidal effects of penicillin. This has been demonstrated in vitro; however, the clinical significance of the interaction is not well documented).
No products indexed under this heading.

Minocycline Hydrochloride (May interfere with bactericidal effects of penicillin. This has been demonstrated in vitro; however, the clinical significance of the interaction is not well documented). Products include:
Solodyn Extended Release Tablets **1890**

Oxytetracycline Hydrochloride (May interfere with bactericidal effects of penicillin. This has been demonstrated in vitro; however, the clinical significance of the interaction is not well documented).
No products indexed under this heading.

Probenecid (Decreases the renal tubular secretion of amoxicillin; concurrent use may result in increased and prolonged blood levels).
No products indexed under this heading.

Sulfamethoxazole (May interfere with bactericidal effects of penicillin. This has been demonstrated in vitro; however, the clinical significance of the interaction is not well documented).
No products indexed under this heading.

Sulfisoxazole Acetyl (May interfere with bactericidal effects of penicillin. This has been demonstrated in vitro; however, the clinical significance of the interaction is not well documented).
No products indexed under this heading.

Tetracycline Hydrochloride (May interfere with bactericidal effects of penicillin. This has been demonstrated in vitro; however, the clinical significance of the interaction is not well documented).
No products indexed under this heading.

Troleandomycin (May interfere with bactericidal effects of penicillin. This has been demonstrated in vitro; however, the clinical significance of the interaction is not well documented).
No products indexed under this heading.

ANALPRAM HC CREAM, 1% AND 2.5%
(Hydrocortisone Acetate, Pramoxine Hydrochloride) **1159**
None cited in PDR database.

ANALPRAM HC LOTION, 2.5%
(Hydrocortisone Acetate, Pramoxine Hydrochloride) **1159**
None cited in PDR database.

ANAPROX TABLETS
(Naproxen Sodium) **2761**
See EC-Naprosyn Delayed-Release Tablets

ANAPROX DS TABLETS
(Naproxen Sodium) **2761**
See EC-Naprosyn Delayed-Release Tablets

ANBESOL COLD SORE THERAPY OINTMENT
(Allantoin, Benzocaine, Camphor, Petrolatum, White) **710**
None cited in PDR database.

BABY ANBESOL GEL
(Benzocaine) **713**
None cited in PDR database.

JUNIOR ANBESOL GEL
(Benzocaine) **713**
None cited in PDR database.

MAXIMUM STRENGTH ANBESOL GEL
(Benzocaine) **713**
None cited in PDR database.

MAXIMUM STRENGTH ANBESOL LIQUID
(Benzocaine) **713**
None cited in PDR database.

ANDROGEL
(Testosterone) **3329**
May interact with corticosteroids, insulin, and certain other agents. Compounds in these categories include:

ACTH (Co-administration of testosterone with ACTH may enhance edema formation).
No products indexed under this heading.

Betamethasone Acetate (Co-administration of testosterone with corticosteroids may enhance edema formation).
No products indexed under this heading.

Betamethasone Sodium Phosphate (Co-administration of testosterone with corticosteroids may enhance edema formation).
No products indexed under this heading.

Cortisone Acetate (Co-administration of testosterone with corticosteroids may enhance edema formation).
No products indexed under this heading.

Dexamethasone (Co-administration of testosterone with corticosteroids may enhance edema formation). Products include:
Ciprodex Otic Suspension **559**
Decadron Tablets **1951**
TobraDex Ophthalmic Ointment **562**
TobraDex Ophthalmic Suspension **563**

Dexamethasone Acetate (Co-administration of testosterone with corticosteroids may enhance edema formation).
No products indexed under this heading.

Dexamethasone Sodium Phosphate (Co-administration of testosterone with corticosteroids may enhance edema formation).
No products indexed under this heading.

Fludrocortisone Acetate (Co-administration of testosterone with corticosteroids may enhance edema formation).
No products indexed under this heading.

Hydrocortisone (Co-administration of testosterone with corticosteroids may enhance edema formation). Products include:
Colocort Rectal Suspension, USP (Retention) 100 mg/60 mL **2476**
Hydrocortone Tablets **1989**
Preparation H Hydrocortisone Cream **646**

Hydrocortisone Acetate (Co-administration of testosterone with corticosteroids may enhance edema formation). Products include:
Analpram-HC **1159**
Pramosone **1161**
ProctoFoam-HC **3099**

Hydrocortisone Sodium Phosphate (Co-administration of testosterone with corticosteroids may enhance edema formation).
No products indexed under this heading.

Hydrocortisone Sodium Succinate (Co-administration of testosterone with corticosteroids may enhance edema formation).
No products indexed under this heading.

Insulin, Human, Zinc Suspension (In diabetic patients, the metabolic effects of androgens may decrease blood glucose and, therefore, insulin requirements). Products include:
Humulin L, 100 Units **1794**
Humulin U, 100 Units **1800**

Insulin, Human NPH (In diabetic patients, the metabolic effects of androgens may decrease blood glucose and, therefore, insulin requirements). Products include:
Humulin N, 100 Units **1795**
Humulin N Pen **1797**

Insulin, Human Regular (In diabetic patients, the metabolic effects of androgens may decrease blood glucose and, therefore, insulin requirements). Products include:
Humulin R, 100 Units **1798**

Insulin, Human Regular and Human NPH Mixture (In diabetic patients, the metabolic effects of androgens may decrease blood glucose and, therefore, insulin requirements). Products include:
Humulin 50/50, 100 Units **1791**
Humulin 70/30 Pen **1793**

Insulin, NPH (In diabetic patients, the metabolic effects of androgens may decrease blood glucose and, therefore, insulin requirements).
No products indexed under this heading.

Insulin, Regular (In diabetic patients, the metabolic effects of androgens may decrease blood glucose and, therefore, insulin requirements).
No products indexed under this heading.

Insulin, Zinc Crystals (In diabetic patients, the metabolic effects of androgens may decrease blood glucose and, therefore, insulin requirements).
No products indexed under this heading.

Insulin, Zinc Suspension (In diabetic patients, the metabolic effects of androgens may decrease blood glucose and, therefore, insulin requirements).
No products indexed under this heading.

Insulin Aspart, Human Regular (In diabetic patients, the metabolic effects of androgens may decrease blood glucose and, therefore, insulin requirements). Products include:
NovoLog Injection **2326**

Insulin glargine (In diabetic patients, the metabolic effects of androgens may decrease blood glucose and, therefore, insulin requirements). Products include:
Lantus Injection **2909**

Insulin Lispro, Human (In diabetic patients, the metabolic effects of androgens may decrease blood glucose and, therefore, insulin requirements). Products include:
Humalog-Pen **1781**
Humalog Mix 50/50-Pen **1783**
Humalog Mix 75/25-Pen **1785**

Insulin Lispro Protamine, Human (In diabetic patients, the metabolic effects of androgens may decrease blood glucose and, therefore, insulin requirements). Products include:

IMPORTANT NOTE: Always consult each drug listing in the patient's regimen for possible interactions.

Humalog Mix 50/50-Pen 1783
Humalog Mix 75/25-Pen 1785

Methylprednisolone Acetate (Co-administration of testosterone with corticosteroids may enhance edema formation). Products include:
Depo-Medrol Injectable
Suspension 2617
Depo-Medrol Single-Dose Vial 2619

Methylprednisolone Sodium Succinate (Co-administration of testosterone with corticosteroids may enhance edema formation).
No products indexed under this heading.

Oxyphenbutazone (Co-administration of androgens and oxyphenbutazone may result in elevated serum levels of oxyphenbutazone).
No products indexed under this heading.

Prednisolone Acetate (Co-administration of testosterone with corticosteroids may enhance edema formation). Products include:
Blephamide Ophthalmic Ointment 568
Blephamide Ophthalmic
Suspension.................................. 569
Poly-Pred Ophthalmic
Suspension............................. ⊙ 233
Pred Forte Ophthalmic
Suspension............................. ⊙ 235
Pred Mild Ophthalmic
Suspension............................. ⊙ 238
Pred-G Ophthalmic Ointment ⊙ 237
Pred-G Ophthalmic Suspension ⊙ 236

Prednisolone Sodium Phosphate (Co-administration of testosterone with corticosteroids may enhance edema formation).
No products indexed under this heading.

Prednisolone Tebutate (Co-administration of testosterone with corticosteroids may enhance edema formation).
No products indexed under this heading.

Prednisone (Co-administration of testosterone with corticosteroids may enhance edema formation).
No products indexed under this heading.

Propranolol Hydrochloride (Co-administration of injectable testosterone cypionate has resulted in an increased clearance of propranolol). Products include:
Inderal LA Long-Acting Capsules 3429
InnoPran XL Capsules 2723

Triamcinolone (Co-administration of testosterone with corticosteroids may enhance edema formation).
No products indexed under this heading.

Triamcinolone Acetonide (Co-administration of testosterone with corticosteroids may enhance edema formation). Products include:
Azmacort Inhalation Aerosol 1726
Nasacort AQ Nasal Spray 2922

Triamcinolone Diacetate (Co-administration of testosterone with corticosteroids may enhance edema formation).
No products indexed under this heading.

Triamcinolone Hexacetonide (Co-administration of testosterone with corticosteroids may enhance edema formation).
No products indexed under this heading.

ANDROXY TABLETS

(Fluoxymesterone) 3335
May interact with corticosteroids, parenterally administered corticosteroids, oral anticoagulants, oral hypoglycemic agents, insulin, potassium-depleting corticosteroids, and certain other agents. Compounds in these categories include:

Acarbose (In diabetic patients, the metabolic effects of androgens may decrease blood glucose and insulin requirements). Products include:
Precose Tablets 751

Adrenocorticotropic Hormone (Enhanced tendency towards edema. Use caution when giving these drugs together, especially in patients with hepatic or cardiac disease).
No products indexed under this heading.

Anisindione (C-17 substituted derivatives of testosterone, such as methandrostenolone, have been reported to decrease the anticoagulant requirement. Patients receiving oral anticoagulant therapy require close monitoring especially when androgens are started or stopped). Products include:
Miradon Tablets 3042

Betamethasone Acetate (Enhanced tendency towards edema. Use caution when giving these drugs together, especially in patients with hepatic or cardiac disease).
No products indexed under this heading.

Betamethasone Sodium Phosphate (Enhanced tendency towards edema. Use caution when giving these drugs together, especially in patients with hepatic or cardiac disease).
No products indexed under this heading.

Chlorpropamide (In diabetic patients, the metabolic effects of androgens may decrease blood glucose and insulin requirements).
No products indexed under this heading.

Cortisone Acetate (Enhanced tendency towards edema. Use caution when giving these drugs together, especially in patients with hepatic or cardiac disease).
No products indexed under this heading.

Dexamethasone (Enhanced tendency towards edema. Use caution when giving these drugs together, especially in patients with hepatic or cardiac disease). Products include:
Ciprodex Otic Suspension 559
Decadron Tablets 1951
TobraDex Ophthalmic Ointment 562
TobraDex Ophthalmic Suspension ... 563

Dexamethasone Acetate (Enhanced tendency towards edema. Use caution when giving these drugs together, especially in patients with hepatic or cardiac disease).
No products indexed under this heading.

Dexamethasone Sodium Phosphate (Enhanced tendency towards edema. Use caution when giving these drugs together, especially in patients with hepatic or cardiac disease).
No products indexed under this heading.

Dicumarol (C-17 substituted derivatives of testosterone, such as methandrostenolone, have been reported to decrease the anticoagulant requirement. Patients receiving oral anticoagulant therapy require close monitoring especially when androgens are started or stopped).
No products indexed under this heading.

Fludrocortisone Acetate (Enhanced tendency towards edema. Use caution when giving these drugs together, especially in patients with hepatic or cardiac disease).
No products indexed under this heading.

Glimepiride (In diabetic patients, the metabolic effects of androgens may decrease blood glucose and insulin requirements). Products include:
Avandaryl Tablets 1379
Duetact Tablets 3226

Glipizide (In diabetic patients, the metabolic effects of androgens may decrease blood glucose and insulin requirements).
No products indexed under this heading.

Glyburide (In diabetic patients, the metabolic effects of androgens may decrease blood glucose and insulin requirements).
No products indexed under this heading.

Hydrocortisone (Enhanced tendency towards edema. Use caution when giving these drugs together, especially in patients with hepatic or cardiac disease). Products include:
Colocort Rectal Suspension, USP
(Retention) 100 mg/60 mL........... 2476
Hydrocortone Tablets 1989
Preparation H Hydrocortisone
Cream ▣▣ 646

Hydrocortisone Acetate (Enhanced tendency towards edema. Use caution when giving these drugs together, especially in patients with hepatic or cardiac disease). Products include:
Analpram-HC 1159
Pramosone 1161
ProctoFoam-HC 3099

Hydrocortisone Sodium Phosphate (Enhanced tendency towards edema. Use caution when giving these drugs together, especially in patients with hepatic or cardiac disease).
No products indexed under this heading.

Hydrocortisone Sodium Succinate (Enhanced tendency towards edema. Use caution when giving these drugs together, especially in patients with hepatic or cardiac disease).
No products indexed under this heading.

Insulin, Human, Zinc Suspension (In diabetic patients, the metabolic effects of androgens may decrease blood glucose and insulin requirements). Products include:
Humulin L, 100 Units 1794
Humulin U, 100 Units 1800

Insulin, Human NPH (In diabetic patients, the metabolic effects of androgens may decrease blood glucose and insulin requirements). Products include:
Humulin N, 100 Units 1795
Humulin N Pen 1797

Insulin, Human Regular (In diabetic patients, the metabolic effects of

androgens may decrease blood glucose and insulin requirements).
Products include:
Humulin R, 100 Units 1798

Insulin, Human Regular and Human NPH Mixture (In diabetic patients, the metabolic effects of androgens may decrease blood glucose and insulin requirements).
Products include:
Humulin 50/50, 100 Units 1791
Humulin 70/30 Pen 1793

Insulin, NPH (In diabetic patients, the metabolic effects of androgens may decrease blood glucose and insulin requirements).
No products indexed under this heading.

Insulin, Regular (In diabetic patients, the metabolic effects of androgens may decrease blood glucose and insulin requirements).
No products indexed under this heading.

Insulin, Zinc Crystals (In diabetic patients, the metabolic effects of androgens may decrease blood glucose and insulin requirements).
No products indexed under this heading.

Insulin, Zinc Suspension (In diabetic patients, the metabolic effects of androgens may decrease blood glucose and insulin requirements).
No products indexed under this heading.

Insulin Aspart, Human Regular (In diabetic patients, the metabolic effects of androgens may decrease blood glucose and insulin requirements). Products include:
NovoLog Injection 2326

Insulin glargine (In diabetic patients, the metabolic effects of androgens may decrease blood glucose and insulin requirements). Products include:
Lantus Injection 2909

Insulin Lispro, Human (In diabetic patients, the metabolic effects of androgens may decrease blood glucose and insulin requirements). Products include:
Humalog-Pen 1781
Humalog Mix 50/50-Pen 1783
Humalog Mix 75/25-Pen 1785

Insulin Lispro Protamine, Human (In diabetic patients, the metabolic effects of androgens may decrease blood glucose and insulin requirements). Products include:
Humalog Mix 50/50-Pen 1783
Humalog Mix 75/25-Pen 1785

Metformin Hydrochloride (In diabetic patients, the metabolic effects of androgens may decrease blood glucose and insulin requirements).
Products include:
ActoPlus Met Tablets 3214
Avandamet Tablets 1373
Fortamet Extended-Release
Tablets 3115

Methylprednisolone Acetate (Enhanced tendency towards edema. Use caution when giving these drugs together, especially in patients with hepatic or cardiac disease).
Products include:
Depo-Medrol Injectable
Suspension 2617
Depo-Medrol Single-Dose Vial 2619

Methylprednisolone Sodium Succinate (Enhanced tendency towards edema. Use caution when giving these drugs together, especially in patients with hepatic or cardiac disease).
No products indexed under this heading.

Miglitol (In diabetic patients, the metabolic effects of androgens may decrease blood glucose and insulin requirements).
No products indexed under this heading.

Oxyphenbutazone (May result in elevated serum levels of oxyphenbutazone).
No products indexed under this heading.

Pioglitazone Hydrochloride (In diabetic patients, the metabolic effects of androgens may decrease blood glucose and insulin requirements). Products include:
ActoPlus Met Tablets ... 3214
Actos Tablets ... 3219
Duetact Tablets ... 3226

Prednisolone Acetate (Enhanced tendency towards edema. Use caution when giving these drugs together, especially in patients with hepatic or cardiac disease). Products include:
Blephamide Ophthalmic Ointment ... 568
Blephamide Ophthalmic Suspension ... 569
Poly-Pred Ophthalmic Suspension ... ⊙233
Pred Forte Ophthalmic Suspension ... ⊙235
Pred Mild Ophthalmic Suspension ... ⊙238
Pred-G Ophthalmic Ointment ... ⊙237
Pred-G Ophthalmic Suspension ... ⊙236

Prednisolone Sodium Phosphate (Enhanced tendency towards edema. Use caution when giving these drugs together, especially in patients with hepatic or cardiac disease).
No products indexed under this heading.

Prednisolone Tebutate (Enhanced tendency towards edema. Use caution when giving these drugs together, especially in patients with hepatic or cardiac disease).
No products indexed under this heading.

Prednisone (Enhanced tendency towards edema. Use caution when giving these drugs together, especially in patients with hepatic or cardiac disease).
No products indexed under this heading.

Repaglinide (In diabetic patients, the metabolic effects of androgens may decrease blood glucose and insulin requirements).
No products indexed under this heading.

Rosiglitazone Maleate (In diabetic patients, the metabolic effects of androgens may decrease blood glucose and insulin requirements). Products include:
Avandamet Tablets ... 1373
Avandaryl Tablets ... 1379
Avandia Tablets ... 1384

Tolazamide (In diabetic patients, the metabolic effects of androgens may decrease blood glucose and insulin requirements).
No products indexed under this heading.

Tolbutamide (In diabetic patients, the metabolic effects of androgens may decrease blood glucose and insulin requirements).
No products indexed under this heading.

Triamcinolone (Enhanced tendency towards edema. Use caution when giving these drugs together, especially in patients with hepatic or cardiac disease).
No products indexed under this heading.

Triamcinolone Acetonide (Enhanced tendency towards edema. Use caution when giving these drugs together, especially in patients with hepatic or cardiac disease). Products include:
Azmacort Inhalation Aerosol ... 1726
Nasacort AQ Nasal Spray ... 2922

Triamcinolone Diacetate (Enhanced tendency towards edema. Use caution when giving these drugs together, especially in patients with hepatic or cardiac disease).
No products indexed under this heading.

Triamcinolone Hexacetonide (Enhanced tendency towards edema. Use caution when giving these drugs together, especially in patients with hepatic or cardiac disease).
No products indexed under this heading.

Troglitazone (In diabetic patients, the metabolic effects of androgens may decrease blood glucose and insulin requirements).
No products indexed under this heading.

Warfarin Sodium (C-17 substituted derivatives of testosterone, such as methandrostenolone, have been reported to decrease the anticoagulant requirement. Patients receiving oral anticoagulant therapy require close monitoring especially when androgens are started or stopped). Products include:
Coumadin for Injection ... 898
Coumadin Tablets ... 898

ANGELIQ TABLETS

(Drospirenone, Estradiol) ... 762

May interact with ACE inhibitors, angiotensin-II receptor antagonists, cytochrome p450 3a4 inducers (selected), cytochrome p450 3a4 inhibitors (selected), and non-steroidal anti-inflammatory agents. Compounds in these categories include:

Acetazolamide (Inhibitors of CYP3A4 such as erythromycin, clarithromycin, ketoconazole, itraconazole, ritonavir and grapefruit juice may increase plasma concentrations of estrogens and may result in side effects).
No products indexed under this heading.

Allium sativum (Inducers of CYP3A4, such as St. John's Wort preparations (Hypericum perforatum), phenobarbital, carbamazepine, and rifampin, may reduce plasma concentrations of estrogens, possibly resulting in a decrease in therapeutic effects and/or changes in the uterine bleeding profile).
No products indexed under this heading.

Amiodarone Hydrochloride (Inhibitors of CYP3A4 such as erythromycin, clarithromycin, ketoconazole, itraconazole, ritonavir and grapefruit juice may increase plasma concentrations of estrogens and may result in side effects).
No products indexed under this heading.

Amprenavir (Inhibitors of CYP3A4 such as erythromycin, clarithromycin, ketoconazole, itraconazole, ritonavir and grapefruit juice may increase plasma concentrations of estrogens and may result in side effects). Products include:
Agenerase Capsules ... 1327
Agenerase Oral Solution ... 1332

Anastrozole (Inhibitors of CYP3A4 such as erythromycin, clarithromycin, ketoconazole, itraconazole, ritonavir and grapefruit juice may increase plasma concentrations of estrogens and may result in side effects). Products include:
Arimidex Tablets ... 673

Aprepitant (Inhibitors of CYP3A4 such as erythromycin, clarithromycin, ketoconazole, itraconazole, ritonavir and grapefruit juice may increase plasma concentrations of estrogens and may result in side effects). Products include:
Emend Capsules ... 1963

Benazepril Hydrochloride (There is potential for an increase in serum potassium in women taking drospirenone with other drugs that may affect electrolytes). Products include:
Lotensin Tablets ... 2243
Lotensin HCT Tablets ... 2246
Lotrel Capsules ... 2249

Betamethasone Acetate (Inducers of CYP3A4, such as St. John's Wort preparations (Hypericum perforatum), phenobarbital, carbamazepine, and rifampin, may reduce plasma concentrations of estrogens, possibly resulting in a decrease in therapeutic effects and/or changes in the uterine bleeding profile).
No products indexed under this heading.

Betamethasone Sodium Phosphate (Inducers of CYP3A4, such as St. John's Wort preparations (Hypericum perforatum), phenobarbital, carbamazepine, and rifampin, may reduce plasma concentrations of estrogens, possibly resulting in a decrease in therapeutic effects and/or changes in the uterine bleeding profile).
No products indexed under this heading.

Candesartan Cilexetil (There is potential for an increase in serum potassium in women taking drospirenone with other drugs that may affect electrolytes). Products include:
Atacand Tablets ... 649
Atacand HCT ... 651

Captopril (There is potential for an increase in serum potassium in women taking drospirenone with other drugs that may affect electrolytes). Products include:
Captopril Tablets ... 2149

Carbamazepine (Inducers of CYP3A4, such as St. John's Wort preparations (Hypericum perforatum), phenobarbital, carbamazepine, and rifampin, may reduce plasma concentrations of estrogens, possibly resulting in a decrease in therapeutic effects and/or changes in the uterine bleeding profile). Products include:
Carbatrol Capsules ... 3171
Equetro Extended-Release Capsules ... 3180
Tegretol/Tegretol-XR ... 2295

Celecoxib (There is potential for an increase in serum potassium in women taking drospirenone with other drugs that may affect electrolytes). Products include:
Celebrex Capsules ... 3134

Cimetidine (Inhibitors of CYP3A4 such as erythromycin, clarithromycin, ketoconazole, itraconazole, ritonavir and grapefruit juice may increase plasma concentrations of estrogens and may result in side effects). Products include:
Tagamet HB 200 Tablets ... 664

Cimetidine Hydrochloride (Inhibitors of CYP3A4 such as erythromycin, clarithromycin, ketoconazole, itraconazole, ritonavir and grapefruit juice may increase plasma concentrations of estrogens and may result in side effects).
No products indexed under this heading.

Ciprofloxacin (Inhibitors of CYP3A4 such as erythromycin, clarithromycin, ketoconazole, itraconazole, ritonavir and grapefruit juice may increase plasma concentrations of estrogens and may result in side effects). Products include:
Cipro Oral Suspension ... 2977
Cipro I.V. ... 2984
Cipro XR Tablets ... 2990
Ciprodex Otic Suspension ... 559

Ciprofloxacin Hydrochloride (Inducers of CYP3A4, such as St. John's Wort preparations (Hypericum perforatum), phenobarbital, carbamazepine, and rifampin, may reduce plasma concentrations of estrogens, possibly resulting in a decrease in therapeutic effects and/or changes in the uterine bleeding profile). Products include:
Ciloxan Ophthalmic Ointment ... 559
Ciloxan Ophthalmic Solution ... ⊙206
Cipro Tablets ... 2977
Proquin XR Tablets ... 1153

Cisplatin (Inducers of CYP3A4, such as St. John's Wort preparations (Hypericum perforatum), phenobarbital, carbamazepine, and rifampin, may reduce plasma concentrations of estrogens, possibly resulting in a decrease in therapeutic effects and/or changes in the uterine bleeding profile).
No products indexed under this heading.

Clarithromycin (Inhibitors of CYP3A4 such as erythromycin, clarithromycin, ketoconazole, itraconazole, ritonavir and grapefruit juice may increase plasma concentrations of estrogens and may result in side effects). Products include:
Biaxin/Biaxin XL ... 402
PREVPAC ... 3284

Clotrimazole (Inhibitors of CYP3A4 such as erythromycin, clarithromycin, ketoconazole, itraconazole, ritonavir and grapefruit juice may increase plasma concentrations of estrogens and may result in side effects). Products include:
Desenex Athlete's Foot Cream ... 635
Lotrimin ... 3039
Lotrisone ... 3040

Cortisone Acetate (Inducers of CYP3A4, such as St. John's Wort preparations (Hypericum perforatum), phenobarbital, carbamazepine, and rifampin, may reduce plasma concentrations of estrogens, possibly resulting in a decrease in therapeutic effects and/or changes in the uterine bleeding profile).
No products indexed under this heading.

Cyclosporine (Inhibitors of CYP3A4 such as erythromycin, clarithromycin, ketoconazole, itraconazole, ritonavir and grapefruit juice may increase plasma concentrations of estrogens and may result in side effects). Products include:
Gengraf Capsules 459
Neoral Oral Solution 2259
Neoral Soft Gelatin Capsules 2259
Restasis Ophthalmic Emulsion 575
Sandimmune 2275

Dalfopristin (Inhibitors of CYP3A4 such as erythromycin, clarithromycin, ketoconazole, itraconazole, ritonavir and grapefruit juice may increase plasma concentrations of estrogens and may result in side effects).
No products indexed under this heading.

Danazol (Inhibitors of CYP3A4 such as erythromycin, clarithromycin, ketoconazole, itraconazole, ritonavir and grapefruit juice may increase plasma concentrations of estrogens and may result in side effects).
No products indexed under this heading.

Delavirdine Mesylate (Inhibitors of CYP3A4 such as erythromycin, clarithromycin, ketoconazole, itraconazole, ritonavir and grapefruit juice may increase plasma concentrations of estrogens and may result in side effects). Products include:
Rescriptor Tablets 2551

Dexamethasone (Inducers of CYP3A4, such as St. John's Wort preparations (Hypericum perforatum), phenobarbital, carbamazepine, and rifampin, may reduce plasma concentrations of estrogens, possibly resulting in a decrease in therapeutic effects and/or changes in the uterine bleeding profile). Products include:
Ciprodex Otic Suspension 559
Decadron Tablets 1951
TobraDex Ophthalmic Ointment 562
TobraDex Ophthalmic Suspension ... 563

Dexamethasone Acetate (Inducers of CYP3A4, such as St. John's Wort preparations (Hypericum perforatum), phenobarbital, carbamazepine, and rifampin, may reduce plasma concentrations of estrogens, possibly resulting in a decrease in therapeutic effects and/or changes in the uterine bleeding profile).
No products indexed under this heading.

Dexamethasone Sodium Phosphate (Inducers of CYP3A4, such as St. John's Wort preparations (Hypericum perforatum), phenobarbital, carbamazepine, and rifampin, may reduce plasma concentrations of estrogens, possibly resulting in a decrease in therapeutic effects and/or changes in the uterine bleeding profile).
No products indexed under this heading.

Diclofenac Potassium (There is potential for an increase in serum potassium in women taking drospirenone with other drugs that may affect electrolytes).
No products indexed under this heading.

Diclofenac Sodium (There is potential for an increase in serum potassium in women taking drospirenone with other drugs that may affect electrolytes). Products include:
Arthrotec Tablets 3129
Voltaren Ophthalmic Solution 2309
Voltaren Tablets 2307
Voltaren-XR Tablets 2310

Diltiazem Hydrochloride (Inhibitors of CYP3A4 such as erythromycin, clarithromycin, ketoconazole, itraconazole, ritonavir and grapefruit juice may increase plasma concentrations of estrogens and may result in side effects). Products include:
Cardizem LA Extended Release Tablets 1728
Tiazac Capsules 1201

Diltiazem Maleate (Inhibitors of CYP3A4 such as erythromycin, clarithromycin, ketoconazole, itraconazole, ritonavir and grapefruit juice may increase plasma concentrations of estrogens and may result in side effects).
No products indexed under this heading.

Doxorubicin Hydrochloride (Inducers of CYP3A4, such as St. John's Wort preparations (Hypericum perforatum), phenobarbital, carbamazepine, and rifampin, may reduce plasma concentrations of estrogens, possibly resulting in a decrease in therapeutic effects and/or changes in the uterine bleeding profile).
No products indexed under this heading.

Efavirenz (Inhibitors of CYP3A4 such as erythromycin, clarithromycin, ketoconazole, itraconazole, ritonavir and grapefruit juice may increase plasma concentrations of estrogens and may result in side effects). Products include:
Atripla Tablets 945
Sustiva Capsules 930
Sustiva Tablets 930

Enalapril Maleate (There is potential for an increase in serum potassium in women taking drospirenone with other drugs that may affect electrolytes). Products include:
Vasotec I.V. Injection 2103

Enalaprilat (There is potential for an increase in serum potassium in women taking drospirenone with other drugs that may affect electrolytes).
No products indexed under this heading.

Eprosartan Mesylate (There is potential for an increase in serum potassium in women taking drospirenone with other drugs that may affect electrolytes). Products include:
Teveten Tablets 1735
Teveten HCT Tablets 1737

Erythromycin (Inhibitors of CYP3A4 such as erythromycin, clarithromycin, ketoconazole, itraconazole, ritonavir and grapefruit juice may increase plasma concentrations of estrogens and may result in side effects). Products include:
Ery-Tab Tablets 449
Erythromycin Base Filmtab Tablets 455
Erythromycin Delayed-Release Capsules, USP 457
PCE Dispertab Tablets 515

Erythromycin Estolate (Inhibitors of CYP3A4 such as erythromycin, clarithromycin, ketoconazole, itraconazole, ritonavir and grapefruit juice may increase plasma concentrations of estrogens and may result in side effects).
No products indexed under this heading.

Erythromycin Ethylsuccinate (Inhibitors of CYP3A4 such as erythromycin, clarithromycin, ketoconazole, itraconazole, ritonavir and grapefruit juice may increase plasma concentrations of estrogens and may result in side effects). Products include:
E.E.S. 451
EryPed 447

Erythromycin Gluceptate (Inhibitors of CYP3A4 such as erythromycin, clarithromycin, ketoconazole, itraconazole, ritonavir and grapefruit juice may increase plasma concentrations of estrogens and may result in side effects).
No products indexed under this heading.

Erythromycin Lactobionate (Inhibitors of CYP3A4 such as erythromycin, clarithromycin, ketoconazole, itraconazole, ritonavir and grapefruit juice may increase plasma concentrations of estrogens and may result in side effects).
No products indexed under this heading.

Erythromycin Stearate (Inhibitors of CYP3A4 such as erythromycin, clarithromycin, ketoconazole, itraconazole, ritonavir and grapefruit juice may increase plasma concentrations of estrogens and may result in side effects). Products include:
Erythrocin Stearate Filmtab Tablets 453

Esomeprazole Magnesium (Inhibitors of CYP3A4 such as erythromycin, clarithromycin, ketoconazole, itraconazole, ritonavir and grapefruit juice may increase plasma concentrations of estrogens and may result in side effects). Products include:
Nexium Delayed-Release Capsules 655

Ethosuximide (Inducers of CYP3A4, such as St. John's Wort preparations (Hypericum perforatum), phenobarbital, carbamazepine, and rifampin, may reduce plasma concentrations of estrogens, possibly resulting in a decrease in therapeutic effects and/or changes in the uterine bleeding profile).
No products indexed under this heading.

Etodolac (There is potential for an increase in serum potassium in women taking drospirenone with other drugs that may affect electrolytes).
No products indexed under this heading.

Felbamate (Inducers of CYP3A4, such as St. John's Wort preparations (Hypericum perforatum), phenobarbital, carbamazepine, and rifampin, may reduce plasma concentrations of estrogens, possibly resulting in a decrease in therapeutic effects and/or changes in the uterine bleeding profile).
No products indexed under this heading.

Fenoprofen Calcium (There is potential for an increase in serum potassium in women taking drospirenone with other drugs that may affect electrolytes). Products include:
Nalfon Capsules 2502

Fluconazole (Inhibitors of CYP3A4 such as erythromycin, clarithromycin, ketoconazole, itraconazole, ritonavir and grapefruit juice may increase plasma concentrations of estrogens and may result in side effects).
No products indexed under this heading.

Fludrocortisone Acetate (Inducers of CYP3A4, such as St. John's Wort preparations (Hypericum perforatum), phenobarbital, carbamazepine, and rifampin, may reduce plasma concentrations of estrogens, possibly resulting in a decrease in therapeutic effects and/or changes in the uterine bleeding profile).
No products indexed under this heading.

Fluoxetine Hydrochloride (Inhibitors of CYP3A4 such as erythromycin, clarithromycin, ketoconazole, itraconazole, ritonavir and grapefruit juice may increase plasma concentrations of estrogens and may result in side effects). Products include:
Prozac Pulvules and Liquid 1801
Symbyax Capsules 1819

Flurbiprofen (There is potential for an increase in serum potassium in women taking drospirenone with other drugs that may affect electrolytes).
No products indexed under this heading.

Fluvoxamine Maleate (Inhibitors of CYP3A4 such as erythromycin, clarithromycin, ketoconazole, itraconazole, ritonavir and grapefruit juice may increase plasma concentrations of estrogens and may result in side effects).
No products indexed under this heading.

Fosamprenavir Calcium (Inhibitors of CYP3A4 such as erythromycin, clarithromycin, ketoconazole, itraconazole, ritonavir and grapefruit juice may increase plasma concentrations of estrogens and may result in side effects). Products include:
Lexiva Tablets 1505

Fosinopril Sodium (There is potential for an increase in serum potassium in women taking drospirenone with other drugs that may affect electrolytes).
No products indexed under this heading.

Fosphenytoin Sodium (Inducers of CYP3A4, such as St. John's Wort preparations (Hypericum perforatum), phenobarbital, carbamazepine, and rifampin, may reduce plasma concentrations of estrogens, possibly resulting in a decrease in therapeutic effects and/or changes in the uterine bleeding profile).
No products indexed under this heading.

Garlic Extract (Inducers of CYP3A4, such as St. John's Wort preparations (Hypericum perforatum), phenobarbital, carbamazepine, and rifampin, may reduce plasma concentrations of estrogens, possibly resulting in a decrease in therapeutic effects and/or changes in the uterine bleeding profile).
No products indexed under this heading.

Garlic Oil (Inducers of CYP3A4, such as St. John's Wort preparations (Hypericum perforatum), phenobarbital, carbamazepine, and rifampin, may reduce plasma concentrations of estrogens, possibly resulting in a decrease in therapeutic effects and/or changes in the uterine bleeding profile).
No products indexed under this heading.

Hydrocortisone (Inducers of CYP3A4, such as St. John's Wort preparations (Hypericum perforatum), phenobarbital, carbamazepine, and rifampin, may reduce plasma concentrations of estrogens, possibly resulting in a decrease in therapeutic effects and/or changes in the uterine bleeding profile). Products include:
Colocort Rectal Suspension, USP (Retention) 100 mg/60 mL 2476
Hydrocortone Tablets 1989
Preparation H Hydrocortisone Cream 646

Hydrocortisone Acetate (Inducers of CYP3A4, such as St. John's Wort preparations (Hypericum perforatum), phenobarbital, carbamazepine, and rifampin, may reduce plasma concentrations of estrogens, possibly resulting in a decrease in therapeutic effects and/or changes in the uterine bleeding profile). Products include:
Analpram-HC 1159
Pramosone 1161
ProctoFoam-HC 3099

Hydrocortisone Butyrate (Inducers of CYP3A4, such as St. John's Wort preparations (Hypericum perforatum), phenobarbital, carbamazepine, and rifampin, may reduce plasma concentrations of estrogens, possibly resulting in a decrease in therapeutic effects and/or changes in the uterine bleeding profile). Products include:
Locoid Lipocream Cream 1160

Hydrocortisone Cypionate (Inducers of CYP3A4, such as St. John's Wort preparations (Hypericum perforatum), phenobarbital, carbamazepine, and rifampin, may reduce plasma concentrations of estrogens, possibly resulting in a decrease in therapeutic effects and/or changes in the uterine bleeding profile).
No products indexed under this heading.

Hydrocortisone Hemisuccinate (Inducers of CYP3A4, such as St. John's Wort preparations (Hypericum perforatum), phenobarbital, carbamazepine, and rifampin, may reduce plasma concentrations of estrogens, possibly resulting in a decrease in therapeutic effects and/or changes in the uterine bleeding profile).
No products indexed under this heading.

Hydrocortisone Probutate (Inducers of CYP3A4, such as St. John's Wort preparations (Hypericum perforatum), phenobarbital, carbamazepine, and rifampin, may reduce plasma concentrations of estrogens, possibly resulting in a decrease in therapeutic effects and/or changes in the uterine bleeding profile).
No products indexed under this heading.

Hydrocortisone Sodium Phosphate (Inducers of CYP3A4, such as St. John's Wort preparations (Hypericum perforatum), phenobarbital, carbamazepine, and rifampin, may reduce plasma concentrations of estrogens, possibly resulting in a decrease in therapeutic effects and/or changes in the uterine bleeding profile).
No products indexed under this heading.

Hydrocortisone Sodium Succinate (Inducers of CYP3A4, such as St. John's Wort preparations (Hypericum perforatum), phenobarbital, carbamazepine, and rifampin, may reduce plasma concentrations of estrogens, possibly resulting in a decrease in therapeutic effects and/or changes in the uterine bleeding profile).
No products indexed under this heading.

Hydrocortisone Valerate (Inducers of CYP3A4, such as St. John's Wort preparations (Hypericum perforatum), phenobarbital, carbamazepine, and rifampin, may reduce plasma concentrations of estrogens, possibly resulting in a decrease in therapeutic effects and/or changes in the uterine bleeding profile).
No products indexed under this heading.

Hypericum (Inducers of CYP3A4, such as St. John's Wort preparations (Hypericum perforatum), phenobarbital, carbamazepine, and rifampin, may reduce plasma concentrations of estrogens, possibly resulting in a decrease in therapeutic effects and/or changes in the uterine bleeding profile). Products include:
Satiete Tablets 832

Hypericum Perforatum (Inducers of CYP3A4, such as St. John's Wort preparations (Hypericum perforatum), phenobarbital, carbamazepine, and rifampin, may reduce plasma concentrations of estrogens, possibly resulting in a decrease in therapeutic effects and/or changes in the uterine bleeding profile).
No products indexed under this heading.

Ibuprofen (There is potential for an increase in serum potassium in women taking drospirenone with other drugs that may affect electrolytes). Products include:
Advil Allergy Sinus Caplets 770
Advil 674
Children's Advil Oral Suspension 603
Children's Advil Chewable Tablets 603
Advil Cold & Sinus 723
Infants' Advil Concentrated Drops 604
Infants' Advil Concentrated Drops - White Grape (Dye-Free) 604
Junior Strength Advil Swallow Tablets 605
Advil Migraine Liquigels 608
Advil Multi-Symptom Cold Caplets 770
Advil PM Caplets 615
Motrin IB Tablets and Caplets 1866
Children's Motrin Oral Suspension 1867
Children's Motrin Non-Staining Dye-Free Oral Suspension 1867
Children's Motrin Cold Oral Suspension 1867
Infants' Motrin Concentrated Drops 1867
Infants' Motrin Non-Staining Dye-Free Concentrated Drops 1867
Junior Strength Motrin Caplets and Chewable Tablets 1867
Vicoprofen Tablets 539

Indinavir Sulfate (Inhibitors of CYP3A4 such as erythromycin, clarithromycin, ketoconazole, itraconazole, ritonavir and grapefruit juice may increase plasma concentrations of estrogens and may result in side effects). Products include:
Crixivan Capsules 1940

Indomethacin (There is potential for an increase in serum potassium in women taking drospirenone with other drugs that may affect electrolytes). Products include:
Indocin 1995

Indomethacin Sodium Trihydrate (There is potential for an increase in serum potassium in women taking drospirenone with other drugs that may affect electrolytes). Products include:
Indocin I.V. 2465

Irbesartan (There is potential for an increase in serum potassium in women taking drospirenone with other drugs that may affect electrolytes). Products include:
Avalide Tablets 888
Avalide Tablets 2874
Avapro Tablets 891
Avapro Tablets 2871

Isoniazid (Inhibitors of CYP3A4 such as erythromycin, clarithromycin, ketoconazole, itraconazole, ritonavir and grapefruit juice may increase plasma concentrations of estrogens and may result in side effects).
No products indexed under this heading.

Itraconazole (Inhibitors of CYP3A4 such as erythromycin, clarithromycin, ketoconazole, itraconazole, ritonavir and grapefruit juice may increase plasma concentrations of estrogens and may result in side effects).
No products indexed under this heading.

Ketoconazole (Inhibitors of CYP3A4 such as erythromycin, clarithromycin, ketoconazole, itraconazole, ritonavir and grapefruit juice may increase plasma concentrations of estrogens and may result in side effects). Products include:
Nizoral A-D Shampoo, 1% 1868

Ketoprofen (There is potential for an increase in serum potassium in women taking drospirenone with other drugs that may affect electrolytes).
No products indexed under this heading.

Ketorolac Tromethamine (There is potential for an increase in serum potassium in women taking drospirenone with other drugs that may affect electrolytes). Products include:
Acular Ophthalmic Solution 565
Acular LS Ophthalmic Solution 566

Lisinopril (There is potential for an increase in serum potassium in women taking drospirenone with other drugs that may affect electrolytes). Products include:
Prinivil Tablets 2052
Prinzide Tablets 2056

Lopinavir (Inhibitors of CYP3A4 such as erythromycin, clarithromycin, ketoconazole, itraconazole, ritonavir and grapefruit juice may increase plasma concentrations of estrogens and may result in side effects). Products include:
Kaletra 476

Loratadine (Inhibitors of CYP3A4 such as erythromycin, clarithromycin, ketoconazole, itraconazole, ritonavir and grapefruit juice may increase plasma concentrations of estrogens and may result in side effects). Products include:
Alavert Allergy & Sinus D-12 Hour Tablets 771
Alavert 771
Children's Claritin Allergy Oral Solution 771
Claritin Non-Drowsy 24 Hour Tablets 772
Claritin Reditabs 24 Hour Non-Drowsy Tablets 772
Claritin-D Non-Drowsy 12 Hour Tablets 772
Claritin-D Non-Drowsy 24 Hour Tablets 772

Losartan Potassium (There is potential for an increase in serum potassium in women taking drospirenone with other drugs that may affect electrolytes). Products include:
Cozaar Tablets 1935
Hyzaar 50-12.5 Tablets 1990
Hyzaar 100-12.5 Tablets 1990
Hyzaar 100-25 Tablets 1990

Meclofenamate Sodium (There is potential for an increase in serum potassium in women taking drospirenone with other drugs that may affect electrolytes).
No products indexed under this heading.

Mefenamic Acid (There is potential for an increase in serum potassium in women taking drospirenone with other drugs that may affect electrolytes).
No products indexed under this heading.

Meloxicam (There is potential for an increase in serum potassium in women taking drospirenone with other drugs that may affect electrolytes). Products include:
Mobic Oral Suspension 863
Mobic Tablets 863

Mephenytoin (Inducers of CYP3A4, such as St. John's Wort preparations (Hypericum perforatum), phenobarbital, carbamazepine, and rifampin, may reduce plasma concentrations of estrogens, possibly resulting in a decrease in therapeutic effects and/or changes in the uterine bleeding profile).
No products indexed under this heading.

Methsuximide (Inducers of CYP3A4, such as St. John's Wort preparations (Hypericum perforatum), phenobarbital, carbamazepine, and rifampin, may reduce plasma concentrations of estrogens, possibly resulting in a decrease in therapeutic effects and/or changes in the uterine bleeding profile).
No products indexed under this heading.

Methylprednisolone (Inducers of CYP3A4, such as St. John's Wort preparations (Hypericum perforatum), phenobarbital, carbamazepine, and rifampin, may reduce plasma concentrations of estrogens, possibly resulting in a decrease in therapeutic effects and/or changes in the uterine bleeding profile).
No products indexed under this heading.

Methylprednisolone Acetate (Inducers of CYP3A4, such as St. John's Wort preparations (Hypericum perforatum), phenobarbital, carbamazepine, and rifampin, may reduce

plasma concentrations of estrogens, possibly resulting in a decrease in therapeutic effects and/or changes in the uterine bleeding profile). Products include:

Depo-Medrol Injectable
Suspension 2617
Depo-Medrol Single-Dose Vial 2619

Methylprednisolone Sodium Succinate (Inducers of CYP3A4, such as St. John's Wort preparations (Hypericum perforatum), phenobarbital, carbamazepine, and rifampin, may reduce plasma concentrations of estrogens, possibly resulting in a decrease in therapeutic effects and/or changes in the uterine bleeding profile).

No products indexed under this heading.

Metronidazole (Inhibitors of CYP3A4 such as erythromycin, clarithromycin, ketoconazole, itraconazole, ritonavir and grapefruit juice may increase plasma concentrations of estrogens and may result in side effects). Products include:

Metrogel 1% 1211
MetroGel-Vaginal Gel 1855
Vandazole Vaginal Gel 3338

Metronidazole Benzoate (Inhibitors of CYP3A4 such as erythromycin, clarithromycin, ketoconazole, itraconazole, ritonavir and grapefruit juice may increase plasma concentrations of estrogens and may result in side effects).

No products indexed under this heading.

Metronidazole Hydrochloride (Inhibitors of CYP3A4 such as erythromycin, clarithromycin, ketoconazole, itraconazole, ritonavir and grapefruit juice may increase plasma concentrations of estrogens and may result in side effects).

No products indexed under this heading.

Miconazole (Inhibitors of CYP3A4 such as erythromycin, clarithromycin, ketoconazole, itraconazole, ritonavir and grapefruit juice may increase plasma concentrations of estrogens and may result in side effects).

No products indexed under this heading.

Miconazole Nitrate (Inhibitors of CYP3A4 such as erythromycin, clarithromycin, ketoconazole, itraconazole, ritonavir and grapefruit juice may increase plasma concentrations of estrogens and may result in side effects). Products include:

Desenex ▣635
Desenex Jock Itch Spray Powder ... ▣635

Modafinil (Inducers of CYP3A4, such as St. John's Wort preparations (Hypericum perforatum), phenobarbital, carbamazepine, and rifampin, may reduce plasma concentrations of estrogens, possibly resulting in a decrease in therapeutic effects and/or changes in the uterine bleeding profile). Products include:

Provigil Tablets 988

Moexipril Hydrochloride (There is potential for an increase in serum potassium in women taking drospirenone with other drugs that may affect electrolytes). Products include:

Uniretic Tablets 3100
Univasc Tablets 3104

Nabumetone (There is potential for an increase in serum potassium in women taking drospirenone with other drugs that may affect electrolytes).

No products indexed under this heading.

Naproxen (There is potential for an increase in serum potassium in women taking drospirenone with other drugs that may affect electrolytes). Products include:

EC-Naprosyn Delayed-Release
Tablets 2761
Naprosyn Suspension 2761
Naprosyn Tablets 2761
Prevacid NapraPAC 3280

Naproxen Sodium (There is potential for an increase in serum potassium in women taking drospirenone with other drugs that may affect electrolytes). Products include:

Aleve Caplets 742
Aleve Gelcaps 743
Aleve Tablets 743
Aleve Cold & Sinus Caplets 744
Anaprox Tablets 2761
Anaprox DS Tablets 2761

Nefazodone Hydrochloride (Inhibitors of CYP3A4 such as erythromycin, clarithromycin, ketoconazole, itraconazole, ritonavir and grapefruit juice may increase plasma concentrations of estrogens and may result in side effects).

No products indexed under this heading.

Nelfinavir Mesylate (Inhibitors of CYP3A4 such as erythromycin, clarithromycin, ketoconazole, itraconazole, ritonavir and grapefruit juice may increase plasma concentrations of estrogens and may result in side effects). Products include:

Viracept 2577

Nevirapine (Inhibitors of CYP3A4 such as erythromycin, clarithromycin, ketoconazole, itraconazole, ritonavir and grapefruit juice may increase plasma concentrations of estrogens and may result in side effects). Products include:

Viramune Oral Suspension 873
Viramune Tablets 873

Niacinamide (Inhibitors of CYP3A4 such as erythromycin, clarithromycin, ketoconazole, itraconazole, ritonavir and grapefruit juice may increase plasma concentrations of estrogens and may result in side effects).

No products indexed under this heading.

Nicotinamide (Inhibitors of CYP3A4 such as erythromycin, clarithromycin, ketoconazole, itraconazole, ritonavir and grapefruit juice may increase plasma concentrations of estrogens and may result in side effects). Products include:

Nicomide Tablets 1088

Nifedipine (Inhibitors of CYP3A4 such as erythromycin, clarithromycin, ketoconazole, itraconazole, ritonavir and grapefruit juice may increase plasma concentrations of estrogens and may result in side effects). Products include:

Adalat CC Tablets 2964

Norfloxacin (Inhibitors of CYP3A4 such as erythromycin, clarithromycin, ketoconazole, itraconazole, ritonavir and grapefruit juice may increase plasma concentrations of estrogens and may result in side effects). Products include:

Noroxin Tablets 2032

Omeprazole (Inhibitors of CYP3A4 such as erythromycin, clarithromycin, ketoconazole, itraconazole, ritonavir and grapefruit juice may increase plasma concentrations of estrogens and may result in side effects). Products include:

Zegerid Capsules 2958
Zegerid Powder for Oral Solution 2958

Oxaprozin (There is potential for an increase in serum potassium in women taking drospirenone with other drugs that may affect electrolytes).

No products indexed under this heading.

Oxcarbazepine (Inducers of CYP3A4, such as St. John's Wort preparations (Hypericum perforatum), phenobarbital, carbamazepine, and rifampin, may reduce plasma concentrations of estrogens, possibly resulting in a decrease in therapeutic effects and/or changes in the uterine bleeding profile). Products include:

Trileptal Tablets 2300
Trileptal Oral Suspension 2300

Paroxetine Hydrochloride (Inhibitors of CYP3A4 such as erythromycin, clarithromycin, ketoconazole, itraconazole, ritonavir and grapefruit juice may increase plasma concentrations of estrogens and may result in side effects). Products include:

Paxil CR Controlled-Release
Tablets 1538
Paxil 1530

Perindopril Erbumine (There is potential for an increase in serum potassium in women taking drospirenone with other drugs that may affect electrolytes). Products include:

Aceon Tablets (2 mg, 4 mg,
8 mg) 3194

Phenobarbital (Inducers of CYP3A4, such as St. John's Wort preparations (Hypericum perforatum), phenobarbital, carbamazepine, and rifampin, may reduce plasma concentrations of estrogens, possibly resulting in a decrease in therapeutic effects and/or changes in the uterine bleeding profile). Products include:

Donnatal Extentabs 2493

Phenobarbital Sodium (Inducers of CYP3A4, such as St. John's Wort preparations (Hypericum perforatum), phenobarbital, carbamazepine, and rifampin, may reduce plasma concentrations of estrogens, possibly resulting in a decrease in therapeutic effects and/or changes in the uterine bleeding profile).

No products indexed under this heading.

Phenylbutazone (There is potential for an increase in serum potassium in women taking drospirenone with other drugs that may affect electrolytes).

No products indexed under this heading.

Phenytoin (Inducers of CYP3A4, such as St. John's Wort preparations (Hypericum perforatum), phenobarbital, carbamazepine, and rifampin, may reduce plasma concentrations of estrogens, possibly resulting in a decrease in therapeutic effects and/or changes in the uterine bleeding profile).

No products indexed under this heading.

Phenytoin Sodium (Inducers of CYP3A4, such as St. John's Wort preparations (Hypericum perfora-

tum), phenobarbital, carbamazepine, and rifampin, may reduce plasma concentrations of estrogens, possibly resulting in a decrease in therapeutic effects and/or changes in the uterine bleeding profile). Products include:

Phenytek Capsules 2160

Piroxicam (There is potential for an increase in serum potassium in women taking drospirenone with other drugs that may affect electrolytes).

No products indexed under this heading.

Prednisolone Acetate (Inducers of CYP3A4, such as St. John's Wort preparations (Hypericum perforatum), phenobarbital, carbamazepine, and rifampin, may reduce plasma concentrations of estrogens, possibly resulting in a decrease in therapeutic effects and/or changes in the uterine bleeding profile). Products include:

Blephamide Ophthalmic Ointment 568
Blephamide Ophthalmic
Suspension......................... 569
Poly-Pred Ophthalmic
Suspension......................... ⊙233
Pred Forte Ophthalmic
Suspension......................... ⊙235
Pred Mild Ophthalmic
Suspension......................... ⊙238
Pred-G Ophthalmic Ointment ⊙237
Pred-G Ophthalmic Suspension ⊙236

Prednisolone Sodium Phosphate (Inducers of CYP3A4, such as St. John's Wort preparations (Hypericum perforatum), phenobarbital, carbamazepine, and rifampin, may reduce plasma concentrations of estrogens, possibly resulting in a decrease in therapeutic effects and/or changes in the uterine bleeding profile).

No products indexed under this heading.

Prednisolone Tebutate (Inducers of CYP3A4, such as St. John's Wort preparations (Hypericum perforatum), phenobarbital, carbamazepine, and rifampin, may reduce plasma concentrations of estrogens, possibly resulting in a decrease in therapeutic effects and/or changes in the uterine bleeding profile).

No products indexed under this heading.

Prednisone (Inducers of CYP3A4, such as St. John's Wort preparations (Hypericum perforatum), phenobarbital, carbamazepine, and rifampin, may reduce plasma concentrations of estrogens, possibly resulting in a decrease in therapeutic effects and/or changes in the uterine bleeding profile).

No products indexed under this heading.

Primidone (Inducers of CYP3A4, such as St. John's Wort preparations (Hypericum perforatum), phenobarbital, carbamazepine, and rifampin, may reduce plasma concentrations of estrogens, possibly resulting in a decrease in therapeutic effects and/or changes in the uterine bleeding profile).

No products indexed under this heading.

Propoxyphene Hydrochloride (Inhibitors of CYP3A4 such as erythromycin, clarithromycin, ketoconazole, itraconazole, ritonavir and grapefruit juice may increase plasma concentrations of estrogens and may result in side effects).

No products indexed under this heading.

Propoxyphene Napsylate (Inhibitors of CYP3A4 such as erythromycin, clarithromycin, ketoconazole, itraconazole, ritonavir and grapefruit juice may increase plasma concentrations of estrogens and may result in side effects).
No products indexed under this heading.

Quinapril Hydrochloride (There is potential for an increase in serum potassium in women taking drospirenone with other drugs that may affect electrolytes).
No products indexed under this heading.

Quinidine (Inhibitors of CYP3A4 such as erythromycin, clarithromycin, ketoconazole, itraconazole, ritonavir and grapefruit juice may increase plasma concentrations of estrogens and may result in side effects).
No products indexed under this heading.

Quinidine Hydrochloride (Inhibitors of CYP3A4 such as erythromycin, clarithromycin, ketoconazole, itraconazole, ritonavir and grapefruit juice may increase plasma concentrations of estrogens and may result in side effects).
No products indexed under this heading.

Quinidine Polygalacturonate (Inhibitors of CYP3A4 such as erythromycin, clarithromycin, ketoconazole, itraconazole, ritonavir and grapefruit juice may increase plasma concentrations of estrogens and may result in side effects).
No products indexed under this heading.

Quinidine Sulfate (Inhibitors of CYP3A4 such as erythromycin, clarithromycin, ketoconazole, itraconazole, ritonavir and grapefruit juice may increase plasma concentrations of estrogens and may result in side effects).
No products indexed under this heading.

Quinine (Inhibitors of CYP3A4 such as erythromycin, clarithromycin, ketoconazole, itraconazole, ritonavir and grapefruit juice may increase plasma concentrations of estrogens and may result in side effects).
No products indexed under this heading.

Quinine Sulfate (Inhibitors of CYP3A4 such as erythromycin, clarithromycin, ketoconazole, itraconazole, ritonavir and grapefruit juice may increase plasma concentrations of estrogens and may result in side effects).
No products indexed under this heading.

Quinupristin (Inhibitors of CYP3A4 such as erythromycin, clarithromycin, ketoconazole, itraconazole, ritonavir and grapefruit juice may increase plasma concentrations of estrogens and may result in side effects).
No products indexed under this heading.

Ramipril (There is potential for an increase in serum potassium in women taking drospirenone with other drugs that may affect electrolytes).
Products include:
Altace Capsules 1702

Ranitidine Bismuth Citrate (Inhibitors of CYP3A4 such as erythromycin, clarithromycin, ketoconazole, itraconazole, ritonavir and grapefruit juice may increase plasma concentrations of estrogens and may result in side effects).
No products indexed under this heading.

Ranitidine Hydrochloride (Inhibitors of CYP3A4 such as erythromycin, clarithromycin, ketoconazole, itraconazole, ritonavir and grapefruit juice may increase plasma concentrations of estrogens and may result in side effects). Products include:
Zantac .. 1624
Zantac Injection 1619
Zantac Injection Pharmacy Bulk Package 1622

Rifabutin (Inducers of CYP3A4, such as St. John's Wort preparations (Hypericum perforatum), phenobarbital, carbamazepine, and rifampin, may reduce plasma concentrations of estrogens, possibly resulting in a decrease in therapeutic effects and/or changes in the uterine bleeding profile).
No products indexed under this heading.

Rifampicin (Inducers of CYP3A4, such as St. John's Wort preparations (Hypericum perforatum), phenobarbital, carbamazepine, and rifampin, may reduce plasma concentrations of estrogens, possibly resulting in a decrease in therapeutic effects and/or changes in the uterine bleeding profile).
No products indexed under this heading.

Rifampin (Inducers of CYP3A4, such as St. John's Wort preparations (Hypericum perforatum), phenobarbital, carbamazepine, and rifampin, may reduce plasma concentrations of estrogens, possibly resulting in a decrease in therapeutic effects and/or changes in the uterine bleeding profile).
No products indexed under this heading.

Rifapentine (Inducers of CYP3A4, such as St. John's Wort preparations (Hypericum perforatum), phenobarbital, carbamazepine, and rifampin, may reduce plasma concentrations of estrogens, possibly resulting in a decrease in therapeutic effects and/or changes in the uterine bleeding profile).
No products indexed under this heading.

Ritonavir (Inhibitors of CYP3A4 such as erythromycin, clarithromycin, ketoconazole, itraconazole, ritonavir and grapefruit juice may increase plasma concentrations of estrogens and may result in side effects). Products include:
Kaletra .. 476
Norvir ... 503

Rofecoxib (There is potential for an increase in serum potassium in women taking drospirenone with other drugs that may affect electrolytes).
No products indexed under this heading.

Saquinavir (Inhibitors of CYP3A4 such as erythromycin, clarithromycin, ketoconazole, itraconazole, ritonavir and grapefruit juice may increase plasma concentrations of estrogens and may result in side effects).
No products indexed under this heading.

Saquinavir Mesylate (Inhibitors of CYP3A4 such as erythromycin, clarithromycin, ketoconazole, itraconazole, ritonavir and grapefruit juice may increase plasma concentrations of estrogens and may result in side effects). Products include:
Invirase 2772

Sertraline Hydrochloride (Inhibitors of CYP3A4 such as erythromycin, clarithromycin, ketoconazole, itraconazole, ritonavir and grapefruit juice may increase plasma concentrations of estrogens and may result in side effects). Products include:
Zoloft .. 2586

Spirapril Hydrochloride (There is potential for an increase in serum potassium in women taking drospirenone with other drugs that may affect electrolytes).
No products indexed under this heading.

Sulfinpyrazone (Inducers of CYP3A4, such as St. John's Wort preparations (Hypericum perforatum), phenobarbital, carbamazepine, and rifampin, may reduce plasma concentrations of estrogens, possibly resulting in a decrease in therapeutic effects and/or changes in the uterine bleeding profile).
No products indexed under this heading.

Sulindac (There is potential for an increase in serum potassium in women taking drospirenone with other drugs that may affect electrolytes). Products include:
Clinoril Tablets 1924

Telithromycin (Inhibitors of CYP3A4 such as erythromycin, clarithromycin, ketoconazole, itraconazole, ritonavir and grapefruit juice may increase plasma concentrations of estrogens and may result in side effects). Products include:
Ketek Tablets 2903

Telmisartan (There is potential for an increase in serum potassium in women taking drospirenone with other drugs that may affect electrolytes). Products include:
Micardis Tablets 854
Micardis HCT Tablets 856

Theophylline (Inducers of CYP3A4, such as St. John's Wort preparations (Hypericum perforatum), phenobarbital, carbamazepine, and rifampin, may reduce plasma concentrations of estrogens, possibly resulting in a decrease in therapeutic effects and/or changes in the uterine bleeding profile).
No products indexed under this heading.

Tolmetin Sodium (There is potential for an increase in serum potassium in women taking drospirenone with other drugs that may affect electrolytes).
No products indexed under this heading.

Trandolapril (There is potential for an increase in serum potassium in women taking drospirenone with other drugs that may affect electrolytes). Products include:
Mavik Tablets 486
Tarka Tablets 524

Triamcinolone (Inducers of CYP3A4, such as St. John's Wort preparations (Hypericum perforatum), phenobarbital, carbamazepine, and rifampin, may reduce plasma concentrations of estrogens, possibly resulting in a decrease in therapeutic effects and/or changes in the uterine bleeding profile).
No products indexed under this heading.

Triamcinolone Acetonide (Inducers of CYP3A4, such as St. John's Wort preparations (Hypericum perforatum), phenobarbital, carbamazepine, and rifampin, may reduce plasma concentrations of estrogens, possibly resulting in a decrease in therapeutic effects and/or changes in the uterine bleeding profile). Products include:
Azmacort Inhalation Aerosol 1726
Nasacort AQ Nasal Spray 2922

Triamcinolone Diacetate (Inducers of CYP3A4, such as St. John's Wort preparations (Hypericum perforatum), phenobarbital, carbamazepine, and rifampin, may reduce plasma concentrations of estrogens, possibly resulting in a decrease in therapeutic effects and/or changes in the uterine bleeding profile).
No products indexed under this heading.

Triamcinolone Hexacetonide (Inducers of CYP3A4, such as St. John's Wort preparations (Hypericum perforatum), phenobarbital, carbamazepine, and rifampin, may reduce plasma concentrations of estrogens, possibly resulting in a decrease in therapeutic effects and/or changes in the uterine bleeding profile).
No products indexed under this heading.

Troglitazone (Inhibitors of CYP3A4 such as erythromycin, clarithromycin, ketoconazole, itraconazole, ritonavir and grapefruit juice may increase plasma concentrations of estrogens and may result in side effects).
No products indexed under this heading.

Troleandomycin (Inhibitors of CYP3A4 such as erythromycin, clarithromycin, ketoconazole, itraconazole, ritonavir and grapefruit juice may increase plasma concentrations of estrogens and may result in side effects).
No products indexed under this heading.

Valdecoxib (There is potential for an increase in serum potassium in women taking drospirenone with other drugs that may affect electrolytes).
No products indexed under this heading.

Valproate Sodium (Inhibitors of CYP3A4 such as erythromycin, clarithromycin, ketoconazole, itraconazole, ritonavir and grapefruit juice may increase plasma concentrations of estrogens and may result in side effects). Products include:
Depacon Injection 412

Valsartan (There is potential for an increase in serum potassium in women taking drospirenone with other drugs that may affect electrolytes). Products include:
Diovan Tablets 2193
Diovan HCT Tablets 2196

Verapamil Hydrochloride (Inhibitors of CYP3A4 such as erythromycin, clarithromycin, ketoconazole, itraconazole, ritonavir and grapefruit juice may increase plasma concentrations of estrogens and may result in side effects). Products include:

Covera-HS Tablets 3139
Tarka Tablets 524
Verelan PM Extended-Release Capsules, Controlled-Onset 3106

Voriconazole (Inhibitors of CYP3A4 such as erythromycin, clarithromycin, ketoconazole, itraconazole, ritonavir and grapefruit juice may increase plasma concentrations of estrogens and may result in side effects). Products include:

VFEND I.V. 2564
VFEND Oral Suspension 2564
VFEND Tablets 2564

Zafirlukast (Inhibitors of CYP3A4 such as erythromycin, clarithromycin, ketoconazole, itraconazole, ritonavir and grapefruit juice may increase plasma concentrations of estrogens and may result in side effects). Products include:

Accolate Tablets 671

Zileuton (Inhibitors of CYP3A4 such as erythromycin, clarithromycin, ketoconazole, itraconazole, ritonavir and grapefruit juice may increase plasma concentrations of estrogens and may result in side effects). Products include:

Zyflo Tablets 1023

Food Interactions

Grapefruit (Inhibitors of CYP3A4 such as erythromycin, clarithromycin, ketoconazole, itraconazole, ritonavir and grapefruit juice may increase plasma concentrations of estrogens and may result in side effects).

Grapefruit Juice (Inhibitors of CYP3A4 such as erythromycin, clarithromycin, ketoconazole, itraconazole, ritonavir and grapefruit juice may increase plasma concentrations of estrogens and may result in side effects).

ANIMI-3 CAPSULES

(Docosahexaenoic Acid (DHA), EPA (Eicosapentaenoic Acid), Folic Acid, Vitamin B_{12}, Vitamin B_6) 2492
None cited in PDR database.

ANTIVENIN (BLACK WIDOW SPIDER ANTIVENIN)

(Black Widow Spider Antivenin (Equine)) 1913
None cited in PDR database.

ANTIVENIN (MICRURUS FULVIUS)

(Antivenin (Micrurus Fulvius)) 3407
May interact with beta blockers and narcotic analgesics. Compounds in these categories include:

Acebutolol Hydrochloride (Co-administration with beta-adrenergic blockers has been associated with an increased severity of acute anaphylaxis; anaphylaxis may be resistant and prolonged; altered or larger than usual doses of epinephrine may be required to treat anaphylaxis).

No products indexed under this heading.

Alfentanil Hydrochloride (Co-administration with drugs that depress respiration, such as narcotic analgesics, are contraindicated).

No products indexed under this heading.

Atenolol (Co-administration with beta-adrenergic blockers has been associated with an increased severity of acute anaphylaxis; anaphylaxis may be resistant and prolonged; altered or larger than usual doses of epinephrine may be required to treat anaphylaxis).

No products indexed under this heading.

Betaxolol Hydrochloride (Co-administration with beta-adrenergic blockers has been associated with an increased severity of acute anaphylaxis; anaphylaxis may be resistant and prolonged; altered or larger than usual doses of epinephrine may be required to treat anaphylaxis). Products include:

Betoptic S Ophthalmic Suspension 558

Bisoprolol Fumarate (Co-administration with beta-adrenergic blockers has been associated with an increased severity of acute anaphylaxis; anaphylaxis may be resistant and prolonged; altered or larger than usual doses of epinephrine may be required to treat anaphylaxis).

No products indexed under this heading.

Buprenorphine Hydrochloride (Co-administration with drugs that depress respiration, such as narcotic analgesics, are contraindicated). Products include:

Buprenex Injectable 2716
Suboxone Tablets 2717
Subutex Tablets 2717

Carteolol Hydrochloride (Co-administration with beta-adrenergic blockers has been associated with an increased severity of acute anaphylaxis; anaphylaxis may be resistant and prolonged; altered or larger than usual doses of epinephrine may be required to treat anaphylaxis). Products include:

Carteolol Hydrochloride Ophthalmic Solution USP, 1% .... ⊙249

Codeine Phosphate (Co-administration with drugs that depress respiration, such as narcotic analgesics, are contraindicated). Products include:

Tylenol with Codeine Tablets 2391

Dezocine (Co-administration with drugs that depress respiration, such as narcotic analgesics, are contraindicated).

No products indexed under this heading.

Esmolol Hydrochloride (Co-administration with beta-adrenergic blockers has been associated with an increased severity of acute anaphylaxis; anaphylaxis may be resistant and prolonged; altered or larger than usual doses of epinephrine may be required to treat anaphylaxis).

No products indexed under this heading.

Fentanyl (Co-administration with drugs that depress respiration, such as narcotic analgesics, are contraindicated). Products include:

Duragesic Transdermal System 2373
Ionsys Transdermal System 2379

Fentanyl Citrate (Co-administration with drugs that depress respiration, such as narcotic analgesics, are contraindicated). Products include:

Actiq 979

Hydrocodone Bitartrate (Co-administration with drugs that depress respiration, such as narcotic analgesics, are contraindicated). Products include:

Hycodan 1116
Hycotuss Expectorant Syrup 1117
Vicodin Tablets 535
Vicodin ES Tablets 536
Vicodin HP Tablets 538
Vicoprofen Tablets 539
Zydone Tablets 1139

Hydrocodone Polistirex (Co-administration with drugs that depress respiration, such as narcotic analgesics, are contraindicated). Products include:

Tussionex Pennkinetic Extended-Release Suspension 3327

Hydromorphone Hydrochloride (Co-administration with drugs that depress respiration, such as narcotic analgesics, are contraindicated). Products include:

Dilaudid 440
Dilaudid Non-Sterile Powder 440
Dilaudid Oral Liquid 445
Dilaudid Rectal Suppositories 440
Dilaudid Tablets 440
Dilaudid Tablets - 8 mg 445
Dilaudid-HP 442

Labetalol Hydrochloride (Co-administration with beta-adrenergic blockers has been associated with an increased severity of acute anaphylaxis; anaphylaxis may be resistant and prolonged; altered or larger than usual doses of epinephrine may be required to treat anaphylaxis).

No products indexed under this heading.

Levobunolol Hydrochloride (Co-administration with beta-adrenergic blockers has been associated with an increased severity of acute anaphylaxis; anaphylaxis may be resistant and prolonged; altered or larger than usual doses of epinephrine may be required to treat anaphylaxis). Products include:

Betagan Ophthalmic Solution, USP .... ⊙220

Levorphanol Tartrate (Co-administration with drugs that depress respiration, such as narcotic analgesics, are contraindicated).

No products indexed under this heading.

Meperidine Hydrochloride (Co-administration with drugs that depress respiration, such as narcotic analgesics, are contraindicated).

No products indexed under this heading.

Methadone Hydrochloride (Co-administration with drugs that depress respiration, such as narcotic analgesics, are contraindicated).

No products indexed under this heading.

Metipranolol Hydrochloride (Co-administration with beta-adrenergic blockers has been associated with an increased severity of acute anaphylaxis; anaphylaxis may be resistant and prolonged; altered or larger than usual doses of epinephrine may be required to treat anaphylaxis).

No products indexed under this heading.

Metoprolol Succinate (Co-administration with beta-adrenergic blockers has been associated with an increased severity of acute anaphylaxis; anaphylaxis may be resistant and prolonged; altered or larger than usual doses of epinephrine may be required to treat anaphylaxis). Products include:

Toprol-XL Tablets 668

Metoprolol Tartrate (Co-administration with beta-adrenergic blockers has been associated with an increased severity of acute anaphylaxis; anaphylaxis may be resistant and prolonged; altered or larger than usual doses of epinephrine may be required to treat anaphylaxis). Products include:

Lopressor Injection 2238
Lopressor Tablets 2238
Lopressor HCT 50/25 Tablets 2241
Lopressor HCT 100/25 Tablets 2241
Lopressor HCT 100/50 Tablets 2241

Morphine Sulfate (Co-administration with drugs that depress respiration, such as narcotic analgesics, are contraindicated). Products include:

Avinza Capsules 1741
Kadian Capsules 577
MS Contin Tablets 2701

Nadolol (Co-administration with beta-adrenergic blockers has been associated with an increased severity of acute anaphylaxis; anaphylaxis may be resistant and prolonged; altered or larger than usual doses of epinephrine may be required to treat anaphylaxis). Products include:

Nadolol Tablets 2159

Oxycodone Hydrochloride (Co-administration with drugs that depress respiration, such as narcotic analgesics, are contraindicated). Products include:

OxyContin Tablets 2703
OxyFast Oral Concentrate Solution 2708
OxyIR Capsules 2708
Percocet Tablets 1131
Percodan Tablets 1132

Penbutolol Sulfate (Co-administration with beta-adrenergic blockers has been associated with an increased severity of acute anaphylaxis; anaphylaxis may be resistant and prolonged; altered or larger than usual doses of epinephrine may be required to treat anaphylaxis).

No products indexed under this heading.

Pindolol (Co-administration with beta-adrenergic blockers has been associated with an increased severity of acute anaphylaxis; anaphylaxis may be resistant and prolonged; altered or larger than usual doses of epinephrine may be required to treat anaphylaxis).

No products indexed under this heading.

Propoxyphene Hydrochloride (Co-administration with drugs that depress respiration, such as narcotic analgesics, are contraindicated).

No products indexed under this heading.

Propoxyphene Napsylate (Co-administration with drugs that depress respiration, such as narcotic analgesics, are contraindicated).

No products indexed under this heading.

Propranolol Hydrochloride (Co-administration with beta-adrenergic blockers has been associated with an increased severity of acute anaphylaxis; anaphylaxis may be resistant and prolonged; altered or larger than usual doses of epinephrine may be required to treat anaphylaxis). Products include:

Inderal LA Long-Acting Capsules 3429
InnoPran XL Capsules 2723

Remifentanil Hydrochloride (Co-administration with drugs that depress respiration, such as narcotic analgesics, are contraindicated).
No products indexed under this heading.

Sotalol Hydrochloride (Co-administration with beta-adrenergic blockers has been associated with an increased severity of acute anaphylaxis; anaphylaxis may be resistant and prolonged; altered or larger than usual doses of epinephrine may be required to treat anaphylaxis).
No products indexed under this heading.

Sufentanil Citrate (Co-administration with drugs that depress respiration, such as narcotic analgesics, are contraindicated).
No products indexed under this heading.

Timolol Hemihydrate (Co-administration with beta-adrenergic blockers has been associated with an increased severity of acute anaphylaxis; anaphylaxis may be resistant and prolonged; altered or larger than usual doses of epinephrine may be required to treat anaphylaxis).
Products include:
Betimol Ophthalmic Solution **3382**
Betimol Ophthalmic Solution .... ⊙**295**

Timolol Maleate (Co-administration with beta-adrenergic blockers has been associated with an increased severity of acute anaphylaxis; anaphylaxis may be resistant and prolonged; altered or larger than usual doses of epinephrine may be required to treat anaphylaxis).
Products include:
Blocadren Tablets **1916**
Cosopt Sterile Ophthalmic Solution.. **1931**
Timolide Tablets **2086**
Timoptic Sterile Ophthalmic Solution.. **2088**
Timoptic in Ocudose **2091**
Timoptic-XE Sterile Ophthalmic Gel Forming Solution.................. **2092**

ANTIVENIN POLYVALENT

(Antivenin (Crotalidae) Polyvalent) **3405**
May interact with beta blockers. Compounds in these categories include:

Acebutolol Hydrochloride (Co-administration with beta-adrenergic blockers has been associated with an increased severity of acute anaphylaxis; anaphylaxis may be resistant and prolonged; altered or larger than usual doses of epinephrine may be required to treat anaphylaxis).
No products indexed under this heading.

Atenolol (Co-administration with beta-adrenergic blockers has been associated with an increased severity of acute anaphylaxis; anaphylaxis may be resistant and prolonged; altered or larger than usual doses of epinephrine may be required to treat anaphylaxis).
No products indexed under this heading.

Betaxolol Hydrochloride (Co-administration with beta-adrenergic blockers has been associated with an increased severity of acute anaphylaxis; anaphylaxis may be resistant and prolonged; altered or larger than usual doses of epinephrine may be required to treat anaphylaxis).
Products include:
Betoptic S Ophthalmic Suspension.................................. **558**

Bisoprolol Fumarate (Co-administration with beta-adrenergic blockers has been associated with an increased severity of acute anaphylaxis; anaphylaxis may be resistant and prolonged; altered or larger than usual doses of epinephrine may be required to treat anaphylaxis).
No products indexed under this heading.

Carteolol Hydrochloride (Co-administration with beta-adrenergic blockers has been associated with an increased severity of acute anaphylaxis; anaphylaxis may be resistant and prolonged; altered or larger than usual doses of epinephrine may be required to treat anaphylaxis).
Products include:
Carteolol Hydrochloride Ophthalmic Solution USP, 1%....... ⊙**249**

Esmolol Hydrochloride (Co-administration with beta-adrenergic blockers has been associated with an increased severity of acute anaphylaxis; anaphylaxis may be resistant and prolonged; altered or larger than usual doses of epinephrine may be required to treat anaphylaxis).
No products indexed under this heading.

Labetalol Hydrochloride (Co-administration with beta-adrenergic blockers has been associated with an increased severity of acute anaphylaxis; anaphylaxis may be resistant and prolonged; altered or larger than usual doses of epinephrine may be required to treat anaphylaxis).
No products indexed under this heading.

Levobunolol Hydrochloride (Co-administration with beta-adrenergic blockers has been associated with an increased severity of acute anaphylaxis; anaphylaxis may be resistant and prolonged; altered or larger than usual doses of epinephrine may be required to treat anaphylaxis).
Products include:
Betagan Ophthalmic Solution, USP.. ⊙**220**

Metipranolol Hydrochloride (Co-administration with beta-adrenergic blockers has been associated with an increased severity of acute anaphylaxis; anaphylaxis may be resistant and prolonged; altered or larger than usual doses of epinephrine may be required to treat anaphylaxis).
No products indexed under this heading.

Metoprolol Succinate (Co-administration with beta-adrenergic blockers has been associated with an increased severity of acute anaphylaxis; anaphylaxis may be resistant and prolonged; altered or larger than usual doses of epinephrine may be required to treat anaphylaxis).
Products include:
Toprol-XL Tablets **668**

Metoprolol Tartrate (Co-administration with beta-adrenergic blockers has been associated with an increased severity of acute anaphylaxis; anaphylaxis may be resistant and prolonged; altered or larger than usual doses of epinephrine may be required to treat anaphylaxis).
Products include:
Lopressor Injection **2238**
Lopressor Tablets **2238**
Lopressor HCT 50/25 Tablets **2241**
Lopressor HCT 100/25 Tablets **2241**
Lopressor HCT 100/50 Tablets **2241**

Nadolol (Co-administration with beta-adrenergic blockers has been associated with an increased severity of acute anaphylaxis; anaphylaxis may be resistant and prolonged; altered or larger than usual doses of epinephrine may be required to treat anaphylaxis). Products include:
Nadolol Tablets **2159**

Penbutolol Sulfate (Co-administration with beta-adrenergic blockers has been associated with an increased severity of acute anaphylaxis; anaphylaxis may be resistant and prolonged; altered or larger than usual doses of epinephrine may be required to treat anaphylaxis).
No products indexed under this heading.

Pindolol (Co-administration with beta-adrenergic blockers has been associated with an increased severity of acute anaphylaxis; anaphylaxis may be resistant and prolonged; altered or larger than usual doses of epinephrine may be required to treat anaphylaxis).
No products indexed under this heading.

Propranolol Hydrochloride (Co-administration with beta-adrenergic blockers has been associated with an increased severity of acute anaphylaxis; anaphylaxis may be resistant and prolonged; altered or larger than usual doses of epinephrine may be required to treat anaphylaxis).
Products include:
Inderal LA Long-Acting Capsules **3429**
InnoPran XL Capsules **2723**

Sotalol Hydrochloride (Co-administration with beta-adrenergic blockers has been associated with an increased severity of acute anaphylaxis; anaphylaxis may be resistant and prolonged; altered or larger than usual doses of epinephrine may be required to treat anaphylaxis).
No products indexed under this heading.

Timolol Hemihydrate (Co-administration with beta-adrenergic blockers has been associated with an increased severity of acute anaphylaxis; anaphylaxis may be resistant and prolonged; altered or larger than usual doses of epinephrine may be required to treat anaphylaxis).
Products include:
Betimol Ophthalmic Solution **3382**
Betimol Ophthalmic Solution .... ⊙**295**

Timolol Maleate (Co-administration with beta-adrenergic blockers has been associated with an increased severity of acute anaphylaxis; anaphylaxis may be resistant and prolonged; altered or larger than usual doses of epinephrine may be required to treat anaphylaxis).
Products include:
Blocadren Tablets **1916**
Cosopt Sterile Ophthalmic Solution.. **1931**
Timolide Tablets **2086**
Timoptic Sterile Ophthalmic Solution.. **2088**
Timoptic in Ocudose **2091**
Timoptic-XE Sterile Ophthalmic Gel Forming Solution.................. **2092**

ANZEMET INJECTION

(Dolasetron Mesylate) **2859**
See Anzemet Tablets

ANZEMET TABLETS

(Dolasetron Mesylate) **2862**
May interact with:

Atenolol (Decreases hydrodolasetron clearance by 27%).
No products indexed under this heading.

Cimetidine (Co-administration of dolasetron with cimetidine, a nonselective inhibitor of CYP450, has resulted in increased blood levels of dolasetron by 24%). Products include:
Tagamet HB 200 Tablets .... ▣**664**

Cimetidine Hydrochloride (Co-administration of dolasetron with cimetidine, a nonselective inhibitor of CYP450, has resulted in increased blood levels of dolasetron by 24%).
No products indexed under this heading.

Rifampin (Co-administration of dolasetron with rifampin, a potent inducer of CYP450, has resulted in decreased blood levels of dolasetron by 28%).
No products indexed under this heading.

APEXICON E CREAM

(Diflorasone Diacetate) **2661**
None cited in PDR database.

APIDRA INJECTION

(Insulin Glulisine) **2864**
May interact with ACE inhibitors, atypical antipsychotics, beta blockers, corticosteroids, diuretics, estrogens, fibrates, oral hypoglycemic agents, lithium preparations, monoamine oxidase inhibitors, phenothiazines, progestins, protease inhibitors, salicylates, sulfonamides, sympathomimetics, thyroid preparations, and certain other agents. Compounds in these categories include:

Acarbose (Oral antidiabetic products may increase the blood glucose-lowering effect and susceptibility to hypoglycemia of insulin).
Products include:
Precose Tablets **751**

Acebutolol Hydrochloride (Beta-blockers may either potentiate or weaken the blood glucose-lowering effect of insulin and reduce or hide the signs of hypoglycemia).
No products indexed under this heading.

Albuterol (Sympathomimetic agents may reduce the blood glucose-lowering effect of insulin).
Products include:
Proventil Inhalation Aerosol **3053**

Albuterol Sulfate (Sympathomimetic agents may reduce the blood glucose-lowering effect of insulin).
Products include:
AccuNeb Inhalation Solution **1055**
Combivent Inhalation Aerosol **847**
DuoNeb Inhalation Solution **1058**
ProAir HFA Inhalation Aerosol **3300**
Proventil Inhalation Solution 0.083%....................................... **3055**
Proventil HFA Inhalation Aerosol....... **3056**
Ventolin HFA Inhalation Aerosol **1600**
VoSpire ER Tablets **1052**

Amiloride Hydrochloride (Diuretics may reduce the blood glucose-lowering effect of insulin). Products include:
Midamor Tablets **2026**
Moduretic Tablets **2028**

IMPORTANT NOTE: Always consult each drug listing in the patient's regimen for possible interactions.

Amprenavir (Protease inhibitors may reduce the blood glucose-lowering effect of insulin). Products include:
- Agenerase Capsules 1327
- Agenerase Oral Solution 1332

Aripiprazole (Atypical antipsychotics may reduce the blood glucose-lowering effect of insulin). Products include:
- Abilify Oral Solution 882
- Abilify Oral Solution 2450
- Abilify Discmelt Orally Disintegrating Tablets 882
- Abilify Discmelt Orally Disintegrating Tablets 2450
- Abilify Tablets 882
- Abilify Tablets 2450

Aspirin (Salicylates may increase the blood glucose-lowering effect and susceptibility to hypoglycemia of insulin). Products include:
- Aggrenox Capsules 822
- Bayer Aspirin 744
- BC Allergy Sinus Cold Powder .... ■677
- BC Headache Powder .... ■677
- Arthritis Strength BC Powder .... ■677
- BC Sinus Cold Powder .... ■677
- Excedrin Extra Strength Caplets/Tablets/Geltabs .... ■684
- Excedrin Migraine Caplets/Tablets/Geltabs .... ■609
- Goody's Body Pain Formula Powder .... ■684
- Goody's Extra Strength Headache Powders .... ■611
- Goody's Extra Strength Pain Relief Tablets .... ■685
- Percodan Tablets 1132
- St. Joseph 81 mg Aspirin Chewable and Enteric Coated Tablets 1869

Aspirin, Enteric Coated (Salicylates may increase the blood glucose-lowering effect and susceptibility to hypoglycemia of insulin).
No products indexed under this heading.

Aspirin Buffered (Salicylates may increase the blood glucose-lowering effect and susceptibility to hypoglycemia of insulin). Products include:
- Bufferin Extra Strength Tablets .... ■678
- Bufferin Regular Strength Tablets ... ■678

Atenolol (Beta-blockers may either potentiate or weaken the blood glucose-lowering effect of insulin and reduce or hide the signs of hypoglycemia).
No products indexed under this heading.

Benazepril Hydrochloride (ACE inhibitors may increase the blood glucose-lowering effect and susceptibility to hypoglycemia of insulin). Products include:
- Lotensin Tablets 2243
- Lotensin HCT Tablets 2246
- Lotrel Capsules 2249

Bendroflumethiazide (Diuretics may reduce the blood glucose-lowering effect of insulin).
No products indexed under this heading.

Betamethasone Acetate (Corticosteroids may reduce the blood glucose-lowering effect of insulin).
No products indexed under this heading.

Betamethasone Sodium Phosphate (Corticosteroids may reduce the blood glucose-lowering effect of insulin).
No products indexed under this heading.

Betaxolol Hydrochloride (Beta-blockers may either potentiate or weaken the blood glucose-lowering effect of insulin and reduce or hide the signs of hypoglycemia). Products include:
- Betoptic S Ophthalmic Suspension 558

Bisoprolol Fumarate (Beta-blockers may either potentiate or weaken the blood glucose-lowering effect of insulin and reduce or hide the signs of hypoglycemia).
No products indexed under this heading.

Bumetanide (Diuretics may reduce the blood glucose-lowering effect of insulin). Products include:
- Bumex Tablets 2746

Captopril (ACE inhibitors may increase the blood glucose-lowering effect and susceptibility to hypoglycemia of insulin). Products include:
- Captopril Tablets 2149

Carteolol Hydrochloride (Beta-blockers may either potentiate or weaken the blood glucose-lowering effect of insulin and reduce or hide the signs of hypoglycemia). Products include:
- Carteolol Hydrochloride Ophthalmic Solution USP, 1% .... ⊙249

Chlorothiazide (Diuretics may reduce the blood glucose-lowering effect of insulin). Products include:
- Diuril Oral Suspension 1954

Chlorothiazide Sodium (Diuretics may reduce the blood glucose-lowering effect of insulin). Products include:
- Diuril Sodium Intravenous 2467

Chlorotrianisene (Estrogens may reduce the blood glucose-lowering effect of insulin).
No products indexed under this heading.

Chlorpromazine (Phenothiazine derivatives may reduce the blood glucose-lowering effect of insulin).
No products indexed under this heading.

Chlorpromazine Hydrochloride (Phenothiazine derivatives may reduce the blood glucose-lowering effect of insulin).
No products indexed under this heading.

Chlorpropamide (Oral antidiabetic products may increase the blood glucose-lowering effect and susceptibility to hypoglycemia of insulin).
No products indexed under this heading.

Chlorthalidone (Diuretics may reduce the blood glucose-lowering effect of insulin). Products include:
- Clorpres Tablets 2153

Choline Magnesium Trisalicylate (Salicylates may increase the blood glucose-lowering effect and susceptibility to hypoglycemia of insulin).
No products indexed under this heading.

Clofibrate (Fibrates may increase the blood glucose-lowering effect and susceptibility to hypoglycemia of insulin).
No products indexed under this heading.

Clonidine (Clonidine may either potentiate or weaken the blood glucose-lowering effect of insulin and reduce or hide the signs of hypoglycemia). Products include:
- Catapres-TTS 844

Clonidine Hydrochloride (Clonidine may either potentiate or weaken the blood glucose-lowering effect of insulin and reduce or hide the signs of hypoglycemia). Products include:
- Catapres Tablets 843
- Clorpres Tablets 2153

Clozapine (Atypical antipsychotics may reduce the blood glucose-lowering effect of insulin). Products include:
- Clozaril Tablets 2184
- FazaClo Orally Disintegrating Tablets 551

Cortisone Acetate (Corticosteroids may reduce the blood glucose-lowering effect of insulin).
No products indexed under this heading.

Danazol (Danazol may reduce the blood glucose-lowering effect of insulin).
No products indexed under this heading.

Desogestrel (Progestogens may reduce the blood glucose-lowering effect of insulin). Products include:
- Mircette Tablets 1066

Dexamethasone (Corticosteroids may reduce the blood glucose-lowering effect of insulin). Products include:
- Ciprodex Otic Suspension 559
- Decadron Tablets 1951
- TobraDex Ophthalmic Ointment 562
- TobraDex Ophthalmic Suspension ... 563

Dexamethasone Acetate (Corticosteroids may reduce the blood glucose-lowering effect of insulin).
No products indexed under this heading.

Dexamethasone Sodium Phosphate (Corticosteroids may reduce the blood glucose-lowering effect of insulin).
No products indexed under this heading.

Diazoxide (Diazoxide may reduce the blood glucose-lowering effect of insulin). Products include:
- Hyperstat I.V. 3017

Dienestrol (Estrogens may reduce the blood glucose-lowering effect of insulin).
No products indexed under this heading.

Diethylstilbestrol (Estrogens may reduce the blood glucose-lowering effect of insulin).
No products indexed under this heading.

Diflunisal (Salicylates may increase the blood glucose-lowering effect and susceptibility to hypoglycemia of insulin). Products include:
- Dolobid Tablets 1955

Disopyramide (Disopyramide may increase the blood glucose-lowering effect and susceptibility to hypoglycemia of insulin).
No products indexed under this heading.

Disopyramide Phosphate (Disopyramide may increase the blood glucose-lowering effect and susceptibility to hypoglycemia of insulin).
No products indexed under this heading.

Dobutamine Hydrochloride (Sympathomimetic agents may reduce the blood glucose-lowering effect of insulin).
No products indexed under this heading.

Dopamine Hydrochloride (Sympathomimetic agents may reduce the blood glucose-lowering effect of insulin).
No products indexed under this heading.

Enalapril Maleate (ACE inhibitors may increase the blood glucose-lowering effect and susceptibility to hypoglycemia of insulin). Products include:
- Vasotec I.V. Injection 2103

Enalaprilat (ACE inhibitors may increase the blood glucose-lowering effect and susceptibility to hypoglycemia of insulin).
No products indexed under this heading.

Ephedrine Hydrochloride (Sympathomimetic agents may reduce the blood glucose-lowering effect of insulin).
No products indexed under this heading.

Ephedrine Sulfate (Sympathomimetic agents may reduce the blood glucose-lowering effect of insulin).
No products indexed under this heading.

Ephedrine Tannate (Sympathomimetic agents may reduce the blood glucose-lowering effect of insulin).
No products indexed under this heading.

Epinephrine (Sympathomimetic agents may reduce the blood glucose-lowering effect of insulin). Products include:
- EpiPen 1061
- Primatene Mist .... ■719
- Twinject 0.15 3379
- Twinject 0.3 3378

Epinephrine Bitartrate (Sympathomimetic agents may reduce the blood glucose-lowering effect of insulin).
No products indexed under this heading.

Epinephrine Hydrochloride (Sympathomimetic agents may reduce the blood glucose-lowering effect of insulin).
No products indexed under this heading.

Esmolol Hydrochloride (Beta-blockers may either potentiate or weaken the blood glucose-lowering effect of insulin and reduce or hide the signs of hypoglycemia).
No products indexed under this heading.

Estradiol (Estrogens may reduce the blood glucose-lowering effect of insulin). Products include:
- Angeliq Tablets 762
- Climara Transdermal System 771
- Climara Pro Transdermal System 776
- Estrasorb Topical Emulsion 1147
- Estring Vaginal Ring 2635
- Menostar Transdermal System 782
- Vagifem Tablets 2334

Estrogens, Conjugated (Estrogens may reduce the blood glucose-lowering effect of insulin). Products include:
- Premarin Intravenous 3442
- Premarin Tablets 3446
- Premarin Vaginal Cream 3452
- Premphase Tablets 3456
- Prempro Tablets 3456

Estrogens, Esterified (Estrogens may reduce the blood glucose-lowering effect of insulin). Products include:
- Estratest Tablets 3199
- Estratest H.S. Tablets 3199

Estropipate (Estrogens may reduce the blood glucose-lowering effect of insulin).
No products indexed under this heading.

Ethacrynic Acid (Diuretics may reduce the blood glucose-lowering effect of insulin). Products include:
Edecrin Tablets 1959

Ethinyl Estradiol (Estrogens may reduce the blood glucose-lowering effect of insulin). Products include:
Mircette Tablets 1066
NuvaRing 2340
Ortho-Cyclen/Ortho Tri-Cyclen 2429
Ortho Evra Transdermal System 2417
Ortho Tri-Cyclen Lo Tablets 2436
Seasonique Tablets 1077
Yasmin 28 Tablets 796
Yaz Tablets 803

Fenofibrate (Fibrates may increase the blood glucose-lowering effect and susceptibility to hypoglycemia of insulin). Products include:
Lofibra Tablets 1219
Lofibra Capsules 1216
Tricor Tablets 527
Triglide Tablets 3123

Fludrocortisone Acetate (Corticosteroids may reduce the blood glucose-lowering effect of insulin).
No products indexed under this heading.

Fluoxetine (Fluoxetine may increase the blood glucose-lowering effect and susceptibility to hypoglycemia of insulin).
No products indexed under this heading.

Fluoxetine Hydrochloride (Fluoxetine may increase the blood glucose-lowering effect and susceptibility to hypoglycemia of insulin). Products include:
Prozac Pulvules and Liquid 1801
Symbyax Capsules 1819

Fluphenazine Decanoate (Phenothiazine derivatives may reduce the blood glucose-lowering effect of insulin).
No products indexed under this heading.

Fluphenazine Enanthate (Phenothiazine derivatives may reduce the blood glucose-lowering effect of insulin).
No products indexed under this heading.

Fluphenazine Hydrochloride (Phenothiazine derivatives may reduce the blood glucose-lowering effect of insulin).
No products indexed under this heading.

Fosinopril Sodium (ACE inhibitors may increase the blood glucose-lowering effect and susceptibility to hypoglycemia of insulin).
No products indexed under this heading.

Furosemide (Diuretics may reduce the blood glucose-lowering effect of insulin). Products include:
Furosemide Tablets 2154

Gemfibrozil (Fibrates may increase the blood glucose-lowering effect and susceptibility to hypoglycemia of insulin).
No products indexed under this heading.

Glimepiride (Oral antidiabetic products may increase the blood glucose-lowering effect and susceptibility to hypoglycemia of insulin). Products include:
Avandaryl Tablets 1379
Duetact Tablets 3226

Glipizide (Oral antidiabetic products may increase the blood glucose-lowering effect and susceptibility to hypoglycemia of insulin).
No products indexed under this heading.

Glucagon (Glucagon may reduce the blood glucose-lowering effect of insulin). Products include:
GlucaGen 761
Glucagon for Injection Vials and Emergency Kit 1778

Glyburide (Oral antidiabetic products may increase the blood glucose-lowering effect and susceptibility to hypoglycemia of insulin).
No products indexed under this heading.

Guanethidine (Under the influence of sympatholytic medicinal products, such as guanethidine, the signs of hypoglycemia may be reduced or absent).
No products indexed under this heading.

Guanethidine Monosulfate (Under the influence of sympatholytic medicinal products, such as guanethidine, the signs of hypoglycemia may be reduced or absent).
No products indexed under this heading.

Guanethidine Sulfate (Under the influence of sympatholytic medicinal products, such as guanethidine, the signs of hypoglycemia may be reduced or absent).
No products indexed under this heading.

Hydrochlorothiazide (Diuretics may reduce the blood glucose-lowering effect of insulin). Products include:
Aldoril Tablets 1910
Atacand HCT 651
Avalide Tablets 888
Avalide Tablets 2874
Benicar HCT Tablets 1044
Diovan HCT Tablets 2196
Dyazide Capsules 1423
Hyzaar 50-12.5 Tablets 1990
Hyzaar 100-12.5 Tablets 1990
Hyzaar 100-25 Tablets 1990
Lopressor HCT 50/25 Tablets 2241
Lopressor HCT 100/25 Tablets 2241
Lopressor HCT 100/50 Tablets 2241
Lotensin HCT Tablets 2246
Micardis HCT Tablets 856
Moduretic Tablets 2028
Prinzide Tablets 2056
Teveten HCT Tablets 1737
Timolide Tablets 2086
Uniretic Tablets 3100

Hydrocortisone (Corticosteroids may reduce the blood glucose-lowering effect of insulin). Products include:
Colocort Rectal Suspension, USP (Retention) 100 mg/60 mL 2476
Hydrocortone Tablets 1989
Preparation H Hydrocortisone Cream 646

Hydrocortisone Acetate (Corticosteroids may reduce the blood glucose-lowering effect of insulin). Products include:
Analpram-HC 1159
Pramosone 1161
ProctoFoam-HC 3099

Hydrocortisone Sodium Phosphate (Corticosteroids may reduce the blood glucose-lowering effect of insulin).
No products indexed under this heading.

Hydrocortisone Sodium Succinate (Corticosteroids may reduce the blood glucose-lowering effect of insulin).
No products indexed under this heading.

Hydroflumethiazide (Diuretics may reduce the blood glucose-lowering effect of insulin).
No products indexed under this heading.

Indapamide (Diuretics may reduce the blood glucose-lowering effect of insulin). Products include:
Indapamide Tablets 2156

Indinavir Sulfate (Protease inhibitors may reduce the blood glucose-lowering effect of insulin). Products include:
Crixivan Capsules 1940

Isocarboxazid (MAO inhibitors may increase the blood glucose-lowering effect and susceptibility to hypoglycemia of insulin).
No products indexed under this heading.

Isoniazid (Isoniazid may reduce the blood glucose-lowering effect of insulin).
No products indexed under this heading.

Isoproterenol Hydrochloride (Sympathomimetic agents may reduce the blood glucose-lowering effect of insulin).
No products indexed under this heading.

Isoproterenol Sulfate (Sympathomimetic agents may reduce the blood glucose-lowering effect of insulin).
No products indexed under this heading.

Labetalol Hydrochloride (Beta-blockers may either potentiate or weaken the blood glucose-lowering effect of insulin and reduce or hide the signs of hypoglycemia).
No products indexed under this heading.

Levalbuterol Hydrochloride (Sympathomimetic agents may reduce the blood glucose-lowering effect of insulin). Products include:
Xopenex Inhalation Solution 3146
Xopenex Inhalation Solution Concentrate 3150

Levobunolol Hydrochloride (Beta-blockers may either potentiate or weaken the blood glucose-lowering effect of insulin and reduce or hide the signs of hypoglycemia). Products include:
Betagan Ophthalmic Solution, USP .... ⊙ 220

Levothyroxine Sodium (Thyroid hormones may reduce the blood glucose-lowering effect of insulin). Products include:
Levothroid Tablets 1186
Levoxyl Tablets 1712
Synthroid Tablets 520
Westhroid Tablets 3403

Liothyronine Sodium (Thyroid hormones may reduce the blood glucose-lowering effect of insulin). Products include:
Cytomel Tablets 1710
Westhroid Tablets 3403

Liotrix (Thyroid hormones may reduce the blood glucose-lowering effect of insulin). Products include:
Thyrolar Tablets 1199

Lisinopril (ACE inhibitors may increase the blood glucose-lowering effect and susceptibility to hypoglycemia of insulin). Products include:
Prinivil Tablets 2052
Prinzide Tablets 2056

Lithium (Lithium salts may either potentiate or weaken the blood-glucose-lowering effect of insulin).
No products indexed under this heading.

Lithium Carbonate (Lithium salts may either potentiate or weaken the blood-glucose-lowering effect of insulin). Products include:
Lithobid Tablets 1692

Lithium Citrate (Lithium salts may either potentiate or weaken the blood-glucose-lowering effect of insulin).
No products indexed under this heading.

Lopinavir (Protease inhibitors may reduce the blood glucose-lowering effect of insulin). Products include:
Kaletra 476

Magnesium Salicylate (Salicylates may increase the blood glucose-lowering effect and susceptibility to hypoglycemia of insulin).
No products indexed under this heading.

Medroxyprogesterone Acetate (Progestogens may reduce the blood glucose-lowering effect of insulin). Products include:
Depo-Provera Contraceptive Injection 2622
depo-subQ provera 104 Injectable Suspension 2624
Premphase Tablets 3456
Prempro Tablets 3456

Megestrol Acetate (Progestogens may reduce the blood glucose-lowering effect of insulin). Products include:
Megace ES Oral Suspension 2481

Mesoridazine Besylate (Phenothiazine derivatives may reduce the blood glucose-lowering effect of insulin).
No products indexed under this heading.

Metaproterenol Sulfate (Sympathomimetic agents may reduce the blood glucose-lowering effect of insulin). Products include:
Alupent Inhalation Aerosol 826

Metaraminol Bitartrate (Sympathomimetic agents may reduce the blood glucose-lowering effect of insulin).
No products indexed under this heading.

Metformin Hydrochloride (Oral antidiabetic products may increase the blood glucose-lowering effect and susceptibility to hypoglycemia of insulin). Products include:
ActoPlus Met Tablets 3214
Avandamet Tablets 1373
Fortamet Extended-Release Tablets 3115

Methotrimeprazine (Phenothiazine derivatives may reduce the blood glucose-lowering effect of insulin).
No products indexed under this heading.

Methoxamine Hydrochloride (Sympathomimetic agents may reduce the blood glucose-lowering effect of insulin).
No products indexed under this heading.

IMPORTANT NOTE: Always consult each drug listing in the patient's regimen for possible interactions.

Methyclothiazide (Diuretics may reduce the blood glucose-lowering effect of insulin).
No products indexed under this heading.

Methylprednisolone Acetate (Corticosteroids may reduce the blood glucose-lowering effect of insulin). Products include:
- Depo-Medrol Injectable Suspension 2617
- Depo-Medrol Single-Dose Vial 2619

Methylprednisolone Sodium Succinate (Corticosteroids may reduce the blood glucose-lowering effect of insulin).
No products indexed under this heading.

Metipranolol Hydrochloride (Beta-blockers may either potentiate or weaken the blood glucose-lowering effect of insulin and reduce or hide the signs of hypoglycemia).
No products indexed under this heading.

Metolazone (Diuretics may reduce the blood glucose-lowering effect of insulin).
No products indexed under this heading.

Metoprolol Succinate (Beta-blockers may either potentiate or weaken the blood glucose-lowering effect of insulin and reduce or hide the signs of hypoglycemia). Products include:
- Toprol-XL Tablets 668

Metoprolol Tartrate (Beta-blockers may either potentiate or weaken the blood glucose-lowering effect of insulin and reduce or hide the signs of hypoglycemia). Products include:
- Lopressor Injection 2238
- Lopressor Tablets 2238
- Lopressor HCT 50/25 Tablets 2241
- Lopressor HCT 100/25 Tablets 2241
- Lopressor HCT 100/50 Tablets 2241

Miglitol (Oral antidiabetic products may increase the blood glucose-lowering effect and susceptibility to hypoglycemia of insulin).
No products indexed under this heading.

Moclobemide (MAO inhibitors may increase the blood glucose-lowering effect and susceptibility to hypoglycemia of insulin).
No products indexed under this heading.

Moexipril Hydrochloride (ACE inhibitors may increase the blood glucose-lowering effect and susceptibility to hypoglycemia of insulin). Products include:
- Uniretic Tablets 3100
- Univasc Tablets 3104

Nadolol (Beta-blockers may either potentiate or weaken the blood glucose-lowering effect of insulin and reduce or hide the signs of hypoglycemia). Products include:
- Nadolol Tablets 2159

Nelfinavir Mesylate (Protease inhibitors may reduce the blood glucose-lowering effect of insulin). Products include:
- Viracept 2577

Norepinephrine Bitartrate (Sympathomimetic agents may reduce the blood glucose-lowering effect of insulin).
No products indexed under this heading.

Norgestimate (Progestogens may reduce the blood glucose-lowering effect of insulin). Products include:
- Ortho-Cyclen/Ortho Tri-Cyclen 2429
- Ortho Tri-Cyclen Lo Tablets 2436

Olanzapine (Atypical antipsychotics may reduce the blood glucose-lowering effect of insulin). Products include:
- Symbyax Capsules 1819
- Zyprexa Tablets 1830
- Zyprexa IntraMuscular 1830
- Zyprexa ZYDIS Orally Disintegrating Tablets 1830

Pargyline Hydrochloride (MAO inhibitors may increase the blood glucose-lowering effect and susceptibility to hypoglycemia of insulin).
No products indexed under this heading.

Penbutolol Sulfate (Beta-blockers may either potentiate or weaken the blood glucose-lowering effect of insulin and reduce or hide the signs of hypoglycemia).
No products indexed under this heading.

Pentamidine Isethionate (Pentamidine may cause hypoglycemia, which may sometimes be followed by hyperglycemia).
No products indexed under this heading.

Pentoxifylline (Pentoxifylline may increase the blood glucose-lowering effect and susceptibility to hypoglycemia of insulin).
No products indexed under this heading.

Perindopril Erbumine (ACE inhibitors may increase the blood glucose-lowering effect and susceptibility to hypoglycemia of insulin). Products include:
- Aceon Tablets (2 mg, 4 mg, 8 mg) 3194

Perphenazine (Phenothiazine derivatives may reduce the blood glucose-lowering effect of insulin).
No products indexed under this heading.

Phenelzine Sulfate (MAO inhibitors may increase the blood glucose-lowering effect and susceptibility to hypoglycemia of insulin).
No products indexed under this heading.

Phenylephrine Bitartrate (Sympathomimetic agents may reduce the blood glucose-lowering effect of insulin).
No products indexed under this heading.

Phenylephrine Hydrochloride (Sympathomimetic agents may reduce the blood glucose-lowering effect of insulin). Products include:
- Comtrex Maximum Strength Non-Drowsy Cold & Cough Caplets .... ▣ 725
- Comtrex Maximum Strength Day/Night Severe Cold & Sinus Caplets - Day Formulation .... ▣ 725
- Comtrex Maximum Strength Day/Night Severe Cold & Sinus Caplets - Night Formulation .... ▣ 725
- Contac Cold and Flu Maximum Strength Caplets .... ▣ 728
- Contac Cold and Flu Day and Night Caplets (Day Formulation Only) .... ▣ 727
- Contac Cold and Flu Day and Night Caplets (Night Formulation Only) .... ▣ 727
- Contac Cold and Flu Non-Drowsy Caplets .... ▣ 728
- Contac-D Cold Non-Drowsy Tablets .... ▣ 729
- Children's Dimetapp Cold & Allergy Elixir .... ▣ 730
- Children's Dimetapp Cold & Allergy Chewable Tablets .... ▣ 730
- Children's Dimetapp DM Cold & Cough Elixir .... ▣ 731
- Toddler's Dimetapp Cold and Cough Drops .... ▣ 732
- Excedrin Sinus Headache Caplets/Tablets .... ▣ 610
- 4-Way Fast Acting Nasal Spray .... ▣ 775
- 4-Way Menthol Nasal Spray .... ▣ 775
- Preparation H Maximum Strength Cream .... ▣ 666
- Preparation H Cooling Gel .... ▣ 666
- Preparation H .... ▣ 666
- Refenesen PE Caplets .... ▣ 721
- Robitussin Cough & Allergy Syrup .... ▣ 736
- Robitussin Cough & Cold Nighttime Liquid .... ▣ 736
- Robitussin Cough, Cold & Flu Nighttime Liquid .... ▣ 738
- Robitussin Head & Chest Congestion PE Syrup .... ▣ 739
- Robitussin Pediatric Cough & Cold Nighttime Liquid .... ▣ 736
- TheraFlu Cold & Cough Hot Liquid .... ▣ 740
- TheraFlu Cold & Sore Throat Hot Liquid .... ▣ 741
- TheraFlu Flu & Sore Throat Hot Liquid .... ▣ 742
- TheraFlu Daytime Severe Cold Hot Liquid .... ▣ 742
- TheraFlu Nighttime Severe Cold Hot Liquid .... ▣ 740
- TheraFlu Warming Relief Daytime Severe Cold .... ▣ 743
- TheraFlu Warming Relief Nighttime Severe Cold .... ▣ 743
- Triaminic Chest & Nasal Congestion Liquid .... ▣ 746
- Triaminic Cold & Allergy Liquid .... ▣ 746
- Triaminic Daytime Cold & Cough Liquid .... ▣ 745
- Triaminic Nighttime Cold & Cough Liquid .... ▣ 746
- Triaminic Thin Strips Cold .... ▣ 748
- Triaminic Thin Strips Cold & Cough .... ▣ 778
- Triaminic Infant Thin Strips Decongestant .... ▣ 747
- Triaminic Infant Thin Strips Decongestant Plus Cough .... ▣ 747
- Children's Tylenol Plus Flu Oral Suspension .... ▣ 749
- Tylenol Cold Head Congestion Daytime Caplets with Cool Burst and Gelcaps .... ▣ 750
- Tylenol Cold Multi-Symptom Daytime Liquid .... ▣ 752
- Tylenol Cold Multi-Symptom Severe Daytime Liquid .... ▣ 752
- Concentrated Tylenol Infants' Drops Plus Cold & Cough .... ▣ 754
- Tylenol Allergy Multi-Symptom Caplets with Cool Burst and Gelcaps 1872
- Tylenol Allergy Multi-Symptom Nighttime Caplets with Cool Burst 1872
- Children's Tylenol Plus Cold Suspension Liquid 1879
- Children's Tylenol Plus Cold & Allergy Suspension Liquid 1878
- Children's Tylenol Plus Flu Suspension Liquid 1881
- Children's Tylenol Plus Multi-Symptom Cold Suspension Liquid 1879
- Tylenol Cold Head Congestion Daytime Caplets with Cool Burst 1873
- Tylenol Cold Head Congestion Nighttime Caplets with Cool Burst 1873
- Tylenol Cold Head Congestion Severe Caplets with Cool Burst 1873
- Tylenol Cold Multi-Symptom Daytime Caplets with Cool Burst and Gelcaps 1874
- Tylenol Cold Multi-Symptom Daytime Liquid with Citrus Burst 1874
- Tylenol Cold Multi-Symptom Nighttime Caplets with Cool Burst 1874
- Tylenol Cold Multi-Symptom Nighttime Liquid with Cool Burst 1874
- Tylenol Cold Multi-Symptom Severe Caplets with Cool Burst 1874
- Tylenol Cold Multi-Symptom Severe Daytime Liquid with Citrus Burst 1874
- Tylenol Sinus Congestion & Pain Daytime Caplets with Cool Burst and Gelcaps 1876
- Tylenol Sinus Congestion & Pain Nighttime Caplets with Cool Burst 1876
- Tylenol Sinus Congestion & Pain Severe Caplets with Cool Burst 1876
- Vicks 44D Cough & Head Congestion Relief Liquid .... ▣ 760
- Vicks DayQuil LiquiCaps/Liquid Multi-Symptom Cold/Flu Relief .... ▣ 761
- Zicam Cough Plus D Cough Spray .... ▣ 767

Phenylephrine Tannate (Sympathomimetic agents may reduce the blood glucose-lowering effect of insulin).
No products indexed under this heading.

Phenylpropanolamine Hydrochloride (Sympathomimetic agents may reduce the blood glucose-lowering effect of insulin).
No products indexed under this heading.

Pindolol (Beta-blockers may either potentiate or weaken the blood glucose-lowering effect of insulin and reduce or hide the signs of hypoglycemia).
No products indexed under this heading.

Pioglitazone Hydrochloride (Oral antidiabetic products may increase the blood glucose-lowering effect and susceptibility to hypoglycemia of insulin). Products include:
- ActoPlus Met Tablets 3214
- Actos Tablets 3219
- Duetact Tablets 3226

Pirbuterol Acetate (Sympathomimetic agents may reduce the blood glucose-lowering effect of insulin). Products include:
- Maxair Autohaler 1852

Polyestradiol Phosphate (Estrogens may reduce the blood glucose-lowering effect of insulin).
No products indexed under this heading.

Polythiazide (Diuretics may reduce the blood glucose-lowering effect of insulin).
No products indexed under this heading.

Prednisolone Acetate (Corticosteroids may reduce the blood glucose-lowering effect of insulin). Products include:
- Blephamide Ophthalmic Ointment 568
- Blephamide Ophthalmic Suspension 569
- Poly-Pred Ophthalmic Suspension .... ⊙ 233
- Pred Forte Ophthalmic Suspension .... ⊙ 235
- Pred Mild Ophthalmic Suspension .... ⊙ 238
- Pred-G Ophthalmic Ointment .... ⊙ 237
- Pred-G Ophthalmic Suspension .... ⊙ 236

Prednisolone Sodium Phosphate (Corticosteroids may reduce the blood glucose-lowering effect of insulin).
No products indexed under this heading.

Prednisolone Tebutate (Corticosteroids may reduce the blood glucose-lowering effect of insulin).
No products indexed under this heading.

Prednisone (Corticosteroids may reduce the blood glucose-lowering effect of insulin).
No products indexed under this heading.

Procarbazine Hydrochloride
(MAO inhibitors may increase the blood glucose-lowering effect and susceptibility to hypoglycemia of insulin). Products include:
Matulane Capsules 3191

Prochlorperazine (Phenothiazine derivatives may reduce the blood glucose-lowering effect of insulin).
No products indexed under this heading.

Promethazine Hydrochloride (Phenothiazine derivatives may reduce the blood glucose-lowering effect of insulin). Products include:
Phenergan Tablets and Suppositories 3440

Propoxyphene Hydrochloride (Propoxyphene may increase the blood glucose-lowering effect and susceptibility to hypoglycemia of insulin).
No products indexed under this heading.

Propoxyphene Napsylate (Propoxyphene may increase the blood glucose-lowering effect and susceptibility to hypoglycemia of insulin).
No products indexed under this heading.

Propranolol Hydrochloride (Beta-blockers may either potentiate or weaken the blood glucose-lowering effect of insulin and reduce or hide the signs of hypoglycemia). Products include:
Inderal LA Long-Acting Capsules 3429
InnoPran XL Capsules 2723

Pseudoephedrine Hydrochloride (Sympathomimetic agents may reduce the blood glucose-lowering effect of insulin). Products include:
Advil Allergy Sinus Caplets ▣770
Advil Cold & Sinus ▣723
Advil Multi-Symptom Cold Caplets ▣770
Aleve Cold & Sinus Caplets 744
Allegra-D 12 Hour Extended-Release Tablets............. 2846
Allegra-D 24 Hour Extended-Release Tablets............. 2849
BC Cold Powder ▣677
Comtrex Maximum Strength Cold & Cough Day/Night Caplets - Day Formulation....................... ▣726
Comtrex Maximum Strength Cold & Cough Day/Night Caplets - Night Formulation ▣726
Children's Motrin Cold Oral Suspension 1867
Mucinex D Extended-Release Bi-Layer Tablets........................ ▣776
Robitussin Cough & Cold CF Liquid ▣735
Robitussin Cough & Cold Pediatric Drops ▣735
Tylenol Sinus Congestion & Pain Nighttime Caplets with Cool Burst ▣778
Tylenol Cold Severe Congestion Non-Drowsy Caplets with Cool Burst................................... 1874
Tylenol Sinus Severe Congestion Caplets with Cool Burst 1876
Vicks 44D Cough & Head Congestion Relief Liquid 2679
Vicks 44M Cough, Cold & Flu Relief Liquid......................... 2680
Vicks DayQuil Multi-Symptom Cold/Flu Relief LiquiCaps............. 2678
Vicks DayQuil Multi-Symptom Cold/Flu Relief Liquid.................. 2678
Vicks NyQuil Multi-Symptom Cold/Flu Relief Liquid................. 2681
Vicks NyQuil Multi-Symptom Cold/Flu Relief LiquiCaps............. 2681
Children's Vicks NyQuil Cold/Cough Relief Liquid............. 2680
Zyrtec-D 12 Hour Extended Release Tablets...................... 2597

Pseudoephedrine Sulfate (Sympathomimetic agents may reduce the blood glucose-lowering effect of insulin). Products include:
Alavert Allergy & Sinus D-12 Hour Tablets................................. ▣771
Clarinex-D 24-Hour Extended-Release Tablets............ 2998
Claritin-D Non-Drowsy 12 Hour Tablets................................. ▣772
Claritin-D Non-Drowsy 24 Hour Tablets................................. ▣772

Quetiapine Fumarate (Atypical antipsychotics may reduce the blood glucose-lowering effect of insulin). Products include:
Seroquel Tablets 690

Quinapril Hydrochloride (ACE inhibitors may increase the blood glucose-lowering effect and susceptibility to hypoglycemia of insulin).
No products indexed under this heading.

Quinestrol (Estrogens may reduce the blood glucose-lowering effect of insulin).
No products indexed under this heading.

Ramipril (ACE inhibitors may increase the blood glucose-lowering effect and susceptibility to hypoglycemia of insulin). Products include:
Altace Capsules 1702

Repaglinide (Oral antidiabetic products may increase the blood glucose-lowering effect and susceptibility to hypoglycemia of insulin).
No products indexed under this heading.

Reserpine (Under the influence of sympatholytic medicinal products, such as reserpine, the signs of hypoglycemia may be reduced or absent).
No products indexed under this heading.

Risperidone (Atypical antipsychotics may reduce the blood glucose-lowering effect of insulin). Products include:
Risperdal 1676
Risperdal Consta Long-Acting Injection 1682
Risperdal M-Tab Orally Disintegrating Tablets.................. 1676

Ritonavir (Protease inhibitors may reduce the blood glucose-lowering effect of insulin). Products include:
Kaletra 476
Norvir 503

Rosiglitazone Maleate (Oral antidiabetic products may increase the blood glucose-lowering effect and susceptibility to hypoglycemia of insulin). Products include:
Avandamet Tablets 1373
Avandaryl Tablets 1379
Avandia Tablets 1384

Salmeterol Xinafoate (Sympathomimetic agents may reduce the blood glucose-lowering effect of insulin). Products include:
Advair Diskus 100/50 1308
Advair Diskus 250/50 1308
Advair Diskus 500/50 1308
Advair HFA Inhalation Aerosol 1318
Serevent Diskus 1568

Salsalate (Salicylates may increase the blood glucose-lowering effect and susceptibility to hypoglycemia of insulin).
No products indexed under this heading.

Saquinavir (Protease inhibitors may reduce the blood glucose-lowering effect of insulin).
No products indexed under this heading.

Saquinavir Mesylate (Protease inhibitors may reduce the blood glucose-lowering effect of insulin). Products include:
Invirase 2772

Selegiline Hydrochloride (MAO inhibitors may increase the blood glucose-lowering effect and susceptibility to hypoglycemia of insulin). Products include:
Eldepryl Capsules 3208
Zelapar Tablets 3372

Somatropin (Somatropin may reduce the blood glucose-lowering effect of insulin). Products include:
Genotropin Lyophilized Powder 2638
Humatrope Vials and Cartridges 1787
Norditropin Cartridges 2323
Nutropin for Injection 1239
Nutropin AQ Injection 1243
Nutropin AQ Pen 1243
Nutropin AQ Pen Cartridge 1243

Sotalol Hydrochloride (Beta-blockers may either potentiate or weaken the blood glucose-lowering effect of insulin and reduce or hide the signs of hypoglycemia).
No products indexed under this heading.

Spirapril Hydrochloride (ACE inhibitors may increase the blood glucose-lowering effect and susceptibility to hypoglycemia of insulin).
No products indexed under this heading.

Spironolactone (Diuretics may reduce the blood glucose-lowering effect of insulin).
No products indexed under this heading.

Sulfacytine (Sulfonamide antibiotics may increase the blood glucose-lowering effect and susceptibility to hypoglycemia of insulin).
No products indexed under this heading.

Sulfamethizole (Sulfonamide antibiotics may increase the blood glucose-lowering effect and susceptibility to hypoglycemia of insulin).
No products indexed under this heading.

Sulfamethoxazole (Sulfonamide antibiotics may increase the blood glucose-lowering effect and susceptibility to hypoglycemia of insulin).
No products indexed under this heading.

Sulfasalazine (Sulfonamide antibiotics may increase the blood glucose-lowering effect and susceptibility to hypoglycemia of insulin).
No products indexed under this heading.

Sulfinpyrazone (Sulfonamide antibiotics may increase the blood glucose-lowering effect and susceptibility to hypoglycemia of insulin).
No products indexed under this heading.

Sulfisoxazole Acetyl (Sulfonamide antibiotics may increase the blood glucose-lowering effect and susceptibility to hypoglycemia of insulin).
No products indexed under this heading.

Sulfisoxazole Diolamine (Sulfonamide antibiotics may increase the blood glucose-lowering effect and susceptibility to hypoglycemia of insulin).
No products indexed under this heading.

Terbutaline Sulfate (Sympathomimetic agents may reduce the blood glucose-lowering effect of insulin).
No products indexed under this heading.

Thioridazine Hydrochloride (Phenothiazine derivatives may reduce the blood glucose-lowering effect of insulin). Products include:
Thioridazine Hydrochloride Tablets................................. 2163

Thyroglobulin (Thyroid hormones may reduce the blood glucose-lowering effect of insulin).
No products indexed under this heading.

Thyroid (Thyroid hormones may reduce the blood glucose-lowering effect of insulin).
No products indexed under this heading.

Thyroxine (Thyroid hormones may reduce the blood glucose-lowering effect of insulin).
No products indexed under this heading.

Thyroxine Sodium (Thyroid hormones may reduce the blood glucose-lowering effect of insulin).
No products indexed under this heading.

Timolol Hemihydrate (Beta-blockers may either potentiate or weaken the blood glucose-lowering effect of insulin and reduce or hide the signs of hypoglycemia). Products include:
Betimol Ophthalmic Solution 3382
Betimol Ophthalmic Solution ⊙295

Timolol Maleate (Beta-blockers may either potentiate or weaken the blood glucose-lowering effect of insulin and reduce or hide the signs of hypoglycemia). Products include:
Blocadren Tablets 1916
Cosopt Sterile Ophthalmic Solution............................... 1931
Timolide Tablets 2086
Timoptic Sterile Ophthalmic Solution............................... 2088
Timoptic in Ocudose 2091
Timoptic-XE Sterile Ophthalmic Gel Forming Solution 2092

Tolazamide (Oral antidiabetic products may increase the blood glucose-lowering effect and susceptibility to hypoglycemia of insulin).
No products indexed under this heading.

Tolbutamide (Oral antidiabetic products may increase the blood glucose-lowering effect and susceptibility to hypoglycemia of insulin).
No products indexed under this heading.

Torsemide (Diuretics may reduce the blood glucose-lowering effect of insulin). Products include:
Demadex Injection 2759
Demadex Tablets 2759

Trandolapril (ACE inhibitors may increase the blood glucose-lowering effect and susceptibility to hypoglycemia of insulin). Products include:
Mavik Tablets 486
Tarka Tablets 524

Tranylcypromine Sulfate (MAO inhibitors may increase the blood glucose-lowering effect and susceptibility to hypoglycemia of insulin). Products include:
Parnate Tablets 1527

Triamcinolone (Corticosteroids may reduce the blood glucose-lowering effect of insulin).
No products indexed under this heading.

IMPORTANT NOTE: Always consult each drug listing in the patient's regimen for possible interactions.

Triamcinolone Acetonide (Corticosteroids may reduce the blood glucose-lowering effect of insulin). Products include:
- Azmacort Inhalation Aerosol 1726
- Nasacort AQ Nasal Spray 2922

Triamcinolone Diacetate (Corticosteroids may reduce the blood glucose-lowering effect of insulin).
No products indexed under this heading.

Triamcinolone Hexacetonide (Corticosteroids may reduce the blood glucose-lowering effect of insulin).
No products indexed under this heading.

Triamterene (Diuretics may reduce the blood glucose-lowering effect of insulin). Products include:
- Dyazide Capsules 1423
- Dyrenium Capsules 3400

Trifluoperazine Hydrochloride (Phenothiazine derivatives may reduce the blood glucose-lowering effect of insulin).
No products indexed under this heading.

Troglitazone (Oral antidiabetic products may increase the blood glucose-lowering effect and susceptibility to hypoglycemia of insulin).
No products indexed under this heading.

Ziprasidone Hydrochloride (Atypical antipsychotics may reduce the blood glucose-lowering effect of insulin). Products include:
- Geodon Capsules 2529

Ziprasidone Mesylate (Atypical antipsychotics may reduce the blood glucose-lowering effect of insulin). Products include:
- Geodon for Injection 2529

Food Interactions

Alcohol (Alcohol may either potentiate or weaken the blood glucose-lowering effect of insulin).

APPEAREX TABLETS

(Biotin) 2125

May interact with phenytoin and certain other agents. Compounds in these categories include:

Antibiotics, unspecified (The use of antibiotics may reduce the contribution of biotin made by bacteria within the large intestine).
No products indexed under this heading.

Carbamazepine (May accelerate biotin metabolism, leading to a reduction in available biotin). Products include:
- Carbatrol Capsules 3171
- Equetro Extended-Release Capsules 3180
- Tegretol/Tegretol-XR 2295

Fosphenytoin Sodium (May accelerate biotin metabolism, leading to a reduction in available biotin).
No products indexed under this heading.

Phenobarbital (May accelerate biotin metabolism, leading to a reduction in available biotin). Products include:
- Donnatal Extentabs 2493

Phenytoin (May accelerate biotin metabolism, leading to a reduction in available biotin).
No products indexed under this heading.

Phenytoin Sodium (May accelerate biotin metabolism, leading to a reduction in available biotin). Products include:
- Phenytek Capsules 2160

Primidone (May accelerate biotin metabolism, leading to a reduction in available biotin).
No products indexed under this heading.

APTIVUS CAPSULES

(Tipranavir) 826

May interact with ergot-containing drugs, estrogens, oral contraceptives, quinidine, and certain other agents. Compounds in these categories include:

Abacavir Sulfate (Co-administration may decrease abacavir AUC by approximately 40%. Clinical relevance of reduction in abacavir levels has not been established. Dose adjustment of abacavir cannot be recommended at this time). Products include:
- Epzicom Tablets 1436
- Trizivir Tablets 1589
- Ziagen 1626

Amiodarone Hydrochloride (Co-administration is contraindicated due to potential for serious and/or life-threatening reactions, such as cardiac arrhythmias secondary to increases in plasma concentrations of antiarrhythmics).
No products indexed under this heading.

Amprenavir (Co-administration may decrease amprenavir levels. Combining amprenavir, lopinavir or saquinavir with tipranavir/ritonavir is not recommended). Products include:
- Agenerase Capsules 1327
- Agenerase Oral Solution 1332

Astemizole (Co-administration is contraindicated due to potential for serious and/or life-threatening reactions, such as cardiac arrhythmias).
No products indexed under this heading.

Atorvastatin Calcium (Co-administration may increase tipranavir and/or atorvastatin levels and decrease hydroxy-atorvastatin levels. Start with the lowest possible dose of atorvastatin with careful monitoring or consider other HMG-CoA reductase inhibitors). Products include:
- Caduet Tablets 2508
- Lipitor Tablets 2483

Bepridil Hydrochloride (Co-administration is contraindicated due to potential for serious and/or life-threatening reactions, such as cardiac arrhythmias secondary to increases in plasma concentrations of antiarrhythmics).
No products indexed under this heading.

Chlorotrianisene (Co-administration may decrease ethinyl estradiol concentrations by 50%. Alternative methods of non-hormonal contraception should be used when estrogen-based oral contraceptives are co-administered with tipranavir and 200 mg of ritonavir. Patients using estrogens as hormone replacement therapy should be clinically monitored for signs of estrogen deficiency. Women using estrogens may have an increased risk of non serious rash).
No products indexed under this heading.

Cisapride (Co-administration is contraindicated due to potential for serious and/or life-threatening reactions, such as cardiac arrhythmias).
No products indexed under this heading.

Clarithromycin (Co-administration may increase tipranavir and/or clarithromycin levels and decrease 14-hydroxy-clarithromycin metabolite levels. No dose adjustment of tipranavir or clarithromycin for patients with normal renal function is necessary. For patients with renal impairment the following dosage adjustments should be considered: for patients with CrCl 30 - 60 mL/min the dose of clarithromycin should be reduced by 50%; for patients with CrCl < 30 mL/min the dose of clarithromycin should be decreased by 75%). Products include:
- Biaxin/Biaxin XL 402
- PREVPAC 3284

Cyclosporine (Co-administration may increase or decrease cyclosporine levels. More frequent concentration monitoring is recommended until blood levels have been stabilized). Products include:
- Gengraf Capsules 459
- Neoral Oral Solution 2259
- Neoral Soft Gelatin Capsules 2259
- Restasis Ophthalmic Emulsion 575
- Sandimmune 2275

Desipramine Hydrochloride (Co-administration may lead to increased desipramine levels. Dosage reduction and concentration monitoring of desipramine is recommended).
No products indexed under this heading.

Desogestrel (Alternative methods of non-hormonal contraception should be used when estrogen-based oral contraceptives are co-administered with tipranavir and 200 mg of ritonavir). Products include:
- Mircette Tablets 1066

Didanosine (Co-administration may decrease didanosine levels. Clinical relevance of reduction in didanosine levels has not been established. For optimal absorption, didanosine should be separated from tipranavir/ritonavir dosing by at least 2 hours).
No products indexed under this heading.

Dienestrol (Co-administration may decrease ethinyl estradiol concentrations by 50%. Alternative methods of non-hormonal contraception should be used when estrogen-based oral contraceptives are co-administered with tipranavir and 200 mg of ritonavir. Patients using estrogens as hormone replacement therapy should be clinically monitored for signs of estrogen deficiency. Women using estrogens may have an increased risk of non serious rash).
No products indexed under this heading.

Diethylstilbestrol (Co-administration may decrease ethinyl estradiol concentrations by 50%. Alternative methods of non-hormonal contraception should be used when estrogen-based oral contraceptives are co-administered with tipranavir and 200 mg of ritonavir. Patients using estrogens as hormone replacement therapy should be clinically monitored for signs of estrogen deficiency. Women using estrogens may have an increased risk of non serious rash).
No products indexed under this heading.

Dihydroergotamine Mesylate (Co-administration is contraindicated due to potential for serious and/or life-threatening reactions, such as acute ergot toxicity characterized by peripheral vasospasm and ischemia of the extremities and other tissues). Products include:
- Migranal Nasal Spray 3348

Diltiazem Hydrochloride (Co-administration may increase or decrease diltiazem levels. Caution is warranted and monitoring of patients is recommended). Products include:
- Cardizem LA Extended Release Tablets 1728
- Tiazac Capsules 1201

Diltiazem Maleate (Co-administration may increase or decrease diltiazem levels. Caution is warranted and monitoring of patients is recommended).
No products indexed under this heading.

Disulfiram (Aptivus capsules contain alcohol that can produce disulfiram-like reactions when co-administered with disulfiram or other drugs which produce this reaction).
No products indexed under this heading.

Ergonovine Maleate (Co-administration is contraindicated due to potential for serious and/or life-threatening reactions, such as acute ergot toxicity characterized by peripheral vasospasm and ischemia of the extremities and other tissues).
No products indexed under this heading.

Ergotamine Tartrate (Co-administration is contraindicated due to potential for serious and/or life-threatening reactions, such as acute ergot toxicity characterized by peripheral vasospasm and ischemia of the extremities and other tissues).
No products indexed under this heading.

Estradiol (Co-administration may decrease ethinyl estradiol concentrations by 50%. Alternative methods of non-hormonal contraception should be used when estrogen-based oral contraceptives are co-administered with tipranavir and 200 mg of ritonavir. Patients using estrogens as hormone replacement therapy should be clinically monitored for signs of estrogen deficiency. Women using estrogens may have an increased risk of non serious rash). Products include:
- Angeliq Tablets 762
- Climara Transdermal System 771
- Climara Pro Transdermal System 776
- Estrasorb Topical Emulsion 1147
- Estring Vaginal Ring 2635
- Menostar Transdermal System 782
- Vagifem Tablets 2334

Estrogens, Conjugated (Co-administration may decrease ethinyl estradiol concentrations by 50%. Alternative methods of non-hormonal contraception should be used when estrogen-based oral contraceptives are co-administered with tipranavir and 200 mg of ritonavir. Patients using estrogens as hormone replacement therapy should be clinically monitored for signs of estrogen deficiency. Women using estrogens may have an increased risk of non serious rash). Products include:

Premarin Intravenous 3442
Premarin Tablets 3446
Premarin Vaginal Cream 3452
Premphase Tablets 3456
Prempro Tablets 3456

Estrogens, Esterified (Co-administration may decrease ethinyl estradiol concentrations by 50%. Alternative methods of non-hormonal contraception should be used when estrogen-based oral contraceptives are co-administered with tipranavir and 200 mg of ritonavir. Patients using estrogens as hormone replacement therapy should be clinically monitored for signs of estrogen deficiency. Women using estrogens may have an increased risk of non serious rash). Products include:

Estratest Tablets 3199
Estratest H.S. Tablets 3199

Estropipate (Co-administration may decrease ethinyl estradiol concentrations by 50%. Alternative methods of non-hormonal contraception should be used when estrogen-based oral contraceptives are co-administered with tipranavir and 200 mg of ritonavir. Patients using estrogens as hormone replacement therapy should be clinically monitored for signs of estrogen deficiency. Women using estrogens may have an increased risk of non serious rash).

No products indexed under this heading.

Ethinyl Estradiol (Co-administration may decrease ethinyl estradiol concentrations by 50%. Alternative methods of non-hormonal contraception should be used when estrogen-based oral contraceptives are co-administered with tipranavir and 200 mg of ritonavir. Patients using estrogens as hormone replacement therapy should be clinically monitored for signs of estrogen deficiency. Women using estrogens may have an increased risk of non-serious rash). Products include:

Mircette Tablets 1066
NuvaRing 2340
Ortho-Cyclen/Ortho Tri-Cyclen 2429
Ortho Evra Transdermal System 2417
Ortho Tri-Cyclen Lo Tablets 2436
Seasonique Tablets 1077
Yasmin 28 Tablets 796
Yaz Tablets 803

Ethynodiol Diacetate (Alternative methods of non-hormonal contraception should be used when estrogen-based oral contraceptives are co-administered with tipranavir and 200 mg of ritonavir).

No products indexed under this heading.

Felodipine (Co-administration may increase felodipine levels. Caution is warranted and monitoring of patients is recommended).

No products indexed under this heading.

Flecainide Acetate (Co-administration is contraindicated due to potential for serious and/or life-threatening reactions, such as cardiac arrhythmias secondary to increases in plasma concentrations of antiarrhythmics). Products include:

Tambocor Tablets 1856

Fluconazole (Co-administration may increase tipranavir levels. Fluconazole increases tipranavir concentrations but dose adjustments are not needed. Fluconazole doses greater than 200 mg/day are not recommended).

No products indexed under this heading.

Fluoxetine (Co-administration may increase fluoxetine levels. Fluoxetine doses may need to be adjusted upon initiation of tipranavir/ritonavir therapy).

No products indexed under this heading.

Fluoxetine Hydrochloride (Co-administration may increase fluoxetine levels. Fluoxetine doses may need to be adjusted upon initiation of tipranavir/ritonavir therapy). Products include:

Prozac Pulvules and Liquid 1801
Symbyax Capsules 1819

Fosamprenavir Calcium (Co-administration may decrease amprenavir levels. Combining amprenavir with tipranavir/ritonavir is not recommended). Products include:

Lexiva Tablets 1505

Glimepiride (Co-administration may increase or decrease glimepiride levels. Careful glucose monitoring is warranted). Products include:

Avandaryl Tablets 1379
Duetact Tablets 3226

Glipizide (Co-administration may increase or decrease glipizide levels. Careful glucose monitoring is warranted).

No products indexed under this heading.

Glyburide (Co-administration may increase or decrease glyburide levels. Careful glucose monitoring is warranted).

No products indexed under this heading.

Hypericum (Co-administration may lead to loss of virologic response and possible resistance to tipranavir or to the class of protease inhibitors). Products include:

Satiete Tablets 832

Itraconazole (Co-administration may increase itraconazole levels. Based on theoretical considerations itraconazole should be used with caution. High doses (200 mg/day) are not recommended).

No products indexed under this heading.

Ketoconazole (Co-administration may increase ketoconazole levels. Based on theoretical considerations ketoconazole should be used with caution. High doses (200 mg/day) are not recommended). Products include:

Nizoral A-D Shampoo, 1% 1868

Levonorgestrel (Alternative methods of non-hormonal contraception should be used when estrogen-based oral contraceptives are co-administered with tipranavir and 200 mg of ritonavir). Products include:

Climara Pro Transdermal System 776
Mirena Intrauterine System 787
Plan B Tablets 1076
Seasonique Tablets 1077

Lopinavir (Co-administration may decrease lopinavir levels. Combining lopinavir with tipranavir/ritonavir is not recommended). Products include:

Kaletra 476

Lovastatin (Co-administration may lead to potential for serious reactions, such as risk of myopathy including rhabdomyolysis. Concomitant use of tipranavir, coadministered with 200 mg of ritonavir, with lovastatin is not recommended). Products include:

Advicor Tablets 1722
Altoprev Extended-Release Tablets 3109
Mevacor Tablets 2021

Meperidine Hydrochloride (Co-administration may decrease meperidine levels and increase normeperidine levels. Dosage increase and long-term use of meperidine are not recommended due to increased concentrations of the metabolite normeperidine which has both analgesic activity and CNS stimulant activity (eg, seizures)).

No products indexed under this heading.

Mestranol (Alternative methods of non-hormonal contraception should be used when estrogen-based oral contraceptives are co-administered with tipranavir and 200 mg of ritonavir).

No products indexed under this heading.

Methadone Hydrochloride (Co-administration may decrease methadone levels by 50%. Dosage of methadone may need to be increased when co-administered with tipranavir and 200 mg of ritonavir).

No products indexed under this heading.

Methylergonovine Maleate (Co-administration is contraindicated due to potential for serious and/or life-threatening reactions, such as acute ergot toxicity characterized by peripheral vasospasm and ischemia of the extremities and other tissues).

No products indexed under this heading.

Methysergide Maleate (Co-administration is contraindicated due to potential for serious and/or life-threatening reactions, such as acute ergot toxicity characterized by peripheral vasospasm and ischemia of the extremities and other tissues).

No products indexed under this heading.

Metronidazole (Aptivus capsules contain alcohol that can produce disulfiram-like reactions when co-administered with metronidazole or other drugs which produce this reaction). Products include:

Metrogel 1% 1211
MetroGel-Vaginal Gel 1855
Vandazole Vaginal Gel 3338

Metronidazole Benzoate (Aptivus capsules contain alcohol that can produce disulfiram-like reactions when co-administered with metronidazole or other drugs which produce this reaction).

No products indexed under this heading.

Metronidazole Hydrochloride (Aptivus capsules contain alcohol that can produce disulfiram-like reactions when co-administered with metronidazole or other drugs which produce this reaction).

No products indexed under this heading.

Metronidazole Sodium (Aptivus capsules contain alcohol that can produce disulfiram-like reactions when co-administered with metronidazole or other drugs which produce this reaction).

No products indexed under this heading.

Midazolam Hydrochloride (Co-administration is contraindicated due to potential for serious and/or life-threatening reactions, such as prolonged or increased sedation or respiratory depression).

No products indexed under this heading.

Nicardipine (Co-administration may increase or decrease nicardipine levels. Caution is warranted and monitoring of patients is recommended).

No products indexed under this heading.

Nicardipine Hydrochloride (Co-administration may increase or decrease nicardipine levels. Caution is warranted and monitoring of patients is recommended). Products include:

Cardene I.V. 2497

Nisoldipine (Co-administration may increase or decrease nisoldipine levels. Caution is warranted and monitoring of patients is recommended). Products include:

Sular Tablets 3122

Norethindrone (Alternative methods of non-hormonal contraception should be used when estrogen-based oral contraceptives are co-administered with tipranavir and 200 mg of ritonavir). Products include:

Ortho Micronor Tablets 2426

Norethynodrel (Alternative methods of non-hormonal contraception should be used when estrogen-based oral contraceptives are co-administered with tipranavir and 200 mg of ritonavir).

No products indexed under this heading.

Norgestimate (Alternative methods of non-hormonal contraception should be used when estrogen-based oral contraceptives are co-administered with tipranavir and 200 mg of ritonavir). Products include:

Ortho-Cyclen/Ortho Tri-Cyclen 2429
Ortho Tri-Cyclen Lo Tablets 2436

Norgestrel (Alternative methods of non-hormonal contraception should be used when estrogen-based oral contraceptives are co-administered with tipranavir and 200 mg of ritonavir).

No products indexed under this heading.

Paroxetine Hydrochloride (Co-administration may increase paroxetine levels. Paroxetine doses may need to be adjusted upon initiation of tipranavir/ritonavir therapy). Products include:

Paxil CR Controlled-Release Tablets 1538
Paxil 1530

Paroxetine Mesylate (Co-administration may increase paroxetine levels. Paroxetine doses may need to be adjusted upon initiation of tipranavir/ritonavir therapy). Products include:

Pexeva Tablets 1694

Pimozide (Co-administration is contraindicated due to potential for serious and/or life-threatening reactions, such as cardiac arrhythmias).
No products indexed under this heading.

Pioglitazone Hydrochloride (Co-administration may increase or decrease pioglitazone levels. Careful glucose monitoring is warranted). Products include:
ActoPlus Met Tablets 3214
Actos Tablets 3219
Duetact Tablets 3226

Polyestradiol Phosphate (Co-administration may decrease ethinyl estradiol concentrations by 50%. Alternative methods of non-hormonal contraception should be used when estrogen-based oral contraceptives are co-administered with tipranavir and 200 mg of ritonavir. Patients using estrogens as hormone replacement therapy should be clinically monitored for signs of estrogen deficiency. Women using estrogens may have an increased risk of non serious rash).
No products indexed under this heading.

Propafenone Hydrochloride (Co-administration is contraindicated due to potential for serious and/or life-threatening reactions, such as cardiac arrhythmias secondary to increases in plasma concentrations of antiarrhythmics). Products include:
Rythmol SR Capsules 2727

Quinestrol (Co-administration may decrease ethinyl estradiol concentrations by 50%. Alternative methods of non-hormonal contraception should be used when estrogen-based oral contraceptives are co-administered with tipranavir and 200 mg of ritonavir. Patients using estrogens as hormone replacement therapy should be clinically monitored for signs of estrogen deficiency. Women using estrogens may have an increased risk of non serious rash).
No products indexed under this heading.

Quinidine (Co-administration is contraindicated due to potential for serious and/or life-threatening reactions, such as cardiac arrhythmias secondary to increases in plasma concentrations of antiarrhythmics).
No products indexed under this heading.

Quinidine Gluconate (Co-administration is contraindicated due to potential for serious and/or life-threatening reactions, such as cardiac arrhythmias secondary to increases in plasma concentrations of antiarrhythmics).
No products indexed under this heading.

Quinidine Hydrochloride (Co-administration is contraindicated due to potential for serious and/or life-threatening reactions, such as cardiac arrhythmias secondary to increases in plasma concentrations of antiarrhythmics).
No products indexed under this heading.

Quinidine Polygalacturonate (Co-administration is contraindicated due to potential for serious and/or life-threatening reactions, such as cardiac arrhythmias secondary to increases in plasma concentrations of antiarrhythmics).
No products indexed under this heading.

Quinidine Sulfate (Co-administration is contraindicated due to potential for serious and/or life-threatening reactions, such as cardiac arrhythmias secondary to increases in plasma concentrations of antiarrhythmics).
No products indexed under this heading.

Repaglinide (Co-administration may increase or decrease repaglinide levels. Careful glucose monitoring is warranted).
No products indexed under this heading.

Rifabutin (Co-administration may increase levels of rifabutin and desacetyl-rifabutin. Dosage reductions of rifabutin by 75% are recommended (eg. 150 mg every other day). Increased monitoring for adverse events in patients receiving the combination is warranted. Further dosage reduction may be necessary).
No products indexed under this heading.

Rifampin (Co-administration may lead to loss of virologic response and possible resistance to tipranavir or to the class of protease inhibitors).
No products indexed under this heading.

Saquinavir (Co-administration may decrease saquinavir levels. Combining saquinavir with tipranavir/ritonavir is not recommended).
No products indexed under this heading.

Saquinavir Mesylate (Co-administration may decrease saquinavir levels. Combining saquinavir with tipranavir/ritonavir is not recommended). Products include:
Invirase 2772

Sertraline Hydrochloride (Co-administration may increase sertraline levels. Sertraline doses may need to be adjusted upon initiation of tipranavir/ritonavir therapy). Products include:
Zoloft 2586

Sildenafil Citrate (Co-administration may increase sildenafil levels. Concomitant use of PDE5 inhibitors with tipranavir and ritonavir should be used with caution and in no case should the starting dose of sildenafil exceed 25 mg within 48 hours). Products include:
Revatio Tablets 2557
Viagra Tablets 2573

Simvastatin (Co-administration may lead to potential for serious reactions, such as risk of myopathy including rhabdomyolysis. Concomitant use of tipranavir, co-administered with 200 mg of ritonavir, with simvastatin is not recommended). Products include:
Vytorin 10/10 Tablets 2114
Vytorin 10/10 Tablets 3077
Vytorin 10/20 Tablets 2114
Vytorin 10/20 Tablets 3077
Vytorin 10/40 Tablets 2114
Vytorin 10/40 Tablets 3077
Vytorin 10/80 Tablets 2114
Vytorin 10/80 Tablets 3077
Zocor Tablets 2105

Sirolimus (Co-administration may increase or decrease cyclosporine levels. More frequent concentration monitoring is recommended until blood levels have been stabilized). Products include:
Rapamune Oral Solution and Tablets 3475

Tacrolimus (Co-administration may increase or decrease cyclosporine levels. More frequent concentration monitoring is recommended until blood levels have been stabilized). Products include:
Prograf Capsules and Injection 632
Protopic Ointment 638

Tadalafil (Co-administration may increase tadalafil levels. Concomitant use of PDE5 inhibitors with tipranavir and ritonavir should be used with caution and in no case should the starting dose of tadalafil exceed 10 mg every 72 hours). Products include:
Cialis Tablets 1838

Terfenadine (Co-administration is contraindicated due to potential for serious and/or life-threatening reactions, such as cardiac arrhythmias).
No products indexed under this heading.

Tolbutamide (Co-administration may increase or decrease tolbutamide levels. Careful glucose monitoring is warranted).
No products indexed under this heading.

Tolbutamide Sodium (Co-administration may increase or decrease tolbutamide levels. Careful glucose monitoring is warranted).
No products indexed under this heading.

Triazolam (Co-administration is contraindicated due to potential for serious and/or life-threatening reactions, such as prolonged or increased sedation or respiratory depression).
No products indexed under this heading.

Vardenafil Hydrochloride (Co-administration may increase vardenafil levels. Concomitant use of PDE5 inhibitors with tipranavir and ritonavir should be used with caution and in no case should the starting dose of vardenafil exceed 2.5 mg every 72 hours). Products include:
Levitra Tablets 3034

Verapamil Hydrochloride (Co-administration may increase or decrease verapamil levels. Caution is warranted and monitoring of patients is recommended). Products include:
Covera-HS Tablets 3139
Tarka Tablets 524
Verelan PM Extended-Release Capsules, Controlled-Onset.......... 3106

Voriconazole (Co-administration may increase or decrease voriconazole levels. Due to multiple enzymes involved with voriconazole metabolism, it is difficult to predict the interaction). Products include:
VFEND I.V. 2564
VFEND Oral Suspension 2564
VFEND Tablets 2564

Warfarin Sodium (Frequent INR monitoring upon initiation of tipranavir/ritonavir therapy is recommended). Products include:
Coumadin for Injection 898
Coumadin Tablets 898

Zidovudine (Co-administration may decrease zidovudine AUC by approximately 35%. Clinical relevance of reduction in zidovudine levels has not been established. Dose adjustment of zidovudine cannot be recommended at this time). Products include:
Combivir Tablets 1411
Retrovir 1560
Retrovir IV Infusion 1564
Trizivir Tablets 1589

ARALAST
(Alpha$_1$-Proteinase Inhibitor (Human)) 717
None cited in PDR database.

ARANESP FOR INJECTION
(Darbepoetin alfa) 581
None cited in PDR database.

AREDIA FOR INJECTION
(Pamidronate Disodium) 2179
May interact with:

Nephrotoxic Drugs (Co-administration with nephrotoxic drugs requires caution due to the risk of clinically significant deterioration in renal function with the use of Aredia).
No products indexed under this heading.

ARGATROBAN INJECTION
(Argatroban) 1346
May interact with anticoagulants, thrombolytics, and certain other agents. Compounds in these categories include:

Alteplase (Co-administration with thrombolytic agents may increase the risk of bleeding). Products include:
Activase I.V. 1223
Cathflo Activase 1231

Anisindione (Co-administration with other anticoagulants may increase the risk of bleeding). Products include:
Miradon Tablets 3042

Anistreplase (Co-administration with thrombolytic agents may increase the risk of bleeding).
No products indexed under this heading.

Ardeparin Sodium (Co-administration with other anticoagulants may increase the risk of bleeding).
No products indexed under this heading.

Aspirin (Co-administration with antiplatelet agents, such as aspirin, may increase the risk of bleeding). Products include:
Aggrenox Capsules 822
Bayer Aspirin 744
BC Allergy Sinus Cold Powder .... ■677
BC Headache Powder .... ■677
Arthritis Strength BC Powder .... ■677
BC Sinus Cold Powder .... ■677
Excedrin Extra Strength Caplets/Tablets/Geltabs .... ■684
Excedrin Migraine Caplets/Tablets/Geltabs .... ■609
Goody's Body Pain Formula Powder .... ■684
Goody's Extra Strength Headache Powders .... ■611
Goody's Extra Strength Pain Relief Tablets .... ■685
Percodan Tablets 1132
St. Joseph 81 mg Aspirin Chewable and Enteric Coated Tablets 1869

Clopidogrel Bisulfate (Co-administration with antiplatelet agents may increase the risk of bleeding). Products include:
- Plavix Tablets 917
- Plavix Tablets 2926

Dalteparin Sodium (Co-administration with other anticoagulants may increase the risk of bleeding). Products include:
- Fragmin Injection 1097

Danaparoid Sodium (Co-administration with other anticoagulants may increase the risk of bleeding).
No products indexed under this heading.

Dicumarol (Co-administration with other anticoagulants may increase the risk of bleeding).
No products indexed under this heading.

Dipyridamole (Co-administration with antiplatelet agents may increase the risk of bleeding). Products include:
- Aggrenox Capsules 822
- Persantine Tablets 868

Enoxaparin Sodium (Co-administration with other anticoagulants may increase the risk of bleeding). Products include:
- Lovenox Injection 2915

Fondaparinux Sodium (Co-administration with other anticoagulants may increase the risk of bleeding). Products include:
- Arixtra Injection 1351

Heparin Calcium (Co-administration with other anticoagulants may increase the risk of bleeding).
No products indexed under this heading.

Heparin Sodium (Co-administration with other anticoagulants may increase the risk of bleeding).
No products indexed under this heading.

Low Molecular Weight Heparins (Co-administration with other anticoagulants may increase the risk of bleeding).
No products indexed under this heading.

Reteplase (Co-administration with thrombolytic agents may increase the risk of bleeding). Products include:
- Retavase 2499

Streptokinase (Co-administration with thrombolytic agents may increase the risk of bleeding).
No products indexed under this heading.

Tinzaparin Sodium (Co-administration with other anticoagulants may increase the risk of bleeding).
No products indexed under this heading.

Urokinase (Co-administration with thrombolytic agents may increase the risk of bleeding).
No products indexed under this heading.

Warfarin Sodium (Co-administration with other anticoagulants may increase the risk of bleeding). Products include:
- Coumadin for Injection 898
- Coumadin Tablets 898

ARICEPT TABLETS

(Donepezil Hydrochloride) **1094**
May interact with anticholinergics, cytochrome p450 2d6 inducers (selected), cytochrome p450 3a4 inducers (selected), dexamethasone, non-steroidal anti-inflammatory agents, phenytoin, quinidine, and certain other agents. Compounds in these categories include:

Allium sativum (Inducers of CYP3A4 could increase the rate of elimination of donepezil).
No products indexed under this heading.

Aprepitant (Inducers of CYP3A4 could increase the rate of elimination of donepezil). Products include:
- Emend Capsules 1963

Atropine Sulfate (Donepezil, a cholinesterase inhibitor, has the potential to interfere with the activity of anticholinergic medications). Products include:
- Donnatal Extentabs 2493

Belladonna Alkaloids (Donepezil, a cholinesterase inhibitor, has the potential to interfere with the activity of anticholinergic medications). Products include:
- Hyland's Teething Tablets 830

Benztropine Mesylate (Donepezil, a cholinesterase inhibitor, has the potential to interfere with the activity of anticholinergic medications).
No products indexed under this heading.

Betamethasone Acetate (Inducers of CYP3A4 could increase the rate of elimination of donepezil).
No products indexed under this heading.

Betamethasone Sodium Phosphate (Inducers of CYP3A4 could increase the rate of elimination of donepezil).
No products indexed under this heading.

Bethanechol Chloride (Potential for synergistic effect).
No products indexed under this heading.

Biperiden Hydrochloride (Donepezil, a cholinesterase inhibitor, has the potential to interfere with the activity of anticholinergic medications).
No products indexed under this heading.

Carbamazepine (Inducers of CYP2D6 and CYP3A4, such as carbamazepine, could increase the rate of elimination of donepezil). Products include:
- Carbatrol Capsules 3171
- Equetro Extended-Release Capsules 3180
- Tegretol/Tegretol-XR 2295

Celecoxib (Cholinesterase inhibitors, such as donepezil, may be expected to increase gastric acid secretion due to increased cholinergic activity, therefore, patients on concurrent NSAID therapy should be monitored closely for increased risk of developing ulcers or symptoms of active or occult gastrointestinal bleeding). Products include:
- Celebrex Capsules 3134

Ciprofloxacin Hydrochloride (Inducers of CYP3A4 could increase the rate of elimination of donepezil). Products include:
- Ciloxan Ophthalmic Ointment 559
- Ciloxan Ophthalmic Solution .... ⊙ 206
- Cipro Tablets 2977
- Proquin XR Tablets 1153

Cisplatin (Inducers of CYP3A4 could increase the rate of elimination of donepezil).
No products indexed under this heading.

Clidinium Bromide (Donepezil, a cholinesterase inhibitor, has the potential to interfere with the activity of anticholinergic medications).
No products indexed under this heading.

Cortisone Acetate (Inducers of CYP3A4 could increase the rate of elimination of donepezil).
No products indexed under this heading.

Dexamethasone (Inducers of CYP2D6 and CYP3A4, such as dexamethasone, could increase the rate of elimination of donepezil). Products include:
- Ciprodex Otic Suspension 559
- Decadron Tablets 1951
- TobraDex Ophthalmic Ointment 562
- TobraDex Ophthalmic Suspension ... 563

Dexamethasone Acetate (Inducers of CYP2D6 and CYP3A4, such as dexamethasone, could increase the rate of elimination of donepezil).
No products indexed under this heading.

Dexamethasone Sodium Phosphate (Inducers of CYP2D6 and CYP3A4, such as dexamethasone, could increase the rate of elimination of donepezil).
No products indexed under this heading.

Diclofenac Potassium (Cholinesterase inhibitors, such as donepezil, may be expected to increase gastric acid secretion due to increased cholinergic activity, therefore, patients on concurrent NSAID therapy should be monitored closely for increased risk of developing ulcers or symptoms of active or occult gastrointestinal bleeding).
No products indexed under this heading.

Diclofenac Sodium (Cholinesterase inhibitors, such as donepezil, may be expected to increase gastric acid secretion due to increased cholinergic activity, therefore, patients on concurrent NSAID therapy should be monitored closely for increased risk of developing ulcers or symptoms of active or occult gastrointestinal bleeding). Products include:
- Arthrotec Tablets 3129
- Voltaren Ophthalmic Solution 2309
- Voltaren Tablets 2307
- Voltaren-XR Tablets 2310

Dicyclomine Hydrochloride (Donepezil, a cholinesterase inhibitor, has the potential to interfere with the activity of anticholinergic medications). Products include:
- Bentyl Capsules 697
- Bentyl Injection 697
- Bentyl Syrup 697
- Bentyl Tablets 697

Doxorubicin Hydrochloride (Inducers of CYP3A4 could increase the rate of elimination of donepezil).
No products indexed under this heading.

Efavirenz (Inducers of CYP3A4 could increase the rate of elimination of donepezil). Products include:
- Atripla Tablets 945
- Sustiva Capsules 930
- Sustiva Tablets 930

Ethanol (Inducers of CYP2D6 could increase the rate of elimination of donepezil).
No products indexed under this heading.

Ethosuximide (Inducers of CYP3A4 could increase the rate of elimination of donepezil).
No products indexed under this heading.

Etodolac (Cholinesterase inhibitors, such as donepezil, may be expected to increase gastric acid secretion due to increased cholinergic activity, therefore, patients on concurrent NSAID therapy should be monitored closely for increased risk of developing ulcers or symptoms of active or occult gastrointestinal bleeding).
No products indexed under this heading.

Felbamate (Inducers of CYP3A4 could increase the rate of elimination of donepezil).
No products indexed under this heading.

Fenoprofen Calcium (Cholinesterase inhibitors, such as donepezil, may be expected to increase gastric acid secretion due to increased cholinergic activity, therefore, patients on concurrent NSAID therapy should be monitored closely for increased risk of developing ulcers or symptoms of active or occult gastrointestinal bleeding). Products include:
- Nalfon Capsules 2502

Fludrocortisone Acetate (Inducers of CYP3A4 could increase the rate of elimination of donepezil).
No products indexed under this heading.

Flurbiprofen (Cholinesterase inhibitors, such as donepezil, may be expected to increase gastric acid secretion due to increased cholinergic activity, therefore, patients on concurrent NSAID therapy should be monitored closely for increased risk of developing ulcers or symptoms of active or occult gastrointestinal bleeding).
No products indexed under this heading.

Fosphenytoin Sodium (Inducers of CYP2D6 and CYP3A4, such as phenytoin, could increase the rate of elimination of donepezil).
No products indexed under this heading.

Garlic Extract (Inducers of CYP3A4 could increase the rate of elimination of donepezil).
No products indexed under this heading.

Garlic Oil (Inducers of CYP3A4 could increase the rate of elimination of donepezil).
No products indexed under this heading.

Glycopyrrolate (Donepezil, a cholinesterase inhibitor, has the potential to interfere with the activity of anticholinergic medications).
No products indexed under this heading.

Hydrocortisone (Inducers of CYP3A4 could increase the rate of elimination of donepezil). Products include:
- Colocort Rectal Suspension, USP (Retention) 100 mg/60 mL 2476
- Hydrocortone Tablets 1989
- Preparation H Hydrocortisone Cream 646

Hydrocortisone Acetate (Inducers of CYP3A4 could increase the rate of elimination of donepezil). Products include:
- Analpram-HC 1159
- Pramosone 1161
- ProctoFoam-HC 3099

Hydrocortisone Butyrate (Inducers of CYP3A4 could increase the rate of elimination of donepezil). Products include:
- Locoid Lipocream Cream 1160

Hydrocortisone Cypionate (Inducers of CYP3A4 could increase the rate of elimination of donepezil).
No products indexed under this heading.

Hydrocortisone Hemisuccinate (Inducers of CYP3A4 could increase the rate of elimination of donepezil).
No products indexed under this heading.

Hydrocortisone Probutate (Inducers of CYP3A4 could increase the rate of elimination of donepezil).
No products indexed under this heading.

Hydrocortisone Sodium Phosphate (Inducers of CYP3A4 could increase the rate of elimination of donepezil).
No products indexed under this heading.

Hydrocortisone Sodium Succinate (Inducers of CYP3A4 could increase the rate of elimination of donepezil).
No products indexed under this heading.

Hydrocortisone Valerate (Inducers of CYP3A4 could increase the rate of elimination of donepezil).
No products indexed under this heading.

Hyoscyamine (Donepezil, a cholinesterase inhibitor, has the potential to interfere with the activity of anticholinergic medications).
No products indexed under this heading.

Hyoscyamine Sulfate (Donepezil, a cholinesterase inhibitor, has the potential to interfere with the activity of anticholinergic medications). Products include:
- Donnatal Extentabs 2493
- Prosed/DS Tablets 1157

Hypericum (Inducers of CYP3A4 could increase the rate of elimination of donepezil). Products include:
- Satiete Tablets .... ▣ 832

Hypericum Perforatum (Inducers of CYP3A4 could increase the rate of elimination of donepezil).
No products indexed under this heading.

Ibuprofen (Cholinesterase inhibitors, such as donepezil, may be expected to increase gastric acid secretion due to increased cholinergic activity, therefore, patients on concurrent NSAID therapy should be monitored closely for increased risk of developing ulcers or symptoms of active or occult gastrointestinal bleeding). Products include:
- Advil Allergy Sinus Caplets .... ▣ 770
- Advil .... ▣ 674
- Children's Advil Oral Suspension .... ▣ 603
- Children's Advil Chewable Tablets .... ▣ 603
- Advil Cold & Sinus .... ▣ 723
- Infants' Advil Concentrated Drops .... ▣ 604
- Infants' Advil Concentrated Drops - White Grape (Dye-Free) .... ▣ 604
- Junior Strength Advil Swallow Tablets .... ▣ 605
- Advil Migraine Liquigels .... ▣ 608
- Advil Multi-Symptom Cold Caplets .... ▣ 770
- Advil PM Caplets .... ▣ 615
- Motrin IB Tablets and Caplets 1866
- Children's Motrin Oral Suspension 1867
- Children's Motrin Non-Staining Dye-Free Oral Suspension 1867
- Children's Motrin Cold Oral Suspension 1867
- Infants' Motrin Concentrated Drops 1867
- Infants' Motrin Non-Staining Dye-Free Concentrated Drops 1867
- Junior Strength Motrin Caplets and Chewable Tablets 1867
- Vicoprofen Tablets 539

Indomethacin (Cholinesterase inhibitors, such as donepezil, may be expected to increase gastric acid secretion due to increased cholinergic activity, therefore, patients on concurrent NSAID therapy should be monitored closely for increased risk of developing ulcers or symptoms of active or occult gastrointestinal bleeding). Products include:
- Indocin 1995

Indomethacin Sodium Trihydrate (Cholinesterase inhibitors, such as donepezil, may be expected to increase gastric acid secretion due to increased cholinergic activity, therefore, patients on concurrent NSAID therapy should be monitored closely for increased risk of developing ulcers or symptoms of active or occult gastrointestinal bleeding). Products include:
- Indocin I.V. 2465

Ipratropium Bromide (Donepezil, a cholinesterase inhibitor, has the potential to interfere with the activity of anticholinergic medications). Products include:
- Atrovent Inhalation Solution 835
- Atrovent HFA Inhalation Aerosol 841
- Atrovent Nasal Spray 0.03% 837
- Atrovent Nasal Spray 0.06% 839
- Combivent Inhalation Aerosol 847
- DuoNeb Inhalation Solution 1058

Ketoconazole (Inhibitors of CYP450, 2D6 and 3A4, such as ketoconazole, inhibit donepezil metabolism in vitro. In a crossover study, ketoconazole increased mean donepezil concentrations by 36%; the clinical relevance is unknown). Products include:
- Nizoral A-D Shampoo, 1% 1868

Ketoprofen (Cholinesterase inhibitors, such as donepezil, may be expected to increase gastric acid secretion due to increased cholinergic activity, therefore, patients on concurrent NSAID therapy should be monitored closely for increased risk of developing ulcers or symptoms of active or occult gastrointestinal bleeding).
No products indexed under this heading.

Ketorolac Tromethamine (Cholinesterase inhibitors, such as donepezil, may be expected to increase gastric acid secretion due to increased cholinergic activity, therefore, patients on concurrent NSAID therapy should be monitored closely for increased risk of developing ulcers or symptoms of active or occult gastrointestinal bleeding). Products include:
- Acular Ophthalmic Solution 565
- Acular LS Ophthalmic Solution 566

Meclofenamate Sodium (Cholinesterase inhibitors, such as donepezil, may be expected to increase gastric acid secretion due to increased cholinergic activity, therefore, patients on concurrent NSAID therapy should be monitored closely for increased risk of developing ulcers or symptoms of active or occult gastrointestinal bleeding).
No products indexed under this heading.

Mefenamic Acid (Cholinesterase inhibitors, such as donepezil, may be expected to increase gastric acid secretion due to increased cholinergic activity, therefore, patients on concurrent NSAID therapy should be monitored closely for increased risk of developing ulcers or symptoms of active or occult gastrointestinal bleeding).
No products indexed under this heading.

Meloxicam (Cholinesterase inhibitors, such as donepezil, may be expected to increase gastric acid secretion due to increased cholinergic activity, therefore, patients on concurrent NSAID therapy should be monitored closely for increased risk of developing ulcers or symptoms of active or occult gastrointestinal bleeding). Products include:
- Mobic Oral Suspension 863
- Mobic Tablets 863

Mepenzolate Bromide (Donepezil, a cholinesterase inhibitor, has the potential to interfere with the activity of anticholinergic medications).
No products indexed under this heading.

Mephenytoin (Inducers of CYP3A4 could increase the rate of elimination of donepezil).
No products indexed under this heading.

Methsuximide (Inducers of CYP3A4 could increase the rate of elimination of donepezil).
No products indexed under this heading.

Methylprednisolone (Inducers of CYP3A4 could increase the rate of elimination of donepezil).
No products indexed under this heading.

Methylprednisolone Acetate (Inducers of CYP3A4 could increase the rate of elimination of donepezil). Products include:
- Depo-Medrol Injectable Suspension 2617
- Depo-Medrol Single-Dose Vial 2619

Methylprednisolone Sodium Succinate (Inducers of CYP3A4 could increase the rate of elimination of donepezil).
No products indexed under this heading.

Modafinil (Inducers of CYP3A4 could increase the rate of elimination of donepezil). Products include:
- Provigil Tablets 988

Nabumetone (Cholinesterase inhibitors, such as donepezil, may be expected to increase gastric acid secretion due to increased cholinergic activity, therefore, patients on concurrent NSAID therapy should be monitored closely for increased risk of developing ulcers or symptoms of active or occult gastrointestinal bleeding).
No products indexed under this heading.

Naproxen (Cholinesterase inhibitors, such as donepezil, may be expected to increase gastric acid secretion due to increased cholinergic activity, therefore, patients on concurrent NSAID therapy should be monitored closely for increased risk of developing ulcers or symptoms of active or occult gastrointestinal bleeding). Products include:
- EC-Naprosyn Delayed-Release Tablets 2761
- Naprosyn Suspension 2761
- Naprosyn Tablets 2761
- Prevacid NapraPAC 3280

Naproxen Sodium (Cholinesterase inhibitors, such as donepezil, may be expected to increase gastric acid secretion due to increased cholinergic activity, therefore, patients on concurrent NSAID therapy should be monitored closely for increased risk of developing ulcers or symptoms of active or occult gastrointestinal bleeding). Products include:
- Aleve Caplets 742
- Aleve Gelcaps 743
- Aleve Tablets 743
- Aleve Cold & Sinus Caplets 744
- Anaprox Tablets 2761
- Anaprox DS Tablets 2761

Nevirapine (Inducers of CYP3A4 could increase the rate of elimination of donepezil). Products include:
- Viramune Oral Suspension 873
- Viramune Tablets 873

Oxaprozin (Cholinesterase inhibitors, such as donepezil, may be expected to increase gastric acid secretion due to increased cholinergic activity, therefore, patients on concurrent NSAID therapy should be monitored closely for increased risk of developing ulcers or symptoms of active or occult gastrointestinal bleeding).
No products indexed under this heading.

Oxcarbazepine (Inducers of CYP3A4 could increase the rate of elimination of donepezil). Products include:
- Trileptal Tablets 2300
- Trileptal Oral Suspension 2300

Oxybutynin Chloride (Donepezil, a cholinesterase inhibitor, has the potential to interfere with the activity of anticholinergic medications). Products include:
- Ditropan XL Extended-Release Tablets 2413

Phenobarbital (Inducers of CYP2D6 and CYP3A4, such as phenobarbital, could increase the rate of elimination of donepezil). Products include:
- Donnatal Extentabs 2493

Phenobarbital Sodium (Inducers of CYP3A4 could increase the rate of elimination of donepezil).
No products indexed under this heading.

Phenylbutazone (Cholinesterase inhibitors, such as donepezil, may be expected to increase gastric acid secretion due to increased cholinergic activity, therefore, patients on concurrent NSAID therapy should be monitored closely for increased risk of developing ulcers or symptoms of active or occult gastrointestinal bleeding).
No products indexed under this heading.

Phenytoin (Inducers of CYP2D6 and CYP3A4, such as phenytoin, could increase the rate of elimination of donepezil).
No products indexed under this heading.

Phenytoin Sodium (Inducers of CYP2D6 and CYP3A4, such as phenytoin, could increase the rate of elimination of donepezil). Products include:
Phenytek Capsules 2160

Piroxicam (Cholinesterase inhibitors, such as donepezil, may be expected to increase gastric acid secretion due to increased cholinergic activity, therefore, patients on concurrent NSAID therapy should be monitored closely for increased risk of developing ulcers or symptoms of active or occult gastrointestinal bleeding).
No products indexed under this heading.

Prednisolone Acetate (Inducers of CYP3A4 could increase the rate of elimination of donepezil). Products include:
Blephamide Ophthalmic Ointment 568
Blephamide Ophthalmic Suspension.................................. 569
Poly-Pred Ophthalmic Suspension.................................. ⊙233
Pred Forte Ophthalmic Suspension.................................. ⊙235
Pred Mild Ophthalmic Suspension.................................. ⊙238
Pred-G Ophthalmic Ointment .... ⊙237
Pred-G Ophthalmic Suspension ...... ⊙236

Prednisolone Sodium Phosphate (Inducers of CYP3A4 could increase the rate of elimination of donepezil).
No products indexed under this heading.

Prednisolone Tebutate (Inducers of CYP3A4 could increase the rate of elimination of donepezil).
No products indexed under this heading.

Prednisone (Inducers of CYP3A4 could increase the rate of elimination of donepezil).
No products indexed under this heading.

Primidone (Inducers of CYP3A4 could increase the rate of elimination of donepezil).
No products indexed under this heading.

Procyclidine Hydrochloride (Donepezil, a cholinesterase inhibitor, has the potential to interfere with the activity of anticholinergic medications).
No products indexed under this heading.

Propantheline Bromide (Donepezil, a cholinesterase inhibitor, has the potential to interfere with the activity of anticholinergic medications).
No products indexed under this heading.

Quinidine (Inhibitors of CYP450, 2D6 and 3A4, such as quinidine, inhibit donepezil metabolism in vitro).
No products indexed under this heading.

Quinidine Gluconate (Inhibitors of CYP450, 2D6 and 3A4, such as quinidine, inhibit donepezil metabolism in vitro).
No products indexed under this heading.

Quinidine Hydrochloride (Inhibitors of CYP450, 2D6 and 3A4, such as quinidine, inhibit donepezil metabolism in vitro).
No products indexed under this heading.

Quinidine Polygalacturonate (Inhibitors of CYP450, 2D6 and 3A4, such as quinidine, inhibit donepezil metabolism in vitro).
No products indexed under this heading.

Quinidine Sulfate (Inhibitors of CYP450, 2D6 and 3A4, such as quinidine, inhibit donepezil metabolism in vitro).
No products indexed under this heading.

Rifabutin (Inducers of CYP3A4 could increase the rate of elimination of donepezil).
No products indexed under this heading.

Rifampicin (Inducers of CYP3A4 could increase the rate of elimination of donepezil).
No products indexed under this heading.

Rifampin (Inducers of CYP2D6 and CYP3A4, such as rifampin, could increase the rate of elimination of donepezil).
No products indexed under this heading.

Rifapentine (Inducers of CYP3A4 could increase the rate of elimination of donepezil).
No products indexed under this heading.

Ritonavir (Inducers of CYP2D6 could increase the rate of elimination of donepezil). Products include:
Kaletra 476
Norvir 503

Rofecoxib (Cholinesterase inhibitors, such as donepezil, may be expected to increase gastric acid secretion due to increased cholinergic activity, therefore, patients on concurrent NSAID therapy should be monitored closely for increased risk of developing ulcers or symptoms of active or occult gastrointestinal bleeding).
No products indexed under this heading.

Scopolamine (Donepezil, a cholinesterase inhibitor, has the potential to interfere with the activity of anticholinergic medications). Products include:
Transderm Scōp Transdermal Therapeutic System 2177

Scopolamine Hydrobromide (Donepezil, a cholinesterase inhibitor, has the potential to interfere with the activity of anticholinergic medications). Products include:
Donnatal Extentabs 2493

Succinylcholine Chloride (Potential for synergistic effect).
No products indexed under this heading.

Sulfinpyrazone (Inducers of CYP3A4 could increase the rate of elimination of donepezil).
No products indexed under this heading.

Sulindac (Cholinesterase inhibitors, such as donepezil, may be expected to increase gastric acid secretion due to increased cholinergic activity, therefore, patients on concurrent NSAID therapy should be monitored closely for increased risk of developing ulcers or symptoms of active or occult gastrointestinal bleeding). Products include:
Clinoril Tablets 1924

Theophylline (Inducers of CYP3A4 could increase the rate of elimination of donepezil).
No products indexed under this heading.

Tolmetin Sodium (Cholinesterase inhibitors, such as donepezil, may be expected to increase gastric acid secretion due to increased cholinergic activity, therefore, patients on concurrent NSAID therapy should be monitored closely for increased risk of developing ulcers or symptoms of active or occult gastrointestinal bleeding).
No products indexed under this heading.

Tolterodine Tartrate (Donepezil, a cholinesterase inhibitor, has the potential to interfere with the activity of anticholinergic medications). Products include:
Detrol Tablets 2628
Detrol LA Capsules 2631

Triamcinolone (Inducers of CYP3A4 could increase the rate of elimination of donepezil).
No products indexed under this heading.

Triamcinolone Acetonide (Inducers of CYP3A4 could increase the rate of elimination of donepezil). Products include:
Azmacort Inhalation Aerosol 1726
Nasacort AQ Nasal Spray 2922

Triamcinolone Diacetate (Inducers of CYP3A4 could increase the rate of elimination of donepezil).
No products indexed under this heading.

Triamcinolone Hexacetonide (Inducers of CYP3A4 could increase the rate of elimination of donepezil).
No products indexed under this heading.

Tridihexethyl Chloride (Donepezil, a cholinesterase inhibitor, has the potential to interfere with the activity of anticholinergic medications).
No products indexed under this heading.

Trihexyphenidyl Hydrochloride (Donepezil, a cholinesterase inhibitor, has the potential to interfere with the activity of anticholinergic medications).
No products indexed under this heading.

Troglitazone (Inducers of CYP3A4 could increase the rate of elimination of donepezil).
No products indexed under this heading.

Valdecoxib (Cholinesterase inhibitors, such as donepezil, may be expected to increase gastric acid secretion due to increased cholinergic activity, therefore, patients on concurrent NSAID therapy should be monitored closely for increased risk of developing ulcers or symptoms of active or occult gastrointestinal bleeding).
No products indexed under this heading.

ARICEPT ODT TABLETS

(Donepezil Hydrochloride) 1094
See Aricept Tablets

ARIMIDEX TABLETS

(Anastrozole) 673
May interact with estrogens and certain other agents. Compounds in these categories include:

Chlorotrianisene (Estrogen-containing therapies should not be used with anastrozole as they may diminish its pharmacologic action).
No products indexed under this heading.

Dienestrol (Estrogen-containing therapies should not be used with anastrozole as they may diminish its pharmacologic action).
No products indexed under this heading.

Diethylstilbestrol (Estrogen-containing therapies should not be used with anastrozole as they may diminish its pharmacologic action).
No products indexed under this heading.

Estradiol (Estrogen-containing therapies should not be used with anastrozole as they may diminish its pharmacologic action). Products include:
Angeliq Tablets 762
Climara Transdermal System 771
Climara Pro Transdermal System 776
Estrasorb Topical Emulsion 1147
Estring Vaginal Ring 2635
Menostar Transdermal System 782
Vagifem Tablets 2334

Estrogens, Conjugated (Estrogen-containing therapies should not be used with anastrozole as they may diminish its pharmacologic action). Products include:
Premarin Intravenous 3442
Premarin Tablets 3446
Premarin Vaginal Cream 3452
Premphase Tablets 3456
Prempro Tablets 3456

Estrogens, Esterified (Estrogen-containing therapies should not be used with anastrozole as they may diminish its pharmacologic action). Products include:
Estratest Tablets 3199
Estratest H.S. Tablets 3199

Estropipate (Estrogen-containing therapies should not be used with anastrozole as they may diminish its pharmacologic action).
No products indexed under this heading.

Ethinyl Estradiol (Estrogen-containing therapies should not be used with anastrozole as they may diminish its pharmacologic action). Products include:
Mircette Tablets 1066
NuvaRing 2340
Ortho-Cyclen/Ortho Tri-Cyclen 2429
Ortho Evra Transdermal System 2417
Ortho Tri-Cyclen Lo Tablets 2436
Seasonique Tablets 1077
Yasmin 28 Tablets 796
Yaz Tablets 803

Polyestradiol Phosphate (Estrogen-containing therapies should not be used with anastrozole as they may diminish its pharmacologic action).
No products indexed under this heading.

Quinestrol (Estrogen-containing therapies should not be used with anastrozole as they may diminish its pharmacologic action).
No products indexed under this heading.

Tamoxifen Citrate (Co-administration of tamoxifen and

anastrozole may reduce anastrozole plasma concentration; avoid co-administration). Products include:

Soltamox Oral Solution 3527

ARIXTRA INJECTION

(Fondaparinux Sodium) 1351

May interact with anticoagulants, non-steroidal anti-inflammatory agents, and certain other agents. Compounds in these categories include:

Abciximab (Agents that may enhance the risk of hemorrhage, such as abciximab, should be discontinued prior to initiation of fondaparinux sodium therapy. If co-administration is essential, close monitoring may be appropriate). Products include:

ReoPro Vials 1809

Anisindione (Agents that may enhance the risk of hemorrhage, such as anticoagulants, should be discontinued prior to initiation of fondaparinux sodium therapy. If co-administration is essential, close monitoring may be appropriate). Products include:

Miradon Tablets 3042

Ardeparin Sodium (Agents that may enhance the risk of hemorrhage, such as anticoagulants, should be discontinued prior to initiation of fondaparinux sodium therapy. If co-administration is essential, close monitoring may be appropriate).

No products indexed under this heading.

Aspirin (Agents that may enhance the risk of hemorrhage, such as aspirin, should be discontinued prior to initiation of fondaparinux sodium therapy. If co-administration is essential, close monitoring may be appropriate). Products include:

Aggrenox Capsules 822
Bayer Aspirin 744
BC Allergy Sinus Cold Powder .... ■ 677
BC Headache Powder .... ■ 677
Arthritis Strength BC Powder .... ■ 677
BC Sinus Cold Powder .... ■ 677
Excedrin Extra Strength Caplets/Tablets/Geltabs .... ■ 684
Excedrin Migraine Caplets/Tablets/Geltabs .... ■ 609
Goody's Body Pain Formula Powder .... ■ 684
Goody's Extra Strength Headache Powders .... ■ 611
Goody's Extra Strength Pain Relief Tablets .... ■ 685
Percodan Tablets 1132
St. Joseph 81 mg Aspirin Chewable and Enteric Coated Tablets 1869

Celecoxib (Agents that may enhance the risk of hemorrhage, such as non-steroidal anti-inflammatory agents, should be discontinued prior to initiation of fondaparinux sodium therapy. If co-administration is essential, close monitoring may be appropriate). Products include:

Celebrex Capsules 3134

Clopidogrel Bisulfate (Agents that may enhance the risk of hemorrhage, such as clopidogrel bisulfate, should be discontinued prior to initiation of fondaparinux sodium therapy. If co-administration is essential, close monitoring may be appropriate). Products include:

Plavix Tablets 917
Plavix Tablets 2926

Dalteparin Sodium (Agents that may enhance the risk of hemorrhage, such as anticoagulants, should be discontinued prior to initiation of fondaparinux sodium therapy. If co-administration is essential, close monitoring may be appropriate). Products include:

Fragmin Injection 1097

Danaparoid Sodium (Agents that may enhance the risk of hemorrhage, such as anticoagulants, should be discontinued prior to initiation of fondaparinux sodium therapy. If co-administration is essential, close monitoring may be appropriate).

No products indexed under this heading.

Diclofenac Potassium (Agents that may enhance the risk of hemorrhage, such as non-steroidal anti-inflammatory agents, should be discontinued prior to initiation of fondaparinux sodium therapy. If co-administration is essential, close monitoring may be appropriate).

No products indexed under this heading.

Diclofenac Sodium (Agents that may enhance the risk of hemorrhage, such as non-steroidal anti-inflammatory agents, should be discontinued prior to initiation of fondaparinux sodium therapy. If co-administration is essential, close monitoring may be appropriate). Products include:

Arthrotec Tablets 3129
Voltaren Ophthalmic Solution 2309
Voltaren Tablets 2307
Voltaren-XR Tablets 2310

Dicumarol (Agents that may enhance the risk of hemorrhage, such as anticoagulants, should be discontinued prior to initiation of fondaparinux sodium therapy. If co-administration is essential, close monitoring may be appropriate).

No products indexed under this heading.

Dipyridamole (Agents that may enhance the risk of hemorrhage, such as dipyridamole, should be discontinued prior to initiation of fondaparinux sodium therapy. If co-administration is essential, close monitoring may be appropriate). Products include:

Aggrenox Capsules 822
Persantine Tablets 868

Enoxaparin Sodium (Agents that may enhance the risk of hemorrhage, such as anticoagulants, should be discontinued prior to initiation of fondaparinux sodium therapy. If co-administration is essential, close monitoring may be appropriate). Products include:

Lovenox Injection 2915

Eptifibatide (Agents that may enhance the risk of hemorrhage, such as eptifibatide, should be discontinued prior to initiation of fondaparinux sodium therapy. If co-administration is essential, close monitoring may be appropriate). Products include:

Integrilin Injection 3020

Etodolac (Agents that may enhance the risk of hemorrhage, such as non-steroidal anti-inflammatory agents, should be discontinued prior to initiation of fondaparinux sodium therapy. If co-administration is essential, close monitoring may be appropriate).

No products indexed under this heading.

Fenoprofen Calcium (Agents that may enhance the risk of hemorrhage, such as non-steroidal anti-inflammatory agents, should be discontinued prior to initiation of fondaparinux sodium therapy. If co-administration is essential, close monitoring may be appropriate). Products include:

Nalfon Capsules 2502

Flurbiprofen (Agents that may enhance the risk of hemorrhage, such as non-steroidal anti-inflammatory agents, should be discontinued prior to initiation of fondaparinux sodium therapy. If co-administration is essential, close monitoring may be appropriate).

No products indexed under this heading.

Heparin Calcium (Agents that may enhance the risk of hemorrhage, such as anticoagulants, should be discontinued prior to initiation of fondaparinux sodium therapy. If co-administration is essential, close monitoring may be appropriate).

No products indexed under this heading.

Heparin Sodium (Agents that may enhance the risk of hemorrhage, such as anticoagulants, should be discontinued prior to initiation of fondaparinux sodium therapy. If co-administration is essential, close monitoring may be appropriate).

No products indexed under this heading.

Ibuprofen (Agents that may enhance the risk of hemorrhage, such as non-steroidal anti-inflammatory agents, should be discontinued prior to initiation of fondaparinux sodium therapy. If co-administration is essential, close monitoring may be appropriate). Products include:

Advil Allergy Sinus Caplets .... ■ 770
Advil .... ■ 674
Children's Advil Oral Suspension .... ■ 603
Children's Advil Chewable Tablets .. ■ 603
Advil Cold & Sinus .... ■ 723
Infants' Advil Concentrated Drops .. ■ 604
Infants' Advil Concentrated Drops - White Grape (Dye-Free)............. ■ 604
Junior Strength Advil Swallow Tablets.. ■ 605
Advil Migraine Liquigels .... ■ 608
Advil Multi-Symptom Cold Caplets.. ■ 770
Advil PM Caplets .... ■ 615
Motrin IB Tablets and Caplets 1866
Children's Motrin Oral Suspension ... 1867
Children's Motrin Non-Staining Dye-Free Oral Suspension............ 1867
Children's Motrin Cold Oral Suspension 1867
Infants' Motrin Concentrated Drops 1867
Infants' Motrin Non-Staining Dye-Free Concentrated Drops....... 1867
Junior Strength Motrin Caplets and Chewable Tablets.................. 1867
Vicoprofen Tablets 539

Indomethacin (Agents that may enhance the risk of hemorrhage, such as non-steroidal anti-inflammatory agents, should be discontinued prior to initiation of fondaparinux sodium therapy. If co-administration is essential, close monitoring may be appropriate). Products include:

Indocin 1995

Indomethacin Sodium Trihydrate (Agents that may enhance the risk of hemorrhage, such as non-steroidal anti-inflammatory agents, should be discontinued prior to initiation of fondaparinux sodium therapy. If co-administration is essential, close monitoring may be appropriate). Products include:

Indocin I.V. 2465

Ketoprofen (Agents that may enhance the risk of hemorrhage, such as non-steroidal anti-inflammatory agents, should be discontinued prior to initiation of fondaparinux sodium therapy. If co-administration is essential, close monitoring may be appropriate).

No products indexed under this heading.

Ketorolac Tromethamine (Agents that may enhance the risk of hemorrhage, such as non-steroidal anti-inflammatory agents, should be discontinued prior to initiation of fondaparinux sodium therapy. If co-administration is essential, close monitoring may be appropriate). Products include:

Acular Ophthalmic Solution 565
Acular LS Ophthalmic Solution 566

Low Molecular Weight Heparins (Agents that may enhance the risk of hemorrhage, such as anticoagulants, should be discontinued prior to initiation of fondaparinux sodium therapy. If co-administration is essential, close monitoring may be appropriate).

No products indexed under this heading.

Meclofenamate Sodium (Agents that may enhance the risk of hemorrhage, such as non-steroidal anti-inflammatory agents, should be discontinued prior to initiation of fondaparinux sodium therapy. If co-administration is essential, close monitoring may be appropriate).

No products indexed under this heading.

Mefenamic Acid (Agents that may enhance the risk of hemorrhage, such as non-steroidal anti-inflammatory agents, should be discontinued prior to initiation of fondaparinux sodium therapy. If co-administration is essential, close monitoring may be appropriate).

No products indexed under this heading.

Meloxicam (Agents that may enhance the risk of hemorrhage, such as non-steroidal anti-inflammatory agents, should be discontinued prior to initiation of fondaparinux sodium therapy. If co-administration is essential, close monitoring may be appropriate). Products include:

Mobic Oral Suspension 863
Mobic Tablets 863

Nabumetone (Agents that may enhance the risk of hemorrhage, such as non-steroidal anti-inflammatory agents, should be discontinued prior to initiation of fondaparinux sodium therapy. If co-administration is essential, close monitoring may be appropriate).

No products indexed under this heading.

Naproxen (Agents that may enhance the risk of hemorrhage, such as non-steroidal anti-inflammatory agents, should be discontinued prior to initiation of fondaparinux sodium therapy. If co-administration is essential, close monitoring may be appropriate). Products include:

EC-Naprosyn Delayed-Release Tablets 2761
Naprosyn Suspension 2761
Naprosyn Tablets 2761
Prevacid NapraPAC 3280

Naproxen Sodium (Agents that may enhance the risk of hemorrhage, such as non-steroidal anti-inflammatory agents, should be discontinued prior to initiation of fondaparinux sodium therapy. If co-administration is essential, close monitoring may be appropriate). Products include:

Aleve Caplets 742
Aleve Gelcaps 743
Aleve Tablets 743
Aleve Cold & Sinus Caplets 744
Anaprox Tablets 2761
Anaprox DS Tablets 2761

Oxaprozin (Agents that may enhance the risk of hemorrhage, such as non-steroidal anti-inflammatory agents, should be discontinued prior to initiation of fondaparinux sodium therapy. If co-administration is essential, close monitoring may be appropriate).
No products indexed under this heading.

Phenylbutazone (Agents that may enhance the risk of hemorrhage, such as non-steroidal anti-inflammatory agents, should be discontinued prior to initiation of fondaparinux sodium therapy. If co-administration is essential, close monitoring may be appropriate).
No products indexed under this heading.

Piroxicam (Agents that may enhance the risk of hemorrhage, such as non-steroidal anti-inflammatory agents, should be discontinued prior to initiation of fondaparinux sodium therapy. If co-administration is essential, close monitoring may be appropriate).
No products indexed under this heading.

Rofecoxib (Agents that may enhance the risk of hemorrhage, such as non-steroidal anti-inflammatory agents, should be discontinued prior to initiation of fondaparinux sodium therapy. If co-administration is essential, close monitoring may be appropriate).
No products indexed under this heading.

Sulindac (Agents that may enhance the risk of hemorrhage, such as non-steroidal anti-inflammatory agents, should be discontinued prior to initiation of fondaparinux sodium therapy. If co-administration is essential, close monitoring may be appropriate). Products include:

Clinoril Tablets 1924

Tinzaparin Sodium (Agents that may enhance the risk of hemorrhage, such as anticoagulants, should be discontinued prior to initiation of fondaparinux sodium therapy. If co-administration is essential, close monitoring may be appropriate).
No products indexed under this heading.

Tirofiban Hydrochloride (Agents that may enhance the risk of hemorrhage, such as tirofiban hydrochloride, should be discontinued prior to initiation of fondaparinux sodium therapy. If co-administration is essential, close monitoring may be appropriate). Products include:

Aggrastat 1907

Tolmetin Sodium (Agents that may enhance the risk of hemorrhage, such as non-steroidal anti-inflammatory agents, should be discontinued prior to initiation of fondaparinux sodium therapy. If co-administration is essential, close monitoring may be appropriate).
No products indexed under this heading.

Valdecoxib (Agents that may enhance the risk of hemorrhage, such as non-steroidal anti-inflammatory agents, should be discontinued prior to initiation of fondaparinux sodium therapy. If co-administration is essential, close monitoring may be appropriate).
No products indexed under this heading.

Warfarin Sodium (Agents that may enhance the risk of hemorrhage, such as anticoagulants, should be discontinued prior to initiation of fondaparinux sodium therapy. If co-administration is essential, close monitoring may be appropriate). Products include:

Coumadin for Injection 898
Coumadin Tablets 898

AROMASIN TABLETS

(Exemestane) 2600

May interact with cytochrome p450 3a4 inducers (selected) and certain other agents. Compounds in these categories include:

Allium sativum (Co-medications that induce CYP3A4 may significantly decrease exposure to exemestane. Dose modification is recommended for patients receiving a potent CYP3A4 inducer).
No products indexed under this heading.

Aprepitant (Co-medications that induce CYP3A4 may significantly decrease exposure to exemestane. Dose modification is recommended for patients receiving a potent CYP3A4 inducer). Products include:

Emend Capsules 1963

Betamethasone Acetate (Co-medications that induce CYP3A4 may significantly decrease exposure to exemestane. Dose modification is recommended for patients receiving a potent CYP3A4 inducer).
No products indexed under this heading.

Betamethasone Sodium Phosphate (Co-medications that induce CYP3A4 may significantly decrease exposure to exemestane. Dose modification is recommended for patients receiving a potent CYP3A4 inducer).
No products indexed under this heading.

Carbamazepine (Co-medications that induce CYP3A4 may significantly decrease exposure to exemestane. Dose modification is recommended for patients receiving a potent CYP3A4 inducer). Products include:

Carbatrol Capsules 3171
Equetro Extended-Release Capsules 3180
Tegretol/Tegretol-XR 2295

Ciprofloxacin Hydrochloride (Co-medications that induce CYP3A4 may significantly decrease exposure to exemestane. Dose modification is recommended for patients receiving a potent CYP3A4 inducer). Products include:

Ciloxan Ophthalmic Ointment 559
Ciloxan Ophthalmic Solution .... ⊙206
Cipro Tablets 2977
Proquin XR Tablets 1153

Cisplatin (Co-medications that induce CYP3A4 may significantly decrease exposure to exemestane. Dose modification is recommended for patients receiving a potent CYP3A4 inducer).
No products indexed under this heading.

Cortisone Acetate (Co-medications that induce CYP3A4 may significantly decrease exposure to exemestane. Dose modification is recommended for patients receiving a potent CYP3A4 inducer).
No products indexed under this heading.

Dexamethasone (Co-medications that induce CYP3A4 may significantly decrease exposure to exemestane. Dose modification is recommended for patients receiving a potent CYP3A4 inducer). Products include:

Ciprodex Otic Suspension 559
Decadron Tablets 1951
TobraDex Ophthalmic Ointment 562
TobraDex Ophthalmic Suspension 563

Dexamethasone Acetate (Co-medications that induce CYP3A4 may significantly decrease exposure to exemestane. Dose modification is recommended for patients receiving a potent CYP3A4 inducer).
No products indexed under this heading.

Dexamethasone Sodium Phosphate (Co-medications that induce CYP3A4 may significantly decrease exposure to exemestane. Dose modification is recommended for patients receiving a potent CYP3A4 inducer).
No products indexed under this heading.

Doxorubicin Hydrochloride (Co-medications that induce CYP3A4 may significantly decrease exposure to exemestane. Dose modification is recommended for patients receiving a potent CYP3A4 inducer).
No products indexed under this heading.

Efavirenz (Co-medications that induce CYP3A4 may significantly decrease exposure to exemestane. Dose modification is recommended for patients receiving a potent CYP3A4 inducer). Products include:

Atripla Tablets 945
Sustiva Capsules 930
Sustiva Tablets 930

Ethosuximide (Co-medications that induce CYP3A4 may significantly decrease exposure to exemestane. Dose modification is recommended for patients receiving a potent CYP3A4 inducer).
No products indexed under this heading.

Felbamate (Co-medications that induce CYP3A4 may significantly decrease exposure to exemestane. Dose modification is recommended for patients receiving a potent CYP3A4 inducer).
No products indexed under this heading.

Fludrocortisone Acetate (Co-medications that induce CYP3A4 may significantly decrease exposure to exemestane. Dose modification is recommended for patients receiving a potent CYP3A4 inducer).
No products indexed under this heading.

Fosphenytoin Sodium (Co-medications that induce CYP3A4 may significantly decrease exposure to exemestane. Dose modification is recommended for patients receiving a potent CYP3A4 inducer).
No products indexed under this heading.

Garlic Extract (Co-medications that induce CYP3A4 may significantly decrease exposure to exemestane. Dose modification is recommended for patients receiving a potent CYP3A4 inducer).
No products indexed under this heading.

Garlic Oil (Co-medications that induce CYP3A4 may significantly decrease exposure to exemestane. Dose modification is recommended for patients receiving a potent CYP3A4 inducer).
No products indexed under this heading.

Hydrocortisone (Co-medications that induce CYP3A4 may significantly decrease exposure to exemestane. Dose modification is recommended for patients receiving a potent CYP3A4 inducer). Products include:

Colocort Rectal Suspension, USP (Retention) 100 mg/60 mL 2476
Hydrocortone Tablets 1989
Preparation H Hydrocortisone Cream 646

Hydrocortisone Acetate (Co-medications that induce CYP3A4 may significantly decrease exposure to exemestane. Dose modification is recommended for patients receiving a potent CYP3A4 inducer). Products include:

Analpram-HC 1159
Pramosone 1161
ProctoFoam-HC 3099

Hydrocortisone Butyrate (Co-medications that induce CYP3A4 may significantly decrease exposure to exemestane. Dose modification is recommended for patients receiving a potent CYP3A4 inducer). Products include:

Locoid Lipocream Cream 1160

Hydrocortisone Cypionate (Co-medications that induce CYP3A4 may significantly decrease exposure to exemestane. Dose modification is recommended for patients receiving a potent CYP3A4 inducer).
No products indexed under this heading.

Hydrocortisone Hemisuccinate (Co-medications that induce CYP3A4 may significantly decrease exposure to exemestane. Dose modification is recommended for patients receiving a potent CYP3A4 inducer).
No products indexed under this heading.

Hydrocortisone Probutate (Co-medications that induce CYP3A4 may significantly decrease exposure to exemestane. Dose modification is recommended for patients receiving a potent CYP3A4 inducer).
No products indexed under this heading.

Hydrocortisone Sodium Phosphate (Co-medications that induce CYP3A4 may significantly decrease exposure to exemestane. Dose modification is recommended for patients receiving a potent CYP3A4 inducer).
No products indexed under this heading.

Hydrocortisone Sodium Succinate (Co-medications that induce CYP3A4 may significantly decrease exposure to exemestane. Dose modification is recommended for patients receiving a potent CYP3A4 inducer).
No products indexed under this heading.

Hydrocortisone Valerate (Co-medications that induce CYP3A4 may significantly decrease exposure to exemestane. Dose modification is recommended for patients receiving a potent CYP3A4 inducer).
No products indexed under this heading.

Hypericum (Co-medications that induce CYP3A4 may significantly decrease exposure to exemestane. Dose modification is recommended for patients receiving a potent CYP3A4 inducer). Products include:
Satiete Tablets .... ▣832

Hypericum Perforatum (Co-medications that induce CYP3A4 may significantly decrease exposure to exemestane. Dose modification is recommended for patients receiving a potent CYP3A4 inducer).
No products indexed under this heading.

Mephenytoin (Co-medications that induce CYP3A4 may significantly decrease exposure to exemestane. Dose modification is recommended for patients receiving a potent CYP3A4 inducer).
No products indexed under this heading.

Methsuximide (Co-medications that induce CYP3A4 may significantly decrease exposure to exemestane. Dose modification is recommended for patients receiving a potent CYP3A4 inducer).
No products indexed under this heading.

Methylprednisolone (Co-medications that induce CYP3A4 may significantly decrease exposure to exemestane. Dose modification is recommended for patients receiving a potent CYP3A4 inducer).
No products indexed under this heading.

Methylprednisolone Acetate (Co-medications that induce CYP3A4 may significantly decrease exposure to exemestane. Dose modification is recommended for patients receiving a potent CYP3A4 inducer). Products include:
Depo-Medrol Injectable Suspension 2617
Depo-Medrol Single-Dose Vial 2619

Methylprednisolone Sodium Succinate (Co-medications that induce CYP3A4 may significantly decrease exposure to exemestane. Dose modification is recommended for patients receiving a potent CYP3A4 inducer).
No products indexed under this heading.

Modafinil (Co-medications that induce CYP3A4 may significantly decrease exposure to exemestane. Dose modification is recommended for patients receiving a potent CYP3A4 inducer). Products include:
Provigil Tablets 988

Nevirapine (Co-medications that induce CYP3A4 may significantly decrease exposure to exemestane. Dose modification is recommended for patients receiving a potent CYP3A4 inducer). Products include:
Viramune Oral Suspension 873
Viramune Tablets 873

Oxcarbazepine (Co-medications that induce CYP3A4 may significantly decrease exposure to exemestane. Dose modification is recommended for patients receiving a potent CYP3A4 inducer). Products include:
Trileptal Tablets 2300
Trileptal Oral Suspension 2300

Phenobarbital (Co-medications that induce CYP3A4 may significantly decrease exposure to exemestane. Dose modification is recommended for patients receiving a potent CYP3A4 inducer). Products include:
Donnatal Extentabs 2493

Phenobarbital Sodium (Co-medications that induce CYP3A4 may significantly decrease exposure to exemestane. Dose modification is recommended for patients receiving a potent CYP3A4 inducer).
No products indexed under this heading.

Phenytoin (Co-medications that induce CYP3A4 may significantly decrease exposure to exemestane. Dose modification is recommended for patients receiving a potent CYP3A4 inducer).
No products indexed under this heading.

Phenytoin Sodium (Co-medications that induce CYP3A4 may significantly decrease exposure to exemestane. Dose modification is recommended for patients receiving a potent CYP3A4 inducer). Products include:
Phenytek Capsules 2160

Prednisolone Acetate (Co-medications that induce CYP3A4 may significantly decrease exposure to exemestane. Dose modification is recommended for patients receiving a potent CYP3A4 inducer). Products include:
Blephamide Ophthalmic Ointment 568
Blephamide Ophthalmic Suspension................................ 569
Poly-Pred Ophthalmic Suspension .... ⊙233
Pred Forte Ophthalmic Suspension .... ⊙235
Pred Mild Ophthalmic Suspension .... ⊙238
Pred-G Ophthalmic Ointment .... ⊙237
Pred-G Ophthalmic Suspension ...... ⊙236

Prednisolone Sodium Phosphate (Co-medications that induce CYP3A4 may significantly decrease exposure to exemestane. Dose modification is recommended for patients receiving a potent CYP3A4 inducer).
No products indexed under this heading.

Prednisolone Tebutate (Co-medications that induce CYP3A4 may significantly decrease exposure to exemestane. Dose modification is recommended for patients receiving a potent CYP3A4 inducer).
No products indexed under this heading.

Prednisone (Co-medications that induce CYP3A4 may significantly decrease exposure to exemestane. Dose modification is recommended for patients receiving a potent CYP3A4 inducer).
No products indexed under this heading.

Primidone (Co-medications that induce CYP3A4 may significantly decrease exposure to exemestane. Dose modification is recommended for patients receiving a potent CYP3A4 inducer).
No products indexed under this heading.

Rifabutin (Co-medications that induce CYP3A4 may significantly decrease exposure to exemestane. Dose modification is recommended for patients receiving a potent CYP3A4 inducer).
No products indexed under this heading.

Rifampicin (When patients were pretreated with rifampicin, a potent CYP3A4 inducer, followed by a single dose of exemestane, the mean plasma Cmax and AUC of exemestane were decreased. Dose modification is recommended).
No products indexed under this heading.

Rifampin (Co-medications that induce CYP3A4 may significantly decrease exposure to exemestane. Dose modification is recommended for patients receiving a potent CYP3A4 inducer).
No products indexed under this heading.

Rifapentine (Co-medications that induce CYP3A4 may significantly decrease exposure to exemestane. Dose modification is recommended for patients receiving a potent CYP3A4 inducer).
No products indexed under this heading.

Sulfinpyrazone (Co-medications that induce CYP3A4 may significantly decrease exposure to exemestane. Dose modification is recommended for patients receiving a potent CYP3A4 inducer).
No products indexed under this heading.

Theophylline (Co-medications that induce CYP3A4 may significantly decrease exposure to exemestane. Dose modification is recommended for patients receiving a potent CYP3A4 inducer).
No products indexed under this heading.

Triamcinolone (Co-medications that induce CYP3A4 may significantly decrease exposure to exemestane. Dose modification is recommended for patients receiving a potent CYP3A4 inducer).
No products indexed under this heading.

Triamcinolone Acetonide (Co-medications that induce CYP3A4 may significantly decrease exposure to exemestane. Dose modification is recommended for patients receiving a potent CYP3A4 inducer). Products include:
Azmacort Inhalation Aerosol 1726
Nasacort AQ Nasal Spray 2922

Triamcinolone Diacetate (Co-medications that induce CYP3A4 may significantly decrease exposure to exemestane. Dose modification is recommended for patients receiving a potent CYP3A4 inducer).
No products indexed under this heading.

Triamcinolone Hexacetonide (Co-medications that induce CYP3A4 may significantly decrease exposure to exemestane. Dose modification is recommended for patients receiving a potent CYP3A4 inducer).
No products indexed under this heading.

Troglitazone (Co-medications that induce CYP3A4 may significantly decrease exposure to exemestane. Dose modification is recommended for patients receiving a potent CYP3A4 inducer).
No products indexed under this heading.

Food Interactions

Food, unspecified (Exemestane plasma levels increased approximately 40% after high-fat breakfast).

ARRANON INJECTION

(Nelarabine) 1357
May interact with:

Pentostatin (Co-administration of nelarabine with adenosine deaminase inhibitors, such as pentostatin, is not recommended). Products include:
Nipent for Injection 1863

ARTHROTEC TABLETS

(Diclofenac Sodium, Misoprostol) 3129
May interact with ACE inhibitors, antacids, antihypertensives, aspirin-acetylsalicylic acid, oral hypoglycemic agents, insulin, lithium preparations, potassium sparing diuretics, thiazides, and certain other agents. Compounds in these categories include:

Acarbose (Diclofenac may alter a diabetic patient's response to oral hypoglycemic agents; both hypo- and hyperglycemic effects have been reported). Products include:
Precose Tablets 751

Acebutolol Hydrochloride (NSAIDs can inhibit the activity of antihypertensives).
No products indexed under this heading.

Aluminum Carbonate (Antacids reduce the bioavailability of misoprostol acid. Antacids may also delay absorption of diclofenac sodium. Magnesium-containing antacids exacerbate misoprostol-associated diarrhea. Thus, it is not recommended that Arthrotec be coadministered with magnesium containing antacids).
No products indexed under this heading.

Aluminum Hydroxide (Antacids reduce the bioavailability of misoprostol acid. Antacids may also delay absorption of diclofenac sodium. Magnesium-containing antacids exacerbate misoprostol-associated diarrhea. Thus, it is not recommended that Arthrotec be coadministered with magnesium containing antacids). Products include:
Gaviscon Regular Strength Liquid .. ▣658
Gaviscon Regular Strength Tablets....................................... ▣658
Gaviscon Extra Strength Liquid ...... ▣658

Gaviscon Extra Strength Tablets .... ▣ 658
Maalox Regular Strength Antacid/Antigas Liquid 2175
Maalox Max Maximum Strength Antacid/Anti-Gas Liquid 2176

Amiloride Hydrochloride (Concomitant therapy with potassium-sparing diuretics may be associated with increased serum potassium levels). Products include:
Midamor Tablets 2026
Moduretic Tablets 2028

Amlodipine Besylate (NSAIDs can inhibit the activity of antihypertensives). Products include:
Caduet Tablets 2508
Lotrel Capsules 2249
Norvasc Tablets 2545

Aspirin (When Arthrotec is administered with aspirin, the protein binding of diclofenac is reduced, although the clearance of the free Arthrotec is not altered. The clinical significance of this interaction is not known; however, as with other NSAIDs, concomitant administration of diclofenac sodium and aspirin is not generally recommended because of the potential risk of increased adverse effects). Products include:
Aggrenox Capsules 822
Bayer Aspirin 744
BC Allergy Sinus Cold Powder .... ▣ 677
BC Headache Powder .... ▣ 677
Arthritis Strength BC Powder .... ▣ 677
BC Sinus Cold Powder .... ▣ 677
Excedrin Extra Strength Caplets/Tablets/Geltabs .... ▣ 684
Excedrin Migraine Caplets/Tablets/Geltabs .... ▣ 609
Goody's Body Pain Formula Powder .... ▣ 684
Goody's Extra Strength Headache Powders .... ▣ 611
Goody's Extra Strength Pain Relief Tablets .... ▣ 685
Percodan Tablets 1132
St. Joseph 81 mg Aspirin Chewable and Enteric Coated Tablets 1869

Aspirin, Enteric Coated (When Arthrotec is administered with aspirin, the protein binding of diclofenac is reduced, although the clearance of the free Arthrotec is not altered. The clinical significance of this interaction is not known; however, as with other NSAIDs, concomitant administration of diclofenac sodium and aspirin is not generally recommended because of the potential risk of increased adverse effects).
No products indexed under this heading.

Aspirin Buffered (When Arthrotec is administered with aspirin, the protein binding of diclofenac is reduced, although the clearance of the free Arthrotec is not altered. The clinical significance of this interaction is not known; however, as with other NSAIDs, concomitant administration of diclofenac sodium and aspirin is not generally recommended because of the potential risk of increased adverse effects). Products include:
Bufferin Extra Strength Tablets .... ▣ 678
Bufferin Regular Strength Tablets .... ▣ 678

Atenolol (NSAIDs can inhibit the activity of antihypertensives).
No products indexed under this heading.

Benazepril Hydrochloride (NSAIDs can inhibit the activity of antihypertensives). Products include:
Lotensin Tablets 2243
Lotensin HCT Tablets 2246
Lotrel Capsules 2249

Bendroflumethiazide (Clinical studies, as well as post marketing observations, have shown that Arthrotec can reduce the natriuretic effect of furosemide and thiazides in some patients. This response has been attributed to the inhibition of renal prostaglandin synthesis. During concomitant therapy with NSAIDs, the patient should be observed closely for signs of renal failure as well as to assure diuretic efficacy).
No products indexed under this heading.

Betaxolol Hydrochloride (NSAIDs can inhibit the activity of antihypertensives). Products include:
Betoptic S Ophthalmic Suspension 558

Bisoprolol Fumarate (NSAIDs can inhibit the activity of antihypertensives).
No products indexed under this heading.

Candesartan Cilexetil (NSAIDs can inhibit the activity of antihypertensives). Products include:
Atacand Tablets 649
Atacand HCT 651

Captopril (NSAIDs can inhibit the activity of antihypertensives). Products include:
Captopril Tablets 2149

Carteolol Hydrochloride (NSAIDs can inhibit the activity of antihypertensives). Products include:
Carteolol Hydrochloride Ophthalmic Solution USP, 1% .... ⊙ 249

Chlorothiazide (Clinical studies, as well as post marketing observations, have shown that Arthrotec can reduce the natriuretic effect of furosemide and thiazides in some patients. This response has been attributed to the inhibition of renal prostaglandin synthesis. During concomitant therapy with NSAIDs, the patient should be observed closely for signs of renal failure as well as to assure diuretic efficacy). Products include:
Diuril Oral Suspension 1954

Chlorothiazide Sodium (Clinical studies, as well as post marketing observations, have shown that Arthrotec can reduce the natriuretic effect of furosemide and thiazides in some patients. This response has been attributed to the inhibition of renal prostaglandin synthesis. During concomitant therapy with NSAIDs, the patient should be observed closely for signs of renal failure as well as to assure diuretic efficacy). Products include:
Diuril Sodium Intravenous 2467

Chlorpropamide (Diclofenac may alter a diabetic patient's response to oral hypoglycemic agents; both hypo- and hyperglycemic effects have been reported).
No products indexed under this heading.

Chlorthalidone (NSAIDs can inhibit the activity of antihypertensives). Products include:
Clorpres Tablets 2153

Clonidine (NSAIDs can inhibit the activity of antihypertensives). Products include:
Catapres-TTS 844

Clonidine Hydrochloride (NSAIDs can inhibit the activity of antihypertensives). Products include:
Catapres Tablets 843
Clorpres Tablets 2153

Cyclosporine (Arthrotec, like other NSAID containing products, may affect renal prostaglandins and increase the toxicity of certain drugs. Ingestion of Arthrotec may increase cyclosporine nephrotoxicity. Patients who begin Arthrotec while taking cyclosporine may develop toxicity characteristics of cyclosporine. They should be observed closely, particularly if renal function is impaired). Products include:
Gengraf Capsules 459
Neoral Oral Solution 2259
Neoral Soft Gelatin Capsules 2259
Restasis Ophthalmic Emulsion 575
Sandimmune 2275

Deserpidine (NSAIDs can inhibit the activity of antihypertensives).
No products indexed under this heading.

Diazoxide (NSAIDs can inhibit the activity of antihypertensives). Products include:
Hyperstat I.V. 3017

Digoxin (Co-administration of digoxin with diclofenac has resulted in elevated digoxin levels). Products include:
Lanoxicaps Capsules 1490
Lanoxin Injection 1494
Lanoxin Injection Pediatric 1497
Lanoxin Tablets 1500

Diltiazem Hydrochloride (NSAIDs can inhibit the activity of antihypertensives). Products include:
Cardizem LA Extended Release Tablets 1728
Tiazac Capsules 1201

Doxazosin Mesylate (NSAIDs can inhibit the activity of antihypertensives). Products include:
Cardura XL Tablets 2515

Enalapril Maleate (NSAIDs can inhibit the activity of antihypertensives). Products include:
Vasotec I.V. Injection 2103

Enalaprilat (NSAIDs can inhibit the activity of antihypertensives).
No products indexed under this heading.

Eprosartan Mesylate (NSAIDs can inhibit the activity of antihypertensives). Products include:
Teveten Tablets 1735
Teveten HCT Tablets 1737

Esmolol Hydrochloride (NSAIDs can inhibit the activity of antihypertensives).
No products indexed under this heading.

Felodipine (NSAIDs can inhibit the activity of antihypertensives).
No products indexed under this heading.

Fosinopril Sodium (NSAIDs can inhibit the activity of antihypertensives).
No products indexed under this heading.

Furosemide (Clinical studies, as well as post marketing observations, have shown that Arthrotec can reduce the natriuretic effect of furosemide and thiazides in some patients. This response has been attributed to the inhibition of renal prostaglandin synthesis. During concomitant therapy with NSAIDs, the patient should be observed closely for signs of renal failure as well as to assure diuretic efficacy). Products include:
Furosemide Tablets 2154

Glimepiride (Diclofenac may alter a diabetic patient's response to oral hypoglycemic agents; both hypo- and hyperglycemic effects have been reported). Products include:
Avandaryl Tablets 1379
Duetact Tablets 3226

Glipizide (Diclofenac may alter a diabetic patient's response to oral hypoglycemic agents; both hypo- and hyperglycemic effects have been reported).
No products indexed under this heading.

Glyburide (Diclofenac may alter a diabetic patient's response to oral hypoglycemic agents; both hypo- and hyperglycemic effects have been reported).
No products indexed under this heading.

Guanabenz Acetate (NSAIDs can inhibit the activity of antihypertensives).
No products indexed under this heading.

Guanethidine Monosulfate (NSAIDs can inhibit the activity of antihypertensives).
No products indexed under this heading.

Hydralazine Hydrochloride (NSAIDs can inhibit the activity of antihypertensives). Products include:
BiDil Tablets 2171

Hydrochlorothiazide (Clinical studies, as well as post marketing observations, have shown that Arthrotec can reduce the natriuretic effect of furosemide and thiazides in some patients. This response has been attributed to the inhibition of renal prostaglandin synthesis. During concomitant therapy with NSAIDs, the patient should be observed closely for signs of renal failure as well as to assure diuretic efficacy). Products include:
Aldoril Tablets 1910
Atacand HCT 651
Avalide Tablets 888
Avalide Tablets 2874
Benicar HCT Tablets 1044
Diovan HCT Tablets 2196
Dyazide Capsules 1423
Hyzaar 50-12.5 Tablets 1990
Hyzaar 100-12.5 Tablets 1990
Hyzaar 100-25 Tablets 1990
Lopressor HCT 50/25 Tablets 2241
Lopressor HCT 100/25 Tablets 2241
Lopressor HCT 100/50 Tablets 2241
Lotensin HCT Tablets 2246
Micardis HCT Tablets 856
Moduretic Tablets 2028
Prinzide Tablets 2056
Teveten HCT Tablets 1737
Timolide Tablets 2086
Uniretic Tablets 3100

Hydroflumethiazide (Clinical studies, as well as post marketing observations, have shown that Arthrotec can reduce the natriuretic effect of furosemide and thiazides in some patients. This response has been attributed to the inhibition of renal prostaglandin synthesis. During concomitant therapy with NSAIDs, the patient should be observed closely for signs of renal failure as well as to assure diuretic efficacy).
No products indexed under this heading.

Indapamide (NSAIDs can inhibit the activity of antihypertensives). Products include:
Indapamide Tablets 2156

Insulin, Human, Zinc Suspension (Diclofenac may alter a diabetic patient's response to insulin; both

hypo- and hyperglycemic effects have been reported). Products include:
- Humulin L, 100 Units 1794
- Humulin U, 100 Units 1800

Insulin, Human NPH (Diclofenac may alter a diabetic patient's response to insulin; both hypo- and hyperglycemic effects have been reported). Products include:
- Humulin N, 100 Units 1795
- Humulin N Pen 1797

Insulin, Human Regular (Diclofenac may alter a diabetic patient's response to insulin; both hypo- and hyperglycemic effects have been reported). Products include:
- Humulin R, 100 Units 1798

Insulin, Human Regular and Human NPH Mixture (Diclofenac may alter a diabetic patient's response to insulin; both hypo- and hyperglycemic effects have been reported). Products include:
- Humulin 50/50, 100 Units 1791
- Humulin 70/30 Pen 1793

Insulin, NPH (Diclofenac may alter a diabetic patient's response to insulin; both hypo- and hyperglycemic effects have been reported).
No products indexed under this heading.

Insulin, Regular (Diclofenac may alter a diabetic patient's response to insulin; both hypo- and hyperglycemic effects have been reported).
No products indexed under this heading.

Insulin, Zinc Crystals (Diclofenac may alter a diabetic patient's response to insulin; both hypo- and hyperglycemic effects have been reported).
No products indexed under this heading.

Insulin, Zinc Suspension (Diclofenac may alter a diabetic patient's response to insulin; both hypo- and hyperglycemic effects have been reported).
No products indexed under this heading.

Insulin Aspart, Human Regular (Diclofenac may alter a diabetic patient's response to insulin; both hypo- and hyperglycemic effects have been reported). Products include:
- NovoLog Injection 2326

Insulin glargine (Diclofenac may alter a diabetic patient's response to insulin; both hypo- and hyperglycemic effects have been reported). Products include:
- Lantus Injection 2909

Insulin Lispro, Human (Diclofenac may alter a diabetic patient's response to insulin; both hypo- and hyperglycemic effects have been reported). Products include:
- Humalog-Pen 1781
- Humalog Mix 50/50-Pen 1783
- Humalog Mix 75/25-Pen 1785

Insulin Lispro Protamine, Human (Diclofenac may alter a diabetic patient's response to insulin; both hypo- and hyperglycemic effects have been reported). Products include:
- Humalog Mix 50/50-Pen 1783
- Humalog Mix 75/25-Pen 1785

Irbesartan (NSAIDs can inhibit the activity of antihypertensives). Products include:
- Avalide Tablets 888
- Avalide Tablets 2874
- Avapro Tablets 891
- Avapro Tablets 2871

Isradipine (NSAIDs can inhibit the activity of antihypertensives). Products include:
- DynaCirc CR Tablets 2721

Labetalol Hydrochloride (NSAIDs can inhibit the activity of antihypertensives).
No products indexed under this heading.

Lisinopril (NSAIDs can inhibit the activity of antihypertensives). Products include:
- Prinivil Tablets 2052
- Prinzide Tablets 2056

Lithium (NSAIDs have produced an elevation of plasma lithium levels and a reduction in renal lithium clearance).
No products indexed under this heading.

Lithium Carbonate (NSAIDs have produced an elevation of plasma lithium levels and a reduction in renal lithium clearance). Products include:
- Lithobid Tablets 1692

Lithium Citrate (NSAIDs have produced an elevation of plasma lithium levels and a reduction in renal lithium clearance).
No products indexed under this heading.

Losartan Potassium (NSAIDs can inhibit the activity of antihypertensives). Products include:
- Cozaar Tablets 1935
- Hyzaar 50-12.5 Tablets 1990
- Hyzaar 100-12.5 Tablets 1990
- Hyzaar 100-25 Tablets 1990

Magaldrate (Antacids reduce the bioavailability of misoprostol acid. Antacids may also delay absorption of diclofenac sodium. Magnesium-containing antacids exacerbate misoprostol-associated diarrhea. Thus, it is not recommended that Arthrotec be coadministered with magnesium containing antacids).
No products indexed under this heading.

Magnesium Hydroxide (Antacids reduce the bioavailability of misoprostol acid and may delay absorption of diclofenac; magnesium-containing antacids exacerbate misoprostol-associated diarrhea). Products include:
- Maalox Regular Strength Antacid/Antigas Liquid................. 2175
- Maalox Max Maximum Strength Antacid/Anti-Gas Liquid................ 2176
- Pepcid Complete Chewable Tablets 1701

Magnesium Oxide (Antacids reduce the bioavailability of misoprostol acid and may delay absorption of diclofenac; magnesium-containing antacids exacerbate misoprostol-associated diarrhea). Products include:
- Beelith Tablets 759
- PremCal Light, Regular, and Extra Strength Tablets................ ▣818

Mecamylamine Hydrochloride (NSAIDs can inhibit the activity of antihypertensives).
No products indexed under this heading.

Metformin Hydrochloride (Diclofenac may alter a diabetic patient's response to oral hypoglycemic agents; both hypo- and hyperglycemic effects have been reported). Products include:
- ActoPlus Met Tablets 3214
- Avandamet Tablets 1373
- Fortamet Extended-Release Tablets 3115

Methotrexate Sodium (NSAIDs have been reported to competitively inhibit methotrexate accumulation in rabbit kidney slices. This may indicate that they could enhance the toxicity of methotrexate. Caution should be used when NSAIDs are administered concomitantly with methotrexate).
No products indexed under this heading.

Methyclothiazide (Clinical studies, as well as post marketing observations, have shown that Arthrotec can reduce the natriuretic effect of furosemide and thiazides in some patients. This response has been attributed to the inhibition of renal prostaglandin synthesis. During concomitant therapy with NSAIDs, the patient should be observed closely for signs of renal failure as well as to assure diuretic efficacy).
No products indexed under this heading.

Methyldopa (NSAIDs can inhibit the activity of antihypertensives). Products include:
- Aldoril Tablets 1910

Methyldopate Hydrochloride (NSAIDs can inhibit the activity of antihypertensives).
No products indexed under this heading.

Metolazone (NSAIDs can inhibit the activity of antihypertensives).
No products indexed under this heading.

Metoprolol Succinate (NSAIDs can inhibit the activity of antihypertensives). Products include:
- Toprol-XL Tablets 668

Metoprolol Tartrate (NSAIDs can inhibit the activity of antihypertensives). Products include:
- Lopressor Injection 2238
- Lopressor Tablets 2238
- Lopressor HCT 50/25 Tablets 2241
- Lopressor HCT 100/25 Tablets 2241
- Lopressor HCT 100/50 Tablets 2241

Metyrosine (NSAIDs can inhibit the activity of antihypertensives). Products include:
- Demser Capsules 1953

Mibefradil Dihydrochloride (NSAIDs can inhibit the activity of antihypertensives).
No products indexed under this heading.

Miglitol (Diclofenac may alter a diabetic patient's response to oral hypoglycemic agents; both hypo- and hyperglycemic effects have been reported).
No products indexed under this heading.

Minoxidil (NSAIDs can inhibit the activity of antihypertensives). Products include:
- Men's Rogaine Extra Strength Hair Regrowth Treatment Topical Solution, Ocean Rush Scent and Original Unscented..... ▣633
- Men's Rogaine Foam Hair Regrowth Treatment.................... ▣633
- Women's Rogaine Hair Regrowth Treatment Topical Solution, Spring Bloom Scent and Original Unscented..................... ▣634

Moexipril Hydrochloride (NSAIDs can inhibit the activity of antihypertensives). Products include:
- Uniretic Tablets 3100
- Univasc Tablets 3104

Nadolol (NSAIDs can inhibit the activity of antihypertensives). Products include:
- Nadolol Tablets 2159

Nicardipine Hydrochloride (NSAIDs can inhibit the activity of antihypertensives). Products include:
- Cardene I.V. 2497

Nifedipine (NSAIDs can inhibit the activity of antihypertensives). Products include:
- Adalat CC Tablets 2964

Nisoldipine (NSAIDs can inhibit the activity of antihypertensives). Products include:
- Sular Tablets 3122

Nitroglycerin (NSAIDs can inhibit the activity of antihypertensives). Products include:
- Nitro-Dur Transdermal Infusion System.. 3046
- Nitrolingual Pumpspray 3120

Penbutolol Sulfate (NSAIDs can inhibit the activity of antihypertensives).
No products indexed under this heading.

Perindopril Erbumine (NSAIDs can inhibit the activity of antihypertensives). Products include:
- Aceon Tablets (2 mg, 4 mg, 8 mg)... 3194

Phenobarbital (Co-administration in patients on chronic phenobarbital therapy has resulted in phenobarbital toxicity). Products include:
- Donnatal Extentabs 2493

Phenoxybenzamine Hydrochloride (NSAIDs can inhibit the activity of antihypertensives). Products include:
- Dibenzyline Capsules 3399

Phentolamine Mesylate (NSAIDs can inhibit the activity of antihypertensives).
No products indexed under this heading.

Pindolol (NSAIDs can inhibit the activity of antihypertensives).
No products indexed under this heading.

Pioglitazone Hydrochloride (Diclofenac may alter a diabetic patient's response to oral hypoglycemic agents; both hypo- and hyperglycemic effects have been reported). Products include:
- ActoPlus Met Tablets 3214
- Actos Tablets 3219
- Duetact Tablets 3226

Polythiazide (Clinical studies, as well as post marketing observations, have shown that Arthrotec can reduce the natriuretic effect of furosemide and thiazides in some patients. This response has been attributed to the inhibition of renal prostaglandin synthesis. During concomitant therapy with NSAIDs, the patient should be observed closely for signs of renal failure as well as to assure diuretic efficacy).
No products indexed under this heading.

Prazosin Hydrochloride (NSAIDs can inhibit the activity of antihypertensives).
No products indexed under this heading.

Propranolol Hydrochloride (NSAIDs can inhibit the activity of antihypertensives). Products include:
- Inderal LA Long-Acting Capsules 3429
- InnoPran XL Capsules 2723

Quinapril Hydrochloride (NSAIDs can inhibit the activity of antihypertensives).
No products indexed under this heading.

Ramipril (NSAIDs can inhibit the activity of antihypertensives). Products include:
Altace Capsules 1702

Rauwolfia Serpentina (NSAIDs can inhibit the activity of antihypertensives).
No products indexed under this heading.

Repaglinide (Diclofenac may alter a diabetic patient's response to oral hypoglycemic agents; both hypo- and hyperglycemic effects have been reported).
No products indexed under this heading.

Rescinnamine (NSAIDs can inhibit the activity of antihypertensives).
No products indexed under this heading.

Reserpine (NSAIDs can inhibit the activity of antihypertensives).
No products indexed under this heading.

Rosiglitazone Maleate (Diclofenac may alter a diabetic patient's response to oral hypoglycemic agents; both hypo- and hyperglycemic effects have been reported). Products include:
Avandamet Tablets 1373
Avandaryl Tablets 1379
Avandia Tablets 1384

Sodium Bicarbonate (Antacids reduce the bioavailability of misoprostol acid. Antacids may also delay absorption of diclofenac sodium. Magnesium-containing antacids exacerbate misoprostol-associated diarrhea. Thus, it is not recommended that Arthrotec be coadministered with magnesium containing antacids). Products include:
Colyte with Flavor Packs for Oral Solution 3088
HalfLytely and Bisacodyl Tablets Bowel Prep Kit with Flavors Packs 881
TriLyte with Flavor Packs for Oral Solution 3100

Sodium Nitroprusside (NSAIDs can inhibit the activity of antihypertensives).
No products indexed under this heading.

Sotalol Hydrochloride (NSAIDs can inhibit the activity of antihypertensives).
No products indexed under this heading.

Spirapril Hydrochloride (NSAIDs can inhibit the activity of antihypertensives).
No products indexed under this heading.

Spironolactone (Concomitant therapy with potassium-sparing diuretics may be associated with increased serum potassium levels).
No products indexed under this heading.

Telmisartan (NSAIDs can inhibit the activity of antihypertensives). Products include:
Micardis Tablets 854
Micardis HCT Tablets 856

Terazosin Hydrochloride (NSAIDs can inhibit the activity of antihypertensives). Products include:
Hytrin Capsules 471

Timolol Maleate (NSAIDs can inhibit the activity of antihypertensives). Products include:
Blocadren Tablets 1916
Cosopt Sterile Ophthalmic Solution 1931
Timolide Tablets 2086
Timoptic Sterile Ophthalmic Solution 2088
Timoptic in Ocudose 2091
Timoptic-XE Sterile Ophthalmic Gel Forming Solution 2092

Tolazamide (Diclofenac may alter a diabetic patient's response to oral hypoglycemic agents; both hypo- and hyperglycemic effects have been reported).
No products indexed under this heading.

Tolbutamide (Diclofenac may alter a diabetic patient's response to oral hypoglycemic agents; both hypo- and hyperglycemic effects have been reported).
No products indexed under this heading.

Torsemide (NSAIDs can inhibit the activity of antihypertensives). Products include:
Demadex Injection 2759
Demadex Tablets 2759

Trandolapril (NSAIDs can inhibit the activity of antihypertensives). Products include:
Mavik Tablets 486
Tarka Tablets 524

Triamterene (Concomitant therapy with potassium-sparing diuretics may be associated with increased serum potassium levels). Products include:
Dyazide Capsules 1423
Dyrenium Capsules 3400

Trimethaphan Camsylate (NSAIDs can inhibit the activity of antihypertensives).
No products indexed under this heading.

Troglitazone (Diclofenac may alter a diabetic patient's response to oral hypoglycemic agents; both hypo- and hyperglycemic effects have been reported).
No products indexed under this heading.

Valsartan (NSAIDs can inhibit the activity of antihypertensives). Products include:
Diovan Tablets 2193
Diovan HCT Tablets 2196

Verapamil Hydrochloride (NSAIDs can inhibit the activity of antihypertensives). Products include:
Covera-HS Tablets 3139
Tarka Tablets 524
Verelan PM Extended-Release Capsules, Controlled-Onset........... 3106

Warfarin Sodium (The effects of warfarin and NSAIDs on GI bleeding are synergistic, such that users of both drugs together have a risk of serious bleeding greater than users of either drug alone). Products include:
Coumadin for Injection 898
Coumadin Tablets 898

ASACOL DELAYED-RELEASE TABLETS

(Mesalamine) 2692
None cited in PDR database.

ASMANEX TWISTHALER

(Mometasone Furoate) 2966
May interact with:

Ketoconazole (Ketoconazole may increase plasma levels of mometasone furoate during concomitant dosing. Since mometasone furoate plasma levels appear to increase plasma and cortisol levels appear to decrease upon concomitant administration of ketoconazole, caution should be exercised in the co-administration of these drugs). Products include:
Nizoral A-D Shampoo, 1% 1868

ASTELIN NASAL SPRAY

(Azelastine Hydrochloride) 1904
May interact with antihistamines, central nervous system depressants, and certain other agents. Compounds in these categories include:

Acrivastine (Co-administration may result in additional reduction in alertness and impairment of CNS performance; concurrent use with other antihistamines should be avoided).
No products indexed under this heading.

Alfentanil Hydrochloride (Co-administration may result in additional reduction in alertness and impairment of CNS performance).
No products indexed under this heading.

Alprazolam (Co-administration may result in additional reduction in alertness and impairment of CNS performance). Products include:
Niravam Orally Disintegrating Tablets 3092

Aprobarbital (Co-administration may result in additional reduction in alertness and impairment of CNS performance).
No products indexed under this heading.

Astemizole (Co-administration may result in additional reduction in alertness and impairment of CNS performance; concurrent use with other antihistamines should be avoided).
No products indexed under this heading.

Azatadine Maleate (Co-administration may result in additional reduction in alertness and impairment of CNS performance; concurrent use with other antihistamines should be avoided).
No products indexed under this heading.

Bromodiphenhydramine Hydrochloride (Co-administration may result in additional reduction in alertness and impairment of CNS performance; concurrent use with other antihistamines should be avoided).
No products indexed under this heading.

Brompheniramine Maleate (Co-administration may result in additional reduction in alertness and impairment of CNS performance; concurrent use with other antihistamines should be avoided). Products include:
Children's Dimetapp Cold & Allergy Elixir 730
Children's Dimetapp Cold & Allergy Chewable Tablets............. 730
Children's Dimetapp DM Cold & Cough Elixir 731

Buprenorphine Hydrochloride (Co-administration may result in additional reduction in alertness and impairment of CNS performance). Products include:
Buprenex Injectable 2716
Suboxone Tablets 2717
Subutex Tablets 2717

Buspirone Hydrochloride (Co-administration may result in additional reduction in alertness and impairment of CNS performance).
No products indexed under this heading.

Butabarbital (Co-administration may result in additional reduction in alertness and impairment of CNS performance).
No products indexed under this heading.

Butalbital (Co-administration may result in additional reduction in alertness and impairment of CNS performance).
No products indexed under this heading.

Cetirizine Hydrochloride (Co-administration may result in additional reduction in alertness and impairment of CNS performance; concurrent use with other antihistamines should be avoided). Products include:
Zyrtec Chewable Tablets 2594
Zyrtec 2594
Zyrtec-D 12 Hour Extended Release Tablets 2597

Chlordiazepoxide (Co-administration may result in additional reduction in alertness and impairment of CNS performance).
No products indexed under this heading.

Chlordiazepoxide Hydrochloride (Co-administration may result in additional reduction in alertness and impairment of CNS performance). Products include:
Librium Capsules 3347

Chlorpheniramine Maleate (Co-administration may result in additional reduction in alertness and impairment of CNS performance; concurrent use with other antihistamines should be avoided). Products include:
Advil Allergy Sinus Caplets 770
Advil Multi-Symptom Cold Caplets 770
BC Allergy Sinus Cold Powder 677
Comtrex Maximum Strength Cold & Cough Day/Night Caplets - Night Formulation 726
Comtrex Maximum Strength Day/Night Severe Cold & Sinus Caplets - Night Formulation 725
Contac Cold and Flu Maximum Strength Caplets......................... 728
Contac Cold and Flu Day and Night Caplets (Night Formulation Only)........................ 727
Children's Dimetapp Long Acting Cough Plus Cold Syrup................ 731
Robitussin Cough & Cold Long-Acting Liquid 735
Robitussin Cough & Allergy Syrup .. 736
Robitussin Cough & Cold Nighttime Liquid........................... 736
Robitussin Cough, Cold & Flu Nighttime Liquid.......................... 738
Robitussin Pediatric Cough & Cold Long-Acting Liquid.............. 735
Robitussin Pediatric Cough & Cold Nighttime Liquid.................. 736
Triaminic Cold & Allergy Liquid 746
Triaminic Cough & Runny Nose Softchews 748
Children's Tylenol Plus Flu Oral Suspension.................................. 749
Tylenol Allergy Multi-Symptom Caplets with Cool Burst and Gelcaps.. 1872
Children's Tylenol Plus Cold Suspension Liquid 1879
Children's Tylenol Plus Cough & Runny Nose Suspension Liquid 1879
Children's Tylenol Plus Flu Suspension Liquid 1881

Children's Tylenol Plus Multi-Symptom Cold Suspension Liquid 1879
Tylenol Cold Head Congestion Nighttime Caplets with Cool Burst 1873
Tylenol Cold Multi-Symptom Nighttime Caplets with Cool Burst 1874
Tylenol Sinus Congestion & Pain Nighttime Caplets with Cool Burst 1876
Vicks 44M Cough, Cold & Flu Relief Liquid 2680
Pediatric Vicks 44m Cough & Cold Relief Liquid 2676
Children's Vicks NyQuil Cold/Cough Relief .... ■756
Children's Vicks NyQuil Cold/Cough Relief Liquid 2680
Zicam Maximum Strength Flu Daytime .... ■768

Chlorpheniramine Polistirex (Co-administration may result in additional reduction in alertness and impairment of CNS performance; concurrent use with other antihistamines should be avoided). Products include:
Tussionex Pennkinetic Extended-Release Suspension 3327

Chlorpheniramine Tannate (Co-administration may result in additional reduction in alertness and impairment of CNS performance; concurrent use with other antihistamines should be avoided).
No products indexed under this heading.

Chlorpromazine (Co-administration may result in additional reduction in alertness and impairment of CNS performance).
No products indexed under this heading.

Chlorpromazine Hydrochloride (Co-administration may result in additional reduction in alertness and impairment of CNS performance).
No products indexed under this heading.

Chlorprothixene (Co-administration may result in additional reduction in alertness and impairment of CNS performance).
No products indexed under this heading.

Chlorprothixene Hydrochloride (Co-administration may result in additional reduction in alertness and impairment of CNS performance).
No products indexed under this heading.

Chlorprothixene Lactate (Co-administration may result in additional reduction in alertness and impairment of CNS performance).
No products indexed under this heading.

Cimetidine (Increases the mean Cmax and AUC of orally administered azelastine by approximately 65%). Products include:
Tagamet HB 200 Tablets .... ■664

Cimetidine Hydrochloride (Co-administration of oral azelastine and cimetidine has resulted in increased mean Cmax and AUC of azelastine).
No products indexed under this heading.

Clemastine Fumarate (Co-administration may result in additional reduction in alertness and impairment of CNS performance; concurrent use with other antihistamines should be avoided).
No products indexed under this heading.

Clorazepate Dipotassium (Co-administration may result in additional reduction in alertness and impairment of CNS performance). Products include:
Tranxene 2474

Clozapine (Co-administration may result in additional reduction in alertness and impairment of CNS performance). Products include:
Clozaril Tablets 2184
FazaClo Orally Disintegrating Tablets 551

Codeine Phosphate (Co-administration may result in additional reduction in alertness and impairment of CNS performance). Products include:
Tylenol with Codeine Tablets 2391

Cyproheptadine Hydrochloride (Co-administration may result in additional reduction in alertness and impairment of CNS performance; concurrent use with other antihistamines should be avoided).
No products indexed under this heading.

Desflurane (Co-administration may result in additional reduction in alertness and impairment of CNS performance).
No products indexed under this heading.

Dexchlorpheniramine Maleate (Co-administration may result in additional reduction in alertness and impairment of CNS performance; concurrent use with other antihistamines should be avoided).
No products indexed under this heading.

Dezocine (Co-administration may result in additional reduction in alertness and impairment of CNS performance).
No products indexed under this heading.

Diazepam (Co-administration may result in additional reduction in alertness and impairment of CNS performance). Products include:
Diastat Rectal Delivery System 3343
Valium Tablets 2819

Diphenhydramine Citrate (Co-administration may result in additional reduction in alertness and impairment of CNS performance; concurrent use with other antihistamines should be avoided). Products include:
Advil PM Caplets .... ■615
Excedrin PM Caplets/Tablets/Geltabs .... ■610
Goody's PM Powder for Pain with Sleeplessness .... ■612

Diphenhydramine Hydrochloride (Co-administration may result in additional reduction in alertness and impairment of CNS performance; concurrent use with other antihistamines should be avoided). Products include:
Nytol QuickCaps Caplets .... ■615
Nytol QuickGels Softgels Maximum Strength .... ■616
Simply Sleep Caplets 1868
Sominex Original Formula Tablets .... ■616
TheraFlu Warming Relief Nighttime Severe Cold .... ■743
TheraFlu Thin Strips Multi Symptom .... ■744
Triaminic Nighttime Cold & Cough Liquid .... ■746
Triaminic Thin Strips Cough & Runny Nose .... ■749
Extra Strength Tylenol PM Caplets, Vanilla Caplets, Geltabs, Gelcaps and Liquid 1875

Tylenol Sore Throat Nighttime Liquid with Cool Burst .... ■790
Tylenol Allergy Multi-Symptom Nighttime Caplets with Cool Burst 1872
Tylenol Severe Allergy Caplets 1872
Children's Tylenol Plus Cold & Allergy Suspension Liquid 1878

Diphenylpyraline Hydrochloride (Co-administration may result in additional reduction in alertness and impairment of CNS performance; concurrent use with other antihistamines should be avoided).
No products indexed under this heading.

Droperidol (Co-administration may result in additional reduction in alertness and impairment of CNS performance).
No products indexed under this heading.

Enflurane (Co-administration may result in additional reduction in alertness and impairment of CNS performance).
No products indexed under this heading.

Estazolam (Co-administration may result in additional reduction in alertness and impairment of CNS performance). Products include:
ProSom Tablets 517

Ethanol (Co-administration may result in additional reduction in alertness and impairment of CNS performance).
No products indexed under this heading.

Ethchlorvynol (Co-administration may result in additional reduction in alertness and impairment of CNS performance).
No products indexed under this heading.

Ethinamate (Co-administration may result in additional reduction in alertness and impairment of CNS performance).
No products indexed under this heading.

Ethyl Alcohol (Co-administration may result in additional reduction in alertness and impairment of CNS performance).
No products indexed under this heading.

Fentanyl (Co-administration may result in additional reduction in alertness and impairment of CNS performance). Products include:
Duragesic Transdermal System 2373
Ionsys Transdermal System 2379

Fentanyl Citrate (Co-administration may result in additional reduction in alertness and impairment of CNS performance). Products include:
Actiq 979

Fexofenadine Hydrochloride (Co-administration may result in additional reduction in alertness and impairment of CNS performance; concurrent use with other antihistamines should be avoided). Products include:
Allegra 2844
Allegra-D 12 Hour Extended-Release Tablets 2846
Allegra-D 24 Hour Extended-Release Tablets 2849

Fluphenazine Decanoate (Co-administration may result in additional reduction in alertness and impairment of CNS performance).
No products indexed under this heading.

Fluphenazine Enanthate (Co-administration may result in additional reduction in alertness and impairment of CNS performance).
No products indexed under this heading.

Fluphenazine Hydrochloride (Co-administration may result in additional reduction in alertness and impairment of CNS performance).
No products indexed under this heading.

Flurazepam Hydrochloride (Co-administration may result in additional reduction in alertness and impairment of CNS performance). Products include:
Dalmane Capsules 3342

Glutethimide (Co-administration may result in additional reduction in alertness and impairment of CNS performance).
No products indexed under this heading.

Haloperidol (Co-administration may result in additional reduction in alertness and impairment of CNS performance).
No products indexed under this heading.

Haloperidol Decanoate (Co-administration may result in additional reduction in alertness and impairment of CNS performance).
No products indexed under this heading.

Hydrocodone Bitartrate (Co-administration may result in additional reduction in alertness and impairment of CNS performance). Products include:
Hycodan 1116
Hycotuss Expectorant Syrup 1117
Vicodin Tablets 535
Vicodin ES Tablets 536
Vicodin HP Tablets 538
Vicoprofen Tablets 539
Zydone Tablets 1139

Hydrocodone Polistirex (Co-administration may result in additional reduction in alertness and impairment of CNS performance). Products include:
Tussionex Pennkinetic Extended-Release Suspension 3327

Hydromorphone Hydrochloride (Co-administration may result in additional reduction in alertness and impairment of CNS performance). Products include:
Dilaudid 440
Dilaudid Non-Sterile Powder 440
Dilaudid Oral Liquid 445
Dilaudid Rectal Suppositories 440
Dilaudid Tablets 440
Dilaudid Tablets - 8 mg 445
Dilaudid-HP 442

Hydroxyzine Hydrochloride (Co-administration may result in additional reduction in alertness and impairment of CNS performance).
No products indexed under this heading.

Isoflurane (Co-administration may result in additional reduction in alertness and impairment of CNS performance).
No products indexed under this heading.

Ketamine Hydrochloride (Co-administration may result in additional reduction in alertness and impairment of CNS performance).
No products indexed under this heading.

Ketoconazole (Co-administration of oral azelastine and ketoconazole interfere with the measurement of azelastine plasma concentrations, however, no effects on QTc have been observed). Products include:

Nizoral A-D Shampoo, 1% ... 1868

Levomethadyl Acetate Hydrochloride (Co-administration may result in additional reduction in alertness and impairment of CNS performance).

No products indexed under this heading.

Levorphanol Tartrate (Co-administration may result in additional reduction in alertness and impairment of CNS performance).

No products indexed under this heading.

Loratadine (Co-administration may result in additional reduction in alertness and impairment of CNS performance; concurrent use with other antihistamines should be avoided). Products include:

Alavert Allergy & Sinus D-12 Hour Tablets ... 771
Alavert ... 771
Children's Claritin Allergy Oral Solution ... 771
Claritin Non-Drowsy 24 Hour Tablets ... 772
Claritin Reditabs 24 Hour Non-Drowsy Tablets ... 772
Claritin-D Non-Drowsy 12 Hour Tablets ... 772
Claritin-D Non-Drowsy 24 Hour Tablets ... 772

Lorazepam (Co-administration may result in additional reduction in alertness and impairment of CNS performance).

No products indexed under this heading.

Loxapine Hydrochloride (Co-administration may result in additional reduction in alertness and impairment of CNS performance).

No products indexed under this heading.

Loxapine Succinate (Co-administration may result in additional reduction in alertness and impairment of CNS performance).

No products indexed under this heading.

Meperidine Hydrochloride (Co-administration may result in additional reduction in alertness and impairment of CNS performance).

No products indexed under this heading.

Mephobarbital (Co-administration may result in additional reduction in alertness and impairment of CNS performance).

No products indexed under this heading.

Meprobamate (Co-administration may result in additional reduction in alertness and impairment of CNS performance).

No products indexed under this heading.

Mesoridazine Besylate (Co-administration may result in additional reduction in alertness and impairment of CNS performance).

No products indexed under this heading.

Methadone Hydrochloride (Co-administration may result in additional reduction in alertness and impairment of CNS performance).

No products indexed under this heading.

Methdilazine Hydrochloride (Co-administration may result in additional reduction in alertness and impairment of CNS performance; concurrent use with other antihistamines should be avoided).

No products indexed under this heading.

Methohexital Sodium (Co-administration may result in additional reduction in alertness and impairment of CNS performance).

No products indexed under this heading.

Methotrimeprazine (Co-administration may result in additional reduction in alertness and impairment of CNS performance).

No products indexed under this heading.

Methoxyflurane (Co-administration may result in additional reduction in alertness and impairment of CNS performance).

No products indexed under this heading.

Midazolam Hydrochloride (Co-administration may result in additional reduction in alertness and impairment of CNS performance).

No products indexed under this heading.

Molindone Hydrochloride (Co-administration may result in additional reduction in alertness and impairment of CNS performance). Products include:

Moban Tablets ... 1119

Morphine Sulfate (Co-administration may result in additional reduction in alertness and impairment of CNS performance). Products include:

Avinza Capsules ... 1741
Kadian Capsules ... 577
MS Contin Tablets ... 2701

Olanzapine (Co-administration may result in additional reduction in alertness and impairment of CNS performance). Products include:

Symbyax Capsules ... 1819
Zyprexa Tablets ... 1830
Zyprexa IntraMuscular ... 1830
Zyprexa ZYDIS Orally Disintegrating Tablets ... 1830

Oxazepam (Co-administration may result in additional reduction in alertness and impairment of CNS performance).

No products indexed under this heading.

Oxycodone Hydrochloride (Co-administration may result in additional reduction in alertness and impairment of CNS performance). Products include:

OxyContin Tablets ... 2703
OxyFast Oral Concentrate Solution ... 2708
OxyIR Capsules ... 2708
Percocet Tablets ... 1131
Percodan Tablets ... 1132

Pentobarbital Sodium (Co-administration may result in additional reduction in alertness and impairment of CNS performance). Products include:

Nembutal Sodium Solution, USP ... 2470

Perphenazine (Co-administration may result in additional reduction in alertness and impairment of CNS performance).

No products indexed under this heading.

Phenobarbital (Co-administration may result in additional reduction in alertness and impairment of CNS performance). Products include:

Donnatal Extentabs ... 2493

Prazepam (Co-administration may result in additional reduction in alertness and impairment of CNS performance).

No products indexed under this heading.

Prochlorperazine (Co-administration may result in additional reduction in alertness and impairment of CNS performance).

No products indexed under this heading.

Promethazine Hydrochloride (Co-administration may result in additional reduction in alertness and impairment of CNS performance; concurrent use with other antihistamines should be avoided). Products include:

Phenergan Tablets and Suppositories ... 3440

Propofol (Co-administration may result in additional reduction in alertness and impairment of CNS performance).

No products indexed under this heading.

Propoxyphene Hydrochloride (Co-administration may result in additional reduction in alertness and impairment of CNS performance).

No products indexed under this heading.

Propoxyphene Napsylate (Co-administration may result in additional reduction in alertness and impairment of CNS performance).

No products indexed under this heading.

Pyrilamine Maleate (Co-administration may result in additional reduction in alertness and impairment of CNS performance; concurrent use with other antihistamines should be avoided).

No products indexed under this heading.

Pyrilamine Tannate (Co-administration may result in additional reduction in alertness and impairment of CNS performance; concurrent use with other antihistamines should be avoided).

No products indexed under this heading.

Quazepam (Co-administration may result in additional reduction in alertness and impairment of CNS performance).

No products indexed under this heading.

Quetiapine Fumarate (Co-administration may result in additional reduction in alertness and impairment of CNS performance). Products include:

Seroquel Tablets ... 690

Remifentanil Hydrochloride (Co-administration may result in additional reduction in alertness and impairment of CNS performance).

No products indexed under this heading.

Risperidone (Co-administration may result in additional reduction in alertness and impairment of CNS performance). Products include:

Risperdal ... 1676
Risperdal Consta Long-Acting Injection ... 1682
Risperdal M-Tab Orally Disintegrating Tablets ... 1676

Secobarbital Sodium (Co-administration may result in additional reduction in alertness and impairment of CNS performance).

No products indexed under this heading.

Sevoflurane (Co-administration may result in additional reduction in alertness and impairment of CNS performance). Products include:

Ultane Liquid for Inhalation ... 531

Sufentanil Citrate (Co-administration may result in additional reduction in alertness and impairment of CNS performance).

No products indexed under this heading.

Temazepam (Co-administration may result in additional reduction in alertness and impairment of CNS performance). Products include:

Restoril Capsules ... 1860

Terfenadine (Co-administration may result in additional reduction in alertness and impairment of CNS performance; concurrent use with other antihistamines should be avoided).

No products indexed under this heading.

Thiamylal Sodium (Co-administration may result in additional reduction in alertness and impairment of CNS performance).

No products indexed under this heading.

Thioridazine Hydrochloride (Co-administration may result in additional reduction in alertness and impairment of CNS performance). Products include:

Thioridazine Hydrochloride Tablets ... 2163

Thiothixene (Co-administration may result in additional reduction in alertness and impairment of CNS performance). Products include:

Thiothixene Capsules ... 2165

Triazolam (Co-administration may result in additional reduction in alertness and impairment of CNS performance).

No products indexed under this heading.

Trifluoperazine Hydrochloride (Co-administration may result in additional reduction in alertness and impairment of CNS performance).

No products indexed under this heading.

Trimeprazine Tartrate (Co-administration may result in additional reduction in alertness and impairment of CNS performance; concurrent use with other antihistamines should be avoided).

No products indexed under this heading.

Tripelennamine Hydrochloride (Co-administration may result in additional reduction in alertness and impairment of CNS performance; concurrent use with other antihistamines should be avoided).

No products indexed under this heading.

Triprolidine Hydrochloride (Co-administration may result in additional reduction in alertness and impairment of CNS performance; concurrent use with other antihistamines should be avoided).

No products indexed under this heading.

Zaleplon (Co-administration may result in additional reduction in alertness and impairment of CNS performance). Products include:
Sonata Capsules 1717

Ziprasidone Hydrochloride (Co-administration may result in additional reduction in alertness and impairment of CNS performance). Products include:
Geodon Capsules 2529

Zolpidem Tartrate (Co-administration may result in additional reduction in alertness and impairment of CNS performance). Products include:
Ambien Tablets 2851
Ambien CR Tablets 2855

Food Interactions

Alcohol (Concurrent use may result in additional reduction in alertness and impairment of CNS performance; alcohol intake should be avoided).

ATACAND TABLETS

(Candesartan Cilexetil) 649
May interact with lithium preparations. Compounds in these categories include:

Lithium (An increase in serum lithium concentration has been reported during concomitant administration of lithium with candesartan cilexetil, so careful monitoring of serum lithium levels is recommended during concomitant use).
No products indexed under this heading.

Lithium Carbonate (An increase in serum lithium concentration has been reported during concomitant administration of lithium with candesartan cilexetil, so careful monitoring of serum lithium levels is recommended during concomitant use). Products include:
Lithobid Tablets 1692

Lithium Citrate (An increase in serum lithium concentration has been reported during concomitant administration of lithium with candesartan cilexetil, so careful monitoring of serum lithium levels is recommended during concomitant use).
No products indexed under this heading.

ATACAND HCT 16-12.5 TABLETS

(Candesartan Cilexetil, Hydrochlorothiazide)........................... 651
May interact with antihypertensives, barbiturates, corticosteroids, oral hypoglycemic agents, insulin, lithium preparations, narcotic analgesics, nondepolarizing neuromuscular blocking agents, non-steroidal anti-inflammatory agents, and certain other agents. Compounds in these categories include:

Acarbose (Hyperglycemia may occur with thiazide diuretics; dosage adjustment of the antidiabetic drugs may be required). Products include:
Precose Tablets 751

Acebutolol Hydrochloride (Co-administration with other antihypertensive drugs may result in additive effect or potentiation of the antihypertensive effects with a potential for aggravation of orthostatic hypotension).
No products indexed under this heading.

ACTH (Co-administration with ACTH intensifies the electrolyte depletion, particularly hypokalemia).
No products indexed under this heading.

Alfentanil Hydrochloride (Narcotics may aggravate orthostatic hypotension produced by hydrochlorothiazide).
No products indexed under this heading.

Amlodipine Besylate (Co-administration with other antihypertensive drugs may result in additive effect or potentiation of the antihypertensive effects with a potential for aggravation of orthostatic hypotension). Products include:
Caduet Tablets 2508
Lotrel Capsules 2249
Norvasc Tablets 2545

Aprobarbital (Barbiturates may aggravate orthostatic hypotension produced by hydrochlorothiazide).
No products indexed under this heading.

Atenolol (Co-administration with other antihypertensive drugs may result in additive effect or potentiation of the antihypertensive effects with a potential for aggravation of orthostatic hypotension).
No products indexed under this heading.

Atracurium Besylate (Possible increased responsiveness to the muscle relaxant).
No products indexed under this heading.

Benazepril Hydrochloride (Co-administration with other antihypertensive drugs may result in additive effect or potentiation of the antihypertensive effects with a potential for aggravation of orthostatic hypotension). Products include:
Lotensin Tablets 2243
Lotensin HCT Tablets 2246
Lotrel Capsules 2249

Bendroflumethiazide (Co-administration with other antihypertensive drugs may result in additive effect or potentiation of the antihypertensive effects with a potential for aggravation of orthostatic hypotension).
No products indexed under this heading.

Betamethasone Acetate (Co-administration with corticosteroids intensifies the electrolyte depletion, particularly hypokalemia).
No products indexed under this heading.

Betamethasone Sodium Phosphate (Co-administration with corticosteroids intensifies the electrolyte depletion, particularly hypokalemia).
No products indexed under this heading.

Betaxolol Hydrochloride (Co-administration with other antihypertensive drugs may result in additive effect or potentiation of the antihypertensive effects with a potential for aggravation of orthostatic hypotension). Products include:
Betoptic S Ophthalmic Suspension.................................. 558

Bisoprolol Fumarate (Co-administration with other antihypertensive drugs may result in additive effect or potentiation of the antihypertensive effects with a potential for aggravation of orthostatic hypotension).
No products indexed under this heading.

Buprenorphine Hydrochloride (Narcotics may aggravate orthostatic hypotension produced by hydrochlorothiazide). Products include:
Buprenex Injectable 2716
Suboxone Tablets 2717
Subutex Tablets 2717

Butabarbital (Barbiturates may aggravate orthostatic hypotension produced by hydrochlorothiazide).
No products indexed under this heading.

Butalbital (Barbiturates may aggravate orthostatic hypotension produced by hydrochlorothiazide).
No products indexed under this heading.

Captopril (Co-administration with other antihypertensive drugs may result in additive effect or potentiation of the antihypertensive effects with a potential for aggravation of orthostatic hypotension). Products include:
Captopril Tablets 2149

Carteolol Hydrochloride (Co-administration with other antihypertensive drugs may result in additive effect or potentiation of the antihypertensive effects with a potential for aggravation of orthostatic hypotension). Products include:
Carteolol Hydrochloride Ophthalmic Solution USP, 1%....... ⊙ 249

Celecoxib (Co-administration of non-steroidal anti-inflammatory agents can reduce the diuretic, natriuretic, and antihypertensive effects of thiazide diuretics). Products include:
Celebrex Capsules 3134

Chlorothiazide (Co-administration with other antihypertensive drugs may result in additive effect or potentiation of the antihypertensive effects with a potential for aggravation of orthostatic hypotension). Products include:
Diuril Oral Suspension 1954

Chlorothiazide Sodium (Co-administration with other antihypertensive drugs may result in additive effect or potentiation of the antihypertensive effects with a potential for aggravation of orthostatic hypotension). Products include:
Diuril Sodium Intravenous 2467

Chlorpropamide (Hyperglycemia may occur with thiazide diuretics; dosage adjustment of the antidiabetic drugs may be required).
No products indexed under this heading.

Chlorthalidone (Co-administration with other antihypertensive drugs may result in additive effect or potentiation of the antihypertensive effects with a potential for aggravation of orthostatic hypotension). Products include:
Clorpres Tablets 2153

Cholestyramine (Co-administration with anionic exchange resins, such as cholestyramine, binds the hydrochlorothiazide and reduces its absorption by up to 85 percent).
No products indexed under this heading.

Cisatracurium Besylate (Possible increased responsiveness to the muscle relaxant). Products include:
Nimbex Injection 498

Clonidine (Co-administration with other antihypertensive drugs may result in additive effect or potentiation of the antihypertensive effects with a potential for aggravation of orthostatic hypotension). Products include:
Catapres-TTS 844

Clonidine Hydrochloride (Co-administration with other antihypertensive drugs may result in additive effect or potentiation of the antihypertensive effects with a potential for aggravation of orthostatic hypotension). Products include:
Catapres Tablets 843
Clorpres Tablets 2153

Codeine Phosphate (Narcotics may aggravate orthostatic hypotension produced by hydrochlorothiazide). Products include:
Tylenol with Codeine Tablets 2391

Colestipol Hydrochloride (Co-administration with anionic exchange resins, such as colestipol, binds the hydrochlorothiazide and reduces its absorption by up to 43 percent).
No products indexed under this heading.

Cortisone Acetate (Co-administration with corticosteroids intensifies the electrolyte depletion, particularly hypokalemia).
No products indexed under this heading.

Deserpidine (Co-administration with other antihypertensive drugs may result in additive effect or potentiation of the antihypertensive effects with a potential for aggravation of orthostatic hypotension).
No products indexed under this heading.

Dexamethasone (Co-administration with corticosteroids intensifies the electrolyte depletion, particularly hypokalemia). Products include:
Ciprodex Otic Suspension 559
Decadron Tablets 1951
TobraDex Ophthalmic Ointment 562
TobraDex Ophthalmic Suspension ... 563

Dexamethasone Acetate (Co-administration with corticosteroids intensifies the electrolyte depletion, particularly hypokalemia).
No products indexed under this heading.

Dexamethasone Sodium Phosphate (Co-administration with corticosteroids intensifies the electrolyte depletion, particularly hypokalemia).
No products indexed under this heading.

Dezocine (Narcotics may aggravate orthostatic hypotension produced by hydrochlorothiazide).
No products indexed under this heading.

Diazoxide (Co-administration with other antihypertensive drugs may result in additive effect or potentiation of the antihypertensive effects with a potential for aggravation of orthostatic hypotension). Products include:

Hyperstat I.V. 3017

Diclofenac Potassium (Co-administration of non-steroidal anti-inflammatory agents can reduce the diuretic, natriuretic, and antihypertensive effects of thiazide diuretics).
No products indexed under this heading.

Diclofenac Sodium (Co-administration of non-steroidal anti-inflammatory agents can reduce the diuretic, natriuretic, and antihypertensive effects of thiazide diuretics). Products include:
Arthrotec Tablets 3129
Voltaren Ophthalmic Solution 2309
Voltaren Tablets 2307
Voltaren-XR Tablets 2310

Diltiazem Hydrochloride (Co-administration with other antihypertensive drugs may result in additive effect or potentiation of the antihypertensive effects with a potential for aggravation of orthostatic hypotension). Products include:
Cardizem LA Extended Release Tablets 1728
Tiazac Capsules 1201

Doxazosin Mesylate (Co-administration with other antihypertensive drugs may result in additive effect or potentiation of the antihypertensive effects with a potential for aggravation of orthostatic hypotension). Products include:
Cardura XL Tablets 2515

Enalapril Maleate (Co-administration with other antihypertensive drugs may result in additive effect or potentiation of the antihypertensive effects with a potential for aggravation of orthostatic hypotension). Products include:
Vasotec I.V. Injection 2103

Enalaprilat (Co-administration with other antihypertensive drugs may result in additive effect or potentiation of the antihypertensive effects with a potential for aggravation of orthostatic hypotension).
No products indexed under this heading.

Eprosartan Mesylate (Co-administration with other antihypertensive drugs may result in additive effect or potentiation of the antihypertensive effects with a potential for aggravation of orthostatic hypotension). Products include:
Teveten Tablets 1735
Teveten HCT Tablets 1737

Esmolol Hydrochloride (Co-administration with other antihypertensive drugs may result in additive effect or potentiation of the antihypertensive effects with a potential for aggravation of orthostatic hypotension).
No products indexed under this heading.

Etodolac (Co-administration of non-steroidal anti-inflammatory agents can reduce the diuretic, natriuretic, and antihypertensive effects of thiazide diuretics).
No products indexed under this heading.

Felodipine (Co-administration with other antihypertensive drugs may result in additive effect or potentiation of the antihypertensive effects with a potential for aggravation of orthostatic hypotension).
No products indexed under this heading.

Fenoprofen Calcium (Co-administration of non-steroidal anti-inflammatory agents can reduce the diuretic, natriuretic, and antihypertensive effects of thiazide diuretics). Products include:
Nalfon Capsules 2502

Fentanyl (Narcotics may aggravate orthostatic hypotension produced by hydrochlorothiazide). Products include:
Duragesic Transdermal System 2373
Ionsys Transdermal System 2379

Fentanyl Citrate (Narcotics may aggravate orthostatic hypotension produced by hydrochlorothiazide). Products include:
Actiq 979

Fludrocortisone Acetate (Co-administration with,corticosteroids intensifies the electrolyte depletion, particularly hypokalemia).
No products indexed under this heading.

Flurbiprofen (Co-administration of non-steroidal anti-inflammatory agents can reduce the diuretic, natriuretic, and antihypertensive effects of thiazide diuretics).
No products indexed under this heading.

Fosinopril Sodium (Co-administration with other antihypertensive drugs may result in additive effect or potentiation of the antihypertensive effects with a potential for aggravation of orthostatic hypotension).
No products indexed under this heading.

Furosemide (Co-administration with other antihypertensive drugs may result in additive effect or potentiation of the antihypertensive effects with a potential for aggravation of orthostatic hypotension). Products include:
Furosemide Tablets 2154

Glimepiride (Hyperglycemia may occur with thiazide diuretics; dosage adjustment of the antidiabetic drugs may be required). Products include:
Avandaryl Tablets 1379
Duetact Tablets 3226

Glipizide (Hyperglycemia may occur with thiazide diuretics; dosage adjustment of the antidiabetic drugs may be required).
No products indexed under this heading.

Glyburide (Hyperglycemia may occur with thiazide diuretics; dosage adjustment of the antidiabetic drugs may be required).
No products indexed under this heading.

Guanabenz Acetate (Co-administration with other antihypertensive drugs may result in additive effect or potentiation of the antihypertensive effects with a potential for aggravation of orthostatic hypotension).
No products indexed under this heading.

Guanethidine Monosulfate (Co-administration with other antihypertensive drugs may result in additive effect or potentiation of the antihypertensive effects with a potential for aggravation of orthostatic hypotension).
No products indexed under this heading.

Hydralazine Hydrochloride (Co-administration with other antihypertensive drugs may result in additive effect or potentiation of the antihypertensive effects with a potential for aggravation of orthostatic hypotension). Products include:
BiDil Tablets 2171

Hydrocodone Bitartrate (Narcotics may aggravate orthostatic hypotension produced by hydrochlorothiazide). Products include:
Hycodan 1116
Hycotuss Expectorant Syrup 1117
Vicodin Tablets 535
Vicodin ES Tablets 536
Vicodin HP Tablets 538
Vicoprofen Tablets 539
Zydone Tablets 1139

Hydrocodone Polistirex (Narcotics may aggravate orthostatic hypotension produced by hydrochlorothiazide). Products include:
Tussionex Pennkinetic Extended-Release Suspension 3327

Hydrocortisone (Co-administration with corticosteroids intensifies the electrolyte depletion, particularly hypokalemia). Products include:
Colocort Rectal Suspension, USP (Retention) 100 mg/60 mL 2476
Hydrocortone Tablets 1989
Preparation H Hydrocortisone Cream 646

Hydrocortisone Acetate (Co-administration with corticosteroids intensifies the electrolyte depletion, particularly hypokalemia). Products include:
Analpram-HC 1159
Pramosone 1161
ProctoFoam-HC 3099

Hydrocortisone Sodium Phosphate (Co-administration with corticosteroids intensifies the electrolyte depletion, particularly hypokalemia).
No products indexed under this heading.

Hydrocortisone Sodium Succinate (Co-administration with corticosteroids intensifies the electrolyte depletion, particularly hypokalemia).
No products indexed under this heading.

Hydroflumethiazide (Co-administration with other antihypertensive drugs may result in additive effect or potentiation of the antihypertensive effects with a potential for aggravation of orthostatic hypotension).
No products indexed under this heading.

Hydromorphone Hydrochloride (Narcotics may aggravate orthostatic hypotension produced by hydrochlorothiazide). Products include:
Dilaudid 440
Dilaudid Non-Sterile Powder 440
Dilaudid Oral Liquid 445
Dilaudid Rectal Suppositories 440
Dilaudid Tablets 440
Dilaudid Tablets - 8 mg 445
Dilaudid-HP 442

Ibuprofen (Co-administration of non-steroidal anti-inflammatory agents can reduce the diuretic, natriuretic, and antihypertensive effects of thiazide diuretics). Products include:
Advil Allergy Sinus Caplets 770
Advil 674
Children's Advil Oral Suspension 603
Children's Advil Chewable Tablets 603
Advil Cold & Sinus 723
Infants' Advil Concentrated Drops 604
Infants' Advil Concentrated Drops - White Grape (Dye-Free) 604
Junior Strength Advil Swallow Tablets 605
Advil Migraine Liquigels 608
Advil Multi-Symptom Cold Caplets 770
Advil PM Caplets 615
Motrin IB Tablets and Caplets 1866
Children's Motrin Oral Suspension 1867
Children's Motrin Non-Staining Dye-Free Oral Suspension 1867
Children's Motrin Cold Oral Suspension 1867
Infants' Motrin Concentrated Drops 1867
Infants' Motrin Non-Staining Dye-Free Concentrated Drops 1867
Junior Strength Motrin Caplets and Chewable Tablets 1867
Vicoprofen Tablets 539

Indapamide (Co-administration with other antihypertensive drugs may result in additive effect or potentiation of the antihypertensive effects with a potential for aggravation of orthostatic hypotension). Products include:
Indapamide Tablets 2156

Indomethacin (Co-administration of non-steroidal anti-inflammatory agents can reduce the diuretic, natriuretic, and antihypertensive effects of thiazide diuretics). Products include:
Indocin 1995

Indomethacin Sodium Trihydrate (Co-administration of non-steroidal anti-inflammatory agents can reduce the diuretic, natriuretic, and antihypertensive effects of thiazide diuretics). Products include:
Indocin I.V. 2465

Insulin, Human, Zinc Suspension (Hyperglycemia may occur with thiazide diuretics; dosage adjustment of the insulin may be required). Products include:
Humulin L, 100 Units 1794
Humulin U, 100 Units 1800

Insulin, Human NPH (Hyperglycemia may occur with thiazide diuretics; dosage adjustment of the insulin may be required). Products include:
Humulin N, 100 Units 1795
Humulin N Pen 1797

Insulin, Human Regular (Hyperglycemia may occur with thiazide diuretics; dosage adjustment of the insulin may be required). Products include:
Humulin R, 100 Units 1798

Insulin, Human Regular and Human NPH Mixture (Hyperglycemia may occur with thiazide diuretics; dosage adjustment of the insulin may be required). Products include:
Humulin 50/50, 100 Units 1791
Humulin 70/30 Pen 1793

Insulin, NPH (Hyperglycemia may occur with thiazide diuretics; dosage adjustment of the insulin may be required).
No products indexed under this heading.

Insulin, Regular (Hyperglycemia may occur with thiazide diuretics; dosage adjustment of the insulin may be required).
No products indexed under this heading.

Insulin, Zinc Crystals (Hyperglycemia may occur with thiazide diuretics; dosage adjustment of the insulin may be required).
No products indexed under this heading.

Insulin, Zinc Suspension (Hyperglycemia may occur with thiazide diuretics; dosage adjustment of the insulin may be required).
No products indexed under this heading.

Insulin Aspart, Human Regular (Hyperglycemia may occur with thia-

zide diuretics; dosage adjustment of the insulin may be required). Products include:

Insulin glargine (Hyperglycemia may occur with thiazide diuretics; dosage adjustment of the insulin may be required). Products include:

Insulin Lispro, Human (Hyperglycemia may occur with thiazide diuretics; dosage adjustment of the insulin may be required). Products include:

Insulin Lispro Protamine, Human (Hyperglycemia may occur with thiazide diuretics; dosage adjustment of the insulin may be required). Products include:

Irbesartan (Co-administration with other antihypertensive drugs may result in additive effect or potentiation of the antihypertensive effects with a potential for aggravation of orthostatic hypotension). Products include:

Isradipine (Co-administration with other antihypertensive drugs may result in additive effect or potentiation of the antihypertensive effects with a potential for aggravation of orthostatic hypotension). Products include:

Ketoprofen (Co-administration of non-steroidal anti-inflammatory agents can reduce the diuretic, natriuretic, and antihypertensive effects of thiazide diuretics).
No products indexed under this heading.

Ketorolac Tromethamine (Co-administration of non-steroidal anti-inflammatory agents can reduce the diuretic, natriuretic, and antihypertensive effects of thiazide diuretics). Products include:

Labetalol Hydrochloride (Co-administration with other antihypertensive drugs may result in additive effect or potentiation of the antihypertensive effects with a potential for aggravation of orthostatic hypotension).
No products indexed under this heading.

Levorphanol Tartrate (Narcotics may aggravate orthostatic hypotension produced by hydrochlorothiazide).
No products indexed under this heading.

Lisinopril (Co-administration with other antihypertensive drugs may result in additive effect or potentiation of the antihypertensive effects with a potential for aggravation of orthostatic hypotension). Products include:

Lithium (Hydrochlorothiazide reduces the renal clearance of lithium and can cause a high risk of lithium toxicity; in general, lithium should not be given with diuretics. An increase in serum lithium concentration has been reported during concomitant administration of lithium with candesartan cilexetil; careful monitoring of serum lithium levels is recommended during concomitant use).
No products indexed under this heading.

Lithium Carbonate (Hydrochlorothiazide reduces the renal clearance of lithium and can cause a high risk of lithium toxicity; in general, lithium should not be given with diuretics. An increase in serum lithium concentration has been reported during concomitant administration of lithium with candesartan cilexetil; careful monitoring of serum lithium levels is recommended during concomitant use). Products include:

Lithium Citrate (Hydrochlorothiazide reduces the renal clearance of lithium and can cause a high risk of lithium toxicity; in general, lithium should not be given with diuretics. An increase in serum lithium concentration has been reported during concomitant administration of lithium with candesartan cilexetil; careful monitoring of serum lithium levels is recommended during concomitant use).
No products indexed under this heading.

Losartan Potassium (Co-administration with other antihypertensive drugs may result in additive effect or potentiation of the antihypertensive effects with a potential for aggravation of orthostatic hypotension). Products include:

Mecamylamine Hydrochloride (Co-administration with other antihypertensive drugs may result in additive effect or potentiation of the antihypertensive effects with a potential for aggravation of orthostatic hypotension).
No products indexed under this heading.

Meclofenamate Sodium (Co-administration of non-steroidal anti-inflammatory agents can reduce the diuretic, natriuretic, and antihypertensive effects of thiazide diuretics).
No products indexed under this heading.

Mefenamic Acid (Co-administration of non-steroidal anti-inflammatory agents can reduce the diuretic, natriuretic, and antihypertensive effects of thiazide diuretics).
No products indexed under this heading.

Meloxicam (Co-administration of non-steroidal anti-inflammatory agents can reduce the diuretic, natriuretic, and antihypertensive effects of thiazide diuretics). Products include:

Meperidine Hydrochloride (Narcotics may aggravate orthostatic hypotension produced by hydrochlorothiazide).
No products indexed under this heading.

Mephobarbital (Barbiturates may aggravate orthostatic hypotension produced by hydrochlorothiazide).
No products indexed under this heading.

Metformin Hydrochloride (Hyperglycemia may occur with thiazide diuretics; dosage adjustment of the antidiabetic drugs may be required). Products include:

Methadone Hydrochloride (Narcotics may aggravate orthostatic hypotension produced by hydrochlorothiazide).
No products indexed under this heading.

Methyclothiazide (Co-administration with other antihypertensive drugs may result in additive effect or potentiation of the antihypertensive effects with a potential for aggravation of orthostatic hypotension).
No products indexed under this heading.

Methyldopa (Co-administration with other antihypertensive drugs may result in additive effect or potentiation of the antihypertensive effects with a potential for aggravation of orthostatic hypotension). Products include:

Methyldopate Hydrochloride (Co-administration with other antihypertensive drugs may result in additive effect or potentiation of the antihypertensive effects with a potential for aggravation of orthostatic hypotension).
No products indexed under this heading.

Methylprednisolone Acetate (Co-administration with corticosteroids intensifies the electrolyte depletion, particularly hypokalemia). Products include:

Methylprednisolone Sodium Succinate (Co-administration with corticosteroids intensifies the electrolyte depletion, particularly hypokalemia).
No products indexed under this heading.

Metocurine Iodide (Possible increased responsiveness to the muscle relaxant).
No products indexed under this heading.

Metolazone (Co-administration with other antihypertensive drugs may result in additive effect or potentiation of the antihypertensive effects with a potential for aggravation of orthostatic hypotension).
No products indexed under this heading.

Metoprolol Succinate (Co-administration with other antihypertensive drugs may result in additive effect or potentiation of the antihypertensive effects with a potential for aggravation of orthostatic hypotension). Products include:

Metoprolol Tartrate (Co-administration with other antihypertensive drugs may result in additive effect or potentiation of the antihypertensive effects with a potential for aggravation of orthostatic hypotension). Products include:

Metyrosine (Co-administration with other antihypertensive drugs may result in additive effect or potentiation of the antihypertensive effects with a potential for aggravation of orthostatic hypotension). Products include:

Mibefradil Dihydrochloride (Co-administration with other antihypertensive drugs may result in additive effect or potentiation of the antihypertensive effects with a potential for aggravation of orthostatic hypotension).
No products indexed under this heading.

Miglitol (Hyperglycemia may occur with thiazide diuretics; dosage adjustment of the antidiabetic drugs may be required).
No products indexed under this heading.

Minoxidil (Co-administration with other antihypertensive drugs may result in additive effect or potentiation of the antihypertensive effects with a potential for aggravation of orthostatic hypotension). Products include:

Mivacurium Chloride (Possible increased responsiveness to the muscle relaxant). Products include:

Moexipril Hydrochloride (Co-administration with other antihypertensive drugs may result in additive effect or potentiation of the antihypertensive effects with a potential for aggravation of orthostatic hypotension). Products include:

Morphine Sulfate (Narcotics may aggravate orthostatic hypotension produced by hydrochlorothiazide). Products include:

Nabumetone (Co-administration of non-steroidal anti-inflammatory agents can reduce the diuretic, natriuretic, and antihypertensive effects of thiazide diuretics).
No products indexed under this heading.

Nadolol (Co-administration with other antihypertensive drugs may result in additive effect or potentiation of the antihypertensive effects with a potential for aggravation of orthostatic hypotension). Products include:

Naproxen (Co-administration of non-steroidal anti-inflammatory agents can reduce the diuretic, natriuretic, and antihypertensive effects of thiazide diuretics). Products include:
- EC-Naprosyn Delayed-Release Tablets 2761
- Naprosyn Suspension 2761
- Naprosyn Tablets 2761
- Prevacid NapraPAC 3280

Naproxen Sodium (Co-administration of non-steroidal anti-inflammatory agents can reduce the diuretic, natriuretic, and antihypertensive effects of thiazide diuretics). Products include:
- Aleve Caplets 742
- Aleve Gelcaps 743
- Aleve Tablets 743
- Aleve Cold & Sinus Caplets 744
- Anaprox Tablets 2761
- Anaprox DS Tablets 2761

Nicardipine Hydrochloride (Co-administration with other antihypertensive drugs may result in additive effect or potentiation of the antihypertensive effects with a potential for aggravation of orthostatic hypotension). Products include:
- Cardene I.V. 2497

Nifedipine (Co-administration with other antihypertensive drugs may result in additive effect or potentiation of the antihypertensive effects with a potential for aggravation of orthostatic hypotension). Products include:
- Adalat CC Tablets 2964

Nisoldipine (Co-administration with other antihypertensive drugs may result in additive effect or potentiation of the antihypertensive effects with a potential for aggravation of orthostatic hypotension). Products include:
- Sular Tablets 3122

Nitroglycerin (Co-administration with other antihypertensive drugs may result in additive effect or potentiation of the antihypertensive effects with a potential for aggravation of orthostatic hypotension). Products include:
- Nitro-Dur Transdermal Infusion System 3046
- Nitrolingual Pumpspray 3120

Norepinephrine Bitartrate (Possible decreased response to pressor amines).
No products indexed under this heading.

Oxaprozin (Co-administration of non-steroidal anti-inflammatory agents can reduce the diuretic, natriuretic, and antihypertensive effects of thiazide diuretics).
No products indexed under this heading.

Oxycodone Hydrochloride (Narcotics may aggravate orthostatic hypotension produced by hydrochlorothiazide). Products include:
- OxyContin Tablets 2703
- OxyFast Oral Concentrate Solution 2708
- OxyIR Capsules 2708
- Percocet Tablets 1131
- Percodan Tablets 1132

Pancuronium Bromide (Possible increased responsiveness to the muscle relaxant).
No products indexed under this heading.

Penbutolol Sulfate (Co-administration with other antihypertensive drugs may result in additive effect or potentiation of the antihypertensive effects with a potential for aggravation of orthostatic hypotension).
No products indexed under this heading.

Pentobarbital Sodium (Barbiturates may aggravate orthostatic hypotension produced by hydrochlorothiazide). Products include:
- Nembutal Sodium Solution, USP 2470

Perindopril Erbumine (Co-administration with other antihypertensive drugs may result in additive effect or potentiation of the antihypertensive effects with a potential for aggravation of orthostatic hypotension). Products include:
- Aceon Tablets (2 mg, 4 mg, 8 mg) 3194

Phenobarbital (Barbiturates may aggravate orthostatic hypotension produced by hydrochlorothiazide). Products include:
- Donnatal Extentabs 2493

Phenoxybenzamine Hydrochloride (Co-administration with other antihypertensive drugs may result in additive effect or potentiation of the antihypertensive effects with a potential for aggravation of orthostatic hypotension). Products include:
- Dibenzyline Capsules 3399

Phentolamine Mesylate (Co-administration with other antihypertensive drugs may result in additive effect or potentiation of the antihypertensive effects with a potential for aggravation of orthostatic hypotension).
No products indexed under this heading.

Phenylbutazone (Co-administration of non-steroidal anti-inflammatory agents can reduce the diuretic, natriuretic, and antihypertensive effects of thiazide diuretics).
No products indexed under this heading.

Pindolol (Co-administration with other antihypertensive drugs may result in additive effect or potentiation of the antihypertensive effects with a potential for aggravation of orthostatic hypotension).
No products indexed under this heading.

Pioglitazone Hydrochloride (Hyperglycemia may occur with thiazide diuretics; dosage adjustment of the antidiabetic drugs may be required). Products include:
- ActoPlus Met Tablets 3214
- Actos Tablets 3219
- Duetact Tablets 3226

Piroxicam (Co-administration of non-steroidal anti-inflammatory agents can reduce the diuretic, natriuretic, and antihypertensive effects of thiazide diuretics).
No products indexed under this heading.

Polythiazide (Co-administration with other antihypertensive drugs may result in additive effect or potentiation of the antihypertensive effects with a potential for aggravation of orthostatic hypotension).
No products indexed under this heading.

Prazosin Hydrochloride (Co-administration with other antihypertensive drugs may result in additive effect or potentiation of the antihypertensive effects with a potential for aggravation of orthostatic hypotension).
No products indexed under this heading.

Prednisolone Acetate (Co-administration with corticosteroids intensifies the electrolyte depletion, particularly hypokalemia). Products include:
- Blephamide Ophthalmic Ointment 568
- Blephamide Ophthalmic Suspension 569
- Poly-Pred Ophthalmic Suspension .... ⊙233
- Pred Forte Ophthalmic Suspension .... ⊙235
- Pred Mild Ophthalmic Suspension .... ⊙238
- Pred-G Ophthalmic Ointment .... ⊙237
- Pred-G Ophthalmic Suspension .... ⊙236

Prednisolone Sodium Phosphate (Co-administration with corticosteroids intensifies the electrolyte depletion, particularly hypokalemia).
No products indexed under this heading.

Prednisolone Tebutate (Co-administration with corticosteroids intensifies the electrolyte depletion, particularly hypokalemia).
No products indexed under this heading.

Prednisone (Co-administration with corticosteroids intensifies the electrolyte depletion, particularly hypokalemia).
No products indexed under this heading.

Propoxyphene Hydrochloride (Narcotics may aggravate orthostatic hypotension produced by hydrochlorothiazide).
No products indexed under this heading.

Propoxyphene Napsylate (Narcotics may aggravate orthostatic hypotension produced by hydrochlorothiazide).
No products indexed under this heading.

Propranolol Hydrochloride (Co-administration with other antihypertensive drugs may result in additive effect or potentiation of the antihypertensive effects with a potential for aggravation of orthostatic hypotension). Products include:
- Inderal LA Long-Acting Capsules 3429
- InnoPran XL Capsules 2723

Quinapril Hydrochloride (Co-administration with other antihypertensive drugs may result in additive effect or potentiation of the antihypertensive effects with a potential for aggravation of orthostatic hypotension).
No products indexed under this heading.

Ramipril (Co-administration with other antihypertensive drugs may result in additive effect or potentiation of the antihypertensive effects with a potential for aggravation of orthostatic hypotension). Products include:
- Altace Capsules 1702

Rapacuronium Bromide (Possible increased responsiveness to the muscle relaxant).
No products indexed under this heading.

Rauwolfia Serpentina (Co-administration with other antihypertensive drugs may result in additive effect or potentiation of the antihypertensive effects with a potential for aggravation of orthostatic hypotension).
No products indexed under this heading.

Remifentanil Hydrochloride (Narcotics may aggravate orthostatic hypotension produced by hydrochlorothiazide).
No products indexed under this heading.

Repaglinide (Hyperglycemia may occur with thiazide diuretics; dosage adjustment of the antidiabetic drugs may be required).
No products indexed under this heading.

Rescinnamine (Co-administration with other antihypertensive drugs may result in additive effect or potentiation of the antihypertensive effects with a potential for aggravation of orthostatic hypotension).
No products indexed under this heading.

Reserpine (Co-administration with other antihypertensive drugs may result in additive effect or potentiation of the antihypertensive effects with a potential for aggravation of orthostatic hypotension).
No products indexed under this heading.

Rocuronium Bromide (Possible increased responsiveness to the muscle relaxant). Products include:
- Zemuron Injection 2346

Rofecoxib (Co-administration of non-steroidal anti-inflammatory agents can reduce the diuretic, natriuretic, and antihypertensive effects of thiazide diuretics).
No products indexed under this heading.

Rosiglitazone Maleate (Hyperglycemia may occur with thiazide diuretics; dosage adjustment of the antidiabetic drugs may be required). Products include:
- Avandamet Tablets 1373
- Avandaryl Tablets 1379
- Avandia Tablets 1384

Secobarbital Sodium (Barbiturates may aggravate orthostatic hypotension produced by hydrochlorothiazide).
No products indexed under this heading.

Sodium Nitroprusside (Co-administration with other antihypertensive drugs may result in additive effect or potentiation of the antihypertensive effects with a potential for aggravation of orthostatic hypotension).
No products indexed under this heading.

Sotalol Hydrochloride (Co-administration with other antihypertensive drugs may result in additive effect or potentiation of the antihypertensive effects with a potential for aggravation of orthostatic hypotension).
No products indexed under this heading.

Spirapril Hydrochloride (Co-administration with other antihypertensive drugs may result in additive effect or potentiation of the antihypertensive effects with a potential for aggravation of orthostatic hypotension).
No products indexed under this heading.

Sufentanil Citrate (Narcotics may aggravate orthostatic hypotension produced by hydrochlorothiazide).
No products indexed under this heading.

Sulindac (Co-administration of non-steroidal anti-inflammatory agents can reduce the diuretic, natriuretic, and antihypertensive effects of thiazide diuretics). Products include:
Clinoril Tablets ... 1924

Telmisartan (Co-administration with other antihypertensive drugs may result in additive effect or potentiation of the antihypertensive effects with a potential for aggravation of orthostatic hypotension). Products include:
Micardis Tablets ... 854
Micardis HCT Tablets ... 856

Terazosin Hydrochloride (Co-administration with other antihypertensive drugs may result in additive effect or potentiation of the antihypertensive effects with a potential for aggravation of orthostatic hypotension). Products include:
Hytrin Capsules ... 471

Thiamylal Sodium (Barbiturates may aggravate orthostatic hypotension produced by hydrochlorothiazide).
No products indexed under this heading.

Timolol Maleate (Co-administration with other antihypertensive drugs may result in additive effect or potentiation of the antihypertensive effects with a potential for aggravation of orthostatic hypotension). Products include:
Blocadren Tablets ... 1916
Cosopt Sterile Ophthalmic Solution ... 1931
Timolide Tablets ... 2086
Timoptic Sterile Ophthalmic Solution ... 2088
Timoptic in Ocudose ... 2091
Timoptic-XE Sterile Ophthalmic Gel Forming Solution ... 2092

Tolazamide (Hyperglycemia may occur with thiazide diuretics; dosage adjustment of the antidiabetic drugs may be required).
No products indexed under this heading.

Tolbutamide (Hyperglycemia may occur with thiazide diuretics; dosage adjustment of the antidiabetic drugs may be required).
No products indexed under this heading.

Tolmetin Sodium (Co-administration of non-steroidal anti-inflammatory agents can reduce the diuretic, natriuretic, and antihypertensive effects of thiazide diuretics).
No products indexed under this heading.

Torsemide (Co-administration with other antihypertensive drugs may result in additive effect or potentiation of the antihypertensive effects with a potential for aggravation of orthostatic hypotension). Products include:
Demadex Injection ... 2759
Demadex Tablets ... 2759

Trandolapril (Co-administration with other antihypertensive drugs may result in additive effect or potentiation of the antihypertensive effects with a potential for aggravation of orthostatic hypotension). Products include:
Mavik Tablets ... 486
Tarka Tablets ... 524

Triamcinolone (Co-administration with corticosteroids intensifies the electrolyte depletion, particularly hypokalemia).
No products indexed under this heading.

Triamcinolone Acetonide (Co-administration with corticosteroids intensifies the electrolyte depletion, particularly hypokalemia). Products include:
Azmacort Inhalation Aerosol ... 1726
Nasacort AQ Nasal Spray ... 2922

Triamcinolone Diacetate (Co-administration with corticosteroids intensifies the electrolyte depletion, particularly hypokalemia).
No products indexed under this heading.

Triamcinolone Hexacetonide (Co-administration with corticosteroids intensifies the electrolyte depletion, particularly hypokalemia).
No products indexed under this heading.

Trimethaphan Camsylate (Co-administration with other antihypertensive drugs may result in additive effect or potentiation of the antihypertensive effects with a potential for aggravation of orthostatic hypotension).
No products indexed under this heading.

Troglitazone (Hyperglycemia may occur with thiazide diuretics; dosage adjustment of the antidiabetic drugs may be required).
No products indexed under this heading.

Tubocurarine Chloride (Possible increased responsiveness to the muscle relaxant).
No products indexed under this heading.

Valdecoxib (Co-administration of non-steroidal anti-inflammatory agents can reduce the diuretic, natriuretic, and antihypertensive effects of thiazide diuretics).
No products indexed under this heading.

Valsartan (Co-administration with other antihypertensive drugs may result in additive effect or potentiation of the antihypertensive effects with a potential for aggravation of orthostatic hypotension). Products include:
Diovan Tablets ... 2193
Diovan HCT Tablets ... 2196

Vecuronium Bromide (Possible increased responsiveness to the muscle relaxant).
No products indexed under this heading.

Verapamil Hydrochloride (Co-administration with other antihypertensive drugs may result in additive effect or potentiation of the antihypertensive effects with a potential for aggravation of orthostatic hypotension). Products include:
Covera-HS Tablets ... 3139
Tarka Tablets ... 524
Verelan PM Extended-Release Capsules, Controlled-Onset ... 3106

Food Interactions

Alcohol (May aggravate orthostatic hypotension produced by hydrochlorothiazide).

ATACAND HCT 32-12.5 TABLETS

(Candesartan Cilexetil, Hydrochlorothiazide) ... 651
See Atacand HCT 16-12.5 Tablets

ATHENA 7 MINUTE LIFT CREAM

(Herbals, Multiple) ... ▣827
None cited in PDR database.

ATRIPLA TABLETS

(Efavirenz, Emtricitabine, Tenofovir Disoproxil Fumarate) ... 945
May interact with cytochrome p450 2c19 substrates (selected), cytochrome p450 2c9 substrates (selected), cytochrome p450 3a4 inducers (selected), cytochrome p450 3a4 substrates (selected), and certain other agents. Compounds in these categories include:

Acarbose (In vitro studies have demonstrated that efavirenz inhibits CYP2C9 in the range of observed efavirenz plasma concentrations. Co-administration of efavirenz with drugs primarily metabolized by CYP2C9 may result in altered plasma concentrations of the co-administered drug. Therefore, appropriate dose adjustments may be necessary for these drugs). Products include:
Precose Tablets ... 751

Acyclovir (Since emtricitabine and tenofovir are primarily eliminated by the kidneys, co-administration of ATRIPLA with drugs that reduce renal fuction or compete for active tubular secretion may increase serum concentrations of emtricitabine, tenofovir, and/or other renally eliminated drugs). Products include:
Zovirax ... 1643
Zovirax Cream ... 820
Zovirax Ointment ... 821

Acyclovir Sodium (Since emtricitabine and tenofovir are primarily eliminated by the kidneys, co-administration of ATRIPLA with drugs that reduce renal fuction or compete for active tubular secretion may increase serum concentrations of emtricitabine, tenofovir, and/or other renally eliminated drugs).
No products indexed under this heading.

Adefovir dipivoxil (Since emtricitabine and tenofovir are primarily eliminated by the kidneys, co-administration of ATRIPLA with drugs that reduce renal fuction or compete for active tubular secretion may increase serum concentrations of emtricitabine, tenofovir, and/or other renally eliminated drugs). Products include:
Hepsera Tablets ... 1292

Alfentanil Hydrochloride (Efavirenz has been shown in vivo to induce CYP3A4. Other compounds that are substrates of CYP3A4 may have decreased plasma concentrations when co-administered with efavirenz).
No products indexed under this heading.

Allium sativum (Drugs which induce CYP3A4 activity would be expected to increase the clearance of efavirenz resulting in lower plasma concentrations).
No products indexed under this heading.

Alprazolam (Efavirenz has been shown in vivo to induce CYP3A4. Other compounds that are substrates of CYP3A4 may have decreased plasma concentrations when co-administered with efavirenz). Products include:
Niravam Orally Disintegrating Tablets ... 3092

Amitriptyline Hydrochloride (Efavirenz has been shown in vivo to induce CYP3A4. Other compounds that are substrates of CYP3A4 may have decreased plasma concentrations when co-administered with efavirenz).
No products indexed under this heading.

Amlodipine Besylate (Efavirenz has been shown in vivo to induce CYP3A4. Other compounds that are substrates of CYP3A4 may have decreased plasma concentrations when co-administered with efavirenz). Products include:
Caduet Tablets ... 2508
Lotrel Capsules ... 2249
Norvasc Tablets ... 2545

Amoxapine (In vitro studies have demonstrated that efavirenz inhibits CYP2C19 in the range of observed efavirenz plasma concetrations. Co-administration of efavirenz with drugs primarily metabolized by CYP2C19 may result in altered plasma concentrations of the co-administered drug. Therefore, appropriate dose adjustments may be necesssary for these drugs).
No products indexed under this heading.

Amprenavir (Efavirenz has the potential to decrease serum concentrations of amprenavir). Products include:
Agenerase Capsules ... 1327
Agenerase Oral Solution ... 1332

Aprepitant (Efavirenz has been shown in vivo to induce CYP3A4. Other compounds that are substrates of CYP3A4 may have decreased plasma concentrations when co-administered with efavirenz). Products include:
Emend Capsules ... 1963

Astemizole (Due to the potential for serious and/or life-threatening reactions, such as cardiac arrhythmias with astemizole, concomitant use is contraindicated).
No products indexed under this heading.

Atazanavir (Atazanavir has been shown to increase tenofovir concentrations. The mechanism of this interaction is unknown. Higher tenofovir concentrations could potentiate tenofovir-associated adverse events, including renal disorders. Patients receiving either atazanavir with tenofovir DF should be monitored for tenofovir-associated adverse events. ATRIPLA should be discontinued in patients who develop tenofovir-assocatied adverse events).
No products indexed under this heading.

Atorvastatin Calcium (Plasma concentrations of atorvastatin, pravastatin, and simvastatin decreased with efavirenz. Consult the complete

prescribing information for the HMG-CoA reductase inhibitor for guidance on individualizing the dose).
Products include:
Caduet Tablets ... **2508**
Lipitor Tablets ... **2483**

Belladonna Ergotamine (Efavirenz has been shown in vivo to induce CYP3A4. Other compounds that are substrates of CYP3A4 may have decreased plasma concentrations when co-administered with efavirenz).
No products indexed under this heading.

Betamethasone Acetate (Drugs which induce CYP3A4 activity would be expected to increase the clearance of efavirenz resulting in lower plasma concentrations).
No products indexed under this heading.

Betamethasone Sodium Phosphate (Drugs which induce CYP3A4 activity would be expected to increase the clearance of efavirenz resulting in lower plasma concentrations).
No products indexed under this heading.

Buspirone Hydrochloride (Efavirenz has been shown in vivo to induce CYP3A4. Other compounds that are substrates of CYP3A4 may have decreased plasma concentrations when co-administered with efavirenz).
No products indexed under this heading.

Busulfan (Efavirenz has been shown in vivo to induce CYP3A4. Other compounds that are substrates of CYP3A4 may have decreased plasma concentrations when co-administered with efavirenz).
Products include:
I.V. Busulfex ... **2493**
Myleran Tablets ... **1525**

Candesartan Cilexetil (In vitro studies have demonstrated that efavirenz inhibits CYP2C9 in the range of observed efavirenz plasma concentrations. Co-administration of efavirenz with drugs primarily metabolized by CYP2C9 may result in altered plasma concentrations of the co-administered drug. Therefore, appropriate dose adjustments may be necessary for these drugs).
Products include:
Atacand Tablets ... **649**
Atacand HCT ... **651**

Carbamazepine (Alternative anticonvulsant treatments should be used due to decreases in both carbamazepine and efavirenz concentrations). Products include:
Carbatrol Capsules ... **3171**
Equetro Extended-Release Capsules ... **3180**
Tegretol/Tegretol-XR ... **2295**

Carisoprodol (In vitro studies have demonstrated that efavirenz inhibits CYP2C19 in the range of observed efavirenz plasma concetrations. Co-administration of efavirenz with drugs primarily metabolized by CYP2C19 may result in altered plasma concentrations of the co-administered drug. Therefore, appropriate dose adjustments may be necesssary for these drugs).
No products indexed under this heading.

Carvedilol (In vitro studies have demonstrated that efavirenz inhibits CYP2C9 in the range of observed efavirenz plasma concentrations. Co-administration of efavirenz with drugs primarily metabolized by CYP2C9 may result in altered plasma concentrations of the co-administered drug. Therefore, appropriate dose adjustments may be necessary for these drugs).
Products include:
Coreg Tablets ... **1414**

Celecoxib (In vitro studies have demonstrated that efavirenz inhibits CYP2C9 in the range of observed efavirenz plasma concentrations. Co-administration of efavirenz with drugs primarily metabolized by CYP2C9 may result in altered plasma concentrations of the co-administered drug. Therefore, appropriate dose adjustments may be necessary for these drugs).
Products include:
Celebrex Capsules ... **3134**

Cerivastatin Sodium (Efavirenz has been shown in vivo to induce CYP3A4. Other compounds that are substrates of CYP3A4 may have decreased plasma concentrations when co-administered with efavirenz).
No products indexed under this heading.

Chlorpheniramine (Efavirenz has been shown in vivo to induce CYP3A4. Other compounds that are substrates of CYP3A4 may have decreased plasma concentrations when co-administered with efavirenz).
No products indexed under this heading.

Chlorpheniramine Maleate (Efavirenz has been shown in vivo to induce CYP3A4. Other compounds that are substrates of CYP3A4 may have decreased plasma concentrations when co-administered with efavirenz). Products include:
Advil Allergy Sinus Caplets ... ▣**770**
Advil Multi-Symptom Cold Caplets ... ▣**770**
BC Allergy Sinus Cold Powder ... ▣**677**
Comtrex Maximum Strength Cold & Cough Day/Night Caplets - Night Formulation ... ▣**726**
Comtrex Maximum Strength Day/Night Severe Cold & Sinus Caplets - Night Formulation ... ▣**725**
Contac Cold and Flu Maximum Strength Caplets ... ▣**728**
Contac Cold and Flu Day and Night Caplets (Night Formulation Only) ... ▣**727**
Children's Dimetapp Long Acting Cough Plus Cold Syrup ... ▣**731**
Robitussin Cough & Cold Long-Acting Liquid ... ▣**735**
Robitussin Cough & Allergy Syrup .. ▣**736**
Robitussin Cough & Cold Nighttime Liquid ... ▣**736**
Robitussin Cough, Cold & Flu Nighttime Liquid ... ▣**738**
Robitussin Pediatric Cough & Cold Long-Acting Liquid ... ▣**735**
Robitussin Pediatric Cough & Cold Nighttime Liquid ... ▣**736**
Triaminic Cold & Allergy Liquid ... ▣**746**
Triaminic Cough & Runny Nose Softchews ... ▣**748**
Children's Tylenol Plus Flu Oral Suspension ... ▣**749**
Tylenol Allergy Multi-Symptom Caplets with Cool Burst and Gelcaps ... **1872**
Children's Tylenol Plus Cold Suspension Liquid ... **1879**
Children's Tylenol Plus Cough & Runny Nose Suspension Liquid ... **1879**
Children's Tylenol Plus Flu Suspension Liquid ... **1881**
Children's Tylenol Plus Multi-Symptom Cold Suspension Liquid ... **1879**
Tylenol Cold Head Congestion Nighttime Caplets with Cool Burst ... **1873**
Tylenol Cold Multi-Symptom Nighttime Caplets with Cool Burst ... **1874**
Tylenol Sinus Congestion & Pain Nighttime Caplets with Cool Burst ... **1876**
Vicks 44M Cough, Cold & Flu Relief Liquid ... **2680**
Pediatric Vicks 44m Cough & Cold Relief Liquid ... **2676**
Children's Vicks NyQuil Cold/Cough Relief ... ▣**756**
Children's Vicks NyQuil Cold/Cough Relief Liquid ... **2680**
Zicam Maximum Strength Flu Daytime ... ▣**768**

Chlorpheniramine Polistirex (Efavirenz has been shown in vivo to induce CYP3A4. Other compounds that are substrates of CYP3A4 may have decreased plasma concentrations when co-administered with efavirenz). Products include:
Tussionex Pennkinetic Extended-Release Suspension ... **3327**

Chlorpheniramine Tannate (Efavirenz has been shown in vivo to induce CYP3A4. Other compounds that are substrates of CYP3A4 may have decreased plasma concentrations when co-administered with efavirenz).
No products indexed under this heading.

Chlorpropamide (In vitro studies have demonstrated that efavirenz inhibits CYP2C9 in the range of observed efavirenz plasma concentrations. Co-administration of efavirenz with drugs primarily metabolized by CYP2C9 may result in altered plasma concentrations of the co-administered drug. Therefore, appropriate dose adjustments may be necessary for these drugs).
No products indexed under this heading.

Cidofovir (Since emtricitabine and tenofovir are primarily eliminated by the kidneys, co-administration of ATRIPLA with drugs that reduce renal fuction or compete for active tubular secretion may increase serum concentrations of emtricitabine, tenofovir, and/or other renally eliminated drugs).
No products indexed under this heading.

Cilostazol (In vitro studies have demonstrated that efavirenz inhibits CYP2C19 in the range of observed efavirenz plasma concetrations. Co-administration of efavirenz with drugs primarily metabolized by CYP2C19 may result in altered plasma concentrations of the co-administered drug. Therefore, appropriate dose adjustments may be necesssary for these drugs).
Products include:
Pletal Tablets ... **2455**

Ciprofloxacin Hydrochloride (Drugs which induce CYP3A4 activity would be expected to increase the clearance of efavirenz resulting in lower plasma concentrations).
Products include:
Ciloxan Ophthalmic Ointment ... **559**
Ciloxan Ophthalmic Solution ... ⊙**206**
Cipro Tablets ... **2977**
Proquin XR Tablets ... **1153**

Cisapride (Due to the potential for serious and/or life-threatening reactions, such as cardiac arrhythmias, concomitant use with cisapride is contraindicated).
No products indexed under this heading.

Cisplatin (Drugs which induce CYP3A4 activity would be expected to increase the clearance of efavirenz resulting in lower plasma concentrations).
No products indexed under this heading.

Citalopram Hydrobromide (In vitro studies have demonstrated that efavirenz inhibits CYP2C19 in the range of observed efavirenz plasma concetrations. Co-administration of efavirenz with drugs primarily metabolized by CYP2C19 may result in altered plasma concentrations of the co-administered drug. Therefore, appropriate dose adjustments may be necesssary for these drugs).
Products include:
Celexa ... **1176**

Clarithromycin (In uninfected volunteers, 46% developed a rash while receiving efavirenz and clarithromycin. No dose adjustment of ATRIPLA is recommended when given with clarithromycin. Alternatives to clarithromycin, such as azithromycin, should be considered. Other macrolide antibiotics, such as erythromycin, have not been studied in combination with ATRIPLA). Products include:
Biaxin/Biaxin XL ... **402**
PREVPAC ... **3284**

Clomipramine Hydrochloride (In vitro studies have demonstrated that efavirenz inhibits CYP2C9 in the range of observed efavirenz plasma concentrations. Co-administration of efavirenz with drugs primarily metabolized by CYP2C9 may result in altered plasma concentrations of the co-administered drug. Therefore, appropriate dose adjustments may be necessary for these drugs).
No products indexed under this heading.

Cortisone Acetate (Drugs which induce CYP3A4 activity would be expected to increase the clearance of efavirenz resulting in lower plasma concentrations).
No products indexed under this heading.

Cyclophosphamide (In vitro studies have demonstrated that efavirenz inhibits CYP2C19 in the range of observed efavirenz plasma concetrations. Co-administration of efavirenz with drugs primarily metabolized by CYP2C19 may result in altered plasma concentrations of the co-administered drug. Therefore, appropriate dose adjustments may be necesssary for these drugs).
No products indexed under this heading.

Cyclosporine (Efavirenz has been shown in vivo to induce CYP3A4. Other compounds that are substrates of CYP3A4 may have decreased plasma concentrations when co-administered with efavirenz). Products include:
Gengraf Capsules ... **459**
Neoral Oral Solution ... **2259**
Neoral Soft Gelatin Capsules ... **2259**
Restasis Ophthalmic Emulsion ... **575**
Sandimmune ... **2275**

Desipramine Hydrochloride (In vitro studies have demonstrated that efavirenz inhibits CYP2C19 in the range of observed efavirenz plasma concetrations. Co-administration of efavirenz with drugs primarily metabolized by CYP2C19 may result in altered plasma concentrations of the co-administered drug. Therefore, appropriate dose adjustments may be necesssary for these drugs).
No products indexed under this heading.

Desogestrel (Efavirenz has been shown in vivo to induce CYP3A4. Other compounds that are substrates of CYP3A4 may have decreased plasma concentrations when co-administered with efavirenz). Products include:
Mircette Tablets 1066

Dexamethasone (Drugs which induce CYP3A4 activity would be expected to increase the clearance of efavirenz resulting in lower plasma concentrations). Products include:
Ciprodex Otic Suspension 559
Decadron Tablets 1951
TobraDex Ophthalmic Ointment 562
TobraDex Ophthalmic Suspension 563

Dexamethasone Acetate (Drugs which induce CYP3A4 activity would be expected to increase the clearance of efavirenz resulting in lower plasma concentrations).
No products indexed under this heading.

Dexamethasone Sodium Phosphate (Drugs which induce CYP3A4 activity would be expected to increase the clearance of efavirenz resulting in lower plasma concentrations).
No products indexed under this heading.

Dextromethorphan (In vitro studies have demonstrated that efavirenz inhibits CYP2C9 in the range of observed efavirenz plasma concentrations. Co-administration of efavirenz with drugs primarily metabolized by CYP2C9 may result in altered plasma concentrations of the co-administered drug. Therefore, appropriate dose adjustments may be necessary for these drugs).
No products indexed under this heading.

Dextromethorphan Hydrobromide (In vitro studies have demonstrated that efavirenz inhibits CYP2C19 in the range of observed efavirenz plasma concetrations. Co-administration of efavirenz with drugs primarily metabolized by CYP2C19 may result in altered plasma concentrations of the co-administered drug. Therefore, appropriate dose adjustments may be necesssary for these drugs).
Products include:
Comtrex Maximum Strength Cold & Cough Day/Night Caplets - Day Formulation .... ■726
Comtrex Maximum Strength Cold & Cough Day/Night Caplets - Night Formulation .... ■726
Comtrex Maximum Strength Non-Drowsy Cold & Cough Caplets .... ■725
Children's Dimetapp DM Cold & Cough Elixir .... ■731
Children's Dimetapp Long Acting Cough Plus Cold Syrup .... ■731
Toddler's Dimetapp Cold and Cough Drops .... ■732
Mucinex DM Extended-Release Bi-Layer Tablets .... ■720
Refenesen DM Caplets .... ■721
Robitussin Cough & Cold CF Liquid .... ■735
Robitussin Cough & Cold Long-Acting Liquid .... ■735
Robitussin Cough & Allergy Syrup .... ■736
Robitussin Cough & Cold Nighttime Liquid .... ■736
Robitussin Cough & Cold Pediatric Drops .... ■735
Robitussin Cough, Cold & Flu Nighttime Liquid .... ■738
Robitussin Cough & Congestion Liquid .... ■738
Robitussin Cough Gels Long-Acting .... ■737
Robitussin Cough Long Acting Liquid .... ■739
Robitussin Cough DM Syrup .... ■738
Robitussin Cough DM Infant Drops .... ■738
Robitussin Pediatric Cough Long Acting Liquid .... ■739
Robitussin Pediatric Cough & Cold Long-Acting Liquid .... ■735
Robitussin Pediatric Cough & Cold Nighttime Liquid .... ■736
Robitussin Sugar Free Cough .... ■738
TheraFlu Cold & Cough Hot Liquid .... ■740
TheraFlu Warming Relief Daytime Severe Cold .... ■743
TheraFlu Thin Strips Long Acting Cough .... ■744
Triaminic Daytime Cold & Cough Liquid .... ■745
Triaminic Cough & Sore Throat Liquid .... ■747
Triaminic Cough & Runny Nose Softchews .... ■748
Triaminic Thin Strips Cold & Cough .... ■778
Triaminic Infant Thin Strips Decongestant Plus Cough .... ■747
Children's Tylenol Plus Flu Oral Suspension .... ■749
Tylenol Cold Head Congestion Daytime Caplets with Cool Burst and Gelcaps .... ■750
Tylenol Cold Multi-Symptom Daytime Liquid .... ■752
Tylenol Cold Multi-Symptom Severe Daytime Liquid .... ■752
Concentrated Tylenol Infants' Drops Plus Cold & Cough .... ■754
Children's Tylenol Plus Cough & Runny Nose Suspension Liquid 1879
Children's Tylenol Plus Cough & Sore Throat Suspension Liquid 1879
Children's Tylenol Plus Flu Suspension Liquid 1881
Children's Tylenol Plus Multi-Symptom Cold Suspension Liquid 1879
Tylenol Cold Severe Congestion Non-Drowsy Caplets with Cool Burst 1874
Tylenol Cold Head Congestion Daytime Caplets with Cool Burst 1873
Tylenol Cold Head Congestion Nighttime Caplets with Cool Burst 1873
Tylenol Cold Head Congestion Severe Caplets with Cool Burst 1873
Tylenol Cold Multi-Symptom Daytime Caplets with Cool Burst and Gelcaps 1874
Tylenol Cold Multi-Symptom Daytime Liquid with Citrus Burst 1874
Tylenol Cold Multi-Symptom Nighttime Caplets with Cool Burst 1874
Tylenol Cold Multi-Symptom Nighttime Liquid with Cool Burst 1874
Tylenol Cold Multi-Symptom Severe Caplets with Cool Burst 1874
Tylenol Cold Multi-Symptom Severe Daytime Liquid with Citrus Burst 1874
Tylenol Cough & Sore Throat Daytime Liquid with Cool Burst 1877
Tylenol Cough & Sore Throat Nighttime Liquid with Cool Burst 1877
Concentrated Tylenol Infants' Drops Plus Cold and Cough 1879
Vicks 44 Cough Relief Liquid 2679
Vicks 44D Cough & Head Congestion Relief Liquid 2679
Vicks 44E Cough & Chest Congestion Relief Liquid 2679
Pediatric Vicks 44e Cough & Chest Congestion Relief Liquid 2676
Vicks 44M Cough, Cold & Flu Relief Liquid 2680
Pediatric Vicks 44m Cough & Cold Relief Liquid 2676
Vicks DayQuil LiquiCaps/Liquid Multi-Symptom Cold/Flu Relief .... ■761
Vicks DayQuil Multi-Symptom Cold/Flu Relief LiquiCaps 2678
Vicks DayQuil Multi-Symptom Cold/Flu Relief Liquid 2678
Vicks NyQuil Multi-Symptom Cold/Flu Relief Liquid 2681
Children's Vicks NyQuil Cold/Cough Relief .... ■756
Vicks NyQuil Multi-Symptom Cold/Flu Relief LiquiCaps 2681
Vicks NyQuil LiquiCaps/Liquid Multi-Symptom Cold/Flu Relief .... ■763
Vicks NyQuil Cough Liquid 2680
Children's Vicks NyQuil Cold/Cough Relief Liquid 2680
Zicam Cough Max Nighttime Cough Spray .... ■767
Zicam Cough Max Cough Spray .... ■767
Zicam Cough Max Cough Melts .... ■767
Zicam Cough Plus D Cough Spray .... ■767
Zicam Cough Relief Cough Spray .... ■767
Zicam Maximum Strength Flu Daytime .... ■768
Zicam Maximum Strength Flu Nighttime .... ■768

Diazepam (Efavirenz has been shown in vivo to induce CYP3A4. Other compounds that are substrates of CYP3A4 may have decreased plasma concentrations when co-administered with efavirenz). Products include:
Diastat Rectal Delivery System 3343
Valium Tablets 2819

Diclofenac Potassium (In vitro studies have demonstrated that efavirenz inhibits CYP2C9 in the range of observed efavirenz plasma concentrations. Co-administration of efavirenz with drugs primarily metabolized by CYP2C9 may result in altered plasma concentrations of the co-administered drug. Therefore, appropriate dose adjustments may be necessary for these drugs).
No products indexed under this heading.

Diclofenac Sodium (In vitro studies have demonstrated that efavirenz inhibits CYP2C9 in the range of observed efavirenz plasma concentrations. Co-administration of efavirenz with drugs primarily metabolized by CYP2C9 may result in altered plasma concentrations of the co-administered drug. Therefore, appropriate dose adjustments may be necessary for these drugs).
Products include:
Arthrotec Tablets 3129
Voltaren Ophthalmic Solution 2309
Voltaren Tablets 2307
Voltaren-XR Tablets 2310

Didanosine (Co-administration of tenofovir DF and didanosine should be undertaken with caution and patients receiving this combination should be monitored closely for didanosine-associated adverse events. Didanosine should be discontinued in patients who develop didanosine-associated adverse events).
No products indexed under this heading.

Dihydroergotamine Mesylate (Due to the potential for serious and/or life-threatening reactions, such as acute ergot toxicity characterized by peripheral vasospasm and ischemia of the extremities and other tissues, concomitant use with ergot derivatives is contraindicated). Products include:
Migranal Nasal Spray 3348

Diltiazem Hydrochloride (Efavirenz has been shown in vivo to induce CYP3A4. Other compounds that are substrates of CYP3A4 may have decreased plasma concentrations when co-administered with efavirenz). Products include:
Cardizem LA Extended Release Tablets 1728
Tiazac Capsules 1201

Diltiazem Maleate (Efavirenz has been shown in vivo to induce CYP3A4. Other compounds that are substrates of CYP3A4 may have decreased plasma concentrations when co-administered with efavirenz).
No products indexed under this heading.

Disopyramide (Efavirenz has been shown in vivo to induce CYP3A4. Other compounds that are substrates of CYP3A4 may have decreased plasma concentrations when co-administered with efavirenz).
No products indexed under this heading.

Disopyramide Phosphate (Efavirenz has been shown in vivo to induce CYP3A4. Other compounds that are substrates of CYP3A4 may have decreased plasma concentrations when co-administered with efavirenz).
No products indexed under this heading.

Disulfiram (Efavirenz has been shown in vivo to induce CYP3A4. Other compounds that are substrates of CYP3A4 may have decreased plasma concentrations when co-administered with efavirenz).
No products indexed under this heading.

Divalproex Sodium (In vitro studies have demonstrated that efavirenz inhibits CYP2C19 in the range of observed efavirenz plasma concetrations. Co-administration of efavirenz with drugs primarily metabolized by CYP2C19 may result in altered plasma concentrations of the co-administered drug. Therefore, appropriate dose adjustments may be necesssary for these drugs).
Products include:
Depakote Sprinkle Capsules 422
Depakote Tablets 427
Depakote ER Tablets 434

Doxepin Hydrochloride (In vitro studies have demonstrated that efavirenz inhibits CYP2C19 in the range of observed efavirenz plasma concetrations. Co-administration of efavirenz with drugs primarily metabolized by CYP2C19 may result in altered plasma concentrations of the co-administered drug. Therefore, appropriate dose adjustments may be necesssary for these drugs).
No products indexed under this heading.

Doxorubicin Hydrochloride (Efavirenz has been shown in vivo to induce CYP3A4. Other compounds that are substrates of CYP3A4 may have decreased plasma concentrations when co-administered with efavirenz).
No products indexed under this heading.

Dronabinol (Efavirenz has been shown in vivo to induce CYP3A4. Other compounds that are substrates of CYP3A4 may have decreased plasma concentrations when co-administered with efavirenz). Products include:
Marinol Capsules 3333

Eprosartan Mesylate (In vitro studies have demonstrated that efavirenz inhibits CYP2C9 in the range of observed efavirenz plasma concentrations. Co-administration of efavirenz with drugs primarily metabolized by CYP2C9 may result in altered plasma concentrations of the co-administered drug. Therefore, appropriate dose adjustments may be necessary for these drugs). Products include:
Teveten Tablets 1735
Teveten HCT Tablets 1737

Ergonovine Maleate (Due to the potential for serious and/or life-threatening reactions, such as acute ergot toxicity characterized by peripheral vasospasm and ischemia of the extremities and other tissues, concomitant use with ergot derivatives is contraindicated).
No products indexed under this heading.

Ergotamine Tartrate (Due to the potential for serious and/or life-threatening reactions, such as acute ergot toxicity characterized by peripheral vasospasm and ischemia of the extremities and other tissues, concomitant use with ergot derivatives is contraindicated).
No products indexed under this heading.

Erythromycin (Efavirenz has been shown in vivo to induce CYP3A4. Other compounds that are substrates of CYP3A4 may have decreased plasma concentrations when co-administered with efavirenz). Products include:
Ery-Tab Tablets 449
Erythromycin Base Filmtab Tablets 455
Erythromycin Delayed-Release Capsules, USP............................. 457
PCE Dispertab Tablets 515

Erythromycin Estolate (Efavirenz has been shown in vivo to induce CYP3A4. Other compounds that are substrates of CYP3A4 may have decreased plasma concentrations when co-administered with efavirenz).
No products indexed under this heading.

Erythromycin Ethylsuccinate (Efavirenz has been shown in vivo to induce CYP3A4. Other compounds that are substrates of CYP3A4 may have decreased plasma concentrations when co-administered with efavirenz). Products include:
E.E.S. 451
EryPed 447

Erythromycin Gluceptate (Efavirenz has been shown in vivo to induce CYP3A4. Other compounds that are substrates of CYP3A4 may have decreased plasma concentrations when co-administered with efavirenz).
No products indexed under this heading.

Erythromycin Lactobionate (Efavirenz has been shown in vivo to induce CYP3A4. Other compounds that are substrates of CYP3A4 may have decreased plasma concentrations when co-administered with efavirenz).
No products indexed under this heading.

Erythromycin Stearate (Efavirenz has been shown in vivo to induce CYP3A4. Other compounds that are substrates of CYP3A4 may have decreased plasma concentrations when co-administered with efavirenz). Products include:
Erythrocin Stearate Filmtab Tablets 453

Esomeprazole Magnesium (In vitro studies have demonstrated that efavirenz inhibits CYP2C19 in the range of observed efavirenz plasma concetrations. Co-administration of efavirenz with drugs primarily metabolized by CYP2C19 may result in altered plasma concentrations of the co-administered drug. Therefore, appropriate dose adjustments may be necesssary for these drugs). Products include:
Nexium Delayed-Release Capsules 655

Estradiol (Efavirenz has been shown in vivo to induce CYP3A4. Other compounds that are substrates of CYP3A4 may have decreased plasma concentrations when co-administered with efavirenz). Products include:
Angeliq Tablets 762
Climara Transdermal System 771
Climara Pro Transdermal System 776
Estrasorb Topical Emulsion 1147
Estring Vaginal Ring 2635
Menostar Transdermal System 782
Vagifem Tablets 2334

Estradiol Benzoate (Efavirenz has been shown in vivo to induce CYP3A4. Other compounds that are substrates of CYP3A4 may have decreased plasma concentrations when co-administered with efavirenz).
No products indexed under this heading.

Estradiol Cypionate (Efavirenz has been shown in vivo to induce CYP3A4. Other compounds that are substrates of CYP3A4 may have decreased plasma concentrations when co-administered with efavirenz).
No products indexed under this heading.

Estradiol Valerate (Efavirenz has been shown in vivo to induce CYP3A4. Other compounds that are substrates of CYP3A4 may have decreased plasma concentrations when co-administered with efavirenz).
No products indexed under this heading.

Ethinyl Estradiol (Because the potential interaction of efavirenz with oral contraceptives has not been fully characterized, a reliable method of barrier contraception should be used in addition to oral contraceptives). Products include:
Mircette Tablets 1066
NuvaRing 2340
Ortho-Cyclen/Ortho Tri-Cyclen 2429
Ortho Evra Transdermal System 2417
Ortho Tri-Cyclen Lo Tablets 2436
Seasonique Tablets 1077
Yasmin 28 Tablets 796
Yaz Tablets 803

Ethosuximide (Efavirenz has been shown in vivo to induce CYP3A4. Other compounds that are substrates of CYP3A4 may have decreased plasma concentrations when co-administered with efavirenz).
No products indexed under this heading.

Ethotoin (In vitro studies have demonstrated that efavirenz inhibits CYP2C19 in the range of observed efavirenz plasma concetrations. Co-administration of efavirenz with drugs primarily metabolized by CYP2C19 may result in altered plasma concentrations of the co-administered drug. Therefore, appropriate dose adjustments may be necesssary for these drugs).
No products indexed under this heading.

Ethynodiol Diacetate (Efavirenz has been shown in vivo to induce CYP3A4. Other compounds that are substrates of CYP3A4 may have decreased plasma concentrations when co-administered with efavirenz).
No products indexed under this heading.

Etodolac (In vitro studies have demonstrated that efavirenz inhibits CYP2C9 in the range of observed efavirenz plasma concentrations. Co-administration of efavirenz with drugs primarily metabolized by CYP2C9 may result in altered plasma concentrations of the co-administered drug. Therefore, appropriate dose adjustments may be necessary for these drugs).
No products indexed under this heading.

Etoposide (Efavirenz has been shown in vivo to induce CYP3A4. Other compounds that are substrates of CYP3A4 may have decreased plasma concentrations when co-administered with efavirenz).
No products indexed under this heading.

Etoposide Phosphate (Efavirenz has been shown in vivo to induce CYP3A4. Other compounds that are substrates of CYP3A4 may have decreased plasma concentrations when co-administered with efavirenz).
No products indexed under this heading.

Felbamate (Drugs which induce CYP3A4 activity would be expected to increase the clearance of efavirenz resulting in lower plasma concentrations).
No products indexed under this heading.

Felodipine (Efavirenz has been shown in vivo to induce CYP3A4. Other compounds that are substrates of CYP3A4 may have decreased plasma concentrations when co-administered with efavirenz).
No products indexed under this heading.

Fenoprofen Calcium (In vitro studies have demonstrated that efavirenz inhibits CYP2C9 in the range of observed efavirenz plasma concentrations. Co-administration of efavirenz with drugs primarily metabolized by CYP2C9 may result in altered plasma concentrations of the co-administered drug. Therefore, appropriate dose adjustments may be necessary for these drugs). Products include:
Nalfon Capsules 2502

Fentanyl (Efavirenz has been shown in vivo to induce CYP3A4. Other compounds that are substrates of CYP3A4 may have decreased plasma concentrations when co-administered with efavirenz). Products include:
Duragesic Transdermal System 2373
Ionsys Transdermal System 2379

Fentanyl Citrate (Efavirenz has been shown in vivo to induce CYP3A4. Other compounds that are substrates of CYP3A4 may have decreased plasma concentrations when co-administered with efavirenz). Products include:
Actiq 979

Fludrocortisone Acetate (Drugs which induce CYP3A4 activity would be expected to increase the clearance of efavirenz resulting in lower plasma concentrations).
No products indexed under this heading.

Fluoxetine Hydrochloride (In vitro studies have demonstrated that efavirenz inhibits CYP2C9 in the range of observed efavirenz plasma concentrations. Co-administration of efavirenz with drugs primarily metabolized by CYP2C9 may result in altered plasma concentrations of the co-administered drug. Therefore, appropriate dose adjustments may be necessary for these drugs). Products include:
Prozac Pulvules and Liquid 1801
Symbyax Capsules 1819

Flurbiprofen (In vitro studies have demonstrated that efavirenz inhibits CYP2C9 in the range of observed efavirenz plasma concentrations. Co-administration of efavirenz with drugs primarily metabolized by CYP2C9 may result in altered plasma concentrations of the co-administered drug. Therefore, appropriate dose adjustments may be necessary for these drugs).
No products indexed under this heading.

Flurbiprofen Sodium (In vitro studies have demonstrated that efavirenz inhibits CYP2C9 in the range of observed efavirenz plasma concentrations. Co-administration of efavirenz with drugs primarily metabolized by CYP2C9 may result in altered plasma concentrations of the co-administered drug. Therefore, appropriate dose adjustments may be necessary for these drugs). Products include:
Ocufen Ophthalmic Solution .... ⊙ 232

Fluvastatin Sodium (In vitro studies have demonstrated that efavirenz inhibits CYP2C9 in the range of observed efavirenz plasma concentrations. Co-administration of efavirenz with drugs primarily metabolized by CYP2C9 may result in altered plasma concentrations of the co-administered drug. Therefore, appropriate dose adjustments may be necessary for these drugs). Products include:
Lescol Capsules 2233
Lescol XL Tablets 2233

Formoterol Fumarate (In vitro studies have demonstrated that efavirenz inhibits CYP2C19 in the range of observed efavirenz plasma concetrations. Co-administration of efavirenz with drugs primarily metabolized by CYP2C19 may result in altered plasma concentrations of the co-administered drug. Therefore, appropriate dose adjustments may be necesssary for these drugs). Products include:

Foradil Aerolizer 3010

Fosamprenavir Calcium (An additional 100 mg/day (300 mg total) of ritonavir is recommended when ATRIPLA is administered with fosamprenavir/ritonavir once daily. No change in the ritonavir dose is required when ATRIPLA is administered with fosamprenavir plus ritonavir twice daily). Products include:

Lexiva Tablets 1505

Fosphenytoin (In vitro studies have demonstrated that efavirenz inhibits CYP2C19 in the range of observed efavirenz plasma concetrations. Co-administration of efavirenz with drugs primarily metabolized by CYP2C19 may result in altered plasma concentrations of the co-administered drug. Therefore, appropriate dose adjustments may be necesssary for these drugs).

No products indexed under this heading.

Fosphenytoin Sodium (Drugs which induce CYP3A4 activity would be expected to increase the clearance of efavirenz resulting in lower plasma concentrations).

No products indexed under this heading.

Gabapentin (In vitro studies have demonstrated that efavirenz inhibits CYP2C19 in the range of observed efavirenz plasma concetrations. Co-administration of efavirenz with drugs primarily metabolized by CYP2C19 may result in altered plasma concentrations of the co-administered drug. Therefore, appropriate dose adjustments may be necesssary for these drugs). Products include:

Neurontin Capsules 2487
Neurontin Oral Solution 2487
Neurontin Tablets 2487

Ganciclovir (Since emtricitabine and tenofovir are primarily eliminated by the kidneys, co-administration of ATRIPLA with drugs that reduce renal fuction or compete for active tubular secretion may increase serum concentrations of emtricitabine, tenofovir, and/or other renally eliminated drugs).

No products indexed under this heading.

Ganciclovir Sodium (Since emtricitabine and tenofovir are primarily eliminated by the kidneys, co-administration of ATRIPLA with drugs that reduce renal fuction or compete for active tubular secretion may increase serum concentrations of emtricitabine, tenofovir, and/or other renally eliminated drugs).

No products indexed under this heading.

Garlic Extract (Drugs which induce CYP3A4 activity would be expected to increase the clearance of efavirenz resulting in lower plasma concentrations).

No products indexed under this heading.

Garlic Oil (Drugs which induce CYP3A4 activity would be expected to increase the clearance of efavirenz resulting in lower plasma concentrations).

No products indexed under this heading.

Glimepiride (In vitro studies have demonstrated that efavirenz inhibits CYP2C9 in the range of observed efavirenz plasma concentrations. Co-administration of efavirenz with drugs primarily metabolized by CYP2C9 may result in altered plasma concentrations of the co-administered drug. Therefore, appropriate dose adjustments may be necessary for these drugs). Products include:

Avandaryl Tablets 1379
Duetact Tablets 3226

Glipizide (In vitro studies have demonstrated that efavirenz inhibits CYP2C9 in the range of observed efavirenz plasma concentrations. Co-administration of efavirenz with drugs primarily metabolized by CYP2C9 may result in altered plasma concentrations of the co-administered drug. Therefore, appropriate dose adjustments may be necessary for these drugs).

No products indexed under this heading.

Haloperidol (Efavirenz has been shown in vivo to induce CYP3A4. Other compounds that are substrates of CYP3A4 may have decreased plasma concentrations when co-administered with efavirenz).

No products indexed under this heading.

Haloperidol Decanoate (Efavirenz has been shown in vivo to induce CYP3A4. Other compounds that are substrates of CYP3A4 may have decreased plasma concentrations when co-administered with efavirenz).

No products indexed under this heading.

Haloperidol Lactate (Efavirenz has been shown in vivo to induce CYP3A4. Other compounds that are substrates of CYP3A4 may have decreased plasma concentrations when co-administered with efavirenz).

No products indexed under this heading.

Hydrocortisone (Drugs which induce CYP3A4 activity would be expected to increase the clearance of efavirenz resulting in lower plasma concentrations). Products include:

Colocort Rectal Suspension, USP (Retention) 100 mg/60 mL.......... 2476
Hydrocortone Tablets 1989
Preparation H Hydrocortisone Cream .... ▣646

Hydrocortisone Acetate (Drugs which induce CYP3A4 activity would be expected to increase the clearance of efavirenz resulting in lower plasma concentrations). Products include:

Analpram-HC 1159
Pramosone 1161
ProctoFoam-HC 3099

Hydrocortisone Butyrate (Drugs which induce CYP3A4 activity would be expected to increase the clearance of efavirenz resulting in lower plasma concentrations). Products include:

Locoid Lipocream Cream 1160

Hydrocortisone Cypionate (Drugs which induce CYP3A4 activity would be expected to increase the clearance of efavirenz resulting in lower plasma concentrations).

No products indexed under this heading.

Hydrocortisone Hemisuccinate (Drugs which induce CYP3A4 activity would be expected to increase the clearance of efavirenz resulting in lower plasma concentrations).

No products indexed under this heading.

Hydrocortisone Probutate (Drugs which induce CYP3A4 activity would be expected to increase the clearance of efavirenz resulting in lower plasma concentrations).

No products indexed under this heading.

Hydrocortisone Sodium Phosphate (Drugs which induce CYP3A4 activity would be expected to increase the clearance of efavirenz resulting in lower plasma concentrations).

No products indexed under this heading.

Hydrocortisone Sodium Succinate (Drugs which induce CYP3A4 activity would be expected to increase the clearance of efavirenz resulting in lower plasma concentrations).

No products indexed under this heading.

Hydrocortisone Valerate (Drugs which induce CYP3A4 activity would be expected to increase the clearance of efavirenz resulting in lower plasma concentrations).

No products indexed under this heading.

Hypericum (Drugs which induce CYP3A4 activity would be expected to increase the clearance of efavirenz resulting in lower plasma concentrations). Products include:

Satiete Tablets .... ▣832

Hypericum Perforatum (Hypericum perforatum is expected to substantially decrease plasma levels of efavirenz. It has not been studied in combination with efavirenz, but concomitant use is not recommended).

No products indexed under this heading.

Ibuprofen (In vitro studies have demonstrated that efavirenz inhibits CYP2C9 in the range of observed efavirenz plasma concentrations. Co-administration of efavirenz with drugs primarily metabolized by CYP2C9 may result in altered plasma concentrations of the co-administered drug. Therefore, appropriate dose adjustments may be necessary for these drugs). Products include:

Advil Allergy Sinus Caplets .... ▣770
Advil .... ▣674
Children's Advil Oral Suspension .... ▣603
Children's Advil Chewable Tablets .. ▣603
Advil Cold & Sinus .... ▣723
Infants' Advil Concentrated Drops .. ▣604
Infants' Advil Concentrated Drops - White Grape (Dye-Free)............ ▣604
Junior Strength Advil Swallow Tablets.. ▣605
Advil Migraine Liquigels .... ▣608
Advil Multi-Symptom Cold Caplets.. ▣770
Advil PM Caplets .... ▣615
Motrin IB Tablets and Caplets 1866
Children's Motrin Oral Suspension ... 1867
Children's Motrin Non-Staining Dye-Free Oral Suspension............ 1867
Children's Motrin Cold Oral Suspension 1867
Infants' Motrin Concentrated Drops... 1867
Infants' Motrin Non-Staining Dye-Free Concentrated Drops....... 1867
Junior Strength Motrin Caplets and Chewable Tablets................. 1867
Vicoprofen Tablets 539

Imipramine Hydrochloride (In vitro studies have demonstrated that efavirenz inhibits CYP2C9 in the range of observed efavirenz plasma concentrations. Co-administration of efavirenz with drugs primarily metabolized by CYP2C9 may result in altered plasma concentrations of the co-administered drug. Therefore, appropriate dose adjustments may be necessary for these drugs).

No products indexed under this heading.

Imipramine Pamoate (In vitro studies have demonstrated that efavirenz inhibits CYP2C19 in the range of observed efavirenz plasma concetrations. Co-administration of efavirenz with drugs primarily metabolized by CYP2C19 may result in altered plasma concentrations of the co-administered drug. Therefore, appropriate dose adjustments may be necesssary for these drugs).

No products indexed under this heading.

Indinavir Sulfate (The optimal dose of indinavir, when given in combination with efavirenz, is not known. Increasing the indinavir dose to 1000 mg every 8 hours does not compensate for the increased indinavir metabolism due to efavirenz). Products include:

Crixivan Capsules 1940

Indomethacin (In vitro studies have demonstrated that efavirenz inhibits CYP2C9 in the range of observed efavirenz plasma concentrations. Co-administration of efavirenz with drugs primarily metabolized by CYP2C9 may result in altered plasma concentrations of the co-administered drug. Therefore, appropriate dose adjustments may be necessary for these drugs). Products include:

Indocin 1995

Indomethacin Sodium Trihydrate (In vitro studies have demonstrated that efavirenz inhibits CYP2C9 in the range of observed efavirenz plasma concentrations. Co-administration of efavirenz with drugs primarily metabolized by CYP2C9 may result in altered plasma concentrations of the co-administered drug. Therefore, appropriate dose adjustments may be necessary for these drugs). Products include:

Indocin I.V. 2465

Irbesartan (In vitro studies have demonstrated that efavirenz inhibits CYP2C9 in the range of observed efavirenz plasma concentrations. Co-administration of efavirenz with drugs primarily metabolized by CYP2C9 may result in altered plasma concentrations of the co-administered drug. Therefore, appropriate dose adjustments may be necessary for these drugs). Products include:

Avalide Tablets 888
Avalide Tablets 2874
Avapro Tablets 891
Avapro Tablets 2871

Isradipine (Efavirenz has been shown in vivo to induce CYP3A4. Other compounds that are substrates of CYP3A4 may have decreased plasma concentrations when co-administered with efavirenz). Products include:
DynaCirc CR Tablets 2721

Itraconazole (Drug interaction studies with ATRIPLA and these imidazole and triazole antifungals have not been conducted. Efavirenz has the potential to decrease plasma concentrations of itraconazole and ketoconazole).
No products indexed under this heading.

Ketoconazole (Drug interaction studies with ATRIPLA and these imidazole and triazole antifungals have not been conducted. Efavirenz has the potential to decrease plasma concentrations of itraconazole and ketoconazole). Products include:
Nizoral A-D Shampoo, 1% 1868

Ketoprofen (In vitro studies have demonstrated that efavirenz inhibits CYP2C9 in the range of observed efavirenz plasma concentrations. Co-administration of efavirenz with drugs primarily metabolized by CYP2C9 may result in altered plasma concentrations of the co-administered drug. Therefore, appropriate dose adjustments may be necessary for these drugs).
No products indexed under this heading.

Ketorolac Tromethamine (In vitro studies have demonstrated that efavirenz inhibits CYP2C9 in the range of observed efavirenz plasma concentrations. Co-administration of efavirenz with drugs primarily metabolized by CYP2C9 may result in altered plasma concentrations of the co-administered drug. Therefore, appropriate dose adjustments may be necessary for these drugs).
Products include:
Acular Ophthalmic Solution 565
Acular LS Ophthalmic Solution 566

Lamotrigine (In vitro studies have demonstrated that efavirenz inhibits CYP2C19 in the range of observed efavirenz plasma concetrations. Co-administration of efavirenz with drugs primarily metabolized by CYP2C19 may result in altered plasma concentrations of the co-administered drug. Therefore, appropriate dose adjustments may be necesssary for these drugs).
Products include:
Lamictal 1481

Lansoprazole (In vitro studies have demonstrated that efavirenz inhibits CYP2C9 in the range of observed efavirenz plasma concentrations. Co-administration of efavirenz with drugs primarily metabolized by CYP2C9 may result in altered plasma concentrations of the co-administered drug. Therefore, appropriate dose adjustments may be necessary for these drugs).
Products include:
Prevacid Delayed-Release Capsules 3271
Prevacid for Delayed-Release Oral Suspension 3271
Prevacid SoluTab Delayed-Release Orally Disintegrating Tablets 3271
Prevacid I.V. for Injection 3277
Prevacid NapraPAC 3280
PREVPAC 3284

Levetiracetam (In vitro studies have demonstrated that efavirenz inhibits CYP2C19 in the range of observed efavirenz plasma concetrations. Co-administration of efavirenz with drugs primarily metabolized by CYP2C19 may result in altered plasma concentrations of the co-administered drug. Therefore, appropriate dose adjustments may be necesssary for these drugs).
Products include:
Keppra Injection 3320
Keppra Oral Solution 3314
Keppra Tablets 3314

Levonorgestrel (Efavirenz has been shown in vivo to induce CYP3A4. Other compounds that are substrates of CYP3A4 may have decreased plasma concentrations when co-administered with efavirenz). Products include:
Climara Pro Transdermal System 776
Mirena Intrauterine System 787
Plan B Tablets 1076
Seasonique Tablets 1077

Lidocaine (Efavirenz has been shown in vivo to induce CYP3A4. Other compounds that are substrates of CYP3A4 may have decreased plasma concentrations when co-administered with efavirenz). Products include:
Lidoderm Patch 1118
Synera Topical Patch 1137

Lidocaine Hydrochloride (Efavirenz has been shown in vivo to induce CYP3A4. Other compounds that are substrates of CYP3A4 may have decreased plasma concentrations when co-administered with efavirenz).
No products indexed under this heading.

Lopinavir (Kaletra has been shown to increase tenofovir concentrations. The mechanism of this interaction is unknown. Higher tenofovir concentrations could potentiate tenofovir-associated adverse events, including renal disorders. Patients receiving Kaletra with tenofovir DF should be monitored for tenofovir-associated adverse events. ATRIPLA should be discontinued in patients who develop tenofovir-assocatied adverse events). Products include:
Kaletra 476

Losartan Potassium (In vitro studies have demonstrated that efavirenz inhibits CYP2C9 in the range of observed efavirenz plasma concentrations. Co-administration of efavirenz with drugs primarily metabolized by CYP2C9 may result in altered plasma concentrations of the co-administered drug. Therefore, appropriate dose adjustments may be necessary for these drugs).
Products include:
Cozaar Tablets 1935
Hyzaar 50-12.5 Tablets 1990
Hyzaar 100-12.5 Tablets 1990
Hyzaar 100-25 Tablets 1990

Lovastatin (Efavirenz has been shown in vivo to induce CYP3A4. Other compounds that are substrates of CYP3A4 may have decreased plasma concentrations when co-administered with efavirenz). Products include:
Advicor Tablets 1722
Altoprev Extended-Release Tablets 3109
Mevacor Tablets 2021

Maprotiline Hydrochloride (In vitro studies have demonstrated that efavirenz inhibits CYP2C19 in the range of observed efavirenz plasma concetrations. Co-administration of efavirenz with drugs primarily metabolized by CYP2C19 may result in altered plasma concentrations of the co-administered drug. Therefore, appropriate dose adjustments may be necesssary for these drugs).
No products indexed under this heading.

Meclofenamate Sodium (In vitro studies have demonstrated that efavirenz inhibits CYP2C9 in the range of observed efavirenz plasma concentrations. Co-administration of efavirenz with drugs primarily metabolized by CYP2C9 may result in altered plasma concentrations of the co-administered drug. Therefore, appropriate dose adjustments may be necessary for these drugs).
No products indexed under this heading.

Mefenamic Acid (In vitro studies have demonstrated that efavirenz inhibits CYP2C9 in the range of observed efavirenz plasma concentrations. Co-administration of efavirenz with drugs primarily metabolized by CYP2C9 may result in altered plasma concentrations of the co-administered drug. Therefore, appropriate dose adjustments may be necessary for these drugs).
No products indexed under this heading.

Meloxicam (In vitro studies have demonstrated that efavirenz inhibits CYP2C9 in the range of observed efavirenz plasma concentrations. Co-administration of efavirenz with drugs primarily metabolized by CYP2C9 may result in altered plasma concentrations of the co-administered drug. Therefore, appropriate dose adjustments may be necessary for these drugs).
Products include:
Mobic Oral Suspension 863
Mobic Tablets 863

Mephenytoin (Drugs which induce CYP3A4 activity would be expected to increase the clearance of efavirenz resulting in lower plasma concentrations).
No products indexed under this heading.

Mephobarbital (In vitro studies have demonstrated that efavirenz inhibits CYP2C19 in the range of observed efavirenz plasma concetrations. Co-administration of efavirenz with drugs primarily metabolized by CYP2C19 may result in altered plasma concentrations of the co-administered drug. Therefore, appropriate dose adjustments may be necesssary for these drugs).
No products indexed under this heading.

Meprobamate (In vitro studies have demonstrated that efavirenz inhibits CYP2C19 in the range of observed efavirenz plasma concetrations. Co-administration of efavirenz with drugs primarily metabolized by CYP2C19 may result in altered plasma concentrations of the co-administered drug. Therefore, appropriate dose adjustments may be necesssary for these drugs).
No products indexed under this heading.

Mestranol (Efavirenz has been shown in vivo to induce CYP3A4. Other compounds that are substrates of CYP3A4 may have decreased plasma concentrations when co-administered with efavirenz).
No products indexed under this heading.

Metformin Hydrochloride (In vitro studies have demonstrated that efavirenz inhibits CYP2C9 in the range of observed efavirenz plasma concentrations. Co-administration of efavirenz with drugs primarily metabolized by CYP2C9 may result in altered plasma concentrations of the co-administered drug. Therefore, appropriate dose adjustments may be necessary for these drugs).
Products include:
ActoPlus Met Tablets 3214
Avandamet Tablets 1373
Fortamet Extended-Release Tablets 3115

Methadone Hydrochloride (Co-administration of efavirenz in HIV-infected individuals with a history of injection drug use resulted in decreased plasma levels of methadone and signs of opiate withdrawal. Methadone dose was increased by a mean of 22% to alleviate withdrawal symptoms. Patients should be monitored for signs of withdrawal and their methadone dose increased as required to alleviate withdrawal symptoms).
No products indexed under this heading.

Methsuximide (Drugs which induce CYP3A4 activity would be expected to increase the clearance of efavirenz resulting in lower plasma concentrations).
No products indexed under this heading.

Methylergonovine Maleate (Due to the potential for serious and/or life-threatening reactions, such as acute ergot toxicity characterized by peripheral vasospasm and ischemia of the extremities and other tissues, concomitant use with ergot derivatives is contraindicated).
No products indexed under this heading.

Methylprednisolone (Drugs which induce CYP3A4 activity would be expected to increase the clearance of efavirenz resulting in lower plasma concentrations).
No products indexed under this heading.

Methylprednisolone Acetate (Drugs which induce CYP3A4 activity would be expected to increase the clearance of efavirenz resulting in lower plasma concentrations).
Products include:
Depo-Medrol Injectable Suspension 2617
Depo-Medrol Single-Dose Vial 2619

Methylprednisolone Sodium Succinate (Drugs which induce CYP3A4 activity would be expected to increase the clearance of efavirenz resulting in lower plasma concentrations).
No products indexed under this heading.

IMPORTANT NOTE: Always consult each drug listing in the patient's regimen for possible interactions.

Midazolam Hydrochloride (Due to the potential for serious and/or life-threatening reactions, such as prolonged or increased sedation or respiratory depression, concomitant use with midazolam hydrochloride is contraindicated).
No products indexed under this heading.

Miglitol (In vitro studies have demonstrated that efavirenz inhibits CYP2C9 in the range of observed efavirenz plasma concentrations. Co-administration of efavirenz with drugs primarily metabolized by CYP2C9 may result in altered plasma concentrations of the co-administered drug. Therefore, appropriate dose adjustments may be necessary for these drugs).
No products indexed under this heading.

Mirtazapine (In vitro studies have demonstrated that efavirenz inhibits CYP2C9 in the range of observed efavirenz plasma concentrations. Co-administration of efavirenz with drugs primarily metabolized by CYP2C9 may result in altered plasma concentrations of the co-administered drug. Therefore, appropriate dose adjustments may be necessary for these drugs).
No products indexed under this heading.

Modafinil (Drugs which induce CYP3A4 activity would be expected to increase the clearance of efavirenz resulting in lower plasma concentrations). Products include:
Provigil Tablets ... 988

Montelukast Sodium (In vitro studies have demonstrated that efavirenz inhibits CYP2C9 in the range of observed efavirenz plasma concentrations. Co-administration of efavirenz with drugs primarily metabolized by CYP2C9 may result in altered plasma concentrations of the co-administered drug. Therefore, appropriate dose adjustments may be necessary for these drugs). Products include:
Singulair ... 2077

Nabumetone (In vitro studies have demonstrated that efavirenz inhibits CYP2C9 in the range of observed efavirenz plasma concentrations. Co-administration of efavirenz with drugs primarily metabolized by CYP2C9 may result in altered plasma concentrations of the co-administered drug. Therefore, appropriate dose adjustments may be necessary for these drugs).
No products indexed under this heading.

Naproxen (In vitro studies have demonstrated that efavirenz inhibits CYP2C9 in the range of observed efavirenz plasma concentrations. Co-administration of efavirenz with drugs primarily metabolized by CYP2C9 may result in altered plasma concentrations of the co-administered drug. Therefore, appropriate dose adjustments may be necessary for these drugs). Products include:
EC-Naprosyn Delayed-Release Tablets ... 2761
Naprosyn Suspension ... 2761
Naprosyn Tablets ... 2761
Prevacid NapraPAC ... 3280

Naproxen Sodium (In vitro studies have demonstrated that efavirenz inhibits CYP2C9 in the range of observed efavirenz plasma concentrations. Co-administration of efavirenz with drugs primarily metabolized by CYP2C9 may result in altered plasma concentrations of the co-administered drug. Therefore, appropriate dose adjustments may be necessary for these drugs). Products include:
Aleve Caplets ... 742
Aleve Gelcaps ... 743
Aleve Tablets ... 743
Aleve Cold & Sinus Caplets ... 744
Anaprox Tablets ... 2761
Anaprox DS Tablets ... 2761

Nateglinide (In vitro studies have demonstrated that efavirenz inhibits CYP2C9 in the range of observed efavirenz plasma concentrations. Co-administration of efavirenz with drugs primarily metabolized by CYP2C9 may result in altered plasma concentrations of the co-administered drug. Therefore, appropriate dose adjustments may be necessary for these drugs). Products include:
Starlix Tablets ... 2292

Nefazodone Hydrochloride (Efavirenz has been shown in vivo to induce CYP3A4. Other compounds that are substrates of CYP3A4 may have decreased plasma concentrations when co-administered with efavirenz).
No products indexed under this heading.

Nelfinavir Mesylate (Efavirenz has been shown in vivo to induce CYP3A4. Other compounds that are substrates of CYP3A4 may have decreased plasma concentrations when co-administered with efavirenz). Products include:
Viracept ... 2577

Nevirapine (Drugs which induce CYP3A4 activity would be expected to increase the clearance of efavirenz resulting in lower plasma concentrations). Products include:
Viramune Oral Suspension ... 873
Viramune Tablets ... 873

Nicardipine Hydrochloride (Efavirenz has been shown in vivo to induce CYP3A4. Other compounds that are substrates of CYP3A4 may have decreased plasma concentrations when co-administered with efavirenz). Products include:
Cardene I.V. ... 2497

Nifedipine (Efavirenz has been shown in vivo to induce CYP3A4. Other compounds that are substrates of CYP3A4 may have decreased plasma concentrations when co-administered with efavirenz). Products include:
Adalat CC Tablets ... 2964

Nilutamide (In vitro studies have demonstrated that efavirenz inhibits CYP2C19 in the range of observed efavirenz plasma concetrations. Co-administration of efavirenz with drugs primarily metabolized by CYP2C19 may result in altered plasma concentrations of the co-administered drug. Therefore, appropriate dose adjustments may be necesssary for these drugs).
No products indexed under this heading.

Nimodipine (Efavirenz has been shown in vivo to induce CYP3A4. Other compounds that are substrates of CYP3A4 may have decreased plasma concentrations when co-administered with efavirenz). Products include:
Nimotop Capsules ... 749

Nisoldipine (Efavirenz has been shown in vivo to induce CYP3A4. Other compounds that are substrates of CYP3A4 may have decreased plasma concentrations when co-administered with efavirenz). Products include:
Sular Tablets ... 3122

Nitrendipine (Efavirenz has been shown in vivo to induce CYP3A4. Other compounds that are substrates of CYP3A4 may have decreased plasma concentrations when co-administered with efavirenz).
No products indexed under this heading.

Norethindrone (Efavirenz has been shown in vivo to induce CYP3A4. Other compounds that are substrates of CYP3A4 may have decreased plasma concentrations when co-administered with efavirenz). Products include:
Ortho Micronor Tablets ... 2426

Norethindrone Acetate (Efavirenz has been shown in vivo to induce CYP3A4. Other compounds that are substrates of CYP3A4 may have decreased plasma concentrations when co-administered with efavirenz).
No products indexed under this heading.

Norgestrel (Efavirenz has been shown in vivo to induce CYP3A4. Other compounds that are substrates of CYP3A4 may have decreased plasma concentrations when co-administered with efavirenz).
No products indexed under this heading.

Nortriptyline Hydrochloride (In vitro studies have demonstrated that efavirenz inhibits CYP2C19 in the range of observed efavirenz plasma concetrations. Co-administration of efavirenz with drugs primarily metabolized by CYP2C19 may result in altered plasma concentrations of the co-administered drug. Therefore, appropriate dose adjustments may be necesssary for these drugs).
No products indexed under this heading.

Omeprazole (In vitro studies have demonstrated that efavirenz inhibits CYP2C9 in the range of observed efavirenz plasma concentrations. Co-administration of efavirenz with drugs primarily metabolized by CYP2C9 may result in altered plasma concentrations of the co-administered drug. Therefore, appropriate dose adjustments may be necessary for these drugs). Products include:
Zegerid Capsules ... 2958
Zegerid Powder for Oral Solution ... 2958

Ondansetron (Efavirenz has been shown in vivo to induce CYP3A4. Other compounds that are substrates of CYP3A4 may have decreased plasma concentrations when co-administered with efavirenz). Products include:
Zofran ODT Orally Disintegrating Tablets ... 1639

Ondansetron Hydrochloride (Efavirenz has been shown in vivo to induce CYP3A4. Other compounds that are substrates of CYP3A4 may have decreased plasma concentrations when co-administered with efavirenz). Products include:
Zofran Injection ... 1634
Zofran ... 1639

Oxaprozin (In vitro studies have demonstrated that efavirenz inhibits CYP2C9 in the range of observed efavirenz plasma concentrations. Co-administration of efavirenz with drugs primarily metabolized by CYP2C9 may result in altered plasma concentrations of the co-administered drug. Therefore, appropriate dose adjustments may be necessary for these drugs).
No products indexed under this heading.

Oxcarbazepine (Drugs which induce CYP3A4 activity would be expected to increase the clearance of efavirenz resulting in lower plasma concentrations). Products include:
Trileptal Tablets ... 2300
Trileptal Oral Suspension ... 2300

Paclitaxel (Efavirenz has been shown in vivo to induce CYP3A4. Other compounds that are substrates of CYP3A4 may have decreased plasma concentrations when co-administered with efavirenz).
No products indexed under this heading.

Pantoprazole Sodium (In vitro studies have demonstrated that efavirenz inhibits CYP2C19 in the range of observed efavirenz plasma concetrations. Co-administration of efavirenz with drugs primarily metabolized by CYP2C19 may result in altered plasma concentrations of the co-administered drug. Therefore, appropriate dose adjustments may be necesssary for these drugs). Products include:
Protonix I.V. ... 3472
Protonix Tablets ... 3469

Paramethadione (In vitro studies have demonstrated that efavirenz inhibits CYP2C19 in the range of observed efavirenz plasma concetrations. Co-administration of efavirenz with drugs primarily metabolized by CYP2C19 may result in altered plasma concentrations of the co-administered drug. Therefore, appropriate dose adjustments may be necesssary for these drugs).
No products indexed under this heading.

Pentamidine Isethionate (In vitro studies have demonstrated that efavirenz inhibits CYP2C19 in the range of observed efavirenz plasma concetrations. Co-administration of efavirenz with drugs primarily metabolized by CYP2C19 may result in altered plasma concentrations of the co-administered drug. Therefore, appropriate dose adjustments may be necesssary for these drugs).
No products indexed under this heading.

Phenacemide (In vitro studies have demonstrated that efavirenz inhibits CYP2C19 in the range of observed efavirenz plasma concetrations. Co-administration of efavirenz with drugs primarily metabolized by CYP2C19 may result in altered plasma concentrations of the co-administered drug. Therefore, appropriate dose adjustments may be necesssary for these drugs).
No products indexed under this heading.

Phenobarbital (Potential for reduction in anticonvulsant and/or efavirenz plasma levels; periodic

monitoring of anticonvulsant plasma levels should be conducted).
Products include:
Donnatal Extentabs 2493

Phenobarbital Sodium (Potential for reduction in anticonvulsant and/ or efavirenz plasma levels; periodic monitoring of anticonvulsant plasma levels should be conducted).
No products indexed under this heading.

Phensuximide (In vitro studies have demonstrated that efavirenz inhibits CYP2C19 in the range of observed efavirenz plasma concetrations. Co-administration of efavirenz with drugs primarily metabolized by CYP2C19 may result in altered plasma concentrations of the co-administered drug. Therefore, appropriate dose adjustments may be necesssary for these drugs).
No products indexed under this heading.

Phenylbutazone (In vitro studies have demonstrated that efavirenz inhibits CYP2C9 in the range of observed efavirenz plasma concentrations. Co-administration of efavirenz with drugs primarily metabolized by CYP2C9 may result in altered plasma concentrations of the co-administered drug. Therefore, appropriate dose adjustments may be necessary for these drugs).
No products indexed under this heading.

Phenytoin (Potential for reduction in anticonvulsant and/or efavirenz plasma levels; periodic monitoring of anticonvulsant plasma levels should be conducted).
No products indexed under this heading.

Phenytoin Sodium (Potential for reduction in anticonvulsant and/or efavirenz plasma levels; periodic monitoring of anticonvulsant plasma levels should be conducted).
Products include:
Phenytek Capsules 2160

Pimozide (Efavirenz has been shown in vivo to induce CYP3A4. Other compounds that are substrates of CYP3A4 may have decreased plasma concentrations when co-administered with efavirenz).
No products indexed under this heading.

Pioglitazone Hydrochloride (In vitro studies have demonstrated that efavirenz inhibits CYP2C9 in the range of observed efavirenz plasma concentrations. Co-administration of efavirenz with drugs primarily metabolized by CYP2C9 may result in altered plasma concentrations of the co-administered drug. Therefore, appropriate dose adjustments may be necessary for these drugs).
Products include:
ActoPlus Met Tablets 3214
Actos Tablets 3219
Duetact Tablets 3226

Piroxicam (In vitro studies have demonstrated that efavirenz inhibits CYP2C9 in the range of observed efavirenz plasma concentrations. Co-administration of efavirenz with drugs primarily metabolized by CYP2C9 may result in altered plasma concentrations of the co-administered drug. Therefore, appropriate dose adjustments may be necessary for these drugs).
No products indexed under this heading.

Polyestradiol Phosphate (Efavirenz has been shown in vivo to induce CYP3A4. Other compounds that are substrates of CYP3A4 may have decreased plasma concentrations when co-administered with efavirenz).
No products indexed under this heading.

Pravastatin Sodium (Plasma concentrations of atorvastatin, pravastatin, and simvastatin decreased with efavirenz. Consult the complete prescribing information for the HMGCoA reductase inhibitor for guidance on individualizing the dose).
No products indexed under this heading.

Prednisolone Acetate (Drugs which induce CYP3A4 activity would be expected to increase the clearance of efavirenz resulting in lower plasma concentrations). Products include:
Blephamide Ophthalmic Ointment 568
Blephamide Ophthalmic Suspension 569
Poly-Pred Ophthalmic Suspension .... ⊙233
Pred Forte Ophthalmic Suspension .... ⊙235
Pred Mild Ophthalmic Suspension .... ⊙238
Pred-G Ophthalmic Ointment .... ⊙237
Pred-G Ophthalmic Suspension ...... ⊙236

Prednisolone Sodium Phosphate (Drugs which induce CYP3A4 activity would be expected to increase the clearance of efavirenz resulting in lower plasma concentrations).
No products indexed under this heading.

Prednisolone Tebutate (Drugs which induce CYP3A4 activity would be expected to increase the clearance of efavirenz resulting in lower plasma concentrations).
No products indexed under this heading.

Prednisone (Drugs which induce CYP3A4 activity would be expected to increase the clearance of efavirenz resulting in lower plasma concentrations).
No products indexed under this heading.

Primidone (Drugs which induce CYP3A4 activity would be expected to increase the clearance of efavirenz resulting in lower plasma concentrations).
No products indexed under this heading.

Progesterone (In vitro studies have demonstrated that efavirenz inhibits CYP2C19 in the range of observed efavirenz plasma concetrations. Co-administration of efavirenz with drugs primarily metabolized by CYP2C19 may result in altered plasma concentrations of the co-administered drug. Therefore, appropriate dose adjustments may be necesssary for these drugs).
Products include:
Prochieve 4% Gel 1003
Prochieve 8% Gel 1003
Prometrium Capsules (100 mg, 200 mg) 3203

Proguanil Hydrochloride (In vitro studies have demonstrated that efavirenz inhibits CYP2C19 in the range of observed efavirenz plasma concetrations. Co-administration of efavirenz with drugs primarily metabolized by CYP2C19 may result in altered plasma concentrations of the co-administered drug. Therefore, appropriate dose adjustments may be necesssary for these drugs).
Products include:
Malarone Pediatric Tablets 1517
Malarone Tablets 1517

Propranolol Hydrochloride (In vitro studies have demonstrated that efavirenz inhibits CYP2C19 in the range of observed efavirenz plasma concetrations. Co-administration of efavirenz with drugs primarily metabolized by CYP2C19 may result in altered plasma concentrations of the co-administered drug. Therefore, appropriate dose adjustments may be necesssary for these drugs).
Products include:
Inderal LA Long-Acting Capsules 3429
InnoPran XL Capsules 2723

Protriptyline Hydrochloride (In vitro studies have demonstrated that efavirenz inhibits CYP2C19 in the range of observed efavirenz plasma concetrations. Co-administration of efavirenz with drugs primarily metabolized by CYP2C19 may result in altered plasma concentrations of the co-administered drug. Therefore, appropriate dose adjustments may be necesssary for these drugs).
No products indexed under this heading.

Quinidine Gluconate (Efavirenz has been shown in vivo to induce CYP3A4. Other compounds that are substrates of CYP3A4 may have decreased plasma concentrations when co-administered with efavirenz).
No products indexed under this heading.

Quinidine Polygalacturonate (Efavirenz has been shown in vivo to induce CYP3A4. Other compounds that are substrates of CYP3A4 may have decreased plasma concentrations when co-administered with efavirenz).
No products indexed under this heading.

Quinidine Sulfate (Efavirenz has been shown in vivo to induce CYP3A4. Other compounds that are substrates of CYP3A4 may have decreased plasma concentrations when co-administered with efavirenz).
No products indexed under this heading.

Rabeprazole Sodium (In vitro studies have demonstrated that efavirenz inhibits CYP2C19 in the range of observed efavirenz plasma concetrations. Co-administration of efavirenz with drugs primarily metabolized by CYP2C19 may result in altered plasma concentrations of the co-administered drug. Therefore, appropriate dose adjustments may be necesssary for these drugs).
Products include:
Aciphex Tablets 1090

Repaglinide (In vitro studies have demonstrated that efavirenz inhibits CYP2C9 in the range of observed efavirenz plasma concentrations. Co-administration of efavirenz with drugs primarily metabolized by CYP2C9 may result in altered plasma concentrations of the co-administered drug. Therefore, appropriate dose adjustments may be necessary for these drugs).
No products indexed under this heading.

Rifabutin (Increase daily dose of rifabutin by 50%. Consider doubling the rifabutin dose regimens where rifabutin is given 2 or 3 times a week).
No products indexed under this heading.

Rifampicin (Drugs which induce CYP3A4 activity would be expected to increase the clearance of efavirenz resulting in lower plasma concentrations).
No products indexed under this heading.

Rifampin (Rifampin reduced plasma concentrations of efavirenz).
No products indexed under this heading.

Rifapentine (Drugs which induce CYP3A4 activity would be expected to increase the clearance of efavirenz resulting in lower plasma concentrations).
No products indexed under this heading.

Ritonavir (Kaletra may increase tenofovir concentrations. The mechanism of this interaction is unknown. Higher tenofovir concentrations could potentiate tenofovir-associated adverse events. Patients receiving Kaletra with tenofovir DF should be monitored for tenofovir-associated adverse events. ATRIPLA should be discontinued in patients who develop tenofovir-assocatied adverse events. When ritonavir 500 mg every 12 hours was co-administered with efavirenz 600 mg once daily, the combination was associatedwith a higher frequency of adverse clinical experiences (e.g., dizziness, nausea, paresthesia) and lab abnormalities (elevated liver enzymes). Monitoring of liver enzymes is recommended when ATRIPLA is used with ritonavir). Products include:
Kaletra 476
Norvir 503

Rofecoxib (In vitro studies have demonstrated that efavirenz inhibits CYP2C9 in the range of observed efavirenz plasma concentrations. Co-administration of efavirenz with drugs primarily metabolized by CYP2C9 may result in altered plasma concentrations of the co-administered drug. Therefore, appropriate dose adjustments may be necessary for these drugs).
No products indexed under this heading.

Rosiglitazone Maleate (In vitro studies have demonstrated that efavirenz inhibits CYP2C9 in the range of observed efavirenz plasma concentrations. Co-administration of efavirenz with drugs primarily metabolized by CYP2C9 may result in altered plasma concentrations of the co-administered drug. Therefore, appropriate dose adjustments may be necessary for these drugs).
Products include:
Avandamet Tablets 1373
Avandaryl Tablets 1379
Avandia Tablets 1384

Saquinavir (Due to a decrease in its concentration, saquinavir should not be used as sole protease inhibitor in combination with ATRIPLA).
No products indexed under this heading.

Saquinavir Mesylate (Due to a decrease in its concentration, saquinavir should not be used as sole protease inhibitor in combination with ATTRIPLA). Products include:

Sertraline Hydrochloride (Increases in sertraline dose should be guided by clinical response). Products include:

Sildenafil Citrate (Efavirenz has been shown in vivo to induce CYP3A4. Other compounds that are substrates of CYP3A4 may have decreased plasma concentrations when co-administered with efavirenz). Products include:

Simvastatin (Plasma concentrations of atorvastatin, pravastatin, and simvastatin decreased with efavirenz. Consult the complete prescribing information for the HMGCoA reductase inhibitor for guidance on individualizing the dose). Products include:

Sirolimus (Efavirenz has been shown in vivo to induce CYP3A4. Other compounds that are substrates of CYP3A4 may have decreased plasma concentrations when co-administered with efavirenz). Products include:

Sulfamethoxazole (In vitro studies have demonstrated that efavirenz inhibits CYP2C9 in the range of observed efavirenz plasma concentrations. Co-administration of efavirenz with drugs primarily metabolized by CYP2C9 may result in altered plasma concentrations of the co-administered drug. Therefore, appropriate dose adjustments may be necessary for these drugs).

No products indexed under this heading.

Sulfinpyrazone (Drugs which induce CYP3A4 activity would be expected to increase the clearance of efavirenz resulting in lower plasma concentrations).

No products indexed under this heading.

Sulindac (In vitro studies have demonstrated that efavirenz inhibits CYP2C9 in the range of observed efavirenz plasma concentrations. Co-administration of efavirenz with drugs primarily metabolized by CYP2C9 may result in altered plasma concentrations of the co-administered drug. Therefore, appropriate dose adjustments may be necessary for these drugs). Products include:

Suprofen (In vitro studies have demonstrated that efavirenz inhibits CYP2C9 in the range of observed efavirenz plasma concentrations. Co-administration of efavirenz with drugs primarily metabolized by CYP2C9 may result in altered plasma concentrations of the co-administered drug. Therefore, appropriate dose adjustments may be necessary for these drugs).

No products indexed under this heading.

Tacrolimus (Efavirenz has been shown in vivo to induce CYP3A4. Other compounds that are substrates of CYP3A4 may have decreased plasma concentrations when co-administered with efavirenz). Products include:

Tamoxifen Citrate (Efavirenz has been shown in vivo to induce CYP3A4. Other compounds that are substrates of CYP3A4 may have decreased plasma concentrations when co-administered with efavirenz). Products include:

Telmisartan (In vitro studies have demonstrated that efavirenz inhibits CYP2C9 in the range of observed efavirenz plasma concentrations. Co-administration of efavirenz with drugs primarily metabolized by CYP2C9 may result in altered plasma concentrations of the co-administered drug. Therefore, appropriate dose adjustments may be necessary for these drugs). Products include:

Teniposide (In vitro studies have demonstrated that efavirenz inhibits CYP2C19 in the range of observed efavirenz plasma concetrations. Co-administration of efavirenz with drugs primarily metabolized by CYP2C19 may result in altered plasma concentrations of the co-administered drug. Therefore, appropriate dose adjustments may be necesssary for these drugs).

No products indexed under this heading.

Theophylline (Drugs which induce CYP3A4 activity would be expected to increase the clearance of efavirenz resulting in lower plasma concentrations).

No products indexed under this heading.

Thioridazine (In vitro studies have demonstrated that efavirenz inhibits CYP2C19 in the range of observed efavirenz plasma concetrations. Co-administration of efavirenz with drugs primarily metabolized by CYP2C19 may result in altered plasma concentrations of the co-administered drug. Therefore, appropriate dose adjustments may be necesssary for these drugs).

No products indexed under this heading.

Thioridazine Hydrochloride (In vitro studies have demonstrated that efavirenz inhibits CYP2C19 in the range of observed efavirenz plasma concentrations. Co-administration of efavirenz with drugs primarily metabolized by CYP2C19 may result in altered plasma concentrations of the co-administered drug. Therefore, appropriate dose adjustments may be necesssary for these drugs). Products include:

Tiagabine Hydrochloride (Efavirenz has been shown in vivo to induce CYP3A4. Other compounds that are substrates of CYP3A4 may have decreased plasma concentrations when co-administered with efavirenz). Products include:

Tolazamide (In vitro studies have demonstrated that efavirenz inhibits CYP2C9 in the range of observed efavirenz plasma concentrations. Co-administration of efavirenz with drugs primarily metabolized by CYP2C9 may result in altered plasma concentrations of the co-administered drug. Therefore, appropriate dose adjustments may be necessary for these drugs).

No products indexed under this heading.

Tolbutamide (In vitro studies have demonstrated that efavirenz inhibits CYP2C9 in the range of observed efavirenz plasma concentrations. Co-administration of efavirenz with drugs primarily metabolized by CYP2C9 may result in altered plasma concentrations of the co-administered drug. Therefore, appropriate dose adjustments may be necessary for these drugs).

No products indexed under this heading.

Tolbutamide Sodium (In vitro studies have demonstrated that efavirenz inhibits CYP2C9 in the range of observed efavirenz plasma concentrations. Co-administration of efavirenz with drugs primarily metabolized by CYP2C9 may result in altered plasma concentrations of the co-administered drug. Therefore, appropriate dose adjustments may be necessary for these drugs).

No products indexed under this heading.

Tolmetin Sodium (In vitro studies have demonstrated that efavirenz inhibits CYP2C9 in the range of observed efavirenz plasma concentrations. Co-administration of efavirenz with drugs primarily metabolized by CYP2C9 may result in altered plasma concentrations of the co-administered drug. Therefore, appropriate dose adjustments may be necessary for these drugs).

No products indexed under this heading.

Tolterodine Tartrate (Efavirenz has been shown in vivo to induce CYP3A4. Other compounds that are substrates of CYP3A4 may have decreased plasma concentrations when co-administered with efavirenz). Products include:

Topiramate (In vitro studies have demonstrated that efavirenz inhibits CYP2C19 in the range of observed efavirenz plasma concetrations. Co-administration of efavirenz with drugs primarily metabolized by CYP2C19 may result in altered plasma concentrations of the co-administered drug. Therefore, appropriate dose adjustments may be necesssary for these drugs). Products include:

Torsemide (In vitro studies have demonstrated that efavirenz inhibits CYP2C9 in the range of observed efavirenz plasma concentrations. Co-administration of efavirenz with drugs primarily metabolized by CYP2C9 may result in altered plasma concentrations of the co-administered drug. Therefore, appropriate dose adjustments may be necessary for these drugs). Products include:

Trazodone Hydrochloride (Efavirenz has been shown in vivo to induce CYP3A4. Other compounds that are substrates of CYP3A4 may have decreased plasma concentrations when co-administered with efavirenz).

No products indexed under this heading.

Triamcinolone (Drugs which induce CYP3A4 activity would be expected to increase the clearance of efavirenz resulting in lower plasma concentrations).

No products indexed under this heading.

Triamcinolone Acetonide (Drugs which induce CYP3A4 activity would be expected to increase the clearance of efavirenz resulting in lower plasma concentrations). Products include:

Triamcinolone Diacetate (Drugs which induce CYP3A4 activity would be expected to increase the clearance of efavirenz resulting in lower plasma concentrations).

No products indexed under this heading.

Triamcinolone Hexacetonide (Drugs which induce CYP3A4 activity would be expected to increase the clearance of efavirenz resulting in lower plasma concentrations).

No products indexed under this heading.

Triazolam (Due to the potential for serious and/or life-threatening reactions, such as prolonged or increased sedation or respiratory depression, concomitant use with triazolam is contraindicated).

No products indexed under this heading.

Trimethadione (In vitro studies have demonstrated that efavirenz inhibits CYP2C19 in the range of observed efavirenz plasma concetrations. Co-administration of efavirenz with drugs primarily metabolized by CYP2C19 may result in altered plasma concentrations of the co-administered drug. Therefore, appropriate dose adjustments may be necesssary for these drugs).

No products indexed under this heading.

Trimipramine Maleate (In vitro studies have demonstrated that efavirenz inhibits CYP2C19 in the range of observed efavirenz plasma concetrations. Co-administration of efavirenz with drugs primarily metabolized by CYP2C19 may result in altered plasma concentrations of the co-administered drug. Therefore, appropriate dose adjustments may be necesssary for these drugs).

No products indexed under this heading.

Troglitazone (Drugs which induce CYP3A4 activity would be expected to increase the clearance of efavirenz resulting in lower plasma concentrations).

No products indexed under this heading.

Valacyclovir Hydrochloride (Since emtricitabine and tenofovir are primarily eliminated by the kidneys, co-administration of ATRIPLA with drugs that reduce renal fuction or compete for active tubular secretion may increase serum concentrations of emtricitabine, tenofovir, and/or other renally eliminated drugs). Products include:

Valtrex Caplets 1597

Valdecoxib (In vitro studies have demonstrated that efavirenz inhibits CYP2C9 in the range of observed efavirenz plasma concentrations. Co-administration of efavirenz with drugs primarily metabolized by CYP2C9 may result in altered plasma concentrations of the co-administered drug. Therefore, appropriate dose adjustments may be necessary for these drugs).

No products indexed under this heading.

Valganciclovir Hydrochloride (Since emtricitabine and tenofovir are primarily eliminated by the kidneys, co-administration of ATRIPLA with drugs that reduce renal fuction or compete for active tubular secretion may increase serum concentrations of emtricitabine, tenofovir, and/or other renally eliminated drugs). Products include:

Valcyte Tablets 2813

Valproate Sodium (In vitro studies have demonstrated that efavirenz inhibits CYP2C19 in the range of observed efavirenz plasma concetrations. Co-administration of efavirenz with drugs primarily metabolized by CYP2C19 may result in altered plasma concentrations of the co-administered drug. Therefore, appropriate dose adjustments may be necesssary for these drugs). Products include:

Depacon Injection 412

Valproic Acid (In vitro studies have demonstrated that efavirenz inhibits CYP2C19 in the range of observed efavirenz plasma concetrations. Co-administration of efavirenz with drugs primarily metabolized by CYP2C19 may result in altered plasma concentrations of the co-administered drug. Therefore, appropriate dose adjustments may be necesssary for these drugs). Products include:

Depakene 417

Valsartan (In vitro studies have demonstrated that efavirenz inhibits CYP2C9 in the range of observed efavirenz plasma concentrations. Co-administration of efavirenz with drugs primarily metabolized by CYP2C9 may result in altered plasma concentrations of the co-administered drug. Therefore, appropriate dose adjustments may be necessary for these drugs). Products include:

Diovan Tablets 2193
Diovan HCT Tablets 2196

Verapamil Hydrochloride (Efavirenz has been shown in vivo to induce CYP3A4. Other compounds that are substrates of CYP3A4 may have decreased plasma concentrations when co-administered with efavirenz). Products include:

Covera-HS Tablets 3139
Tarka Tablets 524
Verelan PM Extended-Release Capsules, Controlled-Onset 3106

Vinblastine Sulfate (Efavirenz has been shown in vivo to induce CYP3A4. Other compounds that are substrates of CYP3A4 may have decreased plasma concentrations when co-administered with efavirenz).

No products indexed under this heading.

Vincristine Sulfate (Efavirenz has been shown in vivo to induce CYP3A4. Other compounds that are substrates of CYP3A4 may have decreased plasma concentrations when co-administered with efavirenz).

No products indexed under this heading.

Voriconazole (Efavirenz significantly decreases voriconazole plasma concentrations, and co-administration may decrease the therapeutic effectiveness of voriconazole. Also, voriconazole significantly increases efavirenz plasma concentrations, which may increase the risk of efavirenz-associated side effects. Concomitant use is contraindicated). Products include:

VFEND I.V. 2564
VFEND Oral Suspension 2564
VFEND Tablets 2564

Warfarin Sodium (Plasma concentrations and effects to warfarin sodium potentially increased or decreased by efavirenz). Products include:

Coumadin for Injection 898
Coumadin Tablets 898

Zafirlukast (In vitro studies have demonstrated that efavirenz inhibits CYP2C9 in the range of observed efavirenz plasma concentrations. Co-administration of efavirenz with drugs primarily metabolized by CYP2C9 may result in altered plasma concentrations of the co-administered drug. Therefore, appropriate dose adjustments may be necessary for these drugs). Products include:

Accolate Tablets 671

Zileuton (In vitro studies have demonstrated that efavirenz inhibits CYP2C9 in the range of observed efavirenz plasma concentrations. Co-administration of efavirenz with drugs primarily metabolized by CYP2C9 may result in altered plasma concentrations of the co-administered drug. Therefore, appropriate dose adjustments may be necessary for these drugs). Products include:

Zyflo Tablets 1023

Zonisamide (In vitro studies have demonstrated that efavirenz inhibits CYP2C19 in the range of observed efavirenz plasma concetrations. Co-administration of efavirenz with drugs primarily metabolized by CYP2C19 may result in altered plasma concentrations of the co-administered drug. Therefore, appropriate dose adjustments may be necesssary for these drugs). Products include:

Zonegran Capsules 1101

ATROVENT INHALATION SOLUTION

(Ipratropium Bromide) 835
None cited in PDR database.

ATROVENT HFA INHALATION AEROSOL

(Ipratropium Bromide) 841
May interact with anticholinergics. Compounds in these categories include:

Atropine Sulfate (Although ipratropium bromide is minimally absorbed into the systemic circulation, there is some potential for an additive interaction with concomitantly used anticholinergic medications. Caution is therefore advised in the co-administration of ipratropium bromide HFA Inhalation Aerosol with other anticholinergic-containing drugs). Products include:

Donnatal Extentabs 2493

Belladonna Alkaloids (Although ipratropium bromide is minimally absorbed into the systemic circulation, there is some potential for an additive interaction with concomitantly used anticholinergic medications. Caution is therefore advised in the co-administration of ipratropium bromide HFA Inhalation Aerosol with other anticholinergic-containing drugs). Products include:

Hyland's Teething Tablets 830

Benztropine Mesylate (Although ipratropium bromide is minimally absorbed into the systemic circulation, there is some potential for an additive interaction with concomitantly used anticholinergic medications. Caution is therefore advised in the co-administration of ipratropium bromide HFA Inhalation Aerosol with other anticholinergic-containing drugs).

No products indexed under this heading.

Biperiden Hydrochloride (Although ipratropium bromide is minimally absorbed into the systemic circulation, there is some potential for an additive interaction with concomitantly used anticholinergic medications. Caution is therefore advised in the co-administration of ipratropium bromide HFA Inhalation Aerosol with other anticholinergic-containing drugs).

No products indexed under this heading.

Clidinium Bromide (Although ipratropium bromide is minimally absorbed into the systemic circulation, there is some potential for an additive interaction with concomitantly used anticholinergic medications. Caution is therefore advised in the co-administration of ipratropium bromide HFA Inhalation Aerosol with other anticholinergic-containing drugs).

No products indexed under this heading.

Dicyclomine Hydrochloride (Although ipratropium bromide is minimally absorbed into the systemic circulation, there is some potential for an additive interaction with concomitantly used anticholinergic medications. Caution is therefore advised in the co-administration of ipratropium bromide HFA Inhalation Aerosol with other anticholinergic-containing drugs). Products include:

Bentyl Capsules 697
Bentyl Injection 697
Bentyl Syrup 697
Bentyl Tablets 697

Glycopyrrolate (Although ipratropium bromide is minimally absorbed into the systemic circulation, there is some potential for an additive interaction with concomitantly used anticholinergic medications. Caution is therefore advised in the co-administration of ipratropium bromide HFA Inhalation Aerosol with other anticholinergic-containing drugs).

No products indexed under this heading.

Hyoscyamine (Although ipratropium bromide is minimally absorbed into the systemic circulation, there is some potential for an additive interaction with concomitantly used anticholinergic medications. Caution is therefore advised in the co-administration of ipratropium bromide HFA Inhalation Aerosol with other anticholinergic-containing drugs).

No products indexed under this heading.

Hyoscyamine Sulfate (Although ipratropium bromide is minimally absorbed into the systemic circulation, there is some potential for an additive interaction with concomitantly used anticholinergic medications. Caution is therefore advised in the co-administration of ipratropium bromide HFA Inhalation Aerosol with other anticholinergic-containing drugs). Products include:

Donnatal Extentabs 2493
Prosed/DS Tablets 1157

Mepenzolate Bromide (Although ipratropium bromide is minimally absorbed into the systemic circulation, there is some potential for an additive interaction with concomitantly used anticholinergic medications. Caution is therefore advised in the co-administration of ipratropium bromide HFA Inhalation Aerosol with other anticholinergic-containing drugs).

No products indexed under this heading.

Oxybutynin Chloride (Although ipratropium bromide is minimally absorbed into the systemic circulation, there is some potential for an additive interaction with concomitantly used anticholinergic medications. Caution is therefore advised in the co-administration of ipratropium bromide HFA Inhalation Aerosol with other anticholinergic-containing drugs). Products include:

Ditropan XL Extended-Release Tablets 2413

Procyclidine Hydrochloride (Although ipratropium bromide is minimally absorbed into the systemic circulation, there is some potential for an additive interaction with concomitantly used anticholinergic medications. Caution is therefore advised in the co-administration of ipratropium bromide HFA Inhalation Aerosol with other anticholinergic-containing drugs).

No products indexed under this heading.

Propantheline Bromide (Although ipratropium bromide is minimally absorbed into the systemic circulation, there is some potential for an additive interaction with concomitantly used anticholinergic medications. Caution is therefore advised in the co-administration of ipratropium bromide HFA Inhalation Aerosol with other anticholinergic-containing drugs).

No products indexed under this heading.

Scopolamine (Although ipratropium bromide is minimally absorbed into the systemic circulation, there is some potential for an additive interaction with concomitantly used anticholinergic medications. Caution is therefore advised in the co-administration of ipratropium bro-

mide HFA Inhalation Aerosol with other anticholinergic-containing drugs). Products include:
- Transderm Scōp Transdermal Therapeutic System 2177

Scopolamine Hydrobromide (Although ipratropium bromide is minimally absorbed into the systemic circulation, there is some potential for an additive interaction with concomitantly used anticholinergic medications. Caution is therefore advised in the co-administration of ipratropium bromide HFA Inhalation Aerosol with other anticholinergic-containing drugs). Products include:
- Donnatal Extentabs 2493

Tolterodine Tartrate (Although ipratropium bromide is minimally absorbed into the systemic circulation, there is some potential for an additive interaction with concomitantly used anticholinergic medications. Caution is therefore advised in the co-administration of ipratropium bromide HFA Inhalation Aerosol with other anticholinergic-containing drugs). Products include:
- Detrol Tablets 2628
- Detrol LA Capsules 2631

Tridihexethyl Chloride (Although ipratropium bromide is minimally absorbed into the systemic circulation, there is some potential for an additive interaction with concomitantly used anticholinergic medications. Caution is therefore advised in the co-administration of ipratropium bromide HFA Inhalation Aerosol with other anticholinergic-containing drugs).
No products indexed under this heading.

Trihexyphenidyl Hydrochloride (Although ipratropium bromide is minimally absorbed into the systemic circulation, there is some potential for an additive interaction with concomitantly used anticholinergic medications. Caution is therefore advised in the co-administration of ipratropium bromide HFA Inhalation Aerosol with other anticholinergic-containing drugs).
No products indexed under this heading.

ATROVENT NASAL SPRAY 0.03%

(Ipratropium Bromide) 837
May interact with anticholinergics. Compounds in these categories include:

Atropine Sulfate (Some potential for an additive interaction with other concomitantly administered anticholinergic drugs). Products include:
- Donnatal Extentabs 2493

Belladonna Alkaloids (Some potential for an additive interaction with other concomitantly administered anticholinergic drugs). Products include:
- Hyland's Teething Tablets .... ▣ 830

Benztropine Mesylate (Some potential for an additive interaction with other concomitantly administered anticholinergic drugs).
No products indexed under this heading.

Biperiden Hydrochloride (Some potential for an additive interaction with other concomitantly administered anticholinergic drugs).
No products indexed under this heading.

Clidinium Bromide (Some potential for an additive interaction with other concomitantly administered anticholinergic drugs).
No products indexed under this heading.

Dicyclomine Hydrochloride (Some potential for an additive interaction with other concomitantly administered anticholinergic drugs). Products include:
- Bentyl Capsules 697
- Bentyl Injection 697
- Bentyl Syrup 697
- Bentyl Tablets 697

Glycopyrrolate (Some potential for an additive interaction with other concomitantly administered anticholinergic drugs).
No products indexed under this heading.

Hyoscyamine (Some potential for an additive interaction with other concomitantly administered anticholinergic drugs).
No products indexed under this heading.

Hyoscyamine Sulfate (Some potential for an additive interaction with other concomitantly administered anticholinergic drugs). Products include:
- Donnatal Extentabs 2493
- Prosed/DS Tablets 1157

Mepenzolate Bromide (Some potential for an additive interaction with other concomitantly administered anticholinergic drugs).
No products indexed under this heading.

Oxybutynin Chloride (Some potential for an additive interaction with other concomitantly administered anticholinergic drugs). Products include:
- Ditropan XL Extended-Release Tablets 2413

Procyclidine Hydrochloride (Some potential for an additive interaction with other concomitantly administered anticholinergic drugs).
No products indexed under this heading.

Propantheline Bromide (Some potential for an additive interaction with other concomitantly administered anticholinergic drugs).
No products indexed under this heading.

Scopolamine (Some potential for an additive interaction with other concomitantly administered anticholinergic drugs). Products include:
- Transderm Scōp Transdermal Therapeutic System 2177

Scopolamine Hydrobromide (Some potential for an additive interaction with other concomitantly administered anticholinergic drugs). Products include:
- Donnatal Extentabs 2493

Tolterodine Tartrate (Some potential for an additive interaction with other concomitantly administered anticholinergic drugs). Products include:
- Detrol Tablets 2628
- Detrol LA Capsules 2631

Tridihexethyl Chloride (Some potential for an additive interaction with other concomitantly administered anticholinergic drugs).
No products indexed under this heading.

Trihexyphenidyl Hydrochloride (Some potential for an additive interaction with other concomitantly administered anticholinergic drugs).
No products indexed under this heading.

ATROVENT NASAL SPRAY 0.06%

(Ipratropium Bromide) 839
May interact with anticholinergics. Compounds in these categories include:

Atropine Sulfate (Some potential for an additive interaction with other concomitantly administered anticholinergic drugs). Products include:
- Donnatal Extentabs 2493

Belladonna Alkaloids (Some potential for an additive interaction with other concomitantly administered anticholinergic drugs). Products include:
- Hyland's Teething Tablets .... ▣ 830

Benztropine Mesylate (Some potential for an additive interaction with other concomitantly administered anticholinergic drugs).
No products indexed under this heading.

Biperiden Hydrochloride (Some potential for an additive interaction with other concomitantly administered anticholinergic drugs).
No products indexed under this heading.

Clidinium Bromide (Some potential for an additive interaction with other concomitantly administered anticholinergic drugs).
No products indexed under this heading.

Dicyclomine Hydrochloride (Some potential for an additive interaction with other concomitantly administered anticholinergic drugs). Products include:
- Bentyl Capsules 697
- Bentyl Injection 697
- Bentyl Syrup 697
- Bentyl Tablets 697

Glycopyrrolate (Some potential for an additive interaction with other concomitantly administered anticholinergic drugs).
No products indexed under this heading.

Hyoscyamine (Some potential for an additive interaction with other concomitantly administered anticholinergic drugs).
No products indexed under this heading.

Hyoscyamine Sulfate (Some potential for an additive interaction with other concomitantly administered anticholinergic drugs). Products include:
- Donnatal Extentabs 2493
- Prosed/DS Tablets 1157

Mepenzolate Bromide (Some potential for an additive interaction with other concomitantly administered anticholinergic drugs).
No products indexed under this heading.

Oxybutynin Chloride (Some potential for an additive interaction with other concomitantly administered anticholinergic drugs). Products include:
- Ditropan XL Extended-Release Tablets 2413

Procyclidine Hydrochloride (Some potential for an additive interaction with other concomitantly administered anticholinergic drugs).
No products indexed under this heading.

Propantheline Bromide (Some potential for an additive interaction with other concomitantly administered anticholinergic drugs).
No products indexed under this heading.

Scopolamine (Some potential for an additive interaction with other concomitantly administered anticholinergic drugs). Products include:
- Transderm Scōp Transdermal Therapeutic System 2177

Scopolamine Hydrobromide (Some potential for an additive interaction with other concomitantly administered anticholinergic drugs). Products include:
- Donnatal Extentabs 2493

Tolterodine Tartrate (Some potential for an additive interaction with other concomitantly administered anticholinergic drugs). Products include:
- Detrol Tablets 2628
- Detrol LA Capsules 2631

Tridihexethyl Chloride (Some potential for an additive interaction with other concomitantly administered anticholinergic drugs).
No products indexed under this heading.

Trihexyphenidyl Hydrochloride (Some potential for an additive interaction with other concomitantly administered anticholinergic drugs).
No products indexed under this heading.

ATTENUVAX

(Measles Virus Vaccine Live) 1914
May interact with immunosuppressive agents. Compounds in these categories include:

Azathioprine (Concurrent use in individuals on immunosuppressive therapy is contraindicated).
No products indexed under this heading.

Basiliximab (Concurrent use in individuals on immunosuppressive therapy is contraindicated). Products include:
- Simulect for Injection 2284

Cyclosporine (Concurrent use in individuals on immunosuppressive therapy is contraindicated). Products include:
- Gengraf Capsules 459
- Neoral Oral Solution 2259
- Neoral Soft Gelatin Capsules 2259
- Restasis Ophthalmic Emulsion 575
- Sandimmune 2275

Muromonab-CD3 (Concurrent use in individuals on immunosuppressive therapy is contraindicated). Products include:
- Orthoclone OKT3 Sterile Solution 2360

Mycophenolate Mofetil (Concurrent use in individuals on immunosuppressive therapy is contraindicated). Products include:
- CellCept Capsules 2747
- CellCept Oral Suspension 2747
- CellCept Tablets 2747

Sirolimus (Concurrent use in individuals on immunosuppressive therapy is contraindicated). Products include:
- Rapamune Oral Solution and Tablets 3475

Tacrolimus (Concurrent use in individuals on immunosuppressive therapy is contraindicated). Products include:
Prograf Capsules and Injection 632
Protopic Ointment 638

AUGMENTIN CHEWABLE TABLETS
(Amoxicillin, Clavulanate Potassium)....................................... 1360
See Augmentin ES-600 Powder for Oral Suspension

AUGMENTIN POWDER FOR ORAL SUSPENSION
(Amoxicillin, Clavulanate Potassium)....................................... 1360
See Augmentin ES-600 Powder for Oral Suspension

AUGMENTIN TABLETS
(Amoxicillin, Clavulanate Potassium)....................................... 1363
See Augmentin ES-600 Powder for Oral Suspension

AUGMENTIN XR EXTENDED-RELEASE TABLETS
(Amoxicillin, Clavulanate Potassium)....................................... 1369
See Augmentin ES-600 Powder for Oral Suspension

AUGMENTIN ES-600 POWDER FOR ORAL SUSPENSION
(Amoxicillin, Clavulanate Potassium)....................................... 1366
May interact with anticoagulants, oral contraceptives, and certain other agents. Compounds in these categories include:

Allopurinol (Co-administration of ampicillin with allopurinol substantially increases the incidence of rashes; there are no data with Augmentin and allopurinol administered concurrently).
No products indexed under this heading.

Anisindione (There have been reports of increased prothrombin time in patients receiving Augmentin and anticoagulant therapy concomitantly). Products include:
Miradon Tablets 3042

Ardeparin Sodium (There have been reports of increased prothrombin time in patients receiving Augmentin and anticoagulant therapy concomitantly).
No products indexed under this heading.

Dalteparin Sodium (There have been reports of increased prothrombin time in patients receiving Augmentin and anticoagulant therapy concomitantly). Products include:
Fragmin Injection 1097

Danaparoid Sodium (There have been reports of increased prothrombin time in patients receiving Augmentin and anticoagulant therapy concomitantly).
No products indexed under this heading.

Desogestrel (Potential for reduced efficacy of oral contraceptives). Products include:
Mircette Tablets 1066

Dicumarol (There have been reports of increased prothrombin time in patients receiving Augmentin and anticoagulant therapy concomitantly).
No products indexed under this heading.

Enoxaparin Sodium (There have been reports of increased prothrombin time in patients receiving Augmentin and anticoagulant therapy concomitantly). Products include:
Lovenox Injection 2915

Ethinyl Estradiol (Potential for reduced efficacy of oral contraceptives). Products include:
Mircette Tablets 1066
NuvaRing 2340
Ortho-Cyclen/Ortho Tri-Cyclen 2429
Ortho Evra Transdermal System 2417
Ortho Tri-Cyclen Lo Tablets 2436
Seasonique Tablets 1077
Yasmin 28 Tablets 796
Yaz Tablets 803

Ethynodiol Diacetate (Potential for reduced efficacy of oral contraceptives).
No products indexed under this heading.

Fondaparinux Sodium (There have been reports of increased prothrombin time in patients receiving Augmentin and anticoagulant therapy concomitantly). Products include:
Arixtra Injection 1351

Heparin Calcium (There have been reports of increased prothrombin time in patients receiving Augmentin and anticoagulant therapy concomitantly).
No products indexed under this heading.

Heparin Sodium (There have been reports of increased prothrombin time in patients receiving Augmentin and anticoagulant therapy concomitantly).
No products indexed under this heading.

Levonorgestrel (Potential for reduced efficacy of oral contraceptives). Products include:
Climara Pro Transdermal System 776
Mirena Intrauterine System 787
Plan B Tablets 1076
Seasonique Tablets 1077

Low Molecular Weight Heparins (There have been reports of increased prothrombin time in patients receiving Augmentin and anticoagulant therapy concomitantly).
No products indexed under this heading.

Mestranol (Potential for reduced efficacy of oral contraceptives).
No products indexed under this heading.

Norethindrone (Potential for reduced efficacy of oral contraceptives). Products include:
Ortho Micronor Tablets 2426

Norethynodrel (Potential for reduced efficacy of oral contraceptives).
No products indexed under this heading.

Norgestimate (Potential for reduced efficacy of oral contraceptives). Products include:
Ortho-Cyclen/Ortho Tri-Cyclen 2429
Ortho Tri-Cyclen Lo Tablets 2436

Norgestrel (Potential for reduced efficacy of oral contraceptives).
No products indexed under this heading.

Probenecid (Decreases the renal tubular secretion of amoxicillin; concurrent use may result in increased and prolonged blood levels of amoxicillin; therefore, concomitant use is not recommended).
No products indexed under this heading.

Tinzaparin Sodium (There have been reports of increased prothrombin time in patients receiving Augmentin and anticoagulant therapy concomitantly).
No products indexed under this heading.

Warfarin Sodium (There have been reports of increased prothrombin time in patients receiving Augmentin and anticoagulant therapy concomitantly). Products include:
Coumadin for Injection 898
Coumadin Tablets 898

AUTHIA CREAM
(Thiamine Disulfide, Vitamin B_{12}) 3404
None cited in PDR database.

AVALIDE TABLETS
(Hydrochlorothiazide, Irbesartan) 888
May interact with antihypertensives, barbiturates, corticosteroids, cardiac glycosides, oral hypoglycemic agents, insulin, lithium preparations, narcotic analgesics, nondepolarizing neuromuscular blocking agents, nonsteroidal anti-inflammatory agents, and certain other agents. Compounds in these categories include:

Acarbose (Hydrochlorothiazide may cause hyperglycemia, therefore, dosage adjustment of oral hypoglycemic agent may be required). Products include:
Precose Tablets 751

Acebutolol Hydrochloride (Hydrochlorothiazide may add to or potentiate the therapeutic effect of other antihypertensive drugs).
No products indexed under this heading.

ACTH (Co-administration with ACTH intensifies electrolyte depletion particularly hypokalemia).
No products indexed under this heading.

Alfentanil Hydrochloride (Potentiation of orthostatic hypotension).
No products indexed under this heading.

Amlodipine Besylate (Hydrochlorothiazide may add to or potentiate the therapeutic effect of other antihypertensive drugs). Products include:
Caduet Tablets 2508
Lotrel Capsules 2249
Norvasc Tablets 2545

Aprobarbital (Potentiation of orthostatic hypotension).
No products indexed under this heading.

Atenolol (Hydrochlorothiazide may add to or potentiate the therapeutic effect of other antihypertensive drugs).
No products indexed under this heading.

Atracurium Besylate (Possible increased responsiveness to the muscle relaxants).
No products indexed under this heading.

Benazepril Hydrochloride (Hydrochlorothiazide may add to or potentiate the therapeutic effect of other antihypertensive drugs). Products include:
Lotensin Tablets 2243
Lotensin HCT Tablets 2246
Lotrel Capsules 2249

Bendroflumethiazide (Hydrochlorothiazide may add to or potentiate the therapeutic effect of other antihypertensive drugs).
No products indexed under this heading.

Betamethasone Acetate (Co-administration with corticosteroids intensifies electrolyte depletion particularly hypokalemia).
No products indexed under this heading.

Betamethasone Sodium Phosphate (Co-administration with corticosteroids intensifies electrolyte depletion particularly hypokalemia).
No products indexed under this heading.

Betaxolol Hydrochloride (Hydrochlorothiazide may add to or potentiate the therapeutic effect of other antihypertensive drugs). Products include:
Betoptic S Ophthalmic Suspension.................................... 558

Bisoprolol Fumarate (Hydrochlorothiazide may add to or potentiate the therapeutic effect of other antihypertensive drugs).
No products indexed under this heading.

Buprenorphine Hydrochloride (Potentiation of orthostatic hypotension). Products include:
Buprenex Injectable 2716
Suboxone Tablets 2717
Subutex Tablets 2717

Butabarbital (Potentiation of orthostatic hypotension).
No products indexed under this heading.

Butalbital (Potentiation of orthostatic hypotension).
No products indexed under this heading.

Candesartan Cilexetil (Hydrochlorothiazide may add to or potentiate the therapeutic effect of other antihypertensive drugs). Products include:
Atacand Tablets 649
Atacand HCT 651

Captopril (Hydrochlorothiazide may add to or potentiate the therapeutic effect of other antihypertensive drugs). Products include:
Captopril Tablets 2149

Carteolol Hydrochloride (Hydrochlorothiazide may add to or potentiate the therapeutic effect of other antihypertensive drugs). Products include:
Carteolol Hydrochloride Ophthalmic Solution USP, 1%....... ⊙249

Celecoxib (Co-administration with non-steroidal anti-inflammatory agents may reduce the natriuretic and antihypertensive effects of thiazides). Products include:
Celebrex Capsules 3134

Chlorothiazide (Hydrochlorothiazide may add to or potentiate the therapeutic effect of other antihypertensive drugs). Products include:
Diuril Oral Suspension 1954

Chlorothiazide Sodium (Hydrochlorothiazide may add to or potentiate the therapeutic effect of other antihypertensive drugs). Products include:
Diuril Sodium Intravenous 2467

Chlorpropamide (Hydrochlorothiazide may cause hyperglycemia, therefore, dosage adjustment of oral hypoglycemic agent may be required).
No products indexed under this heading.

Chlorthalidone (Hydrochlorothiazide may add to or potentiate the therapeutic effect of other antihypertensive drugs). Products include:
Clorpres Tablets 2153

Cholestyramine (Absorption of hydrochlorothiazide is impaired in the presence of anionic exchange resins; single dose of cholestyramine binds the hydrochlorothiazide and reduces its absorption from GI tract by 85%).
No products indexed under this heading.

Cisatracurium Besylate (Possible increased responsiveness to the muscle relaxants). Products include:
Nimbex Injection 498

Clonidine (Hydrochlorothiazide may add to or potentiate the therapeutic effect of other antihypertensive drugs). Products include:
Catapres-TTS 844

Clonidine Hydrochloride (Hydrochlorothiazide may add to or potentiate the therapeutic effect of other antihypertensive drugs). Products include:
Catapres Tablets 843
Clorpres Tablets 2153

Codeine Phosphate (Potentiation of orthostatic hypotension). Products include:
Tylenol with Codeine Tablets 2391

Colestipol Hydrochloride (Absorption of hydrochlorothiazide is impaired in the presence of anionic exchange resins; single dose of colestipol binds the hydrochlorothiazide and reduces its absorption from GI tract by 43%).
No products indexed under this heading.

Cortisone Acetate (Co-administration with corticosteroids intensifies electrolyte depletion particularly hypokalemia).
No products indexed under this heading.

Deserpidine (Hydrochlorothiazide may add to or potentiate the therapeutic effect of other antihypertensive drugs).
No products indexed under this heading.

Deslanoside (Concurrent digitalis therapy may exaggerate metabolic effects of hypokalemia, especially myocardial effects, e.g., increased ventricular irritability).
No products indexed under this heading.

Dexamethasone (Co-administration with corticosteroids intensifies electrolyte depletion particularly hypokalemia). Products include:
Ciprodex Otic Suspension 559
Decadron Tablets 1951
TobraDex Ophthalmic Ointment 562
TobraDex Ophthalmic Suspension 563

Dexamethasone Acetate (Co-administration with corticosteroids intensifies electrolyte depletion particularly hypokalemia).
No products indexed under this heading.

Dexamethasone Sodium Phosphate (Co-administration with corticosteroids intensifies electrolyte depletion particularly hypokalemia).
No products indexed under this heading.

Dezocine (Potentiation of orthostatic hypotension).
No products indexed under this heading.

Diazoxide (Hydrochlorothiazide may add to or potentiate the therapeutic effect of other antihypertensive drugs). Products include:
Hyperstat I.V. 3017

Diclofenac Potassium (Co-administration with non-steroidal anti-inflammatory agents may reduce the natriuretic and antihypertensive effects of thiazides).
No products indexed under this heading.

Diclofenac Sodium (Co-administration with non-steroidal anti-inflammatory agents may reduce the natriuretic and antihypertensive effects of thiazides). Products include:
Arthrotec Tablets 3129
Voltaren Ophthalmic Solution 2309
Voltaren Tablets 2307
Voltaren-XR Tablets 2310

Digitalis Glycoside Preparations (Concurrent digitalis therapy may exaggerate metabolic effects of hypokalemia, especially myocardial effects, e.g., increased ventricular irritability).
No products indexed under this heading.

Digitoxin (Concurrent digitalis therapy may exaggerate metabolic effects of hypokalemia, especially myocardial effects, e.g., increased ventricular irritability).
No products indexed under this heading.

Digoxin (Concurrent digitalis therapy may exaggerate metabolic effects of hypokalemia, especially myocardial effects, e.g., increased ventricular irritability). Products include:
Lanoxicaps Capsules 1490
Lanoxin Injection 1494
Lanoxin Injection Pediatric 1497
Lanoxin Tablets 1500

Diltiazem Hydrochloride (Hydrochlorothiazide may add to or potentiate the therapeutic effect of other antihypertensive drugs). Products include:
Cardizem LA Extended Release Tablets 1728
Tiazac Capsules 1201

Doxazosin Mesylate (Hydrochlorothiazide may add to or potentiate the therapeutic effect of other antihypertensive drugs). Products include:
Cardura XL Tablets 2515

Enalapril Maleate (Hydrochlorothiazide may add to or potentiate the therapeutic effect of other antihypertensive drugs). Products include:
Vasotec I.V. Injection 2103

Enalaprilat (Hydrochlorothiazide may add to or potentiate the therapeutic effect of other antihypertensive drugs).
No products indexed under this heading.

Eprosartan Mesylate (Hydrochlorothiazide may add to or potentiate the therapeutic effect of other antihypertensive drugs). Products include:
Teveten Tablets 1735
Teveten HCT Tablets 1737

Esmolol Hydrochloride (Hydrochlorothiazide may add to or potentiate the therapeutic effect of other antihypertensive drugs).
No products indexed under this heading.

Etodolac (Co-administration with non-steroidal anti-inflammatory agents may reduce the natriuretic and antihypertensive effects of thiazides).
No products indexed under this heading.

Felodipine (Hydrochlorothiazide may add to or potentiate the therapeutic effect of other antihypertensive drugs).
No products indexed under this heading.

Fenoprofen Calcium (Co-administration with non-steroidal anti-inflammatory agents may reduce the natriuretic and antihypertensive effects of thiazides). Products include:
Nalfon Capsules 2502

Fentanyl (Potentiation of orthostatic hypotension). Products include:
Duragesic Transdermal System 2373
Ionsys Transdermal System 2379

Fentanyl Citrate (Potentiation of orthostatic hypotension). Products include:
Actiq 979

Fludrocortisone Acetate (Co-administration with corticosteroids intensifies electrolyte depletion particularly hypokalemia).
No products indexed under this heading.

Flurbiprofen (Co-administration with non-steroidal anti-inflammatory agents may reduce the natriuretic and antihypertensive effects of thiazides).
No products indexed under this heading.

Fosinopril Sodium (Hydrochlorothiazide may add to or potentiate the therapeutic effect of other antihypertensive drugs).
No products indexed under this heading.

Furosemide (Hydrochlorothiazide may add to or potentiate the therapeutic effect of other antihypertensive drugs). Products include:
Furosemide Tablets 2154

Glimepiride (Hydrochlorothiazide may cause hyperglycemia, therefore, dosage adjustment of oral hypoglycemic agent may be required). Products include:
Avandaryl Tablets 1379
Duetact Tablets 3226

Glipizide (Hydrochlorothiazide may cause hyperglycemia, therefore, dosage adjustment of oral hypoglycemic agent may be required).
No products indexed under this heading.

Glyburide (Hydrochlorothiazide may cause hyperglycemia, therefore, dosage adjustment of oral hypoglycemic agent may be required).
No products indexed under this heading.

Guanabenz Acetate (Hydrochlorothiazide may add to or potentiate the therapeutic effect of other antihypertensive drugs).
No products indexed under this heading.

Guanethidine Monosulfate (Hydrochlorothiazide may add to or potentiate the therapeutic effect of other antihypertensive drugs).
No products indexed under this heading.

Hydralazine Hydrochloride (Hydrochlorothiazide may add to or potentiate the therapeutic effect of other antihypertensive drugs). Products include:
BiDil Tablets 2171

Hydrocodone Bitartrate (Potentiation of orthostatic hypotension). Products include:
Hycodan 1116
Hycotuss Expectorant Syrup 1117
Vicodin Tablets 535
Vicodin ES Tablets 536
Vicodin HP Tablets 538
Vicoprofen Tablets 539
Zydone Tablets 1139

Hydrocodone Polistirex (Potentiation of orthostatic hypotension). Products include:
Tussionex Pennkinetic Extended-Release Suspension 3327

Hydrocortisone (Co-administration with corticosteroids intensifies electrolyte depletion particularly hypokalemia). Products include:
Colocort Rectal Suspension, USP (Retention) 100 mg/60 mL 2476
Hydrocortone Tablets 1989
Preparation H Hydrocortisone Cream .... ▣646

Hydrocortisone Acetate (Co-administration with corticosteroids intensifies electrolyte depletion particularly hypokalemia). Products include:
Analpram-HC 1159
Pramosone 1161
ProctoFoam-HC 3099

Hydrocortisone Sodium Phosphate (Co-administration with corticosteroids intensifies electrolyte depletion particularly hypokalemia).
No products indexed under this heading.

Hydrocortisone Sodium Succinate (Co-administration with corticosteroids intensifies electrolyte depletion particularly hypokalemia).
No products indexed under this heading.

Hydroflumethiazide (Hydrochlorothiazide may add to or potentiate the therapeutic effect of other antihypertensive drugs).
No products indexed under this heading.

Hydromorphone Hydrochloride (Potentiation of orthostatic hypotension). Products include:
Dilaudid 440
Dilaudid Non-Sterile Powder 440
Dilaudid Oral Liquid 445
Dilaudid Rectal Suppositories 440
Dilaudid Tablets 440
Dilaudid Tablets - 8 mg 445
Dilaudid-HP 442

Ibuprofen (Co-administration with non-steroidal anti-inflammatory agents may reduce the natriuretic and antihypertensive effects of thiazides). Products include:
Advil Allergy Sinus Caplets .... ▣770
Advil .... ▣674
Children's Advil Oral Suspension .... ▣603
Children's Advil Chewable Tablets .... ▣603
Advil Cold & Sinus .... ▣723
Infants' Advil Concentrated Drops .... ▣604
Infants' Advil Concentrated Drops - White Grape (Dye-Free) .... ▣604
Junior Strength Advil Swallow Tablets .... ▣605
Advil Migraine Liquigels .... ▣608

Advil Multi-Symptom Cold Caplets 770
Advil PM Caplets 615
Motrin IB Tablets and Caplets 1866
Children's Motrin Oral Suspension ... 1867
Children's Motrin Non-Staining Dye-Free Oral Suspension 1867
Children's Motrin Cold Oral Suspension 1867
Infants' Motrin Concentrated Drops 1867
Infants' Motrin Non-Staining Dye-Free Concentrated Drops 1867
Junior Strength Motrin Caplets and Chewable Tablets 1867
Vicoprofen Tablets 539

Indapamide (Hydrochlorothiazide may add to or potentiate the therapeutic effect of other antihypertensive drugs). Products include:
Indapamide Tablets 2156

Indomethacin (Co-administration with non-steroidal anti-inflammatory agents may reduce the natriuretic and antihypertensive effects of thiazides). Products include:
Indocin 1995

Indomethacin Sodium Trihydrate (Co-administration with non-steroidal anti-inflammatory agents may reduce the natriuretic and antihypertensive effects of thiazides). Products include:
Indocin I.V. 2465

Insulin, Human, Zinc Suspension (Hydrochlorothiazide may cause hyperglycemia, therefore, dosage adjustment of insulin may be required). Products include:
Humulin L, 100 Units 1794
Humulin U, 100 Units 1800

Insulin, Human NPH (Hydrochlorothiazide may cause hyperglycemia, therefore, dosage adjustment of insulin may be required). Products include:
Humulin N, 100 Units 1795
Humulin N Pen 1797

Insulin, Human Regular (Hydrochlorothiazide may cause hyperglycemia, therefore, dosage adjustment of insulin may be required). Products include:
Humulin R, 100 Units 1798

Insulin, Human Regular and Human NPH Mixture (Hydrochlorothiazide may cause hyperglycemia, therefore, dosage adjustment of insulin may be required). Products include:
Humulin 50/50, 100 Units 1791
Humulin 70/30 Pen 1793

Insulin, NPH (Hydrochlorothiazide may cause hyperglycemia, therefore, dosage adjustment of insulin may be required).
No products indexed under this heading.

Insulin, Regular (Hydrochlorothiazide may cause hyperglycemia, therefore, dosage adjustment of insulin may be required).
No products indexed under this heading.

Insulin, Zinc Crystals (Hydrochlorothiazide may cause hyperglycemia, therefore, dosage adjustment of insulin may be required).
No products indexed under this heading.

Insulin, Zinc Suspension (Hydrochlorothiazide may cause hyperglycemia, therefore, dosage adjustment of insulin may be required).
No products indexed under this heading.

Insulin Aspart, Human Regular (Hydrochlorothiazide may cause hyperglycemia, therefore, dosage adjustment of insulin may be required). Products include:
NovoLog Injection 2326

Insulin glargine (Hydrochlorothiazide may cause hyperglycemia, therefore, dosage adjustment of insulin may be required). Products include:
Lantus Injection 2909

Insulin Lispro, Human (Hydrochlorothiazide may cause hyperglycemia, therefore, dosage adjustment of insulin may be required). Products include:
Humalog-Pen 1781
Humalog Mix 50/50-Pen 1783
Humalog Mix 75/25-Pen 1785

Insulin Lispro Protamine, Human (Hydrochlorothiazide may cause hyperglycemia, therefore, dosage adjustment of insulin may be required). Products include:
Humalog Mix 50/50-Pen 1783
Humalog Mix 75/25-Pen 1785

Isradipine (Hydrochlorothiazide may add to or potentiate the therapeutic effect of other antihypertensive drugs). Products include:
DynaCirc CR Tablets 2721

Ketoprofen (Co-administration with non-steroidal anti-inflammatory agents may reduce the natriuretic and antihypertensive effects of thiazides).
No products indexed under this heading.

Ketorolac Tromethamine (Co-administration with non-steroidal anti-inflammatory agents may reduce the natriuretic and antihypertensive effects of thiazides). Products include:
Acular Ophthalmic Solution 565
Acular LS Ophthalmic Solution 566

Labetalol Hydrochloride (Hydrochlorothiazide may add to or potentiate the therapeutic effect of other antihypertensive drugs).
No products indexed under this heading.

Levorphanol Tartrate (Potentiation of orthostatic hypotension).
No products indexed under this heading.

Lisinopril (Hydrochlorothiazide may add to or potentiate the therapeutic effect of other antihypertensive drugs). Products include:
Prinivil Tablets 2052
Prinzide Tablets 2056

Lithium (Diuretics reduce lithium's renal clearance and add a high risk of lithium toxicity).
No products indexed under this heading.

Lithium Carbonate (Diuretics reduce lithium's renal clearance and add a high risk of lithium toxicity). Products include:
Lithobid Tablets 1692

Lithium Citrate (Diuretics reduce lithium's renal clearance and add a high risk of lithium toxicity).
No products indexed under this heading.

Losartan Potassium (Hydrochlorothiazide may add to or potentiate the therapeutic effect of other antihypertensive drugs). Products include:
Cozaar Tablets 1935
Hyzaar 50-12.5 Tablets 1990
Hyzaar 100-12.5 Tablets 1990
Hyzaar 100-25 Tablets 1990

Mecamylamine Hydrochloride (Hydrochlorothiazide may add to or potentiate the therapeutic effect of other antihypertensive drugs).
No products indexed under this heading.

Meclofenamate Sodium (Co-administration with non-steroidal anti-inflammatory agents may reduce the natriuretic and antihypertensive effects of thiazides).
No products indexed under this heading.

Mefenamic Acid (Co-administration with non-steroidal anti-inflammatory agents may reduce the natriuretic and antihypertensive effects of thiazides).
No products indexed under this heading.

Meloxicam (Co-administration with non-steroidal anti-inflammatory agents may reduce the natriuretic and antihypertensive effects of thiazides). Products include:
Mobic Oral Suspension 863
Mobic Tablets 863

Meperidine Hydrochloride (Potentiation of orthostatic hypotension).
No products indexed under this heading.

Mephobarbital (Potentiation of orthostatic hypotension).
No products indexed under this heading.

Metformin Hydrochloride (Hydrochlorothiazide may cause hyperglycemia, therefore, dosage adjustment of oral hypoglycemic agent may be required). Products include:
ActoPlus Met Tablets 3214
Avandamet Tablets 1373
Fortamet Extended-Release Tablets 3115

Methadone Hydrochloride (Potentiation of orthostatic hypotension).
No products indexed under this heading.

Methyclothiazide (Hydrochlorothiazide may add to or potentiate the therapeutic effect of other antihypertensive drugs).
No products indexed under this heading.

Methyldopa (Hydrochlorothiazide may add to or potentiate the therapeutic effect of other antihypertensive drugs). Products include:
Aldoril Tablets 1910

Methyldopate Hydrochloride (Hydrochlorothiazide may add to or potentiate the therapeutic effect of other antihypertensive drugs).
No products indexed under this heading.

Methylprednisolone Acetate (Co-administration with corticosteroids intensifies electrolyte depletion particularly hypokalemia). Products include:
Depo-Medrol Injectable Suspension 2617
Depo-Medrol Single-Dose Vial 2619

Methylprednisolone Sodium Succinate (Co-administration with corticosteroids intensifies electrolyte depletion particularly hypokalemia).
No products indexed under this heading.

Metocurine Iodide (Possible increased responsiveness to the muscle relaxants).
No products indexed under this heading.

Metolazone (Hydrochlorothiazide may add to or potentiate the therapeutic effect of other antihypertensive drugs).
No products indexed under this heading.

Metoprolol Succinate (Hydrochlorothiazide may add to or potentiate the therapeutic effect of other antihypertensive drugs). Products include:
Toprol-XL Tablets 668

Metoprolol Tartrate (Hydrochlorothiazide may add to or potentiate the therapeutic effect of other antihypertensive drugs). Products include:
Lopressor Injection 2238
Lopressor Tablets 2238
Lopressor HCT 50/25 Tablets 2241
Lopressor HCT 100/25 Tablets 2241
Lopressor HCT 100/50 Tablets 2241

Metyrosine (Hydrochlorothiazide may add to or potentiate the therapeutic effect of other antihypertensive drugs). Products include:
Demser Capsules 1953

Mibefradil Dihydrochloride (Hydrochlorothiazide may add to or potentiate the therapeutic effect of other antihypertensive drugs).
No products indexed under this heading.

Miglitol (Hydrochlorothiazide may cause hyperglycemia, therefore, dosage adjustment of oral hypoglycemic agent may be required).
No products indexed under this heading.

Minoxidil (Hydrochlorothiazide may add to or potentiate the therapeutic effect of other antihypertensive drugs). Products include:
Men's Rogaine Extra Strength Hair Regrowth Treatment Topical Solution, Ocean Rush Scent and Original Unscented 633
Men's Rogaine Foam Hair Regrowth Treatment 633
Women's Rogaine Hair Regrowth Treatment Topical Solution, Spring Bloom Scent and Original Unscented 634

Mivacurium Chloride (Possible increased responsiveness to the muscle relaxants). Products include:
Mivacron Injection 493

Moexipril Hydrochloride (Hydrochlorothiazide may add to or potentiate the therapeutic effect of other antihypertensive drugs). Products include:
Uniretic Tablets 3100
Univasc Tablets 3104

Morphine Sulfate (Potentiation of orthostatic hypotension). Products include:
Avinza Capsules 1741
Kadian Capsules 577
MS Contin Tablets 2701

Nabumetone (Co-administration with non-steroidal anti-inflammatory agents may reduce the natriuretic and antihypertensive effects of thiazides).
No products indexed under this heading.

Nadolol (Hydrochlorothiazide may add to or potentiate the therapeutic effect of other antihypertensive drugs). Products include:
Nadolol Tablets 2159

Naproxen (Co-administration with non-steroidal anti-inflammatory agents may reduce the natriuretic and antihypertensive effects of thiazides). Products include:
EC-Naprosyn Delayed-Release Tablets 2761
Naprosyn Suspension 2761

Naprosyn Tablets 2761
Prevacid NapraPAC 3280

Naproxen Sodium (Co-administration with non-steroidal anti-inflammatory agents may reduce the natriuretic and antihypertensive effects of thiazides). Products include:
Aleve Caplets 742
Aleve Gelcaps 743
Aleve Tablets 743
Aleve Cold & Sinus Caplets 744
Anaprox Tablets 2761
Anaprox DS Tablets 2761

Nicardipine Hydrochloride (Hydrochlorothiazide may add to or potentiate the therapeutic effect of other antihypertensive drugs). Products include:
Cardene I.V. 2497

Nifedipine (In vitro studies show significant inhibition of the formation of oxidized irbesartan metabolites with the known cytochrome CYP 2C9 substrate/inhibitor, nifedipine; the pharmacokinetics of irbesartan were not affected by co-administration of nifedipine; hydrochlorothiazide may add to or potentiate the therapeutic effect of other antihypertensive drugs). Products include:
Adalat CC Tablets 2964

Nisoldipine (Hydrochlorothiazide may add to or potentiate the therapeutic effect of other antihypertensive drugs). Products include:
Sular Tablets 3122

Nitroglycerin (Hydrochlorothiazide may add to or potentiate the therapeutic effect of other antihypertensive drugs). Products include:
Nitro-Dur Transdermal Infusion System .. 3046
Nitrolingual Pumpspray 3120

Norepinephrine Bitartrate (Thiazides may decrease arterial responsiveness to norepinephrine).
No products indexed under this heading.

Oxaprozin (Co-administration with non-steroidal anti-inflammatory agents may reduce the natriuretic and antihypertensive effects of thiazides).
No products indexed under this heading.

Oxycodone Hydrochloride (Potentiation of orthostatic hypotension). Products include:
OxyContin Tablets 2703
OxyFast Oral Concentrate Solution 2708
OxyIR Capsules,.... 2708
Percocet Tablets 1131
Percodan Tablets 1132

Pancuronium Bromide (Possible increased responsiveness to the muscle relaxants).
No products indexed under this heading.

Penbutolol Sulfate (Hydrochlorothiazide may add to or potentiate the therapeutic effect of other antihypertensive drugs).
No products indexed under this heading.

Pentobarbital Sodium (Potentiation of orthostatic hypotension). Products include:
Nembutal Sodium Solution, USP 2470

Perindopril Erbumine (Hydrochlorothiazide may add to or potentiate the therapeutic effect of other antihypertensive drugs). Products include:
Aceon Tablets (2 mg, 4 mg, 8 mg) .. 3194

Phenobarbital (Potentiation of orthostatic hypotension). Products include:
Donnatal Extentabs 2493

Phenoxybenzamine Hydrochloride (Hydrochlorothiazide may add to or potentiate the therapeutic effect of other antihypertensive drugs). Products include:
Dibenzyline Capsules 3399

Phentolamine Mesylate (Hydrochlorothiazide may add to or potentiate the therapeutic effect of other antihypertensive drugs).
No products indexed under this heading.

Phenylbutazone (Co-administration with non-steroidal anti-inflammatory agents may reduce the natriuretic and antihypertensive effects of thiazides).
No products indexed under this heading.

Pindolol (Hydrochlorothiazide may add to or potentiate the therapeutic effect of other antihypertensive drugs).
No products indexed under this heading.

Pioglitazone Hydrochloride (Hydrochlorothiazide may cause hyperglycemia, therefore, dosage adjustment of oral hypoglycemic agent may be required). Products include:
ActoPlus Met Tablets 3214
Actos Tablets 3219
Duetact Tablets 3226

Piroxicam (Co-administration with non-steroidal anti-inflammatory agents may reduce the natriuretic and antihypertensive effects of thiazides).
No products indexed under this heading.

Polythiazide (Hydrochlorothiazide may add to or potentiate the therapeutic effect of other antihypertensive drugs).
No products indexed under this heading.

Prazosin Hydrochloride (Hydrochlorothiazide may add to or potentiate the therapeutic effect of other antihypertensive drugs).
No products indexed under this heading.

Prednisolone Acetate (Co-administration with corticosteroids intensifies electrolyte depletion particularly hypokalemia). Products include:
Blephamide Ophthalmic Ointment 568
Blephamide Ophthalmic Suspension 569
Poly-Pred Ophthalmic Suspension ☉ 233
Pred Forte Ophthalmic Suspension ☉ 235
Pred Mild Ophthalmic Suspension ☉ 238
Pred-G Ophthalmic Ointment ☉ 237
Pred-G Ophthalmic Suspension ☉ 236

Prednisolone Sodium Phosphate (Co-administration with corticosteroids intensifies electrolyte depletion particularly hypokalemia).
No products indexed under this heading.

Prednisolone Tebutate (Co-administration with corticosteroids intensifies electrolyte depletion particularly hypokalemia).
No products indexed under this heading.

Prednisone (Co-administration with corticosteroids intensifies electrolyte depletion particularly hypokalemia).
No products indexed under this heading.

Propoxyphene Hydrochloride (Potentiation of orthostatic hypotension).
No products indexed under this heading.

Propoxyphene Napsylate (Potentiation of orthostatic hypotension).
No products indexed under this heading.

Propranolol Hydrochloride (Hydrochlorothiazide may add to or potentiate the therapeutic effect of other antihypertensive drugs). Products include:
Inderal LA Long-Acting Capsules 3429
InnoPran XL Capsules 2723

Quinapril Hydrochloride (Hydrochlorothiazide may add to or potentiate the therapeutic effect of other antihypertensive drugs).
No products indexed under this heading.

Ramipril (Hydrochlorothiazide may add to or potentiate the therapeutic effect of other antihypertensive drugs). Products include:
Altace Capsules 1702

Rapacuronium Bromide (Possible increased responsiveness to the muscle relaxants).
No products indexed under this heading.

Rauwolfia Serpentina (Hydrochlorothiazide may add to or potentiate the therapeutic effect of other antihypertensive drugs).
No products indexed under this heading.

Remifentanil Hydrochloride (Potentiation of orthostatic hypotension).
No products indexed under this heading.

Repaglinide (Hydrochlorothiazide may cause hyperglycemia, therefore, dosage adjustment of oral hypoglycemic agent may be required).
No products indexed under this heading.

Rescinnamine (Hydrochlorothiazide may add to or potentiate the therapeutic effect of other antihypertensive drugs).
No products indexed under this heading.

Reserpine (Hydrochlorothiazide may add to or potentiate the therapeutic effect of other antihypertensive drugs).
No products indexed under this heading.

Rocuronium Bromide (Possible increased responsiveness to the muscle relaxants). Products include:
Zemuron Injection 2346

Rofecoxib (Co-administration with non-steroidal anti-inflammatory agents may reduce the natriuretic and antihypertensive effects of thiazides).
No products indexed under this heading.

Rosiglitazone Maleate (Hydrochlorothiazide may cause hyperglycemia, therefore, dosage adjustment of oral hypoglycemic agent may be required). Products include:
Avandamet Tablets 1373
Avandaryl Tablets 1379

Avandia Tablets 1384

Secobarbital Sodium (Potentiation of orthostatic hypotension).
No products indexed under this heading.

Sodium Nitroprusside (Hydrochlorothiazide may add to or potentiate the therapeutic effect of other antihypertensive drugs).
No products indexed under this heading.

Sotalol Hydrochloride (Hydrochlorothiazide may add to or potentiate the therapeutic effect of other antihypertensive drugs).
No products indexed under this heading.

Spirapril Hydrochloride (Hydrochlorothiazide may add to or potentiate the therapeutic effect of other antihypertensive drugs).
No products indexed under this heading.

Sufentanil Citrate (Potentiation of orthostatic hypotension).
No products indexed under this heading.

Sulindac (Co-administration with non-steroidal anti-inflammatory agents may reduce the natriuretic and antihypertensive effects of thiazides). Products include:
Clinoril Tablets 1924

Telmisartan (Hydrochlorothiazide may add to or potentiate the therapeutic effect of other antihypertensive drugs). Products include:
Micardis Tablets 854
Micardis HCT Tablets 856

Terazosin Hydrochloride (Hydrochlorothiazide may add to or potentiate the therapeutic effect of other antihypertensive drugs). Products include:
Hytrin Capsules 471

Thiamylal Sodium (Potentiation of orthostatic hypotension).
No products indexed under this heading.

Timolol Maleate (Hydrochlorothiazide may add to or potentiate the therapeutic effect of other antihypertensive drugs). Products include:
Blocadren Tablets 1916
Cosopt Sterile Ophthalmic Solution 1931
Timolide Tablets 2086
Timoptic Sterile Ophthalmic Solution 2088
Timoptic in Ocudose 2091
Timoptic-XE Sterile Ophthalmic Gel Forming Solution 2092

Tolazamide (Hydrochlorothiazide may cause hyperglycemia, therefore, dosage adjustment of oral hypoglycemic agent may be required).
No products indexed under this heading.

Tolbutamide (In vitro studies show significant inhibition of the formation of oxidized irbesartan metabolites with the known cytochrome CYP 2C9 substrate/inhibitor, tolbutamide; hydrochlorothiazide may cause hyperglycemia, therefore dosage adjustment of oral hypoglycemic agent may be required).
No products indexed under this heading.

Tolmetin Sodium (Co-administration with non-steroidal anti-inflammatory agents may reduce the natriuretic and antihypertensive effects of thiazides).
No products indexed under this heading.

Torsemide (Hydrochlorothiazide may add to or potentiate the therapeutic effect of other antihypertensive drugs). Products include:
- Demadex Injection 2759
- Demadex Tablets 2759

Trandolapril (Hydrochlorothiazide may add to or potentiate the therapeutic effect of other antihypertensive drugs). Products include:
- Mavik Tablets 486
- Tarka Tablets 524

Triamcinolone (Co-administration with corticosteroids intensifies electrolyte depletion particularly hypokalemia).
No products indexed under this heading.

Triamcinolone Acetonide (Co-administration with corticosteroids intensifies electrolyte depletion particularly hypokalemia). Products include:
- Azmacort Inhalation Aerosol 1726
- Nasacort AQ Nasal Spray 2922

Triamcinolone Diacetate (Co-administration with corticosteroids intensifies electrolyte depletion particularly hypokalemia).
No products indexed under this heading.

Triamcinolone Hexacetonide (Co-administration with corticosteroids intensifies electrolyte depletion particularly hypokalemia).
No products indexed under this heading.

Trimethaphan Camsylate (Hydrochlorothiazide may add to or potentiate the therapeutic effect of other antihypertensive drugs).
No products indexed under this heading.

Troglitazone (Hydrochlorothiazide may cause hyperglycemia, therefore, dosage adjustment of oral hypoglycemic agent may be required).
No products indexed under this heading.

Tubocurarine Chloride (Possible increased responsiveness to the muscle relaxants).
No products indexed under this heading.

Valdecoxib (Co-administration with non-steroidal anti-inflammatory agents may reduce the natriuretic and antihypertensive effects of thiazides).
No products indexed under this heading.

Valsartan (Hydrochlorothiazide may add to or potentiate the therapeutic effect of other antihypertensive drugs). Products include:
- Diovan Tablets 2193
- Diovan HCT Tablets 2196

Vecuronium Bromide (Possible increased responsiveness to the muscle relaxants).
No products indexed under this heading.

Verapamil Hydrochloride (Hydrochlorothiazide may add to or potentiate the therapeutic effect of other antihypertensive drugs). Products include:
- Covera-HS Tablets 3139
- Tarka Tablets 524
- Verelan PM Extended-Release Capsules, Controlled-Onset 3106

Food Interactions

Alcohol (Potentiation of orthostatic hypotension).

AVALIDE TABLETS

(Hydrochlorothiazide, Irbesartan) 2874
May interact with antihypertensives, barbiturates, corticosteroids, cardiac glycosides, oral hypoglycemic agents, insulin, lithium preparations, narcotic analgesics, nondepolarizing neuromuscular blocking agents, nonsteroidal anti-inflammatory agents, and certain other agents. Compounds in these categories include:

Acarbose (Hydrochlorothiazide may cause hyperglycemia, therefore, dosage adjustment of oral hypoglycemic agent may be required). Products include:
- Precose Tablets 751

Acebutolol Hydrochloride (Hydrochlorothiazide may add to or potentiate the therapeutic effect of other antihypertensive drugs).
No products indexed under this heading.

ACTH (Co-administration with ACTH intensifies electrolyte depletion particularly hypokalemia).
No products indexed under this heading.

Alfentanil Hydrochloride (Potentiation of orthostatic hypotension).
No products indexed under this heading.

Amlodipine Besylate (Hydrochlorothiazide may add to or potentiate the therapeutic effect of other antihypertensive drugs). Products include:
- Caduet Tablets 2508
- Lotrel Capsules 2249
- Norvasc Tablets 2545

Aprobarbital (Potentiation of orthostatic hypotension).
No products indexed under this heading.

Atenolol (Hydrochlorothiazide may add to or potentiate the therapeutic effect of other antihypertensive drugs).
No products indexed under this heading.

Atracurium Besylate (Possible increased responsiveness to the muscle relaxants).
No products indexed under this heading.

Benazepril Hydrochloride (Hydrochlorothiazide may add to or potentiate the therapeutic effect of other antihypertensive drugs). Products include:
- Lotensin Tablets 2243
- Lotensin HCT Tablets 2246
- Lotrel Capsules 2249

Bendroflumethiazide (Hydrochlorothiazide may add to or potentiate the therapeutic effect of other antihypertensive drugs).
No products indexed under this heading.

Betamethasone Acetate (Co-administration with corticosteroids intensifies electrolyte depletion particularly hypokalemia).
No products indexed under this heading.

Betamethasone Sodium Phosphate (Co-administration with corticosteroids intensifies electrolyte depletion particularly hypokalemia).
No products indexed under this heading.

Betaxolol Hydrochloride (Hydrochlorothiazide may add to or potentiate the therapeutic effect of other antihypertensive drugs). Products include:
- Betoptic S Ophthalmic Suspension 558

Bisoprolol Fumarate (Hydrochlorothiazide may add to or potentiate the therapeutic effect of other antihypertensive drugs).
No products indexed under this heading.

Buprenorphine Hydrochloride (Potentiation of orthostatic hypotension). Products include:
- Buprenex Injectable 2716
- Suboxone Tablets 2717
- Subutex Tablets 2717

Butabarbital (Potentiation of orthostatic hypotension).
No products indexed under this heading.

Butalbital (Potentiation of orthostatic hypotension).
No products indexed under this heading.

Candesartan Cilexetil (Hydrochlorothiazide may add to or potentiate the therapeutic effect of other antihypertensive drugs). Products include:
- Atacand Tablets 649
- Atacand HCT 651

Captopril (Hydrochlorothiazide may add to or potentiate the therapeutic effect of other antihypertensive drugs). Products include:
- Captopril Tablets 2149

Carteolol Hydrochloride (Hydrochlorothiazide may add to or potentiate the therapeutic effect of other antihypertensive drugs). Products include:
- Carteolol Hydrochloride Ophthalmic Solution USP, 1% .... ⊙249

Celecoxib (Co-administration with non-steroidal anti-inflammatory agents may reduce the natriuretic and antihypertensive effects of thiazides). Products include:
- Celebrex Capsules 3134

Chlorothiazide (Hydrochlorothiazide may add to or potentiate the therapeutic effect of other antihypertensive drugs). Products include:
- Diuril Oral Suspension 1954

Chlorothiazide Sodium (Hydrochlorothiazide may add to or potentiate the therapeutic effect of other antihypertensive drugs). Products include:
- Diuril Sodium Intravenous 2467

Chlorpropamide (Hydrochlorothiazide may cause hyperglycemia, therefore, dosage adjustment of oral hypoglycemic agent may be required).
No products indexed under this heading.

Chlorthalidone (Hydrochlorothiazide may add to or potentiate the therapeutic effect of other antihypertensive drugs). Products include:
- Clorpres Tablets 2153

Cholestyramine (Absorption of hydrochlorothiazide is impaired in the presence of anionic exchange resins; single dose of cholestyramine binds the hydrochlorothiazide and reduces its absorption from GI tract by 85%).
No products indexed under this heading.

Cisatracurium Besylate (Possible increased responsiveness to the muscle relaxants). Products include:
- Nimbex Injection 498

Clonidine (Hydrochlorothiazide may add to or potentiate the therapeutic effect of other antihypertensive drugs). Products include:
- Catapres-TTS 844

Clonidine Hydrochloride (Hydrochlorothiazide may add to or potentiate the therapeutic effect of other antihypertensive drugs). Products include:
- Catapres Tablets 843
- Clorpres Tablets 2153

Codeine Phosphate (Potentiation of orthostatic hypotension). Products include:
- Tylenol with Codeine Tablets 2391

Colestipol Hydrochloride (Absorption of hydrochlorothiazide is impaired in the presence of anionic exchange resins; single dose of colestipol binds the hydrochlorothiazide and reduces its absorption from GI tract by 43%).
No products indexed under this heading.

Cortisone Acetate (Co-administration with corticosteroids intensifies electrolyte depletion particularly hypokalemia).
No products indexed under this heading.

Deserpidine (Hydrochlorothiazide may add to or potentiate the therapeutic effect of other antihypertensive drugs).
No products indexed under this heading.

Deslanoside (Concurrent digitalis therapy may exaggerate metabolic effects of hypokalemia, especially myocardial effects, e.g., increased ventricular irritability).
No products indexed under this heading.

Dexamethasone (Co-administration with corticosteroids intensifies electrolyte depletion particularly hypokalemia). Products include:
- Ciprodex Otic Suspension 559
- Decadron Tablets 1951
- TobraDex Ophthalmic Ointment 562
- TobraDex Ophthalmic Suspension 563

Dexamethasone Acetate (Co-administration with corticosteroids intensifies electrolyte depletion particularly hypokalemia).
No products indexed under this heading.

Dexamethasone Sodium Phosphate (Co-administration with corticosteroids intensifies electrolyte depletion particularly hypokalemia).
No products indexed under this heading.

Dezocine (Potentiation of orthostatic hypotension).
No products indexed under this heading.

Diazoxide (Hydrochlorothiazide may add to or potentiate the therapeutic effect of other antihypertensive drugs). Products include:
- Hyperstat I.V. 3017

Diclofenac Potassium (Co-administration with non-steroidal anti-inflammatory agents may reduce the natriuretic and antihypertensive effects of thiazides).
No products indexed under this heading.

Diclofenac Sodium (Co-administration with non-steroidal anti-inflammatory agents may reduce the natriuretic and antihypertensive effects of thiazides). Products include:
- Arthrotec Tablets 3129
- Voltaren Ophthalmic Solution 2309
- Voltaren Tablets 2307

Voltaren-XR Tablets 2310

Digitalis Glycoside Preparations (Concurrent digitalis therapy may exaggerate metabolic effects of hypokalemia, especially myocardial effects, e.g., increased ventricular irritability).
No products indexed under this heading.

Digitoxin (Concurrent digitalis therapy may exaggerate metabolic effects of hypokalemia, especially myocardial effects, e.g., increased ventricular irritability).
No products indexed under this heading.

Digoxin (Concurrent digitalis therapy may exaggerate metabolic effects of hypokalemia, especially myocardial effects, e.g., increased ventricular irritability). Products include:
Lanoxicaps Capsules 1490
Lanoxin Injection 1494
Lanoxin Injection Pediatric 1497
Lanoxin Tablets 1500

Diltiazem Hydrochloride (Hydrochlorothiazide may add to or potentiate the therapeutic effect of other antihypertensive drugs). Products include:
Cardizem LA Extended Release Tablets 1728
Tiazac Capsules 1201

Doxazosin Mesylate (Hydrochlorothiazide may add to or potentiate the therapeutic effect of other antihypertensive drugs). Products include:
Cardura XL Tablets 2515

Enalapril Maleate (Hydrochlorothiazide may add to or potentiate the therapeutic effect of other antihypertensive drugs). Products include:
Vasotec I.V. Injection 2103

Enalaprilat (Hydrochlorothiazide may add to or potentiate the therapeutic effect of other antihypertensive drugs).
No products indexed under this heading.

Eprosartan Mesylate (Hydrochlorothiazide may add to or potentiate the therapeutic effect of other antihypertensive drugs). Products include:
Teveten Tablets 1735
Teveten HCT Tablets 1737

Esmolol Hydrochloride (Hydrochlorothiazide may add to or potentiate the therapeutic effect of other antihypertensive drugs).
No products indexed under this heading.

Etodolac (Co-administration with non-steroidal anti-inflammatory agents may reduce the natriuretic and antihypertensive effects of thiazides).
No products indexed under this heading.

Felodipine (Hydrochlorothiazide may add to or potentiate the therapeutic effect of other antihypertensive drugs).
No products indexed under this heading.

Fenoprofen Calcium (Co-administration with non-steroidal anti-inflammatory agents may reduce the natriuretic and antihypertensive effects of thiazides). Products include:
Nalfon Capsules 2502

Fentanyl (Potentiation of orthostatic hypotension). Products include:
Duragesic Transdermal System 2373
Ionsys Transdermal System 2379

Fentanyl Citrate (Potentiation of orthostatic hypotension). Products include:
Actiq 979

Fludrocortisone Acetate (Co-administration with corticosteroids intensifies electrolyte depletion particularly hypokalemia).
No products indexed under this heading.

Flurbiprofen (Co-administration with non-steroidal anti-inflammatory agents may reduce the natriuretic and antihypertensive effects of thiazides).
No products indexed under this heading.

Fosinopril Sodium (Hydrochlorothiazide may add to or potentiate the therapeutic effect of other antihypertensive drugs).
No products indexed under this heading.

Furosemide (Hydrochlorothiazide may add to or potentiate the therapeutic effect of other antihypertensive drugs). Products include:
Furosemide Tablets 2154

Glimepiride (Hydrochlorothiazide may cause hyperglycemia, therefore, dosage adjustment of oral hypoglycemic agent may be required). Products include:
Avandaryl Tablets 1379
Duetact Tablets 3226

Glipizide (Hydrochlorothiazide may cause hyperglycemia, therefore, dosage adjustment of oral hypoglycemic agent may be required).
No products indexed under this heading.

Glyburide (Hydrochlorothiazide may cause hyperglycemia, therefore, dosage adjustment of oral hypoglycemic agent may be required).
No products indexed under this heading.

Guanabenz Acetate (Hydrochlorothiazide may add to or potentiate the therapeutic effect of other antihypertensive drugs).
No products indexed under this heading.

Guanethidine Monosulfate (Hydrochlorothiazide may add to or potentiate the therapeutic effect of other antihypertensive drugs).
No products indexed under this heading.

Hydralazine Hydrochloride (Hydrochlorothiazide may add to or potentiate the therapeutic effect of other antihypertensive drugs). Products include:
BiDil Tablets 2171

Hydrocodone Bitartrate (Potentiation of orthostatic hypotension). Products include:
Hycodan 1116
Hycotuss Expectorant Syrup 1117
Vicodin Tablets 535
Vicodin ES Tablets 536
Vicodin HP Tablets 538
Vicoprofen Tablets 539
Zydone Tablets 1139

Hydrocodone Polistirex (Potentiation of orthostatic hypotension). Products include:
Tussionex Pennkinetic Extended-Release Suspension 3327

Hydrocortisone (Co-administration with corticosteroids intensifies electrolyte depletion particularly hypokalemia). Products include:
Colocort Rectal Suspension, USP (Retention) 100 mg/60 mL 2476
Hydrocortone Tablets 1989
Preparation H Hydrocortisone Cream .... ▣646

Hydrocortisone Acetate (Co-administration with corticosteroids intensifies electrolyte depletion particularly hypokalemia). Products include:
Analpram-HC 1159
Pramosone 1161
ProctoFoam-HC 3099

Hydrocortisone Sodium Phosphate (Co-administration with corticosteroids intensifies electrolyte depletion particularly hypokalemia).
No products indexed under this heading.

Hydrocortisone Sodium Succinate (Co-administration with corticosteroids intensifies electrolyte depletion particularly hypokalemia).
No products indexed under this heading.

Hydroflumethiazide (Hydrochlorothiazide may add to or potentiate the therapeutic effect of other antihypertensive drugs).
No products indexed under this heading.

Hydromorphone Hydrochloride (Potentiation of orthostatic hypotension). Products include:
Dilaudid 440
Dilaudid Non-Sterile Powder 440
Dilaudid Oral Liquid 445
Dilaudid Rectal Suppositories 440
Dilaudid Tablets 440
Dilaudid Tablets - 8 mg 445
Dilaudid-HP 442

Ibuprofen (Co-administration with non-steroidal anti-inflammatory agents may reduce the natriuretic and antihypertensive effects of thiazides). Products include:
Advil Allergy Sinus Caplets .... ▣770
Advil .... ▣674
Children's Advil Oral Suspension .... ▣603
Children's Advil Chewable Tablets .... ▣603
Advil Cold & Sinus .... ▣723
Infants' Advil Concentrated Drops .... ▣604
Infants' Advil Concentrated Drops - White Grape (Dye-Free) .... ▣604
Junior Strength Advil Swallow Tablets .... ▣605
Advil Migraine Liquigels .... ▣608
Advil Multi-Symptom Cold Caplets .... ▣770
Advil PM Caplets .... ▣615
Motrin IB Tablets and Caplets 1866
Children's Motrin Oral Suspension 1867
Children's Motrin Non-Staining Dye-Free Oral Suspension 1867
Children's Motrin Cold Oral Suspension 1867
Infants' Motrin Concentrated Drops 1867
Infants' Motrin Non-Staining Dye-Free Concentrated Drops 1867
Junior Strength Motrin Caplets and Chewable Tablets 1867
Vicoprofen Tablets 539

Indapamide (Hydrochlorothiazide may add to or potentiate the therapeutic effect of other antihypertensive drugs). Products include:
Indapamide Tablets 2156

Indomethacin (Co-administration with non-steroidal anti-inflammatory agents may reduce the natriuretic and antihypertensive effects of thiazides). Products include:
Indocin 1995

Indomethacin Sodium Trihydrate (Co-administration with non-steroidal anti-inflammatory agents may reduce the natriuretic and antihypertensive effects of thiazides). Products include:
Indocin I.V. 2465

Insulin, Human, Zinc Suspension (Hydrochlorothiazide may cause hyperglycemia, therefore, dosage adjustment of insulin may be required). Products include:
Humulin L, 100 Units 1794
Humulin U, 100 Units 1800

Insulin, Human NPH (Hydrochlorothiazide may cause hyperglycemia, therefore, dosage adjustment of insulin may be required). Products include:
Humulin N, 100 Units 1795
Humulin N Pen 1797

Insulin, Human Regular (Hydrochlorothiazide may cause hyperglycemia, therefore, dosage adjustment of insulin may be required). Products include:
Humulin R, 100 Units 1798

Insulin, Human Regular and Human NPH Mixture (Hydrochlorothiazide may cause hyperglycemia, therefore, dosage adjustment of insulin may be required). Products include:
Humulin 50/50, 100 Units 1791
Humulin 70/30 Pen 1793

Insulin, NPH (Hydrochlorothiazide may cause hyperglycemia, therefore, dosage adjustment of insulin may be required).
No products indexed under this heading.

Insulin, Regular (Hydrochlorothiazide may cause hyperglycemia, therefore, dosage adjustment of insulin may be required).
No products indexed under this heading.

Insulin, Zinc Crystals (Hydrochlorothiazide may cause hyperglycemia, therefore, dosage adjustment of insulin may be required).
No products indexed under this heading.

Insulin, Zinc Suspension (Hydrochlorothiazide may cause hyperglycemia, therefore, dosage adjustment of insulin may be required).
No products indexed under this heading.

Insulin Aspart, Human Regular (Hydrochlorothiazide may cause hyperglycemia, therefore, dosage adjustment of insulin may be required). Products include:
NovoLog Injection 2326

Insulin glargine (Hydrochlorothiazide may cause hyperglycemia, therefore, dosage adjustment of insulin may be required). Products include:
Lantus Injection 2909

Insulin Lispro, Human (Hydrochlorothiazide may cause hyperglycemia, therefore, dosage adjustment of insulin may be required). Products include:
Humalog-Pen 1781
Humalog Mix 50/50-Pen 1783
Humalog Mix 75/25-Pen 1785

Insulin Lispro Protamine, Human (Hydrochlorothiazide may cause hyperglycemia, therefore, dosage adjustment of insulin may be required). Products include:
Humalog Mix 50/50-Pen 1783
Humalog Mix 75/25-Pen 1785

Isradipine (Hydrochlorothiazide may add to or potentiate the therapeutic effect of other antihypertensive drugs). Products include:
DynaCirc CR Tablets 2721

Ketoprofen (Co-administration with non-steroidal anti-inflammatory agents may reduce the natriuretic and antihypertensive effects of thiazides).
No products indexed under this heading.

Ketorolac Tromethamine (Co-administration with non-steroidal anti-inflammatory agents may reduce the natriuretic and antihypertensive effects of thiazides). Products include:
- Acular Ophthalmic Solution 565
- Acular LS Ophthalmic Solution 566

Labetalol Hydrochloride (Hydrochlorothiazide may add to or potentiate the therapeutic effect of other antihypertensive drugs).
No products indexed under this heading.

Levorphanol Tartrate (Potentiation of orthostatic hypotension).
No products indexed under this heading.

Lisinopril (Hydrochlorothiazide may add to or potentiate the therapeutic effect of other antihypertensive drugs). Products include:
- Prinivil Tablets 2052
- Prinzide Tablets 2056

Lithium (Diuretics reduce lithium's renal clearance and add a high risk of lithium toxicity).
No products indexed under this heading.

Lithium Carbonate (Diuretics reduce lithium's renal clearance and add a high risk of lithium toxicity). Products include:
- Lithobid Tablets 1692

Lithium Citrate (Diuretics reduce lithium's renal clearance and add a high risk of lithium toxicity).
No products indexed under this heading.

Losartan Potassium (Hydrochlorothiazide may add to or potentiate the therapeutic effect of other antihypertensive drugs). Products include:
- Cozaar Tablets 1935
- Hyzaar 50-12.5 Tablets 1990
- Hyzaar 100-12.5 Tablets 1990
- Hyzaar 100-25 Tablets 1990

Mecamylamine Hydrochloride (Hydrochlorothiazide may add to or potentiate the therapeutic effect of other antihypertensive drugs).
No products indexed under this heading.

Meclofenamate Sodium (Co-administration with non-steroidal anti-inflammatory agents may reduce the natriuretic and antihypertensive effects of thiazides).
No products indexed under this heading.

Mefenamic Acid (Co-administration with non-steroidal anti-inflammatory agents may reduce the natriuretic and antihypertensive effects of thiazides).
No products indexed under this heading.

Meloxicam (Co-administration with non-steroidal anti-inflammatory agents may reduce the natriuretic and antihypertensive effects of thiazides). Products include:
- Mobic Oral Suspension 863
- Mobic Tablets 863

Meperidine Hydrochloride (Potentiation of orthostatic hypotension).
No products indexed under this heading.

Mephobarbital (Potentiation of orthostatic hypotension).
No products indexed under this heading.

Metformin Hydrochloride (Hydrochlorothiazide may cause hyperglycemia, therefore, dosage adjustment of oral hypoglycemic agent may be required). Products include:
- ActoPlus Met Tablets 3214
- Avandamet Tablets 1373
- Fortamet Extended-Release Tablets 3115

Methadone Hydrochloride (Potentiation of orthostatic hypotension).
No products indexed under this heading.

Methyclothiazide (Hydrochlorothiazide may add to or potentiate the therapeutic effect of other antihypertensive drugs).
No products indexed under this heading.

Methyldopa (Hydrochlorothiazide may add to or potentiate the therapeutic effect of other antihypertensive drugs). Products include:
- Aldoril Tablets 1910

Methyldopate Hydrochloride (Hydrochlorothiazide may add to or potentiate the therapeutic effect of other antihypertensive drugs).
No products indexed under this heading.

Methylprednisolone Acetate (Co-administration with corticosteroids intensifies electrolyte depletion particularly hypokalemia). Products include:
- Depo-Medrol Injectable Suspension 2617
- Depo-Medrol Single-Dose Vial 2619

Methylprednisolone Sodium Succinate (Co-administration with corticosteroids intensifies electrolyte depletion particularly hypokalemia).
No products indexed under this heading.

Metocurine Iodide (Possible increased responsiveness to the muscle relaxants).
No products indexed under this heading.

Metolazone (Hydrochlorothiazide may add to or potentiate the therapeutic effect of other antihypertensive drugs).
No products indexed under this heading.

Metoprolol Succinate (Hydrochlorothiazide may add to or potentiate the therapeutic effect of other antihypertensive drugs). Products include:
- Toprol-XL Tablets 668

Metoprolol Tartrate (Hydrochlorothiazide may add to or potentiate the therapeutic effect of other antihypertensive drugs). Products include:
- Lopressor Injection 2238
- Lopressor Tablets 2238
- Lopressor HCT 50/25 Tablets 2241
- Lopressor HCT 100/25 Tablets 2241
- Lopressor HCT 100/50 Tablets 2241

Metyrosine (Hydrochlorothiazide may add to or potentiate the therapeutic effect of other antihypertensive drugs). Products include:
- Demser Capsules 1953

Mibefradil Dihydrochloride (Hydrochlorothiazide may add to or potentiate the therapeutic effect of other antihypertensive drugs).
No products indexed under this heading.

Miglitol (Hydrochlorothiazide may cause hyperglycemia, therefore, dosage adjustment of oral hypoglycemic agent may be required).
No products indexed under this heading.

Minoxidil (Hydrochlorothiazide may add to or potentiate the therapeutic effect of other antihypertensive drugs). Products include:
- Men's Rogaine Extra Strength Hair Regrowth Treatment Topical Solution, Ocean Rush Scent and Original Unscented 633
- Men's Rogaine Foam Hair Regrowth Treatment.................. 633
- Women's Rogaine Hair Regrowth Treatment Topical Solution, Spring Bloom Scent and Original Unscented.............. 634

Mivacurium Chloride (Possible increased responsiveness to the muscle relaxants). Products include:
- Mivacron Injection 493

Moexipril Hydrochloride (Hydrochlorothiazide may add to or potentiate the therapeutic effect of other antihypertensive drugs). Products include:
- Uniretic Tablets 3100
- Univasc Tablets 3104

Morphine Sulfate (Potentiation of orthostatic hypotension). Products include:
- Avinza Capsules 1741
- Kadian Capsules 577
- MS Contin Tablets 2701

Nabumetone (Co-administration with non-steroidal anti-inflammatory agents may reduce the natriuretic and antihypertensive effects of thiazides).
No products indexed under this heading.

Nadolol (Hydrochlorothiazide may add to or potentiate the therapeutic effect of other antihypertensive drugs). Products include:
- Nadolol Tablets 2159

Naproxen (Co-administration with non-steroidal anti-inflammatory agents may reduce the natriuretic and antihypertensive effects of thiazides). Products include:
- EC-Naprosyn Delayed-Release Tablets 2761
- Naprosyn Suspension 2761
- Naprosyn Tablets 2761
- Prevacid NapraPAC 3280

Naproxen Sodium (Co-administration with non-steroidal anti-inflammatory agents may reduce the natriuretic and antihypertensive effects of thiazides). Products include:
- Aleve Caplets 742
- Aleve Gelcaps 743
- Aleve Tablets 743
- Aleve Cold & Sinus Caplets 744
- Anaprox Tablets 2761
- Anaprox DS Tablets 2761

Nicardipine Hydrochloride (Hydrochlorothiazide may add to or potentiate the therapeutic effect of other antihypertensive drugs). Products include:
- Cardene I.V. 2497

Nifedipine (In vitro studies show significant inhibition of the formation of oxidized irbesartan metabolites with the known cytochrome CYP 2C9 substrate/inhibitor, nifedipine; the pharmacokinetics of irbesartan were not affected by co-administration of nifedipine; hydrochlorothiazide may add to or potentiate the therapeutic effect of other antihypertensive drugs). Products include:
- Adalat CC Tablets 2964

Nisoldipine (Hydrochlorothiazide may add to or potentiate the therapeutic effect of other antihypertensive drugs). Products include:
- Sular Tablets 3122

Nitroglycerin (Hydrochlorothiazide may add to or potentiate the therapeutic effect of other antihypertensive drugs). Products include:
- Nitro-Dur Transdermal Infusion System... 3046
- Nitrolingual Pumpspray 3120

Norepinephrine Bitartrate (Thiazides may decrease arterial responsiveness to norepinephrine).
No products indexed under this heading.

Oxaprozin (Co-administration with non-steroidal anti-inflammatory agents may reduce the natriuretic and antihypertensive effects of thiazides).
No products indexed under this heading.

Oxycodone Hydrochloride (Potentiation of orthostatic hypotension). Products include:
- OxyContin Tablets 2703
- OxyFast Oral Concentrate Solution.. 2708
- OxyIR Capsules 2708
- Percocet Tablets 1131
- Percodan Tablets 1132

Pancuronium Bromide (Possible increased responsiveness to the muscle relaxants).
No products indexed under this heading.

Penbutolol Sulfate (Hydrochlorothiazide may add to or potentiate the therapeutic effect of other antihypertensive drugs).
No products indexed under this heading.

Pentobarbital Sodium (Potentiation of orthostatic hypotension). Products include:
- Nembutal Sodium Solution, USP 2470

Perindopril Erbumine (Hydrochlorothiazide may add to or potentiate the therapeutic effect of other antihypertensive drugs). Products include:
- Aceon Tablets (2 mg, 4 mg, 8 mg).. 3194

Phenobarbital (Potentiation of orthostatic hypotension). Products include:
- Donnatal Extentabs 2493

Phenoxybenzamine Hydrochloride (Hydrochlorothiazide may add to or potentiate the therapeutic effect of other antihypertensive drugs). Products include:
- Dibenzyline Capsules 3399

Phentolamine Mesylate (Hydrochlorothiazide may add to or potentiate the therapeutic effect of other antihypertensive drugs).
No products indexed under this heading.

Phenylbutazone (Co-administration with non-steroidal anti-inflammatory agents may reduce the natriuretic and antihypertensive effects of thiazides).
No products indexed under this heading.

Pindolol (Hydrochlorothiazide may add to or potentiate the therapeutic effect of other antihypertensive drugs).
No products indexed under this heading.

Pioglitazone Hydrochloride (Hydrochlorothiazide may cause hyperglycemia, therefore, dosage adjustment of oral hypoglycemic agent may be required). Products include:

ActoPlus Met Tablets 3214
Actos Tablets 3219
Duetact Tablets 3226

Piroxicam (Co-administration with non-steroidal anti-inflammatory agents may reduce the natriuretic and antihypertensive effects of thiazides).

No products indexed under this heading.

Polythiazide (Hydrochlorothiazide may add to or potentiate the therapeutic effect of other antihypertensive drugs).

No products indexed under this heading.

Prazosin Hydrochloride (Hydrochlorothiazide may add to or potentiate the therapeutic effect of other antihypertensive drugs).

No products indexed under this heading.

Prednisolone Acetate (Co-administration with corticosteroids intensifies electrolyte depletion particularly hypokalemia). Products include:

Blephamide Ophthalmic Ointment 568
Blephamide Ophthalmic Suspension.................................. 569
Poly-Pred Ophthalmic Suspension .... ⊙233
Pred Forte Ophthalmic Suspension .... ⊙235
Pred Mild Ophthalmic Suspension .... ⊙238
Pred-G Ophthalmic Ointment .... ⊙237
Pred-G Ophthalmic Suspension ...... ⊙236

Prednisolone Sodium Phosphate (Co-administration with corticosteroids intensifies electrolyte depletion particularly hypokalemia).

No products indexed under this heading.

Prednisolone Tebutate (Co-administration with corticosteroids intensifies electrolyte depletion particularly hypokalemia).

No products indexed under this heading.

Prednisone (Co-administration with corticosteroids intensifies electrolyte depletion particularly hypokalemia).

No products indexed under this heading.

Propoxyphene Hydrochloride (Potentiation of orthostatic hypotension).

No products indexed under this heading.

Propoxyphene Napsylate (Potentiation of orthostatic hypotension).

No products indexed under this heading.

Propranolol Hydrochloride (Hydrochlorothiazide may add to or potentiate the therapeutic effect of other antihypertensive drugs). Products include:

Inderal LA Long-Acting Capsules 3429
InnoPran XL Capsules 2723

Quinapril Hydrochloride (Hydrochlorothiazide may add to or potentiate the therapeutic effect of other antihypertensive drugs).

No products indexed under this heading.

Ramipril (Hydrochlorothiazide may add to or potentiate the therapeutic effect of other antihypertensive drugs). Products include:

Altace Capsules 1702

Rapacuronium Bromide (Possible increased responsiveness to the muscle relaxants).

No products indexed under this heading.

Rauwolfia Serpentina (Hydrochlorothiazide may add to or potentiate the therapeutic effect of other antihypertensive drugs).

No products indexed under this heading.

Remifentanil Hydrochloride (Potentiation of orthostatic hypotension).

No products indexed under this heading.

Repaglinide (Hydrochlorothiazide may cause hyperglycemia, therefore, dosage adjustment of oral hypoglycemic agent may be required).

No products indexed under this heading.

Rescinnamine (Hydrochlorothiazide may add to or potentiate the therapeutic effect of other antihypertensive drugs).

No products indexed under this heading.

Reserpine (Hydrochlorothiazide may add to or potentiate the therapeutic effect of other antihypertensive drugs).

No products indexed under this heading.

Rocuronium Bromide (Possible increased responsiveness to the muscle relaxants). Products include:

Zemuron Injection 2346

Rofecoxib (Co-administration with non-steroidal anti-inflammatory agents may reduce the natriuretic and antihypertensive effects of thiazides).

No products indexed under this heading.

Rosiglitazone Maleate (Hydrochlorothiazide may cause hyperglycemia, therefore, dosage adjustment of oral hypoglycemic agent may be required). Products include:

Avandamet Tablets 1373
Avandaryl Tablets 1379
Avandia Tablets 1384

Secobarbital Sodium (Potentiation of orthostatic hypotension).

No products indexed under this heading.

Sodium Nitroprusside (Hydrochlorothiazide may add to or potentiate the therapeutic effect of other antihypertensive drugs).

No products indexed under this heading.

Sotalol Hydrochloride (Hydrochlorothiazide may add to or potentiate the therapeutic effect of other antihypertensive drugs).

No products indexed under this heading.

Spirapril Hydrochloride (Hydrochlorothiazide may add to or potentiate the therapeutic effect of other antihypertensive drugs).

No products indexed under this heading.

Sufentanil Citrate (Potentiation of orthostatic hypotension).

No products indexed under this heading.

Sulindac (Co-administration with non-steroidal anti-inflammatory agents may reduce the natriuretic and antihypertensive effects of thiazides). Products include:

Clinoril Tablets 1924

Telmisartan (Hydrochlorothiazide may add to or potentiate the therapeutic effect of other antihypertensive drugs). Products include:

Micardis Tablets 854
Micardis HCT Tablets 856

Terazosin Hydrochloride (Hydrochlorothiazide may add to or potentiate the therapeutic effect of other antihypertensive drugs). Products include:

Hytrin Capsules 471

Thiamylal Sodium (Potentiation of orthostatic hypotension).

No products indexed under this heading.

Timolol Maleate (Hydrochlorothiazide may add to or potentiate the therapeutic effect of other antihypertensive drugs). Products include:

Blocadren Tablets 1916
Cosopt Sterile Ophthalmic Solution.. 1931
Timolide Tablets 2086
Timoptic Sterile Ophthalmic Solution.. 2088
Timoptic in Ocudose 2091
Timoptic-XE Sterile Ophthalmic Gel Forming Solution 2092

Tolazamide (Hydrochlorothiazide may cause hyperglycemia, therefore, dosage adjustment of oral hypoglycemic agent may be required).

No products indexed under this heading.

Tolbutamide (In vitro studies show significant inhibition of the formation of oxidized irbesartan metabolites with the known cytochrome CYP 2C9 substrate/inhibitor, tolbutamide; hydrochlorothiazide may cause hyperglycemia, therefore dosage adjustment of oral hypoglycemic agent may be required).

No products indexed under this heading.

Tolmetin Sodium (Co-administration with non-steroidal anti-inflammatory agents may reduce the natriuretic and antihypertensive effects of thiazides).

No products indexed under this heading.

Torsemide (Hydrochlorothiazide may add to or potentiate the therapeutic effect of other antihypertensive drugs). Products include:

Demadex Injection 2759
Demadex Tablets 2759

Trandolapril (Hydrochlorothiazide may add to or potentiate the therapeutic effect of other antihypertensive drugs). Products include:

Mavik Tablets 486
Tarka Tablets 524

Triamcinolone (Co-administration with corticosteroids intensifies electrolyte depletion particularly hypokalemia).

No products indexed under this heading.

Triamcinolone Acetonide (Co-administration with corticosteroids intensifies electrolyte depletion particularly hypokalemia). Products include:

Azmacort Inhalation Aerosol 1726
Nasacort AQ Nasal Spray 2922

Triamcinolone Diacetate (Co-administration with corticosteroids intensifies electrolyte depletion particularly hypokalemia).

No products indexed under this heading.

Triamcinolone Hexacetonide (Co-administration with corticosteroids intensifies electrolyte depletion particularly hypokalemia).

No products indexed under this heading.

Trimethaphan Camsylate (Hydrochlorothiazide may add to or potentiate the therapeutic effect of other antihypertensive drugs).

No products indexed under this heading.

Troglitazone (Hydrochlorothiazide may cause hyperglycemia, therefore, dosage adjustment of oral hypoglycemic agent may be required).

No products indexed under this heading.

Tubocurarine Chloride (Possible increased responsiveness to the muscle relaxants).

No products indexed under this heading.

Valdecoxib (Co-administration with non-steroidal anti-inflammatory agents may reduce the natriuretic and antihypertensive effects of thiazides).

No products indexed under this heading.

Valsartan (Hydrochlorothiazide may add to or potentiate the therapeutic effect of other antihypertensive drugs). Products include:

Diovan Tablets 2193
Diovan HCT Tablets 2196

Vecuronium Bromide (Possible increased responsiveness to the muscle relaxants).

No products indexed under this heading.

Verapamil Hydrochloride (Hydrochlorothiazide may add to or potentiate the therapeutic effect of other antihypertensive drugs). Products include:

Covera-HS Tablets 3139
Tarka Tablets 524
Verelan PM Extended-Release Capsules, Controlled-Onset........... 3106

Food Interactions

Alcohol (Potentiation of orthostatic hypotension).

AVANDAMET TABLETS

(Metformin Hydrochloride, Rosiglitazone Maleate)....................... 1373

May interact with cationic drugs that are eliminated by renal tubular, calcium channel blockers, corticosteroids, cytochrome p450 2c8 inducers (selected), cytochrome p450 2c8 inhibitors (selected), diuretics, estrogens, insulin, oral contraceptives, phenothiazines, phenytoin, quinidine, radiographic iodinated contrast media, sulfonylureas, sympathomimetics, thiazides, thyroid preparations, and certain other agents. Compounds in these categories include:

Albuterol (Certain drugs, such as sympathomimetics, tend to produce hyperglycemia and may lead to loss of glycemic control). Products include:

Proventil Inhalation Aerosol 3053

Albuterol Sulfate (Certain drugs, such as sympathomimetics, tend to produce hyperglycemia and may lead to loss of glycemic control). Products include:

AccuNeb Inhalation Solution 1055
Combivent Inhalation Aerosol 847
DuoNeb Inhalation Solution 1058
ProAir HFA Inhalation Aerosol 3300

Proventil Inhalation Solution 0.083%........ 3055
Proventil HFA Inhalation Aerosol........ 3056
Ventolin HFA Inhalation Aerosol........ 1600
VoSpire ER Tablets........ 1052

Amiloride Hydrochloride (Potential for loss of glycemic control; theoretical potential for interaction with metformin by competing for common renal tubular transport system). Products include:
Midamor Tablets........ 2026
Moduretic Tablets........ 2028

Amlodipine Besylate (Certain drugs, such as calcium channel blockers, tend to produce hyperglycemia and may lead to loss of glycemic control). Products include:
Caduet Tablets........ 2508
Lotrel Capsules........ 2249
Norvasc Tablets........ 2545

Anastrozole (An inhibitor of CYP2C8 may increase the AUC of rosiglitazone). Products include:
Arimidex Tablets........ 673

Bendroflumethiazide (Certain drugs, such as thiazides and other diuretics, tend to produce hyperglycemia and may lead to loss of glycemic control).
No products indexed under this heading.

Bepridil Hydrochloride (Certain drugs, such as calcium channel blockers, tend to produce hyperglycemia and may lead to loss of glycemic control).
No products indexed under this heading.

Betamethasone Acetate (Certain drugs, such as corticosteroids, tend to produce hyperglycemia and may lead to loss of glycemic control).
No products indexed under this heading.

Betamethasone Sodium Phosphate (Certain drugs, such as corticosteroids, tend to produce hyperglycemia and may lead to loss of glycemic control).
No products indexed under this heading.

Bumetanide (Certain drugs, such as diuretics, tend to produce hyperglycemia and may lead to loss of glycemic control). Products include:
Bumex Tablets........ 2746

Carbamazepine (An inducer of CYP2C8 may decrease the AUC of rosiglitazone). Products include:
Carbatrol Capsules........ 3171
Equetro Extended-Release Capsules........ 3180
Tegretol/Tegretol-XR........ 2295

Chlorothiazide (Certain drugs, such as thiazides and other diuretics, tend to produce hyperglycemia and may lead to loss of glycemic control). Products include:
Diuril Oral Suspension........ 1954

Chlorothiazide Sodium (Certain drugs, such as thiazides and other diuretics, tend to produce hyperglycemia and may lead to loss of glycemic control). Products include:
Diuril Sodium Intravenous........ 2467

Chlorotrianisene (Certain drugs, such as estrogens, tend to produce hyperglycemia and may lead to loss of glycemic control).
No products indexed under this heading.

Chlorpromazine (Certain drugs, such as phenothiazines, tend to produce hyperglycemia and may lead to loss of glycemic control).
No products indexed under this heading.

Chlorpromazine Hydrochloride (Certain drugs, such as phenothiazines, tend to produce hyperglycemia and may lead to loss of glycemic control).
No products indexed under this heading.

Chlorpropamide (An increased incidence of heart failure has been observed when rosiglitazone was added to a sulfonylurea or to a sulfonylurea plus metformin).
No products indexed under this heading.

Chlorthalidone (Certain drugs, such as diuretics, tend to produce hyperglycemia and may lead to loss of glycemic control). Products include:
Clorpres Tablets........ 2153

Cimetidine (Co-administered with oral cimetidine may increase peak metformin plasma and whole blood concentrations by 60% and a 40% increase in plasma and whole blood metformin AUC). Products include:
Tagamet HB 200 Tablets........ 664

Cimetidine Hydrochloride (An inhibitor of CYP2C8 may increase the AUC of rosiglitazone).
No products indexed under this heading.

Cortisone Acetate (Certain drugs, such as corticosteroids, tend to produce hyperglycemia and may lead to loss of glycemic control).
No products indexed under this heading.

Desogestrel (Certain drugs, such as oral contraceptives, tend to produce hyperglycemia and may lead to loss of glycemic control). Products include:
Mircette Tablets........ 1066

Dexamethasone (Certain drugs, such as corticosteroids, tend to produce hyperglycemia and may lead to loss of glycemic control). Products include:
Ciprodex Otic Suspension........ 559
Decadron Tablets........ 1951
TobraDex Ophthalmic Ointment........ 562
TobraDex Ophthalmic Suspension........ 563

Dexamethasone Acetate (Certain drugs, such as corticosteroids, tend to produce hyperglycemia and may lead to loss of glycemic control).
No products indexed under this heading.

Dexamethasone Sodium Phosphate (Certain drugs, such as corticosteroids, tend to produce hyperglycemia and may lead to loss of glycemic control).
No products indexed under this heading.

Diatrizoate Meglumine (Potential for acute alteration of renal function; metformin should be temporarily withheld in patients undergoing radiologic studies involving parenteral iodinated contrast material).
No products indexed under this heading.

Diatrizoate Sodium (Potential for acute alteration of renal function; metformin should be temporarily withheld in patients undergoing radiologic studies involving parenteral iodinated contrast material).
No products indexed under this heading.

Dienestrol (Certain drugs, such as estrogens, tend to produce hyperglycemia and may lead to loss of glycemic control).
No products indexed under this heading.

Diethylstilbestrol (Certain drugs, such as estrogens, tend to produce hyperglycemia and may lead to loss of glycemic control).
No products indexed under this heading.

Digoxin (Theoretical potential for interaction with metformin by competing for common renal tubular transport system). Products include:
Lanoxicaps Capsules........ 1490
Lanoxin Injection........ 1494
Lanoxin Injection Pediatric........ 1497
Lanoxin Tablets........ 1500

Diltiazem Hydrochloride (Certain drugs, such as calcium channel blockers, tend to produce hyperglycemia and may lead to loss of glycemic control). Products include:
Cardizem LA Extended Release Tablets........ 1728
Tiazac Capsules........ 1201

Dobutamine Hydrochloride (Certain drugs, such as sympathomimetics, tend to produce hyperglycemia and may lead to loss of glycemic control).
No products indexed under this heading.

Dopamine Hydrochloride (Certain drugs, such as sympathomimetics, tend to produce hyperglycemia and may lead to loss of glycemic control).
No products indexed under this heading.

Ephedrine Hydrochloride (Certain drugs, such as sympathomimetics, tend to produce hyperglycemia and may lead to loss of glycemic control).
No products indexed under this heading.

Ephedrine Sulfate (Certain drugs, such as sympathomimetics, tend to produce hyperglycemia and may lead to loss of glycemic control).
No products indexed under this heading.

Ephedrine Tannate (Certain drugs, such as sympathomimetics, tend to produce hyperglycemia and may lead to loss of glycemic control).
No products indexed under this heading.

Epinephrine (Certain drugs, such as sympathomimetics, tend to produce hyperglycemia and may lead to loss of glycemic control). Products include:
EpiPen........ 1061
Primatene Mist........ 719
Twinject 0.15........ 3379
Twinject 0.3........ 3378

Epinephrine Bitartrate (Certain drugs, such as sympathomimetics, tend to produce hyperglycemia and may lead to loss of glycemic control).
No products indexed under this heading.

Epinephrine Hydrochloride (Certain drugs, such as sympathomimetics, tend to produce hyperglycemia and may lead to loss of glycemic control).
No products indexed under this heading.

Estradiol (Certain drugs, such as estrogens, tend to produce hyperglycemia and may lead to loss of glycemic control). Products include:
Angeliq Tablets........ 762
Climara Transdermal System........ 771
Climara Pro Transdermal System........ 776
Estrasorb Topical Emulsion........ 1147
Estring Vaginal Ring........ 2635
Menostar Transdermal System........ 782
Vagifem Tablets........ 2334

Estrogens, Conjugated (Certain drugs, such as estrogens, tend to produce hyperglycemia and may lead to loss of glycemic control). Products include:
Premarin Intravenous........ 3442
Premarin Tablets........ 3446
Premarin Vaginal Cream........ 3452
Premphase Tablets........ 3456
Prempro Tablets........ 3456

Estrogens, Esterified (Certain drugs, such as estrogens, tend to produce hyperglycemia and may lead to loss of glycemic control). Products include:
Estratest Tablets........ 3199
Estratest H.S. Tablets........ 3199

Estropipate (Certain drugs, such as estrogens, tend to produce hyperglycemia and may lead to loss of glycemic control).
No products indexed under this heading.

Ethacrynic Acid (Certain drugs, such as diuretics, tend to produce hyperglycemia and may lead to loss of glycemic control). Products include:
Edecrin Tablets........ 1959

Ethinyl Estradiol (Certain drugs, such as estrogens, tend to produce hyperglycemia and may lead to loss of glycemic control). Products include:
Mircette Tablets........ 1066
NuvaRing........ 2340
Ortho-Cyclen/Ortho Tri-Cyclen........ 2429
Ortho Evra Transdermal System........ 2417
Ortho Tri-Cyclen Lo Tablets........ 2436
Seasonique Tablets........ 1077
Yasmin 28 Tablets........ 796
Yaz Tablets........ 803

Ethiodized Oil (Potential for acute alteration of renal function; metformin should be temporarily withheld in patients undergoing radiologic studies involving parenteral iodinated contrast material).
No products indexed under this heading.

Ethynodiol Diacetate (Certain drugs, such as oral contraceptives, tend to produce hyperglycemia and may lead to loss of glycemic control).
No products indexed under this heading.

Felodipine (Certain drugs, such as calcium channel blockers, tend to produce hyperglycemia and may lead to loss of glycemic control).
No products indexed under this heading.

Fludrocortisone Acetate (Certain drugs, such as corticosteroids, tend to produce hyperglycemia and may lead to loss of glycemic control).
No products indexed under this heading.

IMPORTANT NOTE: Always consult each drug listing in the patient's regimen for possible interactions.

Fluphenazine Decanoate (Certain drugs, such as phenothiazines, tend to produce hyperglycemia and may lead to loss of glycemic control).
No products indexed under this heading.

Fluphenazine Enanthate (Certain drugs, such as phenothiazines, tend to produce hyperglycemia and may lead to loss of glycemic control).
No products indexed under this heading.

Fluphenazine Hydrochloride (Certain drugs, such as phenothiazines, tend to produce hyperglycemia and may lead to loss of glycemic control).
No products indexed under this heading.

Fosphenytoin Sodium (Certain drugs, such as phenytoin, tend to produce hyperglycemia and may lead to loss of glycemic control).
No products indexed under this heading.

Furosemide (Increases metformin plasma and blood Cmax by 22% and blood AUC by 15%; the Cmax and AUC of furosemide were 31% and 12% smaller when co-administered; potential for loss of glycemic control). Products include:
Furosemide Tablets ... 2154

Gadopentetate Dimeglumine (Potential for acute alteration of renal function; metformin should be temporarily withheld in patients undergoing radiologic studies involving parenteral iodinated contrast material).
No products indexed under this heading.

Gemfibrozil (Concomitant administration of gemfibrozil (600 mg bid), an inhibitor of CYP2C8, and rosiglitazone (4 mg qd) for 7 days increased rosiglitazone AUC by 127%, compared to administration of rosiglitazone (4 mg qd) alone).
No products indexed under this heading.

Glimepiride (An increased incidence of heart failure has been observed when rosiglitazone was added to a sulfonylurea or to a sulfonylurea plus metformin). Products include:
Avandaryl Tablets ... 1379
Duetact Tablets ... 3226

Glipizide (An increased incidence of heart failure has been observed when rosiglitazone was added to a sulfonylurea or to a sulfonylurea plus metformin).
No products indexed under this heading.

Glyburide (Decrease in glyburide AUC and Cmax have been observed, but were highly variable).
No products indexed under this heading.

Hydrochlorothiazide (Certain drugs, such as thiazides and other diuretics, tend to produce hyperglycemia and may lead to loss of glycemic control). Products include:
Aldoril Tablets ... 1910
Atacand HCT ... 651
Avalide Tablets ... 888
Avalide Tablets ... 2874
Benicar HCT Tablets ... 1044
Diovan HCT Tablets ... 2196
Dyazide Capsules ... 1423
Hyzaar 50-12.5 Tablets ... 1990
Hyzaar 100-12.5 Tablets ... 1990
Hyzaar 100-25 Tablets ... 1990
Lopressor HCT 50/25 Tablets ... 2241
Lopressor HCT 100/25 Tablets ... 2241
Lopressor HCT 100/50 Tablets ... 2241
Lotensin HCT Tablets ... 2246
Micardis HCT Tablets ... 856
Moduretic Tablets ... 2028
Prinzide Tablets ... 2056
Teveten HCT Tablets ... 1737
Timolide Tablets ... 2086
Uniretic Tablets ... 3100

Hydrocortisone (Certain drugs, such as corticosteroids, tend to produce hyperglycemia and may lead to loss of glycemic control). Products include:
Colocort Rectal Suspension, USP (Retention) 100 mg/60 mL ... 2476
Hydrocortone Tablets ... 1989
Preparation H Hydrocortisone Cream ... ▣646

Hydrocortisone Acetate (Certain drugs, such as corticosteroids, tend to produce hyperglycemia and may lead to loss of glycemic control). Products include:
Analpram-HC ... 1159
Pramosone ... 1161
ProctoFoam-HC ... 3099

Hydrocortisone Sodium Phosphate (Certain drugs, such as corticosteroids, tend to produce hyperglycemia and may lead to loss of glycemic control).
No products indexed under this heading.

Hydrocortisone Sodium Succinate (Certain drugs, such as corticosteroids, tend to produce hyperglycemia and may lead to loss of glycemic control).
No products indexed under this heading.

Hydroflumethiazide (Certain drugs, such as thiazides and other diuretics, tend to produce hyperglycemia and may lead to loss of glycemic control).
No products indexed under this heading.

Indapamide (Certain drugs, such as diuretics, tend to produce hyperglycemia and may lead to loss of glycemic control). Products include:
Indapamide Tablets ... 2156

Insulin, Human, Zinc Suspension (Co-administration of rosiglitazone with insulin has resulted in increased incidence of cardiac failure and other cardiovascular adverse events). Products include:
Humulin L, 100 Units ... 1794
Humulin U, 100 Units ... 1800

Insulin, Human NPH (Co-administration of rosiglitazone with insulin has resulted in increased incidence of cardiac failure and other cardiovascular adverse events). Products include:
Humulin N, 100 Units ... 1795
Humulin N Pen ... 1797

Insulin, Human Regular (Co-administration of rosiglitazone with insulin has resulted in increased incidence of cardiac failure and other cardiovascular adverse events). Products include:
Humulin R, 100 Units ... 1798

Insulin, Human Regular and Human NPH Mixture (Co-administration of rosiglitazone with insulin has resulted in increased incidence of cardiac failure and other cardiovascular adverse events). Products include:
Humulin 50/50, 100 Units ... 1791
Humulin 70/30 Pen ... 1793

Insulin, NPH (Co-administration of rosiglitazone with insulin has resulted in increased incidence of cardiac failure and other cardiovascular adverse events).
No products indexed under this heading.

Insulin, Regular (Co-administration of rosiglitazone with insulin has resulted in increased incidence of cardiac failure and other cardiovascular adverse events).
No products indexed under this heading.

Insulin, Zinc Crystals (Co-administration of rosiglitazone with insulin has resulted in increased incidence of cardiac failure and other cardiovascular adverse events).
No products indexed under this heading.

Insulin, Zinc Suspension (Co-administration of rosiglitazone with insulin has resulted in increased incidence of cardiac failure and other cardiovascular adverse events).
No products indexed under this heading.

Insulin Aspart, Human Regular (Co-administration of rosiglitazone with insulin has resulted in increased incidence of cardiac failure and other cardiovascular adverse events). Products include:
NovoLog Injection ... 2326

Insulin glargine (Co-administration of rosiglitazone with insulin has resulted in increased incidence of cardiac failure and other cardiovascular adverse events). Products include:
Lantus Injection ... 2909

Insulin Lispro, Human (Co-administration of rosiglitazone with insulin has resulted in increased incidence of cardiac failure and other cardiovascular adverse events). Products include:
Humalog-Pen ... 1781
Humalog Mix 50/50-Pen ... 1783
Humalog Mix 75/25-Pen ... 1785

Insulin Lispro Protamine, Human (Co-administration of rosiglitazone with insulin has resulted in increased incidence of cardiac failure and other cardiovascular adverse events). Products include:
Humalog Mix 50/50-Pen ... 1783
Humalog Mix 75/25-Pen ... 1785

Iodamide Meglumine (Potential for acute alteration of renal function; metformin should be temporarily withheld in patients undergoing radiologic studies involving parenteral iodinated contrast material).
No products indexed under this heading.

Iohexol (Potential for acute alteration of renal function; metformin should be temporarily withheld in patients undergoing radiologic studies involving parenteral iodinated contrast material).
No products indexed under this heading.

Iopamidol (Potential for acute alteration of renal function; metformin should be temporarily withheld in patients undergoing radiologic studies involving parenteral iodinated contrast material).
No products indexed under this heading.

Iopanoic Acid (Potential for acute alteration of renal function; metformin should be temporarily withheld in patients undergoing radiologic studies involving parenteral iodinated contrast material).
No products indexed under this heading.

Iothalamate Meglumine (Potential for acute alteration of renal function; metformin should be temporarily withheld in patients undergoing radiologic studies involving parenteral iodinated contrast material).
No products indexed under this heading.

Ioxaglate Meglumine (Potential for acute alteration of renal function; metformin should be temporarily withheld in patients undergoing radiologic studies involving parenteral iodinated contrast material).
No products indexed under this heading.

Ioxaglate Sodium (Potential for acute alteration of renal function; metformin should be temporarily withheld in patients undergoing radiologic studies involving parenteral iodinated contrast material).
No products indexed under this heading.

Isoniazid (Certain drugs, such as isoniazid, tend to produce hyperglycemia and may lead to loss of glycemic control).
No products indexed under this heading.

Isoproterenol Hydrochloride (Certain drugs, such as sympathomimetics, tend to produce hyperglycemia and may lead to loss of glycemic control).
No products indexed under this heading.

Isoproterenol Sulfate (Certain drugs, such as sympathomimetics, tend to produce hyperglycemia and may lead to loss of glycemic control).
No products indexed under this heading.

Isradipine (Certain drugs, such as calcium channel blockers, tend to produce hyperglycemia and may lead to loss of glycemic control). Products include:
DynaCirc CR Tablets ... 2721

Levalbuterol Hydrochloride (Certain drugs, such as sympathomimetics, tend to produce hyperglycemia and may lead to loss of glycemic control). Products include:
Xopenex Inhalation Solution ... 3146
Xopenex Inhalation Solution Concentrate ... 3150

Levonorgestrel (Certain drugs, such as oral contraceptives, tend to produce hyperglycemia and may lead to loss of glycemic control). Products include:
Climara Pro Transdermal System ... 776
Mirena Intrauterine System ... 787
Plan B Tablets ... 1076
Seasonique Tablets ... 1077

Levothyroxine Sodium (Certain drugs, such as thyroid products, tend to produce hyperglycemia and may lead to loss of glycemic control). Products include:
Levothroid Tablets ... 1186
Levoxyl Tablets ... 1712
Synthroid Tablets ... 520
Westhroid Tablets ... 3403

Liothyronine Sodium (Certain drugs, such as thyroid products, tend to produce hyperglycemia and may lead to loss of glycemic control). Products include:

Liotrix (Certain drugs, such as thyroid products, tend to produce hyperglycemia and may lead to loss of glycemic control). Products include:

Mesoridazine Besylate (Certain drugs, such as phenothiazines, tend to produce hyperglycemia and may lead to loss of glycemic control).

No products indexed under this heading.

Mestranol (Certain drugs, such as oral contraceptives, tend to produce hyperglycemia and may lead to loss of glycemic control).

No products indexed under this heading.

Metaproterenol Sulfate (Certain drugs, such as sympathomimetics, tend to produce hyperglycemia and may lead to loss of glycemic control). Products include:

Metaraminol Bitartrate (Certain drugs, such as sympathomimetics, tend to produce hyperglycemia and may lead to loss of glycemic control).

No products indexed under this heading.

Methotrimeprazine (Certain drugs, such as phenothiazines, tend to produce hyperglycemia and may lead to loss of glycemic control).

No products indexed under this heading.

Methoxamine Hydrochloride (Certain drugs, such as sympathomimetics, tend to produce hyperglycemia and may lead to loss of glycemic control).

No products indexed under this heading.

Methyclothiazide (Certain drugs, such as thiazides and other diuretics, tend to produce hyperglycemia and may lead to loss of glycemic control).

No products indexed under this heading.

Methylprednisolone Acetate (Certain drugs, such as corticosteroids, tend to produce hyperglycemia and may lead to loss of glycemic control). Products include:

Methylprednisolone Sodium Succinate (Certain drugs, such as corticosteroids, tend to produce hyperglycemia and may lead to loss of glycemic control).

No products indexed under this heading.

Metolazone (Certain drugs, such as diuretics, tend to produce hyperglycemia and may lead to loss of glycemic control).

No products indexed under this heading.

Mibefradil Dihydrochloride (Certain drugs, such as calcium channel blockers, tend to produce hyperglycemia and may lead to loss of glycemic control).

No products indexed under this heading.

Morphine Sulfate (Theoretical potential for interaction with met-

formin by competing for common renal tubular transport system). Products include:

Niacin (Certain drugs, such as niacin, tend to produce hyperglycemia and may lead to loss of glycemic control). Products include:

Nicardipine Hydrochloride (Certain drugs, such as calcium channel blockers, tend to produce hyperglycemia and may lead to loss of glycemic control). Products include:

Nicotinic Acid (Potential for loss of glycemic control).

No products indexed under this heading.

Nifedipine (Enhances the absorption of metformin by increasing plasma metformin Cmax and AUC; potential for loss of glycemic control). Products include:

Nimodipine (Certain drugs, such as calcium channel blockers, tend to produce hyperglycemia and may lead to loss of glycemic control). Products include:

Nisoldipine (Certain drugs, such as calcium channel blockers, tend to produce hyperglycemia and may lead to loss of glycemic control). Products include:

Norepinephrine Bitartrate (Certain drugs, such as sympathomimetics, tend to produce hyperglycemia and may lead to loss of glycemic control).

No products indexed under this heading.

Norethindrone (Certain drugs, such as oral contraceptives, tend to produce hyperglycemia and may lead to loss of glycemic control). Products include:

Norethynodrel (Certain drugs, such as oral contraceptives, tend to produce hyperglycemia and may lead to loss of glycemic control).

No products indexed under this heading.

Norgestimate (Certain drugs, such as oral contraceptives, tend to produce hyperglycemia and may lead to loss of glycemic control). Products include:

Norgestrel (Certain drugs, such as oral contraceptives, tend to produce hyperglycemia and may lead to loss of glycemic control).

No products indexed under this heading.

Omeprazole (An inhibitor of CYP2C8 may increase the AUC of rosiglitazone). Products include:

Perphenazine (Certain drugs, such as phenothiazines, tend to produce hyperglycemia and may lead to loss of glycemic control).

No products indexed under this heading.

Phenobarbital (An inducer of CYP2C8 may decrease the AUC of rosiglitazone). Products include:

Phenylephrine Bitartrate (Certain drugs, such as sympathomimetics, tend to produce hyperglycemia and may lead to loss of glycemic control).

No products indexed under this heading.

Phenylephrine Hydrochloride (Certain drugs, such as sympathomimetics, tend to produce hyperglycemia and may lead to loss of glycemic control). Products include:

Phenylephrine Tannate (Certain drugs, such as sympathomimetics, tend to produce hyperglycemia and may lead to loss of glycemic control).

No products indexed under this heading.

Phenylpropanolamine Hydrochloride (Certain drugs, such as sympathomimetics, tend to produce hyperglycemia and may lead to loss of glycemic control).

No products indexed under this heading.

Phenytoin (Certain drugs, such as phenytoin, tend to produce hyperglycemia and may lead to loss of glycemic control).

No products indexed under this heading.

Phenytoin Sodium (Certain drugs, such as phenytoin, tend to produce hyperglycemia and may lead to loss of glycemic control). Products include:

Pirbuterol Acetate (Certain drugs, such as sympathomimetics, tend to produce hyperglycemia and may lead to loss of glycemic control). Products include:

IMPORTANT NOTE: Always consult each drug listing in the patient's regimen for possible interactions.

Polyestradiol Phosphate (Certain drugs, such as estrogens, tend to produce hyperglycemia and may lead to loss of glycemic control).

No products indexed under this heading.

Polythiazide (Certain drugs, such as thiazides and other diuretics, tend to produce hyperglycemia and may lead to loss of glycemic control).

No products indexed under this heading.

Prednisolone Acetate (Certain drugs, such as corticosteroids, tend to produce hyperglycemia and may lead to loss of glycemic control). Products include:

Prednisolone Sodium Phosphate (Certain drugs, such as corticosteroids, tend to produce hyperglycemia and may lead to loss of glycemic control).

No products indexed under this heading.

Prednisolone Tebutate (Certain drugs, such as corticosteroids, tend to produce hyperglycemia and may lead to loss of glycemic control).

No products indexed under this heading.

Prednisone (Certain drugs, such as corticosteroids, tend to produce hyperglycemia and may lead to loss of glycemic control).

No products indexed under this heading.

Primidone (An inducer of CYP2C8 may decrease the AUC of rosiglitazone).

No products indexed under this heading.

Procainamide Hydrochloride (Theoretical potential for interaction with metformin by competing for common renal tubular transport system).

No products indexed under this heading.

Prochlorperazine (Certain drugs, such as phenothiazines, tend to produce hyperglycemia and may lead to loss of glycemic control).

No products indexed under this heading.

Promethazine Hydrochloride (Certain drugs, such as phenothiazines, tend to produce hyperglycemia and may lead to loss of glycemic control). Products include:

Pseudoephedrine Hydrochloride (Certain drugs, such as sympathomimetics, tend to produce hyperglycemia and may lead to loss of glycemic control). Products include:

Pseudoephedrine Sulfate (Certain drugs, such as sympathomimetics, tend to produce hyperglycemia and may lead to loss of glycemic control). Products include:

Quercetin (An inhibitor of CYP2C8 may increase the AUC of rosiglitazone).

No products indexed under this heading.

Quinestrol (Certain drugs, such as estrogens, tend to produce hyperglycemia and may lead to loss of glycemic control).

No products indexed under this heading.

Quinidine (Theoretical potential for interaction with metformin by competing for common renal tubular transport system).

No products indexed under this heading.

Quinidine Gluconate (Theoretical potential for interaction with metformin by competing for common renal tubular transport system).

No products indexed under this heading.

Quinidine Hydrochloride (Theoretical potential for interaction with metformin by competing for common renal tubular transport system).

No products indexed under this heading.

Quinidine Polygalacturonate (Theoretical potential for interaction with metformin by competing for common renal tubular transport system).

No products indexed under this heading.

Quinidine Sulfate (Theoretical potential for interaction with metformin by competing for common renal tubular transport system).

No products indexed under this heading.

Quinine Sulfate (Theoretical potential for interaction with metformin by competing for common renal tubular transport system).

No products indexed under this heading.

Ranitidine Hydrochloride (Theoretical potential for interaction with metformin by competing for common renal tubular transport system). Products include:

Rifabutin (An inducer of CYP2C8 may decrease the AUC of rosiglitazone).

No products indexed under this heading.

Rifampin (Rifampin administration (600 mg qd) an inducer of CYP2C8, for 6 days is reported to decrease rosiglitazone AUC by 66%, compared to administration of rosiglitazone (8 mg) alone).

No products indexed under this heading.

Salmeterol Xinafoate (Certain drugs, such as sympathomimetics, may lead to loss of glycemic control). Products include:

Spironolactone (Certain drugs, such as diuretics, tend to produce hyperglycemia and may lead to loss of glycemic control).

No products indexed under this heading.

Sulfaphenazole (An inhibitor of CYP2C8 may increase the AUC of rosiglitazone).

No products indexed under this heading.

Sulfinpyrazone (An inhibitor of CYP2C8 may increase the AUC of rosiglitazone).

No products indexed under this heading.

Terbutaline Sulfate (Certain drugs, such as sympathomimetics, tend to produce hyperglycemia and may lead to loss of glycemic control).

No products indexed under this heading.

Thioridazine Hydrochloride (Certain drugs, such as phenothiazines, tend to produce hyperglycemia and may lead to loss of glycemic control). Products include:

Thyroglobulin (Certain drugs, such as thyroid products, tend to produce hyperglycemia and may lead to loss of glycemic control).

No products indexed under this heading.

Thyroid (Certain drugs, such as thyroid products, tend to produce hyperglycemia and may lead to loss of glycemic control).

No products indexed under this heading.

Thyroxine (Certain drugs, such as thyroid products, tend to produce hyperglycemia and may lead to loss of glycemic control).

No products indexed under this heading.

Thyroxine Sodium (Certain drugs, such as thyroid products, tend to produce hyperglycemia and may lead to loss of glycemic control).

No products indexed under this heading.

Tolazamide (An increased incidence of heart failure has been observed when rosiglitazone was added to a sulfonylurea or to a sulfonylurea plus metformin).

No products indexed under this heading.

Tolbutamide (An increased incidence of heart failure has been observed when rosiglitazone was added to a sulfonylurea or to a sulfonylurea plus metformin).

No products indexed under this heading.

Torsemide (Certain drugs, such as diuretics, tend to produce hyperglycemia and may lead to loss of glycemic control). Products include:

Triamcinolone (Certain drugs, such as corticosteroids, tend to produce hyperglycemia and may lead to loss of glycemic control).

No products indexed under this heading.

Triamcinolone Acetonide (Certain drugs, such as corticosteroids, tend to produce hyperglycemia and may lead to loss of glycemic control). Products include:

Triamcinolone Diacetate (Certain drugs, such as corticosteroids, tend to produce hyperglycemia and may lead to loss of glycemic control).

No products indexed under this heading.

Triamcinolone Hexacetonide (Certain drugs, such as corticosteroids, tend to produce hyperglycemia and may lead to loss of glycemic control).

No products indexed under this heading.

Triamterene (Potential for loss of glycemic control; theoretical potential for interaction with metformin by competing for common renal tubular transport system). Products include:

Trifluoperazine Hydrochloride (Certain drugs, such as phenothiazines, tend to produce hyperglycemia and may lead to loss of glycemic control).

No products indexed under this heading.

Trimethoprim (An inhibitor of CYP2C8 may increase the AUC of rosiglitazone).

No products indexed under this heading.

Trimethoprim Hydrochloride (An inhibitor of CYP2C8 may increase the AUC of rosiglitazone).

No products indexed under this heading.

Trimethoprim Sulfate (Theoretical potential for interaction with metformin by competing for common renal tubular transport system). Products include:

Polytrim Ophthalmic Solution 574

Tyropanoate Sodium (Potential for acute alteration of renal function; metformin should be temporarily withheld in patients undergoing radiologic studies involving parenteral iodinated contrast material).
No products indexed under this heading.

Vancomycin Hydrochloride (Theoretical potential for interaction with metformin by competing for common renal tubular transport system). Products include:
Vancocin HCl Capsules, USP 3380

Verapamil Hydrochloride (Certain drugs, such as calcium channel blockers, tend to produce hyperglycemia and may lead to loss of glycemic control). Products include:
Covera-HS Tablets 3139
Tarka Tablets 524
Verelan PM Extended-Release Capsules, Controlled-Onset........... 3106

Food Interactions

Alcohol (Alcohol potentiates the effect of metformin on lactate metabolism; patients should be warned against excessive alcohol intake, acute or chronic).

Food, unspecified (Food decreases the extent and slightly delays the absorption of metformin).

AVANDARYL TABLETS

(Glimepiride, Rosiglitazone Maleate).. 1379

May interact with beta blockers, corticosteroids, oral anticoagulants, cytochrome p450 2c8 inducers (selected), cytochrome p450 2c8 inhibitors (selected), diuretics, estrogens, insulin, monoamine oxidase inhibitors, non-steroidal anti-inflammatory agents, oral contraceptives, phenothiazines, salicylates, sulfonamides, sympathomimetics, thiazides, thyroid preparations, and certain other agents. Compounds in these categories include:

Acebutolol Hydrochloride (May potentiate hypoglycemic action).
No products indexed under this heading.

Albuterol (Sympathomimetics tend to produce hyperglycemia and concurrent use may lead to loss of control). Products include:
Proventil Inhalation Aerosol 3053

Albuterol Sulfate (Sympathomimetics tend to produce hyperglycemia and concurrent use may lead to loss of control). Products include:
AccuNeb Inhalation Solution 1055
Combivent Inhalation Aerosol 847
DuoNeb Inhalation Solution 1058
ProAir HFA Inhalation Aerosol 3300
Proventil Inhalation Solution 0.083%...................................... 3055
Proventil HFA Inhalation Aerosol 3056
Ventolin HFA Inhalation Aerosol 1600
VoSpire ER Tablets 1052

Amiloride Hydrochloride (Diuretics tend to produce hyperglycemia and concurrent use may lead to loss of control). Products include:
Midamor Tablets 2026
Moduretic Tablets 2028

Anastrozole (An inhibitor of CYP2C8 may decrease the AUC of rosiglitazone. Therefore, if an inducer of CYP2C8 is started or stopped during treatment with rosiglitazone, changes in diabetes treatment may be needed upon clinical response). Products include:
Arimidex Tablets 673

Anisindione (May potentiate hypoglycemic action). Products include:
Miradon Tablets 3042

Aspirin (Co-administration of aspirin (1 g tid) led to a 34% decrease in the mean glimepiride AUC and, therefore, a 34% increase in the mean CL/f; no hypoglycemic symptoms were reported). Products include:
Aggrenox Capsules 822
Bayer Aspirin 744
BC Allergy Sinus Cold Powder 677
BC Headache Powder 677
Arthritis Strength BC Powder 677
BC Sinus Cold Powder 677
Excedrin Extra Strength Caplets/Tablets/Geltabs............ 684
Excedrin Migraine Caplets/Tablets/Geltabs............ 609
Goody's Body Pain Formula Powder... 684
Goody's Extra Strength Headache Powders.................... 611
Goody's Extra Strength Pain Relief Tablets............................ 685
Percodan Tablets 1132
St. Joseph 81 mg Aspirin Chewable and Enteric Coated Tablets 1869

Aspirin, Enteric Coated (May potentiate hypoglycemic action; clinical trials data indicate no evidence of significant adverse interaction with concurrent use).
No products indexed under this heading.

Aspirin Buffered (May potentiate hypoglycemic action; clinical trials data indicate no evidence of significant adverse interaction with concurrent use). Products include:
Bufferin Extra Strength Tablets 678
Bufferin Regular Strength Tablets ... 678

Atenolol (May potentiate hypoglycemic action).
No products indexed under this heading.

Bendroflumethiazide (Diuretics tend to produce hyperglycemia and concurrent use may lead to loss of control).
No products indexed under this heading.

Betamethasone Acetate (Corticosteroids tend to produce hyperglycemia and concurrent use may lead to loss of control).
No products indexed under this heading.

Betamethasone Sodium Phosphate (Corticosteroids tend to produce hyperglycemia and concurrent use may lead to loss of control).
No products indexed under this heading.

Betaxolol Hydrochloride (May potentiate hypoglycemic action). Products include:
Betoptic S Ophthalmic Suspension.................................. 558

Bisoprolol Fumarate (May potentiate hypoglycemic action).
No products indexed under this heading.

Bumetanide (Diuretics tend to produce hyperglycemia and concurrent use may lead to loss of control). Products include:
Bumex Tablets 2746

Carbamazepine (An inhibitor of CYP2C8 may decrease the AUC of rosiglitazone. Therefore, if an inducer of CYP2C8 is started or stopped during treatment with rosiglitazone, changes in diabetes treatment may be needed upon clinical response). Products include:
Carbatrol Capsules 3171
Equetro Extended-Release Capsules 3180
Tegretol/Tegretol-XR 2295

Carteolol Hydrochloride (May potentiate hypoglycemic action). Products include:
Carteolol Hydrochloride Ophthalmic Solution USP, 1%....... ⊙249

Celecoxib (May potentiate hypoglycemic action). Products include:
Celebrex Capsules 3134

Chloramphenicol (May potentiate hypoglycemic action).
No products indexed under this heading.

Chloramphenicol Palmitate (May potentiate hypoglycemic action).
No products indexed under this heading.

Chloramphenicol Sodium Succinate (May potentiate hypoglycemic action).
No products indexed under this heading.

Chlorothiazide (Diuretics tend to produce hyperglycemia and concurrent use may lead to loss of control). Products include:
Diuril Oral Suspension 1954

Chlorothiazide Sodium (Diuretics tend to produce hyperglycemia and concurrent use may lead to loss of control). Products include:
Diuril Sodium Intravenous 2467

Chlorotrianisene (Estrogens tend to produce hyperglycemia and concurrent use may lead to loss of control).
No products indexed under this heading.

Chlorpromazine (Phenothiazines tend to produce hyperglycemia and concurrent use may lead to loss of control).
No products indexed under this heading.

Chlorpromazine Hydrochloride (Phenothiazines tend to produce hyperglycemia and concurrent use may lead to loss of control).
No products indexed under this heading.

Chlorpropamide (May potentiate hypoglycemic action).
No products indexed under this heading.

Chlorthalidone (Diuretics tend to produce hyperglycemia and concurrent use may lead to loss of control). Products include:
Clorpres Tablets 2153

Choline Magnesium Trisalicylate (May potentiate hypoglycemic action; clinical trials data indicate no evidence of significant adverse interaction with concurrent use).
No products indexed under this heading.

Cimetidine (An inhibitor of CYP2C8 may decrease the AUC of rosiglitazone. Therefore, if an inducer of CYP2C8 is started or stopped during treatment with rosiglitazone, changes in diabetes treatment may be needed upon clinical response). Products include:
Tagamet HB 200 Tablets 664

Cimetidine Hydrochloride (An inhibitor of CYP2C8 may decrease the AUC of rosiglitazone. Therefore, if an inducer of CYP2C8 is started or stopped during treatment with rosiglitazone, changes in diabetes treatment may be needed upon clinical response).
No products indexed under this heading.

Cortisone Acetate (Corticosteroids tend to produce hyperglycemia and concurrent use may lead to loss of control).
No products indexed under this heading.

Desogestrel (Oral contraceptives tend to produce hyperglycemia and concurrent use may lead to loss of control). Products include:
Mircette Tablets 1066

Dexamethasone (Corticosteroids tend to produce hyperglycemia and concurrent use may lead to loss of control). Products include:
Ciprodex Otic Suspension 559
Decadron Tablets 1951
TobraDex Ophthalmic Ointment 562
TobraDex Ophthalmic Suspension ... 563

Dexamethasone Acetate (Corticosteroids tend to produce hyperglycemia and concurrent use may lead to loss of control).
No products indexed under this heading.

Dexamethasone Sodium Phosphate (Corticosteroids tend to produce hyperglycemia and concurrent use may lead to loss of control).
No products indexed under this heading.

Diclofenac Potassium (May potentiate hypoglycemic action).
No products indexed under this heading.

Diclofenac Sodium (May potentiate hypoglycemic action). Products include:
Arthrotec Tablets 3129
Voltaren Ophthalmic Solution 2309
Voltaren Tablets 2307
Voltaren-XR Tablets 2310

Dicumarol (May potentiate hypoglycemic action).
No products indexed under this heading.

Dienestrol (Estrogens tend to produce hyperglycemia and concurrent use may lead to loss of control).
No products indexed under this heading.

Diethylstilbestrol (Estrogens tend to produce hyperglycemia and concurrent use may lead to loss of control).
No products indexed under this heading.

Diflunisal (May potentiate hypoglycemic action; clinical trials data indicate no evidence of significant adverse interaction with concurrent use). Products include:
Dolobid Tablets 1955

Dobutamine Hydrochloride (Sympathomimetics tend to produce hyperglycemia and concurrent use may lead to loss of control).
No products indexed under this heading.

Dopamine Hydrochloride (Sympathomimetics tend to produce hyperglycemia and concurrent use may lead to loss of control).
No products indexed under this heading.

Ephedrine Hydrochloride (Sympathomimetics tend to produce hyperglycemia and concurrent use may lead to loss of control).
No products indexed under this heading.

Ephedrine Sulfate (Sympathomimetics tend to produce hyperglycemia and concurrent use may lead to loss of control).
No products indexed under this heading.

Ephedrine Tannate (Sympathomimetics tend to produce hyperglycemia and concurrent use may lead to loss of control).
No products indexed under this heading.

Epinephrine (Sympathomimetics tend to produce hyperglycemia and concurrent use may lead to loss of control). Products include:
- EpiPen ... 1061
- Primatene Mist ... ▣ 719
- Twinject 0.15 ... 3379
- Twinject 0.3 ... 3378

Epinephrine Bitartrate (Sympathomimetics tend to produce hyperglycemia and concurrent use may lead to loss of control).
No products indexed under this heading.

Epinephrine Hydrochloride (Sympathomimetics tend to produce hyperglycemia and concurrent use may lead to loss of control).
No products indexed under this heading.

Esmolol Hydrochloride (May potentiate hypoglycemic action).
No products indexed under this heading.

Estradiol (Estrogens tend to produce hyperglycemia and concurrent use may lead to loss of control). Products include:
- Angeliq Tablets ... 762
- Climara Transdermal System ... 771
- Climara Pro Transdermal System ... 776
- Estrasorb Topical Emulsion ... 1147
- Estring Vaginal Ring ... 2635
- Menostar Transdermal System ... 782
- Vagifem Tablets ... 2334

Estrogens, Conjugated (Estrogens tend to produce hyperglycemia and concurrent use may lead to loss of control). Products include:
- Premarin Intravenous ... 3442
- Premarin Tablets ... 3446
- Premarin Vaginal Cream ... 3452
- Premphase Tablets ... 3456
- Prempro Tablets ... 3456

Estrogens, Esterified (Estrogens tend to produce hyperglycemia and concurrent use may lead to loss of control). Products include:
- Estratest Tablets ... 3199
- Estratest H.S. Tablets ... 3199

Estropipate (Estrogens tend to produce hyperglycemia and concurrent use may lead to loss of control).
No products indexed under this heading.

Ethacrynic Acid (Diuretics tend to produce hyperglycemia and concurrent use may lead to loss of control). Products include:
- Edecrin Tablets ... 1959

Ethinyl Estradiol (Estrogens tend to produce hyperglycemia and concurrent use may lead to loss of control). Products include:
- Mircette Tablets ... 1066
- NuvaRing ... 2340
- Ortho-Cyclen/Ortho Tri-Cyclen ... 2429
- Ortho Evra Transdermal System ... 2417
- Ortho Tri-Cyclen Lo Tablets ... 2436
- Seasonique Tablets ... 1077
- Yasmin 28 Tablets ... 796
- Yaz Tablets ... 803

Ethynodiol Diacetate (Oral contraceptives tend to produce hyperglycemia and concurrent use may lead to loss of control).
No products indexed under this heading.

Etodolac (May potentiate hypoglycemic action).
No products indexed under this heading.

Fenoprofen Calcium (May potentiate hypoglycemic action). Products include:
- Nalfon Capsules ... 2502

Fludrocortisone Acetate (Corticosteroids tend to produce hyperglycemia and concurrent use may lead to loss of control).
No products indexed under this heading.

Fluphenazine Decanoate (Phenothiazines tend to produce hyperglycemia and concurrent use may lead to loss of control).
No products indexed under this heading.

Fluphenazine Enanthate (Phenothiazines tend to produce hyperglycemia and concurrent use may lead to loss of control).
No products indexed under this heading.

Fluphenazine Hydrochloride (Phenothiazines tend to produce hyperglycemia and concurrent use may lead to loss of control).
No products indexed under this heading.

Flurbiprofen (May potentiate hypoglycemic action).
No products indexed under this heading.

Furosemide (Diuretics tend to produce hyperglycemia and concurrent use may lead to loss of control). Products include:
- Furosemide Tablets ... 2154

Gemfibrozil (Concomitant administration of gemfibrozil (600 mg twice daily), an inhibitor of CYP2C8 and rosiglitazone (4 mg once daily) for 7 days increased rosiglitazone AUC by 127% compared to the administration of rosiglitazone (4 mg once daily) alone. Given the potential for dose-related adverse events with rosiglitazone, a decrease in the dose of rosiglitazone may be needed when gemfibrozil is introduced).
No products indexed under this heading.

Glipizide (May potentiate hypoglycemic action).
No products indexed under this heading.

Glyburide (Rosiglitazone (2 mg twice daily) taken concomitantly with glyburide (3.75 to 10 mg/day) for 7 days did not alter the mean steady-state 24-hour plasma glucose concentrations in diabetic patients stabilized on glyburide therapy. Repeat doses of rosiglitazone (8 mg once daily) for 8 days in healthy adult Caucasian subjects caused a decrease in glyburide AUC (32%) and Cmax (35%). In Japanese subjects, glyburide AUC (14%) and Cmax (31%) slightly increased following co-administration of rosiglitazone).
No products indexed under this heading.

Hydrochlorothiazide (Diuretics tend to produce hyperglycemia and concurrent use may lead to loss of control). Products include:
- Aldoril Tablets ... 1910
- Atacand HCT ... 651
- Avalide Tablets ... 888
- Avalide Tablets ... 2874
- Benicar HCT Tablets ... 1044
- Diovan HCT Tablets ... 2196
- Dyazide Capsules ... 1423
- Hyzaar 50-12.5 Tablets ... 1990
- Hyzaar 100-12.5 Tablets ... 1990
- Hyzaar 100-25 Tablets ... 1990
- Lopressor HCT 50/25 Tablets ... 2241
- Lopressor HCT 100/25 Tablets ... 2241
- Lopressor HCT 100/50 Tablets ... 2241
- Lotensin HCT Tablets ... 2246
- Micardis HCT Tablets ... 856
- Moduretic Tablets ... 2028
- Prinzide Tablets ... 2056
- Teveten HCT Tablets ... 1737
- Timolide Tablets ... 2086
- Uniretic Tablets ... 3100

Hydrocortisone (Corticosteroids tend to produce hyperglycemia and concurrent use may lead to loss of control). Products include:
- Colocort Rectal Suspension, USP (Retention) 100 mg/60 mL ... 2476
- Hydrocortone Tablets ... 1989
- Preparation H Hydrocortisone Cream ... ▣ 646

Hydrocortisone Acetate (Corticosteroids tend to produce hyperglycemia and concurrent use may lead to loss of control). Products include:
- Analpram-HC ... 1159
- Pramosone ... 1161
- ProctoFoam-HC ... 3099

Hydrocortisone Sodium Phosphate (Corticosteroids tend to produce hyperglycemia and concurrent use may lead to loss of control).
No products indexed under this heading.

Hydrocortisone Sodium Succinate (Corticosteroids tend to produce hyperglycemia and concurrent use may lead to loss of control).
No products indexed under this heading.

Hydroflumethiazide (Diuretics tend to produce hyperglycemia and concurrent use may lead to loss of control).
No products indexed under this heading.

Ibuprofen (May potentiate hypoglycemic action). Products include:
- Advil Allergy Sinus Caplets ... ▣ 770
- Advil ... ▣ 674
- Children's Advil Oral Suspension ... ▣ 603
- Children's Advil Chewable Tablets ... ▣ 603
- Advil Cold & Sinus ... ▣ 723
- Infants' Advil Concentrated Drops ... ▣ 604
- Infants' Advil Concentrated Drops - White Grape (Dye-Free) ... ▣ 604
- Junior Strength Advil Swallow Tablets ... ▣ 605
- Advil Migraine Liquigels ... ▣ 608
- Advil Multi-Symptom Cold Caplets ... ▣ 770
- Advil PM Caplets ... ▣ 615
- Motrin IB Tablets and Caplets ... 1866
- Children's Motrin Oral Suspension ... 1867
- Children's Motrin Non-Staining Dye-Free Oral Suspension ... 1867
- Children's Motrin Cold Oral Suspension ... 1867
- Infants' Motrin Concentrated Drops ... 1867
- Infants' Motrin Non-Staining Dye-Free Concentrated Drops ... 1867
- Junior Strength Motrin Caplets and Chewable Tablets ... 1867
- Vicoprofen Tablets ... 539

Indapamide (Diuretics tend to produce hyperglycemia and concurrent use may lead to loss of control). Products include:
- Indapamide Tablets ... 2156

Indomethacin (May potentiate hypoglycemic action). Products include:
- Indocin ... 1995

Indomethacin Sodium Trihydrate (May potentiate hypoglycemic action). Products include:
- Indocin I.V. ... 2465

Insulin, Human, Zinc Suspension (Co-administration of glimepiride with insulin may increase the potential for hypoglycemia. Co-administration of rosiglitazone with insulin has resulted in increased incidence of cardiac failure and other cardiovascular adverse events). Products include:
- Humulin L, 100 Units ... 1794
- Humulin U, 100 Units ... 1800

Insulin, Human NPH (Co-administration of glimepiride with insulin may increase the potential for hypoglycemia. Co-administration of rosiglitazone with insulin has resulted in increased incidence of cardiac failure and other cardiovascular adverse events). Products include:
- Humulin N, 100 Units ... 1795
- Humulin N Pen ... 1797

Insulin, Human Regular (Co-administration of glimepiride with insulin may increase the potential for hypoglycemia. Co-administration of rosiglitazone with insulin has resulted in increased incidence of cardiac failure and other cardiovascular adverse events). Products include:
- Humulin R, 100 Units ... 1798

Insulin, Human Regular and Human NPH Mixture (Co-administration of glimepiride with insulin may increase the potential for hypoglycemia. Co-administration of rosiglitazone with insulin has resulted in increased incidence of cardiac failure and other cardiovascular adverse events). Products include:
- Humulin 50/50, 100 Units ... 1791
- Humulin 70/30 Pen ... 1793

Insulin, NPH (Co-administration of glimepiride with insulin may increase the potential for hypoglycemia. Co-administration of rosiglitazone with insulin has resulted in increased incidence of cardiac failure and other cardiovascular adverse events).
No products indexed under this heading.

Insulin, Regular (Co-administration of glimepiride with insulin may increase the potential for hypoglycemia. Co-administration of rosiglitazone with insulin has resulted in increased incidence of cardiac failure and other cardiovascular adverse events).
No products indexed under this heading.

Insulin, Zinc Crystals (Co-administration of glimepiride with insulin may increase the potential for hypoglycemia. Co-administration of rosiglitazone with insulin has resulted in increased incidence of cardiac failure and other cardiovascular adverse events).
No products indexed under this heading.

Insulin, Zinc Suspension (Co-administration of glimepiride with insulin may increase the potential for hypoglycemia. Co-administration of rosiglitazone with insulin has resulted in increased incidence of cardiac failure and other cardiovascular adverse events).
No products indexed under this heading.

Insulin Aspart, Human Regular (Co-administration of glimepiride with insulin may increase the potential for hypoglycemia. Co-administration of rosiglitazone with insulin has resulted in increased incidence of cardiac failure and other cardiovascular adverse events). Products include:
NovoLog Injection 2326

Insulin glargine (Co-administration of glimepiride with insulin may increase the potential for hypoglycemia. Co-administration of rosiglitazone with insulin has resulted in increased incidence of cardiac failure and other cardiovascular adverse events). Products include:
Lantus Injection 2909

Insulin Lispro, Human (Co-administration of glimepiride with insulin may increase the potential for hypoglycemia. Co-administration of rosiglitazone with insulin has resulted in increased incidence of cardiac failure and other cardiovascular adverse events). Products include:
Humalog-Pen 1781
Humalog Mix 50/50-Pen 1783
Humalog Mix 75/25-Pen 1785

Insulin Lispro Protamine, Human (Co-administration of glimepiride with insulin may increase the potential for hypoglycemia. Co-administration of rosiglitazone with insulin has resulted in increased incidence of cardiac failure and other cardiovascular adverse events). Products include:
Humalog Mix 50/50-Pen 1783
Humalog Mix 75/25-Pen 1785

Isocarboxazid (May potentiate hypoglycemic action).
No products indexed under this heading.

Isoniazid (Isoniazid tends to produce hyperglycemia and concurrent use may lead to loss of control).
No products indexed under this heading.

Isoproterenol Hydrochloride (Sympathomimetics tend to produce hyperglycemia and concurrent use may lead to loss of control).
No products indexed under this heading.

Isoproterenol Sulfate (Sympathomimetics tend to produce hyperglycemia and concurrent use may lead to loss of control).
No products indexed under this heading.

Ketoprofen (May potentiate hypoglycemic action).
No products indexed under this heading.

Ketorolac Tromethamine (May potentiate hypoglycemic action). Products include:
Acular Ophthalmic Solution 565
Acular LS Ophthalmic Solution 566

Labetalol Hydrochloride (May potentiate hypoglycemic action).
No products indexed under this heading.

Levalbuterol Hydrochloride (Sympathomimetics tend to produce hyperglycemia and concurrent use may lead to loss of control). Products include:
Xopenex Inhalation Solution 3146
Xopenex Inhalation Solution Concentrate 3150

Levobunolol Hydrochloride (May potentiate hypoglycemic action). Products include:
Betagan Ophthalmic Solution, USP .. ⊙ 220

Levonorgestrel (Oral contraceptives tend to produce hyperglycemia and concurrent use may lead to loss of control). Products include:
Climara Pro Transdermal System 776
Mirena Intrauterine System 787
Plan B Tablets 1076
Seasonique Tablets 1077

Levothyroxine Sodium (Thyroid products tend to produce hyperglycemia and concurrent use may lead to loss of control). Products include:
Levothroid Tablets 1186
Levoxyl Tablets 1712
Synthroid Tablets 520
Westhroid Tablets 3403

Liothyronine Sodium (Thyroid products tend to produce hyperglycemia and concurrent use may lead to loss of control). Products include:
Cytomel Tablets 1710
Westhroid Tablets 3403

Liotrix (Thyroid products tend to produce hyperglycemia and concurrent use may lead to loss of control). Products include:
Thyrolar Tablets 1199

Magnesium Salicylate (May potentiate hypoglycemic action; clinical trials data indicate no evidence of significant adverse interaction with concurrent use).
No products indexed under this heading.

Meclofenamate Sodium (May potentiate hypoglycemic action).
No products indexed under this heading.

Mefenamic Acid (May potentiate hypoglycemic action).
No products indexed under this heading.

Meloxicam (May potentiate hypoglycemic action). Products include:
Mobic Oral Suspension 863
Mobic Tablets 863

Mesoridazine Besylate (Phenothiazines tend to produce hyperglycemia and concurrent use may lead to loss of control).
No products indexed under this heading.

Mestranol (Oral contraceptives tend to produce hyperglycemia and concurrent use may lead to loss of control).
No products indexed under this heading.

Metaproterenol Sulfate (Sympathomimetics tend to produce hyperglycemia and concurrent use may lead to loss of control). Products include:
Alupent Inhalation Aerosol 826

Metaraminol Bitartrate (Sympathomimetics tend to produce hyperglycemia and concurrent use may lead to loss of control).
No products indexed under this heading.

Metformin Hydrochloride (Co-administration of glimepiride with metformin may increase the potential for hypoglycemia). Products include:
ActoPlus Met Tablets 3214
Avandamet Tablets 1373
Fortamet Extended-Release Tablets 3115

Methotrimeprazine (Phenothiazines tend to produce hyperglycemia and concurrent use may lead to loss of control).
No products indexed under this heading.

Methoxamine Hydrochloride (Sympathomimetics tend to produce hyperglycemia and concurrent use may lead to loss of control).
No products indexed under this heading.

Methyclothiazide (Diuretics tend to produce hyperglycemia and concurrent use may lead to loss of control).
No products indexed under this heading.

Methylprednisolone Acetate (Corticosteroids tend to produce hyperglycemia and concurrent use may lead to loss of control). Products include:
Depo-Medrol Injectable Suspension 2617
Depo-Medrol Single-Dose Vial 2619

Methylprednisolone Sodium Succinate (Corticosteroids tend to produce hyperglycemia and concurrent use may lead to loss of control).
No products indexed under this heading.

Metipranolol Hydrochloride (May potentiate hypoglycemic action).
No products indexed under this heading.

Metolazone (Diuretics tend to produce hyperglycemia and concurrent use may lead to loss of control).
No products indexed under this heading.

Metoprolol Succinate (May potentiate hypoglycemic action). Products include:
Toprol-XL Tablets 668

Metoprolol Tartrate (May potentiate hypoglycemic action). Products include:
Lopressor Injection 2238
Lopressor Tablets 2238
Lopressor HCT 50/25 Tablets 2241
Lopressor HCT 100/25 Tablets 2241
Lopressor HCT 100/50 Tablets 2241

Miconazole (A potential interaction between oral miconazole and oral hypoglycemic agents leading to severe hypoglycemia has been reported).
No products indexed under this heading.

Moclobemide (May potentiate hypoglycemic action).
No products indexed under this heading.

Nabumetone (May potentiate hypoglycemic action).
No products indexed under this heading.

Nadolol (May potentiate hypoglycemic action). Products include:
Nadolol Tablets 2159

Naproxen (May potentiate hypoglycemic action). Products include:
EC-Naprosyn Delayed-Release Tablets 2761
Naprosyn Suspension 2761
Naprosyn Tablets 2761
Prevacid NapraPAC 3280

Naproxen Sodium (May potentiate hypoglycemic action). Products include:
Aleve Caplets 742
Aleve Gelcaps 743
Aleve Tablets 743
Aleve Cold & Sinus Caplets 744
Anaprox Tablets 2761
Anaprox DS Tablets 2761

Nicardipine Hydrochloride (An inhibitor of CYP2C8 may decrease the AUC of rosiglitazone. Therefore, if an inducer of CYP2C8 is started or stopped during treatment with

rosiglitazone, changes in diabetes treatment may be needed upon clinical response). Products include:
Cardene I.V. 2497

Nicotinic Acid (Nicotinic acid tends to produce hyperglycemia and concurrent use may lead to loss of control).
No products indexed under this heading.

Norepinephrine Bitartrate (Sympathomimetics tend to produce hyperglycemia and concurrent use may lead to loss of control).
No products indexed under this heading.

Norethindrone (Oral contraceptives tend to produce hyperglycemia and concurrent use may lead to loss of control). Products include:
Ortho Micronor Tablets 2426

Norethynodrel (Oral contraceptives tend to produce hyperglycemia and concurrent use may lead to loss of control).
No products indexed under this heading.

Norgestimate (Oral contraceptives tend to produce hyperglycemia and concurrent use may lead to loss of control). Products include:
Ortho-Cyclen/Ortho Tri-Cyclen 2429
Ortho Tri-Cyclen Lo Tablets 2436

Norgestrel (Oral contraceptives tend to produce hyperglycemia and concurrent use may lead to loss of control).
No products indexed under this heading.

Omeprazole (An inhibitor of CYP2C8 may decrease the AUC of rosiglitazone. Therefore, if an inducer of CYP2C8 is started or stopped during treatment with rosiglitazone, changes in diabetes treatment may be needed upon clinical response). Products include:
Zegerid Capsules 2958
Zegerid Powder for Oral Solution 2958

Oxaprozin (May potentiate hypoglycemic action).
No products indexed under this heading.

Pargyline Hydrochloride (May potentiate hypoglycemic action).
No products indexed under this heading.

Penbutolol Sulfate (May potentiate hypoglycemic action).
No products indexed under this heading.

Perphenazine (Phenothiazines tend to produce hyperglycemia and concurrent use may lead to loss of control).
No products indexed under this heading.

Phenelzine Sulfate (May potentiate hypoglycemic action).
No products indexed under this heading.

Phenobarbital (An inhibitor of CYP2C8 may decrease the AUC of rosiglitazone. Therefore, if an inducer of CYP2C8 is started or stopped during treatment with rosiglitazone, changes in diabetes treatment may be needed upon clinical response). Products include:
Donnatal Extentabs 2493

Phenylbutazone (May potentiate hypoglycemic action).
No products indexed under this heading.

IMPORTANT NOTE: Always consult each drug listing in the patient's regimen for possible interactions.

Phenylephrine Bitartrate (Sympathomimetics tend to produce hyperglycemia and concurrent use may lead to loss of control).

No products indexed under this heading.

Phenylephrine Hydrochloride (Sympathomimetics tend to produce hyperglycemia and concurrent use may lead to loss of control). Products include:

Phenylephrine Tannate (Sympathomimetics tend to produce hyperglycemia and concurrent use may lead to loss of control).

No products indexed under this heading.

Phenylpropanolamine Hydrochloride (Sympathomimetics tend to produce hyperglycemia and concurrent use may lead to loss of control).

No products indexed under this heading.

Phenytoin (Phenytoin tends to produce hyperglycemia and concurrent use may lead to loss of control).

No products indexed under this heading.

Phenytoin Sodium (Phenytoin tends to produce hyperglycemia and concurrent use may lead to loss of control). Products include:

Pindolol (May potentiate hypoglycemic action).

No products indexed under this heading.

Pirbuterol Acetate (Sympathomimetics tend to produce hyperglycemia and concurrent use may lead to loss of control). Products include:

Piroxicam (May potentiate hypoglycemic action).

No products indexed under this heading.

Polyestradiol Phosphate (Estrogens tend to produce hyperglycemia and concurrent use may lead to loss of control).

No products indexed under this heading.

Polythiazide (Diuretics tend to produce hyperglycemia and concurrent use may lead to loss of control).

No products indexed under this heading.

Prednisolone Acetate (Corticosteroids tend to produce hyperglycemia and concurrent use may lead to loss of control). Products include:

Prednisolone Sodium Phosphate (Corticosteroids tend to produce hyperglycemia and concurrent use may lead to loss of control).

No products indexed under this heading.

Prednisolone Tebutate (Corticosteroids tend to produce hyperglycemia and concurrent use may lead to loss of control).

No products indexed under this heading.

Prednisone (Corticosteroids tend to produce hyperglycemia and concurrent use may lead to loss of control).

No products indexed under this heading.

Primidone (An inhibitor of CYP2C8 may decrease the AUC of rosiglitazone. Therefore, if an inducer of CYP2C8 is started or stopped during treatment with rosiglitazone, changes in diabetes treatment may be needed upon clinical response).

No products indexed under this heading.

Probenecid (May potentiate hypoglycemic action).

No products indexed under this heading.

Procarbazine Hydrochloride (May potentiate hypoglycemic action). Products include:

Prochlorperazine (Phenothiazines tend to produce hyperglycemia and concurrent use may lead to loss of control).

No products indexed under this heading.

Promethazine Hydrochloride (Phenothiazines tend to produce hyperglycemia and concurrent use may lead to loss of control). Products include:

Propranolol Hydrochloride (Coadministration increases Cmax AUC, and T1/2 of glimepiride by 23%, 22% and 15% respectively and it decreased CL/f by 18%; no evidence of clinically significant adverse interactions). Products include:

Pseudoephedrine Hydrochloride (Sympathomimetics tend to produce hyperglycemia and concurrent use may lead to loss of control). Products include:

Pseudoephedrine Sulfate (Sympathomimetics tend to produce hyperglycemia and concurrent use may lead to loss of control). Products include:

Quercetin (An inhibitor of CYP2C8 may decrease the AUC of rosiglitazone. Therefore, if an inducer of CYP2C8 is started or stopped during treatment with rosiglitazone, changes in diabetes treatment may be needed upon clinical response).

No products indexed under this heading.

Quinestrol (Estrogens tend to produce hyperglycemia and concurrent use may lead to loss of control).

No products indexed under this heading.

Rifabutin (An inhibitor of CYP2C8 may decrease the AUC of rosiglitazone. Therefore, if an inducer of CYP2C8 is started or stopped during treatment with rosiglitazone, changes in diabetes treatment may be needed upon clinical response).

No products indexed under this heading.

Rifampin (Rifampin administration (600 mg twice daily), an inducer of CYP2C8, for 6 days is reported to decrease rosiglitazone AUC by 66%, compared to the administration of rosiglitazone (8 mg) alone).
No products indexed under this heading.

Rofecoxib (May potentiate hypoglycemic action).
No products indexed under this heading.

Salmeterol Xinafoate (Sympathomimetics tend to produce hyperglycemia and concurrent use may lead to loss of control). Products include:
Advair Diskus 100/50 1308
Advair Diskus 250/50 1308
Advair Diskus 500/50 1308
Advair HFA Inhalation Aerosol 1318
Serevent Diskus 1568

Salsalate (May potentiate hypoglycemic action; clinical trials data indicate no evidence of significant adverse interaction with concurrent use).
No products indexed under this heading.

Selegiline Hydrochloride (May potentiate hypoglycemic action). Products include:
Eldepryl Capsules 3208
Zelapar Tablets 3372

Sotalol Hydrochloride (May potentiate hypoglycemic action).
No products indexed under this heading.

Spironolactone (Diuretics tend to produce hyperglycemia and concurrent use may lead to loss of control).
No products indexed under this heading.

Sulfacytine (May potentiate hypoglycemic action).
No products indexed under this heading.

Sulfamethizole (May potentiate hypoglycemic action).
No products indexed under this heading.

Sulfamethoxazole (May potentiate hypoglycemic action).
No products indexed under this heading.

Sulfaphenazole (An inhibitor of CYP2C8 may decrease the AUC of rosiglitazone. Therefore, if an inducer of CYP2C8 is started or stopped during treatment with rosiglitazone, changes in diabetes treatment may be needed upon clinical response).
No products indexed under this heading.

Sulfasalazine (May potentiate hypoglycemic action).
No products indexed under this heading.

Sulfinpyrazone (May potentiate hypoglycemic action).
No products indexed under this heading.

Sulfisoxazole Acetyl (May potentiate hypoglycemic action).
No products indexed under this heading.

Sulfisoxazole Diolamine (May potentiate hypoglycemic action).
No products indexed under this heading.

Sulindac (May potentiate hypoglycemic action). Products include:
Clinoril Tablets 1924

Terbutaline Sulfate (Sympathomimetics tend to produce hyperglycemia and concurrent use may lead to loss of control).
No products indexed under this heading.

Thioridazine Hydrochloride (Phenothiazines tend to produce hyperglycemia and concurrent use may lead to loss of control). Products include:
Thioridazine Hydrochloride Tablets 2163

Thyroglobulin (Thyroid products tend to produce hyperglycemia and concurrent use may lead to loss of control).
No products indexed under this heading.

Thyroid (Thyroid products tend to produce hyperglycemia and concurrent use may lead to loss of control).
No products indexed under this heading.

Thyroxine (Thyroid products tend to produce hyperglycemia and concurrent use may lead to loss of control).
No products indexed under this heading.

Thyroxine Sodium (Thyroid products tend to produce hyperglycemia and concurrent use may lead to loss of control).
No products indexed under this heading.

Timolol Hemihydrate (May potentiate hypoglycemic action). Products include:
Betimol Ophthalmic Solution 3382
Betimol Ophthalmic Solution .... ⊙ 295

Timolol Maleate (May potentiate hypoglycemic action). Products include:
Blocadren Tablets 1916
Cosopt Sterile Ophthalmic Solution....................................... 1931
Timolide Tablets 2086
Timoptic Sterile Ophthalmic Solution....................................... 2088
Timoptic in Ocudose 2091
Timoptic-XE Sterile Ophthalmic Gel Forming Solution 2092

Tolazamide (May potentiate hypoglycemic action).
No products indexed under this heading.

Tolbutamide (May potentiate hypoglycemic action).
No products indexed under this heading.

Tolmetin Sodium (May potentiate hypoglycemic action).
No products indexed under this heading.

Torsemide (Diuretics tend to produce hyperglycemia and concurrent use may lead to loss of control). Products include:
Demadex Injection 2759
Demadex Tablets 2759

Tranylcypromine Sulfate (May potentiate hypoglycemic action). Products include:
Parnate Tablets 1527

Triamcinolone (Corticosteroids tend to produce hyperglycemia and concurrent use may lead to loss of control).
No products indexed under this heading.

Triamcinolone Acetonide (Corticosteroids tend to produce hyperglycemia and concurrent use may lead to loss of control). Products include:
Azmacort Inhalation Aerosol 1726
Nasacort AQ Nasal Spray 2922

Triamcinolone Diacetate (Corticosteroids tend to produce hyperglycemia and concurrent use may lead to loss of control).
No products indexed under this heading.

Triamcinolone Hexacetonide (Corticosteroids tend to produce hyperglycemia and concurrent use may lead to loss of control).
No products indexed under this heading.

Triamterene (Diuretics tend to produce hyperglycemia and concurrent use may lead to loss of control). Products include:
Dyazide Capsules 1423
Dyrenium Capsules 3400

Trifluoperazine Hydrochloride (Phenothiazines tend to produce hyperglycemia and concurrent use may lead to loss of control).
No products indexed under this heading.

Trimethoprim (An inhibitor of CYP2C8 may decrease the AUC of rosiglitazone. Therefore, if an inducer of CYP2C8 is started or stopped during treatment with rosiglitazone, changes in diabetes treatment may be needed upon clinical response).
No products indexed under this heading.

Trimethoprim Hydrochloride (An inhibitor of CYP2C8 may decrease the AUC of rosiglitazone. Therefore, if an inducer of CYP2C8 is started or stopped during treatment with rosiglitazone, changes in diabetes treatment may be needed upon clinical response).
No products indexed under this heading.

Valdecoxib (May potentiate hypoglycemic action).
No products indexed under this heading.

Warfarin Sodium (May potentiate hypoglycemic action). Products include:
Coumadin for Injection 898
Coumadin Tablets 898

Food Interactions

Meal, unspecified (When glimepiride is given with meals the mean Tmax is slightly increased (12%) and mean Cmax and AUC are slightly decreased).

AVANDIA TABLETS

(Rosiglitazone Maleate) 1384
May interact with cytochrome p450 2c8 inducers (selected), cytochrome p450 2c8 inhibitors (selected), insulin, sulfonylureas, and certain other agents. Compounds in these categories include:

Anastrozole (An inhibitor of CYP2C8 may increase the AUC of rosiglitazone. Therefore, if an inhibitor of CYP2C8 is started or stopped during treatment with rosiglitazone, changes in diabetes treatment may be needed upon clinical response). Products include:
Arimidex Tablets 673

Carbamazepine (An inducer of CYP2C8 may decrease the AUC of rosiglitazone. Therefore, if an inducer of CYP2C8 is started or stopped during treatment with rosiglitazone, changes in diabetes treatment may be needed upon clinical response). Products include:
Carbatrol Capsules 3171
Equetro Extended-Release Capsules....................................... 3180
Tegretol/Tegretol-XR 2295

Chlorpropamide (An increased incidence of heart failure has been observed when rosiglitazone was added to a sulfonylurea or to a sulfonylurea plus metformin).
No products indexed under this heading.

Cimetidine (An inhibitor of CYP2C8 may increase the AUC of rosiglitazone. Therefore, if an inhibitor of CYP2C8 is started or stopped during treatment with rosiglitazone, changes in diabetes treatment may be needed upon clinical response). Products include:
Tagamet HB 200 Tablets 664

Cimetidine Hydrochloride (An inhibitor of CYP2C8 may increase the AUC of rosiglitazone. Therefore, if an inhibitor of CYP2C8 is started or stopped during treatment with rosiglitazone, changes in diabetes treatment may be needed upon clinical response).
No products indexed under this heading.

Gemfibrozil (Concomitant administration of gemfibrozil (600 mg twice daily), an inhibitor of CYP2C8, and rosiglitazone (4 mg once daily) for 7 days increased rosiglitazone AUC by 127% compared to the administration of rosiglitazone (4 mg once daily) alone. Given the potential for dose-related adverse events with rosiglitazone, a decrease in the dose of rosiglitazone may be needed when gemfibrozil is introduced).
No products indexed under this heading.

Glimepiride (An increased incidence of heart failure has been observed when rosiglitazone was added to a sulfonylurea or to a sulfonylurea plus metformin). Products include:
Avandaryl Tablets 1379
Duetact Tablets 3226

Glipizide (An increased incidence of heart failure has been observed when rosiglitazone was added to a sulfonylurea or to a sulfonylurea plus metformin).
No products indexed under this heading.

Glyburide (Rosiglitazone (2 mg twice daily) taken concomitantly with glyburide (3.75 to 10 mg/day) for 7 days did not alter the mean steady-state 24-hour plasma glucose concentrations in diabetic patients stabilized on glyburide therapy. Repeat doses of rosiglitazone (8 mg once daily) for 8 days in healthy adult Caucasian subjects caused a decrease in glyburide AUC and Cmax of approximately 30%. In Japanese subjects, glyburide AUC (14%) and Cmax (31%) slightly increased following co-administration of rosiglitazone).
No products indexed under this heading.

Insulin, Human, Zinc Suspension (Co-administration of rosiglitazone with insulin has resulted in increased incidence of cardiac failure and other cardiovascular adverse events). Products include:
Humulin L, 100 Units 1794
Humulin U, 100 Units 1800

Insulin, Human NPH (Co-administration of rosiglitazone with insulin has resulted in increased inci-

dence of cardiac failure and other cardiovascular adverse events). Products include:
Humulin N, 100 Units 1795
Humulin N Pen 1797

Insulin, Human Regular (Co-administration of rosiglitazone with insulin has resulted in increased incidence of cardiac failure and other cardiovascular adverse events). Products include:
Humulin R, 100 Units 1798

Insulin, Human Regular and Human NPH Mixture (Co-administration of rosiglitazone with insulin has resulted in increased incidence of cardiac failure and other cardiovascular adverse events). Products include:
Humulin 50/50, 100 Units 1791
Humulin 70/30 Pen 1793

Insulin, NPH (Co-administration of rosiglitazone with insulin has resulted in increased incidence of cardiac failure and other cardiovascular adverse events).
No products indexed under this heading.

Insulin, Regular (Co-administration of rosiglitazone with insulin has resulted in increased incidence of cardiac failure and other cardiovascular adverse events).
No products indexed under this heading.

Insulin, Zinc Crystals (Co-administration of rosiglitazone with insulin has resulted in increased incidence of cardiac failure and other cardiovascular adverse events).
No products indexed under this heading.

Insulin, Zinc Suspension (Co-administration of rosiglitazone with insulin has resulted in increased incidence of cardiac failure and other cardiovascular adverse events).
No products indexed under this heading.

Insulin Aspart, Human Regular (Co-administration of rosiglitazone with insulin has resulted in increased incidence of cardiac failure and other cardiovascular adverse events). Products include:
NovoLog Injection 2326

Insulin glargine (Co-administration of rosiglitazone with insulin has resulted in increased incidence of cardiac failure and other cardiovascular adverse events). Products include:
Lantus Injection 2909

Insulin Lispro, Human (Co-administration of rosiglitazone with insulin has resulted in increased incidence of cardiac failure and other cardiovascular adverse events). Products include:
Humalog-Pen 1781
Humalog Mix 50/50-Pen 1783
Humalog Mix 75/25-Pen 1785

Insulin Lispro Protamine, Human (Co-administration of rosiglitazone with insulin has resulted in increased incidence of cardiac failure and other cardiovascular adverse events). Products include:
Humalog Mix 50/50-Pen 1783
Humalog Mix 75/25-Pen 1785

Nicardipine Hydrochloride (An inhibitor of CYP2C8 may increase the AUC of rosiglitazone. Therefore, if an inhibitor of CYP2C8 is started or stopped during treatment with rosiglitazone, changes in diabetes treatment may be needed upon clinical response). Products include:
Cardene I.V. 2497

Omeprazole (An inhibitor of CYP2C8 may increase the AUC of rosiglitazone. Therefore, if an inhibitor of CYP2C8 is started or stopped during treatment with rosiglitazone, changes in diabetes treatment may be needed upon clinical response). Products include:
Zegerid Capsules 2958
Zegerid Powder for Oral Solution 2958

Phenobarbital (An inducer of CYP2C8 may decrease the AUC of rosiglitazone. Therefore, if an inducer of CYP2C8 is started or stopped during treatment with rosiglitazone, changes in diabetes treatment may be needed upon clinical response). Products include:
Donnatal Extentabs 2493

Primidone (An inducer of CYP2C8 may decrease the AUC of rosiglitazone. Therefore, if an inducer of CYP2C8 is started or stopped during treatment with rosiglitazone, changes in diabetes treatment may be needed upon clinical response).
No products indexed under this heading.

Quercetin (An inhibitor of CYP2C8 may increase the AUC of rosiglitazone. Therefore, if an inhibitor of CYP2C8 is started or stopped during treatment with rosiglitazone, changes in diabetes treatment may be needed upon clinical response).
No products indexed under this heading.

Rifabutin (An inducer of CYP2C8 may decrease the AUC of rosiglitazone. Therefore, if an inducer of CYP2C8 is started or stopped during treatment with rosiglitazone, changes in diabetes treatment may be needed upon clinical response).
No products indexed under this heading.

Rifampin (Rifampin administration (600 mg twice daily), an inducer of CYP2C8, for 6 days is reported to decrease rosiglitazone AUC by 66%, compared to the administration of rosiglitazone (8 mg) alone).
No products indexed under this heading.

Sulfaphenazole (An inhibitor of CYP2C8 may increase the AUC of rosiglitazone. Therefore, if an inhibitor of CYP2C8 is started or stopped during treatment with rosiglitazone, changes in diabetes treatment may be needed upon clinical response).
No products indexed under this heading.

Sulfinpyrazone (An inhibitor of CYP2C8 may increase the AUC of rosiglitazone. Therefore, if an inhibitor of CYP2C8 is started or stopped during treatment with rosiglitazone, changes in diabetes treatment may be needed upon clinical response).
No products indexed under this heading.

Tolazamide (An increased incidence of heart failure has been observed when rosiglitazone was added to a sulfonylurea or to a sulfonylurea plus metformin).
No products indexed under this heading.

Tolbutamide (An increased incidence of heart failure has been observed when rosiglitazone was added to a sulfonylurea or to a sulfonylurea plus metformin).
No products indexed under this heading.

Trimethoprim (An inhibitor of CYP2C8 may increase the AUC of rosiglitazone. Therefore, if an inhibitor of CYP2C8 is started or stopped during treatment with rosiglitazone, changes in diabetes treatment may be needed upon clinical response).
No products indexed under this heading.

Trimethoprim Hydrochloride (An inhibitor of CYP2C8 may increase the AUC of rosiglitazone. Therefore, if an inhibitor of CYP2C8 is started or stopped during treatment with rosiglitazone, changes in diabetes treatment may be needed upon clinical response).
No products indexed under this heading.

AVAPRO TABLETS
(Irbesartan) 891
None cited in PDR database.

AVAPRO TABLETS
(Irbesartan) 2871
None cited in PDR database.

AVAR CLEANSER
(Sodium Sulfacetamide, Sulfur) 1085
None cited in PDR database.

AVAR GEL
(Sodium Sulfacetamide, Sulfur) 1085
None cited in PDR database.

AVAR GREEN GEL
(Sodium Sulfacetamide, Sulfur) 1085
None cited in PDR database.

AVAR-E EMOLLIENT CREAM
(Sodium Sulfacetamide, Sulfur) 1085
None cited in PDR database.

AVAR-E GREEN CREAM
(Sodium Sulfacetamide, Sulfur) 1085
None cited in PDR database.

AVASTIN IV
(Bevacizumab) 1227
None cited in PDR database.

AVELOX I.V.
(Moxifloxacin Hydrochloride) 2970
See Avelox Tablets

AVELOX TABLETS
(Moxifloxacin Hydrochloride) 2970
May interact with antacids containing aluminum, calcium and magnesium, corticosteroids, oral anticoagulants, erythromycin, iron containing oral preparations, non-steroidal anti-inflammatory agents, phenothiazines, quinidine, tricyclic antidepressants, and certain other agents. Compounds in these categories include:

Aluminum Carbonate (Co-administration of quinolones, such as moxifloxacin, with antacids containing magnesium, calcium, or aluminum may substantially interfere with the absorption of quinolones; moxifloxacin should be taken at least 4 hours before or 8 hours after ingestion of antacids).
No products indexed under this heading.

Aluminum Hydroxide (Co-administration of quinolones, such as moxifloxacin, with antacids containing magnesium, calcium, or aluminum may substantially interfere with the absorption of quinolones; moxifloxacin should be taken at least 4 hours before or 8 hours after ingestion of antacids). Products include:
Gaviscon Regular Strength Liquid .. ▣658
Gaviscon Regular Strength Tablets .... ▣658
Gaviscon Extra Strength Liquid ...... ▣658
Gaviscon Extra Strength Tablets .... ▣658
Maalox Regular Strength Antacid/Antigas Liquid 2175
Maalox Max Maximum Strength Antacid/Anti-Gas Liquid 2176

Amiodarone Hydrochloride (Moxifloxacin has been shown to prolong the QT interval; concurrent use with class 1A antiarrhythmic agents, such as amiodarone, should be avoided).
No products indexed under this heading.

Amitriptyline Hydrochloride (Moxifloxacin has been shown to prolong the QT interval; an additive effect with co-administration cannot be excluded).
No products indexed under this heading.

Amoxapine (Moxifloxacin has been shown to prolong the QT interval; an additive effect with co-administration cannot be excluded).
No products indexed under this heading.

Anisindione (Quinolones, including moxifloxacin, have been reported to enhance the anticoagulant effects of warfarin or its derivatives). Products include:
Miradon Tablets 3042

Atenolol (The mean Cmax of single dose atenolol decreased by about 10% following co-administration with a single dose of moxifloxacin).
No products indexed under this heading.

Betamethasone Acetate (Achilles and other tendon rupture have been reported with quinolones; although not reported in clinical trials with moxifloxacin, post market surveillance reports indicate that the risk may be increased in patients on concomitant corticosteroids).
No products indexed under this heading.

Betamethasone Sodium Phosphate (Achilles and other tendon rupture have been reported with quinolones; although not reported in clinical trials with moxifloxacin, post market surveillance reports indicate that the risk may be increased in patients on concomitant corticosteroids).
No products indexed under this heading.

Calcium Carbonate (Co-administration of quinolones, such as moxifloxacin, with antacids containing magnesium, calcium or aluminum may substantially interfere with the absorption of quinolones; moxifloxacin should be taken at least 4 hours before or 8 hours after ingestion of antacids). Products include:
Actonel with Calcium Tablets 2688
Calcet Tablets 2138
Caltrate 600 PLUS .... ▣809
Caltrate 600 + D Tablets .... ▣809
D-Cal Chewable Caplets .... ▣812
Gas-X with Maalox .... ▣656

Maalox Regular Strength Antacid Chewable Tablets 2177
Maalox Max Maximum Strength Antacid/Antigas Chewable Tablets 2176
Maalox Max Maximum Strength Chewable Tablets 660
Os-Cal Chewable Tablets 818
Pepcid Complete Chewable Tablets 1701
Children's Pepto 2674
PremCal Light, Regular, and Extra Strength Tablets 818
Tums 664

Celecoxib (Co-administration of a non-steroidal anti-inflammatory agent with a quinolone may increase the risks of CNS stimulation and convulsions; this interaction has not been observed in moxifloxacin clinical and preclinical trials). Products include:
Celebrex Capsules 3134

Chlorpromazine (Moxifloxacin has been shown to prolong the QT interval; co-administration with antipsychotic phenothiazines cannot be excluded).
No products indexed under this heading.

Chlorpromazine Hydrochloride (Moxifloxacin has been shown to prolong the QT interval; co-administration with antipsychotic phenothiazines cannot be excluded).
No products indexed under this heading.

Cisapride (Moxifloxacin has been shown to prolong the QT interval; an additive effect with co-administration cannot be excluded).
No products indexed under this heading.

Clomipramine Hydrochloride (Moxifloxacin has been shown to prolong the QT interval; an additive effect with co-administration cannot be excluded).
No products indexed under this heading.

Cortisone Acetate (Achilles and other tendon rupture have been reported with quinolones; although not reported in clinical trials with moxifloxacin, post market surveillance reports indicate that the risk may be increased in patients on concomitant corticosteroids).
No products indexed under this heading.

Desipramine Hydrochloride (Moxifloxacin has been shown to prolong the QT interval; an additive effect with co-administration cannot be excluded).
No products indexed under this heading.

Dexamethasone (Achilles and other tendon rupture have been reported with quinolones; although not reported in clinical trials with moxifloxacin, post market surveillance reports indicate that the risk may be increased in patients on concomitant corticosteroids). Products include:
Ciprodex Otic Suspension 559
Decadron Tablets 1951
TobraDex Ophthalmic Ointment 562
TobraDex Ophthalmic Suspension 563

Dexamethasone Acetate (Achilles and other tendon rupture have been reported with quinolones; although not reported in clinical trials with moxifloxacin, post market surveillance reports indicate that the risk may be increased in patients on concomitant corticosteroids).
No products indexed under this heading.

Dexamethasone Sodium Phosphate (Achilles and other tendon rupture have been reported with quinolones; although not reported in clinical trials with moxifloxacin, post market surveillance reports indicate that the risk may be increased in patients on concomitant corticosteroids).
No products indexed under this heading.

Diclofenac Potassium (Co-administration of a non-steroidal anti-inflammatory agent with a quinolone may increase the risks of CNS stimulation and convulsions; this interaction has not been observed in moxifloxacin clinical and preclinical trials).
No products indexed under this heading.

Diclofenac Sodium (Co-administration of a non-steroidal anti-inflammatory agent with a quinolone may increase the risks of CNS stimulation and convulsions; this interaction has not been observed in moxifloxacin clinical and preclinical trials). Products include:
Arthrotec Tablets 3129
Voltaren Ophthalmic Solution 2309
Voltaren Tablets 2307
Voltaren-XR Tablets 2310

Dicumarol (Quinolones, including moxifloxacin, have been reported to enhance the anticoagulant effects of warfarin or its derivatives).
No products indexed under this heading.

Didanosine (Co-administration of quinolones, such as moxifloxacin, with antacids contained in Videx chewable/buffered tablets or the pediatric powder for oral solution may substantially interfere with the absorption of quinolones; moxifloxacin should be taken at least 4 hours before or 8 hours after ingestion of Videx).
No products indexed under this heading.

Digoxin (Co-administration in healthy individuals has resulted in the increase in mean digoxin Cmax by about 50% during the distribution phase of digoxin; this transient increase in digoxin Cmax is not viewed to be clinically significant). Products include:
Lanoxicaps Capsules 1490
Lanoxin Injection 1494
Lanoxin Injection Pediatric 1497
Lanoxin Tablets 1500

Doxepin Hydrochloride (Moxifloxacin has been shown to prolong the QT interval; an additive effect with co-administration cannot be excluded).
No products indexed under this heading.

Erythromycin (Moxifloxacin has been shown to prolong the QT interval; an additive effect with co-administration cannot be excluded). Products include:
Ery-Tab Tablets 449
Erythromycin Base Filmtab Tablets 455
Erythromycin Delayed-Release Capsules, USP 457
PCE Dispertab Tablets 515

Erythromycin Estolate (Moxifloxacin has been shown to prolong the QT interval; an additive effect with co-administration cannot be excluded).
No products indexed under this heading.

Erythromycin Ethylsuccinate (Moxifloxacin has been shown to prolong the QT interval; an additive effect with co-administration cannot be excluded). Products include:
E.E.S. 451
EryPed 447

Erythromycin Gluceptate (Moxifloxacin has been shown to prolong the QT interval; an additive effect with co-administration cannot be excluded).
No products indexed under this heading.

Erythromycin Lactobionate (Moxifloxacin has been shown to prolong the QT interval; an additive effect with co-administration cannot be excluded).
No products indexed under this heading.

Erythromycin Stearate (Moxifloxacin has been shown to prolong the QT interval; an additive effect with co-administration cannot be excluded). Products include:
Erythrocin Stearate Filmtab Tablets 453

Etodolac (Co-administration of a non-steroidal anti-inflammatory agent with a quinolone may increase the risks of CNS stimulation and convulsions; this interaction has not been observed in moxifloxacin clinical and preclinical trials).
No products indexed under this heading.

Fenoprofen Calcium (Co-administration of a non-steroidal anti-inflammatory agent with a quinolone may increase the risks of CNS stimulation and convulsions; this interaction has not been observed in moxifloxacin clinical and preclinical trials). Products include:
Nalfon Capsules 2502

Ferrous Fumarate (Co-administration of quinolones, such as moxifloxacin, with iron-containing products may substantially interfere with the absorption of quinolones; moxifloxacin should be taken at least 4 hours before or 8 hours after ingestion of iron-containing products).
No products indexed under this heading.

Ferrous Gluconate (Co-administration of quinolones, such as moxifloxacin, with iron-containing products may substantially interfere with the absorption of quinolones; moxifloxacin should be taken at least 4 hours before or 8 hours after ingestion of iron-containing products).
No products indexed under this heading.

Ferrous Sulfate (Co-administration of moxifloxacin with ferrous sulfate has resulted in reduced mean AUC (39%) and Cmax (59%) of moxifloxacin; moxifloxacin should be taken at least 4 hours before or 8 hours after ingestion of ferrous sulfate). Products include:
Slow Fe Iron Tablets 818
Slow Fe with Folic Acid Tablets 819

Fludrocortisone Acetate (Achilles and other tendon rupture have been reported with quinolones; although not reported in clinical trials with moxifloxacin, post market surveillance reports indicate that the risk may be increased in patients on concomitant corticosteroids).
No products indexed under this heading.

Fluphenazine Decanoate (Moxifloxacin has been shown to prolong the QT interval; co-administration with antipsychotic phenothiazines cannot be excluded).
No products indexed under this heading.

Fluphenazine Enanthate (Moxifloxacin has been shown to prolong the QT interval; co-administration with antipsychotic phenothiazines cannot be excluded).
No products indexed under this heading.

Fluphenazine Hydrochloride (Moxifloxacin has been shown to prolong the QT interval; co-administration with antipsychotic phenothiazines cannot be excluded).
No products indexed under this heading.

Flurbiprofen (Co-administration of a non-steroidal anti-inflammatory agent with a quinolone may increase the risks of CNS stimulation and convulsions; this interaction has not been observed in moxifloxacin clinical and preclinical trials).
No products indexed under this heading.

Glyburide (Co-administration has resulted in reduced mean AUC and Cmax by 12% and 21%, respectively; blood glucose levels were decreased slightly in patients on concurrent therapy; these interaction results are not viewed as clinically significant).
No products indexed under this heading.

Hydrocortisone (Achilles and other tendon rupture have been reported with quinolones; although not reported in clinical trials with moxifloxacin, post market surveillance reports indicate that the risk may be increased in patients on concomitant corticosteroids). Products include:
Colocort Rectal Suspension, USP (Retention) 100 mg/60 mL 2476
Hydrocortone Tablets 1989
Preparation H Hydrocortisone Cream 646

Hydrocortisone Acetate (Achilles and other tendon rupture have been reported with quinolones; although not reported in clinical trials with moxifloxacin, post market surveillance reports indicate that the risk may be increased in patients on concomitant corticosteroids). Products include:
Analpram-HC 1159
Pramosone 1161
ProctoFoam-HC 3099

Hydrocortisone Sodium Phosphate (Achilles and other tendon rupture have been reported with quinolones; although not reported in clinical trials with moxifloxacin, post market surveillance reports indicate that the risk may be increased in patients on concomitant corticosteroids).
No products indexed under this heading.

Hydrocortisone Sodium Succinate (Achilles and other tendon rupture have been reported with quinolones; although not reported in clinical trials with moxifloxacin, post market surveillance reports indicate that the risk may be increased in patients on concomitant corticosteroids).
No products indexed under this heading.

IMPORTANT NOTE: Always consult each drug listing in the patient's regimen for possible interactions.

Ibuprofen (Co-administration of a non-steroidal anti-inflammatory agent with a quinolone may increase the risks of CNS stimulation and convulsions; this interaction has not been observed in moxifloxacin clinical and preclinical trials). Products include:
- Advil Allergy Sinus Caplets .... ▣770
- Advil .... ▣674
- Children's Advil Oral Suspension .... ▣603
- Children's Advil Chewable Tablets .. ▣603
- Advil Cold & Sinus .... ▣723
- Infants' Advil Concentrated Drops .. ▣604
- Infants' Advil Concentrated Drops - White Grape (Dye-Free) .... ▣604
- Junior Strength Advil Swallow Tablets .... ▣605
- Advil Migraine Liquigels .... ▣608
- Advil Multi-Symptom Cold Caplets .... ▣770
- Advil PM Caplets .... ▣615
- Motrin IB Tablets and Caplets 1866
- Children's Motrin Oral Suspension ... 1867
- Children's Motrin Non-Staining Dye-Free Oral Suspension 1867
- Children's Motrin Cold Oral Suspension 1867
- Infants' Motrin Concentrated Drops 1867
- Infants' Motrin Non-Staining Dye-Free Concentrated Drops 1867
- Junior Strength Motrin Caplets and Chewable Tablets 1867
- Vicoprofen Tablets 539

Imipramine Hydrochloride (Moxifloxacin has been shown to prolong the QT interval; an additive effect with co-administration cannot be excluded).
No products indexed under this heading.

Imipramine Pamoate (Moxifloxacin has been shown to prolong the QT interval; an additive effect with co-administration cannot be excluded).
No products indexed under this heading.

Indomethacin (Co-administration of a non-steroidal anti-inflammatory agent with a quinolone may increase the risks of CNS stimulation and convulsions; this interaction has not been observed in moxifloxacin clinical and preclinical trials). Products include:
- Indocin 1995

Indomethacin Sodium Trihydrate (Co-administration of a non-steroidal anti-inflammatory agent with a quinolone may increase the risks of CNS stimulation and convulsions; this interaction has not been observed in moxifloxacin clinical and preclinical trials). Products include:
- Indocin I.V. 2465

Iron (Co-administration of quinolones, such as moxifloxacin, with iron-containing products may substantially interfere with the absorption of quinolones; moxifloxacin should be taken at least 4 hours before or 8 hours after ingestion of iron-containing products).
No products indexed under this heading.

Ketoprofen (Co-administration of a non-steroidal anti-inflammatory agent with a quinolone may increase the risks of CNS stimulation and convulsions; this interaction has not been observed in moxifloxacin clinical and preclinical trials).
No products indexed under this heading.

Ketorolac Tromethamine (Co-administration of a non-steroidal anti-inflammatory agent with a quinolone may increase the risks of CNS stimulation and convulsions; this interaction has not been observed in moxifloxacin clinical and preclinical trials). Products include:
- Acular Ophthalmic Solution 565
- Acular LS Ophthalmic Solution 566

Magaldrate (Co-administration of quinolones, such as moxifloxacin, with antacids containing magnesium, calcium, or aluminum may substantially interfere with the absorption of quinolones; moxifloxacin should be taken at least 4 hours before or 8 hours after ingestion of antacids).
No products indexed under this heading.

Magnesium Hydroxide (Co-administration of quinolones, such as moxifloxacin, with antacids containing magnesium, calcium, or aluminum may substantially interfere with the absorption of quinolones; moxifloxacin should be taken at least 4 hours before or 8 hours after ingestion of antacids). Products include:
- Maalox Regular Strength Antacid/Antigas Liquid 2175
- Maalox Max Maximum Strength Antacid/Anti-Gas Liquid 2176
- Pepcid Complete Chewable Tablets 1701

Magnesium Oxide (Co-administration of quinolones, such as moxifloxacin, with antacids containing magnesium, calcium, or aluminum may substantially interfere with the absorption of quinolones; moxifloxacin should be taken at least 4 hours before or 8 hours after ingestion of antacids). Products include:
- Beelith Tablets 759
- PremCal Light, Regular, and Extra Strength Tablets .... ▣818

Maprotiline Hydrochloride (Moxifloxacin has been shown to prolong the QT interval; an additive effect with co-administration cannot be excluded).
No products indexed under this heading.

Meclofenamate Sodium (Co-administration of a non-steroidal anti-inflammatory agent with a quinolone may increase the risks of CNS stimulation and convulsions; this interaction has not been observed in moxifloxacin clinical and preclinical trials).
No products indexed under this heading.

Mefenamic Acid (Co-administration of a non-steroidal anti-inflammatory agent with a quinolone may increase the risks of CNS stimulation and convulsions; this interaction has not been observed in moxifloxacin clinical and preclinical trials).
No products indexed under this heading.

Meloxicam (Co-administration of a non-steroidal anti-inflammatory agent with a quinolone may increase the risks of CNS stimulation and convulsions; this interaction has not been observed in moxifloxacin clinical and preclinical trials). Products include:
- Mobic Oral Suspension 863
- Mobic Tablets 863

Mesoridazine Besylate (Moxifloxacin has been shown to prolong the QT interval; co-administration with antipsychotic phenothiazines cannot be excluded).
No products indexed under this heading.

Methotrimeprazine (Moxifloxacin has been shown to prolong the QT interval; co-administration with antipsychotic phenothiazines cannot be excluded).
No products indexed under this heading.

Methylprednisolone Acetate (Achilles and other tendon rupture have been reported with quinolones; although not reported in clinical trials with moxifloxacin, post market surveillance reports indicate that the risk may be increased in patients on concomitant corticosteroids). Products include:
- Depo-Medrol Injectable Suspension 2617
- Depo-Medrol Single-Dose Vial 2619

Methylprednisolone Sodium Succinate (Achilles and other tendon rupture have been reported with quinolones; although not reported in clinical trials with moxifloxacin, post market surveillance reports indicate that the risk may be increased in patients on concomitant corticosteroids).
No products indexed under this heading.

Nabumetone (Co-administration of a non-steroidal anti-inflammatory agent with a quinolone may increase the risks of CNS stimulation and convulsions; this interaction has not been observed in moxifloxacin clinical and preclinical trials).
No products indexed under this heading.

Naproxen (Co-administration of a non-steroidal anti-inflammatory agent with a quinolone may increase the risks of CNS stimulation and convulsions; this interaction has not been observed in moxifloxacin clinical and preclinical trials). Products include:
- EC-Naprosyn Delayed-Release Tablets 2761
- Naprosyn Suspension 2761
- Naprosyn Tablets 2761
- Prevacid NapraPAC 3280

Naproxen Sodium (Co-administration of a non-steroidal anti-inflammatory agent with a quinolone may increase the risks of CNS stimulation and convulsions; this interaction has not been observed in moxifloxacin clinical and preclinical trials). Products include:
- Aleve Caplets 742
- Aleve Gelcaps 743
- Aleve Tablets 743
- Aleve Cold & Sinus Caplets 744
- Anaprox Tablets 2761
- Anaprox DS Tablets 2761

Nortriptyline Hydrochloride (Moxifloxacin has been shown to prolong the QT interval; an additive effect with co-administration cannot be excluded).
No products indexed under this heading.

Oxaprozin (Co-administration of a non-steroidal anti-inflammatory agent with a quinolone may increase the risks of CNS stimulation and convulsions; this interaction has not been observed in moxifloxacin clinical and preclinical trials).
No products indexed under this heading.

Perphenazine (Moxifloxacin has been shown to prolong the QT interval; co-administration with antipsychotic phenothiazines cannot be excluded).
No products indexed under this heading.

Phenylbutazone (Co-administration of a non-steroidal anti-inflammatory agent with a quinolone may increase the risks of CNS stimulation and convulsions; this interaction has not been observed in moxifloxacin clinical and preclinical trials).
No products indexed under this heading.

Piroxicam (Co-administration of a non-steroidal anti-inflammatory agent with a quinolone may increase the risks of CNS stimulation and convulsions; this interaction has not been observed in moxifloxacin clinical and preclinical trials).
No products indexed under this heading.

Polysaccharide Iron Complex (Co-administration of quinolones, such as moxifloxacin, with iron-containing products may substantially interfere with the absorption of quinolones; moxifloxacin should be taken at least 4 hours before or 8 hours after ingestion of iron-containing products). Products include:
- Nu-Iron 150 Capsules 2127

Prednisolone Acetate (Achilles and other tendon rupture have been reported with quinolones; although not reported in clinical trials with moxifloxacin, post market surveillance reports indicate that the risk may be increased in patients on concomitant corticosteroids). Products include:
- Blephamide Ophthalmic Ointment 568
- Blephamide Ophthalmic Suspension 569
- Poly-Pred Ophthalmic Suspension .... ⊙233
- Pred Forte Ophthalmic Suspension .... ⊙235
- Pred Mild Ophthalmic Suspension .... ⊙238
- Pred-G Ophthalmic Ointment .... ⊙237
- Pred-G Ophthalmic Suspension ...... ⊙236

Prednisolone Sodium Phosphate (Achilles and other tendon rupture have been reported with quinolones; although not reported in clinical trials with moxifloxacin, post market surveillance reports indicate that the risk may be increased in patients on concomitant corticosteroids).
No products indexed under this heading.

Prednisolone Tebutate (Achilles and other tendon rupture have been reported with quinolones; although not reported in clinical trials with moxifloxacin, post market surveillance reports indicate that the risk may be increased in patients on concomitant corticosteroids).
No products indexed under this heading.

Prednisone (Achilles and other tendon rupture have been reported with quinolones; although not reported in clinical trials with moxifloxacin, post market surveillance reports indicate that the risk may be increased in patients on concomitant corticosteroids).
No products indexed under this heading.

Procainamide Hydrochloride (Moxifloxacin has been shown to prolong the QT interval; concurrent use with class 1A antiarrhythmic agents, such as procainamide, should be avoided).
No products indexed under this heading.

Prochlorperazine (Moxifloxacin has been shown to prolong the QT interval; co-administration with antipsychotic phenothiazines cannot be excluded).
No products indexed under this heading.

Promethazine Hydrochloride (Moxifloxacin has been shown to prolong the QT interval; co-administration with antipsychotic phenothiazines cannot be excluded). Products include:
Phenergan Tablets and Suppositories 3440

Protriptyline Hydrochloride (Moxifloxacin has been shown to prolong the QT interval; an additive effect with co-administration cannot be excluded).
No products indexed under this heading.

Quinidine (Moxifloxacin has been shown to prolong the QT interval; concurrent use with class 1A antiarrhythmic agents, such as quinidine, should be avoided).
No products indexed under this heading.

Quinidine Gluconate (Moxifloxacin has been shown to prolong the QT interval; concurrent use with class 1A antiarrhythmic agents, such as quinidine, should be avoided).
No products indexed under this heading.

Quinidine Hydrochloride (Moxifloxacin has been shown to prolong the QT interval; concurrent use with class 1A antiarrhythmic agents, such as quinidine, should be avoided).
No products indexed under this heading.

Quinidine Polygalacturonate (Moxifloxacin has been shown to prolong the QT interval; concurrent use with class 1A antiarrhythmic agents, such as quinidine, should be avoided).
No products indexed under this heading.

Quinidine Sulfate (Moxifloxacin has been shown to prolong the QT interval; concurrent use with class 1A antiarrhythmic agents, such as quinidine, should be avoided).
No products indexed under this heading.

Rofecoxib (Co-administration of a non-steroidal anti-inflammatory agent with a quinolone may increase the risks of CNS stimulation and convulsions; this interaction has not been observed in moxifloxacin clinical and preclinical trials).
No products indexed under this heading.

Sotalol Hydrochloride (Moxifloxacin has been shown to prolong the QT interval; concurrent use with class III antiarrhythmic agents, such as sotalol, should be avoided).
No products indexed under this heading.

Sucralfate (Co-administration of quinolones, such as moxifloxacin, with sucralfate may substantially interfere with the absorption of quinolones; moxifloxacin should be taken at least 4 hours before or 8 hours after ingestion of sucralfate). Products include:
Carafate Suspension 701
Carafate Tablets 701

Sulindac (Co-administration of a non-steroidal anti-inflammatory agent with a quinolone may increase the risks of CNS stimulation and convulsions; this interaction has not been observed in moxifloxacin clinical and preclinical trials). Products include:
Clinoril Tablets 1924

Thioridazine Hydrochloride (Moxifloxacin has been shown to prolong the QT interval; co-administration with antipsychotic phenothiazines cannot be excluded). Products include:
Thioridazine Hydrochloride Tablets 2163

Tolmetin Sodium (Co-administration of a non-steroidal anti-inflammatory agent with a quinolone may increase the risks of CNS stimulation and convulsions; this interaction has not been observed in moxifloxacin clinical and preclinical trials).
No products indexed under this heading.

Triamcinolone (Achilles and other tendon rupture have been reported with quinolones; although not reported in clinical trials with moxifloxacin, post market surveillance reports indicate that the risk may be increased in patients on concomitant corticosteroids).
No products indexed under this heading.

Triamcinolone Acetonide (Achilles and other tendon rupture have been reported with quinolones; although not reported in clinical trials with moxifloxacin, post market surveillance reports indicate that the risk may be increased in patients on concomitant corticosteroids). Products include:
Azmacort Inhalation Aerosol 1726
Nasacort AQ Nasal Spray 2922

Triamcinolone Diacetate (Achilles and other tendon rupture have been reported with quinolones; although not reported in clinical trials with moxifloxacin, post market surveillance reports indicate that the risk may be increased in patients on concomitant corticosteroids).
No products indexed under this heading.

Triamcinolone Hexacetonide (Achilles and other tendon rupture have been reported with quinolones; although not reported in clinical trials with moxifloxacin, post market surveillance reports indicate that the risk may be increased in patients on concomitant corticosteroids).
No products indexed under this heading.

Trifluoperazine Hydrochloride (Moxifloxacin has been shown to prolong the QT interval; co-administration with antipsychotic phenothiazines cannot be excluded).
No products indexed under this heading.

Trimipramine Maleate (Moxifloxacin has been shown to prolong the QT interval; an additive effect with co-administration cannot be excluded).
No products indexed under this heading.

Valdecoxib (Co-administration of a non-steroidal anti-inflammatory agent with a quinolone may increase the risks of CNS stimulation and convulsions; this interaction has not been observed in moxifloxacin clinical and preclinical trials).
No products indexed under this heading.

Warfarin Sodium (Quinolones, including moxifloxacin, have been reported to enhance the anticoagulant effects of warfarin or its derivatives). Products include:
Coumadin for Injection 898
Coumadin Tablets 898

Zinc Sulfate (Co-administration of quinolones, such as moxifloxacin, with zinc-containing products may substantially interfere with the absorption of quinolones; moxifloxacin should be taken at least 4 hours before or 8 hours after ingestion of zinc-containing products). Products include:
Visine A.C. Seasonal Itching and Redness Relief Drops .... ⊙289
Zinc-220 Capsules 580

AVINZA CAPSULES
(Morphine Sulfate) 1741

May interact with central nervous system depressants, monoamine oxidase inhibitors, mixed agonist/antagonist opioid analgesics, muscle relaxants, and certain other agents. Compounds in these categories include:

Alfentanil Hydrochloride (Co-administration increases the risk of respiratory depression, hypotension, profound sedation, or coma).
No products indexed under this heading.

Alprazolam (Co-administration increases the risk of respiratory depression, hypotension, profound sedation, or coma). Products include:
Niravam Orally Disintegrating Tablets 3092

Aprobarbital (Co-administration increases the risk of respiratory depression, hypotension, profound sedation, or coma).
No products indexed under this heading.

Atracurium Besylate (Morphine may enhance the neuromuscular blocking action of skeletal muscle relaxants and produce an increased degree of respiratory depression).
No products indexed under this heading.

Baclofen (Morphine may enhance the neuromuscular blocking action of skeletal muscle relaxants and produce an increased degree of respiratory depression).
No products indexed under this heading.

Buprenorphine Hydrochloride (Mixed agonist/antagonist analgesics may reduce the analgesic effect and/or may precipitate withdrawal symptoms; mixed agonist/antagonist analgesics should NOT be administered to patients who have received or are receiving a course of therapy with pure opioid agonist analgesic). Products include:
Buprenex Injectable 2716
Suboxone Tablets 2717
Subutex Tablets 2717

Buspirone Hydrochloride (Co-administration increases the risk of respiratory depression, hypotension, profound sedation, or coma).
No products indexed under this heading.

Butabarbital (Co-administration increases the risk of respiratory depression, hypotension, profound sedation, or coma).
No products indexed under this heading.

Butalbital (Co-administration increases the risk of respiratory depression, hypotension, profound sedation, or coma).
No products indexed under this heading.

Butorphanol Tartrate (Mixed agonist/antagonist analgesics may reduce the analgesic effect and/or may precipitate withdrawal symptoms; mixed agonist/antagonist analgesics should NOT be administered to patients who have received or are receiving a course of therapy with pure opioid agonist analgesic).
No products indexed under this heading.

Carisoprodol (Morphine may enhance the neuromuscular blocking action of skeletal muscle relaxants and produce an increased degree of respiratory depression).
No products indexed under this heading.

Chlordiazepoxide (Co-administration increases the risk of respiratory depression, hypotension, profound sedation, or coma).
No products indexed under this heading.

Chlordiazepoxide Hydrochloride (Co-administration increases the risk of respiratory depression, hypotension, profound sedation, or coma). Products include:
Librium Capsules 3347

Chlorpromazine (Co-administration increases the risk of respiratory depression, hypotension, profound sedation, or coma).
No products indexed under this heading.

Chlorpromazine Hydrochloride (Co-administration increases the risk of respiratory depression, hypotension, profound sedation, or coma).
No products indexed under this heading.

Chlorprothixene (Co-administration increases the risk of respiratory depression, hypotension, profound sedation, or coma).
No products indexed under this heading.

Chlorprothixene Hydrochloride (Co-administration increases the risk of respiratory depression, hypotension, profound sedation, or coma).
No products indexed under this heading.

Chlorprothixene Lactate (Co-administration increases the risk of respiratory depression, hypotension, profound sedation, or coma).
No products indexed under this heading.

Chlorzoxazone (Morphine may enhance the neuromuscular blocking action of skeletal muscle relaxants and produce an increased degree of respiratory depression).
No products indexed under this heading.

Cimetidine (Co-administration has been reported to precipitate apnea, confusion and muscle twitching in an isolated report). Products include:
Tagamet HB 200 Tablets 664

Cisatracurium Besylate (Morphine may enhance the neuromuscular blocking action of skeletal muscle relaxants and produce an increased degree of respiratory depression). Products include:
Nimbex Injection 498

IMPORTANT NOTE: Always consult each drug listing in the patient's regimen for possible interactions.

Clorazepate Dipotassium (Co-administration increases the risk of respiratory depression, hypotension, profound sedation, or coma).
Products include:
Tranxene .. **2474**

Clozapine (Co-administration increases the risk of respiratory depression, hypotension, profound sedation, or coma). Products include:
Clozaril Tablets **2184**
FazaClo Orally Disintegrating Tablets .. **551**

Codeine Phosphate (Co-administration increases the risk of respiratory depression, hypotension, profound sedation, or coma).
Products include:
Tylenol with Codeine Tablets **2391**

Cyclobenzaprine Hydrochloride (Morphine may enhance the neuromuscular blocking action of skeletal muscle relaxants and produce an increased degree of respiratory depression).
No products indexed under this heading.

Dantrolene Sodium (Morphine may enhance the neuromuscular blocking action of skeletal muscle relaxants and produce an increased degree of respiratory depression).
Products include:
Dantrium Capsules **2694**
Dantrium Intravenous **2695**

Desflurane (Co-administration increases the risk of respiratory depression, hypotension, profound sedation, or coma).
No products indexed under this heading.

Dezocine (Co-administration increases the risk of respiratory depression, hypotension, profound sedation, or coma).
No products indexed under this heading.

Diazepam (Co-administration increases the risk of respiratory depression, hypotension, profound sedation, or coma). Products include:
Diastat Rectal Delivery System **3343**
Valium Tablets **2819**

Doxacurium Chloride (Morphine may enhance the neuromuscular blocking action of skeletal muscle relaxants and produce an increased degree of respiratory depression).
No products indexed under this heading.

Droperidol (Co-administration increases the risk of respiratory depression, hypotension, profound sedation, or coma).
No products indexed under this heading.

Enflurane (Co-administration increases the risk of respiratory depression, hypotension, profound sedation, or coma).
No products indexed under this heading.

Estazolam (Co-administration increases the risk of respiratory depression, hypotension, profound sedation, or coma). Products include:
ProSom Tablets **517**

Ethanol (Co-administration increases the risk of respiratory depression, hypotension, profound sedation, or coma).
No products indexed under this heading.

Ethchlorvynol (Co-administration increases the risk of respiratory depression, hypotension, profound sedation, or coma).
No products indexed under this heading.

Ethinamate (Co-administration increases the risk of respiratory depression, hypotension, profound sedation, or coma).
No products indexed under this heading.

Ethyl Alcohol (Co-administration increases the risk of respiratory depression, hypotension, profound sedation, or coma).
No products indexed under this heading.

Fentanyl (Co-administration increases the risk of respiratory depression, hypotension, profound sedation, or coma). Products include:
Duragesic Transdermal System **2373**
Ionsys Transdermal System **2379**

Fentanyl Citrate (Co-administration increases the risk of respiratory depression, hypotension, profound sedation, or coma). Products include:
Actiq ... **979**

Fluphenazine Decanoate (Co-administration increases the risk of respiratory depression, hypotension, profound sedation, or coma).
No products indexed under this heading.

Fluphenazine Enanthate (Co-administration increases the risk of respiratory depression, hypotension, profound sedation, or coma).
No products indexed under this heading.

Fluphenazine Hydrochloride (Co-administration increases the risk of respiratory depression, hypotension, profound sedation, or coma).
No products indexed under this heading.

Flurazepam Hydrochloride (Co-administration increases the risk of respiratory depression, hypotension, profound sedation, or coma).
Products include:
Dalmane Capsules **3342**

Glutethimide (Co-administration increases the risk of respiratory depression, hypotension, profound sedation, or coma).
No products indexed under this heading.

Haloperidol (Co-administration increases the risk of respiratory depression, hypotension, profound sedation, or coma).
No products indexed under this heading.

Haloperidol Decanoate (Co-administration increases the risk of respiratory depression, hypotension, profound sedation, or coma).
No products indexed under this heading.

Hydrocodone Bitartrate (Co-administration increases the risk of respiratory depression, hypotension, profound sedation, or coma).
Products include:
Hycodan ... **1116**
Hycotuss Expectorant Syrup **1117**
Vicodin Tablets **535**
Vicodin ES Tablets **536**
Vicodin HP Tablets **538**
Vicoprofen Tablets **539**
Zydone Tablets **1139**

Hydrocodone Polistirex (Co-administration increases the risk of respiratory depression, hypotension, profound sedation, or coma).
Products include:
Tussionex Pennkinetic Extended-Release Suspension **3327**

Hydromorphone Hydrochloride (Co-administration increases the risk of respiratory depression, hypotension, profound sedation, or coma).
Products include:
Dilaudid ... **440**
Dilaudid Non-Sterile Powder **440**
Dilaudid Oral Liquid **445**
Dilaudid Rectal Suppositories **440**
Dilaudid Tablets **440**
Dilaudid Tablets - 8 mg **445**
Dilaudid-HP **442**

Hydroxyzine Hydrochloride (Co-administration increases the risk of respiratory depression, hypotension, profound sedation, or coma).
No products indexed under this heading.

Isocarboxazid (MAO inhibitors markedly potentiate the action of morphine; concurrent and/or sequential use should be avoided).
No products indexed under this heading.

Isoflurane (Co-administration increases the risk of respiratory depression, hypotension, profound sedation, or coma).
No products indexed under this heading.

Ketamine Hydrochloride (Co-administration increases the risk of respiratory depression, hypotension, profound sedation, or coma).
No products indexed under this heading.

Levomethadyl Acetate Hydrochloride (Co-administration increases the risk of respiratory depression, hypotension, profound sedation, or coma).
No products indexed under this heading.

Levorphanol Tartrate (Co-administration increases the risk of respiratory depression, hypotension, profound sedation, or coma).
No products indexed under this heading.

Lorazepam (Co-administration increases the risk of respiratory depression, hypotension, profound sedation, or coma).
No products indexed under this heading.

Loxapine Hydrochloride (Co-administration increases the risk of respiratory depression, hypotension, profound sedation, or coma).
No products indexed under this heading.

Loxapine Succinate (Co-administration increases the risk of respiratory depression, hypotension, profound sedation, or coma).
No products indexed under this heading.

Meperidine Hydrochloride (Co-administration increases the risk of respiratory depression, hypotension, profound sedation, or coma).
No products indexed under this heading.

Mephobarbital (Co-administration increases the risk of respiratory depression, hypotension, profound sedation, or coma).
No products indexed under this heading.

Meprobamate (Co-administration increases the risk of respiratory depression, hypotension, profound sedation, or coma).
No products indexed under this heading.

Mesoridazine Besylate (Co-administration increases the risk of respiratory depression, hypotension, profound sedation, or coma).
No products indexed under this heading.

Metaxalone (Morphine may enhance the neuromuscular blocking action of skeletal muscle relaxants and produce an increased degree of respiratory depression). Products include:
Skelaxin Tablets **1716**

Methadone Hydrochloride (Co-administration increases the risk of respiratory depression, hypotension, profound sedation, or coma).
No products indexed under this heading.

Methocarbamol (Morphine may enhance the neuromuscular blocking action of skeletal muscle relaxants and produce an increased degree of respiratory depression).
No products indexed under this heading.

Methohexital Sodium (Co-administration increases the risk of respiratory depression, hypotension, profound sedation, or coma).
No products indexed under this heading.

Methotrimeprazine (Co-administration increases the risk of respiratory depression, hypotension, profound sedation, or coma).
No products indexed under this heading.

Methoxyflurane (Co-administration increases the risk of respiratory depression, hypotension, profound sedation, or coma).
No products indexed under this heading.

Metocurine Iodide (Morphine may enhance the neuromuscular blocking action of skeletal muscle relaxants and produce an increased degree of respiratory depression).
No products indexed under this heading.

Midazolam Hydrochloride (Co-administration increases the risk of respiratory depression, hypotension, profound sedation, or coma).
No products indexed under this heading.

Mivacurium Chloride (Morphine may enhance the neuromuscular blocking action of skeletal muscle relaxants and produce an increased degree of respiratory depression).
Products include:
Mivacron Injection **493**

Moclobemide (MAO inhibitors markedly potentiate the action of morphine; concurrent and/or sequential use should be avoided).
No products indexed under this heading.

Molindone Hydrochloride (Co-administration increases the risk of respiratory depression, hypotension, profound sedation, or coma).
Products include:
Moban Tablets **1119**

Nalbuphine Hydrochloride (Mixed agonist/antagonist analgesics may reduce the analgesic effect and/or may precipitate withdrawal symptoms; mixed agonist/antagonist analgesics should NOT be administered to patients who have received or are receiving a course of therapy with pure opioid agonist analgesic).
No products indexed under this heading.

Olanzapine (Co-administration increases the risk of respiratory depression, hypotension, profound sedation, or coma). Products include:
Symbyax Capsules 1819
Zyprexa Tablets 1830
Zyprexa IntraMuscular 1830
Zyprexa ZYDIS Orally
 Disintegrating Tablets 1830

Orphenadrine Citrate (Morphine may enhance the neuromuscular blocking action of skeletal muscle relaxants and produce an increased degree of respiratory depression). Products include:
Norflex Injection 1856

Oxazepam (Co-administration increases the risk of respiratory depression, hypotension, profound sedation, or coma).
No products indexed under this heading.

Oxycodone Hydrochloride (Co-administration increases the risk of respiratory depression, hypotension, profound sedation, or coma). Products include:
OxyContin Tablets 2703
OxyFast Oral Concentrate
 Solution....................................... 2708
OxyIR Capsules 2708
Percocet Tablets 1131
Percodan Tablets 1132

Pancuronium Bromide (Morphine may enhance the neuromuscular blocking action of skeletal muscle relaxants and produce an increased degree of respiratory depression).
No products indexed under this heading.

Pargyline Hydrochloride (MAO inhibitors markedly potentiate the action of morphine; concurrent and/or sequential use should be avoided).
No products indexed under this heading.

Pentazocine Hydrochloride (Mixed agonist/antagonist analgesics may reduce the analgesic effect and/or may precipitate withdrawal symptoms; mixed agonist/antagonist analgesics should NOT be administered to patients who have received or are receiving a course of therapy with pure opioid agonist analgesic).
No products indexed under this heading.

Pentazocine Lactate (Mixed agonist/antagonist analgesics may reduce the analgesic effect and/or may precipitate withdrawal symptoms; mixed agonist/antagonist analgesics should NOT be administered to patients who have received or are receiving a course of therapy with pure opioid agonist analgesic).
No products indexed under this heading.

Pentobarbital Sodium (Co-administration increases the risk of respiratory depression, hypotension, profound sedation, or coma). Products include:

Nembutal Sodium Solution, USP 2470

Perphenazine (Co-administration increases the risk of respiratory depression, hypotension, profound sedation, or coma).
No products indexed under this heading.

Phenelzine Sulfate (MAO inhibitors markedly potentiate the action of morphine; concurrent and/or sequential use should be avoided).
No products indexed under this heading.

Phenobarbital (Co-administration increases the risk of respiratory depression, hypotension, profound sedation, or coma). Products include:
Donnatal Extentabs 2493

Prazepam (Co-administration increases the risk of respiratory depression, hypotension, profound sedation, or coma).
No products indexed under this heading.

Procarbazine Hydrochloride (MAO inhibitors markedly potentiate the action of morphine; concurrent and/or sequential use should be avoided). Products include:
Matulane Capsules 3191

Prochlorperazine (Co-administration increases the risk of respiratory depression, hypotension, profound sedation, or coma).
No products indexed under this heading.

Promethazine Hydrochloride (Co-administration increases the risk of respiratory depression, hypotension, profound sedation, or coma). Products include:
Phenergan Tablets and
 Suppositories.............................. 3440

Propofol (Co-administration increases the risk of respiratory depression, hypotension, profound sedation, or coma).
No products indexed under this heading.

Propoxyphene Hydrochloride (Co-administration increases the risk of respiratory depression, hypotension, profound sedation, or coma).
No products indexed under this heading.

Propoxyphene Napsylate (Co-administration increases the risk of respiratory depression, hypotension, profound sedation, or coma).
No products indexed under this heading.

Quazepam (Co-administration increases the risk of respiratory depression, hypotension, profound sedation, or coma).
No products indexed under this heading.

Quetiapine Fumarate (Co-administration increases the risk of respiratory depression, hypotension, profound sedation, or coma). Products include:
Seroquel Tablets 690

Rapacuronium Bromide (Morphine may enhance the neuromuscular blocking action of skeletal muscle relaxants and produce an increased degree of respiratory depression).
No products indexed under this heading.

Remifentanil Hydrochloride (Co-administration increases the risk of respiratory depression, hypotension, profound sedation, or coma).
No products indexed under this heading.

Risperidone (Co-administration increases the risk of respiratory depression, hypotension, profound sedation, or coma). Products include:
Risperdal 1676
Risperdal Consta Long-Acting
 Injection..................................... 1682
Risperdal M-Tab Orally
 Disintegrating Tablets.................. 1676

Rocuronium Bromide (Morphine may enhance the neuromuscular blocking action of skeletal muscle relaxants and produce an increased degree of respiratory depression). Products include:
Zemuron Injection 2346

Secobarbital Sodium (Co-administration increases the risk of respiratory depression, hypotension, profound sedation, or coma).
No products indexed under this heading.

Selegiline Hydrochloride (MAO inhibitors markedly potentiate the action of morphine; concurrent and/or sequential use should be avoided). Products include:
Eldepryl Capsules 3208
Zelapar Tablets 3372

Sevoflurane (Co-administration increases the risk of respiratory depression, hypotension, profound sedation, or coma). Products include:
Ultane Liquid for Inhalation 531

Sodium Oxybate (Co-administration increases the risk of respiratory depression, hypotension, profound sedation, or coma). Products include:
Xyrem Oral Solution 1688

Succinylcholine Chloride (Morphine may enhance the neuromuscular blocking action of skeletal muscle relaxants and produce an increased degree of respiratory depression).
No products indexed under this heading.

Sufentanil Citrate (Co-administration increases the risk of respiratory depression, hypotension, profound sedation, or coma).
No products indexed under this heading.

Temazepam (Co-administration increases the risk of respiratory depression, hypotension, profound sedation, or coma). Products include:
Restoril Capsules 1860

Thiamylal Sodium (Co-administration increases the risk of respiratory depression, hypotension, profound sedation, or coma).
No products indexed under this heading.

Thioridazine Hydrochloride (Co-administration increases the risk of respiratory depression, hypotension, profound sedation, or coma). Products include:
Thioridazine Hydrochloride
 Tablets....................................... 2163

Thiothixene (Co-administration increases the risk of respiratory depression, hypotension, profound sedation, or coma). Products include:
Thiothixene Capsules 2165

Tranylcypromine Sulfate (MAO inhibitors markedly potentiate the action of morphine; concurrent and/or sequential use should be avoided). Products include:
Parnate Tablets 1527

Triazolam (Co-administration increases the risk of respiratory depression, hypotension, profound sedation, or coma).
No products indexed under this heading.

Trifluoperazine Hydrochloride (Co-administration increases the risk of respiratory depression, hypotension, profound sedation, or coma).
No products indexed under this heading.

Vecuronium Bromide (Morphine may enhance the neuromuscular blocking action of skeletal muscle relaxants and produce an increased degree of respiratory depression).
No products indexed under this heading.

Zaleplon (Co-administration increases the risk of respiratory depression, hypotension, profound sedation, or coma). Products include:
Sonata Capsules 1717

Ziprasidone Hydrochloride (Co-administration increases the risk of respiratory depression, hypotension, profound sedation, or coma). Products include:
Geodon Capsules 2529

Zolpidem Tartrate (Co-administration increases the risk of respiratory depression, hypotension, profound sedation, or coma). Products include:
Ambien Tablets 2851
Ambien CR Tablets 2855

Food Interactions

Alcohol (Patients must not consume alcoholic beverages, prescription or non-prescription medications containing alcohol while on morphine sulfate therapy. Consumption of alcohol while taking morphine sulfate may result in the rapid release and absoption of a potentially fatal dose of morphine).

AVODART SOFT GELATIN CAPSULES

(Dutasteride) 1390
May interact with cytochrome p450 3a4 inhibitors (selected) and certain other agents. Compounds in these categories include:

Acetazolamide (Blood concentrations of dutasteride may increase in the presence of CYP3A4 inhibitors).
No products indexed under this heading.

Amiodarone Hydrochloride (Blood concentrations of dutasteride may increase in the presence of CYP3A4 inhibitors).
No products indexed under this heading.

Amprenavir (Blood concentrations of dutasteride may increase in the presence of CYP3A4 inhibitors). Products include:
Agenerase Capsules 1327
Agenerase Oral Solution 1332

Anastrozole (Blood concentrations of dutasteride may increase in the presence of CYP3A4 inhibitors). Products include:
Arimidex Tablets 673

Aprepitant (Blood concentrations of dutasteride may increase in the presence of CYP3A4 inhibitors). Products include:
Emend Capsules 1963

Cimetidine (Blood concentrations of dutasteride may increase in the presence of CYP3A4 inhibitors). Products include:

IMPORTANT NOTE: Always consult each drug listing in the patient's regimen for possible interactions.

Tagamet HB 200 Tablets .... ▣664

Cimetidine Hydrochloride (Blood concentrations of dutasteride may increase in the presence of CYP3A4 inhibitors).
No products indexed under this heading.

Ciprofloxacin (Blood concentrations of dutasteride may increase in the presence of CYP3A4 inhibitors). Products include:
Cipro Oral Suspension 2977
Cipro I.V. 2984
Cipro XR Tablets 2990
Ciprodex Otic Suspension 559

Clarithromycin (Blood concentrations of dutasteride may increase in the presence of CYP3A4 inhibitors). Products include:
Biaxin/Biaxin XL 402
PREVPAC 3284

Clotrimazole (Blood concentrations of dutasteride may increase in the presence of CYP3A4 inhibitors). Products include:
Desenex Athlete's Foot Cream .... ▣635
Lotrimin 3039
Lotrisone 3040

Cyclosporine (Blood concentrations of dutasteride may increase in the presence of CYP3A4 inhibitors). Products include:
Gengraf Capsules 459
Neoral Oral Solution 2259
Neoral Soft Gelatin Capsules 2259
Restasis Ophthalmic Emulsion 575
Sandimmune 2275

Dalfopristin (Blood concentrations of dutasteride may increase in the presence of CYP3A4 inhibitors).
No products indexed under this heading.

Danazol (Blood concentrations of dutasteride may increase in the presence of CYP3A4 inhibitors).
No products indexed under this heading.

Delavirdine Mesylate (Blood concentrations of dutasteride may increase in the presence of CYP3A4 inhibitors). Products include:
Rescriptor Tablets 2551

Diltiazem Hydrochloride (Blood concentrations of dutasteride may increase in the presence of CYP3A4 inhibitors). Products include:
Cardizem LA Extended Release Tablets 1728
Tiazac Capsules 1201

Diltiazem Maleate (Blood concentrations of dutasteride may increase in the presence of CYP3A4 inhibitors).
No products indexed under this heading.

Efavirenz (Blood concentrations of dutasteride may increase in the presence of CYP3A4 inhibitors). Products include:
Atripla Tablets 945
Sustiva Capsules 930
Sustiva Tablets 930

Erythromycin (Blood concentrations of dutasteride may increase in the presence of CYP3A4 inhibitors). Products include:
Ery-Tab Tablets 449
Erythromycin Base Filmtab Tablets 455
Erythromycin Delayed-Release Capsules, USP 457
PCE Dispertab Tablets 515

Erythromycin Estolate (Blood concentrations of dutasteride may increase in the presence of CYP3A4 inhibitors).
No products indexed under this heading.

Erythromycin Ethylsuccinate (Blood concentrations of dutasteride may increase in the presence of CYP3A4 inhibitors). Products include:
E.E.S. 451
EryPed 447

Erythromycin Gluceptate (Blood concentrations of dutasteride may increase in the presence of CYP3A4 inhibitors).
No products indexed under this heading.

Erythromycin Lactobionate (Blood concentrations of dutasteride may increase in the presence of CYP3A4 inhibitors).
No products indexed under this heading.

Erythromycin Stearate (Blood concentrations of dutasteride may increase in the presence of CYP3A4 inhibitors). Products include:
Erythrocin Stearate Filmtab Tablets 453

Esomeprazole Magnesium (Blood concentrations of dutasteride may increase in the presence of CYP3A4 inhibitors). Products include:
Nexium Delayed-Release Capsules 655

Fluconazole (Blood concentrations of dutasteride may increase in the presence of CYP3A4 inhibitors).
No products indexed under this heading.

Fluoxetine Hydrochloride (Blood concentrations of dutasteride may increase in the presence of CYP3A4 inhibitors). Products include:
Prozac Pulvules and Liquid 1801
Symbyax Capsules 1819

Fluvoxamine Maleate (Blood concentrations of dutasteride may increase in the presence of CYP3A4 inhibitors).
No products indexed under this heading.

Fosamprenavir Calcium (Blood concentrations of dutasteride may increase in the presence of CYP3A4 inhibitors). Products include:
Lexiva Tablets 1505

Indinavir Sulfate (Blood concentrations of dutasteride may increase in the presence of CYP3A4 inhibitors). Products include:
Crixivan Capsules 1940

Isoniazid (Blood concentrations of dutasteride may increase in the presence of CYP3A4 inhibitors).
No products indexed under this heading.

Itraconazole (Blood concentrations of dutasteride may increase in the presence of CYP3A4 inhibitors).
No products indexed under this heading.

Ketoconazole (Blood concentrations of dutasteride may increase in the presence of CYP3A4 inhibitors). Products include:
Nizoral A-D Shampoo, 1% 1868

Lopinavir (Blood concentrations of dutasteride may increase in the presence of CYP3A4 inhibitors). Products include:
Kaletra 476

Loratadine (Blood concentrations of dutasteride may increase in the presence of CYP3A4 inhibitors). Products include:
Alavert Allergy & Sinus D-12 Hour Tablets .... ▣771
Alavert .... ▣771
Children's Claritin Allergy Oral Solution .... ▣771
Claritin Non-Drowsy 24 Hour Tablets .... ▣772
Claritin Reditabs 24 Hour Non-Drowsy Tablets .... ▣772
Claritin-D Non-Drowsy 12 Hour Tablets .... ▣772
Claritin-D Non-Drowsy 24 Hour Tablets .... ▣772

Metronidazole (Blood concentrations of dutasteride may increase in the presence of CYP3A4 inhibitors). Products include:
Metrogel 1% 1211
MetroGel-Vaginal Gel 1855
Vandazole Vaginal Gel 3338

Metronidazole Benzoate (Blood concentrations of dutasteride may increase in the presence of CYP3A4 inhibitors).
No products indexed under this heading.

Metronidazole Hydrochloride (Blood concentrations of dutasteride may increase in the presence of CYP3A4 inhibitors).
No products indexed under this heading.

Miconazole (Blood concentrations of dutasteride may increase in the presence of CYP3A4 inhibitors).
No products indexed under this heading.

Miconazole Nitrate (Blood concentrations of dutasteride may increase in the presence of CYP3A4 inhibitors). Products include:
Desenex .... ▣635
Desenex Jock Itch Spray Powder ... ▣635

Nefazodone Hydrochloride (Blood concentrations of dutasteride may increase in the presence of CYP3A4 inhibitors).
No products indexed under this heading.

Nelfinavir Mesylate (Blood concentrations of dutasteride may increase in the presence of CYP3A4 inhibitors). Products include:
Viracept 2577

Nevirapine (Blood concentrations of dutasteride may increase in the presence of CYP3A4 inhibitors). Products include:
Viramune Oral Suspension 873
Viramune Tablets 873

Niacinamide (Blood concentrations of dutasteride may increase in the presence of CYP3A4 inhibitors).
No products indexed under this heading.

Nicotinamide (Blood concentrations of dutasteride may increase in the presence of CYP3A4 inhibitors). Products include:
Nicomide Tablets 1088

Nifedipine (Blood concentrations of dutasteride may increase in the presence of CYP3A4 inhibitors). Products include:
Adalat CC Tablets 2964

Norfloxacin (Blood concentrations of dutasteride may increase in the presence of CYP3A4 inhibitors). Products include:
Noroxin Tablets 2032

Omeprazole (Blood concentrations of dutasteride may increase in the presence of CYP3A4 inhibitors). Products include:
Zegerid Capsules 2958
Zegerid Powder for Oral Solution 2958

Paroxetine Hydrochloride (Blood concentrations of dutasteride may increase in the presence of CYP3A4 inhibitors). Products include:
Paxil CR Controlled-Release Tablets 1538
Paxil 1530

Propoxyphene Hydrochloride (Blood concentrations of dutasteride may increase in the presence of CYP3A4 inhibitors).
No products indexed under this heading.

Propoxyphene Napsylate (Blood concentrations of dutasteride may increase in the presence of CYP3A4 inhibitors).
No products indexed under this heading.

Quinidine (Blood concentrations of dutasteride may increase in the presence of CYP3A4 inhibitors).
No products indexed under this heading.

Quinidine Hydrochloride (Blood concentrations of dutasteride may increase in the presence of CYP3A4 inhibitors).
No products indexed under this heading.

Quinidine Polygalacturonate (Blood concentrations of dutasteride may increase in the presence of CYP3A4 inhibitors).
No products indexed under this heading.

Quinidine Sulfate (Blood concentrations of dutasteride may increase in the presence of CYP3A4 inhibitors).
No products indexed under this heading.

Quinine (Blood concentrations of dutasteride may increase in the presence of CYP3A4 inhibitors).
No products indexed under this heading.

Quinine Sulfate (Blood concentrations of dutasteride may increase in the presence of CYP3A4 inhibitors).
No products indexed under this heading.

Quinupristin (Blood concentrations of dutasteride may increase in the presence of CYP3A4 inhibitors).
No products indexed under this heading.

Ranitidine Bismuth Citrate (Blood concentrations of dutasteride may increase in the presence of CYP3A4 inhibitors).
No products indexed under this heading.

Ranitidine Hydrochloride (Blood concentrations of dutasteride may increase in the presence of CYP3A4 inhibitors). Products include:
Zantac 1624
Zantac Injection 1619
Zantac Injection Pharmacy Bulk Package 1622

Ritonavir (Blood concentrations of dutasteride may increase in the presence of CYP3A4 inhibitors). Products include:
Kaletra 476
Norvir 503

Saquinavir (Blood concentrations of dutasteride may increase in the presence of CYP3A4 inhibitors).
No products indexed under this heading.

Saquinavir Mesylate (Blood concentrations of dutasteride may increase in the presence of CYP3A4 inhibitors). Products include:
Invirase 2772

Sertraline Hydrochloride (Blood concentrations of dutasteride may increase in the presence of CYP3A4 inhibitors). Products include:
Zoloft 2586

Telithromycin (Blood concentrations of dutasteride may increase in the presence of CYP3A4 inhibitors). Products include:
Ketek Tablets 2903

Troglitazone (Blood concentrations of dutasteride may increase in the presence of CYP3A4 inhibitors).
No products indexed under this heading.

Troleandomycin (Blood concentrations of dutasteride may increase in the presence of CYP3A4 inhibitors).
No products indexed under this heading.

Valproate Sodium (Blood concentrations of dutasteride may increase in the presence of CYP3A4 inhibitors). Products include:
Depacon Injection 412

Verapamil Hydrochloride (Blood concentrations of dutasteride may increase in the presence of CYP3A4 inhibitors). Products include:
Covera-HS Tablets 3139
Tarka Tablets 524
Verelan PM Extended-Release Capsules, Controlled-Onset 3106

Voriconazole (Blood concentrations of dutasteride may increase in the presence of CYP3A4 inhibitors). Products include:
VFEND I.V. 2564
VFEND Oral Suspension 2564
VFEND Tablets 2564

Zafirlukast (Blood concentrations of dutasteride may increase in the presence of CYP3A4 inhibitors). Products include:
Accolate Tablets 671

Zileuton (Blood concentrations of dutasteride may increase in the presence of CYP3A4 inhibitors). Products include:
Zyflo Tablets 1023

Food Interactions

Grapefruit (Blood concentrations of dutasteride may increase in the presence of CYP3A4 inhibitors).

Grapefruit Juice (Blood concentrations of dutasteride may increase in the presence of CYP3A4 inhibitors).

AWARENESS CLEAR CAPSULES

(Herbals, Multiple) 827
None cited in PDR database.

AXERT TABLETS

(Almotriptan Malate) 2396
May interact with 5HT1-receptor agonists, ergot-containing drugs, erythromycin, selective serotonin reuptake inhibitors, and certain other agents. Compounds in these categories include:

Citalopram Hydrobromide (Co-administration of SSRI and 5HT1 agonist have been rarely reported to cause weakness, hyperreflexia, and incoordination). Products include:
Celexa 1176

Dihydroergotamine Mesylate (Ergot-containing drugs have been reported to cause prolonged vasospastic reactions; because there is a theoretical basis that these effects may be additive, use of ergot-type agents and almotriptan within 24 hours is contraindicated). Products include:
Migranal Nasal Spray 3348

Ergonovine Maleate (Ergot-containing drugs have been reported to cause prolonged vasospastic reactions; because there is a theoretical basis that these effects may be additive, use of ergot-type agents and almotriptan within 24 hours is contraindicated).
No products indexed under this heading.

Ergotamine Tartrate (Ergot-containing drugs have been reported to cause prolonged vasospastic reactions; because there is a theoretical basis that these effects may be additive, use of ergot-type agents and almotriptan within 24 hours is contraindicated).
No products indexed under this heading.

Erythromycin (Co-administration with other potent inhibitors of CYP3A4 inhibitors, such as erythromycin, may result in increased exposures to almotriptan). Products include:
Ery-Tab Tablets 449
Erythromycin Base Filmtab Tablets 455
Erythromycin Delayed-Release Capsules, USP 457
PCE Dispertab Tablets 515

Erythromycin Estolate (Co-administration with other potent inhibitors of CYP3A4 inhibitors, such as erythromycin, may result in increased exposures to almotriptan).
No products indexed under this heading.

Erythromycin Ethylsuccinate (Co-administration with other potent inhibitors of CYP3A4 inhibitors, such as erythromycin, may result in increased exposures to almotriptan). Products include:
E.E.S. 451
EryPed 447

Erythromycin Gluceptate (Co-administration with other potent inhibitors of CYP3A4 inhibitors, such as erythromycin, may result in increased exposures to almotriptan).
No products indexed under this heading.

Erythromycin Stearate (Co-administration with other potent inhibitors of CYP3A4 inhibitors, such as erythromycin, may result in increased exposures to almotriptan). Products include:
Erythrocin Stearate Filmtab Tablets 453

Fluoxetine Hydrochloride (Co-administration has resulted in an increase in maximal concentrations of almotriptan by 18%; this difference is not clinically significant; co-administration of SSRI and 5HT1 agonist have been rarely reported to cause weakness, hyperreflexia, and incoordination). Products include:
Prozac Pulvules and Liquid 1801
Symbyax Capsules 1819

Fluvoxamine Maleate (Co-administration of SSRI and 5HT1 agonist have been rarely reported to cause weakness, hyperreflexia, and incoordination).
No products indexed under this heading.

Itraconazole (Co-administration with other potent inhibitors of CYP3A4 inhibitors, such as itraconazole, may result in increased exposures to almotriptan).
No products indexed under this heading.

Ketoconazole (Co-administration has resulted in an approximately 60% increase in the AUC and maximal plasma concentrations of almotriptan). Products include:
Nizoral A-D Shampoo, 1% 1868

Methylergonovine Maleate (Ergot-containing drugs have been reported to cause prolonged vasospastic reactions; because there is a theoretical basis that these effects may be additive, use of ergot-type agents and almotriptan within 24 hours is contraindicated).
No products indexed under this heading.

Methysergide Maleate (Ergot-containing drugs have been reported to cause prolonged vasospastic reactions; because there is a theoretical basis that these effects may be additive, use of ergot-type agents and almotriptan within 24 hours is contraindicated).
No products indexed under this heading.

Moclobemide (Co-administration has resulted in a 27% decrease in almotriptan clearance).
No products indexed under this heading.

Naratriptan Hydrochloride (Co-administration with other 5HT1 agonists within 24 hours of treatment with almotriptan is contraindicated). Products include:
Amerge Tablets 1339

Paroxetine Hydrochloride (Co-administration of SSRI and 5HT1 agonist have been rarely reported to cause weakness, hyperreflexia, and incoordination). Products include:
Paxil CR Controlled-Release Tablets 1538
Paxil 1530

Ritonavir (Co-administration with other potent inhibitors of CYP3A4 inhibitors, such as ritonavir, may result in increased exposures to almotriptan). Products include:
Kaletra 476
Norvir 503

Rizatriptan Benzoate (Co-administration with other 5HT1 agonists within 24 hours of treatment with almotriptan is contraindicated). Products include:
Maxalt Tablets 2008
Maxalt-MLT Orally Disintegrating Tablets 2008

Sertraline Hydrochloride (Co-administration of SSRI and 5HT1 agonist have been rarely reported to cause weakness, hyperreflexia, and incoordination). Products include:
Zoloft 2586

Sumatriptan (Co-administration with other 5HT1 agonists within 24 hours of treatment with almotriptan is contraindicated). Products include:
Imitrex Nasal Spray 1467

Sumatriptan Succinate (Co-administration with other 5HT1 agonists within 24 hours of treatment with almotriptan is contraindicated). Products include:
Imitrex Injection 1463
Imitrex Tablets 1471

Verapamil Hydrochloride (Co-administration has resulted in a 20% increase in AUC and a 24% increase in maximal plasma concentrations of almotriptan; neither of these changes is clinically significant). Products include:
Covera-HS Tablets 3139
Tarka Tablets 524
Verelan PM Extended-Release Capsules, Controlled-Onset 3106

Zolmitriptan (Co-administration with other 5HT1 agonists within 24 hours of treatment with almotriptan is contraindicated). Products include:
Zomig Tablets 3519
Zomig Nasal Spray 3523
Zomig-ZMT Tablets 3519

AXID ORAL SOLUTION

(Nizatidine) 879
May interact with:

Aspirin (Increased serum salicylate levels when nizatidine is given concurrently with very high doses (3,900 mg) of aspirin). Products include:
Aggrenox Capsules 822
Bayer Aspirin 744
BC Allergy Sinus Cold Powder 677
BC Headache Powder 677
Arthritis Strength BC Powder 677
BC Sinus Cold Powder 677
Excedrin Extra Strength Caplets/Tablets/Geltabs 684
Excedrin Migraine Caplets/Tablets/Geltabs 609
Goody's Body Pain Formula Powder 684
Goody's Extra Strength Headache Powders 611
Goody's Extra Strength Pain Relief Tablets 685
Percodan Tablets 1132
St. Joseph 81 mg Aspirin Chewable and Enteric Coated Tablets 1869

AZILECT TABLETS

(Rasagiline mesylate) 3293
May interact with cytochrome p450 1a2 inhibitors (selected), monoamine oxidase inhibitors, nonselective MAO inhibitors, selective serotonin reuptake inhibitors, sympathomimetics, tricyclic antidepressants, and certain other agents. Compounds in these categories include:

Alatrofloxacin Mesylate (Rasagiline plasma concentrations may increase up to 2 fold in patients using concomitant CYP1A2 inhibitors).
No products indexed under this heading.

Albuterol (Severe hypertensive reactions have followed the administration of sympathomimetics and non-selective MAO inhibitors and concomitant use is contraindicated). Products include:
Proventil Inhalation Aerosol 3053

Albuterol Sulfate (Severe hypertensive reactions have followed the administration of sympathomimetics and non-selective MAO inhibitors and concomitant use is contraindicated). Products include:
AccuNeb Inhalation Solution 1055
Combivent Inhalation Aerosol 847
DuoNeb Inhalation Solution 1058
ProAir HFA Inhalation Aerosol 3300
Proventil Inhalation Solution 0.083% 3055
Proventil HFA Inhalation Aerosol 3056
Ventolin HFA Inhalation Aerosol 1600
VoSpire ER Tablets 1052

to 2 fold in patients using concomitant CYP1A2 inhibitors). Products include:

- Mircette Tablets 1066
- NuvaRing 2340
- Ortho-Cyclen/Ortho Tri-Cyclen 2429
- Ortho Evra Transdermal System 2417
- Ortho Tri-Cyclen Lo Tablets 2436
- Seasonique Tablets 1077
- Yasmin 28 Tablets 796
- Yaz Tablets 803

Fluoxetine Hydrochloride (Severe CNS toxicity associated with hyperpyrexia and death has been reported with the combination of SSRIs). Products include:

- Prozac Pulvules and Liquid 1801
- Symbyax Capsules 1819

Fluvoxamine (Rasagiline plasma concentrations may increase up to 2 fold in patients using concomitant CYP1A2 inhibitors).

No products indexed under this heading.

Fluvoxamine Maleate (Rasagiline plasma concentrations may increase up to 2 fold in patients using concomitant CYP1A2 inhibitors).

No products indexed under this heading.

Gatifloxacin (Rasagiline plasma concentrations may increase up to 2 fold in patients using concomitant CYP1A2 inhibitors). Products include:

- Tequin Injection 938
- Tequin Injection in 5% Dextrose 938
- Tequin Tablets 938
- Zymar Ophthalmic Solution 575

Gemifloxacin Mesylate (Rasagiline plasma concentrations may increase up to 2 fold in patients using concomitant CYP1A2 inhibitors).

No products indexed under this heading.

Grepafloxacin Hydrochloride (Rasagiline plasma concentrations may increase up to 2 fold in patients using concomitant CYP1A2 inhibitors).

No products indexed under this heading.

Hypericum (Rasagiline is contraindicated for use with St. John's wort). Products include:

- Satiete Tablets 832

Hypericum Perforatum (Rasagiline is contraindicated for use with St. John's wort).

No products indexed under this heading.

Imipramine Hydrochloride (Severe CNS toxicity associated with hyperpyrexia and death has been reported with the combination of tricyclic antidepressants).

No products indexed under this heading.

Imipramine Pamoate (Severe CNS toxicity associated with hyperpyrexia and death has been reported with the combination of tricyclic antidepressants).

No products indexed under this heading.

Isocarboxazid (Severe CNS toxicity associated with hyperpyrexia and death has been reported with the combination of selective MAO-B inhibitors).

No products indexed under this heading.

Isoniazid (Rasagiline plasma concentrations may increase up to 2 fold in patients using concomitant CYP1A2 inhibitors).

No products indexed under this heading.

Isoproterenol Hydrochloride (Severe hypertensive reactions have followed the administration of sympathomimetics and non-selective MAO inhibitors and concomitant use is contraindicated).

No products indexed under this heading.

Isoproterenol Sulfate (Severe hypertensive reactions have followed the administration of sympathomimetics and non-selective MAO inhibitors and concomitant use is contraindicated).

No products indexed under this heading.

Ketoconazole (Rasagiline plasma concentrations may increase up to 2 fold in patients using concomitant CYP1A2 inhibitors). Products include:

- Nizoral A-D Shampoo, 1% 1868

Levalbuterol Hydrochloride (Severe hypertensive reactions have followed the administration of sympathomimetics and non-selective MAO inhibitors and concomitant use is contraindicated). Products include:

- Xopenex Inhalation Solution 3146
- Xopenex Inhalation Solution Concentrate 3150

Levofloxacin (Rasagiline plasma concentrations may increase up to 2 fold in patients using concomitant CYP1A2 inhibitors). Products include:

- Levaquin 2384
- Levaquin in 5% Dextrose Injection 2384
- Quixin Ophthalmic Solution 3383

Levonorgestrel (Rasagiline plasma concentrations may increase up to 2 fold in patients using concomitant CYP1A2 inhibitors). Products include:

- Climara Pro Transdermal System 776
- Mirena Intrauterine System 787
- Plan B Tablets 1076
- Seasonique Tablets 1077

Lomefloxacin Hydrochloride (Rasagiline plasma concentrations may increase up to 2 fold in patients using concomitant CYP1A2 inhibitors).

No products indexed under this heading.

Maprotiline Hydrochloride (Severe CNS toxicity associated with hyperpyrexia and death has been reported with the combination of tricyclic antidepressants).

No products indexed under this heading.

Meperidine Hydrochloride (Serious, sometimes fatal reactions have been precipitated with concomitant use of meperidine and MAO inhibitors and concomitant use is contraindicated).

No products indexed under this heading.

Mestranol (Rasagiline plasma concentrations may increase up to 2 fold in patients using concomitant CYP1A2 inhibitors).

No products indexed under this heading.

Metaproterenol Sulfate (Severe hypertensive reactions have followed the administration of sympathomimetics and non-selective MAO inhibitors and concomitant use is contraindicated). Products include:

- Alupent Inhalation Aerosol 826

Metaraminol Bitartrate (Severe hypertensive reactions have followed the administration of sympathomimetics and non-selective MAO inhibitors and concomitant use is contraindicated).

No products indexed under this heading.

Methadone Hydrochloride (Serious, sometimes fatal reactions have been precipitated with concomitant use of methadone and MAO inhibitors and concomitant use is contraindicated).

No products indexed under this heading.

Methoxamine Hydrochloride (Severe hypertensive reactions have followed the administration of sympathomimetics and non-selective MAO inhibitors and concomitant use is contraindicated).

No products indexed under this heading.

Methoxsalen (Rasagiline plasma concentrations may increase up to 2 fold in patients using concomitant CYP1A2 inhibitors). Products include:

- Oxsoralen Lotion 1% 3352
- Oxsoralen-Ultra Capsules 3353

Mexiletine Hydrochloride (Rasagiline plasma concentrations may increase up to 2 fold in patients using concomitant CYP1A2 inhibitors).

No products indexed under this heading.

Mibefradil Dihydrochloride (Rasagiline plasma concentrations may increase up to 2 fold in patients using concomitant CYP1A2 inhibitors).

No products indexed under this heading.

Mirtazapine (Rasagiline is contraindicated for use with mirtazapine).

No products indexed under this heading.

Moclobemide (Severe CNS toxicity associated with hyperpyrexia and death has been reported with the combination of selective MAO-B inhibitors).

No products indexed under this heading.

Moxifloxacin Hydrochloride (Rasagiline plasma concentrations may increase up to 2 fold in patients using concomitant CYP1A2 inhibitors). Products include:

- Avelox 2970
- Vigamox Ophthalmic Solution 564

Nalidixic Acid (Rasagiline plasma concentrations may increase up to 2 fold in patients using concomitant CYP1A2 inhibitors).

No products indexed under this heading.

Norepinephrine Bitartrate (Severe hypertensive reactions have followed the administration of sympathomimetics and non-selective MAO inhibitors and concomitant use is contraindicated).

No products indexed under this heading.

Norethindrone (Rasagiline plasma concentrations may increase up to 2 fold in patients using concomitant CYP1A2 inhibitors). Products include:

- Ortho Micronor Tablets 2426

Norfloxacin (Rasagiline plasma concentrations may increase up to 2 fold in patients using concomitant CYP1A2 inhibitors). Products include:

- Noroxin Tablets 2032

Norgestrel (Rasagiline plasma concentrations may increase up to 2 fold in patients using concomitant CYP1A2 inhibitors).

No products indexed under this heading.

Nortriptyline Hydrochloride (Severe CNS toxicity associated with hyperpyrexia and death has been reported with the combination of tricyclic antidepressants).

No products indexed under this heading.

Ofloxacin (Rasagiline plasma concentrations may increase up to 2 fold in patients using concomitant CYP1A2 inhibitors). Products include:

- Floxin Otic Solution 1049

Omeprazole (Rasagiline plasma concentrations may increase up to 2 fold in patients using concomitant CYP1A2 inhibitors). Products include:

- Zegerid Capsules 2958
- Zegerid Powder for Oral Solution 2958

Pargyline Hydrochloride (Severe CNS toxicity associated with hyperpyrexia and death has been reported with the combination of selective MAO-B inhibitors).

No products indexed under this heading.

Paroxetine Hydrochloride (Rasagiline plasma concentrations may increase up to 2 fold in patients using concomitant CYP1A2 inhibitors). Products include:

- Paxil CR Controlled-Release Tablets 1538
- Paxil 1530

Phenelzine Sulfate (Severe CNS toxicity associated with hyperpyrexia and death has been reported with the combination of selective MAO-B inhibitors).

No products indexed under this heading.

Phenylephrine Bitartrate (Severe hypertensive reactions have followed the administration of sympathomimetics and non-selective MAO inhibitors and concomitant use is contraindicated).

No products indexed under this heading.

Phenylephrine Hydrochloride (Severe hypertensive reactions have followed the administration of sympathomimetics and non-selective MAO inhibitors and concomitant use is contraindicated). Products include:

- Comtrex Maximum Strength Non-Drowsy Cold & Cough Caplets 725
- Comtrex Maximum Strength Day/Night Severe Cold & Sinus Caplets - Day Formulation 725
- Comtrex Maximum Strength Day/Night Severe Cold & Sinus Caplets - Night Formulation 725
- Contac Cold and Flu Maximum Strength Caplets 728
- Contac Cold and Flu Day and Night Caplets (Day Formulation Only) 727
- Contac Cold and Flu Day and Night Caplets (Night Formulation Only) 727
- Contac Cold and Flu Non-Drowsy Caplets 728

Contac-D Cold Non-Drowsy Tablets ▣ 729
Children's Dimetapp Cold & Allergy Elixir ▣ 730
Children's Dimetapp Cold & Allergy Chewable Tablets ▣ 730
Children's Dimetapp DM Cold & Cough Elixir ▣ 731
Toddler's Dimetapp Cold and Cough Drops ▣ 732
Excedrin Sinus Headache Caplets/Tablets ▣ 610
4-Way Fast Acting Nasal Spray ▣ 775
4-Way Menthol Nasal Spray ▣ 775
Preparation H Maximum Strength Cream ▣ 666
Preparation H Cooling Gel ▣ 666
Preparation H ▣ 666
Refenesen PE Caplets ▣ 721
Robitussin Cough & Allergy Syrup ▣ 736
Robitussin Cough & Cold Nighttime Liquid ▣ 736
Robitussin Cough, Cold & Flu Nighttime Liquid ▣ 738
Robitussin Head & Chest Congestion PE Syrup ▣ 739
Robitussin Pediatric Cough & Cold Nighttime Liquid ▣ 736
TheraFlu Cold & Cough Hot Liquid ▣ 740
TheraFlu Cold & Sore Throat Hot Liquid ▣ 741
TheraFlu Flu & Sore Throat Hot Liquid ▣ 742
TheraFlu Daytime Severe Cold Hot Liquid ▣ 742
TheraFlu Nighttime Severe Cold Hot Liquid ▣ 740
TheraFlu Warming Relief Daytime Severe Cold ▣ 743
TheraFlu Warming Relief Nighttime Severe Cold ▣ 743
Triaminic Chest & Nasal Congestion Liquid ▣ 746
Triaminic Cold & Allergy Liquid ▣ 746
Triaminic Daytime Cold & Cough Liquid ▣ 745
Triaminic Nighttime Cold & Cough Liquid ▣ 746
Triaminic Thin Strips Cold ▣ 748
Triaminic Thin Strips Cold & Cough ▣ 778
Triaminic Infant Thin Strips Decongestant ▣ 747
Triaminic Infant Thin Strips Decongestant Plus Cough ▣ 747
Children's Tylenol Plus Flu Oral Suspension ▣ 749
Tylenol Cold Head Congestion Daytime Caplets with Cool Burst and Gelcaps ▣ 750
Tylenol Cold Multi-Symptom Daytime Liquid ▣ 752
Tylenol Cold Multi-Symptom Severe Daytime Liquid ▣ 752
Concentrated Tylenol Infants' Drops Plus Cold & Cough ▣ 754
Tylenol Allergy Multi-Symptom Caplets with Cool Burst and Gelcaps 1872
Tylenol Allergy Multi-Symptom Nighttime Caplets with Cool Burst 1872
Children's Tylenol Plus Cold Suspension Liquid 1879
Children's Tylenol Plus Cold & Allergy Suspension Liquid 1878
Children's Tylenol Plus Flu Suspension Liquid 1881
Children's Tylenol Plus Multi-Symptom Cold Suspension Liquid 1879
Tylenol Cold Head Congestion Daytime Caplets with Cool Burst 1873
Tylenol Cold Head Congestion Nighttime Caplets with Cool Burst 1873
Tylenol Cold Head Congestion Severe Caplets with Cool Burst 1873
Tylenol Cold Multi-Symptom Daytime Caplets with Cool Burst and Gelcaps 1874
Tylenol Cold Multi-Symptom Daytime Liquid with Citrus Burst 1874
Tylenol Cold Multi-Symptom Nighttime Caplets with Cool Burst 1874
Tylenol Cold Multi-Symptom Nighttime Liquid with Cool Burst 1874
Tylenol Cold Multi-Symptom Severe Caplets with Cool Burst 1874
Tylenol Cold Multi-Symptom Severe Daytime Liquid with Citrus Burst 1874
Tylenol Sinus Congestion & Pain Daytime Caplets with Cool Burst and Gelcaps 1876
Tylenol Sinus Congestion & Pain Nighttime Caplets with Cool Burst 1876
Tylenol Sinus Congestion & Pain Severe Caplets with Cool Burst 1876
Vicks 44D Cough & Head Congestion Relief Liquid ▣ 760
Vicks DayQuil LiquiCaps/Liquid Multi-Symptom Cold/Flu Relief ▣ 761
Zicam Cough Plus D Cough Spray ▣ 767

Phenylephrine Tannate (Severe hypertensive reactions have followed the administration of sympathomimetics and non-selective MAO inhibitors and concomitant use is contraindicated).
No products indexed under this heading.

Phenylpropanolamine Hydrochloride (Severe hypertensive reactions have followed the administration of sympathomimetics and non-selective MAO inhibitors and concomitant use is contraindicated).
No products indexed under this heading.

Pirbuterol Acetate (Severe hypertensive reactions have followed the administration of sympathomimetics and non-selective MAO inhibitors and concomitant use is contraindicated). Products include:
Maxair Autohaler 1852

Procarbazine Hydrochloride (Severe CNS toxicity associated with hyperpyrexia and death has been reported with the combination of selective MAO-B inhibitors). Products include:
Matulane Capsules 3191

Protriptyline Hydrochloride (Severe CNS toxicity associated with hyperpyrexia and death has been reported with the combination of tricyclic antidepressants).
No products indexed under this heading.

Pseudoephedrine Hydrochloride (Severe hypertensive reactions have followed the administration of sympathomimetics and non-selective MAO inhibitors and concomitant use is contraindicated). Products include:
Advil Allergy Sinus Caplets ▣ 770
Advil Cold & Sinus ▣ 723
Advil Multi-Symptom Cold Caplets ▣ 770
Aleve Cold & Sinus Caplets 744
Allegra-D 12 Hour Extended-Release Tablets 2846
Allegra-D 24 Hour Extended-Release Tablets 2849
BC Cold Powder ▣ 677
Comtrex Maximum Strength Cold & Cough Day/Night Caplets - Day Formulation ▣ 726
Comtrex Maximum Strength Cold & Cough Day/Night Caplets - Night Formulation ▣ 726
Children's Motrin Cold Oral Suspension 1867
Mucinex D Extended-Release Bi-Layer Tablets ▣ 776
Robitussin Cough & Cold CF Liquid ▣ 735
Robitussin Cough & Cold Pediatric Drops ▣ 735
Tylenol Sinus Congestion & Pain Nighttime Caplets with Cool Burst ▣ 778
Tylenol Cold Severe Congestion Non-Drowsy Caplets with Cool Burst 1874
Tylenol Sinus Severe Congestion Caplets with Cool Burst 1876
Vicks 44D Cough & Head Congestion Relief Liquid 2679
Vicks 44M Cough, Cold & Flu Relief Liquid 2680
Vicks DayQuil Multi-Symptom Cold/Flu Relief LiquiCaps 2678
Vicks DayQuil Multi-Symptom Cold/Flu Relief Liquid 2678
Vicks NyQuil Multi-Symptom Cold/Flu Relief Liquid 2681
Vicks NyQuil Multi-Symptom Cold/Flu Relief LiquiCaps 2681
Children's Vicks NyQuil Cold/Cough Relief Liquid 2680
Zyrtec-D 12 Hour Extended Release Tablets 2597

Pseudoephedrine Sulfate (Severe hypertensive reactions have followed the administration of sympathomimetics and non-selective MAO inhibitors and concomitant use is contraindicated). Products include:
Alavert Allergy & Sinus D-12 Hour Tablets ▣ 771
Clarinex-D 24-Hour Extended-Release Tablets 2998
Claritin-D Non-Drowsy 12 Hour Tablets ▣ 772
Claritin-D Non-Drowsy 24 Hour Tablets ▣ 772

Ranitidine Hydrochloride (Rasagiline plasma concentrations may increase up to 2 fold in patients using concomitant CYP1A2 inhibitors). Products include:
Zantac 1624
Zantac Injection 1619
Zantac Injection Pharmacy Bulk Package 1622

Ritonavir (Rasagiline plasma concentrations may increase up to 2 fold in patients using concomitant CYP1A2 inhibitors). Products include:
Kaletra 476
Norvir 503

Salmeterol Xinafoate (Severe hypertensive reactions have followed the administration of sympathomimetics and non-selective MAO inhibitors and concomitant use is contraindicated). Products include:
Advair Diskus 100/50 1308
Advair Diskus 250/50 1308
Advair Diskus 500/50 1308
Advair HFA Inhalation Aerosol 1318
Serevent Diskus 1568

Selegiline Hydrochloride (Severe CNS toxicity associated with hyperpyrexia and death has been reported with the combination of selective MAO-B inhibitors). Products include:
Eldepryl Capsules 3208
Zelapar Tablets 3372

Sertraline Hydrochloride (Severe CNS toxicity associated with hyperpyrexia and death has been reported with the combination of SSRIs). Products include:
Zoloft 2586

Sparfloxacin (Rasagiline plasma concentrations may increase up to 2 fold in patients using concomitant CYP1A2 inhibitors).
No products indexed under this heading.

Tacrine Hydrochloride (Rasagiline plasma concentrations may increase up to 2 fold in patients using concomitant CYP1A2 inhibitors).
No products indexed under this heading.

Terbutaline Sulfate (Severe hypertensive reactions have followed the administration of sympathomimetics and non-selective MAO inhibitors and concomitant use is contraindicated).
No products indexed under this heading.

Ticlopidine Hydrochloride (Rasagiline plasma concentrations may increase up to 2 fold in patients using concomitant CYP1A2 inhibitors). Products include:
Ticlid Tablets 2810

Tramadol Hydrochloride (Serious, sometimes fatal reactions have been precipitated with concomitant use of tramadol and MAO inhibitors and concomitant use is contraindicated). Products include:
Ultram ER Tablets 2392

Tranylcypromine Sulfate (Severe CNS toxicity associated with hyperpyrexia and death has been reported with the combination of selective MAO-B inhibitors). Products include:
Parnate Tablets 1527

Trimipramine Maleate (Severe CNS toxicity associated with hyperpyrexia and death has been reported with the combination of tricyclic antidepressants).
No products indexed under this heading.

Troleandomycin (Rasagiline plasma concentrations may increase up to 2 fold in patients using concomitant CYP1A2 inhibitors).
No products indexed under this heading.

Trovafloxacin Mesylate (Rasagiline plasma concentrations may increase up to 2 fold in patients using concomitant CYP1A2 inhibitors).
No products indexed under this heading.

Zileuton (Rasagiline plasma concentrations may increase up to 2 fold in patients using concomitant CYP1A2 inhibitors). Products include:
Zyflo Tablets 1023

Food Interactions

Beverages with high tyramine (Severe hypertensive reactions have followed the administration of tyramine rich beverages and non-selective MAO inhibitors).

Food high in tyramine (Severe hypertensive reactions have followed the administration of tyramine rich foods and non-selective MAO inhibitors).

Grapefruit Juice (Rasagiline plasma concentrations may increase up to 2 fold in patients using concomitant CYP1A2 inhibitors).

AZMACORT INHALATION AEROSOL

(Triamcinolone Acetonide) 1726
May interact with:

Prednisone (Potential for increased likelihood of HPA suppression).
No products indexed under this heading.

AZOPT OPHTHALMIC SUSPENSION

(Brinzolamide) 557

May interact with carbonic anhydrase inhibitors and salicylates. Compounds in these categories include:

Acetazolamide (There is a potential for an additive effect on the known systemic effects of carbonic anhydrase inhibition in patients receiving an oral carbonic anhydrase inhibitor and brinzolamide; co-administration is not recommended).

No products indexed under this heading.

Aspirin (Co-administration with high dose salicylate and oral carbonic anhydrase inhibitor has resulted in rare instances of drug interactions). Products include:

Aggrenox Capsules 822
Bayer Aspirin 744
BC Allergy Sinus Cold Powder 677
BC Headache Powder 677
Arthritis Strength BC Powder 677
BC Sinus Cold Powder 677
Excedrin Extra Strength Caplets/Tablets/Geltabs 684
Excedrin Migraine Caplets/Tablets/Geltabs 609
Goody's Body Pain Formula Powder 684
Goody's Extra Strength Headache Powders 611
Goody's Extra Strength Pain Relief Tablets 685
Percodan Tablets 1132
St. Joseph 81 mg Aspirin Chewable and Enteric Coated Tablets 1869

Aspirin, Enteric Coated (Co-administration with high dose salicylate and oral carbonic anhydrase inhibitor has resulted in rare instances of drug interactions).

No products indexed under this heading.

Aspirin Buffered (Co-administration with high dose salicylate and oral carbonic anhydrase inhibitor has resulted in rare instances of drug interactions). Products include:

Bufferin Extra Strength Tablets 678
Bufferin Regular Strength Tablets ... 678

Choline Magnesium Trisalicylate (Co-administration with high dose salicylate and oral carbonic anhydrase inhibitor has resulted in rare instances of drug interactions).

No products indexed under this heading.

Dichlorphenamide (There is a potential for an additive effect on the known systemic effects of carbonic anhydrase inhibition in patients receiving an oral carbonic anhydrase inhibitor and brinzolamide; co-administration is not recommended). Products include:

Daranide Tablets 1950

Diflunisal (Co-administration with high dose salicylate and oral carbonic anhydrase inhibitor has resulted in rare instances of drug interactions). Products include:

Dolobid Tablets 1955

Dorzolamide Hydrochloride (There is a potential for an additive effect on the known systemic effects of carbonic anhydrase inhibition in patients receiving an oral carbonic anhydrase inhibitor and brinzolamide; co-administration is not recommended). Products include:

Cosopt Sterile Ophthalmic Solution 1931
Trusopt Sterile Ophthalmic Solution 2095

Magnesium Salicylate (Co-administration with high dose salicylate and oral carbonic anhydrase inhibitor has resulted in rare instances of drug interactions).

No products indexed under this heading.

Methazolamide (There is a potential for an additive effect on the known systemic effects of carbonic anhydrase inhibition in patients receiving an oral carbonic anhydrase inhibitor and brinzolamide; co-administration is not recommended).

No products indexed under this heading.

Salsalate (Co-administration with high dose salicylate and oral carbonic anhydrase inhibitor has resulted in rare instances of drug interactions).

No products indexed under this heading.

BACTROBAN CREAM

(Mupirocin Calcium) 1394
None cited in PDR database.

BACTROBAN NASAL

(Mupirocin Calcium) 1394
None cited in PDR database.

BACTROBAN OINTMENT

(Mupirocin) 1395
None cited in PDR database.

BARACLUDE ORAL SOLUTION

(Entecavir) 894
See Baraclude Tablets

BARACLUDE TABLETS

(Entecavir) 894

May interact with nephrotoxic agents. Compounds in these categories include:

Abacavir Sulfate (Since entecavir is primarily eliminated by the kidneys co-administration of entecavir with drugs that reduce renal function or compete for active tubular secretion may increase serum concentrations of either entecavir or the co-administered drug). Products include:

Epzicom Tablets 1436
Trizivir Tablets 1589
Ziagen 1626

Acyclovir (Since entecavir is primarily eliminated by the kidneys co-administration of entecavir with drugs that reduce renal function or compete for active tubular secretion may increase serum concentrations of either entecavir or the co-administered drug). Products include:

Zovirax 1643
Zovirax Cream 820
Zovirax Ointment 821

Acyclovir Sodium (Since entecavir is primarily eliminated by the kidneys co-administration of entecavir with drugs that reduce renal function or compete for active tubular secretion may increase serum concentrations of either entecavir or the co-administered drug).

No products indexed under this heading.

Alatrofloxacin Mesylate (Since entecavir is primarily eliminated by the kidneys co-administration of entecavir with drugs that reduce renal function or compete for active tubular secretion may increase serum concentrations of either entecavir or the co-administered drug).

No products indexed under this heading.

Aldesleukin (Since entecavir is primarily eliminated by the kidneys co-administration of entecavir with drugs that reduce renal function or compete for active tubular secretion may increase serum concentrations of either entecavir or the co-administered drug). Products include:

Proleukin for Injection 2266

Amikacin Sulfate (Since entecavir is primarily eliminated by the kidneys co-administration of entecavir with drugs that reduce renal function or compete for active tubular secretion may increase serum concentrations of either entecavir or the co-administered drug).

No products indexed under this heading.

Amoxicillin (Since entecavir is primarily eliminated by the kidneys co-administration of entecavir with drugs that reduce renal function or compete for active tubular secretion may increase serum concentrations of either entecavir or the co-administered drug). Products include:

Amoxil Capsules 1343
Amoxil Chewable Tablets 1343
Amoxil Pediatric Drops for Oral Suspension 1343
Amoxil Powder for Oral Suspension 1343
Amoxil Tablets 1343
Augmentin 1360
Augmentin Tablets 1363
Augmentin XR Extended-Release Tablets 1369
Augmentin ES-600 Powder for Oral Suspension 1366
PREVPAC 3284

Amoxicillin Trihydrate (Since entecavir is primarily eliminated by the kidneys co-administration of entecavir with drugs that reduce renal function or compete for active tubular secretion may increase serum concentrations of either entecavir or the co-administered drug).

No products indexed under this heading.

Amphotericin B (Since entecavir is primarily eliminated by the kidneys co-administration of entecavir with drugs that reduce renal function or compete for active tubular secretion may increase serum concentrations of either entecavir or the co-administered drug).

No products indexed under this heading.

Amphotericin B, liposomal (Since entecavir is primarily eliminated by the kidneys co-administration of entecavir with drugs that reduce renal function or compete for active tubular secretion may increase serum concentrations of either entecavir or the co-administered drug). Products include:

AmBisome for Injection 620

Amphotericin B Cholesteryl Sulfate (Since entecavir is primarily eliminated by the kidneys co-administration of entecavir with drugs that reduce renal function or compete for active tubular secretion may increase serum concentrations of either entecavir or the co-administered drug).

No products indexed under this heading.

Amphotericin B Lipid Complex (Since entecavir is primarily eliminated by the kidneys co-administration of entecavir with drugs that reduce renal function or compete for active tubular secretion may increase serum concentrations of either entecavir or the co-administered drug). Products include:

Abelcet Injection 1141

Ampicillin (Since entecavir is primarily eliminated by the kidneys co-administration of entecavir with drugs that reduce renal function or compete for active tubular secretion may increase serum concentrations of either entecavir or the co-administered drug).

No products indexed under this heading.

Ampicillin Sodium (Since entecavir is primarily eliminated by the kidneys co-administration of entecavir with drugs that reduce renal function or compete for active tubular secretion may increase serum concentrations of either entecavir or the co-administered drug).

No products indexed under this heading.

Ampicillin Trihydrate (Since entecavir is primarily eliminated by the kidneys co-administration of entecavir with drugs that reduce renal function or compete for active tubular secretion may increase serum concentrations of either entecavir or the co-administered drug).

No products indexed under this heading.

Amprenavir (Since entecavir is primarily eliminated by the kidneys co-administration of entecavir with drugs that reduce renal function or compete for active tubular secretion may increase serum concentrations of either entecavir or the co-administered drug). Products include:

Agenerase Capsules 1327
Agenerase Oral Solution 1332

Aspirin (Since entecavir is primarily eliminated by the kidneys co-administration of entecavir with drugs that reduce renal function or compete for active tubular secretion may increase serum concentrations of either entecavir or the co-administered drug). Products include:

Aggrenox Capsules 822
Bayer Aspirin 744
BC Allergy Sinus Cold Powder 677
BC Headache Powder 677
Arthritis Strength BC Powder 677
BC Sinus Cold Powder 677
Excedrin Extra Strength Caplets/Tablets/Geltabs 684
Excedrin Migraine Caplets/Tablets/Geltabs 609
Goody's Body Pain Formula Powder 684
Goody's Extra Strength Headache Powders 611
Goody's Extra Strength Pain Relief Tablets 685
Percodan Tablets 1132

St. Joseph 81 mg Aspirin Chewable and Enteric Coated Tablets 1869

Atazanavir (Since entecavir is primarily eliminated by the kidneys co-administration of entecavir with drugs that reduce renal function or compete for active tubular secretion may increase serum concentrations of either entecavir or the co-administered drug).
No products indexed under this heading.

Atorvastatin Calcium (Since entecavir is primarily eliminated by the kidneys co-administration of entecavir with drugs that reduce renal function or compete for active tubular secretion may increase serum concentrations of either entecavir or the co-administered drug). Products include:
Caduet Tablets 2508
Lipitor Tablets 2483

Azithromycin Dihydrate (Since entecavir is primarily eliminated by the kidneys co-administration of entecavir with drugs that reduce renal function or compete for active tubular secretion may increase serum concentrations of either entecavir or the co-administered drug).
No products indexed under this heading.

Azlocillin Sodium (Since entecavir is primarily eliminated by the kidneys co-administration of entecavir with drugs that reduce renal function or compete for active tubular secretion may increase serum concentrations of either entecavir or the co-administered drug).
No products indexed under this heading.

Aztreonam (Since entecavir is primarily eliminated by the kidneys co-administration of entecavir with drugs that reduce renal function or compete for active tubular secretion may increase serum concentrations of either entecavir or the co-administered drug).
No products indexed under this heading.

Bacampicillin Hydrochloride (Since entecavir is primarily eliminated by the kidneys co-administration of entecavir with drugs that reduce renal function or compete for active tubular secretion may increase serum concentrations of either entecavir or the co-administered drug).
No products indexed under this heading.

Balsalazide Disodium (Since entecavir is primarily eliminated by the kidneys co-administration of entecavir with drugs that reduce renal function or compete for active tubular secretion may increase serum concentrations of either entecavir or the co-administered drug). Products include:
Colazal Capsules 2838

Benazepril Hydrochloride (Since entecavir is primarily eliminated by the kidneys co-administration of entecavir with drugs that reduce renal function or compete for active tubular secretion may increase serum concentrations of either entecavir or the co-administered drug). Products include:
Lotensin Tablets 2243
Lotensin HCT Tablets 2246
Lotrel Capsules 2249

Bendroflumethiazide (Since entecavir is primarily eliminated by the kidneys co-administration of entecavir with drugs that reduce renal function or compete for active tubular secretion may increase serum concentrations of either entecavir or the co-administered drug).
No products indexed under this heading.

Caffeine (Since entecavir is primarily eliminated by the kidneys co-administration of entecavir with drugs that reduce renal function or compete for active tubular secretion may increase serum concentrations of either entecavir or the co-administered drug). Products include:
BC Headache Powder .... ▣677
Arthritis Strength BC Powder .... ▣677
Excedrin Extra Strength Caplets/Tablets/Geltabs .... ▣684
Excedrin Migraine Caplets/Tablets/Geltabs .... ▣609
Excedrin Tension Headache Caplets/Tablets/Geltabs .... ▣611
Goody's Extra Strength Headache Powders .... ▣611
Goody's Extra Strength Pain Relief Tablets .... ▣685
Vivarin .... ▣602
Winrgy Dietary Supplement .... ▣823

Captopril (Since entecavir is primarily eliminated by the kidneys co-administration of entecavir with drugs that reduce renal function or compete for active tubular secretion may increase serum concentrations of either entecavir or the co-administered drug). Products include:
Captopril Tablets 2149

Carbenicillin Disodium (Since entecavir is primarily eliminated by the kidneys co-administration of entecavir with drugs that reduce renal function or compete for active tubular secretion may increase serum concentrations of either entecavir or the co-administered drug).
No products indexed under this heading.

Carbenicillin Indanyl Sodium (Since entecavir is primarily eliminated by the kidneys co-administration of entecavir with drugs that reduce renal function or compete for active tubular secretion may increase serum concentrations of either entecavir or the co-administered drug).
No products indexed under this heading.

Carboplatin (Since entecavir is primarily eliminated by the kidneys co-administration of entecavir with drugs that reduce renal function or compete for active tubular secretion may increase serum concentrations of either entecavir or the co-administered drug).
No products indexed under this heading.

Carmustine (BCNU) (Since entecavir is primarily eliminated by the kidneys co-administration of entecavir with drugs that reduce renal function or compete for active tubular secretion may increase serum concentrations of either entecavir or the co-administered drug).
No products indexed under this heading.

Cefaclor (Since entecavir is primarily eliminated by the kidneys co-administration of entecavir with drugs that reduce renal function or compete for active tubular secretion may increase serum concentrations of either entecavir or the co-administered drug).
No products indexed under this heading.

Cefadroxil (Since entecavir is primarily eliminated by the kidneys co-administration of entecavir with drugs that reduce renal function or compete for active tubular secretion may increase serum concentrations of either entecavir or the co-administered drug).
No products indexed under this heading.

Cefamandole Nafate (Since entecavir is primarily eliminated by the kidneys co-administration of entecavir with drugs that reduce renal function or compete for active tubular secretion may increase serum concentrations of either entecavir or the co-administered drug).
No products indexed under this heading.

Cefazolin Sodium (Since entecavir is primarily eliminated by the kidneys co-administration of entecavir with drugs that reduce renal function or compete for active tubular secretion may increase serum concentrations of either entecavir or the co-administered drug).
No products indexed under this heading.

Cefdinir (Since entecavir is primarily eliminated by the kidneys co-administration of entecavir with drugs that reduce renal function or compete for active tubular secretion may increase serum concentrations of either entecavir or the co-administered drug). Products include:
Omnicef Capsules 511
Omnicef for Oral Suspension 511

Cefepime Hydrochloride (Since entecavir is primarily eliminated by the kidneys co-administration of entecavir with drugs that reduce renal function or compete for active tubular secretion may increase serum concentrations of either entecavir or the co-administered drug). Products include:
Maxipime for Injection 1105

Cefixime (Since entecavir is primarily eliminated by the kidneys co-administration of entecavir with drugs that reduce renal function or compete for active tubular secretion may increase serum concentrations of either entecavir or the co-administered drug). Products include:
Suprax 1843

Cefmetazole Sodium (Since entecavir is primarily eliminated by the kidneys co-administration of entecavir with drugs that reduce renal function or compete for active tubular secretion may increase serum concentrations of either entecavir or the co-administered drug).
No products indexed under this heading.

Cefonicid Sodium (Since entecavir is primarily eliminated by the kidneys co-administration of entecavir with drugs that reduce renal function or compete for active tubular secretion may increase serum concentrations of either entecavir or the co-administered drug).
No products indexed under this heading.

Cefoperazone Sodium (Since entecavir is primarily eliminated by the kidneys co-administration of entecavir with drugs that reduce renal function or compete for active tubular secretion may increase serum concentrations of either entecavir or the co-administered drug).
No products indexed under this heading.

Ceforanide (Since entecavir is primarily eliminated by the kidneys co-administration of entecavir with drugs that reduce renal function or compete for active tubular secretion may increase serum concentrations of either entecavir or the co-administered drug).
No products indexed under this heading.

Cefotaxime Sodium (Since entecavir is primarily eliminated by the kidneys co-administration of entecavir with drugs that reduce renal function or compete for active tubular secretion may increase serum concentrations of either entecavir or the co-administered drug).
No products indexed under this heading.

Cefotetan (Since entecavir is primarily eliminated by the kidneys co-administration of entecavir with drugs that reduce renal function or compete for active tubular secretion may increase serum concentrations of either entecavir or the co-administered drug).
No products indexed under this heading.

Cefoxitin Sodium (Since entecavir is primarily eliminated by the kidneys co-administration of entecavir with drugs that reduce renal function or compete for active tubular secretion may increase serum concentrations of either entecavir or the co-administered drug). Products include:
Mefoxin for Injection 2012
Mefoxin Premixed Intravenous Solution 2016

Cefpodoxime Proxetil (Since entecavir is primarily eliminated by the kidneys co-administration of entecavir with drugs that reduce renal function or compete for active tubular secretion may increase serum concentrations of either entecavir or the co-administered drug). Products include:
Vantin Tablets and Oral Suspension 2645

Cefprozil (Since entecavir is primarily eliminated by the kidneys co-administration of entecavir with drugs that reduce renal function or compete for active tubular secretion may increase serum concentrations of either entecavir or the co-administered drug).
No products indexed under this heading.

Ceftazidime (Since entecavir is primarily eliminated by the kidneys co-administration of entecavir with drugs that reduce renal function or compete for active tubular secretion may increase serum concentrations of either entecavir or the co-administered drug). Products include:

Fortaz 1453

Ceftizoxime Sodium (Since entecavir is primarily eliminated by the kidneys co-administration of entecavir with drugs that reduce renal function or compete for active tubular secretion may increase serum concentrations of either entecavir or the co-administered drug).

No products indexed under this heading.

Ceftriaxone Sodium (Since entecavir is primarily eliminated by the kidneys co-administration of entecavir with drugs that reduce renal function or compete for active tubular secretion may increase serum concentrations of either entecavir or the co-administered drug). Products include:

Rocephin Injectable Vials, ADD-Vantage, Galaxy, Bulk 2800

Cefuroxime Axetil (Since entecavir is primarily eliminated by the kidneys co-administration of entecavir with drugs that reduce renal function or compete for active tubular secretion may increase serum concentrations of either entecavir or the co-administered drug). Products include:

Ceftin 1407

Cefuroxime Sodium (Since entecavir is primarily eliminated by the kidneys co-administration of entecavir with drugs that reduce renal function or compete for active tubular secretion may increase serum concentrations of either entecavir or the co-administered drug).

No products indexed under this heading.

Celecoxib (Since entecavir is primarily eliminated by the kidneys co-administration of entecavir with drugs that reduce renal function or compete for active tubular secretion may increase serum concentrations of either entecavir or the co-administered drug). Products include:

Celebrex Capsules 3134

Cephalexin (Since entecavir is primarily eliminated by the kidneys co-administration of entecavir with drugs that reduce renal function or compete for active tubular secretion may increase serum concentrations of either entecavir or the co-administered drug). Products include:

Keflex Capsules 549

Cephalothin Sodium (Since entecavir is primarily eliminated by the kidneys co-administration of entecavir with drugs that reduce renal function or compete for active tubular secretion may increase serum concentrations of either entecavir or the co-administered drug).

No products indexed under this heading.

Cephapirin Sodium (Since entecavir is primarily eliminated by the kidneys co-administration of entecavir with drugs that reduce renal function or compete for active tubular secretion may increase serum concentrations of either entecavir or the co-administered drug).

No products indexed under this heading.

Cephradine (Since entecavir is primarily eliminated by the kidneys co-administration of entecavir with drugs that reduce renal function or compete for active tubular secretion may increase serum concentrations of either entecavir or the co-administered drug).

No products indexed under this heading.

Cerivastatin Sodium (Since entecavir is primarily eliminated by the kidneys co-administration of entecavir with drugs that reduce renal function or compete for active tubular secretion may increase serum concentrations of either entecavir or the co-administered drug).

No products indexed under this heading.

Chlorothiazide (Since entecavir is primarily eliminated by the kidneys co-administration of entecavir with drugs that reduce renal function or compete for active tubular secretion may increase serum concentrations of either entecavir or the co-administered drug). Products include:

Diuril Oral Suspension 1954

Chlorothiazide Sodium (Since entecavir is primarily eliminated by the kidneys co-administration of entecavir with drugs that reduce renal function or compete for active tubular secretion may increase serum concentrations of either entecavir or the co-administered drug). Products include:

Diuril Sodium Intravenous 2467

Chlorpropamide (Since entecavir is primarily eliminated by the kidneys co-administration of entecavir with drugs that reduce renal function or compete for active tubular secretion may increase serum concentrations of either entecavir or the co-administered drug).

No products indexed under this heading.

Cidofovir (Since entecavir is primarily eliminated by the kidneys co-administration of entecavir with drugs that reduce renal function or compete for active tubular secretion may increase serum concentrations of either entecavir or the co-administered drug).

No products indexed under this heading.

Cilastatin Sodium (Since entecavir is primarily eliminated by the kidneys co-administration of entecavir with drugs that reduce renal function or compete for active tubular secretion may increase serum concentrations of either entecavir or the co-administered drug). Products include:

Primaxin I.M. 2045
Primaxin I.V. 2048

Cimetidine (Since entecavir is primarily eliminated by the kidneys co-administration of entecavir with drugs that reduce renal function or compete for active tubular secretion may increase serum concentrations of either entecavir or the co-administered drug). Products include:

Tagamet HB 200 Tablets 664

Cimetidine Hydrochloride (Since entecavir is primarily eliminated by the kidneys co-administration of entecavir with drugs that reduce renal function or compete for active tubular secretion may increase serum concentrations of either entecavir or the co-administered drug).

No products indexed under this heading.

Cisplatin (Since entecavir is primarily eliminated by the kidneys co-administration of entecavir with drugs that reduce renal function or compete for active tubular secretion may increase serum concentrations of either entecavir or the co-administered drug).

No products indexed under this heading.

Cladribine (Since entecavir is primarily eliminated by the kidneys co-administration of entecavir with drugs that reduce renal function or compete for active tubular secretion may increase serum concentrations of either entecavir or the co-administered drug). Products include:

Leustatin Injection 2357

Clozapine (Since entecavir is primarily eliminated by the kidneys co-administration of entecavir with drugs that reduce renal function or compete for active tubular secretion may increase serum concentrations of either entecavir or the co-administered drug). Products include:

Clozaril Tablets 2184
FazaClo Orally Disintegrating Tablets 551

Colistimethate Sodium (Since entecavir is primarily eliminated by the kidneys co-administration of entecavir with drugs that reduce renal function or compete for active tubular secretion may increase serum concentrations of either entecavir or the co-administered drug).

No products indexed under this heading.

Colistin Sulfate (Since entecavir is primarily eliminated by the kidneys co-administration of entecavir with drugs that reduce renal function or compete for active tubular secretion may increase serum concentrations of either entecavir or the co-administered drug).

No products indexed under this heading.

Cyclophosphamide (Since entecavir is primarily eliminated by the kidneys co-administration of entecavir with drugs that reduce renal function or compete for active tubular secretion may increase serum concentrations of either entecavir or the co-administered drug).

No products indexed under this heading.

Cyclosporine (Since entecavir is primarily eliminated by the kidneys co-administration of entecavir with drugs that reduce renal function or compete for active tubular secretion may increase serum concentrations of either entecavir or the co-administered drug). Products include:

Gengraf Capsules 459
Neoral Oral Solution 2259
Neoral Soft Gelatin Capsules 2259
Restasis Ophthalmic Emulsion 575
Sandimmune 2275

Cytarabine (Since entecavir is primarily eliminated by the kidneys co-administration of entecavir with drugs that reduce renal function or compete for active tubular secretion may increase serum concentrations of either entecavir or the co-administered drug).

No products indexed under this heading.

Cytarabine Liposome (Since entecavir is primarily eliminated by the kidneys co-administration of entecavir with drugs that reduce renal function or compete for active tubular secretion may increase serum concentrations of either entecavir or the co-administered drug). Products include:

DepoCyt Injection 1143

Delavirdine Mesylate (Since entecavir is primarily eliminated by the kidneys co-administration of entecavir with drugs that reduce renal function or compete for active tubular secretion may increase serum concentrations of either entecavir or the co-administered drug). Products include:

Rescriptor Tablets 2551

Diatrizoate Meglumine (Since entecavir is primarily eliminated by the kidneys co-administration of entecavir with drugs that reduce renal function or compete for active tubular secretion may increase serum concentrations of either entecavir or the co-administered drug).

No products indexed under this heading.

Diatrizoate Sodium (Since entecavir is primarily eliminated by the kidneys co-administration of entecavir with drugs that reduce renal function or compete for active tubular secretion may increase serum concentrations of either entecavir or the co-administered drug).

No products indexed under this heading.

Diclofenac Potassium (Since entecavir is primarily eliminated by the kidneys co-administration of entecavir with drugs that reduce renal function or compete for active tubular secretion may increase serum concentrations of either entecavir or the co-administered drug).

No products indexed under this heading.

Diclofenac Sodium (Since entecavir is primarily eliminated by the kidneys co-administration of entecavir with drugs that reduce renal function or compete for active tubular secretion may increase serum concentrations of either entecavir or the co-administered drug). Products include:

Arthrotec Tablets 3129
Voltaren Ophthalmic Solution 2309
Voltaren Tablets 2307
Voltaren-XR Tablets 2310

Dicloxacillin Sodium (Since entecavir is primarily eliminated by the kidneys co-administration of entecavir with drugs that reduce renal function or compete for active tubular secretion may increase serum concentrations of either entecavir or the co-administered drug).

No products indexed under this heading.

Didanosine (Since entecavir is primarily eliminated by the kidneys co-administration of entecavir with drugs that reduce renal function or compete for active tubular secretion may increase serum concentrations of either entecavir or the co-administered drug).
No products indexed under this heading.

Efavirenz (Since entecavir is primarily eliminated by the kidneys co-administration of entecavir with drugs that reduce renal function or compete for active tubular secretion may increase serum concentrations of either entecavir or the co-administered drug). Products include:
Atripla Tablets 945
Sustiva Capsules 930
Sustiva Tablets 930

Emtricitabine (Since entecavir is primarily eliminated by the kidneys co-administration of entecavir with drugs that reduce renal function or compete for active tubular secretion may increase serum concentrations of either entecavir or the co-administered drug). Products include:
Atripla Tablets 945
Emtriva Capsules 1287
Emtriva Oral Solution 1287
Truvada Tablets 1296

Enalapril Maleate (Since entecavir is primarily eliminated by the kidneys co-administration of entecavir with drugs that reduce renal function or compete for active tubular secretion may increase serum concentrations of either entecavir or the co-administered drug). Products include:
Vasotec I.V. Injection 2103

Enalaprilat (Since entecavir is primarily eliminated by the kidneys co-administration of entecavir with drugs that reduce renal function or compete for active tubular secretion may increase serum concentrations of either entecavir or the co-administered drug).
No products indexed under this heading.

Enfuvirtide (Since entecavir is primarily eliminated by the kidneys co-administration of entecavir with drugs that reduce renal function or compete for active tubular secretion may increase serum concentrations of either entecavir or the co-administered drug). Products include:
Fuzeon Injection 2767

Ethiodized Oil (Since entecavir is primarily eliminated by the kidneys co-administration of entecavir with drugs that reduce renal function or compete for active tubular secretion may increase serum concentrations of either entecavir or the co-administered drug).
No products indexed under this heading.

Etodolac (Since entecavir is primarily eliminated by the kidneys co-administration of entecavir with drugs that reduce renal function or compete for active tubular secretion may increase serum concentrations of either entecavir or the co-administered drug).
No products indexed under this heading.

Fenoprofen Calcium (Since entecavir is primarily eliminated by the kidneys co-administration of entecavir with drugs that reduce renal function or compete for active tubular secretion may increase serum concentrations of either entecavir or the co-administered drug). Products include:
Nalfon Capsules 2502

Filgrastim (Since entecavir is primarily eliminated by the kidneys co-administration of entecavir with drugs that reduce renal function or compete for active tubular secretion may increase serum concentrations of either entecavir or the co-administered drug). Products include:
Neupogen for Injection 603

Fluorouracil (Since entecavir is primarily eliminated by the kidneys co-administration of entecavir with drugs that reduce renal function or compete for active tubular secretion may increase serum concentrations of either entecavir or the co-administered drug). Products include:
Carac Cream, 0.5% 2879
Efudex 3363

Flurbiprofen (Since entecavir is primarily eliminated by the kidneys co-administration of entecavir with drugs that reduce renal function or compete for active tubular secretion may increase serum concentrations of either entecavir or the co-administered drug).
No products indexed under this heading.

Fluvastatin Sodium (Since entecavir is primarily eliminated by the kidneys co-administration of entecavir with drugs that reduce renal function or compete for active tubular secretion may increase serum concentrations of either entecavir or the co-administered drug). Products include:
Lescol Capsules 2233
Lescol XL Tablets 2233

Foscarnet Sodium (Since entecavir is primarily eliminated by the kidneys co-administration of entecavir with drugs that reduce renal function or compete for active tubular secretion may increase serum concentrations of either entecavir or the co-administered drug).
No products indexed under this heading.

Fosinopril Sodium (Since entecavir is primarily eliminated by the kidneys co-administration of entecavir with drugs that reduce renal function or compete for active tubular secretion may increase serum concentrations of either entecavir or the co-administered drug).
No products indexed under this heading.

Furosemide (Since entecavir is primarily eliminated by the kidneys co-administration of entecavir with drugs that reduce renal function or compete for active tubular secretion may increase serum concentrations of either entecavir or the co-administered drug). Products include:
Furosemide Tablets 2154

Gadopentetate Dimeglumine (Since entecavir is primarily eliminated by the kidneys co-administration of entecavir with drugs that reduce renal function or compete for active tubular secretion may increase serum concentrations of either entecavir or the co-administered drug).
No products indexed under this heading.

Gentamicin (Since entecavir is primarily eliminated by the kidneys co-administration of entecavir with drugs that reduce renal function or compete for active tubular secretion may increase serum concentrations of either entecavir or the co-administered drug).
No products indexed under this heading.

Gentamicin Sulfate (Since entecavir is primarily eliminated by the kidneys co-administration of entecavir with drugs that reduce renal function or compete for active tubular secretion may increase serum concentrations of either entecavir or the co-administered drug). Products include:
Garamycin Injectable 3014
Pred-G Ophthalmic Ointment .... ⊙237
Pred-G Ophthalmic Suspension .... ⊙236

Glipizide (Since entecavir is primarily eliminated by the kidneys co-administration of entecavir with drugs that reduce renal function or compete for active tubular secretion may increase serum concentrations of either entecavir or the co-administered drug).
No products indexed under this heading.

Globulin, Immune (Human) (Since entecavir is primarily eliminated by the kidneys co-administration of entecavir with drugs that reduce renal function or compete for active tubular secretion may increase serum concentrations of either entecavir or the co-administered drug). Products include:
Flebogamma 5%, Immune Globulin Intravenous (Human) 1658
GamaSTAN 3234

Glyburide (Since entecavir is primarily eliminated by the kidneys co-administration of entecavir with drugs that reduce renal function or compete for active tubular secretion may increase serum concentrations of either entecavir or the co-administered drug).
No products indexed under this heading.

Gold Therapy (Since entecavir is primarily eliminated by the kidneys co-administration of entecavir with drugs that reduce renal function or compete for active tubular secretion may increase serum concentrations of either entecavir or the co-administered drug).
No products indexed under this heading.

HMG-CoA Reductase Inhibitors (Since entecavir is primarily eliminated by the kidneys co-administration of entecavir with drugs that reduce renal function or compete for active tubular secretion may increase serum concentrations of either entecavir or the co-administered drug).
No products indexed under this heading.

Hydrochlorothiazide (Since entecavir is primarily eliminated by the kidneys co-administration of entecavir with drugs that reduce renal function or compete for active tubular secretion may increase serum concentrations of either entecavir or the co-administered drug). Products include:
Aldoril Tablets 1910
Atacand HCT 651
Avalide Tablets 888
Avalide Tablets 2874
Benicar HCT Tablets 1044
Diovan HCT Tablets 2196
Dyazide Capsules 1423
Hyzaar 50-12.5 Tablets 1990
Hyzaar 100-12.5 Tablets 1990
Hyzaar 100-25 Tablets 1990
Lopressor HCT 50/25 Tablets 2241
Lopressor HCT 100/25 Tablets 2241
Lopressor HCT 100/50 Tablets 2241
Lotensin HCT Tablets 2246
Micardis HCT Tablets 856
Moduretic Tablets 2028
Prinzide Tablets 2056
Teveten HCT Tablets 1737
Timolide Tablets 2086
Uniretic Tablets 3100

Hydroflumethiazide (Since entecavir is primarily eliminated by the kidneys co-administration of entecavir with drugs that reduce renal function or compete for active tubular secretion may increase serum concentrations of either entecavir or the co-administered drug).
No products indexed under this heading.

Ibuprofen (Since entecavir is primarily eliminated by the kidneys co-administration of entecavir with drugs that reduce renal function or compete for active tubular secretion may increase serum concentrations of either entecavir or the co-administered drug). Products include:
Advil Allergy Sinus Caplets .... ▣770
Advil .... ▣674
Children's Advil Oral Suspension .... ▣603
Children's Advil Chewable Tablets .... ▣603
Advil Cold & Sinus .... ▣723
Infants' Advil Concentrated Drops .... ▣604
Infants' Advil Concentrated Drops - White Grape (Dye-Free) .... ▣604
Junior Strength Advil Swallow Tablets .... ▣605
Advil Migraine Liquigels .... ▣608
Advil Multi-Symptom Cold Caplets .... ▣770
Advil PM Caplets .... ▣615
Motrin IB Tablets and Caplets 1866
Children's Motrin Oral Suspension 1867
Children's Motrin Non-Staining Dye-Free Oral Suspension 1867
Children's Motrin Cold Oral Suspension 1867
Infants' Motrin Concentrated Drops 1867
Infants' Motrin Non-Staining Dye-Free Concentrated Drops 1867
Junior Strength Motrin Caplets and Chewable Tablets 1867
Vicoprofen Tablets 539

Idarubicin Hydrochloride (Since entecavir is primarily eliminated by the kidneys co-administration of entecavir with drugs that reduce renal function or compete for active tubular secretion may increase serum concentrations of either entecavir or the co-administered drug).
No products indexed under this heading.

Ifosfamide (Since entecavir is primarily eliminated by the kidneys co-administration of entecavir with drugs that reduce renal function or compete for active tubular secretion may increase serum concentrations of either entecavir or the co-administered drug).
No products indexed under this heading.

Imipenem (Since entecavir is primarily eliminated by the kidneys co-administration of entecavir with drugs that reduce renal function or compete for active tubular secretion may increase serum concentrations of either entecavir or the co-administered drug). Products include:
Primaxin I.M. 2045

Primaxin I.V. 2048

Immune Globulin Intravenous (Human) (Since entecavir is primarily eliminated by the kidneys co-administration of entecavir with drugs that reduce renal function or compete for active tubular secretion may increase serum concentrations of either entecavir or the co-administered drug). Products include:

Carimune NF 3499
Gammagard Liquid 721
Gammagard S/D 724
Gamunex Immune Globulin I.V., 10% 3235

Indinavir Sulfate (Since entecavir is primarily eliminated by the kidneys co-administration of entecavir with drugs that reduce renal function or compete for active tubular secretion may increase serum concentrations of either entecavir or the co-administered drug). Products include:

Crixivan Capsules 1940

Indomethacin (Since entecavir is primarily eliminated by the kidneys co-administration of entecavir with drugs that reduce renal function or compete for active tubular secretion may increase serum concentrations of either entecavir or the co-administered drug). Products include:

Indocin 1995

Indomethacin Sodium Trihydrate (Since entecavir is primarily eliminated by the kidneys co-administration of entecavir with drugs that reduce renal function or compete for active tubular secretion may increase serum concentrations of either entecavir or the co-administered drug). Products include:

Indocin I.V. 2465

Interferon Beta-1b (Since entecavir is primarily eliminated by the kidneys co-administration of entecavir with drugs that reduce renal function or compete for active tubular secretion may increase serum concentrations of either entecavir or the co-administered drug). Products include:

Betaseron for SC Injection 767

Interleuken-2 (Since entecavir is primarily eliminated by the kidneys co-administration of entecavir with drugs that reduce renal function or compete for active tubular secretion may increase serum concentrations of either entecavir or the co-administered drug).

No products indexed under this heading.

Iodamide Meglumine (Since entecavir is primarily eliminated by the kidneys co-administration of entecavir with drugs that reduce renal function or compete for active tubular secretion may increase serum concentrations of either entecavir or the co-administered drug).

No products indexed under this heading.

Iohexol (Since entecavir is primarily eliminated by the kidneys co-administration of entecavir with drugs that reduce renal function or compete for active tubular secretion may increase serum concentrations of either entecavir or the co-administered drug).

No products indexed under this heading.

Iopamidol (Since entecavir is primarily eliminated by the kidneys co-administration of entecavir with drugs that reduce renal function or compete for active tubular secretion may increase serum concentrations of either entecavir or the co-administered drug).

No products indexed under this heading.

Iopanoic Acid (Since entecavir is primarily eliminated by the kidneys co-administration of entecavir with drugs that reduce renal function or compete for active tubular secretion may increase serum concentrations of either entecavir or the co-administered drug).

No products indexed under this heading.

Iothalamate Meglumine (Since entecavir is primarily eliminated by the kidneys co-administration of entecavir with drugs that reduce renal function or compete for active tubular secretion may increase serum concentrations of either entecavir or the co-administered drug).

No products indexed under this heading.

Ioxaglate Meglumine (Since entecavir is primarily eliminated by the kidneys co-administration of entecavir with drugs that reduce renal function or compete for active tubular secretion may increase serum concentrations of either entecavir or the co-administered drug).

No products indexed under this heading.

Ioxaglate Sodium (Since entecavir is primarily eliminated by the kidneys co-administration of entecavir with drugs that reduce renal function or compete for active tubular secretion may increase serum concentrations of either entecavir or the co-administered drug).

No products indexed under this heading.

Kanamycin Sulfate (Since entecavir is primarily eliminated by the kidneys co-administration of entecavir with drugs that reduce renal function or compete for active tubular secretion may increase serum concentrations of either entecavir or the co-administered drug).

No products indexed under this heading.

Ketoprofen (Since entecavir is primarily eliminated by the kidneys co-administration of entecavir with drugs that reduce renal function or compete for active tubular secretion may increase serum concentrations of either entecavir or the co-administered drug).

No products indexed under this heading.

Ketorolac Tromethamine (Since entecavir is primarily eliminated by the kidneys co-administration of entecavir with drugs that reduce renal function or compete for active tubular secretion may increase serum concentrations of either entecavir or the co-administered drug). Products include:

Acular Ophthalmic Solution 565
Acular LS Ophthalmic Solution 566

Lamium album (Since entecavir is primarily eliminated by the kidneys co-administration of entecavir with drugs that reduce renal function or compete for active tubular secretion may increase serum concentrations of either entecavir or the co-administered drug).

No products indexed under this heading.

Lisinopril (Since entecavir is primarily eliminated by the kidneys co-administration of entecavir with drugs that reduce renal function or compete for active tubular secretion may increase serum concentrations of either entecavir or the co-administered drug). Products include:

Prinivil Tablets 2052
Prinzide Tablets 2056

Lithium (Since entecavir is primarily eliminated by the kidneys co-administration of entecavir with drugs that reduce renal function or compete for active tubular secretion may increase serum concentrations of either entecavir or the co-administered drug).

No products indexed under this heading.

Lithium Carbonate (Since entecavir is primarily eliminated by the kidneys co-administration of entecavir with drugs that reduce renal function or compete for active tubular secretion may increase serum concentrations of either entecavir or the co-administered drug). Products include:

Lithobid Tablets 1692

Lithium Citrate (Since entecavir is primarily eliminated by the kidneys co-administration of entecavir with drugs that reduce renal function or compete for active tubular secretion may increase serum concentrations of either entecavir or the co-administered drug).

No products indexed under this heading.

Lopinavir (Since entecavir is primarily eliminated by the kidneys co-administration of entecavir with drugs that reduce renal function or compete for active tubular secretion may increase serum concentrations of either entecavir or the co-administered drug). Products include:

Kaletra 476

Loracarbef (Since entecavir is primarily eliminated by the kidneys co-administration of entecavir with drugs that reduce renal function or compete for active tubular secretion may increase serum concentrations of either entecavir or the co-administered drug).

No products indexed under this heading.

Lovastatin (Since entecavir is primarily eliminated by the kidneys co-administration of entecavir with drugs that reduce renal function or compete for active tubular secretion may increase serum concentrations of either entecavir or the co-administered drug). Products include:

Advicor Tablets 1722
Altoprev Extended-Release Tablets 3109
Mevacor Tablets 2021

Meclofenamate Sodium (Since entecavir is primarily eliminated by the kidneys co-administration of entecavir with drugs that reduce renal function or compete for active tubular secretion may increase serum concentrations of either entecavir or the co-administered drug).

No products indexed under this heading.

Mefenamic Acid (Since entecavir is primarily eliminated by the kidneys co-administration of entecavir with drugs that reduce renal function or compete for active tubular secretion may increase serum concentrations of either entecavir or the co-administered drug).

No products indexed under this heading.

Meloxicam (Since entecavir is primarily eliminated by the kidneys co-administration of entecavir with drugs that reduce renal function or compete for active tubular secretion may increase serum concentrations of either entecavir or the co-administered drug). Products include:

Mobic Oral Suspension 863
Mobic Tablets 863

Melphalan Hydrochloride (Since entecavir is primarily eliminated by the kidneys co-administration of entecavir with drugs that reduce renal function or compete for active tubular secretion may increase serum concentrations of either entecavir or the co-administered drug). Products include:

Alkeran for Injection 955

Mesalamine (Since entecavir is primarily eliminated by the kidneys co-administration of entecavir with drugs that reduce renal function or compete for active tubular secretion may increase serum concentrations of either entecavir or the co-administered drug). Products include:

Asacol Delayed-Release Tablets 2692
Canasa Rectal Suppositories 699
Pentasa Capsules 3185

Methimazole (Since entecavir is primarily eliminated by the kidneys co-administration of entecavir with drugs that reduce renal function or compete for active tubular secretion may increase serum concentrations of either entecavir or the co-administered drug).

No products indexed under this heading.

Methotrexate (Since entecavir is primarily eliminated by the kidneys co-administration of entecavir with drugs that reduce renal function or compete for active tubular secretion may increase serum concentrations of either entecavir or the co-administered drug).

No products indexed under this heading.

Methotrexate Sodium (Since entecavir is primarily eliminated by the kidneys co-administration of entecavir with drugs that reduce renal function or compete for active tubular secretion may increase serum concentrations of either entecavir or the co-administered drug).

No products indexed under this heading.

Methyclothiazide (Since entecavir is primarily eliminated by the kidneys co-administration of entecavir with drugs that reduce renal function or compete for active tubular secretion may increase serum concentrations of either entecavir or the co-administered drug).

No products indexed under this heading.

Mezlocillin Sodium (Since entecavir is primarily eliminated by the kidneys co-administration of entecavir with drugs that reduce renal function or compete for active tubular secretion may increase serum concentrations of either entecavir or the co-administered drug).

No products indexed under this heading.

Minocycline Hydrochloride (Since entecavir is primarily eliminated by the kidneys co-administration of entecavir with drugs that reduce renal function or compete for active tubular secretion may increase serum concentrations of either entecavir or the co-administered drug). Products include:

Solodyn Extended Release Tablets 1890

Mitomycin (Mitomycin-C) (Since entecavir is primarily eliminated by the kidneys co-administration of entecavir with drugs that reduce renal function or compete for active tubular secretion may increase serum concentrations of either entecavir or the co-administered drug).

No products indexed under this heading.

Moexipril Hydrochloride (Since entecavir is primarily eliminated by the kidneys co-administration of entecavir with drugs that reduce renal function or compete for active tubular secretion may increase serum concentrations of either entecavir or the co-administered drug). Products include:

Uniretic Tablets 3100
Univasc Tablets 3104

Muromonab-CD3 (Since entecavir is primarily eliminated by the kidneys co-administration of entecavir with drugs that reduce renal function or compete for active tubular secretion may increase serum concentrations of either entecavir or the co-administered drug). Products include:

Orthoclone OKT3 Sterile Solution 2360

Nabumetone (Since entecavir is primarily eliminated by the kidneys co-administration of entecavir with drugs that reduce renal function or compete for active tubular secretion may increase serum concentrations of either entecavir or the co-administered drug).

No products indexed under this heading.

Nafcillin Sodium (Since entecavir is primarily eliminated by the kidneys co-administration of entecavir with drugs that reduce renal function or compete for active tubular secretion may increase serum concentrations of either entecavir or the co-administered drug).

No products indexed under this heading.

Naproxen (Since entecavir is primarily eliminated by the kidneys co-administration of entecavir with drugs that reduce renal function or compete for active tubular secretion may increase serum concentrations of either entecavir or the co-administered drug). Products include:

EC-Naprosyn Delayed-Release Tablets 2761
Naprosyn Suspension 2761
Naprosyn Tablets 2761
Prevacid NapraPAC 3280

Naproxen Sodium (Since entecavir is primarily eliminated by the kidneys co-administration of entecavir with drugs that reduce renal function or compete for active tubular secretion may increase serum concentrations of either entecavir or the co-administered drug). Products include:

Aleve Caplets 742
Aleve Gelcaps 743
Aleve Tablets 743
Aleve Cold & Sinus Caplets 744
Anaprox Tablets 2761
Anaprox DS Tablets 2761

Nelfinavir Mesylate (Since entecavir is primarily eliminated by the kidneys co-administration of entecavir with drugs that reduce renal function or compete for active tubular secretion may increase serum concentrations of either entecavir or the co-administered drug). Products include:

Viracept 2577

Neomycin (Since entecavir is primarily eliminated by the kidneys co-administration of entecavir with drugs that reduce renal function or compete for active tubular secretion may increase serum concentrations of either entecavir or the co-administered drug). Products include:

Neosporin Antibiotic Ointment .... ■643
Neosporin + Pain Relief Antibiotic Cream and Ointment (Maximum Strength) .... ■643

Neomycin, oral (Since entecavir is primarily eliminated by the kidneys co-administration of entecavir with drugs that reduce renal function or compete for active tubular secretion may increase serum concentrations of either entecavir or the co-administered drug).

No products indexed under this heading.

Neomycin Sulfate (Since entecavir is primarily eliminated by the kidneys co-administration of entecavir with drugs that reduce renal function or compete for active tubular secretion may increase serum concentrations of either entecavir or the co-administered drug). Products include:

Neosporin Ophthalmic Solution Sterile .... ⊙265
Poly-Pred Ophthalmic Suspension .... ⊙233

Nevirapine (Since entecavir is primarily eliminated by the kidneys co-administration of entecavir with drugs that reduce renal function or compete for active tubular secretion may increase serum concentrations of either entecavir or the co-administered drug). Products include:

Viramune Oral Suspension 873
Viramune Tablets 873

Norfloxacin (Since entecavir is primarily eliminated by the kidneys co-administration of entecavir with drugs that reduce renal function or compete for active tubular secretion may increase serum concentrations of either entecavir or the co-administered drug). Products include:

Noroxin Tablets 2032

Olsalazine Sodium (Since entecavir is primarily eliminated by the kidneys co-administration of entecavir with drugs that reduce renal function or compete for active tubular secretion may increase serum concentrations of either entecavir or the co-administered drug).

No products indexed under this heading.

Omeprazole (Since entecavir is primarily eliminated by the kidneys co-administration of entecavir with drugs that reduce renal function or compete for active tubular secretion may increase serum concentrations of either entecavir or the co-administered drug). Products include:

Zegerid Capsules 2958
Zegerid Powder for Oral Solution 2958

Oxaprozin (Since entecavir is primarily eliminated by the kidneys co-administration of entecavir with drugs that reduce renal function or compete for active tubular secretion may increase serum concentrations of either entecavir or the co-administered drug).

No products indexed under this heading.

Pamidronate Disodium (Since entecavir is primarily eliminated by the kidneys co-administration of entecavir with drugs that reduce renal function or compete for active tubular secretion may increase serum concentrations of either entecavir or the co-administered drug). Products include:

Aredia for Injection 2179

Paroxetine Hydrochloride (Since entecavir is primarily eliminated by the kidneys co-administration of entecavir with drugs that reduce renal function or compete for active tubular secretion may increase serum concentrations of either entecavir or the co-administered drug). Products include:

Paxil CR Controlled-Release Tablets 1538
Paxil 1530

Penicillamine (Since entecavir is primarily eliminated by the kidneys co-administration of entecavir with drugs that reduce renal function or compete for active tubular secretion may increase serum concentrations of either entecavir or the co-administered drug). Products include:

Cuprimine Capsules 1947

Penicillin G Benzathine (Since entecavir is primarily eliminated by the kidneys co-administration of entecavir with drugs that reduce renal function or compete for active tubular secretion may increase serum concentrations of either entecavir or the co-administered drug). Products include:

Bicillin C-R Injectable Suspension 1706

Penicillin G Potassium (Since entecavir is primarily eliminated by the kidneys co-administration of entecavir with drugs that reduce renal function or compete for active tubular secretion may increase serum concentrations of either entecavir or the co-administered drug).

No products indexed under this heading.

Penicillin G Procaine (Since entecavir is primarily eliminated by the kidneys co-administration of entecavir with drugs that reduce renal function or compete for active tubular secretion may increase serum concentrations of either entecavir or the co-administered drug). Products include:

Bicillin C-R Injectable Suspension 1706

Penicillin G Sodium (Since entecavir is primarily eliminated by the kidneys co-administration of entecavir with drugs that reduce renal function or compete for active tubular secretion may increase serum concentrations of either entecavir or the co-administered drug).

No products indexed under this heading.

Penicillin V Potassium (Since entecavir is primarily eliminated by the kidneys co-administration of entecavir with drugs that reduce renal function or compete for active tubular secretion may increase serum concentrations of either entecavir or the co-administered drug).

No products indexed under this heading.

Pentamidine Isethionate (Since entecavir is primarily eliminated by the kidneys co-administration of entecavir with drugs that reduce renal function or compete for active tubular secretion may increase serum concentrations of either entecavir or the co-administered drug).

No products indexed under this heading.

Perindopril Erbumine (Since entecavir is primarily eliminated by the kidneys co-administration of entecavir with drugs that reduce renal function or compete for active tubular secretion may increase serum concentrations of either entecavir or the co-administered drug). Products include:

Aceon Tablets (2 mg, 4 mg, 8 mg) 3194

Phenylbutazone (Since entecavir is primarily eliminated by the kidneys co-administration of entecavir with drugs that reduce renal function or compete for active tubular secretion may increase serum concentrations of either entecavir or the co-administered drug).

No products indexed under this heading.

Piroxicam (Since entecavir is primarily eliminated by the kidneys co-administration of entecavir with drugs that reduce renal function or compete for active tubular secretion may increase serum concentrations of either entecavir or the co-administered drug).

No products indexed under this heading.

Plicamycin (Since entecavir is primarily eliminated by the kidneys co-administration of entecavir with drugs that reduce renal function or compete for active tubular secretion may increase serum concentrations of either entecavir or the co-administered drug).

No products indexed under this heading.

Polymyxin (Since entecavir is primarily eliminated by the kidneys co-administration of entecavir with drugs that reduce renal function or compete for active tubular secretion may increase serum concentrations of either entecavir or the co-administered drug).

No products indexed under this heading.

Polymyxin B Sulfate (Since entecavir is primarily eliminated by the kidneys co-administration of entecavir with drugs that reduce renal function or compete for active tubular secretion may increase serum concentrations of either entecavir or the co-administered drug). Products include:

- Neosporin Antibiotic Ointment 643
- Neosporin Ophthalmic Solution Sterile .... ⊙265
- Neosporin + Pain Relief Antibiotic Cream and Ointment (Maximum Strength) 643
- Poly-Pred Ophthalmic Suspension .... ⊙233
- Polysporin First Aid Antibiotic Ointment 643
- Polytrim Ophthalmic Solution 574

Polythiazide (Since entecavir is primarily eliminated by the kidneys co-administration of entecavir with drugs that reduce renal function or compete for active tubular secretion may increase serum concentrations of either entecavir or the co-administered drug).

No products indexed under this heading.

Pravastatin Sodium (Since entecavir is primarily eliminated by the kidneys co-administration of entecavir with drugs that reduce renal function or compete for active tubular secretion may increase serum concentrations of either entecavir or the co-administered drug).

No products indexed under this heading.

Probenecid (Since entecavir is primarily eliminated by the kidneys co-administration of entecavir with drugs that reduce renal function or compete for active tubular secretion may increase serum concentrations of either entecavir or the co-administered drug).

No products indexed under this heading.

Quinapril Hydrochloride (Since entecavir is primarily eliminated by the kidneys co-administration of entecavir with drugs that reduce renal function or compete for active tubular secretion may increase serum concentrations of either entecavir or the co-administered drug).

No products indexed under this heading.

Rabeprazole Sodium (Since entecavir is primarily eliminated by the kidneys co-administration of entecavir with drugs that reduce renal function or compete for active tubular secretion may increase serum concentrations of either entecavir or the co-administered drug). Products include:

- Aciphex Tablets 1090

Ramipril (Since entecavir is primarily eliminated by the kidneys co-administration of entecavir with drugs that reduce renal function or compete for active tubular secretion may increase serum concentrations of either entecavir or the co-administered drug). Products include:

- Altace Capsules 1702

Rifampin (Since entecavir is primarily eliminated by the kidneys co-administration of entecavir with drugs that reduce renal function or compete for active tubular secretion may increase serum concentrations of either entecavir or the co-administered drug).

No products indexed under this heading.

Riluzole (Since entecavir is primarily eliminated by the kidneys co-administration of entecavir with drugs that reduce renal function or compete for active tubular secretion may increase serum concentrations of either entecavir or the co-administered drug). Products include:

- Rilutek Tablets 2930

Ritonavir (Since entecavir is primarily eliminated by the kidneys co-administration of entecavir with drugs that reduce renal function or compete for active tubular secretion may increase serum concentrations of either entecavir or the co-administered drug). Products include:

- Kaletra 476
- Norvir 503

Rofecoxib (Since entecavir is primarily eliminated by the kidneys co-administration of entecavir with drugs that reduce renal function or compete for active tubular secretion may increase serum concentrations of either entecavir or the co-administered drug).

No products indexed under this heading.

Saquinavir (Since entecavir is primarily eliminated by the kidneys co-administration of entecavir with drugs that reduce renal function or compete for active tubular secretion may increase serum concentrations of either entecavir or the co-administered drug).

No products indexed under this heading.

Sibutramine Hydrochloride Monohydrate (Since entecavir is primarily eliminated by the kidneys co-administration of entecavir with drugs that reduce renal function or compete for active tubular secretion may increase serum concentrations of either entecavir or the co-administered drug). Products include:

- Meridia Capsules 489

Simvastatin (Since entecavir is primarily eliminated by the kidneys co-administration of entecavir with drugs that reduce renal function or compete for active tubular secretion may increase serum concentrations of either entecavir or the co-administered drug). Products include:

- Vytorin 10/10 Tablets 2114
- Vytorin 10/10 Tablets 3077
- Vytorin 10/20 Tablets 2114
- Vytorin 10/20 Tablets 3077
- Vytorin 10/40 Tablets 2114
- Vytorin 10/40 Tablets 3077
- Vytorin 10/80 Tablets 2114
- Vytorin 10/80 Tablets 3077
- Zocor Tablets 2105

Spirapril Hydrochloride (Since entecavir is primarily eliminated by the kidneys co-administration of entecavir with drugs that reduce renal function or compete for active tubular secretion may increase serum concentrations of either entecavir or the co-administered drug).

No products indexed under this heading.

Stavudine (Since entecavir is primarily eliminated by the kidneys co-administration of entecavir with drugs that reduce renal function or compete for active tubular secretion may increase serum concentrations of either entecavir or the co-administered drug).

No products indexed under this heading.

Streptomycin Sulfate (Since entecavir is primarily eliminated by the kidneys co-administration of entecavir with drugs that reduce renal function or compete for active tubular secretion may increase serum concentrations of either entecavir or the co-administered drug).

No products indexed under this heading.

Streptozocin (Since entecavir is primarily eliminated by the kidneys co-administration of entecavir with drugs that reduce renal function or compete for active tubular secretion may increase serum concentrations of either entecavir or the co-administered drug).

No products indexed under this heading.

Sulfacytine (Since entecavir is primarily eliminated by the kidneys co-administration of entecavir with drugs that reduce renal function or compete for active tubular secretion may increase serum concentrations of either entecavir or the co-administered drug).

No products indexed under this heading.

Sulfamethizole (Since entecavir is primarily eliminated by the kidneys co-administration of entecavir with drugs that reduce renal function or compete for active tubular secretion may increase serum concentrations of either entecavir or the co-administered drug).

No products indexed under this heading.

Sulfamethoxazole (Since entecavir is primarily eliminated by the kidneys co-administration of entecavir with drugs that reduce renal function or compete for active tubular secretion may increase serum concentrations of either entecavir or the co-administered drug).

No products indexed under this heading.

Sulfasalazine (Since entecavir is primarily eliminated by the kidneys co-administration of entecavir with drugs that reduce renal function or compete for active tubular secretion may increase serum concentrations of either entecavir or the co-administered drug).

No products indexed under this heading.

Sulfinpyrazone (Since entecavir is primarily eliminated by the kidneys co-administration of entecavir with drugs that reduce renal function or compete for active tubular secretion may increase serum concentrations of either entecavir or the co-administered drug).

No products indexed under this heading.

Sulfisoxazole Acetyl (Since entecavir is primarily eliminated by the kidneys co-administration of entecavir with drugs that reduce renal function or compete for active tubular secretion may increase serum concentrations of either entecavir or the co-administered drug).

No products indexed under this heading.

Sulfisoxazole Diolamine (Since entecavir is primarily eliminated by the kidneys co-administration of entecavir with drugs that reduce renal function or compete for active tubular secretion may increase serum concentrations of either entecavir or the co-administered drug).

No products indexed under this heading.

Sulindac (Since entecavir is primarily eliminated by the kidneys co-administration of entecavir with drugs that reduce renal function or compete for active tubular secretion may increase serum concentrations of either entecavir or the co-administered drug). Products include:

- Clinoril Tablets 1924

Tacrolimus (Since entecavir is primarily eliminated by the kidneys co-administration of entecavir with drugs that reduce renal function or compete for active tubular secretion may increase serum concentrations of either entecavir or the co-administered drug). Products include:

- Prograf Capsules and Injection 632
- Protopic Ointment 638

Tenofovir Disoproxil Fumarate (Since entecavir is primarily eliminated by the kidneys co-administration of entecavir with drugs that reduce renal function or compete for active tubular secretion may increase serum concentrations of either entecavir or the co-administered drug). Products include:

- Atripla Tablets 945
- Truvada Tablets 1296
- Viread Tablets 1301

Thioguanine (Since entecavir is primarily eliminated by the kidneys co-administration of entecavir with drugs that reduce renal function or compete for active tubular secretion may increase serum concentrations of either entecavir or the co-administered drug). Products include:

- Tabloid Tablets 1575

Ticarcillin Disodium (Since entecavir is primarily eliminated by the kidneys co-administration of entecavir with drugs that reduce renal function or compete for active tubular secretion may increase serum concentrations of either entecavir or the co-administered drug). Products include:

- Timentin ADD-Vantage 1580
- Timentin Injection Galaxy Container 1583
- Timentin IV Infusion 1577
- Timentin Pharmacy Bulk Package 1586

Tobramycin (Since entecavir is primarily eliminated by the kidneys co-administration of entecavir with drugs that reduce renal function or compete for active tubular secretion may increase serum concentrations of either entecavir or the co-administered drug). Products include:

- TOBI Solution for Inhalation 2298
- TobraDex Ophthalmic Ointment 562
- TobraDex Ophthalmic Suspension 563
- Zylet Ophthalmic Suspension .... ⊙259

Tobramycin Sulfate (Since entecavir is primarily eliminated by the kidneys co-administration of entecavir with drugs that reduce renal function or compete for active tubular secretion may increase serum concentrations of either entecavir or the co-administered drug).

No products indexed under this heading.

Tolazamide (Since entecavir is primarily eliminated by the kidneys co-administration of entecavir with drugs that reduce renal function or compete for active tubular secretion may increase serum concentrations of either entecavir or the co-administered drug).
No products indexed under this heading.

Tolbutamide (Since entecavir is primarily eliminated by the kidneys co-administration of entecavir with drugs that reduce renal function or compete for active tubular secretion may increase serum concentrations of either entecavir or the co-administered drug).
No products indexed under this heading.

Tolmetin Sodium (Since entecavir is primarily eliminated by the kidneys co-administration of entecavir with drugs that reduce renal function or compete for active tubular secretion may increase serum concentrations of either entecavir or the co-administered drug).
No products indexed under this heading.

Trandolapril (Since entecavir is primarily eliminated by the kidneys co-administration of entecavir with drugs that reduce renal function or compete for active tubular secretion may increase serum concentrations of either entecavir or the co-administered drug). Products include:
Mavik Tablets 486
Tarka Tablets 524

Triamterene (Since entecavir is primarily eliminated by the kidneys co-administration of entecavir with drugs that reduce renal function or compete for active tubular secretion may increase serum concentrations of either entecavir or the co-administered drug). Products include:
Dyazide Capsules 1423
Dyrenium Capsules 3400

Trimethadione (Since entecavir is primarily eliminated by the kidneys co-administration of entecavir with drugs that reduce renal function or compete for active tubular secretion may increase serum concentrations of either entecavir or the co-administered drug).
No products indexed under this heading.

Trovafloxacin Mesylate (Since entecavir is primarily eliminated by the kidneys co-administration of entecavir with drugs that reduce renal function or compete for active tubular secretion may increase serum concentrations of either entecavir or the co-administered drug).
No products indexed under this heading.

Tyropanoate Sodium (Since entecavir is primarily eliminated by the kidneys co-administration of entecavir with drugs that reduce renal function or compete for active tubular secretion may increase serum concentrations of either entecavir or the co-administered drug).
No products indexed under this heading.

Valacyclovir Hydrochloride (Since entecavir is primarily eliminated by the kidneys co-administration of entecavir with drugs that reduce renal function or compete for active tubular secretion may increase serum concentrations of either entecavir or the co-administered drug). Products include:
Valtrex Caplets 1597

Valdecoxib (Since entecavir is primarily eliminated by the kidneys co-administration of entecavir with drugs that reduce renal function or compete for active tubular secretion may increase serum concentrations of either entecavir or the co-administered drug).
No products indexed under this heading.

Vancomycin Hydrochloride (Since entecavir is primarily eliminated by the kidneys co-administration of entecavir with drugs that reduce renal function or compete for active tubular secretion may increase serum concentrations of either entecavir or the co-administered drug). Products include:
Vancocin HCl Capsules, USP 3380

Voriconazole (Since entecavir is primarily eliminated by the kidneys co-administration of entecavir with drugs that reduce renal function or compete for active tubular secretion may increase serum concentrations of either entecavir or the co-administered drug). Products include:
VFEND I.V. 2564
VFEND Oral Suspension 2564
VFEND Tablets 2564

Zalcitabine (Since entecavir is primarily eliminated by the kidneys co-administration of entecavir with drugs that reduce renal function or compete for active tubular secretion may increase serum concentrations of either entecavir or the co-administered drug).
No products indexed under this heading.

Zidovudine (Since entecavir is primarily eliminated by the kidneys co-administration of entecavir with drugs that reduce renal function or compete for active tubular secretion may increase serum concentrations of either entecavir or the co-administered drug). Products include:
Combivir Tablets 1411
Retrovir 1560
Retrovir IV Infusion 1564
Trizivir Tablets 1589

Zoledronic acid (Since entecavir is primarily eliminated by the kidneys co-administration of entecavir with drugs that reduce renal function or compete for active tubular secretion may increase serum concentrations of either entecavir or the co-administered drug). Products include:
Zometa for Intravenous Infusion 2315

BAUSCH & LOMB PRESERVISION AREDS TABLETS

(Vitamins with Minerals) .... ⊙254
None cited in PDR database.

BAUSCH & LOMB PRESERVISION AREDS SOFTGELS

(Vitamins with Minerals) .... ⊙247
None cited in PDR database.

BAUSCH & LOMB PRESERVISION LUTEIN SOFTGELS

(Lutein, Vitamins with Minerals) .... ⊙247
None cited in PDR database.

BAUSCH & LOMB OCUVITE ADULT EYE VITAMIN AND MINERAL SUPPLEMENT SOFT GELS

(Copper, Lutein, Omega-3 Acids, Vitamin C, Vitamin E, Zinc Oxide)...... ▣706
None cited in PDR database.

BAUSCH & LOMB OCUVITE ADULT 50+ EYE VITAMIN AND MINERAL SUPPLEMENT SOFT GELS

(Copper, Lutein, Omega-3 Acids, Vitamin C, Vitamin E, Zinc Oxide)...... ▣706
None cited in PDR database.

BAUSCH & LOMB PRESERVISION AREDS EYE VITAMIN AND MINERAL SUPPLEMENT SOFT GELS

(Vitamins with Minerals) .... ▣806
None cited in PDR database.

BAUSCH & LOMB PRESERVISION LUTEIN EYE VITAMIN AND MINERAL SUPPLEMENT SOFT GELS

(Lutein, Vitamins with Minerals) .... ▣807
None cited in PDR database.

BAYER ASPIRIN

(Aspirin) 744
May interact with ACE inhibitors, beta blockers, anticoagulants, diuretics, oral hypoglycemic agents, non-steroidal anti-inflammatory agents, phenytoin, valproate, and certain other agents. Compounds in these categories include:

Acarbose (Moderate doses of aspirin may increase the effectiveness of oral hypoglycemic drugs, leading to hypoglycemia). Products include:
Precose Tablets 751

Acebutolol Hydrochloride (The hypotensive effects of beta blockers may be diminished by the concomitant administration of aspirin due to inhibition of renal prostaglandins, leading to decreased renal blood flow, and salt and fluid retention).
No products indexed under this heading.

Acetazolamide (Concurrent use of aspirin and acetazolamide can lead to high serum concentrations of acetazolamide (and toxicity) due to competition at the renal tubule for secretion).
No products indexed under this heading.

Acetazolamide Sodium (Concurrent use of aspirin and acetazolamide can lead to high serum concentrations of acetazolamide (and toxicity) due to competition at the renal tubule for secretion).
No products indexed under this heading.

Amiloride Hydrochloride (The effectiveness of diuretics in patients with underlying renal or cardiovascular disease may be diminished by the concomitant administration of aspirin due to inhibition of renal prostaglandins, leading to decreased renal blood flow, and salt and fluidretention). Products include:
Midamor Tablets 2026
Moduretic Tablets 2028

Anisindione (Patients on anticoagulation therapy are at increased risk for bleeding because of drug-drug interactions and the effect on platelets. Aspirin can displace warfarin from protein binding sites, leading to prolongation of both the prothrombin time and bleeding time. Aspirin can increase the anticoagulant activity of heparin, increasing bleeding risk). Products include:
Miradon Tablets 3042

Ardeparin Sodium (Patients on anticoagulation therapy are at increased risk for bleeding because of drug-drug interactions and the effect on platelets. Aspirin can displace warfarin from protein binding sites, leading to prolongation of both the prothrombin time and bleeding time. Aspirin can increase the anticoagulant activity of heparin, increasing bleeding risk).
No products indexed under this heading.

Atenolol (The hypotensive effects of beta blockers may be diminished by the concomitant administration of aspirin due to inhibition of renal prostaglandins, leading to decreased renal blood flow, and salt and fluid retention).
No products indexed under this heading.

Benazepril Hydrochloride (The hyponatremic and hypotensive effects of ACE inhibitors may be diminished by the concomitant administration of aspirin due to its indirect effect on the renin-angiotensin conversion pathway). Products include:
Lotensin Tablets 2243
Lotensin HCT Tablets 2246
Lotrel Capsules 2249

Bendroflumethiazide (The effectiveness of diuretics in patients with underlying renal or cardiovascular disease may be diminished by the concomitant administration of aspirin due to inhibition of renal prostaglandins, leading to decreased renal blood flow, and salt and fluidretention).
No products indexed under this heading.

Betaxolol Hydrochloride (The hypotensive effects of beta blockers may be diminished by the concomitant administration of aspirin due to inhibition of renal prostaglandins, leading to decreased renal blood flow, and salt and fluid retention). Products include:
Betoptic S Ophthalmic Suspension................................ 558

Bisoprolol Fumarate (The hypotensive effects of beta blockers may be diminished by the concomitant administration of aspirin due to inhibition of renal prostaglandins, leading to decreased renal blood flow, and salt and fluid retention).
No products indexed under this heading.

Bumetanide (The effectiveness of diuretics in patients with underlying renal or cardiovascular disease may be diminished by the concomitant administration of aspirin due to inhibition of renal prostaglandins, leading to decreased renal blood flow, and salt and fluidretention). Products include:
Bumex Tablets 2746

Captopril (The hyponatremic and hypotensive effects of ACE inhibitors may be diminished by the concomitant administration of aspirin due to

its indirect effect on the renin-angiotensin conversion pathway). Products include:
Captopril Tablets 2149

Carteolol Hydrochloride (The hypotensive effects of beta blockers may be diminished by the concomitant administration of aspirin due to inhibition of renal prostaglandins, leading to decreased renal blood flow, and salt and fluid retention). Products include:
Carteolol Hydrochloride Ophthalmic Solution USP, 1%....... ⊙249

Celecoxib (The concurrent use of aspirin with other NSAIDs should be avoided because this may increase bleeding or lead to decreased renal function). Products include:
Celebrex Capsules 3134

Chlorothiazide (The effectiveness of diuretics in patients with underlying renal or cardiovascular disease may be diminished by the concomitant administration of aspirin due to inhibition of renal prostaglandins, leading to decreased renal blood flow, and salt and fluidretention). Products include:
Diuril Oral Suspension 1954

Chlorothiazide Sodium (The effectiveness of diuretics in patients with underlying renal or cardiovascular disease may be diminished by the concomitant administration of aspirin due to inhibition of renal prostaglandins, leading to decreased renal blood flow, and salt and fluidretention). Products include:
Diuril Sodium Intravenous 2467

Chlorpropamide (Moderate doses of aspirin may increase the effectiveness of oral hypoglycemic drugs, leading to hypoglycemia).
No products indexed under this heading.

Chlorthalidone (The effectiveness of diuretics in patients with underlying renal or cardiovascular disease may be diminished by the concomitant administration of aspirin due to inhibition of renal prostaglandins, leading to decreased renal blood flow, and salt and fluidretention). Products include:
Clorpres Tablets 2153

Dalteparin Sodium (Patients on anticoagulation therapy are at increased risk for bleeding because of drug-drug interactions and the effect on platelets. Aspirin can displace warfarin from protein binding sites, leading to prolongation of both the prothrombin time and bleeding time. Aspirin can increase the anticoagulant activity of heparin, increasing bleeding risk). Products include:
Fragmin Injection 1097

Danaparoid Sodium (Patients on anticoagulation therapy are at increased risk for bleeding because of drug-drug interactions and the effect on platelets. Aspirin can displace warfarin from protein binding sites, leading to prolongation of both the prothrombin time and bleeding time. Aspirin can increase the anticoagulant activity of heparin, increasing bleeding risk).
No products indexed under this heading.

Diclofenac Potassium (The concurrent use of aspirin with other NSAIDs should be avoided because this may increase bleeding or lead to decreased renal function).
No products indexed under this heading.

Diclofenac Sodium (The concurrent use of aspirin with other NSAIDs should be avoided because this may increase bleeding or lead to decreased renal function). Products include:
Arthrotec Tablets 3129
Voltaren Ophthalmic Solution 2309
Voltaren Tablets 2307
Voltaren-XR Tablets 2310

Dicumarol (Patients on anticoagulation therapy are at increased risk for bleeding because of drug-drug interactions and the effect on platelets. Aspirin can displace warfarin from protein binding sites, leading to prolongation of both the prothrombin time and bleeding time. Aspirin can increase the anticoagulant activity of heparin, increasing bleeding risk).
No products indexed under this heading.

Divalproex Sodium (Salicylate can displace protein-bound valproic acid, leading to an increase in serum valproic acid levels). Products include:
Depakote Sprinkle Capsules 422
Depakote Tablets 427
Depakote ER Tablets 434

Enalapril Maleate (The hyponatremic and hypotensive effects of ACE inhibitors may be diminished by the concomitant administration of aspirin due to its indirect effect on the renin-angiotensin conversion pathway). Products include:
Vasotec I.V. Injection 2103

Enalaprilat (The hyponatremic and hypotensive effects of ACE inhibitors may be diminished by the concomitant administration of aspirin due to its indirect effect on the renin-angiotensin conversion pathway).
No products indexed under this heading.

Enoxaparin Sodium (Patients on anticoagulation therapy are at increased risk for bleeding because of drug-drug interactions and the effect on platelets. Aspirin can displace warfarin from protein binding sites, leading to prolongation of both the prothrombin time and bleeding time. Aspirin can increase the anticoagulant activity of heparin, increasing bleeding risk). Products include:
Lovenox Injection 2915

Esmolol Hydrochloride (The hypotensive effects of beta blockers may be diminished by the concomitant administration of aspirin due to inhibition of renal prostaglandins, leading to decreased renal blood flow, and salt and fluid retention).
No products indexed under this heading.

Ethacrynic Acid (The effectiveness of diuretics in patients with underlying renal or cardiovascular disease may be diminished by the concomitant administration of aspirin due to inhibition of renal prostaglandins, leading to decreased renal blood flow, and salt and fluidretention). Products include:
Edecrin Tablets 1959

Etodolac (The concurrent use of aspirin with other NSAIDs should be avoided because this may increase bleeding or lead to decreased renal function).
No products indexed under this heading.

Fenoprofen Calcium (The concurrent use of aspirin with other NSAIDs should be avoided because this may increase bleeding or lead to decreased renal function). Products include:
Nalfon Capsules 2502

Flurbiprofen (The concurrent use of aspirin with other NSAIDs should be avoided because this may increase bleeding or lead to decreased renal function).
No products indexed under this heading.

Fondaparinux Sodium (Patients on anticoagulation therapy are at increased risk for bleeding because of drug-drug interactions and the effect on platelets. Aspirin can displace warfarin from protein binding sites, leading to prolongation of both the prothrombin time and bleeding time. Aspirin can increase the anticoagulant activity of heparin, increasing bleeding risk). Products include:
Arixtra Injection 1351

Fosinopril Sodium (The hyponatremic and hypotensive effects of ACE inhibitors may be diminished by the concomitant administration of aspirin due to its indirect effect on the renin-angiotensin conversion pathway).
No products indexed under this heading.

Fosphenytoin Sodium (Salicylate can displace protein-bound phenytoin, leading to a decrease in the total concentration of phenytoin).
No products indexed under this heading.

Furosemide (The effectiveness of diuretics in patients with underlying renal or cardiovascular disease may be diminished by the concomitant administration of aspirin due to inhibition of renal prostaglandins, leading to decreased renal blood flow, and salt and fluidretention). Products include:
Furosemide Tablets 2154

Glimepiride (Moderate doses of aspirin may increase the effectiveness of oral hypoglycemic drugs, leading to hypoglycemia). Products include:
Avandaryl Tablets 1379
Duetact Tablets 3226

Glipizide (Moderate doses of aspirin may increase the effectiveness of oral hypoglycemic drugs, leading to hypoglycemia).
No products indexed under this heading.

Glyburide (Moderate doses of aspirin may increase the effectiveness of oral hypoglycemic drugs, leading to hypoglycemia).
No products indexed under this heading.

Heparin Calcium (Patients on anticoagulation therapy are at increased risk for bleeding because of drug-drug interactions and the effect on platelets. Aspirin can displace warfarin from protein binding sites, leading to prolongation of both the prothrombin time and bleeding time. Aspirin can increase the anticoagulant activity of heparin, increasing bleeding risk).
No products indexed under this heading.

Heparin Sodium (Patients on anticoagulation therapy are at increased risk for bleeding because of drug-drug interactions and the effect on platelets. Aspirin can displace warfarin from protein binding sites, leading to prolongation of both the prothrombin time and bleeding time. Aspirin can increase the anticoagulant activity of heparin, increasing bleeding risk).
No products indexed under this heading.

Hydrochlorothiazide (The effectiveness of diuretics in patients with underlying renal or cardiovascular disease may be diminished by the concomitant administration of aspirin due to inhibition of renal prostaglandins, leading to decreased renal blood flow, and salt and fluidretention). Products include:
Aldoril Tablets 1910
Atacand HCT 651
Avalide Tablets 888
Avalide Tablets 2874
Benicar HCT Tablets 1044
Diovan HCT Tablets 2196
Dyazide Capsules 1423
Hyzaar 50-12.5 Tablets 1990
Hyzaar 100-12.5 Tablets 1990
Hyzaar 100-25 Tablets 1990
Lopressor HCT 50/25 Tablets 2241
Lopressor HCT 100/25 Tablets 2241
Lopressor HCT 100/50 Tablets 2241
Lotensin HCT Tablets 2246
Micardis HCT Tablets 856
Moduretic Tablets 2028
Prinzide Tablets 2056
Teveten HCT Tablets 1737
Timolide Tablets 2086
Uniretic Tablets 3100

Hydroflumethiazide (The effectiveness of diuretics in patients with underlying renal or cardiovascular disease may be diminished by the concomitant administration of aspirin due to inhibition of renal prostaglandins, leading to decreased renal blood flow, and salt and fluidretention).
No products indexed under this heading.

Ibuprofen (The concurrent use of aspirin with other NSAIDs should be avoided because this may increase bleeding or lead to decreased renal function). Products include:
Advil Allergy Sinus Caplets 770
Advil 674
Children's Advil Oral Suspension 603
Children's Advil Chewable Tablets 603
Advil Cold & Sinus 723
Infants' Advil Concentrated Drops 604
Infants' Advil Concentrated Drops - White Grape (Dye-Free) 604
Junior Strength Advil Swallow Tablets 605
Advil Migraine Liquigels 608
Advil Multi-Symptom Cold Caplets 770
Advil PM Caplets 615
Motrin IB Tablets and Caplets 1866
Children's Motrin Oral Suspension 1867
Children's Motrin Non-Staining Dye-Free Oral Suspension 1867
Children's Motrin Cold Oral Suspension 1867
Infants' Motrin Concentrated Drops 1867
Infants' Motrin Non-Staining Dye-Free Concentrated Drops 1867
Junior Strength Motrin Caplets and Chewable Tablets 1867
Vicoprofen Tablets 539

Indapamide (The effectiveness of diuretics in patients with underlying renal or cardiovascular disease may be diminished by the concomitant administration of aspirin due to inhibition of renal prostaglandins, leading to decreased renal blood flow, and salt and fluidretention). Products include:

Indapamide Tablets 2156

Indomethacin (The concurrent use of aspirin with other NSAIDs should be avoided because this may increase bleeding or lead to decreased renal function). Products include:

Indocin 1995

Indomethacin Sodium Trihydrate (The concurrent use of aspirin with other NSAIDs should be avoided because this may increase bleeding or lead to decreased renal function). Products include:

Indocin I.V. 2465

Ketoprofen (The concurrent use of aspirin with other NSAIDs should be avoided because this may increase bleeding or lead to decreased renal function).

No products indexed under this heading.

Ketorolac Tromethamine (The concurrent use of aspirin with other NSAIDs should be avoided because this may increase bleeding or lead to decreased renal function). Products include:

Acular Ophthalmic Solution 565
Acular LS Ophthalmic Solution 566

Labetalol Hydrochloride (The hypotensive effects of beta blockers may be diminished by the concomitant administration of aspirin due to inhibition of renal prostaglandins, leading to decreased renal blood flow, and salt and fluid retention).

No products indexed under this heading.

Levobunolol Hydrochloride (The hypotensive effects of beta blockers may be diminished by the concomitant administration of aspirin due to inhibition of renal prostaglandins, leading to decreased renal blood flow, and salt and fluid retention). Products include:

Betagan Ophthalmic Solution,
USP............................... ⊙ 220

Lisinopril (The hyponatremic and hypotensive effects of ACE inhibitors may be diminished by the concomitant administration of aspirin due to its indirect effect on the renin-angiotensin conversion pathway). Products include:

Prinivil Tablets 2052
Prinzide Tablets 2056

Low Molecular Weight Heparins (Patients on anticoagulation therapy are at increased risk for bleeding because of drug-drug interactions and the effect on platelets. Aspirin can displace warfarin from protein binding sites, leading to prolongation of both the prothrombin time and bleeding time. Aspirin can increase the anticoagulant activity of heparin, increasing bleeding risk).

No products indexed under this heading.

Meclofenamate Sodium (The concurrent use of aspirin with other NSAIDs should be avoided because this may increase bleeding or lead to decreased renal function).

No products indexed under this heading.

Mefenamic Acid (The concurrent use of aspirin with other NSAIDs should be avoided because this may increase bleeding or lead to decreased renal function).

No products indexed under this heading.

Meloxicam (The concurrent use of aspirin with other NSAIDs should be avoided because this may increase bleeding or lead to decreased renal function). Products include:

Mobic Oral Suspension 863
Mobic Tablets 863

Metformin Hydrochloride (Moderate doses of aspirin may increase the effectiveness of oral hypoglycemic drugs, leading to hypoglycemia). Products include:

ActoPlus Met Tablets 3214
Avandamet Tablets 1373
Fortamet Extended-Release
Tablets 3115

Methotrexate (Salicylate can inhibit renal clearance of methotrexate, leading to bone marrow toxicity, especially in the elderly or renal-impaired).

No products indexed under this heading.

Methotrexate Sodium (Salicylate can inhibit renal clearance of methotrexate, leading to bone marrow toxicity, especially in the elderly or renal-impaired).

No products indexed under this heading.

Methyclothiazide (The effectiveness of diuretics in patients with underlying renal or cardiovascular disease may be diminished by the concomitant administration of aspirin due to inhibition of renal prostaglandins, leading to decreased renal blood flow, and salt and fluidretention).

No products indexed under this heading.

Metipranolol Hydrochloride (The hypotensive effects of beta blockers may be diminished by the concomitant administration of aspirin due to inhibition of renal prostaglandins, leading to decreased renal blood flow, and salt and fluid retention).

No products indexed under this heading.

Metolazone (The effectiveness of diuretics in patients with underlying renal or cardiovascular disease may be diminished by the concomitant administration of aspirin due to inhibition of renal prostaglandins, leading to decreased renal blood flow, and salt and fluidretention).

No products indexed under this heading.

Metoprolol Succinate (The hypotensive effects of beta blockers may be diminished by the concomitant administration of aspirin due to inhibition of renal prostaglandins, leading to decreased renal blood flow, and salt and fluid retention). Products include:

Toprol-XL Tablets 668

Metoprolol Tartrate (The hypotensive effects of beta blockers may be diminished by the concomitant administration of aspirin due to inhibition of renal prostaglandins, leading to decreased renal blood flow, and salt and fluid retention). Products include:

Lopressor Injection 2238
Lopressor Tablets 2238
Lopressor HCT 50/25 Tablets 2241

Lopressor HCT 100/25 Tablets 2241
Lopressor HCT 100/50 Tablets 2241

Miglitol (Moderate doses of aspirin may increase the effectiveness of oral hypoglycemic drugs, leading to hypoglycemia).

No products indexed under this heading.

Moexipril Hydrochloride (The hyponatremic and hypotensive effects of ACE inhibitors may be diminished by the concomitant administration of aspirin due to its indirect effect on the renin-angiotensin conversion pathway). Products include:

Uniretic Tablets 3100
Univasc Tablets 3104

Nabumetone (The concurrent use of aspirin with other NSAIDs should be avoided because this may increase bleeding or lead to decreased renal function).

No products indexed under this heading.

Nadolol (The hypotensive effects of beta blockers may be diminished by the concomitant administration of aspirin due to inhibition of renal prostaglandins, leading to decreased renal blood flow, and salt and fluid retention). Products include:

Nadolol Tablets 2159

Naproxen (The concurrent use of aspirin with other NSAIDs should be avoided because this may increase bleeding or lead to decreased renal function). Products include:

EC-Naprosyn Delayed-Release
Tablets 2761
Naprosyn Suspension 2761
Naprosyn Tablets 2761
Prevacid NapraPAC 3280

Naproxen Sodium (The concurrent use of aspirin with other NSAIDs should be avoided because this may increase bleeding or lead to decreased renal function). Products include:

Aleve Caplets 742
Aleve Gelcaps 743
Aleve Tablets 743
Aleve Cold & Sinus Caplets 744
Anaprox Tablets 2761
Anaprox DS Tablets 2761

Oxaprozin (The concurrent use of aspirin with other NSAIDs should be avoided because this may increase bleeding or lead to decreased renal function).

No products indexed under this heading.

Penbutolol Sulfate (The hypotensive effects of beta blockers may be diminished by the concomitant administration of aspirin due to inhibition of renal prostaglandins, leading to decreased renal blood flow, and salt and fluid retention).

No products indexed under this heading.

Perindopril Erbumine (The hyponatremic and hypotensive effects of ACE inhibitors may be diminished by the concomitant administration of aspirin due to its indirect effect on the renin-angiotensin conversion pathway). Products include:

Aceon Tablets (2 mg, 4 mg,
8 mg).......................... 3194

Phenylbutazone (The concurrent use of aspirin with other NSAIDs should be avoided because this may increase bleeding or lead to decreased renal function).

No products indexed under this heading.

Phenytoin (Salicylate can displace protein-bound phenytoin, leading to a decrease in the total concentration of phenytoin).

No products indexed under this heading.

Phenytoin Sodium (Salicylate can displace protein-bound phenytoin, leading to a decrease in the total concentration of phenytoin). Products include:

Phenytek Capsules 2160

Pindolol (The hypotensive effects of beta blockers may be diminished by the concomitant administration of aspirin due to inhibition of renal prostaglandins, leading to decreased renal blood flow, and salt and fluid retention).

No products indexed under this heading.

Pioglitazone Hydrochloride (Moderate doses of aspirin may increase the effectiveness of oral hypoglycemic drugs, leading to hypoglycemia). Products include:

ActoPlus Met Tablets 3214
Actos Tablets 3219
Duetact Tablets 3226

Piroxicam (The concurrent use of aspirin with other NSAIDs should be avoided because this may increase bleeding or lead to decreased renal function).

No products indexed under this heading.

Polythiazide (The effectiveness of diuretics in patients with underlying renal or cardiovascular disease may be diminished by the concomitant administration of aspirin due to inhibition of renal prostaglandins, leading to decreased renal blood flow, and salt and fluidretention).

No products indexed under this heading.

Probenecid (Salicylates antagonize the uricosuric action of uricouric agents).

No products indexed under this heading.

Propranolol Hydrochloride (The hypotensive effects of beta blockers may be diminished by the concomitant administration of aspirin due to inhibition of renal prostaglandins, leading to decreased renal blood flow, and salt and fluid retention). Products include:

Inderal LA Long-Acting Capsules 3429
InnoPran XL Capsules 2723

Quinapril Hydrochloride (The hyponatremic and hypotensive effects of ACE inhibitors may be diminished by the concomitant administration of aspirin due to its indirect effect on the renin-angiotensin conversion pathway).

No products indexed under this heading.

Ramipril (The hyponatremic and hypotensive effects of ACE inhibitors may be diminished by the concomitant administration of aspirin due to its indirect effect on the renin-angiotensin conversion pathway). Products include:

Altace Capsules 1702

Repaglinide (Moderate doses of aspirin may increase the effectiveness of oral hypoglycemic drugs, leading to hypoglycemia).

No products indexed under this heading.

Rofecoxib (The concurrent use of aspirin with other NSAIDs should be avoided because this may increase bleeding or lead to decreased renal function).
No products indexed under this heading.

Rosiglitazone Maleate (Moderate doses of aspirin may increase the effectiveness of oral hypoglycemic drugs, leading to hypoglycemia). Products include:
- Avandamet Tablets ... 1373
- Avandaryl Tablets ... 1379
- Avandia Tablets ... 1384

Sotalol Hydrochloride (The hypotensive effects of beta blockers may be diminished by the concomitant administration of aspirin due to inhibition of renal prostaglandins, leading to decreased renal blood flow, and salt and fluid retention).
No products indexed under this heading.

Spirapril Hydrochloride (The hyponatremic and hypotensive effects of ACE inhibitors may be diminished by the concomitant administration of aspirin due to its indirect effect on the renin-angiotensin conversion pathway).
No products indexed under this heading.

Spironolactone (The effectiveness of diuretics in patients with underlying renal or cardiovascular disease may be diminished by the concomitant administration of aspirin due to inhibition of renal prostaglandins, leading to decreased renal blood flow, and salt and fluidretention).
No products indexed under this heading.

Sulfinpyrazone (Salicylates antagonize the uricosuric action of uricouric agents).
No products indexed under this heading.

Sulindac (The concurrent use of aspirin with other NSAIDs should be avoided because this may increase bleeding or lead to decreased renal function). Products include:
- Clinoril Tablets ... 1924

Timolol Hemihydrate (The hypotensive effects of beta blockers may be diminished by the concomitant administration of aspirin due to inhibition of renal prostaglandins, leading to decreased renal blood flow, and salt and fluid retention). Products include:
- Betimol Ophthalmic Solution ... 3382
- Betimol Ophthalmic Solution ... ⊙295

Timolol Maleate (The hypotensive effects of beta blockers may be diminished by the concomitant administration of aspirin due to inhibition of renal prostaglandins, leading to decreased renal blood flow, and salt and fluid retention). Products include:
- Blocadren Tablets ... 1916
- Cosopt Sterile Ophthalmic Solution ... 1931
- Timolide Tablets ... 2086
- Timoptic Sterile Ophthalmic Solution ... 2088
- Timoptic in Ocudose ... 2091
- Timoptic-XE Sterile Ophthalmic Gel Forming Solution ... 2092

Tinzaparin Sodium (Patients on anticoagulation therapy are at increased risk for bleeding because of drug-drug interactions and the effect on platelets. Aspirin can displace warfarin from protein binding sites, leading to prolongation of both the prothrombin time and bleeding time. Aspirin can increase the anticoagulant activity of heparin, increasing bleeding risk).
No products indexed under this heading.

Tolazamide (Moderate doses of aspirin may increase the effectiveness of oral hypoglycemic drugs, leading to hypoglycemia).
No products indexed under this heading.

Tolbutamide (Moderate doses of aspirin may increase the effectiveness of oral hypoglycemic drugs, leading to hypoglycemia).
No products indexed under this heading.

Tolmetin Sodium (The concurrent use of aspirin with other NSAIDs should be avoided because this may increase bleeding or lead to decreased renal function).
No products indexed under this heading.

Torsemide (The effectiveness of diuretics in patients with underlying renal or cardiovascular disease may be diminished by the concomitant administration of aspirin due to inhibition of renal prostaglandins, leading to decreased renal blood flow, and salt and fluidretention). Products include:
- Demadex Injection ... 2759
- Demadex Tablets ... 2759

Trandolapril (The hyponatremic and hypotensive effects of ACE inhibitors may be diminished by the concomitant administration of aspirin due to its indirect effect on the renin-angiotensin conversion pathway). Products include:
- Mavik Tablets ... 486
- Tarka Tablets ... 524

Triamterene (The effectiveness of diuretics in patients with underlying renal or cardiovascular disease may be diminished by the concomitant administration of aspirin due to inhibition of renal prostaglandins, leading to decreased renal blood flow, and salt and fluidretention). Products include:
- Dyazide Capsules ... 1423
- Dyrenium Capsules ... 3400

Troglitazone (Moderate doses of aspirin may increase the effectiveness of oral hypoglycemic drugs, leading to hypoglycemia).
No products indexed under this heading.

Valdecoxib (The concurrent use of aspirin with other NSAIDs should be avoided because this may increase bleeding or lead to decreased renal function).
No products indexed under this heading.

Valproate Sodium (Salicylate can displace protein-bound valproic acid, leading to an increase in serum valproic acid levels). Products include:
- Depacon Injection ... 412

Valproic Acid (Salicylate can displace protein-bound valproic acid, leading to an increase in serum valproic acid levels). Products include:
- Depakene ... 417

Warfarin Sodium (Patients on anticoagulation therapy are at increased risk for bleeding because of drug-drug interactions and the effect on platelets. Aspirin can displace warfarin from protein binding sites, leading to prolongation of both the prothrombin time and bleeding time. Aspirin can increase the anticoagulant activity of heparin, increasing bleeding risk). Products include:
- Coumadin for Injection ... 898
- Coumadin Tablets ... 898

BAYER ASPIRIN COMPREHENSIVE PRESCRIBING INFORMATION

(Aspirin) ... 796

May interact with ACE inhibitors, beta blockers, oral anticoagulants, diuretics, anticonvulsants, antigout agents, oral hypoglycemic agents, non-steroidal anti-inflammatory agents, and certain other agents. Compounds in these categories include:

Acarbose (Concurrent use should be avoided unless directed by a doctor). Products include:
- Precose Tablets ... 751

Acebutolol Hydrochloride (The hypotensive effects of beta-blockers may be diminished by concomitant administration of aspirin).
No products indexed under this heading.

Acetazolamide (Concurrent use of acetazolamide can lead to high serum levels of acetazolamide and toxicity).
No products indexed under this heading.

Acetazolamide Sodium (Concurrent use of acetazolamide can lead to high serum levels of acetazolamide and toxicity).
No products indexed under this heading.

Allopurinol (Salicylates antagonize the uricosuric action of uricosuric agents).
No products indexed under this heading.

Amiloride Hydrochloride (The effectiveness of diuretics in patients with underlying renal or cardiovascular disease may be diminished by the concomitant administration of aspirin). Products include:
- Midamor Tablets ... 2026
- Moduretic Tablets ... 2028

Anisindione (Concurrent use should be avoided unless directed by a doctor). Products include:
- Miradon Tablets ... 3042

Antiarthritic Drugs, unspecified (Concurrent use should be avoided unless directed by a doctor).
No products indexed under this heading.

Atenolol (The hypotensive effects of beta-blockers may be diminished by concomitant administration of aspirin).
No products indexed under this heading.

Benazepril Hydrochloride (Reports suggested that NSAIDs may diminish the hyponatremic and hypotensive effect of ACE inhibitors). Products include:
- Lotensin Tablets ... 2243
- Lotensin HCT Tablets ... 2246
- Lotrel Capsules ... 2249

Bendroflumethiazide (The effectiveness of diuretics in patients with underlying renal or cardiovascular disease may be diminished by the concomitant administration of aspirin).
No products indexed under this heading.

Betaxolol Hydrochloride (The hypotensive effects of beta-blockers may be diminished by concomitant administration of aspirin). Products include:
- Betoptic S Ophthalmic Suspension ... 558

Bisoprolol Fumarate (The hypotensive effects of beta-blockers may be diminished by concomitant administration of aspirin).
No products indexed under this heading.

Bumetanide (The effectiveness of diuretics in patients with underlying renal or cardiovascular disease may be diminished by the concomitant administration of aspirin). Products include:
- Bumex Tablets ... 2746

Captopril (Reports suggested that NSAIDs may diminish the hyponatremic and hypotensive effect of ACE inhibitors). Products include:
- Captopril Tablets ... 2149

Carbamazepine (Salicylate can displace protein-bound phenytoin and valproic acid leading to a decrease in the total concentration of phenytoin and an increase in serum valproic acid levels). Products include:
- Carbatrol Capsules ... 3171
- Equetro Extended-Release Capsules ... 3180
- Tegretol/Tegretol-XR ... 2295

Carteolol Hydrochloride (The hypotensive effects of beta-blockers may be diminished by concomitant administration of aspirin). Products include:
- Carteolol Hydrochloride Ophthalmic Solution USP, 1% ... ⊙249

Celecoxib (The concurrent use of aspirin with other NSAIDs should be avoided because this may increase bleeding or lead to decreased renal function). Products include:
- Celebrex Capsules ... 3134

Chlorothiazide (The effectiveness of diuretics in patients with underlying renal or cardiovascular disease may be diminished by the concomitant administration of aspirin). Products include:
- Diuril Oral Suspension ... 1954

Chlorothiazide Sodium (The effectiveness of diuretics in patients with underlying renal or cardiovascular disease may be diminished by the concomitant administration of aspirin). Products include:
- Diuril Sodium Intravenous ... 2467

Chlorpropamide (Concurrent use should be avoided unless directed by a doctor).
No products indexed under this heading.

Chlorthalidone (The effectiveness of diuretics in patients with underlying renal or cardiovascular disease may be diminished by the concomitant administration of aspirin). Products include:
- Clorpres Tablets ... 2153

Diclofenac Potassium (The concurrent use of aspirin with other NSAIDs should be avoided because this may increase bleeding or lead to decreased renal function).
No products indexed under this heading.

Diclofenac Sodium (The concurrent use of aspirin with other NSAIDs should be avoided because this may increase bleeding or lead to decreased renal function). Products include:

Dicumarol (Concurrent use should be avoided unless directed by a doctor).
No products indexed under this heading.

Divalproex Sodium (Salicylate can displace protein-bound phenytoin and valproic acid leading to a decrease in the total concentration of phenytoin and an increase in serum valproic acid levels). Products include:

Enalapril Maleate (Reports suggested that NSAIDs may diminish the hyponatremic and hypotensive effect of ACE inhibitors). Products include:

Enalaprilat (Reports suggested that NSAIDs may diminish the hyponatremic and hypotensive effect of ACE inhibitors).
No products indexed under this heading.

Esmolol Hydrochloride (The hypotensive effects of beta-blockers may be diminished by concomitant administration of aspirin).
No products indexed under this heading.

Ethacrynic Acid (The effectiveness of diuretics in patients with underlying renal or cardiovascular disease may be diminished by the concomitant administration of aspirin). Products include:

Ethosuximide (Salicylate can displace protein-bound phenytoin and valproic acid leading to a decrease in the total concentration of phenytoin and an increase in serum valproic acid levels).
No products indexed under this heading.

Ethotoin (Salicylate can displace protein-bound phenytoin and valproic acid leading to a decrease in the total concentration of phenytoin and an increase in serum valproic acid levels).
No products indexed under this heading.

Etodolac (The concurrent use of aspirin with other NSAIDs should be avoided because this may increase bleeding or lead to decreased renal function).
No products indexed under this heading.

Felbamate (Salicylate can displace protein-bound phenytoin and valproic acid leading to a decrease in the total concentration of phenytoin and an increase in serum valproic acid levels).
No products indexed under this heading.

Fenoprofen Calcium (The concurrent use of aspirin with other NSAIDs should be avoided because this may increase bleeding or lead to decreased renal function). Products include:

Flurbiprofen (The concurrent use of aspirin with other NSAIDs should be avoided because this may increase bleeding or lead to decreased renal function).
No products indexed under this heading.

Fosinopril Sodium (Reports suggested that NSAIDs may diminish the hyponatremic and hypotensive effect of ACE inhibitors).
No products indexed under this heading.

Fosphenytoin (Salicylate can displace protein-bound phenytoin and valproic acid leading to a decrease in the total concentration of phenytoin and an increase in serum valproic acid levels).
No products indexed under this heading.

Fosphenytoin Sodium (Salicylate can displace protein-bound phenytoin and valproic acid leading to a decrease in the total concentration of phenytoin and an increase in serum valproic acid levels).
No products indexed under this heading.

Furosemide (The effectiveness of diuretics in patients with underlying renal or cardiovascular disease may be diminished by the concomitant administration of aspirin). Products include:

Gabapentin (Salicylate can displace protein-bound phenytoin and valproic acid leading to a decrease in the total concentration of phenytoin and an increase in serum valproic acid levels). Products include:

Glimepiride (Concurrent use should be avoided unless directed by a doctor). Products include:

Glipizide (Concurrent use should be avoided unless directed by a doctor).
No products indexed under this heading.

Glyburide (Concurrent use should be avoided unless directed by a doctor).
No products indexed under this heading.

Hydrochlorothiazide (The effectiveness of diuretics in patients with underlying renal or cardiovascular disease may be diminished by the concomitant administration of aspirin). Products include:

Hydroflumethiazide (The effectiveness of diuretics in patients with underlying renal or cardiovascular disease may be diminished by the concomitant administration of aspirin).
No products indexed under this heading.

Ibuprofen (The concurrent use of aspirin with other NSAIDs should be avoided because this may increase bleeding or lead to decreased renal function). Products include:

Indapamide (The effectiveness of diuretics in patients with underlying renal or cardiovascular disease may be diminished by the concomitant administration of aspirin). Products include:

Indomethacin (The concurrent use of aspirin with other NSAIDs should be avoided because this may increase bleeding or lead to decreased renal function). Products include:

Indomethacin Sodium Trihydrate (The concurrent use of aspirin with other NSAIDs should be avoided because this may increase bleeding or lead to decreased renal function). Products include:

Ketoprofen (The concurrent use of aspirin with other NSAIDs should be avoided because this may increase bleeding or lead to decreased renal function).
No products indexed under this heading.

Ketorolac Tromethamine (The concurrent use of aspirin with other NSAIDs should be avoided because this may increase bleeding or lead to decreased renal function). Products include:

Labetalol Hydrochloride (The hypotensive effects of beta-blockers may be diminished by concomitant administration of aspirin).
No products indexed under this heading.

Lamotrigine (Salicylate can displace protein-bound phenytoin and

valproic acid leading to a decrease in the total concentration of phenytoin and an increase in serum valproic acid levels). Products include:

Levetiracetam (Salicylate can displace protein-bound phenytoin and valproic acid leading to a decrease in the total concentration of phenytoin and an increase in serum valproic acid levels). Products include:

Levobunolol Hydrochloride (The hypotensive effects of beta-blockers may be diminished by concomitant administration of aspirin). Products include:

Lisinopril (Reports suggested that NSAIDs may diminish the hyponatremic and hypotensive effect of ACE inhibitors). Products include:

Meclofenamate Sodium (The concurrent use of aspirin with other NSAIDs should be avoided because this may increase bleeding or lead to decreased renal function).
No products indexed under this heading.

Mefenamic Acid (The concurrent use of aspirin with other NSAIDs should be avoided because this may increase bleeding or lead to decreased renal function).
No products indexed under this heading.

Meloxicam (The concurrent use of aspirin with other NSAIDs should be avoided because this may increase bleeding or lead to decreased renal function). Products include:

Mephenytoin (Salicylate can displace protein-bound phenytoin and valproic acid leading to a decrease in the total concentration of phenytoin and an increase in serum valproic acid levels).
No products indexed under this heading.

Metformin Hydrochloride (Concurrent use should be avoided unless directed by a doctor). Products include:

Methotrexate (Salicylate can inhibit renal clearance of methotrexate leading to bone marrow toxicity, especially in the elderly or renal impaired).
No products indexed under this heading.

Methotrexate Sodium (Salicylate can inhibit renal clearance of methotrexate leading to bone marrow toxicity, especially in the elderly or renal impaired).
No products indexed under this heading.

Methsuximide (Salicylate can displace protein-bound phenytoin and valproic acid leading to a decrease in the total concentration of phenytoin and an increase in serum valproic acid levels).
No products indexed under this heading.

Methyclothiazide (The effectiveness of diuretics in patients with underlying renal or cardiovascular disease may be diminished by the concomitant administration of aspirin).
 No products indexed under this heading.

Metipranolol Hydrochloride (The hypotensive effects of beta-blockers may be diminished by concomitant administration of aspirin).
 No products indexed under this heading.

Metolazone (The effectiveness of diuretics in patients with underlying renal or cardiovascular disease may be diminished by the concomitant administration of aspirin).
 No products indexed under this heading.

Metoprolol Succinate (The hypotensive effects of beta-blockers may be diminished by concomitant administration of aspirin). Products include:

Metoprolol Tartrate (The hypotensive effects of beta-blockers may be diminished by concomitant administration of aspirin). Products include:

Miglitol (Concurrent use should be avoided unless directed by a doctor).
 No products indexed under this heading.

Moexipril Hydrochloride (Reports suggested that NSAIDs may diminish the hyponatremic and hypotensive effect of ACE inhibitors). Products include:

Nabumetone (The concurrent use of aspirin with other NSAIDs should be avoided because this may increase bleeding or lead to decreased renal function).
 No products indexed under this heading.

Nadolol (The hypotensive effects of beta-blockers may be diminished by concomitant administration of aspirin). Products include:

Naproxen (The concurrent use of aspirin with other NSAIDs should be avoided because this may increase bleeding or lead to decreased renal function). Products include:

Naproxen Sodium (The concurrent use of aspirin with other NSAIDs should be avoided because this may increase bleeding or lead to decreased renal function). Products include:

Oxaprozin (The concurrent use of aspirin with other NSAIDs should be avoided because this may increase bleeding or lead to decreased renal function).
 No products indexed under this heading.

Oxcarbazepine (Salicylate can displace protein-bound phenytoin and valproic acid leading to a decrease in the total concentration of phenytoin and an increase in serum valproic acid levels). Products include:

Paramethadione (Salicylate can displace protein-bound phenytoin and valproic acid leading to a decrease in the total concentration of phenytoin and an increase in serum valproic acid levels).
 No products indexed under this heading.

Penbutolol Sulfate (The hypotensive effects of beta-blockers may be diminished by concomitant administration of aspirin).
 No products indexed under this heading.

Perindopril Erbumine (Reports suggested that NSAIDs may diminish the hyponatremic and hypotensive effect of ACE inhibitors). Products include:

Phenacemide (Salicylate can displace protein-bound phenytoin and valproic acid leading to a decrease in the total concentration of phenytoin and an increase in serum valproic acid levels).
 No products indexed under this heading.

Phenobarbital (Salicylate can displace protein-bound phenytoin and valproic acid leading to a decrease in the total concentration of phenytoin and an increase in serum valproic acid levels). Products include:

Phensuximide (Salicylate can displace protein-bound phenytoin and valproic acid leading to a decrease in the total concentration of phenytoin and an increase in serum valproic acid levels).
 No products indexed under this heading.

Phenylbutazone (The concurrent use of aspirin with other NSAIDs should be avoided because this may increase bleeding or lead to decreased renal function).
 No products indexed under this heading.

Phenytoin (Salicylate can displace protein-bound phenytoin and valproic acid leading to a decrease in the total concentration of phenytoin and an increase in serum valproic acid levels).
 No products indexed under this heading.

Phenytoin Sodium (Salicylate can displace protein-bound phenytoin and valproic acid leading to a decrease in the total concentration of phenytoin and an increase in serum valproic acid levels). Products include:

Pindolol (The hypotensive effects of beta-blockers may be diminished by concomitant administration of aspirin).
 No products indexed under this heading.

Pioglitazone Hydrochloride (Concurrent use should be avoided unless directed by a doctor). Products include:

Piroxicam (The concurrent use of aspirin with other NSAIDs should be avoided because this may increase bleeding or lead to decreased renal function).
 No products indexed under this heading.

Polythiazide (The effectiveness of diuretics in patients with underlying renal or cardiovascular disease may be diminished by the concomitant administration of aspirin).
 No products indexed under this heading.

Primidone (Salicylate can displace protein-bound phenytoin and valproic acid leading to a decrease in the total concentration of phenytoin and an increase in serum valproic acid levels).
 No products indexed under this heading.

Probenecid (Salicylates antagonize the uricosuric action of uricosuric agents).
 No products indexed under this heading.

Propranolol Hydrochloride (The hypotensive effects of beta-blockers may be diminished by concomitant administration of aspirin). Products include:

Quinapril Hydrochloride (Reports suggested that NSAIDs may diminish the hyponatremic and hypotensive effect of ACE inhibitors).
 No products indexed under this heading.

Ramipril (Reports suggested that NSAIDs may diminish the hyponatremic and hypotensive effect of ACE inhibitors). Products include:

Repaglinide (Concurrent use should be avoided unless directed by a doctor).
 No products indexed under this heading.

Rofecoxib (The concurrent use of aspirin with other NSAIDs should be avoided because this may increase bleeding or lead to decreased renal function).
 No products indexed under this heading.

Rosiglitazone Maleate (Concurrent use should be avoided unless directed by a doctor). Products include:

Sotalol Hydrochloride (The hypotensive effects of beta-blockers may be diminished by concomitant administration of aspirin).
 No products indexed under this heading.

Spirapril Hydrochloride (Reports suggested that NSAIDs may diminish the hyponatremic and hypotensive effect of ACE inhibitors).
 No products indexed under this heading.

Spironolactone (The effectiveness of diuretics in patients with underlying renal or cardiovascular disease may be diminished by the concomitant administration of aspirin).
 No products indexed under this heading.

Sulfinpyrazone (Salicylates antagonize the uricosuric action of uricosuric agents).
 No products indexed under this heading.

Sulindac (The concurrent use of aspirin with other NSAIDs should be avoided because this may increase bleeding or lead to decreased renal function). Products include:

Tiagabine Hydrochloride (Salicylate can displace protein-bound phenytoin and valproic acid leading to a decrease in the total concentration of phenytoin and an increase in serum valproic acid levels). Products include:

Timolol Hemihydrate (The hypotensive effects of beta-blockers may be diminished by concomitant administration of aspirin). Products include:

Timolol Maleate (The hypotensive effects of beta-blockers may be diminished by concomitant administration of aspirin). Products include:

Tolazamide (Concurrent use should be avoided unless directed by a doctor).
 No products indexed under this heading.

Tolbutamide (Concurrent use should be avoided unless directed by a doctor).
 No products indexed under this heading.

Tolmetin Sodium (The concurrent use of aspirin with other NSAIDs should be avoided because this may increase bleeding or lead to decreased renal function).
 No products indexed under this heading.

Topiramate (Salicylate can displace protein-bound phenytoin and valproic acid leading to a decrease in the total concentration of phenytoin and an increase in serum valproic acid levels). Products include:

Torsemide (The effectiveness of diuretics in patients with underlying renal or cardiovascular disease may be diminished by the concomitant administration of aspirin). Products include:

Trandolapril (Reports suggested that NSAIDs may diminish the

IMPORTANT NOTE: Always consult each drug listing in the patient's regimen for possible interactions.

hyponatremic and hypotensive effect of ACE inhibitors). Products include:

- Mavik Tablets 486
- Tarka Tablets 524

Triamterene (The effectiveness of diuretics in patients with underlying renal or cardiovascular disease may be diminished by the concomitant administration of aspirin). Products include:

- Dyazide Capsules 1423
- Dyrenium Capsules 3400

Trimethadione (Salicylate can displace protein-bound phenytoin and valproic acid leading to a decrease in the total concentration of phenytoin and an increase in serum valproic acid levels).

No products indexed under this heading.

Troglitazone (Concurrent use should be avoided unless directed by a doctor).

No products indexed under this heading.

Valdecoxib (The concurrent use of aspirin with other NSAIDs should be avoided because this may increase bleeding or lead to decreased renal function).

No products indexed under this heading.

Valproate Sodium (Salicylate can displace protein-bound phenytoin and valproic acid leading to a decrease in the total concentration of phenytoin and an increase in serum valproic acid levels). Products include:

- Depacon Injection 412

Valproic Acid (Salicylate can displace protein-bound phenytoin and valproic acid leading to a decrease in the total concentration of phenytoin and an increase in serum valproic acid levels). Products include:

- Depakene 417

Warfarin Sodium (Concurrent use should be avoided unless directed by a doctor). Products include:

- Coumadin for Injection 898
- Coumadin Tablets 898

Zonisamide (Salicylate can displace protein-bound phenytoin and valproic acid leading to a decrease in the total concentration of phenytoin and an increase in serum valproic acid levels). Products include:

- Zonegran Capsules 1101

Food Interactions

Alcohol (Chronic heavy alcohol users, 3 or more drinks per day, should consult their physicians for advice on when and how they should take pain relievers/fever reducers including aspirin).

BC HEADACHE POWDER

(Aspirin, Caffeine, Salicylamide) .... ▣677

See BC Allergy Sinus Cold Powder

BC ALLERGY SINUS COLD POWDER

(Aspirin, Chlorpheniramine Maleate, Pseudoephedrine Hydrochloride)........ ▣677

May interact with oral anticoagulants, oral hypoglycemic agents, monoamine oxidase inhibitors, and certain other agents. Compounds in these categories include:

Acarbose (Concurrent use should be avoided unless directed by a physician). Products include:

- Precose Tablets 751

Anisindione (Concurrent use should be avoided unless directed by a physician). Products include:

- Miradon Tablets 3042

Chlorpropamide (Concurrent use should be avoided unless directed by a physician).

No products indexed under this heading.

Dicumarol (Concurrent use should be avoided unless directed by a physician).

No products indexed under this heading.

Glimepiride (Concurrent use should be avoided unless directed by a physician). Products include:

- Avandaryl Tablets 1379
- Duetact Tablets 3226

Glipizide (Concurrent use should be avoided unless directed by a physician).

No products indexed under this heading.

Glyburide (Concurrent use should be avoided unless directed by a physician).

No products indexed under this heading.

Isocarboxazid (Concurrent use with MAO inhibitors is not recommended; consult your doctor).

No products indexed under this heading.

Metformin Hydrochloride (Concurrent use should be avoided unless directed by a physician). Products include:

- ActoPlus Met Tablets 3214
- Avandamet Tablets 1373
- Fortamet Extended-Release Tablets 3115

Miglitol (Concurrent use should be avoided unless directed by a physician).

No products indexed under this heading.

Moclobemide (Concurrent use with MAO inhibitors is not recommended; consult your doctor).

No products indexed under this heading.

Pargyline Hydrochloride (Concurrent use with MAO inhibitors is not recommended; consult your doctor).

No products indexed under this heading.

Phenelzine Sulfate (Concurrent use with MAO inhibitors is not recommended; consult your doctor).

No products indexed under this heading.

Pioglitazone Hydrochloride (Concurrent use should be avoided unless directed by a physician). Products include:

- ActoPlus Met Tablets 3214
- Actos Tablets 3219
- Duetact Tablets 3226

Procarbazine Hydrochloride (Concurrent use with MAO inhibitors is not recommended; consult your doctor). Products include:

- Matulane Capsules 3191

Repaglinide (Concurrent use should be avoided unless directed by a physician).

No products indexed under this heading.

Rosiglitazone Maleate (Concurrent use should be avoided unless directed by a physician). Products include:

- Avandamet Tablets 1373
- Avandaryl Tablets 1379
- Avandia Tablets 1384

Selegiline Hydrochloride (Concurrent use with MAO inhibitors is not recommended; consult your doctor). Products include:

- Eldepryl Capsules 3208
- Zelapar Tablets 3372

Tolazamide (Concurrent use should be avoided unless directed by a physician).

No products indexed under this heading.

Tolbutamide (Concurrent use should be avoided unless directed by a physician).

No products indexed under this heading.

Tranylcypromine Sulfate (Concurrent use with MAO inhibitors is not recommended; consult your doctor). Products include:

- Parnate Tablets 1527

Troglitazone (Concurrent use should be avoided unless directed by a physician).

No products indexed under this heading.

Warfarin Sodium (Concurrent use should be avoided unless directed by a physician). Products include:

- Coumadin for Injection 898
- Coumadin Tablets 898

Food Interactions

Alcohol (Individuals consuming 3 or more alcohol-containing drinks per day should consult their physician for advice on when and how they should take this product; increases drowsiness; avoid concurrent use).

ARTHRITIS STRENGTH BC POWDER

(Aspirin, Caffeine, Salicylamide) .... ▣677

See BC Allergy Sinus Cold Powder

BC SINUS COLD POWDER

(Aspirin, Pseudoephedrine Hydrochloride)........ ▣677

See BC Allergy Sinus Cold Powder

BECONASE AQ NASAL SPRAY

(Beclomethasone Dipropionate Monohydrate)........ 1396

None cited in PDR database.

BEELITH TABLETS

(Magnesium Oxide, Vitamin B_6) 759

May interact with:

Prescription Drugs, unspecified (Concurrent use should be avoided).

No products indexed under this heading.

BENEFIBER FIBER SUPPLEMENT CAPLETS

(Fiber, dietary) .... ▣808

None cited in PDR database.

BENEFIBER FIBER SUPPLEMENT POWDER

(Fiber, dietary) .... ▣807

None cited in PDR database.

BENEFIBER FIBER SUPPLEMENT CHEWABLE TABLETS

(Fiber, dietary) .... ▣808

None cited in PDR database.

BENEFIX Vials

(Antihemophilic Factor (Recombinant))........ 3408

None cited in PDR database.

BENICAR TABLETS

(Olmesartan Medoxomil) 1043

None cited in PDR database.

BENICAR HCT TABLETS

(Hydrochlorothiazide, Olmesartan Medoxomil)........ 1044

May interact with angiotensin-II receptor antagonists, antihypertensives, barbiturates, corticosteroids, curariform skeletal muscle relaxants, oral hypoglycemic agents, insulin, lithium preparations, narcotic analgesics, non-steroidal anti-inflammatory agents, vasopressors, and certain other agents. Compounds in these categories include:

Acarbose (Co-administration may require a dosage adjustment of the antidiabetic drug). Products include:

- Precose Tablets 751

Acebutolol Hydrochloride (Co-administration could have additive effect or potentiation).

No products indexed under this heading.

ACTH (Co-administration could cause intensified electrolyte depletion, particularly hypokalemia).

No products indexed under this heading.

Alfentanil Hydrochloride (Concurrent administration could cause potentiation of orthostatic hypotension).

No products indexed under this heading.

Amlodipine Besylate (Co-administration could have additive effect or potentiation). Products include:

- Caduet Tablets 2508
- Lotrel Capsules 2249
- Norvasc Tablets 2545

Aprobarbital (Concurrent administration could cause potentiation of orthostatic hypotension).

No products indexed under this heading.

Atenolol (Co-administration could have additive effect or potentiation).

No products indexed under this heading.

Atracurium Besylate (Co-administration could cause possible increased responsiveness to the muscle relaxant).

No products indexed under this heading.

Benazepril Hydrochloride (Co-administration could have additive effect or potentiation). Products include:

- Lotensin Tablets 2243
- Lotensin HCT Tablets 2246
- Lotrel Capsules 2249

Bendroflumethiazide (Co-administration could have additive effect or potentiation).

No products indexed under this heading.

Betamethasone Acetate (Co-administration could cause intensified electrolyte depletion, particularly hypokalemia).

No products indexed under this heading.

Betamethasone Sodium Phosphate (Co-administration could cause intensified electrolyte depletion, particularly hypokalemia).

No products indexed under this heading.

Betaxolol Hydrochloride (Co-administration could have additive effect or potentiation). Products include:

- Betoptic S Ophthalmic Suspension........ 558

Bisoprolol Fumarate (Co-administration could have additive effect or potentiation).
No products indexed under this heading.

Buprenorphine Hydrochloride (Concurrent administration could cause potentiation of orthostatic hypotension). Products include:
Buprenex Injectable 2716
Suboxone Tablets 2717
Subutex Tablets 2717

Butabarbital (Concurrent administration could cause potentiation of orthostatic hypotension).
No products indexed under this heading.

Butalbital (Concurrent administration could cause potentiation of orthostatic hypotension).
No products indexed under this heading.

Candesartan Cilexetil (Co-administration could have additive effect or potentiation). Products include:
Atacand Tablets 649
Atacand HCT 651

Captopril (Co-administration could have additive effect or potentiation). Products include:
Captopril Tablets 2149

Carteolol Hydrochloride (Co-administration could have additive effect or potentiation). Products include:
Carteolol Hydrochloride Ophthalmic Solution USP, 1%........ ⊙ 249

Celecoxib (In some patients the administration of a non-steroidal anti-inflammatory agent can reduce the diuretic, natriuretic and antihypertensive effects of loop, potassium-sparing and thiazide diuretics). Products include:
Celebrex Capsules 3134

Chlorothiazide (Co-administration could have additive effect or potentiation). Products include:
Diuril Oral Suspension 1954

Chlorothiazide Sodium (Co-administration could have additive effect or potentiation). Products include:
Diuril Sodium Intravenous 2467

Chlorpropamide (Co-administration may require a dosage adjustment of the antidiabetic drug).
No products indexed under this heading.

Chlorthalidone (Co-administration could have additive effect or potentiation). Products include:
Clorpres Tablets 2153

Cholestyramine (Absorption of hydrochlorothiazide is impaired in the presence of anionic exchange resins; single doses of cholestyramine bind the hydrochlorothiazide and reduce its absorption from the gastrointestinal tract by 85%).
No products indexed under this heading.

Cisatracurium Besylate (Co-administration could cause possible increased responsiveness to the muscle relaxant). Products include:
Nimbex Injection 498

Clonidine (Co-administration could have additive effect or potentiation). Products include:
Catapres-TTS 844

Clonidine Hydrochloride (Co-administration could have additive effect or potentiation). Products include:
Catapres Tablets 843
Clorpres Tablets 2153

Codeine Phosphate (Concurrent administration could cause potentiation of orthostatic hypotension). Products include:
Tylenol with Codeine Tablets 2391

Colestipol (Absorption of hydrochlorothiazide is impaired in the presence of anionic exchange resins; single doses of colestipol bind the hydrochlorothiazide and reduce its absorption from the gastrointestinal tract by 43%).
No products indexed under this heading.

Colestipol Hydrochloride (Absorption of hydrochlorothiazide is impaired in the presence of anionic exchange resins; single doses of colestipol bind the hydrochlorothiazide and reduce its absorption from the gastrointestinal tract by 43%).
No products indexed under this heading.

Cortisone Acetate (Co-administration could cause intensified electrolyte depletion, particularly hypokalemia).
No products indexed under this heading.

Deserpidine (Co-administration could have additive effect or potentiation).
No products indexed under this heading.

Dexamethasone (Co-administration could cause intensified electrolyte depletion, particularly hypokalemia). Products include:
Ciprodex Otic Suspension 559
Decadron Tablets 1951
TobraDex Ophthalmic Ointment 562
TobraDex Ophthalmic Suspension ... 563

Dexamethasone Acetate (Co-administration could cause intensified electrolyte depletion, particularly hypokalemia).
No products indexed under this heading.

Dexamethasone Sodium Phosphate (Co-administration could cause intensified electrolyte depletion, particularly hypokalemia).
No products indexed under this heading.

Dezocine (Concurrent administration could cause potentiation of orthostatic hypotension).
No products indexed under this heading.

Diazoxide (Co-administration could have additive effect or potentiation). Products include:
Hyperstat I.V. 3017

Diclofenac Potassium (In some patients the administration of a non-steroidal anti-inflammatory agent can reduce the diuretic, natriuretic and antihypertensive effects of loop, potassium-sparing and thiazide diuretics).
No products indexed under this heading.

Diclofenac Sodium (In some patients the administration of a non-steroidal anti-inflammatory agent can reduce the diuretic, natriuretic and antihypertensive effects of loop, potassium-sparing and thiazide diuretics). Products include:
Arthrotec Tablets 3129
Voltaren Ophthalmic Solution 2309
Voltaren Tablets 2307
Voltaren-XR Tablets 2310

Diltiazem Hydrochloride (Co-administration could have additive effect or potentiation). Products include:
Cardizem LA Extended Release Tablets 1728
Tiazac Capsules 1201

Dobutamine (Co-administration could cause possible decreased response to pressor amines but not sufficient to preclude their use).
No products indexed under this heading.

Dobutamine Hydrochloride (Co-administration could cause possible decreased response to pressor amines but not sufficient to preclude their use).
No products indexed under this heading.

Dopamine Hydrochloride (Co-administration could cause possible decreased response to pressor amines but not sufficient to preclude their use).
No products indexed under this heading.

Doxacurium Chloride (Co-administration could cause possible increased responsiveness to the muscle relaxant).
No products indexed under this heading.

Doxazosin Mesylate (Co-administration could have additive effect or potentiation). Products include:
Cardura XL Tablets 2515

Enalapril Maleate (Co-administration could have additive effect or potentiation). Products include:
Vasotec I.V. Injection 2103

Enalaprilat (Co-administration could have additive effect or potentiation).
No products indexed under this heading.

Ephedrine Sulfate (Co-administration could cause possible decreased response to pressor amines but not sufficient to preclude their use).
No products indexed under this heading.

Epinephrine Bitartrate (Co-administration could cause possible decreased response to pressor amines but not sufficient to preclude their use).
No products indexed under this heading.

Epinephrine Hydrochloride (Co-administration could cause possible decreased response to pressor amines but not sufficient to preclude their use).
No products indexed under this heading.

Eprosartan Mesylate (Co-administration could have additive effect or potentiation). Products include:
Teveten Tablets 1735
Teveten HCT Tablets 1737

Esmolol Hydrochloride (Co-administration could have additive effect or potentiation).
No products indexed under this heading.

Etodolac (In some patients the administration of a non-steroidal anti-inflammatory agent can reduce the diuretic, natriuretic and antihypertensive effects of loop, potassium-sparing and thiazide diuretics).
No products indexed under this heading.

Felodipine (Co-administration could have additive effect or potentiation).
No products indexed under this heading.

Fenoprofen Calcium (In some patients the administration of a non-steroidal anti-inflammatory agent can reduce the diuretic, natriuretic and antihypertensive effects of loop, potassium-sparing and thiazide diuretics). Products include:
Nalfon Capsules 2502

Fentanyl (Concurrent administration could cause potentiation of orthostatic hypotension). Products include:
Duragesic Transdermal System 2373
Ionsys Transdermal System 2379

Fentanyl Citrate (Concurrent administration could cause potentiation of orthostatic hypotension). Products include:
Actiq 979

Fludrocortisone Acetate (Co-administration could cause intensified electrolyte depletion, particularly hypokalemia).
No products indexed under this heading.

Flurbiprofen (In some patients the administration of a non-steroidal anti-inflammatory agent can reduce the diuretic, natriuretic and antihypertensive effects of loop, potassium-sparing and thiazide diuretics).
No products indexed under this heading.

Fosinopril Sodium (Co-administration could have additive effect or potentiation).
No products indexed under this heading.

Furosemide (Co-administration could have additive effect or potentiation). Products include:
Furosemide Tablets 2154

Glimepiride (Co-administration may require a dosage adjustment of the antidiabetic drug). Products include:
Avandaryl Tablets 1379
Duetact Tablets 3226

Glipizide (Co-administration may require a dosage adjustment of the antidiabetic drug).
No products indexed under this heading.

Glyburide (Co-administration may require a dosage adjustment of the antidiabetic drug).
No products indexed under this heading.

Guanabenz Acetate (Co-administration could have additive effect or potentiation).
No products indexed under this heading.

Guanethidine Monosulfate (Co-administration could have additive effect or potentiation).
No products indexed under this heading.

Hydralazine Hydrochloride (Co-administration could have additive effect or potentiation). Products include:
BiDil Tablets 2171

Hydrocodone Bitartrate (Concurrent administration could cause potentiation of orthostatic hypotension). Products include:
- Hycodan ... 1116
- Hycotuss Expectorant Syrup ... 1117
- Vicodin Tablets ... 535
- Vicodin ES Tablets ... 536
- Vicodin HP Tablets ... 538
- Vicoprofen Tablets ... 539
- Zydone Tablets ... 1139

Hydrocodone Polistirex (Concurrent administration could cause potentiation of orthostatic hypotension). Products include:
- Tussionex Pennkinetic Extended-Release Suspension ... 3327

Hydrocortisone (Co-administration could cause intensified electrolyte depletion, particularly hypokalemia). Products include:
- Colocort Rectal Suspension, USP (Retention) 100 mg/60 mL ... 2476
- Hydrocortone Tablets ... 1989
- Preparation H Hydrocortisone Cream ... ■ 646

Hydrocortisone Acetate (Co-administration could cause intensified electrolyte depletion, particularly hypokalemia). Products include:
- Analpram-HC ... 1159
- Pramosone ... 1161
- ProctoFoam-HC ... 3099

Hydrocortisone Sodium Phosphate (Co-administration could cause intensified electrolyte depletion, particularly hypokalemia).
- No products indexed under this heading.

Hydrocortisone Sodium Succinate (Co-administration could cause intensified electrolyte depletion, particularly hypokalemia).
- No products indexed under this heading.

Hydroflumethiazide (Co-administration could have additive effect or potentiation).
- No products indexed under this heading.

Hydromorphone Hydrochloride (Concurrent administration could cause potentiation of orthostatic hypotension). Products include:
- Dilaudid ... 440
- Dilaudid Non-Sterile Powder ... 440
- Dilaudid Oral Liquid ... 445
- Dilaudid Rectal Suppositories ... 440
- Dilaudid Tablets ... 440
- Dilaudid Tablets - 8 mg ... 445
- Dilaudid-HP ... 442

Ibuprofen (In some patients the administration of a non-steroidal anti-inflammatory agent can reduce the diuretic, natriuretic and antihypertensive effects of loop, potassium-sparing and thiazide diuretics). Products include:
- Advil Allergy Sinus Caplets ... ■ 770
- Advil ... ■ 674
- Children's Advil Oral Suspension ... ■ 603
- Children's Advil Chewable Tablets ... ■ 603
- Advil Cold & Sinus ... ■ 723
- Infants' Advil Concentrated Drops ... ■ 604
- Infants' Advil Concentrated Drops - White Grape (Dye-Free) ... ■ 604
- Junior Strength Advil Swallow Tablets ... ■ 605
- Advil Migraine Liquigels ... ■ 608
- Advil Multi-Symptom Cold Caplets ... ■ 770
- Advil PM Caplets ... ■ 615
- Motrin IB Tablets and Caplets ... 1866
- Children's Motrin Oral Suspension ... 1867
- Children's Motrin Non-Staining Dye-Free Oral Suspension ... 1867
- Children's Motrin Cold Oral Suspension ... 1867
- Infants' Motrin Concentrated Drops ... 1867
- Infants' Motrin Non-Staining Dye-Free Concentrated Drops ... 1867
- Junior Strength Motrin Caplets and Chewable Tablets ... 1867
- Vicoprofen Tablets ... 539

Indapamide (Co-administration could have additive effect or potentiation). Products include:
- Indapamide Tablets ... 2156

Indomethacin (In some patients the administration of a non-steroidal anti-inflammatory agent can reduce the diuretic, natriuretic and antihypertensive effects of loop, potassium-sparing and thiazide diuretics). Products include:
- Indocin ... 1995

Indomethacin Sodium Trihydrate (In some patients the administration of a non-steroidal anti-inflammatory agent can reduce the diuretic, natriuretic and antihypertensive effects of loop, potassium-sparing and thiazide diuretics). Products include:
- Indocin I.V. ... 2465

Insulin, Human, Zinc Suspension (Co-administration may require a dosage adjustment of the antidiabetic drug). Products include:
- Humulin L, 100 Units ... 1794
- Humulin U, 100 Units ... 1800

Insulin, Human NPH (Co-administration may require a dosage adjustment of the antidiabetic drug). Products include:
- Humulin N, 100 Units ... 1795
- Humulin N Pen ... 1797

Insulin, Human Regular (Co-administration may require a dosage adjustment of the antidiabetic drug). Products include:
- Humulin R, 100 Units ... 1798

Insulin, Human Regular and Human NPH Mixture (Co-administration may require a dosage adjustment of the antidiabetic drug). Products include:
- Humulin 50/50, 100 Units ... 1791
- Humulin 70/30 Pen ... 1793

Insulin, NPH (Co-administration may require a dosage adjustment of the antidiabetic drug).
- No products indexed under this heading.

Insulin, Regular (Co-administration may require a dosage adjustment of the antidiabetic drug).
- No products indexed under this heading.

Insulin, Zinc Crystals (Co-administration may require a dosage adjustment of the antidiabetic drug).
- No products indexed under this heading.

Insulin, Zinc Suspension (Co-administration may require a dosage adjustment of the antidiabetic drug).
- No products indexed under this heading.

Insulin Aspart, Human Regular (Co-administration may require a dosage adjustment of the antidiabetic drug). Products include:
- NovoLog Injection ... 2326

Insulin glargine (Co-administration may require a dosage adjustment of the antidiabetic drug). Products include:
- Lantus Injection ... 2909

Insulin Lispro, Human (Co-administration may require a dosage adjustment of the antidiabetic drug). Products include:
- Humalog-Pen ... 1781
- Humalog Mix 50/50-Pen ... 1783
- Humalog Mix 75/25-Pen ... 1785

Insulin Lispro Protamine, Human (Co-administration may require a dosage adjustment of the antidiabetic drug). Products include:
- Humalog Mix 50/50-Pen ... 1783
- Humalog Mix 75/25-Pen ... 1785

Irbesartan (Co-administration could have additive effect or potentiation). Products include:
- Avalide Tablets ... 888
- Avalide Tablets ... 2874
- Avapro Tablets ... 891
- Avapro Tablets ... 2871

Isoproterenol Hydrochloride (Co-administration could cause possible decreased response to pressor amines but not sufficient to preclude their use).
- No products indexed under this heading.

Isoproterenol Sulfate (Co-administration could cause possible decreased response to pressor amines but not sufficient to preclude their use).
- No products indexed under this heading.

Isradipine (Co-administration could have additive effect or potentiation). Products include:
- DynaCirc CR Tablets ... 2721

Ketoprofen (In some patients the administration of a non-steroidal anti-inflammatory agent can reduce the diuretic, natriuretic and antihypertensive effects of loop, potassium-sparing and thiazide diuretics).
- No products indexed under this heading.

Ketorolac Tromethamine (In some patients the administration of a non-steroidal anti-inflammatory agent can reduce the diuretic, natriuretic and antihypertensive effects of loop, potassium-sparing and thiazide diuretics). Products include:
- Acular Ophthalmic Solution ... 565
- Acular LS Ophthalmic Solution ... 566

Labetalol Hydrochloride (Co-administration could have additive effect or potentiation).
- No products indexed under this heading.

Levorphanol Tartrate (Concurrent administration could cause potentiation of orthostatic hypotension).
- No products indexed under this heading.

Lisinopril (Co-administration could have additive effect or potentiation). Products include:
- Prinivil Tablets ... 2052
- Prinzide Tablets ... 2056

Lithium (Lithium should not generally be given with diuretics; diuretic agents reduce the renal clearance of lithium and add a high risk of lithium toxicity).
- No products indexed under this heading.

Lithium Carbonate (Lithium should not generally be given with diuretics; diuretic agents reduce the renal clearance of lithium and add a high risk of lithium toxicity). Products include:
- Lithobid Tablets ... 1692

Lithium Citrate (Lithium should not generally be given with diuretics; diuretic agents reduce the renal clearance of lithium and add a high risk of lithium toxicity).
- No products indexed under this heading.

Losartan Potassium (Co-administration could have additive effect or potentiation). Products include:
- Cozaar Tablets ... 1935
- Hyzaar 50-12.5 Tablets ... 1990
- Hyzaar 100-12.5 Tablets ... 1990
- Hyzaar 100-25 Tablets ... 1990

Mecamylamine Hydrochloride (Co-administration could have additive effect or potentiation).
- No products indexed under this heading.

Meclofenamate Sodium (In some patients the administration of a non-steroidal anti-inflammatory agent can reduce the diuretic, natriuretic and antihypertensive effects of loop, potassium-sparing and thiazide diuretics).
- No products indexed under this heading.

Mefenamic Acid (In some patients the administration of a non-steroidal anti-inflammatory agent can reduce the diuretic, natriuretic and antihypertensive effects of loop, potassium-sparing and thiazide diuretics).
- No products indexed under this heading.

Meloxicam (In some patients the administration of a non-steroidal anti-inflammatory agent can reduce the diuretic, natriuretic and antihypertensive effects of loop, potassium-sparing and thiazide diuretics). Products include:
- Mobic Oral Suspension ... 863
- Mobic Tablets ... 863

Meperidine Hydrochloride (Concurrent administration could cause potentiation of orthostatic hypotension).
- No products indexed under this heading.

Mephentermine Sulfate (Co-administration could cause possible decreased response to pressor amines but not sufficient to preclude their use).
- No products indexed under this heading.

Mephobarbital (Concurrent administration could cause potentiation of orthostatic hypotension).
- No products indexed under this heading.

Metaraminol Bitartrate (Co-administration could cause possible decreased response to pressor amines but not sufficient to preclude their use).
- No products indexed under this heading.

Metformin Hydrochloride (Co-administration may require a dosage adjustment of the antidiabetic drug). Products include:
- ActoPlus Met Tablets ... 3214
- Avandamet Tablets ... 1373
- Fortamet Extended-Release Tablets ... 3115

Methadone Hydrochloride (Concurrent administration could cause potentiation of orthostatic hypotension).
- No products indexed under this heading.

Methoxamine Hydrochloride (Co-administration could cause possible decreased response to pressor amines but not sufficient to preclude their use).
- No products indexed under this heading.

Methyclothiazide (Co-administration could have additive effect or potentiation).
No products indexed under this heading.

Methyldopa (Co-administration could have additive effect or potentiation). Products include:
Aldoril Tablets 1910

Methyldopate Hydrochloride (Co-administration could have additive effect or potentiation).
No products indexed under this heading.

Methylprednisolone Acetate (Co-administration could cause intensified electrolyte depletion, particularly hypokalemia). Products include:
Depo-Medrol Injectable Suspension 2617
Depo-Medrol Single-Dose Vial 2619

Methylprednisolone Sodium Succinate (Co-administration could cause intensified electrolyte depletion, particularly hypokalemia).
No products indexed under this heading.

Metocurine Iodide (Co-administration could cause possible increased responsiveness to the muscle relaxant).
No products indexed under this heading.

Metolazone (Co-administration could have additive effect or potentiation).
No products indexed under this heading.

Metoprolol Succinate (Co-administration could have additive effect or potentiation). Products include:
Toprol-XL Tablets 668

Metoprolol Tartrate (Co-administration could have additive effect or potentiation). Products include:
Lopressor Injection 2238
Lopressor Tablets 2238
Lopressor HCT 50/25 Tablets 2241
Lopressor HCT 100/25 Tablets 2241
Lopressor HCT 100/50 Tablets 2241

Metyrosine (Co-administration could have additive effect or potentiation). Products include:
Demser Capsules 1953

Mibefradil Dihydrochloride (Co-administration could have additive effect or potentiation).
No products indexed under this heading.

Miglitol (Co-administration may require a dosage adjustment of the antidiabetic drug).
No products indexed under this heading.

Minoxidil (Co-administration could have additive effect or potentiation). Products include:
Men's Rogaine Extra Strength Hair Regrowth Treatment Topical Solution, Ocean Rush Scent and Original Unscented 633
Men's Rogaine Foam Hair Regrowth Treatment 633
Women's Rogaine Hair Regrowth Treatment Topical Solution, Spring Bloom Scent and Original Unscented 634

Mivacurium Chloride (Co-administration could cause possible increased responsiveness to the muscle relaxant). Products include:
Mivacron Injection 493

Moexipril Hydrochloride (Co-administration could have additive effect or potentiation). Products include:
Uniretic Tablets 3100
Univasc Tablets 3104

Morphine Sulfate (Concurrent administration could cause potentiation of orthostatic hypotension). Products include:
Avinza Capsules 1741
Kadian Capsules 577
MS Contin Tablets 2701

Nabumetone (In some patients the administration of a non-steroidal anti-inflammatory agent can reduce the diuretic, natriuretic and antihypertensive effects of loop, potassium-sparing and thiazide diuretics).
No products indexed under this heading.

Nadolol (Co-administration could have additive effect or potentiation). Products include:
Nadolol Tablets 2159

Naproxen (In some patients the administration of a non-steroidal anti-inflammatory agent can reduce the diuretic, natriuretic and antihypertensive effects of loop, potassium-sparing and thiazide diuretics). Products include:
EC-Naprosyn Delayed-Release Tablets 2761
Naprosyn Suspension 2761
Naprosyn Tablets 2761
Prevacid NapraPAC 3280

Naproxen Sodium (In some patients the administration of a non-steroidal anti-inflammatory agent can reduce the diuretic, natriuretic and antihypertensive effects of loop, potassium-sparing and thiazide diuretics). Products include:
Aleve Caplets 742
Aleve Gelcaps 743
Aleve Tablets 743
Aleve Cold & Sinus Caplets 744
Anaprox Tablets 2761
Anaprox DS Tablets 2761

Nicardipine Hydrochloride (Co-administration could have additive effect or potentiation). Products include:
Cardene I.V. 2497

Nifedipine (Co-administration could have additive effect or potentiation). Products include:
Adalat CC Tablets 2964

Nisoldipine (Co-administration could have additive effect or potentiation). Products include:
Sular Tablets 3122

Nitroglycerin (Co-administration could have additive effect or potentiation). Products include:
Nitro-Dur Transdermal Infusion System 3046
Nitrolingual Pumpspray 3120

Norepinephrine Bitartrate (Co-administration could cause possible decreased response to pressor amines but not sufficient to preclude their use).
No products indexed under this heading.

Oxaprozin (In some patients the administration of a non-steroidal anti-inflammatory agent can reduce the diuretic, natriuretic and antihypertensive effects of loop, potassium-sparing and thiazide diuretics).
No products indexed under this heading.

Oxycodone Hydrochloride (Concurrent administration could cause potentiation of orthostatic hypotension). Products include:
OxyContin Tablets 2703
OxyFast Oral Concentrate Solution 2708
OxyIR Capsules 2708
Percocet Tablets 1131
Percodan Tablets 1132

Pancuronium Bromide (Co-administration could cause possible increased responsiveness to the muscle relaxant).
No products indexed under this heading.

Penbutolol Sulfate (Co-administration could have additive effect or potentiation).
No products indexed under this heading.

Pentobarbital Sodium (Concurrent administration could cause potentiation of orthostatic hypotension). Products include:
Nembutal Sodium Solution, USP 2470

Perindopril Erbumine (Co-administration could have additive effect or potentiation). Products include:
Aceon Tablets (2 mg, 4 mg, 8 mg) 3194

Phenobarbital (Concurrent administration could cause potentiation of orthostatic hypotension). Products include:
Donnatal Extentabs 2493

Phenoxybenzamine Hydrochloride (Co-administration could have additive effect or potentiation). Products include:
Dibenzyline Capsules 3399

Phentolamine Mesylate (Co-administration could have additive effect or potentiation).
No products indexed under this heading.

Phenylbutazone (In some patients the administration of a non-steroidal anti-inflammatory agent can reduce the diuretic, natriuretic and antihypertensive effects of loop, potassium-sparing and thiazide diuretics).
No products indexed under this heading.

Phenylephrine Hydrochloride (Co-administration could cause possible decreased response to pressor amines but not sufficient to preclude their use). Products include:
Comtrex Maximum Strength Non-Drowsy Cold & Cough Caplets 725
Comtrex Maximum Strength Day/Night Severe Cold & Sinus Caplets - Day Formulation 725
Comtrex Maximum Strength Day/Night Severe Cold & Sinus Caplets - Night Formulation 725
Contac Cold and Flu Maximum Strength Caplets 728
Contac Cold and Flu Day and Night Caplets (Day Formulation Only) 727
Contac Cold and Flu Day and Night Caplets (Night Formulation Only) 727
Contac Cold and Flu Non-Drowsy Caplets 728
Contac-D Cold Non-Drowsy Tablets 729
Children's Dimetapp Cold & Allergy Elixir 730
Children's Dimetapp Cold & Allergy Chewable Tablets 730
Children's Dimetapp DM Cold & Cough Elixir 731
Toddler's Dimetapp Cold and Cough Drops 732
Excedrin Sinus Headache Caplets/Tablets 610
4-Way Fast Acting Nasal Spray 775
4-Way Menthol Nasal Spray 775
Preparation H Maximum Strength Cream 666
Preparation H Cooling Gel 666
Preparation H 666
Refenesen PE Caplets 721
Robitussin Cough & Allergy Syrup 736
Robitussin Cough & Cold Nighttime Liquid 736
Robitussin Cough, Cold & Flu Nighttime Liquid 738
Robitussin Head & Chest Congestion PE Syrup 739
Robitussin Pediatric Cough & Cold Nighttime Liquid 736
TheraFlu Cold & Cough Hot Liquid 740
TheraFlu Cold & Sore Throat Hot Liquid 741
TheraFlu Flu & Sore Throat Hot Liquid 742
TheraFlu Daytime Severe Cold Hot Liquid 742
TheraFlu Nighttime Severe Cold Hot Liquid 740
TheraFlu Warming Relief Daytime Severe Cold 743
TheraFlu Warming Relief Nighttime Severe Cold 743
Triaminic Chest & Nasal Congestion Liquid 746
Triaminic Cold & Allergy Liquid 746
Triaminic Daytime Cold & Cough Liquid 745
Triaminic Nighttime Cold & Cough Liquid 746
Triaminic Thin Strips Cold 748
Triaminic Thin Strips Cold & Cough 778
Triaminic Infant Thin Strips Decongestant 747
Triaminic Infant Thin Strips Decongestant Plus Cough 747
Children's Tylenol Plus Flu Oral Suspension 749
Tylenol Cold Head Congestion Daytime Caplets with Cool Burst and Gelcaps 750
Tylenol Cold Multi-Symptom Daytime Liquid 752
Tylenol Cold Multi-Symptom Severe Daytime Liquid 752
Concentrated Tylenol Infants' Drops Plus Cold & Cough 754
Tylenol Allergy Multi-Symptom Caplets with Cool Burst and Gelcaps 1872
Tylenol Allergy Multi-Symptom Nighttime Caplets with Cool Burst 1872
Children's Tylenol Plus Cold Suspension Liquid 1879
Children's Tylenol Plus Cold & Allergy Suspension Liquid 1878
Children's Tylenol Plus Flu Suspension Liquid 1881
Children's Tylenol Plus Multi-Symptom Cold Suspension Liquid 1879
Tylenol Cold Head Congestion Daytime Caplets with Cool Burst 1873
Tylenol Cold Head Congestion Nighttime Caplets with Cool Burst 1873
Tylenol Cold Head Congestion Severe Caplets with Cool Burst 1873
Tylenol Cold Multi-Symptom Daytime Caplets with Cool Burst and Gelcaps 1874
Tylenol Cold Multi-Symptom Daytime Liquid with Citrus Burst 1874
Tylenol Cold Multi-Symptom Nighttime Caplets with Cool Burst 1874
Tylenol Cold Multi-Symptom Nighttime Liquid with Cool Burst 1874
Tylenol Cold Multi-Symptom Severe Caplets with Cool Burst 1874
Tylenol Cold Multi-Symptom Severe Daytime Liquid with Citrus Burst 1874
Tylenol Sinus Congestion & Pain Daytime Caplets with Cool Burst and Gelcaps 1876

Pindolol (Co-administration could have additive effect or potentiation).
 No products indexed under this heading.

Pioglitazone Hydrochloride (Co-administration may require a dosage adjustment of the antidiabetic drug). Products include:

Pipecuronium Bromide (Co-administration could cause possible increased responsiveness to the muscle relaxant).
 No products indexed under this heading.

Piroxicam (In some patients the administration of a non-steroidal anti-inflammatory agent can reduce the diuretic, natriuretic and antihypertensive effects of loop, potassium-sparing and thiazide diuretics).
 No products indexed under this heading.

Polythiazide (Co-administration could have additive effect or potentiation).
 No products indexed under this heading.

Prazosin Hydrochloride (Co-administration could have additive effect or potentiation).
 No products indexed under this heading.

Prednisolone Acetate (Co-administration could cause intensified electrolyte depletion, particularly hypokalemia). Products include:

Prednisolone Sodium Phosphate (Co-administration could cause intensified electrolyte depletion, particularly hypokalemia).
 No products indexed under this heading.

Prednisolone Tebutate (Co-administration could cause intensified electrolyte depletion, particularly hypokalemia).
 No products indexed under this heading.

Prednisone (Co-administration could cause intensified electrolyte depletion, particularly hypokalemia).
 No products indexed under this heading.

Propoxyphene Hydrochloride (Concurrent administration could cause potentiation of orthostatic hypotension).
 No products indexed under this heading.

Propoxyphene Napsylate (Concurrent administration could cause potentiation of orthostatic hypotension).
 No products indexed under this heading.

Propranolol Hydrochloride (Co-administration could have additive effect or potentiation). Products include:

Quinapril Hydrochloride (Co-administration could have additive effect or potentiation).
 No products indexed under this heading.

Ramipril (Co-administration could have additive effect or potentiation). Products include:

Rapacuronium Bromide (Co-administration could cause possible increased responsiveness to the muscle relaxant).
 No products indexed under this heading.

Rauwolfia Serpentina (Co-administration could have additive effect or potentiation).
 No products indexed under this heading.

Remifentanil Hydrochloride (Concurrent administration could cause potentiation of orthostatic hypotension).
 No products indexed under this heading.

Repaglinide (Co-administration may require a dosage adjustment of the antidiabetic drug).
 No products indexed under this heading.

Rescinnamine (Co-administration could have additive effect or potentiation).
 No products indexed under this heading.

Reserpine (Co-administration could have additive effect or potentiation).
 No products indexed under this heading.

Rocuronium Bromide (Co-administration could cause possible increased responsiveness to the muscle relaxant). Products include:

Rofecoxib (In some patients the administration of a non-steroidal anti-inflammatory agent can reduce the diuretic, natriuretic and antihypertensive effects of loop, potassium-sparing and thiazide diuretics).
 No products indexed under this heading.

Rosiglitazone Maleate (Co-administration may require a dosage adjustment of the antidiabetic drug). Products include:

Secobarbital Sodium (Concurrent administration could cause potentiation of orthostatic hypotension).
 No products indexed under this heading.

Sodium Nitroprusside (Co-administration could have additive effect or potentiation).
 No products indexed under this heading.

Sotalol Hydrochloride (Co-administration could have additive effect or potentiation).
 No products indexed under this heading.

Spirapril Hydrochloride (Co-administration could have additive effect or potentiation).
 No products indexed under this heading.

Sufentanil Citrate (Concurrent administration could cause potentiation of orthostatic hypotension).
 No products indexed under this heading.

Sulindac (In some patients the administration of a non-steroidal anti-inflammatory agent can reduce the diuretic, natriuretic and antihypertensive effects of loop, potassium-sparing and thiazide diuretics). Products include:

Telmisartan (Co-administration could have additive effect or potentiation). Products include:

Terazosin Hydrochloride (Co-administration could have additive effect or potentiation). Products include:

Thiamylal Sodium (Concurrent administration could cause potentiation of orthostatic hypotension).
 No products indexed under this heading.

Timolol Maleate (Co-administration could have additive effect or potentiation). Products include:

Tolazamide (Co-administration may require a dosage adjustment of the antidiabetic drug).
 No products indexed under this heading.

Tolbutamide (Co-administration may require a dosage adjustment of the antidiabetic drug).
 No products indexed under this heading.

Tolmetin Sodium (In some patients the administration of a non-steroidal anti-inflammatory agent can reduce the diuretic, natriuretic and antihypertensive effects of loop, potassium-sparing and thiazide diuretics).
 No products indexed under this heading.

Torsemide (Co-administration could have additive effect or potentiation). Products include:

Trandolapril (Co-administration could have additive effect or potentiation). Products include:

Triamcinolone (Co-administration could cause intensified electrolyte depletion, particularly hypokalemia).
 No products indexed under this heading.

Triamcinolone Acetonide (Co-administration could cause intensified electrolyte depletion, particularly hypokalemia). Products include:

Triamcinolone Diacetate (Co-administration could cause intensified electrolyte depletion, particularly hypokalemia).
 No products indexed under this heading.

Triamcinolone Hexacetonide (Co-administration could cause intensified electrolyte depletion, particularly hypokalemia).
 No products indexed under this heading.

Trimethaphan Camsylate (Co-administration could have additive effect or potentiation).
 No products indexed under this heading.

Troglitazone (Co-administration may require a dosage adjustment of the antidiabetic drug).
 No products indexed under this heading.

Tubocurarine Chloride (Co-administration could cause possible increased responsiveness to the muscle relaxant).
 No products indexed under this heading.

Valdecoxib (In some patients the administration of a non-steroidal anti-inflammatory agent can reduce the diuretic, natriuretic and antihypertensive effects of loop, potassium-sparing and thiazide diuretics).
 No products indexed under this heading.

Valsartan (Co-administration could have additive effect or potentiation). Products include:

Vecuronium Bromide (Co-administration could cause possible increased responsiveness to the muscle relaxant).
 No products indexed under this heading.

Verapamil Hydrochloride (Co-administration could have additive effect or potentiation). Products include:

Food Interactions

Alcohol (Concurrent administration could cause potentiation of orthostatic hypotension).

BENTYL CAPSULES
(Dicyclomine Hydrochloride) 697
See Bentyl Tablets

BENTYL INJECTION
(Dicyclomine Hydrochloride) 697
See Bentyl Tablets

BENTYL SYRUP
(Dicyclomine Hydrochloride) 697
See Bentyl Tablets

(▣ Described in PDR For Nonprescription Drugs) (⊙ Described in PDR For Ophthalmic Medicines™)

BENTYL TABLETS

(Dicyclomine Hydrochloride) ... 697

May interact with agents used to treat achlorhydria and/or to test gastric secretion, antacids, antiglaucoma agents, antihistamines, benzodiazepines, corticosteroids, monoamine oxidase inhibitors, narcotic analgesics, antipsychotic agents, nitrates and nitrites, sympathomimetics, tricyclic antidepressants, type 1 antiarrhythmic drugs, and certain other agents. Compounds in these categories include:

Acetazolamide (Anticholinergics antagonize the effects of antiglaucoma agents).
No products indexed under this heading.

Acetylcholine Chloride (Anticholinergics antagonize the effects of antiglaucoma agents).
No products indexed under this heading.

Acrivastine (Antihistamines may increase certain actions or side effects of anticholinergic agents).
No products indexed under this heading.

Albuterol (Sympathomimetic agents may increase certain actions or side effects of anticholinergic agents). Products include:
- Proventil Inhalation Aerosol ... 3053

Albuterol Sulfate (Sympathomimetic agents may increase certain actions or side effects of anticholinergic agents). Products include:
- AccuNeb Inhalation Solution ... 1055
- Combivent Inhalation Aerosol ... 847
- DuoNeb Inhalation Solution ... 1058
- ProAir HFA Inhalation Aerosol ... 3300
- Proventil Inhalation Solution 0.083% ... 3055
- Proventil HFA Inhalation Aerosol ... 3056
- Ventolin HFA Inhalation Aerosol ... 1600
- VoSpire ER Tablets ... 1052

Alfentanil Hydrochloride (Narcotic analgesics may increase certain actions or side effects of anticholinergic agents).
No products indexed under this heading.

Alprazolam (Benzodiazepines may increase certain actions or side effects of anticholinergic agents). Products include:
- Niravam Orally Disintegrating Tablets ... 3092

Aluminum Carbonate (Antacids may interfere with the absorption of anticholinergic agents; therefore, simultaneous use of these drugs should be avoided).
No products indexed under this heading.

Aluminum Hydroxide (Antacids may interfere with the absorption of anticholinergic agents; therefore, simultaneous use of these drugs should be avoided). Products include:
- Gaviscon Regular Strength Liquid ... 658
- Gaviscon Regular Strength Tablets ... 658
- Gaviscon Extra Strength Liquid ... 658
- Gaviscon Extra Strength Tablets ... 658
- Maalox Regular Strength Antacid/Antigas Liquid ... 2175
- Maalox Max Maximum Strength Antacid/Anti-Gas Liquid ... 2176

Amantadine Hydrochloride (Amantadine may increase certain actions or side effects of anticholinergic agents). Products include:
- Symmetrel Tablets ... 1135

Amitriptyline Hydrochloride (Tricyclic antidepressants may increase certain actions or side effects of anticholinergic agents).
No products indexed under this heading.

Amoxapine (Tricyclic antidepressants may increase certain actions or side effects of anticholinergic agents).
No products indexed under this heading.

Amyl Nitrite (Nitrates and nitrites may increase certain actions or side effects of anticholinergic agents).
No products indexed under this heading.

Aripiprazole (Antipsychotic agents may increase certain actions or side effects of anticholinergic agents). Products include:
- Abilify Oral Solution ... 882
- Abilify Oral Solution ... 2450
- Abilify Discmelt Orally Disintegrating Tablets ... 882
- Abilify Discmelt Orally Disintegrating Tablets ... 2450
- Abilify Tablets ... 882
- Abilify Tablets ... 2450

Astemizole (Antihistamines may increase certain actions or side effects of anticholinergic agents).
No products indexed under this heading.

Azatadine Maleate (Antihistamines may increase certain actions or side effects of anticholinergic agents).
No products indexed under this heading.

Betamethasone Acetate (Anticholinergic drugs in the presence of increased intraocular pressure may be hazardous when taken concurrently with agents such as corticosteroids).
No products indexed under this heading.

Betamethasone Sodium Phosphate (Anticholinergic drugs in the presence of increased intraocular pressure may be hazardous when taken concurrently with agents such as corticosteroids).
No products indexed under this heading.

Betaxolol Hydrochloride (Anticholinergics antagonize the effects of antiglaucoma agents). Products include:
- Betoptic S Ophthalmic Suspension ... 558

Bromodiphenhydramine Hydrochloride (Antihistamines may increase certain actions or side effects of anticholinergic agents).
No products indexed under this heading.

Brompheniramine Maleate (Antihistamines may increase certain actions or side effects of anticholinergic agents). Products include:
- Children's Dimetapp Cold & Allergy Elixir ... 730
- Children's Dimetapp Cold & Allergy Chewable Tablets ... 730
- Children's Dimetapp DM Cold & Cough Elixir ... 731

Buprenorphine Hydrochloride (Narcotic analgesics may increase certain actions or side effects of anticholinergic agents). Products include:
- Buprenex Injectable ... 2716
- Suboxone Tablets ... 2717
- Subutex Tablets ... 2717

Carbachol (Anticholinergics antagonize the effects of antiglaucoma agents).
No products indexed under this heading.

Cetirizine Hydrochloride (Antihistamines may increase certain actions or side effects of anticholinergic agents). Products include:
- Zyrtec Chewable Tablets ... 2594
- Zyrtec ... 2594
- Zyrtec-D 12 Hour Extended Release Tablets ... 2597

Chlordiazepoxide (Benzodiazepines may increase certain actions or side effects of anticholinergic agents).
No products indexed under this heading.

Chlordiazepoxide Hydrochloride (Benzodiazepines may increase certain actions or side effects of anticholinergic agents). Products include:
- Librium Capsules ... 3347

Chlorpheniramine Maleate (Antihistamines may increase certain actions or side effects of anticholinergic agents). Products include:
- Advil Allergy Sinus Caplets ... 770
- Advil Multi-Symptom Cold Caplets ... 770
- BC Allergy Sinus Cold Powder ... 677
- Comtrex Maximum Strength Cold & Cough Day/Night Caplets - Night Formulation ... 726
- Comtrex Maximum Strength Day/Night Severe Cold & Sinus Caplets - Night Formulation ... 725
- Contac Cold and Flu Maximum Strength Caplets ... 728
- Contac Cold and Flu Day and Night Caplets (Night Formulation Only) ... 727
- Children's Dimetapp Long Acting Cough Plus Cold Syrup ... 731
- Robitussin Cough & Cold Long-Acting Liquid ... 735
- Robitussin Cough & Allergy Syrup ... 736
- Robitussin Cough & Cold Nighttime Liquid ... 736
- Robitussin Cough, Cold & Flu Nighttime Liquid ... 738
- Robitussin Pediatric Cough & Cold Long-Acting Liquid ... 735
- Robitussin Pediatric Cough & Cold Nighttime Liquid ... 736
- Triaminic Cold & Allergy Liquid ... 746
- Triaminic Cough & Runny Nose Softchews ... 748
- Children's Tylenol Plus Flu Oral Suspension ... 749
- Tylenol Allergy Multi-Symptom Caplets with Cool Burst and Gelcaps ... 1872
- Children's Tylenol Plus Cold Suspension Liquid ... 1879
- Children's Tylenol Plus Cough & Runny Nose Suspension Liquid ... 1879
- Children's Tylenol Plus Flu Suspension Liquid ... 1881
- Children's Tylenol Plus Multi-Symptom Cold Suspension Liquid ... 1879
- Tylenol Cold Head Congestion Nighttime Caplets with Cool Burst ... 1873
- Tylenol Cold Multi-Symptom Nighttime Caplets with Cool Burst ... 1874
- Tylenol Sinus Congestion & Pain Nighttime Caplets with Cool Burst ... 1876
- Vicks 44M Cough, Cold & Flu Relief Liquid ... 2680
- Pediatric Vicks 44m Cough & Cold Relief Liquid ... 2676
- Children's Vicks NyQuil Cold/Cough Relief ... 756
- Children's Vicks NyQuil Cold/Cough Relief Liquid ... 2680
- Zicam Maximum Strength Flu Daytime ... 768

Chlorpheniramine Polistirex (Antihistamines may increase certain actions or side effects of anticholinergic agents). Products include:
- Tussionex Pennkinetic Extended-Release Suspension ... 3327

Chlorpheniramine Tannate (Antihistamines may increase certain actions or side effects of anticholinergic agents).
No products indexed under this heading.

Chlorpromazine (Antipsychotic agents may increase certain actions or side effects of anticholinergic agents).
No products indexed under this heading.

Chlorpromazine Hydrochloride (Antipsychotic agents may increase certain actions or side effects of anticholinergic agents).
No products indexed under this heading.

Chlorprothixene (Antipsychotic agents may increase certain actions or side effects of anticholinergic agents).
No products indexed under this heading.

Chlorprothixene Hydrochloride (Antipsychotic agents may increase certain actions or side effects of anticholinergic agents).
No products indexed under this heading.

Cisapride (Anticholinergic drugs may antagonize the effects of drugs that alter gastrointestinal motility).
No products indexed under this heading.

Clemastine Fumarate (Antihistamines may increase certain actions or side effects of anticholinergic agents).
No products indexed under this heading.

Clomipramine Hydrochloride (Tricyclic antidepressants may increase certain actions or side effects of anticholinergic agents).
No products indexed under this heading.

Clorazepate Dipotassium (Benzodiazepines may increase certain actions or side effects of anticholinergic agents). Products include:
- Tranxene ... 2474

Clozapine (Antipsychotic agents may increase certain actions or side effects of anticholinergic agents). Products include:
- Clozaril Tablets ... 2184
- FazaClo Orally Disintegrating Tablets ... 551

Codeine Phosphate (Narcotic analgesics may increase certain actions or side effects of anticholinergic agents). Products include:
- Tylenol with Codeine Tablets ... 2391

Cortisone Acetate (Anticholinergic drugs in the presence of increased intraocular pressure may be hazardous when taken concurrently with agents such as corticosteroids).
No products indexed under this heading.

Cyproheptadine Hydrochloride (Antihistamines may increase certain actions or side effects of anticholinergic agents).
No products indexed under this heading.

Demecarium Bromide (Anticholinergics antagonize the effects of antiglaucoma agents).
No products indexed under this heading.

Desipramine Hydrochloride (Tricyclic antidepressants may increase certain actions or side effects of anticholinergic agents).
No products indexed under this heading.

Dexamethasone (Anticholinergic drugs in the presence of increased intraocular pressure may be hazardous when taken concurrently with agents such as corticosteroids). Products include:
- Ciprodex Otic Suspension 559
- Decadron Tablets 1951
- TobraDex Ophthalmic Ointment 562
- TobraDex Ophthalmic Suspension ... 563

Dexamethasone Acetate (Anticholinergic drugs in the presence of increased intraocular pressure may be hazardous when taken concurrently with agents such as corticosteroids).
No products indexed under this heading.

Dexamethasone Sodium Phosphate (Anticholinergic drugs in the presence of increased intraocular pressure may be hazardous when taken concurrently with agents such as corticosteroids).
No products indexed under this heading.

Dexchlorpheniramine Maleate (Antihistamines may increase certain actions or side effects of anticholinergic agents).
No products indexed under this heading.

Dexpanthenol (Anticholinergic drugs may antagonize the effects of drugs that alter gastrointestinal motility).
No products indexed under this heading.

Dezocine (Narcotic analgesics may increase certain actions or side effects of anticholinergic agents).
No products indexed under this heading.

Diazepam (Benzodiazepines may increase certain actions or side effects of anticholinergic agents). Products include:
- Diastat Rectal Delivery System 3343
- Valium Tablets 2819

Dichlorphenamide (Anticholinergics antagonize the effects of antiglaucoma agents). Products include:
- Daranide Tablets 1950

Digoxin (Anticholinergic agents may affect gastrointestinal absorption of various drugs, such as slowly dissolving dosage forms of digoxin; increased serum digoxin concentrations may result). Products include:
- Lanoxicaps Capsules 1490
- Lanoxin Injection 1494
- Lanoxin Injection Pediatric 1497
- Lanoxin Tablets 1500

Diphenhydramine Citrate (Antihistamines may increase certain actions or side effects of anticholinergic agents). Products include:
- Advil PM Caplets .... ▣ 615
- Excedrin PM Caplets/Tablets/Geltabs .... ▣ 610
- Goody's PM Powder for Pain with Sleeplessness .... ▣ 612

Diphenhydramine Hydrochloride (Antihistamines may increase certain actions or side effects of anticholinergic agents). Products include:
- Nytol QuickCaps Caplets .... ▣ 615
- Nytol QuickGels Softgels Maximum Strength............... ▣ 616
- Simply Sleep Caplets 1868
- Sominex Original Formula Tablets .. ▣ 616
- TheraFlu Warming Relief Nighttime Severe Cold............... ▣ 743
- TheraFlu Thin Strips Multi Symptom............... ▣ 744
- Triaminic Nighttime Cold & Cough Liquid............... ▣ 746
- Triaminic Thin Strips Cough & Runny Nose............... ▣ 749
- Extra Strength Tylenol PM Caplets, Vanilla Caplets, Geltabs, Gelcaps and Liquid.......... 1875
- Tylenol Sore Throat Nighttime Liquid with Cool Burst............... ▣ 790
- Tylenol Allergy Multi-Symptom Nighttime Caplets with Cool Burst............... 1872
- Tylenol Severe Allergy Caplets 1872
- Children's Tylenol Plus Cold & Allergy Suspension Liquid............ 1878

Diphenylpyraline Hydrochloride (Antihistamines may increase certain actions or side effects of anticholinergic agents).
No products indexed under this heading.

Dipivefrin Hydrochloride (Anticholinergics antagonize the effects of antiglaucoma agents). Products include:
- Propine Ophthalmic Solution .... ⊙ 239

Disopyramide Phosphate (Class I antiarrhythmic agents may increase certain actions or side effects of anticholinergic agents).
No products indexed under this heading.

Dobutamine Hydrochloride (Sympathomimetic agents may increase certain actions or side effects of anticholinergic agents).
No products indexed under this heading.

Dopamine Hydrochloride (Sympathomimetic agents may increase certain actions or side effects of anticholinergic agents).
No products indexed under this heading.

Doxepin Hydrochloride (Tricyclic antidepressants may increase certain actions or side effects of anticholinergic agents).
No products indexed under this heading.

Echothiophate Iodide (Anticholinergics antagonize the effects of antiglaucoma agents).
No products indexed under this heading.

Ephedrine Hydrochloride (Sympathomimetic agents may increase certain actions or side effects of anticholinergic agents).
No products indexed under this heading.

Ephedrine Sulfate (Sympathomimetic agents may increase certain actions or side effects of anticholinergic agents).
No products indexed under this heading.

Ephedrine Tannate (Sympathomimetic agents may increase certain actions or side effects of anticholinergic agents).
No products indexed under this heading.

Epinephrine (Sympathomimetic agents may increase certain actions or side effects of anticholinergic agents). Products include:
- EpiPen 1061
- Primatene Mist .... ▣ 719
- Twinject 0.15 3379
- Twinject 0.3 3378

Epinephrine Bitartrate (Sympathomimetic agents may increase certain actions or side effects of anticholinergic agents).
No products indexed under this heading.

Epinephrine Hydrochloride (Sympathomimetic agents may increase certain actions or side effects of anticholinergic agents).
No products indexed under this heading.

Epinephryl Borate (Anticholinergics antagonize the effects of antiglaucoma agents).
No products indexed under this heading.

Erythrityl Tetranitrate (Nitrates and nitrites may increase certain actions or side effects of anticholinergic agents).
No products indexed under this heading.

Estazolam (Benzodiazepines may increase certain actions or side effects of anticholinergic agents). Products include:
- ProSom Tablets 517

Fentanyl (Narcotic analgesics may increase certain actions or side effects of anticholinergic agents). Products include:
- Duragesic Transdermal System 2373
- Ionsys Transdermal System 2379

Fentanyl Citrate (Narcotic analgesics may increase certain actions or side effects of anticholinergic agents). Products include:
- Actiq 979

Fexofenadine Hydrochloride (Antihistamines may increase certain actions or side effects of anticholinergic agents). Products include:
- Allegra 2844
- Allegra-D 12 Hour Extended-Release Tablets............ 2846
- Allegra-D 24 Hour Extended-Release Tablets............ 2849

Fludrocortisone Acetate (Anticholinergic drugs in the presence of increased intraocular pressure may be hazardous when taken concurrently with agents such as corticosteroids).
No products indexed under this heading.

Fluphenazine Decanoate (Antipsychotic agents may increase certain actions or side effects of anticholinergic agents).
No products indexed under this heading.

Fluphenazine Enanthate (Antipsychotic agents may increase certain actions or side effects of anticholinergic agents).
No products indexed under this heading.

Fluphenazine Hydrochloride (Antipsychotic agents may increase certain actions or side effects of anticholinergic agents).
No products indexed under this heading.

Flurazepam Hydrochloride (Benzodiazepines may increase certain actions or side effects of anticholinergic agents). Products include:
- Dalmane Capsules 3342

Glutamic Acid Hydrochloride (The inhibiting effects of anticholinergic drugs on gastric hydrochloric acid secretion are antagonized by agents used to treat achlorhydria and those used to test gastric secretion).
No products indexed under this heading.

Halazepam (Benzodiazepines may increase certain actions or side effects of anticholinergic agents).
No products indexed under this heading.

Haloperidol (Antipsychotic agents may increase certain actions or side effects of anticholinergic agents).
No products indexed under this heading.

Haloperidol Decanoate (Antipsychotic agents may increase certain actions or side effects of anticholinergic agents).
No products indexed under this heading.

Hydrocodone Bitartrate (Narcotic analgesics may increase certain actions or side effects of anticholinergic agents). Products include:
- Hycodan 1116
- Hycotuss Expectorant Syrup 1117
- Vicodin Tablets 535
- Vicodin ES Tablets 536
- Vicodin HP Tablets 538
- Vicoprofen Tablets 539
- Zydone Tablets 1139

Hydrocodone Polistirex (Narcotic analgesics may increase certain actions or side effects of anticholinergic agents). Products include:
- Tussionex Pennkinetic Extended-Release Suspension...... 3327

Hydrocortisone (Anticholinergic drugs in the presence of increased intraocular pressure may be hazardous when taken concurrently with agents such as corticosteroids). Products include:
- Colocort Rectal Suspension, USP (Retention) 100 mg/60 mL........... 2476
- Hydrocortone Tablets 1989
- Preparation H Hydrocortisone Cream............... ▣ 646

Hydrocortisone Acetate (Anticholinergic drugs in the presence of increased intraocular pressure may be hazardous when taken concurrently with agents such as corticosteroids). Products include:
- Analpram-HC 1159
- Pramosone 1161
- ProctoFoam-HC 3099

Hydrocortisone Sodium Phosphate (Anticholinergic drugs in the presence of increased intraocular pressure may be hazardous when taken concurrently with agents such as corticosteroids).
No products indexed under this heading.

Hydrocortisone Sodium Succinate (Anticholinergic drugs in the presence of increased intraocular pressure may be hazardous when taken concurrently with agents such as corticosteroids).
No products indexed under this heading.

Hydromorphone Hydrochloride (Narcotic analgesics may increase certain actions or side effects of anticholinergic agents). Products include:
- Dilaudid............... 440
- Dilaudid Non-Sterile Powder 440
- Dilaudid Oral Liquid 445
- Dilaudid Rectal Suppositories 440
- Dilaudid Tablets 440

Dilaudid Tablets - 8 mg 445
Dilaudid-HP 442

Imipramine Hydrochloride (Tricyclic antidepressants may increase certain actions or side effects of anticholinergic agents).
No products indexed under this heading.

Imipramine Pamoate (Tricyclic antidepressants may increase certain actions or side effects of anticholinergic agents).
No products indexed under this heading.

Isocarboxazid (MAO inhibitors may increase certain actions or side effects of anticholinergic agents).
No products indexed under this heading.

Isoflurophate (Anticholinergics antagonize the effects of antiglaucoma agents).
No products indexed under this heading.

Isoproterenol Hydrochloride (Sympathomimetic agents may increase certain actions or side effects of anticholinergic agents).
No products indexed under this heading.

Isoproterenol Sulfate (Sympathomimetic agents may increase certain actions or side effects of anticholinergic agents).
No products indexed under this heading.

Isosorbide Dinitrate (Nitrates and nitrites may increase certain actions or side effects of anticholinergic agents). Products include:
BiDil Tablets 2171

Isosorbide Mononitrate (Nitrates and nitrites may increase certain actions or side effects of anticholinergic agents). Products include:
Imdur Tablets 3018

Levalbuterol Hydrochloride (Sympathomimetic agents may increase certain actions or side effects of anticholinergic agents). Products include:
Xopenex Inhalation Solution 3146
Xopenex Inhalation Solution Concentrate 3150

Levobunolol Hydrochloride (Anticholinergics antagonize the effects of antiglaucoma agents). Products include:
Betagan Ophthalmic Solution, USP .... ⊙220

Levorphanol Tartrate (Narcotic analgesics may increase certain actions or side effects of anticholinergic agents).
No products indexed under this heading.

Lithium Carbonate (Antipsychotic agents may increase certain actions or side effects of anticholinergic agents). Products include:
Lithobid Tablets 1692

Lithium Citrate (Antipsychotic agents may increase certain actions or side effects of anticholinergic agents).
No products indexed under this heading.

Loratadine (Antihistamines may increase certain actions or side effects of anticholinergic agents). Products include:
Alavert Allergy & Sinus D-12 Hour Tablets.. 771
Alavert 771
Children's Claritin Allergy Oral Solution 771
Claritin Non-Drowsy 24 Hour Tablets.. 772
Claritin Reditabs 24 Hour Non-Drowsy Tablets.......................... 772
Claritin-D Non-Drowsy 12 Hour Tablets.. 772
Claritin-D Non-Drowsy 24 Hour Tablets.. 772

Lorazepam (Benzodiazepines may increase certain actions or side effects of anticholinergic agents).
No products indexed under this heading.

Loxapine Hydrochloride (Antipsychotic agents may increase certain actions or side effects of anticholinergic agents).
No products indexed under this heading.

Loxapine Succinate (Antipsychotic agents may increase certain actions or side effects of anticholinergic agents).
No products indexed under this heading.

Magaldrate (Antacids may interfere with the absorption of anticholinergic agents; therefore, simultaneous use of these drugs should be avoided).
No products indexed under this heading.

Magnesium Hydroxide (Antacids may interfere with the absorption of anticholinergic agents; therefore, simultaneous use of these drugs should be avoided). Products include:
Maalox Regular Strength Antacid/Antigas Liquid................... 2175
Maalox Max Maximum Strength Antacid/Anti-Gas Liquid................. 2176
Pepcid Complete Chewable Tablets 1701

Magnesium Oxide (Antacids may interfere with the absorption of anticholinergic agents; therefore, simultaneous use of these drugs should be avoided). Products include:
Beelith Tablets 759
PremCal Light, Regular, and Extra Strength Tablets................. 818

Maprotiline Hydrochloride (Tricyclic antidepressants may increase certain actions or side effects of anticholinergic agents).
No products indexed under this heading.

Meperidine Hydrochloride (Narcotic analgesics may increase certain actions or side effects of anticholinergic agents).
No products indexed under this heading.

Mesoridazine Besylate (Antipsychotic agents may increase certain actions or side effects of anticholinergic agents).
No products indexed under this heading.

Metaproterenol Sulfate (Sympathomimetic agents may increase certain actions or side effects of anticholinergic agents). Products include:
Alupent Inhalation Aerosol 826

Metaraminol Bitartrate (Sympathomimetic agents may increase certain actions or side effects of anticholinergic agents).
No products indexed under this heading.

Methadone Hydrochloride (Narcotic analgesics may increase certain actions or side effects of anticholinergic agents).
No products indexed under this heading.

Methazolamide (Anticholinergics antagonize the effects of antiglaucoma agents).
No products indexed under this heading.

Methdilazine Hydrochloride (Antihistamines may increase certain actions or side effects of anticholinergic agents).
No products indexed under this heading.

Methotrimeprazine (Antipsychotic agents may increase certain actions or side effects of anticholinergic agents).
No products indexed under this heading.

Methoxamine Hydrochloride (Sympathomimetic agents may increase certain actions or side effects of anticholinergic agents).
No products indexed under this heading.

Methylprednisolone Acetate (Anticholinergic drugs in the presence of increased intraocular pressure may be hazardous when taken concurrently with agents such as corticosteroids). Products include:
Depo-Medrol Injectable Suspension 2617
Depo-Medrol Single-Dose Vial 2619

Methylprednisolone Sodium Succinate (Anticholinergic drugs in the presence of increased intraocular pressure may be hazardous when taken concurrently with agents such as corticosteroids).
No products indexed under this heading.

Metoclopramide Hydrochloride (Anticholinergic drugs may antagonize the effects of drugs that alter gastrointestinal motility).
No products indexed under this heading.

Midazolam Hydrochloride (Benzodiazepines may increase certain actions or side effects of anticholinergic agents).
No products indexed under this heading.

Moclobemide (MAO inhibitors may increase certain actions or side effects of anticholinergic agents).
No products indexed under this heading.

Molindone Hydrochloride (Antipsychotic agents may increase certain actions or side effects of anticholinergic agents). Products include:
Moban Tablets 1119

Moricizine Hydrochloride (Class I antiarrhythmic agents may increase certain actions or side effects of anticholinergic agents).
No products indexed under this heading.

Morphine Sulfate (Narcotic analgesics may increase certain actions or side effects of anticholinergic agents). Products include:
Avinza Capsules 1741
Kadian Capsules 577
MS Contin Tablets 2701

Nitroglycerin (Nitrates and nitrites may increase certain actions or side effects of anticholinergic agents). Products include:
Nitro-Dur Transdermal Infusion System.. 3046
Nitrolingual Pumpspray 3120

Norepinephrine Bitartrate (Sympathomimetic agents may increase certain actions or side effects of anticholinergic agents).
No products indexed under this heading.

Nortriptyline Hydrochloride (Tricyclic antidepressants may increase certain actions or side effects of anticholinergic agents).
No products indexed under this heading.

Olanzapine (Antipsychotic agents may increase certain actions or side effects of anticholinergic agents). Products include:
Symbyax Capsules 1819
Zyprexa Tablets 1830
Zyprexa IntraMuscular 1830
Zyprexa ZYDIS Orally Disintegrating Tablets.................. 1830

Oxazepam (Benzodiazepines may increase certain actions or side effects of anticholinergic agents).
No products indexed under this heading.

Oxycodone Hydrochloride (Narcotic analgesics may increase certain actions or side effects of anticholinergic agents). Products include:
OxyContin Tablets 2703
OxyFast Oral Concentrate Solution.. 2708
OxyIR Capsules 2708
Percocet Tablets 1131
Percodan Tablets 1132

Pargyline Hydrochloride (MAO inhibitors may increase certain actions or side effects of anticholinergic agents).
No products indexed under this heading.

Pentaerythritol Tetranitrate (Nitrates and nitrites may increase certain actions or side effects of anticholinergic agents).
No products indexed under this heading.

Pentagastrin (The inhibiting effects of anticholinergic drugs on gastric hydrochloric acid secretion are antagonized by agents used to treat achlorhydria and those used to test gastric secretion).
No products indexed under this heading.

Perphenazine (Antipsychotic agents may increase certain actions or side effects of anticholinergic agents).
No products indexed under this heading.

Phenelzine Sulfate (MAO inhibitors may increase certain actions or side effects of anticholinergic agents).
No products indexed under this heading.

Phenylephrine Bitartrate (Sympathomimetic agents may increase certain actions or side effects of anticholinergic agents).
No products indexed under this heading.

Phenylephrine Hydrochloride (Sympathomimetic agents may increase certain actions or side effects of anticholinergic agents). Products include:
Comtrex Maximum Strength Non-Drowsy Cold & Cough Caplets.. 725
Comtrex Maximum Strength Day/Night Severe Cold & Sinus Caplets - Day Formulation 725
Comtrex Maximum Strength Day/Night Severe Cold & Sinus Caplets - Night Formulation 725

IMPORTANT NOTE: Always consult each drug listing in the patient's regimen for possible interactions.

Phenylephrine Tannate (Sympathomimetic agents may increase certain actions or side effects of anticholinergic agents).
No products indexed under this heading.

Phenylpropanolamine Hydrochloride (Sympathomimetic agents may increase certain actions or side effects of anticholinergic agents).
No products indexed under this heading.

Pilocarpine (Anticholinergics antagonize the effects of antiglaucoma agents).
No products indexed under this heading.

Pilocarpine Hydrochloride (Anticholinergics antagonize the effects of antiglaucoma agents).
No products indexed under this heading.

Pimozide (Antipsychotic agents may increase certain actions or side effects of anticholinergic agents).
No products indexed under this heading.

Pirbuterol Acetate (Sympathomimetic agents may increase certain actions or side effects of anticholinergic agents). Products include:

Prazepam (Benzodiazepines may increase certain actions or side effects of anticholinergic agents).
No products indexed under this heading.

Prednisolone Acetate (Anticholinergic drugs in the presence of increased intraocular pressure may be hazardous when taken concurrently with agents such as corticosteroids). Products include:

Prednisolone Sodium Phosphate (Anticholinergic drugs in the presence of increased intraocular pressure may be hazardous when taken concurrently with agents such as corticosteroids).
No products indexed under this heading.

Prednisolone Tebutate (Anticholinergic drugs in the presence of increased intraocular pressure may be hazardous when taken concurrently with agents such as corticosteroids).
No products indexed under this heading.

Prednisone (Anticholinergic drugs in the presence of increased intraocular pressure may be hazardous when taken concurrently with agents such as corticosteroids).
No products indexed under this heading.

Procainamide Hydrochloride (Class I antiarrhythmic agents may increase certain actions or side effects of anticholinergic agents).
No products indexed under this heading.

Procarbazine Hydrochloride (MAO inhibitors may increase certain actions or side effects of anticholinergic agents). Products include:

Prochlorperazine (Antipsychotic agents may increase certain actions or side effects of anticholinergic agents).
No products indexed under this heading.

Promethazine Hydrochloride (Antihistamines may increase certain actions or side effects of anticholinergic agents). Products include:

Propafenone Hydrochloride (Class I antiarrhythmic agents may increase certain actions or side effects of anticholinergic agents). Products include:

Propoxyphene Hydrochloride (Narcotic analgesics may increase certain actions or side effects of anticholinergic agents).
No products indexed under this heading.

Propoxyphene Napsylate (Narcotic analgesics may increase certain actions or side effects of anticholinergic agents).
No products indexed under this heading.

Protriptyline Hydrochloride (Tricyclic antidepressants may increase certain actions or side effects of anticholinergic agents).
No products indexed under this heading.

Pseudoephedrine Hydrochloride (Sympathomimetic agents may increase certain actions or side effects of anticholinergic agents). Products include:

Pseudoephedrine Sulfate (Sympathomimetic agents may increase certain actions or side effects of anticholinergic agents). Products include:

Pyrilamine Maleate (Antihistamines may increase certain actions or side effects of anticholinergic agents).
No products indexed under this heading.

Pyrilamine Tannate (Antihistamines may increase certain actions or side effects of anticholinergic agents).
No products indexed under this heading.

Quazepam (Benzodiazepines may increase certain actions or side effects of anticholinergic agents).
No products indexed under this heading.

Quetiapine Fumarate (Antipsychotic agents may increase certain actions or side effects of anticholinergic agents). Products include:

Quinidine Gluconate (Class I antiarrhythmic agents may increase certain actions or side effects of anticholinergic agents).
No products indexed under this heading.

Quinidine Polygalacturonate (Class I antiarrhythmic agents may increase certain actions or side effects of anticholinergic agents).
No products indexed under this heading.

Quinidine Sulfate (Class I antiarrhythmic agents may increase certain actions or side effects of anticholinergic agents).
No products indexed under this heading.

Remifentanil Hydrochloride (Narcotic analgesics may increase certain actions or side effects of anticholinergic agents).
No products indexed under this heading.

Risperidone (Antipsychotic agents may increase certain actions or side effects of anticholinergic agents). Products include:
Risperdal 1676
Risperdal Consta Long-Acting Injection 1682
Risperdal M-Tab Orally Disintegrating Tablets 1676

Salmeterol Xinafoate (Sympathomimetic agents may increase certain actions or side effects of anticholinergic agents). Products include:
Advair Diskus 100/50 1308
Advair Diskus 250/50 1308
Advair Diskus 500/50 1308
Advair HFA Inhalation Aerosol 1318
Serevent Diskus 1568

Selegiline Hydrochloride (MAO inhibitors may increase certain actions or side effects of anticholinergic agents). Products include:
Eldepryl Capsules 3208
Zelapar Tablets 3372

Sodium Bicarbonate (Antacids may interfere with the absorption of anticholinergic agents; therefore, simultaneous use of these drugs should be avoided). Products include:
Colyte with Flavor Packs for Oral Solution 3088
HalfLytely and Bisacodyl Tablets Bowel Prep Kit with Flavors Packs 881
TriLyte with Flavor Packs for Oral Solution 3100

Sufentanil Citrate (Narcotic analgesics may increase certain actions or side effects of anticholinergic agents).
No products indexed under this heading.

Temazepam (Benzodiazepines may increase certain actions or side effects of anticholinergic agents). Products include:
Restoril Capsules 1860

Terbutaline Sulfate (Sympathomimetic agents may increase certain actions or side effects of anticholinergic agents).
No products indexed under this heading.

Terfenadine (Antihistamines may increase certain actions or side effects of anticholinergic agents).
No products indexed under this heading.

Thioridazine Hydrochloride (Antipsychotic agents may increase certain actions or side effects of anticholinergic agents). Products include:
Thioridazine Hydrochloride Tablets 2163

Thiothixene (Antipsychotic agents may increase certain actions or side effects of anticholinergic agents). Products include:
Thiothixene Capsules 2165

Timolol Maleate (Anticholinergics antagonize the effects of antiglaucoma agents). Products include:
Blocadren Tablets 1916
Cosopt Sterile Ophthalmic Solution 1931
Timolide Tablets 2086
Timoptic Sterile Ophthalmic Solution 2088
Timoptic in Ocudose 2091
Timoptic-XE Sterile Ophthalmic Gel Forming Solution 2092

Tranylcypromine Sulfate (MAO inhibitors may increase certain actions or side effects of anticholinergic agents). Products include:
Parnate Tablets 1527

Triamcinolone (Anticholinergic drugs in the presence of increased intraocular pressure may be hazardous when taken concurrently with agents such as corticosteroids).
No products indexed under this heading.

Triamcinolone Acetonide (Anticholinergic drugs in the presence of increased intraocular pressure may be hazardous when taken concurrently with agents such as corticosteroids). Products include:
Azmacort Inhalation Aerosol 1726
Nasacort AQ Nasal Spray 2922

Triamcinolone Diacetate (Anticholinergic drugs in the presence of increased intraocular pressure may be hazardous when taken concurrently with agents such as corticosteroids).
No products indexed under this heading.

Triamcinolone Hexacetonide (Anticholinergic drugs in the presence of increased intraocular pressure may be hazardous when taken concurrently with agents such as corticosteroids).
No products indexed under this heading.

Triazolam (Benzodiazepines may increase certain actions or side effects of anticholinergic agents).
No products indexed under this heading.

Trifluoperazine Hydrochloride (Antipsychotic agents may increase certain actions or side effects of anticholinergic agents).
No products indexed under this heading.

Trimeprazine Tartrate (Antihistamines may increase certain actions or side effects of anticholinergic agents).
No products indexed under this heading.

Trimipramine Maleate (Tricyclic antidepressants may increase certain actions or side effects of anticholinergic agents).
No products indexed under this heading.

Tripelennamine Hydrochloride (Antihistamines may increase certain actions or side effects of anticholinergic agents).
No products indexed under this heading.

Triprolidine Hydrochloride (Antihistamines may increase certain actions or side effects of anticholinergic agents).
No products indexed under this heading.

Ziprasidone Hydrochloride (Antipsychotic agents may increase certain actions or side effects of anticholinergic agents). Products include:
Geodon Capsules 2529

BENZACLIN TOPICAL GEL

(Benzoyl Peroxide, Clindamycin Phosphate) 2877
May interact with peeling/desquamating agents and certain other agents. Compounds in these categories include:

Acitretin (Concomitant topical acne therapy should be used with caution because a possible cumulative irritancy may occur, especially with the use of peeling, desquamating or abrasive agents). Products include:
Soriatane Capsules 1013

Adapalene (Concomitant topical acne therapy should be used with caution because a possible cumulative irritancy may occur, especially with the use of peeling, desquamating or abrasive agents). Products include:
Differin Cream 1210
Differin Gel 1211

Azelaic Acid (Concomitant topical acne therapy should be used with caution because a possible cumulative irritancy may occur, especially with the use of peeling, desquamating or abrasive agents). Products include:
Finacea Gel 1669

Calcipotriene (Concomitant topical acne therapy should be used with caution because a possible cumulative irritancy may occur, especially with the use of peeling, desquamating or abrasive agents).
No products indexed under this heading.

Clindamycin, Topical (Concomitant topical acne therapy should be used with caution because a possible cumulative irritancy may occur, especially with the use of peeling, desquamating or abrasive agents).
No products indexed under this heading.

Clotrimazole, Topical (Concomitant topical acne therapy should be used with caution because a possible cumulative irritancy may occur, especially with the use of peeling, desquamating or abrasive agents).
No products indexed under this heading.

Coal Tar (Concomitant topical acne therapy should be used with caution because a possible cumulative irritancy may occur, especially with the use of peeling, desquamating or abrasive agents).
No products indexed under this heading.

Concomitant Topical Acne Therapy (Possible cumulative irritancy effect may occur, especially with the use of peeling, desquamating, or abrasive agents).
No products indexed under this heading.

Erythromycin, Topical (Concomitant topical acne therapy should be used with caution because a possible cumulative irritancy may occur, especially with the use of peeling, desquamating or abrasive agents).
No products indexed under this heading.

Fluorouracil, Topical (Concomitant topical acne therapy should be used with caution because a possible cumulative irritancy may occur, especially with the use of peeling, desquamating or abrasive agents).
No products indexed under this heading.

Hydroquinone (Concomitant topical acne therapy should be used with caution because a possible cumulative irritancy may occur, especially with the use of peeling, desquamating or abrasive agents). Products include:
Claripel Cream 3211
Lustra Cream 3289
Lustra-AF Cream 3289
Lustra-Ultra Cream 3289
Tri-Luma Cream 1213

Isotretinoin (Concomitant topical acne therapy should be used with caution because a possible cumulative irritancy may occur, especially with the use of peeling, desquamating or abrasive agents). Products include:
Accutane Capsules 2731

Mequinol (Concomitant topical acne therapy should be used with caution because a possible cumulative irritancy may occur, especially with the use of peeling, desquamating or abrasive agents).
No products indexed under this heading.

Podofilox (Concomitant topical acne therapy should be used with caution because a possible cumulative irritancy may occur, especially with the use of peeling, desquamating or abrasive agents).
No products indexed under this heading.

Salicylic Acid (Concomitant topical acne therapy should be used with caution because a possible cumulative irritancy may occur, especially with the use of peeling, desquamating or abrasive agents).
No products indexed under this heading.

Sulfur Preparations (Concomitant topical acne therapy should be used with caution because a possible cumulative irritancy may occur, especially with the use of peeling, desquamating or abrasive agents).
No products indexed under this heading.

Tazarotene (Concomitant topical acne therapy should be used with caution because a possible cumulative irritancy may occur, especially with the use of peeling, desquamating or abrasive agents).
No products indexed under this heading.

Tretinoin (Concomitant topical acne therapy should be used with caution because a possible cumulative irritancy may occur, especially with the use of peeling, desquamating or abrasive agents). Products include:
Tri-Luma Cream 1213
Vesanoid Capsules 2820

Zalcitabine (Concomitant topical acne therapy should be used with caution because a possible cumulative irritancy may occur, especially with the use of peeling, desquamating or abrasive agents).
No products indexed under this heading.

BETADINE 5% OPHTHALMIC SOLUTION

(Povidone Iodine) .... ⊙202
None cited in PDR database.

BETAGAN OPHTHALMIC SOLUTION, USP

(Levobunolol Hydrochloride) .... ⊙220
May interact with beta blockers, cardiac glycosides, phenothiazines, and certain other agents. Compounds in these categories include:

Acebutolol Hydrochloride (Co-administration with oral beta blockers may result in additive effect either on intraocular pressure or on the known systemic effects of beta blockade).
No products indexed under this heading.

Atenolol (Co-administration with oral beta blockers may result in additive effect either on intraocular pressure or on the known systemic effects of beta blockade).
No products indexed under this heading.

Betaxolol Hydrochloride (Co-administration with oral beta blockers may result in additive effect either on intraocular pressure or on the known systemic effects of beta blockade). Products include:
Betoptic S Ophthalmic Suspension................................. 558

Bisoprolol Fumarate (Co-administration with oral beta blockers may result in additive effect either on intraocular pressure or on the known systemic effects of beta blockade).
No products indexed under this heading.

Carteolol Hydrochloride (Co-administration with oral beta blockers may result in additive effect either on intraocular pressure or on the known systemic effects of beta blockade). Products include:
Carteolol Hydrochloride Ophthalmic Solution USP, 1%....... ⊙249

Chlorpromazine (Co-administration with phenothiazine-related compounds may have an additive hypotensive effect due to inhibition of each other's metabolism).
No products indexed under this heading.

Chlorpromazine Hydrochloride (Co-administration with phenothiazine-related compounds may have an additive hypotensive effect due to inhibition of each other's metabolism).
No products indexed under this heading.

Deserpidine (Possible additive effects and production of hypotension and/or bradycardia when beta blocker is concurrently used with catecholamine-depleting drugs).
No products indexed under this heading.

Deslanoside (Co-administration with digitalis and calcium channel blockers may have an additive effect on prolonging atrioventricular conduction time).
No products indexed under this heading.

Digitalis Glycoside Preparations (Co-administration with digitalis and calcium channel blockers may have an additive effect on prolonging atrioventricular conduction time).
No products indexed under this heading.

Digitoxin (Co-administration with digitalis and calcium channel blockers may have an additive effect on prolonging atrioventricular conduction time).
No products indexed under this heading.

Digoxin (Co-administration with digitalis and calcium channel blockers may have an additive effect on prolonging atrioventricular conduction time). Products include:
Lanoxicaps Capsules 1490
Lanoxin Injection 1494
Lanoxin Injection Pediatric 1497
Lanoxin Tablets 1500

Epinephrine (Concurrent use in patients with history of atopy or severe anaphylactic reaction to allergens may be unresponsive to the usual doses of epinephrine used to treat anaphylactic reaction; mydriasis may result with concomitant epinephrine). Products include:
EpiPen 1061
Primatene Mist .... ▣719
Twinject 0.15 3379
Twinject 0.3 3378

Epinephrine Hydrochloride (Concurrent use in patients with history of atopy or severe anaphylactic reaction to allergens may be unresponsive to the usual doses of epinephrine used to treat anaphylactic reaction; mydriasis may result with concomitant epinephrine).
No products indexed under this heading.

Esmolol Hydrochloride (Co-administration with oral beta blockers may result in additive effect either on intraocular pressure or on the known systemic effects of beta blockade).
No products indexed under this heading.

Fluphenazine Decanoate (Co-administration with phenothiazine-related compounds may have an additive hypotensive effect due to inhibition of each other's metabolism).
No products indexed under this heading.

Fluphenazine Enanthate (Co-administration with phenothiazine-related compounds may have an additive hypotensive effect due to inhibition of each other's metabolism).
No products indexed under this heading.

Fluphenazine Hydrochloride (Co-administration with phenothiazine-related compounds may have an additive hypotensive effect due to inhibition of each other's metabolism).
No products indexed under this heading.

Labetalol Hydrochloride (Co-administration with oral beta blockers may result in additive effect either on intraocular pressure or on the known systemic effects of beta blockade).
No products indexed under this heading.

Mesoridazine Besylate (Co-administration with phenothiazine-related compounds may have an additive hypotensive effect due to inhibition of each other's metabolism).
No products indexed under this heading.

Methotrimeprazine (Co-administration with phenothiazine-related compounds may have an additive hypotensive effect due to inhibition of each other's metabolism).
No products indexed under this heading.

Metipranolol Hydrochloride (Co-administration with oral beta blockers may result in additive effect either on intraocular pressure or on the known systemic effects of beta blockade).
No products indexed under this heading.

Metoprolol Succinate (Co-administration with oral beta blockers may result in additive effect either on intraocular pressure or on the known systemic effects of beta blockade). Products include:
Toprol-XL Tablets 668

Metoprolol Tartrate (Co-administration with oral beta blockers may result in additive effect either on intraocular pressure or on the known systemic effects of beta blockade). Products include:
Lopressor Injection 2238
Lopressor Tablets 2238
Lopressor HCT 50/25 Tablets 2241
Lopressor HCT 100/25 Tablets 2241
Lopressor HCT 100/50 Tablets 2241

Nadolol (Co-administration with oral beta blockers may result in additive effect either on intraocular pressure or on the known systemic effects of beta blockade). Products include:
Nadolol Tablets 2159

Penbutolol Sulfate (Co-administration with oral beta blockers may result in additive effect either on intraocular pressure or on the known systemic effects of beta blockade).
No products indexed under this heading.

Perphenazine (Co-administration with phenothiazine-related compounds may have an additive hypotensive effect due to inhibition of each other's metabolism).
No products indexed under this heading.

Pindolol (Co-administration with oral beta blockers may result in additive effect either on intraocular pressure or on the known systemic effects of beta blockade).
No products indexed under this heading.

Prochlorperazine (Co-administration with phenothiazine-related compounds may have an additive hypotensive effect due to inhibition of each other's metabolism).
No products indexed under this heading.

Promethazine Hydrochloride (Co-administration with phenothiazine-related compounds may have an additive hypotensive effect due to inhibition of each other's metabolism). Products include:
Phenergan Tablets and Suppositories.............................. 3440

Propranolol Hydrochloride (Co-administration with oral beta blockers may result in additive effect either on intraocular pressure or on the known systemic effects of beta blockade). Products include:
Inderal LA Long-Acting Capsules 3429
InnoPran XL Capsules 2723

Rauwolfia Serpentina (Possible additive effects and production of hypotension and/or bradycardia when beta blocker is concurrently used with catecholamine-depleting drugs).
No products indexed under this heading.

Rescinnamine (Possible additive effects and production of hypotension and/or bradycardia when beta blocker is concurrently used with catecholamine-depleting drugs).
No products indexed under this heading.

Reserpine (Possible additive effects and production of hypotension and/or bradycardia when beta blocker is concurrently used with catecholamine-depleting drugs).
No products indexed under this heading.

Sotalol Hydrochloride (Co-administration with oral beta blockers may result in additive effect either on intraocular pressure or on the known systemic effects of beta blockade).
No products indexed under this heading.

Thioridazine Hydrochloride (Co-administration with phenothiazine-related compounds may have an additive hypotensive effect due to inhibition of each other's metabolism). Products include:
Thioridazine Hydrochloride Tablets....................................... 2163

Timolol Hemihydrate (Co-administration with oral beta blockers may result in additive effect either on intraocular pressure or on the known systemic effects of beta blockade). Products include:
Betimol Ophthalmic Solution 3382
Betimol Ophthalmic Solution .... ⊙295

Timolol Maleate (Co-administration with oral beta blockers may result in additive effect either on intraocular pressure or on the known systemic effects of beta blockade). Products include:
Blocadren Tablets 1916
Cosopt Sterile Ophthalmic Solution....................................... 1931
Timolide Tablets 2086
Timoptic Sterile Ophthalmic Solution....................................... 2088
Timoptic in Ocudose 2091
Timoptic-XE Sterile Ophthalmic Gel Forming Solution 2092

Trifluoperazine Hydrochloride (Co-administration with phenothiazine-related compounds may have an additive hypotensive effect due to inhibition of each other's metabolism).
No products indexed under this heading.

BETASERON FOR SC INJECTION

(Interferon Beta-1b) 767
None cited in PDR database.

BETIMOL OPHTHALMIC SOLUTION

(Timolol Hemihydrate) 3382

May interact with beta blockers, calcium channel blockers, cardiac glycosides, and certain other agents. Compounds in these categories include:

Acebutolol Hydrochloride (Concurrent use with systemic beta blockers may result in additive effect either on the intraocular pressure or the known systemic effect of beta blockade).
No products indexed under this heading.

Amlodipine Besylate (Possible atrioventricular conduction disturbances, left ventricular failure, and hypotension). Products include:
Caduet Tablets 2508
Lotrel Capsules 2249
Norvasc Tablets 2545

Atenolol (Concurrent use with systemic beta blockers may result in additive effect either on the intraocular pressure or the known systemic effect of beta blockade).
No products indexed under this heading.

Bepridil Hydrochloride (Possible atrioventricular conduction disturbances, left ventricular failure, and hypotension).
No products indexed under this heading.

Betaxolol Hydrochloride (Concurrent use with systemic beta blockers may result in additive effect either on the intraocular pressure or the known systemic effect of beta blockade). Products include:
Betoptic S Ophthalmic Suspension 558

Bisoprolol Fumarate (Concurrent use with systemic beta blockers may result in additive effect either on the intraocular pressure or the known systemic effect of beta blockade).
No products indexed under this heading.

Carteolol Hydrochloride (Concurrent use with systemic beta blockers may result in additive effect either on the intraocular pressure or the known systemic effect of beta blockade). Products include:
Carteolol Hydrochloride Ophthalmic Solution USP, 1%....... ⊙ 249

Deslanoside (Concomitant use of beta blockers with digitalis and calcium antagonist may have additive effects in prolonging atrioventricular conduction time).
No products indexed under this heading.

Digitalis Glycoside Preparations (Concomitant use of beta blockers with digitalis and calcium antagonists may have additive effects in prolonging atrioventricular conduction time).
No products indexed under this heading.

Digitoxin (Concomitant use of beta blockers with digitalis and calcium antagonists may have additive effects in prolonging atrioventricular conduction time).
No products indexed under this heading.

Digoxin (Concomitant use of beta blockers with digitalis and calcium antagonists may have additive effects in prolonging atrioventricular conduction time). Products include:
Lanoxicaps Capsules 1490
Lanoxin Injection 1494
Lanoxin Injection Pediatric 1497
Lanoxin Tablets 1500

Diltiazem Hydrochloride (Possible atrioventricular conduction disturbances, left ventricular failure, and hypotension). Products include:
Cardizem LA Extended Release Tablets 1728
Tiazac Capsules 1201

Epinephrine (Patients with a history of atopy or anaphylactic reactions to a variety of allergens may be unresponsive to the usual dose of injectable epinephrine used to treat allergic reactions). Products include:
EpiPen 1061
Primatene Mist 719
Twinject 0.15 3379
Twinject 0.3 3378

Epinephrine Bitartrate (Patients with a history of atopy or anaphylactic reactions to a variety of allergens may be unresponsive to the usual dose of injectable epinephrine used to treat allergic reactions).
No products indexed under this heading.

Esmolol Hydrochloride (Concurrent use with systemic beta blockers may result in additive effect either on the intraocular pressure or the known systemic effect of beta blockade).
No products indexed under this heading.

Felodipine (Possible atrioventricular conduction disturbances, left ventricular failure, and hypotension).
No products indexed under this heading.

Isradipine (Possible atrioventricular conduction disturbances, left ventricular failure, and hypotension). Products include:
DynaCirc CR Tablets 2721

Labetalol Hydrochloride (Concurrent use with systemic beta blockers may result in additive effect either on the intraocular pressure or the known systemic effect of beta blockade).
No products indexed under this heading.

Levobunolol Hydrochloride (Concurrent use with systemic beta blockers may result in additive effect either on the intraocular pressure or the known systemic effect of beta blockade). Products include:
Betagan Ophthalmic Solution, USP.............................. ⊙ 220

Metipranolol Hydrochloride (Concurrent use with systemic beta blockers may result in additive effect either on the intraocular pressure or the known systemic effect of beta blockade).
No products indexed under this heading.

Metoprolol Succinate (Concurrent use with systemic beta blockers may result in additive effect either on the intraocular pressure or the known systemic effect of beta blockade). Products include:
Toprol-XL Tablets 668

Metoprolol Tartrate (Concurrent use with systemic beta blockers may result in additive effect either on the intraocular pressure or the known systemic effect of beta blockade). Products include:
Lopressor Injection 2238
Lopressor Tablets 2238
Lopressor HCT 50/25 Tablets 2241
Lopressor HCT 100/25 Tablets 2241
Lopressor HCT 100/50 Tablets 2241

Mibefradil Dihydrochloride (Possible atrioventricular conduction disturbances, left ventricular failure, and hypotension).
No products indexed under this heading.

Nadolol (Concurrent use with systemic beta blockers may result in additive effect either on the intraocular pressure or the known systemic effect of beta blockade). Products include:
Nadolol Tablets 2159

Nicardipine Hydrochloride (Possible atrioventricular conduction disturbances, left ventricular failure, and hypotension). Products include:
Cardene I.V. 2497

Nifedipine (Possible atrioventricular conduction disturbances, left ventricular failure, and hypotension). Products include:
Adalat CC Tablets 2964

Nimodipine (Possible atrioventricular conduction disturbances, left ventricular failure, and hypotension). Products include:
Nimotop Capsules 749

Nisoldipine (Possible atrioventricular conduction disturbances, left ventricular failure, and hypotension). Products include:
Sular Tablets 3122

Penbutolol Sulfate (Concurrent use with systemic beta blockers may result in additive effect either on the intraocular pressure or the known systemic effect of beta blockade).
No products indexed under this heading.

Pindolol (Concurrent use with systemic beta blockers may result in additive effect either on the intraocular pressure or the known systemic effect of beta blockade).
No products indexed under this heading.

Propranolol Hydrochloride (Concurrent use with systemic beta blockers may result in additive effect either on the intraocular pressure or the known systemic effect of beta blockade). Products include:
Inderal LA Long-Acting Capsules 3429
InnoPran XL Capsules 2723

Sotalol Hydrochloride (Concurrent use with systemic beta blockers may result in additive effect either on the intraocular pressure or the known systemic effect of beta blockade).
No products indexed under this heading.

Timolol Maleate (Concurrent use with systemic beta blockers may result in additive effect either on the intraocular pressure or the known systemic effect of beta blockade). Products include:
Blocadren Tablets 1916
Cosopt Sterile Ophthalmic Solution.............................. 1931
Timolide Tablets 2086
Timoptic Sterile Ophthalmic Solution.............................. 2088
Timoptic in Ocudose 2091
Timoptic-XE Sterile Ophthalmic Gel Forming Solution 2092

Verapamil Hydrochloride (Possible atrioventricular conduction disturbances, left ventricular failure, and hypotension). Products include:
Covera-HS Tablets 3139
Tarka Tablets 524
Verelan PM Extended-Release Capsules, Controlled-Onset.............................. 3106

BETOPTIC S OPHTHALMIC SUSPENSION

(Betaxolol Hydrochloride) 558

May interact with adrenergic augmenting psychotropics, beta blockers, and certain other agents. Compounds in these categories include:

Acebutolol Hydrochloride (Co-administration with oral beta blockers may result in additive effects either on intraocular pressure or on the known systemic effects of beta blockade).
No products indexed under this heading.

Atenolol (Co-administration with oral beta blockers may result in additive effects either on intraocular pressure or on the known systemic effects of beta blockade).
No products indexed under this heading.

Bisoprolol Fumarate (Co-administration with oral beta blockers may result in additive effects either on intraocular pressure or on the known systemic effects of beta blockade).
No products indexed under this heading.

Carteolol Hydrochloride (Co-administration with oral beta blockers may result in additive effects either on intraocular pressure or on the known systemic effects of beta blockade). Products include:
Carteolol Hydrochloride Ophthalmic Solution USP, 1%....... ⊙ 249

Deserpidine (Possible additive effects and production of hypotension and/or bradycardia when beta blocker is concurrently used with catecholamine depleting drugs).
No products indexed under this heading.

Epinephrine (Concurrent use in patients with history of atopy or severe anaphylactic reaction to allergens may be unresponsive to the usual doses of epinephrine used to treat anaphylactic reaction). Products include:
EpiPen 1061
Primatene Mist 719
Twinject 0.15 3379
Twinject 0.3 3378

Epinephrine Hydrochloride (Concurrent use in patients with history of atopy or severe anaphylactic reaction to allergens may be unresponsive to the usual doses of epinephrine used to treat anaphylactic reaction).
No products indexed under this heading.

Esmolol Hydrochloride (Co-administration with oral beta blockers may result in additive effects either on intraocular pressure or on the known systemic effects of beta blockade).
No products indexed under this heading.

Isocarboxazid (Exercise caution when used concurrently with adrenergic psychotropic drugs).
No products indexed under this heading.

Labetalol Hydrochloride (Co-administration with oral beta blockers may result in additive effects either on intraocular pressure or on the known systemic effects of beta blockade).
No products indexed under this heading.

Levobunolol Hydrochloride (Co-administration with oral beta blockers may result in additive effects either on intraocular pressure or on the known systemic effects of beta blockade). Products include:
Betagan Ophthalmic Solution, USP .... ⊙ 220

Metipranolol Hydrochloride (Co-administration with oral beta blockers may result in additive effects either on intraocular pressure or on the known systemic effects of beta blockade).
No products indexed under this heading.

Metoprolol Succinate (Co-administration with oral beta blockers may result in additive effects either on intraocular pressure or on the known systemic effects of beta blockade). Products include:
Toprol-XL Tablets 668

Metoprolol Tartrate (Co-administration with oral beta blockers may result in additive effects either on intraocular pressure or on the known systemic effects of beta blockade). Products include:
Lopressor Injection 2238
Lopressor Tablets 2238
Lopressor HCT 50/25 Tablets 2241
Lopressor HCT 100/25 Tablets 2241
Lopressor HCT 100/50 Tablets 2241

Nadolol (Co-administration with oral beta blockers may result in additive effects either on intraocular pressure or on the known systemic effects of beta blockade). Products include:
Nadolol Tablets 2159

Pargyline Hydrochloride (Exercise caution when used concurrently with adrenergic psychotropic drugs).
No products indexed under this heading.

Penbutolol Sulfate (Co-administration with oral beta blockers may result in additive effects either on intraocular pressure or on the known systemic effects of beta blockade).
No products indexed under this heading.

Phenelzine Sulfate (Exercise caution when used concurrently with adrenergic psychotropic drugs).
No products indexed under this heading.

Pindolol (Co-administration with oral beta blockers may result in additive effects either on intraocular pressure or on the known systemic effects of beta blockade).
No products indexed under this heading.

Propranolol Hydrochloride (Co-administration with oral beta blockers may result in additive effects either on intraocular pressure or on the known systemic effects of beta blockade). Products include:
Inderal LA Long-Acting Capsules 3429
InnoPran XL Capsules 2723

Rauwolfia Serpentina (Possible additive effects and production of hypotension and/or bradycardia when beta blocker is concurrently used with catecholamine depleting drugs).
No products indexed under this heading.

Rescinnamine (Possible additive effects and production of hypotension and/or bradycardia when beta blocker is concurrently used with catecholamine depleting drugs).
No products indexed under this heading.

Reserpine (Possible additive effects and production of hypotension and/or bradycardia when beta blocker is concurrently used with catecholamine depleting drugs).
No products indexed under this heading.

Sotalol Hydrochloride (Co-administration with oral beta blockers may result in additive effects either on intraocular pressure or on the known systemic effects of beta blockade).
No products indexed under this heading.

Timolol Hemihydrate (Co-administration with oral beta blockers may result in additive effects either on intraocular pressure or on the known systemic effects of beta blockade). Products include:
Betimol Ophthalmic Solution 3382
Betimol Ophthalmic Solution .... ⊙ 295

Timolol Maleate (Co-administration with oral beta blockers may result in additive effects either on intraocular pressure or on the known systemic effects of beta blockade). Products include:
Blocadren Tablets 1916
Cosopt Sterile Ophthalmic Solution 1931
Timolide Tablets 2086
Timoptic Sterile Ophthalmic Solution 2088
Timoptic in Ocudose 2091
Timoptic-XE Sterile Ophthalmic Gel Forming Solution 2092

Tranylcypromine Sulfate (Exercise caution when used concurrently with adrenergic psychotropic drugs). Products include:
Parnate Tablets 1527

BEVITAMEL TABLETS
(Folic Acid, Melatonin, Vitamin B_{12}) 3404
None cited in PDR database.

BEXXAR
(Iodine I 131 Tositumomab, Tositumomab) 1398
May interact with anticoagulants, oral anticoagulants, and platelet inhibitors. Compounds in these categories include:

Anisindione (Due to the frequent occurrence of severe and prolonged thrombocytopenia, the potential benefits of medications that interfere with platelet function and/or anticoagulation should be weighed against the potential increased risk of bleeding and hemorrhage). Products include:
Miradon Tablets 3042

Ardeparin Sodium (Due to the frequent occurrence of severe and prolonged thrombocytopenia, the potential benefits of medications that interfere with platelet function and/or anticoagulation should be weighed against the potential increased risk of bleeding and hemorrhage).
No products indexed under this heading.

Aspirin (Due to the frequent occurrence of severe and prolonged thrombocytopenia, the potential benefits of medications that interfere with platelet function and/or anticoagulation should be weighed against the potential increased risk of bleeding and hemorrhage). Products include:
Aggrenox Capsules 822
Bayer Aspirin 744
BC Allergy Sinus Cold Powder .... ▣ 677
BC Headache Powder .... ▣ 677
Arthritis Strength BC Powder .... ▣ 677
BC Sinus Cold Powder .... ▣ 677
Excedrin Extra Strength Caplets/Tablets/Geltabs .... ▣ 684
Excedrin Migraine Caplets/Tablets/Geltabs .... ▣ 609
Goody's Body Pain Formula Powder .... ▣ 684
Goody's Extra Strength Headache Powders .... ▣ 611
Goody's Extra Strength Pain Relief Tablets .... ▣ 685
Percodan Tablets 1132
St. Joseph 81 mg Aspirin Chewable and Enteric Coated Tablets 1869

Aspirin, Enteric Coated (Due to the frequent occurrence of severe and prolonged thrombocytopenia, the potential benefits of medications that interfere with platelet function and/or anticoagulation should be weighed against the potential increased risk of bleeding and hemorrhage).
No products indexed under this heading.

Aspirin Buffered (Due to the frequent occurrence of severe and prolonged thrombocytopenia, the potential benefits of medications that interfere with platelet function and/or anticoagulation should be weighed against the potential increased risk of bleeding and hemorrhage). Products include:
Bufferin Extra Strength Tablets .... ▣ 678
Bufferin Regular Strength Tablets .... ▣ 678

Azlocillin Sodium (Due to the frequent occurrence of severe and prolonged thrombocytopenia, the potential benefits of medications that interfere with platelet function and/or anticoagulation should be weighed against the potential increased risk of bleeding and hemorrhage).
No products indexed under this heading.

Carbenicillin Indanyl Sodium (Due to the frequent occurrence of severe and prolonged thrombocytopenia, the potential benefits of medications that interfere with platelet function and/or anticoagulation should be weighed against the potential increased risk of bleeding and hemorrhage).
No products indexed under this heading.

Choline Magnesium Trisalicylate (Due to the frequent occurrence of severe and prolonged thrombocytopenia, the potential benefits of medications that interfere with platelet function and/or anticoagulation should be weighed against the potential increased risk of bleeding and hemorrhage).
No products indexed under this heading.

Clopidogrel Bisulfate (Due to the frequent occurrence of severe and prolonged thrombocytopenia, the potential benefits of medications that interfere with platelet function and/or anticoagulation should be weighed against the potential increased risk of bleeding and hemorrhage). Products include:
Plavix Tablets 917
Plavix Tablets 2926

Dalteparin Sodium (Due to the frequent occurrence of severe and prolonged thrombocytopenia, the potential benefits of medications that interfere with platelet function and/or anticoagulation should be weighed against the potential increased risk of bleeding and hemorrhage). Products include:
Fragmin Injection 1097

Danaparoid Sodium (Due to the frequent occurrence of severe and prolonged thrombocytopenia, the potential benefits of medications that interfere with platelet function and/or anticoagulation should be weighed against the potential increased risk of bleeding and hemorrhage).
No products indexed under this heading.

Diclofenac Potassium (Due to the frequent occurrence of severe and prolonged thrombocytopenia, the potential benefits of medications that interfere with platelet function and/or anticoagulation should be weighed against the potential increased risk of bleeding and hemorrhage).
No products indexed under this heading.

Diclofenac Sodium (Due to the frequent occurrence of severe and prolonged thrombocytopenia, the potential benefits of medications that interfere with platelet function and/or anticoagulation should be weighed against the potential increased risk of bleeding and hemorrhage). Products include:
Arthrotec Tablets 3129
Voltaren Ophthalmic Solution 2309
Voltaren Tablets 2307
Voltaren-XR Tablets 2310

Dicumarol (Due to the frequent occurrence of severe and prolonged thrombocytopenia, the potential benefits of medications that interfere with platelet function and/or anticoagulation should be weighed against the potential increased risk of bleeding and hemorrhage).
No products indexed under this heading.

Diflunisal (Due to the frequent occurrence of severe and prolonged thrombocytopenia, the potential benefits of medications that interfere with platelet function and/or anticoagulation should be weighed against the potential increased risk of bleeding and hemorrhage). Products include:
Dolobid Tablets 1955

Dipyridamole (Due to the frequent occurrence of severe and prolonged thrombocytopenia, the potential benefits of medications that interfere with platelet function and/or anticoagulation should be weighed against the potential increased risk of bleeding and hemorrhage). Products include:
Aggrenox Capsules 822
Persantine Tablets 868

Enoxaparin Sodium (Due to the frequent occurrence of severe and prolonged thrombocytopenia, the potential benefits of medications that interfere with platelet function and/or anticoagulation should be weighed against the potential increased risk of bleeding and hemorrhage). Products include:
Lovenox Injection 2915

Fenoprofen Calcium (Due to the frequent occurrence of severe and prolonged thrombocytopenia, the potential benefits of medications that interfere with platelet function and/or anticoagulation should be weighed against the potential increased risk of bleeding and hemorrhage). Products include:

Nalfon Capsules 2502

Flurbiprofen (Due to the frequent occurrence of severe and prolonged thrombocytopenia, the potential benefits of medications that interfere with platelet function and/or anticoagulation should be weighed against the potential increased risk of bleeding and hemorrhage).

No products indexed under this heading.

Fondaparinux Sodium (Due to the frequent occurrence of severe and prolonged thrombocytopenia, the potential benefits of medications that interfere with platelet function and/or anticoagulation should be weighed against the potential increased risk of bleeding and hemorrhage). Products include:

Arixtra Injection 1351

Heparin Calcium (Due to the frequent occurrence of severe and prolonged thrombocytopenia, the potential benefits of medications that interfere with platelet function and/or anticoagulation should be weighed against the potential increased risk of bleeding and hemorrhage).

No products indexed under this heading.

Heparin Sodium (Due to the frequent occurrence of severe and prolonged thrombocytopenia, the potential benefits of medications that interfere with platelet function and/or anticoagulation should be weighed against the potential increased risk of bleeding and hemorrhage).

No products indexed under this heading.

Ibuprofen (Due to the frequent occurrence of severe and prolonged thrombocytopenia, the potential benefits of medications that interfere with platelet function and/or anticoagulation should be weighed against the potential increased risk of bleeding and hemorrhage). Products include:

Advil Allergy Sinus Caplets 770
Advil 674
Children's Advil Oral Suspension 603
Children's Advil Chewable Tablets .. 603
Advil Cold & Sinus 723
Infants' Advil Concentrated Drops .. 604
Infants' Advil Concentrated Drops - White Grape (Dye-Free)............. 604
Junior Strength Advil Swallow Tablets.. 605
Advil Migraine Liquigels 608
Advil Multi-Symptom Cold Caplets 770
Advil PM Caplets 615
Motrin IB Tablets and Caplets 1866
Children's Motrin Oral Suspension ... 1867
Children's Motrin Non-Staining Dye-Free Oral Suspension............ 1867
Children's Motrin Cold Oral Suspension 1867
Infants' Motrin Concentrated Drops... 1867
Infants' Motrin Non-Staining Dye-Free Concentrated Drops....... 1867
Junior Strength Motrin Caplets and Chewable Tablets.................. 1867
Vicoprofen Tablets 539

Indomethacin (Due to the frequent occurrence of severe and prolonged thrombocytopenia, the potential benefits of medications that interfere with platelet function and/or anticoagulation should be weighed against the potential increased risk of bleeding and hemorrhage). Products include:

Indocin 1995

Indomethacin Sodium Trihydrate (Due to the frequent occurrence of severe and prolonged thrombocytopenia, the potential benefits of medications that interfere with platelet function and/or anticoagulation should be weighed against the potential increased risk of bleeding and hemorrhage). Products include:

Indocin I.V. 2465

Ketoprofen (Due to the frequent occurrence of severe and prolonged thrombocytopenia, the potential benefits of medications that interfere with platelet function and/or anticoagulation should be weighed against the potential increased risk of bleeding and hemorrhage).

No products indexed under this heading.

Low Molecular Weight Heparins (Due to the frequent occurrence of severe and prolonged thrombocytopenia, the potential benefits of medications that interfere with platelet function and/or anticoagulation should be weighed against the potential increased risk of bleeding and hemorrhage).

No products indexed under this heading.

Magnesium Salicylate (Due to the frequent occurrence of severe and prolonged thrombocytopenia, the potential benefits of medications that interfere with platelet function and/or anticoagulation should be weighed against the potential increased risk of bleeding and hemorrhage).

No products indexed under this heading.

Meclofenamate Sodium (Due to the frequent occurrence of severe and prolonged thrombocytopenia, the potential benefits of medications that interfere with platelet function and/or anticoagulation should be weighed against the potential increased risk of bleeding and hemorrhage).

No products indexed under this heading.

Mefenamic Acid (Due to the frequent occurrence of severe and prolonged thrombocytopenia, the potential benefits of medications that interfere with platelet function and/or anticoagulation should be weighed against the potential increased risk of bleeding and hemorrhage).

No products indexed under this heading.

Mezlocillin Sodium (Due to the frequent occurrence of severe and prolonged thrombocytopenia, the potential benefits of medications that interfere with platelet function and/or anticoagulation should be weighed against the potential increased risk of bleeding and hemorrhage).

No products indexed under this heading.

Nafcillin Sodium (Due to the frequent occurrence of severe and prolonged thrombocytopenia, the potential benefits of medications that interfere with platelet function and/or anticoagulation should be weighed against the potential increased risk of bleeding and hemorrhage).

No products indexed under this heading.

Naproxen (Due to the frequent occurrence of severe and prolonged thrombocytopenia, the potential benefits of medications that interfere with platelet function and/or anticoagulation should be weighed against the potential increased risk of bleeding and hemorrhage). Products include:

EC-Naprosyn Delayed-Release Tablets....................................... 2761
Naprosyn Suspension 2761
Naprosyn Tablets 2761
Prevacid NapraPAC 3280

Naproxen Sodium (Due to the frequent occurrence of severe and prolonged thrombocytopenia, the potential benefits of medications that interfere with platelet function and/or anticoagulation should be weighed against the potential increased risk of bleeding and hemorrhage). Products include:

Aleve Caplets 742
Aleve Gelcaps 743
Aleve Tablets 743
Aleve Cold & Sinus Caplets 744
Anaprox Tablets 2761
Anaprox DS Tablets 2761

Penicillin G Benzathine (Due to the frequent occurrence of severe and prolonged thrombocytopenia, the potential benefits of medications that interfere with platelet function and/or anticoagulation should be weighed against the potential increased risk of bleeding and hemorrhage). Products include:

Bicillin C-R Injectable Suspension 1706

Penicillin G Procaine (Due to the frequent occurrence of severe and prolonged thrombocytopenia, the potential benefits of medications that interfere with platelet function and/or anticoagulation should be weighed against the potential increased risk of bleeding and hemorrhage). Products include:

Bicillin C-R Injectable Suspension 1706

Phenylbutazone (Due to the frequent occurrence of severe and prolonged thrombocytopenia, the potential benefits of medications that interfere with platelet function and/or anticoagulation should be weighed against the potential increased risk of bleeding and hemorrhage).

No products indexed under this heading.

Piroxicam (Due to the frequent occurrence of severe and prolonged thrombocytopenia, the potential benefits of medications that interfere with platelet function and/or anticoagulation should be weighed against the potential increased risk of bleeding and hemorrhage).

No products indexed under this heading.

Salsalate (Due to the frequent occurrence of severe and prolonged thrombocytopenia, the potential benefits of medications that interfere with platelet function and/or anticoagulation should be weighed against the potential increased risk of bleeding and hemorrhage).

No products indexed under this heading.

Sulindac (Due to the frequent occurrence of severe and prolonged thrombocytopenia, the potential benefits of medications that interfere with platelet function and/or anticoagulation should be weighed against the potential increased risk of bleeding and hemorrhage). Products include:

Clinoril Tablets 1924

Ticarcillin Disodium (Due to the frequent occurrence of severe and prolonged thrombocytopenia, the potential benefits of medications that interfere with platelet function and/or anticoagulation should be weighed against the potential increased risk of bleeding and hemorrhage). Products include:

Timentin ADD-Vantage 1580
Timentin Injection Galaxy Container 1583
Timentin IV Infusion 1577
Timentin Pharmacy Bulk Package 1586

Ticlopidine Hydrochloride (Due to the frequent occurrence of severe and prolonged thrombocytopenia, the potential benefits of medications that interfere with platelet function and/or anticoagulation should be weighed against the potential increased risk of bleeding and hemorrhage). Products include:

Ticlid Tablets 2810

Tinzaparin Sodium (Due to the frequent occurrence of severe and prolonged thrombocytopenia, the potential benefits of medications that interfere with platelet function and/or anticoagulation should be weighed against the potential increased risk of bleeding and hemorrhage).

No products indexed under this heading.

Tolmetin Sodium (Due to the frequent occurrence of severe and prolonged thrombocytopenia, the potential benefits of medications that interfere with platelet function and/or anticoagulation should be weighed against the potential increased risk of bleeding and hemorrhage).

No products indexed under this heading.

Warfarin Sodium (Due to the frequent occurrence of severe and prolonged thrombocytopenia, the potential benefits of medications that interfere with platelet function and/or anticoagulation should be weighed against the potential increased risk of bleeding and hemorrhage). Products include:

Coumadin for Injection 898
Coumadin Tablets 898

BIAXIN FILMTAB TABLETS

(Clarithromycin) 402

May interact with oral anticoagulants, oral hypoglycemic agents, insulin, phenytoin, valproate, xanthines, and certain other agents. Compounds in these categories include:

Acarbose (Clarithromycin, in rare cases, causes hypoglycemia, some

of which have occurred in patients taking oral hypoglycemic agents). Products include:
Precose Tablets 751

Alfentanil Hydrochloride (Concurrent use of erythromycin and/or clarithromycin in patients receiving drugs metabolized by the cytochrome P450 system may be associated with elevation in serum levels of alfentanil).
No products indexed under this heading.

Aminophylline (Co-administration in patients who are receiving high doses of theophylline may be associated with an increase in serum theophylline levels and potential theophylline toxicity).
No products indexed under this heading.

Anisindione (Co-administration may result in the potentiation of oral anticoagulant effects). Products include:
Miradon Tablets 3042

Astemizole (Concurrent use of erythromycin in patients receiving astemizole has resulted in prolonged QT interval and torsade de pointes; because clarithromycin is metabolized by P450, co-administration is contraindicated).
No products indexed under this heading.

Bromocriptine Mesylate (Concurrent use of erythromycin and/or clarithromycin in patients receiving drugs metabolized by the cytochrome P450 system may be associated with elevation in serum levels of bromocriptine).
No products indexed under this heading.

Carbamazepine (Potential for increased serum concentration of carbamazepine). Products include:
Carbatrol Capsules 3171
Equetro Extended-Release Capsules 3180
Tegretol/Tegretol-XR 2295

Chlorpropamide (Clarithromycin, in rare cases, causes hypoglycemia, some of which have occurred in patients taking oral hypoglycemic agents).
No products indexed under this heading.

Cisapride (Concurrent use of erythromycin and/or clarithromycin in patients receiving cisapride has been reported to result in rare cases of cardiovascular adverse events including prolonged QT interval, ventricular tachycardia, ventricular fibrillation, and torsade de pointes, and death have been reported; co-administration is contraindicated).
No products indexed under this heading.

Colchicine (There have been post-marketing reports of colchicine toxicity with concomitant use of clarithromycin and colchicine, especially in the elderly, some of which occurred in patients with renal insufficiency).
No products indexed under this heading.

Cyclosporine (Concurrent use of erythromycin and/or clarithromycin in patients receiving drugs metabolized by the cytochrome P450 system may be associated with elevation in serum levels of cyclosporine). Products include:
Gengraf Capsules 459
Neoral Oral Solution 2259
Neoral Soft Gelatin Capsules 2259
Restasis Ophthalmic Emulsion 575
Sandimmune 2275

Dicumarol (Co-administration may result in the potentiation of oral anticoagulant effects).
No products indexed under this heading.

Digoxin (Concomitant use has resulted in elevated digoxin serum concentrations and some patients have shown signs of digoxin toxicity, including arrhythmias. Serum digoxin concentrations should be carefully monitored during co-administration). Products include:
Lanoxicaps Capsules 1490
Lanoxin Injection 1494
Lanoxin Injection Pediatric 1497
Lanoxin Tablets 1500

Dihydroergotamine Mesylate (Post-marketing reports indicate that co-administration of clarithromycin with dihydroergotamine has been associated with acute ergot toxicity characterized by vasospasm and ischemia of the extremities and other tissues including the central nervous system. Concomitant administration of clarithromycin with dihydroergotamine is contraindicated). Products include:
Migranal Nasal Spray 3348

Disopyramide Phosphate (Concurrent use of erythromycin and/or clarithromycin in patients receiving drugs metabolized by the cytochrome P450 system may be associated with elevation in serum levels of disopyramide).
No products indexed under this heading.

Divalproex Sodium (Concurrent use of erythromycin and/or clarithromycin in patients receiving drugs metabolized by the cytochrome P450 system may be associated with elevation in serum levels of valproate). Products include:
Depakote Sprinkle Capsules 422
Depakote Tablets 427
Depakote ER Tablets 434

Dyphylline (Co-administration in patients who are receiving high doses of theophylline may be associated with an increase in serum theophylline levels and potential theophylline toxicity).
No products indexed under this heading.

Ergotamine Tartrate (Post-marketing reports indicate that co-administration of clarithromycin with ergotamine has been associated with acute ergot toxicity characterized by vasospasm and ischemia of the extremities and other tissues including the central nervous system. Concomitant administration of clarithromycin with ergotamine is contraindicated).
No products indexed under this heading.

Fluconazole (Co-administration has resulted in increases in the mean steady-state clarithromycin Cmin and AUC).
No products indexed under this heading.

Fosphenytoin Sodium (Concurrent use of erythromycin and/or clarithromycin in patients receiving drugs metabolized by the cytochrome P450 system may be associated with elevation in serum levels of phenytoin).
No products indexed under this heading.

Glimepiride (Clarithromycin, in rare cases, causes hypoglycemia, some of which have occurred in patients taking oral hypoglycemic agents). Products include:
Avandaryl Tablets 1379
Duetact Tablets 3226

Glipizide (Clarithromycin, in rare cases, causes hypoglycemia, some of which have occurred in patients taking oral hypoglycemic agents).
No products indexed under this heading.

Glyburide (Clarithromycin, in rare cases, causes hypoglycemia, some of which have occurred in patients taking oral hypoglycemic agents).
No products indexed under this heading.

Hexobarbital (Concurrent use of erythromycin and/or clarithromycin in patients receiving drugs metabolized by the cytochrome P450 system may be associated with elevation in serum levels of hexobarbital).
No products indexed under this heading.

Insulin, Human, Zinc Suspension (Clarithromycin, in rare cases, causes hypoglycemia, some of which have occurred in patients taking insulin). Products include:
Humulin L, 100 Units 1794
Humulin U, 100 Units 1800

Insulin, Human NPH (Clarithromycin, in rare cases, causes hypoglycemia, some of which have occurred in patients taking insulin). Products include:
Humulin N, 100 Units 1795
Humulin N Pen 1797

Insulin, Human Regular (Clarithromycin, in rare cases, causes hypoglycemia, some of which have occurred in patients taking insulin). Products include:
Humulin R, 100 Units 1798

Insulin, Human Regular and Human NPH Mixture (Clarithromycin, in rare cases, causes hypoglycemia, some of which have occurred in patients taking insulin). Products include:
Humulin 50/50, 100 Units 1791
Humulin 70/30 Pen 1793

Insulin, NPH (Clarithromycin, in rare cases, causes hypoglycemia, some of which have occurred in patients taking insulin).
No products indexed under this heading.

Insulin, Regular (Clarithromycin, in rare cases, causes hypoglycemia, some of which have occurred in patients taking insulin).
No products indexed under this heading.

Insulin, Zinc Crystals (Clarithromycin, in rare cases, causes hypoglycemia, some of which have occurred in patients taking insulin).
No products indexed under this heading.

Insulin, Zinc Suspension (Clarithromycin, in rare cases, causes hypoglycemia, some of which have occurred in patients taking insulin).
No products indexed under this heading.

Insulin Aspart, Human Regular (Clarithromycin, in rare cases, causes hypoglycemia, some of which have occurred in patients taking insulin). Products include:
NovoLog Injection 2326

Insulin glargine (Clarithromycin, in rare cases, causes hypoglycemia, some of which have occurred in patients taking insulin). Products include:
Lantus Injection 2909

Insulin Lispro, Human (Clarithromycin, in rare cases, causes hypoglycemia, some of which have occurred in patients taking insulin). Products include:
Humalog-Pen 1781
Humalog Mix 50/50-Pen 1783
Humalog Mix 75/25-Pen 1785

Insulin Lispro Protamine, Human (Clarithromycin, in rare cases, causes hypoglycemia, some of which have occurred in patients taking insulin). Products include:
Humalog Mix 50/50-Pen 1783
Humalog Mix 75/25-Pen 1785

Lovastatin (As with other macrolides, clarithromycin has been reported to increase concentrations of HMG-CoA reductase inhibitors, such as lovastatin, through inhibition of CYP450 metabolism of simvastatin; rare cases of rhabdomyolysis have been reported). Products include:
Advicor Tablets 1722
Altoprev Extended-Release Tablets 3109
Mevacor Tablets 2021

Metformin Hydrochloride (Clarithromycin, in rare cases, causes hypoglycemia, some of which have occurred in patients taking oral hypoglycemic agents). Products include:
ActoPlus Met Tablets 3214
Avandamet Tablets 1373
Fortamet Extended-Release Tablets 3115

Miglitol (Clarithromycin, in rare cases, causes hypoglycemia, some of which have occurred in patients taking oral hypoglycemic agents).
No products indexed under this heading.

Omeprazole (Co-administration increases the steady-state plasma concentrations, Cmax, AUC 0-24, and T 1/2 of omeprazole). Products include:
Zegerid Capsules 2958
Zegerid Powder for Oral Solution 2958

Phenytoin (Concurrent use of erythromycin and/or clarithromycin in patients receiving drugs metabolized by the cytochrome P450 system may be associated with elevation in serum levels of phenytoin).
No products indexed under this heading.

Phenytoin Sodium (Concurrent use of erythromycin and/or clarithromycin in patients receiving drugs metabolized by the cytochrome P450 system may be associated with elevation in serum levels of phenytoin). Products include:
Phenytek Capsules 2160

Pimozide (Concurrent use of erythromycin and/or clarithromycin in patients receiving pimozide has been reported to result in rare cases of cardiovascular adverse events including prolonged QT interval, ventricular tachycardia, ventricular fibrillation, and torsade de pointes, and death; co-administration is contraindicated).
No products indexed under this heading.

Pioglitazone Hydrochloride (Clarithromycin, in rare cases, causes hypoglycemia, some of which have occurred in patients taking oral hypoglycemic agents). Products include:

ActoPlus Met Tablets 3214
Actos Tablets 3219
Duetact Tablets 3226

Ranitidine Bismuth Citrate (Co-administration has resulted in increased plasma ranitidine concentrations (57%), increased plasma bismuth trough concentrations (48%), and increased 14-hydroxy-clarithromycin plasma concentrations (31%); these effects are clinically insignificant).

No products indexed under this heading.

Repaglinide (Clarithromycin, in rare cases, causes hypoglycemia, some of which have occurred in patients taking oral hypoglycemic agents).

No products indexed under this heading.

Ritonavir (Co-administration has resulted in a 77% increase in clarithromycin AUC and a 100% decrease in the AUC of 14-OH clarithromycin; dosage adjustments may be needed if clarithromycin is administered to patients with renal impairment). Products include:

Kaletra 476
Norvir 503

Rosiglitazone Maleate (Clarithromycin, in rare cases, causes hypoglycemia, some of which have occurred in patients taking oral hypoglycemic agents). Products include:

Avandamet Tablets 1373
Avandaryl Tablets 1379
Avandia Tablets 1384

Simvastatin (As with other macrolides, clarithromycin has been reported to increase concentrations of HMG-CoA reductase inhibitors, such as simvastatin, through inhibition of CYP450 metabolism of simvastatin; rare cases of rhabdomyolysis have been reported). Products include:

Vytorin 10/10 Tablets 2114
Vytorin 10/10 Tablets 3077
Vytorin 10/20 Tablets 2114
Vytorin 10/20 Tablets 3077
Vytorin 10/40 Tablets 2114
Vytorin 10/40 Tablets 3077
Vytorin 10/80 Tablets 2114
Vytorin 10/80 Tablets 3077
Zocor Tablets 2105

Tacrolimus (Concurrent use of erythromycin and/or clarithromycin in patients receiving drugs metabolized by the cytochrome P450 system may be associated with elevation in serum levels of tacrolimus). Products include:

Prograf Capsules and Injection 632
Protopic Ointment 638

Terfenadine (Co-administration has resulted in increase in active metabolite of terfenadine by 3-fold; rare cases of cardiovascular adverse events including prolonged QT interval, ventricular tachycardia, ventricular fibrillation, and torsade de pointes, and death have been reported; co-administration is contraindicated).

No products indexed under this heading.

Theophylline (Co-administration in patients who are receiving high doses of theophylline may be associated with an increase in serum theophylline levels and potential theophylline toxicity).

No products indexed under this heading.

Theophylline Anhydrous (Co-administration in patients who are receiving high doses of theophylline may be associated with an increase in serum theophylline levels and potential theophylline toxicity). Products include:

Uniphyl Tablets 2710

Theophylline Calcium Salicylate (Co-administration in patients who are receiving high doses of theophylline may be associated with an increase in serum theophylline levels and potential theophylline toxicity).

No products indexed under this heading.

Theophylline Dihydroxypropyl (Glyceryl) (Co-administration in patients who are receiving high doses of theophylline may be associated with an increase in serum theophylline levels and potential theophylline toxicity).

No products indexed under this heading.

Theophylline Ethylenediamine (Co-administration in patients who are receiving high doses of theophylline may be associated with an increase in serum theophylline levels and potential theophylline toxicity).

No products indexed under this heading.

Theophylline Sodium Glycinate (Co-administration in patients who are receiving high doses of theophylline may be associated with an increase in serum theophylline levels and potential theophylline toxicity).

No products indexed under this heading.

Tolazamide (Clarithromycin, in rare cases, causes hypoglycemia, some of which have occurred in patients taking oral hypoglycemic agents).

No products indexed under this heading.

Tolbutamide (Clarithromycin, in rare cases, causes hypoglycemia, some of which have occurred in patients taking oral hypoglycemic agents).

No products indexed under this heading.

Triazolam (Erythromycin, another macrolide antibiotic, has been reported to decrease the clearance of triazolam and, thus, may increase the pharmacologic effect of the triazolam; concomitant use has resulted in somnolence and confusion).

No products indexed under this heading.

Troglitazone (Clarithromycin, in rare cases, causes hypoglycemia, some of which have occurred in patients taking oral hypoglycemic agents).

No products indexed under this heading.

Valproate Sodium (Concurrent use of erythromycin and/or clarithromycin in patients receiving drugs metabolized by the cytochrome P450 system may be associated with elevation in serum levels of valproate). Products include:

Depacon Injection 412

Valproic Acid (Concurrent use of erythromycin and/or clarithromycin in patients receiving drugs metabolized by the cytochrome P450 system may be associated with elevation in serum levels of valproate). Products include:

Depakene 417

Warfarin Sodium (Co-administration may result in the potentiation of oral anticoagulant effects). Products include:

Coumadin for Injection 898
Coumadin Tablets 898

Zidovudine (Potential for decreased steady-state zidovudine concentration). Products include:

Combivir Tablets 1411
Retrovir 1560
Retrovir IV Infusion 1564
Trizivir Tablets 1589

Food Interactions

Food, unspecified (Food slightly delays both the onset of absorption and the formation of the active metabolite, but does not affect the extent of bioavailability; Biaxin may be administered without regard to food).

BIAXIN XL FILMTAB TABLETS

(Clarithromycin) 402
See Biaxin Filmtab Tablets

BIAXIN GRANULES

(Clarithromycin) 402
See Biaxin Filmtab Tablets

BICILLIN C-R INJECTABLE SUSPENSION

(Penicillin G Benzathine, Penicillin G Procaine) 1706

May interact with bacteriostatic antibiotics, parenteral tetracyclines, tetracyclines, and certain other agents. Compounds in these categories include:

Chloramphenicol (A bacteriostatic antibiotic may antagonize the bactericidal effect of penicillin, and concurrent use of these drugs should be avoided).

No products indexed under this heading.

Chloramphenicol Palmitate (A bacteriostatic antibiotic may antagonize the bactericidal effect of penicillin, and concurrent use of these drugs should be avoided).

No products indexed under this heading.

Chloramphenicol Sodium Succinate (A bacteriostatic antibiotic may antagonize the bactericidal effect of penicillin, and concurrent use of these drugs should be avoided).

No products indexed under this heading.

Demeclocycline Hydrochloride (A bacteriostatic antibiotic may antagonize the bactericidal effect of penicillin, and concurrent use of these drugs should be avoided).

No products indexed under this heading.

Doxycycline Calcium (A bacteriostatic antibiotic may antagonize the bactericidal effect of penicillin, and concurrent use of these drugs should be avoided).

No products indexed under this heading.

Doxycycline Hyclate (A bacteriostatic antibiotic may antagonize the bactericidal effect of penicillin, and concurrent use of these drugs should be avoided).

No products indexed under this heading.

Doxycycline Monohydrate (A bacteriostatic antibiotic may antagonize the bactericidal effect of penicillin, and concurrent use of these drugs should be avoided). Products include:

Oracea Capsules 1000

Erythromycin (A bacteriostatic antibiotic may antagonize the bactericidal effect of penicillin, and concurrent use of these drugs should be avoided). Products include:

Ery-Tab Tablets 449
Erythromycin Base Filmtab Tablets 455
Erythromycin Delayed-Release Capsules, USP 457
PCE Dispertab Tablets 515

Erythromycin Estolate (A bacteriostatic antibiotic may antagonize the bactericidal effect of penicillin, and concurrent use of these drugs should be avoided).

No products indexed under this heading.

Erythromycin Ethylsuccinate (A bacteriostatic antibiotic may antagonize the bactericidal effect of penicillin, and concurrent use of these drugs should be avoided). Products include:

E.E.S. 451
EryPed 447

Erythromycin Gluceptate (A bacteriostatic antibiotic may antagonize the bactericidal effect of penicillin, and concurrent use of these drugs should be avoided).

No products indexed under this heading.

Erythromycin Stearate (A bacteriostatic antibiotic may antagonize the bactericidal effect of penicillin, and concurrent use of these drugs should be avoided). Products include:

Erythrocin Stearate Filmtab Tablets 453

Methacycline Hydrochloride (A bacteriostatic antibiotic may antagonize the bactericidal effect of penicillin, and concurrent use of these drugs should be avoided).

No products indexed under this heading.

Minocycline Hydrochloride (A bacteriostatic antibiotic may antagonize the bactericidal effect of penicillin, and concurrent use of these drugs should be avoided). Products include:

Solodyn Extended Release Tablets 1890

Oxytetracycline (A bacteriostatic antibiotic may antagonize the bactericidal effect of penicillin, and concurrent use of these drugs should be avoided).

No products indexed under this heading.

Oxytetracycline Hydrochloride (A bacteriostatic antibiotic may antagonize the bactericidal effect of penicillin, and concurrent use of these drugs should be avoided).

No products indexed under this heading.

Probenecid (Concurrent administration of penicillin and probenecid increases and prolongs serum penicillin levels by decreasing the apparent volume of distribution and slowing the rate of excretion by competitively inhibiting renal tubular secretion of penicillin).
No products indexed under this heading.

Sulfamethizole (A bacteriostatic antibiotic may antagonize the bactericidal effect of penicillin, and concurrent use of these drugs should be avoided).
No products indexed under this heading.

Sulfamethoxazole (A bacteriostatic antibiotic may antagonize the bactericidal effect of penicillin, and concurrent use of these drugs should be avoided).
No products indexed under this heading.

Sulfisoxazole Acetyl (A bacteriostatic antibiotic may antagonize the bactericidal effect of penicillin, and concurrent use of these drugs should be avoided).
No products indexed under this heading.

Tetracycline Hydrochloride (A bacteriostatic antibiotic may antagonize the bactericidal effect of penicillin, and concurrent use of these drugs should be avoided).
No products indexed under this heading.

BIDIL TABLETS

(Hydralazine Hydrochloride, Isosorbide Dinitrate) 2171
May interact with antihypertensives, monoamine oxidase inhibitors, vasodilators, and certain other agents. Compounds in these categories include:

Acebutolol Hydrochloride (Increased risk of hypotension with concomitant antihypertensive drugs. Patients treated with BiDil who receive any potent parenteral antihypertensive agent should be continuously observed for several hours for excessive fall in blood pressure).
No products indexed under this heading.

Amlodipine Besylate (Increased risk of hypotension with concomitant antihypertensive drugs. Patients treated with BiDil who receive any potent parenteral antihypertensive agent should be continuously observed for several hours for excessive fall in blood pressure). Products include:
Caduet Tablets 2508
Lotrel Capsules 2249
Norvasc Tablets 2545

Amyl Nitrite (The effects of BiDil on vasodilators may be additive).
No products indexed under this heading.

Atenolol (Increased risk of hypotension with concomitant antihypertensive drugs. Patients treated with BiDil who receive any potent parenteral antihypertensive agent should be continuously observed for several hours for excessive fall in blood pressure).
No products indexed under this heading.

Benazepril Hydrochloride (Increased risk of hypotension with concomitant antihypertensive drugs. Patients treated with BiDil who receive any potent parenteral antihypertensive agent should be continuously observed for several hours for excessive fall in blood pressure). Products include:
Lotensin Tablets 2243
Lotensin HCT Tablets 2246
Lotrel Capsules 2249

Bendroflumethiazide (Increased risk of hypotension with concomitant antihypertensive drugs. Patients treated with BiDil who receive any potent parenteral antihypertensive agent should be continuously observed for several hours for excessive fall in blood pressure).
No products indexed under this heading.

Betaxolol Hydrochloride (Increased risk of hypotension with concomitant antihypertensive drugs. Patients treated with BiDil who receive any potent parenteral antihypertensive agent should be continuously observed for several hours for excessive fall in blood pressure). Products include:
Betoptic S Ophthalmic Suspension 558

Bisoprolol Fumarate (Increased risk of hypotension with concomitant antihypertensive drugs. Patients treated with BiDil who receive any potent parenteral antihypertensive agent should be continuously observed for several hours for excessive fall in blood pressure).
No products indexed under this heading.

Candesartan Cilexetil (Increased risk of hypotension with concomitant antihypertensive drugs. Patients treated with BiDil who receive any potent parenteral antihypertensive agent should be continuously observed for several hours for excessive fall in blood pressure). Products include:
Atacand Tablets 649
Atacand HCT 651

Captopril (Increased risk of hypotension with concomitant antihypertensive drugs. Patients treated with BiDil who receive any potent parenteral antihypertensive agent should be continuously observed for several hours for excessive fall in blood pressure). Products include:
Captopril Tablets 2149

Carteolol Hydrochloride (Increased risk of hypotension with concomitant antihypertensive drugs. Patients treated with BiDil who receive any potent parenteral antihypertensive agent should be continuously observed for several hours for excessive fall in blood pressure). Products include:
Carteolol Hydrochloride Ophthalmic Solution USP, 1% .... ⊙249

Chlorothiazide (Increased risk of hypotension with concomitant antihypertensive drugs. Patients treated with BiDil who receive any potent parenteral antihypertensive agent should be continuously observed for several hours for excessive fall in blood pressure). Products include:
Diuril Oral Suspension 1954

Chlorothiazide Sodium (Increased risk of hypotension with concomitant antihypertensive drugs. Patients treated with BiDil who receive any potent parenteral antihypertensive agent should be continuously observed for several hours for excessive fall in blood pressure). Products include:
Diuril Sodium Intravenous 2467

Chlorthalidone (Increased risk of hypotension with concomitant antihypertensive drugs. Patients treated with BiDil who receive any potent parenteral antihypertensive agent should be continuously observed for several hours for excessive fall in blood pressure). Products include:
Clorpres Tablets 2153

Clonidine (Increased risk of hypotension with concomitant antihypertensive drugs. Patients treated with BiDil who receive any potent parenteral antihypertensive agent should be continuously observed for several hours for excessive fall in blood pressure). Products include:
Catapres-TTS 844

Clonidine Hydrochloride (Increased risk of hypotension with concomitant antihypertensive drugs. Patients treated with BiDil who receive any potent parenteral antihypertensive agent should be continuously observed for several hours for excessive fall in blood pressure). Products include:
Catapres Tablets 843
Clorpres Tablets 2153

Deserpidine (Increased risk of hypotension with concomitant antihypertensive drugs. Patients treated with BiDil who receive any potent parenteral antihypertensive agent should be continuously observed for several hours for excessive fall in blood pressure).
No products indexed under this heading.

Diazoxide (Increased risk of hypotension with concomitant antihypertensive drugs. Patients treated with BiDil who receive any potent parenteral antihypertensive agent should be continuously observed for several hours for excessive fall in blood pressure). Products include:
Hyperstat I.V. 3017

Diltiazem Hydrochloride (Increased risk of hypotension with concomitant antihypertensive drugs. Patients treated with BiDil who receive any potent parenteral antihypertensive agent should be continuously observed for several hours for excessive fall in blood pressure). Products include:
Cardizem LA Extended Release Tablets 1728
Tiazac Capsules 1201

Doxazosin Mesylate (Increased risk of hypotension with concomitant antihypertensive drugs. Patients treated with BiDil who receive any potent parenteral antihypertensive agent should be continuously observed for several hours for excessive fall in blood pressure). Products include:
Cardura XL Tablets 2515

Enalapril Maleate (Increased risk of hypotension with concomitant antihypertensive drugs. Patients treated with BiDil who receive any potent parenteral antihypertensive agent should be continuously observed for several hours for excessive fall in blood pressure). Products include:
Vasotec I.V. Injection 2103

Enalaprilat (Increased risk of hypotension with concomitant antihypertensive drugs. Patients treated with BiDil who receive any potent parenteral antihypertensive agent should be continuously observed for several hours for excessive fall in blood pressure).
No products indexed under this heading.

Epoprostenol Sodium (The effects of BiDil on vasodilators may be additive).
No products indexed under this heading.

Eprosartan Mesylate (Increased risk of hypotension with concomitant antihypertensive drugs. Patients treated with BiDil who receive any potent parenteral antihypertensive agent should be continuously observed for several hours for excessive fall in blood pressure). Products include:
Teveten Tablets 1735
Teveten HCT Tablets 1737

Esmolol Hydrochloride (Increased risk of hypotension with concomitant antihypertensive drugs. Patients treated with BiDil who receive any potent parenteral antihypertensive agent should be continuously observed for several hours for excessive fall in blood pressure).
No products indexed under this heading.

Ethanol (The effects of BiDil on vasodilators, including alcohol, may be additive).
No products indexed under this heading.

Ethaverine Hydrochloride (The effects of BiDil on vasodilators may be additive).
No products indexed under this heading.

Felodipine (Increased risk of hypotension with concomitant antihypertensive drugs. Patients treated with BiDil who receive any potent parenteral antihypertensive agent should be continuously observed for several hours for excessive fall in blood pressure).
No products indexed under this heading.

Fosinopril Sodium (Increased risk of hypotension with concomitant antihypertensive drugs. Patients treated with BiDil who receive any potent parenteral antihypertensive agent should be continuously observed for several hours for excessive fall in blood pressure).
No products indexed under this heading.

Furosemide (Increased risk of hypotension with concomitant antihypertensive drugs. Patients treated with BiDil who receive any potent parenteral antihypertensive agent should be continuously observed for several hours for excessive fall in blood pressure). Products include:
Furosemide Tablets 2154

Guanabenz Acetate (Increased risk of hypotension with concomitant antihypertensive drugs. Patients treated with BiDil who receive any potent parenteral antihypertensive agent should be continuously observed for several hours for excessive fall in blood pressure).
No products indexed under this heading.

Guanethidine Monosulfate
(Increased risk of hypotension with concomitant antihypertensive drugs. Patients treated with BiDil who receive any potent parenteral antihypertensive agent should be continuously observed for several hours for excessive fall in blood pressure).
No products indexed under this heading.

Hydrochlorothiazide (Increased risk of hypotension with concomitant antihypertensive drugs. Patients treated with BiDil who receive any potent parenteral antihypertensive agent should be continuously observed for several hours for excessive fall in blood pressure). Products include:

Hydroflumethiazide (Increased risk of hypotension with concomitant antihypertensive drugs. Patients treated with BiDil who receive any potent parenteral antihypertensive agent should be continuously observed for several hours for excessive fall in blood pressure).
No products indexed under this heading.

Indapamide (Increased risk of hypotension with concomitant antihypertensive drugs. Patients treated with BiDil who receive any potent parenteral antihypertensive agent should be continuously observed for several hours for excessive fall in blood pressure). Products include:

Irbesartan (Increased risk of hypotension with concomitant antihypertensive drugs. Patients treated with BiDil who receive any potent parenteral antihypertensive agent should be continuously observed for several hours for excessive fall in blood pressure). Products include:

Isocarboxazid (Due to the hydralazine component of BiDil, monoamine oxidase inhibitors should be used with caution in patients receiving BiDil).
No products indexed under this heading.

Isosorbide Mononitrate (The effects of BiDil on vasodilators may be additive). Products include:

Isoxsuprine Hydrochloride (The effects of BiDil on vasodilators may be additive).
No products indexed under this heading.

Isradipine (Increased risk of hypotension with concomitant antihypertensive drugs. Patients treated with

BiDil who receive any potent parenteral antihypertensive agent should be continuously observed for several hours for excessive fall in blood pressure). Products include:

Labetalol Hydrochloride
(Increased risk of hypotension with concomitant antihypertensive drugs. Patients treated with BiDil who receive any potent parenteral antihypertensive agent should be continuously observed for several hours for excessive fall in blood pressure).
No products indexed under this heading.

Lisinopril (Increased risk of hypotension with concomitant antihypertensive drugs. Patients treated with BiDil who receive any potent parenteral antihypertensive agent should be continuously observed for several hours for excessive fall in blood pressure). Products include:

Losartan Potassium (Increased risk of hypotension with concomitant antihypertensive drugs. Patients treated with BiDil who receive any potent parenteral antihypertensive agent should be continuously observed for several hours for excessive fall in blood pressure). Products include:

Mecamylamine Hydrochloride
(Increased risk of hypotension with concomitant antihypertensive drugs. Patients treated with BiDil who receive any potent parenteral antihypertensive agent should be continuously observed for several hours for excessive fall in blood pressure).
No products indexed under this heading.

Methyclothiazide (Increased risk of hypotension with concomitant antihypertensive drugs. Patients treated with BiDil who receive any potent parenteral antihypertensive agent should be continuously observed for several hours for excessive fall in blood pressure).
No products indexed under this heading.

Methyldopa (Increased risk of hypotension with concomitant antihypertensive drugs. Patients treated with BiDil who receive any potent parenteral antihypertensive agent should be continuously observed for several hours for excessive fall in blood pressure). Products include:

Methyldopate Hydrochloride
(Increased risk of hypotension with concomitant antihypertensive drugs. Patients treated with BiDil who receive any potent parenteral antihypertensive agent should be continuously observed for several hours for excessive fall in blood pressure).
No products indexed under this heading.

Metolazone (Increased risk of hypotension with concomitant antihypertensive drugs. Patients treated with BiDil who receive any potent parenteral antihypertensive agent should be continuously observed for several hours for excessive fall in blood pressure).
No products indexed under this heading.

Metoprolol Succinate (Increased risk of hypotension with concomitant antihypertensive drugs. Patients treated with BiDil who receive any potent parenteral antihypertensive agent should be continuously observed for several hours for excessive fall in blood pressure). Products include:

Metoprolol Tartrate (Increased risk of hypotension with concomitant antihypertensive drugs. Patients treated with BiDil who receive any potent parenteral antihypertensive agent should be continuously observed for several hours for excessive fall in blood pressure). Products include:

Metyrosine (Increased risk of hypotension with concomitant antihypertensive drugs. Patients treated with BiDil who receive any potent parenteral antihypertensive agent should be continuously observed for several hours for excessive fall in blood pressure). Products include:

Mibefradil Dihydrochloride
(Increased risk of hypotension with concomitant antihypertensive drugs. Patients treated with BiDil who receive any potent parenteral antihypertensive agent should be continuously observed for several hours for excessive fall in blood pressure).
No products indexed under this heading.

Minoxidil (Increased risk of hypotension with concomitant antihypertensive drugs. Patients treated with BiDil who receive any potent parenteral antihypertensive agent should be continuously observed for several hours for excessive fall in blood pressure). Products include:

Moclobemide (Due to the hydralazine component of BiDil, monoamine oxidase inhibitors should be used with caution in patients receiving BiDil).
No products indexed under this heading.

Moexipril Hydrochloride
(Increased risk of hypotension with concomitant antihypertensive drugs. Patients treated with BiDil who receive any potent parenteral antihypertensive agent should be continuously observed for several hours for excessive fall in blood pressure). Products include:

Nadolol (Increased risk of hypotension with concomitant antihypertensive drugs. Patients treated with BiDil who receive any potent parenteral antihypertensive agent should be continuously observed for several hours for excessive fall in blood pressure). Products include:

Nicardipine Hydrochloride
(Increased risk of hypotension with concomitant antihypertensive drugs. Patients treated with BiDil who receive any potent parenteral antihypertensive agent should be continuously observed for several hours for excessive fall in blood pressure). Products include:

Nifedipine (Increased risk of hypotension with concomitant antihypertensive drugs. Patients treated with BiDil who receive any potent parenteral antihypertensive agent should be continuously observed for several hours for excessive fall in blood pressure). Products include:

Nisoldipine (Increased risk of hypotension with concomitant antihypertensive drugs. Patients treated with BiDil who receive any potent parenteral antihypertensive agent should be continuously observed for several hours for excessive fall in blood pressure). Products include:

Nitroglycerin (Increased risk of hypotension with concomitant antihypertensive drugs. Patients treated with BiDil who receive any potent parenteral antihypertensive agent should be continuously observed for several hours for excessive fall in blood pressure). Products include:

Nitroglycerin, long-acting formulations (The effects of BiDil on vasodilators may be additive).
No products indexed under this heading.

Nitroglycerin Intravenous (The effects of BiDil on vasodilators may be additive).
No products indexed under this heading.

Papaverine (The effects of BiDil on vasodilators may be additive).
No products indexed under this heading.

Papaverine Hydrochloride (The effects of BiDil on vasodilators may be additive).
No products indexed under this heading.

Pargyline Hydrochloride (Due to the hydralazine component of BiDil, monoamine oxidase inhibitors should be used with caution in patients receiving BiDil).
No products indexed under this heading.

Penbutolol Sulfate (Increased risk of hypotension with concomitant antihypertensive drugs. Patients treated with BiDil who receive any potent parenteral antihypertensive agent should be continuously observed for several hours for excessive fall in blood pressure).
No products indexed under this heading.

Perindopril Erbumine (Increased risk of hypotension with concomitant antihypertensive drugs. Patients treated with BiDil who receive any potent parenteral antihypertensive agent should be continuously observed for several hours for excessive fall in blood pressure). Products include:

Phenelzine Sulfate (Due to the hydralazine component of BiDil, monoamine oxidase inhibitors should be used with caution in patients receiving BiDil).
No products indexed under this heading.

Phenoxybenzamine Hydrochloride (Increased risk of hypotension with concomitant antihypertensive drugs. Patients treated with BiDil who receive any potent parenteral antihypertensive agent should be continuously observed for several hours for excessive fall in blood pressure). Products include:
Dibenzyline Capsules 3399

Phentolamine Mesylate (Increased risk of hypotension with concomitant antihypertensive drugs. Patients treated with BiDil who receive any potent parenteral antihypertensive agent should be continuously observed for several hours for excessive fall in blood pressure).
No products indexed under this heading.

Pindolol (Increased risk of hypotension with concomitant antihypertensive drugs. Patients treated with BiDil who receive any potent parenteral antihypertensive agent should be continuously observed for several hours for excessive fall in blood pressure).
No products indexed under this heading.

Polythiazide (Increased risk of hypotension with concomitant antihypertensive drugs. Patients treated with BiDil who receive any potent parenteral antihypertensive agent should be continuously observed for several hours for excessive fall in blood pressure).
No products indexed under this heading.

Prazosin Hydrochloride (Increased risk of hypotension with concomitant antihypertensive drugs. Patients treated with BiDil who receive any potent parenteral antihypertensive agent should be continuously observed for several hours for excessive fall in blood pressure).
No products indexed under this heading.

Procarbazine Hydrochloride (Due to the hydralazine component of BiDil, monoamine oxidase inhibitors should be used with caution in patients receiving BiDil). Products include:
Matulane Capsules 3191

Propranolol Hydrochloride (Increased risk of hypotension with concomitant antihypertensive drugs. Patients treated with BiDil who receive any potent parenteral antihypertensive agent should be continuously observed for several hours for excessive fall in blood pressure). Products include:
Inderal LA Long-Acting Capsules 3429
InnoPran XL Capsules 2723

Quinapril Hydrochloride (Increased risk of hypotension with concomitant antihypertensive drugs. Patients treated with BiDil who receive any potent parenteral antihypertensive agent should be continuously observed for several hours for excessive fall in blood pressure).
No products indexed under this heading.

Ramipril (Increased risk of hypotension with concomitant antihyperten-

sive drugs. Patients treated with BiDil who receive any potent parenteral antihypertensive agent should be continuously observed for several hours for excessive fall in blood pressure). Products include:
Altace Capsules 1702

Rauwolfia Serpentina (Increased risk of hypotension with concomitant antihypertensive drugs. Patients treated with BiDil who receive any potent parenteral antihypertensive agent should be continuously observed for several hours for excessive fall in blood pressure).
No products indexed under this heading.

Rescinnamine (Increased risk of hypotension with concomitant antihypertensive drugs. Patients treated with BiDil who receive any potent parenteral antihypertensive agent should be continuously observed for several hours for excessive fall in blood pressure).
No products indexed under this heading.

Reserpine (Increased risk of hypotension with concomitant antihypertensive drugs. Patients treated with BiDil who receive any potent parenteral antihypertensive agent should be continuously observed for several hours for excessive fall in blood pressure).
No products indexed under this heading.

Selegiline Hydrochloride (Due to the hydralazine component of BiDil, monoamine oxidase inhibitors should be used with caution in patients receiving BiDil). Products include:
Eldepryl Capsules 3208
Zelapar Tablets 3372

Sildenafil Citrate (Augmentation of the vasodilatory effects of isosorbide dinitrate by phosphodiesterase inhibitors, such as sildenafil, could result in severe hypotension. The time course and dose dependence of this interaction have not been studied. Reasonable supportivecare should consist of those measures used to treat a nitrate overdose with elevation of the extremities and central volume expansion). Products include:
Revatio Tablets 2557
Viagra Tablets 2573

Sodium Nitroprusside (Increased risk of hypotension with concomitant antihypertensive drugs. Patients treated with BiDil who receive any potent parenteral antihypertensive agent should be continuously observed for several hours for excessive fall in blood pressure).
No products indexed under this heading.

Sotalol Hydrochloride (Increased risk of hypotension with concomitant antihypertensive drugs. Patients treated with BiDil who receive any potent parenteral antihypertensive agent should be continuously observed for several hours for excessive fall in blood pressure).
No products indexed under this heading.

Spirapril Hydrochloride (Increased risk of hypotension with concomitant antihypertensive drugs. Patients treated with BiDil who receive any potent parenteral antihypertensive agent should be continuously observed for several hours for excessive fall in blood pressure).
No products indexed under this heading.

Tadalafil (Augmentation of the vasodilatory effects of isosorbide dinitrate by phosphodiesterase inhibitors, such as tadalafil, could result in severe hypotension. The time course and dose dependence of this interaction have not been studied. Reasonable supportive care should consist of those measures used to treat a nitrate overdose with elevation of the extremities and central volume expansion). Products include:
Cialis Tablets 1838

Telmisartan (Increased risk of hypotension with concomitant antihypertensive drugs. Patients treated with BiDil who receive any potent parenteral antihypertensive agent should be continuously observed for several hours for excessive fall in blood pressure). Products include:
Micardis Tablets 854
Micardis HCT Tablets 856

Terazosin Hydrochloride (Increased risk of hypotension with concomitant antihypertensive drugs. Patients treated with BiDil who receive any potent parenteral antihypertensive agent should be continuously observed for several hours for excessive fall in blood pressure). Products include:
Hytrin Capsules 471

Timolol Maleate (Increased risk of hypotension with concomitant antihypertensive drugs. Patients treated with BiDil who receive any potent parenteral antihypertensive agent should be continuously observed for several hours for excessive fall in blood pressure). Products include:
Blocadren Tablets 1916
Cosopt Sterile Ophthalmic
Solution... 1931
Timolide Tablets 2086
Timoptic Sterile Ophthalmic
Solution... 2088
Timoptic in Ocudose 2091
Timoptic-XE Sterile Ophthalmic
Gel Forming Solution 2092

Tolazoline Hydrochloride (The effects of BiDil on vasodilators may be additive).
No products indexed under this heading.

Torsemide (Increased risk of hypotension with concomitant antihypertensive drugs. Patients treated with BiDil who receive any potent parenteral antihypertensive agent should be continuously observed for several hours for excessive fall in blood pressure). Products include:
Demadex Injection 2759
Demadex Tablets 2759

Trandolapril (Increased risk of hypotension with concomitant antihypertensive drugs. Patients treated with BiDil who receive any potent parenteral antihypertensive agent should be continuously observed for several hours for excessive fall in blood pressure). Products include:
Mavik Tablets 486
Tarka Tablets 524

Tranylcypromine Sulfate (Due to the hydralazine component of BiDil, monoamine oxidase inhibitors should be used with caution in patients receiving BiDil). Products include:
Parnate Tablets 1527

Trimethaphan Camsylate (Increased risk of hypotension with concomitant antihypertensive drugs. Patients treated with BiDil who receive any potent parenteral antihypertensive agent should be continuously observed for several hours for excessive fall in blood pressure).
No products indexed under this heading.

Valsartan (Increased risk of hypotension with concomitant antihypertensive drugs. Patients treated with BiDil who receive any potent parenteral antihypertensive agent should be continuously observed for several hours for excessive fall in blood pressure). Products include:
Diovan Tablets 2193
Diovan HCT Tablets 2196

Vardenafil Hydrochloride (Augmentation of the vasodilatory effects of isosorbide dinitrate by phosphodiesterase inhibitors, such as vardenafil, could result in severe hypotension. The time course and dose dependence of this interaction have not been studied. Reasonable supportivecare should consist of those measures used to treat a nitrate overdose with elevation of the extremities and central volume expansion). Products include:
Levitra Tablets 3034

Verapamil Hydrochloride (Increased risk of hypotension with concomitant antihypertensive drugs. Patients treated with BiDil who receive any potent parenteral antihypertensive agent should be continuously observed for several hours for excessive fall in blood pressure). Products include:
Covera-HS Tablets 3139
Tarka Tablets 524
Verelan PM Extended-Release
Capsules, Controlled-Onset........... 3106

Food Interactions

Alcohol (The effects of BiDil on vasodilators, including alcohol, may be additive).

BILTRICIDE TABLETS
(Praziquantel) 2976
May interact with cytochrome p450 1a2 inducers (selected), cytochrome p450 1a2 inhibitors (selected), cytochrome p450 2c19 inducers (selected), cytochrome p450 2c19 inhibitors (selected), cytochrome p450 2c8 inducers (selected), cytochrome p450 2c8 inhibitors (selected), cytochrome p450 2c9 inducers (selected), cytochrome p450 2c9 inhibitors (selected), cytochrome p450 2d6 inducers (selected), cytochrome p450 2d6 inhibitors (selected), cytochrome p450 3a4 inducers (selected), cytochrome p450 3a4 inhibitors (selected), cytochrome p450 3a inducers (selected), cytochrome p450 3a inhibitors (selected), and certain other agents. Compounds in these categories include:

Acetazolamide (Concomitant administration of drugs that decrease the activity of drug metabolizing liver enzymes (Cytochrome P450) may increase plasma levels of praziquantel).
No products indexed under this heading.

Alatrofloxacin Mesylate (Concomitant administration of drugs that decrease the activity of drug metabolizing liver enzymes (Cytochrome P450) may increase plasma levels of praziqua).

No products indexed under this heading.

Allium sativum (Concomitant administration of drugs that increase the activity of drug metabolizing liver enzymes (Cytochrome P450) may reduce plasma levels of praziquantel).

No products indexed under this heading.

Amiodarone Hydrochloride (Concomitant administration of drugs that decrease the activity of drug metabolizing liver enzymes (Cytochrome P450) may increase plasma levels of praziqua).

No products indexed under this heading.

Amitriptyline Hydrochloride (Concomitant administration of drugs that decrease the activity of drug metabolizing liver enzymes (Cytochrome P450) may increase plasma levels of praziquantel).

No products indexed under this heading.

Amoxapine (Concomitant administration of drugs that decrease the activity of drug metabolizing liver enzymes (Cytochrome P450) may increase plasma levels of praziquantel).

No products indexed under this heading.

Amprenavir (Concomitant administration of drugs that decrease the activity of drug metabolizing liver enzymes (Cytochrome P450) may increase plasma levels of praziquantel). Products include:

Agenerase Capsules **1327**
Agenerase Oral Solution **1332**

Anastrozole (Concomitant administration of drugs that decrease the activity of drug metabolizing liver enzymes (Cytochrome P450) may increase plasma levels of praziqua). Products include:

Arimidex Tablets **673**

Aprepitant (Concomitant administration of drugs that increase the activity of drug metabolizing liver enzymes (Cytochrome P450) may reduce plasma levels of praziquantel). Products include:

Emend Capsules **1963**

Bendroflumethiazide (Concomitant administration of drugs that decrease the activity of drug metabolizing liver enzymes (Cytochrome P450) may increase plasma levels of praziquantel).

No products indexed under this heading.

Betamethasone Acetate (Concomitant administration of drugs that increase the activity of drug metabolizing liver enzymes (Cytochrome P450) may reduce plasma levels of praziquantel).

No products indexed under this heading.

Betamethasone Sodium Phosphate (Concomitant administration of drugs that increase the activity of drug metabolizing liver enzymes (Cytochrome P450) may reduce plasma levels of praziquantel).

No products indexed under this heading.

Bupropion Hydrochloride (Concomitant administration of drugs that decrease the activity of drug metabolizing liver enzymes (Cytochrome P450) may increase plasma levels of praziquantel). Products include:

Wellbutrin Tablets **1603**
Wellbutrin SR Sustained-Release Tablets **1607**
Wellbutrin XL Extended-Release Tablets **1613**
Zyban Sustained-Release Tablets **1644**

Carbamazepine (Concomitant administration of drugs that increase the activity of drug metabolizing liver enzymes (Cytochrome P450) may reduce plasma levels of praziquantel). Products include:

Carbatrol Capsules **3171**
Equetro Extended-Release Capsules **3180**
Tegretol/Tegretol-XR **2295**

Celecoxib (Concomitant administration of drugs that decrease the activity of drug metabolizing liver enzymes (Cytochrome P450) may increase plasma levels of praziquantel). Products include:

Celebrex Capsules **3134**

Chloramphenicol (Concomitant administration of drugs that decrease the activity of drug metabolizing liver enzymes (Cytochrome P450) may increase plasma levels of praziquantel).

No products indexed under this heading.

Chloroquine (Co-administration may lead to lower concentrations of praziquantel).

No products indexed under this heading.

Chloroquine Hydrochloride (Co-administration may lead to lower concentrations of praziquantel).

No products indexed under this heading.

Chloroquine Phosphate (Co-administration may lead to lower concentrations of praziquantel).

No products indexed under this heading.

Chlorothiazide (Concomitant administration of drugs that decrease the activity of drug metabolizing liver enzymes (Cytochrome P450) may increase plasma levels of praziquantel). Products include:

Diuril Oral Suspension **1954**

Chlorothiazide Sodium (Concomitant administration of drugs that decrease the activity of drug metabolizing liver enzymes (Cytochrome P450) may increase plasma levels of praziquantel). Products include:

Diuril Sodium Intravenous **2467**

Chlorpheniramine (Concomitant administration of drugs that decrease the activity of drug metabolizing liver enzymes (Cytochrome P450) may increase plasma levels of praziquantel).

No products indexed under this heading.

Chlorpheniramine Maleate (Concomitant administration of drugs that decrease the activity of drug metabolizing liver enzymes (Cytochrome P450) may increase plasma levels of praziquantel). Products include:

Advil Allergy Sinus Caplets .... ■ **770**
Advil Multi-Symptom Cold Caplets .... ■ **770**
BC Allergy Sinus Cold Powder .... ■ **677**
Comtrex Maximum Strength Cold & Cough Day/Night Caplets - Night Formulation .... ■ **726**
Comtrex Maximum Strength Day/Night Severe Cold & Sinus Caplets - Night Formulation .... ■ **725**
Contac Cold and Flu Maximum Strength Caplets .... ■ **728**
Contac Cold and Flu Day and Night Caplets (Night Formulation Only)....................... ■ **727**
Children's Dimetapp Long Acting Cough Plus Cold Syrup................ ■ **731**
Robitussin Cough & Cold Long-Acting Liquid .... ■ **735**
Robitussin Cough & Allergy Syrup .. ■ **736**
Robitussin Cough & Cold Nighttime Liquid............................ ■ **736**
Robitussin Cough, Cold & Flu Nighttime Liquid.......................... ■ **738**
Robitussin Pediatric Cough & Cold Long-Acting Liquid.............. ■ **735**
Robitussin Pediatric Cough & Cold Nighttime Liquid.................. ■ **736**
Triaminic Cold & Allergy Liquid .... ■ **746**
Triaminic Cough & Runny Nose Softchews .... ■ **748**
Children's Tylenol Plus Flu Oral Suspension................................ ■ **749**
Tylenol Allergy Multi-Symptom Caplets with Cool Burst and Gelcaps.. **1872**
Children's Tylenol Plus Cold Suspension Liquid **1879**
Children's Tylenol Plus Cough & Runny Nose Suspension Liquid **1879**
Children's Tylenol Plus Flu Suspension Liquid **1881**
Children's Tylenol Plus Multi-Symptom Cold Suspension Liquid **1879**
Tylenol Cold Head Congestion Nighttime Caplets with Cool Burst... **1873**
Tylenol Cold Multi-Symptom Nighttime Caplets with Cool Burst... **1874**
Tylenol Sinus Congestion & Pain Nighttime Caplets with Cool Burst... **1876**
Vicks 44M Cough, Cold & Flu Relief Liquid................................ **2680**
Pediatric Vicks 44m Cough & Cold Relief Liquid......................... **2676**
Children's Vicks NyQuil Cold/Cough Relief....................... ■ **756**
Children's Vicks NyQuil Cold/Cough Relief Liquid............. **2680**
Zicam Maximum Strength Flu Daytime.................................... ■ **768**

Chlorpheniramine Polistirex (Concomitant administration of drugs that decrease the activity of drug metabolizing liver enzymes (Cytochrome P450) may increase plasma levels of praziquantel). Products include:

Tussionex Pennkinetic Extended-Release Suspension...... **3327**

Chlorpheniramine Tannate (Concomitant administration of drugs that decrease the activity of drug metabolizing liver enzymes (Cytochrome P450) may increase plasma levels of praziquantel).

No products indexed under this heading.

Chlorpropamide (Concomitant administration of drugs that decrease the activity of drug metabolizing liver enzymes (Cytochrome P450) may increase plasma levels of praziquantel).

No products indexed under this heading.

Cimetidine (Concomitant administration of drugs that decrease the activity of drug metabolizing liver enzymes (Cytochrome P450) may increase plasma levels of praziqua). Products include:

Tagamet HB 200 Tablets .... ■ **664**

Cimetidine Hydrochloride (Concomitant administration of drugs that decrease the activity of drug metabolizing liver enzymes (Cytochrome P450) may increase plasma levels of praziqua).

No products indexed under this heading.

Ciprofloxacin (Concomitant administration of drugs that decrease the activity of drug metabolizing liver enzymes (Cytochrome P450) may increase plasma levels of praziqua). Products include:

Cipro Oral Suspension **2977**
Cipro I.V. **2984**
Cipro XR Tablets **2990**
Ciprodex Otic Suspension **559**

Ciprofloxacin Hydrochloride (Concomitant administration of drugs that increase the activity of drug metabolizing liver enzymes (Cytochrome P450) may reduce plasma levels of praziquantel). Products include:

Ciloxan Ophthalmic Ointment **559**
Ciloxan Ophthalmic Solution .... ⊙ **206**
Cipro Tablets **2977**
Proquin XR Tablets **1153**

Cisplatin (Concomitant administration of drugs that increase the activity of drug metabolizing liver enzymes (Cytochrome P450) may reduce plasma levels of praziquantel).

No products indexed under this heading.

Citalopram Hydrobromide (Concomitant administration of drugs that increase the activity of drug metabolizing liver enzymes (Cytochrome P450) may reduce plasma levels of praziquantel). Products include:

Celexa **1176**

Clarithromycin (Concomitant administration of drugs that decrease the activity of drug metabolizing liver enzymes (Cytochrome P450) may increase plasma levels of praziqua). Products include:

Biaxin/Biaxin XL **402**
PREVPAC **3284**

Clomipramine Hydrochloride (Concomitant administration of drugs that decrease the activity of drug metabolizing liver enzymes (Cytochrome P450) may increase plasma levels of praziquantel).

No products indexed under this heading.

Clopidogrel Hydrogen Sulfate (Concomitant administration of drugs that decrease the activity of drug metabolizing liver enzymes (Cytochrome P450) may increase plasma levels of praziquantel).

No products indexed under this heading.

Clotrimazole (Concomitant administration of drugs that decrease the activity of drug metabolizing liver enzymes (Cytochrome P450) may increase plasma levels of praziquantel). Products include:

Desenex Athlete's Foot Cream .... ■ **635**
Lotrimin **3039**
Lotrisone **3040**

Cocaine Hydrochloride (Concomitant administration of drugs that decrease the activity of drug metabolizing liver enzymes (Cytochrome P450) may increase plasma levels of praziquantel).

No products indexed under this heading.

Cortisone Acetate (Concomitant administration of drugs that increase the activity of drug metabolizing liver enzymes (Cytochrome P450) may reduce plasma levels of praziquantel).
No products indexed under this heading.

Cyclosporine (Concomitant administration of drugs that decrease the activity of drug metabolizing liver enzymes (Cytochrome P450) may increase plasma levels of praziquantel). Products include:
Gengraf Capsules 459
Neoral Oral Solution 2259
Neoral Soft Gelatin Capsules 2259
Restasis Ophthalmic Emulsion 575
Sandimmune 2275

Dalfopristin (Concomitant administration of drugs that decrease the activity of drug metabolizing liver enzymes (Cytochrome P450) may increase plasma levels of praziquantel).
No products indexed under this heading.

Danazol (Concomitant administration of drugs that decrease the activity of drug metabolizing liver enzymes (Cytochrome P450) may increase plasma levels of praziquantel).
No products indexed under this heading.

Delavirdine Mesylate (Concomitant administration of drugs that decrease the activity of drug metabolizing liver enzymes (Cytochrome P450) may increase plasma levels of praziquantel). Products include:
Rescriptor Tablets 2551

Desipramine Hydrochloride (Concomitant administration of drugs that decrease the activity of drug metabolizing liver enzymes (Cytochrome P450) may increase plasma levels of praziquantel).
No products indexed under this heading.

Desogestrel (Concomitant administration of drugs that decrease the activity of drug metabolizing liver enzymes (Cytochrome P450) may increase plasma levels of praziqua). Products include:
Mircette Tablets 1066

Dexamethasone (Concomitant administration of drugs that increase the activity of drug metabolizing liver enzymes (Cytochrome P450) may reduce plasma levels of praziquantel). Products include:
Ciprodex Otic Suspension 559
Decadron Tablets 1951
TobraDex Ophthalmic Ointment 562
TobraDex Ophthalmic Suspension 563

Dexamethasone Acetate (Concomitant administration of drugs that increase the activity of drug metabolizing liver enzymes (Cytochrome P450) may reduce plasma levels of praziquantel).
No products indexed under this heading.

Dexamethasone Sodium Phosphate (Concomitant administration of drugs that increase the activity of drug metabolizing liver enzymes (Cytochrome P450) may reduce plasma levels of praziquantel).
No products indexed under this heading.

Diclofenac Potassium (Concomitant administration of drugs that decrease the activity of drug metabolizing liver enzymes (Cytochrome P450) may increase plasma levels of praziquantel).
No products indexed under this heading.

Diclofenac Sodium (Concomitant administration of drugs that decrease the activity of drug metabolizing liver enzymes (Cytochrome P450) may increase plasma levels of praziquantel). Products include:
Arthrotec Tablets 3129
Voltaren Ophthalmic Solution 2309
Voltaren Tablets 2307
Voltaren-XR Tablets 2310

Diltiazem Hydrochloride (Concomitant administration of drugs that increase the activity of drug metabolizing liver enzymes (Cytochrome P450) may reduce plasma levels of praziquantel). Products include:
Cardizem LA Extended Release Tablets 1728
Tiazac Capsules 1201

Diltiazem Maleate (Concomitant administration of drugs that increase the activity of drug metabolizing liver enzymes (Cytochrome P450) may reduce plasma levels of praziquantel).
No products indexed under this heading.

Diphenhydramine (Concomitant administration of drugs that decrease the activity of drug metabolizing liver enzymes (Cytochrome P450) may increase plasma levels of praziquantel). Products include:
Tylenol Sore Throat Nighttime Liquid with Cool Burst 1877

Diphenhydramine Hydrochloride (Concomitant administration of drugs that decrease the activity of drug metabolizing liver enzymes (Cytochrome P450) may increase plasma levels of praziquantel). Products include:
Nytol QuickCaps Caplets .... ■ 615
Nytol QuickGels Softgels Maximum Strength .... ■ 616
Simply Sleep Caplets 1868
Sominex Original Formula Tablets .... ■ 616
TheraFlu Warming Relief Nighttime Severe Cold .... ■ 743
TheraFlu Thin Strips Multi Symptom .... ■ 744
Triaminic Nighttime Cold & Cough Liquid .... ■ 746
Triaminic Thin Strips Cough & Runny Nose .... ■ 749
Extra Strength Tylenol PM Caplets, Vanilla Caplets, Geltabs, Gelcaps and Liquid 1875
Tylenol Sore Throat Nighttime Liquid with Cool Burst .... ■ 790
Tylenol Allergy Multi-Symptom Nighttime Caplets with Cool Burst 1872
Tylenol Severe Allergy Caplets 1872
Children's Tylenol Plus Cold & Allergy Suspension Liquid 1878

Disulfiram (Concomitant administration of drugs that decrease the activity of drug metabolizing liver enzymes (Cytochrome P450) may increase plasma levels of praziquantel).
No products indexed under this heading.

Doxepin Hydrochloride (Concomitant administration of drugs that decrease the activity of drug metabolizing liver enzymes (Cytochrome P450) may increase plasma levels of praziquantel).
No products indexed under this heading.

Doxorubicin Hydrochloride (Concomitant administration of drugs that increase the activity of drug metabolizing liver enzymes (Cytochrome P450) may reduce plasma levels of praziquantel).
No products indexed under this heading.

Efavirenz (Concomitant administration of drugs that increase the activity of drug metabolizing liver enzymes (Cytochrome P450) may reduce plasma levels of praziquantel). Products include:
Atripla Tablets 945
Sustiva Capsules 930
Sustiva Tablets 930

Enoxacin (Concomitant administration of drugs that decrease the activity of drug metabolizing liver enzymes (Cytochrome P450) may increase plasma levels of praziqua).
No products indexed under this heading.

Erythromycin (Concomitant administration of drugs that increase the activity of drug metabolizing liver enzymes (Cytochrome P450) may reduce plasma levels of praziquantel). Products include:
Ery-Tab Tablets 449
Erythromycin Base Filmtab Tablets 455
Erythromycin Delayed-Release Capsules, USP 457
PCE Dispertab Tablets 515

Erythromycin Estolate (Concomitant administration of drugs that increase the activity of drug metabolizing liver enzymes (Cytochrome P450) may reduce plasma levels of praziquantel).
No products indexed under this heading.

Erythromycin Ethylsuccinate (Concomitant administration of drugs that increase the activity of drug metabolizing liver enzymes (Cytochrome P450) may reduce plasma levels of praziquantel). Products include:
E.E.S. 451
EryPed 447

Erythromycin Gluceptate (Concomitant administration of drugs that increase the activity of drug metabolizing liver enzymes (Cytochrome P450) may reduce plasma levels of praziquantel).
No products indexed under this heading.

Erythromycin Lactobionate (Concomitant administration of drugs that increase the activity of drug metabolizing liver enzymes (Cytochrome P450) may reduce plasma levels of praziquantel).
No products indexed under this heading.

Erythromycin Stearate (Concomitant administration of drugs that increase the activity of drug metabolizing liver enzymes (Cytochrome P450) may reduce plasma levels of praziquantel). Products include:
Erythrocin Stearate Filmtab Tablets 453

Escitalopram Oxalate (Concomitant administration of drugs that decrease the activity of drug metabolizing liver enzymes (Cytochrome P450) may increase plasma levels of praziquantel). Products include:
Lexapro Oral Solution 1190
Lexapro Tablets 1190

Esomeprazole Magnesium (Concomitant administration of drugs that decrease the activity of drug metabolizing liver enzymes (Cytochrome P450) may increase plasma levels of praziquantel). Products include:
Nexium Delayed-Release Capsules 655

Ethanol (Concomitant administration of drugs that increase the activity of drug metabolizing liver enzymes (Cytochrome P450) may reduce plasma levels of praziquantel).
No products indexed under this heading.

Ethinyl Estradiol (Concomitant administration of drugs that decrease the activity of drug metabolizing liver enzymes (Cytochrome P450) may increase plasma levels of praziqua). Products include:
Mircette Tablets 1066
NuvaRing 2340
Ortho-Cyclen/Ortho Tri-Cyclen 2429
Ortho Evra Transdermal System 2417
Ortho Tri-Cyclen Lo Tablets 2436
Seasonique Tablets 1077
Yasmin 28 Tablets 796
Yaz Tablets 803

Ethosuximide (Concomitant administration of drugs that increase the activity of drug metabolizing liver enzymes (Cytochrome P450) may reduce plasma levels of praziquantel).
No products indexed under this heading.

Ethynodiol Diacetate (Concomitant administration of drugs that decrease the activity of drug metabolizing liver enzymes (Cytochrome P450) may increase plasma levels of praziquantel).
No products indexed under this heading.

Felbamate (Concomitant administration of drugs that increase the activity of drug metabolizing liver enzymes (Cytochrome P450) may reduce plasma levels of praziquantel).
No products indexed under this heading.

Fenofibrate (Concomitant administration of drugs that decrease the activity of drug metabolizing liver enzymes (Cytochrome P450) may increase plasma levels of praziquantel). Products include:
Lofibra Tablets 1219
Lofibra Capsules 1216
Tricor Tablets 527
Triglide Tablets 3123

Fluconazole (Concomitant administration of drugs that decrease the activity of drug metabolizing liver enzymes (Cytochrome P450) may increase plasma levels of praziquantel).
No products indexed under this heading.

Fludrocortisone Acetate (Concomitant administration of drugs that increase the activity of drug metabolizing liver enzymes (Cytochrome P450) may reduce plasma levels of praziquantel).
No products indexed under this heading.

Fluorouracil (Concomitant administration of drugs that decrease the activity of drug metabolizing liver enzymes (Cytochrome P450) may increase plasma levels of praziquantel). Products include:
Carac Cream, 0.5% 2879
Efudex 3363

Fluoxetine (Concomitant administration of drugs that decrease the activity of drug metabolizing liver enzymes (Cytochrome P450) may increase plasma levels of praziquantel).
No products indexed under this heading.

Fluoxetine Hydrochloride (Concomitant administration of drugs that decrease the activity of drug metabolizing liver enzymes (Cytochrome P450) may increase plasma levels of praziquantel). Products include:
Prozac Pulvules and Liquid 1801
Symbyax Capsules 1819

Fluphenazine Decanoate (Concomitant administration of drugs that decrease the activity of drug metabolizing liver enzymes (Cytochrome P450) may increase plasma levels of praziquantel).
No products indexed under this heading.

Fluphenazine Enanthate (Concomitant administration of drugs that decrease the activity of drug metabolizing liver enzymes (Cytochrome P450) may increase plasma levels of praziquantel).
No products indexed under this heading.

Fluphenazine Hydrochloride (Concomitant administration of drugs that decrease the activity of drug metabolizing liver enzymes (Cytochrome P450) may increase plasma levels of praziquantel).
No products indexed under this heading.

Flurbiprofen (Concomitant administration of drugs that decrease the activity of drug metabolizing liver enzymes (Cytochrome P450) may increase plasma levels of praziquantel).
No products indexed under this heading.

Flurbiprofen Sodium (Concomitant administration of drugs that decrease the activity of drug metabolizing liver enzymes (Cytochrome P450) may increase plasma levels of praziquantel). Products include:
Ocufen Ophthalmic Solution ⊙232

Fluvastatin Sodium (Concomitant administration of drugs that decrease the activity of drug metabolizing liver enzymes (Cytochrome P450) may increase plasma levels of praziquantel). Products include:
Lescol Capsules 2233
Lescol XL Tablets 2233

Fluvoxamine (Concomitant administration of drugs that decrease the activity of drug metabolizing liver enzymes (Cytochrome P450) may increase plasma levels of praziqua).
No products indexed under this heading.

Fluvoxamine Maleate (Concomitant administration of drugs that increase the activity of drug metabolizing liver enzymes (Cytochrome P450) may reduce plasma levels of praziquantel).
No products indexed under this heading.

Fosamprenavir Calcium (Concomitant administration of drugs that decrease the activity of drug metabolizing liver enzymes (Cytochrome P450) may increase plasma levels of praziquantel). Products include:
Lexiva Tablets 1505

Fosphenytoin Sodium (Concomitant administration of drugs that increase the activity of drug metabolizing liver enzymes (Cytochrome P450) may reduce plasma levels of praziquantel).
No products indexed under this heading.

Garlic Extract (Concomitant administration of drugs that increase the activity of drug metabolizing liver enzymes (Cytochrome P450) may reduce plasma levels of praziquantel).
No products indexed under this heading.

Garlic Oil (Concomitant administration of drugs that increase the activity of drug metabolizing liver enzymes (Cytochrome P450) may reduce plasma levels of praziquantel).
No products indexed under this heading.

Gatifloxacin (Concomitant administration of drugs that decrease the activity of drug metabolizing liver enzymes (Cytochrome P450) may increase plasma levels of praziqua). Products include:
Tequin Injection 938
Tequin Injection in 5% Dextrose 938
Tequin Tablets 938
Zymar Ophthalmic Solution 575

Gemfibrozil (Concomitant administration of drugs that decrease the activity of drug metabolizing liver enzymes (Cytochrome P450) may increase plasma levels of praziquantel).
No products indexed under this heading.

Gemifloxacin Mesylate (Concomitant administration of drugs that decrease the activity of drug metabolizing liver enzymes (Cytochrome P450) may increase plasma levels of praziqua).
No products indexed under this heading.

Glipizide (Concomitant administration of drugs that decrease the activity of drug metabolizing liver enzymes (Cytochrome P450) may increase plasma levels of praziquantel).
No products indexed under this heading.

Glyburide (Concomitant administration of drugs that decrease the activity of drug metabolizing liver enzymes (Cytochrome P450) may increase plasma levels of praziquantel).
No products indexed under this heading.

Grepafloxacin Hydrochloride (Concomitant administration of drugs that decrease the activity of drug metabolizing liver enzymes (Cytochrome P450) may increase plasma levels of praziqua).
No products indexed under this heading.

Halofantrine Hydrochloride (Concomitant administration of drugs that decrease the activity of drug metabolizing liver enzymes (Cytochrome P450) may increase plasma levels of praziquantel).
No products indexed under this heading.

Haloperidol (Concomitant administration of drugs that decrease the activity of drug metabolizing liver enzymes (Cytochrome P450) may increase plasma levels of praziquantel).
No products indexed under this heading.

Haloperidol Decanoate (Concomitant administration of drugs that decrease the activity of drug metabolizing liver enzymes (Cytochrome P450) may increase plasma levels of praziquantel).
No products indexed under this heading.

Hydrochlorothiazide (Concomitant administration of drugs that decrease the activity of drug metabolizing liver enzymes (Cytochrome P450) may increase plasma levels of praziquantel). Products include:
Aldoril Tablets 1910
Atacand HCT 651
Avalide Tablets 888
Avalide Tablets 2874
Benicar HCT Tablets 1044
Diovan HCT Tablets 2196
Dyazide Capsules 1423
Hyzaar 50-12.5 Tablets 1990
Hyzaar 100-12.5 Tablets 1990
Hyzaar 100-25 Tablets 1990
Lopressor HCT 50/25 Tablets 2241
Lopressor HCT 100/25 Tablets 2241
Lopressor HCT 100/50 Tablets 2241
Lotensin HCT Tablets 2246
Micardis HCT Tablets 856
Moduretic Tablets 2028
Prinzide Tablets 2056
Teveten HCT Tablets 1737
Timolide Tablets 2086
Uniretic Tablets 3100

Hydrocortisone (Concomitant administration of drugs that increase the activity of drug metabolizing liver enzymes (Cytochrome P450) may reduce plasma levels of praziquantel). Products include:
Colocort Rectal Suspension, USP (Retention) 100 mg/60 mL.......... 2476
Hydrocortone Tablets 1989
Preparation H Hydrocortisone Cream ■□646

Hydrocortisone Acetate (Concomitant administration of drugs that increase the activity of drug metabolizing liver enzymes (Cytochrome P450) may reduce plasma levels of praziquantel). Products include:
Analpram-HC 1159
Pramosone 1161
ProctoFoam-HC 3099

Hydrocortisone Butyrate (Concomitant administration of drugs that increase the activity of drug metabolizing liver enzymes (Cytochrome P450) may reduce plasma levels of praziquantel). Products include:
Locoid Lipocream Cream 1160

Hydrocortisone Cypionate (Concomitant administration of drugs that increase the activity of drug metabolizing liver enzymes (Cytochrome P450) may reduce plasma levels of praziquantel).
No products indexed under this heading.

Hydrocortisone Hemisuccinate (Concomitant administration of drugs that increase the activity of drug metabolizing liver enzymes (Cytochrome P450) may reduce plasma levels of praziquantel).
No products indexed under this heading.

Hydrocortisone Probutate (Concomitant administration of drugs that increase the activity of drug metabolizing liver enzymes (Cytochrome P450) may reduce plasma levels of praziquantel).
No products indexed under this heading.

Hydrocortisone Sodium Phosphate (Concomitant administration of drugs that increase the activity of drug metabolizing liver enzymes (Cytochrome P450) may reduce plasma levels of praziquantel).
No products indexed under this heading.

Hydrocortisone Sodium Succinate (Concomitant administration of drugs that increase the activity of drug metabolizing liver enzymes (Cytochrome P450) may reduce plasma levels of praziquantel).
No products indexed under this heading.

Hydrocortisone Valerate (Concomitant administration of drugs that increase the activity of drug metabolizing liver enzymes (Cytochrome P450) may reduce plasma levels of praziquantel).
No products indexed under this heading.

Hydroflumethiazide (Concomitant administration of drugs that decrease the activity of drug metabolizing liver enzymes (Cytochrome P450) may increase plasma levels of praziquantel).
No products indexed under this heading.

Hydroxychloroquine Sulfate (Concomitant administration of drugs that decrease the activity of drug metabolizing liver enzymes (Cytochrome P450) may increase plasma levels of praziquantel).
No products indexed under this heading.

Hypericum (Concomitant administration of drugs that increase the activity of drug metabolizing liver enzymes (Cytochrome P450) may reduce plasma levels of praziquantel). Products include:
Satiete Tablets ■□832

Hypericum Perforatum (Concomitant administration of drugs that increase the activity of drug metabolizing liver enzymes (Cytochrome P450) may reduce plasma levels of praziquantel).
No products indexed under this heading.

Imatinib Mesylate (Concomitant administration of drugs that decrease the activity of drug metabolizing liver enzymes (Cytochrome P450) may increase plasma levels of praziquantel). Products include:
Gleevec Tablets 2227

Imipramine Hydrochloride (Concomitant administration of drugs that decrease the activity of drug metabolizing liver enzymes (Cytochrome P450) may increase plasma levels of praziquantel).
No products indexed under this heading.

Imipramine Pamoate (Concomitant administration of drugs that decrease the activity of drug metabolizing liver enzymes (Cytochrome P450) may increase plasma levels of praziquantel).
No products indexed under this heading.

IMPORTANT NOTE: Always consult each drug listing in the patient's regimen for possible interactions.

Indinavir Sulfate (Concomitant administration of drugs that decrease the activity of drug metabolizing liver enzymes (Cytochrome P450) may increase plasma levels of praziquantel). Products include:
- Crixivan Capsules 1940

Indomethacin (Concomitant administration of drugs that decrease the activity of drug metabolizing liver enzymes (Cytochrome P450) may increase plasma levels of praziquantel). Products include:
- Indocin 1995

Indomethacin Sodium Trihydrate (Concomitant administration of drugs that decrease the activity of drug metabolizing liver enzymes (Cytochrome P450) may increase plasma levels of praziquantel). Products include:
- Indocin I.V. 2465

Insulin (Concomitant administration of drugs that increase the activity of drug metabolizing liver enzymes (Cytochrome P450) may reduce plasma levels of praziquantel).
No products indexed under this heading.

Isoniazid (Concomitant administration of drugs that decrease the activity of drug metabolizing liver enzymes (Cytochrome P450) may increase plasma levels of praziqua).
No products indexed under this heading.

Itraconazole (Concomitant administration of drugs that decrease the activity of drug metabolizing liver enzymes (Cytochrome P450) may increase plasma levels of praziquantel).
No products indexed under this heading.

Ketoconazole (Concomitant administration of drugs that decrease the activity of drug metabolizing liver enzymes (Cytochrome P450) may increase plasma levels of praziqua). Products include:
- Nizoral A-D Shampoo, 1% 1868

Ketoprofen (Concomitant administration of drugs that decrease the activity of drug metabolizing liver enzymes (Cytochrome P450) may increase plasma levels of praziquantel).
No products indexed under this heading.

Lansoprazole (Concomitant administration of drugs that increase the activity of drug metabolizing liver enzymes (Cytochrome P450) may reduce plasma levels of praziquantel). Products include:
- Prevacid Delayed-Release Capsules 3271
- Prevacid for Delayed-Release Oral Suspension 3271
- Prevacid SoluTab Delayed-Release Orally Disintegrating Tablets 3271
- Prevacid I.V. for Injection 3277
- Prevacid NapraPAC 3280
- PREVPAC 3284

Leflunomide (Concomitant administration of drugs that decrease the activity of drug metabolizing liver enzymes (Cytochrome P450) may increase plasma levels of praziquantel).
No products indexed under this heading.

Letrozole (Concomitant administration of drugs that decrease the activity of drug metabolizing liver enzymes (Cytochrome P450) may increase plasma levels of praziquantel). Products include:
- Femara Tablets 2214

Levofloxacin (Concomitant administration of drugs that decrease the activity of drug metabolizing liver enzymes (Cytochrome P450) may increase plasma levels of praziqua). Products include:
- Levaquin 2384
- Levaquin in 5% Dextrose Injection 2384
- Quixin Ophthalmic Solution 3383

Levonorgestrel (Concomitant administration of drugs that decrease the activity of drug metabolizing liver enzymes (Cytochrome P450) may increase plasma levels of praziqua). Products include:
- Climara Pro Transdermal System 776
- Mirena Intrauterine System 787
- Plan B Tablets 1076
- Seasonique Tablets 1077

Lomefloxacin Hydrochloride (Concomitant administration of drugs that decrease the activity of drug metabolizing liver enzymes (Cytochrome P450) may increase plasma levels of praziqua).
No products indexed under this heading.

Lopinavir (Concomitant administration of drugs that decrease the activity of drug metabolizing liver enzymes (Cytochrome P450) may increase plasma levels of praziquantel). Products include:
- Kaletra 476

Loratadine (Concomitant administration of drugs that decrease the activity of drug metabolizing liver enzymes (Cytochrome P450) may increase plasma levels of praziquantel). Products include:
- Alavert Allergy & Sinus D-12 Hour Tablets .... ■771
- Alavert .... ■771
- Children's Claritin Allergy Oral Solution .... ■771
- Claritin Non-Drowsy 24 Hour Tablets .... ■772
- Claritin Reditabs 24 Hour Non-Drowsy Tablets .... ■772
- Claritin-D Non-Drowsy 12 Hour Tablets .... ■772
- Claritin-D Non-Drowsy 24 Hour Tablets .... ■772

Lovastatin (Concomitant administration of drugs that decrease the activity of drug metabolizing liver enzymes (Cytochrome P450) may increase plasma levels of praziquantel). Products include:
- Advicor Tablets 1722
- Altoprev Extended-Release Tablets 3109
- Mevacor Tablets 2021

Maprotiline Hydrochloride (Concomitant administration of drugs that decrease the activity of drug metabolizing liver enzymes (Cytochrome P450) may increase plasma levels of praziquantel).
No products indexed under this heading.

Mephenytoin (Concomitant administration of drugs that increase the activity of drug metabolizing liver enzymes (Cytochrome P450) may reduce plasma levels of praziquantel).
No products indexed under this heading.

Mestranol (Concomitant administration of drugs that decrease the activity of drug metabolizing liver enzymes (Cytochrome P450) may increase plasma levels of praziqua).
No products indexed under this heading.

Methadone Hydrochloride (Concomitant administration of drugs that decrease the activity of drug metabolizing liver enzymes (Cytochrome P450) may increase plasma levels of praziquantel).
No products indexed under this heading.

Methoxsalen (Concomitant administration of drugs that decrease the activity of drug metabolizing liver enzymes (Cytochrome P450) may increase plasma levels of praziqua). Products include:
- Oxsoralen Lotion 1% 3352
- Oxsoralen-Ultra Capsules 3353

Methsuximide (Concomitant administration of drugs that increase the activity of drug metabolizing liver enzymes (Cytochrome P450) may reduce plasma levels of praziquantel).
No products indexed under this heading.

Methyclothiazide (Concomitant administration of drugs that decrease the activity of drug metabolizing liver enzymes (Cytochrome P450) may increase plasma levels of praziquantel).
No products indexed under this heading.

Methylprednisolone (Concomitant administration of drugs that increase the activity of drug metabolizing liver enzymes (Cytochrome P450) may reduce plasma levels of praziquantel).
No products indexed under this heading.

Methylprednisolone Acetate (Concomitant administration of drugs that increase the activity of drug metabolizing liver enzymes (Cytochrome P450) may reduce plasma levels of praziquantel). Products include:
- Depo-Medrol Injectable Suspension 2617
- Depo-Medrol Single-Dose Vial 2619

Methylprednisolone Sodium Succinate (Concomitant administration of drugs that increase the activity of drug metabolizing liver enzymes (Cytochrome P450) may reduce plasma levels of praziquantel).
No products indexed under this heading.

Metronidazole (Concomitant administration of drugs that decrease the activity of drug metabolizing liver enzymes (Cytochrome P450) may increase plasma levels of praziquantel). Products include:
- Metrogel 1% 1211
- MetroGel-Vaginal Gel 1855
- Vandazole Vaginal Gel 3338

Metronidazole Benzoate (Concomitant administration of drugs that decrease the activity of drug metabolizing liver enzymes (Cytochrome P450) may increase plasma levels of praziquantel).
No products indexed under this heading.

Metronidazole Hydrochloride (Concomitant administration of drugs that decrease the activity of drug metabolizing liver enzymes (Cytochrome P450) may increase plasma levels of praziquantel).
No products indexed under this heading.

Mexiletine Hydrochloride (Concomitant administration of drugs that decrease the activity of drug metabolizing liver enzymes (Cytochrome P450) may increase plasma levels of praziqua).
No products indexed under this heading.

Mibefradil Dihydrochloride (Concomitant administration of drugs that decrease the activity of drug metabolizing liver enzymes (Cytochrome P450) may increase plasma levels of praziqua).
No products indexed under this heading.

Miconazole (Concomitant administration of drugs that decrease the activity of drug metabolizing liver enzymes (Cytochrome P450) may increase plasma levels of praziquantel).
No products indexed under this heading.

Miconazole Nitrate (Concomitant administration of drugs that decrease the activity of drug metabolizing liver enzymes (Cytochrome P450) may increase plasma levels of praziquantel). Products include:
- Desenex .... ■635
- Desenex Jock Itch Spray Powder .... ■635

Moclobemide (Concomitant administration of drugs that decrease the activity of drug metabolizing liver enzymes (Cytochrome P450) may increase plasma levels of praziquantel).
No products indexed under this heading.

Modafinil (Concomitant administration of drugs that increase the activity of drug metabolizing liver enzymes (Cytochrome P450) may reduce plasma levels of praziquantel). Products include:
- Provigil Tablets 988

Moxifloxacin Hydrochloride (Concomitant administration of drugs that decrease the activity of drug metabolizing liver enzymes (Cytochrome P450) may increase plasma levels of praziqua). Products include:
- Avelox 2970
- Vigamox Ophthalmic Solution 564

Nafcillin Sodium (Concomitant administration of drugs that increase the activity of drug metabolizing liver enzymes (Cytochrome P450) may reduce plasma levels of praziquantel).
No products indexed under this heading.

Nalidixic Acid (Concomitant administration of drugs that decrease the activity of drug metabolizing liver enzymes (Cytochrome P450) may increase plasma levels of praziqua).
No products indexed under this heading.

Nefazodone Hydrochloride (Concomitant administration of drugs that decrease the activity of drug metabolizing liver enzymes (Cytochrome P450) may increase plasma levels of praziquantel).
No products indexed under this heading.

Nelfinavir Mesylate (Concomitant administration of drugs that decrease the activity of drug metabolizing liver enzymes (Cytochrome P450) may increase plasma levels of praziquantel). Products include:
Viracept **2577**

Nevirapine (Concomitant administration of drugs that increase the activity of drug metabolizing liver enzymes (Cytochrome P450) may reduce plasma levels of praziquantel). Products include:
Viramune Oral Suspension **873**
Viramune Tablets **873**

Niacinamide (Concomitant administration of drugs that decrease the activity of drug metabolizing liver enzymes (Cytochrome P450) may increase plasma levels of praziquantel).
No products indexed under this heading.

Nicardipine Hydrochloride (Concomitant administration of drugs that decrease the activity of drug metabolizing liver enzymes (Cytochrome P450) may increase plasma levels of praziquantel). Products include:
Cardene I.V. **2497**

Nicotinamide (Concomitant administration of drugs that decrease the activity of drug metabolizing liver enzymes (Cytochrome P450) may increase plasma levels of praziquantel). Products include:
Nicomide Tablets **1088**

Nicotine (Concomitant administration of drugs that increase the activity of drug metabolizing liver enzymes (Cytochrome P450) may reduce plasma levels of praziquantel). Products include:
NicoDerm CQ Clear Patch **622**

Nicotine Polacrilex (Concomitant administration of drugs that increase the activity of drug metabolizing liver enzymes (Cytochrome P450) may reduce plasma levels of praziquantel).
No products indexed under this heading.

Nicotine Salicylate (Concomitant administration of drugs that increase the activity of drug metabolizing liver enzymes (Cytochrome P450) may reduce plasma levels of praziquantel).
No products indexed under this heading.

Nicotine Sulfate (Concomitant administration of drugs that increase the activity of drug metabolizing liver enzymes (Cytochrome P450) may reduce plasma levels of praziquantel).
No products indexed under this heading.

Nifedipine (Concomitant administration of drugs that decrease the activity of drug metabolizing liver enzymes (Cytochrome P450) may increase plasma levels of praziquantel). Products include:
Adalat CC Tablets **2964**

Norethindrone (Concomitant administration of drugs that increase the activity of drug metabolizing liver enzymes (Cytochrome P450) may reduce plasma levels of praziquantel). Products include:
Ortho Micronor Tablets **2426**

Norethindrone Acetate (Concomitant administration of drugs that increase the activity of drug metabolizing liver enzymes (Cytochrome P450) may reduce plasma levels of praziquantel).
No products indexed under this heading.

Norethynodrel (Concomitant administration of drugs that decrease the activity of drug metabolizing liver enzymes (Cytochrome P450) may increase plasma levels of praziquantel).
No products indexed under this heading.

Norfloxacin (Concomitant administration of drugs that decrease the activity of drug metabolizing liver enzymes (Cytochrome P450) may increase plasma levels of praziqua). Products include:
Noroxin Tablets **2032**

Norgestimate (Concomitant administration of drugs that decrease the activity of drug metabolizing liver enzymes (Cytochrome P450) may increase plasma levels of praziquantel). Products include:
Ortho-Cyclen/Ortho Tri-Cyclen **2429**
Ortho Tri-Cyclen Lo Tablets **2436**

Norgestrel (Concomitant administration of drugs that decrease the activity of drug metabolizing liver enzymes (Cytochrome P450) may increase plasma levels of praziqua).
No products indexed under this heading.

Nortriptyline Hydrochloride (Concomitant administration of drugs that decrease the activity of drug metabolizing liver enzymes (Cytochrome P450) may increase plasma levels of praziquantel).
No products indexed under this heading.

Ofloxacin (Concomitant administration of drugs that decrease the activity of drug metabolizing liver enzymes (Cytochrome P450) may increase plasma levels of praziqua). Products include:
Floxin Otic Solution **1049**

Omeprazole (Concomitant administration of drugs that increase the activity of drug metabolizing liver enzymes (Cytochrome P450) may reduce plasma levels of praziquantel). Products include:
Zegerid Capsules **2958**
Zegerid Powder for Oral Solution **2958**

Oxcarbazepine (Concomitant administration of drugs that increase the activity of drug metabolizing liver enzymes (Cytochrome P450) may reduce plasma levels of praziquantel). Products include:
Trileptal Tablets **2300**
Trileptal Oral Suspension **2300**

Oxiconazole Nitrate (Concomitant administration of drugs that decrease the activity of drug metabolizing liver enzymes (Cytochrome P450) may increase plasma levels of praziquantel). Products include:
Oxistat **2667**

Paroxetine Hydrochloride (Concomitant administration of drugs that decrease the activity of drug metabolizing liver enzymes (Cytochrome P450) may increase plasma levels of praziqua). Products include:
Paxil CR Controlled-Release Tablets **1538**
Paxil **1530**

Perphenazine (Concomitant administration of drugs that decrease the activity of drug metabolizing liver enzymes (Cytochrome P450) may increase plasma levels of praziquantel).
No products indexed under this heading.

Phenobarbital (Concomitant administration of drugs that increase the activity of drug metabolizing liver enzymes (Cytochrome P450) may reduce plasma levels of praziquantel). Products include:
Donnatal Extentabs **2493**

Phenobarbital Sodium (Concomitant administration of drugs that increase the activity of drug metabolizing liver enzymes (Cytochrome P450) may reduce plasma levels of praziquantel).
No products indexed under this heading.

Phenylbutazone (Concomitant administration of drugs that decrease the activity of drug metabolizing liver enzymes (Cytochrome P450) may increase plasma levels of praziquantel).
No products indexed under this heading.

Phenytoin (Concomitant administration of drugs that increase the activity of drug metabolizing liver enzymes (Cytochrome P450) may reduce plasma levels of praziquantel).
No products indexed under this heading.

Phenytoin Sodium (Concomitant administration of drugs that increase the activity of drug metabolizing liver enzymes (Cytochrome P450) may reduce plasma levels of praziquantel). Products include:
Phenytek Capsules **2160**

Polythiazide (Concomitant administration of drugs that decrease the activity of drug metabolizing liver enzymes (Cytochrome P450) may increase plasma levels of praziquantel).
No products indexed under this heading.

Prednisolone Acetate (Concomitant administration of drugs that increase the activity of drug metabolizing liver enzymes (Cytochrome P450) may reduce plasma levels of praziquantel). Products include:
Blephamide Ophthalmic Ointment **568**
Blephamide Ophthalmic Suspension................................. **569**
Poly-Pred Ophthalmic Suspension .... ⊙**233**
Pred Forte Ophthalmic Suspension .... ⊙**235**
Pred Mild Ophthalmic Suspension .... ⊙**238**
Pred-G Ophthalmic Ointment .... ⊙**237**
Pred-G Ophthalmic Suspension ...... ⊙**236**

Prednisolone Sodium Phosphate (Concomitant administration of drugs that increase the activity of drug metabolizing liver enzymes (Cytochrome P450) may reduce plasma levels of praziquantel).
No products indexed under this heading.

Prednisolone Tebutate (Concomitant administration of drugs that increase the activity of drug metabolizing liver enzymes (Cytochrome P450) may reduce plasma levels of praziquantel).
No products indexed under this heading.

Prednisone (Concomitant administration of drugs that increase the activity of drug metabolizing liver enzymes (Cytochrome P450) may reduce plasma levels of praziquantel).
No products indexed under this heading.

Primidone (Concomitant administration of drugs that increase the activity of drug metabolizing liver enzymes (Cytochrome P450) may reduce plasma levels of praziquantel).
No products indexed under this heading.

Propafenone Hydrochloride (Concomitant administration of drugs that decrease the activity of drug metabolizing liver enzymes (Cytochrome P450) may increase plasma levels of praziquantel). Products include:
Rythmol SR Capsules **2727**

Propoxyphene Hydrochloride (Concomitant administration of drugs that decrease the activity of drug metabolizing liver enzymes (Cytochrome P450) may increase plasma levels of praziquantel).
No products indexed under this heading.

Propoxyphene Napsylate (Concomitant administration of drugs that decrease the activity of drug metabolizing liver enzymes (Cytochrome P450) may increase plasma levels of praziquantel).
No products indexed under this heading.

Protriptyline Hydrochloride (Concomitant administration of drugs that decrease the activity of drug metabolizing liver enzymes (Cytochrome P450) may increase plasma levels of praziquantel).
No products indexed under this heading.

Quercetin (Concomitant administration of drugs that decrease the activity of drug metabolizing liver enzymes (Cytochrome P450) may increase plasma levels of praziquantel).
No products indexed under this heading.

Quinacrine Hydrochloride (Concomitant administration of drugs that decrease the activity of drug metabolizing liver enzymes (Cytochrome P450) may increase plasma levels of praziquantel).
No products indexed under this heading.

Quinidine (Concomitant administration of drugs that decrease the activity of drug metabolizing liver enzymes (Cytochrome P450) may increase plasma levels of praziquantel).
No products indexed under this heading.

Quinidine Gluconate (Concomitant administration of drugs that decrease the activity of drug metabolizing liver enzymes (Cytochrome P450) may increase plasma levels of praziquantel).
No products indexed under this heading.

Quinidine Hydrochloride (Concomitant administration of drugs that decrease the activity of drug metabolizing liver enzymes (Cytochrome P450) may increase plasma levels of praziquantel).
 No products indexed under this heading.

Quinidine Polygalacturonate (Concomitant administration of drugs that decrease the activity of drug metabolizing liver enzymes (Cytochrome P450) may increase plasma levels of praziquantel).
 No products indexed under this heading.

Quinidine Sulfate (Concomitant administration of drugs that decrease the activity of drug metabolizing liver enzymes (Cytochrome P450) may increase plasma levels of praziquantel).
 No products indexed under this heading.

Quinine (Concomitant administration of drugs that decrease the activity of drug metabolizing liver enzymes (Cytochrome P450) may increase plasma levels of praziquantel).
 No products indexed under this heading.

Quinine Sulfate (Concomitant administration of drugs that decrease the activity of drug metabolizing liver enzymes (Cytochrome P450) may increase plasma levels of praziquantel).
 No products indexed under this heading.

Quinupristin (Concomitant administration of drugs that decrease the activity of drug metabolizing liver enzymes (Cytochrome P450) may increase plasma levels of praziquantel).
 No products indexed under this heading.

Ranitidine Bismuth Citrate (Concomitant administration of drugs that decrease the activity of drug metabolizing liver enzymes (Cytochrome P450) may increase plasma levels of praziquantel).
 No products indexed under this heading.

Ranitidine Hydrochloride (Concomitant administration of drugs that decrease the activity of drug metabolizing liver enzymes (Cytochrome P450) may increase plasma levels of praziqua). Products include:

Rifabutin (Concomitant administration of drugs that increase the activity of drug metabolizing liver enzymes (Cytochrome P450) may reduce plasma levels of praziquantel).
 No products indexed under this heading.

Rifampicin (Concomitant administration of drugs that increase the activity of drug metabolizing liver enzymes (Cytochrome P450) may reduce plasma levels of praziquantel).
 No products indexed under this heading.

Rifampin (Concomitant administration of rifampin should be avoided).
 No products indexed under this heading.

Rifapentine (Concomitant administration of drugs that increase the activity of drug metabolizing liver enzymes (Cytochrome P450) may reduce plasma levels of praziquantel).
 No products indexed under this heading.

Ritonavir (Concomitant administration of drugs that increase the activity of drug metabolizing liver enzymes (Cytochrome P450) may reduce plasma levels of praziquantel). Products include:

Saquinavir (Concomitant administration of drugs that decrease the activity of drug metabolizing liver enzymes (Cytochrome P450) may increase plasma levels of praziquantel).
 No products indexed under this heading.

Saquinavir Mesylate (Concomitant administration of drugs that decrease the activity of drug metabolizing liver enzymes (Cytochrome P450) may increase plasma levels of praziquantel). Products include:

Secobarbital Sodium (Concomitant administration of drugs that increase the activity of drug metabolizing liver enzymes (Cytochrome P450) may reduce plasma levels of praziquantel).
 No products indexed under this heading.

Sertraline Hydrochloride (Concomitant administration of drugs that decrease the activity of drug metabolizing liver enzymes (Cytochrome P450) may increase plasma levels of praziquantel). Products include:

Sparfloxacin (Concomitant administration of drugs that decrease the activity of drug metabolizing liver enzymes (Cytochrome P450) may increase plasma levels of praziqua).
 No products indexed under this heading.

Sulfacytine (Concomitant administration of drugs that decrease the activity of drug metabolizing liver enzymes (Cytochrome P450) may increase plasma levels of praziquantel).
 No products indexed under this heading.

Sulfamethizole (Concomitant administration of drugs that decrease the activity of drug metabolizing liver enzymes (Cytochrome P450) may increase plasma levels of praziquantel).
 No products indexed under this heading.

Sulfamethoxazole (Concomitant administration of drugs that decrease the activity of drug metabolizing liver enzymes (Cytochrome P450) may increase plasma levels of praziquantel).
 No products indexed under this heading.

Sulfaphenazole (Concomitant administration of drugs that decrease the activity of drug metabolizing liver enzymes (Cytochrome P450) may increase plasma levels of praziquantel).
 No products indexed under this heading.

Sulfasalazine (Concomitant administration of drugs that decrease the activity of drug metabolizing liver enzymes (Cytochrome P450) may increase plasma levels of praziquantel).
 No products indexed under this heading.

Sulfinpyrazone (Concomitant administration of drugs that increase the activity of drug metabolizing liver enzymes (Cytochrome P450) may reduce plasma levels of praziquantel).
 No products indexed under this heading.

Sulfisoxazole Acetyl (Concomitant administration of drugs that decrease the activity of drug metabolizing liver enzymes (Cytochrome P450) may increase plasma levels of praziquantel).
 No products indexed under this heading.

Sulfisoxazole Diolamine (Concomitant administration of drugs that decrease the activity of drug metabolizing liver enzymes (Cytochrome P450) may increase plasma levels of praziquantel).
 No products indexed under this heading.

Tacrine Hydrochloride (Concomitant administration of drugs that decrease the activity of drug metabolizing liver enzymes (Cytochrome P450) may increase plasma levels of praziqua).
 No products indexed under this heading.

Telithromycin (Concomitant administration of drugs that decrease the activity of drug metabolizing liver enzymes (Cytochrome P450) may increase plasma levels of praziquantel). Products include:

Telmisartan (Concomitant administration of drugs that decrease the activity of drug metabolizing liver enzymes (Cytochrome P450) may increase plasma levels of praziquantel). Products include:

Terbinafine Hydrochloride (Concomitant administration of drugs that decrease the activity of drug metabolizing liver enzymes (Cytochrome P450) may increase plasma levels of praziquantel). Products include:

Terconazole (Concomitant administration of drugs that decrease the activity of drug metabolizing liver enzymes (Cytochrome P450) may increase plasma levels of praziquantel).
 No products indexed under this heading.

Theophylline (Concomitant administration of drugs that increase the activity of drug metabolizing liver enzymes (Cytochrome P450) may reduce plasma levels of praziquantel).
 No products indexed under this heading.

Thioridazine Hydrochloride (Concomitant administration of drugs that decrease the activity of drug metabolizing liver enzymes (Cytochrome P450) may increase plasma levels of praziquantel). Products include:

Ticlopidine Hydrochloride (Concomitant administration of drugs that decrease the activity of drug metabolizing liver enzymes (Cytochrome P450) may increase plasma levels of praziqua). Products include:

Tobacco (Concomitant administration of drugs that increase the activity of drug metabolizing liver enzymes (Cytochrome P450) may reduce plasma levels of praziquantel).
 No products indexed under this heading.

Tolazamide (Concomitant administration of drugs that decrease the activity of drug metabolizing liver enzymes (Cytochrome P450) may increase plasma levels of praziquantel).
 No products indexed under this heading.

Tolbutamide (Concomitant administration of drugs that decrease the activity of drug metabolizing liver enzymes (Cytochrome P450) may increase plasma levels of praziquantel).
 No products indexed under this heading.

Tolbutamide Sodium (Concomitant administration of drugs that decrease the activity of drug metabolizing liver enzymes (Cytochrome P450) may increase plasma levels of praziquantel).
 No products indexed under this heading.

Topiramate (Concomitant administration of drugs that decrease the activity of drug metabolizing liver enzymes (Cytochrome P450) may increase plasma levels of praziquantel). Products include:

Triamcinolone (Concomitant administration of drugs that increase the activity of drug metabolizing liver enzymes (Cytochrome P450) may reduce plasma levels of praziquantel).
 No products indexed under this heading.

Triamcinolone Acetonide (Concomitant administration of drugs that increase the activity of drug metabolizing liver enzymes (Cytochrome P450) may reduce plasma levels of praziquantel). Products include:

Triamcinolone Diacetate (Concomitant administration of drugs that increase the activity of drug metabolizing liver enzymes (Cytochrome P450) may reduce plasma levels of praziquantel).
 No products indexed under this heading.

Triamcinolone Hexacetonide (Concomitant administration of drugs that increase the activity of drug metabolizing liver enzymes (Cytochrome P450) may reduce plasma levels of praziquantel).
 No products indexed under this heading.

Trimethoprim (Concomitant administration of drugs that decrease the activity of drug metabolizing liver enzymes (Cytochrome P450) may increase plasma levels of praziquantel).
No products indexed under this heading.

Trimethoprim Hydrochloride (Concomitant administration of drugs that decrease the activity of drug metabolizing liver enzymes (Cytochrome P450) may increase plasma levels of praziquantel).
No products indexed under this heading.

Trimipramine Maleate (Concomitant administration of drugs that decrease the activity of drug metabolizing liver enzymes (Cytochrome P450) may increase plasma levels of praziquantel).
No products indexed under this heading.

Troglitazone (Concomitant administration of drugs that increase the activity of drug metabolizing liver enzymes (Cytochrome P450) may reduce plasma levels of praziquantel).
No products indexed under this heading.

Troleandomycin (Concomitant administration of drugs that decrease the activity of drug metabolizing liver enzymes (Cytochrome P450) may increase plasma levels of praziqua).
No products indexed under this heading.

Trovafloxacin Mesylate (Concomitant administration of drugs that decrease the activity of drug metabolizing liver enzymes (Cytochrome P450) may increase plasma levels of praziqua).
No products indexed under this heading.

Valproate Sodium (Concomitant administration of drugs that decrease the activity of drug metabolizing liver enzymes (Cytochrome P450) may increase plasma levels of praziquantel). Products include:
Depacon Injection 412

Venlafaxine Hydrochloride (Concomitant administration of drugs that decrease the activity of drug metabolizing liver enzymes (Cytochrome P450) may increase plasma levels of praziquantel). Products include:
Effexor Tablets 3411
Effexor XR Capsules 3417

Verapamil Hydrochloride (Concomitant administration of drugs that decrease the activity of drug metabolizing liver enzymes (Cytochrome P450) may increase plasma levels of praziquantel). Products include:
Covera-HS Tablets 3139
Tarka Tablets 524
Verelan PM Extended-Release Capsules, Controlled-Onset 3106

Voriconazole (Concomitant administration of drugs that decrease the activity of drug metabolizing liver enzymes (Cytochrome P450) may increase plasma levels of praziquantel). Products include:
VFEND I.V. 2564
VFEND Oral Suspension 2564
VFEND Tablets 2564

Zafirlukast (Concomitant administration of drugs that decrease the activity of drug metabolizing liver enzymes (Cytochrome P450) may increase plasma levels of praziquantel). Products include:
Accolate Tablets 671

Zileuton (Concomitant administration of drugs that decrease the activity of drug metabolizing liver enzymes (Cytochrome P450) may increase plasma levels of praziqua). Products include:
Zyflo Tablets 1023

Food Interactions

Broccoli (Concomitant administration of drugs that increase the activity of drug metabolizing liver enzymes (Cytochrome P450) may reduce plasma levels of praziquantel).

Brussel Sprouts (Concomitant administration of drugs that increase the activity of drug metabolizing liver enzymes (Cytochrome P450) may reduce plasma levels of praziquantel).

Charbroiled Food (Concomitant administration of drugs that increase the activity of drug metabolizing liver enzymes (Cytochrome P450) may reduce plasma levels of praziquantel).

Grapefruit (Grapefruit juice was reported to produce a 1.6-fold increase in the Cmax and a 1.9-fold increase in the AUC of praziquantel).

Grapefruit Juice (Grapefruit juice was reported to produce a 1.6-fold increase in the Cmax and a 1.9-fold increase in the AUC of praziquantel).

BIOFREEZE PAIN RELIEVING ROLL ON/GEL AND CRYOSPRAY

(Menthol) 678
May interact with:

Topical Medications (Do not use with other ointments, creams, sprays or liniments).
No products indexed under this heading.

BIOLEAN ACCELERATOR TABLETS

(Amino Acid Preparations, Herbals, Multiple) 631
None cited in PDR database.

BIOLEAN FREE TABLETS

(Amino Acid Preparations, Ginkgo biloba, Ginseng, Herbals with Vitamins & Minerals) 631
May interact with monoamine oxidase inhibitors and certain other agents. Compounds in these categories include:

Caffeine (Concurrent caffeine intake should be minimized). Products include:
BC Headache Powder 677
Arthritis Strength BC Powder 677
Excedrin Extra Strength Caplets/Tablets/Geltabs 684
Excedrin Migraine Caplets/Tablets/Geltabs 609
Excedrin Tension Headache Caplets/Tablets/Geltabs 611
Goody's Extra Strength Headache Powders 611
Goody's Extra Strength Pain Relief Tablets 685
Vivarin 602
Winrgy Dietary Supplement 823

Caffeine-containing medications (Concurrent caffeine intake should be minimized).
No products indexed under this heading.

Isocarboxazid (Concurrent use with MAO inhibitors is not recommended).
No products indexed under this heading.

Moclobemide (Concurrent use with MAO inhibitors is not recommended).
No products indexed under this heading.

Pargyline Hydrochloride (Concurrent use with MAO inhibitors is not recommended).
No products indexed under this heading.

Phenelzine Sulfate (Concurrent use with MAO inhibitors is not recommended).
No products indexed under this heading.

Procarbazine Hydrochloride (Concurrent use with MAO inhibitors is not recommended). Products include:
Matulane Capsules 3191

Selegiline Hydrochloride (Concurrent use with MAO inhibitors is not recommended). Products include:
Eldepryl Capsules 3208
Zelapar Tablets 3372

Tranylcypromine Sulfate (Concurrent use with MAO inhibitors is not recommended). Products include:
Parnate Tablets 1527

BIOLEAN II TABLETS

(Amino Acid Preparations, Herbals, Multiple) 808
None cited in PDR database.

BIOLEAN LIPOTRIM CAPSULES

(Herbals with Minerals) 631
None cited in PDR database.

BIOLEAN PROXTREME DIETARY SUPPLEMENT

(Amino Acid Preparations, Protein Preparations, Vitamins with Minerals) 808
None cited in PDR database.

BIOS LIFE DRINK MIX

(Fiber, Vitamins with Minerals) 3328
None cited in PDR database.

BLEPH-10 OPHTHALMIC SOLUTION 10%

(Sulfacetamide Sodium) .... ⊙222
May interact with silver preparations. Compounds in these categories include:

Silver Acetate (Incompatible).
No products indexed under this heading.

Silver Nitrate (Incompatible).
No products indexed under this heading.

Silver Sulfadiazine (Incompatible).
No products indexed under this heading.

BLEPHAMIDE OPHTHALMIC OINTMENT

(Prednisolone Acetate, Sulfacetamide Sodium) 568
May interact with para-aminobenzoic acid based local anesthetics and silver preparations. Compounds in these categories include:

Procaine Hydrochloride (May antagonize the action of sulfonamide).
No products indexed under this heading.

Silver Acetate (Blephamide ointment is incompatible with silver preparations).
No products indexed under this heading.

Silver Nitrate (Blephamide ointment is incompatible with silver preparations).
No products indexed under this heading.

Silver Sulfadiazine (Blephamide ointment is incompatible with silver preparations).
No products indexed under this heading.

Tetracaine Hydrochloride (May antagonize the action of sulfonamide). Products include:
Cetacaine Topical Anesthetic 999

BLEPHAMIDE OPHTHALMIC SUSPENSION

(Prednisolone Acetate, Sulfacetamide Sodium) 569
May interact with para-aminobenzoic acid based local anesthetics and certain other agents. Compounds in these categories include:

Procaine Hydrochloride (Local anesthetics related to p-amino benzoic acid may antagonize the action of the sulfonamides).
No products indexed under this heading.

Silver Nitrate (Blephamide ophthalmic suspension is incompatible with silver preparations).
No products indexed under this heading.

Tetracaine Hydrochloride (Local anesthetics related to p-amino benzoic acid may antagonize the action of the sulfonamides). Products include:
Cetacaine Topical Anesthetic 999

BLOCADREN TABLETS

(Timolol Maleate) 1916
May interact with catecholamine depleting drugs, calcium channel blockers, cardiac glycosides, oral hypoglycemic agents, insulin, nonsteroidal anti-inflammatory agents, quinidine, and certain other agents. Compounds in these categories include:

Acarbose (Beta blockers may mask the signs and symptoms of acute hypoglycemia). Products include:
Precose Tablets 751

Amlodipine Besylate (Hypotension, AV conduction disturbances, and left ventricular failure have been reported in some patients receiving beta-adrenergic blocking agents when an oral calcium antagonist was added to the treatment regimen). Products include:
Caduet Tablets 2508
Lotrel Capsules 2249
Norvasc Tablets 2545

Bepridil Hydrochloride (Hypotension, AV conduction disturbances, and left ventricular failure have been reported in some patients receiving beta-adrenergic blocking agents when an oral calcium antagonist was added to the treatment regimen).
No products indexed under this heading.

Celecoxib (NSAIDs reduce the antihypertensive effects of Blocadren). Products include:
Celebrex Capsules 3134

Chlorpropamide (Beta blockers may mask the signs and symptoms of acute hypoglycemia).
No products indexed under this heading.

Clonidine (Beta adrenergic blocking agents may exacerbate the rebound hypertension). Products include:
Catapres-TTS ... 844

Clonidine Hydrochloride (Beta adrenergic blocking agents may exacerbate the rebound hypertension). Products include:
Catapres Tablets ... 843
Clorpres Tablets ... 2153

Deserpidine (Close observation of the patient is recommended when Blocadren is administered to patients receiving catecholamine-depleting drugs such as reserpine, because of possible additive effects and the production of hypotension and/or marked bradycardia, which may produce vertigo, syncope, or postural hypotension).
No products indexed under this heading.

Deslanoside (The concomitant use of beta-adrenergic blocking agents with digitalis and either diltiazem or verapamil may have additive effects in prolonging AV conduction time).
No products indexed under this heading.

Diclofenac Potassium (NSAIDs reduce the antihypertensive effects of Blocadren).
No products indexed under this heading.

Diclofenac Sodium (NSAIDs reduce the antihypertensive effects of Blocadren). Products include:
Arthrotec Tablets ... 3129
Voltaren Ophthalmic Solution ... 2309
Voltaren Tablets ... 2307
Voltaren-XR Tablets ... 2310

Digitalis Glycoside Preparations (The concomitant use of beta-adrenergic blocking agents with digitalis and either diltiazem or verapamil may have additive effects in prolonging AV conduction time).
No products indexed under this heading.

Digitoxin (The concomitant use of beta-adrenergic blocking agents with digitalis and either diltiazem or verapamil may have additive effects in prolonging AV conduction time).
No products indexed under this heading.

Digoxin (The concomitant use of beta-adrenergic blocking agents with digitalis and either diltiazem or verapamil may have additive effects in prolonging AV conduction time). Products include:
Lanoxicaps Capsules ... 1490
Lanoxin Injection ... 1494
Lanoxin Injection Pediatric ... 1497
Lanoxin Tablets ... 1500

Diltiazem Hydrochloride (Hypotension, AV conduction disturbances, and left ventricular failure have been reported in some patients receiving beta-adrenergic blocking agents when an oral calcium antagonist was added to the treatment regimen). Products include:
Cardizem LA Extended Release Tablets ... 1728
Tiazac Capsules ... 1201

Epinephrine (Patients with a history of atopy or severe anaphylactic reaction to a variety of allergens may be unresponsive to the usual dose of epinephrine to treat anaphylactic reactions). Products include:
EpiPen ... 1061
Primatene Mist ... ▣719
Twinject 0.15 ... 3379
Twinject 0.3 ... 3378

Epinephrine Hydrochloride (Patients with a history of atopy or severe anaphylactic reaction to a variety of allergens may be unresponsive to the usual dose of epinephrine to treat anaphylactic reactions).
No products indexed under this heading.

Etodolac (NSAIDs reduce the antihypertensive effects of Blocadren).
No products indexed under this heading.

Felodipine (Hypotension, AV conduction disturbances, and left ventricular failure have been reported in some patients receiving beta-adrenergic blocking agents when an oral calcium antagonist was added to the treatment regimen).
No products indexed under this heading.

Fenoprofen Calcium (NSAIDs reduce the antihypertensive effects of Blocadren). Products include:
Nalfon Capsules ... 2502

Flurbiprofen (NSAIDs reduce the antihypertensive effects of Blocadren).
No products indexed under this heading.

Glimepiride (Beta blockers may mask the signs and symptoms of acute hypoglycemia). Products include:
Avandaryl Tablets ... 1379
Duetact Tablets ... 3226

Glipizide (Beta blockers may mask the signs and symptoms of acute hypoglycemia).
No products indexed under this heading.

Glyburide (Beta blockers may mask the signs and symptoms of acute hypoglycemia).
No products indexed under this heading.

Guanethidine Monosulfate (Close observation of the patient is recommended when Blocadren is administered to patients receiving catecholamine-depleting drugs such as reserpine, because of possible additive effects and the production of hypotension and/or marked bradycardia, which may produce vertigo, syncope, or postural hypotension).
No products indexed under this heading.

Ibuprofen (NSAIDs reduce the antihypertensive effects of Blocadren). Products include:
Advil Allergy Sinus Caplets ... ▣770
Advil ... ▣674
Children's Advil Oral Suspension ... ▣603
Children's Advil Chewable Tablets ... ▣603
Advil Cold & Sinus ... ▣723
Infants' Advil Concentrated Drops ... ▣604
Infants' Advil Concentrated Drops - White Grape (Dye-Free) ... ▣604
Junior Strength Advil Swallow Tablets ... ▣605
Advil Migraine Liquigels ... ▣608
Advil Multi-Symptom Cold Caplets ... ▣770
Advil PM Caplets ... ▣615
Motrin IB Tablets and Caplets ... 1866
Children's Motrin Oral Suspension ... 1867
Children's Motrin Non-Staining Dye-Free Oral Suspension ... 1867
Children's Motrin Cold Oral Suspension ... 1867
Infants' Motrin Concentrated Drops ... 1867
Infants' Motrin Non-Staining Dye-Free Concentrated Drops ... 1867
Junior Strength Motrin Caplets and Chewable Tablets ... 1867
Vicoprofen Tablets ... 539

Indomethacin (NSAIDs reduce the antihypertensive effects of Blocadren). Products include:
Indocin ... 1995

Indomethacin Sodium Trihydrate (NSAIDs reduce the antihypertensive effects of Blocadren). Products include:
Indocin I.V. ... 2465

Insulin, Human, Zinc Suspension (Beta blockers may mask the signs and symptoms of acute hypoglycemia; insulin requirements may be altered). Products include:
Humulin L, 100 Units ... 1794
Humulin U, 100 Units ... 1800

Insulin, Human NPH (Beta blockers may mask the signs and symptoms of acute hypoglycemia; insulin requirements may be altered). Products include:
Humulin N, 100 Units ... 1795
Humulin N Pen ... 1797

Insulin, Human Regular (Beta blockers may mask the signs and symptoms of acute hypoglycemia; insulin requirements may be altered). Products include:
Humulin R, 100 Units ... 1798

Insulin, Human Regular and Human NPH Mixture (Beta blockers may mask the signs and symptoms of acute hypoglycemia; insulin requirements may be altered). Products include:
Humulin 50/50, 100 Units ... 1791
Humulin 70/30 Pen ... 1793

Insulin, NPH (Beta blockers may mask the signs and symptoms of acute hypoglycemia; insulin requirements may be altered).
No products indexed under this heading.

Insulin, Regular (Beta blockers may mask the signs and symptoms of acute hypoglycemia; insulin requirements may be altered).
No products indexed under this heading.

Insulin, Zinc Crystals (Beta blockers may mask the signs and symptoms of acute hypoglycemia; insulin requirements may be altered).
No products indexed under this heading.

Insulin, Zinc Suspension (Beta blockers may mask the signs and symptoms of acute hypoglycemia; insulin requirements may be altered).
No products indexed under this heading.

Insulin Aspart, Human Regular (Beta blockers may mask the signs and symptoms of acute hypoglycemia; insulin requirements may be altered). Products include:
NovoLog Injection ... 2326

Insulin glargine (Beta blockers may mask the signs and symptoms of acute hypoglycemia; insulin requirements may be altered). Products include:
Lantus Injection ... 2909

Insulin Lispro, Human (Beta blockers may mask the signs and symptoms of acute hypoglycemia; insulin requirements may be altered). Products include:
Humalog-Pen ... 1781
Humalog Mix 50/50-Pen ... 1783
Humalog Mix 75/25-Pen ... 1785

Insulin Lispro Protamine, Human (Beta blockers may mask the signs and symptoms of acute hypoglycemia; insulin requirements may be altered). Products include:
Humalog Mix 50/50-Pen ... 1783
Humalog Mix 75/25-Pen ... 1785

Isradipine (Hypotension, AV conduction disturbances, and left ventricular failure have been reported in some patients receiving beta-adrenergic blocking agents when an oral calcium antagonist was added to the treatment regimen). Products include:
DynaCirc CR Tablets ... 2721

Ketoprofen (NSAIDs reduce the antihypertensive effects of Blocadren).
No products indexed under this heading.

Ketorolac Tromethamine (NSAIDs reduce the antihypertensive effects of Blocadren). Products include:
Acular Ophthalmic Solution ... 565
Acular LS Ophthalmic Solution ... 566

Meclofenamate Sodium (NSAIDs reduce the antihypertensive effects of Blocadren).
No products indexed under this heading.

Mefenamic Acid (NSAIDs reduce the antihypertensive effects of Blocadren).
No products indexed under this heading.

Meloxicam (NSAIDs reduce the antihypertensive effects of Blocadren). Products include:
Mobic Oral Suspension ... 863
Mobic Tablets ... 863

Metformin Hydrochloride (Beta blockers may mask the signs and symptoms of acute hypoglycemia). Products include:
ActoPlus Met Tablets ... 3214
Avandamet Tablets ... 1373
Fortamet Extended-Release Tablets ... 3115

Mibefradil Dihydrochloride (Hypotension, AV conduction disturbances, and left ventricular failure have been reported in some patients receiving beta-adrenergic blocking agents when an oral calcium antagonist was added to the treatment regimen).
No products indexed under this heading.

Miglitol (Beta blockers may mask the signs and symptoms of acute hypoglycemia).
No products indexed under this heading.

Nabumetone (NSAIDs reduce the antihypertensive effects of Blocadren).
No products indexed under this heading.

Naproxen (NSAIDs reduce the antihypertensive effects of Blocadren). Products include:
EC-Naprosyn Delayed-Release Tablets ... 2761
Naprosyn Suspension ... 2761
Naprosyn Tablets ... 2761
Prevacid NapraPAC ... 3280

Naproxen Sodium (NSAIDs reduce the antihypertensive effects of Blocadren). Products include:
Aleve Caplets ... 742
Aleve Gelcaps ... 743
Aleve Tablets ... 743
Aleve Cold & Sinus Caplets ... 744

Anaprox Tablets 2761
Anaprox DS Tablets 2761

Nicardipine Hydrochloride (Hypotension, AV conduction disturbances, and left ventricular failure have been reported in some patients receiving beta-adrenergic blocking agents when an oral calcium antagonist was added to the treatment regimen). Products include:
Cardene I.V. 2497

Nifedipine (Hypotension, AV conduction disturbances, and left ventricular failure have been reported in some patients receiving beta-adrenergic blocking agents when an oral calcium antagonist was added to the treatment regimen). Products include:
Adalat CC Tablets 2964

Nimodipine (Hypotension, AV conduction disturbances, and left ventricular failure have been reported in some patients receiving beta-adrenergic blocking agents when an oral calcium antagonist was added to the treatment regimen). Products include:
Nimotop Capsules 749

Nisoldipine (Hypotension, AV conduction disturbances, and left ventricular failure have been reported in some patients receiving beta-adrenergic blocking agents when an oral calcium antagonist was added to the treatment regimen). Products include:
Sular Tablets 3122

Oxaprozin (NSAIDs reduce the antihypertensive effects of Blocadren).
No products indexed under this heading.

Phenylbutazone (NSAIDs reduce the antihypertensive effects of Blocadren).
No products indexed under this heading.

Pioglitazone Hydrochloride (Beta blockers may mask the signs and symptoms of acute hypoglycemia). Products include:
ActoPlus Met Tablets 3214
Actos Tablets 3219
Duetact Tablets 3226

Piroxicam (NSAIDs reduce the antihypertensive effects of Blocadren).
No products indexed under this heading.

Quinidine (Co-administration has resulted in potentiated systemic beta-blockade, such as decreased heart rate).
No products indexed under this heading.

Quinidine Gluconate (Co-administration has resulted in potentiated systemic beta-blockade, such as decreased heart rate).
No products indexed under this heading.

Quinidine Hydrochloride (Co-administration has resulted in potentiated systemic beta-blockade, such as decreased heart rate).
No products indexed under this heading.

Quinidine Polygalacturonate (Co-administration has resulted in potentiated systemic beta-blockade, such as decreased heart rate).
No products indexed under this heading.

Quinidine Sulfate (Co-administration has resulted in potentiated systemic beta-blockade, such as decreased heart rate).
No products indexed under this heading.

Rauwolfia Serpentina (Close observation of the patient is recommended when Blocadren is administered to patients receiving catecholamine-depleting drugs such as reserpine, because of possible additive effects and the production of hypotension and/or marked bradycardia, which may produce vertigo, syncope, or postural hypotension).
No products indexed under this heading.

Repaglinide (Beta blockers may mask the signs and symptoms of acute hypoglycemia).
No products indexed under this heading.

Rescinnamine (Close observation of the patient is recommended when Blocadren is administered to patients receiving catecholamine-depleting drugs such as reserpine, because of possible additive effects and the production of hypotension and/or marked bradycardia, which may produce vertigo, syncope, or postural hypotension).
No products indexed under this heading.

Reserpine (Close observation of the patient is recommended when Blocadren is administered to patients receiving catecholamine-depleting drugs such as reserpine, because of possible additive effects and the production of hypotension and/or marked bradycardia, which may produce vertigo, syncope, or postural hypotension).
No products indexed under this heading.

Rofecoxib (NSAIDs reduce the antihypertensive effects of Blocadren).
No products indexed under this heading.

Rosiglitazone Maleate (Beta blockers may mask the signs and symptoms of acute hypoglycemia). Products include:
Avandamet Tablets 1373
Avandaryl Tablets 1379
Avandia Tablets 1384

Sulindac (NSAIDs reduce the antihypertensive effects of Blocadren). Products include:
Clinoril Tablets 1924

Tolazamide (Beta blockers may mask the signs and symptoms of acute hypoglycemia).
No products indexed under this heading.

Tolbutamide (Beta blockers may mask the signs and symptoms of acute hypoglycemia).
No products indexed under this heading.

Tolmetin Sodium (NSAIDs reduce the antihypertensive effects of Blocadren).
No products indexed under this heading.

Troglitazone (Beta blockers may mask the signs and symptoms of acute hypoglycemia).
No products indexed under this heading.

Valdecoxib (NSAIDs reduce the antihypertensive effects of Blocadren).
No products indexed under this heading.

Verapamil Hydrochloride (Hypotension, AV conduction disturbances, and left ventricular failure have been reported in some patients receiving beta-adrenergic blocking agents when an oral calcium antagonist was added to the treatment regimen). Products include:
Covera-HS Tablets 3139
Tarka Tablets 524
Verelan PM Extended-Release Capsules, Controlled-Onset........... 3106

BONIVA INJECTION

(Ibandronate Sodium) 2738
None cited in PDR database.

BONIVA TABLETS

(Ibandronate Sodium) 2741
May interact with antacids containing aluminum, calcium and magnesium, non-steroidal anti-inflammatory agents, and certain other agents. Compounds in these categories include:

Aluminum Carbonate (Products containing calcium and other multivalent cations (such as aluminum, magnesium, iron) are likely to interfere with absorption of ibandronate sodium. Ibandronate sodium should be taken at least 60 minutes before any oral medications containing multivalent cations (including antacids)).
No products indexed under this heading.

Aluminum Hydroxide (Products containing calcium and other multivalent cations (such as aluminum, magnesium, iron) are likely to interfere with absorption of ibandronate sodium. Ibandronate sodium should be taken at least 60 minutes before any oral medications containing multivalent cations (including antacids)). Products include:
Gaviscon Regular Strength Liquid .. 658
Gaviscon Regular Strength Tablets.. 658
Gaviscon Extra Strength Liquid 658
Gaviscon Extra Strength Tablets 658
Maalox Regular Strength Antacid/Antigas Liquid................. 2175
Maalox Max Maximum Strength Antacid/Anti-Gas Liquid................ 2176

Aspirin (Since aspirin and bisphosphonates are associated with gastrointestinal irritation, caution should be exercised in the concomitant use of aspirin products with ibandronate sodium). Products include:
Aggrenox Capsules 822
Bayer Aspirin 744
BC Allergy Sinus Cold Powder 677
BC Headache Powder 677
Arthritis Strength BC Powder 677
BC Sinus Cold Powder 677
Excedrin Extra Strength Caplets/Tablets/Geltabs............ 684
Excedrin Migraine Caplets/Tablets/Geltabs............ 609
Goody's Body Pain Formula Powder.. 684
Goody's Extra Strength Headache Powders....................... 611
Goody's Extra Strength Pain Relief Tablets 685
Percodan Tablets 1132
St. Joseph 81 mg Aspirin Chewable and Enteric Coated Tablets... 1869

Aspirin, Enteric Coated (Since aspirin and bisphosphonates are associated with gastrointestinal irritation, caution should be exercised in the concomitant use of aspirin products with ibandronate sodium).
No products indexed under this heading.

Aspirin Buffered (Since aspirin and bisphosphonates are associated with gastrointestinal irritation, caution should be exercised in the concomitant use of aspirin products with ibandronate sodium). Products include:
Bufferin Extra Strength Tablets 678
Bufferin Regular Strength Tablets ... 678

Calcium (Products containing calcium and other multivalent cations (such as aluminum, magnesium, iron) are likely to interfere with absorption of ibandronate sodium. Ibandronate sodium should be taken at least 60 minutes before any oral medications containing multivalent cations (including supplements and vitamins)). Products include:
Os-Cal 250 + D Tablets 817
Os-Cal 500 Tablets 817
Os-Cal 500 + D Tablets 817

Calcium (Oyster Shell) (Products containing calcium and other multivalent cations (such as aluminum, magnesium, iron) are likely to interfere with absorption of ibandronate sodium. Ibandronate sodium should be taken at least 60 minutes before any oral medications containing multivalent cations (including supplements and vitamins)).
No products indexed under this heading.

Calcium Carbonate (Products containing calcium and other multivalent cations (such as aluminum, magnesium, iron) are likely to interfere with absorption of ibandronate sodium. Ibandronate sodium should be taken at least 60 minutes before any oral medications containing multivalent cations (including supplements and vitamins)). Products include:
Actonel with Calcium Tablets 2688
Calcet Tablets 2138
Caltrate 600 PLUS 809
Caltrate 600 + D Tablets 809
D-Cal Chewable Caplets 812
Gas-X with Maalox 656
Maalox Regular Strength Antacid Chewable Tablets 2177
Maalox Max Maximum Strength Antacid/Antigas Chewable Tablets.. 2176
Maalox Max Maximum Strength Chewable Tablets....................... 660
Os-Cal Chewable Tablets 818
Pepcid Complete Chewable Tablets.. 1701
Children's Pepto 2674
PremCal Light, Regular, and Extra Strength Tablets................. 818
Tums 664

Calcium Citrate (Products containing calcium and other multivalent cations (such as aluminum, magnesium, iron) are likely to interfere with absorption of ibandronate sodium. Ibandronate sodium should be taken at least 60 minutes before any oral medications containing multivalent cations (including supplements and vitamins)). Products include:
Active Calcium Tablets 3339
Citracal Caplets 703
Citracal Lemon Cream Creamy Bites.. 2139
Citracal Prenatal + DHA Tablets and Capsules.............................. 2139

Celecoxib (Since NSAIDs and bisphosphonates are associated with gastrointestinal irritation, caution should be exercised in the concomitant use of NSAIDs with ibandronate sodium). Products include:

Celebrex Capsules 3134

Diclofenac Potassium (Since NSAIDs and bisphosphonates are associated with gastrointestinal irritation, caution should be exercised in the concomitant use of NSAIDs with ibandronate sodium).

No products indexed under this heading.

Diclofenac Sodium (Since NSAIDs and bisphosphonates are associated with gastrointestinal irritation, caution should be exercised in the concomitant use of NSAIDs with ibandronate sodium). Products include:

Arthrotec Tablets 3129
Voltaren Ophthalmic Solution 2309
Voltaren Tablets 2307
Voltaren-XR Tablets 2310

Etodolac (Since NSAIDs and bisphosphonates are associated with gastrointestinal irritation, caution should be exercised in the concomitant use of NSAIDs with ibandronate sodium).

No products indexed under this heading.

Fenoprofen Calcium (Since NSAIDs and bisphosphonates are associated with gastrointestinal irritation, caution should be exercised in the concomitant use of NSAIDs with ibandronate sodium). Products include:

Nalfon Capsules 2502

Flurbiprofen (Since NSAIDs and bisphosphonates are associated with gastrointestinal irritation, caution should be exercised in the concomitant use of NSAIDs with ibandronate sodium).

No products indexed under this heading.

Ibuprofen (Since NSAIDs and bisphosphonates are associated with gastrointestinal irritation, caution should be exercised in the concomitant use of NSAIDs with ibandronate sodium). Products include:

Advil Allergy Sinus Caplets .... ▣770
Advil .... ▣674
Children's Advil Oral Suspension .... ▣603
Children's Advil Chewable Tablets .. ▣603
Advil Cold & Sinus .... ▣723
Infants' Advil Concentrated Drops .. ▣604
Infants' Advil Concentrated Drops - White Grape (Dye-Free) .... ▣604
Junior Strength Advil Swallow Tablets .... ▣605
Advil Migraine Liquigels .... ▣608
Advil Multi-Symptom Cold Caplets .... ▣770
Advil PM Caplets .... ▣615
Motrin IB Tablets and Caplets 1866
Children's Motrin Oral Suspension ... 1867
Children's Motrin Non-Staining Dye-Free Oral Suspension 1867
Children's Motrin Cold Oral Suspension 1867
Infants' Motrin Concentrated Drops 1867
Infants' Motrin Non-Staining Dye-Free Concentrated Drops 1867
Junior Strength Motrin Caplets and Chewable Tablets 1867
Vicoprofen Tablets 539

Indomethacin (Since NSAIDs and bisphosphonates are associated with gastrointestinal irritation, caution should be exercised in the concomitant use of NSAIDs with ibandronate sodium). Products include:

Indocin 1995

Indomethacin Sodium Trihydrate (Since NSAIDs and bisphosphonates are associated with gastrointestinal irritation, caution should be exercised in the concomitant use of NSAIDs with ibandronate sodium). Products include:

Indocin I.V. 2465

Iron (Products containing calcium and other multivalent cations (such as aluminum, magnesium, iron) are likely to interfere with absorption of ibandronate sodium. Ibandronate sodium should be taken at least 60 minutes before any oral medications containing multivalent cations (including supplements and vitamins)).

No products indexed under this heading.

Iron Supplements (Products containing calcium and other multivalent cations (such as aluminum, magnesium, iron) are likely to interfere with absorption of ibandronate sodium. Ibandronate sodium should be taken at least 60 minutes before any oral medications containing multivalent cations (including supplements and vitamins)).

No products indexed under this heading.

Ketoprofen (Since NSAIDs and bisphosphonates are associated with gastrointestinal irritation, caution should be exercised in the concomitant use of NSAIDs with ibandronate sodium).

No products indexed under this heading.

Ketorolac Tromethamine (Since NSAIDs and bisphosphonates are associated with gastrointestinal irritation, caution should be exercised in the concomitant use of NSAIDs with ibandronate sodium). Products include:

Acular Ophthalmic Solution 565
Acular LS Ophthalmic Solution 566

Magaldrate (Products containing calcium and other multivalent cations (such as aluminum, magnesium, iron) are likely to interfere with absorption of ibandronate sodium. Ibandronate sodium should be taken at least 60 minutes before any oral medications containing multivalent cations (including antacids)).

No products indexed under this heading.

Magnesium Hydroxide (Products containing calcium and other multivalent cations (such as aluminum, magnesium, iron) are likely to interfere with absorption of ibandronate sodium. Ibandronate sodium should be taken at least 60 minutes before any oral medications containing multivalent cations (including antacids)). Products include:

Maalox Regular Strength Antacid/Antigas Liquid 2175
Maalox Max Maximum Strength Antacid/Anti-Gas Liquid 2176
Pepcid Complete Chewable Tablets 1701

Magnesium Oxide (Products containing calcium and other multivalent cations (such as aluminum, magnesium, iron) are likely to interfere with absorption of ibandronate sodium. Ibandronate sodium should be taken at least 60 minutes before any oral medications containing multivalent cations (including antacids)). Products include:

Beelith Tablets 759
PremCal Light, Regular, and Extra Strength Tablets .... ▣818

Meclofenamate Sodium (Since NSAIDs and bisphosphonates are associated with gastrointestinal irritation, caution should be exercised in the concomitant use of NSAIDs with ibandronate sodium).

No products indexed under this heading.

Mefenamic Acid (Since NSAIDs and bisphosphonates are associated with gastrointestinal irritation, caution should be exercised in the concomitant use of NSAIDs with ibandronate sodium).

No products indexed under this heading.

Meloxicam (Since NSAIDs and bisphosphonates are associated with gastrointestinal irritation, caution should be exercised in the concomitant use of NSAIDs with ibandronate sodium). Products include:

Mobic Oral Suspension 863
Mobic Tablets 863

Multivitamins (Products containing calcium and other multivalent cations (such as aluminum, magnesium, iron) are likely to interfere with absorption of ibandronate sodium. Ibandronate sodium should be taken at least 60 minutes before any oral medications containing multivalent cations (including vitamins)).

No products indexed under this heading.

Multivitamins with Minerals (Products containing calcium and other multivalent cations (such as aluminum, magnesium, iron) are likely to interfere with absorption of ibandronate sodium. Ibandronate sodium should be taken at least 60 minutes before any oral medications containing multivalent cations (including vitamins)). Products include:

Citracal Prenatal + DHA Tablets and Capsules 2139
One-A-Day Cholesterol Plus Tablets .... ▣815
One-A-Day Men's Health Formula Tablets .... ▣815

Nabumetone (Since NSAIDs and bisphosphonates are associated with gastrointestinal irritation, caution should be exercised in the concomitant use of NSAIDs with ibandronate sodium).

No products indexed under this heading.

Naproxen (Since NSAIDs and bisphosphonates are associated with gastrointestinal irritation, caution should be exercised in the concomitant use of NSAIDs with ibandronate sodium). Products include:

EC-Naprosyn Delayed-Release Tablets 2761
Naprosyn Suspension 2761
Naprosyn Tablets 2761
Prevacid NapraPAC 3280

Naproxen Sodium (Since NSAIDs and bisphosphonates are associated with gastrointestinal irritation, caution should be exercised in the concomitant use of NSAIDs with ibandronate sodium). Products include:

Aleve Caplets 742
Aleve Gelcaps 743
Aleve Tablets 743
Aleve Cold & Sinus Caplets 744
Anaprox Tablets 2761
Anaprox DS Tablets 2761

Oxaprozin (Since NSAIDs and bisphosphonates are associated with gastrointestinal irritation, caution should be exercised in the concomitant use of NSAIDs with ibandronate sodium).

No products indexed under this heading.

Phenylbutazone (Since NSAIDs and bisphosphonates are associated with gastrointestinal irritation, caution should be exercised in the concomitant use of NSAIDs with ibandronate sodium).

No products indexed under this heading.

Piroxicam (Since NSAIDs and bisphosphonates are associated with gastrointestinal irritation, caution should be exercised in the concomitant use of NSAIDs with ibandronate sodium).

No products indexed under this heading.

Rofecoxib (Since NSAIDs and bisphosphonates are associated with gastrointestinal irritation, caution should be exercised in the concomitant use of NSAIDs with ibandronate sodium).

No products indexed under this heading.

Sulindac (Since NSAIDs and bisphosphonates are associated with gastrointestinal irritation, caution should be exercised in the concomitant use of NSAIDs with ibandronate sodium). Products include:

Clinoril Tablets 1924

Tolmetin Sodium (Since NSAIDs and bisphosphonates are associated with gastrointestinal irritation, caution should be exercised in the concomitant use of NSAIDs with ibandronate sodium).

No products indexed under this heading.

Valdecoxib (Since NSAIDs and bisphosphonates are associated with gastrointestinal irritation, caution should be exercised in the concomitant use of NSAIDs with ibandronate sodium).

No products indexed under this heading.

Vitamins, Multiple (Products containing calcium and other multivalent cations (such as aluminum, magnesium, iron) are likely to interfere with absorption of ibandronate sodium. Ibandronate sodium should be taken at least 60 minutes before any oral medications containing multivalent cations (including vitamins)). Products include:

Flintstones Gummies .... ▣813
Mega Antioxidant Tablets 3339
My First Flintstones Multivitamin Tablets .... ▣814
Vemma Nutrition Program - Mangosteen Plus .... ▣835

Vitamins with Iron (Products containing calcium and other multivalent cations (such as aluminum, magnesium, iron) are likely to interfere with absorption of ibandronate sodium. Ibandronate sodium should be taken at least 60 minutes before any oral medications containing multivalent cations (including vitamins)).

No products indexed under this heading.

BOOSTRIX
(Diphtheria & Tetanus Toxoids and Acellular Pertussis Vaccine Adsorbed) 1404
May interact with alkylating agents, antimetabolites, corticosteroids, cytotoxic drugs, immunosuppressive agents, and certain other agents. Compounds in these categories include:

Azathioprine (May reduce immune response to vaccines. When administered to patients who are receiving immunosuppressive therapy, who have an immunodeficiency disorder, or who have received a recent injection of immune globulin, an adequate immunologic response may not be obtained).
No products indexed under this heading.

Basiliximab (May reduce immune response to vaccines. When administered to patients who are receiving immunosuppressive therapy, who have an immunodeficiency disorder, or who have received a recent injection of immune globulin, an adequate immunologic response may not be obtained). Products include:
Simulect for Injection 2284

Betamethasone Acetate (May reduce immune response to vaccines when used concomitantly with corticosteroids (greater than physiologic doses). When administered to patients who are receiving immunosuppressive therapy, who have an immunodeficiency disorder, or who have received arecent injection of immune globulin, an adequate immunologic response may not be obtained).
No products indexed under this heading.

Betamethasone Sodium Phosphate (May reduce immune response to vaccines when used concomitantly with corticosteroids (greater than physiologic doses). When administered to patients who are receiving immunosuppressive therapy, who have an immunodeficiency disorder, or who have received arecent injection of immune globulin, an adequate immunologic response may not be obtained).
No products indexed under this heading.

Bleomycin Sulfate (May reduce immune response to vaccines. When administered to patients who are receiving immunosuppressive therapy, who have an immunodeficiency disorder, or who have received a recent injection of immune globulin, an adequate immunologic response may not be obtained).
No products indexed under this heading.

Busulfan (May reduce immune response to vaccines. When administered to patients who are receiving immunosuppressive therapy, who have an immunodeficiency disorder, or who have received a recent injection of immune globulin, an adequate immunologic response may not be obtained). Products include:
I.V. Busulfex 2493
Myleran Tablets 1525

Capecitabine (May reduce immune response to vaccines. When administered to patients who are receiving immunosuppressive therapy, who have an immunodeficiency disorder, or who have received a recent injection of immune globulin, an adequate immunologic response may not be obtained). Products include:
Xeloda Tablets 2822

Carmustine (BCNU) (May reduce immune response to vaccines. When administered to patients who are receiving immunosuppressive therapy, who have an immunodeficiency disorder, or who have received a recent injection of immune globulin, an adequate immunologic response may not be obtained).
No products indexed under this heading.

Chlorambucil (May reduce immune response to vaccines. When administered to patients who are receiving immunosuppressive therapy, who have an immunodeficiency disorder, or who have received a recent injection of immune globulin, an adequate immunologic response may not be obtained). Products include:
Leukeran Tablets 1504

Cladribine (May reduce immune response to vaccines. When administered to patients who are receiving immunosuppressive therapy, who have an immunodeficiency disorder, or who have received a recent injection of immune globulin, an adequate immunologic response may not be obtained). Products include:
Leustatin Injection 2357

Cortisone Acetate (May reduce immune response to vaccines when used concomitantly with corticosteroids (greater than physiologic doses). When administered to patients who are receiving immunosuppressive therapy, who have an immunodeficiency disorder, or who have received arecent injection of immune globulin, an adequate immunologic response may not be obtained).
No products indexed under this heading.

Cyclophosphamide (May reduce immune response to vaccines. When administered to patients who are receiving immunosuppressive therapy, who have an immunodeficiency disorder, or who have received a recent injection of immune globulin, an adequate immunologic response may not be obtained).
No products indexed under this heading.

Cyclosporine (May reduce immune response to vaccines. When administered to patients who are receiving immunosuppressive therapy, who have an immunodeficiency disorder, or who have received a recent injection of immune globulin, an adequate immunologic response may not be obtained). Products include:
Gengraf Capsules 459
Neoral Oral Solution 2259
Neoral Soft Gelatin Capsules 2259
Restasis Ophthalmic Emulsion 575
Sandimmune 2275

Cytarabine (May reduce immune response to vaccines. When administered to patients who are receiving immunosuppressive therapy, who have an immunodeficiency disorder, or who have received a recent injection of immune globulin, an adequate immunologic response may not be obtained).
No products indexed under this heading.

Dacarbazine (May reduce immune response to vaccines. When administered to patients who are receiving immunosuppressive therapy, who have an immunodeficiency disorder, or who have received a recent injection of immune globulin, an adequate immunologic response may not be obtained).
No products indexed under this heading.

Daunorubicin Hydrochloride (May reduce immune response to vaccines. When administered to patients who are receiving immunosuppressive therapy, who have an immunodeficiency disorder, or who have received a recent injection of immune globulin, an adequate immunologic response may not be obtained).
No products indexed under this heading.

Dexamethasone (May reduce immune response to vaccines when used concomitantly with corticosteroids (greater than physiologic doses). When administered to patients who are receiving immunosuppressive therapy, who have an immunodeficiency disorder, or who have received arecent injection of immune globulin, an adequate immunologic response may not be obtained). Products include:
Ciprodex Otic Suspension 559
Decadron Tablets 1951
TobraDex Ophthalmic Ointment 562
TobraDex Ophthalmic Suspension 563

Dexamethasone Acetate (May reduce immune response to vaccines when used concomitantly with corticosteroids (greater than physiologic doses). When administered to patients who are receiving immunosuppressive therapy, who have an immunodeficiency disorder, or who have received arecent injection of immune globulin, an adequate immunologic response may not be obtained).
No products indexed under this heading.

Dexamethasone Sodium Phosphate (May reduce immune response to vaccines when used concomitantly with corticosteroids (greater than physiologic doses). When administered to patients who are receiving immunosuppressive therapy, who have an immunodeficiency disorder, or who have received arecent injection of immune globulin, an adequate immunologic response may not be obtained).
No products indexed under this heading.

Doxorubicin Hydrochloride (May reduce immune response to vaccines. When administered to patients who are receiving immunosuppressive therapy, who have an immunodeficiency disorder, or who have received a recent injection of immune globulin, an adequate immunologic response may not be obtained).
No products indexed under this heading.

Epirubicin Hydrochloride (May reduce immune response to vaccines. When administered to patients who are receiving immunosuppressive therapy, who have an immunodeficiency disorder, or who have received a recent injection of immune globulin, an adequate immunologic response may not be obtained).
No products indexed under this heading.

Floxuridine (May reduce immune response to vaccines. When administered to patients who are receiving immunosuppressive therapy, who have an immunodeficiency disorder, or who have received a recent injection of immune globulin, an adequate immunologic response may not be obtained).
No products indexed under this heading.

Fludarabine Phosphate (May reduce immune response to vaccines. When administered to patients who are receiving immunosuppressive therapy, who have an immunodeficiency disorder, or who have received a recent injection of immune globulin, an adequate immunologic response may not be obtained).
No products indexed under this heading.

Fludrocortisone Acetate (May reduce immune response to vaccines when used concomitantly with corticosteroids (greater than physiologic doses). When administered to patients who are receiving immunosuppressive therapy, who have an immunodeficiency disorder, or who have received arecent injection of immune globulin, an adequate immunologic response may not be obtained).
No products indexed under this heading.

Fluorouracil (May reduce immune response to vaccines. When administered to patients who are receiving immunosuppressive therapy, who have an immunodeficiency disorder, or who have received a recent injection of immune globulin, an adequate immunologic response may not be obtained). Products include:
Carac Cream, 0.5% 2879
Efudex 3363

Gemcitabine Hydrochloride (May reduce immune response to vaccines. When administered to patients who are receiving immunosuppressive therapy, who have an immunodeficiency disorder, or who have received a recent injection of immune globulin, an adequate immunologic response may not be obtained). Products include:
Gemzar for Injection 1771

Hydrocortisone (May reduce immune response to vaccines when used concomitantly with corticosteroids (greater than physiologic doses). When administered to patients who are receiving immunosuppressive therapy, who have an immunodeficiency disorder, or who have received arecent injection of immune globulin, an adequate immunologic response may not be obtained). Products include:
Colocort Rectal Suspension, USP (Retention) 100 mg/60 mL 2476
Hydrocortone Tablets 1989
Preparation H Hydrocortisone Cream 646

Hydrocortisone Acetate (May reduce immune response to vaccines when used concomitantly with corticosteroids (greater than physiologic doses). When administered to patients who are receiving immunosuppressive therapy, who have an immunodeficiency disorder, or who have received arecent injection of immune globulin, an adequate immunologic response may not be obtained). Products include:

Analpram-HC 1159
Pramosone 1161
ProctoFoam-HC 3099

Hydrocortisone Sodium Phosphate (May reduce immune response to vaccines when used concomitantly with corticosteroids (greater than physiologic doses). When administered to patients who are receiving immunosuppressive therapy, who have an immunodeficiency disorder, or who have received arecent injection of immune globulin, an adequate immunologic response may not be obtained).

No products indexed under this heading.

Hydrocortisone Sodium Succinate (May reduce immune response to vaccines when used concomitantly with corticosteroids (greater than physiologic doses). When administered to patients who are receiving immunosuppressive therapy, who have an immunodeficiency disorder, or who have received arecent injection of immune globulin, an adequate immunologic response may not be obtained).

No products indexed under this heading.

Hydroxyurea (May reduce immune response to vaccines. When administered to patients who are receiving immunosuppressive therapy, who have an immunodeficiency disorder, or who have received a recent injection of immune globulin, an adequate immunologic response may not be obtained).

No products indexed under this heading.

Immune Globulin Intravenous (Human) (May reduce immune response to vaccines. When administered to patients who are receiving immunosuppressive therapy, who have an immunodeficiency disorder, or who have received a recent injection of immune globulin, an adequate immunologic response may not be obtained). Products include:

Carimune NF 3499
Gammagard Liquid 721
Gammagard S/D 724
Gamunex Immune Globulin I.V., 10% .. 3235

Lomustine (CCNU) (May reduce immune response to vaccines. When administered to patients who are receiving immunosuppressive therapy, who have an immunodeficiency disorder, or who have received a recent injection of immune globulin, an adequate immunologic response may not be obtained).

No products indexed under this heading.

Mechlorethamine Hydrochloride (May reduce immune response to vaccines. When administered to patients who are receiving immunosuppressive therapy, who have an immunodeficiency disorder, or who have received a recent injection of

immune globulin, an adequate immunologic response may not be obtained). Products include:

Mustargen for Injection 2468

Melphalan (May reduce immune response to vaccines. When administered to patients who are receiving immunosuppressive therapy, who have an immunodeficiency disorder, or who have received a recent injection of immune globulin, an adequate immunologic response may not be obtained). Products include:

Alkeran Tablets 956

Mercaptopurine (May reduce immune response to vaccines. When administered to patients who are receiving immunosuppressive therapy, who have an immunodeficiency disorder, or who have received a recent injection of immune globulin, an adequate immunologic response may not be obtained).

No products indexed under this heading.

Methotrexate (May reduce immune response to vaccines. When administered to patients who are receiving immunosuppressive therapy, who have an immunodeficiency disorder, or who have received a recent injection of immune globulin, an adequate immunologic response may not be obtained).

No products indexed under this heading.

Methotrexate Sodium (May reduce immune response to vaccines. When administered to patients who are receiving immunosuppressive therapy, who have an immunodeficiency disorder, or who have received a recent injection of immune globulin, an adequate immunologic response may not be obtained).

No products indexed under this heading.

Methylprednisolone Acetate (May reduce immune response to vaccines when used concomitantly with corticosteroids (greater than physiologic doses). When administered to patients who are receiving immunosuppressive therapy, who have an immunodeficiency disorder, or who have received arecent injection of immune globulin, an adequate immunologic response may not be obtained). Products include:

Depo-Medrol Injectable Suspension 2617
Depo-Medrol Single-Dose Vial 2619

Methylprednisolone Sodium Succinate (May reduce immune response to vaccines when used concomitantly with corticosteroids (greater than physiologic doses). When administered to patients who are receiving immunosuppressive therapy, who have an immunodeficiency disorder, or who have received arecent injection of immune globulin, an adequate immunologic response may not be obtained).

No products indexed under this heading.

Mitotane (May reduce immune response to vaccines. When administered to patients who are receiving immunosuppressive therapy, who have an immunodeficiency disorder, or who have received a recent injection of immune globulin, an adequate immunologic response may not be obtained).

No products indexed under this heading.

Mitoxantrone Hydrochloride (May reduce immune response to vaccines. When administered to patients who are receiving immunosuppressive therapy, who have an immunodeficiency disorder, or who have received a recent injection of immune globulin, an adequate immunologic response may not be obtained).

No products indexed under this heading.

Muromonab-CD3 (May reduce immune response to vaccines. When administered to patients who are receiving immunosuppressive therapy, who have an immunodeficiency disorder, or who have received a recent injection of immune globulin, an adequate immunologic response may not be obtained). Products include:

Orthoclone OKT3 Sterile Solution 2360

Mycophenolate Mofetil (May reduce immune response to vaccines. When administered to patients who are receiving immunosuppressive therapy, who have an immunodeficiency disorder, or who have received a recent injection of immune globulin, an adequate immunologic response may not be obtained). Products include:

CellCept Capsules 2747
CellCept Oral Suspension 2747
CellCept Tablets 2747

Pentostatin (May reduce immune response to vaccines. When administered to patients who are receiving immunosuppressive therapy, who have an immunodeficiency disorder, or who have received a recent injection of immune globulin, an adequate immunologic response may not be obtained). Products include:

Nipent for Injection 1863

Prednisolone Acetate (May reduce immune response to vaccines when used concomitantly with corticosteroids (greater than physiologic doses). When administered to patients who are receiving immunosuppressive therapy, who have an immunodeficiency disorder, or who have received arecent injection of immune globulin, an adequate immunologic response may not be obtained). Products include:

Blephamide Ophthalmic Ointment 568
Blephamide Ophthalmic Suspension 569
Poly-Pred Ophthalmic Suspension ⊙233
Pred Forte Ophthalmic Suspension ⊙235
Pred Mild Ophthalmic Suspension ⊙238
Pred-G Ophthalmic Ointment ⊙237
Pred-G Ophthalmic Suspension ⊙236

Prednisolone Sodium Phosphate (May reduce immune response to vaccines when used concomitantly with corticosteroids (greater than physiologic doses). When administered to patients who are receiving immunosuppressive therapy, who have an immunodeficiency disorder, or who have received arecent injection of immune globulin, an adequate immunologic response may not be obtained).

No products indexed under this heading.

Prednisolone Tebutate (May reduce immune response to vaccines when used concomitantly with corticosteroids (greater than physiologic doses). When administered to patients who are receiving immunosuppressive therapy, who have an immunodeficiency disorder, or who have received arecent injection of immune globulin, an adequate immunologic response may not be obtained).

No products indexed under this heading.

Prednisone (May reduce immune response to vaccines when used concomitantly with corticosteroids (greater than physiologic doses). When administered to patients who are receiving immunosuppressive therapy, who have an immunodeficiency disorder, or who have received arecent injection of immune globulin, an adequate immunologic response may not be obtained).

No products indexed under this heading.

Procarbazine Hydrochloride (May reduce immune response to vaccines. When administered to patients who are receiving immunosuppressive therapy, who have an immunodeficiency disorder, or who have received a recent injection of immune globulin, an adequate immunologic response may not be obtained). Products include:

Matulane Capsules 3191

Sirolimus (May reduce immune response to vaccines. When administered to patients who are receiving immunosuppressive therapy, who have an immunodeficiency disorder, or who have received a recent injection of immune globulin, an adequate immunologic response may not be obtained). Products include:

Rapamune Oral Solution and Tablets 3475

Tacrolimus (May reduce immune response to vaccines. When administered to patients who are receiving immunosuppressive therapy, who have an immunodeficiency disorder, or who have received a recent injection of immune globulin, an adequate immunologic response may not be obtained). Products include:

Prograf Capsules and Injection 632
Protopic Ointment 638

Tamoxifen Citrate (May reduce immune response to vaccines. When administered to patients who are receiving immunosuppressive therapy, who have an immunodeficiency disorder, or who have received a recent injection of immune globulin, an adequate immunologic response may not be obtained). Products include:

Soltamox Oral Solution 3527

Thioguanine (May reduce immune response to vaccines. When administered to patients who are receiving immunosuppressive therapy, who have an immunodeficiency disorder, or who have received a recent injection of immune globulin, an adequate immunologic response may not be obtained). Products include:

Tabloid Tablets 1575

Thiotepa (May reduce immune response to vaccines. When administered to patients who are receiving immunosuppressive therapy, who have an immunodeficiency disorder, or who have received a recent injection of immune globulin, an adequate immunologic response may not be obtained).
No products indexed under this heading.

Triamcinolone (May reduce immune response to vaccines when used concomitantly with corticosteroids (greater than physiologic doses). When administered to patients who are receiving immunosuppressive therapy, who have an immunodeficiency disorder, or who have received arecent injection of immune globulin, an adequate immunologic response may not be obtained).
No products indexed under this heading.

Triamcinolone Acetonide (May reduce immune response to vaccines when used concomitantly with corticosteroids (greater than physiologic doses). When administered to patients who are receiving immunosuppressive therapy, who have an immunodeficiency disorder, or who have received arecent injection of immune globulin, an adequate immunologic response may not be obtained). Products include:
Azmacort Inhalation Aerosol 1726
Nasacort AQ Nasal Spray 2922

Triamcinolone Diacetate (May reduce immune response to vaccines when used concomitantly with corticosteroids (greater than physiologic doses). When administered to patients who are receiving immunosuppressive therapy, who have an immunodeficiency disorder, or who have received arecent injection of immune globulin, an adequate immunologic response may not be obtained).
No products indexed under this heading.

Triamcinolone Hexacetonide (May reduce immune response to vaccines when used concomitantly with corticosteroids (greater than physiologic doses). When administered to patients who are receiving immunosuppressive therapy, who have an immunodeficiency disorder, or who have received arecent injection of immune globulin, an adequate immunologic response may not be obtained).
No products indexed under this heading.

Vincristine Sulfate (May reduce immune response to vaccines. When administered to patients who are receiving immunosuppressive therapy, who have an immunodeficiency disorder, or who have received a recent injection of immune globulin, an adequate immunologic response may not be obtained).
No products indexed under this heading.

BOTOX PURIFIED NEUROTOXIN COMPLEX

(Botulinum Toxin Type A) 570
None cited in PDR database.

BREVOXYL-4 CREAMY WASH

(Benzoyl Peroxide) 3210
None cited in PDR database.

BREVOXYL-4 GEL

(Benzoyl Peroxide) 3210
None cited in PDR database.

BREVOXYL-8 CREAMY WASH

(Benzoyl Peroxide) 3210
None cited in PDR database.

BREVOXYL-8 GEL

(Benzoyl Peroxide) 3210
None cited in PDR database.

BRIMONIDINE TARTRATE OPHTHALMIC SOLUTION 0.2%

(Brimonidine Tartrate) .... ⊙248
May interact with antihypertensives, beta blockers, central nervous system depressants, cardiac glycosides, monoamine oxidase inhibitors, and tricyclic antidepressants. Compounds in these categories include:

Acebutolol Hydrochloride (Caution is advised in concomitant use of beta-blockers and brimonidine).
No products indexed under this heading.

Alfentanil Hydrochloride (There may be an additive or potentiating effect with CNS depressants and brimonidine administered concomitanty).
No products indexed under this heading.

Alprazolam (There may be an additive or potentiating effect with CNS depressants and brimonidine administered concomitanty). Products include:
Niravam Orally Disintegrating Tablets 3092

Amitriptyline Hydrochloride (Caution is advised in concomitant use of tricyclic antidepressants and brimonidine).
No products indexed under this heading.

Amlodipine Besylate (Caution is advised in concomitant use of antihypertensives and brimonidine). Products include:
Caduet Tablets 2508
Lotrel Capsules 2249
Norvasc Tablets 2545

Amoxapine (Caution is advised in concomitant use of tricyclic antidepressants and brimonidine).
No products indexed under this heading.

Aprobarbital (There may be an additive or potentiating effect with CNS depressants and brimonidine administered concomitanty).
No products indexed under this heading.

Atenolol (Caution is advised in concomitant use of beta-blockers and brimonidine).
No products indexed under this heading.

Benazepril Hydrochloride (Caution is advised in concomitant use of antihypertensives and brimonidine). Products include:
Lotensin Tablets 2243
Lotensin HCT Tablets 2246
Lotrel Capsules 2249

Bendroflumethiazide (Caution is advised in concomitant use of antihypertensives and brimonidine).
No products indexed under this heading.

Betaxolol Hydrochloride (Caution is advised in concomitant use of beta-blockers and brimonidine). Products include:
Betoptic S Ophthalmic Suspension.................................. 558

Bisoprolol Fumarate (Caution is advised in concomitant use of beta-blockers and brimonidine).
No products indexed under this heading.

Buprenorphine Hydrochloride (There may be an additive or potentiating effect with CNS depressants and brimonidine administered concomitanty). Products include:
Buprenex Injectable 2716
Suboxone Tablets 2717
Subutex Tablets 2717

Buspirone Hydrochloride (There may be an additive or potentiating effect with CNS depressants and brimonidine administered concomitanty).
No products indexed under this heading.

Butabarbital (There may be an additive or potentiating effect with CNS depressants and brimonidine administered concomitanty).
No products indexed under this heading.

Butalbital (There may be an additive or potentiating effect with CNS depressants and brimonidine administered concomitanty).
No products indexed under this heading.

Candesartan Cilexetil (Caution is advised in concomitant use of antihypertensives and brimonidine). Products include:
Atacand Tablets 649
Atacand HCT 651

Captopril (Caution is advised in concomitant use of antihypertensives and brimonidine). Products include:
Captopril Tablets 2149

Carteolol Hydrochloride (Caution is advised in concomitant use of beta-blockers and brimonidine). Products include:
Carteolol Hydrochloride Ophthalmic Solution USP, 1%....... ⊙249

Chlordiazepoxide (There may be an additive or potentiating effect with CNS depressants and brimonidine administered concomitanty).
No products indexed under this heading.

Chlordiazepoxide Hydrochloride (There may be an additive or potentiating effect with CNS depressants and brimonidine administered concomitanty). Products include:
Librium Capsules 3347

Chlorothiazide (Caution is advised in concomitant use of antihypertensives and brimonidine). Products include:
Diuril Oral Suspension 1954

Chlorothiazide Sodium (Caution is advised in concomitant use of antihypertensives and brimonidine). Products include:
Diuril Sodium Intravenous 2467

Chlorpromazine (There may be an additive or potentiating effect with CNS depressants and brimonidine administered concomitanty).
No products indexed under this heading.

Chlorpromazine Hydrochloride (There may be an additive or potentiating effect with CNS depressants and brimonidine administered concomitanty).
No products indexed under this heading.

Chlorprothixene (There may be an additive or potentiating effect with CNS depressants and brimonidine administered concomitanty).
No products indexed under this heading.

Chlorprothixene Hydrochloride (There may be an additive or potentiating effect with CNS depressants and brimonidine administered concomitanty).
No products indexed under this heading.

Chlorprothixene Lactate (There may be an additive or potentiating effect with CNS depressants and brimonidine administered concomitanty).
No products indexed under this heading.

Chlorthalidone (Caution is advised in concomitant use of antihypertensives and brimonidine). Products include:
Clorpres Tablets 2153

Clomipramine Hydrochloride (Caution is advised in concomitant use of tricyclic antidepressants and brimonidine).
No products indexed under this heading.

Clonidine (Caution is advised in concomitant use of antihypertensives and brimonidine). Products include:
Catapres-TTS 844

Clonidine Hydrochloride (Caution is advised in concomitant use of antihypertensives and brimonidine). Products include:
Catapres Tablets 843
Clorpres Tablets 2153

Clorazepate Dipotassium (There may be an additive or potentiating effect with CNS depressants and brimonidine administered concomitanty). Products include:
Tranxene 2474

Clozapine (There may be an additive or potentiating effect with CNS depressants and brimonidine administered concomitanty). Products include:
Clozaril Tablets 2184
FazaClo Orally Disintegrating Tablets 551

Codeine Phosphate (There may be an additive or potentiating effect with CNS depressants and brimonidine administered concomitanty). Products include:
Tylenol with Codeine Tablets 2391

Deserpidine (Caution is advised in concomitant use of antihypertensives and brimonidine).
No products indexed under this heading.

Desflurane (There may be an additive or potentiating effect with CNS depressants and brimonidine administered concomitanty).
No products indexed under this heading.

Desipramine Hydrochloride (Caution is advised in concomitant use of tricyclic antidepressants and brimonidine).
No products indexed under this heading.

Deslanoside (Caution is advised in concomitant use of cardiac glycosides and brimonidine).
No products indexed under this heading.

Dezocine (There may be an additive or potentiating effect with CNS depressants and brimonidine administered concomitanty).
No products indexed under this heading.

Diazepam (There may be an additive or potentiating effect with CNS depressants and brimonidine administered concomitanty). Products include:
Diastat Rectal Delivery System 3343
Valium Tablets 2819

Diazoxide (Caution is advised in concomitant use of antihypertensives and brimonidine). Products include:
Hyperstat I.V. 3017

Digitalis Glycoside Preparations (Caution is advised in concomitant use of cardiac glycosides and brimonidine).
No products indexed under this heading.

Digitoxin (Caution is advised in concomitant use of cardiac glycosides and brimonidine).
No products indexed under this heading.

Digoxin (Caution is advised in concomitant use of cardiac glycosides and brimonidine). Products include:
Lanoxicaps Capsules 1490
Lanoxin Injection 1494
Lanoxin Injection Pediatric 1497
Lanoxin Tablets 1500

Diltiazem Hydrochloride (Caution is advised in concomitant use of antihypertensives and brimonidine). Products include:
Cardizem LA Extended Release Tablets 1728
Tiazac Capsules 1201

Doxazosin Mesylate (Caution is advised in concomitant use of antihypertensives and brimonidine). Products include:
Cardura XL Tablets 2515

Doxepin Hydrochloride (Caution is advised in concomitant use of tricyclic antidepressants and brimonidine).
No products indexed under this heading.

Droperidol (There may be an additive or potentiating effect with CNS depressants and brimonidine administered concomitanty).
No products indexed under this heading.

Enalapril Maleate (Caution is advised in concomitant use of antihypertensives and brimonidine). Products include:
Vasotec I.V. Injection 2103

Enalaprilat (Caution is advised in concomitant use of antihypertensives and brimonidine).
No products indexed under this heading.

Enflurane (There may be an additive or potentiating effect with CNS depressants and brimonidine administered concomitanty).
No products indexed under this heading.

Eprosartan Mesylate (Caution is advised in concomitant use of antihypertensives and brimonidine). Products include:
Teveten Tablets 1735
Teveten HCT Tablets 1737

Esmolol Hydrochloride (Caution is advised in concomitant use of beta-blockers and brimonidine).
No products indexed under this heading.

Estazolam (There may be an additive or potentiating effect with CNS depressants and brimonidine administered concomitanty). Products include:
ProSom Tablets 517

Ethanol (There may be an additive or potentiating effect with CNS depressants and brimonidine administered concomitanty).
No products indexed under this heading.

Ethchlorvynol (There may be an additive or potentiating effect with CNS depressants and brimonidine administered concomitanty).
No products indexed under this heading.

Ethinamate (There may be an additive or potentiating effect with CNS depressants and brimonidine administered concomitanty).
No products indexed under this heading.

Ethyl Alcohol (There may be an additive or potentiating effect with CNS depressants and brimonidine administered concomitanty).
No products indexed under this heading.

Felodipine (Caution is advised in concomitant use of antihypertensives and brimonidine).
No products indexed under this heading.

Fentanyl (There may be an additive or potentiating effect with CNS depressants and brimonidine administered concomitanty). Products include:
Duragesic Transdermal System 2373
Ionsys Transdermal System 2379

Fentanyl Citrate (There may be an additive or potentiating effect with CNS depressants and brimonidine administered concomitanty). Products include:
Actiq 979

Fluphenazine Decanoate (There may be an additive or potentiating effect with CNS depressants and brimonidine administered concomitanty).
No products indexed under this heading.

Fluphenazine Enanthate (There may be an additive or potentiating effect with CNS depressants and brimonidine administered concomitanty).
No products indexed under this heading.

Fluphenazine Hydrochloride (There may be an additive or potentiating effect with CNS depressants and brimonidine administered concomitanty).
No products indexed under this heading.

Flurazepam Hydrochloride (There may be an additive or potentiating effect with CNS depressants and brimonidine administered concomitanty). Products include:
Dalmane Capsules 3342

Fosinopril Sodium (Caution is advised in concomitant use of antihypertensives and brimonidine).
No products indexed under this heading.

Furosemide (Caution is advised in concomitant use of antihypertensives and brimonidine). Products include:
Furosemide Tablets 2154

Glutethimide (There may be an additive or potentiating effect with CNS depressants and brimonidine administered concomitanty).
No products indexed under this heading.

Guanabenz Acetate (Caution is advised in concomitant use of antihypertensives and brimonidine).
No products indexed under this heading.

Guanethidine Monosulfate (Caution is advised in concomitant use of antihypertensives and brimonidine).
No products indexed under this heading.

Haloperidol (There may be an additive or potentiating effect with CNS depressants and brimonidine administered concomitanty).
No products indexed under this heading.

Haloperidol Decanoate (There may be an additive or potentiating effect with CNS depressants and brimonidine administered concomitanty).
No products indexed under this heading.

Hydralazine Hydrochloride (Caution is advised in concomitant use of antihypertensives and brimonidine). Products include:
BiDil Tablets 2171

Hydrochlorothiazide (Caution is advised in concomitant use of antihypertensives and brimonidine). Products include:
Aldoril Tablets 1910
Atacand HCT 651
Avalide Tablets 888
Avalide Tablets 2874
Benicar HCT Tablets 1044
Diovan HCT Tablets 2196
Dyazide Capsules 1423
Hyzaar 50-12.5 Tablets 1990
Hyzaar 100-12.5 Tablets 1990
Hyzaar 100-25 Tablets 1990
Lopressor HCT 50/25 Tablets 2241
Lopressor HCT 100/25 Tablets 2241
Lopressor HCT 100/50 Tablets 2241
Lotensin HCT Tablets 2246
Micardis HCT Tablets 856
Moduretic Tablets 2028
Prinzide Tablets 2056
Teveten HCT Tablets 1737
Timolide Tablets 2086
Uniretic Tablets 3100

Hydrocodone Bitartrate (There may be an additive or potentiating effect with CNS depressants and brimonidine administered concomitanty). Products include:
Hycodan 1116
Hycotuss Expectorant Syrup 1117
Vicodin Tablets 535
Vicodin ES Tablets 536
Vicodin HP Tablets 538
Vicoprofen Tablets 539
Zydone Tablets 1139

Hydrocodone Polistirex (There may be an additive or potentiating effect with CNS depressants and brimonidine administered concomitanty). Products include:
Tussionex Pennkinetic Extended-Release Suspension 3327

Hydroflumethiazide (Caution is advised in concomitant use of antihypertensives and brimonidine).
No products indexed under this heading.

Hydromorphone Hydrochloride (There may be an additive or potentiating effect with CNS depressants and brimonidine administered concomitanty). Products include:
Dilaudid 440
Dilaudid Non-Sterile Powder 440
Dilaudid Oral Liquid 445
Dilaudid Rectal Suppositories 440
Dilaudid Tablets 440
Dilaudid Tablets - 8 mg 445
Dilaudid-HP 442

Hydroxyzine Hydrochloride (There may be an additive or potentiating effect with CNS depressants and brimonidine administered concomitanty).
No products indexed under this heading.

Imipramine Hydrochloride (Caution is advised in concomitant use of tricyclic antidepressants and brimonidine).
No products indexed under this heading.

Imipramine Pamoate (Caution is advised in concomitant use of tricyclic antidepressants and brimonidine).
No products indexed under this heading.

Indapamide (Caution is advised in concomitant use of antihypertensives and brimonidine). Products include:
Indapamide Tablets 2156

Irbesartan (Caution is advised in concomitant use of antihypertensives and brimonidine). Products include:
Avalide Tablets 888
Avalide Tablets 2874
Avapro Tablets 891
Avapro Tablets 2871

Isocarboxazid (Concurrent administration of monoamine oxidase (MAO) inhibitors and brimonidine is contraindicated).
No products indexed under this heading.

Isoflurane (There may be an additive or potentiating effect with CNS depressants and brimonidine administered concomitanty).
No products indexed under this heading.

Isradipine (Caution is advised in concomitant use of antihypertensives and brimonidine). Products include:
DynaCirc CR Tablets 2721

Ketamine Hydrochloride (There may be an additive or potentiating effect with CNS depressants and brimonidine administered concomitanty).
No products indexed under this heading.

Labetalol Hydrochloride (Caution is advised in concomitant use of beta-blockers and brimonidine).
No products indexed under this heading.

Levobunolol Hydrochloride (Caution is advised in concomitant use of beta-blockers and brimonidine). Products include:
Betagan Ophthalmic Solution, USP .... ⊙220

Levomethadyl Acetate Hydrochloride (There may be an additive or potentiating effect with CNS depressants and brimonidine administered concomitanty).
No products indexed under this heading.

Levorphanol Tartrate (There may be an additive or potentiating effect with CNS depressants and brimonidine administered concomitanty).
No products indexed under this heading.

Lisinopril (Caution is advised in concomitant use of antihypertensives and brimonidine). Products include:
Prinivil Tablets 2052
Prinzide Tablets 2056

Lorazepam (There may be an additive or potentiating effect with CNS depressants and brimonidine administered concomitanty).
No products indexed under this heading.

Losartan Potassium (Caution is advised in concomitant use of antihypertensives and brimonidine).
Products include:
Cozaar Tablets 1935
Hyzaar 50-12.5 Tablets 1990
Hyzaar 100-12.5 Tablets 1990
Hyzaar 100-25 Tablets 1990

Loxapine Hydrochloride (There may be an additive or potentiating effect with CNS depressants and brimonidine administered concomitanty).
No products indexed under this heading.

Loxapine Succinate (There may be an additive or potentiating effect with CNS depressants and brimonidine administered concomitanty).
No products indexed under this heading.

Maprotiline Hydrochloride (Caution is advised in concomitant use of tricyclic antidepressants and brimonidine).
No products indexed under this heading.

Mecamylamine Hydrochloride (Caution is advised in concomitant use of antihypertensives and brimonidine).
No products indexed under this heading.

Meperidine Hydrochloride (There may be an additive or potentiating effect with CNS depressants and brimonidine administered concomitanty).
No products indexed under this heading.

Mephobarbital (There may be an additive or potentiating effect with CNS depressants and brimonidine administered concomitanty).
No products indexed under this heading.

Meprobamate (There may be an additive or potentiating effect with CNS depressants and brimonidine administered concomitanty).
No products indexed under this heading.

Mesoridazine Besylate (There may be an additive or potentiating effect with CNS depressants and brimonidine administered concomitanty).
No products indexed under this heading.

Methadone Hydrochloride (There may be an additive or potentiating effect with CNS depressants and brimonidine administered concomitanty).
No products indexed under this heading.

Methohexital Sodium (There may be an additive or potentiating effect with CNS depressants and brimonidine administered concomitanty).
No products indexed under this heading.

Methotrimeprazine (There may be an additive or potentiating effect with CNS depressants and brimonidine administered concomitanty).
No products indexed under this heading.

Methoxyflurane (There may be an additive or potentiating effect with CNS depressants and brimonidine administered concomitanty).
No products indexed under this heading.

Methyclothiazide (Caution is advised in concomitant use of antihypertensives and brimonidine).
No products indexed under this heading.

Methyldopa (Caution is advised in concomitant use of antihypertensives and brimonidine). Products include:
Aldoril Tablets 1910

Methyldopate Hydrochloride (Caution is advised in concomitant use of antihypertensives and brimonidine).
No products indexed under this heading.

Metipranolol Hydrochloride (Caution is advised in concomitant use of beta-blockers and brimonidine).
No products indexed under this heading.

Metolazone (Caution is advised in concomitant use of antihypertensives and brimonidine).
No products indexed under this heading.

Metoprolol Succinate (Caution is advised in concomitant use of beta-blockers and brimonidine). Products include:
Toprol-XL Tablets 668

Metoprolol Tartrate (Caution is advised in concomitant use of beta-blockers and brimonidine). Products include:
Lopressor Injection 2238
Lopressor Tablets 2238
Lopressor HCT 50/25 Tablets 2241
Lopressor HCT 100/25 Tablets 2241
Lopressor HCT 100/50 Tablets 2241

Metyrosine (Caution is advised in concomitant use of antihypertensives and brimonidine). Products include:
Demser Capsules 1953

Mibefradil Dihydrochloride (Caution is advised in concomitant use of antihypertensives and brimonidine).
No products indexed under this heading.

Midazolam Hydrochloride (There may be an additive or potentiating effect with CNS depressants and brimonidine administered concomitanty).
No products indexed under this heading.

Minoxidil (Caution is advised in concomitant use of antihypertensives and brimonidine). Products include:
Men's Rogaine Extra Strength Hair Regrowth Treatment Topical Solution, Ocean Rush Scent and Original Unscented 633
Men's Rogaine Foam Hair Regrowth Treatment 633
Women's Rogaine Hair Regrowth Treatment Topical Solution, Spring Bloom Scent and Original Unscented 634

Moclobemide (Concurrent administration of monoamine oxidase (MAO) inhibitors and brimonidine is contraindicated).
No products indexed under this heading.

Moexipril Hydrochloride (Caution is advised in concomitant use of antihypertensives and brimonidine).
Products include:
Uniretic Tablets 3100
Univasc Tablets 3104

Molindone Hydrochloride (There may be an additive or potentiating effect with CNS depressants and brimonidine administered concomitanty). Products include:
Moban Tablets 1119

Morphine Sulfate (There may be an additive or potentiating effect with CNS depressants and brimonidine administered concomitanty).
Products include:
Avinza Capsules 1741
Kadian Capsules 577
MS Contin Tablets 2701

Nadolol (Caution is advised in concomitant use of beta-blockers and brimonidine). Products include:
Nadolol Tablets 2159

Nicardipine Hydrochloride (Caution is advised in concomitant use of antihypertensives and brimonidine).
Products include:
Cardene I.V. 2497

Nifedipine (Caution is advised in concomitant use of antihypertensives and brimonidine). Products include:
Adalat CC Tablets 2964

Nisoldipine (Caution is advised in concomitant use of antihypertensives and brimonidine). Products include:
Sular Tablets 3122

Nitroglycerin (Caution is advised in concomitant use of antihypertensives and brimonidine). Products include:
Nitro-Dur Transdermal Infusion System 3046
Nitrolingual Pumpspray 3120

Nortriptyline Hydrochloride (Caution is advised in concomitant use of tricyclic antidepressants and brimonidine).
No products indexed under this heading.

Olanzapine (There may be an additive or potentiating effect with CNS depressants and brimonidine administered concomitanty). Products include:
Symbyax Capsules 1819
Zyprexa Tablets 1830
Zyprexa IntraMuscular 1830
Zyprexa ZYDIS Orally Disintegrating Tablets 1830

Oxazepam (There may be an additive or potentiating effect with CNS depressants and brimonidine administered concomitanty).
No products indexed under this heading.

Oxycodone Hydrochloride (There may be an additive or potentiating effect with CNS depressants and brimonidine administered concomitanty). Products include:
OxyContin Tablets 2703
OxyFast Oral Concentrate Solution 2708
OxyIR Capsules 2708
Percocet Tablets 1131
Percodan Tablets 1132

Pargyline Hydrochloride (Concurrent administration of monoamine oxidase (MAO) inhibitors and brimonidine is contraindicated).
No products indexed under this heading.

Penbutolol Sulfate (Caution is advised in concomitant use of beta-blockers and brimonidine).
No products indexed under this heading.

Pentobarbital Sodium (There may be an additive or potentiating effect with CNS depressants and brimonidine administered concomitanty).
Products include:
Nembutal Sodium Solution, USP 2470

Perindopril Erbumine (Caution is advised in concomitant use of antihypertensives and brimonidine).
Products include:
Aceon Tablets (2 mg, 4 mg, 8 mg) 3194

Perphenazine (There may be an additive or potentiating effect with CNS depressants and brimonidine administered concomitanty).
No products indexed under this heading.

Phenelzine Sulfate (Concurrent administration of monoamine oxidase (MAO) inhibitors and brimonidine is contraindicated).
No products indexed under this heading.

Phenobarbital (There may be an additive or potentiating effect with CNS depressants and brimonidine administered concomitanty).
Products include:
Donnatal Extentabs 2493

Phenoxybenzamine Hydrochloride (Caution is advised in concomitant use of antihypertensives and brimonidine). Products include:
Dibenzyline Capsules 3399

Phentolamine Mesylate (Caution is advised in concomitant use of antihypertensives and brimonidine).
No products indexed under this heading.

Pindolol (Caution is advised in concomitant use of beta-blockers and brimonidine).
No products indexed under this heading.

Polythiazide (Caution is advised in concomitant use of antihypertensives and brimonidine).
No products indexed under this heading.

Prazepam (There may be an additive or potentiating effect with CNS depressants and brimonidine administered concomitanty).
No products indexed under this heading.

Prazosin Hydrochloride (Caution is advised in concomitant use of antihypertensives and brimonidine).
No products indexed under this heading.

Procarbazine Hydrochloride (Concurrent administration of monoamine oxidase (MAO) inhibitors and brimonidine is contraindicated).
Products include:
Matulane Capsules 3191

Prochlorperazine (There may be an additive or potentiating effect with CNS depressants and brimonidine administered concomitanty).
No products indexed under this heading.

Promethazine Hydrochloride
(There may be an additive or potentiating effect with CNS depressants and brimonidine administered concomitantly). Products include:
Phenergan Tablets and Suppositories 3440

Propofol (There may be an additive or potentiating effect with CNS depressants and brimonidine administered concomitantly).
No products indexed under this heading.

Propoxyphene Hydrochloride (There may be an additive or potentiating effect with CNS depressants and brimonidine administered concomitantly).
No products indexed under this heading.

Propoxyphene Napsylate (There may be an additive or potentiating effect with CNS depressants and brimonidine administered concomitantly).
No products indexed under this heading.

Propranolol Hydrochloride (Caution is advised in concomitant use of beta-blockers and brimonidine).
Products include:
Inderal LA Long-Acting Capsules 3429
InnoPran XL Capsules 2723

Protriptyline Hydrochloride (Caution is advised in concomitant use of tricyclic antidepressants and brimonidine).
No products indexed under this heading.

Quazepam (There may be an additive or potentiating effect with CNS depressants and brimonidine administered concomitantly).
No products indexed under this heading.

Quetiapine Fumarate (There may be an additive or potentiating effect with CNS depressants and brimonidine administered concomitantly).
Products include:
Seroquel Tablets 690

Quinapril Hydrochloride (Caution is advised in concomitant use of antihypertensives and brimonidine).
No products indexed under this heading.

Ramipril (Caution is advised in concomitant use of antihypertensives and brimonidine). Products include:
Altace Capsules 1702

Rauwolfia Serpentina (Caution is advised in concomitant use of antihypertensives and brimonidine).
No products indexed under this heading.

Remifentanil Hydrochloride
(There may be an additive or potentiating effect with CNS depressants and brimonidine administered concomitantly).
No products indexed under this heading.

Rescinnamine (Caution is advised in concomitant use of antihypertensives and brimonidine).
No products indexed under this heading.

Reserpine (Caution is advised in concomitant use of antihypertensives and brimonidine).
No products indexed under this heading.

Risperidone (There may be an additive or potentiating effect with CNS depressants and brimonidine administered concomitantly). Products include:

Risperdal .. 1676
Risperdal Consta Long-Acting Injection 1682
Risperdal M-Tab Orally Disintegrating Tablets.................... 1676

Secobarbital Sodium (There may be an additive or potentiating effect with CNS depressants and brimonidine administered concomitantly).
No products indexed under this heading.

Selegiline Hydrochloride (Concurrent administration of monoamine oxidase (MAO) inhibitors and brimonidine is contraindicated). Products include:
Eldepryl Capsules 3208
Zelapar Tablets 3372

Sevoflurane (There may be an additive or potentiating effect with CNS depressants and brimonidine administered concomitantly). Products include:
Ultane Liquid for Inhalation 531

Sodium Nitroprusside (Caution is advised in concomitant use of antihypertensives and brimonidine).
No products indexed under this heading.

Sodium Oxybate (There may be an additive or potentiating effect with CNS depressants and brimonidine administered concomitantly). Products include:
Xyrem Oral Solution 1688

Sotalol Hydrochloride (Caution is advised in concomitant use of beta-blockers and brimonidine).
No products indexed under this heading.

Spirapril Hydrochloride (Caution is advised in concomitant use of antihypertensives and brimonidine).
No products indexed under this heading.

Sufentanil Citrate (There may be an additive or potentiating effect with CNS depressants and brimonidine administered concomitantly).
No products indexed under this heading.

Telmisartan (Caution is advised in concomitant use of antihypertensives and brimonidine). Products include:
Micardis Tablets 854
Micardis HCT Tablets 856

Temazepam (There may be an additive or potentiating effect with CNS depressants and brimonidine administered concomitantly). Products include:
Restoril Capsules 1860

Terazosin Hydrochloride (Caution is advised in concomitant use of antihypertensives and brimonidine). Products include:
Hytrin Capsules 471

Thiamylal Sodium (There may be an additive or potentiating effect with CNS depressants and brimonidine administered concomitantly).
No products indexed under this heading.

Thioridazine Hydrochloride
(There may be an additive or potentiating effect with CNS depressants and brimonidine administered concomitantly). Products include:
Thioridazine Hydrochloride Tablets 2163

Thiothixene (There may be an additive or potentiating effect with CNS depressants and brimonidine administered concomitantly). Products include:

Thiothixene Capsules 2165

Timolol Hemihydrate (Caution is advised in concomitant use of beta-blockers and brimonidine). Products include:
Betimol Ophthalmic Solution 3382
Betimol Ophthalmic Solution ⊙ 295

Timolol Maleate (Caution is advised in concomitant use of beta-blockers and brimonidine). Products include:
Blocadren Tablets 1916
Cosopt Sterile Ophthalmic Solution 1931
Timolide Tablets 2086
Timoptic Sterile Ophthalmic Solution 2088
Timoptic in Ocudose 2091
Timoptic-XE Sterile Ophthalmic Gel Forming Solution 2092

Torsemide (Caution is advised in concomitant use of antihypertensives and brimonidine). Products include:
Demadex Injection 2759
Demadex Tablets 2759

Trandolapril (Caution is advised in concomitant use of antihypertensives and brimonidine). Products include:
Mavik Tablets 486
Tarka Tablets 524

Tranylcypromine Sulfate (Concurrent administration of monoamine oxidase (MAO) inhibitors and brimonidine is contraindicated). Products include:
Parnate Tablets 1527

Triazolam (There may be an additive or potentiating effect with CNS depressants and brimonidine administered concomitantly).
No products indexed under this heading.

Trifluoperazine Hydrochloride
(There may be an additive or potentiating effect with CNS depressants and brimonidine administered concomitantly).
No products indexed under this heading.

Trimethaphan Camsylate (Caution is advised in concomitant use of antihypertensives and brimonidine).
No products indexed under this heading.

Trimipramine Maleate (Caution is advised in concomitant use of tricyclic antidepressants and brimonidine).
No products indexed under this heading.

Valsartan (Caution is advised in concomitant use of antihypertensives and brimonidine). Products include:
Diovan Tablets 2193
Diovan HCT Tablets 2196

Verapamil Hydrochloride (Caution is advised in concomitant use of antihypertensives and brimonidine). Products include:
Covera-HS Tablets 3139
Tarka Tablets 524
Verelan PM Extended-Release Capsules, Controlled-Onset.......... 3106

Zaleplon (There may be an additive or potentiating effect with CNS depressants and brimonidine administered concomitantly). Products include:
Sonata Capsules 1717

Ziprasidone Hydrochloride
(There may be an additive or potentiating effect with CNS depressants and brimonidine administered concomitantly). Products include:

Geodon Capsules 2529

Zolpidem Tartrate (There may be an additive or potentiating effect with CNS depressants and brimonidine administered concomitantly). Products include:
Ambien Tablets 2851
Ambien CR Tablets 2855

BUFFERIN EXTRA STRENGTH TABLETS
(Aspirin Buffered) ▣678

Food Interactions
Alcohol (Concomitant consumption of alcohol may cause liver damage).

BUFFERIN REGULAR STRENGTH TABLETS
(Aspirin Buffered) ▣678
See Bufferin Extra Strength Tablets

BUMEX TABLETS
(Bumetanide) 2746
May interact with aminoglycosides, antihypertensives, ototoxic drugs, and certain other agents. Compounds in these categories include:

Acebutolol Hydrochloride (May potentiate the effect of various antihypertensives, necessitating a reduction in the dosage of these drugs).
No products indexed under this heading.

Amikacin Sulfate (Administration of aminoglycoside antibiotics in patients with impaired renal function receiving parenterally administered bumetanide should be avoided, except in life-threatening conditions).
No products indexed under this heading.

Amlodipine Besylate (May potentiate the effect of various antihypertensives, necessitating a reduction in the dosage of these drugs).
Products include:
Caduet Tablets 2508
Lotrel Capsules 2249
Norvasc Tablets 2545

Atenolol (May potentiate the effect of various antihypertensives, necessitating a reduction in the dosage of these drugs).
No products indexed under this heading.

Benazepril Hydrochloride (May potentiate the effect of various antihypertensives, necessitating a reduction in the dosage of these drugs). Products include:
Lotensin Tablets 2243
Lotensin HCT Tablets 2246
Lotrel Capsules 2249

Bendroflumethiazide (May potentiate the effect of various antihypertensives, necessitating a reduction in the dosage of these drugs).
No products indexed under this heading.

Betaxolol Hydrochloride (May potentiate the effect of various antihypertensives, necessitating a reduction in the dosage of these drugs). Products include:
Betoptic S Ophthalmic Suspension 558

Bisoprolol Fumarate (May potentiate the effect of various antihypertensives, necessitating a reduction in the dosage of these drugs).
No products indexed under this heading.

Candesartan Cilexetil (May potentiate the effect of various antihyper-

tensives, necessitating a reduction in the dosage of these drugs). Products include:
- Atacand Tablets 649
- Atacand HCT 651

Captopril (May potentiate the effect of various antihypertensives, necessitating a reduction in the dosage of these drugs). Products include:
- Captopril Tablets 2149

Carteolol Hydrochloride (May potentiate the effect of various antihypertensives, necessitating a reduction in the dosage of these drugs). Products include:
- Carteolol Hydrochloride Ophthalmic Solution USP, 1%....... ⊙249

Chlorothiazide (May potentiate the effect of various antihypertensives, necessitating a reduction in the dosage of these drugs). Products include:
- Diuril Oral Suspension 1954

Chlorothiazide Sodium (May potentiate the effect of various antihypertensives, necessitating a reduction in the dosage of these drugs). Products include:
- Diuril Sodium Intravenous 2467

Chlorthalidone (May potentiate the effect of various antihypertensives, necessitating a reduction in the dosage of these drugs). Products include:
- Clorpres Tablets 2153

Cisplatin (Administration of aminoglycoside antibiotics in patients with impaired renal function receiving parenterally administered bumetanide should be avoided, except in life-threatening conditions).
No products indexed under this heading.

Clonidine (May potentiate the effect of various antihypertensives, necessitating a reduction in the dosage of these drugs). Products include:
- Catapres-TTS 844

Clonidine Hydrochloride (May potentiate the effect of various antihypertensives, necessitating a reduction in the dosage of these drugs). Products include:
- Catapres Tablets 843
- Clorpres Tablets 2153

Deserpidine (May potentiate the effect of various antihypertensives, necessitating a reduction in the dosage of these drugs).
No products indexed under this heading.

Diazoxide (May potentiate the effect of various antihypertensives, necessitating a reduction in the dosage of these drugs). Products include:
- Hyperstat I.V. 3017

Diltiazem Hydrochloride (May potentiate the effect of various antihypertensives, necessitating a reduction in the dosage of these drugs). Products include:
- Cardizem LA Extended Release Tablets 1728
- Tiazac Capsules 1201

Doxazosin Mesylate (May potentiate the effect of various antihypertensives, necessitating a reduction in the dosage of these drugs). Products include:
- Cardura XL Tablets 2515

Enalapril Maleate (May potentiate the effect of various antihypertensives, necessitating a reduction in the dosage of these drugs). Products include:
- Vasotec I.V. Injection 2103

Enalaprilat (May potentiate the effect of various antihypertensives, necessitating a reduction in the dosage of these drugs).
No products indexed under this heading.

Eprosartan Mesylate (May potentiate the effect of various antihypertensives, necessitating a reduction in the dosage of these drugs). Products include:
- Teveten Tablets 1735
- Teveten HCT Tablets 1737

Esmolol Hydrochloride (May potentiate the effect of various antihypertensives, necessitating a reduction in the dosage of these drugs).
No products indexed under this heading.

Felodipine (May potentiate the effect of various antihypertensives, necessitating a reduction in the dosage of these drugs).
No products indexed under this heading.

Fosinopril Sodium (May potentiate the effect of various antihypertensives, necessitating a reduction in the dosage of these drugs).
No products indexed under this heading.

Furosemide (May potentiate the effect of various antihypertensives, necessitating a reduction in the dosage of these drugs). Products include:
- Furosemide Tablets 2154

Gentamicin Sulfate (Administration of aminoglycoside antibiotics in patients with impaired renal function receiving parenterally administered bumetanide should be avoided, except in life-threatening conditions). Products include:
- Garamycin Injectable 3014
- Pred-G Ophthalmic Ointment .... ⊙237
- Pred-G Ophthalmic Suspension .... ⊙236

Guanabenz Acetate (May potentiate the effect of various antihypertensives, necessitating a reduction in the dosage of these drugs).
No products indexed under this heading.

Guanethidine Monosulfate (May potentiate the effect of various antihypertensives, necessitating a reduction in the dosage of these drugs).
No products indexed under this heading.

Hydralazine Hydrochloride (May potentiate the effect of various antihypertensives, necessitating a reduction in the dosage of these drugs). Products include:
- BiDil Tablets 2171

Hydrochlorothiazide (May potentiate the effect of various antihypertensives, necessitating a reduction in the dosage of these drugs). Products include:
- Aldoril Tablets 1910
- Atacand HCT 651
- Avalide Tablets 888
- Avalide Tablets 2874
- Benicar HCT Tablets 1044
- Diovan HCT Tablets 2196
- Dyazide Capsules 1423
- Hyzaar 50-12.5 Tablets 1990
- Hyzaar 100-12.5 Tablets 1990
- Hyzaar 100-25 Tablets 1990
- Lopressor HCT 50/25 Tablets 2241
- Lopressor HCT 100/25 Tablets 2241
- Lopressor HCT 100/50 Tablets 2241
- Lotensin HCT Tablets 2246
- Micardis HCT Tablets 856
- Moduretic Tablets 2028
- Prinzide Tablets 2056
- Teveten HCT Tablets 1737
- Timolide Tablets 2086
- Uniretic Tablets 3100

Hydroflumethiazide (May potentiate the effect of various antihypertensives, necessitating a reduction in the dosage of these drugs).
No products indexed under this heading.

Indapamide (May potentiate the effect of various antihypertensives, necessitating a reduction in the dosage of these drugs). Products include:
- Indapamide Tablets 2156

Indomethacin (Indomethacin blunts the increase in urine volume and sodium excretion and inhibits the bumetanide-induced increase in plasma renin activity; concurrent therapy is not recommended). Products include:
- Indocin 1995

Indomethacin Sodium Trihydrate (Indomethacin blunts the increase in urine volume and sodium excretion and inhibits the bumetanide-induced increase in plasma renin activity; concurrent therapy is not recommended). Products include:
- Indocin I.V. 2465

Irbesartan (May potentiate the effect of various antihypertensives, necessitating a reduction in the dosage of these drugs). Products include:
- Avalide Tablets 888
- Avalide Tablets 2874
- Avapro Tablets 891
- Avapro Tablets 2871

Isradipine (May potentiate the effect of various antihypertensives, necessitating a reduction in the dosage of these drugs). Products include:
- DynaCirc CR Tablets 2721

Kanamycin Sulfate (Administration of aminoglycoside antibiotics in patients with impaired renal function receiving parenterally administered bumetanide should be avoided, except in life-threatening conditions).
No products indexed under this heading.

Labetalol Hydrochloride (May potentiate the effect of various antihypertensives, necessitating a reduction in the dosage of these drugs).
No products indexed under this heading.

Lisinopril (May potentiate the effect of various antihypertensives, necessitating a reduction in the dosage of these drugs). Products include:
- Prinivil Tablets 2052
- Prinzide Tablets 2056

Lithium (Lithium should generally not be given with diuretics because they reduce its renal clearance and add a high risk of lithium toxicity).
No products indexed under this heading.

Lithium Carbonate (Lithium should generally not be given with diuretics because they reduce its renal clearance and add a high risk of lithium toxicity). Products include:
- Lithobid Tablets 1692

Lithium Citrate (Lithium should generally not be given with diuretics because they reduce its renal clearance and add a high risk of lithium toxicity).
No products indexed under this heading.

Losartan Potassium (May potentiate the effect of various antihypertensives, necessitating a reduction in the dosage of these drugs). Products include:
- Cozaar Tablets 1935
- Hyzaar 50-12.5 Tablets 1990
- Hyzaar 100-12.5 Tablets 1990
- Hyzaar 100-25 Tablets 1990

Mecamylamine Hydrochloride (May potentiate the effect of various antihypertensives, necessitating a reduction in the dosage of these drugs).
No products indexed under this heading.

Methyclothiazide (May potentiate the effect of various antihypertensives, necessitating a reduction in the dosage of these drugs).
No products indexed under this heading.

Methyldopa (May potentiate the effect of various antihypertensives, necessitating a reduction in the dosage of these drugs). Products include:
- Aldoril Tablets 1910

Methyldopate Hydrochloride (May potentiate the effect of various antihypertensives, necessitating a reduction in the dosage of these drugs).
No products indexed under this heading.

Metolazone (May potentiate the effect of various antihypertensives, necessitating a reduction in the dosage of these drugs).
No products indexed under this heading.

Metoprolol Succinate (May potentiate the effect of various antihypertensives, necessitating a reduction in the dosage of these drugs). Products include:
- Toprol-XL Tablets 668

Metoprolol Tartrate (May potentiate the effect of various antihypertensives, necessitating a reduction in the dosage of these drugs). Products include:
- Lopressor Injection 2238
- Lopressor Tablets 2238
- Lopressor HCT 50/25 Tablets 2241
- Lopressor HCT 100/25 Tablets 2241
- Lopressor HCT 100/50 Tablets 2241

Metyrosine (May potentiate the effect of various antihypertensives, necessitating a reduction in the dosage of these drugs). Products include:
- Demser Capsules 1953

Mibefradil Dihydrochloride (May potentiate the effect of various antihypertensives, necessitating a reduction in the dosage of these drugs).
No products indexed under this heading.

Minoxidil (May potentiate the effect of various antihypertensives, necessitating a reduction in the dosage of these drugs). Products include:
- Men's Rogaine Extra Strength Hair Regrowth Treatment Topical Solution, Ocean Rush Scent and Original Unscented............ ▣633
- Men's Rogaine Foam Hair Regrowth Treatment............ ▣633

IMPORTANT NOTE: Always consult each drug listing in the patient's regimen for possible interactions.

Women's Rogaine Hair Regrowth Treatment Topical Solution, Spring Bloom Scent and Original Unscented .... ◙634

Moexipril Hydrochloride (May potentiate the effect of various antihypertensives, necessitating a reduction in the dosage of these drugs). Products include:
Uniretic Tablets 3100
Univasc Tablets 3104

Nadolol (May potentiate the effect of various antihypertensives, necessitating a reduction in the dosage of these drugs). Products include:
Nadolol Tablets 2159

Nicardipine Hydrochloride (May potentiate the effect of various antihypertensives, necessitating a reduction in the dosage of these drugs). Products include:
Cardene I.V. 2497

Nifedipine (May potentiate the effect of various antihypertensives, necessitating a reduction in the dosage of these drugs). Products include:
Adalat CC Tablets 2964

Nisoldipine (May potentiate the effect of various antihypertensives, necessitating a reduction in the dosage of these drugs). Products include:
Sular Tablets 3122

Nitroglycerin (May potentiate the effect of various antihypertensives, necessitating a reduction in the dosage of these drugs). Products include:
Nitro-Dur Transdermal Infusion System 3046
Nitrolingual Pumpspray 3120

Penbutolol Sulfate (May potentiate the effect of various antihypertensives, necessitating a reduction in the dosage of these drugs).
No products indexed under this heading.

Perindopril Erbumine (May potentiate the effect of various antihypertensives, necessitating a reduction in the dosage of these drugs). Products include:
Aceon Tablets (2 mg, 4 mg, 8 mg) 3194

Phenoxybenzamine Hydrochloride (May potentiate the effect of various antihypertensives, necessitating a reduction in the dosage of these drugs). Products include:
Dibenzyline Capsules 3399

Phentolamine Mesylate (May potentiate the effect of various antihypertensives, necessitating a reduction in the dosage of these drugs).
No products indexed under this heading.

Pindolol (May potentiate the effect of various antihypertensives, necessitating a reduction in the dosage of these drugs).
No products indexed under this heading.

Polythiazide (May potentiate the effect of various antihypertensives, necessitating a reduction in the dosage of these drugs).
No products indexed under this heading.

Prazosin Hydrochloride (May potentiate the effect of various antihypertensives, necessitating a reduction in the dosage of these drugs).
No products indexed under this heading.

Probenecid (Secondary to its inhibitory effect on renal tubular secretion, pretreatment with probenecid reduces the natriuresis and hyperreninemia produced by bumetanide. Thus, probenecid should not be administered concurrently with bumetanide.).
No products indexed under this heading.

Propranolol Hydrochloride (May potentiate the effect of various antihypertensives, necessitating a reduction in the dosage of these drugs). Products include:
Inderal LA Long-Acting Capsules 3429
InnoPran XL Capsules 2723

Quinapril Hydrochloride (May potentiate the effect of various antihypertensives, necessitating a reduction in the dosage of these drugs).
No products indexed under this heading.

Ramipril (May potentiate the effect of various antihypertensives, necessitating a reduction in the dosage of these drugs). Products include:
Altace Capsules 1702

Rauwolfia Serpentina (May potentiate the effect of various antihypertensives, necessitating a reduction in the dosage of these drugs).
No products indexed under this heading.

Rescinnamine (May potentiate the effect of various antihypertensives, necessitating a reduction in the dosage of these drugs).
No products indexed under this heading.

Reserpine (May potentiate the effect of various antihypertensives, necessitating a reduction in the dosage of these drugs).
No products indexed under this heading.

Sodium Nitroprusside (May potentiate the effect of various antihypertensives, necessitating a reduction in the dosage of these drugs).
No products indexed under this heading.

Sotalol Hydrochloride (May potentiate the effect of various antihypertensives, necessitating a reduction in the dosage of these drugs).
No products indexed under this heading.

Spirapril Hydrochloride (May potentiate the effect of various antihypertensives, necessitating a reduction in the dosage of these drugs).
No products indexed under this heading.

Streptomycin Sulfate (Administration of aminoglycoside antibiotics in patients with impaired renal function receiving parenterally administered bumetanide should be avoided, except in life-threatening conditions).
No products indexed under this heading.

Telmisartan (May potentiate the effect of various antihypertensives, necessitating a reduction in the dosage of these drugs). Products include:
Micardis Tablets 854
Micardis HCT Tablets 856

Terazosin Hydrochloride (May potentiate the effect of various antihypertensives, necessitating a reduction in the dosage of these drugs). Products include:
Hytrin Capsules 471

Timolol Maleate (May potentiate the effect of various antihypertensives, necessitating a reduction in the dosage of these drugs). Products include:
Blocadren Tablets 1916
Cosopt Sterile Ophthalmic Solution 1931
Timolide Tablets 2086
Timoptic Sterile Ophthalmic Solution 2088
Timoptic in Ocudose 2091
Timoptic-XE Sterile Ophthalmic Gel Forming Solution 2092

Tobramycin (Administration of aminoglycoside antibiotics in patients with impaired renal function receiving parenterally administered bumetanide should be avoided, except in life-threatening conditions). Products include:
TOBI Solution for Inhalation 2298
TobraDex Ophthalmic Ointment 562
TobraDex Ophthalmic Suspension ... 563
Zylet Ophthalmic Suspension .... ⊙259

Tobramycin Sulfate (Administration of aminoglycoside antibiotics in patients with impaired renal function receiving parenterally administered bumetanide should be avoided, except in life-threatening conditions).
No products indexed under this heading.

Torsemide (May potentiate the effect of various antihypertensives, necessitating a reduction in the dosage of these drugs). Products include:
Demadex Injection 2759
Demadex Tablets 2759

Trandolapril (May potentiate the effect of various antihypertensives, necessitating a reduction in the dosage of these drugs). Products include:
Mavik Tablets 486
Tarka Tablets 524

Trimethaphan Camsylate (May potentiate the effect of various antihypertensives, necessitating a reduction in the dosage of these drugs).
No products indexed under this heading.

Valsartan (May potentiate the effect of various antihypertensives, necessitating a reduction in the dosage of these drugs). Products include:
Diovan Tablets 2193
Diovan HCT Tablets 2196

Vancomycin Hydrochloride (Administration of aminoglycoside antibiotics in patients with impaired renal function receiving parenterally administered bumetanide should be avoided, except in life-threatening conditions). Products include:
Vancocin HCl Capsules, USP 3380

Verapamil Hydrochloride (May potentiate the effect of various antihypertensives, necessitating a reduction in the dosage of these drugs). Products include:
Covera-HS Tablets 3139
Tarka Tablets 524
Verelan PM Extended-Release Capsules, Controlled-Onset 3106

BUPRENEX INJECTABLE

(Buprenorphine Hydrochloride) 2716
May interact with antihistamines, benzodiazepines, central nervous system depressants, cytochrome p450 3a4 inducers (selected), cytochrome p450 3a4 inhibitors (selected), general anesthetics, hypnotics and sedatives, monoamine oxidase inhibitors, narcotic analgesics, phenothiazines, tranquilizers, and certain other agents. Compounds in these categories include:

Acetazolamide (Buprenorphine is metabolized by the CYP3A4 isoenzyme; co-administration with inhibitors of CYP3A4 may cause decrease in clearance of buprenorphine).
No products indexed under this heading.

Acrivastine (Increased CNS depression).
No products indexed under this heading.

Alfentanil Hydrochloride (Increased CNS depression).
No products indexed under this heading.

Allium sativum (Buprenorphine is metabolized by the CYP3A4 isoenzyme; co-administration with inducers of CYP3A4 may cause increase in clearance of buprenorphine).
No products indexed under this heading.

Alprazolam (Increased CNS depression). Products include:
Niravam Orally Disintegrating Tablets 3092

Amiodarone Hydrochloride (Buprenorphine is metabolized by the CYP3A4 isoenzyme; co-administration with inhibitors of CYP3A4 may cause decrease in clearance of buprenorphine).
No products indexed under this heading.

Amprenavir (Buprenorphine is metabolized by the CYP3A4 isoenzyme; co-administration with inhibitors of CYP3A4 may cause decrease in clearance of buprenorphine). Products include:
Agenerase Capsules 1327
Agenerase Oral Solution 1332

Anastrozole (Buprenorphine is metabolized by the CYP3A4 isoenzyme; co-administration with inhibitors of CYP3A4 may cause decrease in clearance of buprenorphine). Products include:
Arimidex Tablets 673

Aprepitant (Buprenorphine is metabolized by the CYP3A4 isoenzyme; co-administration with inhibitors of CYP3A4 may cause decrease in clearance of buprenorphine). Products include:
Emend Capsules 1963

Aprobarbital (Increased CNS depression).
No products indexed under this heading.

Astemizole (Increased CNS depression).
No products indexed under this heading.

Azatadine Maleate (Increased CNS depression).
No products indexed under this heading.

Betamethasone Acetate (Buprenorphine is metabolized by the CYP3A4 isoenzyme; co-administration with inducers of CYP3A4 may cause increase in clearance of buprenorphine).
No products indexed under this heading.

Betamethasone Sodium Phosphate (Buprenorphine is metabolized by the CYP3A4 isoenzyme; co-administration with inducers of CYP3A4 may cause increase in clearance of buprenorphine).
No products indexed under this heading.

Bromodiphenhydramine Hydrochloride (Increased CNS depression).
No products indexed under this heading.

Brompheniramine Maleate (Increased CNS depression).
Products include:
Children's Dimetapp Cold & Allergy Elixir ■ 730
Children's Dimetapp Cold & Allergy Chewable Tablets ■ 730
Children's Dimetapp DM Cold & Cough Elixir ■ 731

Buspirone Hydrochloride (Increased CNS depression).
No products indexed under this heading.

Butabarbital (Increased CNS depression).
No products indexed under this heading.

Butalbital (Increased CNS depression).
No products indexed under this heading.

Carbamazepine (Buprenorphine is metabolized by the CYP3A4 isoenzyme; co-administration with inducers of CYP3A4 may cause increase in clearance of buprenorphine).
Products include:
Carbatrol Capsules 3171
Equetro Extended-Release Capsules 3180
Tegretol/Tegretol-XR 2295

Cetirizine Hydrochloride (Increased CNS depression).
Products include:
Zyrtec Chewable Tablets 2594
Zyrtec 2594
Zyrtec-D 12 Hour Extended Release Tablets 2597

Chlordiazepoxide (Increased CNS depression).
No products indexed under this heading.

Chlordiazepoxide Hydrochloride (Increased CNS depression).
Products include:
Librium Capsules 3347

Chlorpheniramine Maleate (Increased CNS depression).
Products include:
Advil Allergy Sinus Caplets ■ 770
Advil Multi-Symptom Cold Caplets ■ 770
BC Allergy Sinus Cold Powder ■ 677
Comtrex Maximum Strength Cold & Cough Day/Night Caplets - Night Formulation ■ 726
Comtrex Maximum Strength Day/Night Severe Cold & Sinus Caplets - Night Formulation ■ 725
Contac Cold and Flu Maximum Strength Caplets ■ 728
Contac Cold and Flu Day and Night Caplets (Night Formulation Only) ■ 727
Children's Dimetapp Long Acting Cough Plus Cold Syrup ■ 731
Robitussin Cough & Cold Long-Acting Liquid ■ 735
Robitussin Cough & Allergy Syrup ■ 736
Robitussin Cough & Cold Nighttime Liquid ■ 736
Robitussin Cough, Cold & Flu Nighttime Liquid ■ 738
Robitussin Pediatric Cough & Cold Long-Acting Liquid ■ 735
Robitussin Pediatric Cough & Cold Nighttime Liquid ■ 736
Triaminic Cold & Allergy Liquid ■ 746
Triaminic Cough & Runny Nose Softchews ■ 748
Children's Tylenol Plus Flu Oral Suspension ■ 749
Tylenol Allergy Multi-Symptom Caplets with Cool Burst and Gelcaps 1872
Children's Tylenol Plus Cold Suspension Liquid 1879
Children's Tylenol Plus Cough & Runny Nose Suspension Liquid 1879
Children's Tylenol Plus Flu Suspension Liquid 1881
Children's Tylenol Plus Multi-Symptom Cold Suspension Liquid 1879
Tylenol Cold Head Congestion Nighttime Caplets with Cool Burst 1873
Tylenol Cold Multi-Symptom Nighttime Caplets with Cool Burst 1874
Tylenol Sinus Congestion & Pain Nighttime Caplets with Cool Burst 1876
Vicks 44M Cough, Cold & Flu Relief Liquid 2680
Pediatric Vicks 44m Cough & Cold Relief Liquid 2676
Children's Vicks NyQuil Cold/Cough Relief ■ 756
Children's Vicks NyQuil Cold/Cough Relief Liquid 2680
Zicam Maximum Strength Flu Daytime ■ 768

Chlorpheniramine Polistirex (Increased CNS depression).
Products include:
Tussionex Pennkinetic Extended-Release Suspension 3327

Chlorpheniramine Tannate (Increased CNS depression).
No products indexed under this heading.

Chlorpromazine (Increased CNS depression).
No products indexed under this heading.

Chlorpromazine Hydrochloride (Increased CNS depression).
No products indexed under this heading.

Chlorprothixene (Increased CNS depression).
No products indexed under this heading.

Chlorprothixene Hydrochloride (Increased CNS depression).
No products indexed under this heading.

Chlorprothixene Lactate (Increased CNS depression).
No products indexed under this heading.

Cimetidine (Buprenorphine is metabolized by the CYP3A4 isoenzyme; co-administration with inhibitors of CYP3A4 may cause decrease in clearance of buprenorphine).
Products include:
Tagamet HB 200 Tablets ■ 664

Cimetidine Hydrochloride (Buprenorphine is metabolized by the CYP3A4 isoenzyme; co-administration with inhibitors of CYP3A4 may cause decrease in clearance of buprenorphine).
No products indexed under this heading.

Ciprofloxacin (Buprenorphine is metabolized by the CYP3A4 isoenzyme; co-administration with inhibitors of CYP3A4 may cause decrease in clearance of buprenorphine).
Products include:
Cipro Oral Suspension 2977
Cipro I.V. 2984
Cipro XR Tablets 2990
Ciprodex Otic Suspension 559

Ciprofloxacin Hydrochloride (Buprenorphine is metabolized by the CYP3A4 isoenzyme; co-administration with inducers of CYP3A4 may cause increase in clearance of buprenorphine).
Products include:
Ciloxan Ophthalmic Ointment 559
Ciloxan Ophthalmic Solution ⊙ 206
Cipro Tablets 2977
Proquin XR Tablets 1153

Cisplatin (Buprenorphine is metabolized by the CYP3A4 isoenzyme; co-administration with inducers of CYP3A4 may cause increase in clearance of buprenorphine).
No products indexed under this heading.

Clarithromycin (Buprenorphine is metabolized by the CYP3A4 isoenzyme; co-administration with inhibitors of CYP3A4 may cause decrease in clearance of buprenorphine).
Products include:
Biaxin/Biaxin XL 402
PREVPAC 3284

Clemastine Fumarate (Increased CNS depression).
No products indexed under this heading.

Clorazepate Dipotassium (Increased CNS depression).
Products include:
Tranxene 2474

Clotrimazole (Buprenorphine is metabolized by the CYP3A4 isoenzyme; co-administration with inhibitors of CYP3A4 may cause decrease in clearance of buprenorphine).
Products include:
Desenex Athlete's Foot Cream ■ 635
Lotrimin 3039
Lotrisone 3040

Clozapine (Increased CNS depression). Products include:
Clozaril Tablets 2184
FazaClo Orally Disintegrating Tablets 551

Codeine Phosphate (Increased CNS depression). Products include:
Tylenol with Codeine Tablets 2391

Cortisone Acetate (Buprenorphine is metabolized by the CYP3A4 isoenzyme; co-administration with inducers of CYP3A4 may cause increase in clearance of buprenorphine).
No products indexed under this heading.

Cyclosporine (Buprenorphine is metabolized by the CYP3A4 isoenzyme; co-administration with inhibitors of CYP3A4 may cause decrease in clearance of buprenorphine).
Products include:
Gengraf Capsules 459
Neoral Oral Solution 2259
Neoral Soft Gelatin Capsules 2259
Restasis Ophthalmic Emulsion 575
Sandimmune 2275

Cyproheptadine Hydrochloride (Increased CNS depression).
No products indexed under this heading.

Dalfopristin (Buprenorphine is metabolized by the CYP3A4 isoenzyme; co-administration with inhibitors of CYP3A4 may cause decrease in clearance of buprenorphine).
No products indexed under this heading.

Danazol (Buprenorphine is metabolized by the CYP3A4 isoenzyme; co-administration with inhibitors of CYP3A4 may cause decrease in clearance of buprenorphine).
No products indexed under this heading.

Delavirdine Mesylate (Buprenorphine is metabolized by the CYP3A4 isoenzyme; co-administration with inhibitors of CYP3A4 may cause decrease in clearance of buprenorphine). Products include:
Rescriptor Tablets 2551

Desflurane (Increased CNS depression).
No products indexed under this heading.

Dexamethasone (Buprenorphine is metabolized by the CYP3A4 isoenzyme; co-administration with inducers of CYP3A4 may cause increase in clearance of buprenorphine).
Products include:
Ciprodex Otic Suspension 559
Decadron Tablets 1951
TobraDex Ophthalmic Ointment 562
TobraDex Ophthalmic Suspension 563

Dexamethasone Acetate (Buprenorphine is metabolized by the CYP3A4 isoenzyme; co-administration with inducers of CYP3A4 may cause increase in clearance of buprenorphine).
No products indexed under this heading.

Dexamethasone Sodium Phosphate (Buprenorphine is metabolized by the CYP3A4 isoenzyme; co-administration with inducers of CYP3A4 may cause increase in clearance of buprenorphine).
No products indexed under this heading.

Dexchlorpheniramine Maleate (Increased CNS depression).
No products indexed under this heading.

Dezocine (Increased CNS depression).
No products indexed under this heading.

Diazepam (Concurrent use has resulted in respiratory and cardiovascular collapse; increased CNS depression). Products include:
Diastat Rectal Delivery System 3343
Valium Tablets 2819

Diltiazem Hydrochloride (Buprenorphine is metabolized by the CYP3A4 isoenzyme; co-administration with inhibitors of CYP3A4 may cause decrease in clearance of buprenorphine).
Products include:
Cardizem LA Extended Release Tablets 1728
Tiazac Capsules 1201

Diltiazem Maleate (Buprenorphine is metabolized by the CYP3A4 isoenzyme; co-administration with inhibitors of CYP3A4 may cause decrease in clearance of buprenorphine).
No products indexed under this heading.

Diphenhydramine Citrate (Increased CNS depression).
Products include:
Advil PM Caplets ■ 615
Excedrin PM Caplets/Tablets/Geltabs ■ 610
Goody's PM Powder for Pain with Sleeplessness ■ 612

Diphenhydramine Hydrochloride (Increased CNS depression).
Products include:
Nytol QuickCaps Caplets ■ 615

IMPORTANT NOTE: Always consult each drug listing in the patient's regimen for possible interactions.

Nytol QuickGels Softgels Maximum Strength .... ■ 616
Simply Sleep Caplets 1868
Sominex Original Formula Tablets .. ■ 616
TheraFlu Warming Relief Nighttime Severe Cold .... ■ 743
TheraFlu Thin Strips Multi Symptom .... ■ 744
Triaminic Nighttime Cold & Cough Liquid .... ■ 746
Triaminic Thin Strips Cough & Runny Nose .... ■ 749
Extra Strength Tylenol PM Caplets, Vanilla Caplets, Geltabs, Gelcaps and Liquid 1875
Tylenol Sore Throat Nighttime Liquid with Cool Burst .... ■ 790
Tylenol Allergy Multi-Symptom Nighttime Caplets with Cool Burst 1872
Tylenol Severe Allergy Caplets 1872
Children's Tylenol Plus Cold & Allergy Suspension Liquid 1878

Diphenylpyraline Hydrochloride (Increased CNS depression).
No products indexed under this heading.

Doxorubicin Hydrochloride (Buprenorphine is metabolized by the CYP3A4 isoenzyme; co-administration with inducers of CYP3A4 may cause increase in clearance of buprenorphine).
No products indexed under this heading.

Droperidol (Increased CNS depression).
No products indexed under this heading.

Efavirenz (Buprenorphine is metabolized by the CYP3A4 isoenzyme; co-administration with inhibitors of CYP3A4 may cause decrease in clearance of buprenorphine).
Products include:
Atripla Tablets 945
Sustiva Capsules 930
Sustiva Tablets 930

Enflurane (Increased CNS depression).
No products indexed under this heading.

Erythromycin (Buprenorphine is metabolized by the CYP3A4 isoenzyme; co-administration with inhibitors of CYP3A4 may cause decrease in clearance of buprenorphine).
Products include:
Ery-Tab Tablets 449
Erythromycin Base Filmtab Tablets 455
Erythromycin Delayed-Release Capsules, USP 457
PCE Dispertab Tablets 515

Erythromycin Estolate (Buprenorphine is metabolized by the CYP3A4 isoenzyme; co-administration with inhibitors of CYP3A4 may cause decrease in clearance of buprenorphine).
No products indexed under this heading.

Erythromycin Ethylsuccinate (Buprenorphine is metabolized by the CYP3A4 isoenzyme; co-administration with inhibitors of CYP3A4 may cause decrease in clearance of buprenorphine).
Products include:
E.E.S. 451
EryPed 447

Erythromycin Gluceptate (Buprenorphine is metabolized by the CYP3A4 isoenzyme; co-administration with inhibitors of CYP3A4 may cause decrease in clearance of buprenorphine).
No products indexed under this heading.

Erythromycin Lactobionate (Buprenorphine is metabolized by the CYP3A4 isoenzyme; co-administration with inhibitors of CYP3A4 may cause decrease in clearance of buprenorphine).
No products indexed under this heading.

Erythromycin Stearate (Buprenorphine is metabolized by the CYP3A4 isoenzyme; co-administration with inhibitors of CYP3A4 may cause decrease in clearance of buprenorphine). Products include:
Erythrocin Stearate Filmtab Tablets 453

Esomeprazole Magnesium (Buprenorphine is metabolized by the CYP3A4 isoenzyme; co-administration with inhibitors of CYP3A4 may cause decrease in clearance of buprenorphine).
Products include:
Nexium Delayed-Release Capsules 655

Estazolam (Increased CNS depression). Products include:
ProSom Tablets 517

Ethanol (Increased CNS depression).
No products indexed under this heading.

Ethchlorvynol (Increased CNS depression).
No products indexed under this heading.

Ethinamate (Increased CNS depression).
No products indexed under this heading.

Ethosuximide (Buprenorphine is metabolized by the CYP3A4 isoenzyme; co-administration with inducers of CYP3A4 may cause increase in clearance of buprenorphine).
No products indexed under this heading.

Ethyl Alcohol (Increased CNS depression).
No products indexed under this heading.

Felbamate (Buprenorphine is metabolized by the CYP3A4 isoenzyme; co-administration with inducers of CYP3A4 may cause increase in clearance of buprenorphine).
No products indexed under this heading.

Fentanyl (Increased CNS depression). Products include:
Duragesic Transdermal System 2373
Ionsys Transdermal System 2379

Fentanyl Citrate (Increased CNS depression). Products include:
Actiq 979

Fexofenadine Hydrochloride (Increased CNS depression).
Products include:
Allegra 2844
Allegra-D 12 Hour Extended-Release Tablets 2846
Allegra-D 24 Hour Extended-Release Tablets 2849

Fluconazole (Buprenorphine is metabolized by the CYP3A4 isoenzyme; co-administration with inhibitors of CYP3A4 may cause decrease in clearance of buprenorphine).
No products indexed under this heading.

Fludrocortisone Acetate (Buprenorphine is metabolized by the CYP3A4 isoenzyme; co-administration with inducers of CYP3A4 may cause increase in clearance of buprenorphine).
No products indexed under this heading.

Fluoxetine Hydrochloride (Buprenorphine is metabolized by the CYP3A4 isoenzyme; co-administration with inhibitors of CYP3A4 may cause decrease in clearance of buprenorphine).
Products include:
Prozac Pulvules and Liquid 1801
Symbyax Capsules 1819

Fluphenazine Decanoate (Increased CNS depression).
No products indexed under this heading.

Fluphenazine Enanthate (Increased CNS depression).
No products indexed under this heading.

Fluphenazine Hydrochloride (Increased CNS depression).
No products indexed under this heading.

Flurazepam Hydrochloride (Increased CNS depression).
Products include:
Dalmane Capsules 3342

Fluvoxamine Maleate (Buprenorphine is metabolized by the CYP3A4 isoenzyme; co-administration with inhibitors of CYP3A4 may cause decrease in clearance of buprenorphine).
No products indexed under this heading.

Fosamprenavir Calcium (Buprenorphine is metabolized by the CYP3A4 isoenzyme; co-administration with inhibitors of CYP3A4 may cause decrease in clearance of buprenorphine).
Products include:
Lexiva Tablets 1505

Fosphenytoin Sodium (Buprenorphine is metabolized by the CYP3A4 isoenzyme; co-administration with inducers of CYP3A4 may cause increase in clearance of buprenorphine).
No products indexed under this heading.

Garlic Extract (Buprenorphine is metabolized by the CYP3A4 isoenzyme; co-administration with inducers of CYP3A4 may cause increase in clearance of buprenorphine).
No products indexed under this heading.

Garlic Oil (Buprenorphine is metabolized by the CYP3A4 isoenzyme; co-administration with inducers of CYP3A4 may cause increase in clearance of buprenorphine).
No products indexed under this heading.

Glutethimide (Increased CNS depression).
No products indexed under this heading.

Halazepam (Increased CNS depression).
No products indexed under this heading.

Haloperidol (Increased CNS depression).
No products indexed under this heading.

Haloperidol Decanoate (Increased CNS depression).
No products indexed under this heading.

Hydrocodone Bitartrate (Increased CNS depression).
Products include:
Hycodan 1116
Hycotuss Expectorant Syrup 1117
Vicodin Tablets 535
Vicodin ES Tablets 536
Vicodin HP Tablets 538
Vicoprofen Tablets 539
Zydone Tablets 1139

Hydrocodone Polistirex (Increased CNS depression).
Products include:
Tussionex Pennkinetic Extended-Release Suspension 3327

Hydrocortisone (Buprenorphine is metabolized by the CYP3A4 isoenzyme; co-administration with inducers of CYP3A4 may cause increase in clearance of buprenorphine).
Products include:
Colocort Rectal Suspension, USP (Retention) 100 mg/60 mL 2476
Hydrocortone Tablets 1989
Preparation H Hydrocortisone Cream .... ■ 646

Hydrocortisone Acetate (Buprenorphine is metabolized by the CYP3A4 isoenzyme; co-administration with inducers of CYP3A4 may cause increase in clearance of buprenorphine).
Products include:
Analpram-HC 1159
Pramosone 1161
ProctoFoam-HC 3099

Hydrocortisone Butyrate (Buprenorphine is metabolized by the CYP3A4 isoenzyme; co-administration with inducers of CYP3A4 may cause increase in clearance of buprenorphine).
Products include:
Locoid Lipocream Cream 1160

Hydrocortisone Cypionate (Buprenorphine is metabolized by the CYP3A4 isoenzyme; co-administration with inducers of CYP3A4 may cause increase in clearance of buprenorphine).
No products indexed under this heading.

Hydrocortisone Hemisuccinate (Buprenorphine is metabolized by the CYP3A4 isoenzyme; co-administration with inducers of CYP3A4 may cause increase in clearance of buprenorphine).
No products indexed under this heading.

Hydrocortisone Probutate (Buprenorphine is metabolized by the CYP3A4 isoenzyme; co-administration with inducers of CYP3A4 may cause increase in clearance of buprenorphine).
No products indexed under this heading.

Hydrocortisone Sodium Phosphate (Buprenorphine is metabolized by the CYP3A4 isoenzyme; co-administration with inducers of CYP3A4 may cause increase in clearance of buprenorphine).
No products indexed under this heading.

Hydrocortisone Sodium Succinate (Buprenorphine is metabolized by the CYP3A4 isoenzyme; co-administration with inducers of CYP3A4 may cause increase in clearance of buprenorphine).
No products indexed under this heading.

Hydrocortisone Valerate
(Buprenorphine is metabolized by the CYP3A4 isoenzyme; co-administration with inducers of CYP3A4 may cause increase in clearance of buprenorphine).
No products indexed under this heading.

Hydromorphone Hydrochloride
(Increased CNS depression). Products include:

Hydroxyzine Hydrochloride
(Increased CNS depression).
No products indexed under this heading.

Hypericum (Buprenorphine is metabolized by the CYP3A4 isoenzyme; co-administration with inducers of CYP3A4 may cause increase in clearance of buprenorphine). Products include:

Hypericum Perforatum
(Buprenorphine is metabolized by the CYP3A4 isoenzyme; co-administration with inducers of CYP3A4 may cause increase in clearance of buprenorphine).
No products indexed under this heading.

Indinavir Sulfate (Buprenorphine is metabolized by the CYP3A4 isoenzyme; co-administration with inhibitors of CYP3A4 may cause decrease in clearance of buprenorphine). Products include:

Isocarboxazid (Effect unspecified; caution should be exercised).
No products indexed under this heading.

Isoflurane (Increased CNS depression).
No products indexed under this heading.

Isoniazid (Buprenorphine is metabolized by the CYP3A4 isoenzyme; co-administration with inhibitors of CYP3A4 may cause decrease in clearance of buprenorphine).
No products indexed under this heading.

Itraconazole (Buprenorphine is metabolized by the CYP3A4 isoenzyme; co-administration with inhibitors of CYP3A4 may cause decrease in clearance of buprenorphine).
No products indexed under this heading.

Ketamine Hydrochloride
(Increased CNS depression).
No products indexed under this heading.

Ketoconazole (Buprenorphine is metabolized by the CYP3A4 isoenzyme; co-administration with inhibitors of CYP3A4 may cause decrease in clearance of buprenorphine). Products include:

Levomethadyl Acetate Hydrochloride (Increased CNS depression).
No products indexed under this heading.

Levorphanol Tartrate (Increased CNS depression).
No products indexed under this heading.

Lopinavir (Buprenorphine is metabolized by the CYP3A4 isoenzyme; co-administration with inhibitors of CYP3A4 may cause decrease in clearance of buprenorphine). Products include:

Loratadine (Increased CNS depression). Products include:

Lorazepam (Increased CNS depression).
No products indexed under this heading.

Loxapine Hydrochloride
(Increased CNS depression).
No products indexed under this heading.

Loxapine Succinate (Increased CNS depression).
No products indexed under this heading.

Meperidine Hydrochloride
(Increased CNS depression).
No products indexed under this heading.

Mephenytoin (Buprenorphine is metabolized by the CYP3A4 isoenzyme; co-administration with inducers of CYP3A4 may cause increase in clearance of buprenorphine).
No products indexed under this heading.

Mephobarbital (Increased CNS depression).
No products indexed under this heading.

Meprobamate (Increased CNS depression).
No products indexed under this heading.

Mesoridazine Besylate (Increased CNS depression).
No products indexed under this heading.

Methadone Hydrochloride
(Increased CNS depression).
No products indexed under this heading.

Methdilazine Hydrochloride
(Increased CNS depression).
No products indexed under this heading.

Methohexital Sodium (Increased CNS depression).
No products indexed under this heading.

Methotrimeprazine (Increased CNS depression).
No products indexed under this heading.

Methoxyflurane (Increased CNS depression).
No products indexed under this heading.

Methsuximide (Buprenorphine is metabolized by the CYP3A4 isoenzyme; co-administration with inducers of CYP3A4 may cause increase in clearance of buprenorphine).
No products indexed under this heading.

Methylprednisolone (Buprenorphine is metabolized by the CYP3A4 isoenzyme; co-administration with inducers of CYP3A4 may cause increase in clearance of buprenorphine).
No products indexed under this heading.

Methylprednisolone Acetate
(Buprenorphine is metabolized by the CYP3A4 isoenzyme; co-administration with inducers of CYP3A4 may cause increase in clearance of buprenorphine). Products include:

Methylprednisolone Sodium Succinate (Buprenorphine is metabolized by the CYP3A4 isoenzyme; co-administration with inducers of CYP3A4 may cause increase in clearance of buprenorphine).
No products indexed under this heading.

Metronidazole (Buprenorphine is metabolized by the CYP3A4 isoenzyme; co-administration with inhibitors of CYP3A4 may cause decrease in clearance of buprenorphine). Products include:

Metronidazole Benzoate
(Buprenorphine is metabolized by the CYP3A4 isoenzyme; co-administration with inhibitors of CYP3A4 may cause decrease in clearance of buprenorphine).
No products indexed under this heading.

Metronidazole Hydrochloride
(Buprenorphine is metabolized by the CYP3A4 isoenzyme; co-administration with inhibitors of CYP3A4 may cause decrease in clearance of buprenorphine).
No products indexed under this heading.

Miconazole (Buprenorphine is metabolized by the CYP3A4 isoenzyme; co-administration with inhibitors of CYP3A4 may cause decrease in clearance of buprenorphine).
No products indexed under this heading.

Miconazole Nitrate (Buprenorphine is metabolized by the CYP3A4 isoenzyme; co-administration with inhibitors of CYP3A4 may cause decrease in clearance of buprenorphine). Products include:

Midazolam Hydrochloride
(Increased CNS depression).
No products indexed under this heading.

Moclobemide (Effect unspecified; caution should be exercised).
No products indexed under this heading.

Modafinil (Buprenorphine is metabolized by the CYP3A4 isoenzyme; co-administration with inducers of CYP3A4 may cause increase in clearance of buprenorphine). Products include:

Molindone Hydrochloride
(Increased CNS depression). Products include:

Morphine Sulfate (Increased CNS depression). Products include:

Nefazodone Hydrochloride
(Buprenorphine is metabolized by the CYP3A4 isoenzyme; co-administration with inhibitors of CYP3A4 may cause decrease in clearance of buprenorphine).
No products indexed under this heading.

Nelfinavir Mesylate (Buprenorphine is metabolized by the CYP3A4 isoenzyme; co-administration with inhibitors of CYP3A4 may cause decrease in clearance of buprenorphine). Products include:

Nevirapine (Buprenorphine is metabolized by the CYP3A4 isoenzyme; co-administration with inhibitors of CYP3A4 may cause decrease in clearance of buprenorphine). Products include:

Niacinamide (Buprenorphine is metabolized by the CYP3A4 isoenzyme; co-administration with inhibitors of CYP3A4 may cause decrease in clearance of buprenorphine).
No products indexed under this heading.

Nicotinamide (Buprenorphine is metabolized by the CYP3A4 isoenzyme; co-administration with inhibitors of CYP3A4 may cause decrease in clearance of buprenorphine). Products include:

Nifedipine (Buprenorphine is metabolized by the CYP3A4 isoenzyme; co-administration with inhibitors of CYP3A4 may cause decrease in clearance of buprenorphine). Products include:

Norfloxacin (Buprenorphine is metabolized by the CYP3A4 isoenzyme; co-administration with inhibitors of CYP3A4 may cause decrease in clearance of buprenorphine). Products include:

Olanzapine (Increased CNS depression). Products include:

Omeprazole (Buprenorphine is metabolized by the CYP3A4 isoenzyme; co-administration with inhibitors of CYP3A4 may cause decrease in clearance of buprenorphine). Products include:

Oxazepam (Increased CNS depression).
No products indexed under this heading.

Oxcarbazepine (Buprenorphine is metabolized by the CYP3A4 isoenzyme; co-administration with inducers of CYP3A4 may cause increase in clearance of buprenorphine). Products include:

Oxycodone Hydrochloride
(Increased CNS depression). Products include:

IMPORTANT NOTE: Always consult each drug listing in the patient's regimen for possible interactions.

Pargyline Hydrochloride (Effect unspecified; caution should be exercised).

No products indexed under this heading.

Paroxetine Hydrochloride (Buprenorphine is metabolized by the CYP3A4 isoenzyme; co-administration with inhibitors of CYP3A4 may cause decrease in clearance of buprenorphine). Products include:

Pentobarbital Sodium (Increased CNS depression). Products include:

Perphenazine (Increased CNS depression).

No products indexed under this heading.

Phenelzine Sulfate (Effect unspecified; caution should be exercised).

No products indexed under this heading.

Phenobarbital (Increased CNS depression). Products include:

Phenobarbital Sodium (Buprenorphine is metabolized by the CYP3A4 isoenzyme; co-administration with inducers of CYP3A4 may cause increase in clearance of buprenorphine).

No products indexed under this heading.

Phenprocoumon (Potential for purpura).

No products indexed under this heading.

Phenytoin (Buprenorphine is metabolized by the CYP3A4 isoenzyme; co-administration with inducers of CYP3A4 may cause increase in clearance of buprenorphine).

No products indexed under this heading.

Phenytoin Sodium (Buprenorphine is metabolized by the CYP3A4 isoenzyme; co-administration with inducers of CYP3A4 may cause increase in clearance of buprenorphine). Products include:

Prazepam (Increased CNS depression).

No products indexed under this heading.

Prednisolone Acetate (Buprenorphine is metabolized by the CYP3A4 isoenzyme; co-administration with inducers of CYP3A4 may cause increase in clearance of buprenorphine). Products include:

Prednisolone Sodium Phosphate (Buprenorphine is metabolized by the CYP3A4 isoenzyme; co-administration with inducers of CYP3A4 may cause increase in clearance of buprenorphine).

No products indexed under this heading.

Prednisolone Tebutate (Buprenorphine is metabolized by the CYP3A4 isoenzyme; co-administration with inducers of CYP3A4 may cause increase in clearance of buprenorphine).

No products indexed under this heading.

Prednisone (Buprenorphine is metabolized by the CYP3A4 isoenzyme; co-administration with inducers of CYP3A4 may cause increase in clearance of buprenorphine).

No products indexed under this heading.

Primidone (Buprenorphine is metabolized by the CYP3A4 isoenzyme; co-administration with inducers of CYP3A4 may cause increase in clearance of buprenorphine).

No products indexed under this heading.

Procarbazine Hydrochloride (Effect unspecified; caution should be exercised). Products include:

Prochlorperazine (Increased CNS depression).

No products indexed under this heading.

Promethazine Hydrochloride (Increased CNS depression). Products include:

Propofol (Increased CNS depression).

No products indexed under this heading.

Propoxyphene Hydrochloride (Increased CNS depression).

No products indexed under this heading.

Propoxyphene Napsylate (Increased CNS depression).

No products indexed under this heading.

Pyrilamine Maleate (Increased CNS depression).

No products indexed under this heading.

Pyrilamine Tannate (Increased CNS depression).

No products indexed under this heading.

Quazepam (Increased CNS depression).

No products indexed under this heading.

Quetiapine Fumarate (Increased CNS depression). Products include:

Quinidine (Buprenorphine is metabolized by the CYP3A4 isoenzyme; co-administration with inhibitors of CYP3A4 may cause decrease in clearance of buprenorphine).

No products indexed under this heading.

Quinidine Hydrochloride (Buprenorphine is metabolized by the CYP3A4 isoenzyme; co-administration with inhibitors of CYP3A4 may cause decrease in clearance of buprenorphine).

No products indexed under this heading.

Quinidine Polygalacturonate (Buprenorphine is metabolized by the CYP3A4 isoenzyme; co-administration with inhibitors of CYP3A4 may cause decrease in clearance of buprenorphine).

No products indexed under this heading.

Quinidine Sulfate (Buprenorphine is metabolized by the CYP3A4 isoenzyme; co-administration with inhibitors of CYP3A4 may cause decrease in clearance of buprenorphine).

No products indexed under this heading.

Quinine (Buprenorphine is metabolized by the CYP3A4 isoenzyme; co-administration with inhibitors of CYP3A4 may cause decrease in clearance of buprenorphine).

No products indexed under this heading.

Quinine Sulfate (Buprenorphine is metabolized by the CYP3A4 isoenzyme; co-administration with inhibitors of CYP3A4 may cause decrease in clearance of buprenorphine).

No products indexed under this heading.

Quinupristin (Buprenorphine is metabolized by the CYP3A4 isoenzyme; co-administration with inhibitors of CYP3A4 may cause decrease in clearance of buprenorphine).

No products indexed under this heading.

Ramelteon (Increased CNS depression). Products include:

Ranitidine Bismuth Citrate (Buprenorphine is metabolized by the CYP3A4 isoenzyme; co-administration with inhibitors of CYP3A4 may cause decrease in clearance of buprenorphine).

No products indexed under this heading.

Ranitidine Hydrochloride (Buprenorphine is metabolized by the CYP3A4 isoenzyme; co-administration with inhibitors of CYP3A4 may cause decrease in clearance of buprenorphine). Products include:

Remifentanil Hydrochloride (Increased CNS depression).

No products indexed under this heading.

Rifabutin (Buprenorphine is metabolized by the CYP3A4 isoenzyme; co-administration with inducers of CYP3A4 may cause increase in clearance of buprenorphine).

No products indexed under this heading.

Rifampicin (Buprenorphine is metabolized by the CYP3A4 isoenzyme; co-administration with inducers of CYP3A4 may cause increase in clearance of buprenorphine).

No products indexed under this heading.

Rifampin (Buprenorphine is metabolized by the CYP3A4 isoenzyme; co-administration with inducers of CYP3A4 may cause increase in clearance of buprenorphine).

No products indexed under this heading.

Rifapentine (Buprenorphine is metabolized by the CYP3A4 isoenzyme; co-administration with inducers of CYP3A4 may cause increase in clearance of buprenorphine).

No products indexed under this heading.

Risperidone (Increased CNS depression). Products include:

Ritonavir (Buprenorphine is metabolized by the CYP3A4 isoenzyme; co-administration with inhibitors of CYP3A4 may cause decrease in clearance of buprenorphine). Products include:

Saquinavir (Buprenorphine is metabolized by the CYP3A4 isoenzyme; co-administration with inhibitors of CYP3A4 may cause decrease in clearance of buprenorphine).

No products indexed under this heading.

Saquinavir Mesylate (Buprenorphine is metabolized by the CYP3A4 isoenzyme; co-administration with inhibitors of CYP3A4 may cause decrease in clearance of buprenorphine). Products include:

Secobarbital Sodium (Increased CNS depression).

No products indexed under this heading.

Selegiline Hydrochloride (Effect unspecified; caution should be exercised). Products include:

Sertraline Hydrochloride (Buprenorphine is metabolized by the CYP3A4 isoenzyme; co-administration with inhibitors of CYP3A4 may cause decrease in clearance of buprenorphine). Products include:

Sevoflurane (Increased CNS depression). Products include:

Sodium Oxybate (Increased CNS depression). Products include:

Sufentanil Citrate (Increased CNS depression).

No products indexed under this heading.

Sulfinpyrazone (Buprenorphine is metabolized by the CYP3A4 isoenzyme; co-administration with inducers of CYP3A4 may cause increase in clearance of buprenorphine).

No products indexed under this heading.

Telithromycin (Buprenorphine is metabolized by the CYP3A4 isoenzyme; co-administration with inhibitors of CYP3A4 may cause decrease in clearance of buprenorphine). Products include:

Temazepam (Increased CNS depression). Products include:

Terfenadine (Increased CNS depression).

No products indexed under this heading.

Theophylline (Buprenorphine is metabolized by the CYP3A4 isoenzyme; co-administration with inducers of CYP3A4 may cause increase in clearance of buprenorphine).
No products indexed under this heading.

Thiamylal Sodium (Increased CNS depression).
No products indexed under this heading.

Thioridazine Hydrochloride (Increased CNS depression). Products include:
Thioridazine Hydrochloride Tablets 2163

Thiothixene (Increased CNS depression). Products include:
Thiothixene Capsules 2165

Tranylcypromine Sulfate (Effect unspecified; caution should be exercised). Products include:
Parnate Tablets 1527

Triamcinolone (Buprenorphine is metabolized by the CYP3A4 isoenzyme; co-administration with inducers of CYP3A4 may cause increase in clearance of buprenorphine).
No products indexed under this heading.

Triamcinolone Acetonide (Buprenorphine is metabolized by the CYP3A4 isoenzyme; co-administration with inducers of CYP3A4 may cause increase in clearance of buprenorphine). Products include:
Azmacort Inhalation Aerosol 1726
Nasacort AQ Nasal Spray 2922

Triamcinolone Diacetate (Buprenorphine is metabolized by the CYP3A4 isoenzyme; co-administration with inducers of CYP3A4 may cause increase in clearance of buprenorphine).
No products indexed under this heading.

Triamcinolone Hexacetonide (Buprenorphine is metabolized by the CYP3A4 isoenzyme; co-administration with inducers of CYP3A4 may cause increase in clearance of buprenorphine).
No products indexed under this heading.

Triazolam (Increased CNS depression).
No products indexed under this heading.

Trifluoperazine Hydrochloride (Increased CNS depression).
No products indexed under this heading.

Trimeprazine Tartrate (Increased CNS depression).
No products indexed under this heading.

Tripelennamine Hydrochloride (Increased CNS depression).
No products indexed under this heading.

Triprolidine Hydrochloride (Increased CNS depression).
No products indexed under this heading.

Troglitazone (Buprenorphine is metabolized by the CYP3A4 isoenzyme; co-administration with inhibitors of CYP3A4 may cause decrease in clearance of buprenorphine).
No products indexed under this heading.

Troleandomycin (Buprenorphine is metabolized by the CYP3A4 isoenzyme; co-administration with inhibitors of CYP3A4 may cause decrease in clearance of buprenorphine).
No products indexed under this heading.

Valproate Sodium (Buprenorphine is metabolized by the CYP3A4 isoenzyme; co-administration with inhibitors of CYP3A4 may cause decrease in clearance of buprenorphine). Products include:
Depacon Injection 412

Verapamil Hydrochloride (Buprenorphine is metabolized by the CYP3A4 isoenzyme; co-administration with inhibitors of CYP3A4 may cause decrease in clearance of buprenorphine). Products include:
Covera-HS Tablets 3139
Tarka Tablets 524
Verelan PM Extended-Release Capsules, Controlled-Onset 3106

Voriconazole (Buprenorphine is metabolized by the CYP3A4 isoenzyme; co-administration with inhibitors of CYP3A4 may cause decrease in clearance of buprenorphine). Products include:
VFEND I.V. 2564
VFEND Oral Suspension 2564
VFEND Tablets 2564

Zafirlukast (Buprenorphine is metabolized by the CYP3A4 isoenzyme; co-administration with inhibitors of CYP3A4 may cause decrease in clearance of buprenorphine). Products include:
Accolate Tablets 671

Zaleplon (Increased CNS depression). Products include:
Sonata Capsules 1717

Zileuton (Buprenorphine is metabolized by the CYP3A4 isoenzyme; co-administration with inhibitors of CYP3A4 may cause decrease in clearance of buprenorphine). Products include:
Zyflo Tablets 1023

Ziprasidone Hydrochloride (Increased CNS depression). Products include:
Geodon Capsules 2529

Zolpidem Tartrate (Increased CNS depression). Products include:
Ambien Tablets 2851
Ambien CR Tablets 2855

Food Interactions

Alcohol (Increased CNS depression).

Grapefruit (Buprenorphine is metabolized by the CYP3A4 isoenzyme; co-administration with inhibitors of CYP3A4 may cause decrease in clearance of buprenorphine).

Grapefruit Juice (Buprenorphine is metabolized by the CYP3A4 isoenzyme; co-administration with inhibitors of CYP3A4 may cause decrease in clearance of buprenorphine).

BYETTA INJECTION

(Exenatide) 611

May interact with bacteriostatic antibiotics, beta-lactams antibiotics, fluoroquinolone antibiotics, macrolide antibiotics, oral contraceptives, penicillins, tetracyclines, and certain other agents. Compounds in these categories include:

Acetaminophen (When 1000 mg acetaminophen exlixir was given with 10 mcg of exenatide (0 h) and 1 h, 2 h, and 4 h after exenatide, acetaminophen AUCs were decreased by 21%, 23%, 24%, and 14%, respectively; Cmax was decreased by 37%, 56%, 54%, and 41%, respectively; Tmaxwas increased from 0.6 h in the control period to 0.9 h, 4.2 h, 3.3 h, and 1.6 h, respectively. Acetaminohpen AUC, Cmax and Tmax were not significantly changed when acetaminophen was given 1 h before exenatide). Products include:
Comtrex Maximum Strength Cold & Cough Day/Night Caplets - Day Formulation 726
Comtrex Maximum Strength Cold & Cough Day/Night Caplets - Night Formulation 726
Comtrex Maximum Strength Non-Drowsy Cold & Cough Caplets 725
Comtrex Maximum Strength Day/Night Severe Cold & Sinus Caplets - Day Formulation 725
Comtrex Maximum Strength Day/Night Severe Cold & Sinus Caplets - Night Formulation 725
Contac Cold and Flu Maximum Strength Caplets 728
Contac Cold and Flu Day and Night Caplets (Day Formulation Only) 727
Contac Cold and Flu Day and Night Caplets (Night Formulation Only) 727
Contac Cold and Flu Non-Drowsy Caplets 728
Excedrin Extra Strength Caplets/Tablets/Geltabs 684
Excedrin Migraine Caplets/Tablets/Geltabs 609
Excedrin PM Caplets/Tablets/Geltabs 610
Excedrin Sinus Headache Caplets/Tablets 610
Excedrin Tension Headache Caplets/Tablets/Geltabs 611
Goody's Body Pain Formula Powder 684
Goody's Extra Strength Headache Powders 611
Goody's Extra Strength Pain Relief Tablets 685
Goody's PM Powder for Pain with Sleeplessness 612
Percocet Tablets 1131
Robitussin Cough, Cold & Flu Nighttime Liquid 738
TheraFlu Cold & Sore Throat Hot Liquid 741
TheraFlu Flu & Chest Congestion Hot Liquid 741
TheraFlu Flu & Sore Throat Hot Liquid 742
TheraFlu Daytime Severe Cold Hot Liquid 742
TheraFlu Nighttime Severe Cold Hot Liquid 740
TheraFlu Warming Relief Daytime Severe Cold 743
TheraFlu Warming Relief Nighttime Severe Cold 743
Triaminic Cough & Sore Throat Liquid 747
Regular Strength Tylenol Tablets 1870
Children's Tylenol with Flavor Creator 679
Children's Tylenol Plus Flu Oral Suspension 749
Tylenol Cold Head Congestion Daytime Caplets with Cool Burst and Gelcaps 750
Tylenol Cold Multi-Symptom Daytime Liquid 752
Tylenol Cold Multi-Symptom Severe Daytime Liquid 752
Tylenol 8 Hour Extended Release Caplets 1870
Tylenol 1870
Extra Strength Tylenol PM Caplets, Vanilla Caplets, Geltabs, Gelcaps and Liquid 1875
Extra Strength Tylenol Rapid Release Gels 1870
Concentrated Tylenol Infants' Drops Plus Cold & Cough 754
Tylenol with Codeine Tablets 2391
Tylenol Allergy Multi-Symptom Caplets with Cool Burst and Gelcaps 1872
Tylenol Allergy Multi-Symptom Nighttime Caplets with Cool Burst 1872
Tylenol Severe Allergy Caplets 1872
Tylenol Arthritis Pain Extended Release Caplets and Geltabs 1870
Tylenol Chest Congestion Caplets with Cool Burst 1872
Tylenol Chest Congestion Liquid with Cool Burst 1872
Children's Tylenol Suspension Liquid and Meltaways 1878
Children's Tylenol Plus Cold Suspension Liquid 1879
Children's Tylenol Plus Cold & Allergy Suspension Liquid 1878
Children's Tylenol Plus Cough & Runny Nose Suspension Liquid 1879
Children's Tylenol Plus Cough & Sore Throat Suspension Liquid 1879
Children's Tylenol Suspension with Flavor Creator 1878
Children's Tylenol Plus Flu Suspension Liquid 1881
Children's Tylenol Plus Multi-Symptom Cold Suspension Liquid 1879
Tylenol Cold Severe Congestion Non-Drowsy Caplets with Cool Burst 1874
Tylenol Cold Head Congestion Daytime Caplets with Cool Burst 1873
Tylenol Cold Head Congestion Nighttime Caplets with Cool Burst 1873
Tylenol Cold Head Congestion Severe Caplets with Cool Burst 1873
Tylenol Cold Multi-Symptom Daytime Caplets with Cool Burst and Gelcaps 1874
Tylenol Cold Multi-Symptom Daytime Liquid with Citrus Burst 1874
Tylenol Cold Multi-Symptom Nighttime Caplets with Cool Burst 1874
Tylenol Cold Multi-Symptom Nighttime Liquid with Cool Burst 1874
Tylenol Cold Multi-Symptom Severe Caplets with Cool Burst 1874
Tylenol Cold Multi-Symptom Severe Daytime Liquid with Citrus Burst 1874
Tylenol Cough & Sore Throat Daytime Liquid with Cool Burst 1877
Tylenol Cough & Sore Throat Nighttime Liquid with Cool Burst 1877
Concentrated Tylenol Infants' Drops 1878
Concentrated Tylenol Infants' Drops Plus Cold 1879
Concentrated Tylenol Infants' Drops Plus Cold and Cough 1879
Jr. Tylenol Meltaways 1878
Tylenol Sinus Severe Congestion Caplets with Cool Burst 1876
Tylenol Sinus Congestion & Pain Daytime Caplets with Cool Burst and Gelcaps 1876
Tylenol Sinus Congestion & Pain Nighttime Caplets with Cool Burst 1876
Tylenol Sinus Congestion & Pain Severe Caplets with Cool Burst 1876
Tylenol Sore Throat Daytime Liquid with Cool Burst 1877
Tylenol Sore Throat Nighttime Liquid with Cool Burst 1877
Women's Tylenol Menstrual Relief Caplets 1877
Vicks 44M Cough, Cold & Flu Relief Liquid 2680
Vicks DayQuil LiquiCaps/Liquid Multi-Symptom Cold/Flu Relief 761
Vicks DayQuil Multi-Symptom Cold/Flu Relief LiquiCaps 2678
Vicks DayQuil Multi-Symptom Cold/Flu Relief Liquid 2678
Vicks NyQuil Multi-Symptom Cold/Flu Relief Liquid 2681
Vicks NyQuil Multi-Symptom Cold/Flu Relief LiquiCaps 2681
Vicks NyQuil LiquiCaps/Liquid Multi-Symptom Cold/Flu Relief 763
Vicodin Tablets 535
Vicodin ES Tablets 536
Vicodin HP Tablets 538

Zicam Maximum Strength Flu Daytime ▣ 768
Zicam Maximum Strength Flu Nighttime ▣ 768
Zydone Tablets 1139

Alatrofloxacin Mesylate (The effect of exenatide to slow gastric emptying may reduce the extent and rate of absorption of orally administered drugs. Exenatide should be used with caution in patients receiving oral medications that require rapid gastrointestinal absorption. For oral medications that are dependent on threshold concentrations for efficacy, such as antibiotics, patients should be advised to take those drugs at least 1 hr before exenatide injection. If such drugs are to be administered with food, patients should be advised to take them with a meal or snack when exenatide is not administered).
No products indexed under this heading.

5-Amino-Salicylic Acid (The effect of exenatide to slow gastric emptying may reduce the extent and rate of absorption of orally administered drugs. Exenatide should be used with caution in patients receiving oral medications that require rapid gastrointestinal absorption. For oral medications that are dependent on threshold concentrations for efficacy, such as antibiotics, patients should be advised to take those drugs at least 1 hr before exenatide injection. If such drugs are to be administered with food, patients should be advised to take them with a meal or snack when exenatide is not administered).
No products indexed under this heading.

Amoxicillin (The effect of exenatide to slow gastric emptying may reduce the extent and rate of absorption of orally administered drugs. Exenatide should be used with caution in patients receiving oral medications that require rapid gastrointestinal absorption. For oral medications that are dependent on threshold concentrations for efficacy, such as antibiotics, patients should be advised to take those drugs at least 1 hr before exenatide injection. If such drugs are to be administered with food, patients should be advised to take them with a meal or snack when exenatide is not administered).
Products include:
Amoxil Capsules 1343
Amoxil Chewable Tablets 1343
Amoxil Pediatric Drops for Oral Suspension 1343
Amoxil Powder for Oral Suspension 1343
Amoxil Tablets 1343
Augmentin 1360
Augmentin Tablets 1363
Augmentin XR Extended-Release Tablets 1369
Augmentin ES-600 Powder for Oral Suspension 1366
PREVPAC 3284

Amoxicillin Trihydrate (The effect of exenatide to slow gastric emptying may reduce the extent and rate of absorption of orally administered drugs. Exenatide should be used with caution in patients receiving oral medications that require rapid gastrointestinal absorption. For oral medications that are dependent on threshold concentrations for efficacy, such as antibiotics, patients should be advised to take those drugs at least 1 hr before exenatide injection. If such drugs are to be administered with food, patients should be advised to take them with a meal or snack when exenatide is not administered).
No products indexed under this heading.

Ampicillin (The effect of exenatide to slow gastric emptying may reduce the extent and rate of absorption of orally administered drugs. Exenatide should be used with caution in patients receiving oral medications that require rapid gastrointestinal absorption. For oral medications that are dependent on threshold concentrations for efficacy, such as antibiotics, patients should be advised to take those drugs at least 1 hr before exenatide injection. If such drugs are to be administered with food, patients should be advised to take them with a meal or snack when exenatide is not administered).
No products indexed under this heading.

Ampicillin Sodium (The effect of exenatide to slow gastric emptying may reduce the extent and rate of absorption of orally administered drugs. Exenatide should be used with caution in patients receiving oral medications that require rapid gastrointestinal absorption. For oral medications that are dependent on threshold concentrations for efficacy, such as antibiotics, patients should be advised to take those drugs at least 1 hr before exenatide injection. If such drugs are to be administered with food, patients should be advised to take them with a meal or snack when exenatide is not administered).
No products indexed under this heading.

Ampicillin Trihydrate (The effect of exenatide to slow gastric emptying may reduce the extent and rate of absorption of orally administered drugs. Exenatide should be used with caution in patients receiving oral medications that require rapid gastrointestinal absorption. For oral medications that are dependent on threshold concentrations for efficacy, such as antibiotics, patients should be advised to take those drugs at least 1 hr before exenatide injection. If such drugs are to be administered with food, patients should be advised to take them with a meal or snack when exenatide is not administered).
No products indexed under this heading.

Azithromycin Dihydrate (The effect of exenatide to slow gastric emptying may reduce the extent and rate of absorption of orally administered drugs. Exenatide should be used with caution in patients receiving oral medications that require rapid gastrointestinal absorption. For oral medications that are dependent on threshold concentrations for efficacy, such as antibiotics, patients should be advised to take those drugs at least 1 hr before exenatide injection. If such drugs are to be administered with food, patients should be advised to take them with a meal or snack when exenatide is not administered).
No products indexed under this heading.

Azlocillin Sodium (The effect of exenatide to slow gastric emptying may reduce the extent and rate of absorption of orally administered drugs. Exenatide should be used with caution in patients receiving oral medications that require rapid gastrointestinal absorption. For oral medications that are dependent on threshold concentrations for efficacy, such as antibiotics, patients should be advised to take those drugs at least 1 hr before exenatide injection. If such drugs are to be administered with food, patients should be advised to take them with a meal or snack when exenatide is not administered).
No products indexed under this heading.

Aztreonam (The effect of exenatide to slow gastric emptying may reduce the extent and rate of absorption of orally administered drugs. Exenatide should be used with caution in patients receiving oral medications that require rapid gastrointestinal absorption. For oral medications that are dependent on threshold concentrations for efficacy, such as antibiotics, patients should be advised to take those drugs at least 1 hr before exenatide injection. If such drugs are to be administered with food, patients should be advised to take them with a meal or snack when exenatide is not administered).
No products indexed under this heading.

Bacampicillin Hydrochloride (The effect of exenatide to slow gastric emptying may reduce the extent and rate of absorption of orally administered drugs. Exenatide should be used with caution in patients receiving oral medications that require rapid gastrointestinal absorption. For oral medications that are dependent on threshold concentrations for efficacy, such as antibiotics, patients should be advised to take those drugs at least 1 hr before exenatide injection. If such drugs are to be administered with food, patients should be advised to take them with a meal or snack when exenatide is not administered).
No products indexed under this heading.

Carbenicillin Disodium (The effect of exenatide to slow gastric emptying may reduce the extent and rate of absorption of orally administered drugs. Exenatide should be used with caution in patients receiving oral medications that require rapid gastrointestinal absorption. For oral medications that are dependent on threshold concentrations for efficacy, such as antibiotics, patients should be advised to take those drugs at least 1 hr before exenatide injection. If such drugs are to be administered with food, patients should be advised to take them with a meal or snack when exenatide is not administered).
No products indexed under this heading.

Carbenicillin Indanyl Sodium (The effect of exenatide to slow gastric emptying may reduce the extent and rate of absorption of orally administered drugs. Exenatide should be used with caution in patients receiving oral medications that require rapid gastrointestinal absorption. For oral medications that are dependent on threshold concentrations for efficacy, such as antibiotics, patients should be advised to take those drugs at least 1 hr before exenatide injection. If such drugs are to be administered with food, patients should be advised to take them with a meal or snack when exenatide is not administered).
No products indexed under this heading.

Cefaclor (The effect of exenatide to slow gastric emptying may reduce the extent and rate of absorption of orally administered drugs. Exenatide should be used with caution in patients receiving oral medications that require rapid gastrointestinal absorption. For oral medications that are dependent on threshold concentrations for efficacy, such as antibiotics, patients should be advised to take those drugs at least 1 hr before exenatide injection. If such drugs are to be administered with food, patients should be advised to take them with a meal or snack when exenatide is not administered).
No products indexed under this heading.

Cefadroxil (The effect of exenatide to slow gastric emptying may reduce the extent and rate of absorption of orally administered drugs. Exenatide should be used with caution in patients receiving oral medications that require rapid gastrointestinal absorption. For oral medications that are dependent on threshold concentrations for efficacy, such as antibiotics, patients should be advised to take those drugs at least 1 hr before exenatide injection. If such drugs are to be administered with food, patients should be advised to take them with a meal or snack when exenatide is not administered).
No products indexed under this heading.

Cefamandole Nafate (The effect of exenatide to slow gastric emptying may reduce the extent and rate of absorption of orally administered drugs. Exenatide should be used with caution in patients receiving oral medications that require rapid gastrointestinal absorption. For oral medications that are dependent on threshold concentrations for efficacy, such as antibiotics, patients should be advised to take those drugs at least 1 hr before exenatide injection. If such drugs are to be administered with food, patients should be advised to take them with a meal or snack when exenatide is not administered).
No products indexed under this heading.

Cefazolin Sodium (The effect of exenatide to slow gastric emptying may reduce the extent and rate of absorption of orally administered drugs. Exenatide should be used with caution in patients receiving oral medications that require rapid gastrointestinal absorption. For oral medications that are dependent on threshold concentrations for efficacy, such as antibiotics, patients should be advised to take those drugs at least 1 hr before exenatide injection. If such drugs are to be administered with food, patients should be advised to take them with a meal or snack when exenatide is not administered).

No products indexed under this heading.

Cefixime (The effect of exenatide to slow gastric emptying may reduce the extent and rate of absorption of orally administered drugs. Exenatide should be used with caution in patients receiving oral medications that require rapid gastrointestinal absorption. For oral medications that are dependent on threshold concentrations for efficacy, such as antibiotics, patients should be advised to take those drugs at least 1 hr before exenatide injection. If such drugs are to be administered with food, patients should be advised to take them with a meal or snack when exenatide is not administered). Products include:
Suprax 1843

Cefmetazole Sodium (The effect of exenatide to slow gastric emptying may reduce the extent and rate of absorption of orally administered drugs. Exenatide should be used with caution in patients receiving oral medications that require rapid gastrointestinal absorption. For oral medications that are dependent on threshold concentrations for efficacy, such as antibiotics, patients should be advised to take those drugs at least 1 hr before exenatide injection. If such drugs are to be administered with food, patients should be advised to take them with a meal or snack when exenatide is not administered).

No products indexed under this heading.

Cefonicid Sodium (The effect of exenatide to slow gastric emptying may reduce the extent and rate of absorption of orally administered drugs. Exenatide should be used with caution in patients receiving oral medications that require rapid gastrointestinal absorption. For oral medications that are dependent on threshold concentrations for efficacy, such as antibiotics, patients should be advised to take those drugs at least 1 hr before exenatide injection. If such drugs are to be administered with food, patients should be advised to take them with a meal or snack when exenatide is not administered).

No products indexed under this heading.

Cefoperazone Sodium (The effect of exenatide to slow gastric emptying may reduce the extent and rate of absorption of orally administered drugs. Exenatide should be used with caution in patients receiving oral medications that require rapid gastrointestinal absorption. For oral medications that are dependent on threshold concentrations for efficacy, such as antibiotics, patients should be advised to take those drugs at least 1 hr before exenatide injection. If such drugs are to be administered with food, patients should be advised to take them with a meal or snack when exenatide is not administered).

No products indexed under this heading.

Ceforanide (The effect of exenatide to slow gastric emptying may reduce the extent and rate of absorption of orally administered drugs. Exenatide should be used with caution in patients receiving oral medications

that require rapid gastrointestinal absorption. For oral medications that are dependent on threshold concentrations for efficacy, such as antibiotics, patients should be advised to take those drugs at least 1 hr before exenatide injection. If such drugs are to be administered with food, patients should be advised to take them with a meal or snack when exenatide is not administered).

No products indexed under this heading.

Cefotaxime Sodium (The effect of exenatide to slow gastric emptying may reduce the extent and rate of absorption of orally administered drugs. Exenatide should be used with caution in patients receiving oral medications that require rapid gastrointestinal absorption. For oral medications that are dependent on threshold concentrations for efficacy, such as antibiotics, patients should be advised to take those drugs at least 1 hr before exenatide injection. If such drugs are to be administered with food, patients should be advised to take them with a meal or snack when exenatide is not administered).

No products indexed under this heading.

Cefotetan (The effect of exenatide to slow gastric emptying may reduce the extent and rate of absorption of orally administered drugs. Exenatide should be used with caution in patients receiving oral medications that require rapid gastrointestinal absorption. For oral medications that are dependent on threshold concentrations for efficacy, such as antibiotics, patients should be advised to take those drugs at least 1 hr before exenatide injection. If such drugs are to be administered with food, patients should be advised to take them with a meal or snack when exenatide is not administered).

No products indexed under this heading.

Cefoxitin Sodium (The effect of exenatide to slow gastric emptying may reduce the extent and rate of absorption of orally administered drugs. Exenatide should be used with caution in patients receiving oral medications that require rapid gastrointestinal absorption. For oral medications that are dependent on threshold concentrations for efficacy, such as antibiotics, patients should be advised to take those drugs at least 1 hr before exenatide injection. If such drugs are to be administered with food, patients should be advised to take them with a meal or snack when exenatide is not administered). Products include:
Mefoxin for Injection 2012
Mefoxin Premixed Intravenous
 Solution 2016

Cefpodoxime Proxetil (The effect of exenatide to slow gastric emptying may reduce the extent and rate of absorption of orally administered drugs. Exenatide should be used with caution in patients receiving oral medications that require rapid gastrointestinal absorption. For oral medications that are dependent on threshold concentrations for efficacy, such as antibiotics, patients should be advised to take those drugs at least 1 hr before exenatide injection. If such drugs are to be administered with food, patients

should be advised to take them with a meal or snack when exenatide is not administered). Products include:
Vantin Tablets and Oral
 Suspension 2645

Cefprozil (The effect of exenatide to slow gastric emptying may reduce the extent and rate of absorption of orally administered drugs. Exenatide should be used with caution in patients receiving oral medications that require rapid gastrointestinal absorption. For oral medications that are dependent on threshold concentrations for efficacy, such as antibiotics, patients should be advised to take those drugs at least 1 hr before exenatide injection. If such drugs are to be administered with food, patients should be advised to take them with a meal or snack when exenatide is not administered).

No products indexed under this heading.

Ceftazidime (The effect of exenatide to slow gastric emptying may reduce the extent and rate of absorption of orally administered drugs. Exenatide should be used with caution in patients receiving oral medications that require rapid gastrointestinal absorption. For oral medications that are dependent on threshold concentrations for efficacy, such as antibiotics, patients should be advised to take those drugs at least 1 hr before exenatide injection. If such drugs are to be administered with food, patients should be advised to take them with a meal or snack when exenatide is not administered). Products include:
Fortaz 1453

Ceftizoxime Sodium (The effect of exenatide to slow gastric emptying may reduce the extent and rate of absorption of orally administered drugs. Exenatide should be used with caution in patients receiving oral medications that require rapid gastrointestinal absorption. For oral medications that are dependent on threshold concentrations for efficacy, such as antibiotics, patients should be advised to take those drugs at least 1 hr before exenatide injection. If such drugs are to be administered with food, patients should be advised to take them with a meal or snack when exenatide is not administered).

No products indexed under this heading.

Ceftriaxone Sodium (The effect of exenatide to slow gastric emptying may reduce the extent and rate of absorption of orally administered drugs. Exenatide should be used with caution in patients receiving oral medications that require rapid gastrointestinal absorption. For oral medications that are dependent on threshold concentrations for efficacy, such as antibiotics, patients should be advised to take those drugs at least 1 hr before exenatide injection. If such drugs are to be administered with food, patients should be advised to take them with a meal or snack when exenatide is not administered). Products include:
Rocephin Injectable Vials,
 ADD-Vantage, Galaxy, Bulk 2800

Cefuroxime Axetil (The effect of exenatide to slow gastric emptying may reduce the extent and rate of absorption of orally administered drugs. Exenatide should be used

with caution in patients receiving oral medications that require rapid gastrointestinal absorption. For oral medications that are dependent on threshold concentrations for efficacy, such as antibiotics, patients should be advised to take those drugs at least 1 hr before exenatide injection. If such drugs are to be administered with food, patients should be advised to take them with a meal or snack when exenatide is not administered). Products include:
Ceftin 1407

Cefuroxime Sodium (The effect of exenatide to slow gastric emptying may reduce the extent and rate of absorption of orally administered drugs. Exenatide should be used with caution in patients receiving oral medications that require rapid gastrointestinal absorption. For oral medications that are dependent on threshold concentrations for efficacy, such as antibiotics, patients should be advised to take those drugs at least 1 hr before exenatide injection. If such drugs are to be administered with food, patients should be advised to take them with a meal or snack when exenatide is not administered).

No products indexed under this heading.

Cephalexin (The effect of exenatide to slow gastric emptying may reduce the extent and rate of absorption of orally administered drugs. Exenatide should be used with caution in patients receiving oral medications that require rapid gastrointestinal absorption. For oral medications that are dependent on threshold concentrations for efficacy, such as antibiotics, patients should be advised to take those drugs at least 1 hr before exenatide injection. If such drugs are to be administered with food, patients should be advised to take them with a meal or snack when exenatide is not administered). Products include:
Keflex Capsules 549

Cephalothin Sodium (The effect of exenatide to slow gastric emptying may reduce the extent and rate of absorption of orally administered drugs. Exenatide should be used with caution in patients receiving oral medications that require rapid gastrointestinal absorption. For oral medications that are dependent on threshold concentrations for efficacy, such as antibiotics, patients should be advised to take those drugs at least 1 hr before exenatide injection. If such drugs are to be administered with food, patients should be advised to take them with a meal or snack when exenatide is not administered).

No products indexed under this heading.

Cephapirin Sodium (The effect of exenatide to slow gastric emptying may reduce the extent and rate of absorption of orally administered drugs. Exenatide should be used with caution in patients receiving oral medications that require rapid gastrointestinal absorption. For oral medications that are dependent on threshold concentrations for efficacy, such as antibiotics, patients should be advised to take those drugs at least 1 hr before exenatide injection. If such drugs are to be administered with food, patients

IMPORTANT NOTE: Always consult each drug listing in the patient's regimen for possible interactions.

should be advised to take them with a meal or snack when exenatide is not administered).

No products indexed under this heading.

Cephradine (The effect of exenatide to slow gastric emptying may reduce the extent and rate of absorption of orally administered drugs. Exenatide should be used with caution in patients receiving oral medications that require rapid gastrointestinal absorption. For oral medications that are dependent on threshold concentrations for efficacy, such as antibiotics, patients should be advised to take those drugs at least 1 hr before exenatide injection. If such drugs are to be administered with food, patients should be advised to take them with a meal or snack when exenatide is not administered).

No products indexed under this heading.

Chloramphenicol (The effect of exenatide to slow gastric emptying may reduce the extent and rate of absorption of orally administered drugs. Exenatide should be used with caution in patients receiving oral medications that require rapid gastrointestinal absorption. For oral medications that are dependent on threshold concentrations for efficacy, such as antibiotics, patients should be advised to take those drugs at least 1 hr before exenatide injection. If such drugs are to be administered with food, patients should be advised to take them with a meal or snack when exenatide is not administered).

No products indexed under this heading.

Chloramphenicol Palmitate (The effect of exenatide to slow gastric emptying may reduce the extent and rate of absorption of orally administered drugs. Exenatide should be used with caution in patients receiving oral medications that require rapid gastrointestinal absorption. For oral medications that are dependent on threshold concentrations for efficacy, such as antibiotics, patients should be advised to take those drugs at least 1 hr before exenatide injection. If such drugs are to be administered with food, patients should be advised to take them with a meal or snack when exenatide is not administered).

No products indexed under this heading.

Chloramphenicol Sodium Succinate (The effect of exenatide to slow gastric emptying may reduce the extent and rate of absorption of orally administered drugs. Exenatide should be used with caution in patients receiving oral medications that require rapid gastrointestinal absorption. For oral medications that are dependent on threshold concentrations for efficacy, such as antibiotics, patients should be advised to take those drugs at least 1 hr before exenatide injection. If such drugs are to be administered with food, patients should be advised to take them with a meal or snack when exenatide is not administered).

No products indexed under this heading.

Cilastatin Sodium (The effect of exenatide to slow gastric emptying may reduce the extent and rate of absorption of orally administered drugs. Exenatide should be used with caution in patients receiving oral medications that require rapid gastrointestinal absorption. For oral medications that are dependent on threshold concentrations for efficacy, such as antibiotics, patients should be advised to take those drugs at least 1 hr before exenatide injection. If such drugs are to be administered with food, patients should be advised to take them with a meal or snack when exenatide is not administered). Products include:

Primaxin I.M. 2045
Primaxin I.V. 2048

Ciprofloxacin (The effect of exenatide to slow gastric emptying may reduce the extent and rate of absorption of orally administered drugs. Exenatide should be used with caution in patients receiving oral medications that require rapid gastrointestinal absorption. For oral medications that are dependent on threshold concentrations for efficacy, such as antibiotics, patients should be advised to take those drugs at least 1 hr before exenatide injection. If such drugs are to be administered with food, patients should be advised to take them with a meal or snack when exenatide is not administered). Products include:

Cipro Oral Suspension 2977
Cipro I.V. 2984
Cipro XR Tablets 2990
Ciprodex Otic Suspension 559

Ciprofloxacin Hydrochloride (The effect of exenatide to slow gastric emptying may reduce the extent and rate of absorption of orally administered drugs. Exenatide should be used with caution in patients receiving oral medications that require rapid gastrointestinal absorption. For oral medications that are dependent on threshold concentrations for efficacy, such as antibiotics, patients should be advised to take those drugs at least 1 hr before exenatide injection. If such drugs are to be administered with food, patients should be advised to take them with a meal or snack when exenatide is not administered). Products include:

Ciloxan Ophthalmic Ointment 559
Ciloxan Ophthalmic Solution .... ⊙206
Cipro Tablets 2977
Proquin XR Tablets 1153

Clarithromycin (The effect of exenatide to slow gastric emptying may reduce the extent and rate of absorption of orally administered drugs. Exenatide should be used with caution in patients receiving oral medications that require rapid gastrointestinal absorption. For oral medications that are dependent on threshold concentrations for efficacy, such as antibiotics, patients should be advised to take those drugs at least 1 hr before exenatide injection. If such drugs are to be administered with food, patients should be advised to take them with a meal or snack when exenatide is not administered). Products include:

Biaxin/Biaxin XL 402
PREVPAC 3284

Demeclocycline Hydrochloride (The effect of exenatide to slow gastric emptying may reduce the extent and rate of absorption of orally administered drugs. Exenatide should be used with caution in patients receiving oral medications that require rapid gastrointestinal absorption. For oral medications that are dependent on threshold concentrations for efficacy, such as antibiotics, patients should be advised to take those drugs at least 1 hr before exenatide injection. If such drugs are to be administered with food, patients should be advised to take them with a meal or snack when exenatide is not administered).

No products indexed under this heading.

Desogestrel (The effect of exenatide to slow gastric emptying may reduce the extent and rate of absorption of orally administered drugs. Exenatide should be used with caution in patients receiving oral medications that require rapid gastrointestinal absorption. For oral medications that are dependent on threshold concentrations for efficacy, such as contraceptives, patients should be advised to take those drugs at least 1 hr before exenatide injection. If such drugs are to be administered with food, patients should be advised to take them with a meal or snack when exenatide is not administered). Products include:

Mircette Tablets 1066

Dicloxacillin Sodium (The effect of exenatide to slow gastric emptying may reduce the extent and rate of absorption of orally administered drugs. Exenatide should be used with caution in patients receiving oral medications that require rapid gastrointestinal absorption. For oral medications that are dependent on threshold concentrations for efficacy, such as antibiotics, patients should be advised to take those drugs at least 1 hr before exenatide injection. If such drugs are to be administered with food, patients should be advised to take them with a meal or snack when exenatide is not administered).

No products indexed under this heading.

Digoxin (Coadministration of repeated doses of exenatide (10 mcg BID) decreased the Cmax of oral digoxin (0.25 mg QD) by 17% and delayed the Tmax by approximately 2.5 h; however, the overall steady-state pharmacokinetic exposure (AUC) was not changed). Products include:

Lanoxicaps Capsules 1490
Lanoxin Injection 1494
Lanoxin Injection Pediatric 1497
Lanoxin Tablets 1500

Dirithromycin (The effect of exenatide to slow gastric emptying may reduce the extent and rate of absorption of orally administered drugs. Exenatide should be used with caution in patients receiving oral medications that require rapid gastrointestinal absorption. For oral medications that are dependent on threshold concentrations for efficacy, such as antibiotics, patients should be advised to take those drugs at least 1 hr before exenatide injection. If such drugs are to be administered with food, patients should be advised to take them with a meal or snack when exenatide is not administered).

No products indexed under this heading.

Doxycycline Calcium (The effect of exenatide to slow gastric emptying may reduce the extent and rate of absorption of orally administered drugs. Exenatide should be used with caution in patients receiving oral medications that require rapid gastrointestinal absorption. For oral medications that are dependent on threshold concentrations for efficacy, such as antibiotics, patients should be advised to take those drugs at least 1 hr before exenatide injection. If such drugs are to be administered with food, patients should be advised to take them with a meal or snack when exenatide is not administered).

No products indexed under this heading.

Doxycycline Hyclate (The effect of exenatide to slow gastric emptying may reduce the extent and rate of absorption of orally administered drugs. Exenatide should be used with caution in patients receiving oral medications that require rapid gastrointestinal absorption. For oral medications that are dependent on threshold concentrations for efficacy, such as antibiotics, patients should be advised to take those drugs at least 1 hr before exenatide injection. If such drugs are to be administered with food, patients should be advised to take them with a meal or snack when exenatide is not administered).

No products indexed under this heading.

Doxycycline Monohydrate (The effect of exenatide to slow gastric emptying may reduce the extent and rate of absorption of orally administered drugs. Exenatide should be used with caution in patients receiving oral medications that require rapid gastrointestinal absorption. For oral medications that are dependent on threshold concentrations for efficacy, such as antibiotics, patients should be advised to take those drugs at least 1 hr before exenatide injection. If such drugs are to be administered with food, patients should be advised to take them with a meal or snack when exenatide is not administered). Products include:

Oracea Capsules 1000

Enoxacin (The effect of exenatide to slow gastric emptying may reduce the extent and rate of absorption of orally administered drugs. Exenatide should be used with caution in patients receiving oral medications that require rapid gastrointestinal absorption. For oral medications that are dependent on threshold concentrations for efficacy, such as antibiotics, patients should be advised to take those drugs at least 1 hr before exenatide injection. If such drugs are to be administered with food, patients should be advised to take them with a meal or snack when exenatide is not administered).

No products indexed under this heading.

Erythromycin (The effect of exenatide to slow gastric emptying may reduce the extent and rate of absorption of orally administered drugs. Exenatide should be used with caution in patients receiving oral medications that require rapid gastrointestinal absorption. For oral medications that are dependent on threshold concentrations for efficacy, such as antibiotics, patients should be advised to take those drugs at least 1 hr before exenatide injection. If such drugs are to be administered with food, patients should be advised to take them with a meal or snack when exenatide is not administered). Products include:

Erythromycin Estolate (The effect of exenatide to slow gastric emptying may reduce the extent and rate of absorption of orally administered drugs. Exenatide should be used with caution in patients receiving oral medications that require rapid gastrointestinal absorption. For oral medications that are dependent on threshold concentrations for efficacy, such as antibiotics, patients should be advised to take those drugs at least 1 hr before exenatide injection. If such drugs are to be administered with food, patients should be advised to take them with a meal or snack when exenatide is not administered).

No products indexed under this heading.

Erythromycin Ethylsuccinate (The effect of exenatide to slow gastric emptying may reduce the extent and rate of absorption of orally administered drugs. Exenatide should be used with caution in patients receiving oral medications that require rapid gastrointestinal absorption. For oral medications that are dependent on threshold concentrations for efficacy, such as antibiotics, patients should be advised to take those drugs at least 1 hr before exenatide injection. If such drugs are to be administered with food, patients should be advised to take them with a meal or snack when exenatide is not administered). Products include:

Erythromycin Gluceptate (The effect of exenatide to slow gastric emptying may reduce the extent and rate of absorption of orally administered drugs. Exenatide should be used with caution in patients receiving oral medications that require rapid gastrointestinal absorption. For oral medications that are dependent on threshold concentrations for efficacy, such as antibiotics, patients should be advised to take those drugs at least 1 hr before exenatide injection. If such drugs are to be administered with food, patients should be advised to take them with a meal or snack when exenatide is not administered).

No products indexed under this heading.

Erythromycin Stearate (The effect of exenatide to slow gastric emptying may reduce the extent and rate of absorption of orally administered drugs. Exenatide should be used with caution in patients receiving oral medications that require rapid gastrointestinal absorption. For oral medications that are dependent on threshold concentrations for efficacy, such as antibiotics, patients should be advised to take those drugs at least 1 hr before exenatide injection. If such drugs are to be administered with food, patients should be advised to take them with a meal or snack when exenatide is not administered). Products include:

Ethinyl Estradiol (The effect of exenatide to slow gastric emptying may reduce the extent and rate of absorption of orally administered drugs. Exenatide should be used with caution in patients receiving oral medications that require rapid gastrointestinal absorption. For oral medications that are dependent on threshold concentrations for efficacy, such as contraceptives, patients should be advised to take those drugs at least 1 hr before exenatide injection. If such drugs are to be administered with food, patients should be advised to take them with a meal or snack when exenatide is not administered). Products include:

Ethynodiol Diacetate (The effect of exenatide to slow gastric emptying may reduce the extent and rate of absorption of orally administered drugs. Exenatide should be used with caution in patients receiving oral medications that require rapid gastrointestinal absorption. For oral medications that are dependent on threshold concentrations for efficacy, such as contraceptives, patients should be advised to take those drugs at least 1 hr before exenatide injection. If such drugs are to be administered with food, patients should be advised to take them with a meal or snack when exenatide is not administered).

No products indexed under this heading.

Grepafloxacin Hydrochloride (The effect of exenatide to slow gastric emptying may reduce the extent and rate of absorption of orally administered drugs. Exenatide should be used with caution in patients receiving oral medications that require rapid gastrointestinal absorption. For oral medications that are dependent on threshold concentrations for efficacy, such as antibiotics, patients should be advised to take those drugs at least 1 hr before exenatide injection. If such drugs are to be administered with food, patients should be advised to take them with a meal or snack when exenatide is not administered).

No products indexed under this heading.

Imipenem (The effect of exenatide to slow gastric emptying may reduce the extent and rate of absorption of orally administered drugs. Exenatide should be used with caution in patients receiving oral medications that require rapid gastrointestinal absorption. For oral medications that are dependent on threshold concentrations for efficacy, such as antibiotics, patients should be advised to take those drugs at least 1 hr before exenatide injection. If such drugs are to be administered with food, patients should be advised to take them with a meal or snack when exenatide is not administered). Products include:

Levonorgestrel (The effect of exenatide to slow gastric emptying may reduce the extent and rate of absorption of orally administered drugs. Exenatide should be used with caution in patients receiving oral medications that require rapid gastrointestinal absorption. For oral medications that are dependent on threshold concentrations for efficacy, such as contraceptives, patients should be advised to take those drugs at least 1 hr before exenatide injection. If such drugs are to be administered with food, patients should be advised to take them with a meal or snack when exenatide is not administered). Products include:

Lisinopril (Lisinopril steady-state Tmax was delayed 2 h). Products include:

Lomefloxacin Hydrochloride (The effect of exenatide to slow gastric emptying may reduce the extent and rate of absorption of orally administered drugs. Exenatide should be used with caution in patients receiving oral medications that require rapid gastrointestinal absorption. For oral medications that are dependent on threshold concentrations for efficacy, such as antibiotics, patients should be advised to take those drugs at least 1 hr before exenatide injection. If such drugs are to be administered with food, patients should be advised to take them with a meal or snack when exenatide is not administered).

No products indexed under this heading.

Loracarbef (The effect of exenatide to slow gastric emptying may reduce the extent and rate of absorption of orally administered drugs. Exenatide should be used with caution in patients receiving oral medications that require rapid gastrointestinal absorption. For oral medications that are dependent on threshold concentrations for efficacy, such as antibiotics, patients should be advised to take those drugs at least 1 hr before exenatide injection. If such drugs are to be administered with food, patients should be advised to take them with a meal or snack when exenatide is not administered).

No products indexed under this heading.

Lovastatin (Lovastatin AUC and Cmax were decreased approximately 40% and 28%, respectively, and Tmax was delayed about 4 h when exenatide was administered concomitantly with a single dose of lovastatin (40 mg) compared with lovastatin administered alone. In the 30-week controlled clinical trials of exenatide, the use of exenatide in patients already receiving HMG CoA reductase inhibitors was not associated with consisten changes in lipid profiles compared to baseline). Products include:

Mestranol (The effect of exenatide to slow gastric emptying may reduce the extent and rate of absorption of

orally administered drugs. Exenatide should be used with caution in patients receiving oral medications that require rapid gastrointestinal absorption. For oral medications that are dependent on threshold concentrations for efficacy, such as contraceptives, patients should be advised to take those drugs at least 1 hr before exenatide injection. If such drugs are to be administered with food, patients should be advised to take them with a meal or snack when exenatide is not administered).

No products indexed under this heading.

Methacycline Hydrochloride (The effect of exenatide to slow gastric emptying may reduce the extent and rate of absorption of orally administered drugs. Exenatide should be used with caution in patients receiving oral medications that require rapid gastrointestinal absorption. For oral medications that are dependent on threshold concentrations for efficacy, such as antibiotics, patients should be advised to take those drugs at least 1 hr before exenatide injection. If such drugs are to be administered with food, patients should be advised to take them with a meal or snack when exenatide is not administered).

No products indexed under this heading.

Mezlocillin Sodium (The effect of exenatide to slow gastric emptying may reduce the extent and rate of absorption of orally administered drugs. Exenatide should be used with caution in patients receiving oral medications that require rapid gastrointestinal absorption. For oral medications that are dependent on threshold concentrations for efficacy, such as antibiotics, patients should be advised to take those drugs at least 1 hr before exenatide injection. If such drugs are to be administered with food, patients should be advised to take them with a meal or snack when exenatide is not administered).

No products indexed under this heading.

Minocycline Hydrochloride (The effect of exenatide to slow gastric emptying may reduce the extent and rate of absorption of orally administered drugs. Exenatide should be used with caution in patients receiving oral medications that require rapid gastrointestinal absorption. For oral medications that are dependent on threshold concentrations for efficacy, such as antibiotics, patients should be advised to take those drugs at least 1 hr before exenatide injection. If such drugs are to be administered with food, patients should be advised to take them with a meal or snack when exenatide is not administered). Products include:

Moxifloxacin Hydrochloride (The effect of exenatide to slow gastric emptying may reduce the extent and rate of absorption of orally administered drugs. Exenatide should be used with caution in patients receiving oral medications that require rapid gastrointestinal absorption. For oral medications that are dependent on threshold concentrations for efficacy, such as antibiotics, patients should be advised to take those drugs at least 1 hr before exenatide injection. If such drugs are to be administered with food, patients should be advised to take them with a meal or snack when exenatide is not administered). Products include:

Avelox 2970
Vigamox Ophthalmic Solution 564

Nafcillin Sodium (The effect of exenatide to slow gastric emptying may reduce the extent and rate of absorption of orally administered drugs. Exenatide should be used with caution in patients receiving oral medications that require rapid gastrointestinal absorption. For oral medications that are dependent on threshold concentrations for efficacy, such as antibiotics, patients should be advised to take those drugs at least 1 hr before exenatide injection. If such drugs are to be administered with food, patients should be advised to take them with a meal or snack when exenatide is not administered).

No products indexed under this heading.

Norethindrone (The effect of exenatide to slow gastric emptying may reduce the extent and rate of absorption of orally administered drugs. Exenatide should be used with caution in patients receiving oral medications that require rapid gastrointestinal absorption. For oral medications that are dependent on threshold concentrations for efficacy, such as contraceptives, patients should be advised to take those drugs at least 1 hr before exenatide injection. If such drugs are to be administered with food, patients should be advised to take them with a meal or snack when exenatide is not administered). Products include:

Ortho Micronor Tablets 2426

Norethynodrel (The effect of exenatide to slow gastric emptying may reduce the extent and rate of absorption of orally administered drugs. Exenatide should be used with caution in patients receiving oral medications that require rapid gastrointestinal absorption. For oral medications that are dependent on threshold concentrations for efficacy, such as contraceptives, patients should be advised to take those drugs at least 1 hr before exenatide injection. If such drugs are to be administered with food, patients should be advised to take them with a meal or snack when exenatide is not administered).

No products indexed under this heading.

Norfloxacin (The effect of exenatide to slow gastric emptying may reduce the extent and rate of absorption of orally administered drugs. Exenatide should be used with caution in patients receiving oral medications that require rapid gastrointestinal absorption. For oral medications that are dependent on threshold concentrations for efficacy, such as antibiotics, patients should be advised to take those drugs at least 1 hr before exenatide injection. If such drugs are to be administered with food, patients should be advised to take them with a meal or snack when exenatide is not administered). Products include:

Noroxin Tablets 2032

Norgestimate (The effect of exenatide to slow gastric emptying may reduce the extent and rate of absorption of orally administered drugs. Exenatide should be used with caution in patients receiving oral medications that require rapid gastrointestinal absorption. For oral medications that are dependent on threshold concentrations for efficacy, such as contraceptives, patients should be advised to take those drugs at least 1 hr before exenatide injection. If such drugs are to be administered with food, patients should be advised to take them with a meal or snack when exenatide is not administered). Products include:

Ortho-Cyclen/Ortho Tri-Cyclen 2429
Ortho Tri-Cyclen Lo Tablets 2436

Norgestrel (The effect of exenatide to slow gastric emptying may reduce the extent and rate of absorption of orally administered drugs. Exenatide should be used with caution in patients receiving oral medications that require rapid gastrointestinal absorption. For oral medications that are dependent on threshold concentrations for efficacy, such as contraceptives, patients should be advised to take those drugs at least 1 hr before exenatide injection. If such drugs are to be administered with food, patients should be advised to take them with a meal or snack when exenatide is not administered).

No products indexed under this heading.

Ofloxacin (The effect of exenatide to slow gastric emptying may reduce the extent and rate of absorption of orally administered drugs. Exenatide should be used with caution in patients receiving oral medications that require rapid gastrointestinal absorption. For oral medications that are dependent on threshold concentrations for efficacy, such as antibiotics, patients should be advised to take those drugs at least 1 hr before exenatide injection. If such drugs are to be administered with food, patients should be advised to take them with a meal or snack when exenatide is not administered). Products include:

Floxin Otic Solution 1049

Oral Medications, unspecified (The effect of exenatide to slow gastric emptying may reduce the extent and rate of absorption of orally administered drugs. Exenatide should be used with caution in patients receiving oral medications that require rapid gastrointestinal absorption).

No products indexed under this heading.

Oxytetracycline Hydrochloride (The effect of exenatide to slow gastric emptying may reduce the extent and rate of absorption of orally administered drugs. Exenatide should be used with caution in patients receiving oral medications that require rapid gastrointestinal absorption. For oral medications that are dependent on threshold concentrations for efficacy, such as antibiotics, patients should be advised to take those drugs at least 1 hr before exenatide injection. If such drugs are to be administered with food, patients should be advised to take them with a meal or snack when exenatide is not administered).

No products indexed under this heading.

Penicillin G Benzathine (The effect of exenatide to slow gastric emptying may reduce the extent and rate of absorption of orally administered drugs. Exenatide should be used with caution in patients receiving oral medications that require rapid gastrointestinal absorption. For oral medications that are dependent on threshold concentrations for efficacy, such as antibiotics, patients should be advised to take those drugs at least 1 hr before exenatide injection. If such drugs are to be administered with food, patients should be advised to take them with a meal or snack when exenatide is not administered). Products include:

Bicillin C-R Injectable Suspension 1706

Penicillin G Potassium (The effect of exenatide to slow gastric emptying may reduce the extent and rate of absorption of orally administered drugs. Exenatide should be used with caution in patients receiving oral medications that require rapid gastrointestinal absorption. For oral medications that are dependent on threshold concentrations for efficacy, such as antibiotics, patients should be advised to take those drugs at least 1 hr before exenatide injection. If such drugs are to be administered with food, patients should be advised to take them with a meal or snack when exenatide is not administered).

No products indexed under this heading.

Penicillin G Procaine (The effect of exenatide to slow gastric emptying may reduce the extent and rate of absorption of orally administered drugs. Exenatide should be used with caution in patients receiving oral medications that require rapid gastrointestinal absorption. For oral medications that are dependent on threshold concentrations for efficacy, such as antibiotics, patients should be advised to take those drugs at least 1 hr before exenatide injection. If such drugs are to be administered with food, patients should be advised to take them with a meal or snack when exenatide is not administered). Products include:

Bicillin C-R Injectable Suspension 1706

Penicillin G Sodium (The effect of exenatide to slow gastric emptying may reduce the extent and rate of absorption of orally administered drugs. Exenatide should be used with caution in patients receiving oral medications that require rapid gastrointestinal absorption. For oral medications that are dependent on threshold concentrations for efficacy, such as antibiotics, patients should be advised to take those drugs at least 1 hr before exenatide injection. If such drugs are to be administered with food, patients should be advised to take them with a meal or snack when exenatide is not administered).

No products indexed under this heading.

Penicillin V Potassium (The effect of exenatide to slow gastric emptying may reduce the extent and rate of absorption of orally administered drugs. Exenatide should be used with caution in patients receiving oral medications that require rapid gastrointestinal absorption. For oral medications that are dependent on threshold concentrations for efficacy, such as antibiotics, patients should be advised to take those drugs at least 1 hr before exenatide injection. If such drugs are to be administered with food, patients should be advised to take them with a meal or snack when exenatide is not administered).

No products indexed under this heading.

Sulfamethizole (The effect of exenatide to slow gastric emptying may reduce the extent and rate of absorption of orally administered drugs. Exenatide should be used with caution in patients receiving oral medications that require rapid gastrointestinal absorption. For oral medications that are dependent on threshold concentrations for efficacy, such as antibiotics, patients should be advised to take those drugs at least 1 hr before exenatide injection. If such drugs are to be administered with food, patients should be advised to take them with a meal or snack when exenatide is not administered).

No products indexed under this heading.

Sulfamethoxazole (The effect of exenatide to slow gastric emptying may reduce the extent and rate of absorption of orally administered drugs. Exenatide should be used with caution in patients receiving oral medications that require rapid gastrointestinal absorption. For oral medications that are dependent on threshold concentrations for efficacy, such as antibiotics, patients should be advised to take those drugs at least 1 hr before exenatide injection. If such drugs are to be administered with food, patients should be advised to take them with a meal or snack when exenatide is not administered).

No products indexed under this heading.

Sulfisoxazole Acetyl (The effect of exenatide to slow gastric emptying may reduce the extent and rate of absorption of orally administered drugs. Exenatide should be used with caution in patients receiving oral medications that require rapid gastrointestinal absorption. For oral medications that are dependent on threshold concentrations for efficacy, such as antibiotics, patients should be advised to take those drugs at least 1 hr before exenatide injection. If such drugs are to be administered with food, patients should be advised to take them with a meal or snack when exenatide is not administered).

No products indexed under this heading.

Tetracycline Hydrochloride (The effect of exenatide to slow gastric emptying may reduce the extent and rate of absorption of orally administered drugs. Exenatide should be used with caution in patients receiving oral medications that require rapid gastrointestinal absorption. For oral medications that are dependent on threshold concentrations for efficacy, such as antibiotics, patients should be advised to take those drugs at least 1 hr before exenatide injection. If such drugs are to be administered with food, patients should be advised to take them with a meal or snack when exenatide is

not administered).
No products indexed under this heading.

Ticarcillin Disodium (The effect of exenatide to slow gastric emptying may reduce the extent and rate of absorption of orally administered drugs. Exenatide should be used with caution in patients receiving oral medications that require rapid gastrointestinal absorption. For oral medications that are dependent on threshold concentrations for efficacy, such as antibiotics, patients should be advised to take those drugs at least 1 hr before exenatide injection. If such drugs are to be administered with food, patients should be advised to take them with a meal or snack when exenatide is not administered). Products include:
Timentin ADD-Vantage **1580**
Timentin Injection Galaxy Container **1583**
Timentin IV Infusion **1577**
Timentin Pharmacy Bulk Package **1586**

Troleandomycin (The effect of exenatide to slow gastric emptying may reduce the extent and rate of absorption of orally administered drugs. Exenatide should be used with caution in patients receiving oral medications that require rapid gastrointestinal absorption. For oral medications that are dependent on threshold concentrations for efficacy, such as antibiotics, patients should be advised to take those drugs at least 1 hr before exenatide injection. If such drugs are to be administered with food, patients should be advised to take them with a meal or snack when exenatide is not administered).
No products indexed under this heading.

Trovafloxacin Mesylate (The effect of exenatide to slow gastric emptying may reduce the extent and rate of absorption of orally administered drugs. Exenatide should be used with caution in patients receiving oral medications that require rapid gastrointestinal absorption. For oral medications that are dependent on threshold concentrations for efficacy, such as antibiotics, patients should be advised to take those drugs at least 1 hr before exenatide injection. If such drugs are to be administered with food, patients should be advised to take them with a meal or snack when exenatide is not administered).
No products indexed under this heading.

CADUET TABLETS

(Amlodipine Besylate, Atorvastatin Calcium).. **2508**
May interact with azole antifungals, erythromycin, fibrates, and certain other agents. Compounds in these categories include:

Aluminum Hydroxide (Co-administration with aluminum hydroxide/magnesium hydroxide antacid has resulted in decreased atorvastatin plasma concentrations by 35%; LDL-C reduction was unaltered). Products include:
Gaviscon Regular Strength Liquid .. **658**
Gaviscon Regular Strength Tablets.. **658**
Gaviscon Extra Strength Liquid **658**
Gaviscon Extra Strength Tablets **658**
Maalox Regular Strength Antacid/Antigas Liquid................. **2175**
Maalox Max Maximum Strength Antacid/Anti-Gas Liquid................. **2176**

Clofibrate (Co-administration with fibric acid derivatives increases the risk of myopathy).
No products indexed under this heading.

Clotrimazole (Co-administration with azole antifungals increases the risk of myopathy). Products include:
Desenex Athlete's Foot Cream **635**
Lotrimin **3039**
Lotrisone **3040**

Colestipol Hydrochloride (Co-administration has resulted in decreased atorvastatin plasma concentrations by 25%, however; LDL-C reduction was greater when these drugs were given together than when either drug was given alone).
No products indexed under this heading.

Cyclosporine (Co-administration increases the risk of myopathy). Products include:
Gengraf Capsules **459**
Neoral Oral Solution **2259**
Neoral Soft Gelatin Capsules **2259**
Restasis Ophthalmic Emulsion **575**
Sandimmune **2275**

Digoxin (Co-administration has resulted in increased steady-state digoxin plasma concentrations by 20%). Products include:
Lanoxicaps Capsules **1490**
Lanoxin Injection **1494**
Lanoxin Injection Pediatric **1497**
Lanoxin Tablets **1500**

Erythromycin (Co-administration increases the risk of myopathy; plasma concentrations of atorvastatin has increased by 40% when co-administered with erythromycin, a known inhibitor of cytochrome P4503A4). Products include:
Ery-Tab Tablets **449**
Erythromycin Base Filmtab Tablets **455**
Erythromycin Delayed-Release Capsules, USP................................. **457**
PCE Dispertab Tablets **515**

Erythromycin Estolate (Co-administration increases the risk of myopathy; plasma concentrations of atorvastatin has increased by 40% when co-administered with erythromycin, a known inhibitor of cytochrome P4503A4).
No products indexed under this heading.

Erythromycin Ethylsuccinate (Co-administration increases the risk of myopathy; plasma concentrations of atorvastatin has increased by 40% when co-administered with erythromycin, a known inhibitor of cytochrome P4503A4). Products include:
E.E.S. **451**
EryPed **447**

Erythromycin Gluceptate (Co-administration increases the risk of myopathy; plasma concentrations of atorvastatin has increased by 40% when co-administered with erythromycin, a known inhibitor of cytochrome P4503A4).
No products indexed under this heading.

Erythromycin Lactobionate (Co-administration increases the risk of myopathy; plasma concentrations of atorvastatin has increased by 40% when co-administered with erythromycin, a known inhibitor of cytochrome P4503A4).
No products indexed under this heading.

Erythromycin Stearate (Co-administration increases the risk of myopathy; plasma concentrations of atorvastatin has increased by 40% when co-administered with erythromycin, a known inhibitor of cytochrome P4503A4). Products include:
Erythrocin Stearate Filmtab Tablets **453**

Ethinyl Estradiol (Co-administration with an oral contraceptive has increased AUC values for norethindrone and ethinyl estradiol by 30% and 20%, respectively). Products include:
Mircette Tablets **1066**
NuvaRing **2340**
Ortho-Cyclen/Ortho Tri-Cyclen **2429**
Ortho Evra Transdermal System **2417**
Ortho Tri-Cyclen Lo Tablets **2436**
Seasonique Tablets **1077**
Yasmin 28 Tablets **796**
Yaz Tablets **803**

Fenofibrate (Co-administration with fibric acid derivatives increases the risk of myopathy). Products include:
Lofibra Tablets **1219**
Lofibra Capsules **1216**
Tricor Tablets **527**
Triglide Tablets **3123**

Fluconazole (Co-administration with azole antifungals increases the risk of myopathy).
No products indexed under this heading.

Gemfibrozil (Co-administration with fibric acid derivatives increases the risk of myopathy).
No products indexed under this heading.

Itraconazole (Co-administration with azole antifungals increases the risk of myopathy).
No products indexed under this heading.

Ketoconazole (Co-administration with azole antifungals increases the risk of myopathy). Products include:
Nizoral A-D Shampoo, 1% **1868**

Miconazole (Co-administration with azole antifungals increases the risk of myopathy).
No products indexed under this heading.

Niacin (Co-administration increases the risk of myopathy). Products include:
Advicor Tablets **1722**
Niaspan Extended-Release Tablets **1730**

Norethindrone (Co-administration with an oral contraceptive has increased AUC values for norethindrone and ethinyl estradiol by 30% and 20%; respectively). Products include:
Ortho Micronor Tablets **2426**

Oxiconazole Nitrate (Co-administration with azole antifungals increases the risk of myopathy). Products include:
Oxistat **2667**

Terconazole (Co-administration with azole antifungals increases the risk of myopathy).
No products indexed under this heading.

CAFCIT INJECTION

(Caffeine Citrate) **1886**
May interact with cytochrome p450 1a2 inducers (selected), cytochrome p450 1a2 inhibitors (selected), cytochrome p450 1a2 substrates (selected), phenytoin, xanthines, and certain other agents. Compounds in these categories include:

Acetaminophen (Caffeine has the potential to interact with drugs that are substrates for CYP1A2). Products include:
Comtrex Maximum Strength Cold & Cough Day/Night Caplets - Day Formulation......................... **726**
Comtrex Maximum Strength Cold & Cough Day/Night Caplets - Night Formulation **726**
Comtrex Maximum Strength Non-Drowsy Cold & Cough Caplets.. **725**
Comtrex Maximum Strength Day/Night Severe Cold & Sinus Caplets - Day Formulation **725**
Comtrex Maximum Strength Day/Night Severe Cold & Sinus Caplets - Night Formulation **725**
Contac Cold and Flu Maximum Strength Caplets......................... **728**
Contac Cold and Flu Day and Night Caplets (Day Formulation Only)... **727**
Contac Cold and Flu Day and Night Caplets (Night Formulation Only)......................... **727**
Contac Cold and Flu Non-Drowsy Caplets.. **728**
Excedrin Extra Strength Caplets/Tablets/Geltabs **684**
Excedrin Migraine Caplets/Tablets/Geltabs **609**
Excedrin PM Caplets/Tablets/Geltabs **610**
Excedrin Sinus Headache Caplets/Tablets **610**
Excedrin Tension Headache Caplets/Tablets/Geltabs **611**
Goody's Body Pain Formula Powder... **684**
Goody's Extra Strength Headache Powders..................... **611**
Goody's Extra Strength Pain Relief Tablets **685**
Goody's PM Powder for Pain with Sleeplessness **612**
Percocet Tablets **1131**
Robitussin Cough, Cold & Flu Nighttime Liquid............................. **738**
TheraFlu Cold & Sore Throat Hot Liquid **741**
TheraFlu Flu & Chest Congestion Hot Liquid **741**
TheraFlu Flu & Sore Throat Hot Liquid **742**
TheraFlu Daytime Severe Cold Hot Liquid...................................... **742**
TheraFlu Nighttime Severe Cold Hot Liquid...................................... **740**
TheraFlu Warming Relief Daytime Severe Cold...................................... **743**
TheraFlu Warming Relief Nighttime Severe Cold................ **743**
Triaminic Cough & Sore Throat Liquid **747**
Regular Strength Tylenol Tablets **1870**
Children's Tylenol with Flavor Creator.. **679**
Children's Tylenol Plus Flu Oral Suspension...................................... **749**
Tylenol Cold Head Congestion Daytime Caplets with Cool Burst and Gelcaps **750**
Tylenol Cold Multi-Symptom Daytime Liquid................................ **752**
Tylenol Cold Multi-Symptom Severe Daytime Liquid **752**
Tylenol 8 Hour Extended Release Caplets.. **1870**
Tylenol **1870**
Extra Strength Tylenol PM Caplets, Vanilla Caplets, Geltabs, Gelcaps and Liquid.......... **1875**
Extra Strength Tylenol Rapid Release Gels **1870**

IMPORTANT NOTE: Always consult each drug listing in the patient's regimen for possible interactions.

Concentrated Tylenol Infants' Drops Plus Cold & Cough .... ▣754
Tylenol with Codeine Tablets 2391
Tylenol Allergy Multi-Symptom Caplets with Cool Burst and Gelcaps 1872
Tylenol Allergy Multi-Symptom Nighttime Caplets with Cool Burst 1872
Tylenol Severe Allergy Caplets 1872
Tylenol Arthritis Pain Extended Release Caplets and Geltabs 1870
Tylenol Chest Congestion Caplets with Cool Burst 1872
Tylenol Chest Congestion Liquid with Cool Burst 1872
Children's Tylenol Suspension Liquid and Meltaways 1878
Children's Tylenol Plus Cold Suspension Liquid 1879
Children's Tylenol Plus Cold & Allergy Suspension Liquid 1878
Children's Tylenol Plus Cough & Runny Nose Suspension Liquid 1879
Children's Tylenol Plus Cough & Sore Throat Suspension Liquid 1879
Children's Tylenol Suspension with Flavor Creator 1878
Children's Tylenol Plus Flu Suspension Liquid 1881
Children's Tylenol Plus Multi-Symptom Cold Suspension Liquid 1879
Tylenol Cold Severe Congestion Non-Drowsy Caplets with Cool Burst 1874
Tylenol Cold Head Congestion Daytime Caplets with Cool Burst 1873
Tylenol Cold Head Congestion Nighttime Caplets with Cool Burst 1873
Tylenol Cold Head Congestion Severe Caplets with Cool Burst 1873
Tylenol Cold Multi-Symptom Daytime Caplets with Cool Burst and Gelcaps 1874
Tylenol Cold Multi-Symptom Daytime Liquid with Citrus Burst 1874
Tylenol Cold Multi-Symptom Nighttime Caplets with Cool Burst 1874
Tylenol Cold Multi-Symptom Nighttime Liquid with Cool Burst 1874
Tylenol Cold Multi-Symptom Severe Caplets with Cool Burst 1874
Tylenol Cold Multi-Symptom Severe Daytime Liquid with Citrus Burst 1874
Tylenol Cough & Sore Throat Daytime Liquid with Cool Burst 1877
Tylenol Cough & Sore Throat Nighttime Liquid with Cool Burst 1877
Concentrated Tylenol Infants' Drops 1878
Concentrated Tylenol Infants' Drops Plus Cold 1879
Concentrated Tylenol Infants' Drops Plus Cold and Cough 1879
Jr. Tylenol Meltaways 1878
Tylenol Sinus Severe Congestion Caplets with Cool Burst 1876
Tylenol Sinus Congestion & Pain Daytime Caplets with Cool Burst and Gelcaps 1876
Tylenol Sinus Congestion & Pain Nighttime Caplets with Cool Burst 1876
Tylenol Sinus Congestion & Pain Severe Caplets with Cool Burst 1876
Tylenol Sore Throat Daytime Liquid with Cool Burst 1877
Tylenol Sore Throat Nighttime Liquid with Cool Burst 1877
Women's Tylenol Menstrual Relief Caplets 1877
Vicks 44M Cough, Cold & Flu Relief Liquid 2680
Vicks DayQuil LiquiCaps/Liquid Multi-Symptom Cold/Flu Relief .... ▣761
Vicks DayQuil Multi-Symptom Cold/Flu Relief LiquiCaps 2678
Vicks DayQuil Multi-Symptom Cold/Flu Relief Liquid 2678
Vicks NyQuil Multi-Symptom Cold/Flu Relief Liquid 2681
Vicks NyQuil Multi-Symptom Cold/Flu Relief LiquiCaps 2681
Vicks NyQuil LiquiCaps/Liquid Multi-Symptom Cold/Flu Relief .... ▣763
Vicodin Tablets 535
Vicodin ES Tablets 536
Vicodin HP Tablets 538
Zicam Maximum Strength Flu Daytime .... ▣768
Zicam Maximum Strength Flu Nighttime .... ▣768
Zydone Tablets 1139

Alatrofloxacin Mesylate (Caffeine has the potential to interact with drugs that inhibit CYP1A2).
No products indexed under this heading.

Aminophylline (Interconversion between caffeine and theophylline has been reported in preterm neonates; the concurrent use of these drugs is not recommended).
No products indexed under this heading.

Amiodarone Hydrochloride (Caffeine has the potential to interact with drugs that inhibit CYP1A2).
No products indexed under this heading.

Amitriptyline Hydrochloride (Caffeine has the potential to interact with drugs that are substrates for CYP1A2).
No products indexed under this heading.

Amoxapine (Caffeine has the potential to interact with drugs that are substrates for CYP1A2).
No products indexed under this heading.

Anagrelide Hydrochloride (Caffeine has the potential to interact with drugs that are substrates for CYP1A2). Products include:
Agrylin Capsules 3169

Anastrozole (Caffeine has the potential to interact with drugs that inhibit CYP1A2). Products include:
Arimidex Tablets 673

Caffeine (Caffeine has the potential to interact with drugs that are substrates for CYP1A2). Products include:
BC Headache Powder .... ▣677
Arthritis Strength BC Powder .... ▣677
Excedrin Extra Strength Caplets/Tablets/Geltabs .... ▣684
Excedrin Migraine Caplets/Tablets/Geltabs .... ▣609
Excedrin Tension Headache Caplets/Tablets/Geltabs .... ▣611
Goody's Extra Strength Headache Powders .... ▣611
Goody's Extra Strength Pain Relief Tablets .... ▣685
Vivarin .... ▣602
Winrgy Dietary Supplement .... ▣823

Caffeine Anhydrous (Caffeine has the potential to interact with drugs that are substrates for CYP1A2).
No products indexed under this heading.

Carbamazepine (Caffeine has the potential to interact with drugs that induce CYP1A2). Products include:
Carbatrol Capsules 3171
Equetro Extended-Release Capsules 3180
Tegretol/Tegretol-XR 2295

Chlordiazepoxide (Caffeine has the potential to interact with drugs that are substrates for CYP1A2).
No products indexed under this heading.

Chlordiazepoxide Hydrochloride (Caffeine has the potential to interact with drugs that are substrates for CYP1A2). Products include:
Librium Capsules 3347

Cimetidine (Co-administration of caffeine with cimetidine may result in reduced caffeine elimination; lower doses of caffeine may be needed). Products include:
Tagamet HB 200 Tablets .... ▣664

Cimetidine Hydrochloride (Co-administration of caffeine with cimetidine may result in reduced caffeine elimination; lower doses of caffeine may be needed).
No products indexed under this heading.

Ciprofloxacin (Caffeine has the potential to interact with drugs that inhibit CYP1A2). Products include:
Cipro Oral Suspension 2977
Cipro I.V. 2984
Cipro XR Tablets 2990
Ciprodex Otic Suspension 559

Ciprofloxacin Hydrochloride (Caffeine has the potential to interact with drugs that inhibit CYP1A2). Products include:
Ciloxan Ophthalmic Ointment 559
Ciloxan Ophthalmic Solution .... ⊙206
Cipro Tablets 2977
Proquin XR Tablets 1153

Citalopram Hydrobromide (Caffeine has the potential to interact with drugs that induce CYP1A2). Products include:
Celexa 1176

Clarithromycin (Caffeine has the potential to interact with drugs that inhibit CYP1A2). Products include:
Biaxin/Biaxin XL 402
PREVPAC 3284

Clomipramine Hydrochloride (Caffeine has the potential to interact with drugs that are substrates for CYP1A2).
No products indexed under this heading.

Clopidogrel Bisulfate (Caffeine has the potential to interact with drugs that are substrates for CYP1A2). Products include:
Plavix Tablets 917
Plavix Tablets 2926

Clozapine (Caffeine has the potential to interact with drugs that are substrates for CYP1A2). Products include:
Clozaril Tablets 2184
FazaClo Orally Disintegrating Tablets 551

Cyclobenzaprine (Caffeine has the potential to interact with drugs that are substrates for CYP1A2).
No products indexed under this heading.

Cyclobenzaprine Hydrochloride (Caffeine has the potential to interact with drugs that are substrates for CYP1A2).
No products indexed under this heading.

Desipramine Hydrochloride (Caffeine has the potential to interact with drugs that are substrates for CYP1A2).
No products indexed under this heading.

Desogestrel (Caffeine has the potential to interact with drugs that inhibit CYP1A2). Products include:
Mircette Tablets 1066

Diazepam (Caffeine has the potential to interact with drugs that are substrates for CYP1A2). Products include:
Diastat Rectal Delivery System 3343
Valium Tablets 2819

Diltiazem Hydrochloride (Caffeine has the potential to interact with drugs that induce CYP1A2). Products include:
Cardizem LA Extended Release Tablets 1728
Tiazac Capsules 1201

Diltiazem Maleate (Caffeine has the potential to interact with drugs that induce CYP1A2).
No products indexed under this heading.

Doxepin Hydrochloride (Caffeine has the potential to interact with drugs that are substrates for CYP1A2).
No products indexed under this heading.

Dyphylline (Interconversion between caffeine and theophylline has been reported in preterm neonates; the concurrent use of these drugs is not recommended).
No products indexed under this heading.

Enoxacin (Caffeine has the potential to interact with drugs that inhibit CYP1A2).
No products indexed under this heading.

Erythromycin (Caffeine has the potential to interact with drugs that induce CYP1A2). Products include:
Ery-Tab Tablets 449
Erythromycin Base Filmtab Tablets 455
Erythromycin Delayed-Release Capsules, USP 457
PCE Dispertab Tablets 515

Erythromycin Estolate (Caffeine has the potential to interact with drugs that induce CYP1A2).
No products indexed under this heading.

Erythromycin Ethylsuccinate (Caffeine has the potential to interact with drugs that induce CYP1A2). Products include:
E.E.S. 451
EryPed 447

Erythromycin Gluceptate (Caffeine has the potential to interact with drugs that induce CYP1A2).
No products indexed under this heading.

Erythromycin Lactobionate (Caffeine has the potential to interact with drugs that induce CYP1A2).
No products indexed under this heading.

Erythromycin Stearate (Caffeine has the potential to interact with drugs that induce CYP1A2). Products include:
Erythrocin Stearate Filmtab Tablets 453

Estradiol (Caffeine has the potential to interact with drugs that are substrates for CYP1A2). Products include:
Angeliq Tablets 762
Climara Transdermal System 771
Climara Pro Transdermal System 776
Estrasorb Topical Emulsion 1147
Estring Vaginal Ring 2635
Menostar Transdermal System 782
Vagifem Tablets 2334

Estradiol Benzoate (Caffeine has the potential to interact with drugs that are substrates for CYP1A2).
No products indexed under this heading.

Estradiol Cypionate (Caffeine has the potential to interact with drugs that are substrates for CYP1A2).
No products indexed under this heading.

Ethinyl Estradiol (Caffeine has the potential to interact with drugs that inhibit CYP1A2). Products include:
Mircette Tablets ... 1066
NuvaRing ... 2340
Ortho-Cyclen/Ortho Tri-Cyclen ... 2429
Ortho Evra Transdermal System ... 2417
Ortho Tri-Cyclen Lo Tablets ... 2436
Seasonique Tablets ... 1077
Yasmin 28 Tablets ... 796
Yaz Tablets ... 803

Flutamide (Caffeine has the potential to interact with drugs that are substrates for CYP1A2). Products include:
Eulexin Capsules ... 3009

Fluticasone Propionate (Caffeine has the potential to interact with drugs that are substrates for CYP1A2). Products include:
Advair Diskus 100/50 ... 1308
Advair Diskus 250/50 ... 1308
Advair Diskus 500/50 ... 1308
Advair HFA Inhalation Aerosol ... 1318
Cutivate Cream ... 2662
Cutivate Lotion 0.05% ... 2664
Cutivate Ointment ... 2665
Flonase Nasal Spray ... 1440
Flovent Diskus ... 1443

Fluvoxamine (Caffeine has the potential to interact with drugs that inhibit CYP1A2).
No products indexed under this heading.

Fluvoxamine Maleate (Caffeine has the potential to interact with drugs that induce CYP1A2).
No products indexed under this heading.

Fosphenytoin Sodium (Co-administration of caffeine with phenytoin may result in increased caffeine elimination; higher doses of caffeine may be needed).
No products indexed under this heading.

Gatifloxacin (Caffeine has the potential to interact with drugs that inhibit CYP1A2). Products include:
Tequin Injection ... 938
Tequin Injection in 5% Dextrose ... 938
Tequin Tablets ... 938
Zymar Ophthalmic Solution ... 575

Gemifloxacin Mesylate (Caffeine has the potential to interact with drugs that inhibit CYP1A2).
No products indexed under this heading.

Grepafloxacin Hydrochloride (Caffeine has the potential to interact with drugs that inhibit CYP1A2).
No products indexed under this heading.

Haloperidol (Caffeine has the potential to interact with drugs that are substrates for CYP1A2).
No products indexed under this heading.

Haloperidol Decanoate (Caffeine has the potential to interact with drugs that are substrates for CYP1A2).
No products indexed under this heading.

Haloperidol Lactate (Caffeine has the potential to interact with drugs that are substrates for CYP1A2).
No products indexed under this heading.

Hypericum (Caffeine has the potential to interact with drugs that induce CYP1A2). Products include:
Satiete Tablets ... ▣832

Imipramine Hydrochloride (Caffeine has the potential to interact with drugs that are substrates for CYP1A2).
No products indexed under this heading.

Imipramine Pamoate (Caffeine has the potential to interact with drugs that are substrates for CYP1A2).
No products indexed under this heading.

Insulin (Caffeine has the potential to interact with drugs that induce CYP1A2).
No products indexed under this heading.

Isoniazid (Caffeine has the potential to interact with drugs that inhibit CYP1A2).
No products indexed under this heading.

Ketoconazole (Co-administration of caffeine with ketoconazole may result in reduced caffeine elimination; lower doses of caffeine may be needed). Products include:
Nizoral A-D Shampoo, 1% ... 1868

Ketoprofen (Co-administration results in reduced urine volume in healthy volunteers).
No products indexed under this heading.

Lansoprazole (Caffeine has the potential to interact with drugs that induce CYP1A2). Products include:
Prevacid Delayed-Release Capsules ... 3271
Prevacid for Delayed-Release Oral Suspension ... 3271
Prevacid SoluTab Delayed-Release Orally Disintegrating Tablets ... 3271
Prevacid I.V. for Injection ... 3277
Prevacid NapraPAC ... 3280
PREVPAC ... 3284

Levobupivacaine Hydrochloride (Caffeine has the potential to interact with drugs that are substrates for CYP1A2).
No products indexed under this heading.

Levofloxacin (Caffeine has the potential to interact with drugs that inhibit CYP1A2). Products include:
Levaquin ... 2384
Levaquin in 5% Dextrose Injection ... 2384
Quixin Ophthalmic Solution ... 3383

Levonorgestrel (Caffeine has the potential to interact with drugs that inhibit CYP1A2). Products include:
Climara Pro Transdermal System ... 776
Mirena Intrauterine System ... 787
Plan B Tablets ... 1076
Seasonique Tablets ... 1077

Lomefloxacin Hydrochloride (Caffeine has the potential to interact with drugs that inhibit CYP1A2).
No products indexed under this heading.

Maprotiline Hydrochloride (Caffeine has the potential to interact with drugs that are substrates for CYP1A2).
No products indexed under this heading.

Mestranol (Caffeine has the potential to interact with drugs that inhibit CYP1A2).
No products indexed under this heading.

Methadone Hydrochloride (Caffeine has the potential to interact with drugs that are substrates for CYP1A2).
No products indexed under this heading.

Methoxsalen (Caffeine has the potential to interact with drugs that inhibit CYP1A2). Products include:
Oxsoralen Lotion 1% ... 3352
Oxsoralen-Ultra Capsules ... 3353

Mexiletine Hydrochloride (Caffeine has the potential to interact with drugs that inhibit CYP1A2).
No products indexed under this heading.

Mibefradil Dihydrochloride (Caffeine has the potential to interact with drugs that inhibit CYP1A2).
No products indexed under this heading.

Mirtazapine (Caffeine has the potential to interact with drugs that are substrates for CYP1A2).
No products indexed under this heading.

Moxifloxacin Hydrochloride (Caffeine has the potential to interact with drugs that inhibit CYP1A2). Products include:
Avelox ... 2970
Vigamox Ophthalmic Solution ... 564

Nafcillin Sodium (Caffeine has the potential to interact with drugs that induce CYP1A2).
No products indexed under this heading.

Nalidixic Acid (Caffeine has the potential to interact with drugs that inhibit CYP1A2).
No products indexed under this heading.

Naproxen (Caffeine has the potential to interact with drugs that are substrates for CYP1A2). Products include:
EC-Naprosyn Delayed-Release Tablets ... 2761
Naprosyn Suspension ... 2761
Naprosyn Tablets ... 2761
Prevacid NapraPAC ... 3280

Naproxen Sodium (Caffeine has the potential to interact with drugs that are substrates for CYP1A2). Products include:
Aleve Caplets ... 742
Aleve Gelcaps ... 743
Aleve Tablets ... 743
Aleve Cold & Sinus Caplets ... 744
Anaprox Tablets ... 2761
Anaprox DS Tablets ... 2761

Nicotine (Caffeine has the potential to interact with drugs that induce CYP1A2). Products include:
NicoDerm CQ Clear Patch ... ▣622

Nicotine Polacrilex (Caffeine has the potential to interact with drugs that induce CYP1A2).
No products indexed under this heading.

Nicotine Salicylate (Caffeine has the potential to interact with drugs that induce CYP1A2).
No products indexed under this heading.

Nicotine Sulfate (Caffeine has the potential to interact with drugs that induce CYP1A2).
No products indexed under this heading.

Norethindrone (Caffeine has the potential to interact with drugs that inhibit CYP1A2). Products include:
Ortho Micronor Tablets ... 2426

Norethindrone Acetate (Caffeine has the potential to interact with drugs that are substrates for CYP1A2).
No products indexed under this heading.

Norfloxacin (Caffeine has the potential to interact with drugs that inhibit CYP1A2). Products include:
Noroxin Tablets ... 2032

Norgestrel (Caffeine has the potential to interact with drugs that inhibit CYP1A2).
No products indexed under this heading.

Nortriptyline Hydrochloride (Caffeine has the potential to interact with drugs that are substrates for CYP1A2).
No products indexed under this heading.

Ofloxacin (Caffeine has the potential to interact with drugs that inhibit CYP1A2). Products include:
Floxin Otic Solution ... 1049

Olanzapine (Caffeine has the potential to interact with drugs that are substrates for CYP1A2). Products include:
Symbyax Capsules ... 1819
Zyprexa Tablets ... 1830
Zyprexa IntraMuscular ... 1830
Zyprexa ZYDIS Orally Disintegrating Tablets ... 1830

Omeprazole (Caffeine has the potential to interact with drugs that induce CYP1A2). Products include:
Zegerid Capsules ... 2958
Zegerid Powder for Oral Solution ... 2958

Ondansetron (Caffeine has the potential to interact with drugs that are substrates for CYP1A2). Products include:
Zofran ODT Orally Disintegrating Tablets ... 1639

Ondansetron Hydrochloride (Caffeine has the potential to interact with drugs that are substrates for CYP1A2). Products include:
Zofran Injection ... 1634
Zofran ... 1639

Paroxetine Hydrochloride (Caffeine has the potential to interact with drugs that inhibit CYP1A2). Products include:
Paxil CR Controlled-Release Tablets ... 1538
Paxil ... 1530

Phenobarbital (Co-administration of caffeine with phenobarbital may result in increased caffeine elimination; higher doses of caffeine may be needed). Products include:
Donnatal Extentabs ... 2493

Phenobarbital Sodium (Caffeine has the potential to interact with drugs that are substrates for CYP1A2).
No products indexed under this heading.

Phenytoin (Co-administration of caffeine with phenytoin may result in increased caffeine elimination; higher doses of caffeine may be needed).
No products indexed under this heading.

Phenytoin Sodium (Co-administration of caffeine with phenytoin may result in increased caffeine elimination; higher doses of caffeine may be needed). Products include:
Phenytek Capsules ... 2160

Primidone (Caffeine has the potential to interact with drugs that induce CYP1A2).
No products indexed under this heading.

Propafenone Hydrochloride (Caffeine has the potential to interact with drugs that are substrates for CYP1A2). Products include:
Rythmol SR Capsules ... 2727

Propranolol Hydrochloride (Caffeine has the potential to interact with drugs that are substrates for CYP1A2). Products include:
- Inderal LA Long-Acting Capsules 3429
- InnoPran XL Capsules 2723

Protriptyline Hydrochloride (Caffeine has the potential to interact with drugs that are substrates for CYP1A2).
No products indexed under this heading.

Ranitidine Hydrochloride (Caffeine has the potential to interact with drugs that inhibit CYP1A2). Products include:
- Zantac 1624
- Zantac Injection 1619
- Zantac Injection Pharmacy Bulk Package 1622

Rifampicin (Caffeine has the potential to interact with drugs that induce CYP1A2).
No products indexed under this heading.

Rifampin (Caffeine has the potential to interact with drugs that induce CYP1A2).
No products indexed under this heading.

Riluzole (Caffeine has the potential to interact with drugs that are substrates for CYP1A2). Products include:
- Rilutek Tablets 2930

Ritonavir (Caffeine has the potential to interact with drugs that induce CYP1A2). Products include:
- Kaletra 476
- Norvir 503

Ropinirole Hydrochloride (Caffeine has the potential to interact with drugs that are substrates for CYP1A2). Products include:
- Requip Tablets 1555

Ropivacaine Hydrochloride (Caffeine has the potential to interact with drugs that are substrates for CYP1A2).
No products indexed under this heading.

Sparfloxacin (Caffeine has the potential to interact with drugs that inhibit CYP1A2).
No products indexed under this heading.

Tacrine Hydrochloride (Caffeine has the potential to interact with drugs that inhibit CYP1A2).
No products indexed under this heading.

Tamoxifen Citrate (Caffeine has the potential to interact with drugs that are substrates for CYP1A2). Products include:
- Soltamox Oral Solution 3527

Theophylline (Interconversion between caffeine and theophylline has been reported in preterm neonates; the concurrent use of these drugs is not recommended).
No products indexed under this heading.

Theophylline Anhydrous (Interconversion between caffeine and theophylline has been reported in preterm neonates; the concurrent use of these drugs is not recommended). Products include:
- Uniphyl Tablets 2710

Theophylline Calcium Salicylate (Interconversion between caffeine and theophylline has been reported in preterm neonates; the concurrent use of these drugs is not recommended).
No products indexed under this heading.

Theophylline Dihydroxypropyl (Glyceryl) (Interconversion between caffeine and theophylline has been reported in preterm neonates; the concurrent use of these drugs is not recommended).
No products indexed under this heading.

Theophylline Ethylenediamine (Interconversion between caffeine and theophylline has been reported in preterm neonates; the concurrent use of these drugs is not recommended).
No products indexed under this heading.

Theophylline Sodium Glycinate (Interconversion between caffeine and theophylline has been reported in preterm neonates; the concurrent use of these drugs is not recommended).
No products indexed under this heading.

Ticlopidine Hydrochloride (Caffeine has the potential to interact with drugs that inhibit CYP1A2). Products include:
- Ticlid Tablets 2810

Tobacco (Caffeine has the potential to interact with drugs that induce CYP1A2).
No products indexed under this heading.

Trimethaphan Camsylate (Caffeine has the potential to interact with drugs that are substrates for CYP1A2).
No products indexed under this heading.

Trimipramine Maleate (Caffeine has the potential to interact with drugs that are substrates for CYP1A2).
No products indexed under this heading.

Troleandomycin (Caffeine has the potential to interact with drugs that inhibit CYP1A2).
No products indexed under this heading.

Trovafloxacin Mesylate (Caffeine has the potential to interact with drugs that inhibit CYP1A2).
No products indexed under this heading.

Verapamil Hydrochloride (Caffeine has the potential to interact with drugs that are substrates for CYP1A2). Products include:
- Covera-HS Tablets 3139
- Tarka Tablets 524
- Verelan PM Extended-Release Capsules, Controlled-Onset........... 3106

Warfarin Sodium (Caffeine has the potential to interact with drugs that are substrates for CYP1A2). Products include:
- Coumadin for Injection 898
- Coumadin Tablets 898

Zileuton (Caffeine has the potential to interact with drugs that inhibit CYP1A2). Products include:
- Zyflo Tablets 1023

Zolmitriptan (Caffeine has the potential to interact with drugs that are substrates for CYP1A2). Products include:
- Zomig Tablets 3519
- Zomig Nasal Spray 3523
- Zomig-ZMT Tablets 3519

Food Interactions

Broccoli (Caffeine has the potential to interact with drugs that induce CYP1A2).

Brussel Sprouts (Caffeine has the potential to interact with drugs that induce CYP1A2).

Charbroiled Food (Caffeine has the potential to interact with drugs that induce CYP1A2).

Grapefruit Juice (Caffeine has the potential to interact with drugs that inhibit CYP1A2).

CAFCIT ORAL SOLUTION

(Caffeine Citrate) 1886
May interact with:

See (Cafcit Injection).
No products indexed under this heading.

CALCET TABLETS

(Calcium Carbonate, Calcium Gluconate, Calcium Lactate, Cholecalciferol)................................. 2138
None cited in PDR database.

CALCIJEX INJECTION

(Calcitriol) 411
May interact with:

Magnesium Carbonate (Co-administration with magnesium-containing antacids may lead to the development of hypermagnesemia; concurrent use should be avoided). Products include:
- Gaviscon Regular Strength Liquid .. ▣658
- Gaviscon Extra Strength Liquid ...... ▣658
- Gaviscon Extra Strength Tablets .... ▣658

Magnesium Hydroxide (Co-administration with magnesium-containing antacids may lead to the development of hypermagnesemia; concurrent use should be avoided). Products include:
- Maalox Regular Strength Antacid/Antigas Liquid.................. 2175
- Maalox Max Maximum Strength Antacid/Anti-Gas Liquid................ 2176
- Pepcid Complete Chewable Tablets 1701

Vitamin D (Since calcitriol is the most potent metabolite of vitamin D available, vitamin D and its derivatives should be withheld during treatment). Products include:
- Active Calcium Tablets 3339
- Caltrate 600 PLUS .... ▣809
- Caltrate 600 + D Tablets .... ▣809
- D-Cal Chewable Caplets .... ▣812
- Os-Cal 250 + D Tablets .... ▣817
- Os-Cal 500 + D Tablets .... ▣817

CALCIUM DISODIUM VERSENATE INJECTION

(Calcium Disodium Edetate) 1851
May interact with:

Insulin, Human, Zinc Suspension (Interference with the action of zinc insulin by chelating the zinc). Products include:
- Humulin L, 100 Units 1794
- Humulin U, 100 Units 1800

Insulin, Zinc Crystals (Interference with the action of zinc insulin by chelating the zinc).
No products indexed under this heading.

Insulin, Zinc Suspension (Interference with the action of zinc insulin by chelating the zinc).
No products indexed under this heading.

Steroids, unspecified (Enhances renal toxicity of edetate calcium disodium in animals).
No products indexed under this heading.

CALTRATE 600 PLUS MINERALS CHEWABLES

(Calcium Carbonate, Minerals, Multiple, Vitamin D)........................... ▣809
None cited in PDR database.

CALTRATE 600 PLUS MINERALS TABLETS

(Calcium Carbonate, Minerals, Multiple, Vitamin D)........................... ▣809
None cited in PDR database.

CALTRATE 600 + D TABLETS

(Calcium Carbonate, Vitamin D) .... ▣809
None cited in PDR database.

CAMPATH AMPULES

(Alemtuzumab) 811
May interact with:

Live Virus Vaccines (Patients who have recently received Campath, should not be immunized with live viral vaccines due to their immunosuppression).
No products indexed under this heading.

CAMPRAL TABLETS

(Acamprosate Calcium) 1174
May interact with antidepressant drugs and certain other agents. Compounds in these categories include:

Amitriptyline Hydrochloride (Patients taking acaprosate calcium concomitantly with antidepressants more commonly reported both weight gain and weight loss, compared with patients taking either medication alone).
No products indexed under this heading.

Amoxapine (Patients taking acaprosate calcium concomitantly with antidepressants more commonly reported both weight gain and weight loss, compared with patients taking either medication alone).
No products indexed under this heading.

Bupropion Hydrochloride (Patients taking acaprosate calcium concomitantly with antidepressants more commonly reported both weight gain and weight loss, compared with patients taking either medication alone). Products include:
- Wellbutrin Tablets 1603
- Wellbutrin SR Sustained-Release Tablets 1607
- Wellbutrin XL Extended-Release Tablets 1613
- Zyban Sustained-Release Tablets 1644

Citalopram Hydrobromide (Patients taking acaprosate calcium concomitantly with antidepressants more commonly reported both weight gain and weight loss, compared with patients taking either medication alone). Products include:
- Celexa 1176

Desipramine Hydrochloride (Patients taking acaprosate calcium concomitantly with antidepressants more commonly reported both weight gain and weight loss, compared with patients taking either medication alone).
No products indexed under this heading.

Doxepin Hydrochloride (Patients taking acaprosate calcium concomitantly with antidepressants more commonly reported both weight gain and weight loss, compared with patients taking either medication alone).
No products indexed under this heading.

Escitalopram Oxalate (Patients taking acaprosate calcium concomitantly with antidepressants more commonly reported both weight gain and weight loss, compared with patients taking either medication alone). Products include:
Lexapro Oral Solution **1190**
Lexapro Tablets **1190**

Fluoxetine Hydrochloride (Patients taking acaprosate calcium concomitantly with antidepressants more commonly reported both weight gain and weight loss, compared with patients taking either medication alone). Products include:
Prozac Pulvules and Liquid **1801**
Symbyax Capsules **1819**

Imipramine Hydrochloride (Patients taking acaprosate calcium concomitantly with antidepressants more commonly reported both weight gain and weight loss, compared with patients taking either medication alone).
No products indexed under this heading.

Imipramine Pamoate (Patients taking acaprosate calcium concomitantly with antidepressants more commonly reported both weight gain and weight loss, compared with patients taking either medication alone).
No products indexed under this heading.

Isocarboxazid (Patients taking acaprosate calcium concomitantly with antidepressants more commonly reported both weight gain and weight loss, compared with patients taking either medication alone).
No products indexed under this heading.

Maprotiline Hydrochloride (Patients taking acaprosate calcium concomitantly with antidepressants more commonly reported both weight gain and weight loss, compared with patients taking either medication alone).
No products indexed under this heading.

Mirtazapine (Patients taking acaprosate calcium concomitantly with antidepressants more commonly reported both weight gain and weight loss, compared with patients taking either medication alone).
No products indexed under this heading.

Naltrexone Hydrochloride (Co-administration of naltrexone with acamprosate calcium produced a 25% increase in AUC and a 33% increase in the Cmax of acamprosate. No adjustment of dosage is recommended in such patients).
No products indexed under this heading.

Nefazodone Hydrochloride (Patients taking acaprosate calcium concomitantly with antidepressants more commonly reported both weight gain and weight loss, compared with patients taking either medication alone).
No products indexed under this heading.

Nortriptyline Hydrochloride (Patients taking acaprosate calcium concomitantly with antidepressants more commonly reported both weight gain and weight loss, compared with patients taking either medication alone).
No products indexed under this heading.

Paroxetine Hydrochloride (Patients taking acaprosate calcium concomitantly with antidepressants more commonly reported both weight gain and weight loss, compared with patients taking either medication alone). Products include:
Paxil CR Controlled-Release Tablets **1538**
Paxil **1530**

Phenelzine Sulfate (Patients taking acaprosate calcium concomitantly with antidepressants more commonly reported both weight gain and weight loss, compared with patients taking either medication alone).
No products indexed under this heading.

Protriptyline Hydrochloride (Patients taking acaprosate calcium concomitantly with antidepressants more commonly reported both weight gain and weight loss, compared with patients taking either medication alone).
No products indexed under this heading.

Sertraline Hydrochloride (Patients taking acaprosate calcium concomitantly with antidepressants more commonly reported both weight gain and weight loss, compared with patients taking either medication alone). Products include:
Zoloft **2586**

Tranylcypromine Sulfate (Patients taking acaprosate calcium concomitantly with antidepressants more commonly reported both weight gain and weight loss, compared with patients taking either medication alone). Products include:
Parnate Tablets **1527**

Trazodone Hydrochloride (Patients taking acaprosate calcium concomitantly with antidepressants more commonly reported both weight gain and weight loss, compared with patients taking either medication alone).
No products indexed under this heading.

Trimipramine Maleate (Patients taking acaprosate calcium concomitantly with antidepressants more commonly reported both weight gain and weight loss, compared with patients taking either medication alone).
No products indexed under this heading.

Venlafaxine Hydrochloride (Patients taking acaprosate calcium concomitantly with antidepressants more commonly reported both weight gain and weight loss, compared with patients taking either medication alone). Products include:
Effexor Tablets **3411**
Effexor XR Capsules **3417**

CAMPTOSAR INJECTION

(Irinotecan Hydrochloride) **2604**
May interact with antineoplastics, dexamethasone, diuretics, oral hypoglycemic agents, insulin, laxatives, phenytoin, and certain other agents. Compounds in these categories include:

Acarbose (Hyperglycemia has been reported in patients receiving irinotecan and it is probable that the administration of dexamethasone as antiemetic prophylaxis may have contributed to hyperglycemia in some patients). Products include:
Precose Tablets **751**

Altretamine (Co-administration may exacerbate the adverse effects of irinotecan, such as myelosuppression and diarrhea).
No products indexed under this heading.

Amiloride Hydrochloride (Co-administration with diuretics may increase the potential risk of dehydration secondary to vomiting and/or diarrhea induced by irinotecan; the physician may wish to withhold diuretics during dosing with Camptosar and, certainly, during periods of active vomiting or diarrhea). Products include:
Midamor Tablets **2026**
Moduretic Tablets **2028**

Anastrozole (Co-administration may exacerbate the adverse effects of irinotecan, such as myelosuppression and diarrhea). Products include:
Arimidex Tablets **673**

Asparaginase (Co-administration may exacerbate the adverse effects of irinotecan, such as myelosuppression and diarrhea). Products include:
Elspar for Injection **2463**
Elspar for Injection **1960**

Bendroflumethiazide (Co-administration with diuretics may increase the potential risk of dehydration secondary to vomiting and/or diarrhea induced by irinotecan; the physician may wish to withhold diuretics during dosing with Camptosar and, certainly, during periods of active vomiting or diarrhea).
No products indexed under this heading.

Bicalutamide (Co-administration may exacerbate the adverse effects of irinotecan, such as myelosuppression and diarrhea).
No products indexed under this heading.

Bisacodyl (Co-administration with laxatives may worsen the incidence or severity of diarrhea). Products include:
Dulcolax Suppositories **648**
Dulcolax Tablets **649**
Fleet Bisacodyl Laxatives **1165**
Fleet Prep Kits **1170**
HalfLytely and Bisacodyl Tablets Bowel Prep Kit with Flavors Packs **881**

Bleomycin Sulfate (Co-administration may exacerbate the adverse effects of irinotecan, such as myelosuppression and diarrhea).
No products indexed under this heading.

Bumetanide (Co-administration with diuretics may increase the potential risk of dehydration secondary to vomiting and/or diarrhea induced by irinotecan; the physician may wish to withhold diuretics during dosing with Camptosar and, certainly, during periods of active vomiting or diarrhea). Products include:
Bumex Tablets **2746**

Busulfan (Co-administration may exacerbate the adverse effects of irinotecan, such as myelosuppression and diarrhea). Products include:
I.V. Busulfex **2493**
Myleran Tablets **1525**

Carbamazepine (Exposure to irinotecan and its active metabolite SN-38 is substantially reduced in adult and pediatric patients concomitantly receiving the CYP3A4 enzyme-inducing anticonvulsants phenytoin, phenobarbital, or carbamazepine. The appropriate starting dose for patients taking these anticonvulsants has not been formally defined. For patients requiring anticonvulsant treatment, consideration should be given to substituting non-enzyme inducing anticonvulsants at least 2 weeks prior to initiation of irinotecan-therapy). Products include:
Carbatrol Capsules **3171**
Equetro Extended-Release Capsules **3180**
Tegretol/Tegretol-XR **2295**

Carboplatin (Co-administration may exacerbate the adverse effects of irinotecan, such as myelosuppression and diarrhea).
No products indexed under this heading.

Carmustine (BCNU) (Co-administration may exacerbate the adverse effects of irinotecan, such as myelosuppression and diarrhea).
No products indexed under this heading.

Cascara Sagrada (Co-administration with laxatives may worsen the incidence or severity of diarrhea).
No products indexed under this heading.

Castor Oil (Co-administration with laxatives may worsen the incidence or severity of diarrhea). Products include:
Xenaderm Ointment **1664**

Chlorambucil (Co-administration may exacerbate the adverse effects of irinotecan, such as myelosuppression and diarrhea). Products include:
Leukeran Tablets **1504**

Chlorothiazide (Co-administration with diuretics may increase the potential risk of dehydration secondary to vomiting and/or diarrhea induced by irinotecan; the physician may wish to withhold diuretics during dosing with Camptosar and, certainly, during periods of active vomiting or diarrhea). Products include:
Diuril Oral Suspension **1954**

Chlorothiazide Sodium (Co-administration with diuretics may increase the potential risk of dehydration secondary to vomiting and/or diarrhea induced by irinotecan; the physician may wish to withhold diuretics during dosing with Camptosar and, certainly, during periods of active vomiting or diarrhea). Products include:

Diuril Sodium Intravenous 2467

Chlorpropamide (Hyperglycemia has been reported in patients receiving irinotecan and it is probable that the administration of dexamethasone as antiemetic prophylaxis may have contributed to hyperglycemia in some patients).

No products indexed under this heading.

Chlorthalidone (Co-administration with diuretics may increase the potential risk of dehydration secondary to vomiting and/or diarrhea induced by irinotecan; the physician may wish to withhold diuretics during dosing with Camptosar and, certainly, during periods of active vomiting or diarrhea). Products include:

Clorpres Tablets 2153

Cisplatin (Co-administration may exacerbate the adverse effects of irinotecan, such as myelosuppression and diarrhea).

No products indexed under this heading.

Cyclophosphamide (Co-administration may exacerbate the adverse effects of irinotecan, such as myelosuppression and diarrhea).

No products indexed under this heading.

Dacarbazine (Co-administration may exacerbate the adverse effects of irinotecan, such as myelosuppression and diarrhea).

No products indexed under this heading.

Daunorubicin Citrate (Co-administration may exacerbate the adverse effects of irinotecan, such as myelosuppression and diarrhea).

No products indexed under this heading.

Daunorubicin Hydrochloride (Co-administration may exacerbate the adverse effects of irinotecan, such as myelosuppression and diarrhea).

No products indexed under this heading.

Denileukin Diftitox (Co-administration may exacerbate the adverse effects of irinotecan, such as myelosuppression and diarrhea). Products include:

Ontak Vials 1745

Dexamethasone (Lymphocytopenia has been reported in patients receiving irinotecan and it is possible that the administration of dexamethasone as antiemetic prophylaxis may have enhanced the likelihood of this effect. Dexamethasone does not appear to alter the pharmacokinetics of irinotecan). Products include:

Ciprodex Otic Suspension 559
Decadron Tablets 1951
TobraDex Ophthalmic Ointment 562
TobraDex Ophthalmic Suspension ... 563

Dexamethasone Acetate (Lymphocytopenia has been reported in patients receiving irinotecan and it is possible that the administration of dexamethasone as antiemetic prophylaxis may have enhanced the likelihood of this effect. Dexamethasone does not appear to alter the pharmacokinetics of irinotecan).

No products indexed under this heading.

Dexamethasone Sodium Phosphate (Lymphocytopenia has been reported in patients receiving irinotecan and it is possible that the administration of dexamethasone as antiemetic prophylaxis may have enhanced the likelihood of this effect. Dexamethasone does not appear to alter the pharmacokinetics of irinotecan).

No products indexed under this heading.

Docetaxel (Co-administration may exacerbate the adverse effects of irinotecan, such as myelosuppression and diarrhea). Products include:

Taxotere Injection Concentrate 2932

Docusate Sodium (Co-administration with laxatives may worsen the incidence or severity of diarrhea). Products include:

Dulcolax Stool Softener .... ▣648

Doxorubicin Hydrochloride (Co-administration may exacerbate the adverse effects of irinotecan, such as myelosuppression and diarrhea).

No products indexed under this heading.

Epirubicin Hydrochloride (Co-administration may exacerbate the adverse effects of irinotecan, such as myelosuppression and diarrhea).

No products indexed under this heading.

Estramustine Phosphate Sodium (Co-administration may exacerbate the adverse effects of irinotecan, such as myelosuppression and diarrhea). Products include:

Emcyt Capsules 2634

Ethacrynic Acid (Co-administration with diuretics may increase the potential risk of dehydration secondary to vomiting and/or diarrhea induced by irinotecan; the physician may wish to withhold diuretics during dosing with Camptosar and, certainly, during periods of active vomiting or diarrhea). Products include:

Edecrin Tablets 1959

Etoposide (Co-administration may exacerbate the adverse effects of irinotecan, such as myelosuppression and diarrhea).

No products indexed under this heading.

Exemestane (Co-administration may exacerbate the adverse effects of irinotecan, such as myelosuppression and diarrhea). Products include:

Aromasin Tablets 2600

Floxuridine (Co-administration may exacerbate the adverse effects of irinotecan, such as myelosuppression and diarrhea).

No products indexed under this heading.

Fluorouracil (Co-administration may exacerbate the adverse effects of irinotecan, such as myelosuppression and diarrhea). Products include:

Carac Cream, 0.5% 2879
Efudex 3363

Flutamide (Co-administration may exacerbate the adverse effects of irinotecan, such as myelosuppression and diarrhea). Products include:

Eulexin Capsules 3009

Fosphenytoin Sodium (Exposure to irinotecan and its active metabolite SN-38 is substantially reduced in adult and pediatric patients concomitantly receiving the CYP3A4 enzyme-inducing anticonvulsants phenytoin, phenobarbital, or carbamazepine. The appropriate starting dose for patients taking these anticonvulsants has not been formally defined. For patients requiring anticonvulsant treatment, consideration should be given to substituting non-enzyme inducing anticonvulsants at least 2 weeks prior to initiation of irinotecantherapy).

No products indexed under this heading.

Furosemide (Co-administration with diuretics may increase the potential risk of dehydration secondary to vomiting and/or diarrhea induced by irinotecan; the physician may wish to withhold diuretics during dosing with Camptosar and, certainly, during periods of active vomiting or diarrhea). Products include:

Furosemide Tablets 2154

Gemcitabine Hydrochloride (Co-administration may exacerbate the adverse effects of irinotecan, such as myelosuppression and diarrhea). Products include:

Gemzar for Injection 1771

Glimepiride (Hyperglycemia has been reported in patients receiving irinotecan and it is probable that the administration of dexamethasone as antiemetic prophylaxis may have contributed to hyperglycemia in some patients). Products include:

Avandaryl Tablets 1379
Duetact Tablets 3226

Glipizide (Hyperglycemia has been reported in patients receiving irinotecan and it is probable that the administration of dexamethasone as antiemetic prophylaxis may have contributed to hyperglycemia in some patients).

No products indexed under this heading.

Glyburide (Hyperglycemia has been reported in patients receiving irinotecan and it is probable that the administration of dexamethasone as antiemetic prophylaxis may have contributed to hyperglycemia in some patients).

No products indexed under this heading.

Hydrochlorothiazide (Co-administration with diuretics may increase the potential risk of dehydration secondary to vomiting and/or diarrhea induced by irinotecan; the physician may wish to withhold diuretics during dosing with Camptosar and, certainly, during periods of active vomiting or diarrhea). Products include:

Aldoril Tablets 1910
Atacand HCT 651
Avalide Tablets 888
Avalide Tablets 2874
Benicar HCT Tablets 1044
Diovan HCT Tablets 2196
Dyazide Capsules 1423
Hyzaar 50-12.5 Tablets 1990
Hyzaar 100-12.5 Tablets 1990
Hyzaar 100-25 Tablets 1990
Lopressor HCT 50/25 Tablets 2241
Lopressor HCT 100/25 Tablets 2241
Lopressor HCT 100/50 Tablets 2241
Lotensin HCT Tablets 2246
Micardis HCT Tablets 856
Moduretic Tablets 2028
Prinzide Tablets 2056
Teveten HCT Tablets 1737
Timolide Tablets 2086
Uniretic Tablets 3100

Hydroflumethiazide (Co-administration with diuretics may increase the potential risk of dehydration secondary to vomiting and/or diarrhea induced by irinotecan; the physician may wish to withhold diuretics during dosing with Camptosar and, certainly, during periods of active vomiting or diarrhea).

No products indexed under this heading.

Hydroxyurea (Co-administration may exacerbate the adverse effects of irinotecan, such as myelosuppression and diarrhea).

No products indexed under this heading.

Hypericum (St. John's Wort is an inducer of CYP2A4 enzymes. Exposure to the active metabolite SN-38 is reduced in patients receiving concomitant St. John's Wort. St. John's Wort should be discontinued at least 2 weeks prior to the first cycle of irinotecan and St. John's Wort is contraindicated during irinotecan therapy). Products include:

Satiete Tablets .... ▣832

Idarubicin Hydrochloride (Co-administration may exacerbate the adverse effects of irinotecan, such as myelosuppression and diarrhea).

No products indexed under this heading.

Ifosfamide (Co-administration may exacerbate the adverse effects of irinotecan, such as myelosuppression and diarrhea).

No products indexed under this heading.

Indapamide (Co-administration with diuretics may increase the potential risk of dehydration secondary to vomiting and/or diarrhea induced by irinotecan; the physician may wish to withhold diuretics during dosing with Camptosar and, certainly, during periods of active vomiting or diarrhea). Products include:

Indapamide Tablets 2156

Insulin, Human, Zinc Suspension (Hyperglycemia has been reported in patients receiving irinotecan and it is probable that the administration of dexamethasone as antiemetic prophylaxis may have contributed to hyperglycemia in some patients). Products include:

Humulin L, 100 Units 1794
Humulin U, 100 Units 1800

Insulin, Human NPH (Hyperglycemia has been reported in patients receiving irinotecan and it is probable that the administration of dexamethasone as antiemetic prophylaxis may have contributed to hyperglycemia in some patients). Products include:

Humulin N, 100 Units 1795
Humulin N Pen 1797

Insulin, Human Regular (Hyperglycemia has been reported in patients receiving irinotecan and it is probable that the administration of dexamethasone as antiemetic prophylaxis may have contributed to hyperglycemia in some patients). Products include:

Humulin R, 100 Units 1798

Insulin, Human Regular and Human NPH Mixture (Hyperglycemia has been reported in patients receiving irinotecan and it is probable that the administration of dexamethasone as antiemetic prophylaxis may have contributed to hyperglycemia in some patients). Products include:

Humulin 50/50, 100 Units 1791
Humulin 70/30 Pen 1793

Insulin, NPH (Hyperglycemia has been reported in patients receiving irinotecan and it is probable that the administration of dexamethasone as antiemetic prophylaxis may have contributed to hyperglycemia in some patients).

No products indexed under this heading.

Insulin, Regular (Hyperglycemia has been reported in patients receiving irinotecan and it is probable that the administration of dexamethasone as antiemetic prophylaxis may have contributed to hyperglycemia in some patients).

No products indexed under this heading.

Insulin, Zinc Crystals (Hyperglycemia has been reported in patients receiving irinotecan and it is probable that the administration of dexamethasone as antiemetic prophylaxis may have contributed to hyperglycemia in some patients).

No products indexed under this heading.

Insulin, Zinc Suspension (Hyperglycemia has been reported in patients receiving irinotecan and it is probable that the administration of dexamethasone as antiemetic prophylaxis may have contributed to hyperglycemia in some patients).

No products indexed under this heading.

Insulin Aspart, Human Regular (Hyperglycemia has been reported in patients receiving irinotecan and it is probable that the administration of dexamethasone as antiemetic prophylaxis may have contributed to hyperglycemia in some patients). Products include:

NovoLog Injection 2326

Insulin glargine (Hyperglycemia has been reported in patients receiving irinotecan and it is probable that the administration of dexamethasone as antiemetic prophylaxis may have contributed to hyperglycemia in some patients). Products include:

Lantus Injection 2909

Insulin Lispro, Human (Hyperglycemia has been reported in patients receiving irinotecan and it is probable that the administration of dexamethasone as antiemetic prophylaxis may have contributed to hyperglycemia in some patients). Products include:

Humalog-Pen 1781
Humalog Mix 50/50-Pen 1783
Humalog Mix 75/25-Pen 1785

Insulin Lispro Protamine, Human (Hyperglycemia has been reported in patients receiving irinotecan and it is probable that the administration of dexamethasone as antiemetic prophylaxis may have contributed to hyperglycemia in some patients). Products include:

Humalog Mix 50/50-Pen 1783
Humalog Mix 75/25-Pen 1785

Interferon alfa-2a, Recombinant (Co-administration may exacerbate the adverse effects of irinotecan, such as myelosuppression and diarrhea).

No products indexed under this heading.

Interferon alfa-2b, Recombinant (Co-administration may exacerbate the adverse effects of irinotecan, such as myelosuppression and diarrhea). Products include:

Intron A for Injection 3024
Rebetron Combination Therapy 3063

Ketoconazole (Ketoconazole is a strong inhibitor of CYP3A4 enzymes. Patients receiving concomitant ketoconazole have increased exposure to irinotecan and its active metabolite SN-38. Patients should discontinue ketoconazole at least 1 week prior to starting irinotecan therapy and ketoconazole is contraindicated during irinotecan therapy). Products include:

Nizoral A-D Shampoo, 1% 1868

Lactulose (Co-administration with laxatives may worsen the incidence or severity of diarrhea). Products include:

Kristalose for Oral Solution 1034

Levamisole Hydrochloride (Co-administration may exacerbate the adverse effects of irinotecan, such as myelosuppression and diarrhea).

No products indexed under this heading.

Lomustine (CCNU) (Co-administration may exacerbate the adverse effects of irinotecan, such as myelosuppression and diarrhea).

No products indexed under this heading.

Mechlorethamine Hydrochloride (Co-administration may exacerbate the adverse effects of irinotecan, such as myelosuppression and diarrhea). Products include:

Mustargen for Injection 2468

Megestrol Acetate (Co-administration may exacerbate the adverse effects of irinotecan, such as myelosuppression and diarrhea). Products include:

Megace ES Oral Suspension 2481

Melphalan (Co-administration may exacerbate the adverse effects of irinotecan, such as myelosuppression and diarrhea). Products include:

Alkeran Tablets 956

Mercaptopurine (Co-administration may exacerbate the adverse effects of irinotecan, such as myelosuppression and diarrhea).

No products indexed under this heading.

Metformin Hydrochloride (Hyperglycemia has been reported in patients receiving irinotecan and it is probable that the administration of dexamethasone as antiemetic prophylaxis may have contributed to hyperglycemia in some patients). Products include:

ActoPlus Met Tablets 3214
Avandamet Tablets 1373
Fortamet Extended-Release Tablets 3115

Methotrexate Sodium (Co-administration may exacerbate the adverse effects of irinotecan, such as myelosuppression and diarrhea).

No products indexed under this heading.

Methyclothiazide (Co-administration with diuretics may increase the potential risk of dehydration secondary to vomiting and/or diarrhea induced by irinotecan; the physician may wish to withhold diuretics during dosing with Camptosar and, certainly, during periods of active vomiting or diarrhea).

No products indexed under this heading.

Methylcellulose (Co-administration with laxatives may worsen the incidence or severity of diarrhea). Products include:

Citrucel Caplets 647
Citrucel Orange Flavor Powder 647
Citrucel Sugar Free Orange Flavor Powder 648

Metolazone (Co-administration with diuretics may increase the potential risk of dehydration secondary to vomiting and/or diarrhea induced by irinotecan; the physician may wish to withhold diuretics during dosing with Camptosar and, certainly, during periods of active vomiting or diarrhea).

No products indexed under this heading.

Miglitol (Hyperglycemia has been reported in patients receiving irinotecan and it is probable that the administration of dexamethasone as antiemetic prophylaxis may have contributed to hyperglycemia in some patients).

No products indexed under this heading.

Mitomycin (Mitomycin-C) (Co-administration may exacerbate the adverse effects of irinotecan, such as myelosuppression and diarrhea).

No products indexed under this heading.

Mitotane (Co-administration may exacerbate the adverse effects of irinotecan, such as myelosuppression and diarrhea).

No products indexed under this heading.

Mitoxantrone Hydrochloride (Co-administration may exacerbate the adverse effects of irinotecan, such as myelosuppression and diarrhea).

No products indexed under this heading.

Oxaliplatin (Co-administration may exacerbate the adverse effects of irinotecan, such as myelosuppression and diarrhea). Products include:

Eloxatin for Injection 2892

Paclitaxel (Co-administration may exacerbate the adverse effects of irinotecan, such as myelosuppression and diarrhea).

No products indexed under this heading.

Phenobarbital (Exposure to irinotecan and its active metabolite SN-38 is substantially reduced in adult and pediatric patients concomitantly receiving the CYP3A4 enzyme-inducing anticonvulsants phenytoin, phenobarbital, or carbamazepine. The appropriate starting dose for patients taking these anticonvulsants has not been formally defined. For patients requiring anticonvulsant treatment, consideration should be given to substituting non-enzyme inducing anticonvulsants at least 2 weeks prior to initiation of irinotecan therapy). Products include:

Donnatal Extentabs 2493

Phenobarbital Sodium (Exposure to irinotecan and its active metabolite SN-38 is substantially reduced in adult and pediatric patients concomitantly receiving the CYP3A4 enzyme-inducing anticonvulsants phenytoin, phenobarbital, or carbamazepine. The appropriate starting dose for patients taking these anticonvulsants has not been formally defined. For patients requiring anticonvulsant treatment, consideration should be given to substituting non-enzyme inducing anticonvulsants at least 2 weeks prior to initiation of irinotecantherapy).

No products indexed under this heading.

Phenolphthalein (Co-administration with laxatives may worsen the incidence or severity of diarrhea).

No products indexed under this heading.

Phenytoin (Exposure to irinotecan and its active metabolite SN-38 is substantially reduced in adult and pediatric patients concomitantly receiving the CYP3A4 enzyme-inducing anticonvulsants phenytoin, phenobarbital, or carbamazepine. The appropriate starting dose for patients taking these anticonvulsants has not been formally defined. For patients requiring anticonvulsant treatment, consideration should be given to substituting non-enzyme inducing anticonvulsants at least 2 weeks prior to initiation of irinotecantherapy).

No products indexed under this heading.

Phenytoin Sodium (Exposure to irinotecan and its active metabolite SN-38 is substantially reduced in adult and pediatric patients concomitantly receiving the CYP3A4 enzyme-inducing anticonvulsants phenytoin, phenobarbital, or carbamazepine. The appropriate starting dose for patients taking these anticonvulsants has not been formally defined. For patients requiring anticonvulsant treatment, consideration should be given to substituting non-enzyme inducing anticonvulsants at least 2 weeks prior to initiation of irinotecan therapy). Products include:

Phenytek Capsules 2160

Pioglitazone Hydrochloride (Hyperglycemia has been reported in patients receiving irinotecan and it is probable that the administration of dexamethasone as antiemetic prophylaxis may have contributed to hyperglycemia in some patients). Products include:

ActoPlus Met Tablets 3214
Actos Tablets 3219
Duetact Tablets 3226

Polythiazide (Co-administration with diuretics may increase the potential risk of dehydration secondary to vomiting and/or diarrhea induced by irinotecan; the physician may wish to withhold diuretics during dosing with Camptosar and, certainly, during periods of active vomiting or diarrhea).

No products indexed under this heading.

Procarbazine Hydrochloride (Co-administration may exacerbate the adverse effects of irinotecan, such as myelosuppression and diarrhea). Products include:

Matulane Capsules 3191

Prochlorperazine (May increase the incidence of akathisia).
No products indexed under this heading.

Psyllium Preparations (Co-administration with laxatives may worsen the incidence or severity of diarrhea). Products include:
Experience Capsules .... ■ 828
Metamucil Capsules 2675
Metamucil 2675
Metamucil Dietary Fiber Supplement .... ■ 650
StePHan Relief Capsules .... ■ 821

Repaglinide (Hyperglycemia has been reported in patients receiving irinotecan and it is probable that the administration of dexamethasone as antiemetic prophylaxis may have contributed to hyperglycemia in some patients).
No products indexed under this heading.

Rosiglitazone Maleate (Hyperglycemia has been reported in patients receiving irinotecan and it is probable that the administration of dexamethasone as antiemetic prophylaxis may have contributed to hyperglycemia in some patients). Products include:
Avandamet Tablets 1373
Avandaryl Tablets 1379
Avandia Tablets 1384

Senna (Co-administration with laxatives may worsen the incidence or severity of diarrhea).
No products indexed under this heading.

Spironolactone (Co-administration with diuretics may increase the potential risk of dehydration secondary to vomiting and/or diarrhea induced by irinotecan; the physician may wish to withhold diuretics during dosing with Camptosar and, certainly, during periods of active vomiting or diarrhea).
No products indexed under this heading.

Streptozocin (Co-administration may exacerbate the adverse effects of irinotecan, such as myelosuppression and diarrhea).
No products indexed under this heading.

Tamoxifen Citrate (Co-administration may exacerbate the adverse effects of irinotecan, such as myelosuppression and diarrhea). Products include:
Soltamox Oral Solution 3527

Teniposide (Co-administration may exacerbate the adverse effects of irinotecan, such as myelosuppression and diarrhea).
No products indexed under this heading.

Thioguanine (Co-administration may exacerbate the adverse effects of irinotecan, such as myelosuppression and diarrhea). Products include:
Tabloid Tablets 1575

Thiotepa (Co-administration may exacerbate the adverse effects of irinotecan, such as myelosuppression and diarrhea).
No products indexed under this heading.

Tolazamide (Hyperglycemia has been reported in patients receiving irinotecan and it is probable that the administration of dexamethasone as antiemetic prophylaxis may have contributed to hyperglycemia in some patients).
No products indexed under this heading.

Tolbutamide (Hyperglycemia has been reported in patients receiving irinotecan and it is probable that the administration of dexamethasone as antiemetic prophylaxis may have contributed to hyperglycemia in some patients).
No products indexed under this heading.

Topotecan Hydrochloride (Co-administration may exacerbate the adverse effects of irinotecan, such as myelosuppression and diarrhea). Products include:
Hycamtin for Injection 1458

Toremifene Citrate (Co-administration may exacerbate the adverse effects of irinotecan, such as myelosuppression and diarrhea).
No products indexed under this heading.

Torsemide (Co-administration with diuretics may increase the potential risk of dehydration secondary to vomiting and/or diarrhea induced by irinotecan; the physician may wish to withhold diuretics during dosing with Camptosar and, certainly, during periods of active vomiting or diarrhea). Products include:
Demadex Injection 2759
Demadex Tablets 2759

Triamterene (Co-administration with diuretics may increase the potential risk of dehydration secondary to vomiting and/or diarrhea induced by irinotecan; the physician may wish to withhold diuretics during dosing with Camptosar and, certainly, during periods of active vomiting or diarrhea). Products include:
Dyazide Capsules 1423
Dyrenium Capsules 3400

Troglitazone (Hyperglycemia has been reported in patients receiving irinotecan and it is probable that the administration of dexamethasone as antiemetic prophylaxis may have contributed to hyperglycemia in some patients).
No products indexed under this heading.

Valrubicin (Co-administration may exacerbate the adverse effects of irinotecan, such as myelosuppression and diarrhea).
No products indexed under this heading.

Vincristine Sulfate (Co-administration may exacerbate the adverse effects of irinotecan, such as myelosuppression and diarrhea).
No products indexed under this heading.

Vinorelbine Tartrate (Co-administration may exacerbate the adverse effects of irinotecan, such as myelosuppression and diarrhea).
No products indexed under this heading.

CANASA RECTAL SUPPOSITORIES

(Mesalamine) 699
May interact with:

Sulfasalazine (Patients on concurrent oral products that contain or release mesalamine should be carefully monitored with urinalysis, BUN and creatinine testing).
No products indexed under this heading.

CANCIDAS FOR INJECTION

(Caspofungin acetate) 1918
May interact with dexamethasone, phenytoin, and certain other agents. Compounds in these categories include:

Carbamazepine (The results from regression analyses of patient pharmacokinetic data suggest that co-administration of inducers of drug clearance and/or mixed inducers/inhibitors with caspofungin may result in clinically meaningful reductions in caspofungin concentrations; an increase in the daily dose of caspofungin to 70 mg, following the usual 70-mg loading dose, should be considered in patients who are not clinically responding during concomitant therapy). Products include:
Carbatrol Capsules 3171
Equetro Extended-Release Capsules 3180
Tegretol/Tegretol-XR 2295

Cyclosporine (Co-administration with cyclosporine results in increased AUC of caspofungin by approximately 35%; there were transient increases in liver ALT and AST during co-administration; concomitant use is not recommended unless the potential benefit outweighs the potential risk to the patient). Products include:
Gengraf Capsules 459
Neoral Oral Solution 2259
Neoral Soft Gelatin Capsules 2259
Restasis Ophthalmic Emulsion 575
Sandimmune 2275

Dexamethasone (The results from regression analyses of patient pharmacokinetic data suggest that co-administration of inducers of drug clearance and/or mixed inducers/inhibitors with caspofungin may result in clinically meaningful reductions in caspofungin concentrations; an increase in the daily dose of caspofungin to 70 mg, following the usual 70-mg loading dose, should be considered in patients who are not clinically responding during concomitant therapy). Products include:
Ciprodex Otic Suspension 559
Decadron Tablets 1951
TobraDex Ophthalmic Ointment 562
TobraDex Ophthalmic Suspension ... 563

Dexamethasone Acetate (The results from regression analyses of patient pharmacokinetic data suggest that co-administration of inducers of drug clearance and/or mixed inducers/inhibitors with caspofungin may result in clinically meaningful reductions in caspofungin concentrations; an increase in the daily dose of caspofungin to 70 mg, following the usual 70-mg loading dose, should be considered in patients who are not clinically responding during concomitant therapy).
No products indexed under this heading.

Dexamethasone Sodium Phosphate (The results from regression analyses of patient pharmacokinetic data suggest that co-administration of inducers of drug clearance and/or mixed inducers/inhibitors with caspofungin may result in clinically meaningful reductions in caspofungin concentrations; an increase in the daily dose of caspofungin to 70 mg, following the usual 70-mg loading dose, should be considered in patients who are not clinically responding during concomitant therapy).
No products indexed under this heading.

Efavirenz (The results from regression analyses of patient pharmacokinetic data suggest that co-administration of inducers of drug clearance and/or mixed inducers/inhibitors with caspofungin may result in clinically meaningful reductions in caspofungin concentrations; an increase in the daily dose of caspofungin to 70 mg, following the usual 70-mg loading dose, should be considered in patients who are not clinically responding during concomitant therapy). Products include:
Atripla Tablets 945
Sustiva Capsules 930
Sustiva Tablets 930

Fosphenytoin Sodium (The results from regression analyses of patient pharmacokinetic data suggest that co-administration of inducers of drug clearance and/or mixed inducers/inhibitors with caspofungin may result in clinically meaningful reductions in caspofungin concentrations; an increase in the daily dose of caspofungin to 70 mg, following the usual 70-mg loading dose, should be considered in patients who are not clinically responding during concomitant therapy).
No products indexed under this heading.

Nelfinavir Mesylate (The results from regression analyses of patient pharmacokinetic data suggest that co-administration of inducers of drug clearance and/or mixed inducers/inhibitors with caspofungin may result in clinically meaningful reductions in caspofungin concentrations; an increase in the daily dose of caspofungin to 70 mg, following the usual 70-mg loading dose, should be considered in patients who are not clinically responding during concomitant therapy). Products include:
Viracept 2577

Nevirapine (The results from regression analyses of patient pharmacokinetic data suggest that co-administration of inducers of drug clearance and/or mixed inducers/inhibitors with caspofungin may result in clinically meaningful reductions in caspofungin concentrations; an increase in the daily dose of caspofungin to 70 mg, following the usual 70-mg loading dose, should be considered in patients who are not clinically responding during concomitant therapy). Products include:
Viramune Oral Suspension 873
Viramune Tablets 873

Phenytoin (The results from regression analyses of patient pharmacokinetic data suggest that co-administration of inducers of drug clearance and/or mixed inducers/inhibitors with caspofungin may result in clinically meaningful reduc-

tions in caspofungin concentrations; an increase in the daily dose of caspofungin to 70 mg, following the usual 70-mg loading dose, should be considered in patients who are not clinically responding during concomitant therapy).
No products indexed under this heading.

Phenytoin Sodium (The results from regression analyses of patient pharmacokinetic data suggest that co-administration of inducers of drug clearance and/or mixed inducers/ inhibitors with caspofungin may result in clinically meaningful reductions in caspofungin concentrations; an increase in the daily dose of caspofungin to 70 mg, following the usual 70-mg loading dose, should be considered in patients who are not clinically responding during concomitant therapy). Products include:
Phenytek Capsules 2160

Rifampin (The results from regression analyses of patient pharmacokinetic data suggest that co-administration of inducers of drug clearance and/or mixed inducers/ inhibitors with caspofungin may result in clinically meaningful reductions in caspofungin concentrations; an increase in the daily dose of caspofungin to 70 mg, following the usual 70-mg loading dose, should be considered in patients who are not clinically responding during concomitant therapy).
No products indexed under this heading.

Tacrolimus (Co-administration with tacrolimus reduces the AUC of tracrolimus by approximately 20%, peak blood concentration by 16% and 12-hour blood concentration by 26%; standard monitoring of tracrolimus blood concentrations and appropriate tracrolimus dosage adjustments are recommended).
Products include:
Prograf Capsules and Injection 632
Protopic Ointment 638

CAPASTAT SULFATE FOR INJECTION

(Capreomycin Sulfate) 1755
May interact with aminoglycosides, antituberculosis drugs, and certain other agents. Compounds in these categories include:

Amikacin Sulfate (Additive ototoxicity and/or nephrotoxicity).
No products indexed under this heading.

Aminosalicylic Acid (Potential for febrile reactions and abnormal liver function tests). Products include:
Paser Granules 1674

p-Aminosalicylic Acid (Potential for febrile reactions and abnormal liver function tests).
No products indexed under this heading.

Colistin Sulfate (Additive ototoxicity and/or nephrotoxicity).
No products indexed under this heading.

Cycloserine (Potential for febrile reactions and abnormal liver function tests). Products include:
Seromycin Capsules 1813

Ethambutol Hydrochloride (Potential for febrile reactions and abnormal liver function tests).
No products indexed under this heading.

Ether (May enhance the partial neuromuscular blockade caused by capreomycin).
No products indexed under this heading.

Gentamicin Sulfate (Additive ototoxicity and/or nephrotoxicity).
Products include:
Garamycin Injectable 3014
Pred-G Ophthalmic Ointment .... ⊙237
Pred-G Ophthalmic Suspension ...... ⊙236

Isoniazid (Potential for febrile reactions and abnormal liver function tests).
No products indexed under this heading.

Kanamycin Sulfate (Additive ototoxicity and/or nephrotoxicity).
No products indexed under this heading.

Neomycin, oral (Additive ototoxicity and/or nephrotoxicity).
No products indexed under this heading.

Neostigmine Bromide (May antagonize the partial neuromuscular blockade caused by capreomycin).
No products indexed under this heading.

Neostigmine Methylsulfate (May antagonize the partial neuromuscular blockade caused by capreomycin).
No products indexed under this heading.

Paromomycin Sulfate (Additive ototoxicity and/or nephrotoxicity).
No products indexed under this heading.

Polymyxin B Sulfate (Additive ototoxicity and/or nephrotoxicity).
Products include:
Neosporin Antibiotic Ointment .... ▣643
Neosporin Ophthalmic Solution Sterile .... ⊙265
Neosporin + Pain Relief Antibiotic Cream and Ointment (Maximum Strength).................... ▣643
Poly-Pred Ophthalmic Suspension .... ⊙233
Polysporin First Aid Antibiotic Ointment.. ▣643
Polytrim Ophthalmic Solution 574

Pyrazinamide (Potential for febrile reactions and abnormal liver function tests).
No products indexed under this heading.

Rifampin (Potential for febrile reactions and abnormal liver function tests).
No products indexed under this heading.

Rifapentine (Potential for febrile reactions and abnormal liver function tests).
No products indexed under this heading.

Streptomycin Sulfate (Additive ototoxicity and/or nephrotoxicity).
No products indexed under this heading.

Tobramycin (Additive ototoxicity and/or nephrotoxicity). Products include:
TOBI Solution for Inhalation 2298
TobraDex Ophthalmic Ointment 562
TobraDex Ophthalmic Suspension ... 563
Zylet Ophthalmic Suspension .... ⊙259

Tobramycin Sulfate (Additive ototoxicity and/or nephrotoxicity).
No products indexed under this heading.

Vancomycin Hydrochloride (Additive ototoxicity and/or nephrotoxicity). Products include:
Vancocin HCl Capsules, USP 3380

Viomycin (Additive ototoxicity and/ or nephrotoxicity).
No products indexed under this heading.

CAPTOPRIL TABLETS

(Captopril) 2149
May interact with beta blockers, diuretics, ganglionic blocking agents, lithium preparations, nitrates and nitrites, non-steroidal anti-inflammatory agents, peripheral adrenergic blockers, potassium preparations, inhibitors of endogenous prostaglandin synthesis, potassium sparing diuretics, agents causing renin release, thiazides, vasodilators, and certain other agents. Compounds in these categories include:

Acebutolol Hydrochloride (Less than additive antihypertensive effect).
No products indexed under this heading.

Amiloride Hydrochloride (Hypotension; increased serum potassium). Products include:
Midamor Tablets 2026
Moduretic Tablets 2028

Amyl Nitrite (Discontinue before starting captopril; if resumed administer at lower dosage).
No products indexed under this heading.

Aspirin (Antihypertensive effects of captopril reduced). Products include:
Aggrenox Capsules 822
Bayer Aspirin 744
BC Allergy Sinus Cold Powder .... ▣677
BC Headache Powder .... ▣677
Arthritis Strength BC Powder .... ▣677
BC Sinus Cold Powder .... ▣677
Excedrin Extra Strength Caplets/Tablets/Geltabs............ ▣684
Excedrin Migraine Caplets/Tablets/Geltabs............ ▣609
Goody's Body Pain Formula Powder.. ▣684
Goody's Extra Strength Headache Powders.......................... ▣611
Goody's Extra Strength Pain Relief Tablets................................ ▣685
Percodan Tablets 1132
St. Joseph 81 mg Aspirin Chewable and Enteric Coated Tablets 1869

Atenolol (Less than additive antihypertensive effect).
No products indexed under this heading.

Bendroflumethiazide (Captopril's effect will be augmented).
No products indexed under this heading.

Betaxolol Hydrochloride (Less than additive antihypertensive effect). Products include:
Betoptic S Ophthalmic Suspension................................. 558

Bisoprolol Fumarate (Less than additive antihypertensive effect).
No products indexed under this heading.

Bumetanide (Captopril's effect will be augmented; hypotension).
Products include:
Bumex Tablets 2746

Carteolol Hydrochloride (Less than additive antihypertensive effect). Products include:
Carteolol Hydrochloride Ophthalmic Solution USP, 1%....... ⊙249

Celecoxib (Antihypertensive effects of captopril reduced). Products include:
Celebrex Capsules 3134

Chlorothiazide (Captopril's effect will be augmented). Products include:
Diuril Oral Suspension 1954

Chlorothiazide Sodium (Captopril's effect will be augmented).
Products include:
Diuril Sodium Intravenous 2467

Chlorthalidone (Captopril's effect will be augmented; hypotension; increased serum potassium).
Products include:
Clorpres Tablets 2153

Deserpidine (Use with caution).
No products indexed under this heading.

Diazoxide (Drugs having vasodilator activity should, if possible, be discontinued before starting captopril). Products include:
Hyperstat I.V. 3017

Diclofenac Potassium (Antihypertensive effects of captopril reduced).
No products indexed under this heading.

Diclofenac Sodium (Antihypertensive effects of captopril reduced).
Products include:
Arthrotec Tablets 3129
Voltaren Ophthalmic Solution 2309
Voltaren Tablets 2307
Voltaren-XR Tablets 2310

Epoprostenol Sodium (Drugs having vasodilator activity should, if possible, be discontinued before starting captopril).
No products indexed under this heading.

Erythrityl Tetranitrate (Discontinue before starting captopril; if resumed administer at lower dosage).
No products indexed under this heading.

Esmolol Hydrochloride (Less than additive antihypertensive effect).
No products indexed under this heading.

Ethacrynic Acid (Captopril's effect will be augmented; hypotension).
Products include:
Edecrin Tablets 1959

Ethaverine Hydrochloride (Drugs having vasodilator activity should, if possible, be discontinued before starting captopril).
No products indexed under this heading.

Etodolac (Antihypertensive effects of captopril reduced).
No products indexed under this heading.

Fenoprofen Calcium (Antihypertensive effects of captopril reduced).
Products include:
Nalfon Capsules 2502

Flurbiprofen (Antihypertensive effects of captopril reduced).
No products indexed under this heading.

Furosemide (Captopril's effect will be augmented; hypotension).
Products include:
Furosemide Tablets 2154

Guanethidine Monosulfate (Use with caution).
No products indexed under this heading.

Hydralazine Hydrochloride (Drugs having vasodilator activity should, if possible, be discontinued before starting captopril). Products include:
BiDil Tablets 2171

IMPORTANT NOTE: Always consult each drug listing in the patient's regimen for possible interactions.

Hydrochlorothiazide (Captopril's effect will be augmented). Products include:
- Aldoril Tablets ... 1910
- Atacand HCT ... 651
- Avalide Tablets ... 888
- Avalide Tablets ... 2874
- Benicar HCT Tablets ... 1044
- Diovan HCT Tablets ... 2196
- Dyazide Capsules ... 1423
- Hyzaar 50-12.5 Tablets ... 1990
- Hyzaar 100-12.5 Tablets ... 1990
- Hyzaar 100-25 Tablets ... 1990
- Lopressor HCT 50/25 Tablets ... 2241
- Lopressor HCT 100/25 Tablets ... 2241
- Lopressor HCT 100/50 Tablets ... 2241
- Lotensin HCT Tablets ... 2246
- Micardis HCT Tablets ... 856
- Moduretic Tablets ... 2028
- Prinzide Tablets ... 2056
- Teveten HCT Tablets ... 1737
- Timolide Tablets ... 2086
- Uniretic Tablets ... 3100

Hydroflumethiazide (Captopril's effect will be augmented).
- No products indexed under this heading.

Ibuprofen (Antihypertensive effects of captopril reduced). Products include:
- Advil Allergy Sinus Caplets ... ▣770
- Advil ... ▣674
- Children's Advil Oral Suspension ... ▣603
- Children's Advil Chewable Tablets ... ▣603
- Advil Cold & Sinus ... ▣723
- Infants' Advil Concentrated Drops ... ▣604
- Infants' Advil Concentrated Drops - White Grape (Dye-Free) ... ▣604
- Junior Strength Advil Swallow Tablets ... ▣605
- Advil Migraine Liquigels ... ▣608
- Advil Multi-Symptom Cold Caplets ... ▣770
- Advil PM Caplets ... ▣615
- Motrin IB Tablets and Caplets ... 1866
- Children's Motrin Oral Suspension ... 1867
- Children's Motrin Non-Staining Dye-Free Oral Suspension ... 1867
- Children's Motrin Cold Oral Suspension ... 1867
- Infants' Motrin Concentrated Drops ... 1867
- Infants' Motrin Non-Staining Dye-Free Concentrated Drops ... 1867
- Junior Strength Motrin Caplets and Chewable Tablets ... 1867
- Vicoprofen Tablets ... 539

Indapamide (Captopril's effect will be augmented; hypotension). Products include:
- Indapamide Tablets ... 2156

Indomethacin (Antihypertensive effects of captopril reduced). Products include:
- Indocin ... 1995

Indomethacin Sodium Trihydrate (Antihypertensive effects of captopril reduced). Products include:
- Indocin I.V. ... 2465

Isosorbide Dinitrate (Discontinue before starting captopril; if resumed administer at lower dosage). Products include:
- BiDil Tablets ... 2171

Isosorbide Mononitrate (Discontinue before starting captopril; if resumed administer at lower dosage). Products include:
- Imdur Tablets ... 3018

Isoxsuprine Hydrochloride (Drugs having vasodilator activity should, if possible, be discontinued before starting captopril).
- No products indexed under this heading.

Ketoprofen (Antihypertensive effects of captopril reduced).
- No products indexed under this heading.

Ketorolac Tromethamine (Antihypertensive effects of captopril reduced). Products include:
- Acular Ophthalmic Solution ... 565
- Acular LS Ophthalmic Solution ... 566

Labetalol Hydrochloride (Less than additive antihypertensive effect).
- No products indexed under this heading.

Levobunolol Hydrochloride (Less than additive antihypertensive effect). Products include:
- Betagan Ophthalmic Solution, USP ... ⊙220

Lithium (Increased serum lithium levels and symptoms of lithium toxicity).
- No products indexed under this heading.

Lithium Carbonate (Increased serum lithium levels and symptoms of lithium toxicity). Products include:
- Lithobid Tablets ... 1692

Lithium Citrate (Increased serum lithium levels and symptoms of lithium toxicity).
- No products indexed under this heading.

Mecamylamine Hydrochloride (Use with caution).
- No products indexed under this heading.

Meclofenamate Sodium (Antihypertensive effects of captopril reduced).
- No products indexed under this heading.

Mefenamic Acid (Antihypertensive effects of captopril reduced).
- No products indexed under this heading.

Meloxicam (Antihypertensive effects of captopril reduced). Products include:
- Mobic Oral Suspension ... 863
- Mobic Tablets ... 863

Methyclothiazide (Captopril's effect will be augmented).
- No products indexed under this heading.

Metipranolol Hydrochloride (Less than additive antihypertensive effect).
- No products indexed under this heading.

Metolazone (Captopril's effect will be augmented; hypotension).
- No products indexed under this heading.

Metoprolol Succinate (Less than additive antihypertensive effect). Products include:
- Toprol-XL Tablets ... 668

Metoprolol Tartrate (Less than additive antihypertensive effect). Products include:
- Lopressor Injection ... 2238
- Lopressor Tablets ... 2238
- Lopressor HCT 50/25 Tablets ... 2241
- Lopressor HCT 100/25 Tablets ... 2241
- Lopressor HCT 100/50 Tablets ... 2241

Minoxidil (Drugs having vasodilator activity should, if possible, be discontinued before starting captopril). Products include:
- Men's Rogaine Extra Strength Hair Regrowth Treatment Topical Solution, Ocean Rush Scent and Original Unscented ... ▣633
- Men's Rogaine Foam Hair Regrowth Treatment ... ▣633
- Women's Rogaine Hair Regrowth Treatment Topical Solution, Spring Bloom Scent and Original Unscented ... ▣634

Nabumetone (Antihypertensive effects of captopril reduced).
- No products indexed under this heading.

Nadolol (Less than additive antihypertensive effect). Products include:
- Nadolol Tablets ... 2159

Naproxen (Antihypertensive effects of captopril reduced). Products include:
- EC-Naprosyn Delayed-Release Tablets ... 2761
- Naprosyn Suspension ... 2761
- Naprosyn Tablets ... 2761
- Prevacid NapraPAC ... 3280

Naproxen Sodium (Antihypertensive effects of captopril reduced). Products include:
- Aleve Caplets ... 742
- Aleve Gelcaps ... 743
- Aleve Tablets ... 743
- Aleve Cold & Sinus Caplets ... 744
- Anaprox Tablets ... 2761
- Anaprox DS Tablets ... 2761

Nitroglycerin (Discontinue before starting captopril; if resumed administer at lower dosage). Products include:
- Nitro-Dur Transdermal Infusion System ... 3046
- Nitrolingual Pumpspray ... 3120

Nitroglycerin, long-acting formulations (Drugs having vasodilator activity should, if possible, be discontinued before starting captopril).
- No products indexed under this heading.

Nitroglycerin Intravenous (Drugs having vasodilator activity should, if possible, be discontinued before starting captopril).
- No products indexed under this heading.

Oxaprozin (Antihypertensive effects of captopril reduced).
- No products indexed under this heading.

Papaverine (Drugs having vasodilator activity should, if possible, be discontinued before starting captopril).
- No products indexed under this heading.

Papaverine Hydrochloride (Drugs having vasodilator activity should, if possible, be discontinued before starting captopril).
- No products indexed under this heading.

Penbutolol Sulfate (Less than additive antihypertensive effect).
- No products indexed under this heading.

Pentaerythritol Tetranitrate (Discontinue before starting captopril; if resumed administer at lower dosage).
- No products indexed under this heading.

Phenylbutazone (Antihypertensive effects of captopril reduced).
- No products indexed under this heading.

Pindolol (Less than additive antihypertensive effect).
- No products indexed under this heading.

Piroxicam (Antihypertensive effects of captopril reduced).
- No products indexed under this heading.

Polythiazide (Captopril's effect will be augmented).
- No products indexed under this heading.

Potassium Acid Phosphate (Potential for significant increase in serum potassium). Products include:
- K-Phos Original (Sodium Free) Tablets ... 760

Potassium Bicarbonate (Potential for significant increase in serum potassium).
- No products indexed under this heading.

Potassium Chloride (Potential for significant increase in serum potassium). Products include:
- Colyte with Flavor Packs for Oral Solution ... 3088
- HalfLytely and Bisacodyl Tablets Bowel Prep Kit with Flavors Packs ... 881
- K-Dur Extended-Relase Tablets ... 3033
- K-Lor Oral Solution ... 474
- K-Tab Tablets ... 475
- MoviPrep Oral Solution ... 2839
- TriLyte with Flavor Packs for Oral Solution ... 3100

Potassium Citrate (Potential for significant increase in serum potassium). Products include:
- Urocit-K Tablets ... 2144

Potassium Gluconate (Potential for significant increase in serum potassium).
- No products indexed under this heading.

Potassium Phosphate (Potential for significant increase in serum potassium). Products include:
- K-Phos Neutral Tablets ... 760

Prazosin Hydrochloride (Use with caution).
- No products indexed under this heading.

Propranolol Hydrochloride (Less than additive antihypertensive effect). Products include:
- Inderal LA Long-Acting Capsules ... 3429
- InnoPran XL Capsules ... 2723

Rauwolfia Serpentina (Use with caution).
- No products indexed under this heading.

Rescinnamine (Use with caution).
- No products indexed under this heading.

Reserpine (Use with caution).
- No products indexed under this heading.

Rofecoxib (Antihypertensive effects of captopril reduced).
- No products indexed under this heading.

Sotalol Hydrochloride (Less than additive antihypertensive effect).
- No products indexed under this heading.

Spironolactone (Captopril's effect will be augmented; hypotension; increased serum potassium).
- No products indexed under this heading.

Sulindac (Antihypertensive effects of captopril reduced). Products include:
- Clinoril Tablets ... 1924

Terazosin Hydrochloride (Use with caution). Products include:
- Hytrin Capsules ... 471

Timolol Hemihydrate (Less than additive antihypertensive effect). Products include:
- Betimol Ophthalmic Solution ... 3382
- Betimol Ophthalmic Solution ... ⊙295

Timolol Maleate (Less than additive antihypertensive effect). Products include:
- Blocadren Tablets ... 1916

Cosopt Sterile Ophthalmic Solution 1931
Timolide Tablets 2086
Timoptic Sterile Ophthalmic Solution 2088
Timoptic in Ocudose 2091
Timoptic-XE Sterile Ophthalmic Gel Forming Solution 2092

Tolazoline Hydrochloride (Drugs having vasodilator activity should, if possible, be discontinued before starting captopril).
No products indexed under this heading.

Tolmetin Sodium (Antihypertensive effects of captopril reduced).
No products indexed under this heading.

Torsemide (Captopril's effect will be augmented; hypotension). Products include:
Demadex Injection 2759
Demadex Tablets 2759

Triamterene (Captopril's effect will be augmented; hypotension; increased serum potassium). Products include:
Dyazide Capsules 1423
Dyrenium Capsules 3400

Trimethaphan Camsylate (Use with caution).
No products indexed under this heading.

Valdecoxib (Antihypertensive effects of captopril reduced).
No products indexed under this heading.

Food Interactions

Alcohol (Drugs having vasodilator activity should, if possible, be discontinued before starting captopril).

Food, unspecified (Reduces absorption by about 30% to 40%; should be given one hour before meals).

CARAC CREAM, 0.5%

(Fluorouracil) 2879
None cited in PDR database.

CARAFATE SUSPENSION

(Sucralfate) 701
May interact with fluoroquinolone antibiotics, quinidine, xanthines, and certain other agents. Compounds in these categories include:

Alatrofloxacin Mesylate (Potential for reduced extent of absorption (bioavailability) with concomitant oral administration; dosing the concomitant medication 2 hours before sucralfate eliminates the interaction).
No products indexed under this heading.

Aluminum Carbonate (Simultaneous administration within one-half hour before or after sucralfate should be avoided; may increase the total body burden of aluminum).
No products indexed under this heading.

Aluminum Hydroxide (Simultaneous administration within one-half hour before or after sucralfate should be avoided; may increase the total body burden of aluminum). Products include:
Gaviscon Regular Strength Liquid 658
Gaviscon Regular Strength Tablets 658
Gaviscon Extra Strength Liquid 658
Gaviscon Extra Strength Tablets 658
Maalox Regular Strength Antacid/Antigas Liquid 2175
Maalox Max Maximum Strength Antacid/Anti-Gas Liquid 2176

Aminophylline (Simultaneous administration results in reduced oral absorption of theophylline).
No products indexed under this heading.

Cimetidine (Simultaneous administration results in reduced oral absorption of oral cimetidine; dosing the concomitant medication 2 hours before sucralfate eliminates the interaction). Products include:
Tagamet HB 200 Tablets 664

Cimetidine Hydrochloride (Simultaneous administration results in reduced oral absorption of oral cimetidine; dosing the concomitant medication 2 hours before sucralfate eliminates the interaction).
No products indexed under this heading.

Ciprofloxacin (Potential for reduced extent of absorption (bioavailability) with concomitant oral administration; dosing the concomitant medication 2 hours before sucralfate eliminates the interaction). Products include:
Cipro Oral Suspension 2977
Cipro I.V. 2984
Cipro XR Tablets 2990
Ciprodex Otic Suspension 559

Ciprofloxacin Hydrochloride (Potential for reduced extent of absorption (bioavailability) with concomitant oral administration; dosing the concomitant medication 2 hours before sucralfate eliminates the interaction). Products include:
Ciloxan Ophthalmic Ointment 559
Ciloxan Ophthalmic Solution .... ⊙ 206
Cipro Tablets 2977
Proquin XR Tablets 1153

Digoxin (Simultaneous administration results in reduced oral absorption of oral digoxin; dosing the concomitant medication 2 hours before sucralfate eliminates the interaction). Products include:
Lanoxicaps Capsules 1490
Lanoxin Injection 1494
Lanoxin Injection Pediatric 1497
Lanoxin Tablets 1500

Dyphylline (Simultaneous administration results in reduced oral absorption of theophylline).
No products indexed under this heading.

Enoxacin (Potential for reduced extent of absorption (bioavailability) with concomitant oral administration; dosing the concomitant medication 2 hours before sucralfate eliminates the interaction).
No products indexed under this heading.

Grepafloxacin Hydrochloride (Potential for reduced extent of absorption (bioavailability) with concomitant oral administration; dosing the concomitant medication 2 hours before sucralfate eliminates the interaction).
No products indexed under this heading.

Ketoconazole (Simultaneous administration results in reduced oral absorption of oral ketoconazole). Products include:
Nizoral A-D Shampoo, 1% 1868

Levothyroxine Sodium (Potential for reduced extent of absorption (bioavailability) with concomitant oral administration). Products include:
Levothroid Tablets 1186
Levoxyl Tablets 1712
Synthroid Tablets 520
Westhroid Tablets 3403

Lomefloxacin Hydrochloride (Potential for reduced extent of absorption (bioavailability) with concomitant oral administration; dosing the concomitant medication 2 hours before sucralfate eliminates the interaction).
No products indexed under this heading.

Magnesium Hydroxide (Simultaneous administration within one-half hour before or after sucralfate should be avoided; may increase the total body burden of aluminum). Products include:
Maalox Regular Strength Antacid/Antigas Liquid 2175
Maalox Max Maximum Strength Antacid/Anti-Gas Liquid 2176
Pepcid Complete Chewable Tablets 1701

Magnesium Oxide (Simultaneous administration within one-half hour before or after sucralfate should be avoided; may increase the total body burden of aluminum). Products include:
Beelith Tablets 759
PremCal Light, Regular, and Extra Strength Tablets 818

Moxifloxacin Hydrochloride (Potential for reduced extent of absorption (bioavailability) with concomitant oral administration; dosing the concomitant medication 2 hours before sucralfate eliminates the interaction). Products include:
Avelox 2970
Vigamox Ophthalmic Solution 564

Norfloxacin (Potential for reduced extent of absorption (bioavailability) with concomitant oral administration; dosing the concomitant medication 2 hours before sucralfate eliminates the interaction). Products include:
Noroxin Tablets 2032

Ofloxacin (Potential for reduced extent of absorption (bioavailability) with concomitant oral administration; dosing the concomitant medication 2 hours before sucralfate eliminates the interaction). Products include:
Floxin Otic Solution 1049

Phenytoin (Simultaneous administration results in reduced oral absorption of oral phenytoin).
No products indexed under this heading.

Phenytoin Sodium (Simultaneous administration results in reduced oral absorption of oral phenytoin). Products include:
Phenytek Capsules 2160

Quinidine (Potential for reduced extent of absorption (bioavailability) with concomitant oral administration).
No products indexed under this heading.

Quinidine Gluconate (Potential for reduced extent of absorption (bioavailability) with concomitant oral administration).
No products indexed under this heading.

Quinidine Hydrochloride (Potential for reduced extent of absorption (bioavailability) with concomitant oral administration).
No products indexed under this heading.

Quinidine Polygalacturonate (Potential for reduced extent of absorption (bioavailability) with concomitant oral administration).
No products indexed under this heading.

Quinidine Sulfate (Potential for reduced extent of absorption (bioavailability) with concomitant oral administration).
No products indexed under this heading.

Ranitidine Hydrochloride (Simultaneous administration results in reduced oral absorption of oral ranitidine; dosing the concomitant medication 2 hours before sucralfate eliminates the interaction). Products include:
Zantac 1624
Zantac Injection 1619
Zantac Injection Pharmacy Bulk Package 1622

Tetracycline Hydrochloride (Simultaneous administration results in reduced oral absorption of oral tetracycline).
No products indexed under this heading.

Theophylline (Simultaneous administration results in reduced oral absorption of theophylline).
No products indexed under this heading.

Theophylline Anhydrous (Simultaneous administration results in reduced oral absorption of theophylline). Products include:
Uniphyl Tablets 2710

Theophylline Calcium Salicylate (Simultaneous administration results in reduced oral absorption of theophylline).
No products indexed under this heading.

Theophylline Dihydroxypropyl (Glyceryl) (Simultaneous administration results in reduced oral absorption of theophylline).
No products indexed under this heading.

Theophylline Ethylenediamine (Simultaneous administration results in reduced oral absorption of theophylline).
No products indexed under this heading.

Theophylline Sodium Glycinate (Simultaneous administration results in reduced oral absorption of theophylline).
No products indexed under this heading.

Trovafloxacin Mesylate (Potential for reduced extent of absorption (bioavailability) with concomitant oral administration; dosing the concomitant medication 2 hours before sucralfate eliminates the interaction).
No products indexed under this heading.

Warfarin Sodium (Subtherapeutic prothrombin times with concomitant warfarin and sucralfate have been reported in spontaneous and published reports; clinical studies have demonstrated no changes in the prothrombin time with the addition of sucralfate to chronic warfarin therapy). Products include:
Coumadin for Injection 898
Coumadin Tablets 898

CARAFATE TABLETS

(Sucralfate) 701
May interact with fluoroquinolone antibiotics, quinidine, xanthines, and certain other agents. Compounds in these categories include:

Alatrofloxacin Mesylate (Potential for reduced extent of absorption (bioavailability) with concomitant oral administration; dosing the concomitant medication 2 hours before sucralfate eliminates the interaction).
No products indexed under this heading.

Aluminum Carbonate (Simultaneous administration within one-half hour before or after sucralfate should be avoided; may increase the total body burden of aluminum).
No products indexed under this heading.

Aluminum Hydroxide (Simultaneous administration within one-half hour before or after sucralfate should be avoided; may increase the total body burden of aluminum).
Products include:
Gaviscon Regular Strength Liquid .. 🔲658
Gaviscon Regular Strength Tablets............................. 🔲658
Gaviscon Extra Strength Liquid 🔲658
Gaviscon Extra Strength Tablets 🔲658
Maalox Regular Strength Antacid/Antigas Liquid................. 2175
Maalox Max Maximum Strength Antacid/Anti-Gas Liquid................. 2176

Aminophylline (Simultaneous administration results in reduced oral absorption of theophylline).
No products indexed under this heading.

Cimetidine (Simultaneous administration results in reduced oral absorption of oral cimetidine; dosing the concomitant medication 2 hours before sucralfate eliminates the interaction). Products include:
Tagamet HB 200 Tablets 🔲664

Cimetidine Hydrochloride (Simultaneous administration results in reduced oral absorption of oral cimetidine; dosing the concomitant medication 2 hours before sucralfate eliminates the interaction).
No products indexed under this heading.

Ciprofloxacin (Potential for reduced extent of absorption (bioavailability) with concomitant oral administration; dosing the concomitant medication 2 hours before sucralfate eliminates the interaction). Products include:
Cipro Oral Suspension 2977
Cipro I.V. 2984
Cipro XR Tablets 2990
Ciprodex Otic Suspension 559

Ciprofloxacin Hydrochloride (Potential for reduced extent of absorption (bioavailability) with concomitant oral administration; dosing the concomitant medication 2 hours before sucralfate eliminates the interaction). Products include:
Ciloxan Ophthalmic Ointment 559
Ciloxan Ophthalmic Solution ⊙206
Cipro Tablets 2977
Proquin XR Tablets 1153

Digoxin (Simultaneous administration results in reduced oral absorption of oral digoxin; dosing the concomitant medication 2 hours before sucralfate eliminates the interaction). Products include:
Lanoxicaps Capsules 1490
Lanoxin Injection 1494
Lanoxin Injection Pediatric 1497

Lanoxin Tablets 1500

Dyphylline (Simultaneous administration results in reduced oral absorption of theophylline).
No products indexed under this heading.

Enoxacin (Potential for reduced extent of absorption (bioavailability) with concomitant oral administration; dosing the concomitant medication 2 hours before sucralfate eliminates the interaction).
No products indexed under this heading.

Grepafloxacin Hydrochloride (Potential for reduced extent of absorption (bioavailability) with concomitant oral administration; dosing the concomitant medication 2 hours before sucralfate eliminates the interaction).
No products indexed under this heading.

Ketoconazole (Simultaneous administration results in reduced oral absorption of oral ketoconazole). Products include:
Nizoral A-D Shampoo, 1% 1868

Levothyroxine Sodium (Potential for reduced extent of absorption (bioavailability) with concomitant oral administration). Products include:
Levothroid Tablets 1186
Levoxyl Tablets 1712
Synthroid Tablets 520
Westhroid Tablets 3403

Lomefloxacin Hydrochloride (Potential for reduced extent of absorption (bioavailability) with concomitant oral administration; dosing the concomitant medication 2 hours before sucralfate eliminates the interaction).
No products indexed under this heading.

Magnesium Hydroxide (Simultaneous administration within one-half hour before or after sucralfate should be avoided; may increase the total body burden of aluminum).
Products include:
Maalox Regular Strength Antacid/Antigas Liquid................. 2175
Maalox Max Maximum Strength Antacid/Anti-Gas Liquid................. 2176
Pepcid Complete Chewable Tablets 1701

Magnesium Oxide (Simultaneous administration within one-half hour before or after sucralfate should be avoided; may increase the total body burden of aluminum). Products include:
Beelith Tablets 759
PremCal Light, Regular, and Extra Strength Tablets................. 🔲818

Moxifloxacin Hydrochloride (Potential for reduced extent of absorption (bioavailability) with concomitant oral administration; dosing the concomitant medication 2 hours before sucralfate eliminates the interaction). Products include:
Avelox ... 2970
Vigamox Ophthalmic Solution 564

Norfloxacin (Potential for reduced extent of absorption (bioavailability) with concomitant oral administration; dosing the concomitant medication 2 hours before sucralfate eliminates the interaction). Products include:
Noroxin Tablets 2032

Ofloxacin (Potential for reduced extent of absorption (bioavailability) with concomitant oral administration;

dosing the concomitant medication 2 hours before sucralfate eliminates the interaction). Products include:
Floxin Otic Solution 1049

Phenytoin (Simultaneous administration results in reduced oral absorption of oral phenytoin).
No products indexed under this heading.

Phenytoin Sodium (Simultaneous administration results in reduced oral absorption of oral phenytoin). Products include:
Phenytek Capsules 2160

Quinidine (Potential for reduced extent of absorption (bioavailability) with concomitant oral administration).
No products indexed under this heading.

Quinidine Gluconate (Potential for reduced extent of absorption (bioavailability) with concomitant oral administration).
No products indexed under this heading.

Quinidine Hydrochloride (Potential for reduced extent of absorption (bioavailability) with concomitant oral administration).
No products indexed under this heading.

Quinidine Polygalacturonate (Potential for reduced extent of absorption (bioavailability) with concomitant oral administration).
No products indexed under this heading.

Quinidine Sulfate (Potential for reduced extent of absorption (bioavailability) with concomitant oral administration).
No products indexed under this heading.

Ranitidine Hydrochloride (Simultaneous administration results in reduced oral absorption of oral ranitidine; dosing the concomitant medication 2 hours before sucralfate eliminates the interaction). Products include:
Zantac ... 1624
Zantac Injection 1619
Zantac Injection Pharmacy Bulk Package 1622

Tetracycline Hydrochloride (Simultaneous administration results in reduced oral absorption of oral tetracycline).
No products indexed under this heading.

Theophylline (Simultaneous administration results in reduced oral absorption of theophylline).
No products indexed under this heading.

Theophylline Anhydrous (Simultaneous administration results in reduced oral absorption of theophylline). Products include:
Uniphyl Tablets 2710

Theophylline Calcium Salicylate (Simultaneous administration results in reduced oral absorption of theophylline).
No products indexed under this heading.

Theophylline Dihydroxypropyl (Glyceryl) (Simultaneous administration results in reduced oral absorption of theophylline).
No products indexed under this heading.

Theophylline Ethylenediamine (Simultaneous administration results in reduced oral absorption of theophylline).
No products indexed under this heading.

Theophylline Sodium Glycinate (Simultaneous administration results in reduced oral absorption of theophylline).
No products indexed under this heading.

Trovafloxacin Mesylate (Potential for reduced extent of absorption (bioavailability) with concomitant oral administration; dosing the concomitant medication 2 hours before sucralfate eliminates the interaction).
No products indexed under this heading.

Warfarin Sodium (Subtherapeutic prothrombin times with concomitant warfarin and sucralfate have been reported in spontaneous and published reports; clinical studies have demonstrated no changes in the prothrombin time with the addition of sucralfate to chronic warfarin therapy). Products include:
Coumadin for Injection 898
Coumadin Tablets 898

CARBATROL CAPSULES

(Carbamazepine) 3171
May interact with antimalarials, cytochrome p450 1a2 substrates (selected), cytochrome p450 3a4 inducers (selected), cytochrome p450 3a4 inhibitors (selected), cytochrome p450 3a4 substrates (selected), doxycycline, anticonvulsants, erythromycin, lithium preparations, macrolide antibiotics, monoamine oxidase inhibitors, antipsychotic agents, oral contraceptives, phenytoin, valproate, xanthines, and certain other agents. Compounds in these categories include:

Acetaminophen (Carbamazepine induces hepatic CYP activity and causes or would be expected to decrease plasma levels of acetaminophen). Products include:
Comtrex Maximum Strength Cold & Cough Day/Night Caplets - Day Formulation.......................... 🔲726
Comtrex Maximum Strength Cold & Cough Day/Night Caplets - Night Formulation 🔲726
Comtrex Maximum Strength Non-Drowsy Cold & Cough Caplets....................................... 🔲725
Comtrex Maximum Strength Day/Night Severe Cold & Sinus Caplets - Day Formulation 🔲725
Comtrex Maximum Strength Day/Night Severe Cold & Sinus Caplets - Night Formulation 🔲725
Contac Cold and Flu Maximum Strength Caplets....................... 🔲728
Contac Cold and Flu Day and Night Caplets (Day Formulation Only).. 🔲727
Contac Cold and Flu Day and Night Caplets (Night Formulation Only)....................... 🔲727
Contac Cold and Flu Non-Drowsy Caplets....................................... 🔲728
Excedrin Extra Strength Caplets/Tablets/Geltabs............... 🔲684
Excedrin Migraine Caplets/Tablets/Geltabs............... 🔲609
Excedrin PM Caplets/Tablets/Geltabs............. 🔲610
Excedrin Sinus Headache Caplets/Tablets.......................... 🔲610
Excedrin Tension Headache Caplets/Tablets/Geltabs............. 🔲611
Goody's Body Pain Formula Powder...................................... 🔲684
Goody's Extra Strength Headache Powders..................... 🔲611

Goody's Extra Strength Pain Relief Tablets .... ■685
Goody's PM Powder for Pain with Sleeplessness .... ■612
Percocet Tablets 1131
Robitussin Cough, Cold & Flu Nighttime Liquid .... ■738
TheraFlu Cold & Sore Throat Hot Liquid .... ■741
TheraFlu Flu & Chest Congestion Hot Liquid .... ■741
TheraFlu Flu & Sore Throat Hot Liquid .... ■742
TheraFlu Daytime Severe Cold Hot Liquid .... ■742
TheraFlu Nighttime Severe Cold Hot Liquid .... ■740
TheraFlu Warming Relief Daytime Severe Cold .... ■743
TheraFlu Warming Relief Nighttime Severe Cold .... ■743
Triaminic Cough & Sore Throat Liquid .... ■747
Regular Strength Tylenol Tablets 1870
Children's Tylenol with Flavor Creator .... ■679
Children's Tylenol Plus Flu Oral Suspension .... ■749
Tylenol Cold Head Congestion Daytime Caplets with Cool Burst and Gelcaps .... ■750
Tylenol Cold Multi-Symptom Daytime Liquid .... ■752
Tylenol Cold Multi-Symptom Severe Daytime Liquid .... ■752
Tylenol 8 Hour Extended Release Caplets 1870
Tylenol 1870
Extra Strength Tylenol PM Caplets, Vanilla Caplets, Geltabs, Gelcaps and Liquid 1875
Extra Strength Tylenol Rapid Release Gels 1870
Concentrated Tylenol Infants' Drops Plus Cold & Cough .... ■754
Tylenol with Codeine Tablets 2391
Tylenol Allergy Multi-Symptom Caplets with Cool Burst and Gelcaps 1872
Tylenol Allergy Multi-Symptom Nighttime Caplets with Cool Burst 1872
Tylenol Severe Allergy Caplets 1872
Tylenol Arthritis Pain Extended Release Caplets and Geltabs 1870
Tylenol Chest Congestion Caplets with Cool Burst 1872
Tylenol Chest Congestion Liquid with Cool Burst 1872
Children's Tylenol Suspension Liquid and Meltaways 1878
Children's Tylenol Plus Cold Suspension Liquid 1879
Children's Tylenol Plus Cold & Allergy Suspension Liquid 1878
Children's Tylenol Plus Cough & Runny Nose Suspension Liquid 1879
Children's Tylenol Plus Cough & Sore Throat Suspension Liquid 1879
Children's Tylenol Suspension with Flavor Creator 1878
Children's Tylenol Plus Flu Suspension Liquid 1881
Children's Tylenol Plus Multi-Symptom Cold Suspension Liquid 1879
Tylenol Cold Severe Congestion Non-Drowsy Caplets with Cool Burst 1874
Tylenol Cold Head Congestion Daytime Caplets with Cool Burst 1873
Tylenol Cold Head Congestion Nighttime Caplets with Cool Burst 1873
Tylenol Cold Head Congestion Severe Caplets with Cool Burst 1873
Tylenol Cold Multi-Symptom Daytime Caplets with Cool Burst and Gelcaps 1874
Tylenol Cold Multi-Symptom Daytime Liquid with Citrus Burst 1874
Tylenol Cold Multi-Symptom Nighttime Caplets with Cool Burst 1874
Tylenol Cold Multi-Symptom Nighttime Liquid with Cool Burst 1874
Tylenol Cold Multi-Symptom Severe Caplets with Cool Burst 1874
Tylenol Cold Multi-Symptom Severe Daytime Liquid with Citrus Burst 1874
Tylenol Cough & Sore Throat Daytime Liquid with Cool Burst 1877
Tylenol Cough & Sore Throat Nighttime Liquid with Cool Burst 1877
Concentrated Tylenol Infants' Drops 1878
Concentrated Tylenol Infants' Drops Plus Cold 1879
Concentrated Tylenol Infants' Drops Plus Cold and Cough 1879
Jr. Tylenol Meltaways 1878
Tylenol Sinus Severe Congestion Caplets with Cool Burst 1876
Tylenol Sinus Congestion & Pain Daytime Caplets with Cool Burst and Gelcaps 1876
Tylenol Sinus Congestion & Pain Nighttime Caplets with Cool Burst 1876
Tylenol Sinus Congestion & Pain Severe Caplets with Cool Burst 1876
Tylenol Sore Throat Daytime Liquid with Cool Burst 1877
Tylenol Sore Throat Nighttime Liquid with Cool Burst 1877
Women's Tylenol Menstrual Relief Caplets 1877
Vicks 44M Cough, Cold & Flu Relief Liquid 2680
Vicks DayQuil LiquiCaps/Liquid Multi-Symptom Cold/Flu Relief .... ■761
Vicks DayQuil Multi-Symptom Cold/Flu Relief LiquiCaps 2678
Vicks DayQuil Multi-Symptom Cold/Flu Relief Liquid 2678
Vicks NyQuil Multi-Symptom Cold/Flu Relief Liquid 2681
Vicks NyQuil Multi-Symptom Cold/Flu Relief LiquiCaps 2681
Vicks NyQuil LiquiCaps/Liquid Multi-Symptom Cold/Flu Relief .... ■763
Vicodin Tablets 535
Vicodin ES Tablets 536
Vicodin HP Tablets 538
Zicam Maximum Strength Flu Daytime .... ■768
Zicam Maximum Strength Flu Nighttime .... ■768
Zydone Tablets 1139

Acetazolamide (Carbamazepine is metabolized mainly by cytochrome P450 (CYP) 3A4 to the active carbamazepine 10,11 -epoxide, which is further metabolized to the trans-diol by epoxide hydrolase. Therefore, the potential exists for interaction between carbamazepine and any agent that inhibits CYP3A4 and/or epoxide hydrolase).
No products indexed under this heading.

Alatrofloxacin Mesylate (Carbamazepine is known to induce CYP1A2 and CYP3A4. Therefore, the potential exists for interaction between carbamazepine and any agent metabolized by one (or more) of these enzymes).
No products indexed under this heading.

Alfentanil Hydrochloride (Carbamazepine is known to induce CYP1A2 and CYP3A4. Therefore, the potential exists for interaction between carbamazepine and any agent metabolized by one (or more) of these enzymes).
No products indexed under this heading.

Allium sativum (Carbamazepine is metabolized by CYP3A4. Therefore, the potential exists for interaction between caramazepine and any agent that induces CYP3A4).
No products indexed under this heading.

Alprazolam (Carbamazepine induces hepatic CYP activity and causes or would be expected to decrease plasma levels of alprazolam). Products include:
Niravam Orally Disintegrating Tablets 3092

Aminophylline (Inducers of CYP3A4, such as theophylline, can increase the rate of carbamazepine metabolism and can thus decrease plasma carbamazepine levels; carbamazepine induces hepatic CYP activity and causes or would be expected to decrease plasma levels of theophylline).
No products indexed under this heading.

Amiodarone Hydrochloride (Carbamazepine is metabolized mainly by cytochrome P450 (CYP) 3A4 to the active carbamazepine 10,11 -epoxide, which is further metabolized to the trans-diol by epoxide hydrolase. Therefore, the potential exists for interaction between carbamazepine and any agent that inhibits CYP3A4 and/or epoxide hydrolase).
No products indexed under this heading.

Amitriptyline Hydrochloride (Carbamazepine is known to induce CYP1A2 and CYP3A4. Therefore, the potential exists for interaction between carbamazepine and any agent metabolized by one (or more) of these enzymes).
No products indexed under this heading.

Amlodipine Besylate (Carbamazepine is known to induce CYP1A2 and CYP3A4. Therefore, the potential exists for interaction between carbamazepine and any agent metabolized by one (or more) of these enzymes). Products include:
Caduet Tablets 2508
Lotrel Capsules 2249
Norvasc Tablets 2545

Amoxapine (Carbamazepine is known to induce CYP1A2 and CYP3A4. Therefore, the potential exists for interaction between carbamazepine and any agent metabolized by one (or more) of these enzymes).
No products indexed under this heading.

Amprenavir (Carbamazepine is metabolized mainly by cytochrome P450 (CYP) 3A4 to the active carbamazepine 10,11 -epoxide, which is further metabolized to the trans-diol by epoxide hydrolase. Therefore, the potential exists for interaction between carbamazepine and any agent that inhibits CYP3A4 and/or epoxide hydrolase). Products include:
Agenerase Capsules 1327
Agenerase Oral Solution 1332

Anagrelide Hydrochloride (Carbamazepine is known to induce CYP1A2 and CYP3A4. Therefore, the potential exists for interaction between carbamazepine and any agent metabolized by one (or more) of these enzymes). Products include:
Agrylin Capsules 3169

Anastrozole (Carbamazepine is metabolized mainly by cytochrome P450 (CYP) 3A4 to the active carbamazepine 10,11 -epoxide, which is further metabolized to the trans-diol by epoxide hydrolase. Therefore, the potential exists for interaction between carbamazepine and any agent that inhibits CYP3A4 and/or epoxide hydrolase). Products include:
Arimidex Tablets 673

Aprepitant (Carbamazepine is metabolized mainly by cytochrome P450 (CYP) 3A4 to the active carbamazepine 10,11 -epoxide, which is further metabolized to the trans-diol by epoxide hydrolase. Therefore, the potential exists for interaction between carbamazepine and any agent that inhibits CYP3A4 and/or epoxide hydrolase). Products include:
Emend Capsules 1963

Aripiprazole (Co-administration with psychotropic agents has resulted in isolated cases of neuroleptic malignant syndrome). Products include:
Abilify Oral Solution 882
Abilify Oral Solution 2450
Abilify Discmelt Orally Disintegrating Tablets 882
Abilify Discmelt Orally Disintegrating Tablets 2450
Abilify Tablets 882
Abilify Tablets 2450

Astemizole (Carbamazepine is known to induce CYP1A2 and CYP3A4. Therefore, the potential exists for interaction between carbamazepine and any agent metabolized by one (or more) of these enzymes).
No products indexed under this heading.

Atorvastatin Calcium (Carbamazepine is known to induce CYP1A2 and CYP3A4. Therefore, the potential exists for interaction between carbamazepine and any agent metabolized by one (or more) of these enzymes). Products include:
Caduet Tablets 2508
Lipitor Tablets 2483

Azithromycin Dihydrate (Inhibitors of CYP3A4, such as macrolides, inhibit carbamazepine metabolism and thus increase plasma carbamazepine levels).
No products indexed under this heading.

Belladonna Ergotamine (Carbamazepine is known to induce CYP1A2 and CYP3A4. Therefore, the potential exists for interaction between carbamazepine and any agent metabolized by one (or more) of these enzymes).
No products indexed under this heading.

Betamethasone Acetate (Carbamazepine is metabolized by CYP3A4. Therefore, the potential exists for interaction between caramazepine and any agent that induces CYP3A4).
No products indexed under this heading.

Betamethasone Sodium Phosphate (Carbamazepine is metabolized by CYP3A4. Therefore, the potential exists for interaction between caramazepine and any agent that induces CYP3A4).
No products indexed under this heading.

Buspirone Hydrochloride (Carbamazepine is known to induce CYP1A2 and CYP3A4. Therefore, the potential exists for interaction between carbamazepine and any agent metabolized by one (or more) of these enzymes).
No products indexed under this heading.

Busulfan (Carbamazepine is known to induce CYP1A2 and CYP3A4. Therefore, the potential exists for interaction between carbamazepine and any agent metabolized by one (or more) of these enzymes). Products include:
- I.V. Busulfex 2493
- Myleran Tablets 1525

Caffeine (Carbamazepine is known to induce CYP1A2 and CYP3A4. Therefore, the potential exists for interaction between carbamazepine and any agent metabolized by one (or more) of these enzymes). Products include:
- BC Headache Powder .... ▣677
- Arthritis Strength BC Powder .... ▣677
- Excedrin Extra Strength Caplets/Tablets/Geltabs .... ▣684
- Excedrin Migraine Caplets/Tablets/Geltabs .... ▣609
- Excedrin Tension Headache Caplets/Tablets/Geltabs .... ▣611
- Goody's Extra Strength Headache Powders .... ▣611
- Goody's Extra Strength Pain Relief Tablets .... ▣685
- Vivarin .... ▣602
- Winrgy Dietary Supplement .... ▣823

Caffeine Anhydrous (Carbamazepine is known to induce CYP1A2 and CYP3A4. Therefore, the potential exists for interaction between carbamazepine and any agent metabolized by one (or more) of these enzymes).
No products indexed under this heading.

Cerivastatin Sodium (Carbamazepine is known to induce CYP1A2 and CYP3A4. Therefore, the potential exists for interaction between carbamazepine and any agent metabolized by one (or more) of these enzymes).
No products indexed under this heading.

Chlordiazepoxide (Carbamazepine is known to induce CYP1A2 and CYP3A4. Therefore, the potential exists for interaction between carbamazepine and any agent metabolized by one (or more) of these enzymes).
No products indexed under this heading.

Chlordiazepoxide Hydrochloride (Carbamazepine is known to induce CYP1A2 and CYP3A4. Therefore, the potential exists for interaction between carbamazepine and any agent metabolized by one (or more) of these enzymes). Products include:
- Librium Capsules 3347

Chloroquine Hydrochloride (Antimalarial drugs, such as chloroquine and mefloquine, may antagonize the activity of carbamazepine).
No products indexed under this heading.

Chloroquine Phosphate (Antimalarial drugs, such as chloroquine and mefloquine, may antagonize the activity of carbamazepine).
No products indexed under this heading.

Chlorpheniramine (Carbamazepine is known to induce CYP1A2 and CYP3A4. Therefore, the potential exists for interaction between carbamazepine and any agent metabolized by one (or more) of these enzymes).
No products indexed under this heading.

Chlorpheniramine Maleate (Carbamazepine is known to induce CYP1A2 and CYP3A4. Therefore, the potential exists for interaction between carbamazepine and any agent metabolized by one (or more) of these enzymes). Products include:
- Advil Allergy Sinus Caplets .... ▣770
- Advil Multi-Symptom Cold Caplets .... ▣770
- BC Allergy Sinus Cold Powder .... ▣677
- Comtrex Maximum Strength Cold & Cough Day/Night Caplets - Night Formulation .... ▣726
- Comtrex Maximum Strength Day/Night Severe Cold & Sinus Caplets - Night Formulation .... ▣725
- Contac Cold and Flu Maximum Strength Caplets .... ▣728
- Contac Cold and Flu Day and Night Caplets (Night Formulation Only) .... ▣727
- Children's Dimetapp Long Acting Cough Plus Cold Syrup .... ▣731
- Robitussin Cough & Cold Long-Acting Liquid .... ▣735
- Robitussin Cough & Allergy Syrup .. ▣736
- Robitussin Cough & Cold Nighttime Liquid .... ▣736
- Robitussin Cough, Cold & Flu Nighttime Liquid .... ▣738
- Robitussin Pediatric Cough & Cold Long-Acting Liquid .... ▣735
- Robitussin Pediatric Cough & Cold Nighttime Liquid .... ▣736
- Triaminic Cold & Allergy Liquid .... ▣746
- Triaminic Cough & Runny Nose Softchews .... ▣748
- Children's Tylenol Plus Flu Oral Suspension .... ▣749
- Tylenol Allergy Multi-Symptom Caplets with Cool Burst and Gelcaps 1872
- Children's Tylenol Plus Cold Suspension Liquid 1879
- Children's Tylenol Plus Cough & Runny Nose Suspension Liquid 1879
- Children's Tylenol Plus Flu Suspension Liquid 1881
- Children's Tylenol Plus Multi-Symptom Cold Suspension Liquid 1879
- Tylenol Cold Head Congestion Nighttime Caplets with Cool Burst 1873
- Tylenol Cold Multi-Symptom Nighttime Caplets with Cool Burst 1874
- Tylenol Sinus Congestion & Pain Nighttime Caplets with Cool Burst 1876
- Vicks 44M Cough, Cold & Flu Relief Liquid 2680
- Pediatric Vicks 44m Cough & Cold Relief Liquid 2676
- Children's Vicks NyQuil Cold/Cough Relief .... ▣756
- Children's Vicks NyQuil Cold/Cough Relief Liquid 2680
- Zicam Maximum Strength Flu Daytime .... ▣768

Chlorpheniramine Polistirex (Carbamazepine is known to induce CYP1A2 and CYP3A4. Therefore, the potential exists for interaction between carbamazepine and any agent metabolized by one (or more) of these enzymes). Products include:
- Tussionex Pennkinetic Extended-Release Suspension 3327

Chlorpheniramine Tannate (Carbamazepine is known to induce CYP1A2 and CYP3A4. Therefore, the potential exists for interaction between carbamazepine and any agent metabolized by one (or more) of these enzymes).
No products indexed under this heading.

Chlorpromazine (Co-administration with psychotropic agents has resulted in isolated cases of neuroleptic malignant syndrome).
No products indexed under this heading.

Chlorpromazine Hydrochloride (Co-administration with psychotropic agents has resulted in isolated cases of neuroleptic malignant syndrome).
No products indexed under this heading.

Chlorprothixene (Co-administration with psychotropic agents has resulted in isolated cases of neuroleptic malignant syndrome).
No products indexed under this heading.

Chlorprothixene Hydrochloride (Co-administration with psychotropic agents has resulted in isolated cases of neuroleptic malignant syndrome).
No products indexed under this heading.

Cimetidine (Inhibitors of CYP3A4, such as cimetidine, inhibit carbamazepine metabolism and thus increase plasma carbamazepine levels). Products include:
- Tagamet HB 200 Tablets .... ▣664

Cimetidine Hydrochloride (Inhibitors of CYP3A4, such as cimetidine, inhibit carbamazepine metabolism and thus increase plasma carbamazepine levels).
No products indexed under this heading.

Ciprofloxacin (Carbamazepine is metabolized mainly by cytochrome P450 (CYP) 3A4 to the active carbamazepine 10,11 -epoxide, which is further metabolized to the trans-diol by epoxide hydrolase. Therefore, the potential exists for interaction between carbamazepine and any agent that inhibits CYP3A4 and/or epoxide hydrolase). Products include:
- Cipro Oral Suspension 2977
- Cipro I.V. 2984
- Cipro XR Tablets 2990
- Ciprodex Otic Suspension 559

Ciprofloxacin Hydrochloride (Carbamazepine is metabolized by CYP3A4. Therefore, the potential exists for interaction between caramazepine and any agent that induces CYP3A4). Products include:
- Ciloxan Ophthalmic Ointment 559
- Ciloxan Ophthalmic Solution .... ⊙206
- Cipro Tablets 2977
- Proquin XR Tablets 1153

Cisapride (Carbamazepine is known to induce CYP1A2 and CYP3A4. Therefore, the potential exists for interaction between carbamazepine and any agent metabolized by one (or more) of these enzymes).
No products indexed under this heading.

Cisplatin (Inducers of CYP3A4, such as cisplatin, can increase the rate of carbamazepine metabolism and can thus decrease plasma carbamazepine levels).
No products indexed under this heading.

Clarithromycin (Inhibitors of CYP3A4, such as clarithromycin, inhibit carbamazepine metabolism and thus increase plasma carbamazepine levels). Products include:
- Biaxin/Biaxin XL 402
- PREVPAC 3284

Clomipramine Hydrochloride (Carbamazepine can increase plasma levels of clomipramine).
No products indexed under this heading.

Clonazepam (Carbamazepine induces hepatic CYP activity and causes or would be expected to decrease plasma levels of clonazepine; alterations of thryoid function have been reported in combination therapy with other anticonvulsants). Products include:
- Klonopin 2778

Clopidogrel Bisulfate (Carbamazepine is known to induce CYP1A2 and CYP3A4. Therefore, the potential exists for interaction between carbamazepine and any agent metabolized by one (or more) of these enzymes). Products include:
- Plavix Tablets 917
- Plavix Tablets 2926

Clotrimazole (Carbamazepine is metabolized mainly by cytochrome P450 (CYP) 3A4 to the active carbamazepine 10,11 -epoxide, which is further metabolized to the trans-diol by epoxide hydrolase. Therefore, the potential exists for interaction between carbamazepine and any agent that inhibits CYP3A4 and/or epoxide hydrolase). Products include:
- Desenex Athlete's Foot Cream .... ▣635
- Lotrimin 3039
- Lotrisone 3040

Clozapine (Carbamazepine induces hepatic CYP activity and causes or would be expected to decrease plasma levels of clozapine). Products include:
- Clozaril Tablets 2184
- FazaClo Orally Disintegrating Tablets 551

Cortisone Acetate (Carbamazepine is metabolized by CYP3A4. Therefore, the potential exists for interaction between caramazepine and any agent that induces CYP3A4).
No products indexed under this heading.

Cyclobenzaprine (Carbamazepine is known to induce CYP1A2 and CYP3A4. Therefore, the potential exists for interaction between carbamazepine and any agent metabolized by one (or more) of these enzymes).
No products indexed under this heading.

Cyclobenzaprine Hydrochloride (Carbamazepine is known to induce CYP1A2 and CYP3A4. Therefore, the potential exists for interaction between carbamazepine and any agent metabolized by one (or more) of these enzymes).
No products indexed under this heading.

Cyclosporine (Carbamazepine is metabolized mainly by cytochrome P450 (CYP) 3A4 to the active carbamazepine 10,11 -epoxide, which is further metabolized to the trans-diol by epoxide hydrolase. Therefore, the potential exists for interaction between carbamazepine and any agent that inhibits CYP3A4 and/or epoxide hydrolase). Products include:
- Gengraf Capsules 459
- Neoral Oral Solution 2259
- Neoral Soft Gelatin Capsules 2259
- Restasis Ophthalmic Emulsion 575
- Sandimmune 2275

Dalfopristin (Carbamazepine is metabolized mainly by cytochrome P450 (CYP) 3A4 to the active carbamazepine 10,11 -epoxide, which is further metabolized to the trans-diol by epoxide hydrolase. Therefore, the potential exists for interaction between carbamazepine and any agent that inhibits CYP3A4 and/or epoxide hydrolase).
No products indexed under this heading.

Danazol (Inhibitors of CYP3A4, such as danazol, inhibit carbamazepine metabolism and thus increase plasma carbamazepine levels).
No products indexed under this heading.

Delavirdine Mesylate (Carbamazepine is metabolized mainly by cytochrome P450 (CYP) 3A4 to the active carbamazepine 10,11 -epoxide, which is further metabolized to the trans-diol by epoxide hydrolase. Therefore, the potential exists for interaction between carbamazepine and any agent that inhibits CYP3A4 and/or epoxide hydrolase). Products include:
Rescriptor Tablets 2551

Desipramine Hydrochloride (Carbamazepine is known to induce CYP1A2 and CYP3A4. Therefore, the potential exists for interaction between carbamazepine and any agent metabolized by one (or more) of these enzymes).
No products indexed under this heading.

Desogestrel (Carbamazepine induces hepatic CYP activity and causes or would be expected to decrease plasma levels of oral contraceptives; breakthrough bleeding has been reported among patients receiving concomitant oral contraceptives and their reliability may be adversely affected). Products include:
Mircette Tablets 1066

Dexamethasone (Carbamazepine is metabolized by CYP3A4. Therefore, the potential exists for interaction between caramazepine and any agent that induces CYP3A4). Products include:
Ciprodex Otic Suspension 559
Decadron Tablets 1951
TobraDex Ophthalmic Ointment 562
TobraDex Ophthalmic Suspension ... 563

Dexamethasone Acetate (Carbamazepine is metabolized by CYP3A4. Therefore, the potential exists for interaction between caramazepine and any agent that induces CYP3A4).
No products indexed under this heading.

Dexamethasone Sodium Phosphate (Carbamazepine is metabolized by CYP3A4. Therefore, the potential exists for interaction between caramazepine and any agent that induces CYP3A4).
No products indexed under this heading.

Diazepam (Carbamazepine is known to induce CYP1A2 and CYP3A4. Therefore, the potential exists for interaction between carbamazepine and any agent metabolized by one (or more) of these enzymes). Products include:
Diastat Rectal Delivery System 3343
Valium Tablets 2819

Dicumarol (Carbamazepine induces hepatic CYP activity and causes or would be expected to decrease plasma levels of dicumarol).
No products indexed under this heading.

Dihydroergotamine Mesylate (Carbamazepine is known to induce CYP1A2 and CYP3A4. Therefore, the potential exists for interaction between carbamazepine and any agent metabolized by one (or more) of these enzymes). Products include:
Migranal Nasal Spray 3348

Diltiazem Hydrochloride (Inhibitors of CYP3A4, such as diltiazem, inhibit carbamazepine metabolism and thus increase plasma carbamazepine levels). Products include:
Cardizem LA Extended Release Tablets ... 1728
Tiazac Capsules 1201

Diltiazem Maleate (Carbamazepine is metabolized mainly by cytochrome P450 (CYP) 3A4 to the active carbamazepine 10,11 -epoxide, which is further metabolized to the trans-diol by epoxide hydrolase. Therefore, the potential exists for interaction between carbamazepine and any agent that inhibits CYP3A4 and/or epoxide hydrolase).
No products indexed under this heading.

Dirithromycin (Inhibitors of CYP3A4, such as macrolides, inhibit carbamazepine metabolism and thus increase plasma carbamazepine levels).
No products indexed under this heading.

Disopyramide (Carbamazepine is known to induce CYP1A2 and CYP3A4. Therefore, the potential exists for interaction between carbamazepine and any agent metabolized by one (or more) of these enzymes).
No products indexed under this heading.

Disopyramide Phosphate (Carbamazepine is known to induce CYP1A2 and CYP3A4. Therefore, the potential exists for interaction between carbamazepine and any agent metabolized by one (or more) of these enzymes).
No products indexed under this heading.

Disulfiram (Carbamazepine is known to induce CYP1A2 and CYP3A4. Therefore, the potential exists for interaction between carbamazepine and any agent metabolized by one (or more) of these enzymes).
No products indexed under this heading.

Divalproex Sodium (Alterations of thyroid function have been reported in combination therapy with other anticonvulsants). Products include:
Depakote Sprinkle Capsules 422
Depakote Tablets 427
Depakote ER Tablets 434

Doxepin Hydrochloride (Carbamazepine is known to induce CYP1A2 and CYP3A4. Therefore, the potential exists for interaction between carbamazepine and any agent metabolized by one (or more) of these enzymes).
No products indexed under this heading.

Doxorubicin Hydrochloride (Inducers of CYP3A4, such as doxorubicin, can increase the rate of carbamazepine metabolism and can thus decrease plasma carbamazepine levels).
No products indexed under this heading.

Doxycycline Calcium (Carbamazepine induces hepatic CYP activity and causes or would be expected to decrease plasma levels of doxycycline).
No products indexed under this heading.

Doxycycline Hyclate (Carbamazepine induces hepatic CYP activity and causes or would be expected to decrease plasma levels of doxycycline).
No products indexed under this heading.

Doxycycline Monohydrate (Carbamazepine induces hepatic CYP activity and causes or would be expected to decrease plasma levels of doxycycline). Products include:
Oracea Capsules 1000

Dronabinol (Carbamazepine is known to induce CYP1A2 and CYP3A4. Therefore, the potential exists for interaction between carbamazepine and any agent metabolized by one (or more) of these enzymes). Products include:
Marinol Capsules 3333

Dyphylline (Inducers of CYP3A4, such as theophylline, can increase the rate of carbamazepine metabolism and can thus decrease plasma carbamazepine levels; carbamazepine induces hepatic CYP activity and causes or would be expected to decrease plasma levels of theophylline).
No products indexed under this heading.

Efavirenz (Carbamazepine is metabolized mainly by cytochrome P450 (CYP) 3A4 to the active carbamazepine 10,11 -epoxide, which is further metabolized to the trans-diol by epoxide hydrolase. Therefore, the potential exists for interaction between carbamazepine and any agent that inhibits CYP3A4 and/or epoxide hydrolase). Products include:
Atripla Tablets 945
Sustiva Capsules 930
Sustiva Tablets 930

Enoxacin (Carbamazepine is known to induce CYP1A2 and CYP3A4. Therefore, the potential exists for interaction between carbamazepine and any agent metabolized by one (or more) of these enzymes).
No products indexed under this heading.

Ergotamine Tartrate (Carbamazepine is known to induce CYP1A2 and CYP3A4. Therefore, the potential exists for interaction between carbamazepine and any agent metabolized by one (or more) of these enzymes).
No products indexed under this heading.

Erythromycin (Inhibitors of CYP3A4, such as erythromycin, inhibit carbamazepine metabolism and thus increase plasma carbamazepine levels). Products include:
Ery-Tab Tablets 449
Erythromycin Base Filmtab Tablets ... 455

Erythromycin Delayed-Release Capsules, USP............................. 457
PCE Dispertab Tablets 515

Erythromycin Estolate (Inhibitors of CYP3A4, such as erythromycin, inhibit carbamazepine metabolism and thus increase plasma carbamazepine levels).
No products indexed under this heading.

Erythromycin Ethylsuccinate (Inhibitors of CYP3A4, such as erythromycin, inhibit carbamazepine metabolism and thus increase plasma carbamazepine levels). Products include:
E.E.S. .. 451
EryPed ... 447

Erythromycin Gluceptate (Inhibitors of CYP3A4, such as erythromycin, inhibit carbamazepine metabolism and thus increase plasma carbamazepine levels).
No products indexed under this heading.

Erythromycin Lactobionate (Inhibitors of CYP3A4, such as erythromycin, inhibit carbamazepine metabolism and thus increase plasma carbamazepine levels).
No products indexed under this heading.

Erythromycin Stearate (Inhibitors of CYP3A4, such as erythromycin, inhibit carbamazepine metabolism and thus increase plasma carbamazepine levels). Products include:
Erythrocin Stearate Filmtab Tablets ... 453

Esomeprazole Magnesium (Carbamazepine is metabolized mainly by cytochrome P450 (CYP) 3A4 to the active carbamazepine 10,11 -epoxide, which is further metabolized to the trans-diol by epoxide hydrolase. Therefore, the potential exists for interaction between carbamazepine and any agent that inhibits CYP3A4 and/or epoxide hydrolase). Products include:
Nexium Delayed-Release Capsules 655

Estradiol (Carbamazepine is known to induce CYP1A2 and CYP3A4. Therefore, the potential exists for interaction between carbamazepine and any agent metabolized by one (or more) of these enzymes). Products include:
Angeliq Tablets 762
Climara Transdermal System 771
Climara Pro Transdermal System 776
Estrasorb Topical Emulsion 1147
Estring Vaginal Ring 2635
Menostar Transdermal System 782
Vagifem Tablets 2334

Estradiol Benzoate (Carbamazepine is known to induce CYP1A2 and CYP3A4. Therefore, the potential exists for interaction between carbamazepine and any agent metabolized by one (or more) of these enzymes).
No products indexed under this heading.

Estradiol Cypionate (Carbamazepine is known to induce CYP1A2 and CYP3A4. Therefore, the potential exists for interaction between carbamazepine and any agent metabolized by one (or more) of these enzymes).
No products indexed under this heading.

IMPORTANT NOTE: Always consult each drug listing in the patient's regimen for possible interactions.

Estradiol Valerate (Carbamazepine is known to induce CYP1A2 and CYP3A4. Therefore, the potential exists for interaction between carbamazepine and any agent metabolized by one (or more) of these enzymes).
No products indexed under this heading.

Ethinyl Estradiol (Carbamazepine induces hepatic CYP activity and causes or would be expected to decrease plasma levels of oral contraceptives; breakthrough bleeding has been reported among patients receiving concomitant oral contraceptives and their reliability may be adversely affected). Products include:
Mircette Tablets ... 1066
NuvaRing ... 2340
Ortho-Cyclen/Ortho Tri-Cyclen ... 2429
Ortho Evra Transdermal System ... 2417
Ortho Tri-Cyclen Lo Tablets ... 2436
Seasonique Tablets ... 1077
Yasmin 28 Tablets ... 796
Yaz Tablets ... 803

Ethosuximide (Carbamazepine induces hepatic CYP activity and causes or would be expected to decrease plasma levels of ethosuximide; alterations of thyroid function have been reported in combination therapy with other anticonvulsants).
No products indexed under this heading.

Ethotoin (Alterations of thyroid function have been reported in combination therapy with other anticonvulsants).
No products indexed under this heading.

Ethynodiol Diacetate (Carbamazepine induces hepatic CYP activity and causes or would be expected to decrease plasma levels of oral contraceptives; breakthrough bleeding has been reported among patients receiving concomitant oral contraceptives and their reliability may be adversely affected).
No products indexed under this heading.

Etoposide (Carbamazepine is known to induce CYP1A2 and CYP3A4. Therefore, the potential exists for interaction between carbamazepine and any agent metabolized by one (or more) of these enzymes).
No products indexed under this heading.

Etoposide Phosphate (Carbamazepine is known to induce CYP1A2 and CYP3A4. Therefore, the potential exists for interaction between carbamazepine and any agent metabolized by one (or more) of these enzymes).
No products indexed under this heading.

Felbamate (Inducers of CYP3A4, such as felbamate, can increase the rate of carbamazepine metabolism and can thus decrease plasma carbamazepine levels; alterations of thyroid function have been reported in combination therapy with other anticonvulsants).
No products indexed under this heading.

Felodipine (Carbamazepine is known to induce CYP1A2 and CYP3A4. Therefore, the potential exists for interaction between carbamazepine and any agent metabolized by one (or more) of these enzymes).
No products indexed under this heading.

Fentanyl (Carbamazepine is known to induce CYP1A2 and CYP3A4. Therefore, the potential exists for interaction between carbamazepine and any agent metabolized by one (or more) of these enzymes). Products include:
Duragesic Transdermal System ... 2373
Ionsys Transdermal System ... 2379

Fentanyl Citrate (Carbamazepine is known to induce CYP1A2 and CYP3A4. Therefore, the potential exists for interaction between carbamazepine and any agent metabolized by one (or more) of these enzymes). Products include:
Actiq ... 979

Fluconazole (Carbamazepine is metabolized mainly by cytochrome P450 (CYP) 3A4 to the active carbamazepine 10,11 -epoxide, which is further metabolized to the transdiol by epoxide hydrolase. Therefore, the potential exists for interaction between carbamazepine and any agent that inhibits CYP3A4 and/or epoxide hydrolase).
No products indexed under this heading.

Fludrocortisone Acetate (Carbamazepine is metabolized by CYP3A4. Therefore, the potential exists for interaction between caramazepine and any agent that induces CYP3A4).
No products indexed under this heading.

Fluoxetine Hydrochloride (Inhibitors of CYP3A4, such as fluoxetine, inhibit carbamazepine metabolism and thus increase plasma carbamazepine levels). Products include:
Prozac Pulvules and Liquid ... 1801
Symbyax Capsules ... 1819

Fluphenazine Decanoate (Coadministration with psychotropic agents has resulted in isolated cases of neuroleptic malignant syndrome).
No products indexed under this heading.

Fluphenazine Enanthate (Coadministration with psychotropic agents has resulted in isolated cases of neuroleptic malignant syndrome).
No products indexed under this heading.

Fluphenazine Hydrochloride (Coadministration with psychotropic agents has resulted in isolated cases of neuroleptic malignant syndrome).
No products indexed under this heading.

Flutamide (Carbamazepine is known to induce CYP1A2 and CYP3A4. Therefore, the potential exists for interaction between carbamazepine and any agent metabolized by one (or more) of these enzymes). Products include:
Eulexin Capsules ... 3009

Fluticasone Propionate (Carbamazepine is known to induce CYP1A2 and CYP3A4. Therefore, the potential exists for interaction between carbamazepine and any agent metabolized by one (or more) of these enzymes). Products include:
Advair Diskus 100/50 ... 1308
Advair Diskus 250/50 ... 1308
Advair Diskus 500/50 ... 1308
Advair HFA Inhalation Aerosol ... 1318
Cutivate Cream ... 2662
Cutivate Lotion 0.05% ... 2664
Cutivate Ointment ... 2665
Flonase Nasal Spray ... 1440
Flovent Diskus ... 1443

Fluvoxamine Maleate (Carbamazepine is metabolized mainly by cytochrome P450 (CYP) 3A4 to the active carbamazepine 10,11 -epoxide, which is further metabolized to the trans-diol by epoxide hydrolase. Therefore, the potential exists for interaction between carbamazepine and any agent that inhibits CYP3A4 and/or epoxide hydrolase).
No products indexed under this heading.

Fosamprenavir Calcium (Carbamazepine is metabolized mainly by cytochrome P450 (CYP) 3A4 to the active carbamazepine 10,11 -epoxide, which is further metabolized to the trans-diol by epoxide hydrolase. Therefore, the potential exists for interaction between carbamazepine and any agent that inhibits CYP3A4 and/or epoxide hydrolase). Products include:
Lexiva Tablets ... 1505

Fosphenytoin (Alterations of thyroid function have been reported in combination therapy with other anticonvulsants).
No products indexed under this heading.

Fosphenytoin Sodium (Alterations of thyroid function have been reported in combination therapy with other anticonvulsants).
No products indexed under this heading.

Gabapentin (Alterations of thyroid function have been reported in combination therapy with other anticonvulsants). Products include:
Neurontin Capsules ... 2487
Neurontin Oral Solution ... 2487
Neurontin Tablets ... 2487

Garlic Extract (Carbamazepine is metabolized by CYP3A4. Therefore, the potential exists for interaction between caramazepine and any agent that induces CYP3A4).
No products indexed under this heading.

Garlic Oil (Carbamazepine is metabolized by CYP3A4. Therefore, the potential exists for interaction between caramazepine and any agent that induces CYP3A4).
No products indexed under this heading.

Grepafloxacin Hydrochloride (Carbamazepine is known to induce CYP1A2 and CYP3A4. Therefore, the potential exists for interaction between carbamazepine and any agent metabolized by one (or more) of these enzymes).
No products indexed under this heading.

Haloperidol (Carbamazepine induces hepatic CYP activity and causes or would be expected to decrease plasma levels of haloperidol).
No products indexed under this heading.

Haloperidol Decanoate (Carbamazepine induces hepatic CYP activity and causes or would be expected to decrease plasma levels of haloperidol).
No products indexed under this heading.

Haloperidol Lactate (Carbamazepine is known to induce CYP1A2 and CYP3A4. Therefore, the potential exists for interaction between carbamazepine and any agent metabolized by one (or more) of these enzymes).
No products indexed under this heading.

Hydrocortisone (Carbamazepine is metabolized by CYP3A4. Therefore, the potential exists for interaction between caramazepine and any agent that induces CYP3A4). Products include:
Colocort Rectal Suspension, USP (Retention) 100 mg/60 mL ... 2476
Hydrocortone Tablets ... 1989
Preparation H Hydrocortisone Cream ... ▣646

Hydrocortisone Acetate (Carbamazepine is metabolized by CYP3A4. Therefore, the potential exists for interaction between caramazepine and any agent that induces CYP3A4). Products include:
Analpram-HC ... 1159
Pramosone ... 1161
ProctoFoam-HC ... 3099

Hydrocortisone Butyrate (Carbamazepine is metabolized by CYP3A4. Therefore, the potential exists for interaction between caramazepine and any agent that induces CYP3A4). Products include:
Locoid Lipocream Cream ... 1160

Hydrocortisone Cypionate (Carbamazepine is metabolized by CYP3A4. Therefore, the potential exists for interaction between caramazepine and any agent that induces CYP3A4).
No products indexed under this heading.

Hydrocortisone Hemisuccinate (Carbamazepine is metabolized by CYP3A4. Therefore, the potential exists for interaction between caramazepine and any agent that induces CYP3A4).
No products indexed under this heading.

Hydrocortisone Probutate (Carbamazepine is metabolized by CYP3A4. Therefore, the potential exists for interaction between caramazepine and any agent that induces CYP3A4).
No products indexed under this heading.

Hydrocortisone Sodium Phosphate (Carbamazepine is metabolized by CYP3A4. Therefore, the potential exists for interaction between caramazepine and any agent that induces CYP3A4).
No products indexed under this heading.

Hydrocortisone Sodium Succinate (Carbamazepine is metabolized by CYP3A4. Therefore, the potential exists for interaction between caramazepine and any agent that induces CYP3A4).
No products indexed under this heading.

Hydrocortisone Valerate (Carbamazepine is metabolized by CYP3A4. Therefore, the potential exists for interaction between caramazepine and any agent that induces CYP3A4).
No products indexed under this heading.

Hypericum (Carbamazepine is metabolized by CYP3A4. Therefore, the potential exists for interaction between caramazepine and any agent that induces CYP3A4). Products include:
Satiete Tablets 832

Hypericum Perforatum (Carbamazepine is metabolized by CYP3A4. Therefore, the potential exists for interaction between caramazepine and any agent that induces CYP3A4).
No products indexed under this heading.

Imipramine Hydrochloride (Carbamazepine is known to induce CYP1A2 and CYP3A4. Therefore, the potential exists for interaction between carbamazepine and any agent metabolized by one (or more) of these enzymes).
No products indexed under this heading.

Imipramine Pamoate (Carbamazepine is known to induce CYP1A2 and CYP3A4. Therefore, the potential exists for interaction between carbamazepine and any agent metabolized by one (or more) of these enzymes).
No products indexed under this heading.

Indinavir Sulfate (Carbamazepine is metabolized mainly by cytochrome P450 (CYP) 3A4 to the active carbamazepine 10,11 -epoxide, which is further metabolized to the trans-diol by epoxide hydrolase. Therefore, the potential exists for interaction between carbamazepine and any agent that inhibits its CYP3A4 and/or epoxide hydrolase). Products include:
Crixivan Capsules 1940

Isocarboxazid (Because of the relationship of carbamazepine to other tricyclic compounds, on theoretical grounds, co-administration with MAO inhibitors is contraindicated).
No products indexed under this heading.

Isoniazid (Inhibitors of CYP3A4, such as isoniazid, inhibit carbamazepine metabolism and thus increase plasma carbamazepine levels).
No products indexed under this heading.

Isradipine (Carbamazepine is known to induce CYP1A2 and CYP3A4. Therefore, the potential exists for interaction between carbamazepine and any agent metabolized by one (or more) of these enzymes). Products include:
DynaCirc CR Tablets 2721

Itraconazole (Inhibitors of CYP3A4, such as itraconazole, inhibit carbamazepine metabolism and thus increase plasma carbamazepine levels).
No products indexed under this heading.

Ketoconazole (Inhibitors of CYP3A4, such as ketoconazole, inhibit carbamazepine metabolism and thus increase plasma carbamazepine levels). Products include:
Nizoral A-D Shampoo, 1% 1868

Lamotrigine (Alterations of thyroid function have been reported in combination therapy with other anticonvulsants). Products include:
Lamictal 1481

Levetiracetam (Alterations of thyroid function have been reported in combination therapy with other anticonvulsants). Products include:
Keppra Injection 3320
Keppra Oral Solution 3314
Keppra Tablets 3314

Levobupivacaine Hydrochloride (Carbamazepine is known to induce CYP1A2 and CYP3A4. Therefore, the potential exists for interaction between carbamazepine and any agent metabolized by one (or more) of these enzymes).
No products indexed under this heading.

Levonorgestrel (Carbamazepine induces hepatic CYP activity and causes or would be expected to decrease plasma levels of oral contraceptives; breakthrough bleeding has been reported among patients receiving concomitant oral contraceptives and their reliability may be adversely affected). Products include:
Climara Pro Transdermal System 776
Mirena Intrauterine System 787
Plan B Tablets 1076
Seasonique Tablets 1077

Lidocaine (Carbamazepine is known to induce CYP1A2 and CYP3A4. Therefore, the potential exists for interaction between carbamazepine and any agent metabolized by one (or more) of these enzymes). Products include:
Lidoderm Patch 1118
Synera Topical Patch 1137

Lidocaine Hydrochloride (Carbamazepine is known to induce CYP1A2 and CYP3A4. Therefore, the potential exists for interaction between carbamazepine and any agent metabolized by one (or more) of these enzymes).
No products indexed under this heading.

Lithium (Co-administration may increase the risk of neurotoxic side effects).
No products indexed under this heading.

Lithium Carbonate (Co-administration with psychotropic agents has resulted in isolated cases of neuroleptic malignant syndrome). Products include:
Lithobid Tablets 1692

Lithium Citrate (Co-administration with psychotropic agents has resulted in isolated cases of neuroleptic malignant syndrome).
No products indexed under this heading.

Lomefloxacin Hydrochloride (Carbamazepine is known to induce CYP1A2 and CYP3A4. Therefore, the potential exists for interaction between carbamazepine and any agent metabolized by one (or more) of these enzymes).
No products indexed under this heading.

Lopinavir (Carbamazepine is metabolized mainly by cytochrome P450 (CYP) 3A4 to the active carbamazepine 10,11 -epoxide, which is further metabolized to the trans-diol by epoxide hydrolase. Therefore, the potential exists for interaction between carbamazepine and any agent that inhibits CYP3A4 and/or epoxide hydrolase). Products include:
Kaletra 476

Loratadine (Inhibitors of CYP3A4, such as loratadine, inhibit carbamazepine metabolism and thus increase plasma carbamazepine levels). Products include:
Alavert Allergy & Sinus D-12 Hour Tablets 771
Alavert 771
Children's Claritin Allergy Oral Solution 771
Claritin Non-Drowsy 24 Hour Tablets 772
Claritin Reditabs 24 Hour Non-Drowsy Tablets 772
Claritin-D Non-Drowsy 12 Hour Tablets 772
Claritin-D Non-Drowsy 24 Hour Tablets 772

Lovastatin (Carbamazepine is known to induce CYP1A2 and CYP3A4. Therefore, the potential exists for interaction between carbamazepine and any agent metabolized by one (or more) of these enzymes). Products include:
Advicor Tablets 1722
Altoprev Extended-Release Tablets 3109
Mevacor Tablets 2021

Loxapine Hydrochloride (Co-administration with psychotropic agents has resulted in isolated cases of neuroleptic malignant syndrome).
No products indexed under this heading.

Loxapine Succinate (Co-administration with psychotropic agents has resulted in isolated cases of neuroleptic malignant syndrome).
No products indexed under this heading.

Maprotiline Hydrochloride (Carbamazepine is known to induce CYP1A2 and CYP3A4. Therefore, the potential exists for interaction between carbamazepine and any agent metabolized by one (or more) of these enzymes).
No products indexed under this heading.

Mefloquine Hydrochloride (Antimalarial drugs, such as chloroquine and mefloquine, may antagonize the activity of carbamazepine). Products include:
Lariam Tablets 2786

Mephenytoin (Alterations of thyroid function have been reported in combination therapy with other anticonvulsants).
No products indexed under this heading.

Mesoridazine Besylate (Co-administration with psychotropic agents has resulted in isolated cases of neuroleptic malignant syndrome).
No products indexed under this heading.

Mestranol (Carbamazepine induces hepatic CYP activity and causes or would be expected to decrease plasma levels of oral contraceptives; breakthrough bleeding has been reported among patients receiving concomitant oral contraceptives and their reliability may be adversely affected).
No products indexed under this heading.

Methadone Hydrochloride (Carbamazepine is known to induce CYP1A2 and CYP3A4. Therefore, the potential exists for interaction between carbamazepine and any agent metabolized by one (or more) of these enzymes).
No products indexed under this heading.

Methotrimeprazine (Co-administration with psychotropic agents has resulted in isolated cases of neuroleptic malignant syndrome).
No products indexed under this heading.

Methsuximide (Carbamezapine induces hepatic CYP activity and causes or would be expected to decrease plasma levels of methsuximide; alterations of thyroid function have been reported in combination therapy with other anticonvulsants).
No products indexed under this heading.

Methylprednisolone (Carbamazepine is metabolized by CYP3A4. Therefore, the potential exists for interaction between caramazepine and any agent that induces CYP3A4).
No products indexed under this heading.

Methylprednisolone Acetate (Carbamazepine is metabolized by CYP3A4. Therefore, the potential exists for interaction between caramazepine and any agent that induces CYP3A4). Products include:
Depo-Medrol Injectable Suspension 2617
Depo-Medrol Single-Dose Vial 2619

Methylprednisolone Sodium Succinate (Carbamazepine is metabolized by CYP3A4. Therefore, the potential exists for interaction between caramazepine and any agent that induces CYP3A4).
No products indexed under this heading.

Metronidazole (Carbamazepine is metabolized mainly by cytochrome P450 (CYP) 3A4 to the active carbamazepine 10,11 -epoxide, which is further metabolized to the trans-diol by epoxide hydrolase. Therefore, the potential exists for interaction between carbamazepine and any agent that inhibits CYP3A4 and/or epoxide hydrolase). Products include:
Metrogel 1% 1211
MetroGel-Vaginal Gel 1855
Vandazole Vaginal Gel 3338

Metronidazole Benzoate (Carbamazepine is metabolized mainly by cytochrome P450 (CYP) 3A4 to the active carbamazepine 10,11 -epoxide, which is further metabolized to the trans-diol by epoxide hydrolase. Therefore, the potential exists for interaction between carbamazepine and any agent that inhibits its CYP3A4 and/or epoxide hydrolase).
No products indexed under this heading.

IMPORTANT NOTE: Always consult each drug listing in the patient's regimen for possible interactions.

Metronidazole Hydrochloride (Carbamazepine is metabolized mainly by cytochrome P450 (CYP) 3A4 to the active carbamazepine 10,11 -epoxide, which is further metabolized to the trans-diol by epoxide hydrolase. Therefore, the potential exists for interaction between carbamazepine and any agent that inhibits CYP3A4 and/or epoxide hydrolase).
No products indexed under this heading.

Mexiletine Hydrochloride (Carbamazepine is known to induce CYP1A2 and CYP3A4. Therefore, the potential exists for interaction between carbamazepine and any agent metabolized by one (or more) of these enzymes).
No products indexed under this heading.

Miconazole (Carbamazepine is metabolized mainly by cytochrome P450 (CYP) 3A4 to the active carbamazepine 10,11 -epoxide, which is further metabolized to the trans-diol by epoxide hydrolase. Therefore, the potential exists for interaction between carbamazepine and any agent that inhibits CYP3A4 and/or epoxide hydrolase).
No products indexed under this heading.

Miconazole Nitrate (Carbamazepine is metabolized mainly by cytochrome P450 (CYP) 3A4 to the active carbamazepine 10,11 -epoxide, which is further metabolized to the trans-diol by epoxide hydrolase. Therefore, the potential exists for interaction between carbamazepine and any agent that inhibits CYP3A4 and/or epoxide hydrolase). Products include:
Desenex .... ▣ 635
Desenex Jock Itch Spray Powder ... ▣ 635

Midazolam Hydrochloride (Carbamazepine is known to induce CYP1A2 and CYP3A4. Therefore, the potential exists for interaction between carbamazepine and any agent metabolized by one (or more) of these enzymes).
No products indexed under this heading.

Mirtazapine (Carbamazepine is known to induce CYP1A2 and CYP3A4. Therefore, the potential exists for interaction between carbamazepine and any agent metabolized by one (or more) of these enzymes).
No products indexed under this heading.

Moclobemide (Because of the relationship of carbamazepine to other tricyclic compounds, on theoretical grounds, co-administration with MAO inhibitors is contraindicated).
No products indexed under this heading.

Modafinil (Carbamazepine is metabolized by CYP3A4. Therefore, the potential exists for interaction between caramazepine and any agent that induces CYP3A4). Products include:
Provigil Tablets 988

Molindone Hydrochloride (Co-administration with psychotropic agents has resulted in isolated cases of neuroleptic malignant syndrome). Products include:
Moban Tablets 1119

Moxifloxacin Hydrochloride (Carbamazepine is known to induce CYP1A2 and CYP3A4. Therefore, the potential exists for interaction between carbamazepine and any agent metabolized by one (or more) of these enzymes). Products include:
Avelox 2970
Vigamox Ophthalmic Solution 564

Nafcillin Sodium (Carbamazepine is known to induce CYP1A2 and CYP3A4. Therefore, the potential exists for interaction between carbamazepine and any agent metabolized by one (or more) of these enzymes).
No products indexed under this heading.

Naproxen (Carbamazepine is known to induce CYP1A2 and CYP3A4. Therefore, the potential exists for interaction between carbamazepine and any agent metabolized by one (or more) of these enzymes). Products include:
EC-Naprosyn Delayed-Release Tablets 2761
Naprosyn Suspension 2761
Naprosyn Tablets 2761
Prevacid NapraPAC 3280

Naproxen Sodium (Carbamazepine is known to induce CYP1A2 and CYP3A4. Therefore, the potential exists for interaction between carbamazepine and any agent metabolized by one (or more) of these enzymes). Products include:
Aleve Caplets 742
Aleve Gelcaps 743
Aleve Tablets 743
Aleve Cold & Sinus Caplets 744
Anaprox Tablets 2761
Anaprox DS Tablets 2761

Nefazodone Hydrochloride (Carbamazepine is metabolized mainly by cytochrome P450 (CYP) 3A4 to the active carbamazepine 10,11 -epoxide, which is further metabolized to the trans-diol by epoxide hydrolase. Therefore, the potential exists for interaction between carbamazepine and any agent that inhibits CYP3A4 and/or epoxide hydrolase).
No products indexed under this heading.

Nelfinavir Mesylate (Carbamazepine is metabolized mainly by cytochrome P450 (CYP) 3A4 to the active carbamazepine 10,11 -epoxide, which is further metabolized to the trans-diol by epoxide hydrolase. Therefore, the potential exists for interaction between carbamazepine and any agent that inhibits CYP3A4 and/or epoxide hydrolase). Products include:
Viracept 2577

Nevirapine (Carbamazepine is metabolized mainly by cytochrome P450 (CYP) 3A4 to the active carbamazepine 10,11 -epoxide, which is further metabolized to the trans-diol by epoxide hydrolase. Therefore, the potential exists for interaction between carbamazepine and any agent that inhibits CYP3A4 and/or epoxide hydrolase). Products include:
Viramune Oral Suspension 873
Viramune Tablets 873

Niacinamide (Inhibitors of CYP3A4, such as niacinamide, inhibit carbamazepine metabolism and thus increase plasma carbamazepine levels).
No products indexed under this heading.

Nicardipine Hydrochloride (Carbamazepine is known to induce CYP1A2 and CYP3A4. Therefore, the potential exists for interaction between carbamazepine and any agent metabolized by one (or more) of these enzymes). Products include:
Cardene I.V. 2497

Nicotinamide (Inhibitors of CYP3A4, such as nicotinamide, inhibit carbamazepine metabolism and thus increase plasma carbamazepine levels). Products include:
Nicomide Tablets 1088

Nicotine Polacrilex (Carbamazepine is known to induce CYP1A2 and CYP3A4. Therefore, the potential exists for interaction between carbamazepine and any agent metabolized by one (or more) of these enzymes).
No products indexed under this heading.

Nicotine Salicylate (Carbamazepine is known to induce CYP1A2 and CYP3A4. Therefore, the potential exists for interaction between carbamazepine and any agent metabolized by one (or more) of these enzymes).
No products indexed under this heading.

Nicotine Sulfate (Carbamazepine is known to induce CYP1A2 and CYP3A4. Therefore, the potential exists for interaction between carbamazepine and any agent metabolized by one (or more) of these enzymes).
No products indexed under this heading.

Nifedipine (Carbamazepine is metabolized mainly by cytochrome P450 (CYP) 3A4 to the active carbamazepine 10,11 -epoxide, which is further metabolized to the trans-diol by epoxide hydrolase. Therefore, the potential exists for interaction between carbamazepine and any agent that inhibits CYP3A4 and/or epoxide hydrolase). Products include:
Adalat CC Tablets 2964

Nimodipine (Carbamazepine is known to induce CYP1A2 and CYP3A4. Therefore, the potential exists for interaction between carbamazepine and any agent metabolized by one (or more) of these enzymes). Products include:
Nimotop Capsules 749

Nisoldipine (Carbamazepine is known to induce CYP1A2 and CYP3A4. Therefore, the potential exists for interaction between carbamazepine and any agent metabolized by one (or more) of these enzymes). Products include:
Sular Tablets 3122

Nitrendipine (Carbamazepine is known to induce CYP1A2 and CYP3A4. Therefore, the potential exists for interaction between carbamazepine and any agent metabolized by one (or more) of these enzymes).
No products indexed under this heading.

Norethindrone (Carbamazepine induces hepatic CYP activity and causes or would be expected to decrease plasma levels of oral contraceptives; breakthrough bleeding has been reported among patients receiving concomitant oral contraceptives and their reliability may be adversely affected). Products include:
Ortho Micronor Tablets 2426

Norethindrone Acetate (Carbamazepine is known to induce CYP1A2 and CYP3A4. Therefore, the potential exists for interaction between carbamazepine and any agent metabolized by one (or more) of these enzymes).
No products indexed under this heading.

Norethynodrel (Carbamazepine induces hepatic CYP activity and causes or would be expected to decrease plasma levels of oral contraceptives; breakthrough bleeding has been reported among patients receiving concomitant oral contraceptives and their reliability may be adversely affected).
No products indexed under this heading.

Norfloxacin (Carbamazepine is metabolized mainly by cytochrome P450 (CYP) 3A4 to the active carbamazepine 10,11 -epoxide, which is further metabolized to the trans-diol by epoxide hydrolase. Therefore, the potential exists for interaction between carbamazepine and any agent that inhibits CYP3A4 and/or epoxide hydrolase). Products include:
Noroxin Tablets 2032

Norgestimate (Carbamazepine induces hepatic CYP activity and causes or would be expected to decrease plasma levels of oral contraceptives; breakthrough bleeding has been reported among patients receiving concomitant oral contraceptives and their reliability may be adversely affected). Products include:
Ortho-Cyclen/Ortho Tri-Cyclen 2429
Ortho Tri-Cyclen Lo Tablets 2436

Norgestrel (Carbamazepine induces hepatic CYP activity and causes or would be expected to decrease plasma levels of oral contraceptives; breakthrough bleeding has been reported among patients receiving concomitant oral contraceptives and their reliability may be adversely affected).
No products indexed under this heading.

Nortriptyline Hydrochloride (Carbamazepine is known to induce CYP1A2 and CYP3A4. Therefore, the potential exists for interaction between carbamazepine and any agent metabolized by one (or more) of these enzymes).
No products indexed under this heading.

Ofloxacin (Carbamazepine is known to induce CYP1A2 and CYP3A4. Therefore, the potential exists for interaction between carbamazepine and any agent metabolized by one (or more) of these enzymes). Products include:
Floxin Otic Solution 1049

Olanzapine (Co-administration with psychotropic agents has resulted in isolated cases of neuroleptic malignant syndrome). Products include:
Symbyax Capsules 1819
Zyprexa Tablets 1830
Zyprexa IntraMuscular 1830
Zyprexa ZYDIS Orally Disintegrating Tablets 1830

Omeprazole (Carbamazepine is metabolized mainly by cytochrome P450 (CYP) 3A4 to the active carbamazepine 10,11 -epoxide, which is further metabolized to the trans-diol by epoxide hydrolase. There-

fore, the potential exists for interaction between carbamazepine and any agent that inhibits CYP3A4 and/or epoxide hydrolase). Products include:
Zegerid Capsules 2958
Zegerid Powder for Oral Solution 2958

Ondansetron (Carbamazepine is known to induce CYP1A2 and CYP3A4. Therefore, the potential exists for interaction between carbamazepine and any agent metabolized by one (or more) of these enzymes). Products include:
Zofran ODT Orally Disintegrating Tablets 1639

Ondansetron Hydrochloride (Carbamazepine is known to induce CYP1A2 and CYP3A4. Therefore, the potential exists for interaction between carbamazepine and any agent metabolized by one (or more) of these enzymes). Products include:
Zofran Injection 1634
Zofran 1639

Oxcarbazepine (Alterations of thyroid function have been reported in combination therapy with other anticonvulsants). Products include:
Trileptal Tablets 2300
Trileptal Oral Suspension 2300

Paclitaxel (Carbamazepine is known to induce CYP1A2 and CYP3A4. Therefore, the potential exists for interaction between carbamazepine and any agent metabolized by one (or more) of these enzymes).
No products indexed under this heading.

Paramethadione (Alterations of thyroid function have been reported in combination therapy with other anticonvulsants).
No products indexed under this heading.

Pargyline Hydrochloride (Because of the relationship of carbamazepine to other tricyclic compounds, on theoretical grounds, co-administration with MAO inhibitors is contraindicated).
No products indexed under this heading.

Paroxetine Hydrochloride (Carbamazepine is metabolized mainly by cytochrome P450 (CYP) 3A4 to the active carbamazepine 10,11 -epoxide, which is further metabolized to the trans-diol by epoxide hydrolase. Therefore, the potential exists for interaction between carbamazepine and any agent that inhibits CYP3A4 and/or epoxide hydrolase). Products include:
Paxil CR Controlled-Release Tablets 1538
Paxil 1530

Perphenazine (Co-administration with psychotropic agents has resulted in isolated cases of neuroleptic malignant syndrome).
No products indexed under this heading.

Phenacemide (Alterations of thyroid function have been reported in combination therapy with other anticonvulsants).
No products indexed under this heading.

Phenelzine Sulfate (Because of the relationship of carbamazepine to other tricyclic compounds, on theoretical grounds, co-administration with MAO inhibitors is contraindicated).
No products indexed under this heading.

Phenobarbital (Inducers of CYP3A4, such as phenobarbital, can increase the rate of carbamazepine metabolism and can thus decrease plasma carbamazepine levels; alterations of thyroid function have been reported in combination therapy with other anticonvulsants). Products include:
Donnatal Extentabs 2493

Phenobarbital Sodium (Carbamazepine is metabolized by CYP3A4. Therefore, the potential exists for interaction between caramazepine and any agent that induces CYP3A4).
No products indexed under this heading.

Phensuximide (Carbamezapine induces hepatic CYP activity and causes or would be expected to decrease plasma levels of phensuximide; alterations of thyroid function have been reported in combination therapy with other anticonvulsants).
No products indexed under this heading.

Phenytoin (Alterations of thyroid function have been reported in combination therapy with other anticonvulsants).
No products indexed under this heading.

Phenytoin Sodium (Alterations of thyroid function have been reported in combination therapy with other anticonvulsants). Products include:
Phenytek Capsules 2160

Pimozide (Co-administration with psychotropic agents has resulted in isolated cases of neuroleptic malignant syndrome).
No products indexed under this heading.

Polyestradiol Phosphate (Carbamazepine is known to induce CYP1A2 and CYP3A4. Therefore, the potential exists for interaction between carbamazepine and any agent metabolized by one (or more) of these enzymes).
No products indexed under this heading.

Prednisolone Acetate (Carbamazepine is metabolized by CYP3A4. Therefore, the potential exists for interaction between caramazepine and any agent that induces CYP3A4). Products include:
Blephamide Ophthalmic Ointment 568
Blephamide Ophthalmic Suspension.................................. 569
Poly-Pred Ophthalmic Suspension .... ⊙233
Pred Forte Ophthalmic Suspension .... ⊙235
Pred Mild Ophthalmic Suspension .... ⊙238
Pred-G Ophthalmic Ointment .... ⊙237
Pred-G Ophthalmic Suspension ...... ⊙236

Prednisolone Sodium Phosphate (Carbamazepine is metabolized by CYP3A4. Therefore, the potential exists for interaction between caramazepine and any agent that induces CYP3A4).
No products indexed under this heading.

Prednisolone Tebutate (Carbamazepine is metabolized by CYP3A4. Therefore, the potential exists for interaction between caramazepine and any agent that induces CYP3A4).
No products indexed under this heading.

Prednisone (Carbamazepine is metabolized by CYP3A4. Therefore, the potential exists for interaction between caramazepine and any agent that induces CYP3A4).
No products indexed under this heading.

Primidone (Inducers of CYP3A4, such as primidone, can increase the rate of carbamazepine metabolism and can thus decrease plasma carbamazepine levels; carbamazepine increases levels of primidone; alterations of thyroid function have been reported in combination therapy with other anticonvulsants).
No products indexed under this heading.

Procarbazine Hydrochloride (Because of the relationship of carbamazepine to other tricyclic compounds, on theoretical grounds, co-administration with MAO inhibitors is contraindicated). Products include:
Matulane Capsules 3191

Prochlorperazine (Co-administration with psychotropic agents has resulted in isolated cases of neuroleptic malignant syndrome).
No products indexed under this heading.

Promethazine Hydrochloride (Co-administration with psychotropic agents has resulted in isolated cases of neuroleptic malignant syndrome). Products include:
Phenergan Tablets and Suppositories.............................. 3440

Propafenone Hydrochloride (Carbamazepine is known to induce CYP1A2 and CYP3A4. Therefore, the potential exists for interaction between carbamazepine and any agent metabolized by one (or more) of these enzymes). Products include:
Rythmol SR Capsules 2727

Propoxyphene Hydrochloride (Inhibitors of CYP3A4, such as propoxyphene, inhibit carbamazepine metabolism and thus increase plasma carbamazepine levels).
No products indexed under this heading.

Propoxyphene Napsylate (Inhibitors of CYP3A4, such as propoxyphene, inhibit carbamazepine metabolism and thus increase plasma carbamazepine levels).
No products indexed under this heading.

Propranolol Hydrochloride (Carbamazepine is known to induce CYP1A2 and CYP3A4. Therefore, the potential exists for interaction between carbamazepine and any agent metabolized by one (or more) of these enzymes). Products include:
Inderal LA Long-Acting Capsules 3429
InnoPran XL Capsules 2723

Protriptyline Hydrochloride (Carbamazepine is known to induce CYP1A2 and CYP3A4. Therefore, the potential exists for interaction between carbamazepine and any agent metabolized by one (or more) of these enzymes).
No products indexed under this heading.

Pyrimethamine (Anti-malarial drugs, such as chloroquine and mefloquine, may antagonize the activity of carbamazepine). Products include:
Daraprim Tablets 1419
Fansidar Tablets 2765

Quetiapine Fumarate (Co-administration with psychotropic agents has resulted in isolated cases of neuroleptic malignant syndrome). Products include:
Seroquel Tablets 690

Quinidine (Carbamazepine is metabolized mainly by cytochrome P450 (CYP) 3A4 to the active carbamazepine 10,11 -epoxide, which is further metabolized to the trans-diol by epoxide hydrolase. Therefore, the potential exists for interaction between carbamazepine and any agent that inhibits CYP3A4 and/or epoxide hydrolase).
No products indexed under this heading.

Quinidine Gluconate (Carbamazepine is known to induce CYP1A2 and CYP3A4. Therefore, the potential exists for interaction between carbamazepine and any agent metabolized by one (or more) of these enzymes).
No products indexed under this heading.

Quinidine Hydrochloride (Carbamazepine is metabolized mainly by cytochrome P450 (CYP) 3A4 to the active carbamazepine 10,11 -epoxide, which is further metabolized to the trans-diol by epoxide hydrolase. Therefore, the potential exists for interaction between carbamazepine and any agent that inhibits CYP3A4 and/or epoxide hydrolase).
No products indexed under this heading.

Quinidine Polygalacturonate (Carbamazepine is metabolized mainly by cytochrome P450 (CYP) 3A4 to the active carbamazepine 10,11 -epoxide, which is further metabolized to the trans-diol by epoxide hydrolase. Therefore, the potential exists for interaction between carbamazepine and any agent that inhibits CYP3A4 and/or epoxide hydrolase).
No products indexed under this heading.

Quinidine Sulfate (Carbamazepine is metabolized mainly by cytochrome P450 (CYP) 3A4 to the active carbamazepine 10,11 -epoxide, which is further metabolized to the trans-diol by epoxide hydrolase. Therefore, the potential exists for interaction between carbamazepine and any agent that inhibits CYP3A4 and/or epoxide hydrolase).
No products indexed under this heading.

Quinine (Carbamazepine is metabolized mainly by cytochrome P450 (CYP) 3A4 to the active carbamazepine 10,11 -epoxide, which is further metabolized to the trans-diol by epoxide hydrolase. Therefore, the potential exists for interaction between carbamazepine and any agent that inhibits CYP3A4 and/or epoxide hydrolase).
No products indexed under this heading.

Quinine Sulfate (Carbamazepine is metabolized mainly by cytochrome P450 (CYP) 3A4 to the active carbamazepine 10,11 -epoxide, which is further metabolized to the trans-diol by epoxide hydrolase. Therefore, the potential exists for interaction between carbamazepine and any agent that inhibits CYP3A4 and/or epoxide hydrolase).

No products indexed under this heading.

Quinupristin (Carbamazepine is metabolized mainly by cytochrome P450 (CYP) 3A4 to the active carbamazepine 10,11 -epoxide, which is further metabolized to the trans-diol by epoxide hydrolase. Therefore, the potential exists for interaction between carbamazepine and any agent that inhibits CYP3A4 and/or epoxide hydrolase).

No products indexed under this heading.

Ranitidine Bismuth Citrate (Carbamazepine is metabolized mainly by cytochrome P450 (CYP) 3A4 to the active carbamazepine 10,11 -epoxide, which is further metabolized to the trans-diol by epoxide hydrolase. Therefore, the potential exists for interaction between carbamazepine and any agent that inhibits CYP3A4 and/or epoxide hydrolase).

No products indexed under this heading.

Ranitidine Hydrochloride (Carbamazepine is metabolized mainly by cytochrome P450 (CYP) 3A4 to the active carbamazepine 10,11 -epoxide, which is further metabolized to the trans-diol by epoxide hydrolase. Therefore, the potential exists for interaction between carbamazepine and any agent that inhibits CYP3A4 and/or epoxide hydrolase). Products include:

Rifabutin (Carbamazepine is metabolized by CYP3A4. Therefore, the potential exists for interaction between caramazepine and any agent that induces CYP3A4).

No products indexed under this heading.

Rifampicin (Carbamazepine is metabolized by CYP3A4. Therefore, the potential exists for interaction between caramazepine and any agent that induces CYP3A4).

No products indexed under this heading.

Rifampin (Inducers of CYP3A4, such as rifampin, can increase the rate of carbamazepine metabolism and can thus decrease plasma carbamazepine levels).

No products indexed under this heading.

Rifapentine (Carbamazepine is metabolized by CYP3A4. Therefore, the potential exists for interaction between caramazepine and any agent that induces CYP3A4).

No products indexed under this heading.

Riluzole (Carbamazepine is known to induce CYP1A2 and CYP3A4. Therefore, the potential exists for interaction between carbamazepine and any agent metabolized by one (or more) of these enzymes). Products include:

Risperidone (Co-administration with psychotropic agents has resulted in isolated cases of neuroleptic malignant syndrome). Products include:

Ritonavir (Carbamazepine is metabolized mainly by cytochrome P450 (CYP) 3A4 to the active carbamazepine 10,11 -epoxide, which is further metabolized to the trans-diol by epoxide hydrolase. Therefore, the potential exists for interaction between carbamazepine and any agent that inhibits CYP3A4 and/or epoxide hydrolase). Products include:

Ropinirole Hydrochloride (Carbamazepine is known to induce CYP1A2 and CYP3A4. Therefore, the potential exists for interaction between carbamazepine and any agent metabolized by one (or more) of these enzymes). Products include:

Ropivacaine Hydrochloride (Carbamazepine is known to induce CYP1A2 and CYP3A4. Therefore, the potential exists for interaction between carbamazepine and any agent metabolized by one (or more) of these enzymes).

No products indexed under this heading.

Saquinavir (Carbamazepine is metabolized mainly by cytochrome P450 (CYP) 3A4 to the active carbamazepine 10,11 -epoxide, which is further metabolized to the trans-diol by epoxide hydrolase. Therefore, the potential exists for interaction between carbamazepine and any agent that inhibits CYP3A4 and/or epoxide hydrolase).

No products indexed under this heading.

Saquinavir Mesylate (Carbamazepine is metabolized mainly by cytochrome P450 (CYP) 3A4 to the active carbamazepine 10,11 -epoxide, which is further metabolized to the trans-diol by epoxide hydrolase. Therefore, the potential exists for interaction between carbamazepine and any agent that inhibits its CYP3A4 and/or epoxide hydrolase). Products include:

Selegiline Hydrochloride (Because of the relationship of carbamazepine to other tricyclic compounds, on theoretical grounds, co-administration with MAO inhibitors is contraindicated). Products include:

Sertraline Hydrochloride (Carbamazepine is metabolized mainly by cytochrome P450 (CYP) 3A4 to the active carbamazepine 10,11 -epoxide, which is further metabolized to the trans-diol by epoxide hydrolase. Therefore, the potential exists for interaction between carbamazepine and any agent that inhibits its CYP3A4 and/or epoxide hydrolase). Products include:

Sildenafil Citrate (Carbamazepine is known to induce CYP1A2 and CYP3A4. Therefore, the potential exists for interaction between car-

bamazepine and any agent metabolized by one (or more) of these enzymes). Products include:

Simvastatin (Carbamazepine is known to induce CYP1A2 and CYP3A4. Therefore, the potential exists for interaction between carbamazepine and any agent metabolized by one (or more) of these enzymes). Products include:

Sirolimus (Carbamazepine is known to induce CYP1A2 and CYP3A4. Therefore, the potential exists for interaction between carbamazepine and any agent metabolized by one (or more) of these enzymes). Products include:

Sulfinpyrazone (Carbamazepine is metabolized by CYP3A4. Therefore, the potential exists for interaction between caramazepine and any agent that induces CYP3A4).

No products indexed under this heading.

Tacrine Hydrochloride (Carbamazepine is known to induce CYP1A2 and CYP3A4. Therefore, the potential exists for interaction between carbamazepine and any agent metabolized by one (or more) of these enzymes).

No products indexed under this heading.

Tacrolimus (Carbamazepine is known to induce CYP1A2 and CYP3A4. Therefore, the potential exists for interaction between carbamazepine and any agent metabolized by one (or more) of these enzymes). Products include:

Tamoxifen Citrate (Carbamazepine is known to induce CYP1A2 and CYP3A4. Therefore, the potential exists for interaction between carbamazepine and any agent metabolized by one (or more) of these enzymes). Products include:

Telithromycin (Carbamazepine is metabolized mainly by cytochrome P450 (CYP) 3A4 to the active carbamazepine 10,11 -epoxide, which is further metabolized to the trans-diol by epoxide hydrolase. Therefore, the potential exists for interaction between carbamazepine and any agent that inhibits CYP3A4 and/or epoxide hydrolase). Products include:

Terfenadine (Inhibitors of CYP3A4, such as terfenadine, inhibit carbamazepine metabolism and thus increase plasma carbamazepine levels).

No products indexed under this heading.

Theophylline (Inducers of CYP3A4, such as theophylline, can increase the rate of carbamazepine metabolism and can thus decrease plasma carbamazepine levels; carbamazepine induces hepatic CYP activity and causes or would be expected to decrease plasma levels of theophylline).

No products indexed under this heading.

Theophylline Anhydrous (Inducers of CYP3A4, such as theophylline, can increase the rate of carbamazepine metabolism and can thus decrease plasma carbamazepine levels; carbamazepine induces hepatic CYP activity and causes or would be expected to decrease plasma levels of theophylline). Products include:

Theophylline Calcium Salicylate (Inducers of CYP3A4, such as theophylline, can increase the rate of carbamazepine metabolism and can thus decrease plasma carbamazepine levels; carbamazepine induces hepatic CYP activity and causes or would be expected to decrease plasma levels of theophylline).

No products indexed under this heading.

Theophylline Dihydroxypropyl (Glyceryl) (Inducers of CYP3A4, such as theophylline, can increase the rate of carbamazepine metabolism and can thus decrease plasma carbamazepine levels; carbamazepine induces hepatic CYP activity and causes or would be expected to decrease plasma levels of theophylline).

No products indexed under this heading.

Theophylline Ethylenediamine (Inducers of CYP3A4, such as theophylline, can increase the rate of carbamazepine metabolism and can thus decrease plasma carbamazepine levels; carbamazepine induces hepatic CYP activity and causes or would be expected to decrease plasma levels of theophylline).

No products indexed under this heading.

Theophylline Sodium Glycinate (Inducers of CYP3A4, such as theophylline, can increase the rate of carbamazepine metabolism and can thus decrease plasma carbamazepine levels; carbamazepine induces hepatic CYP activity and causes or would be expected to decrease plasma levels of theophylline).

No products indexed under this heading.

Thioridazine Hydrochloride (Co-administration with psychotropic agents has resulted in isolated cases of neuroleptic malignant syndrome). Products include:

Thiothixene (Co-administration with psychotropic agents has resulted in isolated cases of neuroleptic malignant syndrome). Products include:

Tiagabine Hydrochloride (Alterations of thyroid function have been reported in combination therapy with other anticonvulsants). Products include:

Tolterodine Tartrate (Carbamazepine is known to induce CYP1A2 and

CYP3A4. Therefore, the potential exists for interaction between carbamazepine and any agent metabolized by one (or more) of these enzymes). Products include:

- Detrol Tablets 2628
- Detrol LA Capsules 2631

Topiramate (Alterations of thyroid function have been reported in combination therapy with other anticonvulsants). Products include:

- Topamax Sprinkle Capsules 2404
- Topamax Tablets 2404

Tranylcypromine Sulfate (Because of the relationship of carbamazepine to other tricyclic compounds, on theoretical grounds, co-administration with MAO inhibitors is contraindicated). Products include:

- Parnate Tablets 1527

Trazodone Hydrochloride (Carbamazepine is known to induce CYP1A2 and CYP3A4. Therefore, the potential exists for interaction between carbamazepine and any agent metabolized by one (or more) of these enzymes).

No products indexed under this heading.

Triamcinolone (Carbamazepine is metabolized by CYP3A4. Therefore, the potential exists for interaction between caramazepine and any agent that induces CYP3A4).

No products indexed under this heading.

Triamcinolone Acetonide (Carbamazepine is metabolized by CYP3A4. Therefore, the potential exists for interaction between caramazepine and any agent that induces CYP3A4). Products include:

- Azmacort Inhalation Aerosol 1726
- Nasacort AQ Nasal Spray 2922

Triamcinolone Diacetate (Carbamazepine is metabolized by CYP3A4. Therefore, the potential exists for interaction between caramazepine and any agent that induces CYP3A4).

No products indexed under this heading.

Triamcinolone Hexacetonide (Carbamazepine is metabolized by CYP3A4. Therefore, the potential exists for interaction between caramazepine and any agent that induces CYP3A4).

No products indexed under this heading.

Triazolam (Carbamazepine is known to induce CYP1A2 and CYP3A4. Therefore, the potential exists for interaction between carbamazepine and any agent metabolized by one (or more) of these enzymes).

No products indexed under this heading.

Trifluoperazine Hydrochloride (Co-administration with psychotropic agents has resulted in isolated cases of neuroleptic malignant syndrome).

No products indexed under this heading.

Trimethadione (Alterations of thyroid function have been reported in combination therapy with other anticonvulsants).

No products indexed under this heading.

Trimethaphan Camsylate (Carbamazepine is known to induce CYP1A2 and CYP3A4. Therefore, the potential exists for interaction between carbamazepine and any agent metabolized by one (or more) of these enzymes).

No products indexed under this heading.

Trimipramine Maleate (Carbamazepine is known to induce CYP1A2 and CYP3A4. Therefore, the potential exists for interaction between carbamazepine and any agent metabolized by one (or more) of these enzymes).

No products indexed under this heading.

Troglitazone (Carbamazepine is metabolized mainly by cytochrome P450 (CYP) 3A4 to the active carbamazepine 10,11 -epoxide, which is further metabolized to the trans-diol by epoxide hydrolase. Therefore, the potential exists for interaction between carbamazepine and any agent that inhibits CYP3A4 and/ or epoxide hydrolase).

No products indexed under this heading.

Troleandomycin (Inhibitors of CYP3A4, such as troleandomycin, inhibit carbamazepine metabolism and thus increase plasma carbamazepine levels).

No products indexed under this heading.

Trovafloxacin Mesylate (Carbamazepine is known to induce CYP1A2 and CYP3A4. Therefore, the potential exists for interaction between carbamazepine and any agent metabolized by one (or more) of these enzymes).

No products indexed under this heading.

Valproate Sodium (Alterations of thyroid function have been reported in combination therapy with other anticonvulsants). Products include:

- Depacon Injection 412

Valproic Acid (Alterations of thyroid function have been reported in combination therapy with other anticonvulsants). Products include:

- Depakene 417

Verapamil Hydrochloride (Inhibitors of CYP3A4, such as verapamil, inhibit carbamazepine metabolism and thus increase plasma carbamazepine levels). Products include:

- Covera-HS Tablets 3139
- Tarka Tablets 524
- Verelan PM Extended-Release Capsules, Controlled-Onset 3106

Vinblastine Sulfate (Carbamazepine is known to induce CYP1A2 and CYP3A4. Therefore, the potential exists for interaction between carbamazepine and any agent metabolized by one (or more) of these enzymes).

No products indexed under this heading.

Vincristine Sulfate (Carbamazepine is known to induce CYP1A2 and CYP3A4. Therefore, the potential exists for interaction between carbamazepine and any agent metabolized by one (or more) of these enzymes).

No products indexed under this heading.

Voriconazole (Carbamazepine is metabolized mainly by cytochrome P450 (CYP) 3A4 to the active carbamazepine 10,11 -epoxide, which is further metabolized to the trans-diol by epoxide hydrolase. Therefore, the potential exists for interaction between carbamazepine and any agent that inhibits CYP3A4 and/ or epoxide hydrolase). Products include:

- VFEND I.V. 2564
- VFEND Oral Suspension 2564
- VFEND Tablets 2564

Warfarin Sodium (Carbamezapine induces hepatic CYP activity and causes or would be expected to decrease plasma levels of warfarin). Products include:

- Coumadin for Injection 898
- Coumadin Tablets 898

Zafirlukast (Carbamazepine is metabolized mainly by cytochrome P450 (CYP) 3A4 to the active carbamazepine 10,11 -epoxide, which is further metabolized to the trans-diol by epoxide hydrolase. Therefore, the potential exists for interaction between carbamazepine and any agent that inhibits CYP3A4 and/ or epoxide hydrolase). Products include:

- Accolate Tablets 671

Zileuton (Carbamazepine is metabolized mainly by cytochrome P450 (CYP) 3A4 to the active carbamazepine 10,11 -epoxide, which is further metabolized to the trans-diol by epoxide hydrolase. Therefore, the potential exists for interaction between carbamazepine and any agent that inhibits CYP3A4 and/or epoxide hydrolase). Products include:

- Zyflo Tablets 1023

Ziprasidone Hydrochloride (Co-administration with psychotropic agents has resulted in isolated cases of neuroleptic malignant syndrome). Products include:

- Geodon Capsules 2529

Zolmitriptan (Carbamazepine is known to induce CYP1A2 and CYP3A4. Therefore, the potential exists for interaction between carbamazepine and any agent metabolized by one (or more) of these enzymes). Products include:

- Zomig Tablets 3519
- Zomig Nasal Spray 3523
- Zomig-ZMT Tablets 3519

Zonisamide (Alterations of thyroid function have been reported in combination therapy with other anticonvulsants). Products include:

- Zonegran Capsules 1101

Food Interactions

Food, unspecified (A high fat meal increased the rat of absorption of a single 400 mg dose but not the AUC; elimination half-life remains unchanged between fasting and fed states).

Grapefruit (Carbamazepine is metabolized mainly by cytochrome P450 (CYP) 3A4 to the active carbamazepine 10,11 -epoxide, which is further metabolized to the trans-diol by epoxide hydrolase. Therefore, the potential exists for interaction between carbamazepine and any agent that inhibits CYP3A4 and/or epoxide hydrolase).

Grapefruit Juice (Carbamazepine is metabolized mainly by cytochrome P450 (CYP) 3A4 to the active carbamazepine 10,11 -epoxide, which is further metabolized to the trans-diol by epoxide hydrolase. Therefore, the potential exists for interaction between carbamazepine and any agent that inhibits CYP3A4 and/or epoxide hydrolase).

CARDENE I.V.

(Nicardipine Hydrochloride) 2497

May interact with beta blockers and certain other agents. Compounds in these categories include:

Acebutolol Hydrochloride (In vitro and in some patients a negative inotropic effect has been observed with Cardene I.V., therefore, caution should be exercised when co-administered with beta blockers in patients with CHF or significant left ventricular dysfunction).

No products indexed under this heading.

Atenolol (In vitro and in some patients a negative inotropic effect has been observed with Cardene I.V., therefore, caution should be exercised when co-administered with beta blockers in patients with CHF or significant left ventricular dysfunction).

No products indexed under this heading.

Beta Blockers (Cardene I.V. may be safely used concomitantly with beta-blockers. However, exercise caution when using Cardene I.V. in combination with a beta-blocker in CHF patients.).

No products indexed under this heading.

Betaxolol Hydrochloride (In vitro and in some patients a negative inotropic effect has been observed with Cardene I.V., therefore, caution should be exercised when co-administered with beta blockers in patients with CHF or significant left ventricular dysfunction). Products include:

- Betoptic S Ophthalmic Suspension 558

Bisoprolol Fumarate (In vitro and in some patients a negative inotropic effect has been observed with Cardene I.V., therefore, caution should be exercised when co-administered with beta blockers in patients with CHF or significant left ventricular dysfunction).

No products indexed under this heading.

Carteolol Hydrochloride (In vitro and in some patients a negative inotropic effect has been observed with Cardene I.V., therefore, caution should be exercised when co-administered with beta blockers in patients with CHF or significant left ventricular dysfunction). Products include:

- Carteolol Hydrochloride Ophthalmic Solution USP, 1% .... ⊙249

Cimetidine (Co-administration of cimetidine with Cardene I.V. increases nicardipine plasma concentration. Carefully monitor). Products include:

- Tagamet HB 200 Tablets .... ▣664

Cimetidine Hydrochloride (Co-administration of cimetidine with Cardene I.V. increases nicardipine plasma concentration).

No products indexed under this heading.

Cyclosporine (Co-administration of Cardene I.V. and cyclosporine results in elevated plasma cyclosporine levels. Closely monitor plasma concentrations of cyclosporine and reduce dose accordingly). Products include:

- Gengraf Capsules 459
- Neoral Oral Solution 2259

Neoral Soft Gelatin Capsules 2259
Restasis Ophthalmic Emulsion 575
Sandimmune 2275

Digoxin (No alteration in digoxin plasma levels, however, as a precaution, digoxin levels should be evaluated when concomitant therapy is initiated). Products include:
Lanoxicaps Capsules 1490
Lanoxin Injection 1494
Lanoxin Injection Pediatric 1497
Lanoxin Tablets 1500

Esmolol Hydrochloride (In vitro and in some patients a negative inotropic effect has been observed with Cardene I.V., therefore, caution should be exercised when co-administered with beta blockers in patients with CHF or significant left ventricular dysfunction).
No products indexed under this heading.

Fentanyl (Potential for hypotension with fentanyl anesthesia when used with calcium channel blockers and beta blockers; such reaction has not been observed with Cardene I.V. during clinical trials). Products include:
Duragesic Transdermal System 2373
Ionsys Transdermal System 2379

Fentanyl Citrate (Potential for hypotension with fentanyl anesthesia when used with calcium channel blockers and beta blockers; such reaction has not been observed with Cardene I.V. during clinical trials). Products include:
Actiq 979

Labetalol Hydrochloride (In vitro and in some patients a negative inotropic effect has been observed with Cardene I.V., therefore, caution should be exercised when co-administered with beta blockers in patients with CHF or significant left ventricular dysfunction).
No products indexed under this heading.

Levobunolol Hydrochloride (In vitro and in some patients a negative inotropic effect has been observed with Cardene I.V., therefore, caution should be exercised when co-administered with beta blockers in patients with CHF or significant left ventricular dysfunction). Products include:
Betagan Ophthalmic Solution, USP.......... ⊙220

Metipranolol Hydrochloride (In vitro and in some patients a negative inotropic effect has been observed with Cardene I.V., therefore, caution should be exercised when co-administered with beta blockers in patients with CHF or significant left ventricular dysfunction).
No products indexed under this heading.

Metoprolol Succinate (In vitro and in some patients a negative inotropic effect has been observed with Cardene I.V., therefore, caution should be exercised when co-administered with beta blockers in patients with CHF or significant left ventricular dysfunction). Products include:
Toprol-XL Tablets 668

Metoprolol Tartrate (In vitro and in some patients a negative inotropic effect has been observed with Cardene I.V., therefore, caution should be exercised when co-administered with beta blockers in patients with CHF or significant left ventricular dysfunction). Products include:
Lopressor Injection 2238
Lopressor Tablets 2238
Lopressor HCT 50/25 Tablets 2241
Lopressor HCT 100/25 Tablets 2241
Lopressor HCT 100/50 Tablets 2241

Nadolol (In vitro and in some patients a negative inotropic effect has been observed with Cardene I.V., therefore, caution should be exercised when co-administered with beta blockers in patients with CHF or significant left ventricular dysfunction). Products include:
Nadolol Tablets 2159

Penbutolol Sulfate (In vitro and in some patients a negative inotropic effect has been observed with Cardene I.V., therefore, caution should be exercised when co-administered with beta blockers in patients with CHF or significant left ventricular dysfunction).
No products indexed under this heading.

Pindolol (In vitro and in some patients a negative inotropic effect has been observed with Cardene I.V., therefore, caution should be exercised when co-administered with beta blockers in patients with CHF or significant left ventricular dysfunction).
No products indexed under this heading.

Propranolol Hydrochloride (In vitro and in some patients a negative inotropic effect has been observed with Cardene I.V., therefore, caution should be exercised when co-administered with beta blockers in patients with CHF or significant left ventricular dysfunction). Products include:
Inderal LA Long-Acting Capsules 3429
InnoPran XL Capsules 2723

Sotalol Hydrochloride (In vitro and in some patients a negative inotropic effect has been observed with Cardene I.V., therefore, caution should be exercised when co-administered with beta blockers in patients with CHF or significant left ventricular dysfunction).
No products indexed under this heading.

Timolol Hemihydrate (In vitro and in some patients a negative inotropic effect has been observed with Cardene I.V., therefore, caution should be exercised when co-administered with beta blockers in patients with CHF or significant left ventricular dysfunction). Products include:
Betimol Ophthalmic Solution 3382
Betimol Ophthalmic Solution .... ⊙295

Timolol Maleate (In vitro and in some patients a negative inotropic effect has been observed with Cardene I.V., therefore, caution should be exercised when co-administered with beta blockers in patients with CHF or significant left ventricular dysfunction). Products include:
Blocadren Tablets 1916
Cosopt Sterile Ophthalmic Solution 1931
Timolide Tablets 2086
Timoptic Sterile Ophthalmic Solution 2088
Timoptic in Ocudose 2091
Timoptic-XE Sterile Ophthalmic Gel Forming Solution 2092

CARDIO ESSENTIALS CAPSULES

(Coenzyme Q-10) 3328
None cited in PDR database.

CARDIZEM LA EXTENDED RELEASE TABLETS

(Diltiazem Hydrochloride) 1728
May interact with anesthetics, antihypertensives, benzodiazepines, beta blockers, cytochrome p450 3a4 inducers (selected), cytochrome p450 3a4 inhibitors (selected), cytochrome p450 3a4 substrates (selected), cardiac glycosides, quinidine, and certain other agents. Compounds in these categories include:

Acebutolol Hydrochloride (Pharmacologic studies indicate that there may be additive effects in prolonging A-V conduction when using beta-blockers or digitalis concomitantly with diltiazem).
No products indexed under this heading.

Acetazolamide (Diltiazem is both a substrate and an inhibitor of the CYP3A4 enzyme system. Other drugs that are specific substrates, inhibitors, or inducers of this enzyme system may have a significant impact on the efficacy and side effect profile of diltiazem).
No products indexed under this heading.

Alfentanil Hydrochloride (The depression of cardiac contractility, conductivity, and automaticity, as well as the vascular dilation associated with anesthetics, may be potentiated by calcium channel blockers).
No products indexed under this heading.

Allium sativum (Diltiazem is both a substrate and an inhibitor of the CYP3A4 enzyme system. Other drugs that are specific substrates, inhibitors, or inducers of this enzyme system may have a significant impact on the efficacy and side effect profile of diltiazem).
No products indexed under this heading.

Alprazolam (Studies showed that diltiazem increased the AUC of midazolam and triazolam by 3- to 4-fold and the Cmax by 2-fold, compared to placebo. The elimination half-life of midazolam and triazolam also increased during co-administration with diltiazem). Products include:
Niravam Orally Disintegrating Tablets 3092

Amiodarone Hydrochloride (Diltiazem is both a substrate and an inhibitor of the CYP3A4 enzyme system. Other drugs that are specific substrates, inhibitors, or inducers of this enzyme system may have a significant impact on the efficacy and side effect profile of diltiazem).
No products indexed under this heading.

Amitriptyline Hydrochloride (Patients taking other drugs that are substrates of CYP450, especially patients with renal and/or hepatic impairment, may require dosage adjustment when starting or stopping concomitantly administered diltiazem in order to maintain optimum therapeutic blood levels).
No products indexed under this heading.

Amlodipine Besylate (Diltiazem has an additive effect when used with other antihypertensive agents. Therefore, the dosage of diltiazem or concomitant antihypertensives may need to be adjusted when adding one to the other). Products include:
Caduet Tablets 2508
Lotrel Capsules 2249
Norvasc Tablets 2545

Amprenavir (Diltiazem is both a substrate and an inhibitor of the CYP3A4 enzyme system. Other drugs that are specific substrates, inhibitors, or inducers of this enzyme system may have a significant impact on the efficacy and side effect profile of diltiazem). Products include:
Agenerase Capsules 1327
Agenerase Oral Solution 1332

Anastrozole (Diltiazem is both a substrate and an inhibitor of the CYP3A4 enzyme system. Other drugs that are specific substrates, inhibitors, or inducers of this enzyme system may have a significant impact on the efficacy and side effect profile of diltiazem). Products include:
Arimidex Tablets 673

Aprepitant (Patients taking other drugs that are substrates of CYP450, especially patients with renal and/or hepatic impairment, may require dosage adjustment when starting or stopping concomitantly administered diltiazem in order to maintain optimum therapeutic blood levels). Products include:
Emend Capsules 1963

Astemizole (Patients taking other drugs that are substrates of CYP450, especially patients with renal and/or hepatic impairment, may require dosage adjustment when starting or stopping concomitantly administered diltiazem in order to maintain optimum therapeutic blood levels).
No products indexed under this heading.

Atenolol (Pharmacologic studies indicate that there may be additive effects in prolonging A-V conduction when using beta-blockers or digitalis concomitantly with diltiazem).
No products indexed under this heading.

Atorvastatin Calcium (Patients taking other drugs that are substrates of CYP450, especially patients with renal and/or hepatic impairment, may require dosage adjustment when starting or stopping concomitantly administered diltiazem in order to maintain optimum therapeutic blood levels). Products include:
Caduet Tablets 2508
Lipitor Tablets 2483

Belladonna Ergotamine (Patients taking other drugs that are substrates of CYP450, especially patients with renal and/or hepatic impairment, may require dosage adjustment when starting or stopping concomitantly administered diltiazem in order to maintain optimum therapeutic blood levels).
No products indexed under this heading.

Benazepril Hydrochloride (Diltiazem has an additive effect when used with other antihypertensive agents. Therefore, the dosage of diltiazem or concomitant antihypertensives may need to be adjusted when adding one to the other). Products include:
Lotensin Tablets 2243
Lotensin HCT Tablets 2246
Lotrel Capsules 2249

Bendroflumethiazide (Diltiazem has an additive effect when used with other antihypertensive agents. Therefore, the dosage of diltiazem or concomitant antihypertensives may need to be adjusted when adding one to the other).
No products indexed under this heading.

Betamethasone Acetate (Diltiazem is both a substrate and an inhibitor of the CYP3A4 enzyme system. Other drugs that are specific substrates, inhibitors, or inducers of this enzyme system may have a significant impact on the efficacy and side effect profile of diltiazem).
No products indexed under this heading.

Betamethasone Sodium Phosphate (Diltiazem is both a substrate and an inhibitor of the CYP3A4 enzyme system. Other drugs that are specific substrates, inhibitors, or inducers of this enzyme system may have a significant impact on the efficacy and side effect profile of diltiazem).
No products indexed under this heading.

Betaxolol Hydrochloride (Pharmacologic studies indicate that there may be additive effects in prolonging A-V conduction when using beta-blockers or digitalis concomitantly with diltiazem). Products include:
Betoptic S Ophthalmic Suspension.................................. 558

Bisoprolol Fumarate (Pharmacologic studies indicate that there may be additive effects in prolonging A-V conduction when using beta-blockers or digitalis concomitantly with diltiazem).
No products indexed under this heading.

Buspirone Hydrochloride (Studies showed that diltiazem increased the AUC of buspirone by 5.5 fold and the Cmax by 4.1 fold. Enhanced effects of buspirone may be possible).
No products indexed under this heading.

Busulfan (Patients taking other drugs that are substrates of CYP450, especially patients with renal and/or hepatic impairment, may require dosage adjustment when starting or stopping concomitantly administered diltiazem in order to maintain optimum therapeutic blood levels). Products include:
I.V. Busulfex 2493
Myleran Tablets 1525

Candesartan Cilexetil (Diltiazem has an additive effect when used with other antihypertensive agents. Therefore, the dosage of diltiazem or concomitant antihypertensives may need to be adjusted when adding one to the other). Products include:
Atacand Tablets 649
Atacand HCT 651

Captopril (Diltiazem has an additive effect when used with other antihypertensive agents. Therefore, the dosage of diltiazem or concomitant antihypertensives may need to be adjusted when adding one to the other). Products include:
Captopril Tablets 2149

Carbamazepine (Concomitant administration of diltiazem with carbamazepine has been reported to result in elevated serum levels of carbamazepine (40% to 72% increase), resulting in toxicity in some cases). Products include:
Carbatrol Capsules 3171
Equetro Extended-Release Capsules.................................... 3180
Tegretol/Tegretol-XR 2295

Carteolol Hydrochloride (Pharmacologic studies indicate that there may be additive effects in prolonging A-V conduction when using beta-blockers or digitalis concomitantly with diltiazem). Products include:
Carteolol Hydrochloride Ophthalmic Solution USP, 1%....... ⊙249

Cerivastatin Sodium (Patients taking other drugs that are substrates of CYP450, especially patients with renal and/or hepatic impairment, may require dosage adjustment when starting or stopping concomitantly administered diltiazem in order to maintain optimum therapeutic blood levels).
No products indexed under this heading.

Chlordiazepoxide (Studies showed that diltiazem increased the AUC of midazolam and triazolam by 3- to 4-fold and the Cmax by 2-fold, compared to placebo. The elimination half-life of midazolam and triazolam also increased during co-administration with diltiazem).
No products indexed under this heading.

Chlordiazepoxide Hydrochloride (Studies showed that diltiazem increased the AUC of midazolam and triazolam by 3- to 4-fold and the Cmax by 2-fold, compared to placebo. The elimination half-life of midazolam and triazolam also increased during co-administration with diltiazem). Products include:
Librium Capsules 3347

Chlorothiazide (Diltiazem has an additive effect when used with other antihypertensive agents. Therefore, the dosage of diltiazem or concomitant antihypertensives may need to be adjusted when adding one to the other). Products include:
Diuril Oral Suspension 1954

Chlorothiazide Sodium (Diltiazem has an additive effect when used with other antihypertensive agents. Therefore, the dosage of diltiazem or concomitant antihypertensives may need to be adjusted when adding one to the other). Products include:
Diuril Sodium Intravenous 2467

Chlorpheniramine (Patients taking other drugs that are substrates of CYP450, especially patients with renal and/or hepatic impairment, may require dosage adjustment when starting or stopping concomitantly administered diltiazem in order to maintain optimum therapeutic blood levels).
No products indexed under this heading.

Chlorpheniramine Maleate (Patients taking other drugs that are substrates of CYP450, especially patients with renal and/or hepatic impairment, may require dosage adjustment when starting or stopping concomitantly administered diltiazem in order to maintain optimum therapeutic blood levels). Products include:
Advil Allergy Sinus Caplets 770
Advil Multi-Symptom Cold Caplets...................................... 770
BC Allergy Sinus Cold Powder 677
Comtrex Maximum Strength Cold & Cough Day/Night Caplets - Night Formulation 726
Comtrex Maximum Strength Day/Night Severe Cold & Sinus Caplets - Night Formulation 725
Contac Cold and Flu Maximum Strength Caplets........................ 728
Contac Cold and Flu Day and Night Caplets (Night Formulation Only)........................ 727
Children's Dimetapp Long Acting Cough Plus Cold Syrup............... 731
Robitussin Cough & Cold Long-Acting Liquid 735
Robitussin Cough & Allergy Syrup .. 736
Robitussin Cough & Cold Nighttime Liquid.......................... 736
Robitussin Cough, Cold & Flu Nighttime Liquid.......................... 738
Robitussin Pediatric Cough & Cold Long-Acting Liquid.............. 735
Robitussin Pediatric Cough & Cold Nighttime Liquid................. 736
Triaminic Cold & Allergy Liquid 746
Triaminic Cough & Runny Nose Softchews 748
Children's Tylenol Plus Flu Oral Suspension............................... 749
Tylenol Allergy Multi-Symptom Caplets with Cool Burst and Gelcaps.. 1872
Children's Tylenol Plus Cold Suspension Liquid 1879
Children's Tylenol Plus Cough & Runny Nose Suspension Liquid..... 1879
Children's Tylenol Plus Flu Suspension Liquid 1881
Children's Tylenol Plus Multi-Symptom Cold Suspension Liquid 1879
Tylenol Cold Head Congestion Nighttime Caplets with Cool Burst.. 1873
Tylenol Cold Multi-Symptom Nighttime Caplets with Cool Burst.. 1874
Tylenol Sinus Congestion & Pain Nighttime Caplets with Cool Burst.. 1876
Vicks 44M Cough, Cold & Flu Relief Liquid.................................. 2680
Pediatric Vicks 44m Cough & Cold Relief Liquid......................... 2676
Children's Vicks NyQuil Cold/Cough Relief........................ 756
Children's Vicks NyQuil Cold/Cough Relief Liquid 2680
Zicam Maximum Strength Flu Daytime.. 768

Chlorpheniramine Polistirex (Patients taking other drugs that are substrates of CYP450, especially patients with renal and/or hepatic impairment, may require dosage adjustment when starting or stopping concomitantly administered diltiazem in order to maintain optimum therapeutic blood levels). Products include:
Tussionex Pennkinetic Extended-Release Suspension...... 3327

Chlorpheniramine Tannate (Patients taking other drugs that are substrates of CYP450, especially patients with renal and/or hepatic impairment, may require dosage adjustment when starting or stopping concomitantly administered diltiazem in order to maintain optimum therapeutic blood levels).
No products indexed under this heading.

Chlorthalidone (Diltiazem has an additive effect when used with other antihypertensive agents. Therefore, the dosage of diltiazem or concomitant antihypertensives may need to be adjusted when adding one to the other). Products include:
Clorpres Tablets 2153

Cimetidine (A study in six healthy volunteers has shown a significant increase in peak diltiazem plasma levels (58%) and AUC (53%) after a 1-week course of cimetidine at 1200 mg per day and a single dose of diltiazem 60 mg). Products include:
Tagamet HB 200 Tablets 664

Cimetidine Hydrochloride (A study in six healthy volunteers has shown a significant increase in peak diltiazem plasma levels (58%) and AUC (53%) after a 1-week course of cimetidine at 1200 mg per day and a single dose of diltiazem 60 mg).
No products indexed under this heading.

Ciprofloxacin (Diltiazem is both a substrate and an inhibitor of the CYP3A4 enzyme system. Other drugs that are specific substrates, inhibitors, or inducers of this enzyme system may have a significant impact on the efficacy and side effect profile of diltiazem). Products include:
Cipro Oral Suspension 2977
Cipro I.V. 2984
Cipro XR Tablets 2990
Ciprodex Otic Suspension 559

Ciprofloxacin Hydrochloride (Diltiazem is both a substrate and an inhibitor of the CYP3A4 enzyme system. Other drugs that are specific substrates, inhibitors, or inducers of this enzyme system may have a significant impact on the efficacy and side effect profile of diltiazem). Products include:
Ciloxan Ophthalmic Ointment 559
Ciloxan Ophthalmic Solution .... ⊙206
Cipro Tablets 2977
Proquin XR Tablets 1153

Cisapride (Patients taking other drugs that are substrates of CYP450, especially patients with renal and/or hepatic impairment, may require dosage adjustment when starting or stopping concomitantly administered diltiazem in order to maintain optimum therapeutic blood levels).
No products indexed under this heading.

Cisplatin (Diltiazem is both a substrate and an inhibitor of the CYP3A4 enzyme system. Other drugs that are specific substrates, inhibitors, or inducers of this enzyme system may have a significant impact on the efficacy and side effect profile of diltiazem).
No products indexed under this heading.

Clarithromycin (Patients taking other drugs that are substrates of CYP450, especially patients with renal and/or hepatic impairment, may require dosage adjustment when starting or stopping concomitantly administered diltiazem in order to maintain optimum therapeutic blood levels). Products include:
Biaxin/Biaxin XL 402
PREVPAC 3284

Clonidine (Diltiazem has an additive effect when used with other antihypertensive agents. Therefore, the dosage of diltiazem or concomitant antihypertensives may need to be adjusted when adding one to the other). Products include:
Catapres-TTS 844

Clonidine Hydrochloride (Diltiazem has an additive effect when used with other antihypertensive agents. Therefore, the dosage of diltiazem or concomitant antihypertensives may need to be adjusted when adding one to the other). Products include:

Catapres Tablets 843
Clorpres Tablets 2153

Clorazepate Dipotassium (Studies showed that diltiazem increased the AUC of midazolam and triazolam by 3- to 4-fold and the Cmax by 2-fold, compared to placebo. The elimination half-life of midazolam and triazolam also increased during co-administration with diltiazem). Products include:

Tranxene 2474

Clotrimazole (Diltiazem is both a substrate and an inhibitor of the CYP3A4 enzyme system. Other drugs that are specific substrates, inhibitors, or inducers of this enzyme system may have a significant impact on the efficacy and side effect profile of diltiazem). Products include:

Desenex Athlete's Foot Cream .... ▣ 635
Lotrimin 3039
Lotrisone 3040

Cortisone Acetate (Diltiazem is both a substrate and an inhibitor of the CYP3A4 enzyme system. Other drugs that are specific substrates, inhibitors, or inducers of this enzyme system may have a significant impact on the efficacy and side effect profile of diltiazem).

No products indexed under this heading.

Cyclosporine (In renal and cardiac transplant recipients, a reduction of cyclosporine dose ranging from 15% to 48% was necessary to maintain cyclosporine trough concentrations similar to those seen prior to the addition of diltiazem. If these agents are to be administered concurrently, cyclosporine concentrations should be monitored, especially when diltiazem therapy is initiated, adjusted or discontinued). Products include:

Gengraf Capsules 459
Neoral Oral Solution 2259
Neoral Soft Gelatin Capsules 2259
Restasis Ophthalmic Emulsion 575
Sandimmune 2275

Dalfopristin (Diltiazem is both a substrate and an inhibitor of the CYP3A4 enzyme system. Other drugs that are specific substrates, inhibitors, or inducers of this enzyme system may have a significant impact on the efficacy and side effect profile of diltiazem).

No products indexed under this heading.

Danazol (Diltiazem is both a substrate and an inhibitor of the CYP3A4 enzyme system. Other drugs that are specific substrates, inhibitors, or inducers of this enzyme system may have a significant impact on the efficacy and side effect profile of diltiazem).

No products indexed under this heading.

Delavirdine Mesylate (Diltiazem is both a substrate and an inhibitor of the CYP3A4 enzyme system. Other drugs that are specific substrates, inhibitors, or inducers of this enzyme system may have a significant impact on the efficacy and side effect profile of diltiazem). Products include:

Rescriptor Tablets 2551

Deserpidine (Diltiazem has an additive effect when used with other antihypertensive agents. Therefore, the dosage of diltiazem or concomitant antihypertensives may need to be adjusted when adding one to the other).

No products indexed under this heading.

Deslanoside (Pharmacologic studies indicate that there may be additive effects in prolonging A-V conduction when using beta-blockers or digitalis concomitantly with diltiazem).

No products indexed under this heading.

Desogestrel (Patients taking other drugs that are substrates of CYP450, especially patients with renal and/or hepatic impairment, may require dosage adjustment when starting or stopping concomitantly administered diltiazem in order to maintain optimum therapeutic blood levels). Products include:

Mircette Tablets 1066

Dexamethasone (Diltiazem is both a substrate and an inhibitor of the CYP3A4 enzyme system. Other drugs that are specific substrates, inhibitors, or inducers of this enzyme system may have a significant impact on the efficacy and side effect profile of diltiazem). Products include:

Ciprodex Otic Suspension 559
Decadron Tablets 1951
TobraDex Ophthalmic Ointment 562
TobraDex Ophthalmic Suspension ... 563

Dexamethasone Acetate (Diltiazem is both a substrate and an inhibitor of the CYP3A4 enzyme system. Other drugs that are specific substrates, inhibitors, or inducers of this enzyme system may have a significant impact on the efficacy and side effect profile of diltiazem).

No products indexed under this heading.

Dexamethasone Sodium Phosphate (Diltiazem is both a substrate and an inhibitor of the CYP3A4 enzyme system. Other drugs that are specific substrates, inhibitors, or inducers of this enzyme system may have a significant impact on the efficacy and side effect profile of diltiazem).

No products indexed under this heading.

Diazepam (Studies showed that diltiazem increased the AUC of midazolam and triazolam by 3- to 4-fold and the Cmax by 2-fold, compared to placebo. The elimination half-life of midazolam and triazolam also increased during co-administration with diltiazem). Products include:

Diastat Rectal Delivery System 3343
Valium Tablets 2819

Diazoxide (Diltiazem has an additive effect when used with other antihypertensive agents. Therefore, the dosage of diltiazem or concomitant antihypertensives may need to be adjusted when adding one to the other). Products include:

Hyperstat I.V. 3017

Digitalis Glycoside Preparations (Pharmacologic studies indicate that there may be additive effects in prolonging A-V conduction when using beta-blockers or digitalis concomitantly with diltiazem).

No products indexed under this heading.

Digitoxin (Pharmacologic studies indicate that there may be additive effects in prolonging A-V conduction when using beta-blockers or digitalis concomitantly with diltiazem).

No products indexed under this heading.

Digoxin (Pharmacologic studies indicate that there may be additive effects in prolonging A-V conduction when using beta-blockers or digitalis concomitantly with diltiazem). Products include:

Lanoxicaps Capsules 1490
Lanoxin Injection 1494
Lanoxin Injection Pediatric 1497
Lanoxin Tablets 1500

Dihydroergotamine Mesylate (Patients taking other drugs that are substrates of CYP450, especially patients with renal and/or hepatic impairment, may require dosage adjustment when starting or stopping concomitantly administered diltiazem in order to maintain optimum therapeutic blood levels). Products include:

Migranal Nasal Spray 3348

Diltiazem Maleate (Patients taking other drugs that are substrates of CYP450, especially patients with renal and/or hepatic impairment, may require dosage adjustment when starting or stopping concomitantly administered diltiazem in order to maintain optimum therapeutic blood levels).

No products indexed under this heading.

Disopyramide (Patients taking other drugs that are substrates of CYP450, especially patients with renal and/or hepatic impairment, may require dosage adjustment when starting or stopping concomitantly administered diltiazem in order to maintain optimum therapeutic blood levels).

No products indexed under this heading.

Disopyramide Phosphate (Patients taking other drugs that are substrates of CYP450, especially patients with renal and/or hepatic impairment, may require dosage adjustment when starting or stopping concomitantly administered diltiazem in order to maintain optimum therapeutic blood levels).

No products indexed under this heading.

Disulfiram (Patients taking other drugs that are substrates of CYP450, especially patients with renal and/or hepatic impairment, may require dosage adjustment when starting or stopping concomitantly administered diltiazem in order to maintain optimum therapeutic blood levels).

No products indexed under this heading.

Doxazosin Mesylate (Diltiazem has an additive effect when used with other antihypertensive agents. Therefore, the dosage of diltiazem or concomitant antihypertensives may need to be adjusted when adding one to the other). Products include:

Cardura XL Tablets 2515

Doxorubicin Hydrochloride (Patients taking other drugs that are substrates of CYP450, especially patients with renal and/or hepatic impairment, may require dosage adjustment when starting or stopping concomitantly administered diltiazem in order to maintain optimum therapeutic blood levels).

No products indexed under this heading.

Dronabinol (Patients taking other drugs that are substrates of CYP450, especially patients with renal and/or hepatic impairment, may require dosage adjustment when starting or stopping concomitantly administered diltiazem in order to maintain optimum therapeutic blood levels). Products include:

Marinol Capsules 3333

Efavirenz (Diltiazem is both a substrate and an inhibitor of the CYP3A4 enzyme system. Other drugs that are specific substrates, inhibitors, or inducers of this enzyme system may have a significant impact on the efficacy and side effect profile of diltiazem). Products include:

Atripla Tablets 945
Sustiva Capsules 930
Sustiva Tablets 930

Enalapril Maleate (Diltiazem has an additive effect when used with other antihypertensive agents. Therefore, the dosage of diltiazem or concomitant antihypertensives may need to be adjusted when adding one to the other). Products include:

Vasotec I.V. Injection 2103

Enalaprilat (Diltiazem has an additive effect when used with other antihypertensive agents. Therefore, the dosage of diltiazem or concomitant antihypertensives may need to be adjusted when adding one to the other).

No products indexed under this heading.

Enflurane (The depression of cardiac contractility, conductivity, and automaticity, as well as the vascular dilation associated with anesthetics, may be potentiated by calcium channel blockers).

No products indexed under this heading.

Eprosartan Mesylate (Diltiazem has an additive effect when used with other antihypertensive agents. Therefore, the dosage of diltiazem or concomitant antihypertensives may need to be adjusted when adding one to the other). Products include:

Teveten Tablets 1735
Teveten HCT Tablets 1737

Ergotamine Tartrate (Patients taking other drugs that are substrates of CYP450, especially patients with renal and/or hepatic impairment, may require dosage adjustment when starting or stopping concomitantly administered diltiazem in order to maintain optimum therapeutic blood levels).

No products indexed under this heading.

Erythromycin (Patients taking other drugs that are substrates of CYP450, especially patients with renal and/or hepatic impairment, may require dosage adjustment when starting or stopping concomitantly administered diltiazem in order to maintain optimum therapeutic blood levels). Products include:

Erythromycin Estolate (Patients taking other drugs that are substrates of CYP450, especially patients with renal and/or hepatic impairment, may require dosage adjustment when starting or stopping concomitantly administered diltiazem in order to maintain optimum therapeutic blood levels).

No products indexed under this heading.

Erythromycin Ethylsuccinate (Patients taking other drugs that are substrates of CYP450, especially patients with renal and/or hepatic impairment, may require dosage adjustment when starting or stopping concomitantly administered diltiazem in order to maintain optimum therapeutic blood levels). Products include:

Erythromycin Gluceptate (Patients taking other drugs that are substrates of CYP450, especially patients with renal and/or hepatic impairment, may require dosage adjustment when starting or stopping concomitantly administered diltiazem in order to maintain optimum therapeutic blood levels).

No products indexed under this heading.

Erythromycin Lactobionate (Patients taking other drugs that are substrates of CYP450, especially patients with renal and/or hepatic impairment, may require dosage adjustment when starting or stopping concomitantly administered diltiazem in order to maintain optimum therapeutic blood levels).

No products indexed under this heading.

Erythromycin Stearate (Patients taking other drugs that are substrates of CYP450, especially patients with renal and/or hepatic impairment, may require dosage adjustment when starting or stopping concomitantly administered diltiazem in order to maintain optimum therapeutic blood levels). Products include:

Esmolol Hydrochloride (Pharmacologic studies indicate that there may be additive effects in prolonging A-V conduction when using beta-blockers or digitalis concomitantly with diltiazem).

No products indexed under this heading.

Esomeprazole Magnesium (Diltiazem is both a substrate and an inhibitor of the CYP3A4 enzyme system. Other drugs that are specific substrates, inhibitors, or inducers of this enzyme system may have a significant impact on the efficacy and side effect profile of diltiazem). Products include:

Estazolam (Studies showed that diltiazem increased the AUC of midazolam and triazolam by 3- to 4-fold and the Cmax by 2-fold, compared to placebo. The elimination half-life

of midazolam and triazolam also increased during co-administration with diltiazem). Products include:

Estradiol (Patients taking other drugs that are substrates of CYP450, especially patients with renal and/or hepatic impairment, may require dosage adjustment when starting or stopping concomitantly administered diltiazem in order to maintain optimum therapeutic blood levels). Products include:

Estradiol Benzoate (Patients taking other drugs that are substrates of CYP450, especially patients with renal and/or hepatic impairment, may require dosage adjustment when starting or stopping concomitantly administered diltiazem in order to maintain optimum therapeutic blood levels).

No products indexed under this heading.

Estradiol Cypionate (Patients taking other drugs that are substrates of CYP450, especially patients with renal and/or hepatic impairment, may require dosage adjustment when starting or stopping concomitantly administered diltiazem in order to maintain optimum therapeutic blood levels).

No products indexed under this heading.

Estradiol Valerate (Patients taking other drugs that are substrates of CYP450, especially patients with renal and/or hepatic impairment, may require dosage adjustment when starting or stopping concomitantly administered diltiazem in order to maintain optimum therapeutic blood levels).

No products indexed under this heading.

Ethinyl Estradiol (Patients taking other drugs that are substrates of CYP450, especially patients with renal and/or hepatic impairment, may require dosage adjustment when starting or stopping concomitantly administered diltiazem in order to maintain optimum therapeutic blood levels). Products include:

Ethosuximide (Patients taking other drugs that are substrates of CYP450, especially patients with renal and/or hepatic impairment, may require dosage adjustment when starting or stopping concomitantly administered diltiazem in order to maintain optimum therapeutic blood levels).

No products indexed under this heading.

Ethynodiol Diacetate (Patients taking other drugs that are substrates of CYP450, especially patients with renal and/or hepatic impairment, may require dosage adjustment when starting or stopping concomitantly administered diltiazem in order to maintain optimum therapeutic blood levels).

No products indexed under this heading.

Etoposide (Patients taking other drugs that are substrates of CYP450, especially patients with renal and/or hepatic impairment, may require dosage adjustment when starting or stopping concomitantly administered diltiazem in order to maintain optimum therapeutic blood levels).

No products indexed under this heading.

Etoposide Phosphate (Patients taking other drugs that are substrates of CYP450, especially patients with renal and/or hepatic impairment, may require dosage adjustment when starting or stopping concomitantly administered diltiazem in order to maintain optimum therapeutic blood levels).

No products indexed under this heading.

Felbamate (Diltiazem is both a substrate and an inhibitor of the CYP3A4 enzyme system. Other drugs that are specific substrates, inhibitors, or inducers of this enzyme system may have a significant impact on the efficacy and side effect profile of diltiazem).

No products indexed under this heading.

Felodipine (Diltiazem has an additive effect when used with other antihypertensive agents. Therefore, the dosage of diltiazem or concomitant antihypertensives may need to be adjusted when adding one to the other).

No products indexed under this heading.

Fentanyl (Patients taking other drugs that are substrates of CYP450, especially patients with renal and/or hepatic impairment, may require dosage adjustment when starting or stopping concomitantly administered diltiazem in order to maintain optimum therapeutic blood levels). Products include:

Fentanyl Citrate (The depression of cardiac contractility, conductivity, and automaticity, as well as the vascular dilation associated with anesthetics, may be potentiated by calcium channel blockers). Products include:

Fluconazole (Diltiazem is both a substrate and an inhibitor of the CYP3A4 enzyme system. Other drugs that are specific substrates, inhibitors, or inducers of this enzyme system may have a significant impact on the efficacy and side effect profile of diltiazem).

No products indexed under this heading.

Fludrocortisone Acetate (Diltiazem is both a substrate and an inhibitor of the CYP3A4 enzyme system. Other drugs that are specific substrates, inhibitors, or inducers of this enzyme system may have a significant impact on the efficacy and side effect profile of diltiazem).

No products indexed under this heading.

Fluoxetine Hydrochloride (Diltiazem is both a substrate and an inhibitor of the CYP3A4 enzyme system. Other drugs that are specific substrates, inhibitors, or inducers of this enzyme system may have a significant impact on the efficacy and side effect profile of diltiazem). Products include:

Flurazepam Hydrochloride (Studies showed that diltiazem increased the AUC of midazolam and triazolam by 3- to 4-fold and the Cmax by 2-fold, compared to placebo. The elimination half-life of midazolam and triazolam also increased during co-administration with diltiazem). Products include:

Fluvoxamine Maleate (Diltiazem is both a substrate and an inhibitor of the CYP3A4 enzyme system. Other drugs that are specific substrates, inhibitors, or inducers of this enzyme system may have a significant impact on the efficacy and side effect profile of diltiazem).

No products indexed under this heading.

Fosamprenavir Calcium (Diltiazem is both a substrate and an inhibitor of the CYP3A4 enzyme system. Other drugs that are specific substrates, inhibitors, or inducers of this enzyme system may have a significant impact on the efficacy and side effect profile of diltiazem). Products include:

Fosinopril Sodium (Diltiazem has an additive effect when used with other antihypertensive agents. Therefore, the dosage of diltiazem or concomitant antihypertensives may need to be adjusted when adding one to the other).

No products indexed under this heading.

Fosphenytoin Sodium (Diltiazem is both a substrate and an inhibitor of the CYP3A4 enzyme system. Other drugs that are specific substrates, inhibitors, or inducers of this enzyme system may have a significant impact on the efficacy and side effect profile of diltiazem).

No products indexed under this heading.

Furosemide (Diltiazem has an additive effect when used with other antihypertensive agents. Therefore, the dosage of diltiazem or concomitant antihypertensives may need to be adjusted when adding one to the other). Products include:

Garlic Extract (Diltiazem is both a substrate and an inhibitor of the CYP3A4 enzyme system. Other drugs that are specific substrates, inhibitors, or inducers of this enzyme system may have a significant impact on the efficacy and side effect profile of diltiazem).

No products indexed under this heading.

IMPORTANT NOTE: Always consult each drug listing in the patient's regimen for possible interactions.

Garlic Oil (Diltiazem is both a substrate and an inhibitor of the CYP3A4 enzyme system. Other drugs that are specific substrates, inhibitors, or inducers of this enzyme system may have a significant impact on the efficacy and side effect profile of diltiazem).

No products indexed under this heading.

Guanabenz Acetate (Diltiazem has an additive effect when used with other antihypertensive agents. Therefore, the dosage of diltiazem or concomitant antihypertensives may need to be adjusted when adding one to the other).

No products indexed under this heading.

Guanethidine Monosulfate (Diltiazem has an additive effect when used with other antihypertensive agents. Therefore, the dosage of diltiazem or concomitant antihypertensives may need to be adjusted when adding one to the other).

No products indexed under this heading.

Halazepam (Studies showed that diltiazem increased the AUC of midazolam and triazolam by 3- to 4-fold and the Cmax by 2-fold, compared to placebo. The elimination half-life of midazolam and triazolam also increased during co-administration with diltiazem).

No products indexed under this heading.

Haloperidol (Patients taking other drugs that are substrates of CYP450, especially patients with renal and/or hepatic impairment, may require dosage adjustment when starting or stopping concomitantly administered diltiazem in order to maintain optimum therapeutic blood levels).

No products indexed under this heading.

Haloperidol Decanoate (Patients taking other drugs that are substrates of CYP450, especially patients with renal and/or hepatic impairment, may require dosage adjustment when starting or stopping concomitantly administered diltiazem in order to maintain optimum therapeutic blood levels).

No products indexed under this heading.

Haloperidol Lactate (Patients taking other drugs that are substrates of CYP450, especially patients with renal and/or hepatic impairment, may require dosage adjustment when starting or stopping concomitantly administered diltiazem in order to maintain optimum therapeutic blood levels).

No products indexed under this heading.

Halothane (The depression of cardiac contractility, conductivity, and automaticity, as well as the vascular dilation associated with anesthetics, may be potentiated by calcium channel blockers).

No products indexed under this heading.

Hydralazine Hydrochloride (Diltiazem has an additive effect when used with other antihypertensive agents. Therefore, the dosage of diltiazem or concomitant antihypertensives may need to be adjusted when adding one to the other). Products include:

- BiDil Tablets **2171**

Hydrochlorothiazide (Diltiazem has an additive effect when used with other antihypertensive agents. Therefore, the dosage of diltiazem or concomitant antihypertensives may need to be adjusted when adding one to the other). Products include:

- Aldoril Tablets **1910**
- Atacand HCT **651**
- Avalide Tablets **888**
- Avalide Tablets **2874**
- Benicar HCT Tablets **1044**
- Diovan HCT Tablets **2196**
- Dyazide Capsules **1423**
- Hyzaar 50-12.5 Tablets **1990**
- Hyzaar 100-12.5 Tablets **1990**
- Hyzaar 100-25 Tablets **1990**
- Lopressor HCT 50/25 Tablets **2241**
- Lopressor HCT 100/25 Tablets **2241**
- Lopressor HCT 100/50 Tablets **2241**
- Lotensin HCT Tablets **2246**
- Micardis HCT Tablets **856**
- Moduretic Tablets **2028**
- Prinzide Tablets **2056**
- Teveten HCT Tablets **1737**
- Timolide Tablets **2086**
- Uniretic Tablets **3100**

Hydrocortisone (Diltiazem is both a substrate and an inhibitor of the CYP3A4 enzyme system. Other drugs that are specific substrates, inhibitors, or inducers of this enzyme system may have a significant impact on the efficacy and side effect profile of diltiazem). Products include:

- Colocort Rectal Suspension, USP (Retention) 100 mg/60 mL **2476**
- Hydrocortone Tablets **1989**
- Preparation H Hydrocortisone Cream .... ▣**646**

Hydrocortisone Acetate (Diltiazem is both a substrate and an inhibitor of the CYP3A4 enzyme system. Other drugs that are specific substrates, inhibitors, or inducers of this enzyme system may have a significant impact on the efficacy and side effect profile of diltiazem). Products include:

- Analpram-HC **1159**
- Pramosone **1161**
- ProctoFoam-HC **3099**

Hydrocortisone Butyrate (Diltiazem is both a substrate and an inhibitor of the CYP3A4 enzyme system. Other drugs that are specific substrates, inhibitors, or inducers of this enzyme system may have a significant impact on the efficacy and side effect profile of diltiazem). Products include:

- Locoid Lipocream Cream **1160**

Hydrocortisone Cypionate (Diltiazem is both a substrate and an inhibitor of the CYP3A4 enzyme system. Other drugs that are specific substrates, inhibitors, or inducers of this enzyme system may have a significant impact on the efficacy and side effect profile of diltiazem).

No products indexed under this heading.

Hydrocortisone Hemisuccinate (Diltiazem is both a substrate and an inhibitor of the CYP3A4 enzyme system. Other drugs that are specific substrates, inhibitors, or inducers of this enzyme system may have a significant impact on the efficacy and side effect profile of diltiazem).

No products indexed under this heading.

Hydrocortisone Probutate (Diltiazem is both a substrate and an inhibitor of the CYP3A4 enzyme system. Other drugs that are specific substrates, inhibitors, or inducers of this enzyme system may have a significant impact on the efficacy and side effect profile of diltiazem).

No products indexed under this heading.

Hydrocortisone Sodium Phosphate (Diltiazem is both a substrate and an inhibitor of the CYP3A4 enzyme system. Other drugs that are specific substrates, inhibitors, or inducers of this enzyme system may have a significant impact on the efficacy and side effect profile of diltiazem).

No products indexed under this heading.

Hydrocortisone Sodium Succinate (Diltiazem is both a substrate and an inhibitor of the CYP3A4 enzyme system. Other drugs that are specific substrates, inhibitors, or inducers of this enzyme system may have a significant impact on the efficacy and side effect profile of diltiazem).

No products indexed under this heading.

Hydrocortisone Valerate (Diltiazem is both a substrate and an inhibitor of the CYP3A4 enzyme system. Other drugs that are specific substrates, inhibitors, or inducers of this enzyme system may have a significant impact on the efficacy and side effect profile of diltiazem).

No products indexed under this heading.

Hydroflumethiazide (Diltiazem has an additive effect when used with other antihypertensive agents. Therefore, the dosage of diltiazem or concomitant antihypertensives may need to be adjusted when adding one to the other).

No products indexed under this heading.

Hypericum (Diltiazem is both a substrate and an inhibitor of the CYP3A4 enzyme system. Other drugs that are specific substrates, inhibitors, or inducers of this enzyme system may have a significant impact on the efficacy and side effect profile of diltiazem). Products include:

- Satiete Tablets .... ▣**832**

Hypericum Perforatum (Diltiazem is both a substrate and an inhibitor of the CYP3A4 enzyme system. Other drugs that are specific substrates, inhibitors, or inducers of this enzyme system may have a significant impact on the efficacy and side effect profile of diltiazem).

No products indexed under this heading.

Indapamide (Diltiazem has an additive effect when used with other antihypertensive agents. Therefore, the dosage of diltiazem or concomitant antihypertensives may need to be adjusted when adding one to the other). Products include:

- Indapamide Tablets **2156**

Indinavir Sulfate (Patients taking other drugs that are substrates of CYP450, especially patients with renal and/or hepatic impairment, may require dosage adjustment when starting or stopping concomitantly administered diltiazem in order to maintain optimum therapeutic blood levels). Products include:

- Crixivan Capsules **1940**

Irbesartan (Diltiazem has an additive effect when used with other antihypertensive agents. Therefore, the dosage of diltiazem or concomitant antihypertensives may need to be adjusted when adding one to the other). Products include:

- Avalide Tablets **888**
- Avalide Tablets **2874**
- Avapro Tablets **891**
- Avapro Tablets **2871**

Isoflurane (The depression of cardiac contractility, conductivity, and automaticity, as well as the vascular dilation associated with anesthetics, may be potentiated by calcium channel blockers).

No products indexed under this heading.

Isoniazid (Diltiazem is both a substrate and an inhibitor of the CYP3A4 enzyme system. Other drugs that are specific substrates, inhibitors, or inducers of this enzyme system may have a significant impact on the efficacy and side effect profile of diltiazem).

No products indexed under this heading.

Isradipine (Diltiazem has an additive effect when used with other antihypertensive agents. Therefore, the dosage of diltiazem or concomitant antihypertensives may need to be adjusted when adding one to the other). Products include:

- DynaCirc CR Tablets **2721**

Itraconazole (Patients taking other drugs that are substrates of CYP450, especially patients with renal and/or hepatic impairment, may require dosage adjustment when starting or stopping concomitantly administered diltiazem in order to maintain optimum therapeutic blood levels).

No products indexed under this heading.

Ketamine Hydrochloride (The depression of cardiac contractility, conductivity, and automaticity, as well as the vascular dilation associated with anesthetics, may be potentiated by calcium channel blockers).

No products indexed under this heading.

Ketoconazole (Patients taking other drugs that are substrates of CYP450, especially patients with renal and/or hepatic impairment, may require dosage adjustment when starting or stopping concomitantly administered diltiazem in order to maintain optimum therapeutic blood levels). Products include:

- Nizoral A-D Shampoo, 1% **1868**

Labetalol Hydrochloride (Pharmacologic studies indicate that there may be additive effects in prolonging A-V conduction when using beta-blockers or digitalis concomitantly with diltiazem).

No products indexed under this heading.

Levobunolol Hydrochloride (Pharmacologic studies indicate that there may be additive effects in prolonging A-V conduction when using beta-blockers or digitalis concomitantly with diltiazem). Products include:

- Betagan Ophthalmic Solution, USP .... ⊙**220**

Levonorgestrel (Patients taking other drugs that are substrates of CYP450, especially patients with renal and/or hepatic impairment, may require dosage adjustment when starting or stopping concomitantly administered diltiazem in order to maintain optimum therapeutic blood levels). Products include:

Climara Pro Transdermal System 776
Mirena Intrauterine System 787
Plan B Tablets 1076
Seasonique Tablets 1077

Lidocaine (Patients taking other drugs that are substrates of CYP450, especially patients with renal and/or hepatic impairment, may require dosage adjustment when starting or stopping concomitantly administered diltiazem in order to maintain optimum therapeutic blood levels). Products include:

Lidoderm Patch 1118
Synera Topical Patch 1137

Lidocaine Hydrochloride (Patients taking other drugs that are substrates of CYP450, especially patients with renal and/or hepatic impairment, may require dosage adjustment when starting or stopping concomitantly administered diltiazem in order to maintain optimum therapeutic blood levels).

No products indexed under this heading.

Lisinopril (Diltiazem has an additive effect when used with other antihypertensive agents. Therefore, the dosage of diltiazem or concomitant antihypertensives may need to be adjusted when adding one to the other). Products include:

Prinivil Tablets 2052
Prinzide Tablets 2056

Lopinavir (Diltiazem is both a substrate and an inhibitor of the CYP3A4 enzyme system. Other drugs that are specific substrates, inhibitors, or inducers of this enzyme system may have a significant impact on the efficacy and side effect profile of diltiazem). Products include:

Kaletra 476

Loratadine (Diltiazem is both a substrate and an inhibitor of the CYP3A4 enzyme system. Other drugs that are specific substrates, inhibitors, or inducers of this enzyme system may have a significant impact on the efficacy and side effect profile of diltiazem). Products include:

Alavert Allergy & Sinus D-12 Hour Tablets 771
Alavert 771
Children's Claritin Allergy Oral Solution 771
Claritin Non-Drowsy 24 Hour Tablets 772
Claritin Reditabs 24 Hour Non-Drowsy Tablets 772
Claritin-D Non-Drowsy 12 Hour Tablets 772
Claritin-D Non-Drowsy 24 Hour Tablets 772

Lorazepam (Studies showed that diltiazem increased the AUC of midazolam and triazolam by 3- to 4-fold and the Cmax by 2-fold, compared to placebo. The elimination half-life of midazolam and triazolam also increased during co-administration with diltiazem).

No products indexed under this heading.

Losartan Potassium (Diltiazem has an additive effect when used with other antihypertensive agents. Therefore, the dosage of diltiazem or concomitant antihypertensives may need to be adjusted when adding one to the other). Products include:

Cozaar Tablets 1935
Hyzaar 50-12.5 Tablets 1990
Hyzaar 100-12.5 Tablets 1990
Hyzaar 100-25 Tablets 1990

Lovastatin (In a ten-subject study, co-administration of diltiazem (120 mg bid diltiazem SR) with lovastatin resulted in a 3-4 times increase in mean lovastatin AUC and Cmax versus lovastatin alone). Products include:

Advicor Tablets 1722
Altoprev Extended-Release Tablets 3109
Mevacor Tablets 2021

Mecamylamine Hydrochloride (Diltiazem has an additive effect when used with other antihypertensive agents. Therefore, the dosage of diltiazem or concomitant antihypertensives may need to be adjusted when adding one to the other).

No products indexed under this heading.

Mephenytoin (Diltiazem is both a substrate and an inhibitor of the CYP3A4 enzyme system. Other drugs that are specific substrates, inhibitors, or inducers of this enzyme system may have a significant impact on the efficacy and side effect profile of diltiazem).

No products indexed under this heading.

Mestranol (Patients taking other drugs that are substrates of CYP450, especially patients with renal and/or hepatic impairment, may require dosage adjustment when starting or stopping concomitantly administered diltiazem in order to maintain optimum therapeutic blood levels).

No products indexed under this heading.

Methadone Hydrochloride (Patients taking other drugs that are substrates of CYP450, especially patients with renal and/or hepatic impairment, may require dosage adjustment when starting or stopping concomitantly administered diltiazem in order to maintain optimum therapeutic blood levels).

No products indexed under this heading.

Methohexital Sodium (The depression of cardiac contractility, conductivity, and automaticity, as well as the vascular dilation associated with anesthetics, may be potentiated by calcium channel blockers).

No products indexed under this heading.

Methsuximide (Diltiazem is both a substrate and an inhibitor of the CYP3A4 enzyme system. Other drugs that are specific substrates, inhibitors, or inducers of this enzyme system may have a significant impact on the efficacy and side effect profile of diltiazem).

No products indexed under this heading.

Methyclothiazide (Diltiazem has an additive effect when used with other antihypertensive agents. Therefore, the dosage of diltiazem or concomitant antihypertensives may need to be adjusted when adding one to the other).

No products indexed under this heading.

Methyldopa (Diltiazem has an additive effect when used with other antihypertensive agents. Therefore, the dosage of diltiazem or concomitant antihypertensives may need to be adjusted when adding one to the other). Products include:

Aldoril Tablets 1910

Methyldopate Hydrochloride (Diltiazem has an additive effect when used with other antihypertensive agents. Therefore, the dosage of diltiazem or concomitant antihypertensives may need to be adjusted when adding one to the other).

No products indexed under this heading.

Methylprednisolone (Diltiazem is both a substrate and an inhibitor of the CYP3A4 enzyme system. Other drugs that are specific substrates, inhibitors, or inducers of this enzyme system may have a significant impact on the efficacy and side effect profile of diltiazem).

No products indexed under this heading.

Methylprednisolone Acetate (Diltiazem is both a substrate and an inhibitor of the CYP3A4 enzyme system. Other drugs that are specific substrates, inhibitors, or inducers of this enzyme system may have a significant impact on the efficacy and side effect profile of diltiazem). Products include:

Depo-Medrol Injectable Suspension 2617
Depo-Medrol Single-Dose Vial 2619

Methylprednisolone Sodium Succinate (Diltiazem is both a substrate and an inhibitor of the CYP3A4 enzyme system. Other drugs that are specific substrates, inhibitors, or inducers of this enzyme system may have a significant impact on the efficacy and side effect profile of diltiazem).

No products indexed under this heading.

Metipranolol Hydrochloride (Pharmacologic studies indicate that there may be additive effects in prolonging A-V conduction when using beta-blockers or digitalis concomitantly with diltiazem).

No products indexed under this heading.

Metolazone (Diltiazem has an additive effect when used with other antihypertensive agents. Therefore, the dosage of diltiazem or concomitant antihypertensives may need to be adjusted when adding one to the other).

No products indexed under this heading.

Metoprolol Succinate (Pharmacologic studies indicate that there may be additive effects in prolonging A-V conduction when using beta-blockers or digitalis concomitantly with diltiazem). Products include:

Toprol-XL Tablets 668

Metoprolol Tartrate (Pharmacologic studies indicate that there may be additive effects in prolonging A-V conduction when using beta-blockers or digitalis concomitantly with diltiazem). Products include:

Lopressor Injection 2238
Lopressor Tablets 2238
Lopressor HCT 50/25 Tablets 2241
Lopressor HCT 100/25 Tablets 2241
Lopressor HCT 100/50 Tablets 2241

Metronidazole (Diltiazem is both a substrate and an inhibitor of the CYP3A4 enzyme system. Other drugs that are specific substrates, inhibitors, or inducers of this enzyme system may have a significant impact on the efficacy and side effect profile of diltiazem). Products include:

Metrogel 1% 1211
MetroGel-Vaginal Gel 1855
Vandazole Vaginal Gel 3338

Metronidazole Benzoate (Diltiazem is both a substrate and an inhibitor of the CYP3A4 enzyme system. Other drugs that are specific substrates, inhibitors, or inducers of this enzyme system may have a significant impact on the efficacy and side effect profile of diltiazem).

No products indexed under this heading.

Metronidazole Hydrochloride (Diltiazem is both a substrate and an inhibitor of the CYP3A4 enzyme system. Other drugs that are specific substrates, inhibitors, or inducers of this enzyme system may have a significant impact on the efficacy and side effect profile of diltiazem).

No products indexed under this heading.

Metyrosine (Diltiazem has an additive effect when used with other antihypertensive agents. Therefore, the dosage of diltiazem or concomitant antihypertensives may need to be adjusted when adding one to the other). Products include:

Demser Capsules 1953

Mibefradil Dihydrochloride (Diltiazem has an additive effect when used with other antihypertensive agents. Therefore, the dosage of diltiazem or concomitant antihypertensives may need to be adjusted when adding one to the other).

No products indexed under this heading.

Miconazole (Diltiazem is both a substrate and an inhibitor of the CYP3A4 enzyme system. Other drugs that are specific substrates, inhibitors, or inducers of this enzyme system may have a significant impact on the efficacy and side effect profile of diltiazem).

No products indexed under this heading.

Miconazole Nitrate (Diltiazem is both a substrate and an inhibitor of the CYP3A4 enzyme system. Other drugs that are specific substrates, inhibitors, or inducers of this enzyme system may have a significant impact on the efficacy and side effect profile of diltiazem). Products include:

Desenex 635
Desenex Jock Itch Spray Powder 635

Midazolam Hydrochloride (The depression of cardiac contractility, conductivity, and automaticity, as well as the vascular dilation associated with anesthetics, may be potentiated by calcium channel blockers).

No products indexed under this heading.

Minoxidil (Diltiazem has an additive effect when used with other antihypertensive agents. Therefore, the dosage of diltiazem or concomitant antihypertensives may need to be adjusted when adding one to the other). Products include:

Men's Rogaine Extra Strength Hair Regrowth Treatment Topical Solution, Ocean Rush Scent and Original Unscented 633
Men's Rogaine Foam Hair Regrowth Treatment 633

Women's Rogaine Hair Regrowth Treatment Topical Solution, Spring Bloom Scent and Original Unscented .... ▣ 634

Modafinil (Diltiazem is both a substrate and an inhibitor of the CYP3A4 enzyme system. Other drugs that are specific substrates, inhibitors, or inducers of this enzyme system may have a significant impact on the efficacy and side effect profile of diltiazem). Products include:

Provigil Tablets 988

Moexipril Hydrochloride (Diltiazem has an additive effect when used with other antihypertensive agents. Therefore, the dosage of diltiazem or concomitant antihypertensives may need to be adjusted when adding one to the other). Products include:

Uniretic Tablets 3100
Univasc Tablets 3104

Nadolol (Pharmacologic studies indicate that there may be additive effects in prolonging A-V conduction when using beta-blockers or digitalis concomitantly with diltiazem). Products include:

Nadolol Tablets 2159

Nefazodone Hydrochloride (Patients taking other drugs that are substrates of CYP450, especially patients with renal and/or hepatic impairment, may require dosage adjustment when starting or stopping concomitantly administered diltiazem in order to maintain optimum therapeutic blood levels).

No products indexed under this heading.

Nelfinavir Mesylate (Patients taking other drugs that are substrates of CYP450, especially patients with renal and/or hepatic impairment, may require dosage adjustment when starting or stopping concomitantly administered diltiazem in order to maintain optimum therapeutic blood levels). Products include:

Viracept 2577

Nevirapine (Diltiazem is both a substrate and an inhibitor of the CYP3A4 enzyme system. Other drugs that are specific substrates, inhibitors, or inducers of this enzyme system may have a significant impact on the efficacy and side effect profile of diltiazem). Products include:

Viramune Oral Suspension 873
Viramune Tablets 873

Niacinamide (Diltiazem is both a substrate and an inhibitor of the CYP3A4 enzyme system. Other drugs that are specific substrates, inhibitors, or inducers of this enzyme system may have a significant impact on the efficacy and side effect profile of diltiazem).

No products indexed under this heading.

Nicardipine Hydrochloride (Diltiazem has an additive effect when used with other antihypertensive agents. Therefore, the dosage of diltiazem or concomitant antihypertensives may need to be adjusted when adding one to the other). Products include:

Cardene I.V. 2497

Nicotinamide (Diltiazem is both a substrate and an inhibitor of the CYP3A4 enzyme system. Other drugs that are specific substrates, inhibitors, or inducers of this enzyme system may have a significant impact on the efficacy and side effect profile of diltiazem). Products include:

Nicomide Tablets 1088

Nifedipine (Diltiazem has an additive effect when used with other antihypertensive agents. Therefore, the dosage of diltiazem or concomitant antihypertensives may need to be adjusted when adding one to the other). Products include:

Adalat CC Tablets 2964

Nimodipine (Patients taking other drugs that are substrates of CYP450, especially patients with renal and/or hepatic impairment, may require dosage adjustment when starting or stopping concomitantly administered diltiazem in order to maintain optimum therapeutic blood levels). Products include:

Nimotop Capsules 749

Nisoldipine (Diltiazem has an additive effect when used with other antihypertensive agents. Therefore, the dosage of diltiazem or concomitant antihypertensives may need to be adjusted when adding one to the other). Products include:

Sular Tablets 3122

Nitrendipine (Patients taking other drugs that are substrates of CYP450, especially patients with renal and/or hepatic impairment, may require dosage adjustment when starting or stopping concomitantly administered diltiazem in order to maintain optimum therapeutic blood levels).

No products indexed under this heading.

Nitroglycerin (Diltiazem has an additive effect when used with other antihypertensive agents. Therefore, the dosage of diltiazem or concomitant antihypertensives may need to be adjusted when adding one to the other). Products include:

Nitro-Dur Transdermal Infusion System 3046
Nitrolingual Pumpspray 3120

Norethindrone (Patients taking other drugs that are substrates of CYP450, especially patients with renal and/or hepatic impairment, may require dosage adjustment when starting or stopping concomitantly administered diltiazem in order to maintain optimum therapeutic blood levels). Products include:

Ortho Micronor Tablets 2426

Norethindrone Acetate (Patients taking other drugs that are substrates of CYP450, especially patients with renal and/or hepatic impairment, may require dosage adjustment when starting or stopping concomitantly administered diltiazem in order to maintain optimum therapeutic blood levels).

No products indexed under this heading.

Norfloxacin (Diltiazem is both a substrate and an inhibitor of the CYP3A4 enzyme system. Other drugs that are specific substrates, inhibitors, or inducers of this enzyme system may have a significant impact on the efficacy and side effect profile of diltiazem). Products include:

Noroxin Tablets 2032

Norgestrel (Patients taking other drugs that are substrates of CYP450, especially patients with renal and/or hepatic impairment, may require dosage adjustment when starting or stopping concomitantly administered diltiazem in order to maintain optimum therapeutic blood levels).

No products indexed under this heading.

Omeprazole (Diltiazem is both a substrate and an inhibitor of the CYP3A4 enzyme system. Other drugs that are specific substrates, inhibitors, or inducers of this enzyme system may have a significant impact on the efficacy and side effect profile of diltiazem). Products include:

Zegerid Capsules 2958
Zegerid Powder for Oral Solution 2958

Ondansetron (Patients taking other drugs that are substrates of CYP450, especially patients with renal and/or hepatic impairment, may require dosage adjustment when starting or stopping concomitantly administered diltiazem in order to maintain optimum therapeutic blood levels). Products include:

Zofran ODT Orally Disintegrating Tablets 1639

Ondansetron Hydrochloride (Patients taking other drugs that are substrates of CYP450, especially patients with renal and/or hepatic impairment, may require dosage adjustment when starting or stopping concomitantly administered diltiazem in order to maintain optimum therapeutic blood levels). Products include:

Zofran Injection 1634
Zofran 1639

Oxazepam (Studies showed that diltiazem increased the AUC of midazolam and triazolam by 3- to 4-fold and the Cmax by 2-fold, compared to placebo. The elimination half-life of midazolam and triazolam also increased during co-administration with diltiazem).

No products indexed under this heading.

Oxcarbazepine (Diltiazem is both a substrate and an inhibitor of the CYP3A4 enzyme system. Other drugs that are specific substrates, inhibitors, or inducers of this enzyme system may have a significant impact on the efficacy and side effect profile of diltiazem). Products include:

Trileptal Tablets 2300
Trileptal Oral Suspension 2300

Paclitaxel (Patients taking other drugs that are substrates of CYP450, especially patients with renal and/or hepatic impairment, may require dosage adjustment when starting or stopping concomitantly administered diltiazem in order to maintain optimum therapeutic blood levels).

No products indexed under this heading.

Paroxetine Hydrochloride (Diltiazem is both a substrate and an inhibitor of the CYP3A4 enzyme system. Other drugs that are specific substrates, inhibitors, or inducers of this enzyme system may have a significant impact on the efficacy and side effect profile of diltiazem). Products include:

Paxil CR Controlled-Release Tablets 1538
Paxil 1530

Penbutolol Sulfate (Pharmacologic studies indicate that there may be additive effects in prolonging A-V conduction when using beta-blockers or digitalis concomitantly with diltiazem).

No products indexed under this heading.

Perindopril Erbumine (Diltiazem has an additive effect when used with other antihypertensive agents. Therefore, the dosage of diltiazem or concomitant antihypertensives may need to be adjusted when adding one to the other). Products include:

Aceon Tablets (2 mg, 4 mg, 8 mg) 3194

Phenobarbital (Diltiazem is both a substrate and an inhibitor of the CYP3A4 enzyme system. Other drugs that are specific substrates, inhibitors, or inducers of this enzyme system may have a significant impact on the efficacy and side effect profile of diltiazem). Products include:

Donnatal Extentabs 2493

Phenobarbital Sodium (Diltiazem is both a substrate and an inhibitor of the CYP3A4 enzyme system. Other drugs that are specific substrates, inhibitors, or inducers of this enzyme system may have a significant impact on the efficacy and side effect profile of diltiazem).

No products indexed under this heading.

Phenoxybenzamine Hydrochloride (Diltiazem has an additive effect when used with other antihypertensive agents. Therefore, the dosage of diltiazem or concomitant antihypertensives may need to be adjusted when adding one to the other). Products include:

Dibenzyline Capsules 3399

Phentolamine Mesylate (Diltiazem has an additive effect when used with other antihypertensive agents. Therefore, the dosage of diltiazem or concomitant antihypertensives may need to be adjusted when adding one to the other).

No products indexed under this heading.

Phenytoin (Diltiazem is both a substrate and an inhibitor of the CYP3A4 enzyme system. Other drugs that are specific substrates, inhibitors, or inducers of this enzyme system may have a significant impact on the efficacy and side effect profile of diltiazem).

No products indexed under this heading.

Phenytoin Sodium (Diltiazem is both a substrate and an inhibitor of the CYP3A4 enzyme system. Other drugs that are specific substrates, inhibitors, or inducers of this enzyme system may have a significant impact on the efficacy and side effect profile of diltiazem). Products include:

Phenytek Capsules 2160

Pimozide (Patients taking other drugs that are substrates of CYP450, especially patients with renal and/or hepatic impairment, may require dosage adjustment when starting or stopping concomitantly administered diltiazem in order to maintain optimum therapeutic blood levels).

No products indexed under this heading.

Pindolol (Pharmacologic studies indicate that there may be additive effects in prolonging A-V conduction when using beta-blockers or digitalis concomitantly with diltiazem).
No products indexed under this heading.

Polyestradiol Phosphate (Patients taking other drugs that are substrates of CYP450, especially patients with renal and/or hepatic impairment, may require dosage adjustment when starting or stopping concomitantly administered diltiazem in order to maintain optimum therapeutic blood levels).
No products indexed under this heading.

Polythiazide (Diltiazem has an additive effect when used with other antihypertensive agents. Therefore, the dosage of diltiazem or concomitant antihypertensives may need to be adjusted when adding one to the other).
No products indexed under this heading.

Prazepam (Studies showed that diltiazem increased the AUC of midazolam and triazolam by 3- to 4-fold and the Cmax by 2-fold, compared to placebo. The elimination half-life of midazolam and triazolam also increased during co-administration with diltiazem).
No products indexed under this heading.

Prazosin Hydrochloride (Diltiazem has an additive effect when used with other antihypertensive agents. Therefore, the dosage of diltiazem or concomitant antihypertensives may need to be adjusted when adding one to the other).
No products indexed under this heading.

Prednisolone Acetate (Diltiazem is both a substrate and an inhibitor of the CYP3A4 enzyme system. Other drugs that are specific substrates, inhibitors, or inducers of this enzyme system may have a significant impact on the efficacy and side effect profile of diltiazem). Products include:

Prednisolone Sodium Phosphate (Diltiazem is both a substrate and an inhibitor of the CYP3A4 enzyme system. Other drugs that are specific substrates, inhibitors, or inducers of this enzyme system may have a significant impact on the efficacy and side effect profile of diltiazem).
No products indexed under this heading.

Prednisolone Tebutate (Diltiazem is both a substrate and an inhibitor of the CYP3A4 enzyme system. Other drugs that are specific substrates, inhibitors, or inducers of this enzyme system may have a significant impact on the efficacy and side effect profile of diltiazem).
No products indexed under this heading.

Prednisone (Diltiazem is both a substrate and an inhibitor of the CYP3A4 enzyme system. Other drugs that are specific substrates, inhibitors, or inducers of this enzyme system may have a significant impact on the efficacy and side effect profile of diltiazem).
No products indexed under this heading.

Primidone (Diltiazem is both a substrate and an inhibitor of the CYP3A4 enzyme system. Other drugs that are specific substrates, inhibitors, or inducers of this enzyme system may have a significant impact on the efficacy and side effect profile of diltiazem).
No products indexed under this heading.

Propofol (The depression of cardiac contractility, conductivity, and automaticity, as well as the vascular dilation associated with anesthetics, may be potentiated by calcium channel blockers).
No products indexed under this heading.

Propoxyphene Hydrochloride (Diltiazem is both a substrate and an inhibitor of the CYP3A4 enzyme system. Other drugs that are specific substrates, inhibitors, or inducers of this enzyme system may have a significant impact on the efficacy and side effect profile of diltiazem).
No products indexed under this heading.

Propoxyphene Napsylate (Diltiazem is both a substrate and an inhibitor of the CYP3A4 enzyme system. Other drugs that are specific substrates, inhibitors, or inducers of this enzyme system may have a significant impact on the efficacy and side effect profile of diltiazem).
No products indexed under this heading.

Propranolol Hydrochloride (Pharmacologic studies indicate that there may be additive effects in prolonging A-V conduction when using beta-blockers or digitalis concomitantly with diltiazem). Products include:

Quazepam (Studies showed that diltiazem increased the AUC of midazolam and triazolam by 3- to 4-fold and the Cmax by 2-fold, compared to placebo. The elimination half-life of midazolam and triazolam also increased during co-administration with diltiazem).
No products indexed under this heading.

Quinapril Hydrochloride (Diltiazem has an additive effect when used with other antihypertensive agents. Therefore, the dosage of diltiazem or concomitant antihypertensives may need to be adjusted when adding one to the other).
No products indexed under this heading.

Quinidine (Diltiazem significantly increases the AUC of quinidine by 51%, t1/2 by 36%, and decreases it Cloral by 33%. Monitoring for quinidine adverse effects may be warranted and the dose adjusted accordingly).
No products indexed under this heading.

Quinidine Gluconate (Diltiazem significantly increases the AUC of quinidine by 51%, t1/2 by 36%, and decreases it Cloral by 33%. Monitoring for quinidine adverse effects may be warranted and the dose adjusted accordingly).
No products indexed under this heading.

Quinidine Hydrochloride (Diltiazem significantly increases the AUC of quinidine by 51%, t1/2 by 36%, and decreases it Cloral by 33%. Monitoring for quinidine adverse effects may be warranted and the dose adjusted accordingly).
No products indexed under this heading.

Quinidine Polygalacturonate (Diltiazem significantly increases the AUC of quinidine by 51%, t1/2 by 36%, and decreases it Cloral by 33%. Monitoring for quinidine adverse effects may be warranted and the dose adjusted accordingly).
No products indexed under this heading.

Quinidine Sulfate (Diltiazem significantly increases the AUC of quinidine by 51%, t1/2 by 36%, and decreases it Cloral by 33%. Monitoring for quinidine adverse effects may be warranted and the dose adjusted accordingly).
No products indexed under this heading.

Quinine (Diltiazem is both a substrate and an inhibitor of the CYP3A4 enzyme system. Other drugs that are specific substrates, inhibitors, or inducers of this enzyme system may have a significant impact on the efficacy and side effect profile of diltiazem).
No products indexed under this heading.

Quinine Sulfate (Diltiazem is both a substrate and an inhibitor of the CYP3A4 enzyme system. Other drugs that are specific substrates, inhibitors, or inducers of this enzyme system may have a significant impact on the efficacy and side effect profile of diltiazem).
No products indexed under this heading.

Quinupristin (Diltiazem is both a substrate and an inhibitor of the CYP3A4 enzyme system. Other drugs that are specific substrates, inhibitors, or inducers of this enzyme system may have a significant impact on the efficacy and side effect profile of diltiazem).
No products indexed under this heading.

Ramipril (Diltiazem has an additive effect when used with other antihypertensive agents. Therefore, the dosage of diltiazem or concomitant antihypertensives may need to be adjusted when adding one to the other). Products include:

Ranitidine Bismuth Citrate (Diltiazem is both a substrate and an inhibitor of the CYP3A4 enzyme system. Other drugs that are specific substrates, inhibitors, or inducers of this enzyme system may have a significant impact on the efficacy and side effect profile of diltiazem).
No products indexed under this heading.

Ranitidine Hydrochloride (Diltiazem is both a substrate and an inhibitor of the CYP3A4 enzyme system. Other drugs that are specific substrates, inhibitors, or inducers of this enzyme system may have a significant impact on the efficacy and side effect profile of diltiazem). Products include:

Rauwolfia Serpentina (Diltiazem has an additive effect when used with other antihypertensive agents. Therefore, the dosage of diltiazem or concomitant antihypertensives may need to be adjusted when adding one to the other).
No products indexed under this heading.

Remifentanil Hydrochloride (The depression of cardiac contractility, conductivity, and automaticity, as well as the vascular dilation associated with anesthetics, may be potentiated by calcium channel blockers).
No products indexed under this heading.

Rescinnamine (Diltiazem has an additive effect when used with other antihypertensive agents. Therefore, the dosage of diltiazem or concomitant antihypertensives may need to be adjusted when adding one to the other).
No products indexed under this heading.

Reserpine (Diltiazem has an additive effect when used with other antihypertensive agents. Therefore, the dosage of diltiazem or concomitant antihypertensives may need to be adjusted when adding one to the other).
No products indexed under this heading.

Rifabutin (Patients taking other drugs that are substrates of CYP450, especially patients with renal and/or hepatic impairment, may require dosage adjustment when starting or stopping concomitantly administered diltiazem in order to maintain optimum therapeutic blood levels).
No products indexed under this heading.

Rifampicin (Diltiazem is both a substrate and an inhibitor of the CYP3A4 enzyme system. Other drugs that are specific substrates, inhibitors, or inducers of this enzyme system may have a significant impact on the efficacy and side effect profile of diltiazem).
No products indexed under this heading.

Rifampin (Co-administration of rifampin with diltiazem lowered the diltiazem plasma concentrations to undetectable levels. Co-administration of diltiazem with rifampin or any known CYP3A4 inducer should be avoided when possible and alternative therapy considered).
No products indexed under this heading.

Rifapentine (Diltiazem is both a substrate and an inhibitor of the CYP3A4 enzyme system. Other drugs that are specific substrates, inhibitors, or inducers of this enzyme system may have a significant impact on the efficacy and side effect profile of diltiazem).
No products indexed under this heading.

Ritonavir (Patients taking other drugs that are substrates of CYP450, especially patients with renal and/or hepatic impairment, may require dosage adjustment when starting or stopping concomitantly administered diltiazem in order to maintain optimum therapeutic blood levels). Products include:

Kaletra 476
Norvir 503

Saquinavir (Patients taking other drugs that are substrates of CYP450, especially patients with renal and/or hepatic impairment, may require dosage adjustment when starting or stopping concomitantly administered diltiazem in order to maintain optimum therapeutic blood levels).

No products indexed under this heading.

Saquinavir Mesylate (Patients taking other drugs that are substrates of CYP450, especially patients with renal and/or hepatic impairment, may require dosage adjustment when starting or stopping concomitantly administered diltiazem in order to maintain optimum therapeutic blood levels). Products include:

Invirase 2772

Sertraline Hydrochloride (Patients taking other drugs that are substrates of CYP450, especially patients with renal and/or hepatic impairment, may require dosage adjustment when starting or stopping concomitantly administered diltiazem in order to maintain optimum therapeutic blood levels). Products include:

Zoloft 2586

Sildenafil Citrate (Patients taking other drugs that are substrates of CYP450, especially patients with renal and/or hepatic impairment, may require dosage adjustment when starting or stopping concomitantly administered diltiazem in order to maintain optimum therapeutic blood levels). Products include:

Revatio Tablets 2557
Viagra Tablets 2573

Simvastatin (Patients taking other drugs that are substrates of CYP450, especially patients with renal and/or hepatic impairment, may require dosage adjustment when starting or stopping concomitantly administered diltiazem in order to maintain optimum therapeutic blood levels). Products include:

Vytorin 10/10 Tablets 2114
Vytorin 10/10 Tablets 3077
Vytorin 10/20 Tablets 2114
Vytorin 10/20 Tablets 3077
Vytorin 10/40 Tablets 2114
Vytorin 10/40 Tablets 3077
Vytorin 10/80 Tablets 2114
Vytorin 10/80 Tablets 3077
Zocor Tablets 2105

Sirolimus (Patients taking other drugs that are substrates of CYP450, especially patients with renal and/or hepatic impairment, may require dosage adjustment when starting or stopping concomitantly administered diltiazem in order to maintain optimum therapeutic blood levels). Products include:

Rapamune Oral Solution and Tablets 3475

Sodium Nitroprusside (Diltiazem has an additive effect when used with other antihypertensive agents. Therefore, the dosage of diltiazem or concomitant antihypertensives may need to be adjusted when adding one to the other).

No products indexed under this heading.

Sotalol Hydrochloride (Pharmacologic studies indicate that there may be additive effects in prolonging A-V conduction when using beta-blockers or digitalis concomitantly with diltiazem).

No products indexed under this heading.

Spirapril Hydrochloride (Diltiazem has an additive effect when used with other antihypertensive agents. Therefore, the dosage of diltiazem or concomitant antihypertensives may need to be adjusted when adding one to the other).

No products indexed under this heading.

Sufentanil Citrate (The depression of cardiac contractility, conductivity, and automaticity, as well as the vascular dilation associated with anesthetics, may be potentiated by calcium channel blockers).

No products indexed under this heading.

Sulfinpyrazone (Diltiazem is both a substrate and an inhibitor of the CYP3A4 enzyme system. Other drugs that are specific substrates, inhibitors, or inducers of this enzyme system may have a significant impact on the efficacy and side effect profile of diltiazem).

No products indexed under this heading.

Tacrolimus (Patients taking other drugs that are substrates of CYP450, especially patients with renal and/or hepatic impairment, may require dosage adjustment when starting or stopping concomitantly administered diltiazem in order to maintain optimum therapeutic blood levels). Products include:

Prograf Capsules and Injection 632
Protopic Ointment 638

Tamoxifen Citrate (Patients taking other drugs that are substrates of CYP450, especially patients with renal and/or hepatic impairment, may require dosage adjustment when starting or stopping concomitantly administered diltiazem in order to maintain optimum therapeutic blood levels). Products include:

Soltamox Oral Solution 3527

Telithromycin (Diltiazem is both a substrate and an inhibitor of the CYP3A4 enzyme system. Other drugs that are specific substrates, inhibitors, or inducers of this enzyme system may have a significant impact on the efficacy and side effect profile of diltiazem). Products include:

Ketek Tablets 2903

Telmisartan (Diltiazem has an additive effect when used with other antihypertensive agents. Therefore, the dosage of diltiazem or concomitant antihypertensives may need to be adjusted when adding one to the other). Products include:

Micardis Tablets 854
Micardis HCT Tablets 856

Temazepam (Studies showed that diltiazem increased the AUC of midazolam and triazolam by 3- to 4-fold and the Cmax by 2-fold, compared to placebo. The elimination half-life of midazolam and triazolam also increased during co-administration with diltiazem). Products include:

Restoril Capsules 1860

Terazosin Hydrochloride (Diltiazem has an additive effect when used with other antihypertensive agents. Therefore, the dosage of diltiazem or concomitant antihypertensives may need to be adjusted when adding one to the other). Products include:

Hytrin Capsules 471

Theophylline (Diltiazem is both a substrate and an inhibitor of the CYP3A4 enzyme system. Other drugs that are specific substrates, inhibitors, or inducers of this enzyme system may have a significant impact on the efficacy and side effect profile of diltiazem).

No products indexed under this heading.

Thiamylal Sodium (The depression of cardiac contractility, conductivity, and automaticity, as well as the vascular dilation associated with anesthetics, may be potentiated by calcium channel blockers).

No products indexed under this heading.

Tiagabine Hydrochloride (Patients taking other drugs that are substrates of CYP450, especially patients with renal and/or hepatic impairment, may require dosage adjustment when starting or stopping concomitantly administered diltiazem in order to maintain optimum therapeutic blood levels). Products include:

Gabitril Tablets 984

Timolol Hemihydrate (Pharmacologic studies indicate that there may be additive effects in prolonging A-V conduction when using beta-blockers or digitalis concomitantly with diltiazem). Products include:

Betimol Ophthalmic Solution 3382
Betimol Ophthalmic Solution .... ⊙295

Timolol Maleate (Pharmacologic studies indicate that there may be additive effects in prolonging A-V conduction when using beta-blockers or digitalis concomitantly with diltiazem). Products include:

Blocadren Tablets 1916
Cosopt Sterile Ophthalmic Solution 1931
Timolide Tablets 2086
Timoptic Sterile Ophthalmic Solution 2088
Timoptic in Ocudose 2091
Timoptic-XE Sterile Ophthalmic Gel Forming Solution 2092

Tolterodine Tartrate (Patients taking other drugs that are substrates of CYP450, especially patients with renal and/or hepatic impairment, may require dosage adjustment when starting or stopping concomitantly administered diltiazem in order to maintain optimum therapeutic blood levels). Products include:

Detrol Tablets 2628
Detrol LA Capsules 2631

Torsemide (Diltiazem has an additive effect when used with other antihypertensive agents. Therefore, the dosage of diltiazem or concomitant antihypertensives may need to be adjusted when adding one to the other). Products include:

Demadex Injection 2759
Demadex Tablets 2759

Trandolapril (Diltiazem has an additive effect when used with other antihypertensive agents. Therefore, the dosage of diltiazem or concomitant antihypertensives may need to be adjusted when adding one to the other). Products include:

Mavik Tablets 486
Tarka Tablets 524

Trazodone Hydrochloride (Patients taking other drugs that are substrates of CYP450, especially patients with renal and/or hepatic impairment, may require dosage adjustment when starting or stopping concomitantly administered diltiazem in order to maintain optimum therapeutic blood levels).

No products indexed under this heading.

Triamcinolone (Diltiazem is both a substrate and an inhibitor of the CYP3A4 enzyme system. Other drugs that are specific substrates, inhibitors, or inducers of this enzyme system may have a significant impact on the efficacy and side effect profile of diltiazem).

No products indexed under this heading.

Triamcinolone Acetonide (Diltiazem is both a substrate and an inhibitor of the CYP3A4 enzyme system. Other drugs that are specific substrates, inhibitors, or inducers of this enzyme system may have a significant impact on the efficacy and side effect profile of diltiazem). Products include:

Azmacort Inhalation Aerosol 1726
Nasacort AQ Nasal Spray 2922

Triamcinolone Diacetate (Diltiazem is both a substrate and an inhibitor of the CYP3A4 enzyme system. Other drugs that are specific substrates, inhibitors, or inducers of this enzyme system may have a significant impact on the efficacy and side effect profile of diltiazem).

No products indexed under this heading.

Triamcinolone Hexacetonide (Diltiazem is both a substrate and an inhibitor of the CYP3A4 enzyme system. Other drugs that are specific substrates, inhibitors, or inducers of this enzyme system may have a significant impact on the efficacy and side effect profile of diltiazem).

No products indexed under this heading.

Triazolam (Studies showed that diltiazem increased the AUC of midazolam and triazolam by 3- to 4-fold and the Cmax by 2-fold, compared to placebo. The elimination half-life of midazolam and triazolam also increased during co-administration with diltiazem).

No products indexed under this heading.

Trimethaphan Camsylate (Diltiazem has an additive effect when used with other antihypertensive agents. Therefore, the dosage of diltiazem or concomitant antihypertensives may need to be adjusted when adding one to the other).

No products indexed under this heading.

(▣ Described in PDR For Nonprescription Drugs) (⊙ Described in PDR For Ophthalmic Medicines™)

Troglitazone (Diltiazem is both a substrate and an inhibitor of the CYP3A4 enzyme system. Other drugs that are specific substrates, inhibitors, or inducers of this enzyme system may have a significant impact on the efficacy and side effect profile of diltiazem).
No products indexed under this heading.

Troleandomycin (Diltiazem is both a substrate and an inhibitor of the CYP3A4 enzyme system. Other drugs that are specific substrates, inhibitors, or inducers of this enzyme system may have a significant impact on the efficacy and side effect profile of diltiazem).
No products indexed under this heading.

Valproate Sodium (Diltiazem is both a substrate and an inhibitor of the CYP3A4 enzyme system. Other drugs that are specific substrates, inhibitors, or inducers of this enzyme system may have a significant impact on the efficacy and side effect profile of diltiazem). Products include:
Depacon Injection 412

Valsartan (Diltiazem has an additive effect when used with other antihypertensive agents. Therefore, the dosage of diltiazem or concomitant antihypertensives may need to be adjusted when adding one to the other). Products include:
Diovan Tablets 2193
Diovan HCT Tablets 2196

Verapamil Hydrochloride (Diltiazem has an additive effect when used with other antihypertensive agents. Therefore, the dosage of diltiazem or concomitant antihypertensives may need to be adjusted when adding one to the other). Products include:
Covera-HS Tablets 3139
Tarka Tablets 524
Verelan PM Extended-Release Capsules, Controlled-Onset 3106

Vinblastine Sulfate (Patients taking other drugs that are substrates of CYP450, especially patients with renal and/or hepatic impairment, may require dosage adjustment when starting or stopping concomitantly administered diltiazem in order to maintain optimum therapeutic blood levels).
No products indexed under this heading.

Vincristine Sulfate (Patients taking other drugs that are substrates of CYP450, especially patients with renal and/or hepatic impairment, may require dosage adjustment when starting or stopping concomitantly administered diltiazem in order to maintain optimum therapeutic blood levels).
No products indexed under this heading.

Voriconazole (Diltiazem is both a substrate and an inhibitor of the CYP3A4 enzyme system. Other drugs that are specific substrates, inhibitors, or inducers of this enzyme system may have a significant impact on the efficacy and side effect profile of diltiazem). Products include:
VFEND I.V. 2564
VFEND Oral Suspension 2564
VFEND Tablets 2564

Warfarin Sodium (Patients taking other drugs that are substrates of CYP450, especially patients with renal and/or hepatic impairment, may require dosage adjustment when starting or stopping concomitantly administered diltiazem in order to maintain optimum therapeutic blood levels). Products include:
Coumadin for Injection 898
Coumadin Tablets 898

Zafirlukast (Diltiazem is both a substrate and an inhibitor of the CYP3A4 enzyme system. Other drugs that are specific substrates, inhibitors, or inducers of this enzyme system may have a significant impact on the efficacy and side effect profile of diltiazem). Products include:
Accolate Tablets 671

Zileuton (Diltiazem is both a substrate and an inhibitor of the CYP3A4 enzyme system. Other drugs that are specific substrates, inhibitors, or inducers of this enzyme system may have a significant impact on the efficacy and side effect profile of diltiazem). Products include:
Zyflo Tablets 1023

Food Interactions

Grapefruit (Diltiazem is both a substrate and an inhibitor of the CYP3A4 enzyme system. Other drugs that are specific substrates, inhibitors, or inducers of this enzyme system may have a significant impact on the efficacy and side effect profile of diltiazem).

Grapefruit Juice (Diltiazem is both a substrate and an inhibitor of the CYP3A4 enzyme system. Other drugs that are specific substrates, inhibitors, or inducers of this enzyme system may have a significant impact on the efficacy and side effect profile of diltiazem).

CARDURA XL TABLETS

(Doxazosin Mesylate) 2515
May interact with cytochrome p450 3a4 inhibitors, potent and certain other agents. Compounds in these categories include:

Amprenavir (Caution should be exercised when concomitantly administering a potent 3A4 inhibitor with doxasozin mesylate). Products include:
Agenerase Capsules 1327
Agenerase Oral Solution 1332

Atazanavir (Caution should be exercised when concomitantly administering a potent 3A4 inhibitor with doxasozin mesylate).
No products indexed under this heading.

Atazanavir sulfate (Caution should be exercised when concomitantly administering a potent 3A4 inhibitor with doxasozin mesylate). Products include:
Reyataz Capsules 921

Cimetidine (Co-administration with oral cimetidine has resulted in a 10% increase in mean AUC of doxazosin and a slight but statistically insignificant increase in mean Cmax and mean half-life of doxazosin). Products include:
Tagamet HB 200 Tablets .... ⊡664

Cimetidine Hydrochloride (Co-administration with oral cimetidine has resulted in a 10% increase in mean AUC of doxazosin and a slight but statistically insignificant increase in mean Cmax and mean half-life of doxazosin).
No products indexed under this heading.

Clarithromycin (Caution should be exercised when concomitantly administering a potent 3A4 inhibitor with doxasozin mesylate). Products include:
Biaxin/Biaxin XL 402
PREVPAC 3284

Fosamprenavir Calcium (Caution should be exercised when concomitantly administering a potent 3A4 inhibitor with doxasozin mesylate). Products include:
Lexiva Tablets 1505

Indinavir Sulfate (Caution should be exercised when concomitantly administering a potent 3A4 inhibitor with doxasozin mesylate). Products include:
Crixivan Capsules 1940

Itraconazole (Caution should be exercised when concomitantly administering a potent 3A4 inhibitor with doxasozin mesylate).
No products indexed under this heading.

Ketoconazole (Caution should be exercised when concomitantly administering a potent 3A4 inhibitor with doxasozin mesylate). Products include:
Nizoral A-D Shampoo, 1% 1868

Lopinavir (Caution should be exercised when concomitantly administering a potent 3A4 inhibitor with doxasozin mesylate). Products include:
Kaletra 476

Nefazodone Hydrochloride (Caution should be exercised when concomitantly administering a potent 3A4 inhibitor with doxasozin mesylate).
No products indexed under this heading.

Nelfinavir Mesylate (Caution should be exercised when concomitantly administering a potent 3A4 inhibitor with doxasozin mesylate). Products include:
Viracept 2577

Ritonavir (Caution should be exercised when concomitantly administering a potent 3A4 inhibitor with doxasozin mesylate). Products include:
Kaletra 476
Norvir 503

Saquinavir (Caution should be exercised when concomitantly administering a potent 3A4 inhibitor with doxasozin mesylate).
No products indexed under this heading.

Saquinavir Mesylate (Caution should be exercised when concomitantly administering a potent 3A4 inhibitor with doxasozin mesylate). Products include:
Invirase 2772

Telithromycin (Caution should be exercised when concomitantly administering a potent 3A4 inhibitor with doxasozin mesylate). Products include:
Ketek Tablets 2903

Troleandomycin (Caution should be exercised when concomitantly administering a potent 3A4 inhibitor with doxasozin mesylate).
No products indexed under this heading.

Voriconazole (Caution should be exercised when concomitantly administering a potent 3A4 inhibitor with doxasozin mesylate). Products include:
VFEND I.V. 2564
VFEND Oral Suspension 2564
VFEND Tablets 2564

CARIMUNE NF

(Immune Globulin Intravenous (Human)) 3499
May interact with:

Measles, Mumps & Rubella Virus Vaccine, Live (Antibodies in immune globulin intravenous (human) may impair the efficacy of live attenuated viral vaccines). Products include:
M-M-R II 2006

Measles & Rubella Virus Vaccine Live (Antibodies in immune globulin intravenous (human) may impair the efficacy of live attenuated viral vaccines).
No products indexed under this heading.

Measles Virus Vaccine Live (Antibodies in immune globulin intravenous (human) may impair the efficacy of live attenuated viral vaccines). Products include:
Attenuvax 1914

Mumps Virus Vaccine, Live (Antibodies in immune globulin intravenous (human) may impair the efficacy of live attenuated viral vaccines). Products include:
Mumpsvax 2031

Rubella & Mumps Virus Vaccine Live (Antibodies in immune globulin intravenous (human) may impair the efficacy of live attenuated viral vaccines).
No products indexed under this heading.

Rubella Virus Vaccine Live (Antibodies in immune globulin intravenous (human) may impair the efficacy of live attenuated viral vaccines). Products include:
Meruvax II 2019

CARNITOR INJECTION

(Levocarnitine) 3188
None cited in PDR database.

CARNITOR TABLETS AND ORAL SOLUTION

(Levocarnitine) 3190
None cited in PDR database.

CARTEOLOL HYDROCHLORIDE OPHTHALMIC SOLUTION USP, 1%

(Carteolol Hydrochloride) .... ⊙249
May interact with beta blockers and certain other agents. Compounds in these categories include:

Acebutolol Hydrochloride (Co-administration with oral beta-adrenergic blocking agents may result in potential additive effects on systemic beta-blockade).
No products indexed under this heading.

Atenolol (Co-administration with oral beta-adrenergic blocking agents may result in potential additive effects on systemic beta-blockade).
No products indexed under this heading.

Betaxolol Hydrochloride (Co-administration with oral beta-adrenergic blocking agents may result in potential additive effects on systemic beta-blockade). Products include:
Betoptic S Ophthalmic Suspension 558

Bisoprolol Fumarate (Co-administration with oral beta-adrenergic blocking agents may result in potential additive effects on systemic beta-blockade).
No products indexed under this heading.

Esmolol Hydrochloride (Co-administration with oral beta-adrenergic blocking agents may result in potential additive effects on systemic beta-blockade).
No products indexed under this heading.

Guanethidine Monosulfate (Co-administration with catecholamine-depleting drugs, such as guanethidine, may result in possible additive effects and production of hypotension and/or marked bradycardia, which may produce vertigo, syncope, or postural hypertension).
No products indexed under this heading.

Labetalol Hydrochloride (Co-administration with oral beta-adrenergic blocking agents may result in potential additive effects on systemic beta-blockade).
No products indexed under this heading.

Levobunolol Hydrochloride (Co-administration with oral beta-adrenergic blocking agents may result in potential additive effects on systemic beta-blockade). Products include:
Betagan Ophthalmic Solution, USP .... ⊙220

Metipranolol Hydrochloride (Co-administration with oral beta-adrenergic blocking agents may result in potential additive effects on systemic beta-blockade).
No products indexed under this heading.

Metoprolol Succinate (Co-administration with oral beta-adrenergic blocking agents may result in potential additive effects on systemic beta-blockade). Products include:
Toprol-XL Tablets 668

Metoprolol Tartrate (Co-administration with oral beta-adrenergic blocking agents may result in potential additive effects on systemic beta-blockade). Products include:
Lopressor Injection 2238
Lopressor Tablets 2238
Lopressor HCT 50/25 Tablets 2241
Lopressor HCT 100/25 Tablets 2241
Lopressor HCT 100/50 Tablets 2241

Nadolol (Co-administration with oral beta-adrenergic blocking agents may result in potential additive effects on systemic beta-blockade). Products include:
Nadolol Tablets 2159

Penbutolol Sulfate (Co-administration with oral beta-adrenergic blocking agents may result in potential additive effects on systemic beta-blockade).
No products indexed under this heading.

Pindolol (Co-administration with oral beta-adrenergic blocking agents may result in potential additive effects on systemic beta-blockade).
No products indexed under this heading.

Propranolol Hydrochloride (Co-administration with oral beta-adrenergic blocking agents may result in potential additive effects on systemic beta-blockade). Products include:
Inderal LA Long-Acting Capsules 3429
InnoPran XL Capsules 2723

Reserpine (Co-administration with catecholamine-depleting drugs, such as reserpine, may result in possible additive effects and production of hypotension and/or marked bradycardia, which may produce vertigo, syncope, or postural hypertension).
No products indexed under this heading.

Sotalol Hydrochloride (Co-administration with oral beta-adrenergic blocking agents may result in potential additive effects on systemic beta-blockade).
No products indexed under this heading.

Timolol Hemihydrate (Co-administration with oral beta-adrenergic blocking agents may result in potential additive effects on systemic beta-blockade). Products include:
Betimol Ophthalmic Solution 3382
Betimol Ophthalmic Solution .... ⊙295

Timolol Maleate (Co-administration with oral beta-adrenergic blocking agents may result in potential additive effects on systemic beta-blockade). Products include:
Blocadren Tablets 1916
Cosopt Sterile Ophthalmic Solution 1931
Timolide Tablets 2086
Timoptic Sterile Ophthalmic Solution 2088
Timoptic in Ocudose 2091
Timoptic-XE Sterile Ophthalmic Gel Forming Solution 2092

CATAPRES TABLETS

(Clonidine Hydrochloride) 843

May interact with barbiturates, beta blockers, calcium channel blockers, cardiac glycosides, hypnotics and sedatives, tricyclic antidepressants, and certain other agents. Compounds in these categories include:

Acebutolol Hydrochloride (Co-administration with agents known to affect sinus node function or AV nodal conduction, such as beta blockers, may result in additive effects such as bradycardia and AV block).
No products indexed under this heading.

Amitriptyline Hydrochloride (Co-administration may reduce the hypotensive effects; dosage adjustment may be necessary; concurrent use has resulted in corneal lesions in rats within 5 days).
No products indexed under this heading.

Amlodipine Besylate (Co-administration with agents known to affect sinus node function or AV nodal conduction, such as calcium channel blockers, may result in additive effects such as bradycardia and AV block). Products include:
Caduet Tablets 2508
Lotrel Capsules 2249
Norvasc Tablets 2545

Amoxapine (Co-administration may reduce the hypotensive effects; dosage adjustment may be necessary).
No products indexed under this heading.

Aprobarbital (Clonidine may potentiate the CNS-depressive effects).
No products indexed under this heading.

Atenolol (Co-administration with agents known to affect sinus node function or AV nodal conduction, such as beta blockers, may result in additive effects such as bradycardia and AV block).
No products indexed under this heading.

Bepridil Hydrochloride (Co-administration with agents known to affect sinus node function or AV nodal conduction, such as calcium channel blockers, may result in additive effects such as bradycardia and AV block).
No products indexed under this heading.

Betaxolol Hydrochloride (Co-administration with agents known to affect sinus node function or AV nodal conduction, such as beta blockers, may result in additive effects such as bradycardia and AV block). Products include:
Betoptic S Ophthalmic Suspension 558

Bisoprolol Fumarate (Co-administration with agents known to affect sinus node function or AV nodal conduction, such as beta blockers, may result in additive effects such as bradycardia and AV block).
No products indexed under this heading.

Butabarbital (Clonidine may potentiate the CNS-depressive effects).
No products indexed under this heading.

Butalbital (Clonidine may potentiate the CNS-depressive effects).
No products indexed under this heading.

Carteolol Hydrochloride (Co-administration with agents known to affect sinus node function or AV nodal conduction, such as beta blockers, may result in additive effects such as bradycardia and AV block). Products include:
Carteolol Hydrochloride Ophthalmic Solution USP, 1% .... ⊙249

Clomipramine Hydrochloride (Co-administration may reduce the hypotensive effects; dosage adjustment may be necessary).
No products indexed under this heading.

Desipramine Hydrochloride (Co-administration may reduce the hypotensive effects; dosage adjustment may be necessary).
No products indexed under this heading.

Deslanoside (Co-administration with agents known to affect sinus node function or AV nodal conduction, such as digitalis, may result in additive effects such as bradycardia and AV block).
No products indexed under this heading.

Digitalis Glycoside Preparations (Co-administration with agents known to affect sinus node function or AV nodal conduction, such as digitalis, may result in additive effects such as bradycardia and AV block).
No products indexed under this heading.

Digitoxin (Co-administration with agents known to affect sinus node function or AV nodal conduction, such as digitalis, may result in additive effects such as bradycardia and AV block).
No products indexed under this heading.

Digoxin (Co-administration with agents known to affect sinus node function or AV nodal conduction, such as digitalis, may result in additive effects such as bradycardia and AV block). Products include:
Lanoxicaps Capsules 1490
Lanoxin Injection 1494
Lanoxin Injection Pediatric 1497
Lanoxin Tablets 1500

Diltiazem Hydrochloride (Co-administration with agents known to affect sinus node function or AV nodal conduction, such as calcium channel blockers, may result in additive effects such as bradycardia and AV block). Products include:
Cardizem LA Extended Release Tablets 1728
Tiazac Capsules 1201

Doxepin Hydrochloride (Co-administration may reduce the hypotensive effects; dosage adjustment may be necessary).
No products indexed under this heading.

Esmolol Hydrochloride (Co-administration with agents known to affect sinus node function or AV nodal conduction, such as beta blockers, may result in additive effects such as bradycardia and AV block).
No products indexed under this heading.

Estazolam (Clonidine may potentiate the CNS-depressive effects). Products include:
ProSom Tablets 517

Ethchlorvynol (Clonidine may potentiate the CNS-depressive effects).
No products indexed under this heading.

Ethinamate (Clonidine may potentiate the CNS-depressive effects).
No products indexed under this heading.

Felodipine (Co-administration with agents known to affect sinus node function or AV nodal conduction, such as calcium channel blockers, may result in additive effects such as bradycardia and AV block).
No products indexed under this heading.

Flurazepam Hydrochloride (Clonidine may potentiate the CNS-depressive effects). Products include:
Dalmane Capsules 3342

Glutethimide (Clonidine may potentiate the CNS-depressive effects).
No products indexed under this heading.

Imipramine Hydrochloride (Co-administration may reduce the hypotensive effects; dosage adjustment may be necessary).
No products indexed under this heading.

Imipramine Pamoate (Co-administration may reduce the hypotensive effects; dosage adjustment may be necessary).
No products indexed under this heading.

Isradipine (Co-administration with agents known to affect sinus node function or AV nodal conduction, such as calcium channel blockers, may result in additive effects such as bradycardia and AV block). Products include:

DynaCirc CR Tablets 2721

Labetalol Hydrochloride (Co-administration with agents known to affect sinus node function or AV nodal conduction, such as beta blockers, may result in additive effects such as bradycardia and AV block).

No products indexed under this heading.

Levobunolol Hydrochloride (Co-administration with agents known to affect sinus node function or AV nodal conduction, such as beta blockers, may result in additive effects such as bradycardia and AV block). Products include:

Betagan Ophthalmic Solution, USP.............................. ⊘ 220

Lorazepam (Clonidine may potentiate the CNS-depressive effects).

No products indexed under this heading.

Maprotiline Hydrochloride (Co-administration may reduce the hypotensive effects; dosage adjustment may be necessary).

No products indexed under this heading.

Mephobarbital (Clonidine may potentiate the CNS-depressive effects).

No products indexed under this heading.

Metipranolol Hydrochloride (Co-administration with agents known to affect sinus node function or AV nodal conduction, such as beta blockers, may result in additive effects such as bradycardia and AV block).

No products indexed under this heading.

Metoprolol Succinate (Co-administration with agents known to affect sinus node function or AV nodal conduction, such as beta blockers, may result in additive effects such as bradycardia and AV block). Products include:

Toprol-XL Tablets 668

Metoprolol Tartrate (Co-administration with agents known to affect sinus node function or AV nodal conduction, such as beta blockers, may result in additive effects such as bradycardia and AV block). Products include:

Lopressor Injection 2238
Lopressor Tablets 2238
Lopressor HCT 50/25 Tablets 2241
Lopressor HCT 100/25 Tablets 2241
Lopressor HCT 100/50 Tablets 2241

Mibefradil Dihydrochloride (Co-administration with agents known to affect sinus node function or AV nodal conduction, such as calcium channel blockers, may result in additive effects such as bradycardia and AV block).

No products indexed under this heading.

Midazolam Hydrochloride (Clonidine may potentiate the CNS-depressive effects).

No products indexed under this heading.

Nadolol (Co-administration with agents known to affect sinus node function or AV nodal conduction,

such as beta blockers, may result in additive effects such as bradycardia and AV block). Products include:

Nadolol Tablets 2159

Nicardipine Hydrochloride (Co-administration with agents known to affect sinus node function or AV nodal conduction, such as calcium channel blockers, may result in additive effects such as bradycardia and AV block). Products include:

Cardene I.V. 2497

Nifedipine (Co-administration with agents known to affect sinus node function or AV nodal conduction, such as calcium channel blockers, may result in additive effects such as bradycardia and AV block). Products include:

Adalat CC Tablets 2964

Nimodipine (Co-administration with agents known to affect sinus node function or AV nodal conduction, such as calcium channel blockers, may result in additive effects such as bradycardia and AV block). Products include:

Nimotop Capsules 749

Nisoldipine (Co-administration with agents known to affect sinus node function or AV nodal conduction, such as calcium channel blockers, may result in additive effects such as bradycardia and AV block). Products include:

Sular Tablets 3122

Nortriptyline Hydrochloride (Co-administration may reduce the hypotensive effects; dosage adjustment may be necessary).

No products indexed under this heading.

Penbutolol Sulfate (Co-administration with agents known to affect sinus node function or AV nodal conduction, such as beta blockers, may result in additive effects such as bradycardia and AV block).

No products indexed under this heading.

Pentobarbital Sodium (Clonidine may potentiate the CNS-depressive effects). Products include:

Nembutal Sodium Solution, USP 2470

Phenobarbital (Clonidine may potentiate the CNS-depressive effects). Products include:

Donnatal Extentabs 2493

Pindolol (Co-administration with agents known to affect sinus node function or AV nodal conduction, such as beta blockers, may result in additive effects such as bradycardia and AV block).

No products indexed under this heading.

Propofol (Clonidine may potentiate the CNS-depressive effects).

No products indexed under this heading.

Propranolol Hydrochloride (Co-administration with agents known to affect sinus node function or AV nodal conduction, such as beta blockers, may result in additive effects such as bradycardia and AV block). Products include:

Inderal LA Long-Acting Capsules 3429
InnoPran XL Capsules 2723

Protriptyline Hydrochloride (Co-administration may reduce the hypotensive effects; dosage adjustment may be necessary).

No products indexed under this heading.

Quazepam (Clonidine may potentiate the CNS-depressive effects).

No products indexed under this heading.

Ramelteon (Clonidine may potentiate the CNS-depressive effects). Products include:

Rozerem Tablets 3231

Secobarbital Sodium (Clonidine may potentiate the CNS-depressive effects).

No products indexed under this heading.

Sotalol Hydrochloride (Co-administration with agents known to affect sinus node function or AV nodal conduction, such as beta blockers, may result in additive effects such as bradycardia and AV block).

No products indexed under this heading.

Temazepam (Clonidine may potentiate the CNS-depressive effects). Products include:

Restoril Capsules 1860

Thiamylal Sodium (Clonidine may potentiate the CNS-depressive effects).

No products indexed under this heading.

Timolol Hemihydrate (Co-administration with agents known to affect sinus node function or AV nodal conduction, such as beta blockers, may result in additive effects such as bradycardia and AV block). Products include:

Betimol Ophthalmic Solution 3382
Betimol Ophthalmic Solution ⊘ 295

Timolol Maleate (Co-administration with agents known to affect sinus node function or AV nodal conduction, such as beta blockers, may result in additive effects such as bradycardia and AV block). Products include:

Blocadren Tablets 1916
Cosopt Sterile Ophthalmic
 Solution....................................... 1931
Timolide Tablets 2086
Timoptic Sterile Ophthalmic
 Solution....................................... 2088
Timoptic in Ocudose 2091
Timoptic-XE Sterile Ophthalmic
 Gel Forming Solution 2092

Triazolam (Clonidine may potentiate the CNS-depressive effects).

No products indexed under this heading.

Trimipramine Maleate (Co-administration may reduce the hypotensive effects; dosage adjustment may be necessary).

No products indexed under this heading.

Verapamil Hydrochloride (Co-administration with agents known to affect sinus node function or AV nodal conduction, such as calcium channel blockers, may result in additive effects such as bradycardia and AV block). Products include:

Covera-HS Tablets 3139
Tarka Tablets 524
Verelan PM Extended-Release
 Capsules, Controlled-Onset.......... 3106

Zaleplon (Clonidine may potentiate the CNS-depressive effects). Products include:

Sonata Capsules 1717

Zolpidem Tartrate (Clonidine may potentiate the CNS-depressive effects). Products include:

Ambien Tablets 2851
Ambien CR Tablets 2855

Food Interactions

Alcohol (Clonidine may potentiate the CNS-depressive effects).

CATAPRES-TTS

(Clonidine) 844

May interact with barbiturates, beta blockers, calcium channel blockers, cardiac glycosides, hypnotics and sedatives, tricyclic antidepressants, and certain other agents. Compounds in these categories include:

Acebutolol Hydrochloride (Co-administration with agents known to affect sinus node function or AV nodal conduction, such as beta blockers, may result in additive effects such as bradycardia and AV block).

No products indexed under this heading.

Amitriptyline Hydrochloride (Co-administration may reduce the hypotensive effects; dosage adjustment may be necessary; concurrent use has resulted in corneal lesions in rats within 5 days).

No products indexed under this heading.

Amlodipine Besylate (Co-administration with agents known to affect sinus node function or AV nodal conduction, such as calcium channel blockers, may result in additive effects such as bradycardia and AV block). Products include:

Caduet Tablets 2508
Lotrel Capsules 2249
Norvasc Tablets 2545

Amoxapine (Co-administration may reduce the hypotensive effects; dosage adjustment may be necessary).

No products indexed under this heading.

Aprobarbital (Clonidine may potentiate the CNS-depressive effects).

No products indexed under this heading.

Atenolol (Co-administration with agents known to affect sinus node function or AV nodal conduction, such as beta blockers, may result in additive effects such as bradycardia and AV block).

No products indexed under this heading.

Bepridil Hydrochloride (Co-administration with agents known to affect sinus node function or AV nodal conduction, such as calcium channel blockers, may result in additive effects such as bradycardia and AV block).

No products indexed under this heading.

Betaxolol Hydrochloride (Co-administration with agents known to affect sinus node function or AV nodal conduction, such as beta blockers, may result in additive effects such as bradycardia and AV block). Products include:

Betoptic S Ophthalmic
 Suspension................................. 558

Bisoprolol Fumarate (Co-administration with agents known to affect sinus node function or AV nodal conduction, such as beta blockers, may result in additive effects such as bradycardia and AV block).

No products indexed under this heading.

Butabarbital (Clonidine may potentiate the CNS-depressive effects).

No products indexed under this heading.

IMPORTANT NOTE: Always consult each drug listing in the patient's regimen for possible interactions.

Butalbital (Clonidine may potentiate the CNS-depressive effects).
No products indexed under this heading.

Carteolol Hydrochloride (Co-administration with agents known to affect sinus node function or AV nodal conduction, such as beta blockers, may result in additive effects such as bradycardia and AV block). Products include:
Carteolol Hydrochloride Ophthalmic Solution USP, 1% .... ⊙249

Clomipramine Hydrochloride (Co-administration may reduce the hypotensive effects; dosage adjustment may be necessary).
No products indexed under this heading.

Desipramine Hydrochloride (Co-administration may reduce the hypotensive effects; dosage adjustment may be necessary).
No products indexed under this heading.

Deslanoside (Co-administration with agents known to affect sinus node function or AV nodal conduction, such as digitalis, may result in additive effects such as bradycardia and AV block).
No products indexed under this heading.

Digitalis Glycoside Preparations (Co-administration with agents known to affect sinus node function or AV nodal conduction, such as digitalis, may result in additive effects such as bradycardia and AV block).
No products indexed under this heading.

Digitoxin (Co-administration with agents known to affect sinus node function or AV nodal conduction, such as digitalis, may result in additive effects such as bradycardia and AV block).
No products indexed under this heading.

Digoxin (Co-administration with agents known to affect sinus node function or AV nodal conduction, such as digitalis, may result in additive effects such as bradycardia and AV block). Products include:
Lanoxicaps Capsules 1490
Lanoxin Injection 1494
Lanoxin Injection Pediatric 1497
Lanoxin Tablets 1500

Diltiazem Hydrochloride (Co-administration with agents known to affect sinus node function or AV nodal conduction, such as calcium channel blockers, may result in additive effects such as bradycardia and AV block). Products include:
Cardizem LA Extended Release Tablets 1728
Tiazac Capsules 1201

Doxepin Hydrochloride (Co-administration may reduce the hypotensive effects; dosage adjustment may be necessary).
No products indexed under this heading.

Esmolol Hydrochloride (Co-administration with agents known to affect sinus node function or AV nodal conduction, such as beta blockers, may result in additive effects such as bradycardia and AV block).
No products indexed under this heading.

Estazolam (Clonidine may potentiate the CNS-depressive effects). Products include:
ProSom Tablets 517

Ethchlorvynol (Clonidine may potentiate the CNS-depressive effects).
No products indexed under this heading.

Ethinamate (Clonidine may potentiate the CNS-depressive effects).
No products indexed under this heading.

Felodipine (Co-administration with agents known to affect sinus node function or AV nodal conduction, such as calcium channel blockers, may result in additive effects such as bradycardia and AV block).
No products indexed under this heading.

Flurazepam Hydrochloride (Clonidine may potentiate the CNS-depressive effects). Products include:
Dalmane Capsules 3342

Glutethimide (Clonidine may potentiate the CNS-depressive effects).
No products indexed under this heading.

Imipramine Hydrochloride (Co-administration may reduce the hypotensive effects; dosage adjustment may be necessary).
No products indexed under this heading.

Imipramine Pamoate (Co-administration may reduce the hypotensive effects; dosage adjustment may be necessary).
No products indexed under this heading.

Isradipine (Co-administration with agents known to affect sinus node function or AV nodal conduction, such as calcium channel blockers, may result in additive effects such as bradycardia and AV block). Products include:
DynaCirc CR Tablets 2721

Labetalol Hydrochloride (Co-administration with agents known to affect sinus node function or AV nodal conduction, such as beta blockers, may result in additive effects such as bradycardia and AV block).
No products indexed under this heading.

Levobunolol Hydrochloride (Co-administration with agents known to affect sinus node function or AV nodal conduction, such as beta blockers, may result in additive effects such as bradycardia and AV block). Products include:
Betagan Ophthalmic Solution, USP .... ⊙220

Lorazepam (Clonidine may potentiate the CNS-depressive effects).
No products indexed under this heading.

Maprotiline Hydrochloride (Co-administration may reduce the hypotensive effects; dosage adjustment may be necessary).
No products indexed under this heading.

Mephobarbital (Clonidine may potentiate the CNS-depressive effects).
No products indexed under this heading.

Metipranolol Hydrochloride (Co-administration with agents known to affect sinus node function or AV nodal conduction, such as beta blockers, may result in additive effects such as bradycardia and AV block).
No products indexed under this heading.

Metoprolol Succinate (Co-administration with agents known to affect sinus node function or AV nodal conduction, such as beta blockers, may result in additive effects such as bradycardia and AV block). Products include:
Toprol-XL Tablets 668

Metoprolol Tartrate (Co-administration with agents known to affect sinus node function or AV nodal conduction, such as beta blockers, may result in additive effects such as bradycardia and AV block). Products include:
Lopressor Injection 2238
Lopressor Tablets 2238
Lopressor HCT 50/25 Tablets 2241
Lopressor HCT 100/25 Tablets 2241
Lopressor HCT 100/50 Tablets 2241

Mibefradil Dihydrochloride (Co-administration with agents known to affect sinus node function or AV nodal conduction, such as calcium channel blockers, may result in additive effects such as bradycardia and AV block).
No products indexed under this heading.

Midazolam Hydrochloride (Clonidine may potentiate the CNS-depressive effects).
No products indexed under this heading.

Nadolol (Co-administration with agents known to affect sinus node function or AV nodal conduction, such as beta blockers, may result in additive effects such as bradycardia and AV block). Products include:
Nadolol Tablets 2159

Nicardipine Hydrochloride (Co-administration with agents known to affect sinus node function or AV nodal conduction, such as calcium channel blockers, may result in additive effects such as bradycardia and AV block). Products include:
Cardene I.V. 2497

Nifedipine (Co-administration with agents known to affect sinus node function or AV nodal conduction, such as calcium channel blockers, may result in additive effects such as bradycardia and AV block). Products include:
Adalat CC Tablets 2964

Nimodipine (Co-administration with agents known to affect sinus node function or AV nodal conduction, such as calcium channel blockers, may result in additive effects such as bradycardia and AV block). Products include:
Nimotop Capsules 749

Nisoldipine (Co-administration with agents known to affect sinus node function or AV nodal conduction, such as calcium channel blockers, may result in additive effects such as bradycardia and AV block). Products include:
Sular Tablets 3122

Nortriptyline Hydrochloride (Co-administration may reduce the hypotensive effects; dosage adjustment may be necessary).
No products indexed under this heading.

Penbutolol Sulfate (Co-administration with agents known to affect sinus node function or AV nodal conduction, such as beta blockers, may result in additive effects such as bradycardia and AV block).
No products indexed under this heading.

Pentobarbital Sodium (Clonidine may potentiate the CNS-depressive effects). Products include:
Nembutal Sodium Solution, USP 2470

Phenobarbital (Clonidine may potentiate the CNS-depressive effects). Products include:
Donnatal Extentabs 2493

Pindolol (Co-administration with agents known to affect sinus node function or AV nodal conduction, such as beta blockers, may result in additive effects such as bradycardia and AV block).
No products indexed under this heading.

Propofol (Clonidine may potentiate the CNS-depressive effects).
No products indexed under this heading.

Propranolol Hydrochloride (Co-administration with agents known to affect sinus node function or AV nodal conduction, such as beta blockers, may result in additive effects such as bradycardia and AV block). Products include:
Inderal LA Long-Acting Capsules 3429
InnoPran XL Capsules 2723

Protriptyline Hydrochloride (Co-administration may reduce the hypotensive effects; dosage adjustment may be necessary).
No products indexed under this heading.

Quazepam (Clonidine may potentiate the CNS-depressive effects).
No products indexed under this heading.

Ramelteon (Clonidine may potentiate the CNS-depressive effects). Products include:
Rozerem Tablets 3231

Secobarbital Sodium (Clonidine may potentiate the CNS-depressive effects).
No products indexed under this heading.

Sotalol Hydrochloride (Co-administration with agents known to affect sinus node function or AV nodal conduction, such as beta blockers, may result in additive effects such as bradycardia and AV block).
No products indexed under this heading.

Temazepam (Clonidine may potentiate the CNS-depressive effects). Products include:
Restoril Capsules 1860

Thiamylal Sodium (Clonidine may potentiate the CNS-depressive effects).
No products indexed under this heading.

Timolol Hemihydrate (Co-administration with agents known to affect sinus node function or AV nodal conduction, such as beta

blockers, may result in additive effects such as bradycardia and AV block). Products include:
- Betimol Ophthalmic Solution 3382
- Betimol Ophthalmic Solution .... ⊙295

Timolol Maleate (Co-administration with agents known to affect sinus node function or AV nodal conduction, such as beta blockers, may result in additive effects such as bradycardia and AV block). Products include:
- Blocadren Tablets 1916
- Cosopt Sterile Ophthalmic Solution 1931
- Timolide Tablets 2086
- Timoptic Sterile Ophthalmic Solution 2088
- Timoptic in Ocudose 2091
- Timoptic-XE Sterile Ophthalmic Gel Forming Solution 2092

Triazolam (Clonidine may potentiate the CNS-depressive effects).
No products indexed under this heading.

Trimipramine Maleate (Co-administration may reduce the hypotensive effects; dosage adjustment may be necessary).
No products indexed under this heading.

Verapamil Hydrochloride (Co-administration with agents known to affect sinus node function or AV nodal conduction, such as calcium channel blockers, may result in additive effects such as bradycardia and AV block). Products include:
- Covera-HS Tablets 3139
- Tarka Tablets 524
- Verelan PM Extended-Release Capsules, Controlled-Onset........... 3106

Zaleplon (Clonidine may potentiate the CNS-depressive effects). Products include:
- Sonata Capsules 1717

Zolpidem Tartrate (Clonidine may potentiate the CNS-depressive effects). Products include:
- Ambien Tablets 2851
- Ambien CR Tablets 2855

Food Interactions

Alcohol (Clonidine may potentiate the CNS-depressive effects).

CATHFLO ACTIVASE

(Alteplase) 1231
See Activase I.V.

CAVERJECT IMPULSE INJECTION

(Alprostadil) 2612
May interact with:

Heparin Sodium (Patients on anticoagulants, such as heparin, may have increased propensity for bleeding after intracavernosal injection).
No products indexed under this heading.

Sildenafil Citrate (The safety and efficacy of combination therapy with other vasoactive agents, such as sildenafil, have not been studied; therefore, such combinations are not recommended). Products include:
- Revatio Tablets 2557
- Viagra Tablets 2573

Warfarin Sodium (Patients on anticoagulants, such as warfarin, may have increased propensity for bleeding after intracavernosal injection). Products include:
- Coumadin for Injection 898
- Coumadin Tablets 898

CEFTIN FOR ORAL SUSPENSION

(Cefuroxime Axetil) 1407
See Ceftin Tablets

CEFTIN TABLETS

(Cefuroxime Axetil) 1407
May interact with oral anticoagulants, drugs that reduce gastric acidity, and certain other agents. Compounds in these categories include:

Aluminum Carbonate (Drugs that reduce gastric acidity may result in a lower bioavailability of Ceftin compared with that of fasting state and tend to cancel the effect of postprandial absorption).
No products indexed under this heading.

Aluminum Hydroxide (Drugs that reduce gastric acidity may result in a lower bioavailability of Ceftin compared with that of fasting state and tend to cancel the effect of postprandial absorption). Products include:
- Gaviscon Regular Strength Liquid .. 658
- Gaviscon Regular Strength Tablets.. 658
- Gaviscon Extra Strength Liquid 658
- Gaviscon Extra Strength Tablets 658
- Maalox Regular Strength Antacid/Antigas Liquid................. 2175
- Maalox Max Maximum Strength Antacid/Anti-Gas Liquid................ 2176

Anisindione (Cephalosporins may be associated with a fall in prothrombin activity; those at risk include patients previously stabilized on anticoagulant therapy). Products include:
- Miradon Tablets 3042

Cimetidine (Drugs that reduce gastric acidity may result in a lower bioavailability of Ceftin compared with that of fasting state and tend to cancel the effect of postprandial absorption). Products include:
- Tagamet HB 200 Tablets 664

Cimetidine Hydrochloride (Drugs that reduce gastric acidity may result in a lower bioavailability of Ceftin compared with that of fasting state and tend to cancel the effect of postprandial absorption).
No products indexed under this heading.

Dicumarol (Cephalosporins may be associated with a fall in prothrombin activity; those at risk include patients previously stabilized on anticoagulant therapy).
No products indexed under this heading.

Esomeprazole Magnesium (Drugs that reduce gastric acidity may result in a lower bioavailability of Ceftin compared with that of fasting state and tend to cancel the effect of postprandial absorption). Products include:
- Nexium Delayed-Release Capsules.................................... 655

Famotidine (Drugs that reduce gastric acidity may result in a lower bioavailability of Ceftin compared with that of fasting state and tend to cancel the effect of postprandial absorption). Products include:
- Pepcid Injection 2040
- Pepcid 2038
- Pepcid AC Gelcaps 1701
- Pepcid AC Tablets 1701
- Maximum Strength Pepcid AC Tablets 1701
- Pepcid Complete Chewable Tablets 1701

Lansoprazole (Drugs that reduce gastric acidity may result in a lower bioavailability of Ceftin compared with that of fasting state and tend to cancel the effect of postprandial absorption). Products include:
- Prevacid Delayed-Release Capsules 3271
- Prevacid for Delayed-Release Oral Suspension 3271
- Prevacid SoluTab Delayed-Release Orally Disintegrating Tablets.................. 3271
- Prevacid I.V. for Injection 3277
- Prevacid NapraPAC 3280
- PREVPAC 3284

Magnesium Hydroxide (Drugs that reduce gastric acidity may result in a lower bioavailability of Ceftin compared with that of fasting state and tend to cancel the effect of postprandial absorption). Products include:
- Maalox Regular Strength Antacid/Antigas Liquid................. 2175
- Maalox Max Maximum Strength Antacid/Anti-Gas Liquid................ 2176
- Pepcid Complete Chewable Tablets 1701

Nizatidine (Drugs that reduce gastric acidity may result in a lower bioavailability of Ceftin compared with that of fasting state and tend to cancel the effect of postprandial absorption). Products include:
- Axid Oral Solution 879

Omeprazole (Drugs that reduce gastric acidity may result in a lower bioavailability of Ceftin compared with that of fasting state and tend to cancel the effect of postprandial absorption). Products include:
- Zegerid Capsules 2958
- Zegerid Powder for Oral Solution..... 2958

Probenecid (Increases serum concentration of cefuroxime).
No products indexed under this heading.

Rabeprazole Sodium (Drugs that reduce gastric acidity may result in a lower bioavailability of Ceftin compared with that of fasting state and tend to cancel the effect of postprandial absorption). Products include:
- Aciphex Tablets 1090

Ranitidine Hydrochloride (Drugs that reduce gastric acidity may result in a lower bioavailability of Ceftin compared with that of fasting state and tend to cancel the effect of postprandial absorption). Products include:
- Zantac 1624
- Zantac Injection 1619
- Zantac Injection Pharmacy Bulk Package... 1622

Warfarin Sodium (Cephalosporins may be associated with a fall in prothrombin activity; those at risk include patients previously stabilized on anticoagulant therapy). Products include:
- Coumadin for Injection 898
- Coumadin Tablets 898

Food Interactions

Food, unspecified (Absorption is greater when taken after food).

CELEBREX CAPSULES

(Celecoxib) 3134
May interact with ACE inhibitors, antacids containing aluminum, calcium and magnesium, oral anticoagulants, lithium preparations, thiazides, and certain other agents. Compounds in these categories include:

Aluminum Carbonate (Co-administration with an aluminum-and-magnesium-containing antacid resulted in a reduction in plasma celecoxib concentration with a decrease of 37% in Cmax and 10% in AUC).
No products indexed under this heading.

Aluminum Hydroxide (Co-administration with an aluminum-and-magnesium-containing antacid resulted in a reduction in plasma celecoxib concentration with a decrease of 37% in Cmax and 10% in AUC). Products include:
- Gaviscon Regular Strength Liquid .. 658
- Gaviscon Regular Strength Tablets.. 658
- Gaviscon Extra Strength Liquid 658
- Gaviscon Extra Strength Tablets 658
- Maalox Regular Strength Antacid/Antigas Liquid................. 2175
- Maalox Max Maximum Strength Antacid/Anti-Gas Liquid................ 2176

Amiodarone Hydrochloride (Co-administration of celecoxib with drugs known to inhibit CYP4502C9, such as amiodarone, may result in increased plasma concentration; caution should be exercised if used concurrently).
No products indexed under this heading.

Anisindione (Serious bleeding events, some of which were fatal, have been reported, predominately in the elderly, in association with increases in prothrombin time in patients receiving celecoxib concurrently with warfarin. Anticoagulant activity should be monitored,particulary in the first few days, after initiating or changing celecoxib therapy in patients receiving warfarin or similar agents, since these patients are at an increased risk of bleeding complications). Products include:
- Miradon Tablets 3042

Aspirin (Co-administration may result in an increased rate of GI ulceration or other complications; low dose of aspirin can be used with celecoxib). Products include:
- Aggrenox Capsules 822
- Bayer Aspirin 744
- BC Allergy Sinus Cold Powder 677
- BC Headache Powder 677
- Arthritis Strength BC Powder 677
- BC Sinus Cold Powder 677
- Excedrin Extra Strength Caplets/Tablets/Geltabs 684
- Excedrin Migraine Caplets/Tablets/Geltabs 609
- Goody's Body Pain Formula Powder.. 684
- Goody's Extra Strength Headache Powders.......................... 611
- Goody's Extra Strength Pain Relief Tablets 685
- Percodan Tablets 1132
- St. Joseph 81 mg Aspirin Chewable and Enteric Coated Tablets 1869

Benazepril Hydrochloride (Co-administration of NSAIDs with ACE inhibitors may result in diminished antihypertensive effect of ACE inhibitors). Products include:
- Lotensin Tablets 2243
- Lotensin HCT Tablets 2246
- Lotrel Capsules 2249

IMPORTANT NOTE: Always consult each drug listing in the patient's regimen for possible interactions.

Bendroflumethiazide (Co-administration of NSAIDs with thiazides may result in reduced natriuretic effect of thiazide diuretics).
No products indexed under this heading.

Captopril (Co-administration of NSAIDs with ACE inhibitors may result in diminished antihypertensive effect of ACE inhibitors). Products include:
Captopril Tablets 2149

Chlorothiazide (Co-administration of NSAIDs with thiazides may result in reduced natriuretic effect of thiazide diuretics). Products include:
Diuril Oral Suspension 1954

Chlorothiazide Sodium (Co-administration of NSAIDs with thiazides may result in reduced natriuretic effect of thiazide diuretics). Products include:
Diuril Sodium Intravenous 2467

Dicumarol (Serious bleeding events, some of which were fatal, have been reported, predominately in the elderly, in association with increases in prothrombin time in patients receiving celecoxib concurrently with warfarin. Anticoagulant activity should be monitored,particulary in the first few days, after initiating or changing celecoxib therapy in patients receiving warfarin or similar agents, since these patients are at an increased risk of bleeding complications).
No products indexed under this heading.

Enalapril Maleate (Co-administration of NSAIDs with ACE inhibitors may result in diminished antihypertensive effect of ACE inhibitors). Products include:
Vasotec I.V. Injection 2103

Enalaprilat (Co-administration of NSAIDs with ACE inhibitors may result in diminished antihypertensive effect of ACE inhibitors).
No products indexed under this heading.

Fluconazole (Co-administration has resulted in a two-fold increase in celecoxib plasma concentration due to inhibition of celecoxib metabolism via P4502C9).
No products indexed under this heading.

Fosinopril Sodium (Co-administration of NSAIDs with ACE inhibitors may result in diminished antihypertensive effect of ACE inhibitors).
No products indexed under this heading.

Furosemide (Co-administration of NSAIDs with thiazides may result in reduced natriuretic effect of furosemide). Products include:
Furosemide Tablets 2154

Hydrochlorothiazide (Co-administration of NSAIDs with thiazides may result in reduced natriuretic effect of thiazide diuretics). Products include:
Aldoril Tablets 1910
Atacand HCT 651
Avalide Tablets 888
Avalide Tablets 2874
Benicar HCT Tablets 1044
Diovan HCT Tablets 2196
Dyazide Capsules 1423
Hyzaar 50-12.5 Tablets 1990
Hyzaar 100-12.5 Tablets 1990
Hyzaar 100-25 Tablets 1990
Lopressor HCT 50/25 Tablets 2241
Lopressor HCT 100/25 Tablets 2241
Lopressor HCT 100/50 Tablets 2241
Lotensin HCT Tablets 2246
Micardis HCT Tablets 856
Moduretic Tablets 2028
Prinzide Tablets 2056
Teveten HCT Tablets 1737
Timolide Tablets 2086
Uniretic Tablets 3100

Hydroflumethiazide (Co-administration of NSAIDs with thiazides may result in reduced natriuretic effect of thiazide diuretics).
No products indexed under this heading.

Itraconazole (Co-administration of celecoxib with drugs known to inhibit CYP4502C9, such as itraconazole, may result in increased plasma concentration; caution should be exercised if used concurrently).
No products indexed under this heading.

Ketoconazole (Co-administration of celecoxib with drugs known to inhibit CYP4502C9, such as ketoconazole, may result in increased plasma concentration; caution should be exercised if used concurrently). Products include:
Nizoral A-D Shampoo, 1% 1868

Lisinopril (Co-administration of NSAIDs with ACE inhibitors may result in diminished antihypertensive effect of ACE inhibitors). Products include:
Prinivil Tablets 2052
Prinzide Tablets 2056

Lithium (Co-administration has resulted in increased steady-state lithium plasma levels).
No products indexed under this heading.

Lithium Carbonate (Co-administration has resulted in increased steady-state lithium plasma levels). Products include:
Lithobid Tablets 1692

Lithium Citrate (Co-administration has resulted in increased steady-state lithium plasma levels).
No products indexed under this heading.

Magaldrate (Co-administration with an aluminum-and-magnesium-containing antacid resulted in a reduction in plasma celecoxib concentration with a decrease of 37% in Cmax and 10% in AUC).
No products indexed under this heading.

Magnesium Hydroxide (Co-administration with an aluminum-and-magnesium-containing antacid resulted in a reduction in plasma celecoxib concentration with a decrease of 37% in Cmax and 10% in AUC). Products include:
Maalox Regular Strength Antacid/Antigas Liquid................. 2175
Maalox Max Maximum Strength Antacid/Anti-Gas Liquid................ 2176
Pepcid Complete Chewable Tablets 1701

Magnesium Oxide (Co-administration with an aluminum-and-magnesium-containing antacid resulted in a reduction in plasma celecoxib concentration with a decrease of 37% in Cmax and 10% in AUC). Products include:
Beelith Tablets 759
PremCal Light, Regular, and Extra Strength Tablets................ ▣818

Methyclothiazide (Co-administration of NSAIDs with thiazides may result in reduced natriuretic effect of thiazide diuretics).
No products indexed under this heading.

Moexipril Hydrochloride (Co-administration of NSAIDs with ACE inhibitors may result in diminished antihypertensive effect of ACE inhibitors). Products include:
Uniretic Tablets 3100
Univasc Tablets 3104

Perindopril Erbumine (Co-administration of NSAIDs with ACE inhibitors may result in diminished antihypertensive effect of ACE inhibitors). Products include:
Aceon Tablets (2 mg, 4 mg, 8 mg)... 3194

Polythiazide (Co-administration of NSAIDs with thiazides may result in reduced natriuretic effect of thiazide diuretics).
No products indexed under this heading.

Quinapril Hydrochloride (Co-administration of NSAIDs with ACE inhibitors may result in diminished antihypertensive effect of ACE inhibitors).
No products indexed under this heading.

Ramipril (Co-administration of NSAIDs with ACE inhibitors may result in diminished antihypertensive effect of ACE inhibitors). Products include:
Altace Capsules 1702

Spirapril Hydrochloride (Co-administration of NSAIDs with ACE inhibitors may result in diminished antihypertensive effect of ACE inhibitors).
No products indexed under this heading.

Trandolapril (Co-administration of NSAIDs with ACE inhibitors may result in diminished antihypertensive effect of ACE inhibitors). Products include:
Mavik Tablets 486
Tarka Tablets 524

Warfarin Sodium (Serious bleeding events, some of which were fatal, have been reported, predominately in the elderly, in association with increases in prothrombin time in patients receiving celecoxib concurrently with warfarin. Anticoagulant activity should be monitored,particulary in the first few days, after initiating or changing celecoxib therapy in patients receiving warfarin or similar agents, since these patients are at an increased risk of bleeding complications). Products include:
Coumadin for Injection 898
Coumadin Tablets 898

Food Interactions

Food, unspecified (Co-administration with a high-fat meal delayed peak plasma levels for about 1 to 2 hours with an increase in total absorption (AUC) of 10% to 20%; Celebrex can be administered without regard to the timing of meals).

CELEXA ORAL SOLUTION

(Citalopram Hydrobromide) 1176
See Celexa Tablets

CELEXA TABLETS

(Citalopram Hydrobromide) 1176
May interact with anticoagulants, erythromycin, lithium preparations, macrolide antibiotics, monoamine oxidase inhibitors, non-steroidal anti-inflammatory agents, tricyclic antidepressants, and certain other agents. Compounds in these categories include:

Amitriptyline Hydrochloride (Co-administration of imipramine with citalopram has resulted in a 50% increase in active metabolite, desipramine concentration; the clinical significance of these findings is unknown; caution is indicated if tricyclic antidepressants are co-administered with citalopram, a relatively weak inhibitor of CYP2D6).
No products indexed under this heading.

Amoxapine (Co-administration of imipramine with citalopram has resulted in a 50% increase in active metabolite, desipramine concentration; the clinical significance of these findings is unknown; caution is indicated if tricyclic antidepressants are co-administered with citalopram, a relatively weak inhibitor of CYP2D6).
No products indexed under this heading.

Anisindione (The combined use of psycotropic drugs that interfere with serotonin reuptake and drugs that affect coagulation has been associated with an increased risk of bleeding). Products include:
Miradon Tablets 3042

Ardeparin Sodium (The combined use of psycotropic drugs that interfere with serotonin reuptake and drugs that affect coagulation has been associated with an increased risk of bleeding).
No products indexed under this heading.

Aspirin (The combined use of psycotropic drugs that interfere with serotonin reuptake and drugs that affect coagulation has been associated with an increased risk of bleeding; use caution when co-administering). Products include:
Aggrenox Capsules 822
Bayer Aspirin 744
BC Allergy Sinus Cold Powder .... ▣677
BC Headache Powder .... ▣677
Arthritis Strength BC Powder .... ▣677
BC Sinus Cold Powder .... ▣677
Excedrin Extra Strength Caplets/Tablets/Geltabs............ ▣684
Excedrin Migraine Caplets/Tablets/Geltabs............ ▣609
Goody's Body Pain Formula Powder.. ▣684
Goody's Extra Strength Headache Powders.................... ▣611
Goody's Extra Strength Pain Relief Tablets .... ▣685
Percodan Tablets 1132
St. Joseph 81 mg Aspirin Chewable and Enteric Coated Tablets 1869

Aspirin, Enteric Coated (The combined use of psycotropic drugs that interfere with serotonin reuptake and drugs that affect coagulation has been associated with an increased risk of bleeding; use caution when co-administering).
No products indexed under this heading.

Aspirin Buffered (The combined use of psycotropic drugs that interfere with serotonin reuptake and drugs that affect coagulation has been associated with an increased risk of bleeding; use caution when co-administering). Products include:

Bufferin Extra Strength Tablets 678
Bufferin Regular Strength Tablets ... 678

Azithromycin Dihydrate (Co-administration with potent inhibitors of CYP3A4, such as macrolide antibiotics, may decrease the clearance of citalopram).

No products indexed under this heading.

Carbamazepine (Given the enzyme inducing properties of carbamazepine, the possibility that carbamazepine might increase the clearance of citalopram should be considered if the two drugs are co-administered; during pharmacokinetic studies, the citalopram levels were unaffected with concurrent use). Products include:

Carbatrol Capsules 3171
Equetro Extended-Release Capsules 3180
Tegretol/Tegretol-XR 2295

Celecoxib (The combined use of psycotropic drugs that interfere with serotonin reuptake and drugs that affect coagulation has been associated with an increased risk of bleeding; use caution when co-administering). Products include:

Celebrex Capsules 3134

Cimetidine (Co-administration has resulted in an increase in citalopram AUC and Cmax by 43% and 39% respectively; the clinical significance of these findings is unknown). Products include:

Tagamet HB 200 Tablets 664

Cimetidine Hydrochloride (Co-administration has resulted in an increase in citalopram AUC and Cmax by 43% and 39% respectively; the clinical significance of these findings is unknown).

No products indexed under this heading.

Clarithromycin (Co-administration with potent inhibitors of CYP3A4, such as macrolide antibiotics, may decrease the clearance of citalopram). Products include:

Biaxin/Biaxin XL 402
PREVPAC 3284

Clomipramine Hydrochloride (Co-administration of imipramine with citalopram has resulted in a 50% increase in active metabolite, desipramine concentration; the clinical significance of these findings is unknown; caution is indicated if tricyclic antidepressants are co-administered with citalopram, a relatively weak inhibitor of CYP2D6).

No products indexed under this heading.

Dalteparin Sodium (The combined use of psycotropic drugs that interfere with serotonin reuptake and drugs that affect coagulation has been associated with an increased risk of bleeding). Products include:

Fragmin Injection 1097

Danaparoid Sodium (The combined use of psycotropic drugs that interfere with serotonin reuptake and drugs that affect coagulation has been associated with an increased risk of bleeding).

No products indexed under this heading.

Desipramine Hydrochloride (Co-administration of imipramine with citalopram has resulted in a 50% increase in active metabolite, desipramine concentration; the clinical significance of these findings is unknown; caution is indicated if tricyclic antidepressants are co-administered with citalopram, a relatively weak inhibitor of CYP2D6).

No products indexed under this heading.

Diclofenac Potassium (The combined use of psycotropic drugs that interfere with serotonin reuptake and drugs that affect coagulation has been associated with an increased risk of bleeding; use caution when co-administering).

No products indexed under this heading.

Diclofenac Sodium (The combined use of psycotropic drugs that interfere with serotonin reuptake and drugs that affect coagulation has been associated with an increased risk of bleeding; use caution when co-administering). Products include:

Arthrotec Tablets 3129
Voltaren Ophthalmic Solution 2309
Voltaren Tablets 2307
Voltaren-XR Tablets 2310

Dicumarol (The combined use of psycotropic drugs that interfere with serotonin reuptake and drugs that affect coagulation has been associated with an increased risk of bleeding).

No products indexed under this heading.

Dirithromycin (Co-administration with potent inhibitors of CYP3A4, such as macrolide antibiotics, may decrease the clearance of citalopram).

No products indexed under this heading.

Doxepin Hydrochloride (Co-administration of imipramine with citalopram has resulted in a 50% increase in active metabolite, desipramine concentration; the clinical significance of these findings is unknown; caution is indicated if tricyclic antidepressants are co-administered with citalopram, a relatively weak inhibitor of CYP2D6).

No products indexed under this heading.

Enoxaparin Sodium (The combined use of psycotropic drugs that interfere with serotonin reuptake and drugs that affect coagulation has been associated with an increased risk of bleeding). Products include:

Lovenox Injection 2915

Erythromycin (Co-administration with potent inhibitors of CYP3A4, such as macrolide antibiotics, may decrease the clearance of citalopram). Products include:

Ery-Tab Tablets 449
Erythromycin Base Filmtab Tablets 455
Erythromycin Delayed-Release Capsules, USP 457
PCE Dispertab Tablets 515

Erythromycin Estolate (Co-administration with potent inhibitors of CYP3A4, such as macrolide antibiotics, may decrease the clearance of citalopram).

No products indexed under this heading.

Erythromycin Ethylsuccinate (Co-administration with potent inhibitors of CYP3A4, such as macrolide antibiotics, may decrease the clearance of citalopram). Products include:

E.E.S. 451
EryPed 447

Erythromycin Gluceptate (Co-administration with potent inhibitors of CYP3A4, such as macrolide antibiotics, may decrease the clearance of citalopram).

No products indexed under this heading.

Erythromycin Lactobionate (Co-administration with potent inhibitors of CYP3A4, such as erythromycin, may decrease the clearance of citalopram).

No products indexed under this heading.

Erythromycin Stearate (Co-administration with potent inhibitors of CYP3A4, such as macrolide antibiotics, may decrease the clearance of citalopram). Products include:

Erythrocin Stearate Filmtab Tablets 453

Etodolac (The combined use of psycotropic drugs that interfere with serotonin reuptake and drugs that affect coagulation has been associated with an increased risk of bleeding; use caution when co-administering).

No products indexed under this heading.

Fenoprofen Calcium (The combined use of psycotropic drugs that interfere with serotonin reuptake and drugs that affect coagulation has been associated with an increased risk of bleeding; use caution when co-administering). Products include:

Nalfon Capsules 2502

Fluconazole (Co-administration with potent inhibitors of CYP3A4, such as fluconazole, may decrease the clearance of citalopram).

No products indexed under this heading.

Flurbiprofen (The combined use of psycotropic drugs that interfere with serotonin reuptake and drugs that affect coagulation has been associated with an increased risk of bleeding; use caution when co-administering).

No products indexed under this heading.

Fondaparinux Sodium (The combined use of psycotropic drugs that interfere with serotonin reuptake and drugs that affect coagulation has been associated with an increased risk of bleeding). Products include:

Arixtra Injection 1351

Heparin Calcium (The combined use of psycotropic drugs that interfere with serotonin reuptake and drugs that affect coagulation has been associated with an increased risk of bleeding).

No products indexed under this heading.

Heparin Sodium (The combined use of psycotropic drugs that interfere with serotonin reuptake and drugs that affect coagulation has been associated with an increased risk of bleeding).

No products indexed under this heading.

Ibuprofen (The combined use of psycotropic drugs that interfere with serotonin reuptake and drugs that affect coagulation has been associated with an increased risk of bleeding; use caution when co-administering). Products include:

Advil Allergy Sinus Caplets 770
Advil 674
Children's Advil Oral Suspension 603
Children's Advil Chewable Tablets .. 603
Advil Cold & Sinus 723
Infants' Advil Concentrated Drops .. 604
Infants' Advil Concentrated Drops - White Grape (Dye-Free) 604
Junior Strength Advil Swallow Tablets 605
Advil Migraine Liquigels 608
Advil Multi-Symptom Cold Caplets 770
Advil PM Caplets 615
Motrin IB Tablets and Caplets 1866
Children's Motrin Oral Suspension ... 1867
Children's Motrin Non-Staining Dye-Free Oral Suspension 1867
Children's Motrin Cold Oral Suspension 1867
Infants' Motrin Concentrated Drops 1867
Infants' Motrin Non-Staining Dye-Free Concentrated Drops 1867
Junior Strength Motrin Caplets and Chewable Tablets 1867
Vicoprofen Tablets 539

Imipramine Hydrochloride (Co-administration of imipramine with citalopram has resulted in a 50% increase in active metabolite, desipramine concentration; the clinical significance of these findings is unknown; caution is indicated if tricyclic antidepressants are co-administered with citalopram, a relatively weak inhibitor of CYP2D6).

No products indexed under this heading.

Imipramine Pamoate (Co-administration of imipramine with citalopram has resulted in a 50% increase in active metabolite, desipramine concentration; the clinical significance of these findings is unknown; caution is indicated if tricyclic antidepressants are co-administered with citalopram, a relatively weak inhibitor of CYP2D6).

No products indexed under this heading.

Indomethacin (The combined use of psycotropic drugs that interfere with serotonin reuptake and drugs that affect coagulation has been associated with an increased risk of bleeding; use caution when co-administering). Products include:

Indocin 1995

Indomethacin Sodium Trihydrate (The combined use of psycotropic drugs that interfere with serotonin reuptake and drugs that affect coagulation has been associated with an increased risk of bleeding; use caution when co-administering). Products include:

Indocin I.V. 2465

Isocarboxazid (Co-administration of serotonin reuptake inhibitors and MAO inhibitors has resulted in serious, sometimes fatal, reactions including hyperthermia, rigidity, myoclonus, and other potentially serious adverse reactions; concurrent and/or sequential use is contraindicated).

No products indexed under this heading.

Itraconazole (Co-administration with potent inhibitors of CYP3A4, such as itraconazole, may decrease the clearance of citalopram).

No products indexed under this heading.

Ketoconazole (Co-administration resulted in decreased Cmax and

AUC of ketoconazole by 21% and 10% respectively, and did not significantly affect the pharmacokinetics of citalopram). Products include:

Nizoral A-D Shampoo, 1% **1868**

Ketoprofen (The combined use of psycotropic drugs that interfere with serotonin reuptake and drugs that affect coagulation has been associated with an increased risk of bleeding; use caution when co-administering).

No products indexed under this heading.

Ketorolac Tromethamine (The combined use of psycotropic drugs that interfere with serotonin reuptake and drugs that affect coagulation has been associated with an increased risk of bleeding; use caution when co-administering). Products include:

Acular Ophthalmic Solution **565**
Acular LS Ophthalmic Solution **566**

Lithium (Plasma lithium levels should be monitored; if used concurrently, lithium may enhance the serotonergic effects of citalopram; co-administration during clinical trials had no significant effect on the pharmacokinetics of either drug).

No products indexed under this heading.

Lithium Carbonate (Plasma lithium levels should be monitored; if used concurrently, lithium may enhance the serotonergic effects of citalopram; co-administration during clinical trials had no significant effect on the pharmacokinetics of either drug). Products include:

Lithobid Tablets **1692**

Lithium Citrate (Plasma lithium levels should be monitored; if used concurrently, lithium may enhance the serotonergic effects of citalopram; co-administration during clinical trials had no significant effect on the pharmacokinetics of either drug).

No products indexed under this heading.

Low Molecular Weight Heparins (The combined use of psycotropic drugs that interfere with serotonin reuptake and drugs that affect coagulation has been associated with an increased risk of bleeding).

No products indexed under this heading.

Maprotiline Hydrochloride (Co-administration of imipramine with citalopram has resulted in a 50% increase in active metabolite, desipramine concentration; the clinical significance of these findings is unknown; caution is indicated if tricyclic antidepressants are co-administered with citalopram, a relatively weak inhibitor of CYP2D6).

No products indexed under this heading.

Meclofenamate Sodium (The combined use of psycotropic drugs that interfere with serotonin reuptake and drugs that affect coagulation has been associated with an increased risk of bleeding; use caution when co-administering).

No products indexed under this heading.

Mefenamic Acid (The combined use of psycotropic drugs that interfere with serotonin reuptake and drugs that affect coagulation has been associated with an increased risk of bleeding; use caution when co-administering).

No products indexed under this heading.

Meloxicam (The combined use of psycotropic drugs that interfere with serotonin reuptake and drugs that affect coagulation has been associated with an increased risk of bleeding; use caution when co-administering). Products include:

Mobic Oral Suspension **863**
Mobic Tablets **863**

Metoprolol Succinate (Co-administration has resulted in a two-fold increase in the plasma levels of metoprolol; increased plasma levels of metoprolol have been associated with decreased cardioselectivity; no clinically significant effects on the blood pressure or heart rate have been reported with concurrent use). Products include:

Toprol-XL Tablets **668**

Metoprolol Tartrate (Co-administration has resulted in a two-fold increase in the plasma levels of metoprolol; increased plasma levels of metoprolol have been associated with decreased cardioselectivity; no clinically significant effects on the blood pressure or heart rate have been reported with concurrent use). Products include:

Lopressor Injection **2238**
Lopressor Tablets **2238**
Lopressor HCT 50/25 Tablets **2241**
Lopressor HCT 100/25 Tablets **2241**
Lopressor HCT 100/50 Tablets **2241**

Moclobemide (Co-administration of serotonin reuptake inhibitors and MAO inhibitors has resulted in serious, sometimes fatal, reactions including hyperthermia, rigidity, myoclonus, and other potentially serious adverse reactions; concurrent and/or sequential use is contraindicated).

No products indexed under this heading.

Nabumetone (The combined use of psycotropic drugs that interfere with serotonin reuptake and drugs that affect coagulation has been associated with an increased risk of bleeding; use caution when co-administering).

No products indexed under this heading.

Naproxen (The combined use of psycotropic drugs that interfere with serotonin reuptake and drugs that affect coagulation has been associated with an increased risk of bleeding; use caution when co-administering). Products include:

EC-Naprosyn Delayed-Release Tablets **2761**
Naprosyn Suspension **2761**
Naprosyn Tablets **2761**
Prevacid NapraPAC **3280**

Naproxen Sodium (The combined use of psycotropic drugs that interfere with serotonin reuptake and drugs that affect coagulation has been associated with an increased risk of bleeding; use caution when co-administering). Products include:

Aleve Caplets **742**
Aleve Gelcaps **743**
Aleve Tablets **743**
Aleve Cold & Sinus Caplets **744**
Anaprox Tablets **2761**
Anaprox DS Tablets **2761**

Nortriptyline Hydrochloride (Co-administration of imipramine with citalopram has resulted in a 50% increase in active metabolite, desipramine concentration; the clinical significance of these findings is unknown; caution is indicated if tricyclic antidepressants are co-administered with citalopram, a relatively weak inhibitor of CYP2D6).

No products indexed under this heading.

Omeprazole (Co-administration with potent inhibitors of CYP2C19, such as omeprazole, may decrease the clearance of citalopram). Products include:

Zegerid Capsules **2958**
Zegerid Powder for Oral Solution **2958**

Oxaprozin (The combined use of psycotropic drugs that interfere with serotonin reuptake and drugs that affect coagulation has been associated with an increased risk of bleeding; use caution when co-administering).

No products indexed under this heading.

Pargyline Hydrochloride (Co-administration of serotonin reuptake inhibitors and MAO inhibitors has resulted in serious, sometimes fatal, reactions including hyperthermia, rigidity, myoclonus, and other potentially serious adverse reactions; concurrent and/or sequential use is contraindicated).

No products indexed under this heading.

Phenelzine Sulfate (Co-administration of serotonin reuptake inhibitors and MAO inhibitors has resulted in serious, sometimes fatal, reactions including hyperthermia, rigidity, myoclonus, and other potentially serious adverse reactions; concurrent and/or sequential use is contraindicated).

No products indexed under this heading.

Phenylbutazone (The combined use of psycotropic drugs that interfere with serotonin reuptake and drugs that affect coagulation has been associated with an increased risk of bleeding; use caution when co-administering).

No products indexed under this heading.

Pimozide (In a controlled study, a single dose of pimozide 2 mg co-administered with citalopram 40 mg given once daily for 11 days was associated with a mean increase in QTc values of approximately 10 msec. compared to pimozide given alone. Concomitant use in patients taking pimozide is contraindicated).

No products indexed under this heading.

Piroxicam (The combined use of psycotropic drugs that interfere with serotonin reuptake and drugs that affect coagulation has been associated with an increased risk of bleeding; use caution when co-administering).

No products indexed under this heading.

Procarbazine Hydrochloride (Co-administration of serotonin reuptake inhibitors and MAO inhibitors has resulted in serious, sometimes fatal, reactions including hyperthermia, rigidity, myoclonus, and other potentially serious adverse reactions; concurrent and/or sequential use is contraindicated). Products include:

Matulane Capsules **3191**

Protriptyline Hydrochloride (Co-administration of imipramine with citalopram has resulted in a 50% increase in active metabolite, desipramine concentration; the clinical significance of these findings is unknown; caution is indicated if tricyclic antidepressants are co-administered with citalopram, a relatively weak inhibitor of CYP2D6).

No products indexed under this heading.

Rofecoxib (The combined use of psycotropic drugs that interfere with serotonin reuptake and drugs that affect coagulation has been associated with an increased risk of bleeding; use caution when co-administering).

No products indexed under this heading.

Selegiline Hydrochloride (Co-administration of serotonin reuptake inhibitors and MAO inhibitors has resulted in serious, sometimes fatal, reactions including hyperthermia, rigidity, myoclonus, and other potentially serious adverse reactions; concurrent and/or sequential use is contraindicated). Products include:

Eldepryl Capsules **3208**
Zelapar Tablets **3372**

Sulindac (The combined use of psycotropic drugs that interfere with serotonin reuptake and drugs that affect coagulation has been associated with an increased risk of bleeding; use caution when co-administering). Products include:

Clinoril Tablets **1924**

Sumatriptan (Co-administration of SSRIs and sumatriptan has resulted in weakness, hyperreflexia, and incoordination). Products include:

Imitrex Nasal Spray **1467**

Sumatriptan Succinate (Co-administration of SSRIs and sumatriptan has resulted in weakness, hyperreflexia, and incoordination). Products include:

Imitrex Injection **1463**
Imitrex Tablets **1471**

Tinzaparin Sodium (The combined use of psycotropic drugs that interfere with serotonin reuptake and drugs that affect coagulation has been associated with an increased risk of bleeding).

No products indexed under this heading.

Tolmetin Sodium (The combined use of psycotropic drugs that interfere with serotonin reuptake and drugs that affect coagulation has been associated with an increased risk of bleeding; use caution when co-administering).

No products indexed under this heading.

Tranylcypromine Sulfate (Co-administration of serotonin reuptake inhibitors and MAO inhibitors has resulted in serious, sometimes fatal, reactions including hyperthermia, rigidity, myoclonus, and other potentially serious adverse reactions; concurrent and/or sequential use is contraindicated). Products include:

Parnate Tablets **1527**

Trimipramine Maleate (Co-administration of imipramine with citalopram has resulted in a 50% increase in active metabolite, desipramine concentration; the clinical significance of these findings is unknown; caution is indicated if tricyclic antidepressants are co-administered with citalopram, a relatively weak inhibitor of CYP2D6).
No products indexed under this heading.

Troleandomycin (Co-administration with potent inhibitors of CYP3A4, such as macrolide antibiotics, may decrease the clearance of citalopram).
No products indexed under this heading.

Valdecoxib (The combined use of psycotropic drugs that interfere with serotonin reuptake and drugs that affect coagulation has been associated with an increased risk of bleeding; use caution when co-administering).
No products indexed under this heading.

Warfarin Sodium (The combined use of psycotropic drugs that interfere with serotonin reuptake and drugs that affect coagulation has been associated with an increased risk of bleeding). Products include:
Coumadin for Injection 898
Coumadin Tablets 898

Food Interactions

Alcohol (Although citalopram did not potentiate cognitive and motor effects of alcohol, concurrent use is not recommended).

CELLCEPT CAPSULES

(Mycophenolate Mofetil) 2747
May interact with:

Acyclovir (Potential for these two drugs to compete for tubular secretion further increasing the concentrations of both drugs; AUCs were increased 10.6% for phenolic glucuronide of mycophenolate mofetil and 21.9% for acyclovir). Products include:
Zovirax 1643
Zovirax Cream 820
Zovirax Ointment 821

Acyclovir Sodium (Potential for these two drugs to compete for tubular secretion further increasing the concentrations of both drugs; AUCs were increased 10.6% for phenolic glucuronide of mycophenolate mofetil and 21.9% for acyclovir).
No products indexed under this heading.

Aluminum Hydroxide (Potential for decreased absorption when CellCept is administered with the antacids containing aluminum and magnesium hydroxide; avoid simultaneous administration). Products include:
Gaviscon Regular Strength Liquid .. 658
Gaviscon Regular Strength Tablets 658
Gaviscon Extra Strength Liquid 658
Gaviscon Extra Strength Tablets 658
Maalox Regular Strength Antacid/Antigas Liquid.................. 2175
Maalox Max Maximum Strength Antacid/Anti-Gas Liquid................. 2176

Antibiotics, unspecified (Drugs that alter gastrointestinal flora may interact with mycophenolate mofetil by disrupting enterohepatic recirculation).
No products indexed under this heading.

Azathioprine (Concomitant administration is not recommended because such co-administration has not been studied clinically).
No products indexed under this heading.

Azathioprine Sodium (Concomitant administration is not recommended because such co-administration has not been studied clinically).
No products indexed under this heading.

Cholestyramine (Decreased AUC of mycophenolate mofetil by approximately 40%; concomitant use with agents that may interfere with enterohepatic circulation should be avoided).
No products indexed under this heading.

Ethinyl Estradiol (Possibility of changes in the pharmacokinetics of the oral contraceptives under long term dosing conditions with CellCept which might adversely affect the efficacy of the oral contraceptive). Products include:
Mircette Tablets 1066
NuvaRing 2340
Ortho-Cyclen/Ortho Tri-Cyclen 2429
Ortho Evra Transdermal System 2417
Ortho Tri-Cyclen Lo Tablets 2436
Seasonique Tablets 1077
Yasmin 28 Tablets 796
Yaz Tablets 803

Ganciclovir Sodium (Potential for these two drugs to compete for tubular secretion further increasing the concentrations of both drugs).
No products indexed under this heading.

Magnesium Hydroxide (Potential for decreased absorption when CellCept is administered with the antacids containing aluminum and magnesium hydroxide; avoid simultaneous administration). Products include:
Maalox Regular Strength Antacid/Antigas Liquid.................. 2175
Maalox Max Maximum Strength Antacid/Anti-Gas Liquid................ 2176
Pepcid Complete Chewable Tablets 1701

Norethindrone (Possibility of changes in the pharmacokinetics of the oral contraceptives under long term dosing conditions with CellCept which might adversely affect the efficacy of the oral contraceptive). Products include:
Ortho Micronor Tablets 2426

Probenecid (Potential for increased plasma concentration of MPA).
No products indexed under this heading.

Valacyclovir Hydrochloride (Potential for these two drugs to compete for tubular secretion further increasing the concentrations of both drugs; AUCs were increased 10.6% for phenolic glucuronide of mycophenolate mofetil and 21.9% for acyclovir). Products include:
Valtrex Caplets 1597

Valganciclovir Hydrochloride (Potential for these two drugs to compete for tubular secretion further increasing the concentrations of both drugs). Products include:
Valcyte Tablets 2813

Food Interactions

Food, unspecified (Food has no effect on MPA AUC, but has been shown to decrease MPA Cmax by 40%; it is recommended that CellCept be administered on an empty stomach).

CELLCEPT INTRAVENOUS

(Mycophenolate Mofetil Hydrochloride)................................... 2747
See CellCept Capsules

CELLCEPT ORAL SUSPENSION

(Mycophenolate Mofetil) 2747
See CellCept Capsules

CELLCEPT TABLETS

(Mycophenolate Mofetil) 2747
See CellCept Capsules

CENTRUM TABLETS

(Vitamins with Minerals) 809
May interact with:

Vitamin A (Concurrent use with other Vitamin A supplements is not recommended). Products include:
Visutein Capsules 3329

CENTRUM KIDS COMPLETE CHILDREN'S CHEWABLES

(Vitamins with Minerals) 810
None cited in PDR database.

CENTRUM PERFORMANCE MULTIVITAMIN/ MULTIMINERAL SUPPLEMENT

(Ginkgo biloba, Ginseng, Herbals with Vitamins & Minerals, Vitamins with Minerals)................................... 811
May interact with:

Vitamin A (Concurrent use with other Vitamin A supplements is not recommended). Products include:
Visutein Capsules 3329

CENTRUM SILVER TABLETS

(Vitamins with Minerals) 811
May interact with:

Vitamin A (Concurrent use with other Vitamin A supplements is not recommended). Products include:
Visutein Capsules 3329

CEREZYME FOR INJECTION

(Imiglucerase) 1270
None cited in PDR database.

CERVIDIL VAGINAL INSERT

(Dinoprostone) 1181
May interact with oxytocic drugs. Compounds in these categories include:

Ergonovine Maleate (Dinoprostone may augment the activity of oxytocic agents and concomitant use is not recommended; a dosing interval of at least 30 minutes is recommended for sequential use).
No products indexed under this heading.

Methylergonovine Maleate (Dinoprostone may augment the activity of oxytocic agents and concomitant use is not recommended; a dosing interval of at least 30 minutes is recommended for sequential use).
No products indexed under this heading.

Oxytocin (Dinoprostone may augment the activity of oxytocic agents and concomitant use is not recommended; a dosing interval of at least 30 minutes is recommended for sequential use).
No products indexed under this heading.

CESAMET CAPSULES

(Nabilone) 3340
May interact with amphetamines, anticholinergics, antihistamines, barbiturates, benzodiazepines, central nervous system depressants, hypnotics and sedatives, lithium preparations, muscle relaxants, highly protein bound drugs (selected), psychotropics, sympathomimetics, theophyllines, tricyclic antidepressants, and certain other agents. Compounds in these categories include:

Acrivastine (Co-administration may cause additive or super-additive tachycardia and drowsiness).
No products indexed under this heading.

Albuterol (Co-administration may cause additive hypertension, tachycardia, and possibly cardiotoxicity). Products include:
Proventil Inhalation Aerosol 3053

Albuterol Sulfate (Co-administration may cause additive hypertension, tachycardia, and possibly cardiotoxicity). Products include:
AccuNeb Inhalation Solution 1055
Combivent Inhalation Aerosol 847
DuoNeb Inhalation Solution 1058
ProAir HFA Inhalation Aerosol 3300
Proventil Inhalation Solution 0.083%.. 3055
Proventil HFA Inhalation Aerosol 3056
Ventolin HFA Inhalation Aerosol 1600
VoSpire ER Tablets 1052

Alfentanil Hydrochloride (Co-administration may cause additive drowsiness and CNS depression).
No products indexed under this heading.

Alprazolam (Co-administration may cause additive drowsiness and CNS depression). Products include:
Niravam Orally Disintegrating Tablets 3092

Amiodarone Hydrochloride (Nabilone is purportedly highly bound to plasma proteins and may displace other protein-bound drugs; patients on concomitant therapy should be monitored for a change in dosage requirements).
No products indexed under this heading.

Amitriptyline Hydrochloride (Co-administration may cause additive tachycardia, hypertension, and drowsiness).
No products indexed under this heading.

Amoxapine (Co-administration may cause additive tachycardia, hypertension, and drowsiness).
No products indexed under this heading.

Amphetamine Resins (Co-administration may cause additive hypertension, tachycardia, and possibly cardiotoxicity).
No products indexed under this heading.

Amphetamine Sulfate (Co-administration may cause additive hypertension, tachycardia, and possibly cardiotoxicity). Products include:
Adderall Tablets 3164
Adderall XR Capsules 3166

Antipyrine (Co-administration may result in decreased clearance of these agents, presumably via competitive inhibition of metabolism).
No products indexed under this heading.

Aprobarbital (Co-administration may cause additive drowsiness and CNS depression; co-administration may also result in decreased clearance of these agents, presumably via competitive inhibition of metabolism).
No products indexed under this heading.

Astemizole (Co-administration may cause additive or super-additive tachycardia and drowsiness).
No products indexed under this heading.

Atovaquone (Nabilone is purportedly highly bound to plasma proteins and may displace other protein-bound drugs; patients on concomitant therapy should be monitored for a change in dosage requirements). Products include:
Malarone Pediatric Tablets 1517
Malarone Tablets 1517
Mepron Suspension 1521

Atracurium Besylate (Co-administration may cause additive drowsiness and CNS depression).
No products indexed under this heading.

Atropine Derivatives (Co-administration may cause additive or super-additive tachycardia and drowsiness).
No products indexed under this heading.

Atropine Nitrate, Methyl (Co-administration may cause additive or super-additive tachycardia and drowsiness).
No products indexed under this heading.

Atropine Sulfate (Co-administration may cause additive or super-additive tachycardia and drowsiness). Products include:
Donnatal Extentabs 2493

Azatadine Maleate (Co-administration may cause additive or super-additive tachycardia and drowsiness).
No products indexed under this heading.

Baclofen (Co-administration may cause additive drowsiness and CNS depression).
No products indexed under this heading.

Belladonna Alkaloids (Co-administration may cause additive or super-additive tachycardia and drowsiness). Products include:
Hyland's Teething Tablets .... ▣830

Benztropine Mesylate (Co-administration may cause additive or super-additive tachycardia and drowsiness).
No products indexed under this heading.

Biperiden Hydrochloride (Co-administration may cause additive or super-additive tachycardia and drowsiness).
No products indexed under this heading.

Bromodiphenhydramine Hydrochloride (Co-administration may cause additive or super-additive tachycardia and drowsiness).
No products indexed under this heading.

Brompheniramine Maleate (Co-administration may cause additive or super-additive tachycardia and drowsiness). Products include:
Children's Dimetapp Cold & Allergy Elixir .... ▣730
Children's Dimetapp Cold & Allergy Chewable Tablets............ ▣730
Children's Dimetapp DM Cold & Cough Elixir .... ▣731

Buprenorphine Hydrochloride (Co-administration may cause additive drowsiness and CNS depression). Products include:
Buprenex Injectable 2716
Suboxone Tablets 2717
Subutex Tablets 2717

Buspirone Hydrochloride (Co-administration may cause additive drowsiness and CNS depression).
No products indexed under this heading.

Butabarbital (Co-administration may cause additive drowsiness and CNS depression; co-administration may also result in decreased clearance of these agents, presumably via competitive inhibition of metabolism).
No products indexed under this heading.

Butalbital (Co-administration may cause additive drowsiness and CNS depression; co-administration may also result in decreased clearance of these agents, presumably via competitive inhibition of metabolism).
No products indexed under this heading.

Carisoprodol (Co-administration may cause additive drowsiness and CNS depression).
No products indexed under this heading.

Cefonicid Sodium (Nabilone is purportedly highly bound to plasma proteins and may displace other protein-bound drugs; patients on concomitant therapy should be monitored for a change in dosage requirements).
No products indexed under this heading.

Celecoxib (Nabilone is purportedly highly bound to plasma proteins and may displace other protein-bound drugs; patients on concomitant therapy should be monitored for a change in dosage requirements). Products include:
Celebrex Capsules 3134

Cetirizine Hydrochloride (Co-administration may cause additive or super-additive tachycardia and drowsiness). Products include:
Zyrtec Chewable Tablets 2594
Zyrtec 2594
Zyrtec-D 12 Hour Extended Release Tablets 2597

Chlordiazepoxide (Co-administration may cause additive drowsiness and CNS depression).
No products indexed under this heading.

Chlordiazepoxide Hydrochloride (Co-administration may cause additive drowsiness and CNS depression). Products include:
Librium Capsules 3347

Chlorpheniramine Maleate (Co-administration may cause additive or super-additive tachycardia and drowsiness). Products include:
Advil Allergy Sinus Caplets .... ▣770
Advil Multi-Symptom Cold Caplets.. ▣770
BC Allergy Sinus Cold Powder .... ▣677
Comtrex Maximum Strength Cold & Cough Day/Night Caplets - Night Formulation .... ▣726
Comtrex Maximum Strength Day/Night Severe Cold & Sinus Caplets - Night Formulation .... ▣725
Contac Cold and Flu Maximum Strength Caplets........................... ▣728
Contac Cold and Flu Day and Night Caplets (Night Formulation Only)......................... ▣727
Children's Dimetapp Long Acting Cough Plus Cold Syrup................ ▣731
Robitussin Cough & Cold Long-Acting Liquid .... ▣735
Robitussin Cough & Allergy Syrup .. ▣736
Robitussin Cough & Cold Nighttime Liquid............................ ▣736
Robitussin Cough, Cold & Flu Nighttime Liquid............................ ▣738
Robitussin Pediatric Cough & Cold Long-Acting Liquid.............. ▣735
Robitussin Pediatric Cough & Cold Nighttime Liquid .... ▣736
Triaminic Cold & Allergy Liquid ...... ▣746
Triaminic Cough & Runny Nose Softchews .... ▣748
Children's Tylenol Plus Flu Oral Suspension.. ▣749
Tylenol Allergy Multi-Symptom Caplets with Cool Burst and Gelcaps.. 1872
Children's Tylenol Plus Cold Suspension Liquid 1879
Children's Tylenol Plus Cough & Runny Nose Suspension Liquid..... 1879
Children's Tylenol Plus Flu Suspension Liquid 1881
Children's Tylenol Plus Multi-Symptom Cold Suspension Liquid 1879
Tylenol Cold Head Congestion Nighttime Caplets with Cool Burst.. 1873
Tylenol Cold Multi-Symptom Nighttime Caplets with Cool Burst.. 1874
Tylenol Sinus Congestion & Pain Nighttime Caplets with Cool Burst.. 1876
Vicks 44M Cough, Cold & Flu Relief Liquid.................................... 2680
Pediatric Vicks 44m Cough & Cold Relief Liquid.......................... 2676
Children's Vicks NyQuil Cold/Cough Relief......................... ▣756
Children's Vicks NyQuil Cold/Cough Relief Liquid 2680
Zicam Maximum Strength Flu Daytime .... ▣768

Chlorpheniramine Polistirex (Co-administration may cause additive or super-additive tachycardia and drowsiness). Products include:
Tussionex Pennkinetic Extended-Release Suspension...... 3327

Chlorpheniramine Tannate (Co-administration may cause additive or super-additive tachycardia and drowsiness).
No products indexed under this heading.

Chlorpromazine (Nabilone is purportedly highly bound to plasma proteins and may displace other protein-bound drugs; patients on concomitant therapy should be monitored for a change in dosage requirements).
No products indexed under this heading.

Chlorpromazine Hydrochloride (Nabilone is purportedly highly bound to plasma proteins and may displace other protein-bound drugs; patients on concomitant therapy should be monitored for a change in dosage requirements).
No products indexed under this heading.

Chlorprothixene (Co-administration is cautioned in individuals receiving concomitant therapy with psychoactive drugs because of the potential for additive or synergistic CNS effects).
No products indexed under this heading.

Chlorprothixene Hydrochloride (Co-administration is cautioned in individuals receiving concomitant therapy with psychoactive drugs because of the potential for additive or synergistic CNS effects).
No products indexed under this heading.

Chlorprothixene Lactate (Co-administration may cause additive drowsiness and CNS depression).
No products indexed under this heading.

Chlorzoxazone (Co-administration may cause additive drowsiness and CNS depression).
No products indexed under this heading.

Cisatracurium Besylate (Co-administration may cause additive drowsiness and CNS depression). Products include:
Nimbex Injection 498

Clemastine Fumarate (Co-administration may cause additive or super-additive tachycardia and drowsiness).
No products indexed under this heading.

Clidinium Bromide (Co-administration may cause additive or super-additive tachycardia and drowsiness).
No products indexed under this heading.

Clomipramine Hydrochloride (Co-administration may cause additive tachycardia, hypertension, and drowsiness).
No products indexed under this heading.

Clorazepate Dipotassium (Co-administration may cause additive drowsiness and CNS depression). Products include:
Tranxene 2474

Clozapine (Nabilone is purportedly highly bound to plasma proteins and may displace other protein-bound drugs; patients on concomitant therapy should be monitored for a change in dosage requirements). Products include:
Clozaril Tablets 2184
FazaClo Orally Disintegrating Tablets.. 551

Cocaine Hydrochloride (Co-administration may cause additive hypertension, tachycardia, and possibly cardiotoxicity).
No products indexed under this heading.

Codeine Phosphate (Co-administration may cause additive drowsiness and CNS depression). Products include:
Tylenol with Codeine Tablets **2391**

Cyclobenzaprine Hydrochloride (Co-administration may cause additive drowsiness and CNS depression).
No products indexed under this heading.

Cyclosporine (Nabilone is purportedly highly bound to plasma proteins and may displace other protein-bound drugs; patients on concomitant therapy should be monitored for a change in dosage requirements). Products include:
Gengraf Capsules **459**
Neoral Oral Solution **2259**
Neoral Soft Gelatin Capsules **2259**
Restasis Ophthalmic Emulsion **575**
Sandimmune **2275**

Cyproheptadine Hydrochloride (Co-administration may cause additive or super-additive tachycardia and drowsiness).
No products indexed under this heading.

Dantrolene Sodium (Co-administration may cause additive drowsiness and CNS depression). Products include:
Dantrium Capsules **2694**
Dantrium Intravenous **2695**

Desflurane (Co-administration may cause additive drowsiness and CNS depression).
No products indexed under this heading.

Desipramine Hydrochloride (Co-administration may cause additive tachycardia, hypertension, and drowsiness).
No products indexed under this heading.

Dexchlorpheniramine Maleate (Co-administration may cause additive or super-additive tachycardia and drowsiness).
No products indexed under this heading.

Dextroamphetamine Sulfate (Co-administration may cause additive hypertension, tachycardia, and possibly cardiotoxicity). Products include:
Adderall Tablets **3164**
Adderall XR Capsules **3166**
Dexedrine **1420**
DextroStat Tablets **3179**

Dezocine (Co-administration may cause additive drowsiness and CNS depression).
No products indexed under this heading.

Diazepam (Co-administration may cause additive drowsiness and CNS depression). Products include:
Diastat Rectal Delivery System **3343**
Valium Tablets **2819**

Diclofenac Potassium (Nabilone is purportedly highly bound to plasma proteins and may displace other protein-bound drugs; patients on concomitant therapy should be monitored for a change in dosage requirements).
No products indexed under this heading.

Diclofenac Sodium (Nabilone is purportedly highly bound to plasma proteins and may displace other protein-bound drugs; patients on concomitant therapy should be monitored for a change in dosage requirements). Products include:
Arthrotec Tablets **3129**
Voltaren Ophthalmic Solution **2309**
Voltaren Tablets **2307**
Voltaren-XR Tablets **2310**

Dicyclomine Hydrochloride (Co-administration may cause additive or super-additive tachycardia and drowsiness). Products include:
Bentyl Capsules **697**
Bentyl Injection **697**
Bentyl Syrup **697**
Bentyl Tablets **697**

Diphenhydramine Citrate (Co-administration may cause additive or super-additive tachycardia and drowsiness). Products include:
Advil PM Caplets .... ■**615**
Excedrin PM Caplets/Tablets/Geltabs .... ■**610**
Goody's PM Powder for Pain with Sleeplessness .... ■**612**

Diphenhydramine Hydrochloride (Co-administration may cause additive or super-additive tachycardia and drowsiness). Products include:
Nytol QuickCaps Caplets .... ■**615**
Nytol QuickGels Softgels Maximum Strength .... ■**616**
Simply Sleep Caplets **1868**
Sominex Original Formula Tablets .... ■**616**
TheraFlu Warming Relief Nighttime Severe Cold .... ■**743**
TheraFlu Thin Strips Multi Symptom .... ■**744**
Triaminic Nighttime Cold & Cough Liquid .... ■**746**
Triaminic Thin Strips Cough & Runny Nose .... ■**749**
Extra Strength Tylenol PM Caplets, Vanilla Caplets, Geltabs, Gelcaps and Liquid **1875**
Tylenol Sore Throat Nighttime Liquid with Cool Burst .... ■**790**
Tylenol Allergy Multi-Symptom Nighttime Caplets with Cool Burst **1872**
Tylenol Severe Allergy Caplets **1872**
Children's Tylenol Plus Cold & Allergy Suspension Liquid **1878**

Diphenylpyraline Hydrochloride (Co-administration may cause additive or super-additive tachycardia and drowsiness).
No products indexed under this heading.

Dipyridamole (Nabilone is purportedly highly bound to plasma proteins and may displace other protein-bound drugs; patients on concomitant therapy should be monitored for a change in dosage requirements). Products include:
Aggrenox Capsules **822**
Persantine Tablets **868**

Disulfiram (Co-administration may result in a reversible hypomaniac reaction).
No products indexed under this heading.

Dobutamine Hydrochloride (Co-administration may cause additive hypertension, tachycardia, and possibly cardiotoxicity).
No products indexed under this heading.

Dopamine Hydrochloride (Co-administration may cause additive hypertension, tachycardia, and possibly cardiotoxicity).
No products indexed under this heading.

Doxacurium Chloride (Co-administration may cause additive drowsiness and CNS depression).
No products indexed under this heading.

Doxepin Hydrochloride (Co-administration may cause additive tachycardia, hypertension, and drowsiness).
No products indexed under this heading.

Droperidol (Co-administration is cautioned in individuals receiving concomitant therapy with psychoactive drugs because of the potential for additive or synergistic CNS effects).
No products indexed under this heading.

Enflurane (Co-administration may cause additive drowsiness and CNS depression).
No products indexed under this heading.

Ephedrine Hydrochloride (Co-administration may cause additive hypertension, tachycardia, and possibly cardiotoxicity).
No products indexed under this heading.

Ephedrine Sulfate (Co-administration may cause additive hypertension, tachycardia, and possibly cardiotoxicity).
No products indexed under this heading.

Ephedrine Tannate (Co-administration may cause additive hypertension, tachycardia, and possibly cardiotoxicity).
No products indexed under this heading.

Epinephrine (Co-administration may cause additive hypertension, tachycardia, and possibly cardiotoxicity). Products include:
EpiPen **1061**
Primatene Mist .... ■**719**
Twinject 0.15 .... **3379**
Twinject 0.3 .... **3378**

Epinephrine Bitartrate (Co-administration may cause additive hypertension, tachycardia, and possibly cardiotoxicity).
No products indexed under this heading.

Epinephrine Hydrochloride (Co-administration may cause additive hypertension, tachycardia, and possibly cardiotoxicity).
No products indexed under this heading.

Estazolam (Co-administration may cause additive drowsiness and CNS depression). Products include:
ProSom Tablets **517**

Ethanol (Co-administration may cause additive drowsiness and CNS depression).
No products indexed under this heading.

Ethchlorvynol (Co-administration is cautioned in individuals receiving concomitant therapy with sedatives and hypnotics because of the potential for additive or synergistic CNS effects).
No products indexed under this heading.

Ethinamate (Co-administration is cautioned in individuals receiving concomitant therapy with sedatives and hypnotics because of the potential for additive or synergistic CNS effects).
No products indexed under this heading.

Ethyl Alcohol (Co-administration may cause additive drowsiness and CNS depression).
No products indexed under this heading.

Fenoprofen Calcium (Nabilone is purportedly highly bound to plasma proteins and may displace other protein-bound drugs; patients on concomitant therapy should be monitored for a change in dosage requirements). Products include:
Nalfon Capsules **2502**

Fentanyl (Co-administration may cause additive drowsiness and CNS depression). Products include:
Duragesic Transdermal System **2373**
Ionsys Transdermal System **2379**

Fentanyl Citrate (Co-administration may cause additive drowsiness and CNS depression). Products include:
Actiq **979**

Fexofenadine Hydrochloride (Co-administration may cause additive or super-additive tachycardia and drowsiness). Products include:
Allegra **2844**
Allegra-D 12 Hour Extended-Release Tablets **2846**
Allegra-D 24 Hour Extended-Release Tablets **2849**

Fluoxetine (Co-administration may result in a reversible hypomaniac reaction).
No products indexed under this heading.

Fluoxetine Hydrochloride (Co-administration may result in a reversible hypomaniac reaction). Products include:
Prozac Pulvules and Liquid **1801**
Symbyax Capsules **1819**

Fluphenazine Decanoate (Co-administration is cautioned in individuals receiving concomitant therapy with psychoactive drugs because of the potential for additive or synergistic CNS effects).
No products indexed under this heading.

Fluphenazine Enanthate (Co-administration is cautioned in individuals receiving concomitant therapy with psychoactive drugs because of the potential for additive or synergistic CNS effects).
No products indexed under this heading.

Fluphenazine Hydrochloride (Co-administration is cautioned in individuals receiving concomitant therapy with psychoactive drugs because of the potential for additive or synergistic CNS effects).
No products indexed under this heading.

Flurazepam Hydrochloride (Co-administration may cause additive drowsiness and CNS depression). Products include:
Dalmane Capsules **3342**

Flurbiprofen (Nabilone is purportedly highly bound to plasma proteins and may displace other protein-bound drugs; patients on concomitant therapy should be monitored for a change in dosage requirements).
No products indexed under this heading.

Glipizide (Nabilone is purportedly highly bound to plasma proteins and may displace other protein-bound drugs; patients on concomitant therapy should be monitored for a change in dosage requirements).
No products indexed under this heading.

Glutethimide (Co-administration is cautioned in individuals receiving concomitant therapy with sedatives and hypnotics because of the potential for additive or synergistic CNS effects).
No products indexed under this heading.

Glycopyrrolate (Co-administration may cause additive or super-additive tachycardia and drowsiness).
No products indexed under this heading.

Halazepam (Co-administration may cause additive drowsiness and CNS depression).
No products indexed under this heading.

Haloperidol (Co-administration is cautioned in individuals receiving concomitant therapy with psychoactive drugs because of the potential for additive or synergistic CNS effects).
No products indexed under this heading.

Haloperidol Decanoate (Co-administration is cautioned in individuals receiving concomitant therapy with psychoactive drugs because of the potential for additive or synergistic CNS effects).
No products indexed under this heading.

Hydrocodone Bitartrate (Co-administration may cause additive drowsiness and CNS depression). Products include:
Hycodan ... 1116
Hycotuss Expectorant Syrup 1117
Vicodin Tablets 535
Vicodin ES Tablets 536
Vicodin HP Tablets 538
Vicoprofen Tablets 539
Zydone Tablets 1139

Hydrocodone Polistirex (Co-administration may cause additive drowsiness and CNS depression). Products include:
Tussionex Pennkinetic
Extended-Release Suspension...... 3327

Hydromorphone Hydrochloride (Co-administration may cause additive drowsiness and CNS depression). Products include:
Dilaudid... 440
Dilaudid Non-Sterile Powder 440
Dilaudid Oral Liquid 445
Dilaudid Rectal Suppositories 440
Dilaudid Tablets 440
Dilaudid Tablets - 8 mg 445
Dilaudid-HP..................................... 442

Hydroxyzine Hydrochloride (Co-administration is cautioned in individuals receiving concomitant therapy with psychoactive drugs because of the potential for additive or synergistic CNS effects).
No products indexed under this heading.

Hyoscyamine (Co-administration may cause additive or super-additive tachycardia and drowsiness).
No products indexed under this heading.

Hyoscyamine Sulfate (Co-administration may cause additive or super-additive tachycardia and drowsiness). Products include:
Donnatal Extentabs 2493
Prosed/DS Tablets 1157

Ibuprofen (Nabilone is purportedly highly bound to plasma proteins and may displace other protein-bound drugs; patients on concomitant ther-

apy should be monitored for a change in dosage requirements). Products include:
Advil Allergy Sinus Caplets ■□770
Advil .. ■□674
Children's Advil Oral Suspension ■□603
Children's Advil Chewable Tablets .. ■□603
Advil Cold & Sinus ■□723
Infants' Advil Concentrated Drops ... ■□604
Infants' Advil Concentrated Drops
- White Grape (Dye-Free).............. ■□604
Junior Strength Advil Swallow
Tablets .. ■□605
Advil Migraine Liquigels ■□608
Advil Multi-Symptom Cold
Caplets.. ■□770
Advil PM Caplets ■□615
Motrin IB Tablets and Caplets 1866
Children's Motrin Oral Suspension ... 1867
Children's Motrin Non-Staining
Dye-Free Oral Suspension............. 1867
Children's Motrin Cold Oral
Suspension................................... 1867
Infants' Motrin Concentrated
Drops.. 1867
Infants' Motrin Non-Staining
Dye-Free Concentrated Drops....... 1867
Junior Strength Motrin Caplets
and Chewable Tablets................... 1867
Vicoprofen Tablets 539

Imipramine Hydrochloride (Co-administration may cause additive tachycardia, hypertension, and drowsiness).
No products indexed under this heading.

Imipramine Pamoate (Co-administration may cause additive tachycardia, hypertension, and drowsiness).
No products indexed under this heading.

Indomethacin (Nabilone is purportedly highly bound to plasma proteins and may displace other protein-bound drugs; patients on concomitant therapy should be monitored for a change in dosage requirements). Products include:
Indocin ... 1995

Indomethacin Sodium Trihydrate (Nabilone is purportedly highly bound to plasma proteins and may displace other protein-bound drugs; patients on concomitant therapy should be monitored for a change in dosage requirements). Products include:
Indocin I.V. 2465

Ipratropium Bromide (Co-administration may cause additive or super-additive tachycardia and drowsiness). Products include:
Atrovent Inhalation Solution 835
Atrovent HFA Inhalation Aerosol 841
Atrovent Nasal Spray 0.03%............ 837
Atrovent Nasal Spray 0.06%............ 839
Combivent Inhalation Aerosol 847
DuoNeb Inhalation Solution 1058

Isocarboxazid (Co-administration is cautioned in individuals receiving concomitant therapy with psychoactive drugs because of the potential for additive or synergistic CNS effects).
No products indexed under this heading.

Isoflurane (Co-administration may cause additive drowsiness and CNS depression).
No products indexed under this heading.

Isoproterenol Hydrochloride (Co-administration may cause additive hypertension, tachycardia, and possibly cardiotoxicity).
No products indexed under this heading.

Isoproterenol Sulfate (Co-administration may cause additive hypertension, tachycardia, and possibly cardiotoxicity).
No products indexed under this heading.

Ketamine Hydrochloride (Co-administration may cause additive drowsiness and CNS depression).
No products indexed under this heading.

Ketoprofen (Nabilone is purportedly highly bound to plasma proteins and may displace other protein-bound drugs; patients on concomitant therapy should be monitored for a change in dosage requirements).
No products indexed under this heading.

Ketorolac Tromethamine (Nabilone is purportedly highly bound to plasma proteins and may displace other protein-bound drugs; patients on concomitant therapy should be monitored for a change in dosage requirements). Products include:
Acular Ophthalmic Solution 565
Acular LS Ophthalmic Solution 566

Levalbuterol Hydrochloride (Co-administration may cause additive hypertension, tachycardia, and possibly cardiotoxicity). Products include:
Xopenex Inhalation Solution 3146
Xopenex Inhalation Solution
Concentrate 3150

Levomethadyl Acetate Hydrochloride (Co-administration may cause additive drowsiness and CNS depression).
No products indexed under this heading.

Levorphanol Tartrate (Co-administration may cause additive drowsiness and CNS depression).
No products indexed under this heading.

Lithium (Co-administration may cause additive drowsiness and CNS depression).
No products indexed under this heading.

Lithium Carbonate (Co-administration may cause additive drowsiness and CNS depression). Products include:
Lithobid Tablets 1692

Lithium Citrate (Co-administration may cause additive drowsiness and CNS depression).
No products indexed under this heading.

Loratadine (Co-administration may cause additive or super-additive tachycardia and drowsiness). Products include:
Alavert Allergy & Sinus D-12 Hour
Tablets.. ■□771
Alavert .. ■□771
Children's Claritin Allergy Oral
Solution....................................... ■□771
Claritin Non-Drowsy 24 Hour
Tablets.. ■□772
Claritin Reditabs 24 Hour
Non-Drowsy Tablets..................... ■□772
Claritin-D Non-Drowsy 12 Hour
Tablets.. ■□772
Claritin-D Non-Drowsy 24 Hour
Tablets.. ■□772

Lorazepam (Co-administration may cause additive drowsiness and CNS depression).
No products indexed under this heading.

Loxapine Hydrochloride (Co-administration is cautioned in individuals receiving concomitant therapy with psychoactive drugs because of the potential for additive or synergistic CNS effects).
No products indexed under this heading.

Loxapine Succinate (Co-administration is cautioned in individuals receiving concomitant therapy with psychoactive drugs because of the potential for additive or synergistic CNS effects).
No products indexed under this heading.

Maprotiline Hydrochloride (Co-administration may cause additive tachycardia, hypertension, and drowsiness).
No products indexed under this heading.

Meclofenamate Sodium (Nabilone is purportedly highly bound to plasma proteins and may displace other protein-bound drugs; patients on concomitant therapy should be monitored for a change in dosage requirements).
No products indexed under this heading.

Mefenamic Acid (Nabilone is purportedly highly bound to plasma proteins and may displace other protein-bound drugs; patients on concomitant therapy should be monitored for a change in dosage requirements).
No products indexed under this heading.

Mepenzolate Bromide (Co-administration may cause additive or super-additive tachycardia and drowsiness).
No products indexed under this heading.

Meperidine Hydrochloride (Co-administration may cause additive drowsiness and CNS depression).
No products indexed under this heading.

Mephobarbital (Co-administration may cause additive drowsiness and CNS depression; co-administration may also result in decreased clearance of these agents, presumably via competitive inhibition of metabolism).
No products indexed under this heading.

Meprobamate (Co-administration is cautioned in individuals receiving concomitant therapy with psychoactive drugs because of the potential for additive or synergistic CNS effects).
No products indexed under this heading.

Mesoridazine Besylate (Co-administration is cautioned in individuals receiving concomitant therapy with psychoactive drugs because of the potential for additive or synergistic CNS effects).
No products indexed under this heading.

Metaproterenol Sulfate (Co-administration may cause additive hypertension, tachycardia, and possibly cardiotoxicity). Products include:
Alupent Inhalation Aerosol 826

Metaraminol Bitartrate (Co-administration may cause additive hypertension, tachycardia, and possibly cardiotoxicity).
No products indexed under this heading.

Metaxalone (Co-administration may cause additive drowsiness and CNS depression). Products include:
Skelaxin Tablets 1716

Methadone Hydrochloride (Co-administration may cause additive drowsiness and CNS depression).
No products indexed under this heading.

Methamphetamine Hydrochloride (Co-administration may cause additive hypertension, tachycardia, and possibly cardiotoxicity).
Products include:
Desoxyn Tablets, USP 2462

Methdilazine Hydrochloride (Co-administration may cause additive or super-additive tachycardia and drowsiness).
No products indexed under this heading.

Methocarbamol (Co-administration may cause additive drowsiness and CNS depression).
No products indexed under this heading.

Methohexital Sodium (Co-administration may cause additive drowsiness and CNS depression).
No products indexed under this heading.

Methotrimeprazine (Co-administration may cause additive drowsiness and CNS depression).
No products indexed under this heading.

Methoxamine Hydrochloride (Co-administration may cause additive hypertension, tachycardia, and possibly cardiotoxicity).
No products indexed under this heading.

Methoxyflurane (Co-administration may cause additive drowsiness and CNS depression).
No products indexed under this heading.

Metocurine Iodide (Co-administration may cause additive drowsiness and CNS depression).
No products indexed under this heading.

Midazolam Hydrochloride (Co-administration may cause additive drowsiness and CNS depression).
No products indexed under this heading.

Mivacurium Chloride (Co-administration may cause additive drowsiness and CNS depression).
Products include:
Mivacron Injection 493

Molindone Hydrochloride (Co-administration is cautioned in individuals receiving concomitant therapy with psychoactive drugs because of the potential for additive or synergistic CNS effects). Products include:
Moban Tablets 1119

Morphine Sulfate (Co-administration may cause additive drowsiness and CNS depression).
Products include:
Avinza Capsules 1741
Kadian Capsules 577
MS Contin Tablets 2701

Naltrexone Hydrochloride (Oral THC effects were enhanced by opioid receptor blockade).
No products indexed under this heading.

Naproxen (Nabilone is purportedly highly bound to plasma proteins and may displace other protein-bound drugs; patients on concomitant therapy should be monitored for a change in dosage requirements).
Products include:
EC-Naprosyn Delayed-Release Tablets 2761
Naprosyn Suspension 2761
Naprosyn Tablets 2761
Prevacid NapraPAC 3280

Naproxen Sodium (Nabilone is purportedly highly bound to plasma proteins and may displace other protein-bound drugs; patients on concomitant therapy should be monitored for a change in dosage requirements). Products include:
Aleve Caplets 742
Aleve Gelcaps 743
Aleve Tablets 743
Aleve Cold & Sinus Caplets 744
Anaprox Tablets 2761
Anaprox DS Tablets 2761

Norepinephrine Bitartrate (Co-administration may cause additive hypertension, tachycardia, and possibly cardiotoxicity).
No products indexed under this heading.

Nortriptyline Hydrochloride (Co-administration may cause additive tachycardia, hypertension, and drowsiness).
No products indexed under this heading.

Olanzapine (Co-administration is cautioned in individuals receiving concomitant therapy with psychoactive drugs because of the potential for additive or synergistic CNS effects). Products include:
Symbyax Capsules 1819
Zyprexa Tablets 1830
Zyprexa IntraMuscular 1830
Zyprexa ZYDIS Orally Disintegrating Tablets 1830

Opioid Analgesics (Co-administration may cause additive drowsiness and CNS depression, as well as, cross-tolerance and mutual potentiation).
No products indexed under this heading.

Orphenadrine Citrate (Co-administration may cause additive drowsiness and CNS depression).
Products include:
Norflex Injection 1856

Oxaprozin (Nabilone is purportedly highly bound to plasma proteins and may displace other protein-bound drugs; patients on concomitant therapy should be monitored for a change in dosage requirements).
No products indexed under this heading.

Oxazepam (Co-administration may cause additive drowsiness and CNS depression).
No products indexed under this heading.

Oxybutynin Chloride (Co-administration may cause additive or super-additive tachycardia and drowsiness). Products include:
Ditropan XL Extended-Release Tablets 2413

Oxycodone Hydrochloride (Co-administration may cause additive drowsiness and CNS depression).
Products include:
OxyContin Tablets 2703
OxyFast Oral Concentrate Solution 2708
OxyIR Capsules 2708
Percocet Tablets 1131
Percodan Tablets 1132

Pancuronium Bromide (Co-administration may cause additive drowsiness and CNS depression).
No products indexed under this heading.

Pentobarbital Sodium (Co-administration may cause additive drowsiness and CNS depression; co-administration may also result in decreased clearance of these agents, presumably via competitive inhibition of metabolism). Products include:
Nembutal Sodium Solution, USP 2470

Perphenazine (Co-administration is cautioned in individuals receiving concomitant therapy with psychoactive drugs because of the potential for additive or synergistic CNS effects).
No products indexed under this heading.

Phenelzine Sulfate (Co-administration is cautioned in individuals receiving concomitant therapy with psychoactive drugs because of the potential for additive or synergistic CNS effects).
No products indexed under this heading.

Phenobarbital (Co-administration may cause additive drowsiness and CNS depression; co-administration may also result in decreased clearance of these agents, presumably via competitive inhibition of metabolism). Products include:
Donnatal Extentabs 2493

Phenylbutazone (Nabilone is purportedly highly bound to plasma proteins and may displace other protein-bound drugs; patients on concomitant therapy should be monitored for a change in dosage requirements).
No products indexed under this heading.

Phenylephrine Bitartrate (Co-administration may cause additive hypertension, tachycardia, and possibly cardiotoxicity).
No products indexed under this heading.

Phenylephrine Hydrochloride (Co-administration may cause additive hypertension, tachycardia, and possibly cardiotoxicity). Products include:
Comtrex Maximum Strength Non-Drowsy Cold & Cough Caplets .... ■ 725
Comtrex Maximum Strength Day/Night Severe Cold & Sinus Caplets - Day Formulation .... ■ 725
Comtrex Maximum Strength Day/Night Severe Cold & Sinus Caplets - Night Formulation .... ■ 725
Contac Cold and Flu Maximum Strength Caplets .... ■ 728
Contac Cold and Flu Day and Night Caplets (Day Formulation Only) .... ■ 727
Contac Cold and Flu Day and Night Caplets (Night Formulation Only) .... ■ 727
Contac Cold and Flu Non-Drowsy Caplets .... ■ 728
Contac-D Cold Non-Drowsy Tablets .... ■ 729
Children's Dimetapp Cold & Allergy Elixir .... ■ 730
Children's Dimetapp Cold & Allergy Chewable Tablets .... ■ 730
Children's Dimetapp DM Cold & Cough Elixir .... ■ 731
Toddler's Dimetapp Cold and Cough Drops .... ■ 732
Excedrin Sinus Headache Caplets/Tablets .... ■ 610
4-Way Fast Acting Nasal Spray ...... ■ 775
4-Way Menthol Nasal Spray .... ■ 775
Preparation H Maximum Strength Cream .... ■ 666
Preparation H Cooling Gel .... ■ 666
Preparation H .... ■ 666
Refenesen PE Caplets .... ■ 721
Robitussin Cough & Allergy Syrup .. ■ 736
Robitussin Cough & Cold Nighttime Liquid .... ■ 736
Robitussin Cough, Cold & Flu Nighttime Liquid .... ■ 738
Robitussin Head & Chest Congestion PE Syrup .... ■ 739
Robitussin Pediatric Cough & Cold Nighttime Liquid .... ■ 736
TheraFlu Cold & Cough Hot Liquid .... ■ 740
TheraFlu Cold & Sore Throat Hot Liquid .... ■ 741
TheraFlu Flu & Sore Throat Hot Liquid .... ■ 742
TheraFlu Daytime Severe Cold Hot Liquid .... ■ 742
TheraFlu Nighttime Severe Cold Hot Liquid .... ■ 740
TheraFlu Warming Relief Daytime Severe Cold .... ■ 743
TheraFlu Warming Relief Nighttime Severe Cold .... ■ 743
Triaminic Chest & Nasal Congestion Liquid .... ■ 746
Triaminic Cold & Allergy Liquid .... ■ 746
Triaminic Daytime Cold & Cough Liquid .... ■ 745
Triaminic Nighttime Cold & Cough Liquid .... ■ 746
Triaminic Thin Strips Cold .... ■ 748
Triaminic Thin Strips Cold & Cough .... ■ 778
Triaminic Infant Thin Strips Decongestant .... ■ 747
Triaminic Infant Thin Strips Decongestant Plus Cough .... ■ 747
Children's Tylenol Plus Flu Oral Suspension .... ■ 749
Tylenol Cold Head Congestion Daytime Caplets with Cool Burst and Gelcaps .... ■ 750
Tylenol Cold Multi-Symptom Daytime Liquid .... ■ 752
Tylenol Cold Multi-Symptom Severe Daytime Liquid .... ■ 752
Concentrated Tylenol Infants' Drops Plus Cold & Cough .... ■ 754
Tylenol Allergy Multi-Symptom Caplets with Cool Burst and Gelcaps 1872
Tylenol Allergy Multi-Symptom Nighttime Caplets with Cool Burst 1872
Children's Tylenol Plus Cold Suspension Liquid 1879
Children's Tylenol Plus Cold & Allergy Suspension Liquid 1878
Children's Tylenol Plus Flu Suspension Liquid 1881
Children's Tylenol Plus Multi-Symptom Cold Suspension Liquid 1879
Tylenol Cold Head Congestion Daytime Caplets with Cool Burst 1873
Tylenol Cold Head Congestion Nighttime Caplets with Cool Burst 1873
Tylenol Cold Head Congestion Severe Caplets with Cool Burst 1873
Tylenol Cold Multi-Symptom Daytime Caplets with Cool Burst and Gelcaps 1874
Tylenol Cold Multi-Symptom Daytime Liquid with Citrus Burst ... 1874
Tylenol Cold Multi-Symptom Nighttime Caplets with Cool Burst 1874
Tylenol Cold Multi-Symptom Nighttime Liquid with Cool Burst ... 1874
Tylenol Cold Multi-Symptom Severe Caplets with Cool Burst 1874

Tylenol Cold Multi-Symptom Severe Daytime Liquid with Citrus Burst.................... 1874
Tylenol Sinus Congestion & Pain Daytime Caplets with Cool Burst and Gelcaps.................... 1876
Tylenol Sinus Congestion & Pain Nighttime Caplets with Cool Burst.................... 1876
Tylenol Sinus Congestion & Pain Severe Caplets with Cool Burst..... 1876
Vicks 44D Cough & Head Congestion Relief Liquid............. ■ 760
Vicks DayQuil LiquiCaps/Liquid Multi-Symptom Cold/Flu Relief..... ■ 761
Zicam Cough Plus D Cough Spray.................... ■ 767

Phenylephrine Tannate (Co-administration may cause additive hypertension, tachycardia, and possibly cardiotoxicity).
No products indexed under this heading.

Phenylpropanolamine Hydrochloride (Co-administration may cause additive hypertension, tachycardia, and possibly cardiotoxicity).
No products indexed under this heading.

Pirbuterol Acetate (Co-administration may cause additive hypertension, tachycardia, and possibly cardiotoxicity). Products include:
Maxair Autohaler.................... 1852

Piroxicam (Nabilone is purportedly highly bound to plasma proteins and may displace other protein-bound drugs; patients on concomitant therapy should be monitored for a change in dosage requirements).
No products indexed under this heading.

Prazepam (Co-administration may cause additive drowsiness and CNS depression).
No products indexed under this heading.

Prochlorperazine (Co-administration is cautioned in individuals receiving concomitant therapy with psychoactive drugs because of the potential for additive or synergistic CNS effects).
No products indexed under this heading.

Procyclidine Hydrochloride (Co-administration may cause additive or super-additive tachycardia and drowsiness).
No products indexed under this heading.

Promethazine Hydrochloride (Co-administration may cause additive or super-additive tachycardia and drowsiness). Products include:
Phenergan Tablets and Suppositories.................... 3440

Propantheline Bromide (Co-administration may cause additive or super-additive tachycardia and drowsiness).
No products indexed under this heading.

Propofol (Co-administration is cautioned in individuals receiving concomitant therapy with sedatives and hypnotics because of the potential for additive or synergistic CNS effects).
No products indexed under this heading.

Propoxyphene Hydrochloride (Co-administration may cause additive drowsiness and CNS depression).
No products indexed under this heading.

Propoxyphene Napsylate (Co-administration may cause additive drowsiness and CNS depression).
No products indexed under this heading.

Propranolol Hydrochloride (Nabilone is purportedly highly bound to plasma proteins and may displace other protein-bound drugs; patients on concomitant therapy should be monitored for a change in dosage requirements). Products include:
Inderal LA Long-Acting Capsules..... 3429
InnoPran XL Capsules.................... 2723

Protriptyline Hydrochloride (Co-administration may cause additive tachycardia, hypertension, and drowsiness).
No products indexed under this heading.

Pseudoephedrine Hydrochloride (Co-administration may cause additive hypertension, tachycardia, and possibly cardiotoxicity). Products include:
Advil Allergy Sinus Caplets............ ■ 770
Advil Cold & Sinus.................... ■ 723
Advil Multi-Symptom Cold Caplets.................... ■ 770
Aleve Cold & Sinus Caplets............ 744
Allegra-D 12 Hour Extended-Release Tablets............ 2846
Allegra-D 24 Hour Extended-Release Tablets............ 2849
BC Cold Powder.................... ■ 677
Comtrex Maximum Strength Cold & Cough Day/Night Caplets - Day Formulation.................... ■ 726
Comtrex Maximum Strength Cold & Cough Day/Night Caplets - Night Formulation.................... ■ 726
Children's Motrin Cold Oral Suspension.................... 1867
Mucinex D Extended-Release Bi-Layer Tablets.................... ■ 776
Robitussin Cough & Cold CF Liquid.................... ■ 735
Robitussin Cough & Cold Pediatric Drops.................... ■ 735
Tylenol Sinus Congestion & Pain Nighttime Caplets with Cool Burst.................... ■ 778
Tylenol Cold Severe Congestion Non-Drowsy Caplets with Cool Burst.................... 1874
Tylenol Sinus Severe Congestion Caplets with Cool Burst............ 1876
Vicks 44D Cough & Head Congestion Relief Liquid............ 2679
Vicks 44M Cough, Cold & Flu Relief Liquid.................... 2680
Vicks DayQuil Multi-Symptom Cold/Flu Relief LiquiCaps............ 2678
Vicks DayQuil Multi-Symptom Cold/Flu Relief Liquid.................... 2678
Vicks NyQuil Multi-Symptom Cold/Flu Relief Liquid.................... 2681
Vicks NyQuil Multi-Symptom Cold/Flu Relief LiquiCaps............ 2681
Children's Vicks NyQuil Cold/Cough Relief Liquid............ 2680
Zyrtec-D 12 Hour Extended Release Tablets.................... 2597

Pseudoephedrine Sulfate (Co-administration may cause additive hypertension, tachycardia, and possibly cardiotoxicity). Products include:
Alavert Allergy & Sinus D-12 Hour Tablets.................... ■ 771
Clarinex-D 24-Hour Extended-Release Tablets............ 2998
Claritin-D Non-Drowsy 12 Hour Tablets.................... ■ 772
Claritin-D Non-Drowsy 24 Hour Tablets.................... ■ 772

Pyrilamine Maleate (Co-administration may cause additive or super-additive tachycardia and drowsiness).
No products indexed under this heading.

Pyrilamine Tannate (Co-administration may cause additive or super-additive tachycardia and drowsiness).
No products indexed under this heading.

Quazepam (Co-administration may cause additive drowsiness and CNS depression).
No products indexed under this heading.

Quetiapine Fumarate (Co-administration is cautioned in individuals receiving concomitant therapy with psychoactive drugs because of the potential for additive or synergistic CNS effects). Products include:
Seroquel Tablets.................... 690

Ramelteon (Co-administration is cautioned in individuals receiving concomitant therapy with sedatives and hypnotics because of the potential for additive or synergistic CNS effects). Products include:
Rozerem Tablets.................... 3231

Rapacuronium Bromide (Co-administration may cause additive drowsiness and CNS depression).
No products indexed under this heading.

Remifentanil Hydrochloride (Co-administration may cause additive drowsiness and CNS depression).
No products indexed under this heading.

Risperidone (Co-administration is cautioned in individuals receiving concomitant therapy with psychoactive drugs because of the potential for additive or synergistic CNS effects). Products include:
Risperdal.................... 1676
Risperdal Consta Long-Acting Injection.................... 1682
Risperdal M-Tab Orally Disintegrating Tablets.................... 1676

Rocuronium Bromide (Co-administration may cause additive drowsiness and CNS depression). Products include:
Zemuron Injection.................... 2346

Salmeterol Xinafoate (Co-administration may cause additive hypertension, tachycardia, and possibly cardiotoxicity). Products include:
Advair Diskus 100/50.................... 1308
Advair Diskus 250/50.................... 1308
Advair Diskus 500/50.................... 1308
Advair HFA Inhalation Aerosol.......... 1318
Serevent Diskus.................... 1568

Scopolamine (Co-administration may cause additive or super-additive tachycardia and drowsiness). Products include:
Transderm Scōp Transdermal Therapeutic System.................... 2177

Scopolamine Hydrobromide (Co-administration may cause additive or super-additive tachycardia and drowsiness). Products include:
Donnatal Extentabs.................... 2493

Secobarbital Sodium (Co-administration may cause additive drowsiness and CNS depression; co-administration may also result in decreased clearance of these agents, presumably via competitive inhibition of metabolism).
No products indexed under this heading.

Sevoflurane (Co-administration may cause additive drowsiness and CNS depression). Products include:
Ultane Liquid for Inhalation.............. 531

Sodium Oxybate (Co-administration may cause additive drowsiness and CNS depression). Products include:
Xyrem Oral Solution.................... 1688

Succinylcholine Chloride (Co-administration may cause additive drowsiness and CNS depression).
No products indexed under this heading.

Sufentanil Citrate (Co-administration may cause additive drowsiness and CNS depression).
No products indexed under this heading.

Sulindac (Nabilone is purportedly highly bound to plasma proteins and may displace other protein-bound drugs; patients on concomitant therapy should be monitored for a change in dosage requirements). Products include:
Clinoril Tablets.................... 1924

Temazepam (Co-administration may cause additive drowsiness and CNS depression). Products include:
Restoril Capsules.................... 1860

Terbutaline Sulfate (Co-administration may cause additive hypertension, tachycardia, and possibly cardiotoxicity).
No products indexed under this heading.

Terfenadine (Co-administration may cause additive or super-additive tachycardia and drowsiness).
No products indexed under this heading.

Theophylline (Increased theophylline metabolism reported with smoking marijuana; effect similar to that following smoking tobacco).
No products indexed under this heading.

Theophylline Anhydrous (Increased theophylline metabolism reported with smoking marijuana; effect similar to that following smoking tobacco). Products include:
Uniphyl Tablets.................... 2710

Theophylline Calcium Salicylate (Increased theophylline metabolism reported with smoking marijuana; effect similar to that following smoking tobacco).
No products indexed under this heading.

Theophylline Dihydroxypropyl (Glyceryl) (Increased theophylline metabolism reported with smoking marijuana; effect similar to that following smoking tobacco).
No products indexed under this heading.

Theophylline Ethylenediamine (Increased theophylline metabolism reported with smoking marijuana; effect similar to that following smoking tobacco).
No products indexed under this heading.

Theophylline Sodium Glycinate (Increased theophylline metabolism reported with smoking marijuana; effect similar to that following smoking tobacco).
No products indexed under this heading.

Thiamylal Sodium (Co-administration may cause additive drowsiness and CNS depression; co-administration may also result in decreased clearance of these agents, presumably via competitive inhibition of metabolism).
No products indexed under this heading.

Thioridazine Hydrochloride (Co-administration is cautioned in individuals receiving concomitant therapy with psychoactive drugs because of the potential for additive or synergistic CNS effects). Products include:
Thioridazine Hydrochloride Tablets 2163

Thiothixene (Co-administration is cautioned in individuals receiving concomitant therapy with psychoactive drugs because of the potential for additive or synergistic CNS effects). Products include:
Thiothixene Capsules 2165

Tolbutamide (Nabilone is purportedly highly bound to plasma proteins and may displace other protein-bound drugs; patients on concomitant therapy should be monitored for a change in dosage requirements).
No products indexed under this heading.

Tolmetin Sodium (Nabilone is purportedly highly bound to plasma proteins and may displace other protein-bound drugs; patients on concomitant therapy should be monitored for a change in dosage requirements).
No products indexed under this heading.

Tolterodine Tartrate (Co-administration may cause additive or super-additive tachycardia and drowsiness). Products include:
Detrol Tablets 2628
Detrol LA Capsules 2631

Tranylcypromine Sulfate (Co-administration is cautioned in individuals receiving concomitant therapy with psychoactive drugs because of the potential for additive or synergistic CNS effects). Products include:
Parnate Tablets 1527

Triazolam (Co-administration may cause additive drowsiness and CNS depression).
No products indexed under this heading.

Tridihexethyl Chloride (Co-administration may cause additive or super-additive tachycardia and drowsiness).
No products indexed under this heading.

Trifluoperazine Hydrochloride (Co-administration is cautioned in individuals receiving concomitant therapy with psychoactive drugs because of the potential for additive or synergistic CNS effects).
No products indexed under this heading.

Trihexyphenidyl Hydrochloride (Co-administration may cause additive or super-additive tachycardia and drowsiness).
No products indexed under this heading.

Trimeprazine Tartrate (Co-administration may cause additive or super-additive tachycardia and drowsiness).
No products indexed under this heading.

Trimipramine Maleate (Co-administration may cause additive tachycardia, hypertension, and drowsiness).
No products indexed under this heading.

Tripelennamine Hydrochloride (Co-administration may cause additive or super-additive tachycardia and drowsiness).
No products indexed under this heading.

Triprolidine Hydrochloride (Co-administration may cause additive or super-additive tachycardia and drowsiness).
No products indexed under this heading.

Vecuronium Bromide (Co-administration may cause additive drowsiness and CNS depression).
No products indexed under this heading.

Warfarin Sodium (Nabilone is purportedly highly bound to plasma proteins and may displace other protein-bound drugs; patients on concomitant therapy should be monitored for a change in dosage requirements). Products include:
Coumadin for Injection 898
Coumadin Tablets 898

Zaleplon (Co-administration is cautioned in individuals receiving concomitant therapy with sedatives and hypnotics because of the potential for additive or synergistic CNS effects). Products include:
Sonata Capsules 1717

Ziprasidone Hydrochloride (Co-administration is cautioned in individuals receiving concomitant therapy with psychoactive drugs because of the potential for additive or synergistic CNS effects). Products include:
Geodon Capsules 2529

Zolpidem Tartrate (Co-administration is cautioned in individuals receiving concomitant therapy with sedatives and hypnotics because of the potential for additive or synergistic CNS effects). Products include:
Ambien Tablets 2851
Ambien CR Tablets 2855

Food Interactions

Alcohol (Co-administration is cautioned in individuals receiving concomitant therapy with alcohol because of the potential for additive or synergistic CNS effects; also reported to increase the positive subjective mood effects of smoked marijuana).

CETACAINE TOPICAL ANESTHETIC

(Benzocaine, Butyl Aminobenzoate, Tetracaine Hydrochloride).................... 999
None cited in PDR database.

CHANTIX TABLETS

(Varenicline Tartrate) 2517
May interact with:

Cimetidine (Co-administration of an OCT2 inhibitor, cimetidine, with varenicline increased the systemic exposure of varenicline due to a reduction in varenicline renal clearance). Products include:
Tagamet HB 200 Tablets 664

Nicotine (Co-administration of varenicline and transdermal nicotine did not affect nicotine pharmacokinetics, the incidence of nausea, headache, vomiting, dizziness, dyspepsia and fatigue was greater for the combination than for nicotine replacement therapy alone). Products include:
NicoDerm CQ Clear Patch 622

Nicotine Polacrilex (Co-administration of varenicline and transdermal nicotine did not affect nicotine pharmacokinetics, the incidence of nausea, headache, vomiting, dizziness, dyspepsia and fatigue was greater for the combination than for nicotine replacement therapy alone).
No products indexed under this heading.

Nicotine Salicylate (Co-administration of varenicline and transdermal nicotine did not affect nicotine pharmacokinetics, the incidence of nausea, headache, vomiting, dizziness, dyspepsia and fatigue was greater for the combination than for nicotine replacement therapy alone).
No products indexed under this heading.

Nicotine Sulfate (Co-administration of varenicline and transdermal nicotine did not affect nicotine pharmacokinetics, the incidence of nausea, headache, vomiting, dizziness, dyspepsia and fatigue was greater for the combination than for nicotine replacement therapy alone).
No products indexed under this heading.

CHELATED MINERAL TABLETS

(Minerals, Multiple) 3339
None cited in PDR database.

CHEMET CAPSULES

(Succimer) 2458
May interact with:

Calcium Disodium Edetate (Concomitant administration is not recommended). Products include:
Calcium Disodium Versenate Injection 1851

CIALIS TABLETS

(Tadalafil) 1838
May interact with alpha adrenergic blockers, angiotensin-II receptor antagonists, antacids, cytochrome p450 3a4 inducers (selected), cytochrome p450 3a4 inhibitors (selected), erythromycin, nitrates and nitrites, phenytoin, protease inhibitors, and certain other agents. Compounds in these categories include:

Acetazolamide (Tadalafil is metabolized predominantly by CYP3A4 in the liver. The dose of tadalafil should be limited to 10 mg no more than once every 72 hours in patients taking potent inhibitors of CYP3A4).
No products indexed under this heading.

Allium sativum (Drugs that induce CYP3A4 can increase tadalafil exposure).
No products indexed under this heading.

Aluminum Carbonate (Simultaneous administration of an antacid (magnesium hydroxide/aluminum hydroxide) and tadalafil reduced the apparent rate of absorption of tadalafil without altering exposure (AUC) to tadalafil).
No products indexed under this heading.

Aluminum Hydroxide (Simultaneous administration of an antacid (magnesium hydroxide/aluminum hydroxide) and tadalafil reduced the apparent rate of absorption of tadalafil without altering exposure (AUC) to tadalafil). Products include:
Gaviscon Regular Strength Liquid 658
Gaviscon Regular Strength Tablets 658
Gaviscon Extra Strength Liquid 658
Gaviscon Extra Strength Tablets 658
Maalox Regular Strength Antacid/Antigas Liquid 2175
Maalox Max Maximum Strength Antacid/Anti-Gas Liquid 2176

Amiodarone Hydrochloride (Tadalafil is metabolized predominantly by CYP3A4 in the liver. The dose of tadalafil should be limited to 10 mg no more than once every 72 hours in patients taking potent inhibitors of CYP3A4).
No products indexed under this heading.

Amlodipine Besylate (A study was conducted to assess the interaction of amlodipine (5mg daily) and tadalafil 10mg. There were no effects of tadalafil on amlodipine blood levels and no effect of amlodipine on tadalafil blood levels. The mean reduction in supine systolic/diastolic blood pressure due to tadalafil 10mg in subjects taking amlodipine was 3/2mm Hg, compare to placebo). Products include:
Caduet Tablets 2508
Lotrel Capsules 2249
Norvasc Tablets 2545

Amprenavir (Tadalafil is metabolized predominantly by CYP3A4 in the liver. The dose of tadalafil should be limited to 10 mg no more than once every 72 hours in patients taking potent inhibitors of CYP3A4). Products include:
Agenerase Capsules 1327
Agenerase Oral Solution 1332

Amyl Nitrite (Administration of tadalafil to patients using any form of organic nitrate, either regularly and/or intermittently, is contraindicated).
No products indexed under this heading.

Anastrozole (Tadalafil is metabolized predominantly by CYP3A4 in the liver. The dose of tadalafil should be limited to 10 mg no more than once every 72 hours in patients taking potent inhibitors of CYP3A4). Products include:
Arimidex Tablets 673

Aprepitant (Tadalafil is metabolized predominantly by CYP3A4 in the liver. The dose of tadalafil should be limited to 10 mg no more than once every 72 hours in patients taking potent inhibitors of CYP3A4). Products include:
Emend Capsules 1963

Bendrofluazide (A study was conducted to assess the interaction of bendrofluazide (2.5mg daily) and tadalafil 10mg. Following dosing, the mean reduction in supine systolic diastolic blood pressure due to tadalafil 10mg in subjects taking bendrofluazide was 6/4mm Hg, compared to placebo).
No products indexed under this heading.

Betamethasone Acetate (Drugs that induce CYP3A4 can increase tadalafil exposure).
No products indexed under this heading.

Betamethasone Sodium Phosphate (Drugs that induce CYP3A4 can increase tadalafil exposure).
No products indexed under this heading.

Candesartan Cilexetil (A study was conducted to assess the interaction of angiotensin II receptor blockers and tadalafil 20mg. Following dosing, ambulatory measurements of blood pressure revealed differences between tadalafil and placebo of 8/4mm Hg in systolic/diastolic blood pressure). Products include:

Carbamazepine (CYP3A4 inducers, such as carbamazepine, may decrease tadalafil exposure. No dose adjustment is warranted). Products include:

Cimetidine (Tadalafil is metabolized predominantly by CYP3A4 in the liver. The dose of tadalafil should be limited to 10 mg no more than once every 72 hours in patients taking potent inhibitors of CYP3A4). Products include:

Cimetidine Hydrochloride (Tadalafil is metabolized predominantly by CYP3A4 in the liver. The dose of tadalafil should be limited to 10 mg no more than once every 72 hours in patients taking potent inhibitors of CYP3A4).

No products indexed under this heading.

Ciprofloxacin (Tadalafil is metabolized predominantly by CYP3A4 in the liver. The dose of tadalafil should be limited to 10 mg no more than once every 72 hours in patients taking potent inhibitors of CYP3A4). Products include:

Ciprofloxacin Hydrochloride (Drugs that induce CYP3A4 can increase tadalafil exposure). Products include:

Cisplatin (Drugs that induce CYP3A4 can increase tadalafil exposure).

No products indexed under this heading.

Clarithromycin (Tadalafil is metabolized predominantly by CYP3A4 in the liver. The dose of tadalafil should be limited to 10 mg no more than once every 72 hours in patients taking potent inhibitors of CYP3A4). Products include:

Clotrimazole (Tadalafil is metabolized predominantly by CYP3A4 in the liver. The dose of tadalafil should be limited to 10 mg no more than once every 72 hours in patients taking potent inhibitors of CYP3A4). Products include:

Cortisone Acetate (Drugs that induce CYP3A4 can increase tadalafil exposure).

No products indexed under this heading.

Cyclosporine (Tadalafil is metabolized predominantly by CYP3A4 in the liver. The dose of tadalafil should be limited to 10 mg no more than

once every 72 hours in patients taking potent inhibitors of CYP3A4). Products include:

Dalfopristin (Tadalafil is metabolized predominantly by CYP3A4 in the liver. The dose of tadalafil should be limited to 10 mg no more than once every 72 hours in patients taking potent inhibitors of CYP3A4).

No products indexed under this heading.

Danazol (Tadalafil is metabolized predominantly by CYP3A4 in the liver. The dose of tadalafil should be limited to 10 mg no more than once every 72 hours in patients taking potent inhibitors of CYP3A4).

No products indexed under this heading.

Delavirdine Mesylate (Tadalafil is metabolized predominantly by CYP3A4 in the liver. The dose of tadalafil should be limited to 10 mg no more than once every 72 hours in patients taking potent inhibitors of CYP3A4). Products include:

Dexamethasone (Drugs that induce CYP3A4 can increase tadalafil exposure). Products include:

Dexamethasone Acetate (Drugs that induce CYP3A4 can increase tadalafil exposure).

No products indexed under this heading.

Dexamethasone Sodium Phosphate (Drugs that induce CYP3A4 can increase tadalafil exposure).

No products indexed under this heading.

Diltiazem Hydrochloride (Tadalafil is metabolized predominantly by CYP3A4 in the liver. The dose of tadalafil should be limited to 10 mg no more than once every 72 hours in patients taking potent inhibitors of CYP3A4). Products include:

Diltiazem Maleate (Tadalafil is metabolized predominantly by CYP3A4 in the liver. The dose of tadalafil should be limited to 10 mg no more than once every 72 hours in patients taking potent inhibitors of CYP3A4).

No products indexed under this heading.

Doxazosin Mesylate (Caution is advised when PDE5 inhibitors are co-administered with alpha-blockers. PDE5 inhibitors, including tadalafil, and alpha-adrenergic blocking agents are both vasodilators with blood-pressure lowering effects. When vasodilators are used in combination, an additive effect on blood pressure may be anticipated. In some patients, concomitant use of these two drug classes can lower blood presure significantly, which may lead to symptomatic hypotension (e.g., fainting)). Products include:

Doxorubicin Hydrochloride (Drugs that induce CYP3A4 can increase tadalafil exposure).

No products indexed under this heading.

Efavirenz (Tadalafil is metabolized predominantly by CYP3A4 in the liver. The dose of tadalafil should be limited to 10 mg no more than once every 72 hours in patients taking potent inhibitors of CYP3A4). Products include:

Enalapril Maleate (Following dosing with enalapril (10-20mg daily) and tadalafil 10mg, the mean reduction in supine systolic/diastolic blood pressure due to tadalafil 10mg in subjects taking analapril was 4/1mm Hg, compared to placebo). Products include:

Enalaprilat (Following dosing with enalapril (10-20mg daily) and tadalafil 10mg, the mean reduction in supine systolic/diastolic blood pressure due to tadalafil 10mg in subjects taking analapril was 4/1mm Hg, compared to placebo).

No products indexed under this heading.

Eprosartan Mesylate (A study was conducted to assess the interaction of angiotensin II receptor blockers and tadalafil 20mg. Following dosing, ambulatory measurements of blood pressure revealed differences between tadalafil and placebo of 8/4mm Hg in systolic/diastolic blood pressure). Products include:

Erythrityl Tetranitrate (Administration of tadalafil to patients using any form of organic nitrate, either regularly and/or intermittently, is contraindicated).

No products indexed under this heading.

Erythromycin (Tadalafil is metabolized predominantly by CYP3A4 in the liver. The dose of tadalafil should be limited to 10 mg no more than once every 72 hours in patients taking potent inhibitors of CYP3A4). Products include:

Erythromycin Estolate (Tadalafil is metabolized predominantly by CYP3A4 in the liver. The dose of tadalafil should be limited to 10 mg no more than once every 72 hours in patients taking potent inhibitors of CYP3A4).

No products indexed under this heading.

Erythromycin Ethylsuccinate (Tadalafil is metabolized predominantly by CYP3A4 in the liver. The dose of tadalafil should be limited to 10 mg no more than once every 72 hours in patients taking potent inhibitors of CYP3A4). Products include:

Erythromycin Gluceptate (Tadalafil is metabolized predominantly by CYP3A4 in the liver. The dose of tadalafil should be limited to 10 mg no more than once every 72 hours in patients taking potent inhibitors of CYP3A4).

No products indexed under this heading.

Erythromycin Lactobionate (Tadalafil is metabolized predominantly by CYP3A4 in the liver. The dose of tadalafil should be limited to 10 mg no more than once every 72 hours in patients taking potent inhibitors of CYP3A4).

No products indexed under this heading.

Erythromycin Stearate (Tadalafil is metabolized predominantly by CYP3A4 in the liver. The dose of tadalafil should be limited to 10 mg no more than once every 72 hours in patients taking potent inhibitors of CYP3A4). Products include:

Esomeprazole Magnesium (Tadalafil is metabolized predominantly by CYP3A4 in the liver. The dose of tadalafil should be limited to 10 mg no more than once every 72 hours in patients taking potent inhibitors of CYP3A4). Products include:

Ethosuximide (Drugs that induce CYP3A4 can increase tadalafil exposure).

No products indexed under this heading.

Felbamate (Drugs that induce CYP3A4 can increase tadalafil exposure).

No products indexed under this heading.

Fluconazole (Tadalafil is metabolized predominantly by CYP3A4 in the liver. The dose of tadalafil should be limited to 10 mg no more than once every 72 hours in patients taking potent inhibitors of CYP3A4).

No products indexed under this heading.

Fludrocortisone Acetate (Drugs that induce CYP3A4 can increase tadalafil exposure).

No products indexed under this heading.

Fluoxetine Hydrochloride (Tadalafil is metabolized predominantly by CYP3A4 in the liver. The dose of tadalafil should be limited to 10 mg no more than once every 72 hours in patients taking potent inhibitors of CYP3A4). Products include:

Fluvoxamine Maleate (Tadalafil is metabolized predominantly by CYP3A4 in the liver. The dose of tadalafil should be limited to 10 mg no more than once every 72 hours in patients taking potent inhibitors of CYP3A4).

No products indexed under this heading.

Fosamprenavir Calcium (Tadalafil is metabolized predominantly by CYP3A4 in the liver. The dose of tadalafil should be limited to 10 mg no more than once every 72 hours in patients taking potent inhibitors of CYP3A4). Products include:

Fosphenytoin Sodium (Drugs that induce CYP3A4 can increase tadalafil exposure).
No products indexed under this heading.

Garlic Extract (Drugs that induce CYP3A4 can increase tadalafil exposure).
No products indexed under this heading.

Garlic Oil (Drugs that induce CYP3A4 can increase tadalafil exposure).
No products indexed under this heading.

Hydrocortisone (Drugs that induce CYP3A4 can increase tadalafil exposure). Products include:
Colocort Rectal Suspension, USP (Retention) 100 mg/60 mL **2476**
Hydrocortone Tablets **1989**
Preparation H Hydrocortisone Cream .... ▣**646**

Hydrocortisone Acetate (Drugs that induce CYP3A4 can increase tadalafil exposure). Products include:
Analpram-HC **1159**
Pramosone **1161**
ProctoFoam-HC **3099**

Hydrocortisone Butyrate (Drugs that induce CYP3A4 can increase tadalafil exposure). Products include:
Locoid Lipocream Cream **1160**

Hydrocortisone Cypionate (Drugs that induce CYP3A4 can increase tadalafil exposure).
No products indexed under this heading.

Hydrocortisone Hemisuccinate (Drugs that induce CYP3A4 can increase tadalafil exposure).
No products indexed under this heading.

Hydrocortisone Probutate (Drugs that induce CYP3A4 can increase tadalafil exposure).
No products indexed under this heading.

Hydrocortisone Sodium Phosphate (Drugs that induce CYP3A4 can increase tadalafil exposure).
No products indexed under this heading.

Hydrocortisone Sodium Succinate (Drugs that induce CYP3A4 can increase tadalafil exposure).
No products indexed under this heading.

Hydrocortisone Valerate (Drugs that induce CYP3A4 can increase tadalafil exposure).
No products indexed under this heading.

Hypericum (Drugs that induce CYP3A4 can increase tadalafil exposure). Products include:
Satiete Tablets .... ▣**832**

Hypericum Perforatum (Drugs that induce CYP3A4 can increase tadalafil exposure).
No products indexed under this heading.

Indinavir Sulfate (Tadalafil is metabolized predominantly by CYP3A4 in the liver. The dose of tadalafil should be limited to 10 mg no more than once every 72 hours in patients taking potent inhibitors of CYP3A4). Products include:
Crixivan Capsules **1940**

Irbesartan (A study was conducted to assess the interaction of angiotensin II receptor blockers and tadalafil 20mg. Following dosing, ambulatory measurements of blood pressure revealed differences between tadalafil and placebo of 8/4mm Hg in systolic/diastolic blood pressure). Products include:
Avalide Tablets **888**
Avalide Tablets **2874**
Avapro Tablets **891**
Avapro Tablets **2871**

Isoniazid (Tadalafil is metabolized predominantly by CYP3A4 in the liver. The dose of tadalafil should be limited to 10 mg no more than once every 72 hours in patients taking potent inhibitors of CYP3A4).
No products indexed under this heading.

Isosorbide Dinitrate (Administration of tadalafil to patients using any form of organic nitrate, either regularly and/or intermittently, is contraindicated). Products include:
BiDil Tablets **2171**

Isosorbide Mononitrate (Administration of tadalafil to patients using any form of organic nitrate, either regularly and/or intermittently, is contraindicated). Products include:
Imdur Tablets **3018**

Itraconazole (CYP3A4 inhibitors such as itraconazole may likely increase tadalafil exposure).
No products indexed under this heading.

Ketoconazole (Ketoconazole increased tadalafil 20mg single dose exposure (AUC) by 312% and Cmax by 22%, relative to the values for tadalafil 20mg alone. Ketoconazole increased tadalafil 10mg single dose exposure (AUC) by 107% and Cmax by 15%, relative to the values for tadalafil 10mg alone. Based on these results, the dose of tadalafil should not exceed 10mg and tadalafil should not be taken more frequently than once in 72 hours). Products include:
Nizoral A-D Shampoo, 1% **1868**

Lopinavir (Tadalafil is metabolized predominantly by CYP3A4 in the liver. The dose of tadalafil should be limited to 10 mg no more than once every 72 hours in patients taking potent inhibitors of CYP3A4). Products include:
Kaletra **476**

Loratadine (Tadalafil is metabolized predominantly by CYP3A4 in the liver. The dose of tadalafil should be limited to 10 mg no more than once every 72 hours in patients taking potent inhibitors of CYP3A4). Products include:
Alavert Allergy & Sinus D-12 Hour Tablets .... ▣**771**
Alavert .... ▣**771**
Children's Claritin Allergy Oral Solution .... ▣**771**
Claritin Non-Drowsy 24 Hour Tablets .... ▣**772**
Claritin Reditabs 24 Hour Non-Drowsy Tablets .... ▣**772**
Claritin-D Non-Drowsy 12 Hour Tablets .... ▣**772**
Claritin-D Non-Drowsy 24 Hour Tablets .... ▣**772**

Losartan Potassium (A study was conducted to assess the interaction of angiotensin II receptor blockers and tadalafil 20mg. Following dosing, ambulatory measurements of blood pressure revealed differences between tadalafil and placebo of 8/4mm Hg in systolic/diastolic blood pressure). Products include:
Cozaar Tablets **1935**
Hyzaar 50-12.5 Tablets **1990**
Hyzaar 100-12.5 Tablets **1990**
Hyzaar 100-25 Tablets **1990**

Magaldrate (Simultaneous administration of an antacid (magnesium hydroxide/aluminum hydroxide) and tadalafil reduced the apparent rate of absorption of tadalafil without altering exposure (AUC) to tadalafil).
No products indexed under this heading.

Magnesium Hydroxide (Simultaneous administration of an antacid (magnesium hydroxide/aluminum hydroxide) and tadalafil reduced the apparent rate of absorption of tadalafil without altering exposure (AUC) to tadalafil). Products include:
Maalox Regular Strength Antacid/Antigas Liquid **2175**
Maalox Max Maximum Strength Antacid/Anti-Gas Liquid **2176**
Pepcid Complete Chewable Tablets **1701**

Magnesium Oxide (Simultaneous administration of an antacid (magnesium hydroxide/aluminum hydroxide) and tadalafil reduced the apparent rate of absorption of tadalafil without altering exposure (AUC) to tadalafil). Products include:
Beelith Tablets **759**
PremCal Light, Regular, and Extra Strength Tablets .... ▣**818**

Mephenytoin (Drugs that induce CYP3A4 can increase tadalafil exposure).
No products indexed under this heading.

Methsuximide (Drugs that induce CYP3A4 can increase tadalafil exposure).
No products indexed under this heading.

Methylprednisolone (Drugs that induce CYP3A4 can increase tadalafil exposure).
No products indexed under this heading.

Methylprednisolone Acetate (Drugs that induce CYP3A4 can increase tadalafil exposure). Products include:
Depo-Medrol Injectable Suspension **2617**
Depo-Medrol Single-Dose Vial **2619**

Methylprednisolone Sodium Succinate (Drugs that induce CYP3A4 can increase tadalafil exposure).
No products indexed under this heading.

Metoprolol Succinate (Following dosing with sustained-release metoprolol (25-200mg daily) and tadalafil 10mg, the mean reduction in supine systolic/diastolic blood pressure due to tadalafil 10mg in subjects taking metoprolol was 5/3mm Hg, compared to placebo). Products include:
Toprol-XL Tablets **668**

Metoprolol Tartrate (Following dosing with sustained-release metoprolol (25-200mg daily) and tadalafil 10mg, the mean reduction in supine systolic/diastolic blood pressure due to tadalafil 10mg in subjects taking metoprolol was 5/3mm Hg, compared to placebo). Products include:
Lopressor Injection **2238**
Lopressor Tablets **2238**
Lopressor HCT 50/25 Tablets **2241**
Lopressor HCT 100/25 Tablets **2241**
Lopressor HCT 100/50 Tablets **2241**

Metronidazole (Tadalafil is metabolized predominantly by CYP3A4 in the liver. The dose of tadalafil should be limited to 10 mg no more than once every 72 hours in patients taking potent inhibitors of CYP3A4). Products include:
Metrogel 1% **1211**
MetroGel-Vaginal Gel **1855**
Vandazole Vaginal Gel **3338**

Metronidazole Benzoate (Tadalafil is metabolized predominantly by CYP3A4 in the liver. The dose of tadalafil should be limited to 10 mg no more than once every 72 hours in patients taking potent inhibitors of CYP3A4).
No products indexed under this heading.

Metronidazole Hydrochloride (Tadalafil is metabolized predominantly by CYP3A4 in the liver. The dose of tadalafil should be limited to 10 mg no more than once every 72 hours in patients taking potent inhibitors of CYP3A4).
No products indexed under this heading.

Miconazole (Tadalafil is metabolized predominantly by CYP3A4 in the liver. The dose of tadalafil should be limited to 10 mg no more than once every 72 hours in patients taking potent inhibitors of CYP3A4).
No products indexed under this heading.

Miconazole Nitrate (Tadalafil is metabolized predominantly by CYP3A4 in the liver. The dose of tadalafil should be limited to 10 mg no more than once every 72 hours in patients taking potent inhibitors of CYP3A4). Products include:
Desenex .... ▣**635**
Desenex Jock Itch Spray Powder .... ▣**635**

Modafinil (Drugs that induce CYP3A4 can increase tadalafil exposure). Products include:
Provigil Tablets **988**

Nefazodone Hydrochloride (Tadalafil is metabolized predominantly by CYP3A4 in the liver. The dose of tadalafil should be limited to 10 mg no more than once every 72 hours in patients taking potent inhibitors of CYP3A4).
No products indexed under this heading.

Nelfinavir Mesylate (Tadalafil is metabolized predominantly by CYP3A4 in the liver. The dose of tadalafil should be limited to 10 mg no more than once every 72 hours in patients taking potent inhibitors of CYP3A4). Products include:
Viracept **2577**

Nevirapine (Tadalafil is metabolized predominantly by CYP3A4 in the liver. The dose of tadalafil should be limited to 10 mg no more than once every 72 hours in patients taking potent inhibitors of CYP3A4). Products include:
Viramune Oral Suspension **873**
Viramune Tablets **873**

Niacinamide (Tadalafil is metabolized predominantly by CYP3A4 in the liver. The dose of tadalafil should be limited to 10 mg no more than once every 72 hours in patients taking potent inhibitors of CYP3A4).
No products indexed under this heading.

Nicotinamide (Tadalafil is metabolized predominantly by CYP3A4 in the liver. The dose of tadalafil should be limited to 10 mg no more than once every 72 hours in patients taking potent inhibitors of CYP3A4). Products include:
Nicomide Tablets **1088**

Nifedipine (Tadalafil is metabolized predominantly by CYP3A4 in the liver. The dose of tadalafil should be

limited to 10 mg no more than once every 72 hours in patients taking potent inhibitors of CYP3A4). Products include:

Adalat CC Tablets 2964

Nitroglycerin (Administration of tadalafil to patients using any form of organic nitrate, either regularly and/or intermittently, is contraindicated). Products include:

Nitro-Dur Transdermal Infusion System... 3046
Nitrolingual Pumpspray 3120

Norfloxacin (Tadalafil is metabolized predominantly by CYP3A4 in the liver. The dose of tadalafil should be limited to 10 mg no more than once every 72 hours in patients taking potent inhibitors of CYP3A4). Products include:

Noroxin Tablets 2032

Omeprazole (Tadalafil is metabolized predominantly by CYP3A4 in the liver. The dose of tadalafil should be limited to 10 mg no more than once every 72 hours in patients taking potent inhibitors of CYP3A4). Products include:

Zegerid Capsules 2958
Zegerid Powder for Oral Solution 2958

Oxcarbazepine (Drugs that induce CYP3A4 can increase tadalafil exposure). Products include:

Trileptal Tablets 2300
Trileptal Oral Suspension 2300

Paroxetine Hydrochloride (Tadalafil is metabolized predominantly by CYP3A4 in the liver. The dose of tadalafil should be limited to 10 mg no more than once every 72 hours in patients taking potent inhibitors of CYP3A4). Products include:

Paxil CR Controlled-Release Tablets... 1538
Paxil ... 1530

Pentaerythritol Tetranitrate (Administration of tadalafil to patients using any form of organic nitrate, either regularly and/or intermittently, is contraindicated). No products indexed under this heading.

Phenobarbital (CYP3A4 inducers, such as phenobarbital, may decrease tadalafil exposure. No dose adjustment is warranted). Products include:

Donnatal Extentabs 2493

Phenobarbital Sodium (CYP3A4 inducers, such as phenobarbital, may decrease tadalafil exposure. No dose adjustment is warranted). No products indexed under this heading.

Phenytoin (Drugs that induce CYP3A4 can increase tadalafil exposure). No products indexed under this heading.

Phenytoin Sodium (Drugs that induce CYP3A4 can increase tadalafil exposure). Products include:

Phenytek Capsules 2160

Prazosin Hydrochloride (Caution is advised when PDE5 inhibitors are co-administered with alpha-blockers. PDE5 inhibitors, including tadalafil, and alpha-adrenergic blocking agents are both vasodilators with blood-pressure lowering effects. When vasodilators are used in combination, an additive effect on blood pressure may be anticipated. In some patients, concomitant use of these two drug classes can lower blood presure significantly, which may lead to symptomatic hypoten-

sion (e.g., fainting)). No products indexed under this heading.

Prednisolone Acetate (Drugs that induce CYP3A4 can increase tadalafil exposure). Products include:

Blephamide Ophthalmic Ointment 568
Blephamide Ophthalmic Suspension................................. 569
Poly-Pred Ophthalmic Suspension............................ ⊙ 233
Pred Forte Ophthalmic Suspension............................ ⊙ 235
Pred Mild Ophthalmic Suspension............................ ⊙ 238
Pred-G Ophthalmic Ointment ⊙ 237
Pred-G Ophthalmic Suspension ⊙ 236

Prednisolone Sodium Phosphate (Drugs that induce CYP3A4 can increase tadalafil exposure). No products indexed under this heading.

Prednisolone Tebutate (Drugs that induce CYP3A4 can increase tadalafil exposure). No products indexed under this heading.

Prednisone (Drugs that induce CYP3A4 can increase tadalafil exposure). No products indexed under this heading.

Primidone (Drugs that induce CYP3A4 can increase tadalafil exposure). No products indexed under this heading.

Propoxyphene Hydrochloride (Tadalafil is metabolized predominantly by CYP3A4 in the liver. The dose of tadalafil should be limited to 10 mg no more than once every 72 hours in patients taking potent inhibitors of CYP3A4). No products indexed under this heading.

Propoxyphene Napsylate (Tadalafil is metabolized predominantly by CYP3A4 in the liver. The dose of tadalafil should be limited to 10 mg no more than once every 72 hours in patients taking potent inhibitors of CYP3A4). No products indexed under this heading.

Quinidine (Tadalafil is metabolized predominantly by CYP3A4 in the liver. The dose of tadalafil should be limited to 10 mg no more than once every 72 hours in patients taking potent inhibitors of CYP3A4). No products indexed under this heading.

Quinidine Hydrochloride (Tadalafil is metabolized predominantly by CYP3A4 in the liver. The dose of tadalafil should be limited to 10 mg no more than once every 72 hours in patients taking potent inhibitors of CYP3A4). No products indexed under this heading.

Quinidine Polygalacturonate (Tadalafil is metabolized predominantly by CYP3A4 in the liver. The dose of tadalafil should be limited to 10 mg no more than once every 72 hours in patients taking potent inhibitors of CYP3A4). No products indexed under this heading.

Quinidine Sulfate (Tadalafil is metabolized predominantly by CYP3A4 in the liver. The dose of tadalafil should be limited to 10 mg no more than once every 72 hours in patients taking potent inhibitors of CYP3A4). No products indexed under this heading.

Quinine (Tadalafil is metabolized predominantly by CYP3A4 in the liver. The dose of tadalafil should be limited to 10 mg no more than once every 72 hours in patients taking potent inhibitors of CYP3A4). No products indexed under this heading.

Quinine Sulfate (Tadalafil is metabolized predominantly by CYP3A4 in the liver. The dose of tadalafil should be limited to 10 mg no more than once every 72 hours in patients taking potent inhibitors of CYP3A4). No products indexed under this heading.

Quinupristin (Tadalafil is metabolized predominantly by CYP3A4 in the liver. The dose of tadalafil should be limited to 10 mg no more than once every 72 hours in patients taking potent inhibitors of CYP3A4). No products indexed under this heading.

Ranitidine Bismuth Citrate (Tadalafil is metabolized predominantly by CYP3A4 in the liver. The dose of tadalafil should be limited to 10 mg no more than once every 72 hours in patients taking potent inhibitors of CYP3A4). No products indexed under this heading.

Ranitidine Hydrochloride (Tadalafil is metabolized predominantly by CYP3A4 in the liver. The dose of tadalafil should be limited to 10 mg no more than once every 72 hours in patients taking potent inhibitors of CYP3A4). Products include:

Zantac ... 1624
Zantac Injection 1619
Zantac Injection Pharmacy Bulk Package.................................... 1622

Rifabutin (Drugs that induce CYP3A4 can increase tadalafil exposure). No products indexed under this heading.

Rifampicin (Drugs that induce CYP3A4 can increase tadalafil exposure). No products indexed under this heading.

Rifampin (Rifampin reduced tadalafil 10mg single dose exposure (AUC) by 88% and Cmax by 46% relative to the values for tadalafil 10mg alone. No dose adjustment is warranted). No products indexed under this heading.

Rifapentine (Drugs that induce CYP3A4 can increase tadalafil exposure). No products indexed under this heading.

Ritonavir (Ritonavir increased tadalafil 20mg single dose exposure (AUC) by 124% with no change in Cmax, relative to the values for tadalafil 20mg alone. Based on these results, the dose of tadalafil should not exceed 10mg and tadalafil should not be taken more frequently than once in 72 hours). Products include:

Kaletra .. 476

Norvir .. 503

Saquinavir (Tadalafil is metabolized predominantly by CYP3A4 in the liver. The dose of tadalafil should be limited to 10 mg no more than once every 72 hours in patients taking potent inhibitors of CYP3A4). No products indexed under this heading.

Saquinavir Mesylate (Tadalafil is metabolized predominantly by CYP3A4 in the liver. The dose of tadalafil should be limited to 10 mg no more than once every 72 hours in patients taking potent inhibitors of CYP3A4). Products include:

Invirase ... 2772

Sertraline Hydrochloride (Tadalafil is metabolized predominantly by CYP3A4 in the liver. The dose of tadalafil should be limited to 10 mg no more than once every 72 hours in patients taking potent inhibitors of CYP3A4). Products include:

Zoloft .. 2586

Sodium Bicarbonate (Simultaneous administration of an antacid (magnesium hydroxide/aluminum hydroxide) and tadalafil reduced the apparent rate of absorption of tadalafil without altering exposure (AUC) to tadalafil). Products include:

Colyte with Flavor Packs for Oral Solution.................................... 3088
HalfLytely and Bisacodyl Tablets Bowel Prep Kit with Flavors Packs....................................... 881
TriLyte with Flavor Packs for Oral Solution.................................... 3100

Sulfinpyrazone (Drugs that induce CYP3A4 can increase tadalafil exposure). No products indexed under this heading.

Tamsulosin Hydrochloride (Caution is advised when PDE5 inhibitors are co-administered with alpha-blockers. PDE5 inhibitors, including tadalafil, and alpha-adrenergic blocking agents are both vasodilators with blood-pressure lowering effects. When vasodilators are used in combination, an additive effect on blood pressure may be anticipated. In some patients, concomitant use of these two drug classes can lower blood presure significantly, which may lead to symptomatic hypotension (e.g., fainting)). Products include:

Flomax Capsules 850

Telithromycin (Tadalafil is metabolized predominantly by CYP3A4 in the liver. The dose of tadalafil should be limited to 10 mg no more than once every 72 hours in patients taking potent inhibitors of CYP3A4). Products include:

Ketek Tablets 2903

Telmisartan (A study was conducted to assess the interaction of angiotensin II receptor blockers and tadalafil 20mg. Following dosing, ambulatory measurements of blood pressure revealed differences between tadalafil and placebo of 8/4mm Hg in systolic/diastolic blood pressure). Products include:

Micardis Tablets 854
Micardis HCT Tablets 856

Terazosin Hydrochloride (Caution is advised when PDE5 inhibitors are co-administered with alpha-blockers. PDE5 inhibitors, including tadalafil, and alpha-adrenergic blocking agents are both vasodilators with blood-pressure lowering effects. When vasodilators are used in com-

bination, an additive effect on blood pressure may be anticipated. In some patients, concomitant use of these two drug classes can lower blood presure significantly, which may lead to symptomatic hypotension (e.g., fainting)). Products include:
Hytrin Capsules 471

Theophylline (Drugs that induce CYP3A4 can increase tadalafil exposure).
No products indexed under this heading.

Triamcinolone (Drugs that induce CYP3A4 can increase tadalafil exposure).
No products indexed under this heading.

Triamcinolone Acetonide (Drugs that induce CYP3A4 can increase tadalafil exposure). Products include:
Azmacort Inhalation Aerosol 1726
Nasacort AQ Nasal Spray 2922

Triamcinolone Diacetate (Drugs that induce CYP3A4 can increase tadalafil exposure).
No products indexed under this heading.

Triamcinolone Hexacetonide (Drugs that induce CYP3A4 can increase tadalafil exposure).
No products indexed under this heading.

Troglitazone (Tadalafil is metabolized predominantly by CYP3A4 in the liver. The dose of tadalafil should be limited to 10 mg no more than once every 72 hours in patients taking potent inhibitors of CYP3A4).
No products indexed under this heading.

Troleandomycin (Tadalafil is metabolized predominantly by CYP3A4 in the liver. The dose of tadalafil should be limited to 10 mg no more than once every 72 hours in patients taking potent inhibitors of CYP3A4).
No products indexed under this heading.

Valproate Sodium (Tadalafil is metabolized predominantly by CYP3A4 in the liver. The dose of tadalafil should be limited to 10 mg no more than once every 72 hours in patients taking potent inhibitors of CYP3A4). Products include:
Depacon Injection 412

Valsartan (A study was conducted to assess the interaction of angiotensin II receptor blockers and tadalafil 20mg. Following dosing, ambulatory measurements of blood pressure revealed differences between tadalafil and placebo of 8/4mm Hg in systolic/diastolic blood pressure). Products include:
Diovan Tablets 2193
Diovan HCT Tablets 2196

Verapamil Hydrochloride (Tadalafil is metabolized predominantly by CYP3A4 in the liver. The dose of tadalafil should be limited to 10 mg no more than once every 72 hours in patients taking potent inhibitors of CYP3A4). Products include:
Covera-HS Tablets 3139
Tarka Tablets 524
Verelan PM Extended-Release Capsules, Controlled-Onset 3106

Voriconazole (Tadalafil is metabolized predominantly by CYP3A4 in the liver. The dose of tadalafil should be limited to 10 mg no more than once every 72 hours in patients taking potent inhibitors of CYP3A4).
Products include:
VFEND I.V. 2564
VFEND Oral Suspension 2564
VFEND Tablets 2564

Zafirlukast (Tadalafil is metabolized predominantly by CYP3A4 in the liver. The dose of tadalafil should be limited to 10 mg no more than once every 72 hours in patients taking potent inhibitors of CYP3A4).
Products include:
Accolate Tablets 671

Zileuton (Tadalafil is metabolized predominantly by CYP3A4 in the liver. The dose of tadalafil should be limited to 10 mg no more than once every 72 hours in patients taking potent inhibitors of CYP3A4).
Products include:
Zyflo Tablets 1023

Food Interactions

Alcohol (Both tadalafil and alcohol act as mild vasodilators. When mild vasodilators are taken in combination, blood-pressure lowering effects of each individual compound may be increased. Substantial consumption of alcohol in combination with tadalafil may increase the potential for orthostatic signs and symptoms, including increase in heart rate, decrease in standing blood pressure, dizziness, and headache).

Grapefruit (Tadalafil is metabolized predominantly by CYP3A4 in the liver. The dose of tadalafil should be limited to 10 mg no more than once every 72 hours in patients taking potent inhibitors of CYP3A4).

Grapefruit Juice (YP3A4 inhibitors such as grapefruit juice may likely increase tadalafil exposure).

CILOXAN OPHTHALMIC OINTMENT

(Ciprofloxacin Hydrochloride) 559
May interact with oral anticoagulants, xanthines, and certain other agents. Compounds in these categories include:

Aminophylline (Systemic administration of quinolones elevates plasma concentrations of theophylline).
No products indexed under this heading.

Anisindione (Enhanced anticoagulant effect with systemic quinolones).
Products include:
Miradon Tablets 3042

Caffeine (Systemic administration of quinolones has shown to interfere with caffeine metabolism). Products include:
BC Headache Powder .... ▣677
Arthritis Strength BC Powder .... ▣677
Excedrin Extra Strength Caplets/Tablets/Geltabs .... ▣684
Excedrin Migraine Caplets/Tablets/Geltabs .... ▣609
Excedrin Tension Headache Caplets/Tablets/Geltabs .... ▣611
Goody's Extra Strength Headache Powders .... ▣611
Goody's Extra Strength Pain Relief Tablets .... ▣685
Vivarin .... ▣602
Winrgy Dietary Supplement .... ▣823

Caffeine Citrate (Systemic administration of quinolones has shown to interfere with caffeine metabolism).
Products include:
Cafcit 1886

Cyclosporine (Concomitant administration with systemic quinolones may result in transient elevations in serum creatinine). Products include:
Gengraf Capsules 459
Neoral Oral Solution 2259
Neoral Soft Gelatin Capsules 2259
Restasis Ophthalmic Emulsion 575
Sandimmune 2275

Dicumarol (Enhanced anticoagulant effect with systemic quinolones).
No products indexed under this heading.

Dyphylline (Systemic administration of quinolones elevates plasma concentrations of theophylline).
No products indexed under this heading.

Theophylline (Systemic administration of quinolones elevates plasma concentrations of theophylline).
No products indexed under this heading.

Theophylline Anhydrous (Systemic administration of quinolones elevates plasma concentrations of theophylline). Products include:
Uniphyl Tablets 2710

Theophylline Calcium Salicylate (Systemic administration of quinolones elevates plasma concentrations of theophylline).
No products indexed under this heading.

Theophylline Dihydroxypropyl (Glyceryl) (Systemic administration of quinolones elevates plasma concentrations of theophylline).
No products indexed under this heading.

Theophylline Ethylenediamine (Systemic administration of quinolones elevates plasma concentrations of theophylline).
No products indexed under this heading.

Theophylline Sodium Glycinate (Systemic administration of quinolones elevates plasma concentrations of theophylline).
No products indexed under this heading.

Warfarin Sodium (Enhanced anticoagulant effect with systemic quinolones). Products include:
Coumadin for Injection 898
Coumadin Tablets 898

CILOXAN OPHTHALMIC SOLUTION

(Ciprofloxacin Hydrochloride) .... ⊙206
May interact with oral anticoagulants, xanthines, and certain other agents. Compounds in these categories include:

Aminophylline (Systemic administration of quinolones elevates plasma concentrations of theophylline).
No products indexed under this heading.

Anisindione (Enhanced anticoagulant effect with systemic quinolones).
Products include:
Miradon Tablets 3042

Caffeine (Systemic administration of quinolones has shown to interfere with caffeine metabolism). Products include:
BC Headache Powder .... ▣677
Arthritis Strength BC Powder .... ▣677
Excedrin Extra Strength Caplets/Tablets/Geltabs .... ▣684
Excedrin Migraine Caplets/Tablets/Geltabs .... ▣609
Excedrin Tension Headache Caplets/Tablets/Geltabs .... ▣611
Goody's Extra Strength Headache Powders .... ▣611
Goody's Extra Strength Pain Relief Tablets .... ▣685
Vivarin .... ▣602
Winrgy Dietary Supplement .... ▣823

Caffeine Citrate (Systemic administration of quinolones has shown to interfere with caffeine metabolism).
Products include:
Cafcit 1886

Cyclosporine (Concomitant administration with systemic quinolones may result in transient elevations in serum creatinine). Products include:
Gengraf Capsules 459
Neoral Oral Solution 2259
Neoral Soft Gelatin Capsules 2259
Restasis Ophthalmic Emulsion 575
Sandimmune 2275

Dicumarol (Enhanced anticoagulant effect with systemic quinolones).
No products indexed under this heading.

Dyphylline (Systemic administration of quinolones elevates plasma concentrations of theophylline).
No products indexed under this heading.

Theophylline (Systemic administration of quinolones elevates plasma concentrations of theophylline).
No products indexed under this heading.

Theophylline Anhydrous (Systemic administration of quinolones elevates plasma concentrations of theophylline). Products include:
Uniphyl Tablets 2710

Theophylline Calcium Salicylate (Systemic administration of quinolones elevates plasma concentrations of theophylline).
No products indexed under this heading.

Theophylline Dihydroxypropyl (Glyceryl) (Systemic administration of quinolones elevates plasma concentrations of theophylline).
No products indexed under this heading.

Theophylline Ethylenediamine (Systemic administration of quinolones elevates plasma concentrations of theophylline).
No products indexed under this heading.

Theophylline Sodium Glycinate (Systemic administration of quinolones elevates plasma concentrations of theophylline).
No products indexed under this heading.

Warfarin Sodium (Enhanced anticoagulant effect with systemic quinolones). Products include:
Coumadin for Injection 898
Coumadin Tablets 898

CIPRO ORAL SUSPENSION

(Ciprofloxacin) 2977
See Cipro Tablets

CIPRO TABLETS

(Ciprofloxacin Hydrochloride) 2977
May interact with antacids containing aluminum, calcium and magnesium, calcium preparations, corticosteroids, oral anticoagulants, cytochrome p450 1a2 substrates (selected), iron containing oral preparations, non-steroidal anti-inflammatory agents, phenytoin, xanthines, and certain other agents. Compounds in these categories include:

Acetaminophen (Ciprofloxacin is an inhibitor of CYP450 1A2 isoenzymes. Co-administration of ciprofloxacin and other drugs primarily metabolized by CYP1A2 results in increased plasma concentrations of the co-administered drug and could lead to clinically significant pharmacodynamic side effects). Products include:

- Comtrex Maximum Strength Cold & Cough Day/Night Caplets - Day Formulation ▣ 726
- Comtrex Maximum Strength Cold & Cough Day/Night Caplets - Night Formulation ▣ 726
- Comtrex Maximum Strength Non-Drowsy Cold & Cough Caplets ▣ 725
- Comtrex Maximum Strength Day/Night Severe Cold & Sinus Caplets - Day Formulation ▣ 725
- Comtrex Maximum Strength Day/Night Severe Cold & Sinus Caplets - Night Formulation ▣ 725
- Contac Cold and Flu Maximum Strength Caplets ▣ 728
- Contac Cold and Flu Day and Night Caplets (Day Formulation Only) ▣ 727
- Contac Cold and Flu Day and Night Caplets (Night Formulation Only) ▣ 727
- Contac Cold and Flu Non-Drowsy Caplets ▣ 728
- Excedrin Extra Strength Caplets/Tablets/Geltabs ▣ 684
- Excedrin Migraine Caplets/Tablets/Geltabs ▣ 609
- Excedrin PM Caplets/Tablets/Geltabs ▣ 610
- Excedrin Sinus Headache Caplets/Tablets ▣ 610
- Excedrin Tension Headache Caplets/Tablets/Geltabs ▣ 611
- Goody's Body Pain Formula Powder ▣ 684
- Goody's Extra Strength Headache Powders ▣ 611
- Goody's Extra Strength Pain Relief Tablets ▣ 685
- Goody's PM Powder for Pain with Sleeplessness ▣ 612
- Percocet Tablets 1131
- Robitussin Cough, Cold & Flu Nighttime Liquid ▣ 738
- TheraFlu Cold & Sore Throat Hot Liquid ▣ 741
- TheraFlu Flu & Chest Congestion Hot Liquid ▣ 741
- TheraFlu Flu & Sore Throat Hot Liquid ▣ 742
- TheraFlu Daytime Severe Cold Hot Liquid ▣ 742
- TheraFlu Nighttime Severe Cold Hot Liquid ▣ 740
- TheraFlu Warming Relief Daytime Severe Cold ▣ 743
- TheraFlu Warming Relief Nighttime Severe Cold ▣ 743
- Triaminic Cough & Sore Throat Liquid ▣ 747
- Regular Strength Tylenol Tablets 1870
- Children's Tylenol with Flavor Creator ▣ 679
- Children's Tylenol Plus Flu Oral Suspension ▣ 749
- Tylenol Cold Head Congestion Daytime Caplets with Cool Burst and Gelcaps ▣ 750
- Tylenol Cold Multi-Symptom Daytime Liquid ▣ 752
- Tylenol Cold Multi-Symptom Severe Daytime Liquid ▣ 752
- Tylenol 8 Hour Extended Release Caplets 1870
- Tylenol 1870
- Extra Strength Tylenol PM Caplets, Vanilla Caplets, Geltabs, Gelcaps and Liquid 1875
- Extra Strength Tylenol Rapid Release Gels 1870
- Concentrated Tylenol Infants' Drops Plus Cold & Cough ▣ 754
- Tylenol with Codeine Tablets 2391
- Tylenol Allergy Multi-Symptom Caplets with Cool Burst and Gelcaps 1872
- Tylenol Allergy Multi-Symptom Nighttime Caplets with Cool Burst 1872
- Tylenol Severe Allergy Caplets 1872
- Tylenol Arthritis Pain Extended Release Caplets and Geltabs 1870
- Tylenol Chest Congestion Caplets with Cool Burst 1872
- Tylenol Chest Congestion Liquid with Cool Burst 1872
- Children's Tylenol Suspension Liquid and Meltaways 1878
- Children's Tylenol Plus Cold Suspension Liquid 1879
- Children's Tylenol Plus Cold & Allergy Suspension Liquid 1878
- Children's Tylenol Plus Cough & Runny Nose Suspension Liquid 1879
- Children's Tylenol Plus Cough & Sore Throat Suspension Liquid 1879
- Children's Tylenol Suspension with Flavor Creator 1878
- Children's Tylenol Plus Flu Suspension Liquid 1881
- Children's Tylenol Plus Multi-Symptom Cold Suspension Liquid 1879
- Tylenol Cold Severe Congestion Non-Drowsy Caplets with Cool Burst 1874
- Tylenol Cold Head Congestion Daytime Caplets with Cool Burst 1873
- Tylenol Cold Head Congestion Nighttime Caplets with Cool Burst 1873
- Tylenol Cold Head Congestion Severe Caplets with Cool Burst 1873
- Tylenol Cold Multi-Symptom Daytime Caplets with Cool Burst and Gelcaps 1874
- Tylenol Cold Multi-Symptom Daytime Liquid with Citrus Burst 1874
- Tylenol Cold Multi-Symptom Nighttime Caplets with Cool Burst 1874
- Tylenol Cold Multi-Symptom Nighttime Liquid with Cool Burst 1874
- Tylenol Cold Multi-Symptom Severe Caplets with Cool Burst 1874
- Tylenol Cold Multi-Symptom Severe Daytime Liquid with Citrus Burst 1874
- Tylenol Cough & Sore Throat Daytime Liquid with Cool Burst 1877
- Tylenol Cough & Sore Throat Nighttime Liquid with Cool Burst 1877
- Concentrated Tylenol Infants' Drops 1878
- Concentrated Tylenol Infants' Drops Plus Cold 1879
- Concentrated Tylenol Infants' Drops Plus Cold and Cough 1879
- Jr. Tylenol Meltaways 1878
- Tylenol Sinus Severe Congestion Caplets with Cool Burst 1876
- Tylenol Sinus Congestion & Pain Daytime Caplets with Cool Burst and Gelcaps 1876
- Tylenol Sinus Congestion & Pain Nighttime Caplets with Cool Burst 1876
- Tylenol Sinus Congestion & Pain Severe Caplets with Cool Burst 1876
- Tylenol Sore Throat Daytime Liquid with Cool Burst 1877
- Tylenol Sore Throat Nighttime Liquid with Cool Burst 1877
- Women's Tylenol Menstrual Relief Caplets 1877
- Vicks 44M Cough, Cold & Flu Relief Liquid 2680
- Vicks DayQuil LiquiCaps/Liquid Multi-Symptom Cold/Flu Relief ▣ 761
- Vicks DayQuil Multi-Symptom Cold/Flu Relief LiquiCaps 2678
- Vicks DayQuil Multi-Symptom Cold/Flu Relief Liquid 2678
- Vicks NyQuil Multi-Symptom Cold/Flu Relief Liquid 2681
- Vicks NyQuil Multi-Symptom Cold/Flu Relief LiquiCaps 2681
- Vicks NyQuil LiquiCaps/Liquid Multi-Symptom Cold/Flu Relief ▣ 763
- Vicodin Tablets 535
- Vicodin ES Tablets 536
- Vicodin HP Tablets 538
- Zicam Maximum Strength Flu Daytime ▣ 768
- Zicam Maximum Strength Flu Nighttime ▣ 768
- Zydone Tablets 1139

Alatrofloxacin Mesylate (Ciprofloxacin is an inhibitor of CYP450 1A2 isoenzymes. Co-administration of ciprofloxacin and other drugs primarily metabolized by CYP1A2 results in increased plasma concentrations of the co-administered drug and could lead to clinically significant pharmacodynamic side effects).

No products indexed under this heading.

Aluminum Carbonate (Concurrent administration of these antacids may substantially interfere with the oral absorption of ciprofloxacin; antacids may be administered either two hours after or six hours before ciprofloxacin dosing without a significant decrease in bioavailability).

No products indexed under this heading.

Aluminum Hydroxide (Concurrent administration of these antacids may substantially interfere with the oral absorption of ciprofloxacin; antacids may be administered either two hours after or six hours before ciprofloxacin dosing without a significant decrease in bioavailability). Products include:

- Gaviscon Regular Strength Liquid ▣ 658
- Gaviscon Regular Strength Tablets ▣ 658
- Gaviscon Extra Strength Liquid ▣ 658
- Gaviscon Extra Strength Tablets ▣ 658
- Maalox Regular Strength Antacid/Antigas Liquid 2175
- Maalox Max Maximum Strength Antacid/Anti-Gas Liquid 2176

Aminophylline (Potential for severe and fatal reactions including cardiac arrest, seizures, respiratory failure and status epilepticus; concurrent use should be avoided or serum levels of theophylline should be monitored carefully).

No products indexed under this heading.

Amiodarone Hydrochloride (Ciprofloxacin is an inhibitor of CYP450 1A2 isoenzymes. Co-administration of ciprofloxacin and other drugs primarily metabolized by CYP1A2 results in increased plasma concentrations of the co-administered drug and could lead to clinically significant pharmacodynamic side effects).

No products indexed under this heading.

Amitriptyline Hydrochloride (Ciprofloxacin is an inhibitor of CYP450 1A2 isoenzymes. Co-administration of ciprofloxacin and other drugs primarily metabolized by CYP1A2 results in increased plasma concentrations of the co-administered drug and could lead to clinically significant pharmacodynamic side effects).

No products indexed under this heading.

Amoxapine (Ciprofloxacin is an inhibitor of CYP450 1A2 isoenzymes. Co-administration of ciprofloxacin and other drugs primarily metabolized by CYP1A2 results in increased plasma concentrations of the co-administered drug and could lead to clinically significant pharmacodynamic side effects).

No products indexed under this heading.

Anagrelide Hydrochloride (Ciprofloxacin is an inhibitor of CYP450 1A2 isoenzymes. Co-administration of ciprofloxacin and other drugs primarily metabolized by CYP1A2 results in increased plasma concentrations of the co-administered drug and could lead to clinically significant pharmacodynamic side effects). Products include:

- Agrylin Capsules 3169

Anisindione (Enhanced effects of anticoagulant). Products include:

- Miradon Tablets 3042

Betamethasone Acetate (Risk of ruptures of the shoulder, hand, Achilles tendon or other tendons may be increased in patients receiving concomitant corticosteroids, especially in the elderly).

No products indexed under this heading.

Betamethasone Sodium Phosphate (Risk of ruptures of the shoulder, hand, Achilles tendon or other tendons may be increased in patients receiving concomitant corticosteroids, especially in the elderly).

No products indexed under this heading.

Caffeine (Co-administration leads to a reduction of caffeine clearance, prolongation of serum half-life, and inhibition of the formation of paraxanthine). Products include:

- BC Headache Powder ▣ 677
- Arthritis Strength BC Powder ▣ 677
- Excedrin Extra Strength Caplets/Tablets/Geltabs ▣ 684
- Excedrin Migraine Caplets/Tablets/Geltabs ▣ 609
- Excedrin Tension Headache Caplets/Tablets/Geltabs ▣ 611
- Goody's Extra Strength Headache Powders ▣ 611
- Goody's Extra Strength Pain Relief Tablets ▣ 685
- Vivarin ▣ 602
- Winrgy Dietary Supplement ▣ 823

Caffeine Anhydrous (Ciprofloxacin is an inhibitor of CYP450 1A2 isoenzymes. Co-administration of ciprofloxacin and other drugs primarily metabolized by CYP1A2 results in increased plasma concentrations of the co-administered drug and could lead to clinically significant pharmacodynamic side effects).

No products indexed under this heading.

Caffeine Citrate (Co-administration leads to a reduction of caffeine clearance, prolongation of serum half-life, and inhibition of the formation of paraxanthine). Products include:

- Cafcit 1886

Calcium Carbonate (Co-administration with calcium-containing products may substantially interfere with the oral absorption of quinolones; these preparations may be taken six hours before or two hours after taking ciprofloxacin). Products include:

- Actonel with Calcium Tablets 2688
- Calcet Tablets 2138
- Caltrate 600 PLUS ▣ 809
- Caltrate 600 + D Tablets ▣ 809
- D-Cal Chewable Caplets ▣ 812
- Gas-X with Maalox ▣ 656
- Maalox Regular Strength Antacid Chewable Tablets 2177
- Maalox Max Maximum Strength Antacid/Antigas Chewable Tablets 2176
- Maalox Max Maximum Strength Chewable Tablets ▣ 660
- Os-Cal Chewable Tablets ▣ 818
- Pepcid Complete Chewable Tablets 1701
- Children's Pepto 2674
- PremCal Light, Regular, and Extra Strength Tablets ▣ 818
- Tums ▣ 664

Calcium Chloride (Co-administration with calcium-containing products may substantially interfere with the oral absorption of quinolones; these preparations may be taken six hours before or two hours after taking ciprofloxacin).
No products indexed under this heading.

Calcium Citrate (Co-administration with calcium-containing products may substantially interfere with the oral absorption of quinolones; these preparations may be taken six hours before or two hours after taking ciprofloxacin). Products include:
Active Calcium Tablets 3339
Citracal Caplets 703
Citracal Lemon Cream Creamy Bites 2139
Citracal Prenatal + DHA Tablets and Capsules 2139

Calcium Glubionate (Co-administration with calcium-containing products may substantially interfere with the oral absorption of quinolones; these preparations may be taken six hours before or two hours after taking ciprofloxacin).
No products indexed under this heading.

Celecoxib (NSAIDs in combination with very high doses of quinolones have been shown to provoke convulsions in pre-clinical trials). Products include:
Celebrex Capsules 3134

Chlordiazepoxide (Ciprofloxacin is an inhibitor of CYP450 1A2 isoenzymes. Co-administration of ciprofloxacin and other drugs primarily metabolized by CYP1A2 results in increased plasma concentrations of the co-administered drug and could lead to clinically significant pharmacodynamic side effects).
No products indexed under this heading.

Chlordiazepoxide Hydrochloride (Ciprofloxacin is an inhibitor of CYP450 1A2 isoenzymes. Co-administration of ciprofloxacin and other drugs primarily metabolized by CYP1A2 results in increased plasma concentrations of the co-administered drug and could lead to clinically significant pharmacodynamic side effects). Products include:
Librium Capsules 3347

Cimetidine Hydrochloride (Ciprofloxacin is an inhibitor of CYP450 1A2 isoenzymes. Co-administration of ciprofloxacin and other drugs primarily metabolized by CYP1A2 results in increased plasma concentrations of the co-administered drug and could lead to clinically significant pharmacodynamic side effects).
No products indexed under this heading.

Ciprofloxacin (Ciprofloxacin is an inhibitor of CYP450 1A2 isoenzymes. Co-administration of ciprofloxacin and other drugs primarily metabolized by CYP1A2 results in increased plasma concentrations of the co-administered drug and could lead to clinically significant pharmacodynamic side effects). Products include:
Cipro Oral Suspension 2977
Cipro I.V. 2984
Cipro XR Tablets 2990
Ciprodex Otic Suspension 559

Clomipramine Hydrochloride (Ciprofloxacin is an inhibitor of CYP450 1A2 isoenzymes. Co-administration of ciprofloxacin and other drugs primarily metabolized by CYP1A2 results in increased plasma concentrations of the co-administered drug and could lead to clinically significant pharmacodynamic side effects).
No products indexed under this heading.

Clopidogrel Bisulfate (Ciprofloxacin is an inhibitor of CYP450 1A2 isoenzymes. Co-administration of ciprofloxacin and other drugs primarily metabolized by CYP1A2 results in increased plasma concentrations of the co-administered drug and could lead to clinically significant pharmacodynamic side effects). Products include:
Plavix Tablets 917
Plavix Tablets 2926

Clozapine (Ciprofloxacin is an inhibitor of CYP450 1A2 isoenzymes. Co-administration of ciprofloxacin and other drugs primarily metabolized by CYP1A2 results in increased plasma concentrations of the co-administered drug and could lead to clinically significant pharmacodynamic side effects). Products include:
Clozaril Tablets 2184
FazaClo Orally Disintegrating Tablets 551

Cortisone Acetate (Risk of ruptures of the shoulder, hand, Achilles tendon or other tendons may be increased in patients receiving concomitant corticosteroids, especially in the elderly).
No products indexed under this heading.

Cyclobenzaprine (Ciprofloxacin is an inhibitor of CYP450 1A2 isoenzymes. Co-administration of ciprofloxacin and other drugs primarily metabolized by CYP1A2 results in increased plasma concentrations of the co-administered drug and could lead to clinically significant pharmacodynamic side effects).
No products indexed under this heading.

Cyclobenzaprine Hydrochloride (Ciprofloxacin is an inhibitor of CYP450 1A2 isoenzymes. Co-administration of ciprofloxacin and other drugs primarily metabolized by CYP1A2 results in increased plasma concentrations of the co-administered drug and could lead to clinically significant pharmacodynamic side effects).
No products indexed under this heading.

Cyclosporine (Transient elevations in serum creatinine). Products include:
Gengraf Capsules 459
Neoral Oral Solution 2259
Neoral Soft Gelatin Capsules 2259
Restasis Ophthalmic Emulsion 575
Sandimmune 2275

Desipramine Hydrochloride (Ciprofloxacin is an inhibitor of CYP450 1A2 isoenzymes. Co-administration of ciprofloxacin and other drugs primarily metabolized by CYP1A2 results in increased plasma concentrations of the co-administered drug and could lead to clinically significant pharmacodynamic side effects).
No products indexed under this heading.

Dexamethasone (Risk of ruptures of the shoulder, hand, Achilles tendon or other tendons may be increased in patients receiving concomitant corticosteroids, especially in the elderly). Products include:
Ciprodex Otic Suspension 559
Decadron Tablets 1951
TobraDex Ophthalmic Ointment 562
TobraDex Ophthalmic Suspension ... 563

Dexamethasone Acetate (Risk of ruptures of the shoulder, hand, Achilles tendon or other tendons may be increased in patients receiving concomitant corticosteroids, especially in the elderly).
No products indexed under this heading.

Dexamethasone Sodium Phosphate (Risk of ruptures of the shoulder, hand, Achilles tendon or other tendons may be increased in patients receiving concomitant corticosteroids, especially in the elderly).
No products indexed under this heading.

Diazepam (Ciprofloxacin is an inhibitor of CYP450 1A2 isoenzymes. Co-administration of ciprofloxacin and other drugs primarily metabolized by CYP1A2 results in increased plasma concentrations of the co-administered drug and could lead to clinically significant pharmacodynamic side effects). Products include:
Diastat Rectal Delivery System 3343
Valium Tablets 2819

Diclofenac Potassium (NSAIDs in combination with very high doses of quinolones have been shown to provoke convulsions in pre-clinical trials).
No products indexed under this heading.

Diclofenac Sodium (NSAIDs in combination with very high doses of quinolones have been shown to provoke convulsions in pre-clinical trials). Products include:
Arthrotec Tablets 3129
Voltaren Ophthalmic Solution 2309
Voltaren Tablets 2307
Voltaren-XR Tablets 2310

Dicumarol (Enhanced effects of anticoagulant).
No products indexed under this heading.

Didanosine (Didanosine (Videx) chewable tablets or pediatric powder for oral solution contains aluminum-magnesium-based antacid; co-administration may interfere with Cipro oral absorption; these preparations may be taken six hours before or two hours after taking ciprofloxacin).
No products indexed under this heading.

Diltiazem Hydrochloride (Ciprofloxacin is an inhibitor of CYP450 1A2 isoenzymes. Co-administration of ciprofloxacin and other drugs primarily metabolized by CYP1A2 results in increased plasma concentrations of the co-administered drug and could lead to clinically significant pharmacodynamic side effects). Products include:
Cardizem LA Extended Release Tablets 1728
Tiazac Capsules 1201

Diltiazem Maleate (Ciprofloxacin is an inhibitor of CYP450 1A2 isoenzymes. Co-administration of ciprofloxacin and other drugs primarily metabolized by CYP1A2 results in increased plasma concentrations of the co-administered drug and could lead to clinically significant pharmacodynamic side effects).
No products indexed under this heading.

Doxepin Hydrochloride (Ciprofloxacin is an inhibitor of CYP450 1A2 isoenzymes. Co-administration of ciprofloxacin and other drugs primarily metabolized by CYP1A2 results in increased plasma concentrations of the co-administered drug and could lead to clinically significant pharmacodynamic side effects).
No products indexed under this heading.

Dyphylline (Potential for severe and fatal reactions including cardiac arrest, seizures, respiratory failure and status epilepticus; concurrent use should be avoided or serum levels of theophylline should be monitored carefully).
No products indexed under this heading.

Enoxacin (Ciprofloxacin is an inhibitor of CYP450 1A2 isoenzymes. Co-administration of ciprofloxacin and other drugs primarily metabolized by CYP1A2 results in increased plasma concentrations of the co-administered drug and could lead to clinically significant pharmacodynamic side effects).
No products indexed under this heading.

Erythromycin (Ciprofloxacin is an inhibitor of CYP450 1A2 isoenzymes. Co-administration of ciprofloxacin and other drugs primarily metabolized by CYP1A2 results in increased plasma concentrations of the co-administered drug and could lead to clinically significant pharmacodynamic side effects). Products include:
Ery-Tab Tablets 449
Erythromycin Base Filmtab Tablets 455
Erythromycin Delayed-Release Capsules, USP 457
PCE Dispertab Tablets 515

Erythromycin Estolate (Ciprofloxacin is an inhibitor of CYP450 1A2 isoenzymes. Co-administration of ciprofloxacin and other drugs primarily metabolized by CYP1A2 results in increased plasma concentrations of the co-administered drug and could lead to clinically significant pharmacodynamic side effects).
No products indexed under this heading.

Erythromycin Ethylsuccinate (Ciprofloxacin is an inhibitor of CYP450 1A2 isoenzymes. Co-administration of ciprofloxacin and other drugs primarily metabolized by CYP1A2 results in increased plasma concentrations of the co-administered drug and could lead to clinically significant pharmacodynamic side effects). Products include:
E.E.S. 451
EryPed 447

Erythromycin Gluceptate (Ciprofloxacin is an inhibitor of CYP450 1A2 isoenzymes. Co-administration of ciprofloxacin and other drugs primarily metabolized by CYP1A2 results in increased plasma concentrations of the co-administered drug and could lead to clinically significant pharmacodynamic side effects).
No products indexed under this heading.

Erythromycin Lactobionate (Ciprofloxacin is an inhibitor of CYP450 1A2 isoenzymes. Co-administration of ciprofloxacin and other drugs primarily metabolized by CYP1A2 results in increased plasma concentrations of the co-administered drug and could lead to clinically significant pharmacodynamic side effects).
No products indexed under this heading.

Erythromycin Stearate (Ciprofloxacin is an inhibitor of CYP450 1A2 isoenzymes. Co-administration of ciprofloxacin and other drugs primarily metabolized by CYP1A2 results in increased plasma concentrations of the co-administered drug and could lead to clinically significant pharmacodynamic side effects). Products include:
Erythrocin Stearate Filmtab Tablets 453

Estradiol (Ciprofloxacin is an inhibitor of CYP450 1A2 isoenzymes. Co-administration of ciprofloxacin and other drugs primarily metabolized by CYP1A2 results in increased plasma concentrations of the co-administered drug and could lead to clinically significant pharmacodynamic side effects). Products include:
Angeliq Tablets 762
Climara Transdermal System 771
Climara Pro Transdermal System 776
Estrasorb Topical Emulsion 1147
Estring Vaginal Ring 2635
Menostar Transdermal System 782
Vagifem Tablets 2334

Estradiol Benzoate (Ciprofloxacin is an inhibitor of CYP450 1A2 isoenzymes. Co-administration of ciprofloxacin and other drugs primarily metabolized by CYP1A2 results in increased plasma concentrations of the co-administered drug and could lead to clinically significant pharmacodynamic side effects).
No products indexed under this heading.

Estradiol Cypionate (Ciprofloxacin is an inhibitor of CYP450 1A2 isoenzymes. Co-administration of ciprofloxacin and other drugs primarily metabolized by CYP1A2 results in increased plasma concentrations of the co-administered drug and could lead to clinically significant pharmacodynamic side effects).
No products indexed under this heading.

Etodolac (NSAIDs in combination with very high doses of quinolones have been shown to provoke convulsions in pre-clinical trials).
No products indexed under this heading.

Fenoprofen Calcium (NSAIDs in combination with very high doses of quinolones have been shown to provoke convulsions in pre-clinical trials). Products include:
Nalfon Capsules 2502

Ferrous Fumarate (Co-administration with iron-containing products may substantially interfere with the oral absorption of quinolones; these preparations may be taken six hours before or two hours after taking ciprofloxacin).
No products indexed under this heading.

Ferrous Gluconate (Co-administration with iron-containing products may substantially interfere with the oral absorption of quinolones; these preparations may be taken six hours before or two hours after taking ciprofloxacin).
No products indexed under this heading.

Ferrous Sulfate (Co-administration with iron-containing products may substantially interfere with the oral absorption of quinolones; these preparations may be taken six hours before or two hours after taking ciprofloxacin). Products include:
Slow Fe Iron Tablets .... ▣ 818
Slow Fe with Folic Acid Tablets .... ▣ 819

Fludrocortisone Acetate (Risk of ruptures of the shoulder, hand, Achilles tendon or other tendons may be increased in patients receiving concomitant corticosteroids, especially in the elderly).
No products indexed under this heading.

Flurbiprofen (NSAIDs in combination with very high doses of quinolones have been shown to provoke convulsions in pre-clinical trials).
No products indexed under this heading.

Flutamide (Ciprofloxacin is an inhibitor of CYP450 1A2 isoenzymes. Co-administration of ciprofloxacin and other drugs primarily metabolized by CYP1A2 results in increased plasma concentrations of the co-administered drug and could lead to clinically significant pharmacodynamic side effects). Products include:
Eulexin Capsules 3009

Fluticasone Propionate (Ciprofloxacin is an inhibitor of CYP450 1A2 isoenzymes. Co-administration of ciprofloxacin and other drugs primarily metabolized by CYP1A2 results in increased plasma concentrations of the co-administered drug and could lead to clinically significant pharmacodynamic side effects). Products include:
Advair Diskus 100/50 1308
Advair Diskus 250/50 1308
Advair Diskus 500/50 1308
Advair HFA Inhalation Aerosol 1318
Cutivate Cream 2662
Cutivate Lotion 0.05% 2664
Cutivate Ointment 2665
Flonase Nasal Spray 1440
Flovent Diskus 1443

Fluvoxamine Maleate (Ciprofloxacin is an inhibitor of CYP450 1A2 isoenzymes. Co-administration of ciprofloxacin and other drugs primarily metabolized by CYP1A2 results in increased plasma concentrations of the co-administered drug and could lead to clinically significant pharmacodynamic side effects).
No products indexed under this heading.

Fosphenytoin Sodium (Potential for change in serum phenytoin levels).
No products indexed under this heading.

Glyburide (Co-administration, on rare occasions, has resulted in severe hypoglycemia).
No products indexed under this heading.

Grepafloxacin Hydrochloride (Ciprofloxacin is an inhibitor of CYP450 1A2 isoenzymes. Co-administration of ciprofloxacin and other drugs primarily metabolized by CYP1A2 results in increased plasma concentrations of the co-administered drug and could lead to clinically significant pharmacodynamic side effects).
No products indexed under this heading.

Haloperidol (Ciprofloxacin is an inhibitor of CYP450 1A2 isoenzymes. Co-administration of ciprofloxacin and other drugs primarily metabolized by CYP1A2 results in increased plasma concentrations of the co-administered drug and could lead to clinically significant pharmacodynamic side effects).
No products indexed under this heading.

Haloperidol Decanoate (Ciprofloxacin is an inhibitor of CYP450 1A2 isoenzymes. Co-administration of ciprofloxacin and other drugs primarily metabolized by CYP1A2 results in increased plasma concentrations of the co-administered drug and could lead to clinically significant pharmacodynamic side effects).
No products indexed under this heading.

Haloperidol Lactate (Ciprofloxacin is an inhibitor of CYP450 1A2 isoenzymes. Co-administration of ciprofloxacin and other drugs primarily metabolized by CYP1A2 results in increased plasma concentrations of the co-administered drug and could lead to clinically significant pharmacodynamic side effects).
No products indexed under this heading.

Hydrocortisone (Risk of ruptures of the shoulder, hand, Achilles tendon or other tendons may be increased in patients receiving concomitant corticosteroids, especially in the elderly). Products include:
Colocort Rectal Suspension, USP (Retention) 100 mg/60 mL 2476
Hydrocortone Tablets 1989
Preparation H Hydrocortisone Cream .... ▣ 646

Hydrocortisone Acetate (Risk of ruptures of the shoulder, hand, Achilles tendon or other tendons may be increased in patients receiving concomitant corticosteroids, especially in the elderly). Products include:
Analpram-HC 1159
Pramosone 1161
ProctoFoam-HC 3099

Hydrocortisone Sodium Phosphate (Risk of ruptures of the shoulder, hand, Achilles tendon or other tendons may be increased in patients receiving concomitant corticosteroids, especially in the elderly).
No products indexed under this heading.

Hydrocortisone Sodium Succinate (Risk of ruptures of the shoulder, hand, Achilles tendon or other tendons may be increased in patients receiving concomitant corticosteroids, especially in the elderly).
No products indexed under this heading.

Ibuprofen (NSAIDs in combination with very high doses of quinolones have been shown to provoke convulsions in pre-clinical trials). Products include:
Advil Allergy Sinus Caplets .... ▣ 770
Advil .... ▣ 674
Children's Advil Oral Suspension .... ▣ 603
Children's Advil Chewable Tablets .... ▣ 603
Advil Cold & Sinus .... ▣ 723
Infants' Advil Concentrated Drops .... ▣ 604
Infants' Advil Concentrated Drops - White Grape (Dye-Free) .... ▣ 604
Junior Strength Advil Swallow Tablets .... ▣ 605
Advil Migraine Liquigels .... ▣ 608
Advil Multi-Symptom Cold Caplets .... ▣ 770
Advil PM Caplets .... ▣ 615
Motrin IB Tablets and Caplets 1866
Children's Motrin Oral Suspension 1867
Children's Motrin Non-Staining Dye-Free Oral Suspension 1867
Children's Motrin Cold Oral Suspension 1867
Infants' Motrin Concentrated Drops 1867
Infants' Motrin Non-Staining Dye-Free Concentrated Drops 1867
Junior Strength Motrin Caplets and Chewable Tablets 1867
Vicoprofen Tablets 539

Imipramine Hydrochloride (Ciprofloxacin is an inhibitor of CYP450 1A2 isoenzymes. Co-administration of ciprofloxacin and other drugs primarily metabolized by CYP1A2 results in increased plasma concentrations of the co-administered drug and could lead to clinically significant pharmacodynamic side effects).
No products indexed under this heading.

Imipramine Pamoate (Ciprofloxacin is an inhibitor of CYP450 1A2 isoenzymes. Co-administration of ciprofloxacin and other drugs primarily metabolized by CYP1A2 results in increased plasma concentrations of the co-administered drug and could lead to clinically significant pharmacodynamic side effects).
No products indexed under this heading.

Indomethacin (NSAIDs in combination with very high doses of quinolones have been shown to provoke convulsions in pre-clinical trials). Products include:
Indocin 1995

Indomethacin Sodium Trihydrate (NSAIDs in combination with very high doses of quinolones have been shown to provoke convulsions in pre-clinical trials). Products include:
Indocin I.V. 2465

Iron (Co-administration with iron-containing products may substantially interfere with the oral absorption of quinolones; these preparations may be taken six hours before or two hours after taking ciprofloxacin).
No products indexed under this heading.

Ketoprofen (NSAIDs in combination with very high doses of quinolones have been shown to provoke convulsions in pre-clinical trials).
No products indexed under this heading.

Ketorolac Tromethamine (NSAIDs in combination with very high doses of quinolones have been shown to provoke convulsions in pre-clinical trials). Products include:
Acular Ophthalmic Solution 565
Acular LS Ophthalmic Solution 566

Levobupivacaine Hydrochloride (Ciprofloxacin is an inhibitor of CYP450 1A2 isoenzymes. Co-administration of ciprofloxacin and other drugs primarily metabolized by CYP1A2 results in increased plasma concentrations of the co-administered drug and could lead to clinically significant pharmacodynamic side effects).
No products indexed under this heading.

Lomefloxacin Hydrochloride (Ciprofloxacin is an inhibitor of CYP450 1A2 isoenzymes. Co-administration of ciprofloxacin and other drugs primarily metabolized by CYP1A2 results in increased plasma concentrations of the co-administered drug and could lead to clinically significant pharmacodynamic side effects).
No products indexed under this heading.

Magaldrate (Concurrent administration of these antacids may substantially interfere with the oral absorption of ciprofloxacin; antacids may be administered either two hours after or six hours before ciprofloxacin dosing without a significant decrease in bioavailability).
No products indexed under this heading.

Magnesium Hydroxide (Concurrent administration of these antacids may substantially interfere with the oral absorption of ciprofloxacin; antacids may be administered either two hours after or six hours before ciprofloxacin dosing without a significant decrease in bioavailability). Products include:
Maalox Regular Strength Antacid/Antigas Liquid.................. 2175
Maalox Max Maximum Strength Antacid/Anti-Gas Liquid................. 2176
Pepcid Complete Chewable Tablets 1701

Magnesium Oxide (Concurrent administration of these antacids may substantially interfere with the oral absorption of ciprofloxacin; antacids may be administered either two hours after or six hours before ciprofloxacin dosing without a significant decrease in bioavailability). Products include:
Beelith Tablets 759
PremCal Light, Regular, and Extra Strength Tablets................. ▣818

Maprotiline Hydrochloride (Ciprofloxacin is an inhibitor of CYP450 1A2 isoenzymes. Co-administration of ciprofloxacin and other drugs primarily metabolized by CYP1A2 results in increased plasma concentrations of the co-administered drug and could lead to clinically significant pharmacodynamic side effects).
No products indexed under this heading.

Meclofenamate Sodium (NSAIDs in combination with very high doses of quinolones have been shown to provoke convulsions in pre-clinical trials).
No products indexed under this heading.

Mefenamic Acid (NSAIDs in combination with very high doses of quinolones have been shown to provoke convulsions in pre-clinical trials).
No products indexed under this heading.

Meloxicam (NSAIDs in combination with very high doses of quinolones

have been shown to provoke convulsions in pre-clinical trials). Products include:
Mobic Oral Suspension 863
Mobic Tablets 863

Methadone Hydrochloride (Ciprofloxacin is an inhibitor of CYP450 1A2 isoenzymes. Co-administration of ciprofloxacin and other drugs primarily metabolized by CYP1A2 results in increased plasma concentrations of the co-administered drug and could lead to clinically significant pharmacodynamic side effects).
No products indexed under this heading.

Methotrexate (Renal tubular transport of methotrexate may be inhibited by concomitant administration of ciprofloxacin potentially leading to increased plasma levels of methotrexate).
No products indexed under this heading.

Methotrexate Sodium (Renal tubular transport of methotrexate may be inhibited by concomitant administration of ciprofloxacin potentially leading to increased plasma levels of methotrexate).
No products indexed under this heading.

Methylprednisolone Acetate (Risk of ruptures of the shoulder, hand, Achilles tendon or other tendons may be increased in patients receiving concomitant corticosteroids, especially in the elderly). Products include:
Depo-Medrol Injectable Suspension 2617
Depo-Medrol Single-Dose Vial 2619

Methylprednisolone Sodium Succinate (Risk of ruptures of the shoulder, hand, Achilles tendon or other tendons may be increased in patients receiving concomitant corticosteroids, especially in the elderly).
No products indexed under this heading.

Metoclopramide Hydrochloride (Metoclopramide significantly accelerates the absorption of oral ciprofloxacin resulting in a shorter time to reach maximum plasma concentrations).
No products indexed under this heading.

Mexiletine Hydrochloride (Ciprofloxacin is an inhibitor of CYP450 1A2 isoenzymes. Co-administration of ciprofloxacin and other drugs primarily metabolized by CYP1A2 results in increased plasma concentrations of the co-administered drug and could lead to clinically significant pharmacodynamic side effects).
No products indexed under this heading.

Mirtazapine (Ciprofloxacin is an inhibitor of CYP450 1A2 isoenzymes. Co-administration of ciprofloxacin and other drugs primarily metabolized by CYP1A2 results in increased plasma concentrations of the co-administered drug and could lead to clinically significant pharmacodynamic side effects).
No products indexed under this heading.

Moxifloxacin Hydrochloride (Ciprofloxacin is an inhibitor of CYP450 1A2 isoenzymes. Co-administration of ciprofloxacin and other drugs primarily metabolized by CYP1A2 results in increased plasma concentrations of the co-

administered drug and could lead to clinically significant pharmacodynamic side effects). Products include:
Avelox .. 2970
Vigamox Ophthalmic Solution 564

Nabumetone (NSAIDs in combination with very high doses of quinolones have been shown to provoke convulsions in pre-clinical trials).
No products indexed under this heading.

Nafcillin Sodium (Ciprofloxacin is an inhibitor of CYP450 1A2 isoenzymes. Co-administration of ciprofloxacin and other drugs primarily metabolized by CYP1A2 results in increased plasma concentrations of the co-administered drug and could lead to clinically significant pharmacodynamic side effects).
No products indexed under this heading.

Naproxen (NSAIDs in combination with very high doses of quinolones have been shown to provoke convulsions in pre-clinical trials). Products include:
EC-Naprosyn Delayed-Release Tablets 2761
Naprosyn Suspension 2761
Naprosyn Tablets 2761
Prevacid NapraPAC 3280

Naproxen Sodium (NSAIDs in combination with very high doses of quinolones have been shown to provoke convulsions in pre-clinical trials). Products include:
Aleve Caplets 742
Aleve Gelcaps 743
Aleve Tablets 743
Aleve Cold & Sinus Caplets 744
Anaprox Tablets 2761
Anaprox DS Tablets 2761

Nicotine Polacrilex (Ciprofloxacin is an inhibitor of CYP450 1A2 isoenzymes. Co-administration of ciprofloxacin and other drugs primarily metabolized by CYP1A2 results in increased plasma concentrations of the co-administered drug and could lead to clinically significant pharmacodynamic side effects).
No products indexed under this heading.

Nicotine Salicylate (Ciprofloxacin is an inhibitor of CYP450 1A2 isoenzymes. Co-administration of ciprofloxacin and other drugs primarily metabolized by CYP1A2 results in increased plasma concentrations of the co-administered drug and could lead to clinically significant pharmacodynamic side effects).
No products indexed under this heading.

Nicotine Sulfate (Ciprofloxacin is an inhibitor of CYP450 1A2 isoenzymes. Co-administration of ciprofloxacin and other drugs primarily metabolized by CYP1A2 results in increased plasma concentrations of the co-administered drug and could lead to clinically significant pharmacodynamic side effects).
No products indexed under this heading.

Norethindrone Acetate (Ciprofloxacin is an inhibitor of CYP450 1A2 isoenzymes. Co-administration of ciprofloxacin and other drugs primarily metabolized by CYP1A2 results in increased plasma concentrations of the co-administered drug and could lead to clinically significant pharmacodynamic side effects).
No products indexed under this heading.

Norfloxacin (Ciprofloxacin is an inhibitor of CYP450 1A2 isoenzymes. Co-administration of ciprofloxacin and other drugs primarily metabolized by CYP1A2 results in increased plasma concentrations of the co-administered drug and could lead to clinically significant pharmacodynamic side effects). Products include:
Noroxin Tablets 2032

Nortriptyline Hydrochloride (Ciprofloxacin is an inhibitor of CYP450 1A2 isoenzymes. Co-administration of ciprofloxacin and other drugs primarily metabolized by CYP1A2 results in increased plasma concentrations of the co-administered drug and could lead to clinically significant pharmacodynamic side effects).
No products indexed under this heading.

Ofloxacin (Ciprofloxacin is an inhibitor of CYP450 1A2 isoenzymes. Co-administration of ciprofloxacin and other drugs primarily metabolized by CYP1A2 results in increased plasma concentrations of the co-administered drug and could lead to clinically significant pharmacodynamic side effects). Products include:
Floxin Otic Solution 1049

Olanzapine (Ciprofloxacin is an inhibitor of CYP450 1A2 isoenzymes. Co-administration of ciprofloxacin and other drugs primarily metabolized by CYP1A2 results in increased plasma concentrations of the co-administered drug and could lead to clinically significant pharmacodynamic side effects). Products include:
Symbyax Capsules 1819
Zyprexa Tablets 1830
Zyprexa IntraMuscular 1830
Zyprexa ZYDIS Orally Disintegrating Tablets.................. 1830

Ondansetron (Ciprofloxacin is an inhibitor of CYP450 1A2 isoenzymes. Co-administration of ciprofloxacin and other drugs primarily metabolized by CYP1A2 results in increased plasma concentrations of the co-administered drug and could lead to clinically significant pharmacodynamic side effects). Products include:
Zofran ODT Orally Disintegrating Tablets... 1639

Ondansetron Hydrochloride (Ciprofloxacin is an inhibitor of CYP450 1A2 isoenzymes. Co-administration of ciprofloxacin and other drugs primarily metabolized by CYP1A2 results in increased plasma concentrations of the co-administered drug and could lead to clinically significant pharmacodynamic side effects). Products include:
Zofran Injection 1634
Zofran .. 1639

Oxaprozin (NSAIDs in combination with very high doses of quinolones have been shown to provoke convulsions in pre-clinical trials).
No products indexed under this heading.

Phenobarbital Sodium (Ciprofloxacin is an inhibitor of CYP450 1A2 isoenzymes. Co-administration of ciprofloxacin and other drugs primarily metabolized by CYP1A2 results in increased plasma concentrations of the co-administered drug and could lead to clinically significant pharmacodynamic side effects).
No products indexed under this heading.

IMPORTANT NOTE: Always consult each drug listing in the patient's regimen for possible interactions.

Phenylbutazone (NSAIDs in combination with very high doses of quinolones have been shown to provoke convulsions in pre-clinical trials).
No products indexed under this heading.

Phenytoin (Potential for change in serum phenytoin levels).
No products indexed under this heading.

Phenytoin Sodium (Potential for change in serum phenytoin levels). Products include:
Phenytek Capsules 2160

Piroxicam (NSAIDs in combination with very high doses of quinolones have been shown to provoke convulsions in pre-clinical trials).
No products indexed under this heading.

Polysaccharide Iron Complex (Co-administration with iron-containing products may substantially interfere with the oral absorption of quinolones; these preparations may be taken six hours before or two hours after taking ciprofloxacin). Products include:
Nu-Iron 150 Capsules 2127

Prednisolone Acetate (Risk of ruptures of the shoulder, hand, Achilles tendon or other tendons may be increased in patients receiving concomitant corticosteroids, especially in the elderly). Products include:
Blephamide Ophthalmic Ointment 568
Blephamide Ophthalmic
Suspension.................................. 569
Poly-Pred Ophthalmic
Suspension.................................. ⊙233
Pred Forte Ophthalmic
Suspension.................................. ⊙235
Pred Mild Ophthalmic
Suspension.................................. ⊙238
Pred-G Ophthalmic Ointment ⊙237
Pred-G Ophthalmic Suspension ⊙236

Prednisolone Sodium Phosphate (Risk of ruptures of the shoulder, hand, Achilles tendon or other tendons may be increased in patients receiving concomitant corticosteroids, especially in the elderly).
No products indexed under this heading.

Prednisolone Tebutate (Risk of ruptures of the shoulder, hand, Achilles tendon or other tendons may be increased in patients receiving concomitant corticosteroids, especially in the elderly).
No products indexed under this heading.

Prednisone (Risk of ruptures of the shoulder, hand, Achilles tendon or other tendons may be increased in patients receiving concomitant corticosteroids, especially in the elderly).
No products indexed under this heading.

Probenecid (Interferes with renal tubular secretion of ciprofloxacin).
No products indexed under this heading.

Propafenone Hydrochloride (Ciprofloxacin is an inhibitor of CYP450 1A2 isoenzymes. Co-administration of ciprofloxacin and other drugs primarily metabolized by CYP1A2 results in increased plasma concentrations of the co-administered drug and could lead to clinically significant pharmacodynamic side effects). Products include:
Rythmol SR Capsules 2727

Propranolol Hydrochloride (Ciprofloxacin is an inhibitor of CYP450 1A2 isoenzymes. Co-

administration of ciprofloxacin and other drugs primarily metabolized by CYP1A2 results in increased plasma concentrations of the co-administered drug and could lead to clinically significant pharmacodynamic side effects). Products include:
Inderal LA Long-Acting Capsules 3429
InnoPran XL Capsules 2723

Protriptyline Hydrochloride (Ciprofloxacin is an inhibitor of CYP450 1A2 isoenzymes. Co-administration of ciprofloxacin and other drugs primarily metabolized by CYP1A2 results in increased plasma concentrations of the co-administered drug and could lead to clinically significant pharmacodynamic side effects).
No products indexed under this heading.

Riluzole (Ciprofloxacin is an inhibitor of CYP450 1A2 isoenzymes. Co-administration of ciprofloxacin and other drugs primarily metabolized by CYP1A2 results in increased plasma concentrations of the co-administered drug and could lead to clinically significant pharmacodynamic side effects). Products include:
Rilutek Tablets 2930

Ritonavir (Ciprofloxacin is an inhibitor of CYP450 1A2 isoenzymes. Co-administration of ciprofloxacin and other drugs primarily metabolized by CYP1A2 results in increased plasma concentrations of the co-administered drug and could lead to clinically significant pharmacodynamic side effects). Products include:
Kaletra .. 476
Norvir ... 503

Rofecoxib (NSAIDs in combination with very high doses of quinolones have been shown to provoke convulsions in pre-clinical trials).
No products indexed under this heading.

Ropinirole Hydrochloride (Ciprofloxacin is an inhibitor of CYP450 1A2 isoenzymes. Co-administration of ciprofloxacin and other drugs primarily metabolized by CYP1A2 results in increased plasma concentrations of the co-administered drug and could lead to clinically significant pharmacodynamic side effects). Products include:
Requip Tablets 1555

Ropivacaine Hydrochloride (Ciprofloxacin is an inhibitor of CYP450 1A2 isoenzymes. Co-administration of ciprofloxacin and other drugs primarily metabolized by CYP1A2 results in increased plasma concentrations of the co-administered drug and could lead to clinically significant pharmacodynamic side effects).
No products indexed under this heading.

Sucralfate (Co-administration with sucralfate may substantially interfere with the oral absorption of quinolones; these preparations may be taken six hours before or two hours after taking ciprofloxacin). Products include:
Carafate Suspension 701
Carafate Tablets 701

Sulindac (NSAIDs in combination with very high doses of quinolones have been shown to provoke convulsions in pre-clinical trials). Products include:
Clinoril Tablets 1924

Tacrine Hydrochloride (Ciprofloxacin is an inhibitor of CYP450 1A2 isoenzymes. Co-administration of ciprofloxacin and other drugs primarily metabolized by CYP1A2 results in increased plasma concentrations of the co-administered drug and could lead to clinically significant pharmacodynamic side effects).
No products indexed under this heading.

Tamoxifen Citrate (Ciprofloxacin is an inhibitor of CYP450 1A2 isoenzymes. Co-administration of ciprofloxacin and other drugs primarily metabolized by CYP1A2 results in increased plasma concentrations of the co-administered drug and could lead to clinically significant pharmacodynamic side effects). Products include:
Soltamox Oral Solution 3527

Theophylline (Potential for severe and fatal reactions including cardiac arrest, seizures, respiratory failure and status epilepticus; concurrent use should be avoided or serum levels of theophylline should be monitored carefully).
No products indexed under this heading.

Theophylline Anhydrous (Potential for severe and fatal reactions including cardiac arrest, seizures, respiratory failure and status epilepticus; concurrent use should be avoided or serum levels of theophylline should be monitored carefully). Products include:
Uniphyl Tablets 2710

Theophylline Calcium Salicylate (Potential for severe and fatal reactions including cardiac arrest, seizures, respiratory failure and status epilepticus; concurrent use should be avoided or serum levels of theophylline should be monitored carefully).
No products indexed under this heading.

Theophylline Dihydroxypropyl (Glyceryl) (Potential for severe and fatal reactions including cardiac arrest, seizures, respiratory failure and status epilepticus; concurrent use should be avoided or serum levels of theophylline should be monitored carefully).
No products indexed under this heading.

Theophylline Ethylenediamine (Potential for severe and fatal reactions including cardiac arrest, seizures, respiratory failure and status epilepticus; concurrent use should be avoided or serum levels of theophylline should be monitored carefully).
No products indexed under this heading.

Theophylline Sodium Glycinate (Potential for severe and fatal reactions including cardiac arrest, seizures, respiratory failure and status epilepticus; concurrent use should be avoided or serum levels of theophylline should be monitored carefully).
No products indexed under this heading.

Tizanidine Hydrochloride (Concomitant administration is contraindicated).
No products indexed under this heading.

Tolmetin Sodium (NSAIDs in combination with very high doses of quinolones have been shown to provoke convulsions in pre-clinical trials).
No products indexed under this heading.

Triamcinolone (Risk of ruptures of the shoulder, hand, Achilles tendon or other tendons may be increased in patients receiving concomitant corticosteroids, especially in the elderly).
No products indexed under this heading.

Triamcinolone Acetonide (Risk of ruptures of the shoulder, hand, Achilles tendon or other tendons may be increased in patients receiving concomitant corticosteroids, especially in the elderly). Products include:
Azmacort Inhalation Aerosol 1726
Nasacort AQ Nasal Spray 2922

Triamcinolone Diacetate (Risk of ruptures of the shoulder, hand, Achilles tendon or other tendons may be increased in patients receiving concomitant corticosteroids, especially in the elderly).
No products indexed under this heading.

Triamcinolone Hexacetonide (Risk of ruptures of the shoulder, hand, Achilles tendon or other tendons may be increased in patients receiving concomitant corticosteroids, especially in the elderly).
No products indexed under this heading.

Trimethaphan Camsylate (Ciprofloxacin is an inhibitor of CYP450 1A2 isoenzymes. Co-administration of ciprofloxacin and other drugs primarily metabolized by CYP1A2 results in increased plasma concentrations of the co-administered drug and could lead to clinically significant pharmacodynamic side effects).
No products indexed under this heading.

Trimipramine Maleate (Ciprofloxacin is an inhibitor of CYP450 1A2 isoenzymes. Co-administration of ciprofloxacin and other drugs primarily metabolized by CYP1A2 results in increased plasma concentrations of the co-administered drug and could lead to clinically significant pharmacodynamic side effects).
No products indexed under this heading.

Trovafloxacin Mesylate (Ciprofloxacin is an inhibitor of CYP450 1A2 isoenzymes. Co-administration of ciprofloxacin and other drugs primarily metabolized by CYP1A2 results in increased plasma concentrations of the co-administered drug and could lead to clinically significant pharmacodynamic side effects).
No products indexed under this heading.

Valdecoxib (NSAIDs in combination with very high doses of quinolones have been shown to provoke convulsions in pre-clinical trials).
No products indexed under this heading.

Verapamil Hydrochloride (Ciprofloxacin is an inhibitor of CYP450 1A2 isoenzymes. Co-administration of ciprofloxacin and other drugs primarily metabolized by CYP1A2 results in increased plasma concentrations of the co-administered drug and could lead to clinically significant pharmacodynamic side effects). Products include:

- Covera-HS Tablets 3139
- Tarka Tablets 524
- Verelan PM Extended-Release Capsules, Controlled-Onset 3106

Warfarin Sodium (Enhanced effects of anticoagulant). Products include:

- Coumadin for Injection 898
- Coumadin Tablets 898

Zileuton (Ciprofloxacin is an inhibitor of CYP450 1A2 isoenzymes. Co-administration of ciprofloxacin and other drugs primarily metabolized by CYP1A2 results in increased plasma concentrations of the co-administered drug and could lead to clinically significant pharmacodynamic side effects). Products include:

- Zyflo Tablets 1023

Zinc Sulfate (Co-administration with zinc-containing products may substantially interfere with the oral absorption of quinolones; these preparations may be taken six hours before or two hours after taking ciprofloxacin). Products include:

- Visine A.C. Seasonal Itching and Redness Relief Drops .... ⊙ 289
- Zinc-220 Capsules 580

Zolmitriptan (Ciprofloxacin is an inhibitor of CYP450 1A2 isoenzymes. Co-administration of ciprofloxacin and other drugs primarily metabolized by CYP1A2 results in increased plasma concentrations of the co-administered drug and could lead to clinically significant pharmacodynamic side effects). Products include:

- Zomig Tablets 3519
- Zomig Nasal Spray 3523
- Zomig-ZMT Tablets 3519

Food Interactions

Dairy products (Oral ciprofloxacin should not be taken concurrently with milk or yogurt alone, since absorption of ciprofloxacin may be significantly reduced; dietary calcium as part of a meal, however, does not significantly affect ciprofloxacin absorption).

Food, unspecified (Delays the oral absorption of the drug resulting in peak concentrations that are closer to two hours after dosing).

CIPRODEX OTIC SUSPENSION

(Ciprofloxacin, Dexamethasone) 559

None cited in PDR database.

CIPRO I.V.

(Ciprofloxacin) 2984

May interact with antacids containing aluminum, calcium and magnesium, calcium preparations, corticosteroids, oral anticoagulants, cytochrome p450 1a2 substrates (selected), iron containing oral preparations, non-steroidal anti-inflammatory agents, phenytoin, xanthines, and certain other agents. Compounds in these categories include:

Acetaminophen (Ciprofloxacin is a moderate inhibitor of CYP450 1A2 isoenzymes. Co-administration of ciprofloxacin and other drugs primarily metabolized by the CYP450 1A2 enzyme pathway may result in increased plasma concentrations of the co-administered drug and couldlead to clinically significant pharmacodynamic side effects). Products include:

- Comtrex Maximum Strength Cold & Cough Day/Night Caplets - Day Formulation 726
- Comtrex Maximum Strength Cold & Cough Day/Night Caplets - Night Formulation 726
- Comtrex Maximum Strength Non-Drowsy Cold & Cough Caplets 725
- Comtrex Maximum Strength Day/Night Severe Cold & Sinus Caplets - Day Formulation 725
- Comtrex Maximum Strength Day/Night Severe Cold & Sinus Caplets - Night Formulation 725
- Contac Cold and Flu Maximum Strength Caplets 728
- Contac Cold and Flu Day and Night Caplets (Day Formulation Only) 727
- Contac Cold and Flu Day and Night Caplets (Night Formulation Only) 727
- Contac Cold and Flu Non-Drowsy Caplets 728
- Excedrin Extra Strength Caplets/Tablets/Geltabs 684
- Excedrin Migraine Caplets/Tablets/Geltabs 609
- Excedrin PM Caplets/Tablets/Geltabs 610
- Excedrin Sinus Headache Caplets/Tablets 610
- Excedrin Tension Headache Caplets/Tablets/Geltabs 611
- Goody's Body Pain Formula Powder 684
- Goody's Extra Strength Headache Powders 611
- Goody's Extra Strength Pain Relief Tablets 685
- Goody's PM Powder for Pain with Sleeplessness 612
- Percocet Tablets 1131
- Robitussin Cough, Cold & Flu Nighttime Liquid 738
- TheraFlu Cold & Sore Throat Hot Liquid 741
- TheraFlu Flu & Chest Congestion Hot Liquid 741
- TheraFlu Flu & Sore Throat Hot Liquid 742
- TheraFlu Daytime Severe Cold Hot Liquid 742
- TheraFlu Nighttime Severe Cold Hot Liquid 740
- TheraFlu Warming Relief Daytime Severe Cold 743
- TheraFlu Warming Relief Nighttime Severe Cold 743
- Triaminic Cough & Sore Throat Liquid 747
- Regular Strength Tylenol Tablets 1870
- Children's Tylenol with Flavor Creator 679
- Children's Tylenol Plus Flu Oral Suspension 749
- Tylenol Cold Head Congestion Daytime Caplets with Cool Burst and Gelcaps 750
- Tylenol Cold Multi-Symptom Daytime Liquid 752
- Tylenol Cold Multi-Symptom Severe Daytime Liquid 752
- Tylenol 8 Hour Extended Release Caplets 1870
- Tylenol 1870
- Extra Strength Tylenol PM Caplets, Vanilla Caplets, Geltabs, Gelcaps and Liquid 1875
- Extra Strength Tylenol Rapid Release Gels 1870
- Concentrated Tylenol Infants' Drops Plus Cold & Cough 754
- Tylenol with Codeine Tablets 2391
- Tylenol Allergy Multi-Symptom Caplets with Cool Burst and Gelcaps 1872
- Tylenol Allergy Multi-Symptom Nighttime Caplets with Cool Burst 1872
- Tylenol Severe Allergy Caplets 1872
- Tylenol Arthritis Pain Extended Release Caplets and Geltabs 1870
- Tylenol Chest Congestion Caplets with Cool Burst 1872
- Tylenol Chest Congestion Liquid with Cool Burst 1872
- Children's Tylenol Suspension Liquid and Meltaways 1878
- Children's Tylenol Plus Cold Suspension Liquid 1879
- Children's Tylenol Plus Cold & Allergy Suspension Liquid 1878
- Children's Tylenol Plus Cough & Runny Nose Suspension Liquid 1879
- Children's Tylenol Plus Cough & Sore Throat Suspension Liquid 1879
- Children's Tylenol Suspension with Flavor Creator 1878
- Children's Tylenol Plus Flu Suspension Liquid 1881
- Children's Tylenol Plus Multi-Symptom Cold Suspension Liquid 1879
- Tylenol Cold Severe Congestion Non-Drowsy Caplets with Cool Burst 1874
- Tylenol Cold Head Congestion Daytime Caplets with Cool Burst 1873
- Tylenol Cold Head Congestion Nighttime Caplets with Cool Burst 1873
- Tylenol Cold Head Congestion Severe Caplets with Cool Burst 1873
- Tylenol Cold Multi-Symptom Daytime Caplets with Cool Burst and Gelcaps 1874
- Tylenol Cold Multi-Symptom Daytime Liquid with Citrus Burst 1874
- Tylenol Cold Multi-Symptom Nighttime Caplets with Cool Burst 1874
- Tylenol Cold Multi-Symptom Nighttime Liquid with Cool Burst 1874
- Tylenol Cold Multi-Symptom Severe Caplets with Cool Burst 1874
- Tylenol Cold Multi-Symptom Severe Daytime Liquid with Citrus Burst 1874
- Tylenol Cough & Sore Throat Daytime Liquid with Cool Burst 1877
- Tylenol Cough & Sore Throat Nighttime Liquid with Cool Burst 1877
- Concentrated Tylenol Infants' Drops 1878
- Concentrated Tylenol Infants' Drops Plus Cold 1879
- Concentrated Tylenol Infants' Drops Plus Cold and Cough 1879
- Jr. Tylenol Meltaways 1878
- Tylenol Sinus Severe Congestion Caplets with Cool Burst 1876
- Tylenol Sinus Congestion & Pain Daytime Caplets with Cool Burst and Gelcaps 1876
- Tylenol Sinus Congestion & Pain Nighttime Caplets with Cool Burst 1876
- Tylenol Sinus Congestion & Pain Severe Caplets with Cool Burst 1876
- Tylenol Sore Throat Daytime Liquid with Cool Burst 1877
- Tylenol Sore Throat Nighttime Liquid with Cool Burst 1877
- Women's Tylenol Menstrual Relief Caplets 1877
- Vicks 44M Cough, Cold & Flu Relief Liquid 2680
- Vicks DayQuil LiquiCaps/Liquid Multi-Symptom Cold/Flu Relief 761
- Vicks DayQuil Multi-Symptom Cold/Flu Relief LiquiCaps 2678
- Vicks DayQuil Multi-Symptom Cold/Flu Relief Liquid 2678
- Vicks NyQuil Multi-Symptom Cold/Flu Relief Liquid 2681
- Vicks NyQuil Multi-Symptom Cold/Flu Relief LiquiCaps 2681
- Vicks NyQuil LiquiCaps/Liquid Multi-Symptom Cold/Flu Relief 763
- Vicodin Tablets 535
- Vicodin ES Tablets 536
- Vicodin HP Tablets 538
- Zicam Maximum Strength Flu Daytime 768
- Zicam Maximum Strength Flu Nighttime 768
- Zydone Tablets 1139

Alatrofloxacin Mesylate (Ciprofloxacin is a moderate inhibitor of CYP450 1A2 isoenzymes. Co-administration of ciprofloxacin and other drugs primarily metabolized by the CYP450 1A2 enzyme pathway may result in increased plasma concentrations of the co-administered drug and couldlead to clinically significant pharmacodynamic side effects).

No products indexed under this heading.

Aluminum Carbonate (Concurrent administration of these antacids may substantially interfere with the oral absorption of ciprofloxacin; antacids may be administered either two hours after or six hours before ciprofloxacin dosing without a significant decrease in bioavailability).

No products indexed under this heading.

Aluminum Hydroxide (Concurrent administration of these antacids may substantially interfere with the oral absorption of ciprofloxacin; antacids may be administered either two hours after or six hours before ciprofloxacin dosing without a significant decrease in bioavailability). Products include:

- Gaviscon Regular Strength Liquid 658
- Gaviscon Regular Strength Tablets 658
- Gaviscon Extra Strength Liquid 658
- Gaviscon Extra Strength Tablets 658
- Maalox Regular Strength Antacid/Antigas Liquid 2175
- Maalox Max Maximum Strength Antacid/Anti-Gas Liquid 2176

Aminophylline (Potential for severe and fatal reactions including cardiac arrest, seizures, respiratory failure and status epilepticus; concurrent use should be avoided or serum levels of theophylline should be monitored carefully).

No products indexed under this heading.

Amiodarone Hydrochloride (Ciprofloxacin is a moderate inhibitor of CYP450 1A2 isoenzymes. Co-administration of ciprofloxacin and other drugs primarily metabolized by the CYP450 1A2 enzyme pathway may result in increased plasma concentrations of the co-administered drug and couldlead to clinically significant pharmacodynamic side effects).

No products indexed under this heading.

Amitriptyline Hydrochloride (Ciprofloxacin is a moderate inhibitor of CYP450 1A2 isoenzymes. Co-administration of ciprofloxacin and other drugs primarily metabolized by the CYP450 1A2 enzyme pathway may result in increased plasma concentrations of the co-administered drug and couldlead to clinically significant pharmacodynamic side effects).

No products indexed under this heading.

Amoxapine (Ciprofloxacin is a moderate inhibitor of CYP450 1A2 isoenzymes. Co-administration of ciprofloxacin and other drugs primarily metabolized by the CYP450 1A2 enzyme pathway may result in increased plasma concentrations of the co-administered drug and couldlead to clinically significant pharmacodynamic side effects).

No products indexed under this heading.

Anagrelide Hydrochloride (Ciprofloxacin is a moderate inhibitor of CYP450 1A2 isoenzymes. Co-administration of ciprofloxacin and other drugs primarily metabolized by the CYP450 1A2 enzyme pathway may result in increased plasma concentrations of the co-administered drug and couldlead to clinically significant pharmacodynamic side effects). Products include:
- Agrylin Capsules **3169**

Anisindione (Enhanced effects of anticoagulant). Products include:
- Miradon Tablets **3042**

Betamethasone Acetate (Risk of ruptures of the shoulder, hand, Achilles tendon or other tendons may be increased in patients receiving concomitant corticosteroids, especially in the elderly).
- No products indexed under this heading.

Betamethasone Sodium Phosphate (Risk of ruptures of the shoulder, hand, Achilles tendon or other tendons may be increased in patients receiving concomitant corticosteroids, especially in the elderly).
- No products indexed under this heading.

Caffeine (Reduced clearance of caffeine and a prolongation of its serum half-life). Products include:
- BC Headache Powder ..... ▣**677**
- Arthritis Strength BC Powder ..... ▣**677**
- Excedrin Extra Strength Caplets/Tablets/Geltabs ..... ▣**684**
- Excedrin Migraine Caplets/Tablets/Geltabs ..... ▣**609**
- Excedrin Tension Headache Caplets/Tablets/Geltabs ..... ▣**611**
- Goody's Extra Strength Headache Powders ..... ▣**611**
- Goody's Extra Strength Pain Relief Tablets ..... ▣**685**
- Vivarin ..... ▣**602**
- Winrgy Dietary Supplement ..... ▣**823**

Caffeine Anhydrous (Ciprofloxacin is a moderate inhibitor of CYP450 1A2 isoenzymes. Co-administration of ciprofloxacin and other drugs primarily metabolized by the CYP450 1A2 enzyme pathway may result in increased plasma concentrations of the co-administered drug and couldlead to clinically significant pharmacodynamic side effects).
- No products indexed under this heading.

Caffeine Citrate (Reduced clearance of caffeine and a prolongation of its serum half-life). Products include:
- Cafcit **1886**

Calcium Carbonate (Co-administration with calcium-containing products may substantially interfere with the oral absorption of quinolones; these preparations may be taken six hours before or two hours after taking ciprofloxacin). Products include:
- Actonel with Calcium Tablets **2688**
- Calcet Tablets **2138**
- Caltrate 600 PLUS ..... ▣**809**
- Caltrate 600 + D Tablets ..... ▣**809**
- D-Cal Chewable Caplets ..... ▣**812**
- Gas-X with Maalox ..... ▣**656**
- Maalox Regular Strength Antacid Chewable Tablets **2177**
- Maalox Max Maximum Strength Antacid/Antigas Chewable Tablets **2176**
- Maalox Max Maximum Strength Chewable Tablets ..... ▣**660**
- Os-Cal Chewable Tablets ..... ▣**818**
- Pepcid Complete Chewable Tablets **1701**
- Children's Pepto **2674**
- PremCal Light, Regular, and Extra Strength Tablets ..... ▣**818**
- Tums ..... ▣**664**

Calcium Chloride (Co-administration with calcium-containing products may substantially interfere with the oral absorption of quinolones; these preparations may be taken six hours before or two hours after taking ciprofloxacin).
- No products indexed under this heading.

Calcium Citrate (Co-administration with calcium-containing products may substantially interfere with the oral absorption of quinolones; these preparations may be taken six hours before or two hours after taking ciprofloxacin). Products include:
- Active Calcium Tablets **3339**
- Citracal Caplets ..... ▣**703**
- Citracal Lemon Cream Creamy Bites **2139**
- Citracal Prenatal + DHA Tablets and Capsules **2139**

Calcium Glubionate (Co-administration with calcium-containing products may substantially interfere with the oral absorption of quinolones; these preparations may be taken six hours before or two hours after taking ciprofloxacin).
- No products indexed under this heading.

Celecoxib (NSAIDs in combination with very high doses of quinolones have been shown to provoke convulsions in pre-clinical trials). Products include:
- Celebrex Capsules **3134**

Chlordiazepoxide (Ciprofloxacin is a moderate inhibitor of CYP450 1A2 isoenzymes. Co-administration of ciprofloxacin and other drugs primarily metabolized by the CYP450 1A2 enzyme pathway may result in increased plasma concentrations of the co-administered drug and couldlead to clinically significant pharmacodynamic side effects).
- No products indexed under this heading.

Chlordiazepoxide Hydrochloride (Ciprofloxacin is a moderate inhibitor of CYP450 1A2 isoenzymes. Co-administration of ciprofloxacin and other drugs primarily metabolized by the CYP450 1A2 enzyme pathway may result in increased plasma concentrations of the co-administered drug and couldlead to clinically significant pharmacodynamic side effects). Products include:
- Librium Capsules **3347**

Cimetidine Hydrochloride (Ciprofloxacin is a moderate inhibitor of CYP450 1A2 isoenzymes. Co-administration of ciprofloxacin and other drugs primarily metabolized by the CYP450 1A2 enzyme pathway may result in increased plasma concentrations of the co-administered drug and couldlead to clinically significant pharmacodynamic side effects).
- No products indexed under this heading.

Ciprofloxacin Hydrochloride (Ciprofloxacin is a moderate inhibitor of CYP450 1A2 isoenzymes. Co-administration of ciprofloxacin and other drugs primarily metabolized by the CYP450 1A2 enzyme pathway may result in increased plasma concentrations of the co-administered drug and couldlead to clinically significant pharmacodynamic side effects). Products include:
- Ciloxan Ophthalmic Ointment **559**
- Ciloxan Ophthalmic Solution ..... ⊙**206**
- Cipro Tablets **2977**
- Proquin XR Tablets **1153**

Clomipramine Hydrochloride (Ciprofloxacin is a moderate inhibitor of CYP450 1A2 isoenzymes. Co-administration of ciprofloxacin and other drugs primarily metabolized by the CYP450 1A2 enzyme pathway may result in increased plasma concentrations of the co-administered drug and couldlead to clinically significant pharmacodynamic side effects).
- No products indexed under this heading.

Clopidogrel Bisulfate (Ciprofloxacin is a moderate inhibitor of CYP450 1A2 isoenzymes. Co-administration of ciprofloxacin and other drugs primarily metabolized by the CYP450 1A2 enzyme pathway may result in increased plasma concentrations of the co-administered drug and couldlead to clinically significant pharmacodynamic side effects). Products include:
- Plavix Tablets **917**
- Plavix Tablets **2926**

Clozapine (Ciprofloxacin is a moderate inhibitor of CYP450 1A2 isoenzymes. Co-administration of ciprofloxacin and other drugs primarily metabolized by the CYP450 1A2 enzyme pathway may result in increased plasma concentrations of the co-administered drug and couldlead to clinically significant pharmacodynamic side effects). Products include:
- Clozaril Tablets **2184**
- FazaClo Orally Disintegrating Tablets **551**

Cortisone Acetate (Risk of ruptures of the shoulder, hand, Achilles tendon or other tendons may be increased in patients receiving concomitant corticosteroids, especially in the elderly).
- No products indexed under this heading.

Cyclobenzaprine (Ciprofloxacin is a moderate inhibitor of CYP450 1A2 isoenzymes. Co-administration of ciprofloxacin and other drugs primarily metabolized by the CYP450 1A2 enzyme pathway may result in increased plasma concentrations of the co-administered drug and couldlead to clinically significant pharmacodynamic side effects).
- No products indexed under this heading.

Cyclobenzaprine Hydrochloride (Ciprofloxacin is a moderate inhibitor of CYP450 1A2 isoenzymes. Co-administration of ciprofloxacin and other drugs primarily metabolized by the CYP450 1A2 enzyme pathway may result in increased plasma concentrations of the co-administered drug and couldlead to clinically significant pharmacodynamic side effects).
- No products indexed under this heading.

Cyclosporine (Transient elevations in serum creatinine). Products include:
- Gengraf Capsules **459**
- Neoral Oral Solution **2259**
- Neoral Soft Gelatin Capsules **2259**
- Restasis Ophthalmic Emulsion **575**
- Sandimmune **2275**

Desipramine Hydrochloride (Ciprofloxacin is a moderate inhibitor of CYP450 1A2 isoenzymes. Co-administration of ciprofloxacin and other drugs primarily metabolized by the CYP450 1A2 enzyme pathway may result in increased plasma concentrations of the co-administered drug and couldlead to clinically significant pharmacodynamic side effects).
- No products indexed under this heading.

Dexamethasone (Risk of ruptures of the shoulder, hand, Achilles tendon or other tendons may be increased in patients receiving concomitant corticosteroids, especially in the elderly). Products include:
- Ciprodex Otic Suspension **559**
- Decadron Tablets **1951**
- TobraDex Ophthalmic Ointment **562**
- TobraDex Ophthalmic Suspension **563**

Dexamethasone Acetate (Risk of ruptures of the shoulder, hand, Achilles tendon or other tendons may be increased in patients receiving concomitant corticosteroids, especially in the elderly).
- No products indexed under this heading.

Dexamethasone Sodium Phosphate (Risk of ruptures of the shoulder, hand, Achilles tendon or other tendons may be increased in patients receiving concomitant corticosteroids, especially in the elderly).
- No products indexed under this heading.

Diazepam (Ciprofloxacin is a moderate inhibitor of CYP450 1A2 isoenzymes. Co-administration of ciprofloxacin and other drugs primarily metabolized by the CYP450 1A2 enzyme pathway may result in increased plasma concentrations of the co-administered drug and couldlead to clinically significant pharmacodynamic side effects). Products include:
- Diastat Rectal Delivery System **3343**
- Valium Tablets **2819**

Diclofenac Potassium (NSAIDs in combination with very high doses of quinolones have been shown to provoke convulsions in pre-clinical trials).
- No products indexed under this heading.

Diclofenac Sodium (NSAIDs in combination with very high doses of quinolones have been shown to provoke convulsions in pre-clinical trials). Products include:
- Arthrotec Tablets **3129**
- Voltaren Ophthalmic Solution **2309**
- Voltaren Tablets **2307**
- Voltaren-XR Tablets **2310**

Dicumarol (Enhanced effects of anticoagulant).
- No products indexed under this heading.

Didanosine (Didanosine (Videx) chewable tablets or pediatric powder for oral solution contains aluminum-magnesium-based antacid; co-administration may interfere with Cipro oral absorption; these preparations may be taken six hours before or two hours after taking ciprofloxacin).
- No products indexed under this heading.

Diltiazem Hydrochloride (Ciprofloxacin is a moderate inhibitor of CYP450 1A2 isoenzymes. Co-administration of ciprofloxacin and other drugs primarily metabolized by the CYP450 1A2 enzyme pathway may result in increased plasma concentrations of the co-administered drug and couldlead to clinically significant pharmacodynamic side effects). Products include:

Cardizem LA Extended Release Tablets 1728
Tiazac Capsules 1201

Diltiazem Maleate (Ciprofloxacin is a moderate inhibitor of CYP450 1A2 isoenzymes. Co-administration of ciprofloxacin and other drugs primarily metabolized by the CYP450 1A2 enzyme pathway may result in increased plasma concentrations of the co-administered drug and could-lead to clinically significant pharmacodynamic side effects).

No products indexed under this heading.

Doxepin Hydrochloride (Ciprofloxacin is a moderate inhibitor of CYP450 1A2 isoenzymes. Co-administration of ciprofloxacin and other drugs primarily metabolized by the CYP450 1A2 enzyme pathway may result in increased plasma concentrations of the co-administered drug and couldlead to clinically significant pharmacodynamic side effects).

No products indexed under this heading.

Dyphylline (Potential for severe and fatal reactions including cardiac arrest, seizures, respiratory failure and status epilepticus; concurrent use should be avoided or serum levels of theophylline should be monitored carefully).

No products indexed under this heading.

Enoxacin (Ciprofloxacin is a moderate inhibitor of CYP450 1A2 isoenzymes. Co-administration of ciprofloxacin and other drugs primarily metabolized by the CYP450 1A2 enzyme pathway may result in increased plasma concentrations of the co-administered drug and could-lead to clinically significant pharmacodynamic side effects).

No products indexed under this heading.

Erythromycin (Ciprofloxacin is a moderate inhibitor of CYP450 1A2 isoenzymes. Co-administration of ciprofloxacin and other drugs primarily metabolized by the CYP450 1A2 enzyme pathway may result in increased plasma concentrations of the co-administered drug and could-lead to clinically significant pharmacodynamic side effects). Products include:

Ery-Tab Tablets 449
Erythromycin Base Filmtab Tablets 455
Erythromycin Delayed-Release Capsules, USP 457
PCE Dispertab Tablets 515

Erythromycin Estolate (Ciprofloxacin is a moderate inhibitor of CYP450 1A2 isoenzymes. Co-administration of ciprofloxacin and other drugs primarily metabolized by the CYP450 1A2 enzyme pathway may result in increased plasma concentrations of the co-administered drug and couldlead to clinically significant pharmacodynamic side effects).

No products indexed under this heading.

Erythromycin Ethylsuccinate (Ciprofloxacin is a moderate inhibitor of CYP450 1A2 isoenzymes. Co-administration of ciprofloxacin and other drugs primarily metabolized by the CYP450 1A2 enzyme pathway may result in increased plasma concentrations of the co-administered drug and couldlead to clinically significant pharmacodynamic side effects). Products include:

E.E.S. 451
EryPed 447

Erythromycin Gluceptate (Ciprofloxacin is a moderate inhibitor of CYP450 1A2 isoenzymes. Co-administration of ciprofloxacin and other drugs primarily metabolized by the CYP450 1A2 enzyme pathway may result in increased plasma concentrations of the co-administered drug and couldlead to clinically significant pharmacodynamic side effects).

No products indexed under this heading.

Erythromycin Lactobionate (Ciprofloxacin is a moderate inhibitor of CYP450 1A2 isoenzymes. Co-administration of ciprofloxacin and other drugs primarily metabolized by the CYP450 1A2 enzyme pathway may result in increased plasma concentrations of the co-administered drug and couldlead to clinically significant pharmacodynamic side effects).

No products indexed under this heading.

Erythromycin Stearate (Ciprofloxacin is a moderate inhibitor of CYP450 1A2 isoenzymes. Co-administration of ciprofloxacin and other drugs primarily metabolized by the CYP450 1A2 enzyme pathway may result in increased plasma concentrations of the co-administered drug and couldlead to clinically significant pharmacodynamic side effects). Products include:

Erythrocin Stearate Filmtab Tablets 453

Estradiol (Ciprofloxacin is a moderate inhibitor of CYP450 1A2 isoenzymes. Co-administration of ciprofloxacin and other drugs primarily metabolized by the CYP450 1A2 enzyme pathway may result in increased plasma concentrations of the co-administered drug and could-lead to clinically significant pharmacodynamic side effects). Products include:

Angeliq Tablets 762
Climara Transdermal System 771
Climara Pro Transdermal System 776
Estrasorb Topical Emulsion 1147
Estring Vaginal Ring 2635
Menostar Transdermal System 782
Vagifem Tablets 2334

Estradiol Benzoate (Ciprofloxacin is a moderate inhibitor of CYP450 1A2 isoenzymes. Co-administration of ciprofloxacin and other drugs primarily metabolized by the CYP450 1A2 enzyme pathway may result in increased plasma concentrations of the co-administered drug and could-lead to clinically significant pharmacodynamic side effects).

No products indexed under this heading.

Estradiol Cypionate (Ciprofloxacin is a moderate inhibitor of CYP450 1A2 isoenzymes. Co-administration of ciprofloxacin and other drugs primarily metabolized by the CYP450 1A2 enzyme pathway may result in increased plasma concentrations of the co-administered drug and could-lead to clinically significant pharmacodynamic side effects).

No products indexed under this heading.

Etodolac (NSAIDs in combination with very high doses of quinolones have been shown to provoke convulsions in pre-clinical trials).

No products indexed under this heading.

Fenoprofen Calcium (NSAIDs in combination with very high doses of quinolones have been shown to provoke convulsions in pre-clinical trials). Products include:

Nalfon Capsules 2502

Ferrous Fumarate (Co-administration with iron-containing products may substantially interfere with the oral absorption of quinolones; these preparations may be taken six hours before or two hours after taking ciprofloxacin).

No products indexed under this heading.

Ferrous Gluconate (Co-administration with iron-containing products may substantially interfere with the oral absorption of quinolones; these preparations may be taken six hours before or two hours after taking ciprofloxacin).

No products indexed under this heading.

Ferrous Sulfate (Co-administration with iron-containing products may substantially interfere with the oral absorption of quinolones; these preparations may be taken six hours before or two hours after taking ciprofloxacin). Products include:

Slow Fe Iron Tablets 818
Slow Fe with Folic Acid Tablets 819

Fludrocortisone Acetate (Risk of ruptures of the shoulder, hand, Achilles tendon or other tendons may be increased in patients receiving concomitant corticosteroids, especially in the elderly).

No products indexed under this heading.

Flurbiprofen (NSAIDs in combination with very high doses of quinolones have been shown to provoke convulsions in pre-clinical trial[illegible]

No products indexed [illegible] this heading.

Flutamide (Ciproflo[illegible] a moderate inhibitor of [illegible] 1A2 isoenzymes. Co-adm[illegible]ation of ciprofloxacin and [illegible]rugs primarily metaboli[illegible]he CYP450 1A2 enzyme [illegible]way may result in increased plasma concentrations of the co-administered drug and could-lead to clinically significant pharmacodynamic side effects). Products include:

Eulexin Capsules 3009

Fluticasone Propionate (Ciprofloxacin is a moderate inhibitor of CYP450 1A2 isoenzymes. Co-administration of ciprofloxacin and other drugs primarily metabolized by the CYP450 1A2 enzyme pathway may result in increased plasma concentrations of the co-administered drug and couldlead to clinically significant pharmacodynamic side effects). Products include:

Advair Diskus 100/50 1308
Advair Diskus 250/50 1308
Advair Diskus 500/50 1308
Advair HFA Inhalation Aerosol 1318
Cutivate Cream 2662
Cutivate Lotion 0.05% 2664
Cutivate Ointment 2665
Flonase Nasal Spray 1440
Flovent Diskus 1443

Fluvoxamine Maleate (Ciprofloxacin is a moderate inhibitor of CYP450 1A2 isoenzymes. Co-administration of ciprofloxacin and other drugs primarily metabolized by the CYP450 1A2 enzyme pathway may result in increased plasma concentrations of the co-administered drug and couldlead to clinically significant pharmacodynamic side effects).

No products indexed under this heading.

Fosphenytoin Sodium (Potential for change in serum phenytoin levels).

No products indexed under this heading.

Glyburide (Co-administration, on rare occasions, has resulted in severe hypoglycemia).

No products indexed under this heading.

Grepafloxacin Hydrochloride (Ciprofloxacin is a moderate inhibitor of CYP450 1A2 isoenzymes. Co-administration of ciprofloxacin and other drugs primarily metabolized by the CYP450 1A2 enzyme pathway may result in increased plasma concentrations of the co-administered drug and couldlead to clinically significant pharmacodynamic side effects).

No products indexed under t[illegible] heading.

Haloperidol (Ciprofloxacin is [illegible] moderate inhibitor of CYP4[illegible] isoenzymes. Co-administ[illegible] ciprofloxacin and othe[illegible] primarily metabolized by [illegible]450 1A2 enzyme pathwa[illegible]esult in increased pla[illegible]ncentrations of the co-adm[illegible]ed drug and could-lead to c[illegible]y significant pharmacody[illegible]ide effects).

N[illegible]oducts indexed under this [illegible]ading.

[illegible]operidol Decanoate (Ciprof-[illegible]oxacin is a moderate inhibitor of CYP450 1A2 isoenzymes. Co-administration of ciprofloxacin and other drugs primarily metabolized by the CYP450 1A2 enzyme pathway may result in increased plasma concentrations of the co-administered drug and couldlead to clinically significant pharmacodynamic side effects).

No products indexed under this heading.

Haloperidol Lactate (Ciprofloxacin is a moderate inhibitor of CYP450 1A2 isoenzymes. Co-administration of ciprofloxacin and other drugs primarily metabolized by the CYP450 1A2 enzyme pathway may result in increased plasma concentrations of the co-administered drug and could-lead to clinically significant pharmacodynamic side effects).

No products indexed under this heading.

Hydrocortisone (Risk of ruptures of the shoulder, hand, Achilles tendon or other tendons may be increased in patients receiving concomitant corticosteroids, especially in the elderly). Products include:

- Colocort Rectal Suspension, USP (Retention) 100 mg/60 mL 2476
- Hydrocortone Tablets 1989
- Preparation H Hydrocortisone Cream .... ■646

Hydrocortisone Acetate (Risk of ruptures of the shoulder, hand, Achilles tendon or other tendons may be increased in patients receiving concomitant corticosteroids, especially in the elderly). Products include:

- Analpram-HC 1159
- Pramosone 1161
- ProctoFoam-HC 3099

Hydrocortisone Sodium Phosphate (Risk of ruptures of the shoulder, hand, Achilles tendon or other tendons may be increased in patients receiving concomitant corticosteroids, especially in the elderly).

No products indexed under this heading.

Hydrocortisone Sodium Succinate (Risk of ruptures of the shoulder, hand, Achilles tendon or other tendons may be increased in patients receiving concomitant corticosteroids, especially in the elderly).

No products indexed under this heading.

Ibuprofen (NSAIDs in combination with very high doses of quinolones have been shown to provoke convulsions in pre-clinical trials). Products include:

- Advil Allergy Sinus Caplets .... ■770
- Advil .... ■674
- Children's Advil Oral Suspension .... ■603
- Children's Advil Chewable Tablets .. ■603
- Advil Cold & Sinus .... ■723
- Infants' Advil Concentrated Drops .. ■604
- Infants' Advil Concentrated Drops - White Grape (Dye-Free) .... ■604
- Junior Strength Advil Swallow Tablets .... ■605
- Advil Migraine Liquigels .... ■608
- Advil Multi-Symptom Cold Caplets .... ■770
- Advil PM Caplets .... ■615
- Motrin IB Tablets and Caplets 1866
- Children's Motrin Oral Suspension ... 1867
- Children's Motrin Non-Staining Dye-Free Oral Suspension 1867
- Children's Motrin Cold Oral Suspension 1867
- Infants' Motrin Concentrated Drops 1867
- Infants' Motrin Non-Staining Dye-Free Concentrated Drops 1867
- Junior Strength Motrin Caplets and Chewable Tablets 1867
- Vicoprofen Tablets 539

Imipramine Hydrochloride (Ciprofloxacin is a moderate inhibitor of CYP450 1A2 isoenzymes. Co-administration of ciprofloxacin and other drugs primarily metabolized by the CYP450 1A2 enzyme pathway may result in increased plasma concentrations of the co-administered drug and couldlead to clinically significant pharmacodynamic side effects).

No products indexed under this heading.

Imipramine Pamoate (Ciprofloxacin is a moderate inhibitor of CYP450 1A2 isoenzymes. Co-administration of ciprofloxacin and other drugs primarily metabolized by the CYP450 1A2 enzyme pathway may result in increased plasma concentrations of the co-administered drug and couldlead to clinically significant pharmacodynamic side effects).

No products indexed under this heading.

Indomethacin (NSAIDs in combination with very high doses of quinolones have been shown to provoke convulsions in pre-clinical trials). Products include:

- Indocin 1995

Indomethacin Sodium Trihydrate (NSAIDs in combination with very high doses of quinolones have been shown to provoke convulsions in pre-clinical trials). Products include:

- Indocin I.V. 2465

Iron (Co-administration with iron-containing products may substantially interfere with the oral absorption of quinolones; these preparations may be taken six hours before or two hours after taking ciprofloxacin).

No products indexed under this heading.

Ketoprofen (NSAIDs in combination with very high doses of quinolones have been shown to provoke convulsions in pre-clinical trials).

No products indexed under this heading.

Ketorolac Tromethamine (NSAIDs in combination with very high doses of quinolones have been shown to provoke convulsions in pre-clinical trials). Products include:

- Acular Ophthalmic Solution 565
- Acular LS Ophthalmic Solution 566

Levobupivacaine Hydrochloride (Ciprofloxacin is a moderate inhibitor of CYP450 1A2 isoenzymes. Co-administration of ciprofloxacin and other drugs primarily metabolized by the CYP450 1A2 enzyme pathway may result in increased plasma concentrations of the co-administered drug and couldlead to clinically significant pharmacodynamic side effects).

No products indexed under this heading.

Lomefloxacin Hydrochloride (Ciprofloxacin is a moderate inhibitor of CYP450 1A2 isoenzymes. Co-administration of ciprofloxacin and other drugs primarily metabolized by the CYP450 1A2 enzyme pathway may result in increased plasma concentrations of the co-administered drug and couldlead to clinically significant pharmacodynamic side effects).

No products indexed under this heading.

Magaldrate (Concurrent administration of these antacids may substantially interfere with the oral absorption of ciprofloxacin; antacids may be administered either two hours after or six hours before ciprofloxacin dosing without a significant decrease in bioavailability).

No products indexed under this heading.

Magnesium Hydroxide (Concurrent administration of these antacids may substantially interfere with the oral absorption of ciprofloxacin; antacids may be administered either two hours after or six hours before ciprofloxacin dosing without a significant decrease in bioavailability). Products include:

- Maalox Regular Strength Antacid/Antigas Liquid 2175
- Maalox Max Maximum Strength Antacid/Anti-Gas Liquid 2176
- Pepcid Complete Chewable Tablets 1701

Magnesium Oxide (Concurrent administration of these antacids may substantially interfere with the oral absorption of ciprofloxacin; antacids may be administered either two hours after or six hours before ciprofloxacin dosing without a significant decrease in bioavailability). Products include:

- Beelith Tablets 759
- PremCal Light, Regular, and Extra Strength Tablets .... ■818

Maprotiline Hydrochloride (Ciprofloxacin is a moderate inhibitor of CYP450 1A2 isoenzymes. Co-administration of ciprofloxacin and other drugs primarily metabolized by the CYP450 1A2 enzyme pathway may result in increased plasma concentrations of the co-administered drug and couldlead to clinically significant pharmacodynamic side effects).

No products indexed under this heading.

Meclofenamate Sodium (NSAIDs in combination with very high doses of quinolones have been shown to provoke convulsions in pre-clinical trials).

No products indexed under this heading.

Mefenamic Acid (NSAIDs in combination with very high doses of quinolones have been shown to provoke convulsions in pre-clinical trials).

No products indexed under this heading.

Meloxicam (NSAIDs in combination with very high doses of quinolones have been shown to provoke convulsions in pre-clinical trials). Products include:

- Mobic Oral Suspension 863
- Mobic Tablets 863

Methadone Hydrochloride (Ciprofloxacin is a moderate inhibitor of CYP450 1A2 isoenzymes. Co-administration of ciprofloxacin and other drugs primarily metabolized by the CYP450 1A2 enzyme pathway may result in increased plasma concentrations of the co-administered drug and couldlead to clinically significant pharmacodynamic side effects).

No products indexed under this heading.

Methotrexate (Renal tubular transport of methotrexate may be inhibited by concomitant administration of ciprofloxacin potentially leading to increased plasma levels of methotrexate).

No products indexed under this heading.

Methotrexate Sodium (Renal tubular transport of methotrexate may be inhibited by concomitant administration of ciprofloxacin potentially leading to increased plasma levels of methotrexate).

No products indexed under this heading.

Methylprednisolone Acetate (Risk of ruptures of the shoulder, hand, Achilles tendon or other tendons may be increased in patients receiving concomitant corticosteroids, especially in the elderly). Products include:

- Depo-Medrol Injectable Suspension 2617
- Depo-Medrol Single-Dose Vial 2619

Methylprednisolone Sodium Succinate (Risk of ruptures of the shoulder, hand, Achilles tendon or other tendons may be increased in patients receiving concomitant corticosteroids, especially in the elderly).

No products indexed under this heading.

Metoclopramide Hydrochloride (Metoclopramide significantly accelerates the absorption of oral ciprofloxacin resulting in a shorter time to reach maximum plasma concentrations).

No products indexed under this heading.

Mexiletine Hydrochloride (Ciprofloxacin is a moderate inhibitor of CYP450 1A2 isoenzymes. Co-administration of ciprofloxacin and other drugs primarily metabolized by the CYP450 1A2 enzyme pathway may result in increased plasma concentrations of the co-administered drug and couldlead to clinically significant pharmacodynamic side effects).

No products indexed under this heading.

Mirtazapine (Ciprofloxacin is a moderate inhibitor of CYP450 1A2 isoenzymes. Co-administration of ciprofloxacin and other drugs primarily metabolized by the CYP450 1A2 enzyme pathway may result in increased plasma concentrations of the co-administered drug and couldlead to clinically significant pharmacodynamic side effects).

No products indexed under this heading.

Moxifloxacin Hydrochloride (Ciprofloxacin is a moderate inhibitor of CYP450 1A2 isoenzymes. Co-administration of ciprofloxacin and other drugs primarily metabolized by the CYP450 1A2 enzyme pathway may result in increased plasma concentrations of the co-administered drug and couldlead to clinically significant pharmacodynamic side effects). Products include:

- Avelox 2970
- Vigamox Ophthalmic Solution 564

Nabumetone (NSAIDs in combination with very high doses of quinolones have been shown to provoke convulsions in pre-clinical trials).

No products indexed under this heading.

Nafcillin Sodium (Ciprofloxacin is a moderate inhibitor of CYP450 1A2 isoenzymes. Co-administration of ciprofloxacin and other drugs primarily metabolized by the CYP450 1A2 enzyme pathway may result in increased plasma concentrations of the co-administered drug and couldlead to clinically significant pharmacodynamic side effects).

No products indexed under this heading.

Naproxen (NSAIDs in combination with very high doses of quinolones have been shown to provoke convulsions in pre-clinical trials). Products include:

- EC-Naprosyn Delayed-Release Tablets 2761
- Naprosyn Suspension 2761
- Naprosyn Tablets 2761
- Prevacid NapraPAC 3280

Naproxen Sodium (NSAIDs in combination with very high doses of quinolones have been shown to provoke convulsions in pre-clinical trials). Products include:

Aleve Caplets **742**
Aleve Gelcaps **743**
Aleve Tablets **743**
Aleve Cold & Sinus Caplets **744**
Anaprox Tablets **2761**
Anaprox DS Tablets **2761**

Nicotine Polacrilex (Ciprofloxacin is a moderate inhibitor of CYP450 1A2 isoenzymes. Co-administration of ciprofloxacin and other drugs primarily metabolized by the CYP450 1A2 enzyme pathway may result in increased plasma concentrations of the co-administered drug and couldlead to clinically significant pharmacodynamic side effects).
No products indexed under this heading.

Nicotine Salicylate (Ciprofloxacin is a moderate inhibitor of CYP450 1A2 isoenzymes. Co-administration of ciprofloxacin and other drugs primarily metabolized by the CYP450 1A2 enzyme pathway may result in increased plasma concentrations of the co-administered drug and couldlead to clinically significant pharmacodynamic side effects).
No products indexed under this heading.

Nicotine Sulfate (Ciprofloxacin is a moderate inhibitor of CYP450 1A2 isoenzymes. Co-administration of ciprofloxacin and other drugs primarily metabolized by the CYP450 1A2 enzyme pathway may result in increased plasma concentrations of the co-administered drug and couldlead to clinically significant pharmacodynamic side effects).
No products indexed under this heading.

Norethindrone Acetate (Ciprofloxacin is a moderate inhibitor of CYP450 1A2 isoenzymes. Co-administration of ciprofloxacin and other drugs primarily metabolized by the CYP450 1A2 enzyme pathway may result in increased plasma concentrations of the co-administered drug and couldlead to clinically significant pharmacodynamic side effects).
No products indexed under this heading.

Norfloxacin (Ciprofloxacin is a moderate inhibitor of CYP450 1A2 isoenzymes. Co-administration of ciprofloxacin and other drugs primarily metabolized by the CYP450 1A2 enzyme pathway may result in increased plasma concentrations of the co-administered drug and couldlead to clinically significant pharmacodynamic side effects). Products include:
Noroxin Tablets **2032**

Nortriptyline Hydrochloride (Ciprofloxacin is a moderate inhibitor of CYP450 1A2 isoenzymes. Co-administration of ciprofloxacin and other drugs primarily metabolized by the CYP450 1A2 enzyme pathway may result in increased plasma concentrations of the co-administered drug and couldlead to clinically significant pharmacodynamic side effects).
No products indexed under this heading.

Ofloxacin (Ciprofloxacin is a moderate inhibitor of CYP450 1A2 isoenzymes. Co-administration of ciprofloxacin and other drugs primarily metabolized by the CYP450 1A2 enzyme pathway may result in increased plasma concentrations of the co-administered drug and couldlead to clinically significant pharmacodynamic side effects). Products include:
Floxin Otic Solution **1049**

Olanzapine (Ciprofloxacin is a moderate inhibitor of CYP450 1A2 isoenzymes. Co-administration of ciprofloxacin and other drugs primarily metabolized by the CYP450 1A2 enzyme pathway may result in increased plasma concentrations of the co-administered drug and couldlead to clinically significant pharmacodynamic side effects). Products include:
Symbyax Capsules **1819**
Zyprexa Tablets **1830**
Zyprexa IntraMuscular **1830**
Zyprexa ZYDIS Orally Disintegrating Tablets **1830**

Ondansetron (Ciprofloxacin is a moderate inhibitor of CYP450 1A2 isoenzymes. Co-administration of ciprofloxacin and other drugs primarily metabolized by the CYP450 1A2 enzyme pathway may result in increased plasma concentrations of the co-administered drug and couldlead to clinically significant pharmacodynamic side effects). Products include:
Zofran ODT Orally Disintegrating Tablets **1639**

Ondansetron Hydrochloride (Ciprofloxacin is a moderate inhibitor of CYP450 1A2 isoenzymes. Co-administration of ciprofloxacin and other drugs primarily metabolized by the CYP450 1A2 enzyme pathway may result in increased plasma concentrations of the co-administered drug and couldlead to clinically significant pharmacodynamic side effects). Products include:
Zofran Injection **1634**
Zofran **1639**

Oxaprozin (NSAIDs in combination with very high doses of quinolones have been shown to provoke convulsions in pre-clinical trials).
No products indexed under this heading.

Phenobarbital Sodium (Ciprofloxacin is a moderate inhibitor of CYP450 1A2 isoenzymes. Co-administration of ciprofloxacin and other drugs primarily metabolized by the CYP450 1A2 enzyme pathway may result in increased plasma concentrations of the co-administered drug and couldlead to clinically significant pharmacodynamic side effects).
No products indexed under this heading.

Phenylbutazone (NSAIDs in combination with very high doses of quinolones have been shown to provoke convulsions in pre-clinical trials).
No products indexed under this heading.

Phenytoin (Potential for change in serum phenytoin levels).
No products indexed under this heading.

Phenytoin Sodium (Potential for change in serum phenytoin levels). Products include:
Phenytek Capsules **2160**

Piroxicam (NSAIDs in combination with very high doses of quinolones have been shown to provoke convulsions in pre-clinical trials).
No products indexed under this heading.

Polysaccharide Iron Complex (Co-administration with iron-containing products may substantially interfere with the oral absorption of quinolones; these preparations may be taken six hours before or two hours after taking ciprofloxacin). Products include:
Nu-Iron 150 Capsules **2127**

Prednisolone Acetate (Risk of ruptures of the shoulder, hand, Achilles tendon or other tendons may be increased in patients receiving concomitant corticosteroids, especially in the elderly). Products include:
Blephamide Ophthalmic Ointment **568**
Blephamide Ophthalmic Suspension................................. **569**
Poly-Pred Ophthalmic Suspension .... ⊙**233**
Pred Forte Ophthalmic Suspension .... ⊙**235**
Pred Mild Ophthalmic Suspension .... ⊙**238**
Pred-G Ophthalmic Ointment .... ⊙**237**
Pred-G Ophthalmic Suspension ...... ⊙**236**

Prednisolone Sodium Phosphate (Risk of ruptures of the shoulder, hand, Achilles tendon or other tendons may be increased in patients receiving concomitant corticosteroids, especially in the elderly).
No products indexed under this heading.

Prednisolone Tebutate (Risk of ruptures of the shoulder, hand, Achilles tendon or other tendons may be increased in patients receiving concomitant corticosteroids, especially in the elderly).
No products indexed under this heading.

Prednisone (Risk of ruptures of the shoulder, hand, Achilles tendon or other tendons may be increased in patients receiving concomitant corticosteroids, especially in the elderly).
No products indexed under this heading.

Probenecid (Interferes with renal tubular secretion of ciprofloxacin).
No products indexed under this heading.

Propafenone Hydrochloride (Ciprofloxacin is a moderate inhibitor of CYP450 1A2 isoenzymes. Co-administration of ciprofloxacin and other drugs primarily metabolized by the CYP450 1A2 enzyme pathway may result in increased plasma concentrations of the co-administered drug and couldlead to clinically significant pharmacodynamic side effects). Products include:
Rythmol SR Capsules **2727**

Propranolol Hydrochloride (Ciprofloxacin is a moderate inhibitor of CYP450 1A2 isoenzymes. Co-administration of ciprofloxacin and other drugs primarily metabolized by the CYP450 1A2 enzyme pathway may result in increased plasma concentrations of the co-administered drug and couldlead to clinically significant pharmacodynamic side effects). Products include:
Inderal LA Long-Acting Capsules **3429**
InnoPran XL Capsules **2723**

Protriptyline Hydrochloride (Ciprofloxacin is a moderate inhibitor of CYP450 1A2 isoenzymes. Co-administration of ciprofloxacin and other drugs primarily metabolized by the CYP450 1A2 enzyme pathway may result in increased plasma concentrations of the co-administered drug and couldlead to clinically significant pharmacodynamic side effects).
No products indexed under this heading.

Riluzole (Ciprofloxacin is a moderate inhibitor of CYP450 1A2 isoenzymes. Co-administration of ciprofloxacin and other drugs primarily metabolized by the CYP450 1A2 enzyme pathway may result in increased plasma concentrations of the co-administered drug and couldlead to clinically significant pharmacodynamic side effects). Products include:
Rilutek Tablets **2930**

Ritonavir (Ciprofloxacin is a moderate inhibitor of CYP450 1A2 isoenzymes. Co-administration of ciprofloxacin and other drugs primarily metabolized by the CYP450 1A2 enzyme pathway may result in increased plasma concentrations of the co-administered drug and couldlead to clinically significant pharmacodynamic side effects). Products include:
Kaletra **476**
Norvir **503**

Rofecoxib (NSAIDs in combination with very high doses of quinolones have been shown to provoke convulsions in pre-clinical trials).
No products indexed under this heading.

Ropinirole Hydrochloride (Ciprofloxacin is a moderate inhibitor of CYP450 1A2 isoenzymes. Co-administration of ciprofloxacin and other drugs primarily metabolized by the CYP450 1A2 enzyme pathway may result in increased plasma concentrations of the co-administered drug and couldlead to clinically significant pharmacodynamic side effects). Products include:
Requip Tablets **1555**

Ropivacaine Hydrochloride (Ciprofloxacin is a moderate inhibitor of CYP450 1A2 isoenzymes. Co-administration of ciprofloxacin and other drugs primarily metabolized by the CYP450 1A2 enzyme pathway may result in increased plasma concentrations of the co-administered drug and couldlead to clinically significant pharmacodynamic side effects).
No products indexed under this heading.

Sucralfate (Co-administration with sucralfate may substantially interfere with the oral absorption of quinolones; these preparations may be taken six hours before or two hours after taking ciprofloxacin). Products include:
Carafate Suspension **701**
Carafate Tablets **701**

Sulindac (NSAIDs in combination with very high doses of quinolones have been shown to provoke convulsions in pre-clinical trials). Products include:
Clinoril Tablets **1924**

Tacrine Hydrochloride (Ciprofloxacin is a moderate inhibitor of CYP450 1A2 isoenzymes. Co-administration of ciprofloxacin and other drugs primarily metabolized by the CYP450 1A2 enzyme pathway may result in increased plasma concentrations of the co-administered drug and couldlead to clinically significant pharmacodynamic side effects).
No products indexed under this heading.

Tamoxifen Citrate (Ciprofloxacin is a moderate inhibitor of CYP450 1A2 isoenzymes. Co-administration of ciprofloxacin and other drugs primarily metabolized by the CYP450 1A2 enzyme pathway may result in increased plasma concentrations of the co-administered drug and couldlead to clinically significant pharmacodynamic side effects). Products include:

Soltamox Oral Solution 3527

Theophylline (Potential for severe and fatal reactions including cardiac arrest, seizures, respiratory failure and status epilepticus; concurrent use should be avoided or serum levels of theophylline should be monitored carefully).

No products indexed under this heading.

Theophylline Anhydrous (Potential for severe and fatal reactions including cardiac arrest, seizures, respiratory failure and status epilepticus; concurrent use should be avoided or serum levels of theophylline should be monitored carefully). Products include:

Uniphyl Tablets 2710

Theophylline Calcium Salicylate (Potential for severe and fatal reactions including cardiac arrest, seizures, respiratory failure and status epilepticus; concurrent use should be avoided or serum levels of theophylline should be monitored carefully).

No products indexed under this heading.

Theophylline Dihydroxypropyl (Glyceryl) (Potential for severe and fatal reactions including cardiac arrest, seizures, respiratory failure and status epilepticus; concurrent use should be avoided or serum levels of theophylline should be monitored carefully).

No products indexed under this heading.

Theophylline Ethylenediamine (Potential for severe and fatal reactions including cardiac arrest, seizures, respiratory failure and status epilepticus; concurrent use should be avoided or serum levels of theophylline should be monitored carefully).

No products indexed under this heading.

Theophylline Sodium Glycinate (Potential for severe and fatal reactions including cardiac arrest, seizures, respiratory failure and status epilepticus; concurrent use should be avoided or serum levels of theophylline should be monitored carefully).

No products indexed under this heading.

Tizanidine Hydrochloride (Concomitant administration is contraindicated).

No products indexed under this heading.

Tolmetin Sodium (NSAIDs in combination with very high doses of quinolones have been shown to provoke convulsions in pre-clinical trials).

No products indexed under this heading.

Triamcinolone (Risk of ruptures of the shoulder, hand, Achilles tendon or other tendons may be increased in patients receiving concomitant corticosteroids, especially in the elderly).

No products indexed under this heading.

Triamcinolone Acetonide (Risk of ruptures of the shoulder, hand, Achilles tendon or other tendons may be increased in patients receiving concomitant corticosteroids, especially in the elderly). Products include:

Azmacort Inhalation Aerosol 1726
Nasacort AQ Nasal Spray 2922

Triamcinolone Diacetate (Risk of ruptures of the shoulder, hand, Achilles tendon or other tendons may be increased in patients receiving concomitant corticosteroids, especially in the elderly).

No products indexed under this heading.

Triamcinolone Hexacetonide (Risk of ruptures of the shoulder, hand, Achilles tendon or other tendons may be increased in patients receiving concomitant corticosteroids, especially in the elderly).

No products indexed under this heading.

Trimethaphan Camsylate (Ciprofloxacin is a moderate inhibitor of CYP450 1A2 isoenzymes. Co-administration of ciprofloxacin and other drugs primarily metabolized by the CYP450 1A2 enzyme pathway may result in increased plasma concentrations of the co-administered drug and couldlead to clinically significant pharmacodynamic side effects).

No products indexed under this heading.

Trimipramine Maleate (Ciprofloxacin is a moderate inhibitor of CYP450 1A2 isoenzymes. Co-administration of ciprofloxacin and other drugs primarily metabolized by the CYP450 1A2 enzyme pathway may result in increased plasma concentrations of the co-administered drug and couldlead to clinically significant pharmacodynamic side effects).

No products indexed under this heading.

Trovafloxacin Mesylate (Ciprofloxacin is a moderate inhibitor of CYP450 1A2 isoenzymes. Co-administration of ciprofloxacin and other drugs primarily metabolized by the CYP450 1A2 enzyme pathway may result in increased plasma concentrations of the co-administered drug and couldlead to clinically significant pharmacodynamic side effects).

No products indexed under this heading.

Valdecoxib (NSAIDs in combination with very high doses of quinolones have been shown to provoke convulsions in pre-clinical trials).

No products indexed under this heading.

Verapamil Hydrochloride (Ciprofloxacin is a moderate inhibitor of CYP450 1A2 isoenzymes. Co-administration of ciprofloxacin and other drugs primarily metabolized by the CYP450 1A2 enzyme pathway may result in increased plasma concentrations of the co-administered drug and couldlead to clinically significant pharmacodynamic side effects). Products include:

Covera-HS Tablets 3139
Tarka Tablets 524
Verelan PM Extended-Release Capsules, Controlled-Onset 3106

Warfarin Sodium (Enhanced effects of anticoagulant). Products include:

Coumadin for Injection 898
Coumadin Tablets 898

Zileuton (Ciprofloxacin is a moderate inhibitor of CYP450 1A2 isoenzymes. Co-administration of ciprofloxacin and other drugs primarily metabolized by the CYP450 1A2 enzyme pathway may result in increased plasma concentrations of the co-administered drug and couldlead to clinically significant pharmacodynamic side effects). Products include:

Zyflo Tablets 1023

Zinc Sulfate (Co-administration with zinc-containing products may substantially interfere with the oral absorption of quinolones; these preparations may be taken six hours before or two hours after taking ciprofloxacin). Products include:

Visine A.C. Seasonal Itching and Redness Relief Drops .... ⊙289
Zinc-220 Capsules 580

Zolmitriptan (Ciprofloxacin is a moderate inhibitor of CYP450 1A2 isoenzymes. Co-administration of ciprofloxacin and other drugs primarily metabolized by the CYP450 1A2 enzyme pathway may result in increased plasma concentrations of the co-administered drug and couldlead to clinically significant pharmacodynamic side effects). Products include:

Zomig Tablets 3519
Zomig Nasal Spray 3523
Zomig-ZMT Tablets 3519

Food Interactions

Dairy products (Oral ciprofloxacin should not be taken concurrently with milk or yogurt alone, since absorption of ciprofloxacin may be significantly reduced; dietary calcium as part of a meal; however, does not significantly affect ciprofloxacin absorption).

Food, unspecified (Delays the oral absorption of the drug resulting in peak concentrations that are closer to two hours after dosing).

CIPRO XR TABLETS

(Ciprofloxacin) 2990

May interact with antacids containing aluminum, calcium and magnesium, nonabsorbable antacids, calcium preparations, cations, corticosteroids, oral anticoagulants, cytochrome p450 1a2 substrates (selected), iron containing oral preparations, non-steroidal anti-inflammatory agents, phenytoin, xanthines, and certain other agents. Compounds in these categories include:

Acetaminophen (Ciprofloxacin is an inhibitor of CYP450 1A2 isoenzymes. Co-administration of ciprofloxacin and other drugs primarily metabolized by CYP1A2 results in increased plasma concentrations of the co-administered drug and could lead to clinically significant pharmacodynamic side effects). Products include:

Comtrex Maximum Strength Cold & Cough Day/Night Caplets - Day Formulation .... ■726
Comtrex Maximum Strength Cold & Cough Day/Night Caplets - Night Formulation .... ■726
Comtrex Maximum Strength Non-Drowsy Cold & Cough Caplets .... ■725
Comtrex Maximum Strength Day/Night Severe Cold & Sinus Caplets - Day Formulation .... ■725
Comtrex Maximum Strength Day/Night Severe Cold & Sinus Caplets - Night Formulation .... ■725
Contac Cold and Flu Maximum Strength Caplets .... ■728
Contac Cold and Flu Day and Night Caplets (Day Formulation Only) .... ■727
Contac Cold and Flu Day and Night Caplets (Night Formulation Only) .... ■727
Contac Cold and Flu Non-Drowsy Caplets .... ■728
Excedrin Extra Strength Caplets/Tablets/Geltabs .... ■684
Excedrin Migraine Caplets/Tablets/Geltabs .... ■609
Excedrin PM Caplets/Tablets/Geltabs .... ■610
Excedrin Sinus Headache Caplets/Tablets .... ■610
Excedrin Tension Headache Caplets/Tablets/Geltabs .... ■611
Goody's Body Pain Formula Powder .... ■684
Goody's Extra Strength Headache Powders .... ■611
Goody's Extra Strength Pain Relief Tablets .... ■685
Goody's PM Powder for Pain with Sleeplessness .... ■612
Percocet Tablets 1131
Robitussin Cough, Cold & Flu Nighttime Liquid .... ■738
TheraFlu Cold & Sore Throat Hot Liquid .... ■741
TheraFlu Flu & Chest Congestion Hot Liquid .... ■741
TheraFlu Flu & Sore Throat Hot Liquid .... ■742
TheraFlu Daytime Severe Cold Hot Liquid .... ■742
TheraFlu Nighttime Severe Cold Hot Liquid .... ■740
TheraFlu Warming Relief Daytime Severe Cold .... ■743
TheraFlu Warming Relief Nighttime Severe Cold .... ■743
Triaminic Cough & Sore Throat Liquid .... ■747
Regular Strength Tylenol Tablets 1870
Children's Tylenol with Flavor Creator .... ■679
Children's Tylenol Plus Flu Oral Suspension .... ■749
Tylenol Cold Head Congestion Daytime Caplets with Cool Burst and Gelcaps .... ■750
Tylenol Cold Multi-Symptom Daytime Liquid .... ■752
Tylenol Cold Multi-Symptom Severe Daytime Liquid .... ■752
Tylenol 8 Hour Extended Release Caplets 1870
Tylenol 1870
Extra Strength Tylenol PM Caplets, Vanilla Caplets, Geltabs, Gelcaps and Liquid 1875
Extra Strength Tylenol Rapid Release Gels 1870
Concentrated Tylenol Infants' Drops Plus Cold & Cough .... ■754
Tylenol with Codeine Tablets 2391
Tylenol Allergy Multi-Symptom Caplets with Cool Burst and Gelcaps 1872
Tylenol Allergy Multi-Symptom Nighttime Caplets with Cool Burst 1872
Tylenol Severe Allergy Caplets 1872
Tylenol Arthritis Pain Extended Release Caplets and Geltabs 1870
Tylenol Chest Congestion Caplets with Cool Burst 1872
Tylenol Chest Congestion Liquid with Cool Burst 1872
Children's Tylenol Suspension Liquid and Meltaways 1878
Children's Tylenol Plus Cold Suspension Liquid 1879
Children's Tylenol Plus Cold & Allergy Suspension Liquid 1878
Children's Tylenol Plus Cough & Runny Nose Suspension Liquid 1879
Children's Tylenol Plus Cough & Sore Throat Suspension Liquid 1879
Children's Tylenol Suspension with Flavor Creator 1878

Children's Tylenol Plus Flu Suspension Liquid 1881
Children's Tylenol Plus Multi-Symptom Cold Suspension Liquid 1879
Tylenol Cold Severe Congestion Non-Drowsy Caplets with Cool Burst 1874
Tylenol Cold Head Congestion Daytime Caplets with Cool Burst 1873
Tylenol Cold Head Congestion Nighttime Caplets with Cool Burst 1873
Tylenol Cold Head Congestion Severe Caplets with Cool Burst 1873
Tylenol Cold Multi-Symptom Daytime Caplets with Cool Burst and Gelcaps 1874
Tylenol Cold Multi-Symptom Daytime Liquid with Citrus Burst ... 1874
Tylenol Cold Multi-Symptom Nighttime Caplets with Cool Burst 1874
Tylenol Cold Multi-Symptom Nighttime Liquid with Cool Burst ... 1874
Tylenol Cold Multi-Symptom Severe Caplets with Cool Burst 1874
Tylenol Cold Multi-Symptom Severe Daytime Liquid with Citrus Burst 1874
Tylenol Cough & Sore Throat Daytime Liquid with Cool Burst 1877
Tylenol Cough & Sore Throat Nighttime Liquid with Cool Burst ... 1877
Concentrated Tylenol Infants' Drops 1878
Concentrated Tylenol Infants' Drops Plus Cold 1879
Concentrated Tylenol Infants' Drops Plus Cold and Cough 1879
Jr. Tylenol Meltaways 1878
Tylenol Sinus Severe Congestion Caplets with Cool Burst 1876
Tylenol Sinus Congestion & Pain Daytime Caplets with Cool Burst and Gelcaps 1876
Tylenol Sinus Congestion & Pain Nighttime Caplets with Cool Burst 1876
Tylenol Sinus Congestion & Pain Severe Caplets with Cool Burst 1876
Tylenol Sore Throat Daytime Liquid with Cool Burst 1877
Tylenol Sore Throat Nighttime Liquid with Cool Burst 1877
Women's Tylenol Menstrual Relief Caplets 1877
Vicks 44M Cough, Cold & Flu Relief Liquid 2680
Vicks DayQuil LiquiCaps/Liquid Multi-Symptom Cold/Flu Relief 761
Vicks DayQuil Multi-Symptom Cold/Flu Relief LiquiCaps 2678
Vicks DayQuil Multi-Symptom Cold/Flu Relief Liquid 2678
Vicks NyQuil Multi-Symptom Cold/Flu Relief Liquid 2681
Vicks NyQuil Multi-Symptom Cold/Flu Relief LiquiCaps 2681
Vicks NyQuil LiquiCaps/Liquid Multi-Symptom Cold/Flu Relief 763
Vicodin Tablets 535
Vicodin ES Tablets 536
Vicodin HP Tablets 538
Zicam Maximum Strength Flu Daytime 768
Zicam Maximum Strength Flu Nighttime 768
Zydone Tablets 1139

Alatrofloxacin Mesylate (Ciprofloxacin is an inhibitor of CYP450 1A2 isoenzymes. Co-administration of ciprofloxacin and other drugs primarily metabolized by CYP1A2 results in increased plasma concentrations of the co-administered drug and could lead to clinically significant pharmacodynamic side effects).
No products indexed under this heading.

Aluminum Carbonate (Concurrent administration may substantially interfere with the absorption of ciprofloxacin, resulting in serum and urine levels of ciprofloxacin considerably lower than desired. Ciprofloxacin extended-release tablets should be administered at least 2 hours before or 6 hours after antacids containing magnesium or aluminum.).
No products indexed under this heading.

Aluminum-containing Compounds, unspecified (Concurrent administration may substantially interfere with the absorption of ciprofloxacin, resulting in serum and urine levels of ciprofloxacin considerably lower than desired. Ciprofloxacin extended-release tablets should be administered at least 2 hours before or 6 hours after metal cations.).
No products indexed under this heading.

Aluminum Hydroxide (Concurrent administration may substantially interfere with the absorption of ciprofloxacin, resulting in serum and urine levels of ciprofloxacin considerably lower than desired. Ciprofloxacin extended-release tablets should be administered at least 2 hours before or 6 hours after antacids containing magnesium or aluminum). Products include:
Gaviscon Regular Strength Liquid .. 658
Gaviscon Regular Strength Tablets 658
Gaviscon Extra Strength Liquid 658
Gaviscon Extra Strength Tablets 658
Maalox Regular Strength Antacid/Antigas Liquid 2175
Maalox Max Maximum Strength Antacid/Anti-Gas Liquid 2176

Aminophylline (Concurrent administration of ciprofloxacin and theophylline may lead to elevated serum concentrations of theophylline and prolongation of its elimination half-life. Serious and fatal reactions have been reported in patients receiving concurrent administration. These reactions have included cardiac arrest, seizure, status epilepticus, and respiratory failure.).
No products indexed under this heading.

Amiodarone Hydrochloride (Ciprofloxacin is an inhibitor of CYP450 1A2 isoenzymes. Co-administration of ciprofloxacin and other drugs primarily metabolized by CYP1A2 results in increased plasma concentrations of the co-administered drug and could lead to clinically significant pharmacodynamic side effects).
No products indexed under this heading.

Amitriptyline Hydrochloride (Ciprofloxacin is an inhibitor of CYP450 1A2 isoenzymes. Co-administration of ciprofloxacin and other drugs primarily metabolized by CYP1A2 results in increased plasma concentrations of the co-administered drug and could lead to clinically significant pharmacodynamic side effects).
No products indexed under this heading.

Amoxapine (Ciprofloxacin is an inhibitor of CYP450 1A2 isoenzymes. Co-administration of ciprofloxacin and other drugs primarily metabolized by CYP1A2 results in increased plasma concentrations of the co-administered drug and could lead to clinically significant pharmacodynamic side effects).
No products indexed under this heading.

Anagrelide Hydrochloride (Ciprofloxacin is an inhibitor of CYP450 1A2 isoenzymes. Co-administration of ciprofloxacin and other drugs primarily metabolized by CYP1A2 results in increased plasma concentrations of the co-administered drug and could lead to clinically significant pharmacodynamic side effects). Products include:
Agrylin Capsules 3169

Anisindione (Quinolones have been reported to enhance the effects of the oral anticoagulant warfarin or its derivatives). Products include:
Miradon Tablets 3042

Betamethasone Acetate (Risk of ruptures of the shoulder, hand, Achilles tendon or other tendons may be increased in patients receiving concomitant corticosteroids, especially in the elderly).
No products indexed under this heading.

Betamethasone Sodium Phosphate (Risk of ruptures of the shoulder, hand, Achilles tendon or other tendons may be increased in patients receiving concomitant corticosteroids, especially in the elderly).
No products indexed under this heading.

Caffeine (Co-administration leads to a reduction of caffeine clearance, prolongation of serum half-life, and inhibition of the formation of paraxanthine). Products include:
BC Headache Powder 677
Arthritis Strength BC Powder 677
Excedrin Extra Strength Caplets/Tablets/Geltabs 684
Excedrin Migraine Caplets/Tablets/Geltabs 609
Excedrin Tension Headache Caplets/Tablets/Geltabs 611
Goody's Extra Strength Headache Powders 611
Goody's Extra Strength Pain Relief Tablets 685
Vivarin 602
Winrgy Dietary Supplement 823

Caffeine Anhydrous (Ciprofloxacin is an inhibitor of CYP450 1A2 isoenzymes. Co-administration of ciprofloxacin and other drugs primarily metabolized by CYP1A2 results in increased plasma concentrations of the co-administered drug and could lead to clinically significant pharmacodynamic side effects).
No products indexed under this heading.

Caffeine Citrate (Co-administration leads to a reduction of caffeine clearance, prolongation of serum half-life, and inhibition of the formation of paraxanthine). Products include:
Cafcit 1886

Calcium (Concurrent administration may substantially interfere with the absorption of ciprofloxacin, resulting in serum and urine levels of ciprofloxacin considerably lower than desired. Ciprofloxacin extended-release tablets should be administered at least 2 hours before or 6 hours after metal cations). Products include:
Os-Cal 250 + D Tablets 817
Os-Cal 500 Tablets 817
Os-Cal 500 + D Tablets 817

Calcium Carbonate (Concurrent administration may substantially interfere with the absorption of ciprofloxacin, resulting in serum and urine levels of ciprofloxacin considerably lower than desired). Products include:
Actonel with Calcium Tablets 2688
Calcet Tablets 2138
Caltrate 600 PLUS 809
Caltrate 600 + D Tablets 809
D-Cal Chewable Caplets 812
Gas-X with Maalox 656
Maalox Regular Strength Antacid Chewable Tablets 2177
Maalox Max Maximum Strength Antacid/Antigas Chewable Tablets 2176
Maalox Max Maximum Strength Chewable Tablets 660
Os-Cal Chewable Tablets 818
Pepcid Complete Chewable Tablets 1701
Children's Pepto 2674
PremCal Light, Regular, and Extra Strength Tablets 818
Tums 664

Calcium Chloride (Concurrent administration may substantially interfere with the absorption of ciprofloxacin, resulting in serum and urine levels of ciprofloxacin considerably lower than desired).
No products indexed under this heading.

Calcium Citrate (Concurrent administration may substantially interfere with the absorption of ciprofloxacin, resulting in serum and urine levels of ciprofloxacin considerably lower than desired). Products include:
Active Calcium Tablets 3339
Citracal Caplets 703
Citracal Lemon Cream Creamy Bites 2139
Citracal Prenatal + DHA Tablets and Capsules 2139

Calcium Glubionate (Concurrent administration may substantially interfere with the absorption of ciprofloxacin, resulting in serum and urine levels of ciprofloxacin considerably lower than desired).
No products indexed under this heading.

Celecoxib (NSAIDs in combination with very high doses of quinolones have been shown to provoke convulsions in pre-clinical trials). Products include:
Celebrex Capsules 3134

Chlordiazepoxide (Ciprofloxacin is an inhibitor of CYP450 1A2 isoenzymes. Co-administration of ciprofloxacin and other drugs primarily metabolized by CYP1A2 results in increased plasma concentrations of the co-administered drug and could lead to clinically significant pharmacodynamic side effects).
No products indexed under this heading.

Chlordiazepoxide Hydrochloride (Ciprofloxacin is an inhibitor of CYP450 1A2 isoenzymes. Co-administration of ciprofloxacin and other drugs primarily metabolized by CYP1A2 results in increased plasma concentrations of the co-administered drug and could lead to clinically significant pharmacodynamic side effects). Products include:

Librium Capsules 3347

Cimetidine Hydrochloride (Ciprofloxacin is an inhibitor of CYP450 1A2 isoenzymes. Co-administration of ciprofloxacin and other drugs primarily metabolized by CYP1A2 results in increased plasma concentrations of the co-administered drug and could lead to clinically significant pharmacodynamic side effects).
No products indexed under this heading.

Ciprofloxacin Hydrochloride (Ciprofloxacin is an inhibitor of CYP450 1A2 isoenzymes. Co-administration of ciprofloxacin and other drugs primarily metabolized by CYP1A2 results in increased plasma concentrations of the co-administered drug and could lead to clinically significant pharmacodynamic side effects). Products include:
Ciloxan Ophthalmic Ointment 559
Ciloxan Ophthalmic Solution .... ⊙ 206
Cipro Tablets 2977
Proquin XR Tablets 1153

Clomipramine Hydrochloride (Ciprofloxacin is an inhibitor of CYP450 1A2 isoenzymes. Co-administration of ciprofloxacin and other drugs primarily metabolized by CYP1A2 results in increased plasma concentrations of the co-administered drug and could lead to clinically significant pharmacodynamic side effects).
No products indexed under this heading.

Clopidogrel Bisulfate (Ciprofloxacin is an inhibitor of CYP450 1A2 isoenzymes. Co-administration of ciprofloxacin and other drugs primarily metabolized by CYP1A2 results in increased plasma concentrations of the co-administered drug and could lead to clinically significant pharmacodynamic side effects). Products include:
Plavix Tablets 917
Plavix Tablets 2926

Clozapine (Ciprofloxacin is an inhibitor of CYP450 1A2 isoenzymes. Co-administration of ciprofloxacin and other drugs primarily metabolized by CYP1A2 results in increased plasma concentrations of the co-administered drug and could lead to clinically significant pharmacodynamic side effects). Products include:
Clozaril Tablets 2184
FazaClo Orally Disintegrating Tablets 551

Cortisone Acetate (Risk of ruptures of the shoulder, hand, Achilles tendon or other tendons may be increased in patients receiving concomitant corticosteroids, especially in the elderly).
No products indexed under this heading.

Cyclobenzaprine (Ciprofloxacin is an inhibitor of CYP450 1A2 isoenzymes. Co-administration of ciprofloxacin and other drugs primarily metabolized by CYP1A2 results in increased plasma concentrations of the co-administered drug and could lead to clinically significant pharmacodynamic side effects).
No products indexed under this heading.

Cyclobenzaprine Hydrochloride (Ciprofloxacin is an inhibitor of CYP450 1A2 isoenzymes. Co-administration of ciprofloxacin and other drugs primarily metabolized by CYP1A2 results in increased plasma concentrations of the co-administered drug and could lead to clinically significant pharmacodynamic side effects).
No products indexed under this heading.

Cyclosporine (Transient elevations in serum creatinine have been reported in patients receiving ciprofloxacin and cyclosporine concomitantly). Products include:
Gengraf Capsules 459
Neoral Oral Solution 2259
Neoral Soft Gelatin Capsules 2259
Restasis Ophthalmic Emulsion 575
Sandimmune 2275

Desipramine Hydrochloride (Ciprofloxacin is an inhibitor of CYP450 1A2 isoenzymes. Co-administration of ciprofloxacin and other drugs primarily metabolized by CYP1A2 results in increased plasma concentrations of the co-administered drug and could lead to clinically significant pharmacodynamic side effects).
No products indexed under this heading.

Dexamethasone (Risk of ruptures of the shoulder, hand, Achilles tendon or other tendons may be increased in patients receiving concomitant corticosteroids, especially in the elderly). Products include:
Ciprodex Otic Suspension 559
Decadron Tablets 1951
TobraDex Ophthalmic Ointment 562
TobraDex Ophthalmic Suspension ... 563

Dexamethasone Acetate (Risk of ruptures of the shoulder, hand, Achilles tendon or other tendons may be increased in patients receiving concomitant corticosteroids, especially in the elderly).
No products indexed under this heading.

Dexamethasone Sodium Phosphate (Risk of ruptures of the shoulder, hand, Achilles tendon or other tendons may be increased in patients receiving concomitant corticosteroids, especially in the elderly).
No products indexed under this heading.

Diazepam (Ciprofloxacin is an inhibitor of CYP450 1A2 isoenzymes. Co-administration of ciprofloxacin and other drugs primarily metabolized by CYP1A2 results in increased plasma concentrations of the co-administered drug and could lead to clinically significant pharmacodynamic side effects). Products include:
Diastat Rectal Delivery System 3343
Valium Tablets 2819

Diclofenac Potassium (NSAIDs in combination with very high doses of quinolones have been shown to provoke convulsions in pre-clinical trials).
No products indexed under this heading.

Diclofenac Sodium (NSAIDs in combination with very high doses of quinolones have been shown to provoke convulsions in pre-clinical trials). Products include:
Arthrotec Tablets 3129
Voltaren Ophthalmic Solution 2309
Voltaren Tablets 2307
Voltaren-XR Tablets 2310

Dicumarol (Quinolones have been reported to enhance the effects of the oral anticoagulant warfarin or its derivatives).
No products indexed under this heading.

Didanosine (Concurrent administration may substantially interfere with the absorption of ciprofloxacin, resulting in serum and urine levels of ciprofloxacin considerably lower than desired. Ciprofloxacin extended-release tablets should be administered at least 2 hours before or 6 hours after didanosine chewable/buffered tablets or pediatric powder).
No products indexed under this heading.

Diltiazem Hydrochloride (Ciprofloxacin is an inhibitor of CYP450 1A2 isoenzymes. Co-administration of ciprofloxacin and other drugs primarily metabolized by CYP1A2 results in increased plasma concentrations of the co-administered drug and could lead to clinically significant pharmacodynamic side effects). Products include:
Cardizem LA Extended Release Tablets 1728
Tiazac Capsules 1201

Diltiazem Maleate (Ciprofloxacin is an inhibitor of CYP450 1A2 isoenzymes. Co-administration of ciprofloxacin and other drugs primarily metabolized by CYP1A2 results in increased plasma concentrations of the co-administered drug and could lead to clinically significant pharmacodynamic side effects).
No products indexed under this heading.

Doxepin Hydrochloride (Ciprofloxacin is an inhibitor of CYP450 1A2 isoenzymes. Co-administration of ciprofloxacin and other drugs primarily metabolized by CYP1A2 results in increased plasma concentrations of the co-administered drug and could lead to clinically significant pharmacodynamic side effects).
No products indexed under this heading.

Dyphylline (Concurrent administration of ciprofloxacin and theophylline may lead to elevated serum concentrations of theophylline and prolongation of its elimination half-life. Serious and fatal reactions have been reported in patients receiving concurrent administration. These reactions have included cardiac arrest, seizure, status epilepticus, and respiratory failure.).
No products indexed under this heading.

Enoxacin (Ciprofloxacin is an inhibitor of CYP450 1A2 isoenzymes. Co-administration of ciprofloxacin and other drugs primarily metabolized by CYP1A2 results in increased plasma concentrations of the co-administered drug and could lead to clinically significant pharmacodynamic side effects).
No products indexed under this heading.

Erythromycin (Ciprofloxacin is an inhibitor of CYP450 1A2 isoenzymes. Co-administration of ciprofloxacin and other drugs primarily metabolized by CYP1A2 results in increased plasma concentrations of the co-administered drug and could lead to clinically significant pharmacodynamic side effects). Products include:
Ery-Tab Tablets 449
Erythromycin Base Filmtab Tablets 455
Erythromycin Delayed-Release Capsules, USP 457
PCE Dispertab Tablets 515

Erythromycin Estolate (Ciprofloxacin is an inhibitor of CYP450 1A2 isoenzymes. Co-administration of ciprofloxacin and other drugs primarily metabolized by CYP1A2 results in increased plasma concentrations of the co-administered drug and could lead to clinically significant pharmacodynamic side effects).
No products indexed under this heading.

Erythromycin Ethylsuccinate (Ciprofloxacin is an inhibitor of CYP450 1A2 isoenzymes. Co-administration of ciprofloxacin and other drugs primarily metabolized by CYP1A2 results in increased plasma concentrations of the co-administered drug and could lead to clinically significant pharmacodynamic side effects). Products include:
E.E.S. 451
EryPed 447

Erythromycin Gluceptate (Ciprofloxacin is an inhibitor of CYP450 1A2 isoenzymes. Co-administration of ciprofloxacin and other drugs primarily metabolized by CYP1A2 results in increased plasma concentrations of the co-administered drug and could lead to clinically significant pharmacodynamic side effects).
No products indexed under this heading.

Erythromycin Lactobionate (Ciprofloxacin is an inhibitor of CYP450 1A2 isoenzymes. Co-administration of ciprofloxacin and other drugs primarily metabolized by CYP1A2 results in increased plasma concentrations of the co-administered drug and could lead to clinically significant pharmacodynamic side effects).
No products indexed under this heading.

Erythromycin Stearate (Ciprofloxacin is an inhibitor of CYP450 1A2 isoenzymes. Co-administration of ciprofloxacin and other drugs primarily metabolized by CYP1A2 results in increased plasma concentrations of the co-administered drug and could lead to clinically significant pharmacodynamic side effects). Products include:
Erythrocin Stearate Filmtab Tablets 453

Estradiol (Ciprofloxacin is an inhibitor of CYP450 1A2 isoenzymes. Co-administration of ciprofloxacin and other drugs primarily metabolized by CYP1A2 results in increased plasma concentrations of the co-administered drug and could lead to clinically significant pharmacodynamic side effects). Products include:
Angeliq Tablets 762
Climara Transdermal System 771
Climara Pro Transdermal System 776
Estrasorb Topical Emulsion 1147
Estring Vaginal Ring 2635
Menostar Transdermal System 782
Vagifem Tablets 2334

Estradiol Benzoate (Ciprofloxacin is an inhibitor of CYP450 1A2 isoenzymes. Co-administration of ciprofloxacin and other drugs primarily metabolized by CYP1A2 results in increased plasma concentrations of the co-administered drug and could lead to clinically significant pharmacodynamic side effects).
No products indexed under this heading.

Estradiol Cypionate (Ciprofloxacin is an inhibitor of CYP450 1A2 isoenzymes. Co-administration of ciprofloxacin and other drugs primarily metabolized by CYP1A2 results in increased plasma concentrations of the co-administered drug and could lead to clinically significant pharmacodynamic side effects).
No products indexed under this heading.

Etodolac (NSAIDs in combination with very high doses of quinolones have been shown to provoke convulsions in pre-clinical trials).
No products indexed under this heading.

Fenoprofen Calcium (NSAIDs in combination with very high doses of quinolones have been shown to provoke convulsions in pre-clinical trials). Products include:
Nalfon Capsules **2502**

Ferrous Fumarate (Concurrent administration may substantially interfere with the absorption of ciprofloxacin, resulting in serum and urine levels of ciprofloxacin considerably lower than desired. Ciprofloxacin extended-release tablets should be administered at least 2 hours before or 6 hours after metal cations, such as iron.).
No products indexed under this heading.

Ferrous Gluconate (Concurrent administration may substantially interfere with the absorption of ciprofloxacin, resulting in serum and urine levels of ciprofloxacin considerably lower than desired. Ciprofloxacin extended-release tablets should be administered at least 2 hours before or 6 hours after metal cations, such as iron.).
No products indexed under this heading.

Ferrous Sulfate (Concurrent administration may substantially interfere with the absorption of ciprofloxacin, resulting in serum and urine levels of ciprofloxacin considerably lower than desired. Ciprofloxacin extended-release tablets should be administered at least 2 hours before or 6 hours after metal cations, such as iron). Products include:
Slow Fe Iron Tablets **818**
Slow Fe with Folic Acid Tablets **819**

Fludrocortisone Acetate (Risk of ruptures of the shoulder, hand, Achilles tendon or other tendons may be increased in patients receiving concomitant corticosteroids, especially in the elderly).
No products indexed under this heading.

Flurbiprofen (NSAIDs in combination with very high doses of quinolones have been shown to provoke convulsions in pre-clinical trials).
No products indexed under this heading.

Flutamide (Ciprofloxacin is an inhibitor of CYP450 1A2 isoenzymes. Co-administration of ciprofloxacin and other drugs primarily metabolized by CYP1A2 results in increased plasma concentrations of the co-administered drug and could lead to clinically significant pharmacodynamic side effects). Products include:
Eulexin Capsules **3009**

Fluticasone Propionate (Ciprofloxacin is an inhibitor of CYP450 1A2 isoenzymes. Co-administration of ciprofloxacin and other drugs primarily metabolized by CYP1A2 results in increased plasma concentrations of the co-administered drug and could lead to clinically significant pharmacodynamic side effects). Products include:
Advair Diskus 100/50 .... **1308**
Advair Diskus 250/50 .... **1308**
Advair Diskus 500/50 .... **1308**
Advair HFA Inhalation Aerosol **1318**
Cutivate Cream **2662**
Cutivate Lotion 0.05% **2664**
Cutivate Ointment **2665**
Flonase Nasal Spray **1440**
Flovent Diskus **1443**

Fluvoxamine Maleate (Ciprofloxacin is an inhibitor of CYP450 1A2 isoenzymes. Co-administration of ciprofloxacin and other drugs primarily metabolized by CYP1A2 results in increased plasma concentrations of the co-administered drug and could lead to clinically significant pharmacodynamic side effects).
No products indexed under this heading.

Fosphenytoin Sodium (Altered serum levels of phenytoin (increased and decreased) have been reported in patients receiving concomitant ciprofloxacin).
No products indexed under this heading.

Glyburide (The concomitant administration of ciprofloxacin with glyburide has, on rare occasions, resulted in severe hypoglycemia).
No products indexed under this heading.

Grepafloxacin Hydrochloride (Ciprofloxacin is an inhibitor of CYP450 1A2 isoenzymes. Co-administration of ciprofloxacin and other drugs primarily metabolized by CYP1A2 results in increased plasma concentrations of the co-administered drug and could lead to clinically significant pharmacodynamic side effects).
No products indexed under this heading.

Haloperidol (Ciprofloxacin is an inhibitor of CYP450 1A2 isoenzymes. Co-administration of ciprofloxacin and other drugs primarily metabolized by CYP1A2 results in increased plasma concentrations of the co-administered drug and could lead to clinically significant pharmacodynamic side effects).
No products indexed under this heading.

Haloperidol Decanoate (Ciprofloxacin is an inhibitor of CYP450 1A2 isoenzymes. Co-administration of ciprofloxacin and other drugs primarily metabolized by CYP1A2 results in increased plasma concentrations of the co-administered drug and could lead to clinically significant pharmacodynamic side effects).
No products indexed under this heading.

Haloperidol Lactate (Ciprofloxacin is an inhibitor of CYP450 1A2 isoenzymes. Co-administration of ciprofloxacin and other drugs primarily metabolized by CYP1A2 results in increased plasma concentrations of the co-administered drug and could lead to clinically significant pharmacodynamic side effects).
No products indexed under this heading.

Hydrocortisone (Risk of ruptures of the shoulder, hand, Achilles tendon or other tendons may be increased in patients receiving concomitant corticosteroids, especially in the elderly). Products include:
Colocort Rectal Suspension, USP (Retention) 100 mg/60 mL **2476**
Hydrocortone Tablets **1989**
Preparation H Hydrocortisone Cream **646**

Hydrocortisone Acetate (Risk of ruptures of the shoulder, hand, Achilles tendon or other tendons may be increased in patients receiving concomitant corticosteroids, especially in the elderly). Products include:
Analpram-HC **1159**
Pramosone **1161**
ProctoFoam-HC **3099**

Hydrocortisone Sodium Phosphate (Risk of ruptures of the shoulder, hand, Achilles tendon or other tendons may be increased in patients receiving concomitant corticosteroids, especially in the elderly).
No products indexed under this heading.

Hydrocortisone Sodium Succinate (Risk of ruptures of the shoulder, hand, Achilles tendon or other tendons may be increased in patients receiving concomitant corticosteroids, especially in the elderly).
No products indexed under this heading.

Ibuprofen (NSAIDs in combination with very high doses of quinolones have been shown to provoke convulsions in pre-clinical trials). Products include:
Advil Allergy Sinus Caplets **770**
Advil **674**
Children's Advil Oral Suspension **603**
Children's Advil Chewable Tablets **603**
Advil Cold & Sinus **723**
Infants' Advil Concentrated Drops **604**
Infants' Advil Concentrated Drops - White Grape (Dye-Free) **604**
Junior Strength Advil Swallow Tablets **605**
Advil Migraine Liquigels **608**
Advil Multi-Symptom Cold Caplets **770**
Advil PM Caplets **615**
Motrin IB Tablets and Caplets **1866**
Children's Motrin Oral Suspension **1867**
Children's Motrin Non-Staining Dye-Free Oral Suspension **1867**
Children's Motrin Cold Oral Suspension **1867**
Infants' Motrin Concentrated Drops **1867**
Infants' Motrin Non-Staining Dye-Free Concentrated Drops **1867**
Junior Strength Motrin Caplets and Chewable Tablets **1867**
Vicoprofen Tablets **539**

Imipramine Hydrochloride (Ciprofloxacin is an inhibitor of CYP450 1A2 isoenzymes. Co-administration of ciprofloxacin and other drugs primarily metabolized by CYP1A2 results in increased plasma concentrations of the co-administered drug and could lead to clinically significant pharmacodynamic side effects).
No products indexed under this heading.

Imipramine Pamoate (Ciprofloxacin is an inhibitor of CYP450 1A2 isoenzymes. Co-administration of ciprofloxacin and other drugs primarily metabolized by CYP1A2 results in increased plasma concentrations of the co-administered drug and could lead to clinically significant pharmacodynamic side effects).
No products indexed under this heading.

Indomethacin (NSAIDs in combination with very high doses of quinolones have been shown to provoke convulsions in pre-clinical trials). Products include:
Indocin **1995**

Indomethacin Sodium Trihydrate (NSAIDs in combination with very high doses of quinolones have been shown to provoke convulsions in pre-clinical trials). Products include:
Indocin I.V. **2465**

Iron (Concurrent administration may substantially interfere with the absorption of ciprofloxacin, resulting in serum and urine levels of ciprofloxacin considerably lower than desired. Ciprofloxacin extended-release tablets should be administered at least 2 hours before or 6 hours after metal cations, such as iron.).
No products indexed under this heading.

Ketoprofen (NSAIDs in combination with very high doses of quinolones have been shown to provoke convulsions in pre-clinical trials).
No products indexed under this heading.

Ketorolac Tromethamine (NSAIDs in combination with very high doses of quinolones have been shown to provoke convulsions in pre-clinical trials). Products include:
Acular Ophthalmic Solution **565**
Acular LS Ophthalmic Solution **566**

Levobupivacaine Hydrochloride (Ciprofloxacin is an inhibitor of CYP450 1A2 isoenzymes. Co-administration of ciprofloxacin and other drugs primarily metabolized by CYP1A2 results in increased plasma concentrations of the co-administered drug and could lead to clinically significant pharmacodynamic side effects).
No products indexed under this heading.

Lomefloxacin Hydrochloride (Ciprofloxacin is an inhibitor of CYP450 1A2 isoenzymes. Co-administration of ciprofloxacin and other drugs primarily metabolized by CYP1A2 results in increased plasma concentrations of the co-administered drug and could lead to clinically significant pharmacodynamic side effects).
No products indexed under this heading.

Magaldrate (Concurrent administration may substantially interfere with the absorption of ciprofloxacin, resulting in serum and urine levels of ciprofloxacin considerably lower than desired. Ciprofloxacin extended-release tablets should be administered at least 2 hours before or 6 hours after antacids containing magnesium or aluminum.).
No products indexed under this heading.

Magnesium (Concurrent administration may substantially interfere with the absorption of ciprofloxacin, resulting in serum and urine levels of ciprofloxacin considerably lower than desired. Ciprofloxacin extended-release tablets should be administered at least 2 hours before or 6 hours after metal cations.).
No products indexed under this heading.

Magnesium Carbonate (Concurrent administration may substantially interfere with the absorption of ciprofloxacin, resulting in serum and urine levels of ciprofloxacin considerably lower than desired). Products include:
Gaviscon Regular Strength Liquid .. ■ 658
Gaviscon Extra Strength Liquid ...... ■ 658
Gaviscon Extra Strength Tablets .... ■ 658

Magnesium Hydroxide (Concurrent administration may substantially interfere with the absorption of ciprofloxacin, resulting in serum and urine levels of ciprofloxacin considerably lower than desired. Ciprofloxacin extended-release tablets should be administered at least 2 hours before or 6 hours after antacids containing magnesium or aluminum). Products include:
Maalox Regular Strength Antacid/Antigas Liquid................. 2175
Maalox Max Maximum Strength Antacid/Anti-Gas Liquid................. 2176
Pepcid Complete Chewable Tablets.. 1701

Magnesium Oxide (Concurrent administration may substantially interfere with the absorption of ciprofloxacin, resulting in serum and urine levels of ciprofloxacin considerably lower than desired. Ciprofloxacin extended-release tablets should be administered at least 2 hours before or 6 hours after antacids containing magnesium or aluminum). Products include:
Beelith Tablets 759
PremCal Light, Regular, and Extra Strength Tablets................ ■ 818

Maprotiline Hydrochloride (Ciprofloxacin is an inhibitor of CYP450 1A2 isoenzymes. Co-administration of ciprofloxacin and other drugs primarily metabolized by CYP1A2 results in increased plasma concentrations of the co-administered drug and could lead to clinically significant pharmacodynamic side effects).
No products indexed under this heading.

Meclofenamate Sodium (NSAIDs in combination with very high doses of quinolones have been shown to provoke convulsions in pre-clinical trials).
No products indexed under this heading.

Mefenamic Acid (NSAIDs in combination with very high doses of quinolones have been shown to provoke convulsions in pre-clinical trials).
No products indexed under this heading.

Meloxicam (NSAIDs in combination with very high doses of quinolones have been shown to provoke convulsions in pre-clinical trials). Products include:
Mobic Oral Suspension 863
Mobic Tablets 863

Methadone Hydrochloride (Ciprofloxacin is an inhibitor of CYP450 1A2 isoenzymes. Co-administration of ciprofloxacin and other drugs primarily metabolized by CYP1A2 results in increased plasma concentrations of the co-administered drug and could lead to clinically significant pharmacodynamic side effects).
No products indexed under this heading.

Methotrexate (Renal tubular transport of methotrexate may be inhibited by concomitant administration of ciprofloxacin potentially leading to increased plasma levels of methotrexate).
No products indexed under this heading.

Methotrexate Sodium (Renal tubular transport of methotrexate may be inhibited by concomitant administration of ciprofloxacin potentially leading to increased plasma levels of methotrexate).
No products indexed under this heading.

Methylprednisolone Acetate (Risk of ruptures of the shoulder, hand, Achilles tendon or other tendons may be increased in patients receiving concomitant corticosteroids, especially in the elderly). Products include:
Depo-Medrol Injectable Suspension 2617
Depo-Medrol Single-Dose Vial 2619

Methylprednisolone Sodium Succinate (Risk of ruptures of the shoulder, hand, Achilles tendon or other tendons may be increased in patients receiving concomitant corticosteroids, especially in the elderly).
No products indexed under this heading.

Metoclopramide Hydrochloride (Metoclopramide significantly accelerates the absorption of oral ciprofloxacin resulting in a shorter time to reach maximum plasma concentrations).
No products indexed under this heading.

Mexiletine Hydrochloride (Ciprofloxacin is an inhibitor of CYP450 1A2 isoenzymes. Co-administration of ciprofloxacin and other drugs primarily metabolized by CYP1A2 results in increased plasma concentrations of the co-administered drug and could lead to clinically significant pharmacodynamic side effects).
No products indexed under this heading.

Mirtazapine (Ciprofloxacin is an inhibitor of CYP450 1A2 isoenzymes. Co-administration of ciprofloxacin and other drugs primarily metabolized by CYP1A2 results in increased plasma concentrations of the co-administered drug and could lead to clinically significant pharmacodynamic side effects).
No products indexed under this heading.

Moxifloxacin Hydrochloride (Ciprofloxacin is an inhibitor of CYP450 1A2 isoenzymes. Co-administration of ciprofloxacin and other drugs primarily metabolized by CYP1A2 results in increased plasma concentrations of the co-administered drug and could lead to clinically significant pharmacodynamic side effects). Products include:
Avelox 2970
Vigamox Ophthalmic Solution 564

Nabumetone (NSAIDs in combination with very high doses of quinolones have been shown to provoke convulsions in pre-clinical trials).
No products indexed under this heading.

Nafcillin Sodium (Ciprofloxacin is an inhibitor of CYP450 1A2 isoenzymes. Co-administration of ciprofloxacin and other drugs primarily metabolized by CYP1A2 results in increased plasma concentrations of the co-administered drug and could lead to clinically significant pharmacodynamic side effects).
No products indexed under this heading.

Naproxen (NSAIDs in combination with very high doses of quinolones have been shown to provoke convulsions in pre-clinical trials). Products include:
EC-Naprosyn Delayed-Release Tablets.. 2761
Naprosyn Suspension 2761
Naprosyn Tablets 2761
Prevacid NapraPAC 3280

Naproxen Sodium (NSAIDs in combination with very high doses of quinolones have been shown to provoke convulsions in pre-clinical trials). Products include:
Aleve Caplets 742
Aleve Gelcaps 743
Aleve Tablets 743
Aleve Cold & Sinus Caplets 744
Anaprox Tablets 2761
Anaprox DS Tablets 2761

Nicotine Polacrilex (Ciprofloxacin is an inhibitor of CYP450 1A2 isoenzymes. Co-administration of ciprofloxacin and other drugs primarily metabolized by CYP1A2 results in increased plasma concentrations of the co-administered drug and could lead to clinically significant pharmacodynamic side effects).
No products indexed under this heading.

Nicotine Salicylate (Ciprofloxacin is an inhibitor of CYP450 1A2 isoenzymes. Co-administration of ciprofloxacin and other drugs primarily metabolized by CYP1A2 results in increased plasma concentrations of the co-administered drug and could lead to clinically significant pharmacodynamic side effects).
No products indexed under this heading.

Nicotine Sulfate (Ciprofloxacin is an inhibitor of CYP450 1A2 isoenzymes. Co-administration of ciprofloxacin and other drugs primarily metabolized by CYP1A2 results in increased plasma concentrations of the co-administered drug and could lead to clinically significant pharmacodynamic side effects).
No products indexed under this heading.

Norethindrone Acetate (Ciprofloxacin is an inhibitor of CYP450 1A2 isoenzymes. Co-administration of ciprofloxacin and other drugs primarily metabolized by CYP1A2 results in increased plasma concentrations of the co-administered drug and could lead to clinically significant pharmacodynamic side effects).
No products indexed under this heading.

Norfloxacin (Ciprofloxacin is an inhibitor of CYP450 1A2 isoenzymes. Co-administration of ciprofloxacin and other drugs primarily metabolized by CYP1A2 results in increased plasma concentrations of the co-administered drug and could lead to clinically significant pharmacodynamic side effects). Products include:
Noroxin Tablets 2032

Nortriptyline Hydrochloride (Ciprofloxacin is an inhibitor of CYP450 1A2 isoenzymes. Co-administration of ciprofloxacin and other drugs primarily metabolized by CYP1A2 results in increased plasma concentrations of the co-administered drug and could lead to clinically significant pharmacodynamic side effects).
No products indexed under this heading.

Ofloxacin (Ciprofloxacin is an inhibitor of CYP450 1A2 isoenzymes. Co-administration of ciprofloxacin and other drugs primarily metabolized by CYP1A2 results in increased plasma concentrations of the co-administered drug and could lead to clinically significant pharmacodynamic side effects). Products include:
Floxin Otic Solution 1049

Olanzapine (Ciprofloxacin is an inhibitor of CYP450 1A2 isoenzymes. Co-administration of ciprofloxacin and other drugs primarily metabolized by CYP1A2 results in increased plasma concentrations of the co-administered drug and could lead to clinically significant pharmacodynamic side effects). Products include:
Symbyax Capsules 1819
Zyprexa Tablets 1830
Zyprexa IntraMuscular 1830
Zyprexa ZYDIS Orally Disintegrating Tablets.................. 1830

Omeprazole (Absorption of the Cipro XR tablet was slightly diminished (20%) when given concomitantly with omeprazole). Products include:
Zegerid Capsules 2958
Zegerid Powder for Oral Solution 2958

Ondansetron (Ciprofloxacin is an inhibitor of CYP450 1A2 isoenzymes. Co-administration of ciprofloxacin and other drugs primarily metabolized by CYP1A2 results in increased plasma concentrations of the co-administered drug and could lead to clinically significant pharmacodynamic side effects). Products include:
Zofran ODT Orally Disintegrating Tablets.. 1639

Ondansetron Hydrochloride (Ciprofloxacin is an inhibitor of CYP450 1A2 isoenzymes. Co-administration of ciprofloxacin and other drugs primarily metabolized by CYP1A2 results in increased plasma concentrations of the co-administered drug and could lead to clinically significant pharmacodynamic side effects). Products include:
Zofran Injection 1634
Zofran 1639

Oxaprozin (NSAIDs in combination with very high doses of quinolones have been shown to provoke convulsions in pre-clinical trials).
No products indexed under this heading.

Phenobarbital Sodium (Ciprofloxacin is an inhibitor of CYP450 1A2 isoenzymes. Co-administration of ciprofloxacin and other drugs primarily metabolized by CYP1A2 results in increased plasma concentrations of the co-administered drug and could lead to clinically significant pharmacodynamic side effects).
No products indexed under this heading.

Phenylbutazone (NSAIDs in combination with very high doses of quinolones have been shown to provoke convulsions in pre-clinical trials).
No products indexed under this heading.

Phenytoin (Altered serum levels of phenytoin (increased and decreased) have been reported in patients receiving concomitant ciprofloxacin).
No products indexed under this heading.

Phenytoin Sodium (Altered serum levels of phenytoin (increased and decreased) have been reported in patients receiving concomitant ciprofloxacin). Products include:
Phenytek Capsules **2160**

Piroxicam (NSAIDs in combination with very high doses of quinolones have been shown to provoke convulsions in pre-clinical trials).
No products indexed under this heading.

Polysaccharide Iron Complex (Concurrent administration may substantially interfere with the absorption of ciprofloxacin, resulting in serum and urine levels of ciprofloxacin considerably lower than desired. Ciprofloxacin extended-release tablets should be administered at least 2 hours before or 6 hours after metal cations, such as iron). Products include:
Nu-Iron 150 Capsules **2127**

Prednisolone Acetate (Risk of ruptures of the shoulder, hand, Achilles tendon or other tendons may be increased in patients receiving concomitant corticosteroids, especially in the elderly). Products include:
Blephamide Ophthalmic Ointment **568**
Blephamide Ophthalmic Suspension **569**
Poly-Pred Ophthalmic Suspension .... **⊙233**
Pred Forte Ophthalmic Suspension .... **⊙235**
Pred Mild Ophthalmic Suspension .... **⊙238**
Pred-G Ophthalmic Ointment .... **⊙237**
Pred-G Ophthalmic Suspension .... **⊙236**

Prednisolone Sodium Phosphate (Risk of ruptures of the shoulder, hand, Achilles tendon or other tendons may be increased in patients receiving concomitant corticosteroids, especially in the elderly).
No products indexed under this heading.

Prednisolone Tebutate (Risk of ruptures of the shoulder, hand, Achilles tendon or other tendons may be increased in patients receiving concomitant corticosteroids, especially in the elderly).
No products indexed under this heading.

Prednisone (Risk of ruptures of the shoulder, hand, Achilles tendon or other tendons may be increased in patients receiving concomitant corticosteroids, especially in the elderly).
No products indexed under this heading.

Probenecid (Probenecid interferes with renal tubular secretion of ciprofloxacin and produces an increase in the level of ciprofloxacin in the serum).
No products indexed under this heading.

Propafenone Hydrochloride (Ciprofloxacin is an inhibitor of CYP450 1A2 isoenzymes. Co-administration of ciprofloxacin and other drugs primarily metabolized by CYP1A2 results in increased plasma concentrations of the co-administered drug and could lead to clinically significant pharmacodynamic side effects). Products include:
Rythmol SR Capsules **2727**

Propranolol Hydrochloride (Ciprofloxacin is an inhibitor of CYP450 1A2 isoenzymes. Co-administration of ciprofloxacin and other drugs primarily metabolized by CYP1A2 results in increased plasma concentrations of the co-administered drug and could lead to clinically significant pharmacodynamic side effects). Products include:
Inderal LA Long-Acting Capsules **3429**
InnoPran XL Capsules **2723**

Protriptyline Hydrochloride (Ciprofloxacin is an inhibitor of CYP450 1A2 isoenzymes. Co-administration of ciprofloxacin and other drugs primarily metabolized by CYP1A2 results in increased plasma concentrations of the co-administered drug and could lead to clinically significant pharmacodynamic side effects).
No products indexed under this heading.

Riluzole (Ciprofloxacin is an inhibitor of CYP450 1A2 isoenzymes. Co-administration of ciprofloxacin and other drugs primarily metabolized by CYP1A2 results in increased plasma concentrations of the co-administered drug and could lead to clinically significant pharmacodynamic side effects). Products include:
Rilutek Tablets **2930**

Ritonavir (Ciprofloxacin is an inhibitor of CYP450 1A2 isoenzymes. Co-administration of ciprofloxacin and other drugs primarily metabolized by CYP1A2 results in increased plasma concentrations of the co-administered drug and could lead to clinically significant pharmacodynamic side effects). Products include:
Kaletra **476**
Norvir **503**

Rofecoxib (NSAIDs in combination with very high doses of quinolones have been shown to provoke convulsions in pre-clinical trials).
No products indexed under this heading.

Ropinirole Hydrochloride (Ciprofloxacin is an inhibitor of CYP450 1A2 isoenzymes. Co-administration of ciprofloxacin and other drugs primarily metabolized by CYP1A2 results in increased plasma concentrations of the co-administered drug and could lead to clinically significant pharmacodynamic side effects). Products include:
Requip Tablets **1555**

Ropivacaine Hydrochloride (Ciprofloxacin is an inhibitor of CYP450 1A2 isoenzymes. Co-administration of ciprofloxacin and other drugs primarily metabolized by CYP1A2 results in increased plasma concentrations of the co-administered drug and could lead to clinically significant pharmacodynamic side effects).
No products indexed under this heading.

Sucralfate (Concurrent administration may substantially interfere with the absorption of ciprofloxacin, resulting in serum and urine levels of ciprofloxacin considerably lower than desired. Ciprofloxacin extended-release tablets should be administered at least 2 hours before or 6 hours after sucralfate). Products include:
Carafate Suspension **701**
Carafate Tablets **701**

Sulindac (NSAIDs in combination with very high doses of quinolones have been shown to provoke convulsions in pre-clinical trials). Products include:
Clinoril Tablets **1924**

Tacrine Hydrochloride (Ciprofloxacin is an inhibitor of CYP450 1A2 isoenzymes. Co-administration of ciprofloxacin and other drugs primarily metabolized by CYP1A2 results in increased plasma concentrations of the co-administered drug and could lead to clinically significant pharmacodynamic side effects).
No products indexed under this heading.

Tamoxifen Citrate (Ciprofloxacin is an inhibitor of CYP450 1A2 isoenzymes. Co-administration of ciprofloxacin and other drugs primarily metabolized by CYP1A2 results in increased plasma concentrations of the co-administered drug and could lead to clinically significant pharmacodynamic side effects). Products include:
Soltamox Oral Solution **3527**

Theophylline (Concurrent administration of ciprofloxacin and theophylline may lead to elevated serum concentrations of theophylline and prolongation of its elimination half-life. Serious and fatal reactions have been reported in patients receiving concurrent administration. These reactions have included cardiac arrest, seizure, status epilepticus, and respiratory failure.).
No products indexed under this heading.

Theophylline Anhydrous (Concurrent administration of ciprofloxacin and theophylline may lead to elevated serum concentrations of theophylline and prolongation of its elimination half-life. Serious and fatal reactions have been reported in patients receiving concurrent administration. These reactions have included cardiac arrest, seizure, status epilepticus, and respiratory failure). Products include:
Uniphyl Tablets **2710**

Theophylline Calcium Salicylate (Concurrent administration of ciprofloxacin and theophylline may lead to elevated serum concentrations of theophylline and prolongation of its elimination half-life. Serious and fatal reactions have been reported in patients receiving concurrent administration. These reactions have included cardiac arrest, seizure, status epilepticus, and respiratory failure).
No products indexed under this heading.

Theophylline Dihydroxypropyl (Glyceryl) (Concurrent administration of ciprofloxacin and theophylline may lead to elevated serum concentrations of theophylline and prolongation of its elimination half-life. Serious and fatal reactions have been reported in patients receiving concurrent administration. These reactions have included cardiac arrest, seizure, status epilepticus, and respiratory failure).
No products indexed under this heading.

Theophylline Ethylenediamine (Concurrent administration of ciprofloxacin and theophylline may lead to elevated serum concentrations of theophylline and prolongation of its elimination half-life. Serious and fatal reactions have been reported in patients receiving concurrent administration. These reactions have included cardiac arrest, seizure, status epilepticus, and respiratory failure).
No products indexed under this heading.

Theophylline Sodium Glycinate (Concurrent administration of ciprofloxacin and theophylline may lead to elevated serum concentrations of theophylline and prolongation of its elimination half-life. Serious and fatal reactions have been reported in patients receiving concurrent administration. These reactions have included cardiac arrest, seizure, status epilepticus, and respiratory failure).
No products indexed under this heading.

Tizanidine Hydrochloride (Concomitant administration is contraindicated).
No products indexed under this heading.

Tolmetin Sodium (NSAIDs in combination with very high doses of quinolones have been shown to provoke convulsions in pre-clinical trials).
No products indexed under this heading.

Triamcinolone (Risk of ruptures of the shoulder, hand, Achilles tendon or other tendons may be increased in patients receiving concomitant corticosteroids, especially in the elderly).
No products indexed under this heading.

Triamcinolone Acetonide (Risk of ruptures of the shoulder, hand, Achilles tendon or other tendons may be increased in patients receiving concomitant corticosteroids, especially in the elderly). Products include:
Azmacort Inhalation Aerosol **1726**
Nasacort AQ Nasal Spray **2922**

Triamcinolone Diacetate (Risk of ruptures of the shoulder, hand, Achilles tendon or other tendons may be increased in patients receiving concomitant corticosteroids, especially in the elderly).
No products indexed under this heading.

Triamcinolone Hexacetonide (Risk of ruptures of the shoulder, hand, Achilles tendon or other tendons may be increased in patients receiving concomitant corticosteroids, especially in the elderly).
No products indexed under this heading.

Trimethaphan Camsylate (Ciprofloxacin is an inhibitor of CYP450 1A2 isoenzymes. Co-administration of ciprofloxacin and other drugs primarily metabolized by CYP1A2 results in increased plasma concentrations of the co-administered drug and could lead to clinically significant pharmacodynamic side effects).
No products indexed under this heading.

Trimipramine Maleate (Ciprofloxacin is an inhibitor of CYP450 1A2 isoenzymes. Co-administration of ciprofloxacin and other drugs primarily metabolized by CYP1A2 results in increased plasma concentrations of the co-administered drug and could lead to clinically significant pharmacodynamic side effects).
No products indexed under this heading.

Trovafloxacin Mesylate (Ciprofloxacin is an inhibitor of CYP450 1A2 isoenzymes. Co-administration of ciprofloxacin and other drugs primarily metabolized by CYP1A2 results in increased plasma concentrations of the co-administered drug and could lead to clinically significant pharmacodynamic side effects).
No products indexed under this heading.

Valdecoxib (NSAIDs in combination with very high doses of quinolones have been shown to provoke convulsions in pre-clinical trials).
No products indexed under this heading.

Verapamil Hydrochloride (Ciprofloxacin is an inhibitor of CYP450 1A2 isoenzymes. Co-administration of ciprofloxacin and other drugs primarily metabolized by CYP1A2 results in increased plasma concentrations of the co-administered drug and could lead to clinically significant pharmacodynamic side effects). Products include:
- Covera-HS Tablets 3139
- Tarka Tablets 524
- Verelan PM Extended-Release Capsules, Controlled-Onset 3106

Warfarin Sodium (Quinolones have been reported to enhance the effects of the oral anticoagulant warfarin or its derivatives). Products include:
- Coumadin for Injection 898
- Coumadin Tablets 898

Zileuton (Ciprofloxacin is an inhibitor of CYP450 1A2 isoenzymes. Co-administration of ciprofloxacin and other drugs primarily metabolized by CYP1A2 results in increased plasma concentrations of the co-administered drug and could lead to clinically significant pharmacodynamic side effects). Products include:
- Zyflo Tablets 1023

Zinc (Concurrent administration may substantially interfere with the absorption of ciprofloxacin, resulting in serum and urine levels of ciprofloxacin considerably lower than desired. Ciprofloxacin extended-release tablets should be administered at least 2 hours before or 6 hours after zinc-containing products). Products include:
- Visutein Capsules 3329

Zinc Acetate (Concurrent administration may substantially interfere with the absorption of ciprofloxacin, resulting in serum and urine levels of ciprofloxacin considerably lower than desired. Ciprofloxacin extended-release tablets should be administered at least 2 hours before or 6 hours after zinc-containing products).
No products indexed under this heading.

Zinc Chloride (Concurrent administration may substantially interfere with the absorption of ciprofloxacin, resulting in serum and urine levels of ciprofloxacin considerably lower than desired. Ciprofloxacin extended-release tablets should be administered at least 2 hours before or 6 hours after zinc-containing products).
No products indexed under this heading.

Zinc Citrate (Concurrent administration may substantially interfere with the absorption of ciprofloxacin, resulting in serum and urine levels of ciprofloxacin considerably lower than desired. Ciprofloxacin extended-release tablets should be administered at least 2 hours before or 6 hours after zinc-containing products).
No products indexed under this heading.

Zinc-Containing Multivitamins (Concurrent administration may substantially interfere with the absorption of ciprofloxacin, resulting in serum and urine levels of ciprofloxacin considerably lower than desired. Ciprofloxacin extended-release tablets should be administered at least 2 hours before or 6 hours after multivitamin preparations with zinc).
No products indexed under this heading.

Zinc Gluconate (Concurrent administration may substantially interfere with the absorption of ciprofloxacin, resulting in serum and urine levels of ciprofloxacin considerably lower than desired. Ciprofloxacin extended-release tablets should be administered at least 2 hours before or 6 hours after zinc-containing products).
No products indexed under this heading.

Zinc Oxide (Concurrent administration may substantially interfere with the absorption of ciprofloxacin, resulting in serum and urine levels of ciprofloxacin considerably lower than desired. Ciprofloxacin extended-release tablets should be administered at least 2 hours before or 6 hours after zinc-containing products). Products include:
- Bausch & Lomb Ocuvite Adult Eye Vitamin and Mineral Supplement Soft Gels .... ■□706
- Bausch & Lomb Ocuvite Adult 50+ Eye Vitamin and Mineral Supplement Soft Gels .... ■□706
- Nicomide Tablets 1088
- Ocuvite Adult Vitamin and Mineral Supplement .... ⊙253
- Ocuvite Adult 50+ Vitamin and Mineral Supplement .... ⊙253

Zinc Phenosulfonate (Concurrent administration may substantially interfere with the absorption of ciprofloxacin, resulting in serum and urine levels of ciprofloxacin considerably lower than desired. Ciprofloxacin extended-release tablets should be administered at least 2 hours before or 6 hours after zinc-containing products).
No products indexed under this heading.

Zinc Pyrithione (Concurrent administration may substantially interfere with the absorption of ciprofloxacin, resulting in serum and urine levels of ciprofloxacin considerably lower than desired. Ciprofloxacin extended-release tablets should be administered at least 2 hours before or 6 hours after zinc-containing products).
No products indexed under this heading.

Zinc Sulfate (Concurrent administration may substantially interfere with the absorption of ciprofloxacin, resulting in serum and urine levels of ciprofloxacin considerably lower than desired. Ciprofloxacin extended-release tablets should be administered at least 2 hours before or 6 hours after zinc-containing products). Products include:
- Visine A.C. Seasonal Itching and Redness Relief Drops .... ⊙289
- Zinc-220 Capsules 580

Zinc Undecylenate (Concurrent administration may substantially interfere with the absorption of ciprofloxacin, resulting in serum and urine levels of ciprofloxacin considerably lower than desired. Ciprofloxacin extended-release tablets should be administered at least 2 hours before or 6 hours after zinc-containing products).
No products indexed under this heading.

Zolmitriptan (Ciprofloxacin is an inhibitor of CYP450 1A2 isoenzymes. Co-administration of ciprofloxacin and other drugs primarily metabolized by CYP1A2 results in increased plasma concentrations of the co-administered drug and could lead to clinically significant pharmacodynamic side effects). Products include:
- Zomig Tablets 3519
- Zomig Nasal Spray 3523
- Zomig-ZMT Tablets 3519

Food Interactions

Dairy products (Concurrent administration of ciprofloxacin with dairy products should be avoided since decreased absorption of ciprofloxacin is possible).

Food, calcium-rich (Concurrent administration of ciprofloxacin with calcium-fortified juices should be avoided since decreased absorption of ciprofloxacin is possible).

CITRACAL CAPLETS
(Calcium Citrate) .... ■□703
None cited in PDR database.

CITRACAL LEMON CREAM CREAMY BITES
(Calcium Citrate) 2139
None cited in PDR database.

CITRACAL PRENATAL + DHA TABLETS AND CAPSULES
(Calcium Citrate, Docosahexaenoic Acid (DHA), Multivitamins with Minerals) 2139
None cited in PDR database.

CITRACAL PRENATAL RX TABLETS
(Vitamins, Prenatal) 2139
None cited in PDR database.

CITRUCEL CAPLETS
(Methylcellulose) .... ■□647
None cited in PDR database.

CITRUCEL ORANGE FLAVOR POWDER
(Methylcellulose) .... ■□647
None cited in PDR database.

CITRUCEL SUGAR FREE ORANGE FLAVOR POWDER
(Methylcellulose) .... ■□648
None cited in PDR database.

CLARINEX SYRUP
(Desloratadine) 2995
See Clarinex Tablets

CLARINEX TABLETS
(Desloratadine) 2995
May interact with erythromycin and certain other agents. Compounds in these categories include:

Azithromycin Dihydrate (Co-administration resulted in increased Cmax and AUC of desloratadine by 15% and 5% respectively; Cmax and AUC of 3-hydroxydesloratadine increased by 15% and 4% respectively; there were no clinically relevant changes in the safety profile of desloratadine).
No products indexed under this heading.

Cimetidine (Co-administration resulted in increased Cmax and AUC of desloratadine by 12% and 19% respectively; Cmax and AUC of 3-hydroxydesloratadine decreased by 11% and 3% respectively; there were no clinically relevant changes in the safety profile of desloratadine). Products include:
- Tagamet HB 200 Tablets .... ■□664

Cimetidine Hydrochloride (Co-administration resulted in increased Cmax and AUC of desloratadine by 12% and 19% respectively; Cmax and AUC of 3-hydroxydesloratadine decreased by 11% and 3% respectively; there were no clinically relevant changes in the safety profile of desloratadine).
No products indexed under this heading.

Erythromycin (Co-administration resulted in increased Cmax and AUC of desloratadine by 24% and 14% respectively; Cmax and AUC of 3-hydroxydesloratadine increased by 43% and 40% respectively; there were no clinically relevant changes in the safety profile of desloratadine). Products include:
- Ery-Tab Tablets 449
- Erythromycin Base Filmtab Tablets 455
- Erythromycin Delayed-Release Capsules, USP 457
- PCE Dispertab Tablets 515

Erythromycin Estolate (Co-administration resulted in increased Cmax and AUC of desloratadine by 24% and 14% respectively; Cmax and AUC of 3-hydroxydesloratadine increased by 43% and 40% respectively; there were no clinically relevant changes in the safety profile of desloratadine).
No products indexed under this heading.

Erythromycin Ethylsuccinate (Co-administration resulted in increased Cmax and AUC of desloratadine by 24% and 14% respectively; Cmax and AUC of 3-hydroxydesloratadine increased by 43% and 40% respectively; there were no clinically relevant changes in the safety profile of desloratadine). Products include:
E.E.S. 451
EryPed 447

Erythromycin Gluceptate (Co-administration resulted in increased Cmax and AUC of desloratadine by 24% and 14% respectively; Cmax and AUC of 3-hydroxydesloratadine increased by 43% and 40% respectively; there were no clinically relevant changes in the safety profile of desloratadine).
No products indexed under this heading.

Erythromycin Lactobionate (Co-administration resulted in increased Cmax and AUC of desloratadine by 24% and 14% respectively; Cmax and AUC of 3-hydroxydesloratadine increased by 43% and 40% respectively; there were no clinically relevant changes in the safety profile of desloratadine).
No products indexed under this heading.

Erythromycin Stearate (Co-administration resulted in increased Cmax and AUC of desloratadine by 24% and 14% respectively; Cmax and AUC of 3-hydroxydesloratadine increased by 43% and 40% respectively; there were no clinically relevant changes in the safety profile of desloratadine). Products include:
Erythrocin Stearate Filmtab Tablets 453

Fluoxetine Hydrochloride (Co-administration resulted in increased Cmax of desloratadine by 15%; Cmax and AUC of 3-hydroxydesloratadine increased by 17% and 13% respectively; there were no clinically relevant changes in the safety profile of desloratadine). Products include:
Prozac Pulvules and Liquid 1801
Symbyax Capsules 1819

Ketoconazole (Co-administration resulted in increased Cmax and AUC of desloratadine by 45% and 39% respectively; Cmax and AUC of 3-hydroxydesloratadine increased by 43% and 72% respectively; there were no clinically relevant changes in the safety profile of desloratadine). Products include:
Nizoral A-D Shampoo, 1% 1868

CLARINEX REDITABS TABLETS

(Desloratadine) 2995
See Clarinex Tablets

CLARINEX-D 24-HOUR EXTENDED-RELEASE TABLETS

(Desloratadine, Pseudoephedrine Sulfate) 2998
May interact with beta blockers, cardiac glycosides, monoamine oxidase inhibitors, veratrum alkaloids, and certain other agents. Compounds in these categories include:

Acebutolol Hydrochloride (The antihypertensive effects of beta-adrenergic blocking agents may be reduced by sympathomimetics).
No products indexed under this heading.

Atenolol (The antihypertensive effects of beta-adrenergic blocking agents may be reduced by sympathomimetics).
No products indexed under this heading.

Betaxolol Hydrochloride (The antihypertensive effects of beta-adrenergic blocking agents may be reduced by sympathomimetics). Products include:
Betoptic S Ophthalmic Suspension 558

Bisoprolol Fumarate (The antihypertensive effects of beta-adrenergic blocking agents may be reduced by sympathomimetics).
No products indexed under this heading.

Carteolol Hydrochloride (The antihypertensive effects of beta-adrenergic blocking agents may be reduced by sympathomimetics). Products include:
Carteolol Hydrochloride Ophthalmic Solution USP, 1% .... ⊙249

Cryptenamine Preparations (The antihypertensive effects of veratrum alkaloids may be reduced by sympathomimetics).
No products indexed under this heading.

Deslanoside (Increased ectopic pacemaker activity can occur when pseudoephedrine is used concomitantly with digitalis).
No products indexed under this heading.

Digitalis Glycoside Preparations (Increased ectopic pacemaker activity can occur when pseudoephedrine is used concomitantly with digitalis).
No products indexed under this heading.

Digitoxin (Increased ectopic pacemaker activity can occur when pseudoephedrine is used concomitantly with digitalis).
No products indexed under this heading.

Digoxin (Increased ectopic pacemaker activity can occur when pseudoephedrine is used concomitantly with digitalis). Products include:
Lanoxicaps Capsules 1490
Lanoxin Injection 1494
Lanoxin Injection Pediatric 1497
Lanoxin Tablets 1500

Esmolol Hydrochloride (The antihypertensive effects of beta-adrenergic blocking agents may be reduced by sympathomimetics).
No products indexed under this heading.

Isocarboxazid (Due to the pseudoephedrine component, Clarinex-D 24 Hour extended-release tablets should not be used by patients taking monoamine oxidase inhibitors or within 14 days after stopping such treatment).
No products indexed under this heading.

Labetalol Hydrochloride (The antihypertensive effects of beta-adrenergic blocking agents may be reduced by sympathomimetics).
No products indexed under this heading.

Levobunolol Hydrochloride (The antihypertensive effects of beta-adrenergic blocking agents may be reduced by sympathomimetics). Products include:
Betagan Ophthalmic Solution, USP .... ⊙220

Mecamylamine Hydrochloride (The antihypertensive effects of mecamylamine may be reduced by sympathomimetics).
No products indexed under this heading.

Methyldopa (The antihypertensive effects of methyldopa may be reduced by sympathomimetics). Products include:
Aldoril Tablets 1910

Methyldopate Hydrochloride (The antihypertensive effects of methyldopa may be reduced by sympathomimetics.).
No products indexed under this heading.

Metipranolol Hydrochloride (The antihypertensive effects of beta-adrenergic blocking agents may be reduced by sympathomimetics).
No products indexed under this heading.

Metoprolol Succinate (The antihypertensive effects of beta-adrenergic blocking agents may be reduced by sympathomimetics). Products include:
Toprol-XL Tablets 668

Metoprolol Tartrate (The antihypertensive effects of beta-adrenergic blocking agents may be reduced by sympathomimetics). Products include:
Lopressor Injection 2238
Lopressor Tablets 2238
Lopressor HCT 50/25 Tablets 2241
Lopressor HCT 100/25 Tablets 2241
Lopressor HCT 100/50 Tablets 2241

Moclobemide (Due to the pseudoephedrine component, Clarinex-D 24 Hour extended-release tablets should not be used by patients taking monoamine oxidase inhibitors or within 14 days after stopping such treatment).
No products indexed under this heading.

Nadolol (The antihypertensive effects of beta-adrenergic blocking agents may be reduced by sympathomimetics). Products include:
Nadolol Tablets 2159

Pargyline Hydrochloride (Due to the pseudoephedrine component, Clarinex-D 24 Hour extended-release tablets should not be used by patients taking monoamine oxidase inhibitors or within 14 days after stopping such treatment).
No products indexed under this heading.

Penbutolol Sulfate (The antihypertensive effects of beta-adrenergic blocking agents may be reduced by sympathomimetics).
No products indexed under this heading.

Phenelzine Sulfate (Due to the pseudoephedrine component, Clarinex-D 24 Hour extended-release tablets should not be used by patients taking monoamine oxidase inhibitors or within 14 days after stopping such treatment).
No products indexed under this heading.

Pindolol (The antihypertensive effects of beta-adrenergic blocking agents may be reduced by sympathomimetics).
No products indexed under this heading.

Procarbazine Hydrochloride (Due to the pseudoephedrine component, Clarinex-D 24 Hour extended-release tablets should not be used by patients taking monoamine oxidase inhibitors or within 14 days after stopping such treatment). Products include:
Matulane Capsules 3191

Propranolol Hydrochloride (The antihypertensive effects of beta-adrenergic blocking agents may be reduced by sympathomimetics). Products include:
Inderal LA Long-Acting Capsules 3429
InnoPran XL Capsules 2723

Reserpine (The antihypertensive effects of reserpine may be reduced by sympathomimetics).
No products indexed under this heading.

Selegiline Hydrochloride (Due to the pseudoephedrine component, Clarinex-D 24 Hour extended-release tablets should not be used by patients taking monoamine oxidase inhibitors or within 14 days after stopping such treatment). Products include:
Eldepryl Capsules 3208
Zelapar Tablets 3372

Sotalol Hydrochloride (The antihypertensive effects of beta-adrenergic blocking agents may be reduced by sympathomimetics).
No products indexed under this heading.

Timolol Hemihydrate (The antihypertensive effects of beta-adrenergic blocking agents may be reduced by sympathomimetics). Products include:
Betimol Ophthalmic Solution 3382
Betimol Ophthalmic Solution .... ⊙295

Timolol Maleate (The antihypertensive effects of beta-adrenergic blocking agents may be reduced by sympathomimetics). Products include:
Blocadren Tablets 1916
Cosopt Sterile Ophthalmic Solution 1931
Timolide Tablets 2086
Timoptic Sterile Ophthalmic Solution 2088
Timoptic in Ocudose 2091
Timoptic-XE Sterile Ophthalmic Gel Forming Solution 2092

Tranylcypromine Sulfate (Due to the pseudoephedrine component, Clarinex-D 24 Hour extended-release tablets should not be used by patients taking monoamine oxidase inhibitors or within 14 days after stopping such treatment). Products include:
Parnate Tablets 1527

CLARIPEL CREAM
(Hydroquinone) 3211
None cited in PDR database.

CHILDREN'S CLARITIN ALLERGY ORAL SOLUTION
(Loratadine) .... ▣771
None cited in PDR database.

CLARITIN NON-DROWSY 24 HOUR TABLETS
(Loratadine) .... ▣772
None cited in PDR database.

CLARITIN REDITABS 24 HOUR NON-DROWSY TABLETS
(Loratadine) .... ▣772
None cited in PDR database.

CLARITIN-D NON-DROWSY 12 HOUR TABLETS
(Loratadine, Pseudoephedrine Sulfate) .... ▣772
May interact with monoamine oxidase inhibitors. Compounds in these categories include:

Isocarboxazid (Concurrent and/or sequential use with MAO inhibitors is not recommended).
No products indexed under this heading.

Moclobemide (Concurrent and/or sequential use with MAO inhibitors is not recommended).
No products indexed under this heading.

Pargyline Hydrochloride (Concurrent and/or sequential use with MAO inhibitors is not recommended).
No products indexed under this heading.

Phenelzine Sulfate (Concurrent and/or sequential use with MAO inhibitors is not recommended).
No products indexed under this heading.

Procarbazine Hydrochloride (Concurrent and/or sequential use with MAO inhibitors is not recommended). Products include:
Matulane Capsules 3191

Selegiline Hydrochloride (Concurrent and/or sequential use with MAO inhibitors is not recommended). Products include:
Eldepryl Capsules 3208
Zelapar Tablets 3372

Tranylcypromine Sulfate (Concurrent and/or sequential use with MAO inhibitors is not recommended). Products include:
Parnate Tablets 1527

CLARITIN-D NON-DROWSY 24 HOUR TABLETS
(Loratadine, Pseudoephedrine Sulfate) .... ▣772
See Claritin-D Non-Drowsy 12 Hour Tablets

CLEOCIN VAGINAL OVULES
(Clindamycin Hydrochloride) 2616
May interact with erythromycin, neuromuscular blocking agents, and certain other agents. Compounds in these categories include:

Atracurium Besylate (Co-administration with clindamycin will enhance the action of other neuromuscular blocking agents).
No products indexed under this heading.

Cisatracurium Besylate (Co-administration with clindamycin will enhance the action of other neuromuscular blocking agents). Products include:
Nimbex Injection 498

Diphenoxylate Hydrochloride (May prolong and/or worsen colitis).
No products indexed under this heading.

Doxacurium Chloride (Co-administration with clindamycin will enhance the action of other neuromuscular blocking agents).
No products indexed under this heading.

Erythromycin (Antagonism has been demonstrated between clindamycin and erythromycin in vitro because of possible clinical significance; these two drugs should not be administered concurrently). Products include:
Ery-Tab Tablets 449
Erythromycin Base Filmtab Tablets 455
Erythromycin Delayed-Release Capsules, USP 457
PCE Dispertab Tablets 515

Erythromycin Estolate (Antagonism has been demonstrated between clindamycin and erythromycin in vitro because of possible clinical significance; these two drugs should not be administered concurrently).
No products indexed under this heading.

Erythromycin Ethylsuccinate (Antagonism has been demonstrated between clindamycin and erythromycin in vitro because of possible clinical significance; these two drugs should not be administered concurrently). Products include:
E.E.S. 451
EryPed 447

Erythromycin Gluceptate (Antagonism has been demonstrated between clindamycin and erythromycin in vitro because of possible clinical significance; these two drugs should not be administered concurrently).
No products indexed under this heading.

Erythromycin Lactobionate (Antagonism has been demonstrated between clindamycin and erythromycin in vitro because of possible clinical significance; these two drugs should not be administered concurrently).
No products indexed under this heading.

Erythromycin Stearate (Antagonism has been demonstrated between clindamycin and erythromycin in vitro because of possible clinical significance; these two drugs should not be administered concurrently). Products include:
Erythrocin Stearate Filmtab Tablets 453

Metocurine Iodide (Co-administration with clindamycin will enhance the action of other neuromuscular blocking agents).
No products indexed under this heading.

Mivacurium Chloride (Co-administration with clindamycin will enhance the action of other neuromuscular blocking agents). Products include:
Mivacron Injection 493

Pancuronium Bromide (Co-administration with clindamycin will enhance the action of other neuromuscular blocking agents).
No products indexed under this heading.

Rapacuronium Bromide (Co-administration with clindamycin will enhance the action of other neuromuscular blocking agents).
No products indexed under this heading.

Rocuronium Bromide (Co-administration with clindamycin will enhance the action of other neuromuscular blocking agents). Products include:
Zemuron Injection 2346

Succinylcholine Chloride (Co-administration with clindamycin will enhance the action of other neuromuscular blocking agents).
No products indexed under this heading.

Vecuronium Bromide (Co-administration with clindamycin will enhance the action of other neuromuscular blocking agents).
No products indexed under this heading.

CLIMARA TRANSDERMAL SYSTEM
(Estradiol) 771
May interact with cytochrome p450 3a4 inducers (selected), cytochrome p450 3a4 inhibitors (selected), and certain other agents. Compounds in these categories include:

Acetazolamide (Inhibitors of CYP3A4 such as erythromycin, clarithromycin, ketoconazole, itraconazole, ritonavir and grapefruit juice may increase plasma concentrations of estrogens and may result in side effects).
No products indexed under this heading.

Allium sativum (Inducers of CYP3A4 may reduce plasma concentrations of estrogens, possibly resulting in a decrease in therapeutic effects and/or changes in the uterine bleeding profile).
No products indexed under this heading.

Amiodarone Hydrochloride (Inhibitors of CYP3A4 such as erythromycin, clarithromycin, ketoconazole, itraconazole, ritonavir and grapefruit juice may increase plasma concentrations of estrogens and may result in side effects).
No products indexed under this heading.

Amprenavir (Inhibitors of CYP3A4 such as erythromycin, clarithromycin, ketoconazole, itraconazole, ritonavir and grapefruit juice may increase plasma concentrations of estrogens and may result in side effects). Products include:
Agenerase Capsules 1327
Agenerase Oral Solution 1332

Anastrozole (Inhibitors of CYP3A4 such as erythromycin, clarithromycin, ketoconazole, itraconazole, ritonavir and grapefruit juice may increase plasma concentrations of estrogens and may result in side effects). Products include:
Arimidex Tablets 673

Aprepitant (Inducers of CYP3A4 may reduce plasma concentrations of estrogens, possibly resulting in a decrease in therapeutic effects and/or changes in the uterine bleeding profile). Products include:
Emend Capsules 1963

Betamethasone Acetate (Inducers of CYP3A4 may reduce plasma concentrations of estrogens, possibly resulting in a decrease in therapeutic effects and/or changes in the uterine bleeding profile).
No products indexed under this heading.

Betamethasone Sodium Phosphate (Inducers of CYP3A4 may reduce plasma concentrations of estrogens, possibly resulting in a decrease in therapeutic effects and/or changes in the uterine bleeding profile).
No products indexed under this heading.

Carbamazepine (Inducers of CYP3A4, such as carbamazepine, may be reduce plasma concentrations of estrogens, possibly resulting in a decrease in therapeutic effects and/or changes in uterine bleeding profile). Products include:
Carbatrol Capsules 3171
Equetro Extended-Release Capsules 3180
Tegretol/Tegretol-XR 2295

Cimetidine (Inhibitors of CYP3A4 such as erythromycin, clarithromycin, ketoconazole, itraconazole, ritonavir and grapefruit juice may increase plasma concentrations of estrogens and may result in side effects). Products include:
Tagamet HB 200 Tablets .... ▣664

Cimetidine Hydrochloride (Inhibitors of CYP3A4 such as erythromycin, clarithromycin, ketoconazole, itraconazole, ritonavir and grapefruit juice may increase plasma concentrations of estrogens and may result in side effects).
No products indexed under this heading.

Ciprofloxacin (Inhibitors of CYP3A4 such as erythromycin, clarithromycin, ketoconazole, itraconazole, ritonavir and grapefruit juice may increase plasma concentrations of estrogens and may result in side effects). Products include:
Cipro Oral Suspension 2977
Cipro I.V. 2984
Cipro XR Tablets 2990
Ciprodex Otic Suspension 559

Ciprofloxacin Hydrochloride (Inducers of CYP3A4 may reduce plasma concentrations of estrogens, possibly resulting in a decrease in therapeutic effects and/or changes in the uterine bleeding profile). Products include:
Ciloxan Ophthalmic Ointment 559
Ciloxan Ophthalmic Solution .... ⊙206
Cipro Tablets 2977
Proquin XR Tablets 1153

Cisplatin (Inducers of CYP3A4 may reduce plasma concentrations of estrogens, possibly resulting in a decrease in therapeutic effects and/or changes in the uterine bleeding profile).
No products indexed under this heading.

Clarithromycin (Inducers of CYP3A4, such as clarithromycin, may increase plasma concentrations of estrogens and may result in side effects). Products include:
Biaxin/Biaxin XL 402
PREVPAC 3284

Clotrimazole (Inhibitors of CYP3A4 such as erythromycin, clarithromycin, ketoconazole, itraconazole, ritonavir and grapefruit juice may increase plasma concentrations of estrogens and may result in side effects). Products include:
- Desenex Athlete's Foot Cream 635
- Lotrimin 3039
- Lotrisone 3040

Cortisone Acetate (Inducers of CYP3A4 may reduce plasma concentrations of estrogens, possibly resulting in a decrease in therapeutic effects and/or changes in the uterine bleeding profile).
No products indexed under this heading.

Cyclosporine (Inhibitors of CYP3A4 such as erythromycin, clarithromycin, ketoconazole, itraconazole, ritonavir and grapefruit juice may increase plasma concentrations of estrogens and may result in side effects). Products include:
- Gengraf Capsules 459
- Neoral Oral Solution 2259
- Neoral Soft Gelatin Capsules 2259
- Restasis Ophthalmic Emulsion 575
- Sandimmune 2275

Dalfopristin (Inhibitors of CYP3A4 such as erythromycin, clarithromycin, ketoconazole, itraconazole, ritonavir and grapefruit juice may increase plasma concentrations of estrogens and may result in side effects).
No products indexed under this heading.

Danazol (Inhibitors of CYP3A4 such as erythromycin, clarithromycin, ketoconazole, itraconazole, ritonavir and grapefruit juice may increase plasma concentrations of estrogens and may result in side effects).
No products indexed under this heading.

Delavirdine Mesylate (Inhibitors of CYP3A4 such as erythromycin, clarithromycin, ketoconazole, itraconazole, ritonavir and grapefruit juice may increase plasma concentrations of estrogens and may result in side effects). Products include:
- Rescriptor Tablets 2551

Dexamethasone (Inducers of CYP3A4 may reduce plasma concentrations of estrogens, possibly resulting in a decrease in therapeutic effects and/or changes in the uterine bleeding profile). Products include:
- Ciprodex Otic Suspension 559
- Decadron Tablets 1951
- TobraDex Ophthalmic Ointment 562
- TobraDex Ophthalmic Suspension ... 563

Dexamethasone Acetate (Inducers of CYP3A4 may reduce plasma concentrations of estrogens, possibly resulting in a decrease in therapeutic effects and/or changes in the uterine bleeding profile).
No products indexed under this heading.

Dexamethasone Sodium Phosphate (Inducers of CYP3A4 may reduce plasma concentrations of estrogens, possibly resulting in a decrease in therapeutic effects and/or changes in the uterine bleeding profile).
No products indexed under this heading.

Diltiazem Hydrochloride (Inhibitors of CYP3A4 such as erythromycin, clarithromycin, ketoconazole, itraconazole, ritonavir and grapefruit juice may increase plasma concentrations of estrogens and may result in side effects). Products include:
- Cardizem LA Extended Release Tablets 1728
- Tiazac Capsules 1201

Diltiazem Maleate (Inhibitors of CYP3A4 such as erythromycin, clarithromycin, ketoconazole, itraconazole, ritonavir and grapefruit juice may increase plasma concentrations of estrogens and may result in side effects).
No products indexed under this heading.

Doxorubicin Hydrochloride (Inducers of CYP3A4 may reduce plasma concentrations of estrogens, possibly resulting in a decrease in therapeutic effects and/or changes in the uterine bleeding profile).
No products indexed under this heading.

Efavirenz (Inducers of CYP3A4 may reduce plasma concentrations of estrogens, possibly resulting in a decrease in therapeutic effects and/or changes in the uterine bleeding profile). Products include:
- Atripla Tablets 945
- Sustiva Capsules 930
- Sustiva Tablets 930

Erythromycin (Inhibitors of CYP3A4 such as erythromycin, clarithromycin, ketoconazole, itraconazole, ritonavir and grapefruit juice may increase plasma concentrations of estrogens and may result in side effects). Products include:
- Ery-Tab Tablets 449
- Erythromycin Base Filmtab Tablets 455
- Erythromycin Delayed-Release Capsules, USP 457
- PCE Dispertab Tablets 515

Erythromycin Estolate (Inhibitors of CYP3A4 such as erythromycin, clarithromycin, ketoconazole, itraconazole, ritonavir and grapefruit juice may increase plasma concentrations of estrogens and may result in side effects).
No products indexed under this heading.

Erythromycin Ethylsuccinate (Inhibitors of CYP3A4 such as erythromycin, clarithromycin, ketoconazole, itraconazole, ritonavir and grapefruit juice may increase plasma concentrations of estrogens and may result in side effects). Products include:
- E.E.S. 451
- EryPed 447

Erythromycin Gluceptate (Inhibitors of CYP3A4 such as erythromycin, clarithromycin, ketoconazole, itraconazole, ritonavir and grapefruit juice may increase plasma concentrations of estrogens and may result in side effects).
No products indexed under this heading.

Erythromycin Lactobionate (Inhibitors of CYP3A4 such as erythromycin, clarithromycin, ketoconazole, itraconazole, ritonavir and grapefruit juice may increase plasma concentrations of estrogens and may result in side effects).
No products indexed under this heading.

Erythromycin Stearate (Inhibitors of CYP3A4 such as erythromycin, clarithromycin, ketoconazole, itraconazole, ritonavir and grapefruit juice may increase plasma concentrations of estrogens and may result in side effects). Products include:
- Erythrocin Stearate Filmtab Tablets 453

Esomeprazole Magnesium (Inhibitors of CYP3A4 such as erythromycin, clarithromycin, ketoconazole, itraconazole, ritonavir and grapefruit juice may increase plasma concentrations of estrogens and may result in side effects). Products include:
- Nexium Delayed-Release Capsules 655

Ethosuximide (Inducers of CYP3A4 may reduce plasma concentrations of estrogens, possibly resulting in a decrease in therapeutic effects and/or changes in the uterine bleeding profile).
No products indexed under this heading.

Felbamate (Inducers of CYP3A4 may reduce plasma concentrations of estrogens, possibly resulting in a decrease in therapeutic effects and/or changes in the uterine bleeding profile).
No products indexed under this heading.

Fluconazole (Inhibitors of CYP3A4 such as erythromycin, clarithromycin, ketoconazole, itraconazole, ritonavir and grapefruit juice may increase plasma concentrations of estrogens and may result in side effects).
No products indexed under this heading.

Fludrocortisone Acetate (Inducers of CYP3A4 may reduce plasma concentrations of estrogens, possibly resulting in a decrease in therapeutic effects and/or changes in the uterine bleeding profile).
No products indexed under this heading.

Fluoxetine Hydrochloride (Inhibitors of CYP3A4 such as erythromycin, clarithromycin, ketoconazole, itraconazole, ritonavir and grapefruit juice may increase plasma concentrations of estrogens and may result in side effects). Products include:
- Prozac Pulvules and Liquid 1801
- Symbyax Capsules 1819

Fluvoxamine Maleate (Inhibitors of CYP3A4 such as erythromycin, clarithromycin, ketoconazole, itraconazole, ritonavir and grapefruit juice may increase plasma concentrations of estrogens and may result in side effects).
No products indexed under this heading.

Fosamprenavir Calcium (Inhibitors of CYP3A4 such as erythromycin, clarithromycin, ketoconazole, itraconazole, ritonavir and grapefruit juice may increase plasma concentrations of estrogens and may result in side effects). Products include:
- Lexiva Tablets 1505

Fosphenytoin Sodium (Inducers of CYP3A4 may reduce plasma concentrations of estrogens, possibly resulting in a decrease in therapeutic effects and/or changes in the uterine bleeding profile).
No products indexed under this heading.

Garlic Extract (Inducers of CYP3A4 may reduce plasma concentrations of estrogens, possibly resulting in a decrease in therapeutic effects and/or changes in the uterine bleeding profile).
No products indexed under this heading.

Garlic Oil (Inducers of CYP3A4 may reduce plasma concentrations of estrogens, possibly resulting in a decrease in therapeutic effects and/or changes in the uterine bleeding profile).
No products indexed under this heading.

Hydrocortisone (Inducers of CYP3A4 may reduce plasma concentrations of estrogens, possibly resulting in a decrease in therapeutic effects and/or changes in the uterine bleeding profile). Products include:
- Colocort Rectal Suspension, USP (Retention) 100 mg/60 mL 2476
- Hydrocortone Tablets 1989
- Preparation H Hydrocortisone Cream 646

Hydrocortisone Acetate (Inducers of CYP3A4 may reduce plasma concentrations of estrogens, possibly resulting in a decrease in therapeutic effects and/or changes in the uterine bleeding profile). Products include:
- Analpram-HC 1159
- Pramosone 1161
- ProctoFoam-HC 3099

Hydrocortisone Butyrate (Inducers of CYP3A4 may reduce plasma concentrations of estrogens, possibly resulting in a decrease in therapeutic effects and/or changes in the uterine bleeding profile). Products include:
- Locoid Lipocream Cream 1160

Hydrocortisone Cypionate (Inducers of CYP3A4 may reduce plasma concentrations of estrogens, possibly resulting in a decrease in therapeutic effects and/or changes in the uterine bleeding profile).
No products indexed under this heading.

Hydrocortisone Hemisuccinate (Inducers of CYP3A4 may reduce plasma concentrations of estrogens, possibly resulting in a decrease in therapeutic effects and/or changes in the uterine bleeding profile).
No products indexed under this heading.

Hydrocortisone Probutate (Inducers of CYP3A4 may reduce plasma concentrations of estrogens, possibly resulting in a decrease in therapeutic effects and/or changes in the uterine bleeding profile).
No products indexed under this heading.

Hydrocortisone Sodium Phosphate (Inducers of CYP3A4 may reduce plasma concentrations of estrogens, possibly resulting in a decrease in therapeutic effects and/or changes in the uterine bleeding profile).
No products indexed under this heading.

Hydrocortisone Sodium Succinate (Inducers of CYP3A4 may reduce plasma concentrations of estrogens, possibly resulting in a decrease in therapeutic effects and/or changes in the uterine bleeding profile).
No products indexed under this heading.

Hydrocortisone Valerate (Inducers of CYP3A4 may reduce plasma concentrations of estrogens, possibly resulting in a decrease in therapeutic effects and/or changes in the uterine bleeding profile).
No products indexed under this heading.

Hypericum (Inducers of CYP3A4 may reduce plasma concentrations of estrogens, possibly resulting in a decrease in therapeutic effects and/or changes in the uterine bleeding profile). Products include:
Satiete Tablets .... ◙832

Hypericum Perforatum (Inducers of CYP3A4, such as St. John's Wort preparations (Hypericum perforatum) may reduce plasma concentrations of estrogens, possibly resulting in a decrease in therapuetic effects and/or changes in uterine bleeding profile).
No products indexed under this heading.

Indinavir Sulfate (Inhibitors of CYP3A4 such as erythromycin, clarithromycin, ketoconazole, itraconazole, ritonavir and grapefruit juice may increase plasma concentrations of estrogens and may result in side effects). Products include:
Crixivan Capsules 1940

Isoniazid (Inhibitors of CYP3A4 such as erythromycin, clarithromycin, ketoconazole, itraconazole, ritonavir and grapefruit juice may increase plasma concentrations of estrogens and may result in side effects).
No products indexed under this heading.

Itraconazole (Inducers of CYP3A4, such as itraconazole, may increase plasma concentrations of estrogens and may result in side effects).
No products indexed under this heading.

Ketoconazole (Inducers of CYP3A4, such as ketoconazole, may increase plasma concentrations of estrogens and may result in side effects). Products include:
Nizoral A-D Shampoo, 1% 1868

Lopinavir (Inhibitors of CYP3A4 such as erythromycin, clarithromycin, ketoconazole, itraconazole, ritonavir and grapefruit juice may increase plasma concentrations of estrogens and may result in side effects). Products include:
Kaletra 476

Loratadine (Inhibitors of CYP3A4 such as erythromycin, clarithromycin, ketoconazole, itraconazole, ritonavir and grapefruit juice may increase plasma concentrations of estrogens and may result in side effects). Products include:
Alavert Allergy & Sinus D-12 Hour Tablets .... ◙771
Alavert .... ◙771
Children's Claritin Allergy Oral Solution .... ◙771
Claritin Non-Drowsy 24 Hour Tablets .... ◙772
Claritin Reditabs 24 Hour Non-Drowsy Tablets .... ◙772
Claritin-D Non-Drowsy 12 Hour Tablets .... ◙772
Claritin-D Non-Drowsy 24 Hour Tablets .... ◙772

Mephenytoin (Inducers of CYP3A4 may reduce plasma concentrations of estrogens, possibly resulting in a decrease in therapeutic effects and/or changes in the uterine bleeding profile).
No products indexed under this heading.

Methsuximide (Inducers of CYP3A4 may reduce plasma concentrations of estrogens, possibly resulting in a decrease in therapeutic effects and/or changes in the uterine bleeding profile).
No products indexed under this heading.

Methylprednisolone (Inducers of CYP3A4 may reduce plasma concentrations of estrogens, possibly resulting in a decrease in therapeutic effects and/or changes in the uterine bleeding profile).
No products indexed under this heading.

Methylprednisolone Acetate (Inducers of CYP3A4 may reduce plasma concentrations of estrogens, possibly resulting in a decrease in therapeutic effects and/or changes in the uterine bleeding profile). Products include:
Depo-Medrol Injectable Suspension 2617
Depo-Medrol Single-Dose Vial 2619

Methylprednisolone Sodium Succinate (Inducers of CYP3A4 may reduce plasma concentrations of estrogens, possibly resulting in a decrease in therapeutic effects and/or changes in the uterine bleeding profile).
No products indexed under this heading.

Metronidazole (Inhibitors of CYP3A4 such as erythromycin, clarithromycin, ketoconazole, itraconazole, ritonavir and grapefruit juice may increase plasma concentrations of estrogens and may result in side effects). Products include:
Metrogel 1% 1211
MetroGel-Vaginal Gel 1855
Vandazole Vaginal Gel 3338

Metronidazole Benzoate (Inhibitors of CYP3A4 such as erythromycin, clarithromycin, ketoconazole, itraconazole, ritonavir and grapefruit juice may increase plasma concentrations of estrogens and may result in side effects).
No products indexed under this heading.

Metronidazole Hydrochloride (Inhibitors of CYP3A4 such as erythromycin, clarithromycin, ketoconazole, itraconazole, ritonavir and grapefruit juice may increase plasma concentrations of estrogens and may result in side effects).
No products indexed under this heading.

Miconazole (Inhibitors of CYP3A4 such as erythromycin, clarithromycin, ketoconazole, itraconazole, ritonavir and grapefruit juice may increase plasma concentrations of estrogens and may result in side effects).
No products indexed under this heading.

Miconazole Nitrate (Inhibitors of CYP3A4 such as erythromycin, clarithromycin, ketoconazole, itraconazole, ritonavir and grapefruit juice may increase plasma concentrations of estrogens and may result in side effects). Products include:
Desenex .... ◙635
Desenex Jock Itch Spray Powder ... ◙635

Modafinil (Inducers of CYP3A4 may reduce plasma concentrations of estrogens, possibly resulting in a decrease in therapeutic effects and/or changes in the uterine bleeding profile). Products include:
Provigil Tablets 988

Nefazodone Hydrochloride (Inhibitors of CYP3A4 such as erythromycin, clarithromycin, ketoconazole, itraconazole, ritonavir and grapefruit juice may increase plasma concentrations of estrogens and may result in side effects).
No products indexed under this heading.

Nelfinavir Mesylate (Inhibitors of CYP3A4 such as erythromycin, clarithromycin, ketoconazole, itraconazole, ritonavir and grapefruit juice may increase plasma concentrations of estrogens and may result in side effects). Products include:
Viracept 2577

Nevirapine (Inducers of CYP3A4 may reduce plasma concentrations of estrogens, possibly resulting in a decrease in therapeutic effects and/or changes in the uterine bleeding profile). Products include:
Viramune Oral Suspension 873
Viramune Tablets 873

Niacinamide (Inhibitors of CYP3A4 such as erythromycin, clarithromycin, ketoconazole, itraconazole, ritonavir and grapefruit juice may increase plasma concentrations of estrogens and may result in side effects).
No products indexed under this heading.

Nicotinamide (Inhibitors of CYP3A4 such as erythromycin, clarithromycin, ketoconazole, itraconazole, ritonavir and grapefruit juice may increase plasma concentrations of estrogens and may result in side effects). Products include:
Nicomide Tablets 1088

Nifedipine (Inhibitors of CYP3A4 such as erythromycin, clarithromycin, ketoconazole, itraconazole, ritonavir and grapefruit juice may increase plasma concentrations of estrogens and may result in side effects). Products include:
Adalat CC Tablets 2964

Norfloxacin (Inhibitors of CYP3A4 such as erythromycin, clarithromycin, ketoconazole, itraconazole, ritonavir and grapefruit juice may increase plasma concentrations of estrogens and may result in side effects). Products include:
Noroxin Tablets 2032

Omeprazole (Inhibitors of CYP3A4 such as erythromycin, clarithromycin, ketoconazole, itraconazole, ritonavir and grapefruit juice may increase plasma concentrations of estrogens and may result in side effects). Products include:
Zegerid Capsules 2958
Zegerid Powder for Oral Solution 2958

Oxcarbazepine (Inducers of CYP3A4 may reduce plasma concentrations of estrogens, possibly resulting in a decrease in therapeutic effects and/or changes in the uterine bleeding profile). Products include:
Trileptal Tablets 2300
Trileptal Oral Suspension 2300

Paroxetine Hydrochloride (Inhibitors of CYP3A4 such as erythromycin, clarithromycin, ketoconazole, itraconazole, ritonavir and grapefruit juice may increase plasma concentrations of estrogens and may result in side effects). Products include:
Paxil CR Controlled-Release Tablets 1538
Paxil 1530

Phenobarbital (Inducers of CYP3A4, such as phenobarbital, may be reduce plasma concentrations of estrogens, possibly resulting in a decrease in therapeutic effects and/or changes in uterine bleeding profile). Products include:
Donnatal Extentabs 2493

Phenobarbital Sodium (Inducers of CYP3A4 may reduce plasma concentrations of estrogens, possibly resulting in a decrease in therapeutic effects and/or changes in the uterine bleeding profile).
No products indexed under this heading.

Phenytoin (Inducers of CYP3A4 may reduce plasma concentrations of estrogens, possibly resulting in a decrease in therapeutic effects and/or changes in the uterine bleeding profile).
No products indexed under this heading.

Phenytoin Sodium (Inducers of CYP3A4 may reduce plasma concentrations of estrogens, possibly resulting in a decrease in therapeutic effects and/or changes in the uterine bleeding profile). Products include:
Phenytek Capsules 2160

Prednisolone Acetate (Inducers of CYP3A4 may reduce plasma concentrations of estrogens, possibly resulting in a decrease in therapeutic effects and/or changes in the uterine bleeding profile). Products include:
Blephamide Ophthalmic Ointment 568
Blephamide Ophthalmic Suspension 569
Poly-Pred Ophthalmic Suspension .... ⊙233
Pred Forte Ophthalmic Suspension .... ⊙235
Pred Mild Ophthalmic Suspension .... ⊙238
Pred-G Ophthalmic Ointment .... ⊙237
Pred-G Ophthalmic Suspension ...... ⊙236

Prednisolone Sodium Phosphate (Inducers of CYP3A4 may reduce plasma concentrations of estrogens, possibly resulting in a decrease in therapeutic effects and/or changes in the uterine bleeding profile).
No products indexed under this heading.

Prednisolone Tebutate (Inducers of CYP3A4 may reduce plasma concentrations of estrogens, possibly resulting in a decrease in therapeutic effects and/or changes in the uterine bleeding profile).
No products indexed under this heading.

Prednisone (Inducers of CYP3A4 may reduce plasma concentrations of estrogens, possibly resulting in a decrease in therapeutic effects and/or changes in the uterine bleeding profile).
No products indexed under this heading.

Primidone (Inducers of CYP3A4 may reduce plasma concentrations of estrogens, possibly resulting in a decrease in therapeutic effects and/or changes in the uterine bleeding profile).
No products indexed under this heading.

Propoxyphene Hydrochloride (Inhibitors of CYP3A4 such as erythromycin, clarithromycin, ketoconazole, itraconazole, ritonavir and grapefruit juice may increase plasma concentrations of estrogens and may result in side effects).
No products indexed under this heading.

Propoxyphene Napsylate (Inhibitors of CYP3A4 such as erythromycin, clarithromycin, ketoconazole, itraconazole, ritonavir and grapefruit juice may increase plasma concentrations of estrogens and may result in side effects).
No products indexed under this heading.

Quinidine (Inhibitors of CYP3A4 such as erythromycin, clarithromycin, ketoconazole, itraconazole, ritonavir and grapefruit juice may increase plasma concentrations of estrogens and may result in side effects).
No products indexed under this heading.

Quinidine Hydrochloride (Inhibitors of CYP3A4 such as erythromycin, clarithromycin, ketoconazole, itraconazole, ritonavir and grapefruit juice may increase plasma concentrations of estrogens and may result in side effects).
No products indexed under this heading.

Quinidine Polygalacturonate (Inhibitors of CYP3A4 such as erythromycin, clarithromycin, ketoconazole, itraconazole, ritonavir and grapefruit juice may increase plasma concentrations of estrogens and may result in side effects).
No products indexed under this heading.

Quinidine Sulfate (Inhibitors of CYP3A4 such as erythromycin, clarithromycin, ketoconazole, itraconazole, ritonavir and grapefruit juice may increase plasma concentrations of estrogens and may result in side effects).
No products indexed under this heading.

Quinine (Inhibitors of CYP3A4 such as erythromycin, clarithromycin, ketoconazole, itraconazole, ritonavir and grapefruit juice may increase plasma concentrations of estrogens and may result in side effects).
No products indexed under this heading.

Quinine Sulfate (Inhibitors of CYP3A4 such as erythromycin, clarithromycin, ketoconazole, itraconazole, ritonavir and grapefruit juice may increase plasma concentrations of estrogens and may result in side effects).
No products indexed under this heading.

Quinupristin (Inhibitors of CYP3A4 such as erythromycin, clarithromycin, ketoconazole, itraconazole, ritonavir and grapefruit juice may increase plasma concentrations of estrogens and may result in side effects).
No products indexed under this heading.

Ranitidine Bismuth Citrate (Inhibitors of CYP3A4 such as erythromycin, clarithromycin, ketoconazole, itraconazole, ritonavir and grapefruit juice may increase plasma concentrations of estrogens and may result in side effects).
No products indexed under this heading.

Ranitidine Hydrochloride (Inhibitors of CYP3A4 such as erythromycin, clarithromycin, ketoconazole, itraconazole, ritonavir and grapefruit juice may increase plasma concentrations of estrogens and may result in side effects). Products include:

Rifabutin (Inducers of CYP3A4 may reduce plasma concentrations of estrogens, possibly resulting in a decrease in therapeutic effects and/or changes in the uterine bleeding profile).
No products indexed under this heading.

Rifampicin (Inducers of CYP3A4 may reduce plasma concentrations of estrogens, possibly resulting in a decrease in therapeutic effects and/or changes in the uterine bleeding profile).
No products indexed under this heading.

Rifampin (Inducers of CYP3A4, such as rifampin, may reduce plasma concentrations of estrogens, possibly resulting in a decrease in therapeutic effects and/or changes in uterine bleeding profile).
No products indexed under this heading.

Rifapentine (Inducers of CYP3A4 may reduce plasma concentrations of estrogens, possibly resulting in a decrease in therapeutic effects and/or changes in the uterine bleeding profile).
No products indexed under this heading.

Ritonavir (Inducers of CYP3A4, such as ritonavir, may increase plasma concentrations of estrogens and may result in side effects). Products include:

Saquinavir (Inhibitors of CYP3A4 such as erythromycin, clarithromycin, ketoconazole, itraconazole, ritonavir and grapefruit juice may increase plasma concentrations of estrogens and may result in side effects).
No products indexed under this heading.

Saquinavir Mesylate (Inhibitors of CYP3A4 such as erythromycin, clarithromycin, ketoconazole, itraconazole, ritonavir and grapefruit juice may increase plasma concentrations of estrogens and may result in side effects). Products include:

Sertraline Hydrochloride (Inhibitors of CYP3A4 such as erythromycin, clarithromycin, ketoconazole, itraconazole, ritonavir and grapefruit juice may increase plasma concentrations of estrogens and may result in side effects). Products include:

Sulfinpyrazone (Inducers of CYP3A4 may reduce plasma concentrations of estrogens, possibly resulting in a decrease in therapeutic effects and/or changes in the uterine bleeding profile).
No products indexed under this heading.

Telithromycin (Inhibitors of CYP3A4 such as erythromycin, clarithromycin, ketoconazole, itraconazole, ritonavir and grapefruit juice may increase plasma concentrations of estrogens and may result in side effects). Products include:

Theophylline (Inducers of CYP3A4 may reduce plasma concentrations of estrogens, possibly resulting in a decrease in therapeutic effects and/or changes in the uterine bleeding profile).
No products indexed under this heading.

Triamcinolone (Inducers of CYP3A4 may reduce plasma concentrations of estrogens, possibly resulting in a decrease in therapeutic effects and/or changes in the uterine bleeding profile).
No products indexed under this heading.

Triamcinolone Acetonide (Inducers of CYP3A4 may reduce plasma concentrations of estrogens, possibly resulting in a decrease in therapeutic effects and/or changes in the uterine bleeding profile). Products include:

Triamcinolone Diacetate (Inducers of CYP3A4 may reduce plasma concentrations of estrogens, possibly resulting in a decrease in therapeutic effects and/or changes in the uterine bleeding profile).
No products indexed under this heading.

Triamcinolone Hexacetonide (Inducers of CYP3A4 may reduce plasma concentrations of estrogens, possibly resulting in a decrease in therapeutic effects and/or changes in the uterine bleeding profile).
No products indexed under this heading.

Troglitazone (Inducers of CYP3A4 may reduce plasma concentrations of estrogens, possibly resulting in a decrease in therapeutic effects and/or changes in the uterine bleeding profile).
No products indexed under this heading.

Troleandomycin (Inhibitors of CYP3A4 such as erythromycin, clarithromycin, ketoconazole, itraconazole, ritonavir and grapefruit juice may increase plasma concentrations of estrogens and may result in side effects).
No products indexed under this heading.

Valproate Sodium (Inhibitors of CYP3A4 such as erythromycin, clarithromycin, ketoconazole, itraconazole, ritonavir and grapefruit juice may increase plasma concentrations of estrogens and may result in side effects). Products include:

cin, clarithromycin, ketoconazole, itraconazole, ritonavir and grapefruit juice may increase plasma concentrations of estrogens and may result in side effects). Products include:

Verapamil Hydrochloride (Inhibitors of CYP3A4 such as erythromycin, clarithromycin, ketoconazole, itraconazole, ritonavir and grapefruit juice may increase plasma concentrations of estrogens and may result in side effects). Products include:

Voriconazole (Inhibitors of CYP3A4 such as erythromycin, clarithromycin, ketoconazole, itraconazole, ritonavir and grapefruit juice may increase plasma concentrations of estrogens and may result in side effects). Products include:

Zafirlukast (Inhibitors of CYP3A4 such as erythromycin, clarithromycin, ketoconazole, itraconazole, ritonavir and grapefruit juice may increase plasma concentrations of estrogens and may result in side effects). Products include:

Zileuton (Inhibitors of CYP3A4 such as erythromycin, clarithromycin, ketoconazole, itraconazole, ritonavir and grapefruit juice may increase plasma concentrations of estrogens and may result in side effects). Products include:

Food Interactions

Grapefruit (Inhibitors of CYP3A4 such as erythromycin, clarithromycin, ketoconazole, itraconazole, ritonavir and grapefruit juice may increase plasma concentrations of estrogens and may result in side effects).

Grapefruit Juice (Inducers of CYP3A4, such as grapefruit juice, may increase plasma concentrations of estrogens and may result in side effects).

CLIMARA PRO TRANSDERMAL SYSTEM

May interact with cytochrome p450 2c18 inhibitors (selected), cytochrome p450 2c19 inducers (selected), cytochrome p450 2c19 inhibitors (selected), cytochrome p450 2c8 inducers (selected), cytochrome p450 2c8 inhibitors (selected), cytochrome p450 2c9 inducers (selected), cytochrome p450 2c9 inhibitors (selected), cytochrome p450 3a4 inducers (selected), and cytochrome p450 3a4 inhibitors (selected). Compounds in these categories include:

Acetazolamide (Inhibitors of CYP3A4 such as erythromycin, clarithromycin, ketoconazole, itraconazole, ritonavir and grapefruit juice may increase plasma concentrations of estrogens and may result in side effects).
No products indexed under this heading.

Allium sativum (Inducers of CYP3A4 may reduce plasma concentrations of estrogens, possibly resulting in a decrease in therapeutic effects and/or changes in the uterine bleeding profile).
No products indexed under this heading.

IMPORTANT NOTE: Always consult each drug listing in the patient's regimen for possible interactions.

Amiodarone Hydrochloride (Inhibitors of CYP3A4 such as erythromycin, clarithromycin, ketoconazole, itraconazole, ritonavir and grapefruit juice may increase plasma concentrations of estrogens and may result in side effects).
 No products indexed under this heading.

Amprenavir (Inhibitors of CYP3A4 such as erythromycin, clarithromycin, ketoconazole, itraconazole, ritonavir and grapefruit juice may increase plasma concentrations of estrogens and may result in side effects). Products include:
 Agenerase Capsules 1327
 Agenerase Oral Solution 1332

Anastrozole (Inhibitors of CYP3A4 such as erythromycin, clarithromycin, ketoconazole, itraconazole, ritonavir and grapefruit juice may increase plasma concentrations of estrogens and may result in side effects). Products include:
 Arimidex Tablets 673

Aprepitant (Inducers of CYP3A4 may reduce plasma concentrations of estrogens, possibly resulting in a decrease in therapeutic effects and/or changes in the uterine bleeding profile). Products include:
 Emend Capsules 1963

Bendroflumethiazide (Based on in-vitro and in-vivo studies, it can be assumed that CYP3A, CYP2E and CYP2C are involved in the metabolism of levonorgestrel. Likewise, inducers or inhibitors of these enzymes may either, respectively, decrease the therapeutic effects or resultin side effects).
 No products indexed under this heading.

Betamethasone Acetate (Inducers of CYP3A4 may reduce plasma concentrations of estrogens, possibly resulting in a decrease in therapeutic effects and/or changes in the uterine bleeding profile).
 No products indexed under this heading.

Betamethasone Sodium Phosphate (Inducers of CYP3A4 may reduce plasma concentrations of estrogens, possibly resulting in a decrease in therapeutic effects and/or changes in the uterine bleeding profile).
 No products indexed under this heading.

Carbamazepine (Inducers of CYP3A4 may reduce plasma concentrations of estrogens, possibly resulting in a decrease in therapeutic effects and/or changes in the uterine bleeding profile). Products include:
 Carbatrol Capsules 3171
 Equetro Extended-Release Capsules ... 3180
 Tegretol/Tegretol-XR 2295

Chloramphenicol (Based on in-vitro and in-vivo studies, it can be assumed that CYP3A, CYP2E and CYP2C are involved in the metabolism of levonorgestrel. Likewise, inducers or inhibitors of these enzymes may either, respectively, decrease the therapeutic effects or resultin side effects).
 No products indexed under this heading.

Chlorothiazide (Based on in-vitro and in-vivo studies, it can be assumed that CYP3A, CYP2E and CYP2C are involved in the metabolism of levonorgestrel. Likewise,

inducers or inhibitors of these enzymes may either, respectively, decrease the therapeutic effects or resultin side effects). Products include:
 Diuril Oral Suspension 1954

Chlorothiazide Sodium (Based on in-vitro and in-vivo studies, it can be assumed that CYP3A, CYP2E and CYP2C are involved in the metabolism of levonorgestrel. Likewise, inducers or inhibitors of these enzymes may either, respectively, decrease the therapeutic effects or resultin side effects). Products include:
 Diuril Sodium Intravenous 2467

Chlorpropamide (Based on in-vitro and in-vivo studies, it can be assumed that CYP3A, CYP2E and CYP2C are involved in the metabolism of levonorgestrel. Likewise, inducers or inhibitors of these enzymes may either, respectively, decrease the therapeutic effects or resultin side effects).
 No products indexed under this heading.

Cimetidine (Inhibitors of CYP3A4 such as erythromycin, clarithromycin, ketoconazole, itraconazole, ritonavir and grapefruit juice may increase plasma concentrations of estrogens and may result in side effects). Products include:
 Tagamet HB 200 Tablets ▣⊙664

Cimetidine Hydrochloride (Inhibitors of CYP3A4 such as erythromycin, clarithromycin, ketoconazole, itraconazole, ritonavir and grapefruit juice may increase plasma concentrations of estrogens and may result in side effects).
 No products indexed under this heading.

Ciprofloxacin (Inhibitors of CYP3A4 such as erythromycin, clarithromycin, ketoconazole, itraconazole, ritonavir and grapefruit juice may increase plasma concentrations of estrogens and may result in side effects). Products include:
 Cipro Oral Suspension 2977
 Cipro I.V. ... 2984
 Cipro XR Tablets 2990
 Ciprodex Otic Suspension 559

Ciprofloxacin Hydrochloride (Inducers of CYP3A4 may reduce plasma concentrations of estrogens, possibly resulting in a decrease in therapeutic effects and/or changes in the uterine bleeding profile). Products include:
 Ciloxan Ophthalmic Ointment 559
 Ciloxan Ophthalmic Solution ⊙206
 Cipro Tablets 2977
 Proquin XR Tablets 1153

Cisplatin (Inducers of CYP3A4 may reduce plasma concentrations of estrogens, possibly resulting in a decrease in therapeutic effects and/or changes in the uterine bleeding profile).
 No products indexed under this heading.

Citalopram Hydrobromide (Based on in-vitro and in-vivo studies, it can be assumed that CYP3A, CYP2E and CYP2C are involved in the metabolism of levonorgestrel. Likewise, inducers or inhibitors of these enzymes may either, respectively, decrease the therapeutic effects or resultin side effects). Products include:
 Celexa ... 1176

Clarithromycin (Inhibitors of CYP3A4 such as erythromycin, clarithromycin, ketoconazole, itraconazole, ritonavir and grapefruit juice may increase plasma concentrations of estrogens and may result in side effects). Products include:
 Biaxin/Biaxin XL 402
 PREVPAC 3284

Clopidogrel Hydrogen Sulfate (Based on in-vitro and in-vivo studies, it can be assumed that CYP3A, CYP2E and CYP2C are involved in the metabolism of levonorgestrel. Likewise, inducers or inhibitors of these enzymes may either, respectively, decrease the therapeutic effects or resultin side effects).
 No products indexed under this heading.

Clotrimazole (Inhibitors of CYP3A4 such as erythromycin, clarithromycin, ketoconazole, itraconazole, ritonavir and grapefruit juice may increase plasma concentrations of estrogens and may result in side effects). Products include:
 Desenex Athlete's Foot Cream ▣⊙635
 Lotrimin ... 3039
 Lotrisone ... 3040

Cortisone Acetate (Inducers of CYP3A4 may reduce plasma concentrations of estrogens, possibly resulting in a decrease in therapeutic effects and/or changes in the uterine bleeding profile).
 No products indexed under this heading.

Cyclosporine (Inhibitors of CYP3A4 such as erythromycin, clarithromycin, ketoconazole, itraconazole, ritonavir and grapefruit juice may increase plasma concentrations of estrogens and may result in side effects). Products include:
 Gengraf Capsules 459
 Neoral Oral Solution 2259
 Neoral Soft Gelatin Capsules 2259
 Restasis Ophthalmic Emulsion 575
 Sandimmune 2275

Dalfopristin (Inhibitors of CYP3A4 such as erythromycin, clarithromycin, ketoconazole, itraconazole, ritonavir and grapefruit juice may increase plasma concentrations of estrogens and may result in side effects).
 No products indexed under this heading.

Danazol (Inhibitors of CYP3A4 such as erythromycin, clarithromycin, ketoconazole, itraconazole, ritonavir and grapefruit juice may increase plasma concentrations of estrogens and may result in side effects).
 No products indexed under this heading.

Delavirdine Mesylate (Inhibitors of CYP3A4 such as erythromycin, clarithromycin, ketoconazole, itraconazole, ritonavir and grapefruit juice may increase plasma concentrations of estrogens and may result in side effects). Products include:
 Rescriptor Tablets 2551

Desogestrel (Based on in-vitro and in-vivo studies, it can be assumed that CYP3A, CYP2E and CYP2C are involved in the metabolism of levonorgestrel. Likewise, inducers or inhibitors of these enzymes may either, respectively, decrease the therapeutic effects or resultin side effects). Products include:
 Mircette Tablets 1066

Dexamethasone (Inducers of CYP3A4 may reduce plasma concen-

trations of estrogens, possibly resulting in a decrease in therapeutic effects and/or changes in the uterine bleeding profile). Products include:
 Ciprodex Otic Suspension 559
 Decadron Tablets 1951
 TobraDex Ophthalmic Ointment 562
 TobraDex Ophthalmic Suspension ... 563

Dexamethasone Acetate (Inducers of CYP3A4 may reduce plasma concentrations of estrogens, possibly resulting in a decrease in therapeutic effects and/or changes in the uterine bleeding profile).
 No products indexed under this heading.

Dexamethasone Sodium Phosphate (Inducers of CYP3A4 may reduce plasma concentrations of estrogens, possibly resulting in a decrease in therapeutic effects and/or changes in the uterine bleeding profile).
 No products indexed under this heading.

Diclofenac Potassium (Based on in-vitro and in-vivo studies, it can be assumed that CYP3A, CYP2E and CYP2C are involved in the metabolism of levonorgestrel. Likewise, inducers or inhibitors of these enzymes may either, respectively, decrease the therapeutic effects or resultin side effects).
 No products indexed under this heading.

Diclofenac Sodium (Based on in-vitro and in-vivo studies, it can be assumed that CYP3A, CYP2E and CYP2C are involved in the metabolism of levonorgestrel. Likewise, inducers or inhibitors of these enzymes may either, respectively, decrease the therapeutic effects or resultin side effects). Products include:
 Arthrotec Tablets 3129
 Voltaren Ophthalmic Solution 2309
 Voltaren Tablets 2307
 Voltaren-XR Tablets 2310

Diltiazem Hydrochloride (Inhibitors of CYP3A4 such as erythromycin, clarithromycin, ketoconazole, itraconazole, ritonavir and grapefruit juice may increase plasma concentrations of estrogens and may result in side effects). Products include:
 Cardizem LA Extended Release Tablets ... 1728
 Tiazac Capsules 1201

Diltiazem Maleate (Inhibitors of CYP3A4 such as erythromycin, clarithromycin, ketoconazole, itraconazole, ritonavir and grapefruit juice may increase plasma concentrations of estrogens and may result in side effects).
 No products indexed under this heading.

Disulfiram (Based on in-vitro and in-vivo studies, it can be assumed that CYP3A, CYP2E and CYP2C are involved in the metabolism of levonorgestrel. Likewise, inducers or inhibitors of these enzymes may either, respectively, decrease the therapeutic effects or resultin side effects).
 No products indexed under this heading.

Doxorubicin Hydrochloride (Inducers of CYP3A4 may reduce plasma concentrations of estrogens, possibly resulting in a decrease in therapeutic effects and/or changes in the uterine bleeding profile).
No products indexed under this heading.

Efavirenz (Inducers of CYP3A4 may reduce plasma concentrations of estrogens, possibly resulting in a decrease in therapeutic effects and/or changes in the uterine bleeding profile). Products include:
Atripla Tablets 945
Sustiva Capsules 930
Sustiva Tablets 930

Erythromycin (Inhibitors of CYP3A4 such as erythromycin, clarithromycin, ketoconazole, itraconazole, ritonavir and grapefruit juice may increase plasma concentrations of estrogens and may result in side effects). Products include:
Ery-Tab Tablets 449
Erythromycin Base Filmtab Tablets 455
Erythromycin Delayed-Release Capsules, USP 457
PCE Dispertab Tablets 515

Erythromycin Estolate (Inhibitors of CYP3A4 such as erythromycin, clarithromycin, ketoconazole, itraconazole, ritonavir and grapefruit juice may increase plasma concentrations of estrogens and may result in side effects).
No products indexed under this heading.

Erythromycin Ethylsuccinate (Inhibitors of CYP3A4 such as erythromycin, clarithromycin, ketoconazole, itraconazole, ritonavir and grapefruit juice may increase plasma concentrations of estrogens and may result in side effects). Products include:
E.E.S. 451
EryPed 447

Erythromycin Gluceptate (Inhibitors of CYP3A4 such as erythromycin, clarithromycin, ketoconazole, itraconazole, ritonavir and grapefruit juice may increase plasma concentrations of estrogens and may result in side effects).
No products indexed under this heading.

Erythromycin Lactobionate (Inhibitors of CYP3A4 such as erythromycin, clarithromycin, ketoconazole, itraconazole, ritonavir and grapefruit juice may increase plasma concentrations of estrogens and may result in side effects).
No products indexed under this heading.

Erythromycin Stearate (Inhibitors of CYP3A4 such as erythromycin, clarithromycin, ketoconazole, itraconazole, ritonavir and grapefruit juice may increase plasma concentrations of estrogens and may result in side effects). Products include:
Erythrocin Stearate Filmtab Tablets 453

Esomeprazole Magnesium (Inhibitors of CYP3A4 such as erythromycin, clarithromycin, ketoconazole, itraconazole, ritonavir and grapefruit juice may increase plasma concentrations of estrogens and may result in side effects). Products include:
Nexium Delayed-Release Capsules 655

Ethinyl Estradiol (Based on in-vitro and in-vivo studies, it can be assumed that CYP3A, CYP2E and CYP2C are involved in the metabolism of levonorgestrel. Likewise, inducers or inhibitors of these enzymes may either, respectively, decrease the therapeutic effects or resultin side effects). Products include:
Mircette Tablets 1066
NuvaRing 2340
Ortho-Cyclen/Ortho Tri-Cyclen 2429
Ortho Evra Transdermal System 2417
Ortho Tri-Cyclen Lo Tablets 2436
Seasonique Tablets 1077
Yasmin 28 Tablets 796
Yaz Tablets 803

Ethosuximide (Inducers of CYP3A4 may reduce plasma concentrations of estrogens, possibly resulting in a decrease in therapeutic effects and/or changes in the uterine bleeding profile).
No products indexed under this heading.

Ethynodiol Diacetate (Based on in-vitro and in-vivo studies, it can be assumed that CYP3A, CYP2E and CYP2C are involved in the metabolism of levonorgestrel. Likewise, inducers or inhibitors of these enzymes may either, respectively, decrease the therapeutic effects or resultin side effects).
No products indexed under this heading.

Felbamate (Inducers of CYP3A4 may reduce plasma concentrations of estrogens, possibly resulting in a decrease in therapeutic effects and/or changes in the uterine bleeding profile).
No products indexed under this heading.

Fenofibrate (Based on in-vitro and in-vivo studies, it can be assumed that CYP3A, CYP2E and CYP2C are involved in the metabolism of levonorgestrel. Likewise, inducers or inhibitors of these enzymes may either, respectively, decrease the therapeutic effects or resultin side effects). Products include:
Lofibra Tablets 1219
Lofibra Capsules 1216
Tricor Tablets 527
Triglide Tablets 3123

Fluconazole (Inhibitors of CYP3A4 such as erythromycin, clarithromycin, ketoconazole, itraconazole, ritonavir and grapefruit juice may increase plasma concentrations of estrogens and may result in side effects).
No products indexed under this heading.

Fludrocortisone Acetate (Inducers of CYP3A4 may reduce plasma concentrations of estrogens, possibly resulting in a decrease in therapeutic effects and/or changes in the uterine bleeding profile).
No products indexed under this heading.

Fluorouracil (Based on in-vitro and in-vivo studies, it can be assumed that CYP3A, CYP2E and CYP2C are involved in the metabolism of levonorgestrel. Likewise, inducers or inhibitors of these enzymes may either, respectively, decrease the therapeutic effects or resultin side effects). Products include:
Carac Cream, 0.5% 2879
Efudex 3363

Fluoxetine (Based on in-vitro and in-vivo studies, it can be assumed that CYP3A, CYP2E and CYP2C are involved in the metabolism of levonorgestrel. Likewise, inducers or inhibitors of these enzymes may either, respectively, decrease the therapeutic effects or resultin side effects).
No products indexed under this heading.

Fluoxetine Hydrochloride (Inhibitors of CYP3A4 such as erythromycin, clarithromycin, ketoconazole, itraconazole, ritonavir and grapefruit juice may increase plasma concentrations of estrogens and may result in side effects). Products include:
Prozac Pulvules and Liquid 1801
Symbyax Capsules 1819

Flurbiprofen (Based on in-vitro and in-vivo studies, it can be assumed that CYP3A, CYP2E and CYP2C are involved in the metabolism of levonorgestrel. Likewise, inducers or inhibitors of these enzymes may either, respectively, decrease the therapeutic effects or resultin side effects).
No products indexed under this heading.

Flurbiprofen Sodium (Based on in-vitro and in-vivo studies, it can be assumed that CYP3A, CYP2E and CYP2C are involved in the metabolism of levonorgestrel. Likewise, inducers or inhibitors of these enzymes may either, respectively, decrease the therapeutic effects or resultin side effects). Products include:
Ocufen Ophthalmic Solution .... ⊙232

Fluvastatin Sodium (Based on in-vitro and in-vivo studies, it can be assumed that CYP3A, CYP2E and CYP2C are involved in the metabolism of levonorgestrel. Likewise, inducers or inhibitors of these enzymes may either, respectively, decrease the therapeutic effects or resultin side effects). Products include:
Lescol Capsules 2233
Lescol XL Tablets 2233

Fluvoxamine (Based on in-vitro and in-vivo studies, it can be assumed that CYP3A, CYP2E and CYP2C are involved in the metabolism of levonorgestrel. Likewise, inducers or inhibitors of these enzymes may either, respectively, decrease the therapeutic effects or resultin side effects).
No products indexed under this heading.

Fluvoxamine Maleate (Inhibitors of CYP3A4 such as erythromycin, clarithromycin, ketoconazole, itraconazole, ritonavir and grapefruit juice may increase plasma concentrations of estrogens and may result in side effects).
No products indexed under this heading.

Fosamprenavir Calcium (Inhibitors of CYP3A4 such as erythromycin, clarithromycin, ketoconazole, itraconazole, ritonavir and grapefruit juice may increase plasma concentrations of estrogens and may result in side effects). Products include:
Lexiva Tablets 1505

Fosphenytoin Sodium (Inducers of CYP3A4 may reduce plasma concentrations of estrogens, possibly resulting in a decrease in therapeutic effects and/or changes in the uterine bleeding profile).
No products indexed under this heading.

Garlic Extract (Inducers of CYP3A4 may reduce plasma concentrations of estrogens, possibly resulting in a decrease in therapeutic effects and/or changes in the uterine bleeding profile).
No products indexed under this heading.

Garlic Oil (Inducers of CYP3A4 may reduce plasma concentrations of estrogens, possibly resulting in a decrease in therapeutic effects and/or changes in the uterine bleeding profile).
No products indexed under this heading.

Gemfibrozil (Based on in-vitro and in-vivo studies, it can be assumed that CYP3A, CYP2E and CYP2C are involved in the metabolism of levonorgestrel. Likewise, inducers or inhibitors of these enzymes may either, respectively, decrease the therapeutic effects or resultin side effects).
No products indexed under this heading.

Glipizide (Based on in-vitro and in-vivo studies, it can be assumed that CYP3A, CYP2E and CYP2C are involved in the metabolism of levonorgestrel. Likewise, inducers or inhibitors of these enzymes may either, respectively, decrease the therapeutic effects or resultin side effects).
No products indexed under this heading.

Glyburide (Based on in-vitro and in-vivo studies, it can be assumed that CYP3A, CYP2E and CYP2C are involved in the metabolism of levonorgestrel. Likewise, inducers or inhibitors of these enzymes may either, respectively, decrease the therapeutic effects or resultin side effects).
No products indexed under this heading.

Hydrochlorothiazide (Based on in-vitro and in-vivo studies, it can be assumed that CYP3A, CYP2E and CYP2C are involved in the metabolism of levonorgestrel. Likewise, inducers or inhibitors of these enzymes may either, respectively, decrease the therapeutic effects or resultin side effects). Products include:
Aldoril Tablets 1910
Atacand HCT 651
Avalide Tablets 888
Avalide Tablets 2874
Benicar HCT Tablets 1044
Diovan HCT Tablets 2196
Dyazide Capsules 1423
Hyzaar 50-12.5 Tablets 1990
Hyzaar 100-12.5 Tablets 1990
Hyzaar 100-25 Tablets 1990
Lopressor HCT 50/25 Tablets 2241
Lopressor HCT 100/25 Tablets 2241
Lopressor HCT 100/50 Tablets 2241
Lotensin HCT Tablets 2246
Micardis HCT Tablets 856
Moduretic Tablets 2028
Prinzide Tablets 2056
Teveten HCT Tablets 1737
Timolide Tablets 2086
Uniretic Tablets 3100

Hydrocortisone (Inducers of CYP3A4 may reduce plasma concentrations of estrogens, possibly resulting in a decrease in therapeutic effects and/or changes in the uterine bleeding profile). Products include:

Colocort Rectal Suspension, USP (Retention) 100 mg/60 mL 2476
Hydrocortone Tablets 1989
Preparation H Hydrocortisone Cream .... ■ 646

Hydrocortisone Acetate (Inducers of CYP3A4 may reduce plasma concentrations of estrogens, possibly resulting in a decrease in therapeutic effects and/or changes in the uterine bleeding profile). Products include:

Analpram-HC 1159
Pramosone 1161
ProctoFoam-HC 3099

Hydrocortisone Butyrate (Inducers of CYP3A4 may reduce plasma concentrations of estrogens, possibly resulting in a decrease in therapeutic effects and/or changes in the uterine bleeding profile). Products include:

Locoid Lipocream Cream 1160

Hydrocortisone Cypionate (Inducers of CYP3A4 may reduce plasma concentrations of estrogens, possibly resulting in a decrease in therapeutic effects and/or changes in the uterine bleeding profile).

No products indexed under this heading.

Hydrocortisone Hemisuccinate (Inducers of CYP3A4 may reduce plasma concentrations of estrogens, possibly resulting in a decrease in therapeutic effects and/or changes in the uterine bleeding profile).

No products indexed under this heading.

Hydrocortisone Probutate (Inducers of CYP3A4 may reduce plasma concentrations of estrogens, possibly resulting in a decrease in therapeutic effects and/or changes in the uterine bleeding profile).

No products indexed under this heading.

Hydrocortisone Sodium Phosphate (Inducers of CYP3A4 may reduce plasma concentrations of estrogens, possibly resulting in a decrease in therapeutic effects and/or changes in the uterine bleeding profile).

No products indexed under this heading.

Hydrocortisone Sodium Succinate (Inducers of CYP3A4 may reduce plasma concentrations of estrogens, possibly resulting in a decrease in therapeutic effects and/or changes in the uterine bleeding profile).

No products indexed under this heading.

Hydrocortisone Valerate (Inducers of CYP3A4 may reduce plasma concentrations of estrogens, possibly resulting in a decrease in therapeutic effects and/or changes in the uterine bleeding profile).

No products indexed under this heading.

Hydroflumethiazide (Based on in-vitro and in-vivo studies, it can be assumed that CYP3A, CYP2E and CYP2C are involved in the metabolism of levonorgestrel. Likewise, inducers or inhibitors of these enzymes may either, respectively, decrease the therapeutic effects or resultin side effects).

No products indexed under this heading.

Hypericum (Inducers of CYP3A4 may reduce plasma concentrations of estrogens, possibly resulting in a decrease in therapeutic effects and/or changes in the uterine bleeding profile). Products include:

Satiete Tablets .... ■ 832

Hypericum Perforatum (Inducers of CYP3A4 may reduce plasma concentrations of estrogens, possibly resulting in a decrease in therapeutic effects and/or changes in the uterine bleeding profile).

No products indexed under this heading.

Imatinib Mesylate (Based on in-vitro and in-vivo studies, it can be assumed that CYP3A, CYP2E and CYP2C are involved in the metabolism of levonorgestrel. Likewise, inducers or inhibitors of these enzymes may either, respectively, decrease the therapeutic effects or resultin side effects). Products include:

Gleevec Tablets 2227

Indinavir Sulfate (Inhibitors of CYP3A4 such as erythromycin, clarithromycin, ketoconazole, itraconazole, ritonavir and grapefruit juice may increase plasma concentrations of estrogens and may result in side effects). Products include:

Crixivan Capsules 1940

Indomethacin (Based on in-vitro and in-vivo studies, it can be assumed that CYP3A, CYP2E and CYP2C are involved in the metabolism of levonorgestrel. Likewise, inducers or inhibitors of these enzymes may either, respectively, decrease the therapeutic effects or resultin side effects). Products include:

Indocin 1995

Indomethacin Sodium Trihydrate (Based on in-vitro and in-vivo studies, it can be assumed that CYP3A, CYP2E and CYP2C are involved in the metabolism of levonorgestrel. Likewise, inducers or inhibitors of these enzymes may either, respectively, decrease the therapeutic effects or resultin side effects). Products include:

Indocin I.V. 2465

Isoniazid (Inhibitors of CYP3A4 such as erythromycin, clarithromycin, ketoconazole, itraconazole, ritonavir and grapefruit juice may increase plasma concentrations of estrogens and may result in side effects).

No products indexed under this heading.

Itraconazole (Inhibitors of CYP3A4 such as erythromycin, clarithromycin, ketoconazole, itraconazole, ritonavir and grapefruit juice may increase plasma concentrations of estrogens and may result in side effects).

No products indexed under this heading.

Ketoconazole (Inhibitors of CYP3A4 such as erythromycin, clarithromycin, ketoconazole, itraconazole, ritonavir and grapefruit juice may increase plasma concentrations of estrogens and may result in side effects). Products include:

Nizoral A-D Shampoo, 1% 1868

Ketoprofen (Based on in-vitro and in-vivo studies, it can be assumed that CYP3A, CYP2E and CYP2C are involved in the metabolism of levonorgestrel. Likewise, inducers or inhibitors of these enzymes may either, respectively, decrease the therapeutic effects or resultin side effects).

No products indexed under this heading.

Lansoprazole (Based on in-vitro and in-vivo studies, it can be assumed that CYP3A, CYP2E and CYP2C are involved in the metabolism of levonorgestrel. Likewise, inducers or inhibitors of these enzymes may either, respectively, decrease the therapeutic effects or resultin side effects). Products include:

Prevacid Delayed-Release Capsules 3271
Prevacid for Delayed-Release Oral Suspension 3271
Prevacid SoluTab Delayed-Release Orally Disintegrating Tablets 3271
Prevacid I.V. for Injection 3277
Prevacid NapraPAC 3280
PREVPAC 3284

Leflunomide (Based on in-vitro and in-vivo studies, it can be assumed that CYP3A, CYP2E and CYP2C are involved in the metabolism of levonorgestrel. Likewise, inducers or inhibitors of these enzymes may either, respectively, decrease the therapeutic effects or resultin side effects).

No products indexed under this heading.

Letrozole (Based on in-vitro and in-vivo studies, it can be assumed that CYP3A, CYP2E and CYP2C are involved in the metabolism of levonorgestrel. Likewise, inducers or inhibitors of these enzymes may either, respectively, decrease the therapeutic effects or resultin side effects). Products include:

Femara Tablets 2214

Lopinavir (Inhibitors of CYP3A4 such as erythromycin, clarithromycin, ketoconazole, itraconazole, ritonavir and grapefruit juice may increase plasma concentrations of estrogens and may result in side effects). Products include:

Kaletra 476

Loratadine (Inhibitors of CYP3A4 such as erythromycin, clarithromycin, ketoconazole, itraconazole, ritonavir and grapefruit juice may increase plasma concentrations of estrogens and may result in side effects). Products include:

Alavert Allergy & Sinus D-12 Hour Tablets.. ■ 771
Alavert .... ■ 771
Children's Claritin Allergy Oral Solution .... ■ 771
Claritin Non-Drowsy 24 Hour Tablets... ■ 772
Claritin Reditabs 24 Hour Non-Drowsy Tablets .... ■ 772
Claritin-D Non-Drowsy 12 Hour Tablets... ■ 772
Claritin-D Non-Drowsy 24 Hour Tablets... ■ 772

Lovastatin (Based on in-vitro and in-vivo studies, it can be assumed that CYP3A, CYP2E and CYP2C are involved in the metabolism of levonorgestrel. Likewise, inducers or inhibitors of these enzymes may either, respectively, decrease the therapeutic effects or resultin side effects). Products include:

Advicor Tablets 1722
Altoprev Extended-Release Tablets 3109
Mevacor Tablets 2021

Mephenytoin (Inducers of CYP3A4 may reduce plasma concentrations of estrogens, possibly resulting in a decrease in therapeutic effects and/or changes in the uterine bleeding profile).

No products indexed under this heading.

Mestranol (Based on in-vitro and in-vivo studies, it can be assumed that CYP3A, CYP2E and CYP2C are involved in the metabolism of levonorgestrel. Likewise, inducers or inhibitors of these enzymes may either, respectively, decrease the therapeutic effects or resultin side effects).

No products indexed under this heading.

Methsuximide (Inducers of CYP3A4 may reduce plasma concentrations of estrogens, possibly resulting in a decrease in therapeutic effects and/or changes in the uterine bleeding profile).

No products indexed under this heading.

Methyclothiazide (Based on in-vitro and in-vivo studies, it can be assumed that CYP3A, CYP2E and CYP2C are involved in the metabolism of levonorgestrel. Likewise, inducers or inhibitors of these enzymes may either, respectively, decrease the therapeutic effects or resultin side effects).

No products indexed under this heading.

Methylprednisolone (Inducers of CYP3A4 may reduce plasma concentrations of estrogens, possibly resulting in a decrease in therapeutic effects and/or changes in the uterine bleeding profile).

No products indexed under this heading.

Methylprednisolone Acetate (Inducers of CYP3A4 may reduce plasma concentrations of estrogens, possibly resulting in a decrease in therapeutic effects and/or changes in the uterine bleeding profile). Products include:

Depo-Medrol Injectable Suspension 2617
Depo-Medrol Single-Dose Vial 2619

Methylprednisolone Sodium Succinate (Inducers of CYP3A4 may reduce plasma concentrations of estrogens, possibly resulting in a decrease in therapeutic effects and/or changes in the uterine bleeding profile).

No products indexed under this heading.

Metronidazole (Inhibitors of CYP3A4 such as erythromycin, clarithromycin, ketoconazole, itraconazole, ritonavir and grapefruit juice may increase plasma concentrations of estrogens and may result in side effects). Products include:

Metrogel 1% 1211
MetroGel-Vaginal Gel 1855
Vandazole Vaginal Gel 3338

Metronidazole Benzoate (Inhibitors of CYP3A4 such as erythromycin, clarithromycin, ketoconazole, itraconazole, ritonavir and grapefruit juice may increase plasma concentrations of estrogens and may result in side effects).

No products indexed under this heading.

Metronidazole Hydrochloride (Inhibitors of CYP3A4 such as erythromycin, clarithromycin, ketoconazole, itraconazole, ritonavir and grapefruit juice may increase plasma concentrations of estrogens and may result in side effects).

No products indexed under this heading.

Miconazole (Inhibitors of CYP3A4 such as erythromycin, clarithromycin, ketoconazole, itraconazole, ritonavir and grapefruit juice may increase plasma concentrations of estrogens and may result in side effects).

No products indexed under this heading.

Miconazole Nitrate (Inhibitors of CYP3A4 such as erythromycin, clarithromycin, ketoconazole, itraconazole, ritonavir and grapefruit juice may increase plasma concentrations of estrogens and may result in side effects). Products include:
Desenex ... ▣635
Desenex Jock Itch Spray Powder ... ▣635

Modafinil (Inducers of CYP3A4 may reduce plasma concentrations of estrogens, possibly resulting in a decrease in therapeutic effects and/or changes in the uterine bleeding profile). Products include:
Provigil Tablets 988

Nefazodone Hydrochloride (Inhibitors of CYP3A4 such as erythromycin, clarithromycin, ketoconazole, itraconazole, ritonavir and grapefruit juice may increase plasma concentrations of estrogens and may result in side effects).

No products indexed under this heading.

Nelfinavir Mesylate (Inhibitors of CYP3A4 such as erythromycin, clarithromycin, ketoconazole, itraconazole, ritonavir and grapefruit juice may increase plasma concentrations of estrogens and may result in side effects). Products include:
Viracept .. 2577

Nevirapine (Inducers of CYP3A4 may reduce plasma concentrations of estrogens, possibly resulting in a decrease in therapeutic effects and/or changes in the uterine bleeding profile). Products include:
Viramune Oral Suspension 873
Viramune Tablets 873

Niacinamide (Inhibitors of CYP3A4 such as erythromycin, clarithromycin, ketoconazole, itraconazole, ritonavir and grapefruit juice may increase plasma concentrations of estrogens and may result in side effects).

No products indexed under this heading.

Nicardipine Hydrochloride (Based on in-vitro and in-vivo studies, it can be assumed that CYP3A, CYP2E and CYP2C are involved in the metabolism of levonorgestrel. Likewise, inducers or inhibitors of these enzymes may either, respectively, decrease the therapeutic effects or resultin side effects). Products include:

Cardene I.V. 2497

Nicotinamide (Inhibitors of CYP3A4 such as erythromycin, clarithromycin, ketoconazole, itraconazole, ritonavir and grapefruit juice may increase plasma concentrations of estrogens and may result in side effects). Products include:
Nicomide Tablets 1088

Nifedipine (Inhibitors of CYP3A4 such as erythromycin, clarithromycin, ketoconazole, itraconazole, ritonavir and grapefruit juice may increase plasma concentrations of estrogens and may result in side effects). Products include:
Adalat CC Tablets 2964

Norethindrone (Based on in-vitro and in-vivo studies, it can be assumed that CYP3A, CYP2E and CYP2C are involved in the metabolism of levonorgestrel. Likewise, inducers or inhibitors of these enzymes may either, respectively, decrease the therapeutic effects or resultin side effects). Products include:
Ortho Micronor Tablets 2426

Norethindrone Acetate (Based on in-vitro and in-vivo studies, it can be assumed that CYP3A, CYP2E and CYP2C are involved in the metabolism of levonorgestrel. Likewise, inducers or inhibitors of these enzymes may either, respectively, decrease the therapeutic effects or resultin side effects).

No products indexed under this heading.

Norethynodrel (Based on in-vitro and in-vivo studies, it can be assumed that CYP3A, CYP2E and CYP2C are involved in the metabolism of levonorgestrel. Likewise, inducers or inhibitors of these enzymes may either, respectively, decrease the therapeutic effects or resultin side effects).

No products indexed under this heading.

Norfloxacin (Inhibitors of CYP3A4 such as erythromycin, clarithromycin, ketoconazole, itraconazole, ritonavir and grapefruit juice may increase plasma concentrations of estrogens and may result in side effects). Products include:
Noroxin Tablets 2032

Norgestimate (Based on in-vitro and in-vivo studies, it can be assumed that CYP3A, CYP2E and CYP2C are involved in the metabolism of levonorgestrel. Likewise, inducers or inhibitors of these enzymes may either, respectively, decrease the therapeutic effects or resultin side effects). Products include:
Ortho-Cyclen/Ortho Tri-Cyclen 2429
Ortho Tri-Cyclen Lo Tablets 2436

Norgestrel (Based on in-vitro and in-vivo studies, it can be assumed that CYP3A, CYP2E and CYP2C are involved in the metabolism of levonorgestrel. Likewise, inducers or inhibitors of these enzymes may either, respectively, decrease the therapeutic effects or resultin side effects).

No products indexed under this heading.

Omeprazole (Inhibitors of CYP3A4 such as erythromycin, clarithromycin, ketoconazole, itraconazole, ritonavir and grapefruit juice may

increase plasma concentrations of estrogens and may result in side effects). Products include:
Zegerid Capsules 2958
Zegerid Powder for Oral Solution 2958

Oxcarbazepine (Inducers of CYP3A4 may reduce plasma concentrations of estrogens, possibly resulting in a decrease in therapeutic effects and/or changes in the uterine bleeding profile). Products include:
Trileptal Tablets 2300
Trileptal Oral Suspension 2300

Oxiconazole Nitrate (Based on in-vitro and in-vivo studies, it can be assumed that CYP3A, CYP2E and CYP2C are involved in the metabolism of levonorgestrel. Likewise, inducers or inhibitors of these enzymes may either, respectively, decrease the therapeutic effects or resultin side effects). Products include:
Oxistat .. 2667

Paroxetine Hydrochloride (Inhibitors of CYP3A4 such as erythromycin, clarithromycin, ketoconazole, itraconazole, ritonavir and grapefruit juice may increase plasma concentrations of estrogens and may result in side effects). Products include:
Paxil CR Controlled-Release
Tablets 1538
Paxil .. 1530

Phenobarbital (Inducers of CYP3A4 may reduce plasma concentrations of estrogens, possibly resulting in a decrease in therapeutic effects and/or changes in the uterine bleeding profile). Products include:
Donnatal Extentabs 2493

Phenobarbital Sodium (Inducers of CYP3A4 may reduce plasma concentrations of estrogens, possibly resulting in a decrease in therapeutic effects and/or changes in the uterine bleeding profile).

No products indexed under this heading.

Phenylbutazone (Based on in-vitro and in-vivo studies, it can be assumed that CYP3A, CYP2E and CYP2C are involved in the metabolism of levonorgestrel. Likewise, inducers or inhibitors of these enzymes may either, respectively, decrease the therapeutic effects or resultin side effects).

No products indexed under this heading.

Phenytoin (Inducers of CYP3A4 may reduce plasma concentrations of estrogens, possibly resulting in a decrease in therapeutic effects and/or changes in the uterine bleeding profile).

No products indexed under this heading.

Phenytoin Sodium (Inducers of CYP3A4 may reduce plasma concentrations of estrogens, possibly resulting in a decrease in therapeutic effects and/or changes in the uterine bleeding profile). Products include:
Phenytek Capsules 2160

Polythiazide (Based on in-vitro and in-vivo studies, it can be assumed that CYP3A, CYP2E and CYP2C are involved in the metabolism of levonorgestrel. Likewise, inducers or inhibitors of these enzymes may either, respectively, decrease the therapeutic effects or resultin side effects).

No products indexed under this heading.

Prednisolone Acetate (Inducers of CYP3A4 may reduce plasma concentrations of estrogens, possibly resulting in a decrease in therapeutic effects and/or changes in the uterine bleeding profile). Products include:
Blephamide Ophthalmic Ointment 568
Blephamide Ophthalmic
Suspension 569
Poly-Pred Ophthalmic
Suspension ⊙233
Pred Forte Ophthalmic
Suspension ⊙235
Pred Mild Ophthalmic
Suspension ⊙238
Pred-G Ophthalmic Ointment ⊙237
Pred-G Ophthalmic Suspension ⊙236

Prednisolone Sodium Phosphate (Inducers of CYP3A4 may reduce plasma concentrations of estrogens, possibly resulting in a decrease in therapeutic effects and/or changes in the uterine bleeding profile).

No products indexed under this heading.

Prednisolone Tebutate (Inducers of CYP3A4 may reduce plasma concentrations of estrogens, possibly resulting in a decrease in therapeutic effects and/or changes in the uterine bleeding profile).

No products indexed under this heading.

Prednisone (Inducers of CYP3A4 may reduce plasma concentrations of estrogens, possibly resulting in a decrease in therapeutic effects and/or changes in the uterine bleeding profile).

No products indexed under this heading.

Primidone (Inducers of CYP3A4 may reduce plasma concentrations of estrogens, possibly resulting in a decrease in therapeutic effects and/or changes in the uterine bleeding profile).

No products indexed under this heading.

Propoxyphene Hydrochloride (Inhibitors of CYP3A4 such as erythromycin, clarithromycin, ketoconazole, itraconazole, ritonavir and grapefruit juice may increase plasma concentrations of estrogens and may result in side effects).

No products indexed under this heading.

Propoxyphene Napsylate (Inhibitors of CYP3A4 such as erythromycin, clarithromycin, ketoconazole, itraconazole, ritonavir and grapefruit juice may increase plasma concentrations of estrogens and may result in side effects).

No products indexed under this heading.

Quercetin (Based on in-vitro and in-vivo studies, it can be assumed that CYP3A, CYP2E and CYP2C are involved in the metabolism of levonorgestrel. Likewise, inducers or inhibitors of these enzymes may either, respectively, decrease the therapeutic effects or resultin side effects).

No products indexed under this heading.

Quinidine (Inhibitors of CYP3A4 such as erythromycin, clarithromycin, ketoconazole, itraconazole, ritonavir and grapefruit juice may increase plasma concentrations of estrogens and may result in side effects).

No products indexed under this heading.

IMPORTANT NOTE: Always consult each drug listing in the patient's regimen for possible interactions.

Quinidine Hydrochloride (Inhibitors of CYP3A4 such as erythromycin, clarithromycin, ketoconazole, itraconazole, ritonavir and grapefruit juice may increase plasma concentrations of estrogens and may result in side effects).
 No products indexed under this heading.

Quinidine Polygalacturonate (Inhibitors of CYP3A4 such as erythromycin, clarithromycin, ketoconazole, itraconazole, ritonavir and grapefruit juice may increase plasma concentrations of estrogens and may result in side effects).
 No products indexed under this heading.

Quinidine Sulfate (Inhibitors of CYP3A4 such as erythromycin, clarithromycin, ketoconazole, itraconazole, ritonavir and grapefruit juice may increase plasma concentrations of estrogens and may result in side effects).
 No products indexed under this heading.

Quinine (Inhibitors of CYP3A4 such as erythromycin, clarithromycin, ketoconazole, itraconazole, ritonavir and grapefruit juice may increase plasma concentrations of estrogens and may result in side effects).
 No products indexed under this heading.

Quinine Sulfate (Inhibitors of CYP3A4 such as erythromycin, clarithromycin, ketoconazole, itraconazole, ritonavir and grapefruit juice may increase plasma concentrations of estrogens and may result in side effects).
 No products indexed under this heading.

Quinupristin (Inhibitors of CYP3A4 such as erythromycin, clarithromycin, ketoconazole, itraconazole, ritonavir and grapefruit juice may increase plasma concentrations of estrogens and may result in side effects).
 No products indexed under this heading.

Ranitidine Bismuth Citrate (Inhibitors of CYP3A4 such as erythromycin, clarithromycin, ketoconazole, itraconazole, ritonavir and grapefruit juice may increase plasma concentrations of estrogens and may result in side effects).
 No products indexed under this heading.

Ranitidine Hydrochloride (Inhibitors of CYP3A4 such as erythromycin, clarithromycin, ketoconazole, itraconazole, ritonavir and grapefruit juice may increase plasma concentrations of estrogens and may result in side effects). Products include:

Rifabutin (Inducers of CYP3A4 may reduce plasma concentrations of estrogens, possibly resulting in a decrease in therapeutic effects and/or changes in the uterine bleeding profile).
 No products indexed under this heading.

Rifampicin (Inducers of CYP3A4 may reduce plasma concentrations of estrogens, possibly resulting in a decrease in therapeutic effects and/or changes in the uterine bleeding profile).
 No products indexed under this heading.

Rifampin (Inducers of CYP3A4 may reduce plasma concentrations of estrogens, possibly resulting in a decrease in therapeutic effects and/or changes in the uterine bleeding profile).
 No products indexed under this heading.

Rifapentine (Inducers of CYP3A4 may reduce plasma concentrations of estrogens, possibly resulting in a decrease in therapeutic effects and/or changes in the uterine bleeding profile).
 No products indexed under this heading.

Ritonavir (Inhibitors of CYP3A4 such as erythromycin, clarithromycin, ketoconazole, itraconazole, ritonavir and grapefruit juice may increase plasma concentrations of estrogens and may result in side effects). Products include:

Saquinavir (Inhibitors of CYP3A4 such as erythromycin, clarithromycin, ketoconazole, itraconazole, ritonavir and grapefruit juice may increase plasma concentrations of estrogens and may result in side effects).
 No products indexed under this heading.

Saquinavir Mesylate (Inhibitors of CYP3A4 such as erythromycin, clarithromycin, ketoconazole, itraconazole, ritonavir and grapefruit juice may increase plasma concentrations of estrogens and may result in side effects). Products include:

Secobarbital Sodium (Based on in-vitro and in-vivo studies, it can be assumed that CYP3A, CYP2E and CYP2C are involved in the metabolism of levonorgestrel. Likewise, inducers or inhibitors of these enzymes may either, respectively, decrease the therapeutic effects or resultin side effects).
 No products indexed under this heading.

Sertraline Hydrochloride (Inhibitors of CYP3A4 such as erythromycin, clarithromycin, ketoconazole, itraconazole, ritonavir and grapefruit juice may increase plasma concentrations of estrogens and may result in side effects). Products include:

Sulfacytine (Based on in-vitro and in-vivo studies, it can be assumed that CYP3A, CYP2E and CYP2C are involved in the metabolism of levonorgestrel. Likewise, inducers or inhibitors of these enzymes may either, respectively, decrease the therapeutic effects or resultin side effects).
 No products indexed under this heading.

Sulfamethizole (Based on in-vitro and in-vivo studies, it can be assumed that CYP3A, CYP2E and CYP2C are involved in the metabolism of levonorgestrel. Likewise, inducers or inhibitors of these enzymes may either, respectively, decrease the therapeutic effects or resultin side effects).
 No products indexed under this heading.

Sulfamethoxazole (Based on in-vitro and in-vivo studies, it can be assumed that CYP3A, CYP2E and CYP2C are involved in the metabolism of levonorgestrel. Likewise, inducers or inhibitors of these enzymes may either, respectively, decrease the therapeutic effects or resultin side effects).
 No products indexed under this heading.

Sulfaphenazole (Based on in-vitro and in-vivo studies, it can be assumed that CYP3A, CYP2E and CYP2C are involved in the metabolism of levonorgestrel. Likewise, inducers or inhibitors of these enzymes may either, respectively, decrease the therapeutic effects or resultin side effects).
 No products indexed under this heading.

Sulfasalazine (Based on in-vitro and in-vivo studies, it can be assumed that CYP3A, CYP2E and CYP2C are involved in the metabolism of levonorgestrel. Likewise, inducers or inhibitors of these enzymes may either, respectively, decrease the therapeutic effects or resultin side effects).
 No products indexed under this heading.

Sulfinpyrazone (Inducers of CYP3A4 may reduce plasma concentrations of estrogens, possibly resulting in a decrease in therapeutic effects and/or changes in the uterine bleeding profile).
 No products indexed under this heading.

Sulfisoxazole Acetyl (Based on in-vitro and in-vivo studies, it can be assumed that CYP3A, CYP2E and CYP2C are involved in the metabolism of levonorgestrel. Likewise, inducers or inhibitors of these enzymes may either, respectively, decrease the therapeutic effects or resultin side effects).
 No products indexed under this heading.

Sulfisoxazole Diolamine (Based on in-vitro and in-vivo studies, it can be assumed that CYP3A, CYP2E and CYP2C are involved in the metabolism of levonorgestrel. Likewise, inducers or inhibitors of these enzymes may either, respectively, decrease the therapeutic effects or resultin side effects).
 No products indexed under this heading.

Telithromycin (Inhibitors of CYP3A4 such as erythromycin, clarithromycin, ketoconazole, itraconazole, ritonavir and grapefruit juice may increase plasma concentrations of estrogens and may result in side effects). Products include:

Telmisartan (Based on in-vitro and in-vivo studies, it can be assumed that CYP3A, CYP2E and CYP2C are involved in the metabolism of levonorgestrel. Likewise, inducers or

inhibitors of these enzymes may either, respectively, decrease the therapeutic effects or resultin side effects). Products include:

Terconazole (Based on in-vitro and in-vivo studies, it can be assumed that CYP3A, CYP2E and CYP2C are involved in the metabolism of levonorgestrel. Likewise, inducers or inhibitors of these enzymes may either, respectively, decrease the therapeutic effects or resultin side effects).
 No products indexed under this heading.

Theophylline (Inducers of CYP3A4 may reduce plasma concentrations of estrogens, possibly resulting in a decrease in therapeutic effects and/or changes in the uterine bleeding profile).
 No products indexed under this heading.

Ticlopidine Hydrochloride (Based on in-vitro and in-vivo studies, it can be assumed that CYP3A, CYP2E and CYP2C are involved in the metabolism of levonorgestrel. Likewise, inducers or inhibitors of these enzymes may either, respectively, decrease the therapeutic effects or resultin side effects). Products include:

Tolazamide (Based on in-vitro and in-vivo studies, it can be assumed that CYP3A, CYP2E and CYP2C are involved in the metabolism of levonorgestrel. Likewise, inducers or inhibitors of these enzymes may either, respectively, decrease the therapeutic effects or resultin side effects).
 No products indexed under this heading.

Tolbutamide (Based on in-vitro and in-vivo studies, it can be assumed that CYP3A, CYP2E and CYP2C are involved in the metabolism of levonorgestrel. Likewise, inducers or inhibitors of these enzymes may either, respectively, decrease the therapeutic effects or resultin side effects).
 No products indexed under this heading.

Tolbutamide Sodium (Based on in-vitro and in-vivo studies, it can be assumed that CYP3A, CYP2E and CYP2C are involved in the metabolism of levonorgestrel. Likewise, inducers or inhibitors of these enzymes may either, respectively, decrease the therapeutic effects or resultin side effects).
 No products indexed under this heading.

Topiramate (Based on in-vitro and in-vivo studies, it can be assumed that CYP3A, CYP2E and CYP2C are involved in the metabolism of levonorgestrel. Likewise, inducers or inhibitors of these enzymes may either, respectively, decrease the therapeutic effects or resultin side effects). Products include:

Triamcinolone (Inducers of CYP3A4 may reduce plasma concentrations of estrogens, possibly resulting in a decrease in therapeutic effects and/or changes in the uterine bleeding profile).
No products indexed under this heading.

Triamcinolone Acetonide (Inducers of CYP3A4 may reduce plasma concentrations of estrogens, possibly resulting in a decrease in therapeutic effects and/or changes in the uterine bleeding profile). Products include:
Azmacort Inhalation Aerosol **1726**
Nasacort AQ Nasal Spray **2922**

Triamcinolone Diacetate (Inducers of CYP3A4 may reduce plasma concentrations of estrogens, possibly resulting in a decrease in therapeutic effects and/or changes in the uterine bleeding profile).
No products indexed under this heading.

Triamcinolone Hexacetonide (Inducers of CYP3A4 may reduce plasma concentrations of estrogens, possibly resulting in a decrease in therapeutic effects and/or changes in the uterine bleeding profile).
No products indexed under this heading.

Trimethoprim (Based on in-vitro and in-vivo studies, it can be assumed that CYP3A, CYP2E and CYP2C are involved in the metabolism of levonorgestrel. Likewise, inducers or inhibitors of these enzymes may either, respectively, decrease the therapeutic effects or resultin side effects).
No products indexed under this heading.

Trimethoprim Hydrochloride (Based on in-vitro and in-vivo studies, it can be assumed that CYP3A, CYP2E and CYP2C are involved in the metabolism of levonorgestrel. Likewise, inducers or inhibitors of these enzymes may either, respectively, decrease the therapeutic effects or resultin side effects).
No products indexed under this heading.

Troglitazone (Inducers of CYP3A4 may reduce plasma concentrations of estrogens, possibly resulting in a decrease in therapeutic effects and/ or changes in the uterine bleeding profile).
No products indexed under this heading.

Troleandomycin (Inhibitors of CYP3A4 such as erythromycin, clarithromycin, ketoconazole, itraconazole, ritonavir and grapefruit juice may increase plasma concentrations of estrogens and may result in side effects).
No products indexed under this heading.

Valproate Sodium (Inhibitors of CYP3A4 such as erythromycin, clarithromycin, ketoconazole, itraconazole, ritonavir and grapefruit juice may increase plasma concentrations of estrogens and may result in side effects). Products include:
Depacon Injection **412**

Verapamil Hydrochloride (Inhibitors of CYP3A4 such as erythromycin, clarithromycin, ketoconazole, itraconazole, ritonavir and grapefruit juice may increase plasma concentrations of estrogens and may result in side effects). Products include:
Covera-HS Tablets **3139**
Tarka Tablets **524**
Verelan PM Extended-Release Capsules, Controlled-Onset........... **3106**

Voriconazole (Inhibitors of CYP3A4 such as erythromycin, clarithromycin, ketoconazole, itraconazole, ritonavir and grapefruit juice may increase plasma concentrations of estrogens and may result in side effects). Products include:
VFEND I.V. **2564**
VFEND Oral Suspension **2564**
VFEND Tablets **2564**

Zafirlukast (Inhibitors of CYP3A4 such as erythromycin, clarithromycin, ketoconazole, itraconazole, ritonavir and grapefruit juice may increase plasma concentrations of estrogens and may result in side effects). Products include:
Accolate Tablets **671**

Zileuton (Inhibitors of CYP3A4 such as erythromycin, clarithromycin, ketoconazole, itraconazole, ritonavir and grapefruit juice may increase plasma concentrations of estrogens and may result in side effects). Products include:
Zyflo Tablets **1023**

Food Interactions

Grapefruit (Inhibitors of CYP3A4 such as erythromycin, clarithromycin, ketoconazole, itraconazole, ritonavir and grapefruit juice may increase plasma concentrations of estrogens and may result in side effects).

Grapefruit Juice (Inhibitors of CYP3A4 such as erythromycin, clarithromycin, ketoconazole, itraconazole, ritonavir and grapefruit juice may increase plasma concentrations of estrogens and may result in side effects).

CLINDAGEL

(Clindamycin Phosphate) **1203**
May interact with neuromuscular blocking agents. Compounds in these categories include:

Atracurium Besylate (Clindamycin has neuromuscular blocking properties that may enhance the action of other neuromuscular blocking agents).
No products indexed under this heading.

Cisatracurium Besylate (Clindamycin has neuromuscular blocking properties that may enhance the action of other neuromuscular blocking agents). Products include:
Nimbex Injection **498**

Doxacurium Chloride (Clindamycin has neuromuscular blocking properties that may enhance the action of other neuromuscular blocking agents).
No products indexed under this heading.

Metocurine Iodide (Clindamycin has neuromuscular blocking properties that may enhance the action of other neuromuscular blocking agents).
No products indexed under this heading.

Mivacurium Chloride (Clindamycin has neuromuscular blocking properties that may enhance the action of other neuromuscular blocking agents). Products include:
Mivacron Injection **493**

Pancuronium Bromide (Clindamycin has neuromuscular blocking properties that may enhance the action of other neuromuscular blocking agents).
No products indexed under this heading.

Rapacuronium Bromide (Clindamycin has neuromuscular blocking properties that may enhance the action of other neuromuscular blocking agents).
No products indexed under this heading.

Rocuronium Bromide (Clindamycin has neuromuscular blocking properties that may enhance the action of other neuromuscular blocking agents). Products include:
Zemuron Injection **2346**

Succinylcholine Chloride (Clindamycin has neuromuscular blocking properties that may enhance the action of other neuromuscular blocking agents).
No products indexed under this heading.

Vecuronium Bromide (Clindamycin has neuromuscular blocking properties that may enhance the action of other neuromuscular blocking agents).
No products indexed under this heading.

CLINORIL TABLETS

(Sulindac) **1924**
May interact with ACE inhibitors, angiotensin-II receptor antagonists, oral anticoagulants, diuretics, oral hypoglycemic agents, lithium preparations, non-steroidal anti-inflammatory agents, and certain other agents. Compounds in these categories include:

Acarbose (Special attention should be paid to patients taking higher doses than those recommended and to patients with renal or metabolic impairment). Products include:
Precose Tablets **751**

Amiloride Hydrochloride (Sulindac can reduce the natriuretic effect of furosemide and thiazides in some patients. This response has been attributed to inhibition of renal prostaglandin synthesis. During concomitant therapy with NSAIDs, the patient should be observed closely for signs of renal failure, as well as to assure diuretic efficacy). Products include:
Midamor Tablets **2026**
Moduretic Tablets **2028**

Anisindione (Special attention should be paid to patients taking higher doses than those recommended and to patients with renal or metabolic impairment). Products include:
Miradon Tablets **3042**

Aspirin (Increased gastrointestinal reactions). Products include:
Aggrenox Capsules **822**
Bayer Aspirin **744**
BC Allergy Sinus Cold Powder **677**
BC Headache Powder **677**
Arthritis Strength BC Powder **677**
BC Sinus Cold Powder **677**
Excedrin Extra Strength Caplets/Tablets/Geltabs............ **684**
Excedrin Migraine Caplets/Tablets/Geltabs............ **609**
Goody's Body Pain Formula Powder....................................... **684**
Goody's Extra Strength Headache Powders..................... **611**
Goody's Extra Strength Pain Relief Tablets............................ **685**
Percodan Tablets **1132**
St. Joseph 81 mg Aspirin Chewable and Enteric Coated Tablets.. **1869**

Aspirin, Enteric Coated (Increased gastrointestinal reactions).
No products indexed under this heading.

Benazepril Hydrochloride (Reports suggest that NSAIDs may diminish the antihypertensive effect of ACE-inhibitors and angiotensin II antagonists. These interactions should be given consideration in patients taking NSAIDs concomitantly with ACE-inhibitors or angiotensin II antagonists. In some patients with compromised renal function, the co-administration of an NSAID and an ACE-inhibitor or an angiotensin II antagonist may result in further deterioration of renal function, including possible acute renal failure, which is usually reversible). Products include:
Lotensin Tablets **2243**
Lotensin HCT Tablets **2246**
Lotrel Capsules **2249**

Bendroflumethiazide (Sulindac can reduce the natriuretic effect of furosemide and thiazides in some patients. This response has been attributed to inhibition of renal prostaglandin synthesis. During concomitant therapy with NSAIDs, the patient should be observed closely for signs of renal failure, as well as to assure diuretic efficacy).
No products indexed under this heading.

Bumetanide (Sulindac can reduce the natriuretic effect of furosemide and thiazides in some patients. This response has been attributed to inhibition of renal prostaglandin synthesis. During concomitant therapy with NSAIDs, the patient should be observed closely for signs of renal failure, as well as to assure diuretic efficacy). Products include:
Bumex Tablets **2746**

Candesartan Cilexetil (Reports suggest that NSAIDs may diminish the antihypertensive effect of ACE-inhibitors and angiotensin II antagonists. These interactions should be given consideration in patients taking NSAIDs concomitantly with ACE-inhibitors or angiotensin II antagonists. In some patients with compromised renal function, the co-administration of an NSAID and an ACE-inhibitor or an angiotensin II antagonist may result in further deterioration of renal function, including possible acute renal failure, which is usually reversible). Products include:
Atacand Tablets **649**
Atacand HCT **651**

Captopril (Reports suggest that NSAIDs may diminish the antihypertensive effect of ACE-inhibitors and angiotensin II antagonists. These interactions should be given consideration in patients taking NSAIDs concomitantly with ACE-inhibitors or angiotensin II antagonists. In some patients with compromised renal function, the co-administration of an NSAID and an ACE-inhibitor or an angiotensin II antagonist may result in further deterioration of renal function, including possible acute renal failure, which is usually reversible). Products include:
Captopril Tablets **2149**

Celecoxib (Concomitant use is not recommended due to the increased possibility of gastrointestinal toxicity, with little or no increase in efficacy). Products include:

Celebrex Capsules 3134

Chlorothiazide (Sulindac can reduce the natriuretic effect of furosemide and thiazides in some patients. This response has been attributed to inhibition of renal prostaglandin synthesis. During concomitant therapy with NSAIDs, the patient should be observed closely for signs of renal failure, as well as to assure diuretic efficacy). Products include:

Diuril Oral Suspension 1954

Chlorothiazide Sodium (Sulindac can reduce the natriuretic effect of furosemide and thiazides in some patients. This response has been attributed to inhibition of renal prostaglandin synthesis. During concomitant therapy with NSAIDs, the patient should be observed closely for signs of renal failure, as well as to assure diuretic efficacy). Products include:

Diuril Sodium Intravenous 2467

Chlorpropamide (Special attention should be paid to patients taking higher doses than those recommended and to patients with renal or metabolic impairment).

No products indexed under this heading.

Chlorthalidone (Sulindac can reduce the natriuretic effect of furosemide and thiazides in some patients. This response has been attributed to inhibition of renal prostaglandin synthesis. During concomitant therapy with NSAIDs, the patient should be observed closely for signs of renal failure, as well as to assure diuretic efficacy). Products include:

Clorpres Tablets 2153

Cyclosporine (Increased cyclosporine-induced toxicity). Products include:

Gengraf Capsules 459
Neoral Oral Solution 2259
Neoral Soft Gelatin Capsules 2259
Restasis Ophthalmic Emulsion 575
Sandimmune 2275

Diclofenac Potassium (Concomitant use is not recommended due to the increased possibility of gastrointestinal toxicity, with little or no increase in efficacy).

No products indexed under this heading.

Diclofenac Sodium (Concomitant use is not recommended due to the increased possibility of gastrointestinal toxicity, with little or no increase in efficacy). Products include:

Arthrotec Tablets 3129
Voltaren Ophthalmic Solution 2309
Voltaren Tablets 2307
Voltaren-XR Tablets 2310

Dicumarol (Special attention should be paid to patients taking higher doses than those recommended and to patients with renal or metabolic impairment).

No products indexed under this heading.

Diflunisal (Decreased plasma levels of sulindac). Products include:

Dolobid Tablets 1955

DMSO (Reduced efficacy of sulindac; peripheral neuropathy).

No products indexed under this heading.

Enalapril Maleate (Reports suggest that NSAIDs may diminish the antihypertensive effect of ACE-inhibitors and angiotensin II antagonists. These interactions should be

given consideration in patients taking NSAIDs concomitantly with ACE-inhibitors or angiotensin II antagonists. In some patients with compromised renal function, the co-administration of an NSAID and an ACE-inhibitor or an angiotensin II antagonist may result in further deterioration of renal function, including possible acute renal failure, which is usually reversible). Products include:

Vasotec I.V. Injection 2103

Enalaprilat (Reports suggest that NSAIDs may diminish the antihypertensive effect of ACE-inhibitors and angiotensin II antagonists. These interactions should be given consideration in patients taking NSAIDs concomitantly with ACE-inhibitors or angiotensin II antagonists. In some patients with compromised renal function, the co-administration of an NSAID and an ACE-inhibitor or an angiotensin II antagonist may result in further deterioration of renal function, including possible acute renal failure, which is usually reversible).

No products indexed under this heading.

Eprosartan Mesylate (Reports suggest that NSAIDs may diminish the antihypertensive effect of ACE-inhibitors and angiotensin II antagonists. These interactions should be given consideration in patients taking NSAIDs concomitantly with ACE-inhibitors or angiotensin II antagonists. In some patients with compromised renal function, the co-administration of an NSAID and an ACE-inhibitor or an angiotensin II antagonist may result in further deterioration of renal function, including possible acute renal failure, which is usually reversible). Products include:

Teveten Tablets 1735
Teveten HCT Tablets 1737

Ethacrynic Acid (Sulindac can reduce the natriuretic effect of furosemide and thiazides in some patients. This response has been attributed to inhibition of renal prostaglandin synthesis. During concomitant therapy with NSAIDs, the patient should be observed closely for signs of renal failure, as well as to assure diuretic efficacy). Products include:

Edecrin Tablets 1959

Etodolac (Concomitant use is not recommended due to the increased possibility of gastrointestinal toxicity, with little or no increase in efficacy).

No products indexed under this heading.

Fenoprofen Calcium (Concomitant use is not recommended due to the increased possibility of gastrointestinal toxicity, with little or no increase in efficacy). Products include:

Nalfon Capsules 2502

Flurbiprofen (Concomitant use is not recommended due to the increased possibility of gastrointestinal toxicity, with little or no increase in efficacy).

No products indexed under this heading.

Fosinopril Sodium (Reports suggest that NSAIDs may diminish the antihypertensive effect of ACE-inhibitors or angiotensin II antagonists. These interactions should be given consideration in patients taking NSAIDs concomitantly with ACE-inhibitors or angiotensin II antagonists. In some patients with compromised renal function, the co-administration of an NSAID and an

ACE-inhibitor or an angiotensin II antagonist may result in further deterioration of renal function, including possible acute renal failure, which is usually reversible).

No products indexed under this heading.

Furosemide (Clinoril may blunt the renal response to I.V. furosemide). Products include:

Furosemide Tablets 2154

Glimepiride (Special attention should be paid to patients taking higher doses than those recommended and to patients with renal or metabolic impairment). Products include:

Avandaryl Tablets 1379
Duetact Tablets 3226

Glipizide (Special attention should be paid to patients taking higher doses than those recommended and to patients with renal or metabolic impairment).

No products indexed under this heading.

Glyburide (Special attention should be paid to patients taking higher doses than those recommended and to patients with renal or metabolic impairment).

No products indexed under this heading.

Hydrochlorothiazide (Sulindac can reduce the natriuretic effect of furosemide and thiazides in some patients. This response has been attributed to inhibition of renal prostaglandin synthesis. During concomitant therapy with NSAIDs, the patient should be observed closely for signs of renal failure, as well as to assure diuretic efficacy). Products include:

Aldoril Tablets 1910
Atacand HCT 651
Avalide Tablets 888
Avalide Tablets 2874
Benicar HCT Tablets 1044
Diovan HCT Tablets 2196
Dyazide Capsules 1423
Hyzaar 50-12.5 Tablets 1990
Hyzaar 100-12.5 Tablets 1990
Hyzaar 100-25 Tablets 1990
Lopressor HCT 50/25 Tablets 2241
Lopressor HCT 100/25 Tablets 2241
Lopressor HCT 100/50 Tablets 2241
Lotensin HCT Tablets 2246
Micardis HCT Tablets 856
Moduretic Tablets 2028
Prinzide Tablets 2056
Teveten HCT Tablets 1737
Timolide Tablets 2086
Uniretic Tablets 3100

Hydroflumethiazide (Sulindac can reduce the natriuretic effect of furosemide and thiazides in some patients. This response has been attributed to inhibition of renal prostaglandin synthesis. During concomitant therapy with NSAIDs, the patient should be observed closely for signs of renal failure, as well as to assure diuretic efficacy).

No products indexed under this heading.

Ibuprofen (Concomitant use is not recommended due to the increased possibility of gastrointestinal toxicity, with little or no increase in efficacy). Products include:

Advil Allergy Sinus Caplets ⬛770
Advil .. ⬛674
Children's Advil Oral Suspension ⬛603
Children's Advil Chewable Tablets .. ⬛603
Advil Cold & Sinus ⬛723
Infants' Advil Concentrated Drops .. ⬛604
Infants' Advil Concentrated Drops
- White Grape (Dye-Free).............. ⬛604

Junior Strength Advil Swallow
Tablets ... ⬛605
Advil Migraine Liquigels ⬛608
Advil Multi-Symptom Cold
Caplets.. ⬛770
Advil PM Caplets............................. ⬛615
Motrin IB Tablets and Caplets 1866
Children's Motrin Oral Suspension ... 1867
Children's Motrin Non-Staining
Dye-Free Oral Suspension 1867
Children's Motrin Cold Oral
Suspension 1867
Infants' Motrin Concentrated
Drops.. 1867
Infants' Motrin Non-Staining
Dye-Free Concentrated Drops....... 1867
Junior Strength Motrin Caplets
and Chewable Tablets................... 1867
Vicoprofen Tablets 539

Indapamide (Sulindac can reduce the natriuretic effect of furosemide and thiazides in some patients. This response has been attributed to inhibition of renal prostaglandin synthesis. During concomitant therapy with NSAIDs, the patient should be observed closely for signs of renal failure, as well as to assure diuretic efficacy). Products include:

Indapamide Tablets 2156

Indomethacin (Concomitant use is not recommended due to the increased possibility of gastrointestinal toxicity, with little or no increase in efficacy). Products include:

Indocin .. 1995

Indomethacin Sodium Trihydrate (Concomitant use is not recommended due to the increased possibility of gastrointestinal toxicity, with little or no increase in efficacy). Products include:

Indocin I.V. 2465

Irbesartan (Reports suggest that NSAIDs may diminish the antihypertensive effect of ACE-inhibitors and angiotensin II antagonists. These interactions should be given consideration in patients taking NSAIDs concomitantly with ACE-inhibitors or angiotensin II antagonists. In some patients with compromised renal function, the co-administration of an NSAID and an ACE-inhibitor or an angiotensin II antagonist may result in further deterioration of renal function, including possible acute renal failure, which is usually reversible). Products include:

Avalide Tablets 888
Avalide Tablets 2874
Avapro Tablets 891
Avapro Tablets 2871

Ketoprofen (Concomitant use is not recommended due to the increased possibility of gastrointestinal toxicity, with little or no increase in efficacy).

No products indexed under this heading.

Ketorolac Tromethamine (Concomitant use is not recommended due to the increased possibility of gastrointestinal toxicity, with little or no increase in efficacy). Products include:

Acular Ophthalmic Solution 565
Acular LS Ophthalmic Solution 566

Lisinopril (Reports suggest that NSAIDs may diminish the antihypertensive effect of ACE-inhibitors and angiotensin II antagonists. These interactions should be given consideration in patients taking NSAIDs concomitantly with ACE-inhibitors or angiotensin II antagonists. In some patients with compromised renal function, the co-administration of an NSAID and an ACE-inhibitor or an angiotensin II antagonist may result

in further deterioration of renal function, including possible acute renal failure, which is usually reversible). Products include:
- Prinivil Tablets ... **2052**
- Prinzide Tablets ... **2056**

Lithium (NSAIDs have produced an elevation of plasma lithium levels and a reduction in renal lithium clearance. The mean minimum lithium concentration increased 15% and the renal clearance was decreased by approximately 20%. These effects have been attributed to inhibition of renal prostaglandin synthesis by the NSAID. Thus, when NSAIDs and lithium are administered concurrently, subject should be observed carefully for signs of lithium toxicity).
No products indexed under this heading.

Lithium Carbonate (NSAIDs have produced an elevation of plasma lithium levels and a reduction in renal lithium clearance. The mean minimum lithium concentration increased 15% and the renal clearance was decreased by approximately 20%. These effects have been attributed to inhibition of renal prostaglandin synthesis by the NSAID. Thus, when NSAIDs and lithium are administered concurrently, subject should be observed carefully for signs of lithium toxicity). Products include:
- Lithobid Tablets ... **1692**

Lithium Citrate (NSAIDs have produced an elevation of plasma lithium levels and a reduction in renal lithium clearance. The mean minimum lithium concentration increased 15% and the renal clearance was decreased by approximately 20%. These effects have been attributed to inhibition of renal prostaglandin synthesis by the NSAID. Thus, when NSAIDs and lithium are administered concurrently, subject should be observed carefully for signs of lithium toxicity).
No products indexed under this heading.

Losartan Potassium (Reports suggest that NSAIDs may diminish the antihypertensive effect of ACE-inhibitors and angiotensin II antagonists. These interactions should be given consideration in patients taking NSAIDs concomitantly with ACE-inhibitors or angiotensin II antagonists. In some patients with compromised renal function, the co-administration of an NSAID and an ACE-inhibitor or an angiotensin II antagonist may result in further deterioration of renal function, including possible acute renal failure, which is usually reversible). Products include:
- Cozaar Tablets ... **1935**
- Hyzaar 50-12.5 Tablets ... **1990**
- Hyzaar 100-12.5 Tablets ... **1990**
- Hyzaar 100-25 Tablets ... **1990**

Meclofenamate Sodium (Concomitant use is not recommended due to the increased possibility of gastrointestinal toxicity, with little or no increase in efficacy).
No products indexed under this heading.

Mefenamic Acid (Concomitant use is not recommended due to the increased possibility of gastrointestinal toxicity, with little or no increase in efficacy).
No products indexed under this heading.

Meloxicam (Concomitant use is not recommended due to the increased possibility of gastrointestinal toxicity, with little or no increase in efficacy). Products include:
- Mobic Oral Suspension ... **863**
- Mobic Tablets ... **863**

Metformin Hydrochloride (Special attention should be paid to patients taking higher doses than those recommended and to patients with renal or metabolic impairment). Products include:
- ActoPlus Met Tablets ... **3214**
- Avandamet Tablets ... **1373**
- Fortamet Extended-Release Tablets ... **3115**

Methotrexate Sodium (Decreased tubular secretion of methotrexate and potentiation of its toxicity).
No products indexed under this heading.

Methyclothiazide (Sulindac can reduce the natriuretic effect of furosemide and thiazides in some patients. This response has been attributed to inhibition of renal prostaglandin synthesis. During concomitant therapy with NSAIDs, the patient should be observed closely for signs of renal failure, as well as to assure diuretic efficacy).
No products indexed under this heading.

Metolazone (Sulindac can reduce the natriuretic effect of furosemide and thiazides in some patients. This response has been attributed to inhibition of renal prostaglandin synthesis. During concomitant therapy with NSAIDs, the patient should be observed closely for signs of renal failure, as well as to assure diuretic efficacy).
No products indexed under this heading.

Miglitol (Special attention should be paid to patients taking higher doses than those recommended and to patients with renal or metabolic impairment).
No products indexed under this heading.

Moexipril Hydrochloride (Reports suggest that NSAIDs may diminish the antihypertensive effect of ACE-inhibitors and angiotensin II antagonists. These interactions should be given consideration in patients taking NSAIDs concomitantly with ACE-inhibitors or angiotensin II antagonists. In some patients with compromised renal function, the co-administration of an NSAID and an ACE-inhibitor or an angiotensin II antagonist may result in further deterioration of renal function, including possible acute renal failure, which is usually reversible). Products include:
- Uniretic Tablets ... **3100**
- Univasc Tablets ... **3104**

Nabumetone (Concomitant use is not recommended due to the increased possibility of gastrointestinal toxicity, with little or no increase in efficacy).
No products indexed under this heading.

Naproxen (Concomitant use is not recommended due to the increased possibility of gastrointestinal toxicity, with little or no increase in efficacy). Products include:
- EC-Naprosyn Delayed-Release Tablets ... **2761**
- Naprosyn Suspension ... **2761**
- Naprosyn Tablets ... **2761**
- Prevacid NapraPAC ... **3280**

Naproxen Sodium (Concomitant use is not recommended due to the increased possibility of gastrointestinal toxicity, with little or no increase in efficacy). Products include:
- Aleve Caplets ... **742**
- Aleve Gelcaps ... **743**
- Aleve Tablets ... **743**
- Aleve Cold & Sinus Caplets ... **744**
- Anaprox Tablets ... **2761**
- Anaprox DS Tablets ... **2761**

Oxaprozin (Concomitant use is not recommended due to the increased possibility of gastrointestinal toxicity, with little or no increase in efficacy).
No products indexed under this heading.

Perindopril Erbumine (Reports suggest that NSAIDs may diminish the antihypertensive effect of ACE-inhibitors and angiotensin II antagonists. These interactions should be given consideration in patients taking NSAIDs concomitantly with ACE-inhibitors or angiotensin II antagonists. In some patients with compromised renal function, the co-administration of an NSAID and an ACE-inhibitor or an angiotensin II antagonist may result in further deterioration of renal function, including possible acute renal failure, which is usually reversible). Products include:
- Aceon Tablets (2 mg, 4 mg, 8 mg) ... **3194**

Phenylbutazone (Concomitant use is not recommended due to the increased possibility of gastrointestinal toxicity, with little or no increase in efficacy).
No products indexed under this heading.

Pioglitazone Hydrochloride (Special attention should be paid to patients taking higher doses than those recommended and to patients with renal or metabolic impairment). Products include:
- ActoPlus Met Tablets ... **3214**
- Actos Tablets ... **3219**
- Duetact Tablets ... **3226**

Piroxicam (Concomitant use is not recommended due to the increased possibility of gastrointestinal toxicity, with little or no increase in efficacy).
No products indexed under this heading.

Polythiazide (Sulindac can reduce the natriuretic effect of furosemide and thiazides in some patients. This response has been attributed to inhibition of renal prostaglandin synthesis. During concomitant therapy with NSAIDs, the patient should be observed closely for signs of renal failure, as well as to assure diuretic efficacy).
No products indexed under this heading.

Probenecid (Increased plasma levels of sulindac; modest reduction in uricosuric action of probenecid).
No products indexed under this heading.

Quinapril Hydrochloride (Reports suggest that NSAIDs may diminish the antihypertensive effect of ACE-inhibitors and angiotensin II antagonists. These interactions should be given consideration in patients taking NSAIDs concomitantly with ACE-inhibitors or angiotensin II antagonists. In some patients with compromised renal function, the co-administration of an NSAID and an ACE-inhibitor or an angiotensin II antagonist may result in further deterioration of renal function, including possible acute renal failure, which is usually reversible).
No products indexed under this heading.

Ramipril (Reports suggest that NSAIDs may diminish the antihypertensive effect of ACE-inhibitors and angiotensin II antagonists. These interactions should be given consideration in patients taking NSAIDs concomitantly with ACE-inhibitors or angiotensin II antagonists. In some patients with compromised renal function, the co-administration of an NSAID and an ACE-inhibitor or an angiotensin II antagonist may result in further deterioration of renal function, including possible acute renal failure, which is usually reversible). Products include:
- Altace Capsules ... **1702**

Repaglinide (Special attention should be paid to patients taking higher doses than those recommended and to patients with renal or metabolic impairment).
No products indexed under this heading.

Rofecoxib (Concomitant use is not recommended due to the increased possibility of gastrointestinal toxicity, with little or no increase in efficacy).
No products indexed under this heading.

Rosiglitazone Maleate (Special attention should be paid to patients taking higher doses than those recommended and to patients with renal or metabolic impairment). Products include:
- Avandamet Tablets ... **1373**
- Avandaryl Tablets ... **1379**
- Avandia Tablets ... **1384**

Spirapril Hydrochloride (Reports suggest that NSAIDs may diminish the antihypertensive effect of ACE-inhibitors and angiotensin II antagonists. These interactions should be given consideration in patients taking NSAIDs concomitantly with ACE-inhibitors or angiotensin II antagonists. In some patients with compromised renal function, the co-administration of an NSAID and an ACE-inhibitor or an angiotensin II antagonist may result in further deterioration of renal function, including possible acute renal failure, which is usually reversible).
No products indexed under this heading.

Spironolactone (Sulindac can reduce the natriuretic effect of furosemide and thiazides in some patients. This response has been attributed to inhibition of renal prostaglandin synthesis. During concomitant therapy with NSAIDs, the patient should be observed closely for signs of renal failure, as well as to assure diuretic efficacy).
No products indexed under this heading.

Telmisartan (Reports suggest that NSAIDs may diminish the antihypertensive effect of ACE-inhibitors and angiotensin II antagonists. These interactions should be given consideration in patients taking NSAIDs concomitantly with ACE-inhibitors or angiotensin II antagonists. In some patients with compromised renal function, the co-administration of an NSAID and an ACE-inhibitor or an angiotensin II antagonist may result in further deterioration of renal func-

tion, including possible acute renal failure, which is usually reversible). Products include:
Micardis Tablets 854
Micardis HCT Tablets 856
Tolazamide (Special attention should be paid to patients taking higher doses than those recommended and to patients with renal or metabolic impairment).
No products indexed under this heading.
Tolbutamide (Special attention should be paid to patients taking higher doses than those recommended and to patients with renal or metabolic impairment).
No products indexed under this heading.
Tolmetin Sodium (Concomitant use is not recommended due to the increased possibility of gastrointestinal toxicity, with little or no increase in efficacy).
No products indexed under this heading.
Torsemide (Sulindac can reduce the natriuretic effect of furosemide and thiazides in some patients. This response has been attributed to inhibition of renal prostaglandin synthesis. During concomitant therapy with NSAIDs, the patient should be observed closely for signs of renal failure, as well as to assure diuretic efficacy). Products include:
Demadex Injection 2759
Demadex Tablets 2759
Trandolapril (Reports suggest that NSAIDs may diminish the antihypertensive effect of ACE-inhibitors and angiotensin II antagonists. These interactions should be given consideration in patients taking NSAIDs concomitantly with ACE-inhibitors or angiotensin II antagonists. In some patients with compromised renal function, the co-administration of an NSAID and an ACE-inhibitor or an angiotensin II antagonist may result in further deterioration of renal function, including possible acute renal failure, which is usually reversible). Products include:
Mavik Tablets 486
Tarka Tablets 524
Triamterene (Sulindac can reduce the natriuretic effect of furosemide and thiazides in some patients. This response has been attributed to inhibition of renal prostaglandin synthesis. During concomitant therapy with NSAIDs, the patient should be observed closely for signs of renal failure, as well as to assure diuretic efficacy). Products include:
Dyazide Capsules 1423
Dyrenium Capsules 3400
Troglitazone (Special attention should be paid to patients taking higher doses than those recommended and to patients with renal or metabolic impairment).
No products indexed under this heading.
Valdecoxib (Concomitant use is not recommended due to the increased possibility of gastrointestinal toxicity, with little or no increase in efficacy).
No products indexed under this heading.
Valsartan (Reports suggest that NSAIDs may diminish the antihypertensive effect of ACE-inhibitors and angiotensin II antagonists. These interactions should be given consideration in patients taking NSAIDs concomitantly with ACE-inhibitors or angiotensin II antagonists. In some patients with compromised renal function, the co-administration of an NSAID and an ACE-inhibitor or an angiotensin II antagonist may result in further deterioration of renal function, including possible acute renal failure, which is usually reversible). Products include:
Diovan Tablets 2193
Diovan HCT Tablets 2196
Warfarin Sodium (Special attention should be paid to patients taking higher doses than those recommended and to patients with renal or metabolic impairment). Products include:
Coumadin for Injection 898
Coumadin Tablets 898

Food Interactions

Food, unspecified (The peak plasma concentrations of biologically active sulfide metabolite is delayed slightly in the presence of food).

CLOBEVATE GEL

(Clobetasol Propionate) 3211
None cited in PDR database.

CLOBEX LOTION

(Clobetasol Propionate) 1204
None cited in PDR database.

CLOBEX SHAMPOO

(Clobetasol Propionate) 1206
None cited in PDR database.

CLOBEX SPRAY

(Clobetasol Propionate) 1208
None cited in PDR database.

CLOLAR FOR INTRAVENOUS INFUSION

(Clofarabine) 1271
None cited in PDR database.

CLORPACTIN WCS-90

(Sodium Oxychlorosene) 1662
None cited in PDR database.

CLORPRES TABLETS

(Chlorthalidone, Clonidine Hydrochloride)................................... 2153
May interact with antihypertensives, barbiturates, beta blockers, cardiac glycosides, oral hypoglycemic agents, hypnotics and sedatives, insulin, lithium preparations, narcotic analgesics, tricyclic antidepressants, and certain other agents. Compounds in these categories include:
Acarbose (Chlorthalidone causes hyperglycemia; higher dosage of oral hypoglycemic agents may be required). Products include:
Precose Tablets 751
Acebutolol Hydrochloride (Chlorthalidone may add to or potentiate the action of other antihypertensives; if therapy is to be discontinued in patients receiving clonidine and beta blockers concurrently, beta blockers should be discontinued several days before the gradual withdrawal of clonidine).
No products indexed under this heading.
Alfentanil Hydrochloride (Orthostatic hypotension may be aggravated by narcotics; orthostatic hypotension may be aggravated by barbiturates).
No products indexed under this heading.
Amitriptyline Hydrochloride (Co-administration of clonidine with tricyclic antidepressants may result in reduced effect of clonidine, necessitating an increase in dosage; concurrent use enhances the manifestation of corneal lesions in rats).
No products indexed under this heading.
Amlodipine Besylate (Chlorthalidone may add to or potentiate the action of other antihypertensives). Products include:
Caduet Tablets 2508
Lotrel Capsules 2249
Norvasc Tablets 2545
Amoxapine (Co-administration of clonidine with tricyclic antidepressants may result in reduced effect of clonidine, necessitating an increase in dosage).
No products indexed under this heading.
Aprobarbital (Clonidine may enhance the CNS-depressive effects of barbiturates; orthostatic hypotension may be aggravated by barbiturates).
No products indexed under this heading.
Atenolol (Chlorthalidone may add to or potentiate the action of other antihypertensives; if therapy is to be discontinued in patients receiving clonidine and beta blockers concurrently, beta blockers should be discontinued several days before the gradual withdrawal of clonidine).
No products indexed under this heading.
Benazepril Hydrochloride (Chlorthalidone may add to or potentiate the action of other antihypertensives). Products include:
Lotensin Tablets 2243
Lotensin HCT Tablets 2246
Lotrel Capsules 2249
Bendroflumethiazide (Chlorthalidone may add to or potentiate the action of other antihypertensives).
No products indexed under this heading.
Betaxolol Hydrochloride (Chlorthalidone may add to or potentiate the action of other antihypertensives; if therapy is to be discontinued in patients receiving clonidine and beta blockers concurrently, beta blockers should be discontinued several days before the gradual withdrawal of clonidine). Products include:
Betoptic S Ophthalmic Suspension.................................... 558
Bisoprolol Fumarate (Chlorthalidone may add to or potentiate the action of other antihypertensives; if therapy is to be discontinued in patients receiving clonidine and beta blockers concurrently, beta blockers should be discontinued several days before the gradual withdrawal of clonidine).
No products indexed under this heading.
Buprenorphine Hydrochloride (Orthostatic hypotension may be aggravated by narcotics; orthostatic hypotension may be aggravated by barbiturates). Products include:
Buprenex Injectable 2716
Suboxone Tablets 2717
Subutex Tablets 2717
Butabarbital (Clonidine may enhance the CNS-depressive effects of barbiturates; orthostatic hypotension may be aggravated by barbiturates).
No products indexed under this heading.
Butalbital (Clonidine may enhance the CNS-depressive effects of barbiturates; orthostatic hypotension may be aggravated by barbiturates).
No products indexed under this heading.
Candesartan Cilexetil (Chlorthalidone may add to or potentiate the action of other antihypertensives). Products include:
Atacand Tablets 649
Atacand HCT 651
Captopril (Chlorthalidone may add to or potentiate the action of other antihypertensives). Products include:
Captopril Tablets 2149
Carteolol Hydrochloride (Chlorthalidone may add to or potentiate the action of other antihypertensives; if therapy is to be discontinued in patients receiving clonidine and beta blockers concurrently, beta blockers should be discontinued several days before the gradual withdrawal of clonidine). Products include:
Carteolol Hydrochloride Ophthalmic Solution USP, 1%....... ⊙249
Chlorothiazide (Chlorthalidone may add to or potentiate the action of other antihypertensives). Products include:
Diuril Oral Suspension 1954
Chlorothiazide Sodium (Chlorthalidone may add to or potentiate the action of other antihypertensives). Products include:
Diuril Sodium Intravenous 2467
Chlorpropamide (Chlorthalidone causes hyperglycemia; higher dosage of oral hypoglycemic agents may be required).
No products indexed under this heading.
Clomipramine Hydrochloride (Co-administration of clonidine with tricyclic antidepressants may result in reduced effect of clonidine, necessitating an increase in dosage).
No products indexed under this heading.
Clonidine (Chlorthalidone may add to or potentiate the action of other antihypertensives). Products include:
Catapres-TTS 844
Codeine Phosphate (Orthostatic hypotension may be aggravated by narcotics; orthostatic hypotension may be aggravated by barbiturates). Products include:
Tylenol with Codeine Tablets 2391
Deserpidine (Chlorthalidone may add to or potentiate the action of other antihypertensives).
No products indexed under this heading.
Desipramine Hydrochloride (Co-administration of clonidine with tricyclic antidepressants may result in reduced effect of clonidine, necessitating an increase in dosage).
No products indexed under this heading.
Deslanoside (Digitalis therapy may exaggerate the metabolic effects of hypokalemia especially with reference to myocardial activity).
No products indexed under this heading.

Dezocine (Orthostatic hypotension may be aggravated by narcotics; orthostatic hypotension may be aggravated by barbiturates).
No products indexed under this heading.

Diazoxide (Chlorthalidone may add to or potentiate the action of other antihypertensives). Products include:
Hyperstat I.V. ... 3017

Digitalis Glycoside Preparations (Digitalis therapy may exaggerate the metabolic effects of hypokalemia especially with reference to myocardial activity).
No products indexed under this heading.

Digitoxin (Digitalis therapy may exaggerate the metabolic effects of hypokalemia especially with reference to myocardial activity).
No products indexed under this heading.

Digoxin (Digitalis therapy may exaggerate the metabolic effects of hypokalemia especially with reference to myocardial activity). Products include:
Lanoxicaps Capsules ... 1490
Lanoxin Injection ... 1494
Lanoxin Injection Pediatric ... 1497
Lanoxin Tablets ... 1500

Diltiazem Hydrochloride (Chlorthalidone may add to or potentiate the action of other antihypertensives). Products include:
Cardizem LA Extended Release Tablets ... 1728
Tiazac Capsules ... 1201

Doxazosin Mesylate (Chlorthalidone may add to or potentiate the action of other antihypertensives). Products include:
Cardura XL Tablets ... 2515

Doxepin Hydrochloride (Co-administration of clonidine with tricyclic antidepressants may result in reduced effect of clonidine, necessitating an increase in dosage).
No products indexed under this heading.

Enalapril Maleate (Chlorthalidone may add to or potentiate the action of other antihypertensives). Products include:
Vasotec I.V. Injection ... 2103

Enalaprilat (Chlorthalidone may add to or potentiate the action of other antihypertensives).
No products indexed under this heading.

Eprosartan Mesylate (Chlorthalidone may add to or potentiate the action of other antihypertensives). Products include:
Teveten Tablets ... 1735
Teveten HCT Tablets ... 1737

Esmolol Hydrochloride (Chlorthalidone may add to or potentiate the action of other antihypertensives; if therapy is to be discontinued in patients receiving clonidine and beta blockers concurrently, beta blockers should be discontinued several days before the gradual withdrawal of clonidine).
No products indexed under this heading.

Estazolam (Clonidine may enhance the CNS-depressive effects of other sedatives). Products include:
ProSom Tablets ... 517

Ethchlorvynol (Clonidine may enhance the CNS-depressive effects of other sedatives).
No products indexed under this heading.

Ethinamate (Clonidine may enhance the CNS-depressive effects of other sedatives).
No products indexed under this heading.

Felodipine (Chlorthalidone may add to or potentiate the action of other antihypertensives).
No products indexed under this heading.

Fentanyl (Orthostatic hypotension may be aggravated by narcotics; orthostatic hypotension may be aggravated by barbiturates). Products include:
Duragesic Transdermal System ... 2373
Ionsys Transdermal System ... 2379

Fentanyl Citrate (Orthostatic hypotension may be aggravated by narcotics; orthostatic hypotension may be aggravated by barbiturates). Products include:
Actiq ... 979

Flurazepam Hydrochloride (Clonidine may enhance the CNS-depressive effects of other sedatives). Products include:
Dalmane Capsules ... 3342

Fosinopril Sodium (Chlorthalidone may add to or potentiate the action of other antihypertensives).
No products indexed under this heading.

Furosemide (Chlorthalidone may add to or potentiate the action of other antihypertensives). Products include:
Furosemide Tablets ... 2154

Glimepiride (Chlorthalidone causes hyperglycemia; higher dosage of oral hypoglycemic agents may be required). Products include:
Avandaryl Tablets ... 1379
Duetact Tablets ... 3226

Glipizide (Chlorthalidone causes hyperglycemia; higher dosage of oral hypoglycemic agents may be required).
No products indexed under this heading.

Glutethimide (Clonidine may enhance the CNS-depressive effects of other sedatives).
No products indexed under this heading.

Glyburide (Chlorthalidone causes hyperglycemia; higher dosage of oral hypoglycemic agents may be required).
No products indexed under this heading.

Guanabenz Acetate (Chlorthalidone may add to or potentiate the action of other antihypertensives).
No products indexed under this heading.

Guanethidine Monosulfate (Chlorthalidone may add to or potentiate the action of other antihypertensives).
No products indexed under this heading.

Hydralazine Hydrochloride (Chlorthalidone may add to or potentiate the action of other antihypertensives). Products include:
BiDil Tablets ... 2171

Hydrochlorothiazide (Chlorthalidone may add to or potentiate the action of other antihypertensives). Products include:
Aldoril Tablets ... 1910
Atacand HCT ... 651
Avalide Tablets ... 888
Avalide Tablets ... 2874
Benicar HCT Tablets ... 1044
Diovan HCT Tablets ... 2196
Dyazide Capsules ... 1423
Hyzaar 50-12.5 Tablets ... 1990
Hyzaar 100-12.5 Tablets ... 1990
Hyzaar 100-25 Tablets ... 1990
Lopressor HCT 50/25 Tablets ... 2241
Lopressor HCT 100/25 Tablets ... 2241
Lopressor HCT 100/50 Tablets ... 2241
Lotensin HCT Tablets ... 2246
Micardis HCT Tablets ... 856
Moduretic Tablets ... 2028
Prinzide Tablets ... 2056
Teveten HCT Tablets ... 1737
Timolide Tablets ... 2086
Uniretic Tablets ... 3100

Hydrocodone Bitartrate (Orthostatic hypotension may be aggravated by narcotics; orthostatic hypotension may be aggravated by barbiturates). Products include:
Hycodan ... 1116
Hycotuss Expectorant Syrup ... 1117
Vicodin Tablets ... 535
Vicodin ES Tablets ... 536
Vicodin HP Tablets ... 538
Vicoprofen Tablets ... 539
Zydone Tablets ... 1139

Hydrocodone Polistirex (Orthostatic hypotension may be aggravated by narcotics; orthostatic hypotension may be aggravated by barbiturates). Products include:
Tussionex Pennkinetic Extended-Release Suspension ... 3327

Hydroflumethiazide (Chlorthalidone may add to or potentiate the action of other antihypertensives).
No products indexed under this heading.

Hydromorphone Hydrochloride (Orthostatic hypotension may be aggravated by narcotics; orthostatic hypotension may be aggravated by barbiturates). Products include:
Dilaudid ... 440
Dilaudid Non-Sterile Powder ... 440
Dilaudid Oral Liquid ... 445
Dilaudid Rectal Suppositories ... 440
Dilaudid Tablets ... 440
Dilaudid Tablets - 8 mg ... 445
Dilaudid-HP ... 442

Imipramine Hydrochloride (Co-administration of clonidine with tricyclic antidepressants may result in reduced effect of clonidine, necessitating an increase in dosage).
No products indexed under this heading.

Imipramine Pamoate (Co-administration of clonidine with tricyclic antidepressants may result in reduced effect of clonidine, necessitating an increase in dosage).
No products indexed under this heading.

Indapamide (Chlorthalidone may add to or potentiate the action of other antihypertensives). Products include:
Indapamide Tablets ... 2156

Insulin, Human, Zinc Suspension (Chlorthalidone causes hyperglycemia; insulin requirements may be increased, decreased, or unchanged). Products include:
Humulin L, 100 Units ... 1794
Humulin U, 100 Units ... 1800

Insulin, Human NPH (Chlorthalidone causes hyperglycemia; insulin requirements may be increased, decreased, or unchanged). Products include:
Humulin N, 100 Units ... 1795
Humulin N Pen ... 1797

Insulin, Human Regular (Chlorthalidone causes hyperglycemia; insulin requirements may be increased, decreased, or unchanged). Products include:
Humulin R, 100 Units ... 1798

Insulin, Human Regular and Human NPH Mixture (Chlorthalidone causes hyperglycemia; insulin requirements may be increased, decreased, or unchanged). Products include:
Humulin 50/50, 100 Units ... 1791
Humulin 70/30 Pen ... 1793

Insulin, NPH (Chlorthalidone causes hyperglycemia; insulin requirements may be increased, decreased, or unchanged).
No products indexed under this heading.

Insulin, Regular (Chlorthalidone causes hyperglycemia; insulin requirements may be increased, decreased, or unchanged).
No products indexed under this heading.

Insulin, Zinc Crystals (Chlorthalidone causes hyperglycemia; insulin requirements may be increased, decreased, or unchanged).
No products indexed under this heading.

Insulin, Zinc Suspension (Chlorthalidone causes hyperglycemia; insulin requirements may be increased, decreased, or unchanged).
No products indexed under this heading.

Insulin Aspart, Human Regular (Chlorthalidone causes hyperglycemia; insulin requirements may be increased, decreased, or unchanged). Products include:
NovoLog Injection ... 2326

Insulin glargine (Chlorthalidone causes hyperglycemia; insulin requirements may be increased, decreased, or unchanged). Products include:
Lantus Injection ... 2909

Insulin Lispro, Human (Chlorthalidone causes hyperglycemia; insulin requirements may be increased, decreased, or unchanged). Products include:
Humalog-Pen ... 1781
Humalog Mix 50/50-Pen ... 1783
Humalog Mix 75/25-Pen ... 1785

Insulin Lispro Protamine, Human (Chlorthalidone causes hyperglycemia; insulin requirements may be increased, decreased, or unchanged). Products include:
Humalog Mix 50/50-Pen ... 1783
Humalog Mix 75/25-Pen ... 1785

Irbesartan (Chlorthalidone may add to or potentiate the action of other antihypertensives). Products include:
Avalide Tablets ... 888
Avalide Tablets ... 2874
Avapro Tablets ... 891
Avapro Tablets ... 2871

Isradipine (Chlorthalidone may add to or potentiate the action of other antihypertensives). Products include:
DynaCirc CR Tablets ... 2721

Labetalol Hydrochloride (Chlorthalidone may add to or potentiate the action of other antihypertensives; if therapy is to be discontinued in patients receiving clonidine and beta blockers concurrently, beta blockers should be discontinued several days before the gradual withdrawal of clonidine).
No products indexed under this heading.

Levobunolol Hydrochloride (Chlorthalidone may add to or potentiate the action of other antihypertensives; if therapy is to be discontinued in patients receiving clonidine and beta blockers concurrently, beta blockers should be discontinued several days before the gradual withdrawal of clonidine). Products include:

Betagan Ophthalmic Solution, USP.............................⊙220

Levorphanol Tartrate (Orthostatic hypotension may be aggravated by narcotics; orthostatic hypotension may be aggravated by barbiturates).

No products indexed under this heading.

Lisinopril (Chlorthalidone may add to or potentiate the action of other antihypertensives). Products include:

Prinivil Tablets2052
Prinzide Tablets2056

Lithium (Chlorthalidone reduces renal clearance of lithium, increasing the risk of lithium toxicity).

No products indexed under this heading.

Lithium Carbonate (Chlorthalidone reduces renal clearance of lithium, increasing the risk of lithium toxicity). Products include:

Lithobid Tablets1692

Lithium Citrate (Chlorthalidone reduces renal clearance of lithium, increasing the risk of lithium toxicity).

No products indexed under this heading.

Lorazepam (Clonidine may enhance the CNS-depressive effects of other sedatives).

No products indexed under this heading.

Losartan Potassium (Chlorthalidone may add to or potentiate the action of other antihypertensives). Products include:

Cozaar Tablets1935
Hyzaar 50-12.5 Tablets1990
Hyzaar 100-12.5 Tablets1990
Hyzaar 100-25 Tablets1990

Maprotiline Hydrochloride (Coadministration of clonidine with tricyclic antidepressants may result in reduced effect of clonidine, necessitating an increase in dosage).

No products indexed under this heading.

Mecamylamine Hydrochloride (Chlorthalidone may add to or potentiate the action of other antihypertensives).

No products indexed under this heading.

Meperidine Hydrochloride (Orthostatic hypotension may be aggravated by narcotics; orthostatic hypotension may be aggravated by barbiturates).

No products indexed under this heading.

Mephobarbital (Clonidine may enhance the CNS-depressive effects of barbiturates; orthostatic hypotension may be aggravated by barbiturates).

No products indexed under this heading.

Metformin Hydrochloride (Chlorthalidone causes hyperglycemia; higher dosage of oral hypoglycemic agents may be required) Products include:

ActoPlus Met Tablets3214
Avandamet Tablets1373
Fortamet Extended-Release Tablets...................................3115

Methadone Hydrochloride (Orthostatic hypotension may be aggravated by narcotics; orthostatic hypotension may be aggravated by barbiturates).

No products indexed under this heading.

Methyclothiazide (Chlorthalidone may add to or potentiate the action of other antihypertensives).

No products indexed under this heading.

Methyldopa (Chlorthalidone may add to or potentiate the action of other antihypertensives). Products include:

Aldoril Tablets1910

Methyldopate Hydrochloride (Chlorthalidone may add to or potentiate the action of other antihypertensives).

No products indexed under this heading.

Metipranolol Hydrochloride (Chlorthalidone may add to or potentiate the action of other antihypertensives; if therapy is to be discontinued in patients receiving clonidine and beta blockers concurrently, beta blockers should be discontinued several days before the gradual withdrawal of clonidine).

No products indexed under this heading.

Metolazone (Chlorthalidone may add to or potentiate the action of other antihypertensives).

No products indexed under this heading.

Metoprolol Succinate (Chlorthalidone may add to or potentiate the action of other antihypertensives; if therapy is to be discontinued in patients receiving clonidine and beta blockers concurrently, beta blockers should be discontinued several days before the gradual withdrawal of clonidine). Products include:

Toprol-XL Tablets668

Metoprolol Tartrate (Chlorthalidone may add to or potentiate the action of other antihypertensives; if therapy is to be discontinued in patients receiving clonidine and beta blockers concurrently, beta blockers should be discontinued several days before the gradual withdrawal of clonidine). Products include:

Lopressor Injection2238
Lopressor Tablets2238
Lopressor HCT 50/25 Tablets2241
Lopressor HCT 100/25 Tablets2241
Lopressor HCT 100/50 Tablets2241

Metyrosine (Chlorthalidone may add to or potentiate the action of other antihypertensives). Products include:

Demser Capsules1953

Mibefradil Dihydrochloride (Chlorthalidone may add to or potentiate the action of other antihypertensives).

No products indexed under this heading.

Midazolam Hydrochloride (Clonidine may enhance the CNS-depressive effects of other sedatives).

No products indexed under this heading.

Miglitol (Chlorthalidone causes hyperglycemia; higher dosage of oral hypoglycemic agents may be required).

No products indexed under this heading.

Minoxidil (Chlorthalidone may add to or potentiate the action of other antihypertensives). Products include:

Men's Rogaine Extra Strength Hair Regrowth Treatment Topical Solution, Ocean Rush Scent and Original Unscented..... ▣◻633
Men's Rogaine Foam Hair Regrowth Treatment....................▣◻633
Women's Rogaine Hair Regrowth Treatment Topical Solution, Spring Bloom Scent and Original Unscented.....................▣◻634

Moexipril Hydrochloride (Chlorthalidone may add to or potentiate the action of other antihypertensives). Products include:

Uniretic Tablets3100
Univasc Tablets3104

Morphine Sulfate (Orthostatic hypotension may be aggravated by narcotics; orthostatic hypotension may be aggravated by barbiturates). Products include:

Avinza Capsules1741
Kadian Capsules577
MS Contin Tablets2701

Nadolol (Chlorthalidone may add to or potentiate the action of other antihypertensives; if therapy is to be discontinued in patients receiving clonidine and beta blockers concurrently, beta blockers should be discontinued several days before the gradual withdrawal of clonidine). Products include:

Nadolol Tablets2159

Nicardipine Hydrochloride (Chlorthalidone may add to or potentiate the action of other antihypertensives). Products include:

Cardene I.V.2497

Nifedipine (Chlorthalidone may add to or potentiate the action of other antihypertensives). Products include:

Adalat CC Tablets2964

Nisoldipine (Chlorthalidone may add to or potentiate the action of other antihypertensives). Products include:

Sular Tablets3122

Nitroglycerin (Chlorthalidone may add to or potentiate the action of other antihypertensives). Products include:

Nitro-Dur Transdermal Infusion System.......................................3046
Nitrolingual Pumpspray3120

Norepinephrine Bitartrate (Chlorthalidone may decrease arterial responsiveness to norepinephrine).

No products indexed under this heading.

Nortriptyline Hydrochloride (Coadministration of clonidine with tricyclic antidepressants may result in reduced effect of clonidine, necessitating an increase in dosage).

No products indexed under this heading.

Oxycodone Hydrochloride (Orthostatic hypotension may be aggravated by narcotics; orthostatic hypotension may be aggravated by barbiturates). Products include:

OxyContin Tablets2703
OxyFast Oral Concentrate Solution.......................................2708
OxyIR Capsules2708
Percocet Tablets1131
Percodan Tablets1132

Penbutolol Sulfate (Chlorthalidone may add to or potentiate the action of other antihypertensives; if therapy is to be discontinued in patients receiving clonidine and beta blockers concurrently, beta blockers should be discontinued several days before the gradual withdrawal of clonidine).

No products indexed under this heading.

Pentobarbital Sodium (Clonidine may enhance the CNS-depressive effects of barbiturates; orthostatic hypotension may be aggravated by barbiturates). Products include:

Nembutal Sodium Solution, USP 2470

Perindopril Erbumine (Chlorthalidone may add to or potentiate the action of other antihypertensives). Products include:

Aceon Tablets (2 mg, 4 mg, 8 mg)....................................3194

Phenobarbital (Clonidine may enhance the CNS-depressive effects of barbiturates; orthostatic hypotension may be aggravated by barbiturates). Products include:

Donnatal Extentabs2493

Phenoxybenzamine Hydrochloride (Chlorthalidone may add to or potentiate the action of other antihypertensives). Products include:

Dibenzyline Capsules3399

Phentolamine Mesylate (Chlorthalidone may add to or potentiate the action of other antihypertensives).

No products indexed under this heading.

Pindolol (Chlorthalidone may add to or potentiate the action of other antihypertensives; if therapy is to be discontinued in patients receiving clonidine and beta blockers concurrently, beta blockers should be discontinued several days before the gradual withdrawal of clonidine).

No products indexed under this heading.

Pioglitazone Hydrochloride (Chlorthalidone causes hyperglycemia; higher dosage of oral hypoglycemic agents may be required). Products include:

ActoPlus Met Tablets3214
Actos Tablets3219
Duetact Tablets3226

Polythiazide (Chlorthalidone may add to or potentiate the action of other antihypertensives).

No products indexed under this heading.

Prazosin Hydrochloride (Chlorthalidone may add to or potentiate the action of other antihypertensives).

No products indexed under this heading.

Propofol (Clonidine may enhance the CNS-depressive effects of other sedatives).

No products indexed under this heading.

Propoxyphene Hydrochloride (Orthostatic hypotension may be aggravated by narcotics; orthostatic hypotension may be aggravated by barbiturates).

No products indexed under this heading.

(▣◻ Described in PDR For Nonprescription Drugs) (⊙ Described in PDR For Ophthalmic Medicines™)

Propoxyphene Napsylate (Orthostatic hypotension may be aggravated by narcotics; orthostatic hypotension may be aggravated by barbiturates).
No products indexed under this heading.

Propranolol Hydrochloride (Chlorthalidone may add to or potentiate the action of other antihypertensives; if therapy is to be discontinued in patients receiving clonidine and beta blockers concurrently, beta blockers should be discontinued several days before the gradual withdrawal of clonidine). Products include:
Inderal LA Long-Acting Capsules 3429
InnoPran XL Capsules 2723

Protriptyline Hydrochloride (Coadministration of clonidine with tricyclic antidepressants may result in reduced effect of clonidine, necessitating an increase in dosage).
No products indexed under this heading.

Quazepam (Clonidine may enhance the CNS-depressive effects of other sedatives).
No products indexed under this heading.

Quinapril Hydrochloride (Chlorthalidone may add to or potentiate the action of other antihypertensives).
No products indexed under this heading.

Ramelteon (Clonidine may enhance the CNS-depressive effects of other sedatives). Products include:
Rozerem Tablets 3231

Ramipril (Chlorthalidone may add to or potentiate the action of other antihypertensives). Products include:
Altace Capsules 1702

Rauwolfia Serpentina (Chlorthalidone may add to or potentiate the action of other antihypertensives).
No products indexed under this heading.

Remifentanil Hydrochloride (Orthostatic hypotension may be aggravated by narcotics; orthostatic hypotension may be aggravated by barbiturates).
No products indexed under this heading.

Repaglinide (Chlorthalidone causes hyperglycemia; higher dosage of oral hypoglycemic agents may be required).
No products indexed under this heading.

Rescinnamine (Chlorthalidone may add to or potentiate the action of other antihypertensives).
No products indexed under this heading.

Reserpine (Chlorthalidone may add to or potentiate the action of other antihypertensives).
No products indexed under this heading.

Rosiglitazone Maleate (Chlorthalidone causes hyperglycemia; higher dosage of oral hypoglycemic agents may be required). Products include:
Avandamet Tablets 1373
Avandaryl Tablets 1379
Avandia Tablets 1384

Secobarbital Sodium (Clonidine may enhance the CNS-depressive effects of barbiturates; orthostatic hypotension may be aggravated by barbiturates).
No products indexed under this heading.

Sodium Nitroprusside (Chlorthalidone may add to or potentiate the action of other antihypertensives).
No products indexed under this heading.

Sotalol Hydrochloride (Chlorthalidone may add to or potentiate the action of other antihypertensives; if therapy is to be discontinued in patients receiving clonidine and beta blockers concurrently, beta blockers should be discontinued several days before the gradual withdrawal of clonidine).
No products indexed under this heading.

Spirapril Hydrochloride (Chlorthalidone may add to or potentiate the action of other antihypertensives).
No products indexed under this heading.

Sufentanil Citrate (Orthostatic hypotension may be aggravated by narcotics; orthostatic hypotension may be aggravated by barbiturates).
No products indexed under this heading.

Telmisartan (Chlorthalidone may add to or potentiate the action of other antihypertensives). Products include:
Micardis Tablets 854
Micardis HCT Tablets 856

Temazepam (Clonidine may enhance the CNS-depressive effects of other sedatives). Products include:
Restoril Capsules 1860

Terazosin Hydrochloride (Chlorthalidone may add to or potentiate the action of other antihypertensives). Products include:
Hytrin Capsules 471

Thiamylal Sodium (Clonidine may enhance the CNS-depressive effects of barbiturates; orthostatic hypotension may be aggravated by barbiturates).
No products indexed under this heading.

Timolol Hemihydrate (Chlorthalidone may add to or potentiate the action of other antihypertensives; if therapy is to be discontinued in patients receiving clonidine and beta blockers concurrently, beta blockers should be discontinued several days before the gradual withdrawal of clonidine). Products include:
Betimol Ophthalmic Solution 3382
Betimol Ophthalmic Solution .... ⊙295

Timolol Maleate (Chlorthalidone may add to or potentiate the action of other antihypertensives; if therapy is to be discontinued in patients receiving clonidine and beta blockers concurrently, beta blockers should be discontinued several days before the gradual withdrawal of clonidine). Products include:
Blocadren Tablets 1916
Cosopt Sterile Ophthalmic Solution 1931
Timolide Tablets 2086
Timoptic Sterile Ophthalmic Solution 2088
Timoptic in Ocudose 2091
Timoptic-XE Sterile Ophthalmic Gel Forming Solution 2092

Tolazamide (Chlorthalidone causes hyperglycemia; higher dosage of oral hypoglycemic agents may be required).
No products indexed under this heading.

Tolbutamide (Chlorthalidone causes hyperglycemia; higher dosage of oral hypoglycemic agents may be required).
No products indexed under this heading.

Torsemide (Chlorthalidone may add to or potentiate the action of other antihypertensives). Products include:
Demadex Injection 2759
Demadex Tablets 2759

Trandolapril (Chlorthalidone may add to or potentiate the action of other antihypertensives). Products include:
Mavik Tablets 486
Tarka Tablets 524

Triazolam (Clonidine may enhance the CNS-depressive effects of other sedatives).
No products indexed under this heading.

Trimethaphan Camsylate (Chlorthalidone may add to or potentiate the action of other antihypertensives).
No products indexed under this heading.

Trimipramine Maleate (Coadministration of clonidine with tricyclic antidepressants may result in reduced effect of clonidine, necessitating an increase in dosage).
No products indexed under this heading.

Troglitazone (Chlorthalidone causes hyperglycemia; higher dosage of oral hypoglycemic agents may be required).
No products indexed under this heading.

Tubocurarine Chloride (Chlorthalidone may increase responsiveness to tubocurarine).
No products indexed under this heading.

Valsartan (Chlorthalidone may add to or potentiate the action of other antihypertensives). Products include:
Diovan Tablets 2193
Diovan HCT Tablets 2196

Verapamil Hydrochloride (Chlorthalidone may add to or potentiate the action of other antihypertensives). Products include:
Covera-HS Tablets 3139
Tarka Tablets 524
Verelan PM Extended-Release Capsules, Controlled-Onset.......... 3106

Zaleplon (Clonidine may enhance the CNS-depressive effects of other sedatives). Products include:
Sonata Capsules 1717

Zolpidem Tartrate (Clonidine may enhance the CNS-depressive effects of other sedatives). Products include:
Ambien Tablets 2851
Ambien CR Tablets 2855

Food Interactions

Alcohol (Clonidine may enhance the CNS-depressive effects of alcohol; orthostatic hypotension may be aggravated by alcohol).

CLOZARIL TABLETS

(Clozapine) 2184
May interact with anticholinergics, antihypertensives, benzodiazepines, central nervous system depressants, antidepressant drugs, erythromycin, general anesthetics, phenothiazines, phenytoin, psychotropics, quinidine, and certain other agents. Compounds in these categories include:

Acebutolol Hydrochloride (Clozapine may potentiate the hypotensive effects of antihypertensive drugs).
No products indexed under this heading.

Alfentanil Hydrochloride (Given the primary CNS effect of clozapine, caution is advised in using it concomitantly with CNS-active drugs).
No products indexed under this heading.

Alprazolam (Co-administration with benzodiazepines or other psychotropic agents may be accompanied by orthostatic hypotension leading to profound collapse and respiratory and/or cardiac arrest; caution is advised if used concurrently). Products include:
Niravam Orally Disintegrating Tablets 3092

Amitriptyline Hydrochloride (Concomitant use of clozapine with other drugs metabolized by CYP4502D6 may require lower than usual doses for either drug).
No products indexed under this heading.

Amlodipine Besylate (Clozapine may potentiate the hypotensive effects of antihypertensive drugs). Products include:
Caduet Tablets 2508
Lotrel Capsules 2249
Norvasc Tablets 2545

Amoxapine (Concomitant use of clozapine with other drugs metabolized by CYP4502D6 may require lower than usual doses for either drug).
No products indexed under this heading.

Aprobarbital (Given the primary CNS effect of clozapine, caution is advised in using it concomitantly with CNS-active drugs).
No products indexed under this heading.

Atenolol (Clozapine may potentiate the hypotensive effects of antihypertensive drugs).
No products indexed under this heading.

Atropine Sulfate (Clozapine may potentiate anticholinergic effects). Products include:
Donnatal Extentabs 2493

Belladonna Alkaloids (Clozapine may potentiate anticholinergic effects). Products include:
Hyland's Teething Tablets .... ▣830

Benazepril Hydrochloride (Clozapine may potentiate the hypotensive effects of antihypertensive drugs). Products include:
Lotensin Tablets 2243
Lotensin HCT Tablets 2246
Lotrel Capsules 2249

Bendroflumethiazide (Clozapine may potentiate the hypotensive effects of antihypertensive drugs).
No products indexed under this heading.

IMPORTANT NOTE: Always consult each drug listing in the patient's regimen for possible interactions.

Benztropine Mesylate (Clozapine may potentiate anticholinergic effects).
No products indexed under this heading.

Betaxolol Hydrochloride (Clozapine may potentiate the hypotensive effects of antihypertensive drugs). Products include:
Betoptic S Ophthalmic Suspension 558

Biperiden Hydrochloride (Clozapine may potentiate anticholinergic effects).
No products indexed under this heading.

Bisoprolol Fumarate (Clozapine may potentiate the hypotensive effects of antihypertensive drugs).
No products indexed under this heading.

Bone Marrow Depressants, unspecified (Clozapine should not be used with agents having a well-known potential to suppress bone-marrow function. Co-administration may increase the risk and/or severity of bone marrow suppression).
No products indexed under this heading.

Buprenorphine Hydrochloride (Given the primary CNS effect of clozapine, caution is advised in using it concomitantly with CNS-active drugs). Products include:
Buprenex Injectable 2716
Suboxone Tablets 2717
Subutex Tablets 2717

Bupropion Hydrochloride (Concomitant use of clozapine with other drugs metabolized by CYP4502D6 may require lower than usual doses for either drug). Products include:
Wellbutrin Tablets 1603
Wellbutrin SR Sustained-Release Tablets 1607
Wellbutrin XL Extended-Release Tablets 1613
Zyban Sustained-Release Tablets 1644

Buspirone Hydrochloride (Co-administration with benzodiazepines or other psychotropic agents may be accompanied by orthostatic hypotension leading to profound collapse and respiratory and/or cardiac arrest; caution is advised if used concurrently).
No products indexed under this heading.

Butabarbital (Given the primary CNS effect of clozapine, caution is advised in using it concomitantly with CNS-active drugs).
No products indexed under this heading.

Butalbital (Given the primary CNS effect of clozapine, caution is advised in using it concomitantly with CNS-active drugs).
No products indexed under this heading.

Caffeine (May increase plasma levels of clozapine, potentially resulting in adverse effects). Products include:
BC Headache Powder .... ◘677
Arthritis Strength BC Powder .... ◘677
Excedrin Extra Strength Caplets/Tablets/Geltabs .... ◘684
Excedrin Migraine Caplets/Tablets/Geltabs .... ◘609
Excedrin Tension Headache Caplets/Tablets/Geltabs .... ◘611
Goody's Extra Strength Headache Powders .... ◘611
Goody's Extra Strength Pain Relief Tablets .... ◘685
Vivarin .... ◘602
Winrgy Dietary Supplement .... ◘823

Caffeine Citrate (May increase plasma levels of clozapine, potentially resulting in adverse effects). Products include:
Cafcit 1886

Candesartan Cilexetil (Clozapine may potentiate the hypotensive effects of antihypertensive drugs). Products include:
Atacand Tablets 649
Atacand HCT 651

Captopril (Clozapine may potentiate the hypotensive effects of antihypertensive drugs). Products include:
Captopril Tablets 2149

Carbamazepine (Concomitant use is not recommended; discontinuation of concomitant carbamazepine administration may result in increase in clozapine levels). Products include:
Carbatrol Capsules 3171
Equetro Extended-Release Capsules 3180
Tegretol/Tegretol-XR 2295

Carteolol Hydrochloride (Clozapine may potentiate the hypotensive effects of antihypertensive drugs). Products include:
Carteolol Hydrochloride Ophthalmic Solution USP, 1% .... ⊙249

Chlordiazepoxide (Co-administration with benzodiazepines or other psychotropic agents may be accompanied by orthostatic hypotension leading to profound collapse and respiratory and/or cardiac arrest; caution is advised if used concurrently).
No products indexed under this heading.

Chlordiazepoxide Hydrochloride (Co-administration with benzodiazepines or other psychotropic agents may be accompanied by orthostatic hypotension leading to profound collapse and respiratory and/or cardiac arrest; caution is advised if used concurrently). Products include:
Librium Capsules 3347

Chlorothiazide (Clozapine may potentiate the hypotensive effects of antihypertensive drugs). Products include:
Diuril Oral Suspension 1954

Chlorothiazide Sodium (Clozapine may potentiate the hypotensive effects of antihypertensive drugs). Products include:
Diuril Sodium Intravenous 2467

Chlorpromazine (Co-administration with benzodiazepines or other psychotropic agents may be accompanied by orthostatic hypotension leading to profound collapse and respiratory and/or cardiac arrest; caution is advised if used concurrently).
No products indexed under this heading.

Chlorpromazine Hydrochloride (Co-administration with benzodiazepines or other psychotropic agents may be accompanied by orthostatic hypotension leading to profound collapse and respiratory and/or cardiac arrest; caution is advised if used concurrently).
No products indexed under this heading.

Chlorprothixene (Co-administration with benzodiazepines or other psychotropic agents may be accompanied by orthostatic hypotension leading to profound collapse and respiratory and/or cardiac arrest; caution is advised if used concurrently).
No products indexed under this heading.

Chlorprothixene Hydrochloride (Co-administration with benzodiazepines or other psychotropic agents may be accompanied by orthostatic hypotension leading to profound collapse and respiratory and/or cardiac arrest; caution is advised if used concurrently).
No products indexed under this heading.

Chlorprothixene Lactate (Given the primary CNS effect of clozapine, caution is advised in using it concomitantly with CNS-active drugs).
No products indexed under this heading.

Chlorthalidone (Clozapine may potentiate the hypotensive effects of antihypertensive drugs). Products include:
Clorpres Tablets 2153

Cimetidine (May increase plasma levels of clozapine, potentially resulting in adverse effects). Products include:
Tagamet HB 200 Tablets .... ◘664

Cimetidine Hydrochloride (May increase plasma levels of clozapine, potentially resulting in adverse effects).
No products indexed under this heading.

Citalopram Hydrobromide (May increase plasma levels of clozaril, potentially resulting in adverse effects). Products include:
Celexa 1176

Clidinium Bromide (Clozapine may potentiate anticholinergic effects).
No products indexed under this heading.

Clonidine (Clozapine may potentiate the hypotensive effects of antihypertensive drugs). Products include:
Catapres-TTS 844

Clonidine Hydrochloride (Clozapine may potentiate the hypotensive effects of antihypertensive drugs). Products include:
Catapres Tablets 843
Clorpres Tablets 2153

Clorazepate Dipotassium (Co-administration with benzodiazepines or other psychotropic agents may be accompanied by orthostatic hypotension leading to profound collapse and respiratory and/or cardiac arrest; caution is advised if used concurrently). Products include:
Tranxene 2474

Codeine Phosphate (Given the primary CNS effect of clozapine, caution is advised in using it concomitantly with CNS-active drugs). Products include:
Tylenol with Codeine Tablets 2391

Deserpidine (Clozapine may potentiate the hypotensive effects of antihypertensive drugs).
No products indexed under this heading.

Desflurane (Given the primary CNS effect of clozapine, caution is advised in using it concomitantly with CNS-active drugs).
No products indexed under this heading.

Desipramine Hydrochloride (Concomitant use of clozapine with other drugs metabolized by CYP4502D6 may require lower than usual doses for either drug).
No products indexed under this heading.

Dezocine (Given the primary CNS effect of clozapine, caution is advised in using it concomitantly with CNS-active drugs).
No products indexed under this heading.

Diazepam (Co-administration with benzodiazepines or other psychotropic agents may be accompanied by orthostatic hypotension leading to profound collapse and respiratory and/or cardiac arrest; caution is advised if used concurrently). Products include:
Diastat Rectal Delivery System 3343
Valium Tablets 2819

Diazoxide (Clozapine may potentiate the hypotensive effects of antihypertensive drugs). Products include:
Hyperstat I.V. 3017

Dicyclomine Hydrochloride (Clozapine may potentiate anticholinergic effects). Products include:
Bentyl Capsules 697
Bentyl Injection 697
Bentyl Syrup 697
Bentyl Tablets 697

Diltiazem Hydrochloride (Clozapine may potentiate the hypotensive effects of antihypertensive drugs). Products include:
Cardizem LA Extended Release Tablets 1728
Tiazac Capsules 1201

Doxazosin Mesylate (Clozapine may potentiate the hypotensive effects of antihypertensive drugs). Products include:
Cardura XL Tablets 2515

Doxepin Hydrochloride (Concomitant use of clozapine with other drugs metabolized by CYP4502D6 may require lower than usual doses for either drug).
No products indexed under this heading.

Droperidol (Co-administration with benzodiazepines or other psychotropic agents may be accompanied by orthostatic hypotension leading to profound collapse and respiratory and/or cardiac arrest; caution is advised if used concurrently).
No products indexed under this heading.

Enalapril Maleate (Clozapine may potentiate the hypotensive effects of antihypertensive drugs). Products include:
Vasotec I.V. Injection 2103

Enalaprilat (Clozapine may potentiate the hypotensive effects of antihypertensive drugs).
No products indexed under this heading.

Encainide Hydrochloride (Concomitant use of clozapine with other drugs metabolized by CYP4502D6 may require lower than usual doses for either drug).
No products indexed under this heading.

Enflurane (Given the primary CNS effect of clozapine, caution is advised in using it concomitantly with CNS-active drugs).
No products indexed under this heading.

Epinephrine (The administration of epinephrine should be avoided in the

treatment of clozapine-induced hypotension because of a possible reverse epinephrine effect).
Products include:

EpiPen **1061**
Primatene Mist **719**
Twinject 0.15 .... **3379**
Twinject 0.3 .... **3378**

Epinephrine Hydrochloride (The administration of epinephrine should be avoided in the treatment of clozapine-induced hypotension because of a possible reverse epinephrine effect).
No products indexed under this heading.

Eprosartan Mesylate (Clozapine may potentiate the hypotensive effects of antihypertensive drugs).
Products include:

Teveten Tablets **1735**
Teveten HCT Tablets **1737**

Erythromycin (May increase plasma levels of clozapine, potentially resulting in adverse effects).
Products include:

Ery-Tab Tablets **449**
Erythromycin Base Filmtab Tablets **455**
Erythromycin Delayed-Release Capsules, USP **457**
PCE Dispertab Tablets **515**

Erythromycin Estolate (May increase plasma levels of clozapine, potentially resulting in adverse effects).
No products indexed under this heading.

Erythromycin Ethylsuccinate (May increase plasma levels of clozapine, potentially resulting in adverse effects). Products include:

E.E.S. **451**
EryPed **447**

Erythromycin Gluceptate (May increase plasma levels of clozapine, potentially resulting in adverse effects).
No products indexed under this heading.

Erythromycin Lactobionate (May increase plasma levels of clozapine, potentially resulting in adverse effects).
No products indexed under this heading.

Erythromycin Stearate (May increase plasma levels of clozapine, potentially resulting in adverse effects). Products include:

Erythrocin Stearate Filmtab Tablets **453**

Escitalopram Oxalate (Concomitant use of clozapine with other drugs metabolized by CYP4502D6 may require lower than usual doses for either drug). Products include:

Lexapro Oral Solution **1190**
Lexapro Tablets **1190**

Esmolol Hydrochloride (Clozapine may potentiate the hypotensive effects of antihypertensive drugs).
No products indexed under this heading.

Estazolam (Co-administration with benzodiazepines or other psychotropic agents may be accompanied by orthostatic hypotension leading to profound collapse and respiratory and/or cardiac arrest; caution is advised if used concurrently).
Products include:

ProSom Tablets **517**

Ethanol (Given the primary CNS effect of clozapine, caution is advised in using it concomitantly with CNS-active drugs).
No products indexed under this heading.

Ethchlorvynol (Given the primary CNS effect of clozapine, caution is advised in using it concomitantly with CNS-active drugs).
No products indexed under this heading.

Ethinamate (Given the primary CNS effect of clozapine, caution is advised in using it concomitantly with CNS-active drugs).
No products indexed under this heading.

Ethyl Alcohol (Given the primary CNS effect of clozapine, caution is advised in using it concomitantly with CNS-active drugs).
No products indexed under this heading.

Felodipine (Clozapine may potentiate the hypotensive effects of antihypertensive drugs).
No products indexed under this heading.

Fentanyl (Given the primary CNS effect of clozapine, caution is advised in using it concomitantly with CNS-active drugs). Products include:

Duragesic Transdermal System **2373**
Ionsys Transdermal System **2379**

Fentanyl Citrate (Given the primary CNS effect of clozapine, caution is advised in using it concomitantly with CNS-active drugs). Products include:

Actiq **979**

Flecainide Acetate (Concomitant use of clozapine with other drugs metabolized by CYP4502D6 may require lower than usual doses for either drug). Products include:

Tambocor Tablets **1856**

Fluoxetine Hydrochloride (Co-administration in schizophrenic patients has resulted in elevated mean trough concentrations of clozapine and its metabolites by less than two-fold compared to baseline concentrations; a reduced clozapine dose should be considered).
Products include:

Prozac Pulvules and Liquid **1801**
Symbyax Capsules **1819**

Fluphenazine Decanoate (Co-administration with benzodiazepines or other psychotropic agents may be accompanied by orthostatic hypotension leading to profound collapse and respiratory and/or cardiac arrest; caution is advised if used concurrently).
No products indexed under this heading.

Fluphenazine Enanthate (Co-administration with benzodiazepines or other psychotropic agents may be accompanied by orthostatic hypotension leading to profound collapse and respiratory and/or cardiac arrest; caution is advised if used concurrently).
No products indexed under this heading.

Fluphenazine Hydrochloride (Co-administration with benzodiazepines or other psychotropic agents may be accompanied by orthostatic hypotension leading to profound collapse and respiratory and/or cardiac arrest; caution is advised if used concurrently).
No products indexed under this heading.

Flurazepam Hydrochloride (Co-administration with benzodiazepines or other psychotropic agents may be accompanied by orthostatic hypotension leading to profound collapse and respiratory and/or cardiac arrest; caution is advised if used concurrently). Products include:

Dalmane Capsules **3342**

Fluvoxamine Maleate (Co-administration in schizophrenic patients has resulted in elevated mean trough concentrations of clozapine and its metabolites by about three-fold compared to baseline concentrations; a reduced clozapine dose should be considered).
No products indexed under this heading.

Fosinopril Sodium (Clozapine may potentiate the hypotensive effects of antihypertensive drugs).
No products indexed under this heading.

Fosphenytoin Sodium (May decrease clozapine plasma levels resulting in a decrease in effectiveness of a previously effective clozapine dose).
No products indexed under this heading.

Furosemide (Clozapine may potentiate the hypotensive effects of antihypertensive drugs). Products include:

Furosemide Tablets **2154**

Glutethimide (Given the primary CNS effect of clozapine, caution is advised in using it concomitantly with CNS-active drugs).
No products indexed under this heading.

Glycopyrrolate (Clozapine may potentiate anticholinergic effects).
No products indexed under this heading.

Guanabenz Acetate (Clozapine may potentiate the hypotensive effects of antihypertensive drugs).
No products indexed under this heading.

Guanethidine Monosulfate (Clozapine may potentiate the hypotensive effects of antihypertensive drugs).
No products indexed under this heading.

Halazepam (Co-administration with benzodiazepines or other psychotropic agents may be accompanied by orthostatic hypotension leading to profound collapse and respiratory and/or cardiac arrest; caution is advised if used concurrently).
No products indexed under this heading.

Haloperidol (Co-administration with benzodiazepines or other psychotropic agents may be accompanied by orthostatic hypotension leading to profound collapse and respiratory and/or cardiac arrest; caution is advised if used concurrently).
No products indexed under this heading.

Haloperidol Decanoate (Co-administration with benzodiazepines or other psychotropic agents may be accompanied by orthostatic hypotension leading to profound collapse and respiratory and/or cardiac arrest; caution is advised if used concurrently).
No products indexed under this heading.

Hydralazine Hydrochloride (Clozapine may potentiate the hypotensive effects of antihypertensive drugs). Products include:

BiDil Tablets **2171**

Hydrochlorothiazide (Clozapine may potentiate the hypotensive effects of antihypertensive drugs).
Products include:

Aldoril Tablets **1910**
Atacand HCT **651**
Avalide Tablets **888**
Avalide Tablets **2874**
Benicar HCT Tablets **1044**
Diovan HCT Tablets **2196**
Dyazide Capsules **1423**
Hyzaar 50-12.5 Tablets **1990**
Hyzaar 100-12.5 Tablets **1990**
Hyzaar 100-25 Tablets **1990**
Lopressor HCT 50/25 Tablets **2241**
Lopressor HCT 100/25 Tablets **2241**
Lopressor HCT 100/50 Tablets **2241**
Lotensin HCT Tablets **2246**
Micardis HCT Tablets **856**
Moduretic Tablets **2028**
Prinzide Tablets **2056**
Teveten HCT Tablets **1737**
Timolide Tablets **2086**
Uniretic Tablets **3100**

Hydrocodone Bitartrate (Given the primary CNS effect of clozapine, caution is advised in using it concomitantly with CNS-active drugs).
Products include:

Hycodan **1116**
Hycotuss Expectorant Syrup **1117**
Vicodin Tablets **535**
Vicodin ES Tablets **536**
Vicodin HP Tablets **538**
Vicoprofen Tablets **539**
Zydone Tablets **1139**

Hydrocodone Polistirex (Given the primary CNS effect of clozapine, caution is advised in using it concomitantly with CNS-active drugs).
Products include:

Tussionex Pennkinetic Extended-Release Suspension **3327**

Hydroflumethiazide (Clozapine may potentiate the hypotensive effects of antihypertensive drugs).
No products indexed under this heading.

Hydromorphone Hydrochloride (Given the primary CNS effect of clozapine, caution is advised in using it concomitantly with CNS-active drugs). Products include:

Dilaudid **440**
Dilaudid Non-Sterile Powder **440**
Dilaudid Oral Liquid **445**
Dilaudid Rectal Suppositories **440**
Dilaudid Tablets **440**
Dilaudid Tablets - 8 mg **445**
Dilaudid-HP **442**

Hydroxyzine Hydrochloride (Co-administration with benzodiazepines or other psychotropic agents may be accompanied by orthostatic hypotension leading to profound collapse and respiratory and/or cardiac arrest; caution is advised if used concurrently).
No products indexed under this heading.

Hyoscyamine (Clozapine may potentiate anticholinergic effects).
No products indexed under this heading.

IMPORTANT NOTE: Always consult each drug listing in the patient's regimen for possible interactions.

Nifedipine (Clozapine may potentiate the hypotensive effects of antihypertensive drugs). Products include:
Adalat CC Tablets 2964
Nisoldipine (Clozapine may potentiate the hypotensive effects of antihypertensive drugs). Products include:
Sular Tablets 3122
Nitroglycerin (Clozapine may potentiate the hypotensive effects of antihypertensive drugs). Products include:
Nitro-Dur Transdermal Infusion System 3046
Nitrolingual Pumpspray 3120
Nortriptyline Hydrochloride (Concomitant use of clozapine with other drugs metabolized by CYP4502D6 may require lower than usual doses for either drug).
No products indexed under this heading.
Olanzapine (Co-administration with benzodiazepines or other psychotropic agents may be accompanied by orthostatic hypotension leading to profound collapse and respiratory and/or cardiac arrest; caution is advised if used concurrently). Products include:
Symbyax Capsules 1819
Zyprexa Tablets 1830
Zyprexa IntraMuscular 1830
Zyprexa ZYDIS Orally Disintegrating Tablets 1830
Oxazepam (Co-administration with benzodiazepines or other psychotropic agents may be accompanied by orthostatic hypotension leading to profound collapse and respiratory and/or cardiac arrest; caution is advised if used concurrently).
No products indexed under this heading.
Oxybutynin Chloride (Clozapine may potentiate anticholinergic effects). Products include:
Ditropan XL Extended-Release Tablets 2413
Oxycodone Hydrochloride (Given the primary CNS effect of clozapine, caution is advised in using it concomitantly with CNS-active drugs). Products include:
OxyContin Tablets 2703
OxyFast Oral Concentrate Solution 2708
OxyIR Capsules 2708
Percocet Tablets 1131
Percodan Tablets 1132
Paroxetine Hydrochloride (Co-administration in schizophrenic patients has resulted in elevated mean trough concentrations of clozapine and its metabolites by less than two-fold compared to baseline concentrations; a reduced clozapine dose should be considered). Products include:
Paxil CR Controlled-Release Tablets 1538
Paxil 1530
Penbutolol Sulfate (Clozapine may potentiate the hypotensive effects of antihypertensive drugs).
No products indexed under this heading.
Pentobarbital Sodium (Given the primary CNS effect of clozapine, caution is advised in using it concomitantly with CNS-active drugs). Products include:
Nembutal Sodium Solution, USP 2470
Perindopril Erbumine (Clozapine may potentiate the hypotensive effects of antihypertensive drugs). Products include:
Aceon Tablets (2 mg, 4 mg, 8 mg) 3194
Perphenazine (Co-administration with benzodiazepines or other psychotropic agents may be accompanied by orthostatic hypotension leading to profound collapse and respiratory and/or cardiac arrest; caution is advised if used concurrently).
No products indexed under this heading.
Phenelzine Sulfate (Concomitant use of clozapine with other drugs metabolized by CYP4502D6 may require lower than usual doses for either drug).
No products indexed under this heading.
Phenobarbital (Given the primary CNS effect of clozapine, caution is advised in using it concomitantly with CNS-active drugs). Products include:
Donnatal Extentabs 2493
Phenoxybenzamine Hydrochloride (Clozapine may potentiate the hypotensive effects of antihypertensive drugs). Products include:
Dibenzyline Capsules 3399
Phentolamine Mesylate (Clozapine may potentiate the hypotensive effects of antihypertensive drugs).
No products indexed under this heading.
Phenytoin (May decrease clozapine plasma levels resulting in a decrease in effectiveness of a previously effective clozapine dose).
No products indexed under this heading.
Phenytoin Sodium (May decrease clozapine plasma levels resulting in a decrease in effectiveness of a previously effective clozapine dose). Products include:
Phenytek Capsules 2160
Pindolol (Clozapine may potentiate the hypotensive effects of antihypertensive drugs).
No products indexed under this heading.
Polythiazide (Clozapine may potentiate the hypotensive effects of antihypertensive drugs).
No products indexed under this heading.
Prazepam (Co-administration with benzodiazepines or other psychotropic agents may be accompanied by orthostatic hypotension leading to profound collapse and respiratory and/or cardiac arrest; caution is advised if used concurrently).
No products indexed under this heading.
Prazosin Hydrochloride (Clozapine may potentiate the hypotensive effects of antihypertensive drugs).
No products indexed under this heading.
Prochlorperazine (Co-administration with benzodiazepines or other psychotropic agents may be accompanied by orthostatic hypotension leading to profound collapse and respiratory and/or cardiac arrest; caution is advised if used concurrently).
No products indexed under this heading.
Procyclidine Hydrochloride (Clozapine may potentiate anticholinergic effects).
No products indexed under this heading.
Promethazine Hydrochloride (Co-administration with benzodiazepines or other psychotropic agents may be accompanied by orthostatic hypotension leading to profound collapse and respiratory and/or cardiac arrest; caution is advised if used concurrently). Products include:
Phenergan Tablets and Suppositories 3440
Propafenone Hydrochloride (Concomitant use of clozapine with other drugs metabolized by CYP4502D6 may require lower than usual doses for either drug). Products include:
Rythmol SR Capsules 2727
Propantheline Bromide (Clozapine may potentiate anticholinergic effects).
No products indexed under this heading.
Propofol (Given the primary CNS effect of clozapine, caution is advised in using it concomitantly with CNS-active drugs).
No products indexed under this heading.
Propoxyphene Hydrochloride (Given the primary CNS effect of clozapine, caution is advised in using it concomitantly with CNS-active drugs).
No products indexed under this heading.
Propoxyphene Napsylate (Given the primary CNS effect of clozapine, caution is advised in using it concomitantly with CNS-active drugs).
No products indexed under this heading.
Propranolol Hydrochloride (Clozapine may potentiate the hypotensive effects of antihypertensive drugs). Products include:
Inderal LA Long-Acting Capsules 3429
InnoPran XL Capsules 2723
Protriptyline Hydrochloride (Concomitant use of clozapine with other drugs metabolized by CYP4502D6 may require lower than usual doses for either drug).
No products indexed under this heading.
Quazepam (Co-administration with benzodiazepines or other psychotropic agents may be accompanied by orthostatic hypotension leading to profound collapse and respiratory and/or cardiac arrest; caution is advised if used concurrently).
No products indexed under this heading.
Quetiapine Fumarate (Co-administration with benzodiazepines or other psychotropic agents may be accompanied by orthostatic hypotension leading to profound collapse and respiratory and/or cardiac arrest; caution is advised if used concurrently). Products include:
Seroquel Tablets 690
Quinapril Hydrochloride (Clozapine may potentiate the hypotensive effects of antihypertensive drugs).
No products indexed under this heading.
Quinidine (Co-administration of drugs that inhibit CYP4502D6, such as quinidine, should be approached with caution).
No products indexed under this heading.
Quinidine Gluconate (Co-administration of drugs that inhibit CYP4502D6, such as quinidine, should be approached with caution).
No products indexed under this heading.
Quinidine Hydrochloride (Co-administration of drugs that inhibit CYP4502D6, such as quinidine, should be approached with caution).
No products indexed under this heading.
Quinidine Polygalacturonate (Co-administration of drugs that inhibit CYP4502D6, such as quinidine, should be approached with caution).
No products indexed under this heading.
Quinidine Sulfate (Co-administration of drugs that inhibit CYP4502D6, such as quinidine, should be approached with caution).
No products indexed under this heading.
Ramipril (Clozapine may potentiate the hypotensive effects of antihypertensive drugs). Products include:
Altace Capsules 1702
Rauwolfia Serpentina (Clozapine may potentiate the hypotensive effects of antihypertensive drugs).
No products indexed under this heading.
Remifentanil Hydrochloride (Given the primary CNS effect of clozapine, caution is advised in using it concomitantly with CNS-active drugs).
No products indexed under this heading.
Rescinnamine (Clozapine may potentiate the hypotensive effects of antihypertensive drugs).
No products indexed under this heading.
Reserpine (Clozapine may potentiate the hypotensive effects of antihypertensive drugs).
No products indexed under this heading.
Rifampin (May decrease clozapine plasma levels resulting in a decrease in effectiveness of a previously effective clozapine dose).
No products indexed under this heading.
Risperidone (Co-administration with benzodiazepines or other psychotropic agents may be accompanied by orthostatic hypotension leading to profound collapse and respiratory and/or cardiac arrest; caution is advised if used concurrently). Products include:
Risperdal 1676
Risperdal Consta Long-Acting Injection 1682
Risperdal M-Tab Orally Disintegrating Tablets 1676
Scopolamine (Clozapine may potentiate anticholinergic effects). Products include:
Transderm Scōp Transdermal Therapeutic System 2177
Scopolamine Hydrobromide (Clozapine may potentiate anticholinergic effects). Products include:
Donnatal Extentabs 2493
Secobarbital Sodium (Given the primary CNS effect of clozapine, caution is advised in using it concomitantly with CNS-active drugs).
No products indexed under this heading.
Sertraline Hydrochloride (Co-administration in schizophrenic patients has resulted in elevated mean trough concentrations of

clozapine and its metabolites by less than two-fold compared to baseline concentrations; a reduced clozapine dose should be considered). Products include:
- Zoloft 2586

Sevoflurane (Given the primary CNS effect of clozapine, caution is advised in using it concomitantly with CNS-active drugs). Products include:
- Ultane Liquid for Inhalation 531

Sodium Nitroprusside (Clozapine may potentiate the hypotensive effects of antihypertensive drugs).
- No products indexed under this heading.

Sodium Oxybate (Given the primary CNS effect of clozapine, caution is advised in using it concomitantly with CNS-active drugs). Products include:
- Xyrem Oral Solution 1688

Sotalol Hydrochloride (Clozapine may potentiate the hypotensive effects of antihypertensive drugs).
- No products indexed under this heading.

Spirapril Hydrochloride (Clozapine may potentiate the hypotensive effects of antihypertensive drugs).
- No products indexed under this heading.

Sufentanil Citrate (Given the primary CNS effect of clozapine, caution is advised in using it concomitantly with CNS-active drugs).
- No products indexed under this heading.

Telmisartan (Clozapine may potentiate the hypotensive effects of antihypertensive drugs). Products include:
- Micardis Tablets 854
- Micardis HCT Tablets 856

Temazepam (Co-administration with benzodiazepines or other psychotropic agents may be accompanied by orthostatic hypotension leading to profound collapse and respiratory and/or cardiac arrest; caution is advised if used concurrently). Products include:
- Restoril Capsules 1860

Terazosin Hydrochloride (Clozapine may potentiate the hypotensive effects of antihypertensive drugs). Products include:
- Hytrin Capsules 471

Thiamylal Sodium (Given the primary CNS effect of clozapine, caution is advised in using it concomitantly with CNS-active drugs).
- No products indexed under this heading.

Thioridazine Hydrochloride (Co-administration with benzodiazepines or other psychotropic agents may be accompanied by orthostatic hypotension leading to profound collapse and respiratory and/or cardiac arrest; caution is advised if used concurrently). Products include:
- Thioridazine Hydrochloride Tablets 2163

Thiothixene (Co-administration with benzodiazepines or other psychotropic agents may be accompanied by orthostatic hypotension leading to profound collapse and respiratory and/or cardiac arrest; caution is advised if used concurrently). Products include:
- Thiothixene Capsules 2165

Timolol Maleate (Clozapine may potentiate the hypotensive effects of antihypertensive drugs). Products include:
- Blocadren Tablets 1916
- Cosopt Sterile Ophthalmic Solution 1931
- Timolide Tablets 2086
- Timoptic Sterile Ophthalmic Solution 2088
- Timoptic in Ocudose 2091
- Timoptic-XE Sterile Ophthalmic Gel Forming Solution 2092

Tolterodine Tartrate (Clozapine may potentiate anticholinergic effects). Products include:
- Detrol Tablets 2628
- Detrol LA Capsules 2631

Torsemide (Clozapine may potentiate the hypotensive effects of antihypertensive drugs). Products include:
- Demadex Injection 2759
- Demadex Tablets 2759

Trandolapril (Clozapine may potentiate the hypotensive effects of antihypertensive drugs). Products include:
- Mavik Tablets 486
- Tarka Tablets 524

Tranylcypromine Sulfate (Concomitant use of clozapine with other drugs metabolized by CYP4502D6 may require lower than usual doses for either drug). Products include:
- Parnate Tablets 1527

Trazodone Hydrochloride (Concomitant use of clozapine with other drugs metabolized by CYP4502D6 may require lower than usual doses for either drug).
- No products indexed under this heading.

Triazolam (Co-administration with benzodiazepines or other psychotropic agents may be accompanied by orthostatic hypotension leading to profound collapse and respiratory and/or cardiac arrest; caution is advised if used concurrently).
- No products indexed under this heading.

Tridihexethyl Chloride (Clozapine may potentiate anticholinergic effects).
- No products indexed under this heading.

Trifluoperazine Hydrochloride (Co-administration with benzodiazepines or other psychotropic agents may be accompanied by orthostatic hypotension leading to profound collapse and respiratory and/or cardiac arrest; caution is advised if used concurrently).
- No products indexed under this heading.

Trihexyphenidyl Hydrochloride (Clozapine may potentiate anticholinergic effects).
- No products indexed under this heading.

Trimethaphan Camsylate (Clozapine may potentiate the hypotensive effects of antihypertensive drugs).
- No products indexed under this heading.

Trimipramine Maleate (Concomitant use of clozapine with other drugs metabolized by CYP4502D6 may require lower than usual doses for either drug).
- No products indexed under this heading.

Valsartan (Clozapine may potentiate the hypotensive effects of antihypertensive drugs). Products include:
- Diovan Tablets 2193
- Diovan HCT Tablets 2196

Venlafaxine Hydrochloride (Concomitant use of clozapine with other drugs metabolized by CYP4502D6 may require lower than usual doses for either drug). Products include:
- Effexor Tablets 3411
- Effexor XR Capsules 3417

Verapamil Hydrochloride (Clozapine may potentiate the hypotensive effects of antihypertensive drugs). Products include:
- Covera-HS Tablets 3139
- Tarka Tablets 524
- Verelan PM Extended-Release Capsules, Controlled-Onset 3106

Zaleplon (Given the primary CNS effect of clozapine, caution is advised in using it concomitantly with CNS-active drugs). Products include:
- Sonata Capsules 1717

Ziprasidone Hydrochloride (Co-administration with benzodiazepines or other psychotropic agents may be accompanied by orthostatic hypotension leading to profound collapse and respiratory and/or cardiac arrest; caution is advised if used concurrently). Products include:
- Geodon Capsules 2529

Zolpidem Tartrate (Given the primary CNS effect of clozapine, caution is advised in using it concomitantly with CNS-active drugs). Products include:
- Ambien Tablets 2851
- Ambien CR Tablets 2855

Food Interactions

Alcohol (Given the primary CNS effect of clozapine, caution is advised in using it concomitantly with alcohol).

CM PLEX CREAM

(Cetyl Myristate, Cetyl Myristoleate, Fatty Acids) 3329

None cited in PDR database.

CM PLEX SOFTGELS

(Cetyl Myristate, Cetyl Myristoleate, Fatty Acids) 3329

None cited in PDR database.

COLAZAL CAPSULES

(Balsalazide Disodium) 2838

May interact with:

Antibiotics, unspecified (Use of orally administered antibiotics could, theoretically, interfere with the release of mesalamine in the colon).
- No products indexed under this heading.

COLD-FX CAPSULES

(Dietary Supplement) 1000

None cited in PDR database.

COLOCORT RECTAL SUSPENSION, USP (RETENTION) 100 MG/ 60 ML

(Hydrocortisone) 2476

May interact with vaccines, live and certain other agents. Compounds in these categories include:

Aspirin (Aspirin should be used cautiously in conjunction with corticosteroids in hypoprothrombinemia). Products include:
- Aggrenox Capsules 822
- Bayer Aspirin 744
- BC Allergy Sinus Cold Powder ..... ■□677
- BC Headache Powder ..... ■□677
- Arthritis Strength BC Powder ..... ■□677
- BC Sinus Cold Powder ..... ■□677
- Excedrin Extra Strength Caplets/Tablets/Geltabs ..... ■□684
- Excedrin Migraine Caplets/Tablets/Geltabs ..... ■□609
- Goody's Body Pain Formula Powder ..... ■□684
- Goody's Extra Strength Headache Powders ..... ■□611
- Goody's Extra Strength Pain Relief Tablets ..... ■□685
- Percodan Tablets 1132
- St. Joseph 81 mg Aspirin Chewable and Enteric Coated Tablets 1869

Aspirin, Enteric Coated (Aspirin should be used cautiously in conjunction with corticosteroids in hypoprothrombinemia).
- No products indexed under this heading.

Aspirin Buffered (Aspirin should be used cautiously in conjunction with corticosteroids in hypoprothrombinemia). Products include:
- Bufferin Extra Strength Tablets ..... ■□678
- Bufferin Regular Strength Tablets ..... ■□678

BCG Vaccine (Immunization procedures should not be undertaken in patients who are on corticosteroids, especially on high dose, because of possible hazards of neurological complications and a lack of antibody response).
- No products indexed under this heading.

Live Virus Vaccines; Smallpox (While on corticosteroid therapy patients should not be vaccinated against smallpox).
- No products indexed under this heading.

Measles, Mumps, Rubella and Varicella Virus Vaccine Live (Immunization procedures should not be undertaken in patients who are on corticosteroids, especially on high dose, because of possible hazards of neurological complications and a lack of antibody response). Products include:
- ProQuad 2064

Measles, Mumps & Rubella Virus Vaccine, Live (Immunization procedures should not be undertaken in patients who are on corticosteroids, especially on high dose, because of possible hazards of neurological complications and a lack of antibody response). Products include:
- M-M-R II 2006

Measles & Rubella Virus Vaccine Live (Immunization procedures should not be undertaken in patients who are on corticosteroids, especially on high dose, because of possible hazards of neurological complications and a lack of antibody response).
- No products indexed under this heading.

Measles Virus Vaccine Live (Immunization procedures should not be undertaken in patients who are on corticosteroids, especially on high dose, because of possible hazards of neurological complications and a lack of antibody response). Products include:
- Attenuvax 1914

Mumps Virus Vaccine, Live (Immunization procedures should not be undertaken in patients who are on corticosteroids, especially on high dose, because of possible hazards of neurological complications and a lack of antibody response). Products include:

Mumpsvax 2031

Poliovirus Vaccine, Live, Oral, Trivalent, Types 1,2,3 (Sabin) (Immunization procedures should not be undertaken in patients who are on corticosteroids, especially on high dose, because of possible hazards of neurological complications and a lack of antibody response).
No products indexed under this heading.

Rotavirus Vaccine, Live, Oral, Tetravalent (Immunization procedures should not be undertaken in patients who are on corticosteroids, especially on high dose, because of possible hazards of neurological complications and a lack of antibody response).
No products indexed under this heading.

Rubella & Mumps Virus Vaccine Live (Immunization procedures should not be undertaken in patients who are on corticosteroids, especially on high dose, because of possible hazards of neurological complications and a lack of antibody response).
No products indexed under this heading.

Rubella Virus Vaccine Live (Immunization procedures should not be undertaken in patients who are on corticosteroids, especially on high dose, because of possible hazards of neurological complications and a lack of antibody response). Products include:
Meruvax II 2019

Smallpox Vaccine (Immunization procedures should not be undertaken in patients who are on corticosteroids, especially on high dose, because of possible hazards of neurological complications and a lack of antibody response).
No products indexed under this heading.

Typhoid Vaccine (Immunization procedures should not be undertaken in patients who are on corticosteroids, especially on high dose, because of possible hazards of neurological complications and a lack of antibody response).
No products indexed under this heading.

Varicella Virus Vaccine Live (Immunization procedures should not be undertaken in patients who are on corticosteroids, especially on high dose, because of possible hazards of neurological complications and a lack of antibody response). Products include:
Varivax 2100

Yellow Fever Vaccine (Immunization procedures should not be undertaken in patients who are on corticosteroids, especially on high dose, because of possible hazards of neurological complications and a lack of antibody response).
No products indexed under this heading.

COLYTE WITH FLAVOR PACKS FOR ORAL SOLUTION

(Polyethylene Glycol, Potassium Chloride, Sodium Bicarbonate, Sodium Chloride, Sodium Sulfate)....... 3088
May interact with:

Oral Medications, unspecified (Those administered within one hour of Colyte usage may be flushed from the gastrointestinal tract and not absorbed).
No products indexed under this heading.

COMBIVENT INHALATION AEROSOL

(Albuterol Sulfate, Ipratropium Bromide) 847
May interact with anticholinergics, beta blockers, monoamine oxidase inhibitors, potassium-depleting diuretics, sympathomimetics, and tricyclic antidepressants. Compounds in these categories include:

Acebutolol Hydrochloride (Co-administration with beta blockers inhibits the effects of each other).
No products indexed under this heading.

Albuterol (Co-administration with other sympathomimetic agents increases the risk of adverse cardiovascular effects). Products include:
Proventil Inhalation Aerosol 3053

Amitriptyline Hydrochloride (Co-administration with tricyclic antidepressant can potentiate the action of albuterol on the cardiovascular system).
No products indexed under this heading.

Amoxapine (Co-administration with tricyclic antidepressant can potentiate the action of albuterol on the cardiovascular system).
No products indexed under this heading.

Atenolol (Co-administration with beta blockers inhibits the effects of each other).
No products indexed under this heading.

Atropine Sulfate (Co-administration has some potential for additive anticholinergic effects; caution is advised). Products include:
Donnatal Extentabs 2493

Belladonna Alkaloids (Co-administration has some potential for additive anticholinergic effects; caution is advised). Products include:
Hyland's Teething Tablets .... ▣830

Bendroflumethiazide (Co-administration with non-potassium-sparing diuretics can result in acute worsening of ECG changes and/or hypokalemia, especially when recommended dose of the beta agonist is exceeded; clinical significance of this interaction is unknown).
No products indexed under this heading.

Benztropine Mesylate (Co-administration has some potential for additive anticholinergic effects; caution is advised).
No products indexed under this heading.

Betaxolol Hydrochloride (Co-administration with beta blockers inhibits the effects of each other). Products include:
Betoptic S Ophthalmic Suspension.................................. 558

Biperiden Hydrochloride (Co-administration has some potential for additive anticholinergic effects; caution is advised).
No products indexed under this heading.

Bisoprolol Fumarate (Co-administration with beta blockers inhibits the effects of each other).
No products indexed under this heading.

Bumetanide (Co-administration with non-potassium-sparing diuretics can result in acute worsening of ECG changes and/or hypokalemia, especially when recommended dose of the beta agonist is exceeded; clinical significance of this interaction is unknown). Products include:
Bumex Tablets 2746

Carteolol Hydrochloride (Co-administration with beta blockers inhibits the effects of each other). Products include:
Carteolol Hydrochloride Ophthalmic Solution USP, 1%....... ⊙249

Chlorothiazide (Co-administration with non-potassium-sparing diuretics can result in acute worsening of ECG changes and/or hypokalemia, especially when recommended dose of the beta agonist is exceeded; clinical significance of this interaction is unknown). Products include:
Diuril Oral Suspension 1954

Chlorothiazide Sodium (Co-administration with non-potassium-sparing diuretics can result in acute worsening of ECG changes and/or hypokalemia, especially when recommended dose of the beta agonist is exceeded; clinical significance of this interaction is unknown). Products include:
Diuril Sodium Intravenous 2467

Clidinium Bromide (Co-administration has some potential for additive anticholinergic effects; caution is advised).
No products indexed under this heading.

Clomipramine Hydrochloride (Co-administration with tricyclic antidepressant can potentiate the action of albuterol on the cardiovascular system).
No products indexed under this heading.

Desipramine Hydrochloride (Co-administration with tricyclic antidepressant can potentiate the action of albuterol on the cardiovascular system).
No products indexed under this heading.

Dicyclomine Hydrochloride (Co-administration has some potential for additive anticholinergic effects; caution is advised). Products include:
Bentyl Capsules 697
Bentyl Injection 697
Bentyl Syrup 697
Bentyl Tablets 697

Dobutamine Hydrochloride (Co-administration with other sympathomimetic agents increases the risk of adverse cardiovascular effects).
No products indexed under this heading.

Dopamine Hydrochloride (Co-administration with other sympathomimetic agents increases the risk of adverse cardiovascular effects).
No products indexed under this heading.

Doxepin Hydrochloride (Co-administration with tricyclic antidepressant can potentiate the action of albuterol on the cardiovascular system).
No products indexed under this heading.

Ephedrine Hydrochloride (Co-administration with other sympathomimetic agents increases the risk of adverse cardiovascular effects).
No products indexed under this heading.

Ephedrine Sulfate (Co-administration with other sympathomimetic agents increases the risk of adverse cardiovascular effects).
No products indexed under this heading.

Ephedrine Tannate (Co-administration with other sympathomimetic agents increases the risk of adverse cardiovascular effects).
No products indexed under this heading.

Epinephrine (Co-administration with other sympathomimetic agents increases the risk of adverse cardiovascular effects). Products include:
EpiPen 1061
Primatene Mist .... ▣719
Twinject 0.15 3379
Twinject 0.3 3378

Epinephrine Bitartrate (Co-administration with other sympathomimetic agents increases the risk of adverse cardiovascular effects).
No products indexed under this heading.

Epinephrine Hydrochloride (Co-administration with other sympathomimetic agents increases the risk of adverse cardiovascular effects).
No products indexed under this heading.

Esmolol Hydrochloride (Co-administration with beta blockers inhibits the effects of each other).
No products indexed under this heading.

Ethacrynic Acid (Co-administration with non-potassium-sparing diuretics can result in acute worsening of ECG changes and/or hypokalemia, especially when recommended dose of the beta agonist is exceeded; clinical significance of this interaction is unknown). Products include:
Edecrin Tablets 1959

Furosemide (Co-administration with non-potassium-sparing diuretics can result in acute worsening of ECG changes and/or hypokalemia, especially when recommended dose of the beta agonist is exceeded; clinical significance of this interaction is unknown). Products include:
Furosemide Tablets 2154

Glycopyrrolate (Co-administration has some potential for additive anticholinergic effects; caution is advised).
No products indexed under this heading.

Hydrochlorothiazide (Co-administration with non-potassium-sparing diuretics can result in acute worsening of ECG changes and/or hypokalemia, especially when recommended dose of the beta agonist is

exceeded; clinical significance of this interaction is unknown).
Products include:
- Aldoril Tablets ... 1910
- Atacand HCT ... 651
- Avalide Tablets ... 888
- Avalide Tablets ... 2874
- Benicar HCT Tablets ... 1044
- Diovan HCT Tablets ... 2196
- Dyazide Capsules ... 1423
- Hyzaar 50-12.5 Tablets ... 1990
- Hyzaar 100-12.5 Tablets ... 1990
- Hyzaar 100-25 Tablets ... 1990
- Lopressor HCT 50/25 Tablets ... 2241
- Lopressor HCT 100/25 Tablets ... 2241
- Lopressor HCT 100/50 Tablets ... 2241
- Lotensin HCT Tablets ... 2246
- Micardis HCT Tablets ... 856
- Moduretic Tablets ... 2028
- Prinzide Tablets ... 2056
- Teveten HCT Tablets ... 1737
- Timolide Tablets ... 2086
- Uniretic Tablets ... 3100

Hydroflumethiazide (Co-administration with non-potassium-sparing diuretics can result in acute worsening of ECG changes and/or hypokalemia, especially when recommended dose of the beta agonist is exceeded; clinical significance of this interaction is unknown).
No products indexed under this heading.

Hyoscyamine (Co-administration has some potential for additive anticholinergic effects; caution is advised).
No products indexed under this heading.

Hyoscyamine Sulfate (Co-administration has some potential for additive anticholinergic effects; caution is advised). Products include:
- Donnatal Extentabs ... 2493
- Prosed/DS Tablets ... 1157

Imipramine Hydrochloride (Co-administration with tricyclic antidepressant can potentiate the action of albuterol on the cardiovascular system).
No products indexed under this heading.

Imipramine Pamoate (Co-administration with tricyclic antidepressant can potentiate the action of albuterol on the cardiovascular system).
No products indexed under this heading.

Isocarboxazid (Co-administration with MAO inhibitors can potentiate the action of albuterol on the cardiovascular system).
No products indexed under this heading.

Isoproterenol Hydrochloride (Co-administration with other sympathomimetic agents increases the risk of adverse cardiovascular effects).
No products indexed under this heading.

Isoproterenol Sulfate (Co-administration with other sympathomimetic agents increases the risk of adverse cardiovascular effects).
No products indexed under this heading.

Labetalol Hydrochloride (Co-administration with beta blockers inhibits the effects of each other).
No products indexed under this heading.

Levalbuterol Hydrochloride (Co-administration with other sympathomimetic agents increases the risk of adverse cardiovascular effects).
Products include:
- Xopenex Inhalation Solution ... 3146
- Xopenex Inhalation Solution Concentrate ... 3150

Levobunolol Hydrochloride (Co-administration with beta blockers inhibits the effects of each other).
Products include:
- Betagan Ophthalmic Solution, USP ... ⊙ 220

Maprotiline Hydrochloride (Co-administration with tricyclic antidepressant can potentiate the action of albuterol on the cardiovascular system).
No products indexed under this heading.

Mepenzolate Bromide (Co-administration has some potential for additive anticholinergic effects; caution is advised).
No products indexed under this heading.

Metaproterenol Sulfate (Co-administration with other sympathomimetic agents increases the risk of adverse cardiovascular effects).
Products include:
- Alupent Inhalation Aerosol ... 826

Metaraminol Bitartrate (Co-administration with other sympathomimetic agents increases the risk of adverse cardiovascular effects).
No products indexed under this heading.

Methoxamine Hydrochloride (Co-administration with other sympathomimetic agents increases the risk of adverse cardiovascular effects).
No products indexed under this heading.

Methyclothiazide (Co-administration with non-potassium-sparing diuretics can result in acute worsening of ECG changes and/or hypokalemia, especially when recommended dose of the beta agonist is exceeded; clinical significance of this interaction is unknown).
No products indexed under this heading.

Metipranolol Hydrochloride (Co-administration with beta blockers inhibits the effects of each other).
No products indexed under this heading.

Metoprolol Succinate (Co-administration with beta blockers inhibits the effects of each other).
Products include:
- Toprol-XL Tablets ... 668

Metoprolol Tartrate (Co-administration with beta blockers inhibits the effects of each other).
Products include:
- Lopressor Injection ... 2238
- Lopressor Tablets ... 2238
- Lopressor HCT 50/25 Tablets ... 2241
- Lopressor HCT 100/25 Tablets ... 2241
- Lopressor HCT 100/50 Tablets ... 2241

Moclobemide (Co-administration with MAO inhibitors can potentiate the action of albuterol on the cardiovascular system).
No products indexed under this heading.

Nadolol (Co-administration with beta blockers inhibits the effects of each other). Products include:
- Nadolol Tablets ... 2159

Norepinephrine Bitartrate (Co-administration with other sympathomimetic agents increases the risk of adverse cardiovascular effects).
No products indexed under this heading.

Nortriptyline Hydrochloride (Co-administration with tricyclic antidepressant can potentiate the action of albuterol on the cardiovascular system).
No products indexed under this heading.

Oxybutynin Chloride (Co-administration has some potential for additive anticholinergic effects; caution is advised). Products include:
- Ditropan XL Extended-Release Tablets ... 2413

Pargyline Hydrochloride (Co-administration with MAO inhibitors can potentiate the action of albuterol on the cardiovascular system).
No products indexed under this heading.

Penbutolol Sulfate (Co-administration with beta blockers inhibits the effects of each other).
No products indexed under this heading.

Phenelzine Sulfate (Co-administration with MAO inhibitors can potentiate the action of albuterol on the cardiovascular system).
No products indexed under this heading.

Phenylephrine Bitartrate (Co-administration with other sympathomimetic agents increases the risk of adverse cardiovascular effects).
No products indexed under this heading.

Phenylephrine Hydrochloride (Co-administration with other sympathomimetic agents increases the risk of adverse cardiovascular effects).
Products include:
- Comtrex Maximum Strength Non-Drowsy Cold & Cough Caplets ... ▣ 725
- Comtrex Maximum Strength Day/Night Severe Cold & Sinus Caplets - Day Formulation ... ▣ 725
- Comtrex Maximum Strength Day/Night Severe Cold & Sinus Caplets - Night Formulation ... ▣ 725
- Contac Cold and Flu Maximum Strength Caplets ... ▣ 728
- Contac Cold and Flu Day and Night Caplets (Day Formulation Only) ... ▣ 727
- Contac Cold and Flu Day and Night Caplets (Night Formulation Only) ... ▣ 727
- Contac Cold and Flu Non-Drowsy Caplets ... ▣ 728
- Contac-D Cold Non-Drowsy Tablets ... ▣ 729
- Children's Dimetapp Cold & Allergy Elixir ... ▣ 730
- Children's Dimetapp Cold & Allergy Chewable Tablets ... ▣ 730
- Children's Dimetapp DM Cold & Cough Elixir ... ▣ 731
- Toddler's Dimetapp Cold and Cough Drops ... ▣ 732
- Excedrin Sinus Headache Caplets/Tablets ... ▣ 610
- 4-Way Fast Acting Nasal Spray ... ▣ 775
- 4-Way Menthol Nasal Spray ... ▣ 775
- Preparation H Maximum Strength Cream ... ▣ 666
- Preparation H Cooling Gel ... ▣ 666
- Preparation H ... ▣ 666
- Refenesen PE Caplets ... ▣ 721
- Robitussin Cough & Allergy Syrup ... ▣ 736
- Robitussin Cough & Cold Nighttime Liquid ... ▣ 736
- Robitussin Cough, Cold & Flu Nighttime Liquid ... ▣ 738
- Robitussin Head & Chest Congestion PE Syrup ... ▣ 739
- Robitussin Pediatric Cough & Cold Nighttime Liquid ... ▣ 736
- TheraFlu Cold & Cough Hot Liquid ... ▣ 740
- TheraFlu Cold & Sore Throat Hot Liquid ... ▣ 741
- TheraFlu Flu & Sore Throat Hot Liquid ... ▣ 742
- TheraFlu Daytime Severe Cold Hot Liquid ... ▣ 742
- TheraFlu Nighttime Severe Cold Hot Liquid ... ▣ 740
- TheraFlu Warming Relief Daytime Severe Cold ... ▣ 743
- TheraFlu Warming Relief Nighttime Severe Cold ... ▣ 743
- Triaminic Chest & Nasal Congestion Liquid ... ▣ 746
- Triaminic Cold & Allergy Liquid ... ▣ 746
- Triaminic Daytime Cold & Cough Liquid ... ▣ 745
- Triaminic Nighttime Cold & Cough Liquid ... ▣ 746
- Triaminic Thin Strips Cold ... ▣ 748
- Triaminic Thin Strips Cold & Cough ... ▣ 778
- Triaminic Infant Thin Strips Decongestant ... ▣ 747
- Triaminic Infant Thin Strips Decongestant Plus Cough ... ▣ 747
- Children's Tylenol Plus Flu Oral Suspension ... ▣ 749
- Tylenol Cold Head Congestion Daytime Caplets with Cool Burst and Gelcaps ... ▣ 750
- Tylenol Cold Multi-Symptom Daytime Liquid ... ▣ 752
- Tylenol Cold Multi-Symptom Severe Daytime Liquid ... ▣ 752
- Concentrated Tylenol Infants' Drops Plus Cold & Cough ... ▣ 754
- Tylenol Allergy Multi-Symptom Caplets with Cool Burst and Gelcaps ... 1872
- Tylenol Allergy Multi-Symptom Nighttime Caplets with Cool Burst ... 1872
- Children's Tylenol Plus Cold Suspension Liquid ... 1879
- Children's Tylenol Plus Cold & Allergy Suspension Liquid ... 1878
- Children's Tylenol Plus Flu Suspension Liquid ... 1881
- Children's Tylenol Plus Multi-Symptom Cold Suspension Liquid ... 1879
- Tylenol Cold Head Congestion Daytime Caplets with Cool Burst ... 1873
- Tylenol Cold Head Congestion Nighttime Caplets with Cool Burst ... 1873
- Tylenol Cold Head Congestion Severe Caplets with Cool Burst ... 1873
- Tylenol Cold Multi-Symptom Daytime Caplets with Cool Burst and Gelcaps ... 1874
- Tylenol Cold Multi-Symptom Daytime Liquid with Citrus Burst ... 1874
- Tylenol Cold Multi-Symptom Nighttime Caplets with Cool Burst ... 1874
- Tylenol Cold Multi-Symptom Nighttime Liquid with Cool Burst ... 1874
- Tylenol Cold Multi-Symptom Severe Caplets with Cool Burst ... 1874
- Tylenol Cold Multi-Symptom Severe Daytime Liquid with Citrus Burst ... 1874
- Tylenol Sinus Congestion & Pain Daytime Caplets with Cool Burst and Gelcaps ... 1876
- Tylenol Sinus Congestion & Pain Nighttime Caplets with Cool Burst ... 1876
- Tylenol Sinus Congestion & Pain Severe Caplets with Cool Burst ... 1876
- Vicks 44D Cough & Head Congestion Relief Liquid ... ▣ 760
- Vicks DayQuil LiquiCaps/Liquid Multi-Symptom Cold/Flu Relief ... ▣ 761
- Zicam Cough Plus D Cough Spray ... ▣ 767

Phenylephrine Tannate (Co-administration with other sympathomimetic agents increases the risk of adverse cardiovascular effects).
No products indexed under this heading.

Phenylpropanolamine Hydrochloride (Co-administration with other sympathomimetic agents increases the risk of adverse cardiovascular effects).
No products indexed under this heading.

Pindolol (Co-administration with beta blockers inhibits the effects of each other).
No products indexed under this heading.

Pirbuterol Acetate (Co-administration with other sympathomimetic agents increases the risk of adverse cardiovascular effects). Products include:
Maxair Autohaler 1852

Polythiazide (Co-administration with non-potassium-sparing diuretics can result in acute worsening of ECG changes and/or hypokalemia, especially when recommended dose of the beta agonist is exceeded; clinical significance of this interaction is unknown).
No products indexed under this heading.

Procarbazine Hydrochloride (Co-administration with MAO inhibitors can potentiate the action of albuterol on the cardiovascular system). Products include:
Matulane Capsules 3191

Procyclidine Hydrochloride (Co-administration has some potential for additive anticholinergic effects; caution is advised).
No products indexed under this heading.

Propantheline Bromide (Co-administration has some potential for additive anticholinergic effects; caution is advised).
No products indexed under this heading.

Propranolol Hydrochloride (Co-administration with beta blockers inhibits the effects of each other). Products include:
Inderal LA Long-Acting Capsules 3429
InnoPran XL Capsules 2723

Protriptyline Hydrochloride (Co-administration with tricyclic antidepressant can potentiate the action of albuterol on the cardiovascular system).
No products indexed under this heading.

Pseudoephedrine Hydrochloride (Co-administration with other sympathomimetic agents increases the risk of adverse cardiovascular effects). Products include:
Advil Allergy Sinus Caplets 770
Advil Cold & Sinus 723
Advil Multi-Symptom Cold Caplets 770
Aleve Cold & Sinus Caplets 744
Allegra-D 12 Hour Extended-Release Tablets 2846
Allegra-D 24 Hour Extended-Release Tablets 2849
BC Cold Powder 677
Comtrex Maximum Strength Cold & Cough Day/Night Caplets - Day Formulation 726
Comtrex Maximum Strength Cold & Cough Day/Night Caplets - Night Formulation 726
Children's Motrin Cold Oral Suspension 1867
Mucinex D Extended-Release Bi-Layer Tablets 776
Robitussin Cough & Cold CF Liquid 735
Robitussin Cough & Cold Pediatric Drops 735
Tylenol Sinus Congestion & Pain Nighttime Caplets with Cool Burst 778
Tylenol Cold Severe Congestion Non-Drowsy Caplets with Cool Burst 1874
Tylenol Sinus Severe Congestion Caplets with Cool Burst 1876
Vicks 44D Cough & Head Congestion Relief Liquid 2679
Vicks 44M Cough, Cold & Flu Relief Liquid 2680
Vicks DayQuil Multi-Symptom Cold/Flu Relief LiquiCaps 2678
Vicks DayQuil Multi-Symptom Cold/Flu Relief Liquid 2678
Vicks NyQuil Multi-Symptom Cold/Flu Relief Liquid 2681
Vicks NyQuil Multi-Symptom Cold/Flu Relief LiquiCaps 2681
Children's Vicks NyQuil Cold/Cough Relief Liquid 2680
Zyrtec-D 12 Hour Extended Release Tablets 2597

Pseudoephedrine Sulfate (Co-administration with other sympathomimetic agents increases the risk of adverse cardiovascular effects). Products include:
Alavert Allergy & Sinus D-12 Hour Tablets 771
Clarinex-D 24-Hour Extended-Release Tablets 2998
Claritin-D Non-Drowsy 12 Hour Tablets 772
Claritin-D Non-Drowsy 24 Hour Tablets 772

Salmeterol Xinafoate (Co-administration with other sympathomimetic agents increases the risk of adverse cardiovascular effects). Products include:
Advair Diskus 100/50 1308
Advair Diskus 250/50 1308
Advair Diskus 500/50 1308
Advair HFA Inhalation Aerosol 1318
Serevent Diskus 1568

Scopolamine (Co-administration has some potential for additive anticholinergic effects; caution is advised). Products include:
Transderm Scōp Transdermal Therapeutic System 2177

Scopolamine Hydrobromide (Co-administration has some potential for additive anticholinergic effects; caution is advised). Products include:
Donnatal Extentabs 2493

Selegiline Hydrochloride (Co-administration with MAO inhibitors can potentiate the action of albuterol on the cardiovascular system). Products include:
Eldepryl Capsules 3208
Zelapar Tablets 3372

Sotalol Hydrochloride (Co-administration with beta blockers inhibits the effects of each other).
No products indexed under this heading.

Terbutaline Sulfate (Co-administration with other sympathomimetic agents increases the risk of adverse cardiovascular effects).
No products indexed under this heading.

Timolol Hemihydrate (Co-administration with beta blockers inhibits the effects of each other). Products include:
Betimol Ophthalmic Solution 3382
Betimol Ophthalmic Solution .... ⊙295

Timolol Maleate (Co-administration with beta blockers inhibits the effects of each other). Products include:
Blocadren Tablets 1916
Cosopt Sterile Ophthalmic Solution 1931
Timolide Tablets 2086
Timoptic Sterile Ophthalmic Solution 2088
Timoptic in Ocudose 2091
Timoptic-XE Sterile Ophthalmic Gel Forming Solution 2092

Tolterodine Tartrate (Co-administration has some potential for additive anticholinergic effects; caution is advised). Products include:
Detrol Tablets 2628
Detrol LA Capsules 2631

Torsemide (Co-administration with non-potassium-sparing diuretics can result in acute worsening of ECG changes and/or hypokalemia, especially when recommended dose of the beta agonist is exceeded; clinical significance of this interaction is unknown). Products include:
Demadex Injection 2759
Demadex Tablets 2759

Tranylcypromine Sulfate (Co-administration with MAO inhibitors can potentiate the action of albuterol on the cardiovascular system). Products include:
Parnate Tablets 1527

Tridihexethyl Chloride (Co-administration has some potential for additive anticholinergic effects; caution is advised).
No products indexed under this heading.

Trihexyphenidyl Hydrochloride (Co-administration has some potential for additive anticholinergic effects; caution is advised).
No products indexed under this heading.

Trimipramine Maleate (Co-administration with tricyclic antidepressant can potentiate the action of albuterol on the cardiovascular system).
No products indexed under this heading.

COMBIVIR TABLETS

(Lamivudine, Zidovudine) 1411

May interact with cytotoxic drugs, interferon alpha, and certain other agents. Compounds in these categories include:

Bleomycin Sulfate (May increase the hematologic toxicity of zidovudine).
No products indexed under this heading.

Bone Marrow Depressants, unspecified (May increase the hematologic toxicity of zidovudine).
No products indexed under this heading.

Cyclophosphamide (May increase the hematologic toxicity of zidovudine).
No products indexed under this heading.

Daunorubicin Hydrochloride (May increase the hematologic toxicity of zidovudine).
No products indexed under this heading.

Doxorubicin Hydrochloride (Co-administration should be avoided since an antagonistic relationship with zidovudine has been demonstrated in vitro; may increase the hematologic toxicity of zidovudine).
No products indexed under this heading.

Epirubicin Hydrochloride (May increase the hematologic toxicity of zidovudine).
No products indexed under this heading.

Fluorouracil (May increase the hematologic toxicity of zidovudine). Products include:
Carac Cream, 0.5% 2879
Efudex 3363

Ganciclovir Sodium (May increase the hematologic toxicity of zidovudine).
No products indexed under this heading.

Hydroxyurea (May increase the hematologic toxicity of zidovudine).
No products indexed under this heading.

Interferon alfa-2a, Recombinant (Hepatic decompensation has occurred in HIV/HCV co-infected patients receiving combination antiretroviral therapy for HIV and interferon alpha with or without ribavirin. Patients receiving interferon alpha with or without ribavirin and Combivir should be closely monitored for treatment-associated toxicities, especially hepatic decompensation, neutropenia, and anemia. Discontinuation of Combivir should be considered as medically appropriate. Discontinuation of interferon alpha, ribavirin, or both should also be considered if worsening clinical toxicities are observed, including hepatic decompensation (e.g., Childs Pugh greater than 6)).
No products indexed under this heading.

Interferon alfa-2b, Recombinant (Hepatic decompensation has occurred in HIV/HCV co-infected patients receiving combination antiretroviral therapy for HIV and interferon alpha with or without ribavirin. Patients receiving interferon alpha with or without ribavirin and Combivir should be closely monitored for treatment-associated toxicities, especially hepatic decompensation, neutropenia, and anemia. Discontinuation of Combivir should be considered as medically appropriate. Discontinuation of interferon alpha, ribavirin, or both should also be considered if worsening clinical toxicities are observed, including hepatic decompensation (e.g., Childs Pugh greater than 6)). Products include:
Intron A for Injection 3024
Rebetron Combination Therapy 3063

Interferon alfa-N3 (Human Leukocyte Derived) (Hepatic decompensation has occurred in HIV/HCV co-infected patients receiving combination antiretroviral therapy for HIV and interferon alpha with or without ribavirin. Patients receiving interferon alpha with or without ribavirin and Combivir should be closely monitored for treatment-associated toxicities, especially hepatic decompensation, neutropenia, and anemia. Discontinuation of Combivir should be considered as medically appropriate. Discontinuation of interferon alpha, ribavirin, or both should also be considered if worsening clinical toxicities are observed, including hepatic decompensation (e.g., Childs Pugh greater than 6)). Products include:
Alferon N Injection 1665

Methotrexate Sodium (May increase the hematologic toxicity of zidovudine).
No products indexed under this heading.

Mitotane (May increase the hematologic toxicity of zidovudine).
No products indexed under this heading.

Mitoxantrone Hydrochloride (May increase the hematologic toxicity of zidovudine).
No products indexed under this heading.

Peginterferon Alfa-2b (Hepatic decompensation has occurred in HIV/HCV co-infected patients receiving combination antiretroviral therapy for HIV and interferon alpha with or without ribavirin. Patients receiving interferon alpha with or without ribavirin and Combivir should be closely monitored for treatment-associated toxicities, especially hepatic decompensation, neutropenia, and anemia. Discontinuation of Combivir should be considered as medically appropriate. Discontinuation of interferon alpha, ribavirin, or both should also be considered if worsening clinical toxicities are observed, including hepatic decompensation (e.g., Childs Pugh greater than 6)). Products include:
PEG-Intron Powder for Injection 3048

Procarbazine Hydrochloride (May increase the hematologic toxicity of zidovudine). Products include:
Matulane Capsules 3191

Ribavirin (Co-administration should be avoided since an antagonistic relationship with zidovudine has been demonstrated in vitro). Products include:
Copegus Tablets 2754
Rebetol 3058
Rebetron Combination Therapy 3063
Ribavirin, USP Capsules 3068
Virazole for Inhalation Solution 3370

Stavudine (Co-administration should be avoided since an antagonistic relationship with zidovudine has been demonstrated in vitro).
No products indexed under this heading.

Sulfamethoxazole (Co-administration with TMP/SMX has been shown to increase lamivudine exposure).
No products indexed under this heading.

Tamoxifen Citrate (May increase the hematologic toxicity of zidovudine). Products include:
Soltamox Oral Solution 3527

Trimethoprim (Co-administration with TMP/SMX has been shown to increase lamivudine exposure).
No products indexed under this heading.

Vincristine Sulfate (May increase the hematologic toxicity of zidovudine).
No products indexed under this heading.

Zalacitabine (Lamivudine and zalacitabine may inhibit the intracellular phosphorylation of one another; combination therapy is not recommended).
No products indexed under this heading.

COMTAN TABLETS

(Entacapone) 2189

May interact with central nervous system depressants, drugs metabolized by Catechol-O-methyltransferase, erythromycin, nonselective MAO inhibitors, and certain other agents. Compounds in these categories include:

Alfentanil Hydrochloride (Possible additive sedative effects).
No products indexed under this heading.

Alprazolam (Possible additive sedative effects). Products include:
Niravam Orally Disintegrating Tablets 3092

Ampicillin Sodium (As most entacapone excretion is via bile, co-administration with drugs known to interfere with biliary excretion, glucuronidation, and intestinal beta-glucuronidation, such as ampicillin, requires caution).
No products indexed under this heading.

Apomorphine (Co-administration of drugs that are metabolized by catechol-O-methyltransferase (COMT) may result in increased heart rates, possibly arrhythmias, and excessive changes in blood pressure).
No products indexed under this heading.

Aprobarbital (Possible additive sedative effects).
No products indexed under this heading.

Bitolterol Mesylate (Co-administration of drugs that are metabolized by catechol-O-methyltransferase (COMT) may result in increased heart rates, possibly arrhythmias, and excessive changes in blood pressure).
No products indexed under this heading.

Buprenorphine Hydrochloride (Possible additive sedative effects). Products include:
Buprenex Injectable 2716
Suboxone Tablets 2717
Subutex Tablets 2717

Buspirone Hydrochloride (Possible additive sedative effects).
No products indexed under this heading.

Butabarbital (Possible additive sedative effects).
No products indexed under this heading.

Butalbital (Possible additive sedative effects).
No products indexed under this heading.

Chloramphenicol Sodium Succinate (As most entacapone excretion is via bile, co-administration with drugs known to interfere with biliary excretion, glucuronidation, and intestinal beta-glucuronidation, such as chloramphenicol, requires caution).
No products indexed under this heading.

Chlordiazepoxide (Possible additive sedative effects).
No products indexed under this heading.

Chlordiazepoxide Hydrochloride (Possible additive sedative effects). Products include:
Librium Capsules 3347

Chlorpromazine (Possible additive sedative effects).
No products indexed under this heading.

Chlorpromazine Hydrochloride (Possible additive sedative effects).
No products indexed under this heading.

Chlorprothixene (Possible additive sedative effects).
No products indexed under this heading.

Chlorprothixene Hydrochloride (Possible additive sedative effects).
No products indexed under this heading.

Chlorprothixene Lactate (Possible additive sedative effects).
No products indexed under this heading.

Cholestyramine (As most entacapone excretion is via bile, co-administration with drugs known to interfere with biliary excretion, glucuronidation, and intestinal beta-glucuronidation, such as cholestyramine, requires caution).
No products indexed under this heading.

Clorazepate Dipotassium (Possible additive sedative effects). Products include:
Tranxene 2474

Clozapine (Possible additive sedative effects). Products include:
Clozaril Tablets 2184
FazaClo Orally Disintegrating Tablets 551

Codeine Phosphate (Possible additive sedative effects). Products include:
Tylenol with Codeine Tablets 2391

Desflurane (Possible additive sedative effects).
No products indexed under this heading.

Dezocine (Possible additive sedative effects).
No products indexed under this heading.

Diazepam (Possible additive sedative effects). Products include:
Diastat Rectal Delivery System 3343
Valium Tablets 2819

Dobutamine Hydrochloride (Co-administration of drugs that are metabolized by catechol-O-methyltransferase (COMT) may result in increased heart rates, possibly arrhythmias, and excessive changes in blood pressure).
No products indexed under this heading.

Dopamine Hydrochloride (Co-administration of drugs that are metabolized by catechol-O-methyltransferase (COMT) may result in increased heart rates, possibly arrhythmias, and excessive changes in blood pressure).
No products indexed under this heading.

Droperidol (Possible additive sedative effects).
No products indexed under this heading.

Enflurane (Possible additive sedative effects).
No products indexed under this heading.

Epinephrine (Co-administration of drugs that are metabolized by catechol-O-methyltransferase (COMT) may result in increased heart rates, possibly arrhythmias, and excessive changes in blood pressure; concurrent use of epinephrine infusion has resulted in a case report of ventricular tachycardia). Products include:
EpiPen 1061
Primatene Mist .... ▣ 719
Twinject 0.15 3379
Twinject 0.3 3378

Epinephrine Bitartrate (Co-administration of drugs that are metabolized by catechol-O-methyltransferase (COMT) may result in increased heart rates, possibly arrhythmias, and excessive changes in blood pressure; concurrent use of epinephrine infusion has resulted in a case report of ventricular tachycardia).
No products indexed under this heading.

Epinephrine Hydrochloride (Co-administration of drugs that are metabolized by catechol-O-methyltransferase (COMT) may result in increased heart rates, possibly arrhythmias, and excessive changes in blood pressure; concurrent use of epinephrine infusion has resulted in a case report of ventricular tachycardia).
No products indexed under this heading.

Erythromycin (As most entacapone excretion is via bile, co-administration with drugs known to interfere with biliary excretion, glucuronidation, and intestinal beta-glucuronidation, such as erythromycin, requires caution). Products include:
Ery-Tab Tablets 449
Erythromycin Base Filmtab Tablets 455
Erythromycin Delayed-Release Capsules, USP 457
PCE Dispertab Tablets 515

Erythromycin Estolate (As most entacapone excretion is via bile, co-administration with drugs known to interfere with biliary excretion, glucuronidation, and intestinal beta-glucuronidation, such as erythromycin, requires caution).
No products indexed under this heading.

Erythromycin Ethylsuccinate (As most entacapone excretion is via bile, co-administration with drugs known to interfere with biliary excretion, glucuronidation, and intestinal beta-glucuronidation, such as erythromycin, requires caution). Products include:
E.E.S. 451
EryPed 447

Erythromycin Gluceptate (As most entacapone excretion is via bile, co-administration with drugs known to interfere with biliary excretion, glucuronidation, and intestinal beta-glucuronidation, such as erythromycin, requires caution).
No products indexed under this heading.

Erythromycin Lactobionate (As most entacapone excretion is via bile, co-administration with drugs known to interfere with biliary excretion, glucuronidation, and intestinal beta-glucuronidation, such as erythromycin, requires caution).
No products indexed under this heading.

Erythromycin Stearate (As most entacapone excretion is via bile, co-administration with drugs known to interfere with biliary excretion, glucuronidation, and intestinal beta-glucuronidation, such as erythromycin, requires caution). Products include:
Erythrocin Stearate Filmtab Tablets 453

Estazolam (Possible additive sedative effects). Products include:

ProSom Tablets 517

Ethanol (Possible additive sedative effects).
No products indexed under this heading.

Ethchlorvynol (Possible additive sedative effects).
No products indexed under this heading.

Ethinamate (Possible additive sedative effects).
No products indexed under this heading.

Ethyl Alcohol (Possible additive sedative effects).
No products indexed under this heading.

Fentanyl (Possible additive sedative effects). Products include:
Duragesic Transdermal System 2373
Ionsys Transdermal System 2379

Fentanyl Citrate (Possible additive sedative effects). Products include:
Actiq 979

Fluphenazine Decanoate (Possible additive sedative effects).
No products indexed under this heading.

Fluphenazine Enanthate (Possible additive sedative effects).
No products indexed under this heading.

Fluphenazine Hydrochloride (Possible additive sedative effects).
No products indexed under this heading.

Flurazepam Hydrochloride (Possible additive sedative effects). Products include:
Dalmane Capsules 3342

Glutethimide (Possible additive sedative effects).
No products indexed under this heading.

Haloperidol (Possible additive sedative effects).
No products indexed under this heading.

Haloperidol Decanoate (Possible additive sedative effects).
No products indexed under this heading.

Hydrocodone Bitartrate (Possible additive sedative effects). Products include:
Hycodan 1116
Hycotuss Expectorant Syrup 1117
Vicodin Tablets 535
Vicodin ES Tablets 536
Vicodin HP Tablets 538
Vicoprofen Tablets 539
Zydone Tablets 1139

Hydrocodone Polistirex (Possible additive sedative effects). Products include:
Tussionex Pennkinetic Extended-Release Suspension 3327

Hydromorphone Hydrochloride (Possible additive sedative effects). Products include:
Dilaudid 440
Dilaudid Non-Sterile Powder 440
Dilaudid Oral Liquid 445
Dilaudid Rectal Suppositories 440
Dilaudid Tablets 440
Dilaudid Tablets - 8 mg 445
Dilaudid-HP 442

Hydroxyzine Hydrochloride (Possible additive sedative effects).
No products indexed under this heading.

Isocarboxazid (Co-administration of non-selective MAO inhibitors with entacapone would result in inhibition of the majority of the pathways responsible for normal catecholamine metabolism; concurrent use should be avoided).
No products indexed under this heading.

Isoetharine (Co-administration of drugs that are metabolized by catechol-O-methyltransferase (COMT) may result in increased heart rates, possibly arrhythmias, and excessive changes in blood pressure).
No products indexed under this heading.

Isoflurane (Possible additive sedative effects).
No products indexed under this heading.

Isoproterenol Hydrochloride (Co-administration of drugs that are metabolized by catechol-O-methyltransferase (COMT) may result in increased heart rates, possibly arrhythmias, and excessive changes in blood pressure).
No products indexed under this heading.

Isoproterenol Sulfate (Co-administration of drugs that are metabolized by catechol-O-methyltransferase (COMT) may result in increased heart rates, possibly arrhythmias, and excessive changes in blood pressure).
No products indexed under this heading.

Ketamine Hydrochloride (Possible additive sedative effects).
No products indexed under this heading.

Levodopa (Entacapone enhances levodopa bioavailability and, therefore, might be expected to increase the occurence of orthostatic hypotension). Products include:
Parcopa Orally Disintegrating Tablets 3097
Stalevo Tablets 2287

Levomethadyl Acetate Hydrochloride (Possible additive sedative effects).
No products indexed under this heading.

Levorphanol Tartrate (Possible additive sedative effects).
No products indexed under this heading.

Lorazepam (Possible additive sedative effects).
No products indexed under this heading.

Loxapine Hydrochloride (Possible additive sedative effects).
No products indexed under this heading.

Loxapine Succinate (Possible additive sedative effects).
No products indexed under this heading.

Meperidine Hydrochloride (Possible additive sedative effects).
No products indexed under this heading.

Mephobarbital (Possible additive sedative effects).
No products indexed under this heading.

Meprobamate (Possible additive sedative effects).
No products indexed under this heading.

Mesoridazine Besylate (Possible additive sedative effects).
No products indexed under this heading.

Methadone Hydrochloride (Possible additive sedative effects).
No products indexed under this heading.

Methohexital Sodium (Possible additive sedative effects).
No products indexed under this heading.

Methotrimeprazine (Possible additive sedative effects).
No products indexed under this heading.

Methoxyflurane (Possible additive sedative effects).
No products indexed under this heading.

Methyldopa (Co-administration of drugs that are metabolized by catechol-O-methyltransferase (COMT) may result in increased heart rates, possibly arrhythmias, and excessive changes in blood pressure). Products include:
Aldoril Tablets 1910

Midazolam Hydrochloride (Possible additive sedative effects).
No products indexed under this heading.

Molindone Hydrochloride (Possible additive sedative effects). Products include:
Moban Tablets 1119

Morphine Sulfate (Possible additive sedative effects). Products include:
Avinza Capsules 1741
Kadian Capsules 577
MS Contin Tablets 2701

Norepinephrine Bitartrate (Co-administration of drugs that are metabolized by catechol-O-methyltransferase (COMT) may result in increased heart rates, possibly arrhythmias, and excessive changes in blood pressure).
No products indexed under this heading.

Olanzapine (Possible additive sedative effects). Products include:
Symbyax Capsules 1819
Zyprexa Tablets 1830
Zyprexa IntraMuscular 1830
Zyprexa ZYDIS Orally Disintegrating Tablets 1830

Oxazepam (Possible additive sedative effects).
No products indexed under this heading.

Oxycodone Hydrochloride (Possible additive sedative effects). Products include:
OxyContin Tablets 2703
OxyFast Oral Concentrate Solution 2708
OxyIR Capsules 2708
Percocet Tablets 1131
Percodan Tablets 1132

Pargyline Hydrochloride (Co-administration of non-selective MAO inhibitors with entacapone would result in inhibition of the majority of the pathways responsible for normal catecholamine metabolism; concurrent use should be avoided).
No products indexed under this heading.

Pentobarbital Sodium (Possible additive sedative effects). Products include:
Nembutal Sodium Solution, USP 2470

Perphenazine (Possible additive sedative effects).
No products indexed under this heading.

Phenelzine Sulfate (Co-administration of non-selective MAO inhibitors with entacapone would result in inhibition of the majority of the pathways responsible for normal catecholamine metabolism; concurrent use should be avoided).
No products indexed under this heading.

Phenobarbital (Possible additive sedative effects). Products include:
Donnatal Extentabs 2493

Prazepam (Possible additive sedative effects).
No products indexed under this heading.

Probenecid (As most entacapone excretion is via bile, co-administration with drugs known to interfere with biliary excretion, glucuronidation, and intestinal beta-glucuronidation, such as probenecid, requires caution).
No products indexed under this heading.

Procarbazine Hydrochloride (Co-administration of non-selective MAO inhibitors with entacapone would result in inhibition of the majority of the pathways responsible for normal catecholamine metabolism; concurrent use should be avoided). Products include:
Matulane Capsules 3191

Prochlorperazine (Possible additive sedative effects).
No products indexed under this heading.

Promethazine Hydrochloride (Possible additive sedative effects). Products include:
Phenergan Tablets and Suppositories.............................. 3440

Propofol (Possible additive sedative effects).
No products indexed under this heading.

Propoxyphene Hydrochloride (Possible additive sedative effects).
No products indexed under this heading.

Propoxyphene Napsylate (Possible additive sedative effects).
No products indexed under this heading.

Quazepam (Possible additive sedative effects).
No products indexed under this heading.

Quetiapine Fumarate (Possible additive sedative effects). Products include:
Seroquel Tablets 690

Remifentanil Hydrochloride (Possible additive sedative effects).
No products indexed under this heading.

Rifampin (As most entacapone excretion is via bile, co-administration with drugs known to interfere with biliary excretion, glucuronidation, and intestinal beta-glucuronidation, such as rifampin, requires caution).
No products indexed under this heading.

Risperidone (Possible additive sedative effects). Products include:
Risperdal 1676
Risperdal Consta Long-Acting Injection 1682

Risperdal M-Tab Orally Disintegrating Tablets **1676**

Secobarbital Sodium (Possible additive sedative effects).
No products indexed under this heading.

Sevoflurane (Possible additive sedative effects). Products include:
Ultane Liquid for Inhalation **531**

Sufentanil Citrate (Possible additive sedative effects).
No products indexed under this heading.

Temazepam (Possible additive sedative effects). Products include:
Restoril Capsules **1860**

Thiamylal Sodium (Possible additive sedative effects).
No products indexed under this heading.

Thioridazine Hydrochloride (Possible additive sedative effects). Products include:
Thioridazine Hydrochloride Tablets **2163**

Thiothixene (Possible additive sedative effects). Products include:
Thiothixene Capsules **2165**

Tranylcypromine Sulfate (Co-administration of non-selective MAO inhibitors with entacapone would result in inhibition of the majority of the pathways responsible for normal catecholamine metabolism; concurrent use should be avoided). Products include:
Parnate Tablets **1527**

Triazolam (Possible additive sedative effects).
No products indexed under this heading.

Trifluoperazine Hydrochloride (Possible additive sedative effects).
No products indexed under this heading.

Zaleplon (Possible additive sedative effects). Products include:
Sonata Capsules **1717**

Ziprasidone Hydrochloride (Possible additive sedative effects). Products include:
Geodon Capsules **2529**

Zolpidem Tartrate (Possible additive sedative effects). Products include:
Ambien Tablets **2851**
Ambien CR Tablets **2855**

Food Interactions

Alcohol (Possible additive sedative effects).

COMTREX MAXIMUM STRENGTH COLD & COUGH DAY/NIGHT CAPLETS - DAY FORMULATION

(Acetaminophen, Dextromethorphan Hydrobromide, Pseudoephedrine Hydrochloride)....... ■□**726**

May interact with hypnotics and sedatives, monoamine oxidase inhibitors, and certain other agents. Compounds in these categories include:

Estazolam (Concurrent use may increase drowsiness). Products include:
ProSom Tablets **517**

Ethchlorvynol (Concurrent use may increase drowsiness).
No products indexed under this heading.

Ethinamate (Concurrent use may increase drowsiness).
No products indexed under this heading.

Flurazepam Hydrochloride (Concurrent use may increase drowsiness). Products include:
Dalmane Capsules **3342**

Glutethimide (Concurrent use may increase drowsiness).
No products indexed under this heading.

Isocarboxazid (Avoid with MAO inhibitors, or for 2 weeks after stopping MAO inhibitors).
No products indexed under this heading.

Lorazepam (Concurrent use may increase drowsiness).
No products indexed under this heading.

Midazolam Hydrochloride (Concurrent use may increase drowsiness).
No products indexed under this heading.

Moclobemide (Avoid with MAO inhibitors, or for 2 weeks after stopping MAO inhibitors).
No products indexed under this heading.

Pargyline Hydrochloride (Avoid with MAO inhibitors, or for 2 weeks after stopping MAO inhibitors).
No products indexed under this heading.

Phenelzine Sulfate (Avoid with MAO inhibitors, or for 2 weeks after stopping MAO inhibitors).
No products indexed under this heading.

Procarbazine Hydrochloride (Avoid with MAO inhibitors, or for 2 weeks after stopping MAO inhibitors). Products include:
Matulane Capsules **3191**

Propofol (Concurrent use may increase drowsiness).
No products indexed under this heading.

Quazepam (Concurrent use may increase drowsiness).
No products indexed under this heading.

Ramelteon (Concurrent use may increase drowsiness). Products include:
Rozerem Tablets **3231**

Secobarbital Sodium (Concurrent use may increase drowsiness).
No products indexed under this heading.

Selegiline Hydrochloride (Avoid with MAO inhibitors, or for 2 weeks after stopping MAO inhibitors). Products include:
Eldepryl Capsules **3208**
Zelapar Tablets **3372**

Temazepam (Concurrent use may increase drowsiness). Products include:
Restoril Capsules **1860**

Tranylcypromine Sulfate (Avoid with MAO inhibitors, or for 2 weeks after stopping MAO inhibitors). Products include:
Parnate Tablets **1527**

Triazolam (Concurrent use may increase drowsiness).
No products indexed under this heading.

Zaleplon (Concurrent use may increase drowsiness). Products include:
Sonata Capsules **1717**

Zolpidem Tartrate (Concurrent use may increase drowsiness). Products include:
Ambien Tablets **2851**
Ambien CR Tablets **2855**

Food Interactions

Alcohol (Concurrent use may increase drowsiness).

COMTREX MAXIMUM STRENGTH COLD & COUGH DAY/NIGHT CAPLETS - NIGHT FORMULATION

(Acetaminophen, Chlorpheniramine Maleate, Dextromethorphan Hydrobromide, Pseudoephedrine Hydrochloride)....... ■□**726**

May interact with hypnotics and sedatives, monoamine oxidase inhibitors, and certain other agents. Compounds in these categories include:

Estazolam (Concurrent use may increase drowsiness). Products include:
ProSom Tablets **517**

Ethchlorvynol (Concurrent use may increase drowsiness).
No products indexed under this heading.

Ethinamate (Concurrent use may increase drowsiness).
No products indexed under this heading.

Flurazepam Hydrochloride (Concurrent use may increase drowsiness). Products include:
Dalmane Capsules **3342**

Glutethimide (Concurrent use may increase drowsiness).
No products indexed under this heading.

Isocarboxazid (Avoid with MAO inhibitors, or for 2 weeks after stopping MAO inhibitors).
No products indexed under this heading.

Lorazepam (Concurrent use may increase drowsiness).
No products indexed under this heading.

Midazolam Hydrochloride (Concurrent use may increase drowsiness).
No products indexed under this heading.

Moclobemide (Avoid with MAO inhibitors, or for 2 weeks after stopping MAO inhibitors).
No products indexed under this heading.

Pargyline Hydrochloride (Avoid with MAO inhibitors, or for 2 weeks after stopping MAO inhibitors).
No products indexed under this heading.

Phenelzine Sulfate (Avoid with MAO inhibitors, or for 2 weeks after stopping MAO inhibitors).
No products indexed under this heading.

Procarbazine Hydrochloride (Avoid with MAO inhibitors, or for 2 weeks after stopping MAO inhibitors). Products include:
Matulane Capsules **3191**

Propofol (Concurrent use may increase drowsiness).
No products indexed under this heading.

Quazepam (Concurrent use may increase drowsiness).
No products indexed under this heading.

Ramelteon (Concurrent use may increase drowsiness). Products include:
Rozerem Tablets **3231**

Secobarbital Sodium (Concurrent use may increase drowsiness).
No products indexed under this heading.

Selegiline Hydrochloride (Avoid with MAO inhibitors, or for 2 weeks after stopping MAO inhibitors). Products include:
Eldepryl Capsules **3208**
Zelapar Tablets **3372**

Temazepam (Concurrent use may increase drowsiness). Products include:
Restoril Capsules **1860**

Tranylcypromine Sulfate (Avoid with MAO inhibitors, or for 2 weeks after stopping MAO inhibitors). Products include:
Parnate Tablets **1527**

Triazolam (Concurrent use may increase drowsiness).
No products indexed under this heading.

Zaleplon (Concurrent use may increase drowsiness). Products include:
Sonata Capsules **1717**

Zolpidem Tartrate (Concurrent use may increase drowsiness). Products include:
Ambien Tablets **2851**
Ambien CR Tablets **2855**

Food Interactions

Alcohol (Concurrent use may increase drowsiness).

COMTREX MAXIMUM STRENGTH NON-DROWSY COLD & COUGH CAPLETS

(Acetaminophen, Dextromethorphan Hydrobromide, Phenylephrine Hydrochloride)........... ■□**725**

May interact with monoamine oxidase inhibitors and certain other agents. Compounds in these categories include:

Isocarboxazid (Do not use while taking, or 2 weeks after stopping, MAO inhibitors).
No products indexed under this heading.

Moclobemide (Do not use while taking, or 2 weeks after stopping, MAO inhibitors).
No products indexed under this heading.

Pargyline Hydrochloride (Do not use while taking, or 2 weeks after stopping, MAO inhibitors).
No products indexed under this heading.

Phenelzine Sulfate (Do not use while taking, or 2 weeks after stopping, MAO inhibitors).
No products indexed under this heading.

Procarbazine Hydrochloride (Do not use while taking, or 2 weeks after stopping, MAO inhibitors). Products include:
Matulane Capsules **3191**

Selegiline Hydrochloride (Do not use while taking, or 2 weeks after stopping, MAO inhibitors). Products include:
Eldepryl Capsules **3208**
Zelapar Tablets **3372**

Tranylcypromine Sulfate (Do not use while taking, or 2 weeks after stopping, MAO inhibitors). Products include:

Parnate Tablets 1527

Food Interactions

Alcohol (Chronic heavy alcohol users, 3 or more alcoholic drinks per day, should consult their physicians for advice on when and how to use pain relievers including acetaminophen).

COMTREX MAXIMUM STRENGTH DAY/NIGHT SEVERE COLD & SINUS CAPLETS - DAY FORMULATION

(Acetaminophen, Phenylephrine Hydrochloride)............................ 🔲 725
May interact with monoamine oxidase inhibitors and certain other agents. Compounds in these categories include:

Isocarboxazid (Do not use while taking, or 2 weeks after stopping, MAO inhibitors).
No products indexed under this heading.

Moclobemide (Do not use while taking, or 2 weeks after stopping, MAO inhibitors).
No products indexed under this heading.

Pargyline Hydrochloride (Do not use while taking, or 2 weeks after stopping, MAO inhibitors).
No products indexed under this heading.

Phenelzine Sulfate (Do not use while taking, or 2 weeks after stopping, MAO inhibitors).
No products indexed under this heading.

Procarbazine Hydrochloride (Do not use while taking, or 2 weeks after stopping, MAO inhibitors).
Products include:
Matulane Capsules 3191

Selegiline Hydrochloride (Do not use while taking, or 2 weeks after stopping, MAO inhibitors). Products include:
Eldepryl Capsules 3208
Zelapar Tablets 3372

Tranylcypromine Sulfate (Do not use while taking, or 2 weeks after stopping, MAO inhibitors). Products include:
Parnate Tablets 1527

Food Interactions

Alcohol (Chronic heavy alcohol users, 3 or more alcoholic drinks per day, should consult their physicians for advice on when and how to use pain relievers including acetaminophen).

COMTREX MAXIMUM STRENGTH DAY/NIGHT SEVERE COLD & SINUS CAPLETS - NIGHT FORMULATION

(Acetaminophen, Chlorpheniramine Maleate, Phenylephrine Hydrochloride)............ 🔲 725
May interact with hypnotics and sedatives, monoamine oxidase inhibitors, tranquilizers, and certain other agents. Compounds in these categories include:

Alprazolam (Concurrent use may increase drowsiness effect). Products include:
Niravam Orally Disintegrating Tablets 3092

Buspirone Hydrochloride (Concurrent use may increase drowsiness effect).
No products indexed under this heading.

Chlordiazepoxide (Concurrent use may increase drowsiness effect).
No products indexed under this heading.

Chlordiazepoxide Hydrochloride (Concurrent use may increase drowsiness effect). Products include:
Librium Capsules 3347

Chlorpromazine (Concurrent use may increase drowsiness effect).
No products indexed under this heading.

Chlorpromazine Hydrochloride (Concurrent use may increase drowsiness effect).
No products indexed under this heading.

Chlorprothixene (Concurrent use may increase drowsiness effect).
No products indexed under this heading.

Chlorprothixene Hydrochloride (Concurrent use may increase drowsiness effect).
No products indexed under this heading.

Clorazepate Dipotassium (Concurrent use may increase drowsiness effect). Products include:
Tranxene .. 2474

Diazepam (Concurrent use may increase drowsiness effect). Products include:
Diastat Rectal Delivery System 3343
Valium Tablets 2819

Droperidol (Concurrent use may increase drowsiness effect).
No products indexed under this heading.

Estazolam (Concurrent use may increase drowsiness effect). Products include:
ProSom Tablets 517

Ethchlorvynol (Concurrent use may increase drowsiness effect).
No products indexed under this heading.

Ethinamate (Concurrent use may increase drowsiness effect).
No products indexed under this heading.

Fluphenazine Decanoate (Concurrent use may increase drowsiness effect).
No products indexed under this heading.

Fluphenazine Enanthate (Concurrent use may increase drowsiness effect).
No products indexed under this heading.

Fluphenazine Hydrochloride (Concurrent use may increase drowsiness effect).
No products indexed under this heading.

Flurazepam Hydrochloride (Concurrent use may increase drowsiness effect). Products include:
Dalmane Capsules 3342

Glutethimide (Concurrent use may increase drowsiness effect).
No products indexed under this heading.

Haloperidol (Concurrent use may increase drowsiness effect).
No products indexed under this heading.

Haloperidol Decanoate (Concurrent use may increase drowsiness effect).
No products indexed under this heading.

Hydroxyzine Hydrochloride (Concurrent use may increase drowsiness effect).
No products indexed under this heading.

Isocarboxazid (Do not use while taking, or 2 weeks after stopping, MAO inhibitors).
No products indexed under this heading.

Lorazepam (Concurrent use may increase drowsiness effect).
No products indexed under this heading.

Loxapine Hydrochloride (Concurrent use may increase drowsiness effect).
No products indexed under this heading.

Loxapine Succinate (Concurrent use may increase drowsiness effect).
No products indexed under this heading.

Meprobamate (Concurrent use may increase drowsiness effect).
No products indexed under this heading.

Mesoridazine Besylate (Concurrent use may increase drowsiness effect).
No products indexed under this heading.

Midazolam Hydrochloride (Concurrent use may increase drowsiness effect).
No products indexed under this heading.

Moclobemide (Do not use while taking, or 2 weeks after stopping, MAO inhibitors).
No products indexed under this heading.

Molindone Hydrochloride (Concurrent use may increase drowsiness effect). Products include:
Moban Tablets 1119

Oxazepam (Concurrent use may increase drowsiness effect).
No products indexed under this heading.

Pargyline Hydrochloride (Do not use while taking, or 2 weeks after stopping, MAO inhibitors).
No products indexed under this heading.

Perphenazine (Concurrent use may increase drowsiness effect).
No products indexed under this heading.

Phenelzine Sulfate (Do not use while taking, or 2 weeks after stopping, MAO inhibitors).
No products indexed under this heading.

Prazepam (Concurrent use may increase drowsiness effect).
No products indexed under this heading.

Procarbazine Hydrochloride (Do not use while taking, or 2 weeks after stopping, MAO inhibitors).
Products include:
Matulane Capsules 3191

Prochlorperazine (Concurrent use may increase drowsiness effect).
No products indexed under this heading.

Promethazine Hydrochloride (Concurrent use may increase drowsiness effect). Products include:
Phenergan Tablets and Suppositories 3440

Propofol (Concurrent use may increase drowsiness effect).
No products indexed under this heading.

Quazepam (Concurrent use may increase drowsiness effect).
No products indexed under this heading.

Ramelteon (Concurrent use may increase drowsiness effect). Products include:
Rozerem Tablets 3231

Secobarbital Sodium (Concurrent use may increase drowsiness effect).
No products indexed under this heading.

Selegiline Hydrochloride (Do not use while taking, or 2 weeks after stopping, MAO inhibitors). Products include:
Eldepryl Capsules 3208
Zelapar Tablets 3372

Temazepam (Concurrent use may increase drowsiness effect). Products include:
Restoril Capsules 1860

Thioridazine Hydrochloride (Concurrent use may increase drowsiness effect). Products include:
Thioridazine Hydrochloride Tablets .. 2163

Thiothixene (Concurrent use may increase drowsiness effect). Products include:
Thiothixene Capsules 2165

Tranylcypromine Sulfate (Do not use while taking, or 2 weeks after stopping, MAO inhibitors). Products include:
Parnate Tablets 1527

Triazolam (Concurrent use may increase drowsiness effect).
No products indexed under this heading.

Trifluoperazine Hydrochloride (Concurrent use may increase drowsiness effect).
No products indexed under this heading.

Zaleplon (Concurrent use may increase drowsiness effect). Products include:
Sonata Capsules 1717

Zolpidem Tartrate (Concurrent use may increase drowsiness effect). Products include:
Ambien Tablets 2851
Ambien CR Tablets 2855

Food Interactions

Alcohol (Chronic heavy alcohol users, 3 or more alcoholic drinks per day, should consult their physicians for advice on when and how to use pain relievers including acetaminophen; concurrent use may increase drowsiness effect).

COMVAX

(Haemophilus B Conjugate Vaccine, Hepatitis B Vaccine, Recombinant)................................. 1928
May interact with immunosuppressive agents. Compounds in these categories include:

Azathioprine (Deferral of immunization may be considered in individuals receiving immunosuppresive therapy).
No products indexed under this heading.

Basiliximab (Deferral of immunization may be considered in individuals receiving immunosuppresive therapy). Products include:

Simulect for Injection 2284

Cyclosporine (Deferral of immunization may be considered in individuals receiving immunosuppresive therapy). Products include:
Gengraf Capsules 459
Neoral Oral Solution 2259
Neoral Soft Gelatin Capsules 2259
Restasis Ophthalmic Emulsion 575
Sandimmune 2275

Muromonab-CD3 (Deferral of immunization may be considered in individuals receiving immunosuppresive therapy). Products include:
Orthoclone OKT3 Sterile Solution 2360

Mycophenolate Mofetil (Deferral of immunization may be considered in individuals receiving immunosuppresive therapy). Products include:
CellCept Capsules 2747
CellCept Oral Suspension 2747
CellCept Tablets 2747

Sirolimus (Deferral of immunization may be considered in individuals receiving immunosuppresive therapy). Products include:
Rapamune Oral Solution and Tablets 3475

Tacrolimus (Deferral of immunization may be considered in individuals receiving immunosuppresive therapy). Products include:
Prograf Capsules and Injection 632
Protopic Ointment 638

CONCERTA EXTENDED-RELEASE TABLETS

(Methylphenidate Hydrochloride) 1881

May interact with oral anticoagulants, monoamine oxidase inhibitors, phenytoin, selective serotonin reuptake inhibitors, tricyclic antidepressants, vasopressors, and certain other agents. Compounds in these categories include:

Amitriptyline Hydrochloride (Methylphenidate may inhibit the metabolism of certain tricyclic antidepressants; downward dosage adjustment of tricyclic antidepressants may be required).
No products indexed under this heading.

Amoxapine (Methylphenidate may inhibit the metabolism of certain tricyclic antidepressants; downward dosage adjustment of tricyclic antidepressants may be required).
No products indexed under this heading.

Anisindione (Methylphenidate may inhibit the metabolism of coumarin anticoagulants; downward dosage adjustment of anticoagulants may be required). Products include:
Miradon Tablets 3042

Citalopram Hydrobromide (Methylphenidate may inhibit the metabolism of certain selective serotonin reuptake inhibitors; downward dosage adjustment of these drugs may be required). Products include:
Celexa 1176

Clomipramine Hydrochloride (Methylphenidate may inhibit the metabolism of certain tricyclic antidepressants; downward dosage adjustment of tricyclic antidepressants may be required).
No products indexed under this heading.

Clonidine (Serious adverse events have been reported in concomitant use with clonidine, although no causality for the combination has been established). Products include:
Catapres-TTS 844

Clonidine Hydrochloride (Serious adverse events have been reported in concomitant use with clonidine, although no causality for the combination has been established). Products include:
Catapres Tablets 843
Clorpres Tablets 2153

Desipramine Hydrochloride (Methylphenidate may inhibit the metabolism of certain tricyclic antidepressants; downward dosage adjustment of tricyclic antidepressants may be required).
No products indexed under this heading.

Dicumarol (Methylphenidate may inhibit the metabolism of coumarin anticoagulants; downward dosage adjustment of anticoagulants may be required).
No products indexed under this heading.

Dobutamine (Methylphenidate causes a rise in blood pressure; co-administration with other pressor agents should be undertaken with caution).
No products indexed under this heading.

Dobutamine Hydrochloride (Methylphenidate causes a rise in blood pressure; co-administration with other pressor agents should be undertaken with caution).
No products indexed under this heading.

Dopamine Hydrochloride (Methylphenidate causes a rise in blood pressure; co-administration with other pressor agents should be undertaken with caution).
No products indexed under this heading.

Doxepin Hydrochloride (Methylphenidate may inhibit the metabolism of certain tricyclic antidepressants; downward dosage adjustment of tricyclic antidepressants may be required).
No products indexed under this heading.

Ephedrine Sulfate (Methylphenidate causes a rise in blood pressure; co-administration with other pressor agents should be undertaken with caution).
No products indexed under this heading.

Epinephrine Bitartrate (Methylphenidate causes a rise in blood pressure; co-administration with other pressor agents should be undertaken with caution).
No products indexed under this heading.

Epinephrine Hydrochloride (Methylphenidate causes a rise in blood pressure; co-administration with other pressor agents should be undertaken with caution).
No products indexed under this heading.

Escitalopram Oxalate (Methylphenidate may inhibit the metabolism of certain selective serotonin reuptake inhibitors; downward dosage adjustment of these drugs may be required). Products include:
Lexapro Oral Solution 1190
Lexapro Tablets 1190

Fluoxetine Hydrochloride (Methylphenidate may inhibit the metabolism of certain selective serotonin reuptake inhibitors; downward dosage adjustment of these drugs may be required). Products include:
Prozac Pulvules and Liquid 1801
Symbyax Capsules 1819

Fluvoxamine Maleate (Methylphenidate may inhibit the metabolism of certain selective serotonin reuptake inhibitors; downward dosage adjustment of these drugs may be required).
No products indexed under this heading.

Fosphenytoin Sodium (Methylphenidate may inhibit the metabolism of phenytoin; downward dosage adjustment of phenytoin may be required).
No products indexed under this heading.

Imipramine Hydrochloride (Methylphenidate may inhibit the metabolism of certain tricyclic antidepressants; downward dosage adjustment of tricyclic antidepressants may be required).
No products indexed under this heading.

Imipramine Pamoate (Methylphenidate may inhibit the metabolism of certain tricyclic antidepressants; downward dosage adjustment of tricyclic antidepressants may be required).
No products indexed under this heading.

Isocarboxazid (Co-administration with MAO inhibitors may result in hypertensive crises; concurrent and/or sequential use is contraindicated).
No products indexed under this heading.

Isoproterenol Hydrochloride (Methylphenidate causes a rise in blood pressure; co-administration with other pressor agents should be undertaken with caution).
No products indexed under this heading.

Isoproterenol Sulfate (Methylphenidate causes a rise in blood pressure; co-administration with other pressor agents should be undertaken with caution).
No products indexed under this heading.

Maprotiline Hydrochloride (Methylphenidate may inhibit the metabolism of certain tricyclic antidepressants; downward dosage adjustment of tricyclic antidepressants may be required).
No products indexed under this heading.

Mephentermine Sulfate (Methylphenidate causes a rise in blood pressure; co-administration with other pressor agents should be undertaken with caution).
No products indexed under this heading.

Metaraminol Bitartrate (Methylphenidate causes a rise in blood pressure; co-administration with other pressor agents should be undertaken with caution).
No products indexed under this heading.

Methoxamine Hydrochloride (Methylphenidate causes a rise in blood pressure; co-administration with other pressor agents should be undertaken with caution).
No products indexed under this heading.

Moclobemide (Co-administration with MAO inhibitors may result in hypertensive crises; concurrent and/or sequential use is contraindicated).
No products indexed under this heading.

Norepinephrine Bitartrate (Methylphenidate causes a rise in blood pressure; co-administration with other pressor agents should be undertaken with caution).
No products indexed under this heading.

Nortriptyline Hydrochloride (Methylphenidate may inhibit the metabolism of certain tricyclic antidepressants; downward dosage adjustment of tricyclic antidepressants may be required).
No products indexed under this heading.

Pargyline Hydrochloride (Co-administration with MAO inhibitors may result in hypertensive crises; concurrent and/or sequential use is contraindicated).
No products indexed under this heading.

Paroxetine Hydrochloride (Methylphenidate may inhibit the metabolism of certain selective serotonin reuptake inhibitors; downward dosage adjustment of these drugs may be required). Products include:
Paxil CR Controlled-Release Tablets 1538
Paxil 1530

Phenelzine Sulfate (Co-administration with MAO inhibitors may result in hypertensive crises; concurrent and/or sequential use is contraindicated).
No products indexed under this heading.

Phenobarbital (Methylphenidate may inhibit the metabolism of phenobarbital; downward dosage adjustment of phenobarbital may be required). Products include:
Donnatal Extentabs 2493

Phenylephrine Hydrochloride (Methylphenidate causes a rise in blood pressure; co-administration with other pressor agents should be undertaken with caution). Products include:
Comtrex Maximum Strength Non-Drowsy Cold & Cough Caplets .... ■ 725
Comtrex Maximum Strength Day/Night Severe Cold & Sinus Caplets - Day Formulation .... ■ 725
Comtrex Maximum Strength Day/Night Severe Cold & Sinus Caplets - Night Formulation .... ■ 725
Contac Cold and Flu Maximum Strength Caplets .... ■ 728
Contac Cold and Flu Day and Night Caplets (Day Formulation Only) .... ■ 727
Contac Cold and Flu Day and Night Caplets (Night Formulation Only) .... ■ 727
Contac Cold and Flu Non-Drowsy Caplets .... ■ 728
Contac-D Cold Non-Drowsy Tablets .... ■ 729
Children's Dimetapp Cold & Allergy Elixir .... ■ 730
Children's Dimetapp Cold & Allergy Chewable Tablets .... ■ 730
Children's Dimetapp DM Cold & Cough Elixir .... ■ 731
Toddler's Dimetapp Cold and Cough Drops .... ■ 732
Excedrin Sinus Headache Caplets/Tablets .... ■ 610
4-Way Fast Acting Nasal Spray ...... ■ 775
4-Way Menthol Nasal Spray .... ■ 775

Preparation H Maximum Strength Cream 666
Preparation H Cooling Gel 666
Preparation H 666
Refenesen PE Caplets 721
Robitussin Cough & Allergy Syrup .. 736
Robitussin Cough & Cold Nighttime Liquid 736
Robitussin Cough, Cold & Flu Nighttime Liquid 738
Robitussin Head & Chest Congestion PE Syrup 739
Robitussin Pediatric Cough & Cold Nighttime Liquid 736
TheraFlu Cold & Cough Hot Liquid 740
TheraFlu Cold & Sore Throat Hot Liquid 741
TheraFlu Flu & Sore Throat Hot Liquid 742
TheraFlu Daytime Severe Cold Hot Liquid 742
TheraFlu Nighttime Severe Cold Hot Liquid 740
TheraFlu Warming Relief Daytime Severe Cold 743
TheraFlu Warming Relief Nighttime Severe Cold 743
Triaminic Chest & Nasal Congestion Liquid 746
Triaminic Cold & Allergy Liquid 746
Triaminic Daytime Cold & Cough Liquid 745
Triaminic Nighttime Cold & Cough Liquid 746
Triaminic Thin Strips Cold 748
Triaminic Thin Strips Cold & Cough 778
Triaminic Infant Thin Strips Decongestant 747
Triaminic Infant Thin Strips Decongestant Plus Cough 747
Children's Tylenol Plus Flu Oral Suspension 749
Tylenol Cold Head Congestion Daytime Caplets with Cool Burst and Gelcaps 750
Tylenol Cold Multi-Symptom Daytime Liquid 752
Tylenol Cold Multi-Symptom Severe Daytime Liquid 752
Concentrated Tylenol Infants' Drops Plus Cold & Cough 754
Tylenol Allergy Multi-Symptom Caplets with Cool Burst and Gelcaps 1872
Tylenol Allergy Multi-Symptom Nighttime Caplets with Cool Burst 1872
Children's Tylenol Plus Cold Suspension Liquid 1879
Children's Tylenol Plus Cold & Allergy Suspension Liquid 1878
Children's Tylenol Plus Flu Suspension Liquid 1881
Children's Tylenol Plus Multi-Symptom Cold Suspension Liquid 1879
Tylenol Cold Head Congestion Daytime Caplets with Cool Burst 1873
Tylenol Cold Head Congestion Nighttime Caplets with Cool Burst 1873
Tylenol Cold Head Congestion Severe Caplets with Cool Burst 1873
Tylenol Cold Multi-Symptom Daytime Caplets with Cool Burst and Gelcaps 1874
Tylenol Cold Multi-Symptom Daytime Liquid with Citrus Burst ... 1874
Tylenol Cold Multi-Symptom Nighttime Caplets with Cool Burst 1874
Tylenol Cold Multi-Symptom Nighttime Liquid with Cool Burst ... 1874
Tylenol Cold Multi-Symptom Severe Caplets with Cool Burst 1874
Tylenol Cold Multi-Symptom Severe Daytime Liquid with Citrus Burst 1874
Tylenol Sinus Congestion & Pain Daytime Caplets with Cool Burst and Gelcaps 1876
Tylenol Sinus Congestion & Pain Nighttime Caplets with Cool Burst 1876
Tylenol Sinus Congestion & Pain Severe Caplets with Cool Burst 1876
Vicks 44D Cough & Head Congestion Relief Liquid 760
Vicks DayQuil LiquiCaps/Liquid Multi-Symptom Cold/Flu Relief 761
Zicam Cough Plus D Cough Spray 767

Phenytoin (Methylphenidate may inhibit the metabolism of phenytoin; downward dosage adjustment of phenytoin may be required).
No products indexed under this heading.

Phenytoin Sodium (Methylphenidate may inhibit the metabolism of phenytoin; downward dosage adjustment of phenytoin may be required). Products include:
Phenytek Capsules 2160

Primidone (Methylphenidate may inhibit the metabolism of primidone; downward dosage adjustment of primidone may be required).
No products indexed under this heading.

Procarbazine Hydrochloride (Coadministration with MAO inhibitors may result in hypertensive crises; concurrent and/or sequential use is contraindicated). Products include:
Matulane Capsules 3191

Protriptyline Hydrochloride (Methylphenidate may inhibit the metabolism of certain tricyclic antidepressants; downward dosage adjustment of tricyclic antidepressants may be required).
No products indexed under this heading.

Selegiline Hydrochloride (Coadministration with MAO inhibitors may result in hypertensive crises; concurrent and/or sequential use is contraindicated). Products include:
Eldepryl Capsules 3208
Zelapar Tablets 3372

Sertraline Hydrochloride (Methylphenidate may inhibit the metabolism of certain selective serotonin reuptake inhibitors; downward dosage adjustment of these drugs may be required). Products include:
Zoloft 2586

Tranylcypromine Sulfate (Coadministration with MAO inhibitors may result in hypertensive crises; concurrent and/or sequential use is contraindicated). Products include:
Parnate Tablets 1527

Trimipramine Maleate (Methylphenidate may inhibit the metabolism of certain tricyclic antidepressants; downward dosage adjustment of tricyclic antidepressants may be required).
No products indexed under this heading.

Warfarin Sodium (Methylphenidate may inhibit the metabolism of coumarin anticoagulants; downward dosage adjustment of anticoagulants may be required). Products include:
Coumadin for Injection 898
Coumadin Tablets 898

CONTAC COLD AND FLU MAXIMUM STRENGTH CAPLETS

(Acetaminophen, Chlorpheniramine Maleate, Phenylephrine Hydrochloride) 728
May interact with hypnotics and sedatives, monoamine oxidase inhibitors, tranquilizers, and certain other agents. Compounds in these categories include:

Alprazolam (May increase drowsiness effect). Products include:
Niravam Orally Disintegrating Tablets 3092

Buspirone Hydrochloride (May increase drowsiness effect).
No products indexed under this heading.

Chlordiazepoxide (May increase drowsiness effect).
No products indexed under this heading.

Chlordiazepoxide Hydrochloride (May increase drowsiness effect). Products include:
Librium Capsules 3347

Chlorpromazine (May increase drowsiness effect).
No products indexed under this heading.

Chlorpromazine Hydrochloride (May increase drowsiness effect).
No products indexed under this heading.

Chlorprothixene (May increase drowsiness effect).
No products indexed under this heading.

Chlorprothixene Hydrochloride (May increase drowsiness effect).
No products indexed under this heading.

Clorazepate Dipotassium (May increase drowsiness effect). Products include:
Tranxene 2474

Diazepam (May increase drowsiness effect). Products include:
Diastat Rectal Delivery System 3343
Valium Tablets 2819

Droperidol (May increase drowsiness effect).
No products indexed under this heading.

Estazolam (May increase drowsiness effect). Products include:
ProSom Tablets 517

Ethchlorvynol (May increase drowsiness effect).
No products indexed under this heading.

Ethinamate (May increase drowsiness effect).
No products indexed under this heading.

Fluphenazine Decanoate (May increase drowsiness effect).
No products indexed under this heading.

Fluphenazine Enanthate (May increase drowsiness effect).
No products indexed under this heading.

Fluphenazine Hydrochloride (May increase drowsiness effect).
No products indexed under this heading.

Flurazepam Hydrochloride (May increase drowsiness effect). Products include:
Dalmane Capsules 3342

Glutethimide (May increase drowsiness effect).
No products indexed under this heading.

Haloperidol (May increase drowsiness effect).
No products indexed under this heading.

Haloperidol Decanoate (May increase drowsiness effect).
No products indexed under this heading.

Hydroxyzine Hydrochloride (May increase drowsiness effect).
No products indexed under this heading.

Isocarboxazid (Concurrent and/or sequential use with MAO inhibitors is not recommended).
No products indexed under this heading.

Lorazepam (May increase drowsiness effect).
No products indexed under this heading.

Loxapine Hydrochloride (May increase drowsiness effect).
No products indexed under this heading.

Loxapine Succinate (May increase drowsiness effect).
No products indexed under this heading.

Meprobamate (May increase drowsiness effect).
No products indexed under this heading.

Mesoridazine Besylate (May increase drowsiness effect).
No products indexed under this heading.

Midazolam Hydrochloride (May increase drowsiness effect).
No products indexed under this heading.

Moclobemide (Concurrent and/or sequential use with MAO inhibitors is not recommended).
No products indexed under this heading.

Molindone Hydrochloride (May increase drowsiness effect). Products include:
Moban Tablets 1119

Oxazepam (May increase drowsiness effect).
No products indexed under this heading.

Pargyline Hydrochloride (Concurrent and/or sequential use with MAO inhibitors is not recommended).
No products indexed under this heading.

Perphenazine (May increase drowsiness effect).
No products indexed under this heading.

Phenelzine Sulfate (Concurrent and/or sequential use with MAO inhibitors is not recommended).
No products indexed under this heading.

Prazepam (May increase drowsiness effect).
No products indexed under this heading.

Procarbazine Hydrochloride (Concurrent and/or sequential use with MAO inhibitors is not recommended). Products include:
Matulane Capsules 3191

Prochlorperazine (May increase drowsiness effect).
No products indexed under this heading.

Promethazine Hydrochloride (May increase drowsiness effect). Products include:
Phenergan Tablets and Suppositories 3440

Propofol (May increase drowsiness effect).
No products indexed under this heading.

Quazepam (May increase drowsiness effect).
No products indexed under this heading.

Ramelteon (May increase drowsiness effect). Products include:

Rozerem Tablets 3231

Secobarbital Sodium (May increase drowsiness effect).
No products indexed under this heading.

Selegiline Hydrochloride (Concurrent and/or sequential use with MAO inhibitors is not recommended).
Products include:
Eldepryl Capsules 3208
Zelapar Tablets 3372

Temazepam (May increase drowsiness effect). Products include:
Restoril Capsules 1860

Thioridazine Hydrochloride (May increase drowsiness effect).
Products include:
Thioridazine Hydrochloride Tablets 2163

Thiothixene (May increase drowsiness effect). Products include:
Thiothixene Capsules 2165

Tranylcypromine Sulfate (Concurrent and/or sequential use with MAO inhibitors is not recommended).
Products include:
Parnate Tablets 1527

Triazolam (May increase drowsiness effect).
No products indexed under this heading.

Trifluoperazine Hydrochloride (May increase drowsiness effect).
No products indexed under this heading.

Zaleplon (May increase drowsiness effect). Products include:
Sonata Capsules 1717

Zolpidem Tartrate (May increase drowsiness effect). Products include:
Ambien Tablets 2851
Ambien CR Tablets 2855

Food Interactions

Alcohol (Concomitant consumption of alcohol may cause liver damage; may increase drowsiness effect).

CONTAC COLD AND FLU DAY AND NIGHT CAPLETS (DAY FORMULATION ONLY)

(Acetaminophen, Phenylephrine Hydrochloride) .... ▣ 727
May interact with hypnotics and sedatives, monoamine oxidase inhibitors, tranquilizers, and certain other agents. Compounds in these categories include:

Alprazolam (May increase drowsiness effect). Products include:
Niravam Orally Disintegrating Tablets 3092

Buspirone Hydrochloride (May increase drowsiness effect).
No products indexed under this heading.

Chlordiazepoxide (May increase drowsiness effect).
No products indexed under this heading.

Chlordiazepoxide Hydrochloride (May increase drowsiness effect).
Products include:
Librium Capsules 3347

Chlorpromazine (May increase drowsiness effect).
No products indexed under this heading.

Chlorpromazine Hydrochloride (May increase drowsiness effect).
No products indexed under this heading.

Chlorprothixene (May increase drowsiness effect).
No products indexed under this heading.

Chlorprothixene Hydrochloride (May increase drowsiness effect).
No products indexed under this heading.

Clorazepate Dipotassium (May increase drowsiness effect).
Products include:
Tranxene 2474

Diazepam (May increase drowsiness effect). Products include:
Diastat Rectal Delivery System 3343
Valium Tablets 2819

Droperidol (May increase drowsiness effect).
No products indexed under this heading.

Estazolam (May increase drowsiness effect). Products include:
ProSom Tablets 517

Ethchlorvynol (May increase drowsiness effect).
No products indexed under this heading.

Ethinamate (May increase drowsiness effect).
No products indexed under this heading.

Fluphenazine Decanoate (May increase drowsiness effect).
No products indexed under this heading.

Fluphenazine Enanthate (May increase drowsiness effect).
No products indexed under this heading.

Fluphenazine Hydrochloride (May increase drowsiness effect).
No products indexed under this heading.

Flurazepam Hydrochloride (May increase drowsiness effect).
Products include:
Dalmane Capsules 3342

Glutethimide (May increase drowsiness effect).
No products indexed under this heading.

Haloperidol (May increase drowsiness effect).
No products indexed under this heading.

Haloperidol Decanoate (May increase drowsiness effect).
No products indexed under this heading.

Hydroxyzine Hydrochloride (May increase drowsiness effect).
No products indexed under this heading.

Isocarboxazid (Concurrent and/or sequential use with MAO inhibitors is not recommended).
No products indexed under this heading.

Lorazepam (May increase drowsiness effect).
No products indexed under this heading.

Loxapine Hydrochloride (May increase drowsiness effect).
No products indexed under this heading.

Loxapine Succinate (May increase drowsiness effect).
No products indexed under this heading.

Meprobamate (May increase drowsiness effect).
No products indexed under this heading.

Mesoridazine Besylate (May increase drowsiness effect).
No products indexed under this heading.

Midazolam Hydrochloride (May increase drowsiness effect).
No products indexed under this heading.

Moclobemide (Concurrent and/or sequential use with MAO inhibitors is not recommended).
No products indexed under this heading.

Molindone Hydrochloride (May increase drowsiness effect).
Products include:
Moban Tablets 1119

Oxazepam (May increase drowsiness effect).
No products indexed under this heading.

Pargyline Hydrochloride (Concurrent and/or sequential use with MAO inhibitors is not recommended).
No products indexed under this heading.

Perphenazine (May increase drowsiness effect).
No products indexed under this heading.

Phenelzine Sulfate (Concurrent and/or sequential use with MAO inhibitors is not recommended).
No products indexed under this heading.

Prazepam (May increase drowsiness effect).
No products indexed under this heading.

Procarbazine Hydrochloride (Concurrent and/or sequential use with MAO inhibitors is not recommended). Products include:
Matulane Capsules 3191

Prochlorperazine (May increase drowsiness effect).
No products indexed under this heading.

Promethazine Hydrochloride (May increase drowsiness effect).
Products include:
Phenergan Tablets and Suppositories 3440

Propofol (May increase drowsiness effect).
No products indexed under this heading.

Quazepam (May increase drowsiness effect).
No products indexed under this heading.

Ramelteon (May increase drowsiness effect). Products include:
Rozerem Tablets 3231

Secobarbital Sodium (May increase drowsiness effect).
No products indexed under this heading.

Selegiline Hydrochloride (Concurrent and/or sequential use with MAO inhibitors is not recommended).
Products include:
Eldepryl Capsules 3208
Zelapar Tablets 3372

Temazepam (May increase drowsiness effect). Products include:
Restoril Capsules 1860

Thioridazine Hydrochloride (May increase drowsiness effect).
Products include:
Thioridazine Hydrochloride Tablets 2163

Thiothixene (May increase drowsiness effect). Products include:
Thiothixene Capsules 2165

Tranylcypromine Sulfate (Concurrent and/or sequential use with MAO inhibitors is not recommended).
Products include:
Parnate Tablets 1527

Triazolam (May increase drowsiness effect).
No products indexed under this heading.

Trifluoperazine Hydrochloride (May increase drowsiness effect).
No products indexed under this heading.

Zaleplon (May increase drowsiness effect). Products include:
Sonata Capsules 1717

Zolpidem Tartrate (May increase drowsiness effect). Products include:
Ambien Tablets 2851
Ambien CR Tablets 2855

Food Interactions

Alcohol (Concomitant consumption of alcohol may cause liver damage; may increase drowsiness effect).

CONTAC COLD AND FLU DAY AND NIGHT CAPLETS (NIGHT FORMULATION ONLY)

(Acetaminophen, Chlorpheniramine Maleate, Phenylephrine Hydrochloride) .... ▣ 727
May interact with hypnotics and sedatives, monoamine oxidase inhibitors, tranquilizers, and certain other agents. Compounds in these categories include:

Alprazolam (May increase drowsiness effect). Products include:
Niravam Orally Disintegrating Tablets 3092

Buspirone Hydrochloride (May increase drowsiness effect).
No products indexed under this heading.

Chlordiazepoxide (May increase drowsiness effect).
No products indexed under this heading.

Chlordiazepoxide Hydrochloride (May increase drowsiness effect).
Products include:
Librium Capsules 3347

Chlorpromazine (May increase drowsiness effect).
No products indexed under this heading.

Chlorpromazine Hydrochloride (May increase drowsiness effect).
No products indexed under this heading.

Chlorprothixene (May increase drowsiness effect).
No products indexed under this heading.

Chlorprothixene Hydrochloride (May increase drowsiness effect).
No products indexed under this heading.

Clorazepate Dipotassium (May increase drowsiness effect).
Products include:
Tranxene 2474

Diazepam (May increase drowsiness effect). Products include:
Diastat Rectal Delivery System 3343
Valium Tablets 2819

Droperidol (May increase drowsiness effect).
No products indexed under this heading.

Estazolam (May increase drowsiness effect). Products include:

ProSom Tablets 517

Ethchlorvynol (May increase drowsiness effect).
No products indexed under this heading.

Ethinamate (May increase drowsiness effect).
No products indexed under this heading.

Fluphenazine Decanoate (May increase drowsiness effect).
No products indexed under this heading.

Fluphenazine Enanthate (May increase drowsiness effect).
No products indexed under this heading.

Fluphenazine Hydrochloride (May increase drowsiness effect).
No products indexed under this heading.

Flurazepam Hydrochloride (May increase drowsiness effect).
Products include:
Dalmane Capsules 3342

Glutethimide (May increase drowsiness effect).
No products indexed under this heading.

Haloperidol (May increase drowsiness effect).
No products indexed under this heading.

Haloperidol Decanoate (May increase drowsiness effect).
No products indexed under this heading.

Hydroxyzine Hydrochloride (May increase drowsiness effect).
No products indexed under this heading.

Isocarboxazid (Concurrent and/or sequential use with MAO inhibitors is not recommended).
No products indexed under this heading.

Lorazepam (May increase drowsiness effect).
No products indexed under this heading.

Loxapine Hydrochloride (May increase drowsiness effect).
No products indexed under this heading.

Loxapine Succinate (May increase drowsiness effect).
No products indexed under this heading.

Meprobamate (May increase drowsiness effect).
No products indexed under this heading.

Mesoridazine Besylate (May increase drowsiness effect).
No products indexed under this heading.

Midazolam Hydrochloride (May increase drowsiness effect).
No products indexed under this heading.

Moclobemide (Concurrent and/or sequential use with MAO inhibitors is not recommended).
No products indexed under this heading.

Molindone Hydrochloride (May increase drowsiness effect).
Products include:
Moban Tablets 1119

Oxazepam (May increase drowsiness effect).
No products indexed under this heading.

Pargyline Hydrochloride (Concurrent and/or sequential use with MAO inhibitors is not recommended).
No products indexed under this heading.

Perphenazine (May increase drowsiness effect).
No products indexed under this heading.

Phenelzine Sulfate (Concurrent and/or sequential use with MAO inhibitors is not recommended).
No products indexed under this heading.

Prazepam (May increase drowsiness effect).
No products indexed under this heading.

Procarbazine Hydrochloride (Concurrent and/or sequential use with MAO inhibitors is not recommended). Products include:
Matulane Capsules 3191

Prochlorperazine (May increase drowsiness effect).
No products indexed under this heading.

Promethazine Hydrochloride (May increase drowsiness effect).
Products include:
Phenergan Tablets and Suppositories 3440

Propofol (May increase drowsiness effect).
No products indexed under this heading.

Quazepam (May increase drowsiness effect).
No products indexed under this heading.

Ramelteon (May increase drowsiness effect). Products include:
Rozerem Tablets 3231

Secobarbital Sodium (May increase drowsiness effect).
No products indexed under this heading.

Selegiline Hydrochloride (Concurrent and/or sequential use with MAO inhibitors is not recommended).
Products include:
Eldepryl Capsules 3208
Zelapar Tablets 3372

Temazepam (May increase drowsiness effect). Products include:
Restoril Capsules 1860

Thioridazine Hydrochloride (May increase drowsiness effect).
Products include:
Thioridazine Hydrochloride Tablets 2163

Thiothixene (May increase drowsiness effect). Products include:
Thiothixene Capsules 2165

Tranylcypromine Sulfate (Concurrent and/or sequential use with MAO inhibitors is not recommended).
Products include:
Parnate Tablets 1527

Triazolam (May increase drowsiness effect).
No products indexed under this heading.

Trifluoperazine Hydrochloride (May increase drowsiness effect).
No products indexed under this heading.

Zaleplon (May increase drowsiness effect). Products include:
Sonata Capsules 1717

Zolpidem Tartrate (May increase drowsiness effect). Products include:
Ambien Tablets 2851
Ambien CR Tablets 2855

Food Interactions

Alcohol (Concomitant consumption of alcohol may cause liver damage; may increase drowsiness effect).

CONTAC COLD AND FLU NON-DROWSY CAPLETS

(Acetaminophen, Phenylephrine Hydrochloride)................................. 728
May interact with monoamine oxidase inhibitors. Compounds in these categories include:

Isocarboxazid (Concurrent and/or sequential use with MAO inhibitors is not recommended).
No products indexed under this heading.

Moclobemide (Concurrent and/or sequential use with MAO inhibitors is not recommended).
No products indexed under this heading.

Pargyline Hydrochloride (Concurrent and/or sequential use with MAO inhibitors is not recommended).
No products indexed under this heading.

Phenelzine Sulfate (Concurrent and/or sequential use with MAO inhibitors is not recommended).
No products indexed under this heading.

Procarbazine Hydrochloride (Concurrent and/or sequential use with MAO inhibitors is not recommended). Products include:
Matulane Capsules 3191

Selegiline Hydrochloride (Concurrent and/or sequential use with MAO inhibitors is not recommended).
Products include:
Eldepryl Capsules 3208
Zelapar Tablets 3372

Tranylcypromine Sulfate (Concurrent and/or sequential use with MAO inhibitors is not recommended).
Products include:
Parnate Tablets 1527

Food Interactions

Alcohol (Concomitant consumption of alcohol may cause liver damage; may increase drowsiness effect).

CONTAC-D COLD NON-DROWSY TABLETS

(Phenylephrine Hydrochloride) 729
May interact with monoamine oxidase inhibitors. Compounds in these categories include:

Isocarboxazid (Concurrent and/or sequential use with MAO inhibitors is not recommended).
No products indexed under this heading.

Moclobemide (Concurrent and/or sequential use with MAO inhibitors is not recommended).
No products indexed under this heading.

Pargyline Hydrochloride (Concurrent and/or sequential use with MAO inhibitors is not recommended).
No products indexed under this heading.

Phenelzine Sulfate (Concurrent and/or sequential use with MAO inhibitors is not recommended).
No products indexed under this heading.

Procarbazine Hydrochloride (Concurrent and/or sequential use with MAO inhibitors is not recommended). Products include:
Matulane Capsules 3191

Selegiline Hydrochloride (Concurrent and/or sequential use with MAO inhibitors is not recommended).
Products include:
Eldepryl Capsules 3208
Zelapar Tablets 3372

Tranylcypromine Sulfate (Concurrent and/or sequential use with MAO inhibitors is not recommended).
Products include:
Parnate Tablets 1527

COPAXONE FOR INJECTION

(Glatiramer Acetate) 3297
None cited in PDR database.

COPEGUS TABLETS

(Ribavirin) 2754
May interact with nucleoside analogue reverse transcriptase inhibitors and certain other agents. Compounds in these categories include:

Didanosine (Co-administration of ribavirin and didanosine is not recommended. Reports of fatal kepatic failure, as well as peripheral neuropathy, pancreatitis, and symptomatic hyperlactatemia/lactic acidosis have been reported).
No products indexed under this heading.

Lamivudine (Co-administration of ribavirin and nucleoside analogue reverse transcriptase inhibitors should be closely monitored for treatment associated toxicities. In addition, dose reduction or discontinuation of ribavirin or both should also be considered if worsening of toxicities are observed). Products include:
Combivir Tablets 1411
Epivir 1427
Epivir-HBV 1432
Epzicom Tablets 1436
Trizivir Tablets 1589

Stavudine (Ribavirin can antagonize the in-vitro antiviral activity of stavudine against HIV. Therefore, concomitant use of ribavirin with stavudine should be avoided).
No products indexed under this heading.

Zalcitabine (Co-administration of ribavirin and nucleoside analogue reverse transcriptase inhibitors should be closely monitored for treatment associated toxicities. In addition, dose reduction or discontinuation of ribavirin or both should also be considered if worsening of toxicities are observed).
No products indexed under this heading.

Zidovudine (Ribavirin can antagonize the in-vitro antiviral activity of zidovudine against HIV. Therefore, concomitant use of ribavirin with zidovudine should be avoided).
Products include:
Combivir Tablets 1411
Retrovir 1560
Retrovir IV Infusion 1564
Trizivir Tablets 1589

COQUINONE CAPSULES

(Coenzyme Q-10, Lipoic Acid) 3339
None cited in PDR database.

CORDYMAX CS-4 CAPSULES
(Herbals, Multiple) 2672
May interact with oral anticoagulants and monoamine oxidase inhibitors. Compounds in these categories include:

Anisindione (Concurrent use with anticoagulants requires consultation with a physician). Products include:
Miradon Tablets 3042

Dicumarol (Concurrent use with anticoagulants requires consultation with a physician).
No products indexed under this heading.

Isocarboxazid (Concurrent use with MAO inhibitors requires consultation with a physician).
No products indexed under this heading.

Moclobemide (Concurrent use with MAO inhibitors requires consultation with a physician).
No products indexed under this heading.

Pargyline Hydrochloride (Concurrent use with MAO inhibitors requires consultation with a physician).
No products indexed under this heading.

Phenelzine Sulfate (Concurrent use with MAO inhibitors requires consultation with a physician).
No products indexed under this heading.

Procarbazine Hydrochloride (Concurrent use with MAO inhibitors requires consultation with a physician). Products include:
Matulane Capsules 3191

Selegiline Hydrochloride (Concurrent use with MAO inhibitors requires consultation with a physician).
Products include:
Eldepryl Capsules 3208
Zelapar Tablets 3372

Tranylcypromine Sulfate (Concurrent use with MAO inhibitors requires consultation with a physician).
Products include:
Parnate Tablets 1527

Warfarin Sodium (Concurrent use with anticoagulants requires consultation with a physician). Products include:
Coumadin for Injection 898
Coumadin Tablets 898

COREG TABLETS
(Carvedilol) 1414
May interact with catecholamine depleting drugs, cytochrome p450 2d6 inhibitors (selected), epinephrine-containing products, oral hypoglycemic agents, insulin, monoamine oxidase inhibitors, quinidine, and certain other agents. Compounds in these categories include:

Acarbose (Beta-blockers may mask some of the manifestations of hypoglycemia, particularly tachycardia; nonselective beta-blockers may potentiate insulin-induced hypoglycemia and delay recovery of serum glucose levels; in congestive heart failure patients with diabetes, carvedilol therapy may lead to worsening of hyperglycemia, which responds to intensification of hypoglycemia). Products include:
Precose Tablets 751

Amiodarone Hydrochloride (Interactions of carvedilol with strong inhibitors of CYP2D6, such as quinidine, have not been studied, but these drugs would be expected to increase blood levels of the R(+) enantiomer of carvedilol. Analysis of side effects showed that poor 2D6 metabolizers had a higher rate of dizziness during up-titration, presumably resulting from vasodilating effects of the higher concentrations of the alpha-blocking R(+) enantiomer).
No products indexed under this heading.

Amitriptyline Hydrochloride (Interactions of carvedilol with strong inhibitors of CYP2D6, such as quinidine, have not been studied, but these drugs would be expected to increase blood levels of the R(+) enantiomer of carvedilol. Analysis of side effects showed that poor 2D6 metabolizers had a higher rate of dizziness during up-titration, presumably resulting from vasodilating effects of the higher concentrations of the alpha-blocking R(+) enantiomer).
No products indexed under this heading.

Amoxapine (Interactions of carvedilol with strong inhibitors of CYP2D6, such as quinidine, have not been studied, but these drugs would be expected to increase blood levels of the R(+) enantiomer of carvedilol. Analysis of side effects showed that poor 2D6 metabolizers had a higher rate of dizziness during up-titration, presumably resulting from vasodilating effects of the higher concentrations of the alpha-blocking R(+) enantiomer).
No products indexed under this heading.

Bupropion Hydrochloride (Interactions of carvedilol with strong inhibitors of CYP2D6, such as quinidine, have not been studied, but these drugs would be expected to increase blood levels of the R(+) enantiomer of carvedilol. Analysis of side effects showed that poor 2D6 metabolizers had a higher rate of dizziness during up-titration, presumably resulting from vasodilating effects of the higher concentrations of the alpha-blocking R(+) enantiomer). Products include:
Wellbutrin Tablets 1603
Wellbutrin SR Sustained-Release Tablets 1607
Wellbutrin XL Extended-Release Tablets 1613
Zyban Sustained-Release Tablets 1644

Celecoxib (Interactions of carvedilol with strong inhibitors of CYP2D6, such as quinidine, have not been studied, but these drugs would be expected to increase blood levels of the R(+) enantiomer of carvedilol. Analysis of side effects showed that poor 2D6 metabolizers had a higher rate of dizziness during up-titration, presumably resulting from vasodilating effects of the higher concentrations of the alpha-blocking R(+) enantiomer). Products include:
Celebrex Capsules 3134

Chloroquine Hydrochloride (Interactions of carvedilol with strong inhibitors of CYP2D6, such as quinidine, have not been studied, but these drugs would be expected to increase blood levels of the R(+) enantiomer of carvedilol. Analysis of side effects showed that poor 2D6 metabolizers had a higher rate of dizziness during up-titration, presumably resulting from vasodilating effects of the higher concentrations of the alpha-blocking R(+) enantiomer).
No products indexed under this heading.

Chloroquine Phosphate (Interactions of carvedilol with strong inhibitors of CYP2D6, such as quinidine, have not been studied, but these drugs would be expected to increase blood levels of the R(+) enantiomer of carvedilol. Analysis of side effects showed that poor 2D6 metabolizers had a higher rate of dizziness during up-titration, presumably resulting from vasodilating effects of the higher concentrations of the alpha-blocking R(+) enantiomer).
No products indexed under this heading.

Chlorpheniramine (Interactions of carvedilol with strong inhibitors of CYP2D6, such as quinidine, have not been studied, but these drugs would be expected to increase blood levels of the R(+) enantiomer of carvedilol. Analysis of side effects showed that poor 2D6 metabolizers had a higher rate of dizziness during up-titration, presumably resulting from vasodilating effects of the higher concentrations of the alpha-blocking R(+) enantiomer).
No products indexed under this heading.

Chlorpheniramine Maleate (Interactions of carvedilol with strong inhibitors of CYP2D6, such as quinidine, have not been studied, but these drugs would be expected to increase blood levels of the R(+) enantiomer of carvedilol. Analysis of side effects showed that poor 2D6 metabolizers had a higher rate of dizziness during up-titration, presumably resulting from vasodilating effects of the higher concentrations of the alpha-blocking R(+) enantiomer). Products include:
Advil Allergy Sinus Caplets .... ▣ 770
Advil Multi-Symptom Cold Caplets .... ▣ 770
BC Allergy Sinus Cold Powder .... ▣ 677
Comtrex Maximum Strength Cold & Cough Day/Night Caplets - Night Formulation .... ▣ 726
Comtrex Maximum Strength Day/Night Severe Cold & Sinus Caplets - Night Formulation .... ▣ 725
Contac Cold and Flu Maximum Strength Caplets .... ▣ 728
Contac Cold and Flu Day and Night Caplets (Night Formulation Only) .... ▣ 727
Children's Dimetapp Long Acting Cough Plus Cold Syrup .... ▣ 731
Robitussin Cough & Cold Long-Acting Liquid .... ▣ 735
Robitussin Cough & Allergy Syrup .... ▣ 736
Robitussin Cough & Cold Nighttime Liquid .... ▣ 736
Robitussin Cough, Cold & Flu Nighttime Liquid .... ▣ 738
Robitussin Pediatric Cough & Cold Long-Acting Liquid .... ▣ 735
Robitussin Pediatric Cough & Cold Nighttime Liquid .... ▣ 736
Triaminic Cold & Allergy Liquid .... ▣ 746
Triaminic Cough & Runny Nose Softchews .... ▣ 748
Children's Tylenol Plus Flu Oral Suspension .... ▣ 749
Tylenol Allergy Multi-Symptom Caplets with Cool Burst and Gelcaps 1872
Children's Tylenol Plus Cold Suspension Liquid 1879
Children's Tylenol Plus Cough & Runny Nose Suspension Liquid 1879
Children's Tylenol Plus Flu Suspension Liquid 1881
Children's Tylenol Plus Multi-Symptom Cold Suspension Liquid 1879
Tylenol Cold Head Congestion Nighttime Caplets with Cool Burst 1873
Tylenol Cold Multi-Symptom Nighttime Caplets with Cool Burst 1874
Tylenol Sinus Congestion & Pain Nighttime Caplets with Cool Burst 1876
Vicks 44M Cough, Cold & Flu Relief Liquid 2680
Pediatric Vicks 44m Cough & Cold Relief Liquid 2676
Children's Vicks NyQuil Cold/Cough Relief .... ▣ 756
Children's Vicks NyQuil Cold/Cough Relief Liquid 2680
Zicam Maximum Strength Flu Daytime .... ▣ 768

Chlorpheniramine Polistirex (Interactions of carvedilol with strong inhibitors of CYP2D6, such as quinidine, have not been studied, but these drugs would be expected to increase blood levels of the R(+) enantiomer of carvedilol. Analysis of side effects showed that poor 2D6 metabolizers had a higher rate of dizziness during up-titration, presumably resulting from vasodilating effects of the higher concentrations of the alpha-blocking R(+) enantiomer). Products include:
Tussionex Pennkinetic Extended-Release Suspension 3327

Chlorpheniramine Tannate (Interactions of carvedilol with strong inhibitors of CYP2D6, such as quinidine, have not been studied, but these drugs would be expected to increase blood levels of the R(+) enantiomer of carvedilol. Analysis of side effects showed that poor 2D6 metabolizers had a higher rate of dizziness during up-titration, presumably resulting from vasodilating effects of the higher concentrations of the alpha-blocking R(+) enantiomer).
No products indexed under this heading.

Chlorpropamide (Beta-blockers may mask some of the manifestations of hypoglycemia, particularly tachycardia; nonselective beta-blockers may potentiate insulin-induced hypoglycemia and delay recovery of serum glucose levels; in congestive heart failure patients with diabetes, carvedilol therapy may lead to worsening of hyperglycemia, which responds to intensification of hypoglycemia).
No products indexed under this heading.

Cimetidine (Carvedilol undergoes substantial oxidative metabolism; co-administration has resulted in increased steady-state AUC of carvedilol by about 30% with no change in Cmax). Products include:
Tagamet HB 200 Tablets .... ▣ 664

Cimetidine Hydrochloride (Carvedilol undergoes substantial oxidative metabolism; co-administration has resulted in increased steady-state AUC of carvedilol by about 30% with no change in Cmax).
No products indexed under this heading.

Citalopram Hydrobromide (Interactions of carvedilol with strong inhibitors of CYP2D6, such as quinidine, have not been studied, but these drugs would be expected to increase blood levels of the R(+)

enantiomer of carvedilol. Analysis of side effects showed that poor 2D6 metabolizers had a higher rate of dizziness during up-titration, presumably resulting from vasodilating effects of the higher concentrations of the alpha-blocking R(+) enantiomer). Products include:

Celexa 1176

Clomipramine Hydrochloride (Interactions of carvedilol with strong inhibitors of CYP2D6, such as quinidine, have not been studied, but these drugs would be expected to increase blood levels of the R(+) enantiomer of carvedilol. Analysis of side effects showed that poor 2D6 metabolizers had a higher rate of dizziness during up-titration, presumably resulting from vasodilating effects of the higher concentrations of the alpha-blocking R(+) enantiomer).

No products indexed under this heading.

Clonidine (Co-administration of clonidine with agents with β-blocking properties may potentiate blood pressure- and heart rate-lowering effects). Products include:

Catapres-TTS 844

Clonidine Hydrochloride (Co-administration of clonidine with agents with β-blocking properties may potentiate blood pressure- and heart rate-lowering effects). Products include:

Catapres Tablets 843
Clorpres Tablets 2153

Cocaine Hydrochloride (Interactions of carvedilol with strong inhibitors of CYP2D6, such as quinidine, have not been studied, but these drugs would be expected to increase blood levels of the R(+) enantiomer of carvedilol. Analysis of side effects showed that poor 2D6 metabolizers had a higher rate of dizziness during up-titration, presumably resulting from vasodilating effects of the higher concentrations of the alpha-blocking R(+) enantiomer).

No products indexed under this heading.

Cyclosporine (Co-administration in renal transplant patients has resulted in a modest increase in mean trough cyclosporine concentrations; dose of cyclosporine may need to be reduced in some patients). Products include:

Gengraf Capsules 459
Neoral Oral Solution 2259
Neoral Soft Gelatin Capsules 2259
Restasis Ophthalmic Emulsion 575
Sandimmune 2275

Deserpidine (Patients receiving agents with beta-blocking properties and a drug that may deplete catecholamines should be observed closely for signs of hypotension and/or severe bradycardia).

No products indexed under this heading.

Desipramine Hydrochloride (Interactions of carvedilol with strong inhibitors of CYP2D6, such as quinidine, have not been studied, but these drugs would be expected to increase blood levels of the R(+) enantiomer of carvedilol. Analysis of side effects showed that poor 2D6 metabolizers had a higher rate of dizziness during up-titration, presumably resulting from vasodilating effects of the higher concentrations of the alpha-blocking R(+) enantiomer).

No products indexed under this heading.

Digoxin (Co-administration increases digoxin concentraton by 15%. Both digoxin and carvedilol slow AV conduction. Therefore, increased monitoring of digoxin is recommended when initiating, adjusting or discontinuing carvedilol). Products include:

Lanoxicaps Capsules 1490
Lanoxin Injection 1494
Lanoxin Injection Pediatric 1497
Lanoxin Tablets 1500

Diltiazem Hydrochloride (Co-administration has resulted in isolated cases of conduction disturbances, rarely with hemodynamic. Monitoring of ECG and blood pressure is recommended). Products include:

Cardizem LA Extended Release Tablets 1728
Tiazac Capsules 1201

Diphenhydramine (Interactions of carvedilol with strong inhibitors of CYP2D6, such as quinidine, have not been studied, but these drugs would be expected to increase blood levels of the R(+) enantiomer of carvedilol. Analysis of side effects showed that poor 2D6 metabolizers had a higher rate of dizziness during up-titration, presumably resulting from vasodilating effects of the higher concentrations of the alpha-blocking R(+) enantiomer). Products include:

Tylenol Sore Throat Nighttime Liquid with Cool Burst 1877

Diphenhydramine Hydrochloride (Interactions of carvedilol with strong inhibitors of CYP2D6, such as quinidine, have not been studied, but these drugs would be expected to increase blood levels of the R(+) enantiomer of carvedilol. Analysis of side effects showed that poor 2D6 metabolizers had a higher rate of dizziness during up-titration, presumably resulting from vasodilating effects of the higher concentrations of the alpha-blocking R(+) enantiomer). Products include:

Nytol QuickCaps Caplets .... ■615
Nytol QuickGels Softgels Maximum Strength .... ■616
Simply Sleep Caplets 1868
Sominex Original Formula Tablets .. ■616
TheraFlu Warming Relief Nighttime Severe Cold .... ■743
TheraFlu Thin Strips Multi Symptom .... ■744
Triaminic Nighttime Cold & Cough Liquid .... ■746
Triaminic Thin Strips Cough & Runny Nose .... ■749
Extra Strength Tylenol PM Caplets, Vanilla Caplets, Geltabs, Gelcaps and Liquid 1875
Tylenol Sore Throat Nighttime Liquid with Cool Burst .... ■790
Tylenol Allergy Multi-Symptom Nighttime Caplets with Cool Burst 1872
Tylenol Severe Allergy Caplets 1872
Children's Tylenol Plus Cold & Allergy Suspension Liquid 1878

Doxepin Hydrochloride (Interactions of carvedilol with strong inhibitors of CYP2D6, such as quinidine, have not been studied, but these drugs would be expected to increase blood levels of the R(+) enantiomer of carvedilol. Analysis of side effects showed that poor 2D6 metabolizers had a higher rate of dizziness during up-titration, presumably resulting from vasodilating effects of the higher concentrations of the alpha-blocking R(+) enantiomer).

No products indexed under this heading.

Epinephrine (Patients on beta-blocker therapy and with a history of severe anaphylactic reactions to a variety of allergens may be unresponsive to the usual doses of epinephrine used to treat allergic reactions). Products include:

EpiPen 1061
Primatene Mist .... ■719
Twinject 0.15 3379
Twinject 0.3 3378

Epinephrine Bitartrate (Patients on beta-blocker therapy and with a history of severe anaphylactic reactions to a variety of allergens may be unresponsive to the usual doses of epinephrine used to treat allergic reactions).

No products indexed under this heading.

Epinephrine Hydrochloride (Potential for unresponsiveness to the usual dose of epinephrine used to treat allergic reactions).

No products indexed under this heading.

Escitalopram Oxalate (Interactions of carvedilol with strong inhibitors of CYP2D6, such as quinidine, have not been studied, but these drugs would be expected to increase blood levels of the R(+) enantiomer of carvedilol. Analysis of side effects showed that poor 2D6 metabolizers had a higher rate of dizziness during up-titration, presumably resulting from vasodilating effects of the higher concentrations of the alpha-blocking R(+) enantiomer). Products include:

Lexapro Oral Solution 1190
Lexapro Tablets 1190

Fluoxetine (Interactions of carvedilol with strong inhibitors of CYP2D6, such as quinidine, have not been studied, but these drugs would be expected to increase blood levels of the R(+) enantiomer of carvedilol. Analysis of side effects showed that poor 2D6 metabolizers had a higher rate of dizziness during up-titration, presumably resulting from vasodilating effects of the higher concentrations of the alpha-blocking R(+) enantiomer).

No products indexed under this heading.

Fluoxetine Hydrochloride (Interactions of carvedilol with strong inhibitors of CYP2D6, such as fluoxetine, have not been studied, but these drugs would be expected to increase blood levels of the R(+) enantiomer of carvedilol. Analysis of side effects showed that poor 2D6 metabolizers had a higher rate of dizziness during up-titration, presumably resulting from vasodilating effects of the higher concentrations of the alpha-blocking R(+) enantiomer). Products include:

Prozac Pulvules and Liquid 1801
Symbyax Capsules 1819

Fluphenazine Decanoate (Interactions of carvedilol with strong inhibitors of CYP2D6, such as quinidine, have not been studied, but these drugs would be expected to increase blood levels of the R(+) enantiomer of carvedilol. Analysis of side effects showed that poor 2D6 metabolizers had a higher rate of dizziness during up-titration, presumably resulting from vasodilating effects of the higher concentrations of the alpha-blocking R(+) enantiomer).

No products indexed under this heading.

Fluphenazine Enanthate (Interactions of carvedilol with strong inhibitors of CYP2D6, such as quinidine, have not been studied, but these drugs would be expected to increase blood levels of the R(+) enantiomer of carvedilol. Analysis of side effects showed that poor 2D6 metabolizers had a higher rate of dizziness during up-titration, presumably resulting from vasodilating effects of the higher concentrations of the alpha-blocking R(+) enantiomer).

No products indexed under this heading.

Fluphenazine Hydrochloride (Interactions of carvedilol with strong inhibitors of CYP2D6, such as quinidine, have not been studied, but these drugs would be expected to increase blood levels of the R(+) enantiomer of carvedilol. Analysis of side effects showed that poor 2D6 metabolizers had a higher rate of dizziness during up-titration, presumably resulting from vasodilating effects of the higher concentrations of the alpha-blocking R(+) enantiomer).

No products indexed under this heading.

Fluvoxamine Maleate (Interactions of carvedilol with strong inhibitors of CYP2D6, such as quinidine, have not been studied, but these drugs would be expected to increase blood levels of the R(+) enantiomer of carvedilol. Analysis of side effects showed that poor 2D6 metabolizers had a higher rate of dizziness during up-titration, presumably resulting from vasodilating effects of the higher concentrations of the alpha-blocking R(+) enantiomer).

No products indexed under this heading.

Glimepiride (Beta-blockers may mask some of the manifestations of hypoglycemia, particularly tachycardia; nonselective beta-blockers may potentiate insulin-induced hypoglycemia and delay recovery of serum glucose levels; in congestive heart failure patients with diabetes, carvedilol therapy may lead to worsening of hyperglycemia, which responds to intensification of hypoglycemia). Products include:

Avandaryl Tablets 1379
Duetact Tablets 3226

Glipizide (Beta-blockers may mask some of the manifestations of hypoglycemia, particularly tachycardia; nonselective beta-blockers may potentiate insulin-induced hypoglycemia and delay recovery of serum glucose levels; in congestive heart failure patients with diabetes, carvedilol therapy may lead to worsening of hyperglycemia, which responds to intensification of hypoglycemia).

No products indexed under this heading.

Glyburide (Beta-blockers may mask some of the manifestations of hypoglycemia, particularly tachycardia; nonselective beta-blockers may potentiate insulin-induced hypoglycemia and delay recovery of serum glucose levels; in congestive heart failure patients with diabetes, carvedilol therapy may lead to worsening of hyperglycemia, which responds to intensification of hypoglycemia).

No products indexed under this heading.

Guanethidine Monosulfate (Patients receiving agents with beta-blocking properties and a drug that may deplete catecholamines should be observed closely for signs of hypotension and/or severe bradycardia).

No products indexed under this heading.

Halofantrine Hydrochloride (Interactions of carvedilol with strong inhibitors of CYP2D6, such as quinidine, have not been studied, but these drugs would be expected to increase blood levels of the R(+) enantiomer of carvedilol. Analysis of side effects showed that poor 2D6 metabolizers had a higher rate of dizziness during up-titration, presumably resulting from vasodilating effects of the higher concentrations of the alpha-blocking R(+) enantiomer).

No products indexed under this heading.

Haloperidol (Interactions of carvedilol with strong inhibitors of CYP2D6, such as quinidine, have not been studied, but these drugs would be expected to increase blood levels of the R(+) enantiomer of carvedilol. Analysis of side effects showed that poor 2D6 metabolizers had a higher rate of dizziness during up-titration, presumably resulting from vasodilating effects of the higher concentrations of the alpha-blocking R(+) enantiomer).

No products indexed under this heading.

Haloperidol Decanoate (Interactions of carvedilol with strong inhibitors of CYP2D6, such as quinidine, have not been studied, but these drugs would be expected to increase blood levels of the R(+) enantiomer of carvedilol. Analysis of side effects showed that poor 2D6 metabolizers had a higher rate of dizziness during up-titration, presumably resulting from vasodilating effects of the higher concentrations of the alpha-blocking R(+) enantiomer).

No products indexed under this heading.

Hydroxychloroquine Sulfate (Interactions of carvedilol with strong inhibitors of CYP2D6, such as quinidine, have not been studied, but these drugs would be expected to increase blood levels of the R(+) enantiomer of carvedilol. Analysis of side effects showed that poor 2D6 metabolizers had a higher rate of dizziness during up-titration, presumably resulting from vasodilating effects of the higher concentrations of the alpha-blocking R(+) enantiomer).

No products indexed under this heading.

Imatinib Mesylate (Interactions of carvedilol with strong inhibitors of

CYP2D6, such as quinidine, have not been studied, but these drugs would be expected to increase blood levels of the R(+) enantiomer of carvedilol. Analysis of side effects showed that poor 2D6 metabolizers had a higher rate of dizziness during up-titration, presumably resulting from vasodilating effects of the alpha-blocking R(+) enantiomer). Products include:

Gleevec Tablets 2227

Imipramine Hydrochloride (Interactions of carvedilol with strong inhibitors of CYP2D6, such as quinidine, have not been studied, but these drugs would be expected to increase blood levels of the R(+) enantiomer of carvedilol. Analysis of side effects showed that poor 2D6 metabolizers had a higher rate of dizziness during up-titration, presumably resulting from vasodilating effects of the higher concentrations of the alpha-blocking R(+) enantiomer).

No products indexed under this heading.

Imipramine Pamoate (Interactions of carvedilol with strong inhibitors of CYP2D6, such as quinidine, have not been studied, but these drugs would be expected to increase blood levels of the R(+) enantiomer of carvedilol. Analysis of side effects showed that poor 2D6 metabolizers had a higher rate of dizziness during up-titration, presumably resulting from vasodilating effects of the alpha-blocking R(+) enantiomer).

No products indexed under this heading.

Insulin, Human, Zinc Suspension (Beta-blockers may mask some of the manifestations of hypoglycemia, particularly tachycardia; nonselective beta-blockers may potentiate insulin-induced hypoglycemia and delay recovery of serum glucose levels; in congestive heart failure patients with diabetes, carvedilol therapy may lead to worsening of hyperglycemia, which responds to intensification of hypoglycemia). Products include:

Humulin L, 100 Units 1794
Humulin U, 100 Units 1800

Insulin, Human NPH (Beta-blockers may mask some of the manifestations of hypoglycemia, particularly tachycardia; nonselective beta-blockers may potentiate insulin-induced hypoglycemia and delay recovery of serum glucose levels; in congestive heart failure patients with diabetes, carvedilol therapy may lead to worsening of hyperglycemia, which responds to intensification of hypoglycemia). Products include:

Humulin N, 100 Units 1795
Humulin N Pen 1797

Insulin, Human Regular (Beta-blockers may mask some of the manifestations of hypoglycemia, particularly tachycardia; nonselective beta-blockers may potentiate insulin-induced hypoglycemia and delay recovery of serum glucose levels; in congestive heart failure patients with diabetes, carvedilol therapy may lead to worsening of hyperglycemia, which responds to intensification of hypoglycemia). Products include:

Humulin R, 100 Units 1798

Insulin, Human Regular and Human NPH Mixture (Beta-blockers may mask some of the manifestations of hypoglycemia, particularly tachycardia; nonselective beta-blockers may potentiate insulin-induced hypoglycemia and delay recovery of serum glucose levels; in congestive heart failure patients with diabetes, carvedilol therapy may lead to worsening of hyperglycemia, which responds to intensification of hypoglycemia). Products include:

Humulin 50/50, 100 Units 1791
Humulin 70/30 Pen 1793

Insulin, NPH (Beta-blockers may mask some of the manifestations of hypoglycemia, particularly tachycardia; nonselective beta-blockers may potentiate insulin-induced hypoglycemia and delay recovery of serum glucose levels; in congestive heart failure patients with diabetes, carvedilol therapy may lead to worsening of hyperglycemia, which responds to intensification of hypoglycemia).

No products indexed under this heading.

Insulin, Regular (Beta-blockers may mask some of the manifestations of hypoglycemia, particularly tachycardia; nonselective beta-blockers may potentiate insulin-induced hypoglycemia and delay recovery of serum glucose levels; in congestive heart failure patients with diabetes, carvedilol therapy may lead to worsening of hyperglycemia, which responds to intensification of hypoglycemia).

No products indexed under this heading.

Insulin, Zinc Crystals (Beta-blockers may mask some of the manifestations of hypoglycemia, particularly tachycardia; nonselective beta-blockers may potentiate insulin-induced hypoglycemia and delay recovery of serum glucose levels; in congestive heart failure patients with diabetes, carvedilol therapy may lead to worsening of hyperglycemia, which responds to intensification of hypoglycemia).

No products indexed under this heading.

Insulin, Zinc Suspension (Beta-blockers may mask some of the manifestations of hypoglycemia, particularly tachycardia; nonselective beta-blockers may potentiate insulin-induced hypoglycemia and delay recovery of serum glucose levels; in congestive heart failure patients with diabetes, carvedilol therapy may lead to worsening of hyperglycemia, which responds to intensification of hypoglycemia).

No products indexed under this heading.

Insulin Aspart, Human Regular (Beta-blockers may mask some of the manifestations of hypoglycemia, particularly tachycardia; nonselective beta-blockers may potentiate insulin-induced hypoglycemia and delay recovery of serum glucose levels; in congestive heart failure patients with diabetes, carvedilol therapy may lead to worsening of hyperglycemia, which responds to intensification of hypoglycemia). Products include:

NovoLog Injection 2326

Insulin glargine (Beta-blockers may mask some of the manifesta-

tions of hypoglycemia, particularly tachycardia; nonselective beta-blockers may potentiate insulin-induced hypoglycemia and delay recovery of serum glucose levels; in congestive heart failure patients with diabetes, carvedilol therapy may lead to worsening of hyperglycemia, which responds to intensification of hypoglycemia). Products include:

Lantus Injection 2909

Insulin Lispro, Human (Beta-blockers may mask some of the manifestations of hypoglycemia, particularly tachycardia; nonselective beta-blockers may potentiate insulin-induced hypoglycemia and delay recovery of serum glucose levels; in congestive heart failure patients with diabetes, carvedilol therapy may lead to worsening of hyperglycemia, which responds to intensification of hypoglycemia). Products include:

Humalog-Pen 1781
Humalog Mix 50/50-Pen 1783
Humalog Mix 75/25-Pen 1785

Insulin Lispro Protamine, Human (Beta-blockers may mask some of the manifestations of hypoglycemia, particularly tachycardia; nonselective beta-blockers may potentiate insulin-induced hypoglycemia and delay recovery of serum glucose levels; in congestive heart failure patients with diabetes, carvedilol therapy may lead to worsening of hyperglycemia, which responds to intensification of hypoglycemia). Products include:

Humalog Mix 50/50-Pen 1783
Humalog Mix 75/25-Pen 1785

Isocarboxazid (Patients receiving agents with beta-blocking properties and a drug that may deplete catecholamines should be observed closely for signs of hypotension and/or severe bradycardia).

No products indexed under this heading.

Maprotiline Hydrochloride (Interactions of carvedilol with strong inhibitors of CYP2D6, such as quinidine, have not been studied, but these drugs would be expected to increase blood levels of the R(+) enantiomer of carvedilol. Analysis of side effects showed that poor 2D6 metabolizers had a higher rate of dizziness during up-titration, presumably resulting from vasodilating effects of the higher concentrations of the alpha-blocking R(+) enantiomer).

No products indexed under this heading.

Metformin Hydrochloride (Beta-blockers may mask some of the manifestations of hypoglycemia, particularly tachycardia; nonselective beta-blockers may potentiate insulin-induced hypoglycemia and delay recovery of serum glucose levels; in congestive heart failure patients with diabetes, carvedilol therapy may lead to worsening of hyperglycemia, which responds to intensification of hypoglycemia). Products include:

ActoPlus Met Tablets 3214
Avandamet Tablets 1373
Fortamet Extended-Release
 Tablets .. 3115

Methadone Hydrochloride (Interactions of carvedilol with strong inhibitors of CYP2D6, such as quinidine, have not been studied, but these drugs would be expected to increase blood levels of the R(+) enantiomer of carvedilol. Analysis of side effects showed that poor 2D6 metabolizers had a higher rate of dizziness during up-titration, presumably resulting from vasodilating effects of the higher concentrations of the alpha-blocking R(+) enantiomer).

No products indexed under this heading.

Mibefradil Dihydrochloride (Interactions of carvedilol with strong inhibitors of CYP2D6, such as quinidine, have not been studied, but these drugs would be expected to increase blood levels of the R(+) enantiomer of carvedilol. Analysis of side effects showed that poor 2D6 metabolizers had a higher rate of dizziness during up-titration, presumably resulting from vasodilating effects of the higher concentrations of the alpha-blocking R(+) enantiomer).

No products indexed under this heading.

Miglitol (Beta-blockers may mask some of the manifestations of hypoglycemia, particularly tachycardia; nonselective beta-blockers may potentiate insulin-induced hypoglycemia and delay recovery of serum glucose levels; in congestive heart failure patients with diabetes, carvedilol therapy may lead to worsening of hyperglycemia, which responds to intensification of hypoglycemia).

No products indexed under this heading.

Moclobemide (Patients receiving agents with beta-blocking properties and a drug that may deplete catecholamines should be observed closely for signs of hypotension and/or severe bradycardia).

No products indexed under this heading.

Nortriptyline Hydrochloride (Interactions of carvedilol with strong inhibitors of CYP2D6, such as quinidine, have not been studied, but these drugs would be expected to increase blood levels of the R(+) enantiomer of carvedilol. Analysis of side effects showed that poor 2D6 metabolizers had a higher rate of dizziness during up-titration, presumably resulting from vasodilating effects of the higher concentrations of the alpha-blocking R(+) enantiomer).

No products indexed under this heading.

Pargyline Hydrochloride (Patients receiving agents with beta-blocking properties and a drug that may deplete catecholamines should be observed closely for signs of hypotension and/or severe bradycardia).

No products indexed under this heading.

Paroxetine Hydrochloride (Interactions of carvedilol with strong inhibitors of CYP2D6, such as paroxetine, have not been studied, but these drugs would be expected to increase blood levels of the R(+) enantiomer of carvedilol. Analysis of side effects showed that poor 2D6 metabolizers had a higher rate of dizziness during up-titration, presumably resulting from vasodilating effects of the higher concentrations of the alpha-blocking R(+) enantiomer). Products include:

Perphenazine (Interactions of carvedilol with strong inhibitors of CYP2D6, such as quinidine, have not been studied, but these drugs would be expected to increase blood levels of the R(+) enantiomer of carvedilol. Analysis of side effects showed that poor 2D6 metabolizers had a higher rate of dizziness during up-titration, presumably resulting from vasodilating effects of the higher concentrations of the alpha-blocking R(+) enantiomer).

No products indexed under this heading.

Phenelzine Sulfate (Patients receiving agents with beta-blocking properties and a drug that may deplete catecholamines should be observed closely for signs of hypotension and/or severe bradycardia).

No products indexed under this heading.

Pioglitazone Hydrochloride (Beta-blockers may mask some of the manifestations of hypoglycemia, particularly tachycardia; nonselective beta-blockers may potentiate insulin-induced hypoglycemia and delay recovery of serum glucose levels; in congestive heart failure patients with diabetes, carvedilol therapy may lead to worsening of hyperglycemia, which responds to intensification of hypoglycemia). Products include:

Procarbazine Hydrochloride (Patients receiving agents with beta-blocking properties and a drug that may deplete catecholamines should be observed closely for signs of hypotension and/or severe bradycardia). Products include:

Propafenone Hydrochloride (Interactions of carvedilol with strong inhibitors of CYP2D6, such as propafenone, have not been studied, but these drugs would be expected to increase blood levels of the R(+) enantiomer of carvedilol. Analysis of side effects showed that poor 2D6 metabolizers had a higher rate of dizziness during up-titration, presumably resulting from vasodilating effects of the higher concentrations of the alpha-blocking R(+) enantiomer). Products include:

Propoxyphene Hydrochloride (Interactions of carvedilol with strong inhibitors of CYP2D6, such as quinidine, have not been studied, but these drugs would be expected to increase blood levels of the R(+) enantiomer of carvedilol. Analysis of side effects showed that poor 2D6 metabolizers had a higher rate of dizziness during up-titration, presumably resulting from vasodilating effects of the higher concentrations of the alpha-blocking R(+) enantiomer).

No products indexed under this heading.

Propoxyphene Napsylate (Interactions of carvedilol with strong inhibitors of CYP2D6, such as quinidine, have not been studied, but these drugs would be expected to increase blood levels of the R(+) enantiomer of carvedilol. Analysis of

side effects showed that poor 2D6 metabolizers had a higher rate of dizziness during up-titration, presumably resulting from vasodilating effects of the higher concentrations of the alpha-blocking R(+) enantiomer).

No products indexed under this heading.

Protriptyline Hydrochloride (Interactions of carvedilol with strong inhibitors of CYP2D6, such as quinidine, have not been studied, but these drugs would be expected to increase blood levels of the R(+) enantiomer of carvedilol. Analysis of side effects showed that poor 2D6 metabolizers had a higher rate of dizziness during up-titration, presumably resulting from vasodilating effects of the higher concentrations of the alpha-blocking R(+) enantiomer).

No products indexed under this heading.

Quinacrine Hydrochloride (Interactions of carvedilol with strong inhibitors of CYP2D6, such as quinidine, have not been studied, but these drugs would be expected to increase blood levels of the R(+) enantiomer of carvedilol. Analysis of side effects showed that poor 2D6 metabolizers had a higher rate of dizziness during up-titration, presumably resulting from vasodilating effects of the higher concentrations of the alpha-blocking R(+) enantiomer).

No products indexed under this heading.

Quinidine (Co-administration of carvedilol with strong inhibitors of CYP2D6, such as quinidine, have not been studied, but quinidine would be expected to increase blood levels).

No products indexed under this heading.

Quinidine Gluconate (Co-administration of carvedilol with strong inhibitors of CYP2D6, such as quinidine, have not been studied, but quinidine would be expected to increase blood levels).

No products indexed under this heading.

Quinidine Hydrochloride (Co-administration of carvedilol with strong inhibitors of CYP2D6, such as quinidine, have not been studied, but quinidine would be expected to increase blood levels).

No products indexed under this heading.

Quinidine Polygalacturonate (Co-administration of carvedilol with strong inhibitors of CYP2D6, such as quinidine, have not been studied, but quinidine would be expected to increase blood levels).

No products indexed under this heading.

Quinidine Sulfate (Co-administration of carvedilol with strong inhibitors of CYP2D6, such as quinidine, have not been studied, but quinidine would be expected to increase blood levels).

No products indexed under this heading.

Ranitidine Bismuth Citrate (Interactions of carvedilol with strong inhibitors of CYP2D6, such as quinidine, have not been studied, but these drugs would be expected to increase blood levels of the R(+) enantiomer of carvedilol. Analysis of

side effects showed that poor 2D6 metabolizers had a higher rate of dizziness during up-titration, presumably resulting from vasodilating effects of the higher concentrations of the alpha-blocking R(+) enantiomer).

No products indexed under this heading.

Ranitidine Hydrochloride (Interactions of carvedilol with strong inhibitors of CYP2D6, such as quinidine, have not been studied, but these drugs would be expected to increase blood levels of the R(+) enantiomer of carvedilol. Analysis of side effects showed that poor 2D6 metabolizers had a higher rate of dizziness during up-titration, presumably resulting from vasodilating effects of the higher concentrations of the alpha-blocking R(+) enantiomer). Products include:

Rauwolfia Serpentina (Patients receiving agents with beta-blocking properties and a drug that may deplete catecholamines should be observed closely for signs of hypotension and/or severe bradycardia).

No products indexed under this heading.

Repaglinide (Beta-blockers may mask some of the manifestations of hypoglycemia, particularly tachycardia; nonselective beta-blockers may potentiate insulin-induced hypoglycemia and delay recovery of serum glucose levels; in congestive heart failure patients with diabetes, carvedilol therapy may lead to worsening of hyperglycemia, which responds to intensification of hypoglycemia).

No products indexed under this heading.

Rescinnamine (Patients receiving agents with beta-blocking properties and a drug that may deplete catecholamines should be observed closely for signs of hypotension and/or severe bradycardia).

No products indexed under this heading.

Reserpine (Co-administration of agents with beta-blocking properties and a drug that can deplete catecholamines, such as reserpine, may result in hypotension and/or severe bradycardia).

No products indexed under this heading.

Rifampin (Carvedilol undergoes substantial oxidative metabolism, co-administration has resulted in decreased AUC and Cmax of carvedilol by about 70%).

No products indexed under this heading.

Ritonavir (Interactions of carvedilol with strong inhibitors of CYP2D6, such as quinidine, have not been studied, but these drugs would be expected to increase blood levels of the R(+) enantiomer of carvedilol. Analysis of side effects showed that poor 2D6 metabolizers had a higher rate of dizziness during up-titration, presumably resulting from vasodilating effects of the higher concentrations of the alpha-blocking R(+) enantiomer). Products include:

IMPORTANT NOTE: Always consult each drug listing in the patient's regimen for possible interactions.

Rosiglitazone Maleate (Beta-blockers may mask some of the manifestations of hypoglycemia, particularly tachycardia; nonselective beta-blockers may potentiate insulin-induced hypoglycemia and delay recovery of serum glucose levels; in congestive heart failure patients with diabetes, carvedilol therapy may lead to worsening of hyperglycemia, which responds to intensification of hypoglycemia). Products include:

Avandamet Tablets … 1373
Avandaryl Tablets … 1379
Avandia Tablets … 1384

Selegiline Hydrochloride (Patients receiving agents with beta-blocking properties and a drug that may deplete catecholamines should be observed closely for signs of hypotension and/or severe bradycardia). Products include:

Eldepryl Capsules … 3208
Zelapar Tablets … 3372

Sertraline Hydrochloride (Interactions of carvedilol with strong inhibitors of CYP2D6, such as quinidine, have not been studied, but these drugs would be expected to increase blood levels of the R(+) enantiomer of carvedilol. Analysis of side effects showed that poor 2D6 metabolizers had a higher rate of dizziness during up-titration, presumably resulting from vasodilating effects of the higher concentrations of the alpha-blocking R(+) enantiomer). Products include:

Zoloft … 2586

Terbinafine Hydrochloride (Interactions of carvedilol with strong inhibitors of CYP2D6, such as quinidine, have not been studied, but these drugs would be expected to increase blood levels of the R(+) enantiomer of carvedilol. Analysis of side effects showed that poor 2D6 metabolizers had a higher rate of dizziness during up-titration, presumably resulting from vasodilating effects of the higher concentrations of the alpha-blocking R(+) enantiomer). Products include:

Lamisil Tablets … 2232
Lamisil AT Creams (Athlete's Foot & Jock Itch) … ▣ 636

Thioridazine Hydrochloride (Interactions of carvedilol with strong inhibitors of CYP2D6, such as quinidine, have not been studied, but these drugs would be expected to increase blood levels of the R(+) enantiomer of carvedilol. Analysis of side effects showed that poor 2D6 metabolizers had a higher rate of dizziness during up-titration, presumably resulting from vasodilating effects of the higher concentrations of the alpha-blocking R(+) enantiomer). Products include:

Thioridazine Hydrochloride Tablets … 2163

Tolazamide (Beta-blockers may mask some of the manifestations of hypoglycemia, particularly tachycardia; nonselective beta-blockers may potentiate insulin-induced hypoglycemia and delay recovery of serum glucose levels; in congestive heart failure patients with diabetes, carvedilol therapy may lead to worsening of hyperglycemia, which responds to intensification of hypoglycemia).

No products indexed under this heading.

Tolbutamide (Beta-blockers may mask some of the manifestations of hypoglycemia, particularly tachycardia; nonselective beta-blockers may potentiate insulin-induced hypoglycemia and delay recovery of serum glucose levels; in congestive heart failure patients with diabetes, carvedilol therapy may lead to worsening of hyperglycemia, which responds to intensification of hypoglycemia).

No products indexed under this heading.

Tranylcypromine Sulfate (Patients receiving agents with beta-blocking properties and a drug that may deplete catecholamines should be observed closely for signs of hypotension and/or severe bradycardia). Products include:

Parnate Tablets … 1527

Trimipramine Maleate (Interactions of carvedilol with strong inhibitors of CYP2D6, such as quinidine, have not been studied, but these drugs would be expected to increase blood levels of the R(+) enantiomer of carvedilol. Analysis of side effects showed that poor 2D6 metabolizers had a higher rate of dizziness during up-titration, presumably resulting from vasodilating effects of the higher concentrations of the alpha-blocking R(+) enantiomer).

No products indexed under this heading.

Troglitazone (Beta-blockers may mask some of the manifestations of hypoglycemia, particularly tachycardia; nonselective beta-blockers may potentiate insulin-induced hypoglycemia and delay recovery of serum glucose levels; in congestive heart failure patients with diabetes, carvedilol therapy may lead to worsening of hyperglycemia, which responds to intensification of hypoglycemia).

No products indexed under this heading.

Verapamil Hydrochloride (Co-administration has resulted in isolated cases of conduction disturbances, rarely with hemodynamic. Monitoring of ECG and blood pressure is recommended). Products include:

Covera-HS Tablets … 3139
Tarka Tablets … 524
Verelan PM Extended-Release Capsules, Controlled-Onset … 3106

Food Interactions

Food, unspecified (When carvedilol is administered with food, the rate of absorption is slowed, as evidenced by a delay in the time to reach peak plasma levels, with no significant difference in extent of bioavailability; patients should be instructed to take Coreg with food in order to minimize the risk of hypotension).

COSMEGEN FOR INJECTION

(Dactinomycin) … 2459

May interact with vaccines, live. Compounds in these categories include:

BCG Vaccine (Live virus vaccines should not be administered during drug therapy with dactinomycin).

No products indexed under this heading.

Measles, Mumps, Rubella and Varicella Virus Vaccine Live (Live virus vaccines should not be administered during drug therapy with dactinomycin). Products include:

ProQuad … 2064

Measles, Mumps & Rubella Virus Vaccine, Live (Live virus vaccines should not be administered during drug therapy with dactinomycin). Products include:

M-M-R II … 2006

Measles & Rubella Virus Vaccine Live (Live virus vaccines should not be administered during drug therapy with dactinomycin).

No products indexed under this heading.

Measles Virus Vaccine Live (Live virus vaccines should not be administered during drug therapy with dactinomycin). Products include:

Attenuvax … 1914

Mumps Virus Vaccine, Live (Live virus vaccines should not be administered during drug therapy with dactinomycin). Products include:

Mumpsvax … 2031

Poliovirus Vaccine, Live, Oral, Trivalent, Types 1,2,3 (Sabin) (Live virus vaccines should not be administered during drug therapy with dactinomycin).

No products indexed under this heading.

Rotavirus Vaccine, Live, Oral, Tetravalent (Live virus vaccines should not be administered during drug therapy with dactinomycin).

No products indexed under this heading.

Rubella & Mumps Virus Vaccine Live (Live virus vaccines should not be administered during drug therapy with dactinomycin).

No products indexed under this heading.

Rubella Virus Vaccine Live (Live virus vaccines should not be administered during drug therapy with dactinomycin). Products include:

Meruvax II … 2019

Smallpox Vaccine (Live virus vaccines should not be administered during drug therapy with dactinomycin).

No products indexed under this heading.

Typhoid Vaccine (Live virus vaccines should not be administered during drug therapy with dactinomycin).

No products indexed under this heading.

Varicella Virus Vaccine Live (Live virus vaccines should not be administered during drug therapy with dactinomycin). Products include:

Varivax … 2100

Yellow Fever Vaccine (Live virus vaccines should not be administered during drug therapy with dactinomycin).

No products indexed under this heading.

COSOPT STERILE OPHTHALMIC SOLUTION

(Dorzolamide Hydrochloride, Timolol Maleate) … 1931

May interact with beta blockers, carbonic anhydrase inhibitors, calcium channel blockers, cardiac glycosides, quinidine, salicylates, and certain other agents. Compounds in these categories include:

Acebutolol Hydrochloride (Co-administration of oral beta-adrenergic blockers and Cosopt may result in potential additive effects of beta-blockade, both systemic and on intraocular pressure).

No products indexed under this heading.

Acetazolamide (Co-administration with oral carbonic anhydrase inhibitor may result in additive carbonic anhydrase inhibition).

No products indexed under this heading.

Amlodipine Besylate (Co-administration of beta-adrenergic blockers and calcium channel blockers may result in possible atrioventricular conduction disturbances, left ventricular failure, and hypotension). Products include:

Caduet Tablets … 2508
Lotrel Capsules … 2249
Norvasc Tablets … 2545

Aspirin (Potential for acid-base and electrolyte disturbances with high-dose salicylate therapy). Products include:

Aggrenox Capsules … 822
Bayer Aspirin … 744
BC Allergy Sinus Cold Powder … ▣ 677
BC Headache Powder … ▣ 677
Arthritis Strength BC Powder … ▣ 677
BC Sinus Cold Powder … ▣ 677
Excedrin Extra Strength Caplets/Tablets/Geltabs … ▣ 684
Excedrin Migraine Caplets/Tablets/Geltabs … ▣ 609
Goody's Body Pain Formula Powder … ▣ 684
Goody's Extra Strength Headache Powders … ▣ 611
Goody's Extra Strength Pain Relief Tablets … ▣ 685
Percodan Tablets … 1132
St. Joseph 81 mg Aspirin Chewable and Enteric Coated Tablets … 1869

Aspirin, Enteric Coated (Potential for acid-base and electrolyte disturbances with high-dose salicylate therapy).

No products indexed under this heading.

Aspirin Buffered (Potential for acid-base and electrolyte disturbances with high-dose salicylate therapy). Products include:

Bufferin Extra Strength Tablets … ▣ 678
Bufferin Regular Strength Tablets … ▣ 678

Atenolol (Co-administration of oral beta-adrenergic blockers and Cosopt may result in potential additive effects of beta-blockade, both systemic and on intraocular pressure).

No products indexed under this heading.

Bepridil Hydrochloride (Co-administration of beta-adrenergic blockers and calcium channel blockers may result in possible atrioventricular conduction disturbances, left ventricular failure, and hypotension).

No products indexed under this heading.

Betaxolol Hydrochloride (Co-administration of oral beta-adrenergic blockers and Cosopt may result in potential additive effects of beta-

blockade, both systemic and on intraocular pressure; the concomitant use of two topical beta-adrenergic agents is not recommended). Products include:
Betoptic S Ophthalmic Suspension 558

Carteolol Hydrochloride (Co-administration of oral beta-adrenergic blockers and Cosopt may result in potential additive effects of beta-blockade, both systemic and on intraocular pressure; the concomitant use of two topical beta-adrenergic agents is not recommended). Products include:
Carteolol Hydrochloride Ophthalmic Solution USP, 1% .... ⊙249

Choline Magnesium Trisalicylate (Potential for acid-base and electrolyte disturbances with high-dose salicylate therapy).
No products indexed under this heading.

Clonidine (Oral beta-adrenergic blocking agents may exacerbate the rebound hypertension which can follow withdrawal of clonidine; there have been no reports of exacerbation of rebound hypertension with ophthalmic timolol). Products include:
Catapres-TTS 844

Clonidine Hydrochloride (Oral beta-adrenergic blocking agents may exacerbate the rebound hypertension which can follow withdrawal of clonidine; there have been no reports of exacerbation of rebound hypertension with ophthalmic timolol). Products include:
Catapres Tablets 843
Clorpres Tablets 2153

Deslanoside (The concomitant use of beta-adrenergic blocking agents with digitalis and calcium antagonists may have additive effects in prolonging atrioventricular conduction time).
No products indexed under this heading.

Dichlorphenamide (Co-administration with oral carbonic anhydrase inhibitor may result in additive carbonic anhydrase inhibition). Products include:
Daranide Tablets 1950

Diflunisal (Potential for acid-base and electrolyte disturbances with high-dose salicylate therapy). Products include:
Dolobid Tablets 1955

Digitalis Glycoside Preparations (The concomitant use of beta-adrenergic blocking agents with digitalis and calcium antagonists may have additive effects in prolonging atrioventricular conduction time).
No products indexed under this heading.

Digitoxin (The concomitant use of beta-adrenergic blocking agents with digitalis and calcium antagonists may have additive effects in prolonging atrioventricular conduction time).
No products indexed under this heading.

Digoxin (The concomitant use of beta-adrenergic blocking agents with digitalis and calcium antagonists may have additive effects in prolonging atrioventricular conduction time). Products include:
Lanoxicaps Capsules 1490
Lanoxin Injection 1494
Lanoxin Injection Pediatric 1497
Lanoxin Tablets 1500

Diltiazem Hydrochloride (Co-administration of beta-adrenergic blockers and calcium channel blockers may result in possible atrioventricular conduction disturbances, left ventricular failure, and hypotension). Products include:
Cardizem LA Extended Release Tablets 1728
Tiazac Capsules 1201

Epinephrine (Patients with a history of atopy or anaphylactic reactions to a variety of allergens may be unresponsive to the usual dose of injectable epinephrine used to treat allergic reactions). Products include:
EpiPen 1061
Primatene Mist .... ▣719
Twinject 0.15 3379
Twinject 0.3 3378

Epinephrine Hydrochloride (Patients with a history of atopy or anaphylactic reactions to a variety of allergens may be unresponsive to the usual dose of injectable epinephrine used to treat allergic reactions).
No products indexed under this heading.

Felodipine (Co-administration of beta-adrenergic blockers and calcium channel blockers may result in possible atrioventricular conduction disturbances, left ventricular failure, and hypotension).
No products indexed under this heading.

Isradipine (Co-administration of beta-adrenergic blockers and calcium channel blockers may result in possible atrioventricular conduction disturbances, left ventricular failure, and hypotension). Products include:
DynaCirc CR Tablets 2721

Levobunolol Hydrochloride (Co-administration of oral beta-adrenergic blockers and Cosopt may result in potential additive effects of beta-blockade, both systemic and on intraocular pressure; the concomitant use of two topical beta-adrenergic agents is not recommended). Products include:
Betagan Ophthalmic Solution, USP .... ⊙220

Magnesium Salicylate (Potential for acid-base and electrolyte disturbances with high-dose salicylate therapy).
No products indexed under this heading.

Methazolamide (Co-administration with oral carbonic anhydrase inhibitor may result in additive carbonic anhydrase inhibition).
No products indexed under this heading.

Metipranolol Hydrochloride (Co-administration of oral beta-adrenergic blockers and Cosopt may result in potential additive effects of beta-blockade, both systemic and on intraocular pressure; the concomitant use of two topical beta-adrenergic agents is not recommended).
No products indexed under this heading.

Mibefradil Dihydrochloride (Co-administration of beta-adrenergic blockers and calcium channel blockers may result in possible atrioventricular conduction disturbances, left ventricular failure, and hypotension).
No products indexed under this heading.

Nicardipine Hydrochloride (Co-administration of beta-adrenergic blockers and calcium channel blockers may result in possible atrioventricular conduction disturbances, left ventricular failure, and hypotension). Products include:
Cardene I.V. 2497

Nifedipine (Co-administration of beta-adrenergic blockers and calcium channel blockers may result in possible atrioventricular conduction disturbances, left ventricular failure, and hypotension). Products include:
Adalat CC Tablets 2964

Nimodipine (Co-administration of beta-adrenergic blockers and calcium channel blockers may result in possible atrioventricular conduction disturbances, left ventricular failure, and hypotension). Products include:
Nimotop Capsules 749

Nisoldipine (Co-administration of beta-adrenergic blockers and calcium channel blockers may result in possible atrioventricular conduction disturbances, left ventricular failure, and hypotension). Products include:
Sular Tablets 3122

Quinidine (Potentiated systemic beta-blockade has been reported during combined treatment with quinidine and timolol).
No products indexed under this heading.

Quinidine Gluconate (Potentiated systemic beta-blockade has been reported during combined treatment with quinidine and timolol).
No products indexed under this heading.

Quinidine Hydrochloride (Potentiated systemic beta-blockade has been reported during combined treatment with quinidine and timolol).
No products indexed under this heading.

Quinidine Polygalacturonate (Potentiated systemic beta-blockade has been reported during combined treatment with quinidine and timolol).
No products indexed under this heading.

Quinidine Sulfate (Potentiated systemic beta-blockade has been reported during combined treatment with quinidine and timolol).
No products indexed under this heading.

Reserpine (Co-administration of catecholamine-depleting drugs and beta-adrenergic blocker may result in possible additive effects and the production of hypotension and/or marked bradycardia).
No products indexed under this heading.

Salsalate (Potential for acid-base and electrolyte disturbances with high-dose salicylate therapy).
No products indexed under this heading.

Timolol Hemihydrate (Co-administration of oral beta-adrenergic blockers and Cosopt may result in potential additive effects of beta-blockade, both systemic and on intraocular pressure; the concomitant use of two topical beta-adrenergic agents is not recommended). Products include:
Betimol Ophthalmic Solution 3382
Betimol Ophthalmic Solution .... ⊙295

Verapamil Hydrochloride (Co-administration of beta-adrenergic blockers and calcium channel blockers may result in possible atrioventricular conduction disturbances, left ventricular failure, and hypotension). Products include:
Covera-HS Tablets 3139
Tarka Tablets 524
Verelan PM Extended-Release Capsules, Controlled-Onset 3106

COUMADIN FOR INJECTION

(Warfarin Sodium) 898
See Coumadin Tablets

COUMADIN TABLETS

(Warfarin Sodium) 898
May interact with 5-lipoxygenase inhibitors, oral aminoglycosides, androgens, antacids, antihistamines, antiandrogens, barbiturates, corticosteroids, diuretics, erythromycin, fluoroquinolone antibiotics, inhalant anesthetics, leukotriene receptor antagonists, monoamine oxidase inhibitors, narcotic analgesics, nonsteroidal anti-inflammatory agents, oral contraceptives, pyrazolon derivatives, salicylates, selective serotonin reuptake inhibitors, sulfonamides, thyroid preparations, and certain other agents. Compounds in these categories include:

Acetaminophen (May be responsible for increased prothrombin time response). Products include:
Comtrex Maximum Strength Cold & Cough Day/Night Caplets - Day Formulation .... ▣726
Comtrex Maximum Strength Cold & Cough Day/Night Caplets - Night Formulation .... ▣726
Comtrex Maximum Strength Non-Drowsy Cold & Cough Caplets .... ▣725
Comtrex Maximum Strength Day/Night Severe Cold & Sinus Caplets - Day Formulation .... ▣725
Comtrex Maximum Strength Day/Night Severe Cold & Sinus Caplets - Night Formulation .... ▣725
Contac Cold and Flu Maximum Strength Caplets .... ▣728
Contac Cold and Flu Day and Night Caplets (Day Formulation Only) .... ▣727
Contac Cold and Flu Day and Night Caplets (Night Formulation Only) .... ▣727
Contac Cold and Flu Non-Drowsy Caplets .... ▣728
Excedrin Extra Strength Caplets/Tablets/Geltabs .... ▣684
Excedrin Migraine Caplets/Tablets/Geltabs .... ▣609
Excedrin PM Caplets/Tablets/Geltabs .... ▣610
Excedrin Sinus Headache Caplets/Tablets .... ▣610
Excedrin Tension Headache Caplets/Tablets/Geltabs .... ▣611
Goody's Body Pain Formula Powder .... ▣684
Goody's Extra Strength Headache Powders .... ▣611
Goody's Extra Strength Pain Relief Tablets .... ▣685
Goody's PM Powder for Pain with Sleeplessness .... ▣612
Percocet Tablets 1131
Robitussin Cough, Cold & Flu Nighttime Liquid .... ▣738
TheraFlu Cold & Sore Throat Hot Liquid .... ▣741
TheraFlu Flu & Chest Congestion Hot Liquid .... ▣741
TheraFlu Flu & Sore Throat Hot Liquid .... ▣742
TheraFlu Daytime Severe Cold Hot Liquid .... ▣742
TheraFlu Nighttime Severe Cold Hot Liquid .... ▣740
TheraFlu Warming Relief Daytime Severe Cold .... ▣743
TheraFlu Warming Relief Nighttime Severe Cold .... ▣743
Triaminic Cough & Sore Throat Liquid .... ▣747
Regular Strength Tylenol Tablets 1870
Children's Tylenol with Flavor Creator .... ▣679

Children's Tylenol Plus Flu Oral Suspension .... ▣749
Tylenol Cold Head Congestion Daytime Caplets with Cool Burst and Gelcaps .... ▣750
Tylenol Cold Multi-Symptom Daytime Liquid .... ▣752
Tylenol Cold Multi-Symptom Severe Daytime Liquid .... ▣752
Tylenol 8 Hour Extended Release Caplets 1870
Tylenol 1870
Extra Strength Tylenol PM Caplets, Vanilla Caplets, Geltabs, Gelcaps and Liquid 1875
Extra Strength Tylenol Rapid Release Gels 1870
Concentrated Tylenol Infants' Drops Plus Cold & Cough .... ▣754
Tylenol with Codeine Tablets 2391
Tylenol Allergy Multi-Symptom Caplets with Cool Burst and Gelcaps 1872
Tylenol Allergy Multi-Symptom Nighttime Caplets with Cool Burst 1872
Tylenol Severe Allergy Caplets 1872
Tylenol Arthritis Pain Extended Release Caplets and Geltabs 1870
Tylenol Chest Congestion Caplets with Cool Burst 1872
Tylenol Chest Congestion Liquid with Cool Burst 1872
Children's Tylenol Suspension Liquid and Meltaways 1878
Children's Tylenol Plus Cold Suspension Liquid 1879
Children's Tylenol Plus Cold & Allergy Suspension Liquid 1878
Children's Tylenol Plus Cough & Runny Nose Suspension Liquid 1879
Children's Tylenol Plus Cough & Sore Throat Suspension Liquid 1879
Children's Tylenol Suspension with Flavor Creator 1878
Children's Tylenol Plus Flu Suspension Liquid 1881
Children's Tylenol Plus Multi-Symptom Cold Suspension Liquid 1879
Tylenol Cold Severe Congestion Non-Drowsy Caplets with Cool Burst 1874
Tylenol Cold Head Congestion Daytime Caplets with Cool Burst 1873
Tylenol Cold Head Congestion Nighttime Caplets with Cool Burst 1873
Tylenol Cold Head Congestion Severe Caplets with Cool Burst 1873
Tylenol Cold Multi-Symptom Daytime Caplets with Cool Burst and Gelcaps 1874
Tylenol Cold Multi-Symptom Daytime Liquid with Citrus Burst 1874
Tylenol Cold Multi-Symptom Nighttime Caplets with Cool Burst 1874
Tylenol Cold Multi-Symptom Nighttime Liquid with Cool Burst 1874
Tylenol Cold Multi-Symptom Severe Caplets with Cool Burst 1874
Tylenol Cold Multi-Symptom Severe Daytime Liquid with Citrus Burst 1874
Tylenol Cough & Sore Throat Daytime Liquid with Cool Burst 1877
Tylenol Cough & Sore Throat Nighttime Liquid with Cool Burst 1877
Concentrated Tylenol Infants' Drops 1878
Concentrated Tylenol Infants' Drops Plus Cold 1879
Concentrated Tylenol Infants' Drops Plus Cold and Cough 1879
Jr. Tylenol Meltaways 1878
Tylenol Sinus Severe Congestion Caplets with Cool Burst 1876
Tylenol Sinus Congestion & Pain Daytime Caplets with Cool Burst and Gelcaps 1876
Tylenol Sinus Congestion & Pain Nighttime Caplets with Cool Burst 1876
Tylenol Sinus Congestion & Pain Severe Caplets with Cool Burst 1876
Tylenol Sore Throat Daytime Liquid with Cool Burst 1877
Tylenol Sore Throat Nighttime Liquid with Cool Burst 1877
Women's Tylenol Menstrual Relief Caplets 1877
Vicks 44M Cough, Cold & Flu Relief Liquid 2680
Vicks DayQuil LiquiCaps/Liquid Multi-Symptom Cold/Flu Relief .... ▣761
Vicks DayQuil Multi-Symptom Cold/Flu Relief LiquiCaps 2678
Vicks DayQuil Multi-Symptom Cold/Flu Relief Liquid 2678
Vicks NyQuil Multi-Symptom Cold/Flu Relief Liquid 2681
Vicks NyQuil Multi-Symptom Cold/Flu Relief LiquiCaps 2681
Vicks NyQuil LiquiCaps/Liquid Multi-Symptom Cold/Flu Relief .... ▣763
Vicodin Tablets 535
Vicodin ES Tablets 536
Vicodin HP Tablets 538
Zicam Maximum Strength Flu Daytime .... ▣768
Zicam Maximum Strength Flu Nighttime .... ▣768
Zydone Tablets 1139

Achillea millefolium (Co-administration with botanicals with coagulant properties, such as yarrow, may affect the anticoagulant effects of warfarin).
No products indexed under this heading.

Acrivastine (Decreased prothrombin time response).
No products indexed under this heading.

ACTH (Decreased prothrombin time response).
No products indexed under this heading.

Agrimonia eupatoria (Co-administration with botanicals that contain salicylate and/or have antiplatelet properties, such as agrimony, may result in increased anticoagulant effects; agrimony contains salicylate and has coagulant properties).
No products indexed under this heading.

Alatrofloxacin Mesylate (Increased prothrombin time response).
No products indexed under this heading.

Alfentanil Hydrochloride (Increased prothrombin time response with prolonged use).
No products indexed under this heading.

Allium cepa (Co-administration with botanicals that contain salicylate and/or have antiplatelet or fibrinolytic properties, such as onion, may result in increased anticoagulant effects). Products include:
Mederma Topical Gel 2126
Mederma for Kids Topical Gel 2126

Allium sativum (Co-administration is associated most often with increases in the effects of warfarin; garlic may cause bleeding events when taken alone and may have anticoagulant, antiplatelet, and/or fibrinolytic properties).
No products indexed under this heading.

Allopurinol (Increased prothrombin time response).
No products indexed under this heading.

Aloe Gel (Co-administration with botanicals that contain salicylate and/or have antiplatelet properties, such as aloe gel, may result in increased anticoagulant effects).
No products indexed under this heading.

Alteplase (Increased prothrombin time response). Products include:
Activase I.V. 1223
Cathflo Activase 1231

Aluminum Carbonate (Decreased prothrombin time response).
No products indexed under this heading.

Aluminum Hydroxide (Decreased prothrombin time response). Products include:
Gaviscon Regular Strength Liquid .... ▣658
Gaviscon Regular Strength Tablets .... ▣658
Gaviscon Extra Strength Liquid .... ▣658
Gaviscon Extra Strength Tablets .... ▣658
Maalox Regular Strength Antacid/Antigas Liquid 2175
Maalox Max Maximum Strength Antacid/Anti-Gas Liquid 2176

Amiloride Hydrochloride (Decreased or increased prothrombin time response). Products include:
Midamor Tablets 2026
Moduretic Tablets 2028

Aminoglutethimide (Decreased prothrombin time response).
No products indexed under this heading.

p-Aminosalicylic Acid (Increased prothrombin time response).
No products indexed under this heading.

Amiodarone Hydrochloride (Increased prothrombin time response).
No products indexed under this heading.

Amobarbital (Decreased prothrombin time response).
No products indexed under this heading.

Aniseed (Co-administration with botanicals that contain coumarins, such as aniseed, may result in increased anticoagulant effects).
No products indexed under this heading.

Anistreplase (Increased prothrombin time response).
No products indexed under this heading.

Antibiotics, unspecified (Decreased or increased prothrombin time response).
No products indexed under this heading.

Antipyrine (Increased prothrombin time response).
No products indexed under this heading.

Apium graveolens (Co-administration with botanicals that contain coumarins, such as celery, may result in increased anticoagulant effects).
No products indexed under this heading.

Aprobarbital (Decreased prothrombin time response).
No products indexed under this heading.

Ardeparin Sodium (Co-administration has resulted in cases of venous limb ischemia, necrosis, and gangrene in patients with heparin-induced thrombocytopenia and deep venous thrombosis when heparin treatment was discontinued and warfarin therapy was started or continued; sequelae have included amputation of the involved area and/or death).
No products indexed under this heading.

Armoracia rusticana (Co-administration with botanicals that contain coumarins, such as horseradish, may result in increased anticoagulant effects).
No products indexed under this heading.

Arnica montana (Co-administration with botanicals that contain coumarins, such as arnica, may result in increased anticoagulant effects). Products include:
Zeel Solution 1665

Aspen (Co-administration with botanicals that contain salicylate and/or have antiplatelet properties, such as aspen, may result in increased anticoagulant effects).
No products indexed under this heading.

Aspirin (Increased prothrombin time response; caution should be observed when used concurrently). Products include:
Aggrenox Capsules 822
Bayer Aspirin 744
BC Allergy Sinus Cold Powder .... ▣677
BC Headache Powder .... ▣677
Arthritis Strength BC Powder .... ▣677
BC Sinus Cold Powder .... ▣677
Excedrin Extra Strength Caplets/Tablets/Geltabs .... ▣684
Excedrin Migraine Caplets/Tablets/Geltabs .... ▣609
Goody's Body Pain Formula Powder .... ▣684
Goody's Extra Strength Headache Powders .... ▣611
Goody's Extra Strength Pain Relief Tablets .... ▣685
Percodan Tablets 1132
St. Joseph 81 mg Aspirin Chewable and Enteric Coated Tablets 1869

Aspirin, Enteric Coated (Increased prothrombin time response; caution should be observed when used concurrently).
No products indexed under this heading.

Aspirin Buffered (Increased prothrombin time response; caution should be observed when used concurrently). Products include:
Bufferin Extra Strength Tablets .... ▣678
Bufferin Regular Strength Tablets .... ▣678

Astemizole (Decreased prothrombin time response).
No products indexed under this heading.

Atorvastatin Calcium (Decreased prothrombin time response). Products include:
Caduet Tablets 2508
Lipitor Tablets 2483

Azatadine Maleate (Decreased prothrombin time response).
No products indexed under this heading.

Azathioprine (Decreased prothrombin time response).
No products indexed under this heading.

Azithromycin Dihydrate (Increased prothrombin time response).
No products indexed under this heading.

Bendroflumethiazide (Decreased or increased prothrombin time response).
No products indexed under this heading.

Betamethasone Acetate (Decreased or increased prothrombin time response).
No products indexed under this heading.

Betamethasone Sodium Phosphate (Decreased or increased prothrombin time response).
No products indexed under this heading.

Bicalutamide (May be responsible, alone or in combination, for increased prothrombin time/ international normalized ratio (PT/ INR) response).
No products indexed under this heading.

Black Cohosh (Co-administration with botanicals that contain salicylate and/or have antiplatelet properties, such as black cohosh, may result in increased anticoagulant effects).
No products indexed under this heading.

Bromelains (Co-administration is associated most often with increases in the effects of warfarin).
No products indexed under this heading.

Bromodiphenhydramine Hydrochloride (Decreased prothrombin time response).
No products indexed under this heading.

Brompheniramine Maleate (Decreased prothrombin time response). Products include:
Children's Dimetapp Cold & Allergy Elixir ■ 730
Children's Dimetapp Cold & Allergy Chewable Tablets ■ 730
Children's Dimetapp DM Cold & Cough Elixir ■ 731

Buchu (Co-administration with botanicals that contain coumarins, such as buchu, may result in increased anticoagulant effects).
No products indexed under this heading.

Bumetanide (Decreased or increased prothrombin time response). Products include:
Bumex Tablets 2746

Buprenorphine Hydrochloride (Increased prothrombin time response with prolonged use). Products include:
Buprenex Injectable 2716
Suboxone Tablets 2717
Subutex Tablets 2717

Butabarbital (Decreased prothrombin time response).
No products indexed under this heading.

Butalbital (Decreased prothrombin time response).
No products indexed under this heading.

Capecitabine (Increased prothrombin time response). Products include:
Xeloda Tablets 2822

Capsicum annuum (Co-administration with botanicals that contain coumarins, such as capsicum, may result in increased anticoagulant effects; capsicum also has fibrinolytic properties).
No products indexed under this heading.

Carbamazepine (Decreased prothrombin time response). Products include:
Carbatrol Capsules 3171
Equetro Extended-Release Capsules 3180
Tegretol/Tegretol-XR 2295

Cassia angustifolia (Co-administration with botanicals that contain coumarins, such as cassia, may result in increased anticoagulant effects).
No products indexed under this heading.

Cassia fistula (Co-administration with botanicals that contain coumarins, such as cassia, may result in increased anticoagulant effects).
No products indexed under this heading.

Cassia senna (Co-administration with botanicals that contain coumarins, such as cassia, may result in increased anticoagulant effects).
No products indexed under this heading.

Cefamandole Nafate (Increased prothrombin time response).
No products indexed under this heading.

Cefazolin Sodium (Increased prothrombin time response).
No products indexed under this heading.

Cefoperazone Sodium (Increased prothrombin time response).
No products indexed under this heading.

Cefotetan (Increased prothrombin time response).
No products indexed under this heading.

Cefoxitin Sodium (Increased prothrombin time response). Products include:
Mefoxin for Injection 2012
Mefoxin Premixed Intravenous Solution 2016

Ceftriaxone Sodium (Increased prothrombin time response). Products include:
Rocephin Injectable Vials, ADD-Vantage, Galaxy, Bulk 2800

Celecoxib (Increased prothrombin time response; caution should be observed when used concurrently). Products include:
Celebrex Capsules 3134

Cerivastatin Sodium (May be responsible, alone or in combination, for increased prothrombin time/ international normalized ratio (PT/ INR) response).
No products indexed under this heading.

Cetirizine Hydrochloride (Decreased prothrombin time response). Products include:
Zyrtec Chewable Tablets 2594
Zyrtec 2594
Zyrtec-D 12 Hour Extended Release Tablets 2597

Chenodiol (Increased prothrombin time response).
No products indexed under this heading.

Chloral Hydrate (Decreased or increased prothrombin time response).
No products indexed under this heading.

Chloramphenicol (Increased prothrombin time response).
No products indexed under this heading.

Chloramphenicol Palmitate (Increased prothrombin time response).
No products indexed under this heading.

Chloramphenicol Sodium Succinate (Increased prothrombin time response).
No products indexed under this heading.

Chlordiazepoxide (Decreased prothrombin time response).
No products indexed under this heading.

Chlordiazepoxide Hydrochloride (Decreased prothrombin time response). Products include:
Librium Capsules 3347

Chlorothiazide (Decreased or increased prothrombin time response). Products include:
Diuril Oral Suspension 1954

Chlorothiazide Sodium (Decreased or increased prothrombin time response). Products include:
Diuril Sodium Intravenous 2467

Chlorpheniramine Maleate (Decreased prothrombin time response). Products include:
Advil Allergy Sinus Caplets ■ 770
Advil Multi-Symptom Cold Caplets ■ 770
BC Allergy Sinus Cold Powder ■ 677
Comtrex Maximum Strength Cold & Cough Day/Night Caplets - Night Formulation ■ 726
Comtrex Maximum Strength Day/Night Severe Cold & Sinus Caplets - Night Formulation ■ 725
Contac Cold and Flu Maximum Strength Caplets ■ 728
Contac Cold and Flu Day and Night Caplets (Night Formulation Only) ■ 727
Children's Dimetapp Long Acting Cough Plus Cold Syrup ■ 731
Robitussin Cough & Cold Long-Acting Liquid ■ 735
Robitussin Cough & Allergy Syrup ■ 736
Robitussin Cough & Cold Nighttime Liquid ■ 736
Robitussin Cough, Cold & Flu Nighttime Liquid ■ 738
Robitussin Pediatric Cough & Cold Long-Acting Liquid ■ 735
Robitussin Pediatric Cough & Cold Nighttime Liquid ■ 736
Triaminic Cold & Allergy Liquid ■ 746
Triaminic Cough & Runny Nose Softchews ■ 748
Children's Tylenol Plus Flu Oral Suspension ■ 749
Tylenol Allergy Multi-Symptom Caplets with Cool Burst and Gelcaps 1872
Children's Tylenol Plus Cold Suspension Liquid 1879
Children's Tylenol Plus Cough & Runny Nose Suspension Liquid 1879
Children's Tylenol Plus Flu Suspension Liquid 1881
Children's Tylenol Plus Multi-Symptom Cold Suspension Liquid 1879
Tylenol Cold Head Congestion Nighttime Caplets with Cool Burst 1873
Tylenol Cold Multi-Symptom Nighttime Caplets with Cool Burst 1874
Tylenol Sinus Congestion & Pain Nighttime Caplets with Cool Burst 1876
Vicks 44M Cough, Cold & Flu Relief Liquid 2680
Pediatric Vicks 44m Cough & Cold Relief Liquid 2676
Children's Vicks NyQuil Cold/Cough Relief ■ 756
Children's Vicks NyQuil Cold/Cough Relief Liquid 2680
Zicam Maximum Strength Flu Daytime ■ 768

Chlorpheniramine Polistirex (Decreased prothrombin time response). Products include:
Tussionex Pennkinetic Extended-Release Suspension 3327

Chlorpheniramine Tannate (Decreased prothrombin time response).
No products indexed under this heading.

Chlorpropamide (Increased prothrombin time response; accumulation of chlorpropamide).
No products indexed under this heading.

Chlorthalidone (Decreased or increased prothrombin time response). Products include:
Clorpres Tablets 2153

Cholestyramine (Decreased or increased prothrombin time response).
No products indexed under this heading.

Choline Magnesium Trisalicylate (Increased prothrombin time response; caution should be observed when used concurrently).
No products indexed under this heading.

Cimetidine (Increased prothrombin time response). Products include:
Tagamet HB 200 Tablets ■ 664

Cimetidine Hydrochloride (Increased prothrombin time response).
No products indexed under this heading.

Ciprofloxacin (Increased prothrombin time response). Products include:
Cipro Oral Suspension 2977
Cipro I.V. 2984
Cipro XR Tablets 2990
Ciprodex Otic Suspension 559

Ciprofloxacin Hydrochloride (Increased prothrombin time response). Products include:
Ciloxan Ophthalmic Ointment 559
Ciloxan Ophthalmic Solution ⊙ 206
Cipro Tablets 2977
Proquin XR Tablets 1153

Cisapride (Increased prothrombin time response).
No products indexed under this heading.

Citalopram Hydrobromide (Increased prothrombin time response). Products include:
Celexa 1176

Clarithromycin (Increased prothrombin time response). Products include:
Biaxin/Biaxin XL 402
PREVPAC 3284

Clemastine Fumarate (Decreased prothrombin time response).
No products indexed under this heading.

Clofibrate (Increased prothrombin time response).
No products indexed under this heading.

Clozapine (May be responsible, alone or in combination, for

decreased prothrombin time/international normalized ratio (PT/INR) response). Products include:
Clozaril Tablets 2184
FazaClo Orally Disintegrating Tablets 551

Codeine Phosphate (Increased prothrombin time response with prolonged use). Products include:
Tylenol with Codeine Tablets 2391

Coenzyme Q-10 (Co-administration is associated most often with decreases in the effects of warfarin). Products include:
Cardio Essentials Capsules 3328
CoQuinone Capsules 3339

Cortisone Acetate (Decreased or increased prothrombin time response).
No products indexed under this heading.

Cyclophosphamide (Increased or decreased prothrombin time response).
No products indexed under this heading.

Cyproheptadine Hydrochloride (Decreased prothrombin time response).
No products indexed under this heading.

Dalteparin Sodium (Co-administration has resulted in cases of venous limb ischemia, necrosis, and gangrene in patients with heparin-induced thrombocytopenia and deep venous thrombosis when heparin treatment was discontinued and warfarin therapy was started or continued; sequelae have included amputation of the involved area and/or death). Products include:
Fragmin Injection 1097

Danazol (Increased prothrombin time response).
No products indexed under this heading.

Danshen (Increased prothrombin time response).
No products indexed under this heading.

Daucus carota (Co-administration with botanicals that contain coumarins, such as wild carrots, may result in increased anticoagulant effects).
No products indexed under this heading.

Desflurane (Increased prothrombin time response).
No products indexed under this heading.

Desogestrel (Decreased prothrombin time response). Products include:
Mircette Tablets 1066

Dexamethasone (Decreased or increased prothrombin time response). Products include:
Ciprodex Otic Suspension 559
Decadron Tablets 1951
TobraDex Ophthalmic Ointment 562
TobraDex Ophthalmic Suspension 563

Dexamethasone Acetate (Decreased or increased prothrombin time response).
No products indexed under this heading.

Dexamethasone Sodium Phosphate (Decreased or increased prothrombin time response).
No products indexed under this heading.

Dexchlorpheniramine Maleate (Decreased prothrombin time response).
No products indexed under this heading.

Dextrans (Low Molecular Weight) (Increased prothrombin time response).
No products indexed under this heading.

Dextrothyroxine Sodium (Increased prothrombin time response).
No products indexed under this heading.

Dezocine (Increased prothrombin time response with prolonged use).
No products indexed under this heading.

Diazoxide (Increased prothrombin time response). Products include:
Hyperstat I.V. 3017

Diclofenac Potassium (Increased prothrombin time response; caution should be observed when used concurrently).
No products indexed under this heading.

Diclofenac Sodium (Increased prothrombin time response; caution should be observed when used concurrently). Products include:
Arthrotec Tablets 3129
Voltaren Ophthalmic Solution 2309
Voltaren Tablets 2307
Voltaren-XR Tablets 2310

Dicloxacillin Sodium (Decreased prothrombin time response).
No products indexed under this heading.

Dicumarol (Increased prothrombin time response).
No products indexed under this heading.

Diflunisal (Increased prothrombin time response; caution should be observed when used concurrently). Products include:
Dolobid Tablets 1955

Diphenhydramine Citrate (Decreased prothrombin time response). Products include:
Advil PM Caplets .... ▣615
Excedrin PM Caplets/Tablets/Geltabs .... ▣610
Goody's PM Powder for Pain with Sleeplessness .... ▣612

Diphenhydramine Hydrochloride (Decreased prothrombin time response). Products include:
Nytol QuickCaps Caplets .... ▣615
Nytol QuickGels Softgels Maximum Strength .... ▣616
Simply Sleep Caplets 1868
Sominex Original Formula Tablets .... ▣616
TheraFlu Warming Relief Nighttime Severe Cold .... ▣743
TheraFlu Thin Strips Multi Symptom .... ▣744
Triaminic Nighttime Cold & Cough Liquid .... ▣746
Triaminic Thin Strips Cough & Runny Nose .... ▣749
Extra Strength Tylenol PM Caplets, Vanilla Caplets, Geltabs, Gelcaps and Liquid 1875
Tylenol Sore Throat Nighttime Liquid with Cool Burst .... ▣790
Tylenol Allergy Multi-Symptom Nighttime Caplets with Cool Burst 1872
Tylenol Severe Allergy Caplets 1872
Children's Tylenol Plus Cold & Allergy Suspension Liquid 1878

Diphenylpyraline Hydrochloride (Decreased prothrombin time response).
No products indexed under this heading.

Dipteryx odorata (Co-administration with botanicals that contain coumarins, such as tonka beans, may result in increased anticoagulant effects).
No products indexed under this heading.

Disulfiram (Increased prothrombin time response).
No products indexed under this heading.

Divalproex Sodium (Increased prothrombin time response). Products include:
Depakote Sprinkle Capsules 422
Depakote Tablets 427
Depakote ER Tablets 434

Dong Quai (Co-administration with botanicals that contain coumarins, such as dong quai (angelica), may result in increased anticoagulant effects).
No products indexed under this heading.

Doxycycline Calcium (Increased prothrombin time response).
No products indexed under this heading.

Doxycycline Hyclate (Increased prothrombin time response).
No products indexed under this heading.

Doxycycline Monohydrate (Increased prothrombin time response). Products include:
Oracea Capsules 1000

Enflurane (Increased prothrombin time response).
No products indexed under this heading.

Enoxacin (Increased prothrombin time response).
No products indexed under this heading.

Enoxaparin Sodium (Co-administration has resulted in cases of venous limb ischemia, necrosis, and gangrene in patients with heparin-induced thrombocytopenia and deep venous thrombosis when heparin treatment was discontinued and warfarin therapy was started or continued; sequelae have included amputation of the involved area and/or death). Products include:
Lovenox Injection 2915

Erythromycin (Increased prothrombin time response). Products include:
Ery-Tab Tablets 449
Erythromycin Base Filmtab Tablets 455
Erythromycin Delayed-Release Capsules, USP 457
PCE Dispertab Tablets 515

Erythromycin Estolate (Increased prothrombin time response).
No products indexed under this heading.

Erythromycin Ethylsuccinate (Increased prothrombin time response). Products include:
E.E.S. 451
EryPed 447

Erythromycin Gluceptate (Increased prothrombin time response).
No products indexed under this heading.

Erythromycin Lactobionate (Increased prothrombin time response).
No products indexed under this heading.

Erythromycin Stearate (Increased prothrombin time response). Products include:
Erythrocin Stearate Filmtab Tablets 453

Escitalopram Oxalate (Increased prothrombin time response). Products include:
Lexapro Oral Solution 1190
Lexapro Tablets 1190

Ethacrynic Acid (Decreased or increased prothrombin time response). Products include:
Edecrin Tablets 1959

Ethchlorvynol (Decreased prothrombin time response).
No products indexed under this heading.

Ethinyl Estradiol (Decreased prothrombin time response). Products include:
Mircette Tablets 1066
NuvaRing 2340
Ortho-Cyclen/Ortho Tri-Cyclen 2429
Ortho Evra Transdermal System 2417
Ortho Tri-Cyclen Lo Tablets 2436
Seasonique Tablets 1077
Yasmin 28 Tablets 796
Yaz Tablets 803

Ethynodiol Diacetate (Decreased prothrombin time response).
No products indexed under this heading.

Etodolac (Increased prothrombin time response; caution should be observed when used concurrently).
No products indexed under this heading.

Fenofibrate (Increased prothrombin time response). Products include:
Lofibra Tablets 1219
Lofibra Capsules 1216
Tricor Tablets 527
Triglide Tablets 3123

Fenoprofen Calcium (Increased prothrombin time response; caution should be observed when used concurrently). Products include:
Nalfon Capsules 2502

Fentanyl (Increased prothrombin time response with prolonged use). Products include:
Duragesic Transdermal System 2373
Ionsys Transdermal System 2379

Fentanyl Citrate (Increased prothrombin time response with prolonged use). Products include:
Actiq 979

Ferula foetida (Co-administration with botanicals that contain coumarins, such as asafoetida, may result in increased anticoagulant effects).
No products indexed under this heading.

Fexofenadine Hydrochloride (Decreased prothrombin time response). Products include:
Allegra 2844
Allegra-D 12 Hour Extended-Release Tablets 2846
Allegra-D 24 Hour Extended-Release Tablets 2849

Filipendula ulmaria (Co-administration with botanicals that contain coumarins and salicylate, such as meadowsweet, may result in increased anticoagulant effects).
No products indexed under this heading.

Fluconazole (Increased prothrombin time response).
No products indexed under this heading.

Fludrocortisone Acetate (Decreased or increased prothrombin time response).
No products indexed under this heading.

Fluorouracil (Increased prothrombin time response). Products include:
- Carac Cream, 0.5% 2879
- Efudex 3363

Fluoxetine Hydrochloride (Increased prothrombin time response). Products include:
- Prozac Pulvules and Liquid 1801
- Symbyax Capsules 1819

Fluoxymesterone (Increased prothrombin time response). Products include:
- Androxy Tablets 3335

Flurbiprofen (Increased prothrombin time response; caution should be observed when used concurrently).
No products indexed under this heading.

Flutamide (May be responsible, alone or in combination, for increased prothrombin time/international normalized ratio (PT/INR) response). Products include:
- Eulexin Capsules 3009

Fluvastatin Sodium (Increased prothrombin time response). Products include:
- Lescol Capsules 2233
- Lescol XL Tablets 2233

Fluvoxamine Maleate (Increased prothrombin time response).
No products indexed under this heading.

Fosphenytoin Sodium (Accumulation of phenytoin; decreased or increased prothrombin time response).
No products indexed under this heading.

Fucus vesiculosus (Concurrent use may result in increased anticoagulant effects).
No products indexed under this heading.

Furosemide (Decreased or increased prothrombin time response). Products include:
- Furosemide Tablets 2154

Galium odoratum (Co-administration with botanicals that contain coumarins, such as sweet woodruff, may result in increased anticoagulant effects).
No products indexed under this heading.

Garlic Extract (Co-administration is associated most often with increases in the effects of warfarin; garlic may cause bleeding events when taken alone and may have anticoagulant, antiplatelet, and/or fibrinolytic properties).
No products indexed under this heading.

Garlic Oil (Co-administration is associated most often with increases in the effects of warfarin; garlic may cause bleeding events when taken alone and may have anticoagulant, antiplatelet, and/or fibrinolytic properties).
No products indexed under this heading.

Gaultheria procumbens (Co-administration with botanicals that contain salicylate and/or have antiplatelet properties, such as wintergreen, may result in increased anticoagulant effects).
No products indexed under this heading.

Gefitinib (Increased prothrombin time response). Products include:
- Iressa Tablets 684

Gemfibrozil (May be responsible, alone or in combination, for increased prothrombin time/international normalized ratio (PT/INR) response).
No products indexed under this heading.

Ginger (Co-administration with botanicals that contain salicylate and/or have antiplatelet properties, such as ginger, may result in increased anticoagulant effects).
No products indexed under this heading.

Ginkgo biloba (Co-administration is associated most often with increases in the effects of warfarin; Gingko biloba may cause bleeding events when taken alone and may have anticoagulant, antiplatelet, and/or fibrinolytic properties). Products include:
- BioLean Free Tablets 631
- Centrum Performance Multivitamin/Multimineral Supplement 811
- DHEA Plus Capsules 827
- Phyto-Vite Tablets 831
- Satiete Tablets 832
- StePHan Clarity Capsules 819
- StePHan Elixir Capsules 814

Ginseng (Co-administration with botanicals that contain salicylate and/or have antiplatelet properties, such as ginseng (Panax) may result in increased anticoagulant effects). Products include:
- BioLean Free Tablets 631
- Centrum Performance Multivitamin/Multimineral Supplement 811

Glipizide (Increased prothrombin time response).
No products indexed under this heading.

Glucagon (Increased prothrombin time response). Products include:
- GlucaGen 761
- Glucagon for Injection Vials and Emergency Kit 1778

Glutethimide (Decreased prothrombin time response).
No products indexed under this heading.

Glyburide (Increased prothrombin time response).
No products indexed under this heading.

Grepafloxacin Hydrochloride (Increased prothrombin time response).
No products indexed under this heading.

Griseofulvin (Decreased prothrombin time response). Products include:
- Gris-PEG Tablets 2502

Haloperidol (Decreased prothrombin time response).
No products indexed under this heading.

Haloperidol Decanoate (Decreased prothrombin time response).
No products indexed under this heading.

Halothane (Increased prothrombin time response).
No products indexed under this heading.

Heparin Sodium (Co-administration has resulted in cases of venous limb ischemia, necrosis, and gangrene in patients with heparin-induced thrombocytopenia and deep venous thrombosis when heparin treatment was discontinued and warfarin therapy was started or continued; sequelae have included amputation of the involved area and/or death).
No products indexed under this heading.

Hepatotoxic Drugs, unspecified (Increased prothrombin time response).
No products indexed under this heading.

Horse Chestnut Seed Extract (Co-administration with botanicals that contain coumarins, such as horse chestnut, may result in increased anticoagulant effects).
No products indexed under this heading.

Hydrastis canadensis (Co-administration with botanicals with coagulant properties, such as goldenseal, may affect the anticoagulant effects of warfarin).
No products indexed under this heading.

Hydrochlorothiazide (Decreased or increased prothrombin time response). Products include:
- Aldoril Tablets 1910
- Atacand HCT 651
- Avalide Tablets 888
- Avalide Tablets 2874
- Benicar HCT Tablets 1044
- Diovan HCT Tablets 2196
- Dyazide Capsules 1423
- Hyzaar 50-12.5 Tablets 1990
- Hyzaar 100-12.5 Tablets 1990
- Hyzaar 100-25 Tablets 1990
- Lopressor HCT 50/25 Tablets 2241
- Lopressor HCT 100/25 Tablets 2241
- Lopressor HCT 100/50 Tablets 2241
- Lotensin HCT Tablets 2246
- Micardis HCT Tablets 856
- Moduretic Tablets 2028
- Prinzide Tablets 2056
- Teveten HCT Tablets 1737
- Timolide Tablets 2086
- Uniretic Tablets 3100

Hydrocodone Bitartrate (Increased prothrombin time response with prolonged use). Products include:
- Hycodan 1116
- Hycotuss Expectorant Syrup 1117
- Vicodin Tablets 535
- Vicodin ES Tablets 536
- Vicodin HP Tablets 538
- Vicoprofen Tablets 539
- Zydone Tablets 1139

Hydrocodone Polistirex (Increased prothrombin time response with prolonged use). Products include:
- Tussionex Pennkinetic Extended-Release Suspension 3327

Hydrocortisone (Decreased or increased prothrombin time response). Products include:
- Colocort Rectal Suspension, USP (Retention) 100 mg/60 mL 2476
- Hydrocortone Tablets 1989
- Preparation H Hydrocortisone Cream 646

Hydrocortisone Acetate (Decreased or increased prothrombin time response). Products include:
- Analpram-HC 1159
- Pramosone 1161
- ProctoFoam-HC 3099

Hydrocortisone Sodium Phosphate (Decreased or increased prothrombin time response).
No products indexed under this heading.

Hydrocortisone Sodium Succinate (Decreased or increased prothrombin time response).
No products indexed under this heading.

Hydroflumethiazide (Decreased or increased prothrombin time response).
No products indexed under this heading.

Hydromorphone Hydrochloride (Increased prothrombin time response with prolonged use). Products include:
- Dilaudid 440
- Dilaudid Non-Sterile Powder 440
- Dilaudid Oral Liquid 445
- Dilaudid Rectal Suppositories 440
- Dilaudid Tablets 440
- Dilaudid Tablets - 8 mg 445
- Dilaudid-HP 442

Hypericum (Co-administration is associated most often with decreases in the effects of warfarin). Products include:
- Satiete Tablets 832

Ibuprofen (Increased prothrombin time response; caution should be observed when used concurrently). Products include:
- Advil Allergy Sinus Caplets 770
- Advil 674
- Children's Advil Oral Suspension 603
- Children's Advil Chewable Tablets 603
- Advil Cold & Sinus 723
- Infants' Advil Concentrated Drops 604
- Infants' Advil Concentrated Drops - White Grape (Dye-Free) 604
- Junior Strength Advil Swallow Tablets 605
- Advil Migraine Liquigels 608
- Advil Multi-Symptom Cold Caplets 770
- Advil PM Caplets 615
- Motrin IB Tablets and Caplets 1866
- Children's Motrin Oral Suspension 1867
- Children's Motrin Non-Staining Dye-Free Oral Suspension 1867
- Children's Motrin Cold Oral Suspension 1867
- Infants' Motrin Concentrated Drops 1867
- Infants' Motrin Non-Staining Dye-Free Concentrated Drops 1867
- Junior Strength Motrin Caplets and Chewable Tablets 1867
- Vicoprofen Tablets 539

Ifosfamide (Increased prothrombin time response).
No products indexed under this heading.

Indapamide (Decreased or increased prothrombin time response). Products include:
- Indapamide Tablets 2156

Indomethacin (Increased prothrombin time response; caution should be observed when used concurrently). Products include:
- Indocin 1995

Indomethacin Sodium Trihydrate (Increased prothrombin time response; caution should be observed when used concurrently). Products include:
- Indocin I.V. 2465

Influenza Virus Vaccine (Increased prothrombin time response). Products include:
- Fluarix 1451
- Flumist Vaccine 1901

Inositol Nicotinate (Co-administration with botanicals that contain salicylate and/or have antiplatelet properties, such as inositol nicotinate, may result in increased anticoagulant effects).
No products indexed under this heading.

Isocarboxazid (Increased prothrombin time response).
No products indexed under this heading.

Isoflurane (Increased prothrombin time response).
No products indexed under this heading.

Itraconazole (Increased prothrombin time response).
No products indexed under this heading.

Kanamycin Sulfate (Increased prothrombin time response with oral aminoglycosides).
No products indexed under this heading.

Ketoprofen (Increased prothrombin time response; caution should be observed when used concurrently).
No products indexed under this heading.

Ketorolac Tromethamine (Increased prothrombin time response; caution should be observed when used concurrently). Products include:
Acular Ophthalmic Solution 565
Acular LS Ophthalmic Solution 566

Lansoprazole (Increased prothrombin time response). Products include:
Prevacid Delayed-Release Capsules 3271
Prevacid for Delayed-Release Oral Suspension 3271
Prevacid SoluTab Delayed-Release Orally Disintegrating Tablets 3271
Prevacid I.V. for Injection 3277
Prevacid NapraPAC 3280
PREVPAC 3284

Levamisole Hydrochloride (Increased prothrombin time response).
No products indexed under this heading.

Levonorgestrel (Decreased prothrombin time response). Products include:
Climara Pro Transdermal System 776
Mirena Intrauterine System 787
Plan B Tablets 1076
Seasonique Tablets 1077

Levorphanol Tartrate (Increased prothrombin time response with prolonged use).
No products indexed under this heading.

Levothyroxine Sodium (Decreased or increased prothrombin time response). Products include:
Levothroid Tablets 1186
Levoxyl Tablets 1712
Synthroid Tablets 520
Westhroid Tablets 3403

Licorice (Co-administration with botanicals that contain coumarins, such as licorice, may result in increased anticoagulant effects; licorice also has antiplatelet properties).
No products indexed under this heading.

Liothyronine Sodium (Decreased or increased prothrombin time response). Products include:
Cytomel Tablets 1710
Westhroid Tablets 3403

Liotrix (Decreased or increased prothrombin time response). Products include:
Thyrolar Tablets 1199

Lomefloxacin Hydrochloride (Increased prothrombin time response).
No products indexed under this heading.

Loratadine (Decreased prothrombin time response). Products include:
Alavert Allergy & Sinus D-12 Hour Tablets .... ▣771
Alavert .... ▣771
Children's Claritin Allergy Oral Solution .... ▣771
Claritin Non-Drowsy 24 Hour Tablets .... ▣772
Claritin Reditabs 24 Hour Non-Drowsy Tablets .... ▣772
Claritin-D Non-Drowsy 12 Hour Tablets .... ▣772
Claritin-D Non-Drowsy 24 Hour Tablets .... ▣772

Lovastatin (Increased prothrombin time response). Products include:
Advicor Tablets 1722
Altoprev Extended-Release Tablets 3109
Mevacor Tablets 2021

Magaldrate (Decreased prothrombin time response).
No products indexed under this heading.

Magnesium Hydroxide (Decreased prothrombin time response). Products include:
Maalox Regular Strength Antacid/Antigas Liquid................. 2175
Maalox Max Maximum Strength Antacid/Anti-Gas Liquid................ 2176
Pepcid Complete Chewable Tablets 1701

Magnesium Oxide (Decreased prothrombin time response). Products include:
Beelith Tablets 759
PremCal Light, Regular, and Extra Strength Tablets................. ▣818

Magnesium Salicylate (Increased prothrombin time response; caution should be observed when used concurrently).
No products indexed under this heading.

Matricaria recutita (Co-administration with botanicals that contain coumarins, such as chamomile, may result in increased anticoagulant effects).
No products indexed under this heading.

Meclofenamate Sodium (Increased prothrombin time response; caution should be observed when used concurrently).
No products indexed under this heading.

Medicago sativa (Co-administration with botanicals that contain coumarins, such as alfalfa, may result in increased anticoagulant effects).
No products indexed under this heading.

Mefenamic Acid (Increased prothrombin time response; caution should be observed when used concurrently).
No products indexed under this heading.

Melilotus officinalis (Co-administration with botanicals that contain coumarins, such as sweet clover, may result in increased anticoagulant effects).
No products indexed under this heading.

Meloxicam (Increased prothrombin time response; caution should be observed when used concurrently). Products include:
Mobic Oral Suspension 863
Mobic Tablets 863

Menyanthes trifoliata (Co-administration with botanicals that contain coumarins, such as bogbean, may result in increased anticoagulant effects).
No products indexed under this heading.

Meperidine Hydrochloride (Increased prothrombin time response with prolonged use).
No products indexed under this heading.

Mephobarbital (Decreased prothrombin time response).
No products indexed under this heading.

Meprobamate (Decreased prothrombin time response).
No products indexed under this heading.

Mercaptopurine (Decreased prothrombin time response).
No products indexed under this heading.

Mestranol (Decreased prothrombin time response).
No products indexed under this heading.

Methadone Hydrochloride (Increased prothrombin time response with prolonged use).
No products indexed under this heading.

Methdilazine Hydrochloride (Decreased prothrombin time response).
No products indexed under this heading.

Methimazole (Increased or decreased prothrombin time response).
No products indexed under this heading.

Methoxyflurane (Increased or decreased prothrombin time response).
No products indexed under this heading.

Methyclothiazide (Decreased or increased prothrombin time response).
No products indexed under this heading.

Methyl Salicylate (Increased prothrombin time response with topical methyl salicylate ointment). Products include:
Thera-Gesic Creme 2141

Methyldopa (Increased prothrombin time response). Products include:
Aldoril Tablets 1910

Methyldopate Hydrochloride (Increased prothrombin time response).
No products indexed under this heading.

Methylphenidate Hydrochloride (Increased prothrombin time response). Products include:
Concerta Extended-Release Tablets 1881
Metadate CD Capsules 3323
Ritalin Hydrochloride Tablets 2269
Ritalin LA Capsules 2271
Ritalin-SR Tablets 2269

Methylprednisolone Acetate (Decreased or increased prothrombin time response). Products include:
Depo-Medrol Injectable Suspension 2617
Depo-Medrol Single-Dose Vial 2619

Methylprednisolone Sodium Succinate (Decreased or increased prothrombin time response).
No products indexed under this heading.

Methyltestosterone (Increased prothrombin time response). Products include:
Estratest Tablets 3199
Estratest H.S. Tablets 3199

Metolazone (Decreased or increased prothrombin time response).
No products indexed under this heading.

Metronidazole (Increased prothrombin time response). Products include:
Metrogel 1% 1211
MetroGel-Vaginal Gel 1855
Vandazole Vaginal Gel 3338

Metronidazole Hydrochloride (Increased prothrombin time response).
No products indexed under this heading.

Miconazole (Increased prothrombin time response).
No products indexed under this heading.

Mistletoe (Co-administration with botanicals with coagulant properties, such as mistletoe, may affect the anticoagulant effects of warfarin).
No products indexed under this heading.

Moclobemide (Increased prothrombin time response).
No products indexed under this heading.

Montelukast Sodium (May be responsible, alone or in combination, for increased prothrombin time/international normalized ratio (PT/INR) response). Products include:
Singulair 2077

Moricizine Hydrochloride (Decreased or increased prothrombin time response).
No products indexed under this heading.

Morphine Sulfate (Increased prothrombin time response with prolonged use). Products include:
Avinza Capsules 1741
Kadian Capsules 577
MS Contin Tablets 2701

Moxifloxacin Hydrochloride (Increased prothrombin time response). Products include:
Avelox 2970
Vigamox Ophthalmic Solution 564

Nabumetone (Increased prothrombin time response; caution should be observed when used concurrently).
No products indexed under this heading.

Nafcillin Sodium (Decreased prothrombin time response).
No products indexed under this heading.

Nalidixic Acid (Increased prothrombin time response).
No products indexed under this heading.

Naproxen (Increased prothrombin time response; caution should be observed when used concurrently). Products include:

EC-Naprosyn Delayed-Release Tablets 2761
Naprosyn Suspension 2761
Naprosyn Tablets 2761
Prevacid NapraPAC 3280

Naproxen Sodium (Increased prothrombin time response; caution should be observed when used concurrently). Products include:
Aleve Caplets 742
Aleve Gelcaps 743
Aleve Tablets 743
Aleve Cold & Sinus Caplets 744
Anaprox Tablets 2761
Anaprox DS Tablets 2761

Neomycin, oral (Increased prothrombin time response with oral aminoglycosides).
No products indexed under this heading.

Nettle (Co-administration with botanicals that contain coumarins, such as nettle, may result in increased anticoagulant effects).
No products indexed under this heading.

Nilutamide (May be responsible, alone or in combination, for increased prothrombin time/international normalized ratio (PT/INR) response).
No products indexed under this heading.

Norethindrone (Decreased prothrombin time response). Products include:
Ortho Micronor Tablets 2426

Norethynodrel (Decreased prothrombin time response).
No products indexed under this heading.

Norfloxacin (Increased prothrombin time response). Products include:
Noroxin Tablets 2032

Norgestimate (Decreased prothrombin time response). Products include:
Ortho-Cyclen/Ortho Tri-Cyclen 2429
Ortho Tri-Cyclen Lo Tablets 2436

Norgestrel (Decreased prothrombin time response).
No products indexed under this heading.

Ofloxacin (Increased prothrombin time response). Products include:
Floxin Otic Solution 1049

Olsalazine Sodium (Increased prothrombin time response).
No products indexed under this heading.

Omeprazole (Increased prothrombin time response). Products include:
Zegerid Capsules 2958
Zegerid Powder for Oral Solution 2958

Oxandrolone (Increased prothrombin time response). Products include:
Oxandrin Tablets 2962

Oxaprozin (Increased prothrombin time response; caution should be observed when used concurrently).
No products indexed under this heading.

Oxycodone Hydrochloride (Increased prothrombin time response with prolonged use). Products include:
OxyContin Tablets 2703
OxyFast Oral Concentrate Solution 2708
OxyIR Capsules 2708
Percocet Tablets 1131
Percodan Tablets 1132

Oxymetholone (Increased prothrombin time response).
No products indexed under this heading.

Oxyphenbutazone (Increased prothrombin time response).
No products indexed under this heading.

Pantoprazole Sodium (Increased prothrombin time response). Products include:
Protonix I.V. 3472
Protonix Tablets 3469

Paraldehyde (Decreased prothrombin time response).
No products indexed under this heading.

Pargyline Hydrochloride (Increased prothrombin time response).
No products indexed under this heading.

Paromomycin Sulfate (Increased prothrombin time response with oral aminoglycosides).
No products indexed under this heading.

Paroxetine Hydrochloride (Increased prothrombin time response). Products include:
Paxil CR Controlled-Release Tablets 1538
Paxil 1530

Passiflora incarnata (Co-administration with botanicals that contain coumarins, such as passion flower, may result in increased anticoagulant effects).
No products indexed under this heading.

Pau d'arco (Concurrent use may result in increased anticoagulant effects).
No products indexed under this heading.

Penicillin G Potassium (Increased prothrombin time response with intravenous penicillin G).
No products indexed under this heading.

Penicillin G Sodium (Increased prothrombin time response with intravenous penicillin G).
No products indexed under this heading.

Pentobarbital Sodium (Decreased prothrombin time response). Products include:
Nembutal Sodium Solution, USP 2470

Pentoxifylline (Increased prothrombin time response).
No products indexed under this heading.

Petroselinum crispum (Co-administration with botanicals that contain coumarins, such as parsley, may result in increased anticoagulant effects).
No products indexed under this heading.

Peumus boldus (Co-administration with botanicals that contain coumarins, such as boldo, may result in increased anticoagulant effects).
No products indexed under this heading.

Phenelzine Sulfate (Increased prothrombin time response).
No products indexed under this heading.

Phenobarbital (Decreased prothrombin time response; accumulation of phenobarbital). Products include:
Donnatal Extentabs 2493

Phenylbutazone (Increased prothrombin time response; caution should be observed when used concurrently).
No products indexed under this heading.

Phenytoin (Accumulation of phenytoin; decreased or increased prothrombin time response).
No products indexed under this heading.

Phenytoin Sodium (Accumulation of phenytoin; decreased or increased prothrombin time response). Products include:
Phenytek Capsules 2160

Phytonadione (Decreased prothrombin time response).
No products indexed under this heading.

Piperacillin Sodium (Increased prothrombin time response). Products include:
Zosyn 3492

Piroxicam (Increased prothrombin time response; caution should be observed when used concurrently).
No products indexed under this heading.

Policosanol (Co-administration with botanicals that contain salicylate and/or have antiplatelet properties, such as policosanol, may result in increased anticoagulant effects).
No products indexed under this heading.

Polythiazide (Decreased or increased prothrombin time response).
No products indexed under this heading.

Populus species (Co-administration with botanicals that contain salicylate and/or have antiplatelet properties, such as poplar, may result in increased anticoagulant effects).
No products indexed under this heading.

Prednisolone Acetate (Decreased or increased prothrombin time response). Products include:
Blephamide Ophthalmic Ointment 568
Blephamide Ophthalmic Suspension 569
Poly-Pred Ophthalmic Suspension .... ⊙233
Pred Forte Ophthalmic Suspension .... ⊙235
Pred Mild Ophthalmic Suspension .... ⊙238
Pred-G Ophthalmic Ointment .... ⊙237
Pred-G Ophthalmic Suspension .... ⊙236

Prednisolone Sodium Phosphate (Decreased or increased prothrombin time response).
No products indexed under this heading.

Prednisolone Tebutate (Decreased or increased prothrombin time response).
No products indexed under this heading.

Prednisone (Decreased or increased prothrombin time response).
No products indexed under this heading.

Prickly Ash (Co-administration with botanicals that contain coumarins, such as prickly ash, may result in increased anticoagulant effects).
No products indexed under this heading.

Primidone (Decreased prothrombin time response).
No products indexed under this heading.

Procarbazine Hydrochloride (Increased prothrombin time response). Products include:
Matulane Capsules 3191

Promethazine Hydrochloride (Decreased prothrombin time response). Products include:
Phenergan Tablets and Suppositories 3440

Propafenone Hydrochloride (Increased prothrombin time response). Products include:
Rythmol SR Capsules 2727

Propoxyphene Hydrochloride (Increased prothrombin time response with prolonged use).
No products indexed under this heading.

Propoxyphene Napsylate (Increased prothrombin time response with prolonged use).
No products indexed under this heading.

Propranolol Hydrochloride (Increased prothrombin time response). Products include:
Inderal LA Long-Acting Capsules 3429
InnoPran XL Capsules 2723

Propylthiouracil (Increased or decreased prothrombin time response).
No products indexed under this heading.

Pyrazolones (Increased prothrombin time response).
No products indexed under this heading.

Pyrilamine Maleate (Decreased prothrombin time response).
No products indexed under this heading.

Pyrilamine Tannate (Decreased prothrombin time response).
No products indexed under this heading.

Quassia amara (Co-administration with botanicals that contain coumarins, such as quassia, may result in increased anticoagulant effects).
No products indexed under this heading.

Quinidine Gluconate (Increased prothrombin time response).
No products indexed under this heading.

Quinidine Polygalacturonate (Increased prothrombin time response).
No products indexed under this heading.

Quinidine Sulfate (Increased prothrombin time response).
No products indexed under this heading.

Quinine Sulfate (Increased prothrombin time response).
No products indexed under this heading.

Raloxifene Hydrochloride (May be responsible, alone or in combination, for decreased prothrombin time/international normalized ratio (PT/INR) response). Products include:
Evista Tablets 1763

Ranitidine Hydrochloride (Decreased or increased prothrombin time response). Products include:
Zantac 1624
Zantac Injection 1619
Zantac Injection Pharmacy Bulk Package 1622

Remifentanil Hydrochloride (Increased prothrombin time response with prolonged use).
No products indexed under this heading.

Rifampin (Decreased prothrombin time response).
No products indexed under this heading.

Rofecoxib (Increased prothrombin time response; caution should be observed when used concurrently).
No products indexed under this heading.

Salsalate (Increased prothrombin time response; caution should be observed when used concurrently).
No products indexed under this heading.

Sarsaparilla, German (Co-administration with botanicals that contain salicylate and/or have antiplatelet properties, such as German sarsaparilla, may result in increased anticoagulant effects).
No products indexed under this heading.

Secobarbital Sodium (Decreased prothrombin time response).
No products indexed under this heading.

Selegiline Hydrochloride (Increased prothrombin time response). Products include:
- Eldepryl Capsules 3208
- Zelapar Tablets 3372

Senega (Co-administration with botanicals that contain salicylate and/or have antiplatelet properties, such as senega, may result in increased anticoagulant effects).
No products indexed under this heading.

Sertraline Hydrochloride (Increased prothrombin time response). Products include:
- Zoloft 2586

Simvastatin (Increased prothrombin time response). Products include:
- Vytorin 10/10 Tablets 2114
- Vytorin 10/10 Tablets 3077
- Vytorin 10/20 Tablets 2114
- Vytorin 10/20 Tablets 3077
- Vytorin 10/40 Tablets 2114
- Vytorin 10/40 Tablets 3077
- Vytorin 10/80 Tablets 2114
- Vytorin 10/80 Tablets 3077
- Zocor Tablets 2105

Sodium Bicarbonate (Decreased prothrombin time response). Products include:
- Colyte with Flavor Packs for Oral Solution 3088
- HalfLytely and Bisacodyl Tablets Bowel Prep Kit with Flavors Packs 881
- TriLyte with Flavor Packs for Oral Solution 3100

Spironolactone (Decreased or increased prothrombin time response).
No products indexed under this heading.

Stanozolol (Increased prothrombin time response).
No products indexed under this heading.

Streptokinase (Concurrent use is not recommended and may be hazardous; increased prothrombin time response).
No products indexed under this heading.

Sucralfate (Decreased prothrombin time response). Products include:
- Carafate Suspension 701
- Carafate Tablets 701

Sufentanil Citrate (Increased prothrombin time response with prolonged use).
No products indexed under this heading.

Sulfacytine (Increased prothrombin time response).
No products indexed under this heading.

Sulfamethizole (Increased prothrombin time response).
No products indexed under this heading.

Sulfamethoxazole (Increased prothrombin time response).
No products indexed under this heading.

Sulfasalazine (Increased prothrombin time response).
No products indexed under this heading.

Sulfinpyrazone (Increased prothrombin time response).
No products indexed under this heading.

Sulfisoxazole Acetyl (Increased prothrombin time response).
No products indexed under this heading.

Sulfisoxazole Diolamine (Increased prothrombin time response).
No products indexed under this heading.

Sulindac (Increased prothrombin time response; caution should be observed when used concurrently). Products include:
- Clinoril Tablets 1924

Syzygium aromaticum (Co-administration with botanicals that contain salicylate and/or have antiplatelet properties, such as clove, may result in increased anticoagulant effects).
No products indexed under this heading.

Tamarindus indica (Co-administration with botanicals that contain salicylate and/or have antiplatelet properties, such as tamarind, may result in increased anticoagulant effects).
No products indexed under this heading.

Tamoxifen Citrate (Increased prothrombin time response). Products include:
- Soltamox Oral Solution 3527

Tanacetum parthenium (Co-administration with botanicals that contain salicylate and/or have antiplatelet properties, such as feverfew, may result in increased anticoagulant effects).
No products indexed under this heading.

Taraxacum officinale (Co-administration with botanicals that contain coumarins, such as dandelion, may result in increased anticoagulant effects; dandelion also has antiplatelet properties).
No products indexed under this heading.

Terfenadine (Decreased prothrombin time response).
No products indexed under this heading.

Tetracycline Hydrochloride (Increased prothrombin time response).
No products indexed under this heading.

Thiamylal Sodium (Decreased prothrombin time response).
No products indexed under this heading.

Thyroglobulin (Decreased or increased prothrombin time response).
No products indexed under this heading.

Thyroid (Decreased or increased prothrombin time response).
No products indexed under this heading.

Thyroxine (Decreased or increased prothrombin time response).
No products indexed under this heading.

Thyroxine Sodium (Decreased or increased prothrombin time response).
No products indexed under this heading.

Ticarcillin Disodium (Increased prothrombin time response). Products include:
- Timentin ADD-Vantage 1580
- Timentin Injection Galaxy Container 1583
- Timentin IV Infusion 1577
- Timentin Pharmacy Bulk Package 1586

Ticlopidine Hydrochloride (Concomitant administration may be associated with cholestatic hepatitis; increased prothrombin time response). Products include:
- Ticlid Tablets 2810

Tolazamide (Increased prothrombin time response).
No products indexed under this heading.

Tolbutamide (Increased prothrombin time response; accumulation of tolbutamide).
No products indexed under this heading.

Tolmetin Sodium (Increased prothrombin time response; caution should be observed when used concurrently).
No products indexed under this heading.

Torsemide (Decreased or increased prothrombin time response). Products include:
- Demadex Injection 2759
- Demadex Tablets 2759

Tramadol Hydrochloride (Increased prothrombin time response). Products include:
- Ultram ER Tablets 2392

Tranylcypromine Sulfate (Increased prothrombin time response). Products include:
- Parnate Tablets 1527

Trazodone Hydrochloride (Decreased prothrombin time response).
No products indexed under this heading.

Triamcinolone (Decreased or increased prothrombin time response).
No products indexed under this heading.

Triamcinolone Acetonide (Decreased or increased prothrombin time response). Products include:
- Azmacort Inhalation Aerosol 1726
- Nasacort AQ Nasal Spray 2922

Triamcinolone Diacetate (Decreased or increased prothrombin time response).
No products indexed under this heading.

Triamcinolone Hexacetonide (Decreased or increased prothrombin time response).
No products indexed under this heading.

Triamterene (Decreased or increased prothrombin time response). Products include:
- Dyazide Capsules 1423
- Dyrenium Capsules 3400

Trifolium pratense (Co-administration with botanicals that contain coumarins, such as red clover, may result in increased anticoagulant effects).
No products indexed under this heading.

Trigonella foenum-graecum (Co-administration with botanicals that contain coumarins, such as fenugreek, may result in increased anticoagulant effects).
No products indexed under this heading.

Trimeprazine Tartrate (Decreased prothrombin time response).
No products indexed under this heading.

Trimethoprim (Increased prothrombin time response).
No products indexed under this heading.

Tripelennamine Hydrochloride (Decreased prothrombin time response).
No products indexed under this heading.

Triprolidine Hydrochloride (Decreased prothrombin time response).
No products indexed under this heading.

Trovafloxacin Mesylate (Increased prothrombin time response).
No products indexed under this heading.

Urokinase (Concurrent use is not recommended and may be hazardous).
No products indexed under this heading.

Valdecoxib (Increased prothrombin time response; caution should be observed when used concurrently).
No products indexed under this heading.

Valproic Acid (Increased prothrombin time response). Products include:
- Depakene 417

Viburnum prunifolium (Co-administration with botanicals that contain salicylate and/or have antiplatelet properties, such as black haw, may result in increased anticoagulant effects).
No products indexed under this heading.

Vitamin C (Decreased prothrombin time response (with high dose)). Products include:
- Bausch & Lomb Ocuvite Adult Eye Vitamin and Mineral Supplement Soft Gels .... ▣706
- Bausch & Lomb Ocuvite Adult 50+ Eye Vitamin and Mineral Supplement Soft Gels .... ▣706
- Ocuvite Adult Vitamin and Mineral Supplement .... ⊙253
- Ocuvite Adult 50+ Vitamin and Mineral Supplement .... ⊙253
- Peridin-C Vitamin C Supplement .... ▣818

Vitamin E (Increased prothrombin time response). Products include:

Bausch & Lomb Ocuvite Adult Eye Vitamin and Mineral Supplement Soft Gels 706
Bausch & Lomb Ocuvite Adult 50+ Eye Vitamin and Mineral Supplement Soft Gels 706
MarineOmega Softgel Capsules 2672
Ocuvite Adult Vitamin and Mineral Supplement .... ⊙ 253
Ocuvite Adult 50+ Vitamin and Mineral Supplement .... ⊙ 253

Wild Lettuce (Co-administration with botanicals that contain coumarins, such as wild lettuce, may result in increased anticoagulant effects).
No products indexed under this heading.

Willow (Co-administration with botanicals that contain salicylate and/or have antiplatelet properties, such as willow, may result in increased anticoagulant effects).
No products indexed under this heading.

Zafirlukast (May be responsible, alone or in combination, for increased prothrombin time/international normalized ratio (PT/INR) response). Products include:
Accolate Tablets 671

Zileuton (May be responsible, alone or in combination, for increased prothrombin time/international normalized ratio (PT/INR) response). Products include:
Zyflo Tablets 1023

Food Interactions

Alcohol (Decreased or increased prothrombin time response).

Diet high in vitamin K (Decreased prothrombin time).

Vegetables, green leafy (Large amounts of green leafy vegetables may affect warfarin therapy).

COVERA-HS TABLETS

(Verapamil Hydrochloride) 3139
May interact with ACE inhibitors, antihypertensives, beta blockers, cytochrome p450 3a4 inducers (selected), cytochrome p450 3a4 inhibitors (selected), diuretics, cardiac glycosides, inhalant anesthetics, lithium preparations, nondepolarizing neuromuscular blocking agents, vasodilators, xanthines, and certain other agents. Compounds in these categories include:

Acebutolol Hydrochloride (Concomitant therapy may result in additive negative effects on heart rate, atrioventricular conduction and/or cardiac contractility; excessive bradycardia and AV block, including complete heart block).
No products indexed under this heading.

Acetazolamide (Clinically significant interactions have been reported with inhibitors of CYP3A4 causing elevation of plasma levels of verapamil while inducers of CYP3A4 have caused a lowering of plasma levels of verapamil).
No products indexed under this heading.

Allium sativum (Clinically significant interactions have been reported with inhibitors of CYP3A4 causing elevation of plasma levels of verapamil while inducers of CYP3A4 have caused a lowering of plasma levels of verapamil).
No products indexed under this heading.

Amiloride Hydrochloride (Possible additive effect on lowering of blood pressure). Products include:
Midamor Tablets 2026
Moduretic Tablets 2028

Aminophylline (Verapamil may inhibit the clearance and increase plasma levels of theophylline).
No products indexed under this heading.

Amiodarone Hydrochloride (Clinically significant interactions have been reported with inhibitors of CYP3A4 causing elevation of plasma levels of verapamil while inducers of CYP3A4 have caused a lowering of plasma levels of verapamil).
No products indexed under this heading.

Amlodipine Besylate (Possible additive effect on lowering of blood pressure). Products include:
Caduet Tablets 2508
Lotrel Capsules 2249
Norvasc Tablets 2545

Amprenavir (Clinically significant interactions have been reported with inhibitors of CYP3A4 causing elevation of plasma levels of verapamil while inducers of CYP3A4 have caused a lowering of plasma levels of verapamil). Products include:
Agenerase Capsules 1327
Agenerase Oral Solution 1332

Amyl Nitrite (Possible additive effect on lowering of blood pressure).
No products indexed under this heading.

Anastrozole (Clinically significant interactions have been reported with inhibitors of CYP3A4 causing elevation of plasma levels of verapamil while inducers of CYP3A4 have caused a lowering of plasma levels of verapamil). Products include:
Arimidex Tablets 673

Aprepitant (Clinically significant interactions have been reported with inhibitors of CYP3A4 causing elevation of plasma levels of verapamil while inducers of CYP3A4 have caused a lowering of plasma levels of verapamil). Products include:
Emend Capsules 1963

Aspirin (In a few reported cases, co-administration of verapamil with aspirin has led to increased bleeding times greater than observed with aspirin alone). Products include:
Aggrenox Capsules 822
Bayer Aspirin 744
BC Allergy Sinus Cold Powder 677
BC Headache Powder 677
Arthritis Strength BC Powder 677
BC Sinus Cold Powder 677
Excedrin Extra Strength Caplets/Tablets/Geltabs 684
Excedrin Migraine Caplets/Tablets/Geltabs 609
Goody's Body Pain Formula Powder 684
Goody's Extra Strength Headache Powders 611
Goody's Extra Strength Pain Relief Tablets 685
Percodan Tablets 1132
St. Joseph 81 mg Aspirin Chewable and Enteric Coated Tablets 1869

Atenolol (Concomitant therapy may result in additive negative effects on heart rate, atrioventricular conduction and/or cardiac contractility; excessive bradycardia and AV block, including complete heart block; a variable effect on atenolol clearance has been observed with concomitant use).
No products indexed under this heading.

Atracurium Besylate (Verapamil may potentiate the activity of neuromuscular blocking agents).
No products indexed under this heading.

Benazepril Hydrochloride (Possible additive effect on lowering of blood pressure). Products include:
Lotensin Tablets 2243
Lotensin HCT Tablets 2246
Lotrel Capsules 2249

Bendroflumethiazide (Possible additive effect on lowering of blood pressure).
No products indexed under this heading.

Betamethasone Acetate (Clinically significant interactions have been reported with inhibitors of CYP3A4 causing elevation of plasma levels of verapamil while inducers of CYP3A4 have caused a lowering of plasma levels of verapamil).
No products indexed under this heading.

Betamethasone Sodium Phosphate (Clinically significant interactions have been reported with inhibitors of CYP3A4 causing elevation of plasma levels of verapamil while inducers of CYP3A4 have caused a lowering of plasma levels of verapamil).
No products indexed under this heading.

Betaxolol Hydrochloride (Concomitant therapy may result in additive negative effects on heart rate, atrioventricular conduction and/or cardiac contractility; excessive bradycardia and AV block, including complete heart block). Products include:
Betoptic S Ophthalmic Suspension.................................. 558

Bisoprolol Fumarate (Concomitant therapy may result in additive negative effects on heart rate, atrioventricular conduction and/or cardiac contractility; excessive bradycardia and AV block, including complete heart block).
No products indexed under this heading.

Bumetanide (Possible additive effect on lowering of blood pressure). Products include:
Bumex Tablets 2746

Candesartan Cilexetil (Possible additive effect on lowering of blood pressure). Products include:
Atacand Tablets 649
Atacand HCT 651

Captopril (Possible additive effect on lowering of blood pressure). Products include:
Captopril Tablets 2149

Carbamazepine (Co-administration may increase carbamazepine concentrations and this may produce side effects such as diplopia, headache, ataxia, or dizziness). Products include:
Carbatrol Capsules 3171
Equetro Extended-Release Capsules.................................... 3180
Tegretol/Tegretol-XR 2295

Carteolol Hydrochloride (Concomitant therapy may result in additive negative effects on heart rate, atrioventricular conduction and/or cardiac contractility; excessive bradycardia and AV block, including complete heart block). Products include:
Carteolol Hydrochloride Ophthalmic Solution USP, 1%...... ⊙ 249

Chlorothiazide (Possible additive effect on lowering of blood pressure). Products include:
Diuril Oral Suspension 1954

Chlorothiazide Sodium (Possible additive effect on lowering of blood pressure). Products include:
Diuril Sodium Intravenous 2467

Chlorthalidone (Possible additive effect on lowering of blood pressure). Products include:
Clorpres Tablets 2153

Cimetidine (Variable results on verapamil clearance). Products include:
Tagamet HB 200 Tablets 664

Cimetidine Hydrochloride (Variable results on verapamil clearance).
No products indexed under this heading.

Ciprofloxacin (Clinically significant interactions have been reported with inhibitors of CYP3A4 causing elevation of plasma levels of verapamil while inducers of CYP3A4 have caused a lowering of plasma levels of verapamil). Products include:
Cipro Oral Suspension 2977
Cipro I.V. 2984
Cipro XR Tablets 2990
Ciprodex Otic Suspension 559

Ciprofloxacin Hydrochloride (Clinically significant interactions have been reported with inhibitors of CYP3A4 causing elevation of plasma levels of verapamil while inducers of CYP3A4 have caused a lowering of plasma levels of verapamil). Products include:
Ciloxan Ophthalmic Ointment 559
Ciloxan Ophthalmic Solution .... ⊙ 206
Cipro Tablets 2977
Proquin XR Tablets 1153

Cisatracurium Besylate (Verapamil may potentiate the activity of neuromuscular blocking agents). Products include:
Nimbex Injection 498

Cisplatin (Clinically significant interactions have been reported with inhibitors of CYP3A4 causing elevation of plasma levels of verapamil while inducers of CYP3A4 have caused a lowering of plasma levels of verapamil).
No products indexed under this heading.

Clarithromycin (Clinically significant interactions have been reported with inhibitors of CYP3A4 causing elevation of plasma levels of verapamil while inducers of CYP3A4 have caused a lowering of plasma levels of verapamil). Products include:
Biaxin/Biaxin XL 402
PREVPAC 3284

Clonidine (Possible additive effect on lowering of blood pressure). Products include:
Catapres-TTS 844

Clonidine Hydrochloride (Possible additive effect on lowering of blood pressure). Products include:
Catapres Tablets 843
Clorpres Tablets 2153

Clotrimazole (Clinically significant interactions have been reported with inhibitors of CYP3A4 causing elevation of plasma levels of verapamil while inducers of CYP3A4 have caused a lowering of plasma levels of verapamil). Products include:
Desenex Athlete's Foot Cream 635
Lotrimin 3039
Lotrisone 3040

Cortisone Acetate (Clinically significant interactions have been reported with inhibitors of CYP3A4 causing elevation of plasma levels of verapamil while inducers of CYP3A4 have caused a lowering of plasma levels of verapamil).

No products indexed under this heading.

Cyclosporine (Increased serum levels of cyclosporine). Products include:

Dalfopristin (Clinically significant interactions have been reported with inhibitors of CYP3A4 causing elevation of plasma levels of verapamil while inducers of CYP3A4 have caused a lowering of plasma levels of verapamil).

No products indexed under this heading.

Danazol (Clinically significant interactions have been reported with inhibitors of CYP3A4 causing elevation of plasma levels of verapamil while inducers of CYP3A4 have caused a lowering of plasma levels of verapamil).

No products indexed under this heading.

Delavirdine Mesylate (Clinically significant interactions have been reported with inhibitors of CYP3A4 causing elevation of plasma levels of verapamil while inducers of CYP3A4 have caused a lowering of plasma levels of verapamil). Products include:

Deserpidine (Possible additive effect on lowering of blood pressure).

No products indexed under this heading.

Desflurane (Potential for excessive cardiovascular depression).

No products indexed under this heading.

Deslanoside (Chronic verapamil treatment can increase serum digoxin levels by 50% to 75% and this can result in digitalis toxicity).

No products indexed under this heading.

Dexamethasone (Clinically significant interactions have been reported with inhibitors of CYP3A4 causing elevation of plasma levels of verapamil while inducers of CYP3A4 have caused a lowering of plasma levels of verapamil). Products include:

Dexamethasone Acetate (Clinically significant interactions have been reported with inhibitors of CYP3A4 causing elevation of plasma levels of verapamil while inducers of CYP3A4 have caused a lowering of plasma levels of verapamil).

No products indexed under this heading.

Dexamethasone Sodium Phosphate (Clinically significant interactions have been reported with inhibitors of CYP3A4 causing elevation of plasma levels of verapamil while inducers of CYP3A4 have caused a lowering of plasma levels of verapamil).

No products indexed under this heading.

Diazoxide (Possible additive effect on lowering of blood pressure). Products include:

Digitalis Glycoside Preparations (Chronic verapamil treatment can increase serum digoxin levels by 50% to 75% and this can result in digitalis toxicity).

No products indexed under this heading.

Digitoxin (Chronic verapamil treatment can increase serum digoxin levels by 50% to 75% and this can result in digitalis toxicity).

No products indexed under this heading.

Digoxin (Chronic verapamil treatment can increase serum digoxin levels by 50% to 75% and this can result in digitalis toxicity). Products include:

Diltiazem Hydrochloride (Possible additive effect on lowering of blood pressure). Products include:

Diltiazem Maleate (Clinically significant interactions have been reported with inhibitors of CYP3A4 causing elevation of plasma levels of verapamil while inducers of CYP3A4 have caused a lowering of plasma levels of verapamil).

No products indexed under this heading.

Disopyramide Phosphate (Concurrent use within 48 hours before or 24 hours after verapamil administration is not recommended).

No products indexed under this heading.

Doxazosin Mesylate (Possible additive effect on lowering of blood pressure). Products include:

Doxorubicin Hydrochloride (Clinically significant interactions have been reported with inhibitors of CYP3A4 causing elevation of plasma levels of verapamil while inducers of CYP3A4 have caused a lowering of plasma levels of verapamil).

No products indexed under this heading.

Dyphylline (Verapamil may inhibit the clearance and increase plasma levels of theophylline).

No products indexed under this heading.

Efavirenz (Clinically significant interactions have been reported with inhibitors of CYP3A4 causing elevation of plasma levels of verapamil while inducers of CYP3A4 have caused a lowering of plasma levels of verapamil). Products include:

Enalapril Maleate (Possible additive effect on lowering of blood pressure). Products include:

Enalaprilat (Possible additive effect on lowering of blood pressure).

No products indexed under this heading.

Enflurane (Potential for excessive cardiovascular depression).

No products indexed under this heading.

Epoprostenol Sodium (Possible additive effect on lowering of blood pressure).

No products indexed under this heading.

Eprosartan Mesylate (Possible additive effect on lowering of blood pressure). Products include:

Erythromycin (Clinically significant interactions have been reported with inhibitors of CYP3A4 causing elevation of plasma levels of verapamil while inducers of CYP3A4 have caused a lowering of plasma levels of verapamil). Products include:

Erythromycin Estolate (Clinically significant interactions have been reported with inhibitors of CYP3A4 causing elevation of plasma levels of verapamil while inducers of CYP3A4 have caused a lowering of plasma levels of verapamil).

No products indexed under this heading.

Erythromycin Ethylsuccinate (Clinically significant interactions have been reported with inhibitors of CYP3A4 causing elevation of plasma levels of verapamil while inducers of CYP3A4 have caused a lowering of plasma levels of verapamil). Products include:

Erythromycin Gluceptate (Clinically significant interactions have been reported with inhibitors of CYP3A4 causing elevation of plasma levels of verapamil while inducers of CYP3A4 have caused a lowering of plasma levels of verapamil).

No products indexed under this heading.

Erythromycin Lactobionate (Clinically significant interactions have been reported with inhibitors of CYP3A4 causing elevation of plasma levels of verapamil while inducers of CYP3A4 have caused a lowering of plasma levels of verapamil).

No products indexed under this heading.

Erythromycin Stearate (Clinically significant interactions have been reported with inhibitors of CYP3A4 causing elevation of plasma levels of verapamil while inducers of CYP3A4 have caused a lowering of plasma levels of verapamil). Products include:

Esmolol Hydrochloride (Concomitant therapy may result in additive negative effects on heart rate, atrioventricular conduction and/or cardiac contractility; excessive bradycardia and AV block, including complete heart block).

No products indexed under this heading.

Esomeprazole Magnesium (Clinically significant interactions have been reported with inhibitors of CYP3A4 causing elevation of plasma levels of verapamil while inducers of CYP3A4 have caused a lowering of plasma levels of verapamil). Products include:

Ethacrynic Acid (Possible additive effect on lowering of blood pressure). Products include:

Ethaverine Hydrochloride (Possible additive effect on lowering of blood pressure).

No products indexed under this heading.

Ethosuximide (Clinically significant interactions have been reported with inhibitors of CYP3A4 causing elevation of plasma levels of verapamil while inducers of CYP3A4 have caused a lowering of plasma levels of verapamil).

No products indexed under this heading.

Felbamate (Clinically significant interactions have been reported with inhibitors of CYP3A4 causing elevation of plasma levels of verapamil while inducers of CYP3A4 have caused a lowering of plasma levels of verapamil).

No products indexed under this heading.

Felodipine (Possible additive effect on lowering of blood pressure).

No products indexed under this heading.

Flecainide Acetate (Potential for additive effects on myocardial contractility, AV conduction, and repolarization). Products include:

Fluconazole (Clinically significant interactions have been reported with inhibitors of CYP3A4 causing elevation of plasma levels of verapamil while inducers of CYP3A4 have caused a lowering of plasma levels of verapamil).

No products indexed under this heading.

Fludrocortisone Acetate (Clinically significant interactions have been reported with inhibitors of CYP3A4 causing elevation of plasma levels of verapamil while inducers of CYP3A4 have caused a lowering of plasma levels of verapamil).

No products indexed under this heading.

Fluoxetine Hydrochloride (Clinically significant interactions have been reported with inhibitors of CYP3A4 causing elevation of plasma levels of verapamil while inducers of CYP3A4 have caused a lowering of plasma levels of verapamil). Products include:

Fluvoxamine Maleate (Clinically significant interactions have been reported with inhibitors of CYP3A4 causing elevation of plasma levels of verapamil while inducers of CYP3A4 have caused a lowering of plasma levels of verapamil).
No products indexed under this heading.

Fosamprenavir Calcium (Clinically significant interactions have been reported with inhibitors of CYP3A4 causing elevation of plasma levels of verapamil while inducers of CYP3A4 have caused a lowering of plasma levels of verapamil). Products include:
Lexiva Tablets 1505

Fosinopril Sodium (Possible additive effect on lowering of blood pressure).
No products indexed under this heading.

Fosphenytoin Sodium (Clinically significant interactions have been reported with inhibitors of CYP3A4 causing elevation of plasma levels of verapamil while inducers of CYP3A4 have caused a lowering of plasma levels of verapamil).
No products indexed under this heading.

Furosemide (Possible additive effect on lowering of blood pressure). Products include:
Furosemide Tablets 2154

Garlic Extract (Clinically significant interactions have been reported with inhibitors of CYP3A4 causing elevation of plasma levels of verapamil while inducers of CYP3A4 have caused a lowering of plasma levels of verapamil).
No products indexed under this heading.

Garlic Oil (Clinically significant interactions have been reported with inhibitors of CYP3A4 causing elevation of plasma levels of verapamil while inducers of CYP3A4 have caused a lowering of plasma levels of verapamil).
No products indexed under this heading.

Guanabenz Acetate (Possible additive effect on lowering of blood pressure).
No products indexed under this heading.

Guanethidine Monosulfate (Possible additive effect on lowering of blood pressure).
No products indexed under this heading.

Halothane (Potential for excessive cardiovascular depression).
No products indexed under this heading.

Hydralazine Hydrochloride (Possible additive effect on lowering of blood pressure). Products include:
BiDil Tablets 2171

Hydrochlorothiazide (Possible additive effect on lowering of blood pressure). Products include:
Aldoril Tablets 1910
Atacand HCT 651
Avalide Tablets 888
Avalide Tablets 2874
Benicar HCT Tablets 1044
Diovan HCT Tablets 2196
Dyazide Capsules 1423
Hyzaar 50-12.5 Tablets 1990
Hyzaar 100-12.5 Tablets 1990
Hyzaar 100-25 Tablets 1990
Lopressor HCT 50/25 Tablets 2241
Lopressor HCT 100/25 Tablets 2241

Lopressor HCT 100/50 Tablets 2241
Lotensin HCT Tablets 2246
Micardis HCT Tablets 856
Moduretic Tablets 2028
Prinzide Tablets 2056
Teveten HCT Tablets 1737
Timolide Tablets 2086
Uniretic Tablets 3100

Hydrocortisone (Clinically significant interactions have been reported with inhibitors of CYP3A4 causing elevation of plasma levels of verapamil while inducers of CYP3A4 have caused a lowering of plasma levels of verapamil). Products include:
Colocort Rectal Suspension, USP (Retention) 100 mg/60 mL 2476
Hydrocortone Tablets 1989
Preparation H Hydrocortisone Cream ▧□646

Hydrocortisone Acetate (Clinically significant interactions have been reported with inhibitors of CYP3A4 causing elevation of plasma levels of verapamil while inducers of CYP3A4 have caused a lowering of plasma levels of verapamil). Products include:
Analpram-HC 1159
Pramosone 1161
ProctoFoam-HC 3099

Hydrocortisone Butyrate (Clinically significant interactions have been reported with inhibitors of CYP3A4 causing elevation of plasma levels of verapamil while inducers of CYP3A4 have caused a lowering of plasma levels of verapamil). Products include:
Locoid Lipocream Cream 1160

Hydrocortisone Cypionate (Clinically significant interactions have been reported with inhibitors of CYP3A4 causing elevation of plasma levels of verapamil while inducers of CYP3A4 have caused a lowering of plasma levels of verapamil).
No products indexed under this heading.

Hydrocortisone Hemisuccinate (Clinically significant interactions have been reported with inhibitors of CYP3A4 causing elevation of plasma levels of verapamil while inducers of CYP3A4 have caused a lowering of plasma levels of verapamil).
No products indexed under this heading.

Hydrocortisone Probutate (Clinically significant interactions have been reported with inhibitors of CYP3A4 causing elevation of plasma levels of verapamil while inducers of CYP3A4 have caused a lowering of plasma levels of verapamil).
No products indexed under this heading.

Hydrocortisone Sodium Phosphate (Clinically significant interactions have been reported with inhibitors of CYP3A4 causing elevation of plasma levels of verapamil while inducers of CYP3A4 have caused a lowering of plasma levels of verapamil).
No products indexed under this heading.

Hydrocortisone Sodium Succinate (Clinically significant interactions have been reported with inhibitors of CYP3A4 causing elevation of plasma levels of verapamil while inducers of CYP3A4 have caused a lowering of plasma levels of verapamil).
No products indexed under this heading.

Hydrocortisone Valerate (Clinically significant interactions have been reported with inhibitors of CYP3A4 causing elevation of plasma levels of verapamil while inducers of CYP3A4 have caused a lowering of plasma levels of verapamil).
No products indexed under this heading.

Hydroflumethiazide (Possible additive effect on lowering of blood pressure).
No products indexed under this heading.

Hypericum (Clinically significant interactions have been reported with inhibitors of CYP3A4 causing elevation of plasma levels of verapamil while inducers of CYP3A4 have caused a lowering of plasma levels of verapamil). Products include:
Satiete Tablets ▧□832

Hypericum Perforatum (Clinically significant interactions have been reported with inhibitors of CYP3A4 causing elevation of plasma levels of verapamil while inducers of CYP3A4 have caused a lowering of plasma levels of verapamil).
No products indexed under this heading.

Indapamide (Possible additive effect on lowering of blood pressure). Products include:
Indapamide Tablets 2156

Indinavir Sulfate (Clinically significant interactions have been reported with inhibitors of CYP3A4 causing elevation of plasma levels of verapamil while inducers of CYP3A4 have caused a lowering of plasma levels of verapamil). Products include:
Crixivan Capsules 1940

Irbesartan (Possible additive effect on lowering of blood pressure). Products include:
Avalide Tablets 888
Avalide Tablets 2874
Avapro Tablets 891
Avapro Tablets 2871

Isoflurane (Potential for excessive cardiovascular depression).
No products indexed under this heading.

Isoniazid (Clinically significant interactions have been reported with inhibitors of CYP3A4 causing elevation of plasma levels of verapamil while inducers of CYP3A4 have caused a lowering of plasma levels of verapamil).
No products indexed under this heading.

Isosorbide Dinitrate (Possible additive effect on lowering of blood pressure). Products include:
BiDil Tablets 2171

Isosorbide Mononitrate (Possible additive effect on lowering of blood pressure). Products include:
Imdur Tablets 3018

Isoxsuprine Hydrochloride (Possible additive effect on lowering of blood pressure).
No products indexed under this heading.

Isradipine (Possible additive effect on lowering of blood pressure). Products include:
DynaCirc CR Tablets 2721

Itraconazole (Clinically significant interactions have been reported with inhibitors of CYP3A4 causing elevation of plasma levels of verapamil while inducers of CYP3A4 have caused a lowering of plasma levels of verapamil).
No products indexed under this heading.

Ketoconazole (Clinically significant interactions have been reported with inhibitors of CYP3A4 causing elevation of plasma levels of verapamil while inducers of CYP3A4 have caused a lowering of plasma levels of verapamil). Products include:
Nizoral A-D Shampoo, 1% 1868

Labetalol Hydrochloride (Concomitant therapy may result in additive negative effects on heart rate, atrioventricular conduction and/or cardiac contractility; excessive bradycardia and AV block, including complete heart block).
No products indexed under this heading.

Levobunolol Hydrochloride (Concomitant therapy may result in additive negative effects on heart rate, atrioventricular conduction and/or cardiac contractility; excessive bradycardia and AV block, including complete heart block). Products include:
Betagan Ophthalmic Solution, USP .. ⊙220

Lisinopril (Possible additive effect on lowering of blood pressure). Products include:
Prinivil Tablets 2052
Prinzide Tablets 2056

Lithium (Co-administration has resulted in increased sensitivity to the effects of lithium neurotoxicity; lithium levels have been observed sometimes to increase, decrease, or remain unchanged).
No products indexed under this heading.

Lithium Carbonate (Co-administration has resulted in increased sensitivity to the effects of lithium neurotoxicity; lithium levels have been observed sometimes to increase, decrease, or remain unchanged). Products include:
Lithobid Tablets 1692

Lithium Citrate (Co-administration has resulted in increased sensitivity to the effects of lithium neurotoxicity; lithium levels have been observed sometimes to increase, decrease, or remain unchanged).
No products indexed under this heading.

Lopinavir (Clinically significant interactions have been reported with inhibitors of CYP3A4 causing elevation of plasma levels of verapamil while inducers of CYP3A4 have caused a lowering of plasma levels of verapamil). Products include:
Kaletra ... 476

Loratadine (Clinically significant interactions have been reported with inhibitors of CYP3A4 causing elevation of plasma levels of verapamil while inducers of CYP3A4 have caused a lowering of plasma levels of verapamil). Products include:
Alavert Allergy & Sinus D-12 Hour Tablets.................................... ▧□771
Alavert ▧□771
Children's Claritin Allergy Oral Solution ▧□771
Claritin Non-Drowsy 24 Hour Tablets.................................... ▧□772

Losartan Potassium (Possible additive effect on lowering of blood pressure). Products include:

Mecamylamine Hydrochloride (Possible additive effect on lowering of blood pressure).
No products indexed under this heading.

Mephenytoin (Clinically significant interactions have been reported with inhibitors of CYP3A4 causing elevation of plasma levels of verapamil while inducers of CYP3A4 have caused a lowering of plasma levels of verapamil).
No products indexed under this heading.

Methoxyflurane (Potential for excessive cardiovascular depression).
No products indexed under this heading.

Methsuximide (Clinically significant interactions have been reported with inhibitors of CYP3A4 causing elevation of plasma levels of verapamil while inducers of CYP3A4 have caused a lowering of plasma levels of verapamil).
No products indexed under this heading.

Methyclothiazide (Possible additive effect on lowering of blood pressure).
No products indexed under this heading.

Methyldopa (Possible additive effect on lowering of blood pressure). Products include:

Methyldopate Hydrochloride (Possible additive effect on lowering of blood pressure).
No products indexed under this heading.

Methylprednisolone (Clinically significant interactions have been reported with inhibitors of CYP3A4 causing elevation of plasma levels of verapamil while inducers of CYP3A4 have caused a lowering of plasma levels of verapamil).
No products indexed under this heading.

Methylprednisolone Acetate (Clinically significant interactions have been reported with inhibitors of CYP3A4 causing elevation of plasma levels of verapamil while inducers of CYP3A4 have caused a lowering of plasma levels of verapamil). Products include:

Methylprednisolone Sodium Succinate (Clinically significant interactions have been reported with inhibitors of CYP3A4 causing elevation of plasma levels of verapamil while inducers of CYP3A4 have caused a lowering of plasma levels of verapamil).
No products indexed under this heading.

Metipranolol Hydrochloride (Concomitant therapy may result in additive negative effects on heart rate, atrioventricular conduction and/or cardiac contractility; excessive bradycardia and AV block, including complete heart block).
No products indexed under this heading.

Metocurine Iodide (Verapamil may potentiate the activity of neuromuscular blocking agents).
No products indexed under this heading.

Metolazone (Possible additive effect on lowering of blood pressure).
No products indexed under this heading.

Metoprolol Succinate (Concomitant therapy may result in additive negative effects on heart rate, atrioventricular conduction and/or cardiac contractility; excessive bradycardia and AV block, including complete heart block; a decrease in metoprolol clearance has been observed with concomitant use). Products include:

Metoprolol Tartrate (Concomitant therapy may result in additive negative effects on heart rate, atrioventricular conduction and/or cardiac contractility; excessive bradycardia and AV block, including complete heart block; a decrease in metoprolol clearance has been observed with concomitant use). Products include:

Metronidazole (Clinically significant interactions have been reported with inhibitors of CYP3A4 causing elevation of plasma levels of verapamil while inducers of CYP3A4 have caused a lowering of plasma levels of verapamil). Products include:

Metronidazole Benzoate (Clinically significant interactions have been reported with inhibitors of CYP3A4 causing elevation of plasma levels of verapamil while inducers of CYP3A4 have caused a lowering of plasma levels of verapamil).
No products indexed under this heading.

Metronidazole Hydrochloride (Clinically significant interactions have been reported with inhibitors of CYP3A4 causing elevation of plasma levels of verapamil while inducers of CYP3A4 have caused a lowering of plasma levels of verapamil).
No products indexed under this heading.

Metyrosine (Possible additive effect on lowering of blood pressure). Products include:

Mibefradil Dihydrochloride (Possible additive effect on lowering of blood pressure).
No products indexed under this heading.

Miconazole (Clinically significant interactions have been reported with inhibitors of CYP3A4 causing elevation of plasma levels of verapamil while inducers of CYP3A4 have caused a lowering of plasma levels of verapamil).
No products indexed under this heading.

Miconazole Nitrate (Clinically significant interactions have been reported with inhibitors of CYP3A4 causing elevation of plasma levels of verapamil while inducers of CYP3A4 have caused a lowering of plasma levels of verapamil). Products include:

Minoxidil (Possible additive effect on lowering of blood pressure). Products include:

Mivacurium Chloride (Verapamil may potentiate the activity of neuromuscular blocking agents). Products include:

Modafinil (Clinically significant interactions have been reported with inhibitors of CYP3A4 causing elevation of plasma levels of verapamil while inducers of CYP3A4 have caused a lowering of plasma levels of verapamil). Products include:

Moexipril Hydrochloride (Possible additive effect on lowering of blood pressure). Products include:

Nadolol (Concomitant therapy may result in additive negative effects on heart rate, atrioventricular conduction and/or cardiac contractility; excessive bradycardia and AV block, including complete heart block). Products include:

Nefazodone Hydrochloride (Clinically significant interactions have been reported with inhibitors of CYP3A4 causing elevation of plasma levels of verapamil while inducers of CYP3A4 have caused a lowering of plasma levels of verapamil).
No products indexed under this heading.

Nelfinavir Mesylate (Clinically significant interactions have been reported with inhibitors of CYP3A4 causing elevation of plasma levels of verapamil while inducers of CYP3A4 have caused a lowering of plasma levels of verapamil). Products include:

Nevirapine (Clinically significant interactions have been reported with inhibitors of CYP3A4 causing elevation of plasma levels of verapamil while inducers of CYP3A4 have caused a lowering of plasma levels of verapamil). Products include:

Niacinamide (Clinically significant interactions have been reported with inhibitors of CYP3A4 causing elevation of plasma levels of verapamil while inducers of CYP3A4 have caused a lowering of plasma levels of verapamil).
No products indexed under this heading.

Nicardipine Hydrochloride (Possible additive effect on lowering of blood pressure). Products include:

Nicotinamide (Clinically significant interactions have been reported with inhibitors of CYP3A4 causing elevation of plasma levels of verapamil while inducers of CYP3A4 have caused a lowering of plasma levels of verapamil). Products include:

Nifedipine (Possible additive effect on lowering of blood pressure). Products include:

Nisoldipine (Possible additive effect on lowering of blood pressure). Products include:

Nitroglycerin (Possible additive effect on lowering of blood pressure). Products include:

Nitroglycerin, long-acting formulations (Possible additive effect on lowering of blood pressure).
No products indexed under this heading.

Nitroglycerin Intravenous (Possible additive effect on lowering of blood pressure).
No products indexed under this heading.

Norfloxacin (Clinically significant interactions have been reported with inhibitors of CYP3A4 causing elevation of plasma levels of verapamil while inducers of CYP3A4 have caused a lowering of plasma levels of verapamil). Products include:

Omeprazole (Clinically significant interactions have been reported with inhibitors of CYP3A4 causing elevation of plasma levels of verapamil while inducers of CYP3A4 have caused a lowering of plasma levels of verapamil). Products include:

Oxcarbazepine (Clinically significant interactions have been reported with inhibitors of CYP3A4 causing elevation of plasma levels of verapamil while inducers of CYP3A4 have caused a lowering of plasma levels of verapamil). Products include:

Pancuronium Bromide (Verapamil may potentiate the activity of neuromuscular blocking agents).
No products indexed under this heading.

Papaverine (Possible additive effect on lowering of blood pressure).
No products indexed under this heading.

Papaverine Hydrochloride (Possible additive effect on lowering of blood pressure).
No products indexed under this heading.

Paroxetine Hydrochloride (Clinically significant interactions have been reported with inhibitors of CYP3A4 causing elevation of plasma levels of verapamil while inducers of CYP3A4 have caused a lowering of plasma levels of verapamil). Products include:
- Paxil CR Controlled-Release Tablets **1538**
- Paxil **1530**

Penbutolol Sulfate (Concomitant therapy may result in additive negative effects on heart rate, atrioventricular conduction and/or cardiac contractility; excessive bradycardia and AV block, including complete heart block).
- No products indexed under this heading.

Perindopril Erbumine (Possible additive effect on lowering of blood pressure). Products include:
- Aceon Tablets (2 mg, 4 mg, 8 mg) **3194**

Phenobarbital (May increase verapamil clearance). Products include:
- Donnatal Extentabs **2493**

Phenobarbital Sodium (Clinically significant interactions have been reported with inhibitors of CYP3A4 causing elevation of plasma levels of verapamil while inducers of CYP3A4 have caused a lowering of plasma levels of verapamil).
- No products indexed under this heading.

Phenoxybenzamine Hydrochloride (Possible additive effect on lowering of blood pressure). Products include:
- Dibenzyline Capsules **3399**

Phentolamine Mesylate (Possible additive effect on lowering of blood pressure).
- No products indexed under this heading.

Phenytoin (Clinically significant interactions have been reported with inhibitors of CYP3A4 causing elevation of plasma levels of verapamil while inducers of CYP3A4 have caused a lowering of plasma levels of verapamil).
- No products indexed under this heading.

Phenytoin Sodium (Clinically significant interactions have been reported with inhibitors of CYP3A4 causing elevation of plasma levels of verapamil while inducers of CYP3A4 have caused a lowering of plasma levels of verapamil). Products include:
- Phenytek Capsules **2160**

Pindolol (Concomitant therapy may result in additive negative effects on heart rate, atrioventricular conduction and/or cardiac contractility; excessive bradycardia and AV block, including complete heart block).
- No products indexed under this heading.

Polythiazide (Possible additive effect on lowering of blood pressure).
- No products indexed under this heading.

Prazosin Hydrochloride (Possible additive effect on lowering of blood pressure).
- No products indexed under this heading.

Prednisolone Acetate (Clinically significant interactions have been reported with inhibitors of CYP3A4 causing elevation of plasma levels of verapamil while inducers of CYP3A4 have caused a lowering of plasma levels of verapamil). Products include:
- Blephamide Ophthalmic Ointment **568**
- Blephamide Ophthalmic Suspension **569**
- Poly-Pred Ophthalmic Suspension .... ⊙**233**
- Pred Forte Ophthalmic Suspension .... ⊙**235**
- Pred Mild Ophthalmic Suspension .... ⊙**238**
- Pred-G Ophthalmic Ointment .... ⊙**237**
- Pred-G Ophthalmic Suspension .... ⊙**236**

Prednisolone Sodium Phosphate (Clinically significant interactions have been reported with inhibitors of CYP3A4 causing elevation of plasma levels of verapamil while inducers of CYP3A4 have caused a lowering of plasma levels of verapamil).
- No products indexed under this heading.

Prednisolone Tebutate (Clinically significant interactions have been reported with inhibitors of CYP3A4 causing elevation of plasma levels of verapamil while inducers of CYP3A4 have caused a lowering of plasma levels of verapamil).
- No products indexed under this heading.

Prednisone (Clinically significant interactions have been reported with inhibitors of CYP3A4 causing elevation of plasma levels of verapamil while inducers of CYP3A4 have caused a lowering of plasma levels of verapamil).
- No products indexed under this heading.

Primidone (Clinically significant interactions have been reported with inhibitors of CYP3A4 causing elevation of plasma levels of verapamil while inducers of CYP3A4 have caused a lowering of plasma levels of verapamil).
- No products indexed under this heading.

Propoxyphene Hydrochloride (Clinically significant interactions have been reported with inhibitors of CYP3A4 causing elevation of plasma levels of verapamil while inducers of CYP3A4 have caused a lowering of plasma levels of verapamil).
- No products indexed under this heading.

Propoxyphene Napsylate (Clinically significant interactions have been reported with inhibitors of CYP3A4 causing elevation of plasma levels of verapamil while inducers of CYP3A4 have caused a lowering of plasma levels of verapamil).
- No products indexed under this heading.

Propranolol Hydrochloride (Concomitant therapy may result in additive negative effects on heart rate, atrioventricular conduction and/or cardiac contractility; excessive bradycardia and AV block, including complete heart block; a decrease in propranolol clearance has been observed with concomitant use). Products include:
- Inderal LA Long-Acting Capsules **3429**
- InnoPran XL Capsules **2723**

Quinapril Hydrochloride (Possible additive effect on lowering of blood pressure).
- No products indexed under this heading.

Quinidine (Clinically significant interactions have been reported with inhibitors of CYP3A4 causing elevation of plasma levels of verapamil while inducers of CYP3A4 have caused a lowering of plasma levels of verapamil).
- No products indexed under this heading.

Quinidine Gluconate (Concomitant use may result in significant hypertension; verapamil significantly counteracts the effects of quinidine on AV conduction; potential for increased quinidine levels with co-administration).
- No products indexed under this heading.

Quinidine Hydrochloride (Clinically significant interactions have been reported with inhibitors of CYP3A4 causing elevation of plasma levels of verapamil while inducers of CYP3A4 have caused a lowering of plasma levels of verapamil).
- No products indexed under this heading.

Quinidine Polygalacturonate (Concomitant use may result in significant hypertension; verapamil significantly counteracts the effects of quinidine on AV conduction; potential for increased quinidine levels with co-administration).
- No products indexed under this heading.

Quinidine Sulfate (Concomitant use may result in significant hypertension; verapamil significantly counteracts the effects of quinidine on AV conduction; potential for increased quinidine levels with co-administration).
- No products indexed under this heading.

Quinine (Clinically significant interactions have been reported with inhibitors of CYP3A4 causing elevation of plasma levels of verapamil while inducers of CYP3A4 have caused a lowering of plasma levels of verapamil).
- No products indexed under this heading.

Quinine Sulfate (Clinically significant interactions have been reported with inhibitors of CYP3A4 causing elevation of plasma levels of verapamil while inducers of CYP3A4 have caused a lowering of plasma levels of verapamil).
- No products indexed under this heading.

Quinupristin (Clinically significant interactions have been reported with inhibitors of CYP3A4 causing elevation of plasma levels of verapamil while inducers of CYP3A4 have caused a lowering of plasma levels of verapamil).
- No products indexed under this heading.

Ramipril (Possible additive effect on lowering of blood pressure). Products include:
- Altace Capsules **1702**

Ranitidine Bismuth Citrate (Clinically significant interactions have been reported with inhibitors of CYP3A4 causing elevation of plasma levels of verapamil while inducers of CYP3A4 have caused a lowering of plasma levels of verapamil).
- No products indexed under this heading.

Ranitidine Hydrochloride (Clinically significant interactions have been reported with inhibitors of CYP3A4 causing elevation of plasma levels of verapamil while inducers of CYP3A4 have caused a lowering of plasma levels of verapamil). Products include:
- Zantac **1624**
- Zantac Injection **1619**
- Zantac Injection Pharmacy Bulk Package **1622**

Rapacuronium Bromide (Verapamil may potentiate the activity of neuromuscular blocking agents).
- No products indexed under this heading.

Rauwolfia Serpentina (Possible additive effect on lowering of blood pressure).
- No products indexed under this heading.

Rescinnamine (Possible additive effect on lowering of blood pressure).
- No products indexed under this heading.

Reserpine (Possible additive effect on lowering of blood pressure).
- No products indexed under this heading.

Rifabutin (Clinically significant interactions have been reported with inhibitors of CYP3A4 causing elevation of plasma levels of verapamil while inducers of CYP3A4 have caused a lowering of plasma levels of verapamil).
- No products indexed under this heading.

Rifampicin (Clinically significant interactions have been reported with inhibitors of CYP3A4 causing elevation of plasma levels of verapamil while inducers of CYP3A4 have caused a lowering of plasma levels of verapamil).
- No products indexed under this heading.

Rifampin (Therapy with rifampin may markedly reduce oral verapamil bioavailability).
- No products indexed under this heading.

Rifapentine (Clinically significant interactions have been reported with inhibitors of CYP3A4 causing elevation of plasma levels of verapamil while inducers of CYP3A4 have caused a lowering of plasma levels of verapamil).
- No products indexed under this heading.

Ritonavir (Clinically significant interactions have been reported with inhibitors of CYP3A4 causing elevation of plasma levels of verapamil while inducers of CYP3A4 have caused a lowering of plasma levels of verapamil). Products include:
- Kaletra **476**
- Norvir **503**

Rocuronium Bromide (Verapamil may potentiate the activity of neuromuscular blocking agents). Products include:
- Zemuron Injection **2346**

Saquinavir (Clinically significant interactions have been reported with inhibitors of CYP3A4 causing elevation of plasma levels of verapamil while inducers of CYP3A4 have caused a lowering of plasma levels of verapamil).
- No products indexed under this heading.

Saquinavir Mesylate (Clinically significant interactions have been reported with inhibitors of CYP3A4

causing elevation of plasma levels of verapamil while inducers of CYP3A4 have caused a lowering of plasma levels of verapamil). Products include:
Invirase 2772

Sertraline Hydrochloride (Clinically significant interactions have been reported with inhibitors of CYP3A4 causing elevation of plasma levels of verapamil while inducers of CYP3A4 have caused a lowering of plasma levels of verapamil). Products include:
Zoloft 2586

Sodium Nitroprusside (Possible additive effect on lowering of blood pressure).
No products indexed under this heading.

Sotalol Hydrochloride (Concomitant therapy may result in additive negative effects on heart rate, atrioventricular conduction and/or cardiac contractility; excessive bradycardia and AV block, including complete heart block).
No products indexed under this heading.

Spirapril Hydrochloride (Possible additive effect on lowering of blood pressure).
No products indexed under this heading.

Spironolactone (Possible additive effect on lowering of blood pressure).
No products indexed under this heading.

Sulfinpyrazone (Clinically significant interactions have been reported with inhibitors of CYP3A4 causing elevation of plasma levels of verapamil while inducers of CYP3A4 have caused a lowering of plasma levels of verapamil).
No products indexed under this heading.

Telithromycin (Clinically significant interactions have been reported with inhibitors of CYP3A4 causing elevation of plasma levels of verapamil while inducers of CYP3A4 have caused a lowering of plasma levels of verapamil). Products include:
Ketek Tablets 2903

Telmisartan (Possible additive effect on lowering of blood pressure). Products include:
Micardis Tablets 854
Micardis HCT Tablets 856

Terazosin Hydrochloride (Possible additive effect on lowering of blood pressure). Products include:
Hytrin Capsules 471

Theophylline (Verapamil may inhibit the clearance and increase plasma levels of theophylline).
No products indexed under this heading.

Theophylline Anhydrous (Verapamil may inhibit the clearance and increase plasma levels of theophylline). Products include:
Uniphyl Tablets 2710

Theophylline Calcium Salicylate (Verapamil may inhibit the clearance and increase plasma levels of theophylline).
No products indexed under this heading.

Theophylline Dihydroxypropyl (Glyceryl) (Verapamil may inhibit the clearance and increase plasma levels of theophylline).
No products indexed under this heading.

Theophylline Ethylenediamine (Verapamil may inhibit the clearance and increase plasma levels of theophylline).
No products indexed under this heading.

Theophylline Sodium Glycinate (Verapamil may inhibit the clearance and increase plasma levels of theophylline).
No products indexed under this heading.

Timolol Hemihydrate (Concomitant therapy may result in additive negative effects on heart rate, atrioventricular conduction and/or cardiac contractility; excessive bradycardia and AV block, including complete heart block; one case of asymptomatic bradycardia with a wandering atrial pacemaker has been observed with timolol eye drops and oral verapamil). Products include:
Betimol Ophthalmic Solution 3382
Betimol Ophthalmic Solution .... ⊙ 295

Timolol Maleate (Concomitant therapy may result in additive negative effects on heart rate, atrioventricular conduction and/or cardiac contractility; excessive bradycardia and AV block, including complete heart block; one case of asymptomatic bradycardia with a wandering atrial pacemaker has been observed with timolol eye drops and oral verapamil). Products include:
Blocadren Tablets 1916
Cosopt Sterile Ophthalmic Solution 1931
Timolide Tablets 2086
Timoptic Sterile Ophthalmic Solution 2088
Timoptic in Ocudose 2091
Timoptic-XE Sterile Ophthalmic Gel Forming Solution 2092

Tolazoline Hydrochloride (Possible additive effect on lowering of blood pressure).
No products indexed under this heading.

Torsemide (Possible additive effect on lowering of blood pressure). Products include:
Demadex Injection 2759
Demadex Tablets 2759

Trandolapril (Possible additive effect on lowering of blood pressure). Products include:
Mavik Tablets 486
Tarka Tablets 524

Triamcinolone (Clinically significant interactions have been reported with inhibitors of CYP3A4 causing elevation of plasma levels of verapamil while inducers of CYP3A4 have caused a lowering of plasma levels of verapamil).
No products indexed under this heading.

Triamcinolone Acetonide (Clinically significant interactions have been reported with inhibitors of CYP3A4 causing elevation of plasma levels of verapamil while inducers of CYP3A4 have caused a lowering of plasma levels of verapamil). Products include:
Azmacort Inhalation Aerosol 1726
Nasacort AQ Nasal Spray 2922

Triamcinolone Diacetate (Clinically significant interactions have been reported with inhibitors of CYP3A4 causing elevation of plasma levels of verapamil while inducers of CYP3A4 have caused a lowering of plasma levels of verapamil).
No products indexed under this heading.

Triamcinolone Hexacetonide (Clinically significant interactions have been reported with inhibitors of CYP3A4 causing elevation of plasma levels of verapamil while inducers of CYP3A4 have caused a lowering of plasma levels of verapamil).
No products indexed under this heading.

Triamterene (Possible additive effect on lowering of blood pressure). Products include:
Dyazide Capsules 1423
Dyrenium Capsules 3400

Trimethaphan Camsylate (Possible additive effect on lowering of blood pressure).
No products indexed under this heading.

Troglitazone (Clinically significant interactions have been reported with inhibitors of CYP3A4 causing elevation of plasma levels of verapamil while inducers of CYP3A4 have caused a lowering of plasma levels of verapamil).
No products indexed under this heading.

Troleandomycin (Clinically significant interactions have been reported with inhibitors of CYP3A4 causing elevation of plasma levels of verapamil while inducers of CYP3A4 have caused a lowering of plasma levels of verapamil).
No products indexed under this heading.

Valproate Sodium (Clinically significant interactions have been reported with inhibitors of CYP3A4 causing elevation of plasma levels of verapamil while inducers of CYP3A4 have caused a lowering of plasma levels of verapamil). Products include:
Depacon Injection 412

Valsartan (Possible additive effect on lowering of blood pressure). Products include:
Diovan Tablets 2193
Diovan HCT Tablets 2196

Vecuronium Bromide (Verapamil may potentiate the activity of neuromuscular blocking agents).
No products indexed under this heading.

Voriconazole (Clinically significant interactions have been reported with inhibitors of CYP3A4 causing elevation of plasma levels of verapamil while inducers of CYP3A4 have caused a lowering of plasma levels of verapamil). Products include:
VFEND I.V. 2564
VFEND Oral Suspension 2564
VFEND Tablets 2564

Zafirlukast (Clinically significant interactions have been reported with inhibitors of CYP3A4 causing elevation of plasma levels of verapamil while inducers of CYP3A4 have caused a lowering of plasma levels of verapamil). Products include:
Accolate Tablets 671

Zileuton (Clinically significant interactions have been reported with inhibitors of CYP3A4 causing elevation of plasma levels of verapamil while inducers of CYP3A4 have caused a lowering of plasma levels of verapamil). Products include:
Zyflo Tablets 1023

Food Interactions

Alcohol (Verapamil may increase blood alcohol concentrations and prolong its effect).

Grapefruit (Clinically significant interactions have been reported with inhibitors of CYP3A4 causing elevation of plasma levels of verapamil while inducers of CYP3A4 have caused a lowering of plasma levels of verapamil).

Grapefruit Juice (Grapefruit juice may significantly increase concentrations of verapamil).

COZAAR TABLETS

(Losartan Potassium) 1935

May interact with lithium preparations, non-steroidal anti-inflammatory agents, potassium preparations, potassium sparing diuretics, and certain other agents. Compounds in these categories include:

Amiloride Hydrochloride (Concomitant use with potassium-sparing diuretics may lead to hyperkalemia). Products include:
Midamor Tablets 2026
Moduretic Tablets 2028

Celecoxib (In some patients with compromised renal function who are being treated with non-steroidal anti-inflammatory drugs (NSAIDs), including those that selectively inhibit cyclooxygenase-2 inhibitors (COX-2 inhibitors), the co-administration of angiotensin II receptor antagonists including losartan may result in a further deterioration of renal function. These effects are usually reversible. Reports suggest that NSAIDs, including selective COX-2 inhibitors, may diminish the antihypertensive effect of angiotensin II receptor antagonists, including losartan. This interaction should be given consideration in patients taking NSAIDs, including selective COX-2 inhibitors, concomitantly with angiotensin II receptor antagonists). Products include:
Celebrex Capsules 3134

Cimetidine (Co-administration leads to an increase of about 18% in AUC of losartan with no effect on pharmacokinetics of its active metabolites). Products include:
Tagamet HB 200 Tablets .... ▣ 664

Cimetidine Hydrochloride (Co-administration leads to an increase of about 18% in AUC of losartan with no effect on pharmacokinetics of its active metabolites).
No products indexed under this heading.

Diclofenac Potassium (In some patients with compromised renal function who are being treated with non-steroidal anti-inflammatory drugs (NSAIDs), including those that selectively inhibit cyclooxygenase-2 inhibitors (COX-2 inhibitors), the co-administration of angiotensin II receptor antagonists including losartan may result in a further deterioration of renal function. These effects are usually reversible. Reports suggest that NSAIDs, including selective COX-2 inhibitors, may diminish the antihypertensive effect of angiotensin II receptor antagonists, including losartan. This interaction should be given consideration in patients taking NSAIDs, including selective COX-2 inhibitors, concomitantly with angiotensin II receptor antagonists).
No products indexed under this heading.

Diclofenac Sodium (In some patients with compromised renal function who are being treated with non-steroidal anti-inflammatory drugs

(NSAIDs), including those that selectively inhibit cyclooxygenase-2 inhibitors (COX-2 inhibitors), the co-administration of angiotensin II receptor antagonists including losartan may result in a further deterioration of renal function. These effects are usually reversible. Reports suggest that NSAIDs, including selective COX-2 inhibitors, may diminish the antihypertensive effect of angiotensin II receptor antagonists, including losartan. This interaction should be given consideration in patients taking NSAIDs, including selective COX-2 inhibitors, concomitantly with angiotensin II receptor antagonists). Products include:

Arthrotec Tablets ... **3129**
Voltaren Ophthalmic Solution ... **2309**
Voltaren Tablets ... **2307**
Voltaren-XR Tablets ... **2310**

Etodolac (In some patients with compromised renal function who are being treated with non-steroidal anti-inflammatory drugs (NSAIDs), including those that selectively inhibit cyclooxygenase-2 inhibitors (COX-2 inhibitors), the co-administration of angiotensin II receptor antagonists including losartan may result in a further deterioration of renal function. These effects are usually reversible. Reports suggest that NSAIDs, including selective COX-2 inhibitors, may diminish the antihypertensive effect of angiotensin II receptor antagonists, including losartan. This interaction should be given consideration in patients taking NSAIDs, including selective COX-2 inhibitors, concomitantly with angiotensin II receptor antagonists).

No products indexed under this heading.

Fenoprofen Calcium (In some patients with compromised renal function who are being treated with non-steroidal anti-inflammatory drugs (NSAIDs), including those that selectively inhibit cyclooxygenase-2 inhibitors (COX-2 inhibitors), the co-administration of angiotensin II receptor antagonists including losartan may result in a further deterioration of renal function. These effects are usually reversible. Reports suggest that NSAIDs, including selective COX-2 inhibitors, may diminish the antihypertensive effect of angiotensin II receptor antagonists, including losartan. This interaction should be given consideration in patients taking NSAIDs, including selective COX-2 inhibitors, concomitantly with angiotensin II receptor antagonists). Products include:

Nalfon Capsules ... **2502**

Fluconazole (Fluconazole, an inhibitor of cytochrome P450 2C, decreased the AUC of the active metabolite by approximately 40%, but increased the AUC of losartan by approximately 70% following multiple doses).

No products indexed under this heading.

Flurbiprofen (In some patients with compromised renal function who are being treated with non-steroidal anti-inflammatory drugs (NSAIDs), including those that selectively inhibit cyclooxygenase-2 inhibitors (COX-2 inhibitors), the co-administration of angiotensin II receptor antagonists including losartan may result in a further deterioration of renal function. These effects are usually reversible. Reports suggest that NSAIDs, including selective COX-2 inhibitors, may diminish the antihypertensive effect of angiotensin II receptor antagonists, including losartan. This interaction should be given consideration in patients taking NSAIDs, including selective COX-2 inhibitors, concomitantly with angiotensin II receptor antagonists).

No products indexed under this heading.

Gestodene (In vitro studies show significant inhibition of the formation of the active metabolite by inhibitors of P450 3A4 such as gestodene; pharmacodynamic consequences of concomitant use is undefined).

No products indexed under this heading.

Ibuprofen (In some patients with compromised renal function who are being treated with non-steroidal anti-inflammatory drugs (NSAIDs), including those that selectively inhibit cyclooxygenase-2 inhibitors (COX-2 inhibitors), the co-administration of angiotensin II receptor antagonists including losartan may result in a further deterioration of renal function. These effects are usually reversible. Reports suggest that NSAIDs, including selective COX-2 inhibitors, may diminish the antihypertensive effect of angiotensin II receptor antagonists, including losartan. This interaction should be given consideration in patients taking NSAIDs, including selective COX-2 inhibitors, concomitantly with angiotensin II receptor antagonists). Products include:

Advil Allergy Sinus Caplets ... **770**
Advil ... **674**
Children's Advil Oral Suspension ... **603**
Children's Advil Chewable Tablets ... **603**
Advil Cold & Sinus ... **723**
Infants' Advil Concentrated Drops ... **604**
Infants' Advil Concentrated Drops - White Grape (Dye-Free) ... **604**
Junior Strength Advil Swallow Tablets ... **605**
Advil Migraine Liquigels ... **608**
Advil Multi-Symptom Cold Caplets ... **770**
Advil PM Caplets ... **615**
Motrin IB Tablets and Caplets ... **1866**
Children's Motrin Oral Suspension ... **1867**
Children's Motrin Non-Staining Dye-Free Oral Suspension ... **1867**
Children's Motrin Cold Oral Suspension ... **1867**
Infants' Motrin Concentrated Drops ... **1867**
Infants' Motrin Non-Staining Dye-Free Concentrated Drops ... **1867**
Junior Strength Motrin Caplets and Chewable Tablets ... **1867**
Vicoprofen Tablets ... **539**

Indomethacin (Antihypertensive effect of losartan may be blunted by indomethacin). Products include:

Indocin ... **1995**

Indomethacin Sodium Trihydrate (Antihypertensive effect of losartan may be blunted by indomethacin). Products include:

Indocin I.V. ... **2465**

Ketoconazole (In vitro studies show significant inhibition of the formation of the active metabolite by inhibitors of P450 3A4 such as ketoconazole or complete inhibition by the combination of ketoconazole and sulfaphenazole; pharmacodynamic consequences of concomitant use is undefined). Products include:

Nizoral A-D Shampoo, 1% ... **1868**

Ketoprofen (In some patients with compromised renal function who are being treated with non-steroidal anti-inflammatory drugs (NSAIDs), including those that selectively inhibit cyclooxygenase-2 inhibitors (COX-2 inhibitors), the co-administration of angiotensin II receptor antagonists including losartan may result in a further deterioration of renal function. These effects are usually reversible. Reports suggest that NSAIDs, including selective COX-2 inhibitors, may diminish the antihypertensive effect of angiotensin II receptor antagonists, including losartan. This interaction should be given consideration in patients taking NSAIDs, including selective COX-2 inhibitors, concomitantly with angiotensin II receptor antagonists).

No products indexed under this heading.

Ketorolac Tromethamine (In some patients with compromised renal function who are being treated with non-steroidal anti-inflammatory drugs (NSAIDs), including those that selectively inhibit cyclooxygenase-2 inhibitors (COX-2 inhibitors), the co-administration of angiotensin II receptor antagonists including losartan may result in a further deterioration of renal function. These effects are usually reversible. Reports suggest that NSAIDs, including selective COX-2 inhibitors, may diminish the antihypertensive effect of angiotensin II receptor antagonists, including losartan. This interaction should be given consideration in patients taking NSAIDs, including selective COX-2 inhibitors, concomitantly with angiotensin II receptor antagonists). Products include:

Acular Ophthalmic Solution ... **565**
Acular LS Ophthalmic Solution ... **566**

Lithium (As with other drugs which affect the excretion of sodium, lithium excretion may be reduced. Therefore, serum lithium levels should be monitored carefully if lithium salts are to be co-administered with angiotensin II receptor antagonists).

No products indexed under this heading.

Lithium Carbonate (As with other drugs which affect the excretion of sodium, lithium excretion may be reduced. Therefore, serum lithium levels should be monitored carefully if lithium salts are to be co-administered with angiotensin II receptor antagonists). Products include:

Lithobid Tablets ... **1692**

Lithium Citrate (As with other drugs which affect the excretion of sodium, lithium excretion may be reduced. Therefore, serum lithium levels should be monitored carefully if lithium salts are to be co-administered with angiotensin II receptor antagonists).

No products indexed under this heading.

Meclofenamate Sodium (In some patients with compromised renal function who are being treated with non-steroidal anti-inflammatory drugs (NSAIDs), including those that selectively inhibit cyclooxygenase-2 inhibitors (COX-2 inhibitors), the co-administration of angiotensin II receptor antagonists including losartan may result in a further deterioration of renal function. These effects are usually reversible. Reports suggest that NSAIDs, including selective COX-2 inhibitors, may diminish the antihypertensive effect of angiotensin II receptor antagonists, including losartan. This interaction should be given consideration in patients taking NSAIDs, including selective COX-2 inhibitors, concomitantly with angiotensin II receptor antagonists).

No products indexed under this heading.

Mefenamic Acid (In some patients with compromised renal function who are being treated with non-steroidal anti-inflammatory drugs (NSAIDs), including those that selectively inhibit cyclooxygenase-2 inhibitors (COX-2 inhibitors), the co-administration of angiotensin II receptor antagonists including losartan may result in a further deterioration of renal function. These effects are usually reversible. Reports suggest that NSAIDs, including selective COX-2 inhibitors, may diminish the antihypertensive effect of angiotensin II receptor antagonists, including losartan. This interaction should be given consideration in patients taking NSAIDs, including selective COX-2 inhibitors, concomitantly with angiotensin II receptor antagonists).

No products indexed under this heading.

Meloxicam (In some patients with compromised renal function who are being treated with non-steroidal anti-inflammatory drugs (NSAIDs), including those that selectively inhibit cyclooxygenase-2 inhibitors (COX-2 inhibitors), the co-administration of angiotensin II receptor antagonists including losartan may result in a further deterioration of renal function. These effects are usually reversible. Reports suggest that NSAIDs, including selective COX-2 inhibitors, may diminish the antihypertensive effect of angiotensin II receptor antagonists, including losartan. This interaction should be given consideration in patients taking NSAIDs, including selective COX-2 inhibitors, concomitantly with angiotensin II receptor antagonists). Products include:

Mobic Oral Suspension ... **863**
Mobic Tablets ... **863**

Nabumetone (In some patients with compromised renal function who are being treated with non-steroidal anti-inflammatory drugs (NSAIDs), including those that selectively inhibit cyclooxygenase-2 inhibitors (COX-2 inhibitors), the co-administration of angiotensin II receptor antagonists including losartan may result in a further deterioration of renal function. These effects are usually reversible. Reports suggest that NSAIDs, including selective COX-2 inhibitors, may diminish the antihypertensive effect of angiotensin II receptor antagonists, including losartan. This interaction should be given consideration in patients taking NSAIDs, including selective COX-2 inhibitors, concomitantly with angiotensin II receptor antagonists).

No products indexed under this heading.

Naproxen (In some patients with compromised renal function who are being treated with non-steroidal anti-inflammatory drugs (NSAIDs), including those that selectively inhibit cyclooxygenase-2 inhibitors (COX-2 inhibitors), the co-administration of angiotensin II receptor antagonists including losartan may result in a further deterioration of renal function. These effects are usually reversible. Reports suggest that NSAIDs, including selective COX-2 inhibitors, may diminish the antihypertensive effect of angiotensin II receptor antagonists, including losartan. This interaction should be given consideration in patients taking NSAIDs, including selective COX-2 inhibitors, concomitantly with angiotensin II receptor antagonists). Products include:

- EC-Naprosyn Delayed-Release Tablets **2761**
- Naprosyn Suspension **2761**
- Naprosyn Tablets **2761**
- Prevacid NapraPAC **3280**

Naproxen Sodium (In some patients with compromised renal function who are being treated with non-steroidal anti-inflammatory drugs (NSAIDs), including those that selectively inhibit cyclooxygenase-2 inhibitors (COX-2 inhibitors), the co-administration of angiotensin II receptor antagonists including losartan may result in a further deterioration of renal function. These effects are usually reversible. Reports suggest that NSAIDs, including selective COX-2 inhibitors, may diminish the antihypertensive effect of angiotensin II receptor antagonists, including losartan. This interaction should be given consideration in patients taking NSAIDs, including selective COX-2 inhibitors, concomitantly with angiotensin II receptor antagonists). Products include:

- Aleve Caplets **742**
- Aleve Gelcaps **743**
- Aleve Tablets **743**
- Aleve Cold & Sinus Caplets **744**
- Anaprox Tablets **2761**
- Anaprox DS Tablets **2761**

Oxaprozin (In some patients with compromised renal function who are being treated with non-steroidal anti-inflammatory drugs (NSAIDs), including those that selectively inhibit cyclooxygenase-2 inhibitors (COX-2 inhibitors), the co-administration of angiotensin II receptor antagonists including losartan may result in a further deterioration of renal function. These effects are usually reversible. Reports suggest that NSAIDs, including selective COX-2 inhibitors, may diminish the antihypertensive effect of angiotensin II receptor antagonists, including losartan. This interaction should be given consideration in patients taking NSAIDs, including selective COX-2 inhibitors, concomitantly with angiotensin II receptor antagonists).

No products indexed under this heading.

Phenobarbital (Co-administration leads to a reduction of about 20% in AUC of losartan and that of its active metabolites). Products include:

- Donnatal Extentabs **2493**

Phenylbutazone (In some patients with compromised renal function who are being treated with non-steroidal anti-inflammatory drugs (NSAIDs), including those that selectively inhibit cyclooxygenase-2 inhibitors (COX-2 inhibitors), the co-administration of angiotensin II receptor antagonists including losartan may result in a further deterioration of renal function. These effects are usually reversible. Reports suggest that NSAIDs, including selective COX-2 inhibitors, may diminish the antihypertensive effect of angiotensin II receptor antagonists, including losartan. This interaction should be given consideration in patients taking NSAIDs, including selective COX-2 inhibitors, concomitantly with angiotensin II receptor antagonists).

No products indexed under this heading.

Piroxicam (In some patients with compromised renal function who are being treated with non-steroidal anti-inflammatory drugs (NSAIDs), including those that selectively inhibit cyclooxygenase-2 inhibitors (COX-2 inhibitors), the co-administration of angiotensin II receptor antagonists including losartan may result in a further deterioration of renal function. These effects are usually reversible. Reports suggest that NSAIDs, including selective COX-2 inhibitors, may diminish the antihypertensive effect of angiotensin II receptor antagonists, including losartan. This interaction should be given consideration in patients taking NSAIDs, including selective COX-2 inhibitors, concomitantly with angiotensin II receptor antagonists).

No products indexed under this heading.

Potassium Acid Phosphate (Concomitant use with potassium supplements or salt substitute containing potassium may lead to hyperkalemia; patients should be advised to avoid these potassium-containing preparations). Products include:

- K-Phos Original (Sodium Free) Tablets **760**

Potassium Bicarbonate (Concomitant use with potassium supplements or salt substitute containing potassium may lead to hyperkalemia; patients should be advised to avoid these potassium-containing preparations).

No products indexed under this heading.

Potassium Chloride (Concomitant use with potassium supplements or salt substitute containing potassium may lead to hyperkalemia; patients should be advised to avoid these potassium-containing preparations). Products include:

- Colyte with Flavor Packs for Oral Solution **3088**
- HalfLytely and Bisacodyl Tablets Bowel Prep Kit with Flavors Packs **881**
- K-Dur Extended-Relase Tablets **3033**
- K-Lor Oral Solution **474**
- K-Tab Tablets **475**
- MoviPrep Oral Solution **2839**
- TriLyte with Flavor Packs for Oral Solution **3100**

Potassium Citrate (Concomitant use with potassium supplements or salt substitute containing potassium may lead to hyperkalemia; patients should be advised to avoid these potassium-containing preparations). Products include:

- Urocit-K Tablets **2144**

Potassium Gluconate (Concomitant use with potassium supplements or salt substitute containing potassium may lead to hyperkalemia; patients should be advised to avoid these potassium-containing preparations).

No products indexed under this heading.

Potassium Phosphate (Concomitant use with potassium supplements or salt substitute containing potassium may lead to hyperkalemia; patients should be advised to avoid these potassium-containing preparations). Products include:

- K-Phos Neutral Tablets **760**

Rifampin (Approximately 40% reduction in the AUC of losartan has been reported with rifampin).

No products indexed under this heading.

Rofecoxib (In some patients with compromised renal function who are being treated with non-steroidal anti-inflammatory drugs (NSAIDs), including those that selectively inhibit cyclooxygenase-2 inhibitors (COX-2 inhibitors), the co-administration of angiotensin II receptor antagonists including losartan may result in a further deterioration of renal function. These effects are usually reversible. Reports suggest that NSAIDs, including selective COX-2 inhibitors, may diminish the antihypertensive effect of angiotensin II receptor antagonists, including losartan. This interaction should be given consideration in patients taking NSAIDs, including selective COX-2 inhibitors, concomitantly with angiotensin II receptor antagonists).

No products indexed under this heading.

Salt Substitutes (Concomitant use with salt substitutes may lead to hyperkalemia).

No products indexed under this heading.

Spironolactone (Concomitant use with potassium-sparing diuretics may lead to hyperkalemia).

No products indexed under this heading.

Sulfaphenazole (In vitro studies show significant inhibition of the formation of the active metabolite by inhibitors of P450 3A4 such as sulfaphenazole; pharmacodynamic consequences of concomitant use is undefined).

No products indexed under this heading.

Sulindac (In some patients with compromised renal function who are being treated with non-steroidal anti-inflammatory drugs (NSAIDs), including those that selectively inhibit cyclooxygenase-2 inhibitors (COX-2 inhibitors), the co-administration of angiotensin II receptor antagonists including losartan may result in a further deterioration of renal function. These effects are usually reversible. Reports suggest that NSAIDs, including selective COX-2 inhibitors, may diminish the antihypertensive effect of angiotensin II receptor antagonists, including losartan. This interaction should be given consideration in patients taking NSAIDs, including selective COX-2 inhibitors, concomitantly with angiotensin II receptor antagonists). Products include:

- Clinoril Tablets **1924**

Tolmetin Sodium (In some patients with compromised renal function who are being treated with non-steroidal anti-inflammatory drugs (NSAIDs), including those that selectively inhibit cyclooxygenase-2 inhibitors (COX-2 inhibitors), the co-administration of angiotensin II receptor antagonists including losartan may result in a further deterioration of renal function. These effects are usually reversible. Reports suggest that NSAIDs, including selective COX-2 inhibitors, may diminish the antihypertensive effect of angiotensin II receptor antagonists, including losartan. This interaction should be given consideration in patients taking NSAIDs, including selective COX-2 inhibitors, concomitantly with angiotensin II receptor antagonists).

No products indexed under this heading.

Triamterene (Concomitant use with potassium-sparing diuretics may lead to hyperkalemia). Products include:

- Dyazide Capsules **1423**
- Dyrenium Capsules **3400**

Troleandomycin (In vitro studies show significant inhibition of the formation of the active metabolite by inhibitors of P450 3A4 such as troleandomycin; pharmacodynamic consequences of concomitant use is undefined).

No products indexed under this heading.

Valdecoxib (In some patients with compromised renal function who are being treated with non-steroidal anti-inflammatory drugs (NSAIDs), including those that selectively inhibit cyclooxygenase-2 inhibitors (COX-2 inhibitors), the co-administration of angiotensin II receptor antagonists including losartan may result in a further deterioration of renal function. These effects are usually reversible. Reports suggest that NSAIDs, including selective COX-2 inhibitors, may diminish the antihypertensive effect of angiotensin II receptor antagonists, including losartan. This interaction should be given consideration in patients taking NSAIDs, including selective COX-2 inhibitors, concomitantly with angiotensin II receptor antagonists).

No products indexed under this heading.

Food Interactions

Meal, unspecified (A meal slows absorption and decreases Cmax, but has minor effects on losartan AUC or on the AUC of the metabolite).

CREON 5 CAPSULES

(Pancrelipase) **3198**

Food Interactions

Food having a pH greater than 5.5 (Can dissolve the protective coating resulting in early release of enzymes, irritation of oral mucosa, and/or loss of enzyme activity).

CREON 10 CAPSULES

(Pancrelipase) **3198**

See Creon 5 Capsules

CREON 20 CAPSULES

(Pancrelipase) **3199**

See Creon 5 Capsules

CRESTOR TABLETS

(Rosuvastatin Calcium) **678**

May interact with oral anticoagulants, erythromycin, fibrates, oral contraceptives, and certain other agents. Compounds in these categories include:

Anisindione (Co-administration of rosuvastatin to patients on stable warfarin therapy resulted in clinically significant rises in INR. In patients taking coumarin anticoagulants and rosuvastatin concomitantly, INR should be monitored). Products include:

Miradon Tablets ... 3042

Antacids, unspecified (Co-administration of an antacid (aluminum and magnesium hydroxide combination) with rosuvastatin resulted in a decrease in plasma concentrations of rosuvastatin by 54%. However, when the antacid was given 2 hours after rosuvastatin, there were no clinically significant changes in plasma concentrations of rosuvastatin).
No products indexed under this heading.

Cimetidine (Caution should be exercised if any HMG-CoA reductase inhibitor is administered concomitantly with drugs that may decrease the levels or activity of endogenous steroid hormones, such as cimetidine). Products include:
Tagamet HB 200 Tablets ... 664

Cimetidine Hydrochloride (Caution should be exercised if any HMG-CoA reductase inhibitor is administered concomitantly with drugs that may decrease the levels or activity of endogenous steroid hormones, such as cimetidine).
No products indexed under this heading.

Clofibrate (The risk of myopathy during treatment with rosuvastatin may be increased with concurrent administration of other lipid-lowering therapies. The benefit of further alterations in lipid levels by the combined use of rosuvastatin with fibrates should be carefully weighed against the potential risks of this combination).
No products indexed under this heading.

Cyclosporine (Co-administration of cyclosporine with rosuvastatin resulted in no significant changes in cyclosporine concentrations. However, Cmax and AUC of rosuvastatin increased 11- and 7-fold, respectively, compared with historical data in healthy subjects. These increases are considered to be clinically significant. The risk of myopathy during treatment with rosuvastatin may be increased with concurrent administration of cyclosporine). Products include:
Gengraf Capsules ... 459
Neoral Oral Solution ... 2259
Neoral Soft Gelatin Capsules ... 2259
Restasis Ophthalmic Emulsion ... 575
Sandimmune ... 2275

Desogestrel (Co-administration of oral contraceptives (ethinyl estradiol and norgestrel) with rosuvastatin resulted in an increase in plasma concentrations of ethinyl estradiol and norgestrel by 26% and 34%, respectively). Products include:
Mircette Tablets ... 1066

Dicumarol (Co-administration of rosuvastatin to patients on stable warfarin therapy resulted in clinically significant rises in INR. In patients taking coumarin anticoagulants and rosuvastatin concomitantly, INR should be monitored).
No products indexed under this heading.

Erythromycin (Co-administration of erythromycin and rosuvastatin decreased AUC and Cmax of rosuvastatin by 20% and 31%, respectively. These reductions are not considered clinically significant). Products include:
Ery-Tab Tablets ... 449
Erythromycin Base Filmtab Tablets ... 455
Erythromycin Delayed-Release Capsules, USP ... 457
PCE Dispertab Tablets ... 515

Erythromycin Estolate (Co-administration of erythromycin and rosuvastatin decreased AUC and Cmax of rosuvastatin by 20% and 31%, respectively. These reductions are not considered clinically significant).
No products indexed under this heading.

Erythromycin Ethylsuccinate (Co-administration of erythromycin and rosuvastatin decreased AUC and Cmax of rosuvastatin by 20% and 31%, respectively. These reductions are not considered clinically significant). Products include:
E.E.S. ... 451
EryPed ... 447

Erythromycin Gluceptate (Co-administration of erythromycin and rosuvastatin decreased AUC and Cmax of rosuvastatin by 20% and 31%, respectively. These reductions are not considered clinically significant).
No products indexed under this heading.

Erythromycin Lactobionate (Co-administration of erythromycin and rosuvastatin decreased AUC and Cmax of rosuvastatin by 20% and 31%, respectively. These reductions are not considered clinically significant).
No products indexed under this heading.

Erythromycin Stearate (Co-administration of erythromycin and rosuvastatin decreased AUC and Cmax of rosuvastatin by 20% and 31%, respectively. These reductions are not considered clinically significant). Products include:
Erythrocin Stearate Filmtab Tablets ... 453

Ethinyl Estradiol (Co-administration of oral contraceptives (ethinyl estradiol and norgestrel) with rosuvastatin resulted in an increase in plasma concentrations of ethinyl estradiol and norgestrel by 26% and 34%, respectively). Products include:
Mircette Tablets ... 1066
NuvaRing ... 2340
Ortho-Cyclen/Ortho Tri-Cyclen ... 2429
Ortho Evra Transdermal System ... 2417
Ortho Tri-Cyclen Lo Tablets ... 2436
Seasonique Tablets ... 1077
Yasmin 28 Tablets ... 796
Yaz Tablets ... 803

Ethynodiol Diacetate (Co-administration of oral contraceptives (ethinyl estradiol and norgestrel) with rosuvastatin resulted in an increase in plasma concentrations of ethinyl estradiol and norgestrel by 26% and 34%, respectively).
No products indexed under this heading.

Fenofibrate (The risk of myopathy during treatment with rosuvastatin may be increased with concurrent administration of other lipid-lowering therapies. The benefit of further alterations in lipid levels by the combined use of rosuvastatin with fibrates should be carefully weighed against the potential risks of this combination). Products include:
Lofibra Tablets ... 1219
Lofibra Capsules ... 1216
Tricor Tablets ... 527
Triglide Tablets ... 3123

Fluconazole (Co-administration of fluconazole with rosuvastatin resulted in a 14% increase in AUC of rosuvastatin. This increase is not considered clinically significant).
No products indexed under this heading.

Gemfibrozil (Co-administration of gemfibrozil with rosuvastatin resulted in a 90% and 120% increase for AUC and Cmax of rosuvastatin, respectively. This increase is considered to be clinically significant; combination therapy with rosuvastatin and gemfibrozil should generally be avoided).
No products indexed under this heading.

Itraconazole (Itraconazole resulted in a 39% and 28% increase in AUC of rosuvastatin after 10mg and 80mg dosing, respectively. These increases are not considered clinically significant).
No products indexed under this heading.

Ketoconazole (Caution should be exercised if any HMG-CoA reductase inhibitor is administered concomitantly with drugs that may decrease the levels or activity of endogenous steroid hormones, such as ketoconazole). Products include:
Nizoral A-D Shampoo, 1% ... 1868

Levonorgestrel (Co-administration of oral contraceptives (ethinyl estradiol and norgestrel) with rosuvastatin resulted in an increase in plasma concentrations of ethinyl estradiol and norgestrel by 26% and 34%, respectively). Products include:
Climara Pro Transdermal System ... 776
Mirena Intrauterine System ... 787
Plan B Tablets ... 1076
Seasonique Tablets ... 1077

Mestranol (Co-administration of oral contraceptives (ethinyl estradiol and norgestrel) with rosuvastatin resulted in an increase in plasma concentrations of ethinyl estradiol and norgestrel by 26% and 34%, respectively).
No products indexed under this heading.

Niacin (The risk of myopathy during treatment with rosuvastatin may be increased with concurrent administration of other lipid-lowering therapies. The benefit of further alterations in lipid levels by the combined use of rosuvastatin with niacin should be carefully weighed against the potential risks of this combination). Products include:
Advicor Tablets ... 1722
Niaspan Extended-Release Tablets ... 1730

Niacinamide (The risk of myopathy during treatment with rosuvastatin may be increased with concurrent administration of other lipid-lowering therapies. The benefit of further alterations in lipid levels by the combined use of rosuvastatin with niacin should be carefully weighed against the potential risks of this combination).
No products indexed under this heading.

Norethindrone (Co-administration of oral contraceptives (ethinyl estradiol and norgestrel) with rosuvastatin resulted in an increase in plasma concentrations of ethinyl estradiol and norgestrel by 26% and 34%, respectively). Products include:
Ortho Micronor Tablets ... 2426

Norethynodrel (Co-administration of oral contraceptives (ethinyl estradiol and norgestrel) with rosuvastatin resulted in an increase in plasma concentrations of ethinyl estradiol and norgestrel by 26% and 34%, respectively).
No products indexed under this heading.

Norgestimate (Co-administration of oral contraceptives (ethinyl estradiol and norgestrel) with rosuvastatin resulted in an increase in plasma concentrations of ethinyl estradiol and norgestrel by 26% and 34%, respectively). Products include:
Ortho-Cyclen/Ortho Tri-Cyclen ... 2429
Ortho Tri-Cyclen Lo Tablets ... 2436

Norgestrel (Co-administration of oral contraceptives (ethinyl estradiol and norgestrel) with rosuvastatin resulted in an increase in plasma concentrations of ethinyl estradiol and norgestrel by 26% and 34%, respectively).
No products indexed under this heading.

Spironolactone (Caution should be exercised if any HMG-CoA reductase inhibitor is administered concomitantly with drugs that may decrease the levels or activity of endogenous steroid hormones, such as spironolactone).
No products indexed under this heading.

Warfarin Sodium (Co-administration of rosuvastatin to patients on stable warfarin therapy resulted in clinically significant rises in INR. In patients taking coumarin anticoagulants and rosuvastatin concomitantly, INR should be monitored). Products include:
Coumadin for Injection ... 898
Coumadin Tablets ... 898

CRIXIVAN CAPSULES

(Indinavir Sulfate) ... 1940

May interact with calcium channel blockers, cytochrome p450 3a4 inducers (selected), cytochrome p450 3a4 inhibitors (selected), cytochrome p450 3a4 substrates (selected), dexamethasone, ergot-containing drugs, phenytoin, and certain other agents. Compounds in these categories include:

Acetazolamide (Co-administration of indinavir and other drugs that inhibit CYP3A4 may decrease the clearance of indinavir and may result in increased plasma concentrations of indinavir).
No products indexed under this heading.

Alfentanil Hydrochloride (Co-administration of indinavir and drugs primarily metabolized by CYP3A4 may result in increased plasma concentrations of the other drug, which could increase or prolong its therapeutic and adverse effects).
No products indexed under this heading.

Allium sativum (Drugs that induce CYP3A4 activity would be expected to increase the clearance of indinavir, resulting in lowered plasma concentrations of indinavir).
No products indexed under this heading.

Alprazolam (Co-administration of indinavir and drugs primarily metabolized by CYP3A4 may result in increased plasma concentrations of the other drug, which could increase or prolong its therapeutic and adverse effects). Products include:

Niravam Orally Disintegrating Tablets 3092

Amiodarone Hydrochloride (Inhibition of CYP3A4 by indinavir could result in elevated plasma concentrations of amiodarone potentially causing serious or life-threatening reactions; co-administration is contraindicated).
No products indexed under this heading.

Amitriptyline Hydrochloride (Co-administration of indinavir and drugs primarily metabolized by CYP3A4 may result in increased plasma concentrations of the other drug, which could increase or prolong its therapeutic and adverse effects).
No products indexed under this heading.

Amlodipine Besylate (Co-administration of calcium channel blockers with indinavir may result in increased plasma concentrations of the dihydropyridine calcium channel blockers which could increase or prolong their therapeutic and adverse effects. Caution is warranted and clinical monitoring is recommended). Products include:
Caduet Tablets 2508
Lotrel Capsules 2249
Norvasc Tablets 2545

Amprenavir (Co-administration of indinavir and other drugs that inhibit CYP3A4 may decrease the clearance of indinavir and may result in increased plasma concentrations of indinavir). Products include:
Agenerase Capsules 1327
Agenerase Oral Solution 1332

Anastrozole (Co-administration of indinavir and other drugs that inhibit CYP3A4 may decrease the clearance of indinavir and may result in increased plasma concentrations of indinavir). Products include:
Arimidex Tablets 673

Aprepitant (Co-administration of indinavir and drugs primarily metabolized by CYP3A4 may result in increased plasma concentrations of the other drug, which could increase or prolong its therapeutic and adverse effects). Products include:
Emend Capsules 1963

Astemizole (Inhibition of CYP3A4 by indinavir could result in elevated plasma concentrations of astemizole potentially causing serious or life-threatening reactions; co-administration is contraindicated).
No products indexed under this heading.

Atazanavir (Both indinavir sulfate and atazanavir are associated with indirect (unconjugated) hyperbilirubinemia. Combinations of these drugs have not been studied and co-administration of indinavir sulfate and atazanavir is not recommended).
No products indexed under this heading.

Atazanavir sulfate (Both indinavir sulfate and atazanavir are associated with indirect (unconjugated) hyperbilirubinemia. Combinations of these drugs have not been studied and coadministration of indinavir sulfate and atazanavir is not recommended). Products include:
Reyataz Capsules 921

Atorvastatin Calcium (Co-administration of indinavir and atorvastatin may lead to increased astorvastatin concentrations. The risk of myopathy, including rhabdomyolysis, may be increased when protease inhibitors, including indinavir, are used in combination with HMG-CoA inhibitors that are metabolized by the CYP3A4 pathway. Use lowest possible dose of atorvastatin with careful monitoring, or consider HMG-CoA reduuctase inhibitors that are not primarily metabolized by CYP3A, such as pravastatin, fluvastatin, or rosuvastain in combination with indinavir). Products include:
Caduet Tablets 2508
Lipitor Tablets 2483

Belladonna Ergotamine (Co-administration of indinavir and drugs primarily metabolized by CYP3A4 may result in increased plasma concentrations of the other drug, which could increase or prolong its therapeutic and adverse effects).
No products indexed under this heading.

Bepridil Hydrochloride (Co-administration may lead to increased bepridil concentrations. Caution is warranted and therapeutic concentration monitoring is recommended for antiarrhythmics when co-administered with indinavir).
No products indexed under this heading.

Betamethasone Acetate (Drugs that induce CYP3A4 activity would be expected to increase the clearance of indinavir, resulting in lowered plasma concentrations of indinavir).
No products indexed under this heading.

Betamethasone Sodium Phosphate (Drugs that induce CYP3A4 activity would be expected to increase the clearance of indinavir, resulting in lowered plasma concentrations of indinavir).
No products indexed under this heading.

Buspirone Hydrochloride (Co-administration of indinavir and drugs primarily metabolized by CYP3A4 may result in increased plasma concentrations of the other drug, which could increase or prolong its therapeutic and adverse effects).
No products indexed under this heading.

Busulfan (Co-administration of indinavir and drugs primarily metabolized by CYP3A4 may result in increased plasma concentrations of the other drug, which could increase or prolong its therapeutic and adverse effects). Products include:
I.V. Busulfex 2493
Myleran Tablets 1525

Carbamazepine (Could diminish plasma concentrations of indinavir because carbamazepine is an inducer of P450 3A4; caution is advised if co-administered). Products include:
Carbatrol Capsules 3171
Equetro Extended-Release Capsules 3180
Tegretol/Tegretol-XR 2295

Cerivastatin Sodium (The risk of myopathy including rhabdomyolysis may be increased when protease inhibitors, including indinavir, are used in combination with HMG-CoA inhibitors that are metabolized by the CYP3A4 pathway).
No products indexed under this heading.

Chlorpheniramine (Co-administration of indinavir and drugs primarily metabolized by CYP3A4 may result in increased plasma concentrations of the other drug, which could increase or prolong its therapeutic and adverse effects).
No products indexed under this heading.

Chlorpheniramine Maleate (Co-administration of indinavir and drugs primarily metabolized by CYP3A4 may result in increased plasma concentrations of the other drug, which could increase or prolong its therapeutic and adverse effects). Products include:
Advil Allergy Sinus Caplets .... ▣770
Advil Multi-Symptom Cold Caplets .... ▣770
BC Allergy Sinus Cold Powder .... ▣677
Comtrex Maximum Strength Cold & Cough Day/Night Caplets - Night Formulation .... ▣726
Comtrex Maximum Strength Day/Night Severe Cold & Sinus Caplets - Night Formulation .... ▣725
Contac Cold and Flu Maximum Strength Caplets .... ▣728
Contac Cold and Flu Day and Night Caplets (Night Formulation Only) .... ▣727
Children's Dimetapp Long Acting Cough Plus Cold Syrup .... ▣731
Robitussin Cough & Cold Long-Acting Liquid .... ▣735
Robitussin Cough & Allergy Syrup .... ▣736
Robitussin Cough & Cold Nighttime Liquid .... ▣736
Robitussin Cough, Cold & Flu Nighttime Liquid .... ▣738
Robitussin Pediatric Cough & Cold Long-Acting Liquid .... ▣735
Robitussin Pediatric Cough & Cold Nighttime Liquid .... ▣736
Triaminic Cold & Allergy Liquid .... ▣746
Triaminic Cough & Runny Nose Softchews .... ▣748
Children's Tylenol Plus Flu Oral Suspension .... ▣749
Tylenol Allergy Multi-Symptom Caplets with Cool Burst and Gelcaps 1872
Children's Tylenol Plus Cold Suspension Liquid 1879
Children's Tylenol Plus Cough & Runny Nose Suspension Liquid 1879
Children's Tylenol Plus Flu Suspension Liquid 1881
Children's Tylenol Plus Multi-Symptom Cold Suspension Liquid 1879
Tylenol Cold Head Congestion Nighttime Caplets with Cool Burst 1873
Tylenol Cold Multi-Symptom Nighttime Caplets with Cool Burst 1874
Tylenol Sinus Congestion & Pain Nighttime Caplets with Cool Burst 1876
Vicks 44M Cough, Cold & Flu Relief Liquid 2680
Pediatric Vicks 44m Cough & Cold Relief Liquid 2676
Children's Vicks NyQuil Cold/Cough Relief .... ▣756
Children's Vicks NyQuil Cold/Cough Relief Liquid 2680
Zicam Maximum Strength Flu Daytime .... ▣768

Chlorpheniramine Polistirex (Co-administration of indinavir and drugs primarily metabolized by CYP3A4 may result in increased plasma concentrations of the other drug, which could increase or prolong its therapeutic and adverse effects). Products include:
Tussionex Pennkinetic Extended-Release Suspension 3327

Chlorpheniramine Tannate (Co-administration of indinavir and drugs primarily metabolized by CYP3A4 may result in increased plasma concentrations of the other drug, which could increase or prolong its therapeutic and adverse effects).
No products indexed under this heading.

Cimetidine (Co-administration of indinavir and other drugs that inhibit CYP3A4 may decrease the clearance of indinavir and may result in increased plasma concentrations of indinavir). Products include:
Tagamet HB 200 Tablets .... ▣664

Cimetidine Hydrochloride (Co-administration of indinavir and other drugs that inhibit CYP3A4 may decrease the clearance of indinavir and may result in increased plasma concentrations of indinavir).
No products indexed under this heading.

Ciprofloxacin (Co-administration of indinavir and other drugs that inhibit CYP3A4 may decrease the clearance of indinavir and may result in increased plasma concentrations of indinavir). Products include:
Cipro Oral Suspension 2977
Cipro I.V. 2984
Cipro XR Tablets 2990
Ciprodex Otic Suspension 559

Ciprofloxacin Hydrochloride (Drugs that induce CYP3A4 activity would be expected to increase the clearance of indinavir, resulting in lowered plasma concentrations of indinavir). Products include:
Ciloxan Ophthalmic Ointment 559
Ciloxan Ophthalmic Solution .... ⊙206
Cipro Tablets 2977
Proquin XR Tablets 1153

Cisapride (Inhibition of CYP3A4 by indinavir could result in elevated plasma concentrations of cisapride, potentially causing serious or life-threatening reactions; co-administration is contraindicated).
No products indexed under this heading.

Cisplatin (Drugs that induce CYP3A4 activity would be expected to increase the clearance of indinavir, resulting in lowered plasma concentrations of indinavir).
No products indexed under this heading.

Clarithromycin (Co-administration of indinavir and clarithromycin may lead to increased clarithromycin and indinvair concentrations. The appropriate doses for this combination, with respect to safety and efficacy, have not been established). Products include:
Biaxin/Biaxin XL 402
PREVPAC 3284

Clotrimazole (Co-administration of indinavir and other drugs that inhibit CYP3A4 may decrease the clearance of indinavir and may result in increased plasma concentrations of indinavir). Products include:
Desenex Athlete's Foot Cream .... ▣635
Lotrimin 3039
Lotrisone 3040

Cortisone Acetate (Drugs that induce CYP3A4 activity would be expected to increase the clearance of indinavir, resulting in lowered plasma concentrations of indinavir).
No products indexed under this heading.

(▣ Described in PDR For Nonprescription Drugs) (⊙ Described in PDR For Ophthalmic Medicines™)

Cyclosporine (Co-administration of indinavir and cyclosporine may lead to increased cyclosporine concentrations). Products include:

Dalfopristin (Co-administration of indinavir and other drugs that inhibit CYP3A4 may decrease the clearance of indinavir and may result in increased plasma concentrations of indinavir).

No products indexed under this heading.

Danazol (Co-administration of indinavir and other drugs that inhibit CYP3A4 may decrease the clearance of indinavir and may result in increased plasma concentrations of indinavir).

No products indexed under this heading.

Delavirdine Mesylate (Co-administration results in inhibition of indinavir metabolism producing an increase in indinavir concentrations; a reduction of indinavir dosage should be considered when used concurrently). Products include:

Desogestrel (Co-administration of indinavir and drugs primarily metabolized by CYP3A4 may result in increased plasma concentrations of the other drug, which could increase or prolong its therapeutic and adverse effects). Products include:

Dexamethasone (Could diminish plasma concentrations of indinavir because dexamethasone is an inducer of P450 3A4; caution is advised if co-administered). Products include:

Dexamethasone Acetate (Could diminish plasma concentrations of indinavir because dexamethasone is an inducer of P450 3A4; caution is advised if co-administered).

No products indexed under this heading.

Dexamethasone Sodium Phosphate (Could diminish plasma concentrations of indinavir because dexamethasone is an inducer of P450 3A4; caution is advised if co-administered).

No products indexed under this heading.

Diazepam (Co-administration of indinavir and drugs primarily metabolized by CYP3A4 may result in increased plasma concentrations of the other drug, which could increase or prolong its therapeutic and adverse effects). Products include:

Didanosine (Gastric acid rapidly degrades didanosine and a normal (acidic) gastric pH may be necessary for the optimum absorption of indinavir; if administered concomitantly, they should be administered at least one hour apart on an empty stomach).

No products indexed under this heading.

Dihydroergotamine Mesylate (Inhibition of CYP3A4 by indinavir could result in elevated plasma concentrations of ergot derivatives,

potentially causing serious or life-threatening reactions; co-administration is contraindicated). Products include:

Diltiazem Hydrochloride (Co-administration of calcium channel blockers with indinavir may result in increased plasma concentrations of the dihydropyridine calcium channel blockers which could increase or prolong their therapeutic and adverse effects. Caution is warranted and clinical monitoring is recommended). Products include:

Diltiazem Maleate (Co-administration of indinavir and drugs primarily metabolized by CYP3A4 may result in increased plasma concentrations of the other drug, which could increase or prolong its therapeutic and adverse effects).

No products indexed under this heading.

Disopyramide (Co-administration of indinavir and drugs primarily metabolized by CYP3A4 may result in increased plasma concentrations of the other drug, which could increase or prolong its therapeutic and adverse effects).

No products indexed under this heading.

Disopyramide Phosphate (Co-administration of indinavir and drugs primarily metabolized by CYP3A4 may result in increased plasma concentrations of the other drug, which could increase or prolong its therapeutic and adverse effects).

No products indexed under this heading.

Disulfiram (Co-administration of indinavir and drugs primarily metabolized by CYP3A4 may result in increased plasma concentrations of the other drug, which could increase or prolong its therapeutic and adverse effects).

No products indexed under this heading.

Doxorubicin Hydrochloride (Co-administration of indinavir and drugs primarily metabolized by CYP3A4 may result in increased plasma concentrations of the other drug, which could increase or prolong its therapeutic and adverse effects).

No products indexed under this heading.

Dronabinol (Co-administration of indinavir and drugs primarily metabolized by CYP3A4 may result in increased plasma concentrations of the other drug, which could increase or prolong its therapeutic and adverse effects). Products include:

Efavirenz (Co-administration results in a decrease in the plasma concentrations of indinavir; a dosage increase of indinavir is recommended when used concurrently). Products include:

Ergonovine Maleate (Inhibition of CYP3A4 by indinavir could result in elevated plasma concentrations of ergot derivatives, potentially causing serious or life-threatening reactions; co-administration is contraindicated).

No products indexed under this heading.

Ergotamine Tartrate (Inhibition of CYP3A4 by indinavir could result in elevated plasma concentrations of ergot derivatives, potentially causing serious or life-threatening reactions; co-administration is contraindicated).

No products indexed under this heading.

Erythromycin (Co-administration of indinavir and drugs primarily metabolized by CYP3A4 may result in increased plasma concentrations of the other drug, which could increase or prolong its therapeutic and adverse effects). Products include:

Erythromycin Estolate (Co-administration of indinavir and drugs primarily metabolized by CYP3A4 may result in increased plasma concentrations of the other drug, which could increase or prolong its therapeutic and adverse effects).

No products indexed under this heading.

Erythromycin Ethylsuccinate (Co-administration of indinavir and drugs primarily metabolized by CYP3A4 may result in increased plasma concentrations of the other drug, which could increase or prolong its therapeutic and adverse effects). Products include:

Erythromycin Gluceptate (Co-administration of indinavir and drugs primarily metabolized by CYP3A4 may result in increased plasma concentrations of the other drug, which could increase or prolong its therapeutic and adverse effects).

No products indexed under this heading.

Erythromycin Lactobionate (Co-administration of indinavir and drugs primarily metabolized by CYP3A4 may result in increased plasma concentrations of the other drug, which could increase or prolong its therapeutic and adverse effects).

No products indexed under this heading.

Erythromycin Stearate (Co-administration of indinavir and drugs primarily metabolized by CYP3A4 may result in increased plasma concentrations of the other drug, which could increase or prolong its therapeutic and adverse effects). Products include:

Esomeprazole Magnesium (Co-administration of indinavir and other drugs that inhibit CYP3A4 may decrease the clearance of indinavir and may result in increased plasma concentrations of indinavir). Products include:

Estradiol (Co-administration of indinavir and drugs primarily metabolized by CYP3A4 may result in

increased plasma concentrations of the other drug, which could increase or prolong its therapeutic and adverse effects). Products include:

Estradiol Benzoate (Co-administration of indinavir and drugs primarily metabolized by CYP3A4 may result in increased plasma concentrations of the other drug, which could increase or prolong its therapeutic and adverse effects).

No products indexed under this heading.

Estradiol Cypionate (Co-administration of indinavir and drugs primarily metabolized by CYP3A4 may result in increased plasma concentrations of the other drug, which could increase or prolong its therapeutic and adverse effects).

No products indexed under this heading.

Estradiol Valerate (Co-administration of indinavir and drugs primarily metabolized by CYP3A4 may result in increased plasma concentrations of the other drug, which could increase or prolong its therapeutic and adverse effects).

No products indexed under this heading.

Ethinyl Estradiol (Co-administration with Ortho-Novum 1/35 has resulted in an increase in ethinyl estradiol AUC). Products include:

Ethosuximide (Co-administration of indinavir and drugs primarily metabolized by CYP3A4 may result in increased plasma concentrations of the other drug, which could increase or prolong its therapeutic and adverse effects).

No products indexed under this heading.

Ethynodiol Diacetate (Co-administration of indinavir and drugs primarily metabolized by CYP3A4 may result in increased plasma concentrations of the other drug, which could increase or prolong its therapeutic and adverse effects).

No products indexed under this heading.

Etoposide (Co-administration of indinavir and drugs primarily metabolized by CYP3A4 may result in increased plasma concentrations of the other drug, which could increase or prolong its therapeutic and adverse effects).

No products indexed under this heading.

Etoposide Phosphate (Co-administration of indinavir and drugs primarily metabolized by CYP3A4 may result in increased plasma concentrations of the other drug, which could increase or prolong its therapeutic and adverse effects).

No products indexed under this heading.

Felbamate (Drugs that induce CYP3A4 activity would be expected to increase the clearance of indinavir, resulting in lowered plasma concentrations of indinavir).

No products indexed under this heading.

Felodipine (Co-administration of calcium channel blockers with indinavir may result in increased plasma concentrations of the dihydropyridine calcium channel blockers which could increase or prolong their therapeutic and adverse effects. Caution is warranted and clinical monitoring is recommended).

No products indexed under this heading.

Fentanyl (Co-administration of indinavir and drugs primarily metabolized by CYP3A4 may result in increased plasma concentrations of the other drug, which could increase or prolong its therapeutic and adverse effects. Products include:

| Duragesic Transdermal System | 2373 |
| Ionsys Transdermal System | 2379 |

Fentanyl Citrate (Co-administration of indinavir and drugs primarily metabolized by CYP3A4 may result in increased plasma concentrations of the other drug, which could increase or prolong its therapeutic and adverse effects). Products include:

| Actiq | 979 |

Fluconazole (Co-administration has resulted in a 19% ± 33% decrease in indinavir AUC).

No products indexed under this heading.

Fludrocortisone Acetate (Drugs that induce CYP3A4 activity would be expected to increase the clearance of indinavir, resulting in lowered plasma concentrations of indinavir).

No products indexed under this heading.

Fluoxetine Hydrochloride (Co-administration of indinavir and other drugs that inhibit CYP3A4 may decrease the clearance of indinavir and may result in increased plasma concentrations of indinavir). Products include:

| Prozac Pulvules and Liquid | 1801 |
| Symbyax Capsules | 1819 |

Fluticasone Propionate (Concomitant use of fluticasone propionate and indinavir sulfate may increase plasma concentrations of fluticasone propionate; co-administer with caution. Consider alternatives to fluticasone propionate, particularly for long-term use). Products include:

Advair Diskus 100/50	1308
Advair Diskus 250/50	1308
Advair Diskus 500/50	1308
Advair HFA Inhalation Aerosol	1318
Cutivate Cream	2662
Cutivate Lotion 0.05%	2664
Cutivate Ointment	2665
Flonase Nasal Spray	1440
Flovent Diskus	1443

Fluticasone Propionate HFA (Concomitant use of fluticasone propionate and indinavir sulfate may increase plasma concentrations of fluticasone propionate; co-administer with caution. Consider alternatives to fluticasone propionate, particularly for long-term use). Products include:

| Flovent HFA | 1447 |

Fluvoxamine Maleate (Co-administration of indinavir and other drugs that inhibit CYP3A4 may decrease the clearance of indinavir and may result in increased plasma concentrations of indinavir).

No products indexed under this heading.

Fosamprenavir Calcium (Co-administration of indinavir and other drugs that inhibit CYP3A4 may decrease the clearance of indinavir and may result in increased plasma concentrations of indinavir). Products include:

| Lexiva Tablets | 1505 |

Fosphenytoin Sodium (Could diminish plasma concentrations of indinavir because phenytoin is an inducer of P450 3A4; caution is advised if co-administered).

No products indexed under this heading.

Garlic Extract (Drugs that induce CYP3A4 activity would be expected to increase the clearance of indinavir, resulting in lowered plasma concentrations of indinavir).

No products indexed under this heading.

Garlic Oil (Drugs that induce CYP3A4 activity would be expected to increase the clearance of indinavir, resulting in lowered plasma concentrations of indinavir).

No products indexed under this heading.

Haloperidol (Co-administration of indinavir and drugs primarily metabolized by CYP3A4 may result in increased plasma concentrations of the other drug, which could increase or prolong its therapeutic and adverse effects).

No products indexed under this heading.

Haloperidol Decanoate (Co-administration of indinavir and drugs primarily metabolized by CYP3A4 may result in increased plasma concentrations of the other drug, which could increase or prolong its therapeutic and adverse effects).

No products indexed under this heading.

Haloperidol Lactate (Co-administration of indinavir and drugs primarily metabolized by CYP3A4 may result in increased plasma concentrations of the other drug, which could increase or prolong its therapeutic and adverse effects).

No products indexed under this heading.

Hydrocortisone (Drugs that induce CYP3A4 activity would be expected to increase the clearance of indinavir, resulting in lowered plasma concentrations of indinavir). Products include:

Colocort Rectal Suspension, USP (Retention) 100 mg/60 mL	2476
Hydrocortone Tablets	1989
Preparation H Hydrocortisone Cream	▣ 646

Hydrocortisone Acetate (Drugs that induce CYP3A4 activity would be expected to increase the clearance of indinavir, resulting in lowered plasma concentrations of indinavir). Products include:

Analpram-HC	1159
Pramosone	1161
ProctoFoam-HC	3099

Hydrocortisone Butyrate (Drugs that induce CYP3A4 activity would be expected to increase the clear-

ance of indinavir, resulting in lowered plasma concentrations of indinavir). Products include:

| Locoid Lipocream Cream | 1160 |

Hydrocortisone Cypionate (Drugs that induce CYP3A4 activity would be expected to increase the clearance of indinavir, resulting in lowered plasma concentrations of indinavir).

No products indexed under this heading.

Hydrocortisone Hemisuccinate (Drugs that induce CYP3A4 activity would be expected to increase the clearance of indinavir, resulting in lowered plasma concentrations of indinavir).

No products indexed under this heading.

Hydrocortisone Probutate (Drugs that induce CYP3A4 activity would be expected to increase the clearance of indinavir, resulting in lowered plasma concentrations of indinavir).

No products indexed under this heading.

Hydrocortisone Sodium Phosphate (Drugs that induce CYP3A4 activity would be expected to increase the clearance of indinavir, resulting in lowered plasma concentrations of indinavir).

No products indexed under this heading.

Hydrocortisone Sodium Succinate (Drugs that induce CYP3A4 activity would be expected to increase the clearance of indinavir, resulting in lowered plasma concentrations of indinavir).

No products indexed under this heading.

Hydrocortisone Valerate (Drugs that induce CYP3A4 activity would be expected to increase the clearance of indinavir, resulting in lowered plasma concentrations of indinavir).

No products indexed under this heading.

Hypericum (Co-administration of indinavir and St. John's Wort (hypericum perforatum) or products containing St. John's Wort has been shown to substantially decrease indinavir concentrations and may lead to loss of virologic response and possible resistance to indinavir or to the class of protease inhibitors; co-administration is not recommended). Products include:

| Satiete Tablets | ▣ 832 |

Hypericum Perforatum (Drugs that induce CYP3A4 activity would be expected to increase the clearance of indinavir, resulting in lowered plasma concentrations of indinavir).

No products indexed under this heading.

Isoniazid (Co-administration has resulted in a 13% ± 15% increase in isoniazid AUC).

No products indexed under this heading.

Isradipine (Co-administration of calcium channel blockers with indinavir may result in increased plasma concentrations of the dihydropyridine calcium channel blockers which could increase or prolong their therapeutic and adverse effects. Caution is warranted and clinical monitoring is recommended). Products include:

| DynaCirc CR Tablets | 2721 |

Itraconazole (Co-administration of indinavir and itraconzole may lead to increased indinvair concentrations. Dose reduction of indinavir to 600 mg every 8 hours is recommended when administering itraconzole concomitantly).

No products indexed under this heading.

Ketoconazole (Co-administration of indinavir and ketoconazole may lead to increased indinvair concentrations. Dose reduction of indinavir to 600 mg every 8 hours is recommended when administering ketoconazole concomitantly). Products include:

| Nizoral A-D Shampoo, 1% | 1868 |

Levonorgestrel (Co-administration of indinavir and drugs primarily metabolized by CYP3A4 may result in increased plasma concentrations of the other drug, which could increase or prolong its therapeutic and adverse effects). Products include:

Climara Pro Transdermal System	776
Mirena Intrauterine System	787
Plan B Tablets	1076
Seasonique Tablets	1077

Lidocaine (Co-administration may lead to increased lidocaine concentrations. Caution is warranted and therapeutic concentration monitoring is recommended for antiarrhythmics when co-administered with indinavir). Products include:

| Lidoderm Patch | 1118 |
| Synera Topical Patch | 1137 |

Lidocaine Hydrochloride (Co-administration may lead to increased lidocaine concentrations. Caution is warranted and therapeutic concentration monitoring is recommended for antiarrhythmics when co-administered with indinavir).

No products indexed under this heading.

Lopinavir (Co-administration of indinavir and other drugs that inhibit CYP3A4 may decrease the clearance of indinavir and may result in increased plasma concentrations of indinavir). Products include:

| Kaletra | 476 |

Loratadine (Co-administration of indinavir and other drugs that inhibit CYP3A4 may decrease the clearance of indinavir and may result in increased plasma concentrations of indinavir). Products include:

Alavert Allergy & Sinus D-12 Hour Tablets	▣ 771
Alavert	▣ 771
Children's Claritin Allergy Oral Solution	▣ 771
Claritin Non-Drowsy 24 Hour Tablets	▣ 772
Claritin Reditabs 24 Hour Non-Drowsy Tablets	▣ 772
Claritin-D Non-Drowsy 12 Hour Tablets	▣ 772
Claritin-D Non-Drowsy 24 Hour Tablets	▣ 772

Lovastatin (The risk of myopathy including rhabdomyolysis may be increased when protease inhibitors, including indinavir, are used in combination with HMG-CoA inhibitors that are metabolized by the CYP3A4 pathway; concomitant use is not recommended). Products include:

Advicor Tablets	1722
Altoprev Extended-Release Tablets	3109
Mevacor Tablets	2021

Mephenytoin (Drugs that induce CYP3A4 activity would be expected to increase the clearance of indinavir, resulting in lowered plasma concentrations of indinavir).

No products indexed under this heading.

Mestranol (Co-administration of indinavir and drugs primarily metabolized by CYP3A4 may result in increased plasma concentrations of the other drug, which could increase or prolong its therapeutic and adverse effects).

No products indexed under this heading.

Methadone Hydrochloride (Co-administration of indinavir and drugs primarily metabolized by CYP3A4 may result in increased plasma concentrations of the other drug, which could increase or prolong its therapeutic and adverse effects).

No products indexed under this heading.

Methsuximide (Drugs that induce CYP3A4 activity would be expected to increase the clearance of indinavir, resulting in lowered plasma concentrations of indinavir).

No products indexed under this heading.

Methylergonovine Maleate (Inhibition of CYP3A4 by indinavir could result in elevated plasma concentrations of ergot derivatives, potentially causing serious or life-threatening reactions; co-administration is contraindicated).

No products indexed under this heading.

Methylprednisolone (Drugs that induce CYP3A4 activity would be expected to increase the clearance of indinavir, resulting in lowered plasma concentrations of indinavir).

No products indexed under this heading.

Methylprednisolone Acetate (Drugs that induce CYP3A4 activity would be expected to increase the clearance of indinavir, resulting in lowered plasma concentrations of indinavir). Products include:

Depo-Medrol Injectable
Suspension 2617
Depo-Medrol Single-Dose Vial 2619

Methylprednisolone Sodium Succinate (Drugs that induce CYP3A4 activity would be expected to increase the clearance of indinavir, resulting in lowered plasma concentrations of indinavir).

No products indexed under this heading.

Methysergide Maleate (Inhibition of CYP3A4 by indinavir could result in elevated plasma concentrations of ergot derivatives, potentially causing serious or life-threatening reactions; co-administration is contraindicated).

No products indexed under this heading.

Metronidazole (Co-administration of indinavir and other drugs that inhibit CYP3A4 may decrease the clearance of indinavir and may result in increased plasma concentrations of indinavir). Products include:

Metrogel 1% 1211
MetroGel-Vaginal Gel 1855
Vandazole Vaginal Gel 3338

Metronidazole Benzoate (Co-administration of indinavir and other drugs that inhibit CYP3A4 may decrease the clearance of indinavir and may result in increased plasma concentrations of indinavir).

No products indexed under this heading.

Metronidazole Hydrochloride (Co-administration of indinavir and other drugs that inhibit CYP3A4 may decrease the clearance of indinavir and may result in increased plasma concentrations of indinavir).

No products indexed under this heading.

Mibefradil Dihydrochloride (Co-administration of calcium channel blockers with indinavir may result in increased plasma concentrations of the dihydropyridine calcium channel blockers which could increase or prolong their therapeutic and adverse effects. Caution is warranted and clinical monitoring is recommended).

No products indexed under this heading.

Miconazole (Co-administration of indinavir and other drugs that inhibit CYP3A4 may decrease the clearance of indinavir and may result in increased plasma concentrations of indinavir).

No products indexed under this heading.

Miconazole Nitrate (Co-administration of indinavir and other drugs that inhibit CYP3A4 may decrease the clearance of indinavir and may result in increased plasma concentrations of indinavir). Products include:

Desenex .. ▣635
Desenex Jock Itch Spray Powder ... ▣635

Midazolam Hydrochloride (Inhibition of CYP3A4 by indinavir could result in elevated plasma concentrations of midazolam potentially causing serious or life-threatening reactions; co-administration is contraindicated).

No products indexed under this heading.

Modafinil (Drugs that induce CYP3A4 activity would be expected to increase the clearance of indinavir, resulting in lowered plasma concentrations of indinavir). Products include:

Provigil Tablets 988

Nefazodone Hydrochloride (Co-administration of indinavir and drugs primarily metabolized by CYP3A4 may result in increased plasma concentrations of the other drug, which could increase or prolong its therapeutic and adverse effects).

No products indexed under this heading.

Nelfinavir Mesylate (Co-administration of indinavir and nelfinavir may lead to increased indinavir concentrations. The appropriate doses for this combination, with respect to safety and efficacy, have not been established). Products include:

Viracept .. 2577

Nevirapine (Co-administration of indinavir and nevirapine may lead to decreased indinavir concentrations. The appropriate doses for this combination, with respect to saftey and efficacy, have not been established). Products include:

Viramune Oral Suspension 873

Viramune Tablets 873

Niacinamide (Co-administration of indinavir and other drugs that inhibit CYP3A4 may decrease the clearance of indinavir and may result in increased plasma concentrations of indinavir).

No products indexed under this heading.

Nicardipine Hydrochloride (Co-administration of calcium channel blockers with indinavir may result in increased plasma concentrations of the dihydropyridine calcium channel blockers which could increase or prolong their therapeutic and adverse effects. Caution is warranted and clinical monitoring is recommended). Products include:

Cardene I.V. 2497

Nicotinamide (Co-administration of indinavir and other drugs that inhibit CYP3A4 may decrease the clearance of indinavir and may result in increased plasma concentrations of indinavir). Products include:

Nicomide Tablets 1088

Nifedipine (Co-administration of calcium channel blockers with indinavir may result in increased plasma concentrations of the dihydropyridine calcium channel blockers which could increase or prolong their therapeutic and adverse effects. Caution is warranted and clinical monitoring is recommended). Products include:

Adalat CC Tablets 2964

Nimodipine (Co-administration of calcium channel blockers with indinavir may result in increased plasma concentrations of the dihydropyridine calcium channel blockers which could increase or prolong their therapeutic and adverse effects. Caution is warranted and clinical monitoring is recommended). Products include:

Nimotop Capsules 749

Nisoldipine (Co-administration of calcium channel blockers with indinavir may result in increased plasma concentrations of the dihydropyridine calcium channel blockers which could increase or prolong their therapeutic and adverse effects. Caution is warranted and clinical monitoring is recommended). Products include:

Sular Tablets 3122

Nitrendipine (Co-administration of indinavir and drugs primarily metabolized by CYP3A4 may result in increased plasma concentrations of the other drug, which could increase or prolong its therapeutic and adverse effects).

No products indexed under this heading.

Norethindrone (Co-administration with Ortho-Novum 1/35 has resulted in an increase in norethindrone AUC). Products include:

Ortho Micronor Tablets 2426

Norethindrone Acetate (Co-administration of indinavir and drugs primarily metabolized by CYP3A4 may result in increased plasma concentrations of the other drug, which could increase or prolong its therapeutic and adverse effects).

No products indexed under this heading.

Norfloxacin (Co-administration of indinavir and other drugs that inhibit CYP3A4 may decrease the clearance of indinavir and may result in increased plasma concentrations of indinavir). Products include:

Noroxin Tablets 2032

Norgestrel (Co-administration of indinavir and drugs primarily metabolized by CYP3A4 may result in increased plasma concentrations of the other drug, which could increase or prolong its therapeutic and adverse effects).

No products indexed under this heading.

Omeprazole (Co-administration of indinavir and other drugs that inhibit CYP3A4 may decrease the clearance of indinavir and may result in increased plasma concentrations of indinavir). Products include:

Zegerid Capsules 2958
Zegerid Powder for Oral Solution 2958

Ondansetron (Co-administration of indinavir and drugs primarily metabolized by CYP3A4 may result in increased plasma concentrations of the other drug, which could increase or prolong its therapeutic and adverse effects). Products include:

Zofran ODT Orally Disintegrating
Tablets .. 1639

Ondansetron Hydrochloride (Co-administration of indinavir and drugs primarily metabolized by CYP3A4 may result in increased plasma concentrations of the other drug, which could increase or prolong its therapeutic and adverse effects). Products include:

Zofran Injection 1634
Zofran ... 1639

Oxcarbazepine (Drugs that induce CYP3A4 activity would be expected to increase the clearance of indinavir, resulting in lowered plasma concentrations of indinavir). Products include:

Trileptal Tablets 2300
Trileptal Oral Suspension 2300

Paclitaxel (Co-administration of indinavir and drugs primarily metabolized by CYP3A4 may result in increased plasma concentrations of the other drug, which could increase or prolong its therapeutic and adverse effects).

No products indexed under this heading.

Paroxetine Hydrochloride (Co-administration of indinavir and other drugs that inhibit CYP3A4 may decrease the clearance of indinavir and may result in increased plasma concentrations of indinavir). Products include:

Paxil CR Controlled-Release
Tablets .. 1538
Paxil ... 1530

Phenobarbital (Could diminish plasma concentrations of indinavir because phenobarbital is an inducer of P450 3A4; caution is advised if co-administered). Products include:

Donnatal Extentabs 2493

Phenobarbital Sodium (Drugs that induce CYP3A4 activity would be expected to increase the clearance of indinavir, resulting in lowered plasma concentrations of indinavir).

No products indexed under this heading.

Phenytoin (Could diminish plasma concentrations of indinavir because phenytoin is an inducer of P450 3A4; caution is advised if co-administered).

No products indexed under this heading.

Phenytoin Sodium (Could diminish plasma concentrations of indinavir because phenytoin is an inducer of P450 3A4; caution is advised if co-administered). Products include:

Pimozide (Inhibition of CYP3A4 by indinavir could result in elevated plasma concentrations of pimozide potentially causing serious or life-threatening reactions; co-administration is contraindicated).
No products indexed under this heading.

Polyestradiol Phosphate (Co-administration of indinavir and drugs primarily metabolized by CYP3A4 may result in increased plasma concentrations of the other drug, which could increase or prolong its therapeutic and adverse effects).
No products indexed under this heading.

Prednisolone Acetate (Drugs that induce CYP3A4 activity would be expected to increase the clearance of indinavir, resulting in lowered plasma concentrations of indinavir).
Products include:

Prednisolone Sodium Phosphate (Drugs that induce CYP3A4 activity would be expected to increase the clearance of indinavir, resulting in lowered plasma concentrations of indinavir).
No products indexed under this heading.

Prednisolone Tebutate (Drugs that induce CYP3A4 activity would be expected to increase the clearance of indinavir, resulting in lowered plasma concentrations of indinavir).
No products indexed under this heading.

Prednisone (Drugs that induce CYP3A4 activity would be expected to increase the clearance of indinavir, resulting in lowered plasma concentrations of indinavir).
No products indexed under this heading.

Primidone (Drugs that induce CYP3A4 activity would be expected to increase the clearance of indinavir, resulting in lowered plasma concentrations of indinavir).
No products indexed under this heading.

Propoxyphene Hydrochloride (Co-administration of indinavir and other drugs that inhibit CYP3A4 may decrease the clearance of indinavir and may result in increased plasma concentrations of indinavir).
No products indexed under this heading.

Propoxyphene Napsylate (Co-administration of indinavir and other drugs that inhibit CYP3A4 may decrease the clearance of indinavir and may result in increased plasma concentrations of indinavir).
No products indexed under this heading.

Quinidine (Co-administration of indinavir and quinidine may lead to increased quinidine concentrations. Caution is warranted and therapeutic concentration monitoring is recommended for antiarrhythmics when co-administered with indinavir).
No products indexed under this heading.

Quinidine Gluconate (Co-administration of indinavir and quinidine may lead to increased quinidine concentrations. Caution is warranted and therapeutic concentration monitoring is recommended for antiarrhythmics when co-administered with indinavir).
No products indexed under this heading.

Quinidine Hydrochloride (Co-administration of indinavir and quinidine may lead to increased quinidine concentrations. Caution is warranted and therapeutic concentration monitoring is recommended for antiarrhythmics when co-administered with indinavir).
No products indexed under this heading.

Quinidine Polygalacturonate (Co-administration of indinavir and quinidine lead to increased quinidine, concentrations. Caution is warranted and therapeutic concentration monitoring is recommended for antiarrhythmics when co-administered with indinavir).
No products indexed under this heading.

Quinidine Sulfate (Co-administration of indinavir and quinidine lead to increased quinidine, concentrations. Caution is warranted and therapeutic concentration monitoring is recommended for antiarrhythmics when co-administered with indinavir).
No products indexed under this heading.

Quinine (Co-administration of indinavir and other drugs that inhibit CYP3A4 may decrease the clearance of indinavir and may result in increased plasma concentrations of indinavir).
No products indexed under this heading.

Quinine Sulfate (Co-administration of indinavir and other drugs that inhibit CYP3A4 may decrease the clearance of indinavir and may result in increased plasma concentrations of indinavir).
No products indexed under this heading.

Quinupristin (Co-administration of indinavir and other drugs that inhibit CYP3A4 may decrease the clearance of indinavir and may result in increased plasma concentrations of indinavir).
No products indexed under this heading.

Ranitidine Bismuth Citrate (Co-administration of indinavir and other drugs that inhibit CYP3A4 may decrease the clearance of indinavir and may result in increased plasma concentrations of indinavir).
No products indexed under this heading.

Ranitidine Hydrochloride (Co-administration of indinavir and other drugs that inhibit CYP3A4 may decrease the clearance of indinavir

and may result in increased plasma concentrations of indinavir).
Products include:

Rifabutin (Co-administration of indinavir and rifabutin may lead to decreased indinavir and increased rifabutin concentrations. Dose reduction of rifabutin to half the standard dose and a dose increase of indinavir to 1000 mg (three 333-mg capsules) every 8 hours are recommended when rifabutin and indinavir are co-administered).
No products indexed under this heading.

Rifampicin (Drugs that induce CYP3A4 activity would be expected to increase the clearance of indinavir, resulting in lowered plasma concentrations of indinavir).
No products indexed under this heading.

Rifampin (Markedly diminishes plasma concentrations of indinavir because rifampin is a potent inducer of P450 3A4; co-administration is not recommended).
No products indexed under this heading.

Rifapentine (Drugs that induce CYP3A4 activity would be expected to increase the clearance of indinavir, resulting in lowered plasma concentrations of indinavir).
No products indexed under this heading.

Ritonavir (Co-administration of indinavir and ritonavir may lead to increased indinavir and ritonavir concentrations. The appropriate doses for this combination, with respect to saftey and efficacy, have not been established. Preliminary clinical data suggest that the incidence of nephrolithiasis is higher in patients receiving indinavir in combination with ritonavir than those receiving indinavir 800 mg q8h). Products include:

Saquinavir (Co-administration of indinavir and saquinavir may lead to increased saquinavir concentrations).
No products indexed under this heading.

Saquinavir Mesylate (Co-administration of indinavir and saquinavir may lead to increased saquinavir concentrations). Products include:

Sertraline Hydrochloride (Co-administration of indinavir and drugs primarily metabolized by CYP3A4 may result in increased plasma concentrations of the other drug, which could increase or prolong its therapeutic and adverse effects).
Products include:

Sildenafil Citrate (Co-administration has resulted in increased sildenafil AUC by 340%; this may result in an increase in sildenafil-associated adverse events, including hypotension, priapism, and visual changes; based on this result the dose of sildenafil should not exceed 25 mg in a 48-hour period).
Products include:

Simvastatin (The risk of myopathy including rhabdomyolysis may be increased when protease inhibitors, including indinavir, are used in combination with HMG-CoA inhibitors that are metabolized by the CYP3A4 pathway; concomitant use is not recommended). Products include:

Sirolimus (Co-administration of indinavir and sirolimus may lead to increased sirolimus concentrations). Products include:

Stavudine (Co-administration has resulted in a 25% ± 26% increase in stavudine AUC and no change in indinavir AUC; co-administration does not require dose modification).
No products indexed under this heading.

Sulfinpyrazone (Drugs that induce CYP3A4 activity would be expected to increase the clearance of indinavir, resulting in lowered plasma concentrations of indinavir).
No products indexed under this heading.

Tacrolimus (Co-administration of indinavir and tacrolimus may lead to increased tacrolimus concentrations). Products include:

Tadalafil (Co-administration of indinavir and tadalafil is expected to substantially increase plasma concentrations of tadalafil and may result in an increase in adverse events. Tadalafil dose should not exceed a maximum of 10 mg in a 72-hour period in patients receiving concomitant indinavir therapy). Products include:

Tamoxifen Citrate (Co-administration of indinavir and drugs primarily metabolized by CYP3A4 may result in increased plasma concentrations of the other drug, which could increase or prolong its therapeutic and adverse effects). Products include:

Telithromycin (Co-administration of indinavir and other drugs that inhibit CYP3A4 may decrease the clearance of indinavir and may result in increased plasma concentrations of indinavir). Products include:

Terfenadine (Inhibition of CYP3A4 by indinavir could result in elevated plasma concentrations of terfenadine potentially causing serious or life-threatening reactions; co-administration is contraindicated).
No products indexed under this heading.

Theophylline (Drugs that induce CYP3A4 activity would be expected to increase the clearance of indinavir, resulting in lowered plasma concentrations of indinavir).
No products indexed under this heading.

Tiagabine Hydrochloride (Co-administration of indinavir and drugs

primarily metabolized by CYP3A4 may result in increased plasma concentrations of the other drug, which could increase or prolong its therapeutic and adverse effects). Products include:
Gabitril Tablets 984

Tolterodine Tartrate (Co-administration of indinavir and drugs primarily metabolized by CYP3A4 may result in increased plasma concentrations of the other drug, which could increase or prolong its therapeutic and adverse effects). Products include:
Detrol Tablets 2628
Detrol LA Capsules 2631

Trazodone Hydrochloride (Concomitant use of trazodone hydrochloride and indinavir sulfate may increase plasma concentrations of trazodone. If trazodone is used with a CYP3A4 inhibitor such as indinavir sulfate, the combinatin should be used with caution and a lower dose of trazodone should be considered).
No products indexed under this heading.

Triamcinolone (Drugs that induce CYP3A4 activity would be expected to increase the clearance of indinavir, resulting in lowered plasma concentrations of indinavir).
No products indexed under this heading.

Triamcinolone Acetonide (Drugs that induce CYP3A4 activity would be expected to increase the clearance of indinavir, resulting in lowered plasma concentrations of indinavir). Products include:
Azmacort Inhalation Aerosol 1726
Nasacort AQ Nasal Spray 2922

Triamcinolone Diacetate (Drugs that induce CYP3A4 activity would be expected to increase the clearance of indinavir, resulting in lowered plasma concentrations of indinavir).
No products indexed under this heading.

Triamcinolone Hexacetonide (Drugs that induce CYP3A4 activity would be expected to increase the clearance of indinavir, resulting in lowered plasma concentrations of indinavir).
No products indexed under this heading.

Triazolam (Inhibition of CYP3A4 by indinavir could result in elevated plasma concentrations of triazolam potentially causing serious or life-threatening reactions; co-administration is contraindicated).
No products indexed under this heading.

Trimethoprim (Co-administration with trimethoprim/sulfamethoxazole tablets has resulted in a 19% ± 31% increase in trimethoprim AUC).
No products indexed under this heading.

Troglitazone (Drugs that induce CYP3A4 activity would be expected to increase the clearance of indinavir, resulting in lowered plasma concentrations of indinavir).
No products indexed under this heading.

Troleandomycin (Co-administration of indinavir and other drugs that inhibit CYP3A4 may decrease the clearance of indinavir and may result in increased plasma concentrations of indinavir).
No products indexed under this heading.

Valproate Sodium (Co-administration of indinavir and other drugs that inhibit CYP3A4 may decrease the clearance of indinavir and may result in increased plasma concentrations of indinavir). Products include:
Depacon Injection 412

Vardenafil Hydrochloride (Co-administration of indinavir and vardenafil is expected to substantially increase plasma concentrations of vardenafil and may result in an increase in adverse events. Vardenafil dose should not exceed a maximum of 2.5 mg in a 24-hour period in patient receiving concomitant indinavir therapy). Products include:
Levitra Tablets 3034

Venlafaxine Hydrochloride (In a study, venlafaxine administered under steady-state conditions at 150 mg/day resulted in a 28% decrease in the AUC of a single 800 mg oral dose of indinavir and a 36% decrease in indinavir Cmax. Indinavir did not affect the pharmacokinetics of venlafaxine). Products include:
Effexor Tablets 3411
Effexor XR Capsules 3417

Verapamil Hydrochloride (Co-administration of calcium channel blockers with indinavir may result in increased plasma concentrations of the dihydropyridine calcium channel blockers which could increase or prolong their therapeutic and adverse effects. Caution is warranted and clinical monitoring is recommended). Products include:
Covera-HS Tablets 3139
Tarka Tablets 524
Verelan PM Extended-Release Capsules, Controlled-Onset 3106

Vinblastine Sulfate (Co-administration of indinavir and drugs primarily metabolized by CYP3A4 may result in increased plasma concentrations of the other drug, which could increase or prolong its therapeutic and adverse effects).
No products indexed under this heading.

Vincristine Sulfate (Co-administration of indinavir and drugs primarily metabolized by CYP3A4 may result in increased plasma concentrations of the other drug, which could increase or prolong its therapeutic and adverse effects).
No products indexed under this heading.

Voriconazole (Co-administration of indinavir and other drugs that inhibit CYP3A4 may decrease the clearance of indinavir and may result in increased plasma concentrations of indinavir). Products include:
VFEND I.V. 2564
VFEND Oral Suspension 2564
VFEND Tablets 2564

Warfarin Sodium (Co-administration of indinavir and drugs primarily metabolized by CYP3A4 may result in increased plasma concentrations of the other drug, which could increase or prolong its therapeutic and adverse effects). Products include:
Coumadin for Injection 898
Coumadin Tablets 898

Zafirlukast (Co-administration of indinavir and other drugs that inhibit CYP3A4 may decrease the clearance of indinavir and may result in increased plasma concentrations of indinavir). Products include:
Accolate Tablets 671

Zidovudine (Co-administration has resulted in a 13% ± 48% increase in indinavir AUC and a 17% +/- 23% increase in zidovudine AUC; co-administration does not require dose modification). Products include:
Combivir Tablets 1411
Retrovir 1560
Retrovir IV Infusion 1564
Trizivir Tablets 1589

Zileuton (Co-administration of indinavir and other drugs that inhibit CYP3A4 may decrease the clearance of indinavir and may result in increased plasma concentrations of indinavir). Products include:
Zyflo Tablets 1023

Food Interactions

Food, unspecified (Co-administration with a meal high in calories, fat, and protein has resulted in a 77% ± 8% reduction in AUC and an 84% +/- 7% reduction in Cmax; administer without food 1 hour before or 2 hours after a meal).

Grapefruit (Co-administration of indinavir and other drugs that inhibit CYP3A4 may decrease the clearance of indinavir and may result in increased plasma concentrations of indinavir).

Grapefruit Juice (Potential for decrease in indinavir AUC).

CUBICIN FOR INJECTION

(Daptomycin) 1026

May interact with aminoglycosides, beta-lactams antibiotics, HMG-CoA reductase inhibitors, and certain other agents. Compounds in these categories include:

Amikacin Sulfate (In vitro synergistic interactions of daptomycin with aminoglycosides, beta-lactam antibiotics, and rifampin have been shown against some isolates of staphylococci and enterococci).
No products indexed under this heading.

Atorvastatin Calcium (Experience with co-administration of HMG-CoA reductase inhibitors and Cubicin is limited, therefore, considerations should be given to temporarily suspending use of HMG-CoA reductase inhibitors in patients recieving Cubicin). Products include:
Caduet Tablets 2508
Lipitor Tablets 2483

Aztreonam (In vitro synergistic interactions of daptomycin with aminoglycosides, beta-lactam antibiotics, and rifampin have been shown against some isolates of staphylococci and enterococci).
No products indexed under this heading.

Cefaclor (In vitro synergistic interactions of daptomycin with aminoglycosides, beta-lactam antibiotics, and rifampin have been shown against some isolates of staphylococci and enterococci).
No products indexed under this heading.

Cefadroxil (In vitro synergistic interactions of daptomycin with aminoglycosides, beta-lactam antibiotics, and rifampin have been shown against some isolates of staphylococci and enterococci).
No products indexed under this heading.

Cefamandole Nafate (In vitro synergistic interactions of daptomycin with aminoglycosides, beta-lactam antibiotics, and rifampin have been shown against some isolates of staphylococci and enterococci).
No products indexed under this heading.

Cefazolin Sodium (In vitro synergistic interactions of daptomycin with aminoglycosides, beta-lactam antibiotics, and rifampin have been shown against some isolates of staphylococci and enterococci).
No products indexed under this heading.

Cefixime (In vitro synergistic interactions of daptomycin with aminoglycosides, beta-lactam antibiotics, and rifampin have been shown against some isolates of staphylococci and enterococci). Products include:
Suprax 1843

Cefmetazole Sodium (In vitro synergistic interactions of daptomycin with aminoglycosides, beta-lactam antibiotics, and rifampin have been shown against some isolates of staphylococci and enterococci).
No products indexed under this heading.

Cefonicid Sodium (In vitro synergistic interactions of daptomycin with aminoglycosides, beta-lactam antibiotics, and rifampin have been shown against some isolates of staphylococci and enterococci).
No products indexed under this heading.

Cefoperazone Sodium (In vitro synergistic interactions of daptomycin with aminoglycosides, beta-lactam antibiotics, and rifampin have been shown against some isolates of staphylococci and enterococci).
No products indexed under this heading.

Ceforanide (In vitro synergistic interactions of daptomycin with aminoglycosides, beta-lactam antibiotics, and rifampin have been shown against some isolates of staphylococci and enterococci).
No products indexed under this heading.

Cefotaxime Sodium (In vitro synergistic interactions of daptomycin with aminoglycosides, beta-lactam antibiotics, and rifampin have been shown against some isolates of staphylococci and enterococci).
No products indexed under this heading.

Cefotetan (In vitro synergistic interactions of daptomycin with aminoglycosides, beta-lactam antibiotics, and rifampin have been shown against some isolates of staphylococci and enterococci).
No products indexed under this heading.

Cefoxitin Sodium (In vitro synergistic interactions of daptomycin with aminoglycosides, beta-lactam antibiotics, and rifampin have been shown against some isolates of staphylococci and enterococci). Products include:
Mefoxin for Injection 2012
Mefoxin Premixed Intravenous Solution 2016

Cefpodoxime Proxetil (In vitro synergistic interactions of daptomycin with aminoglycosides, beta-lactam antibiotics, and rifampin have been shown against some isolates of staphylococci and enterococci). Products include:

Vantin Tablets and Oral Suspension 2645

Cefprozil (In vitro synergistic interactions of daptomycin with aminoglycosides, beta-lactam antibiotics, and rifampin have been shown against some isolates of staphylococci and enterococci).

No products indexed under this heading.

Ceftazidime (In vitro synergistic interactions of daptomycin with aminoglycosides, beta-lactam antibiotics, and rifampin have been shown against some isolates of staphylococci and enterococci). Products include:

Fortaz 1453

Ceftizoxime Sodium (In vitro synergistic interactions of daptomycin with aminoglycosides, beta-lactam antibiotics, and rifampin have been shown against some isolates of staphylococci and enterococci).

No products indexed under this heading.

Ceftriaxone Sodium (In vitro synergistic interactions of daptomycin with aminoglycosides, beta-lactam antibiotics, and rifampin have been shown against some isolates of staphylococci and enterococci). Products include:

Rocephin Injectable Vials, ADD-Vantage, Galaxy, Bulk........ 2800

Cefuroxime Axetil (In vitro synergistic interactions of daptomycin with aminoglycosides, beta-lactam antibiotics, and rifampin have been shown against some isolates of staphylococci and enterococci). Products include:

Ceftin 1407

Cefuroxime Sodium (In vitro synergistic interactions of daptomycin with aminoglycosides, beta-lactam antibiotics, and rifampin have been shown against some isolates of staphylococci and enterococci).

No products indexed under this heading.

Cephalexin (In vitro synergistic interactions of daptomycin with aminoglycosides, beta-lactam antibiotics, and rifampin have been shown against some isolates of staphylococci and enterococci). Products include:

Keflex Capsules 549

Cephalothin Sodium (In vitro synergistic interactions of daptomycin with aminoglycosides, beta-lactam antibiotics, and rifampin have been shown against some isolates of staphylococci and enterococci).

No products indexed under this heading.

Cephapirin Sodium (In vitro synergistic interactions of daptomycin with aminoglycosides, beta-lactam antibiotics, and rifampin have been shown against some isolates of staphylococci and enterococci).

No products indexed under this heading.

Cephradine (In vitro synergistic interactions of daptomycin with aminoglycosides, beta-lactam antibiotics, and rifampin have been shown against some isolates of staphylococci and enterococci).

No products indexed under this heading.

Cerivastatin Sodium (Experience with co-administration of HMG-CoA reductase inhibitors and Cubicin is limited, therefore, considerations should be given to temporarily suspending use of HMG-CoA reductase inhibitors in patients recieving Cubicin).

No products indexed under this heading.

Cilastatin Sodium (In vitro synergistic interactions of daptomycin with aminoglycosides, beta-lactam antibiotics, and rifampin have been shown against some isolates of staphylococci and enterococci). Products include:

Primaxin I.M. 2045
Primaxin I.V. 2048

Fluvastatin Sodium (Experience with co-administration of HMG-CoA reductase inhibitors and Cubicin is limited, therefore, considerations should be given to temporarily suspending use of HMG-CoA reductase inhibitors in patients recieving Cubicin). Products include:

Lescol Capsules 2233
Lescol XL Tablets 2233

Gentamicin Sulfate (In vitro synergistic interactions of daptomycin with aminoglycosides, beta-lactam antibiotics, and rifampin have been shown against some isolates of staphylococci and enterococci). Products include:

Garamycin Injectable 3014
Pred-G Ophthalmic Ointment .... ⊙237
Pred-G Ophthalmic Suspension .... ⊙236

Imipenem (In vitro synergistic interactions of daptomycin with aminoglycosides, beta-lactam antibiotics, and rifampin have been shown against some isolates of staphylococci and enterococci). Products include:

Primaxin I.M. 2045
Primaxin I.V. 2048

Kanamycin Sulfate (In vitro synergistic interactions of daptomycin with aminoglycosides, beta-lactam antibiotics, and rifampin have been shown against some isolates of staphylococci and enterococci).

No products indexed under this heading.

Loracarbef (In vitro synergistic interactions of daptomycin with aminoglycosides, beta-lactam antibiotics, and rifampin have been shown against some isolates of staphylococci and enterococci).

No products indexed under this heading.

Lovastatin (Experience with co-administration of HMG-CoA reductase inhibitors and Cubicin is limited, therefore, considerations should be given to temporarily suspending use of HMG-CoA reductase inhibitors in patients recieving Cubicin). Products include:

Advicor Tablets 1722
Altoprev Extended-Release Tablets 3109
Mevacor Tablets 2021

Pravastatin Sodium (Experience with co-administration of HMG-CoA reductase inhibitors and Cubicin is limited, therefore, considerations should be given to temporarily suspending use of HMG-CoA reductase inhibitors in patients recieving Cubicin).

No products indexed under this heading.

Rifampin (In vitro synergistic interactions of daptomycin with aminoglycosides, beta-lactam antibiotics, and rifampin have been shown against some isolates of staphylococci and enterococci).

No products indexed under this heading.

Simvastatin (Experience with co-administration of HMG-CoA reductase inhibitors and Cubicin is limited, therefore, considerations should be given to temporarily suspending use of HMG-CoA reductase inhibitors in patients recieving Cubicin). Products include:

Vytorin 10/10 Tablets 2114
Vytorin 10/10 Tablets 3077
Vytorin 10/20 Tablets 2114
Vytorin 10/20 Tablets 3077
Vytorin 10/40 Tablets 2114
Vytorin 10/40 Tablets 3077
Vytorin 10/80 Tablets 2114
Vytorin 10/80 Tablets 3077
Zocor Tablets 2105

Streptomycin Sulfate (In vitro synergistic interactions of daptomycin with aminoglycosides, beta-lactam antibiotics, and rifampin have been shown against some isolates of staphylococci and enterococci).

No products indexed under this heading.

Tobramycin (In vitro synergistic interactions of daptomycin with aminoglycosides, beta-lactam antibiotics, and rifampin have been shown against some isolates of staphylococci and enterococci). Products include:

TOBI Solution for Inhalation 2298
TobraDex Ophthalmic Ointment 562
TobraDex Ophthalmic Suspension ... 563
Zylet Ophthalmic Suspension .... ⊙259

Tobramycin Sulfate (Mean Cmax and AUC 0-8 of daptomycin increased when administered with tobramycin, and the mean Cmax and AUC 0-8 of tobramycin decreased when administered with daptomycin. Therefore, caution is warranted when daptomycin is co-administered with tobramycin).

No products indexed under this heading.

CUPRIMINE CAPSULES

(Penicillamine) 1947

May interact with antacids, antimalarials, cytotoxic drugs, iron containing oral preparations, and certain other agents. Compounds in these categories include:

Aluminum Carbonate (Antacids reduce the absorption of penicillamine. In all patients receiving penicillamine, it is important that penicillamine be given at least one hour apart from any antacid. This permits maximum strength absorption and reduces the likelihood of inactivation by metal binding in the gastrointestinal tract).

No products indexed under this heading.

Aluminum Hydroxide (Antacids reduce the absorption of penicillamine. In all patients receiving penicillamine, it is important that penicillamine be given at least one hour apart from any antacid. This permits maximum strength absorption and reduces the likelihood of inactivation by metal binding in the gastrointestinal tract). Products include:

Gaviscon Regular Strength Liquid .. ▣658
Gaviscon Regular Strength Tablets .... ▣658
Gaviscon Extra Strength Liquid .... ▣658
Gaviscon Extra Strength Tablets .... ▣658
Maalox Regular Strength Antacid/Antigas Liquid 2175
Maalox Max Maximum Strength Antacid/Anti-Gas Liquid 2176

Auranofin (Concurrent use not recommended).

No products indexed under this heading.

Aurothioglucose (Concurrent use not recommended).

No products indexed under this heading.

Bleomycin Sulfate (Concurrent use not recommended).

No products indexed under this heading.

Chloroquine Hydrochloride (Concurrent use not recommended).

No products indexed under this heading.

Chloroquine Phosphate (Concurrent use not recommended).

No products indexed under this heading.

Cyclophosphamide (Concurrent use not recommended).

No products indexed under this heading.

Daunorubicin Hydrochloride (Concurrent use not recommended).

No products indexed under this heading.

Doxorubicin Hydrochloride (Concurrent use not recommended).

No products indexed under this heading.

Epirubicin Hydrochloride (Concurrent use not recommended).

No products indexed under this heading.

Ferrous Fumarate (In all patients receiving penicillamine, it is important that penicillamine be given at least one hour apart from any iron-containing preparation. This permits maximum abορtion and reduces the likelihood of inactivation by metal binding in the gastrointestinal tract).

No products indexed under this heading.

Ferrous Gluconate (In all patients receiving penicillamine, it is important that penicillamine be given at least one hour apart from any iron-containing preparation. This permits maximum aborption and reduces the likelihood of inactivation by metal binding in the gastrointestinal tract).

No products indexed under this heading.

Ferrous Sulfate (In all patients receiving penicillamine, it is important that penicillamine be given at least one hour apart from any iron-containing preparation. This permits maximum aborption and reduces the likelihood of inactivation by metal binding in the gastrointestinal tract). Products include:

Slow Fe Iron Tablets .... ▣818
Slow Fe with Folic Acid Tablets .... ▣819

Fluorouracil (Concurrent use not recommended). Products include:

Carac Cream, 0.5% 2879
Efudex 3363

Hydroxychloroquine Sulfate (Concurrent use not recommended).

No products indexed under this heading.

Hydroxyurea (Concurrent use not recommended).

No products indexed under this heading.

Iron (In all patients receiving penicillamine, it is important that penicillamine be given at least one hour apart from any iron-containing preparation. This permits maximum aborption and reduces the likelihood of inactivation by metal binding in the gastrointestinal tract).
No products indexed under this heading.

Magaldrate (Antacids reduce the absorption of penicillamine. In all patients receiving penicillamine, it is important that penicillamine be given at least one hour apart from any antacid. This permits maximum strength absorption and reduces the likelihood of inactivation by metal binding in the gastrointestinal tract).
No products indexed under this heading.

Magnesium Hydroxide (Antacids reduce the absorption of penicillamine. In all patients receiving penicillamine, it is important that penicillamine be given at least one hour apart from any antacid. This permits maximum strength absorption and reduces the likelihood of inactivation by metal binding in the gastrointestinal tract). Products include:
Maalox Regular Strength Antacid/Antigas Liquid.................. 2175
Maalox Max Maximum Strength Antacid/Anti-Gas Liquid................ 2176
Pepcid Complete Chewable Tablets.. 1701

Magnesium Oxide (Antacids reduce the absorption of penicillamine. In all patients receiving penicillamine, it is important that penicillamine be given at least one hour apart from any antacid. This permits maximum strength absorption and reduces the likelihood of inactivation by metal binding in the gastrointestinal tract). Products include:
Beelith Tablets.................................. 759
PremCal Light, Regular, and Extra Strength Tablets................ 818

Mefloquine Hydrochloride (Concurrent use not recommended). Products include:
Lariam Tablets 2786

Methotrexate Sodium (Concurrent use not recommended).
No products indexed under this heading.

Mineral Supplements (Block response).
No products indexed under this heading.

Mitotane (Concurrent use not recommended).
No products indexed under this heading.

Mitoxantrone Hydrochloride (Concurrent use not recommended).
No products indexed under this heading.

Oxyphenbutazone (Concurrent use not recommended).
No products indexed under this heading.

Phenylbutazone (Concurrent use not recommended).
No products indexed under this heading.

Polysaccharide Iron Complex (In all patients receiving penicillamine, it is important that penicillamine be given at least one hour apart from any iron-containing preparation. This permits maximum aborption and reduces the likelihood of inactivation by metal binding in the gastrointestinal tract). Products include:
Nu-Iron 150 Capsules 2127

Procarbazine Hydrochloride (Concurrent use not recommended). Products include:
Matulane Capsules 3191

Pyridoxine (Penicillamine increases pyridoxine requirement).
No products indexed under this heading.

Pyrimethamine (Concurrent use not recommended). Products include:
Daraprim Tablets 1419
Fansidar Tablets 2765

Sodium Bicarbonate (Antacids reduce the absorption of penicillamine. In all patients receiving penicillamine, it is important that penicillamine be given at least one hour apart from any antacid. This permits maximum strength absorption and reduces the likelihood of inactivation by metal binding in the gastrointestinal tract). Products include:
Colyte with Flavor Packs for Oral Solution....................................... 3088
HalfLytely and Bisacodyl Tablets Bowel Prep Kit with Flavors Packs... 881
TriLyte with Flavor Packs for Oral Solution....................................... 3100

Tamoxifen Citrate (Concurrent use not recommended). Products include:
Soltamox Oral Solution 3527

Vincristine Sulfate (Concurrent use not recommended).
No products indexed under this heading.

Zinc-Containing Multivitamins (In all patients receiving penicillamine, it is important that penicillamine be given at least one hour apart from any iron-containing preparation. This permits maximim absorption and reduces the likelihood of inactivation by metal binding in the gastrointestinal tract).
No products indexed under this heading.

Zinc Gluconate (In all patients receiving penicillamine, it is important that penicillamine be given at least one hour apart from any iron-containing preparation. This permits maximim absorption and reduces the likelihood of inactivation by metal binding in the gastrointestinal tract).
No products indexed under this heading.

Zinc Sulfate (In all patients receiving penicillamine, it is important that penicillamine be given at least one hour apart from any iron-containing preparation. This permits maximim absorption and reduces the likelihood of inactivation by metal binding in the gastrointestinal tract). Products include:
Visine A.C. Seasonal Itching and Redness Relief Drops................. ⊙289
Zinc-220 Capsules 580

Food Interactions

Dairy products (In all patients receiving penicillamine, it is important that penicillamine be given at least one hour apart from milk. This permits maximim absorption and reduces the likelihood of inactivation by metal binding in the gastrointestinal tract).

Food, unspecified (Food reduces the absorption of penicillamine. In all patients receiving penicillamine, it is important that penicillamine be given on an empty stomach, at least one hour before meals or two hours after meals. This permits maximum absorption and reduces the likelihood of inactivation by metal binding in the gastrointestinal tract).

CUROSURF INTRATRACHEAL SUSPENSION

(Poractant alfa) 1057
None cited in PDR database.

CUTIVATE CREAM

(Fluticasone Propionate) 2662
None cited in PDR database.

CUTIVATE LOTION 0.05%

(Fluticasone Propionate) 2664
None cited in PDR database.

CUTIVATE OINTMENT

(Fluticasone Propionate) 2665
None cited in PDR database.

CYMBALTA DELAYED-RELEASE CAPSULES

(Duloxetine Hydrochloride) 1757
May interact with central nervous system depressants, central nervous system stimulants, cytochrome p450 1a2 inhibitors (selected), cytochrome p450 2d6 inhibitors (selected), cytochrome p450 2d6 substrates (selected), drugs that reduce gastric acidity, monoamine oxidase inhibitors, phenothiazines, quinolones, serotoninergic agents, tricyclic antidepressants, triptans, and certain other agents. Compounds in these categories include:

Alatrofloxacin Mesylate (Concomitant use of duloxetine with fluvoxamine, an inhibitor of CYP1A2, results in a 6-fold increase in AUC, about 2.5-fold increase in Cmax, and an approximately 3-fold increase in t1/2 of duloxetine. Since duloxetine is metabolized in part by CYP1A2, concomitant use of duloxetine with other inhibitors of CYP1A2, would be expected to have the same effects; these combinations should be avoided).
No products indexed under this heading.

Alfentanil Hydrochloride (Given the primary CNS effects of duloxetine, it should be used with caution when it is taken in combination with or substituted for other centrally acting drugs, including those with a similar mechanism of action).
No products indexed under this heading.

Almotriptan Malate (Development of a potentially life-threatening serotonin syndrome may occur with concomitant use of duloxetine HCl and triptans. If concomitant treatment is clinically warranted, careful observation of the patient is advised, particularly during treatment initiation and dose increases). Products include:
Axert Tablets 2396

Alprazolam (Given the primary CNS effects of duloxetine, it should be used with caution when it is taken in combination with or substituted for other centrally acting drugs, including those with a similar mechanism of action). Products include:
Niravam Orally Disintegrating Tablets....................................... 3092

Aluminum Carbonate (Duloxetine has an enteric coating that resists dissolution until reaching a segment of the gastrointestinal tract where the pH exceeds 5.5. Drugs that raise the gastrointestinal pH may lead to an earlier release of duloxetine).
No products indexed under this heading.

Aluminum Hydroxide (Duloxetine has an enteric coating that resists dissolution until reaching a segment of the gastrointestinal tract where the pH exceeds 5.5. Drugs that raise the gastrointestinal pH may lead to an earlier release of duloxetine). Products include:
Gaviscon Regular Strength Liquid .. 658
Gaviscon Regular Strength Tablets.. 658
Gaviscon Extra Strength Liquid 658
Gaviscon Extra Strength Tablets 658
Maalox Regular Strength Antacid/Antigas Liquid................. 2175
Maalox Max Maximum Strength Antacid/Anti-Gas Liquid................. 2176

Amiodarone Hydrochloride (Concomitant use of duloxetine with fluvoxamine, an inhibitor of CYP1A2, results in a 6-fold increase in AUC, about 2.5-fold increase in Cmax, and an approximately 3-fold increase in t1/2 of duloxetine. Since duloxetine is metabolized in part by CYP1A2, concomitant use of duloxetine with other inhibitors of CYP1A2, would be expected to have the same effects; these combinations should be avoided).
No products indexed under this heading.

Amitriptyline Hydrochloride (Duloxetine is a moderate inhibitor of CYP2D6. Co-administration of duloxetine with other drugs that are extensively metabolized by this isoenzyme, and which have a narrow therapeutic window, should be approached with caution. Plasma tricyclic antidepressant (TCA) concentrations may need to be monitored, and the dose of the TCA may need to be reduced, if a TCA is co-administered with duloxetine).
No products indexed under this heading.

Amoxapine (Duloxetine is a moderate inhibitor of CYP2D6. Co-administration of duloxetine with other drugs that are extensively metabolized by this isoenzyme, and which have a narrow therapeutic window, should be approached with caution. Plasma tricyclic antidepressant (TCA) concentrations may need to be monitored, and the dose of the TCA may need to be reduced, if a TCA is co-administered with duloxetine).
No products indexed under this heading.

Amphetamine Aspartate (Duloxetine is a moderate inhibitor of CYP2D6. Co-administration of duloxetine with other drugs that are extensively metabolized by this isoenzyme, and which have a narrow therapeutic window, should be approached with caution). Products include:
Adderall Tablets 3164
Adderall XR Capsules 3166

Amphetamine Aspartate Monohydrate (Duloxetine is a moderate inhibitor of CYP2D6. Co-administration of duloxetine with other drugs that are extensively metabolized by this isoenzyme, and which have a narrow therapeutic window, should be approached with caution).
No products indexed under this heading.

Amphetamine Resins (Given the primary CNS effects of duloxetine, it should be used with caution when it is taken in combination with or substituted for other centrally acting drugs, including those with a similar mechanism of action).
No products indexed under this heading.

Amphetamine Sulfate (Duloxetine is a moderate inhibitor of CYP2D6. Co-administration of duloxetine with other drugs that are extensively metabolized by this isoenzyme, and which have a narrow therapeutic window, should be approached with caution). Products include:
Adderall Tablets 3164
Adderall XR Capsules 3166

Anastrozole (Concomitant use of duloxetine with fluvoxamine, an inhibitor of CYP1A2, results in a 6-fold increase in AUC, about 2.5-fold increase in Cmax, and an approximately 3-fold increase in t1/2 of duloxetine. Since duloxetine is metabolized in part by CYP1A2, concomitant use of duloxetine with other inhibitors of CYP1A2, would be expected to have the same effects; these combinations should be avoided). Products include:
Arimidex Tablets 673

Aprobarbital (Given the primary CNS effects of duloxetine, it should be used with caution when it is taken in combination with or substituted for other centrally acting drugs, including those with a similar mechanism of action).
No products indexed under this heading.

Atomoxetine Hydrochloride (Duloxetine is a moderate inhibitor of CYP2D6. Co-administration of duloxetine with other drugs that are extensively metabolized by this isoenzyme, and which have a narrow therapeutic window, should be approached with caution). Products include:
Strattera Capsules 1814

Bisoprolol Fumarate (Duloxetine is a moderate inhibitor of CYP2D6. Co-administration of duloxetine with other drugs that are extensively metabolized by this isoenzyme, and which have a narrow therapeutic window, should be approached with caution).
No products indexed under this heading.

Buprenorphine Hydrochloride (Given the primary CNS effects of duloxetine, it should be used with caution when it is taken in combination with or substituted for other centrally acting drugs, including those with a similar mechanism of action). Products include:
Buprenex Injectable 2716
Suboxone Tablets 2717
Subutex Tablets 2717

Bupropion Hydrochloride (Because CYP2D6 is involved in duloxetine metabolism, concomitant use of duloxetine with potent inhibitors of CYP2D6 would be expected to, and does, result in higher concentrations of duloxetine). Products include:
Wellbutrin Tablets 1603
Wellbutrin SR Sustained-Release Tablets 1607
Wellbutrin XL Extended-Release Tablets 1613
Zyban Sustained-Release Tablets 1644

Buspirone Hydrochloride (Given the primary CNS effects of duloxetine, it should be used with caution when it is taken in combination with or substituted for other centrally acting drugs, including those with a similar mechanism of action).
No products indexed under this heading.

Butabarbital (Given the primary CNS effects of duloxetine, it should be used with caution when it is taken in combination with or substituted for other centrally acting drugs, including those with a similar mechanism of action).
No products indexed under this heading.

Butalbital (Given the primary CNS effects of duloxetine, it should be used with caution when it is taken in combination with or substituted for other centrally acting drugs, including those with a similar mechanism of action).
No products indexed under this heading.

Captopril (Duloxetine is a moderate inhibitor of CYP2D6. Co-administration of duloxetine with other drugs that are extensively metabolized by this isoenzyme, and which have a narrow therapeutic window, should be approached with caution). Products include:
Captopril Tablets 2149

Carvedilol (Duloxetine is a moderate inhibitor of CYP2D6. Co-administration of duloxetine with other drugs that are extensively metabolized by this isoenzyme, and which have a narrow therapeutic window, should be approached with caution). Products include:
Coreg Tablets 1414

Celecoxib (Because CYP2D6 is involved in duloxetine metabolism, concomitant use of duloxetine with potent inhibitors of CYP2D6 would be expected to, and does, result in higher concentrations of duloxetine). Products include:
Celebrex Capsules 3134

Cevimeline Hydrochloride (Duloxetine is a moderate inhibitor of CYP2D6. Co-administration of duloxetine with other drugs that are extensively metabolized by this isoenzyme, and which have a narrow therapeutic window, should be approached with caution). Products include:
Evoxac Capsules 1047

Chlordiazepoxide (Given the primary CNS effects of duloxetine, it should be used with caution when it is taken in combination with or substituted for other centrally acting drugs, including those with a similar mechanism of action).
No products indexed under this heading.

Chlordiazepoxide Hydrochloride (Given the primary CNS effects of duloxetine, it should be used with caution when it is taken in combination with or substituted for other centrally acting drugs, including those with a similar mechanism of action). Products include:
Librium Capsules 3347

Chloroquine Hydrochloride (Because CYP2D6 is involved in duloxetine metabolism, concomitant use of duloxetine with potent inhibitors of CYP2D6 would be expected to, and does, result in higher concentrations of duloxetine).
No products indexed under this heading.

Chloroquine Phosphate (Because CYP2D6 is involved in duloxetine metabolism, concomitant use of duloxetine with potent inhibitors of CYP2D6 would be expected to, and does, result in higher concentrations of duloxetine).
No products indexed under this heading.

Chlorpheniramine (Because CYP2D6 is involved in duloxetine metabolism, concomitant use of duloxetine with potent inhibitors of CYP2D6 would be expected to, and does, result in higher concentrations of duloxetine).
No products indexed under this heading.

Chlorpheniramine Maleate (Because CYP2D6 is involved in duloxetine metabolism, concomitant use of duloxetine with potent inhibitors of CYP2D6 would be expected to, and does, result in higher concentrations of duloxetine). Products include:
Advil Allergy Sinus Caplets .... ▣ 770
Advil Multi-Symptom Cold Caplets .... ▣ 770
BC Allergy Sinus Cold Powder .... ▣ 677
Comtrex Maximum Strength Cold & Cough Day/Night Caplets - Night Formulation .... ▣ 726
Comtrex Maximum Strength Day/Night Severe Cold & Sinus Caplets - Night Formulation .... ▣ 725
Contac Cold and Flu Maximum Strength Caplets .... ▣ 728
Contac Cold and Flu Day and Night Caplets (Night Formulation Only) .... ▣ 727
Children's Dimetapp Long Acting Cough Plus Cold Syrup .... ▣ 731
Robitussin Cough & Cold Long-Acting Liquid .... ▣ 735
Robitussin Cough & Allergy Syrup .. ▣ 736
Robitussin Cough & Cold Nighttime Liquid .... ▣ 736
Robitussin Cough, Cold & Flu Nighttime Liquid .... ▣ 738
Robitussin Pediatric Cough & Cold Long-Acting Liquid .... ▣ 735
Robitussin Pediatric Cough & Cold Nighttime Liquid .... ▣ 736
Triaminic Cold & Allergy Liquid .... ▣ 746
Triaminic Cough & Runny Nose Softchews .... ▣ 748
Children's Tylenol Plus Flu Oral Suspension .... ▣ 749
Tylenol Allergy Multi-Symptom Caplets with Cool Burst and Gelcaps 1872
Children's Tylenol Plus Cold Suspension Liquid 1879
Children's Tylenol Plus Cough & Runny Nose Suspension Liquid 1879
Children's Tylenol Plus Flu Suspension Liquid 1881
Children's Tylenol Plus Multi-Symptom Cold Suspension Liquid 1879
Tylenol Cold Head Congestion Nighttime Caplets with Cool Burst 1873
Tylenol Cold Multi-Symptom Nighttime Caplets with Cool Burst 1874
Tylenol Sinus Congestion & Pain Nighttime Caplets with Cool Burst 1876
Vicks 44M Cough, Cold & Flu Relief Liquid 2680
Pediatric Vicks 44m Cough & Cold Relief Liquid 2676
Children's Vicks NyQuil Cold/Cough Relief .... ▣ 756
Children's Vicks NyQuil Cold/Cough Relief Liquid 2680
Zicam Maximum Strength Flu Daytime .... ▣ 768

Chlorpheniramine Polistirex (Because CYP2D6 is involved in duloxetine metabolism, concomitant use of duloxetine with potent inhibitors of CYP2D6 would be expected to, and does, result in higher concentrations of duloxetine). Products include:
Tussionex Pennkinetic Extended-Release Suspension 3327

Chlorpheniramine Tannate (Because CYP2D6 is involved in duloxetine metabolism, concomitant use of duloxetine with potent inhibitors of CYP2D6 would be expected to, and does, result in higher concentrations of duloxetine).
No products indexed under this heading.

Chlorpromazine (Duloxetine is a moderate inhibitor of CYP2D6. Co-administration of duloxetine with other drugs that are extensively metabolized by this isoenzyme, and which have a narrow therapeutic window, should be approached with caution).
No products indexed under this heading.

Chlorpromazine Hydrochloride (Duloxetine is a moderate inhibitor of CYP2D6. Co-administration of duloxetine with other drugs that are extensively metabolized by this isoenzyme, and which have a narrow therapeutic window, should be approached with caution).
No products indexed under this heading.

Chlorpropamide (Duloxetine is a moderate inhibitor of CYP2D6. Co-administration of duloxetine with other drugs that are extensively metabolized by this isoenzyme, and which have a narrow therapeutic window, should be approached with caution).
No products indexed under this heading.

Chlorprothixene (Given the primary CNS effects of duloxetine, it should be used with caution when it is taken in combination with or substituted for other centrally acting drugs, including those with a similar mechanism of action).
No products indexed under this heading.

Chlorprothixene Hydrochloride (Given the primary CNS effects of duloxetine, it should be used with caution when it is taken in combination with or substituted for other centrally acting drugs, including those with a similar mechanism of action).
No products indexed under this heading.

Chlorprothixene Lactate (Given the primary CNS effects of duloxetine, it should be used with caution when it is taken in combination with or substituted for other centrally acting drugs, including those with a similar mechanism of action).
No products indexed under this heading.

Cimetidine (Duloxetine has an enteric coating that resists dissolution until reaching a segment of the gastrointestinal tract where the pH exceeds 5.5. Drugs that raise the gastrointestinal pH may lead to an earlier release of duloxetine). Products include:

Tagamet HB 200 Tablets 664

Cimetidine Hydrochloride (Duloxetine has an enteric coating that resists dissolution until reaching a segment of the gastrointestinal tract where the pH exceeds 5.5. Drugs that raise the gastrointestinal pH may lead to an earlier release of duloxetine).

No products indexed under this heading.

Ciprofloxacin (Concomitant use of duloxetine with fluvoxamine, an inhibitor of CYP1A2, results in a 6-fold increase in AUC, about 2.5-fold increase in Cmax, and an approximately 3-fold increase in t1/2 of duloxetine. Since duloxetine is metabolized in part by CYP1A2, concomitant use of duloxetine with other inhibitors of CYP1A2, would be expected to have the same effects; these combinations should be avoided). Products include:

Cipro Oral Suspension 2977
Cipro I.V. 2984
Cipro XR Tablets 2990
Ciprodex Otic Suspension 559

Ciprofloxacin Hydrochloride (Concomitant use of duloxetine with fluvoxamine, an inhibitor of CYP1A2, results in a 6-fold increase in AUC, about 2.5-fold increase in Cmax, and an approximately 3-fold increase in t1/2 of duloxetine. Since duloxetine is metabolized in part by CYP1A2, concomitant use of duloxetine with other inhibitors of CYP1A2, would be expected to have the same effects; these combinations should be avoided). Products include:

Ciloxan Ophthalmic Ointment 559
Ciloxan Ophthalmic Solution .... ⊙206
Cipro Tablets 2977
Proquin XR Tablets 1153

Citalopram Hydrobromide (Development of a potentially life-threatening serotonin syndrome may occur with concomitant use of duloxetine HCl and serotonergic drugs). Products include:

Celexa 1176

Clarithromycin (Concomitant use of duloxetine with fluvoxamine, an inhibitor of CYP1A2, results in a 6-fold increase in AUC, about 2.5-fold increase in Cmax, and an approximately 3-fold increase in t1/2 of duloxetine. Since duloxetine is metabolized in part by CYP1A2, concomitant use of duloxetine with other inhibitors of CYP1A2, would be expected to have the same effects; these combinations should be avoided). Products include:

Biaxin/Biaxin XL 402
PREVPAC 3284

Clomipramine Hydrochloride (Duloxetine is a moderate inhibitor of CYP2D6. Co-administration of duloxetine with other drugs that are extensively metabolized by this isoenzyme, and which have a narrow therapeutic window, should be approached with caution. Plasma tricyclic antidepressant (TCA) concentrations may need to be monitored, and the dose of the TCA may need to be reduced, if a TCA is co-administered with duloxetine).

No products indexed under this heading.

Clorazepate Dipotassium (Given the primary CNS effects of duloxetine, it should be used with caution when it is taken in combination with or substituted for other centrally acting drugs, including those with a similar mechanism of action). Products include:

Tranxene 2474

Clozapine (Duloxetine is a moderate inhibitor of CYP2D6. Co-administration of duloxetine with other drugs that are extensively metabolized by this isoenzyme, and which have a narrow therapeutic window, should be approached with caution). Products include:

Clozaril Tablets 2184
FazaClo Orally Disintegrating Tablets 551

Cocaine Hydrochloride (Because CYP2D6 is involved in duloxetine metabolism, concomitant use of duloxetine with potent inhibitors of CYP2D6 would be expected to, and does, result in higher concentrations of duloxetine).

No products indexed under this heading.

Codeine Phosphate (Duloxetine is a moderate inhibitor of CYP2D6. Co-administration of duloxetine with other drugs that are extensively metabolized by this isoenzyme, and which have a narrow therapeutic window, should be approached with caution). Products include:

Tylenol with Codeine Tablets 2391

Codeine Sulfate (Duloxetine is a moderate inhibitor of CYP2D6. Co-administration of duloxetine with other drugs that are extensively metabolized by this isoenzyme, and which have a narrow therapeutic window, should be approached with caution).

No products indexed under this heading.

Cyclobenzaprine Hydrochloride (Duloxetine is a moderate inhibitor of CYP2D6. Co-administration of duloxetine with other drugs that are extensively metabolized by this isoenzyme, and which have a narrow therapeutic window, should be approached with caution).

No products indexed under this heading.

Desflurane (Given the primary CNS effects of duloxetine, it should be used with caution when it is taken in combination with or substituted for other centrally acting drugs, including those with a similar mechanism of action).

No products indexed under this heading.

Desipramine Hydrochloride (Duloxetine is a moderate inhibitor of CYP2D6. Co-administration of duloxetine with other drugs that are extensively metabolized by this isoenzyme, and which have a narrow therapeutic window, should be approached with caution. Plasma tricyclic antidepressant (TCA) concentrations may need to be monitored, and the dose of the TCA may need to be reduced, if a TCA is co-administered with duloxetine).

No products indexed under this heading.

Desogestrel (Concomitant use of duloxetine with fluvoxamine, an inhibitor of CYP1A2, results in a 6-fold increase in AUC, about 2.5-fold increase in Cmax, and an approximately 3-fold increase in t1/2 of duloxetine. Since duloxetine is metabolized in part by CYP1A2, concomitant use of duloxetine with other inhibitors of CYP1A2, would be expected to have the same effects; these combinations should be avoided). Products include:

Mircette Tablets 1066

Dexfenfluramine Hydrochloride (Duloxetine is a moderate inhibitor of CYP2D6. Co-administration of duloxetine with other drugs that are extensively metabolized by this isoenzyme, and which have a narrow therapeutic window, should be approached with caution).

No products indexed under this heading.

Dextroamphetamine Sulfate (Given the primary CNS effects of duloxetine, it should be used with caution when it is taken in combination with or substituted for other centrally acting drugs, including those with a similar mechanism of action). Products include:

Adderall Tablets 3164
Adderall XR Capsules 3166
Dexedrine 1420
DextroStat Tablets 3179

Dextromethorphan Hydrobromide (Duloxetine is a moderate inhibitor of CYP2D6. Co-administration of duloxetine with other drugs that are extensively metabolized by this isoenzyme, and which have a narrow therapeutic window, should be approached with caution). Products include:

Comtrex Maximum Strength Cold & Cough Day/Night Caplets - Day Formulation 726
Comtrex Maximum Strength Cold & Cough Day/Night Caplets - Night Formulation 726
Comtrex Maximum Strength Non-Drowsy Cold & Cough Caplets 725
Children's Dimetapp DM Cold & Cough Elixir 731
Children's Dimetapp Long Acting Cough Plus Cold Syrup.............. 731
Toddler's Dimetapp Cold and Cough Drops 732
Mucinex DM Extended-Release Bi-Layer Tablets 720
Refenesen DM Caplets 721
Robitussin Cough & Cold CF Liquid 735
Robitussin Cough & Cold Long-Acting Liquid 735
Robitussin Cough & Allergy Syrup .. 736
Robitussin Cough & Cold Nighttime Liquid.......................... 736
Robitussin Cough & Cold Pediatric Drops............................. 735
Robitussin Cough, Cold & Flu Nighttime Liquid.......................... 738
Robitussin Cough & Congestion Liquid 738
Robitussin Cough Gels Long-Acting 737
Robitussin Cough Long Acting Liquid 739
Robitussin Cough DM Syrup 738
Robitussin Cough DM Infant Drops 738
Robitussin Pediatric Cough Long Acting Liquid 739
Robitussin Pediatric Cough & Cold Long-Acting Liquid.............. 735
Robitussin Pediatric Cough & Cold Nighttime Liquid................. 736
Robitussin Sugar Free Cough 738
TheraFlu Cold & Cough Hot Liquid 740
TheraFlu Warming Relief Daytime Severe Cold................................ 743
TheraFlu Thin Strips Long Acting Cough.. 744
Triaminic Daytime Cold & Cough Liquid 745
Triaminic Cough & Sore Throat Liquid 747
Triaminic Cough & Runny Nose Softchews 748
Triaminic Thin Strips Cold & Cough.. 778
Triaminic Infant Thin Strips Decongestant Plus Cough........... 747
Children's Tylenol Plus Flu Oral Suspension.................................... 749
Tylenol Cold Head Congestion Daytime Caplets with Cool Burst and Gelcaps 750
Tylenol Cold Multi-Symptom Daytime Liquid 752
Tylenol Cold Multi-Symptom Severe Daytime Liquid 752
Concentrated Tylenol Infants' Drops Plus Cold & Cough.......... 754
Children's Tylenol Plus Cough & Runny Nose Suspension Liquid..... 1879
Children's Tylenol Plus Cough & Sore Throat Suspension Liquid..... 1879
Children's Tylenol Plus Flu Suspension Liquid 1881
Children's Tylenol Plus Multi-Symptom Cold Suspension Liquid 1879
Tylenol Cold Severe Congestion Non-Drowsy Caplets with Cool Burst.. 1874
Tylenol Cold Head Congestion Daytime Caplets with Cool Burst.. 1873
Tylenol Cold Head Congestion Nighttime Caplets with Cool Burst.. 1873
Tylenol Cold Head Congestion Severe Caplets with Cool Burst..... 1873
Tylenol Cold Multi-Symptom Daytime Caplets with Cool Burst and Gelcaps 1874
Tylenol Cold Multi-Symptom Daytime Liquid with Citrus Burst... 1874
Tylenol Cold Multi-Symptom Nighttime Caplets with Cool Burst.. 1874
Tylenol Cold Multi-Symptom Nighttime Liquid with Cool Burst... 1874
Tylenol Cold Multi-Symptom Severe Caplets with Cool Burst..... 1874
Tylenol Cold Multi-Symptom Severe Daytime Liquid with Citrus Burst..................................... 1874
Tylenol Cough & Sore Throat Daytime Liquid with Cool Burst...... 1877
Tylenol Cough & Sore Throat Nighttime Liquid with Cool Burst... 1877
Concentrated Tylenol Infants' Drops Plus Cold and Cough.......... 1879
Vicks 44 Cough Relief Liquid 2679
Vicks 44D Cough & Head Congestion Relief Liquid.............. 2679
Vicks 44E Cough & Chest Congestion Relief Liquid.............. 2679
Pediatric Vicks 44e Cough & Chest Congestion Relief Liquid...... 2676
Vicks 44M Cough, Cold & Flu Relief Liquid.................................... 2680
Pediatric Vicks 44m Cough & Cold Relief Liquid........................ 2676
Vicks DayQuil LiquiCaps/Liquid Multi-Symptom Cold/Flu Relief..... 761
Vicks DayQuil Multi-Symptom Cold/Flu Relief LiquiCaps............. 2678
Vicks DayQuil Multi-Symptom Cold/Flu Relief Liquid.................. 2678
Vicks NyQuil Multi-Symptom Cold/Flu Relief Liquid.................. 2681
Children's Vicks NyQuil Cold/Cough Relief............................ 756
Vicks NyQuil Multi-Symptom Cold/Flu Relief LiquiCaps............. 2681
Vicks NyQuil LiquiCaps/Liquid Multi-Symptom Cold/Flu Relief..... 763
Vicks NyQuil Cough Liquid 2680
Children's Vicks NyQuil Cold/Cough Relief Liquid 2680
Zicam Cough Max Nighttime Cough Spray.................................. 767
Zicam Cough Max Cough Spray 767
Zicam Cough Max Cough Melts 767
Zicam Cough Plus D Cough Spray.. 767
Zicam Cough Relief Cough Spray ... 767
Zicam Maximum Strength Flu Daytime.. 768
Zicam Maximum Strength Flu Nighttime.................................... 768

Dextromethorphan Polistirex (Duloxetine is a moderate inhibitor of

CYP2D6. Co-administration of duloxetine with other drugs that are extensively metabolized by this isoenzyme, and which have a narrow therapeutic window, should be approached with caution). Products include:

- Delsym Extended-Release Suspension 12 Hour Cough Suppressant .... ■611

Dezocine (Given the primary CNS effects of duloxetine, it should be used with caution when it is taken in combination with or substituted for other centrally acting drugs, including those with a similar mechanism of action).

No products indexed under this heading.

Diazepam (Given the primary CNS effects of duloxetine, it should be used with caution when it is taken in combination with or substituted for other centrally acting drugs, including those with a similar mechanism of action). Products include:

- Diastat Rectal Delivery System 3343
- Valium Tablets 2819

Diphenhydramine (Because CYP2D6 is involved in duloxetine metabolism, concomitant use of duloxetine with potent inhibitors of CYP2D6 would be expected to, and does, result in higher concentrations of duloxetine). Products include:

- Tylenol Sore Throat Nighttime Liquid with Cool Burst 1877

Diphenhydramine Hydrochloride (Because CYP2D6 is involved in duloxetine metabolism, concomitant use of duloxetine with potent inhibitors of CYP2D6 would be expected to, and does, result in higher concentrations of duloxetine). Products include:

- Nytol QuickCaps Caplets .... ■615
- Nytol QuickGels Softgels Maximum Strength .... ■616
- Simply Sleep Caplets 1868
- Sominex Original Formula Tablets .. ■616
- TheraFlu Warming Relief Nighttime Severe Cold .... ■743
- TheraFlu Thin Strips Multi Symptom .... ■744
- Triaminic Nighttime Cold & Cough Liquid .... ■746
- Triaminic Thin Strips Cough & Runny Nose .... ■749
- Extra Strength Tylenol PM Caplets, Vanilla Caplets, Geltabs, Gelcaps and Liquid 1875
- Tylenol Sore Throat Nighttime Liquid with Cool Burst .... ■790
- Tylenol Allergy Multi-Symptom Nighttime Caplets with Cool Burst 1872
- Tylenol Severe Allergy Caplets 1872
- Children's Tylenol Plus Cold & Allergy Suspension Liquid 1878

Dolasetron Mesylate (Duloxetine is a moderate inhibitor of CYP2D6. Co-administration of duloxetine with other drugs that are extensively metabolized by this isoenzyme, and which have a narrow therapeutic window, should be approached with caution). Products include:

- Anzemet Injection 2859
- Anzemet Tablets 2862

Donepezil Hydrochloride (Duloxetine is a moderate inhibitor of CYP2D6. Co-administration of duloxetine with other drugs that are extensively metabolized by this isoenzyme, and which have a narrow therapeutic window, should be approached with caution). Products include:

- Aricept Tablets 1094
- Aricept ODT Tablets 1094

Doxepin Hydrochloride (Duloxetine is a moderate inhibitor of CYP2D6. Co-administration of duloxetine with other drugs that are extensively metabolized by this isoenzyme, and which have a narrow therapeutic window, should be approached with caution. Plasma tricyclic antidepressant (TCA) concentrations may need to be monitored, and the dose of the TCA may need to be reduced, if a TCA is co-administered with duloxetine).

No products indexed under this heading.

Droperidol (Given the primary CNS effects of duloxetine, it should be used with caution when it is taken in combination with or substituted for other centrally acting drugs, including those with a similar mechanism of action).

No products indexed under this heading.

Eletriptan Hydrobromide (Development of a potentially life-threatening serotonin syndrome may occur with concomitant use of duloxetine HCl and triptans. If concomitant treatment is clinically warranted, careful observation of the patient is advised, particularly during treatment initiation and dose increases). Products include:

- Relpax Tablets 2548

Encainide Hydrochloride (Duloxetine is a moderate inhibitor of CYP2D6. Co-administration of duloxetine with other drugs that are extensively metabolized by this isoenzyme, and which have a narrow therapeutic window, should be approached with caution).

No products indexed under this heading.

Enflurane (Given the primary CNS effects of duloxetine, it should be used with caution when it is taken in combination with or substituted for other centrally acting drugs, including those with a similar mechanism of action).

No products indexed under this heading.

Enoxacin (Concomitant use of duloxetine with fluvoxamine, an inhibitor of CYP1A2, results in a 6-fold increase in AUC, about 2.5-fold increase in Cmax, and an approximately 3-fold increase in t1/2 of duloxetine. Since duloxetine is metabolized in part by CYP1A2, concomitant use of duloxetine with other inhibitors of CYP1A2, would be expected to have the same effects; these combinations should be avoided).

No products indexed under this heading.

Escitalopram Oxalate (Development of a potentially life-threatening serotonin syndrome may occur with concomitant use of duloxetine HCl and serotonergic drugs). Products include:

- Lexapro Oral Solution 1190
- Lexapro Tablets 1190

Esomeprazole Magnesium (Duloxetine has an enteric coating that resists dissolution until reaching a segment of the gastrointestinal tract where the pH exceeds 5.5. Drugs that raise the gastrointestinal pH may lead to an earlier release of duloxetine). Products include:

- Nexium Delayed-Release Capsules 655

Estazolam (Given the primary CNS effects of duloxetine, it should be used with caution when it is taken in combination with or substituted for other centrally acting drugs, including those with a similar mechanism of action). Products include:

- ProSom Tablets 517

Ethanol (Given the primary CNS effects of duloxetine, it should be used with caution when it is taken in combination with or substituted for other centrally acting drugs, including those with a similar mechanism of action).

No products indexed under this heading.

Ethchlorvynol (Given the primary CNS effects of duloxetine, it should be used with caution when it is taken in combination with or substituted for other centrally acting drugs, including those with a similar mechanism of action).

No products indexed under this heading.

Ethinamate (Given the primary CNS effects of duloxetine, it should be used with caution when it is taken in combination with or substituted for other centrally acting drugs, including those with a similar mechanism of action).

No products indexed under this heading.

Ethinyl Estradiol (Concomitant use of duloxetine with fluvoxamine, an inhibitor of CYP1A2, results in a 6-fold increase in AUC, about 2.5-fold increase in Cmax, and an approximately 3-fold increase in t1/2 of duloxetine. Since duloxetine is metabolized in part by CYP1A2, concomitant use of duloxetine with other inhibitors of CYP1A2, would be expected to have the same effects; these combinations should be avoided). Products include:

- Mircette Tablets 1066
- NuvaRing 2340
- Ortho-Cyclen/Ortho Tri-Cyclen 2429
- Ortho Evra Transdermal System 2417
- Ortho Tri-Cyclen Lo Tablets 2436
- Seasonique Tablets 1077
- Yasmin 28 Tablets 796
- Yaz Tablets 803

Ethyl Alcohol (Given the primary CNS effects of duloxetine, it should be used with caution when it is taken in combination with or substituted for other centrally acting drugs, including those with a similar mechanism of action).

No products indexed under this heading.

Famotidine (Duloxetine has an enteric coating that resists dissolution until reaching a segment of the gastrointestinal tract where the pH exceeds 5.5. Drugs that raise the gastrointestinal pH may lead to an earlier release of duloxetine). Products include:

- Pepcid Injection 2040
- Pepcid 2038
- Pepcid AC Gelcaps 1701
- Pepcid AC Tablets 1701
- Maximum Strength Pepcid AC Tablets 1701
- Pepcid Complete Chewable Tablets 1701

Fentanyl (Duloxetine is a moderate inhibitor of CYP2D6. Co-administration of duloxetine with other drugs that are extensively metabolized by this isoenzyme, and which have a narrow therapeutic window, should be approached with caution). Products include:

- Duragesic Transdermal System 2373
- Ionsys Transdermal System 2379

Fentanyl Citrate (Duloxetine is a moderate inhibitor of CYP2D6. Co-administration of duloxetine with other drugs that are extensively metabolized by this isoenzyme, and which have a narrow therapeutic window, should be approached with caution). Products include:

- Actiq 979

Flecainide Acetate (Duloxetine is a moderate inhibitor of CYP2D6. Co-administration of duloxetine with other drugs that are extensively metabolized by this isoenzyme, and which have a narrow therapeutic window, should be approached with caution). Products include:

- Tambocor Tablets 1856

Fluoxetine (Duloxetine is a moderate inhibitor of CYP2D6. Co-administration of duloxetine with other drugs that are extensively metabolized by this isoenzyme, and which have a narrow therapeutic window, should be approached with caution).

No products indexed under this heading.

Fluoxetine Hydrochloride (Development of a potentially life-threatening serotonin syndrome may occur with concomitant use of duloxetine HCl and serotonergic drugs). Products include:

- Prozac Pulvules and Liquid 1801
- Symbyax Capsules 1819

Fluphenazine Decanoate (Duloxetine is a moderate inhibitor of CYP2D6. Co-administration of duloxetine with other drugs that are extensively metabolized by this isoenzyme, and which have a narrow therapeutic window, should be approached with caution).

No products indexed under this heading.

Fluphenazine Enanthate (Duloxetine is a moderate inhibitor of CYP2D6. Co-administration of duloxetine with other drugs that are extensively metabolized by this isoenzyme, and which have a narrow therapeutic window, should be approached with caution).

No products indexed under this heading.

Fluphenazine Hydrochloride (Duloxetine is a moderate inhibitor of CYP2D6. Co-administration of duloxetine with other drugs that are extensively metabolized by this isoenzyme, and which have a narrow therapeutic window, should be approached with caution).

No products indexed under this heading.

Flurazepam Hydrochloride (Given the primary CNS effects of duloxetine, it should be used with caution when it is taken in combination with or substituted for other centrally acting drugs, including those with a similar mechanism of action). Products include:

- Dalmane Capsules 3342

Fluvoxamine (Concomitant use of duloxetine with fluvoxamine, an inhibitor of CYP1A2, results in approximately a 6-fold increase in AUC and about a 2.5-fold increase in Cmax of duloxetine; co-administration should be avoided).
No products indexed under this heading.

Fluvoxamine Maleate (Concomitant use of duloxetine with fluvoxamine, an inhibitor of CYP1A2, results in approximately a 6-fold increase in AUC and about a 2.5-fold increase in Cmax of duloxetine; co-administration should be avoided).
No products indexed under this heading.

Formoterol Fumarate (Duloxetine is a moderate inhibitor of CYP2D6. Co-administration of duloxetine with other drugs that are extensively metabolized by this isoenzyme, and which have a narrow therapeutic window, should be approached with caution). Products include:
Foradil Aerolizer 3010

Frovatriptan Succinate (Development of a potentially life-threatening serotonin syndrome may occur with concomitant use of duloxetine HCl and triptans. If concomitant treatment is clinically warranted, careful observation of the patient is advised, particularly during treatment initiation and dose increases). Products include:
Frova Tablets 1113

Galantamine Hydrobromide (Duloxetine is a moderate inhibitor of CYP2D6. Co-administration of duloxetine with other drugs that are extensively metabolized by this isoenzyme, and which have a narrow therapeutic window, should be approached with caution). Products include:
Razadyne 2399
Razadyne ER Extended-Release Capsules 2399

Gatifloxacin (Concomitant use of duloxetine with fluvoxamine, an inhibitor of CYP1A2, results in a 6-fold increase in AUC, about 2.5-fold increase in Cmax, and an approximately 3-fold increase in t1/2 of duloxetine. Since duloxetine is metabolized in part by CYP1A2, concomitant use of duloxetine with other inhibitors of CYP1A2, would be expected to have the same effects; these combinations should be avoided). Products include:
Tequin Injection 938
Tequin Injection in 5% Dextrose 938
Tequin Tablets 938
Zymar Ophthalmic Solution 575

Gemifloxacin Mesylate (Concomitant use of duloxetine with fluvoxamine, an inhibitor of CYP1A2, results in a 6-fold increase in AUC, about 2.5-fold increase in Cmax, and an approximately 3-fold increase in t1/2 of duloxetine. Since duloxetine is metabolized in part by CYP1A2, concomitant use of duloxetine with other inhibitors of CYP1A2, would be expected to have the same effects; these combinations should be avoided).
No products indexed under this heading.

Glutethimide (Given the primary CNS effects of duloxetine, it should be used with caution when it is taken in combination with or substituted for other centrally acting drugs, including those with a similar mechanism of action).
No products indexed under this heading.

Grepafloxacin Hydrochloride (Concomitant use of duloxetine with fluvoxamine, an inhibitor of CYP1A2, results in a 6-fold increase in AUC, about 2.5-fold increase in Cmax, and an approximately 3-fold increase in t1/2 of duloxetine. Since duloxetine is metabolized in part by CYP1A2, concomitant use of duloxetine with other inhibitors of CYP1A2, would be expected to have the same effects; these combinations should be avoided).
No products indexed under this heading.

Halofantrine Hydrochloride (Because CYP2D6 is involved in duloxetine metabolism, concomitant use of duloxetine with potent inhibitors of CYP2D6 would be expected to, and does, result in higher concentrations of duloxetine).
No products indexed under this heading.

Haloperidol (Duloxetine is a moderate inhibitor of CYP2D6. Co-administration of duloxetine with other drugs that are extensively metabolized by this isoenzyme, and which have a narrow therapeutic window, should be approached with caution).
No products indexed under this heading.

Haloperidol Decanoate (Duloxetine is a moderate inhibitor of CYP2D6. Co-administration of duloxetine with other drugs that are extensively metabolized by this isoenzyme, and which have a narrow therapeutic window, should be approached with caution).
No products indexed under this heading.

Hydrocodone Bitartrate (Duloxetine is a moderate inhibitor of CYP2D6. Co-administration of duloxetine with other drugs that are extensively metabolized by this isoenzyme, and which have a narrow therapeutic window, should be approached with caution). Products include:
Hycodan 1116
Hycotuss Expectorant Syrup 1117
Vicodin Tablets 535
Vicodin ES Tablets 536
Vicodin HP Tablets 538
Vicoprofen Tablets 539
Zydone Tablets 1139

Hydrocodone Polistirex (Given the primary CNS effects of duloxetine, it should be used with caution when it is taken in combination with or substituted for other centrally acting drugs, including those with a similar mechanism of action). Products include:
Tussionex Pennkinetic Extended-Release Suspension 3327

Hydromorphone Hydrochloride (Given the primary CNS effects of duloxetine, it should be used with caution when it is taken in combination with or substituted for other centrally acting drugs, including those with a similar mechanism of action). Products include:
Dilaudid 440
Dilaudid Non-Sterile Powder 440
Dilaudid Oral Liquid 445
Dilaudid Rectal Suppositories 440
Dilaudid Tablets 440
Dilaudid Tablets - 8 mg 445
Dilaudid-HP 442

Hydroxychloroquine Sulfate (Because CYP2D6 is involved in duloxetine metabolism, concomitant use of duloxetine with potent inhibitors of CYP2D6 would be expected to, and does, result in higher concentrations of duloxetine).
No products indexed under this heading.

Hydroxyzine Hydrochloride (Given the primary CNS effects of duloxetine, it should be used with caution when it is taken in combination with or substituted for other centrally acting drugs, including those with a similar mechanism of action).
No products indexed under this heading.

Hypericum (Caution is advised with co-administration of duloxetine with drugs that may affect the serotonergic neurotransmitter systems such as St. John's Wort because of potential development of serotonin syndrome). Products include:
Satiete Tablets 832

Imatinib Mesylate (Because CYP2D6 is involved in duloxetine metabolism, concomitant use of duloxetine with potent inhibitors of CYP2D6 would be expected to, and does, result in higher concentrations of duloxetine). Products include:
Gleevec Tablets 2227

Imipramine Hydrochloride (Duloxetine is a moderate inhibitor of CYP2D6. Co-administration of duloxetine with other drugs that are extensively metabolized by this isoenzyme, and which have a narrow therapeutic window, should be approached with caution. Plasma tricyclic antidepressant (TCA) concentrations may need to be monitored, and the dose of the TCA may need to be reduced, if a TCA is co-administered with duloxetine).
No products indexed under this heading.

Imipramine Pamoate (Duloxetine is a moderate inhibitor of CYP2D6. Co-administration of duloxetine with other drugs that are extensively metabolized by this isoenzyme, and which have a narrow therapeutic window, should be approached with caution. Plasma tricyclic antidepressant (TCA) concentrations may need to be monitored, and the dose of the TCA may need to be reduced, if a TCA is co-administered with duloxetine).
No products indexed under this heading.

Indoramin Hydrochloride (Duloxetine is a moderate inhibitor of CYP2D6. Co-administration of duloxetine with other drugs that are extensively metabolized by this isoenzyme, and which have a narrow therapeutic window, should be approached with caution).
No products indexed under this heading.

Isocarboxazid (There have been reports of serious, sometimes fatal, reactions in patients receiving a serotonin reuptake inhibitor in combination with a monoamine oxidase inhibitor (MAOI). These reactions have also been reported in patients who have recently discontinued serotonin reuptake inhibitors and are started on an MAOI. Therefore, duloxetine use is contraindicated in combination with an MAOI, or within at least 14 days of discontinuing treatment with an MAOI. Based on the half-life of duloxetine, at least 5 days should be allowed after stopping duloxetine before starting an MAOI. Development of a potentially life-threatening serotonin syndrome may occur with concomitant use of duloxetine HCl and drugs which impair the metabolism of serotonin (e.g., MAOIs)).
No products indexed under this heading.

Isoflurane (Given the primary CNS effects of duloxetine, it should be used with caution when it is taken in combination with or substituted for other centrally acting drugs, including those with a similar mechanism of action).
No products indexed under this heading.

Isoniazid (Concomitant use of duloxetine with fluvoxamine, an inhibitor of CYP1A2, results in a 6-fold increase in AUC, about 2.5-fold increase in Cmax, and an approximately 3-fold increase in t1/2 of duloxetine. Since duloxetine is metabolized in part by CYP1A2, concomitant use of duloxetine with other inhibitors of CYP1A2, would be expected to have the same effects; these combinations should be avoided).
No products indexed under this heading.

Ketamine Hydrochloride (Given the primary CNS effects of duloxetine, it should be used with caution when it is taken in combination with or substituted for other centrally acting drugs, including those with a similar mechanism of action).
No products indexed under this heading.

Ketoconazole (Concomitant use of duloxetine with fluvoxamine, an inhibitor of CYP1A2, results in a 6-fold increase in AUC, about 2.5-fold increase in Cmax, and an approximately 3-fold increase in t1/2 of duloxetine. Since duloxetine is metabolized in part by CYP1A2, concomitant use of duloxetine with other inhibitors of CYP1A2, would be expected to have the same effects; these combinations should be avoided). Products include:
Nizoral A-D Shampoo, 1% 1868

Labetalol Hydrochloride (Duloxetine is a moderate inhibitor of CYP2D6. Co-administration of duloxetine with other drugs that are extensively metabolized by this isoenzyme, and which have a narrow therapeutic window, should be approached with caution).
No products indexed under this heading.

Lansoprazole (Duloxetine has an enteric coating that resists dissolution until reaching a segment of the gastrointestinal tract where the pH exceeds 5.5. Drugs that raise the gastrointestinal pH may lead to an earlier release of duloxetine). Products include:
Prevacid Delayed-Release Capsules 3271
Prevacid for Delayed-Release Oral Suspension 3271

Prevacid SoluTab Delayed-Release Orally Disintegrating Tablets 3271
Prevacid I.V. for Injection 3277
Prevacid NapraPAC 3280
PREVPAC 3284

Levofloxacin (Concomitant use of duloxetine with fluvoxamine, an inhibitor of CYP1A2, results in a 6-fold increase in AUC, about 2.5-fold increase in Cmax, and an approximately 3-fold increase in t1/2 of duloxetine. Since duloxetine is metabolized in part by CYP1A2, concomitant use of duloxetine with other inhibitors of CYP1A2, would be expected to have the same effects; these combinations should be avoided). Products include:
Levaquin 2384
Levaquin in 5% Dextrose Injection 2384
Quixin Ophthalmic Solution 3383

Levomethadyl Acetate Hydrochloride (Given the primary CNS effects of duloxetine, it should be used with caution when it is taken in combination with or substituted for other centrally acting drugs, including those with a similar mechanism of action).
No products indexed under this heading.

Levonorgestrel (Concomitant use of duloxetine with fluvoxamine, an inhibitor of CYP1A2, results in a 6-fold increase in AUC, about 2.5-fold increase in Cmax, and an approximately 3-fold increase in t1/2 of duloxetine. Since duloxetine is metabolized in part by CYP1A2, concomitant use of duloxetine with other inhibitors of CYP1A2, would be expected to have the same effects; these combinations should be avoided). Products include:
Climara Pro Transdermal System 776
Mirena Intrauterine System 787
Plan B Tablets 1076
Seasonique Tablets 1077

Levorphanol Tartrate (Given the primary CNS effects of duloxetine, it should be used with caution when it is taken in combination with or substituted for other centrally acting drugs, including those with a similar mechanism of action).
No products indexed under this heading.

Lidocaine (Duloxetine is a moderate inhibitor of CYP2D6. Co-administration of duloxetine with other drugs that are extensively metabolized by this isoenzyme, and which have a narrow therapeutic window, should be approached with caution). Products include:
Lidoderm Patch 1118
Synera Topical Patch 1137

Lidocaine Hydrochloride (Duloxetine is a moderate inhibitor of CYP2D6. Co-administration of duloxetine with other drugs that are extensively metabolized by this isoenzyme, and which have a narrow therapeutic window, should be approached with caution).
No products indexed under this heading.

Lithium (Caution is advised with co-administration of duloxetine with drugs that may affect the serotonergic neurotransmitter systems such as tramadol because of potential development of serotonin syndrome).
No products indexed under this heading.

Lomefloxacin Hydrochloride (Concomitant use of duloxetine with fluvoxamine, an inhibitor of CYP1A2, results in a 6-fold increase in AUC, about 2.5-fold increase in Cmax, and an approximately 3-fold increase in t1/2 of duloxetine. Since duloxetine is metabolized in part by CYP1A2, concomitant use of duloxetine with other inhibitors of CYP1A2, would be expected to have the same effects; these combinations should be avoided).
No products indexed under this heading.

Lorazepam (Given the primary CNS effects of duloxetine, it should be used with caution when it is taken in combination with or substituted for other centrally acting drugs, including those with a similar mechanism of action).
No products indexed under this heading.

Loxapine Hydrochloride (Given the primary CNS effects of duloxetine, it should be used with caution when it is taken in combination with or substituted for other centrally acting drugs, including those with a similar mechanism of action).
No products indexed under this heading.

Loxapine Succinate (Given the primary CNS effects of duloxetine, it should be used with caution when it is taken in combination with or substituted for other centrally acting drugs, including those with a similar mechanism of action).
No products indexed under this heading.

Magnesium Hydroxide (Duloxetine has an enteric coating that resists dissolution until reaching a segment of the gastrointestinal tract where the pH exceeds 5.5. Drugs that raise the gastrointestinal pH may lead to an earlier release of duloxetine). Products include:
Maalox Regular Strength Antacid/Antigas Liquid 2175
Maalox Max Maximum Strength Antacid/Anti-Gas Liquid 2176
Pepcid Complete Chewable Tablets 1701

Maprotiline Hydrochloride (Duloxetine is a moderate inhibitor of CYP2D6. Co-administration of duloxetine with other drugs that are extensively metabolized by this isoenzyme, and which have a narrow therapeutic window, should be approached with caution. Plasma tricyclic antidepressant (TCA) concentrations may need to be monitored, and the dose of the TCA may need to be reduced, if a TCA is co-administered with duloxetine).
No products indexed under this heading.

Meperidine Hydrochloride (Duloxetine is a moderate inhibitor of CYP2D6. Co-administration of duloxetine with other drugs that are extensively metabolized by this isoenzyme, and which have a narrow therapeutic window, should be approached with caution).
No products indexed under this heading.

Mephobarbital (Given the primary CNS effects of duloxetine, it should be used with caution when it is taken in combination with or substituted for other centrally acting drugs, including those with a similar mechanism of action).
No products indexed under this heading.

Meprobamate (Given the primary CNS effects of duloxetine, it should be used with caution when it is taken in combination with or substituted for other centrally acting drugs, including those with a similar mechanism of action).
No products indexed under this heading.

Mesoridazine Besylate (Duloxetine is a moderate inhibitor of CYP2D6. Co-administration of duloxetine with other drugs that are extensively metabolized by this isoenzyme, and which have a narrow therapeutic window, should be approached with caution).
No products indexed under this heading.

Mestranol (Concomitant use of duloxetine with fluvoxamine, an inhibitor of CYP1A2, results in a 6-fold increase in AUC, about 2.5-fold increase in Cmax, and an approximately 3-fold increase in t1/2 of duloxetine. Since duloxetine is metabolized in part by CYP1A2, concomitant use of duloxetine with other inhibitors of CYP1A2, would be expected to have the same effects; these combinations should be avoided).
No products indexed under this heading.

Methadone Hydrochloride (Duloxetine is a moderate inhibitor of CYP2D6. Co-administration of duloxetine with other drugs that are extensively metabolized by this isoenzyme, and which have a narrow therapeutic window, should be approached with caution).
No products indexed under this heading.

Methamphetamine Hydrochloride (Duloxetine is a moderate inhibitor of CYP2D6. Co-administration of duloxetine with other drugs that are extensively metabolized by this isoenzyme, and which have a narrow therapeutic window, should be approached with caution). Products include:
Desoxyn Tablets, USP 2462

Methohexital Sodium (Given the primary CNS effects of duloxetine, it should be used with caution when it is taken in combination with or substituted for other centrally acting drugs, including those with a similar mechanism of action).
No products indexed under this heading.

Methotrimeprazine (Duloxetine is a moderate inhibitor of CYP2D6. Co-administration of duloxetine with other drugs that are extensively metabolized by this isoenzyme, and which have a narrow therapeutic window, should be approached with caution).
No products indexed under this heading.

Methoxsalen (Concomitant use of duloxetine with fluvoxamine, an inhibitor of CYP1A2, results in a 6-fold increase in AUC, about 2.5-fold increase in Cmax, and an approximately 3-fold increase in t1/2 of duloxetine. Since duloxetine is metabolized in part by CYP1A2, concomitant use of duloxetine with other inhibitors of CYP1A2, would be expected to have the same effects; these combinations should be avoided). Products include:
Oxsoralen Lotion 1% 3352
Oxsoralen-Ultra Capsules 3353

Methoxyflurane (Given the primary CNS effects of duloxetine, it should be used with caution when it is taken in combination with or substituted for other centrally acting drugs, including those with a similar mechanism of action).
No products indexed under this heading.

Methylphenidate (Given the primary CNS effects of duloxetine, it should be used with caution when it is taken in combination with or substituted for other centrally acting drugs, including those with a similar mechanism of action). Products include:
Daytrana Transdermal Patch 3174

Methylphenidate Hydrochloride (Given the primary CNS effects of duloxetine, it should be used with caution when it is taken in combination with or substituted for other centrally acting drugs, including those with a similar mechanism of action). Products include:
Concerta Extended-Release Tablets 1881
Metadate CD Capsules 3323
Ritalin Hydrochloride Tablets 2269
Ritalin LA Capsules 2271
Ritalin-SR Tablets 2269

Metoprolol Succinate (Duloxetine is a moderate inhibitor of CYP2D6. Co-administration of duloxetine with other drugs that are extensively metabolized by this isoenzyme, and which have a narrow therapeutic window, should be approached with caution). Products include:
Toprol-XL Tablets 668

Metoprolol Tartrate (Duloxetine is a moderate inhibitor of CYP2D6. Co-administration of duloxetine with other drugs that are extensively metabolized by this isoenzyme, and which have a narrow therapeutic window, should be approached with caution). Products include:
Lopressor Injection 2238
Lopressor Tablets 2238
Lopressor HCT 50/25 Tablets 2241
Lopressor HCT 100/25 Tablets 2241
Lopressor HCT 100/50 Tablets 2241

Mexiletine Hydrochloride (Duloxetine is a moderate inhibitor of CYP2D6. Co-administration of duloxetine with other drugs that are extensively metabolized by this isoenzyme, and which have a narrow therapeutic window, should be approached with caution).
No products indexed under this heading.

Mibefradil Dihydrochloride (Concomitant use of duloxetine with fluvoxamine, an inhibitor of CYP1A2, results in a 6-fold increase in AUC, about 2.5-fold increase in Cmax, and an approximately 3-fold increase in t1/2 of duloxetine. Since duloxetine is metabolized in part by CYP1A2, concomitant use of duloxetine with other inhibitors of CYP1A2, would be expected to have the same effects; these combinations should be avoided).

No products indexed under this heading.

Midazolam Hydrochloride (Given the primary CNS effects of duloxetine, it should be used with caution when it is taken in combination with or substituted for other centrally acting drugs, including those with a similar mechanism of action).

No products indexed under this heading.

Mirtazapine (Duloxetine is a moderate inhibitor of CYP2D6. Co-administration of duloxetine with other drugs that are extensively metabolized by this isoenzyme, and which have a narrow therapeutic window, should be approached with caution).

No products indexed under this heading.

Moclobemide (There have been reports of serious, sometimes fatal, reactions in patients receiving a serotonin reuptake inhibitor in combination with a monoamine oxidase inhibitor (MAOI). These reactions have also been reported in patients who have recently discontinued serotonin reuptake inhibitors and are started on an MAOI. Therefore, duloxetine use is contraindicated in combination with an MAOI, or within at least 14 days of discontinuing treatment with an MAOI. Based on the half-life of duloxetine, at least 5 days should be allowed after stopping duloxetine before starting an MAOI. Development of a potentially life-threatening serotonin syndrome may occur with concomitant use of duloxetine HCl and drugs which impair the metabolism of serotonin (e.g., MAOIs)).

No products indexed under this heading.

Molindone Hydrochloride (Given the primary CNS effects of duloxetine, it should be used with caution when it is taken in combination with or substituted for other centrally acting drugs, including those with a similar mechanism of action).
Products include:
Moban Tablets 1119

Morphine Sulfate (Duloxetine is a moderate inhibitor of CYP2D6. Co-administration of duloxetine with other drugs that are extensively metabolized by this isoenzyme, and which have a narrow therapeutic window, should be approached with caution).
Products include:
Avinza Capsules 1741
Kadian Capsules 577
MS Contin Tablets 2701

Moxifloxacin Hydrochloride (Concomitant use of duloxetine with fluvoxamine, an inhibitor of CYP1A2, results in a 6-fold increase in AUC, about 2.5-fold increase in Cmax, and an approximately 3-fold increase in t1/2 of duloxetine. Since duloxetine is metabolized in part by CYP1A2, concomitant use of duloxetine with other inhibitors of CYP1A2, would be expected to have the same effects; these combinations should be avoided). Products include:
Avelox ... 2970
Vigamox Ophthalmic Solution 564

Nalidixic Acid (Concomitant use of duloxetine with fluvoxamine, an inhibitor of CYP1A2, results in a 6-fold increase in AUC, about 2.5-fold increase in Cmax, and an approximately 3-fold increase in t1/2 of

duloxetine. Since duloxetine is metabolized in part by CYP1A2, concomitant use of duloxetine with other inhibitors of CYP1A2, would be expected to have the same effects; these combinations should be avoided).

No products indexed under this heading.

Naratriptan Hydrochloride (Development of a potentially life-threatening serotonin syndrome may occur with concomitant use of duloxetine HCl and triptans. If concomitant treatment is clinically warranted, careful observation of the patient is advised, particularly during treatment initiation and dose increases).
Products include:
Amerge Tablets 1339

Nelfinavir Mesylate (Duloxetine is a moderate inhibitor of CYP2D6. Co-administration of duloxetine with other drugs that are extensively metabolized by this isoenzyme, and which have a narrow therapeutic window, should be approached with caution). Products include:
Viracept ... 2577

Nizatidine (Duloxetine has an enteric coating that resists dissolution until reaching a segment of the gastrointestinal tract where the pH exceeds 5.5. Drugs that raise the gastrointestinal pH may lead to an earlier release of duloxetine).
Products include:
Axid Oral Solution 879

Norethindrone (Concomitant use of duloxetine with fluvoxamine, an inhibitor of CYP1A2, results in a 6-fold increase in AUC, about 2.5-fold increase in Cmax, and an approximately 3-fold increase in t1/2 of duloxetine. Since duloxetine is metabolized in part by CYP1A2, concomitant use of duloxetine with other inhibitors of CYP1A2, would be expected to have the same effects; these combinations should be avoided). Products include:
Ortho Micronor Tablets 2426

Norfloxacin (Concomitant use of duloxetine with fluvoxamine, an inhibitor of CYP1A2, results in a 6-fold increase in AUC, about 2.5-fold increase in Cmax, and an approximately 3-fold increase in t1/2 of duloxetine. Since duloxetine is metabolized in part by CYP1A2, concomitant use of duloxetine with other inhibitors of CYP1A2, would be expected to have the same effects; these combinations should be avoided). Products include:
Noroxin Tablets 2032

Norgestrel (Concomitant use of duloxetine with fluvoxamine, an inhibitor of CYP1A2, results in a 6-fold increase in AUC, about 2.5-fold increase in Cmax, and an approximately 3-fold increase in t1/2 of duloxetine. Since duloxetine is metabolized in part by CYP1A2, concomitant use of duloxetine with other inhibitors of CYP1A2, would be expected to have the same effects; these combinations should be avoided).

No products indexed under this heading.

Nortriptyline Hydrochloride (Duloxetine is a moderate inhibitor of CYP2D6. Co-administration of duloxetine with other drugs that are extensively metabolized by this isoenzyme, and which have a narrow therapeutic window, should be

approached with caution. Plasma tricyclic antidepressant (TCA) concentrations may need to be monitored, and the dose of the TCA may need to be reduced, if a TCA is co-administered with duloxetine).

No products indexed under this heading.

Ofloxacin (Concomitant use of duloxetine with fluvoxamine, an inhibitor of CYP1A2, results in a 6-fold increase in AUC, about 2.5-fold increase in Cmax, and an approximately 3-fold increase in t1/2 of duloxetine. Since duloxetine is metabolized in part by CYP1A2, concomitant use of duloxetine with other inhibitors of CYP1A2, would be expected to have the same effects; these combinations should be avoided). Products include:
Floxin Otic Solution 1049

Olanzapine (Duloxetine is a moderate inhibitor of CYP2D6. Co-administration of duloxetine with other drugs that are extensively metabolized by this isoenzyme, and which have a narrow therapeutic window, should be approached with caution). Products include:
Symbyax Capsules 1819
Zyprexa Tablets 1830
Zyprexa IntraMuscular 1830
Zyprexa ZYDIS Orally
 Disintegrating Tablets 1830

Omeprazole (Duloxetine is a moderate inhibitor of CYP2D6. Co-administration of duloxetine with other drugs that are extensively metabolized by this isoenzyme, and which have a narrow therapeutic window, should be approached with caution). Products include:
Zegerid Capsules 2958
Zegerid Powder for Oral Solution 2958

Ondansetron (Duloxetine is a moderate inhibitor of CYP2D6. Co-administration of duloxetine with other drugs that are extensively metabolized by this isoenzyme, and which have a narrow therapeutic window, should be approached with caution). Products include:
Zofran ODT Orally Disintegrating
 Tablets 1639

Ondansetron Hydrochloride (Duloxetine is a moderate inhibitor of CYP2D6. Co-administration of duloxetine with other drugs that are extensively metabolized by this isoenzyme, and which have a narrow therapeutic window, should be approached with caution). Products include:
Zofran Injection 1634
Zofran .. 1639

Oxazepam (Given the primary CNS effects of duloxetine, it should be used with caution when it is taken in combination with or substituted for other centrally acting drugs, including those with a similar mechanism of action).

No products indexed under this heading.

Oxycodone Hydrochloride (Duloxetine is a moderate inhibitor of CYP2D6. Co-administration of duloxetine with other drugs that are extensively metabolized by this isoenzyme, and which have a narrow therapeutic window, should be approached with caution). Products include:
OxyContin Tablets 2703
OxyFast Oral Concentrate
 Solution 2708
OxyIR Capsules 2708

Percocet Tablets 1131
Percodan Tablets 1132

Paclitaxel (Duloxetine is a moderate inhibitor of CYP2D6. Co-administration of duloxetine with other drugs that are extensively metabolized by this isoenzyme, and which have a narrow therapeutic window, should be approached with caution).

No products indexed under this heading.

Pargyline Hydrochloride (There have been reports of serious, sometimes fatal, reactions in patients receiving a serotonin reuptake inhibitor in combination with a monoamine oxidase inhibitor (MAOI). These reactions have also been reported in patients who have recently discontinued serotonin reuptake inhibitors and are started on an MAOI. Therefore, duloxetine use is contraindicated in combination with an MAOI, or within at least 14 days of discontinuing treatment with an MAOI. Based on the half-life of duloxetine, at least 5 days should be allowed after stopping duloxetine before starting an MAOI. Development of a potentially life-threatening serotonin syndrome may occur with concomitant use of duloxetine HCl and drugs which impair the metabolism of serotonin (e.g., MAOIs)).

No products indexed under this heading.

Paroxetine Hydrochloride (Paroxetine (20mg qd) increased the concentration of duloxetine (40mg qd) by about 60% and greater degrees of inhibition are expected with higher doses of paroxetine). Products include:
Paxil CR Controlled-Release
 Tablets 1538
Paxil ... 1530

Pemoline (Given the primary CNS effects of duloxetine, it should be used with caution when it is taken in combination with or substituted for other centrally acting drugs, including those with a similar mechanism of action).

No products indexed under this heading.

Pentobarbital Sodium (Given the primary CNS effects of duloxetine, it should be used with caution when it is taken in combination with or substituted for other centrally acting drugs, including those with a similar mechanism of action). Products include:
Nembutal Sodium Solution, USP 2470

Perphenazine (Duloxetine is a moderate inhibitor of CYP2D6. Co-administration of duloxetine with other drugs that are extensively metabolized by this isoenzyme, and which have a narrow therapeutic window, should be approached with caution).

No products indexed under this heading.

Phenelzine Sulfate (There have been reports of serious, sometimes fatal, reactions in patients receiving a serotonin reuptake inhibitor in combination with a monoamine oxidase inhibitor (MAOI). These reactions have also been reported in patients who have recently discontinued serotonin reuptake inhibitors and are started on an MAOI. Therefore, duloxetine use is contraindicated in combination with an MAOI, or within at least 14 days of discontinuing treatment with an MAOI. Based on

IMPORTANT NOTE: Always consult each drug listing in the patient's regimen for possible interactions.

the half-life of duloxetine, at least 5 days should be allowed after stopping duloxetine before starting an MAOI. Development of a potentially life-threatening serotonin syndrome may occur with concomitant use of duloxetine HCl and drugs which impair the metabolism of serotonin (e.g., MAOIs)).

No products indexed under this heading.

Phenobarbital (Given the primary CNS effects of duloxetine, it should be used with caution when it is taken in combination with or substituted for other centrally acting drugs, including those with a similar mechanism of action). Products include:

Donnatal Extentabs 2493

Pindolol (Duloxetine is a moderate inhibitor of CYP2D6. Co-administration of duloxetine with other drugs that are extensively metabolized by this isoenzyme, and which have a narrow therapeutic window, should be approached with caution).

No products indexed under this heading.

Prazepam (Given the primary CNS effects of duloxetine, it should be used with caution when it is taken in combination with or substituted for other centrally acting drugs, including those with a similar mechanism of action).

No products indexed under this heading.

Procarbazine Hydrochloride (There have been reports of serious, sometimes fatal, reactions in patients receiving a serotonin reuptake inhibitor in combination with a monoamine oxidase inhibitor (MAOI). These reactions have also been reported in patients who have recently discontinued serotonin reuptake inhibitors and are started on an MAOI. Therefore, duloxetine use is contraindicated in combination with an MAOI, or within at least 14 days of discontinuing treatment with an MAOI. Based on the half-life of duloxetine, at least 5 days should be allowed after stopping duloxetine before starting an MAOI. Development of a potentially life-threatening serotonin syndrome may occur with concomitant use of duloxetine HCl and drugs which impair the metabolism of serotonin (e.g., MAOIs)). Products include:

Matulane Capsules 3191

Prochlorperazine (Duloxetine is a moderate inhibitor of CYP2D6. Co-administration of duloxetine with other drugs that are extensively metabolized by this isoenzyme, and which have a narrow therapeutic window, should be approached with caution).

No products indexed under this heading.

Promethazine Hydrochloride (Duloxetine is a moderate inhibitor of CYP2D6. Co-administration of duloxetine with other drugs that are extensively metabolized by this isoenzyme, and which have a narrow therapeutic window, should be approached with caution). Products include:

Phenergan Tablets and Suppositories 3440

Propafenone Hydrochloride (Duloxetine is a moderate inhibitor of CYP2D6. Co-administration of duloxetine with other drugs that are extensively metabolized by this isoenzyme, and which have a narrow therapeutic window, should be approached with caution). Products include:

Rythmol SR Capsules 2727

Propofol (Given the primary CNS effects of duloxetine, it should be used with caution when it is taken in combination with or substituted for other centrally acting drugs, including those with a similar mechanism of action).

No products indexed under this heading.

Propoxyphene Hydrochloride (Duloxetine is a moderate inhibitor of CYP2D6. Co-administration of duloxetine with other drugs that are extensively metabolized by this isoenzyme, and which have a narrow therapeutic window, should be approached with caution).

No products indexed under this heading.

Propoxyphene Napsylate (Duloxetine is a moderate inhibitor of CYP2D6. Co-administration of duloxetine with other drugs that are extensively metabolized by this isoenzyme, and which have a narrow therapeutic window, should be approached with caution).

No products indexed under this heading.

Propranolol Hydrochloride (Duloxetine is a moderate inhibitor of CYP2D6. Co-administration of duloxetine with other drugs that are extensively metabolized by this isoenzyme, and which have a narrow therapeutic window, should be approached with caution). Products include:

Inderal LA Long-Acting Capsules 3429

InnoPran XL Capsules 2723

Protriptyline Hydrochloride (Duloxetine is a moderate inhibitor of CYP2D6. Co-administration of duloxetine with other drugs that are extensively metabolized by this isoenzyme, and which have a narrow therapeutic window, should be approached with caution. Plasma tricyclic antidepressant (TCA) concentrations may need to be monitored, and the dose of the TCA may need to be reduced, if a TCA is co-administered with duloxetine).

No products indexed under this heading.

Quazepam (Given the primary CNS effects of duloxetine, it should be used with caution when it is taken in combination with or substituted for other centrally acting drugs, including those with a similar mechanism of action).

No products indexed under this heading.

Quetiapine Fumarate (Duloxetine is a moderate inhibitor of CYP2D6. Co-administration of duloxetine with other drugs that are extensively metabolized by this isoenzyme, and which have a narrow therapeutic window, should be approached with caution). Products include:

Seroquel Tablets 690

Quinacrine Hydrochloride (Because CYP2D6 is involved in duloxetine metabolism, concomitant use of duloxetine with potent inhibitors of CYP2D6 would be expected to, and does, result in higher concentrations of duloxetine).

No products indexed under this heading.

Quinidine Gluconate (Duloxetine is a moderate inhibitor of CYP2D6. Co-administration of duloxetine with other drugs that are extensively metabolized by this isoenzyme, and which have a narrow therapeutic window, should be approached with caution).

No products indexed under this heading.

Quinidine Hydrochloride (Duloxetine is a moderate inhibitor of CYP2D6. Co-administration of duloxetine with other drugs that are extensively metabolized by this isoenzyme, and which have a narrow therapeutic window, should be approached with caution).

No products indexed under this heading.

Quinidine Polygalacturonate (Duloxetine is a moderate inhibitor of CYP2D6. Co-administration of duloxetine with other drugs that are extensively metabolized by this isoenzyme, and which have a narrow therapeutic window, should be approached with caution).

No products indexed under this heading.

Quinidine Sulfate (Duloxetine is a moderate inhibitor of CYP2D6. Co-administration of duloxetine with other drugs that are extensively metabolized by this isoenzyme, and which have a narrow therapeutic window, should be approached with caution).

No products indexed under this heading.

Rabeprazole Sodium (Duloxetine has an enteric coating that resists dissolution until reaching a segment of the gastrointestinal tract where the pH exceeds 5.5. Drugs that raise the gastrointestinal pH may lead to an earlier release of duloxetine). Products include:

Aciphex Tablets 1090

Ranitidine Bismuth Citrate (Because CYP2D6 is involved in duloxetine metabolism, concomitant use of duloxetine with potent inhibitors of CYP2D6 would be expected to, and does, result in higher concentrations of duloxetine).

No products indexed under this heading.

Ranitidine Hydrochloride (Duloxetine has an enteric coating that resists dissolution until reaching a segment of the gastrointestinal tract where the pH exceeds 5.5. Drugs that raise the gastrointestinal pH may lead to an earlier release of duloxetine). Products include:

Zantac 1624

Zantac Injection 1619

Zantac Injection Pharmacy Bulk Package 1622

Remifentanil Hydrochloride (Given the primary CNS effects of duloxetine, it should be used with caution when it is taken in combination with or substituted for other centrally acting drugs, including those with a similar mechanism of action).

No products indexed under this heading.

Risperidone (Duloxetine is a moderate inhibitor of CYP2D6. Co-administration of duloxetine with other drugs that are extensively metabolized by this isoenzyme, and which have a narrow therapeutic window, should be approached with caution). Products include:

Risperdal 1676

Risperdal Consta Long-Acting Injection 1682

Risperdal M-Tab Orally Disintegrating Tablets 1676

Ritonavir (Duloxetine is a moderate inhibitor of CYP2D6. Co-administration of duloxetine with other drugs that are extensively metabolized by this isoenzyme, and which have a narrow therapeutic window, should be approached with caution). Products include:

Kaletra 476

Norvir 503

Rizatriptan Benzoate (Development of a potentially life-threatening serotonin syndrome may occur with concomitant use of duloxetine HCl and triptans. If concomitant treatment is clinically warranted, careful observation of the patient is advised, particularly during treatment initiation and dose increases). Products include:

Maxalt Tablets 2008

Maxalt-MLT Orally Disintegrating Tablets 2008

Secobarbital Sodium (Given the primary CNS effects of duloxetine, it should be used with caution when it is taken in combination with or substituted for other centrally acting drugs, including those with a similar mechanism of action).

No products indexed under this heading.

Selegiline Hydrochloride (There have been reports of serious, sometimes fatal, reactions in patients receiving a serotonin reuptake inhibitor in combination with a monoamine oxidase inhibitor (MAOI). These reactions have also been reported in patients who have recently discontinued serotonin reuptake inhibitors and are started on an MAOI. Therefore, duloxetine use is contraindicated in combination with an MAOI, or within at least 14 days of discontinuing treatment with an MAOI. Based on the half-life of duloxetine, at least 5 days should be allowed after stopping duloxetine before starting an MAOI. Development of a potentially life-threatening serotonin syndrome may occur with concomitant use of duloxetine HCl and drugs which impair the metabolism of serotonin (e.g., MAOIs)). Products include:

Eldepryl Capsules 3208

Zelapar Tablets 3372

Sertraline Hydrochloride (Development of a potentially life-threatening serotonin syndrome may occur with concomitant use of duloxetine HCl and serotonergic drugs). Products include:

Zoloft 2586

Sevoflurane (Given the primary CNS effects of duloxetine, it should be used with caution when it is taken in combination with or substituted for other centrally acting drugs, including those with a similar mechanism of action). Products include:

Ultane Liquid for Inhalation 531

Sodium Oxybate (Given the primary CNS effects of duloxetine, it should be used with caution when it is taken in combination with or substituted for other centrally acting drugs, including those with a similar mechanism of action). Products include:

Xyrem Oral Solution 1688

Sparfloxacin (Concomitant use of duloxetine with fluvoxamine, an inhib-

itor of CYP1A2, results in a 6-fold increase in AUC, about 2.5-fold increase in Cmax, and an approximately 3-fold increase in t1/2 of duloxetine. Since duloxetine is metabolized in part by CYP1A2, concomitant use of duloxetine with other inhibitors of CYP1A2, would be expected to have the same effects; these combinations should be avoided).
No products indexed under this heading.

Sufentanil Citrate (Given the primary CNS effects of duloxetine, it should be used with caution when it is taken in combination with or substituted for other centrally acting drugs, including those with a similar mechanism of action).
No products indexed under this heading.

Sumatriptan (Development of a potentially life-threatening serotonin syndrome may occur with concomitant use of duloxetine HCl and triptans. If concomitant treatment is clinically warranted, careful observation of the patient is advised, particularly during treatment initiation and dose increases). Products include:
Imitrex Nasal Spray 1467

Sumatriptan Succinate (Development of a potentially life-threatening serotonin syndrome may occur with concomitant use of duloxetine HCl and triptans. If concomitant treatment is clinically warranted, careful observation of the patient is advised, particularly during treatment initiation and dose increases). Products include:
Imitrex Injection 1463
Imitrex Tablets 1471

Tacrine Hydrochloride (Concomitant use of duloxetine with fluvoxamine, an inhibitor of CYP1A2, results in a 6-fold increase in AUC, about 2.5-fold increase in Cmax, and an approximately 3-fold increase in t1/2 of duloxetine. Since duloxetine is metabolized in part by CYP1A2, concomitant use of duloxetine with other inhibitors of CYP1A2, would be expected to have the same effects; these combinations should be avoided).
No products indexed under this heading.

Tamoxifen Citrate (Duloxetine is a moderate inhibitor of CYP2D6. Co-administration of duloxetine with other drugs that are extensively metabolized by this isoenzyme, and which have a narrow therapeutic window, should be approached with caution). Products include:
Soltamox Oral Solution 3527

Temazepam (Given the primary CNS effects of duloxetine, it should be used with caution when it is taken in combination with or substituted for other centrally acting drugs, including those with a similar mechanism of action). Products include:
Restoril Capsules 1860

Teniposide (Duloxetine is a moderate inhibitor of CYP2D6. Co-administration of duloxetine with other drugs that are extensively metabolized by this isoenzyme, and which have a narrow therapeutic window, should be approached with caution).
No products indexed under this heading.

Terbinafine Hydrochloride (Because CYP2D6 is involved in duloxetine metabolism, concomitant use of duloxetine with potent inhibitors of CYP2D6 would be expected to, and does, result in higher concentrations of duloxetine). Products include:
Lamisil Tablets 2232
Lamisil AT Creams (Athlete's Foot & Jock Itch) 636

Testosterone (Duloxetine is a moderate inhibitor of CYP2D6. Co-administration of duloxetine with other drugs that are extensively metabolized by this isoenzyme, and which have a narrow therapeutic window, should be approached with caution). Products include:
AndroGel 3329
Striant Mucoadhesive 1007
Testim 1% Gel 695

Testosterone Cypionate (Duloxetine is a moderate inhibitor of CYP2D6. Co-administration of duloxetine with other drugs that are extensively metabolized by this isoenzyme, and which have a narrow therapeutic window, should be approached with caution).
No products indexed under this heading.

Testosterone Enanthate (Duloxetine is a moderate inhibitor of CYP2D6. Co-administration of duloxetine with other drugs that are extensively metabolized by this isoenzyme, and which have a narrow therapeutic window, should be approached with caution).
No products indexed under this heading.

Testosterone Propionate (Duloxetine is a moderate inhibitor of CYP2D6. Co-administration of duloxetine with other drugs that are extensively metabolized by this isoenzyme, and which have a narrow therapeutic window, should be approached with caution).
No products indexed under this heading.

Thiamylal Sodium (Given the primary CNS effects of duloxetine, it should be used with caution when it is taken in combination with or substituted for other centrally acting drugs, including those with a similar mechanism of action).
No products indexed under this heading.

Thioridazine (Duloxetine is a moderate inhibitor of CYP2D6. Co-administration of duloxetine with other drugs that are extensively metabolized by this isoenzyme, and which have a narrow therapeutic window, should be approached with caution. Because of the risk of serious ventricular arrhythmias and sudden death potentially associated with elevated plasma levels of thioridazine, duloxetine and thioridazine should not be co-administered).
No products indexed under this heading.

Thioridazine Hydrochloride (Duloxetine is a moderate inhibitor of CYP2D6. Co-administration of duloxetine with other drugs that are extensively metabolized by this isoenzyme, and which have a narrow therapeutic window, should be approached with caution. Because of the risk of serious ventricular arrhythmias and sudden death potentially associated with elevated plasma levels of thioridazine, duloxetine and thioridazine should not be co-administered). Products include:
Thioridazine Hydrochloride Tablets 2163

Thiothixene (Given the primary CNS effects of duloxetine, it should be used with caution when it is taken in combination with or substituted for other centrally acting drugs, including those with a similar mechanism of action). Products include:
Thiothixene Capsules 2165

Ticlopidine Hydrochloride (Concomitant use of duloxetine with fluvoxamine, an inhibitor of CYP1A2, results in a 6-fold increase in AUC, about 2.5-fold increase in Cmax, and an approximately 3-fold increase in t1/2 of duloxetine. Since duloxetine is metabolized in part by CYP1A2, concomitant use of duloxetine with other inhibitors of CYP1A2, would be expected to have the same effects; these combinations should be avoided). Products include:
Ticlid Tablets 2810

Timolol Maleate (Duloxetine is a moderate inhibitor of CYP2D6. Co-administration of duloxetine with other drugs that are extensively metabolized by this isoenzyme, and which have a narrow therapeutic window, should be approached with caution). Products include:
Blocadren Tablets 1916
Cosopt Sterile Ophthalmic Solution 1931
Timolide Tablets 2086
Timoptic Sterile Ophthalmic Solution 2088
Timoptic in Ocudose 2091
Timoptic-XE Sterile Ophthalmic Gel Forming Solution 2092

Tolterodine Tartrate (Duloxetine is a moderate inhibitor of CYP2D6. Co-administration of duloxetine with other drugs that are extensively metabolized by this isoenzyme, and which have a narrow therapeutic window, should be approached with caution). Products include:
Detrol Tablets 2628
Detrol LA Capsules 2631

Tramadol Hydrochloride (Caution is advised with co-administration of duloxetine with drugs that may affect the serotonergic neurotransmitter systems such as lithium because of potential development of serotonin syndrome). Products include:
Ultram ER Tablets 2392

Tranylcypromine Sulfate (There have been reports of serious, sometimes fatal, reactions in patients receiving a serotonin reuptake inhibitor in combination with a monoamine oxidase inhibitor (MAOI). These reactions have also been reported in patients who have recently discontinued serotonin reuptake inhibitors and are started on an MAOI. Therefore, duloxetine use is contraindicated in combination with an MAOI, or within at least 14 days of discontinuing treatment with an MAOI. Based on the half-life of duloxetine, at least 5 days should be allowed after stopping duloxetine before starting an MAOI. Development of a potentially life-threatening serotonin syndrome may occur with concomitant use of duloxetine HCl and drugs which impair the metabolism of serotonin (e.g., MAOIs)). Products include:
Parnate Tablets 1527

Trazodone Hydrochloride (Duloxetine is a moderate inhibitor of CYP2D6. Co-administration of duloxetine with other drugs that are extensively metabolized by this isoenzyme, and which have a narrow therapeutic window, should be approached with caution).
No products indexed under this heading.

Triazolam (Duloxetine is a moderate inhibitor of CYP2D6. Co-administration of duloxetine with other drugs that are extensively metabolized by this isoenzyme, and which have a narrow therapeutic window, should be approached with caution).
No products indexed under this heading.

Trifluoperazine Hydrochloride (Duloxetine is a moderate inhibitor of CYP2D6. Co-administration of duloxetine with other drugs that are extensively metabolized by this isoenzyme, and which have a narrow therapeutic window, should be approached with caution).
No products indexed under this heading.

Trimipramine Maleate (Duloxetine is a moderate inhibitor of CYP2D6. Co-administration of duloxetine with other drugs that are extensively metabolized by this isoenzyme, and which have a narrow therapeutic window, should be approached with caution. Plasma tricyclic antidepressant (TCA) concentrations may need to be monitored, and the dose of the TCA may need to be reduced, if a TCA is co-administered with duloxetine).
No products indexed under this heading.

Troleandomycin (Concomitant use of duloxetine with fluvoxamine, an inhibitor of CYP1A2, results in a 6-fold increase in AUC, about 2.5-fold increase in Cmax, and an approximately 3-fold increase in t1/2 of duloxetine. Since duloxetine is metabolized in part by CYP1A2, concomitant use of duloxetine with other inhibitors of CYP1A2, would be expected to have the same effects; these combinations should be avoided).
No products indexed under this heading.

Trovafloxacin Mesylate (Concomitant use of duloxetine with fluvoxamine, an inhibitor of CYP1A2, results in a 6-fold increase in AUC, about 2.5-fold increase in Cmax, and an approximately 3-fold increase in t1/2 of duloxetine. Since duloxetine is metabolized in part by CYP1A2, concomitant use of duloxetine with other inhibitors of CYP1A2, would be expected to have the same effects; these combinations should be avoided).
No products indexed under this heading.

Tryptophan (Concomitant use of duloxetine with serotonin precursors (e.g., tryptophan) is not recommended).
No products indexed under this heading.

Venlafaxine Hydrochloride (Development of a potentially life-threatening serotonin syndrome may occur with concomitant use of duloxetine HCl and serotonergic drugs). Products include:

Effexor Tablets **3411**
Effexor XR Capsules **3417**

Vinblastine Sulfate (Duloxetine is a moderate inhibitor of CYP2D6. Co-administration of duloxetine with other drugs that are extensively metabolized by this isoenzyme, and which have a narrow therapeutic window, should be approached with caution).
No products indexed under this heading.

Zaleplon (Given the primary CNS effects of duloxetine, it should be used with caution when it is taken in combination with or substituted for other centrally acting drugs, including those with a similar mechanism of action). Products include:
Sonata Capsules **1717**

Zileuton (Concomitant use of duloxetine with fluvoxamine, an inhibitor of CYP1A2, results in a 6-fold increase in AUC, about 2.5-fold increase in Cmax, and an approximately 3-fold increase in t1/2 of duloxetine. Since duloxetine is metabolized in part by CYP1A2, concomitant use of duloxetine with other inhibitors of CYP1A2, would be expected to have the same effects; these combinations should be avoided). Products include:
Zyflo Tablets **1023**

Ziprasidone Hydrochloride (Given the primary CNS effects of duloxetine, it should be used with caution when it is taken in combination with or substituted for other centrally acting drugs, including those with a similar mechanism of action). Products include:
Geodon Capsules **2529**

Zolmitriptan (Development of a potentially life-threatening serotonin syndrome may occur with concomitant use of duloxetine HCl and triptans. If concomitant treatment is clinically warranted, careful observation of the patient is advised, particularly during treatment initiation and dose increases). Products include:
Zomig Tablets **3519**
Zomig Nasal Spray **3523**
Zomig-ZMT Tablets **3519**

Zolpidem Tartrate (Given the primary CNS effects of duloxetine, it should be used with caution when it is taken in combination with or substituted for other centrally acting drugs, including those with a similar mechanism of action). Products include:
Ambien Tablets **2851**
Ambien CR Tablets **2855**

Zonisamide (Duloxetine is a moderate inhibitor of CYP2D6. Co-administration of duloxetine with other drugs that are extensively metabolized by this isoenzyme, and which have a narrow therapeutic window, should be approached with caution). Products include:
Zonegran Capsules **1101**

Food Interactions

Alcohol (Use of duloxetine concomitantly with heavy alcohol intake may be associated with severe liver injury; therefore, duloxetine should ordinarily not be prescribed for patients with substantial alcohol use).

Grapefruit Juice (Concomitant use of duloxetine with fluvoxamine, an inhibitor of CYP1A2, results in a 6-fold increase in AUC, about 2.5-fold increase in Cmax, and an approximately 3-fold increase in t1/2 of duloxetine. Since duloxetine is metabolized in part by CYP1A2, concomitant use of duloxetine with other inhibitors of CYP1A2, would be expected to have the same effects; these combinations should be avoided).

CYTOGAM INTRAVENOUS

(Cytomegalovirus Immune Globulin) ... **1895**
May interact with:

Measles, Mumps & Rubella Virus Vaccine, Live (May interfere with the immune response to live virus vaccine). Products include:
M-M-R II **2006**

CYTOMEL TABLETS

(Liothyronine Sodium) **1710**
May interact with estrogens, cardiac glycosides, oral hypoglycemic agents, insulin, tricyclic antidepressants, and certain other agents. Compounds in these categories include:

Acarbose (Initiating thyroid replacement therapy may cause increases in oral hypoglycemic requirements). Products include:
Precose Tablets **751**

Amitriptyline Hydrochloride (Use of thyroid hormones may increase receptor sensitivity and enhance antidepressant activity; transient cardiac arrhythmias; thyroid hormone activity may also be enhanced).
No products indexed under this heading.

Amoxapine (Use of thyroid hormones may increase receptor sensitivity and enhance antidepressant activity; transient cardiac arrhythmias; thyroid hormone activity may also be enhanced).
No products indexed under this heading.

Anisindione (Thyroid hormones appear to increase catabolism of vitamin K-dependent clotting factor; if oral anticoagulants are also given compensatory increases in clotting factor synthesis are impaired). Products include:
Miradon Tablets **3042**

Chlorotrianisene (Estrogens tend to increase serum thyroxine-binding globulin in a patient with a nonfunctioning thyroid gland who is receiving thyroid replacement therapy; patients without functioning thyroid gland who are on thyroid replacement therapy may need to increase their thyroid dose if estrogens or estrogen-containing oral contraceptives are given).
No products indexed under this heading.

Chlorpropamide (Initiating thyroid replacement therapy may cause increases in oral hypoglycemic requirements).
No products indexed under this heading.

Cholestyramine (Binds both T4 and T3 in the intestine thus impairing absorption of thyroid hormones; 4 to 5 hours should elapse between administration of thyroid hormone and cholestyramine).
No products indexed under this heading.

Clomipramine Hydrochloride (Use of thyroid hormones may increase receptor sensitivity and enhance antidepressant activity; transient cardiac arrhythmias; thyroid hormone activity may also be enhanced).
No products indexed under this heading.

Desipramine Hydrochloride (Use of thyroid hormones may increase receptor sensitivity and enhance antidepressant activity; transient cardiac arrhythmias; thyroid hormone activity may also be enhanced).
No products indexed under this heading.

Deslanoside (Thyroid preparations may potentiate the toxic effects of digitalis; thyroid hormone increase metabolic rate which requires an increase in digitalis dosage).
No products indexed under this heading.

Dicumarol (Thyroid hormones appear to increase catabolism of vitamin K-dependent clotting factor; if oral anticoagulants are also given compensatory increases in clotting factor synthesis are impaired).
No products indexed under this heading.

Dienestrol (Estrogens tend to increase serum thyroxine-binding globulin in a patient with a nonfunctioning thyroid gland who is receiving thyroid replacement therapy; patients without functioning thyroid gland who are on thyroid replacement therapy may need to increase their thyroid dose if estrogens or estrogen-containing oral contraceptives are given).
No products indexed under this heading.

Diethylstilbestrol (Estrogens tend to increase serum thyroxine-binding globulin in a patient with a nonfunctioning thyroid gland who is receiving thyroid replacement therapy; patients without functioning thyroid gland who are on thyroid replacement therapy may need to increase their thyroid dose if estrogens or estrogen-containing oral contraceptives are given).
No products indexed under this heading.

Digitalis Glycoside Preparations (Thyroid preparations may potentiate the toxic effects of digitalis; thyroid hormone increase metabolic rate which requires an increase in digitalis dosage).
No products indexed under this heading.

Digitoxin (Thyroid preparations may potentiate the toxic effects of digitalis; thyroid hormone increase metabolic rate which requires an increase in digitalis dosage).
No products indexed under this heading.

Digoxin (Thyroid preparations may potentiate the toxic effects of digitalis; thyroid hormone increase metabolic rate which requires an increase in digitalis dosage). Products include:
Lanoxicaps Capsules **1490**
Lanoxin Injection **1494**
Lanoxin Injection Pediatric **1497**
Lanoxin Tablets **1500**

Doxepin Hydrochloride (Use of thyroid hormones may increase receptor sensitivity and enhance antidepressant activity; transient cardiac arrhythmias; thyroid hormone activity may also be enhanced).
No products indexed under this heading.

Epinephrine (Thyroxine increases the adrenergic effect of catecholamines, such as epinephrine). Products include:
EpiPen **1061**
Primatene Mist .... ▣ **719**
Twinject 0.15 .... **3379**
Twinject 0.3 .... **3378**

Epinephrine Bitartrate (Thyroxine increases the adrenergic effect of catecholamines, such as epinephrine).
No products indexed under this heading.

Epinephrine Hydrochloride (Thyroxine increases the adrenergic effect of catecholamines, such as epinephrine).
No products indexed under this heading.

Estradiol (Estrogens tend to increase serum thyroxine-binding globulin in a patient with a nonfunctioning thyroid gland who is receiving thyroid replacement therapy; patients without functioning thyroid gland who are on thyroid replacement therapy may need to increase their thyroid dose if estrogens or estrogen-containing oral contraceptives are given). Products include:
Angeliq Tablets **762**
Climara Transdermal System **771**
Climara Pro Transdermal System **776**
Estrasorb Topical Emulsion **1147**
Estring Vaginal Ring **2635**
Menostar Transdermal System **782**
Vagifem Tablets **2334**

Estrogens, Conjugated (Estrogens tend to increase serum thyroxine-binding globulin in a patient with a nonfunctioning thyroid gland who is receiving thyroid replacement therapy; patients without functioning thyroid gland who are on thyroid replacement therapy may need to increase their thyroid dose if estrogens or estrogen-containing oral contraceptives are given). Products include:
Premarin Intravenous **3442**
Premarin Tablets **3446**
Premarin Vaginal Cream **3452**
Premphase Tablets **3456**
Prempro Tablets **3456**

Estrogens, Esterified (Estrogens tend to increase serum thyroxine-binding globulin in a patient with a nonfunctioning thyroid gland who is receiving thyroid replacement therapy; patients without functioning thyroid gland who are on thyroid replacement therapy may need to increase their thyroid dose if estrogens or estrogen-containing oral contraceptives are given). Products include:
Estratest Tablets **3199**
Estratest H.S. Tablets **3199**

Estropipate (Estrogens tend to increase serum thyroxine-binding globulin in a patient with a nonfunctioning thyroid gland who is receiving thyroid replacement therapy; patients without functioning thyroid gland who are on thyroid replacement therapy may need to increase their thyroid dose if estrogens or estrogen-containing oral contraceptives are given).
No products indexed under this heading.

Ethinyl Estradiol (Estrogens tend to increase serum thyroxine-binding globulin in a patient with a nonfunctioning thyroid gland who is receiving thyroid replacement therapy; patients without functioning thyroid gland who are on thyroid replacement therapy may need to increase their thyroid dose if estrogens or estrogen-containing oral contraceptives are given). Products include:
Mircette Tablets ... **1066**
NuvaRing ... **2340**
Ortho-Cyclen/Ortho Tri-Cyclen ... **2429**
Ortho Evra Transdermal System ... **2417**
Ortho Tri-Cyclen Lo Tablets ... **2436**
Seasonique Tablets ... **1077**
Yasmin 28 Tablets ... **796**
Yaz Tablets ... **803**

Glimepiride (Initiating thyroid replacement therapy may cause increases in oral hypoglycemic requirements). Products include:
Avandaryl Tablets ... **1379**
Duetact Tablets ... **3226**

Glipizide (Initiating thyroid replacement therapy may cause increases in oral hypoglycemic requirements).
No products indexed under this heading.

Glyburide (Initiating thyroid replacement therapy may cause increases in oral hypoglycemic requirements).
No products indexed under this heading.

Imipramine Hydrochloride (Use of thyroid hormones may increase receptor sensitivity and enhance antidepressant activity; transient cardiac arrhythmias; thyroid hormone activity may also be enhanced).
No products indexed under this heading.

Imipramine Pamoate (Use of thyroid hormones may increase receptor sensitivity and enhance antidepressant activity; transient cardiac arrhythmias; thyroid hormone activity may also be enhanced).
No products indexed under this heading.

Insulin, Human, Zinc Suspension (Initiating thyroid replacement therapy may cause increases in insulin requirements). Products include:
Humulin L, 100 Units ... **1794**
Humulin U, 100 Units ... **1800**

Insulin, Human NPH (Initiating thyroid replacement therapy may cause increases in insulin requirements). Products include:
Humulin N, 100 Units ... **1795**
Humulin N Pen ... **1797**

Insulin, Human Regular (Initiating thyroid replacement therapy may cause increases in insulin requirements). Products include:
Humulin R, 100 Units ... **1798**

Insulin, Human Regular and Human NPH Mixture (Initiating thyroid replacement therapy may cause increases in insulin requirements). Products include:
Humulin 50/50, 100 Units ... **1791**
Humulin 70/30 Pen ... **1793**

Insulin, NPH (Initiating thyroid replacement therapy may cause increases in insulin requirements).
No products indexed under this heading.

Insulin, Regular (Initiating thyroid replacement therapy may cause increases in insulin requirements).
No products indexed under this heading.

Insulin, Zinc Crystals (Initiating thyroid replacement therapy may cause increases in insulin requirements).
No products indexed under this heading.

Insulin, Zinc Suspension (Initiating thyroid replacement therapy may cause increases in insulin requirements).
No products indexed under this heading.

Insulin Aspart, Human Regular (Initiating thyroid replacement therapy may cause increases in insulin requirements). Products include:
NovoLog Injection ... **2326**

Insulin glargine (Initiating thyroid replacement therapy may cause increases in insulin requirements). Products include:
Lantus Injection ... **2909**

Insulin Lispro, Human (Initiating thyroid replacement therapy may cause increases in insulin requirements). Products include:
Humalog-Pen ... **1781**
Humalog Mix 50/50-Pen ... **1783**
Humalog Mix 75/25-Pen ... **1785**

Insulin Lispro Protamine, Human (Initiating thyroid replacement therapy may cause increases in insulin requirements). Products include:
Humalog Mix 50/50-Pen ... **1783**
Humalog Mix 75/25-Pen ... **1785**

Ketamine Hydrochloride (Co-administration may cause hypertension and tachycardia).
No products indexed under this heading.

Maprotiline Hydrochloride (Use of thyroid hormones may increase receptor sensitivity and enhance antidepressant activity; transient cardiac arrhythmias; thyroid hormone activity may also be enhanced).
No products indexed under this heading.

Metformin Hydrochloride (Initiating thyroid replacement therapy may cause increases in oral hypoglycemic requirements). Products include:
ActoPlus Met Tablets ... **3214**
Avandamet Tablets ... **1373**
Fortamet Extended-Release Tablets ... **3115**

Miglitol (Initiating thyroid replacement therapy may cause increases in oral hypoglycemic requirements).
No products indexed under this heading.

Norepinephrine Hydrochloride (Thyroxine increases the adrenergic effect of catecholamines, such as norepinephrine).
No products indexed under this heading.

Nortriptyline Hydrochloride (Use of thyroid hormones may increase receptor sensitivity and enhance antidepressant activity; transient cardiac arrhythmias; thyroid hormone activity may also be enhanced).
No products indexed under this heading.

Pioglitazone Hydrochloride (Initiating thyroid replacement therapy may cause increases in oral hypoglycemic requirements). Products include:
ActoPlus Met Tablets ... **3214**
Actos Tablets ... **3219**
Duetact Tablets ... **3226**

Polyestradiol Phosphate (Estrogens tend to increase serum thyroxine-binding globulin in a patient with a nonfunctioning thyroid gland who is receiving thyroid replacement therapy; patients without functioning thyroid gland who are on thyroid replacement therapy may need to increase their thyroid dose if estrogens or estrogen-containing oral contraceptives are given).
No products indexed under this heading.

Protriptyline Hydrochloride (Use of thyroid hormones may increase receptor sensitivity and enhance antidepressant activity; transient cardiac arrhythmias; thyroid hormone activity may also be enhanced).
No products indexed under this heading.

Quinestrol (Estrogens tend to increase serum thyroxine-binding globulin in a patient with a nonfunctioning thyroid gland who is receiving thyroid replacement therapy; patients without functioning thyroid gland who are on thyroid replacement therapy may need to increase their thyroid dose if estrogens or estrogen-containing oral contraceptives are given).
No products indexed under this heading.

Repaglinide (Initiating thyroid replacement therapy may cause increases in oral hypoglycemic requirements).
No products indexed under this heading.

Rosiglitazone Maleate (Initiating thyroid replacement therapy may cause increases in oral hypoglycemic requirements). Products include:
Avandamet Tablets ... **1373**
Avandaryl Tablets ... **1379**
Avandia Tablets ... **1384**

Tolazamide (Initiating thyroid replacement therapy may cause increases in oral hypoglycemic requirements).
No products indexed under this heading.

Tolbutamide (Initiating thyroid replacement therapy may cause increases in oral hypoglycemic requirements).
No products indexed under this heading.

Trimipramine Maleate (Use of thyroid hormones may increase receptor sensitivity and enhance antidepressant activity; transient cardiac arrhythmias; thyroid hormone activity may also be enhanced).
No products indexed under this heading.

Troglitazone (Initiating thyroid replacement therapy may cause increases in oral hypoglycemic requirements).
No products indexed under this heading.

Warfarin Sodium (Thyroid hormones appear to increase catabolism of vitamin K-dependent clotting factor; if oral anticoagulants are also given compensatory increases in clotting factor synthesis are impaired). Products include:
Coumadin for Injection ... **898**
Coumadin Tablets ... **898**

DACOGEN INJECTION

(Decitabine) ... **2129**
None cited in PDR database.

DAILY COMPLETE LIQUID

(Aloe vera, Amino Acid Preparations, Antioxidants, Herbals with Vitamins & Minerals) ... **827**
None cited in PDR database.

DALMANE CAPSULES

(Flurazepam Hydrochloride) ... **3342**
None cited in PDR database.

DANTRIUM CAPSULES

(Dantrolene Sodium) ... **2694**
May interact with calcium channel blockers, central nervous system depressants, estrogens, hypnotics and sedatives, tranquilizers, and certain other agents. Compounds in these categories include:

Alfentanil Hydrochloride (Co-administration may result in increased drowsiness; caution should be exercised).
No products indexed under this heading.

Alprazolam (Co-administration may result in increased drowsiness; caution should be exercised). Products include:
Niravam Orally Disintegrating Tablets ... **3092**

Amlodipine Besylate (Due to interaction between verapamil and dantrolene, combination of dantrolene and calcium channel blockers is not recommended during the management of malignant hyperthermia). Products include:
Caduet Tablets ... **2508**
Lotrel Capsules ... **2249**
Norvasc Tablets ... **2545**

Aprobarbital (Co-administration may result in increased drowsiness; caution should be exercised).
No products indexed under this heading.

Bepridil Hydrochloride (Due to interaction between verapamil and dantrolene, combination of dantrolene and calcium channel blockers is not recommended during the management of malignant hyperthermia).
No products indexed under this heading.

Buprenorphine Hydrochloride (Co-administration may result in increased drowsiness; caution should be exercised). Products include:
Buprenex Injectable ... **2716**
Suboxone Tablets ... **2717**
Subutex Tablets ... **2717**

Buspirone Hydrochloride (Co-administration may result in increased drowsiness; caution should be exercised).
No products indexed under this heading.

IMPORTANT NOTE: Always consult each drug listing in the patient's regimen for possible interactions.

Butabarbital (Co-administration may result in increased drowsiness; caution should be exercised).
No products indexed under this heading.

Butalbital (Co-administration may result in increased drowsiness; caution should be exercised).
No products indexed under this heading.

Chlordiazepoxide (Co-administration may result in increased drowsiness; caution should be exercised).
No products indexed under this heading.

Chlordiazepoxide Hydrochloride (Co-administration may result in increased drowsiness; caution should be exercised). Products include:
Librium Capsules 3347

Chlorotrianisene (Hepatotoxicity has occurred more often in women over 35 years of age receiving concomitant estrogen therapy).
No products indexed under this heading.

Chlorpromazine (Co-administration may result in increased drowsiness; caution should be exercised).
No products indexed under this heading.

Chlorpromazine Hydrochloride (Co-administration may result in increased drowsiness; caution should be exercised).
No products indexed under this heading.

Chlorprothixene (Co-administration may result in increased drowsiness; caution should be exercised).
No products indexed under this heading.

Chlorprothixene Hydrochloride (Co-administration may result in increased drowsiness; caution should be exercised).
No products indexed under this heading.

Chlorprothixene Lactate (Co-administration may result in increased drowsiness; caution should be exercised).
No products indexed under this heading.

Clorazepate Dipotassium (Co-administration may result in increased drowsiness; caution should be exercised). Products include:
Tranxene 2474

Clozapine (Co-administration may result in increased drowsiness; caution should be exercised). Products include:
Clozaril Tablets 2184
FazaClo Orally Disintegrating Tablets 551

Codeine Phosphate (Co-administration may result in increased drowsiness; caution should be exercised). Products include:
Tylenol with Codeine Tablets 2391

Desflurane (Co-administration may result in increased drowsiness; caution should be exercised).
No products indexed under this heading.

Dezocine (Co-administration may result in increased drowsiness; caution should be exercised).
No products indexed under this heading.

Diazepam (Co-administration may result in increased drowsiness; caution should be exercised). Products include:
Diastat Rectal Delivery System 3343
Valium Tablets 2819

Dienestrol (Hepatotoxicity has occurred more often in women over 35 years of age receiving concomitant estrogen therapy).
No products indexed under this heading.

Diethylstilbestrol (Hepatotoxicity has occurred more often in women over 35 years of age receiving concomitant estrogen therapy).
No products indexed under this heading.

Diltiazem Hydrochloride (Due to interaction between verapamil and dantrolene, combination of dantrolene and calcium channel blockers is not recommended during the management of malignant hyperthermia). Products include:
Cardizem LA Extended Release Tablets 1728
Tiazac Capsules 1201

Droperidol (Co-administration may result in increased drowsiness; caution should be exercised).
No products indexed under this heading.

Enflurane (Co-administration may result in increased drowsiness; caution should be exercised).
No products indexed under this heading.

Estazolam (Co-administration may result in increased drowsiness; caution should be exercised). Products include:
ProSom Tablets 517

Estradiol (Hepatotoxicity has occurred more often in women over 35 years of age receiving concomitant estrogen therapy). Products include:
Angeliq Tablets 762
Climara Transdermal System 771
Climara Pro Transdermal System 776
Estrasorb Topical Emulsion 1147
Estring Vaginal Ring 2635
Menostar Transdermal System 782
Vagifem Tablets 2334

Estrogens, Conjugated (Hepatotoxicity has occurred more often in women over 35 years of age receiving concomitant estrogen therapy). Products include:
Premarin Intravenous 3442
Premarin Tablets 3446
Premarin Vaginal Cream 3452
Premphase Tablets 3456
Prempro Tablets 3456

Estrogens, Esterified (Hepatotoxicity has occurred more often in women over 35 years of age receiving concomitant estrogen therapy). Products include:
Estratest Tablets 3199
Estratest H.S. Tablets 3199

Estropipate (Hepatotoxicity has occurred more often in women over 35 years of age receiving concomitant estrogen therapy).
No products indexed under this heading.

Ethanol (Co-administration may result in increased drowsiness; caution should be exercised).
No products indexed under this heading.

Ethchlorvynol (Co-administration may result in increased drowsiness; caution should be exercised).
No products indexed under this heading.

Ethinamate (Co-administration may result in increased drowsiness; caution should be exercised).
No products indexed under this heading.

Ethinyl Estradiol (Hepatotoxicity has occurred more often in women over 35 years of age receiving concomitant estrogen therapy). Products include:
Mircette Tablets 1066
NuvaRing 2340
Ortho-Cyclen/Ortho Tri-Cyclen 2429
Ortho Evra Transdermal System 2417
Ortho Tri-Cyclen Lo Tablets 2436
Seasonique Tablets 1077
Yasmin 28 Tablets 796
Yaz Tablets 803

Ethyl Alcohol (Co-administration may result in increased drowsiness; caution should be exercised).
No products indexed under this heading.

Felodipine (Due to interaction between verapamil and dantrolene, combination of dantrolene and calcium channel blockers is not recommended during the management of malignant hyperthermia).
No products indexed under this heading.

Fentanyl (Co-administration may result in increased drowsiness; caution should be exercised). Products include:
Duragesic Transdermal System 2373
Ionsys Transdermal System 2379

Fentanyl Citrate (Co-administration may result in increased drowsiness; caution should be exercised). Products include:
Actiq 979

Fluphenazine Decanoate (Co-administration may result in increased drowsiness; caution should be exercised).
No products indexed under this heading.

Fluphenazine Enanthate (Co-administration may result in increased drowsiness; caution should be exercised).
No products indexed under this heading.

Fluphenazine Hydrochloride (Co-administration may result in increased drowsiness; caution should be exercised).
No products indexed under this heading.

Flurazepam Hydrochloride (Co-administration may result in increased drowsiness; caution should be exercised). Products include:
Dalmane Capsules 3342

Glutethimide (Co-administration may result in increased drowsiness; caution should be exercised).
No products indexed under this heading.

Haloperidol (Co-administration may result in increased drowsiness; caution should be exercised).
No products indexed under this heading.

Haloperidol Decanoate (Co-administration may result in increased drowsiness; caution should be exercised).
No products indexed under this heading.

Hydrocodone Bitartrate (Co-administration may result in increased drowsiness; caution should be exercised). Products include:
Hycodan 1116
Hycotuss Expectorant Syrup 1117
Vicodin Tablets 535
Vicodin ES Tablets 536
Vicodin HP Tablets 538
Vicoprofen Tablets 539
Zydone Tablets 1139

Hydrocodone Polistirex (Co-administration may result in increased drowsiness; caution should be exercised). Products include:
Tussionex Pennkinetic Extended-Release Suspension 3327

Hydromorphone Hydrochloride (Co-administration may result in increased drowsiness; caution should be exercised). Products include:
Dilaudid 440
Dilaudid Non-Sterile Powder 440
Dilaudid Oral Liquid 445
Dilaudid Rectal Suppositories 440
Dilaudid Tablets 440
Dilaudid Tablets - 8 mg 445
Dilaudid-HP 442

Hydroxyzine Hydrochloride (Co-administration may result in increased drowsiness; caution should be exercised).
No products indexed under this heading.

Isoflurane (Co-administration may result in increased drowsiness; caution should be exercised).
No products indexed under this heading.

Isradipine (Due to interaction between verapamil and dantrolene, combination of dantrolene and calcium channel blockers is not recommended during the management of malignant hyperthermia). Products include:
DynaCirc CR Tablets 2721

Ketamine Hydrochloride (Co-administration may result in increased drowsiness; caution should be exercised).
No products indexed under this heading.

Levomethadyl Acetate Hydrochloride (Co-administration may result in increased drowsiness; caution should be exercised).
No products indexed under this heading.

Levorphanol Tartrate (Co-administration may result in increased drowsiness; caution should be exercised).
No products indexed under this heading.

Lorazepam (Co-administration may result in increased drowsiness; caution should be exercised).
No products indexed under this heading.

Loxapine Hydrochloride (Co-administration may result in increased drowsiness; caution should be exercised).
No products indexed under this heading.

Loxapine Succinate (Co-administration may result in increased drowsiness; caution should be exercised).
No products indexed under this heading.

Meperidine Hydrochloride (Co-administration may result in increased drowsiness; caution should be exercised).
No products indexed under this heading.

Mephobarbital (Co-administration may result in increased drowsiness; caution should be exercised).
No products indexed under this heading.

Meprobamate (Co-administration may result in increased drowsiness; caution should be exercised).
No products indexed under this heading.

Mesoridazine Besylate (Co-administration may result in increased drowsiness; caution should be exercised).
No products indexed under this heading.

Methadone Hydrochloride (Co-administration may result in increased drowsiness; caution should be exercised).
No products indexed under this heading.

Methohexital Sodium (Co-administration may result in increased drowsiness; caution should be exercised).
No products indexed under this heading.

Methotrimeprazine (Co-administration may result in increased drowsiness; caution should be exercised).
No products indexed under this heading.

Methoxyflurane (Co-administration may result in increased drowsiness; caution should be exercised).
No products indexed under this heading.

Mibefradil Dihydrochloride (Due to interaction between verapamil and dantrolene, combination of dantrolene and calcium channel blockers is not recommended during the management of malignant hyperthermia).
No products indexed under this heading.

Midazolam Hydrochloride (Co-administration may result in increased drowsiness; caution should be exercised).
No products indexed under this heading.

Molindone Hydrochloride (Co-administration may result in increased drowsiness; caution should be exercised). Products include:
Moban Tablets 1119

Morphine Sulfate (Co-administration may result in increased drowsiness; caution should be exercised). Products include:
Avinza Capsules 1741
Kadian Capsules 577
MS Contin Tablets 2701

Nicardipine Hydrochloride (Due to interaction between verapamil and dantrolene, combination of dantrolene and calcium channel blockers is not recommended during the management of malignant hyperthermia). Products include:
Cardene I.V. 2497

Nifedipine (Due to interaction between verapamil and dantrolene, combination of dantrolene and calcium channel blockers is not recommended during the management of malignant hyperthermia). Products include:
Adalat CC Tablets 2964

Nimodipine (Due to interaction between verapamil and dantrolene, combination of dantrolene and calcium channel blockers is not recommended during the management of malignant hyperthermia). Products include:
Nimotop Capsules 749

Nisoldipine (Due to interaction between verapamil and dantrolene, combination of dantrolene and calcium channel blockers is not recommended during the management of malignant hyperthermia). Products include:
Sular Tablets 3122

Olanzapine (Co-administration may result in increased drowsiness; caution should be exercised). Products include:
Symbyax Capsules 1819
Zyprexa Tablets 1830
Zyprexa IntraMuscular 1830
Zyprexa ZYDIS Orally
Disintegrating Tablets.................. 1830

Oxazepam (Co-administration may result in increased drowsiness; caution should be exercised).
No products indexed under this heading.

Oxycodone Hydrochloride (Co-administration may result in increased drowsiness; caution should be exercised). Products include:
OxyContin Tablets 2703
OxyFast Oral Concentrate
Solution 2708
OxyIR Capsules 2708
Percocet Tablets 1131
Percodan Tablets 1132

Pentobarbital Sodium (Co-administration may result in increased drowsiness; caution should be exercised). Products include:
Nembutal Sodium Solution, USP 2470

Perphenazine (Co-administration may result in increased drowsiness; caution should be exercised).
No products indexed under this heading.

Phenobarbital (Co-administration may result in increased drowsiness; caution should be exercised). Products include:
Donnatal Extentabs 2493

Polyestradiol Phosphate (Hepatotoxicity has occurred more often in women over 35 years of age receiving concomitant estrogen therapy).
No products indexed under this heading.

Prazepam (Co-administration may result in increased drowsiness; caution should be exercised).
No products indexed under this heading.

Prochlorperazine (Co-administration may result in increased drowsiness; caution should be exercised).
No products indexed under this heading.

Promethazine Hydrochloride (Co-administration may result in increased drowsiness; caution should be exercised). Products include:
Phenergan Tablets and
Suppositories.............................. 3440

Propofol (Co-administration may result in increased drowsiness; caution should be exercised).
No products indexed under this heading.

Propoxyphene Hydrochloride (Co-administration may result in increased drowsiness; caution should be exercised).
No products indexed under this heading.

Propoxyphene Napsylate (Co-administration may result in increased drowsiness; caution should be exercised).
No products indexed under this heading.

Quazepam (Co-administration may result in increased drowsiness; caution should be exercised).
No products indexed under this heading.

Quetiapine Fumarate (Co-administration may result in increased drowsiness; caution should be exercised). Products include:
Seroquel Tablets 690

Quinestrol (Hepatotoxicity has occurred more often in women over 35 years of age receiving concomitant estrogen therapy).
No products indexed under this heading.

Ramelteon (Co-administration may result in increased drowsiness; caution should be exercised). Products include:
Rozerem Tablets 3231

Remifentanil Hydrochloride (Co-administration may result in increased drowsiness; caution should be exercised).
No products indexed under this heading.

Risperidone (Co-administration may result in increased drowsiness; caution should be exercised). Products include:
Risperdal 1676
Risperdal Consta Long-Acting
Injection 1682
Risperdal M-Tab Orally
Disintegrating Tablets.................. 1676

Secobarbital Sodium (Co-administration may result in increased drowsiness; caution should be exercised).
No products indexed under this heading.

Sevoflurane (Co-administration may result in increased drowsiness; caution should be exercised). Products include:
Ultane Liquid for Inhalation 531

Sufentanil Citrate (Co-administration may result in increased drowsiness; caution should be exercised).
No products indexed under this heading.

Temazepam (Co-administration may result in increased drowsiness; caution should be exercised). Products include:
Restoril Capsules 1860

Thiamylal Sodium (Co-administration may result in increased drowsiness; caution should be exercised).
No products indexed under this heading.

Thioridazine Hydrochloride (Co-administration may result in increased drowsiness; caution should be exercised). Products include:
Thioridazine Hydrochloride
Tablets............................... 2163

Thiothixene (Co-administration may result in increased drowsiness; caution should be exercised). Products include:
Thiothixene Capsules 2165

Triazolam (Co-administration may result in increased drowsiness; caution should be exercised).
No products indexed under this heading.

Trifluoperazine Hydrochloride (Co-administration may result in increased drowsiness; caution should be exercised).
No products indexed under this heading.

Vecuronium Bromide (Co-administration may result in potentiation of vecuronium-induced neuromuscular block).
No products indexed under this heading.

Verapamil Hydrochloride (Simultaneous use has resulted in rare cases of cardiovascular collapse). Products include:
Covera-HS Tablets 3139
Tarka Tablets 524
Verelan PM Extended-Release
Capsules, Controlled-Onset........... 3106

Zaleplon (Co-administration may result in increased drowsiness; caution should be exercised). Products include:
Sonata Capsules 1717

Ziprasidone Hydrochloride (Co-administration may result in increased drowsiness; caution should be exercised). Products include:
Geodon Capsules 2529

Zolpidem Tartrate (Co-administration may result in increased drowsiness; caution should be exercised). Products include:
Ambien Tablets 2851
Ambien CR Tablets 2855

Food Interactions

Alcohol (Co-administration may result in increased drowsiness; caution should be exercised).

DANTRIUM INTRAVENOUS
(Dantrolene Sodium) 2695
May interact with:

Clofibrate (Reduces binding of dantrolene to plasma proteins).
No products indexed under this heading.

Tolbutamide (Increases binding of dantrolene to plasma proteins).
No products indexed under this heading.

Vecuronium Bromide (Administration of dantrolene may potentiate vecuronium-induced neuromuscular block).
No products indexed under this heading.

Verapamil Hydrochloride (The combination of therapeutic doses of intravenous dantrolene sodium and verapamil in halothane/alpha-chloralose anesthetized swine has resulted in ventricular fibrillation and cardiovascular collapse in association with hyperkalemia; it is recommended that this combination should not be used during the management of malignant hyperthermia crisis until the human data is available). Products include:

IMPORTANT NOTE: Always consult each drug listing in the patient's regimen for possible interactions.

Covera-HS Tablets 3139
Tarka Tablets 524
Verelan PM Extended-Release Capsules, Controlled-Onset 3106

Warfarin Sodium (Reduces binding of dantrolene to plasma proteins). Products include:
Coumadin for Injection 898
Coumadin Tablets 898

DAPSONE TABLETS USP
(Dapsone) 1673
May interact with:

Pyrimethamine (Agranulocytosis; increased likelihood of hematological reactions). Products include:
Daraprim Tablets 1419
Fansidar Tablets 2765

Rifampin (Lowered Dapsone levels).
No products indexed under this heading.

Trimethoprim (Mutual interaction between Dapsone and trimethoprim in which each raises the level of the other about 1.5 times).
No products indexed under this heading.

DAPTACEL VACCINE
(Diphtheria & Tetanus Toxoids and Acellular Pertussis Vaccine Adsorbed) 2950
May interact with alkylating agents, antimetabolites, antineoplastics, corticosteroids, oral anticoagulants, and cytotoxic drugs. Compounds in these categories include:

Altretamine (May reduce the immune response to vaccine).
No products indexed under this heading.

Anastrozole (May reduce the immune response to vaccine). Products include:
Arimidex Tablets 673

Anisindione (Intra-muscular injection should be used with caution in patients on anticoagulant therapy). Products include:
Miradon Tablets 3042

Asparaginase (May reduce the immune response to vaccine). Products include:
Elspar for Injection 2463
Elspar for Injection 1960

Betamethasone Acetate (May reduce the immune response to vaccine when corticosteroids are used in greater than physiologic doses).
No products indexed under this heading.

Betamethasone Sodium Phosphate (May reduce the immune response to vaccine when corticosteroids are used in greater than physiologic doses).
No products indexed under this heading.

Bicalutamide (May reduce the immune response to vaccine).
No products indexed under this heading.

Bleomycin Sulfate (May reduce the immune response to vaccine).
No products indexed under this heading.

Busulfan (May reduce the immune response to vaccine). Products include:
I.V. Busulfex 2493
Myleran Tablets 1525

Capecitabine (Immunosuppressive therapies may reduce the immune response to vaccines). Products include:
Xeloda Tablets 2822

Carboplatin (May reduce the immune response to vaccine).
No products indexed under this heading.

Carmustine (BCNU) (May reduce the immune response to vaccine).
No products indexed under this heading.

Chlorambucil (May reduce the immune response to vaccine). Products include:
Leukeran Tablets 1504

Cisplatin (May reduce the immune response to vaccine).
No products indexed under this heading.

Cladribine (Immunosuppressive therapies may reduce the immune response to vaccines). Products include:
Leustatin Injection 2357

Cortisone Acetate (May reduce the immune response to vaccine when corticosteroids are used in greater than physiologic doses).
No products indexed under this heading.

Cyclophosphamide (May reduce the immune response to vaccine).
No products indexed under this heading.

Cytarabine (Immunosuppressive therapies may reduce the immune response to vaccines).
No products indexed under this heading.

Dacarbazine (May reduce the immune response to vaccine).
No products indexed under this heading.

Daunorubicin Citrate (May reduce the immune response to vaccine).
No products indexed under this heading.

Daunorubicin Hydrochloride (May reduce the immune response to vaccine).
No products indexed under this heading.

Denileukin Diftitox (May reduce the immune response to vaccine). Products include:
Ontak Vials 1745

Dexamethasone (May reduce the immune response to vaccine when corticosteroids are used in greater than physiologic doses). Products include:
Ciprodex Otic Suspension 559
Decadron Tablets 1951
TobraDex Ophthalmic Ointment 562
TobraDex Ophthalmic Suspension ... 563

Dexamethasone Acetate (May reduce the immune response to vaccine when corticosteroids are used in greater than physiologic doses).
No products indexed under this heading.

Dexamethasone Sodium Phosphate (May reduce the immune response to vaccine when corticosteroids are used in greater than physiologic doses).
No products indexed under this heading.

Dicumarol (Intra-muscular injection should be used with caution in patients on anticoagulant therapy).
No products indexed under this heading.

Docetaxel (May reduce the immune response to vaccine). Products include:
Taxotere Injection Concentrate 2932

Doxorubicin Hydrochloride (May reduce the immune response to vaccine).
No products indexed under this heading.

Epirubicin Hydrochloride (May reduce the immune response to vaccine).
No products indexed under this heading.

Estramustine Phosphate Sodium (May reduce the immune response to vaccine). Products include:
Emcyt Capsules 2634

Etoposide (May reduce the immune response to vaccine).
No products indexed under this heading.

Exemestane (May reduce the immune response to vaccine). Products include:
Aromasin Tablets 2600

Floxuridine (May reduce the immune response to vaccine).
No products indexed under this heading.

Fludarabine Phosphate (Immunosuppressive therapies may reduce the immune response to vaccines).
No products indexed under this heading.

Fludrocortisone Acetate (May reduce the immune response to vaccine when corticosteroids are used in greater than physiologic doses).
No products indexed under this heading.

Fluorouracil (May reduce the immune response to vaccine). Products include:
Carac Cream, 0.5% 2879
Efudex 3363

Flutamide (May reduce the immune response to vaccine). Products include:
Eulexin Capsules 3009

Gemcitabine Hydrochloride (May reduce the immune response to vaccine). Products include:
Gemzar for Injection 1771

Hydrocortisone (May reduce the immune response to vaccine when corticosteroids are used in greater than physiologic doses). Products include:
Colocort Rectal Suspension, USP (Retention) 100 mg/60 mL 2476
Hydrocortone Tablets 1989
Preparation H Hydrocortisone Cream .... ▣646

Hydrocortisone Acetate (May reduce the immune response to vaccine when corticosteroids are used in greater than physiologic doses). Products include:
Analpram-HC 1159
Pramosone 1161
ProctoFoam-HC 3099

Hydrocortisone Sodium Phosphate (May reduce the immune response to vaccine when corticosteroids are used in greater than physiologic doses).
No products indexed under this heading.

Hydrocortisone Sodium Succinate (May reduce the immune response to vaccine when corticosteroids are used in greater than physiologic doses).
No products indexed under this heading.

Hydroxyurea (May reduce the immune response to vaccine).
No products indexed under this heading.

Idarubicin Hydrochloride (May reduce the immune response to vaccine).
No products indexed under this heading.

Ifosfamide (May reduce the immune response to vaccine).
No products indexed under this heading.

Interferon alfa-2a, Recombinant (May reduce the immune response to vaccine).
No products indexed under this heading.

Interferon alfa-2b, Recombinant (May reduce the immune response to vaccine). Products include:
Intron A for Injection 3024
Rebetron Combination Therapy 3063

Irinotecan Hydrochloride (May reduce the immune response to vaccine). Products include:
Camptosar Injection 2604

Levamisole Hydrochloride (May reduce the immune response to vaccine).
No products indexed under this heading.

Lomustine (CCNU) (May reduce the immune response to vaccine).
No products indexed under this heading.

Mechlorethamine Hydrochloride (May reduce the immune response to vaccine). Products include:
Mustargen for Injection 2468

Megestrol Acetate (May reduce the immune response to vaccine). Products include:
Megace ES Oral Suspension 2481

Melphalan (May reduce the immune response to vaccine). Products include:
Alkeran Tablets 956

Mercaptopurine (May reduce the immune response to vaccine).
No products indexed under this heading.

Methotrexate (Immunosuppressive therapies may reduce the immune response to vaccines).
No products indexed under this heading.

Methotrexate Sodium (May reduce the immune response to vaccine).
No products indexed under this heading.

Methylprednisolone Acetate (May reduce the immune response to vaccine when corticosteroids are used in greater than physiologic doses). Products include:
Depo-Medrol Injectable Suspension 2617
Depo-Medrol Single-Dose Vial 2619

Methylprednisolone Sodium Succinate (May reduce the immune response to vaccine when corticosteroids are used in greater than physiologic doses).
No products indexed under this heading.

Mitomycin (Mitomycin-C) (May reduce the immune response to vaccine).
No products indexed under this heading.

Mitotane (May reduce the immune response to vaccine).
No products indexed under this heading.

Mitoxantrone Hydrochloride (May reduce the immune response to vaccine).
No products indexed under this heading.

Oxaliplatin (May reduce the immune response to vaccine). Products include:
Eloxatin for Injection 2892

Paclitaxel (May reduce the immune response to vaccine).
No products indexed under this heading.

Pentostatin (Immunosuppressive therapies may reduce the immune response to vaccines). Products include:
Nipent for Injection 1863

Prednisolone Acetate (May reduce the immune response to vaccine when corticosteroids are used in greater than physiologic doses). Products include:
Blephamide Ophthalmic Ointment 568
Blephamide Ophthalmic Suspension.................................. 569
Poly-Pred Ophthalmic Suspension .... ⊙233
Pred Forte Ophthalmic Suspension .... ⊙235
Pred Mild Ophthalmic Suspension .... ⊙238
Pred-G Ophthalmic Ointment .... ⊙237
Pred-G Ophthalmic Suspension ...... ⊙236

Prednisolone Sodium Phosphate (May reduce the immune response to vaccine when corticosteroids are used in greater than physiologic doses).
No products indexed under this heading.

Prednisolone Tebutate (May reduce the immune response to vaccine when corticosteroids are used in greater than physiologic doses).
No products indexed under this heading.

Prednisone (May reduce the immune response to vaccine when corticosteroids are used in greater than physiologic doses).
No products indexed under this heading.

Procarbazine Hydrochloride (May reduce the immune response to vaccine). Products include:
Matulane Capsules 3191

Streptozocin (May reduce the immune response to vaccine).
No products indexed under this heading.

Tamoxifen Citrate (May reduce the immune response to vaccine). Products include:
Soltamox Oral Solution 3527

Teniposide (May reduce the immune response to vaccine).
No products indexed under this heading.

Thioguanine (May reduce the immune response to vaccine). Products include:
Tabloid Tablets 1575

Thiotepa (May reduce the immune response to vaccine).
No products indexed under this heading.

Topotecan Hydrochloride (May reduce the immune response to vaccine). Products include:
Hycamtin for Injection 1458

Toremifene Citrate (May reduce the immune response to vaccine).
No products indexed under this heading.

Triamcinolone (May reduce the immune response to vaccine when corticosteroids are used in greater than physiologic doses).
No products indexed under this heading.

Triamcinolone Acetonide (May reduce the immune response to vaccine when corticosteroids are used in greater than physiologic doses). Products include:
Azmacort Inhalation Aerosol 1726
Nasacort AQ Nasal Spray 2922

Triamcinolone Diacetate (May reduce the immune response to vaccine when corticosteroids are used in greater than physiologic doses).
No products indexed under this heading.

Triamcinolone Hexacetonide (May reduce the immune response to vaccine when corticosteroids are used in greater than physiologic doses).
No products indexed under this heading.

Valrubicin (May reduce the immune response to vaccine).
No products indexed under this heading.

Vincristine Sulfate (May reduce the immune response to vaccine).
No products indexed under this heading.

Vinorelbine Tartrate (May reduce the immune response to vaccine).
No products indexed under this heading.

Warfarin Sodium (Intra-muscular injection should be used with caution in patients on anticoagulant therapy). Products include:
Coumadin for Injection 898
Coumadin Tablets 898

DARANIDE TABLETS

(Dichlorphenamide) 1950
May interact with corticosteroids and certain other agents. Compounds in these categories include:

ACTH (Hypokalemia may develop).
No products indexed under this heading.

Aspirin (Concomitant high-dose aspirin may produce anorexia, tachypnea, lethargy and coma). Products include:
Aggrenox Capsules 822
Bayer Aspirin 744
BC Allergy Sinus Cold Powder .... ▣677
BC Headache Powder .... ▣677
Arthritis Strength BC Powder .... ▣677
BC Sinus Cold Powder .... ▣677
Excedrin Extra Strength Caplets/Tablets/Geltabs .... ▣684
Excedrin Migraine Caplets/Tablets/Geltabs .... ▣609
Goody's Body Pain Formula Powder.. ▣684
Goody's Extra Strength Headache Powders.................... ▣611
Goody's Extra Strength Pain Relief Tablets .... ▣685
Percodan Tablets 1132
St. Joseph 81 mg Aspirin Chewable and Enteric Coated Tablets 1869

Aspirin, Enteric Coated (Concomitant high-dose aspirin may produce anorexia, tachypnea, lethargy and coma).
No products indexed under this heading.

Betamethasone Acetate (Hypokalemia may develop).
No products indexed under this heading.

Betamethasone Sodium Phosphate (Hypokalemia may develop).
No products indexed under this heading.

Cortisone Acetate (Hypokalemia may develop).
No products indexed under this heading.

Dexamethasone (Hypokalemia may develop). Products include:
Ciprodex Otic Suspension 559
Decadron Tablets 1951
TobraDex Ophthalmic Ointment 562
TobraDex Ophthalmic Suspension ... 563

Dexamethasone Acetate (Hypokalemia may develop).
No products indexed under this heading.

Dexamethasone Sodium Phosphate (Hypokalemia may develop).
No products indexed under this heading.

Fludrocortisone Acetate (Hypokalemia may develop).
No products indexed under this heading.

Hydrocortisone (Hypokalemia may develop). Products include:
Colocort Rectal Suspension, USP (Retention) 100 mg/60 mL.......... 2476
Hydrocortone Tablets 1989
Preparation H Hydrocortisone Cream .... ▣646

Hydrocortisone Acetate (Hypokalemia may develop). Products include:
Analpram-HC 1159
Pramosone 1161
ProctoFoam-HC 3099

Hydrocortisone Sodium Phosphate (Hypokalemia may develop).
No products indexed under this heading.

Hydrocortisone Sodium Succinate (Hypokalemia may develop).
No products indexed under this heading.

Methylprednisolone Acetate (Hypokalemia may develop). Products include:
Depo-Medrol Injectable Suspension 2617
Depo-Medrol Single-Dose Vial 2619

Methylprednisolone Sodium Succinate (Hypokalemia may develop).
No products indexed under this heading.

Prednisolone Acetate (Hypokalemia may develop). Products include:
Blephamide Ophthalmic Ointment 568
Blephamide Ophthalmic Suspension.................................. 569
Poly-Pred Ophthalmic Suspension .... ⊙233
Pred Forte Ophthalmic Suspension .... ⊙235
Pred Mild Ophthalmic Suspension .... ⊙238
Pred-G Ophthalmic Ointment .... ⊙237
Pred-G Ophthalmic Suspension ...... ⊙236

Prednisolone Sodium Phosphate (Hypokalemia may develop).
No products indexed under this heading.

Prednisolone Tebutate (Hypokalemia may develop).
No products indexed under this heading.

Prednisone (Hypokalemia may develop).
No products indexed under this heading.

Triamcinolone (Hypokalemia may develop).
No products indexed under this heading.

Triamcinolone Acetonide (Hypokalemia may develop). Products include:
Azmacort Inhalation Aerosol 1726
Nasacort AQ Nasal Spray 2922

Triamcinolone Diacetate (Hypokalemia may develop).
No products indexed under this heading.

Triamcinolone Hexacetonide (Hypokalemia may develop).
No products indexed under this heading.

DARAPRIM TABLETS

(Pyrimethamine) 1419
May interact with cytotoxic drugs, dihydrofolate reductase inhibitors, agents associated with myelosuppression, phenytoin, sulfonamides, and certain other agents. Compounds in these categories include:

Altretamine (The concomitant use of other antifolic drugs or agents associated with myelosuppression including cytostatic agents while the patient is receiving pyrimethamine, may increase the risk of bone marrow suppression).
No products indexed under this heading.

Bendroflumethiazide (Co-administration of other antifolic drugs, such as sulfonamides, may increase the risk of bone marrow suppression; potential for hypersensitivity reactions such as Stevens-Johnson syndrome, toxic epidermal necrolysis, erythema multiforme, and anaphylaxis).
No products indexed under this heading.

Bleomycin Sulfate (The concomitant use of other antifolic drugs or agents associated with myelosuppression including cytostatic agents while the patient is receiving pyrimethamine, may increase the risk of bone marrow suppression).
No products indexed under this heading.

Busulfan (The concomitant use of other antifolic drugs or agents associated with myelosuppression including cytostatic agents while the patient is receiving pyrimethamine, may increase the risk of bone marrow suppression). Products include:
I.V. Busulfex 2493
Myleran Tablets 1525

Chlorambucil (The concomitant use of other antifolic drugs or agents associated with myelosuppression including cytostatic agents while the patient is receiving pyrimethamine, may increase the risk of bone marrow suppression). Products include:
Leukeran Tablets 1504

Chlorothiazide (Co-administration of other antifolic drugs, such as sulfonamides, may increase the risk of bone marrow suppression; potential for hypersensitivity reactions such as Stevens-Johnson syndrome, toxic epidermal necrolysis, erythema multiforme, and anaphylaxis). Products include:
Diuril Oral Suspension 1954

Chlorothiazide Sodium (Co-administration of other antifolic drugs, such as sulfonamides, may increase the risk of bone marrow suppression; potential for hypersensitivity reactions such as Stevens-

Johnson syndrome, toxic epidermal necrolysis, erythema multiforme, and anaphylaxis). Products include:

Diuril Sodium Intravenous 2467

Chlorpropamide (Co-administration of other antifolic drugs, such as sulfonamides, may increase the risk of bone marrow suppression; potential for hypersensitivity reactions such as Stevens-Johnson syndrome, toxic epidermal necrolysis, erythema multiforme, and anaphylaxis).

No products indexed under this heading.

Cladribine (The concomitant use of other antifolic drugs or agents associated with myelosuppression including cytostatic agents while the patient is receiving pyrimethamine, may increase the risk of bone marrow suppression). Products include:

Leustatin Injection 2357

Cyclophosphamide (The concomitant use of other antifolic drugs or agents associated with myelosuppression including cytostatic agents while the patient is receiving pyrimethamine, may increase the risk of bone marrow suppression).

No products indexed under this heading.

Daunorubicin Citrate Liposome (The concomitant use of other antifolic drugs or agents associated with myelosuppression including cytostatic agents while the patient is receiving pyrimethamine, may increase the risk of bone marrow suppression).

No products indexed under this heading.

Daunorubicin Hydrochloride (The concomitant use of other antifolic drugs or agents associated with myelosuppression including cytostatic agents while the patient is receiving pyrimethamine, may increase the risk of bone marrow suppression).

No products indexed under this heading.

Dexrazoxane (The concomitant use of other antifolic drugs or agents associated with myelosuppression including cytostatic agents while the patient is receiving pyrimethamine, may increase the risk of bone marrow suppression). Products include:

Zinecard for Injection 2650

Doxorubicin Hydrochloride (The concomitant use of other antifolic drugs or agents associated with myelosuppression including cytostatic agents while the patient is receiving pyrimethamine, may increase the risk of bone marrow suppression).

No products indexed under this heading.

Doxorubicin Hydrochloride Liposome (The concomitant use of other antifolic drugs or agents associated with myelosuppression including cytostatic agents while the patient is receiving pyrimethamine, may increase the risk of bone marrow suppression). Products include:

Doxil Injection 2351

Epirubicin Hydrochloride (The concomitant use of other antifolic drugs or agents associated with myelosuppression including cytostatic agents while the patient is receiving pyrimethamine, may increase the risk of bone marrow suppression).

No products indexed under this heading.

Fludarabine Phosphate (The concomitant use of other antifolic drugs or agents associated with myelosuppression including cytostatic agents while the patient is receiving pyrimethamine, may increase the risk of bone marrow suppression).

No products indexed under this heading.

Fluorouracil (The concomitant use of other antifolic drugs or agents associated with myelosuppression including cytostatic agents while the patient is receiving pyrimethamine, may increase the risk of bone marrow suppression). Products include:

Carac Cream, 0.5% 2879
Efudex 3363

Fosphenytoin Sodium (Co-administration with agents that affect folate levels, such as phenytoin, should be undertaken with caution).

No products indexed under this heading.

Gemcitabine Hydrochloride (The concomitant use of other antifolic drugs or agents associated with myelosuppression including cytostatic agents while the patient is receiving pyrimethamine, may increase the risk of bone marrow suppression). Products include:

Gemzar for Injection 1771

Gemtuzumab Ozogamicin (The concomitant use of other antifolic drugs or agents associated with myelosuppression including cytostatic agents while the patient is receiving pyrimethamine, may increase the risk of bone marrow suppression). Products include:

Mylotarg for Injection 3431

Glipizide (Co-administration of other antifolic drugs, such as sulfonamides, may increase the risk of bone marrow suppression; potential for hypersensitivity reactions such as Stevens-Johnson syndrome, toxic epidermal necrolysis, erythema multiforme, and anaphylaxis).

No products indexed under this heading.

Glyburide (Co-administration of other antifolic drugs, such as sulfonamides, may increase the risk of bone marrow suppression; potential for hypersensitivity reactions such as Stevens-Johnson syndrome, toxic epidermal necrolysis, erythema multiforme, and anaphylaxis).

No products indexed under this heading.

Hydrochlorothiazide (Co-administration of other antifolic drugs, such as sulfonamides, may increase the risk of bone marrow suppression; potential for hypersensitivity reactions such as Stevens-Johnson syndrome, toxic epidermal necrolysis, erythema multiforme, and anaphylaxis). Products include:

Aldoril Tablets 1910
Atacand HCT 651
Avalide Tablets 888
Avalide Tablets 2874
Benicar HCT Tablets 1044
Diovan HCT Tablets 2196
Dyazide Capsules 1423
Hyzaar 50-12.5 Tablets 1990
Hyzaar 100-12.5 Tablets 1990
Hyzaar 100-25 Tablets 1990
Lopressor HCT 50/25 Tablets 2241
Lopressor HCT 100/25 Tablets 2241
Lopressor HCT 100/50 Tablets 2241
Lotensin HCT Tablets 2246
Micardis HCT Tablets 856
Moduretic Tablets 2028
Prinzide Tablets 2056
Teveten HCT Tablets 1737
Timolide Tablets 2086
Uniretic Tablets 3100

Hydroflumethiazide (Co-administration of other antifolic drugs, such as sulfonamides, may increase the risk of bone marrow suppression; potential for hypersensitivity reactions such as Stevens-Johnson syndrome, toxic epidermal necrolysis, erythema multiforme, and anaphylaxis).

No products indexed under this heading.

Hydroxyurea (The concomitant use of other antifolic drugs or agents associated with myelosuppression including cytostatic agents while the patient is receiving pyrimethamine, may increase the risk of bone marrow suppression).

No products indexed under this heading.

Idarubicin Hydrochloride (The concomitant use of other antifolic drugs or agents associated with myelosuppression including cytostatic agents while the patient is receiving pyrimethamine, may increase the risk of bone marrow suppression).

No products indexed under this heading.

Interferon alfa-2a, Recombinant (The concomitant use of other antifolic drugs or agents associated with myelosuppression including cytostatic agents while the patient is receiving pyrimethamine, may increase the risk of bone marrow suppression).

No products indexed under this heading.

Irinotecan Hydrochloride (The concomitant use of other antifolic drugs or agents associated with myelosuppression including cytostatic agents while the patient is receiving pyrimethamine, may increase the risk of bone marrow suppression). Products include:

Camptosar Injection 2604

Lamotrigine (The concomitant use of other antifolic drugs, while the patient is receiving pyrimethamine, may increase the risk of bone marrow suppression). Products include:

Lamictal 1481

Lorazepam (Concomitant therapy may result in mild hepatotoxicity).

No products indexed under this heading.

Melphalan Hydrochloride (The concomitant use of other antifolic drugs or agents associated with myelosuppression including cytostatic agents while the patient is receiving pyrimethamine, may increase the risk of bone marrow suppression). Products include:

Alkeran for Injection 955

Mercaptopurine (The concomitant use of other antifolic drugs or agents associated with myelosuppression including cytostatic agents while the patient is receiving pyrimethamine, may increase the risk of bone marrow suppression).

No products indexed under this heading.

Methotrexate Sodium (The concomitant use of other antifolic drugs or agents associated with myelosuppression including cytostatic agents while the patient is receiving pyrimethamine, may increase the risk of bone marrow suppression).

No products indexed under this heading.

Methyclothiazide (Co-administration of other antifolic drugs, such as sulfonamides, may increase the risk of bone marrow suppression; potential for hypersensitivity reactions such as Stevens-Johnson syndrome, toxic epidermal necrolysis, erythema multiforme, and anaphylaxis).

No products indexed under this heading.

Mitotane (The concomitant use of other antifolic drugs or agents associated with myelosuppression including cytostatic agents while the patient is receiving pyrimethamine, may increase the risk of bone marrow suppression).

No products indexed under this heading.

Mitoxantrone Hydrochloride (The concomitant use of other antifolic drugs or agents associated with myelosuppression including cytostatic agents while the patient is receiving pyrimethamine, may increase the risk of bone marrow suppression).

No products indexed under this heading.

Phenytoin (Co-administration with agents that affect folate levels, such as phenytoin, should be undertaken with caution).

No products indexed under this heading.

Phenytoin Sodium (Co-administration with agents that affect folate levels, such as phenytoin, should be undertaken with caution). Products include:

Phenytek Capsules 2160

Polythiazide (Co-administration of other antifolic drugs, such as sulfonamides, may increase the risk of bone marrow suppression; potential for hypersensitivity reactions such as Stevens-Johnson syndrome, toxic epidermal necrolysis, erythema multiforme, and anaphylaxis).

No products indexed under this heading.

Procarbazine Hydrochloride (The concomitant use of other antifolic drugs or agents associated with myelosuppression including cytostatic agents while the patient is receiving pyrimethamine, may increase the risk of bone marrow suppression). Products include:

Matulane Capsules 3191

Proguanil (May increase risk of bone marrow suppression).

No products indexed under this heading.

Sulfacytine (Co-administration of other antifolic drugs, such as sulfonamides, may increase the risk of bone marrow suppression; potential for hypersensitivity reactions such as Stevens-Johnson syndrome, toxic epidermal necrolysis, erythema multiforme, and anaphylaxis).

No products indexed under this heading.

Sulfamethizole (Co-administration of other antifolic drugs, such as sulfonamides, may increase the risk of bone marrow suppression; potential for hypersensitivity reactions such as Stevens-Johnson syndrome, toxic epidermal necrolysis, erythema multiforme, and anaphylaxis).
No products indexed under this heading.

Sulfamethoxazole (Co-administration of other antifolic drugs, such as sulfonamides, may increase the risk of bone marrow suppression; potential for hypersensitivity reactions such as Stevens-Johnson syndrome, toxic epidermal necrolysis, erythema multiforme, and anaphylaxis).
No products indexed under this heading.

Sulfasalazine (Co-administration of other antifolic drugs, such as sulfonamides, may increase the risk of bone marrow suppression; potential for hypersensitivity reactions such as Stevens-Johnson syndrome, toxic epidermal necrolysis, erythema multiforme, and anaphylaxis).
No products indexed under this heading.

Sulfinpyrazone (Co-administration of other antifolic drugs, such as sulfonamides, may increase the risk of bone marrow suppression; potential for hypersensitivity reactions such as Stevens-Johnson syndrome, toxic epidermal necrolysis, erythema multiforme, and anaphylaxis).
No products indexed under this heading.

Sulfisoxazole Acetyl (Co-administration of other antifolic drugs, such as sulfonamides, may increase the risk of bone marrow suppression; potential for hypersensitivity reactions such as Stevens-Johnson syndrome, toxic epidermal necrolysis, erythema multiforme, and anaphylaxis).
No products indexed under this heading.

Sulfisoxazole Diolamine (Co-administration of other antifolic drugs, such as sulfonamides, may increase the risk of bone marrow suppression; potential for hypersensitivity reactions such as Stevens-Johnson syndrome, toxic epidermal necrolysis, erythema multiforme, and anaphylaxis).
No products indexed under this heading.

Tamoxifen Citrate (The concomitant use of other antifolic drugs or agents associated with myelosuppression including cytostatic agents while the patient is receiving pyrimethamine, may increase the risk of bone marrow suppression). Products include:
Soltamox Oral Solution 3527

Temozolomide (The concomitant use of other antifolic drugs or agents associated with myelosuppression including cytostatic agents while the patient is receiving pyrimethamine, may increase the risk of bone marrow suppression). Products include:
Temodar Capsules 3073

Thioguanine (The concomitant use of other antifolic drugs or agents associated with myelosuppression including cytostatic agents while the patient is receiving pyrimethamine, may increase the risk of bone marrow suppression). Products include:
Tabloid Tablets 1575

Tolazamide (Co-administration of other antifolic drugs, such as sulfonamides, may increase the risk of bone marrow suppression; potential for hypersensitivity reactions such as Stevens-Johnson syndrome, toxic epidermal necrolysis, erythema multiforme, and anaphylaxis).
No products indexed under this heading.

Tolbutamide (Co-administration of other antifolic drugs, such as sulfonamides, may increase the risk of bone marrow suppression; potential for hypersensitivity reactions such as Stevens-Johnson syndrome, toxic epidermal necrolysis, erythema multiforme, and anaphylaxis).
No products indexed under this heading.

Trimethoprim (Co-administration of other antifolic drugs, such as sulfonamides or trimethoprim-sulfamethoxazole combinations, may increase the risk of bone marrow suppression; potential for hypersensitivity reactions such as Stevens-Johnson syndrome, toxic epidermal necrolysis, erythema multiforme, and anaphylaxis).
No products indexed under this heading.

Trimetrexate Glucuronate (The concomitant use of other antifolic drugs, while the patient is receiving pyrimethamine, may increase the risk of bone marrow suppression).
No products indexed under this heading.

Vincristine Sulfate (The concomitant use of other antifolic drugs or agents associated with myelosuppression including cytostatic agents while the patient is receiving pyrimethamine, may increase the risk of bone marrow suppression).
No products indexed under this heading.

Vinorelbine Tartrate (The concomitant use of other antifolic drugs or agents associated with myelosuppression including cytostatic agents while the patient is receiving pyrimethamine, may increase the risk of bone marrow suppression).
No products indexed under this heading.

Zidovudine (May increase risk of bone marrow suppression). Products include:
Combivir Tablets 1411
Retrovir 1560
Retrovir IV Infusion 1564
Trizivir Tablets 1589

DAYTRANA TRANSDERMAL PATCH

(Methylphenidate) 3174
May interact with antihypertensives, oral anticoagulants, anticonvulsants, monoamine oxidase inhibitors, selective serotonin reuptake inhibitors, tricyclic antidepressants, vasopressors, and certain other agents. Compounds in these categories include:

Acebutolol Hydrochloride (Methylphenidate may decrease the effectiveness of drugs used to treat hypertension).
No products indexed under this heading.

Amitriptyline Hydrochloride (Human pharmacologic studies have shown that methylphenidate may inhibit the metabolism of some tricyclic drugs (eg, imipramine, clomipramine, desipramine). Downward dose adjustments of these drugs may be required when given concomitantly with methylphenidate. It may be necessary to adjust the dosage and monitor plasma drug concentrations when initiating or discontinuing methylphenidate).
No products indexed under this heading.

Amlodipine Besylate (Methylphenidate may decrease the effectiveness of drugs used to treat hypertension). Products include:
Caduet Tablets 2508
Lotrel Capsules 2249
Norvasc Tablets 2545

Amoxapine (Human pharmacologic studies have shown that methylphenidate may inhibit the metabolism of some tricyclic drugs (eg, imipramine, clomipramine, desipramine). Downward dose adjustments of these drugs may be required when given concomitantly with methylphenidate. It may be necessary to adjust the dosage and monitor plasma drug concentrations when initiating or discontinuing methylphenidate).
No products indexed under this heading.

Anisindione (Human pharmacologic studies have shown that methylphenidate may inhibit the metabolism of coumarin anticoagulants. Downward dose adjustments of these drugs may be required when given concomitantly with methylphenidate. It may be necessary to adjust the dosage and monitor plasma drug concentrations or coagulation times when initiating or discontinuing methylphenidate). Products include:
Miradon Tablets 3042

Atenolol (Methylphenidate may decrease the effectiveness of drugs used to treat hypertension).
No products indexed under this heading.

Benazepril Hydrochloride (Methylphenidate may decrease the effectiveness of drugs used to treat hypertension). Products include:
Lotensin Tablets 2243
Lotensin HCT Tablets 2246
Lotrel Capsules 2249

Bendroflumethiazide (Methylphenidate may decrease the effectiveness of drugs used to treat hypertension).
No products indexed under this heading.

Betaxolol Hydrochloride (Methylphenidate may decrease the effectiveness of drugs used to treat hypertension). Products include:
Betoptic S Ophthalmic Suspension 558

Bisoprolol Fumarate (Methylphenidate may decrease the effectiveness of drugs used to treat hypertension).
No products indexed under this heading.

Candesartan Cilexetil (Methylphenidate may decrease the effectiveness of drugs used to treat hypertension). Products include:
Atacand Tablets 649
Atacand HCT 651

Captopril (Methylphenidate may decrease the effectiveness of drugs used to treat hypertension). Products include:
Captopril Tablets 2149

Carbamazepine (Human pharmacologic studies have shown that methylphenidate may inhibit the metabolism of anticonvulsants (eg, phenobarbital, phenytoin, primidone). Downward dose adjustments of these drugs may be required when given concomitantly with methylphenidate. It may be necessary to adjust the dosage and monitor plasma drug concentrations when initiating or discontinuing methylphenidate). Products include:
Carbatrol Capsules 3171
Equetro Extended-Release Capsules 3180
Tegretol/Tegretol-XR 2295

Carteolol Hydrochloride (Methylphenidate may decrease the effectiveness of drugs used to treat hypertension). Products include:
Carteolol Hydrochloride Ophthalmic Solution USP, 1%....... ⊙ 249

Chlorothiazide (Methylphenidate may decrease the effectiveness of drugs used to treat hypertension). Products include:
Diuril Oral Suspension 1954

Chlorothiazide Sodium (Methylphenidate may decrease the effectiveness of drugs used to treat hypertension). Products include:
Diuril Sodium Intravenous 2467

Chlorthalidone (Methylphenidate may decrease the effectiveness of drugs used to treat hypertension). Products include:
Clorpres Tablets 2153

Citalopram Hydrobromide (Human pharmacologic studies have shown that methylphenidate may inhibit the metabolism of selective serotonin reuptake inhibitors. Downward dose adjustments of these drugs may be required when given concomitantly with methylphenidate. It may be necessary to adjust the dosage and monitor plasma drug concentrations when initiating or discontinuing methylphenidate). Products include:
Celexa 1176

Clomipramine Hydrochloride (Human pharmacologic studies have shown that methylphenidate may inhibit the metabolism of some tricyclic drugs (eg, imipramine, clomipramine, desipramine). Downward dose adjustments of these drugs may be required when given concomitantly with methylphenidate. It may be necessary to adjust the dosage and monitor plasma drug concentrations when initiating or discontinuing methylphenidate).
No products indexed under this heading.

Clonidine (Serious adverse events have been reported in concomitant use of methylphenidate with clonidine, although no causality for the combination has been established). Products include:
Catapres-TTS 844

Clonidine Hydrochloride (Serious adverse events have been reported in concomitant use of methylphenidate with clonidine, although no causality for the combination has been established). Products include:
Catapres Tablets 843
Clorpres Tablets 2153

Deserpidine (Methylphenidate may decrease the effectiveness of drugs used to treat hypertension).
No products indexed under this heading.

Desipramine Hydrochloride
(Human pharmacologic studies have shown that methylphenidate may inhibit the metabolism of some tricyclic drugs (eg, imipramine, clomipramine, desipramine). Downward dose adjustments of these drugs may be required when given concomitantly with methylphenidate. It may be necessary to adjust the dosage and monitor plasma drug concentrations when initiating or discontinuing methylphenidate).

No products indexed under this heading.

Diazoxide (Methylphenidate may decrease the effectiveness of drugs used to treat hypertension).
Products include:
Hyperstat I.V. 3017

Dicumarol (Human pharmacologic studies have shown that methylphenidate may inhibit the metabolism of coumarin anticoagulants. Downward dose adjustments of these drugs may be required when given concomitantly with methylphenidate. It may be necessary to adjust the dosage and monitor plasma drug concentrations or coagulation times when initiating or discontinuing methylphenidate).

No products indexed under this heading.

Diltiazem Hydrochloride (Methylphenidate may decrease the effectiveness of drugs used to treat hypertension). Products include:
Cardizem LA Extended Release Tablets 1728
Tiazac Capsules 1201

Divalproex Sodium (Human pharmacologic studies have shown that methylphenidate may inhibit the metabolism of anticonvulsants (eg, phenobarbital, phenytoin, primidone). Downward dose adjustments of these drugs may be required when given concomitantly with methylphenidate. It may be necessary to adjust the dosage and monitor plasma drug concentrations when initiating or discontinuing methylphenidate). Products include:
Depakote Sprinkle Capsules 422
Depakote Tablets 427
Depakote ER Tablets 434

Dobutamine (Because of a possible effect on blood pressure, methylphenidate transdermal system should be used cautiously with pressor agents).
No products indexed under this heading.

Dobutamine Hydrochloride (Because of a possible effect on blood pressure, methylphenidate transdermal system should be used cautiously with pressor agents).
No products indexed under this heading.

Dopamine Hydrochloride (Because of a possible effect on blood pressure, methylphenidate transdermal system should be used cautiously with pressor agents).
No products indexed under this heading.

Doxazosin Mesylate (Methylphenidate may decrease the effectiveness of drugs used to treat hypertension).
Products include:
Cardura XL Tablets 2515

Doxepin Hydrochloride (Human pharmacologic studies have shown that methylphenidate may inhibit the metabolism of some tricyclic drugs (eg, imipramine, clomipramine, desipramine). Downward dose adjustments of these drugs may be required when given concomitantly with methylphenidate. It may be necessary to adjust the dosage and monitor plasma drug concentrations when initiating or discontinuing methylphenidate).
No products indexed under this heading.

Enalapril Maleate (Methylphenidate may decrease the effectiveness of drugs used to treat hypertension).
Products include:
Vasotec I.V. Injection 2103

Enalaprilat (Methylphenidate may decrease the effectiveness of drugs used to treat hypertension).
No products indexed under this heading.

Ephedrine Sulfate (Because of a possible effect on blood pressure, methylphenidate transdermal system should be used cautiously with pressor agents).
No products indexed under this heading.

Epinephrine Bitartrate (Because of a possible effect on blood pressure, methylphenidate transdermal system should be used cautiously with pressor agents).
No products indexed under this heading.

Epinephrine Hydrochloride (Because of a possible effect on blood pressure, methylphenidate transdermal system should be used cautiously with pressor agents).
No products indexed under this heading.

Eprosartan Mesylate (Methylphenidate may decrease the effectiveness of drugs used to treat hypertension). Products include:
Teveten Tablets 1735
Teveten HCT Tablets 1737

Escitalopram Oxalate (Human pharmacologic studies have shown that methylphenidate may inhibit the metabolism of selective serotonin reuptake inhibitors. Downward dose adjustments of these drugs may be required when given concomitantly with methylphenidate. It may be necessary to adjust the dosage and monitor plasma drug concentrations when initiating or discontinuing methylphenidate). Products include:
Lexapro Oral Solution 1190
Lexapro Tablets 1190

Esmolol Hydrochloride (Methylphenidate may decrease the effectiveness of drugs used to treat hypertension).
No products indexed under this heading.

Ethosuximide (Human pharmacologic studies have shown that methylphenidate may inhibit the metabolism of anticonvulsants (eg, phenobarbital, phenytoin, primidone). Downward dose adjustments of these drugs may be required when given concomitantly with methylphenidate. It may be necessary to adjust the dosage and monitor plasma drug concentrations when initiating or discontinuing methylphenidate).
No products indexed under this heading.

Ethotoin (Human pharmacologic studies have shown that methylphenidate may inhibit the metabolism of anticonvulsants (eg, phenobarbital,

phenytoin, primidone). Downward dose adjustments of these drugs may be required when given concomitantly with methylphenidate. It may be necessary to adjust the dosage and monitor plasma drug concentrations when initiating or discontinuing methylphenidate).
No products indexed under this heading.

Felbamate (Human pharmacologic studies have shown that methylphenidate may inhibit the metabolism of anticonvulsants (eg, phenobarbital, phenytoin, primidone). Downward dose adjustments of these drugs may be required when given concomitantly with methylphenidate. It may be necessary to adjust the dosage and monitor plasma drug concentrations when initiating or discontinuing methylphenidate).
No products indexed under this heading.

Felodipine (Methylphenidate may decrease the effectiveness of drugs used to treat hypertension).
No products indexed under this heading.

Fluoxetine Hydrochloride (Human pharmacologic studies have shown that methylphenidate may inhibit the metabolism of selective serotonin reuptake inhibitors. Downward dose adjustments of these drugs may be required when given concomitantly with methylphenidate. It may be necessary to adjust the dosage and monitor plasma drug concentrations when initiating or discontinuing methylphenidate). Products include:
Prozac Pulvules and Liquid 1801
Symbyax Capsules 1819

Fluvoxamine Maleate (Human pharmacologic studies have shown that methylphenidate may inhibit the metabolism of selective serotonin reuptake inhibitors. Downward dose adjustments of these drugs may be required when given concomitantly with methylphenidate. It may be necessary to adjust the dosage and monitor plasma drug concentrations when initiating or discontinuing methylphenidate).
No products indexed under this heading.

Fosinopril Sodium (Methylphenidate may decrease the effectiveness of drugs used to treat hypertension).
No products indexed under this heading.

Fosphenytoin (Human pharmacologic studies have shown that methylphenidate may inhibit the metabolism of anticonvulsants (eg, phenobarbital, phenytoin, primidone). Downward dose adjustments of these drugs may be required when given concomitantly with methylphenidate. It may be necessary to adjust the dosage and monitor plasma drug concentrations when initiating or discontinuing methylphenidate).
No products indexed under this heading.

Fosphenytoin Sodium (Human pharmacologic studies have shown that methylphenidate may inhibit the metabolism of anticonvulsants (eg, phenobarbital, phenytoin, primidone). Downward dose adjustments of these drugs may be required when given concomitantly with methylphenidate. It may be necessary to adjust the dosage and monitor plasma drug concentrations when initiat-

ing or discontinuing methylphenidate).
No products indexed under this heading.

Furosemide (Methylphenidate may decrease the effectiveness of drugs used to treat hypertension).
Products include:
Furosemide Tablets 2154

Gabapentin (Human pharmacologic studies have shown that methylphenidate may inhibit the metabolism of anticonvulsants (eg, phenobarbital, phenytoin, primidone). Downward dose adjustments of these drugs may be required when given concomitantly with methylphenidate. It may be necessary to adjust the dosage and monitor plasma drug concentrations when initiating or discontinuing methylphenidate). Products include:
Neurontin Capsules 2487
Neurontin Oral Solution 2487
Neurontin Tablets 2487

Guanabenz Acetate (Methylphenidate may decrease the effectiveness of drugs used to treat hypertension).
No products indexed under this heading.

Guanethidine Monosulfate (Methylphenidate may decrease the effectiveness of drugs used to treat hypertension).
No products indexed under this heading.

Hydralazine Hydrochloride (Methylphenidate may decrease the effectiveness of drugs used to treat hypertension). Products include:
BiDil Tablets 2171

Hydrochlorothiazide (Methylphenidate may decrease the effectiveness of drugs used to treat hypertension). Products include:
Aldoril Tablets 1910
Atacand HCT 651
Avalide Tablets 888
Avalide Tablets 2874
Benicar HCT Tablets 1044
Diovan HCT Tablets 2196
Dyazide Capsules 1423
Hyzaar 50-12.5 Tablets 1990
Hyzaar 100-12.5 Tablets 1990
Hyzaar 100-25 Tablets 1990
Lopressor HCT 50/25 Tablets 2241
Lopressor HCT 100/25 Tablets 2241
Lopressor HCT 100/50 Tablets 2241
Lotensin HCT Tablets 2246
Micardis HCT Tablets 856
Moduretic Tablets 2028
Prinzide Tablets 2056
Teveten HCT Tablets 1737
Timolide Tablets 2086
Uniretic Tablets 3100

Hydroflumethiazide (Methylphenidate may decrease the effectiveness of drugs used to treat hypertension).
No products indexed under this heading.

Imipramine Hydrochloride (Human pharmacologic studies have shown that methylphenidate may inhibit the metabolism of some tricyclic drugs (eg, imipramine, clomipramine, desipramine). Downward dose adjustments of these drugs may be required when given concomitantly with methylphenidate. It may be necessary to adjust the dosage and monitor plasma drug concentrations when initiating or discontinuing methylphenidate).
No products indexed under this heading.

Imipramine Pamoate (Human pharmacologic studies have shown that methylphenidate may inhibit the

metabolism of some tricyclic drugs (eg, imipramine, clomipramine, desipramine). Downward dose adjustments of these drugs may be required when given concomitantly with methylphenidate. It may be necessary to adjust the dosage and monitor plasma drug concentrations when initiating or discontinuing methylphenidate).
No products indexed under this heading.

Indapamide (Methylphenidate may decrease the effectiveness of drugs used to treat hypertension).
Products include:
Indapamide Tablets 2156

Irbesartan (Methylphenidate may decrease the effectiveness of drugs used to treat hypertension).
Products include:
Avalide Tablets 888
Avalide Tablets 2874
Avapro Tablets 891
Avapro Tablets 2871

Isocarboxazid (Methylphenidate transdermal system is contraindicated during treatment with monoamine oxidase inhibitors and also within a minimum of 14 days following discontinuation of treatment with a MAO inhibitor (hypertensive crises may occur)).
No products indexed under this heading.

Isoproterenol Hydrochloride (Because of a possible effect on blood pressure, methylphenidate transdermal system should be used cautiously with pressor agents).
No products indexed under this heading.

Isoproterenol Sulfate (Because of a possible effect on blood pressure, methylphenidate transdermal system should be used cautiously with pressor agents).
No products indexed under this heading.

Isradipine (Methylphenidate may decrease the effectiveness of drugs used to treat hypertension).
Products include:
DynaCirc CR Tablets 2721

Labetalol Hydrochloride (Methylphenidate may decrease the effectiveness of drugs used to treat hypertension).
No products indexed under this heading.

Lamotrigine (Human pharmacologic studies have shown that methylphenidate may inhibit the metabolism of anticonvulsants (eg, phenobarbital, phenytoin, primidone). Downward dose adjustments of these drugs may be required when given concomitantly with methylphenidate. It may be necessary to adjust the dosage and monitor plasma drug concentrations when initiating or discontinuing methylphenidate). Products include:
Lamictal 1481

Levetiracetam (Human pharmacologic studies have shown that methylphenidate may inhibit the metabolism of anticonvulsants (eg, phenobarbital, phenytoin, primidone). Downward dose adjustments of these drugs may be required when given concomitantly with methylphenidate. It may be necessary to adjust the dosage and monitor plasma drug concentrations when initiating or discontinuing methylphenidate). Products include:
Keppra Injection 3320
Keppra Oral Solution 3314
Keppra Tablets 3314

Lisinopril (Methylphenidate may decrease the effectiveness of drugs used to treat hypertension).
Products include:
Prinivil Tablets 2052
Prinzide Tablets 2056

Losartan Potassium (Methylphenidate may decrease the effectiveness of drugs used to treat hypertension).
Products include:
Cozaar Tablets 1935
Hyzaar 50-12.5 Tablets 1990
Hyzaar 100-12.5 Tablets 1990
Hyzaar 100-25 Tablets 1990

Maprotiline Hydrochloride (Human pharmacologic studies have shown that methylphenidate may inhibit the metabolism of some tricyclic drugs (eg, imipramine, clomipramine, desipramine). Downward dose adjustments of these drugs may be required when given concomitantly with methylphenidate. It may be necessary to adjust the dosage and monitor plasma drug concentrations when initiating or discontinuing methylphenidate).
No products indexed under this heading.

Mecamylamine Hydrochloride (Methylphenidate may decrease the effectiveness of drugs used to treat hypertension).
No products indexed under this heading.

Mephentermine Sulfate (Because of a possible effect on blood pressure, methylphenidate transdermal system should be used cautiously with pressor agents).
No products indexed under this heading.

Mephenytoin (Human pharmacologic studies have shown that methylphenidate may inhibit the metabolism of anticonvulsants (eg, phenobarbital, phenytoin, primidone). Downward dose adjustments of these drugs may be required when given concomitantly with methylphenidate. It may be necessary to adjust the dosage and monitor plasma drug concentrations when initiating or discontinuing methylphenidate).
No products indexed under this heading.

Metaraminol Bitartrate (Because of a possible effect on blood pressure, methylphenidate transdermal system should be used cautiously with pressor agents).
No products indexed under this heading.

Methoxamine Hydrochloride (Because of a possible effect on blood pressure, methylphenidate transdermal system should be used cautiously with pressor agents).
No products indexed under this heading.

Methsuximide (Human pharmacologic studies have shown that methylphenidate may inhibit the metabolism of anticonvulsants (eg, phenobarbital, phenytoin, primidone). Downward dose adjustments of these drugs may be required when given concomitantly with methylphenidate. It may be necessary to adjust the dosage and monitor plasma drug concentrations when initiating or discontinuing methylphenidate).
No products indexed under this heading.

Methyclothiazide (Methylphenidate may decrease the effectiveness of drugs used to treat hypertension).
No products indexed under this heading.

Methyldopa (Methylphenidate may decrease the effectiveness of drugs used to treat hypertension).
Products include:
Aldoril Tablets 1910

Methyldopate Hydrochloride (Methylphenidate may decrease the effectiveness of drugs used to treat hypertension).
No products indexed under this heading.

Metolazone (Methylphenidate may decrease the effectiveness of drugs used to treat hypertension).
No products indexed under this heading.

Metoprolol Succinate (Methylphenidate may decrease the effectiveness of drugs used to treat hypertension). Products include:
Toprol-XL Tablets 668

Metoprolol Tartrate (Methylphenidate may decrease the effectiveness of drugs used to treat hypertension).
Products include:
Lopressor Injection 2238
Lopressor Tablets 2238
Lopressor HCT 50/25 Tablets 2241
Lopressor HCT 100/25 Tablets 2241
Lopressor HCT 100/50 Tablets 2241

Metyrosine (Methylphenidate may decrease the effectiveness of drugs used to treat hypertension).
Products include:
Demser Capsules 1953

Mibefradil Dihydrochloride (Methylphenidate may decrease the effectiveness of drugs used to treat hypertension).
No products indexed under this heading.

Minoxidil (Methylphenidate may decrease the effectiveness of drugs used to treat hypertension).
Products include:
Men's Rogaine Extra Strength Hair Regrowth Treatment Topical Solution, Ocean Rush Scent and Original Unscented 633
Men's Rogaine Foam Hair Regrowth Treatment 633
Women's Rogaine Hair Regrowth Treatment Topical Solution, Spring Bloom Scent and Original Unscented 634

Moclobemide (Methylphenidate transdermal system is contraindicated during treatment with monoamine oxidase inhibitors and also within a minimum of 14 days following discontinuation of treatment with a MAO inhibitor (hypertensive crises may occur)).
No products indexed under this heading.

Moexipril Hydrochloride (Methylphenidate may decrease the effectiveness of drugs used to treat hypertension). Products include:
Uniretic Tablets 3100
Univasc Tablets 3104

Nadolol (Methylphenidate may decrease the effectiveness of drugs used to treat hypertension).
Products include:
Nadolol Tablets 2159

Nicardipine Hydrochloride (Methylphenidate may decrease the effectiveness of drugs used to treat hypertension). Products include:
Cardene I.V. 2497

Nifedipine (Methylphenidate may decrease the effectiveness of drugs used to treat hypertension).
Products include:
Adalat CC Tablets 2964

Nisoldipine (Methylphenidate may decrease the effectiveness of drugs used to treat hypertension).
Products include:
Sular Tablets 3122

Nitroglycerin (Methylphenidate may decrease the effectiveness of drugs used to treat hypertension).
Products include:
Nitro-Dur Transdermal Infusion System 3046
Nitrolingual Pumpspray 3120

Norepinephrine Bitartrate (Because of a possible effect on blood pressure, methylphenidate transdermal system should be used cautiously with pressor agents).
No products indexed under this heading.

Nortriptyline Hydrochloride (Human pharmacologic studies have shown that methylphenidate may inhibit the metabolism of some tricyclic drugs (eg, imipramine, clomipramine, desipramine). Downward dose adjustments of these drugs may be required when given concomitantly with methylphenidate. It may be necessary to adjust the dosage and monitor plasma drug concentrations when initiating or discontinuing methylphenidate).
No products indexed under this heading.

Oxcarbazepine (Human pharmacologic studies have shown that methylphenidate may inhibit the metabolism of anticonvulsants (eg, phenobarbital, phenytoin, primidone). Downward dose adjustments of these drugs may be required when given concomitantly with methylphenidate. It may be necessary to adjust the dosage and monitor plasma drug concentrations when initiating or discontinuing methylphenidate). Products include:
Trileptal Tablets 2300
Trileptal Oral Suspension 2300

Paramethadione (Human pharmacologic studies have shown that methylphenidate may inhibit the metabolism of anticonvulsants (eg, phenobarbital, phenytoin, primidone). Downward dose adjustments of these drugs may be required when given concomitantly with methylphenidate. It may be necessary to adjust the dosage and monitor plasma drug concentrations when initiating or discontinuing methylphenidate).
No products indexed under this heading.

Pargyline Hydrochloride (Methylphenidate transdermal system is contraindicated during treatment with monoamine oxidase inhibitors and also within a minimum of 14 days following discontinuation of treatment with a MAO inhibitor (hypertensive crises may occur)).
No products indexed under this heading.

Paroxetine Hydrochloride (Human pharmacologic studies have shown that methylphenidate may inhibit the metabolism of selective serotonin reuptake inhibitors. Downward dose adjustments of these drugs may be required when given concomitantly with methylphenidate. It may be necessary to adjust the dosage and monitor plasma drug concentrations when initiating or discontinuing methylphenidate). Products include:

Paxil CR Controlled-Release Tablets 1538
Paxil 1530

Penbutolol Sulfate (Methylphenidate may decrease the effectiveness of drugs used to treat hypertension).
No products indexed under this heading.

Perindopril Erbumine (Methylphenidate may decrease the effectiveness of drugs used to treat hypertension). Products include:

Aceon Tablets (2 mg, 4 mg, 8 mg) 3194

Phenacemide (Human pharmacologic studies have shown that methylphenidate may inhibit the metabolism of anticonvulsants (eg, phenobarbital, phenytoin, primidone). Downward dose adjustments of these drugs may be required when given concomitantly with methylphenidate. It may be necessary to adjust the dosage and monitor plasma drug concentrations when initiating or discontinuing methylphenidate).
No products indexed under this heading.

Phenelzine Sulfate (Methylphenidate transdermal system is contraindicated during treatment with monoamine oxidase inhibitors and also within a minimum of 14 days following discontinuation of treatment with a MAO inhibitor (hypertensive crises may occur)).
No products indexed under this heading.

Phenobarbital (Human pharmacologic studies have shown that methylphenidate may inhibit the metabolism of anticonvulsants (eg, phenobarbital, phenytoin, primidone). Downward dose adjustments of these drugs may be required when given concomitantly with methylphenidate. It may be necessary to adjust the dosage and monitor plasma drug concentrations when initiating or discontinuing methylphenidate). Products include:

Donnatal Extentabs 2493

Phenoxybenzamine Hydrochloride (Methylphenidate may decrease the effectiveness of drugs used to treat hypertension). Products include:

Dibenzyline Capsules 3399

Phensuximide (Human pharmacologic studies have shown that methylphenidate may inhibit the metabolism of anticonvulsants (eg, phenobarbital, phenytoin, primidone). Downward dose adjustments of these drugs may be required when given concomitantly with methylphenidate. It may be necessary to adjust the dosage and monitor plasma drug concentrations when initiating or discontinuing methylphenidate).
No products indexed under this heading.

Phentolamine Mesylate (Methylphenidate may decrease the effectiveness of drugs used to treat hypertension).
No products indexed under this heading.

Phenylephrine Hydrochloride (Because of a possible effect on blood pressure, methylphenidate transdermal system should be used cautiously with pressor agents). Products include:

Comtrex Maximum Strength Non-Drowsy Cold & Cough Caplets .... ▣725
Comtrex Maximum Strength Day/Night Severe Cold & Sinus Caplets - Day Formulation .... ▣725
Comtrex Maximum Strength Day/Night Severe Cold & Sinus Caplets - Night Formulation .... ▣725
Contac Cold and Flu Maximum Strength Caplets .... ▣728
Contac Cold and Flu Day and Night Caplets (Day Formulation Only) .... ▣727
Contac Cold and Flu Day and Night Caplets (Night Formulation Only) .... ▣727
Contac Cold and Flu Non-Drowsy Caplets .... ▣728
Contac-D Cold Non-Drowsy Tablets .... ▣729
Children's Dimetapp Cold & Allergy Elixir .... ▣730
Children's Dimetapp Cold & Allergy Chewable Tablets .... ▣730
Children's Dimetapp DM Cold & Cough Elixir .... ▣731
Toddler's Dimetapp Cold and Cough Drops .... ▣732
Excedrin Sinus Headache Caplets/Tablets .... ▣610
4-Way Fast Acting Nasal Spray .... ▣775
4-Way Menthol Nasal Spray .... ▣775
Preparation H Maximum Strength Cream .... ▣666
Preparation H Cooling Gel .... ▣666
Preparation H .... ▣666
Refenesen PE Caplets .... ▣721
Robitussin Cough & Allergy Syrup .... ▣736
Robitussin Cough & Cold Nighttime Liquid .... ▣736
Robitussin Cough, Cold & Flu Nighttime Liquid .... ▣738
Robitussin Head & Chest Congestion PE Syrup .... ▣739
Robitussin Pediatric Cough & Cold Nighttime Liquid .... ▣736
TheraFlu Cold & Cough Hot Liquid .... ▣740
TheraFlu Cold & Sore Throat Hot Liquid .... ▣741
TheraFlu Flu & Sore Throat Hot Liquid .... ▣742
TheraFlu Daytime Severe Cold Hot Liquid .... ▣742
TheraFlu Nighttime Severe Cold Hot Liquid .... ▣740
TheraFlu Warming Relief Daytime Severe Cold .... ▣743
TheraFlu Warming Relief Nighttime Severe Cold .... ▣743
Triaminic Chest & Nasal Congestion Liquid .... ▣746
Triaminic Cold & Allergy Liquid .... ▣746
Triaminic Daytime Cold & Cough Liquid .... ▣745
Triaminic Nighttime Cold & Cough Liquid .... ▣746
Triaminic Thin Strips Cold .... ▣748
Triaminic Thin Strips Cold & Cough .... ▣778
Triaminic Infant Thin Strips Decongestant .... ▣747
Triaminic Infant Thin Strips Decongestant Plus Cough .... ▣747
Children's Tylenol Plus Flu Oral Suspension .... ▣749
Tylenol Cold Head Congestion Daytime Caplets with Cool Burst and Gelcaps .... ▣750
Tylenol Cold Multi-Symptom Daytime Liquid .... ▣752
Tylenol Cold Multi-Symptom Severe Daytime Liquid .... ▣752
Concentrated Tylenol Infants' Drops Plus Cold & Cough .... ▣754
Tylenol Allergy Multi-Symptom Caplets with Cool Burst and Gelcaps 1872
Tylenol Allergy Multi-Symptom Nighttime Caplets with Cool Burst 1872
Children's Tylenol Plus Cold Suspension Liquid 1879
Children's Tylenol Plus Cold & Allergy Suspension Liquid 1878
Children's Tylenol Plus Flu Suspension Liquid 1881
Children's Tylenol Plus Multi-Symptom Cold Suspension Liquid 1879
Tylenol Cold Head Congestion Daytime Caplets with Cool Burst 1873
Tylenol Cold Head Congestion Nighttime Caplets with Cool Burst 1873
Tylenol Cold Head Congestion Severe Caplets with Cool Burst 1873
Tylenol Cold Multi-Symptom Daytime Caplets with Cool Burst and Gelcaps 1874
Tylenol Cold Multi-Symptom Daytime Liquid with Citrus Burst 1874
Tylenol Cold Multi-Symptom Nighttime Caplets with Cool Burst 1874
Tylenol Cold Multi-Symptom Nighttime Liquid with Cool Burst 1874
Tylenol Cold Multi-Symptom Severe Caplets with Cool Burst 1874
Tylenol Cold Multi-Symptom Severe Daytime Liquid with Citrus Burst 1874
Tylenol Sinus Congestion & Pain Daytime Caplets with Cool Burst and Gelcaps 1876
Tylenol Sinus Congestion & Pain Nighttime Caplets with Cool Burst 1876
Tylenol Sinus Congestion & Pain Severe Caplets with Cool Burst 1876
Vicks 44D Cough & Head Congestion Relief Liquid .... ▣760
Vicks DayQuil LiquiCaps/Liquid Multi-Symptom Cold/Flu Relief .... ▣761
Zicam Cough Plus D Cough Spray .... ▣767

Phenytoin (Human pharmacologic studies have shown that methylphenidate may inhibit the metabolism of anticonvulsants (eg, phenobarbital, phenytoin, primidone). Downward dose adjustments of these drugs may be required when given concomitantly with methylphenidate. It may be necessary to adjust the dosage and monitor plasma drug concentrations when initiating or discontinuing methylphenidate).
No products indexed under this heading.

Phenytoin Sodium (Human pharmacologic studies have shown that methylphenidate may inhibit the metabolism of anticonvulsants (eg, phenobarbital, phenytoin, primidone). Downward dose adjustments of these drugs may be required when given concomitantly with methylphenidate. It may be necessary to adjust the dosage and monitor plasma drug concentrations when initiating or discontinuing methylphenidate). Products include:

Phenytek Capsules 2160

Pindolol (Methylphenidate may decrease the effectiveness of drugs used to treat hypertension).
No products indexed under this heading.

Polythiazide (Methylphenidate may decrease the effectiveness of drugs used to treat hypertension).
No products indexed under this heading.

Prazosin Hydrochloride (Methylphenidate may decrease the effectiveness of drugs used to treat hypertension).
No products indexed under this heading.

Primidone (Human pharmacologic studies have shown that methylphenidate may inhibit the metabolism of anticonvulsants (eg, phenobarbital, phenytoin, primidone). Downward dose adjustments of these drugs may be required when given concomitantly with methylphenidate. It may be necessary to adjust the dosage and monitor plasma drug concentrations when initiating or discontinuing methylphenidate).
No products indexed under this heading.

Procarbazine Hydrochloride (Methylphenidate transdermal system is contraindicated during treatment with monoamine oxidase inhibitors and also within a minimum of 14 days following discontinuation of treatment with a MAO inhibitor (hypertensive crises may occur)). Products include:

Matulane Capsules 3191

Propranolol Hydrochloride (Methylphenidate may decrease the effectiveness of drugs used to treat hypertension). Products include:

Inderal LA Long-Acting Capsules 3429
InnoPran XL Capsules 2723

Protriptyline Hydrochloride (Human pharmacologic studies have shown that methylphenidate may inhibit the metabolism of some tricyclic drugs (eg, imipramine, clomipramine, desipramine). Downward dose adjustments of these drugs may be required when given concomitantly with methylphenidate. It may be necessary to adjust the dosage and monitor plasma drug concentrations when initiating or discontinuing methylphenidate).
No products indexed under this heading.

Quinapril Hydrochloride (Methylphenidate may decrease the effectiveness of drugs used to treat hypertension).
No products indexed under this heading.

Ramipril (Methylphenidate may decrease the effectiveness of drugs used to treat hypertension). Products include:

Altace Capsules 1702

Rauwolfia Serpentina (Methylphenidate may decrease the effectiveness of drugs used to treat hypertension).
No products indexed under this heading.

Rescinnamine (Methylphenidate may decrease the effectiveness of drugs used to treat hypertension).
No products indexed under this heading.

Reserpine (Methylphenidate may decrease the effectiveness of drugs used to treat hypertension).
No products indexed under this heading.

Selegiline Hydrochloride (Methylphenidate transdermal system is contraindicated during treatment with monoamine oxidase inhibitors and also within a minimum of 14 days following discontinuation of treatment with a MAO inhibitor (hypertensive crises may occur)). Products include:

Eldepryl Capsules 3208
Zelapar Tablets 3372

Sertraline Hydrochloride (Human pharmacologic studies have shown that methylphenidate may inhibit the metabolism of selective serotonin reuptake inhibitors. Downward dose adjustments of these drugs may be required when given concomitantly with methylphenidate. It may be necessary to adjust the dosage and monitor plasma drug concentrations when initiating or discontinuing methylphenidate). Products include:
Zoloft 2586

Sodium Nitroprusside (Methylphenidate may decrease the effectiveness of drugs used to treat hypertension).
No products indexed under this heading.

Sotalol Hydrochloride (Methylphenidate may decrease the effectiveness of drugs used to treat hypertension).
No products indexed under this heading.

Spirapril Hydrochloride (Methylphenidate may decrease the effectiveness of drugs used to treat hypertension).
No products indexed under this heading.

Telmisartan (Methylphenidate may decrease the effectiveness of drugs used to treat hypertension). Products include:
Micardis Tablets 854
Micardis HCT Tablets 856

Terazosin Hydrochloride (Methylphenidate may decrease the effectiveness of drugs used to treat hypertension). Products include:
Hytrin Capsules 471

Tiagabine Hydrochloride (Human pharmacologic studies have shown that methylphenidate may inhibit the metabolism of anticonvulsants (eg, phenobarbital, phenytoin, primidone). Downward dose adjustments of these drugs may be required when given concomitantly with methylphenidate. It may be necessary to adjust the dosage and monitor plasma drug concentrations when initiating or discontinuing methylphenidate). Products include:
Gabitril Tablets 984

Timolol Maleate (Methylphenidate may decrease the effectiveness of drugs used to treat hypertension). Products include:
Blocadren Tablets 1916
Cosopt Sterile Ophthalmic Solution.. 1931
Timolide Tablets 2086
Timoptic Sterile Ophthalmic Solution.. 2088
Timoptic in Ocudose 2091
Timoptic-XE Sterile Ophthalmic Gel Forming Solution 2092

Topiramate (Human pharmacologic studies have shown that methylphenidate may inhibit the metabolism of anticonvulsants (eg, phenobarbital, phenytoin, primidone). Downward dose adjustments of these drugs may be required when given concomitantly with methylphenidate. It may be necessary to adjust the dosage and monitor plasma drug concentrations when initiating or discontinuing methylphenidate). Products include:
Topamax Sprinkle Capsules 2404
Topamax Tablets 2404

Torsemide (Methylphenidate may decrease the effectiveness of drugs used to treat hypertension). Products include:
Demadex Injection 2759
Demadex Tablets 2759

Trandolapril (Methylphenidate may decrease the effectiveness of drugs used to treat hypertension). Products include:
Mavik Tablets 486
Tarka Tablets 524

Tranylcypromine Sulfate (Methylphenidate transdermal system is contraindicated during treatment with monoamine oxidase inhibitors and also within a minimum of 14 days following discontinuation of treatment with a MAO inhibitor (hypertensive crises may occur)). Products include:
Parnate Tablets 1527

Trimethadione (Human pharmacologic studies have shown that methylphenidate may inhibit the metabolism of anticonvulsants (eg, phenobarbital, phenytoin, primidone). Downward dose adjustments of these drugs may be required when given concomitantly with methylphenidate. It may be necessary to adjust the dosage and monitor plasma drug concentrations when initiating or discontinuing methylphenidate).
No products indexed under this heading.

Trimethaphan Camsylate (Methylphenidate may decrease the effectiveness of drugs used to treat hypertension).
No products indexed under this heading.

Trimipramine Maleate (Human pharmacologic studies have shown that methylphenidate may inhibit the metabolism of some tricyclic drugs (eg, imipramine, clomipramine, desipramine). Downward dose adjustments of these drugs may be required when given concomitantly with methylphenidate. It may be necessary to adjust the dosage and monitor plasma drug concentrations when initiating or discontinuing methylphenidate).
No products indexed under this heading.

Valproate Sodium (Human pharmacologic studies have shown that methylphenidate may inhibit the metabolism of anticonvulsants (eg, phenobarbital, phenytoin, primidone). Downward dose adjustments of these drugs may be required when given concomitantly with methylphenidate. It may be necessary to adjust the dosage and monitor plasma drug concentrations when initiating or discontinuing methylphenidate). Products include:
Depacon Injection 412

Valproic Acid (Human pharmacologic studies have shown that methylphenidate may inhibit the metabolism of anticonvulsants (eg, phenobarbital, phenytoin, primidone). Downward dose adjustments of these drugs may be required when given concomitantly with methylphenidate. It may be necessary to adjust the dosage and monitor plasma drug concentrations when initiating or discontinuing methylphenidate). Products include:
Depakene 417

Valsartan (Methylphenidate may decrease the effectiveness of drugs used to treat hypertension). Products include:
Diovan Tablets 2193
Diovan HCT Tablets 2196

Verapamil Hydrochloride (Methylphenidate may decrease the effectiveness of drugs used to treat hypertension). Products include:
Covera-HS Tablets 3139
Tarka Tablets 524
Verelan PM Extended-Release Capsules, Controlled-Onset........... 3106

Warfarin Sodium (Human pharmacologic studies have shown that methylphenidate may inhibit the metabolism of coumarin anticoagulants. Downward dose adjustments of these drugs may be required when given concomitantly with methylphenidate. It may be necessary to adjust the dosage and monitor plasma drug concentrations or coagulation times when initiating or discontinuing methylphenidate). Products include:
Coumadin for Injection 898
Coumadin Tablets 898

Zonisamide (Human pharmacologic studies have shown that methylphenidate may inhibit the metabolism of anticonvulsants (eg, phenobarbital, phenytoin, primidone). Downward dose adjustments of these drugs may be required when given concomitantly with methylphenidate. It may be necessary to adjust the dosage and monitor plasma drug concentrations when initiating or discontinuing methylphenidate). Products include:
Zonegran Capsules 1101

D-CAL CHEWABLE CAPLETS
(Calcium Carbonate, Vitamin D) 812

DDS-ACIDOPHILUS CAPSULES, TABLETS, AND POWDER
(Lactobacillus Acidophilus) 812
None cited in PDR database.

DEBROX DROPS
(Carbamide Peroxide) 715
None cited in PDR database.

DECADRON TABLETS
(Dexamethasone) 1951
May interact with anticholinesterase drugs, barbiturates, oral anticoagulants, cytochrome p450 3a4 inducers (selected), cytochrome p450 3a4 inhibitors (selected), cytochrome p450 3a4 substrates (selected), estrogens, cardiac glycosides, oral hypoglycemic agents, insulin, macrolide antibiotics, nonsteroidal anti-inflammatory agents, oral contraceptives, phenytoin, potassium-depleting diuretics, vaccines, live, and certain other agents. Compounds in these categories include:

Acarbose (Because corticosteroids may increase blood glucose concentrations, dosage adjustments of antidiabetic agents may be required). Products include:
Precose Tablets 751

Acetazolamide (Drugs which inhibit cytochrome P450 3A4 enzyme activity have the potential to result in increased plasma concentrations of corticosteroids).
No products indexed under this heading.

Alfentanil Hydrochloride (Dexamethasone is a moderate inducer of the cytochrome P450 3A4 enzyme system. Co-administration with other drugs that are metabolized by CYP 3A4 may increase their clearance, resulting in decreased plasma concentrations).
No products indexed under this heading.

Allium sativum (Drugs which induce cytochrome P450 3A4 enzyme activity may enhance the metabolism of corticosteroids and require that the dosage of the corticosteroid be increased).
No products indexed under this heading.

Alprazolam (Dexamethasone is a moderate inducer of the cytochrome P450 3A4 enzyme system. Co-administration with other drugs that are metabolized by CYP 3A4 may increase their clearance, resulting in decreased plasma concentrations). Products include:
Niravam Orally Disintegrating Tablets.. 3092

Aminoglutethimide (Aminoglutethimide may diminish adrenal suppression by corticosteroids).
No products indexed under this heading.

Amiodarone Hydrochloride (Drugs which inhibit cytochrome P450 3A4 enzyme activity have the potential to result in increased plasma concentrations of corticosteroids).
No products indexed under this heading.

Amitriptyline Hydrochloride (Dexamethasone is a moderate inducer of the cytochrome P450 3A4 enzyme system. Co-administration with other drugs that are metabolized by CYP 3A4 may increase their clearance, resulting in decreased plasma concentrations).
No products indexed under this heading.

Amlodipine Besylate (Dexamethasone is a moderate inducer of the cytochrome P450 3A4 enzyme system. Co-administration with other drugs that are metabolized by CYP 3A4 may increase their clearance, resulting in decreased plasma concentrations). Products include:
Caduet Tablets 2508
Lotrel Capsules 2249
Norvasc Tablets 2545

Amphotericin B (When corticosteroids are administered with potassium-depleting agents (eg, amphotericin B), patients should be observed closely for development of hypokalemia. In addition, there have been cases reported in which concomitant use of amphotericin B and hydrocortisone was followed by cardiac enlargement and congestive heart failure).
No products indexed under this heading.

Amphotericin B, liposomal (When corticosteroids are administered with potassium-depleting agents (eg, amphotericin B), patients should be observed closely for development of hypokalemia. In addition, there have been cases reported in which concomitant use of amphotericin B and hydrocortisone was followed by cardiac enlargement and congestive heart failure). Products include:
AmBisome for Injection 620

Amphotericin B Cholesteryl Sulfate (When corticosteroids are administered with potassium-depleting agents (eg, amphotericin B), patients should be observed closely for development of hypokalemia. In addition, there have been cases reported in which concomitant use of amphotericin B and hydrocortisone was followed by cardiac enlargement and congestive heart failure).

No products indexed under this heading.

Amphotericin B Lipid Complex (When corticosteroids are administered with potassium-depleting agents (eg, amphotericin B), patients should be observed closely for development of hypokalemia. In addition, there have been cases reported in which concomitant use of amphotericin B and hydrocortisone was followed by cardiac enlargement and congestive heart failure). Products include:

Abelcet Injection 1141

Amprenavir (Drugs which inhibit cytochrome P450 3A4 enzyme activity have the potential to result in increased plasma concentrations of corticosteroids). Products include:

Agenerase Capsules 1327
Agenerase Oral Solution 1332

Anastrozole (Drugs which inhibit cytochrome P450 3A4 enzyme activity have the potential to result in increased plasma concentrations of corticosteroids). Products include:

Arimidex Tablets 673

Anisindione (Co-administration of corticosteroids and warfarin usually results in inhibition of response to warfarin, although there have been some conflicting reports. Therefore, coagulation indices should be monitored frequently to maintain the desired anticoagulant effect). Products include:

Miradon Tablets 3042

Aprepitant (Drugs which inhibit cytochrome P450 3A4 enzyme activity have the potential to result in increased plasma concentrations of corticosteroids). Products include:

Emend Capsules 1963

Aprobarbital (Drugs which induce cytochrome P450 3A4 enzyme activity (eg, barbiturates) may enhance the metabolism of corticosteroids and require that the dosage of the corticosteroid be increased).

No products indexed under this heading.

Astemizole (Dexamethasone is a moderate inducer of the cytochrome P450 3A4 enzyme system. Co-administration with other drugs that are metabolized by CYP 3A4 may increase their clearance, resulting in decreased plasma concentrations).

No products indexed under this heading.

Atorvastatin Calcium (Dexamethasone is a moderate inducer of the cytochrome P450 3A4 enzyme system. Co-administration with other drugs that are metabolized by CYP 3A4 may increase their clearance, resulting in decreased plasma concentrations). Products include:

Caduet Tablets 2508
Lipitor Tablets 2483

Azithromycin Dihydrate (Macrolide antibiotics have been reported to cause a significant decrease in corticosteroid clearance. Drugs which inhibit cytochrome P450 3A4 enzyme activity (eg, macrolide antibiotics) have the potential to result in increased plasma concentrations of corticosteroids. Dexamethasone is a moderate inducer of the cytochrome P450 3A4 enzyme system. Co-administration with other drugs that are metabolized by CYP 3A4 (eg, erythromycin) may increase their clearance, resulting in decreased plasma concentrations).

No products indexed under this heading.

BCG Vaccine (Patients on corticosteroid therapy may exhibit a diminished response to toxoids and live or inactivated vaccines due to inhibition of antibody response. Corticosteroids may also potentiate the replication of some organisms contained in live attenuated vaccines. Routine administration of vaccines or toxoids should be deferred until corticosteroid therapy is discontinued if possible. Administration of live or live, attenuated vaccines is contraindicated in patients receiving immunosuppressive doses of corticosteroids).

No products indexed under this heading.

Belladonna Ergotamine (Dexamethasone is a moderate inducer of the cytochrome P450 3A4 enzyme system. Co-administration with other drugs that are metabolized by CYP 3A4 may increase their clearance, resulting in decreased plasma concentrations).

No products indexed under this heading.

Bendroflumethiazide (When corticosteroids are administered with potassium-depleting agents (eg, diuretics), patients should be observed closely for development of hypokalemia).

No products indexed under this heading.

Betamethasone Acetate (Drugs which induce cytochrome P450 3A4 enzyme activity may enhance the metabolism of corticosteroids and require that the dosage of the corticosteroid be increased).

No products indexed under this heading.

Betamethasone Sodium Phosphate (Drugs which induce cytochrome P450 3A4 enzyme activity may enhance the metabolism of corticosteroids and require that the dosage of the corticosteroid be increased).

No products indexed under this heading.

Bumetanide (When corticosteroids are administered with potassium-depleting agents (eg, diuretics), patients should be observed closely for development of hypokalemia). Products include:

Bumex Tablets 2746

Buspirone Hydrochloride (Dexamethasone is a moderate inducer of the cytochrome P450 3A4 enzyme system. Co-administration with other drugs that are metabolized by CYP 3A4 may increase their clearance, resulting in decreased plasma concentrations).

No products indexed under this heading.

Busulfan (Dexamethasone is a moderate inducer of the cytochrome P450 3A4 enzyme system. Co-administration with other drugs that are metabolized by CYP 3A4 may increase their clearance, resulting in decreased plasma concentrations). Products include:

I.V. Busulfex 2493
Myleran Tablets 1525

Butabarbital (Drugs which induce cytochrome P450 3A4 enzyme activity (eg, barbiturates) may enhance the metabolism of corticosteroids and require that the dosage of the corticosteroid be increased).

No products indexed under this heading.

Butalbital (Drugs which induce cytochrome P450 3A4 enzyme activity (eg, barbiturates) may enhance the metabolism of corticosteroids and require that the dosage of the corticosteroid be increased).

No products indexed under this heading.

Carbamazepine (Dexamethasone is a moderate inducer of the cytochrome P450 3A4 enzyme system. Co-administration with other drugs that are metabolized by CYP 3A4 may increase their clearance, resulting in decreased plasma concentrations). Products include:

Carbatrol Capsules 3171
Equetro Extended-Release Capsules 3180
Tegretol/Tegretol-XR 2295

Celecoxib (Concomitant use of non-steroidal anti-inflammatory agents and corticosteroids increases the risk of gastrointestinal side effects). Products include:

Celebrex Capsules 3134

Cerivastatin Sodium (Dexamethasone is a moderate inducer of the cytochrome P450 3A4 enzyme system. Co-administration with other drugs that are metabolized by CYP 3A4 may increase their clearance, resulting in decreased plasma concentrations).

No products indexed under this heading.

Chlorothiazide (When corticosteroids are administered with potassium-depleting agents (eg, diuretics), patients should be observed closely for development of hypokalemia). Products include:

Diuril Oral Suspension 1954

Chlorothiazide Sodium (When corticosteroids are administered with potassium-depleting agents (eg, diuretics), patients should be observed closely for development of hypokalemia). Products include:

Diuril Sodium Intravenous 2467

Chlorotrianisene (Estrogens may decrease the hepatic metabolism of certain corticosteroids, thereby increasing their effect).

No products indexed under this heading.

Chlorpheniramine (Dexamethasone is a moderate inducer of the cytochrome P450 3A4 enzyme system. Co-administration with other drugs that are metabolized by CYP 3A4 may increase their clearance, resulting in decreased plasma concentrations).

No products indexed under this heading.

Chlorpheniramine Maleate (Dexamethasone is a moderate inducer of the cytochrome P450 3A4 enzyme system. Co-administration with other drugs that are metabolized by CYP 3A4 may increase their clearance, resulting in decreased plasma concentrations). Products include:

Advil Allergy Sinus Caplets .... ▣770
Advil Multi-Symptom Cold Caplets .... ▣770
BC Allergy Sinus Cold Powder .... ▣677
Comtrex Maximum Strength Cold & Cough Day/Night Caplets - Night Formulation .... ▣726
Comtrex Maximum Strength Day/Night Severe Cold & Sinus Caplets - Night Formulation .... ▣725
Contac Cold and Flu Maximum Strength Caplets .... ▣728
Contac Cold and Flu Day and Night Caplets (Night Formulation Only) .... ▣727
Children's Dimetapp Long Acting Cough Plus Cold Syrup .... ▣731
Robitussin Cough & Cold Long-Acting Liquid .... ▣735
Robitussin Cough & Allergy Syrup .. ▣736
Robitussin Cough & Cold Nighttime Liquid .... ▣736
Robitussin Cough, Cold & Flu Nighttime Liquid .... ▣738
Robitussin Pediatric Cough & Cold Long-Acting Liquid .... ▣735
Robitussin Pediatric Cough & Cold Nighttime Liquid .... ▣736
Triaminic Cold & Allergy Liquid .... ▣746
Triaminic Cough & Runny Nose Softchews .... ▣748
Children's Tylenol Plus Flu Oral Suspension .... ▣749
Tylenol Allergy Multi-Symptom Caplets with Cool Burst and Gelcaps 1872
Children's Tylenol Plus Cold Suspension Liquid 1879
Children's Tylenol Plus Cough & Runny Nose Suspension Liquid 1879
Children's Tylenol Plus Flu Suspension Liquid 1881
Children's Tylenol Plus Multi-Symptom Cold Suspension Liquid 1879
Tylenol Cold Head Congestion Nighttime Caplets with Cool Burst 1873
Tylenol Cold Multi-Symptom Nighttime Caplets with Cool Burst 1874
Tylenol Sinus Congestion & Pain Nighttime Caplets with Cool Burst 1876
Vicks 44M Cough, Cold & Flu Relief Liquid 2680
Pediatric Vicks 44m Cough & Cold Relief Liquid 2676
Children's Vicks NyQuil Cold/Cough Relief .... ▣756
Children's Vicks NyQuil Cold/Cough Relief Liquid 2680
Zicam Maximum Strength Flu Daytime .... ▣768

Chlorpheniramine Polistirex (Dexamethasone is a moderate inducer of the cytochrome P450 3A4 enzyme system. Co-administration with other drugs that are metabolized by CYP 3A4 may increase their clearance, resulting in decreased plasma concentrations). Products include:

Tussionex Pennkinetic Extended-Release Suspension 3327

Chlorpheniramine Tannate (Dexamethasone is a moderate inducer of the cytochrome P450 3A4 enzyme system. Co-administration with other drugs that are metabolized by CYP 3A4 may increase their clearance, resulting in decreased plasma concentrations).

No products indexed under this heading.

Chlorpropamide (Because corticosteroids may increase blood glucose concentrations, dosage adjustments of antidiabetic agents may be required).

No products indexed under this heading.

Cholestyramine (Cholestyramine may increase the clearance of corticosteroids).

No products indexed under this heading.

Cimetidine (Drugs which inhibit cytochrome P450 3A4 enzyme activity have the potential to result in increased plasma concentrations of corticosteroids). Products include:

Cimetidine Hydrochloride (Drugs which inhibit cytochrome P450 3A4 enzyme activity have the potential to result in increased plasma concentrations of corticosteroids).

No products indexed under this heading.

Ciprofloxacin (Drugs which inhibit cytochrome P450 3A4 enzyme activity have the potential to result in increased plasma concentrations of corticosteroids). Products include:

Ciprofloxacin Hydrochloride (Drugs which induce cytochrome P450 3A4 enzyme activity may enhance the metabolism of corticosteroids and require that the dosage of the corticosteroid be increased). Products include:

Cisapride (Dexamethasone is a moderate inducer of the cytochrome P450 3A4 enzyme system. Co-administration with other drugs that are metabolized by CYP 3A4 may increase their clearance, resulting in decreased plasma concentrations).

No products indexed under this heading.

Cisplatin (Drugs which induce cytochrome P450 3A4 enzyme activity may enhance the metabolism of corticosteroids and require that the dosage of the corticosteroid be increased).

No products indexed under this heading.

Clarithromycin (Macrolide antibiotics have been reported to cause a significant decrease in corticosteroid clearance. Drugs which inhibit cytochrome P450 3A4 enzyme activity (eg, macrolide antibiotics) have the potential to result in increased plasma concentrations of corticosteroids. Dexamethasone is a moderate inducer of the cytochrome P450 3A4 enzyme system. Co-administration with other drugs that are metabolized by CYP 3A4 (eg, erythromycin) may increase their clearance, resulting in decreased plasma concentrations). Products include:

Clotrimazole (Drugs which inhibit cytochrome P450 3A4 enzyme activity have the potential to result in increased plasma concentrations of corticosteroids). Products include:

Cortisone Acetate (Drugs which induce cytochrome P450 3A4 enzyme activity may enhance the metabolism of corticosteroids and require that the dosage of the corticosteroid be increased).

No products indexed under this heading.

Cyclosporine (Increased activity of both cyclosporine and corticosteroids may occur when the two are used concurrently. Convulsions have been reported with this concurrent use). Products include:

Dalfopristin (Drugs which inhibit cytochrome P450 3A4 enzyme activity have the potential to result in increased plasma concentrations of corticosteroids).

No products indexed under this heading.

Danazol (Drugs which inhibit cytochrome P450 3A4 enzyme activity have the potential to result in increased plasma concentrations of corticosteroids).

No products indexed under this heading.

Delavirdine Mesylate (Drugs which inhibit cytochrome P450 3A4 enzyme activity have the potential to result in increased plasma concentrations of corticosteroids). Products include:

Deslanoside (Patients on digitalis glycosides may be at increased risk of arrhythmias due to hypokalemia).

No products indexed under this heading.

Desogestrel (Estrogens may decrease the hepatic metabolism of certain corticosteroids, thereby increasing their effect). Products include:

Dexamethasone Acetate (Drugs which induce cytochrome P450 3A4 enzyme activity may enhance the metabolism of corticosteroids and require that the dosage of the corticosteroid be increased).

No products indexed under this heading.

Dexamethasone Sodium Phosphate (Drugs which induce cytochrome P450 3A4 enzyme activity may enhance the metabolism of corticosteroids and require that the dosage of the corticosteroid be increased).

No products indexed under this heading.

Diazepam (Dexamethasone is a moderate inducer of the cytochrome P450 3A4 enzyme system. Co-administration with other drugs that are metabolized by CYP 3A4 may increase their clearance, resulting in decreased plasma concentrations). Products include:

Diclofenac Potassium (Concomitant use of non-steroidal anti-inflammatory agents and corticosteroids increases the risk of gastrointestinal side effects).

No products indexed under this heading.

Diclofenac Sodium (Concomitant use of non-steroidal anti-inflammato-

ry agents and corticosteroids increases the risk of gastrointestinal side effects). Products include:

Dicumarol (Co-administration of corticosteroids and warfarin usually results in inhibition of response to warfarin, although there have been some conflicting reports. Therefore, coagulation indices should be monitored frequently to maintain the desired anticoagulant effect).

No products indexed under this heading.

Dienestrol (Estrogens may decrease the hepatic metabolism of certain corticosteroids, thereby increasing their effect).

No products indexed under this heading.

Diethylstilbestrol (Estrogens may decrease the hepatic metabolism of certain corticosteroids, thereby increasing their effect).

No products indexed under this heading.

Digitalis Glycoside Preparations (Patients on digitalis glycosides may be at increased risk of arrhythmias due to hypokalemia).

No products indexed under this heading.

Digitoxin (Patients on digitalis glycosides may be at increased risk of arrhythmias due to hypokalemia).

No products indexed under this heading.

Digoxin (Patients on digitalis glycosides may be at increased risk of arrhythmias due to hypokalemia). Products include:

Dihydroergotamine Mesylate (Dexamethasone is a moderate inducer of the cytochrome P450 3A4 enzyme system. Co-administration with other drugs that are metabolized by CYP 3A4 may increase their clearance, resulting in decreased plasma concentrations). Products include:

Diltiazem Hydrochloride (Drugs which inhibit cytochrome P450 3A4 enzyme activity have the potential to result in increased plasma concentrations of corticosteroids). Products include:

Diltiazem Maleate (Drugs which inhibit cytochrome P450 3A4 enzyme activity have the potential to result in increased plasma concentrations of corticosteroids).

No products indexed under this heading.

Dirithromycin (Macrolide antibiotics have been reported to cause a significant decrease in corticosteroid clearance. Drugs which inhibit cytochrome P450 3A4 enzyme activity (eg, macrolide antibiotics) have the potential to result in increased plasma concentrations of corticosteroids. Dexamethasone is a moderate inducer of the cytochrome P450 3A4 enzyme system. Co-administration with other drugs that are metabolized by CYP 3A4 (eg, erythromycin) may increase their

clearance, resulting in decreased plasma concentrations).

No products indexed under this heading.

Disopyramide (Dexamethasone is a moderate inducer of the cytochrome P450 3A4 enzyme system. Co-administration with other drugs that are metabolized by CYP 3A4 may increase their clearance, resulting in decreased plasma concentrations).

No products indexed under this heading.

Disopyramide Phosphate (Dexamethasone is a moderate inducer of the cytochrome P450 3A4 enzyme system. Co-administration with other drugs that are metabolized by CYP 3A4 may increase their clearance, resulting in decreased plasma concentrations).

No products indexed under this heading.

Disulfiram (Dexamethasone is a moderate inducer of the cytochrome P450 3A4 enzyme system. Co-administration with other drugs that are metabolized by CYP 3A4 may increase their clearance, resulting in decreased plasma concentrations).

No products indexed under this heading.

Donepezil Hydrochloride (Concomitant use of anticholinesterase agents and corticosteroids may produce severe weakness in patients with myasthenia gravis. If possible, anticholinesterase agents should be withdrawn at least 24 hours before initiating corticosteroid therapy). Products include:

Doxorubicin Hydrochloride (Dexamethasone is a moderate inducer of the cytochrome P450 3A4 enzyme system. Co-administration with other drugs that are metabolized by CYP 3A4 may increase their clearance, resulting in decreased plasma concentrations).

No products indexed under this heading.

Dronabinol (Dexamethasone is a moderate inducer of the cytochrome P450 3A4 enzyme system. Co-administration with other drugs that are metabolized by CYP 3A4 may increase their clearance, resulting in decreased plasma concentrations). Products include:

Efavirenz (Drugs which inhibit cytochrome P450 3A4 enzyme activity have the potential to result in increased plasma concentrations of corticosteroids). Products include:

Ephedrine Hydrochloride (Ephedrine may enhance the metabolic clearance of corticosteroids, resulting in decreased blood levels and lessened physiologic activity, thus requiring an increase in corticosteroid dosage).

No products indexed under this heading.

IMPORTANT NOTE: Always consult each drug listing in the patient's regimen for possible interactions.

Ephedrine Sulfate (Ephedrine may enhance the metabolic clearance of corticosteroids, resulting in decreased blood levels and lessened physiologic activity, thus requiring an increase in corticosteroid dosage).
No products indexed under this heading.

Ephedrine Tannate (Ephedrine may enhance the metabolic clearance of corticosteroids, resulting in decreased blood levels and lessened physiologic activity, thus requiring an increase in corticosteroid dosage).
No products indexed under this heading.

Ergotamine Tartrate (Dexamethasone is a moderate inducer of the cytochrome P450 3A4 enzyme system. Co-administration with other drugs that are metabolized by CYP 3A4 may increase their clearance, resulting in decreased plasma concentrations).
No products indexed under this heading.

Erythromycin (Macrolide antibiotics have been reported to cause a significant decrease in corticosteroid clearance. Drugs which inhibit cytochrome P450 3A4 enzyme activity (eg, macrolide antibiotics) have the potential to result in increased plasma concentrations of corticosteroids. Dexamethasone is a moderate inducer of the cytochrome P450 3A4 enzyme system. Co-administration with other drugs that are metabolized by CYP 3A4 (eg, erythromycin) may increase their clearance, resulting in decreased plasma concentrations). Products include:

Erythromycin Estolate (Macrolide antibiotics have been reported to cause a significant decrease in corticosteroid clearance. Drugs which inhibit cytochrome P450 3A4 enzyme activity (eg, macrolide antibiotics) have the potential to result in increased plasma concentrations of corticosteroids. Dexamethasone is a moderate inducer of the cytochrome P450 3A4 enzyme system. Co-administration with other drugs that are metabolized by CYP 3A4 (eg, erythromycin) may increase their clearance, resulting in decreased plasma concentrations).
No products indexed under this heading.

Erythromycin Ethylsuccinate (Macrolide antibiotics have been reported to cause a significant decrease in corticosteroid clearance. Drugs which inhibit cytochrome P450 3A4 enzyme activity (eg, macrolide antibiotics) have the potential to result in increased plasma concentrations of corticosteroids. Dexamethasone is a moderate inducer of the cytochrome P450 3A4 enzyme system. Co-administration with other drugs that are metabolized by CYP 3A4 (eg, erythromycin) may increase their clearance, resulting in decreased plasma concentrations). Products include:

Erythromycin Gluceptate (Macrolide antibiotics have been reported to cause a significant decrease in corticosteroid clearance. Drugs which inhibit cytochrome P450 3A4 enzyme activity (eg, macrolide antibiotics) have the potential to result in increased plasma concentrations of corticosteroids. Dexamethasone is a moderate inducer of the cytochrome P450 3A4 enzyme system. Co-administration with other drugs that are metabolized by CYP 3A4 (eg, erythromycin) may increase their clearance, resulting in decreased plasma concentrations).
No products indexed under this heading.

Erythromycin Lactobionate (Drugs which inhibit cytochrome P450 3A4 enzyme activity have the potential to result in increased plasma concentrations of corticosteroids).
No products indexed under this heading.

Erythromycin Stearate (Macrolide antibiotics have been reported to cause a significant decrease in corticosteroid clearance. Drugs which inhibit cytochrome P450 3A4 enzyme activity (eg, macrolide antibiotics) have the potential to result in increased plasma concentrations of corticosteroids. Dexamethasone is a moderate inducer of the cytochrome P450 3A4 enzyme system. Co-administration with other drugs that are metabolized by CYP 3A4 (eg, erythromycin) may increase their clearance, resulting in decreased plasma concentrations). Products include:

Esomeprazole Magnesium (Drugs which inhibit cytochrome P450 3A4 enzyme activity have the potential to result in increased plasma concentrations of corticosteroids). Products include:

Estradiol (Estrogens may decrease the hepatic metabolism of certain corticosteroids, thereby increasing their effect). Products include:

Estradiol Benzoate (Dexamethasone is a moderate inducer of the cytochrome P450 3A4 enzyme system. Co-administration with other drugs that are metabolized by CYP 3A4 may increase their clearance, resulting in decreased plasma concentrations).
No products indexed under this heading.

Estradiol Cypionate (Dexamethasone is a moderate inducer of the cytochrome P450 3A4 enzyme system. Co-administration with other drugs that are metabolized by CYP 3A4 may increase their clearance, resulting in decreased plasma concentrations).
No products indexed under this heading.

Estradiol Valerate (Dexamethasone is a moderate inducer of the cytochrome P450 3A4 enzyme system. Co-administration with other drugs that are metabolized by CYP 3A4 may increase their clearance, resulting in decreased plasma concentrations).
No products indexed under this heading.

Estrogens, Conjugated (Estrogens may decrease the hepatic metabolism of certain corticosteroids, thereby increasing their effect). Products include:

Estrogens, Esterified (Estrogens may decrease the hepatic metabolism of certain corticosteroids, thereby increasing their effect). Products include:

Estropipate (Estrogens may decrease the hepatic metabolism of certain corticosteroids, thereby increasing their effect).
No products indexed under this heading.

Ethacrynic Acid (When corticosteroids are administered with potassium-depleting agents (eg, diuretics), patients should be observed closely for development of hypokalemia). Products include:

Ethinyl Estradiol (Estrogens may decrease the hepatic metabolism of certain corticosteroids, thereby increasing their effect). Products include:

Ethosuximide (Dexamethasone is a moderate inducer of the cytochrome P450 3A4 enzyme system. Co-administration with other drugs that are metabolized by CYP 3A4 may increase their clearance, resulting in decreased plasma concentrations).
No products indexed under this heading.

Ethynodiol Diacetate (Estrogens may decrease the hepatic metabolism of certain corticosteroids, thereby increasing their effect).
No products indexed under this heading.

Etodolac (Concomitant use of non-steroidal anti-inflammatory agents and corticosteroids increases the risk of gastrointestinal side effects).
No products indexed under this heading.

Etoposide (Dexamethasone is a moderate inducer of the cytochrome P450 3A4 enzyme system. Co-administration with other drugs that are metabolized by CYP 3A4 may increase their clearance, resulting in decreased plasma concentrations).
No products indexed under this heading.

Etoposide Phosphate (Dexamethasone is a moderate inducer of the cytochrome P450 3A4 enzyme system. Co-administration with other drugs that are metabolized by CYP 3A4 may increase their clearance, resulting in decreased plasma concentrations).
No products indexed under this heading.

Felbamate (Drugs which induce cytochrome P450 3A4 enzyme activity may enhance the metabolism of corticosteroids and require that the dosage of the corticosteroid be increased).
No products indexed under this heading.

Felodipine (Dexamethasone is a moderate inducer of the cytochrome P450 3A4 enzyme system. Co-administration with other drugs that are metabolized by CYP 3A4 may increase their clearance, resulting in decreased plasma concentrations).
No products indexed under this heading.

Fenoprofen Calcium (Concomitant use of non-steroidal anti-inflammatory agents and corticosteroids increases the risk of gastrointestinal side effects). Products include:

Fentanyl (Dexamethasone is a moderate inducer of the cytochrome P450 3A4 enzyme system. Co-administration with other drugs that are metabolized by CYP 3A4 may increase their clearance, resulting in decreased plasma concentrations). Products include:

Fentanyl Citrate (Dexamethasone is a moderate inducer of the cytochrome P450 3A4 enzyme system. Co-administration with other drugs that are metabolized by CYP 3A4 may increase their clearance, resulting in decreased plasma concentrations). Products include:

Fluconazole (Drugs which inhibit cytochrome P450 3A4 enzyme activity have the potential to result in increased plasma concentrations of corticosteroids).
No products indexed under this heading.

Fludrocortisone Acetate (Drugs which induce cytochrome P450 3A4 enzyme activity may enhance the metabolism of corticosteroids and require that the dosage of the corticosteroid be increased).
No products indexed under this heading.

Fluoxetine Hydrochloride (Drugs which inhibit cytochrome P450 3A4 enzyme activity have the potential to result in increased plasma concentrations of corticosteroids). Products include:

Flurbiprofen (Concomitant use of non-steroidal anti-inflammatory agents and corticosteroids increases the risk of gastrointestinal side effects).
No products indexed under this heading.

(**⚏** Described in PDR For Nonprescription Drugs)

(⊙ Described in PDR For Ophthalmic Medicines™)

Fluvoxamine Maleate (Drugs which inhibit cytochrome P450 3A4 enzyme activity have the potential to result in increased plasma concentrations of corticosteroids).
No products indexed under this heading.

Fosamprenavir Calcium (Drugs which inhibit cytochrome P450 3A4 enzyme activity have the potential to result in increased plasma concentrations of corticosteroids). Products include:
Lexiva Tablets 1505

Fosphenytoin Sodium (Drugs which induce cytochrome P450 3A4 enzyme activity (eg, phenytoin) may enhance the metabolism of corticosteroids and require that the dosage of the corticosteroid be increased. In post-marketing experience, there have been reports of both increases and decreases in phenytoin levels with dexamethsone co-administration, leading to alterations in seizure control).
No products indexed under this heading.

Furosemide (When corticosteroids are administered with potassium-depleting agents (eg, diuretics), patients should be observed closely for development of hypokalemia). Products include:
Furosemide Tablets 2154

Galantamine Hydrobromide (Concomitant use of anticholinesterase agents and corticosteroids may produce severe weakness in patients with myasthenia gravis. If possible, anticholinesterase agents should be withdrawn at least 24 hours before initiating corticosteroid therapy). Products include:
Razadyne 2399
Razadyne ER Extended-Release Capsules 2399

Garlic Extract (Drugs which induce cytochrome P450 3A4 enzyme activity may enhance the metabolism of corticosteroids and require that the dosage of the corticosteroid be increased).
No products indexed under this heading.

Garlic Oil (Drugs which induce cytochrome P450 3A4 enzyme activity may enhance the metabolism of corticosteroids and require that the dosage of the corticosteroid be increased).
No products indexed under this heading.

Glimepiride (Because corticosteroids may increase blood glucose concentrations, dosage adjustments of antidiabetic agents may be required). Products include:
Avandaryl Tablets 1379
Duetact Tablets 3226

Glipizide (Because corticosteroids may increase blood glucose concentrations, dosage adjustments of antidiabetic agents may be required).
No products indexed under this heading.

Glyburide (Because corticosteroids may increase blood glucose concentrations, dosage adjustments of antidiabetic agents may be required).
No products indexed under this heading.

Haloperidol (Dexamethasone is a moderate inducer of the cytochrome P450 3A4 enzyme system. Co-administration with other drugs that are metabolized by CYP 3A4 may increase their clearance, resulting in decreased plasma concentrations).
No products indexed under this heading.

Haloperidol Decanoate (Dexamethasone is a moderate inducer of the cytochrome P450 3A4 enzyme system. Co-administration with other drugs that are metabolized by CYP 3A4 may increase their clearance, resulting in decreased plasma concentrations).
No products indexed under this heading.

Haloperidol Lactate (Dexamethasone is a moderate inducer of the cytochrome P450 3A4 enzyme system. Co-administration with other drugs that are metabolized by CYP 3A4 may increase their clearance, resulting in decreased plasma concentrations).
No products indexed under this heading.

Hydrochlorothiazide (When corticosteroids are administered with potassium-depleting agents (eg, diuretics), patients should be observed closely for development of hypokalemia). Products include:
Aldoril Tablets 1910
Atacand HCT 651
Avalide Tablets 888
Avalide Tablets 2874
Benicar HCT Tablets 1044
Diovan HCT Tablets 2196
Dyazide Capsules 1423
Hyzaar 50-12.5 Tablets 1990
Hyzaar 100-12.5 Tablets 1990
Hyzaar 100-25 Tablets 1990
Lopressor HCT 50/25 Tablets 2241
Lopressor HCT 100/25 Tablets 2241
Lopressor HCT 100/50 Tablets 2241
Lotensin HCT Tablets 2246
Micardis HCT Tablets 856
Moduretic Tablets 2028
Prinzide Tablets 2056
Teveten HCT Tablets 1737
Timolide Tablets 2086
Uniretic Tablets 3100

Hydrocortisone (Drugs which induce cytochrome P450 3A4 enzyme activity may enhance the metabolism of corticosteroids and require that the dosage of the corticosteroid be increased). Products include:
Colocort Rectal Suspension, USP (Retention) 100 mg/60 mL........... 2476
Hydrocortone Tablets 1989
Preparation H Hydrocortisone Cream 646

Hydrocortisone Acetate (Drugs which induce cytochrome P450 3A4 enzyme activity may enhance the metabolism of corticosteroids and require that the dosage of the corticosteroid be increased). Products include:
Analpram-HC 1159
Pramosone 1161
ProctoFoam-HC 3099

Hydrocortisone Butyrate (Drugs which induce cytochrome P450 3A4 enzyme activity may enhance the metabolism of corticosteroids and require that the dosage of the corticosteroid be increased). Products include:
Locoid Lipocream Cream 1160

Hydrocortisone Cypionate (Drugs which induce cytochrome P450 3A4 enzyme activity may enhance the metabolism of corticosteroids and require that the dosage of the corticosteroid be increased).
No products indexed under this heading.

Hydrocortisone Hemisuccinate (Drugs which induce cytochrome P450 3A4 enzyme activity may enhance the metabolism of corticosteroids and require that the dosage of the corticosteroid be increased).
No products indexed under this heading.

Hydrocortisone Probutate (Drugs which induce cytochrome P450 3A4 enzyme activity may enhance the metabolism of corticosteroids and require that the dosage of the corticosteroid be increased).
No products indexed under this heading.

Hydrocortisone Sodium Phosphate (Drugs which induce cytochrome P450 3A4 enzyme activity may enhance the metabolism of corticosteroids and require that the dosage of the corticosteroid be increased).
No products indexed under this heading.

Hydrocortisone Sodium Succinate (Drugs which induce cytochrome P450 3A4 enzyme activity may enhance the metabolism of corticosteroids and require that the dosage of the corticosteroid be increased).
No products indexed under this heading.

Hydrocortisone Valerate (Drugs which induce cytochrome P450 3A4 enzyme activity may enhance the metabolism of corticosteroids and require that the dosage of the corticosteroid be increased).
No products indexed under this heading.

Hydroflumethiazide (When corticosteroids are administered with potassium-depleting agents (eg, diuretics), patients should be observed closely for development of hypokalemia).
No products indexed under this heading.

Hypericum (Drugs which induce cytochrome P450 3A4 enzyme activity may enhance the metabolism of corticosteroids and require that the dosage of the corticosteroid be increased). Products include:
Satiete Tablets 832

Hypericum Perforatum (Drugs which induce cytochrome P450 3A4 enzyme activity may enhance the metabolism of corticosteroids and require that the dosage of the corticosteroid be increased).
No products indexed under this heading.

Ibuprofen (Concomitant use of non-steroidal anti-inflammatory agents and corticosteroids increases the risk of gastrointestinal side effects). Products include:
Advil Allergy Sinus Caplets 770
Advil 674
Children's Advil Oral Suspension 603
Children's Advil Chewable Tablets .. 603
Advil Cold & Sinus 723
Infants' Advil Concentrated Drops .. 604
Infants' Advil Concentrated Drops - White Grape (Dye-Free)............. 604
Junior Strength Advil Swallow Tablets.. 605
Advil Migraine Liquigels 608
Advil Multi-Symptom Cold Caplets.. 770
Advil PM Caplets 615
Motrin IB Tablets and Caplets 1866
Children's Motrin Oral Suspension ... 1867
Children's Motrin Non-Staining Dye-Free Oral Suspension............ 1867
Children's Motrin Cold Oral Suspension 1867
Infants' Motrin Concentrated Drops.. 1867
Infants' Motrin Non-Staining Dye-Free Concentrated Drops....... 1867
Junior Strength Motrin Caplets and Chewable Tablets................. 1867
Vicoprofen Tablets 539

Indinavir Sulfate (Drugs which inhibit cytochrome P450 3A4 enzyme activity have the potential to result in increased plasma concentrations of corticosteroids). Products include:
Crixivan Capsules 1940

Indomethacin (Concomitant use of non-steroidal anti-inflammatory agents and corticosteroids increases the risk of gastrointestinal side effects). Products include:
Indocin 1995

Indomethacin Sodium Trihydrate (Concomitant use of non-steroidal anti-inflammatory agents and corticosteroids increases the risk of gastrointestinal side effects). Products include:
Indocin I.V. 2465

Insulin, Human, Zinc Suspension (Because corticosteroids may increase blood glucose concentrations, dosage adjustments of antidiabetic agents may be required). Products include:
Humulin L, 100 Units 1794
Humulin U, 100 Units 1800

Insulin, Human NPH (Because corticosteroids may increase blood glucose concentrations, dosage adjustments of antidiabetic agents may be required). Products include:
Humulin N, 100 Units 1795
Humulin N Pen 1797

Insulin, Human Regular (Because corticosteroids may increase blood glucose concentrations, dosage adjustments of antidiabetic agents may be required). Products include:
Humulin R, 100 Units...................... 1798

Insulin, Human Regular and Human NPH Mixture (Because corticosteroids may increase blood glucose concentrations, dosage adjustments of antidiabetic agents may be required). Products include:
Humulin 50/50, 100 Units 1791
Humulin 70/30 Pen 1793

Insulin, NPH (Because corticosteroids may increase blood glucose concentrations, dosage adjustments of antidiabetic agents may be required).
No products indexed under this heading.

Insulin, Regular (Because corticosteroids may increase blood glucose concentrations, dosage adjustments of antidiabetic agents may be required).
No products indexed under this heading.

Insulin, Zinc Crystals (Because corticosteroids may increase blood glucose concentrations, dosage adjustments of antidiabetic agents may be required).
No products indexed under this heading.

Insulin, Zinc Suspension (Because corticosteroids may increase blood glucose concentrations, dosage adjustments of antidiabetic agents may be required).
No products indexed under this heading.

Insulin Aspart, Human Regular (Because corticosteroids may increase blood glucose concentrations, dosage adjustments of antidiabetic agents may be required).
Products include:
NovoLog Injection 2326

Insulin glargine (Because corticosteroids may increase blood glucose concentrations, dosage adjustments of antidiabetic agents may be required). Products include:
Lantus Injection 2909

Insulin Lispro, Human (Because corticosteroids may increase blood glucose concentrations, dosage adjustments of antidiabetic agents may be required). Products include:
Humalog-Pen 1781
Humalog Mix 50/50-Pen 1783
Humalog Mix 75/25-Pen 1785

Insulin Lispro Protamine, Human (Because corticosteroids may increase blood glucose concentrations, dosage adjustments of antidiabetic agents may be required).
Products include:
Humalog Mix 50/50-Pen 1783
Humalog Mix 75/25-Pen 1785

Isoniazid (Serum concentrations of isoniazid may be decreased).
No products indexed under this heading.

Isradipine (Dexamethasone is a moderate inducer of the cytochrome P450 3A4 enzyme system. Co-administration with other drugs that are metabolized by CYP 3A4 may increase their clearance, resulting in decreased plasma concentrations).
Products include:
DynaCirc CR Tablets 2721

Itraconazole (Drugs which inhibit cytochrome P450 3A4 enzyme activity have the potential to result in increased plasma concentrations of corticosteroids).
No products indexed under this heading.

Ketoconazole (Drugs which inhibit cytochrome P450 3A4 enzyme activity (eg, ketoconazole) have the potential to result in increased plasma concentrations of corticosteroids. Ketoconazole has been reported to decrease the metabolism of certain corticosteroids by up to 60%, leading to increased risk of corticosteroid side effects. In addition, ketoconazole alone can inhibit adrenal corticosteroid synthesis and may cause adrenal insufficiency during corticosteroid withdrawal).
Products include:
Nizoral A-D Shampoo, 1% 1868

Ketoprofen (Concomitant use of non-steroidal anti-inflammatory agents and corticosteroids increases the risk of gastrointestinal side effects).
No products indexed under this heading.

Ketorolac Tromethamine (Concomitant use of non-steroidal anti-inflammatory agents and corticosteroids increases the risk of gastrointestinal side effects).
Products include:
Acular Ophthalmic Solution 565
Acular LS Ophthalmic Solution 566

Levonorgestrel (Estrogens may decrease the hepatic metabolism of certain corticosteroids, thereby increasing their effect). Products include:
Climara Pro Transdermal System 776
Mirena Intrauterine System 787
Plan B Tablets 1076
Seasonique Tablets 1077

Lidocaine (Dexamethasone is a moderate inducer of the cytochrome P450 3A4 enzyme system. Co-administration with other drugs that are metabolized by CYP 3A4 may increase their clearance, resulting in decreased plasma concentrations).
Products include:
Lidoderm Patch 1118
Synera Topical Patch 1137

Lidocaine Hydrochloride (Dexamethasone is a moderate inducer of the cytochrome P450 3A4 enzyme system. Co-administration with other drugs that are metabolized by CYP 3A4 may increase their clearance, resulting in decreased plasma concentrations).
No products indexed under this heading.

Lopinavir (Drugs which inhibit cytochrome P450 3A4 enzyme activity have the potential to result in increased plasma concentrations of corticosteroids). Products include:
Kaletra 476

Loratadine (Drugs which inhibit cytochrome P450 3A4 enzyme activity have the potential to result in increased plasma concentrations of corticosteroids). Products include:
Alavert Allergy & Sinus D-12 Hour Tablets .... ▣771
Alavert .... ▣771
Children's Claritin Allergy Oral Solution .... ▣771
Claritin Non-Drowsy 24 Hour Tablets .... ▣772
Claritin Reditabs 24 Hour Non-Drowsy Tablets .... ▣772
Claritin-D Non-Drowsy 12 Hour Tablets .... ▣772
Claritin-D Non-Drowsy 24 Hour Tablets .... ▣772

Lovastatin (Dexamethasone is a moderate inducer of the cytochrome P450 3A4 enzyme system. Co-administration with other drugs that are metabolized by CYP 3A4 may increase their clearance, resulting in decreased plasma concentrations).
Products include:
Advicor Tablets 1722
Altoprev Extended-Release Tablets 3109
Mevacor Tablets 2021

Measles, Mumps, Rubella and Varicella Virus Vaccine Live (Patients on corticosteroid therapy may exhibit a diminished response to toxoids and live or inactivated vaccines due to inhibition of antibody response. Corticosteroids may also potentiate the replication of some organisms contained in live attenuated vaccines. Routine administration of vaccines or toxoids should be deferred until corticosteroid therapy is discontinued if possible. Administration of live or live, attenuated vaccines is contraindicated in patients receiving immunosuppressive doses of corticosteroids). Products include:
ProQuad 2064

Measles, Mumps & Rubella Virus Vaccine, Live (Patients on corticosteroid therapy may exhibit a diminished response to toxoids and live or inactivated vaccines due to inhibition of antibody response. Corticosteroids may also potentiate the replication of some organisms contained in live attenuated vaccines. Routine administration of vaccines or toxoids should be deferred until corticosteroid therapy is discontinued if possible. Administration of live or live, attenuated vaccines is contraindicated in patients receiving immunosuppressive doses of corticosteroids). Products include:
M-M-R II 2006

Measles & Rubella Virus Vaccine Live (Patients on corticosteroid therapy may exhibit a diminished response to toxoids and live or inactivated vaccines due to inhibition of antibody response. Corticosteroids may also potentiate the replication of some organisms contained in live attenuated vaccines. Routine administration of vaccines or toxoids should be deferred until corticosteroid therapy is discontinued if possible. Administration of live or live, attenuated vaccines is contraindicated in patients receiving immunosuppressive doses of corticosteroids).
No products indexed under this heading.

Measles Virus Vaccine Live (Patients on corticosteroid therapy may exhibit a diminished response to toxoids and live or inactivated vaccines due to inhibition of antibody response. Corticosteroids may also potentiate the replication of some organisms contained in live attenuated vaccines. Routine administration of vaccines or toxoids should be deferred until corticosteroid therapy is discontinued if possible. Administration of live or live, attenuated vaccines is contraindicated in patients receiving immunosuppressive doses of corticosteroids). Products include:
Attenuvax 1914

Meclofenamate Sodium (Concomitant use of non-steroidal anti-inflammatory agents and corticosteroids increases the risk of gastrointestinal side effects).
No products indexed under this heading.

Mefenamic Acid (Concomitant use of non-steroidal anti-inflammatory agents and corticosteroids increases the risk of gastrointestinal side effects).
No products indexed under this heading.

Meloxicam (Concomitant use of non-steroidal anti-inflammatory agents and corticosteroids increases the risk of gastrointestinal side effects). Products include:
Mobic Oral Suspension 863
Mobic Tablets 863

Mephenytoin (Drugs which induce cytochrome P450 3A4 enzyme activity may enhance the metabolism of corticosteroids and require that the dosage of the corticosteroid be increased).
No products indexed under this heading.

Mephobarbital (Drugs which induce cytochrome P450 3A4 enzyme activity (eg, barbiturates) may enhance the metabolism of corticosteroids and require that the dosage of the corticosteroid be increased).
No products indexed under this heading.

Mestranol (Estrogens may decrease the hepatic metabolism of certain corticosteroids, thereby increasing their effect).
No products indexed under this heading.

Metformin Hydrochloride (Because corticosteroids may increase blood glucose concentrations, dosage adjustments of antidiabetic agents may be required).
Products include:
ActoPlus Met Tablets 3214
Avandamet Tablets 1373
Fortamet Extended-Release Tablets 3115

Methadone Hydrochloride (Dexamethasone is a moderate inducer of the cytochrome P450 3A4 enzyme system. Co-administration with other drugs that are metabolized by CYP 3A4 may increase their clearance, resulting in decreased plasma concentrations).
No products indexed under this heading.

Methsuximide (Drugs which induce cytochrome P450 3A4 enzyme activity may enhance the metabolism of corticosteroids and require that the dosage of the corticosteroid be increased).
No products indexed under this heading.

Methyclothiazide (When corticosteroids are administered with potassium-depleting agents (eg, diuretics), patients should be observed closely for development of hypokalemia).
No products indexed under this heading.

Methylprednisolone (Drugs which induce cytochrome P450 3A4 enzyme activity may enhance the metabolism of corticosteroids and require that the dosage of the corticosteroid be increased).
No products indexed under this heading.

Methylprednisolone Acetate (Drugs which induce cytochrome P450 3A4 enzyme activity may enhance the metabolism of corticosteroids and require that the dosage of the corticosteroid be increased).
Products include:
Depo-Medrol Injectable Suspension 2617
Depo-Medrol Single-Dose Vial 2619

Methylprednisolone Sodium Succinate (Drugs which induce cytochrome P450 3A4 enzyme activity may enhance the metabolism of corticosteroids and require that the dosage of the corticosteroid be increased).
No products indexed under this heading.

Metronidazole (Drugs which inhibit cytochrome P450 3A4 enzyme activity have the potential to result in increased plasma concentrations of corticosteroids). Products include:
Metrogel 1% 1211
MetroGel-Vaginal Gel 1855
Vandazole Vaginal Gel 3338

Metronidazole Benzoate (Drugs which inhibit cytochrome P450 3A4 enzyme activity have the potential to result in increased plasma concentrations of corticosteroids).
No products indexed under this heading.

Metronidazole Hydrochloride (Drugs which inhibit cytochrome P450 3A4 enzyme activity have the potential to result in increased plasma concentrations of corticosteroids).
No products indexed under this heading.

Miconazole (Drugs which inhibit cytochrome P450 3A4 enzyme activity have the potential to result in increased plasma concentrations of corticosteroids).
No products indexed under this heading.

Miconazole Nitrate (Drugs which inhibit cytochrome P450 3A4 enzyme activity have the potential to result in increased plasma concentrations of corticosteroids). Products include:
Desenex 635
Desenex Jock Itch Spray Powder 635

Midazolam Hydrochloride (Dexamethasone is a moderate inducer of the cytochrome P450 3A4 enzyme system. Co-administration with other drugs that are metabolized by CYP 3A4 may increase their clearance, resulting in decreased plasma concentrations).
No products indexed under this heading.

Miglitol (Because corticosteroids may increase blood glucose concentrations, dosage adjustments of antidiabetic agents may be required).
No products indexed under this heading.

Modafinil (Drugs which induce cytochrome P450 3A4 enzyme activity may enhance the metabolism of corticosteroids and require that the dosage of the corticosteroid be increased). Products include:
Provigil Tablets 988

Mumps Virus Vaccine, Live (Patients on corticosteroid therapy may exhibit a diminished response to toxoids and live or inactivated vaccines due to inhibition of antibody response. Corticosteroids may also potentiate the replication of some organisms contained in live attenuated vaccines. Routine administration of vaccines or toxoids should be deferred until corticosteroid therapy is discontinued if possible. Administration of live or live, attenuated vaccines is contraindicated in patients receiving immunosuppressive doses of corticosteroids). Products include:
Mumpsvax 2031

Nabumetone (Concomitant use of non-steroidal anti-inflammatory agents and corticosteroids increases the risk of gastrointestinal side effects).
No products indexed under this heading.

Naproxen (Concomitant use of non-steroidal anti-inflammatory agents and corticosteroids increases the risk of gastrointestinal side effects). Products include:
EC-Naprosyn Delayed-Release Tablets 2761
Naprosyn Suspension 2761
Naprosyn Tablets 2761
Prevacid NapraPAC 3280

Naproxen Sodium (Concomitant use of non-steroidal anti-inflammatory agents and corticosteroids increases the risk of gastrointestinal side effects). Products include:
Aleve Caplets 742
Aleve Gelcaps 743
Aleve Tablets 743
Aleve Cold & Sinus Caplets 744
Anaprox Tablets 2761
Anaprox DS Tablets 2761

Nefazodone Hydrochloride (Drugs which inhibit cytochrome P450 3A4 enzyme activity have the potential to result in increased plasma concentrations of corticosteroids).
No products indexed under this heading.

Nelfinavir Mesylate (Drugs which inhibit cytochrome P450 3A4 enzyme activity have the potential to result in increased plasma concentrations of corticosteroids). Products include:
Viracept 2577

Neostigmine Bromide (Concomitant use of anticholinesterase agents and corticosteroids may produce severe weakness in patients with myasthenia gravis. If possible, anticholinesterase agents should be withdrawn at least 24 hours before initiating corticosteroid therapy).
No products indexed under this heading.

Neostigmine Methylsulfate (Concomitant use of anticholinesterase agents and corticosteroids may produce severe weakness in patients with myasthenia gravis. If possible, anticholinesterase agents should be withdrawn at least 24 hours before initiating corticosteroid therapy).
No products indexed under this heading.

Nevirapine (Drugs which inhibit cytochrome P450 3A4 enzyme activity have the potential to result in increased plasma concentrations of corticosteroids). Products include:
Viramune Oral Suspension 873
Viramune Tablets 873

Niacinamide (Drugs which inhibit cytochrome P450 3A4 enzyme activity have the potential to result in increased plasma concentrations of corticosteroids).
No products indexed under this heading.

Nicardipine Hydrochloride (Dexamethasone is a moderate inducer of the cytochrome P450 3A4 enzyme system. Co-administration with other drugs that are metabolized by CYP 3A4 may increase their clearance, resulting in decreased plasma concentrations). Products include:
Cardene I.V. 2497

Nicotinamide (Drugs which inhibit cytochrome P450 3A4 enzyme activity have the potential to result in increased plasma concentrations of corticosteroids). Products include:
Nicomide Tablets 1088

Nifedipine (Drugs which inhibit cytochrome P450 3A4 enzyme activity have the potential to result in increased plasma concentrations of corticosteroids). Products include:
Adalat CC Tablets 2964

Nimodipine (Dexamethasone is a moderate inducer of the cytochrome P450 3A4 enzyme system. Co-administration with other drugs that are metabolized by CYP 3A4 may increase their clearance, resulting in decreased plasma concentrations). Products include:
Nimotop Capsules 749

Nisoldipine (Dexamethasone is a moderate inducer of the cytochrome P450 3A4 enzyme system. Co-administration with other drugs that are metabolized by CYP 3A4 may increase their clearance, resulting in decreased plasma concentrations). Products include:
Sular Tablets 3122

Nitrendipine (Dexamethasone is a moderate inducer of the cytochrome P450 3A4 enzyme system. Co-administration with other drugs that are metabolized by CYP 3A4 may increase their clearance, resulting in decreased plasma concentrations).
No products indexed under this heading.

Norethindrone (Estrogens may decrease the hepatic metabolism of certain corticosteroids, thereby increasing their effect). Products include:
Ortho Micronor Tablets 2426

Norethindrone Acetate (Dexamethasone is a moderate inducer of the cytochrome P450 3A4 enzyme system. Co-administration with other drugs that are metabolized by CYP 3A4 may increase their clearance, resulting in decreased plasma concentrations).
No products indexed under this heading.

Norethynodrel (Estrogens may decrease the hepatic metabolism of certain corticosteroids, thereby increasing their effect).
No products indexed under this heading.

Norfloxacin (Drugs which inhibit cytochrome P450 3A4 enzyme activity have the potential to result in increased plasma concentrations of corticosteroids). Products include:
Noroxin Tablets 2032

Norgestimate (Estrogens may decrease the hepatic metabolism of certain corticosteroids, thereby increasing their effect). Products include:
Ortho-Cyclen/Ortho Tri-Cyclen 2429
Ortho Tri-Cyclen Lo Tablets 2436

Norgestrel (Estrogens may decrease the hepatic metabolism of certain corticosteroids, thereby increasing their effect).
No products indexed under this heading.

Omeprazole (Drugs which inhibit cytochrome P450 3A4 enzyme activity have the potential to result in increased plasma concentrations of corticosteroids). Products include:
Zegerid Capsules 2958
Zegerid Powder for Oral Solution 2958

Ondansetron (Dexamethasone is a moderate inducer of the cytochrome P450 3A4 enzyme system. Co-administration with other drugs that are metabolized by CYP 3A4 may increase their clearance, resulting in decreased plasma concentrations). Products include:
Zofran ODT Orally Disintegrating Tablets 1639

Ondansetron Hydrochloride (Dexamethasone is a moderate inducer of the cytochrome P450 3A4 enzyme system. Co-administration with other drugs that are metabolized by CYP 3A4 may increase their clearance, resulting in decreased plasma concentrations). Products include:
Zofran Injection 1634
Zofran 1639

Oxaprozin (Concomitant use of non-steroidal anti-inflammatory agents and corticosteroids increases the risk of gastrointestinal side effects).
No products indexed under this heading.

Oxcarbazepine (Drugs which induce cytochrome P450 3A4 enzyme activity may enhance the metabolism of corticosteroids and require that the dosage of the corticosteroid be increased). Products include:
Trileptal Tablets 2300
Trileptal Oral Suspension 2300

Paclitaxel (Dexamethasone is a moderate inducer of the cytochrome P450 3A4 enzyme system. Co-administration with other drugs that are metabolized by CYP 3A4 may increase their clearance, resulting in decreased plasma concentrations).
No products indexed under this heading.

Paroxetine Hydrochloride (Drugs which inhibit cytochrome P450 3A4 enzyme activity have the potential to result in increased plasma concentrations of corticosteroids). Products include:
Paxil CR Controlled-Release Tablets 1538
Paxil 1530

Pentobarbital Sodium (Drugs which induce cytochrome P450 3A4 enzyme activity (eg, barbiturates) may enhance the metabolism of corticosteroids and require that the dosage of the corticosteroid be increased). Products include:
Nembutal Sodium Solution, USP 2470

Phenobarbital (Drugs which induce cytochrome P450 3A4 enzyme activity (eg, barbiturates) may enhance the metabolism of corticosteroids and require that the dosage of the corticosteroid be increased). Products include:
Donnatal Extentabs 2493

Phenobarbital Sodium (Drugs which induce cytochrome P450 3A4 enzyme activity may enhance the metabolism of corticosteroids and require that the dosage of the corticosteroid be increased).
No products indexed under this heading.

Phenylbutazone (Concomitant use of non-steroidal anti-inflammatory agents and corticosteroids increases the risk of gastrointestinal side effects).
No products indexed under this heading.

Phenytoin (Drugs which induce cytochrome P450 3A4 enzyme activity (eg, phenytoin) may enhance the metabolism of corticosteroids and require that the dosage of the corticosteroid be increased. In post-marketing experience, there have been reports of both increases and decreases in phenytoin levels with dexamethsone co-administration, leading to alterations in seizure control).
No products indexed under this heading.

Phenytoin Sodium (Drugs which induce cytochrome P450 3A4 enzyme activity (eg, phenytoin) may enhance the metabolism of corticosteroids and require that the dosage of the corticosteroid be increased. In post-marketing experience, there have been reports of both increases

and decreases in phenytoin levels with dexamethsone co-administration, leading to alterations in seizure control). Products include:

Phenytek Capsules 2160

Pimozide (Dexamethasone is a moderate inducer of the cytochrome P450 3A4 enzyme system. Co-administration with other drugs that are metabolized by CYP 3A4 may increase their clearance, resulting in decreased plasma concentrations).

No products indexed under this heading.

Pioglitazone Hydrochloride (Because corticosteroids may increase blood glucose concentrations, dosage adjustments of antidiabetic agents may be required). Products include:

ActoPlus Met Tablets 3214
Actos Tablets 3219
Duetact Tablets 3226

Piroxicam (Concomitant use of non-steroidal anti-inflammatory agents and corticosteroids increases the risk of gastrointestinal side effects).

No products indexed under this heading.

Poliovirus Vaccine, Live, Oral, Trivalent, Types 1,2,3 (Sabin) (Patients on corticosteroid therapy may exhibit a diminished response to toxoids and live or inactivated vaccines due to inhibition of antibody response. Corticosteroids may also potentiate the replication of some organisms contained in live attenuated vaccines. Routine administration of vaccines or toxoids should be deferred until corticosteroid therapy is discontinued if possible. Administration of live or live, attenuated vaccines is contraindicated in patients receiving immunosuppressive doses of corticosteroids).

No products indexed under this heading.

Polyestradiol Phosphate (Estrogens may decrease the hepatic metabolism of certain corticosteroids, thereby increasing their effect).

No products indexed under this heading.

Polythiazide (When corticosteroids are administered with potassium-depleting agents (eg, diuretics), patients should be observed closely for development of hypokalemia).

No products indexed under this heading.

Prednisolone Acetate (Drugs which induce cytochrome P450 3A4 enzyme activity may enhance the metabolism of corticosteroids and require that the dosage of the corticosteroid be increased). Products include:

Blephamide Ophthalmic Ointment 568
Blephamide Ophthalmic Suspension 569
Poly-Pred Ophthalmic Suspension .... ⊙233
Pred Forte Ophthalmic Suspension .... ⊙235
Pred Mild Ophthalmic Suspension .... ⊙238
Pred-G Ophthalmic Ointment .... ⊙237
Pred-G Ophthalmic Suspension ...... ⊙236

Prednisolone Sodium Phosphate (Drugs which induce cytochrome P450 3A4 enzyme activity may enhance the metabolism of corticosteroids and require that the dosage of the corticosteroid be increased).

No products indexed under this heading.

Prednisolone Tebutate (Drugs which induce cytochrome P450 3A4 enzyme activity may enhance the metabolism of corticosteroids and require that the dosage of the corticosteroid be increased).

No products indexed under this heading.

Prednisone (Drugs which induce cytochrome P450 3A4 enzyme activity may enhance the metabolism of corticosteroids and require that the dosage of the corticosteroid be increased).

No products indexed under this heading.

Primidone (Drugs which induce cytochrome P450 3A4 enzyme activity may enhance the metabolism of corticosteroids and require that the dosage of the corticosteroid be increased).

No products indexed under this heading.

Propoxyphene Hydrochloride (Drugs which inhibit cytochrome P450 3A4 enzyme activity have the potential to result in increased plasma concentrations of corticosteroids).

No products indexed under this heading.

Propoxyphene Napsylate (Drugs which inhibit cytochrome P450 3A4 enzyme activity have the potential to result in increased plasma concentrations of corticosteroids).

No products indexed under this heading.

Pyridostigmine Bromide (Concomitant use of anticholinesterase agents and corticosteroids may produce severe weakness in patients with myasthenia gravis. If possible, anticholinesterase agents should be withdrawn at least 24 hours before initiating corticosteroid therapy).

No products indexed under this heading.

Quinestrol (Estrogens may decrease the hepatic metabolism of certain corticosteroids, thereby increasing their effect).

No products indexed under this heading.

Quinidine (Drugs which inhibit cytochrome P450 3A4 enzyme activity have the potential to result in increased plasma concentrations of corticosteroids).

No products indexed under this heading.

Quinidine Gluconate (Dexamethasone is a moderate inducer of the cytochrome P450 3A4 enzyme system. Co-administration with other drugs that are metabolized by CYP 3A4 may increase their clearance, resulting in decreased plasma concentrations).

No products indexed under this heading.

Quinidine Hydrochloride (Drugs which inhibit cytochrome P450 3A4 enzyme activity have the potential to result in increased plasma concentrations of corticosteroids).

No products indexed under this heading.

Quinidine Polygalacturonate (Drugs which inhibit cytochrome P450 3A4 enzyme activity have the potential to result in increased plasma concentrations of corticosteroids).

No products indexed under this heading.

Quinidine Sulfate (Drugs which inhibit cytochrome P450 3A4 enzyme activity have the potential to result in increased plasma concentrations of corticosteroids).

No products indexed under this heading.

Quinine (Drugs which inhibit cytochrome P450 3A4 enzyme activity have the potential to result in increased plasma concentrations of corticosteroids).

No products indexed under this heading.

Quinine Sulfate (Drugs which inhibit cytochrome P450 3A4 enzyme activity have the potential to result in increased plasma concentrations of corticosteroids).

No products indexed under this heading.

Quinupristin (Drugs which inhibit cytochrome P450 3A4 enzyme activity have the potential to result in increased plasma concentrations of corticosteroids).

No products indexed under this heading.

Ranitidine Bismuth Citrate (Drugs which inhibit cytochrome P450 3A4 enzyme activity have the potential to result in increased plasma concentrations of corticosteroids).

No products indexed under this heading.

Ranitidine Hydrochloride (Drugs which inhibit cytochrome P450 3A4 enzyme activity have the potential to result in increased plasma concentrations of corticosteroids). Products include:

Zantac 1624
Zantac Injection 1619
Zantac Injection Pharmacy Bulk Package 1622

Repaglinide (Because corticosteroids may increase blood glucose concentrations, dosage adjustments of antidiabetic agents may be required).

No products indexed under this heading.

Rifabutin (Dexamethasone is a moderate inducer of the cytochrome P450 3A4 enzyme system. Co-administration with other drugs that are metabolized by CYP 3A4 may increase their clearance, resulting in decreased plasma concentrations).

No products indexed under this heading.

Rifampicin (Drugs which induce cytochrome P450 3A4 enzyme activity may enhance the metabolism of corticosteroids and require that the dosage of the corticosteroid be increased).

No products indexed under this heading.

Rifampin (Drugs which induce cytochrome P450 3A4 enzyme activity may enhance the metabolism of corticosteroids and require that the dosage of the corticosteroid be increased).

No products indexed under this heading.

Rifapentine (Drugs which induce cytochrome P450 3A4 enzyme activity may enhance the metabolism of corticosteroids and require that the dosage of the corticosteroid be increased).

No products indexed under this heading.

Ritonavir (Drugs which inhibit cytochrome P450 3A4 enzyme activity have the potential to result in increased plasma concentrations of corticosteroids). Products include:

Kaletra 476
Norvir 503

Rivastigmine Tartrate (Concomitant use of anticholinesterase agents and corticosteroids may produce severe weakness in patients with myasthenia gravis. If possible, anticholinesterase agents should be withdrawn at least 24 hours before initiating corticosteroid therapy). Products include:

Exelon Capsules 2206
Exelon Oral Solution 2206

Rofecoxib (Concomitant use of non-steroidal anti-inflammatory agents and corticosteroids increases the risk of gastrointestinal side effects).

No products indexed under this heading.

Rosiglitazone Maleate (Because corticosteroids may increase blood glucose concentrations, dosage adjustments of antidiabetic agents may be required). Products include:

Avandamet Tablets 1373
Avandaryl Tablets 1379
Avandia Tablets 1384

Rotavirus Vaccine, Live, Oral, Tetravalent (Patients on corticosteroid therapy may exhibit a diminished response to toxoids and live or inactivated vaccines due to inhibition of antibody response. Corticosteroids may also potentiate the replication of some organisms contained in live attenuated vaccines. Routine administration of vaccines or toxoids should be deferred until corticosteroid therapy is discontinued if possible. Administration of live or live, attenuated vaccines is contraindicated in patients receiving immunosuppressive doses of corticosteroids).

No products indexed under this heading.

Rubella & Mumps Virus Vaccine Live (Patients on corticosteroid therapy may exhibit a diminished response to toxoids and live or inactivated vaccines due to inhibition of antibody response. Corticosteroids may also potentiate the replication of some organisms contained in live attenuated vaccines. Routine administration of vaccines or toxoids should be deferred until corticosteroid therapy is discontinued if possible. Administration of live or live, attenuated vaccines is contraindicated in patients receiving immunosuppressive doses of corticosteroids).

No products indexed under this heading.

Rubella Virus Vaccine Live (Patients on corticosteroid therapy may exhibit a diminished response to toxoids and live or inactivated vaccines due to inhibition of antibody response. Corticosteroids may also potentiate the replication of some organisms contained in live attenuated vaccines. Routine administration of vaccines or toxoids should be deferred until corticosteroid therapy is discontinued if possible. Administration of live or live, attenuated vaccines is contraindicated in patients receiving immunosuppressive doses of corticosteroids). Products include:

Meruvax II 2019

Saquinavir (Drugs which inhibit cytochrome P450 3A4 enzyme activity have the potential to result in increased plasma concentrations of corticosteroids).
 No products indexed under this heading.

Saquinavir Mesylate (Drugs which inhibit cytochrome P450 3A4 enzyme activity have the potential to result in increased plasma concentrations of corticosteroids). Products include:
 Invirase ... 2772

Secobarbital Sodium (Drugs which induce cytochrome P450 3A4 enzyme activity (eg, barbiturates) may enhance the metabolism of corticosteroids and require that the dosage of the corticosteroid be increased).
 No products indexed under this heading.

Sertraline Hydrochloride (Drugs which inhibit cytochrome P450 3A4 enzyme activity have the potential to result in increased plasma concentrations of corticosteroids). Products include:
 Zoloft ... 2586

Sildenafil Citrate (Dexamethasone is a moderate inducer of the cytochrome P450 3A4 enzyme system. Co-administration with other drugs that are metabolized by CYP 3A4 may increase their clearance, resulting in decreased plasma concentrations). Products include:
 Revatio Tablets 2557
 Viagra Tablets 2573

Simvastatin (Dexamethasone is a moderate inducer of the cytochrome P450 3A4 enzyme system. Co-administration with other drugs that are metabolized by CYP 3A4 may increase their clearance, resulting in decreased plasma concentrations). Products include:
 Vytorin 10/10 Tablets 2114
 Vytorin 10/10 Tablets 3077
 Vytorin 10/20 Tablets 2114
 Vytorin 10/20 Tablets 3077
 Vytorin 10/40 Tablets 2114
 Vytorin 10/40 Tablets 3077
 Vytorin 10/80 Tablets 2114
 Vytorin 10/80 Tablets 3077
 Zocor Tablets 2105

Sirolimus (Dexamethasone is a moderate inducer of the cytochrome P450 3A4 enzyme system. Co-administration with other drugs that are metabolized by CYP 3A4 may increase their clearance, resulting in decreased plasma concentrations). Products include:
 Rapamune Oral Solution and
 Tablets 3475

Smallpox Vaccine (Patients on corticosteroid therapy may exhibit a diminished response to toxoids and live or inactivated vaccines due to inhibition of antibody response. Corticosteroids may also potentiate the replication of some organisms contained in live attenuated vaccines. Routine administration of vaccines or toxoids should be deferred until corticosteroid therapy is discontinued if possible. Administration of live or live, attenuated vaccines is contraindicated in patients receiving immunosuppressive doses of corticosteroids).
 No products indexed under this heading.

Sulfinpyrazone (Drugs which induce cytochrome P450 3A4 enzyme activity may enhance the metabolism of corticosteroids and require that the dosage of the corticosteroid be increased).
 No products indexed under this heading.

Sulindac (Concomitant use of non-steroidal anti-inflammatory agents and corticosteroids increases the risk of gastrointestinal side effects). Products include:
 Clinoril Tablets 1924

Tacrine Hydrochloride (Concomitant use of anticholinesterase agents and corticosteroids may produce severe weakness in patients with myasthenia gravis. If possible, anticholinesterase agents should be withdrawn at least 24 hours before initiating corticosteroid therapy).
 No products indexed under this heading.

Tacrolimus (Dexamethasone is a moderate inducer of the cytochrome P450 3A4 enzyme system. Co-administration with other drugs that are metabolized by CYP 3A4 may increase their clearance, resulting in decreased plasma concentrations). Products include:
 Prograf Capsules and Injection 632
 Protopic Ointment 638

Tamoxifen Citrate (Dexamethasone is a moderate inducer of the cytochrome P450 3A4 enzyme system. Co-administration with other drugs that are metabolized by CYP 3A4 may increase their clearance, resulting in decreased plasma concentrations). Products include:
 Soltamox Oral Solution 3527

Telithromycin (Drugs which inhibit cytochrome P450 3A4 enzyme activity have the potential to result in increased plasma concentrations of corticosteroids). Products include:
 Ketek Tablets 2903

Thalidomide (Co-administration with thalidomide should be employed cautiously, as toxic epidermal necrolysis has been reported with concomitant use). Products include:
 Thalomid Capsules 965

Theophylline (Drugs which induce cytochrome P450 3A4 enzyme activity may enhance the metabolism of corticosteroids and require that the dosage of the corticosteroid be increased).
 No products indexed under this heading.

Thiamylal Sodium (Drugs which induce cytochrome P450 3A4 enzyme activity (eg, barbiturates) may enhance the metabolism of corticosteroids and require that the dosage of the corticosteroid be increased).
 No products indexed under this heading.

Tiagabine Hydrochloride (Dexamethasone is a moderate inducer of the cytochrome P450 3A4 enzyme system. Co-administration with other drugs that are metabolized by CYP 3A4 may increase their clearance, resulting in decreased plasma concentrations). Products include:
 Gabitril Tablets 984

Tolazamide (Because corticosteroids may increase blood glucose concentrations, dosage adjustments of antidiabetic agents may be required).
 No products indexed under this heading.

Tolbutamide (Because corticosteroids may increase blood glucose concentrations, dosage adjustments of antidiabetic agents may be required).
 No products indexed under this heading.

Tolmetin Sodium (Concomitant use of non-steroidal anti-inflammatory agents and corticosteroids increases the risk of gastrointestinal side effects).
 No products indexed under this heading.

Tolterodine Tartrate (Dexamethasone is a moderate inducer of the cytochrome P450 3A4 enzyme system. Co-administration with other drugs that are metabolized by CYP 3A4 may increase their clearance, resulting in decreased plasma concentrations). Products include:
 Detrol Tablets 2628
 Detrol LA Capsules 2631

Torsemide (When corticosteroids are administered with potassium-depleting agents (eg, diuretics), patients should be observed closely for development of hypokalemia). Products include:
 Demadex Injection 2759
 Demadex Tablets 2759

Trazodone Hydrochloride (Dexamethasone is a moderate inducer of the cytochrome P450 3A4 enzyme system. Co-administration with other drugs that are metabolized by CYP 3A4 may increase their clearance, resulting in decreased plasma concentrations).
 No products indexed under this heading.

Triamcinolone (Drugs which induce cytochrome P450 3A4 enzyme activity may enhance the metabolism of corticosteroids and require that the dosage of the corticosteroid be increased).
 No products indexed under this heading.

Triamcinolone Acetonide (Drugs which induce cytochrome P450 3A4 enzyme activity may enhance the metabolism of corticosteroids and require that the dosage of the corticosteroid be increased). Products include:
 Azmacort Inhalation Aerosol 1726
 Nasacort AQ Nasal Spray 2922

Triamcinolone Diacetate (Drugs which induce cytochrome P450 3A4 enzyme activity may enhance the metabolism of corticosteroids and require that the dosage of the corticosteroid be increased).
 No products indexed under this heading.

Triamcinolone Hexacetonide (Drugs which induce cytochrome P450 3A4 enzyme activity may enhance the metabolism of corticosteroids and require that the dosage of the corticosteroid be increased).
 No products indexed under this heading.

Triazolam (Dexamethasone is a moderate inducer of the cytochrome P450 3A4 enzyme system. Co-administration with other drugs that are metabolized by CYP 3A4 may increase their clearance, resulting in decreased plasma concentrations).
 No products indexed under this heading.

Troglitazone (Because corticosteroids may increase blood glucose concentrations, dosage adjustments of antidiabetic agents may be required).
 No products indexed under this heading.

Troleandomycin (Macrolide antibiotics have been reported to cause a significant decrease in corticosteroid clearance. Drugs which inhibit cytochrome P450 3A4 enzyme activity (eg, macrolide antibiotics) have the potential to result in increased plasma concentrations of corticosteroids. Dexamethasone is a moderate inducer of the cytochrome P450 3A4 enzyme system. Co-administration with other drugs that are metabolized by CYP 3A4 (eg, erythromycin) may increase their clearance, resulting in decreased plasma concentrations).
 No products indexed under this heading.

Typhoid Vaccine (Patients on corticosteroid therapy may exhibit a diminished response to toxoids and live or inactivated vaccines due to inhibition of antibody response. Corticosteroids may also potentiate the replication of some organisms contained in live attenuated vaccines. Routine administration of vaccines or toxoids should be deferred until corticosteroid therapy is discontinued if possible. Administration of live or live, attenuated vaccines is contraindicated in patients receiving immunosuppressive doses of corticosteroids).
 No products indexed under this heading.

Valdecoxib (Concomitant use of non-steroidal anti-inflammatory agents and corticosteroids increases the risk of gastrointestinal side effects).
 No products indexed under this heading.

Valproate Sodium (Drugs which inhibit cytochrome P450 3A4 enzyme activity have the potential to result in increased plasma concentrations of corticosteroids). Products include:
 Depacon Injection 412

Varicella Virus Vaccine Live (Patients on corticosteroid therapy may exhibit a diminished response to toxoids and live or inactivated vaccines due to inhibition of antibody response. Corticosteroids may also potentiate the replication of some organisms contained in live attenuated vaccines. Routine administration of vaccines or toxoids should be deferred until corticosteroid therapy is discontinued if possible. Administration of live or live, attenuated vaccines is contraindicated in patients receiving immunosuppressive doses of corticosteroids). Products include:
 Varivax ... 2100

Verapamil Hydrochloride (Drugs which inhibit cytochrome P450 3A4 enzyme activity have the potential to

IMPORTANT NOTE: Always consult each drug listing in the patient's regimen for possible interactions.

result in increased plasma concentrations of corticosteroids). Products include:
- Covera-HS Tablets ... 3139
- Tarka Tablets ... 524
- Verelan PM Extended-Release Capsules, Controlled-Onset ... 3106

Vinblastine Sulfate (Dexamethasone is a moderate inducer of the cytochrome P450 3A4 enzyme system. Co-administration with other drugs that are metabolized by CYP 3A4 may increase their clearance, resulting in decreased plasma concentrations).
No products indexed under this heading.

Vincristine Sulfate (Dexamethasone is a moderate inducer of the cytochrome P450 3A4 enzyme system. Co-administration with other drugs that are metabolized by CYP 3A4 may increase their clearance, resulting in decreased plasma concentrations).
No products indexed under this heading.

Voriconazole (Drugs which inhibit cytochrome P450 3A4 enzyme activity have the potential to result in increased plasma concentrations of corticosteroids). Products include:
- VFEND I.V. ... 2564
- VFEND Oral Suspension ... 2564
- VFEND Tablets ... 2564

Warfarin Sodium (Co-administration of corticosteroids and warfarin usually results in inhibition of response to warfarin, although there have been some conflicting reports. Therefore, coagulation indices should be monitored frequently to maintain the desired anticoagulant effect). Products include:
- Coumadin for Injection ... 898
- Coumadin Tablets ... 898

Yellow Fever Vaccine (Patients on corticosteroid therapy may exhibit a diminished response to toxoids and live or inactivated vaccines due to inhibition of antibody response. Corticosteroids may also potentiate the replication of some organisms contained in live attenuated vaccines. Routine administration of vaccines or toxoids should be deferred until corticosteroid therapy is discontinued if possible. Administration of live or live, attenuated vaccines is contraindicated in patients receiving immunosuppressive doses of corticosteroids).
No products indexed under this heading.

Zafirlukast (Drugs which inhibit cytochrome P450 3A4 enzyme activity have the potential to result in increased plasma concentrations of corticosteroids). Products include:
- Accolate Tablets ... 671

Zileuton (Drugs which inhibit cytochrome P450 3A4 enzyme activity have the potential to result in increased plasma concentrations of corticosteroids). Products include:
- Zyflo Tablets ... 1023

Food Interactions

Grapefruit (Drugs which inhibit cytochrome P450 3A4 enzyme activity have the potential to result in increased plasma concentrations of corticosteroids).

Grapefruit Juice (Drugs which inhibit cytochrome P450 3A4 enzyme activity have the potential to result in increased plasma concentrations of corticosteroids).

DELSYM EXTENDED-RELEASE SUSPENSION 12 HOUR COUGH SUPPRESSANT

(Dextromethorphan Polistirex) ... ▣611

May interact with monoamine oxidase inhibitors. Compounds in these categories include:

Isocarboxazid (Concurrent and/or sequential use is not recommended).
No products indexed under this heading.

Moclobemide (Concurrent and/or sequential use is not recommended).
No products indexed under this heading.

Pargyline Hydrochloride (Concurrent and/or sequential use is not recommended).
No products indexed under this heading.

Phenelzine Sulfate (Concurrent and/or sequential use is not recommended).
No products indexed under this heading.

Procarbazine Hydrochloride (Concurrent and/or sequential use is not recommended). Products include:
- Matulane Capsules ... 3191

Selegiline Hydrochloride (Concurrent and/or sequential use is not recommended). Products include:
- Eldepryl Capsules ... 3208
- Zelapar Tablets ... 3372

Tranylcypromine Sulfate (Concurrent and/or sequential use is not recommended). Products include:
- Parnate Tablets ... 1527

DEMADEX INJECTION

(Torsemide) ... 2759

See Demadex Tablets

DEMADEX TABLETS

(Torsemide) ... 2759

May interact with aminoglycosides, lithium preparations, non-steroidal anti-inflammatory agents, salicylates, and certain other agents. Compounds in these categories include:

Amikacin Sulfate (Co-administration of other diuretics has been reported to increase the ototoxic potential of aminoglycoside antibiotics, especially in the presence of impaired renal function; concurrent use of aminoglycoside and torsemide has not been studied, however, such combined therapy should be undertaken with great caution).
No products indexed under this heading.

Aspirin (Co-administration in patients receiving high dose of salicylates may be associated with salicylate toxicity due to competition for secretion by renal tubule). Products include:
- Aggrenox Capsules ... 822
- Bayer Aspirin ... 744
- BC Allergy Sinus Cold Powder ... ▣677
- BC Headache Powder ... ▣677
- Arthritis Strength BC Powder ... ▣677
- BC Sinus Cold Powder ... ▣677
- Excedrin Extra Strength Caplets/Tablets/Geltabs ... ▣684
- Excedrin Migraine Caplets/Tablets/Geltabs ... ▣609
- Goody's Body Pain Formula Powder ... ▣684
- Goody's Extra Strength Headache Powders ... ▣611
- Goody's Extra Strength Pain Relief Tablets ... ▣685
- Percodan Tablets ... 1132
- St. Joseph 81 mg Aspirin Chewable and Enteric Coated Tablets ... 1869

Aspirin, Enteric Coated (Co-administration in patients receiving high dose of salicylates may be associated with salicylate toxicity due to competition for secretion by renal tubule).
No products indexed under this heading.

Aspirin Buffered (Co-administration in patients receiving high dose of salicylates may be associated with salicylate toxicity due to competition for secretion by renal tubule). Products include:
- Bufferin Extra Strength Tablets ... ▣678
- Bufferin Regular Strength Tablets ... ▣678

Celecoxib (Co-administration of another loop diuretic and nonsteroidal anti-inflammatory agents has been associated with renal dysfunction; concurrent use of torsemide and these agents has not been studied, however, such combined therapy should be undertaken with great caution). Products include:
- Celebrex Capsules ... 3134

Cholestyramine (Possibility of decreased oral absorption of torsemide; simultaneous administration is not recommended).
No products indexed under this heading.

Choline Magnesium Trisalicylate (Co-administration in patients receiving high dose of salicylates may be associated with salicylate toxicity due to competition for secretion by renal tubule).
No products indexed under this heading.

Diclofenac Potassium (Co-administration of another loop diuretic and nonsteroidal anti-inflammatory agents has been associated with renal dysfunction; concurrent use of torsemide and these agents has not been studied, however, such combined therapy should be undertaken with great caution).
No products indexed under this heading.

Diclofenac Sodium (Co-administration of another loop diuretic and nonsteroidal anti-inflammatory agents has been associated with renal dysfunction; concurrent use of torsemide and these agents has not been studied, however, such combined therapy should be undertaken with great caution). Products include:
- Arthrotec Tablets ... 3129
- Voltaren Ophthalmic Solution ... 2309
- Voltaren Tablets ... 2307
- Voltaren-XR Tablets ... 2310

Diflunisal (Co-administration in patients receiving high dose of salicylates may be associated with salicylate toxicity due to competition for secretion by renal tubule). Products include:
- Dolobid Tablets ... 1955

Digoxin (Co-administration of digoxin is reported to increase the AUC for torsemide by 50%, but dose adjustment of torsemide is not necessary). Products include:
- Lanoxicaps Capsules ... 1490
- Lanoxin Injection ... 1494
- Lanoxin Injection Pediatric ... 1497
- Lanoxin Tablets ... 1500

Etodolac (Co-administration of another loop diuretic and nonsteroidal anti-inflammatory agents has been associated with renal dysfunction; concurrent use of torsemide and these agents has not been studied, however, such combined therapy should be undertaken with great caution).
No products indexed under this heading.

Fenoprofen Calcium (Co-administration of another loop diuretic and nonsteroidal anti-inflammatory agents has been associated with renal dysfunction; concurrent use of torsemide and these agents has not been studied, however, such combined therapy should be undertaken with great caution). Products include:
- Nalfon Capsules ... 2502

Flurbiprofen (Co-administration of another loop diuretic and nonsteroidal anti-inflammatory agents has been associated with renal dysfunction; concurrent use of torsemide and these agents has not been studied, however, such combined therapy should be undertaken with great caution).
No products indexed under this heading.

Gentamicin Sulfate (Co-administration of other diuretics has been reported to increase the ototoxic potential of aminoglycoside antibiotics, especially in the presence of impaired renal function; concurrent use of aminoglycoside and torsemide has not been studied, however, such combined therapy should be undertaken with great caution). Products include:
- Garamycin Injectable ... 3014
- Pred-G Ophthalmic Ointment ... ⊙237
- Pred-G Ophthalmic Suspension ... ⊙236

Ibuprofen (Co-administration of another loop diuretic and nonsteroidal anti-inflammatory agents has been associated with renal dysfunction; concurrent use of torsemide and these agents has not been studied, however, such combined therapy should be undertaken with great caution). Products include:
- Advil Allergy Sinus Caplets ... ▣770
- Advil ... ▣674
- Children's Advil Oral Suspension ... ▣603
- Children's Advil Chewable Tablets ... ▣603
- Advil Cold & Sinus ... ▣723
- Infants' Advil Concentrated Drops ... ▣604
- Infants' Advil Concentrated Drops - White Grape (Dye-Free) ... ▣604
- Junior Strength Advil Swallow Tablets ... ▣605
- Advil Migraine Liquigels ... ▣608
- Advil Multi-Symptom Cold Caplets ... ▣770
- Advil PM Caplets ... ▣615
- Motrin IB Tablets and Caplets ... 1866
- Children's Motrin Oral Suspension ... 1867
- Children's Motrin Non-Staining Dye-Free Oral Suspension ... 1867
- Children's Motrin Cold Oral Suspension ... 1867
- Infants' Motrin Concentrated Drops ... 1867
- Infants' Motrin Non-Staining Dye-Free Concentrated Drops ... 1867
- Junior Strength Motrin Caplets and Chewable Tablets ... 1867
- Vicoprofen Tablets ... 539

Indomethacin (The natriuretic effect of torsemide is partially inhibited by the concomitant administration of indomethacin). Products include:
- Indocin ... 1995

Indomethacin Sodium Trihydrate (The natriuretic effect of torsemide is partially inhibited by the concomitant administration of indomethacin). Products include:

Indocin I.V. 2465

Kanamycin Sulfate (Co-administration of other diuretics has been reported to increase the ototoxic potential of aminoglycoside antibiotics, especially in the presence of impaired renal function; concurrent use of aminoglycoside and torsemide has not been studied, however, such combined therapy should be undertaken with great caution).

No products indexed under this heading.

Ketoprofen (Co-administration of another loop diuretic and nonsteroidal anti-inflammatory agents has been associated with renal dysfunction; concurrent use of torsemide and these agents has not been studied, however, such combined therapy should be undertaken with great caution).

No products indexed under this heading.

Ketorolac Tromethamine (Co-administration of another loop diuretic and nonsteroidal anti-inflammatory agents has been associated with renal dysfunction; concurrent use of torsemide and these agents has not been studied, however, such combined therapy should be undertaken with great caution). Products include:

Acular Ophthalmic Solution 565
Acular LS Ophthalmic Solution 566

Lithium (Co-administration of other diuretics are known to reduce the renal clearance of lithium, inducing a high risk of lithium toxicity; concurrent use of lithium and torsemide has not been studied, however, such combined therapy should be undertaken with great caution).

No products indexed under this heading.

Lithium Carbonate (Co-administration of other diuretics are known to reduce the renal clearance of lithium, inducing a high risk of lithium toxicity; concurrent use of lithium and torsemide has not been studied, however, such combined therapy should be undertaken with great caution). Products include:

Lithobid Tablets 1692

Lithium Citrate (Co-administration of other diuretics are known to reduce the renal clearance of lithium, inducing a high risk of lithium toxicity; concurrent use of lithium and torsemide has not been studied, however, such combined therapy should be undertaken with great caution).

No products indexed under this heading.

Magnesium Salicylate (Co-administration in patients receiving high dose of salicylates may be associated with salicylate toxicity due to competition for secretion by renal tubule).

No products indexed under this heading.

Meclofenamate Sodium (Co-administration of another loop diuretic and nonsteroidal anti-inflammatory agents has been associated with renal dysfunction; concurrent use of torsemide and these agents has not been studied, however, such combined therapy should be undertaken with great caution).

No products indexed under this heading.

Mefenamic Acid (Co-administration of another loop diuretic and nonsteroidal anti-inflammatory agents has been associated with renal dysfunction; concurrent use of torsemide and these agents has not been studied, however, such combined therapy should be undertaken with great caution).

No products indexed under this heading.

Meloxicam (Co-administration of another loop diuretic and nonsteroidal anti-inflammatory agents has been associated with renal dysfunction; concurrent use of torsemide and these agents has not been studied, however, such combined therapy should be undertaken with great caution). Products include:

Mobic Oral Suspension 863
Mobic Tablets 863

Nabumetone (Co-administration of another loop diuretic and nonsteroidal anti-inflammatory agents has been associated with renal dysfunction; concurrent use of torsemide and these agents has not been studied, however, such combined therapy should be undertaken with great caution).

No products indexed under this heading.

Naproxen (Co-administration of another loop diuretic and nonsteroidal anti-inflammatory agents has been associated with renal dysfunction; concurrent use of torsemide and these agents has not been studied, however, such combined therapy should be undertaken with great caution). Products include:

EC-Naprosyn Delayed-Release Tablets 2761
Naprosyn Suspension 2761
Naprosyn Tablets 2761
Prevacid NapraPAC 3280

Naproxen Sodium (Co-administration of another loop diuretic and nonsteroidal anti-inflammatory agents has been associated with renal dysfunction; concurrent use of torsemide and these agents has not been studied, however, such combined therapy should be undertaken with great caution). Products include:

Aleve Caplets 742
Aleve Gelcaps 743
Aleve Tablets 743
Aleve Cold & Sinus Caplets 744
Anaprox Tablets 2761
Anaprox DS Tablets 2761

Oxaprozin (Co-administration of another loop diuretic and nonsteroidal anti-inflammatory agents has been associated with renal dysfunction; concurrent use of torsemide and these agents has not been studied, however, such combined therapy should be undertaken with great caution).

No products indexed under this heading.

Phenylbutazone (Co-administration of another loop diuretic and nonsteroidal anti-inflammatory agents has been associated with renal dysfunction; concurrent use of torsemide and these agents has not been studied, however, such combined therapy should be undertaken with great caution).

No products indexed under this heading.

Piroxicam (Co-administration of another loop diuretic and nonsteroidal anti-inflammatory agents has been associated with renal dysfunction; concurrent use of torsemide and these agents has not been studied, however, such combined therapy should be undertaken with great caution).

No products indexed under this heading.

Probenecid (Reduces secretion of torsemide into the proximal tubule and thereby decreases diuretic effect).

No products indexed under this heading.

Rofecoxib (Co-administration of another loop diuretic and nonsteroidal anti-inflammatory agents has been associated with renal dysfunction; concurrent use of torsemide and these agents has not been studied, however, such combined therapy should be undertaken with great caution).

No products indexed under this heading.

Salsalate (Co-administration in patients receiving high dose of salicylates may be associated with salicylate toxicity due to competition for secretion by renal tubule).

No products indexed under this heading.

Spironolactone (Co-administration may be associated with significant reduction in the renal clearance of spironolactone, with corresponding increase in the AUC).

No products indexed under this heading.

Streptomycin Sulfate (Co-administration of other diuretics has been reported to increase the ototoxic potential of aminoglycoside antibiotics, especially in the presence of impaired renal function; concurrent use of aminoglycoside and torsemide has not been studied, however, such combined therapy should be undertaken with great caution).

No products indexed under this heading.

Sulindac (Co-administration of another loop diuretic and nonsteroidal anti-inflammatory agents has been associated with renal dysfunction; concurrent use of torsemide and these agents has not been studied, however, such combined therapy should be undertaken with great caution). Products include:

Clinoril Tablets 1924

Tobramycin (Co-administration of other diuretics has been reported to increase the ototoxic potential of aminoglycoside antibiotics, especially in the presence of impaired renal function; concurrent use of aminoglycoside and torsemide has not been studied, however, such combined therapy should be undertaken with great caution). Products include:

TOBI Solution for Inhalation 2298
TobraDex Ophthalmic Ointment 562
TobraDex Ophthalmic Suspension ... 563
Zylet Ophthalmic Suspension .... ⊙ 259

Tobramycin Sulfate (Co-administration of other diuretics has been reported to increase the ototoxic potential of aminoglycoside antibiotics, especially in the presence of impaired renal function; concurrent use of aminoglycoside and torsemide has not been studied, however, such combined therapy should be undertaken with great caution).

No products indexed under this heading.

Tolmetin Sodium (Co-administration of another loop diuretic and nonsteroidal anti-inflammatory agents has been associated with renal dysfunction; concurrent use of torsemide and these agents has not been studied, however, such combined therapy should be undertaken with great caution).

No products indexed under this heading.

Valdecoxib (Co-administration of another loop diuretic and nonsteroidal anti-inflammatory agents has been associated with renal dysfunction; concurrent use of torsemide and these agents has not been studied, however, such combined therapy should be undertaken with great caution).

No products indexed under this heading.

Food Interactions

Food, unspecified (Simultaneous food intake delays the time to Cmax by about 30 minutes, but overall bioavailability (AUC) and diuretic activity are unchanged).

DEMSER CAPSULES

(Metyrosine) 1953

May interact with central nervous system depressants, phenothiazines, and certain other agents. Compounds in these categories include:

Alfentanil Hydrochloride (Additive sedative effects).

No products indexed under this heading.

Alprazolam (Additive sedative effects). Products include:

Niravam Orally Disintegrating Tablets 3092

Aprobarbital (Additive sedative effects).

No products indexed under this heading.

Buprenorphine Hydrochloride (Additive sedative effects). Products include:

Buprenex Injectable 2716
Suboxone Tablets 2717
Subutex Tablets 2717

Buspirone Hydrochloride (Additive sedative effects).

No products indexed under this heading.

Butabarbital (Additive sedative effects).

No products indexed under this heading.

Butalbital (Additive sedative effects).

No products indexed under this heading.

Chlordiazepoxide (Additive sedative effects).

No products indexed under this heading.

Chlordiazepoxide Hydrochloride (Additive sedative effects). Products include:
Librium Capsules 3347

Chlorpromazine (Possible potentiation of extrapyramidal effects; additive sedative effects).
No products indexed under this heading.

Chlorpromazine Hydrochloride (Possible potentiation of extrapyramidal effects; additive sedative effects).
No products indexed under this heading.

Chlorprothixene (Additive sedative effects).
No products indexed under this heading.

Chlorprothixene Hydrochloride (Additive sedative effects).
No products indexed under this heading.

Chlorprothixene Lactate (Additive sedative effects).
No products indexed under this heading.

Clorazepate Dipotassium (Additive sedative effects). Products include:
Tranxene .. 2474

Clozapine (Additive sedative effects). Products include:
Clozaril Tablets 2184
FazaClo Orally Disintegrating
Tablets .. 551

Codeine Phosphate (Additive sedative effects). Products include:
Tylenol with Codeine Tablets 2391

Desflurane (Additive sedative effects).
No products indexed under this heading.

Dezocine (Additive sedative effects).
No products indexed under this heading.

Diazepam (Additive sedative effects). Products include:
Diastat Rectal Delivery System 3343
Valium Tablets 2819

Droperidol (Additive sedative effects).
No products indexed under this heading.

Enflurane (Additive sedative effects).
No products indexed under this heading.

Estazolam (Additive sedative effects). Products include:
ProSom Tablets 517

Ethanol (Additive sedative effects).
No products indexed under this heading.

Ethchlorvynol (Additive sedative effects).
No products indexed under this heading.

Ethinamate (Additive sedative effects).
No products indexed under this heading.

Ethyl Alcohol (Additive sedative effects).
No products indexed under this heading.

Fentanyl (Additive sedative effects). Products include:
Duragesic Transdermal System 2373
Ionsys Transdermal System 2379

Fentanyl Citrate (Additive sedative effects). Products include:
Actiq .. 979

Fluphenazine Decanoate (Possible potentiation of extrapyramidal effects; additive sedative effects).
No products indexed under this heading.

Fluphenazine Enanthate (Possible potentiation of extrapyramidal effects; additive sedative effects).
No products indexed under this heading.

Fluphenazine Hydrochloride (Possible potentiation of extrapyramidal effects; additive sedative effects).
No products indexed under this heading.

Flurazepam Hydrochloride (Additive sedative effects). Products include:
Dalmane Capsules 3342

Glutethimide (Additive sedative effects).
No products indexed under this heading.

Haloperidol (Possible potentiation of extrapyramidal effects; additive sedative effects).
No products indexed under this heading.

Haloperidol Decanoate (Possible potentiation of extrapyramidal effects; additive sedative effects).
No products indexed under this heading.

Hydrocodone Bitartrate (Additive sedative effects). Products include:
Hycodan 1116
Hycotuss Expectorant Syrup 1117
Vicodin Tablets 535
Vicodin ES Tablets 536
Vicodin HP Tablets 538
Vicoprofen Tablets 539
Zydone Tablets 1139

Hydrocodone Polistirex (Additive sedative effects). Products include:
Tussionex Pennkinetic
Extended-Release Suspension 3327

Hydromorphone Hydrochloride (Additive sedative effects). Products include:
Dilaudid 440
Dilaudid Non-Sterile Powder 440
Dilaudid Oral Liquid 445
Dilaudid Rectal Suppositories 440
Dilaudid Tablets 440
Dilaudid Tablets - 8 mg 445
Dilaudid-HP 442

Hydroxyzine Hydrochloride (Additive sedative effects).
No products indexed under this heading.

Isoflurane (Additive sedative effects).
No products indexed under this heading.

Ketamine Hydrochloride (Additive sedative effects).
No products indexed under this heading.

Levomethadyl Acetate Hydrochloride (Additive sedative effects).
No products indexed under this heading.

Levorphanol Tartrate (Additive sedative effects).
No products indexed under this heading.

Lorazepam (Additive sedative effects).
No products indexed under this heading.

Loxapine Hydrochloride (Additive sedative effects).
No products indexed under this heading.

Loxapine Succinate (Additive sedative effects).
No products indexed under this heading.

Meperidine Hydrochloride (Additive sedative effects).
No products indexed under this heading.

Mephobarbital (Additive sedative effects).
No products indexed under this heading.

Meprobamate (Additive sedative effects).
No products indexed under this heading.

Mesoridazine Besylate (Possible potentiation of extrapyramidal effects; additive sedative effects).
No products indexed under this heading.

Methadone Hydrochloride (Additive sedative effects).
No products indexed under this heading.

Methohexital Sodium (Additive sedative effects).
No products indexed under this heading.

Methotrimeprazine (Possible potentiation of extrapyramidal effects; additive sedative effects).
No products indexed under this heading.

Methoxyflurane (Additive sedative effects).
No products indexed under this heading.

Midazolam Hydrochloride (Additive sedative effects).
No products indexed under this heading.

Molindone Hydrochloride (Additive sedative effects). Products include:
Moban Tablets 1119

Morphine Sulfate (Additive sedative effects). Products include:
Avinza Capsules 1741
Kadian Capsules 577
MS Contin Tablets 2701

Olanzapine (Additive sedative effects). Products include:
Symbyax Capsules 1819
Zyprexa Tablets 1830
Zyprexa IntraMuscular 1830
Zyprexa ZYDIS Orally
Disintegrating Tablets 1830

Oxazepam (Additive sedative effects).
No products indexed under this heading.

Oxycodone Hydrochloride (Additive sedative effects). Products include:
OxyContin Tablets 2703
OxyFast Oral Concentrate
Solution 2708
OxyIR Capsules 2708
Percocet Tablets 1131
Percodan Tablets 1132

Pentobarbital Sodium (Additive sedative effects). Products include:
Nembutal Sodium Solution, USP 2470

Perphenazine (Possible potentiation of extrapyramidal effects of perphenazine; additive sedative effects).
No products indexed under this heading.

Phenobarbital (Additive sedative effects). Products include:
Donnatal Extentabs 2493

Prazepam (Additive sedative effects).
No products indexed under this heading.

Prochlorperazine (Possible potentiation of extrapyramidal effects; additive sedative effects).
No products indexed under this heading.

Promethazine Hydrochloride (Possible potentiation of extrapyramidal effects; additive sedative effects). Products include:
Phenergan Tablets and
Suppositories 3440

Propofol (Additive sedative effects).
No products indexed under this heading.

Propoxyphene Hydrochloride (Additive sedative effects).
No products indexed under this heading.

Propoxyphene Napsylate (Additive sedative effects).
No products indexed under this heading.

Quazepam (Additive sedative effects).
No products indexed under this heading.

Quetiapine Fumarate (Additive sedative effects). Products include:
Seroquel Tablets 690

Remifentanil Hydrochloride (Additive sedative effects).
No products indexed under this heading.

Risperidone (Additive sedative effects). Products include:
Risperdal 1676
Risperdal Consta Long-Acting
Injection 1682
Risperdal M-Tab Orally
Disintegrating Tablets 1676

Secobarbital Sodium (Additive sedative effects).
No products indexed under this heading.

Sevoflurane (Additive sedative effects). Products include:
Ultane Liquid for Inhalation 531

Sufentanil Citrate (Additive sedative effects).
No products indexed under this heading.

Temazepam (Additive sedative effects). Products include:
Restoril Capsules 1860

Thiamylal Sodium (Additive sedative effects).
No products indexed under this heading.

Thioridazine Hydrochloride (Possible potentiation of extrapyramidal effects; additive sedative effects). Products include:
Thioridazine Hydrochloride
Tablets 2163

Thiothixene (Additive sedative effects). Products include:
Thiothixene Capsules 2165

Triazolam (Additive sedative effects).
No products indexed under this heading.

Trifluoperazine Hydrochloride (Possible potentiation of extrapyramidal effects; additive sedative effects).
No products indexed under this heading.

Zaleplon (Additive sedative effects). Products include:
Sonata Capsules 1717

Ziprasidone Hydrochloride (Additive sedative effects). Products include:
Geodon Capsules 2529

Zolpidem Tartrate (Additive sedative effects). Products include:
Ambien Tablets 2851
Ambien CR Tablets 2855

Food Interactions

Alcohol (Additive sedative effects).

DENAVIR CREAM

(Penciclovir) 2174
None cited in PDR database.

DEPACON INJECTION

(Valproate Sodium) 412
May interact with central nervous system depressants, phenytoin, and certain other agents. Compounds in these categories include:

Alfentanil Hydrochloride (Co-administration may result in additive CNS depression).
No products indexed under this heading.

Alprazolam (Co-administration may result in additive CNS depression). Products include:
Niravam Orally Disintegrating Tablets 3092

Amitriptyline Hydrochloride (Co-administration has resulted in a 21% decrease in plasma clearance of amitriptyline; this interaction is likely to be clinically unimportant).
No products indexed under this heading.

Aprobarbital (Co-administration may result in additive CNS depression).
No products indexed under this heading.

Aspirin (Co-administration has resulted in decreased protein binding and an inhibition of metabolism of valproate). Products include:
Aggrenox Capsules 822
Bayer Aspirin 744
BC Allergy Sinus Cold Powder ⊞677
BC Headache Powder ⊞677
Arthritis Strength BC Powder ⊞677
BC Sinus Cold Powder ⊞677
Excedrin Extra Strength Caplets/Tablets/Geltabs.............. ⊞684
Excedrin Migraine Caplets/Tablets/Geltabs........... ⊞609
Goody's Body Pain Formula Powder ⊞684
Goody's Extra Strength Headache Powders ⊞611
Goody's Extra Strength Pain Relief Tablets.......................... ⊞685
Percodan Tablets 1132
St. Joseph 81 mg Aspirin Chewable and Enteric Coated Tablets.................................. 1869

Buprenorphine Hydrochloride (Co-administration may result in additive CNS depression). Products include:
Buprenex Injectable 2716
Suboxone Tablets 2717
Subutex Tablets 2717

Buspirone Hydrochloride (Co-administration may result in additive CNS depression).
No products indexed under this heading.

Butabarbital (Co-administration may result in additive CNS depression).
No products indexed under this heading.

Butalbital (Co-administration may result in additive CNS depression).
No products indexed under this heading.

Carbamazepine (Can double the clearance of valproate; co-administration has resulted in decreased carbamazepine and increased carbamazepine 10,11-epoxide serum levels). Products include:
Carbatrol Capsules 3171
Equetro Extended-Release Capsules........................... 3180
Tegretol/Tegretol-XR 2295

Chlordiazepoxide (Co-administration may result in additive CNS depression).
No products indexed under this heading.

Chlordiazepoxide Hydrochloride (Co-administration may result in additive CNS depression). Products include:
Librium Capsules 3347

Chlorpromazine (Co-administration has resulted in a 15% increase in trough plasma levels of valproate; concurrent use may result in additive CNS depression).
No products indexed under this heading.

Chlorpromazine Hydrochloride (Co-administration has resulted in a 15% increase in trough plasma levels of valproate; concurrent use may result in additive CNS depression).
No products indexed under this heading.

Chlorprothixene (Co-administration may result in additive CNS depression).
No products indexed under this heading.

Chlorprothixene Hydrochloride (Co-administration may result in additive CNS depression).
No products indexed under this heading.

Chlorprothixene Lactate (Co-administration may result in additive CNS depression).
No products indexed under this heading.

Clonazepam (Co-administration may induce absence status in patients with a history of absence-type seizures). Products include:
Klonopin 2778

Clorazepate Dipotassium (Co-administration may result in additive CNS depression). Products include:
Tranxene 2474

Clozapine (Co-administration may result in additive CNS depression). Products include:
Clozaril Tablets 2184
FazaClo Orally Disintegrating Tablets 551

Codeine Phosphate (Co-administration may result in additive CNS depression). Products include:
Tylenol with Codeine Tablets 2391

Desflurane (Co-administration may result in additive CNS depression).
No products indexed under this heading.

Dezocine (Co-administration may result in additive CNS depression).
No products indexed under this heading.

Diazepam (Valproate displaces diazepam from its plasma albumin binding sites and inhibits its metabolism; plasma clearance and volume of distribution for free diazepam may be reduced; concurrent use may result in additive CNS depression). Products include:
Diastat Rectal Delivery System 3343

Valium Tablets 2819

Droperidol (Co-administration may result in additive CNS depression).
No products indexed under this heading.

Enflurane (Co-administration may result in additive CNS depression).
No products indexed under this heading.

Estazolam (Co-administration may result in additive CNS depression). Products include:
ProSom Tablets 517

Ethanol (Co-administration may result in additive CNS depression).
No products indexed under this heading.

Ethchlorvynol (Co-administration may result in additive CNS depression).
No products indexed under this heading.

Ethinamate (Co-administration may result in additive CNS depression).
No products indexed under this heading.

Ethosuximide (Valproate inhibits the metabolism of ethosuximide).
No products indexed under this heading.

Ethyl Alcohol (Co-administration may result in additive CNS depression).
No products indexed under this heading.

Felbamate (Co-administration has resulted in an increase in mean valproate peak concentration; a reduction in valproate dosage may be necessary).
No products indexed under this heading.

Fentanyl (Co-administration may result in additive CNS depression). Products include:
Duragesic Transdermal System 2373
Ionsys Transdermal System 2379

Fentanyl Citrate (Co-administration may result in additive CNS depression). Products include:
Actiq 979

Fluphenazine Decanoate (Co-administration may result in additive CNS depression).
No products indexed under this heading.

Fluphenazine Enanthate (Co-administration may result in additive CNS depression).
No products indexed under this heading.

Fluphenazine Hydrochloride (Co-administration may result in additive CNS depression).
No products indexed under this heading.

Flurazepam Hydrochloride (Co-administration may result in additive CNS depression). Products include:
Dalmane Capsules 3342

Fosphenytoin Sodium (Can double the clearance of valproate; valproate displaces phenytoin from its plasma albumin binding sites and inhibits its hepatic metabolism; co-administration has resulted in breakthrough seizures).
No products indexed under this heading.

Glutethimide (Co-administration may result in additive CNS depression).
No products indexed under this heading.

Haloperidol (Co-administration may result in additive CNS depression).
No products indexed under this heading.

Haloperidol Decanoate (Co-administration may result in additive CNS depression).
No products indexed under this heading.

Hydrocodone Bitartrate (Co-administration may result in additive CNS depression). Products include:
Hycodan 1116
Hycotuss Expectorant Syrup 1117
Vicodin Tablets 535
Vicodin ES Tablets 536
Vicodin HP Tablets 538
Vicoprofen Tablets 539
Zydone Tablets 1139

Hydrocodone Polistirex (Co-administration may result in additive CNS depression). Products include:
Tussionex Pennkinetic Extended-Release Suspension...... 3327

Hydromorphone Hydrochloride (Co-administration may result in additive CNS depression). Products include:
Dilaudid 440
Dilaudid Non-Sterile Powder 440
Dilaudid Oral Liquid 445
Dilaudid Rectal Suppositories 440
Dilaudid Tablets 440
Dilaudid Tablets - 8 mg 445
Dilaudid-HP 442

Hydroxyzine Hydrochloride (Co-administration may result in additive CNS depression).
No products indexed under this heading.

Isoflurane (Co-administration may result in additive CNS depression).
No products indexed under this heading.

Ketamine Hydrochloride (Co-administration may result in additive CNS depression).
No products indexed under this heading.

Lamotrigine (Co-administration has resulted in increased elimination half-life of lamotrigine, and serious skin reactions, such as Stevens-Johnson syndrome and toxic epidermal necrolysis; the dose of lamotrigine should be reduced if used concurrently). Products include:
Lamictal 1481

Levomethadyl Acetate Hydrochloride (Co-administration may result in additive CNS depression).
No products indexed under this heading.

Levorphanol Tartrate (Co-administration may result in additive CNS depression).
No products indexed under this heading.

Lorazepam (Co-administration was accompanied by a 17% decrease in the plasma clearance of lorazepam; this pharmacokinetic interaction is likely to be clinically unimportant; concurrent use may result in additive CNS depression).
No products indexed under this heading.

Loxapine Hydrochloride (Co-administration may result in additive CNS depression).
No products indexed under this heading.

Loxapine Succinate (Co-administration may result in additive CNS depression).
No products indexed under this heading.

IMPORTANT NOTE: Always consult each drug listing in the patient's regimen for possible interactions.

Meperidine Hydrochloride (Co-administration may result in additive CNS depression).
No products indexed under this heading.

Mephobarbital (Co-administration may result in additive CNS depression).
No products indexed under this heading.

Meprobamate (Co-administration may result in additive CNS depression).
No products indexed under this heading.

Meropenem (Sub-therapeutic valproic acid levels have been reported when meropenem was co-administered). Products include:
Merrem I.V. 686

Mesoridazine Besylate (Co-administration may result in additive CNS depression).
No products indexed under this heading.

Methadone Hydrochloride (Co-administration may result in additive CNS depression).
No products indexed under this heading.

Methohexital Sodium (Co-administration may result in additive CNS depression).
No products indexed under this heading.

Methotrimeprazine (Co-administration may result in additive CNS depression).
No products indexed under this heading.

Methoxyflurane (Co-administration may result in additive CNS depression).
No products indexed under this heading.

Midazolam Hydrochloride (Co-administration may result in additive CNS depression).
No products indexed under this heading.

Molindone Hydrochloride (Co-administration may result in additive CNS depression). Products include:
Moban Tablets 1119

Morphine Sulfate (Co-administration may result in additive CNS depression). Products include:
Avinza Capsules 1741
Kadian Capsules 577
MS Contin Tablets 2701

Nortriptyline Hydrochloride (Co-administration has resulted in a 34% decrease in the net clearance of nortriptyline; this interaction is likely to be clinically unimportant).
No products indexed under this heading.

Olanzapine (Co-administration may result in additive CNS depression). Products include:
Symbyax Capsules 1819
Zyprexa Tablets 1830
Zyprexa IntraMuscular 1830
Zyprexa ZYDIS Orally Disintegrating Tablets 1830

Oxazepam (Co-administration may result in additive CNS depression).
No products indexed under this heading.

Oxycodone Hydrochloride (Co-administration may result in additive CNS depression). Products include:
OxyContin Tablets 2703
OxyFast Oral Concentrate Solution 2708
OxyIR Capsules 2708
Percocet Tablets 1131
Percodan Tablets 1132

Pentobarbital Sodium (Co-administration may result in additive CNS depression). Products include:
Nembutal Sodium Solution, USP 2470

Perphenazine (Co-administration may result in additive CNS depression).
No products indexed under this heading.

Phenobarbital (Can double the clearance of valproate; co-administration has resulted in inhibition of the metabolism of phenobarbital resulting in increased half-life and decreased plasma clearance; concurrent use may result in additive CNS depression). Products include:
Donnatal Extentabs 2493

Phenytoin (Can double the clearance of valproate; valproate displaces phenytoin from its plasma albumin binding sites and inhibits its hepatic metabolism; co-administration has resulted in breakthrough seizures).
No products indexed under this heading.

Phenytoin Sodium (Can double the clearance of valproate; valproate displaces phenytoin from its plasma albumin binding sites and inhibits its hepatic metabolism; co-administration has resulted in breakthrough seizures). Products include:
Phenytek Capsules 2160

Prazepam (Co-administration may result in additive CNS depression).
No products indexed under this heading.

Primidone (Can double the clearance of valproate; primidone is metabolized to a barbiturate; therefore, co-administration may result in inhibition of the metabolism of primidone resulting in increased half-life and decreased plasma clearance).
No products indexed under this heading.

Prochlorperazine (Co-administration may result in additive CNS depression).
No products indexed under this heading.

Promethazine Hydrochloride (Co-administration may result in additive CNS depression). Products include:
Phenergan Tablets and Suppositories 3440

Propofol (Co-administration may result in additive CNS depression).
No products indexed under this heading.

Propoxyphene Hydrochloride (Co-administration may result in additive CNS depression).
No products indexed under this heading.

Propoxyphene Napsylate (Co-administration may result in additive CNS depression).
No products indexed under this heading.

Quazepam (Co-administration may result in additive CNS depression).
No products indexed under this heading.

Quetiapine Fumarate (Co-administration may result in additive CNS depression). Products include:
Seroquel Tablets 690

Remifentanil Hydrochloride (Co-administration may result in additive CNS depression).
No products indexed under this heading.

Rifampin (Co-administration has resulted in a 40% increase in oral clearance of valproate).
No products indexed under this heading.

Risperidone (Co-administration may result in additive CNS depression). Products include:
Risperdal 1676
Risperdal Consta Long-Acting Injection 1682
Risperdal M-Tab Orally Disintegrating Tablets 1676

Secobarbital Sodium (Co-administration may result in additive CNS depression).
No products indexed under this heading.

Sevoflurane (Co-administration may result in additive CNS depression). Products include:
Ultane Liquid for Inhalation 531

Sufentanil Citrate (Co-administration may result in additive CNS depression).
No products indexed under this heading.

Temazepam (Co-administration may result in additive CNS depression). Products include:
Restoril Capsules 1860

Thiamylal Sodium (Co-administration may result in additive CNS depression).
No products indexed under this heading.

Thioridazine Hydrochloride (Co-administration may result in additive CNS depression). Products include:
Thioridazine Hydrochloride Tablets 2163

Thiothixene (Co-administration may result in additive CNS depression). Products include:
Thiothixene Capsules 2165

Tolbutamide (Co-administration in in vitro studies has resulted in an increase in unbound fraction of tolbutamide; the clinical relevance of this displacement is unknown).
No products indexed under this heading.

Topiramate (Concomitant administration of valproic acid and topiramate has been associated with hyperammonemia with and without encephalopathy). Products include:
Topamax Sprinkle Capsules 2404
Topamax Tablets 2404

Triazolam (Co-administration may result in additive CNS depression).
No products indexed under this heading.

Trifluoperazine Hydrochloride (Co-administration may result in additive CNS depression).
No products indexed under this heading.

Warfarin Sodium (In an *in vitro* study, valproate increased the unbound fraction of warfarin by up to 32.6%; therapeutic relevance of this is unknown). Products include:
Coumadin for Injection 898
Coumadin Tablets 898

Zaleplon (Co-administration may result in additive CNS depression). Products include:
Sonata Capsules 1717

Ziprasidone Hydrochloride (Co-administration may result in additive CNS depression). Products include:
Geodon Capsules 2529

Zolpidem Tartrate (Co-administration may result in additive CNS depression). Products include:
Ambien Tablets 2851
Ambien CR Tablets 2855

Food Interactions

Alcohol (Co-administration may result in additive CNS depression).

DEPAKENE CAPSULES

(Valproic Acid) 417
May interact with central nervous system depressants, phenytoin, and certain other agents. Compounds in these categories include:

Alfentanil Hydrochloride (Valproate produces CNS depression, especially when combined with another CNS depressant).
No products indexed under this heading.

Alprazolam (Valproate produces CNS depression, especially when combined with another CNS depressant). Products include:
Niravam Orally Disintegrating Tablets 3092

Amitriptyline Hydrochloride (Co-administration has resulted in a decrease in plasma clearance of amitriptyline; rare postmarketing reports of increased amitriptyline levels).
No products indexed under this heading.

Aprobarbital (Valproate produces CNS depression, especially when combined with another CNS depressant).
No products indexed under this heading.

Aspirin (Co-administration has resulted in a decrease in protein binding and an inhibition of metabolism of valproate; valproate free fraction was increased 4-fold in the presence of aspirin compared to valproate alone). Products include:
Aggrenox Capsules 822
Bayer Aspirin 744
BC Allergy Sinus Cold Powder .... ▣677
BC Headache Powder .... ▣677
Arthritis Strength BC Powder .... ▣677
BC Sinus Cold Powder .... ▣677
Excedrin Extra Strength Caplets/Tablets/Geltabs .... ▣684
Excedrin Migraine Caplets/Tablets/Geltabs .... ▣609
Goody's Body Pain Formula Powder .... ▣684
Goody's Extra Strength Headache Powders .... ▣611
Goody's Extra Strength Pain Relief Tablets .... ▣685
Percodan Tablets 1132
St. Joseph 81 mg Aspirin Chewable and Enteric Coated Tablets 1869

Buprenorphine Hydrochloride (Valproate produces CNS depression, especially when combined with another CNS depressant). Products include:
Buprenex Injectable 2716
Suboxone Tablets 2717
Subutex Tablets 2717

Buspirone Hydrochloride (Valproate produces CNS depression, especially when combined with another CNS depressant).
No products indexed under this heading.

Butabarbital (Valproate produces CNS depression, especially when combined with another CNS depressant).

No products indexed under this heading.

Butalbital (Valproate produces CNS depression, especially when combined with another CNS depressant).

No products indexed under this heading.

Carbamazepine (Co-administration has resulted in decreased serum levels of carbamazepine and increased serum levels of carbamazepine 10, 11-epoxide; drugs that affect the levels of expression of hepatic enzymes, particularly those that elevate levels of glucuronosyltransferases, such as carbamazepine, may increase the clearance of valproate). Products include:

Chlordiazepoxide (Valproate produces CNS depression, especially when combined with another CNS depressant).

No products indexed under this heading.

Chlordiazepoxide Hydrochloride (Valproate produces CNS depression, especially when combined with another CNS depressant). Products include:

Chlorpromazine (Co-administration has resulted in an increase in trough plasma levels of valproate).

No products indexed under this heading.

Chlorpromazine Hydrochloride (Co-administration has resulted in an increase in trough plasma levels of valproate).

No products indexed under this heading.

Chlorprothixene (Valproate produces CNS depression, especially when combined with another CNS depressant).

No products indexed under this heading.

Chlorprothixene Hydrochloride (Valproate produces CNS depression, especially when combined with another CNS depressant).

No products indexed under this heading.

Chlorprothixene Lactate (Valproate produces CNS depression, especially when combined with another CNS depressant).

No products indexed under this heading.

Clonazepam (Co-administration may induce absence status in patients with a history of absence type seizures). Products include:

Clorazepate Dipotassium (Valproate produces CNS depression, especially when combined with another CNS depressant). Products include:

Clozapine (Valproate produces CNS depression, especially when combined with another CNS depressant). Products include:

Codeine Phosphate (Valproate produces CNS depression, especially when combined with another CNS depressant). Products include:

Desflurane (Valproate produces CNS depression, especially when combined with another CNS depressant).

No products indexed under this heading.

Dezocine (Valproate produces CNS depression, especially when combined with another CNS depressant).

No products indexed under this heading.

Diazepam (Co-administration increases the free fraction of diazepam by 90% in healthy volunteers; plasma clearance and volume of distribution for diazepam were reduced by 25% and 20%, respectively, in the presence of valproate). Products include:

Droperidol (Valproate produces CNS depression, especially when combined with another CNS depressant).

No products indexed under this heading.

Enflurane (Valproate produces CNS depression, especially when combined with another CNS depressant).

No products indexed under this heading.

Estazolam (Valproate produces CNS depression, especially when combined with another CNS depressant). Products include:

Ethanol (Valproate produces CNS depression, especially when combined with another CNS depressant).

No products indexed under this heading.

Ethchlorvynol (Valproate produces CNS depression, especially when combined with another CNS depressant).

No products indexed under this heading.

Ethinamate (Valproate produces CNS depression, especially when combined with another CNS depressant).

No products indexed under this heading.

Ethosuximide (Valproate inhibits the metabolism of ethosuximide; co-administration was accompanied by a 25% increase in elimination half-life of ethosuximide and a 15% decrease in its total clearance as compared to ethosuximide alone).

No products indexed under this heading.

Ethyl Alcohol (Valproate produces CNS depression, especially when combined with another CNS depressant).

No products indexed under this heading.

Felbamate (Co-administration has resulted in an increase in mean valproate peak concentration).

No products indexed under this heading.

Fentanyl (Valproate produces CNS depression, especially when combined with another CNS depressant). Products include:

Fentanyl Citrate (Valproate produces CNS depression, especially when combined with another CNS depressant). Products include:

Fluphenazine Decanoate (Valproate produces CNS depression, especially when combined with another CNS depressant).

No products indexed under this heading.

Fluphenazine Enanthate (Valproate produces CNS depression, especially when combined with another CNS depressant).

No products indexed under this heading.

Fluphenazine Hydrochloride (Valproate produces CNS depression, especially when combined with another CNS depressant).

No products indexed under this heading.

Flurazepam Hydrochloride (Valproate produces CNS depression, especially when combined with another CNS depressant). Products include:

Fosphenytoin Sodium (Co-administration with drugs that affect the levels of expression of hepatic enzymes, particularly those that elevate levels of glucuronosyltransferases, such as phenytoin, may increase the clearance of valproate; valproate displaces phenytoin from its plasma binding sites and inhibits its hepatic metabolism; concurrent use has resulted in breakthrough seizures).

No products indexed under this heading.

Glutethimide (Valproate produces CNS depression, especially when combined with another CNS depressant).

No products indexed under this heading.

Haloperidol (Valproate produces CNS depression, especially when combined with another CNS depressant).

No products indexed under this heading.

Haloperidol Decanoate (Valproate produces CNS depression, especially when combined with another CNS depressant).

No products indexed under this heading.

Hydrocodone Bitartrate (Valproate produces CNS depression, especially when combined with another CNS depressant). Products include:

Hydrocodone Polistirex (Valproate produces CNS depression, especially when combined with another CNS depressant). Products include:

Hydromorphone Hydrochloride (Valproate produces CNS depression, especially when combined with another CNS depressant). Products include:

Hydroxyzine Hydrochloride (Valproate produces CNS depression, especially when combined with another CNS depressant).

No products indexed under this heading.

Isoflurane (Valproate produces CNS depression, especially when combined with another CNS depressant).

No products indexed under this heading.

Ketamine Hydrochloride (Valproate produces CNS depression, especially when combined with another CNS depressant).

No products indexed under this heading.

Lamotrigine (Co-administration has resulted in increased elimination half-life of lamotrigine from 26 to 72 hours and serious skin reactions, such as Stevens-Johnson syndrome and toxic epidermal necrolysis). Products include:

Levomethadyl Acetate Hydrochloride (Valproate produces CNS depression, especially when combined with another CNS depressant).

No products indexed under this heading.

Levorphanol Tartrate (Valproate produces CNS depression, especially when combined with another CNS depressant).

No products indexed under this heading.

Lorazepam (Co-administration was accompanied by a 17% decrease in the plasma clearance of lorazepam).

No products indexed under this heading.

Loxapine Hydrochloride (Valproate produces CNS depression, especially when combined with another CNS depressant).

No products indexed under this heading.

Loxapine Succinate (Valproate produces CNS depression, especially when combined with another CNS depressant).

No products indexed under this heading.

Meperidine Hydrochloride (Valproate produces CNS depression, especially when combined with another CNS depressant).

No products indexed under this heading.

Mephobarbital (Valproate produces CNS depression, especially when combined with another CNS depressant).

No products indexed under this heading.

Meprobamate (Valproate produces CNS depression, especially when combined with another CNS depressant).

No products indexed under this heading.

Meropenem (Sub-therapeutic valproic acid levels have been reported when meropenem was co-administered). Products include:

IMPORTANT NOTE: Always consult each drug listing in the patient's regimen for possible interactions.

Mesoridazine Besylate (Valproate produces CNS depression, especially when combined with another CNS depressant).
No products indexed under this heading.

Methadone Hydrochloride (Valproate produces CNS depression, especially when combined with another CNS depressant).
No products indexed under this heading.

Methohexital Sodium (Valproate produces CNS depression, especially when combined with another CNS depressant).
No products indexed under this heading.

Methotrimeprazine (Valproate produces CNS depression, especially when combined with another CNS depressant).
No products indexed under this heading.

Methoxyflurane (Valproate produces CNS depression, especially when combined with another CNS depressant).
No products indexed under this heading.

Midazolam Hydrochloride (Valproate produces CNS depression, especially when combined with another CNS depressant).
No products indexed under this heading.

Molindone Hydrochloride (Valproate produces CNS depression, especially when combined with another CNS depressant). Products include:
Moban Tablets **1119**

Morphine Sulfate (Valproate produces CNS depression, especially when combined with another CNS depressant). Products include:
Avinza Capsules **1741**
Kadian Capsules **577**
MS Contin Tablets **2701**

Nortriptyline Hydrochloride (Co-administration has resulted in a decrease in the net clearance of nortriptyline).
No products indexed under this heading.

Olanzapine (Valproate produces CNS depression, especially when combined with another CNS depressant). Products include:
Symbyax Capsules **1819**
Zyprexa Tablets **1830**
Zyprexa IntraMuscular **1830**
Zyprexa ZYDIS Orally Disintegrating Tablets **1830**

Oxazepam (Valproate produces CNS depression, especially when combined with another CNS depressant).
No products indexed under this heading.

Oxycodone Hydrochloride (Valproate produces CNS depression, especially when combined with another CNS depressant). Products include:
OxyContin Tablets **2703**
OxyFast Oral Concentrate Solution **2708**
OxyIR Capsules **2708**
Percocet Tablets **1131**
Percodan Tablets **1132**

Pentobarbital Sodium (Valproate produces CNS depression, especially when combined with another CNS depressant). Products include:
Nembutal Sodium Solution, USP **2470**

Perphenazine (Valproate produces CNS depression, especially when combined with another CNS depressant).
No products indexed under this heading.

Phenobarbital (Co-administration with drugs that affect the levels of expression of hepatic enzymes, particularly those that elevate levels of glucuronosyltransferases, such as phenobarbital, may increase the clearance of valproate; valproate inhibits the metabolism of phenobarbital; co-administration has resulted in an increase in half-life and decrease in plasma clearance of phenobarbital; all patients should be monitored for neurological toxicity because of severe CNS depression). Products include:
Donnatal Extentabs **2493**

Phenytoin (Co-administration with drugs that affect the levels of expression of hepatic enzymes, particularly those that elevate levels of glucuronosyltransferases, such as phenytoin, may increase the clearance of valproate; valproate displaces phenytoin from its plasma binding sites and inhibits its hepatic metabolism; concurrent use has resulted in breakthrough seizures).
No products indexed under this heading.

Phenytoin Sodium (Co-administration with drugs that affect the levels of expression of hepatic enzymes, particularly those that elevate levels of glucuronosyltransferases, such as phenytoin, may increase the clearance of valproate; valproate displaces phenytoin from its plasma binding sites and inhibits its hepatic metabolism; concurrent use has resulted in breakthrough seizures). Products include:
Phenytek Capsules **2160**

Prazepam (Valproate produces CNS depression, especially when combined with another CNS depressant).
No products indexed under this heading.

Primidone (Co-administraion may result in severe CNS depression because primidone is metabolized to a barbiturate; potential for same interaction as phenobarbital and valproate).
No products indexed under this heading.

Prochlorperazine (Valproate produces CNS depression, especially when combined with another CNS depressant).
No products indexed under this heading.

Promethazine Hydrochloride (Valproate produces CNS depression, especially when combined with another CNS depressant). Products include:
Phenergan Tablets and Suppositories **3440**

Propofol (Valproate produces CNS depression, especially when combined with another CNS depressant).
No products indexed under this heading.

Propoxyphene Hydrochloride (Valproate produces CNS depression, especially when combined with another CNS depressant).
No products indexed under this heading.

Propoxyphene Napsylate (Valproate produces CNS depression, especially when combined with another CNS depressant).
No products indexed under this heading.

Quazepam (Valproate produces CNS depression, especially when combined with another CNS depressant).
No products indexed under this heading.

Quetiapine Fumarate (Valproate produces CNS depression, especially when combined with another CNS depressant). Products include:
Seroquel Tablets **690**

Remifentanil Hydrochloride (Valproate produces CNS depression, especially when combined with another CNS depressant).
No products indexed under this heading.

Rifampin (Co-administration has resulted in an increase in the oral clearance of valproate).
No products indexed under this heading.

Risperidone (Valproate produces CNS depression, especially when combined with another CNS depressant). Products include:
Risperdal **1676**
Risperdal Consta Long-Acting Injection **1682**
Risperdal M-Tab Orally Disintegrating Tablets **1676**

Secobarbital Sodium (Valproate produces CNS depression, especially when combined with another CNS depressant).
No products indexed under this heading.

Sevoflurane (Valproate produces CNS depression, especially when combined with another CNS depressant). Products include:
Ultane Liquid for Inhalation **531**

Sufentanil Citrate (Valproate produces CNS depression, especially when combined with another CNS depressant).
No products indexed under this heading.

Temazepam (Valproate produces CNS depression, especially when combined with another CNS depressant). Products include:
Restoril Capsules **1860**

Thiamylal Sodium (Valproate produces CNS depression, especially when combined with another CNS depressant).
No products indexed under this heading.

Thioridazine Hydrochloride (Valproate produces CNS depression, especially when combined with another CNS depressant). Products include:
Thioridazine Hydrochloride Tablets **2163**

Thiothixene (Valproate produces CNS depression, especially when combined with another CNS depressant). Products include:
Thiothixene Capsules **2165**

Tolbutamide (Co-administration in in vitro experiments has resulted in increased unbound fraction of tolbutamide).
No products indexed under this heading.

Topiramate (Concomitant administration of valproic acid and topiramate has been associated with hyperammonemia with and without encephalopathy). Products include:
Topamax Sprinkle Capsules **2404**
Topamax Tablets **2404**

Triazolam (Valproate produces CNS depression, especially when combined with another CNS depressant).
No products indexed under this heading.

Trifluoperazine Hydrochloride (Valproate produces CNS depression, especially when combined with another CNS depressant).
No products indexed under this heading.

Warfarin Sodium (Co-administration in in vitro experiments has resulted in increased unbound fraction of warfarin). Products include:
Coumadin for Injection **898**
Coumadin Tablets **898**

Zaleplon (Valproate produces CNS depression, especially when combined with another CNS depressant). Products include:
Sonata Capsules **1717**

Zidovudine (Co-administration has resulted in decreased clearance of zidovudine; the half-life of zidovudine was unaffected). Products include:
Combivir Tablets **1411**
Retrovir **1560**
Retrovir IV Infusion **1564**
Trizivir Tablets **1589**

Ziprasidone Hydrochloride (Valproate produces CNS depression, especially when combined with another CNS depressant). Products include:
Geodon Capsules **2529**

Zolpidem Tartrate (Valproate produces CNS depression, especially when combined with another CNS depressant). Products include:
Ambien Tablets **2851**
Ambien CR Tablets **2855**

Food Interactions

Alcohol (Valproate produces CNS depression, especially when combined with another CNS depressant, such as alcohol).

DEPAKENE ORAL SOLUTION

(Valproic Acid) **417**

See Depakene Capsules

DEPAKOTE SPRINKLE CAPSULES

(Divalproex Sodium) **422**

See Depakote Tablets

DEPAKOTE TABLETS

(Divalproex Sodium) **427**

May interact with central nervous system depressants, phenytoin, and certain other agents. Compounds in these categories include:

Alfentanil Hydrochloride (Valproate produces CNS depression, especially when combined with another CNS depressant).
No products indexed under this heading.

Alprazolam (Valproate produces CNS depression, especially when combined with another CNS depressant). Products include:
Niravam Orally Disintegrating Tablets **3092**

Amitriptyline Hydrochloride (Co-administration has resulted in a decrease in plasma clearance of amitriptyline; rare postmarketing reports of increased amitriptyline levels).

No products indexed under this heading.

Aprobarbital (Valproate produces CNS depression, especially when combined with another CNS depressant).

No products indexed under this heading.

Aspirin (Co-administration has resulted in a decrease in protein binding and an inhibition of metabolism of valproate; valproate free fraction was increased 4-fold in the presence of aspirin compared to valproate alone). Products include:

Aggrenox Capsules	822
Bayer Aspirin	744
BC Allergy Sinus Cold Powder	▣◑677
BC Headache Powder	▣◑677
Arthritis Strength BC Powder	▣◑677
BC Sinus Cold Powder	▣◑677
Excedrin Extra Strength Caplets/Tablets/Geltabs	▣◑684
Excedrin Migraine Caplets/Tablets/Geltabs	▣◑609
Goody's Body Pain Formula Powder	▣◑684
Goody's Extra Strength Headache Powders	▣◑611
Goody's Extra Strength Pain Relief Tablets	▣◑685
Percodan Tablets	1132
St. Joseph 81 mg Aspirin Chewable and Enteric Coated Tablets	1869

Buprenorphine Hydrochloride (Valproate produces CNS depression, especially when combined with another CNS depressant). Products include:

Buprenex Injectable	2716
Suboxone Tablets	2717
Subutex Tablets	2717

Buspirone Hydrochloride (Valproate produces CNS depression, especially when combined with another CNS depressant).

No products indexed under this heading.

Butabarbital (Valproate produces CNS depression, especially when combined with another CNS depressant).

No products indexed under this heading.

Butalbital (Valproate produces CNS depression, especially when combined with another CNS depressant).

No products indexed under this heading.

Carbamazepine (Co-administration has resulted in decreased serum levels of carbamazepine and increased serum levels of carbamazepine 10,11-epoxide; drugs that affect the levels of expression of hepatic enzymes, particularly those that elevate levels of glucuronosyltransferases, such as carbamazepine, may increase the clearance of valproate). Products include:

Carbatrol Capsules	3171
Equetro Extended-Release Capsules	3180
Tegretol/Tegretol-XR	2295

Chlordiazepoxide (Valproate produces CNS depression, especially when combined with another CNS depressant).

No products indexed under this heading.

Chlordiazepoxide Hydrochloride (Valproate produces CNS depression, especially when combined with another CNS depressant). Products include:

Librium Capsules	3347

Chlorpromazine (Co-administration has resulted in an increase in trough plasma levels of valproate).

No products indexed under this heading.

Chlorpromazine Hydrochloride (Co-administration has resulted in an increase in trough plasma levels of valproate).

No products indexed under this heading.

Chlorprothixene (Valproate produces CNS depression, especially when combined with another CNS depressant).

No products indexed under this heading.

Chlorprothixene Hydrochloride (Valproate produces CNS depression, especially when combined with another CNS depressant).

No products indexed under this heading.

Chlorprothixene Lactate (Valproate produces CNS depression, especially when combined with another CNS depressant).

No products indexed under this heading.

Clonazepam (Co-administration may induce absence status in patients with a history of absence type seizures). Products include:

Klonopin	2778

Clorazepate Dipotassium (Valproate produces CNS depression, especially when combined with another CNS depressant). Products include:

Tranxene	2474

Clozapine (Valproate produces CNS depression, especially when combined with another CNS depressant). Products include:

Clozaril Tablets	2184
FazaClo Orally Disintegrating Tablets	551

Codeine Phosphate (Valproate produces CNS depression, especially when combined with another CNS depressant). Products include:

Tylenol with Codeine Tablets	2391

Desflurane (Valproate produces CNS depression, especially when combined with another CNS depressant).

No products indexed under this heading.

Dezocine (Valproate produces CNS depression, especially when combined with another CNS depressant).

No products indexed under this heading.

Diazepam (Co-administration increases the free fraction of diazepam by 90% in healthy volunteers; plasma clearance and volume of distribution for diazepam were reduced by 25% and 20%, respectively, in the presence of valproate). Products include:

Diastat Rectal Delivery System	3343
Valium Tablets	2819

Droperidol (Valproate produces CNS depression, especially when combined with another CNS depressant).

No products indexed under this heading.

Enflurane (Valproate produces CNS depression, especially when combined with another CNS depressant).

No products indexed under this heading.

Estazolam (Valproate produces CNS depression, especially when combined with another CNS depressant). Products include:

ProSom Tablets	517

Ethanol (Valproate produces CNS depression, especially when combined with another CNS depressant).

No products indexed under this heading.

Ethchlorvynol (Valproate produces CNS depression, especially when combined with another CNS depressant).

No products indexed under this heading.

Ethinamate (Valproate produces CNS depression, especially when combined with another CNS depressant).

No products indexed under this heading.

Ethosuximide (Valproate inhibits the metabolism of ethosuximide; co-administration was accompanied by a 25% increase in elimination half-life of ethosuximide and a 15% decrease in its total clearance as compared to ethosuximide alone).

No products indexed under this heading.

Ethyl Alcohol (Valproate produces CNS depression, especially when combined with another CNS depressant).

No products indexed under this heading.

Felbamate (Co-administration has resulted in an increase in mean valproate peak concentration).

No products indexed under this heading.

Fentanyl (Valproate produces CNS depression, especially when combined with another CNS depressant). Products include:

Duragesic Transdermal System	2373
Ionsys Transdermal System	2379

Fentanyl Citrate (Valproate produces CNS depression, especially when combined with another CNS depressant). Products include:

Actiq	979

Fluphenazine Decanoate (Valproate produces CNS depression, especially when combined with another CNS depressant).

No products indexed under this heading.

Fluphenazine Enanthate (Valproate produces CNS depression, especially when combined with another CNS depressant).

No products indexed under this heading.

Fluphenazine Hydrochloride (Valproate produces CNS depression, especially when combined with another CNS depressant).

No products indexed under this heading.

Flurazepam Hydrochloride (Valproate produces CNS depression, especially when combined with another CNS depressant). Products include:

Dalmane Capsules	3342

Fosphenytoin Sodium (Co-administration with drugs that affect the levels of expression of hepatic enzymes, particularly those that elevate levels of glucuronosyltransferases, such as phenytoin, may increase the clearance of valproate; valproate displaces phenytoin from its plasma binding sites and inhibits its hepatic metabolism; concurrent use has resulted in breakthrough seizures).

No products indexed under this heading.

Glutethimide (Valproate produces CNS depression, especially when combined with another CNS depressant).

No products indexed under this heading.

Haloperidol (Valproate produces CNS depression, especially when combined with another CNS depressant).

No products indexed under this heading.

Haloperidol Decanoate (Valproate produces CNS depression, especially when combined with another CNS depressant).

No products indexed under this heading.

Hydrocodone Bitartrate (Valproate produces CNS depression, especially when combined with another CNS depressant). Products include:

Hycodan	1116
Hycotuss Expectorant Syrup	1117
Vicodin Tablets	535
Vicodin ES Tablets	536
Vicodin HP Tablets	538
Vicoprofen Tablets	539
Zydone Tablets	1139

Hydrocodone Polistirex (Valproate produces CNS depression, especially when combined with another CNS depressant). Products include:

Tussionex Pennkinetic Extended-Release Suspension	3327

Hydromorphone Hydrochloride (Valproate produces CNS depression, especially when combined with another CNS depressant). Products include:

Dilaudid	440
Dilaudid Non-Sterile Powder	440
Dilaudid Oral Liquid	445
Dilaudid Rectal Suppositories	440
Dilaudid Tablets	440
Dilaudid Tablets - 8 mg	445
Dilaudid-HP	442

Hydroxyzine Hydrochloride (Valproate produces CNS depression, especially when combined with another CNS depressant).

No products indexed under this heading.

Isoflurane (Valproate produces CNS depression, especially when combined with another CNS depressant).

No products indexed under this heading.

Ketamine Hydrochloride (Valproate produces CNS depression, especially when combined with another CNS depressant).

No products indexed under this heading.

Lamotrigine (Co-administration has resulted in increased elimination half-life of lamotrigine from 26 to 72 hours and serious skin reactions, such as Stevens-Johnson syndrome and toxic epidermal necrolysis). Products include:

IMPORTANT NOTE: Always consult each drug listing in the patient's regimen for possible interactions.

Zaleplon (Valproate produces CNS depression, especially when combined with another CNS depressant). Products include:
Sonata Capsules 1717

Zidovudine (Co-administration has resulted in decreased clearance of zidovudine; the half-life of zidovudine was unaffected). Products include:
Combivir Tablets 1411
Retrovir 1560
Retrovir IV Infusion 1564
Trizivir Tablets 1589

Ziprasidone Hydrochloride (Valproate produces CNS depression, especially when combined with another CNS depressant). Products include:
Geodon Capsules 2529

Zolpidem Tartrate (Valproate produces CNS depression, especially when combined with another CNS depressant). Products include:
Ambien Tablets 2851
Ambien CR Tablets 2855

Food Interactions

Alcohol (Valproate produces CNS depression, especially when combined with another CNS depressant, such as alcohol).

DEPAKOTE ER TABLETS

(Divalproex Sodium) 434

May interact with central nervous system depressants, phenytoin, and certain other agents. Compounds in these categories include:

Alfentanil Hydrochloride (Valproate produces CNS depression, especially when combined with another CNS depressant).
No products indexed under this heading.

Alprazolam (Valproate produces CNS depression, especially when combined with another CNS depressant). Products include:
Niravam Orally Disintegrating Tablets 3092

Amitriptyline Hydrochloride (Co-administration has resulted in a decrease in plasma clearance of amitriptyline; rare postmarketing reports of increased amitriptyline levels).
No products indexed under this heading.

Aprobarbital (Valproate produces CNS depression, especially when combined with another CNS depressant).
No products indexed under this heading.

Aspirin (Co-administration has resulted in a decrease in protein binding and an inhibition of metabolism of valproate; valproate free fraction was increased 4-fold in the presence of aspirin compared to valproate alone). Products include:
Aggrenox Capsules 822
Bayer Aspirin 744
BC Allergy Sinus Cold Powder 677
BC Headache Powder 677
Arthritis Strength BC Powder 677
BC Sinus Cold Powder 677
Excedrin Extra Strength Caplets/Tablets/Geltabs 684
Excedrin Migraine Caplets/Tablets/Geltabs 609
Goody's Body Pain Formula Powder 684
Goody's Extra Strength Headache Powders 611
Goody's Extra Strength Pain Relief Tablets 685
Percodan Tablets 1132
St. Joseph 81 mg Aspirin Chewable and Enteric Coated Tablets 1869

Buprenorphine Hydrochloride (Valproate produces CNS depression, especially when combined with another CNS depressant). Products include:
Buprenex Injectable 2716
Suboxone Tablets 2717
Subutex Tablets 2717

Buspirone Hydrochloride (Valproate produces CNS depression, especially when combined with another CNS depressant).
No products indexed under this heading.

Butabarbital (Valproate produces CNS depression, especially when combined with another CNS depressant).
No products indexed under this heading.

Butalbital (Valproate produces CNS depression, especially when combined with another CNS depressant).
No products indexed under this heading.

Carbamazepine (Co-administration has resulted in decreased serum levels of carbamazepine and increased serum levels of carbamazepine 10,11-epoxide; drugs that affect the levels of expression of hepatic enzymes, particularly those that elevate levels of glucuronosyltransferases, such as carbamazepine, may increase the clearance of valproate). Products include:
Carbatrol Capsules 3171
Equetro Extended-Release Capsules 3180
Tegretol/Tegretol-XR 2295

Chlordiazepoxide (Valproate produces CNS depression, especially when combined with another CNS depressant).
No products indexed under this heading.

Chlordiazepoxide Hydrochloride (Valproate produces CNS depression, especially when combined with another CNS depressant). Products include:
Librium Capsules 3347

Chlorpromazine (Co-administration has resulted in an increase in trough plasma levels of valproate).
No products indexed under this heading.

Chlorpromazine Hydrochloride (Co-administration has resulted in an increase in trough plasma levels of valproate).
No products indexed under this heading.

Chlorprothixene (Valproate produces CNS depression, especially when combined with another CNS depressant).
No products indexed under this heading.

Chlorprothixene Hydrochloride (Valproate produces CNS depression, especially when combined with another CNS depressant).
No products indexed under this heading.

Chlorprothixene Lactate (Valproate produces CNS depression, especially when combined with another CNS depressant).
No products indexed under this heading.

Clonazepam (Co-administration may induce absence status in patients with a history of absence type seizures). Products include:
Klonopin 2778

Clorazepate Dipotassium (Valproate produces CNS depression, especially when combined with another CNS depressant). Products include:
Tranxene 2474

Clozapine (Valproate produces CNS depression, especially when combined with another CNS depressant). Products include:
Clozaril Tablets 2184
FazaClo Orally Disintegrating Tablets 551

Codeine Phosphate (Valproate produces CNS depression, especially when combined with another CNS depressant). Products include:
Tylenol with Codeine Tablets 2391

Desflurane (Valproate produces CNS depression, especially when combined with another CNS depressant).
No products indexed under this heading.

Dezocine (Valproate produces CNS depression, especially when combined with another CNS depressant).
No products indexed under this heading.

Diazepam (Co-administration increases the free fraction of diazepam by 90% in healthy volunteers; plasma clearance and volume of distribution for diazepam were reduced by 25% and 20%, respectively, in the presence of valproate). Products include:
Diastat Rectal Delivery System 3343
Valium Tablets 2819

Droperidol (Valproate produces CNS depression, especially when combined with another CNS depressant).
No products indexed under this heading.

Enflurane (Valproate produces CNS depression, especially when combined with another CNS depressant).
No products indexed under this heading.

Estazolam (Valproate produces CNS depression, especially when combined with another CNS depressant). Products include:
ProSom Tablets 517

Ethanol (Valproate produces CNS depression, especially when combined with another CNS depressant).
No products indexed under this heading.

Ethchlorvynol (Valproate produces CNS depression, especially when combined with another CNS depressant).
No products indexed under this heading.

Ethinamate (Valproate produces CNS depression, especially when combined with another CNS depressant).
No products indexed under this heading.

Ethosuximide (Valproate inhibits the metabolism of ethosuximide; co-administration was accompanied by a 25% increase in elimination half-life of ethosuximide and a 15% decrease in its total clearance as compared to ethosuximide alone).
No products indexed under this heading.

Ethyl Alcohol (Valproate produces CNS depression, especially when combined with another CNS depressant).
No products indexed under this heading.

Felbamate (Co-administration has resulted in an increase in mean valproate peak concentration).
No products indexed under this heading.

Fentanyl (Valproate produces CNS depression, especially when combined with another CNS depressant). Products include:
Duragesic Transdermal System 2373
Ionsys Transdermal System 2379

Fentanyl Citrate (Valproate produces CNS depression, especially when combined with another CNS depressant). Products include:
Actiq 979

Fluphenazine Decanoate (Valproate produces CNS depression, especially when combined with another CNS depressant).
No products indexed under this heading.

Fluphenazine Enanthate (Valproate produces CNS depression, especially when combined with another CNS depressant).
No products indexed under this heading.

Fluphenazine Hydrochloride (Valproate produces CNS depression, especially when combined with another CNS depressant).
No products indexed under this heading.

Flurazepam Hydrochloride (Valproate produces CNS depression, especially when combined with another CNS depressant). Products include:
Dalmane Capsules 3342

Fosphenytoin Sodium (Co-administration with drugs that affect the levels of expression of hepatic enzymes, particularly those that elevate levels of glucuronosyltransferases, such as phenytoin, may increase the clearance of valproate; valproate displaces phenytoin from its plasma binding sites and inhibits its hepatic metabolism; concurrent use has resulted in breakthrough seizures).
No products indexed under this heading.

Glutethimide (Valproate produces CNS depression, especially when combined with another CNS depressant).
No products indexed under this heading.

Haloperidol (Valproate produces CNS depression, especially when combined with another CNS depressant).
No products indexed under this heading.

Haloperidol Decanoate (Valproate produces CNS depression, especially when combined with another CNS depressant).
No products indexed under this heading.

Hydrocodone Bitartrate (Valproate produces CNS depression, especially when combined with another CNS depressant). Products include:
Hycodan 1116
Hycotuss Expectorant Syrup 1117
Vicodin Tablets 535

Thiamylal Sodium (Valproate produces CNS depression, especially when combined with another CNS depressant).
No products indexed under this heading.

Thioridazine Hydrochloride (Valproate produces CNS depression, especially when combined with another CNS depressant). Products include:
Thioridazine Hydrochloride Tablets 2163

Thiothixene (Valproate produces CNS depression, especially when combined with another CNS depressant). Products include:
Thiothixene Capsules 2165

Tolbutamide (Co-administration in in vitro experiments has resulted in increased unbound fraction of tolbutamide).
No products indexed under this heading.

Topiramate (Concomitant administration of topiramate and valproic acid has been associated with hyperammonemia with or without encephalopathy in patients who have tolerated either drug alone). Products include:
Topamax Sprinkle Capsules 2404
Topamax Tablets 2404

Triazolam (Valproate produces CNS depression, especially when combined with another CNS depressant).
No products indexed under this heading.

Trifluoperazine Hydrochloride (Valproate produces CNS depression, especially when combined with another CNS depressant).
No products indexed under this heading.

Warfarin Sodium (Co-administration in in vitro experiments has resulted in increased unbound fraction of warfarin). Products include:
Coumadin for Injection 898
Coumadin Tablets 898

Zaleplon (Valproate produces CNS depression, especially when combined with another CNS depressant). Products include:
Sonata Capsules 1717

Zidovudine (Co-administration has resulted in decreased clearance of zidovudine; the half-life of zidovudine was unaffected). Products include:
Combivir Tablets 1411
Retrovir 1560
Retrovir IV Infusion 1564
Trizivir Tablets 1589

Ziprasidone Hydrochloride (Valproate produces CNS depression, especially when combined with another CNS depressant). Products include:
Geodon Capsules 2529

Zolpidem Tartrate (Valproate produces CNS depression, especially when combined with another CNS depressant). Products include:
Ambien Tablets 2851
Ambien CR Tablets 2855

Food Interactions

Alcohol (Valproate produces CNS depression, especially when combined with another CNS depressant, such as alcohol).

DEPOCYT INJECTION

(Cytarabine Liposome) 1143
May interact with cytotoxic drugs. Compounds in these categories include:

Bleomycin Sulfate (Co-administration of intrathecal cytarabine and other cytotoxic agents administered intrathecally may enhance neurotoxicity).
No products indexed under this heading.

Cyclophosphamide (Co-administration of intrathecal cytarabine and other cytotoxic agents administered intrathecally may enhance neurotoxicity).
No products indexed under this heading.

Daunorubicin Hydrochloride (Co-administration of intrathecal cytarabine and other cytotoxic agents administered intrathecally may enhance neurotoxicity).
No products indexed under this heading.

Doxorubicin Hydrochloride (Co-administration of intrathecal cytarabine and other cytotoxic agents administered intrathecally may enhance neurotoxicity).
No products indexed under this heading.

Epirubicin Hydrochloride (Co-administration of intrathecal cytarabine and other cytotoxic agents administered intrathecally may enhance neurotoxicity).
No products indexed under this heading.

Fluorouracil (Co-administration of intrathecal cytarabine and other cytotoxic agents administered intrathecally may enhance neurotoxicity). Products include:
Carac Cream, 0.5% 2879
Efudex 3363

Hydroxyurea (Co-administration of intrathecal cytarabine and other cytotoxic agents administered intrathecally may enhance neurotoxicity).
No products indexed under this heading.

Methotrexate Sodium (Co-administration of intrathecal cytarabine and other cytotoxic agents administered intrathecally may enhance neurotoxicity).
No products indexed under this heading.

Mitotane (Co-administration of intrathecal cytarabine and other cytotoxic agents administered intrathecally may enhance neurotoxicity).
No products indexed under this heading.

Mitoxantrone Hydrochloride (Co-administration of intrathecal cytarabine and other cytotoxic agents administered intrathecally may enhance neurotoxicity).
No products indexed under this heading.

Procarbazine Hydrochloride (Co-administration of intrathecal cytarabine and other cytotoxic agents administered intrathecally may enhance neurotoxicity). Products include:
Matulane Capsules 3191

Tamoxifen Citrate (Co-administration of intrathecal cytarabine and other cytotoxic agents administered intrathecally may enhance neurotoxicity). Products include:
Soltamox Oral Solution 3527

Vincristine Sulfate (Co-administration of intrathecal cytarabine and other cytotoxic agents administered intrathecally may enhance neurotoxicity).
No products indexed under this heading.

DEPODUR EXTENDED-RELEASE INJECTION

(Morphine sulfate, liposomal) 1110
May interact with central nervous system depressants, general anesthetics, hypnotics and sedatives, monoamine oxidase inhibitors, neuromuscular blocking agents, phenothiazines, tranquilizers, and certain other agents. Compounds in these categories include:

Alfentanil Hydrochloride (The concurrent use of other central nervous system (CNS) depressants increases the risk of respiratory depression, hypotension, profound sedation or coma. Use with caution and with vigilant monitoring in patients taking these agents).
No products indexed under this heading.

Alprazolam (The concurrent use of other central nervous system (CNS) depressants, including tranquilizers, increases the risk of respiratory depression, hypotension, profound sedation or coma. Use with caution and with vigilant monitoring in patients taking these agents). Products include:
Niravam Orally Disintegrating Tablets 3092

Aprobarbital (The concurrent use of other central nervous system (CNS) depressants increases the risk of respiratory depression, hypotension, profound sedation or coma. Use with caution and with vigilant monitoring in patients taking these agents).
No products indexed under this heading.

Atracurium Besylate (Respiratory depression associated with morphine may delay recovery of spontaneous pulmonary ventilation when neuromuscular blocking agents are co-administered).
No products indexed under this heading.

Buprenorphine Hydrochloride (The concurrent use of other central nervous system (CNS) depressants increases the risk of respiratory depression, hypotension, profound sedation or coma. Use with caution and with vigilant monitoring in patients taking these agents). Products include:
Buprenex Injectable 2716
Suboxone Tablets 2717
Subutex Tablets 2717

Buspirone Hydrochloride (The concurrent use of other central nervous system (CNS) depressants, including tranquilizers, increases the risk of respiratory depression, hypotension, profound sedation or coma. Use with caution and with vigilant monitoring in patients taking these agents).
No products indexed under this heading.

Butabarbital (The concurrent use of other central nervous system (CNS) depressants increases the risk of respiratory depression, hypotension, profound sedation or coma. Use with caution and with vigilant monitoring in patients taking these agents).
No products indexed under this heading.

Butalbital (The concurrent use of other central nervous system (CNS) depressants increases the risk of respiratory depression, hypotension, profound sedation or coma. Use with caution and with vigilant monitoring in patients taking these agents).
No products indexed under this heading.

Chlordiazepoxide (The concurrent use of other central nervous system (CNS) depressants, including tranquilizers, increases the risk of respiratory depression, hypotension, profound sedation or coma. Use with caution and with vigilant monitoring in patients taking these agents).
No products indexed under this heading.

Chlordiazepoxide Hydrochloride (The concurrent use of other central nervous system (CNS) depressants, including tranquilizers, increases the risk of respiratory depression, hypotension, profound sedation or coma. Use with caution and with vigilant monitoring in patients taking these agents). Products include:
Librium Capsules 3347

Chlorpromazine (The concurrent use of other central nervous system (CNS) depressants, including phenothiazines, increases the risk of respiratory depression, hypotension, profound sedation or coma. Use with caution and with vigilant monitoring in patients taking these agents).
No products indexed under this heading.

Chlorpromazine Hydrochloride (The concurrent use of other central nervous system (CNS) depressants, including phenothiazines, increases the risk of respiratory depression, hypotension, profound sedation or coma. Use with caution and with vigilant monitoring in patients taking these agents).
No products indexed under this heading.

Chlorprothixene (The concurrent use of other central nervous system (CNS) depressants, including tranquilizers, increases the risk of respiratory depression, hypotension, profound sedation or coma. Use with caution and with vigilant monitoring in patients taking these agents).
No products indexed under this heading.

Chlorprothixene Hydrochloride (The concurrent use of other central nervous system (CNS) depressants, including tranquilizers, increases the risk of respiratory depression, hypotension, profound sedation or coma. Use with caution and with vigilant monitoring in patients taking these agents).
No products indexed under this heading.

Chlorprothixene Lactate (The concurrent use of other central nervous system (CNS) depressants increases the risk of respiratory depression, hypotension, profound sedation or coma. Use with caution and with vigilant monitoring in patients taking these agents).

 No products indexed under this heading.

Cisatracurium Besylate (Respiratory depression associated with morphine may delay recovery of spontaneous pulmonary ventilation when neuromuscular blocking agents are co-administered). Products include:

 Nimbex Injection **498**

Clorazepate Dipotassium (The concurrent use of other central nervous system (CNS) depressants, including tranquilizers, increases the risk of respiratory depression, hypotension, profound sedation or coma. Use with caution and with vigilant monitoring in patients taking these agents). Products include:

 Tranxene **2474**

Clozapine (The concurrent use of other central nervous system (CNS) depressants increases the risk of respiratory depression, hypotension, profound sedation or coma. Use with caution and with vigilant monitoring in patients taking these agents). Products include:

 Clozaril Tablets **2184**
 FazaClo Orally Disintegrating Tablets **551**

Codeine Phosphate (The concurrent use of other central nervous system (CNS) depressants increases the risk of respiratory depression, hypotension, profound sedation or coma. Use with caution and with vigilant monitoring in patients taking these agents). Products include:

 Tylenol with Codeine Tablets **2391**

Desflurane (The concurrent use of other central nervous system (CNS) depressants increases the risk of respiratory depression, hypotension, profound sedation or coma. Use with caution and with vigilant monitoring in patients taking these agents).

 No products indexed under this heading.

Dezocine (The concurrent use of other central nervous system (CNS) depressants increases the risk of respiratory depression, hypotension, profound sedation or coma. Use with caution and with vigilant monitoring in patients taking these agents).

 No products indexed under this heading.

Diazepam (The concurrent use of other central nervous system (CNS) depressants, including tranquilizers, increases the risk of respiratory depression, hypotension, profound sedation or coma. Use with caution and with vigilant monitoring in patients taking these agents). Products include:

 Diastat Rectal Delivery System **3343**
 Valium Tablets **2819**

Doxacurium Chloride (Respiratory depression associated with morphine may delay recovery of spontaneous pulmonary ventilation when neuromuscular blocking agents are co-administered).

 No products indexed under this heading.

Droperidol (The concurrent use of other central nervous system (CNS) depressants, including droperidol, increases the risk of respiratory depression, hypotension, profound sedation or coma. Use with caution and with vigilant monitoring in patients taking these agents).

 No products indexed under this heading.

Enflurane (The concurrent use of other central nervous system (CNS) depressants increases the risk of respiratory depression, hypotension, profound sedation or coma. Use with caution and with vigilant monitoring in patients taking these agents).

 No products indexed under this heading.

Estazolam (The concurrent use of other central nervous system (CNS) depressants, including sedatives and hypnotics, increases the risk of respiratory depression, hypotension, profound sedation or coma. Use with caution and with vigilant monitoring in patients taking these agents). Products include:

 ProSom Tablets **517**

Ethanol (The concurrent use of other central nervous system (CNS) depressants increases the risk of respiratory depression, hypotension, profound sedation or coma. Use with caution and with vigilant monitoring in patients taking these agents).

 No products indexed under this heading.

Ethchlorvynol (The concurrent use of other central nervous system (CNS) depressants, including sedatives and hypnotics, increases the risk of respiratory depression, hypotension, profound sedation or coma. Use with caution and with vigilant monitoring in patients taking these agents).

 No products indexed under this heading.

Ethinamate (The concurrent use of other central nervous system (CNS) depressants, including sedatives and hypnotics, increases the risk of respiratory depression, hypotension, profound sedation or coma. Use with caution and with vigilant monitoring in patients taking these agents).

 No products indexed under this heading.

Ethyl Alcohol (The concurrent use of other central nervous system (CNS) depressants increases the risk of respiratory depression, hypotension, profound sedation or coma. Use with caution and with vigilant monitoring in patients taking these agents).

 No products indexed under this heading.

Fentanyl (The concurrent use of other central nervous system (CNS) depressants increases the risk of respiratory depression, hypotension, profound sedation or coma. Use with caution and with vigilant monitoring in patients taking these agents). Products include:

 Duragesic Transdermal System **2373**
 Ionsys Transdermal System **2379**

Fentanyl Citrate (The concurrent use of other central nervous system (CNS) depressants increases the risk of respiratory depression, hypotension, profound sedation or coma. Use with caution and with vigilant monitoring in patients taking these agents). Products include:

 Actiq ... **979**

Fluphenazine Decanoate (The concurrent use of other central nervous system (CNS) depressants, including phenothiazines, increases the risk of respiratory depression, hypotension, profound sedation or coma. Use with caution and with vigilant monitoring in patients taking these agents).

 No products indexed under this heading.

Fluphenazine Enanthate (The concurrent use of other central nervous system (CNS) depressants, including phenothiazines, increases the risk of respiratory depression, hypotension, profound sedation or coma. Use with caution and with vigilant monitoring in patients taking these agents).

 No products indexed under this heading.

Fluphenazine Hydrochloride (The concurrent use of other central nervous system (CNS) depressants, including phenothiazines, increases the risk of respiratory depression, hypotension, profound sedation or coma. Use with caution and with vigilant monitoring in patients taking these agents).

 No products indexed under this heading.

Flurazepam Hydrochloride (The concurrent use of other central nervous system (CNS) depressants, including sedatives and hypnotics, increases the risk of respiratory depression, hypotension, profound sedation or coma. Use with caution and with vigilant monitoring in patients taking these agents). Products include:

 Dalmane Capsules **3342**

Glutethimide (The concurrent use of other central nervous system (CNS) depressants, including sedatives and hypnotics, increases the risk of respiratory depression, hypotension, profound sedation or coma. Use with caution and with vigilant monitoring in patients taking these agents).

 No products indexed under this heading.

Haloperidol (The concurrent use of other central nervous system (CNS) depressants, including tranquilizers, increases the risk of respiratory depression, hypotension, profound sedation or coma. Use with caution and with vigilant monitoring in patients taking these agents).

 No products indexed under this heading.

Haloperidol Decanoate (The concurrent use of other central nervous system (CNS) depressants, including tranquilizers, increases the risk of respiratory depression, hypotension, profound sedation or coma. Use with caution and with vigilant monitoring in patients taking these agents).

 No products indexed under this heading.

Hydrocodone Bitartrate (The concurrent use of other central nervous system (CNS) depressants increases the risk of respiratory depression, hypotension, profound sedation or coma. Use with caution and with vigilant monitoring in patients taking these agents). Products include:

 Hycodan **1116**
 Hycotuss Expectorant Syrup **1117**
 Vicodin Tablets **535**
 Vicodin ES Tablets **536**
 Vicodin HP Tablets **538**
 Vicoprofen Tablets **539**
 Zydone Tablets **1139**

Hydrocodone Polistirex (The concurrent use of other central nervous system (CNS) depressants increases the risk of respiratory depression, hypotension, profound sedation or coma. Use with caution and with vigilant monitoring in patients taking these agents). Products include:

 Tussionex Pennkinetic Extended-Release Suspension **3327**

Hydromorphone Hydrochloride (The concurrent use of other central nervous system (CNS) depressants increases the risk of respiratory depression, hypotension, profound sedation or coma. Use with caution and with vigilant monitoring in patients taking these agents). Products include:

 Dilaudid **440**
 Dilaudid Non-Sterile Powder **440**
 Dilaudid Oral Liquid **445**
 Dilaudid Rectal Suppositories **440**
 Dilaudid Tablets **440**
 Dilaudid Tablets - 8 mg **445**
 Dilaudid-HP **442**

Hydroxyzine Hydrochloride (The concurrent use of other central nervous system (CNS) depressants, including tranquilizers, increases the risk of respiratory depression, hypotension, profound sedation or coma. Use with caution and with vigilant monitoring in patients taking these agents).

 No products indexed under this heading.

Isocarboxazid (MAOIs markedly potentiate the action of morphine. DepoDur should not be used in patients taking MAOIs, or within 14 days of stopping such treatment).

 No products indexed under this heading.

Isoflurane (The concurrent use of other central nervous system (CNS) depressants increases the risk of respiratory depression, hypotension, profound sedation or coma. Use with caution and with vigilant monitoring in patients taking these agents).

 No products indexed under this heading.

Ketamine Hydrochloride (The concurrent use of other central nervous system (CNS) depressants increases the risk of respiratory depression, hypotension, profound sedation or coma. Use with caution and with vigilant monitoring in patients taking these agents).

 No products indexed under this heading.

Levomethadyl Acetate Hydrochloride (The concurrent use of other central nervous system (CNS) depressants increases the risk of respiratory depression, hypotension, profound sedation or coma. Use with caution and with vigilant monitoring in patients taking these agents).

 No products indexed under this heading.

Levorphanol Tartrate (The concurrent use of other central nervous system (CNS) depressants increases the risk of respiratory depression, hypotension, profound sedation or coma. Use with caution and with vigilant monitoring in patients taking these agents).

 No products indexed under this heading.

Lorazepam (The concurrent use of other central nervous system (CNS) depressants, including sedatives and hypnotics, increases the risk of respiratory depression, hypotension, profound sedation or coma. Use with caution and with vigilant monitoring in patients taking these agents).
No products indexed under this heading.

Loxapine Hydrochloride (The concurrent use of other central nervous system (CNS) depressants, including tranquilizers, increases the risk of respiratory depression, hypotension, profound sedation or coma. Use with caution and with vigilant monitoring in patients taking these agents).
No products indexed under this heading.

Loxapine Succinate (The concurrent use of other central nervous system (CNS) depressants, including tranquilizers, increases the risk of respiratory depression, hypotension, profound sedation or coma. Use with caution and with vigilant monitoring in patients taking these agents).
No products indexed under this heading.

Meperidine Hydrochloride (The concurrent use of other central nervous system (CNS) depressants increases the risk of respiratory depression, hypotension, profound sedation or coma. Use with caution and with vigilant monitoring in patients taking these agents).
No products indexed under this heading.

Mephobarbital (The concurrent use of other central nervous system (CNS) depressants increases the risk of respiratory depression, hypotension, profound sedation or coma. Use with caution and with vigilant monitoring in patients taking these agents).
No products indexed under this heading.

Meprobamate (The concurrent use of other central nervous system (CNS) depressants, including tranquilizers, increases the risk of respiratory depression, hypotension, profound sedation or coma. Use with caution and with vigilant monitoring in patients taking these agents).
No products indexed under this heading.

Mesoridazine Besylate (The concurrent use of other central nervous system (CNS) depressants, including phenothiazines, increases the risk of respiratory depression, hypotension, profound sedation or coma. Use with caution and with vigilant monitoring in patients taking these agents).
No products indexed under this heading.

Methadone Hydrochloride (The concurrent use of other central nervous system (CNS) depressants increases the risk of respiratory depression, hypotension, profound sedation or coma. Use with caution and with vigilant monitoring in patients taking these agents).
No products indexed under this heading.

Methohexital Sodium (The concurrent use of other central nervous system (CNS) depressants increases the risk of respiratory depression, hypotension, profound sedation or coma. Use with caution and with vigilant monitoring in patients taking these agents).
No products indexed under this heading.

Methotrimeprazine (The concurrent use of other central nervous system (CNS) depressants, including phenothiazines, increases the risk of respiratory depression, hypotension, profound sedation or coma. Use with caution and with vigilant monitoring in patients taking these agents).
No products indexed under this heading.

Methoxyflurane (The concurrent use of other central nervous system (CNS) depressants increases the risk of respiratory depression, hypotension, profound sedation or coma. Use with caution and with vigilant monitoring in patients taking these agents).
No products indexed under this heading.

Metocurine Iodide (Respiratory depression associated with morphine may delay recovery of spontaneous pulmonary ventilation when neuromuscular blocking agents are co-administered).
No products indexed under this heading.

Midazolam Hydrochloride (The concurrent use of other central nervous system (CNS) depressants, including sedatives and hypnotics, increases the risk of respiratory depression, hypotension, profound sedation or coma. Use with caution and with vigilant monitoring in patients taking these agents).
No products indexed under this heading.

Mivacurium Chloride (Respiratory depression associated with morphine may delay recovery of spontaneous pulmonary ventilation when neuromuscular blocking agents are co-administered). Products include:
Mivacron Injection **493**

Moclobemide (MAOIs markedly potentiate the action of morphine. DepoDur should not be used in patients taking MAOIs, or within 14 days of stopping such treatment).
No products indexed under this heading.

Molindone Hydrochloride (The concurrent use of other central nervous system (CNS) depressants, including tranquilizers, increases the risk of respiratory depression, hypotension, profound sedation or coma. Use with caution and with vigilant monitoring in patients taking these agents). Products include:
Moban Tablets **1119**

Morphine Sulfate (The concurrent use of other central nervous system (CNS) depressants increases the risk of respiratory depression, hypotension, profound sedation or coma. Use with caution and with vigilant monitoring in patients taking these agents). Products include:
Avinza Capsules **1741**
Kadian Capsules **577**
MS Contin Tablets **2701**

Olanzapine (The concurrent use of other central nervous system (CNS) depressants increases the risk of

respiratory depression, hypotension, profound sedation or coma. Use with caution and with vigilant monitoring in patients taking these agents). Products include:
Symbyax Capsules **1819**
Zyprexa Tablets **1830**
Zyprexa IntraMuscular **1830**
Zyprexa ZYDIS Orally
Disintegrating Tablets.................. **1830**

Oxazepam (The concurrent use of other central nervous system (CNS) depressants, including tranquilizers, increases the risk of respiratory depression, hypotension, profound sedation or coma. Use with caution and with vigilant monitoring in patients taking these agents).
No products indexed under this heading.

Oxycodone Hydrochloride (The concurrent use of other central nervous system (CNS) depressants increases the risk of respiratory depression, hypotension, profound sedation or coma. Use with caution and with vigilant monitoring in patients taking these agents). Products include:
OxyContin Tablets **2703**
OxyFast Oral Concentrate
Solution **2708**
OxyIR Capsules **2708**
Percocet Tablets **1131**
Percodan Tablets **1132**

Pancuronium Bromide (Respiratory depression associated with morphine may delay recovery of spontaneous pulmonary ventilation when neuromuscular blocking agents are co-administered).
No products indexed under this heading.

Pargyline Hydrochloride (MAOIs markedly potentiate the action of morphine. DepoDur should not be used in patients taking MAOIs, or within 14 days of stopping such treatment).
No products indexed under this heading.

Pentobarbital Sodium (The concurrent use of other central nervous system (CNS) depressants increases the risk of respiratory depression, hypotension, profound sedation or coma. Use with caution and with vigilant monitoring in patients taking these agents). Products include:
Nembutal Sodium Solution, USP **2470**

Perphenazine (The concurrent use of other central nervous system (CNS) depressants, including phenothiazines, increases the risk of respiratory depression, hypotension, profound sedation or coma. Use with caution and with vigilant monitoring in patients taking these agents).
No products indexed under this heading.

Phenelzine Sulfate (MAOIs markedly potentiate the action of morphine. DepoDur should not be used in patients taking MAOIs, or within 14 days of stopping such treatment).
No products indexed under this heading.

Phenobarbital (The concurrent use of other central nervous system (CNS) depressants increases the risk of respiratory depression, hypotension, profound sedation or coma. Use with caution and with vigilant monitoring in patients taking these agents). Products include:
Donnatal Extentabs **2493**

Prazepam (The concurrent use of other central nervous system (CNS) depressants, including tranquilizers, increases the risk of respiratory depression, hypotension, profound sedation or coma. Use with caution and with vigilant monitoring in patients taking these agents).
No products indexed under this heading.

Procarbazine Hydrochloride (MAOIs markedly potentiate the action of morphine. DepoDur should not be used in patients taking MAOIs, or within 14 days of stopping such treatment). Products include:
Matulane Capsules **3191**

Prochlorperazine (The concurrent use of other central nervous system (CNS) depressants, including phenothiazines, increases the risk of respiratory depression, hypotension, profound sedation or coma. Use with caution and with vigilant monitoring in patients taking these agents).
No products indexed under this heading.

Promethazine Hydrochloride (The concurrent use of other central nervous system (CNS) depressants, including phenothiazines, increases the risk of respiratory depression, hypotension, profound sedation or coma. Use with caution and with vigilant monitoring in patients taking these agents). Products include:
Phenergan Tablets and
Suppositories................................ **3440**

Propofol (The concurrent use of other central nervous system (CNS) depressants, including sedatives and hypnotics, increases the risk of respiratory depression, hypotension, profound sedation or coma. Use with caution and with vigilant monitoring in patients taking these agents).
No products indexed under this heading.

Propoxyphene Hydrochloride (The concurrent use of other central nervous system (CNS) depressants increases the risk of respiratory depression, hypotension, profound sedation or coma. Use with caution and with vigilant monitoring in patients taking these agents).
No products indexed under this heading.

Propoxyphene Napsylate (The concurrent use of other central nervous system (CNS) depressants increases the risk of respiratory depression, hypotension, profound sedation or coma. Use with caution and with vigilant monitoring in patients taking these agents).
No products indexed under this heading.

Quazepam (The concurrent use of other central nervous system (CNS) depressants, including sedatives and hypnotics, increases the risk of respiratory depression, hypotension, profound sedation or coma. Use with caution and with vigilant monitoring in patients taking these agents).
No products indexed under this heading.

Quetiapine Fumarate (The concurrent use of other central nervous system (CNS) depressants increases the risk of respiratory depression, hypotension, profound sedation or coma. Use with caution and with vigilant monitoring in patients taking these agents). Products include:
Seroquel Tablets **690**

Ramelteon (The concurrent use of other central nervous system (CNS) depressants, including sedatives and hypnotics, increases the risk of respiratory depression, hypotension, profound sedation or coma. Use with caution and with vigilant monitoring in patients taking these agents). Products include:

Rozerem Tablets 3231

Rapacuronium Bromide (Respiratory depression associated with morphine may delay recovery of spontaneous pulmonary ventilation when neuromuscular blocking agents are co-administered).

No products indexed under this heading.

Remifentanil Hydrochloride (The concurrent use of other central nervous system (CNS) depressants increases the risk of respiratory depression, hypotension, profound sedation or coma. Use with caution and with vigilant monitoring in patients taking these agents).

No products indexed under this heading.

Risperidone (The concurrent use of other central nervous system (CNS) depressants increases the risk of respiratory depression, hypotension, profound sedation or coma. Use with caution and with vigilant monitoring in patients taking these agents). Products include:

Risperdal 1676
Risperdal Consta Long-Acting Injection 1682
Risperdal M-Tab Orally Disintegrating Tablets 1676

Rocuronium Bromide (Respiratory depression associated with morphine may delay recovery of spontaneous pulmonary ventilation when neuromuscular blocking agents are co-administered). Products include:

Zemuron Injection 2346

Secobarbital Sodium (The concurrent use of other central nervous system (CNS) depressants, including sedatives and hypnotics, increases the risk of respiratory depression, hypotension, profound sedation or coma. Use with caution and with vigilant monitoring in patients taking these agents).

No products indexed under this heading.

Selegiline Hydrochloride (MAOIs markedly potentiate the action of morphine. DepoDur should not be used in patients taking MAOIs, or within 14 days of stopping such treatment). Products include:

Eldepryl Capsules 3208
Zelapar Tablets 3372

Sevoflurane (The concurrent use of other central nervous system (CNS) depressants increases the risk of respiratory depression, hypotension, profound sedation or coma. Use with caution and with vigilant monitoring in patients taking these agents). Products include:

Ultane Liquid for Inhalation 531

Sodium Oxybate (The concurrent use of other central nervous system (CNS) depressants increases the risk of respiratory depression, hypotension, profound sedation or coma. Use with caution and with vigilant monitoring in patients taking these agents). Products include:

Xyrem Oral Solution 1688

Succinylcholine Chloride (Respiratory depression associated with morphine may delay recovery of spontaneous pulmonary ventilation when neuromuscular blocking agents are co-administered).

No products indexed under this heading.

Sufentanil Citrate (The concurrent use of other central nervous system (CNS) depressants increases the risk of respiratory depression, hypotension, profound sedation or coma. Use with caution and with vigilant monitoring in patients taking these agents).

No products indexed under this heading.

Temazepam (The concurrent use of other central nervous system (CNS) depressants, including sedatives and hypnotics, increases the risk of respiratory depression, hypotension, profound sedation or coma. Use with caution and with vigilant monitoring in patients taking these agents). Products include:

Restoril Capsules 1860

Thiamylal Sodium (The concurrent use of other central nervous system (CNS) depressants increases the risk of respiratory depression, hypotension, profound sedation or coma. Use with caution and with vigilant monitoring in patients taking these agents).

No products indexed under this heading.

Thioridazine Hydrochloride (The concurrent use of other central nervous system (CNS) depressants, including phenothiazines, increases the risk of respiratory depression, hypotension, profound sedation or coma. Use with caution and with vigilant monitoring in patients taking these agents). Products include:

Thioridazine Hydrochloride Tablets 2163

Thiothixene (The concurrent use of other central nervous system (CNS) depressants, including tranquilizers, increases the risk of respiratory depression, hypotension, profound sedation or coma. Use with caution and with vigilant monitoring in patients taking these agents). Products include:

Thiothixene Capsules 2165

Tranylcypromine Sulfate (MAOIs markedly potentiate the action of morphine. DepoDur should not be used in patients taking MAOIs, or within 14 days of stopping such treatment). Products include:

Parnate Tablets 1527

Triazolam (The concurrent use of other central nervous system (CNS) depressants, including sedatives and hypnotics, increases the risk of respiratory depression, hypotension, profound sedation or coma. Use with caution and with vigilant monitoring in patients taking these agents).

No products indexed under this heading.

Trifluoperazine Hydrochloride (The concurrent use of other central nervous system (CNS) depressants, including phenothiazines, increases the risk of respiratory depression, hypotension, profound sedation or coma. Use with caution and with vigilant monitoring in patients taking these agents).

No products indexed under this heading.

Vecuronium Bromide (Respiratory depression associated with morphine may delay recovery of spontaneous pulmonary ventilation when neuromuscular blocking agents are co-administered).

No products indexed under this heading.

Zaleplon (The concurrent use of other central nervous system (CNS) depressants, including sedatives and hypnotics, increases the risk of respiratory depression, hypotension, profound sedation or coma. Use with caution and with vigilant monitoring in patients taking these agents). Products include:

Sonata Capsules 1717

Ziprasidone Hydrochloride (The concurrent use of other central nervous system (CNS) depressants increases the risk of respiratory depression, hypotension, profound sedation or coma. Use with caution and with vigilant monitoring in patients taking these agents). Products include:

Geodon Capsules 2529

Zolpidem Tartrate (The concurrent use of other central nervous system (CNS) depressants, including sedatives and hypnotics, increases the risk of respiratory depression, hypotension, profound sedation or coma. Use with caution and with vigilant monitoring in patients taking these agents). Products include:

Ambien Tablets 2851
Ambien CR Tablets 2855

Food Interactions

Alcohol (The concurrent use of other central nervous system (CNS) depressants, including alcohol, increases the risk of respiratory depression, hypotension, profound sedation or coma. Use with caution and with vigilant monitoring in patients taking these agents).

DEPO-MEDROL INJECTABLE SUSPENSION

(Methylprednisolone Acetate) 2617

May interact with oral anticoagulants, phenytoin, killed/inactivated vaccines, vaccines, live, and certain other agents. Compounds in these categories include:

Anisindione (The effect of methylprednisolone on oral anticoagulants is variable; there are reports of enhanced as well as diminished effects of anticoagulants when given concurrently with corticosteroids). Products include:

Miradon Tablets 3042

Aspirin (Methylprednisolone may increase the clearance of chronic high dose aspirin resulting in decreased salicylate serum levels or increased risk of salicylate toxicity when methylprednisolone is withdrawn; aspirin should be used cautiously in conjunction withcorticosteroids in patients suffering from hypoprothrombinemia). Products include:

Aggrenox Capsules 822
Bayer Aspirin 744
BC Allergy Sinus Cold Powder .... ▣677
BC Headache Powder .... ▣677
Arthritis Strength BC Powder .... ▣677
BC Sinus Cold Powder .... ▣677
Excedrin Extra Strength Caplets/Tablets/Geltabs .... ▣684
Excedrin Migraine Caplets/Tablets/Geltabs .... ▣609
Goody's Body Pain Formula Powder .... ▣684
Goody's Extra Strength Headache Powders .... ▣611
Goody's Extra Strength Pain Relief Tablets .... ▣685
Percodan Tablets 1132
St. Joseph 81 mg Aspirin Chewable and Enteric Coated Tablets 1869

BCG Vaccine (Administration of live or live, attenuated vaccines is contraindicated in patients receiving immunosuppressive doses of corticosteroids).

No products indexed under this heading.

Cyclosporine (Co-administration results in mutual inhibition of metabolism, therefore, it is possible that adverse events associated with the individual use of either drug may be more apt to occur; convulsions have been reported with concurrent use). Products include:

Gengraf Capsules 459
Neoral Oral Solution 2259
Neoral Soft Gelatin Capsules 2259
Restasis Ophthalmic Emulsion 575
Sandimmune 2275

Dicumarol (The effect of methylprednisolone on oral anticoagulants is variable; there are reports of enhanced as well as diminished effects of anticoagulants when given concurrently with corticosteroids).

No products indexed under this heading.

Diphtheria & Tetanus Toxoids and Acellular Pertussis Vaccine Adsorbed, Hepatitis B (recombinant) and Inactivated Poliovirus Vaccine Combined (Killed or inactivated vaccines may be administered to patients receiving immunosuppressive doses of corticosteroids; however, the response to such vaccines may be diminished).

No products indexed under this heading.

Fosphenytoin Sodium (Co-administration with drugs that induce hepatic metabolism, such as phenytoin, may increase the clearance of methylprednisolone and may require increases in methylprednisolone dose to achieve the desired response).

No products indexed under this heading.

Hepatitis A Vaccine, Inactivated (Killed or inactivated vaccines may be administered to patients receiving immunosuppressive doses of corticosteroids; however, the response to such vaccines may be diminished). Products include:

Havrix Vaccine 1456
Twinrix Vaccine 1595
Vaqta 2097

Influenza Virus Vaccine (Killed or inactivated vaccines may be administered to patients receiving immunosuppressive doses of corticosteroids; however, the response to such vaccines may be diminished). Products include:

Fluarix 1451
Flumist Vaccine 1901

Japanese Encephalitis Vaccine Inactivated (Killed or inactivated vaccines may be administered to patients receiving immunosuppressive doses of corticosteroids; however, the response to such vaccines may be diminished).

No products indexed under this heading.

Ketoconazole (Co-administration with drugs that inhibit the metabolism of methylprednisolone, such as ketoconazole, may decrease the clearance of methylprednisolone and may require dose titration to avoid steroid toxicity). Products include:
- Nizoral A-D Shampoo, 1% 1868

Measles, Mumps, Rubella and Varicella Virus Vaccine Live (Administration of live or live, attenuated vaccines is contraindicated in patients receiving immunosuppressive doses of corticosteroids). Products include:
- ProQuad 2064

Measles, Mumps & Rubella Virus Vaccine, Live (Administration of live or live, attenuated vaccines is contraindicated in patients receiving immunosuppressive doses of corticosteroids). Products include:
- M-M-R II 2006

Measles & Rubella Virus Vaccine Live (Administration of live or live, attenuated vaccines is contraindicated in patients receiving immunosuppressive doses of corticosteroids).
No products indexed under this heading.

Measles Virus Vaccine Live (Administration of live or live, attenuated vaccines is contraindicated in patients receiving immunosuppressive doses of corticosteroids). Products include:
- Attenuvax 1914

Mumps Virus Vaccine, Live (Administration of live or live, attenuated vaccines is contraindicated in patients receiving immunosuppressive doses of corticosteroids). Products include:
- Mumpsvax 2031

Phenobarbital (Co-administration with drugs that induce hepatic metabolism, such as phenobarbital, may increase the clearance of methylprednisolone and may require increases in methylprednisolone dose to achieve the desired response). Products include:
- Donnatal Extentabs 2493

Phenytoin (Co-administration with drugs that induce hepatic metabolism, such as phenytoin, may increase the clearance of methylprednisolone and may require increases in methylprednisolone dose to achieve the desired response).
No products indexed under this heading.

Phenytoin Sodium (Co-administration with drugs that induce hepatic metabolism, such as phenytoin, may increase the clearance of methylprednisolone and may require increases in methylprednisolone dose to achieve the desired response). Products include:
- Phenytek Capsules 2160

Poliovirus Vaccine, Live, Oral, Trivalent, Types 1,2,3 (Sabin) (Administration of live or live, attenuated vaccines is contraindicated in patients receiving immunosuppressive doses of corticosteroids).
No products indexed under this heading.

Poliovirus Vaccine Inactivated, Trivalent Types 1,2,3 (Killed or inactivated vaccines may be administered to patients receiving immunosuppressive doses of corticosteroids; however, the response to such vaccines may be diminished). Products include:
- Pediarix Vaccine 1548

Rifampin (Co-administration with drugs that induce hepatic metabolism, such as rifampin, may increase the clearance of methylprednisolone and may require increases in methylprednisolone dose to achieve the desired response).
No products indexed under this heading.

Rotavirus Vaccine, Live, Oral, Tetravalent (Administration of live or live, attenuated vaccines is contraindicated in patients receiving immunosuppressive doses of corticosteroids).
No products indexed under this heading.

Rubella & Mumps Virus Vaccine Live (Administration of live or live, attenuated vaccines is contraindicated in patients receiving immunosuppressive doses of corticosteroids).
No products indexed under this heading.

Rubella Virus Vaccine Live (Administration of live or live, attenuated vaccines is contraindicated in patients receiving immunosuppressive doses of corticosteroids). Products include:
- Meruvax II 2019

Smallpox Vaccine (Administration of live or live, attenuated vaccines is contraindicated in patients receiving immunosuppressive doses of corticosteroids).
No products indexed under this heading.

Troleandomycin (Co-administration with drugs that inhibit the metabolism of methylprednisolone, such as troleandomycin, may decrease the clearance of methylprednisolone and may require dose titration to avoid steroid toxicity).
No products indexed under this heading.

Typhoid Vaccine (Administration of live or live, attenuated vaccines is contraindicated in patients receiving immunosuppressive doses of corticosteroids).
No products indexed under this heading.

Varicella Virus Vaccine Live (Administration of live or live, attenuated vaccines is contraindicated in patients receiving immunosuppressive doses of corticosteroids). Products include:
- Varivax 2100

Warfarin Sodium (The effect of methylprednisolone on oral anticoagulants is variable; there are reports of enhanced as well as diminished effects of anticoagulants when given concurrently with corticosteroids). Products include:
- Coumadin for Injection 898
- Coumadin Tablets 898

Yellow Fever Vaccine (Administration of live or live, attenuated vaccines is contraindicated in patients receiving immunosuppressive doses of corticosteroids).
No products indexed under this heading.

DEPO-MEDROL SINGLE-DOSE VIAL

(Methylprednisolone Acetate) 2619

May interact with oral anticoagulants, hepatic microsomal enzyme inducers, killed/inactivated vaccines, vaccines, live, and certain other agents. Compounds in these categories include:

Anisindione (There are reports of enhanced as well as diminished effects of anticoagulant when given concurrently with corticosteroids. Therefore, coagulation indices should be monitored to maintain the desired anticoagulant effect). Products include:
- Miradon Tablets 3042

Aspirin (Methylprednisolone may increase the clearance of chronic high dose aspirin. This could lead to decreased salicylate serum levels or increase the risk of salicylate toxicity when methylprednisolone is withdrawn. Aspirin should be used cautiously in conjunction with corticosteroids in patients suffering from hypoprothrombinemia). Products include:
- Aggrenox Capsules 822
- Bayer Aspirin 744
- BC Allergy Sinus Cold Powder 677
- BC Headache Powder 677
- Arthritis Strength BC Powder 677
- BC Sinus Cold Powder 677
- Excedrin Extra Strength Caplets/Tablets/Geltabs 684
- Excedrin Migraine Caplets/Tablets/Geltabs 609
- Goody's Body Pain Formula Powder 684
- Goody's Extra Strength Headache Powders 611
- Goody's Extra Strength Pain Relief Tablets 685
- Percodan Tablets 1132
- St. Joseph 81 mg Aspirin Chewable and Enteric Coated Tablets 1869

BCG Vaccine (Administration of live or live, attenuated vaccines is contraindicated in patients receiving immunosuppressive doses of corticosteroids).
No products indexed under this heading.

Carbamazepine (Drugs that induce hepatic enzymes such as phenobarbital, phenytoin and rifampin may increase the clearance of methylprednisolone and may require increases in methylprednisolone dose to achieve the desired response). Products include:
- Carbatrol Capsules 3171
- Equetro Extended-Release Capsules 3180
- Tegretol/Tegretol-XR 2295

Chlorpropamide (Drugs that induce hepatic enzymes such as phenobarbital, phenytoin and rifampin may increase the clearance of methylprednisolone and may require increases in methylprednisolone dose to achieve the desired response).
No products indexed under this heading.

Cyclosporine (Mutual inhibition of metabolism occurs with concurrent use of cyclosporine and methylprednisolone; therefore, it is possible that adverse events associated with the individual use of either drug may be more apt to occur. Convulsions have been reported with concurrent use of methylprednisolone and cyclosporine). Products include:
- Gengraf Capsules 459
- Neoral Oral Solution 2259
- Neoral Soft Gelatin Capsules 2259
- Restasis Ophthalmic Emulsion 575
- Sandimmune 2275

Dicumarol (There are reports of enhanced as well as diminished effects of anticoagulant when given concurrently with corticosteroids. Therefore, coagulation indices should be monitored to maintain the desired anticoagulant effect.).
No products indexed under this heading.

Diphtheria & Tetanus Toxoids and Acellular Pertussis Vaccine Adsorbed, Hepatitis B (recombinant) and Inactivated Poliovirus Vaccine Combined (Killed or inactivated vaccines may be administered to patients receiving immunosuppressive doses of corticosteroids; however, the response to such vaccines may be diminished).
No products indexed under this heading.

Ethanol (Drugs that induce hepatic enzymes such as phenobarbital, phenytoin and rifampin may increase the clearance of methylprednisolone and may require increases in methylprednisolone dose to achieve the desired response).
No products indexed under this heading.

Fosphenytoin Sodium (Drugs that induce hepatic enzymes such as phenobarbital, phenytoin and rifampin may increase the clearance of methylprednisolone and may require increases in methylprednisolone dose to achieve the desired response).
No products indexed under this heading.

Glipizide (Drugs that induce hepatic enzymes such as phenobarbital, phenytoin and rifampin may increase the clearance of methylprednisolone and may require increases in methylprednisolone dose to achieve the desired response).
No products indexed under this heading.

Glyburide (Drugs that induce hepatic enzymes such as phenobarbital, phenytoin and rifampin may increase the clearance of methylprednisolone and may require increases in methylprednisolone dose to achieve the desired response).
No products indexed under this heading.

Hepatitis A Vaccine, Inactivated (Killed or inactivated vaccines may be administered to patients receiving immunosuppressive doses of corticosteroids; however, the response to such vaccines may be diminished). Products include:
- Havrix Vaccine 1456
- Twinrix Vaccine 1595
- Vaqta 2097

Influenza Virus Vaccine (Killed or inactivated vaccines may be administered to patients receiving immunosuppressive doses of corticosteroids; however, the response to such vaccines may be diminished). Products include:
- Fluarix 1451
- Flumist Vaccine 1901

Japanese Encephalitis Vaccine Inactivated (Killed or inactivated vaccines may be administered to patients receiving immunosuppressive doses of corticosteroids; however, the response to such vaccines may be diminished).
No products indexed under this heading.

Ketoconazole (Drugs such as ketoconazole may inhibit the metabolism of methylprednisolone and decrease its clearance; therefore, the dose of methylprednisolone should be titrated to avoid steroid toxicity). Products include:
Nizoral A-D Shampoo, 1% 1868

Measles, Mumps, Rubella and Varicella Virus Vaccine Live (Administration of live or live, attenuated vaccines is contraindicated in patients receiving immunosuppressive doses of corticosteroids). Products include:
ProQuad 2064

Measles, Mumps & Rubella Virus Vaccine, Live (Administration of live or live, attenuated vaccines is contraindicated in patients receiving immunosuppressive doses of corticosteroids). Products include:
M-M-R II 2006

Measles & Rubella Virus Vaccine Live (Administration of live or live, attenuated vaccines is contraindicated in patients receiving immunosuppressive doses of corticosteroids).
No products indexed under this heading.

Measles Virus Vaccine Live (Administration of live or live, attenuated vaccines is contraindicated in patients receiving immunosuppressive doses of corticosteroids). Products include:
Attenuvax 1914

Mumps Virus Vaccine, Live (Administration of live or live, attenuated vaccines is contraindicated in patients receiving immunosuppressive doses of corticosteroids). Products include:
Mumpsvax 2031

Phenobarbital (Drugs that induce hepatic enzymes such as phenobarbital, phenytoin and rifampin may increase the clearance of methylprednisolone and may require increases in methylprednisolone dose to achieve the desired response). Products include:
Donnatal Extentabs 2493

Phenylbutazone (Drugs that induce hepatic enzymes such as phenobarbital, phenytoin and rifampin may increase the clearance of methylprednisolone and may require increases in methylprednisolone dose to achieve the desired response).
No products indexed under this heading.

Phenytoin (Drugs that induce hepatic enzymes such as phenobarbital, phenytoin and rifampin may increase the clearance of methylprednisolone and may require increases in methylprednisolone dose to achieve the desired response).
No products indexed under this heading.

Phenytoin Sodium (Drugs that induce hepatic enzymes such as phenobarbital, phenytoin and rifampin may increase the clearance of methylprednisolone and may require increases in methylprednisolone dose to achieve the desired response). Products include:
Phenytek Capsules 2160

Poliovirus Vaccine, Live, Oral, Trivalent, Types 1,2,3 (Sabin) (Administration of live or live, attenuated vaccines is contraindicated in patients receiving immunosuppressive doses of corticosteroids).
No products indexed under this heading.

Poliovirus Vaccine Inactivated, Trivalent Types 1,2,3 (Killed or inactivated vaccines may be administered to patients receiving immunosuppressive doses of corticosteroids; however, the response to such vaccines may be diminished). Products include:
Pediarix Vaccine 1548

Rifampin (Drugs that induce hepatic enzymes such as phenobarbital, phenytoin and rifampin may increase the clearance of methylprednisolone and may require increases in methylprednisolone dose to achieve the desired response).
No products indexed under this heading.

Rifapentine (Drugs that induce hepatic enzymes such as phenobarbital, phenytoin and rifampin may increase the clearance of methylprednisolone and may require increases in methylprednisolone dose to achieve the desired response).
No products indexed under this heading.

Rotavirus Vaccine, Live, Oral, Tetravalent (Administration of live or live, attenuated vaccines is contraindicated in patients receiving immunosuppressive doses of corticosteroids).
No products indexed under this heading.

Rubella & Mumps Virus Vaccine Live (Administration of live or live, attenuated vaccines is contraindicated in patients receiving immunosuppressive doses of corticosteroids).
No products indexed under this heading.

Rubella Virus Vaccine Live (Administration of live or live, attenuated vaccines is contraindicated in patients receiving immunosuppressive doses of corticosteroids). Products include:
Meruvax II 2019

Smallpox Vaccine (Administration of live or live, attenuated vaccines is contraindicated in patients receiving immunosuppressive doses of corticosteroids).
No products indexed under this heading.

Tolazamide (Drugs that induce hepatic enzymes such as phenobarbital, phenytoin and rifampin may increase the clearance of methylprednisolone and may require increases in methylprednisolone dose to achieve the desired response).
No products indexed under this heading.

Tolbutamide (Drugs that induce hepatic enzymes such as phenobarbital, phenytoin and rifampin may increase the clearance of methylprednisolone and may require increases in methylprednisolone dose to achieve the desired response).
No products indexed under this heading.

Troleandomycin (Drugs such as troleandomycin may inhibit the metabolism of methylprednisolone and decrease its clearance; therefore, the dose of methylprednisolone should be titrated to avoid steroid toxicity.).
No products indexed under this heading.

Typhoid Vaccine (Administration of live or live, attenuated vaccines is contraindicated in patients receiving immunosuppressive doses of corticosteroids).
No products indexed under this heading.

Varicella Virus Vaccine Live (Administration of live or live, attenuated vaccines is contraindicated in patients receiving immunosuppressive doses of corticosteroids). Products include:
Varivax 2100

Warfarin Sodium (There are reports of enhanced as well as diminished effects of anticoagulant when given concurrently with corticosteroids. Therefore, coagulation indices should be monitored to maintain the desired anticoagulant effect). Products include:
Coumadin for Injection 898
Coumadin Tablets 898

Yellow Fever Vaccine (Administration of live or live, attenuated vaccines is contraindicated in patients receiving immunosuppressive doses of corticosteroids).
No products indexed under this heading.

DEPO-PROVERA CONTRACEPTIVE INJECTION

(Medroxyprogesterone Acetate) 2622
May interact with:

Aminoglutethimide (Aminoglutethimide may significantly depress the serum concentrations of medroxyprogesterone acetate).
No products indexed under this heading.

DEPO-SUBQ PROVERA 104 INJECTABLE SUSPENSION

(Medroxyprogesterone Acetate) 2624
May interact with:

Aminoglutethimide (Aminoglutethimide may significantly decrease the serum concentrations of medroxyprogesterone acetate).
No products indexed under this heading.

DESENEX ATHLETE'S FOOT CREAM

(Clotrimazole) .... ▣635
None cited in PDR database.

DESENEX ATHLETE'S FOOT LIQUID SPRAY

(Miconazole Nitrate) .... ▣635
None cited in PDR database.

DESENEX ATHLETE'S FOOT SHAKE POWDER

(Miconazole Nitrate) .... ▣635
None cited in PDR database.

DESENEX ATHLETE'S FOOT SPRAY POWDER

(Miconazole Nitrate) .... ▣635
None cited in PDR database.

DESENEX JOCK ITCH SPRAY POWDER

(Miconazole Nitrate) .... ▣635
None cited in PDR database.

DESOXYN TABLETS, USP

(Methamphetamine Hydrochloride) 2462
May interact with insulin, monoamine oxidase inhibitors, phenothiazines, tricyclic antidepressants, and certain other agents. Compounds in these categories include:

Amitriptyline Hydrochloride (Co-administration of tricyclic antidepressants and indirect-acting sympathomimetic amines such as amphetamines should be closely supervised and dosage carefully adjusted).
No products indexed under this heading.

Amoxapine (Co-administration of tricyclic antidepressants and indirect-acting sympathomimetic amines such as amphetamines should be closely supervised and dosage carefully adjusted).
No products indexed under this heading.

Chlorpromazine (May antagonize the CNS stimulant action of the amphetamine).
No products indexed under this heading.

Chlorpromazine Hydrochloride (May antagonize the CNS stimulant action of the amphetamine).
No products indexed under this heading.

Clomipramine Hydrochloride (Co-administration of tricyclic antidepressants and indirect-acting sympathomimetic amines such as amphetamines should be closely supervised and dosage carefully adjusted).
No products indexed under this heading.

Desipramine Hydrochloride (Co-administration of tricyclic antidepressants and indirect-acting sympathomimetic amines such as amphetamines should be closely supervised and dosage carefully adjusted).
No products indexed under this heading.

Doxepin Hydrochloride (Co-administration of tricyclic antidepressants and indirect-acting sympathomimetic amines such as amphetamines should be closely supervised and dosage carefully adjusted).
No products indexed under this heading.

Fluphenazine Decanoate (May antagonize the CNS stimulant action of the amphetamine).
No products indexed under this heading.

Fluphenazine Enanthate (May antagonize the CNS stimulant action of the amphetamine).
No products indexed under this heading.

Fluphenazine Hydrochloride (May antagonize the CNS stimulant action of the amphetamine).
No products indexed under this heading.

Guanethidine Monosulfate (Decreased hypotensive effect).
No products indexed under this heading.

Imipramine Hydrochloride (Co-administration of tricyclic antidepressants and indirect-acting sympathomimetic amines such as amphetamines should be closely supervised and dosage carefully adjusted).
No products indexed under this heading.

Imipramine Pamoate (Co-administration of tricyclic antidepressants and indirect-acting sympathomimetic amines such as amphetamines should be closely supervised and dosage carefully adjusted).
No products indexed under this heading.

Insulin, Human, Zinc Suspension (Insulin requirement in diabetics may be altered). Products include:
Humulin L, 100 Units 1794
Humulin U, 100 Units 1800

Insulin, Human NPH (Insulin requirement in diabetics may be altered). Products include:
Humulin N, 100 Units 1795
Humulin N Pen 1797

Insulin, Human Regular (Insulin requirement in diabetics may be altered). Products include:
Humulin R, 100 Units 1798

Insulin, Human Regular and Human NPH Mixture (Insulin requirement in diabetics may be altered). Products include:
Humulin 50/50, 100 Units 1791
Humulin 70/30 Pen 1793

Insulin, NPH (Insulin requirement in diabetics may be altered).
No products indexed under this heading.

Insulin, Regular (Insulin requirement in diabetics may be altered).
No products indexed under this heading.

Insulin, Zinc Crystals (Insulin requirement in diabetics may be altered).
No products indexed under this heading.

Insulin, Zinc Suspension (Insulin requirement in diabetics may be altered).
No products indexed under this heading.

Insulin Aspart, Human Regular (Insulin requirement in diabetics may be altered). Products include:
NovoLog Injection 2326

Insulin glargine (Insulin requirement in diabetics may be altered). Products include:
Lantus Injection 2909

Insulin Lispro, Human (Insulin requirement in diabetics may be altered). Products include:
Humalog-Pen 1781
Humalog Mix 50/50-Pen 1783
Humalog Mix 75/25-Pen 1785

Insulin Lispro Protamine, Human (Insulin requirement in diabetics may be altered). Products include:
Humalog Mix 50/50-Pen 1783
Humalog Mix 75/25-Pen 1785

Isocarboxazid (Co-administration may result in hypertensive crises; concurrent and/or sequential use is contraindicated).
No products indexed under this heading.

Maprotiline Hydrochloride (Co-administration of tricyclic antidepressants and indirect-acting sympathomimetic amines such as amphetamines should be closely supervised and dosage carefully adjusted).
No products indexed under this heading.

Mesoridazine Besylate (May antagonize the CNS stimulant action of the amphetamine).
No products indexed under this heading.

Methotrimeprazine (May antagonize the CNS stimulant action of the amphetamine).
No products indexed under this heading.

Moclobemide (Co-administration may result in hypertensive crises; concurrent and/or sequential use is contraindicated).
No products indexed under this heading.

Nortriptyline Hydrochloride (Co-administration of tricyclic antidepressants and indirect-acting sympathomimetic amines such as amphetamines should be closely supervised and dosage carefully adjusted).
No products indexed under this heading.

Pargyline Hydrochloride (Co-administration may result in hypertensive crises; concurrent and/or sequential use is contraindicated).
No products indexed under this heading.

Perphenazine (May antagonize the CNS stimulant action of the amphetamine).
No products indexed under this heading.

Phenelzine Sulfate (Co-administration may result in hypertensive crises; concurrent and/or sequential use is contraindicated).
No products indexed under this heading.

Procarbazine Hydrochloride (Co-administration may result in hypertensive crises; concurrent and/or sequential use is contraindicated). Products include:
Matulane Capsules 3191

Prochlorperazine (May antagonize the CNS stimulant action of the amphetamine).
No products indexed under this heading.

Promethazine Hydrochloride (May antagonize the CNS stimulant action of the amphetamine). Products include:
Phenergan Tablets and Suppositories 3440

Protriptyline Hydrochloride (Co-administration of tricyclic antidepressants and indirect-acting sympathomimetic amines such as amphetamines should be closely supervised and dosage carefully adjusted).
No products indexed under this heading.

Selegiline Hydrochloride (Co-administration may result in hypertensive crises; concurrent and/or sequential use is contraindicated). Products include:
Eldepryl Capsules 3208
Zelapar Tablets 3372

Thioridazine Hydrochloride (May antagonize the CNS stimulant action of the amphetamine). Products include:
Thioridazine Hydrochloride Tablets 2163

Tranylcypromine Sulfate (Co-administration may result in hypertensive crises; concurrent and/or sequential use is contraindicated). Products include:
Parnate Tablets 1527

Trifluoperazine Hydrochloride (May antagonize the CNS stimulant action of the amphetamine).
No products indexed under this heading.

Trimipramine Maleate (Co-administration of tricyclic antidepressants and indirect-acting sympathomimetic amines such as amphetamines should be closely supervised and dosage carefully adjusted).
No products indexed under this heading.

DETROL TABLETS

(Tolterodine Tartrate) 2628
See Detrol LA Capsules

DETROL LA CAPSULES

(Tolterodine Tartrate) 2631
May interact with class 1A antiarrhythmics, class III antiarrhythmics, cytochrome p450 3a4 inhibitors, potent, erythromycin, and certain other agents. Compounds in these categories include:

Amiodarone Hydrochloride (Caution with concomitant use).
No products indexed under this heading.

Amprenavir (Co-administration with potent CYP3A4 inhibitors may lead to increased plasma concentrations of tolterodine; for patients receiving potent CYP3A4 inhibitirs, the recommended dose of Detrol LA is 2 mg). Products include:
Agenerase Capsules 1327
Agenerase Oral Solution 1332

Atazanavir (Co-administration with potent CYP3A4 inhibitors may lead to increased plasma concentrations of tolterodine; for patients receiving potent CYP3A4 inhibitirs, the recommended dose of Detrol LA is 2 mg).
No products indexed under this heading.

Atazanavir sulfate (Co-administration with potent CYP3A4 inhibitors may lead to increased plasma concentrations of tolterodine; for patients receiving potent CYP3A4 inhibitirs, the recommended dose of Detrol LA is 2 mg). Products include:
Reyataz Capsules 921

Bretylium Tosylate (Caution with concomitant use).
No products indexed under this heading.

Clarithromycin (Co-administration with potent inhibitors of CYP3A4, such as clarithromycin, may lead to increase of tolterodine plasma concentrations; for patients receiving concomitant erythromycin, the recommended dose of Detrol LA is 2 mg). Products include:
Biaxin/Biaxin XL 402
PREVPAC 3284

Cyclosporine (Co-administration with potent inhibitors of CYP3A4, such as cyclosporine, may lead to increase of tolterodine plasma concentrations; for patients receiving concomitant cyclosporine, the recommended dose of Detrol LA is 2 mg). Products include:
Gengraf Capsules 459
Neoral Oral Solution 2259
Neoral Soft Gelatin Capsules 2259
Restasis Ophthalmic Emulsion 575
Sandimmune 2275

Disopyramide (Caution with concomitant use).
No products indexed under this heading.

Erythromycin (Co-administration with potent inhibitors of CYP3A4, such as erythromycin, may lead to increase of tolterodine plasma concentrations; for patients receiving concomitant erythromycin, the recommended dose of Detrol LA is 2 mg). Products include:
Ery-Tab Tablets 449
Erythromycin Base Filmtab Tablets 455
Erythromycin Delayed-Release Capsules, USP 457
PCE Dispertab Tablets 515

Erythromycin Estolate (Co-administration with potent inhibitors of CYP3A4, such as erythromycin, may lead to increase of tolterodine plasma concentrations; for patients receiving concomitant erythromycin, the recommended dose of Detrol LA is 2 mg).
No products indexed under this heading.

Erythromycin Ethylsuccinate (Co-administration with potent inhibitors of CYP3A4, such as erythromycin, may lead to increase of tolterodine plasma concentrations; for patients receiving concomitant erythromycin, the recommended dose of Detrol LA is 2 mg). Products include:
E.E.S. 451
EryPed 447

Erythromycin Gluceptate (Co-administration with potent inhibitors of CYP3A4, such as erythromycin, may lead to increase of tolterodine plasma concentrations; for patients receiving concomitant erythromycin, the recommended dose of Detrol LA is 2 mg).
No products indexed under this heading.

Erythromycin Lactobionate (Co-administration with potent inhibitors of CYP3A4, such as erythromycin, may lead to increase of tolterodine plasma concentrations; for patients receiving concomitant erythromycin, the recommended dose of Detrol LA is 2 mg).
No products indexed under this heading.

Erythromycin Stearate (Co-administration with potent inhibitors of CYP3A4, such as erythromycin, may lead to increase of tolterodine plasma concentrations; for patients receiving concomitant erythromycin, the recommended dose of Detrol LA is 2 mg). Products include:
Erythrocin Stearate Filmtab Tablets 453

Fluoxetine Hydrochloride (Co-administration with a potent inhibitor of CYP2D6, such as fluoxetine, significantly inhibits the metabolism of tolterodine immediate release formulation in extensive metabolizers, resulting in a 4.8-fold increase in tolterodine AUC; the sums of unbound serum concentrations of tolterodine and the 5-hydroxymethyl metabolite are only 25% higher during the interaction; no dose adjustment is required). Products include:

Prozac Pulvules and Liquid 1801
Symbyax Capsules 1819

Fosamprenavir Calcium (Co-administration with potent CYP3A4 inhibitors may lead to increased plasma concentrations of tolterodine; for patients receiving potent CYP3A4 inhibitirs, the recommended dose of Detrol LA is 2 mg). Products include:

Lexiva Tablets 1505

Indinavir Sulfate (Co-administration with potent CYP3A4 inhibitors may lead to increased plasma concentrations of tolterodine; for patients receiving potent CYP3A4 inhibitirs, the recommended dose of Detrol LA is 2 mg). Products include:

Crixivan Capsules 1940

Itraconazole (Co-administration with potent inhibitors of CYP3A4, such as itraconazole, may lead to increase of tolterodine plasma concentrations; for patients receiving concomitant itraconazole, the recommended dose of Detrol LA is 2 mg).

No products indexed under this heading.

Ketoconazole (Co-administration of ketoconazole, an inhibitor of CYP3A4, significantly increased plasma concentrations of tolterodine to subjects who were poor metabolizers; for patients receiving concomitant ketoconazole, the recommended dose of Detrol LA is 2 mg). Products include:

Nizoral A-D Shampoo, 1% 1868

Lopinavir (Co-administration with potent CYP3A4 inhibitors may lead to increased plasma concentrations of tolterodine; for patients receiving potent CYP3A4 inhibitirs, the recommended dose of Detrol LA is 2 mg). Products include:

Kaletra 476

Miconazole (Co-administration with potent inhibitors of CYP3A4, such as miconazole, may lead to increase of tolterodine plasma concentrations; for patients receiving concomitant miconazole, the recommended dose of Detrol LA is 2 mg).

No products indexed under this heading.

Moricizine Hydrochloride (Caution with concomitant use).

No products indexed under this heading.

Nefazodone Hydrochloride (Co-administration with potent CYP3A4 inhibitors may lead to increased plasma concentrations of tolterodine; for patients receiving potent CYP3A4 inhibitirs, the recommended dose of Detrol LA is 2 mg).

No products indexed under this heading.

Nelfinavir Mesylate (Co-administration with potent CYP3A4 inhibitors may lead to increased plasma concentrations of tolterodine; for patients receiving potent CYP3A4 inhibitirs, the recommended dose of Detrol LA is 2 mg). Products include:

Viracept 2577

Procainamide (Caution with concomitant use).

No products indexed under this heading.

Quinidine (Caution with concomitant use).

No products indexed under this heading.

Quinidine Gluconate (Caution with concomitant use).

No products indexed under this heading.

Ritonavir (Co-administration with potent CYP3A4 inhibitors may lead to increased plasma concentrations of tolterodine; for patients receiving potent CYP3A4 inhibitirs, the recommended dose of Detrol LA is 2 mg). Products include:

Kaletra 476
Norvir 503

Saquinavir (Co-administration with potent CYP3A4 inhibitors may lead to increased plasma concentrations of tolterodine; for patients receiving potent CYP3A4 inhibitirs, the recommended dose of Detrol LA is 2 mg).

No products indexed under this heading.

Saquinavir Mesylate (Co-administration with potent CYP3A4 inhibitors may lead to increased plasma concentrations of tolterodine; for patients receiving potent CYP3A4 inhibitirs, the recommended dose of Detrol LA is 2 mg). Products include:

Invirase 2772

Sotalol Hydrochloride (Caution with concomitant use).

No products indexed under this heading.

Telithromycin (Co-administration with potent CYP3A4 inhibitors may lead to increased plasma concentrations of tolterodine; for patients receiving potent CYP3A4 inhibitirs, the recommended dose of Detrol LA is 2 mg). Products include:

Ketek Tablets 2903

Troleandomycin (Co-administration with potent CYP3A4 inhibitors may lead to increased plasma concentrations of tolterodine; for patients receiving potent CYP3A4 inhibitirs, the recommended dose of Detrol LA is 2 mg).

No products indexed under this heading.

Vinblastine Sulfate (Co-administration with potent inhibitors of CYP3A4, such as vinblastine, may lead to increase of tolterodine plasma concentrations; for patients receiving concomitant vinblastine, the recommended dose of Detrol LA is 2 mg).

No products indexed under this heading.

Voriconazole (Co-administration with potent CYP3A4 inhibitors may lead to increased plasma concentrations of tolterodine; for patients receiving potent CYP3A4 inhibitirs, the recommended dose of Detrol LA is 2 mg). Products include:

VFEND I.V. 2564
VFEND Oral Suspension 2564
VFEND Tablets 2564

DEXEDRINE SPANSULE CAPSULES

(Dextroamphetamine Sulfate) 1420

May interact with antihistamines, antihypertensives, beta blockers, monoamine oxidase inhibitors, phenytoin, thiazides, tricyclic antidepressants, urinary alkalinizing agents, veratrum alkaloids, and certain other agents. Compounds in these categories include:

Acebutolol Hydrochloride (Amphetamine may antagonize the hypotensive effects of antihypertensives; adrenergic blockers are inhibited by amphetamines).

No products indexed under this heading.

Acetazolamide (Increases the concentration of the non-ionized species of the amphetamine molecule, thereby decreasing urinary excretion; increases amphetamines blood levels and thereby potentiates the actions of amphetamines).

No products indexed under this heading.

Acetazolamide Sodium (Increases the concentration of the non-ionized species of the amphetamine molecule, thereby decreasing urinary excretion; increases amphetamines blood levels and thereby potentiates the actions of amphetamines).

No products indexed under this heading.

Acrivastine (Amphetamines may counteract the sedative effect of antihistamine).

No products indexed under this heading.

Amitriptyline Hydrochloride (Enhanced activity of tricyclic or sympathomimetics; possible increases in the brain concentration of d-amphetamine in the brain; cardiovascular effect may be potentiated).

No products indexed under this heading.

Amlodipine Besylate (Amphetamine may antagonize the hypotensive effects of antihypertensives). Products include:

Caduet Tablets 2508
Lotrel Capsules 2249
Norvasc Tablets 2545

Ammonium Chloride (Increases the concentration of the ionized species of the amphetamine molecule, thereby increasing urinary excretion; lowers amphetamines blood levels and efficacy).

No products indexed under this heading.

Amoxapine (Enhanced activity of tricyclic or sympathomimetics; possible increases in the brain concentration of d-amphetamine in the brain; cardiovascular effect may be potentiated).

No products indexed under this heading.

Astemizole (Amphetamines may counteract the sedative effect of antihistamine).

No products indexed under this heading.

Atenolol (Amphetamine may antagonize the hypotensive effects of antihypertensives; adrenergic blockers are inhibited by amphetamines).

No products indexed under this heading.

Azatadine Maleate (Amphetamines may counteract the sedative effect of antihistamine).

No products indexed under this heading.

Benazepril Hydrochloride (Amphetamine may antagonize the hypotensive effects of antihypertensives). Products include:

Lotensin Tablets 2243
Lotensin HCT Tablets 2246
Lotrel Capsules 2249

Bendroflumethiazide (Increases the concentration of the non-ionized species of the amphetamine molecule, thereby decreasing urinary excretion; increases amphetamines blood levels and thereby potentiates the actions of amphetamines).

No products indexed under this heading.

Betaxolol Hydrochloride (Amphetamine may antagonize the hypotensive effects of antihypertensives; adrenergic blockers are inhibited by amphetamines). Products include:

Betoptic S Ophthalmic Suspension.................................. 558

Bisoprolol Fumarate (Amphetamine may antagonize the hypotensive effects of antihypertensives; adrenergic blockers are inhibited by amphetamines).

No products indexed under this heading.

Bromodiphenhydramine Hydrochloride (Amphetamines may counteract the sedative effect of antihistamine).

No products indexed under this heading.

Brompheniramine Maleate (Amphetamines may counteract the sedative effect of antihistamine). Products include:

Children's Dimetapp Cold & Allergy Elixir .... ■□730
Children's Dimetapp Cold & Allergy Chewable Tablets............. ■□730
Children's Dimetapp DM Cold & Cough Elixir .... ■□731

Candesartan Cilexetil (Amphetamine may antagonize the hypotensive effects of antihypertensives). Products include:

Atacand Tablets 649
Atacand HCT 651

Captopril (Amphetamine may antagonize the hypotensive effects of antihypertensives). Products include:

Captopril Tablets 2149

Carteolol Hydrochloride (Amphetamine may antagonize the hypotensive effects of antihypertensives; adrenergic blockers are inhibited by amphetamines). Products include:

Carteolol Hydrochloride Ophthalmic Solution USP, 1%....... ⊙249

Cetirizine Hydrochloride (Amphetamines may counteract the sedative effect of antihistamine). Products include:

Zyrtec Chewable Tablets 2594
Zyrtec 2594
Zyrtec-D 12 Hour Extended Release Tablets........................... 2597

Chlorothiazide (Increases the concentration of the non-ionized species of the amphetamine molecule, thereby decreasing urinary excretion; increases amphetamines blood levels and thereby potentiates the actions of amphetamines). Products include:

Diuril Oral Suspension 1954

Chlorothiazide Sodium (Increases the concentration of the non-ionized species of the amphetamine molecule, thereby decreasing urinary excretion; increases amphetamines blood levels and thereby potentiates the actions of amphetamines). Products include:

Diuril Sodium Intravenous 2467

Chlorpheniramine Maleate (Amphetamines may counteract the sedative effect of antihistamine). Products include:

Advil Allergy Sinus Caplets 770
Advil Multi-Symptom Cold Caplets 770
BC Allergy Sinus Cold Powder 677
Comtrex Maximum Strength Cold & Cough Day/Night Caplets - Night Formulation 726
Comtrex Maximum Strength Day/Night Severe Cold & Sinus Caplets - Night Formulation 725
Contac Cold and Flu Maximum Strength Caplets 728
Contac Cold and Flu Day and Night Caplets (Night Formulation Only) 727
Children's Dimetapp Long Acting Cough Plus Cold Syrup 731
Robitussin Cough & Cold Long-Acting Liquid 735
Robitussin Cough & Allergy Syrup .. 736
Robitussin Cough & Cold Nighttime Liquid 736
Robitussin Cough, Cold & Flu Nighttime Liquid 738
Robitussin Pediatric Cough & Cold Long-Acting Liquid 735
Robitussin Pediatric Cough & Cold Nighttime Liquid 736
Triaminic Cold & Allergy Liquid 746
Triaminic Cough & Runny Nose Softchews 748
Children's Tylenol Plus Flu Oral Suspension 749
Tylenol Allergy Multi-Symptom Caplets with Cool Burst and Gelcaps 1872
Children's Tylenol Plus Cold Suspension Liquid 1879
Children's Tylenol Plus Cough & Runny Nose Suspension Liquid 1879
Children's Tylenol Plus Flu Suspension Liquid 1881
Children's Tylenol Plus Multi-Symptom Cold Suspension Liquid 1879
Tylenol Cold Head Congestion Nighttime Caplets with Cool Burst 1873
Tylenol Cold Multi-Symptom Nighttime Caplets with Cool Burst 1874
Tylenol Sinus Congestion & Pain Nighttime Caplets with Cool Burst 1876
Vicks 44M Cough, Cold & Flu Relief Liquid 2680
Pediatric Vicks 44m Cough & Cold Relief Liquid 2676
Children's Vicks NyQuil Cold/Cough Relief 756
Children's Vicks NyQuil Cold/Cough Relief Liquid 2680
Zicam Maximum Strength Flu Daytime 768

Chlorpheniramine Polistirex (Amphetamines may counteract the sedative effect of antihistamine). Products include:

Tussionex Pennkinetic Extended-Release Suspension 3327

Chlorpheniramine Tannate (Amphetamines may counteract the sedative effect of antihistamine).

No products indexed under this heading.

Chlorpromazine (Blocks dopamine and norepinephrine reuptake resulting in inhibition of central stimulating effects).

No products indexed under this heading.

Chlorpromazine Hydrochloride (Blocks dopamine and norepinephrine reuptake resulting in inhibition of central stimulating effects).

No products indexed under this heading.

Chlorthalidone (Amphetamine may antagonize the hypotensive effects of antihypertensives). Products include:

Clorpres Tablets 2153

Clemastine Fumarate (Amphetamines may counteract the sedative effect of antihistamine).

No products indexed under this heading.

Clomipramine Hydrochloride (Enhanced activity of tricyclic or sympathomimetics; possible increases in the brain concentration of d-amphetamine in the brain; cardiovascular effect may be potentiated).

No products indexed under this heading.

Clonidine (Amphetamine may antagonize the hypotensive effects of antihypertensives). Products include:

Catapres-TTS 844

Clonidine Hydrochloride (Amphetamine may antagonize the hypotensive effects of antihypertensives). Products include:

Catapres Tablets 843
Clorpres Tablets 2153

Cryptenamine Preparations (Amphetamines inhibit the hypotensive effect of veratrum alkaloids).

No products indexed under this heading.

Cyproheptadine Hydrochloride (Amphetamines may counteract the sedative effect of antihistamine).

No products indexed under this heading.

Deserpidine (Amphetamine may antagonize the hypotensive effects of antihypertensives).

No products indexed under this heading.

Desipramine Hydrochloride (Enhanced activity of tricyclic or sympathomimetics; possible increases in the brain concentration of d-amphetamine in the brain; cardiovascular effect may be potentiated).

No products indexed under this heading.

Dexchlorpheniramine Maleate (Amphetamines may counteract the sedative effect of antihistamine).

No products indexed under this heading.

Diazoxide (Amphetamine may antagonize the hypotensive effects of antihypertensives). Products include:

Hyperstat I.V. 3017

Diltiazem Hydrochloride (Amphetamine may antagonize the hypotensive effects of antihypertensives). Products include:

Cardizem LA Extended Release Tablets 1728
Tiazac Capsules 1201

Diphenhydramine Citrate (Amphetamines may counteract the sedative effect of antihistamine). Products include:

Advil PM Caplets 615
Excedrin PM Caplets/Tablets/Geltabs 610
Goody's PM Powder for Pain with Sleeplessness 612

Diphenhydramine Hydrochloride (Amphetamines may counteract the sedative effect of antihistamine). Products include:

Nytol QuickCaps Caplets 615
Nytol QuickGels Softgels Maximum Strength 616
Simply Sleep Caplets 1868
Sominex Original Formula Tablets .. 616
TheraFlu Warming Relief Nighttime Severe Cold 743
TheraFlu Thin Strips Multi Symptom 744
Triaminic Nighttime Cold & Cough Liquid 746
Triaminic Thin Strips Cough & Runny Nose 749
Extra Strength Tylenol PM Caplets, Vanilla Caplets, Geltabs, Gelcaps and Liquid 1875
Tylenol Sore Throat Nighttime Liquid with Cool Burst 790
Tylenol Allergy Multi-Symptom Nighttime Caplets with Cool Burst 1872
Tylenol Severe Allergy Caplets 1872
Children's Tylenol Plus Cold & Allergy Suspension Liquid 1878

Diphenylpyraline Hydrochloride (Amphetamines may counteract the sedative effect of antihistamine).

No products indexed under this heading.

Doxazosin Mesylate (Amphetamine may antagonize the hypotensive effects of antihypertensives). Products include:

Cardura XL Tablets 2515

Doxepin Hydrochloride (Enhanced activity of tricyclic or sympathomimetics; possible increases in the brain concentration of d-amphetamine in the brain; cardiovascular effect may be potentiated).

No products indexed under this heading.

Enalapril Maleate (Amphetamine may antagonize the hypotensive effects of antihypertensives). Products include:

Vasotec I.V. Injection 2103

Enalaprilat (Amphetamine may antagonize the hypotensive effects of antihypertensives).

No products indexed under this heading.

Eprosartan Mesylate (Amphetamine may antagonize the hypotensive effects of antihypertensives). Products include:

Teveten Tablets 1735
Teveten HCT Tablets 1737

Esmolol Hydrochloride (Amphetamine may antagonize the hypotensive effects of antihypertensives; adrenergic blockers are inhibited by amphetamines).

No products indexed under this heading.

Ethosuximide (Amphetamine may delay intestinal absorption of ethosuximide).

No products indexed under this heading.

Felodipine (Amphetamine may antagonize the hypotensive effects of antihypertensives).

No products indexed under this heading.

Fexofenadine Hydrochloride (Amphetamines may counteract the sedative effect of antihistamine). Products include:

Allegra 2844
Allegra-D 12 Hour Extended-Release Tablets 2846
Allegra-D 24 Hour Extended-Release Tablets 2849

Fosinopril Sodium (Amphetamine may antagonize the hypotensive effects of antihypertensives).

No products indexed under this heading.

Fosphenytoin Sodium (Amphetamine delays intestinal absorption of phenytoin; co-administration may produce synergestic anticonvulsant action).

No products indexed under this heading.

Furosemide (Amphetamine may antagonize the hypotensive effects of antihypertensives). Products include:

Furosemide Tablets 2154

Glutamic Acid Hydrochloride (Lowers absorption of amphetamines).

No products indexed under this heading.

Guanabenz Acetate (Amphetamine may antagonize the hypotensive effects of antihypertensives).

No products indexed under this heading.

Guanethidine Monosulfate (Lowers absorption of amphetamines).

No products indexed under this heading.

Haloperidol (Blocks dopamine and norepinephrine reuptake resulting in inhibition of central stimulating effects).

No products indexed under this heading.

Haloperidol Decanoate (Blocks dopamine and norepinephrine reuptake resulting in inhibition of central stimulating effects).

No products indexed under this heading.

Hydralazine Hydrochloride (Amphetamine may antagonize the hypotensive effects of antihypertensives). Products include:

BiDil Tablets 2171

Hydrochlorothiazide (Increases the concentration of the non-ionized species of the amphetamine molecule, thereby decreasing urinary excretion; increases amphetamines blood levels and thereby potentiates the actions of amphetamines). Products include:

Aldoril Tablets 1910
Atacand HCT 651
Avalide Tablets 888
Avalide Tablets 2874
Benicar HCT Tablets 1044
Diovan HCT Tablets 2196
Dyazide Capsules 1423
Hyzaar 50-12.5 Tablets 1990
Hyzaar 100-12.5 Tablets 1990
Hyzaar 100-25 Tablets 1990
Lopressor HCT 50/25 Tablets 2241
Lopressor HCT 100/25 Tablets 2241
Lopressor HCT 100/50 Tablets 2241
Lotensin HCT Tablets 2246
Micardis HCT Tablets 856
Moduretic Tablets 2028
Prinzide Tablets 2056
Teveten HCT Tablets 1737
Timolide Tablets 2086
Uniretic Tablets 3100

Hydroflumethiazide (Increases the concentration of the non-ionized species of the amphetamine molecule, thereby decreasing urinary excretion; increases amphetamines blood levels and thereby potentiates the actions of amphetamines).

No products indexed under this heading.

Imipramine Hydrochloride
(Enhanced activity of tricyclic or sympathomimetics; possible increases in the brain concentration of d-amphetamine in the brain; cardiovascular effect may be potentiated).
 No products indexed under this heading.

Imipramine Pamoate (Enhanced activity of tricyclic or sympathomimetics; possible increases in the brain concentration of d-amphetamine in the brain; cardiovascular effect may be potentiated).
 No products indexed under this heading.

Indapamide (Amphetamine may antagonize the hypotensive effects of antihypertensives). Products include:
 Indapamide Tablets 2156

Irbesartan (Amphetamine may antagonize the hypotensive effects of antihypertensives). Products include:
 Avalide Tablets 888
 Avalide Tablets 2874
 Avapro Tablets 891
 Avapro Tablets 2871

Isocarboxazid (Concurrent and/or sequential use with MAO inhibitors is contraindicated; hypertensive crisis may occur).
 No products indexed under this heading.

Isradipine (Amphetamine may antagonize the hypotensive effects of antihypertensives). Products include:
 DynaCirc CR Tablets 2721

Labetalol Hydrochloride (Amphetamine may antagonize the hypotensive effects of antihypertensives; adrenergic blockers are inhibited by amphetamines).
 No products indexed under this heading.

Levobunolol Hydrochloride (Amphetamine may antagonize the hypotensive effects of antihypertensives; adrenergic blockers are inhibited by amphetamines). Products include:
 Betagan Ophthalmic Solution, USP............................... ⊙ 220

Lisinopril (Amphetamine may antagonize the hypotensive effects of antihypertensives). Products include:
 Prinivil Tablets 2052
 Prinzide Tablets 2056

Lithium Carbonate (Inhibits stimulatory effects of amphetamines). Products include:
 Lithobid Tablets 1692

Loratadine (Amphetamines may counteract the sedative effect of antihistamine). Products include:
 Alavert Allergy & Sinus D-12 Hour Tablets............................... ▥ 771
 Alavert ▥ 771
 Children's Claritin Allergy Oral Solution ▥ 771
 Claritin Non-Drowsy 24 Hour Tablets............................... ▥ 772
 Claritin Reditabs 24 Hour Non-Drowsy Tablets............... ▥ 772
 Claritin-D Non-Drowsy 12 Hour Tablets............................... ▥ 772
 Claritin-D Non-Drowsy 24 Hour Tablets............................... ▥ 772

Losartan Potassium (Amphetamine may antagonize the hypotensive effects of antihypertensives). Products include:
 Cozaar Tablets 1935
 Hyzaar 50-12.5 Tablets 1990
 Hyzaar 100-12.5 Tablets 1990

 Hyzaar 100-25 Tablets 1990

Maprotiline Hydrochloride (Enhanced activity of tricyclic or sympathomimetics; possible increases in the brain concentration of d-amphetamine in the brain; cardiovascular effect may be potentiated).
 No products indexed under this heading.

Mecamylamine Hydrochloride (Amphetamine may antagonize the hypotensive effects of antihypertensives).
 No products indexed under this heading.

Meperidine Hydrochloride (Amphetamine potentiates the analgesic effect of meperidine).
 No products indexed under this heading.

Methdilazine Hydrochloride (Amphetamines may counteract the sedative effect of antihistamine).
 No products indexed under this heading.

Methenamine (Acidifying agents used in methenamine therapy increases the urinary excretion and reduces the efficacy of amphetamine). Products include:
 Prosed/DS Tablets 1157

Methenamine Hippurate (Acidifying agents used in methenamine therapy increases the urinary excretion and reduces the efficacy of amphetamine).
 No products indexed under this heading.

Methenamine Mandelate (Acidifying agents used in methenamine therapy increases the urinary excretion and reduces the efficacy of amphetamine). Products include:
 Uroqid-Acid No. 2 Tablets 760

Methyclothiazide (Increases the concentration of the non-ionized species of the amphetamine molecule, thereby decreasing urinary excretion; increases amphetamines blood levels and thereby potentiates the actions of amphetamines).
 No products indexed under this heading.

Methyldopa (Amphetamine may antagonize the hypotensive effects of antihypertensives). Products include:
 Aldoril Tablets 1910

Methyldopate Hydrochloride (Amphetamine may antagonize the hypotensive effects of antihypertensives).
 No products indexed under this heading.

Metipranolol Hydrochloride (Amphetamine may antagonize the hypotensive effects of antihypertensives; adrenergic blockers are inhibited by amphetamines).
 No products indexed under this heading.

Metolazone (Amphetamine may antagonize the hypotensive effects of antihypertensives).
 No products indexed under this heading.

Metoprolol Succinate (Amphetamine may antagonize the hypotensive effects of antihypertensives; adrenergic blockers are inhibited by amphetamines). Products include:
 Toprol-XL Tablets 668

Metoprolol Tartrate (Amphetamine may antagonize the hypotensive

effects of antihypertensives; adrenergic blockers are inhibited by amphetamines). Products include:
 Lopressor Injection 2238
 Lopressor Tablets 2238
 Lopressor HCT 50/25 Tablets 2241
 Lopressor HCT 100/25 Tablets 2241
 Lopressor HCT 100/50 Tablets 2241

Metyrosine (Amphetamine may antagonize the hypotensive effects of antihypertensives). Products include:
 Demser Capsules 1953

Mibefradil Dihydrochloride (Amphetamine may antagonize the hypotensive effects of antihypertensives).
 No products indexed under this heading.

Minoxidil (Amphetamine may antagonize the hypotensive effects of antihypertensives). Products include:
 Men's Rogaine Extra Strength Hair Regrowth Treatment Topical Solution, Ocean Rush Scent and Original Unscented ▥ 633
 Men's Rogaine Foam Hair Regrowth Treatment.................... ▥ 633
 Women's Rogaine Hair Regrowth Treatment Topical Solution, Spring Bloom Scent and Original Unscented.................... ▥ 634

Moclobemide (Concurrent and/or sequential use with MAO inhibitors is contraindicated; hypertensive crisis may occur).
 No products indexed under this heading.

Moexipril Hydrochloride (Amphetamine may antagonize the hypotensive effects of antihypertensives). Products include:
 Uniretic Tablets 3100
 Univasc Tablets 3104

Nadolol (Amphetamine may antagonize the hypotensive effects of antihypertensives; adrenergic blockers are inhibited by amphetamines). Products include:
 Nadolol Tablets 2159

Nicardipine Hydrochloride (Amphetamine may antagonize the hypotensive effects of antihypertensives). Products include:
 Cardene I.V. 2497

Nifedipine (Amphetamine may antagonize the hypotensive effects of antihypertensives). Products include:
 Adalat CC Tablets 2964

Nisoldipine (Amphetamine may antagonize the hypotensive effects of antihypertensives). Products include:
 Sular Tablets 3122

Nitroglycerin (Amphetamine may antagonize the hypotensive effects of antihypertensives). Products include:
 Nitro-Dur Transdermal Infusion System............................... 3046
 Nitrolingual Pumpspray 3120

Norepinephrine Hydrochloride (Enhances adenergic effect of norepinephrine).
 No products indexed under this heading.

Nortriptyline Hydrochloride (Enhanced activity of tricyclic or sympathomimetics; possible increases in the brain concentration of d-amphetamine in the brain; cardiovascular effect may be potentiated).
 No products indexed under this heading.

Pargyline Hydrochloride (Concurrent and/or sequential use with MAO inhibitors is contraindicated; hypertensive crisis may occur).
 No products indexed under this heading.

Penbutolol Sulfate (Amphetamine may antagonize the hypotensive effects of antihypertensives; adrenergic blockers are inhibited by amphetamines).
 No products indexed under this heading.

Perindopril Erbumine (Amphetamine may antagonize the hypotensive effects of antihypertensives). Products include:
 Aceon Tablets (2 mg, 4 mg, 8 mg)............................... 3194

Phenelzine Sulfate (Concurrent and/or sequential use with MAO inhibitors is contraindicated; hypertensive crisis may occur).
 No products indexed under this heading.

Phenobarbital (Amphetamine delays intestinal absorption of phenobarbital; co-administration may produce synergistic anticonvulsant action). Products include:
 Donnatal Extentabs 2493

Phenoxybenzamine Hydrochloride (Amphetamine may antagonize the hypotensive effects of antihypertensives). Products include:
 Dibenzyline Capsules 3399

Phentolamine Mesylate (Amphetamine may antagonize the hypotensive effects of antihypertensives).
 No products indexed under this heading.

Phenytoin (Amphetamine delays intestinal absorption of phenytoin; co-administration may produce synergistic anticonvulsant action).
 No products indexed under this heading.

Phenytoin Sodium (Amphetamine delays intestinal absorption of phenytoin; co-administration may produce synergistic anticonvulsant action). Products include:
 Phenytek Capsules 2160

Pindolol (Amphetamine may antagonize the hypotensive effects of antihypertensives; adrenergic blockers are inhibited by amphetamines).
 No products indexed under this heading.

Polythiazide (Increases the concentration of the non-ionized species of the amphetamine molecule, thereby decreasing urinary excretion; increases amphetamines blood levels and thereby potentiates the actions of amphetamines).
 No products indexed under this heading.

Potassium Citrate (Increases the concentration of the non-ionized species of the amphetamine molecule, thereby decreasing urinary excretion; increases amphetamines blood levels and thereby potentiates the actions of amphetamines). Products include:
 Urocit-K Tablets 2144

Prazosin Hydrochloride (Amphetamine may antagonize the hypotensive effects of antihypertensives).
 No products indexed under this heading.

Procarbazine Hydrochloride (Concurrent and/or sequential use with MAO inhibitors is contraindicated; hypertensive crisis may occur). Products include:

Matulane Capsules 3191

Promethazine Hydrochloride (Amphetamines may counteract the sedative effect of antihistamine). Products include:
Phenergan Tablets and Suppositories 3440

Propoxyphene Hydrochloride (In cases of propoxyphene overdosage, amphetamine CNS stimulation is potentiated and fatal convulsions can occur).
No products indexed under this heading.

Propoxyphene Napsylate (In cases of propoxyphene overdosage, amphetamine CNS stimulation is potentiated and fatal convulsions can occur).
No products indexed under this heading.

Propranolol Hydrochloride (Amphetamine may antagonize the hypotensive effects of antihypertensives; adrenergic blockers are inhibited by amphetamines). Products include:
Inderal LA Long-Acting Capsules 3429
InnoPran XL Capsules 2723

Protriptyline Hydrochloride (Enhanced activity of tricyclic or sympathomimetics; possible increases in the brain concentration of d-amphetamine in the brain; cardiovascular effect may be potentiated).
No products indexed under this heading.

Pyrilamine Maleate (Amphetamines may counteract the sedative effect of antihistamine).
No products indexed under this heading.

Pyrilamine Tannate (Amphetamines may counteract the sedative effect of antihistamine).
No products indexed under this heading.

Quinapril Hydrochloride (Amphetamine may antagonize the hypotensive effects of antihypertensives).
No products indexed under this heading.

Ramipril (Amphetamine may antagonize the hypotensive effects of antihypertensives). Products include:
Altace Capsules 1702

Rauwolfia Serpentina (Amphetamine may antagonize the hypotensive effects of antihypertensives).
No products indexed under this heading.

Rescinnamine (Amphetamine may antagonize the hypotensive effects of antihypertensives).
No products indexed under this heading.

Reserpine (Lowers absorption of amphetamines).
No products indexed under this heading.

Selegiline Hydrochloride (Concurrent and/or sequential use with MAO inhibitors is contraindicated; hypertensive crisis may occur). Products include:
Eldepryl Capsules 3208
Zelapar Tablets 3372

Sodium Acid Phosphate (Increases the concentration of the ionized species of the amphetamine molecule, thereby increasing urinary excretion; lowers amphetamines blood levels and efficacy). Products include:
Uroqid-Acid No. 2 Tablets 760

Sodium Bicarbonate (Increases absorption of amphetamines). Products include:
Colyte with Flavor Packs for Oral Solution 3088
HalfLytely and Bisacodyl Tablets Bowel Prep Kit with Flavors Packs 881
TriLyte with Flavor Packs for Oral Solution 3100

Sodium Citrate (Increases the concentration of the non-ionized species of the amphetamine molecule, thereby decreasing urinary excretion; increases amphetamines blood levels and thereby potentiates the actions of amphetamines).
No products indexed under this heading.

Sodium Nitroprusside (Amphetamine may antagonize the hypotensive effects of antihypertensives).
No products indexed under this heading.

Sotalol Hydrochloride (Amphetamine may antagonize the hypotensive effects of antihypertensives; adrenergic blockers are inhibited by amphetamines).
No products indexed under this heading.

Spirapril Hydrochloride (Amphetamine may antagonize the hypotensive effects of antihypertensives).
No products indexed under this heading.

Telmisartan (Amphetamine may antagonize the hypotensive effects of antihypertensives). Products include:
Micardis Tablets 854
Micardis HCT Tablets 856

Terazosin Hydrochloride (Amphetamine may antagonize the hypotensive effects of antihypertensives). Products include:
Hytrin Capsules 471

Terfenadine (Amphetamines may counteract the sedative effect of antihistamine).
No products indexed under this heading.

Timolol Hemihydrate (Amphetamine may antagonize the hypotensive effects of antihypertensives; adrenergic blockers are inhibited by amphetamines). Products include:
Betimol Ophthalmic Solution 3382
Betimol Ophthalmic Solution .... ⊙295

Timolol Maleate (Amphetamine may antagonize the hypotensive effects of antihypertensives; adrenergic blockers are inhibited by amphetamines). Products include:
Blocadren Tablets 1916
Cosopt Sterile Ophthalmic Solution 1931
Timolide Tablets 2086
Timoptic Sterile Ophthalmic Solution 2088
Timoptic in Ocudose 2091
Timoptic-XE Sterile Ophthalmic Gel Forming Solution 2092

Torsemide (Amphetamine may antagonize the hypotensive effects of antihypertensives). Products include:
Demadex Injection 2759
Demadex Tablets 2759

Trandolapril (Amphetamine may antagonize the hypotensive effects of antihypertensives). Products include:
Mavik Tablets 486
Tarka Tablets 524

Tranylcypromine Sulfate (Concurrent and/or sequential use with MAO inhibitors is contraindicated; hypertensive crisis may occur). Products include:
Parnate Tablets 1527

Trimeprazine Tartrate (Amphetamines may counteract the sedative effect of antihistamine).
No products indexed under this heading.

Trimethaphan Camsylate (Amphetamine may antagonize the hypotensive effects of antihypertensives).
No products indexed under this heading.

Trimipramine Maleate (Enhanced activity of tricyclic or sympathomimetics; possible increases in the brain concentration of d-amphetamine in the brain; cardiovascular effect may be potentiated).
No products indexed under this heading.

Tripelennamine Hydrochloride (Amphetamines may counteract the sedative effect of antihistamine).
No products indexed under this heading.

Triprolidine Hydrochloride (Amphetamines may counteract the sedative effect of antihistamine).
No products indexed under this heading.

Valsartan (Amphetamine may antagonize the hypotensive effects of antihypertensives). Products include:
Diovan Tablets 2193
Diovan HCT Tablets 2196

Verapamil Hydrochloride (Amphetamine may antagonize the hypotensive effects of antihypertensives). Products include:
Covera-HS Tablets 3139
Tarka Tablets 524
Verelan PM Extended-Release Capsules, Controlled-Onset........... 3106

Vitamin C (Lowers absorption of amphetamines). Products include:
Bausch & Lomb Ocuvite Adult Eye Vitamin and Mineral Supplement Soft Gels 706
Bausch & Lomb Ocuvite Adult 50+ Eye Vitamin and Mineral Supplement Soft Gels 706
Ocuvite Adult Vitamin and Mineral Supplement................................ ⊙253
Ocuvite Adult 50+ Vitamin and Mineral Supplement..................... ⊙253
Peridin-C Vitamin C Supplement 818

Food Interactions

Fruit juices, unspecified (Lowers absorption of amphetamines).

DEXEDRINE TABLETS

(Dextroamphetamine Sulfate) 1420
See Dexedrine Spansule Capsules

DEXTROSTAT TABLETS

(Dextroamphetamine Sulfate) 3179
May interact with alpha adrenergic blockers, antihistamines, antihypertensives, beta blockers, monoamine oxidase inhibitors, sympathomimetics, thiazides, tricyclic antidepressants, urinary alkalinizing agents, veratrum alkaloids, and certain other agents. Compounds in these categories include:

Acebutolol Hydrochloride (Adrenergic blockers are inhibited by amphetamines; amphetamines may antagonize the hypotensive effects of antihypertensives).
No products indexed under this heading.

Acetazolamide (Increases the concentration of the non-ionized species of the amphetamine molecule thereby decreasing urinary excretion; increases blood levels and potentiates the action of amphetamines).
No products indexed under this heading.

Acetazolamide Sodium (Increases the concentration of the non-ionized species of the amphetamine molecule thereby decreasing urinary excretion; increases blood levels and potentiates the action of amphetamines).
No products indexed under this heading.

Acrivastine (Amphetamines may counteract the sedative effect of antihistamines).
No products indexed under this heading.

Albuterol (Enhanced activity of sympathomimetics). Products include:
Proventil Inhalation Aerosol 3053

Albuterol Sulfate (Enhanced activity of sympathomimetics). Products include:
AccuNeb Inhalation Solution 1055
Combivent Inhalation Aerosol 847
DuoNeb Inhalation Solution 1058
ProAir HFA Inhalation Aerosol 3300
Proventil Inhalation Solution 0.083%...................................... 3055
Proventil HFA Inhalation Aerosol 3056
Ventolin HFA Inhalation Aerosol 1600
VoSpire ER Tablets 1052

Amitriptyline Hydrochloride (Enhanced activity of tricyclic antidepressants; cardiovascular effects can be potentiated).
No products indexed under this heading.

Amlodipine Besylate (Amphetamines may antagonize the hypotensive effects of antihypertensives). Products include:
Caduet Tablets 2508
Lotrel Capsules 2249
Norvasc Tablets 2545

Ammonium Chloride (Increases the concentration of ionized species of the amphetamine molecule thereby increasing urinary excretion; lowers blood levels and efficacy of amphetamines).
No products indexed under this heading.

Amoxapine (Enhanced activity of tricyclic antidepressants; cardiovascular effects can be potentiated).
No products indexed under this heading.

Astemizole (Amphetamines may counteract the sedative effect of antihistamines).
No products indexed under this heading.

Atenolol (Adrenergic blockers are inhibited by amphetamines; amphetamines may antagonize the hypotensive effects of antihypertensives).
No products indexed under this heading.

Azatadine Maleate (Amphetamines may counteract the sedative effect of antihistamines).
No products indexed under this heading.

Benazepril Hydrochloride (Amphetamines may antagonize the hypotensive effects of antihypertensives). Products include:
Lotensin Tablets 2243
Lotensin HCT Tablets 2246
Lotrel Capsules 2249

Teveten Tablets 1735
Teveten HCT Tablets 1737

Esmolol Hydrochloride (Adrenergic blockers are inhibited by amphetamines; amphetamines may antagonize the hypotensive effects of antihypertensives).
No products indexed under this heading.

Ethosuximide (Delayed intestinal absorption of ethosuximide).
No products indexed under this heading.

Felodipine (Amphetamines may antagonize the hypotensive effects of antihypertensives).
No products indexed under this heading.

Fexofenadine Hydrochloride (Amphetamines may counteract the sedative effect of antihistamines). Products include:
Allegra 2844
Allegra-D 12 Hour Extended-Release Tablets 2846
Allegra-D 24 Hour Extended-Release Tablets 2849

Fosinopril Sodium (Amphetamines may antagonize the hypotensive effects of antihypertensives).
No products indexed under this heading.

Fosphenytoin Sodium (Co-administration may produce synergistic anticonvulsant action).
No products indexed under this heading.

Furosemide (Amphetamines may antagonize the hypotensive effects of antihypertensives). Products include:
Furosemide Tablets 2154

Glutamic Acid Hydrochloride (Lowers absorption of amphetamines by acting as gastrointestinal acidifying agent).
No products indexed under this heading.

Guanabenz Acetate (Amphetamines may antagonize the hypotensive effects of antihypertensives).
No products indexed under this heading.

Guanethidine Monosulfate (Lowers absorption of amphetamines by acting as gastrointestinal acidifying agent; amphetamines may antagonize the hypotensive effects of antihypertensives).
No products indexed under this heading.

Haloperidol (Inhibits central stimulant effects of amphetamines).
No products indexed under this heading.

Haloperidol Decanoate (Inhibits central stimulant effects of amphetamines).
No products indexed under this heading.

Hydralazine Hydrochloride (Amphetamines may antagonize the hypotensive effects of antihypertensives). Products include:
BiDil Tablets 2171

Hydrochlorothiazide (Some thiazide diuretics increase concentration of the non-ionized species of the amphetamine molecule thereby decreasing urinary excretion; increases blood levels and potentiates the action of amphetamines; amphetamines may antagonize the hypotensive effects of antihypertensives). Products include:
Aldoril Tablets 1910
Atacand HCT 651
Avalide Tablets 888
Avalide Tablets 2874
Benicar HCT Tablets 1044
Diovan HCT Tablets 2196
Dyazide Capsules 1423
Hyzaar 50-12.5 Tablets 1990
Hyzaar 100-12.5 Tablets 1990
Hyzaar 100-25 Tablets 1990
Lopressor HCT 50/25 Tablets 2241
Lopressor HCT 100/25 Tablets 2241
Lopressor HCT 100/50 Tablets 2241
Lotensin HCT Tablets 2246
Micardis HCT Tablets 856
Moduretic Tablets 2028
Prinzide Tablets 2056
Teveten HCT Tablets 1737
Timolide Tablets 2086
Uniretic Tablets 3100

Hydroflumethiazide (Some thiazide diuretics increase concentration of the non-ionized species of the amphetamine molecule thereby decreasing urinary excretion; increases blood levels and potentiates the action of amphetamines; amphetamines may antagonize the hypotensive effects of antihypertensives).
No products indexed under this heading.

Imipramine Hydrochloride (Enhanced activity of tricyclic antidepressants; cardiovascular effects can be potentiated).
No products indexed under this heading.

Imipramine Pamoate (Enhanced activity of tricyclic antidepressants; cardiovascular effects can be potentiated).
No products indexed under this heading.

Indapamide (Amphetamines may antagonize the hypotensive effects of antihypertensives). Products include:
Indapamide Tablets 2156

Irbesartan (Amphetamines may antagonize the hypotensive effects of antihypertensives). Products include:
Avalide Tablets 888
Avalide Tablets 2874
Avapro Tablets 891
Avapro Tablets 2871

Isocarboxazid (Potential for hypertensive crisis; slows amphetamine metabolism; concurrent and/or sequential use is contraindicated).
No products indexed under this heading.

Isoproterenol Hydrochloride (Enhanced activity of sympathomimetics).
No products indexed under this heading.

Isoproterenol Sulfate (Enhanced activity of sympathomimetics).
No products indexed under this heading.

Isradipine (Amphetamines may antagonize the hypotensive effects of antihypertensives). Products include:
DynaCirc CR Tablets 2721

Labetalol Hydrochloride (Adrenergic blockers are inhibited by amphetamines; amphetamines may antagonize the hypotensive effects of antihypertensives).
No products indexed under this heading.

Levalbuterol Hydrochloride (Enhanced activity of sympathomimetics). Products include:
Xopenex Inhalation Solution 3146
Xopenex Inhalation Solution Concentrate 3150

Levobunolol Hydrochloride (Adrenergic blockers are inhibited by amphetamines; amphetamines may antagonize the hypotensive effects of antihypertensives). Products include:
Betagan Ophthalmic Solution, USP .... ⊙ 220

Lisinopril (Amphetamines may antagonize the hypotensive effects of antihypertensives). Products include:
Prinivil Tablets 2052
Prinzide Tablets 2056

Lithium Carbonate (Inhibits stimulatory effects of amphetamines). Products include:
Lithobid Tablets 1692

Loratadine (Amphetamines may counteract the sedative effect of antihistamines). Products include:
Alavert Allergy & Sinus D-12 Hour Tablets .... ▣ 771
Alavert .... ▣ 771
Children's Claritin Allergy Oral Solution .... ▣ 771
Claritin Non-Drowsy 24 Hour Tablets .... ▣ 772
Claritin Reditabs 24 Hour Non-Drowsy Tablets .... ▣ 772
Claritin-D Non-Drowsy 12 Hour Tablets .... ▣ 772
Claritin-D Non-Drowsy 24 Hour Tablets .... ▣ 772

Losartan Potassium (Amphetamines may antagonize the hypotensive effects of antihypertensives). Products include:
Cozaar Tablets 1935
Hyzaar 50-12.5 Tablets 1990
Hyzaar 100-12.5 Tablets 1990
Hyzaar 100-25 Tablets 1990

Maprotiline Hydrochloride (Enhanced activity of tricyclic antidepressants; cardiovascular effects can be potentiated).
No products indexed under this heading.

Mecamylamine Hydrochloride (Amphetamines may antagonize the hypotensive effects of antihypertensives).
No products indexed under this heading.

Meperidine Hydrochloride (Analgesic effect of meperidine potentiated).
No products indexed under this heading.

Metaproterenol Sulfate (Enhanced activity of sympathomimetics). Products include:
Alupent Inhalation Aerosol 826

Metaraminol Bitartrate (Enhanced activity of sympathomimetics).
No products indexed under this heading.

Methdilazine Hydrochloride (Amphetamines may counteract the sedative effect of antihistamines).
No products indexed under this heading.

Methenamine (Increases urinary excretion and efficacy is reduced by acidifying agents used in methenamine therapy). Products include:
Prosed/DS Tablets 1157

Methenamine Hippurate (Increases urinary excretion and efficacy is reduced by acidifying agents used in methenamine therapy).
No products indexed under this heading.

Methenamine Mandelate (Increases urinary excretion and efficacy is reduced by acidifying agents used in methenamine therapy). Products include:
Uroqid-Acid No. 2 Tablets 760

Methoxamine Hydrochloride (Enhanced activity of sympathomimetics).
No products indexed under this heading.

Methyclothiazide (Some thiazide diuretics increase concentration of the non-ionized species of the amphetamine molecule thereby decreasing urinary excretion; increases blood levels and potentiates the action of amphetamines; amphetamines may antagonize the hypotensive effects of antihypertensives).
No products indexed under this heading.

Methyldopa (Amphetamines may antagonize the hypotensive effects of antihypertensives). Products include:
Aldoril Tablets 1910

Methyldopate Hydrochloride (Amphetamines may antagonize the hypotensive effects of antihypertensives).
No products indexed under this heading.

Metipranolol Hydrochloride (Adrenergic blockers are inhibited by amphetamines; amphetamines may antagonize the hypotensive effects of antihypertensives).
No products indexed under this heading.

Metolazone (Amphetamines may antagonize the hypotensive effects of antihypertensives).
No products indexed under this heading.

Metoprolol Succinate (Adrenergic blockers are inhibited by amphetamines; amphetamines may antagonize the hypotensive effects of antihypertensives). Products include:
Toprol-XL Tablets 668

Metoprolol Tartrate (Adrenergic blockers are inhibited by amphetamines; amphetamines may antagonize the hypotensive effects of antihypertensives). Products include:
Lopressor Injection 2238
Lopressor Tablets 2238
Lopressor HCT 50/25 Tablets 2241
Lopressor HCT 100/25 Tablets 2241
Lopressor HCT 100/50 Tablets 2241

Metyrosine (Amphetamines may antagonize the hypotensive effects of antihypertensives). Products include:
Demser Capsules 1953

Mibefradil Dihydrochloride (Amphetamines may antagonize the hypotensive effects of antihypertensives).
No products indexed under this heading.

Minoxidil (Amphetamines may antagonize the hypotensive effects of antihypertensives). Products include:
Men's Rogaine Extra Strength Hair Regrowth Treatment Topical Solution, Ocean Rush Scent and Original Unscented ..... ▣ 633
Men's Rogaine Foam Hair Regrowth Treatment .... ▣ 633
Women's Rogaine Hair Regrowth Treatment Topical Solution, Spring Bloom Scent and Original Unscented .... ▣ 634

Moclobemide (Potential for hypertensive crisis; slows amphetamine metabolism; concurrent and/or sequential use is contraindicated).
No products indexed under this heading.

Moexipril Hydrochloride (Amphetamines may antagonize the hypotensive effects of antihypertensives). Products include:
Uniretic Tablets 3100
Univasc Tablets 3104

Nadolol (Adrenergic blockers are inhibited by amphetamines; amphetamines may antagonize the hypotensive effects of antihypertensives). Products include:
Nadolol Tablets 2159

Nicardipine Hydrochloride (Amphetamines may antagonize the hypotensive effects of antihypertensives). Products include:
Cardene I.V. 2497

Nifedipine (Amphetamines may antagonize the hypotensive effects of antihypertensives). Products include:
Adalat CC Tablets 2964

Nisoldipine (Amphetamines may antagonize the hypotensive effects of antihypertensives). Products include:
Sular Tablets 3122

Nitroglycerin (Amphetamines may antagonize the hypotensive effects of antihypertensives). Products include:
Nitro-Dur Transdermal Infusion System 3046
Nitrolingual Pumpspray 3120

Norepinephrine Bitartrate (Enhanced activity of sympathomimetics).
No products indexed under this heading.

Norepinephrine Hydrochloride (Enhanced adrenergic effect of norepinephrine).
No products indexed under this heading.

Nortriptyline Hydrochloride (Enhanced activity of tricyclic antidepressants; cardiovascular effects can be potentiated).
No products indexed under this heading.

Pargyline Hydrochloride (Potential for hypertensive crisis; slows amphetamine metabolism; concurrent and/or sequential use is contraindicated).
No products indexed under this heading.

Penbutolol Sulfate (Adrenergic blockers are inhibited by amphetamines; amphetamines may antagonize the hypotensive effects of antihypertensives).
No products indexed under this heading.

Perindopril Erbumine (Amphetamines may antagonize the hypotensive effects of antihypertensives). Products include:
Aceon Tablets (2 mg, 4 mg, 8 mg) 3194

Phenelzine Sulfate (Potential for hypertensive crisis; slows amphetamine metabolism; concurrent and/or sequential use is contraindicated).
No products indexed under this heading.

Phenobarbital (Delayed intestinal absorption of phenobarbital; synergistic anticonvulsant action may be produced). Products include:
Donnatal Extentabs 2493

Phenoxybenzamine Hydrochloride (Amphetamines may antagonize the hypotensive effects of antihypertensives). Products include:
Dibenzyline Capsules 3399

Phentolamine Mesylate (Amphetamines may antagonize the hypotensive effects of antihypertensives).
No products indexed under this heading.

Phenylephrine Bitartrate (Enhanced activity of sympathomimetics).
No products indexed under this heading.

Phenylephrine Hydrochloride (Enhanced activity of sympathomimetics). Products include:
Comtrex Maximum Strength Non-Drowsy Cold & Cough Caplets .... ■ 725
Comtrex Maximum Strength Day/Night Severe Cold & Sinus Caplets - Day Formulation .... ■ 725
Comtrex Maximum Strength Day/Night Severe Cold & Sinus Caplets - Night Formulation .... ■ 725
Contac Cold and Flu Maximum Strength Caplets .... ■ 728
Contac Cold and Flu Day and Night Caplets (Day Formulation Only) .... ■ 727
Contac Cold and Flu Day and Night Caplets (Night Formulation Only) .... ■ 727
Contac Cold and Flu Non-Drowsy Caplets .... ■ 728
Contac-D Cold Non-Drowsy Tablets .... ■ 729
Children's Dimetapp Cold & Allergy Elixir .... ■ 730
Children's Dimetapp Cold & Allergy Chewable Tablets .... ■ 730
Children's Dimetapp DM Cold & Cough Elixir .... ■ 731
Toddler's Dimetapp Cold and Cough Drops .... ■ 732
Excedrin Sinus Headache Caplets/Tablets .... ■ 610
4-Way Fast Acting Nasal Spray .... ■ 775
4-Way Menthol Nasal Spray .... ■ 775
Preparation H Maximum Strength Cream .... ■ 666
Preparation H Cooling Gel .... ■ 666
Preparation H .... ■ 666
Refenesen PE Caplets .... ■ 721
Robitussin Cough & Allergy Syrup .. ■ 736
Robitussin Cough & Cold Nighttime Liquid .... ■ 736
Robitussin Cough, Cold & Flu Nighttime Liquid .... ■ 738
Robitussin Head & Chest Congestion PE Syrup .... ■ 739
Robitussin Pediatric Cough & Cold Nighttime Liquid .... ■ 736
TheraFlu Cold & Cough Hot Liquid .... ■ 740
TheraFlu Cold & Sore Throat Hot Liquid .... ■ 741
TheraFlu Flu & Sore Throat Hot Liquid .... ■ 742
TheraFlu Daytime Severe Cold Hot Liquid .... ■ 742
TheraFlu Nighttime Severe Cold Hot Liquid .... ■ 740
TheraFlu Warming Relief Daytime Severe Cold .... ■ 743
TheraFlu Warming Relief Nighttime Severe Cold .... ■ 743
Triaminic Chest & Nasal Congestion Liquid .... ■ 746
Triaminic Cold & Allergy Liquid .... ■ 746
Triaminic Daytime Cold & Cough Liquid .... ■ 745
Triaminic Nighttime Cold & Cough Liquid .... ■ 746
Triaminic Thin Strips Cold .... ■ 748
Triaminic Thin Strips Cold & Cough .... ■ 778
Triaminic Infant Thin Strips Decongestant .... ■ 747
Triaminic Infant Thin Strips Decongestant Plus Cough .... ■ 747
Children's Tylenol Plus Flu Oral Suspension .... ■ 749
Tylenol Cold Head Congestion Daytime Caplets with Cool Burst and Gelcaps .... ■ 750
Tylenol Cold Multi-Symptom Daytime Liquid .... ■ 752
Tylenol Cold Multi-Symptom Severe Daytime Liquid .... ■ 752
Concentrated Tylenol Infants' Drops Plus Cold & Cough .... ■ 754
Tylenol Allergy Multi-Symptom Caplets with Cool Burst and Gelcaps 1872
Tylenol Allergy Multi-Symptom Nighttime Caplets with Cool Burst 1872
Children's Tylenol Plus Cold Suspension Liquid 1879
Children's Tylenol Plus Cold & Allergy Suspension Liquid 1878
Children's Tylenol Plus Flu Suspension Liquid 1881
Children's Tylenol Plus Multi-Symptom Cold Suspension Liquid 1879
Tylenol Cold Head Congestion Daytime Caplets with Cool Burst 1873
Tylenol Cold Head Congestion Nighttime Caplets with Cool Burst 1873
Tylenol Cold Head Congestion Severe Caplets with Cool Burst 1873
Tylenol Cold Multi-Symptom Daytime Caplets with Cool Burst and Gelcaps 1874
Tylenol Cold Multi-Symptom Daytime Liquid with Citrus Burst ... 1874
Tylenol Cold Multi-Symptom Nighttime Caplets with Cool Burst 1874
Tylenol Cold Multi-Symptom Nighttime Liquid with Cool Burst ... 1874
Tylenol Cold Multi-Symptom Severe Caplets with Cool Burst 1874
Tylenol Cold Multi-Symptom Severe Daytime Liquid with Citrus Burst 1874
Tylenol Sinus Congestion & Pain Daytime Caplets with Cool Burst and Gelcaps 1876
Tylenol Sinus Congestion & Pain Nighttime Caplets with Cool Burst 1876
Tylenol Sinus Congestion & Pain Severe Caplets with Cool Burst 1876
Vicks 44D Cough & Head Congestion Relief Liquid .... ■ 760
Vicks DayQuil LiquiCaps/Liquid Multi-Symptom Cold/Flu Relief ..... ■ 761
Zicam Cough Plus D Cough Spray .... ■ 767

Phenylephrine Tannate (Enhanced activity of sympathomimetics).
No products indexed under this heading.

Phenylpropanolamine Hydrochloride (Enhanced activity of sympathomimetics).
No products indexed under this heading.

Phenytoin (Delayed intestinal absorption of phenobarbital; synergistic anticonvulsant action may be produced).
No products indexed under this heading.

Phenytoin Sodium (Delayed intestinal absorption of phenobarbital; synergistic anticonvulsant action may be produced). Products include:
Phenytek Capsules 2160

Pindolol (Adrenergic blockers are inhibited by amphetamines; amphetamines may antagonize the hypotensive effects of antihypertensives).
No products indexed under this heading.

Pirbuterol Acetate (Enhanced activity of sympathomimetics). Products include:
Maxair Autohaler 1852

Polythiazide (Some thiazide diuretics increase concentration of the non-ionized species of the amphetamine molecule thereby decreasing urinary excretion; increases blood levels and potentiates the action of amphetamines; amphetamines may antagonize the hypotensive effects of antihypertensives).
No products indexed under this heading.

Potassium Citrate (Increases the concentration of the non-ionized species of the amphetamine molecule thereby decreasing urinary excretion; increases blood levels and potentiates the action of amphetamines). Products include:
Urocit-K Tablets 2144

Prazosin Hydrochloride (Adrenergic blockers are inhibited by amphetamines; amphetamines may antagonize the hypotensive effects of antihypertensives).
No products indexed under this heading.

Procarbazine Hydrochloride (Potential for hypertensive crisis; slows amphetamine metabolism; concurrent and/or sequential use is contraindicated). Products include:
Matulane Capsules 3191

Promethazine Hydrochloride (Amphetamines may counteract the sedative effect of antihistamines). Products include:
Phenergan Tablets and Suppositories 3440

Propoxyphene Hydrochloride (In cases of propoxyphene overdosage, amphetamine CNS stimulation is potentiated and fatal convulsions can occur).
No products indexed under this heading.

Propoxyphene Napsylate (In cases of propoxyphene overdosage, amphetamine CNS stimulation is potentiated and fatal convulsions can occur).
No products indexed under this heading.

Propranolol Hydrochloride (Adrenergic blockers are inhibited by amphetamines; amphetamines may antagonize the hypotensive effects of antihypertensives). Products include:
Inderal LA Long-Acting Capsules 3429
InnoPran XL Capsules 2723

Protriptyline Hydrochloride (Enhanced activity of tricyclic antidepressants; cardiovascular effects can be potentiated).
No products indexed under this heading.

Pseudoephedrine Hydrochloride (Enhanced activity of sympathomimetics). Products include:
Advil Allergy Sinus Caplets .... ■ 770
Advil Cold & Sinus .... ■ 723
Advil Multi-Symptom Cold Caplets .... ■ 770
Aleve Cold & Sinus Caplets 744
Allegra-D 12 Hour Extended-Release Tablets 2846
Allegra-D 24 Hour Extended-Release Tablets 2849
BC Cold Powder .... ■ 677
Comtrex Maximum Strength Cold & Cough Day/Night Caplets - Day Formulation .... ■ 726
Comtrex Maximum Strength Cold & Cough Day/Night Caplets - Night Formulation .... ■ 726
Children's Motrin Cold Oral Suspension 1867

Mucinex D Extended-Release Bi-Layer Tablets 776
Robitussin Cough & Cold CF Liquid 735
Robitussin Cough & Cold Pediatric Drops 735
Tylenol Sinus Congestion & Pain Nighttime Caplets with Cool Burst 778
Tylenol Cold Severe Congestion Non-Drowsy Caplets with Cool Burst **1874**
Tylenol Sinus Severe Congestion Caplets with Cool Burst **1876**
Vicks 44D Cough & Head Congestion Relief Liquid **2679**
Vicks 44M Cough, Cold & Flu Relief Liquid **2680**
Vicks DayQuil Multi-Symptom Cold/Flu Relief LiquiCaps **2678**
Vicks DayQuil Multi-Symptom Cold/Flu Relief Liquid **2678**
Vicks NyQuil Multi-Symptom Cold/Flu Relief Liquid **2681**
Vicks NyQuil Multi-Symptom Cold/Flu Relief LiquiCaps **2681**
Children's Vicks NyQuil Cold/Cough Relief Liquid **2680**
Zyrtec-D 12 Hour Extended Release Tablets **2597**

Pseudoephedrine Sulfate (Enhanced activity of sympathomimetics). Products include:
Alavert Allergy & Sinus D-12 Hour Tablets 771
Clarinex-D 24-Hour Extended-Release Tablets **2998**
Claritin-D Non-Drowsy 12 Hour Tablets 772
Claritin-D Non-Drowsy 24 Hour Tablets 772

Pyrilamine Maleate (Amphetamines may counteract the sedative effect of antihistamines).
No products indexed under this heading.

Pyrilamine Tannate (Amphetamines may counteract the sedative effect of antihistamines).
No products indexed under this heading.

Quinapril Hydrochloride (Amphetamines may antagonize the hypotensive effects of antihypertensives).
No products indexed under this heading.

Ramipril (Amphetamines may antagonize the hypotensive effects of antihypertensives). Products include:
Altace Capsules **1702**

Rauwolfia Serpentina (Amphetamines may antagonize the hypotensive effects of antihypertensives).
No products indexed under this heading.

Rescinnamine (Amphetamines may antagonize the hypotensive effects of antihypertensives).
No products indexed under this heading.

Reserpine (Lowers absorption of amphetamines by acting as gastrointestinal acidifying agent; amphetamines may antagonize the hypotensive effects of antihypertensives).
No products indexed under this heading.

Salmeterol Xinafoate (Enhanced activity of sympathomimetics). Products include:
Advair Diskus 100/50 .... **1308**
Advair Diskus 250/50 .... **1308**
Advair Diskus 500/50 .... **1308**
Advair HFA Inhalation Aerosol **1318**
Serevent Diskus **1568**

Selegiline Hydrochloride (Potential for hypertensive crisis; slows amphetamine metabolism; concurrent and/or sequential use is contraindicated). Products include:
Eldepryl Capsules **3208**
Zelapar Tablets **3372**

Sodium Acid Phosphate (Increases the concentration of ionized species of the amphetamine molecule thereby increasing urinary excretion; lowers blood levels and efficacy of amphetamines). Products include:
Uroqid-Acid No. 2 Tablets **760**

Sodium Bicarbonate (Increases absorption of amphetamines; increases blood levels and potentiates the action of amphetamines). Products include:
Colyte with Flavor Packs for Oral Solution **3088**
HalfLytely and Bisacodyl Tablets Bowel Prep Kit with Flavors Packs **881**
TriLyte with Flavor Packs for Oral Solution **3100**

Sodium Citrate (Increases the concentration of the non-ionized species of the amphetamine molecule thereby decreasing urinary excretion; increases blood levels and potentiates the action of amphetamines).
No products indexed under this heading.

Sodium Nitroprusside (Amphetamines may antagonize the hypotensive effects of antihypertensives).
No products indexed under this heading.

Sotalol Hydrochloride (Adrenergic blockers are inhibited by amphetamines; amphetamines may antagonize the hypotensive effects of antihypertensives).
No products indexed under this heading.

Spirapril Hydrochloride (Amphetamines may antagonize the hypotensive effects of antihypertensives).
No products indexed under this heading.

Tamsulosin Hydrochloride (Adrenergic blockers are inhibited by amphetamines; amphetamines may antagonize the hypotensive effects of antihypertensives). Products include:
Flomax Capsules **850**

Telmisartan (Amphetamines may antagonize the hypotensive effects of antihypertensives). Products include:
Micardis Tablets **854**
Micardis HCT Tablets **856**

Terazosin Hydrochloride (Adrenergic blockers are inhibited by amphetamines; amphetamines may antagonize the hypotensive effects of antihypertensives). Products include:
Hytrin Capsules **471**

Terbutaline Sulfate (Enhanced activity of sympathomimetics).
No products indexed under this heading.

Terfenadine (Amphetamines may counteract the sedative effect of antihistamines).
No products indexed under this heading.

Timolol Hemihydrate (Adrenergic blockers are inhibited by amphetamines; amphetamines may antagonize the hypotensive effects of antihypertensives). Products include:
Betimol Ophthalmic Solution **3382**
Betimol Ophthalmic Solution .... ⊙**295**

Timolol Maleate (Adrenergic blockers are inhibited by amphetamines; amphetamines may antagonize the hypotensive effects of antihypertensives). Products include:
Blocadren Tablets **1916**
Cosopt Sterile Ophthalmic Solution **1931**
Timolide Tablets **2086**
Timoptic Sterile Ophthalmic Solution **2088**
Timoptic in Ocudose **2091**
Timoptic-XE Sterile Ophthalmic Gel Forming Solution **2092**

Torsemide (Amphetamines may antagonize the hypotensive effects of antihypertensives). Products include:
Demadex Injection **2759**
Demadex Tablets **2759**

Trandolapril (Amphetamines may antagonize the hypotensive effects of antihypertensives). Products include:
Mavik Tablets **486**
Tarka Tablets **524**

Tranylcypromine Sulfate (Potential for hypertensive crisis; slows amphetamine metabolism; concurrent and/or sequential use is contraindicated). Products include:
Parnate Tablets **1527**

Trimeprazine Tartrate (Amphetamines may counteract the sedative effect of antihistamines).
No products indexed under this heading.

Trimethaphan Camsylate (Amphetamines may antagonize the hypotensive effects of antihypertensives).
No products indexed under this heading.

Trimipramine Maleate (Enhanced activity of tricyclic antidepressants; cardiovascular effects can be potentiated).
No products indexed under this heading.

Tripelennamine Hydrochloride (Amphetamines may counteract the sedative effect of antihistamines).
No products indexed under this heading.

Triprolidine Hydrochloride (Amphetamines may counteract the sedative effect of antihistamines).
No products indexed under this heading.

Valsartan (Amphetamines may antagonize the hypotensive effects of antihypertensives). Products include:
Diovan Tablets **2193**
Diovan HCT Tablets **2196**

Verapamil Hydrochloride (Amphetamines may antagonize the hypotensive effects of antihypertensives). Products include:
Covera-HS Tablets **3139**
Tarka Tablets **524**
Verelan PM Extended-Release Capsules, Controlled-Onset **3106**

Vitamin C (Lowers absorption of amphetamines by acting as gastrointestinal acidifying agent). Products include:
Bausch & Lomb Ocuvite Adult Eye Vitamin and Mineral Supplement Soft Gels **706**
Bausch & Lomb Ocuvite Adult 50+ Eye Vitamin and Mineral Supplement Soft Gels **706**
Ocuvite Adult Vitamin and Mineral Supplement .... ⊙**253**
Ocuvite Adult 50+ Vitamin and Mineral Supplement .... ⊙**253**
Peridin-C Vitamin C Supplement **818**

Food Interactions

Fruit juices, unspecified (Lowers absorption of amphetamines by acting as gastrointestinal acidifying agent).

DHEA PLUS CAPSULES

(Dihydroepiandrosterone (DHEA), Ginkgo biloba) **827**
None cited in PDR database.

DIASTAT RECTAL DELIVERY SYSTEM

(Diazepam) **3343**
May interact with barbiturates, central nervous system depressants, cytochrome p450 2c19 inducers (selected), cytochrome p450 2c19 inhibitors (selected), cytochrome p450 2c19 substrates (selected), cytochrome p450 3a4 inducers (selected), cytochrome p450 3a4 inhibitors (selected), cytochrome p450 3a4 substrates (selected), antidepressant drugs, dexamethasone, monoamine oxidase inhibitors, narcotic analgesics, phenothiazines, phenytoin, quinidine, valproate, xanthines, and certain other agents. Compounds in these categories include:

Acetazolamide (Studies suggest that CYP2C19 and CYP3A4 are the principal enzymes involved in the initial oxidative metabolism of diazepam. Therefore, potential interactions may occur when diazepam is given concurrently with agents that affect CYP2C19 and CYP3A4 activity. Potential inhibitors of CYP3A4 could decrease the rate of diazepam elimination).
No products indexed under this heading.

Alfentanil Hydrochloride (Potential for synergistic CNS-depressant effect).
No products indexed under this heading.

Allium sativum (Studies suggest that CYP2C19 and CYP3A4 are the principal enzymes involved in the initial oxidative metabolism of diazepam. Therefore, potential interactions may occur when diazepam is given concurrently with agents that affect CYP2C19 and CYP3A4 activity. Potential inducers of CYP3A4 could increase the rate of diazepam elimination).
No products indexed under this heading.

Alprazolam (Potential for synergistic CNS-depressant effect). Products include:
Niravam Orally Disintegrating Tablets **3092**

Aminophylline (Diazepam is a substrate of CYP2C19 and CYP3A4, it is possible that diazepam may interfere with the metabolism of drugs which are substrates for CYP3A4, such as theophylline).
No products indexed under this heading.

Amiodarone Hydrochloride (Studies suggest that CYP2C19 and CYP3A4 are the principal enzymes involved in the initial oxidative metabolism of diazepam. Therefore, potential interactions may occur when diazepam is given concurrently with agents that affect CYP2C19 and CYP3A4 activity. Potential inhibitors of CYP3A4 could decrease the rate of diazepam elimination).
No products indexed under this heading.

Amitriptyline Hydrochloride (Potential for synergistic CNS-depressant effect).
No products indexed under this heading.

Amlodipine Besylate (There are no reports as to which isoenzymes could be inhibited or induced by diazepam. But based on the fact that diazepam is a substrate for CYP2C19 and CYP3A4, it is possible that diazepam may interfere with the metabolism of drugs which are substrates for CYP2C19 and CYP3A4 leading to a potential drug-drug interaction). Products include:
Caduet Tablets 2508
Lotrel Capsules 2249
Norvasc Tablets 2545

Amoxapine (Potential for synergistic CNS-depressant effect).
No products indexed under this heading.

Amprenavir (Studies suggest that CYP2C19 and CYP3A4 are the principal enzymes involved in the initial oxidative metabolism of diazepam. Therefore, potential interactions may occur when diazepam is given concurrently with agents that affect CYP2C19 and CYP3A4 activity. Potential inhibitors of CYP3A4 could decrease the rate of diazepam elimination). Products include:
Agenerase Capsules 1327
Agenerase Oral Solution 1332

Anastrozole (Studies suggest that CYP2C19 and CYP3A4 are the principal enzymes involved in the initial oxidative metabolism of diazepam. Therefore, potential interactions may occur when diazepam is given concurrently with agents that affect CYP2C19 and CYP3A4 activity. Potential inhibitors of CYP3A4 could decrease the rate of diazepam elimination). Products include:
Arimidex Tablets 673

Aprepitant (Studies suggest that CYP2C19 and CYP3A4 are the principal enzymes involved in the initial oxidative metabolism of diazepam. Therefore, potential interactions may occur when diazepam is given concurrently with agents that affect CYP2C19 and CYP3A4 activity. Potential inhibitors of CYP3A4 could decrease the rate of diazepam elimination). Products include:
Emend Capsules 1963

Aprobarbital (Potential for synergistic CNS-depressant effect).
No products indexed under this heading.

Astemizole (There are no reports as to which isoenzymes could be inhibited or induced by diazepam. But based on the fact that diazepam is a substrate for CYP2C19 and CYP3A4, it is possible that diazepam may interfere with the metabolism of drugs which are substrates for CYP2C19 and CYP3A4 leading to a potential drug-drug interaction).
No products indexed under this heading.

Atorvastatin Calcium (There are no reports as to which isoenzymes could be inhibited or induced by diazepam. But based on the fact that diazepam is a substrate for CYP2C19 and CYP3A4, it is possible that diazepam may interfere with the metabolism of drugs which are substrates for CYP2C19 and CYP3A4 leading to a potential drug-drug interaction). Products include:
Caduet Tablets 2508
Lipitor Tablets 2483

Belladonna Ergotamine (There are no reports as to which isoenzymes could be inhibited or induced by diazepam. But based on the fact that diazepam is a substrate for CYP2C19 and CYP3A4, it is possible that diazepam may interfere with the metabolism of drugs which are substrates for CYP2C19 and CYP3A4 leading to a potential drug-drug interaction).
No products indexed under this heading.

Betamethasone Acetate (Studies suggest that CYP2C19 and CYP3A4 are the principal enzymes involved in the initial oxidative metabolism of diazepam. Therefore, potential interactions may occur when diazepam is given concurrently with agents that affect CYP2C19 and CYP3A4 activity. Potential inducers of CYP3A4 could increase the rate of diazepam elimination).
No products indexed under this heading.

Betamethasone Sodium Phosphate (Studies suggest that CYP2C19 and CYP3A4 are the principal enzymes involved in the initial oxidative metabolism of diazepam. Therefore, potential interactions may occur when diazepam is given concurrently with agents that affect CYP2C19 and CYP3A4 activity. Potential inducers of CYP3A4 could increase the rate of diazepam elimination).
No products indexed under this heading.

Buprenorphine Hydrochloride (Potential for synergistic CNS-depressant effect). Products include:
Buprenex Injectable 2716
Suboxone Tablets 2717
Subutex Tablets 2717

Bupropion Hydrochloride (Potential for synergistic CNS-depressant effect). Products include:
Wellbutrin Tablets 1603
Wellbutrin SR Sustained-Release Tablets 1607
Wellbutrin XL Extended-Release Tablets 1613
Zyban Sustained-Release Tablets 1644

Buspirone Hydrochloride (Potential for synergistic CNS-depressant effect).
No products indexed under this heading.

Busulfan (There are no reports as to which isoenzymes could be inhibited or induced by diazepam. But based on the fact that diazepam is a substrate for CYP2C19 and CYP3A4, it is possible that diazepam may interfere with the metabolism of drugs which are substrates for CYP2C19 and CYP3A4 leading to a potential drug-drug interaction). Products include:
I.V. Busulfex 2493
Myleran Tablets 1525

Butabarbital (Potential for synergistic CNS-depressant effect).
No products indexed under this heading.

Butalbital (Potential for synergistic CNS-depressant effect).
No products indexed under this heading.

Carbamazepine (Inducers of CYP3A4, such as carbamazepine, could increase the rate of elimination of diazepam). Products include:
Carbatrol Capsules 3171
Equetro Extended-Release Capsules 3180
Tegretol/Tegretol-XR 2295

Carisoprodol (There are no reports as to which isoenzymes could be inhibited or induced by diazepam. But based on the fact that diazepam is a substrate for CYP2C19 and CYP3A4, it is possible that diazepam may interfere with the metabolism of drugs which are substrates for CYP2C19 and CYP3A4 leading to a potential drug-drug interaction).
No products indexed under this heading.

Cerivastatin Sodium (There are no reports as to which isoenzymes could be inhibited or induced by diazepam. But based on the fact that diazepam is a substrate for CYP2C19 and CYP3A4, it is possible that diazepam may interfere with the metabolism of drugs which are substrates for CYP2C19 and CYP3A4 leading to a potential drug-drug interaction).
No products indexed under this heading.

Chlordiazepoxide (Potential for synergistic CNS-depressant effect).
No products indexed under this heading.

Chlordiazepoxide Hydrochloride (Potential for synergistic CNS-depressant effect). Products include:
Librium Capsules 3347

Chlorpheniramine (There are no reports as to which isoenzymes could be inhibited or induced by diazepam. But based on the fact that diazepam is a substrate for CYP2C19 and CYP3A4, it is possible that diazepam may interfere with the metabolism of drugs which are substrates for CYP2C19 and CYP3A4 leading to a potential drug-drug interaction).
No products indexed under this heading.

Chlorpheniramine Maleate (There are no reports as to which isoenzymes could be inhibited or induced by diazepam. But based on the fact that diazepam is a substrate for CYP2C19 and CYP3A4, it is possible that diazepam may interfere with the metabolism of drugs which are substrates for CYP2C19 and CYP3A4 leading to a potential drug-drug interaction). Products include:
Advil Allergy Sinus Caplets .... ▣ 770
Advil Multi-Symptom Cold Caplets .... ▣ 770
BC Allergy Sinus Cold Powder .... ▣ 677
Comtrex Maximum Strength Cold & Cough Day/Night Caplets - Night Formulation .... ▣ 726
Comtrex Maximum Strength Day/Night Severe Cold & Sinus Caplets - Night Formulation .... ▣ 725
Contac Cold and Flu Maximum Strength Caplets .... ▣ 728
Contac Cold and Flu Day and Night Caplets (Night Formulation Only) .... ▣ 727
Children's Dimetapp Long Acting Cough Plus Cold Syrup .... ▣ 731
Robitussin Cough & Cold Long-Acting Liquid .... ▣ 735
Robitussin Cough & Allergy Syrup .... ▣ 736
Robitussin Cough & Cold Nighttime Liquid .... ▣ 736
Robitussin Cough, Cold & Flu Nighttime Liquid .... ▣ 738
Robitussin Pediatric Cough & Cold Long-Acting Liquid .... ▣ 735
Robitussin Pediatric Cough & Cold Nighttime Liquid .... ▣ 736
Triaminic Cold & Allergy Liquid .... ▣ 746
Triaminic Cough & Runny Nose Softchews .... ▣ 748
Children's Tylenol Plus Flu Oral Suspension .... ▣ 749
Tylenol Allergy Multi-Symptom Caplets with Cool Burst and Gelcaps 1872
Children's Tylenol Plus Cold Suspension Liquid 1879
Children's Tylenol Plus Cough & Runny Nose Suspension Liquid 1879
Children's Tylenol Plus Flu Suspension Liquid 1881
Children's Tylenol Plus Multi-Symptom Cold Suspension Liquid 1879
Tylenol Cold Head Congestion Nighttime Caplets with Cool Burst 1873
Tylenol Cold Multi-Symptom Nighttime Caplets with Cool Burst 1874
Tylenol Sinus Congestion & Pain Nighttime Caplets with Cool Burst 1876
Vicks 44M Cough, Cold & Flu Relief Liquid 2680
Pediatric Vicks 44m Cough & Cold Relief Liquid 2676
Children's Vicks NyQuil Cold/Cough Relief .... ▣ 756
Children's Vicks NyQuil Cold/Cough Relief Liquid 2680
Zicam Maximum Strength Flu Daytime .... ▣ 768

Chlorpheniramine Polistirex (There are no reports as to which isoenzymes could be inhibited or induced by diazepam. But based on the fact that diazepam is a substrate for CYP2C19 and CYP3A4, it is possible that diazepam may interfere with the metabolism of drugs which are substrates for CYP2C19 and CYP3A4 leading to a potential drug-drug interaction). Products include:
Tussionex Pennkinetic Extended-Release Suspension 3327

Chlorpheniramine Tannate (There are no reports as to which isoenzymes could be inhibited or induced by diazepam. But based on the fact that diazepam is a substrate for CYP2C19 and CYP3A4, it is possible that diazepam may interfere with the metabolism of drugs which are substrates for CYP2C19 and CYP3A4 leading to a potential drug-drug interaction).
No products indexed under this heading.

Chlorpromazine (Potential for synergistic CNS-depressant effect).
No products indexed under this heading.

Chlorpromazine Hydrochloride (Potential for synergistic CNS-depressant effect).
No products indexed under this heading.

Chlorprothixene (Potential for synergistic CNS-depressant effect).
No products indexed under this heading.

Chlorprothixene Hydrochloride (Potential for synergistic CNS-depressant effect).
No products indexed under this heading.

Chlorprothixene Lactate (Potential for synergistic CNS-depressant effect).
No products indexed under this heading.

Cilostazol (There are no reports as to which isoenzymes could be inhibited or induced by diazepam. But based on the fact that diazepam is a substrate for CYP2C19 and CYP3A4, it is possible that diazepam may interfere with the metabolism of drugs which are substrates for CYP2C19 and CYP3A4 leading to a potential drug-drug interaction). Products include:

Pletal Tablets 2455

Cimetidine (Potential inhibitors of CYP2C19, such as cimetidine, could decrease the rate of diazepam elimination). Products include:

Tagamet HB 200 Tablets 664

Cimetidine Hydrochloride (Potential inhibitors of CYP2C19, such as cimetidine, could decrease the rate of diazepam elimination).

No products indexed under this heading.

Ciprofloxacin (Studies suggest that CYP2C19 and CYP3A4 are the principal enzymes involved in the initial oxidative metabolism of diazepam. Therefore, potential interactions may occur when diazepam is given concurrently with agents that affect CYP2C19 and CYP3A4 activity. Potential inhibitors of CYP3A4 could decrease the rate of diazepam elimination). Products include:

Cipro Oral Suspension 2977
Cipro I.V. 2984
Cipro XR Tablets 2990
Ciprodex Otic Suspension 559

Ciprofloxacin Hydrochloride (Studies suggest that CYP2C19 and CYP3A4 are the principal enzymes involved in the initial oxidative metabolism of diazepam. Therefore, potential interactions may occur when diazepam is given concurrently with agents that affect CYP2C19 and CYP3A4 activity. Potential inducers of CYP3A4 could increase the rate of diazepam elimination). Products include:

Ciloxan Ophthalmic Ointment 559
Ciloxan Ophthalmic Solution 206
Cipro Tablets 2977
Proquin XR Tablets 1153

Cisapride (There are no reports as to which isoenzymes could be inhibited or induced by diazepam. But based on the fact that diazepam is a substrate for CYP2C19 and CYP3A4, it is possible that diazepam may interfere with the metabolism of drugs which are substrates for CYP2C19 and CYP3A4 leading to a potential drug-drug interaction).

No products indexed under this heading.

Cisplatin (Studies suggest that CYP2C19 and CYP3A4 are the principal enzymes involved in the initial oxidative metabolism of diazepam. Therefore, potential interactions may occur when diazepam is given concurrently with agents that affect CYP2C19 and CYP3A4 activity. Potential inducers of CYP3A4 could increase the rate of diazepam elimination).

No products indexed under this heading.

Citalopram Hydrobromide (Potential for synergistic CNS-depressant effect). Products include:

Celexa 1176

Clarithromycin (Studies suggest that CYP2C19 and CYP3A4 are the principal enzymes involved in the initial oxidative metabolism of diazepam. Therefore, potential interactions may occur when diazepam is given concurrently with agents that affect CYP2C19 and CYP3A4 activity. Potential inhibitors of CYP3A4 could decrease the rate of diazepam elimination). Products include:

Biaxin/Biaxin XL 402
PREVPAC 3284

Clomipramine Hydrochloride (There are no reports as to which isoenzymes could be inhibited or induced by diazepam. But based on the fact that diazepam is a substrate for CYP2C19 and CYP3A4, it is possible that diazepam may interfere with the metabolism of drugs which are substrates for CYP2C19 and CYP3A4 leading to a potential drug-drug interaction).

No products indexed under this heading.

Clorazepate Dipotassium (Potential for synergistic CNS-depressant effect). Products include:

Tranxene 2474

Clotrimazole (Potential inhibitors of CYP3A4, such as clotrimazole, could decrease the rate of diazepam elimination). Products include:

Desenex Athlete's Foot Cream 635
Lotrimin 3039
Lotrisone 3040

Clozapine (Potential for synergistic CNS-depressant effect). Products include:

Clozaril Tablets 2184
FazaClo Orally Disintegrating Tablets 551

Codeine Phosphate (Potential for synergistic CNS-depressant effect). Products include:

Tylenol with Codeine Tablets 2391

Cortisone Acetate (Studies suggest that CYP2C19 and CYP3A4 are the principal enzymes involved in the initial oxidative metabolism of diazepam. Therefore, potential interactions may occur when diazepam is given concurrently with agents that affect CYP2C19 and CYP3A4 activity. Potential inducers of CYP3A4 could increase the rate of diazepam elimination).

No products indexed under this heading.

Cyclophosphamide (There are no reports as to which isoenzymes could be inhibited or induced by diazepam. But based on the fact that diazepam is a substrate for CYP2C19 and CYP3A4, it is possible that diazepam may interfere with the metabolism of drugs which are substrates for CYP2C19 and CYP3A4 leading to a potential drug-drug interaction).

No products indexed under this heading.

Cyclosporine (Diazepam is a substrate of CYP2C19 and CYP3A4, it is possible that diazepam may interfere with the metabolism of drugs which are substrates for CYP3A4, such as cyclosporine). Products include:

Gengraf Capsules 459
Neoral Oral Solution 2259
Neoral Soft Gelatin Capsules 2259
Restasis Ophthalmic Emulsion 575
Sandimmune 2275

Dalfopristin (Studies suggest that CYP2C19 and CYP3A4 are the principal enzymes involved in the initial oxidative metabolism of diazepam. Therefore, potential interactions may occur when diazepam is given concurrently with agents that affect CYP2C19 and CYP3A4 activity. Potential inhibitors of CYP3A4 could decrease the rate of diazepam elimination).

No products indexed under this heading.

Danazol (Studies suggest that CYP2C19 and CYP3A4 are the principal enzymes involved in the initial oxidative metabolism of diazepam. Therefore, potential interactions may occur when diazepam is given concurrently with agents that affect CYP2C19 and CYP3A4 activity. Potential inhibitors of CYP3A4 could decrease the rate of diazepam elimination).

No products indexed under this heading.

Delavirdine Mesylate (Studies suggest that CYP2C19 and CYP3A4 are the principal enzymes involved in the initial oxidative metabolism of diazepam. Therefore, potential interactions may occur when diazepam is given concurrently with agents that affect CYP2C19 and CYP3A4 activity. Potential inhibitors of CYP2C19 could decrease the rate of diazepam elimination). Products include:

Rescriptor Tablets 2551

Desflurane (Potential for synergistic CNS-depressant effect).

No products indexed under this heading.

Desipramine Hydrochloride (Potential for synergistic CNS-depressant effect).

No products indexed under this heading.

Desogestrel (Studies suggest that CYP2C19 and CYP3A4 are the principal enzymes involved in the initial oxidative metabolism of diazepam. Therefore, potential interactions may occur when diazepam is given concurrently with agents that affect CYP2C19 and CYP3A4 activity. Potential inhibitors of CYP2C19 could decrease the rate of diazepam elimination). Products include:

Mircette Tablets 1066

Dexamethasone (Potential inducers of CYP3A4, such as dexamethasone, could increase the rate of elimination of diazepam). Products include:

Ciprodex Otic Suspension 559
Decadron Tablets 1951
TobraDex Ophthalmic Ointment 562
TobraDex Ophthalmic Suspension 563

Dexamethasone Acetate (Potential inducers of CYP3A4, such as dexamethasone, could increase the rate of elimination of diazepam).

No products indexed under this heading.

Dexamethasone Sodium Phosphate (Potential inducers of CYP3A4, such as dexamethasone, could increase the rate of elimination of diazepam).

No products indexed under this heading.

Dextromethorphan (There are no reports as to which isoenzymes could be inhibited or induced by diazepam. But based on the fact that diazepam is a substrate for CYP2C19 and CYP3A4, it is possible that diazepam may interfere with the metabolism of drugs which are substrates for CYP2C19 and CYP3A4 leading to a potential drug-drug interaction).

No products indexed under this heading.

Dextromethorphan Hydrobromide (There are no reports as to which isoenzymes could be inhibited or induced by diazepam. But based on the fact that diazepam is a substrate for CYP2C19 and CYP3A4, it is possible that diazepam may interfere with the metabolism of drugs which are substrates for CYP2C19 and CYP3A4 leading to a potential drug-drug interaction). Products include:

Comtrex Maximum Strength Cold & Cough Day/Night Caplets - Day Formulation 726
Comtrex Maximum Strength Cold & Cough Day/Night Caplets - Night Formulation 726
Comtrex Maximum Strength Non-Drowsy Cold & Cough Caplets 725
Children's Dimetapp DM Cold & Cough Elixir 731
Children's Dimetapp Long Acting Cough Plus Cold Syrup 731
Toddler's Dimetapp Cold and Cough Drops 732
Mucinex DM Extended-Release Bi-Layer Tablets 720
Refenesen DM Caplets 721
Robitussin Cough & Cold CF Liquid 735
Robitussin Cough & Cold Long-Acting Liquid 735
Robitussin Cough & Allergy Syrup 736
Robitussin Cough & Cold Nighttime Liquid 736
Robitussin Cough & Cold Pediatric Drops 735
Robitussin Cough, Cold & Flu Nighttime Liquid 738
Robitussin Cough & Congestion Liquid 738
Robitussin Cough Gels Long-Acting 737
Robitussin Cough Long Acting Liquid 739
Robitussin Cough DM Syrup 738
Robitussin Cough DM Infant Drops 738
Robitussin Pediatric Cough Long Acting Liquid 739
Robitussin Pediatric Cough & Cold Long-Acting Liquid 735
Robitussin Pediatric Cough & Cold Nighttime Liquid 736
Robitussin Sugar Free Cough 738
TheraFlu Cold & Cough Hot Liquid 740
TheraFlu Warming Relief Daytime Severe Cold 743
TheraFlu Thin Strips Long Acting Cough 744
Triaminic Daytime Cold & Cough Liquid 745
Triaminic Cough & Sore Throat Liquid 747
Triaminic Cough & Runny Nose Softchews 748
Triaminic Thin Strips Cold & Cough 778
Triaminic Infant Thin Strips Decongestant Plus Cough 747
Children's Tylenol Plus Flu Oral Suspension 749
Tylenol Cold Head Congestion Daytime Caplets with Cool Burst and Gelcaps 750
Tylenol Cold Multi-Symptom Daytime Liquid 752
Tylenol Cold Multi-Symptom Severe Daytime Liquid 752
Concentrated Tylenol Infants' Drops Plus Cold & Cough 754
Children's Tylenol Plus Cough & Runny Nose Suspension Liquid 1879
Children's Tylenol Plus Cough & Sore Throat Suspension Liquid 1879
Children's Tylenol Plus Flu Suspension Liquid 1881
Children's Tylenol Plus Multi-Symptom Cold Suspension Liquid 1879
Tylenol Cold Severe Congestion Non-Drowsy Caplets with Cool Burst 1874
Tylenol Cold Head Congestion Daytime Caplets with Cool Burst 1873
Tylenol Cold Head Congestion Nighttime Caplets with Cool Burst 1873

Dezocine (Potential for synergistic CNS-depressant effect).
　No products indexed under this heading.

Dihydroergotamine Mesylate (There are no reports as to which isoenzymes could be inhibited or induced by diazepam. But based on the fact that diazepam is a substrate for CYP2C19 and CYP3A4, it is possible that diazepam may interfere with the metabolism of drugs which are substrates for CYP2C19 and CYP3A4 leading to a potential drug-drug interaction). Products include:

Diltiazem Hydrochloride (Studies suggest that CYP2C19 and CYP3A4 are the principal enzymes involved in the initial oxidative metabolism of diazepam. Therefore, potential interactions may occur when diazepam is given concurrently with agents that affect CYP2C19 and CYP3A4 activity. Potential inhibitors of CYP3A4 could decrease the rate of diazepam elimination). Products include:

Diltiazem Maleate (Studies suggest that CYP2C19 and CYP3A4 are the principal enzymes involved in the initial oxidative metabolism of diazepam. Therefore, potential interactions may occur when diazepam is given concurrently with agents that affect CYP2C19 and CYP3A4 activity. Potential inhibitors of CYP3A4 could decrease the rate of diazepam elimination).
　No products indexed under this heading.

Disopyramide (There are no reports as to which isoenzymes could be inhibited or induced by diazepam. But based on the fact that diazepam is a substrate for CYP2C19 and CYP3A4, it is possible that diazepam may interfere with the metabolism of drugs which are substrates for CYP2C19 and CYP3A4 leading to a potential drug-drug interaction).
　No products indexed under this heading.

Disopyramide Phosphate (There are no reports as to which isoenzymes could be inhibited or induced by diazepam. But based on the fact that diazepam is a substrate for CYP2C19 and CYP3A4, it is possible that diazepam may interfere with the metabolism of drugs which are substrates for CYP2C19 and CYP3A4 leading to a potential drug-drug interaction).
　No products indexed under this heading.

Disulfiram (There are no reports as to which isoenzymes could be inhibited or induced by diazepam. But based on the fact that diazepam is a substrate for CYP2C19 and CYP3A4, it is possible that diazepam may interfere with the metabolism of drugs which are substrates for CYP2C19 and CYP3A4 leading to a potential drug-drug interaction).
　No products indexed under this heading.

Divalproex Sodium (Valproate may potentiate the CNS-depressant effect). Products include:

Doxepin Hydrochloride (Potential for synergistic CNS-depressant effect).
　No products indexed under this heading.

Doxorubicin Hydrochloride (Studies suggest that CYP2C19 and CYP3A4 are the principal enzymes involved in the initial oxidative metabolism of diazepam. Therefore, potential interactions may occur when diazepam is given concurrently with agents that affect CYP2C19 and CYP3A4 activity. Potential inducers of CYP3A4 could increase the rate of diazepam elimination).
　No products indexed under this heading.

Dronabinol (There are no reports as to which isoenzymes could be inhibited or induced by diazepam. But based on the fact that diazepam is a substrate for CYP2C19 and CYP3A4, it is possible that diazepam may interfere with the metabolism of drugs which are substrates for CYP2C19 and CYP3A4 leading to a potential drug-drug interaction). Products include:

Droperidol (Potential for synergistic CNS-depressant effect).
　No products indexed under this heading.

Dyphylline (Diazepam is a substrate of CYP2C19 and CYP3A4, it is possible that diazepam may interfere with the metabolism of drugs which are substrates for CYP3A4, such as theophylline).
　No products indexed under this heading.

Efavirenz (Studies suggest that CYP2C19 and CYP3A4 are the principal enzymes involved in the initial oxidative metabolism of diazepam. Therefore, potential interactions may occur when diazepam is given concurrently with agents that affect CYP2C19 and CYP3A4 activity. Potential inhibitors of CYP2C19 could decrease the rate of diazepam elimination). Products include:

Enflurane (Potential for synergistic CNS-depressant effect).
　No products indexed under this heading.

Ergotamine Tartrate (There are no reports as to which isoenzymes could be inhibited or induced by diazepam. But based on the fact that diazepam is a substrate for CYP2C19 and CYP3A4, it is possible that diazepam may interfere with the metabolism of drugs which are substrates for CYP2C19 and CYP3A4 leading to a potential drug-drug interaction).
　No products indexed under this heading.

Erythromycin (Studies suggest that CYP2C19 and CYP3A4 are the principal enzymes involved in the initial oxidative metabolism of diazepam. Therefore, potential interactions may occur when diazepam is given concurrently with agents that affect CYP2C19 and CYP3A4 activity. Potential inhibitors of CYP3A4 could decrease the rate of diazepam elimination). Products include:

Erythromycin Estolate (Studies suggest that CYP2C19 and CYP3A4 are the principal enzymes involved in the initial oxidative metabolism of diazepam. Therefore, potential interactions may occur when diazepam is given concurrently with agents that affect CYP2C19 and CYP3A4 activity. Potential inhibitors of CYP3A4 could decrease the rate of diazepam elimination).
　No products indexed under this heading.

Erythromycin Ethylsuccinate (Studies suggest that CYP2C19 and CYP3A4 are the principal enzymes involved in the initial oxidative metabolism of diazepam. Therefore, potential interactions may occur when diazepam is given concurrently with agents that affect CYP2C19 and CYP3A4 activity. Potential inhibitors of CYP3A4 could decrease the rate of diazepam elimination). Products include:

Erythromycin Gluceptate (Studies suggest that CYP2C19 and CYP3A4 are the principal enzymes involved in the initial oxidative metabolism of diazepam. Therefore, potential interactions may occur when diazepam is given concurrently with agents that affect CYP2C19 and CYP3A4 activity. Potential inhibitors of CYP3A4 could decrease the rate of diazepam elimination).
　No products indexed under this heading.

Erythromycin Lactobionate (Studies suggest that CYP2C19 and CYP3A4 are the principal enzymes involved in the initial oxidative metabolism of diazepam. Therefore, potential interactions may occur when diazepam is given concurrently with agents that affect CYP2C19 and CYP3A4 activity. Potential inhibitors of CYP3A4 could decrease the rate of diazepam elimination).
　No products indexed under this heading.

Erythromycin Stearate (Studies suggest that CYP2C19 and CYP3A4 are the principal enzymes involved in the initial oxidative metabolism of diazepam. Therefore, potential interactions may occur when diazepam is given concurrently with agents that affect CYP2C19 and CYP3A4 activity. Potential inhibitors of CYP3A4 could decrease the rate of diazepam elimination). Products include:

Escitalopram Oxalate (Potential for synergistic CNS-depressant effect). Products include:

Esomeprazole Magnesium (Studies suggest that CYP2C19 and CYP3A4 are the principal enzymes involved in the initial oxidative metabolism of diazepam. Therefore, potential interactions may occur when diazepam is given concurrently with agents that affect CYP2C19 and CYP3A4 activity. Potential inhibitors of CYP3A4 could decrease the rate of diazepam elimination). Products include:

Estazolam (Potential for synergistic CNS-depressant effect). Products include:

Estradiol (There are no reports as to which isoenzymes could be inhibited or induced by diazepam. But based on the fact that diazepam is a substrate for CYP2C19 and CYP3A4, it is possible that diazepam may interfere with the metabolism of drugs which are substrates for CYP2C19 and CYP3A4 leading to a potential drug-drug interaction). Products include:

Estradiol Benzoate (There are no reports as to which isoenzymes could be inhibited or induced by diazepam. But based on the fact that diazepam is a substrate for CYP2C19 and CYP3A4, it is possible that diazepam may interfere with the metabolism of drugs which are substrates for CYP2C19 and CYP3A4 leading to a potential drug-drug interaction).
No products indexed under this heading.

Estradiol Cypionate (There are no reports as to which isoenzymes could be inhibited or induced by diazepam. But based on the fact that diazepam is a substrate for CYP2C19 and CYP3A4, it is possible that diazepam may interfere with the metabolism of drugs which are substrates for CYP2C19 and CYP3A4 leading to a potential drug-drug interaction).
No products indexed under this heading.

Estradiol Valerate (There are no reports as to which isoenzymes could be inhibited or induced by diazepam. But based on the fact that diazepam is a substrate for CYP2C19 and CYP3A4, it is possible that diazepam may interfere with the metabolism of drugs which are substrates for CYP2C19 and CYP3A4 leading to a potential drug-drug interaction).
No products indexed under this heading.

Ethanol (Potential for synergistic CNS-depressant effect).
No products indexed under this heading.

Ethchlorvynol (Potential for synergistic CNS-depressant effect).
No products indexed under this heading.

Ethinamate (Potential for synergistic CNS-depressant effect).
No products indexed under this heading.

Ethinyl Estradiol (Studies suggest that CYP2C19 and CYP3A4 are the principal enzymes involved in the initial oxidative metabolism of diazepam. Therefore, potential interactions may occur when diazepam is given concurrently with agents that affect CYP2C19 and CYP3A4 activity. Potential inhibitors of CYP2C19 could decrease the rate of diazepam elimination). Products include:

Ethosuximide (Studies suggest that CYP2C19 and CYP3A4 are the principal enzymes involved in the initial oxidative metabolism of diazepam. Therefore, potential interactions may occur when diazepam is given concurrently with agents that affect CYP2C19 and CYP3A4 activity. Potential inducers of CYP3A4 could increase the rate of diazepam elimination).
No products indexed under this heading.

Ethotoin (There are no reports as to which isoenzymes could be inhibited or induced by diazepam. But based on the fact that diazepam is a substrate for CYP2C19 and CYP3A4, it is possible that diazepam may interfere with the metabolism of drugs which are substrates for CYP2C19 and CYP3A4 leading to a potential drug-drug interaction).
No products indexed under this heading.

Ethyl Alcohol (Potential for synergistic CNS-depressant effect).
No products indexed under this heading.

Ethynodiol Diacetate (Studies suggest that CYP2C19 and CYP3A4 are the principal enzymes involved in the initial oxidative metabolism of diazepam. Therefore, potential interactions may occur when diazepam is given concurrently with agents that affect CYP2C19 and CYP3A4 activity. Potential inhibitors of CYP2C19 could decrease the rate of diazepam elimination).
No products indexed under this heading.

Etoposide (There are no reports as to which isoenzymes could be inhibited or induced by diazepam. But based on the fact that diazepam is a substrate for CYP2C19 and CYP3A4, it is possible that diazepam may interfere with the metabolism of drugs which are substrates for CYP2C19 and CYP3A4 leading to a potential drug-drug interaction).
No products indexed under this heading.

Etoposide Phosphate (There are no reports as to which isoenzymes could be inhibited or induced by diazepam. But based on the fact that diazepam is a substrate for CYP2C19 and CYP3A4, it is possible that diazepam may interfere with the metabolism of drugs which are substrates for CYP2C19 and CYP3A4 leading to a potential drug-drug interaction).
No products indexed under this heading.

Felbamate (Studies suggest that CYP2C19 and CYP3A4 are the principal enzymes involved in the initial oxidative metabolism of diazepam. Therefore, potential interactions may occur when diazepam is given concurrently with agents that affect CYP2C19 and CYP3A4 activity. Potential inhibitors of CYP2C19 could decrease the rate of diazepam elimination).
No products indexed under this heading.

Felodipine (There are no reports as to which isoenzymes could be inhibited or induced by diazepam. But based on the fact that diazepam is a substrate for CYP2C19 and CYP3A4, it is possible that diazepam may interfere with the metabolism of drugs which are substrates for CYP2C19 and CYP3A4 leading to a potential drug-drug interaction).
No products indexed under this heading.

Fentanyl (Potential for synergistic CNS-depressant effect). Products include:

Fentanyl Citrate (Potential for synergistic CNS-depressant effect).
Products include:

Fluconazole (Studies suggest that CYP2C19 and CYP3A4 are the principal enzymes involved in the initial oxidative metabolism of diazepam. Therefore, potential interactions may occur when diazepam is given concurrently with agents that affect CYP2C19 and CYP3A4 activity. Potential inhibitors of CYP3A4 could decrease the rate of diazepam elimination).
No products indexed under this heading.

Fludrocortisone Acetate (Studies suggest that CYP2C19 and CYP3A4 are the principal enzymes involved in the initial oxidative metabolism of diazepam. Therefore, potential interactions may occur when diazepam is given concurrently with agents that affect CYP2C19 and CYP3A4 activity. Potential inducers of CYP3A4 could increase the rate of diazepam elimination).
No products indexed under this heading.

Fluoxetine (Studies suggest that CYP2C19 and CYP3A4 are the principal enzymes involved in the initial oxidative metabolism of diazepam. Therefore, potential interactions may occur when diazepam is given concurrently with agents that affect CYP2C19 and CYP3A4 activity. Potential inhibitors of CYP2C19 could decrease the rate of diazepam elimination).
No products indexed under this heading.

Fluoxetine Hydrochloride (Potential for synergistic CNS-depressant effect). Products include:

Fluphenazine Decanoate (Potential for synergistic CNS-depressant effect).
No products indexed under this heading.

Fluphenazine Enanthate (Potential for synergistic CNS-depressant effect).
No products indexed under this heading.

Fluphenazine Hydrochloride (Potential for synergistic CNS-depressant effect).
No products indexed under this heading.

Flurazepam Hydrochloride (Potential for synergistic CNS-depressant effect). Products include:

Fluvastatin Sodium (Studies suggest that CYP2C19 and CYP3A4 are the principal enzymes involved in the initial oxidative metabolism of diazepam. Therefore, potential interactions may occur when diazepam is given concurrently with agents that affect CYP2C19 and CYP3A4 activity. Potential inhibitors of CYP2C19 could decrease the rate of diazepam elimination). Products include:

Fluvoxamine (Studies suggest that CYP2C19 and CYP3A4 are the principal enzymes involved in the initial oxidative metabolism of diazepam. Therefore, potential interactions may occur when diazepam is given concurrently with agents that affect CYP2C19 and CYP3A4 activity. Potential inhibitors of CYP2C19 could decrease the rate of diazepam elimination).
No products indexed under this heading.

Fluvoxamine Maleate (Studies suggest that CYP2C19 and CYP3A4 are the principal enzymes involved in the initial oxidative metabolism of diazepam. Therefore, potential interactions may occur when diazepam is given concurrently with agents that affect CYP2C19 and CYP3A4 activity. Potential inhibitors of CYP2C19 could decrease the rate of diazepam elimination).
No products indexed under this heading.

Formoterol Fumarate (There are no reports as to which isoenzymes could be inhibited or induced by diazepam. But based on the fact that diazepam is a substrate for CYP2C19 and CYP3A4, it is possible that diazepam may interfere with the metabolism of drugs which are substrates for CYP2C19 and CYP3A4 leading to a potential drug-drug interaction). Products include:

Fosamprenavir Calcium (Studies suggest that CYP2C19 and CYP3A4 are the principal enzymes involved in the initial oxidative metabolism of diazepam. Therefore, potential interactions may occur when diazepam is given concurrently with agents that affect CYP2C19 and CYP3A4 activity. Potential inhibitors of CYP2C19 could decrease the rate of diazepam elimination). Products include:

Fosphenytoin (There are no reports as to which isoenzymes could be inhibited or induced by diazepam. But based on the fact that diazepam is a substrate for CYP2C19 and CYP3A4, it is possible that diazepam may interfere with the metabolism of drugs which are substrates for CYP2C19 and CYP3A4 leading to a potential drug-drug interaction).
No products indexed under this heading.

Fosphenytoin Sodium (Inducers of CYP3A4, such as phenytoin, could increase the rate of elimination of diazepam).
No products indexed under this heading.

Gabapentin (There are no reports as to which isoenzymes could be inhibited or induced by diazepam. But based on the fact that diazepam is a substrate for CYP2C19 and CYP3A4, it is possible that diazepam may interfere with the metabolism of drugs which are substrates for CYP2C19 and CYP3A4 leading to a potential drug-drug interaction). Products include:

IMPORTANT NOTE: Always consult each drug listing in the patient's regimen for possible interactions.

Garlic Extract (Studies suggest that CYP2C19 and CYP3A4 are the principal enzymes involved in the initial oxidative metabolism of diazepam. Therefore, potential interactions may occur when diazepam is given concurrently with agents that affect CYP2C19 and CYP3A4 activity. Potential inducers of CYP3A4 could increase the rate of diazepam elimination).
No products indexed under this heading.

Garlic Oil (Studies suggest that CYP2C19 and CYP3A4 are the principal enzymes involved in the initial oxidative metabolism of diazepam. Therefore, potential interactions may occur when diazepam is given concurrently with agents that affect CYP2C19 and CYP3A4 activity. Potential inducers of CYP3A4 could increase the rate of diazepam elimination).
No products indexed under this heading.

Glutethimide (Potential for synergistic CNS-depressant effect).
No products indexed under this heading.

Haloperidol (Potential for synergistic CNS-depressant effect).
No products indexed under this heading.

Haloperidol Decanoate (Potential for synergistic CNS-depressant effect).
No products indexed under this heading.

Haloperidol Lactate (There are no reports as to which isoenzymes could be inhibited or induced by diazepam. But based on the fact that diazepam is a substrate for CYP2C19 and CYP3A4, it is possible that diazepam may interfere with the metabolism of drugs which are substrates for CYP2C19 and CYP3A4 leading to a potential drug-drug interaction).
No products indexed under this heading.

Hydrocodone Bitartrate (Potential for synergistic CNS-depressant effect). Products include:
Hycodan **1116**
Hycotuss Expectorant Syrup **1117**
Vicodin Tablets **535**
Vicodin ES Tablets **536**
Vicodin HP Tablets **538**
Vicoprofen Tablets **539**
Zydone Tablets **1139**

Hydrocodone Polistirex (Potential for synergistic CNS-depressant effect). Products include:
Tussionex Pennkinetic Extended-Release Suspension...... **3327**

Hydrocortisone (Studies suggest that CYP2C19 and CYP3A4 are the principal enzymes involved in the initial oxidative metabolism of diazepam. Therefore, potential interactions may occur when diazepam is given concurrently with agents that affect CYP2C19 and CYP3A4 activity. Potential inducers of CYP3A4 could increase the rate of diazepam elimination). Products include:
Colocort Rectal Suspension, USP (Retention) 100 mg/60 mL.......... **2476**
Hydrocortone Tablets **1989**
Preparation H Hydrocortisone Cream.......... ▣**646**

Hydrocortisone Acetate (Studies suggest that CYP2C19 and CYP3A4 are the principal enzymes involved in the initial oxidative metabolism of diazepam. Therefore, potential interactions may occur when diazepam is given concurrently with agents that affect CYP2C19 and CYP3A4 activity. Potential inducers of CYP3A4 could increase the rate of diazepam elimination). Products include:
Analpram-HC **1159**
Pramosone **1161**
ProctoFoam-HC **3099**

Hydrocortisone Butyrate (Studies suggest that CYP2C19 and CYP3A4 are the principal enzymes involved in the initial oxidative metabolism of diazepam. Therefore, potential interactions may occur when diazepam is given concurrently with agents that affect CYP2C19 and CYP3A4 activity. Potential inducers of CYP3A4 could increase the rate of diazepam elimination). Products include:
Locoid Lipocream Cream **1160**

Hydrocortisone Cypionate (Studies suggest that CYP2C19 and CYP3A4 are the principal enzymes involved in the initial oxidative metabolism of diazepam. Therefore, potential interactions may occur when diazepam is given concurrently with agents that affect CYP2C19 and CYP3A4 activity. Potential inducers of CYP3A4 could increase the rate of diazepam elimination).
No products indexed under this heading.

Hydrocortisone Hemisuccinate (Studies suggest that CYP2C19 and CYP3A4 are the principal enzymes involved in the initial oxidative metabolism of diazepam. Therefore, potential interactions may occur when diazepam is given concurrently with agents that affect CYP2C19 and CYP3A4 activity. Potential inducers of CYP3A4 could increase the rate of diazepam elimination).
No products indexed under this heading.

Hydrocortisone Probutate (Studies suggest that CYP2C19 and CYP3A4 are the principal enzymes involved in the initial oxidative metabolism of diazepam. Therefore, potential interactions may occur when diazepam is given concurrently with agents that affect CYP2C19 and CYP3A4 activity. Potential inducers of CYP3A4 could increase the rate of diazepam elimination).
No products indexed under this heading.

Hydrocortisone Sodium Phosphate (Studies suggest that CYP2C19 and CYP3A4 are the principal enzymes involved in the initial oxidative metabolism of diazepam. Therefore, potential interactions may occur when diazepam is given concurrently with agents that affect CYP2C19 and CYP3A4 activity. Potential inducers of CYP3A4 could increase the rate of diazepam elimination).
No products indexed under this heading.

Hydrocortisone Sodium Succinate (Studies suggest that CYP2C19 and CYP3A4 are the principal enzymes involved in the initial oxidative metabolism of diazepam. Therefore, potential interactions may occur when diazepam is given concurrently with agents that affect CYP2C19 and CYP3A4 activity. Potential inducers of CYP3A4 could increase the rate of diazepam elimination).
No products indexed under this heading.

Hydrocortisone Valerate (Studies suggest that CYP2C19 and CYP3A4 are the principal enzymes involved in the initial oxidative metabolism of diazepam. Therefore, potential interactions may occur when diazepam is given concurrently with agents that affect CYP2C19 and CYP3A4 activity. Potential inducers of CYP3A4 could increase the rate of diazepam elimination).
No products indexed under this heading.

Hydromorphone Hydrochloride (Potential for synergistic CNS-depressant effect). Products include:
Dilaudid **440**
Dilaudid Non-Sterile Powder **440**
Dilaudid Oral Liquid **445**
Dilaudid Rectal Suppositories **440**
Dilaudid Tablets **440**
Dilaudid Tablets - 8 mg **445**
Dilaudid-HP **442**

Hydroxyzine Hydrochloride (Potential for synergistic CNS-depressant effect).
No products indexed under this heading.

Hypericum (Studies suggest that CYP2C19 and CYP3A4 are the principal enzymes involved in the initial oxidative metabolism of diazepam. Therefore, potential interactions may occur when diazepam is given concurrently with agents that affect CYP2C19 and CYP3A4 activity. Potential inducers of CYP3A4 could increase the rate of diazepam elimination). Products include:
Satiete Tablets .... ▣**832**

Hypericum Perforatum (Studies suggest that CYP2C19 and CYP3A4 are the principal enzymes involved in the initial oxidative metabolism of diazepam. Therefore, potential interactions may occur when diazepam is given concurrently with agents that affect CYP2C19 and CYP3A4 activity. Potential inducers of CYP3A4 could increase the rate of diazepam elimination).
No products indexed under this heading.

Imipramine Hydrochloride (Diazepam is a substrate of CYP2C19 and CYP3A4, it is possible that diazepam may interfere with the metabolism of drugs which are substrates for CYP2C19, such as imipramine; potential for synergistic CNS-depressant effect).
No products indexed under this heading.

Imipramine Pamoate (Diazepam is a substrate of CYP2C19 and CYP3A4, it is possible that diazepam may interfere with the metabolism of drugs which are substrates for CYP2C19, such as imipramine; potential for synergistic CNS-depressant effect).
No products indexed under this heading.

Indinavir Sulfate (Studies suggest that CYP2C19 and CYP3A4 are the principal enzymes involved in the initial oxidative metabolism of diazepam. Therefore, potential interactions may occur when diazepam is given concurrently with agents that affect CYP2C19 and CYP3A4 activity. Potential inhibitors of CYP3A4 could decrease the rate of diazepam elimination). Products include:
Crixivan Capsules **1940**

Indomethacin (Studies suggest that CYP2C19 and CYP3A4 are the principal enzymes involved in the initial oxidative metabolism of diazepam. Therefore, potential interactions may occur when diazepam is given concurrently with agents that affect CYP2C19 and CYP3A4 activity. Potential inhibitors of CYP2C19 could decrease the rate of diazepam elimination). Products include:
Indocin **1995**

Indomethacin Sodium Trihydrate (Studies suggest that CYP2C19 and CYP3A4 are the principal enzymes involved in the initial oxidative metabolism of diazepam. Therefore, potential interactions may occur when diazepam is given concurrently with agents that affect CYP2C19 and CYP3A4 activity. Potential inhibitors of CYP2C19 could decrease the rate of diazepam elimination). Products include:
Indocin I.V. **2465**

Isocarboxazid (Potential for synergistic CNS-depressant effect).
No products indexed under this heading.

Isoflurane (Potential for synergistic CNS-depressant effect).
No products indexed under this heading.

Isoniazid (Studies suggest that CYP2C19 and CYP3A4 are the principal enzymes involved in the initial oxidative metabolism of diazepam. Therefore, potential interactions may occur when diazepam is given concurrently with agents that affect CYP2C19 and CYP3A4 activity. Potential inhibitors of CYP2C19 could decrease the rate of diazepam elimination).
No products indexed under this heading.

Isradipine (There are no reports as to which isoenzymes could be inhibited or induced by diazepam. But based on the fact that diazepam is a substrate for CYP2C19 and CYP3A4, it is possible that diazepam may interfere with the metabolism of drugs which are substrates for CYP2C19 and CYP3A4 leading to a potential drug-drug interaction). Products include:
DynaCirc CR Tablets **2721**

Itraconazole (Studies suggest that CYP2C19 and CYP3A4 are the principal enzymes involved in the initial oxidative metabolism of diazepam. Therefore, potential interactions may occur when diazepam is given concurrently with agents that affect CYP2C19 and CYP3A4 activity. Potential inhibitors of CYP3A4 could decrease the rate of diazepam elimination).
No products indexed under this heading.

Ketamine Hydrochloride (Potential for synergistic CNS-depressant effect).
No products indexed under this heading.

Ketoconazole (Potential inhibitors of CYP3A4, such as ketoconazole, could decrease the rate of diazepam elimination). Products include:
Nizoral A-D Shampoo, 1% **1868**

Lamotrigine (There are no reports as to which isoenzymes could be inhibited or induced by diazepam. But based on the fact that diazepam is a substrate for CYP2C19 and CYP3A4, it is possible that diazepam may interfere with the metabolism of drugs which are substrates for

CYP2C19 and CYP3A4 leading to a potential drug-drug interaction). Products include:

Lamictal 1481

Lansoprazole (Studies suggest that CYP2C19 and CYP3A4 are the principal enzymes involved in the initial oxidative metabolism of diazepam. Therefore, potential interactions may occur when diazepam is given concurrently with agents that affect CYP2C19 and CYP3A4 activity. Potential inhibitors of CYP2C19 could decrease the rate of diazepam elimination). Products include:

Prevacid Delayed-Release Capsules 3271
Prevacid for Delayed-Release Oral Suspension 3271
Prevacid SoluTab Delayed-Release Orally Disintegrating Tablets 3271
Prevacid I.V. for Injection 3277
Prevacid NapraPAC 3280
PREVPAC 3284

Letrozole (Studies suggest that CYP2C19 and CYP3A4 are the principal enzymes involved in the initial oxidative metabolism of diazepam. Therefore, potential interactions may occur when diazepam is given concurrently with agents that affect CYP2C19 and CYP3A4 activity. Potential inhibitors of CYP2C19 could decrease the rate of diazepam elimination). Products include:

Femara Tablets 2214

Levetiracetam (There are no reports as to which isoenzymes could be inhibited or induced by diazepam. But based on the fact that diazepam is a substrate for CYP2C19 and CYP3A4, it is possible that diazepam may interfere with the metabolism of drugs which are substrates for CYP2C19 and CYP3A4 leading to a potential drug-drug interaction). Products include:

Keppra Injection 3320
Keppra Oral Solution 3314
Keppra Tablets 3314

Levomethadyl Acetate Hydrochloride (Potential for synergistic CNS-depressant effect).

No products indexed under this heading.

Levonorgestrel (Studies suggest that CYP2C19 and CYP3A4 are the principal enzymes involved in the initial oxidative metabolism of diazepam. Therefore, potential interactions may occur when diazepam is given concurrently with agents that affect CYP2C19 and CYP3A4 activity. Potential inhibitors of CYP2C19 could decrease the rate of diazepam elimination). Products include:

Climara Pro Transdermal System 776
Mirena Intrauterine System 787
Plan B Tablets 1076
Seasonique Tablets 1077

Levorphanol Tartrate (Potential for synergistic CNS-depressant effect).

No products indexed under this heading.

Lidocaine (There are no reports as to which isoenzymes could be inhibited or induced by diazepam. But based on the fact that diazepam is a substrate for CYP2C19 and CYP3A4, it is possible that diazepam may interfere with the metabolism of drugs which are substrates for CYP2C19 and CYP3A4 leading to a potential drug-drug interaction). Products include:

Lidoderm Patch 1118
Synera Topical Patch 1137

Lidocaine Hydrochloride (There are no reports as to which isoenzymes could be inhibited or induced by diazepam. But based on the fact that diazepam is a substrate for CYP2C19 and CYP3A4, it is possible that diazepam may interfere with the metabolism of drugs which are substrates for CYP2C19 and CYP3A4 leading to a potential drug-drug interaction).

No products indexed under this heading.

Lopinavir (Studies suggest that CYP2C19 and CYP3A4 are the principal enzymes involved in the initial oxidative metabolism of diazepam. Therefore, potential interactions may occur when diazepam is given concurrently with agents that affect CYP2C19 and CYP3A4 activity. Potential inhibitors of CYP3A4 could decrease the rate of diazepam elimination). Products include:

Kaletra 476

Loratadine (Studies suggest that CYP2C19 and CYP3A4 are the principal enzymes involved in the initial oxidative metabolism of diazepam. Therefore, potential interactions may occur when diazepam is given concurrently with agents that affect CYP2C19 and CYP3A4 activity. Potential inhibitors of CYP3A4 could decrease the rate of diazepam elimination). Products include:

Alavert Allergy & Sinus D-12 Hour Tablets 771
Alavert 771
Children's Claritin Allergy Oral Solution 771
Claritin Non-Drowsy 24 Hour Tablets 772
Claritin Reditabs 24 Hour Non-Drowsy Tablets 772
Claritin-D Non-Drowsy 12 Hour Tablets 772
Claritin-D Non-Drowsy 24 Hour Tablets 772

Lorazepam (Potential for synergistic CNS-depressant effect).

No products indexed under this heading.

Lovastatin (There are no reports as to which isoenzymes could be inhibited or induced by diazepam. But based on the fact that diazepam is a substrate for CYP2C19 and CYP3A4, it is possible that diazepam may interfere with the metabolism of drugs which are substrates for CYP2C19 and CYP3A4 leading to a potential drug-drug interaction). Products include:

Advicor Tablets 1722
Altoprev Extended-Release Tablets 3109
Mevacor Tablets 2021

Loxapine Hydrochloride (Potential for synergistic CNS-depressant effect).

No products indexed under this heading.

Loxapine Succinate (Potential for synergistic CNS-depressant effect).

No products indexed under this heading.

Maprotiline Hydrochloride (Potential for synergistic CNS-depressant effect).

No products indexed under this heading.

Meperidine Hydrochloride (Potential for synergistic CNS-depressant effect).

No products indexed under this heading.

Mephenytoin (Studies suggest that CYP2C19 and CYP3A4 are the principal enzymes involved in the initial oxidative metabolism of diazepam. Therefore, potential interactions may occur when diazepam is given concurrently with agents that affect CYP2C19 and CYP3A4 activity. Potential inducers of CYP3A4 could increase the rate of diazepam elimination).

No products indexed under this heading.

Mephobarbital (Potential for synergistic CNS-depressant effect).

No products indexed under this heading.

Meprobamate (Potential for synergistic CNS-depressant effect).

No products indexed under this heading.

Mesoridazine Besylate (Potential for synergistic CNS-depressant effect).

No products indexed under this heading.

Mestranol (Studies suggest that CYP2C19 and CYP3A4 are the principal enzymes involved in the initial oxidative metabolism of diazepam. Therefore, potential interactions may occur when diazepam is given concurrently with agents that affect CYP2C19 and CYP3A4 activity. Potential inhibitors of CYP2C19 could decrease the rate of diazepam elimination).

No products indexed under this heading.

Methadone Hydrochloride (Potential for synergistic CNS-depressant effect).

No products indexed under this heading.

Methohexital Sodium (Potential for synergistic CNS-depressant effect).

No products indexed under this heading.

Methotrimeprazine (Potential for synergistic CNS-depressant effect).

No products indexed under this heading.

Methoxyflurane (Potential for synergistic CNS-depressant effect).

No products indexed under this heading.

Methsuximide (Studies suggest that CYP2C19 and CYP3A4 are the principal enzymes involved in the initial oxidative metabolism of diazepam. Therefore, potential interactions may occur when diazepam is given concurrently with agents that affect CYP2C19 and CYP3A4 activity. Potential inducers of CYP3A4 could increase the rate of diazepam elimination).

No products indexed under this heading.

Methylprednisolone (Studies suggest that CYP2C19 and CYP3A4 are the principal enzymes involved in the initial oxidative metabolism of diazepam. Therefore, potential interactions may occur when diazepam is given concurrently with agents that affect CYP2C19 and CYP3A4 activity. Potential inducers of CYP3A4 could increase the rate of diazepam elimination).

No products indexed under this heading.

Methylprednisolone Acetate (Studies suggest that CYP2C19 and CYP3A4 are the principal enzymes involved in the initial oxidative metabolism of diazepam. Therefore, potential interactions may occur when diazepam is given concurrently with agents that affect CYP2C19 and CYP3A4 activity. Potential inducers of CYP3A4 could increase the rate of diazepam elimination). Products include:

Depo-Medrol Injectable Suspension 2617
Depo-Medrol Single-Dose Vial 2619

Methylprednisolone Sodium Succinate (Studies suggest that CYP2C19 and CYP3A4 are the principal enzymes involved in the initial oxidative metabolism of diazepam. Therefore, potential interactions may occur when diazepam is given concurrently with agents that affect CYP2C19 and CYP3A4 activity. Potential inducers of CYP3A4 could increase the rate of diazepam elimination).

No products indexed under this heading.

Metronidazole (Studies suggest that CYP2C19 and CYP3A4 are the principal enzymes involved in the initial oxidative metabolism of diazepam. Therefore, potential interactions may occur when diazepam is given concurrently with agents that affect CYP2C19 and CYP3A4 activity. Potential inhibitors of CYP3A4 could decrease the rate of diazepam elimination). Products include:

Metrogel 1% 1211
MetroGel-Vaginal Gel 1855
Vandazole Vaginal Gel 3338

Metronidazole Benzoate (Studies suggest that CYP2C19 and CYP3A4 are the principal enzymes involved in the initial oxidative metabolism of diazepam. Therefore, potential interactions may occur when diazepam is given concurrently with agents that affect CYP2C19 and CYP3A4 activity. Potential inhibitors of CYP3A4 could decrease the rate of diazepam elimination).

No products indexed under this heading.

Metronidazole Hydrochloride (Studies suggest that CYP2C19 and CYP3A4 are the principal enzymes involved in the initial oxidative metabolism of diazepam. Therefore, potential interactions may occur when diazepam is given concurrently with agents that affect CYP2C19 and CYP3A4 activity. Potential inhibitors of CYP3A4 could decrease the rate of diazepam elimination).

No products indexed under this heading.

Miconazole (Studies suggest that CYP2C19 and CYP3A4 are the principal enzymes involved in the initial oxidative metabolism of diazepam. Therefore, potential interactions may occur when diazepam is given concurrently with agents that affect CYP2C19 and CYP3A4 activity. Potential inhibitors of CYP3A4 could decrease the rate of diazepam elimination).

No products indexed under this heading.

Miconazole Nitrate (Studies suggest that CYP2C19 and CYP3A4 are the principal enzymes involved in the initial oxidative metabolism of diazepam. Therefore, potential interactions may occur when diazepam is given concurrently with agents that affect CYP2C19 and CYP3A4 activity. Potential inhibitors of CYP3A4 could decrease the rate of diazepam elimination). Products include:

Desenex .... ◘ 635
Desenex Jock Itch Spray Powder ... ◘ 635

Midazolam Hydrochloride (Potential for synergistic CNS-depressant effect).

No products indexed under this heading.

Mirtazapine (Potential for synergistic CNS-depressant effect).

No products indexed under this heading.

Moclobemide (Potential for synergistic CNS-depressant effect).

No products indexed under this heading.

Modafinil (Studies suggest that CYP2C19 and CYP3A4 are the principal enzymes involved in the initial oxidative metabolism of diazepam. Therefore, potential interactions may occur when diazepam is given concurrently with agents that affect CYP2C19 and CYP3A4 activity. Potential inhibitors of CYP2C19 could decrease the rate of diazepam elimination). Products include:

Provigil Tablets 988

Molindone Hydrochloride (Potential for synergistic CNS-depressant effect). Products include:

Moban Tablets 1119

Morphine Sulfate (Potential for synergistic CNS-depressant effect). Products include:

Avinza Capsules 1741
Kadian Capsules 577
MS Contin Tablets 2701

Nefazodone Hydrochloride (Potential for synergistic CNS-depressant effect).

No products indexed under this heading.

Nelfinavir Mesylate (Studies suggest that CYP2C19 and CYP3A4 are the principal enzymes involved in the initial oxidative metabolism of diazepam. Therefore, potential interactions may occur when diazepam is given concurrently with agents that affect CYP2C19 and CYP3A4 activity. Potential inhibitors of CYP3A4 could decrease the rate of diazepam elimination). Products include:

Viracept 2577

Nevirapine (Studies suggest that CYP2C19 and CYP3A4 are the principal enzymes involved in the initial oxidative metabolism of diazepam. Therefore, potential interactions may occur when diazepam is given concurrently with agents that affect CYP2C19 and CYP3A4 activity. Potential inhibitors of CYP3A4 could decrease the rate of diazepam elimination). Products include:

Viramune Oral Suspension 873
Viramune Tablets 873

Niacinamide (Studies suggest that CYP2C19 and CYP3A4 are the principal enzymes involved in the initial oxidative metabolism of diazepam. Therefore, potential interactions may occur when diazepam is given concurrently with agents that affect CYP2C19 and CYP3A4 activity. Potential inhibitors of CYP3A4 could decrease the rate of diazepam elimination).

No products indexed under this heading.

Nicardipine Hydrochloride (There are no reports as to which isoenzymes could be inhibited or induced by diazepam. But based on the fact that diazepam is a substrate for CYP2C19 and CYP3A4, it is possible that diazepam may interfere with the metabolism of drugs which are substrates for CYP2C19 and CYP3A4 leading to a potential drug-drug interaction). Products include:

Cardene I.V. 2497

Nicotinamide (Studies suggest that CYP2C19 and CYP3A4 are the principal enzymes involved in the initial oxidative metabolism of diazepam. Therefore, potential interactions may occur when diazepam is given concurrently with agents that affect CYP2C19 and CYP3A4 activity. Potential inhibitors of CYP3A4 could decrease the rate of diazepam elimination). Products include:

Nicomide Tablets 1088

Nifedipine (Studies suggest that CYP2C19 and CYP3A4 are the principal enzymes involved in the initial oxidative metabolism of diazepam. Therefore, potential interactions may occur when diazepam is given concurrently with agents that affect CYP2C19 and CYP3A4 activity. Potential inhibitors of CYP3A4 could decrease the rate of diazepam elimination). Products include:

Adalat CC Tablets 2964

Nilutamide (There are no reports as to which isoenzymes could be inhibited or induced by diazepam. But based on the fact that diazepam is a substrate for CYP2C19 and CYP3A4, it is possible that diazepam may interfere with the metabolism of drugs which are substrates for CYP2C19 and CYP3A4 leading to a potential drug-drug interaction).

No products indexed under this heading.

Nimodipine (There are no reports as to which isoenzymes could be inhibited or induced by diazepam. But based on the fact that diazepam is a substrate for CYP2C19 and CYP3A4, it is possible that diazepam may interfere with the metabolism of drugs which are substrates for CYP2C19 and CYP3A4 leading to a potential drug-drug interaction). Products include:

Nimotop Capsules 749

Nisoldipine (There are no reports as to which isoenzymes could be inhibited or induced by diazepam. But based on the fact that diazepam is a substrate for CYP2C19 and CYP3A4, it is possible that diazepam may interfere with the metabolism of drugs which are substrates for CYP2C19 and CYP3A4 leading to a potential drug-drug interaction). Products include:

Sular Tablets 3122

Nitrendipine (There are no reports as to which isoenzymes could be inhibited or induced by diazepam. But based on the fact that diazepam is a substrate for CYP2C19 and CYP3A4, it is possible that diazepam may interfere with the metabolism of drugs which are substrates for CYP2C19 and CYP3A4 leading to a potential drug-drug interaction).

No products indexed under this heading.

Norethindrone (Studies suggest that CYP2C19 and CYP3A4 are the principal enzymes involved in the initial oxidative metabolism of diazepam. Therefore, potential interactions may occur when diazepam is given concurrently with agents that affect CYP2C19 and CYP3A4 activity. Potential inhibitors of CYP2C19 could decrease the rate of diazepam elimination). Products include:

Ortho Micronor Tablets 2426

Norethindrone Acetate (Studies suggest that CYP2C19 and CYP3A4 are the principal enzymes involved in the initial oxidative metabolism of diazepam. Therefore, potential inter actions may occur when diazepam is given concurrently with agents that affect CYP2C19 and CYP3A4 activity. Potential inducers of CYP2C19 could increase the rate of diazepam elimination).

No products indexed under this heading.

Norethynodrel (Studies suggest that CYP2C19 and CYP3A4 are the principal enzymes involved in the initial oxidative metabolism of diazepam. Therefore, potential interactions may occur when diazepam is given concurrently with agents that affect CYP2C19 and CYP3A4 activity. Potential inhibitors of CYP2C19 could decrease the rate of diazepam elimination).

No products indexed under this heading.

Norfloxacin (Studies suggest that CYP2C19 and CYP3A4 are the principal enzymes involved in the initial oxidative metabolism of diazepam. Therefore, potential interactions may occur when diazepam is given concurrently with agents that affect CYP2C19 and CYP3A4 activity. Potential inhibitors of CYP3A4 could decrease the rate of diazepam elimination). Products include:

Noroxin Tablets 2032

Norgestimate (Studies suggest that CYP2C19 and CYP3A4 are the principal enzymes involved in the initial oxidative metabolism of diazepam. Therefore, potential interactions may occur when diazepam is given concurrently with agents that affect CYP2C19 and CYP3A4 activity. Potential inhibitors of CYP2C19 could decrease the rate of diazepam elimination). Products include:

Ortho-Cyclen/Ortho Tri-Cyclen 2429
Ortho Tri-Cyclen Lo Tablets 2436

Norgestrel (Studies suggest that CYP2C19 and CYP3A4 are the principal enzymes involved in the initial oxidative metabolism of diazepam. Therefore, potential interactions may occur when diazepam is given concurrently with agents that affect CYP2C19 and CYP3A4 activity. Potential inhibitors of CYP2C19 could decrease the rate of diazepam elimination).

No products indexed under this heading.

Nortriptyline Hydrochloride (Potential for synergistic CNS-depressant effect).

No products indexed under this heading.

Olanzapine (Potential for synergistic CNS-depressant effect). Products include:

Symbyax Capsules 1819
Zyprexa Tablets 1830
Zyprexa IntraMuscular 1830
Zyprexa ZYDIS Orally Disintegrating Tablets 1830

Omeprazole (Diazepam is a substrate of CYP2C19 and CYP3A4, it is possible that diazepam may interfere with the metabolism of drugs which are substrates for CYP2C19, such as omeprazole). Products include:

Zegerid Capsules 2958
Zegerid Powder for Oral Solution 2958

Ondansetron (There are no reports as to which isoenzymes could be inhibited or induced by diazepam. But based on the fact that diazepam is a substrate for CYP2C19 and CYP3A4, it is possible that diazepam may interfere with the metabolism of drugs which are substrates for CYP2C19 and CYP3A4 leading to a potential drug-drug interaction). Products include:

Zofran ODT Orally Disintegrating Tablets 1639

Ondansetron Hydrochloride (There are no reports as to which isoenzymes could be inhibited or induced by diazepam. But based on the fact that diazepam is a substrate for CYP2C19 and CYP3A4, it is possible that diazepam may interfere with the metabolism of drugs which are substrates for CYP2C19 and CYP3A4 leading to a potential drug-drug interaction). Products include:

Zofran Injection 1634
Zofran 1639

Oxazepam (Potential for synergistic CNS-depressant effect).

No products indexed under this heading.

Oxcarbazepine (Studies suggest that CYP2C19 and CYP3A4 are the principal enzymes involved in the initial oxidative metabolism of diazepam. Therefore, potential interactions may occur when diazepam is given concurrently with agents that affect CYP2C19 and CYP3A4 activity. Potential inhibitors of CYP2C19 could decrease the rate of diazepam elimination). Products include:

Trileptal Tablets 2300
Trileptal Oral Suspension 2300

Oxycodone Hydrochloride (Potential for synergistic CNS-depressant effect). Products include:

OxyContin Tablets 2703
OxyFast Oral Concentrate Solution 2708
OxyIR Capsules 2708
Percocet Tablets 1131
Percodan Tablets 1132

Paclitaxel (Diazepam is a substrate of CYP2C19 and CYP3A4, it is possible that diazepam may interfere with the metabolism of drugs which are substrates for CYP3A4, such as paclitaxel).

No products indexed under this heading.

Pantoprazole Sodium (There are no reports as to which isoenzymes could be inhibited or induced by diazepam. But based on the fact that diazepam is a substrate for CYP2C19 and CYP3A4, it is possible that diazepam may interfere with the metabolism of drugs which are substrates for CYP2C19 and CYP3A4 leading to a potential drug-drug interaction). Products include:

Protonix I.V. 3472
Protonix Tablets 3469

Paramethadione (There are no reports as to which isoenzymes could be inhibited or induced by diazepam. But based on the fact that diazepam is a substrate for CYP2C19 and CYP3A4, it is possible that diazepam may interfere with the metabolism of drugs which are substrates for CYP2C19 and CYP3A4 leading to a potential drug-drug interaction).
No products indexed under this heading.

Pargyline Hydrochloride (Potential for synergistic CNS-depressant effect).
No products indexed under this heading.

Paroxetine Hydrochloride (Potential for synergistic CNS-depressant effect). Products include:
Paxil CR Controlled-Release Tablets **1538**
Paxil **1530**

Pentamidine Isethionate (There are no reports as to which isoenzymes could be inhibited or induced by diazepam. But based on the fact that diazepam is a substrate for CYP2C19 and CYP3A4, it is possible that diazepam may interfere with the metabolism of drugs which are substrates for CYP2C19 and CYP3A4 leading to a potential drug-drug interaction).
No products indexed under this heading.

Pentobarbital Sodium (Potential for synergistic CNS-depressant effect). Products include:
Nembutal Sodium Solution, USP **2470**

Perphenazine (Potential for synergistic CNS-depressant effect).
No products indexed under this heading.

Phenacemide (There are no reports as to which isoenzymes could be inhibited or induced by diazepam. But based on the fact that diazepam is a substrate for CYP2C19 and CYP3A4, it is possible that diazepam may interfere with the metabolism of drugs which are substrates for CYP2C19 and CYP3A4 leading to a potential drug-drug interaction).
No products indexed under this heading.

Phenelzine Sulfate (Potential for synergistic CNS-depressant effect).
No products indexed under this heading.

Phenobarbital (Potential inducers of CYP3A4, such as phenobarbital, could increase the rate of elimination of diazepam; potential for synergistic CNS-depressant effect). Products include:
Donnatal Extentabs **2493**

Phenobarbital Sodium (Studies suggest that CYP2C19 and CYP3A4 are the principal enzymes involved in the initial oxidative metabolism of diazepam. Therefore, potential interactions may occur when diazepam is given concurrently with agents that affect CYP2C19 and CYP3A4 activity. Potential inducers of CYP2C19 could increase the rate of diazepam elimination).
No products indexed under this heading.

Phensuximide (There are no reports as to which isoenzymes could be inhibited or induced by diazepam. But based on the fact that diazepam is a substrate for CYP2C19 and CYP3A4, it is possible that diazepam may interfere with the metabolism of drugs which are substrates for CYP2C19 and CYP3A4 leading to a potential drug-drug interaction).
No products indexed under this heading.

Phenytoin (Inducers of CYP3A4, such as phenytoin, could increase the rate of elimination of diazepam).
No products indexed under this heading.

Phenytoin Sodium (Inducers of CYP3A4, such as phenytoin, could increase the rate of elimination of diazepam). Products include:
Phenytek Capsules **2160**

Pimozide (There are no reports as to which isoenzymes could be inhibited or induced by diazepam. But based on the fact that diazepam is a substrate for CYP2C19 and CYP3A4, it is possible that diazepam may interfere with the metabolism of drugs which are substrates for CYP2C19 and CYP3A4 leading to a potential drug-drug interaction).
No products indexed under this heading.

Polyestradiol Phosphate (There are no reports as to which isoenzymes could be inhibited or induced by diazepam. But based on the fact that diazepam is a substrate for CYP2C19 and CYP3A4, it is possible that diazepam may interfere with the metabolism of drugs which are substrates for CYP2C19 and CYP3A4 leading to a potential drug-drug interaction).
No products indexed under this heading.

Prazepam (Potential for synergistic CNS-depressant effect).
No products indexed under this heading.

Prednisolone Acetate (Studies suggest that CYP2C19 and CYP3A4 are the principal enzymes involved in the initial oxidative metabolism of diazepam. Therefore, potential interactions may occur when diazepam is given concurrently with agents that affect CYP2C19 and CYP3A4 activity. Potential inducers of CYP3A4 could increase the rate of diazepam elimination). Products include:
Blephamide Ophthalmic Ointment **568**
Blephamide Ophthalmic Suspension **569**
Poly-Pred Ophthalmic Suspension .... ⊙**233**
Pred Forte Ophthalmic Suspension .... ⊙**235**
Pred Mild Ophthalmic Suspension .... ⊙**238**
Pred-G Ophthalmic Ointment .... ⊙**237**
Pred-G Ophthalmic Suspension .... ⊙**236**

Prednisolone Sodium Phosphate (Studies suggest that CYP2C19 and CYP3A4 are the principal enzymes involved in the initial oxidative metabolism of diazepam. Therefore, potential interactions may occur when diazepam is given concurrently with agents that affect CYP2C19 and CYP3A4 activity. Potential inducers of CYP3A4 could increase the rate of diazepam elimination).
No products indexed under this heading.

Prednisolone Tebutate (Studies suggest that CYP2C19 and CYP3A4 are the principal enzymes involved in the initial oxidative metabolism of diazepam. Therefore, potential interactions may occur when diazepam is given concurrently with agents that affect CYP2C19 and CYP3A4 activity. Potential inducers of CYP3A4 could increase the rate of diazepam elimination).
No products indexed under this heading.

Prednisone (Studies suggest that CYP2C19 and CYP3A4 are the principal enzymes involved in the initial oxidative metabolism of diazepam. Therefore, potential interactions may occur when diazepam is given concurrently with agents that affect CYP2C19 and CYP3A4 activity. Potential inducers of CYP2C19 could increase the rate of diazepam elimination).
No products indexed under this heading.

Primidone (Studies suggest that CYP2C19 and CYP3A4 are the principal enzymes involved in the initial oxidative metabolism of diazepam. Therefore, potential interactions may occur when diazepam is given concurrently with agents that affect CYP2C19 and CYP3A4 activity. Potential inducers of CYP3A4 could increase the rate of diazepam elimination).
No products indexed under this heading.

Procarbazine Hydrochloride (Potential for synergistic CNS-depressant effect). Products include:
Matulane Capsules **3191**

Prochlorperazine (Potential for synergistic CNS-depressant effect).
No products indexed under this heading.

Progesterone (There are no reports as to which isoenzymes could be inhibited or induced by diazepam. But based on the fact that diazepam is a substrate for CYP2C19 and CYP3A4, it is possible that diazepam may interfere with the metabolism of drugs which are substrates for CYP2C19 and CYP3A4 leading to a potential drug-drug interaction). Products include:
Prochieve 4% Gel **1003**
Prochieve 8% Gel **1003**
Prometrium Capsules (100 mg, 200 mg) **3203**

Proguanil Hydrochloride (There are no reports as to which isoenzymes could be inhibited or induced by diazepam. But based on the fact that diazepam is a substrate for CYP2C19 and CYP3A4, it is possible that diazepam may interfere with the metabolism of drugs which are substrates for CYP2C19 and CYP3A4 leading to a potential drug-drug interaction). Products include:
Malarone Pediatric Tablets **1517**
Malarone Tablets **1517**

Promethazine Hydrochloride (Potential for synergistic CNS-depressant effect). Products include:
Phenergan Tablets and Suppositories **3440**

Propofol (Potential for synergistic CNS-depressant effect).
No products indexed under this heading.

Propoxyphene Hydrochloride (Potential for synergistic CNS-depressant effect).
No products indexed under this heading.

Propoxyphene Napsylate (Potential for synergistic CNS-depressant effect).
No products indexed under this heading.

Propranolol Hydrochloride (Diazepam is a substrate of CYP2C19 and CYP3A4; it is possible that diazepam may interfere with the metabolism of drugs which are substrates for CYP2C19, such as propranolol). Products include:
Inderal LA Long-Acting Capsules **3429**
InnoPran XL Capsules **2723**

Protriptyline Hydrochloride (Potential for synergistic CNS-depressant effect).
No products indexed under this heading.

Quazepam (Potential for synergistic CNS-depressant effect).
No products indexed under this heading.

Quetiapine Fumarate (Potential for synergistic CNS-depressant effect). Products include:
Seroquel Tablets **690**

Quinidine (Potential inhibitors of CYP2C19, such as quinidine, could decrease the rate of diazepam elimination).
No products indexed under this heading.

Quinidine Gluconate (Potential inhibitors of CYP2C19, such as quinidine, could decrease the rate of diazepam elimination).
No products indexed under this heading.

Quinidine Hydrochloride (Potential inhibitors of CYP2C19, such as quinidine, could decrease the rate of diazepam elimination).
No products indexed under this heading.

Quinidine Polygalacturonate (Potential inhibitors of CYP2C19, such as quinidine, could decrease the rate of diazepam elimination).
No products indexed under this heading.

Quinidine Sulfate (Potential inhibitors of CYP2C19, such as quinidine, could decrease the rate of diazepam elimination).
No products indexed under this heading.

Quinine (Studies suggest that CYP2C19 and CYP3A4 are the principal enzymes involved in the initial oxidative metabolism of diazepam. Therefore, potential interactions may occur when diazepam is given concurrently with agents that affect CYP2C19 and CYP3A4 activity. Potential inhibitors of CYP3A4 could decrease the rate of diazepam elimination).
No products indexed under this heading.

Quinine Sulfate (Studies suggest that CYP2C19 and CYP3A4 are the principal enzymes involved in the initial oxidative metabolism of diazepam. Therefore, potential interactions may occur when diazepam is given concurrently with agents that affect CYP2C19 and CYP3A4 activity. Potential inhibitors of CYP3A4 could decrease the rate of diazepam elimination).
No products indexed under this heading.

Quinupristin (Studies suggest that CYP2C19 and CYP3A4 are the principal enzymes involved in the initial oxidative metabolism of diazepam. Therefore, potential interactions may occur when diazepam is given concurrently with agents that affect CYP2C19 and CYP3A4 activity. Potential inhibitors of CYP3A4 could decrease the rate of diazepam elimination).
No products indexed under this heading.

Rabeprazole Sodium (There are no reports as to which isoenzymes could be inhibited or induced by diazepam. But based on the fact that diazepam is a substrate for CYP2C19 and CYP3A4, it is possible that diazepam may interfere with the metabolism of drugs which are substrates for CYP2C19 and CYP3A4 leading to a potential drug-drug interaction). Products include:
Aciphex Tablets **1090**

Ranitidine Bismuth Citrate (Studies suggest that CYP2C19 and CYP3A4 are the principal enzymes involved in the initial oxidative metabolism of diazepam. Therefore, potential interactions may occur when diazepam is given concurrently with agents that affect CYP2C19 and CYP3A4 activity. Potential inhibitors of CYP3A4 could decrease the rate of diazepam elimination).
No products indexed under this heading.

Ranitidine Hydrochloride (Studies suggest that CYP2C19 and CYP3A4 are the principal enzymes involved in the initial oxidative metabolism of diazepam. Therefore, potential interactions may occur when diazepam is given concurrently with agents that affect CYP2C19 and CYP3A4 activity. Potential inhibitors of CYP3A4 could decrease the rate of diazepam elimination). Products include:
Zantac **1624**
Zantac Injection **1619**
Zantac Injection Pharmacy Bulk Package **1622**

Remifentanil Hydrochloride (Potential for synergistic CNS-depressant effect).
No products indexed under this heading.

Rifabutin (Studies suggest that CYP2C19 and CYP3A4 are the principal enzymes involved in the initial oxidative metabolism of diazepam. Therefore, potential interactions may occur when diazepam is given concurrently with agents that affect CYP2C19 and CYP3A4 activity. Potential inducers of CYP3A4 could increase the rate of diazepam elimination).
No products indexed under this heading.

Rifampicin (Studies suggest that CYP2C19 and CYP3A4 are the principal enzymes involved in the initial oxidative metabolism of diazepam. Therefore, potential interactions may occur when diazepam is given concurrently with agents that affect CYP2C19 and CYP3A4 activity. Potential inducers of CYP3A4 could increase the rate of diazepam elimination).
No products indexed under this heading.

Rifampin (Inducers of CYP3A4, such as rifampin, could increase the rate of elimination of diazepam)..
No products indexed under this heading.

Rifapentine (Studies suggest that CYP2C19 and CYP3A4 are the principal enzymes involved in the initial oxidative metabolism of diazepam. Therefore, potential interactions may occur when diazepam is given concurrently with agents that affect CYP2C19 and CYP3A4 activity. Potential inducers of CYP3A4 could increase the rate of diazepam elimination).
No products indexed under this heading.

Risperidone (Potential for synergistic CNS-depressant effect). Products include:
Risperdal **1676**
Risperdal Consta Long-Acting Injection **1682**
Risperdal M-Tab Orally Disintegrating Tablets **1676**

Ritonavir (Studies suggest that CYP2C19 and CYP3A4 are the principal enzymes involved in the initial oxidative metabolism of diazepam. Therefore, potential interactions may occur when diazepam is given concurrently with agents that affect CYP2C19 and CYP3A4 activity. Potential inhibitors of CYP2C19 could decrease the rate of diazepam elimination). Products include:
Kaletra **476**
Norvir **503**

Saquinavir (Studies suggest that CYP2C19 and CYP3A4 are the principal enzymes involved in the initial oxidative metabolism of diazepam. Therefore, potential interactions may occur when diazepam is given concurrently with agents that affect CYP2C19 and CYP3A4 activity. Potential inhibitors of CYP3A4 could decrease the rate of diazepam elimination).
No products indexed under this heading.

Saquinavir Mesylate (Studies suggest that CYP2C19 and CYP3A4 are the principal enzymes involved in the initial oxidative metabolism of diazepam. Therefore, potential interactions may occur when diazepam is given concurrently with agents that affect CYP2C19 and CYP3A4 activity. Potential inhibitors of CYP3A4 could decrease the rate of diazepam elimination). Products include:
Invirase **2772**

Secobarbital Sodium (Potential for synergistic CNS-depressant effect).
No products indexed under this heading.

Selegiline Hydrochloride (Potential for synergistic CNS-depressant effect). Products include:
Eldepryl Capsules **3208**
Zelapar Tablets **3372**

Sertraline Hydrochloride (Potential for synergistic CNS-depressant effect). Products include:
Zoloft **2586**

Sevoflurane (Potential for synergistic CNS-depressant effect). Products include:
Ultane Liquid for Inhalation **531**

Sildenafil Citrate (There are no reports as to which isoenzymes could be inhibited or induced by diazepam. But based on the fact that diazepam is a substrate for CYP2C19 and CYP3A4, it is possible that diazepam may interfere with the metabolism of drugs which are substrates for CYP2C19 and CYP3A4 leading to a potential drug-drug interaction). Products include:
Revatio Tablets **2557**
Viagra Tablets **2573**

Simvastatin (There are no reports as to which isoenzymes could be inhibited or induced by diazepam. But based on the fact that diazepam is a substrate for CYP2C19 and CYP3A4, it is possible that diazepam may interfere with the metabolism of drugs which are substrates for CYP2C19 and CYP3A4 leading to a potential drug-drug interaction). Products include:
Vytorin 10/10 Tablets **2114**
Vytorin 10/10 Tablets **3077**
Vytorin 10/20 Tablets **2114**
Vytorin 10/20 Tablets **3077**
Vytorin 10/40 Tablets **2114**
Vytorin 10/40 Tablets **3077**
Vytorin 10/80 Tablets **2114**
Vytorin 10/80 Tablets **3077**
Zocor Tablets **2105**

Sirolimus (There are no reports as to which isoenzymes could be inhibited or induced by diazepam. But based on the fact that diazepam is a substrate for CYP2C19 and CYP3A4, it is possible that diazepam may interfere with the metabolism of drugs which are substrates for CYP2C19 and CYP3A4 leading to a potential drug-drug interaction). Products include:
Rapamune Oral Solution and Tablets **3475**

Sodium Oxybate (Potential for synergistic CNS-depressant effect). Products include:
Xyrem Oral Solution **1688**

Sufentanil Citrate (Potential for synergistic CNS-depressant effect).
No products indexed under this heading.

Sulfaphenazole (Studies suggest that CYP2C19 and CYP3A4 are the principal enzymes involved in the initial oxidative metabolism of diazepam. Therefore, potential interactions may occur when diazepam is given concurrently with agents that affect CYP2C19 and CYP3A4 activity. Potential inhibitors of CYP2C19 could decrease the rate of diazepam elimination).
No products indexed under this heading.

Sulfinpyrazone (Studies suggest that CYP2C19 and CYP3A4 are the principal enzymes involved in the initial oxidative metabolism of diazepam. Therefore, potential interactions may occur when diazepam is given concurrently with agents that affect CYP2C19 and CYP3A4 activity. Potential inducers of CYP3A4 could increase the rate of diazepam elimination).
No products indexed under this heading.

Tacrolimus (There are no reports as to which isoenzymes could be inhibited or induced by diazepam. But based on the fact that diazepam is a substrate for CYP2C19 and CYP3A4, it is possible that diazepam may interfere with the metabolism of drugs which are substrates for CYP2C19 and CYP3A4 leading to a potential drug-drug interaction). Products include:
Prograf Capsules and Injection **632**
Protopic Ointment **638**

Tamoxifen Citrate (There are no reports as to which isoenzymes could be inhibited or induced by diazepam. But based on the fact that diazepam is a substrate for CYP2C19 and CYP3A4, it is possible that diazepam may interfere with the metabolism of drugs which are substrates for CYP2C19 and CYP3A4 leading to a potential drug-drug interaction). Products include:
Soltamox Oral Solution **3527**

Telithromycin (Studies suggest that CYP2C19 and CYP3A4 are the principal enzymes involved in the initial oxidative metabolism of diazepam. Therefore, potential interactions may occur when diazepam is given concurrently with agents that affect CYP2C19 and CYP3A4 activity. Potential inhibitors of CYP3A4 could decrease the rate of diazepam elimination). Products include:
Ketek Tablets **2903**

Telmisartan (Studies suggest that CYP2C19 and CYP3A4 are the principal enzymes involved in the initial oxidative metabolism of diazepam. Therefore, potential interactions may occur when diazepam is given concurrently with agents that affect CYP2C19 and CYP3A4 activity. Potential inhibitors of CYP2C19 could decrease the rate of diazepam elimination). Products include:
Micardis Tablets **854**
Micardis HCT Tablets **856**

Temazepam (Potential for synergistic CNS-depressant effect). Products include:
Restoril Capsules **1860**

Teniposide (There are no reports as to which isoenzymes could be inhibited or induced by diazepam. But based on the fact that diazepam is a substrate for CYP2C19 and CYP3A4, it is possible that diazepam may interfere with the metabolism of drugs which are substrates for CYP2C19 and CYP3A4 leading to a potential drug-drug interaction).
No products indexed under this heading.

Terfenadine (Diazepam is a substrate of CYP2C19 and CYP3A4; it is possible that diazepam may interfere with the metabolism of drugs which are substrates for CYP3A4, such as terfenadine).
No products indexed under this heading.

Theophylline (Diazepam is a substrate of CYP2C19 and CYP3A4, it is possible that diazepam may interfere with the metabolism of drugs which are substrates for CYP3A4, such as theophylline).
No products indexed under this heading.

Theophylline Anhydrous (Diazepam is a substrate of CYP2C19 and CYP3A4, it is possible that diazepam may interfere with the metabolism of drugs which are substrates for CYP3A4, such as theophylline). Products include:
Uniphyl Tablets **2710**

Theophylline Calcium Salicylate (Diazepam is a substrate of CYP2C19 and CYP3A4, it is possible that diazepam may interfere with the metabolism of drugs which are substrates for CYP3A4, such as theophylline).
No products indexed under this heading.

Theophylline Dihydroxypropyl (Glyceryl) (Diazepam is a substrate of CYP2C19 and CYP3A4, it is possible that diazepam may interfere with the metabolism of drugs which are substrates for CYP3A4, such as theophylline).
No products indexed under this heading.

Theophylline Ethylenediamine (Diazepam is a substrate of CYP2C19 and CYP3A4, it is possible that diazepam may interfere with the metabolism of drugs which are substrates for CYP3A4, such as theophylline).
No products indexed under this heading.

Theophylline Sodium Glycinate (Diazepam is a substrate of CYP2C19 and CYP3A4, it is possible that diazepam may interfere with the metabolism of drugs which are substrates for CYP3A4, such as theophylline).
No products indexed under this heading.

Thiamylal Sodium (Potential for synergistic CNS-depressant effect).
No products indexed under this heading.

Thioridazine (There are no reports as to which isoenzymes could be inhibited or induced by diazepam. But based on the fact that diazepam is a substrate for CYP2C19 and CYP3A4, it is possible that diazepam may interfere with the metabolism of drugs which are substrates for CYP2C19 and CYP3A4 leading to a potential drug-drug interaction).
No products indexed under this heading.

Thioridazine Hydrochloride (Potential for synergistic CNS-depressant effect). Products include:
Thioridazine Hydrochloride
Tablets 2163

Thiothixene (Potential for synergistic CNS-depressant effect). Products include:
Thiothixene Capsules 2165

Tiagabine Hydrochloride (There are no reports as to which isoenzymes could be inhibited or induced by diazepam. But based on the fact that diazepam is a substrate for CYP2C19 and CYP3A4, it is possible that diazepam may interfere with the metabolism of drugs which are substrates for CYP2C19 and CYP3A4 leading to a potential drug-drug interaction). Products include:
Gabitril Tablets 984

Ticlopidine Hydrochloride (Studies suggest that CYP2C19 and CYP3A4 are the principal enzymes involved in the initial oxidative metabolism of diazepam. Therefore, potential interactions may occur when diazepam is given concurrently with agents that affect CYP2C19 and CYP3A4 activity. Potential inhibitors of CYP2C19 could decrease the rate of diazepam elimination). Products include:
Ticlid Tablets 2810

Tolbutamide (Studies suggest that CYP2C19 and CYP3A4 are the principal enzymes involved in the initial oxidative metabolism of diazepam. Therefore, potential interactions may occur when diazepam is given concurrently with agents that affect CYP2C19 and CYP3A4 activity. Potential inhibitors of CYP2C19 could decrease the rate of diazepam elimination).
No products indexed under this heading.

Tolbutamide Sodium (Studies suggest that CYP2C19 and CYP3A4 are the principal enzymes involved in the initial oxidative metabolism of diazepam. Therefore, potential interactions may occur when diazepam is given concurrently with agents that affect CYP2C19 and CYP3A4 activity. Potential inhibitors of CYP2C19 could decrease the rate of diazepam elimination).
No products indexed under this heading.

Tolterodine Tartrate (There are no reports as to which isoenzymes could be inhibited or induced by diazepam. But based on the fact that diazepam is a substrate for CYP2C19 and CYP3A4, it is possible that diazepam may interfere with the metabolism of drugs which are substrates for CYP2C19 and CYP3A4 leading to a potential drug-drug interaction). Products include:
Detrol Tablets 2628
Detrol LA Capsules 2631

Topiramate (Studies suggest that CYP2C19 and CYP3A4 are the principal enzymes involved in the initial oxidative metabolism of diazepam. Therefore, potential interactions may occur when diazepam is given concurrently with agents that affect CYP2C19 and CYP3A4 activity. Potential inhibitors of CYP2C19 could decrease the rate of diazepam elimination). Products include:
Topamax Sprinkle Capsules 2404
Topamax Tablets 2404

Tranylcypromine Sulfate (Potential inhibitors of CYP2C19, such as tranylcypromine, could decrease the rate of diazepam elimination; potential for synergistic CNS-depressant effect). Products include:
Parnate Tablets 1527

Trazodone Hydrochloride (Potential for synergistic CNS-depressant effect).
No products indexed under this heading.

Triamcinolone (Studies suggest that CYP2C19 and CYP3A4 are the principal enzymes involved in the initial oxidative metabolism of diazepam. Therefore, potential interactions may occur when diazepam is given concurrently with agents that affect CYP2C19 and CYP3A4 activity. Potential inducers of CYP3A4 could increase the rate of diazepam elimination).
No products indexed under this heading.

Triamcinolone Acetonide (Studies suggest that CYP2C19 and CYP3A4 are the principal enzymes involved in the initial oxidative metabolism of diazepam. Therefore, potential interactions may occur when diazepam is given concurrently with agents that affect CYP2C19 and CYP3A4 activity. Potential inducers of CYP3A4 could increase the rate of diazepam elimination). Products include:

Azmacort Inhalation Aerosol 1726
Nasacort AQ Nasal Spray 2922

Triamcinolone Diacetate (Studies suggest that CYP2C19 and CYP3A4 are the principal enzymes involved in the initial oxidative metabolism of diazepam. Therefore, potential interactions may occur when diazepam is given concurrently with agents that affect CYP2C19 and CYP3A4 activity. Potential inducers of CYP3A4 could increase the rate of diazepam elimination).
No products indexed under this heading.

Triamcinolone Hexacetonide (Studies suggest that CYP2C19 and CYP3A4 are the principal enzymes involved in the initial oxidative metabolism of diazepam. Therefore, potential interactions may occur when diazepam is given concurrently with agents that affect CYP2C19 and CYP3A4 activity. Potential inducers of CYP3A4 could increase the rate of diazepam elimination).
No products indexed under this heading.

Triazolam (Potential for synergistic CNS-depressant effect).
No products indexed under this heading.

Trifluoperazine Hydrochloride (Potential for synergistic CNS-depressant effect).
No products indexed under this heading.

Trimethadione (There are no reports as to which isoenzymes could be inhibited or induced by diazepam. But based on the fact that diazepam is a substrate for CYP2C19 and CYP3A4, it is possible that diazepam may interfere with the metabolism of drugs which are substrates for CYP2C19 and CYP3A4 leading to a potential drug-drug interaction).
No products indexed under this heading.

Trimipramine Maleate (Potential for synergistic CNS-depressant effect).
No products indexed under this heading.

Troglitazone (Studies suggest that CYP2C19 and CYP3A4 are the principal enzymes involved in the initial oxidative metabolism of diazepam. Therefore, potential interactions may occur when diazepam is given concurrently with agents that affect CYP2C19 and CYP3A4 activity. Potential inhibitors of CYP3A4 could decrease the rate of diazepam elimination).
No products indexed under this heading.

Troleandomycin (Potential inhibitors of CYP3A4, such as troleandomycin, could decrease the rate of diazepam elimination).
No products indexed under this heading.

Valproate Sodium (Valproate may potentiate the CNS-depressant effect). Products include:
Depacon Injection 412

Valproic Acid (Valproate may potentiate the CNS-depressant effect). Products include:
Depakene 417

Venlafaxine Hydrochloride (Potential for synergistic CNS-depressant effect). Products include:
Effexor Tablets 3411

Effexor XR Capsules 3417

Verapamil Hydrochloride (Studies suggest that CYP2C19 and CYP3A4 are the principal enzymes involved in the initial oxidative metabolism of diazepam. Therefore, potential interactions may occur when diazepam is given concurrently with agents that affect CYP2C19 and CYP3A4 activity. Potential inhibitors of CYP3A4 could decrease the rate of diazepam elimination). Products include:
Covera-HS Tablets 3139
Tarka Tablets 524
Verelan PM Extended-Release
Capsules, Controlled-Onset.......... 3106

Vinblastine Sulfate (There are no reports as to which isoenzymes could be inhibited or induced by diazepam. But based on the fact that diazepam is a substrate for CYP2C19 and CYP3A4, it is possible that diazepam may interfere with the metabolism of drugs which are substrates for CYP2C19 and CYP3A4 leading to a potential drug-drug interaction).
No products indexed under this heading.

Vincristine Sulfate (There are no reports as to which isoenzymes could be inhibited or induced by diazepam. But based on the fact that diazepam is a substrate for CYP2C19 and CYP3A4, it is possible that diazepam may interfere with the metabolism of drugs which are substrates for CYP2C19 and CYP3A4 leading to a potential drug-drug interaction).
No products indexed under this heading.

Voriconazole (Studies suggest that CYP2C19 and CYP3A4 are the principal enzymes involved in the initial oxidative metabolism of diazepam. Therefore, potential interactions may occur when diazepam is given concurrently with agents that affect CYP2C19 and CYP3A4 activity. Potential inhibitors of CYP2C19 could decrease the rate of diazepam elimination). Products include:
VFEND I.V. 2564
VFEND Oral Suspension 2564
VFEND Tablets 2564

Warfarin Sodium (Diazepam is a substrate of CYP2C19 and CYP3A4, it is possible that diazepam may interfere with the metabolism of drugs which are substrates for CYP3A4, such as warfarin). Products include:
Coumadin for Injection 898
Coumadin Tablets 898

Zafirlukast (Studies suggest that CYP2C19 and CYP3A4 are the principal enzymes involved in the initial oxidative metabolism of diazepam. Therefore, potential interactions may occur when diazepam is given concurrently with agents that affect CYP2C19 and CYP3A4 activity. Potential inhibitors of CYP3A4 could decrease the rate of diazepam elimination). Products include:
Accolate Tablets 671

Zaleplon (Potential for synergistic CNS-depressant effect). Products include:
Sonata Capsules 1717

Zileuton (Studies suggest that CYP2C19 and CYP3A4 are the principal enzymes involved in the initial oxidative metabolism of diazepam. Therefore, potential interactions may occur when diazepam is given con-

IMPORTANT NOTE: Always consult each drug listing in the patient's regimen for possible interactions.

currently with agents that affect CYP2C19 and CYP3A4 activity. Potential inhibitors of CYP3A4 could decrease the rate of diazepam elimination). Products include:
Zyflo Tablets 1023

Ziprasidone Hydrochloride (Potential for synergistic CNS-depressant effect). Products include:
Geodon Capsules 2529

Zolpidem Tartrate (Potential for synergistic CNS-depressant effect). Products include:
Ambien Tablets 2851
Ambien CR Tablets 2855

Zonisamide (There are no reports as to which isoenzymes could be inhibited or induced by diazepam. But based on the fact that diazepam is a substrate for CYP2C19 and CYP3A4, it is possible that diazepam may interfere with the metabolism of drugs which are substrates for CYP2C19 and CYP3A4 leading to a potential drug-drug interaction). Products include:
Zonegran Capsules 1101

Food Interactions

Alcohol (Potential for synergistic CNS-depressant effect).

Grapefruit (Studies suggest that CYP2C19 and CYP3A4 are the principal enzymes involved in the initial oxidative metabolism of diazepam. Therefore, potential interactions may occur when diazepam is given concurrently with agents that affect CYP2C19 and CYP3A4 activity. Potential inhibitors of CYP3A4 could decrease the rate of diazepam elimination).

Grapefruit Juice (Studies suggest that CYP2C19 and CYP3A4 are the principal enzymes involved in the initial oxidative metabolism of diazepam. Therefore, potential interactions may occur when diazepam is given concurrently with agents that affect CYP2C19 and CYP3A4 activity. Potential inhibitors of CYP3A4 could decrease the rate of diazepam elimination).

DIBENZYLINE CAPSULES

(Phenoxybenzamine Hydrochloride) ... 3399
May interact with:

Alpha and Beta Adrenergic Stimulators (Exaggerated hypotensive response; tachycardia).
No products indexed under this heading.

Epinephrine (Exaggerated hypotensive response; tachycardia). Products include:
EpiPen 1061
Primatene Mist .... ■719
Twinject 0.15 3379
Twinject 0.3 3378

Epinephrine Bitartrate (Exaggerated hypotensive response; tachycardia).
No products indexed under this heading.

Norepinephrine Bitartrate (Hyperthermia production of levarterenol blocked by dibenzyline).
No products indexed under this heading.

Reserpine (Hypothermia production of reserpine blocked by dibenzyline).
No products indexed under this heading.

DIDRONEL TABLETS

(Etidronate Disodium) 2697
May interact with:

Warfarin Sodium (Co-administration has resulted in isolated reports of increase in prothrombin time without clinically significant sequelae). Products include:
Coumadin for Injection 898
Coumadin Tablets 898

DIFFERIN CREAM

(Adapalene) 1210
See Differin Gel

DIFFERIN GEL

(Adapalene) 1211
May interact with:

Resorcinol (Increased potential for local irritation).
No products indexed under this heading.

Salicylic Acid (Increased potential for local irritation).
No products indexed under this heading.

Sulfur (Increased potential for local irritation). Products include:
Avar Cleanser 1085
Avar Gel 1085
Avar Green Gel 1085
Avar-e Emollient Cream 1085
Avar-e Green Cream 1085
Hyland's Calm Forte 4 Kids Tablets .... ■828
Plexion 1889
Rosac Cream with Sunscreens 3213
Zeel Solution 1665
Zicam Allergy Relief .... ■774

DIGIBIND FOR INJECTION

(Digoxin Immune Fab (Ovine)) 1421
None cited in PDR database.

DILAUDID AMPULES

(Hydromorphone Hydrochloride) 440
May interact with central nervous system depressants, neuromuscular blocking agents, tricyclic antidepressants, and certain other agents. Compounds in these categories include:

Alfentanil Hydrochloride (Additive CNS depression).
No products indexed under this heading.

Alprazolam (Additive CNS depression). Products include:
Niravam Orally Disintegrating Tablets 3092

Amitriptyline Hydrochloride (Additive CNS depression).
No products indexed under this heading.

Amoxapine (Additive CNS depression).
No products indexed under this heading.

Aprobarbital (Additive CNS depression).
No products indexed under this heading.

Atracurium Besylate (Opioid analgesics including Dilaudid may enhance the action of neuromuscular blocking agents and produce an excessive degree of respiratory depression).
No products indexed under this heading.

Buprenorphine Hydrochloride (Additive CNS depression). Products include:
Buprenex Injectable 2716
Suboxone Tablets 2717
Subutex Tablets 2717

Buspirone Hydrochloride (Additive CNS depression).
No products indexed under this heading.

Butabarbital (Additive CNS depression).
No products indexed under this heading.

Butalbital (Additive CNS depression).
No products indexed under this heading.

Chlordiazepoxide (Additive CNS depression).
No products indexed under this heading.

Chlordiazepoxide Hydrochloride (Additive CNS depression). Products include:
Librium Capsules 3347

Chlorpromazine (Additive CNS depression).
No products indexed under this heading.

Chlorpromazine Hydrochloride (Additive CNS depression).
No products indexed under this heading.

Chlorprothixene (Additive CNS depression).
No products indexed under this heading.

Chlorprothixene Hydrochloride (Additive CNS depression).
No products indexed under this heading.

Chlorprothixene Lactate (Additive CNS depression).
No products indexed under this heading.

Cisatracurium Besylate (Opioid analgesics including Dilaudid may enhance the action of neuromuscular blocking agents and produce an excessive degree of respiratory depression). Products include:
Nimbex Injection 498

Clomipramine Hydrochloride (Additive CNS depression).
No products indexed under this heading.

Clorazepate Dipotassium (Additive CNS depression). Products include:
Tranxene 2474

Clozapine (Additive CNS depression). Products include:
Clozaril Tablets 2184
FazaClo Orally Disintegrating Tablets 551

Codeine Phosphate (Additive CNS depression). Products include:
Tylenol with Codeine Tablets 2391

Desflurane (Additive CNS depression).
No products indexed under this heading.

Desipramine Hydrochloride (Additive CNS depression).
No products indexed under this heading.

Dezocine (Additive CNS depression).
No products indexed under this heading.

Diazepam (Additive CNS depression). Products include:
Diastat Rectal Delivery System 3343
Valium Tablets 2819

Doxacurium Chloride (Opioid analgesics including Dilaudid may enhance the action of neuromuscular blocking agents and produce an excessive degree of respiratory depression).
No products indexed under this heading.

Doxepin Hydrochloride (Additive CNS depression).
No products indexed under this heading.

Droperidol (Additive CNS depression).
No products indexed under this heading.

Enflurane (Additive CNS depression).
No products indexed under this heading.

Estazolam (Additive CNS depression). Products include:
ProSom Tablets 517

Ethanol (Additive CNS depression).
No products indexed under this heading.

Ethchlorvynol (Additive CNS depression).
No products indexed under this heading.

Ethinamate (Additive CNS depression).
No products indexed under this heading.

Ethyl Alcohol (Additive CNS depression).
No products indexed under this heading.

Fentanyl (Additive CNS depression). Products include:
Duragesic Transdermal System 2373
Ionsys Transdermal System 2379

Fentanyl Citrate (Additive CNS depression). Products include:
Actiq 979

Fluphenazine Decanoate (Additive CNS depression).
No products indexed under this heading.

Fluphenazine Enanthate (Additive CNS depression).
No products indexed under this heading.

Fluphenazine Hydrochloride (Additive CNS depression).
No products indexed under this heading.

Flurazepam Hydrochloride (Additive CNS depression). Products include:
Dalmane Capsules 3342

Glutethimide (Additive CNS depression).
No products indexed under this heading.

Haloperidol (Additive CNS depression).
No products indexed under this heading.

Haloperidol Decanoate (Additive CNS depression).
No products indexed under this heading.

Hydrocodone Bitartrate (Additive CNS depression). Products include:
Hycodan 1116
Hycotuss Expectorant Syrup 1117
Vicodin Tablets 535
Vicodin ES Tablets 536
Vicodin HP Tablets 538
Vicoprofen Tablets 539
Zydone Tablets 1139

Hydrocodone Polistirex (Additive CNS depression). Products include:
Tussionex Pennkinetic Extended-Release Suspension 3327

Hydroxyzine Hydrochloride (Additive CNS depression).
No products indexed under this heading.

Imipramine Hydrochloride (Additive CNS depression).
No products indexed under this heading.

Imipramine Pamoate (Additive CNS depression).
No products indexed under this heading.

Isoflurane (Additive CNS depression).
No products indexed under this heading.

Ketamine Hydrochloride (Additive CNS depression).
No products indexed under this heading.

Levomethadyl Acetate Hydrochloride (Additive CNS depression).
No products indexed under this heading.

Levorphanol Tartrate (Additive CNS depression).
No products indexed under this heading.

Lorazepam (Additive CNS depression).
No products indexed under this heading.

Loxapine Hydrochloride (Additive CNS depression).
No products indexed under this heading.

Loxapine Succinate (Additive CNS depression).
No products indexed under this heading.

Maprotiline Hydrochloride (Additive CNS depression).
No products indexed under this heading.

Meperidine Hydrochloride (Additive CNS depression).
No products indexed under this heading.

Mephobarbital (Additive CNS depression).
No products indexed under this heading.

Meprobamate (Additive CNS depression).
No products indexed under this heading.

Mesoridazine Besylate (Additive CNS depression).
No products indexed under this heading.

Methadone Hydrochloride (Additive CNS depression).
No products indexed under this heading.

Methohexital Sodium (Additive CNS depression).
No products indexed under this heading.

Methotrimeprazine (Additive CNS depression).
No products indexed under this heading.

Methoxyflurane (Additive CNS depression).
No products indexed under this heading.

Metocurine Iodide (Opioid analgesics including Dilaudid may enhance the action of neuromuscular blocking agents and produce an excessive degree of respiratory depression).
No products indexed under this heading.

Midazolam Hydrochloride (Additive CNS depression).
No products indexed under this heading.

Mivacurium Chloride (Opioid analgesics including Dilaudid may enhance the action of neuromuscular blocking agents and produce an excessive degree of respiratory depression). Products include:
Mivacron Injection 493

Molindone Hydrochloride (Additive CNS depression). Products include:
Moban Tablets 1119

Morphine Sulfate (Additive CNS depression). Products include:
Avinza Capsules 1741
Kadian Capsules 577
MS Contin Tablets 2701

Nortriptyline Hydrochloride (Additive CNS depression).
No products indexed under this heading.

Olanzapine (Additive CNS depression). Products include:
Symbyax Capsules 1819
Zyprexa Tablets 1830
Zyprexa IntraMuscular 1830
Zyprexa ZYDIS Orally Disintegrating Tablets 1830

Oxazepam (Additive CNS depression).
No products indexed under this heading.

Oxycodone Hydrochloride (Additive CNS depression). Products include:
OxyContin Tablets 2703
OxyFast Oral Concentrate Solution 2708
OxyIR Capsules 2708
Percocet Tablets 1131
Percodan Tablets 1132

Pancuronium Bromide (Opioid analgesics including Dilaudid may enhance the action of neuromuscular blocking agents and produce an excessive degree of respiratory depression).
No products indexed under this heading.

Pentobarbital Sodium (Additive CNS depression). Products include:
Nembutal Sodium Solution, USP 2470

Perphenazine (Additive CNS depression).
No products indexed under this heading.

Phenobarbital (Additive CNS depression). Products include:
Donnatal Extentabs 2493

Prazepam (Additive CNS depression).
No products indexed under this heading.

Prochlorperazine (Additive CNS depression).
No products indexed under this heading.

Promethazine Hydrochloride (Additive CNS depression). Products include:
Phenergan Tablets and Suppositories 3440

Propofol (Additive CNS depression).
No products indexed under this heading.

Propoxyphene Hydrochloride (Additive CNS depression).
No products indexed under this heading.

Propoxyphene Napsylate (Additive CNS depression).
No products indexed under this heading.

Protriptyline Hydrochloride (Additive CNS depression).
No products indexed under this heading.

Quazepam (Additive CNS depression).
No products indexed under this heading.

Quetiapine Fumarate (Additive CNS depression). Products include:
Seroquel Tablets 690

Rapacuronium Bromide (Opioid analgesics including Dilaudid may enhance the action of neuromuscular blocking agents and produce an excessive degree of respiratory depression).
No products indexed under this heading.

Remifentanil Hydrochloride (Additive CNS depression).
No products indexed under this heading.

Risperidone (Additive CNS depression). Products include:
Risperdal 1676
Risperdal Consta Long-Acting Injection 1682
Risperdal M-Tab Orally Disintegrating Tablets 1676

Rocuronium Bromide (Opioid analgesics including Dilaudid may enhance the action of neuromuscular blocking agents and produce an excessive degree of respiratory depression). Products include:
Zemuron Injection 2346

Secobarbital Sodium (Additive CNS depression).
No products indexed under this heading.

Sevoflurane (Additive CNS depression). Products include:
Ultane Liquid for Inhalation 531

Sodium Oxybate (Additive CNS depression). Products include:
Xyrem Oral Solution 1688

Succinylcholine Chloride (Opioid analgesics including Dilaudid may enhance the action of neuromuscular blocking agents and produce an excessive degree of respiratory depression).
No products indexed under this heading.

Sufentanil Citrate (Additive CNS depression).
No products indexed under this heading.

Temazepam (Additive CNS depression). Products include:
Restoril Capsules 1860

Thiamylal Sodium (Additive CNS depression).
No products indexed under this heading.

Thioridazine Hydrochloride (Additive CNS depression). Products include:
Thioridazine Hydrochloride Tablets 2163

Thiothixene (Additive CNS depression). Products include:
Thiothixene Capsules 2165

Triazolam (Additive CNS depression).
No products indexed under this heading.

Trifluoperazine Hydrochloride (Additive CNS depression).
No products indexed under this heading.

Trimipramine Maleate (Additive CNS depression).
No products indexed under this heading.

Vecuronium Bromide (Opioid analgesics including Dilaudid may enhance the action of neuromuscular blocking agents and produce an excessive degree of respiratory depression).
No products indexed under this heading.

Zaleplon (Additive CNS depression). Products include:
Sonata Capsules 1717

Ziprasidone Hydrochloride (Additive CNS depression). Products include:
Geodon Capsules 2529

Zolpidem Tartrate (Additive CNS depression). Products include:
Ambien Tablets 2851
Ambien CR Tablets 2855

Food Interactions

Alcohol (Additive CNS depression).

DILAUDID MULTIPLE DOSE VIALS

(Hydromorphone Hydrochloride) 440
See Dilaudid Ampules

DILAUDID NON-STERILE POWDER

(Hydromorphone Hydrochloride) 440
See Dilaudid Ampules

DILAUDID ORAL LIQUID

(Hydromorphone Hydrochloride) 445
May interact with central nervous system depressants, general anesthetics, hypnotics and sedatives, neuromuscular blocking agents, phenothiazines, tranquilizers, and certain other agents. Compounds in these categories include:

Alfentanil Hydrochloride (May produce additive depressant effects; respiratory depression, hypotension and profound sedation or coma may occur; the dose of one or both agents should be reduced).
No products indexed under this heading.

Alprazolam (May produce additive depressant effects; respiratory depression, hypotension and profound sedation or coma may occur; the dose of one or both agents should be reduced). Products include:
Niravam Orally Disintegrating Tablets 3092

Aprobarbital (May produce additive depressant effects; respiratory depression, hypotension and profound sedation or coma may occur; the dose of one or both agents should be reduced).
No products indexed under this heading.

Atracurium Besylate (Enhanced action of neuromuscular blocking agents and produce an excessive degree of respiratory depression).
No products indexed under this heading.

Buprenorphine Hydrochloride (May produce additive depressant effects; respiratory depression, hypotension and profound sedation or coma may occur; the dose of one or both agents should be reduced). Products include:
Buprenex Injectable 2716
Suboxone Tablets 2717
Subutex Tablets 2717

Buspirone Hydrochloride (May produce additive depressant effects; respiratory depression, hypotension and profound sedation or coma may occur; the dose of one or both agents should be reduced).
No products indexed under this heading.

Butabarbital (May produce additive depressant effects; respiratory depression, hypotension and profound sedation or coma may occur; the dose of one or both agents should be reduced).
No products indexed under this heading.

Butalbital (May produce additive depressant effects; respiratory depression, hypotension and profound sedation or coma may occur; the dose of one or both agents should be reduced).
No products indexed under this heading.

Chlordiazepoxide (May produce additive depressant effects; respiratory depression, hypotension and profound sedation or coma may occur; the dose of one or both agents should be reduced).
No products indexed under this heading.

Chlordiazepoxide Hydrochloride (May produce additive depressant effects; respiratory depression, hypotension and profound sedation or coma may occur; the dose of one or both agents should be reduced). Products include:
Librium Capsules 3347

Chlorpromazine (May produce additive depressant effects; respiratory depression, hypotension and profound sedation or coma may occur; the dose of one or both agents should be reduced).
No products indexed under this heading.

Chlorpromazine Hydrochloride (May produce additive depressant effects; respiratory depression, hypotension and profound sedation or coma may occur; the dose of one or both agents should be reduced).
No products indexed under this heading.

Chlorprothixene (May produce additive depressant effects; respiratory depression, hypotension and profound sedation or coma may occur; the dose of one or both agents should be reduced).
No products indexed under this heading.

Chlorprothixene Hydrochloride (May produce additive depressant effects; respiratory depression, hypotension and profound sedation or coma may occur; the dose of one or both agents should be reduced).
No products indexed under this heading.

Chlorprothixene Lactate (May produce additive depressant effects; respiratory depression, hypotension and profound sedation or coma may occur; the dose of one or both agents should be reduced).
No products indexed under this heading.

Cisatracurium Besylate (Enhanced action of neuromuscular blocking agents and produce an excessive degree of respiratory depression). Products include:
Nimbex Injection 498

Clorazepate Dipotassium (May produce additive depressant effects; respiratory depression, hypotension and profound sedation or coma may occur; the dose of one or both agents should be reduced). Products include:
Tranxene 2474

Clozapine (May produce additive depressant effects; respiratory depression, hypotension and profound sedation or coma may occur; the dose of one or both agents should be reduced). Products include:
Clozaril Tablets 2184
FazaClo Orally Disintegrating Tablets .. 551

Codeine Phosphate (May produce additive depressant effects; respiratory depression, hypotension and profound sedation or coma may occur; the dose of one or both agents should be reduced). Products include:
Tylenol with Codeine Tablets 2391

Desflurane (May produce additive depressant effects; respiratory depression, hypotension and profound sedation or coma may occur; the dose of one or both agents should be reduced).
No products indexed under this heading.

Dezocine (May produce additive depressant effects; respiratory depression, hypotension and profound sedation or coma may occur; the dose of one or both agents should be reduced).
No products indexed under this heading.

Diazepam (May produce additive depressant effects; respiratory depression, hypotension and profound sedation or coma may occur; the dose of one or both agents should be reduced). Products include:
Diastat Rectal Delivery System 3343
Valium Tablets 2819

Doxacurium Chloride (Enhanced action of neuromuscular blocking agents and produce an excessive degree of respiratory depression).
No products indexed under this heading.

Droperidol (May produce additive depressant effects; respiratory depression, hypotension and profound sedation or coma may occur; the dose of one or both agents should be reduced).
No products indexed under this heading.

Enflurane (May produce additive depressant effects; respiratory depression, hypotension and profound sedation or coma may occur; the dose of one or both agents should be reduced).
No products indexed under this heading.

Estazolam (May produce additive depressant effects; respiratory depression, hypotension and profound sedation or coma may occur; the dose of one or both agents should be reduced). Products include:
ProSom Tablets 517

Ethanol (May produce additive depressant effects; respiratory depression, hypotension and profound sedation or coma may occur; the dose of one or both agents should be reduced).
No products indexed under this heading.

Ethchlorvynol (May produce additive depressant effects; respiratory depression, hypotension and profound sedation or coma may occur; the dose of one or both agents should be reduced).
No products indexed under this heading.

Ethinamate (May produce additive depressant effects; respiratory depression, hypotension and profound sedation or coma may occur; the dose of one or both agents should be reduced).
No products indexed under this heading.

Ethyl Alcohol (May produce additive depressant effects; respiratory depression, hypotension and profound sedation or coma may occur; the dose of one or both agents should be reduced).
No products indexed under this heading.

Fentanyl (May produce additive depressant effects; respiratory depression, hypotension and profound sedation or coma may occur; the dose of one or both agents should be reduced). Products include:
Duragesic Transdermal System 2373
Ionsys Transdermal System 2379

Fentanyl Citrate (May produce additive depressant effects; respiratory depression, hypotension and profound sedation or coma may occur; the dose of one or both agents should be reduced). Products include:
Actiq .. 979

Fluphenazine Decanoate (May produce additive depressant effects; respiratory depression, hypotension and profound sedation or coma may occur; the dose of one or both agents should be reduced).
No products indexed under this heading.

Fluphenazine Enanthate (May produce additive depressant effects; respiratory depression, hypotension and profound sedation or coma may occur; the dose of one or both agents should be reduced).
No products indexed under this heading.

Fluphenazine Hydrochloride (May produce additive depressant effects; respiratory depression, hypotension and profound sedation or coma may occur; the dose of one or both agents should be reduced).
No products indexed under this heading.

Flurazepam Hydrochloride (May produce additive depressant effects; respiratory depression, hypotension and profound sedation or coma may occur; the dose of one or both agents should be reduced). Products include:
Dalmane Capsules 3342

Glutethimide (May produce additive depressant effects; respiratory depression, hypotension and profound sedation or coma may occur; the dose of one or both agents should be reduced).
No products indexed under this heading.

Haloperidol (May produce additive depressant effects; respiratory depression, hypotension and profound sedation or coma may occur; the dose of one or both agents should be reduced).
No products indexed under this heading.

Haloperidol Decanoate (May produce additive depressant effects; respiratory depression, hypotension and profound sedation or coma may occur; the dose of one or both agents should be reduced).
No products indexed under this heading.

Hydrocodone Bitartrate (May produce additive depressant effects; respiratory depression, hypotension and profound sedation or coma may occur; the dose of one or both agents should be reduced). Products include:
Hycodan ... 1116
Hycotuss Expectorant Syrup 1117
Vicodin Tablets 535
Vicodin ES Tablets 536
Vicodin HP Tablets 538
Vicoprofen Tablets 539
Zydone Tablets 1139

Hydrocodone Polistirex (May produce additive depressant effects; respiratory depression, hypotension and profound sedation or coma may occur; the dose of one or both agents should be reduced). Products include:
Tussionex Pennkinetic Extended-Release Suspension 3327

Hydroxyzine Hydrochloride (May produce additive depressant effects; respiratory depression, hypotension and profound sedation or coma may occur; the dose of one or both agents should be reduced).
No products indexed under this heading.

Isoflurane (May produce additive depressant effects; respiratory depression, hypotension and profound sedation or coma may occur; the dose of one or both agents should be reduced).
No products indexed under this heading.

Ketamine Hydrochloride (May produce additive depressant effects; respiratory depression, hypotension and profound sedation or coma may occur; the dose of one or both agents should be reduced).
No products indexed under this heading.

Levomethadyl Acetate Hydrochloride (May produce additive depressant effects; respiratory depression, hypotension and profound sedation or coma may occur; the dose of one or both agents should be reduced).
No products indexed under this heading.

Levorphanol Tartrate (May produce additive depressant effects; respiratory depression, hypotension and profound sedation or coma may occur; the dose of one or both agents should be reduced).
No products indexed under this heading.

Lorazepam (May produce additive depressant effects; respiratory depression, hypotension and profound sedation or coma may occur; the dose of one or both agents should be reduced).

No products indexed under this heading.

Loxapine Hydrochloride (May produce additive depressant effects; respiratory depression, hypotension and profound sedation or coma may occur; the dose of one or both agents should be reduced).

No products indexed under this heading.

Loxapine Succinate (May produce additive depressant effects; respiratory depression, hypotension and profound sedation or coma may occur; the dose of one or both agents should be reduced).

No products indexed under this heading.

Meperidine Hydrochloride (May produce additive depressant effects; respiratory depression, hypotension and profound sedation or coma may occur; the dose of one or both agents should be reduced).

No products indexed under this heading.

Mephobarbital (May produce additive depressant effects; respiratory depression, hypotension and profound sedation or coma may occur; the dose of one or both agents should be reduced).

No products indexed under this heading.

Meprobamate (May produce additive depressant effects; respiratory depression, hypotension and profound sedation or coma may occur; the dose of one or both agents should be reduced).

No products indexed under this heading.

Mesoridazine Besylate (May produce additive depressant effects; respiratory depression, hypotension and profound sedation or coma may occur; the dose of one or both agents should be reduced).

No products indexed under this heading.

Methadone Hydrochloride (May produce additive depressant effects; respiratory depression, hypotension and profound sedation or coma may occur; the dose of one or both agents should be reduced).

No products indexed under this heading.

Methohexital Sodium (May produce additive depressant effects; respiratory depression, hypotension and profound sedation or coma may occur; the dose of one or both agents should be reduced).

No products indexed under this heading.

Methotrimeprazine (May produce additive depressant effects; respiratory depression, hypotension and profound sedation or coma may occur; the dose of one or both agents should be reduced).

No products indexed under this heading.

Methoxyflurane (May produce additive depressant effects; respiratory depression, hypotension and profound sedation or coma may occur; the dose of one or both agents should be reduced).

No products indexed under this heading.

Metocurine Iodide (Enhanced action of neuromuscular blocking agents and produce an excessive degree of respiratory depression).

No products indexed under this heading.

Midazolam Hydrochloride (May produce additive depressant effects; respiratory depression, hypotension and profound sedation or coma may occur; the dose of one or both agents should be reduced).

No products indexed under this heading.

Mivacurium Chloride (Enhanced action of neuromuscular blocking agents and produce an excessive degree of respiratory depression). Products include:

Mivacron Injection 493

Molindone Hydrochloride (May produce additive depressant effects; respiratory depression, hypotension and profound sedation or coma may occur; the dose of one or both agents should be reduced). Products include:

Moban Tablets 1119

Morphine Sulfate (May produce additive depressant effects; respiratory depression, hypotension and profound sedation or coma may occur; the dose of one or both agents should be reduced). Products include:

Avinza Capsules 1741
Kadian Capsules 577
MS Contin Tablets 2701

Olanzapine (May produce additive depressant effects; respiratory depression, hypotension and profound sedation or coma may occur; the dose of one or both agents should be reduced). Products include:

Symbyax Capsules 1819
Zyprexa Tablets 1830
Zyprexa IntraMuscular 1830
Zyprexa ZYDIS Orally Disintegrating Tablets.................. 1830

Oxazepam (May produce additive depressant effects; respiratory depression, hypotension and profound sedation or coma may occur; the dose of one or both agents should be reduced).

No products indexed under this heading.

Oxycodone Hydrochloride (May produce additive depressant effects; respiratory depression, hypotension and profound sedation or coma may occur; the dose of one or both agents should be reduced). Products include:

OxyContin Tablets 2703
OxyFast Oral Concentrate Solution....................................... 2708
OxyIR Capsules 2708
Percocet Tablets 1131
Percodan Tablets 1132

Pancuronium Bromide (Enhanced action of neuromuscular blocking agents and produce an excessive degree of respiratory depression).

No products indexed under this heading.

Pentobarbital Sodium (May produce additive depressant effects; respiratory depression, hypotension

and profound sedation or coma may occur; the dose of one or both agents should be reduced). Products include:

Nembutal Sodium Solution, USP 2470

Perphenazine (May produce additive depressant effects; respiratory depression, hypotension and profound sedation or coma may occur; the dose of one or both agents should be reduced).

No products indexed under this heading.

Phenobarbital (May produce additive depressant effects; respiratory depression, hypotension and profound sedation or coma may occur; the dose of one or both agents should be reduced). Products include:

Donnatal Extentabs 2493

Prazepam (May produce additive depressant effects; respiratory depression, hypotension and profound sedation or coma may occur; the dose of one or both agents should be reduced).

No products indexed under this heading.

Prochlorperazine (May produce additive depressant effects; respiratory depression, hypotension and profound sedation or coma may occur; the dose of one or both agents should be reduced).

No products indexed under this heading.

Promethazine Hydrochloride (May produce additive depressant effects; respiratory depression, hypotension and profound sedation or coma may occur; the dose of one or both agents should be reduced). Products include:

Phenergan Tablets and Suppositories................................. 3440

Propofol (May produce additive depressant effects; respiratory depression, hypotension and profound sedation or coma may occur; the dose of one or both agents should be reduced).

No products indexed under this heading.

Propoxyphene Hydrochloride (May produce additive depressant effects; respiratory depression, hypotension and profound sedation or coma may occur; the dose of one or both agents should be reduced).

No products indexed under this heading.

Propoxyphene Napsylate (May produce additive depressant effects; respiratory depression, hypotension and profound sedation or coma may occur; the dose of one or both agents should be reduced).

No products indexed under this heading.

Quazepam (May produce additive depressant effects; respiratory depression, hypotension and profound sedation or coma may occur; the dose of one or both agents should be reduced).

No products indexed under this heading.

Quetiapine Fumarate (May produce additive depressant effects; respiratory depression, hypotension and profound sedation or coma may occur; the dose of one or both agents should be reduced). Products include:

Seroquel Tablets 690

Ramelteon (May produce additive depressant effects; respiratory depression, hypotension and profound sedation or coma may occur; the dose of one or both agents should be reduced). Products include:

Rozerem Tablets 3231

Rapacuronium Bromide (Enhanced action of neuromuscular blocking agents and produce an excessive degree of respiratory depression).

No products indexed under this heading.

Remifentanil Hydrochloride (May produce additive depressant effects; respiratory depression, hypotension and profound sedation or coma may occur; the dose of one or both agents should be reduced).

No products indexed under this heading.

Risperidone (May produce additive depressant effects; respiratory depression, hypotension and profound sedation or coma may occur; the dose of one or both agents should be reduced). Products include:

Risperdal ... 1676
Risperdal Consta Long-Acting Injection 1682
Risperdal M-Tab Orally Disintegrating Tablets.................. 1676

Rocuronium Bromide (Enhanced action of neuromuscular blocking agents and produce an excessive degree of respiratory depression). Products include:

Zemuron Injection 2346

Secobarbital Sodium (May produce additive depressant effects; respiratory depression, hypotension and profound sedation or coma may occur; the dose of one or both agents should be reduced).

No products indexed under this heading.

Sevoflurane (May produce additive depressant effects; respiratory depression, hypotension and profound sedation or coma may occur; the dose of one or both agents should be reduced). Products include:

Ultane Liquid for Inhalation 531

Succinylcholine Chloride (Enhanced action of neuromuscular blocking agents and produce an excessive degree of respiratory depression).

No products indexed under this heading.

Sufentanil Citrate (May produce additive depressant effects; respiratory depression, hypotension and profound sedation or coma may occur; the dose of one or both agents should be reduced).

No products indexed under this heading.

Temazepam (May produce additive depressant effects; respiratory depression, hypotension and profound sedation or coma may occur; the dose of one or both agents should be reduced). Products include:

Restoril Capsules 1860

IMPORTANT NOTE: Always consult each drug listing in the patient's regimen for possible interactions.

Thiamylal Sodium (May produce additive depressant effects; respiratory depression, hypotension and profound sedation or coma may occur; the dose of one or both agents should be reduced).
No products indexed under this heading.

Thioridazine Hydrochloride (May produce additive depressant effects; respiratory depression, hypotension and profound sedation or coma may occur; the dose of one or both agents should be reduced). Products include:
Thioridazine Hydrochloride Tablets 2163

Thiothixene (May produce additive depressant effects; respiratory depression, hypotension and profound sedation or coma may occur; the dose of one or both agents should be reduced). Products include:
Thiothixene Capsules 2165

Triazolam (May produce additive depressant effects; respiratory depression, hypotension and profound sedation or coma may occur; the dose of one or both agents should be reduced).
No products indexed under this heading.

Trifluoperazine Hydrochloride (May produce additive depressant effects; respiratory depression, hypotension and profound sedation or coma may occur; the dose of one or both agents should be reduced).
No products indexed under this heading.

Vecuronium Bromide (Enhanced action of neuromuscular blocking agents and produce an excessive degree of respiratory depression).
No products indexed under this heading.

Zaleplon (May produce additive depressant effects; respiratory depression, hypotension and profound sedation or coma may occur; the dose of one or both agents should be reduced). Products include:
Sonata Capsules 1717

Ziprasidone Hydrochloride (May produce additive depressant effects; respiratory depression, hypotension and profound sedation or coma may occur; the dose of one or both agents should be reduced). Products include:
Geodon Capsules 2529

Zolpidem Tartrate (May produce additive depressant effects; respiratory depression, hypotension and profound sedation or coma may occur; the dose of one or both agents should be reduced). Products include:
Ambien Tablets 2851
Ambien CR Tablets 2855

Food Interactions

Alcohol (May exhibit an additive CNS depression).

DILAUDID RECTAL SUPPOSITORIES

(Hydromorphone Hydrochloride) 440
See Dilaudid Ampules

DILAUDID TABLETS

(Hydromorphone Hydrochloride) 440
See Dilaudid Ampules

DILAUDID TABLETS - 8 MG

(Hydromorphone Hydrochloride) 445
See Dilaudid Oral Liquid

DILAUDID-HP INJECTION

(Hydromorphone Hydrochloride) 442
See Dilaudid Oral Liquid

DILAUDID-HP LYOPHILIZED POWDER 250 MG

(Hydromorphone Hydrochloride) 442
See Dilaudid Oral Liquid

CHILDREN'S DIMETAPP COLD & ALLERGY ELIXIR

(Brompheniramine Maleate, Phenylephrine Hydrochloride)........ ▣730
May interact with hypnotics and sedatives, monoamine oxidase inhibitors, tranquilizers, and certain other agents. Compounds in these categories include:

Alprazolam (May increase drowsiness effect). Products include:
Niravam Orally Disintegrating Tablets 3092

Buspirone Hydrochloride (May increase drowsiness effect).
No products indexed under this heading.

Chlordiazepoxide (May increase drowsiness effect).
No products indexed under this heading.

Chlordiazepoxide Hydrochloride (May increase drowsiness effect). Products include:
Librium Capsules 3347

Chlorpromazine (May increase drowsiness effect).
No products indexed under this heading.

Chlorpromazine Hydrochloride (May increase drowsiness effect).
No products indexed under this heading.

Chlorprothixene (May increase drowsiness effect).
No products indexed under this heading.

Chlorprothixene Hydrochloride (May increase drowsiness effect).
No products indexed under this heading.

Clorazepate Dipotassium (May increase drowsiness effect). Products include:
Tranxene 2474

Diazepam (May increase drowsiness effect). Products include:
Diastat Rectal Delivery System 3343
Valium Tablets 2819

Droperidol (May increase drowsiness effect).
No products indexed under this heading.

Estazolam (May increase drowsiness effect). Products include:
ProSom Tablets 517

Ethchlorvynol (May increase drowsiness effect).
No products indexed under this heading.

Ethinamate (May increase drowsiness effect).
No products indexed under this heading.

Fluphenazine Decanoate (May increase drowsiness effect).
No products indexed under this heading.

Fluphenazine Enanthate (May increase drowsiness effect).
No products indexed under this heading.

Fluphenazine Hydrochloride (May increase drowsiness effect).
No products indexed under this heading.

Flurazepam Hydrochloride (May increase drowsiness effect). Products include:
Dalmane Capsules 3342

Glutethimide (May increase drowsiness effect).
No products indexed under this heading.

Haloperidol (May increase drowsiness effect).
No products indexed under this heading.

Haloperidol Decanoate (May increase drowsiness effect).
No products indexed under this heading.

Hydroxyzine Hydrochloride (May increase drowsiness effect).
No products indexed under this heading.

Isocarboxazid (Concurrent and/or sequential use with MAO inhibitors is not recommended).
No products indexed under this heading.

Lorazepam (May increase drowsiness effect).
No products indexed under this heading.

Loxapine Hydrochloride (May increase drowsiness effect).
No products indexed under this heading.

Loxapine Succinate (May increase drowsiness effect).
No products indexed under this heading.

Meprobamate (May increase drowsiness effect).
No products indexed under this heading.

Mesoridazine Besylate (May increase drowsiness effect).
No products indexed under this heading.

Midazolam Hydrochloride (May increase drowsiness effect).
No products indexed under this heading.

Moclobemide (Concurrent and/or sequential use with MAO inhibitors is not recommended).
No products indexed under this heading.

Molindone Hydrochloride (May increase drowsiness effect). Products include:
Moban Tablets 1119

Oxazepam (May increase drowsiness effect).
No products indexed under this heading.

Pargyline Hydrochloride (Concurrent and/or sequential use with MAO inhibitors is not recommended).
No products indexed under this heading.

Perphenazine (May increase drowsiness effect).
No products indexed under this heading.

Phenelzine Sulfate (Concurrent and/or sequential use with MAO inhibitors is not recommended).
No products indexed under this heading.

Prazepam (May increase drowsiness effect).
No products indexed under this heading.

Procarbazine Hydrochloride (Concurrent and/or sequential use with MAO inhibitors is not recommended). Products include:
Matulane Capsules 3191

Prochlorperazine (May increase drowsiness effect).
No products indexed under this heading.

Promethazine Hydrochloride (May increase drowsiness effect). Products include:
Phenergan Tablets and Suppositories 3440

Propofol (May increase drowsiness effect).
No products indexed under this heading.

Quazepam (May increase drowsiness effect).
No products indexed under this heading.

Ramelteon (May increase drowsiness effect). Products include:
Rozerem Tablets 3231

Secobarbital Sodium (May increase drowsiness effect).
No products indexed under this heading.

Selegiline Hydrochloride (Concurrent and/or sequential use with MAO inhibitors is not recommended). Products include:
Eldepryl Capsules 3208
Zelapar Tablets 3372

Temazepam (May increase drowsiness effect). Products include:
Restoril Capsules 1860

Thioridazine Hydrochloride (May increase drowsiness effect). Products include:
Thioridazine Hydrochloride Tablets 2163

Thiothixene (May increase drowsiness effect). Products include:
Thiothixene Capsules 2165

Tranylcypromine Sulfate (Concurrent and/or sequential use with MAO inhibitors is not recommended). Products include:
Parnate Tablets 1527

Triazolam (May increase drowsiness effect).
No products indexed under this heading.

Trifluoperazine Hydrochloride (May increase drowsiness effect).
No products indexed under this heading.

Zaleplon (May increase drowsiness effect). Products include:
Sonata Capsules 1717

Zolpidem Tartrate (May increase drowsiness effect). Products include:
Ambien Tablets 2851
Ambien CR Tablets 2855

Food Interactions

Alcohol (May increase drowsiness effect).

CHILDREN'S DIMETAPP COLD & ALLERGY CHEWABLE TABLETS

(Brompheniramine Maleate, Phenylephrine Hydrochloride)........ ▣730
May interact with hypnotics and sedatives, monoamine oxidase inhibitors, and tranquilizers. Compounds in these categories include:

Alprazolam (May increase drowsiness effect). Products include:
Niravam Orally Disintegrating Tablets 3092

Buspirone Hydrochloride (May increase drowsiness effect).
No products indexed under this heading.

Chlordiazepoxide (May increase drowsiness effect).
No products indexed under this heading.

Chlordiazepoxide Hydrochloride (May increase drowsiness effect). Products include:
Librium Capsules 3347

Chlorpromazine (May increase drowsiness effect).
No products indexed under this heading.

Chlorpromazine Hydrochloride (May increase drowsiness effect).
No products indexed under this heading.

Chlorprothixene (May increase drowsiness effect).
No products indexed under this heading.

Chlorprothixene Hydrochloride (May increase drowsiness effect).
No products indexed under this heading.

Clorazepate Dipotassium (May increase drowsiness effect). Products include:
Tranxene 2474

Diazepam (May increase drowsiness effect). Products include:
Diastat Rectal Delivery System 3343
Valium Tablets 2819

Droperidol (May increase drowsiness effect).
No products indexed under this heading.

Estazolam (May increase drowsiness effect). Products include:
ProSom Tablets 517

Ethchlorvynol (May increase drowsiness effect).
No products indexed under this heading.

Ethinamate (May increase drowsiness effect).
No products indexed under this heading.

Fluphenazine Decanoate (May increase drowsiness effect).
No products indexed under this heading.

Fluphenazine Enanthate (May increase drowsiness effect).
No products indexed under this heading.

Fluphenazine Hydrochloride (May increase drowsiness effect).
No products indexed under this heading.

Flurazepam Hydrochloride (May increase drowsiness effect). Products include:
Dalmane Capsules 3342

Glutethimide (May increase drowsiness effect).
No products indexed under this heading.

Haloperidol (May increase drowsiness effect).
No products indexed under this heading.

Haloperidol Decanoate (May increase drowsiness effect).
No products indexed under this heading.

Hydroxyzine Hydrochloride (May increase drowsiness effect).
No products indexed under this heading.

Isocarboxazid (Concurrent or sequential use with MAO inhibitors is not recommended).
No products indexed under this heading.

Lorazepam (May increase drowsiness effect).
No products indexed under this heading.

Loxapine Hydrochloride (May increase drowsiness effect).
No products indexed under this heading.

Loxapine Succinate (May increase drowsiness effect).
No products indexed under this heading.

Meprobamate (May increase drowsiness effect).
No products indexed under this heading.

Mesoridazine Besylate (May increase drowsiness effect).
No products indexed under this heading.

Midazolam Hydrochloride (May increase drowsiness effect).
No products indexed under this heading.

Moclobemide (Concurrent or sequential use with MAO inhibitors is not recommended).
No products indexed under this heading.

Molindone Hydrochloride (May increase drowsiness effect). Products include:
Moban Tablets 1119

Oxazepam (May increase drowsiness effect).
No products indexed under this heading.

Pargyline Hydrochloride (Concurrent or sequential use with MAO inhibitors is not recommended).
No products indexed under this heading.

Perphenazine (May increase drowsiness effect).
No products indexed under this heading.

Phenelzine Sulfate (Concurrent or sequential use with MAO inhibitors is not recommended).
No products indexed under this heading.

Prazepam (May increase drowsiness effect).
No products indexed under this heading.

Procarbazine Hydrochloride (Concurrent or sequential use with MAO inhibitors is not recommended). Products include:
Matulane Capsules 3191

Prochlorperazine (May increase drowsiness effect).
No products indexed under this heading.

Promethazine Hydrochloride (May increase drowsiness effect). Products include:
Phenergan Tablets and
Suppositories 3440

Propofol (May increase drowsiness effect).
No products indexed under this heading.

Quazepam (May increase drowsiness effect).
No products indexed under this heading.

Ramelteon (May increase drowsiness effect). Products include:

Rozerem Tablets 3231

Secobarbital Sodium (May increase drowsiness effect).
No products indexed under this heading.

Selegiline Hydrochloride (Concurrent or sequential use with MAO inhibitors is not recommended). Products include:
Eldepryl Capsules 3208
Zelapar Tablets 3372

Temazepam (May increase drowsiness effect). Products include:
Restoril Capsules 1860

Thioridazine Hydrochloride (May increase drowsiness effect). Products include:
Thioridazine Hydrochloride
Tablets 2163

Thiothixene (May increase drowsiness effect). Products include:
Thiothixene Capsules 2165

Tranylcypromine Sulfate (Concurrent or sequential use with MAO inhibitors is not recommended). Products include:
Parnate Tablets 1527

Triazolam (May increase drowsiness effect).
No products indexed under this heading.

Trifluoperazine Hydrochloride (May increase drowsiness effect).
No products indexed under this heading.

Zaleplon (May increase drowsiness effect). Products include:
Sonata Capsules 1717

Zolpidem Tartrate (May increase drowsiness effect). Products include:
Ambien Tablets 2851
Ambien CR Tablets 2855

CHILDREN'S DIMETAPP DM COLD & COUGH ELIXIR

(Brompheniramine Maleate, Dextromethorphan Hydrobromide, Phenylephrine Hydrochloride)............ 731
May interact with hypnotics and sedatives, monoamine oxidase inhibitors, tranquilizers, and certain other agents. Compounds in these categories include:

Alprazolam (Increases drowsiness effect). Products include:
Niravam Orally Disintegrating
Tablets 3092

Buspirone Hydrochloride (Increases drowsiness effect).
No products indexed under this heading.

Chlordiazepoxide (Increases drowsiness effect).
No products indexed under this heading.

Chlordiazepoxide Hydrochloride (Increases drowsiness effect). Products include:
Librium Capsules 3347

Chlorpromazine (Increases drowsiness effect).
No products indexed under this heading.

Chlorpromazine Hydrochloride (Increases drowsiness effect).
No products indexed under this heading.

Chlorprothixene (Increases drowsiness effect).
No products indexed under this heading.

Chlorprothixene Hydrochloride (Increases drowsiness effect).
No products indexed under this heading.

Clorazepate Dipotassium (Increases drowsiness effect). Products include:
Tranxene 2474

Diazepam (Increases drowsiness effect). Products include:
Diastat Rectal Delivery System 3343
Valium Tablets 2819

Droperidol (Increases drowsiness effect).
No products indexed under this heading.

Estazolam (Increases drowsiness effect). Products include:
ProSom Tablets 517

Ethchlorvynol (Increases drowsiness effect).
No products indexed under this heading.

Ethinamate (Increases drowsiness effect).
No products indexed under this heading.

Fluphenazine Decanoate (Increases drowsiness effect).
No products indexed under this heading.

Fluphenazine Enanthate (Increases drowsiness effect).
No products indexed under this heading.

Fluphenazine Hydrochloride (Increases drowsiness effect).
No products indexed under this heading.

Flurazepam Hydrochloride (Increases drowsiness effect). Products include:
Dalmane Capsules 3342

Glutethimide (Increases drowsiness effect).
No products indexed under this heading.

Haloperidol (Increases drowsiness effect).
No products indexed under this heading.

Haloperidol Decanoate (Increases drowsiness effect).
No products indexed under this heading.

Hydroxyzine Hydrochloride (Increases drowsiness effect).
No products indexed under this heading.

Isocarboxazid (Concurrent and/or sequential use with MAO inhibitors is not recommended).
No products indexed under this heading.

Lorazepam (Increases drowsiness effect).
No products indexed under this heading.

Loxapine Hydrochloride (Increases drowsiness effect).
No products indexed under this heading.

Loxapine Succinate (Increases drowsiness effect).
No products indexed under this heading.

Meprobamate (Increases drowsiness effect).
No products indexed under this heading.

Mesoridazine Besylate (Increases drowsiness effect).
No products indexed under this heading.

Midazolam Hydrochloride (Increases drowsiness effect).
No products indexed under this heading.

IMPORTANT NOTE: Always consult each drug listing in the patient's regimen for possible interactions.

Moclobemide (Concurrent and/or sequential use with MAO inhibitors is not recommended).
No products indexed under this heading.

Molindone Hydrochloride (Increases drowsiness effect). Products include:
Moban Tablets 1119

Oxazepam (Increases drowsiness effect).
No products indexed under this heading.

Pargyline Hydrochloride (Concurrent and/or sequential use with MAO inhibitors is not recommended).
No products indexed under this heading.

Perphenazine (Increases drowsiness effect).
No products indexed under this heading.

Phenelzine Sulfate (Concurrent and/or sequential use with MAO inhibitors is not recommended).
No products indexed under this heading.

Prazepam (Increases drowsiness effect).
No products indexed under this heading.

Procarbazine Hydrochloride (Concurrent and/or sequential use with MAO inhibitors is not recommended). Products include:
Matulane Capsules 3191

Prochlorperazine (Increases drowsiness effect).
No products indexed under this heading.

Promethazine Hydrochloride (Increases drowsiness effect). Products include:
Phenergan Tablets and
Suppositories................................ 3440

Propofol (Increases drowsiness effect).
No products indexed under this heading.

Quazepam (Increases drowsiness effect).
No products indexed under this heading.

Ramelteon (Increases drowsiness effect). Products include:
Rozerem Tablets 3231

Secobarbital Sodium (Increases drowsiness effect).
No products indexed under this heading.

Selegiline Hydrochloride (Concurrent and/or sequential use with MAO inhibitors is not recommended). Products include:
Eldepryl Capsules 3208
Zelapar Tablets 3372

Temazepam (Increases drowsiness effect). Products include:
Restoril Capsules 1860

Thioridazine Hydrochloride (Increases drowsiness effect). Products include:
Thioridazine Hydrochloride
Tablets 2163

Thiothixene (Increases drowsiness effect). Products include:
Thiothixene Capsules 2165

Tranylcypromine Sulfate (Concurrent and/or sequential use with MAO inhibitors is not recommended). Products include:
Parnate Tablets 1527

Triazolam (Increases drowsiness effect).
No products indexed under this heading.

Trifluoperazine Hydrochloride (Increases drowsiness effect).
No products indexed under this heading.

Zaleplon (Increases drowsiness effect). Products include:
Sonata Capsules 1717

Zolpidem Tartrate (Increases drowsiness effect). Products include:
Ambien Tablets 2851
Ambien CR Tablets 2855

Food Interactions

Alcohol (Increases drowsiness effect; avoid concurrent use).

CHILDREN'S DIMETAPP LONG ACTING COUGH PLUS COLD SYRUP

(Chlorpheniramine Maleate, Dextromethorphan Hydrobromide).... ▣731
May interact with hypnotics and sedatives, monoamine oxidase inhibitors, and tranquilizers. Compounds in these categories include:

Alprazolam (May increase drowsiness). Products include:
Niravam Orally Disintegrating
Tablets .. 3092

Buspirone Hydrochloride (May increase drowsiness).
No products indexed under this heading.

Chlordiazepoxide (May increase drowsiness).
No products indexed under this heading.

Chlordiazepoxide Hydrochloride (May increase drowsiness). Products include:
Librium Capsules 3347

Chlorpromazine (May increase drowsiness).
No products indexed under this heading.

Chlorpromazine Hydrochloride (May increase drowsiness).
No products indexed under this heading.

Chlorprothixene (May increase drowsiness).
No products indexed under this heading.

Chlorprothixene Hydrochloride (May increase drowsiness).
No products indexed under this heading.

Clorazepate Dipotassium (May increase drowsiness). Products include:
Tranxene 2474

Diazepam (May increase drowsiness). Products include:
Diastat Rectal Delivery System 3343
Valium Tablets 2819

Droperidol (May increase drowsiness).
No products indexed under this heading.

Estazolam (May increase drowsiness). Products include:
ProSom Tablets 517

Ethchlorvynol (May increase drowsiness).
No products indexed under this heading.

Ethinamate (May increase drowsiness).
No products indexed under this heading.

Fluphenazine Decanoate (May increase drowsiness).
No products indexed under this heading.

Fluphenazine Enanthate (May increase drowsiness).
No products indexed under this heading.

Fluphenazine Hydrochloride (May increase drowsiness).
No products indexed under this heading.

Flurazepam Hydrochloride (May increase drowsiness). Products include:
Dalmane Capsules 3342

Glutethimide (May increase drowsiness).
No products indexed under this heading.

Haloperidol (May increase drowsiness).
No products indexed under this heading.

Haloperidol Decanoate (May increase drowsiness).
No products indexed under this heading.

Hydroxyzine Hydrochloride (May increase drowsiness).
No products indexed under this heading.

Isocarboxazid (Do not use while taking, or for up to two weeks after stopping, MAO inhibitors.).
No products indexed under this heading.

Lorazepam (May increase drowsiness).
No products indexed under this heading.

Loxapine Hydrochloride (May increase drowsiness).
No products indexed under this heading.

Loxapine Succinate (May increase drowsiness).
No products indexed under this heading.

Meprobamate (May increase drowsiness).
No products indexed under this heading.

Mesoridazine Besylate (May increase drowsiness).
No products indexed under this heading.

Midazolam Hydrochloride (May increase drowsiness).
No products indexed under this heading.

Moclobemide (Do not use while taking, or for up to two weeks after stopping, MAO inhibitors.).
No products indexed under this heading.

Molindone Hydrochloride (May increase drowsiness). Products include:
Moban Tablets 1119

Oxazepam (May increase drowsiness).
No products indexed under this heading.

Pargyline Hydrochloride (Do not use while taking, or for up to two weeks after stopping, MAO inhibitors.).
No products indexed under this heading.

Perphenazine (May increase drowsiness).
No products indexed under this heading.

Phenelzine Sulfate (Do not use while taking, or for up to two weeks after stopping, MAO inhibitors.).
No products indexed under this heading.

Prazepam (May increase drowsiness).
No products indexed under this heading.

Procarbazine Hydrochloride (Do not use while taking, or for up to two weeks after stopping, MAO inhibitors). Products include:
Matulane Capsules 3191

Prochlorperazine (May increase drowsiness).
No products indexed under this heading.

Promethazine Hydrochloride (May increase drowsiness). Products include:
Phenergan Tablets and
Suppositories................................ 3440

Propofol (May increase drowsiness).
No products indexed under this heading.

Quazepam (May increase drowsiness).
No products indexed under this heading.

Ramelteon (May increase drowsiness). Products include:
Rozerem Tablets 3231

Secobarbital Sodium (May increase drowsiness).
No products indexed under this heading.

Selegiline Hydrochloride (Do not use while taking, or for up to two weeks after stopping, MAO inhibitors). Products include:
Eldepryl Capsules 3208
Zelapar Tablets 3372

Temazepam (May increase drowsiness). Products include:
Restoril Capsules 1860

Thioridazine Hydrochloride (May increase drowsiness). Products include:
Thioridazine Hydrochloride
Tablets 2163

Thiothixene (May increase drowsiness). Products include:
Thiothixene Capsules 2165

Tranylcypromine Sulfate (Do not use while taking, or for up to two weeks after stopping, MAO inhibitors). Products include:
Parnate Tablets 1527

Triazolam (May increase drowsiness).
No products indexed under this heading.

Trifluoperazine Hydrochloride (May increase drowsiness).
No products indexed under this heading.

Zaleplon (May increase drowsiness). Products include:
Sonata Capsules 1717

Zolpidem Tartrate (May increase drowsiness). Products include:
Ambien Tablets 2851
Ambien CR Tablets 2855

TODDLER'S DIMETAPP COLD AND COUGH DROPS
(Dextromethorphan Hydrobromide, Phenylephrine Hydrochloride) 732
May interact with monoamine oxidase inhibitors. Compounds in these categories include:

Isocarboxazid (Concurrent and/or sequential use with MAO inhibitors is not recommended).
No products indexed under this heading.

Moclobemide (Concurrent and/or sequential use with MAO inhibitors is not recommended).
No products indexed under this heading.

Pargyline Hydrochloride (Concurrent and/or sequential use with MAO inhibitors is not recommended).
No products indexed under this heading.

Phenelzine Sulfate (Concurrent and/or sequential use with MAO inhibitors is not recommended).
No products indexed under this heading.

Procarbazine Hydrochloride (Concurrent and/or sequential use with MAO inhibitors is not recommended). Products include:
Matulane Capsules 3191

Selegiline Hydrochloride (Concurrent and/or sequential use with MAO inhibitors is not recommended). Products include:
Eldepryl Capsules 3208
Zelapar Tablets 3372

Tranylcypromine Sulfate (Concurrent and/or sequential use with MAO inhibitors is not recommended). Products include:
Parnate Tablets 1527

DIOVAN TABLETS
(Valsartan) 2193
May interact with potassium preparations, potassium sparing diuretics, and certain other agents. Compounds in these categories include:

Amiloride Hydrochloride (Concurrent use may lead to hyperkalemia; potential for increase in serum creatinine in heart failure patients if used concurrently). Products include:
Midamor Tablets 2026
Moduretic Tablets 2028

Atenolol (Combination therapy is more antihypertensive than either component, but does not lower the heart rate more than atenolol alone).
No products indexed under this heading.

Potassium Acid Phosphate (Concurrent use may lead to hyperkalemia; potential for increase in serum creatinine in heart failure patients if used concurrently). Products include:
K-Phos Original (Sodium Free) Tablets 760

Potassium Bicarbonate (Concurrent use may lead to hyperkalemia; potential for increase in serum creatinine in heart failure patients if used concurrently).
No products indexed under this heading.

Potassium Chloride (Concurrent use may lead to hyperkalemia; potential for increase in serum creatinine in heart failure patients if used concurrently). Products include:
Colyte with Flavor Packs for Oral Solution 3088
HalfLytely and Bisacodyl Tablets Bowel Prep Kit with Flavors Packs 881
K-Dur Extended-Relase Tablets 3033
K-Lor Oral Solution 474
K-Tab Tablets 475
MoviPrep Oral Solution 2839
TriLyte with Flavor Packs for Oral Solution 3100

Potassium Citrate (Concurrent use may lead to hyperkalemia; potential for increase in serum creatinine in heart failure patients if used concurrently). Products include:
Urocit-K Tablets 2144

Potassium Gluconate (Concurrent use may lead to hyperkalemia; potential for increase in serum creatinine in heart failure patients if used concurrently).
No products indexed under this heading.

Potassium Phosphate (Concurrent use may lead to hyperkalemia; potential for increase in serum creatinine in heart failure patients if used concurrently). Products include:
K-Phos Neutral Tablets 760

Salt Substitutes (Concurrent use may lead to hyperkalemia; potential for increase in serum creatinine in heart failure patients if used concurrently).
No products indexed under this heading.

Spironolactone (Concurrent use may lead to hyperkalemia; potential for increase in serum creatinine in heart failure patients if used concurrently).
No products indexed under this heading.

Triamterene (Concurrent use may lead to hyperkalemia; potential for increase in serum creatinine in heart failure patients if used concurrently). Products include:
Dyazide Capsules 1423
Dyrenium Capsules 3400

Food Interactions

Food, unspecified (Decreases the exposure (as measured by AUC) to valsartan about 40% and peak plasma concentration by about 50%).

DIOVAN HCT TABLETS
(Hydrochlorothiazide, Valsartan) 2196
May interact with antihypertensives, barbiturates, corticosteroids, cardiac glycosides, oral hypoglycemic agents, insulin, lithium preparations, narcotic analgesics, nondepolarizing neuromuscular blocking agents, nonsteroidal anti-inflammatory agents, potassium preparations, and certain other agents. Compounds in these categories include:

Acarbose (Dosage adjustment of the antidiabetic drug may be required). Products include:
Precose Tablets 751

Acebutolol Hydrochloride (Co-administration with other antihypertensives may result in additive effect or potentiation).
No products indexed under this heading.

ACTH (Co-administration of thiazide diuretics and ACTH may intensify electrolyte depletion, particularly hypokalemia).
No products indexed under this heading.

Alfentanil Hydrochloride (Co-administration of thiazide diuretics and narcotics may result in potentiation of orthostatic hypotension).
No products indexed under this heading.

Amlodipine Besylate (Co-administration with other antihypertensives may result in additive effect or potentiation). Products include:
Caduet Tablets 2508
Lotrel Capsules 2249
Norvasc Tablets 2545

Aprobarbital (Co-administration of thiazide diuretics and barbiturates may result in potentiation of orthostatic hypotension).
No products indexed under this heading.

Atenolol (Co-administration with other antihypertensives may result in additive effect or potentiation).
No products indexed under this heading.

Atracurium Besylate (Co-administration of thiazide diuretics and nondepolarizing skeletal muscle relaxants increases responsiveness to the muscle relaxants).
No products indexed under this heading.

Benazepril Hydrochloride (Co-administration with other antihypertensives may result in additive effect or potentiation). Products include:
Lotensin Tablets 2243
Lotensin HCT Tablets 2246
Lotrel Capsules 2249

Bendroflumethiazide (Co-administration with other antihypertensives may result in additive effect or potentiation).
No products indexed under this heading.

Betamethasone Acetate (Co-administration of thiazide diuretics and corticosteroids may intensify electrolyte depletion, particularly hypokalemia).
No products indexed under this heading.

Betamethasone Sodium Phosphate (Co-administration of thiazide diuretics and corticosteroids may intensify electrolyte depletion, particularly hypokalemia).
No products indexed under this heading.

Betaxolol Hydrochloride (Co-administration with other antihypertensives may result in additive effect or potentiation). Products include:
Betoptic S Ophthalmic Suspension 558

Bisoprolol Fumarate (Co-administration with other antihypertensives may result in additive effect or potentiation).
No products indexed under this heading.

Buprenorphine Hydrochloride (Co-administration of thiazide diuretics and narcotics may result in potentiation of orthostatic hypotension). Products include:
Buprenex Injectable 2716
Suboxone Tablets 2717
Subutex Tablets 2717

Butabarbital (Co-administration of thiazide diuretics and barbiturates may result in potentiation of orthostatic hypotension).
No products indexed under this heading.

Butalbital (Co-administration of thiazide diuretics and barbiturates may result in potentiation of orthostatic hypotension).
No products indexed under this heading.

Candesartan Cilexetil (Co-administration with other antihypertensives may result in additive effect or potentiation). Products include:
Atacand Tablets 649
Atacand HCT 651

Captopril (Co-administration with other antihypertensives may result in additive effect or potentiation). Products include:
Captopril Tablets 2149

Carteolol Hydrochloride (Co-administration with other antihypertensives may result in additive effect or potentiation). Products include:
Carteolol Hydrochloride Ophthalmic Solution USP, 1% .... ⊙249

Celecoxib (Co-administration of thiazide diuretics and non-steroidal anti-inflammatory agents can reduce the diuretic, natiuretic, and antihypertensive effects). Products include:
Celebrex Capsules 3134

Chlorothiazide (Co-administration with other antihypertensives may result in additive effect or potentiation). Products include:
Diuril Oral Suspension 1954

Chlorothiazide Sodium (Co-administration with other antihypertensives may result in additive effect or potentiation). Products include:
Diuril Sodium Intravenous 2467

Chlorpropamide (Dosage adjustment of the antidiabetic drug may be required).
No products indexed under this heading.

Chlorthalidone (Co-administration with other antihypertensives may result in additive effect or potentiation). Products include:
Clorpres Tablets 2153

Cholestyramine (Absorption of hydrochlorothiazide is impaired in the presence of anionic exchange resins, such as cholestyramine resulting in binding of the hydrochlorothiazide resulting in reduced absorption from GI tract by 85%).
No products indexed under this heading.

Cisatracurium Besylate (Co-administration of thiazide diuretics and nondepolarizing skeletal muscle relaxants increases responsiveness to the muscle relaxants). Products include:
Nimbex Injection 498

Clonidine (Co-administration with other antihypertensives may result in additive effect or potentiation). Products include:
Catapres-TTS 844

Clonidine Hydrochloride (Co-administration with other antihypertensives may result in additive effect or potentiation). Products include:
Catapres Tablets 843
Clorpres Tablets 2153

Codeine Phosphate (Co-administration of thiazide diuretics and narcotics may result in potentiation of orthostatic hypotension). Products include:
Tylenol with Codeine Tablets 2391

Colestipol Hydrochloride (Absorption of hydrochlorothiazide is impaired in the presence of anionic exchange resins, such as colestipol resulting in binding of the hydrochlorothiazide resulting in reduced absorption from GI tract by 43%).
No products indexed under this heading.

Cortisone Acetate (Co-administration of thiazide diuretics and corticosteroids may intensify electrolyte depletion, particularly hypokalemia).
No products indexed under this heading.

Deserpidine (Co-administration with other antihypertensives may result in additive effect or potentiation).
No products indexed under this heading.

Deslanoside (Hypokalemia induced by thiazides may cause cardiac arrhythmia and may sensitize or exaggerate the response of the heart to the toxic effects of digitalis, such as increased ventricular irritability).
No products indexed under this heading.

Dexamethasone (Co-administration of thiazide diuretics and corticosteroids may intensify electrolyte depletion, particularly hypokalemia). Products include:
Ciprodex Otic Suspension 559
Decadron Tablets 1951
TobraDex Ophthalmic Ointment 562
TobraDex Ophthalmic Suspension 563

Dexamethasone Acetate (Co-administration of thiazide diuretics and corticosteroids may intensify electrolyte depletion, particularly hypokalemia).
No products indexed under this heading.

Dexamethasone Sodium Phosphate (Co-administration of thiazide diuretics and corticosteroids may intensify electrolyte depletion, particularly hypokalemia).
No products indexed under this heading.

Dezocine (Co-administration of thiazide diuretics and narcotics may result in potentiation of orthostatic hypotension).
No products indexed under this heading.

Diazoxide (Co-administration with other antihypertensives may result in additive effect or potentiation). Products include:
Hyperstat I.V. 3017

Diclofenac Potassium (Co-administration of thiazide diuretics and non-steroidal anti-inflammatory agents can reduce the diuretic, natiuretic, and antihypertensive effects).
No products indexed under this heading.

Diclofenac Sodium (Co-administration of thiazide diuretics and non-steroidal anti-inflammatory agents can reduce the diuretic, natiuretic, and antihypertensive effects). Products include:
Arthrotec Tablets 3129
Voltaren Ophthalmic Solution 2309
Voltaren Tablets 2307
Voltaren-XR Tablets 2310

Digitalis Glycoside Preparations (Hypokalemia induced by thiazides may cause cardiac arrhythmia and may sensitize or exaggerate the response of the heart to the toxic effects of digitalis, such as increased ventricular irritability).
No products indexed under this heading.

Digitoxin (Hypokalemia induced by thiazides may cause cardiac arrhythmia and may sensitize or exaggerate the response of the heart to the toxic effects of digitalis, such as increased ventricular irritability).
No products indexed under this heading.

Digoxin (Hypokalemia induced by thiazides may cause cardiac arrhythmia and may sensitize or exaggerate the response of the heart to the toxic effects of digitalis, such as increased ventricular irritability). Products include:
Lanoxicaps Capsules 1490
Lanoxin Injection 1494
Lanoxin Injection Pediatric 1497
Lanoxin Tablets 1500

Diltiazem Hydrochloride (Co-administration with other antihypertensives may result in additive effect or potentiation). Products include:
Cardizem LA Extended Release Tablets 1728
Tiazac Capsules 1201

Doxazosin Mesylate (Co-administration with other antihypertensives may result in additive effect or potentiation). Products include:
Cardura XL Tablets 2515

Enalapril Maleate (Co-administration with other antihypertensives may result in additive effect or potentiation). Products include:
Vasotec I.V. Injection 2103

Enalaprilat (Co-administration with other antihypertensives may result in additive effect or potentiation).
No products indexed under this heading.

Eprosartan Mesylate (Co-administration with other antihypertensives may result in additive effect or potentiation). Products include:
Teveten Tablets 1735
Teveten HCT Tablets 1737

Esmolol Hydrochloride (Co-administration with other antihypertensives may result in additive effect or potentiation).
No products indexed under this heading.

Etodolac (Co-administration of thiazide diuretics and non-steroidal anti-inflammatory agents can reduce the diuretic, natiuretic, and antihypertensive effects).
No products indexed under this heading.

Felodipine (Co-administration with other antihypertensives may result in additive effect or potentiation).
No products indexed under this heading.

Fenoprofen Calcium (Co-administration of thiazide diuretics and non-steroidal anti-inflammatory agents can reduce the diuretic, natiuretic, and antihypertensive effects). Products include:
Nalfon Capsules 2502

Fentanyl (Co-administration of thiazide diuretics and narcotics may result in potentiation of orthostatic hypotension). Products include:
Duragesic Transdermal System 2373
Ionsys Transdermal System 2379

Fentanyl Citrate (Co-administration of thiazide diuretics and narcotics may result in potentiation of orthostatic hypotension). Products include:
Actiq 979

Fludrocortisone Acetate (Co-administration of thiazide diuretics and corticosteroids may intensify electrolyte depletion, particularly hypokalemia).
No products indexed under this heading.

Flurbiprofen (Co-administration of thiazide diuretics and non-steroidal anti-inflammatory agents can reduce the diuretic, natiuretic, and antihypertensive effects).
No products indexed under this heading.

Fosinopril Sodium (Co-administration with other antihypertensives may result in additive effect or potentiation).
No products indexed under this heading.

Furosemide (Co-administration with other antihypertensives may result in additive effect or potentiation). Products include:
Furosemide Tablets 2154

Glimepiride (Dosage adjustment of the antidiabetic drug may be required). Products include:
Avandaryl Tablets 1379
Duetact Tablets 3226

Glipizide (Dosage adjustment of the antidiabetic drug may be required).
No products indexed under this heading.

Glyburide (Dosage adjustment of the antidiabetic drug may be required).
No products indexed under this heading.

Guanabenz Acetate (Co-administration with other antihypertensives may result in additive effect or potentiation).
No products indexed under this heading.

Guanethidine Monosulfate (Co-administration with other antihypertensives may result in additive effect or potentiation).
No products indexed under this heading.

Hydralazine Hydrochloride (Co-administration with other antihypertensives may result in additive effect or potentiation). Products include:
BiDil Tablets 2171

Hydrocodone Bitartrate (Co-administration of thiazide diuretics and narcotics may result in potentiation of orthostatic hypotension). Products include:
Hycodan 1116
Hycotuss Expectorant Syrup 1117
Vicodin Tablets 535
Vicodin ES Tablets 536
Vicodin HP Tablets 538
Vicoprofen Tablets 539
Zydone Tablets 1139

Hydrocodone Polistirex (Co-administration of thiazide diuretics and narcotics may result in potentiation of orthostatic hypotension). Products include:
Tussionex Pennkinetic Extended-Release Suspension 3327

Hydrocortisone (Co-administration of thiazide diuretics and corticosteroids may intensify electrolyte depletion, particularly hypokalemia). Products include:
Colocort Rectal Suspension, USP (Retention) 100 mg/60 mL 2476
Hydrocortone Tablets 1989
Preparation H Hydrocortisone Cream .... ■□ 646

Hydrocortisone Acetate (Co-administration of thiazide diuretics and corticosteroids may intensify electrolyte depletion, particularly hypokalemia). Products include:
Analpram-HC 1159
Pramosone 1161
ProctoFoam-HC 3099

Hydrocortisone Sodium Phosphate (Co-administration of thiazide diuretics and corticosteroids may intensify electrolyte depletion, particularly hypokalemia).
No products indexed under this heading.

Hydrocortisone Sodium Succinate (Co-administration of thiazide diuretics and corticosteroids may intensify electrolyte depletion, particularly hypokalemia).
No products indexed under this heading.

Hydroflumethiazide (Co-administration with other antihypertensives may result in additive effect or potentiation).
No products indexed under this heading.

Hydromorphone Hydrochloride (Co-administration of thiazide diuretics and narcotics may result in potentiation of orthostatic hypotension). Products include:
Dilaudid 440
Dilaudid Non-Sterile Powder 440
Dilaudid Oral Liquid 445
Dilaudid Rectal Suppositories 440
Dilaudid Tablets 440
Dilaudid Tablets - 8 mg 445
Dilaudid-HP 442

Ibuprofen (Co-administration of thiazide diuretics and non-steroidal anti-inflammatory agents can reduce the diuretic, natiuretic, and antihypertensive effects). Products include:
Advil Allergy Sinus Caplets .... ■□ 770
Advil .... ■□ 674
Children's Advil Oral Suspension .... ■□ 603
Children's Advil Chewable Tablets .... ■□ 603
Advil Cold & Sinus .... ■□ 723
Infants' Advil Concentrated Drops .... ■□ 604
Infants' Advil Concentrated Drops - White Grape (Dye-Free) .... ■□ 604
Junior Strength Advil Swallow Tablets .... ■□ 605
Advil Migraine Liquigels .... ■□ 608
Advil Multi-Symptom Cold Caplets .... ■□ 770
Advil PM Caplets .... ■□ 615
Motrin IB Tablets and Caplets 1866
Children's Motrin Oral Suspension 1867
Children's Motrin Non-Staining Dye-Free Oral Suspension 1867
Children's Motrin Cold Oral Suspension 1867
Infants' Motrin Concentrated Drops 1867
Infants' Motrin Non-Staining Dye-Free Concentrated Drops 1867
Junior Strength Motrin Caplets and Chewable Tablets 1867
Vicoprofen Tablets 539

Indapamide (Co-administration with other antihypertensives may result in additive effect or potentiation). Products include:
Indapamide Tablets 2156

Indomethacin (Co-administration of thiazide diuretics and non-steroidal anti-inflammatory agents can reduce the diuretic, natiuretic, and antihypertensive effects). Products include:

Indocin 1995

Indomethacin Sodium Trihydrate (Co-administration of thiazide diuretics and non-steroidal anti-inflammatory agents can reduce the diuretic, natiuretic, and antihypertensive effects). Products include:
Indocin I.V. 2465

Insulin, Human, Zinc Suspension (Dosage adjustment of the antidiabetic drug may be required). Products include:
Humulin L, 100 Units 1794
Humulin U, 100 Units 1800

Insulin, Human NPH (Dosage adjustment of the antidiabetic drug may be required). Products include:
Humulin N, 100 Units 1795
Humulin N Pen 1797

Insulin, Human Regular (Dosage adjustment of the antidiabetic drug may be required). Products include:
Humulin R, 100 Units 1798

Insulin, Human Regular and Human NPH Mixture (Dosage adjustment of the antidiabetic drug may be required). Products include:
Humulin 50/50, 100 Units 1791
Humulin 70/30 Pen 1793

Insulin, NPH (Dosage adjustment of the antidiabetic drug may be required).
No products indexed under this heading.

Insulin, Regular (Dosage adjustment of the antidiabetic drug may be required).
No products indexed under this heading.

Insulin, Zinc Crystals (Dosage adjustment of the antidiabetic drug may be required).
No products indexed under this heading.

Insulin, Zinc Suspension (Dosage adjustment of the antidiabetic drug may be required).
No products indexed under this heading.

Insulin Aspart, Human Regular (Dosage adjustment of the antidiabetic drug may be required). Products include:
NovoLog Injection 2326

Insulin glargine (Dosage adjustment of the antidiabetic drug may be required). Products include:
Lantus Injection 2909

Insulin Lispro, Human (Dosage adjustment of the antidiabetic drug may be required). Products include:
Humalog-Pen 1781
Humalog Mix 50/50-Pen 1783
Humalog Mix 75/25-Pen 1785

Insulin Lispro Protamine, Human (Dosage adjustment of the antidiabetic drug may be required). Products include:
Humalog Mix 50/50-Pen 1783
Humalog Mix 75/25-Pen 1785

Irbesartan (Co-administration with other antihypertensives may result in additive effect or potentiation). Products include:
Avalide Tablets 888
Avalide Tablets 2874
Avapro Tablets 891
Avapro Tablets 2871

Isradipine (Co-administration with other antihypertensives may result in additive effect or potentiation). Products include:
DynaCirc CR Tablets 2721

Ketoprofen (Co-administration of thiazide diuretics and non-steroidal anti-inflammatory agents can reduce the diuretic, natiuretic, and antihypertensive effects).
No products indexed under this heading.

Ketorolac Tromethamine (Co-administration of thiazide diuretics and non-steroidal anti-inflammatory agents can reduce the diuretic, natiuretic, and antihypertensive effects). Products include:
Acular Ophthalmic Solution 565
Acular LS Ophthalmic Solution 566

Labetalol Hydrochloride (Co-administration with other antihypertensives may result in additive effect or potentiation).
No products indexed under this heading.

Levorphanol Tartrate (Co-administration of thiazide diuretics and narcotics may result in potentiation of orthostatic hypotension).
No products indexed under this heading.

Lisinopril (Co-administration with other antihypertensives may result in additive effect or potentiation). Products include:
Prinivil Tablets 2052
Prinzide Tablets 2056

Lithium (Diuretics reduce the renal clearance of lithium and add a high risk of lithium toxicity; concurrent use should be avoided).
No products indexed under this heading.

Lithium Carbonate (Diuretics reduce the renal clearance of lithium and add a high risk of lithium toxicity; concurrent use should be avoided). Products include:
Lithobid Tablets 1692

Lithium Citrate (Diuretics reduce the renal clearance of lithium and add a high risk of lithium toxicity; concurrent use should be avoided).
No products indexed under this heading.

Losartan Potassium (Co-administration with other antihypertensives may result in additive effect or potentiation). Products include:
Cozaar Tablets 1935
Hyzaar 50-12.5 Tablets 1990
Hyzaar 100-12.5 Tablets 1990
Hyzaar 100-25 Tablets 1990

Mecamylamine Hydrochloride (Co-administration with other antihypertensives may result in additive effect or potentiation).
No products indexed under this heading.

Meclofenamate Sodium (Co-administration of thiazide diuretics and non-steroidal anti-inflammatory agents can reduce the diuretic, natiuretic, and antihypertensive effects).
No products indexed under this heading.

Mefenamic Acid (Co-administration of thiazide diuretics and non-steroidal anti-inflammatory agents can reduce the diuretic, natiuretic, and antihypertensive effects).
No products indexed under this heading.

Meloxicam (Co-administration of thiazide diuretics and non-steroidal anti-inflammatory agents can reduce the diuretic, natiuretic, and antihypertensive effects). Products include:
Mobic Oral Suspension 863
Mobic Tablets 863

Meperidine Hydrochloride (Co-administration of thiazide diuretics and narcotics may result in potentiation of orthostatic hypotension).
No products indexed under this heading.

Mephobarbital (Co-administration of thiazide diuretics and barbiturates may result in potentiation of orthostatic hypotension).
No products indexed under this heading.

Metformin Hydrochloride (Dosage adjustment of the antidiabetic drug may be required). Products include:
ActoPlus Met Tablets 3214
Avandamet Tablets 1373
Fortamet Extended-Release Tablets 3115

Methadone Hydrochloride (Co-administration of thiazide diuretics and narcotics may result in potentiation of orthostatic hypotension).
No products indexed under this heading.

Methyclothiazide (Co-administration with other antihypertensives may result in additive effect or potentiation).
No products indexed under this heading.

Methyldopa (Co-administration with other antihypertensives may result in additive effect or potentiation). Products include:
Aldoril Tablets 1910

Methyldopate Hydrochloride (Co-administration with other antihypertensives may result in additive effect or potentiation).
No products indexed under this heading.

Methylprednisolone Acetate (Co-administration of thiazide diuretics and corticosteroids may intensify electrolyte depletion, particularly hypokalemia). Products include:
Depo-Medrol Injectable Suspension 2617
Depo-Medrol Single-Dose Vial 2619

Methylprednisolone Sodium Succinate (Co-administration of thiazide diuretics and corticosteroids may intensify electrolyte depletion, particularly hypokalemia).
No products indexed under this heading.

Metocurine Iodide (Co-administration of thiazide diuretics and nondepolarizing skeletal muscle relaxants increases responsiveness to the muscle relaxants).
No products indexed under this heading.

Metolazone (Co-administration with other antihypertensives may result in additive effect or potentiation).
No products indexed under this heading.

Metoprolol Succinate (Co-administration with other antihypertensives may result in additive effect or potentiation). Products include:
Toprol-XL Tablets 668

Metoprolol Tartrate (Co-administration with other antihypertensives may result in additive effect or potentiation). Products include:
Lopressor Injection 2238
Lopressor Tablets 2238
Lopressor HCT 50/25 Tablets 2241
Lopressor HCT 100/25 Tablets 2241
Lopressor HCT 100/50 Tablets 2241

Metyrosine (Co-administration with other antihypertensives may result in additive effect or potentiation). Products include:
Demser Capsules 1953

Mibefradil Dihydrochloride (Co-administration with other antihypertensives may result in additive effect or potentiation).
No products indexed under this heading.

Miglitol (Dosage adjustment of the antidiabetic drug may be required).
No products indexed under this heading.

Minoxidil (Co-administration with other antihypertensives may result in additive effect or potentiation). Products include:
Men's Rogaine Extra Strength Hair Regrowth Treatment Topical Solution, Ocean Rush Scent and Original Unscented 633
Men's Rogaine Foam Hair Regrowth Treatment 633
Women's Rogaine Hair Regrowth Treatment Topical Solution, Spring Bloom Scent and Original Unscented 634

Mivacurium Chloride (Co-administration of thiazide diuretics and nondepolarizing skeletal muscle relaxants increases responsiveness to the muscle relaxants). Products include:
Mivacron Injection 493

Moexipril Hydrochloride (Co-administration with other antihypertensives may result in additive effect or potentiation). Products include:
Uniretic Tablets 3100
Univasc Tablets 3104

Morphine Sulfate (Co-administration of thiazide diuretics and narcotics may result in potentiation of orthostatic hypotension). Products include:
Avinza Capsules 1741
Kadian Capsules 577
MS Contin Tablets 2701

Nabumetone (Co-administration of thiazide diuretics and non-steroidal anti-inflammatory agents can reduce the diuretic, natiuretic, and antihypertensive effects).
No products indexed under this heading.

Nadolol (Co-administration with other antihypertensives may result in additive effect or potentiation). Products include:
Nadolol Tablets 2159

Naproxen (Co-administration of thiazide diuretics and non-steroidal anti-inflammatory agents can reduce the diuretic, natiuretic, and antihypertensive effects). Products include:
EC-Naprosyn Delayed-Release Tablets 2761
Naprosyn Suspension 2761
Naprosyn Tablets 2761
Prevacid NapraPAC 3280

Naproxen Sodium (Co-administration of thiazide diuretics and non-steroidal anti-inflammatory agents can reduce the diuretic, natiuretic, and antihypertensive effects). Products include:
Aleve Caplets 742
Aleve Gelcaps 743
Aleve Tablets 743
Aleve Cold & Sinus Caplets 744
Anaprox Tablets 2761
Anaprox DS Tablets 2761

Nicardipine Hydrochloride (Co-administration with other antihypertensives may result in additive effect or potentiation). Products include:

Cardene I.V. 2497

Nifedipine (Co-administration with other antihypertensives may result in additive effect or potentiation). Products include:

Adalat CC Tablets 2964

Nisoldipine (Co-administration with other antihypertensives may result in additive effect or potentiation). Products include:

Sular Tablets 3122

Nitroglycerin (Co-administration with other antihypertensives may result in additive effect or potentiation). Products include:

Nitro-Dur Transdermal Infusion System.. 3046
Nitrolingual Pumpspray 3120

Norepinephrine Bitartrate (Possible decreased response to pressor amines but not sufficient to preclude their use).

No products indexed under this heading.

Oxaprozin (Co-administration of thiazide diuretics and non-steroidal anti-inflammatory agents can reduce the diuretic, natiuretic, and antihypertensive effects).

No products indexed under this heading.

Oxycodone Hydrochloride (Co-administration of thiazide diuretics and narcotics may result in potentiation of orthostatic hypotension). Products include:

OxyContin Tablets 2703
OxyFast Oral Concentrate Solution.. 2708
OxyIR Capsules 2708
Percocet Tablets 1131
Percodan Tablets 1132

Pancuronium Bromide (Co-administration of thiazide diuretics and nondepolarizing skeletal muscle relaxants increases responsiveness to the muscle relaxants).

No products indexed under this heading.

Penbutolol Sulfate (Co-administration with other antihypertensives may result in additive effect or potentiation).

No products indexed under this heading.

Pentobarbital Sodium (Co-administration of thiazide diuretics and barbiturates may result in potentiation of orthostatic hypotension). Products include:

Nembutal Sodium Solution, USP 2470

Perindopril Erbumine (Co-administration with other antihypertensives may result in additive effect or potentiation). Products include:

Aceon Tablets (2 mg, 4 mg, 8 mg)... 3194

Phenobarbital (Co-administration of thiazide diuretics and barbiturates may result in potentiation of orthostatic hypotension). Products include:

Donnatal Extentabs 2493

Phenoxybenzamine Hydrochloride (Co-administration with other antihypertensives may result in additive effect or potentiation). Products include:

Dibenzyline Capsules 3399

Phentolamine Mesylate (Co-administration with other antihypertensives may result in additive effect or potentiation).

No products indexed under this heading.

Phenylbutazone (Co-administration of thiazide diuretics and non-steroidal anti-inflammatory agents can reduce the diuretic, natiuretic, and antihypertensive effects).

No products indexed under this heading.

Pindolol (Co-administration with other antihypertensives may result in additive effect or potentiation).

No products indexed under this heading.

Pioglitazone Hydrochloride (Dosage adjustment of the antidiabetic drug may be required). Products include:

ActoPlus Met Tablets 3214
Actos Tablets 3219
Duetact Tablets 3226

Piroxicam (Co-administration of thiazide diuretics and non-steroidal anti-inflammatory agents can reduce the diuretic, natiuretic, and antihypertensive effects).

No products indexed under this heading.

Polythiazide (Co-administration with other antihypertensives may result in additive effect or potentiation).

No products indexed under this heading.

Potassium Acid Phosphate (Concurrent use with potassium salt substitutes or potassium supplements should be avoided unless directed by a prescriber). Products include:

K-Phos Original (Sodium Free) Tablets 760

Potassium Bicarbonate (Concurrent use with potassium salt substitutes or potassium supplements should be avoided unless directed by a prescriber).

No products indexed under this heading.

Potassium Chloride (Concurrent use with potassium salt substitutes or potassium supplements should be avoided unless directed by a prescriber). Products include:

Colyte with Flavor Packs for Oral Solution.. 3088
HalfLytely and Bisacodyl Tablets Bowel Prep Kit with Flavors Packs.. 881
K-Dur Extended-Relase Tablets 3033
K-Lor Oral Solution 474
K-Tab Tablets 475
MoviPrep Oral Solution 2839
TriLyte with Flavor Packs for Oral Solution.. 3100

Potassium Citrate (Concurrent use with potassium salt substitutes or potassium supplements should be avoided unless directed by a prescriber). Products include:

Urocit-K Tablets 2144

Potassium Gluconate (Concurrent use with potassium salt substitutes or potassium supplements should be avoided unless directed by a prescriber).

No products indexed under this heading.

Potassium Phosphate (Concurrent use with potassium salt substitutes or potassium supplements should be avoided unless directed by a prescriber). Products include:

K-Phos Neutral Tablets 760

Prazosin Hydrochloride (Co-administration with other antihypertensives may result in additive effect or potentiation).

No products indexed under this heading.

Prednisolone Acetate (Co-administration of thiazide diuretics and corticosteroids may intensify electrolyte depletion, particularly hypokalemia). Products include:

Blephamide Ophthalmic Ointment 568
Blephamide Ophthalmic Suspension.. 569
Poly-Pred Ophthalmic Suspension .... ⊙233
Pred Forte Ophthalmic Suspension .... ⊙235
Pred Mild Ophthalmic Suspension .... ⊙238
Pred-G Ophthalmic Ointment .... ⊙237
Pred-G Ophthalmic Suspension ...... ⊙236

Prednisolone Sodium Phosphate (Co-administration of thiazide diuretics and corticosteroids may intensify electrolyte depletion, particularly hypokalemia).

No products indexed under this heading.

Prednisolone Tebutate (Co-administration of thiazide diuretics and corticosteroids may intensify electrolyte depletion, particularly hypokalemia).

No products indexed under this heading.

Prednisone (Co-administration of thiazide diuretics and corticosteroids may intensify electrolyte depletion, particularly hypokalemia).

No products indexed under this heading.

Propoxyphene Hydrochloride (Co-administration of thiazide diuretics and narcotics may result in potentiation of orthostatic hypotension).

No products indexed under this heading.

Propoxyphene Napsylate (Co-administration of thiazide diuretics and narcotics may result in potentiation of orthostatic hypotension).

No products indexed under this heading.

Propranolol Hydrochloride (Co-administration with other antihypertensives may result in additive effect or potentiation). Products include:

Inderal LA Long-Acting Capsules 3429
InnoPran XL Capsules 2723

Quinapril Hydrochloride (Co-administration with other antihypertensives may result in additive effect or potentiation).

No products indexed under this heading.

Ramipril (Co-administration with other antihypertensives may result in additive effect or potentiation). Products include:

Altace Capsules 1702

Rapacuronium Bromide (Co-administration of thiazide diuretics and nondepolarizing skeletal muscle relaxants increases responsiveness to the muscle relaxants).

No products indexed under this heading.

Rauwolfia Serpentina (Co-administration with other antihypertensives may result in additive effect or potentiation).

No products indexed under this heading.

Remifentanil Hydrochloride (Co-administration of thiazide diuretics and narcotics may result in potentiation of orthostatic hypotension).

No products indexed under this heading.

Repaglinide (Dosage adjustment of the antidiabetic drug may be required).

No products indexed under this heading.

Rescinnamine (Co-administration with other antihypertensives may result in additive effect or potentiation).

No products indexed under this heading.

Reserpine (Co-administration with other antihypertensives may result in additive effect or potentiation).

No products indexed under this heading.

Rocuronium Bromide (Co-administration of thiazide diuretics and nondepolarizing skeletal muscle relaxants increases responsiveness to the muscle relaxants). Products include:

Zemuron Injection 2346

Rofecoxib (Co-administration of thiazide diuretics and non-steroidal anti-inflammatory agents can reduce the diuretic, natiuretic, and antihypertensive effects).

No products indexed under this heading.

Rosiglitazone Maleate (Dosage adjustment of the antidiabetic drug may be required). Products include:

Avandamet Tablets 1373
Avandaryl Tablets 1379
Avandia Tablets 1384

Secobarbital Sodium (Co-administration of thiazide diuretics and barbiturates may result in potentiation of orthostatic hypotension).

No products indexed under this heading.

Sodium Nitroprusside (Co-administration with other antihypertensives may result in additive effect or potentiation).

No products indexed under this heading.

Sotalol Hydrochloride (Co-administration with other antihypertensives may result in additive effect or potentiation).

No products indexed under this heading.

Spirapril Hydrochloride (Co-administration with other antihypertensives may result in additive effect or potentiation).

No products indexed under this heading.

Sufentanil Citrate (Co-administration of thiazide diuretics and narcotics may result in potentiation of orthostatic hypotension).

No products indexed under this heading.

Sulindac (Co-administration of thiazide diuretics and non-steroidal anti-inflammatory agents can reduce the diuretic, natiuretic, and antihypertensive effects). Products include:

Clinoril Tablets 1924

Telmisartan (Co-administration with other antihypertensives may result in additive effect or potentiation). Products include:

Micardis Tablets 854
Micardis HCT Tablets 856

Terazosin Hydrochloride (Co-administration with other antihypertensives may result in additive effect or potentiation). Products include:

Hytrin Capsules 471

Thiamylal Sodium (Co-administration of thiazide diuretics and barbiturates may result in potentiation of orthostatic hypotension).
No products indexed under this heading.

Timolol Maleate (Co-administration with other antihypertensives may result in additive effect or potentiation). Products include:
- Blocadren Tablets 1916
- Cosopt Sterile Ophthalmic Solution 1931
- Timolide Tablets 2086
- Timoptic Sterile Ophthalmic Solution 2088
- Timoptic in Ocudose 2091
- Timoptic-XE Sterile Ophthalmic Gel Forming Solution 2092

Tolazamide (Dosage adjustment of the antidiabetic drug may be required).
No products indexed under this heading.

Tolbutamide (Dosage adjustment of the antidiabetic drug may be required).
No products indexed under this heading.

Tolmetin Sodium (Co-administration of thiazide diuretics and non-steroidal anti-inflammatory agents can reduce the diuretic, natiuretic, and antihypertensive effects).
No products indexed under this heading.

Torsemide (Co-administration with other antihypertensives may result in additive effect or potentiation). Products include:
- Demadex Injection 2759
- Demadex Tablets 2759

Trandolapril (Co-administration with other antihypertensives may result in additive effect or potentiation). Products include:
- Mavik Tablets 486
- Tarka Tablets 524

Triamcinolone (Co-administration of thiazide diuretics and corticosteroids may intensify electrolyte depletion, particularly hypokalemia).
No products indexed under this heading.

Triamcinolone Acetonide (Co-administration of thiazide diuretics and corticosteroids may intensify electrolyte depletion, particularly hypokalemia). Products include:
- Azmacort Inhalation Aerosol 1726
- Nasacort AQ Nasal Spray 2922

Triamcinolone Diacetate (Co-administration of thiazide diuretics and corticosteroids may intensify electrolyte depletion, particularly hypokalemia).
No products indexed under this heading.

Triamcinolone Hexacetonide (Co-administration of thiazide diuretics and corticosteroids may intensify electrolyte depletion, particularly hypokalemia).
No products indexed under this heading.

Trimethaphan Camsylate (Co-administration with other antihypertensives may result in additive effect or potentiation).
No products indexed under this heading.

Troglitazone (Dosage adjustment of the antidiabetic drug may be required).
No products indexed under this heading.

Tubocurarine Chloride (Co-administration of thiazide diuretics and nondepolarizing skeletal muscle relaxants increases responsiveness to the muscle relaxants).
No products indexed under this heading.

Valdecoxib (Co-administration of thiazide diuretics and non-steroidal anti-inflammatory agents can reduce the diuretic, natiuretic, and antihypertensive effects).
No products indexed under this heading.

Vecuronium Bromide (Co-administration of thiazide diuretics and nondepolarizing skeletal muscle relaxants increases responsiveness to the muscle relaxants).
No products indexed under this heading.

Verapamil Hydrochloride (Co-administration with other antihypertensives may result in additive effect or potentiation). Products include:
- Covera-HS Tablets 3139
- Tarka Tablets 524
- Verelan PM Extended-Release Capsules, Controlled-Onset 3106

Food Interactions

Alcohol (Co-administration of thiazide diuretics and alcohol may result in potentiation of orthostatic hypotension).

DIPROLENE GEL 0.05%

(Betamethasone Dipropionate) 3001
None cited in PDR database.

DIPROLENE LOTION 0.05%

(Betamethasone Dipropionate) 3002
None cited in PDR database.

DIPROLENE OINTMENT 0.05%

(Betamethasone Dipropionate) 3003
None cited in PDR database.

DIPROLENE AF CREAM 0.05%

(Betamethasone Dipropionate) 3000
None cited in PDR database.

DIPROSONE CREAM, USP 0.05%

(Betamethasone Dipropionate) 3004
None cited in PDR database.

DITROPAN XL EXTENDED-RELEASE TABLETS

(Oxybutynin Chloride) 2413
May interact with anticholinergics, bisphosphonates, erythromycin, and certain other agents. Compounds in these categories include:

Alendronate Sodium (Concurrent use with drugs that can cause or exacerbate esophagitis, such as biphosphonates, should be undertaken with caution). Products include:
- Fosamax 1969
- Fosamax Plus D Tablets 1977

Atropine Sulfate (Co-administration of oxybutynin with other anticholinergic drugs may increase the frequency and/or severity of anticholinergic side effects such as dry mouth, constipation, drowsiness and others). Products include:
- Donnatal Extentabs 2493

Belladonna Alkaloids (Co-administration of oxybutynin with other anticholinergic drugs may increase the frequency and/or severity of anticholinergic side effects such as dry mouth, constipation, drowsiness and others). Products include:
- Hyland's Teething Tablets 830

Benztropine Mesylate (Co-administration of oxybutynin with other anticholinergic drugs may increase the frequency and/or severity of anticholinergic side effects such as dry mouth, constipation, drowsiness and others).
No products indexed under this heading.

Biperiden Hydrochloride (Co-administration of oxybutynin with other anticholinergic drugs may increase the frequency and/or severity of anticholinergic side effects such as dry mouth, constipation, drowsiness and others).
No products indexed under this heading.

Cisapride (Co-administration of cisapride with anticholinergic agents would be expected to compromise the beneficial effects of cisapride).
No products indexed under this heading.

Clarithromycin (Clarythromycin, a CYP3A4 inhibitor, may alter mean pharmacokinetic parameters (ie, Cmax, AUC). The clinical relevance of such potential interaction is not known; caution should be used when co-administered). Products include:
- Biaxin/Biaxin XL 402
- PREVPAC 3284

Clidinium Bromide (Co-administration of oxybutynin with other anticholinergic drugs may increase the frequency and/or severity of anticholinergic side effects such as dry mouth, constipation, drowsiness and others).
No products indexed under this heading.

Dicyclomine Hydrochloride (Co-administration of oxybutynin with other anticholinergic drugs may increase the frequency and/or severity of anticholinergic side effects such as dry mouth, constipation, drowsiness and others). Products include:
- Bentyl Capsules 697
- Bentyl Injection 697
- Bentyl Syrup 697
- Bentyl Tablets 697

Erythromycin (Erythromycin, a CYP3A4 inhibitor, may alter mean pharmacokinetic parameters (ie, Cmax, AUC). The clinical relevance of such potential interaction is not known, caution should be used when co-administered). Products include:
- Ery-Tab Tablets 449
- Erythromycin Base Filmtab Tablets 455
- Erythromycin Delayed-Release Capsules, USP 457
- PCE Dispertab Tablets 515

Erythromycin Estolate (Erythromycin, a CYP3A4 inhibitor, may alter mean pharmacokinetic parameters (ie, Cmax, AUC). The clinical relevance of such potential interaction is not known, caution should be used when co-administered).
No products indexed under this heading.

Erythromycin Ethylsuccinate (Erythromycin, a CYP3A4 inhibitor, may alter mean pharmacokinetic parameters (ie, Cmax, AUC). The clinical relevance of such potential interaction is not known, caution should be used when co-administered). Products include:
- E.E.S. 451
- EryPed 447

Erythromycin Gluceptate (Erythromycin, a CYP3A4 inhibitor, may alter mean pharmacokinetic parameters (ie, Cmax, AUC). The clinical relevance of such potential interaction is not known, caution should be used when co-administered).
No products indexed under this heading.

Erythromycin Lactobionate (Erythromycin, a CYP3A4 inhibitor, may alter mean pharmacokinetic parameters (ie, Cmax, AUC). The clinical relevance of such potential interaction is not known, caution should be used when co-administered).
No products indexed under this heading.

Erythromycin Stearate (Erythromycin, a CYP3A4 inhibitor, may alter mean pharmacokinetic parameters (ie, Cmax, AUC). The clinical relevance of such potential interaction is not known, caution should be used when co-administered). Products include:
- Erythrocin Stearate Filmtab Tablets 453

Etidronate Disodium (Concurrent use with drugs that can cause or exacerbate esophagitis, such as biphosphonates, should be undertaken with caution). Products include:
- Didronel Tablets 2697

Glycopyrrolate (Co-administration of oxybutynin with other anticholinergic drugs may increase the frequency and/or severity of anticholinergic side effects such as dry mouth, constipation, drowsiness and others).
No products indexed under this heading.

Hyoscyamine (Co-administration of oxybutynin with other anticholinergic drugs may increase the frequency and/or severity of anticholinergic side effects such as dry mouth, constipation, drowsiness and others).
No products indexed under this heading.

Hyoscyamine Sulfate (Co-administration of oxybutynin with other anticholinergic drugs may increase the frequency and/or severity of anticholinergic side effects such as dry mouth, constipation, drowsiness and others). Products include:
- Donnatal Extentabs 2493
- Prosed/DS Tablets 1157

Ipratropium Bromide (Co-administration of oxybutynin with other anticholinergic drugs may increase the frequency and/or severity of anticholinergic side effects such as dry mouth, constipation, drowsiness and others). Products include:
- Atrovent Inhalation Solution 835
- Atrovent HFA Inhalation Aerosol 841
- Atrovent Nasal Spray 0.03% 837
- Atrovent Nasal Spray 0.06% 839
- Combivent Inhalation Aerosol 847
- DuoNeb Inhalation Solution 1058

Itraconazole (Itraconazole, a CYP3A4 inhibitor, may alter mean pharmacokinetic parameters (ie, Cmax, AUC). The clinical relevance of such potential interaction is not known; caution should be used when co-administered).
No products indexed under this heading.

Ketoconazole (Mean oxybutynin plasma concentrations were approximately 2-fold higher when oxybutynin was administered with ketoconazole, a potent CYP3A4 inhibitor). Products include:
Nizoral A-D Shampoo, 1% **1868**

Mepenzolate Bromide (Co-administration of oxybutynin with other anticholinergic drugs may increase the frequency and/or severity of anticholinergic side effects such as dry mouth, constipation, drowsiness and others).
No products indexed under this heading.

Miconazole (Miconazole, a CYP3A4 inhibitor, may alter mean pharmacokinetic parameters (ie, Cmax, AUC). The clinical relevance of such potential interaction is not known; caution should be used when co-administered).
No products indexed under this heading.

Oxybutynin Chloride (Co-administration of oxybutynin with other anticholinergic drugs may increase the frequency and/or severity of anticholinergic side effects such as dry mouth, constipation, drowsiness and others). Products include:
Ditropan XL Extended-Release Tablets **2413**

Procyclidine Hydrochloride (Co-administration of oxybutynin with other anticholinergic drugs may increase the frequency and/or severity of anticholinergic side effects such as dry mouth, constipation, drowsiness and others).
No products indexed under this heading.

Propantheline Bromide (Co-administration of oxybutynin with other anticholinergic drugs may increase the frequency and/or severity of anticholinergic side effects such as dry mouth, constipation, drowsiness and others).
No products indexed under this heading.

Risedronate Sodium (Concurrent use with drugs that can cause or exacerbate esophagitis, such as biphosphonates, should be undertaken with caution). Products include:
Actonel Tablets **2683**
Actonel with Calcium Tablets **2688**

Scopolamine (Co-administration of oxybutynin with other anticholinergic drugs may increase the frequency and/or severity of anticholinergic side effects such as dry mouth, constipation, drowsiness and others). Products include:
Transderm Scōp Transdermal Therapeutic System **2177**

Scopolamine Hydrobromide (Co-administration of oxybutynin with other anticholinergic drugs may increase the frequency and/or severity of anticholinergic side effects such as dry mouth, constipation, drowsiness and others). Products include:
Donnatal Extentabs **2493**

Tiludronate Disodium (Concurrent use with drugs that can cause or exacerbate esophagitis, such as biphosphonates, should be undertaken with caution).
No products indexed under this heading.

Tolterodine Tartrate (Co-administration of oxybutynin with other anticholinergic drugs may increase the frequency and/or severity of anticholinergic side effects such as dry mouth, constipation, drowsiness and others). Products include:
Detrol Tablets **2628**
Detrol LA Capsules **2631**

Tridihexethyl Chloride (Co-administration of oxybutynin with other anticholinergic drugs may increase the frequency and/or severity of anticholinergic side effects such as dry mouth, constipation, drowsiness and others).
No products indexed under this heading.

Trihexyphenidyl Hydrochloride (Co-administration of oxybutynin with other anticholinergic drugs may increase the frequency and/or severity of anticholinergic side effects such as dry mouth, constipation, drowsiness and others).
No products indexed under this heading.

Food Interactions

Alcohol (Enhances the drowsiness effect caused by anticholinergic agents such as oxybutynin).

DIURIL ORAL SUSPENSION

(Chlorothiazide) **1954**
May interact with antihypertensives, barbiturates, bile acid sequestering agents, corticosteroids, cardiac glycosides, oral hypoglycemic agents, insulin, lithium preparations, narcotic analgesics, nondepolarizing neuromuscular blocking agents, non-steroidal anti-inflammatory agents, and certain other agents. Compounds in these categories include:

Acarbose (Thiazide-induced hyperglycemia may require dosage adjustment of hypoglycemic agents). Products include:
Precose Tablets **751**

Acebutolol Hydrochloride (Concurrent use with other antihypertensive agents may result in additive effect or potentiation).
No products indexed under this heading.

ACTH (Intensified electrolyte depletion particularly hypokalemia).
No products indexed under this heading.

Alfentanil Hydrochloride (Potentiation of orthostatic hypotension may occur).
No products indexed under this heading.

Amlodipine Besylate (Concurrent use with other antihypertensive agents may result in additive effect or potentiation). Products include:
Caduet Tablets **2508**
Lotrel Capsules **2249**
Norvasc Tablets **2545**

Aprobarbital (Potentiation of orthostatic hypotension may occur).
No products indexed under this heading.

Atenolol (Concurrent use with other antihypertensive agents may result in additive effect or potentiation).
No products indexed under this heading.

Atracurium Besylate (Possible increased responsiveness to the muscle relaxants).
No products indexed under this heading.

Benazepril Hydrochloride (Concurrent use with other antihypertensive agents may result in additive effect or potentiation). Products include:
Lotensin Tablets **2243**
Lotensin HCT Tablets **2246**
Lotrel Capsules **2249**

Bendroflumethiazide (Concurrent use with other antihypertensive agents may result in additive effect or potentiation).
No products indexed under this heading.

Betamethasone Acetate (Intensified electrolyte depletion particularly hypokalemia).
No products indexed under this heading.

Betamethasone Sodium Phosphate (Intensified electrolyte depletion particularly hypokalemia).
No products indexed under this heading.

Betaxolol Hydrochloride (Concurrent use with other antihypertensive agents may result in additive effect or potentiation). Products include:
Betoptic S Ophthalmic Suspension................................. **558**

Bisoprolol Fumarate (Concurrent use with other antihypertensive agents may result in additive effect or potentiation).
No products indexed under this heading.

Buprenorphine Hydrochloride (Potentiation of orthostatic hypotension may occur). Products include:
Buprenex Injectable **2716**
Suboxone Tablets **2717**
Subutex Tablets **2717**

Butabarbital (Potentiation of orthostatic hypotension may occur).
No products indexed under this heading.

Butalbital (Potentiation of orthostatic hypotension may occur).
No products indexed under this heading.

Candesartan Cilexetil (Concurrent use with other antihypertensive agents may result in additive effect or potentiation). Products include:
Atacand Tablets **649**
Atacand HCT **651**

Captopril (Concurrent use with other antihypertensive agents may result in additive effect or potentiation). Products include:
Captopril Tablets **2149**

Carteolol Hydrochloride (Concurrent use with other antihypertensive agents may result in additive effect or potentiation). Products include:
Carteolol Hydrochloride Ophthalmic Solution USP, 1%...... ⊙ **249**

Celecoxib (Reduces diuretic, natriuretic, and antihypertensive effects). Products include:
Celebrex Capsules **3134**

Chlorothiazide Sodium (Concurrent use with other antihypertensive agents may result in additive effect or potentiation). Products include:
Diuril Sodium Intravenous **2467**

Chlorpropamide (Thiazide-induced hyperglycemia may require dosage adjustment of hypoglycemic agents).
No products indexed under this heading.

Chlorthalidone (Concurrent use with other antihypertensive agents may result in additive effect or potentiation). Products include:
Clorpres Tablets **2153**

Cholestyramine (Resins have potential to bind thiazide diuretics and reduce their absorption from the gastrointestinal tract).
No products indexed under this heading.

Cisatracurium Besylate (Possible increased responsiveness to the muscle relaxants). Products include:
Nimbex Injection **498**

Clonidine (Concurrent use with other antihypertensive agents may result in additive effect or potentiation). Products include:
Catapres-TTS **844**

Clonidine Hydrochloride (Concurrent use with other antihypertensive agents may result in additive effect or potentiation). Products include:
Catapres Tablets **843**
Clorpres Tablets **2153**

Codeine Phosphate (Potentiation of orthostatic hypotension may occur). Products include:
Tylenol with Codeine Tablets **2391**

Colesevelam Hydrochloride (Resins have potential to bind thiazide diuretics and reduce their absorption from the gastrointestinal tract). Products include:
WelChol Tablets **1050**

Colestipol Hydrochloride (Resins have potential to bind thiazide diuretics and reduce their absorption from the gastrointestinal tract).
No products indexed under this heading.

Cortisone Acetate (Intensified electrolyte depletion particularly hypokalemia).
No products indexed under this heading.

Deserpidine (Concurrent use with other antihypertensive agents may result in additive effect or potentiation).
No products indexed under this heading.

Deslanoside (Thiazide-induced hypokalemia may sensitize or exaggerate the response of the heart to the toxic effects of digitalis).
No products indexed under this heading.

Dexamethasone (Intensified electrolyte depletion particularly hypokalemia). Products include:
Ciprodex Otic Suspension **559**
Decadron Tablets **1951**
TobraDex Ophthalmic Ointment **562**
TobraDex Ophthalmic Suspension ... **563**

Dexamethasone Acetate (Intensified electrolyte depletion particularly hypokalemia).
No products indexed under this heading.

Dexamethasone Sodium Phosphate (Intensified electrolyte depletion particularly hypokalemia).
No products indexed under this heading.

Dezocine (Potentiation of orthostatic hypotension may occur).
No products indexed under this heading.

Diazoxide (Concurrent use with other antihypertensive agents may result in additive effect or potentiation). Products include:
Hyperstat I.V. ... 3017

Diclofenac Potassium (Reduces diuretic, natriuretic, and antihypertensive effects).
No products indexed under this heading.

Diclofenac Sodium (Reduces diuretic, natriuretic, and antihypertensive effects). Products include:
Arthrotec Tablets ... 3129
Voltaren Ophthalmic Solution ... 2309
Voltaren Tablets ... 2307
Voltaren-XR Tablets ... 2310

Digitalis Glycoside Preparations (Thiazide-induced hypokalemia may sensitize or exaggerate the response of the heart to the toxic effects of digitalis).
No products indexed under this heading.

Digitoxin (Thiazide-induced hypokalemia may sensitize or exaggerate the response of the heart to the toxic effects of digitalis).
No products indexed under this heading.

Digoxin (Thiazide-induced hypokalemia may sensitize or exaggerate the response of the heart to the toxic effects of digitalis). Products include:
Lanoxicaps Capsules ... 1490
Lanoxin Injection ... 1494
Lanoxin Injection Pediatric ... 1497
Lanoxin Tablets ... 1500

Diltiazem Hydrochloride (Concurrent use with other antihypertensive agents may result in additive effect or potentiation). Products include:
Cardizem LA Extended Release Tablets ... 1728
Tiazac Capsules ... 1201

Doxazosin Mesylate (Concurrent use with other antihypertensive agents may result in additive effect or potentiation). Products include:
Cardura XL Tablets ... 2515

Enalapril Maleate (Concurrent use with other antihypertensive agents may result in additive effect or potentiation). Products include:
Vasotec I.V. Injection ... 2103

Enalaprilat (Concurrent use with other antihypertensive agents may result in additive effect or potentiation).
No products indexed under this heading.

Eprosartan Mesylate (Concurrent use with other antihypertensive agents may result in additive effect or potentiation). Products include:
Teveten Tablets ... 1735
Teveten HCT Tablets ... 1737

Esmolol Hydrochloride (Concurrent use with other antihypertensive agents may result in additive effect or potentiation).
No products indexed under this heading.

Etodolac (Reduces diuretic, natriuretic, and antihypertensive effects).
No products indexed under this heading.

Felodipine (Concurrent use with other antihypertensive agents may result in additive effect or potentiation).
No products indexed under this heading.

Fenoprofen Calcium (Reduces diuretic, natriuretic, and antihypertensive effects). Products include:
Nalfon Capsules ... 2502

Fentanyl (Potentiation of orthostatic hypotension may occur). Products include:
Duragesic Transdermal System ... 2373
Ionsys Transdermal System ... 2379

Fentanyl Citrate (Potentiation of orthostatic hypotension may occur). Products include:
Actiq ... 979

Fludrocortisone Acetate (Intensified electrolyte depletion particularly hypokalemia).
No products indexed under this heading.

Flurbiprofen (Reduces diuretic, natriuretic, and antihypertensive effects).
No products indexed under this heading.

Fosinopril Sodium (Concurrent use with other antihypertensive agents may result in additive effect or potentiation).
No products indexed under this heading.

Furosemide (Concurrent use with other antihypertensive agents may result in additive effect or potentiation). Products include:
Furosemide Tablets ... 2154

Glimepiride (Thiazide-induced hyperglycemia may require dosage adjustment of hypoglycemic agents). Products include:
Avandaryl Tablets ... 1379
Duetact Tablets ... 3226

Glipizide (Thiazide-induced hyperglycemia may require dosage adjustment of hypoglycemic agents).
No products indexed under this heading.

Glyburide (Thiazide-induced hyperglycemia may require dosage adjustment of hypoglycemic agents).
No products indexed under this heading.

Guanabenz Acetate (Concurrent use with other antihypertensive agents may result in additive effect or potentiation).
No products indexed under this heading.

Guanethidine Monosulfate (Concurrent use with other antihypertensive agents may result in additive effect or potentiation).
No products indexed under this heading.

Hydralazine Hydrochloride (Concurrent use with other antihypertensive agents may result in additive effect or potentiation). Products include:
BiDil Tablets ... 2171

Hydrochlorothiazide (Concurrent use with other antihypertensive agents may result in additive effect or potentiation). Products include:
Aldoril Tablets ... 1910
Atacand HCT ... 651
Avalide Tablets ... 888
Avalide Tablets ... 2874
Benicar HCT Tablets ... 1044
Diovan HCT Tablets ... 2196
Dyazide Capsules ... 1423
Hyzaar 50-12.5 Tablets ... 1990
Hyzaar 100-12.5 Tablets ... 1990
Hyzaar 100-25 Tablets ... 1990
Lopressor HCT 50/25 Tablets ... 2241
Lopressor HCT 100/25 Tablets ... 2241
Lopressor HCT 100/50 Tablets ... 2241
Lotensin HCT Tablets ... 2246
Micardis HCT Tablets ... 856
Moduretic Tablets ... 2028
Prinzide Tablets ... 2056
Teveten HCT Tablets ... 1737
Timolide Tablets ... 2086
Uniretic Tablets ... 3100

Hydrocodone Bitartrate (Potentiation of orthostatic hypotension may occur). Products include:
Hycodan ... 1116
Hycotuss Expectorant Syrup ... 1117
Vicodin Tablets ... 535
Vicodin ES Tablets ... 536
Vicodin HP Tablets ... 538
Vicoprofen Tablets ... 539
Zydone Tablets ... 1139

Hydrocodone Polistirex (Potentiation of orthostatic hypotension may occur). Products include:
Tussionex Pennkinetic Extended-Release Suspension ... 3327

Hydrocortisone (Intensified electrolyte depletion particularly hypokalemia). Products include:
Colocort Rectal Suspension, USP (Retention) 100 mg/60 mL ... 2476
Hydrocortone Tablets ... 1989
Preparation H Hydrocortisone Cream ... 646

Hydrocortisone Acetate (Intensified electrolyte depletion particularly hypokalemia). Products include:
Analpram-HC ... 1159
Pramosone ... 1161
ProctoFoam-HC ... 3099

Hydrocortisone Sodium Phosphate (Intensified electrolyte depletion particularly hypokalemia).
No products indexed under this heading.

Hydrocortisone Sodium Succinate (Intensified electrolyte depletion particularly hypokalemia).
No products indexed under this heading.

Hydroflumethiazide (Concurrent use with other antihypertensive agents may result in additive effect or potentiation).
No products indexed under this heading.

Hydromorphone Hydrochloride (Potentiation of orthostatic hypotension may occur). Products include:
Dilaudid ... 440
Dilaudid Non-Sterile Powder ... 440
Dilaudid Oral Liquid ... 445
Dilaudid Rectal Suppositories ... 440
Dilaudid Tablets ... 440
Dilaudid Tablets - 8 mg ... 445
Dilaudid-HP ... 442

Ibuprofen (Reduces diuretic, natriuretic, and antihypertensive effects). Products include:
Advil Allergy Sinus Caplets ... 770
Advil ... 674
Children's Advil Oral Suspension ... 603
Children's Advil Chewable Tablets ... 603
Advil Cold & Sinus ... 723
Infants' Advil Concentrated Drops ... 604
Infants' Advil Concentrated Drops - White Grape (Dye-Free) ... 604
Junior Strength Advil Swallow Tablets ... 605
Advil Migraine Liquigels ... 608
Advil Multi-Symptom Cold Caplets ... 770
Advil PM Caplets ... 615
Motrin IB Tablets and Caplets ... 1866
Children's Motrin Oral Suspension ... 1867
Children's Motrin Non-Staining Dye-Free Oral Suspension ... 1867
Children's Motrin Cold Oral Suspension ... 1867
Infants' Motrin Concentrated Drops ... 1867
Infants' Motrin Non-Staining Dye-Free Concentrated Drops ... 1867
Junior Strength Motrin Caplets and Chewable Tablets ... 1867
Vicoprofen Tablets ... 539

Indapamide (Concurrent use with other antihypertensive agents may result in additive effect or potentiation). Products include:
Indapamide Tablets ... 2156

Indomethacin (Reduces diuretic, natriuretic, and antihypertensive effects). Products include:
Indocin ... 1995

Indomethacin Sodium Trihydrate (Reduces diuretic, natriuretic, and antihypertensive effects). Products include:
Indocin I.V. ... 2465

Insulin, Human, Zinc Suspension (Thiazide-induce hyperglycemia may require dosage adjustment of hypoglycemic agents). Products include:
Humulin L, 100 Units ... 1794
Humulin U, 100 Units ... 1800

Insulin, Human NPH (Thiazide-induce hyperglycemia may require dosage adjustment of hypoglycemic agents). Products include:
Humulin N, 100 Units ... 1795
Humulin N Pen ... 1797

Insulin, Human Regular (Thiazide-induce hyperglycemia may require dosage adjustment of hypoglycemic agents). Products include:
Humulin R, 100 Units ... 1798

Insulin, Human Regular and Human NPH Mixture (Thiazide-induce hyperglycemia may require dosage adjustment of hypoglycemic agents). Products include:
Humulin 50/50, 100 Units ... 1791
Humulin 70/30 Pen ... 1793

Insulin, NPH (Thiazide-induce hyperglycemia may require dosage adjustment of hypoglycemic agents).
No products indexed under this heading.

Insulin, Regular (Thiazide-induce hyperglycemia may require dosage adjustment of hypoglycemic agents).
No products indexed under this heading.

Insulin, Zinc Crystals (Thiazide-induce hyperglycemia may require dosage adjustment of hypoglycemic agents).
No products indexed under this heading.

Insulin, Zinc Suspension (Thiazide-induce hyperglycemia may require dosage adjustment of hypoglycemic agents).
No products indexed under this heading.

Insulin Aspart, Human Regular (Thiazide-induce hyperglycemia may require dosage adjustment of hypoglycemic agents). Products include:
NovoLog Injection ... 2326

Insulin glargine (Thiazide-induce hyperglycemia may require dosage adjustment of hypoglycemic agents). Products include:
Lantus Injection ... 2909

Insulin Lispro, Human (Thiazide-induce hyperglycemia may require dosage adjustment of hypoglycemic agents). Products include:
Humalog-Pen ... 1781
Humalog Mix 50/50-Pen ... 1783
Humalog Mix 75/25-Pen ... 1785

Insulin Lispro Protamine, Human (Thiazide-induce hyperglycemia may require dosage adjustment of hypoglycemic agents). Products include:
Humalog Mix 50/50-Pen ... 1783
Humalog Mix 75/25-Pen ... 1785

IMPORTANT NOTE: Always consult each drug listing in the patient's regimen for possible interactions.

Irbesartan (Concurrent use with other antihypertensive agents may result in additive effect or potentiation). Products include:
- Avalide Tablets ... 888
- Avalide Tablets ... 2874
- Avapro Tablets ... 891
- Avapro Tablets ... 2871

Isradipine (Concurrent use with other antihypertensive agents may result in additive effect or potentiation). Products include:
- DynaCirc CR Tablets ... 2721

Ketoprofen (Reduces diuretic, natriuretic, and antihypertensive effects).
No products indexed under this heading.

Ketorolac Tromethamine (Reduces diuretic, natriuretic, and antihypertensive effects). Products include:
- Acular Ophthalmic Solution ... 565
- Acular LS Ophthalmic Solution ... 566

Labetalol Hydrochloride (Concurrent use with other antihypertensive agents may result in additive effect or potentiation).
No products indexed under this heading.

Levorphanol Tartrate (Potentiation of orthostatic hypotension may occur).
No products indexed under this heading.

Lisinopril (Concurrent use with other antihypertensive agents may result in additive effect or potentiation). Products include:
- Prinivil Tablets ... 2052
- Prinzide Tablets ... 2056

Lithium (Diuretics reduce the renal clearance of lithium and this may lead to lithium toxicity).
No products indexed under this heading.

Lithium Carbonate (Diuretics reduce the renal clearance of lithium and this may lead to lithium toxicity). Products include:
- Lithobid Tablets ... 1692

Lithium Citrate (Diuretics reduce the renal clearance of lithium and this may lead to lithium toxicity).
No products indexed under this heading.

Losartan Potassium (Concurrent use with other antihypertensive agents may result in additive effect or potentiation). Products include:
- Cozaar Tablets ... 1935
- Hyzaar 50-12.5 Tablets ... 1990
- Hyzaar 100-12.5 Tablets ... 1990
- Hyzaar 100-25 Tablets ... 1990

Mecamylamine Hydrochloride (Concurrent use with other antihypertensive agents may result in additive effect or potentiation).
No products indexed under this heading.

Meclofenamate Sodium (Reduces diuretic, natriuretic, and antihypertensive effects).
No products indexed under this heading.

Mefenamic Acid (Reduces diuretic, natriuretic, and antihypertensive effects).
No products indexed under this heading.

Meloxicam (Reduces diuretic, natriuretic, and antihypertensive effects). Products include:
- Mobic Oral Suspension ... 863
- Mobic Tablets ... 863

Meperidine Hydrochloride (Potentiation of orthostatic hypotension may occur).
No products indexed under this heading.

Mephobarbital (Potentiation of orthostatic hypotension may occur).
No products indexed under this heading.

Metformin Hydrochloride (Thiazide-induced hyperglycemia may require dosage adjustment of hypoglycemic agents). Products include:
- ActoPlus Met Tablets ... 3214
- Avandamet Tablets ... 1373
- Fortamet Extended-Release Tablets ... 3115

Methadone Hydrochloride (Potentiation of orthostatic hypotension may occur).
No products indexed under this heading.

Methyclothiazide (Concurrent use with other antihypertensive agents may result in additive effect or potentiation).
No products indexed under this heading.

Methyldopa (Concurrent use with other antihypertensive agents may result in additive effect or potentiation). Products include:
- Aldoril Tablets ... 1910

Methyldopate Hydrochloride (Concurrent use with other antihypertensive agents may result in additive effect or potentiation).
No products indexed under this heading.

Methylprednisolone Acetate (Intensified electrolyte depletion particularly hypokalemia). Products include:
- Depo-Medrol Injectable Suspension ... 2617
- Depo-Medrol Single-Dose Vial ... 2619

Methylprednisolone Sodium Succinate (Intensified electrolyte depletion particularly hypokalemia).
No products indexed under this heading.

Metipranolol Hydrochloride (Concurrent use with other antihypertensive agents may result in additive effect or potentiation).
No products indexed under this heading.

Metocurine Iodide (Possible increased responsiveness to the muscle relaxants).
No products indexed under this heading.

Metolazone (Concurrent use with other antihypertensive agents may result in additive effect or potentiation).
No products indexed under this heading.

Metoprolol Succinate (Concurrent use with other antihypertensive agents may result in additive effect or potentiation). Products include:
- Toprol-XL Tablets ... 668

Metoprolol Tartrate (Concurrent use with other antihypertensive agents may result in additive effect or potentiation). Products include:
- Lopressor Injection ... 2238
- Lopressor Tablets ... 2238
- Lopressor HCT 50/25 Tablets ... 2241
- Lopressor HCT 100/25 Tablets ... 2241
- Lopressor HCT 100/50 Tablets ... 2241

Metyrosine (Concurrent use with other antihypertensive agents may result in additive effect or potentiation). Products include:
- Demser Capsules ... 1953

Mibefradil Dihydrochloride (Concurrent use with other antihypertensive agents may result in additive effect or potentiation).
No products indexed under this heading.

Miglitol (Thiazide-induced hyperglycemia may require dosage adjustment of hypoglycemic agents).
No products indexed under this heading.

Minoxidil (Concurrent use with other antihypertensive agents may result in additive effect or potentiation). Products include:
- Men's Rogaine Extra Strength Hair Regrowth Treatment Topical Solution, Ocean Rush Scent and Original Unscented ... ▣633
- Men's Rogaine Foam Hair Regrowth Treatment ... ▣633
- Women's Rogaine Hair Regrowth Treatment Topical Solution, Spring Bloom Scent and Original Unscented ... ▣634

Mivacurium Chloride (Possible increased responsiveness to the muscle relaxants). Products include:
- Mivacron Injection ... 493

Moexipril Hydrochloride (Concurrent use with other antihypertensive agents may result in additive effect or potentiation). Products include:
- Uniretic Tablets ... 3100
- Univasc Tablets ... 3104

Morphine Sulfate (Potentiation of orthostatic hypotension may occur). Products include:
- Avinza Capsules ... 1741
- Kadian Capsules ... 577
- MS Contin Tablets ... 2701

Nabumetone (Reduces diuretic, natriuretic, and antihypertensive effects).
No products indexed under this heading.

Nadolol (Concurrent use with other antihypertensive agents may result in additive effect or potentiation). Products include:
- Nadolol Tablets ... 2159

Naproxen (Reduces diuretic, natriuretic, and antihypertensive effects). Products include:
- EC-Naprosyn Delayed-Release Tablets ... 2761
- Naprosyn Suspension ... 2761
- Naprosyn Tablets ... 2761
- Prevacid NapraPAC ... 3280

Naproxen Sodium (Reduces diuretic, natriuretic, and antihypertensive effects). Products include:
- Aleve Caplets ... 742
- Aleve Gelcaps ... 743
- Aleve Tablets ... 743
- Aleve Cold & Sinus Caplets ... 744
- Anaprox Tablets ... 2761
- Anaprox DS Tablets ... 2761

Nicardipine Hydrochloride (Concurrent use with other antihypertensive agents may result in additive effect or potentiation). Products include:
- Cardene I.V. ... 2497

Nifedipine (Concurrent use with other antihypertensive agents may result in additive effect or potentiation). Products include:
- Adalat CC Tablets ... 2964

Nisoldipine (Concurrent use with other antihypertensive agents may result in additive effect or potentiation). Products include:
- Sular Tablets ... 3122

Nitroglycerin (Concurrent use with other antihypertensive agents may result in additive effect or potentiation). Products include:
- Nitro-Dur Transdermal Infusion System ... 3046
- Nitrolingual Pumpspray ... 3120

Norepinephrine Hydrochloride (Decreased arterial responsiveness to pressor amine).
No products indexed under this heading.

Oxaprozin (Reduces diuretic, natriuretic, and antihypertensive effects).
No products indexed under this heading.

Oxycodone Hydrochloride (Potentiation of orthostatic hypotension may occur). Products include:
- OxyContin Tablets ... 2703
- OxyFast Oral Concentrate Solution ... 2708
- OxyIR Capsules ... 2708
- Percocet Tablets ... 1131
- Percodan Tablets ... 1132

Pancuronium Bromide (Possible increased responsiveness to the muscle relaxants).
No products indexed under this heading.

Penbutolol Sulfate (Concurrent use with other antihypertensive agents may result in additive effect or potentiation).
No products indexed under this heading.

Pentobarbital Sodium (Potentiation of orthostatic hypotension may occur). Products include:
- Nembutal Sodium Solution, USP ... 2470

Perindopril Erbumine (Concurrent use with other antihypertensive agents may result in additive effect or potentiation). Products include:
- Aceon Tablets (2 mg, 4 mg, 8 mg) ... 3194

Phenobarbital (Potentiation of orthostatic hypotension may occur). Products include:
- Donnatal Extentabs ... 2493

Phenoxybenzamine Hydrochloride (Concurrent use with other antihypertensive agents may result in additive effect or potentiation). Products include:
- Dibenzyline Capsules ... 3399

Phentolamine Mesylate (Concurrent use with other antihypertensive agents may result in additive effect or potentiation).
No products indexed under this heading.

Phenylbutazone (Reduces diuretic, natriuretic, and antihypertensive effects).
No products indexed under this heading.

Pindolol (Concurrent use with other antihypertensive agents may result in additive effect or potentiation).
No products indexed under this heading.

Pioglitazone Hydrochloride (Thiazide-induced hyperglycemia may require dosage adjustment of hypoglycemic agents). Products include:
- ActoPlus Met Tablets ... 3214
- Actos Tablets ... 3219
- Duetact Tablets ... 3226

Piroxicam (Reduces diuretic, natriuretic, and antihypertensive effects).
No products indexed under this heading.

Polythiazide (Concurrent use with other antihypertensive agents may result in additive effect or potentiation).
No products indexed under this heading.

Prazosin Hydrochloride (Concurrent use with other antihypertensive agents may result in additive effect or potentiation).
No products indexed under this heading.

Prednisolone Acetate (Intensified electrolyte depletion particularly hypokalemia). Products include:
Blephamide Ophthalmic Ointment 568
Blephamide Ophthalmic
Suspension 569
Poly-Pred Ophthalmic
Suspension ⊙233
Pred Forte Ophthalmic
Suspension ⊙235
Pred Mild Ophthalmic
Suspension ⊙238
Pred-G Ophthalmic Ointment ⊙237
Pred-G Ophthalmic Suspension ⊙236

Prednisolone Sodium Phosphate (Intensified electrolyte depletion particularly hypokalemia).
No products indexed under this heading.

Prednisolone Tebutate (Intensified electrolyte depletion particularly hypokalemia).
No products indexed under this heading.

Prednisone (Intensified electrolyte depletion particularly hypokalemia).
No products indexed under this heading.

Propoxyphene Hydrochloride (Potentiation of orthostatic hypotension may occur).
No products indexed under this heading.

Propoxyphene Napsylate (Potentiation of orthostatic hypotension may occur).
No products indexed under this heading.

Propranolol Hydrochloride (Concurrent use with other antihypertensive agents may result in additive effect or potentiation). Products include:
Inderal LA Long-Acting Capsules 3429
InnoPran XL Capsules 2723

Quinapril Hydrochloride (Concurrent use with other antihypertensive agents may result in additive effect or potentiation).
No products indexed under this heading.

Ramipril (Concurrent use with other antihypertensive agents may result in additive effect or potentiation). Products include:
Altace Capsules 1702

Rapacuronium Bromide (Possible increased responsiveness to the muscle relaxants).
No products indexed under this heading.

Rauwolfia Serpentina (Concurrent use with other antihypertensive agents may result in additive effect or potentiation).
No products indexed under this heading.

Remifentanil Hydrochloride (Potentiation of orthostatic hypotension may occur).
No products indexed under this heading.

Repaglinide (Thiazide-induced hyperglycemia may require dosage adjustment of hypoglycemic agents).
No products indexed under this heading.

Rescinnamine (Concurrent use with other antihypertensive agents may result in additive effect or potentiation).
No products indexed under this heading.

Reserpine (Concurrent use with other antihypertensive agents may result in additive effect or potentiation).
No products indexed under this heading.

Rocuronium Bromide (Possible increased responsiveness to the muscle relaxants). Products include:
Zemuron Injection 2346

Rofecoxib (Reduces diuretic, natriuretic, and antihypertensive effects).
No products indexed under this heading.

Rosiglitazone Maleate (Thiazide-induced hyperglycemia may require dosage adjustment of hypoglycemic agents). Products include:
Avandamet Tablets 1373
Avandaryl Tablets 1379
Avandia Tablets 1384

Secobarbital Sodium (Potentiation of orthostatic hypotension may occur).
No products indexed under this heading.

Sodium Nitroprusside (Concurrent use with other antihypertensive agents may result in additive effect or potentiation).
No products indexed under this heading.

Sotalol Hydrochloride (Concurrent use with other antihypertensive agents may result in additive effect or potentiation).
No products indexed under this heading.

Spirapril Hydrochloride (Concurrent use with other antihypertensive agents may result in additive effect or potentiation).
No products indexed under this heading.

Sufentanil Citrate (Potentiation of orthostatic hypotension may occur).
No products indexed under this heading.

Sulindac (Reduces diuretic, natriuretic, and antihypertensive effects). Products include:
Clinoril Tablets 1924

Telmisartan (Concurrent use with other antihypertensive agents may result in additive effect or potentiation). Products include:
Micardis Tablets 854
Micardis HCT Tablets 856

Terazosin Hydrochloride (Concurrent use with other antihypertensive agents may result in additive effect or potentiation). Products include:
Hytrin Capsules 471

Thiamylal Sodium (Potentiation of orthostatic hypotension may occur).
No products indexed under this heading.

Timolol Maleate (Concurrent use with other antihypertensive agents may result in additive effect or potentiation). Products include:
Blocadren Tablets 1916
Cosopt Sterile Ophthalmic
Solution..................................... 1931
Timolide Tablets 2086

Timoptic Sterile Ophthalmic
Solution..................................... 2088
Timoptic in Ocudose 2091
Timoptic-XE Sterile Ophthalmic
Gel Forming Solution 2092

Tolazamide (Thiazide-induced hyperglycemia may require dosage adjustment of hypoglycemic agents).
No products indexed under this heading.

Tolbutamide (Thiazide-induced hyperglycemia may require dosage adjustment of hypoglycemic agents).
No products indexed under this heading.

Tolmetin Sodium (Reduces diuretic, natriuretic, and antihypertensive effects).
No products indexed under this heading.

Torsemide (Concurrent use with other antihypertensive agents may result in additive effect or potentiation). Products include:
Demadex Injection 2759
Demadex Tablets 2759

Trandolapril (Concurrent use with other antihypertensive agents may result in additive effect or potentiation). Products include:
Mavik Tablets 486
Tarka Tablets 524

Triamcinolone (Intensified electrolyte depletion particularly hypokalemia).
No products indexed under this heading.

Triamcinolone Acetonide (Intensified electrolyte depletion particularly hypokalemia). Products include:
Azmacort Inhalation Aerosol 1726
Nasacort AQ Nasal Spray 2922

Triamcinolone Diacetate (Intensified electrolyte depletion particularly hypokalemia).
No products indexed under this heading.

Triamcinolone Hexacetonide (Intensified electrolyte depletion particularly hypokalemia).
No products indexed under this heading.

Trimethaphan Camsylate (Concurrent use with other antihypertensive agents may result in additive effect or potentiation).
No products indexed under this heading.

Troglitazone (Thiazide-induced hyperglycemia may require dosage adjustment of hypoglycemic agents).
No products indexed under this heading.

Tubocurarine Chloride (Possible increased responsiveness to the muscle relaxants).
No products indexed under this heading.

Valdecoxib (Reduces diuretic, natriuretic, and antihypertensive effects).
No products indexed under this heading.

Valsartan (Concurrent use with other antihypertensive agents may result in additive effect or potentiation). Products include:
Diovan Tablets 2193
Diovan HCT Tablets 2196

Vecuronium Bromide (Possible increased responsiveness to the muscle relaxants).
No products indexed under this heading.

Verapamil Hydrochloride (Concurrent use with other antihyperten-

sive agents may result in additive effect or potentiation). Products include:
Covera-HS Tablets 3139
Tarka Tablets 524
Verelan PM Extended-Release
Capsules, Controlled-Onset........... 3106

Food Interactions

Alcohol (Potentiation of orthostatic hypotension may occur).

DIURIL SODIUM INTRAVENOUS

(Chlorothiazide Sodium) 2467
May interact with antihypertensives, barbiturates, corticosteroids, cardiac glycosides, oral hypoglycemic agents, insulin, lithium preparations, narcotic analgesics, nondepolarizing neuromuscular blocking agents, nonsteroidal anti-inflammatory agents, and certain other agents. Compounds in these categories include:

Acarbose (Thiazide-induced hyperglycemia may require dosage adjustment of hypoglycemic agents). Products include:
Precose Tablets 751

Acebutolol Hydrochloride (Concurrent use with other antihypertensive agents may result in additive effect or potentiation).
No products indexed under this heading.

ACTH (Intensified electrolyte depletion particularly hypokalemia).
No products indexed under this heading.

Alfentanil Hydrochloride (Potentiation of orthostatic hypotension may occur).
No products indexed under this heading.

Amlodipine Besylate (Concurrent use with other antihypertensive agents may result in additive effect or potentiation). Products include:
Caduet Tablets 2508
Lotrel Capsules 2249
Norvasc Tablets 2545

Aprobarbital (Potentiation of orthostatic hypotension may occur).
No products indexed under this heading.

Atenolol (Concurrent use with other antihypertensive agents may result in additive effect or potentiation).
No products indexed under this heading.

Atracurium Besylate (Possible increased responsiveness to the muscle relaxants).
No products indexed under this heading.

Benazepril Hydrochloride (Concurrent use with other antihypertensive agents may result in additive effect or potentiation). Products include:
Lotensin Tablets 2243
Lotensin HCT Tablets 2246
Lotrel Capsules 2249

Bendroflumethiazide (Concurrent use with other antihypertensive agents may result in additive effect or potentiation).
No products indexed under this heading.

Betamethasone Acetate (Intensified electrolyte depletion particularly hypokalemia).
No products indexed under this heading.

IMPORTANT NOTE: Always consult each drug listing in the patient's regimen for possible interactions.

Betamethasone Sodium Phosphate (Intensified electrolyte depletion particularly hypokalemia).
No products indexed under this heading.

Betaxolol Hydrochloride (Concurrent use with other antihypertensive agents may result in additive effect or potentiation). Products include:
Betoptic S Ophthalmic Suspension 558

Bisoprolol Fumarate (Concurrent use with other antihypertensive agents may result in additive effect or potentiation).
No products indexed under this heading.

Buprenorphine Hydrochloride (Potentiation of orthostatic hypotension may occur). Products include:
Buprenex Injectable 2716
Suboxone Tablets 2717
Subutex Tablets 2717

Butabarbital (Potentiation of orthostatic hypotension may occur).
No products indexed under this heading.

Butalbital (Potentiation of orthostatic hypotension may occur).
No products indexed under this heading.

Candesartan Cilexetil (Concurrent use with other antihypertensive agents may result in additive effect or potentiation). Products include:
Atacand Tablets 649
Atacand HCT 651

Captopril (Concurrent use with other antihypertensive agents may result in additive effect or potentiation). Products include:
Captopril Tablets 2149

Carteolol Hydrochloride (Concurrent use with other antihypertensive agents may result in additive effect or potentiation). Products include:
Carteolol Hydrochloride Ophthalmic Solution USP, 1% .... ⊙249

Celecoxib (Reduces diuretic, natriuretic, and antihypertensive effects). Products include:
Celebrex Capsules 3134

Chlorothiazide (Concurrent use with other antihypertensive agents may result in additive effect or potentiation). Products include:
Diuril Oral Suspension 1954

Chlorpropamide (Thiazide-induced hyperglycemia may require dosage adjustment of hypoglycemic agents).
No products indexed under this heading.

Chlorthalidone (Concurrent use with other antihypertensive agents may result in additive effect or potentiation). Products include:
Clorpres Tablets 2153

Cisatracurium Besylate (Possible increased responsiveness to the muscle relaxants). Products include:
Nimbex Injection 498

Clonidine (Concurrent use with other antihypertensive agents may result in additive effect or potentiation). Products include:
Catapres-TTS 844

Clonidine Hydrochloride (Concurrent use with other antihypertensive agents may result in additive effect or potentiation). Products include:
Catapres Tablets 843
Clorpres Tablets 2153

Codeine Phosphate (Potentiation of orthostatic hypotension may occur). Products include:
Tylenol with Codeine Tablets 2391

Cortisone Acetate (Intensified electrolyte depletion particularly hypokalemia).
No products indexed under this heading.

Deserpidine (Concurrent use with other antihypertensive agents may result in additive effect or potentiation).
No products indexed under this heading.

Deslanoside (Thiazide-induced hypokalemia may sensitize or exaggerate the response of the heart to the toxic effects of digitalis).
No products indexed under this heading.

Dexamethasone (Intensified electrolyte depletion particularly hypokalemia). Products include:
Ciprodex Otic Suspension 559
Decadron Tablets 1951
TobraDex Ophthalmic Ointment 562
TobraDex Ophthalmic Suspension 563

Dexamethasone Acetate (Intensified electrolyte depletion particularly hypokalemia).
No products indexed under this heading.

Dexamethasone Sodium Phosphate (Intensified electrolyte depletion particularly hypokalemia).
No products indexed under this heading.

Dezocine (Potentiation of orthostatic hypotension may occur).
No products indexed under this heading.

Diazoxide (Concurrent use with other antihypertensive agents may result in additive effect or potentiation). Products include:
Hyperstat I.V. 3017

Diclofenac Potassium (Reduces diuretic, natriuretic, and antihypertensive effects).
No products indexed under this heading.

Diclofenac Sodium (Reduces diuretic, natriuretic, and antihypertensive effects). Products include:
Arthrotec Tablets 3129
Voltaren Ophthalmic Solution 2309
Voltaren Tablets 2307
Voltaren-XR Tablets 2310

Digitalis Glycoside Preparations (Thiazide-induced hypokalemia may sensitize or exaggerate the response of the heart to the toxic effects of digitalis).
No products indexed under this heading.

Digitoxin (Thiazide-induced hypokalemia may sensitize or exaggerate the response of the heart to the toxic effects of digitalis).
No products indexed under this heading.

Digoxin (Thiazide-induced hypokalemia may sensitize or exaggerate the response of the heart to the toxic effects of digitalis). Products include:
Lanoxicaps Capsules 1490
Lanoxin Injection 1494
Lanoxin Injection Pediatric 1497
Lanoxin Tablets 1500

Diltiazem Hydrochloride (Concurrent use with other antihypertensive agents may result in additive effect or potentiation). Products include:
Cardizem LA Extended Release Tablets 1728
Tiazac Capsules 1201

Doxazosin Mesylate (Concurrent use with other antihypertensive agents may result in additive effect or potentiation). Products include:
Cardura XL Tablets 2515

Enalapril Maleate (Concurrent use with other antihypertensive agents may result in additive effect or potentiation). Products include:
Vasotec I.V. Injection 2103

Enalaprilat (Concurrent use with other antihypertensive agents may result in additive effect or potentiation).
No products indexed under this heading.

Eprosartan Mesylate (Concurrent use with other antihypertensive agents may result in additive effect or potentiation). Products include:
Teveten Tablets 1735
Teveten HCT Tablets 1737

Esmolol Hydrochloride (Concurrent use with other antihypertensive agents may result in additive effect or potentiation).
No products indexed under this heading.

Etodolac (Reduces diuretic, natriuretic, and antihypertensive effects).
No products indexed under this heading.

Felodipine (Concurrent use with other antihypertensive agents may result in additive effect or potentiation).
No products indexed under this heading.

Fenoprofen Calcium (Reduces diuretic, natriuretic, and antihypertensive effects). Products include:
Nalfon Capsules 2502

Fentanyl (Potentiation of orthostatic hypotension may occur). Products include:
Duragesic Transdermal System 2373
Ionsys Transdermal System 2379

Fentanyl Citrate (Potentiation of orthostatic hypotension may occur). Products include:
Actiq 979

Fludrocortisone Acetate (Intensified electrolyte depletion particularly hypokalemia).
No products indexed under this heading.

Flurbiprofen (Reduces diuretic, natriuretic, and antihypertensive effects).
No products indexed under this heading.

Fosinopril Sodium (Concurrent use with other antihypertensive agents may result in additive effect or potentiation).
No products indexed under this heading.

Furosemide (Concurrent use with other antihypertensive agents may result in additive effect or potentiation). Products include:
Furosemide Tablets 2154

Glimepiride (Thiazide-induced hyperglycemia may require dosage adjustment of hypoglycemic agents). Products include:
Avandaryl Tablets 1379
Duetact Tablets 3226

Glipizide (Thiazide-induced hyperglycemia may require dosage adjustment of hypoglycemic agents).
No products indexed under this heading.

Glyburide (Thiazide-induced hyperglycemia may require dosage adjustment of hypoglycemic agents).
No products indexed under this heading.

Guanabenz Acetate (Concurrent use with other antihypertensive agents may result in additive effect or potentiation).
No products indexed under this heading.

Guanethidine Monosulfate (Concurrent use with other antihypertensive agents may result in additive effect or potentiation).
No products indexed under this heading.

Hydralazine Hydrochloride (Concurrent use with other antihypertensive agents may result in additive effect or potentiation). Products include:
BiDil Tablets 2171

Hydrochlorothiazide (Concurrent use with other antihypertensive agents may result in additive effect or potentiation). Products include:
Aldoril Tablets 1910
Atacand HCT 651
Avalide Tablets 888
Avalide Tablets 2874
Benicar HCT Tablets 1044
Diovan HCT Tablets 2196
Dyazide Capsules 1423
Hyzaar 50-12.5 Tablets 1990
Hyzaar 100-12.5 Tablets 1990
Hyzaar 100-25 Tablets 1990
Lopressor HCT 50/25 Tablets 2241
Lopressor HCT 100/25 Tablets 2241
Lopressor HCT 100/50 Tablets 2241
Lotensin HCT Tablets 2246
Micardis HCT Tablets 856
Moduretic Tablets 2028
Prinzide Tablets 2056
Teveten HCT Tablets 1737
Timolide Tablets 2086
Uniretic Tablets 3100

Hydrocodone Bitartrate (Potentiation of orthostatic hypotension may occur). Products include:
Hycodan 1116
Hycotuss Expectorant Syrup 1117
Vicodin Tablets 535
Vicodin ES Tablets 536
Vicodin HP Tablets 538
Vicoprofen Tablets 539
Zydone Tablets 1139

Hydrocodone Polistirex (Potentiation of orthostatic hypotension may occur). Products include:
Tussionex Pennkinetic Extended-Release Suspension 3327

Hydrocortisone (Intensified electrolyte depletion particularly hypokalemia). Products include:
Colocort Rectal Suspension, USP (Retention) 100 mg/60 mL 2476
Hydrocortone Tablets 1989
Preparation H Hydrocortisone Cream .... ▣646

Hydrocortisone Acetate (Intensified electrolyte depletion particularly hypokalemia). Products include:
Analpram-HC 1159
Pramosone 1161
ProctoFoam-HC 3099

Hydrocortisone Sodium Phosphate (Intensified electrolyte depletion particularly hypokalemia).
No products indexed under this heading.

Hydrocortisone Sodium Succinate (Intensified electrolyte depletion particularly hypokalemia).
No products indexed under this heading.

Hydroflumethiazide (Concurrent use with other antihypertensive agents may result in additive effect or potentiation).
 No products indexed under this heading.

Hydromorphone Hydrochloride (Potentiation of orthostatic hypotension may occur). Products include:
Dilaudid 440
Dilaudid Non-Sterile Powder 440
Dilaudid Oral Liquid 445
Dilaudid Rectal Suppositories 440
Dilaudid Tablets 440
Dilaudid Tablets - 8 mg 445
Dilaudid-HP 442

Ibuprofen (Reduces diuretic, natriuretic, and antihypertensive effects). Products include:
Advil Allergy Sinus Caplets ▣770
Advil ▣674
Children's Advil Oral Suspension ▣603
Children's Advil Chewable Tablets .. ▣603
Advil Cold & Sinus ▣723
Infants' Advil Concentrated Drops .. ▣604
Infants' Advil Concentrated Drops
 - White Grape (Dye-Free)............... ▣604
Junior Strength Advil Swallow
 Tablets.. ▣605
Advil Migraine Liquigels ▣608
Advil Multi-Symptom Cold
 Caplets.................................... ▣770
Advil PM Caplets ▣615
Motrin IB Tablets and Caplets 1866
Children's Motrin Oral Suspension ... 1867
Children's Motrin Non-Staining
 Dye-Free Oral Suspension............. 1867
Children's Motrin Cold Oral
 Suspension................................ 1867
Infants' Motrin Concentrated
 Drops.. 1867
Infants' Motrin Non-Staining
 Dye-Free Concentrated Drops....... 1867
Junior Strength Motrin Caplets
 and Chewable Tablets.................. 1867
Vicoprofen Tablets 539

Indapamide (Concurrent use with other antihypertensive agents may result in additive effect or potentiation). Products include:
Indapamide Tablets 2156

Indomethacin (Reduces diuretic, natriuretic, and antihypertensive effects). Products include:
Indocin 1995

Indomethacin Sodium Trihydrate (Reduces diuretic, natriuretic, and antihypertensive effects). Products include:
Indocin I.V. 2465

Insulin, Human, Zinc Suspension (Thiazide-induced hyperglycemia may require dosage adjustment of hypoglycemic agents). Products include:
Humulin L, 100 Units 1794
Humulin U, 100 Units 1800

Insulin, Human NPH (Thiazide-induced hyperglycemia may require dosage adjustment of hypoglycemic agents). Products include:
Humulin N, 100 Units 1795
Humulin N Pen 1797

Insulin, Human Regular (Thiazide-induced hyperglycemia may require dosage adjustment of hypoglycemic agents). Products include:
Humulin R, 100 Units 1798

Insulin, Human Regular and Human NPH Mixture (Thiazide-induced hyperglycemia may require dosage adjustment of hypoglycemic agents). Products include:
Humulin 50/50, 100 Units 1791
Humulin 70/30 Pen 1793

Insulin, NPH (Thiazide-induced hyperglycemia may require dosage adjustment of hypoglycemic agents).
 No products indexed under this heading.

Insulin, Regular (Thiazide-induced hyperglycemia may require dosage adjustment of hypoglycemic agents).
 No products indexed under this heading.

Insulin, Zinc Crystals (Thiazide-induced hyperglycemia may require dosage adjustment of hypoglycemic agents).
 No products indexed under this heading.

Insulin, Zinc Suspension (Thiazide-induced hyperglycemia may require dosage adjustment of hypoglycemic agents).
 No products indexed under this heading.

Insulin Aspart, Human Regular (Thiazide-induced hyperglycemia may require dosage adjustment of hypoglycemic agents). Products include:
NovoLog Injection 2326

Insulin glargine (Thiazide-induced hyperglycemia may require dosage adjustment of hypoglycemic agents). Products include:
Lantus Injection 2909

Insulin Lispro, Human (Thiazide-induced hyperglycemia may require dosage adjustment of hypoglycemic agents). Products include:
Humalog-Pen 1781
Humalog Mix 50/50-Pen 1783
Humalog Mix 75/25-Pen 1785

Insulin Lispro Protamine, Human (Thiazide-induced hyperglycemia may require dosage adjustment of hypoglycemic agents). Products include:
Humalog Mix 50/50-Pen 1783
Humalog Mix 75/25-Pen 1785

Irbesartan (Concurrent use with other antihypertensive agents may result in additive effect or potentiation). Products include:
Avalide Tablets 888
Avalide Tablets 2874
Avapro Tablets 891
Avapro Tablets 2871

Isradipine (Concurrent use with other antihypertensive agents may result in additive effect or potentiation). Products include:
DynaCirc CR Tablets 2721

Ketoprofen (Reduces diuretic, natriuretic, and antihypertensive effects).
 No products indexed under this heading.

Ketorolac Tromethamine (Reduces diuretic, natriuretic, and antihypertensive effects). Products include:
Acular Ophthalmic Solution 565
Acular LS Ophthalmic Solution 566

Labetalol Hydrochloride (Concurrent use with other antihypertensive agents may result in additive effect or potentiation).
 No products indexed under this heading.

Levobunolol Hydrochloride (Concurrent use with other antihypertensive agents may result in additive effect or potentiation). Products include:
Betagan Ophthalmic Solution,
 USP.................................... ⊙220

Levorphanol Tartrate (Potentiation of orthostatic hypotension may occur).
 No products indexed under this heading.

Lisinopril (Concurrent use with other antihypertensive agents may result in additive effect or potentiation). Products include:

Prinivil Tablets 2052
Prinzide Tablets 2056

Lithium (Diuretics reduce the renal clearance of lithium and this may lead to lithium toxicity).
 No products indexed under this heading.

Lithium Carbonate (Diuretics reduce the renal clearance of lithium and this may lead to lithium toxicity). Products include:
Lithobid Tablets 1692

Lithium Citrate (Diuretics reduce the renal clearance of lithium and this may lead to lithium toxicity).
 No products indexed under this heading.

Losartan Potassium (Concurrent use with other antihypertensive agents may result in additive effect or potentiation). Products include:
Cozaar Tablets 1935
Hyzaar 50-12.5 Tablets 1990
Hyzaar 100-12.5 Tablets 1990
Hyzaar 100-25 Tablets 1990

Mecamylamine Hydrochloride (Concurrent use with other antihypertensive agents may result in additive effect or potentiation).
 No products indexed under this heading.

Meclofenamate Sodium (Reduces diuretic, natriuretic, and antihypertensive effects).
 No products indexed under this heading.

Mefenamic Acid (Reduces diuretic, natriuretic, and antihypertensive effects).
 No products indexed under this heading.

Meloxicam (Reduces diuretic, natriuretic, and antihypertensive effects). Products include:
Mobic Oral Suspension 863
Mobic Tablets 863

Meperidine Hydrochloride (Potentiation of orthostatic hypotension may occur).
 No products indexed under this heading.

Mephobarbital (Potentiation of orthostatic hypotension may occur).
 No products indexed under this heading.

Metformin Hydrochloride (Thiazide-induced hyperglycemia may require dosage adjustment of hypoglycemic agents). Products include:
ActoPlus Met Tablets 3214
Avandamet Tablets 1373
Fortamet Extended-Release
 Tablets.. 3115

Methadone Hydrochloride (Potentiation of orthostatic hypotension may occur).
 No products indexed under this heading.

Methyclothiazide (Concurrent use with other antihypertensive agents may result in additive effect or potentiation).
 No products indexed under this heading.

Methyldopa (Concurrent use with other antihypertensive agents may result in additive effect or potentiation). Products include:
Aldoril Tablets 1910

Methyldopate Hydrochloride (Concurrent use with other antihypertensive agents may result in additive effect or potentiation).
 No products indexed under this heading.

Methylprednisolone Acetate (Intensified electrolyte depletion particularly hypokalemia). Products include:
Depo-Medrol Injectable
 Suspension 2617
Depo-Medrol Single-Dose Vial 2619

Methylprednisolone Sodium Succinate (Intensified electrolyte depletion particularly hypokalemia).
 No products indexed under this heading.

Metipranolol Hydrochloride (Concurrent use with other antihypertensive agents may result in additive effect or potentiation).
 No products indexed under this heading.

Metocurine Iodide (Possible increased responsiveness to the muscle relaxants).
 No products indexed under this heading.

Metolazone (Concurrent use with other antihypertensive agents may result in additive effect or potentiation).
 No products indexed under this heading.

Metoprolol Succinate (Concurrent use with other antihypertensive agents may result in additive effect or potentiation). Products include:
Toprol-XL Tablets 668

Metoprolol Tartrate (Concurrent use with other antihypertensive agents may result in additive effect or potentiation). Products include:
Lopressor Injection 2238
Lopressor Tablets 2238
Lopressor HCT 50/25 Tablets 2241
Lopressor HCT 100/25 Tablets 2241
Lopressor HCT 100/50 Tablets 2241

Metyrosine (Concurrent use with other antihypertensive agents may result in additive effect or potentiation). Products include:
Demser Capsules 1953

Mibefradil Dihydrochloride (Concurrent use with other antihypertensive agents may result in additive effect or potentiation).
 No products indexed under this heading.

Miglitol (Thiazide-induced hyperglycemia may require dosage adjustment of hypoglycemic agents).
 No products indexed under this heading.

Minoxidil (Concurrent use with other antihypertensive agents may result in additive effect or potentiation). Products include:
Men's Rogaine Extra Strength
 Hair Regrowth Treatment
 Topical Solution, Ocean Rush
 Scent and Original Unscented..... ▣633
Men's Rogaine Foam Hair
 Regrowth Treatment.................... ▣633
Women's Rogaine Hair Regrowth
 Treatment Topical Solution,
 Spring Bloom Scent and
 Original Unscented..................... ▣634

Mivacurium Chloride (Possible increased responsiveness to the muscle relaxants). Products include:
Mivacron Injection 493

Moexipril Hydrochloride (Concurrent use with other antihypertensive agents may result in additive effect or potentiation). Products include:
Uniretic Tablets 3100
Univasc Tablets 3104

Morphine Sulfate (Potentiation of orthostatic hypotension may occur). Products include:
Avinza Capsules 1741

IMPORTANT NOTE: Always consult each drug listing in the patient's regimen for possible interactions.

Kadian Capsules 577
MS Contin Tablets 2701

Nabumetone (Reduces diuretic, natriuretic, and antihypertensive effects).
No products indexed under this heading.

Nadolol (Concurrent use with other antihypertensive agents may result in additive effect or potentiation). Products include:
Nadolol Tablets 2159

Naproxen (Reduces diuretic, natriuretic, and antihypertensive effects). Products include:
EC-Naprosyn Delayed-Release Tablets 2761
Naprosyn Suspension 2761
Naprosyn Tablets 2761
Prevacid NapraPAC 3280

Naproxen Sodium (Reduces diuretic, natriuretic, and antihypertensive effects). Products include:
Aleve Caplets 742
Aleve Gelcaps 743
Aleve Tablets 743
Aleve Cold & Sinus Caplets 744
Anaprox Tablets 2761
Anaprox DS Tablets 2761

Nicardipine Hydrochloride (Concurrent use with other antihypertensive agents may result in additive effect or potentiation). Products include:
Cardene I.V. 2497

Nifedipine (Concurrent use with other antihypertensive agents may result in additive effect or potentiation). Products include:
Adalat CC Tablets 2964

Nisoldipine (Concurrent use with other antihypertensive agents may result in additive effect or potentiation). Products include:
Sular Tablets 3122

Nitroglycerin (Concurrent use with other antihypertensive agents may result in additive effect or potentiation). Products include:
Nitro-Dur Transdermal Infusion System 3046
Nitrolingual Pumpspray 3120

Norepinephrine Hydrochloride (Decreased arterial responsiveness to pressor amine).
No products indexed under this heading.

Oxaprozin (Reduces diuretic, natriuretic, and antihypertensive effects).
No products indexed under this heading.

Oxycodone Hydrochloride (Potentiation of orthostatic hypotension may occur). Products include:
OxyContin Tablets 2703
OxyFast Oral Concentrate Solution 2708
OxyIR Capsules 2708
Percocet Tablets 1131
Percodan Tablets 1132

Pancuronium Bromide (Possible increased responsiveness to the muscle relaxants).
No products indexed under this heading.

Penbutolol Sulfate (Concurrent use with other antihypertensive agents may result in additive effect or potentiation).
No products indexed under this heading.

Pentobarbital Sodium (Potentiation of orthostatic hypotension may occur). Products include:
Nembutal Sodium Solution, USP 2470

Perindopril Erbumine (Concurrent use with other antihypertensive agents may result in additive effect or potentiation). Products include:
Aceon Tablets (2 mg, 4 mg, 8 mg) 3194

Phenobarbital (Potentiation of orthostatic hypotension may occur). Products include:
Donnatal Extentabs 2493

Phenoxybenzamine Hydrochloride (Concurrent use with other antihypertensive agents may result in additive effect or potentiation). Products include:
Dibenzyline Capsules 3399

Phentolamine Mesylate (Concurrent use with other antihypertensive agents may result in additive effect or potentiation).
No products indexed under this heading.

Phenylbutazone (Reduces diuretic, natriuretic, and antihypertensive effects).
No products indexed under this heading.

Pindolol (Concurrent use with other antihypertensive agents may result in additive effect or potentiation).
No products indexed under this heading.

Pioglitazone Hydrochloride (Thiazide-induced hyperglycemia may require dosage adjustment of hypoglycemic agents). Products include:
ActoPlus Met Tablets 3214
Actos Tablets 3219
Duetact Tablets 3226

Piroxicam (Reduces diuretic, natriuretic, and antihypertensive effects).
No products indexed under this heading.

Polythiazide (Concurrent use with other antihypertensive agents may result in additive effect or potentiation).
No products indexed under this heading.

Prazosin Hydrochloride (Concurrent use with other antihypertensive agents may result in additive effect or potentiation).
No products indexed under this heading.

Prednisolone Acetate (Intensified electrolyte depletion particularly hypokalemia). Products include:
Blephamide Ophthalmic Ointment 568
Blephamide Ophthalmic Suspension 569
Poly-Pred Ophthalmic Suspension .... ⊙ 233
Pred Forte Ophthalmic Suspension .... ⊙ 235
Pred Mild Ophthalmic Suspension .... ⊙ 238
Pred-G Ophthalmic Ointment .... ⊙ 237
Pred-G Ophthalmic Suspension ...... ⊙ 236

Prednisolone Sodium Phosphate (Intensified electrolyte depletion particularly hypokalemia).
No products indexed under this heading.

Prednisolone Tebutate (Intensified electrolyte depletion particularly hypokalemia).
No products indexed under this heading.

Prednisone (Intensified electrolyte depletion particularly hypokalemia).
No products indexed under this heading.

Propoxyphene Hydrochloride (Potentiation of orthostatic hypotension may occur).
No products indexed under this heading.

Propoxyphene Napsylate (Potentiation of orthostatic hypotension may occur).
No products indexed under this heading.

Propranolol Hydrochloride (Concurrent use with other antihypertensive agents may result in additive effect or potentiation). Products include:
Inderal LA Long-Acting Capsules 3429
InnoPran XL Capsules 2723

Quinapril Hydrochloride (Concurrent use with other antihypertensive agents may result in additive effect or potentiation).
No products indexed under this heading.

Ramipril (Concurrent use with other antihypertensive agents may result in additive effect or potentiation). Products include:
Altace Capsules 1702

Rapacuronium Bromide (Possible increased responsiveness to the muscle relaxants).
No products indexed under this heading.

Rauwolfia Serpentina (Concurrent use with other antihypertensive agents may result in additive effect or potentiation).
No products indexed under this heading.

Remifentanil Hydrochloride (Potentiation of orthostatic hypotension may occur).
No products indexed under this heading.

Repaglinide (Thiazide-induced hyperglycemia may require dosage adjustment of hypoglycemic agents).
No products indexed under this heading.

Rescinnamine (Concurrent use with other antihypertensive agents may result in additive effect or potentiation).
No products indexed under this heading.

Reserpine (Concurrent use with other antihypertensive agents may result in additive effect or potentiation).
No products indexed under this heading.

Rocuronium Bromide (Possible increased responsiveness to the muscle relaxants). Products include:
Zemuron Injection 2346

Rofecoxib (Reduces diuretic, natriuretic, and antihypertensive effects).
No products indexed under this heading.

Rosiglitazone Maleate (Thiazide-induced hyperglycemia may require dosage adjustment of hypoglycemic agents). Products include:
Avandamet Tablets 1373
Avandaryl Tablets 1379
Avandia Tablets 1384

Secobarbital Sodium (Potentiation of orthostatic hypotension may occur).
No products indexed under this heading.

Sodium Nitroprusside (Concurrent use with other antihypertensive agents may result in additive effect or potentiation).
No products indexed under this heading.

Sotalol Hydrochloride (Concurrent use with other antihypertensive agents may result in additive effect or potentiation).
No products indexed under this heading.

Spirapril Hydrochloride (Concurrent use with other antihypertensive agents may result in additive effect or potentiation).
No products indexed under this heading.

Sufentanil Citrate (Potentiation of orthostatic hypotension may occur).
No products indexed under this heading.

Sulindac (Reduces diuretic, natriuretic, and antihypertensive effects). Products include:
Clinoril Tablets 1924

Telmisartan (Concurrent use with other antihypertensive agents may result in additive effect or potentiation). Products include:
Micardis Tablets 854
Micardis HCT Tablets 856

Terazosin Hydrochloride (Concurrent use with other antihypertensive agents may result in additive effect or potentiation). Products include:
Hytrin Capsules 471

Thiamylal Sodium (Potentiation of orthostatic hypotension may occur).
No products indexed under this heading.

Timolol Maleate (Concurrent use with other antihypertensive agents may result in additive effect or potentiation). Products include:
Blocadren Tablets 1916
Cosopt Sterile Ophthalmic Solution 1931
Timolide Tablets 2086
Timoptic Sterile Ophthalmic Solution 2088
Timoptic in Ocudose 2091
Timoptic-XE Sterile Ophthalmic Gel Forming Solution 2092

Tolazamide (Thiazide-induced hyperglycemia may require dosage adjustment of hypoglycemic agents).
No products indexed under this heading.

Tolbutamide (Thiazide-induced hyperglycemia may require dosage adjustment of hypoglycemic agents).
No products indexed under this heading.

Tolmetin Sodium (Reduces diuretic, natriuretic, and antihypertensive effects).
No products indexed under this heading.

Torsemide (Concurrent use with other antihypertensive agents may result in additive effect or potentiation). Products include:
Demadex Injection 2759
Demadex Tablets 2759

Trandolapril (Concurrent use with other antihypertensive agents may result in additive effect or potentiation). Products include:
Mavik Tablets 486
Tarka Tablets 524

Triamcinolone (Intensified electrolyte depletion particularly hypokalemia).
No products indexed under this heading.

Triamcinolone Acetonide (Intensified electrolyte depletion particularly hypokalemia). Products include:

Azmacort Inhalation Aerosol **1726**
Nasacort AQ Nasal Spray **2922**

Triamcinolone Diacetate (Intensified electrolyte depletion particularly hypokalemia).

No products indexed under this heading.

Triamcinolone Hexacetonide (Intensified electrolyte depletion particularly hypokalemia).

No products indexed under this heading.

Trimethaphan Camsylate (Concurrent use with other antihypertensive agents may result in additive effect or potentiation).

No products indexed under this heading.

Troglitazone (Thiazide-induced hyperglycemia may require dosage adjustment of hypoglycemic agents).

No products indexed under this heading.

Tubocurarine Chloride (Possible increased responsiveness to the muscle relaxants).

No products indexed under this heading.

Valdecoxib (Reduces diuretic, natriuretic, and antihypertensive effects).

No products indexed under this heading.

Valsartan (Concurrent use with other antihypertensive agents may result in additive effect or potentiation). Products include:

Diovan Tablets **2193**
Diovan HCT Tablets **2196**

Vecuronium Bromide (Possible increased responsiveness to the muscle relaxants).

No products indexed under this heading.

Verapamil Hydrochloride (Concurrent use with other antihypertensive agents may result in additive effect or potentiation). Products include:

Covera-HS Tablets **3139**
Tarka Tablets **524**
Verelan PM Extended-Release Capsules, Controlled-Onset **3106**

Food Interactions

Alcohol (Potentiation of orthostatic hypotension may occur).

DOLOBID TABLETS

(Diflunisal) **1955**

May interact with antacids, aspirin-acetylsalicylic acid, oral anticoagulants, lithium preparations, non-steroidal anti-inflammatory agents, thiazides, and certain other agents. Compounds in these categories include:

Acetaminophen (Concomitant administraton of diflunisal and acetaminophen has resulted in an approximate 50% increase in plasma levels of acetaminophen. Acetaminophen had no effect on plasma levels of diflunisal. Since acetaminophen in high doses has been associated with hepatotoxicity, concomitant administration of diflunisal and acetaminophen should be used cautiously, with careful monitoring of patients). Products include:

Comtrex Maximum Strength Cold & Cough Day/Night Caplets - Day Formulation .... ■ **726**
Comtrex Maximum Strength Cold & Cough Day/Night Caplets - Night Formulation .... ■ **726**
Comtrex Maximum Strength Non-Drowsy Cold & Cough Caplets .... ■ **725**
Comtrex Maximum Strength Day/Night Severe Cold & Sinus Caplets - Day Formulation .... ■ **725**
Comtrex Maximum Strength Day/Night Severe Cold & Sinus Caplets - Night Formulation .... ■ **725**
Contac Cold and Flu Maximum Strength Caplets .... ■ **728**
Contac Cold and Flu Day and Night Caplets (Day Formulation Only) .... ■ **727**
Contac Cold and Flu Day and Night Caplets (Night Formulation Only) .... ■ **727**
Contac Cold and Flu Non-Drowsy Caplets .... ■ **728**
Excedrin Extra Strength Caplets/Tablets/Geltabs .... ■ **684**
Excedrin Migraine Caplets/Tablets/Geltabs .... ■ **609**
Excedrin PM Caplets/Tablets/Geltabs .... ■ **610**
Excedrin Sinus Headache Caplets/Tablets .... ■ **610**
Excedrin Tension Headache Caplets/Tablets/Geltabs .... ■ **611**
Goody's Body Pain Formula Powder .... ■ **684**
Goody's Extra Strength Headache Powders .... ■ **611**
Goody's Extra Strength Pain Relief Tablets .... ■ **685**
Goody's PM Powder for Pain with Sleeplessness .... ■ **612**
Percocet Tablets **1131**
Robitussin Cough, Cold & Flu Nighttime Liquid .... ■ **738**
TheraFlu Cold & Sore Throat Hot Liquid .... ■ **741**
TheraFlu Flu & Chest Congestion Hot Liquid .... ■ **741**
TheraFlu Flu & Sore Throat Hot Liquid .... ■ **742**
TheraFlu Daytime Severe Cold Hot Liquid .... ■ **742**
TheraFlu Nighttime Severe Cold Hot Liquid .... ■ **740**
TheraFlu Warming Relief Daytime Severe Cold .... ■ **743**
TheraFlu Warming Relief Nighttime Severe Cold .... ■ **743**
Triaminic Cough & Sore Throat Liquid .... ■ **747**
Regular Strength Tylenol Tablets **1870**
Children's Tylenol with Flavor Creator .... ■ **679**
Children's Tylenol Plus Flu Oral Suspension .... ■ **749**
Tylenol Cold Head Congestion Daytime Caplets with Cool Burst and Gelcaps .... ■ **750**
Tylenol Cold Multi-Symptom Daytime Liquid .... ■ **752**
Tylenol Cold Multi-Symptom Severe Daytime Liquid .... ■ **752**
Tylenol 8 Hour Extended Release Caplets **1870**
Tylenol **1870**
Extra Strength Tylenol PM Caplets, Vanilla Caplets, Geltabs, Gelcaps and Liquid **1875**
Extra Strength Tylenol Rapid Release Gels **1870**
Concentrated Tylenol Infants' Drops Plus Cold & Cough .... ■ **754**
Tylenol with Codeine Tablets **2391**
Tylenol Allergy Multi-Symptom Caplets with Cool Burst and Gelcaps **1872**
Tylenol Allergy Multi-Symptom Nighttime Caplets with Cool Burst **1872**
Tylenol Severe Allergy Caplets **1872**
Tylenol Arthritis Pain Extended Release Caplets and Geltabs **1870**
Tylenol Chest Congestion Caplets with Cool Burst **1872**
Tylenol Chest Congestion Liquid with Cool Burst **1872**
Children's Tylenol Suspension Liquid and Meltaways **1878**
Children's Tylenol Plus Cold Suspension Liquid **1879**
Children's Tylenol Plus Cold & Allergy Suspension Liquid **1878**
Children's Tylenol Plus Cough & Runny Nose Suspension Liquid **1879**
Children's Tylenol Plus Cough & Sore Throat Suspension Liquid **1879**
Children's Tylenol Suspension with Flavor Creator **1878**
Children's Tylenol Plus Flu Suspension Liquid **1881**
Children's Tylenol Plus Multi-Symptom Cold Suspension Liquid **1879**
Tylenol Cold Severe Congestion Non-Drowsy Caplets with Cool Burst **1874**
Tylenol Cold Head Congestion Daytime Caplets with Cool Burst **1873**
Tylenol Cold Head Congestion Nighttime Caplets with Cool Burst **1873**
Tylenol Cold Head Congestion Severe Caplets with Cool Burst **1873**
Tylenol Cold Multi-Symptom Daytime Caplets with Cool Burst and Gelcaps **1874**
Tylenol Cold Multi-Symptom Daytime Liquid with Citrus Burst **1874**
Tylenol Cold Multi-Symptom Nighttime Caplets with Cool Burst **1874**
Tylenol Cold Multi-Symptom Nighttime Liquid with Cool Burst **1874**
Tylenol Cold Multi-Symptom Severe Caplets with Cool Burst **1874**
Tylenol Cold Multi-Symptom Severe Daytime Liquid with Citrus Burst **1874**
Tylenol Cough & Sore Throat Daytime Liquid with Cool Burst **1877**
Tylenol Cough & Sore Throat Nighttime Liquid with Cool Burst **1877**
Concentrated Tylenol Infants' Drops **1878**
Concentrated Tylenol Infants' Drops Plus Cold **1879**
Concentrated Tylenol Infants' Drops Plus Cold and Cough **1879**
Jr. Tylenol Meltaways **1878**
Tylenol Sinus Severe Congestion Caplets with Cool Burst **1876**
Tylenol Sinus Congestion & Pain Daytime Caplets with Cool Burst and Gelcaps **1876**
Tylenol Sinus Congestion & Pain Nighttime Caplets with Cool Burst **1876**
Tylenol Sinus Congestion & Pain Severe Caplets with Cool Burst **1876**
Tylenol Sore Throat Daytime Liquid with Cool Burst **1877**
Tylenol Sore Throat Nighttime Liquid with Cool Burst **1877**
Women's Tylenol Menstrual Relief Caplets **1877**
Vicks 44M Cough, Cold & Flu Relief Liquid **2680**
Vicks DayQuil LiquiCaps/Liquid Multi-Symptom Cold/Flu Relief .... ■ **761**
Vicks DayQuil Multi-Symptom Cold/Flu Relief LiquiCaps **2678**
Vicks DayQuil Multi-Symptom Cold/Flu Relief Liquid **2678**
Vicks NyQuil Multi-Symptom Cold/Flu Relief Liquid **2681**
Vicks NyQuil Multi-Symptom Cold/Flu Relief LiquiCaps **2681**
Vicks NyQuil LiquiCaps/Liquid Multi-Symptom Cold/Flu Relief .... ■ **763**
Vicodin Tablets **535**
Vicodin ES Tablets **536**
Vicodin HP Tablets **538**
Zicam Maximum Strength Flu Daytime .... ■ **768**
Zicam Maximum Strength Flu Nighttime .... ■ **768**
Zydone Tablets **1139**

Aluminum Carbonate (Concomitant administration of antacids may reduce plasma levels of diflunisal. This effect is small with occasional doses of antacids, but may be clinically significant when antacids are used on a continuous schedule).

No products indexed under this heading.

Aluminum Hydroxide (Concomitant administration of antacids may reduce plasma levels of diflunisal. This effect is small with occasional doses of antacids, but may be clinically significant when antacids are used on a continuous schedule). Products include:

Gaviscon Regular Strength Liquid .. ■ **658**
Gaviscon Regular Strength Tablets .... ■ **658**
Gaviscon Extra Strength Liquid ...... ■ **658**
Gaviscon Extra Strength Tablets .... ■ **658**
Maalox Regular Strength Antacid/Antigas Liquid **2175**
Maalox Max Maximum Strength Antacid/Anti-Gas Liquid **2176**

Anisindione (In normal volunteers, the concomitant administration of diflunisal and warfarin, acenocoumarol or phenprocoumon resulted in prolongation of prothrombin time. This may occur because diflunisal competitively displaces coumarins from protein binding sites. Accordingly, when diflunisal is administered with oral anticoagulants, the prothrombin time should be closely monitored during, and for several days after, concomitant drug administration. Adjustment of dosage of oral anticoagulants may be required. The effects of warfarin and NSAIDs on GI bleeding are synergistic, such that users of both drugs together have a risk of serious GI bleeding higher than users of either drug alone). Products include:

Miradon Tablets **3042**

Aspirin (When diflunisal is administered with aspirin, its protein binding is reduced, although the clearance of free diflunisal is not altered. The clinical significance of this interaction is not known, however, as with other NSAIDs, concomitant administrationof diflunisal and aspirin is not generally recommended because of the potential of increased adverse effects). Products include:

Aggrenox Capsules **822**
Bayer Aspirin **744**
BC Allergy Sinus Cold Powder .... ■ **677**
BC Headache Powder .... ■ **677**
Arthritis Strength BC Powder .... ■ **677**
BC Sinus Cold Powder .... ■ **677**
Excedrin Extra Strength Caplets/Tablets/Geltabs .... ■ **684**
Excedrin Migraine Caplets/Tablets/Geltabs .... ■ **609**
Goody's Body Pain Formula Powder .... ■ **684**
Goody's Extra Strength Headache Powders .... ■ **611**
Goody's Extra Strength Pain Relief Tablets .... ■ **685**
Percodan Tablets **1132**
St. Joseph 81 mg Aspirin Chewable and Enteric Coated Tablets **1869**

Aspirin, Enteric Coated (When diflunisal is administered with aspirin, its protein binding is reduced, although the clearance of free diflunisal is not altered. The clinical significance of this interaction is not known, however, as with other NSAIDs, concomitant administrationof diflunisal and aspirin is not generally recommended because of the potential of increased adverse effects).

No products indexed under this heading.

Aspirin Buffered (When diflunisal is administered with aspirin, its protein binding is reduced, although the clearance of free diflunisal is not altered. The clinical significance of this interaction is not known, however, as with other NSAIDs, concomitant administrationof diflunisal and aspirin is not generally recommended because of the potential of increased adverse effects). Products include:

- Bufferin Extra Strength Tablets ...... ▣678
- Bufferin Regular Strength Tablets ... ▣678

Bendroflumethiazide (Clinical studies, as well as post-marketing observations, have shown that diflunisal can reduce the natriuretic effect of thiazides in some patients. This response has been attributed to inhibition of renal prostaglandin synthesis. In normal volunteers, concomitant administration of diflunisal and hydrochlorothiazide (HCTZ) resulted in significantly increased plasma levels of HCTZ. Diflunisal also decreased the hyperiuricemic effect of HCTZ. During concomitant therapy with NSAIDs, the patients shouldbe observed closely for signs of renal failure, as well as to assure diuretic efficacy).

No products indexed under this heading.

Celecoxib (The concomitant use of diflunisal and other NSAIDs is not recommended due to the increased possibility of gastrointestinal toxicity, with little or no increase in efficacy). Products include:

- Celebrex Capsules 3134

Chlorothiazide (Clinical studies, as well as post-marketing observations, have shown that diflunisal can reduce the natriuretic effect of thiazides in some patients. This response has been attributed to inhibition of renal prostaglandin synthesis. In normal volunteers, concomitant administration of diflunisal and hydrochlorothiazide (HCTZ) resulted in significantly increased plasma levels of HCTZ. Diflunisal also decreased the hyperiuricemic effect of HCTZ. During concomitant therapy with NSAIDs, the patients shouldbe observed closely for signs of renal failure, as well as to assure diuretic efficacy). Products include:

- Diuril Oral Suspension 1954

Chlorothiazide Sodium (Clinical studies, as well as post-marketing observations, have shown that diflunisal can reduce the natriuretic effect of thiazides in some patients. This response has been attributed to inhibition of renal prostaglandin synthesis. In normal volunteers, concomitant administration of diflunisal and hydrochlorothiazide (HCTZ) resulted in significantly increased plasma levels of HCTZ. Diflunisal also decreased the hyperiuricemic effect of HCTZ. During concomitant therapy with NSAIDs, the patients shouldbe observed closely for signs of renal failure, as well as to assure diuretic efficacy). Products include:

- Diuril Sodium Intravenous 2467

Cyclosporine (Administration of non-steroidal anti-inflamatory drugs concomitantly with cyclosporine has been associated with an increase in cyclosporine-induced toxicity, possibly due to decreased synthesis of renal prostacyclin. NSAIDs should be used with caution in patients taking cyclosporine, and renal function should be carefully monitored). Products include:

- Gengraf Capsules 459
- Neoral Oral Solution 2259
- Neoral Soft Gelatin Capsules 2259
- Restasis Ophthalmic Emulsion 575
- Sandimmune 2275

Diclofenac Potassium (The concomitant use of diflunisal and other NSAIDs is not recommended due to the increased possibility of gastrointestinal toxicity, with little or no increase in efficacy).

No products indexed under this heading.

Diclofenac Sodium (The concomitant use of diflunisal and other NSAIDs is not recommended due to the increased possibility of gastrointestinal toxicity, with little or no increase in efficacy). Products include:

- Arthrotec Tablets 3129
- Voltaren Ophthalmic Solution 2309
- Voltaren Tablets 2307
- Voltaren-XR Tablets 2310

Dicumarol (In normal volunteers, the concomitant administration of diflunisal and warfarin, acenocoumarol or phenprocoumon resulted in prolongation of prothrombin time. This may occur because diflunisal competitively displaces coumarins from protein binding sites. Accordingly, when diflunisal is administered with oral anticoagulants, the prothrombin time should be closely monitored during, and for several days after, concomitant drug administration. Adjustment of dosage of oral anticoagulants may be required. The effects of warfarin and NSAIDs on GI bleeding are synergistic, such that users of both drugs together have a risk of serious GI bleeding higher than users of either drug alone).

No products indexed under this heading.

Etodolac (The concomitant use of diflunisal and other NSAIDs is not recommended due to the increased possibility of gastrointestinal toxicity, with little or no increase in efficacy).

No products indexed under this heading.

Fenoprofen Calcium (The concomitant use of diflunisal and other NSAIDs is not recommended due to the increased possibility of gastrointestinal toxicity, with little or no increase in efficacy). Products include:

- Nalfon Capsules 2502

Flurbiprofen (The concomitant use of diflunisal and other NSAIDs is not recommended due to the increased possibility of gastrointestinal toxicity, with little or no increase in efficacy).

No products indexed under this heading.

Furosemide (Decreased hyperuricemic effect). Products include:

- Furosemide Tablets 2154

Hydrochlorothiazide (Decreased hyperuricemic effect; increased plasma levels). Products include:

- Aldoril Tablets 1910
- Atacand HCT 651
- Avalide Tablets 888
- Avalide Tablets 2874
- Benicar HCT Tablets 1044
- Diovan HCT Tablets 2196
- Dyazide Capsules 1423
- Hyzaar 50-12.5 Tablets 1990
- Hyzaar 100-12.5 Tablets 1990
- Hyzaar 100-25 Tablets 1990
- Lopressor HCT 50/25 Tablets 2241
- Lopressor HCT 100/25 Tablets 2241
- Lopressor HCT 100/50 Tablets 2241
- Lotensin HCT Tablets 2246
- Micardis HCT Tablets 856
- Moduretic Tablets 2028
- Prinzide Tablets 2056
- Teveten HCT Tablets 1737
- Timolide Tablets 2086
- Uniretic Tablets 3100

Hydroflumethiazide (Clinical studies, as well as post-marketing observations, have shown that diflunisal can reduce the natriuretic effect of thiazides in some patients. This response has been attributed to inhibition of renal prostaglandin synthesis. In normal volunteers, concomitant administration of diflunisal and hydrochlorothiazide (HCTZ) resulted in significantly increased plasma levels of HCTZ. Diflunisal also decreased the hyperiuricemic effect of HCTZ. During concomitant therapy with NSAIDs, the patients shouldbe observed closely for signs of renal failure, as well as to assure diuretic efficacy).

No products indexed under this heading.

Ibuprofen (The concomitant use of diflunisal and other NSAIDs is not recommended due to the increased possibility of gastrointestinal toxicity, with little or no increase in efficacy). Products include:

- Advil Allergy Sinus Caplets .... ▣770
- Advil .... ▣674
- Children's Advil Oral Suspension .... ▣603
- Children's Advil Chewable Tablets .. ▣603
- Advil Cold & Sinus .... ▣723
- Infants' Advil Concentrated Drops .. ▣604
- Infants' Advil Concentrated Drops - White Grape (Dye-Free)............. ▣604
- Junior Strength Advil Swallow Tablets.. ▣605
- Advil Migraine Liquigels .... ▣608
- Advil Multi-Symptom Cold Caplets.. ▣770
- Advil PM Caplets .... ▣615
- Motrin IB Tablets and Caplets 1866
- Children's Motrin Oral Suspension ... 1867
- Children's Motrin Non-Staining Dye-Free Oral Suspension............ 1867
- Children's Motrin Cold Oral Suspension 1867
- Infants' Motrin Concentrated Drops... 1867
- Infants' Motrin Non-Staining Dye-Free Concentrated Drops....... 1867
- Junior Strength Motrin Caplets and Chewable Tablets.................. 1867
- Vicoprofen Tablets 539

Indomethacin (The administration of diflunisal to normal volunteers receiving indomethacin decreased the renal clearance and significantly increased the plasma levels of indomethacin. In some patients the combined use of indomethacin and diflunisal has been associated with fatal gastrointestinal hemorrhage. Therefore, indomethacin and diflunisal should not be used concomitantly). Products include:

- Indocin 1995

Indomethacin Sodium Trihydrate (The administration of diflunisal to normal volunteers receiving indomethacin decreased the renal clearance and significantly increased the plasma levels of indomethacin. In some patients the combined use of indomethacin and diflunisal has been associated with fatal gastrointestinal hemorrhage. Therefore, indomethacin and diflunisal should not be used concomitantly). Products include:

- Indocin I.V. 2465

Ketoprofen (The concomitant use of diflunisal and other NSAIDs is not recommended due to the increased possibility of gastrointestinal toxicity, with little or no increase in efficacy).

No products indexed under this heading.

Ketorolac Tromethamine (The concomitant use of diflunisal and other NSAIDs is not recommended due to the increased possibility of gastrointestinal toxicity, with little or no increase in efficacy). Products include:

- Acular Ophthalmic Solution 565
- Acular LS Ophthalmic Solution 566

Lithium (NSAIDs have produced an elevation of plasma lithium levels and a reduction in renal lithium clearance. The mean minimum lithium concentration increased 15% and the renal clearance was decreased by approximately 20%. These effects have been attributed to the inhibition of renal prostaglandin synthesis by the NSAID. Thus, when NSAIDs and lithium are administered concurrently, subjects should be observed carefully for signs of lithium toxicity).

No products indexed under this heading.

Lithium Carbonate (NSAIDs have produced an elevation of plasma lithium levels and a reduction in renal lithium clearance. The mean minimum lithium concentration increased 15% and the renal clearance was decreased by approximately 20%. These effects have been attributed to the inhibition of renal prostaglandin synthesis by the NSAID. Thus, when NSAIDs and lithium are administered concurrently, subjects should be observed carefully for signs of lithium toxicity). Products include:

- Lithobid Tablets 1692

Lithium Citrate (NSAIDs have produced an elevation of plasma lithium levels and a reduction in renal lithium clearance. The mean minimum lithium concentration increased 15% and the renal clearance was decreased by approximately 20%. These effects have been attributed to the inhibition of renal prostaglandin synthesis by the NSAID. Thus, when NSAIDs and lithium are administered concurrently, subjects should be observed carefully for signs of lithium toxicity).

No products indexed under this heading.

Magaldrate (Concomitant administration of antacids may reduce plasma levels of diflunisal. This effect is small with occasional doses of antacids, but may be clinically significant when antacids are used on a continuous schedule).

No products indexed under this heading.

Magnesium Hydroxide (Concomitant administration of antacids may reduce plasma levels of diflunisal. This effect is small with occasional doses of antacids, but may be clinically significant when antacids are used on a continuous schedule). Products include:

- Maalox Regular Strength Antacid/Antigas Liquid................. 2175
- Maalox Max Maximum Strength Antacid/Anti-Gas Liquid................ 2176
- Pepcid Complete Chewable Tablets 1701

Magnesium Oxide (Concomitant administration of antacids may reduce plasma levels of diflunisal. This effect is small with occasional doses of antacids, but may be clinically significant when antacids are used on a continuous schedule). Products include:

- Beelith Tablets 759

PremCal Light, Regular, and Extra Strength Tablets 818

Meclofenamate Sodium (The concomitant use of diflunisal and other NSAIDs is not recommended due to the increased possibility of gastrointestinal toxicity, with little or no increase in efficacy).
No products indexed under this heading.

Mefenamic Acid (The concomitant use of diflunisal and other NSAIDs is not recommended due to the increased possibility of gastrointestinal toxicity, with little or no increase in efficacy).
No products indexed under this heading.

Meloxicam (The concomitant use of diflunisal and other NSAIDs is not recommended due to the increased possibility of gastrointestinal toxicity, with little or no increase in efficacy). Products include:
Mobic Oral Suspension 863
Mobic Tablets 863

Methotrexate Sodium (NSAIDs have been reported to competitively inhibit methotrexate accumulation in rabbit kidney slices. This may indicate that they could enhance the toxicity of methotrexate. Caution should be used when NSAIDs are administered concomitantly with methotrexate.).
No products indexed under this heading.

Methyclothiazide (Clinical studies, as well as post-marketing observations, have shown that diflunisal can reduce the natriuretic effect of thiazides in some patients. This response has been attributed to inhibition of renal prostaglandin synthesis. In normal volunteers, concomitant administration of diflunisal and hydrochlorothiazide (HCTZ) resulted in significantly increased plasma levels of HCTZ. Diflunisal also decreased the hyperiuricemic effect of HCTZ. During concomitant therapy with NSAIDs, the patients shouldbe observed closely for signs of renal failure, as well as to assure diuretic efficacy).
No products indexed under this heading.

Nabumetone (The concomitant use of diflunisal and other NSAIDs is not recommended due to the increased possibility of gastrointestinal toxicity, with little or no increase in efficacy).
No products indexed under this heading.

Naproxen (The concomitant administration of diflunisal and naproxen in normal volunteers had no effect on plasma levels of naproxen, but significantly decreased the urinary excretion of naproxen and its glucuronide metabolite. Naproxen had no effect on plasma levels of diflunisal). Products include:
EC-Naprosyn Delayed-Release Tablets 2761
Naprosyn Suspension 2761
Naprosyn Tablets 2761
Prevacid NapraPAC 3280

Naproxen Sodium (The concomitant administration of diflunisal and naproxen in normal volunteers had no effect on plasma levels of naproxen, but significantly decreased the urinary excretion of naproxen and its glucuronide metabolite. Naproxen had no effect on plasma levels of diflunisal). Products include:
Aleve Caplets 742
Aleve Gelcaps 743
Aleve Tablets 743
Aleve Cold & Sinus Caplets 744
Anaprox Tablets 2761
Anaprox DS Tablets 2761

Nephrotoxic Drugs (Overt renal decompensation).
No products indexed under this heading.

Oxaprozin (The concomitant use of diflunisal and other NSAIDs is not recommended due to the increased possibility of gastrointestinal toxicity, with little or no increase in efficacy).
No products indexed under this heading.

Phenprocoumon (Prolonged prothrombin time).
No products indexed under this heading.

Phenylbutazone (The concomitant use of diflunisal and other NSAIDs is not recommended due to the increased possibility of gastrointestinal toxicity, with little or no increase in efficacy).
No products indexed under this heading.

Piroxicam (The concomitant use of diflunisal and other NSAIDs is not recommended due to the increased possibility of gastrointestinal toxicity, with little or no increase in efficacy).
No products indexed under this heading.

Polythiazide (Clinical studies, as well as post-marketing observations, have shown that diflunisal can reduce the natriuretic effect of thiazides in some patients. This response has been attributed to inhibition of renal prostaglandin synthesis. In normal volunteers, concomitant administration of diflunisal and hydrochlorothiazide (HCTZ) resulted in significantly increased plasma levels of HCTZ. Diflunisal also decreased the hyperiuricemic effect of HCTZ. During concomitant therapy with NSAIDs, the patients shouldbe observed closely for signs of renal failure, as well as to assure diuretic efficacy).
No products indexed under this heading.

Rofecoxib (The concomitant use of diflunisal and other NSAIDs is not recommended due to the increased possibility of gastrointestinal toxicity, with little or no increase in efficacy).
No products indexed under this heading.

Sodium Bicarbonate (Concomitant administration of antacids may reduce plasma levels of diflunisal. This effect is small with occasional doses of antacids, but may be clinically significant when antacids are used on a continuous schedule). Products include:
Colyte with Flavor Packs for Oral Solution 3088
HalfLytely and Bisacodyl Tablets Bowel Prep Kit with Flavors Packs 881
TriLyte with Flavor Packs for Oral Solution 3100

Sulindac (The concomitant administration of diflunisal and sulindac in normal volunteers resulted in lowering of the plasma levels of the active sulindac sulfide metabolite by approximately one-third). Products include:
Clinoril Tablets 1924

Tolmetin Sodium (The concomitant use of diflunisal and other NSAIDs is not recommended due to the increased possibility of gastrointestinal toxicity, with little or no increase in efficacy).
No products indexed under this heading.

Valdecoxib (The concomitant use of diflunisal and other NSAIDs is not recommended due to the increased possibility of gastrointestinal toxicity, with little or no increase in efficacy).
No products indexed under this heading.

Warfarin Sodium (In normal volunteers, the concomitant administration of diflunisal and warfarin, acenocoumarol or phenprocoumon resulted in prolongation of prothrombin time. This may occur because diflunisal competitively displaces coumarins from protein binding sites. Accordingly, when diflunisal is administered with oral anticoagulants, the prothrombin time should be closely monitored during, and for several days after, concomitant drug administration. Adjustment of dosage of oral anticoagulants may be required. The effects of warfarin and NSAIDs on GI bleeding are synergistic, such that users of both drugs together have a risk of serious GI bleeding higher than users of either drug alone). Products include:
Coumadin for Injection 898
Coumadin Tablets 898

DONNATAL EXTENTABS

(Atropine Sulfate, Hyoscyamine Sulfate, Phenobarbital, Scopolamine Hydrobromide) 2493
May interact with anticoagulants. Compounds in these categories include:

Anisindione (Phenobarbital may decrease the effect of anticoagulants and necessitate larger doses of the anticoagulant for optimal effect. When phenobarbital is discontinued, the dose of the anticoagulant may have to be decreased). Products include:
Miradon Tablets 3042

Ardeparin Sodium (Phenobarbital may decrease the effect of anticoagulants and necessitate larger doses of the anticoagulant for optimal effect. When phenobarbital is discontinued, the dose of the anticoagulant may have to be decreased).
No products indexed under this heading.

Dalteparin Sodium (Phenobarbital may decrease the effect of anticoagulants and necessitate larger doses of the anticoagulant for optimal effect. When phenobarbital is discontinued, the dose of the anticoagulant may have to be decreased). Products include:
Fragmin Injection 1097

Danaparoid Sodium (Phenobarbital may decrease the effect of anticoagulants and necessitate larger doses of the anticoagulant for optimal effect. When phenobarbital is discontinued, the dose of the anticoagulant may have to be decreased).
No products indexed under this heading.

Dicumarol (Phenobarbital may decrease the effect of anticoagulants and necessitate larger doses of the anticoagulant for optimal effect. When phenobarbital is discontinued, the dose of the anticoagulant may have to be decreased).
No products indexed under this heading.

Enoxaparin Sodium (Phenobarbital may decrease the effect of anticoagulants and necessitate larger doses of the anticoagulant for optimal effect. When phenobarbital is discontinued, the dose of the anticoagulant may have to be decreased). Products include:
Lovenox Injection 2915

Fondaparinux Sodium (Phenobarbital may decrease the effect of anticoagulants and necessitate larger doses of the anticoagulant for optimal effect. When phenobarbital is discontinued, the dose of the anticoagulant may have to be decreased). Products include:
Arixtra Injection 1351

Heparin Calcium (Phenobarbital may decrease the effect of anticoagulants and necessitate larger doses of the anticoagulant for optimal effect. When phenobarbital is discontinued, the dose of the anticoagulant may have to be decreased).
No products indexed under this heading.

Heparin Sodium (Phenobarbital may decrease the effect of anticoagulants and necessitate larger doses of the anticoagulant for optimal effect. When phenobarbital is discontinued, the dose of the anticoagulant may have to be decreased).
No products indexed under this heading.

Low Molecular Weight Heparins (Phenobarbital may decrease the effect of anticoagulants and necessitate larger doses of the anticoagulant for optimal effect. When phenobarbital is discontinued, the dose of the anticoagulant may have to be decreased).
No products indexed under this heading.

Tinzaparin Sodium (Phenobarbital may decrease the effect of anticoagulants and necessitate larger doses of the anticoagulant for optimal effect. When phenobarbital is discontinued, the dose of the anticoagulant may have to be decreased).
No products indexed under this heading.

Warfarin Sodium (Phenobarbital may decrease the effect of anticoagulants and necessitate larger doses of the anticoagulant for optimal effect. When phenobarbital is discontinued, the dose of the anticoagulant may have to be decreased). Products include:
Coumadin for Injection 898
Coumadin Tablets 898

DOXIL INJECTION

(Doxorubicin Hydrochloride Liposome) 2351
May interact with antineoplastics and certain other agents. Compounds in these categories include:

Altretamine (Co-administration with the conventional formulation of doxorubicin results in potentiation of the toxicity of other anticancer therapies; this interaction may occur with Doxil).
No products indexed under this heading.

Anastrozole (Co-administration with the conventional formulation of doxorubicin results in potentiation of the toxicity of other anticancer therapies; this interaction may occur with Doxil). Products include:
Arimidex Tablets 673

Asparaginase (Co-administration with the conventional formulation of doxorubicin results in potentiation of the toxicity of other anticancer therapies; this interaction may occur with Doxil). Products include:

Bicalutamide (Co-administration with the conventional formulation of doxorubicin results in potentiation of the toxicity of other anticancer therapies; this interaction may occur with Doxil).

No products indexed under this heading.

Bleomycin Sulfate (Co-administration with the conventional formulation of doxorubicin results in potentiation of the toxicity of other anticancer therapies; this interaction may occur with Doxil).

No products indexed under this heading.

Busulfan (Co-administration with the conventional formulation of doxorubicin results in potentiation of the toxicity of other anticancer therapies; this interaction may occur with Doxil). Products include:

Carboplatin (Co-administration with the conventional formulation of doxorubicin results in potentiation of the toxicity of other anticancer therapies; this interaction may occur with Doxil).

No products indexed under this heading.

Carmustine (BCNU) (Co-administration with the conventional formulation of doxorubicin results in potentiation of the toxicity of other anticancer therapies; this interaction may occur with Doxil).

No products indexed under this heading.

Chlorambucil (Co-administration with the conventional formulation of doxorubicin results in potentiation of the toxicity of other anticancer therapies; this interaction may occur with Doxil). Products include:

Cisplatin (Co-administration with the conventional formulation of doxorubicin results in potentiation of the toxicity of other anticancer therapies; this interaction may occur with Doxil).

No products indexed under this heading.

Cyclophosphamide (Co-administration of conventional formulation of doxorubicin with cyclophosphamide has resulted in exacerbation of cyclophosphamide-induced hemorrhagic cystitis; cardiac toxicity may occur at lower cumulative doses in patients who are receiving cyclophosphamide).

No products indexed under this heading.

Cyclosporine (Co-administration of conventional formulation of doxorubicin may result in increases in AUC for both doxorubicin and doxorubicinol possibly due to a decrease in clearance of parent drug and a decrease in metabolism of doxorubicin; potential for more profound and prolonged hematologic toxicity is associated with combined use; coma and seizures have also been reported). Products include:

Dacarbazine (Co-administration with the conventional formulation of doxorubicin results in potentiation of the toxicity of other anticancer therapies; this interaction may occur with Doxil).

No products indexed under this heading.

Daunorubicin Citrate (Co-administration with the conventional formulation of doxorubicin results in potentiation of the toxicity of other anticancer therapies; this interaction may occur with Doxil).

No products indexed under this heading.

Daunorubicin Hydrochloride (Co-administration with the conventional formulation of doxorubicin results in potentiation of the toxicity of other anticancer therapies; this interaction may occur with Doxil).

No products indexed under this heading.

Denileukin Diftitox (Co-administration with the conventional formulation of doxorubicin results in potentiation of the toxicity of other anticancer therapies; this interaction may occur with Doxil). Products include:

Docetaxel (Co-administration with the conventional formulation of doxorubicin results in potentiation of the toxicity of other anticancer therapies; this interaction may occur with Doxil). Products include:

Doxorubicin Hydrochloride (Co-administration with the conventional formulation of doxorubicin results in potentiation of the toxicity of other anticancer therapies; this interaction may occur with Doxil).

No products indexed under this heading.

Epirubicin Hydrochloride (Co-administration with the conventional formulation of doxorubicin results in potentiation of the toxicity of other anticancer therapies; this interaction may occur with Doxil).

No products indexed under this heading.

Estramustine Phosphate Sodium (Co-administration with the conventional formulation of doxorubicin results in potentiation of the toxicity of other anticancer therapies; this interaction may occur with Doxil). Products include:

Etoposide (Co-administration with the conventional formulation of doxorubicin results in potentiation of the toxicity of other anticancer therapies; this interaction may occur with Doxil).

No products indexed under this heading.

Exemestane (Co-administration with the conventional formulation of doxorubicin results in potentiation of the toxicity of other anticancer therapies; this interaction may occur with Doxil). Products include:

Floxuridine (Co-administration with the conventional formulation of doxorubicin results in potentiation of the toxicity of other anticancer therapies; this interaction may occur with Doxil).

No products indexed under this heading.

Fluorouracil (Co-administration with the conventional formulation of doxorubicin results in potentiation of the toxicity of other anticancer therapies; this interaction may occur with Doxil). Products include:

Flutamide (Co-administration with the conventional formulation of doxorubicin results in potentiation of the toxicity of other anticancer therapies; this interaction may occur with Doxil). Products include:

Gemcitabine Hydrochloride (Co-administration with the conventional formulation of doxorubicin results in potentiation of the toxicity of other anticancer therapies; this interaction may occur with Doxil). Products include:

Hydroxyurea (Co-administration with the conventional formulation of doxorubicin results in potentiation of the toxicity of other anticancer therapies; this interaction may occur with Doxil).

No products indexed under this heading.

Idarubicin Hydrochloride (Co-administration with the conventional formulation of doxorubicin results in potentiation of the toxicity of other anticancer therapies; this interaction may occur with Doxil).

No products indexed under this heading.

Ifosfamide (Co-administration with the conventional formulation of doxorubicin results in potentiation of the toxicity of other anticancer therapies; this interaction may occur with Doxil).

No products indexed under this heading.

Interferon alfa-2a, Recombinant (Co-administration with the conventional formulation of doxorubicin results in potentiation of the toxicity of other anticancer therapies; this interaction may occur with Doxil).

No products indexed under this heading.

Interferon alfa-2b, Recombinant (Co-administration with the conventional formulation of doxorubicin results in potentiation of the toxicity of other anticancer therapies; this interaction may occur with Doxil). Products include:

Irinotecan Hydrochloride (Co-administration with the conventional formulation of doxorubicin results in potentiation of the toxicity of other anticancer therapies; this interaction may occur with Doxil). Products include:

Levamisole Hydrochloride (Co-administration with the conventional formulation of doxorubicin results in potentiation of the toxicity of other anticancer therapies; this interaction may occur with Doxil).

No products indexed under this heading.

Lomustine (CCNU) (Co-administration with the conventional formulation of doxorubicin results in potentiation of the toxicity of other anticancer therapies; this interaction may occur with Doxil).

No products indexed under this heading.

Mechlorethamine Hydrochloride (Co-administration with the conventional formulation of doxorubicin results in potentiation of the toxicity of other anticancer therapies; this interaction may occur with Doxil). Products include:

Medroxyprogesterone Acetate (Co-administration of intravenous progesterone to patients with advanced malignancies at high doses with conventional formulation of fixed doxorubicin dose via bolus enhances doxorubicin-induced neutropenia and thrombocytopenia; this interaction may occur with Doxil). Products include:

Megestrol Acetate (Co-administration with the conventional formulation of doxorubicin results in potentiation of the toxicity of other anticancer therapies; this interaction may occur with Doxil). Products include:

Melphalan (Co-administration with the conventional formulation of doxorubicin results in potentiation of the toxicity of other anticancer therapies; this interaction may occur with Doxil). Products include:

Mercaptopurine (Co-administration of conventional formulation of doxorubicin with 6-mercaptopurine has resulted in enhancement of hepatotoxicity of 6-mercaptopurine).

No products indexed under this heading.

Methotrexate Sodium (Co-administration with the conventional formulation of doxorubicin results in potentiation of the toxicity of other anticancer therapies; this interaction may occur with Doxil).

No products indexed under this heading.

Mitomycin (Mitomycin-C) (Co-administration with the conventional formulation of doxorubicin results in potentiation of the toxicity of other anticancer therapies; this interaction may occur with Doxil).

No products indexed under this heading.

Mitotane (Co-administration with the conventional formulation of doxorubicin results in potentiation of the toxicity of other anticancer therapies; this interaction may occur with Doxil).

No products indexed under this heading.

Mitoxantrone Hydrochloride (Co-administration with the conventional formulation of doxorubicin results in potentiation of the toxicity of other anticancer therapies; this interaction may occur with Doxil).
No products indexed under this heading.

Oxaliplatin (Co-administration with the conventional formulation of doxorubicin results in potentiation of the toxicity of other anticancer therapies; this interaction may occur with Doxil). Products include:
Eloxatin for Injection 2892

Paclitaxel (Administration of paclitaxel infused over 24 hours followed by conventional formulation of doxorubicin administered over 48 hours resulted in a significant decrease in doxorubicin clearance with more profound neutropenic and stomatitis episodes than the reverse sequence of administration; this interaction may occur with Doxil).
No products indexed under this heading.

Phenobarbital (Co-administration with the conventional formulation of doxorubicin results in increased elimination of doxorubicin; this interaction may occur with Doxil). Products include:
Donnatal Extentabs 2493

Phenytoin (Co-administration with the conventional formulation of doxorubicin results in decreased phenytoin levels; this interaction may occur with Doxil).
No products indexed under this heading.

Phenytoin Sodium (Co-administration with the conventional formulation of doxorubicin results in decreased phenytoin levels; this interaction may occur with Doxil). Products include:
Phenytek Capsules 2160

Procarbazine Hydrochloride (Co-administration with the conventional formulation of doxorubicin results in potentiation of the toxicity of other anticancer therapies; this interaction may occur with Doxil). Products include:
Matulane Capsules 3191

Progesterone (Co-administration of intravenous progesterone to patients with advanced malignancies at high doses with conventional formulation of fixed doxorubicin dose via bolus enhances doxorubicin-induced neutropenia and thrombocytopenia; this interaction may occur with Doxil). Products include:
Prochieve 4% Gel 1003
Prochieve 8% Gel 1003
Prometrium Capsules (100 mg, 200 mg) 3203

Streptozocin (Co-administration with the conventional formulation of doxorubicin results in inhibition of hepatic metabolism; this interaction may occur with Doxil).
No products indexed under this heading.

Tamoxifen Citrate (Co-administration with the conventional formulation of doxorubicin results in potentiation of the toxicity of other anticancer therapies; this interaction may occur with Doxil). Products include:
Soltamox Oral Solution 3527

Teniposide (Co-administration with the conventional formulation of doxorubicin results in potentiation of the toxicity of other anticancer therapies; this interaction may occur with Doxil).
No products indexed under this heading.

Thioguanine (Co-administration with the conventional formulation of doxorubicin results in potentiation of the toxicity of other anticancer therapies; this interaction may occur with Doxil). Products include:
Tabloid Tablets 1575

Thiotepa (Co-administration with the conventional formulation of doxorubicin results in potentiation of the toxicity of other anticancer therapies; this interaction may occur with Doxil).
No products indexed under this heading.

Topotecan Hydrochloride (Co-administration with the conventional formulation of doxorubicin results in potentiation of the toxicity of other anticancer therapies; this interaction may occur with Doxil). Products include:
Hycamtin for Injection 1458

Toremifene Citrate (Co-administration with the conventional formulation of doxorubicin results in potentiation of the toxicity of other anticancer therapies; this interaction may occur with Doxil).
No products indexed under this heading.

Valrubicin (Co-administration with the conventional formulation of doxorubicin results in potentiation of the toxicity of other anticancer therapies; this interaction may occur with Doxil).
No products indexed under this heading.

Verapamil Hydrochloride (Co-administration of conventional formulation of doxorubicin in animal studies has resulted in higher initial peak concentrations of doxorubicin in the heart with a higher incidence and severity of degenerative changes in cardiac tissue resulting in a shorter survival; this interaction may occur with Doxil). Products include:
Covera-HS Tablets 3139
Tarka Tablets 524
Verelan PM Extended-Release Capsules, Controlled-Onset 3106

Vincristine Sulfate (Co-administration with the conventional formulation of doxorubicin results in potentiation of the toxicity of other anticancer therapies; this interaction may occur with Doxil).
No products indexed under this heading.

Vinorelbine Tartrate (Co-administration with the conventional formulation of doxorubicin results in potentiation of the toxicity of other anticancer therapies; this interaction may occur with Doxil).
No products indexed under this heading.

DRYSOL SOLUTION
(Aluminum Chloride) 2507
None cited in PDR database.

DUAC TOPICAL GEL
(Benzoyl Peroxide, Clindamycin) 3212
May interact with:

Concomitant Topical Acne Therapy (Possible cumulative irritancy effect may occur, especially with the use of peeling, desquamating, or abrasive agents).
No products indexed under this heading.

DUETACT TABLETS
(Glimepiride, Pioglitazone Hydrochloride) 3226
None cited in PDR database.

DULCOLAX STOOL SOFTENER
(Docusate Sodium) 648
None cited in PDR database.

DULCOLAX SUPPOSITORIES
(Bisacodyl) 648
None cited in PDR database.

DULCOLAX TABLETS
(Bisacodyl) 649
May interact with antacids and certain other agents. Compounds in these categories include:

Aluminum Carbonate (Dulcolax should not be taken within one hour of taking an antacid).
No products indexed under this heading.

Aluminum Hydroxide (Dulcolax should not be taken within one hour of taking an antacid). Products include:
Gaviscon Regular Strength Liquid .. 658
Gaviscon Regular Strength Tablets 658
Gaviscon Extra Strength Liquid 658
Gaviscon Extra Strength Tablets 658
Maalox Regular Strength Antacid/Antigas Liquid 2175
Maalox Max Maximum Strength Antacid/Anti-Gas Liquid 2176

Magaldrate (Dulcolax should not be taken within one hour of taking an antacid).
No products indexed under this heading.

Magnesium Hydroxide (Dulcolax should not be taken within one hour of taking an antacid). Products include:
Maalox Regular Strength Antacid/Antigas Liquid 2175
Maalox Max Maximum Strength Antacid/Anti-Gas Liquid 2176
Pepcid Complete Chewable Tablets 1701

Magnesium Oxide (Dulcolax should not be taken within one hour of taking an antacid). Products include:
Beelith Tablets 759
PremCal Light, Regular, and Extra Strength Tablets 818

Sodium Bicarbonate (Dulcolax should not be taken within one hour of taking an antacid). Products include:
Colyte with Flavor Packs for Oral Solution 3088
HalfLytely and Bisacodyl Tablets Bowel Prep Kit with Flavors Packs 881
TriLyte with Flavor Packs for Oral Solution 3100

Food Interactions

Dairy products (Dulcolax should not be taken within one hour of taking milk).

DUONEB INHALATION SOLUTION
(Albuterol Sulfate, Ipratropium Bromide) 1058
May interact with anticholinergics, beta blockers, monoamine oxidase inhibitors, potassium-depleting diuretics, sympathomimetics, and tricyclic antidepressants. Compounds in these categories include:

Acebutolol Hydrochloride (Co-administration with beta blockers inhibits the effects of each other).
No products indexed under this heading.

Albuterol (Co-administration with other sympathomimetic agents increases the risk of adverse cardiovascular effects). Products include:
Proventil Inhalation Aerosol 3053

Amitriptyline Hydrochloride (Co-administration with tricyclic antidepressants can potentiate the action of albuterol on the cardiovascular system).
No products indexed under this heading.

Amoxapine (Co-administration with tricyclic antidepressants can potentiate the action of albuterol on the cardiovascular system).
No products indexed under this heading.

Atenolol (Co-administration with beta blockers inhibits the effects of each other).
No products indexed under this heading.

Atropine Sulfate (Co-administration has some potential for additive anticholinergic effects; caution is advised). Products include:
Donnatal Extentabs 2493

Belladonna Alkaloids (Co-administration has some potential for additive anticholinergic effects; caution is advised). Products include:
Hyland's Teething Tablets 830

Bendroflumethiazide (Co-administration with non-potassium sparing diuretics can result in acute worsening of ECG changes and/or hypokalemia, especially when recommended dose of the beta agonist is exceeded; clinical significance of this interaction is unknown).
No products indexed under this heading.

Benztropine Mesylate (Co-administration has some potential for additive anticholinergic effects; caution is advised).
No products indexed under this heading.

Betaxolol Hydrochloride (Co-administration with beta blockers inhibits the effects of each other). Products include:
Betoptic S Ophthalmic Suspension 558

Biperiden Hydrochloride (Co-administration has some potential for additive anticholinergic effects; caution is advised).
No products indexed under this heading.

Bisoprolol Fumarate (Co-administration with beta blockers inhibits the effects of each other).
No products indexed under this heading.

Bumetanide (Co-administration with non-potassium sparing diuretics can result in acute worsening of ECG changes and/or hypokalemia, espe-

cially when recommended dose of the beta agonist is exceeded; clinical significance of this interaction is unknown). Products include:
Bumex Tablets 2746

Carteolol Hydrochloride (Co-administration with beta blockers inhibits the effects of each other). Products include:
Carteolol Hydrochloride Ophthalmic Solution USP, 1% ..... ⊙249

Chlorothiazide (Co-administration with non-potassium sparing diuretics can result in acute worsening of ECG changes and/or hypokalemia, especially when recommended dose of the beta agonist is exceeded; clinical significance of this interaction is unknown). Products include:
Diuril Oral Suspension 1954

Chlorothiazide Sodium (Co-administration with non-potassium sparing diuretics can result in acute worsening of ECG changes and/or hypokalemia, especially when recommended dose of the beta agonist is exceeded; clinical significance of this interaction is unknown). Products include:
Diuril Sodium Intravenous 2467

Clidinium Bromide (Co-administration has some potential for additive anticholinergic effects; caution is advised).
No products indexed under this heading.

Clomipramine Hydrochloride (Co-administration with tricyclic antidepressants can potentiate the action of albuterol on the cardiovascular system).
No products indexed under this heading.

Desipramine Hydrochloride (Co-administration with tricyclic antidepressants can potentiate the action of albuterol on the cardiovascular system).
No products indexed under this heading.

Dicyclomine Hydrochloride (Co-administration has some potential for additive anticholinergic effects; caution is advised). Products include:
Bentyl Capsules 697
Bentyl Injection 697
Bentyl Syrup 697
Bentyl Tablets 697

Dobutamine Hydrochloride (Co-administration with other sympathomimetic agents increases the risk of adverse cardiovascular effects).
No products indexed under this heading.

Dopamine Hydrochloride (Co-administration with other sympathomimetic agents increases the risk of adverse cardiovascular effects).
No products indexed under this heading.

Doxepin Hydrochloride (Co-administration with tricyclic antidepressants can potentiate the action of albuterol on the cardiovascular system).
No products indexed under this heading.

Ephedrine Hydrochloride (Co-administration with other sympathomimetic agents increases the risk of adverse cardiovascular effects).
No products indexed under this heading.

Ephedrine Sulfate (Co-administration with other sympathomimetic agents increases the risk of adverse cardiovascular effects).
No products indexed under this heading.

Ephedrine Tannate (Co-administration with other sympathomimetic agents increases the risk of adverse cardiovascular effects).
No products indexed under this heading.

Epinephrine (Co-administration with other sympathomimetic agents increases the risk of adverse cardiovascular effects). Products include:
EpiPen 1061
Primatene Mist ..... ▣719
Twinject 0.15 3379
Twinject 0.3 3378

Epinephrine Bitartrate (Co-administration with other sympathomimetic agents increases the risk of adverse cardiovascular effects).
No products indexed under this heading.

Epinephrine Hydrochloride (Co-administration with other sympathomimetic agents increases the risk of adverse cardiovascular effects).
No products indexed under this heading.

Esmolol Hydrochloride (Co-administration with beta blockers inhibits the effects of each other).
No products indexed under this heading.

Ethacrynic Acid (Co-administration with non-potassium sparing diuretics can result in acute worsening of ECG changes and/or hypokalemia, especially when recommended dose of the beta agonist is exceeded; clinical significance of this interaction is unknown). Products include:
Edecrin Tablets 1959

Furosemide (Co-administration with non-potassium sparing diuretics can result in acute worsening of ECG changes and/or hypokalemia, especially when recommended dose of the beta agonist is exceeded; clinical significance of this interaction is unknown). Products include:
Furosemide Tablets 2154

Glycopyrrolate (Co-administration has some potential for additive anticholinergic effects; caution is advised).
No products indexed under this heading.

Hydrochlorothiazide (Co-administration with non-potassium sparing diuretics can result in acute worsening of ECG changes and/or hypokalemia, especially when recommended dose of the beta agonist is exceeded; clinical significance of this interaction is unknown). Products include:
Aldoril Tablets 1910
Atacand HCT 651
Avalide Tablets 888
Avalide Tablets 2874
Benicar HCT Tablets 1044
Diovan HCT Tablets 2196
Dyazide Capsules 1423
Hyzaar 50-12.5 Tablets 1990
Hyzaar 100-12.5 Tablets 1990
Hyzaar 100-25 Tablets 1990
Lopressor HCT 50/25 Tablets 2241
Lopressor HCT 100/25 Tablets 2241
Lopressor HCT 100/50 Tablets 2241
Lotensin HCT Tablets 2246
Micardis HCT Tablets 856
Moduretic Tablets 2028
Prinzide Tablets 2056
Teveten HCT Tablets 1737
Timolide Tablets 2086
Uniretic Tablets 3100

Hydroflumethiazide (Co-administration with non-potassium sparing diuretics can result in acute worsening of ECG changes and/or hypokalemia, especially when recommended dose of the beta agonist is exceeded; clinical significance of this interaction is unknown).
No products indexed under this heading.

Hyoscyamine (Co-administration has some potential for additive anticholinergic effects; caution is advised).
No products indexed under this heading.

Hyoscyamine Sulfate (Co-administration has some potential for additive anticholinergic effects; caution is advised). Products include:
Donnatal Extentabs 2493
Prosed/DS Tablets 1157

Imipramine Hydrochloride (Co-administration with tricyclic antidepressants can potentiate the action of albuterol on the cardiovascular system).
No products indexed under this heading.

Imipramine Pamoate (Co-administration with tricyclic antidepressants can potentiate the action of albuterol on the cardiovascular system).
No products indexed under this heading.

Isocarboxazid (Co-administration with MAO inhibitors can potentiate the action of albuterol on the cardiovascular system).
No products indexed under this heading.

Isoproterenol Hydrochloride (Co-administration with other sympathomimetic agents increases the risk of adverse cardiovascular effects).
No products indexed under this heading.

Isoproterenol Sulfate (Co-administration with other sympathomimetic agents increases the risk of adverse cardiovascular effects).
No products indexed under this heading.

Labetalol Hydrochloride (Co-administration with beta blockers inhibits the effects of each other).
No products indexed under this heading.

Levalbuterol Hydrochloride (Co-administration with other sympathomimetic agents increases the risk of adverse cardiovascular effects). Products include:
Xopenex Inhalation Solution 3146
Xopenex Inhalation Solution Concentrate 3150

Levobunolol Hydrochloride (Co-administration with beta blockers inhibits the effects of each other). Products include:
Betagan Ophthalmic Solution, USP ..... ⊙220

Maprotiline Hydrochloride (Co-administration with tricyclic antidepressants can potentiate the action of albuterol on the cardiovascular system).
No products indexed under this heading.

Mepenzolate Bromide (Co-administration has some potential for additive anticholinergic effects; caution is advised).
No products indexed under this heading.

Metaproterenol Sulfate (Co-administration with other sympathomimetic agents increases the risk of adverse cardiovascular effects). Products include:
Alupent Inhalation Aerosol 826

Metaraminol Bitartrate (Co-administration with other sympathomimetic agents increases the risk of adverse cardiovascular effects).
No products indexed under this heading.

Methoxamine Hydrochloride (Co-administration with other sympathomimetic agents increases the risk of adverse cardiovascular effects).
No products indexed under this heading.

Methyclothiazide (Co-administration with non-potassium sparing diuretics can result in acute worsening of ECG changes and/or hypokalemia, especially when recommended dose of the beta agonist is exceeded; clinical significance of this interaction is unknown).
No products indexed under this heading.

Metipranolol Hydrochloride (Co-administration with beta blockers inhibits the effects of each other).
No products indexed under this heading.

Metoprolol Succinate (Co-administration with beta blockers inhibits the effects of each other). Products include:
Toprol-XL Tablets 668

Metoprolol Tartrate (Co-administration with beta blockers inhibits the effects of each other). Products include:
Lopressor Injection 2238
Lopressor Tablets 2238
Lopressor HCT 50/25 Tablets 2241
Lopressor HCT 100/25 Tablets 2241
Lopressor HCT 100/50 Tablets 2241

Moclobemide (Co-administration with MAO inhibitors can potentiate the action of albuterol on the cardiovascular system).
No products indexed under this heading.

Nadolol (Co-administration with beta blockers inhibits the effects of each other). Products include:
Nadolol Tablets 2159

Norepinephrine Bitartrate (Co-administration with other sympathomimetic agents increases the risk of adverse cardiovascular effects).
No products indexed under this heading.

Nortriptyline Hydrochloride (Co-administration with tricyclic antidepressants can potentiate the action of albuterol on the cardiovascular system).
No products indexed under this heading.

Oxybutynin Chloride (Co-administration has some potential for additive anticholinergic effects; caution is advised). Products include:
Ditropan XL Extended-Release Tablets 2413

the beta agonist is exceeded; clinical significance of this interaction is unknown). Products include:
Demadex Injection 2759
Demadex Tablets 2759

Tranylcypromine Sulfate (Co-administration with MAO inhibitors can potentiate the action of albuterol on the cardiovascular system). Products include:
Parnate Tablets 1527

Tridihexethyl Chloride (Co-administration has some potential for additive anticholinergic effects; caution is advised).
No products indexed under this heading.

Trihexyphenidyl Hydrochloride (Co-administration has some potential for additive anticholinergic effects; caution is advised).
No products indexed under this heading.

Trimipramine Maleate (Co-administration with tricyclic antidepressants can potentiate the action of albuterol on the cardiovascular system).
No products indexed under this heading.

DURAGESIC TRANSDERMAL SYSTEM

(Fentanyl) 2373

May interact with central nervous system depressants, cytochrome p450 3a4 inducers (selected), cytochrome p450 3a4 inhibitors (selected), cytochrome p450 3a4 inhibitors, potent, general anesthetics, hypnotics and sedatives, monoamine oxidase inhibitors, narcotic analgesics, phenothiazines, skeletal muscle relaxants, tranquilizers, and certain other agents. Compounds in these categories include:

Acetazolamide (The concurrent use of CYP3A4 inhibitors with transdermal fentanyl may result in an increase in fentanyl plasma concentrations, which could increase or prolong adverse drug effects and may cause serious respiratory depression. In this situation, special patient care and observation are appropriate).
No products indexed under this heading.

Alfentanil Hydrochloride (The comcomitant use of fentanyl with other CNS depressants may cause respiratory depression, hypotension, and profound sedation or potentially result in coma. When such combined therapy is contemplated, the dose of one or both agents should be significantly reduced).
No products indexed under this heading.

Allium sativum (Fentanyl is metabolized mainly via the human cytochrome P450 3A4 isoenzyme system (CYP3A4). Co-administration with agents that induce CYP 3A4 activity may reduce the efficacy of fentanyl).
No products indexed under this heading.

Alprazolam (The comcomitant use of fentanyl with other CNS depressants may cause respiratory depression, hypotension, and profound sedation or potentially result in coma. When such combined therapy is contemplated, the dose of one or both agents should be significantly reduced). Products include:
Niravam Orally Disintegrating Tablets 3092

Amiodarone Hydrochloride (The concurrent use of CYP3A4 inhibitors with transdermal fentanyl may result in an increase in fentanyl plasma concentrations, which could increase or prolong adverse drug effects and may cause serious respiratory depression. In this situation, special patient care and observation are appropriate).
No products indexed under this heading.

Amprenavir (The concomitant use of fentanyl with potent cytochrome P450 3A4 inhibitors may result in an increase in fentanyl plasma concentrations, which could increase or prolong adverse drug effects and may cause potentially fatal respiratory depression. Patients receiving fentanyl and potent CYP3A4 inhibitors should be carefully monitored for an extended period of time and dosage adjustments should be made if warranted). Products include:
Agenerase Capsules 1327
Agenerase Oral Solution 1332

Anastrozole (The concurrent use of CYP3A4 inhibitors with transdermal fentanyl may result in an increase in fentanyl plasma concentrations, which could increase or prolong adverse drug effects and may cause serious respiratory depression. In this situation, special patient care and observation are appropriate). Products include:
Arimidex Tablets 673

Aprepitant (The concurrent use of CYP3A4 inhibitors with transdermal fentanyl may result in an increase in fentanyl plasma concentrations, which could increase or prolong adverse drug effects and may cause serious respiratory depression. In this situation, special patient care and observation are appropriate). Products include:
Emend Capsules 1963

Aprobarbital (The comcomitant use of fentanyl with other CNS depressants may cause respiratory depression, hypotension, and profound sedation or potentially result in coma. When such combined therapy is contemplated, the dose of one or both agents should be significantly reduced).
No products indexed under this heading.

Atazanavir (The concomitant use of fentanyl with potent cytochrome P450 3A4 inhibitors may result in an increase in fentanyl plasma concentrations, which could increase or prolong adverse drug effects and may cause potentially fatal respiratory depression. Patients receiving fentanyl and potent CYP3A4 inhibitors should be carefully monitored for an extended period of time and dosage adjustments should be made if warranted).
No products indexed under this heading.

Atazanavir sulfate (The concomitant use of fentanyl with potent cytochrome P450 3A4 inhibitors may result in an increase in fentanyl plasma concentrations, which could increase or prolong adverse drug effects and may cause potentially fatal respiratory depression. Patients receiving fentanyl and potent CYP3A4 inhibitors should be carefully monitored for an extended period of time and dosage adjustments should be made if warranted). Products include:
Reyataz Capsules 921

Baclofen (The concomitant use of fentanyl with other CNS depressants, including skeletal muscle relaxants, may cause respiratory depression, hypotension, and profound sedation or potentially result in coma. When such combined therapy is contemplated, the dose of one or both agents should be significantly reduced).
No products indexed under this heading.

Betamethasone Acetate (Fentanyl is metabolized mainly via the human cytochrome P450 3A4 isoenzyme system (CYP3A4). Co-administration with agents that induce CYP 3A4 activity may reduce the efficacy of fentanyl).
No products indexed under this heading.

Betamethasone Sodium Phosphate (Fentanyl is metabolized mainly via the human cytochrome P450 3A4 isoenzyme system (CYP3A4). Co-administration with agents that induce CYP 3A4 activity may reduce the efficacy of fentanyl).
No products indexed under this heading.

Buprenorphine Hydrochloride (The comcomitant use of fentanyl with other CNS depressants may cause respiratory depression, hypotension, and profound sedation or potentially result in coma. When such combined therapy is contemplated, the dose of one or both agents should be significantly reduced). Products include:
Buprenex Injectable 2716
Suboxone Tablets 2717
Subutex Tablets 2717

Buspirone Hydrochloride (The comcomitant use of fentanyl with other CNS depressants may cause respiratory depression, hypotension, and profound sedation or potentially result in coma. When such combined therapy is contemplated, the dose of one or both agents should be significantly reduced).
No products indexed under this heading.

Butabarbital (The comcomitant use of fentanyl with other CNS depressants may cause respiratory depression, hypotension, and profound sedation or potentially result in coma. When such combined therapy is contemplated, the dose of one or both agents should be significantly reduced).
No products indexed under this heading.

Butalbital (The comcomitant use of fentanyl with other CNS depressants may cause respiratory depression, hypotension, and profound sedation or potentially result in coma. When such combined therapy is contemplated, the dose of one or both agents should be significantly reduced).
No products indexed under this heading.

Carbamazepine (Fentanyl is metabolized mainly via the human cytochrome P450 3A4 isoenzyme system (CYP3A4). Co-administration with agents that induce CYP 3A4 activity may reduce the efficacy of fentanyl). Products include:
Carbatrol Capsules 3171
Equetro Extended-Release Capsules 3180
Tegretol/Tegretol-XR 2295

Carisoprodol (The comcomitant use of fentanyl with other CNS depressants, including skeletal muscle relaxants, may cause respiratory depression, hypotension, and profound sedation or potentially result in coma. When such combined therapy is contemplated, the dose of one or both agents should be significantly reduced).
No products indexed under this heading.

Chlordiazepoxide (The comcomitant use of fentanyl with other CNS depressants may cause respiratory depression, hypotension, and profound sedation or potentially result in coma. When such combined therapy is contemplated, the dose of one or both agents should be significantly reduced).
No products indexed under this heading.

Chlordiazepoxide Hydrochloride (The comcomitant use of fentanyl with other CNS depressants may cause respiratory depression, hypotension, and profound sedation or potentially result in coma. When such combined therapy is contemplated, the dose of one or both agents should be significantly reduced). Products include:
Librium Capsules 3347

Chlorpromazine (The comcomitant use of fentanyl with other CNS depressants may cause respiratory depression, hypotension, and profound sedation or potentially result in coma. When such combined therapy is contemplated, the dose of one or both agents should be significantly reduced).
No products indexed under this heading.

Chlorpromazine Hydrochloride (The comcomitant use of fentanyl with other CNS depressants may cause respiratory depression, hypotension, and profound sedation or potentially result in coma. When such combined therapy is contemplated, the dose of one or both agents should be significantly reduced).
No products indexed under this heading.

Chlorprothixene (The comcomitant use of fentanyl with other CNS depressants may cause respiratory depression, hypotension, and profound sedation or potentially result in coma. When such combined therapy is contemplated, the dose of one or both agents should be significantly reduced).
No products indexed under this heading.

Chlorprothixene Hydrochloride (The comcomitant use of fentanyl with other CNS depressants may cause respiratory depression, hypotension, and profound sedation or potentially result in coma. When such combined therapy is contemplated, the dose of one or both agents should be significantly reduced).
No products indexed under this heading.

Chlorprothixene Lactate (The comcomitant use of fentanyl with other CNS depressants may cause respiratory depression, hypotension, and profound sedation or potentially result in coma. When such combined therapy is contemplated, the dose of one or both agents should be significantly reduced).
No products indexed under this heading.

Chlorzoxazone (The concomitant use of fentanyl with other CNS depressants, including skeletal muscle relaxants, may cause respiratory depression, hypotension, and profound sedation or potentially result in coma. When such combined therapy is contemplated, the dose of one or both agents should be significantly reduced).
No products indexed under this heading.

Cimetidine (The concurrent use of CYP3A4 inhibitors with transdermal fentanyl may result in an increase in fentanyl plasma concentrations, which could increase or prolong adverse drug effects and may cause serious respiratory depression. In this situation, special patient care and observation are appropriate). Products include:
Tagamet HB 200 Tablets .... ▣664

Cimetidine Hydrochloride (The concurrent use of CYP3A4 inhibitors with transdermal fentanyl may result in an increase in fentanyl plasma concentrations, which could increase or prolong adverse drug effects and may cause serious respiratory depression. In this situation, special patient care and observation are appropriate).
No products indexed under this heading.

Ciprofloxacin (The concurrent use of CYP3A4 inhibitors with transdermal fentanyl may result in an increase in fentanyl plasma concentrations, which could increase or prolong adverse drug effects and may cause serious respiratory depression. In this situation, special patient care and observation are appropriate). Products include:
Cipro Oral Suspension **2977**
Cipro I.V. **2984**
Cipro XR Tablets **2990**
Ciprodex Otic Suspension **559**

Ciprofloxacin Hydrochloride (Fentanyl is metabolized mainly via the human cytochrome P450 3A4 isoenzyme system (CYP3A4). Co-administration with agents that induce CYP 3A4 activity may reduce the efficacy of fentanyl). Products include:
Ciloxan Ophthalmic Ointment **559**
Ciloxan Ophthalmic Solution .... ⊙**206**
Cipro Tablets **2977**
Proquin XR Tablets **1153**

Cisplatin (Fentanyl is metabolized mainly via the human cytochrome P450 3A4 isoenzyme system (CYP3A4). Co-administration with agents that induce CYP 3A4 activity may reduce the efficacy of fentanyl).
No products indexed under this heading.

Clarithromycin (The concomitant use of fentanyl with potent cytochrome P450 3A4 inhibitors may result in an increase in fentanyl plasma concentrations, which could increase or prolong adverse drug effects and may cause potentially fatal respiratory depression. Patients receiving fentanyl and potent CYP3A4 inhibitors should be carefully monitored for an extended period of time and dosage adjustments should be made if warranted). Products include:
Biaxin/Biaxin XL **402**
PREVPAC **3284**

Clorazepate Dipotassium (The comcomitant use of fentanyl with other CNS depressants may cause respiratory depression, hypotension, and profound sedation or potentially result in coma. When such combined therapy is contemplated, the dose of one or both agents should be significantly reduced). Products include:
Tranxene **2474**

Clotrimazole (The concurrent use of CYP3A4 inhibitors with transdermal fentanyl may result in an increase in fentanyl plasma concentrations, which could increase or prolong adverse drug effects and may cause serious respiratory depression. In this situation, special patient care and observation are appropriate). Products include:
Desenex Athlete's Foot Cream .... ▣**635**
Lotrimin **3039**
Lotrisone **3040**

Clozapine (The comcomitant use of fentanyl with other CNS depressants may cause respiratory depression, hypotension, and profound sedation or potentially result in coma. When such combined therapy is contemplated, the dose of one or both agents should be significantly reduced). Products include:
Clozaril Tablets **2184**
FazaClo Orally Disintegrating Tablets **551**

Codeine Phosphate (The comcomitant use of fentanyl with other CNS depressants may cause respiratory depression, hypotension, and profound sedation or potentially result in coma. When such combined therapy is contemplated, the dose of one or both agents should be significantly reduced). Products include:
Tylenol with Codeine Tablets **2391**

Cortisone Acetate (Fentanyl is metabolized mainly via the human cytochrome P450 3A4 isoenzyme system (CYP3A4). Co-administration with agents that induce CYP 3A4 activity may reduce the efficacy of fentanyl).
No products indexed under this heading.

Cyclobenzaprine Hydrochloride (The concomitant use of fentanyl with other CNS depressants, including skeletal muscle relaxants, may cause respiratory depression, hypotension, and profound sedation or potentially result in coma. When such combined therapy is contemplated, the dose of one or both agents should be significantly reduced).
No products indexed under this heading.

Cyclosporine (The concurrent use of CYP3A4 inhibitors with transdermal fentanyl may result in an increase in fentanyl plasma concentrations, which could increase or prolong adverse drug effects and may cause serious respiratory depression. In this situation, special patient care and observation are appropriate). Products include:
Gengraf Capsules **459**
Neoral Oral Solution **2259**
Neoral Soft Gelatin Capsules **2259**
Restasis Ophthalmic Emulsion **575**
Sandimmune **2275**

Dalfopristin (The concurrent use of CYP3A4 inhibitors with transdermal fentanyl may result in an increase in fentanyl plasma concentrations, which could increase or prolong adverse drug effects and may cause serious respiratory depression. In this situation, special patient care and observation are appropriate).
No products indexed under this heading.

Danazol (The concurrent use of CYP3A4 inhibitors with transdermal fentanyl may result in an increase in fentanyl plasma concentrations, which could increase or prolong adverse drug effects and may cause serious respiratory depression. In this situation, special patient care and observation are appropriate).
No products indexed under this heading.

Dantrolene Sodium (The concomitant use of fentanyl with other CNS depressants, including skeletal muscle relaxants, may cause respiratory depression, hypotension, and profound sedation or potentially result in coma. When such combined therapy is contemplated, the dose of one or both agents should be significantly reduced). Products include:
Dantrium Capsules **2694**
Dantrium Intravenous **2695**

Delavirdine Mesylate (The concurrent use of CYP3A4 inhibitors with transdermal fentanyl may result in an increase in fentanyl plasma concentrations, which could increase or prolong adverse drug effects and may cause serious respiratory depression. In this situation, special patient care and observation are appropriate). Products include:
Rescriptor Tablets **2551**

Desflurane (The comcomitant use of fentanyl with other CNS depressants may cause respiratory depression, hypotension, and profound sedation or potentially result in coma. When such combined therapy is contemplated, the dose of one or both agents should be significantly reduced).
No products indexed under this heading.

Dexamethasone (Fentanyl is metabolized mainly via the human cytochrome P450 3A4 isoenzyme system (CYP3A4). Co-administration with agents that induce CYP 3A4 activity may reduce the efficacy of fentanyl). Products include:
Ciprodex Otic Suspension **559**
Decadron Tablets **1951**
TobraDex Ophthalmic Ointment **562**
TobraDex Ophthalmic Suspension ... **563**

Dexamethasone Acetate (Fentanyl is metabolized mainly via the human cytochrome P450 3A4 isoenzyme system (CYP3A4). Co-administration with agents that induce CYP 3A4 activity may reduce the efficacy of fentanyl).
No products indexed under this heading.

Dexamethasone Sodium Phosphate (Fentanyl is metabolized mainly via the human cytochrome P450 3A4 isoenzyme system (CYP3A4). Co-administration with agents that induce CYP 3A4 activity may reduce the efficacy of fentanyl).
No products indexed under this heading.

Dezocine (The comcomitant use of fentanyl with other CNS depressants may cause respiratory depression, hypotension, and profound sedation or potentially result in coma. When such combined therapy is contemplated, the dose of one or both agents should be significantly reduced).
No products indexed under this heading.

Diazepam (The comcomitant use of fentanyl with other CNS depressants may cause respiratory depression, hypotension, and profound sedation or potentially result in coma. When such combined therapy is contemplated, the dose of one or both agents should be significantly reduced). Products include:
Diastat Rectal Delivery System **3343**
Valium Tablets **2819**

Diltiazem Hydrochloride (The concurrent use of CYP3A4 inhibitors with transdermal fentanyl may result in an increase in fentanyl plasma concentrations, which could increase or prolong adverse drug effects and may cause serious respiratory depression. In this situation, special patient care and observation are appropriate). Products include:
Cardizem LA Extended Release Tablets **1728**
Tiazac Capsules **1201**

Diltiazem Maleate (The concurrent use of CYP3A4 inhibitors with transdermal fentanyl may result in an increase in fentanyl plasma concentrations, which could increase or prolong adverse drug effects and may cause serious respiratory depression. In this situation, special patient care and observation are appropriate).
No products indexed under this heading.

Doxorubicin Hydrochloride (Fentanyl is metabolized mainly via the human cytochrome P450 3A4 isoenzyme system (CYP3A4). Co-administration with agents that induce CYP 3A4 activity may reduce the efficacy of fentanyl).
No products indexed under this heading.

Droperidol (The comcomitant use of fentanyl with other CNS depressants may cause respiratory depression, hypotension, and profound sedation or potentially result in coma. When such combined therapy is contemplated, the dose of one or both agents should be significantly reduced).
No products indexed under this heading.

Efavirenz (The concurrent use of CYP3A4 inhibitors with transdermal fentanyl may result in an increase in fentanyl plasma concentrations, which could increase or prolong adverse drug effects and may cause serious respiratory depression. In this situation, special patient care and observation are appropriate). Products include:
Atripla Tablets **945**
Sustiva Capsules **930**
Sustiva Tablets **930**

Enflurane (The comcomitant use of fentanyl with other CNS depressants may cause respiratory depression, hypotension, and profound sedation or potentially result in coma. When such combined therapy is contemplated, the dose of one or both agents should be significantly reduced).

No products indexed under this heading.

Erythromycin (The concurrent use of CYP3A4 inhibitors with transdermal fentanyl may result in an increase in fentanyl plasma concentrations, which could increase or prolong adverse drug effects and may cause serious respiratory depression. In this situation, special patient care and observation are appropriate). Products include:

Ery-Tab Tablets 449
Erythromycin Base Filmtab
Tablets 455
Erythromycin Delayed-Release
Capsules, USP 457
PCE Dispertab Tablets 515

Erythromycin Estolate (The concurrent use of CYP3A4 inhibitors with transdermal fentanyl may result in an increase in fentanyl plasma concentrations, which could increase or prolong adverse drug effects and may cause serious respiratory depression. In this situation, special patient care and observation are appropriate).

No products indexed under this heading.

Erythromycin Ethylsuccinate (The concurrent use of CYP3A4 inhibitors with transdermal fentanyl may result in an increase in fentanyl plasma concentrations, which could increase or prolong adverse drug effects and may cause serious respiratory depression. In this situation, special patient care and observation are appropriate). Products include:

E.E.S. 451
EryPed 447

Erythromycin Gluceptate (The concurrent use of CYP3A4 inhibitors with transdermal fentanyl may result in an increase in fentanyl plasma concentrations, which could increase or prolong adverse drug effects and may cause serious respiratory depression. In this situation, special patient care and observation are appropriate).

No products indexed under this heading.

Erythromycin Lactobionate (The concurrent use of CYP3A4 inhibitors with transdermal fentanyl may result in an increase in fentanyl plasma concentrations, which could increase or prolong adverse drug effects and may cause serious respiratory depression. In this situation, special patient care and observation are appropriate).

No products indexed under this heading.

Erythromycin Stearate (The concurrent use of CYP3A4 inhibitors with transdermal fentanyl may result in an increase in fentanyl plasma concentrations, which could increase or prolong adverse drug effects and may cause serious respiratory depression. In this situation, special patient care and observation are appropriate). Products include:

Erythrocin Stearate Filmtab
Tablets 453

Esomeprazole Magnesium (The concurrent use of CYP3A4 inhibitors with transdermal fentanyl may result in an increase in fentanyl plasma concentrations, which could increase or prolong adverse drug effects and may cause serious respiratory depression. In this situation, special patient care and observation are appropriate). Products include:

Nexium Delayed-Release
Capsules 655

Estazolam (The comcomitant use of fentanyl with other CNS depressants may cause respiratory depression, hypotension, and profound sedation or potentially result in coma. When such combined therapy is contemplated, the dose of one or both agents should be significantly reduced). Products include:

ProSom Tablets 517

Ethanol (The comcomitant use of fentanyl with other CNS depressants may cause respiratory depression, hypotension, and profound sedation or potentially result in coma. When such combined therapy is contemplated, the dose of one or both agents should be significantly reduced).

No products indexed under this heading.

Ethchlorvynol (The comcomitant use of fentanyl with other CNS depressants may cause respiratory depression, hypotension, and profound sedation or potentially result in coma. When such combined therapy is contemplated, the dose of one or both agents should be significantly reduced).

No products indexed under this heading.

Ethinamate (The comcomitant use of fentanyl with other CNS depressants may cause respiratory depression, hypotension, and profound sedation or potentially result in coma. When such combined therapy is contemplated, the dose of one or both agents should be significantly reduced).

No products indexed under this heading.

Ethosuximide (Fentanyl is metabolized mainly via the human cytochrome P450 3A4 isoenzyme system (CYP3A4). Co-administration with agents that induce CYP 3A4 activity may reduce the efficacy of fentanyl).

No products indexed under this heading.

Ethyl Alcohol (The comcomitant use of fentanyl with other CNS depressants may cause respiratory depression, hypotension, and profound sedation or potentially result in coma. When such combined therapy is contemplated, the dose of one or both agents should be significantly reduced).

No products indexed under this heading.

Felbamate (Fentanyl is metabolized mainly via the human cytochrome P450 3A4 isoenzyme system (CYP3A4). Co-administration with agents that induce CYP 3A4 activity may reduce the efficacy of fentanyl).

No products indexed under this heading.

Fentanyl Citrate (The comcomitant use of fentanyl with other CNS depressants may cause respiratory depression, hypotension, and pro-

found sedation or potentially result in coma. When such combined therapy is contemplated, the dose of one or both agents should be significantly reduced). Products include:

Actiq ... 979

Fluconazole (The concurrent use of CYP3A4 inhibitors with transdermal fentanyl may result in an increase in fentanyl plasma concentrations, which could increase or prolong adverse drug effects and may cause serious respiratory depression. In this situation, special patient care and observation are appropriate).

No products indexed under this heading.

Fludrocortisone Acetate (Fentanyl is metabolized mainly via the human cytochrome P450 3A4 isoenzyme system (CYP3A4). Co-administration with agents that induce CYP 3A4 activity may reduce the efficacy of fentanyl).

No products indexed under this heading.

Fluoxetine Hydrochloride (The concurrent use of CYP3A4 inhibitors with transdermal fentanyl may result in an increase in fentanyl plasma concentrations, which could increase or prolong adverse drug effects and may cause serious respiratory depression. In this situation, special patient care and observation are appropriate). Products include:

Prozac Pulvules and Liquid 1801
Symbyax Capsules 1819

Fluphenazine Decanoate (The comcomitant use of fentanyl with other CNS depressants may cause respiratory depression, hypotension, and profound sedation or potentially result in coma. When such combined therapy is contemplated, the dose of one or both agents should be significantly reduced).

No products indexed under this heading.

Fluphenazine Enanthate (The comcomitant use of fentanyl with other CNS depressants may cause respiratory depression, hypotension, and profound sedation or potentially result in coma. When such combined therapy is contemplated, the dose of one or both agents should be significantly reduced).

No products indexed under this heading.

Fluphenazine Hydrochloride (The comcomitant use of fentanyl with other CNS depressants may cause respiratory depression, hypotension, and profound sedation or potentially result in coma. When such combined therapy is contemplated, the dose of one or both agents should be significantly reduced).

No products indexed under this heading.

Flurazepam Hydrochloride (The comcomitant use of fentanyl with other CNS depressants may cause respiratory depression, hypotension, and profound sedation or potentially result in coma. When such combined therapy is contemplated, the dose of one or both agents should be significantly reduced). Products include:

Dalmane Capsules 3342

Fluvoxamine Maleate (The concurrent use of CYP3A4 inhibitors with transdermal fentanyl may result in an increase in fentanyl plasma concentrations, which could increase or prolong adverse drug effects and may cause serious respiratory depression. In this situation, special patient care and observation are appropriate).

No products indexed under this heading.

Fosamprenavir Calcium (The comcomitant use of fentanyl with potent cytochrome P450 3A4 inhibitors may result in an increase in fentanyl plasma concentrations, which could increase or prolong adverse drug effects and may cause potentially fatal respiratory depression. Patients receiving fentanyl and potent CYP3A4 inhibitors should be carefully monitored for an extended period of time and dosage adjustments should be made if warranted). Products include:

Lexiva Tablets 1505

Fosphenytoin Sodium (Fentanyl is metabolized mainly via the human cytochrome P450 3A4 isoenzyme system (CYP3A4). Co-administration with agents that induce CYP 3A4 activity may reduce the efficacy of fentanyl).

No products indexed under this heading.

Garlic Extract (Fentanyl is metabolized mainly via the human cytochrome P450 3A4 isoenzyme system (CYP3A4). Co-administration with agents that induce CYP 3A4 activity may reduce the efficacy of fentanyl).

No products indexed under this heading.

Garlic Oil (Fentanyl is metabolized mainly via the human cytochrome P450 3A4 isoenzyme system (CYP3A4). Co-administration with agents that induce CYP 3A4 activity may reduce the efficacy of fentanyl).

No products indexed under this heading.

Glutethimide (The comcomitant use of fentanyl with other CNS depressants may cause respiratory depression, hypotension, and profound sedation or potentially result in coma. When such combined therapy is contemplated, the dose of one or both agents should be significantly reduced).

No products indexed under this heading.

Haloperidol (The comcomitant use of fentanyl with other CNS depressants may cause respiratory depression, hypotension, and profound sedation or potentially result in coma. When such combined therapy is contemplated, the dose of one or both agents should be significantly reduced).

No products indexed under this heading.

Haloperidol Decanoate (The comcomitant use of fentanyl with other CNS depressants may cause respiratory depression, hypotension, and profound sedation or potentially result in coma. When such combined therapy is contemplated, the dose of one or both agents should be significantly reduced).

No products indexed under this heading.

Hydrocodone Bitartrate (The comcomitant use of fentanyl with other CNS depressants may cause respiratory depression, hypotension, and profound sedation or potentially result in coma. When such combined therapy is contemplated, the dose of one or both agents should be significantly reduced). Products include:

Hycodan 1116
Hycotuss Expectorant Syrup 1117
Vicodin Tablets 535
Vicodin ES Tablets 536
Vicodin HP Tablets 538
Vicoprofen Tablets 539
Zydone Tablets 1139

Hydrocodone Polistirex (The comcomitant use of fentanyl with other CNS depressants may cause respiratory depression, hypotension, and profound sedation or potentially result in coma. When such combined therapy is contemplated, the dose of one or both agents should be significantly reduced). Products include:

Tussionex Pennkinetic Extended-Release Suspension 3327

Hydrocortisone (Fentanyl is metabolized mainly via the human cytochrome P450 3A4 isoenzyme system (CYP3A4). Co-administration with agents that induce CYP 3A4 activity may reduce the efficacy of fentanyl). Products include:

Colocort Rectal Suspension, USP (Retention) 100 mg/60 mL 2476
Hydrocortone Tablets 1989
Preparation H Hydrocortisone Cream 646

Hydrocortisone Acetate (Fentanyl is metabolized mainly via the human cytochrome P450 3A4 isoenzyme system (CYP3A4). Co-administration with agents that induce CYP 3A4 activity may reduce the efficacy of fentanyl). Products include:

Analpram-HC 1159
Pramosone 1161
ProctoFoam-HC 3099

Hydrocortisone Butyrate (Fentanyl is metabolized mainly via the human cytochrome P450 3A4 isoenzyme system (CYP3A4). Co-administration with agents that induce CYP 3A4 activity may reduce the efficacy of fentanyl). Products include:

Locoid Lipocream Cream 1160

Hydrocortisone Cypionate (Fentanyl is metabolized mainly via the human cytochrome P450 3A4 isoenzyme system (CYP3A4). Co-administration with agents that induce CYP 3A4 activity may reduce the efficacy of fentanyl).

No products indexed under this heading.

Hydrocortisone Hemisuccinate (Fentanyl is metabolized mainly via the human cytochrome P450 3A4 isoenzyme system (CYP3A4). Co-administration with agents that induce CYP 3A4 activity may reduce the efficacy of fentanyl).

No products indexed under this heading.

Hydrocortisone Probutate (Fentanyl is metabolized mainly via the human cytochrome P450 3A4 isoenzyme system (CYP3A4). Co-administration with agents that induce CYP 3A4 activity may reduce the efficacy of fentanyl).

No products indexed under this heading.

Hydrocortisone Sodium Phosphate (Fentanyl is metabolized mainly via the human cytochrome P450 3A4 isoenzyme system (CYP3A4). Co-administration with agents that induce CYP 3A4 activity may reduce the efficacy of fentanyl).

No products indexed under this heading.

Hydrocortisone Sodium Succinate (Fentanyl is metabolized mainly via the human cytochrome P450 3A4 isoenzyme system (CYP3A4). Co-administration with agents that induce CYP 3A4 activity may reduce the efficacy of fentanyl).

No products indexed under this heading.

Hydrocortisone Valerate (Fentanyl is metabolized mainly via the human cytochrome P450 3A4 isoenzyme system (CYP3A4). Co-administration with agents that induce CYP 3A4 activity may reduce the efficacy of fentanyl).

No products indexed under this heading.

Hydromorphone Hydrochloride (The comcomitant use of fentanyl with other CNS depressants may cause respiratory depression, hypotension, and profound sedation or potentially result in coma. When such combined therapy is contemplated, the dose of one or both agents should be significantly reduced). Products include:

Dilaudid 440
Dilaudid Non-Sterile Powder 440
Dilaudid Oral Liquid 445
Dilaudid Rectal Suppositories 440
Dilaudid Tablets 440
Dilaudid Tablets - 8 mg 445
Dilaudid-HP 442

Hydroxyzine Hydrochloride (The comcomitant use of fentanyl with other CNS depressants may cause respiratory depression, hypotension, and profound sedation or potentially result in coma. When such combined therapy is contemplated, the dose of one or both agents should be significantly reduced).

No products indexed under this heading.

Hypericum (Fentanyl is metabolized mainly via the human cytochrome P450 3A4 isoenzyme system (CYP3A4). Co-administration with agents that induce CYP 3A4 activity may reduce the efficacy of fentanyl). Products include:

Satiete Tablets 832

Hypericum Perforatum (Fentanyl is metabolized mainly via the human cytochrome P450 3A4 isoenzyme system (CYP3A4). Co-administration with agents that induce CYP 3A4 activity may reduce the efficacy of fentanyl).

No products indexed under this heading.

Indinavir Sulfate (The concomitant use of fentanyl with potent cytochrome P450 3A4 inhibitors may result in an increase in fentanyl plasma concentrations, which could increase or prolong adverse drug effects and may cause potentially fatal respiratory depression. Patients receiving fentanyl and potent CYP3A4 inhibitors should be carefully monitored for an extended period of time and dosage adjustments should be made if warranted). Products include:

Crixivan Capsules 1940

Isocarboxazid (Fentanyl is not recommended for use in patients who have received monoamine oxidase (MAO) inhibitors within 14 days because severe and unpredictable potentiation by MAO inhibitors has been reported with opioid analgesics).

No products indexed under this heading.

Isoflurane (The comcomitant use of fentanyl with other CNS depressants may cause respiratory depression, hypotension, and profound sedation or potentially result in coma. When such combined therapy is contemplated, the dose of one or both agents should be significantly reduced).

No products indexed under this heading.

Isoniazid (The concurrent use of CYP3A4 inhibitors with transdermal fentanyl may result in an increase in fentanyl plasma concentrations, which could increase or prolong adverse drug effects and may cause serious respiratory depression. In this situation, special patient care and observation are appropriate).

No products indexed under this heading.

Itraconazole (The concomitant use of fentanyl with potent cytochrome P450 3A4 inhibitors may result in an increase in fentanyl plasma concentrations, which could increase or prolong adverse drug effects and may cause potentially fatal respiratory depression. Patients receiving fentanyl and potent CYP3A4 inhibitors should be carefully monitored for an extended period of time and dosage adjustments should be made if warranted).

No products indexed under this heading.

Ketamine Hydrochloride (The comcomitant use of fentanyl with other CNS depressants may cause respiratory depression, hypotension, and profound sedation or potentially result in coma. When such combined therapy is contemplated, the dose of one or both agents should be significantly reduced).

No products indexed under this heading.

Ketoconazole (The concomitant use of fentanyl with potent cytochrome P450 3A4 inhibitors may result in an increase in fentanyl plasma concentrations, which could increase or prolong adverse drug effects and may cause potentially fatal respiratory depression. Patients receiving fentanyl and potent CYP3A4 inhibitors should be carefully monitored for an extended period of time and dosage adjustments should be made if warranted). Products include:

Nizoral A-D Shampoo, 1% 1868

Levomethadyl Acetate Hydrochloride (The comcomitant use of fentanyl with other CNS depressants may cause respiratory depression, hypotension, and profound sedation or potentially result in coma. When such combined therapy is contemplated, the dose of one or both agents should be significantly reduced).

No products indexed under this heading.

Levorphanol Tartrate (The comcomitant use of fentanyl with other CNS depressants may cause respiratory depression, hypotension, and profound sedation or potentially result in coma. When such combined therapy is contemplated, the dose of one or both agents should be significantly reduced).

No products indexed under this heading.

Lopinavir (The concomitant use of fentanyl with potent cytochrome P450 3A4 inhibitors may result in an increase in fentanyl plasma concentrations, which could increase or prolong adverse drug effects and may cause potentially fatal respiratory depression. Patients receiving fentanyl and potent CYP3A4 inhibitors should be carefully monitored for an extended period of time and dosage adjustments should be made if warranted). Products include:

Kaletra 476

Loratadine (The concurrent use of CYP3A4 inhibitors with transdermal fentanyl may result in an increase in fentanyl plasma concentrations, which could increase or prolong adverse drug effects and may cause serious respiratory depression. In this situation, special patient care and observation are appropriate). Products include:

Alavert Allergy & Sinus D-12 Hour Tablets 771
Alavert 771
Children's Claritin Allergy Oral Solution 771
Claritin Non-Drowsy 24 Hour Tablets 772
Claritin Reditabs 24 Hour Non-Drowsy Tablets 772
Claritin-D Non-Drowsy 12 Hour Tablets 772
Claritin-D Non-Drowsy 24 Hour Tablets 772

Lorazepam (The comcomitant use of fentanyl with other CNS depressants may cause respiratory depression, hypotension, and profound sedation or potentially result in coma. When such combined therapy is contemplated, the dose of one or both agents should be significantly reduced).

No products indexed under this heading.

Loxapine Hydrochloride (The comcomitant use of fentanyl with other CNS depressants may cause respiratory depression, hypotension, and profound sedation or potentially result in coma. When such combined therapy is contemplated, the dose of one or both agents should be significantly reduced).

No products indexed under this heading.

Loxapine Succinate (The comcomitant use of fentanyl with other CNS depressants may cause respiratory depression, hypotension, and profound sedation or potentially result in coma. When such combined therapy is contemplated, the dose of one or both agents should be significantly reduced).

No products indexed under this heading.

Meperidine Hydrochloride (The comcomitant use of fentanyl with other CNS depressants may cause respiratory depression, hypotension, and profound sedation or potentially result in coma. When such combined therapy is contemplated, the dose of one or both agents should be significantly reduced).
No products indexed under this heading.

Mephenytoin (Fentanyl is metabolized mainly via the human cytochrome P450 3A4 isoenzyme system (CYP3A4). Co-administration with agents that induce CYP 3A4 activity may reduce the efficacy of fentanyl).
No products indexed under this heading.

Mephobarbital (The comcomitant use of fentanyl with other CNS depressants may cause respiratory depression, hypotension, and profound sedation or potentially result in coma. When such combined therapy is contemplated, the dose of one or both agents should be significantly reduced).
No products indexed under this heading.

Meprobamate (The comcomitant use of fentanyl with other CNS depressants may cause respiratory depression, hypotension, and profound sedation or potentially result in coma. When such combined therapy is contemplated, the dose of one or both agents should be significantly reduced).
No products indexed under this heading.

Mesoridazine Besylate (The comcomitant use of fentanyl with other CNS depressants may cause respiratory depression, hypotension, and profound sedation or potentially result in coma. When such combined therapy is contemplated, the dose of one or both agents should be significantly reduced).
No products indexed under this heading.

Metaxalone (The concomitant use of fentanyl with other CNS depressants, including skeletal muscle relaxants, may cause respiratory depression, hypotension, and profound sedation or potentially result in coma. When such combined therapy is contemplated, the dose of one or both agents should be significantly reduced). Products include:
Skelaxin Tablets **1716**

Methadone Hydrochloride (The comcomitant use of fentanyl with other CNS depressants may cause respiratory depression, hypotension, and profound sedation or potentially result in coma. When such combined therapy is contemplated, the dose of one or both agents should be significantly reduced).
No products indexed under this heading.

Methocarbamol (The concomitant use of fentanyl with other CNS depressants, including skeletal muscle relaxants, may cause respiratory depression, hypotension, and profound sedation or potentially result in coma. When such combined therapy is contemplated, the dose of one or both agents should be significantly reduced).
No products indexed under this heading.

Methohexital Sodium (The comcomitant use of fentanyl with other CNS depressants may cause respiratory depression, hypotension, and profound sedation or potentially result in coma. When such combined therapy is contemplated, the dose of one or both agents should be significantly reduced).
No products indexed under this heading.

Methotrimeprazine (The comcomitant use of fentanyl with other CNS depressants may cause respiratory depression, hypotension, and profound sedation or potentially result in coma. When such combined therapy is contemplated, the dose of one or both agents should be significantly reduced).
No products indexed under this heading.

Methoxyflurane (The comcomitant use of fentanyl with other CNS depressants may cause respiratory depression, hypotension, and profound sedation or potentially result in coma. When such combined therapy is contemplated, the dose of one or both agents should be significantly reduced).
No products indexed under this heading.

Methsuximide (Fentanyl is metabolized mainly via the human cytochrome P450 3A4 isoenzyme system (CYP3A4). Co-administration with agents that induce CYP 3A4 activity may reduce the efficacy of fentanyl).
No products indexed under this heading.

Methylprednisolone (Fentanyl is metabolized mainly via the human cytochrome P450 3A4 isoenzyme system (CYP3A4). Co-administration with agents that induce CYP 3A4 activity may reduce the efficacy of fentanyl).
No products indexed under this heading.

Methylprednisolone Acetate (Fentanyl is metabolized mainly via the human cytochrome P450 3A4 isoenzyme system (CYP3A4). Co-administration with agents that induce CYP 3A4 activity may reduce the efficacy of fentanyl). Products include:
Depo-Medrol Injectable Suspension **2617**
Depo-Medrol Single-Dose Vial **2619**

Methylprednisolone Sodium Succinate (Fentanyl is metabolized mainly via the human cytochrome P450 3A4 isoenzyme system (CYP3A4). Co-administration with agents that induce CYP 3A4 activity may reduce the efficacy of fentanyl).
No products indexed under this heading.

Metronidazole (The concurrent use of CYP3A4 inhibitors with transdermal fentanyl may result in an increase in fentanyl plasma concentrations, which could increase or prolong adverse drug effects and may cause serious respiratory depression. In this situation, special patient care and observation are appropriate). Products include:
Metrogel 1% **1211**
MetroGel-Vaginal Gel **1855**
Vandazole Vaginal Gel **3338**

Metronidazole Benzoate (The concurrent use of CYP3A4 inhibitors with transdermal fentanyl may result in an increase in fentanyl plasma concentrations, which could increase or prolong adverse drug effects and may cause serious respiratory depression. In this situation, special patient care and observation are appropriate).
No products indexed under this heading.

Metronidazole Hydrochloride (The concurrent use of CYP3A4 inhibitors with transdermal fentanyl may result in an increase in fentanyl plasma concentrations, which could increase or prolong adverse drug effects and may cause serious respiratory depression. In this situation, special patient care and observation are appropriate).
No products indexed under this heading.

Miconazole (The concurrent use of CYP3A4 inhibitors with transdermal fentanyl may result in an increase in fentanyl plasma concentrations, which could increase or prolong adverse drug effects and may cause serious respiratory depression. In this situation, special patient care and observation are appropriate).
No products indexed under this heading.

Miconazole Nitrate (The concurrent use of CYP3A4 inhibitors with transdermal fentanyl may result in an increase in fentanyl plasma concentrations, which could increase or prolong adverse drug effects and may cause serious respiratory depression. In this situation, special patient care and observation are appropriate). Products include:
Desenex .... ▣**635**
Desenex Jock Itch Spray Powder ... ▣**635**

Midazolam Hydrochloride (The comcomitant use of fentanyl with other CNS depressants may cause respiratory depression, hypotension, and profound sedation or potentially result in coma. When such combined therapy is contemplated, the dose of one or both agents should be significantly reduced).
No products indexed under this heading.

Moclobemide (Fentanyl is not recommended for use in patients who have received monoamine oxidase (MAO) inhibitors within 14 days because severe and unpredictable potentiation by MAO inhibitors has been reported with opioid analgesics).
No products indexed under this heading.

Modafinil (Fentanyl is metabolized mainly via the human cytochrome P450 3A4 isoenzyme system (CYP3A4). Co-administration with agents that induce CYP 3A4 activity may reduce the efficacy of fentanyl). Products include:
Provigil Tablets **988**

Molindone Hydrochloride (The comcomitant use of fentanyl with other CNS depressants may cause respiratory depression, hypotension, and profound sedation or potentially result in coma. When such combined therapy is contemplated, the dose of one or both agents should be significantly reduced). Products include:
Moban Tablets **1119**

Morphine Sulfate (The comcomitant use of fentanyl with other CNS depressants may cause respiratory depression, hypotension, and profound sedation or potentially result in coma. When such combined therapy is contemplated, the dose of one or both agents should be significantly reduced). Products include:
Avinza Capsules **1741**
Kadian Capsules **577**
MS Contin Tablets **2701**

Nefazodone Hydrochloride (The concomitant use of fentanyl with potent cytochrome P450 3A4 inhibitors may result in an increase in fentanyl plasma concentrations, which could increase or prolong adverse drug effects and may cause potentially fatal respiratory depression. Patients receiving fentanyl and potent CYP3A4 inhibitors should be carefully monitored for an extended period of time and dosage adjustments should be made if warranted).
No products indexed under this heading.

Nelfinavir Mesylate (The concomitant use of fentanyl with potent cytochrome P450 3A4 inhibitors may result in an increase in fentanyl plasma concentrations, which could increase or prolong adverse drug effects and may cause potentially fatal respiratory depression. Patients receiving fentanyl and potent CYP3A4 inhibitors should be carefully monitored for an extended period of time and dosage adjustments should be made if warranted). Products include:
Viracept **2577**

Nevirapine (The concurrent use of CYP3A4 inhibitors with transdermal fentanyl may result in an increase in fentanyl plasma concentrations, which could increase or prolong adverse drug effects and may cause serious respiratory depression. In this situation, special patient care and observation are appropriate). Products include:
Viramune Oral Suspension **873**
Viramune Tablets **873**

Niacinamide (The concurrent use of CYP3A4 inhibitors with transdermal fentanyl may result in an increase in fentanyl plasma concentrations, which could increase or prolong adverse drug effects and may cause serious respiratory depression. In this situation, special patient care and observation are appropriate).
No products indexed under this heading.

Nicotinamide (The concurrent use of CYP3A4 inhibitors with transdermal fentanyl may result in an increase in fentanyl plasma concentrations, which could increase or prolong adverse drug effects and may cause serious respiratory depression. In this situation, special patient care and observation are appropriate). Products include:
Nicomide Tablets **1088**

Nifedipine (The concurrent use of CYP3A4 inhibitors with transdermal fentanyl may result in an increase in fentanyl plasma concentrations, which could increase or prolong adverse drug effects and may cause serious respiratory depression. In this situation, special patient care and observation are appropriate). Products include:
Adalat CC Tablets **2964**

Norfloxacin (The concurrent use of CYP3A4 inhibitors with transdermal fentanyl may result in an increase in fentanyl plasma concentrations, which could increase or prolong adverse drug effects and may cause serious respiratory depression. In this situation, special patient care and observation are appropriate). Products include:
Noroxin Tablets **2032**

Olanzapine (The comcomitant use of fentanyl with other CNS depressants may cause respiratory depression, hypotension, and profound sedation or potentially result in coma. When such combined therapy is contemplated, the dose of one or both agents should be significantly reduced). Products include:
Symbyax Capsules **1819**
Zyprexa Tablets **1830**
Zyprexa IntraMuscular **1830**
Zyprexa ZYDIS Orally Disintegrating Tablets **1830**

Omeprazole (The concurrent use of CYP3A4 inhibitors with transdermal fentanyl may result in an increase in fentanyl plasma concentrations, which could increase or prolong adverse drug effects and may cause serious respiratory depression. In this situation, special patient care and observation are appropriate). Products include:
Zegerid Capsules **2958**
Zegerid Powder for Oral Solution **2958**

Orphenadrine Citrate (The concomitant use of fentanyl with other CNS depressants, including skeletal muscle relaxants, may cause respiratory depression, hypotension, and profound sedation or potentially result in coma. When such combined therapy is contemplated, the dose of one or both agents should be significantly reduced). Products include:
Norflex Injection **1856**

Oxazepam (The comcomitant use of fentanyl with other CNS depressants may cause respiratory depression, hypotension, and profound sedation or potentially result in coma. When such combined therapy is contemplated, the dose of one or both agents should be significantly reduced).
No products indexed under this heading.

Oxcarbazepine (Fentanyl is metabolized mainly via the human cytochrome P450 3A4 isoenzyme system (CYP3A4). Co-administration with agents that induce CYP 3A4 activity may reduce the efficacy of fentanyl). Products include:
Trileptal Tablets **2300**
Trileptal Oral Suspension **2300**

Oxycodone Hydrochloride (The comcomitant use of fentanyl with other CNS depressants may cause respiratory depression, hypotension, and profound sedation or potentially result in coma. When such combined therapy is contemplated, the dose of one or both agents should be significantly reduced). Products include:
OxyContin Tablets **2703**
OxyFast Oral Concentrate Solution **2708**
OxyIR Capsules **2708**
Percocet Tablets **1131**
Percodan Tablets **1132**

Pargyline Hydrochloride (Fentanyl is not recommended for use in patients who have received monoamine oxidase (MAO) inhibitors within 14 days because severe and unpredictable potentiation by MAO inhibitors has been reported with opioid analgesics).
No products indexed under this heading.

Paroxetine Hydrochloride (The concurrent use of CYP3A4 inhibitors with transdermal fentanyl may result in an increase in fentanyl plasma concentrations, which could increase or prolong adverse drug effects and may cause serious respiratory depression. In this situation, special patient care and observation are appropriate). Products include:
Paxil CR Controlled-Release Tablets **1538**
Paxil **1530**

Pentobarbital Sodium (The comcomitant use of fentanyl with other CNS depressants may cause respiratory depression, hypotension, and profound sedation or potentially result in coma. When such combined therapy is contemplated, the dose of one or both agents should be significantly reduced). Products include:
Nembutal Sodium Solution, USP **2470**

Perphenazine (The comcomitant use of fentanyl with other CNS depressants may cause respiratory depression, hypotension, and profound sedation or potentially result in coma. When such combined therapy is contemplated, the dose of one or both agents should be significantly reduced).
No products indexed under this heading.

Phenelzine Sulfate (Fentanyl is not recommended for use in patients who have received monoamine oxidase (MAO) inhibitors within 14 days because severe and unpredictable potentiation by MAO inhibitors has been reported with opioid analgesics).
No products indexed under this heading.

Phenobarbital (The comcomitant use of fentanyl with other CNS depressants may cause respiratory depression, hypotension, and profound sedation or potentially result in coma. When such combined therapy is contemplated, the dose of one or both agents should be significantly reduced). Products include:
Donnatal Extentabs **2493**

Phenobarbital Sodium (Fentanyl is metabolized mainly via the human cytochrome P450 3A4 isoenzyme system (CYP3A4). Co-administration with agents that induce CYP 3A4 activity may reduce the efficacy of fentanyl).
No products indexed under this heading.

Phenytoin (Fentanyl is metabolized mainly via the human cytochrome P450 3A4 isoenzyme system (CYP3A4). Co-administration with agents that induce CYP 3A4 activity may reduce the efficacy of fentanyl).
No products indexed under this heading.

Phenytoin Sodium (Fentanyl is metabolized mainly via the human cytochrome P450 3A4 isoenzyme system (CYP3A4). Co-administration with agents that induce CYP 3A4 activity may reduce the efficacy of fentanyl). Products include:
Phenytek Capsules **2160**

Prazepam (The comcomitant use of fentanyl with other CNS depressants may cause respiratory depression, hypotension, and profound sedation or potentially result in coma. When such combined therapy is contemplated, the dose of one or both agents should be significantly reduced).
No products indexed under this heading.

Prednisolone Acetate (Fentanyl is metabolized mainly via the human cytochrome P450 3A4 isoenzyme system (CYP3A4). Co-administration with agents that induce CYP 3A4 activity may reduce the efficacy of fentanyl). Products include:
Blephamide Ophthalmic Ointment **568**
Blephamide Ophthalmic Suspension **569**
Poly-Pred Ophthalmic Suspension .... ⊙**233**
Pred Forte Ophthalmic Suspension .... ⊙**235**
Pred Mild Ophthalmic Suspension .... ⊙**238**
Pred-G Ophthalmic Ointment .... ⊙**237**
Pred-G Ophthalmic Suspension ...... ⊙**236**

Prednisolone Sodium Phosphate (Fentanyl is metabolized mainly via the human cytochrome P450 3A4 isoenzyme system (CYP3A4). Co-administration with agents that induce CYP 3A4 activity may reduce the efficacy of fentanyl).
No products indexed under this heading.

Prednisolone Tebutate (Fentanyl is metabolized mainly via the human cytochrome P450 3A4 isoenzyme system (CYP3A4). Co-administration with agents that induce CYP 3A4 activity may reduce the efficacy of fentanyl).
No products indexed under this heading.

Prednisone (Fentanyl is metabolized mainly via the human cytochrome P450 3A4 isoenzyme system (CYP3A4). Co-administration with agents that induce CYP 3A4 activity may reduce the efficacy of fentanyl).
No products indexed under this heading.

Primidone (Fentanyl is metabolized mainly via the human cytochrome P450 3A4 isoenzyme system (CYP3A4). Co-administration with agents that induce CYP 3A4 activity may reduce the efficacy of fentanyl).
No products indexed under this heading.

Procarbazine Hydrochloride (Fentanyl is not recommended for use in patients who have received monoamine oxidase (MAO) inhibitors within 14 days because severe and unpredictable potentiation by MAO inhibitors has been reported with opioid analgesics). Products include:
Matulane Capsules **3191**

Prochlorperazine (The comcomitant use of fentanyl with other CNS depressants may cause respiratory depression, hypotension, and profound sedation or potentially result in coma. When such combined therapy is contemplated, the dose of one or both agents should be significantly reduced).
No products indexed under this heading.

Promethazine Hydrochloride (The comcomitant use of fentanyl with other CNS depressants may cause respiratory depression, hypotension, and profound sedation or potentially result in coma. When such combined therapy is contemplated, the dose of one or both agents should be significantly reduced). Products include:
Phenergan Tablets and Suppositories **3440**

Propofol (The comcomitant use of fentanyl with other CNS depressants may cause respiratory depression, hypotension, and profound sedation or potentially result in coma. When such combined therapy is contemplated, the dose of one or both agents should be significantly reduced).
No products indexed under this heading.

Propoxyphene Hydrochloride (The comcomitant use of fentanyl with other CNS depressants may cause respiratory depression, hypotension, and profound sedation or potentially result in coma. When such combined therapy is contemplated, the dose of one or both agents should be significantly reduced).
No products indexed under this heading.

Propoxyphene Napsylate (The comcomitant use of fentanyl with other CNS depressants may cause respiratory depression, hypotension, and profound sedation or potentially result in coma. When such combined therapy is contemplated, the dose of one or both agents should be significantly reduced).
No products indexed under this heading.

Quazepam (The comcomitant use of fentanyl with other CNS depressants may cause respiratory depression, hypotension, and profound sedation or potentially result in coma. When such combined therapy is contemplated, the dose of one or both agents should be significantly reduced).
No products indexed under this heading.

Quetiapine Fumarate (The comcomitant use of fentanyl with other CNS depressants may cause respiratory depression, hypotension, and profound sedation or potentially result in coma. When such combined therapy is contemplated, the dose of one or both agents should be significantly reduced). Products include:
Seroquel Tablets **690**

Quinidine (The concurrent use of CYP3A4 inhibitors with transdermal fentanyl may result in an increase in fentanyl plasma concentrations, which could increase or prolong adverse drug effects and may cause serious respiratory depression. In this situation, special patient care and observation are appropriate).
No products indexed under this heading.

Quinidine Hydrochloride (The concurrent use of CYP3A4 inhibitors with transdermal fentanyl may result in an increase in fentanyl plasma concentrations, which could increase or prolong adverse drug effects and may cause serious respiratory depression. In this situation, special patient care and observation are appropriate).
No products indexed under this heading.

Quinidine Polygalacturonate (The concurrent use of CYP3A4 inhibitors with transdermal fentanyl may result in an increase in fentanyl plasma concentrations, which could increase or prolong adverse drug effects and may cause serious respiratory depression. In this situation, special patient care and observation are appropriate).

No products indexed under this heading.

Quinidine Sulfate (The concurrent use of CYP3A4 inhibitors with transdermal fentanyl may result in an increase in fentanyl plasma concentrations, which could increase or prolong adverse drug effects and may cause serious respiratory depression. In this situation, special patient care and observation are appropriate).

No products indexed under this heading.

Quinine (The concurrent use of CYP3A4 inhibitors with transdermal fentanyl may result in an increase in fentanyl plasma concentrations, which could increase or prolong adverse drug effects and may cause serious respiratory depression. In this situation, special patient care and observation are appropriate).

No products indexed under this heading.

Quinine Sulfate (The concurrent use of CYP3A4 inhibitors with transdermal fentanyl may result in an increase in fentanyl plasma concentrations, which could increase or prolong adverse drug effects and may cause serious respiratory depression. In this situation, special patient care and observation are appropriate).

No products indexed under this heading.

Quinupristin (The concurrent use of CYP3A4 inhibitors with transdermal fentanyl may result in an increase in fentanyl plasma concentrations, which could increase or prolong adverse drug effects and may cause serious respiratory depression. In this situation, special patient care and observation are appropriate).

No products indexed under this heading.

Ramelteon (The concomitant use of fentanyl with other CNS depressants, including sedatives and hypnotics, may cause respiratory depression, hypotension, and profound sedation or potentially result in coma. When such combined therapy is contemplated, the dose of oneor both agents should be significantly reduced). Products include:

Rozerem Tablets 3231

Ranitidine Bismuth Citrate (The concurrent use of CYP3A4 inhibitors with transdermal fentanyl may result in an increase in fentanyl plasma concentrations, which could increase or prolong adverse drug effects and may cause serious respiratory depression. In this situation, special patient care and observation are appropriate).

No products indexed under this heading.

Ranitidine Hydrochloride (The concurrent use of CYP3A4 inhibitors with transdermal fentanyl may result in an increase in fentanyl plasma concentrations, which could increase or prolong adverse drug effects and may cause serious respiratory depression. In this situation, special patient care and observation are appropriate). Products include:

Zantac 1624
Zantac Injection 1619
Zantac Injection Pharmacy Bulk Package 1622

Remifentanil Hydrochloride (The comcomitant use of fentanyl with other CNS depressants may cause respiratory depression, hypotension, and profound sedation or potentially result in coma. When such combined therapy is contemplated, the dose of one or both agents should be significantly reduced).

No products indexed under this heading.

Rifabutin (Fentanyl is metabolized mainly via the human cytochrome P450 3A4 isoenzyme system (CYP3A4). Co-administration with agents that induce CYP 3A4 activity may reduce the efficacy of fentanyl).

No products indexed under this heading.

Rifampicin (Fentanyl is metabolized mainly via the human cytochrome P450 3A4 isoenzyme system (CYP3A4). Co-administration with agents that induce CYP 3A4 activity may reduce the efficacy of fentanyl).

No products indexed under this heading.

Rifampin (Fentanyl is metabolized mainly via the human cytochrome P450 3A4 isoenzyme system (CYP3A4). Co-administration with agents that induce CYP 3A4 activity may reduce the efficacy of fentanyl).

No products indexed under this heading.

Rifapentine (Fentanyl is metabolized mainly via the human cytochrome P450 3A4 isoenzyme system (CYP3A4). Co-administration with agents that induce CYP 3A4 activity may reduce the efficacy of fentanyl).

No products indexed under this heading.

Risperidone (The comcomitant use of fentanyl with other CNS depressants may cause respiratory depression, hypotension, and profound sedation or potentially result in coma. When such combined therapy is contemplated, the dose of one or both agents should be significantly reduced). Products include:

Risperdal 1676
Risperdal Consta Long-Acting Injection 1682
Risperdal M-Tab Orally Disintegrating Tablets 1676

Ritonavir (The concomitant use of fentanyl with potent cytochrome P450 3A4 inhibitors may result in an increase in fentanyl plasma concentrations, which could increase or prolong adverse drug effects and may cause potentially fatal respiratory depression. Patients receiving fentanyl and potent CYP3A4 inhibitors should be carefully monitored for an extended period of time and dosage adjustments should be made if warranted). Products include:

Kaletra 476
Norvir 503

Saquinavir (The concomitant use of fentanyl with potent cytochrome P450 3A4 inhibitors may result in an increase in fentanyl plasma concentrations, which could increase or prolong adverse drug effects and may cause potentially fatal respiratory depression. Patients receiving fentanyl and potent CYP3A4 inhibitors should be carefully monitored for an extended period of time and dosage adjustments should be made if warranted).

No products indexed under this heading.

Saquinavir Mesylate (The concomitant use of fentanyl with potent cytochrome P450 3A4 inhibitors may result in an increase in fentanyl plasma concentrations, which could increase or prolong adverse drug effects and may cause potentially fatal respiratory depression. Patients receiving fentanyl and potent CYP3A4 inhibitors should be carefully monitored for an extended period of time and dosage adjustments should be made if warranted). Products include:

Invirase 2772

Secobarbital Sodium (The comcomitant use of fentanyl with other CNS depressants may cause respiratory depression, hypotension, and profound sedation or potentially result in coma. When such combined therapy is contemplated, the dose of one or both agents should be significantly reduced).

No products indexed under this heading.

Selegiline Hydrochloride (Fentanyl is not recommended for use in patients who have received monoamine oxidase (MAO) inhibitors within 14 days because severe and unpredictable potentiation by MAO inhibitors has been reported with opioid analgesics). Products include:

Eldepryl Capsules 3208
Zelapar Tablets 3372

Sertraline Hydrochloride (The concurrent use of CYP3A4 inhibitors with transdermal fentanyl may result in an increase in fentanyl plasma concentrations, which could increase or prolong adverse drug effects and may cause serious respiratory depression. In this situation, special patient care and observation are appropriate). Products include:

Zoloft 2586

Sevoflurane (The comcomitant use of fentanyl with other CNS depressants may cause respiratory depression, hypotension, and profound sedation or potentially result in coma. When such combined therapy is contemplated, the dose of one or both agents should be significantly reduced). Products include:

Ultane Liquid for Inhalation 531

Sodium Oxybate (The comcomitant use of fentanyl with other CNS depressants may cause respiratory depression, hypotension, and profound sedation or potentially result in coma. When such combined therapy is contemplated, the dose of one or both agents should be significantly reduced). Products include:

Xyrem Oral Solution 1688

Sufentanil Citrate (The comcomitant use of fentanyl with other CNS depressants may cause respiratory depression, hypotension, and profound sedation or potentially result in coma. When such combined therapy is contemplated, the dose of one or both agents should be significantly reduced).

No products indexed under this heading.

Sulfinpyrazone (Fentanyl is metabolized mainly via the human cytochrome P450 3A4 isoenzyme system (CYP3A4). Co-administration with agents that induce CYP 3A4 activity may reduce the efficacy of fentanyl).

No products indexed under this heading.

Telithromycin (The concomitant use of fentanyl with potent cytochrome P450 3A4 inhibitors may result in an increase in fentanyl plasma concentrations, which could increase or prolong adverse drug effects and may cause potentially fatal respiratory depression. Patients receiving fentanyl and potent CYP3A4 inhibitors should be carefully monitored for an extended period of time and dosage adjustments should be made if warranted). Products include:

Ketek Tablets 2903

Temazepam (The comcomitant use of fentanyl with other CNS depressants may cause respiratory depression, hypotension, and profound sedation or potentially result in coma. When such combined therapy is contemplated, the dose of one or both agents should be significantly reduced). Products include:

Restoril Capsules 1860

Theophylline (Fentanyl is metabolized mainly via the human cytochrome P450 3A4 isoenzyme system (CYP3A4). Co-administration with agents that induce CYP 3A4 activity may reduce the efficacy of fentanyl).

No products indexed under this heading.

Thiamylal Sodium (The comcomitant use of fentanyl with other CNS depressants may cause respiratory depression, hypotension, and profound sedation or potentially result in coma. When such combined therapy is contemplated, the dose of one or both agents should be significantly reduced).

No products indexed under this heading.

Thioridazine Hydrochloride (The comcomitant use of fentanyl with other CNS depressants may cause respiratory depression, hypotension, and profound sedation or potentially result in coma. When such combined therapy is contemplated, the dose of one or both agents should be significantly reduced). Products include:

Thioridazine Hydrochloride Tablets 2163

Thiothixene (The comcomitant use of fentanyl with other CNS depressants may cause respiratory depression, hypotension, and profound sedation or potentially result in coma. When such combined therapy is contemplated, the dose of one or both agents should be significantly reduced). Products include:

Thiothixene Capsules 2165

Tranylcypromine Sulfate (Fentanyl is not recommended for use in patients who have received monoamine oxidase (MAO) inhibitors within 14 days because severe and unpredictable potentiation by MAO inhibitors has been reported with opioid analgesics). Products include:

Parnate Tablets 1527

Triamcinolone (Fentanyl is metabolized mainly via the human cytochrome P450 3A4 isoenzyme system (CYP3A4). Co-administration with agents that induce CYP 3A4 activity may reduce the efficacy of fentanyl).
No products indexed under this heading.

Triamcinolone Acetonide (Fentanyl is metabolized mainly via the human cytochrome P450 3A4 isoenzyme system (CYP3A4). Co-administration with agents that induce CYP 3A4 activity may reduce the efficacy of fentanyl). Products include:
Azmacort Inhalation Aerosol **1726**
Nasacort AQ Nasal Spray **2922**

Triamcinolone Diacetate (Fentanyl is metabolized mainly via the human cytochrome P450 3A4 isoenzyme system (CYP3A4). Co-administration with agents that induce CYP 3A4 activity may reduce the efficacy of fentanyl).
No products indexed under this heading.

Triamcinolone Hexacetonide (Fentanyl is metabolized mainly via the human cytochrome P450 3A4 isoenzyme system (CYP3A4). Co-administration with agents that induce CYP 3A4 activity may reduce the efficacy of fentanyl).
No products indexed under this heading.

Triazolam (The comcomitant use of fentanyl with other CNS depressants may cause respiratory depression, hypotension, and profound sedation or potentially result in coma. When such combined therapy is contemplated, the dose of one or both agents should be significantly reduced).
No products indexed under this heading.

Trifluoperazine Hydrochloride (The comcomitant use of fentanyl with other CNS depressants may cause respiratory depression, hypotension, and profound sedation or potentially result in coma. When such combined therapy is contemplated, the dose of one or both agents should be significantly reduced).
No products indexed under this heading.

Troglitazone (The concurrent use of CYP3A4 inhibitors with transdermal fentanyl may result in an increase in fentanyl plasma concentrations, which could increase or prolong adverse drug effects and may cause serious respiratory depression. In this situation, special patient care and observation are appropriate).
No products indexed under this heading.

Troleandomycin (The concomitant use of fentanyl with potent cytochrome P450 3A4 inhibitors may result in an increase in fentanyl plasma concentrations, which could increase or prolong adverse drug effects and may cause potentially fatal respiratory depression. Patients receiving fentanyl and potent CYP3A4 inhibitors should be carefully monitored for an extended period of time and dosage adjustments should be made if warranted).
No products indexed under this heading.

Valproate Sodium (The concurrent use of CYP3A4 inhibitors with transdermal fentanyl may result in an increase in fentanyl plasma concentrations, which could increase or prolong adverse drug effects and may cause serious respiratory depression. In this situation, special patient care and observation are appropriate). Products include:
Depacon Injection **412**

Verapamil Hydrochloride (The concurrent use of CYP3A4 inhibitors with transdermal fentanyl may result in an increase in fentanyl plasma concentrations, which could increase or prolong adverse drug effects and may cause serious respiratory depression. In this situation, special patient care and observation are appropriate). Products include:
Covera-HS Tablets **3139**
Tarka Tablets **524**
Verelan PM Extended-Release Capsules, Controlled-Onset........... **3106**

Voriconazole (The concomitant use of fentanyl with potent cytochrome P450 3A4 inhibitors may result in an increase in fentanyl plasma concentrations, which could increase or prolong adverse drug effects and may cause potentially fatal respiratory depression. Patients receiving fentanyl and potent CYP3A4 inhibitors should be carefully monitored for an extended period of time and dosage adjustments should be made if warranted). Products include:
VFEND I.V. **2564**
VFEND Oral Suspension **2564**
VFEND Tablets **2564**

Zafirlukast (The concurrent use of CYP3A4 inhibitors with transdermal fentanyl may result in an increase in fentanyl plasma concentrations, which could increase or prolong adverse drug effects and may cause serious respiratory depression. In this situation, special patient care and observation are appropriate). Products include:
Accolate Tablets **671**

Zaleplon (The comcomitant use of fentanyl with other CNS depressants may cause respiratory depression, hypotension, and profound sedation or potentially result in coma. When such combined therapy is contemplated, the dose of one or both agents should be significantly reduced). Products include:
Sonata Capsules **1717**

Zileuton (The concurrent use of CYP3A4 inhibitors with transdermal fentanyl may result in an increase in fentanyl plasma concentrations, which could increase or prolong adverse drug effects and may cause serious respiratory depression. In this situation, special patient care and observation are appropriate). Products include:
Zyflo Tablets **1023**

Ziprasidone Hydrochloride (The comcomitant use of fentanyl with other CNS depressants may cause respiratory depression, hypotension, and profound sedation or potentially result in coma. When such combined therapy is contemplated, the dose of one or both agents should be significantly reduced). Products include:
Geodon Capsules **2529**

Zolpidem Tartrate (The comcomitant use of fentanyl with other CNS depressants may cause respiratory depression, hypotension, and profound sedation or potentially result in coma. When such combined therapy is contemplated, the dose of one or both agents should be significantly reduced). Products include:
Ambien Tablets **2851**
Ambien CR Tablets **2855**

Food Interactions

Alcohol (The concomitant use of fentanyl with other CNS depressants, including alcohol, may cause respiratory depression, hypotension, and profound sedation or potentially result in coma. When such combined therapy is contemplated, the dose of one or both agents should be significantly reduced).

Grapefruit (The concurrent use of CYP3A4 inhibitors with transdermal fentanyl may result in an increase in fentanyl plasma concentrations, which could increase or prolong adverse drug effects and may cause serious respiratory depression. In this situation, special patient care and observation are appropriate).

Grapefruit Juice (The concurrent use of CYP3A4 inhibitors with transdermal fentanyl may result in an increase in fentanyl plasma concentrations, which could increase or prolong adverse drug effects and may cause serious respiratory depression. In this situation, special patient care and observation are appropriate).

DYAZIDE CAPSULES

(Hydrochlorothiazide, Triamterene) **1423**
May interact with ACE inhibitors, antihypertensives, corticosteroids, oral anticoagulants, antigout agents, oral hypoglycemic agents, insulin, lithium preparations, nondepolarizing neuromuscular blocking agents, nonsteroidal anti-inflammatory agents, potassium preparations, potassium sparing diuretics, and certain other agents. Compounds in these categories include:

Acarbose (Increased risk of severe hyponatremia). Products include:
Precose Tablets **751**

Acebutolol Hydrochloride (May add to potentiate the action of other hypertensives).
No products indexed under this heading.

ACTH (May intensify electrolyte imbalance, particularly hypokalemia).
No products indexed under this heading.

Allopurinol (Dyazide may raise the level of blood uric acid; may require dosage adjustment of antigout agent).
No products indexed under this heading.

Amiloride Hydrochloride (Concurrent use is contraindicated). Products include:
Midamor Tablets **2026**
Moduretic Tablets **2028**

Amlodipine Besylate (May add to potentiate the action of other hypertensives). Products include:
Caduet Tablets **2508**
Lotrel Capsules **2249**
Norvasc Tablets **2545**

Amphotericin B (May intensify electrolyte imbalance, particularly hypokalemia).
No products indexed under this heading.

Anisindione (Effects of oral anticoagulants may be decreased). Products include:
Miradon Tablets **3042**

Atenolol (May add to potentiate the action of other hypertensives).
No products indexed under this heading.

Atracurium Besylate (Increased paralyzing effect).
No products indexed under this heading.

Benazepril Hydrochloride (May add to potentiate the action of other hypertensives; increased risk of hyperkalemia). Products include:
Lotensin Tablets **2243**
Lotensin HCT Tablets **2246**
Lotrel Capsules **2249**

Bendroflumethiazide (May add to potentiate the action of other hypertensives).
No products indexed under this heading.

Betamethasone Acetate (May intensify electrolyte imbalance, particularly hypokalemia).
No products indexed under this heading.

Betamethasone Sodium Phosphate (May intensify electrolyte imbalance, particularly hypokalemia).
No products indexed under this heading.

Betaxolol Hydrochloride (May add to potentiate the action of other hypertensives). Products include:
Betoptic S Ophthalmic Suspension.................................. **558**

Bisoprolol Fumarate (May add to potentiate the action of other hypertensives).
No products indexed under this heading.

Blood, whole (Concurrent use of whole blood from blood bank with triamterene may result in hyperkalemia, especially in patients with renal insufficiency).
No products indexed under this heading.

Candesartan Cilexetil (May add to potentiate the action of other hypertensives). Products include:
Atacand Tablets **649**
Atacand HCT **651**

Captopril (May add to potentiate the action of other hypertensives; increased risk of hyperkalemia). Products include:
Captopril Tablets **2149**

Carteolol Hydrochloride (May add to potentiate the action of other hypertensives). Products include:
Carteolol Hydrochloride Ophthalmic Solution USP, 1%....... ⊙**249**

Celecoxib (Potential for acute renal failure). Products include:
Celebrex Capsules **3134**

Chlorothiazide (May add to potentiate the action of other hypertensives). Products include:
Diuril Oral Suspension **1954**

Chlorothiazide Sodium (May add to potentiate the action of other hypertensives). Products include:
Diuril Sodium Intravenous **2467**

Chlorpropamide (Increased risk of severe hyponatremia).
No products indexed under this heading.

Chlorthalidone (May add to potentiate the action of other hypertensives). Products include:
Clorpres Tablets **2153**

Cisatracurium Besylate (Increased paralyzing effect). Products include:
Nimbex Injection **498**

Clonidine (May add to potentiate the action of other hypertensives). Products include:
Catapres-TTS ... 844

Clonidine Hydrochloride (May add to potentiate the action of other hypertensives). Products include:
Catapres Tablets ... 843
Clorpres Tablets ... 2153

Cortisone Acetate (May intensify electrolyte imbalance, particularly hypokalemia).
No products indexed under this heading.

Deserpidine (May add to potentiate the action of other hypertensives).
No products indexed under this heading.

Dexamethasone (May intensify electrolyte imbalance, particularly hypokalemia). Products include:
Ciprodex Otic Suspension ... 559
Decadron Tablets ... 1951
TobraDex Ophthalmic Ointment ... 562
TobraDex Ophthalmic Suspension ... 563

Dexamethasone Acetate (May intensify electrolyte imbalance, particularly hypokalemia).
No products indexed under this heading.

Dexamethasone Sodium Phosphate (May intensify electrolyte imbalance, particularly hypokalemia).
No products indexed under this heading.

Diazoxide (May add to potentiate the action of other hypertensives). Products include:
Hyperstat I.V. ... 3017

Diclofenac Potassium (Potential for acute renal failure).
No products indexed under this heading.

Diclofenac Sodium (Potential for acute renal failure). Products include:
Arthrotec Tablets ... 3129
Voltaren Ophthalmic Solution ... 2309
Voltaren Tablets ... 2307
Voltaren-XR Tablets ... 2310

Dicumarol (Effects of oral anticoagulants may be decreased).
No products indexed under this heading.

Diltiazem Hydrochloride (May add to potentiate the action of other hypertensives). Products include:
Cardizem LA Extended Release Tablets ... 1728
Tiazac Capsules ... 1201

Doxazosin Mesylate (May add to potentiate the action of other hypertensives). Products include:
Cardura XL Tablets ... 2515

Enalapril Maleate (May add to potentiate the action of other hypertensives; increased risk of hyperkalemia). Products include:
Vasotec I.V. Injection ... 2103

Enalaprilat (May add to potentiate the action of other hypertensives; increased risk of hyperkalemia).
No products indexed under this heading.

Eprosartan Mesylate (May add to potentiate the action of other hypertensives). Products include:
Teveten Tablets ... 1735
Teveten HCT Tablets ... 1737

Esmolol Hydrochloride (May add to potentiate the action of other hypertensives).
No products indexed under this heading.

Etodolac (Potential for acute renal failure).
No products indexed under this heading.

Felodipine (May add to potentiate the action of other hypertensives).
No products indexed under this heading.

Fenoprofen Calcium (Potential for acute renal failure). Products include:
Nalfon Capsules ... 2502

Fludrocortisone Acetate (May intensify electrolyte imbalance, particularly hypokalemia).
No products indexed under this heading.

Flurbiprofen (Potential for acute renal failure).
No products indexed under this heading.

Fosinopril Sodium (May add to potentiate the action of other hypertensives; increased risk of hyperkalemia).
No products indexed under this heading.

Furosemide (May add to potentiate the action of other hypertensives). Products include:
Furosemide Tablets ... 2154

Glimepiride (Thiazides may cause hyperglycemia and glycosuria; dosage alteration of oral antidiabetic agents may be required). Products include:
Avandaryl Tablets ... 1379
Duetact Tablets ... 3226

Glipizide (Thiazides may cause hyperglycemia and glycosuria; dosage alteration of oral antidiabetic agents may be required).
No products indexed under this heading.

Glyburide (Thiazides may cause hyperglycemia and glycosuria; dosage alteration of oral antidiabetic agents may be required).
No products indexed under this heading.

Guanabenz Acetate (May add to potentiate the action of other hypertensives).
No products indexed under this heading.

Guanethidine Monosulfate (May add to potentiate the action of other hypertensives).
No products indexed under this heading.

Hydralazine Hydrochloride (May add to potentiate the action of other hypertensives). Products include:
BiDil Tablets ... 2171

Hydrocortisone (May intensify electrolyte imbalance, particularly hypokalemia). Products include:
Colocort Rectal Suspension, USP (Retention) 100 mg/60 mL ... 2476
Hydrocortone Tablets ... 1989
Preparation H Hydrocortisone Cream ... ▣646

Hydrocortisone Acetate (May intensify electrolyte imbalance, particularly hypokalemia). Products include:
Analpram-HC ... 1159
Pramosone ... 1161
ProctoFoam-HC ... 3099

Hydrocortisone Sodium Phosphate (May intensify electrolyte imbalance, particularly hypokalemia).
No products indexed under this heading.

Hydrocortisone Sodium Succinate (May intensify electrolyte imbalance, particularly hypokalemia).
No products indexed under this heading.

Hydroflumethiazide (May add to potentiate the action of other hypertensives).
No products indexed under this heading.

Ibuprofen (Potential for acute renal failure). Products include:
Advil Allergy Sinus Caplets ... ▣770
Advil ... ▣674
Children's Advil Oral Suspension ... ▣603
Children's Advil Chewable Tablets ... ▣603
Advil Cold & Sinus ... ▣723
Infants' Advil Concentrated Drops ... ▣604
Infants' Advil Concentrated Drops - White Grape (Dye-Free) ... ▣604
Junior Strength Advil Swallow Tablets ... ▣605
Advil Migraine Liquigels ... ▣608
Advil Multi-Symptom Cold Caplets ... ▣770
Advil PM Caplets ... ▣615
Motrin IB Tablets and Caplets ... 1866
Children's Motrin Oral Suspension ... 1867
Children's Motrin Non-Staining Dye-Free Oral Suspension ... 1867
Children's Motrin Cold Oral Suspension ... 1867
Infants' Motrin Concentrated Drops ... 1867
Infants' Motrin Non-Staining Dye-Free Concentrated Drops ... 1867
Junior Strength Motrin Caplets and Chewable Tablets ... 1867
Vicoprofen Tablets ... 539

Indapamide (May add to potentiate the action of other hypertensives). Products include:
Indapamide Tablets ... 2156

Indomethacin (Potential for acute renal failure). Products include:
Indocin ... 1995

Indomethacin Sodium Trihydrate (Potential for acute renal failure). Products include:
Indocin I.V. ... 2465

Insulin, Human, Zinc Suspension (Thiazides may cause hyperglycemia, glycosuria and alter insulin requirements in diabetes; diabetes mellitus may become manifest during thiazide administration). Products include:
Humulin L, 100 Units ... 1794
Humulin U, 100 Units ... 1800

Insulin, Human NPH (Thiazides may cause hyperglycemia, glycosuria and alter insulin requirements in diabetes; diabetes mellitus may become manifest during thiazide administration). Products include:
Humulin N, 100 Units ... 1795
Humulin N Pen ... 1797

Insulin, Human Regular (Thiazides may cause hyperglycemia, glycosuria and alter insulin requirements in diabetes; diabetes mellitus may become manifest during thiazide administration). Products include:
Humulin R, 100 Units ... 1798

Insulin, Human Regular and Human NPH Mixture (Thiazides may cause hyperglycemia, glycosuria and alter insulin requirements in diabetes; diabetes mellitus may become manifest during thiazide administration). Products include:
Humulin 50/50, 100 Units ... 1791
Humulin 70/30 Pen ... 1793

Insulin, NPH (Thiazides may cause hyperglycemia, glycosuria and alter insulin requirements in diabetes; diabetes mellitus may become manifest during thiazide administration).
No products indexed under this heading.

Insulin, Regular (Thiazides may cause hyperglycemia, glycosuria and alter insulin requirements in diabetes; diabetes mellitus may become manifest during thiazide administration).
No products indexed under this heading.

Insulin, Zinc Crystals (Thiazides may cause hyperglycemia, glycosuria and alter insulin requirements in diabetes; diabetes mellitus may become manifest during thiazide administration).
No products indexed under this heading.

Insulin, Zinc Suspension (Thiazides may cause hyperglycemia, glycosuria and alter insulin requirements in diabetes; diabetes mellitus may become manifest during thiazide administration).
No products indexed under this heading.

Insulin Aspart, Human Regular (Thiazides may cause hyperglycemia, glycosuria and alter insulin requirements in diabetes; diabetes mellitus may become manifest during thiazide administration). Products include:
NovoLog Injection ... 2326

Insulin glargine (Thiazides may cause hyperglycemia, glycosuria and alter insulin requirements in diabetes; diabetes mellitus may become manifest during thiazide administration). Products include:
Lantus Injection ... 2909

Insulin Lispro, Human (Thiazides may cause hyperglycemia, glycosuria and alter insulin requirements in diabetes; diabetes mellitus may become manifest during thiazide administration). Products include:
Humalog-Pen ... 1781
Humalog Mix 50/50-Pen ... 1783
Humalog Mix 75/25-Pen ... 1785

Insulin Lispro Protamine, Human (Thiazides may cause hyperglycemia, glycosuria and alter insulin requirements in diabetes; diabetes mellitus may become manifest during thiazide administration). Products include:
Humalog Mix 50/50-Pen ... 1783
Humalog Mix 75/25-Pen ... 1785

Irbesartan (May add to potentiate the action of other hypertensives). Products include:
Avalide Tablets ... 888
Avalide Tablets ... 2874
Avapro Tablets ... 891
Avapro Tablets ... 2871

Isradipine (May add to potentiate the action of other hypertensives). Products include:
DynaCirc CR Tablets ... 2721

Ketoprofen (Potential for acute renal failure).
No products indexed under this heading.

Ketorolac Tromethamine (Potential for acute renal failure). Products include:
Acular Ophthalmic Solution ... 565
Acular LS Ophthalmic Solution ... 566

Labetalol Hydrochloride (May add to potentiate the action of other hypertensives).
No products indexed under this heading.

Laxatives, unspecified (Interferes with the potassium-retaining effects of triamterene; chronic or overuse of laxatives may reduce serum potassium).
No products indexed under this heading.

Lisinopril (May add to potentiate the action of other hypertensives; increased risk of hyperkalemia). Products include:
Prinivil Tablets **2052**
Prinzide Tablets **2056**

Lithium (Reduced renal clearance and increased risk of lithium toxicity).
No products indexed under this heading.

Lithium Carbonate (Reduced renal clearance and increased risk of lithium toxicity). Products include:
Lithobid Tablets **1692**

Lithium Citrate (Reduced renal clearance and increased risk of lithium toxicity).
No products indexed under this heading.

Losartan Potassium (May add to potentiate the action of other hypertensives). Products include:
Cozaar Tablets **1935**
Hyzaar 50-12.5 Tablets **1990**
Hyzaar 100-12.5 Tablets **1990**
Hyzaar 100-25 Tablets **1990**

Mecamylamine Hydrochloride (May add to potentiate the action of other hypertensives).
No products indexed under this heading.

Meclofenamate Sodium (Potential for acute renal failure).
No products indexed under this heading.

Mefenamic Acid (Potential for acute renal failure).
No products indexed under this heading.

Meloxicam (Potential for acute renal failure). Products include:
Mobic Oral Suspension **863**
Mobic Tablets **863**

Metformin Hydrochloride (Increased risk of severe hyponatremia). Products include:
ActoPlus Met Tablets **3214**
Avandamet Tablets **1373**
Fortamet Extended-Release Tablets **3115**

Methenamine (Decreased effectiveness of methenamine due to alkalinization of urine). Products include:
Prosed/DS Tablets **1157**

Methenamine Hippurate (Decreased effectiveness of methenamine due to alkalinization of urine).
No products indexed under this heading.

Methenamine Mandelate (Decreased effectiveness of methenamine due to alkalinization of urine). Products include:
Uroqid-Acid No. 2 Tablets **760**

Methyclothiazide (May add to potentiate the action of other hypertensives).
No products indexed under this heading.

Methyldopa (May add to potentiate the action of other hypertensives). Products include:
Aldoril Tablets **1910**

Methyldopate Hydrochloride (May add to potentiate the action of other hypertensives).
No products indexed under this heading.

Methylprednisolone Acetate (May intensify electrolyte imbalance, particularly hypokalemia). Products include:
Depo-Medrol Injectable Suspension **2617**
Depo-Medrol Single-Dose Vial **2619**

Methylprednisolone Sodium Succinate (May intensify electrolyte imbalance, particularly hypokalemia).
No products indexed under this heading.

Metocurine Iodide (Increased paralyzing effect).
No products indexed under this heading.

Metolazone (May add to potentiate the action of other hypertensives).
No products indexed under this heading.

Metoprolol Succinate (May add to potentiate the action of other hypertensives). Products include:
Toprol-XL Tablets **668**

Metoprolol Tartrate (May add to potentiate the action of other hypertensives). Products include:
Lopressor Injection **2238**
Lopressor Tablets **2238**
Lopressor HCT 50/25 Tablets **2241**
Lopressor HCT 100/25 Tablets **2241**
Lopressor HCT 100/50 Tablets **2241**

Metyrosine (May add to potentiate the action of other hypertensives). Products include:
Demser Capsules **1953**

Mibefradil Dihydrochloride (May add to potentiate the action of other hypertensives).
No products indexed under this heading.

Miglitol (Thiazides may cause hyperglycemia and glycosuria; dosage alteration of oral antidiabetic agents may be required).
No products indexed under this heading.

Minoxidil (May add to potentiate the action of other hypertensives). Products include:
Men's Rogaine Extra Strength Hair Regrowth Treatment Topical Solution, Ocean Rush Scent and Original Unscented .... ▣**633**
Men's Rogaine Foam Hair Regrowth Treatment .... ▣**633**
Women's Rogaine Hair Regrowth Treatment Topical Solution, Spring Bloom Scent and Original Unscented .... ▣**634**

Mivacurium Chloride (Increased paralyzing effect). Products include:
Mivacron Injection **493**

Moexipril Hydrochloride (May add to potentiate the action of other hypertensives; increased risk of hyperkalemia). Products include:
Uniretic Tablets **3100**
Univasc Tablets **3104**

Nabumetone (Potential for acute renal failure).
No products indexed under this heading.

Nadolol (May add to potentiate the action of other hypertensives). Products include:
Nadolol Tablets **2159**

Naproxen (Potential for acute renal failure). Products include:
EC-Naprosyn Delayed-Release Tablets **2761**
Naprosyn Suspension **2761**
Naprosyn Tablets **2761**
Prevacid NapraPAC **3280**

Naproxen Sodium (Potential for acute renal failure). Products include:
Aleve Caplets **742**
Aleve Gelcaps **743**
Aleve Tablets **743**
Aleve Cold & Sinus Caplets **744**
Anaprox Tablets **2761**
Anaprox DS Tablets **2761**

Nicardipine Hydrochloride (May add to potentiate the action of other hypertensives). Products include:
Cardene I.V. **2497**

Nifedipine (May add to potentiate the action of other hypertensives). Products include:
Adalat CC Tablets **2964**

Nisoldipine (May add to potentiate the action of other hypertensives). Products include:
Sular Tablets **3122**

Nitroglycerin (May add to potentiate the action of other hypertensives). Products include:
Nitro-Dur Transdermal Infusion System **3046**
Nitrolingual Pumpspray **3120**

Norepinephrine Bitartrate (Decreased arterial responsiveness to norepinephrine).
No products indexed under this heading.

Oxaprozin (Potential for acute renal failure).
No products indexed under this heading.

Pancuronium Bromide (Increased paralyzing effect).
No products indexed under this heading.

Penbutolol Sulfate (May add to potentiate the action of other hypertensives).
No products indexed under this heading.

Penicillin G Potassium (Concurrent use of parenteral penicillin G potassium with triamterene may result in hyperkalemia, especially in patients with renal insufficiency).
No products indexed under this heading.

Perindopril Erbumine (May add to potentiate the action of other hypertensives; increased risk of hyperkalemia). Products include:
Aceon Tablets (2 mg, 4 mg, 8 mg) **3194**

Phenoxybenzamine Hydrochloride (May add to potentiate the action of other hypertensives). Products include:
Dibenzyline Capsules **3399**

Phentolamine Mesylate (May add to potentiate the action of other hypertensives).
No products indexed under this heading.

Phenylbutazone (Potential for acute renal failure).
No products indexed under this heading.

Pindolol (May add to potentiate the action of other hypertensives).
No products indexed under this heading.

Pioglitazone Hydrochloride (Thiazides may cause hyperglycemia and glycosuria; dosage alteration of oral antidiabetic agents may be required). Products include:
ActoPlus Met Tablets **3214**
Actos Tablets **3219**
Duetact Tablets **3226**

Piroxicam (Potential for acute renal failure).
No products indexed under this heading.

Polythiazide (May add to potentiate the action of other hypertensives).
No products indexed under this heading.

Potassium Acid Phosphate (Potential for hyperkalemia; concomitant use should be avoided). Products include:
K-Phos Original (Sodium Free) Tablets **760**

Potassium Bicarbonate (Potential for hyperkalemia; concomitant use should be avoided).
No products indexed under this heading.

Potassium Chloride (Potential for hyperkalemia; concomitant use should be avoided). Products include:
Colyte with Flavor Packs for Oral Solution **3088**
HalfLytely and Bisacodyl Tablets Bowel Prep Kit with Flavors Packs **881**
K-Dur Extended-Relase Tablets **3033**
K-Lor Oral Solution **474**
K-Tab Tablets **475**
MoviPrep Oral Solution **2839**
TriLyte with Flavor Packs for Oral Solution **3100**

Potassium Citrate (Potential for hyperkalemia; concomitant use should be avoided). Products include:
Urocit-K Tablets **2144**

Potassium Gluconate (Potential for hyperkalemia; concomitant use should be avoided).
No products indexed under this heading.

Potassium Phosphate (Potential for hyperkalemia; concomitant use should be avoided). Products include:
K-Phos Neutral Tablets **760**

Prazosin Hydrochloride (May add to potentiate the action of other hypertensives).
No products indexed under this heading.

Prednisolone Acetate (May intensify electrolyte imbalance, particularly hypokalemia). Products include:
Blephamide Ophthalmic Ointment **568**
Blephamide Ophthalmic Suspension **569**
Poly-Pred Ophthalmic Suspension .... ⊙**233**
Pred Forte Ophthalmic Suspension .... ⊙**235**
Pred Mild Ophthalmic Suspension .... ⊙**238**
Pred-G Ophthalmic Ointment .... ⊙**237**
Pred-G Ophthalmic Suspension .... ⊙**236**

Prednisolone Sodium Phosphate (May intensify electrolyte imbalance, particularly hypokalemia).
No products indexed under this heading.

Prednisolone Tebutate (May intensify electrolyte imbalance, particularly hypokalemia).
No products indexed under this heading.

Prednisone (May intensify electrolyte imbalance, particularly hypokalemia).
No products indexed under this heading.

Probenecid (Dyazide may raise the level of blood uric acid; may require dosage adjustment of antigout agent).
No products indexed under this heading.

Propranolol Hydrochloride (May add to potentiate the action of other hypertensives). Products include:
Inderal LA Long-Acting Capsules 3429
InnoPran XL Capsules 2723

Quinapril Hydrochloride (May add to potentiate the action of other hypertensives; increased risk of hyperkalemia).
No products indexed under this heading.

Ramipril (May add to potentiate the action of other hypertensives; increased risk of hyperkalemia). Products include:
Altace Capsules 1702

Rapacuronium Bromide (Increased paralyzing effect).
No products indexed under this heading.

Rauwolfia Serpentina (May add to potentiate the action of other hypertensives).
No products indexed under this heading.

Repaglinide (Thiazides may cause hyperglycemia and glycosuria; dosage alteration of oral antidiabetic agents may be required).
No products indexed under this heading.

Rescinnamine (May add to potentiate the action of other hypertensives).
No products indexed under this heading.

Reserpine (May add to potentiate the action of other hypertensives).
No products indexed under this heading.

Rocuronium Bromide (Increased paralyzing effect). Products include:
Zemuron Injection 2346

Rofecoxib (Potential for acute renal failure).
No products indexed under this heading.

Rosiglitazone Maleate (Thiazides may cause hyperglycemia and glycosuria; dosage alteration of oral antidiabetic agents may be required). Products include:
Avandamet Tablets 1373
Avandaryl Tablets 1379
Avandia Tablets 1384

Salt Substitutes (Concurrent use of salt substitutes with triamterene may result in hyperkalemia, especially in patients with renal insufficiency).
No products indexed under this heading.

Sodium Nitroprusside (May add to potentiate the action of other hypertensives).
No products indexed under this heading.

Sodium Polystyrene Sulfonate (May result in fluid retention).
No products indexed under this heading.

Sotalol Hydrochloride (May add to potentiate the action of other hypertensives).
No products indexed under this heading.

Spirapril Hydrochloride (May add to potentiate the action of other hypertensives; increased risk of hyperkalemia).
No products indexed under this heading.

Spironolactone (Concurrent use is contraindicated).
No products indexed under this heading.

Sulfinpyrazone (Dyazide may raise the level of blood uric acid; may require dosage adjustment of antigout agent).
No products indexed under this heading.

Sulindac (Potential for acute renal failure). Products include:
Clinoril Tablets 1924

Telmisartan (May add to potentiate the action of other hypertensives). Products include:
Micardis Tablets 854
Micardis HCT Tablets 856

Terazosin Hydrochloride (May add to potentiate the action of other hypertensives). Products include:
Hytrin Capsules 471

Timolol Maleate (May add to potentiate the action of other hypertensives). Products include:
Blocadren Tablets 1916
Cosopt Sterile Ophthalmic Solution 1931
Timolide Tablets 2086
Timoptic Sterile Ophthalmic Solution 2088
Timoptic in Ocudose 2091
Timoptic-XE Sterile Ophthalmic Gel Forming Solution 2092

Tolazamide (Thiazides may cause hyperglycemia and glycosuria; dosage alteration of oral antidiabetic agents may be required).
No products indexed under this heading.

Tolbutamide (Thiazides may cause hyperglycemia and glycosuria; dosage alteration of oral antidiabetic agents may be required).
No products indexed under this heading.

Tolmetin Sodium (Potential for acute renal failure).
No products indexed under this heading.

Torsemide (May add to potentiate the action of other hypertensives). Products include:
Demadex Injection 2759
Demadex Tablets 2759

Trandolapril (May add to potentiate the action of other hypertensives; increased risk of hyperkalemia). Products include:
Mavik Tablets 486
Tarka Tablets 524

Triamcinolone (May intensify electrolyte imbalance, particularly hypokalemia).
No products indexed under this heading.

Triamcinolone Acetonide (May intensify electrolyte imbalance, particularly hypokalemia). Products include:
Azmacort Inhalation Aerosol 1726
Nasacort AQ Nasal Spray 2922

Triamcinolone Diacetate (May intensify electrolyte imbalance, particularly hypokalemia).
No products indexed under this heading.

Triamcinolone Hexacetonide (May intensify electrolyte imbalance, particularly hypokalemia).
No products indexed under this heading.

Trimethaphan Camsylate (May add to potentiate the action of other hypertensives).
No products indexed under this heading.

Troglitazone (Thiazides may cause hyperglycemia and glycosuria; dosage alteration of oral antidiabetic agents may be required).
No products indexed under this heading.

Tubocurarine Chloride (Increased paralyzing effect).
No products indexed under this heading.

Valdecoxib (Potential for acute renal failure).
No products indexed under this heading.

Valsartan (May add to potentiate the action of other hypertensives). Products include:
Diovan Tablets 2193
Diovan HCT Tablets 2196

Vecuronium Bromide (Increased paralyzing effect).
No products indexed under this heading.

Verapamil Hydrochloride (May add to potentiate the action of other hypertensives). Products include:
Covera-HS Tablets 3139
Tarka Tablets 524
Verelan PM Extended-Release Capsules, Controlled-Onset 3106

Warfarin Sodium (Effects of oral anticoagulants may be decreased). Products include:
Coumadin for Injection 898
Coumadin Tablets 898

Food Interactions

Milk, low fat (Concurrent use of low-salt milk with triamterene may result in hyperkalemia, especially in patients with renal insufficiency).

DYNACIRC CR TABLETS

(Isradipine) 2721
May interact with:

Cimetidine (Co-administration has resulted in increase in isradipine mean peak plasma concentrations and significant increase in the AUC). Products include:
Tagamet HB 200 Tablets ..... ▣ 664

Cimetidine Hydrochloride (Co-administration has resulted in increase in isradipine mean peak plasma concentrations and significant increase in the AUC).
No products indexed under this heading.

Fentanyl (Severe hypotension has been reported during fentanyl anesthesia with concomitant use of beta-blocker and a calcium channel blocker). Products include:
Duragesic Transdermal System 2373
Ionsys Transdermal System 2379

Fentanyl Citrate (Severe hypotension has been reported during fentanyl anesthesia with concomitant use of beta-blocker and a calcium channel blocker). Products include:
Actiq 979

Hydrochlorothiazide (Additive antihypertensive effect). Products include:
Aldoril Tablets 1910
Atacand HCT 651
Avalide Tablets 888
Avalide Tablets 2874
Benicar HCT Tablets 1044
Diovan HCT Tablets 2196
Dyazide Capsules 1423
Hyzaar 50-12.5 Tablets 1990
Hyzaar 100-12.5 Tablets 1990
Hyzaar 100-25 Tablets 1990
Lopressor HCT 50/25 Tablets 2241
Lopressor HCT 100/25 Tablets 2241
Lopressor HCT 100/50 Tablets 2241
Lotensin HCT Tablets 2246
Micardis HCT Tablets 856
Moduretic Tablets 2028
Prinzide Tablets 2056
Teveten HCT Tablets 1737
Timolide Tablets 2086
Uniretic Tablets 3100

Propranolol Hydrochloride (Co-administration has resulted in a small effect on the rate but no effect on the extent of isradipine bioavailability; significant increases in AUC and Cmax and decreases in tmax of propranolol were noted). Products include:
Inderal LA Long-Acting Capsules 3429
InnoPran XL Capsules 2723

Rifampin (Co-administration has resulted in increased metabolism and higher clearance of isradipine; a reduction in isradipine levels to below the detectable limits has been noted).
No products indexed under this heading.

DYRENIUM CAPSULES

(Triamterene) 3400
May interact with ACE inhibitors, anesthetics, antihypertensives, diuretics, oral hypoglycemic agents, lithium preparations, nondepolarizing neuromuscular blocking agents, potassium preparations, preanesthetic medications, potassium sparing diuretics, and certain other agents. Compounds in these categories include:

Acarbose (Triamterene may raise blood glucose levels; for adult onset diabetes, dosage adjustments of hypoglycemic agents may be necessary during and after therapy). Products include:
Precose Tablets 751

Acebutolol Hydrochloride (The effects of antihypertensive agents may be potentiated when given concurrently).
No products indexed under this heading.

Alfentanil Hydrochloride (The effects of anesthetics may be potentiated when given concurrently).
No products indexed under this heading.

Amiloride Hydrochloride (Co-administration with other potassium-sparing agents has resulted in fatalities; these agents should not be given concomitantly). Products include:
Midamor Tablets 2026
Moduretic Tablets 2028

Amlodipine Besylate (The effects of antihypertensive agents may be potentiated when given concurrently). Products include:
Caduet Tablets 2508
Lotrel Capsules 2249
Norvasc Tablets 2545

Atenolol (The effects of antihypertensive agents may be potentiated when given concurrently).
No products indexed under this heading.

Atracurium Besylate (The effects of nondepolarizing skeletal muscle relaxants may be potentiated when given concurrently).
No products indexed under this heading.

Benazepril Hydrochloride (Co-administration with potassium-sparing agents and angiotensin-coverting enzyme inhibitors increases the risk of hyperkalemia). Products include:
Lotensin Tablets ... 2243
Lotensin HCT Tablets ... 2246
Lotrel Capsules ... 2249

Bendroflumethiazide (The effects of other diuretics may be potentiated when given concurrently).
No products indexed under this heading.

Betaxolol Hydrochloride (The effects of antihypertensive agents may be potentiated when given concurrently). Products include:
Betoptic S Ophthalmic Suspension ... 558

Bisoprolol Fumarate (The effects of antihypertensive agents may be potentiated when given concurrently).
No products indexed under this heading.

Blood, whole (Co-administration with blood from blood banks may promote serum potassium accumulation and possibly result in hyperkalemia).
No products indexed under this heading.

Bumetanide (The effects of other diuretics may be potentiated when given concurrently). Products include:
Bumex Tablets ... 2746

Candesartan Cilexetil (The effects of antihypertensive agents may be potentiated when given concurrently). Products include:
Atacand Tablets ... 649
Atacand HCT ... 651

Captopril (Co-administration with potassium-sparing agents and angiotensin-coverting enzyme inhibitors increases the risk of hyperkalemia). Products include:
Captopril Tablets ... 2149

Carteolol Hydrochloride (The effects of antihypertensive agents may be potentiated when given concurrently). Products include:
Carteolol Hydrochloride Ophthalmic Solution USP, 1% ... ⊙249

Chlorothiazide (The effects of other diuretics may be potentiated when given concurrently). Products include:
Diuril Oral Suspension ... 1954

Chlorothiazide Sodium (The effects of other diuretics may be potentiated when given concurrently). Products include:
Diuril Sodium Intravenous ... 2467

Chlorpropamide (Triamterene may raise blood glucose levels; for adult onset diabetes, dosage adjustments of hypoglycemic agents may be necessary during and after therapy; increased risk of severe hyponatremia with concurrent use).
No products indexed under this heading.

Chlorthalidone (The effects of other diuretics may be potentiated when given concurrently). Products include:
Clorpres Tablets ... 2153

Cisatracurium Besylate (The effects of nondepolarizing skeletal muscle relaxants may be potentiated when given concurrently). Products include:
Nimbex Injection ... 498

Clonidine (The effects of antihypertensive agents may be potentiated when given concurrently). Products include:
Catapres-TTS ... 844

Clonidine Hydrochloride (The effects of antihypertensive agents may be potentiated when given concurrently). Products include:
Catapres Tablets ... 843
Clorpres Tablets ... 2153

Deserpidine (The effects of antihypertensive agents may be potentiated when given concurrently).
No products indexed under this heading.

Diazepam (The effects of pre-anesthetic agents may be potentiated when given concurrently). Products include:
Diastat Rectal Delivery System ... 3343
Valium Tablets ... 2819

Diazoxide (The effects of antihypertensive agents may be potentiated when given concurrently). Products include:
Hyperstat I.V. ... 3017

Diltiazem Hydrochloride (The effects of antihypertensive agents may be potentiated when given concurrently). Products include:
Cardizem LA Extended Release Tablets ... 1728
Tiazac Capsules ... 1201

Doxazosin Mesylate (The effects of antihypertensive agents may be potentiated when given concurrently). Products include:
Cardura XL Tablets ... 2515

Droperidol (The effects of pre-anesthetic agents may be potentiated when given concurrently).
No products indexed under this heading.

Enalapril Maleate (Co-administration with potassium-sparing agents and angiotensin-coverting enzyme inhibitors increases the risk of hyperkalemia). Products include:
Vasotec I.V. Injection ... 2103

Enalaprilat (Co-administration with potassium-sparing agents and angiotensin-coverting enzyme inhibitors increases the risk of hyperkalemia).
No products indexed under this heading.

Enflurane (The effects of anesthetics may be potentiated when given concurrently).
No products indexed under this heading.

Eprosartan Mesylate (The effects of antihypertensive agents may be potentiated when given concurrently). Products include:
Teveten Tablets ... 1735
Teveten HCT Tablets ... 1737

Esmolol Hydrochloride (The effects of antihypertensive agents may be potentiated when given concurrently).
No products indexed under this heading.

Ethacrynic Acid (The effects of other diuretics may be potentiated when given concurrently). Products include:
Edecrin Tablets ... 1959

Felodipine (The effects of antihypertensive agents may be potentiated when given concurrently).
No products indexed under this heading.

Fentanyl Citrate (The effects of anesthetics may be potentiated when given concurrently). Products include:
Actiq ... 979

Fosinopril Sodium (Co-administration with potassium-sparing agents and angiotensin-coverting enzyme inhibitors increases the risk of hyperkalemia).
No products indexed under this heading.

Furosemide (The effects of other diuretics may be potentiated when given concurrently). Products include:
Furosemide Tablets ... 2154

Glimepiride (Triamterene may raise blood glucose levels; for adult onset diabetes, dosage adjustments of hypoglycemic agents may be necessary during and after therapy). Products include:
Avandaryl Tablets ... 1379
Duetact Tablets ... 3226

Glipizide (Triamterene may raise blood glucose levels; for adult onset diabetes, dosage adjustments of hypoglycemic agents may be necessary during and after therapy).
No products indexed under this heading.

Glyburide (Triamterene may raise blood glucose levels; for adult onset diabetes, dosage adjustments of hypoglycemic agents may be necessary during and after therapy).
No products indexed under this heading.

Guanabenz Acetate (The effects of antihypertensive agents may be potentiated when given concurrently).
No products indexed under this heading.

Guanethidine Monosulfate (The effects of antihypertensive agents may be potentiated when given concurrently).
No products indexed under this heading.

Halothane (The effects of anesthetics may be potentiated when given concurrently).
No products indexed under this heading.

Hydralazine Hydrochloride (The effects of antihypertensive agents may be potentiated when given concurrently). Products include:
BiDil Tablets ... 2171

Hydrochlorothiazide (The effects of other diuretics may be potentiated when given concurrently). Products include:
Aldoril Tablets ... 1910
Atacand HCT ... 651
Avalide Tablets ... 888
Avalide Tablets ... 2874
Benicar HCT Tablets ... 1044
Diovan HCT Tablets ... 2196
Dyazide Capsules ... 1423
Hyzaar 50-12.5 Tablets ... 1990
Hyzaar 100-12.5 Tablets ... 1990
Hyzaar 100-25 Tablets ... 1990
Lopressor HCT 50/25 Tablets ... 2241
Lopressor HCT 100/25 Tablets ... 2241
Lopressor HCT 100/50 Tablets ... 2241
Lotensin HCT Tablets ... 2246
Micardis HCT Tablets ... 856
Moduretic Tablets ... 2028
Prinzide Tablets ... 2056
Teveten HCT Tablets ... 1737
Timolide Tablets ... 2086
Uniretic Tablets ... 3100

Hydroflumethiazide (The effects of other diuretics may be potentiated when given concurrently).
No products indexed under this heading.

Hydroxyzine Hydrochloride (The effects of pre-anesthetic agents may be potentiated when given concurrently).
No products indexed under this heading.

Indapamide (The effects of other diuretics may be potentiated when given concurrently). Products include:
Indapamide Tablets ... 2156

Indomethacin (Co-administration has resulted in acute renal failure). Products include:
Indocin ... 1995

Irbesartan (The effects of antihypertensive agents may be potentiated when given concurrently). Products include:
Avalide Tablets ... 888
Avalide Tablets ... 2874
Avapro Tablets ... 891
Avapro Tablets ... 2871

Isoflurane (The effects of anesthetics may be potentiated when given concurrently).
No products indexed under this heading.

Isradipine (The effects of antihypertensive agents may be potentiated when given concurrently). Products include:
DynaCirc CR Tablets ... 2721

Ketamine Hydrochloride (The effects of anesthetics may be potentiated when given concurrently).
No products indexed under this heading.

Labetalol Hydrochloride (The effects of antihypertensive agents may be potentiated when given concurrently).
No products indexed under this heading.

Lisinopril (Co-administration with potassium-sparing agents and angiotensin-coverting enzyme inhibitors increases the risk of hyperkalemia). Products include:
Prinivil Tablets ... 2052
Prinzide Tablets ... 2056

Lithium (Co-administration of lithium and diuretics results in diuretic-induced sodium loss that may reduce renal clearance of lithium and increase serum lithium levels with risk of lithium toxicity).
No products indexed under this heading.

Lithium Carbonate (Co-administration of lithium and diuretics results in diuretic-induced sodium loss that may reduce renal clearance of lithium and increase serum lithium levels with risk of lithium toxicity). Products include:
Lithobid Tablets ... 1692

Lithium Citrate (Co-administration of lithium and diuretics results in diuretic-induced sodium loss that may reduce renal clearance of lithium and increase serum lithium levels with risk of lithium toxicity).
No products indexed under this heading.

Lorazepam (The effects of pre-anesthetic agents may be potentiated when given concurrently).
No products indexed under this heading.

Losartan Potassium (The effects of antihypertensive agents may be potentiated when given concurrently). Products include:
Cozaar Tablets **1935**
Hyzaar 50-12.5 Tablets **1990**
Hyzaar 100-12.5 Tablets **1990**
Hyzaar 100-25 Tablets **1990**

Mecamylamine Hydrochloride (The effects of antihypertensive agents may be potentiated when given concurrently).
No products indexed under this heading.

Meperidine Hydrochloride (The effects of pre-anesthetic agents may be potentiated when given concurrently).
No products indexed under this heading.

Metformin Hydrochloride (Triamterene may raise blood glucose levels; for adult onset diabetes, dosage adjustments of hypoglycemic agents may be necessary during and after therapy). Products include:
ActoPlus Met Tablets **3214**
Avandamet Tablets **1373**
Fortamet Extended-Release Tablets **3115**

Methohexital Sodium (The effects of anesthetics may be potentiated when given concurrently).
No products indexed under this heading.

Methyclothiazide (The effects of other diuretics may be potentiated when given concurrently).
No products indexed under this heading.

Methyldopa (The effects of antihypertensive agents may be potentiated when given concurrently). Products include:
Aldoril Tablets **1910**

Methyldopate Hydrochloride (The effects of antihypertensive agents may be potentiated when given concurrently).
No products indexed under this heading.

Metocurine Iodide (The effects of nondepolarizing skeletal muscle relaxants may be potentiated when given concurrently).
No products indexed under this heading.

Metolazone (The effects of other diuretics may be potentiated when given concurrently).
No products indexed under this heading.

Metoprolol Succinate (The effects of antihypertensive agents may be potentiated when given concurrently). Products include:
Toprol-XL Tablets **668**

Metoprolol Tartrate (The effects of antihypertensive agents may be potentiated when given concurrently). Products include:
Lopressor Injection **2238**
Lopressor Tablets **2238**
Lopressor HCT 50/25 Tablets **2241**
Lopressor HCT 100/25 Tablets **2241**
Lopressor HCT 100/50 Tablets **2241**

Metyrosine (The effects of antihypertensive agents may be potentiated when given concurrently). Products include:
Demser Capsules **1953**

Mibefradil Dihydrochloride (The effects of antihypertensive agents may be potentiated when given concurrently).
No products indexed under this heading.

Midazolam Hydrochloride (The effects of anesthetics may be potentiated when given concurrently).
No products indexed under this heading.

Miglitol (Triamterene may raise blood glucose levels; for adult onset diabetes, dosage adjustments of hypoglycemic agents may be necessary during and after therapy).
No products indexed under this heading.

Minoxidil (The effects of antihypertensive agents may be potentiated when given concurrently). Products include:
Men's Rogaine Extra Strength Hair Regrowth Treatment Topical Solution, Ocean Rush Scent and Original Unscented ..... ■ **633**
Men's Rogaine Foam Hair Regrowth Treatment.................. ■ **633**
Women's Rogaine Hair Regrowth Treatment Topical Solution, Spring Bloom Scent and Original Unscented................... ■ **634**

Mivacurium Chloride (The effects of nondepolarizing skeletal muscle relaxants may be potentiated when given concurrently). Products include:
Mivacron Injection **493**

Moexipril Hydrochloride (Co-administration with potassium-sparing agents and angiotensin-coverting enzyme inhibitors increases the risk of hyperkalemia). Products include:
Uniretic Tablets **3100**
Univasc Tablets **3104**

Morphine Sulfate (The effects of pre-anesthetic agents may be potentiated when given concurrently). Products include:
Avinza Capsules **1741**
Kadian Capsules **577**
MS Contin Tablets **2701**

Nadolol (The effects of antihypertensive agents may be potentiated when given concurrently). Products include:
Nadolol Tablets **2159**

Nicardipine Hydrochloride (The effects of antihypertensive agents may be potentiated when given concurrently). Products include:
Cardene I.V. **2497**

Nifedipine (The effects of antihypertensive agents may be potentiated when given concurrently). Products include:
Adalat CC Tablets **2964**

Nisoldipine (The effects of antihypertensive agents may be potentiated when given concurrently). Products include:
Sular Tablets **3122**

Nitroglycerin (The effects of antihypertensive agents may be potentiated when given concurrently). Products include:
Nitro-Dur Transdermal Infusion System.. **3046**
Nitrolingual Pumpspray **3120**

Pancuronium Bromide (The effects of nondepolarizing skeletal muscle relaxants may be potentiated when given concurrently).
No products indexed under this heading.

Penbutolol Sulfate (The effects of antihypertensive agents may be potentiated when given concurrently).
No products indexed under this heading.

Penicillin G Potassium (Co-administration may promote serum potassium accumulation and possibly result in hyperkalemia).
No products indexed under this heading.

Pentobarbital Sodium (The effects of pre-anesthetic agents may be potentiated when given concurrently). Products include:
Nembutal Sodium Solution, USP **2470**

Perindopril Erbumine (Co-administration with potassium-sparing agents and angiotensin-coverting enzyme inhibitors increases the risk of hyperkalemia). Products include:
Aceon Tablets (2 mg, 4 mg, 8 mg)... **3194**

Phenoxybenzamine Hydrochloride (The effects of antihypertensive agents may be potentiated when given concurrently). Products include:
Dibenzyline Capsules **3399**

Phentolamine Mesylate (The effects of antihypertensive agents may be potentiated when given concurrently).
No products indexed under this heading.

Pindolol (The effects of antihypertensive agents may be potentiated when given concurrently).
No products indexed under this heading.

Pioglitazone Hydrochloride (Triamterene may raise blood glucose levels; for adult onset diabetes, dosage adjustments of hypoglycemic agents may be necessary during and after therapy). Products include:
ActoPlus Met Tablets **3214**
Actos Tablets **3219**
Duetact Tablets **3226**

Polythiazide (The effects of other diuretics may be potentiated when given concurrently).
No products indexed under this heading.

Potassium Acid Phosphate (Co-administration with dietary potassium supplements increases the risk of hyperkalemia; concurrent use is contraindicated). Products include:
K-Phos Original (Sodium Free) Tablets **760**

Potassium Bicarbonate (Co-administration with dietary potassium supplements increases the risk of hyperkalemia; concurrent use is contraindicated).
No products indexed under this heading.

Potassium Chloride (Co-administration with dietary potassium supplements increases the risk of hyperkalemia; concurrent use is contraindicated). Products include:
Colyte with Flavor Packs for Oral Solution... **3088**
HalfLytely and Bisacodyl Tablets Bowel Prep Kit with Flavors Packs.. **881**
K-Dur Extended-Relase Tablets **3033**
K-Lor Oral Solution **474**
K-Tab Tablets **475**
MoviPrep Oral Solution **2839**
TriLyte with Flavor Packs for Oral Solution... **3100**

Potassium Citrate (Co-administration with dietary potassium supplements increases the risk of hyperkalemia; concurrent use is contraindicated). Products include:
Urocit-K Tablets **2144**

Potassium Gluconate (Co-administration with dietary potassium supplements increases the risk of hyperkalemia; concurrent use is contraindicated).
No products indexed under this heading.

Potassium Phosphate (Co-administration with dietary potassium supplements increases the risk of hyperkalemia; concurrent use is contraindicated). Products include:
K-Phos Neutral Tablets **760**

Prazosin Hydrochloride (The effects of antihypertensive agents may be potentiated when given concurrently).
No products indexed under this heading.

Promethazine Hydrochloride (The effects of pre-anesthetic agents may be potentiated when given concurrently). Products include:
Phenergan Tablets and Suppositories................................. **3440**

Propofol (The effects of anesthetics may be potentiated when given concurrently).
No products indexed under this heading.

Propranolol Hydrochloride (The effects of antihypertensive agents may be potentiated when given concurrently). Products include:
Inderal LA Long-Acting Capsules **3429**
InnoPran XL Capsules **2723**

Quinapril Hydrochloride (Co-administration with potassium-sparing agents and angiotensin-coverting enzyme inhibitors increases the risk of hyperkalemia).
No products indexed under this heading.

Ramipril (Co-administration with potassium-sparing agents and angiotensin-coverting enzyme inhibitors increases the risk of hyperkalemia). Products include:
Altace Capsules **1702**

Rapacuronium Bromide (The effects of nondepolarizing skeletal muscle relaxants may be potentiated when given concurrently).
No products indexed under this heading.

Rauwolfia Serpentina (The effects of antihypertensive agents may be potentiated when given concurrently).
No products indexed under this heading.

Remifentanil Hydrochloride (The effects of anesthetics may be potentiated when given concurrently).
No products indexed under this heading.

Repaglinide (Triamterene may raise blood glucose levels; for adult onset diabetes, dosage adjustments of hypoglycemic agents may be necessary during and after therapy).
No products indexed under this heading.

Rescinnamine (The effects of antihypertensive agents may be potentiated when given concurrently).
No products indexed under this heading.

Reserpine (The effects of antihypertensive agents may be potentiated when given concurrently).
No products indexed under this heading.

Rocuronium Bromide (The effects of nondepolarizing skeletal muscle relaxants may be potentiated when given concurrently). Products include:
Zemuron Injection 2346

Rosiglitazone Maleate (Triamterene may raise blood glucose levels; for adult onset diabetes, dosage adjustments of hypoglycemic agents may be necessary during and after therapy). Products include:
Avandamet Tablets 1373
Avandaryl Tablets 1379
Avandia Tablets 1384

Secobarbital Sodium (The effects of pre-anesthetic agents may be potentiated when given concurrently).
No products indexed under this heading.

Sodium Nitroprusside (The effects of antihypertensive agents may be potentiated when given concurrently).
No products indexed under this heading.

Sotalol Hydrochloride (The effects of antihypertensive agents may be potentiated when given concurrently).
No products indexed under this heading.

Spirapril Hydrochloride (Co-administration with potassium-sparing agents and angiotensin-coverting enzyme inhibitors increases the risk of hyperkalemia).
No products indexed under this heading.

Spironolactone (Co-administration with other potassium-sparing agents has resulted in fatalities; these agents should not be given concomitantly).
No products indexed under this heading.

Sufentanil Citrate (The effects of anesthetics may be potentiated when given concurrently).
No products indexed under this heading.

Telmisartan (The effects of antihypertensive agents may be potentiated when given concurrently). Products include:
Micardis Tablets 854
Micardis HCT Tablets 856

Terazosin Hydrochloride (The effects of antihypertensive agents may be potentiated when given concurrently). Products include:
Hytrin Capsules 471

Thiamylal Sodium (The effects of anesthetics may be potentiated when given concurrently).
No products indexed under this heading.

Timolol Maleate (The effects of antihypertensive agents may be potentiated when given concurrently). Products include:
Blocadren Tablets 1916
Cosopt Sterile Ophthalmic Solution 1931
Timolide Tablets 2086
Timoptic Sterile Ophthalmic Solution 2088
Timoptic in Ocudose 2091
Timoptic-XE Sterile Ophthalmic Gel Forming Solution 2092

Tolazamide (Triamterene may raise blood glucose levels; for adult onset diabetes, dosage adjustments of hypoglycemic agents may be necessary during and after therapy).
No products indexed under this heading.

Tolbutamide (Triamterene may raise blood glucose levels; for adult onset diabetes, dosage adjustments of hypoglycemic agents may be necessary during and after therapy).
No products indexed under this heading.

Torsemide (The effects of other diuretics may be potentiated when given concurrently). Products include:
Demadex Injection 2759
Demadex Tablets 2759

Trandolapril (Co-administration with potassium-sparing agents and angiotensin-coverting enzyme inhibitors increases the risk of hyperkalemia). Products include:
Mavik Tablets 486
Tarka Tablets 524

Trimethaphan Camsylate (The effects of antihypertensive agents may be potentiated when given concurrently).
No products indexed under this heading.

Troglitazone (Triamterene may raise blood glucose levels; for adult onset diabetes, dosage adjustments of hypoglycemic agents may be necessary during and after therapy).
No products indexed under this heading.

Valsartan (The effects of antihypertensive agents may be potentiated when given concurrently). Products include:
Diovan Tablets 2193
Diovan HCT Tablets 2196

Vecuronium Bromide (The effects of nondepolarizing skeletal muscle relaxants may be potentiated when given concurrently).
No products indexed under this heading.

Verapamil Hydrochloride (The effects of antihypertensive agents may be potentiated when given concurrently). Products include:
Covera-HS Tablets 3139
Tarka Tablets 524
Verelan PM Extended-Release Capsules, Controlled-Onset 3106

Food Interactions

Milk, low salt (Co-administration may promote serum potassium accumulation and possibly result in hyperkalemia).

EC-NAPROSYN DELAYED-RELEASE TABLETS

(Naproxen) 2761
May interact with ACE inhibitors, antacids containing aluminum, calcium and magnesium, beta blockers, oral anticoagulants, diuretics, histamine H2-receptor antagonists, hydantoin anticonvulsants, lithium preparations, sulfonylureas, and certain other agents. Compounds in these categories include:

Acebutolol Hydrochloride (Reduced antihypertensive effect of beta blockers).
No products indexed under this heading.

Aluminum Carbonate (Due to the gastric pH elevating effects of intensive antacids therapy, concomitant administration of EC-Naprosyn is not recommended).
No products indexed under this heading.

Aluminum Hydroxide (Due to the gastric pH elevating effects of intensive antacids therapy, concomitant administration of EC-Naprosyn is not recommended). Products include:
Gaviscon Regular Strength Liquid 658
Gaviscon Regular Strength Tablets 658
Gaviscon Extra Strength Liquid 658
Gaviscon Extra Strength Tablets 658
Maalox Regular Strength Antacid/Antigas Liquid 2175
Maalox Max Maximum Strength Antacid/Anti-Gas Liquid 2176

Amiloride Hydrochloride (Clinical sutdies, as well as postmarketing ovservations, have shown that Naproxen can reduce the natriuretic effect of furosemide and thiazides in some patients. Response has been attributed to inhibition of renal prostaglandin sythensis. Patients should be observed closely for signs of renal failure, as well as to assure diuretic efficacy). Products include:
Midamor Tablets 2026
Moduretic Tablets 2028

Anisindione (Short-term studies have failed to show any significant effect of concurrent use on prothrombin time; caution is advised since interactions have been seen with other NSAIDs). Products include:
Miradon Tablets 3042

Aspirin (Naproxen is displaced from its binding sites during the concomitant administration of aspirin resulting in lower plasma concentrations and peak plasma levels; concurrent use is not recommended). Products include:
Aggrenox Capsules 822
Bayer Aspirin 744
BC Allergy Sinus Cold Powder 677
BC Headache Powder 677
Arthritis Strength BC Powder 677
BC Sinus Cold Powder 677
Excedrin Extra Strength Caplets/Tablets/Geltabs 684
Excedrin Migraine Caplets/Tablets/Geltabs 609
Goody's Body Pain Formula Powder 684
Goody's Extra Strength Headache Powders 611
Goody's Extra Strength Pain Relief Tablets 685
Percodan Tablets 1132
St. Joseph 81 mg Aspirin Chewable and Enteric Coated Tablets 1869

Atenolol (Reduced antihypertensive effect of beta blockers).
No products indexed under this heading.

Benazepril Hydrochloride (Reports suggest that NSAIDs may diminish the antihypertensive effect of ACE-inhibitors. The use of NSAIDs in patients who are receiving ACE-inhibitors may potentiate renal dise states). Products include:
Lotensin Tablets 2243
Lotensin HCT Tablets 2246
Lotrel Capsules 2249

Bendroflumethiazide (Clinical sutdies, as well as postmarketing ovservations, have shown that Naproxen can reduce the natriuretic effect of furosemide and thiazides in some patients. Response has been attributed to inhibition of renal prostaglandin sythensis. Patients should be observed closely for signs of renal failure, as well as to assure diuretic efficacy).
No products indexed under this heading.

Betaxolol Hydrochloride (Reduced antihypertensive effect of beta blockers). Products include:
Betoptic S Ophthalmic Suspension 558

Bisoprolol Fumarate (Reduced antihypertensive effect of beta blockers).
No products indexed under this heading.

Bumetanide (Clinical sutdies, as well as postmarketing ovservations, have shown that Naproxen can reduce the natriuretic effect of furosemide and thiazides in some patients. Response has been attributed to inhibition of renal prostaglandin sythensis. Patients should be observed closely for signs of renal failure, as well as to assure diuretic efficacy). Products include:
Bumex Tablets 2746

Captopril (Reports suggest that NSAIDs may diminish the antihypertensive effect of ACE-inhibitors. The use of NSAIDs in patients who are receiving ACE-inhibitors may potentiate renal dise states). Products include:
Captopril Tablets 2149

Carteolol Hydrochloride (Reduced antihypertensive effect of beta blockers). Products include:
Carteolol Hydrochloride Ophthalmic Solution USP, 1% .... ⊙ 249

Chlorothiazide (Clinical sutdies, as well as postmarketing ovservations, have shown that Naproxen can reduce the natriuretic effect of furosemide and thiazides in some patients. Response has been attributed to inhibition of renal prostaglandin sythensis. Patients should be observed closely for signs of renal failure, as well as to assure diuretic efficacy). Products include:
Diuril Oral Suspension 1954

Chlorothiazide Sodium (Clinical sutdies, as well as postmarketing ovservations, have shown that Naproxen can reduce the natriuretic effect of furosemide and thiazides in some patients. Response has been attributed to inhibition of renal prostaglandin sythensis. Patients should be observed closely for signs of renal failure, as well as to assure diuretic efficacy). Products include:
Diuril Sodium Intravenous 2467

Chlorpropamide (Potential for sulfonylurea toxicity).
No products indexed under this heading.

Chlorthalidone (Clinical sutdies, as well as postmarketing ovservations, have shown that Naproxen can reduce the natriuretic effect of furosemide and thiazides in some patients. Response has been attributed to inhibition of renal prostaglandin sythensis. Patients should be observed closely for signs of renal failure, as well as to assure diuretic efficacy). Products include:

Clorpres Tablets 2153

Cholestyramine (Concomitant administration of cholestyramine can delay the absorption of naproxen).
No products indexed under this heading.

Cimetidine (Due to the gastric pH elevating effects of H_2-blockers concomitant administration of EC-Naprosyn is not recommended). Products include:
Tagamet HB 200 Tablets .... ▣664

Cimetidine Hydrochloride (Due to the gastric pH elevating effects of H_2-blockers concomitant administration of EC-Naprosyn is not recommended).
No products indexed under this heading.

Dicumarol (Short-term studies have failed to show any significant effect of concurrent use on prothrombin time; caution is advised since interactions have been seen with other NSAIDs).
No products indexed under this heading.

Enalapril Maleate (Reports suggest that NSAIDs may diminish the antihypertensive effect of ACE-inhibitors. The use of NSAIDs in patients who are receiving ACE-inhibitors may potentiate renal dise states). Products include:
Vasotec I.V. Injection 2103

Enalaprilat (Reports suggest that NSAIDs may diminish the antihypertensive effect of ACE-inhibitors. The use of NSAIDs in patients who are receiving ACE-inhibitors may potentiate renal dise states).
No products indexed under this heading.

Esmolol Hydrochloride (Reduced antihypertensive effect of beta blockers).
No products indexed under this heading.

Ethacrynic Acid (Clinical sutdies, as well as postmarketing ovservations, have shown that Naproxen can reduce the natriuretic effect of furosemide and thiazides in some patients. Response has been attributed to inhibition of renal prostaglandin sythensis. Patients should be observed closely for signs of renal failure, as well as to assure diuretic efficacy). Products include:
Edecrin Tablets 1959

Ethotoin (Potential for hydantoin toxicity).
No products indexed under this heading.

Famotidine (Due to the gastric pH elevating effects of H_2-blockers concomitant administration of EC-Naprosyn is not recommended). Products include:
Pepcid Injection 2040
Pepcid 2038
Pepcid AC Gelcaps 1701
Pepcid AC Tablets 1701
Maximum Strength Pepcid AC Tablets 1701
Pepcid Complete Chewable Tablets 1701

Fosinopril Sodium (Reports suggest that NSAIDs may diminish the antihypertensive effect of ACE-inhibitors. The use of NSAIDs in patients who are receiving ACE-inhibitors may potentiate renal dise states).
No products indexed under this heading.

Fosphenytoin Sodium (Potential for hydantoin toxicity).
No products indexed under this heading.

Furosemide (Inhibition of natriuretic effect of furosemide). Products include:
Furosemide Tablets 2154

Glimepiride (Potential for sulfonylurea toxicity). Products include:
Avandaryl Tablets 1379
Duetact Tablets 3226

Glipizide (Potential for sulfonylurea toxicity).
No products indexed under this heading.

Glyburide (Potential for sulfonylurea toxicity).
No products indexed under this heading.

Hydrochlorothiazide (Clinical sutdies, as well as postmarketing ovservations, have shown that Naproxen can reduce the natriuretic effect of furosemide and thiazides in some patients. Response has been attributed to inhibition of renal prostaglandin sythensis. Patients should be observed closely for signs of renal failure, as well as to assure diuretic efficacy). Products include:
Aldoril Tablets 1910
Atacand HCT 651
Avalide Tablets 888
Avalide Tablets 2874
Benicar HCT Tablets 1044
Diovan HCT Tablets 2196
Dyazide Capsules 1423
Hyzaar 50-12.5 Tablets 1990
Hyzaar 100-12.5 Tablets 1990
Hyzaar 100-25 Tablets 1990
Lopressor HCT 50/25 Tablets 2241
Lopressor HCT 100/25 Tablets 2241
Lopressor HCT 100/50 Tablets 2241
Lotensin HCT Tablets 2246
Micardis HCT Tablets 856
Moduretic Tablets 2028
Prinzide Tablets 2056
Teveten HCT Tablets 1737
Timolide Tablets 2086
Uniretic Tablets 3100

Hydroflumethiazide (Clinical sutdies, as well as postmarketing ovservations, have shown that Naproxen can reduce the natriuretic effect of furosemide and thiazides in some patients. Response has been attributed to inhibition of renal prostaglandin sythensis. Patients should be observed closely for signs of renal failure, as well as to assure diuretic efficacy).
No products indexed under this heading.

Indapamide (Clinical sutdies, as well as postmarketing ovservations, have shown that Naproxen can reduce the natriuretic effect of furosemide and thiazides in some patients. Response has been attributed to inhibition of renal prostaglandin sythensis. Patients should be observed closely for signs of renal failure, as well as to assure diuretic efficacy). Products include:
Indapamide Tablets 2156

Labetalol Hydrochloride (Reduced antihypertensive effect of beta blockers).
No products indexed under this heading.

Levobunolol Hydrochloride (Reduced antihypertensive effect of beta blockers). Products include:
Betagan Ophthalmic Solution, USP .... ⊙220

Lisinopril (Reports suggest that NSAIDs may diminish the antihypertensive effect of ACE-inhibitors. The use of NSAIDs in patients who are receiving ACE-inhibitors may potentiate renal dise states). Products include:
Prinivil Tablets 2052
Prinzide Tablets 2056

Lithium (Inhibition of lithium renal clearance leading to increase in plasma lithium concentrations).
No products indexed under this heading.

Lithium Carbonate (Inhibition of lithium renal clearance leading to increase in plasma lithium concentrations). Products include:
Lithobid Tablets 1692

Lithium Citrate (Inhibition of lithium renal clearance leading to increase in plasma lithium concentrations).
No products indexed under this heading.

Magaldrate (Due to the gastric pH elevating effects of intensive antacids therapy, concomitant administration of EC-Naprosyn is not recommended).
No products indexed under this heading.

Magnesium Hydroxide (Due to the gastric pH elevating effects of intensive antacids therapy, concomitant administration of EC-Naprosyn is not recommended). Products include:
Maalox Regular Strength Antacid/Antigas Liquid................. 2175
Maalox Max Maximum Strength Antacid/Anti-Gas Liquid................ 2176
Pepcid Complete Chewable Tablets 1701

Magnesium Oxide (Due to the gastric pH elevating effects of intensive antacids therapy, concomitant administration of EC-Naprosyn is not recommended). Products include:
Beelith Tablets 759
PremCal Light, Regular, and Extra Strength Tablets................ ▣818

Mephenytoin (Potential for hydantoin toxicity).
No products indexed under this heading.

Methotrexate Sodium (Potential for reduced tubular secretion of methotrexate and possible increased methotrexate toxicity as shown in animal model; caution is recommended).
No products indexed under this heading.

Methyclothiazide (Clinical sutdies, as well as postmarketing ovservations, have shown that Naproxen can reduce the natriuretic effect of furosemide and thiazides in some patients. Response has been attributed to inhibition of renal prostaglandin sythensis. Patients should be observed closely for signs of renal failure, as well as to assure diuretic efficacy).
No products indexed under this heading.

Metipranolol Hydrochloride (Reduced antihypertensive effect of beta blockers).
No products indexed under this heading.

Metolazone (Clinical sutdies, as well as postmarketing ovservations, have shown that Naproxen can reduce the natriuretic effect of furosemide and thiazides in some patients. Response has been attributed to inhibition of renal prostaglandin sythensis. Patients should be observed closely for signs of renal failure, as well as to assure diuretic efficacy).
No products indexed under this heading.

Metoprolol Succinate (Reduced antihypertensive effect of beta blockers). Products include:
Toprol-XL Tablets 668

Metoprolol Tartrate (Reduced antihypertensive effect of beta blockers). Products include:
Lopressor Injection 2238
Lopressor Tablets 2238
Lopressor HCT 50/25 Tablets 2241
Lopressor HCT 100/25 Tablets 2241
Lopressor HCT 100/50 Tablets 2241

Moexipril Hydrochloride (Reports suggest that NSAIDs may diminish the antihypertensive effect of ACE-inhibitors. The use of NSAIDs in patients who are receiving ACE-inhibitors may potentiate renal dise states). Products include:
Uniretic Tablets 3100
Univasc Tablets 3104

Nadolol (Reduced antihypertensive effect of beta blockers). Products include:
Nadolol Tablets 2159

Naproxen Sodium (Concurrent use of naproxen or naproxen sodium in any dosage form is not recommended since they all circulate in the plasma as the naproxen anion). Products include:
Aleve Caplets 742
Aleve Gelcaps 743
Aleve Tablets 743
Aleve Cold & Sinus Caplets 744
Anaprox Tablets 2761
Anaprox DS Tablets 2761

Nizatidine (Due to the gastric pH elevating effects of H_2-blockers concomitant administration of EC-Naprosyn is not recommended). Products include:
Axid Oral Solution 879

Penbutolol Sulfate (Reduced antihypertensive effect of beta blockers).
No products indexed under this heading.

Perindopril Erbumine (Reports suggest that NSAIDs may diminish the antihypertensive effect of ACE-inhibitors. The use of NSAIDs in patients who are receiving ACE-inhibitors may potentiate renal dise states). Products include:
Aceon Tablets (2 mg, 4 mg, 8 mg).. 3194

Phenytoin (Potential for hydantoin toxicity).
No products indexed under this heading.

Phenytoin Sodium (Potential for hydantoin toxicity). Products include:
Phenytek Capsules 2160

Pindolol (Reduced antihypertensive effect of beta blockers).
No products indexed under this heading.

Polythiazide (Clinical sutdies, as well as postmarketing ovservations, have shown that Naproxen can reduce the natriuretic effect of furosemide and thiazides in some patients. Response has been attributed to inhibition of renal prostaglandin sythensis. Patients should be observed closely for signs of renal failure, as well as to assure diuretic efficacy).

No products indexed under this heading.

Probenecid (Probenecid given concurrently increases naproxen anion plasma levels and extends its plasma half-life significantly).

No products indexed under this heading.

Propranolol Hydrochloride (Reduced antihypertensive effect of beta blockers). Products include:

Inderal LA Long-Acting Capsules 3429
InnoPran XL Capsules 2723

Quinapril Hydrochloride (Reports suggest that NSAIDs may diminish the antihypertensive effect of ACE-inhibitors. The use of NSAIDs in patients who are receiving ACE-inhibitors may potentiate renal dise states).

No products indexed under this heading.

Ramipril (Reports suggest that NSAIDs may diminish the antihypertensive effect of ACE-inhibitors. The use of NSAIDs in patients who are receiving ACE-inhibitors may potentiate renal dise states). Products include:

Altace Capsules 1702

Ranitidine Bismuth Citrate (Due to the gastric pH elevating effects of H_2-blockers concomitant administration of EC-Naprosyn is not recommended).

No products indexed under this heading.

Ranitidine Hydrochloride (Due to the gastric pH elevating effects of H_2-blockers concomitant administration of EC-Naprosyn is not recommended). Products include:

Zantac 1624
Zantac Injection 1619
Zantac Injection Pharmacy Bulk Package 1622

Sotalol Hydrochloride (Reduced antihypertensive effect of beta blockers).

No products indexed under this heading.

Spirapril Hydrochloride (Reports suggest that NSAIDs may diminish the antihypertensive effect of ACE-inhibitors. The use of NSAIDs in patients who are receiving ACE-inhibitors may potentiate renal dise states).

No products indexed under this heading.

Spironolactone (Clinical sutdies, as well as postmarketing ovservations, have shown that Naproxen can reduce the natriuretic effect of furosemide and thiazides in some patients. Response has been attributed to inhibition of renal prostaglandin sythensis. Patients should be observed closely for signs of renal failure, as well as to assure diuretic efficacy).

No products indexed under this heading.

Sucralfate (Due to the gastric pH elevating effects of sucralfate, concomitant administration of EC-Naprosyn is not recommended). Products include:

Carafate Suspension 701
Carafate Tablets 701

Sulfamethoxazole (Potential for sulfonamide toxicity).

No products indexed under this heading.

Sulfisoxazole Acetyl (Potential for sulfonamide toxicity).

No products indexed under this heading.

Timolol Hemihydrate (Reduced antihypertensive effect of beta blockers). Products include:

Betimol Ophthalmic Solution 3382
Betimol Ophthalmic Solution .... ⊙295

Timolol Maleate (Reduced antihypertensive effect of beta blockers). Products include:

Blocadren Tablets 1916
Cosopt Sterile Ophthalmic Solution 1931
Timolide Tablets 2086
Timoptic Sterile Ophthalmic Solution 2088
Timoptic in Ocudose 2091
Timoptic-XE Sterile Ophthalmic Gel Forming Solution 2092

Tolazamide (Potential for sulfonylurea toxicity).

No products indexed under this heading.

Tolbutamide (Potential for sulfonylurea toxicity).

No products indexed under this heading.

Torsemide (Clinical sutdies, as well as postmarketing ovservations, have shown that Naproxen can reduce the natriuretic effect of furosemide and thiazides in some patients. Response has been attributed to inhibition of renal prostaglandin sythensis. Patients should be observed closely for signs of renal failure, as well as to assure diuretic efficacy). Products include:

Demadex Injection 2759
Demadex Tablets 2759

Trandolapril (Co-administration of NSAIDs and ACE inhibitors may potentiate renal disease states). Products include:

Mavik Tablets 486
Tarka Tablets 524

Triamterene (Clinical sutdies, as well as postmarketing ovservations, have shown that Naproxen can reduce the natriuretic effect of furosemide and thiazides in some patients. Response has been attributed to inhibition of renal prostaglandin sythensis. Patients should be observed closely for signs of renal failure, as well as to assure diuretic efficacy). Products include:

Dyazide Capsules 1423
Dyrenium Capsules 3400

Warfarin Sodium (Short-term studies have failed to show any significant effect of concurrent use on prothrombin time; caution is advised since interactions have been seen with other NSAIDs). Products include:

Coumadin for Injection 898
Coumadin Tablets 898

Food Interactions

Food, unspecified (The presence of food prolonged the time the EC-Naprosyn remained in the stomach, time to first detectable serum naproxen levels, and time to maximal naproxen levels (Tmax), but did not affect peak naproxen levels (Cmax)).

EDECRIN TABLETS

(Ethacrynic Acid) 1959

See Edecrin Sodium Intravenous

EDECRIN SODIUM INTRAVENOUS

(Ethacrynate Sodium) 1959

May interact with aminoglycosides, cephalosporins, cardiac glycosides, non-steroidal anti-inflammatory agents, and certain other agents. Compounds in these categories include:

Amikacin Sulfate (Increased ototoxic potential of aminoglycosides).

No products indexed under this heading.

Cefaclor (Increased ototoxic potential of cephalosporins).

No products indexed under this heading.

Cefadroxil (Increased ototoxic potential of cephalosporins).

No products indexed under this heading.

Cefamandole Nafate (Increased ototoxic potential of cephalosporins).

No products indexed under this heading.

Cefazolin Sodium (Increased ototoxic potential of cephalosporins).

No products indexed under this heading.

Cefdinir (Increased ototoxic potential of cephalosporins). Products include:

Omnicef Capsules 511
Omnicef for Oral Suspension 511

Cefepime Hydrochloride (Increased ototoxic potential of cephalosporins). Products include:

Maxipime for Injection 1105

Cefixime (Increased ototoxic potential of cephalosporins). Products include:

Suprax 1843

Cefmetazole Sodium (Increased ototoxic potential of cephalosporins).

No products indexed under this heading.

Cefonicid Sodium (Increased ototoxic potential of cephalosporins).

No products indexed under this heading.

Cefoperazone Sodium (Increased ototoxic potential of cephalosporins).

No products indexed under this heading.

Ceforanide (Increased ototoxic potential of cephalosporins).

No products indexed under this heading.

Cefotaxime Sodium (Increased ototoxic potential of cephalosporins).

No products indexed under this heading.

Cefotetan (Increased ototoxic potential of cephalosporins).

No products indexed under this heading.

Cefoxitin Sodium (Increased ototoxic potential of cephalosporins). Products include:

Mefoxin for Injection 2012
Mefoxin Premixed Intravenous Solution 2016

Cefpodoxime Proxetil (Increased ototoxic potential of cephalosporins). Products include:

Vantin Tablets and Oral Suspension 2645

Cefprozil (Increased ototoxic potential of cephalosporins).

No products indexed under this heading.

Ceftazidime (Increased ototoxic potential of cephalosporins). Products include:

Fortaz 1453

Ceftizoxime Sodium (Increased ototoxic potential of cephalosporins).

No products indexed under this heading.

Ceftriaxone Sodium (Increased ototoxic potential of cephalosporins). Products include:

Rocephin Injectable Vials, ADD-Vantage, Galaxy, Bulk............ 2800

Cefuroxime Axetil (Increased ototoxic potential of cephalosporins). Products include:

Ceftin 1407

Cefuroxime Sodium (Increased ototoxic potential of cephalosporins).

No products indexed under this heading.

Celecoxib (Reduces diuretic, natriuretic, and antihypertensive effects). Products include:

Celebrex Capsules 3134

Cephalexin (Increased ototoxic potential of cephalosporins). Products include:

Keflex Capsules 549

Cephalothin Sodium (Increased ototoxic potential of cephalosporins).

No products indexed under this heading.

Cephapirin Sodium (Increased ototoxic potential of cephalosporins).

No products indexed under this heading.

Cephradine (Increased ototoxic potential of cephalosporins).

No products indexed under this heading.

Deslanoside (Excessive potassium loss may precipitate digitalis toxicity).

No products indexed under this heading.

Diclofenac Potassium (Reduces diuretic, natriuretic, and antihypertensive effects).

No products indexed under this heading.

Diclofenac Sodium (Reduces diuretic, natriuretic, and antihypertensive effects). Products include:

Arthrotec Tablets 3129
Voltaren Ophthalmic Solution 2309
Voltaren Tablets 2307
Voltaren-XR Tablets 2310

Digitalis Glycoside Preparations (Excessive potassium loss may precipitate digitalis toxicity).

No products indexed under this heading.

Digitoxin (Excessive potassium loss may precipitate digitalis toxicity).

No products indexed under this heading.

Digoxin (Excessive potassium loss may precipitate digitalis toxicity). Products include:

Lanoxicaps Capsules 1490
Lanoxin Injection 1494
Lanoxin Injection Pediatric 1497
Lanoxin Tablets 1500

Etodolac (Reduces diuretic, natriuretic, and antihypertensive effects).

No products indexed under this heading.

IMPORTANT NOTE: Always consult each drug listing in the patient's regimen for possible interactions.

Fenoprofen Calcium (Reduces diuretic, natriuretic, and antihypertensive effects). Products include:
- Nalfon Capsules 2502

Flurbiprofen (Reduces diuretic, natriuretic, and antihypertensive effects).
- No products indexed under this heading.

Gentamicin Sulfate (Increased ototoxic potential of aminoglycosides). Products include:
- Garamycin Injectable 3014
- Pred-G Ophthalmic Ointment .... ⊙237
- Pred-G Ophthalmic Suspension .... ⊙236

Ibuprofen (Reduces diuretic, natriuretic, and antihypertensive effects). Products include:
- Advil Allergy Sinus Caplets .... ▣770
- Advil .... ▣674
- Children's Advil Oral Suspension .... ▣603
- Children's Advil Chewable Tablets .... ▣603
- Advil Cold & Sinus .... ▣723
- Infants' Advil Concentrated Drops .... ▣604
- Infants' Advil Concentrated Drops - White Grape (Dye-Free) .... ▣604
- Junior Strength Advil Swallow Tablets .... ▣605
- Advil Migraine Liquigels .... ▣608
- Advil Multi-Symptom Cold Caplets .... ▣770
- Advil PM Caplets .... ▣615
- Motrin IB Tablets and Caplets 1866
- Children's Motrin Oral Suspension 1867
- Children's Motrin Non-Staining Dye-Free Oral Suspension 1867
- Children's Motrin Cold Oral Suspension 1867
- Infants' Motrin Concentrated Drops 1867
- Infants' Motrin Non-Staining Dye-Free Concentrated Drops 1867
- Junior Strength Motrin Caplets and Chewable Tablets 1867
- Vicoprofen Tablets 539

Indomethacin (Reduces diuretic, natriuretic, and antihypertensive effects). Products include:
- Indocin 1995

Indomethacin Sodium Trihydrate (Reduces diuretic, natriuretic, and antihypertensive effects). Products include:
- Indocin I.V. 2465

Isoproterenol Hydrochloride (Careful adjustment of dosages required).
- No products indexed under this heading.

Kanamycin Sulfate (Increased ototoxic potential of aminoglycosides).
- No products indexed under this heading.

Ketoprofen (Reduces diuretic, natriuretic, and antihypertensive effects).
- No products indexed under this heading.

Ketorolac Tromethamine (Reduces diuretic, natriuretic, and antihypertensive effects). Products include:
- Acular Ophthalmic Solution 565
- Acular LS Ophthalmic Solution 566

Lithium Carbonate (High risk of lithium toxicity). Products include:
- Lithobid Tablets 1692

Lithium Citrate (High risk of lithium toxicity).
- No products indexed under this heading.

Loracarbef (Increased ototoxic potential of cephalosporins).
- No products indexed under this heading.

Meclofenamate Sodium (Reduces diuretic, natriuretic, and antihypertensive effects).
- No products indexed under this heading.

Mefenamic Acid (Reduces diuretic, natriuretic, and antihypertensive effects).
- No products indexed under this heading.

Meloxicam (Reduces diuretic, natriuretic, and antihypertensive effects). Products include:
- Mobic Oral Suspension 863
- Mobic Tablets 863

Nabumetone (Reduces diuretic, natriuretic, and antihypertensive effects).
- No products indexed under this heading.

Naproxen (Reduces diuretic, natriuretic, and antihypertensive effects). Products include:
- EC-Naprosyn Delayed-Release Tablets 2761
- Naprosyn Suspension 2761
- Naprosyn Tablets 2761
- Prevacid NapraPAC 3280

Naproxen Sodium (Reduces diuretic, natriuretic, and antihypertensive effects). Products include:
- Aleve Caplets 742
- Aleve Gelcaps 743
- Aleve Tablets 743
- Aleve Cold & Sinus Caplets 744
- Anaprox Tablets 2761
- Anaprox DS Tablets 2761

Oxaprozin (Reduces diuretic, natriuretic, and antihypertensive effects).
- No products indexed under this heading.

Phenylbutazone (Reduces diuretic, natriuretic, and antihypertensive effects).
- No products indexed under this heading.

Piroxicam (Reduces diuretic, natriuretic, and antihypertensive effects).
- No products indexed under this heading.

Rofecoxib (Reduces diuretic, natriuretic, and antihypertensive effects).
- No products indexed under this heading.

Streptomycin Sulfate (Increased ototoxic potential of aminoglycosides).
- No products indexed under this heading.

Sulindac (Reduces diuretic, natriuretic, and antihypertensive effects). Products include:
- Clinoril Tablets 1924

Tobramycin (Increased ototoxic potential of aminoglycosides). Products include:
- TOBI Solution for Inhalation 2298
- TobraDex Ophthalmic Ointment 562
- TobraDex Ophthalmic Suspension 563
- Zylet Ophthalmic Suspension .... ⊙259

Tobramycin Sulfate (Increased ototoxic potential of aminoglycosides).
- No products indexed under this heading.

Tolmetin Sodium (Reduces diuretic, natriuretic, and antihypertensive effects).
- No products indexed under this heading.

Valdecoxib (Reduces diuretic, natriuretic, and antihypertensive effects).
- No products indexed under this heading.

Warfarin Sodium (Warfarin displaced from plasma protein; reduction in warfarin dosage may be required). Products include:
- Coumadin for Injection 898
- Coumadin Tablets 898

EDEX INJECTION

(Alprostadil) 3089

May interact with:

Heparin Calcium (The pharmacodynamic interaction between heparin and alprostadil intravenous infusion was investigated. The results indicate significant changes in partial thromboplastin time (140% increase) and thrombin time (120% increase). Therefore, caution should be exercised with concomitant administration of heparin and alprostadil).
- No products indexed under this heading.

Heparin Sodium (The pharmacodynamic interaction between heparin and alprostadil intravenous infusion was investigated. The results indicate significant changes in partial thromboplastin time (140% increase) and thrombin time (120% increase). Therefore, caution should be exercised with concomitant administration of heparin and alprostadil).
- No products indexed under this heading.

E.E.S. 200 LIQUID

(Erythromycin Ethylsuccinate) 451

See E.E.S. 400 Filmtab Tablets

E.E.S. 400 LIQUID

(Erythromycin Ethylsuccinate) 451

See E.E.S. 400 Filmtab Tablets

E.E.S. 400 FILMTAB TABLETS

(Erythromycin Ethylsuccinate) 451

May interact with oral anticoagulants, HMG-CoA reductase inhibitors, phenytoin, triazolobenzodiazepines, valproate, xanthines, and certain other agents. Compounds in these categories include:

Alfentanil Hydrochloride (Concurrent use of erythromycin in patients receiving drugs metabolized by the cytochrome P450 system may be associated with elevation in serum levels of alfentanil).
- No products indexed under this heading.

Alprazolam (Erythromycin has been reported to decrease the clearance of triazolam and midazolam; may increase the pharmacologic effect of these benzodiazepines). Products include:
- Niravam Orally Disintegrating Tablets 3092

Aminophylline (Co-administration in patients who are receiving high doses of theophylline may be associated with an increase in serum theophylline levels and potential theophylline toxicity).
- No products indexed under this heading.

Anisindione (Co-administration has resulted in increased anticoagulant effects). Products include:
- Miradon Tablets 3042

Astemizole (Concurrent use of erythromycin in patients receiving astemizole has been reported to significantly alter the metabolism of astemizole; rare cases of cardiovascular adverse events, including prolonged QT interval, cardiac arrest, torsade de pointes, and other ventricular arrhythmias have been reported; co-administration is contraindicated).
- No products indexed under this heading.

Atorvastatin Calcium (Erythromycin has been reported to increase concentrations of HMG-CoA reductase inhibitors (e.g. lovastatin and simvastatin); rare reports of rhabdomyolysis have been reported in patients taking these drugs concomitantly). Products include:
- Caduet Tablets 2508
- Lipitor Tablets 2483

Bromocriptine Mesylate (Concurrent use of erythromycin in patients receiving drugs metabolized by the cytochrome P450 system may be associated with elevation in serum levels of bromocriptine).
- No products indexed under this heading.

Carbamazepine (Concurrent use of erythromycin in patients receiving drugs metabolized by the cytochrome P450 system may be associated with elevation in serum levels of carbamazepine). Products include:
- Carbatrol Capsules 3171
- Equetro Extended-Release Capsules 3180
- Tegretol/Tegretol-XR 2295

Cerivastatin Sodium (Erythromycin has been reported to increase concentrations of HMG-CoA reductase inhibitors (e.g. lovastatin and simvastatin); rare reports of rhabdomyolysis have been reported in patients taking these drugs concomitantly).
- No products indexed under this heading.

Cisapride (Concurrent use of erythromycin in patients receiving cisapride has been reported to inhibit the metabolism of cisapride; cases of cardiovascular adverse events, including prolonged QT interval, torsade de pointes, ventricular tachycardia, and ventricular fibrillation have been reported; co-administration is contraindicated).
- No products indexed under this heading.

Cyclosporine (Concurrent use of erythromycin in patients receiving drugs metabolized by the cytochrome P450 system may be associated with elevation in serum levels of cyclosporine). Products include:
- Gengraf Capsules 459
- Neoral Oral Solution 2259
- Neoral Soft Gelatin Capsules 2259
- Restasis Ophthalmic Emulsion 575
- Sandimmune 2275

Dicumarol (Co-administration has resulted in increased anticoagulant effects).
- No products indexed under this heading.

Digoxin (Co-administration has been reported to result in elevated digoxin serum levels). Products include:
- Lanoxicaps Capsules 1490
- Lanoxin Injection 1494
- Lanoxin Injection Pediatric 1497
- Lanoxin Tablets 1500

Dihydroergotamine Mesylate (Co-administration has been associated in some patients with acute ergot toxicity characterized by severe peripheral vasospasm and dysesthesia). Products include:
Migranal Nasal Spray 3348

Disopyramide Phosphate (Concurrent use of erythromycin in patients receiving drugs metabolized by the cytochrome P450 system may be associated with elevation in serum levels of disopyramide).
No products indexed under this heading.

Divalproex Sodium (There have been reports of interactions of erythromycin with drugs not thought to be metabolized by CYP3A, including valproate). Products include:
Depakote Sprinkle Capsules 422
Depakote Tablets 427
Depakote ER Tablets 434

Dyphylline (Co-administration in patients who are receiving high doses of theophylline may be associated with an increase in serum theophylline levels and potential theophylline toxicity).
No products indexed under this heading.

Ergotamine Tartrate (Co-administration has been associated in some patients with acute ergot toxicity characterized by severe peripheral vasospasm and dysesthesia).
No products indexed under this heading.

Fluvastatin Sodium (Erythromycin has been reported to increase concentrations of HMG-CoA reductase inhibitors (e.g. lovastatin and simvastatin); rare reports of rhabdomyolysis have been reported in patients taking these drugs concomitantly). Products include:
Lescol Capsules 2233
Lescol XL Tablets 2233

Fosphenytoin Sodium (There have been reports of interactions of erythromycin with drugs not thought to be metabolized by CYP3A, including phenytoin).
No products indexed under this heading.

Hexobarbital (There have been reports of interactions of erythromycin with drugs not thought to be metabolized by CYP3A, including hexobarbital).
No products indexed under this heading.

Lovastatin (Erythromycin has been reported to increase concentrations of HMG-CoA reductase inhibitors (e.g. lovastatin and simvastatin); rare reports of rhabdomyolysis have been reported in patients taking these drugs concomitantly). Products include:
Advicor Tablets 1722
Altoprev Extended-Release Tablets 3109
Mevacor Tablets 2021

Midazolam Hydrochloride (Erythromycin has been reported to decrease the clearance of triazolam and midazolam; may increase the pharmacologic effect of these benzodiazepines).
No products indexed under this heading.

Phenytoin (There have been reports of interactions of erythromycin with drugs not thought to be metabolized by CYP3A, including phenytoin).
No products indexed under this heading.

Phenytoin Sodium (There have been reports of interactions of erythromycin with drugs not thought to be metabolized by CYP3A, including phenytoin). Products include:
Phenytek Capsules 2160

Pimozide (Concurrent use of erythromycin in patients receiving drugs metabolized by the cytochrome P450 system may be associated with elevation in serum levels of pimozide; co-administration is contraindicated).
No products indexed under this heading.

Pravastatin Sodium (Erythromycin has been reported to increase concentrations of HMG-CoA reductase inhibitors (e.g. lovastatin and simvastatin); rare reports of rhabdomyolysis have been reported in patients taking these drugs concomitantly).
No products indexed under this heading.

Sildenafil Citrate (Erythromycin has been reported to increase the systemic exposure (AUC) of sildenafil). Products include:
Revatio Tablets 2557
Viagra Tablets 2573

Simvastatin (Erythromycin has been reported to increase concentrations of HMG-CoA reductase inhibitors (e.g. lovastatin and simvastatin); rare reports of rhabdomyolysis have been reported in patients taking these drugs concomitantly). Products include:
Vytorin 10/10 Tablets 2114
Vytorin 10/10 Tablets 3077
Vytorin 10/20 Tablets 2114
Vytorin 10/20 Tablets 3077
Vytorin 10/40 Tablets 2114
Vytorin 10/40 Tablets 3077
Vytorin 10/80 Tablets 2114
Vytorin 10/80 Tablets 3077
Zocor Tablets 2105

Tacrolimus (Concurrent use of erythromycin in patients receiving drugs metabolized by the cytochrome P450 system may be associated with elevation in serum levels of tacrolimus). Products include:
Prograf Capsules and Injection 632
Protopic Ointment 638

Terfenadine (Concurrent use of erythromycin in patients receiving terfenadine has been reported to significantly alter the metabolism of terfenadine; rare cases of cardiovascular adverse events, including prolonged QT interval, cardiac arrest, torsade de pointes, other ventricular arrhythmias, and death have been reported; co-administration is contraindicated).
No products indexed under this heading.

Theophylline (Co-administration in patients who are receiving high doses of theophylline may be associated with an increase in serum theophylline levels and potential theophylline toxicity).
No products indexed under this heading.

Theophylline Anhydrous (Co-administration in patients who are receiving high doses of theophylline may be associated with an increase in serum theophylline levels and potential theophylline toxicity). Products include:
Uniphyl Tablets 2710

Theophylline Calcium Salicylate (Co-administration in patients who are receiving high doses of theophylline may be associated with an increase in serum theophylline levels and potential theophylline toxicity).
No products indexed under this heading.

Theophylline Dihydroxypropyl (Glyceryl) (Co-administration in patients who are receiving high doses of theophylline may be associated with an increase in serum theophylline levels and potential theophylline toxicity).
No products indexed under this heading.

Theophylline Ethylenediamine (Co-administration in patients who are receiving high doses of theophylline may be associated with an increase in serum theophylline levels and potential theophylline toxicity).
No products indexed under this heading.

Theophylline Sodium Glycinate (Co-administration in patients who are receiving high doses of theophylline may be associated with an increase in serum theophylline levels and potential theophylline toxicity).
No products indexed under this heading.

Triazolam (Erythromycin has been reported to decrease the clearance of triazolam and, thus, may increase the pharmacologic effect of the benzodiazepine).
No products indexed under this heading.

Valproate Sodium (There have been reports of interactions of erythromycin with drugs not thought to be metabolized by CYP3A, including valproate). Products include:
Depacon Injection 412

Valproic Acid (There have been reports of interactions of erythromycin with drugs not thought to be metabolized by CYP3A, including valproate). Products include:
Depakene 417

Warfarin Sodium (Co-administration has resulted in increased anticoagulant effects). Products include:
Coumadin for Injection 898
Coumadin Tablets 898

E.E.S. GRANULES

(Erythromycin Ethylsuccinate) 451
See E.E.S. 400 Filmtab Tablets

EFFEXOR TABLETS

(Venlafaxine Hydrochloride) 3411
See Effexor XR Capsules

EFFEXOR XR CAPSULES

(Venlafaxine Hydrochloride) 3417
May interact with 5HT1-receptor agonists, central nervous system depressants, central nervous system stimulants, monoamine oxidase inhibitors, quinidine, selective serotonin reuptake inhibitors, and certain other agents. Compounds in these categories include:

5-hydroxytryptophan (Caution is advised when velafaxine is coadministered with other drugs that may affect serotonergic neurotransmitter systems).
No products indexed under this heading.

Alfentanil Hydrochloride (Caution is advised if the concomitant administration of venlafaxine and CNS-active drugs is required).
No products indexed under this heading.

Alprazolam (Caution is advised if the concomitant administration of venlafaxine and CNS-active drugs is required). Products include:
Niravam Orally Disintegrating Tablets 3092

Amphetamine Resins (Caution is advised if the concomitant administration of venlafaxine and CNS-active drugs is required).
No products indexed under this heading.

Aprobarbital (Caution is advised if the concomitant administration of venlafaxine and CNS-active drugs is required).
No products indexed under this heading.

Buprenorphine Hydrochloride (Caution is advised if the concomitant administration of venlafaxine and CNS-active drugs is required). Products include:
Buprenex Injectable 2716
Suboxone Tablets 2717
Subutex Tablets 2717

Buspirone Hydrochloride (Caution is advised if the concomitant administration of venlafaxine and CNS-active drugs is required).
No products indexed under this heading.

Butabarbital (Caution is advised if the concomitant administration of venlafaxine and CNS-active drugs is required).
No products indexed under this heading.

Butalbital (Caution is advised if the concomitant administration of venlafaxine and CNS-active drugs is required).
No products indexed under this heading.

Chlordiazepoxide (Caution is advised if the concomitant administration of venlafaxine and CNS-active drugs is required).
No products indexed under this heading.

Chlordiazepoxide Hydrochloride (Caution is advised if the concomitant administration of venlafaxine and CNS-active drugs is required). Products include:
Librium Capsules 3347

Chlorpromazine (Caution is advised if the concomitant administration of venlafaxine and CNS-active drugs is required).
No products indexed under this heading.

Chlorpromazine Hydrochloride (Caution is advised if the concomitant administration of venlafaxine and CNS-active drugs is required).
No products indexed under this heading.

Chlorprothixene (Caution is advised if the concomitant administration of venlafaxine and CNS-active drugs is required).
No products indexed under this heading.

Chlorprothixene Hydrochloride (Caution is advised if the concomitant administration of venlafaxine and CNS-active drugs is required).
No products indexed under this heading.

Chlorprothixene Lactate (Caution is advised if the concomitant administration of venlafaxine and CNS-active drugs is required).
No products indexed under this heading.

Cimetidine (Co-administration in a steady-state study for both drugs has resulted in inhibition of first-pass metabolism of venlafaxine; the oral clearance of venlafaxine was reduced by 43% and AUC and Cmax were increased by about 60%). Products include:
Tagamet HB 200 Tablets ▩**664**

Cimetidine Hydrochloride (Co-administration in a steady-state study for both drugs has resulted in inhibition of first-pass metabolism of venlafaxine; the oral clearance of venlafaxine was reduced by 43% and AUC and Cmax were increased by about 60%).
No products indexed under this heading.

Citalopram Hydrobromide (Based on the mechanism of action of venlafaxine and the potential for serotonin syndrome, caution is advised when velafaxine is co-administered with other drugs that may affect the serotonergic neurotransmitter systems, such as serotonin reuptake inhibitors). Products include:
Celexa **1176**

Clorazepate Dipotassium (Caution is advised if the concomitant administration of venlafaxine and CNS-active drugs is required). Products include:
Tranxene **2474**

Clozapine (There have been reports of elevated clozapine levels that were temporarily associated with adverse events including seizures, following the addition of venlafaxine). Products include:
Clozaril Tablets **2184**
FazaClo Orally Disintegrating Tablets **551**

Codeine Phosphate (Caution is advised if the concomitant administration of venlafaxine and CNS-active drugs is required). Products include:
Tylenol with Codeine Tablets **2391**

Desflurane (Caution is advised if the concomitant administration of venlafaxine and CNS-active drugs is required).
No products indexed under this heading.

Desipramine Hydrochloride (Based on the mechanism of action of venlafaxine and the potential for serotonin syndrome, caution is advised when venlafaxine is co-administered with other drugs that may affect serotonergic neurotransmitter systems, such as serotonin-norepinephrine reuptake inhibitors).
No products indexed under this heading.

Dextroamphetamine Sulfate (Caution is advised if the concomitant administration of venlafaxine and CNS-active drugs is required). Products include:
Adderall Tablets **3164**
Adderall XR Capsules **3166**
Dexedrine **1420**
DextroStat Tablets **3179**

Dezocine (Caution is advised if the concomitant administration of venlafaxine and CNS-active drugs is required).
No products indexed under this heading.

Diazepam (Caution is advised if the concomitant administration of venlafaxine and CNS-active drugs is required). Products include:
Diastat Rectal Delivery System **3343**
Valium Tablets **2819**

3-Diphenylacrylate (Based on the mechanism of action of venlafaxine and the potential for serotonin syndrome, caution is advised when velafaxine is co-administered with other drugs that may affect the serotonergic neurotransmitter systems, such as triptans).
No products indexed under this heading.

Droperidol (Caution is advised if the concomitant administration of venlafaxine and CNS-active drugs is required).
No products indexed under this heading.

Duloxetine Hydrochloride (Based on the mechanism of action of venlafaxine and the potential for serotonin syndrome, caution is advised when venlafaxine is co-administered with other drugs that may affect serotonergic neurotransmitter systems, such as serotonin-norepinephrine reuptake inhibitors). Products include:
Cymbalta Delayed-Release Capsules **1757**

Enflurane (Caution is advised if the concomitant administration of venlafaxine and CNS-active drugs is required).
No products indexed under this heading.

Escitalopram Oxalate (Based on the mechanism of action of venlafaxine and the potential for serotonin syndrome, caution is advised when velafaxine is co-administered with other drugs that may affect the serotonergic neurotransmitter systems, such as serotonin reuptake inhibitors). Products include:
Lexapro Oral Solution **1190**
Lexapro Tablets **1190**

Estazolam (Caution is advised if the concomitant administration of venlafaxine and CNS-active drugs is required). Products include:
ProSom Tablets **517**

Ethanol (Caution is advised if the concomitant administration of venlafaxine and CNS-active drugs is required).
No products indexed under this heading.

Ethchlorvynol (Caution is advised if the concomitant administration of venlafaxine and CNS-active drugs is required).
No products indexed under this heading.

Ethinamate (Caution is advised if the concomitant administration of venlafaxine and CNS-active drugs is required).
No products indexed under this heading.

Ethyl Alcohol (Caution is advised if the concomitant administration of venlafaxine and CNS-active drugs is required).
No products indexed under this heading.

Fentanyl (Caution is advised if the concomitant administration of venlafaxine and CNS-active drugs is required). Products include:
Duragesic Transdermal System **2373**
Ionsys Transdermal System **2379**

Fentanyl Citrate (Caution is advised if the concomitant administration of venlafaxine and CNS-active drugs is required). Products include:
Actiq **979**

Fluoxetine Hydrochloride (Based on the mechanism of action of venlafaxine and the potential for serotonin syndrome, caution is advised when velafaxine is co-administered with other drugs that may affect the serotonergic neurotransmitter systems, such as serotonin reuptake inhibitors). Products include:
Prozac Pulvules and Liquid **1801**
Symbyax Capsules **1819**

Fluphenazine Decanoate (Caution is advised if the concomitant administration of venlafaxine and CNS-active drugs is required).
No products indexed under this heading.

Fluphenazine Enanthate (Caution is advised if the concomitant administration of venlafaxine and CNS-active drugs is required).
No products indexed under this heading.

Fluphenazine Hydrochloride (Caution is advised if the concomitant administration of venlafaxine and CNS-active drugs is required).
No products indexed under this heading.

Flurazepam Hydrochloride (Caution is advised if the concomitant administration of venlafaxine and CNS-active drugs is required). Products include:
Dalmane Capsules **3342**

Fluvoxamine Maleate (Based on the mechanism of action of venlafaxine and the potential for serotonin syndrome, caution is advised when velafaxine is co-administered with other drugs that may affect the serotonergic neurotransmitter systems, such as serotonin reuptake inhibitors).
No products indexed under this heading.

Glutethimide (Caution is advised if the concomitant administration of venlafaxine and CNS-active drugs is required).
No products indexed under this heading.

Haloperidol (Venlafaxine administered under steady-state conditions in healthy subjects decreased total oral-dose clearance of a single dose of haloperidol by 42%, which resulted in a 70% increase in haloperidol AUC and an 88% increase in Cmax).
No products indexed under this heading.

Haloperidol Decanoate (Venlafaxine administered under steady-state conditions in healthy subjects decreased total oral-dose clearance of a single dose of haloperidol by 42%, which resulted in a 70% increase in haloperidol AUC and an 88% increase in Cmax).
No products indexed under this heading.

Hydrocodone Bitartrate (Caution is advised if the concomitant administration of venlafaxine and CNS-active drugs is required). Products include:

Hycodan **1116**
Hycotuss Expectorant Syrup **1117**
Vicodin Tablets **535**
Vicodin ES Tablets **536**
Vicodin HP Tablets **538**
Vicoprofen Tablets **539**
Zydone Tablets **1139**

Hydrocodone Polistirex (Caution is advised if the concomitant administration of venlafaxine and CNS-active drugs is required). Products include:
Tussionex Pennkinetic Extended-Release Suspension **3327**

Hydromorphone Hydrochloride (Caution is advised if the concomitant administration of venlafaxine and CNS-active drugs is required). Products include:
Dilaudid **440**
Dilaudid Non-Sterile Powder **440**
Dilaudid Oral Liquid **445**
Dilaudid Rectal Suppositories **440**
Dilaudid Tablets **440**
Dilaudid Tablets - 8 mg **445**
Dilaudid-HP **442**

Hydroxyzine Hydrochloride (Caution is advised if the concomitant administration of venlafaxine and CNS-active drugs is required).
No products indexed under this heading.

Hypericum (Caution is advised when velafaxine is coadministered with other drugs that may affect serotonergic neurotransmitter systems). Products include:
Satiete Tablets ▩**832**

Hypericum Perforatum (Caution is advised when velafaxine is coadministered with other drugs that may affect serotonergic neurotransmitter systems).
No products indexed under this heading.

Indinavir Sulfate (Co-administration has resulted in a 28% decrease in the AUC and 36% decrease in the indinavir Cmax; the clinical significance of these findings is unknown). Products include:
Crixivan Capsules **1940**

Isocarboxazid (Adverse reactions, some of which were serious, have been reported in patients who have recently been discontinued from an MAO inhibitor and started on venlafaxine, or who have recently had venlafaxine therapy discontinued prior to initiation of an MAO inhibitor; concurrent and/or sequential use is contraindicated).
No products indexed under this heading.

Isoflurane (Caution is advised if the concomitant administration of venlafaxine and CNS-active drugs is required).
No products indexed under this heading.

Ketamine Hydrochloride (Caution is advised if the concomitant administration of venlafaxine and CNS-active drugs is required).
No products indexed under this heading.

Levomethadyl Acetate Hydrochloride (Caution is advised if the concomitant administration of venlafaxine and CNS-active drugs is required).
No products indexed under this heading.

(▩ Described in PDR For Nonprescription Drugs) (⊙ Described in PDR For Ophthalmic Medicines™)

Levorphanol Tartrate (Caution is advised if the concomitant administration of venlafaxine and CNS-active drugs is required).

No products indexed under this heading.

Lithium Carbonate (Based on the mechanism of action of venlafaxine and the potential for serotonin syndrome, caution is advised when velafaxine is co-administered with other drugs that may affect the serotonergic neurotransmitter systems, such as lithium). Products include:

Lithobid Tablets 1692

Lithium Citrate (Based on the mechanism of action of venlafaxine and the potential for serotonin syndrome, caution is advised when velafaxine is co-administered with other drugs that may affect the serotonergic neurotransmitter systems, such as lithium).

No products indexed under this heading.

Lorazepam (Caution is advised if the concomitant administration of venlafaxine and CNS-active drugs is required).

No products indexed under this heading.

Loxapine Hydrochloride (Caution is advised if the concomitant administration of venlafaxine and CNS-active drugs is required).

No products indexed under this heading.

Loxapine Succinate (Caution is advised if the concomitant administration of venlafaxine and CNS-active drugs is required).

No products indexed under this heading.

Meperidine Hydrochloride (Caution is advised if the concomitant administration of venlafaxine and CNS-active drugs is required).

No products indexed under this heading.

Mephobarbital (Caution is advised if the concomitant administration of venlafaxine and CNS-active drugs is required).

No products indexed under this heading.

Meprobamate (Caution is advised if the concomitant administration of venlafaxine and CNS-active drugs is required).

No products indexed under this heading.

Mesoridazine Besylate (Caution is advised if the concomitant administration of venlafaxine and CNS-active drugs is required).

No products indexed under this heading.

Methadone Hydrochloride (Caution is advised if the concomitant administration of venlafaxine and CNS-active drugs is required).

No products indexed under this heading.

Methamphetamine Hydrochloride (Caution is advised if the concomitant administration of venlafaxine and CNS-active drugs is required). Products include:

Desoxyn Tablets, USP 2462

Methohexital Sodium (Caution is advised if the concomitant administration of venlafaxine and CNS-active drugs is required).

No products indexed under this heading.

Methotrimeprazine (Caution is advised if the concomitant administration of venlafaxine and CNS-active drugs is required).

No products indexed under this heading.

Methoxyflurane (Caution is advised if the concomitant administration of venlafaxine and CNS-active drugs is required).

No products indexed under this heading.

Methylphenidate (Caution is advised if the concomitant administration of venlafaxine and CNS-active drugs is required). Products include:

Daytrana Transdermal Patch 3174

Methylphenidate Hydrochloride (Caution is advised if the concomitant administration of venlafaxine and CNS-active drugs is required). Products include:

Concerta Extended-Release Tablets .. 1881
Metadate CD Capsules 3323
Ritalin Hydrochloride Tablets 2269
Ritalin LA Capsules 2271
Ritalin-SR Tablets 2269

Midazolam Hydrochloride (Caution is advised if the concomitant administration of venlafaxine and CNS-active drugs is required).

No products indexed under this heading.

Moclobemide (Adverse reactions, some of which were serious, have been reported in patients who have recently been discontinued from an MAO inhibitor and started on venlafaxine, or who have recently had venlafaxine therapy discontinued prior to initiation of an MAO inhibitor; concurrent and/or sequential use is contraindicated).

No products indexed under this heading.

Molindone Hydrochloride (Caution is advised if the concomitant administration of venlafaxine and CNS-active drugs is required). Products include:

Moban Tablets 1119

Morphine Sulfate (Caution is advised if the concomitant administration of venlafaxine and CNS-active drugs is required). Products include:

Avinza Capsules 1741
Kadian Capsules 577
MS Contin Tablets 2701

Naratriptan Hydrochloride (Based on the mechanism of action of venlafaxine and the potential for serotonin syndrome, caution is advised when velafaxine is co-administered with other drugs that may affect the serotonergic neurotransmitter systems, such as triptans). Products include:

Amerge Tablets 1339

Nefazodone Hydrochloride (Based on the mechanism of action of venlafaxine and the potential for serotonin syndrome, caution is advised when venlafaxine is co-administered with other drugs that may affect serotonergic neurotransmitter systems, such as serotonin-norepinephrine reuptake inhibitors).

No products indexed under this heading.

Olanzapine (Caution is advised if the concomitant administration of venlafaxine and CNS-active drugs is required). Products include:

Symbyax Capsules 1819
Zyprexa Tablets 1830
Zyprexa IntraMuscular 1830

Zyprexa ZYDIS Orally Disintegrating Tablets.................. 1830

Oxazepam (Caution is advised if the concomitant administration of venlafaxine and CNS-active drugs is required).

No products indexed under this heading.

Oxycodone Hydrochloride (Caution is advised if the concomitant administration of venlafaxine and CNS-active drugs is required). Products include:

OxyContin Tablets 2703
OxyFast Oral Concentrate Solution..................................... 2708
OxyIR Capsules 2708
Percocet Tablets 1131
Percodan Tablets 1132

Pargyline Hydrochloride (Adverse reactions, some of which were serious, have been reported in patients who have recently been discontinued from an MAO inhibitor and started on venlafaxine, or who have recently had venlafaxine therapy discontinued prior to initiation of an MAO inhibitor; concurrent and/or sequential use is contraindicated).

No products indexed under this heading.

Paroxetine Hydrochloride (Based on the mechanism of action of venlafaxine and the potential for serotonin syndrome, caution is advised when velafaxine is co-administered with other drugs that may affect the serotonergic neurotransmitter systems, such as serotonin reuptake inhibitors). Products include:

Paxil CR Controlled-Release Tablets .. 1538
Paxil .. 1530

Pemoline (Caution is advised if the concomitant administration of venlafaxine and CNS-active drugs is required).

No products indexed under this heading.

Pentobarbital Sodium (Caution is advised if the concomitant administration of venlafaxine and CNS-active drugs is required). Products include:

Nembutal Sodium Solution, USP 2470

Perphenazine (Caution is advised if the concomitant administration of venlafaxine and CNS-active drugs is required).

No products indexed under this heading.

Phenelzine Sulfate (Adverse reactions, some of which were serious, have been reported in patients who have recently been discontinued from an MAO inhibitor and started on venlafaxine, or who have recently had venlafaxine therapy discontinued prior to initiation of an MAO inhibitor; concurrent and/or sequential use is contraindicated).

No products indexed under this heading.

Phenobarbital (Caution is advised if the concomitant administration of venlafaxine and CNS-active drugs is required). Products include:

Donnatal Extentabs 2493

Prazepam (Caution is advised if the concomitant administration of venlafaxine and CNS-active drugs is required).

No products indexed under this heading.

Procarbazine Hydrochloride (Adverse reactions, some of which were serious, have been reported in patients who have recently been discontinued from an MAO inhibitor and

started on venlafaxine, or who have recently had venlafaxine therapy discontinued prior to initiation of an MAO inhibitor; concurrent and/or sequential use is contraindicated). Products include:

Matulane Capsules 3191

Prochlorperazine (Caution is advised if the concomitant administration of venlafaxine and CNS-active drugs is required).

No products indexed under this heading.

Promethazine Hydrochloride (Caution is advised if the concomitant administration of venlafaxine and CNS-active drugs is required). Products include:

Phenergan Tablets and Suppositories.............................. 3440

Propofol (Caution is advised if the concomitant administration of venlafaxine and CNS-active drugs is required).

No products indexed under this heading.

Propoxyphene Hydrochloride (Caution is advised if the concomitant administration of venlafaxine and CNS-active drugs is required).

No products indexed under this heading.

Propoxyphene Napsylate (Caution is advised if the concomitant administration of venlafaxine and CNS-active drugs is required).

No products indexed under this heading.

Quazepam (Caution is advised if the concomitant administration of venlafaxine and CNS-active drugs is required).

No products indexed under this heading.

Quetiapine Fumarate (Caution is advised if the concomitant administration of venlafaxine and CNS-active drugs is required). Products include:

Seroquel Tablets 690

Quinidine (Venlafaxine is metabolized to its active metabolite, ODV, by CYP2D6; therefore, the potential exists for a drug interaction between the inhibitors of CYP2D6, such as quinidine and venlafaxine, resulting in increased plasma concentrations of venlafaxine and decreased concentrations of the active metabolite).

No products indexed under this heading.

Quinidine Gluconate (Venlafaxine is metabolized to its active metabolite, ODV, by CYP2D6; therefore, the potential exists for a drug interaction between the inhibitors of CYP2D6, such as quinidine and venlafaxine, resulting in increased plasma concentrations of venlafaxine and decreased concentrations of the active metabolite).

No products indexed under this heading.

Quinidine Hydrochloride (Venlafaxine is metabolized to its active metabolite, ODV, by CYP2D6; therefore, the potential exists for a drug interaction between the inhibitors of CYP2D6, such as quinidine and venlafaxine, resulting in increased plasma concentrations of venlafaxine and decreased concentrations of the active metabolite).

No products indexed under this heading.

IMPORTANT NOTE: Always consult each drug listing in the patient's regimen for possible interactions.

Quinidine Polygalacturonate (Venlafaxine is metabolized to its active metabolite, ODV, by CYP2D6; therefore, the potential exists for a drug interaction between the inhibitors of CYP2D6, such as quinidine and venlafaxine, resulting in increased plasma concentrations of venlafaxine and decreased concentrations of the active metabolite).
No products indexed under this heading.

Quinidine Sulfate (Venlafaxine is metabolized to its active metabolite, ODV, by CYP2D6; therefore, the potential exists for a drug interaction between the inhibitors of CYP2D6, such as quinidine and venlafaxine, resulting in increased plasma concentrations of venlafaxine and decreased concentrations of the active metabolite).
No products indexed under this heading.

Remifentanil Hydrochloride (Caution is advised if the concomitant administration of venlafaxine and CNS-active drugs is required).
No products indexed under this heading.

Risperidone (Venlafaxine slightly inhibits the CYP2D6-mediated metabolism of risperidone resulting in an approximate 32% increase in risperidone AUC). Products include:
Risperdal 1676
Risperdal Consta Long-Acting Injection 1682
Risperdal M-Tab Orally Disintegrating Tablets 1676

Rizatriptan Benzoate (Based on the mechanism of action of venlafaxine and the potential for serotonin syndrome, caution is advised when velafaxine is co-administered with other drugs that may affect the serotonergic neurotransmitter systems, such as triptans). Products include:
Maxalt Tablets 2008
Maxalt-MLT Orally Disintegrating Tablets 2008

Secobarbital Sodium (Caution is advised if the concomitant administration of venlafaxine and CNS-active drugs is required).
No products indexed under this heading.

Selegiline Hydrochloride (Adverse reactions, some of which were serious, have been reported in patients who have recently been discontinued from an MAO inhibitor and started on venlafaxine, or who have recently had venlafaxine therapy discontinued prior to initiation of an MAO inhibitor; concurrent and/or sequential use is contraindicated). Products include:
Eldepryl Capsules 3208
Zelapar Tablets 3372

Sertraline Hydrochloride (Based on the mechanism of action of venlafaxine and the potential for serotonin syndrome, caution is advised when velafaxine is co-administered with other drugs that may affect the serotonergic neurotransmitter systems, such as serotonin reuptake inhibitors). Products include:
Zoloft 2586

Sevoflurane (Caution is advised if the concomitant administration of venlafaxine and CNS-active drugs is required). Products include:
Ultane Liquid for Inhalation 531

Sodium Oxybate (Caution is advised if the concomitant administration of venlafaxine and CNS-active drugs is required). Products include:
Xyrem Oral Solution 1688

Sufentanil Citrate (Caution is advised if the concomitant administration of venlafaxine and CNS-active drugs is required).
No products indexed under this heading.

Sumatriptan (Based on the mechanism of action of venlafaxine and the potential for serotonin syndrome, caution is advised when velafaxine is co-administered with other drugs that may affect the serotonergic neurotransmitter systems, such as triptans). Products include:
Imitrex Nasal Spray 1467

Sumatriptan Succinate (Based on the mechanism of action of venlafaxine and the potential for serotonin syndrome, caution is advised when velafaxine is co-administered with other drugs that may affect the serotonergic neurotransmitter systems, such as triptans). Products include:
Imitrex Injection 1463
Imitrex Tablets 1471

Temazepam (Caution is advised if the concomitant administration of venlafaxine and CNS-active drugs is required). Products include:
Restoril Capsules 1860

Thiamylal Sodium (Caution is advised if the concomitant administration of venlafaxine and CNS-active drugs is required).
No products indexed under this heading.

Thioridazine Hydrochloride (Caution is advised if the concomitant administration of venlafaxine and CNS-active drugs is required). Products include:
Thioridazine Hydrochloride Tablets 2163

Thiothixene (Caution is advised if the concomitant administration of venlafaxine and CNS-active drugs is required). Products include:
Thiothixene Capsules 2165

Tramadol Hydrochloride (Caution is advised when velafaxine is coadministered with other drugs that may affect serotonergic neurotransmitter systems). Products include:
Ultram ER Tablets 2392

Tranylcypromine Sulfate (Adverse reactions, some of which were serious, have been reported in patients who have recently been discontinued from an MAO inhibitor and started on venlafaxine, or who have recently had venlafaxine therapy discontinued prior to initiation of an MAO inhibitor; concurrent and/or sequential use is contraindicated). Products include:
Parnate Tablets 1527

Triazolam (Caution is advised if the concomitant administration of venlafaxine and CNS-active drugs is required).
No products indexed under this heading.

Trifluoperazine Hydrochloride (Caution is advised if the concomitant administration of venlafaxine and CNS-active drugs is required).
No products indexed under this heading.

Tryptophan (Caution is advised when velafaxine is coadministered with other drugs that may affect serotonergic neurotransmitter systems).
No products indexed under this heading.

L-Tryptophan (Caution is advised when velafaxine is coadministered with other drugs that may affect serotonergic neurotransmitter systems). Products include:
L-Tryptophan Capsules 2145

Warfarin Sodium (There have been reports of increases in prothrombin time, partial thromboplastin time, or INR when venlafaxine was given to patients receiving warfarin therapy). Products include:
Coumadin for Injection 898
Coumadin Tablets 898

Zaleplon (Caution is advised if the concomitant administration of venlafaxine and CNS-active drugs is required). Products include:
Sonata Capsules 1717

Ziprasidone Hydrochloride (Caution is advised if the concomitant administration of venlafaxine and CNS-active drugs is required). Products include:
Geodon Capsules 2529

Zolmitriptan (Based on the mechanism of action of venlafaxine and the potential for serotonin syndrome, caution is advised when velafaxine is co-administered with other drugs that may affect the serotonergic neurotransmitter systems, such as triptans). Products include:
Zomig Tablets 3519
Zomig Nasal Spray 3523
Zomig-ZMT Tablets 3519

Zolpidem Tartrate (Caution is advised if the concomitant administration of venlafaxine and CNS-active drugs is required). Products include:
Ambien Tablets 2851
Ambien CR Tablets 2855

Food Interactions

Alcohol (Co-administration of venlafaxine as a stable regimen did not exaggerate the psychomotor and psychometric effects of alcohol; however, patients should be advised to avoid alcohol while taking venlafaxine).

EFUDEX TOPICAL CREAM

(Fluorouracil) 3363
None cited in PDR database.

EFUDEX TOPICAL SOLUTIONS

(Fluorouracil) 3363
None cited in PDR database.

ELDEPRYL CAPSULES

(Selegiline Hydrochloride) 3208
May interact with narcotic analgesics, selective serotonin reuptake inhibitors, tricyclic antidepressants, and certain other agents. Compounds in these categories include:

Alfentanil Hydrochloride (Contraindication warning for meperidine is extended to other opioids).
No products indexed under this heading.

Amitriptyline Hydrochloride (Co-administraton has resulted in severe CNS toxicity associated with hyperpyrexia and fatality; concurrent use in some patients may result in hypertension, syncope, asystole, diaphoresis seizures, changes in behavioral and mental status, and muscular rigidity; concurrent and/or sequential use is not recommended).
No products indexed under this heading.

Amoxapine (Co-administration may result in hypertension, syncope, asystole, diaphoresis seizures, changes in behavioral and mental status, and muscular rigidity; concurrent and/or sequential use is not recommended).
No products indexed under this heading.

Buprenorphine Hydrochloride (Contraindication warning for meperidine is extended to other opioids). Products include:
Buprenex Injectable 2716
Suboxone Tablets 2717
Subutex Tablets 2717

Citalopram Hydrobromide (Potential for serious, sometimes fatal, reactions including hyperthermia, rigidity, myoclonus, autonomic instability, extreme agitation progressing to delirium and coma; concurrent and/or sequential use is not recommended). Products include:
Celexa 1176

Clomipramine Hydrochloride (Co-administration may result in hypertension, syncope, asystole, diaphoresis seizures, changes in behavioral and mental status, and muscular rigidity; concurrent and/or sequential use is not recommended).
No products indexed under this heading.

Codeine Phosphate (Contraindication warning for meperidine is extended to other opioids). Products include:
Tylenol with Codeine Tablets 2391

Desipramine Hydrochloride (Co-administration may result in hypertension, syncope, asystole, diaphoresis seizures, changes in behavioral and mental status, and muscular rigidity; concurrent and/or sequential use is not recommended).
No products indexed under this heading.

Dezocine (Contraindication warning for meperidine is extended to other opioids).
No products indexed under this heading.

Doxepin Hydrochloride (Co-administration may result in hypertension, syncope, asystole, diaphoresis seizures, changes in behavioral and mental status, and muscular rigidity; concurrent and/or sequential use is not recommended).
No products indexed under this heading.

Ephedrine Hydrochloride (Co-administration has resulted in one case of hypertensive crisis).
No products indexed under this heading.

Ephedrine Sulfate (Co-administration has resulted in one case of hypertensive crisis).
No products indexed under this heading.

Ephedrine Tannate (Co-administration has resulted in one case of hypertensive crisis).
No products indexed under this heading.

Fentanyl (Contraindication warning for meperidine is extended to other opioids). Products include:
- Duragesic Transdermal System **2373**
- Ionsys Transdermal System **2379**

Fentanyl Citrate (Contraindication warning for meperidine is extended to other opioids). Products include:
- Actiq **979**

Fluoxetine Hydrochloride (Co-administration has resulted in serious, sometimes fatal, reactions including hyperthermia, rigidity, myoclonus, autonomic instability, extreme agitation progressing to delirium and coma; concurrent and/or sequential use is not recommended; because of long half-life of fluoxetine, at least 5 weeks or longer should elapse between discontinuation of fluoxetine and initiation of Eldepryl). Products include:
- Prozac Pulvules and Liquid **1801**
- Symbyax Capsules **1819**

Fluvoxamine Maleate (Potential for serious, sometimes fatal, reactions including hyperthermia, rigidity, myoclonus, autonomic instability, extreme agitation progressing to delirium and coma; concurrent and/or sequential use is not recommended).
No products indexed under this heading.

Hydrocodone Bitartrate (Contraindication warning for meperidine is extended to other opioids). Products include:
- Hycodan **1116**
- Hycotuss Expectorant Syrup **1117**
- Vicodin Tablets **535**
- Vicodin ES Tablets **536**
- Vicodin HP Tablets **538**
- Vicoprofen Tablets **539**
- Zydone Tablets **1139**

Hydrocodone Polistirex (Contraindication warning for meperidine is extended to other opioids). Products include:
- Tussionex Pennkinetic Extended-Release Suspension...... **3327**

Hydromorphone Hydrochloride (Contraindication warning for meperidine is extended to other opioids). Products include:
- Dilaudid **440**
- Dilaudid Non-Sterile Powder **440**
- Dilaudid Oral Liquid **445**
- Dilaudid Rectal Suppositories **440**
- Dilaudid Tablets **440**
- Dilaudid Tablets - 8 mg **445**
- Dilaudid-HP **442**

Imipramine Hydrochloride (Co-administration may result in hypertension, syncope, asystole, diaphoresis seizures, changes in behavioral and mental status, and muscular rigidity; concurrent and/or sequential use is not recommended).
No products indexed under this heading.

Imipramine Pamoate (Co-administration may result in hypertension, syncope, asystole, diaphoresis seizures, changes in behavioral and mental status, and muscular rigidity; concurrent and/or sequential use is not recommended).
No products indexed under this heading.

Levodopa (Co-administration in some patients may exacerbate levodopa-associated side effects). Products include:
- Parcopa Orally Disintegrating Tablets **3097**
- Stalevo Tablets **2287**

Levorphanol Tartrate (Contraindication warning for meperidine is extended to other opioids).
No products indexed under this heading.

Maprotiline Hydrochloride (Co-administration may result in hypertension, syncope, asystole, diaphoresis seizures, changes in behavioral and mental status, and muscular rigidity; concurrent and/or sequential use is not recommended).
No products indexed under this heading.

Meperidine Hydrochloride (Co-administration has resulted in stupor, muscular rigidity, severe agitation, hallucination, and hyperpyrexia; concurrent use is contraindicated).
No products indexed under this heading.

Methadone Hydrochloride (Contraindication warning for meperidine is extended to other opioids).
No products indexed under this heading.

Morphine Sulfate (Contraindication warning for meperidine is extended to other opioids). Products include:
- Avinza Capsules **1741**
- Kadian Capsules **577**
- MS Contin Tablets **2701**

Nortriptyline Hydrochloride (Co-administration may result in hypertension, syncope, asystole, diaphoresis seizures, changes in behavioral and mental status, and muscular rigidity; concurrent and/or sequential use is not recommended).
No products indexed under this heading.

Oxycodone Hydrochloride (Contraindication warning for meperidine is extended to other opioids). Products include:
- OxyContin Tablets **2703**
- OxyFast Oral Concentrate Solution....................................... **2708**
- OxyIR Capsules **2708**
- Percocet Tablets **1131**
- Percodan Tablets **1132**

Paroxetine Hydrochloride (Potential for serious, sometimes fatal, reactions including hyperthermia, rigidity, myoclonus, autonomic instability, extreme agitation progressing to delirium and coma; concurrent and/or sequential use is not recommended). Products include:
- Paxil CR Controlled-Release Tablets **1538**
- Paxil **1530**

Propoxyphene Hydrochloride (Contraindication warning for meperidine is extended to other opioids).
No products indexed under this heading.

Propoxyphene Napsylate (Contraindication warning for meperidine is extended to other opioids).
No products indexed under this heading.

Protriptyline Hydrochloride (Co-administration has resulted in tremors, agitation, and restlessness followed by unresponsiveness and fatality; concurrent use in some patients may result in hypertension, syncope, asystole, diaphoresis seizures, changes in behavioral and mental status, and muscular rigidity; concurrent and/or sequential use is not recommended).
No products indexed under this heading.

Sertraline Hydrochloride (Potential for serious, sometimes fatal, reactions including hyperthermia, rigidity, myoclonus, autonomic instability, extreme agitation progressing to delirium and coma; concurrent and/or sequential use is not recommended). Products include:
- Zoloft **2586**

Sufentanil Citrate (Contraindication warning for meperidine is extended to other opioids).
No products indexed under this heading.

Trimipramine Maleate (Co-administration may result in hypertension, syncope, asystole, diaphoresis seizures, changes in behavioral and mental status, and muscular rigidity; concurrent and/or sequential use is not recommended).
No products indexed under this heading.

Venlafaxine Hydrochloride (Potential for serious, sometimes fatal, reactions including hyperthermia, rigidity, myoclonus, autonomic instability, extreme agitation progressing to delirium and coma; concurrent and/or sequential use is not recommended). Products include:
- Effexor Tablets **3411**
- Effexor XR Capsules **3417**

Food Interactions

Food, unspecified (The bioavailability of selegiline is increased 3 to 4 fold when it is taken with food).

ELDERTONIC
(Vitamins with Minerals) **2126**
None cited in PDR database.

ELESTAT OPHTHALMIC SOLUTION
(Epinastine Hydrochloride) **1669**
None cited in PDR database.

ELIDEL CREAM 1%
(Pimecrolimus) **2200**
None cited in PDR database.

ELIGARD 7.5 MG
(Leuprolide Acetate) **2880**
None cited in PDR database.

ELIGARD 22.5 MG
(Leuprolide Acetate) **2883**
None cited in PDR database.

ELIGARD 30 MG
(Leuprolide Acetate) **2885**
None cited in PDR database.

ELIGARD 45 MG
(Leuprolide Acetate) **2888**
None cited in PDR database.

ELITEK
(Rasburicase) **2890**
None cited in PDR database.

ELMIRON CAPSULES
(Pentosan Polysulfate Sodium) **2415**
May interact with anticoagulants, thrombolytics, and certain other agents. Compounds in these categories include:

Alteplase (Pentosan polysulfate sodium is a weak anticoagulant and bleeding complications of ecchymosis, epistaxis and gum hemorrhage have been reported with its use; caution should be exercised in patients with increased risk of bleeding due to other concomitant therapies, such as thrombolytics). Products include:
- Activase I.V. **1223**
- Cathflo Activase **1231**

Anisindione (Pentosan polysulfate sodium is a weak anticoagulant and bleeding complications of ecchymosis, epistaxis and gum hemorrhage have been reported with its use; caution should be exercised in patients with increased risk of bleeding due to other concomitant therapies, such as anticoagulants). Products include:
- Miradon Tablets **3042**

Anistreplase (Pentosan polysulfate sodium is a weak anticoagulant and bleeding complications of ecchymosis, epistaxis and gum hemorrhage have been reported with its use; caution should be exercised in patients with increased risk of bleeding due to other concomitant therapies, such as thrombolytics).
No products indexed under this heading.

Ardeparin Sodium (Pentosan polysulfate sodium is a weak anticoagulant and bleeding complications of ecchymosis, epistaxis and gum hemorrhage have been reported with its use; caution should be exercised in patients with increased risk of bleeding due to other concomitant therapies, such as anticoagulants).
No products indexed under this heading.

Aspirin (Pentosan polysulfate sodium is a weak anticoagulant and bleeding complications of ecchymosis, epistaxis and gum hemorrhage have been reported with its use; caution should be exercised in patients with increased risk of bleeding due to other concomitant therapies, such as high dose aspirin). Products include:
- Aggrenox Capsules **822**
- Bayer Aspirin **744**
- BC Allergy Sinus Cold Powder **677**
- BC Headache Powder **677**
- Arthritis Strength BC Powder **677**
- BC Sinus Cold Powder **677**
- Excedrin Extra Strength Caplets/Tablets/Geltabs............ **684**
- Excedrin Migraine Caplets/Tablets/Geltabs............ **609**
- Goody's Body Pain Formula Powder... **684**
- Goody's Extra Strength Headache Powders.................... **611**
- Goody's Extra Strength Pain Relief Tablets **685**
- Percodan Tablets **1132**
- St. Joseph 81 mg Aspirin Chewable and Enteric Coated Tablets **1869**

Dalteparin Sodium (Pentosan polysulfate sodium is a weak anticoagulant and bleeding complications of ecchymosis, epistaxis and gum hemorrhage have been reported with its use; caution should be exercised in patients with increased risk of bleeding due to other concomitant therapies, such as anticoagulants). Products include:

Fragmin Injection 1097

Danaparoid Sodium (Pentosan polysulfate sodium is a weak anticoagulant and bleeding complications of ecchymosis, epistaxis and gum hemorrhage have been reported with its use; caution should be exercised in patients with increased risk of bleeding due to other concomitant therapies, such as anticoagulants).
No products indexed under this heading.

Dicumarol (Pentosan polysulfate sodium is a weak anticoagulant and bleeding complications of ecchymosis, epistaxis and gum hemorrhage have been reported with its use; caution should be exercised in patients with increased risk of bleeding due to other concomitant therapies, such as anticoagulants).
No products indexed under this heading.

Enoxaparin Sodium (Pentosan polysulfate sodium is a weak anticoagulant and bleeding complications of ecchymosis, epistaxis and gum hemorrhage have been reported with its use; caution should be exercised in patients with increased risk of bleeding due to other concomitant therapies, such as anticoagulants). Products include:
Lovenox Injection 2915

Fondaparinux Sodium (Pentosan polysulfate sodium is a weak anticoagulant and bleeding complications of ecchymosis, epistaxis and gum hemorrhage have been reported with its use; caution should be exercised in patients with increased risk of bleeding due to other concomitant therapies, such as anticoagulants). Products include:
Arixtra Injection 1351

Heparin Calcium (Pentosan polysulfate sodium is a weak anticoagulant and bleeding complications of ecchymosis, epistaxis and gum hemorrhage have been reported with its use; caution should be exercised in patients with increased risk of bleeding due to other concomitant therapies, such as anticoagulants).
No products indexed under this heading.

Heparin Sodium (Pentosan polysulfate sodium is a weak anticoagulant and bleeding complications of ecchymosis, epistaxis and gum hemorrhage have been reported with its use; caution should be exercised in patients with increased risk of bleeding due to other concomitant therapies, such as anticoagulants).
No products indexed under this heading.

Low Molecular Weight Heparins (Pentosan polysulfate sodium is a weak anticoagulant and bleeding complications of ecchymosis, epistaxis and gum hemorrhage have been reported with its use; caution should be exercised in patients with increased risk of bleeding due to other concomitant therapies, such as anticoagulants).
No products indexed under this heading.

Reteplase (Pentosan polysulfate sodium is a weak anticoagulant and bleeding complications of ecchymosis, epistaxis and gum hemorrhage have been reported with its use; caution should be exercised in patients with increased risk of bleeding due to other concomitant therapies, such as thrombolytics). Products include:
Retavase 2499

Streptokinase (Pentosan polysulfate sodium is a weak anticoagulant and bleeding complications of ecchymosis, epistaxis and gum hemorrhage have been reported with its use; caution should be exercised in patients with increased risk of bleeding due to other concomitant therapies, such as thrombolytics).
No products indexed under this heading.

Tinzaparin Sodium (Pentosan polysulfate sodium is a weak anticoagulant and bleeding complications of ecchymosis, epistaxis and gum hemorrhage have been reported with its use; caution should be exercised in patients with increased risk of bleeding due to other concomitant therapies, such as anticoagulants).
No products indexed under this heading.

Urokinase (Pentosan polysulfate sodium is a weak anticoagulant and bleeding complications of ecchymosis, epistaxis and gum hemorrhage have been reported with its use; caution should be exercised in patients with increased risk of bleeding due to other concomitant therapies, such as thrombolytics).
No products indexed under this heading.

Warfarin Sodium (Pentosan polysulfate sodium is a weak anticoagulant and bleeding complications of ecchymosis, epistaxis and gum hemorrhage have been reported with its use; caution should be exercised in patients with increased risk of bleeding due to other concomitant therapies, such as anticoagulants). Products include:
Coumadin for Injection 898
Coumadin Tablets 898

ELOCON CREAM 0.1%

(Mometasone Furoate) 3005
None cited in PDR database.

ELOCON LOTION 0.1%

(Mometasone Furoate) 3006
None cited in PDR database.

ELOCON OINTMENT 0.1%

(Mometasone Furoate) 3007
None cited in PDR database.

ELOXATIN FOR INJECTION

(Oxaliplatin) 2892
May interact with anticoagulants and certain other agents. Compounds in these categories include:

Anisindione (Prolongation of prothrombin time and of INR occasionally associated with hemorrhage in patients receiving anticoagulants has been reported with oxaliplatin plus 5-FU/LV). Products include:
Miradon Tablets 3042

Ardeparin Sodium (Prolongation of prothrombin time and of INR occasionally associated with hemorrhage in patients receiving anticoagulants has been reported with oxaliplatin plus 5-FU/LV).
No products indexed under this heading.

Dalteparin Sodium (Prolongation of prothrombin time and of INR occasionally associated with hemorrhage in patients receiving anticoagulants has been reported with oxaliplatin plus 5-FU/LV). Products include:
Fragmin Injection 1097

Danaparoid Sodium (Prolongation of prothrombin time and of INR occasionally associated with hemorrhage in patients receiving anticoagulants has been reported with oxaliplatin plus 5-FU/LV).
No products indexed under this heading.

Dicumarol (Prolongation of prothrombin time and of INR occasionally associated with hemorrhage in patients receiving anticoagulants has been reported with oxaliplatin plus 5-FU/LV).
No products indexed under this heading.

Enoxaparin Sodium (Prolongation of prothrombin time and of INR occasionally associated with hemorrhage in patients receiving anticoagulants has been reported with oxaliplatin plus 5-FU/LV). Products include:
Lovenox Injection 2915

Fondaparinux Sodium (Prolongation of prothrombin time and of INR occasionally associated with hemorrhage in patients receiving anticoagulants has been reported with oxaliplatin plus 5-FU/LV). Products include:
Arixtra Injection 1351

Heparin Calcium (Prolongation of prothrombin time and of INR occasionally associated with hemorrhage in patients receiving anticoagulants has been reported with oxaliplatin plus 5-FU/LV).
No products indexed under this heading.

Heparin Sodium (Prolongation of prothrombin time and of INR occasionally associated with hemorrhage in patients receiving anticoagulants has been reported with oxaliplatin plus 5-FU/LV).
No products indexed under this heading.

Low Molecular Weight Heparins (Prolongation of prothrombin time and of INR occasionally associated with hemorrhage in patients receiving anticoagulants has been reported with oxaliplatin plus 5-FU/LV).
No products indexed under this heading.

Nephrotoxic Drugs (Co-administration with nephrotoxic drugs may decrease renal clearance although this has not been studied).
No products indexed under this heading.

Tinzaparin Sodium (Prolongation of prothrombin time and of INR occasionally associated with hemorrhage in patients receiving anticoagulants has been reported with oxaliplatin plus 5-FU/LV).
No products indexed under this heading.

Warfarin Sodium (Prolongation of prothrombin time and of INR occasionally associated with hemorrhage in patients receiving anticoagulants has been reported with oxaliplatin plus 5-FU/LV). Products include:
Coumadin for Injection 898
Coumadin Tablets 898

ELSPAR FOR INJECTION

(Asparaginase) 2463
May interact with:

Methotrexate Sodium (Tissue culture and animal studies indicate that asparaginase can diminish or abolish the effect of methotrexate on malignant cells).
No products indexed under this heading.

Prednisone (The administration of asparaginase intravenously and concurrently with or immediately before a course of prednisone may be associated with increased toxicity).
No products indexed under this heading.

Vincristine Sulfate (The administration of asparaginase intravenously and concurrently with or immediately before a course of prednisone may be associated with increased toxicity).
No products indexed under this heading.

ELSPAR FOR INJECTION

(Asparaginase) 1960
May interact with:

Methotrexate Sodium (Tissue culture and animal studies indicate that asparaginase can diminish or abolish the effect of methotrexate on malignant cells).
No products indexed under this heading.

Prednisone (The administration of asparaginase intravenously and concurrently with or immediately before a course of prednisone may be associated with increased toxicity).
No products indexed under this heading.

Vincristine Sulfate (The administration of asparaginase intravenously and concurrently with or immediately before a course of prednisone may be associated with increased toxicity).
No products indexed under this heading.

EMCYT CAPSULES

(Estramustine Phosphate Sodium) 2634
May interact with calcium preparations and certain other agents. Compounds in these categories include:

Calcium Carbonate (Calcium-rich drugs may impair the absorption of estramustine). Products include:
Actonel with Calcium Tablets 2688
Calcet Tablets 2138
Caltrate 600 PLUS .... ▣809
Caltrate 600 + D Tablets .... ▣809
D-Cal Chewable Caplets .... ▣812
Gas-X with Maalox .... ▣656
Maalox Regular Strength Antacid Chewable Tablets 2177
Maalox Max Maximum Strength Antacid/Antigas Chewable Tablets 2176
Maalox Max Maximum Strength Chewable Tablets .... ▣660
Os-Cal Chewable Tablets .... ▣818
Pepcid Complete Chewable Tablets 1701
Children's Pepto 2674
PremCal Light, Regular, and Extra Strength Tablets .... ▣818
Tums .... ▣664

Calcium Chloride (Calcium-rich drugs may impair the absorption of estramustine).
No products indexed under this heading.

Calcium Citrate (Calcium-rich drugs may impair the absorption of estramustine). Products include:
- Active Calcium Tablets 3339
- Citracal Caplets .... ◙ 703
- Citracal Lemon Cream Creamy Bites 2139
- Citracal Prenatal + DHA Tablets and Capsules 2139

Calcium Glubionate (Calcium-rich drugs may impair the absorption of estramustine).
No products indexed under this heading.

Food Interactions

Dairy products (Calcium-rich foods may impair the absorption of estramustine).

Food, calcium-rich (Calcium-rich foods may impair the absorption of estramustine).

EMEND CAPSULES

(Aprepitant) 1963

May interact with benzodiazepine that are metabolized by CYP3A4, cytochrome p450 3a4 inducers (selected), cytochrome p450 3a4 inhibitors (selected), dexamethasone, methylprednisolone, oral contraceptives, phenytoin, and certain other agents. Compounds in these categories include:

Acetazolamide (Co-administration of EMEND with drugs that inhibit CYP3A4 activity may result in increased plasma concentrations of aprepitant and should be approached with caution).
No products indexed under this heading.

Allium sativum (Co-administration of EMEND with drugs that strongly induce CYP3A4 activity may result in reduced plasma concentrations of aprepitant that may result in decreased efficacy of EMEND).
No products indexed under this heading.

Alprazolam (The potential effects of increased plasma concentrations of midazolam or other benzodiazepines metabolized via CYP3A4 (alprazolam, triazolam) should be considered when co-administering these agents with EMEND). Products include:
- Niravam Orally Disintegrating Tablets 3092

Amiodarone Hydrochloride (Co-administration of EMEND with drugs that inhibit CYP3A4 activity may result in increased plasma concentrations of aprepitant and should be approached with caution).
No products indexed under this heading.

Amprenavir (Co-administration of EMEND with drugs that inhibit CYP3A4 activity may result in increased plasma concentrations of aprepitant and should be approached with caution). Products include:
- Agenerase Capsules 1327
- Agenerase Oral Solution 1332

Anastrozole (Co-administration of EMEND with drugs that inhibit CYP3A4 activity may result in increased plasma concentrations of aprepitant and should be approached with caution). Products include:
- Arimidex Tablets 673

Astemizole (EMEND is a moderate CYP3A4 inhibitor; concurrent use with EMEND could result in elevated plasma concentrations of astemizole, potentially causing serious or life-threatening reactions, and is contraindicated).
No products indexed under this heading.

Betamethasone Acetate (Co-administration of EMEND with drugs that strongly induce CYP3A4 activity may result in reduced plasma concentrations of aprepitant that may result in decreased efficacy of EMEND).
No products indexed under this heading.

Betamethasone Sodium Phosphate (Co-administration of EMEND with drugs that strongly induce CYP3A4 activity may result in reduced plasma concentrations of aprepitant that may result in decreased efficacy of EMEND).
No products indexed under this heading.

Carbamazepine (Co-administration of EMEND with drugs that strongly induce CYP3A4 activity may result in reduced plasma concentrations of aprepitant that may result in decreased efficacy of EMEND). Products include:
- Carbatrol Capsules 3171
- Equetro Extended-Release Capsules 3180
- Tegretol/Tegretol-XR 2295

Cimetidine (Co-administration of EMEND with drugs that inhibit CYP3A4 activity may result in increased plasma concentrations of aprepitant and should be approached with caution). Products include:
- Tagamet HB 200 Tablets .... ◙ 664

Cimetidine Hydrochloride (Co-administration of EMEND with drugs that inhibit CYP3A4 activity may result in increased plasma concentrations of aprepitant and should be approached with caution).
No products indexed under this heading.

Ciprofloxacin (Co-administration of EMEND with drugs that inhibit CYP3A4 activity may result in increased plasma concentrations of aprepitant and should be approached with caution). Products include:
- Cipro Oral Suspension 2977
- Cipro I.V. 2984
- Cipro XR Tablets 2990
- Ciprodex Otic Suspension 559

Ciprofloxacin Hydrochloride (Co-administration of EMEND with drugs that strongly induce CYP3A4 activity may result in reduced plasma concentrations of aprepitant that may result in decreased efficacy of EMEND). Products include:
- Ciloxan Ophthalmic Ointment 559
- Ciloxan Ophthalmic Solution .... ⊙ 206
- Cipro Tablets 2977
- Proquin XR Tablets 1153

Cisapride (EMEND is a moderate CYP3A4 inhibitor; concurrent use with EMEND could result in elevated plasma concentrations of cisapride, potentially causing serious or life-threatening reactions, and is contraindicated).
No products indexed under this heading.

Cisplatin (Co-administration of EMEND with drugs that strongly induce CYP3A4 activity may result in reduced plasma concentrations of aprepitant that may result in decreased efficacy of EMEND).
No products indexed under this heading.

Clarithromycin (Co-administration of EMEND with drugs that inhibit CYP3A4 activity may result in increased plasma concentrations of aprepitant and should be approached with caution). Products include:
- Biaxin/Biaxin XL 402
- PREVPAC 3284

Clotrimazole (Co-administration of EMEND with drugs that inhibit CYP3A4 activity may result in increased plasma concentrations of aprepitant and should be approached with caution). Products include:
- Desenex Athlete's Foot Cream .... ◙ 635
- Lotrimin 3039
- Lotrisone 3040

Cortisone Acetate (Co-administration of EMEND with drugs that strongly induce CYP3A4 activity may result in reduced plasma concentrations of aprepitant that may result in decreased efficacy of EMEND).
No products indexed under this heading.

Cyclosporine (Co-administration of EMEND with drugs that inhibit CYP3A4 activity may result in increased plasma concentrations of aprepitant and should be approached with caution). Products include:
- Gengraf Capsules 459
- Neoral Oral Solution 2259
- Neoral Soft Gelatin Capsules 2259
- Restasis Ophthalmic Emulsion 575
- Sandimmune 2275

Dalfopristin (Co-administration of EMEND with drugs that inhibit CYP3A4 activity may result in increased plasma concentrations of aprepitant and should be approached with caution).
No products indexed under this heading.

Danazol (Co-administration of EMEND with drugs that inhibit CYP3A4 activity may result in increased plasma concentrations of aprepitant and should be approached with caution).
No products indexed under this heading.

Delavirdine Mesylate (Co-administration of EMEND with drugs that inhibit CYP3A4 activity may result in increased plasma concentrations of aprepitant and should be approached with caution). Products include:
- Rescriptor Tablets 2551

Desogestrel (The co-administration of aprepitant may reduce the efficacy of hormonal contraceptives during and for 28 days after administration of the last dose of aprepitant. Alternative or back-up methods of contraception should be used during treatment with aprepitant and for one month following the last dose of aprepitant). Products include:
- Mircette Tablets 1066

Dexamethasone (The oral dexamethasone doses should be reduced by approximately 50% when co-administered with EMEND to achieve exposures of dexamethasone similar to those obtained when it is given without EMEND). Products include:
- Ciprodex Otic Suspension 559
- Decadron Tablets 1951
- TobraDex Ophthalmic Ointment 562
- TobraDex Ophthalmic Suspension 563

Dexamethasone Acetate (The oral dexamethasone doses should be reduced by approximately 50% when co-administered with EMEND to achieve exposures of dexamethasone similar to those obtained when it is given without EMEND).
No products indexed under this heading.

Dexamethasone Sodium Phosphate (The oral dexamethasone doses should be reduced by approximately 50% when co-administered with EMEND to achieve exposures of dexamethasone similar to those obtained when it is given without EMEND).
No products indexed under this heading.

Diazepam (The potential effects of increased plasma concentrations of midazolam or other benzodiazepines metabolized via CYP3A4 (alprazolam, triazolam) should be considered when co-administering these agents with EMEND). Products include:
- Diastat Rectal Delivery System 3343
- Valium Tablets 2819

Diltiazem Hydrochloride (Co-administration of EMEND with drugs that inhibit CYP3A4 activity may result in increased plasma concentrations of aprepitant and should be approached with caution). Products include:
- Cardizem LA Extended Release Tablets 1728
- Tiazac Capsules 1201

Diltiazem Maleate (Co-administration of EMEND with drugs that inhibit CYP3A4 activity may result in increased plasma concentrations of aprepitant and should be approached with caution).
No products indexed under this heading.

Doxorubicin Hydrochloride (Co-administration of EMEND with drugs that strongly induce CYP3A4 activity may result in reduced plasma concentrations of aprepitant that may result in decreased efficacy of EMEND).
No products indexed under this heading.

Efavirenz (Co-administration of EMEND with drugs that inhibit CYP3A4 activity may result in increased plasma concentrations of aprepitant and should be approached with caution). Products include:
- Atripla Tablets 945
- Sustiva Capsules 930
- Sustiva Tablets 930

Erythromycin (Co-administration of EMEND with drugs that inhibit CYP3A4 activity may result in increased plasma concentrations of aprepitant and should be approached with caution). Products include:
- Ery-Tab Tablets 449
- Erythromycin Base Filmtab Tablets 455
- Erythromycin Delayed-Release Capsules, USP 457
- PCE Dispertab Tablets 515

Erythromycin Estolate (Co-administration of EMEND with drugs that inhibit CYP3A4 activity may result in increased plasma concentrations of aprepitant and should be approached with caution).
No products indexed under this heading.

Erythromycin Ethylsuccinate (Co-administration of EMEND with drugs that inhibit CYP3A4 activity may result in increased plasma concentrations of aprepitant and should be approached with caution). Products include:
E.E.S. 451
EryPed 447

Erythromycin Gluceptate (Co-administration of EMEND with drugs that inhibit CYP3A4 activity may result in increased plasma concentrations of aprepitant and should be approached with caution).
No products indexed under this heading.

Erythromycin Lactobionate (Co-administration of EMEND with drugs that inhibit CYP3A4 activity may result in increased plasma concentrations of aprepitant and should be approached with caution).
No products indexed under this heading.

Erythromycin Stearate (Co-administration of EMEND with drugs that inhibit CYP3A4 activity may result in increased plasma concentrations of aprepitant and should be approached with caution). Products include:
Erythrocin Stearate Filmtab Tablets 453

Esomeprazole Magnesium (Co-administration of EMEND with drugs that inhibit CYP3A4 activity may result in increased plasma concentrations of aprepitant and should be approached with caution). Products include:
Nexium Delayed-Release Capsules 655

Ethinyl Estradiol (The co-administration of aprepitant may reduce the efficacy of hormonal contraceptives during and for 28 days after administration of the last dose of aprepitant. Alternative or back-up methods of contraception should be used during treatment with aprepitant and for one month following the last dose of aprepitant). Products include:
Mircette Tablets 1066
NuvaRing 2340
Ortho-Cyclen/Ortho Tri-Cyclen 2429
Ortho Evra Transdermal System 2417
Ortho Tri-Cyclen Lo Tablets 2436
Seasonique Tablets 1077
Yasmin 28 Tablets 796
Yaz Tablets 803

Ethosuximide (Co-administration of EMEND with drugs that strongly induce CYP3A4 activity may result in reduced plasma concentrations of aprepitant that may result in decreased efficacy of EMEND).
No products indexed under this heading.

Ethynodiol Diacetate (The co-administration of aprepitant may reduce the efficacy of hormonal contraceptives during and for 28 days after administration of the last dose of aprepitant. Alternative or back-up methods of contraception should be used during treatment with aprepitant and for one month following the last dose of aprepitant).
No products indexed under this heading.

Etoposide (Particular caution and careful monitoring are advised in patients receiving chemotherapy agents metabolized primarily by CYP3A4, like etoposide).
No products indexed under this heading.

Felbamate (Co-administration of EMEND with drugs that strongly induce CYP3A4 activity may result in reduced plasma concentrations of aprepitant that may result in decreased efficacy of EMEND).
No products indexed under this heading.

Fluconazole (Co-administration of EMEND with drugs that inhibit CYP3A4 activity may result in increased plasma concentrations of aprepitant and should be approached with caution).
No products indexed under this heading.

Fludrocortisone Acetate (Co-administration of EMEND with drugs that strongly induce CYP3A4 activity may result in reduced plasma concentrations of aprepitant that may result in decreased efficacy of EMEND).
No products indexed under this heading.

Fluoxetine Hydrochloride (Co-administration of EMEND with drugs that inhibit CYP3A4 activity may result in increased plasma concentrations of aprepitant and should be approached with caution). Products include:
Prozac Pulvules and Liquid 1801
Symbyax Capsules 1819

Fluvoxamine Maleate (Co-administration of EMEND with drugs that inhibit CYP3A4 activity may result in increased plasma concentrations of aprepitant and should be approached with caution).
No products indexed under this heading.

Fosamprenavir Calcium (Co-administration of EMEND with drugs that inhibit CYP3A4 activity may result in increased plasma concentrations of aprepitant and should be approached with caution). Products include:
Lexiva Tablets 1505

Fosphenytoin Sodium (Aprepitant is an inducer of CYP2C9; co-administration has been shown to induce the metabolism of tolbutamide which is metabolized through CYP2C9).
No products indexed under this heading.

Garlic Extract (Co-administration of EMEND with drugs that strongly induce CYP3A4 activity may result in reduced plasma concentrations of aprepitant that may result in decreased efficacy of EMEND).
No products indexed under this heading.

Garlic Oil (Co-administration of EMEND with drugs that strongly induce CYP3A4 activity may result in reduced plasma concentrations of aprepitant that may result in decreased efficacy of EMEND).
No products indexed under this heading.

Hydrocortisone (Co-administration of EMEND with drugs that strongly induce CYP3A4 activity may result in reduced plasma concentrations of aprepitant that may result in decreased efficacy of EMEND). Products include:
Colocort Rectal Suspension, USP (Retention) 100 mg/60 mL 2476
Hydrocortone Tablets 1989
Preparation H Hydrocortisone Cream .... ▣646

Hydrocortisone Acetate (Co-administration of EMEND with drugs that strongly induce CYP3A4 activity may result in reduced plasma concentrations of aprepitant that may result in decreased efficacy of EMEND). Products include:
Analpram-HC 1159
Pramosone 1161
ProctoFoam-HC 3099

Hydrocortisone Butyrate (Co-administration of EMEND with drugs that strongly induce CYP3A4 activity may result in reduced plasma concentrations of aprepitant that may result in decreased efficacy of EMEND). Products include:
Locoid Lipocream Cream 1160

Hydrocortisone Cypionate (Co-administration of EMEND with drugs that strongly induce CYP3A4 activity may result in reduced plasma concentrations of aprepitant that may result in decreased efficacy of EMEND).
No products indexed under this heading.

Hydrocortisone Hemisuccinate (Co-administration of EMEND with drugs that strongly induce CYP3A4 activity may result in reduced plasma concentrations of aprepitant that may result in decreased efficacy of EMEND).
No products indexed under this heading.

Hydrocortisone Probutate (Co-administration of EMEND with drugs that strongly induce CYP3A4 activity may result in reduced plasma concentrations of aprepitant that may result in decreased efficacy of EMEND).
No products indexed under this heading.

Hydrocortisone Sodium Phosphate (Co-administration of EMEND with drugs that strongly induce CYP3A4 activity may result in reduced plasma concentrations of aprepitant that may result in decreased efficacy of EMEND).
No products indexed under this heading.

Hydrocortisone Sodium Succinate (Co-administration of EMEND with drugs that strongly induce CYP3A4 activity may result in reduced plasma concentrations of aprepitant that may result in decreased efficacy of EMEND).
No products indexed under this heading.

Hydrocortisone Valerate (Co-administration of EMEND with drugs that strongly induce CYP3A4 activity may result in reduced plasma concentrations of aprepitant that may result in decreased efficacy of EMEND).
No products indexed under this heading.

Hypericum (Co-administration of EMEND with drugs that strongly induce CYP3A4 activity may result in reduced plasma concentrations of aprepitant that may result in decreased efficacy of EMEND). Products include:
Satiete Tablets .... ▣832

Hypericum Perforatum (Co-administration of EMEND with drugs that strongly induce CYP3A4 activity may result in reduced plasma concentrations of aprepitant that may result in decreased efficacy of EMEND).
No products indexed under this heading.

Ifosfamide (Particular caution and careful monitoring are advised in patients receiving chemotherapy agents metabolized primarily by CYP3A4, like ifosfamide).
No products indexed under this heading.

Imatinib Mesylate (Particular caution and careful monitoring are advised in patients receiving chemotherapy agents metabolized primarily by CYP3A4, like imatinib). Products include:
Gleevec Tablets 2227

Indinavir Sulfate (Co-administration of EMEND with drugs that inhibit CYP3A4 activity may result in increased plasma concentrations of aprepitant and should be approached with caution). Products include:
Crixivan Capsules 1940

Irinotecan Hydrochloride (Particular caution and careful monitoring are advised in patients receiving chemotherapy agents metabolized primarily by CYP3A4, like irinotecan). Products include:
Camptosar Injection 2604

Isoniazid (Co-administration of EMEND with drugs that inhibit CYP3A4 activity may result in increased plasma concentrations of aprepitant and should be approached with caution).
No products indexed under this heading.

Itraconazole (Co-administration of EMEND with drugs that inhibit CYP3A4 activity may result in increased plasma concentrations of aprepitant and should be approached with caution).
No products indexed under this heading.

Ketoconazole (Co-administration of EMEND with drugs that inhibit CYP3A4 activity may result in increased plasma concentrations of aprepitant and should be approached with caution). Products include:
Nizoral A-D Shampoo, 1% 1868

Levonorgestrel (The co-administration of aprepitant may reduce the efficacy of hormonal contraceptives during and for 28 days after administration of the last dose of aprepitant. Alternative or back-up methods of contraception should be used during treatment with aprepitant and for one month following the last dose of aprepitant). Products include:
Climara Pro Transdermal System 776
Mirena Intrauterine System 787
Plan B Tablets 1076
Seasonique Tablets 1077

Lopinavir (Co-administration of EMEND with drugs that inhibit CYP3A4 activity may result in increased plasma concentrations of aprepitant and should be approached with caution). Products include:
Kaletra 476

Loratadine (Co-administration of EMEND with drugs that inhibit CYP3A4 activity may result in increased plasma concentrations of aprepitant and should be approached with caution). Products include:

- Alavert Allergy & Sinus D-12 Hour Tablets 771
- Alavert 771
- Children's Claritin Allergy Oral Solution 771
- Claritin Non-Drowsy 24 Hour Tablets 772
- Claritin Reditabs 24 Hour Non-Drowsy Tablets 772
- Claritin-D Non-Drowsy 12 Hour Tablets 772
- Claritin-D Non-Drowsy 24 Hour Tablets 772

Mephenytoin (Co-administration of EMEND with drugs that strongly induce CYP3A4 activity may result in reduced plasma concentrations of aprepitant that may result in decreased efficacy of EMEND).

No products indexed under this heading.

Mestranol (The co-administration of aprepitant may reduce the efficacy of hormonal contraceptives during and for 28 days after administration of the last dose of aprepitant. Alternative or back-up methods of contraception should be used during treatment with aprepitant and for one month following the last dose of aprepitant).

No products indexed under this heading.

Methsuximide (Co-administration of EMEND with drugs that strongly induce CYP3A4 activity may result in reduced plasma concentrations of aprepitant that may result in decreased efficacy of EMEND).

No products indexed under this heading.

Methylprednisolone (The IV methylprednisolone doses should be reduced by approximately 25% and the oral methylprednisolone dose should be reduced by approximately 50% when co-administered with EMEND to achieve exposures of methylprednisolone similar to those obtained when it is given without EMEND).

No products indexed under this heading.

Methylprednisolone Acetate (The IV methylprednisolone doses should be reduced by approximately 25% and the oral methylprednisolone dose should be reduced by approximately 50% when co-administered with EMEND to achieve exposures of methylprednisolone similar to those obtained when it is given without EMEND). Products include:

- Depo-Medrol Injectable Suspension 2617
- Depo-Medrol Single-Dose Vial 2619

Methylprednisolone Sodium Succinate (The IV methylprednisolone doses should be reduced by approximately 25% and the oral methylprednisolone dose should be reduced by approximately 50% when co-administered with EMEND to achieve exposures of methylprednisolone similar to those obtained when it is given without EMEND).

No products indexed under this heading.

Metronidazole (Co-administration of EMEND with drugs that inhibit CYP3A4 activity may result in increased plasma concentrations of aprepitant and should be approached with caution). Products include:

- Metrogel 1% 1211
- MetroGel-Vaginal Gel 1855
- Vandazole Vaginal Gel 3338

Metronidazole Benzoate (Co-administration of EMEND with drugs that inhibit CYP3A4 activity may result in increased plasma concentrations of aprepitant and should be approached with caution).

No products indexed under this heading.

Metronidazole Hydrochloride (Co-administration of EMEND with drugs that inhibit CYP3A4 activity may result in increased plasma concentrations of aprepitant and should be approached with caution).

No products indexed under this heading.

Miconazole (Co-administration of EMEND with drugs that inhibit CYP3A4 activity may result in increased plasma concentrations of aprepitant and should be approached with caution).

No products indexed under this heading.

Miconazole Nitrate (Co-administration of EMEND with drugs that inhibit CYP3A4 activity may result in increased plasma concentrations of aprepitant and should be approached with caution). Products include:

- Desenex 635
- Desenex Jock Itch Spray Powder ... 635

Midazolam Hydrochloride (The potential effects of increased plasma concentrations of midazolam or other benzodiazepines metabolized via CYP3A4 (alprazolam, triazolam) should be considered when co-administering these agents with EMEND).

No products indexed under this heading.

Modafinil (Co-administration of EMEND with drugs that strongly induce CYP3A4 activity may result in reduced plasma concentrations of aprepitant that may result in decreased efficacy of EMEND). Products include:

- Provigil Tablets 988

Nefazodone Hydrochloride (Co-administration of EMEND with drugs that inhibit CYP3A4 activity may result in increased plasma concentrations of aprepitant and should be approached with caution).

No products indexed under this heading.

Nelfinavir Mesylate (Co-administration of EMEND with drugs that inhibit CYP3A4 activity may result in increased plasma concentrations of aprepitant and should be approached with caution). Products include:

- Viracept 2577

Nevirapine (Co-administration of EMEND with drugs that inhibit CYP3A4 activity may result in increased plasma concentrations of aprepitant and should be approached with caution). Products include:

- Viramune Oral Suspension 873
- Viramune Tablets 873

Niacinamide (Co-administration of EMEND with drugs that inhibit CYP3A4 activity may result in increased plasma concentrations of aprepitant and should be approached with caution).

No products indexed under this heading.

Nicotinamide (Co-administration of EMEND with drugs that inhibit CYP3A4 activity may result in increased plasma concentrations of aprepitant and should be approached with caution). Products include:

- Nicomide Tablets 1088

Nifedipine (Co-administration of EMEND with drugs that inhibit CYP3A4 activity may result in increased plasma concentrations of aprepitant and should be approached with caution). Products include:

- Adalat CC Tablets 2964

Norethindrone (The co-administration of aprepitant may reduce the efficacy of hormonal contraceptives during and for 28 days after administration of the last dose of aprepitant. Alternative or back-up methods of contraception should be used during treatment with aprepitant and for one month following the last dose of aprepitant). Products include:

- Ortho Micronor Tablets 2426

Norethynodrel (The co-administration of aprepitant may reduce the efficacy of hormonal contraceptives during and for 28 days after administration of the last dose of aprepitant. Alternative or back-up methods of contraception should be used during treatment with aprepitant and for one month following the last dose of aprepitant).

No products indexed under this heading.

Norfloxacin (Co-administration of EMEND with drugs that inhibit CYP3A4 activity may result in increased plasma concentrations of aprepitant and should be approached with caution). Products include:

- Noroxin Tablets 2032

Norgestimate (The co-administration of aprepitant may reduce the efficacy of hormonal contraceptives during and for 28 days after administration of the last dose of aprepitant. Alternative or back-up methods of contraception should be used during treatment with aprepitant and for one month following the last dose of aprepitant). Products include:

- Ortho-Cyclen/Ortho Tri-Cyclen 2429
- Ortho Tri-Cyclen Lo Tablets 2436

Norgestrel (The co-administration of aprepitant may reduce the efficacy of hormonal contraceptives during and for 28 days after administration of the last dose of aprepitant. Alternative or back-up methods of contraception should be used during treatment with aprepitant and for one month following the last dose of aprepitant).

No products indexed under this heading.

Omeprazole (Co-administration of EMEND with drugs that inhibit CYP3A4 activity may result in increased plasma concentrations of aprepitant and should be approached with caution). Products include:

- Zegerid Capsules 2958
- Zegerid Powder for Oral Solution 2958

Oxcarbazepine (Co-administration of EMEND with drugs that strongly induce CYP3A4 activity may result in reduced plasma concentrations of aprepitant that may result in decreased efficacy of EMEND). Products include:

- Trileptal Tablets 2300
- Trileptal Oral Suspension 2300

Paclitaxel (Particular caution and careful monitoring are advised in patients receiving chemotherapy agents metabolized primarily by CYP3A4, like paclitaxel).

No products indexed under this heading.

Paroxetine Hydrochloride (Co-administration resulted in a decrease in AUC by approximately 25% and Cmax by approximately 20% of both aprepitant and paroxetine). Products include:

- Paxil CR Controlled-Release Tablets 1538
- Paxil 1530

Phenobarbital (Co-administration of EMEND with drugs that strongly induce CYP3A4 activity may result in reduced plasma concentrations of aprepitant that may result in decreased efficacy of EMEND). Products include:

- Donnatal Extentabs 2493

Phenobarbital Sodium (Co-administration of EMEND with drugs that strongly induce CYP3A4 activity may result in reduced plasma concentrations of aprepitant that may result in decreased efficacy of EMEND).

No products indexed under this heading.

Phenytoin (Aprepitant is an inducer of CYP2C9; co-administration has been shown to induce the metabolism of tolbutamide which is metabolized through CYP2C9).

No products indexed under this heading.

Phenytoin Sodium (Aprepitant is an inducer of CYP2C9; co-administration has been shown to induce the metabolism of tolbutamide which is metabolized through CYP2C9). Products include:

- Phenytek Capsules 2160

Pimozide (EMEND is a moderate CYP3A4 inhibitor; concurrent use with EMEND could result in elevated plasma concentrations of pimozide, potentially causing serious or life-threatening reactions, and is contraindicated).

No products indexed under this heading.

Prednisolone Acetate (Co-administration of EMEND with drugs that strongly induce CYP3A4 activity may result in reduced plasma concentrations of aprepitant that may result in decreased efficacy of EMEND). Products include:

- Blephamide Ophthalmic Ointment 568
- Blephamide Ophthalmic Suspension 569
- Poly-Pred Ophthalmic Suspension .... ⊙233
- Pred Forte Ophthalmic Suspension .... ⊙235
- Pred Mild Ophthalmic Suspension .... ⊙238
- Pred-G Ophthalmic Ointment .... ⊙237
- Pred-G Ophthalmic Suspension .... ⊙236

Prednisolone Sodium Phosphate (Co-administration of EMEND with drugs that strongly induce CYP3A4 activity may result in reduced plasma concentrations of aprepitant that may result in decreased efficacy of EMEND).
No products indexed under this heading.

Prednisolone Tebutate (Co-administration of EMEND with drugs that strongly induce CYP3A4 activity may result in reduced plasma concentrations of aprepitant that may result in decreased efficacy of EMEND).
No products indexed under this heading.

Prednisone (Co-administration of EMEND with drugs that strongly induce CYP3A4 activity may result in reduced plasma concentrations of aprepitant that may result in decreased efficacy of EMEND).
No products indexed under this heading.

Primidone (Co-administration of EMEND with drugs that strongly induce CYP3A4 activity may result in reduced plasma concentrations of aprepitant that may result in decreased efficacy of EMEND).
No products indexed under this heading.

Propoxyphene Hydrochloride (Co-administration of EMEND with drugs that inhibit CYP3A4 activity may result in increased plasma concentrations of aprepitant and should be approached with caution).
No products indexed under this heading.

Propoxyphene Napsylate (Co-administration of EMEND with drugs that inhibit CYP3A4 activity may result in increased plasma concentrations of aprepitant and should be approached with caution).
No products indexed under this heading.

Quinidine (Co-administration of EMEND with drugs that inhibit CYP3A4 activity may result in increased plasma concentrations of aprepitant and should be approached with caution).
No products indexed under this heading.

Quinidine Hydrochloride (Co-administration of EMEND with drugs that inhibit CYP3A4 activity may result in increased plasma concentrations of aprepitant and should be approached with caution).
No products indexed under this heading.

Quinidine Polygalacturonate (Co-administration of EMEND with drugs that inhibit CYP3A4 activity may result in increased plasma concentrations of aprepitant and should be approached with caution).
No products indexed under this heading.

Quinidine Sulfate (Co-administration of EMEND with drugs that inhibit CYP3A4 activity may result in increased plasma concentrations of aprepitant and should be approached with caution).
No products indexed under this heading.

Quinine (Co-administration of EMEND with drugs that inhibit CYP3A4 activity may result in increased plasma concentrations of aprepitant and should be approached with caution).
No products indexed under this heading.

Quinine Sulfate (Co-administration of EMEND with drugs that inhibit CYP3A4 activity may result in increased plasma concentrations of aprepitant and should be approached with caution).
No products indexed under this heading.

Quinupristin (Co-administration of EMEND with drugs that inhibit CYP3A4 activity may result in increased plasma concentrations of aprepitant and should be approached with caution).
No products indexed under this heading.

Ranitidine Bismuth Citrate (Co-administration of EMEND with drugs that inhibit CYP3A4 activity may result in increased plasma concentrations of aprepitant and should be approached with caution).
No products indexed under this heading.

Ranitidine Hydrochloride (Co-administration of EMEND with drugs that inhibit CYP3A4 activity may result in increased plasma concentrations of aprepitant and should be approached with caution). Products include:
Zantac 1624
Zantac Injection 1619
Zantac Injection Pharmacy Bulk Package 1622

Rifabutin (Co-administration of EMEND with drugs that strongly induce CYP3A4 activity may result in reduced plasma concentrations of aprepitant that may result in decreased efficacy of EMEND).
No products indexed under this heading.

Rifampicin (Co-administration of EMEND with drugs that strongly induce CYP3A4 activity may result in reduced plasma concentrations of aprepitant that may result in decreased efficacy of EMEND).
No products indexed under this heading.

Rifampin (Co-administration of EMEND with drugs that strongly induce CYP3A4 activity may result in reduced plasma concentrations of aprepitant that may result in decreased efficacy of EMEND).
No products indexed under this heading.

Rifapentine (Co-administration of EMEND with drugs that strongly induce CYP3A4 activity may result in reduced plasma concentrations of aprepitant that may result in decreased efficacy of EMEND).
No products indexed under this heading.

Ritonavir (Co-administration of EMEND with drugs that inhibit CYP3A4 activity may result in increased plasma concentrations of aprepitant and should be approached with caution). Products include:
Kaletra 476
Norvir 503

Saquinavir (Co-administration of EMEND with drugs that inhibit CYP3A4 activity may result in increased plasma concentrations of aprepitant and should be approached with caution).
No products indexed under this heading.

Saquinavir Mesylate (Co-administration of EMEND with drugs that inhibit CYP3A4 activity may result in increased plasma concentrations of aprepitant and should be approached with caution). Products include:
Invirase 2772

Sertraline Hydrochloride (Co-administration of EMEND with drugs that inhibit CYP3A4 activity may result in increased plasma concentrations of aprepitant and should be approached with caution). Products include:
Zoloft 2586

Sulfinpyrazone (Co-administration of EMEND with drugs that strongly induce CYP3A4 activity may result in reduced plasma concentrations of aprepitant that may result in decreased efficacy of EMEND).
No products indexed under this heading.

Telithromycin (Co-administration of EMEND with drugs that inhibit CYP3A4 activity may result in increased plasma concentrations of aprepitant and should be approached with caution). Products include:
Ketek Tablets 2903

Terfenadine (EMEND is a moderate CYP3A4 inhibitor; concurrent use with EMEND could result in elevated plasma concentrations of terfenadine, potentially causing serious or life-threatening reactions, and is contraindicated).
No products indexed under this heading.

Theophylline (Co-administration of EMEND with drugs that strongly induce CYP3A4 activity may result in reduced plasma concentrations of aprepitant that may result in decreased efficacy of EMEND).
No products indexed under this heading.

Tolbutamide (Aprepitant is an inducer of CYP2C9; co-administration has been shown to induce the metabolism of tolbutamide which is metabolized through CYP2C9).
No products indexed under this heading.

Triamcinolone (Co-administration of EMEND with drugs that strongly induce CYP3A4 activity may result in reduced plasma concentrations of aprepitant that may result in decreased efficacy of EMEND).
No products indexed under this heading.

Triamcinolone Acetonide (Co-administration of EMEND with drugs that strongly induce CYP3A4 activity may result in reduced plasma concentrations of aprepitant that may result in decreased efficacy of EMEND). Products include:
Azmacort Inhalation Aerosol 1726
Nasacort AQ Nasal Spray 2922

Triamcinolone Diacetate (Co-administration of EMEND with drugs that strongly induce CYP3A4 activity may result in reduced plasma concentrations of aprepitant that may result in decreased efficacy of EMEND).
No products indexed under this heading.

Triamcinolone Hexacetonide (Co-administration of EMEND with drugs that strongly induce CYP3A4 activity may result in reduced plasma concentrations of aprepitant that may result in decreased efficacy of EMEND).
No products indexed under this heading.

Triazolam (The potential effects of increased plasma concentrations of midazolam or other benzodiazepines metabolized via CYP3A4 (alprazolam, triazolam) should be considered when co-administering these agents with EMEND).
No products indexed under this heading.

Troglitazone (Co-administration of EMEND with drugs that inhibit CYP3A4 activity may result in increased plasma concentrations of aprepitant and should be approached with caution).
No products indexed under this heading.

Troleandomycin (Co-administration of EMEND with drugs that inhibit CYP3A4 activity may result in increased plasma concentrations of aprepitant and should be approached with caution).
No products indexed under this heading.

Valproate Sodium (Co-administration of EMEND with drugs that inhibit CYP3A4 activity may result in increased plasma concentrations of aprepitant and should be approached with caution). Products include:
Depacon Injection 412

Verapamil Hydrochloride (Co-administration of EMEND with drugs that inhibit CYP3A4 activity may result in increased plasma concentrations of aprepitant and should be approached with caution). Products include:
Covera-HS Tablets 3139
Tarka Tablets 524
Verelan PM Extended-Release Capsules, Controlled-Onset 3106

Vinblastine Sulfate (Particular caution and careful monitoring are advised in patients receiving chemotherapy agents metabolized primarily by CYP3A4, like vinblastine).
No products indexed under this heading.

Vincristine Sulfate (Particular caution and careful monitoring are advised in patients receiving chemotherapy agents metabolized primarily by CYP3A4, like vincristine).
No products indexed under this heading.

Vinorelbine Tartrate (Particular caution and careful monitoring are advised in patients receiving chemotherapy agents metabolized primarily by CYP3A4, like vinorelbine).
No products indexed under this heading.

Voriconazole (Co-administration of EMEND with drugs that inhibit CYP3A4 activity may result in increased plasma concentrations of

aprepitant and should be approached with caution). Products include:
- VFEND I.V. 2564
- VFEND Oral Suspension 2564
- VFEND Tablets 2564

Warfarin Sodium (Aprepitant is an inducer of CYP2C9; co-administration has been shown to induce the metabolism of S(-) warfarin which is metabolized through CYP2C9; may result in a clinically significant decrease in INR of prothrombin time). Products include:
- Coumadin for Injection 898
- Coumadin Tablets 898

Zafirlukast (Co-administration of EMEND with drugs that inhibit CYP3A4 activity may result in increased plasma concentrations of aprepitant and should be approached with caution). Products include:
- Accolate Tablets 671

Zileuton (Co-administration of EMEND with drugs that inhibit CYP3A4 activity may result in increased plasma concentrations of aprepitant and should be approached with caution). Products include:
- Zyflo Tablets 1023

Food Interactions

Grapefruit (Co-administration of EMEND with drugs that inhibit CYP3A4 activity may result in increased plasma concentrations of aprepitant and should be approached with caution).

Grapefruit Juice (Co-administration of EMEND with drugs that inhibit CYP3A4 activity may result in increased plasma concentrations of aprepitant and should be approached with caution).

EMSAM TRANSDERMAL SYSTEM

(Selegiline) 903

May interact with amphetamines, general anesthetics, local anesthetics, monoamine oxidase inhibitors, narcotic analgesics, selective serotonin reuptake inhibitors, sympathomimetics, tricyclic antidepressants, and certain other agents. Compounds in these categories include:

Albuterol (Avoid concomitant use of sympathomimetic agents with selegiline transdermal system). Products include:
- Proventil Inhalation Aerosol 3053

Albuterol Sulfate (Avoid concomitant use of sympathomimetic agents with selegiline transdermal system). Products include:
- AccuNeb Inhalation Solution 1055
- Combivent Inhalation Aerosol 847
- DuoNeb Inhalation Solution 1058
- ProAir HFA Inhalation Aerosol 3300
- Proventil Inhalation Solution 0.083% 3055
- Proventil HFA Inhalation Aerosol 3056
- Ventolin HFA Inhalation Aerosol 1600
- VoSpire ER Tablets 1052

Alfentanil Hydrochloride (Selegiline transdermal system is contraindicated with analgesic agents such as tramadol, methadone, and propoxyphene).
No products indexed under this heading.

Amitriptyline Hydrochloride (Selegiline transdermal system is contraindicated with tricyclic antidepressants).
No products indexed under this heading.

Amoxapine (Selegiline transdermal system is contraindicated with tricyclic antidepressants).
No products indexed under this heading.

Amphetamine Resins (Selegiline transdermal system is contraindicated for use with sympathomimetic amines, including amphetamines).
No products indexed under this heading.

Amphetamine Sulfate (Selegiline transdermal system is contraindicated for use with sympathomimetic amines, including amphetamines). Products include:
- Adderall Tablets 3164
- Adderall XR Capsules 3166

Bupivacaine Hydrochloride (Patients taking selegiline transdermal system should not be given local anesthesia containing sympathomimetic vasoconstrictors).
No products indexed under this heading.

Buprenorphine Hydrochloride (Selegiline transdermal system is contraindicated with analgesic agents such as tramadol, methadone, and propoxyphene). Products include:
- Buprenex Injectable 2716
- Suboxone Tablets 2717
- Subutex Tablets 2717

Bupropion (Selegiline transdermal system is contraindicated with bupropion hydrochloride. Concomitant use of selegiline transdermal system and buspirone hydrochloride is not advised since several cases of elevated blood pressure have been reported in patients taking MAO inhibitors who were then given buspirone hydrochloride).
No products indexed under this heading.

Bupropion Hydrochloride (Selegiline transdermal system is contraindicated with bupropion hydrochloride. Concomitant use of selegiline transdermal system and buspirone hydrochloride is not advised since several cases of elevated blood pressure have been reported in patients taking MAO inhibitors who were then given buspirone hydrochloride). Products include:
- Wellbutrin Tablets 1603
- Wellbutrin SR Sustained-Release Tablets 1607
- Wellbutrin XL Extended-Release Tablets 1613
- Zyban Sustained-Release Tablets 1644

Carbamazepine (Carbamazepine is contraindicated in patients taking selegiline). Products include:
- Carbatrol Capsules 3171
- Equetro Extended-Release Capsules 3180
- Tegretol/Tegretol-XR 2295

Chloroprocaine Hydrochloride (Patients taking selegiline transdermal system should not be given local anesthesia containing sympathomimetic vasoconstrictors).
No products indexed under this heading.

Citalopram Hydrobromide (Selegiline transdermal system is contraindicated with selective serotonin reuptake inhibitors). Products include:
- Celexa 1176

Clomipramine Hydrochloride (Selegiline transdermal system is contraindicated with tricyclic antidepressants).
No products indexed under this heading.

Cocaine Hydrochloride (Patients taking selegiline transdermal system should not be given cocaine).
No products indexed under this heading.

Codeine Phosphate (Selegiline transdermal system is contraindicated with analgesic agents such as tramadol, methadone, and propoxyphene). Products include:
- Tylenol with Codeine Tablets 2391

Cyclobenzaprine (Selegiline transdermal system is contraindicated with cyclobenzaprine).
No products indexed under this heading.

Cyclobenzaprine Hydrochloride (Selegiline transdermal system is contraindicated with cyclobenzaprine).
No products indexed under this heading.

Desipramine Hydrochloride (Selegiline transdermal system is contraindicated with tricyclic antidepressants).
No products indexed under this heading.

Dextroamphetamine Sulfate (Selegiline transdermal system is contraindicated for use with sympathomimetic amines, including amphetamines). Products include:
- Adderall Tablets 3164
- Adderall XR Capsules 3166
- Dexedrine 1420
- DextroStat Tablets 3179

Dextromethorphan (Selegiline transdermal system is contraindicated with the antitussive agent dextromethorphan).
No products indexed under this heading.

Dextromethorphan Hydrobromide (Selegiline transdermal system is contraindicated with the antitussive agent dextromethorphan). Products include:
- Comtrex Maximum Strength Cold & Cough Day/Night Caplets - Day Formulation 726
- Comtrex Maximum Strength Cold & Cough Day/Night Caplets - Night Formulation 726
- Comtrex Maximum Strength Non-Drowsy Cold & Cough Caplets 725
- Children's Dimetapp DM Cold & Cough Elixir 731
- Children's Dimetapp Long Acting Cough Plus Cold Syrup 731
- Toddler's Dimetapp Cold and Cough Drops 732
- Mucinex DM Extended-Release Bi-Layer Tablets 720
- Refenesen DM Caplets 721
- Robitussin Cough & Cold CF Liquid 735
- Robitussin Cough & Cold Long-Acting Liquid 735
- Robitussin Cough & Allergy Syrup .. 736
- Robitussin Cough & Cold Nighttime Liquid 736
- Robitussin Cough & Cold Pediatric Drops 735
- Robitussin Cough, Cold & Flu Nighttime Liquid 738
- Robitussin Cough & Congestion Liquid 738
- Robitussin Cough Gels Long-Acting 737
- Robitussin Cough Long Acting Liquid 739
- Robitussin Cough DM Syrup 738
- Robitussin Cough DM Infant Drops 738
- Robitussin Pediatric Cough Long Acting Liquid 739
- Robitussin Pediatric Cough & Cold Long-Acting Liquid 735
- Robitussin Pediatric Cough & Cold Nighttime Liquid 736
- Robitussin Sugar Free Cough 738
- TheraFlu Cold & Cough Hot Liquid 740
- TheraFlu Warming Relief Daytime Severe Cold 743
- TheraFlu Thin Strips Long Acting Cough 744
- Triaminic Daytime Cold & Cough Liquid 745
- Triaminic Cough & Sore Throat Liquid 747
- Triaminic Cough & Runny Nose Softchews 748
- Triaminic Thin Strips Cold & Cough 778
- Triaminic Infant Thin Strips Decongestant Plus Cough 747
- Children's Tylenol Plus Flu Oral Suspension 749
- Tylenol Cold Head Congestion Daytime Caplets with Cool Burst and Gelcaps 750
- Tylenol Cold Multi-Symptom Daytime Liquid 752
- Tylenol Cold Multi-Symptom Severe Daytime Liquid 752
- Concentrated Tylenol Infants' Drops Plus Cold & Cough 754
- Children's Tylenol Plus Cough & Runny Nose Suspension Liquid 1879
- Children's Tylenol Plus Cough & Sore Throat Suspension Liquid 1879
- Children's Tylenol Plus Flu Suspension Liquid 1881
- Children's Tylenol Plus Multi-Symptom Cold Suspension Liquid 1879
- Tylenol Cold Severe Congestion Non-Drowsy Caplets with Cool Burst 1874
- Tylenol Cold Head Congestion Daytime Caplets with Cool Burst 1873
- Tylenol Cold Head Congestion Nighttime Caplets with Cool Burst 1873
- Tylenol Cold Head Congestion Severe Caplets with Cool Burst 1873
- Tylenol Cold Multi-Symptom Daytime Caplets with Cool Burst and Gelcaps 1874
- Tylenol Cold Multi-Symptom Daytime Liquid with Citrus Burst 1874
- Tylenol Cold Multi-Symptom Nighttime Caplets with Cool Burst 1874
- Tylenol Cold Multi-Symptom Nighttime Liquid with Cool Burst 1874
- Tylenol Cold Multi-Symptom Severe Caplets with Cool Burst 1874
- Tylenol Cold Multi-Symptom Severe Daytime Liquid with Citrus Burst 1874
- Tylenol Cough & Sore Throat Daytime Liquid with Cool Burst 1877
- Tylenol Cough & Sore Throat Nighttime Liquid with Cool Burst 1877
- Concentrated Tylenol Infants' Drops Plus Cold and Cough 1879
- Vicks 44 Cough Relief Liquid 2679
- Vicks 44D Cough & Head Congestion Relief Liquid 2679
- Vicks 44E Cough & Chest Congestion Relief Liquid 2679
- Pediatric Vicks 44e Cough & Chest Congestion Relief Liquid 2676
- Vicks 44M Cough, Cold & Flu Relief Liquid 2680
- Pediatric Vicks 44m Cough & Cold Relief Liquid 2676
- Vicks DayQuil LiquiCaps/Liquid Multi-Symptom Cold/Flu Relief 761
- Vicks DayQuil Multi-Symptom Cold/Flu Relief LiquiCaps 2678
- Vicks DayQuil Multi-Symptom Cold/Flu Relief Liquid 2678
- Vicks NyQuil Multi-Symptom Cold/Flu Relief Liquid 2681
- Children's Vicks NyQuil Cold/Cough Relief 756

Pseudoephedrine Tannate (Selegiline transdermal system is contraindicated for use with pseudoephedrine).
No products indexed under this heading.

Remifentanil Hydrochloride (Selegiline transdermal system is contraindicated with analgesic agents such as tramadol, methadone, and propoxyphene).
No products indexed under this heading.

Salmeterol Xinafoate (Avoid concomitant use of sympathomimetic agents with selegiline transdermal system). Products include:
Advair Diskus 100/50 1308
Advair Diskus 250/50 1308
Advair Diskus 500/50 1308
Advair HFA Inhalation Aerosol 1318
Serevent Diskus 1568

Selegiline Hydrochloride (Selegiline transdermal system should not be used with oral selegiline or other MAO inhibitors). Products include:
Eldepryl Capsules 3208
Zelapar Tablets 3372

Sertraline Hydrochloride (Selegiline transdermal system is contraindicated with selective serotonin reuptake inhibitors). Products include:
Zoloft 2586

Sevoflurane (Patients taking selegiline transdermal system should not undergo elective surgery requiring general anesthesia). Products include:
Ultane Liquid for Inhalation 531

Sufentanil Citrate (Selegiline transdermal system is contraindicated with analgesic agents such as tramadol, methadone, and propoxyphene).
No products indexed under this heading.

Terbutaline Sulfate (Avoid concomitant use of sympathomimetic agents with selegiline transdermal system).
No products indexed under this heading.

Tetracaine Hydrochloride (Patients taking selegiline transdermal system should not be given local anesthesia containing sympathomimetic vasoconstrictors). Products include:
Cetacaine Topical Anesthetic 999

Tramadol Hydrochloride (Selegiline transdermal system is contraindicated with analgesic agents such as tramadol, methadone, and propoxyphene). Products include:
Ultram ER Tablets 2392

Tranylcypromine Sulfate (Selegiline transdermal system should not be used with oral selegiline or other MAO inhibitors). Products include:
Parnate Tablets 1527

Trimipramine Maleate (Selegiline transdermal system is contraindicated with tricyclic antidepressants).
No products indexed under this heading.

Tyramine (As a class, MAO inhibitors have been associated with hypertensive crises caused by the ingestion of foods with a high concentration of tyramine).
No products indexed under this heading.

Venlafaxine Hydrochloride (Selegiline transdermal system is contraindicated with dual serotonin and norepinephrine reuptake inhibitors). Products include:
Effexor Tablets 3411
Effexor XR Capsules 3417

Food Interactions

Alcohol (The use of alcohol is not recommended while using selegiline transdermal system).

Beverages with high tyramine (As a class, MAO inhibitors have been associated with hypertensive crises caused by the ingestion of foods with a high concentration of tyramine).

Food high in tyramine (As a class, MAO inhibitors have been associated with hypertensive crises caused by the ingestion of foods with a high concentration of tyramine).

Food with high concentration of tyramine (As a class, MAO inhibitors have been associated with hypertensive crises caused by the ingestion of foods with a high concentration of tyramine).

EMTRIVA CAPSULES
(Emtricitabine) 1287
None cited in PDR database.

EMTRIVA ORAL SOLUTION
(Emtricitabine) 1287
None cited in PDR database.

ENABLEX EXTENDED-RELEASE TABLETS
(Darifenacin) 2203
May interact with anticholinergics, cytochrome p450 2d6 substrates (selected), cytochrome p450 3a4 inhibitors, potent, and certain other agents. Compounds in these categories include:

Amitriptyline Hydrochloride (Caution should be taken when darifenacin is used concomitantly with medications that are predominantly metabolized by CYP2D6 and which have a narrow therapeutic window).
No products indexed under this heading.

Amphetamine Aspartate (Caution should be taken when darifenacin is used concomitantly with medications that are predominantly metabolized by CYP2D6 and which have a narrow therapeutic window). Products include:
Adderall Tablets 3164
Adderall XR Capsules 3166

Amphetamine Aspartate Monohydrate (Caution should be taken when darifenacin is used concomitantly with medications that are predominantly metabolized by CYP2D6 and which have a narrow therapeutic window).
No products indexed under this heading.

Amphetamine Sulfate (Caution should be taken when darifenacin is used concomitantly with medications that are predominantly metabolized by CYP2D6 and which have a narrow therapeutic window). Products include:
Adderall Tablets 3164
Adderall XR Capsules 3166

Amprenavir (The daily dose of darifenacin should not exceed 7.5 mg when co-administered with potent CYP3A4 inhibitors). Products include:
Agenerase Capsules 1327
Agenerase Oral Solution 1332

Atazanavir (The daily dose of darifenacin should not exceed 7.5 mg when co-administered with potent CYP3A4 inhibitors).
No products indexed under this heading.

Atazanavir sulfate (The daily dose of darifenacin should not exceed 7.5 mg when co-administered with potent CYP3A4 inhibitors). Products include:
Reyataz Capsules 921

Atomoxetine Hydrochloride (Caution should be taken when darifenacin is used concomitantly with medications that are predominantly metabolized by CYP2D6 and which have a narrow therapeutic window). Products include:
Strattera Capsules 1814

Atropine Sulfate (The concomitant use of darifenacin with other anticholinergic agents may increase the frequency and/or severity of dry mouth, constipation, blurred vision and other anticholinergic pharmacolgical effects. Anticholinergic agents may potentially alter the absorption of some concomitantly administered drugs due to effects on gastrointestinal motility). Products include:
Donnatal Extentabs 2493

Belladonna Alkaloids (The concomitant use of darifenacin with other anticholinergic agents may increase the frequency and/or severity of dry mouth, constipation, blurred vision and other anticholinergic pharmacolgical effects. Anticholinergic agents may potentially alter the absorption of some concomitantly administered drugs due to effects on gastrointestinal motility). Products include:
Hyland's Teething Tablets .... ▣830

Benztropine Mesylate (The concomitant use of darifenacin with other anticholinergic agents may increase the frequency and/or severity of dry mouth, constipation, blurred vision and other anticholinergic pharmacolgical effects. Anticholinergic agents may potentially alter the absorption of some concomitantly administered drugs due to effects on gastrointestinal motility).
No products indexed under this heading.

Biperiden Hydrochloride (The concomitant use of darifenacin with other anticholinergic agents may increase the frequency and/or severity of dry mouth, constipation, blurred vision and other anticholinergic pharmacolgical effects. Anticholinergic agents may potentially alter the absorption of some concomitantly administered drugs due to effects on gastrointestinal motility).
No products indexed under this heading.

Bisoprolol Fumarate (Caution should be taken when darifenacin is used concomitantly with medications that are predominantly metabolized by CYP2D6 and which have a narrow therapeutic window).
No products indexed under this heading.

Captopril (Caution should be taken when darifenacin is used concomitantly with medications that are predominantly metabolized by CYP2D6 and which have a narrow therapeutic window). Products include:
Captopril Tablets 2149

Carvedilol (Caution should be taken when darifenacin is used concomitantly with medications that are predominantly metabolized by CYP2D6 and which have a narrow therapeutic window). Products include:
Coreg Tablets 1414

Cevimeline Hydrochloride (Caution should be taken when darifenacin is used concomitantly with medications that are predominantly metabolized by CYP2D6 and which have a narrow therapeutic window). Products include:
Evoxac Capsules 1047

Chlorpromazine (Caution should be taken when darifenacin is used concomitantly with medications that are predominantly metabolized by CYP2D6 and which have a narrow therapeutic window).
No products indexed under this heading.

Chlorpromazine Hydrochloride (Caution should be taken when darifenacin is used concomitantly with medications that are predominantly metabolized by CYP2D6 and which have a narrow therapeutic window).
No products indexed under this heading.

Chlorpropamide (Caution should be taken when darifenacin is used concomitantly with medications that are predominantly metabolized by CYP2D6 and which have a narrow therapeutic window).
No products indexed under this heading.

Clarithromycin (The daily dose of darifenacin should not exceed 7.5 mg when co-administered with potent CYP3A4 inhibitors). Products include:
Biaxin/Biaxin XL 402
PREVPAC 3284

Clidinium Bromide (The concomitant use of darifenacin with other anticholinergic agents may increase the frequency and/or severity of dry mouth, constipation, blurred vision and other anticholinergic pharmacolgical effects. Anticholinergic agents may potentially alter the absorption of some concomitantly administered drugs due to effects on gastrointestinal motility).
No products indexed under this heading.

Clomipramine Hydrochloride (Caution should be taken when darifenacin is used concomitantly with medications that are predominantly metabolized by CYP2D6 and which have a narrow therapeutic window).
No products indexed under this heading.

Clozapine (Caution should be taken when darifenacin is used concomitantly with medications that are predominantly metabolized by CYP2D6 and which have a narrow therapeutic window). Products include:
Clozaril Tablets 2184
FazaClo Orally Disintegrating Tablets 551

Codeine Phosphate (Caution should be taken when darifenacin is used concomitantly with medications that are predominantly metabolized

by CYP2D6 and which have a narrow therapeutic window). Products include:
Tylenol with Codeine Tablets 2391

Codeine Sulfate (Caution should be taken when darifenacin is used concomitantly with medications that are predominantly metabolized by CYP2D6 and which have a narrow therapeutic window).
No products indexed under this heading.

Cyclobenzaprine Hydrochloride (Caution should be taken when darifenacin is used concomitantly with medications that are predominantly metabolized by CYP2D6 and which have a narrow therapeutic window).
No products indexed under this heading.

Desipramine Hydrochloride (Caution should be taken when darifenacin is used concomitantly with medications that are predominantly metabolized by CYP2D6 and which have a narrow therapeutic window).
No products indexed under this heading.

Dexfenfluramine Hydrochloride (Caution should be taken when darifenacin is used concomitantly with medications that are predominantly metabolized by CYP2D6 and which have a narrow therapeutic window).
No products indexed under this heading.

Dextromethorphan Hydrobromide (Caution should be taken when darifenacin is used concomitantly with medications that are predominantly metabolized by CYP2D6 and which have a narrow therapeutic window). Products include:
Comtrex Maximum Strength Cold & Cough Day/Night Caplets - Day Formulation 726
Comtrex Maximum Strength Cold & Cough Day/Night Caplets - Night Formulation 726
Comtrex Maximum Strength Non-Drowsy Cold & Cough Caplets 725
Children's Dimetapp DM Cold & Cough Elixir 731
Children's Dimetapp Long Acting Cough Plus Cold Syrup 731
Toddler's Dimetapp Cold and Cough Drops 732
Mucinex DM Extended-Release Bi-Layer Tablets 720
Refenesen DM Caplets 721
Robitussin Cough & Cold CF Liquid 735
Robitussin Cough & Cold Long-Acting Liquid 735
Robitussin Cough & Allergy Syrup .. 736
Robitussin Cough & Cold Nighttime Liquid 736
Robitussin Cough & Cold Pediatric Drops 735
Robitussin Cough, Cold & Flu Nighttime Liquid 738
Robitussin Cough & Congestion Liquid 738
Robitussin Cough Gels Long-Acting 737
Robitussin Cough Long Acting Liquid 739
Robitussin Cough DM Syrup 738
Robitussin Cough DM Infant Drops 738
Robitussin Pediatric Cough Long Acting Liquid 739
Robitussin Pediatric Cough & Cold Long-Acting Liquid 735
Robitussin Pediatric Cough & Cold Nighttime Liquid 736
Robitussin Sugar Free Cough 738
TheraFlu Cold & Cough Hot Liquid 740
TheraFlu Warming Relief Daytime Severe Cold 743
TheraFlu Thin Strips Long Acting Cough 744
Triaminic Daytime Cold & Cough Liquid 745
Triaminic Cough & Sore Throat Liquid 747
Triaminic Cough & Runny Nose Softchews 748
Triaminic Thin Strips Cold & Cough 778
Triaminic Infant Thin Strips Decongestant Plus Cough 747
Children's Tylenol Plus Flu Oral Suspension 749
Tylenol Cold Head Congestion Daytime Caplets with Cool Burst and Gelcaps 750
Tylenol Cold Multi-Symptom Daytime Liquid 752
Tylenol Cold Multi-Symptom Severe Daytime Liquid 752
Concentrated Tylenol Infants' Drops Plus Cold & Cough 754
Children's Tylenol Plus Cough & Runny Nose Suspension Liquid 1879
Children's Tylenol Plus Cough & Sore Throat Suspension Liquid 1879
Children's Tylenol Plus Flu Suspension Liquid 1881
Children's Tylenol Plus Multi-Symptom Cold Suspension Liquid 1879
Tylenol Cold Severe Congestion Non-Drowsy Caplets with Cool Burst 1874
Tylenol Cold Head Congestion Daytime Caplets with Cool Burst 1873
Tylenol Cold Head Congestion Nighttime Caplets with Cool Burst 1873
Tylenol Cold Head Congestion Severe Caplets with Cool Burst 1873
Tylenol Cold Multi-Symptom Daytime Caplets with Cool Burst and Gelcaps 1874
Tylenol Cold Multi-Symptom Daytime Liquid with Citrus Burst ... 1874
Tylenol Cold Multi-Symptom Nighttime Caplets with Cool Burst 1874
Tylenol Cold Multi-Symptom Nighttime Liquid with Cool Burst ... 1874
Tylenol Cold Multi-Symptom Severe Caplets with Cool Burst 1874
Tylenol Cold Multi-Symptom Severe Daytime Liquid with Citrus Burst 1874
Tylenol Cough & Sore Throat Daytime Liquid with Cool Burst 1877
Tylenol Cough & Sore Throat Nighttime Liquid with Cool Burst ... 1877
Concentrated Tylenol Infants' Drops Plus Cold and Cough 1879
Vicks 44 Cough Relief Liquid 2679
Vicks 44D Cough & Head Congestion Relief Liquid 2679
Vicks 44E Cough & Chest Congestion Relief Liquid 2679
Pediatric Vicks 44e Cough & Chest Congestion Relief Liquid 2676
Vicks 44M Cough, Cold & Flu Relief Liquid 2680
Pediatric Vicks 44m Cough & Cold Relief Liquid 2676
Vicks DayQuil LiquiCaps/Liquid Multi-Symptom Cold/Flu Relief 761
Vicks DayQuil Multi-Symptom Cold/Flu Relief LiquiCaps 2678
Vicks DayQuil Multi-Symptom Cold/Flu Relief Liquid 2678
Vicks NyQuil Multi-Symptom Cold/Flu Relief Liquid 2681
Children's Vicks NyQuil Cold/Cough Relief 756
Vicks NyQuil Multi-Symptom Cold/Flu Relief LiquiCaps 2681
Vicks NyQuil LiquiCaps/Liquid Multi-Symptom Cold/Flu Relief 763
Vicks NyQuil Cough Liquid 2680
Children's Vicks NyQuil Cold/Cough Relief Liquid 2680
Zicam Cough Max Nighttime Cough Spray 767
Zicam Cough Max Cough Spray 767
Zicam Cough Max Cough Melts 767
Zicam Cough Plus D Cough Spray 767
Zicam Cough Relief Cough Spray 767
Zicam Maximum Strength Flu Daytime 768
Zicam Maximum Strength Flu Nighttime 768

Dextromethorphan Polistirex (Caution should be taken when darifenacin is used concomitantly with medications that are predominantly metabolized by CYP2D6 and which have a narrow therapeutic window). Products include:
Delsym Extended-Release Suspension 12 Hour Cough Suppressant 611

Dicyclomine Hydrochloride (The concomitant use of darifenacin with other anticholinergic agents may increase the frequency and/or severity of dry mouth, constipation, blurred vision and other anticholinergic pharmacolgical effects. Anticholinergic agents may potentially alter the absorption of some concomitantly administered drugs due to effects on gastrointestinal motility). Products include:
Bentyl Capsules 697
Bentyl Injection 697
Bentyl Syrup 697
Bentyl Tablets 697

Digoxin (Darifenacin (30 mg daily) co-administered with digoxin (0.25 mg) at steady state resulted in a 16% increase in digoxin exposure. Routine therapeutic drug monitoring for digoxin should be continued). Products include:
Lanoxicaps Capsules 1490
Lanoxin Injection 1494
Lanoxin Injection Pediatric 1497
Lanoxin Tablets 1500

Dolasetron Mesylate (Caution should be taken when darifenacin is used concomitantly with medications that are predominantly metabolized by CYP2D6 and which have a narrow therapeutic window). Products include:
Anzemet Injection 2859
Anzemet Tablets 2862

Donepezil Hydrochloride (Caution should be taken when darifenacin is used concomitantly with medications that are predominantly metabolized by CYP2D6 and which have a narrow therapeutic window). Products include:
Aricept Tablets 1094
Aricept ODT Tablets 1094

Doxepin Hydrochloride (Caution should be taken when darifenacin is used concomitantly with medications that are predominantly metabolized by CYP2D6 and which have a narrow therapeutic window).
No products indexed under this heading.

Encainide Hydrochloride (Caution should be taken when darifenacin is used concomitantly with medications that are predominantly metabolized by CYP2D6 and which have a narrow therapeutic window).
No products indexed under this heading.

Fentanyl (Caution should be taken when darifenacin is used concomitantly with medications that are predominantly metabolized by CYP2D6 and which have a narrow therapeutic window). Products include:
Duragesic Transdermal System 2373
Ionsys Transdermal System 2379

Fentanyl Citrate (Caution should be taken when darifenacin is used concomitantly with medications that are predominantly metabolized by CYP2D6 and which have a narrow therapeutic window). Products include:
Actiq 979

Flecainide Acetate (Caution should be taken when darifenacin is used concomitantly with medications that are predominantly metabolized by CYP2D6 and which have a narrow therapeutic window). Products include:
Tambocor Tablets 1856

Fluoxetine (Caution should be taken when darifenacin is used concomitantly with medications that are predominantly metabolized by CYP2D6 and which have a narrow therapeutic window).
No products indexed under this heading.

Fluoxetine Hydrochloride (Caution should be taken when darifenacin is used concomitantly with medications that are predominantly metabolized by CYP2D6 and which have a narrow therapeutic window). Products include:
Prozac Pulvules and Liquid 1801
Symbyax Capsules 1819

Fluphenazine Decanoate (Caution should be taken when darifenacin is used concomitantly with medications that are predominantly metabolized by CYP2D6 and which have a narrow therapeutic window).
No products indexed under this heading.

Fluphenazine Enanthate (Caution should be taken when darifenacin is used concomitantly with medications that are predominantly metabolized by CYP2D6 and which have a narrow therapeutic window).
No products indexed under this heading.

Fluphenazine Hydrochloride (Caution should be taken when darifenacin is used concomitantly with medications that are predominantly metabolized by CYP2D6 and which have a narrow therapeutic window).
No products indexed under this heading.

Fluvoxamine Maleate (Caution should be taken when darifenacin is used concomitantly with medications that are predominantly metabolized by CYP2D6 and which have a narrow therapeutic window).
No products indexed under this heading.

Formoterol Fumarate (Caution should be taken when darifenacin is used concomitantly with medications that are predominantly metabolized by CYP2D6 and which have a narrow therapeutic window). Products include:
Foradil Aerolizer 3010

Fosamprenavir Calcium (The daily dose of darifenacin should not exceed 7.5 mg when co-administered with potent CYP3A4 inhibitors). Products include:
Lexiva Tablets 1505

Galantamine Hydrobromide (Caution should be taken when darifenacin is used concomitantly with medications that are predominantly metabolized by CYP2D6 and which have a narrow therapeutic window). Products include:
Razadyne 2399
Razadyne ER Extended-Release Capsules 2399

Glycopyrrolate (The concomitant use of darifenacin with other anticholinergic agents may increase the frequency and/or severity of dry mouth, constipation, blurred vision and other anticholinergic pharmacolgical effects. Anticholinergic agents may potentially alter the absorption of some concomitantly administered drugs due to effects on gastrointestinal motility).
No products indexed under this heading.

Haloperidol (Caution should be taken when darifenacin is used concomitantly with medications that are predominantly metabolized by CYP2D6 and which have a narrow therapeutic window).
No products indexed under this heading.

Haloperidol Decanoate (Caution should be taken when darifenacin is used concomitantly with medications that are predominantly metabolized by CYP2D6 and which have a narrow therapeutic window).
No products indexed under this heading.

Hydrocodone Bitartrate (Caution should be taken when darifenacin is used concomitantly with medications that are predominantly metabolized by CYP2D6 and which have a narrow therapeutic window). Products include:
Hycodan **1116**
Hycotuss Expectorant Syrup **1117**
Vicodin Tablets **535**
Vicodin ES Tablets **536**
Vicodin HP Tablets **538**
Vicoprofen Tablets **539**
Zydone Tablets **1139**

Hyoscyamine (The concomitant use of darifenacin with other anticholinergic agents may increase the frequency and/or severity of dry mouth, constipation, blurred vision and other anticholinergic pharmacolgical effects. Anticholinergic agents may potentially alter the absorption of some concomitantly administered drugs due to effects on gastrointestinal motility).
No products indexed under this heading.

Hyoscyamine Sulfate (The concomitant use of darifenacin with other anticholinergic agents may increase the frequency and/or severity of dry mouth, constipation, blurred vision and other anticholinergic pharmacolgical effects. Anticholinergic agents may potentially alter the absorption of some concomitantly administered drugs due to effects on gastrointestinal motility). Products include:
Donnatal Extentabs **2493**
Prosed/DS Tablets **1157**

Imipramine Hydrochloride (The mean Cmax and AUC of imipramine, a CYP2D6 substrate, were increased 57% and 70%, respectively, in the presence of steady state darifenacin 30 mg once daily. This was accompanied by a 3.6 fold increase in the mean Cmax and AUC of desipramine, the active metabolite of imipramine. Caution should be taken when darifenacin is used concomitantly with medications that are predominantly metabolized by CYP2D6 and which have a narrow therapeutic window).
No products indexed under this heading.

Imipramine Pamoate (The mean Cmax and AUC of imipramine, a CYP2D6 substrate, were increased 57% and 70%, respectively, in the presence of steady state darifenacin 30 mg once daily. This was accompanied by a 3.6 fold increase in the mean Cmax and AUC of desipramine, the active metabolite of imipramine. Caution should be taken when darifenacin is used concomitantly with medications that are predominantly metabolized by CYP2D6 and which have a narrow therapeutic window).
No products indexed under this heading.

Indinavir Sulfate (The daily dose of darifenacin should not exceed 7.5 mg when co-administered with potent CYP3A4 inhibitors). Products include:
Crixivan Capsules **1940**

Indoramin Hydrochloride (Caution should be taken when darifenacin is used concomitantly with medications that are predominantly metabolized by CYP2D6 and which have a narrow therapeutic window).
No products indexed under this heading.

Ipratropium Bromide (The concomitant use of darifenacin with other anticholinergic agents may increase the frequency and/or severity of dry mouth, constipation, blurred vision and other anticholinergic pharmacolgical effects. Anticholinergic agents may potentially alter the absorption of some concomitantly administered drugs due to effects on gastrointestinal motility). Products include:
Atrovent Inhalation Solution **835**
Atrovent HFA Inhalation Aerosol **841**
Atrovent Nasal Spray 0.03% **837**
Atrovent Nasal Spray 0.06% **839**
Combivent Inhalation Aerosol **847**
DuoNeb Inhalation Solution **1058**

Itraconazole (The daily dose of darifenacin should not exceed 7.5 mg when co-administered with potent CYP3A4 inhibitors).
No products indexed under this heading.

Ketoconazole (The daily dose of darifenacin should not exceed 7.5 mg when co-administered with potent CYP3A4 inhibitors). Products include:
Nizoral A-D Shampoo, 1% **1868**

Labetalol Hydrochloride (Caution should be taken when darifenacin is used concomitantly with medications that are predominantly metabolized by CYP2D6 and which have a narrow therapeutic window).
No products indexed under this heading.

Lidocaine (Caution should be taken when darifenacin is used concomitantly with medications that are predominantly metabolized by CYP2D6 and which have a narrow therapeutic window). Products include:
Lidoderm Patch **1118**
Synera Topical Patch **1137**

Lidocaine Hydrochloride (Caution should be taken when darifenacin is used concomitantly with medications that are predominantly metabolized by CYP2D6 and which have a narrow therapeutic window).
No products indexed under this heading.

Lopinavir (The daily dose of darifenacin should not exceed 7.5 mg when co-administered with potent CYP3A4 inhibitors). Products include:
Kaletra **476**

Maprotiline Hydrochloride (Caution should be taken when darifenacin is used concomitantly with medications that are predominantly metabolized by CYP2D6 and which have a narrow therapeutic window).
No products indexed under this heading.

Mepenzolate Bromide (The concomitant use of darifenacin with other anticholinergic agents may increase the frequency and/or severity of dry mouth, constipation, blurred vision and other anticholinergic pharmacolgical effects. Anticholinergic agents may potentially alter the absorption of some concomitantly administered drugs due to effects on gastrointestinal motility).
No products indexed under this heading.

Meperidine Hydrochloride (Caution should be taken when darifenacin is used concomitantly with medications that are predominantly metabolized by CYP2D6 and which have a narrow therapeutic window).
No products indexed under this heading.

Methadone Hydrochloride (Caution should be taken when darifenacin is used concomitantly with medications that are predominantly metabolized by CYP2D6 and which have a narrow therapeutic window).
No products indexed under this heading.

Methamphetamine Hydrochloride (Caution should be taken when darifenacin is used concomitantly with medications that are predominantly metabolized by CYP2D6 and which have a narrow therapeutic window). Products include:
Desoxyn Tablets, USP **2462**

Metoprolol Succinate (Caution should be taken when darifenacin is used concomitantly with medications that are predominantly metabolized by CYP2D6 and which have a narrow therapeutic window). Products include:
Toprol-XL Tablets **668**

Metoprolol Tartrate (Caution should be taken when darifenacin is used concomitantly with medications that are predominantly metabolized by CYP2D6 and which have a narrow therapeutic window). Products include:
Lopressor Injection **2238**
Lopressor Tablets **2238**
Lopressor HCT 50/25 Tablets **2241**
Lopressor HCT 100/25 Tablets **2241**
Lopressor HCT 100/50 Tablets **2241**

Mexiletine Hydrochloride (Caution should be taken when darifenacin is used concomitantly with medications that are predominantly metabolized by CYP2D6 and which have a narrow therapeutic window).
No products indexed under this heading.

Midazolam Hydrochloride (Darifenacin (30 mg daily) co-administered with a single oral dose of midazolam 7.5 mg resulted in a 17% increase in midazolam exposure).
No products indexed under this heading.

Mirtazapine (Caution should be taken when darifenacin is used concomitantly with medications that are predominantly metabolized by CYP2D6 and which have a narrow therapeutic window).
No products indexed under this heading.

Morphine Sulfate (Caution should be taken when darifenacin is used concomitantly with medications that are predominantly metabolized by CYP2D6 and which have a narrow therapeutic window). Products include:
Avinza Capsules **1741**
Kadian Capsules **577**
MS Contin Tablets **2701**

Nefazodone Hydrochloride (The daily dose of darifenacin should not exceed 7.5 mg when co-administered with potent CYP3A4 inhibitors).
No products indexed under this heading.

Nelfinavir Mesylate (The daily dose of darifenacin should not exceed 7.5 mg when co-administered with potent CYP3A4 inhibitors). Products include:
Viracept **2577**

Nortriptyline Hydrochloride (Caution should be taken when darifenacin is used concomitantly with medications that are predominantly metabolized by CYP2D6 and which have a narrow therapeutic window).
No products indexed under this heading.

Olanzapine (Caution should be taken when darifenacin is used concomitantly with medications that are predominantly metabolized by CYP2D6 and which have a narrow therapeutic window). Products include:
Symbyax Capsules **1819**
Zyprexa Tablets **1830**
Zyprexa IntraMuscular **1830**
Zyprexa ZYDIS Orally Disintegrating Tablets **1830**

Omeprazole (Caution should be taken when darifenacin is used concomitantly with medications that are predominantly metabolized by CYP2D6 and which have a narrow therapeutic window). Products include:
Zegerid Capsules **2958**
Zegerid Powder for Oral Solution **2958**

Ondansetron (Caution should be taken when darifenacin is used concomitantly with medications that are predominantly metabolized by CYP2D6 and which have a narrow therapeutic window). Products include:
Zofran ODT Orally Disintegrating Tablets **1639**

Ondansetron Hydrochloride (Caution should be taken when darifenacin is used concomitantly with medications that are predominantly metabolized by CYP2D6 and which have a narrow therapeutic window). Products include:
Zofran Injection **1634**
Zofran **1639**

Oxybutynin Chloride (The concomitant use of darifenacin with other anticholinergic agents may increase the frequency and/or severity of dry mouth, constipation, blurred vision and other anticholinergic pharmacolgical effects. Anticholinergic agents may potentially alter the absorption of some concomitantly administered drugs due to effects on gastrointestinal motility). Products include:

Ditropan XL Extended-Release
Tablets ... **2413**

Oxycodone Hydrochloride (Caution should be taken when darifenacin is used concomitantly with medications that are predominantly metabolized by CYP2D6 and which have a narrow therapeutic window). Products include:

OxyContin Tablets **2703**
OxyFast Oral Concentrate
Solution **2708**
OxyIR Capsules **2708**
Percocet Tablets **1131**
Percodan Tablets **1132**

Paclitaxel (Caution should be taken when darifenacin is used concomitantly with medications that are predominantly metabolized by CYP2D6 and which have a narrow therapeutic window).

No products indexed under this heading.

Paroxetine Hydrochloride (Caution should be taken when darifenacin is used concomitantly with medications that are predominantly metabolized by CYP2D6 and which have a narrow therapeutic window). Products include:

Paxil CR Controlled-Release
Tablets ... **1538**
Paxil .. **1530**

Pindolol (Caution should be taken when darifenacin is used concomitantly with medications that are predominantly metabolized by CYP2D6 and which have a narrow therapeutic window).

No products indexed under this heading.

Procyclidine Hydrochloride (The concomitant use of darifenacin with other anticholinergic agents may increase the frequency and/or severity of dry mouth, constipation, blurred vision and other anticholinergic pharmacolgical effects. Anticholinergic agents may potentially alter the absorption of some concomitantly administered drugs due to effects on gastrointestinal motility).

No products indexed under this heading.

Propafenone Hydrochloride (Caution should be taken when darifenacin is used concomitantly with medications that are predominantly metabolized by CYP2D6 and which have a narrow therapeutic window). Products include:

Rythmol SR Capsules **2727**

Propantheline Bromide (The concomitant use of darifenacin with other anticholinergic agents may increase the frequency and/or severity of dry mouth, constipation, blurred vision and other anticholinergic pharmacolgical effects. Anticholinergic agents may potentially alter the absorption of some concomitantly administered drugs due to effects on gastrointestinal motility).

No products indexed under this heading.

Propoxyphene Hydrochloride
(Caution should be taken when darifenacin is used concomitantly with medications that are predominantly metabolized by CYP2D6 and which have a narrow therapeutic window).

No products indexed under this heading.

Propoxyphene Napsylate (Caution should be taken when darifenacin is used concomitantly with medications that are predominantly metabolized by CYP2D6 and which have a narrow therapeutic window).

No products indexed under this heading.

Propranolol Hydrochloride (Caution should be taken when darifenacin is used concomitantly with medications that are predominantly metabolized by CYP2D6 and which have a narrow therapeutic window). Products include:

Inderal LA Long-Acting Capsules **3429**
InnoPran XL Capsules **2723**

Quetiapine Fumarate (Caution should be taken when darifenacin is used concomitantly with medications that are predominantly metabolized by CYP2D6 and which have a narrow therapeutic window). Products include:

Seroquel Tablets **690**

Quinidine Gluconate (Caution should be taken when darifenacin is used concomitantly with medications that are predominantly metabolized by CYP2D6 and which have a narrow therapeutic window).

No products indexed under this heading.

Quinidine Hydrochloride (Caution should be taken when darifenacin is used concomitantly with medications that are predominantly metabolized by CYP2D6 and which have a narrow therapeutic window).

No products indexed under this heading.

Quinidine Polygalacturonate
(Caution should be taken when darifenacin is used concomitantly with medications that are predominantly metabolized by CYP2D6 and which have a narrow therapeutic window).

No products indexed under this heading.

Quinidine Sulfate (Caution should be taken when darifenacin is used concomitantly with medications that are predominantly metabolized by CYP2D6 and which have a narrow therapeutic window).

No products indexed under this heading.

Risperidone (Caution should be taken when darifenacin is used concomitantly with medications that are predominantly metabolized by CYP2D6 and which have a narrow therapeutic window). Products include:

Risperdal **1676**
Risperdal Consta Long-Acting
Injection **1682**
Risperdal M-Tab Orally
Disintegrating Tablets.................... **1676**

Ritonavir (The daily dose of darifenacin should not exceed 7.5 mg when co-administered with potent CYP3A4 inhibitors). Products include:

Kaletra ... **476**
Norvir .. **503**

Saquinavir (The daily dose of darifenacin should not exceed 7.5 mg when co-administered with potent CYP3A4 inhibitors).

No products indexed under this heading.

Saquinavir Mesylate (The daily dose of darifenacin should not exceed 7.5 mg when co-administered with potent CYP3A4 inhibitors). Products include:

Invirase ... **2772**

Scopolamine (The concomitant use of darifenacin with other anticholinergic agents may increase the frequency and/or severity of dry mouth, constipation, blurred vision and other anticholinergic pharmacolgical effects. Anticholinergic agents may potentially alter the absorption of some concomitantly administered drugs due to effects on gastrointestinal motility). Products include:

Transderm Scōp Transdermal
Therapeutic System **2177**

Scopolamine Hydrobromide (The concomitant use of darifenacin with other anticholinergic agents may increase the frequency and/or severity of dry mouth, constipation, blurred vision and other anticholinergic pharmacolgical effects. Anticholinergic agents may potentially alter the absorption of some concomitantly administered drugs due to effects on gastrointestinal motility). Products include:

Donnatal Extentabs **2493**

Tamoxifen Citrate (Caution should be taken when darifenacin is used concomitantly with medications that are predominantly metabolized by CYP2D6 and which have a narrow therapeutic window). Products include:

Soltamox Oral Solution **3527**

Telithromycin (The daily dose of darifenacin should not exceed 7.5 mg when co-administered with potent CYP3A4 inhibitors). Products include:

Ketek Tablets **2903**

Teniposide (Caution should be taken when darifenacin is used concomitantly with medications that are predominantly metabolized by CYP2D6 and which have a narrow therapeutic window).

No products indexed under this heading.

Testosterone (Caution should be taken when darifenacin is used concomitantly with medications that are predominantly metabolized by CYP2D6 and which have a narrow therapeutic window). Products include:

AndroGel **3329**
Striant Mucoadhesive **1007**
Testim 1% Gel **695**

Testosterone Cypionate (Caution should be taken when darifenacin is used concomitantly with medications that are predominantly metabolized by CYP2D6 and which have a narrow therapeutic window).

No products indexed under this heading.

Testosterone Enanthate (Caution should be taken when darifenacin is used concomitantly with medications that are predominantly metabolized by CYP2D6 and which have a narrow therapeutic window).

No products indexed under this heading.

Testosterone Propionate (Caution should be taken when darifenacin is used concomitantly with medications that are predominantly metabolized by CYP2D6 and which have a narrow therapeutic window).

No products indexed under this heading.

Thioridazine (Caution should be taken when darifenacin is used concomitantly with medications that are predominantly metabolized by CYP2D6 and which have a narrow therapeutic window).

No products indexed under this heading.

Thioridazine Hydrochloride (Caution should be taken when darifenacin is used concomitantly with medications that are predominantly metabolized by CYP2D6 and which have a narrow therapeutic window). Products include:

Thioridazine Hydrochloride
Tablets ... **2163**

Timolol Maleate (Caution should be taken when darifenacin is used concomitantly with medications that are predominantly metabolized by CYP2D6 and which have a narrow therapeutic window). Products include:

Blocadren Tablets **1916**
Cosopt Sterile Ophthalmic
Solution...................................... **1931**
Timolide Tablets **2086**
Timoptic Sterile Ophthalmic
Solution...................................... **2088**
Timoptic in Ocudose **2091**
Timoptic-XE Sterile Ophthalmic
Gel Forming Solution **2092**

Tolterodine Tartrate (Caution should be taken when darifenacin is used concomitantly with medications that are predominantly metabolized by CYP2D6 and which have a narrow therapeutic window). Products include:

Detrol Tablets **2628**
Detrol LA Capsules **2631**

Tramadol Hydrochloride (Caution should be taken when darifenacin is used concomitantly with medications that are predominantly metabolized by CYP2D6 and which have a narrow therapeutic window). Products include:

Ultram ER Tablets **2392**

Trazodone Hydrochloride (Caution should be taken when darifenacin is used concomitantly with medications that are predominantly metabolized by CYP2D6 and which have a narrow therapeutic window).

No products indexed under this heading.

Triazolam (Caution should be taken when darifenacin is used concomitantly with medications that are predominantly metabolized by CYP2D6 and which have a narrow therapeutic window).

No products indexed under this heading.

Tridihexethyl Chloride (The concomitant use of darifenacin with other anticholinergic agents may increase the frequency and/or severity of dry mouth, constipation, blurred vision and other anticholinergic pharmacolgical effects. Anticholinergic agents may potentially alter the absorption of some concomitantly administered drugs due to effects on gastrointestinal motility).

No products indexed under this heading.

IMPORTANT NOTE: Always consult each drug listing in the patient's regimen for possible interactions.

Trihexyphenidyl Hydrochloride (The concomitant use of darifenacin with other anticholinergic agents may increase the frequency and/or severity of dry mouth, constipation, blurred vision and other anticholinergic pharmacolgical effects. Anticholinergic agents may potentially alter the absorption of some concomitantly administered drugs due to effects on gastrointestinal motility).
No products indexed under this heading.

Trimipramine Maleate (Caution should be taken when darifenacin is used concomitantly with medications that are predominantly metabolized by CYP2D6 and which have a narrow therapeutic window).
No products indexed under this heading.

Troleandomycin (The daily dose of darifenacin should not exceed 7.5 mg when co-administered with potent CYP3A4 inhibitors).
No products indexed under this heading.

Venlafaxine Hydrochloride (Caution should be taken when darifenacin is used concomitantly with medications that are predominantly metabolized by CYP2D6 and which have a narrow therapeutic window). Products include:
Effexor Tablets **3411**
Effexor XR Capsules **3417**

Vinblastine Sulfate (Caution should be taken when darifenacin is used concomitantly with medications that are predominantly metabolized by CYP2D6 and which have a narrow therapeutic window).
No products indexed under this heading.

Voriconazole (The daily dose of darifenacin should not exceed 7.5 mg when co-administered with potent CYP3A4 inhibitors). Products include:
VFEND I.V. **2564**
VFEND Oral Suspension **2564**
VFEND Tablets **2564**

Zonisamide (Caution should be taken when darifenacin is used concomitantly with medications that are predominantly metabolized by CYP2D6 and which have a narrow therapeutic window). Products include:
Zonegran Capsules **1101**

ENBREL FOR INJECTION

(Etanercept) **584**
May interact with vaccines, live and certain other agents. Compounds in these categories include:

Anakinra (Co-administration results in a 7% rate of serious infections and 2% of the patients develop neutropenia). Products include:
Kineret Injection **599**

BCG Vaccine (Patients receiving etanercept may receive concurrent vaccinations, except for live vaccines).
No products indexed under this heading.

Cyclophosphamide (Concurrent cyclophosphamide therapy is not recommended).
No products indexed under this heading.

Measles, Mumps, Rubella and Varicella Virus Vaccine Live (Patients receiving etanercept may receive concurrent vaccinations, except for live vaccines). Products include:
ProQuad **2064**

Measles, Mumps & Rubella Virus Vaccine, Live (Patients receiving etanercept may receive concurrent vaccinations, except for live vaccines). Products include:
M-M-R II **2006**

Measles & Rubella Virus Vaccine Live (Patients receiving etanercept may receive concurrent vaccinations, except for live vaccines).
No products indexed under this heading.

Measles Virus Vaccine Live (Patients receiving etanercept may receive concurrent vaccinations, except for live vaccines). Products include:
Attenuvax **1914**

Mumps Virus Vaccine, Live (Patients receiving etanercept may receive concurrent vaccinations, except for live vaccines). Products include:
Mumpsvax **2031**

Poliovirus Vaccine, Live, Oral, Trivalent, Types 1,2,3 (Sabin) (Patients receiving etanercept may receive concurrent vaccinations, except for live vaccines).
No products indexed under this heading.

Rotavirus Vaccine, Live, Oral, Tetravalent (Patients receiving etanercept may receive concurrent vaccinations, except for live vaccines).
No products indexed under this heading.

Rubella & Mumps Virus Vaccine Live (Patients receiving etanercept may receive concurrent vaccinations, except for live vaccines).
No products indexed under this heading.

Rubella Virus Vaccine Live (Patients receiving etanercept may receive concurrent vaccinations, except for live vaccines). Products include:
Meruvax II **2019**

Smallpox Vaccine (Patients receiving etanercept may receive concurrent vaccinations, except for live vaccines).
No products indexed under this heading.

Sulfasalazine (Co-administration results in a mild decrease in mean neutrophil count).
No products indexed under this heading.

Typhoid Vaccine (Patients receiving etanercept may receive concurrent vaccinations, except for live vaccines).
No products indexed under this heading.

Varicella Virus Vaccine Live (Patients receiving etanercept may receive concurrent vaccinations, except for live vaccines). Products include:
Varivax **2100**

Yellow Fever Vaccine (Patients receiving etanercept may receive concurrent vaccinations, except for live vaccines).
No products indexed under this heading.

ENGERIX-B VACCINE

(Hepatitis B Vaccine, Recombinant) ... **1425**
None cited in PDR database.

ENJUVIA TABLETS

(Estrogens, Conjugated, Synthetic B).. **1062**
May interact with cytochrome p450 3a4 inducers (selected), cytochrome p450 3a4 inhibitors (selected), and thyroid preparations. Compounds in these categories include:

Acetazolamide (Inhibitors of CYP3A4 such as erythromycin, clarithromycin, ketoconazole, itraconazole, ritonavir and grapefruit juice may increase plasma concentrations of estrogens and may result in side effects).
No products indexed under this heading.

Allium sativum (Inducers of CYP3A4 such as St. John's Wort preparations (hypericum perforatum), phenobarbital, carbamazepine and rifampin may reduce plasma concentrations of estrogens, possibly resulting in a decrease in therapeutic effects and/or changes in the uterine bleeding profile).
No products indexed under this heading.

Amiodarone Hydrochloride (Inhibitors of CYP3A4 such as erythromycin, clarithromycin, ketoconazole, itraconazole, ritonavir and grapefruit juice may increase plasma concentrations of estrogens and may result in side effects).
No products indexed under this heading.

Amprenavir (Inhibitors of CYP3A4 such as erythromycin, clarithromycin, ketoconazole, itraconazole, ritonavir and grapefruit juice may increase plasma concentrations of estrogens and may result in side effects). Products include:
Agenerase Capsules **1327**
Agenerase Oral Solution **1332**

Anastrozole (Inhibitors of CYP3A4 such as erythromycin, clarithromycin, ketoconazole, itraconazole, ritonavir and grapefruit juice may increase plasma concentrations of estrogens and may result in side effects). Products include:
Arimidex Tablets **673**

Aprepitant (Inducers of CYP3A4 such as St. John's Wort preparations (hypericum perforatum), phenobarbital, carbamazepine and rifampin may reduce plasma concentrations of estrogens, possibly resulting in a decrease in therapeutic effects and/or changes in the uterine bleeding profile). Products include:
Emend Capsules **1963**

Betamethasone Acetate (Inducers of CYP3A4 such as St. John's Wort preparations (hypericum perforatum), phenobarbital, carbamazepine and rifampin may reduce plasma concentrations of estrogens, possibly resulting in a decrease in therapeutic effects and/or changes in the uterine bleeding profile).
No products indexed under this heading.

Betamethasone Sodium Phosphate (Inducers of CYP3A4 such as St. John's Wort preparations (hypericum perforatum), phenobarbital, carbamazepine and rifampin may reduce plasma concentrations of estrogens, possibly resulting in a decrease in therapeutic effects and/or changes in the uterine bleeding profile).
No products indexed under this heading.

Carbamazepine (Inducers of CYP3A4 such as St. John's Wort preparations (hypericum perforatum), phenobarbital, carbamazepine and rifampin may reduce plasma concentrations of estrogens, possibly resulting in a decrease in therapeutic effects and/or changes in the uterine bleeding profile). Products include:
Carbatrol Capsules **3171**
Equetro Extended-Release Capsules **3180**
Tegretol/Tegretol-XR **2295**

Cimetidine (Inhibitors of CYP3A4 such as erythromycin, clarithromycin, ketoconazole, itraconazole, ritonavir and grapefruit juice may increase plasma concentrations of estrogens and may result in side effects). Products include:
Tagamet HB 200 Tablets .... ▣**664**

Cimetidine Hydrochloride (Inhibitors of CYP3A4 such as erythromycin, clarithromycin, ketoconazole, itraconazole, ritonavir and grapefruit juice may increase plasma concentrations of estrogens and may result in side effects).
No products indexed under this heading.

Ciprofloxacin (Inhibitors of CYP3A4 such as erythromycin, clarithromycin, ketoconazole, itraconazole, ritonavir and grapefruit juice may increase plasma concentrations of estrogens and may result in side effects). Products include:
Cipro Oral Suspension **2977**
Cipro I.V. **2984**
Cipro XR Tablets **2990**
Ciprodex Otic Suspension **559**

Ciprofloxacin Hydrochloride (Inducers of CYP3A4 such as St. John's Wort preparations (hypericum perforatum), phenobarbital, carbamazepine and rifampin may reduce plasma concentrations of estrogens, possibly resulting in a decrease in therapeutic effects and/or changes in the uterine bleeding profile). Products include:
Ciloxan Ophthalmic Ointment **559**
Ciloxan Ophthalmic Solution .... ⊙**206**
Cipro Tablets **2977**
Proquin XR Tablets **1153**

Cisplatin (Inducers of CYP3A4 such as St. John's Wort preparations (hypericum perforatum), phenobarbital, carbamazepine and rifampin may reduce plasma concentrations of estrogens, possibly resulting in a decrease in therapeutic effects and/or changes in the uterine bleeding profile).
No products indexed under this heading.

Clarithromycin (Inhibitors of CYP3A4 such as erythromycin, clarithromycin, ketoconazole, itraconazole, ritonavir and grapefruit juice may increase plasma concentrations of estrogens and may result in side effects). Products include:
Biaxin/Biaxin XL **402**
PREVPAC **3284**

Clotrimazole (Inhibitors of CYP3A4 such as erythromycin, clarithromycin, ketoconazole, itraconazole, ritonavir and grapefruit juice may increase plasma concentrations of estrogens and may result in side effects). Products include:
Desenex Athlete's Foot Cream .... ▣**635**
Lotrimin **3039**
Lotrisone **3040**

Cortisone Acetate (Inducers of CYP3A4 such as St. John's Wort preparations (hypericum perforatum), phenobarbital, carbamazepine and rifampin may reduce plasma concentrations of estrogens, possibly resulting in a decrease in therapeutic effects and/or changes in the uterine bleeding profile).

No products indexed under this heading.

Cyclosporine (Inhibitors of CYP3A4 such as erythromycin, clarithromycin, ketoconazole, itraconazole, ritonavir and grapefruit juice may increase plasma concentrations of estrogens and may result in side effects). Products include:

Dalfopristin (Inhibitors of CYP3A4 such as erythromycin, clarithromycin, ketoconazole, itraconazole, ritonavir and grapefruit juice may increase plasma concentrations of estrogens and may result in side effects).

No products indexed under this heading.

Danazol (Inhibitors of CYP3A4 such as erythromycin, clarithromycin, ketoconazole, itraconazole, ritonavir and grapefruit juice may increase plasma concentrations of estrogens and may result in side effects).

No products indexed under this heading.

Delavirdine Mesylate (Inhibitors of CYP3A4 such as erythromycin, clarithromycin, ketoconazole, itraconazole, ritonavir and grapefruit juice may increase plasma concentrations of estrogens and may result in side effects). Products include:

Dexamethasone (Inducers of CYP3A4 such as St. John's Wort preparations (hypericum perforatum), phenobarbital, carbamazepine and rifampin may reduce plasma concentrations of estrogens, possibly resulting in a decrease in therapeutic effects and/or changes in the uterine bleeding profile). Products include:

Dexamethasone Acetate (Inducers of CYP3A4 such as St. John's Wort preparations (hypericum perforatum), phenobarbital, carbamazepine and rifampin may reduce plasma concentrations of estrogens, possibly resulting in a decrease in therapeutic effects and/or changes in the uterine bleeding profile).

No products indexed under this heading.

Dexamethasone Sodium Phosphate (Inducers of CYP3A4 such as St. John's Wort preparations (hypericum perforatum), phenobarbital, carbamazepine and rifampin may reduce plasma concentrations of estrogens, possibly resulting in a decrease in therapeutic effects and/or changes in the uterine bleeding profile).

No products indexed under this heading.

Diltiazem Hydrochloride (Inhibitors of CYP3A4 such as erythromycin, clarithromycin, ketoconazole,

itraconazole, ritonavir and grapefruit juice may increase plasma concentrations of estrogens and may result in side effects). Products include:

Diltiazem Maleate (Inhibitors of CYP3A4 such as erythromycin, clarithromycin, ketoconazole, itraconazole, ritonavir and grapefruit juice may increase plasma concentrations of estrogens and may result in side effects).

No products indexed under this heading.

Doxorubicin Hydrochloride (Inducers of CYP3A4 such as St. John's Wort preparations (hypericum perforatum), phenobarbital, carbamazepine and rifampin may reduce plasma concentrations of estrogens, possibly resulting in a decrease in therapeutic effects and/or changes in the uterine bleeding profile).

No products indexed under this heading.

Efavirenz (Inducers of CYP3A4 such as St. John's Wort preparations (hypericum perforatum), phenobarbital, carbamazepine and rifampin may reduce plasma concentrations of estrogens, possibly resulting in a decrease in therapeutic effects and/or changes in the uterine bleeding profile). Products include:

Erythromycin (Inhibitors of CYP3A4 such as erythromycin, clarithromycin, ketoconazole, itraconazole, ritonavir and grapefruit juice may increase plasma concentrations of estrogens and may result in side effects). Products include:

Erythromycin Estolate (Inhibitors of CYP3A4 such as erythromycin, clarithromycin, ketoconazole, itraconazole, ritonavir and grapefruit juice may increase plasma concentrations of estrogens and may result in side effects).

No products indexed under this heading.

Erythromycin Ethylsuccinate (Inhibitors of CYP3A4 such as erythromycin, clarithromycin, ketoconazole, itraconazole, ritonavir and grapefruit juice may increase plasma concentrations of estrogens and may result in side effects). Products include:

Erythromycin Gluceptate (Inhibitors of CYP3A4 such as erythromycin, clarithromycin, ketoconazole, itraconazole, ritonavir and grapefruit juice may increase plasma concentrations of estrogens and may result in side effects).

No products indexed under this heading.

Erythromycin Lactobionate (Inhibitors of CYP3A4 such as erythromycin, clarithromycin, ketoconazole, itraconazole, ritonavir and grapefruit juice may increase plasma concentrations of estrogens and may result in side effects).

No products indexed under this heading.

Erythromycin Stearate (Inhibitors of CYP3A4 such as erythromycin, clarithromycin, ketoconazole, itraconazole, ritonavir and grapefruit juice may increase plasma concentrations of estrogens and may result in side effects). Products include:

Esomeprazole Magnesium (Inhibitors of CYP3A4 such as erythromycin, clarithromycin, ketoconazole, itraconazole, ritonavir and grapefruit juice may increase plasma concentrations of estrogens and may result in side effects). Products include:

Ethosuximide (Inducers of CYP3A4 such as St. John's Wort preparations (hypericum perforatum), phenobarbital, carbamazepine and rifampin may reduce plasma concentrations of estrogens, possibly resulting in a decrease in therapeutic effects and/or changes in the uterine bleeding profile).

No products indexed under this heading.

Felbamate (Inducers of CYP3A4 such as St. John's Wort preparations (hypericum perforatum), phenobarbital, carbamazepine and rifampin may reduce plasma concentrations of estrogens, possibly resulting in a decrease in therapeutic effects and/or changes in the uterine bleeding profile).

No products indexed under this heading.

Fluconazole (Inhibitors of CYP3A4 such as erythromycin, clarithromycin, ketoconazole, itraconazole, ritonavir and grapefruit juice may increase plasma concentrations of estrogens and may result in side effects).

No products indexed under this heading.

Fludrocortisone Acetate (Inducers of CYP3A4 such as St. John's Wort preparations (hypericum perforatum), phenobarbital, carbamazepine and rifampin may reduce plasma concentrations of estrogens, possibly resulting in a decrease in therapeutic effects and/or changes in the uterine bleeding profile).

No products indexed under this heading.

Fluoxetine Hydrochloride (Inhibitors of CYP3A4 such as erythromycin, clarithromycin, ketoconazole, itraconazole, ritonavir and grapefruit juice may increase plasma concentrations of estrogens and may result in side effects). Products include:

Fluvoxamine Maleate (Inhibitors of CYP3A4 such as erythromycin, clarithromycin, ketoconazole, itraconazole, ritonavir and grapefruit juice may increase plasma concen-

trations of estrogens and may result in side effects).

No products indexed under this heading.

Fosamprenavir Calcium (Inhibitors of CYP3A4 such as erythromycin, clarithromycin, ketoconazole, itraconazole, ritonavir and grapefruit juice may increase plasma concentrations of estrogens and may result in side effects). Products include:

Fosphenytoin Sodium (Inducers of CYP3A4 such as St. John's Wort preparations (hypericum perforatum), phenobarbital, carbamazepine and rifampin may reduce plasma concentrations of estrogens, possibly resulting in a decrease in therapeutic effects and/or changes in the uterine bleeding profile).

No products indexed under this heading.

Garlic Extract (Inducers of CYP3A4 such as St. John's Wort preparations (hypericum perforatum), phenobarbital, carbamazepine and rifampin may reduce plasma concentrations of estrogens, possibly resulting in a decrease in therapeutic effects and/or changes in the uterine bleeding profile).

No products indexed under this heading.

Garlic Oil (Inducers of CYP3A4 such as St. John's Wort preparations (hypericum perforatum), phenobarbital, carbamazepine and rifampin may reduce plasma concentrations of estrogens, possibly resulting in a decrease in therapeutic effects and/or changes in the uterine bleeding profile).

No products indexed under this heading.

Hydrocortisone (Inducers of CYP3A4 such as St. John's Wort preparations (hypericum perforatum), phenobarbital, carbamazepine and rifampin may reduce plasma concentrations of estrogens, possibly resulting in a decrease in therapeutic effects and/or changes in the uterine bleeding profile). Products include:

Hydrocortisone Acetate (Inducers of CYP3A4 such as St. John's Wort preparations (hypericum perforatum), phenobarbital, carbamazepine and rifampin may reduce plasma concentrations of estrogens, possibly resulting in a decrease in therapeutic effects and/or changes in the uterine bleeding profile). Products include:

Hydrocortisone Butyrate (Inducers of CYP3A4 such as St. John's Wort preparations (hypericum perforatum), phenobarbital, carbamazepine and rifampin may reduce plasma concentrations of estrogens, possibly resulting in a decrease in therapeutic effects and/or changes in the uterine bleeding profile). Products include:

IMPORTANT NOTE: Always consult each drug listing in the patient's regimen for possible interactions.

Hydrocortisone Cypionate (Inducers of CYP3A4 such as St. John's Wort preparations (hypericum perforatum), phenobarbital, carbamazepine and rifampin may reduce plasma concentrations of estrogens, possibly resulting in a decrease in therapeutic effects and/or changes in the uterine bleeding profile).
No products indexed under this heading.

Hydrocortisone Hemisuccinate (Inducers of CYP3A4 such as St. John's Wort preparations (hypericum perforatum), phenobarbital, carbamazepine and rifampin may reduce plasma concentrations of estrogens, possibly resulting in a decrease in therapeutic effects and/or changes in the uterine bleeding profile).
No products indexed under this heading.

Hydrocortisone Probutate (Inducers of CYP3A4 such as St. John's Wort preparations (hypericum perforatum), phenobarbital, carbamazepine and rifampin may reduce plasma concentrations of estrogens, possibly resulting in a decrease in therapeutic effects and/or changes in the uterine bleeding profile).
No products indexed under this heading.

Hydrocortisone Sodium Phosphate (Inducers of CYP3A4 such as St. John's Wort preparations (hypericum perforatum), phenobarbital, carbamazepine and rifampin may reduce plasma concentrations of estrogens, possibly resulting in a decrease in therapeutic effects and/or changes in the uterine bleeding profile).
No products indexed under this heading.

Hydrocortisone Sodium Succinate (Inducers of CYP3A4 such as St. John's Wort preparations (hypericum perforatum), phenobarbital, carbamazepine and rifampin may reduce plasma concentrations of estrogens, possibly resulting in a decrease in therapeutic effects and/or changes in the uterine bleeding profile).
No products indexed under this heading.

Hydrocortisone Valerate (Inducers of CYP3A4 such as St. John's Wort preparations (hypericum perforatum), phenobarbital, carbamazepine and rifampin may reduce plasma concentrations of estrogens, possibly resulting in a decrease in therapeutic effects and/or changes in the uterine bleeding profile).
No products indexed under this heading.

Hypericum (Inducers of CYP3A4 such as St. John's Wort preparations (hypericum perforatum), phenobarbital, carbamazepine and rifampin may reduce plasma concentrations of estrogens, possibly resulting in a decrease in therapeutic effects and/or changes in the uterine bleeding profile). Products include:
Satiete Tablets .... ▣**832**

Hypericum Perforatum (Inducers of CYP3A4 such as St. John's Wort preparations (hypericum perforatum), phenobarbital, carbamazepine and rifampin may reduce plasma concentrations of estrogens, possibly resulting in a decrease in therapeutic effects and/or changes in the uterine bleeding profile).
No products indexed under this heading.

Indinavir Sulfate (Inhibitors of CYP3A4 such as erythromycin, clarithromycin, ketoconazole, itraconazole, ritonavir and grapefruit juice may increase plasma concentrations of estrogens and may result in side effects). Products include:
Crixivan Capsules **1940**

Isoniazid (Inhibitors of CYP3A4 such as erythromycin, clarithromycin, ketoconazole, itraconazole, ritonavir and grapefruit juice may increase plasma concentrations of estrogens and may result in side effects).
No products indexed under this heading.

Itraconazole (Inhibitors of CYP3A4 such as erythromycin, clarithromycin, ketoconazole, itraconazole, ritonavir and grapefruit juice may increase plasma concentrations of estrogens and may result in side effects).
No products indexed under this heading.

Ketoconazole (Inhibitors of CYP3A4 such as erythromycin, clarithromycin, ketoconazole, itraconazole, ritonavir and grapefruit juice may increase plasma concentrations of estrogens and may result in side effects). Products include:
Nizoral A-D Shampoo, 1% **1868**

Levothyroxine Sodium (Patients on thyroid replacement therapy may require higher doses of thryoid hormone). Products include:
Levothroid Tablets **1186**
Levoxyl Tablets **1712**
Synthroid Tablets **520**
Westhroid Tablets **3403**

Liothyronine Sodium (Patients on thyroid replacement therapy may require higher doses of thryoid hormone). Products include:
Cytomel Tablets **1710**
Westhroid Tablets **3403**

Liotrix (Patients on thyroid replacement therapy may require higher doses of thyroid hormone). Products include:
Thyrolar Tablets **1199**

Lopinavir (Inhibitors of CYP3A4 such as erythromycin, clarithromycin, ketoconazole, itraconazole, ritonavir and grapefruit juice may increase plasma concentrations of estrogens and may result in side effects). Products include:
Kaletra **476**

Loratadine (Inhibitors of CYP3A4 such as erythromycin, clarithromycin, ketoconazole, itraconazole, ritonavir and grapefruit juice may increase plasma concentrations of estrogens and may result in side effects). Products include:
Alavert Allergy & Sinus D-12 Hour Tablets .... ▣**771**
Alavert .... ▣**771**
Children's Claritin Allergy Oral Solution .... ▣**771**
Claritin Non-Drowsy 24 Hour Tablets .... ▣**772**
Claritin Reditabs 24 Hour Non-Drowsy Tablets .... ▣**772**
Claritin-D Non-Drowsy 12 Hour Tablets .... ▣**772**
Claritin-D Non-Drowsy 24 Hour Tablets .... ▣**772**

Mephenytoin (Inducers of CYP3A4 such as St. John's Wort preparations (hypericum perforatum), phenobarbital, carbamazepine and rifampin may reduce plasma concentrations of estrogens, possibly resulting in a decrease in therapeutic effects and/or changes in the uterine bleeding profile).
No products indexed under this heading.

Methsuximide (Inducers of CYP3A4 such as St. John's Wort preparations (hypericum perforatum), phenobarbital, carbamazepine and rifampin may reduce plasma concentrations of estrogens, possibly resulting in a decrease in therapeutic effects and/or changes in the uterine bleeding profile).
No products indexed under this heading.

Methylprednisolone (Inducers of CYP3A4 such as St. John's Wort preparations (hypericum perforatum), phenobarbital, carbamazepine and rifampin may reduce plasma concentrations of estrogens, possibly resulting in a decrease in therapeutic effects and/or changes in the uterine bleeding profile).
No products indexed under this heading.

Methylprednisolone Acetate (Inducers of CYP3A4 such as St. John's Wort preparations (hypericum perforatum), phenobarbital, carbamazepine and rifampin may reduce plasma concentrations of estrogens, possibly resulting in a decrease in therapeutic effects and/or changes in the uterine bleeding profile). Products include:
Depo-Medrol Injectable Suspension **2617**
Depo-Medrol Single-Dose Vial **2619**

Methylprednisolone Sodium Succinate (Inducers of CYP3A4 such as St. John's Wort preparations (hypericum perforatum), phenobarbital, carbamazepine and rifampin may reduce plasma concentrations of estrogens, possibly resulting in a decrease in therapeutic effects and/or changes in the uterine bleeding profile).
No products indexed under this heading.

Metronidazole (Inhibitors of CYP3A4 such as erythromycin, clarithromycin, ketoconazole, itraconazole, ritonavir and grapefruit juice may increase plasma concentrations of estrogens and may result in side effects). Products include:
Metrogel 1% **1211**
MetroGel-Vaginal Gel **1855**
Vandazole Vaginal Gel **3338**

Metronidazole Benzoate (Inhibitors of CYP3A4 such as erythromycin, clarithromycin, ketoconazole, itraconazole, ritonavir and grapefruit juice may increase plasma concentrations of estrogens and may result in side effects).
No products indexed under this heading.

Metronidazole Hydrochloride (Inhibitors of CYP3A4 such as erythromycin, clarithromycin, ketoconazole, itraconazole, ritonavir and grapefruit juice may increase plasma concentrations of estrogens and may result in side effects).
No products indexed under this heading.

Miconazole (Inhibitors of CYP3A4 such as erythromycin, clarithromycin, ketoconazole, itraconazole, ritonavir and grapefruit juice may increase plasma concentrations of estrogens and may result in side effects).
No products indexed under this heading.

Miconazole Nitrate (Inhibitors of CYP3A4 such as erythromycin, clarithromycin, ketoconazole, itraconazole, ritonavir and grapefruit juice may increase plasma concentrations of estrogens and may result in side effects). Products include:
Desenex .... ▣**635**
Desenex Jock Itch Spray Powder ... ▣**635**

Modafinil (Inducers of CYP3A4 such as St. John's Wort preparations (hypericum perforatum), phenobarbital, carbamazepine and rifampin may reduce plasma concentrations of estrogens, possibly resulting in a decrease in therapeutic effects and/or changes in the uterine bleeding profile). Products include:
Provigil Tablets **988**

Nefazodone Hydrochloride (Inhibitors of CYP3A4 such as erythromycin, clarithromycin, ketoconazole, itraconazole, ritonavir and grapefruit juice may increase plasma concentrations of estrogens and may result in side effects).
No products indexed under this heading.

Nelfinavir Mesylate (Inhibitors of CYP3A4 such as erythromycin, clarithromycin, ketoconazole, itraconazole, ritonavir and grapefruit juice may increase plasma concentrations of estrogens and may result in side effects). Products include:
Viracept **2577**

Nevirapine (Inducers of CYP3A4 such as St. John's Wort preparations (hypericum perforatum), phenobarbital, carbamazepine and rifampin may reduce plasma concentrations of estrogens, possibly resulting in a decrease in therapeutic effects and/or changes in the uterine bleeding profile). Products include:
Viramune Oral Suspension **873**
Viramune Tablets **873**

Niacinamide (Inhibitors of CYP3A4 such as erythromycin, clarithromycin, ketoconazole, itraconazole, ritonavir and grapefruit juice may increase plasma concentrations of estrogens and may result in side effects).
No products indexed under this heading.

Nicotinamide (Inhibitors of CYP3A4 such as erythromycin, clarithromycin, ketoconazole, itraconazole, ritonavir and grapefruit juice may increase plasma concentrations of estrogens and may result in side effects). Products include:
Nicomide Tablets **1088**

Nifedipine (Inhibitors of CYP3A4 such as erythromycin, clarithromycin, ketoconazole, itraconazole, ritonavir and grapefruit juice may increase plasma concentrations of estrogens and may result in side effects). Products include:
Adalat CC Tablets **2964**

Norfloxacin (Inhibitors of CYP3A4 such as erythromycin, clarithromycin, ketoconazole, itraconazole, ritonavir and grapefruit juice may increase plasma concentrations of estrogens and may result in side effects). Products include:

Noroxin Tablets 2032

Omeprazole (Inhibitors of CYP3A4 such as erythromycin, clarithromycin, ketoconazole, itraconazole, ritonavir and grapefruit juice may increase plasma concentrations of estrogens and may result in side effects). Products include:

Zegerid Capsules 2958
Zegerid Powder for Oral Solution 2958

Oxcarbazepine (Inducers of CYP3A4 such as St. John's Wort preparations (hypericum perforatum), phenobarbital, carbamazepine and rifampin may reduce plasma concentrations of estrogens, possibly resulting in a decrease in therapeutic effects and/or changes in the uterine bleeding profile). Products include:

Trileptal Tablets 2300
Trileptal Oral Suspension 2300

Paroxetine Hydrochloride (Inhibitors of CYP3A4 such as erythromycin, clarithromycin, ketoconazole, itraconazole, ritonavir and grapefruit juice may increase plasma concentrations of estrogens and may result in side effects). Products include:

Paxil CR Controlled-Release Tablets 1538
Paxil 1530

Phenobarbital (Inducers of CYP3A4 such as St. John's Wort preparations (hypericum perforatum), phenobarbital, carbamazepine and rifampin may reduce plasma concentrations of estrogens, possibly resulting in a decrease in therapeutic effects and/or changes in the uterine bleeding profile). Products include:

Donnatal Extentabs 2493

Phenobarbital Sodium (Inducers of CYP3A4 such as St. John's Wort preparations (hypericum perforatum), phenobarbital, carbamazepine and rifampin may reduce plasma concentrations of estrogens, possibly resulting in a decrease in therapeutic effects and/or changes in the uterine bleeding profile).

No products indexed under this heading.

Phenytoin (Inducers of CYP3A4 such as St. John's Wort preparations (hypericum perforatum), phenobarbital, carbamazepine and rifampin may reduce plasma concentrations of estrogens, possibly resulting in a decrease in therapeutic effects and/or changes in the uterine bleeding profile).

No products indexed under this heading.

Phenytoin Sodium (Inducers of CYP3A4 such as St. John's Wort preparations (hypericum perforatum), phenobarbital, carbamazepine and rifampin may reduce plasma concentrations of estrogens, possibly resulting in a decrease in therapeutic effects and/or changes in the uterine bleeding profile). Products include:

Phenytek Capsules 2160

Prednisolone Acetate (Inducers of CYP3A4 such as St. John's Wort preparations (hypericum perforatum), phenobarbital, carbamazepine and rifampin may reduce plasma concentrations of estrogens, possibly resulting in a decrease in therapeutic effects and/or changes in the uterine bleeding profile). Products include:

Blephamide Ophthalmic Ointment 568
Blephamide Ophthalmic Suspension 569
Poly-Pred Ophthalmic Suspension .... ⊙233
Pred Forte Ophthalmic Suspension .... ⊙235
Pred Mild Ophthalmic Suspension .... ⊙238
Pred-G Ophthalmic Ointment .... ⊙237
Pred-G Ophthalmic Suspension ...... ⊙236

Prednisolone Sodium Phosphate (Inducers of CYP3A4 such as St. John's Wort preparations (hypericum perforatum), phenobarbital, carbamazepine and rifampin may reduce plasma concentrations of estrogens, possibly resulting in a decrease in therapeutic effects and/or changes in the uterine bleeding profile).

No products indexed under this heading.

Prednisolone Tebutate (Inducers of CYP3A4 such as St. John's Wort preparations (hypericum perforatum), phenobarbital, carbamazepine and rifampin may reduce plasma concentrations of estrogens, possibly resulting in a decrease in therapeutic effects and/or changes in the uterine bleeding profile).

No products indexed under this heading.

Prednisone (Inducers of CYP3A4 such as St. John's Wort preparations (hypericum perforatum), phenobarbital, carbamazepine and rifampin may reduce plasma concentrations of estrogens, possibly resulting in a decrease in therapeutic effects and/or changes in the uterine bleeding profile).

No products indexed under this heading.

Primidone (Inducers of CYP3A4 such as St. John's Wort preparations (hypericum perforatum), phenobarbital, carbamazepine and rifampin may reduce plasma concentrations of estrogens, possibly resulting in a decrease in therapeutic effects and/or changes in the uterine bleeding profile).

No products indexed under this heading.

Propoxyphene Hydrochloride (Inhibitors of CYP3A4 such as erythromycin, clarithromycin, ketoconazole, itraconazole, ritonavir and grapefruit juice may increase plasma concentrations of estrogens and may result in side effects).

No products indexed under this heading.

Propoxyphene Napsylate (Inhibitors of CYP3A4 such as erythromycin, clarithromycin, ketoconazole, itraconazole, ritonavir and grapefruit juice may increase plasma concentrations of estrogens and may result in side effects).

No products indexed under this heading.

Quinidine (Inhibitors of CYP3A4 such as erythromycin, clarithromycin, ketoconazole, itraconazole, ritonavir and grapefruit juice may increase plasma concentrations of estrogens and may result in side effects).

No products indexed under this heading.

Quinidine Hydrochloride (Inhibitors of CYP3A4 such as erythromycin, clarithromycin, ketoconazole, itraconazole, ritonavir and grapefruit juice may increase plasma concentrations of estrogens and may result in side effects).

No products indexed under this heading.

Quinidine Polygalacturonate (Inhibitors of CYP3A4 such as erythromycin, clarithromycin, ketoconazole, itraconazole, ritonavir and grapefruit juice may increase plasma concentrations of estrogens and may result in side effects).

No products indexed under this heading.

Quinidine Sulfate (Inhibitors of CYP3A4 such as erythromycin, clarithromycin, ketoconazole, itraconazole, ritonavir and grapefruit juice may increase plasma concentrations of estrogens and may result in side effects).

No products indexed under this heading.

Quinine (Inhibitors of CYP3A4 such as erythromycin, clarithromycin, ketoconazole, itraconazole, ritonavir and grapefruit juice may increase plasma concentrations of estrogens and may result in side effects).

No products indexed under this heading.

Quinine Sulfate (Inhibitors of CYP3A4 such as erythromycin, clarithromycin, ketoconazole, itraconazole, ritonavir and grapefruit juice may increase plasma concentrations of estrogens and may result in side effects).

No products indexed under this heading.

Quinupristin (Inhibitors of CYP3A4 such as erythromycin, clarithromycin, ketoconazole, itraconazole, ritonavir and grapefruit juice may increase plasma concentrations of estrogens and may result in side effects).

No products indexed under this heading.

Ranitidine Bismuth Citrate (Inhibitors of CYP3A4 such as erythromycin, clarithromycin, ketoconazole, itraconazole, ritonavir and grapefruit juice may increase plasma concentrations of estrogens and may result in side effects).

No products indexed under this heading.

Ranitidine Hydrochloride (Inhibitors of CYP3A4 such as erythromycin, clarithromycin, ketoconazole, itraconazole, ritonavir and grapefruit juice may increase plasma concentrations of estrogens and may result in side effects). Products include:

Zantac 1624
Zantac Injection 1619
Zantac Injection Pharmacy Bulk Package 1622

Rifabutin (Inducers of CYP3A4 such as St. John's Wort preparations (hypericum perforatum), phenobarbital, carbamazepine and rifampin may reduce plasma concentrations of estrogens, possibly resulting in a decrease in therapeutic effects and/or changes in the uterine bleeding profile).

No products indexed under this heading.

Rifampicin (Inducers of CYP3A4 such as St. John's Wort preparations (hypericum perforatum), phenobarbital, carbamazepine and rifampin may reduce plasma concentrations of estrogens, possibly resulting in a decrease in therapeutic effects and/or changes in the uterine bleeding profile).

No products indexed under this heading.

Rifampin (Inducers of CYP3A4 such as St. John's Wort preparations (hypericum perforatum), phenobarbital, carbamazepine and rifampin may reduce plasma concentrations of estrogens, possibly resulting in a decrease in therapeutic effects and/or changes in the uterine bleeding profile).

No products indexed under this heading.

Rifapentine (Inducers of CYP3A4 such as St. John's Wort preparations (hypericum perforatum), phenobarbital, carbamazepine and rifampin may reduce plasma concentrations of estrogens, possibly resulting in a decrease in therapeutic effects and/or changes in the uterine bleeding profile).

No products indexed under this heading.

Ritonavir (Inhibitors of CYP3A4 such as erythromycin, clarithromycin, ketoconazole, itraconazole, ritonavir and grapefruit juice may increase plasma concentrations of estrogens and may result in side effects). Products include:

Kaletra 476
Norvir 503

Saquinavir (Inhibitors of CYP3A4 such as erythromycin, clarithromycin, ketoconazole, itraconazole, ritonavir and grapefruit juice may increase plasma concentrations of estrogens and may result in side effects).

No products indexed under this heading.

Saquinavir Mesylate (Inhibitors of CYP3A4 such as erythromycin, clarithromycin, ketoconazole, itraconazole, ritonavir and grapefruit juice may increase plasma concentrations of estrogens and may result in side effects). Products include:

Invirase 2772

Sertraline Hydrochloride (Inhibitors of CYP3A4 such as erythromycin, clarithromycin, ketoconazole, itraconazole, ritonavir and grapefruit juice may increase plasma concentrations of estrogens and may result in side effects). Products include:

Zoloft 2586

Sulfinpyrazone (Inducers of CYP3A4 such as St. John's Wort preparations (hypericum perforatum), phenobarbital, carbamazepine and rifampin may reduce plasma concentrations of estrogens, possibly resulting in a decrease in therapeutic effects and/or changes in the uterine bleeding profile).

No products indexed under this heading.

Telithromycin (Inhibitors of CYP3A4 such as erythromycin, clarithromycin, ketoconazole, itraconazole, ritonavir and grapefruit juice may increase plasma concentrations of estrogens and may result in side effects). Products include:

Ketek Tablets 2903

Theophylline (Inducers of CYP3A4 such as St. John's Wort preparations (hypericum perforatum), phenobarbital, carbamazepine and rifampin may reduce plasma concentrations of estrogens, possibly resulting in a decrease in therapeutic effects and/or changes in the uterine bleeding profile).
No products indexed under this heading.

Thyroglobulin (Patients on thyroid replacement therapy may require higher doses of thryoid hormone).
No products indexed under this heading.

Thyroid (Patients on thyroid replacement therapy may require higher doses of thryoid hormone).
No products indexed under this heading.

Thyroxine (Patients on thyroid replacement therapy may require higher doses of thryoid hormone).
No products indexed under this heading.

Thyroxine Sodium (Patients on thyroid replacement therapy may require higher doses of thryoid hormone).
No products indexed under this heading.

Triamcinolone (Inducers of CYP3A4 such as St. John's Wort preparations (hypericum perforatum), phenobarbital, carbamazepine and rifampin may reduce plasma concentrations of estrogens, possibly resulting in a decrease in therapeutic effects and/or changes in the uterine bleeding profile).
No products indexed under this heading.

Triamcinolone Acetonide (Inducers of CYP3A4 such as St. John's Wort preparations (hypericum perforatum), phenobarbital, carbamazepine and rifampin may reduce plasma concentrations of estrogens, possibly resulting in a decrease in therapeutic effects and/or changes in the uterine bleeding profile). Products include:
Azmacort Inhalation Aerosol **1726**
Nasacort AQ Nasal Spray **2922**

Triamcinolone Diacetate (Inducers of CYP3A4 such as St. John's Wort preparations (hypericum perforatum), phenobarbital, carbamazepine and rifampin may reduce plasma concentrations of estrogens, possibly resulting in a decrease in therapeutic effects and/or changes in the uterine bleeding profile).
No products indexed under this heading.

Triamcinolone Hexacetonide (Inducers of CYP3A4 such as St. John's Wort preparations (hypericum perforatum), phenobarbital, carbamazepine and rifampin may reduce plasma concentrations of estrogens, possibly resulting in a decrease in therapeutic effects and/or changes in the uterine bleeding profile).
No products indexed under this heading.

Troglitazone (Inducers of CYP3A4 such as St. John's Wort preparations (hypericum perforatum), phenobarbital, carbamazepine and rifampin may reduce plasma concentrations of estrogens, possibly resulting in a decrease in therapeutic effects and/or changes in the uterine bleeding profile).
No products indexed under this heading.

Troleandomycin (Inhibitors of CYP3A4 such as erythromycin, clarithromycin, ketoconazole, itraconazole, ritonavir and grapefruit juice may increase plasma concentrations of estrogens and may result in side effects).
No products indexed under this heading.

Valproate Sodium (Inhibitors of CYP3A4 such as erythromycin, clarithromycin, ketoconazole, itraconazole, ritonavir and grapefruit juice may increase plasma concentrations of estrogens and may result in side effects). Products include:
Depacon Injection **412**

Verapamil Hydrochloride (Inhibitors of CYP3A4 such as erythromycin, clarithromycin, ketoconazole, itraconazole, ritonavir and grapefruit juice may increase plasma concentrations of estrogens and may result in side effects). Products include:
Covera-HS Tablets **3139**
Tarka Tablets **524**
Verelan PM Extended-Release Capsules, Controlled-Onset........... **3106**

Voriconazole (Inhibitors of CYP3A4 such as erythromycin, clarithromycin, ketoconazole, itraconazole, ritonavir and grapefruit juice may increase plasma concentrations of estrogens and may result in side effects). Products include:
VFEND I.V. **2564**
VFEND Oral Suspension **2564**
VFEND Tablets **2564**

Zafirlukast (Inhibitors of CYP3A4 such as erythromycin, clarithromycin, ketoconazole, itraconazole, ritonavir and grapefruit juice may increase plasma concentrations of estrogens and may result in side effects). Products include:
Accolate Tablets **671**

Zileuton (Inhibitors of CYP3A4 such as erythromycin, clarithromycin, ketoconazole, itraconazole, ritonavir and grapefruit juice may increase plasma concentrations of estrogens and may result in side effects). Products include:
Zyflo Tablets **1023**

Food Interactions

Grapefruit (Inhibitors of CYP3A4 such as erythromycin, clarithromycin, ketoconazole, itraconazole, ritonavir and grapefruit juice may increase plasma concentrations of estrogens and may result in side effects).

Grapefruit Juice (Inhibitors of CYP3A4 such as erythromycin, clarithromycin, ketoconazole, itraconazole, ritonavir and grapefruit juice may increase plasma concentrations of estrogens and may result in side effects).

ENTOCORT EC CAPSULES

(Budesonide) **2698**
May interact with cytochrome p450 3a4 inducers (selected), cytochrome p450 3a4 inhibitors (selected), erythromycin, and certain other agents. Compounds in these categories include:

Acetazolamide (Co-administration with known inhibitors of CYP3A4 may increase the plasma levels of budesonide several-fold).
No products indexed under this heading.

Allium sativum (Induction of CYP3A4 can result in the lowering of budesonide plasma levels).
No products indexed under this heading.

Amiodarone Hydrochloride (Co-administration with known inhibitors of CYP3A4 may increase the plasma levels of budesonide several-fold).
No products indexed under this heading.

Amprenavir (Co-administration with known inhibitors of CYP3A4 may increase the plasma levels of budesonide several-fold). Products include:
Agenerase Capsules **1327**
Agenerase Oral Solution **1332**

Anastrozole (Co-administration with known inhibitors of CYP3A4 may increase the plasma levels of budesonide several-fold). Products include:
Arimidex Tablets **673**

Aprepitant (Co-administration with known inhibitors of CYP3A4 may increase the plasma levels of budesonide several-fold). Products include:
Emend Capsules **1963**

Betamethasone Acetate (Induction of CYP3A4 can result in the lowering of budesonide plasma levels).
No products indexed under this heading.

Betamethasone Sodium Phosphate (Induction of CYP3A4 can result in the lowering of budesonide plasma levels).
No products indexed under this heading.

Carbamazepine (Induction of CYP3A4 can result in the lowering of budesonide plasma levels). Products include:
Carbatrol Capsules **3171**
Equetro Extended-Release Capsules.. **3180**
Tegretol/Tegretol-XR **2295**

Cimetidine (Co-administration with known inhibitors of CYP3A4 may increase the plasma levels of budesonide several-fold). Products include:
Tagamet HB 200 Tablets .... ■**664**

Cimetidine Hydrochloride (Co-administration with known inhibitors of CYP3A4 may increase the plasma levels of budesonide several-fold).
No products indexed under this heading.

Ciprofloxacin (Co-administration with known inhibitors of CYP3A4 may increase the plasma levels of budesonide several-fold). Products include:
Cipro Oral Suspension **2977**
Cipro I.V. **2984**
Cipro XR Tablets **2990**
Ciprodex Otic Suspension **559**

Ciprofloxacin Hydrochloride (Induction of CYP3A4 can result in the lowering of budesonide plasma levels). Products include:
Ciloxan Ophthalmic Ointment **559**
Ciloxan Ophthalmic Solution .... ⊙**206**
Cipro Tablets **2977**
Proquin XR Tablets **1153**

Cisplatin (Induction of CYP3A4 can result in the lowering of budesonide plasma levels).
No products indexed under this heading.

Clarithromycin (Co-administration with known inhibitors of CYP3A4 may increase the plasma levels of budesonide several-fold). Products include:
Biaxin/Biaxin XL **402**
PREVPAC **3284**

Clotrimazole (Co-administration with known inhibitors of CYP3A4 may increase the plasma levels of budesonide several-fold). Products include:
Desenex Athlete's Foot Cream .... ■**635**
Lotrimin **3039**
Lotrisone **3040**

Cortisone Acetate (Induction of CYP3A4 can result in the lowering of budesonide plasma levels).
No products indexed under this heading.

Cyclosporine (Co-administration with known inhibitors of CYP3A4 may increase the plasma levels of budesonide several-fold). Products include:
Gengraf Capsules **459**
Neoral Oral Solution **2259**
Neoral Soft Gelatin Capsules **2259**
Restasis Ophthalmic Emulsion **575**
Sandimmune **2275**

Dalfopristin (Co-administration with known inhibitors of CYP3A4 may increase the plasma levels of budesonide several-fold).
No products indexed under this heading.

Danazol (Co-administration with known inhibitors of CYP3A4 may increase the plasma levels of budesonide several-fold).
No products indexed under this heading.

Delavirdine Mesylate (Co-administration with known inhibitors of CYP3A4 may increase the plasma levels of budesonide several-fold). Products include:
Rescriptor Tablets **2551**

Dexamethasone (Induction of CYP3A4 can result in the lowering of budesonide plasma levels). Products include:
Ciprodex Otic Suspension **559**
Decadron Tablets **1951**
TobraDex Ophthalmic Ointment **562**
TobraDex Ophthalmic Suspension ... **563**

Dexamethasone Acetate (Induction of CYP3A4 can result in the lowering of budesonide plasma levels).
No products indexed under this heading.

Dexamethasone Sodium Phosphate (Induction of CYP3A4 can result in the lowering of budesonide plasma levels).
No products indexed under this heading.

Diltiazem Hydrochloride (Co-administration with known inhibitors of CYP3A4 may increase the plasma levels of budesonide several-fold). Products include:
Cardizem LA Extended Release Tablets.. **1728**
Tiazac Capsules **1201**

Diltiazem Maleate (Co-administration with known inhibitors of CYP3A4 may increase the plasma levels of budesonide several-fold).
No products indexed under this heading.

Doxorubicin Hydrochloride (Induction of CYP3A4 can result in the lowering of budesonide plasma levels).
No products indexed under this heading.

Efavirenz (Co-administration with known inhibitors of CYP3A4 may increase the plasma levels of budesonide several-fold). Products include:
Atripla Tablets **945**
Sustiva Capsules **930**
Sustiva Tablets **930**

Erythromycin (Co-administration with known inhibitors of CYP3A4 may cause rise in systemic exposure to oral budesonide; reduction in budesonide dosage should be considered). Products include:

Erythromycin Estolate (Co-administration with known inhibitors of CYP3A4 may cause rise in systemic exposure to oral budesonide; reduction in budesonide dosage should be considered).
 No products indexed under this heading.

Erythromycin Ethylsuccinate (Co-administration with known inhibitors of CYP3A4 may cause rise in systemic exposure to oral budesonide; reduction in budesonide dosage should be considered). Products include:

Erythromycin Gluceptate (Co-administration with known inhibitors of CYP3A4 may cause rise in systemic exposure to oral budesonide; reduction in budesonide dosage should be considered).
 No products indexed under this heading.

Erythromycin Lactobionate (Co-administration with known inhibitors of CYP3A4 may cause rise in systemic exposure to oral budesonide; reduction in budesonide dosage should be considered).
 No products indexed under this heading.

Erythromycin Stearate (Co-administration with known inhibitors of CYP3A4 may cause rise in systemic exposure to oral budesonide; reduction in budesonide dosage should be considered). Products include:

Esomeprazole Magnesium (Co-administration with known inhibitors of CYP3A4 may increase the plasma levels of budesonide several-fold). Products include:

Ethosuximide (Induction of CYP3A4 can result in the lowering of budesonide plasma levels).
 No products indexed under this heading.

Felbamate (Induction of CYP3A4 can result in the lowering of budesonide plasma levels).
 No products indexed under this heading.

Fluconazole (Co-administration with known inhibitors of CYP3A4 may increase the plasma levels of budesonide several-fold).
 No products indexed under this heading.

Fludrocortisone Acetate (Induction of CYP3A4 can result in the lowering of budesonide plasma levels).
 No products indexed under this heading.

Fluoxetine Hydrochloride (Co-administration with known inhibitors of CYP3A4 may increase the plasma levels of budesonide several-fold). Products include:

Fluvoxamine Maleate (Co-administration with known inhibitors of CYP3A4 may increase the plasma levels of budesonide several-fold).
 No products indexed under this heading.

Fosamprenavir Calcium (Co-administration with known inhibitors of CYP3A4 may increase the plasma levels of budesonide several-fold). Products include:

Fosphenytoin Sodium (Induction of CYP3A4 can result in the lowering of budesonide plasma levels).
 No products indexed under this heading.

Garlic Extract (Induction of CYP3A4 can result in the lowering of budesonide plasma levels).
 No products indexed under this heading.

Garlic Oil (Induction of CYP3A4 can result in the lowering of budesonide plasma levels).
 No products indexed under this heading.

Hydrocortisone (Induction of CYP3A4 can result in the lowering of budesonide plasma levels). Products include:

Hydrocortisone Acetate (Induction of CYP3A4 can result in the lowering of budesonide plasma levels). Products include:

Hydrocortisone Butyrate (Induction of CYP3A4 can result in the lowering of budesonide plasma levels). Products include:

Hydrocortisone Cypionate (Induction of CYP3A4 can result in the lowering of budesonide plasma levels).
 No products indexed under this heading.

Hydrocortisone Hemisuccinate (Induction of CYP3A4 can result in the lowering of budesonide plasma levels).
 No products indexed under this heading.

Hydrocortisone Probutate (Induction of CYP3A4 can result in the lowering of budesonide plasma levels).
 No products indexed under this heading.

Hydrocortisone Sodium Phosphate (Induction of CYP3A4 can result in the lowering of budesonide plasma levels).
 No products indexed under this heading.

Hydrocortisone Sodium Succinate (Induction of CYP3A4 can result in the lowering of budesonide plasma levels).
 No products indexed under this heading.

Hydrocortisone Valerate (Induction of CYP3A4 can result in the lowering of budesonide plasma levels).
 No products indexed under this heading.

Hypericum (Induction of CYP3A4 can result in the lowering of budesonide plasma levels). Products include:

Hypericum Perforatum (Induction of CYP3A4 can result in the lowering of budesonide plasma levels).
 No products indexed under this heading.

Indinavir Sulfate (Co-administration with known inhibitors of CYP3A4 may cause rise in systemic exposure to oral budesonide; reduction in budesonide dosage should be considered). Products include:

Isoniazid (Co-administration with known inhibitors of CYP3A4 may increase the plasma levels of budesonide several-fold).
 No products indexed under this heading.

Itraconazole (Co-administration with known inhibitors of CYP3A4 may cause rise in systemic exposure to oral budesonide; reduction in budesonide dosage should be considered).
 No products indexed under this heading.

Ketoconazole (Co-administration caused an eight-fold increase of the systemic exposure to oral budesonide; reduction in budesonide dosage should be considered). Products include:

Lopinavir (Co-administration with known inhibitors of CYP3A4 may increase the plasma levels of budesonide several-fold). Products include:

Loratadine (Co-administration with known inhibitors of CYP3A4 may increase the plasma levels of budesonide several-fold). Products include:

Mephenytoin (Induction of CYP3A4 can result in the lowering of budesonide plasma levels).
 No products indexed under this heading.

Methsuximide (Induction of CYP3A4 can result in the lowering of budesonide plasma levels).
 No products indexed under this heading.

Methylprednisolone (Induction of CYP3A4 can result in the lowering of budesonide plasma levels).
 No products indexed under this heading.

Methylprednisolone Acetate (Induction of CYP3A4 can result in the lowering of budesonide plasma levels). Products include:

Methylprednisolone Sodium Succinate (Induction of CYP3A4 can result in the lowering of budesonide plasma levels).
 No products indexed under this heading.

Metronidazole (Co-administration with known inhibitors of CYP3A4

may increase the plasma levels of budesonide several-fold). Products include:

Metronidazole Benzoate (Co-administration with known inhibitors of CYP3A4 may increase the plasma levels of budesonide several-fold).
 No products indexed under this heading.

Metronidazole Hydrochloride (Co-administration with known inhibitors of CYP3A4 may increase the plasma levels of budesonide several-fold).
 No products indexed under this heading.

Miconazole (Co-administration with known inhibitors of CYP3A4 may increase the plasma levels of budesonide several-fold).
 No products indexed under this heading.

Miconazole Nitrate (Co-administration with known inhibitors of CYP3A4 may increase the plasma levels of budesonide several-fold). Products include:

Modafinil (Induction of CYP3A4 can result in the lowering of budesonide plasma levels). Products include:

Nefazodone Hydrochloride (Co-administration with known inhibitors of CYP3A4 may increase the plasma levels of budesonide several-fold).
 No products indexed under this heading.

Nelfinavir Mesylate (Co-administration with known inhibitors of CYP3A4 may increase the plasma levels of budesonide several-fold). Products include:

Nevirapine (Co-administration with known inhibitors of CYP3A4 may increase the plasma levels of budesonide several-fold). Products include:

Niacinamide (Co-administration with known inhibitors of CYP3A4 may increase the plasma levels of budesonide several-fold).
 No products indexed under this heading.

Nicotinamide (Co-administration with known inhibitors of CYP3A4 may increase the plasma levels of budesonide several-fold). Products include:

Nifedipine (Co-administration with known inhibitors of CYP3A4 may increase the plasma levels of budesonide several-fold). Products include:

Norfloxacin (Co-administration with known inhibitors of CYP3A4 may increase the plasma levels of budesonide several-fold). Products include:

Omeprazole (Co-administration with known inhibitors of CYP3A4 may increase the plasma levels of budesonide several-fold). Products include:

IMPORTANT NOTE: Always consult each drug listing in the patient's regimen for possible interactions.

Oxcarbazepine (Induction of CYP3A4 can result in the lowering of budesonide plasma levels). Products include:

Paroxetine Hydrochloride (Co-administration with known inhibitors of CYP3A4 may increase the plasma levels of budesonide several-fold). Products include:

Phenobarbital (Induction of CYP3A4 can result in the lowering of budesonide plasma levels). Products include:

Phenobarbital Sodium (Induction of CYP3A4 can result in the lowering of budesonide plasma levels).
No products indexed under this heading.

Phenytoin (Induction of CYP3A4 can result in the lowering of budesonide plasma levels).
No products indexed under this heading.

Phenytoin Sodium (Induction of CYP3A4 can result in the lowering of budesonide plasma levels). Products include:

Prednisolone Acetate (Induction of CYP3A4 can result in the lowering of budesonide plasma levels). Products include:

Prednisolone Sodium Phosphate (Induction of CYP3A4 can result in the lowering of budesonide plasma levels).
No products indexed under this heading.

Prednisolone Tebutate (Induction of CYP3A4 can result in the lowering of budesonide plasma levels).
No products indexed under this heading.

Prednisone (Induction of CYP3A4 can result in the lowering of budesonide plasma levels).
No products indexed under this heading.

Primidone (Induction of CYP3A4 can result in the lowering of budesonide plasma levels).
No products indexed under this heading.

Propoxyphene Hydrochloride (Co-administration with known inhibitors of CYP3A4 may increase the plasma levels of budesonide several-fold).
No products indexed under this heading.

Propoxyphene Napsylate (Co-administration with known inhibitors of CYP3A4 may increase the plasma levels of budesonide several-fold).
No products indexed under this heading.

Quinidine (Co-administration with known inhibitors of CYP3A4 may increase the plasma levels of budes-onide several-fold).
No products indexed under this heading.

Quinidine Hydrochloride (Co-administration with known inhibitors of CYP3A4 may increase the plasma levels of budesonide several-fold).
No products indexed under this heading.

Quinidine Polygalacturonate (Co-administration with known inhibitors of CYP3A4 may increase the plasma levels of budesonide several-fold).
No products indexed under this heading.

Quinidine Sulfate (Co-administration with known inhibitors of CYP3A4 may increase the plasma levels of budesonide several-fold).
No products indexed under this heading.

Quinine (Co-administration with known inhibitors of CYP3A4 may increase the plasma levels of budes-onide several-fold).
No products indexed under this heading.

Quinine Sulfate (Co-administration with known inhibitors of CYP3A4 may increase the plasma levels of budesonide several-fold).
No products indexed under this heading.

Quinupristin (Co-administration with known inhibitors of CYP3A4 may increase the plasma levels of budesonide several-fold).
No products indexed under this heading.

Ranitidine Bismuth Citrate (Co-administration with known inhibitors of CYP3A4 may increase the plasma levels of budesonide several-fold).
No products indexed under this heading.

Ranitidine Hydrochloride (Co-administration with known inhibitors of CYP3A4 may increase the plasma levels of budesonide several-fold). Products include:

Rifabutin (Induction of CYP3A4 can result in the lowering of budesonide plasma levels).
No products indexed under this heading.

Rifampicin (Induction of CYP3A4 can result in the lowering of budes-onide plasma levels).
No products indexed under this heading.

Rifampin (Induction of CYP3A4 can result in the lowering of budesonide plasma levels).
No products indexed under this heading.

Rifapentine (Induction of CYP3A4 can result in the lowering of budes-onide plasma levels).
No products indexed under this heading.

Ritonavir (Co-administration with known inhibitors of CYP3A4 may cause rise in systemic exposure to oral budesonide; reduction in budes-onide dosage should be considered). Products include:

Saquinavir (Co-administration with known inhibitors of CYP3A4 may cause rise in systemic exposure to oral budesonide; reduction in budes-onide dosage should be considered).
No products indexed under this heading.

Saquinavir Mesylate (Co-administration with known inhibitors of CYP3A4 may cause rise in sys-temic exposure to oral budesonide; reduction in budesonide dosage should be considered). Products include:

Sertraline Hydrochloride (Co-administration with known inhibitors of CYP3A4 may increase the plasma levels of budesonide several-fold). Products include:

Sulfinpyrazone (Induction of CYP3A4 can result in the lowering of budesonide plasma levels).
No products indexed under this heading.

Telithromycin (Co-administration with known inhibitors of CYP3A4 may increase the plasma levels of budesonide several-fold). Products include:

Theophylline (Induction of CYP3A4 can result in the lowering of budes-onide plasma levels).
No products indexed under this heading.

Triamcinolone (Induction of CYP3A4 can result in the lowering of budesonide plasma levels).
No products indexed under this heading.

Triamcinolone Acetonide (Induc-tion of CYP3A4 can result in the low-ering of budesonide plasma levels). Products include:

Triamcinolone Diacetate (Induc-tion of CYP3A4 can result in the low-ering of budesonide plasma levels).
No products indexed under this heading.

Triamcinolone Hexacetonide (Induction of CYP3A4 can result in the lowering of budesonide plasma levels).
No products indexed under this heading.

Troglitazone (Co-administration with known inhibitors of CYP3A4 may increase the plasma levels of budesonide several-fold).
No products indexed under this heading.

Troleandomycin (Co-administration with known inhibitors of CYP3A4 may increase the plasma levels of budesonide several-fold).
No products indexed under this heading.

Valproate Sodium (Co-administration with known inhibitors of CYP3A4 may increase the plasma levels of budesonide several-fold). Products include:

Verapamil Hydrochloride (Co-administration with known inhibitors of CYP3A4 may increase the plasma levels of budesonide several-fold). Products include:

Voriconazole (Co-administration with known inhibitors of CYP3A4 may increase the plasma levels of budesonide several-fold). Products include:

Zafirlukast (Co-administration with known inhibitors of CYP3A4 may increase the plasma levels of budes-onide several-fold). Products include:

Zileuton (Co-administration with known inhibitors of CYP3A4 may increase the plasma levels of budes-onide several-fold). Products include:

Food Interactions

Grapefruit (Concurrent use with exten-sive intake of grapefruit juice has caused rise in systemic exposure of budesonide by two-fold; ingestion of grapefruit should be avoided).

Grapefruit Juice (Concurrent use with extensive intake of grapefruit juice has caused rise in systemic exposure of budesonide by two-fold; ingestion of grapefruit juice should be avoided).

EPIPEN AUTO-INJECTOR
(Epinephrine) 1061
May interact with cardiac glyco-sides, monoamine oxidase inhibi-tors, quinidine, tricyclic antidepres-sants, and certain other agents. Compounds in these categories in-clude:

Amitriptyline Hydrochloride (Co-administration with tricylcic antide-pressants may potentiate the effects of epinephrine).
No products indexed under this heading.

Amoxapine (Co-administration with tricylcic antidepressants may poten-tiate the effects of epinephrine).
No products indexed under this heading.

Clomipramine Hydrochloride (Co-administration with tricylcic anti-depressants may potentiate the effects of epinephrine).
No products indexed under this heading.

Desipramine Hydrochloride (Co-administration with tricylcic antide-pressants may potentiate the effects of epinephrine).
No products indexed under this heading.

Deslanoside (Co-administration with drugs that may sensitize the heart to arrhythmias, such as digita-lis, is not recommended).
No products indexed under this heading.

Digitalis Glycoside Preparations (Co-administration with drugs that may sensitize the heart to arrhyth-mias, such as digitalis, is not recommended).
No products indexed under this heading.

Digitoxin (Co-administration with drugs that may sensitize the heart to arrhythmias, such as digitalis, is not recommended).
No products indexed under this heading.

Digoxin (Co-administration with drugs that may sensitize the heart to arrhythmias, such as digitalis, is not recommended). Products include:

Lanoxin Injection 1494
Lanoxin Injection Pediatric 1497
Lanoxin Tablets 1500

Doxepin Hydrochloride (Co-administration with tricylcic antidepressants may potentiate the effects of epinephrine).
No products indexed under this heading.

Imipramine Hydrochloride (Co-administration with tricylcic antidepressants may potentiate the effects of epinephrine).
No products indexed under this heading.

Imipramine Pamoate (Co-administration with tricylcic antidepressants may potentiate the effects of epinephrine).
No products indexed under this heading.

Isocarboxazid (Co-administration with MAO inhibitors may potentiate the effects of epinephrine).
No products indexed under this heading.

Maprotiline Hydrochloride (Co-administration with tricylcic antidepressants may potentiate the effects of epinephrine).
No products indexed under this heading.

Mercurial Diuretics (Co-administration with drugs that may sensitize the heart to arrhythmias, such as mercurial diuretics, is not recommended).
No products indexed under this heading.

Moclobemide (Co-administration with MAO inhibitors may potentiate the effects of epinephrine).
No products indexed under this heading.

Nortriptyline Hydrochloride (Co-administration with tricylcic antidepressants may potentiate the effects of epinephrine).
No products indexed under this heading.

Pargyline Hydrochloride (Co-administration with MAO inhibitors may potentiate the effects of epinephrine).
No products indexed under this heading.

Phenelzine Sulfate (Co-administration with MAO inhibitors may potentiate the effects of epinephrine).
No products indexed under this heading.

Procarbazine Hydrochloride (Co-administration with MAO inhibitors may potentiate the effects of epinephrine). Products include:
Matulane Capsules 3191

Protriptyline Hydrochloride (Co-administration with tricylcic antidepressants may potentiate the effects of epinephrine).
No products indexed under this heading.

Quinidine (Co-administration with drugs that may sensitize the heart to arrhythmias, such as quinidine, is not recommended).
No products indexed under this heading.

Quinidine Gluconate (Co-administration with drugs that may sensitize the heart to arrhythmias, such as quinidine, is not recommended).
No products indexed under this heading.

Quinidine Hydrochloride (Co-administration with drugs that may sensitize the heart to arrhythmias, such as quinidine, is not recommended).
No products indexed under this heading.

Quinidine Polygalacturonate (Co-administration with drugs that may sensitize the heart to arrhythmias, such as quinidine, is not recommended).
No products indexed under this heading.

Quinidine Sulfate (Co-administration with drugs that may sensitize the heart to arrhythmias, such as quinidine, is not recommended).
No products indexed under this heading.

Selegiline Hydrochloride (Co-administration with MAO inhibitors may potentiate the effects of epinephrine). Products include:
Eldepryl Capsules 3208
Zelapar Tablets 3372

Tranylcypromine Sulfate (Co-administration with MAO inhibitors may potentiate the effects of epinephrine). Products include:
Parnate Tablets 1527

Trimipramine Maleate (Co-administration with tricylcic antidepressants may potentiate the effects of epinephrine).
No products indexed under this heading.

EPIPEN JR. AUTO-INJECTOR

(Epinephrine) 1061
See EpiPen Auto-Injector

EPIVIR ORAL SOLUTION

(Lamivudine) 1427
See Epivir Tablets

EPIVIR TABLETS

(Lamivudine) 1427
May interact with cationic drugs that are eliminated by renal tubular, Interferon alpha, and certain other agents. Compounds in these categories include:

Amiloride Hydrochloride (Lamivudine is predominantly eliminated in the urine by active organic secretion; therefore, the possibility of interactions with other drugs whose main route of elimination is active renal secretion via the organic cationic transport system should be considered). Products include:
Midamor Tablets 2026
Moduretic Tablets 2028

Digoxin (Lamivudine is predominantly eliminated in the urine by active organic secretion; therefore, the possibility of interactions with other drugs whose main route of elimination is active renal secretion via the organic cationic transport system should be considered). Products include:
Lanoxicaps Capsules 1490
Lanoxin Injection 1494
Lanoxin Injection Pediatric 1497
Lanoxin Tablets 1500

Interferon alfa-2a, Recombinant (Hepatic decompensation has occurred in HIV/HCV co-infected patients receiving combination antiretroviral therapy for HIV and interferon alpha with or withour ribavirin. Patients receiving interferon alpha with or without ribavirin and lamivudine should be closely monitored for treatment-associated toxicities, especially hepatic decompensation. Discontinuation of lamivudine should be considered as medically appropriate. Discontinuation of interferon alpha, ribavirin, or both should also be considered if worsening clinical toxicities are observed, including hepatic decompensation (e.g., Childs Pugh greater than 6)).
No products indexed under this heading.

Interferon alfa-2b, Recombinant (Hepatic decompensation has occurred in HIV/HCV co-infected patients receiving combination antiretroviral therapy for HIV and interferon alpha with or withour ribavirin. Patients receiving interferon alpha with or without ribavirin and lamivudine should be closely monitored for treatment-associated toxicities, especially hepatic decompensation. Discontinuation of lamivudine should be considered as medically appropriate. Discontinuation of interferon alpha, ribavirin, or both should also be considered if worsening clinical toxicities are observed, including hepatic decompensation (e.g., Childs Pugh greater than 6)). Products include:
Intron A for Injection 3024
Rebetron Combination Therapy 3063

Interferon alfa-N3 (Human Leukocyte Derived) (Hepatic decompensation has occurred in HIV/HCV co-infected patients receiving combination antiretroviral therapy for HIV and interferon alpha with or withour ribavirin. Patients receiving interferon alpha with or without ribavirin and lamivudine should be closely monitored for treatment-associated toxicities, especially hepatic decompensation. Discontinuation of lamivudine should be considered as medically appropriate. Discontinuation of interferon alpha, ribavirin, or both should also be considered if worsening clinical toxicities are observed, including hepatic decompensation (e.g., Childs Pugh greater than 6)). Products include:
Alferon N Injection 1665

Morphine Sulfate (Lamivudine is predominantly eliminated in the urine by active organic secretion; therefore, the possibility of interactions with other drugs whose main route of elimination is active renal secretion via the organic cationic transport system should be considered). Products include:
Avinza Capsules 1741
Kadian Capsules 577
MS Contin Tablets 2701

Peginterferon Alfa-2b (Hepatic decompensation has occurred in HIV/HCV co-infected patients receiving combination antiretroviral therapy for HIV and interferon alpha with or withour ribavirin. Patients receiving interferon alpha with or without ribavirin and lamivudine should be closely monitored for treatment-associated toxicities, especially hepatic decompensation. Discontinuation of lamivudine should be considered as medically appropriate. Discontinuation of interferon alpha, ribavirin, or both should also be considered if worsening clinical toxicities are observed, including hepatic decompensation (e.g., Childs Pugh greater than 6)). Products include:
PEG-Intron Powder for Injection 3048

Procainamide Hydrochloride (Lamivudine is predominantly eliminated in the urine by active organic secretion; therefore, the possibility of interactions with other drugs whose main route of elimination is active renal secretion via the organic cationic transport system should be considered).
No products indexed under this heading.

Quinidine Gluconate (Lamivudine is predominantly eliminated in the urine by active organic secretion; therefore, the possibility of interactions with other drugs whose main route of elimination is active renal secretion via the organic cationic transport system should be considered).
No products indexed under this heading.

Quinidine Polygalacturonate (Lamivudine is predominantly eliminated in the urine by active organic secretion; therefore, the possibility of interactions with other drugs whose main route of elimination is active renal secretion via the organic cationic transport system should be considered).
No products indexed under this heading.

Quinidine Sulfate (Lamivudine is predominantly eliminated in the urine by active organic secretion; therefore, the possibility of interactions with other drugs whose main route of elimination is active renal secretion via the organic cationic transport system should be considered).
No products indexed under this heading.

Quinine Sulfate (Lamivudine is predominantly eliminated in the urine by active organic secretion; therefore, the possibility of interactions with other drugs whose main route of elimination is active renal secretion via the organic cationic transport system should be considered).
No products indexed under this heading.

Ranitidine Hydrochloride (Lamivudine is predominantly eliminated in the urine by active organic secretion; therefore, the possibility of interactions with other drugs whose main route of elimination is active renal secretion via the organic cationic transport system should be considered). Products include:
Zantac 1624
Zantac Injection 1619
Zantac Injection Pharmacy Bulk Package 1622

Sulfamethoxazole (Co-administration of lamivudine with 160 mg of trimethoprim and 800 mg of sulfamethoxazole once daily has been shown to increase lamivudine exposure (AUC); the effect of higher doses of TMP/SMX on lamivudine pharmacokinetics has not been investigated; no change in dose of either drug is recommended).
No products indexed under this heading.

Triamterene (Lamivudine is predominantly eliminated in the urine by active organic secretion; therefore, the possibility of interactions with other drugs whose main route of elimination is active renal secretion via the organic cationic transport system should be considered). Products include:

Trimethoprim (Co-administration of lamivudine with 160 mg of trimethoprim and 800 mg of sulfamethoxazole once daily has been shown to increase lamivudine exposure (AUC); the effect of higher doses of TMP/SMX on lamivudine pharmacokinetics has not been investigated; no change in dose of either drug is recommended).

No products indexed under this heading.

Trimethoprim Sulfate (Lamivudine is predominantly eliminated in the urine by active organic secretion; therefore, the possibility of interactions with other drugs whose main route of elimination is active renal secretion via the organic cationic transport system should be considered). Products include:

Vancomycin Hydrochloride (Lamivudine is predominantly eliminated in the urine by active organic secretion; therefore, the possibility of interactions with other drugs whose main route of elimination is active renal secretion via the organic cationic transport system should be considered). Products include:

Zalcitabine (Lamivudine and zalcitabine may inhibit the intracellular phosphorylation of one another; concurrent use is not recommended).

No products indexed under this heading.

Food Interactions

Food, unspecified (Absorption of lamivudine was slower in the fed state compared with fasted state; there was no significant difference in systemic exposure in the fed state and fasted states; Epivir may be given with or without food).

EPIVIR-HBV ORAL SOLUTION

See Epivir-HBV Tablets

EPIVIR-HBV TABLETS

May interact with cationic drugs that are eliminated by renal tubular and certain other agents. Compounds in these categories include:

Amiloride Hydrochloride (Lamivudine is predominantly eliminated in the urine by active organic secretion; therefore, the possibility of interactions with other drugs whose main route of elimination is active renal secretion via the organic cationic transport system should be considered). Products include:

Digoxin (Lamivudine is predominantly eliminated in the urine by active organic secretion; therefore, the possibility of interactions with other drugs whose main route of elimination is active renal secretion via the organic cationic transport system should be considered). Products include:

Morphine Sulfate (Lamivudine is predominantly eliminated in the urine by active organic secretion; there-

fore, the possibility of interactions with other drugs whose main route of elimination is active renal secretion via the organic cationic transport system should be considered). Products include:

Procainamide Hydrochloride (Lamivudine is predominantly eliminated in the urine by active organic secretion; therefore, the possibility of interactions with other drugs whose main route of elimination is active renal secretion via the organic cationic transport system should be considered).

No products indexed under this heading.

Quinidine Gluconate (Lamivudine is predominantly eliminated in the urine by active organic secretion; therefore, the possibility of interactions with other drugs whose main route of elimination is active renal secretion via the organic cationic transport system should be considered).

No products indexed under this heading.

Quinidine Polygalacturonate (Lamivudine is predominantly eliminated in the urine by active organic secretion; therefore, the possibility of interactions with other drugs whose main route of elimination is active renal secretion via the organic cationic transport system should be considered).

No products indexed under this heading.

Quinidine Sulfate (Lamivudine is predominantly eliminated in the urine by active organic secretion; therefore, the possibility of interactions with other drugs whose main route of elimination is active renal secretion via the organic cationic transport system should be considered).

No products indexed under this heading.

Quinine Sulfate (Lamivudine is predominantly eliminated in the urine by active organic secretion; therefore, the possibility of interactions with other drugs whose main route of elimination is active renal secretion via the organic cationic transport system should be considered).

No products indexed under this heading.

Ranitidine Hydrochloride (Lamivudine is predominantly eliminated in the urine by active organic secretion; therefore, the possibility of interactions with other drugs whose main route of elimination is active renal secretion via the organic cationic transport system should be considered). Products include:

Sulfamethoxazole (Co-administration of lamivudine with 160 mg of trimethoprim and 800 mg of sulfamethoxazole once daily has been shown to increase lamivudine exposure (AUC); the effect of higher doses of TMP/SMX on lamivudine pharmacokinetics has not been investigated; no change in

dose of either drug is recommended).

No products indexed under this heading.

Triamterene (Lamivudine is predominantly eliminated in the urine by active organic secretion; therefore, the possibility of interactions with other drugs whose main route of elimination is active renal secretion via the organic cationic transport system should be considered). Products include:

Trimethoprim (Co-administration of lamivudine with 160 mg of trimethoprim and 800 mg of sulfamethoxazole once daily has been shown to increase lamivudine exposure (AUC); the effect of higher doses of TMP/SMX on lamivudine pharmacokinetics has not been investigated; no change in dose of either drug is recommended).

No products indexed under this heading.

Trimethoprim Sulfate (Lamivudine is predominantly eliminated in the urine by active organic secretion; therefore, the possibility of interactions with other drugs whose main route of elimination is active renal secretion via the organic cationic transport system should be considered). Products include:

Vancomycin Hydrochloride (Lamivudine is predominantly eliminated in the urine by active organic secretion; therefore, the possibility of interactions with other drugs whose main route of elimination is active renal secretion via the organic cationic transport system should be considered). Products include:

Zalacitabine (Lamivudine and zalcitabine may inhibit the intracellular phosphorylation of one another; co-administration is not recommended).

No products indexed under this heading.

EPOGEN FOR INJECTION

None cited in PDR database.

EPZICOM TABLETS

May interact with Interferon alpha and certain other agents. Compounds in these categories include:

Ethanol (Ethanol decreased the elimination of abacavir causing an increase in overall exposure).

No products indexed under this heading.

Interferon alfa-2a, Recombinant (Hepatic decompensation has occurred in HIV/HCV co-infected patients receiving combination antiretroviral therapy for HIV and interferon alpha with or without ribavirin. Patients receiving interferon alpha with or without ribavirin and Epzicom should be closely monitored for treatment-associated toxicities, especially hepatic decompensation. Discontinuation of Epzicom should be considered as medically appropriate. Discontinuation of interferon alpha, ribavirin, or both should also be considered if worsening clinical toxicities are observed, including

hepatic decompensation (e.g., Childs Pugh greater than 6)).

No products indexed under this heading.

Interferon alfa-2b, Recombinant (Hepatic decompensation has occurred in HIV/HCV co-infected patients receiving combination antiretroviral therapy for HIV and interferon alpha with or without ribavirin. Patients receiving interferon alpha with or without ribavirin and Epzicom should be closely monitored for treatment-associated toxicities, especially hepatic decompensation. Discontinuation of Epzicom should be considered as medically appropriate. Discontinuation of interferon alpha, ribavirin, or both should also be considered if worsening clinical toxicities are observed, including hepatic decompensation (e.g., Childs Pugh greater than 6)). Products include:

Interferon alfa-N3 (Human Leukocyte Derived) (Hepatic decompensation has occurred in HIV/HCV co-infected patients receiving combination antiretroviral therapy for HIV and interferon alpha with or without ribavirin. Patients receiving interferon alpha with or without ribavirin and Epzicom should be closely monitored for treatment-associated toxicities, especially hepatic decompensation. Discontinuation of Epzicom should be considered as medically appropriate. Discontinuation of interferon alpha, ribavirin, or both should also be considered if worsening clinical toxicities are observed, including hepatic decompensation (e.g., Childs Pugh greater than 6)). Products include:

Methadone Hydrochloride (Co-administration in patients on methadone-maintenance therapy had increased methadone clearance by 22%. This alteration will not result in a methadone dose modification in the majority of patients; however, an increased methadone dose may be required in a small number of patients).

No products indexed under this heading.

Nelfinavir Mesylate (Co-administration of lamivudine with nelfinavir has been shown to increase the AUC of lamivudine by 10%). Products include:

Peginterferon Alfa-2b (Hepatic decompensation has occurred in HIV/HCV co-infected patients receiving combination antiretroviral therapy for HIV and interferon alpha with or without ribavirin. Patients receiving interferon alpha with or without ribavirin and Epzicom should be closely monitored for treatment-associated toxicities, especially hepatic decompensation. Discontinuation of Epzicom should be considered as medically appropriate. Discontinuation of interferon alpha, ribavirin, or both should also be considered if worsening clinical toxicities are observed, including hepatic decompensation (e.g., Childs Pugh greater than 6)). Products include:

Sulfamethoxazole (Co-administration of lamivudine with 160mg of trimethoprim and 800mg of sulfamethoxazole once daily has been shown to increase lamivudine exposure (AUC). The effect of higher doses of TMP/SMX on lamivudine pharmacokinetics has not been investigated; no change in dose of either drug is recommended).

No products indexed under this heading.

Trimethoprim (Co-administration of lamivudine with 160mg of trimethoprim and 800mg of sulfamethoxazole once daily has been shown to increase lamivudine exposure (AUC). The effect of higher doses of TMP/SMX on lamivudine pharmacokinetics has not been investigated; no change in dose of either drug is recommended).

No products indexed under this heading.

Zalcitabine (Lamivudine and zalcitabine may inhibit the intracellular phosphorylation of one another; concurrent use is not recommended).

No products indexed under this heading.

EQUETRO EXTENDED-RELEASE CAPSULES

(Carbamazepine) ... **3180**

May interact with antimalarials, central nervous system depressants, cytochrome p450 1a2 substrates (selected), cytochrome p450 3a4 inducers (selected), cytochrome p450 3a4 inhibitors (selected), cytochrome p450 3a4 substrates (selected), oral contraceptives, phenytoin, and certain other agents. Compounds in these categories include:

Acetaminophen (Carbamazepine is known to induce CYP1A2 and CYP3A4. Therefore, the potential exists for interaction between carbamazepine and any agent metabolized by one (or more) of these enzymes. Agents that are metabolized by CYP1A2 and CYP3A4 may have decreased plasma levels when administered concomitantly with carbamazepine. Thus, if a patient has been titrated to a stable dosage on one of the agents in these categories, and then begins a course of treatment with carbamazepine, it is reasonable to expect that a dose increase for the concomitant agent may be necessary). Products include:

Comtrex Maximum Strength Cold & Cough Day/Night Caplets - Day Formulation ... **726**
Comtrex Maximum Strength Cold & Cough Day/Night Caplets - Night Formulation ... **726**
Comtrex Maximum Strength Non-Drowsy Cold & Cough Caplets ... **725**
Comtrex Maximum Strength Day/Night Severe Cold & Sinus Caplets - Day Formulation ... **725**
Comtrex Maximum Strength Day/Night Severe Cold & Sinus Caplets - Night Formulation ... **725**
Contac Cold and Flu Maximum Strength Caplets ... **728**
Contac Cold and Flu Day and Night Caplets (Day Formulation Only) ... **727**
Contac Cold and Flu Day and Night Caplets (Night Formulation Only) ... **727**
Contac Cold and Flu Non-Drowsy Caplets ... **728**
Excedrin Extra Strength Caplets/Tablets/Geltabs ... **684**
Excedrin Migraine Caplets/Tablets/Geltabs ... **609**
Excedrin PM Caplets/Tablets/Geltabs ... **610**
Excedrin Sinus Headache Caplets/Tablets ... **610**
Excedrin Tension Headache Caplets/Tablets/Geltabs ... **611**
Goody's Body Pain Formula Powder ... **684**
Goody's Extra Strength Headache Powders ... **611**
Goody's Extra Strength Pain Relief Tablets ... **685**
Goody's PM Powder for Pain with Sleeplessness ... **612**
Percocet Tablets ... **1131**
Robitussin Cough, Cold & Flu Nighttime Liquid ... **738**
TheraFlu Cold & Sore Throat Hot Liquid ... **741**
TheraFlu Flu & Chest Congestion Hot Liquid ... **741**
TheraFlu Flu & Sore Throat Hot Liquid ... **742**
TheraFlu Daytime Severe Cold Hot Liquid ... **742**
TheraFlu Nighttime Severe Cold Hot Liquid ... **740**
TheraFlu Warming Relief Daytime Severe Cold ... **743**
TheraFlu Warming Relief Nighttime Severe Cold ... **743**
Triaminic Cough & Sore Throat Liquid ... **747**
Regular Strength Tylenol Tablets ... **1870**
Children's Tylenol with Flavor Creator ... **679**
Children's Tylenol Plus Flu Oral Suspension ... **749**
Tylenol Cold Head Congestion Daytime Caplets with Cool Burst and Gelcaps ... **750**
Tylenol Cold Multi-Symptom Daytime Liquid ... **752**
Tylenol Cold Multi-Symptom Severe Daytime Liquid ... **752**
Tylenol 8 Hour Extended Release Caplets ... **1870**
Tylenol ... **1870**
Extra Strength Tylenol PM Caplets, Vanilla Caplets, Geltabs, Gelcaps and Liquid ... **1875**
Extra Strength Tylenol Rapid Release Gels ... **1870**
Concentrated Tylenol Infants' Drops Plus Cold & Cough ... **754**
Tylenol with Codeine Tablets ... **2391**
Tylenol Allergy Multi-Symptom Caplets with Cool Burst and Gelcaps ... **1872**
Tylenol Allergy Multi-Symptom Nighttime Caplets with Cool Burst ... **1872**
Tylenol Severe Allergy Caplets ... **1872**
Tylenol Arthritis Pain Extended Release Caplets and Geltabs ... **1870**
Tylenol Chest Congestion Caplets with Cool Burst ... **1872**
Tylenol Chest Congestion Liquid with Cool Burst ... **1872**
Children's Tylenol Suspension Liquid and Meltaways ... **1878**
Children's Tylenol Plus Cold Suspension Liquid ... **1879**
Children's Tylenol Plus Cold & Allergy Suspension Liquid ... **1878**
Children's Tylenol Plus Cough & Runny Nose Suspension Liquid ... **1879**
Children's Tylenol Plus Cough & Sore Throat Suspension Liquid ... **1879**
Children's Tylenol Suspension with Flavor Creator ... **1878**
Children's Tylenol Plus Flu Suspension Liquid ... **1881**
Children's Tylenol Plus Multi-Symptom Cold Suspension Liquid ... **1879**
Tylenol Cold Severe Congestion Non-Drowsy Caplets with Cool Burst ... **1874**
Tylenol Cold Head Congestion Daytime Caplets with Cool Burst ... **1873**
Tylenol Cold Head Congestion Nighttime Caplets with Cool Burst ... **1873**
Tylenol Cold Head Congestion Severe Caplets with Cool Burst ... **1873**
Tylenol Cold Multi-Symptom Daytime Caplets with Cool Burst and Gelcaps ... **1874**
Tylenol Cold Multi-Symptom Daytime Liquid with Citrus Burst ... **1874**
Tylenol Cold Multi-Symptom Nighttime Caplets with Cool Burst ... **1874**
Tylenol Cold Multi-Symptom Nighttime Liquid with Cool Burst ... **1874**
Tylenol Cold Multi-Symptom Severe Caplets with Cool Burst ... **1874**
Tylenol Cold Multi-Symptom Severe Daytime Liquid with Citrus Burst ... **1874**
Tylenol Cough & Sore Throat Daytime Liquid with Cool Burst ... **1877**
Tylenol Cough & Sore Throat Nighttime Liquid with Cool Burst ... **1877**
Concentrated Tylenol Infants' Drops ... **1878**
Concentrated Tylenol Infants' Drops Plus Cold ... **1879**
Concentrated Tylenol Infants' Drops Plus Cold and Cough ... **1879**
Jr. Tylenol Meltaways ... **1878**
Tylenol Sinus Severe Congestion Caplets with Cool Burst ... **1876**
Tylenol Sinus Congestion & Pain Daytime Caplets with Cool Burst and Gelcaps ... **1876**
Tylenol Sinus Congestion & Pain Nighttime Caplets with Cool Burst ... **1876**
Tylenol Sinus Congestion & Pain Severe Caplets with Cool Burst ... **1876**
Tylenol Sore Throat Daytime Liquid with Cool Burst ... **1877**
Tylenol Sore Throat Nighttime Liquid with Cool Burst ... **1877**
Women's Tylenol Menstrual Relief Caplets ... **1877**
Vicks 44M Cough, Cold & Flu Relief Liquid ... **2680**
Vicks DayQuil LiquiCaps/Liquid Multi-Symptom Cold/Flu Relief ... **761**
Vicks DayQuil Multi-Symptom Cold/Flu Relief LiquiCaps ... **2678**
Vicks DayQuil Multi-Symptom Cold/Flu Relief Liquid ... **2678**
Vicks NyQuil Multi-Symptom Cold/Flu Relief Liquid ... **2681**
Vicks NyQuil Multi-Symptom Cold/Flu Relief LiquiCaps ... **2681**
Vicks NyQuil LiquiCaps/Liquid Multi-Symptom Cold/Flu Relief ... **763**
Vicodin Tablets ... **535**
Vicodin ES Tablets ... **536**
Vicodin HP Tablets ... **538**
Zicam Maximum Strength Flu Daytime ... **768**
Zicam Maximum Strength Flu Nighttime ... **768**
Zydone Tablets ... **1139**

Acetazolamide (Carbamazepine is metabolized mainly by CYP3A4 the active carbamazepine 10,11-epoxide, which is futher metabolized to the trans-diol by epoxide hydrolase. Therefore, the potential exists for interaction between carbamazepine and any agent that inhibits CYP3A4 and/or epoxide hydrolase. Agents that are CYP3A4 inhibitors may increase the plasma levels of carbamazepine. Thus, if a patient has been titrated to a stable dosage of carbamazepine, and then begins a course of treatment with a CYP3A4 or epoxide hydrolase inhibitor, it is reasonable to expect that a dose reduction for carbamazepine may be necessary).

No products indexed under this heading.

Alatrofloxacin Mesylate (Carbamazepine is known to induce CYP1A2 and CYP3A4. Therefore, the potential exists for interaction between carbamazepine and any agent metabolized by one (or more) of these enzymes. Agents that are metabolized by CYP1A2 and CYP3A4 may have decreased plasma levels when administered concomitantly with carbamazepine. Thus, if a patient has been titrated to a stable dosage on one of the agents in these categories, and then begins a course of treatment with carbamazepine, it is reasonable to expect that a dose increase for the concomitant agent may be necessary).

No products indexed under this heading.

Alfentanil Hydrochloride (Carbamazepine is known to induce CYP1A2 and CYP3A4. Therefore, the potential exists for interaction between carbamazepine and any agent metabolized by one (or more) of these enzymes. Agents that are metabolized by CYP1A2 and CYP3A4 may have decreased plasma levels when administered concomitantly with carbamazepine. Thus, if a patient has been titrated to a stable dosage on one of the agents in these categories, and then begins a course of treatment with carbamazepine, it is reasonable to expect that a dose increase for the concomitant agent may be necessary).

No products indexed under this heading.

Allium sativum (Carbamazepine is metabolized by CYP3A4. Therefore, the potential exists for interaction between carbamazepine and any agent that induces CYP3A4. Agents that are CYP3A4 inducers may decrease plasma levels of carbamazepine. Thus, if a patient has been titrated to a stable dosage on carbamazepine, and then begins a course of treatment with a CYP3A4 inducers, it is reasonable to expect that a dose increase for carbamazepine may be necessary).

No products indexed under this heading.

Alprazolam (Carbamazepine is known to induce CYP1A2 and CYP3A4. Therefore, the potential exists for interaction between carbamazepine and any agent metabolized by one (or more) of these enzymes. Agents that are metabolized by CYP1A2 and CYP3A4 may have decreased plasma levels when administered concomitantly with carbamazepine. Thus, if a patient has been titrated to a stable dosage on one of the agents in these categories, and then begins a course of treatment with carbamazepine, it is reasonable to expect that a dose increase for the concomitant agent may be necessary). Products include:

Niravam Orally Disintegrating Tablets ... **3092**

Amiodarone Hydrochloride (Carbamazepine is metabolized mainly by CYP3A4 the active carbamazepine 10,11-epoxide, which is futher metabolized to the trans-diol by epoxide hydrolase. Therefore, the potential exists for interaction between carbamazepine and any agent that inhibits CYP3A4 and/or epoxide hydrolase. Agents that are CYP3A4 inhibitors may increase the plasma levels of carbamazepine. Thus, if a patient has been titrated to a stable dosage of carbamazepine, and then begins a course of treatment with a CYP3A4 or epoxide hydrolase inhibitor, it is reasonable

IMPORTANT NOTE: Always consult each drug listing in the patient's regimen for possible interactions.

to expect that a dose reduction for carbamazepine may be necessary).

No products indexed under this heading.

Amitriptyline Hydrochloride (Carbamazepine is known to induce CYP1A2 and CYP3A4. Therefore, the potential exists for interaction between carbamazepine and any agent metabolized by one (or more) of these enzymes. Agents that are metabolized by CYP1A2 and CYP3A4 may have decreased plasma levels when administered concomitantly with carbamazepine. Thus, if a patient has been titrated to a stable dosage on one of the agents in these categories, and then begins a course of treatment with carbamazepine, it is reasonable to expect that a dose increase for the concomitant agent may be necessary).

No products indexed under this heading.

Amlodipine Besylate (Carbamazepine is known to induce CYP1A2 and CYP3A4. Therefore, the potential exists for interaction between carbamazepine and any agent metabolized by one (or more) of these enzymes. Agents that are metabolized by CYP1A2 and CYP3A4 may have decreased plasma levels when administered concomitantly with carbamazepine. Thus, if a patient has been titrated to a stable dosage on one of the agents in these categories, and then begins a course of treatment with carbamazepine, it is reasonable to expect that a dose increase for the concomitant agent may be necessary). Products include:

Caduet Tablets **2508**
Lotrel Capsules **2249**
Norvasc Tablets **2545**

Amoxapine (Carbamazepine is known to induce CYP1A2 and CYP3A4. Therefore, the potential exists for interaction between carbamazepine and any agent metabolized by one (or more) of these enzymes. Agents that are metabolized by CYP1A2 and CYP3A4 may have decreased plasma levels when administered concomitantly with carbamazepine. Thus, if a patient has been titrated to a stable dosage on one of the agents in these categories, and then begins a course of treatment with carbamazepine, it is reasonable to expect that a dose increase for the concomitant agent may be necessary).

No products indexed under this heading.

Amprenavir (Carbamazepine is metabolized mainly by CYP3A4 the active carbamazepine 10,11-epoxide, which is futher metabolized to the trans-diol by epoxide hydrolase. Therefore, the potential exists for interaction between carbamazepine and any agent that inhibits CYP3A4 and/or epoxide hydrolase. Agents that are CYP3A4 inhibitors may increase the plasma levels of carbamazepine. Thus, if a patient has been titrated to a stable dosage of carbamazepine, and then begins a course of treatment with a CYP3A4 or epoxide hydrolase inhibitor, it is reasonable to expect that a dose reduction for carbamazepine may be necessary). Products include:

Agenerase Capsules **1327**
Agenerase Oral Solution **1332**

Anagrelide Hydrochloride (Carbamazepine is known to induce CYP1A2 and CYP3A4. Therefore, the potential exists for interaction between carbamazepine and any agent metabolized by one (or more) of these enzymes. Agents that are metabolized by CYP1A2 and CYP3A4 may have decreased plasma levels when administered concomitantly with carbamazepine. Thus, if a patient has been titrated to a stable dosage on one of the agents in these categories, and then begins a course of treatment with carbamazepine, it is reasonable to expect that a dose increase for the concomitant agent may be necessary). Products include:

Agrylin Capsules **3169**

Anastrozole (Carbamazepine is metabolized mainly by CYP3A4 the active carbamazepine 10,11-epoxide, which is futher metabolized to the trans-diol by epoxide hydrolase. Therefore, the potential exists for interaction between carbamazepine and any agent that inhibits CYP3A4 and/or epoxide hydrolase. Agents that are CYP3A4 inhibitors may increase the plasma levels of carbamazepine. Thus, if a patient has been titrated to a stable dosage of carbamazepine, and then begins a course of treatment with a CYP3A4 or epoxide hydrolase inhibitor, it is reasonable to expect that a dose reduction for carbamazepine may be necessary). Products include:

Arimidex Tablets **673**

Aprepitant (Carbamazepine is metabolized mainly by CYP3A4 the active carbamazepine 10,11-epoxide, which is futher metabolized to the trans-diol by epoxide hydrolase. Therefore, the potential exists for interaction between carbamazepine and any agent that inhibits CYP3A4 and/or epoxide hydrolase. Agents that are CYP3A4 inhibitors may increase the plasma levels of carbamazepine. Thus, if a patient has been titrated to a stable dosage of carbamazepine, and then begins a course of treatment with a CYP3A4 or epoxide hydrolase inhibitor, it is reasonable to expect that a dose reduction for carbamazepine may be necessary). Products include:

Emend Capsules **1963**

Aprobarbital (Because of its primary CNS effect, caution should be used when carbamazepine is taken with other centrally-acting drugs).

No products indexed under this heading.

Astemizole (Carbamazepine is known to induce CYP1A2 and CYP3A4. Therefore, the potential exists for interaction between carbamazepine and any agent metabolized by one (or more) of these enzymes. Agents that are metabolized by CYP1A2 and CYP3A4 may have decreased plasma levels when administered concomitantly with carbamazepine. Thus, if a patient has been titrated to a stable dosage on one of the agents in these categories, and then begins a course of treatment with carbamazepine, it is reasonable to expect that a dose increase for the concomitant agent may be necessary).

No products indexed under this heading.

Atorvastatin Calcium (Carbamazepine is known to induce CYP1A2 and CYP3A4. Therefore, the potential exists for interaction between carbamazepine and any agent metabolized by one (or more) of these enzymes. Agents that are metabolized by CYP1A2 and CYP3A4 may have decreased plasma levels when administered concomitantly with carbamazepine. Thus, if a patient has been titrated to a stable dosage on one of the agents in these categories, and then begins a course of treatment with carbamazepine, it is reasonable to expect that a dose increase for the concomitant agent may be necessary). Products include:

Caduet Tablets **2508**
Lipitor Tablets **2483**

Belladonna Ergotamine (Carbamazepine is known to induce CYP1A2 and CYP3A4. Therefore, the potential exists for interaction between carbamazepine and any agent metabolized by one (or more) of these enzymes. Agents that are metabolized by CYP1A2 and CYP3A4 may have decreased plasma levels when administered concomitantly with carbamazepine. Thus, if a patient has been titrated to a stable dosage on one of the agents in these categories, and then begins a course of treatment with carbamazepine, it is reasonable to expect that a dose increase for the concomitant agent may be necessary).

No products indexed under this heading.

Betamethasone Acetate (Carbamazepine is metabolized by CYP3A4. Therefore, the potential exists for interaction between carbamazepine and any agent that induces CYP3A4. Agents that are CYP3A4 inducers may decrease plasma levels of carbamazepine. Thus, if a patient has been titrated to a stable dosage on carbamazepine, and then begins a course of treatment with a CYP3A4 inducers, it is reasonable to expect that a dose increase for carbamazepine may be necessary).

No products indexed under this heading.

Betamethasone Sodium Phosphate (Carbamazepine is metabolized by CYP3A4. Therefore, the potential exists for interaction between carbamazepine and any agent that induces CYP3A4. Agents that are CYP3A4 inducers may decrease plasma levels of carbamazepine. Thus, if a patient has been titrated to a stable dosage on carbamazepine, and then begins a course of treatment with a CYP3A4 inducers, it is reasonable to expect that a dose increase for carbamazepine may be necessary).

No products indexed under this heading.

Buprenorphine Hydrochloride (Because of its primary CNS effect, caution should be used when carbamazepine is taken with other centrally-acting drugs). Products include:

Buprenex Injectable **2716**
Suboxone Tablets **2717**
Subutex Tablets **2717**

Buspirone Hydrochloride (Carbamazepine is known to induce CYP1A2 and CYP3A4. Therefore, the potential exists for interaction between carbamazepine and any agent metabolized by one (or more) of these enzymes. Agents that are metabolized by CYP1A2 and CYP3A4 may have decreased plasma levels when administered concomitantly with carbamazepine. Thus, if a patient has been titrated to a stable dosage on one of the agents in these categories, and then begins a course of treatment with carbamazepine, it is reasonable to expect that a dose increase for the concomitant agent may be necessary).

No products indexed under this heading.

Busulfan (Carbamazepine is known to induce CYP1A2 and CYP3A4. Therefore, the potential exists for interaction between carbamazepine and any agent metabolized by one (or more) of these enzymes. Agents that are metabolized by CYP1A2 and CYP3A4 may have decreased plasma levels when administered concomitantly with carbamazepine. Thus, if a patient has been titrated to a stable dosage on one of the agents in these categories, and then begins a course of treatment with carbamazepine, it is reasonable to expect that a dose increase for the concomitant agent may be necessary). Products include:

I.V. Busulfex **2493**
Myleran Tablets **1525**

Butabarbital (Because of its primary CNS effect, caution should be used when carbamazepine is taken with other centrally-acting drugs).

No products indexed under this heading.

Butalbital (Because of its primary CNS effect, caution should be used when carbamazepine is taken with other centrally-acting drugs).

No products indexed under this heading.

Caffeine (Carbamazepine is known to induce CYP1A2 and CYP3A4. Therefore, the potential exists for interaction between carbamazepine and any agent metabolized by one (or more) of these enzymes. Agents that are metabolized by CYP1A2 and CYP3A4 may have decreased plasma levels when administered concomitantly with carbamazepine. Thus, if a patient has been titrated to a stable dosage on one of the agents in these categories, and then begins a course of treatment with carbamazepine, it is reasonable to expect that a dose increase for the concomitant agent may be necessary). Products include:

BC Headache Powder .... ■ **677**
Arthritis Strength BC Powder .... ■ **677**
Excedrin Extra Strength Caplets/Tablets/Geltabs .... ■ **684**
Excedrin Migraine Caplets/Tablets/Geltabs .... ■ **609**
Excedrin Tension Headache Caplets/Tablets/Geltabs .... ■ **611**
Goody's Extra Strength Headache Powders .... ■ **611**
Goody's Extra Strength Pain Relief Tablets .... ■ **685**
Vivarin .... ■ **602**
Winrgy Dietary Supplement .... ■ **823**

Caffeine Anhydrous (Carbamazepine is known to induce CYP1A2 and CYP3A4. Therefore, the potential exists for interaction between car-

bamazepine and any agent metabolized by one (or more) of these enzymes. Agents that are metabolized by CYP1A2 and CYP3A4 may have decreased plasma levels when administered concomitantly with carbamazepine. Thus, if a patient has been titrated to a stable dosage on one of the agents in these categories, and then begins a course of treatment with carbamazepine, it is reasonable to expect that a dose increase for the concomitant agent may be necessary).
No products indexed under this heading.

Cerivastatin Sodium (Carbamazepine is known to induce CYP1A2 and CYP3A4. Therefore, the potential exists for interaction between carbamazepine and any agent metabolized by one (or more) of these enzymes. Agents that are metabolized by CYP1A2 and CYP3A4 may have decreased plasma levels when administered concomitantly with carbamazepine. Thus, if a patient has been titrated to a stable dosage on one of the agents in these categories, and then begins a course of treatment with carbamazepine, it is reasonable to expect that a dose increase for the concomitant agent may be necessary).
No products indexed under this heading.

Chlordiazepoxide (Carbamazepine is known to induce CYP1A2 and CYP3A4. Therefore, the potential exists for interaction between carbamazepine and any agent metabolized by one (or more) of these enzymes. Agents that are metabolized by CYP1A2 and CYP3A4 may have decreased plasma levels when administered concomitantly with carbamazepine. Thus, if a patient has been titrated to a stable dosage on one of the agents in these categories, and then begins a course of treatment with carbamazepine, it is reasonable to expect that a dose increase for the concomitant agent may be necessary).
No products indexed under this heading.

Chlordiazepoxide Hydrochloride (Carbamazepine is known to induce CYP1A2 and CYP3A4. Therefore, the potential exists for interaction between carbamazepine and any agent metabolized by one (or more) of these enzymes. Agents that are metabolized by CYP1A2 and CYP3A4 may have decreased plasma levels when administered concomitantly with carbamazepine. Thus, if a patient has been titrated to a stable dosage on one of the agents in these categories, and then begins a course of treatment with carbamazepine, it is reasonable to expect that a dose increase for the concomitant agent may be necessary). Products include:
Librium Capsules ... **3347**

Chloroquine Hydrochloride (Antimalarial drugs, such as chloroquine and mefloquine, may antagonize the activity of carbamazepine).
No products indexed under this heading.

Chloroquine Phosphate (Antimalarial drugs, such as chloroquine and mefloquine, may antagonize the activity of carbamazepine).
No products indexed under this heading.

Chlorpheniramine (Carbamazepine is known to induce CYP1A2 and CYP3A4. Therefore, the potential exists for interaction between carbamazepine and any agent metabolized by one (or more) of these enzymes. Agents that are metabolized by CYP1A2 and CYP3A4 may have decreased plasma levels when administered concomitantly with carbamazepine. Thus, if a patient has been titrated to a stable dosage on one of the agents in these categories, and then begins a course of treatment with carbamazepine, it is reasonable to expect that a dose increase for the concomitant agent may be necessary).
No products indexed under this heading.

Chlorpheniramine Maleate (Carbamazepine is known to induce CYP1A2 and CYP3A4. Therefore, the potential exists for interaction between carbamazepine and any agent metabolized by one (or more) of these enzymes. Agents that are metabolized by CYP1A2 and CYP3A4 may have decreased plasma levels when administered concomitantly with carbamazepine. Thus, if a patient has been titrated to a stable dosage on one of the agents in these categories, and then begins a course of treatment with carbamazepine, it is reasonable to expect that a dose increase for the concomitant agent may be necessary). Products include:
Advil Allergy Sinus Caplets ... ■**770**
Advil Multi-Symptom Cold Caplets ... ■**770**
BC Allergy Sinus Cold Powder ... ■**677**
Comtrex Maximum Strength Cold & Cough Day/Night Caplets - Night Formulation ... ■**726**
Comtrex Maximum Strength Day/Night Severe Cold & Sinus Caplets - Night Formulation ... ■**725**
Contac Cold and Flu Maximum Strength Caplets ... ■**728**
Contac Cold and Flu Day and Night Caplets (Night Formulation Only) ... ■**727**
Children's Dimetapp Long Acting Cough Plus Cold Syrup ... ■**731**
Robitussin Cough & Cold Long-Acting Liquid ... ■**735**
Robitussin Cough & Allergy Syrup .. ■**736**
Robitussin Cough & Cold Nighttime Liquid ... ■**736**
Robitussin Cough, Cold & Flu Nighttime Liquid ... ■**738**
Robitussin Pediatric Cough & Cold Long-Acting Liquid ... ■**735**
Robitussin Pediatric Cough & Cold Nighttime Liquid ... ■**736**
Triaminic Cold & Allergy Liquid ... ■**746**
Triaminic Cough & Runny Nose Softchews ... ■**748**
Children's Tylenol Plus Flu Oral Suspension ... ■**749**
Tylenol Allergy Multi-Symptom Caplets with Cool Burst and Gelcaps ... **1872**
Children's Tylenol Plus Cold Suspension Liquid ... **1879**
Children's Tylenol Plus Cough & Runny Nose Suspension Liquid ... **1879**
Children's Tylenol Plus Flu Suspension Liquid ... **1881**
Children's Tylenol Plus Multi-Symptom Cold Suspension Liquid ... **1879**
Tylenol Cold Head Congestion Nighttime Caplets with Cool Burst ... **1873**
Tylenol Cold Multi-Symptom Nighttime Caplets with Cool Burst ... **1874**
Tylenol Sinus Congestion & Pain Nighttime Caplets with Cool Burst ... **1876**
Vicks 44M Cough, Cold & Flu Relief Liquid ... **2680**
Pediatric Vicks 44m Cough & Cold Relief Liquid ... **2676**
Children's Vicks NyQuil Cold/Cough Relief ... ■**756**
Children's Vicks NyQuil Cold/Cough Relief Liquid ... **2680**
Zicam Maximum Strength Flu Daytime ... ■**768**

Chlorpheniramine Polistirex (Carbamazepine is known to induce CYP1A2 and CYP3A4. Therefore, the potential exists for interaction between carbamazepine and any agent metabolized by one (or more) of these enzymes. Agents that are metabolized by CYP1A2 and CYP3A4 may have decreased plasma levels when administered concomitantly with carbamazepine. Thus, if a patient has been titrated to a stable dosage on one of the agents in these categories, and then begins a course of treatment with carbamazepine, it is reasonable to expect that a dose increase for the concomitant agent may be necessary). Products include:
Tussionex Pennkinetic Extended-Release Suspension ... **3327**

Chlorpheniramine Tannate (Carbamazepine is known to induce CYP1A2 and CYP3A4. Therefore, the potential exists for interaction between carbamazepine and any agent metabolized by one (or more) of these enzymes. Agents that are metabolized by CYP1A2 and CYP3A4 may have decreased plasma levels when administered concomitantly with carbamazepine. Thus, if a patient has been titrated to a stable dosage on one of the agents in these categories, and then begins a course of treatment with carbamazepine, it is reasonable to expect that a dose increase for the concomitant agent may be necessary).
No products indexed under this heading.

Chlorpromazine (Because of its primary CNS effect, caution should be used when carbamazepine is taken with other centrally-acting drugs).
No products indexed under this heading.

Chlorpromazine Hydrochloride (Because of its primary CNS effect, caution should be used when carbamazepine is taken with other centrally-acting drugs).
No products indexed under this heading.

Chlorprothixene (Because of its primary CNS effect, caution should be used when carbamazepine is taken with other centrally-acting drugs).
No products indexed under this heading.

Chlorprothixene Hydrochloride (Because of its primary CNS effect, caution should be used when carbamazepine is taken with other centrally-acting drugs).
No products indexed under this heading.

Chlorprothixene Lactate (Because of its primary CNS effect, caution should be used when carbamazepine is taken with other centrally-acting drugs).
No products indexed under this heading.

Cimetidine (Carbamazepine is metabolized mainly by CYP3A4 the active carbamazepine 10,11-epoxide, which is futher metabolized to the trans-diol by epoxide hydrolase. Therefore, the potential exists for interaction between carbamazepine and any agent that inhibits CYP3A4 and/or epoxide hydrolase. Agents that are CYP3A4 inhibitors may increase the plasma levels of carbamazepine. Thus, if a patient has been titrated to a stable dosage of carbamazepine, and then begins a course of treatment with a CYP3A4 or epoxide hydrolase inhibitor, it is reasonable to expect that a dose reduction for carbamazepine may be necessary). Products include:
Tagamet HB 200 Tablets ... ■**664**

Cimetidine Hydrochloride (Carbamazepine is metabolized mainly by CYP3A4 the active carbamazepine 10,11-epoxide, which is futher metabolized to the trans-diol by epoxide hydrolase. Therefore, the potential exists for interaction between carbamazepine and any agent that inhibits CYP3A4 and/or epoxide hydrolase. Agents that are CYP3A4 inhibitors may increase the plasma levels of carbamazepine. Thus, if a patient has been titrated to a stable dosage of carbamazepine, and then begins a course of treatment with a CYP3A4 or epoxide hydrolase inhibitor, it is reasonable to expect that a dose reduction for carbamazepine may be necessary).
No products indexed under this heading.

Ciprofloxacin (Carbamazepine is metabolized mainly by CYP3A4 the active carbamazepine 10,11-epoxide, which is futher metabolized to the trans-diol by epoxide hydrolase. Therefore, the potential exists for interaction between carbamazepine and any agent that inhibits CYP3A4 and/or epoxide hydrolase. Agents that are CYP3A4 inhibitors may increase the plasma levels of carbamazepine. Thus, if a patient has been titrated to a stable dosage of carbamazepine, and then begins a course of treatment with a CYP3A4 or epoxide hydrolase inhibitor, it is reasonable to expect that a dose reduction for carbamazepine may be necessary). Products include:
Cipro Oral Suspension ... **2977**
Cipro I.V. ... **2984**
Cipro XR Tablets ... **2990**
Ciprodex Otic Suspension ... **559**

Ciprofloxacin Hydrochloride (Carbamazepine is metabolized by CYP3A4. Therefore, the potential exists for interaction between carbamazepine and any agent that induces CYP3A4. Agents that are CYP3A4 inducers may decrease plasma levels of carbamazepine. Thus, if a patient has been titrated to a stable dosage on carbamazepine, and then begins a course of treatment with a CYP3A4 inducers, it is reasonable to expect that a dose increase for carbamazepine may be necessary). Products include:
Ciloxan Ophthalmic Ointment ... **559**
Ciloxan Ophthalmic Solution ... ⊙**206**
Cipro Tablets ... **2977**
Proquin XR Tablets ... **1153**

Cisapride (Carbamazepine is known to induce CYP1A2 and CYP3A4. Therefore, the potential exists for interaction between carbamazepine and any agent metabo-

lized by one (or more) of these enzymes. Agents that are metabolized by CYP1A2 and CYP3A4 may have decreased plasma levels when administered concomitantly with carbamazepine. Thus, if a patient has been titrated to a stable dosage on one of the agents in these categories, and then begins a course of treatment with carbamazepine, it is reasonable to expect that a dose increase for the concomitant agent may be necessary).
No products indexed under this heading.

Cisplatin (Carbamazepine is metabolized by CYP3A4. Therefore, the potential exists for interaction between carbamazepine and any agent that induces CYP3A4. Agents that are CYP3A4 inducers may decrease plasma levels of carbamazepine. Thus, if a patient has been titrated to a stable dosage on carbamazepine, and then begins a course of treatment with a CYP3A4 inducers, it is reasonable to expect that a dose increase for carbamazepine may be necessary).
No products indexed under this heading.

Clarithromycin (Carbamazepine is metabolized mainly by CYP3A4 the active carbamazepine 10,11-epoxide, which is futher metabolized to the trans-diol by epoxide hydrolase. Therefore, the potential exists for interaction between carbamazepine and any agent that inhibits CYP3A4 and/or epoxide hydrolase. Agents that are CYP3A4 inhibitors may increase the plasma levels of carbamazepine. Thus, if a patient has been titrated to a stable dosage of carbamazepine, and then begins a course of treatment with a CYP3A4 or epoxide hydrolase inhibitor, it is reasonable to expect that a dose reduction for carbamazepine may be necessary). Products include:
Biaxin/Biaxin XL 402
PREVPAC 3284

Clomipramine Hydrochloride (Carbamazepine increases the plasma levels of clomipramine HCl).
No products indexed under this heading.

Clopidogrel Bisulfate (Carbamazepine is known to induce CYP1A2 and CYP3A4. Therefore, the potential exists for interaction between carbamazepine and any agent metabolized by one (or more) of these enzymes. Agents that are metabolized by CYP1A2 and CYP3A4 may have decreased plasma levels when administered concomitantly with carbamazepine. Thus, if a patient has been titrated to a stable dosage on one of the agents in these categories, and then begins a course of treatment with carbamazepine, it is reasonable to expect that a dose increase for the concomitant agent may be necessary). Products include:
Plavix Tablets 917
Plavix Tablets 2926

Clorazepate Dipotassium (Because of its primary CNS effect, caution should be used when carbamazepine is taken with other centrally-acting drugs). Products include:
Tranxene 2474

Clotrimazole (Carbamazepine is metabolized mainly by CYP3A4 the active carbamazepine 10,11-epoxide, which is futher metabolized to the trans-diol by epoxide hydrolase. Therefore, the potential exists for interaction between carbamazepine and any agent that inhibits CYP3A4 and/or epoxide hydrolase. Agents that are CYP3A4 inhibitors may increase the plasma levels of carbamazepine. Thus, if a patient has been titrated to a stable dosage of carbamazepine, and then begins a course of treatment with a CYP3A4 or epoxide hydrolase inhibitor, it is reasonable to expect that a dose reduction for carbamazepine may be necessary). Products include:
Desenex Athlete's Foot Cream .... ⊡ 635
Lotrimin 3039
Lotrisone 3040

Clozapine (Carbamazepine is known to induce CYP1A2 and CYP3A4. Therefore, the potential exists for interaction between carbamazepine and any agent metabolized by one (or more) of these enzymes. Agents that are metabolized by CYP1A2 and CYP3A4 may have decreased plasma levels when administered concomitantly with carbamazepine. Thus, if a patient has been titrated to a stable dosage on one of the agents in these categories, and then begins a course of treatment with carbamazepine, it is reasonable to expect that a dose increase for the concomitant agent may be necessary). Products include:
Clozaril Tablets 2184
FazaClo Orally Disintegrating Tablets 551

Codeine Phosphate (Because of its primary CNS effect, caution should be used when carbamazepine is taken with other centrally-acting drugs). Products include:
Tylenol with Codeine Tablets 2391

Cortisone Acetate (Carbamazepine is metabolized by CYP3A4. Therefore, the potential exists for interaction between carbamazepine and any agent that induces CYP3A4. Agents that are CYP3A4 inducers may decrease plasma levels of carbamazepine. Thus, if a patient has been titrated to a stable dosage on carbamazepine, and then begins a course of treatment with a CYP3A4 inducers, it is reasonable to expect that a dose increase for carbamazepine may be necessary).
No products indexed under this heading.

Cyclobenzaprine (Carbamazepine is known to induce CYP1A2 and CYP3A4. Therefore, the potential exists for interaction between carbamazepine and any agent metabolized by one (or more) of these enzymes. Agents that are metabolized by CYP1A2 and CYP3A4 may have decreased plasma levels when administered concomitantly with carbamazepine. Thus, if a patient has been titrated to a stable dosage on one of the agents in these categories, and then begins a course of treatment with carbamazepine, it is reasonable to expect that a dose increase for the concomitant agent may be necessary).
No products indexed under this heading.

Cyclobenzaprine Hydrochloride (Carbamazepine is known to induce CYP1A2 and CYP3A4. Therefore, the potential exists for interaction between carbamazepine and any agent metabolized by one (or more) of these enzymes. Agents that are metabolized by CYP1A2 and CYP3A4 may have decreased plasma levels when administered concomitantly with carbamazepine. Thus, if a patient has been titrated to a stable dosage on one of the agents in these categories, and then begins a course of treatment with carbamazepine, it is reasonable to expect that a dose increase for the concomitant agent may be necessary).
No products indexed under this heading.

Cyclosporine (Carbamazepine is metabolized mainly by CYP3A4 the active carbamazepine 10,11-epoxide, which is futher metabolized to the trans-diol by epoxide hydrolase. Therefore, the potential exists for interaction between carbamazepine and any agent that inhibits CYP3A4 and/or epoxide hydrolase. Agents that are CYP3A4 inhibitors may increase the plasma levels of carbamazepine. Thus, if a patient has been titrated to a stable dosage of carbamazepine, and then begins a course of treatment with a CYP3A4 or epoxide hydrolase inhibitor, it is reasonable to expect that a dose reduction for carbamazepine may be necessary). Products include:
Gengraf Capsules 459
Neoral Oral Solution 2259
Neoral Soft Gelatin Capsules 2259
Restasis Ophthalmic Emulsion 575
Sandimmune 2275

Dalfopristin (Carbamazepine is metabolized mainly by CYP3A4 the active carbamazepine 10,11-epoxide, which is futher metabolized to the trans-diol by epoxide hydrolase. Therefore, the potential exists for interaction between carbamazepine and any agent that inhibits CYP3A4 and/or epoxide hydrolase. Agents that are CYP3A4 inhibitors may increase the plasma levels of carbamazepine. Thus, if a patient has been titrated to a stable dosage of carbamazepine, and then begins a course of treatment with a CYP3A4 or epoxide hydrolase inhibitor, it is reasonable to expect that a dose reduction for carbamazepine may be necessary).
No products indexed under this heading.

Danazol (Carbamazepine is metabolized mainly by CYP3A4 the active carbamazepine 10,11-epoxide, which is futher metabolized to the trans-diol by epoxide hydrolase. Therefore, the potential exists for interaction between carbamazepine and any agent that inhibits CYP3A4 and/or epoxide hydrolase. Agents that are CYP3A4 inhibitors may increase the plasma levels of carbamazepine. Thus, if a patient has been titrated to a stable dosage of carbamazepine, and then begins a course of treatment with a CYP3A4 or epoxide hydrolase inhibitor, it is reasonable to expect that a dose reduction for carbamazepine may be necessary).
No products indexed under this heading.

Delavirdine Mesylate (Carbamazepine is metabolized mainly by CYP3A4 the active carbamazepine 10,11-epoxide, which is futher metabolized to the trans-diol by epoxide hydrolase. Therefore, the potential exists for interaction between carbamazepine and any agent that inhibits CYP3A4 and/or epoxide hydrolase. Agents that are CYP3A4 inhibitors may increase the plasma levels of carbamazepine. Thus, if a patient has been titrated to a stable dosage of carbamazepine, and then begins a course of treatment with a CYP3A4 or epoxide hydrolase inhibitor, it is reasonable to expect that a dose reduction for carbamazepine may be necessary). Products include:
Rescriptor Tablets 2551

Desflurane (Because of its primary CNS effect, caution should be used when carbamazepine is taken with other centrally-acting drugs).
No products indexed under this heading.

Desipramine Hydrochloride (Carbamazepine is known to induce CYP1A2 and CYP3A4. Therefore, the potential exists for interaction between carbamazepine and any agent metabolized by one (or more) of these enzymes. Agents that are metabolized by CYP1A2 and CYP3A4 may have decreased plasma levels when administered concomitantly with carbamazepine. Thus, if a patient has been titrated to a stable dosage on one of the agents in these categories, and then begins a course of treatment with carbamazepine, it is reasonable to expect that a dose increase for the concomitant agent may be necessary).
No products indexed under this heading.

Desogestrel (Carbamazepine is known to induce CYP1A2 and CYP3A4. Therefore, the potential exists for interaction between carbamazepine and any agent metabolized by one (or more) of these enzymes. Agents that are metabolized by CYP1A2 or CYP3A4 may have decreased plasma levels when administered concomitantly with carbamazepine. Breakthrough bleeding has been reported among patients receiving concomitant oral contraceptives and their reliability may be adversely affected). Products include:
Mircette Tablets 1066

Dexamethasone (Carbamazepine is metabolized by CYP3A4. Therefore, the potential exists for interaction between carbamazepine and any agent that induces CYP3A4. Agents that are CYP3A4 inducers may decrease plasma levels of carbamazepine. Thus, if a patient has been titrated to a stable dosage on carbamazepine, and then begins a course of treatment with a CYP3A4 inducers, it is reasonable to expect that a dose increase for carbamazepine may be necessary). Products include:
Ciprodex Otic Suspension 559
Decadron Tablets 1951
TobraDex Ophthalmic Ointment 562
TobraDex Ophthalmic Suspension 563

Dexamethasone Acetate (Carbamazepine is metabolized by CYP3A4. Therefore, the potential exists for interaction between carbamazepine and any agent that induces CYP3A4. Agents that are CYP3A4 inducers may decrease plasma levels of carbamazepine. Thus, if a patient has been titrated to a stable dosage on carbamazepine, and then begins a course of treatment with a CYP3A4 inducers, it is reasonable to expect that a dose increase for carbamazepine may be necessary).

No products indexed under this heading.

Dexamethasone Sodium Phosphate (Carbamazepine is metabolized by CYP3A4. Therefore, the potential exists for interaction between carbamazepine and any agent that induces CYP3A4. Agents that are CYP3A4 inducers may decrease plasma levels of carbamazepine. Thus, if a patient has been titrated to a stable dosage on carbamazepine, and then begins a course of treatment with a CYP3A4 inducers, it is reasonable to expect that a dose increase for carbamazepine may be necessary).

No products indexed under this heading.

Dezocine (Because of its primary CNS effect, caution should be used when carbamazepine is taken with other centrally-acting drugs).

No products indexed under this heading.

Diazepam (Carbamazepine is known to induce CYP1A2 and CYP3A4. Therefore, the potential exists for interaction between carbamazepine and any agent metabolized by one (or more) of these enzymes. Agents that are metabolized by CYP1A2 and CYP3A4 may have decreased plasma levels when administered concomitantly with carbamazepine. Thus, if a patient has been titrated to a stable dosage on one of the agents in these categories, and then begins a course of treatment with carbamazepine, it is reasonable to expect that a dose increase for the concomitant agent may be necessary). Products include:

- Diastat Rectal Delivery System **3343**
- Valium Tablets **2819**

Dihydroergotamine Mesylate (Carbamazepine is known to induce CYP1A2 and CYP3A4. Therefore, the potential exists for interaction between carbamazepine and any agent metabolized by one (or more) of these enzymes. Agents that are metabolized by CYP1A2 and CYP3A4 may have decreased plasma levels when administered concomitantly with carbamazepine. Thus, if a patient has been titrated to a stable dosage on one of the agents in these categories, and then begins a course of treatment with carbamazepine, it is reasonable to expect that a dose increase for the concomitant agent may be necessary). Products include:

- Migranal Nasal Spray **3348**

Diltiazem Hydrochloride (Carbamazepine is metabolized mainly by CYP3A4 the active carbamazepine 10,11-epoxide, which is futher metabolized to the trans-diol by epoxide hydrolase. Therefore, the potential exists for interaction between carbamazepine and any agent that inhibits CYP3A4 and/or epoxide hydrolase. Agents that are CYP3A4 inhibitors may increase the plasma levels of carbamazepine. Thus, if a patient has been titrated to a stable dosage of carbamazepine, and then begins a course of treatment with a CYP3A4 or epoxide hydrolase inhibitor, it is reasonable to expect that a dose reduction for carbamazepine may be necessary). Products include:

- Cardizem LA Extended Release Tablets **1728**
- Tiazac Capsules **1201**

Diltiazem Maleate (Carbamazepine is metabolized mainly by CYP3A4 the active carbamazepine 10,11-epoxide, which is futher metabolized to the trans-diol by epoxide hydrolase. Therefore, the potential exists for interaction between carbamazepine and any agent that inhibits CYP3A4 and/or epoxide hydrolase. Agents that are CYP3A4 inhibitors may increase the plasma levels of carbamazepine. Thus, if a patient has been titrated to a stable dosage of carbamazepine, and then begins a course of treatment with a CYP3A4 or epoxide hydrolase inhibitor, it is reasonable to expect that a dose reduction for carbamazepine may be necessary).

No products indexed under this heading.

Disopyramide (Carbamazepine is known to induce CYP1A2 and CYP3A4. Therefore, the potential exists for interaction between carbamazepine and any agent metabolized by one (or more) of these enzymes. Agents that are metabolized by CYP1A2 and CYP3A4 may have decreased plasma levels when administered concomitantly with carbamazepine. Thus, if a patient has been titrated to a stable dosage on one of the agents in these categories, and then begins a course of treatment with carbamazepine, it is reasonable to expect that a dose increase for the concomitant agent may be necessary).

No products indexed under this heading.

Disopyramide Phosphate (Carbamazepine is known to induce CYP1A2 and CYP3A4. Therefore, the potential exists for interaction between carbamazepine and any agent metabolized by one (or more) of these enzymes. Agents that are metabolized by CYP1A2 and CYP3A4 may have decreased plasma levels when administered concomitantly with carbamazepine. Thus, if a patient has been titrated to a stable dosage on one of the agents in these categories, and then begins a course of treatment with carbamazepine, it is reasonable to expect that a dose increase for the concomitant agent may be necessary).

No products indexed under this heading.

Disulfiram (Carbamazepine is known to induce CYP1A2 and CYP3A4. Therefore, the potential exists for interaction between carbamazepine and any agent metabolized by one (or more) of these enzymes. Agents that are metabolized by CYP1A2 and CYP3A4 may have decreased plasma levels when administered concomitantly with carbamazepine. Thus, if a patient has been titrated to a stable dosage on one of the agents in these categories, and then begins a course of treatment with carbamazepine, it is reasonable to expect that a dose increase for the concomitant agent may be necessary).

No products indexed under this heading.

Doxepin Hydrochloride (Carbamazepine is known to induce CYP1A2 and CYP3A4. Therefore, the potential exists for interaction between carbamazepine and any agent metabolized by one (or more) of these enzymes. Agents that are metabolized by CYP1A2 and CYP3A4 may have decreased plasma levels when administered concomitantly with carbamazepine. Thus, if a patient has been titrated to a stable dosage on one of the agents in these categories, and then begins a course of treatment with carbamazepine, it is reasonable to expect that a dose increase for the concomitant agent may be necessary).

No products indexed under this heading.

Doxorubicin Hydrochloride (Carbamazepine is metabolized by CYP3A4. Therefore, the potential exists for interaction between carbamazepine and any agent that induces CYP3A4. Agents that are CYP3A4 inducers may decrease plasma levels of carbamazepine. Thus, if a patient has been titrated to a stable dosage on carbamazepine, and then begins a course of treatment with a CYP3A4 inducers, it is reasonable to expect that a dose increase for carbamazepine may be necessary).

No products indexed under this heading.

Dronabinol (Carbamazepine is known to induce CYP1A2 and CYP3A4. Therefore, the potential exists for interaction between carbamazepine and any agent metabolized by one (or more) of these enzymes. Agents that are metabolized by CYP1A2 and CYP3A4 may have decreased plasma levels when administered concomitantly with carbamazepine. Thus, if a patient has been titrated to a stable dosage on one of the agents in these categories, and then begins a course of treatment with carbamazepine, it is reasonable to expect that a dose increase for the concomitant agent may be necessary). Products include:

- Marinol Capsules **3333**

Droperidol (Because of its primary CNS effect, caution should be used when carbamazepine is taken with other centrally-acting drugs).

No products indexed under this heading.

Efavirenz (Carbamazepine is metabolized mainly by CYP3A4 the active carbamazepine 10,11-epoxide, which is futher metabolized to the trans-diol by epoxide hydrolase. Therefore, the potential exists for interaction between carbamazepine and any agent that inhibits CYP3A4 and/or epoxide hydrolase. Agents that are CYP3A4 inhibitors may increase the plasma levels of carbamazepine. Thus, if a patient has been titrated to a stable dosage of carbamazepine, and then begins a course of treatment with a CYP3A4 or epoxide hydrolase inhibitor, it is reasonable to expect that a dose reduction for carbamazepine may be necessary). Products include:

- Atripla Tablets **945**
- Sustiva Capsules **930**
- Sustiva Tablets **930**

Enflurane (Because of its primary CNS effect, caution should be used when carbamazepine is taken with other centrally-acting drugs).

No products indexed under this heading.

Enoxacin (Carbamazepine is known to induce CYP1A2 and CYP3A4. Therefore, the potential exists for interaction between carbamazepine and any agent metabolized by one (or more) of these enzymes. Agents that are metabolized by CYP1A2 and CYP3A4 may have decreased plasma levels when administered concomitantly with carbamazepine. Thus, if a patient has been titrated to a stable dosage on one of the agents in these categories, and then begins a course of treatment with carbamazepine, it is reasonable to expect that a dose increase for the concomitant agent may be necessary).

No products indexed under this heading.

Ergotamine Tartrate (Carbamazepine is known to induce CYP1A2 and CYP3A4. Therefore, the potential exists for interaction between carbamazepine and any agent metabolized by one (or more) of these enzymes. Agents that are metabolized by CYP1A2 and CYP3A4 may have decreased plasma levels when administered concomitantly with carbamazepine. Thus, if a patient has been titrated to a stable dosage on one of the agents in these categories, and then begins a course of treatment with carbamazepine, it is reasonable to expect that a dose increase for the concomitant agent may be necessary).

No products indexed under this heading.

Erythromycin (Carbamazepine is metabolized mainly by CYP3A4 the active carbamazepine 10,11-epoxide, which is futher metabolized to the trans-diol by epoxide hydrolase. Therefore, the potential exists for interaction between carbamazepine and any agent that inhibits CYP3A4 and/or epoxide hydrolase. Agents that are CYP3A4 inhibitors may increase the plasma levels of carbamazepine. Thus, if a patient has been titrated to a stable dosage of carbamazepine, and then begins a course of treatment with a CYP3A4 or epoxide hydrolase inhibitor, it is reasonable to expect that a dose reduction for carbamazepine may be necessary). Products include:

- Ery-Tab Tablets **449**
- Erythromycin Base Filmtab Tablets **455**
- Erythromycin Delayed-Release Capsules, USP **457**
- PCE Dispertab Tablets **515**

Erythromycin Estolate (Carbamazepine is metabolized mainly by CYP3A4 the active carbamazepine 10,11-epoxide, which is futher metabolized to the trans-diol by epoxide hydrolase. Therefore, the potential exists for interaction between carbamazepine and any agent that inhibits CYP3A4 and/or epoxide hydrolase. Agents that are CYP3A4 inhibitors may increase the plasma levels of carbamazepine. Thus, if a patient has been titrated to a stable dosage of carbamazepine, and then begins a course of treatment with a CYP3A4 or epoxide hydrolase inhibitor, it is reasonable to expect that a dose reduction for carbamazepine may be necessary).

No products indexed under this heading.

Erythromycin Ethylsuccinate (Carbamazepine is metabolized mainly by CYP3A4 the active carbamazepine 10,11-epoxide, which is futher metabolized to the trans-diol by epoxide hydrolase. Therefore, the potential exists for interaction between carbamazepine and any agent that inhibits CYP3A4 and/or epoxide hydrolase. Agents that are CYP3A4 inhibitors may increase the plasma levels of carbamazepine. Thus, if a patient has been titrated to a stable dosage of carbamazepine, and then begins a course of treatment with a CYP3A4 or epoxide hydrolase inhibitor, it is reasonable to expect that a dose reduction for carbamazepine may be necessary). Products include:

Erythromycin Gluceptate (Carbamazepine is metabolized mainly by CYP3A4 the active carbamazepine 10,11-epoxide, which is futher metabolized to the trans-diol by epoxide hydrolase. Therefore, the potential exists for interaction between carbamazepine and any agent that inhibits CYP3A4 and/or epoxide hydrolase. Agents that are CYP3A4 inhibitors may increase the plasma levels of carbamazepine. Thus, if a patient has been titrated to a stable dosage of carbamazepine, and then begins a course of treatment with a CYP3A4 or epoxide hydrolase inhibitor, it is reasonable to expect that a dose reduction for carbamazepine may be necessary).

No products indexed under this heading.

Erythromycin Lactobionate (Carbamazepine is metabolized mainly by CYP3A4 the active carbamazepine 10,11-epoxide, which is futher metabolized to the trans-diol by epoxide hydrolase. Therefore, the potential exists for interaction between carbamazepine and any agent that inhibits CYP3A4 and/or epoxide hydrolase. Agents that are CYP3A4 inhibitors may increase the plasma levels of carbamazepine. Thus, if a patient has been titrated to a stable dosage of carbamazepine, and then begins a course of treatment with a CYP3A4 or epoxide hydrolase inhibitor, it is reasonable to expect that a dose reduction for carbamazepine may be necessary).

No products indexed under this heading.

Erythromycin Stearate (Carbamazepine is metabolized mainly by CYP3A4 the active carbamazepine 10,11-epoxide, which is futher metabolized to the trans-diol by epoxide hydrolase. Therefore, the potential exists for interaction between carbamazepine and any agent that inhibits CYP3A4 and/or epoxide hydrolase. Agents that are CYP3A4 inhibitors may increase the plasma levels of carbamazepine. Thus, if a patient has been titrated to a stable dosage of carbamazepine, and then begins a course of treatment with a CYP3A4 or epoxide

hydrolase inhibitor, it is reasonable to expect that a dose reduction for carbamazepine may be necessary). Products include:

Esomeprazole Magnesium (Carbamazepine is metabolized mainly by CYP3A4 the active carbamazepine 10,11-epoxide, which is futher metabolized to the trans-diol by epoxide hydrolase. Therefore, the potential exists for interaction between carbamazepine and any agent that inhibits CYP3A4 and/or epoxide hydrolase. Agents that are CYP3A4 inhibitors may increase the plasma levels of carbamazepine. Thus, if a patient has been titrated to a stable dosage of carbamazepine, and then begins a course of treatment with a CYP3A4 or epoxide hydrolase inhibitor, it is reasonable to expect that a dose reduction for carbamazepine may be necessary). Products include:

Estazolam (Because of its primary CNS effect, caution should be used when carbamazepine is taken with other centrally-acting drugs). Products include:

Estradiol (Carbamazepine is known to induce CYP1A2 and CYP3A4. Therefore, the potential exists for interaction between carbamazepine and any agent metabolized by one (or more) of these enzymes. Agents that are metabolized by CYP1A2 and CYP3A4 may have decreased plasma levels when administered concomitantly with carbamazepine. Thus, if a patient has been titrated to a stable dosage on one of the agents in these categories, and then begins a course of treatment with carbamazepine, it is reasonable to expect that a dose increase for the concomitant agent may be necessary). Products include:

Estradiol Benzoate (Carbamazepine is known to induce CYP1A2 and CYP3A4. Therefore, the potential exists for interaction between carbamazepine and any agent metabolized by one (or more) of these enzymes. Agents that are metabolized by CYP1A2 and CYP3A4 may have decreased plasma levels when administered concomitantly with carbamazepine. Thus, if a patient has been titrated to a stable dosage on one of the agents in these categories, and then begins a course of treatment with carbamazepine, it is reasonable to expect that a dose increase for the concomitant agent may be necessary).

No products indexed under this heading.

Estradiol Cypionate (Carbamazepine is known to induce CYP1A2 and CYP3A4. Therefore, the potential exists for interaction between carbamazepine and any agent metabolized by one (or more) of these enzymes. Agents that are metabolized by CYP1A2 and CYP3A4 may have decreased plasma levels when administered concomitantly with car-

bamazepine. Thus, if a patient has been titrated to a stable dosage on one of the agents in these categories, and then begins a course of treatment with carbamazepine, it is reasonable to expect that a dose increase for the concomitant agent may be necessary).

No products indexed under this heading.

Estradiol Valerate (Carbamazepine is known to induce CYP1A2 and CYP3A4. Therefore, the potential exists for interaction between carbamazepine and any agent metabolized by one (or more) of these enzymes. Agents that are metabolized by CYP1A2 and CYP3A4 may have decreased plasma levels when administered concomitantly with carbamazepine. Thus, if a patient has been titrated to a stable dosage on one of the agents in these categories, and then begins a course of treatment with carbamazepine, it is reasonable to expect that a dose increase for the concomitant agent may be necessary).

No products indexed under this heading.

Ethanol (Because of its primary CNS effect, caution should be used when carbamazepine is taken with alcohol).

No products indexed under this heading.

Ethchlorvynol (Because of its primary CNS effect, caution should be used when carbamazepine is taken with other centrally-acting drugs).

No products indexed under this heading.

Ethinamate (Because of its primary CNS effect, caution should be used when carbamazepine is taken with other centrally-acting drugs).

No products indexed under this heading.

Ethinyl Estradiol (Carbamazepine is known to induce CYP1A2 and CYP3A4. Therefore, the potential exists for interaction between carbamazepine and any agent metabolized by one (or more) of these enzymes. Agents that are metabolized by CYP1A2 or CYP3A4 may have decreased plasma levels when administered concomitantly with carbamazepine. Breakthrough bleeding has been reported among patients receiving concomitant oral contraceptives and their reliability may be adversely affected). Products include:

Ethosuximide (Carbamazepine is metabolized by CYP3A4. Therefore, the potential exists for interaction between carbamazepine and any agent that induces CYP3A4. Agents that are CYP3A4 inducers may decrease plasma levels of carbamazepine. Thus, if a patient has been titrated to a stable dosage on carbamazepine, and then begins a course of treatment with a CYP3A4 inducers, it is reasonable to expect that a dose increase for carbamazepine may be necessary).

No products indexed under this heading.

Ethyl Alcohol (Because of its primary CNS effect, caution should be used when carbamazepine is taken with other centrally-acting drugs).

No products indexed under this heading.

Ethynodiol Diacetate (Carbamazepine is known to induce CYP1A2 and CYP3A4. Therefore, the potential exists for interaction between carbamazepine and any agent metabolized by one (or more) of these enzymes. Agents that are metabolized by CYP1A2 or CYP3A4 may have decreased plasma levels when administered concomitantly with carbamazepine. Breakthrough bleeding has been reported among patients receiving concomitant oral contraceptives and their reliability may be adversely affected).

No products indexed under this heading.

Etoposide (Carbamazepine is known to induce CYP1A2 and CYP3A4. Therefore, the potential exists for interaction between carbamazepine and any agent metabolized by one (or more) of these enzymes. Agents that are metabolized by CYP1A2 and CYP3A4 may have decreased plasma levels when administered concomitantly with carbamazepine. Thus, if a patient has been titrated to a stable dosage on one of the agents in these categories, and then begins a course of treatment with carbamazepine, it is reasonable to expect that a dose increase for the concomitant agent may be necessary).

No products indexed under this heading.

Etoposide Phosphate (Carbamazepine is known to induce CYP1A2 and CYP3A4. Therefore, the potential exists for interaction between carbamazepine and any agent metabolized by one (or more) of these enzymes. Agents that are metabolized by CYP1A2 and CYP3A4 may have decreased plasma levels when administered concomitantly with carbamazepine. Thus, if a patient has been titrated to a stable dosage on one of the agents in these categories, and then begins a course of treatment with carbamazepine, it is reasonable to expect that a dose increase for the concomitant agent may be necessary).

No products indexed under this heading.

Felbamate (Carbamazepine is metabolized by CYP3A4. Therefore, the potential exists for interaction between carbamazepine and any agent that induces CYP3A4. Agents that are CYP3A4 inducers may decrease plasma levels of carbamazepine. Thus, if a patient has been titrated to a stable dosage on carbamazepine, and then begins a course of treatment with a CYP3A4 inducers, it is reasonable to expect that a dose increase for carbamazepine may be necessary).

No products indexed under this heading.

Felodipine (Carbamazepine is known to induce CYP1A2 and CYP3A4. Therefore, the potential exists for interaction between carbamazepine and any agent metabolized by one (or more) of these enzymes. Agents that are metabolized by CYP1A2 and CYP3A4 may have decreased plasma levels when administered concomitantly with carbamazepine. Thus, if a patient has been titrated to a stable dosage on one of the agents in these categories, and then begins a course of treatment with carbamazepine, it is reasonable to expect that a dose increase for the concomitant agent may be necessary).

No products indexed under this heading.

Fentanyl (Carbamazepine is known to induce CYP1A2 and CYP3A4. Therefore, the potential exists for interaction between carbamazepine and any agent metabolized by one (or more) of these enzymes. Agents that are metabolized by CYP1A2 and CYP3A4 may have decreased plasma levels when administered concomitantly with carbamazepine. Thus, if a patient has been titrated to a stable dosage on one of the agents in these categories, and then begins a course of treatment with carbamazepine, it is reasonable to expect that a dose increase for the concomitant agent may be necessary). Products include:

Duragesic Transdermal System **2373**
Ionsys Transdermal System **2379**

Fentanyl Citrate (Carbamazepine is known to induce CYP1A2 and CYP3A4. Therefore, the potential exists for interaction between carbamazepine and any agent metabolized by one (or more) of these enzymes. Agents that are metabolized by CYP1A2 and CYP3A4 may have decreased plasma levels when administered concomitantly with carbamazepine. Thus, if a patient has been titrated to a stable dosage on one of the agents in these categories, and then begins a course of treatment with carbamazepine, it is reasonable to expect that a dose increase for the concomitant agent may be necessary). Products include:

Actiq **979**

Fluconazole (Carbamazepine is metabolized mainly by CYP3A4 the active carbamazepine 10,11-epoxide, which is futher metabolized to the trans-diol by epoxide hydrolase. Therefore, the potential exists for interaction between carbamazepine and any agent that inhibits CYP3A4 and/or epoxide hydrolase. Agents that are CYP3A4 inhibitors may increase the plasma levels of carbamazepine. Thus, if a patient has been titrated to a stable dosage of carbamazepine, and then begins a course of treatment with a CYP3A4 or epoxide hydrolase inhibitor, it is reasonable to expect that a dose reduction for carbamazepine may be necessary).

No products indexed under this heading.

Fludrocortisone Acetate (Carbamazepine is metabolized by CYP3A4. Therefore, the potential exists for interaction between carbamazepine and any agent that induces CYP3A4. Agents that are CYP3A4 inducers may decrease plasma levels of carbamazepine. Thus, if a patient has been titrated to a stable dosage on carbamazepine, and then begins a course of treatment with a CYP3A4 inducers, it is reasonable to expect that a dose increase for carbamazepine may be

necessary).

No products indexed under this heading.

Fluoxetine Hydrochloride (Carbamazepine is metabolized mainly by CYP3A4 the active carbamazepine 10,11-epoxide, which is futher metabolized to the trans-diol by epoxide hydrolase. Therefore, the potential exists for interaction between carbamazepine and any agent that inhibits CYP3A4 and/or epoxide hydrolase. Agents that are CYP3A4 inhibitors may increase the plasma levels of carbamazepine. Thus, if a patient has been titrated to a stable dosage of carbamazepine, and then begins a course of treatment with a CYP3A4 or epoxide hydrolase inhibitor, it is reasonable to expect that a dose reduction for carbamazepine may be necessary). Products include:

Prozac Pulvules and Liquid **1801**
Symbyax Capsules **1819**

Fluphenazine Decanoate (Because of its primary CNS effect, caution should be used when carbamazepine is taken with other centrally-acting drugs).

No products indexed under this heading.

Fluphenazine Enanthate (Because of its primary CNS effect, caution should be used when carbamazepine is taken with other centrally-acting drugs).

No products indexed under this heading.

Fluphenazine Hydrochloride (Because of its primary CNS effect, caution should be used when carbamazepine is taken with other centrally-acting drugs).

No products indexed under this heading.

Flurazepam Hydrochloride (Because of its primary CNS effect, caution should be used when carbamazepine is taken with other centrally-acting drugs). Products include:

Dalmane Capsules **3342**

Flutamide (Carbamazepine is known to induce CYP1A2 and CYP3A4. Therefore, the potential exists for interaction between carbamazepine and any agent metabolized by one (or more) of these enzymes. Agents that are metabolized by CYP1A2 and CYP3A4 may have decreased plasma levels when administered concomitantly with carbamazepine. Thus, if a patient has been titrated to a stable dosage on one of the agents in these categories, and then begins a course of treatment with carbamazepine, it is reasonable to expect that a dose increase for the concomitant agent may be necessary). Products include:

Eulexin Capsules **3009**

Fluticasone Propionate (Carbamazepine is known to induce CYP1A2 and CYP3A4. Therefore, the potential exists for interaction between carbamazepine and any agent metabolized by one (or more) of these enzymes. Agents that are metabolized by CYP1A2 and CYP3A4 may have decreased plasma levels when administered concomitantly with carbamazepine. Thus, if a patient has been titrated to a stable dosage on one of the agents in these categories, and then begins a course of treatment with

carbamazepine, it is reasonable to expect that a dose increase for the concomitant agent may be necessary). Products include:

Advair Diskus 100/50 **1308**
Advair Diskus 250/50 **1308**
Advair Diskus 500/50 **1308**
Advair HFA Inhalation Aerosol **1318**
Cutivate Cream **2662**
Cutivate Lotion 0.05% **2664**
Cutivate Ointment **2665**
Flonase Nasal Spray **1440**
Flovent Diskus **1443**

Fluvoxamine Maleate (Carbamazepine is metabolized mainly by CYP3A4 the active carbamazepine 10,11-epoxide, which is futher metabolized to the trans-diol by epoxide hydrolase. Therefore, the potential exists for interaction between carbamazepine and any agent that inhibits CYP3A4 and/or epoxide hydrolase. Agents that are CYP3A4 inhibitors may increase the plasma levels of carbamazepine. Thus, if a patient has been titrated to a stable dosage of carbamazepine, and then begins a course of treatment with a CYP3A4 or epoxide hydrolase inhibitor, it is reasonable to expect that a dose reduction for carbamazepine may be necessary).

No products indexed under this heading.

Fosamprenavir Calcium (Carbamazepine is metabolized mainly by CYP3A4 the active carbamazepine 10,11-epoxide, which is futher metabolized to the trans-diol by epoxide hydrolase. Therefore, the potential exists for interaction between carbamazepine and any agent that inhibits CYP3A4 and/or epoxide hydrolase. Agents that are CYP3A4 inhibitors may increase the plasma levels of carbamazepine. Thus, if a patient has been titrated to a stable dosage of carbamazepine, and then begins a course of treatment with a CYP3A4 or epoxide hydrolase inhibitor, it is reasonable to expect that a dose reduction for carbamazepine may be necessary). Products include:

Lexiva Tablets **1505**

Fosphenytoin Sodium (Carbamazepine is metabolized by CYP3A4. Therefore, the potential exists for interaction between carbamazepine and any agent that induces CYP3A4. Agents that are CYP3A4 inducers may decrease plasma levels of carbamazepine. Thus, if a patient has been titrated to a stable dosage on carbamazepine, and then begins a course of treatment with a CYP3A4 inducers, it is reasonable to expect that a dose increase for carbamazepine may be necessary).

No products indexed under this heading.

Garlic Extract (Carbamazepine is metabolized by CYP3A4. Therefore, the potential exists for interaction between carbamazepine and any agent that induces CYP3A4. Agents that are CYP3A4 inducers may decrease plasma levels of carbamazepine. Thus, if a patient has been titrated to a stable dosage on carbamazepine, and then begins a course of treatment with a CYP3A4 inducers, it is reasonable to expect that a dose increase for carbamazepine may be necessary).

No products indexed under this heading.

Garlic Oil (Carbamazepine is metabolized by CYP3A4. Therefore, the potential exists for interaction between carbamazepine and any agent that induces CYP3A4. Agents that are CYP3A4 inducers may decrease plasma levels of carbamazepine. Thus, if a patient has been titrated to a stable dosage on carbamazepine, and then begins a course of treatment with a CYP3A4 inducers, it is reasonable to expect that a dose increase for carbamazepine may be necessary).

No products indexed under this heading.

Glutethimide (Because of its primary CNS effect, caution should be used when carbamazepine is taken with other centrally-acting drugs).

No products indexed under this heading.

Grepafloxacin Hydrochloride (Carbamazepine is known to induce CYP1A2 and CYP3A4. Therefore, the potential exists for interaction between carbamazepine and any agent metabolized by one (or more) of these enzymes. Agents that are metabolized by CYP1A2 and CYP3A4 may have decreased plasma levels when administered concomitantly with carbamazepine. Thus, if a patient has been titrated to a stable dosage on one of the agents in these categories, and then begins a course of treatment with carbamazepine, it is reasonable to expect that a dose increase for the concomitant agent may be necessary).

No products indexed under this heading.

Haloperidol (Carbamazepine is known to induce CYP1A2 and CYP3A4. Therefore, the potential exists for interaction between carbamazepine and any agent metabolized by one (or more) of these enzymes. Agents that are metabolized by CYP1A2 and CYP3A4 may have decreased plasma levels when administered concomitantly with carbamazepine. Thus, if a patient has been titrated to a stable dosage on one of the agents in these categories, and then begins a course of treatment with carbamazepine, it is reasonable to expect that a dose increase for the concomitant agent may be necessary).

No products indexed under this heading.

Haloperidol Decanoate (Carbamazepine is known to induce CYP1A2 and CYP3A4. Therefore, the potential exists for interaction between carbamazepine and any agent metabolized by one (or more) of these enzymes. Agents that are metabolized by CYP1A2 and CYP3A4 may have decreased plasma levels when administered concomitantly with carbamazepine. Thus, if a patient has been titrated to a stable dosage on one of the agents in these categories, and then begins a course of treatment with carbamazepine, it is reasonable to expect that a dose increase for the concomitant agent may be necessary).

No products indexed under this heading.

Haloperidol Lactate (Carbamazepine is known to induce CYP1A2 and CYP3A4. Therefore, the potential exists for interaction between car-

bamazepine and any agent metabolized by one (or more) of these enzymes. Agents that are metabolized by CYP1A2 and CYP3A4 may have decreased plasma levels when administered concomitantly with carbamazepine. Thus, if a patient has been titrated to a stable dosage on one of the agents in these categories, and then begins a course of treatment with carbamazepine, it is reasonable to expect that a dose increase for the concomitant agent may be necessary).
No products indexed under this heading.

Hydrocodone Bitartrate (Because of its primary CNS effect, caution should be used when carbamazepine is taken with other centrally-acting drugs). Products include:
Hycodan **1116**
Hycotuss Expectorant Syrup **1117**
Vicodin Tablets **535**
Vicodin ES Tablets **536**
Vicodin HP Tablets **538**
Vicoprofen Tablets **539**
Zydone Tablets **1139**

Hydrocodone Polistirex (Because of its primary CNS effect, caution should be used when carbamazepine is taken with other centrally-acting drugs). Products include:
Tussionex Pennkinetic Extended-Release Suspension **3327**

Hydrocortisone (Carbamazepine is metabolized by CYP3A4. Therefore, the potential exists for interaction between carbamazepine and any agent that induces CYP3A4. Agents that are CYP3A4 inducers may decrease plasma levels of carbamazepine. Thus, if a patient has been titrated to a stable dosage on carbamazepine, and then begins a course of treatment with a CYP3A4 inducers, it is reasonable to expect that a dose increase for carbamazepine may be necessary). Products include:
Colocort Rectal Suspension, USP (Retention) 100 mg/60 mL.......... **2476**
Hydrocortone Tablets **1989**
Preparation H Hydrocortisone Cream .... ▣**646**

Hydrocortisone Acetate (Carbamazepine is metabolized by CYP3A4. Therefore, the potential exists for interaction between carbamazepine and any agent that induces CYP3A4. Agents that are CYP3A4 inducers may decrease plasma levels of carbamazepine. Thus, if a patient has been titrated to a stable dosage on carbamazepine, and then begins a course of treatment with a CYP3A4 inducers, it is reasonable to expect that a dose increase for carbamazepine may be necessary). Products include:
Analpram-HC **1159**
Pramosone **1161**
ProctoFoam-HC **3099**

Hydrocortisone Butyrate (Carbamazepine is metabolized by CYP3A4. Therefore, the potential exists for interaction between carbamazepine and any agent that induces CYP3A4. Agents that are CYP3A4 inducers may decrease plasma levels of carbamazepine. Thus, if a patient has been titrated to a stable dosage on carbamazepine, and then begins a course of treatment with a CYP3A4 inducers, it is reasonable to expect that a dose increase for carbamazepine may be necessary). Products include:
Locoid Lipocream Cream **1160**

Hydrocortisone Cypionate (Carbamazepine is metabolized by CYP3A4. Therefore, the potential exists for interaction between carbamazepine and any agent that induces CYP3A4. Agents that are CYP3A4 inducers may decrease plasma levels of carbamazepine. Thus, if a patient has been titrated to a stable dosage on carbamazepine, and then begins a course of treatment with a CYP3A4 inducers, it is reasonable to expect that a dose increase for carbamazepine may be necessary).
No products indexed under this heading.

Hydrocortisone Hemisuccinate (Carbamazepine is metabolized by CYP3A4. Therefore, the potential exists for interaction between carbamazepine and any agent that induces CYP3A4. Agents that are CYP3A4 inducers may decrease plasma levels of carbamazepine. Thus, if a patient has been titrated to a stable dosage on carbamazepine, and then begins a course of treatment with a CYP3A4 inducers, it is reasonable to expect that a dose increase for carbamazepine may be necessary).
No products indexed under this heading.

Hydrocortisone Probutate (Carbamazepine is metabolized by CYP3A4. Therefore, the potential exists for interaction between carbamazepine and any agent that induces CYP3A4. Agents that are CYP3A4 inducers may decrease plasma levels of carbamazepine. Thus, if a patient has been titrated to a stable dosage on carbamazepine, and then begins a course of treatment with a CYP3A4 inducers, it is reasonable to expect that a dose increase for carbamazepine may be necessary).
No products indexed under this heading.

Hydrocortisone Sodium Phosphate (Carbamazepine is metabolized by CYP3A4. Therefore, the potential exists for interaction between carbamazepine and any agent that induces CYP3A4. Agents that are CYP3A4 inducers may decrease plasma levels of carbamazepine. Thus, if a patient has been titrated to a stable dosage on carbamazepine, and then begins a course of treatment with a CYP3A4 inducers, it is reasonable to expect that a dose increase for carbamazepine may be necessary).
No products indexed under this heading.

Hydrocortisone Sodium Succinate (Carbamazepine is metabolized by CYP3A4. Therefore, the potential exists for interaction between carbamazepine and any agent that induces CYP3A4. Agents that are CYP3A4 inducers may decrease plasma levels of carbamazepine. Thus, if a patient has been titrated to a stable dosage on carbamazepine, and then begins a course of treatment with a CYP3A4 inducers, it is reasonable to expect that a dose increase for carbamazepine may be necessary).
No products indexed under this heading.

Hydrocortisone Valerate (Carbamazepine is metabolized by CYP3A4. Therefore, the potential exists for interaction between carbamazepine and any agent that induces CYP3A4. Agents that are CYP3A4 inducers may decrease plasma levels of carbamazepine. Thus, if a patient has been titrated to a stable dosage on carbamazepine, and then begins a course of treatment with a CYP3A4 inducers, it is reasonable to expect that a dose increase for carbamazepine may be necessary).
No products indexed under this heading.

Hydromorphone Hydrochloride (Because of its primary CNS effect, caution should be used when carbamazepine is taken with other centrally-acting drugs). Products include:
Dilaudid **440**
Dilaudid Non-Sterile Powder **440**
Dilaudid Oral Liquid **445**
Dilaudid Rectal Suppositories **440**
Dilaudid Tablets **440**
Dilaudid Tablets - 8 mg **445**
Dilaudid-HP **442**

Hydroxyzine Hydrochloride (Because of its primary CNS effect, caution should be used when carbamazepine is taken with other centrally-acting drugs).
No products indexed under this heading.

Hypericum (Carbamazepine is metabolized by CYP3A4. Therefore, the potential exists for interaction between carbamazepine and any agent that induces CYP3A4. Agents that are CYP3A4 inducers may decrease plasma levels of carbamazepine. Thus, if a patient has been titrated to a stable dosage on carbamazepine, and then begins a course of treatment with a CYP3A4 inducers, it is reasonable to expect that a dose increase for carbamazepine may be necessary). Products include:
Satiete Tablets .... ▣**832**

Hypericum Perforatum (Carbamazepine is metabolized by CYP3A4. Therefore, the potential exists for interaction between carbamazepine and any agent that induces CYP3A4. Agents that are CYP3A4 inducers may decrease plasma levels of carbamazepine. Thus, if a patient has been titrated to a stable dosage on carbamazepine, and then begins a course of treatment with a CYP3A4 inducers, it is reasonable to expect that a dose increase for carbamazepine may be necessary).
No products indexed under this heading.

Imipramine Hydrochloride (Carbamazepine is known to induce CYP1A2 and CYP3A4. Therefore, the potential exists for interaction between carbamazepine and any agent metabolized by one (or more) of these enzymes. Agents that are metabolized by CYP1A2 and CYP3A4 may have decreased plasma levels when administered concomitantly with carbamazepine. Thus, if a patient has been titrated to a stable dosage on one of the agents in these categories, and then begins a course of treatment with carbamazepine, it is reasonable to expect that a dose increase for the concomitant agent may be necessary).
No products indexed under this heading.

Imipramine Pamoate (Carbamazepine is known to induce CYP1A2 and CYP3A4. Therefore, the potential exists for interaction between carbamazepine and any agent metabolized by one (or more) of these enzymes. Agents that are metabolized by CYP1A2 and CYP3A4 may have decreased plasma levels when administered concomitantly with carbamazepine. Thus, if a patient has been titrated to a stable dosage on one of the agents in these categories, and then begins a course of treatment with carbamazepine, it is reasonable to expect that a dose increase for the concomitant agent may be necessary).
No products indexed under this heading.

Indinavir Sulfate (Carbamazepine is metabolized mainly by CYP3A4 the active carbamazepine 10,11-epoxide, which is futher metabolized to the trans-diol by epoxide hydrolase. Therefore, the potential exists for interaction between carbamazepine and any agent that inhibits CYP3A4 and/or epoxide hydrolase. Agents that are CYP3A4 inhibitors may increase the plasma levels of carbamazepine. Thus, if a patient has been titrated to a stable dosage of carbamazepine, and then begins a course of treatment with a CYP3A4 or epoxide hydrolase inhibitor, it is reasonable to expect that a dose reduction for carbamazepine may be necessary). Products include:
Crixivan Capsules **1940**

Isoflurane (Because of its primary CNS effect, caution should be used when carbamazepine is taken with other centrally-acting drugs).
No products indexed under this heading.

Isoniazid (Carbamazepine is metabolized mainly by CYP3A4 the active carbamazepine 10,11-epoxide, which is futher metabolized to the trans-diol by epoxide hydrolase. Therefore, the potential exists for interaction between carbamazepine and any agent that inhibits CYP3A4 and/or epoxide hydrolase. Agents that are CYP3A4 inhibitors may increase the plasma levels of carbamazepine. Thus, if a patient has been titrated to a stable dosage of carbamazepine, and then begins a course of treatment with a CYP3A4 or epoxide hydrolase inhibitor, it is reasonable to expect that a dose reduction for carbamazepine may be necessary).
No products indexed under this heading.

Isradipine (Carbamazepine is known to induce CYP1A2 and CYP3A4. Therefore, the potential exists for interaction between carbamazepine and any agent metabolized by one (or more) of these enzymes. Agents that are metabolized by CYP1A2 and CYP3A4 may have decreased plasma levels when administered concomitantly with carbamazepine. Thus, if a patient has been titrated to a stable dosage on one of the agents in these categories, and then begins a course of treatment with carbamazepine, it is reasonable to expect that a dose increase for the concomitant agent may be necessary). Products include:

DynaCirc CR Tablets 2721

Itraconazole (Carbamazepine is metabolized mainly by CYP3A4 the active carbamazepine 10,11-epoxide, which is futher metabolized to the trans-diol by epoxide hydrolase. Therefore, the potential exists for interaction between carbamazepine and any agent that inhibits CYP3A4 and/or epoxide hydrolase. Agents that are CYP3A4 inhibitors may increase the plasma levels of carbamazepine. Thus, if a patient has been titrated to a stable dosage of carbamazepine, and then begins a course of treatment with a CYP3A4 or epoxide hydrolase inhibitor, it is reasonable to expect that a dose reduction for carbamazepine may be necessary).

No products indexed under this heading.

Ketamine Hydrochloride (Because of its primary CNS effect, caution should be used when carbamazepine is taken with other centrally-acting drugs).

No products indexed under this heading.

Ketoconazole (Carbamazepine is metabolized mainly by CYP3A4 the active carbamazepine 10,11-epoxide, which is futher metabolized to the trans-diol by epoxide hydrolase. Therefore, the potential exists for interaction between carbamazepine and any agent that inhibits CYP3A4 and/or epoxide hydrolase. Agents that are CYP3A4 inhibitors may increase the plasma levels of carbamazepine. Thus, if a patient has been titrated to a stable dosage of carbamazepine, and then begins a course of treatment with a CYP3A4 or epoxide hydrolase inhibitor, it is reasonable to expect that a dose reduction for carbamazepine may be necessary). Products include:

Nizoral A-D Shampoo, 1% 1868

Levobupivacaine Hydrochloride (Carbamazepine is known to induce CYP1A2 and CYP3A4. Therefore, the potential exists for interaction between carbamazepine and any agent metabolized by one (or more) of these enzymes. Agents that are metabolized by CYP1A2 and CYP3A4 may have decreased plasma levels when administered concomitantly with carbamazepine. Thus, if a patient has been titrated to a stable dosage on one of the agents in these categories, and then begins a course of treatment with carbamazepine, it is reasonable to expect that a dose increase for the concomitant agent may be necessary).

No products indexed under this heading.

Levomethadyl Acetate Hydrochloride (Because of its primary CNS effect, caution should be used when carbamazepine is taken with other centrally-acting drugs).

No products indexed under this heading.

Levonorgestrel (Carbamazepine is known to induce CYP1A2 and CYP3A4. Therefore, the potential exists for interaction between carbamazepine and any agent metabolized by one (or more) of these enzymes. Agents that are metabolized by CYP1A2 or CYP3A4 may have decreased plasma levels when administered concomitantly with carbamazepine. Breakthrough bleeding has been reported among patients receiving concomitant oral contraceptives and their reliability may be adversely affected). Products include:

Climara Pro Transdermal System 776
Mirena Intrauterine System 787
Plan B Tablets 1076
Seasonique Tablets 1077

Levorphanol Tartrate (Because of its primary CNS effect, caution should be used when carbamazepine is taken with other centrally-acting drugs).

No products indexed under this heading.

Lidocaine (Carbamazepine is known to induce CYP1A2 and CYP3A4. Therefore, the potential exists for interaction between carbamazepine and any agent metabolized by one (or more) of these enzymes. Agents that are metabolized by CYP1A2 and CYP3A4 may have decreased plasma levels when administered concomitantly with carbamazepine. Thus, if a patient has been titrated to a stable dosage on one of the agents in these categories, and then begins a course of treatment with carbamazepine, it is reasonable to expect that a dose increase for the concomitant agent may be necessary). Products include:

Lidoderm Patch 1118
Synera Topical Patch 1137

Lidocaine Hydrochloride (Carbamazepine is known to induce CYP1A2 and CYP3A4. Therefore, the potential exists for interaction between carbamazepine and any agent metabolized by one (or more) of these enzymes. Agents that are metabolized by CYP1A2 and CYP3A4 may have decreased plasma levels when administered concomitantly with carbamazepine. Thus, if a patient has been titrated to a stable dosage on one of the agents in these categories, and then begins a course of treatment with carbamazepine, it is reasonable to expect that a dose increase for the concomitant agent may be necessary).

No products indexed under this heading.

Lithium (Concomitant administration of carbamazepine and lithium may increase the risk of neurotoxic side effects).

No products indexed under this heading.

Lithium Carbonate (Concomitant administration of carbamazepine and lithium may increase the risk of neurotoxic side effects). Products include:

Lithobid Tablets 1692

Lithium Citrate (Concomitant administration of carbamazepine and lithium may increase the risk of neurotoxic side effects).

No products indexed under this heading.

Lomefloxacin Hydrochloride (Carbamazepine is known to induce CYP1A2 and CYP3A4. Therefore, the potential exists for interaction between carbamazepine and any agent metabolized by one (or more) of these enzymes. Agents that are metabolized by CYP1A2 and CYP3A4 may have decreased plasma levels when administered concomitantly with carbamazepine. Thus, if a patient has been titrated to a stable dosage on one of the agents in these categories, and then begins a course of treatment with carbamazepine, it is reasonable to expect that a dose increase for the concomitant agent may be necessary).

No products indexed under this heading.

Lopinavir (Carbamazepine is metabolized mainly by CYP3A4 the active carbamazepine 10,11-epoxide, which is futher metabolized to the trans-diol by epoxide hydrolase. Therefore, the potential exists for interaction between carbamazepine and any agent that inhibits CYP3A4 and/or epoxide hydrolase. Agents that are CYP3A4 inhibitors may increase the plasma levels of carbamazepine. Thus, if a patient has been titrated to a stable dosage of carbamazepine, and then begins a course of treatment with a CYP3A4 or epoxide hydrolase inhibitor, it is reasonable to expect that a dose reduction for carbamazepine may be necessary). Products include:

Kaletra 476

Loratadine (Carbamazepine is metabolized mainly by CYP3A4 the active carbamazepine 10,11-epoxide, which is futher metabolized to the trans-diol by epoxide hydrolase. Therefore, the potential exists for interaction between carbamazepine and any agent that inhibits CYP3A4 and/or epoxide hydrolase. Agents that are CYP3A4 inhibitors may increase the plasma levels of carbamazepine. Thus, if a patient has been titrated to a stable dosage of carbamazepine, and then begins a course of treatment with a CYP3A4 or epoxide hydrolase inhibitor, it is reasonable to expect that a dose reduction for carbamazepine may be necessary). Products include:

Alavert Allergy & Sinus D-12 Hour Tablets.. 771
Alavert 771
Children's Claritin Allergy Oral Solution 771
Claritin Non-Drowsy 24 Hour Tablets.. 772
Claritin Reditabs 24 Hour Non-Drowsy Tablets 772
Claritin-D Non-Drowsy 12 Hour Tablets.. 772
Claritin-D Non-Drowsy 24 Hour Tablets.. 772

Lorazepam (Because of its primary CNS effect, caution should be used when carbamazepine is taken with other centrally-acting drugs).

No products indexed under this heading.

Lovastatin (Carbamazepine is known to induce CYP1A2 and CYP3A4. Therefore, the potential exists for interaction between carbamazepine and any agent metabolized by one (or more) of these enzymes. Agents that are metabolized by CYP1A2 and CYP3A4 may have decreased plasma levels when administered concomitantly with carbamazepine. Thus, if a patient has been titrated to a stable dosage on one of the agents in these categories, and then begins a course of treatment with carbamazepine, it is reasonable to expect that a dose increase for the concomitant agent may be necessary). Products include:

Advicor Tablets 1722
Altoprev Extended-Release Tablets 3109
Mevacor Tablets 2021

Loxapine Hydrochloride (Because of its primary CNS effect, caution should be used when carbamazepine is taken with other centrally-acting drugs).

No products indexed under this heading.

Loxapine Succinate (Because of its primary CNS effect, caution should be used when carbamazepine is taken with other centrally-acting drugs).

No products indexed under this heading.

Maprotiline Hydrochloride (Carbamazepine is known to induce CYP1A2 and CYP3A4. Therefore, the potential exists for interaction between carbamazepine and any agent metabolized by one (or more) of these enzymes. Agents that are metabolized by CYP1A2 and CYP3A4 may have decreased plasma levels when administered concomitantly with carbamazepine. Thus, if a patient has been titrated to a stable dosage on one of the agents in these categories, and then begins a course of treatment with carbamazepine, it is reasonable to expect that a dose increase for the concomitant agent may be necessary).

No products indexed under this heading.

Mefloquine Hydrochloride (Antimalarial drugs, such as chloroquine and mefloquine, may antagonize the activity of carbamazepine). Products include:

Lariam Tablets 2786

Meperidine Hydrochloride (Because of its primary CNS effect, caution should be used when carbamazepine is taken with other centrally-acting drugs).

No products indexed under this heading.

Mephenytoin (Carbamazepine is metabolized by CYP3A4. Therefore, the potential exists for interaction between carbamazepine and any agent that induces CYP3A4. Agents that are CYP3A4 inducers may decrease plasma levels of carbamazepine. Thus, if a patient has been titrated to a stable dosage on carbamazepine, and then begins a course of treatment with a CYP3A4 inducers, it is reasonable to expect that a dose increase for carbamazepine may be necessary).

No products indexed under this heading.

Mephobarbital (Because of its primary CNS effect, caution should be used when carbamazepine is taken with other centrally-acting drugs).

No products indexed under this heading.

Meprobamate (Because of its primary CNS effect, caution should be used when carbamazepine is taken with other centrally-acting drugs).

No products indexed under this heading.

Mesoridazine Besylate (Because of its primary CNS effect, caution should be used when carbamazepine is taken with other centrally-acting drugs).

No products indexed under this heading.

Mestranol (Carbamazepine is known to induce CYP1A2 and CYP3A4. Therefore, the potential exists for interaction between carbamazepine and any agent metabolized by one (or more) of these enzymes. Agents that are metabolized by CYP1A2 or CYP3A4 may have decreased plasma levels when administered concomitantly with carbamazepine. Breakthrough bleeding has been reported among patients receiving concomitant oral contraceptives and their reliability may be adversely affected).
No products indexed under this heading.

Methadone Hydrochloride (Carbamazepine is known to induce CYP1A2 and CYP3A4. Therefore, the potential exists for interaction between carbamazepine and any agent metabolized by one (or more) of these enzymes. Agents that are metabolized by CYP1A2 and CYP3A4 may have decreased plasma levels when administered concomitantly with carbamazepine. Thus, if a patient has been titrated to a stable dosage on one of the agents in these categories, and then begins a course of treatment with carbamazepine, it is reasonable to expect that a dose increase for the concomitant agent may be necessary).
No products indexed under this heading.

Methohexital Sodium (Because of its primary CNS effect, caution should be used when carbamazepine is taken with other centrally-acting drugs).
No products indexed under this heading.

Methotrimeprazine (Because of its primary CNS effect, caution should be used when carbamazepine is taken with other centrally-acting drugs).
No products indexed under this heading.

Methoxyflurane (Because of its primary CNS effect, caution should be used when carbamazepine is taken with other centrally-acting drugs).
No products indexed under this heading.

Methsuximide (Carbamazepine is metabolized by CYP3A4. Therefore, the potential exists for interaction between carbamazepine and any agent that induces CYP3A4. Agents that are CYP3A4 inducers may decrease plasma levels of carbamazepine. Thus, if a patient has been titrated to a stable dosage on carbamazepine, and then begins a course of treatment with a CYP3A4 inducers, it is reasonable to expect that a dose increase for carbamazepine may be necessary).
No products indexed under this heading.

Methylprednisolone (Carbamazepine is metabolized by CYP3A4. Therefore, the potential exists for interaction between carbamazepine and any agent that induces CYP3A4. Agents that are CYP3A4 inducers may decrease plasma levels of carbamazepine. Thus, if a patient has been titrated to a stable dosage on carbamazepine, and then begins a course of treatment with a CYP3A4 inducers, it is reasonable to expect that a dose increase for carbamazepine may be necessary).
No products indexed under this heading.

Methylprednisolone Acetate (Carbamazepine is metabolized by CYP3A4. Therefore, the potential exists for interaction between carbamazepine and any agent that induces CYP3A4. Agents that are CYP3A4 inducers may decrease plasma levels of carbamazepine. Thus, if a patient has been titrated to a stable dosage on carbamazepine, and then begins a course of treatment with a CYP3A4 inducers, it is reasonable to expect that a dose increase for carbamazepine may be necessary). Products include:
Depo-Medrol Injectable Suspension 2617
Depo-Medrol Single-Dose Vial 2619

Methylprednisolone Sodium Succinate (Carbamazepine is metabolized by CYP3A4. Therefore, the potential exists for interaction between carbamazepine and any agent that induces CYP3A4. Agents that are CYP3A4 inducers may decrease plasma levels of carbamazepine. Thus, if a patient has been titrated to a stable dosage on carbamazepine, and then begins a course of treatment with a CYP3A4 inducers, it is reasonable to expect that a dose increase for carbamazepine may be necessary).
No products indexed under this heading.

Metronidazole (Carbamazepine is metabolized mainly by CYP3A4 the active carbamazepine 10,11-epoxide, which is futher metabolized to the trans-diol by epoxide hydrolase. Therefore, the potential exists for interaction between carbamazepine and any agent that inhibits CYP3A4 and/or epoxide hydrolase. Agents that are CYP3A4 inhibitors may increase the plasma levels of carbamazepine. Thus, if a patient has been titrated to a stable dosage of carbamazepine, and then begins a course of treatment with a CYP3A4 or epoxide hydrolase inhibitor, it is reasonable to expect that a dose reduction for carbamazepine may be necessary). Products include:
Metrogel 1% 1211
MetroGel-Vaginal Gel 1855
Vandazole Vaginal Gel 3338

Metronidazole Benzoate (Carbamazepine is metabolized mainly by CYP3A4 the active carbamazepine 10,11-epoxide, which is futher metabolized to the trans-diol by epoxide hydrolase. Therefore, the potential exists for interaction between carbamazepine and any agent that inhibits CYP3A4 and/or epoxide hydrolase. Agents that are CYP3A4 inhibitors may increase the plasma levels of carbamazepine. Thus, if a patient has been titrated to a stable dosage of carbamazepine, and then begins a course of treatment with a CYP3A4 or epoxide hydrolase inhibitor, it is reasonable to expect that a dose reduction for carbamazepine may be necessary).
No products indexed under this heading.

Metronidazole Hydrochloride (Carbamazepine is metabolized mainly by CYP3A4 the active carbamazepine 10,11-epoxide, which is futher metabolized to the trans-diol by epoxide hydrolase. Therefore, the potential exists for interaction between carbamazepine and any agent that inhibits CYP3A4 and/or epoxide hydrolase. Agents that are CYP3A4 inhibitors may increase the plasma levels of carbamazepine. Thus, if a patient has been titrated to a stable dosage of carbamazepine, and then begins a course of treatment with a CYP3A4 or epoxide hydrolase inhibitor, it is reasonable to expect that a dose reduction for carbamazepine may be necessary).
No products indexed under this heading.

Mexiletine Hydrochloride (Carbamazepine is known to induce CYP1A2 and CYP3A4. Therefore, the potential exists for interaction between carbamazepine and any agent metabolized by one (or more) of these enzymes. Agents that are metabolized by CYP1A2 and CYP3A4 may have decreased plasma levels when administered concomitantly with carbamazepine. Thus, if a patient has been titrated to a stable dosage on one of the agents in these categories, and then begins a course of treatment with carbamazepine, it is reasonable to expect that a dose increase for the concomitant agent may be necessary).
No products indexed under this heading.

Miconazole (Carbamazepine is metabolized mainly by CYP3A4 the active carbamazepine 10,11-epoxide, which is futher metabolized to the trans-diol by epoxide hydrolase. Therefore, the potential exists for interaction between carbamazepine and any agent that inhibits CYP3A4 and/or epoxide hydrolase. Agents that are CYP3A4 inhibitors may increase the plasma levels of carbamazepine. Thus, if a patient has been titrated to a stable dosage of carbamazepine, and then begins a course of treatment with a CYP3A4 or epoxide hydrolase inhibitor, it is reasonable to expect that a dose reduction for carbamazepine may be necessary).
No products indexed under this heading.

Miconazole Nitrate (Carbamazepine is metabolized mainly by CYP3A4 the active carbamazepine 10,11-epoxide, which is futher metabolized to the trans-diol by epoxide hydrolase. Therefore, the potential exists for interaction between carbamazepine and any agent that inhibits CYP3A4 and/or epoxide hydrolase. Agents that are CYP3A4 inhibitors may increase the plasma levels of carbamazepine. Thus, if a patient has been titrated to a stable dosage of carbamazepine, and then begins a course of treatment with a CYP3A4 or epoxide hydrolase inhibitor, it is reasonable to expect that a dose reduction for carbamazepine may be necessary). Products include:
Desenex .... ▣635
Desenex Jock Itch Spray Powder ... ▣635

Midazolam Hydrochloride (Carbamazepine is known to induce CYP1A2 and CYP3A4. Therefore, the potential exists for interaction between carbamazepine and any agent metabolized by one (or more) of these enzymes. Agents that are metabolized by CYP1A2 and CYP3A4 may have decreased plasma levels when administered concomitantly with carbamazepine. Thus, if a patient has been titrated to a stable dosage on one of the agents in these categories, and then begins a course of treatment with carbamazepine, it is reasonable to expect that a dose increase for the concomitant agent may be necessary).
No products indexed under this heading.

Mirtazapine (Carbamazepine is known to induce CYP1A2 and CYP3A4. Therefore, the potential exists for interaction between carbamazepine and any agent metabolized by one (or more) of these enzymes. Agents that are metabolized by CYP1A2 and CYP3A4 may have decreased plasma levels when administered concomitantly with carbamazepine. Thus, if a patient has been titrated to a stable dosage on one of the agents in these categories, and then begins a course of treatment with carbamazepine, it is reasonable to expect that a dose increase for the concomitant agent may be necessary).
No products indexed under this heading.

Modafinil (Carbamazepine is metabolized by CYP3A4. Therefore, the potential exists for interaction between carbamazepine and any agent that induces CYP3A4. Agents that are CYP3A4 inducers may decrease plasma levels of carbamazepine. Thus, if a patient has been titrated to a stable dosage on carbamazepine, and then begins a course of treatment with a CYP3A4 inducers, it is reasonable to expect that a dose increase for carbamazepine may be necessary). Products include:
Provigil Tablets 988

Molindone Hydrochloride (Because of its primary CNS effect, caution should be used when carbamazepine is taken with other centrally-acting drugs). Products include:
Moban Tablets 1119

Morphine Sulfate (Because of its primary CNS effect, caution should be used when carbamazepine is taken with other centrally-acting drugs). Products include:
Avinza Capsules 1741
Kadian Capsules 577
MS Contin Tablets 2701

Moxifloxacin Hydrochloride (Carbamazepine is known to induce CYP1A2 and CYP3A4. Therefore, the potential exists for interaction between carbamazepine and any agent metabolized by one (or more) of these enzymes. Agents that are metabolized by CYP1A2 and CYP3A4 may have decreased plasma levels when administered concomitantly with carbamazepine. Thus, if a patient has been titrated to a stable dosage on one of the agents in these categories, and then begins a course of treatment with carbamazepine, it is reasonable to expect that a dose increase for the concomitant agent may be necessary). Products include:
Avelox 2970
Vigamox Ophthalmic Solution 564

Nafcillin Sodium (Carbamazepine is known to induce CYP1A2 and CYP3A4. Therefore, the potential exists for interaction between car-

bamazepine and any agent metabolized by one (or more) of these enzymes. Agents that are metabolized by CYP1A2 and CYP3A4 may have decreased plasma levels when administered concomitantly with carbamazepine. Thus, if a patient has been titrated to a stable dosage on one of the agents in these categories, and then begins a course of treatment with carbamazepine, it is reasonable to expect that a dose increase for the concomitant agent may be necessary).

No products indexed under this heading.

Naproxen (Carbamazepine is known to induce CYP1A2 and CYP3A4. Therefore, the potential exists for interaction between carbamazepine and any agent metabolized by one (or more) of these enzymes. Agents that are metabolized by CYP1A2 and CYP3A4 may have decreased plasma levels when administered concomitantly with carbamazepine. Thus, if a patient has been titrated to a stable dosage on one of the agents in these categories, and then begins a course of treatment with carbamazepine, it is reasonable to expect that a dose increase for the concomitant agent may be necessary). Products include:

Naproxen Sodium (Carbamazepine is known to induce CYP1A2 and CYP3A4. Therefore, the potential exists for interaction between carbamazepine and any agent metabolized by one (or more) of these enzymes. Agents that are metabolized by CYP1A2 and CYP3A4 may have decreased plasma levels when administered concomitantly with carbamazepine. Thus, if a patient has been titrated to a stable dosage on one of the agents in these categories, and then begins a course of treatment with carbamazepine, it is reasonable to expect that a dose increase for the concomitant agent may be necessary). Products include:

Nefazodone Hydrochloride (Carbamazepine is metabolized mainly by CYP3A4 the active carbamazepine 10,11-epoxide, which is futher metabolized to the trans-diol by epoxide hydrolase. Therefore, the potential exists for interaction between carbamazepine and any agent that inhibits CYP3A4 and/or epoxide hydrolase. Agents that are CYP3A4 inhibitors may increase the plasma levels of carbamazepine. Thus, if a patient has been titrated to a stable dosage of carbamazepine, and then begins a course of treatment with a CYP3A4 or epoxide hydrolase inhibitor, it is reasonable to expect that a dose reduction for carbamazepine may be necessary).

No products indexed under this heading.

Nelfinavir Mesylate (Carbamazepine is metabolized mainly by CYP3A4 the active carbamazepine

10,11-epoxide, which is futher metabolized to the trans-diol by epoxide hydrolase. Therefore, the potential exists for interaction between carbamazepine and any agent that inhibits CYP3A4 and/or epoxide hydrolase. Agents that are CYP3A4 inhibitors may increase the plasma levels of carbamazepine. Thus, if a patient has been titrated to a stable dosage of carbamazepine, and then begins a course of treatment with a CYP3A4 or epoxide hydrolase inhibitor, it is reasonable to expect that a dose reduction for carbamazepine may be necessary). Products include:

Nevirapine (Carbamazepine is metabolized mainly by CYP3A4 the active carbamazepine 10,11-epoxide, which is futher metabolized to the trans-diol by epoxide hydrolase. Therefore, the potential exists for interaction between carbamazepine and any agent that inhibits CYP3A4 and/or epoxide hydrolase. Agents that are CYP3A4 inhibitors may increase the plasma levels of carbamazepine. Thus, if a patient has been titrated to a stable dosage of carbamazepine, and then begins a course of treatment with a CYP3A4 or epoxide hydrolase inhibitor, it is reasonable to expect that a dose reduction for carbamazepine may be necessary). Products include:

Niacinamide (Carbamazepine is metabolized mainly by CYP3A4 the active carbamazepine 10,11-epoxide, which is futher metabolized to the trans-diol by epoxide hydrolase. Therefore, the potential exists for interaction between carbamazepine and any agent that inhibits CYP3A4 and/or epoxide hydrolase. Agents that are CYP3A4 inhibitors may increase the plasma levels of carbamazepine. Thus, if a patient has been titrated to a stable dosage of carbamazepine, and then begins a course of treatment with a CYP3A4 or epoxide hydrolase inhibitor, it is reasonable to expect that a dose reduction for carbamazepine may be necessary).

No products indexed under this heading.

Nicardipine Hydrochloride (Carbamazepine is known to induce CYP1A2 and CYP3A4. Therefore, the potential exists for interaction between carbamazepine and any agent metabolized by one (or more) of these enzymes. Agents that are metabolized by CYP1A2 and CYP3A4 may have decreased plasma levels when administered concomitantly with carbamazepine. Thus, if a patient has been titrated to a stable dosage on one of the agents in these categories, and then begins a course of treatment with carbamazepine, it is reasonable to expect that a dose increase for the concomitant agent may be necessary). Products include:

Nicotinamide (Carbamazepine is metabolized mainly by CYP3A4 the active carbamazepine 10,11-epoxide, which is futher metabolized to the trans-diol by epoxide hydrolase. Therefore, the potential exists for interaction

between carbamazepine and any agent that inhibits CYP3A4 and/or epoxide hydrolase. Agents that are CYP3A4 inhibitors may increase the plasma levels of carbamazepine. Thus, if a patient has been titrated to a stable dosage of carbamazepine, and then begins a course of treatment with a CYP3A4 or epoxide hydrolase inhibitor, it is reasonable to expect that a dose reduction for carbamazepine may be necessary). Products include:

Nicotine Polacrilex (Carbamazepine is known to induce CYP1A2 and CYP3A4. Therefore, the potential exists for interaction between carbamazepine and any agent metabolized by one (or more) of these enzymes. Agents that are metabolized by CYP1A2 and CYP3A4 may have decreased plasma levels when administered concomitantly with carbamazepine. Thus, if a patient has been titrated to a stable dosage on one of the agents in these categories, and then begins a course of treatment with carbamazepine, it is reasonable to expect that a dose increase for the concomitant agent may be necessary).

No products indexed under this heading.

Nicotine Salicylate (Carbamazepine is known to induce CYP1A2 and CYP3A4. Therefore, the potential exists for interaction between carbamazepine and any agent metabolized by one (or more) of these enzymes. Agents that are metabolized by CYP1A2 and CYP3A4 may have decreased plasma levels when administered concomitantly with carbamazepine. Thus, if a patient has been titrated to a stable dosage on one of the agents in these categories, and then begins a course of treatment with carbamazepine, it is reasonable to expect that a dose increase for the concomitant agent may be necessary).

No products indexed under this heading.

Nicotine Sulfate (Carbamazepine is known to induce CYP1A2 and CYP3A4. Therefore, the potential exists for interaction between carbamazepine and any agent metabolized by one (or more) of these enzymes. Agents that are metabolized by CYP1A2 and CYP3A4 may have decreased plasma levels when administered concomitantly with carbamazepine. Thus, if a patient has been titrated to a stable dosage on one of the agents in these categories, and then begins a course of treatment with carbamazepine, it is reasonable to expect that a dose increase for the concomitant agent may be necessary).

No products indexed under this heading.

Nifedipine (Carbamazepine is metabolized mainly by CYP3A4 the active carbamazepine 10,11-epoxide, which is futher metabolized to the trans-diol by epoxide hydrolase. Therefore, the potential exists for interaction between carbamazepine and any agent that inhibits CYP3A4 and/or epoxide hydrolase. Agents that are CYP3A4 inhibitors may increase the plasma levels of carbamazepine. Thus, if a patient has been titrated to a stable dosage of carbamazepine,

and then begins a course of treatment with a CYP3A4 or epoxide hydrolase inhibitor, it is reasonable to expect that a dose reduction for carbamazepine may be necessary). Products include:

Nimodipine (Carbamazepine is known to induce CYP1A2 and CYP3A4. Therefore, the potential exists for interaction between carbamazepine and any agent metabolized by one (or more) of these enzymes. Agents that are metabolized by CYP1A2 and CYP3A4 may have decreased plasma levels when administered concomitantly with carbamazepine. Thus, if a patient has been titrated to a stable dosage on one of the agents in these categories, and then begins a course of treatment with carbamazepine, it is reasonable to expect that a dose increase for the concomitant agent may be necessary). Products include:

Nisoldipine (Carbamazepine is known to induce CYP1A2 and CYP3A4. Therefore, the potential exists for interaction between carbamazepine and any agent metabolized by one (or more) of these enzymes. Agents that are metabolized by CYP1A2 and CYP3A4 may have decreased plasma levels when administered concomitantly with carbamazepine. Thus, if a patient has been titrated to a stable dosage on one of the agents in these categories, and then begins a course of treatment with carbamazepine, it is reasonable to expect that a dose increase for the concomitant agent may be necessary). Products include:

Nitrendipine (Carbamazepine is known to induce CYP1A2 and CYP3A4. Therefore, the potential exists for interaction between carbamazepine and any agent metabolized by one (or more) of these enzymes. Agents that are metabolized by CYP1A2 and CYP3A4 may have decreased plasma levels when administered concomitantly with carbamazepine. Thus, if a patient has been titrated to a stable dosage on one of the agents in these categories, and then begins a course of treatment with carbamazepine, it is reasonable to expect that a dose increase for the concomitant agent may be necessary).

No products indexed under this heading.

Norethindrone (Carbamazepine is known to induce CYP1A2 and CYP3A4. Therefore, the potential exists for interaction between carbamazepine and any agent metabolized by one (or more) of these enzymes. Agents that are metabolized by CYP1A2 or CYP3A4 may have decreased plasma levels when administered concomitantly with carbamazepine. Breakthrough bleeding has been reported among patients receiving concomitant oral contraceptives and their reliability may be adversely affected). Products include:

Norethindrone Acetate (Carbamazepine is known to induce CYP1A2 and CYP3A4. Therefore, the potential exists for interaction between carbamazepine and any agent metabolized by one (or more) of these enzymes. Agents that are metabolized by CYP1A2 and CYP3A4 may have decreased plasma levels when administered concomitantly with carbamazepine. Thus, if a patient has been titrated to a stable dosage on one of the agents in these categories, and then begins a course of treatment with carbamazepine, it is reasonable to expect that a dose increase for the concomitant agent may be necessary).

No products indexed under this heading.

Norethynodrel (Carbamazepine is known to induce CYP1A2 and CYP3A4. Therefore, the potential exists for interaction between carbamazepine and any agent metabolized by one (or more) of these enzymes. Agents that are metabolized by CYP1A2 or CYP3A4 may have decreased plasma levels when administered concomitantly with carbamazepine. Breakthrough bleeding has been reported among patients receiving concomitant oral contraceptives and their reliability may be adversely affected).

No products indexed under this heading.

Norfloxacin (Carbamazepine is metabolized mainly by CYP3A4 the active carbamazepine 10,11-epoxide, which is futher metabolized to the trans-diol by epoxide hydrolase. Therefore, the potential exists for interaction between carbamazepine and any agent that inhibits CYP3A4 and/or epoxide hydrolase. Agents that are CYP3A4 inhibitors may increase the plasma levels of carbamazepine. Thus, if a patient has been titrated to a stable dosage of carbamazepine, and then begins a course of treatment with a CYP3A4 or epoxide hydrolase inhibitor, it is reasonable to expect that a dose reduction for carbamazepine may be necessary). Products include:

Noroxin Tablets ... **2032**

Norgestimate (Carbamazepine is known to induce CYP1A2 and CYP3A4. Therefore, the potential exists for interaction between carbamazepine and any agent metabolized by one (or more) of these enzymes. Agents that are metabolized by CYP1A2 or CYP3A4 may have decreased plasma levels when administered concomitantly with carbamazepine. Breakthrough bleeding has been reported among patients receiving concomitant oral contraceptives and their reliability may be adversely affected). Products include:

Ortho-Cyclen/Ortho Tri-Cyclen ... **2429**
Ortho Tri-Cyclen Lo Tablets ... **2436**

Norgestrel (Carbamazepine is known to induce CYP1A2 and CYP3A4. Therefore, the potential exists for interaction between carbamazepine and any agent metabolized by one (or more) of these enzymes. Agents that are metabolized by CYP1A2 or CYP3A4 may have decreased plasma levels when administered concomitantly with carbamazepine. Breakthrough bleeding has been reported among patients receiving concomitant oral contraceptives and their reliability may be adversely affected).

No products indexed under this heading.

Nortriptyline Hydrochloride (Carbamazepine is known to induce CYP1A2 and CYP3A4. Therefore, the potential exists for interaction between carbamazepine and any agent metabolized by one (or more) of these enzymes. Agents that are metabolized by CYP1A2 and CYP3A4 may have decreased plasma levels when administered concomitantly with carbamazepine. Thus, if a patient has been titrated to a stable dosage on one of the agents in these categories, and then begins a course of treatment with carbamazepine, it is reasonable to expect that a dose increase for the concomitant agent may be necessary).

No products indexed under this heading.

Ofloxacin (Carbamazepine is known to induce CYP1A2 and CYP3A4. Therefore, the potential exists for interaction between carbamazepine and any agent metabolized by one (or more) of these enzymes. Agents that are metabolized by CYP1A2 and CYP3A4 may have decreased plasma levels when administered concomitantly with carbamazepine. Thus, if a patient has been titrated to a stable dosage on one of the agents in these categories, and then begins a course of treatment with carbamazepine, it is reasonable to expect that a dose increase for the concomitant agent may be necessary). Products include:

Floxin Otic Solution ... **1049**

Olanzapine (Carbamazepine is known to induce CYP1A2 and CYP3A4. Therefore, the potential exists for interaction between carbamazepine and any agent metabolized by one (or more) of these enzymes. Agents that are metabolized by CYP1A2 and CYP3A4 may have decreased plasma levels when administered concomitantly with carbamazepine. Thus, if a patient has been titrated to a stable dosage on one of the agents in these categories, and then begins a course of treatment with carbamazepine, it is reasonable to expect that a dose increase for the concomitant agent may be necessary). Products include:

Symbyax Capsules ... **1819**
Zyprexa Tablets ... **1830**
Zyprexa IntraMuscular ... **1830**
Zyprexa ZYDIS Orally Disintegrating Tablets ... **1830**

Omeprazole (Carbamazepine is metabolized mainly by CYP3A4 the active carbamazepine 10,11-epoxide, which is futher metabolized to the trans-diol by epoxide hydrolase. Therefore, the potential exists for interaction between carbamazepine and any agent that inhibits CYP3A4 and/or epoxide hydrolase. Agents that are CYP3A4 inhibitors may increase the plasma levels of carbamazepine. Thus, if a patient has been titrated to a stable dosage of carbamazepine, and then begins a course of treatment with a CYP3A4 or epoxide hydrolase inhibitor, it is reasonable to expect that a dose reduction for carbamazepine may be necessary). Products include:

Zegerid Capsules ... **2958**
Zegerid Powder for Oral Solution ... **2958**

Ondansetron (Carbamazepine is known to induce CYP1A2 and CYP3A4. Therefore, the potential exists for interaction between carbamazepine and any agent metabolized by one (or more) of these enzymes. Agents that are metabolized by CYP1A2 and CYP3A4 may have decreased plasma levels when administered concomitantly with carbamazepine. Thus, if a patient has been titrated to a stable dosage on one of the agents in these categories, and then begins a course of treatment with carbamazepine, it is reasonable to expect that a dose increase for the concomitant agent may be necessary). Products include:

Zofran ODT Orally Disintegrating Tablets ... **1639**

Ondansetron Hydrochloride (Carbamazepine is known to induce CYP1A2 and CYP3A4. Therefore, the potential exists for interaction between carbamazepine and any agent metabolized by one (or more) of these enzymes. Agents that are metabolized by CYP1A2 and CYP3A4 may have decreased plasma levels when administered concomitantly with carbamazepine. Thus, if a patient has been titrated to a stable dosage on one of the agents in these categories, and then begins a course of treatment with carbamazepine, it is reasonable to expect that a dose increase for the concomitant agent may be necessary). Products include:

Zofran Injection ... **1634**
Zofran ... **1639**

Oxazepam (Because of its primary CNS effect, caution should be used when carbamazepine is taken with other centrally-acting drugs).

No products indexed under this heading.

Oxcarbazepine (Carbamazepine is metabolized by CYP3A4. Therefore, the potential exists for interaction between carbamazepine and any agent that induces CYP3A4. Agents that are CYP3A4 inducers may decrease plasma levels of carbamazepine. Thus, if a patient has been titrated to a stable dosage on carbamazepine, and then begins a course of treatment with a CYP3A4 inducers, it is reasonable to expect that a dose increase for carbamazepine may be necessary). Products include:

Trileptal Tablets ... **2300**
Trileptal Oral Suspension ... **2300**

Oxycodone Hydrochloride (Because of its primary CNS effect, caution should be used when carbamazepine is taken with other centrally-acting drugs). Products include:

OxyContin Tablets ... **2703**
OxyFast Oral Concentrate Solution ... **2708**
OxyIR Capsules ... **2708**
Percocet Tablets ... **1131**
Percodan Tablets ... **1132**

Paclitaxel (Carbamazepine is known to induce CYP1A2 and CYP3A4. Therefore, the potential exists for interaction between carbamazepine and any agent metabolized by one (or more) of these enzymes. Agents that are metabolized by CYP1A2 and CYP3A4 may have decreased plasma levels when administered concomitantly with carbamazepine. Thus, if a patient has been titrated to a stable dosage on one of the agents in these categories, and then begins a course of treatment with carbamazepine, it is reasonable to expect that a dose increase for the concomitant agent may be necessary).

No products indexed under this heading.

Paroxetine Hydrochloride (Carbamazepine is metabolized mainly by CYP3A4 the active carbamazepine 10,11-epoxide, which is futher metabolized to the trans-diol by epoxide hydrolase. Therefore, the potential exists for interaction between carbamazepine and any agent that inhibits CYP3A4 and/or epoxide hydrolase. Agents that are CYP3A4 inhibitors may increase the plasma levels of carbamazepine. Thus, if a patient has been titrated to a stable dosage of carbamazepine, and then begins a course of treatment with a CYP3A4 or epoxide hydrolase inhibitor, it is reasonable to expect that a dose reduction for carbamazepine may be necessary). Products include:

Paxil CR Controlled-Release Tablets ... **1538**
Paxil ... **1530**

Pentobarbital Sodium (Because of its primary CNS effect, caution should be used when carbamazepine is taken with other centrally-acting drugs). Products include:

Nembutal Sodium Solution, USP ... **2470**

Perphenazine (Because of its primary CNS effect, caution should be used when carbamazepine is taken with other centrally-acting drugs).

No products indexed under this heading.

Phenobarbital (Carbamazepine is metabolized by CYP3A4. Therefore, the potential exists for interaction between carbamazepine and any agent that induces CYP3A4. Agents that are CYP3A4 inducers may decrease plasma levels of carbamazepine. Thus, if a patient has been titrated to a stable dosage on carbamazepine, and then begins a course of treatment with a CYP3A4 inducers, it is reasonable to expect that a dose increase for carbamazepine may be necessary). Products include:

Donnatal Extentabs ... **2493**

Phenobarbital Sodium (Carbamazepine is metabolized by CYP3A4. Therefore, the potential exists for interaction between carbamazepine and any agent that induces CYP3A4. Agents that are CYP3A4 inducers may decrease plasma levels of carbamazepine. Thus, if a patient has been titrated to a stable dosage on carbamazepine, and then begins a course of treatment with a CYP3A4 inducers, it is reasonable to expect that a dose increase for carbamazepine may be necessary).

No products indexed under this heading.

Phenytoin (Carbamazepine is metabolized by CYP3A4. Therefore, the potential exists for interaction between carbamazepine and any agent that induces CYP3A4. Agents that are CYP3A4 inducers may decrease plasma levels of carbamazepine. Thus, if a patient has been titrated to a stable dosage on carbamazepine, and then begins a course of treatment with a CYP3A4 inducers, it is reasonable to expect that a dose increase for carbamazepine may be necessary).

No products indexed under this heading.

Phenytoin Sodium (Carbamazepine is metabolized by CYP3A4. Therefore, the potential exists for interaction between carbamazepine and any agent that induces CYP3A4. Agents that are CYP3A4 inducers may decrease plasma levels of carbamazepine. Thus, if a patient has been titrated to a stable dosage on carbamazepine, and then begins a course of treatment with a CYP3A4 inducers, it is reasonable to expect that a dose increase for carbamazepine may be necessary). Products include:

Phenytek Capsules 2160

Pimozide (Carbamazepine is known to induce CYP1A2 and CYP3A4. Therefore, the potential exists for interaction between carbamazepine and any agent metabolized by one (or more) of these enzymes. Agents that are metabolized by CYP1A2 and CYP3A4 may have decreased plasma levels when administered concomitantly with carbamazepine. Thus, if a patient has been titrated to a stable dosage on one of the agents in these categories, and then begins a course of treatment with carbamazepine, it is reasonable to expect that a dose increase for the concomitant agent may be necessary).

No products indexed under this heading.

Polyestradiol Phosphate (Carbamazepine is known to induce CYP1A2 and CYP3A4. Therefore, the potential exists for interaction between carbamazepine and any agent metabolized by one (or more) of these enzymes. Agents that are metabolized by CYP1A2 and CYP3A4 may have decreased plasma levels when administered concomitantly with carbamazepine. Thus, if a patient has been titrated to a stable dosage on one of the agents in these categories, and then begins a course of treatment with carbamazepine, it is reasonable to expect that a dose increase for the concomitant agent may be necessary).

No products indexed under this heading.

Prazepam (Because of its primary CNS effect, caution should be used when carbamazepine is taken with other centrally-acting drugs).

No products indexed under this heading.

Prednisolone Acetate (Carbamazepine is metabolized by CYP3A4. Therefore, the potential exists for interaction between carbamazepine and any agent that induces CYP3A4. Agents that are CYP3A4 inducers may decrease plasma levels of carbamazepine. Thus, if a patient has been titrated to a stable dosage on carbamazepine, and then begins a course of treatment with a CYP3A4 inducers, it is reasonable to expect that a dose increase for carbamazepine may be necessary). Products include:

Blephamide Ophthalmic Ointment 568
Blephamide Ophthalmic Suspension 569
Poly-Pred Ophthalmic Suspension .... ⊙233
Pred Forte Ophthalmic Suspension .... ⊙235
Pred Mild Ophthalmic Suspension .... ⊙238
Pred-G Ophthalmic Ointment .... ⊙237
Pred-G Ophthalmic Suspension ...... ⊙236

Prednisolone Sodium Phosphate (Carbamazepine is metabolized by CYP3A4. Therefore, the potential exists for interaction between carbamazepine and any agent that induces CYP3A4. Agents that are CYP3A4 inducers may decrease plasma levels of carbamazepine. Thus, if a patient has been titrated to a stable dosage on carbamazepine, and then begins a course of treatment with a CYP3A4 inducers, it is reasonable to expect that a dose increase for carbamazepine may be necessary).

No products indexed under this heading.

Prednisolone Tebutate (Carbamazepine is metabolized by CYP3A4. Therefore, the potential exists for interaction between carbamazepine and any agent that induces CYP3A4. Agents that are CYP3A4 inducers may decrease plasma levels of carbamazepine. Thus, if a patient has been titrated to a stable dosage on carbamazepine, and then begins a course of treatment with a CYP3A4 inducers, it is reasonable to expect that a dose increase for carbamazepine may be necessary).

No products indexed under this heading.

Prednisone (Carbamazepine is metabolized by CYP3A4. Therefore, the potential exists for interaction between carbamazepine and any agent that induces CYP3A4. Agents that are CYP3A4 inducers may decrease plasma levels of carbamazepine. Thus, if a patient has been titrated to a stable dosage on carbamazepine, and then begins a course of treatment with a CYP3A4 inducers, it is reasonable to expect that a dose increase for carbamazepine may be necessary).

No products indexed under this heading.

Primidone (Carbamazepine increases the plasma levels of primidone).

No products indexed under this heading.

Prochlorperazine (Because of its primary CNS effect, caution should be used when carbamazepine is taken with other centrally-acting drugs).

No products indexed under this heading.

Promethazine Hydrochloride (Because of its primary CNS effect, caution should be used when carbamazepine is taken with other centrally-acting drugs). Products include:

Phenergan Tablets and Suppositories 3440

Propafenone Hydrochloride (Carbamazepine is known to induce CYP1A2 and CYP3A4. Therefore, the potential exists for interaction between carbamazepine and any agent metabolized by one (or more) of these enzymes. Agents that are metabolized by CYP1A2 and CYP3A4 may have decreased plasma levels when administered concomitantly with carbamazepine. Thus, if a patient has been titrated to a stable dosage on one of the agents in these categories, and then begins a course of treatment with carbamazepine, it is reasonable to expect that a dose increase for the concomitant agent may be necessary). Products include:

Rythmol SR Capsules 2727

Propofol (Because of its primary CNS effect, caution should be used when carbamazepine is taken with other centrally-acting drugs).

No products indexed under this heading.

Propoxyphene Hydrochloride (Carbamazepine is metabolized mainly by CYP3A4 the active carbamazepine 10,11-epoxide, which is futher metabolized to the trans-diol by epoxide hydrolase. Therefore, the potential exists for interaction between carbamazepine and any agent that inhibits CYP3A4 and/or epoxide hydrolase. Agents that are CYP3A4 inhibitors may increase the plasma levels of carbamazepine. Thus, if a patient has been titrated to a stable dosage of carbamazepine, and then begins a course of treatment with a CYP3A4 or epoxide hydrolase inhibitor, it is reasonable to expect that a dose reduction for carbamazepine may be necessary).

No products indexed under this heading.

Propoxyphene Napsylate (Carbamazepine is metabolized mainly by CYP3A4 the active carbamazepine 10,11-epoxide, which is futher metabolized to the trans-diol by epoxide hydrolase. Therefore, the potential exists for interaction between carbamazepine and any agent that inhibits CYP3A4 and/or epoxide hydrolase. Agents that are CYP3A4 inhibitors may increase the plasma levels of carbamazepine. Thus, if a patient has been titrated to a stable dosage of carbamazepine, and then begins a course of treatment with a CYP3A4 or epoxide hydrolase inhibitor, it is reasonable to expect that a dose reduction for carbamazepine may be necessary).

No products indexed under this heading.

Propranolol Hydrochloride (Carbamazepine is known to induce CYP1A2 and CYP3A4. Therefore, the potential exists for interaction between carbamazepine and any agent metabolized by one (or more) of these enzymes. Agents that are metabolized by CYP1A2 and CYP3A4 may have decreased plasma levels when administered concomitantly with carbamazepine. Thus, if a patient has been titrated to a stable dosage on one of the agents in these categories, and then begins a course of treatment with carbamazepine, it is reasonable to expect that a dose increase for the concomitant agent may be necessary). Products include:

Inderal LA Long-Acting Capsules 3429
InnoPran XL Capsules 2723

Protriptyline Hydrochloride (Carbamazepine is known to induce CYP1A2 and CYP3A4. Therefore, the potential exists for interaction between carbamazepine and any agent metabolized by one (or more) of these enzymes. Agents that are metabolized by CYP1A2 and CYP3A4 may have decreased plasma levels when administered concomitantly with carbamazepine. Thus, if a patient has been titrated to a stable dosage on one of the agents in these categories, and then begins a course of treatment with carbamazepine, it is reasonable to expect that a dose increase for the concomitant agent may be necessary).

No products indexed under this heading.

Pyrimethamine (Anti-malarial drugs, such as chloroquine and mefloquine, may antagonize the activity of carbamazepine). Products include:

Daraprim Tablets 1419
Fansidar Tablets 2765

Quazepam (Because of its primary CNS effect, caution should be used when carbamazepine is taken with other centrally-acting drugs).

No products indexed under this heading.

Quetiapine Fumarate (Because of its primary CNS effect, caution should be used when carbamazepine is taken with other centrally-acting drugs). Products include:

Seroquel Tablets 690

Quinidine (Carbamazepine is metabolized mainly by CYP3A4 the active carbamazepine 10,11-epoxide, which is futher metabolized to the trans-diol by epoxide hydrolase. Therefore, the potential exists for interaction between carbamazepine and any agent that inhibits CYP3A4 and/or epoxide hydrolase. Agents that are CYP3A4 inhibitors may increase the plasma levels of carbamazepine. Thus, if a patient has been titrated to a stable dosage of carbamazepine, and then begins a course of treatment with a CYP3A4 or epoxide hydrolase inhibitor, it is reasonable to expect that a dose reduction for carbamazepine may be necessary).

No products indexed under this heading.

Quinidine Gluconate (Carbamazepine is known to induce CYP1A2 and CYP3A4. Therefore, the potential exists for interaction between carbamazepine and any agent metabolized by one (or more) of these enzymes. Agents that are metabolized by CYP1A2 and CYP3A4 may have decreased plasma levels when administered concomitantly with carbamazepine. Thus, if a patient has been titrated to a stable dosage on one of the agents in these categories, and then begins a course of treatment with carbamazepine, it is reasonable to expect that a dose increase for the concomitant agent may be necessary).

No products indexed under this heading.

Quinidine Hydrochloride (Carbamazepine is metabolized mainly by CYP3A4 the active carbamazepine 10,11-epoxide, which is futher metabolized to the trans-diol by epoxide hydrolase. Therefore, the potential exists for interaction between carbamazepine and any agent that inhibits CYP3A4 and/or epoxide hydrolase. Agents that are CYP3A4 inhibitors may increase the plasma levels of carbamazepine. Thus, if a patient has been titrated to a stable dosage of carbamazepine, and then begins a course of treatment with a CYP3A4 or epoxide hydrolase inhibitor, it is reasonable to expect that a dose reduction for

carbamazepine may be necessary).
No products indexed under this heading.

Quinidine Polygalacturonate (Carbamazepine is metabolized mainly by CYP3A4 the active carbamazepine 10,11-epoxide, which is futher metabolized to the trans-diol by epoxide hydrolase. Therefore, the potential exists for interaction between carbamazepine and any agent that inhibits CYP3A4 and/or epoxide hydrolase. Agents that are CYP3A4 inhibitors may increase the plasma levels of carbamazepine. Thus, if a patient has been titrated to a stable dosage of carbamazepine, and then begins a course of treatment with a CYP3A4 or epoxide hydrolase inhibitor, it is reasonable to expect that a dose reduction for carbamazepine may be necessary).
No products indexed under this heading.

Quinidine Sulfate (Carbamazepine is metabolized mainly by CYP3A4 the active carbamazepine 10,11-epoxide, which is futher metabolized to the trans-diol by epoxide hydrolase. Therefore, the potential exists for interaction between carbamazepine and any agent that inhibits CYP3A4 and/or epoxide hydrolase. Agents that are CYP3A4 inhibitors may increase the plasma levels of carbamazepine. Thus, if a patient has been titrated to a stable dosage of carbamazepine, and then begins a course of treatment with a CYP3A4 or epoxide hydrolase inhibitor, it is reasonable to expect that a dose reduction for carbamazepine may be necessary).
No products indexed under this heading.

Quinine (Carbamazepine is metabolized mainly by CYP3A4 the active carbamazepine 10,11-epoxide, which is futher metabolized to the trans-diol by epoxide hydrolase. Therefore, the potential exists for interaction between carbamazepine and any agent that inhibits CYP3A4 and/or epoxide hydrolase. Agents that are CYP3A4 inhibitors may increase the plasma levels of carbamazepine. Thus, if a patient has been titrated to a stable dosage of carbamazepine, and then begins a course of treatment with a CYP3A4 or epoxide hydrolase inhibitor, it is reasonable to expect that a dose reduction for carbamazepine may be necessary).
No products indexed under this heading.

Quinine Sulfate (Carbamazepine is metabolized mainly by CYP3A4 the active carbamazepine 10,11-epoxide, which is futher metabolized to the trans-diol by epoxide hydrolase. Therefore, the potential exists for interaction between carbamazepine and any agent that inhibits CYP3A4 and/or epoxide hydrolase. Agents that are CYP3A4 inhibitors may increase the plasma levels of carbamazepine. Thus, if a patient has been titrated to a stable dosage of carbamazepine, and then begins a course of treatment with a CYP3A4 or epoxide hydrolase inhibitor, it is reasonable to expect that a dose reduction for carbamazepine may be necessary).
No products indexed under this heading.

Quinupristin (Carbamazepine is metabolized mainly by CYP3A4 the active carbamazepine 10,11-epoxide, which is futher metabolized to the trans-diol by epoxide hydrolase. Therefore, the potential exists for interaction between carbamazepine and any agent that inhibits CYP3A4 and/or epoxide hydrolase. Agents that are CYP3A4 inhibitors may increase the plasma levels of carbamazepine. Thus, if a patient has been titrated to a stable dosage of carbamazepine, and then begins a course of treatment with a CYP3A4 or epoxide hydrolase inhibitor, it is reasonable to expect that a dose reduction for carbamazepine may be necessary).
No products indexed under this heading.

Ranitidine Bismuth Citrate (Carbamazepine is metabolized mainly by CYP3A4 the active carbamazepine 10,11-epoxide, which is futher metabolized to the trans-diol by epoxide hydrolase. Therefore, the potential exists for interaction between carbamazepine and any agent that inhibits CYP3A4 and/or epoxide hydrolase. Agents that are CYP3A4 inhibitors may increase the plasma levels of carbamazepine. Thus, if a patient has been titrated to a stable dosage of carbamazepine, and then begins a course of treatment with a CYP3A4 or epoxide hydrolase inhibitor, it is reasonable to expect that a dose reduction for carbamazepine may be necessary).
No products indexed under this heading.

Ranitidine Hydrochloride (Carbamazepine is metabolized mainly by CYP3A4 the active carbamazepine 10,11-epoxide, which is futher metabolized to the trans-diol by epoxide hydrolase. Therefore, the potential exists for interaction between carbamazepine and any agent that inhibits CYP3A4 and/or epoxide hydrolase. Agents that are CYP3A4 inhibitors may increase the plasma levels of carbamazepine. Thus, if a patient has been titrated to a stable dosage of carbamazepine, and then begins a course of treatment with a CYP3A4 or epoxide hydrolase inhibitor, it is reasonable to expect that a dose reduction for carbamazepine may be necessary). Products include:
Zantac 1624
Zantac Injection 1619
Zantac Injection Pharmacy Bulk Package.. 1622

Remifentanil Hydrochloride (Because of its primary CNS effect, caution should be used when carbamazepine is taken with other centrally-acting drugs).
No products indexed under this heading.

Rifabutin (Carbamazepine is metabolized by CYP3A4. Therefore, the potential exists for interaction between carbamazepine and any agent that induces CYP3A4. Agents that are CYP3A4 inducers may decrease plasma levels of carbamazepine. Thus, if a patient has been titrated to a stable dosage on carbamazepine, and then begins a course of treatment with a CYP3A4 inducers, it is reasonable to expect that a dose increase for carbamazepine may be necessary).
No products indexed under this heading.

Rifampicin (Carbamazepine is metabolized by CYP3A4. Therefore, the potential exists for interaction between carbamazepine and any agent that induces CYP3A4. Agents that are CYP3A4 inducers may decrease plasma levels of carbamazepine. Thus, if a patient has been titrated to a stable dosage on carbamazepine, and then begins a course of treatment with a CYP3A4 inducers, it is reasonable to expect that a dose increase for carbamazepine may be necessary).
No products indexed under this heading.

Rifampin (Carbamazepine is metabolized by CYP3A4. Therefore, the potential exists for interaction between carbamazepine and any agent that induces CYP3A4. Agents that are CYP3A4 inducers may decrease plasma levels of carbamazepine. Thus, if a patient has been titrated to a stable dosage on carbamazepine, and then begins a course of treatment with a CYP3A4 inducers, it is reasonable to expect that a dose increase for carbamazepine may be necessary).
No products indexed under this heading.

Rifapentine (Carbamazepine is metabolized by CYP3A4. Therefore, the potential exists for interaction between carbamazepine and any agent that induces CYP3A4. Agents that are CYP3A4 inducers may decrease plasma levels of carbamazepine. Thus, if a patient has been titrated to a stable dosage on carbamazepine, and then begins a course of treatment with a CYP3A4 inducers, it is reasonable to expect that a dose increase for carbamazepine may be necessary).
No products indexed under this heading.

Riluzole (Carbamazepine is known to induce CYP1A2 and CYP3A4. Therefore, the potential exists for interaction between carbamazepine and any agent metabolized by one (or more) of these enzymes. Agents that are metabolized by CYP1A2 and CYP3A4 may have decreased plasma levels when administered concomitantly with carbamazepine. Thus, if a patient has been titrated to a stable dosage on one of the agents in these categories, and then begins a course of treatment with carbamazepine, it is reasonable to expect that a dose increase for the concomitant agent may be necessary). Products include:
Rilutek Tablets 2930

Risperidone (Because of its primary CNS effect, caution should be used when carbamazepine is taken with other centrally-acting drugs). Products include:
Risperdal 1676
Risperdal Consta Long-Acting Injection 1682
Risperdal M-Tab Orally Disintegrating Tablets.. 1676

Ritonavir (Carbamazepine is metabolized mainly by CYP3A4 the active carbamazepine 10,11-epoxide, which is futher metabolized to the trans-diol by epoxide hydrolase. Therefore, the potential exists for interaction between carbamazepine and any agent that inhibits CYP3A4 and/or epoxide hydrolase. Agents that are CYP3A4 inhibitors may increase the plasma levels of carbamazepine. Thus, if a patient has been titrated to a stable dosage of carbamazepine, and then begins a course of treatment with a CYP3A4 or epoxide hydrolase inhibitor, it is reasonable to expect that a dose reduction for carbamazepine may be necessary). Products include:
Kaletra 476
Norvir 503

Ropinirole Hydrochloride (Carbamazepine is known to induce CYP1A2 and CYP3A4. Therefore, the potential exists for interaction between carbamazepine and any agent metabolized by one (or more) of these enzymes. Agents that are metabolized by CYP1A2 and CYP3A4 may have decreased plasma levels when administered concomitantly with carbamazepine. Thus, if a patient has been titrated to a stable dosage on one of the agents in these categories, and then begins a course of treatment with carbamazepine, it is reasonable to expect that a dose increase for the concomitant agent may be necessary). Products include:
Requip Tablets 1555

Ropivacaine Hydrochloride (Carbamazepine is known to induce CYP1A2 and CYP3A4. Therefore, the potential exists for interaction between carbamazepine and any agent metabolized by one (or more) of these enzymes. Agents that are metabolized by CYP1A2 and CYP3A4 may have decreased plasma levels when administered concomitantly with carbamazepine. Thus, if a patient has been titrated to a stable dosage on one of the agents in these categories, and then begins a course of treatment with carbamazepine, it is reasonable to expect that a dose increase for the concomitant agent may be necessary).
No products indexed under this heading.

Saquinavir (Carbamazepine is metabolized mainly by CYP3A4 the active carbamazepine 10,11-epoxide, which is futher metabolized to the trans-diol by epoxide hydrolase. Therefore, the potential exists for interaction between carbamazepine and any agent that inhibits CYP3A4 and/or epoxide hydrolase. Agents that are CYP3A4 inhibitors may increase the plasma levels of carbamazepine. Thus, if a patient has been titrated to a stable dosage of carbamazepine, and then begins a course of treatment with a CYP3A4 or epoxide hydrolase inhibitor, it is reasonable to expect that a dose reduction for carbamazepine may be necessary).
No products indexed under this heading.

Saquinavir Mesylate (Carbamazepine is metabolized mainly by CYP3A4 the active carbamazepine 10,11-epoxide, which is futher metabolized to the trans-diol by epoxide hydrolase. Therefore, the potential exists for interaction between carbamazepine and any agent that inhibits CYP3A4 and/or epoxide hydrolase. Agents that are CYP3A4 inhibitors may increase the plasma levels of carbamazepine. Thus, if a patient has been titrated to a stable dosage of carbamazepine, and then begins a course of treatment with a CYP3A4 or epoxide hydrolase inhibitor, it is reasonable to expect that a dose reduction for carbamazepine may be necessary). Products include:

Secobarbital Sodium (Because of its primary CNS effect, caution should be used when carbamazepine is taken with other centrally-acting drugs).

No products indexed under this heading.

Sertraline Hydrochloride (Carbamazepine is metabolized mainly by CYP3A4 the active carbamazepine 10,11-epoxide, which is futher metabolized to the trans-diol by epoxide hydrolase. Therefore, the potential exists for interaction between carbamazepine and any agent that inhibits CYP3A4 and/or epoxide hydrolase. Agents that are CYP3A4 inhibitors may increase the plasma levels of carbamazepine. Thus, if a patient has been titrated to a stable dosage of carbamazepine, and then begins a course of treatment with a CYP3A4 or epoxide hydrolase inhibitor, it is reasonable to expect that a dose reduction for carbamazepine may be necessary). Products include:

Sevoflurane (Because of its primary CNS effect, caution should be used when carbamazepine is taken with other centrally-acting drugs). Products include:

Sildenafil Citrate (Carbamazepine is known to induce CYP1A2 and CYP3A4. Therefore, the potential exists for interaction between carbamazepine and any agent metabolized by one (or more) of these enzymes. Agents that are metabolized by CYP1A2 and CYP3A4 may have decreased plasma levels when administered concomitantly with carbamazepine. Thus, if a patient has been titrated to a stable dosage on one of the agents in these categories, and then begins a course of treatment with carbamazepine, it is reasonable to expect that a dose increase for the concomitant agent may be necessary). Products include:

Simvastatin (Carbamazepine is known to induce CYP1A2 and CYP3A4. Therefore, the potential exists for interaction between carbamazepine and any agent metabolized by one (or more) of these enzymes. Agents that are metabolized by CYP1A2 and CYP3A4 may have decreased plasma levels when administered concomitantly with carbamazepine. Thus, if a patient has been titrated to a stable dosage on one of the agents in these categories, and then begins a course of treatment with carbamazepine, it is reasonable to expect that a dose increase for the concomitant agent may be necessary). Products include:

Sirolimus (Carbamazepine is known to induce CYP1A2 and CYP3A4. Therefore, the potential exists for interaction between carbamazepine and any agent metabolized by one (or more) of these enzymes. Agents that are metabolized by CYP1A2 and CYP3A4 may have decreased plasma levels when administered concomitantly with carbamazepine. Thus, if a patient has been titrated to a stable dosage on one of the agents in these categories, and then begins a course of treatment with carbamazepine, it is reasonable to expect that a dose increase for the concomitant agent may be necessary). Products include:

Sodium Oxybate (Because of its primary CNS effect, caution should be used when carbamazepine is taken with other centrally-acting drugs). Products include:

Sufentanil Citrate (Because of its primary CNS effect, caution should be used when carbamazepine is taken with other centrally-acting drugs).

No products indexed under this heading.

Sulfinpyrazone (Carbamazepine is metabolized by CYP3A4. Therefore, the potential exists for interaction between carbamazepine and any agent that induces CYP3A4. Agents that are CYP3A4 inducers may decrease plasma levels of carbamazepine. Thus, if a patient has been titrated to a stable dosage on carbamazepine, and then begins a course of treatment with a CYP3A4 inducers, it is reasonable to expect that a dose increase for carbamazepine may be necessary).

No products indexed under this heading.

Tacrine Hydrochloride (Carbamazepine is known to induce CYP1A2 and CYP3A4. Therefore, the potential exists for interaction between carbamazepine and any agent metabolized by one (or more) of these enzymes. Agents that are metabolized by CYP1A2 and CYP3A4 may have decreased plasma levels when administered concomitantly with carbamazepine. Thus, if a patient has been titrated to a stable dosage on one of the agents in these categories, and then begins a course of treatment with carbamazepine, it is reasonable to expect that a dose increase for the concomitant agent may be necessary).

No products indexed under this heading.

Tacrolimus (Carbamazepine is known to induce CYP1A2 and CYP3A4. Therefore, the potential exists for interaction between carbamazepine and any agent metabolized by one (or more) of these enzymes. Agents that are metabolized by CYP1A2 and CYP3A4 may have decreased plasma levels when administered concomitantly with carbamazepine. Thus, if a patient has been titrated to a stable dosage on one of the agents in these categories, and then begins a course of treatment with carbamazepine, it is

reasonable to expect that a dose increase for the concomitant agent may be necessary). Products include:

Tamoxifen Citrate (Carbamazepine is known to induce CYP1A2 and CYP3A4. Therefore, the potential exists for interaction between carbamazepine and any agent metabolized by one (or more) of these enzymes. Agents that are metabolized by CYP1A2 and CYP3A4 may have decreased plasma levels when administered concomitantly with carbamazepine. Thus, if a patient has been titrated to a stable dosage on one of the agents in these categories, and then begins a course of treatment with carbamazepine, it is reasonable to expect that a dose increase for the concomitant agent may be necessary). Products include:

Telithromycin (Carbamazepine is metabolized mainly by CYP3A4 the active carbamazepine 10,11-epoxide, which is futher metabolized to the trans-diol by epoxide hydrolase. Therefore, the potential exists for interaction between carbamazepine and any agent that inhibits CYP3A4 and/or epoxide hydrolase. Agents that are CYP3A4 inhibitors may increase the plasma levels of carbamazepine. Thus, if a patient has been titrated to a stable dosage of carbamazepine, and then begins a course of treatment with a CYP3A4 or epoxide hydrolase inhibitor, it is reasonable to expect that a dose reduction for carbamazepine may be necessary). Products include:

Temazepam (Because of its primary CNS effect, caution should be used when carbamazepine is taken with other centrally-acting drugs). Products include:

Theophylline (Carbamazepine is metabolized by CYP3A4. Therefore, the potential exists for interaction between carbamazepine and any agent that induces CYP3A4. Agents that are CYP3A4 inducers may decrease plasma levels of carbamazepine. Thus, if a patient has been titrated to a stable dosage on carbamazepine, and then begins a course of treatment with a CYP3A4 inducers, it is reasonable to expect that a dose increase for carbamazepine may be necessary).

No products indexed under this heading.

Theophylline Anhydrous (Carbamazepine is known to induce CYP1A2 and CYP3A4. Therefore, the potential exists for interaction between carbamazepine and any agent metabolized by one (or more) of these enzymes. Agents that are metabolized by CYP1A2 and CYP3A4 may have decreased plasma levels when administered concomitantly with carbamazepine. Thus, if a patient has been titrated to a stable dosage on one of the agents in these categories, and then begins a course of treatment with carbamazepine, it is reasonable to expect that a dose increase for the concomitant agent may be necessary). Products include:

Thiamylal Sodium (Because of its primary CNS effect, caution should be used when carbamazepine is taken with other centrally-acting drugs).

No products indexed under this heading.

Thioridazine Hydrochloride (Because of its primary CNS effect, caution should be used when carbamazepine is taken with other centrally-acting drugs). Products include:

Thiothixene (Because of its primary CNS effect, caution should be used when carbamazepine is taken with other centrally-acting drugs). Products include:

Tiagabine Hydrochloride (Carbamazepine is known to induce CYP1A2 and CYP3A4. Therefore, the potential exists for interaction between carbamazepine and any agent metabolized by one (or more) of these enzymes. Agents that are metabolized by CYP1A2 and CYP3A4 may have decreased plasma levels when administered concomitantly with carbamazepine. Thus, if a patient has been titrated to a stable dosage on one of the agents in these categories, and then begins a course of treatment with carbamazepine, it is reasonable to expect that a dose increase for the concomitant agent may be necessary). Products include:

Tolterodine Tartrate (Carbamazepine is known to induce CYP1A2 and CYP3A4. Therefore, the potential exists for interaction between carbamazepine and any agent metabolized by one (or more) of these enzymes. Agents that are metabolized by CYP1A2 and CYP3A4 may have decreased plasma levels when administered concomitantly with carbamazepine. Thus, if a patient has been titrated to a stable dosage on one of the agents in these categories, and then begins a course of treatment with carbamazepine, it is reasonable to expect that a dose increase for the concomitant agent may be necessary). Products include:

Trazodone Hydrochloride (Carbamazepine is known to induce CYP1A2 and CYP3A4. Therefore, the potential exists for interaction between carbamazepine and any agent metabolized by one (or more) of these enzymes. Agents that are metabolized by CYP1A2 and CYP3A4 may have decreased plasma levels when administered concomitantly with carbamazepine. Thus, if a patient has been titrated to a stable dosage on one of the agents in these categories, and then begins a course of treatment with carbamazepine, it is reasonable to expect that a dose increase for the concomitant agent may be necessary).

No products indexed under this heading.

Triamcinolone (Carbamazepine is metabolized by CYP3A4. Therefore, the potential exists for interaction between carbamazepine and any agent that induces CYP3A4. Agents that are CYP3A4 inducers may decrease plasma levels of carbamazepine. Thus, if a patient has been titrated to a stable dosage on carbamazepine, and then begins a course of treatment with a CYP3A4 inducers, it is reasonable to expect that a dose increase for carbamazepine may be necessary).

No products indexed under this heading.

Triamcinolone Acetonide (Carbamazepine is metabolized by CYP3A4. Therefore, the potential exists for interaction between carbamazepine and any agent that induces CYP3A4. Agents that are CYP3A4 inducers may decrease plasma levels of carbamazepine. Thus, if a patient has been titrated to a stable dosage on carbamazepine, and then begins a course of treatment with a CYP3A4 inducers, it is reasonable to expect that a dose increase for carbamazepine may be necessary). Products include:

Azmacort Inhalation Aerosol 1726
Nasacort AQ Nasal Spray 2922

Triamcinolone Diacetate (Carbamazepine is metabolized by CYP3A4. Therefore, the potential exists for interaction between carbamazepine and any agent that induces CYP3A4. Agents that are CYP3A4 inducers may decrease plasma levels of carbamazepine. Thus, if a patient has been titrated to a stable dosage on carbamazepine, and then begins a course of treatment with a CYP3A4 inducers, it is reasonable to expect that a dose increase for carbamazepine may be necessary).

No products indexed under this heading.

Triamcinolone Hexacetonide (Carbamazepine is metabolized by CYP3A4. Therefore, the potential exists for interaction between carbamazepine and any agent that induces CYP3A4. Agents that are CYP3A4 inducers may decrease plasma levels of carbamazepine. Thus, if a patient has been titrated to a stable dosage on carbamazepine, and then begins a course of treatment with a CYP3A4 inducers, it is reasonable to expect that a dose increase for carbamazepine may be necessary).

No products indexed under this heading.

Triazolam (Carbamazepine is known to induce CYP1A2 and CYP3A4. Therefore, the potential exists for interaction between carbamazepine and any agent metabolized by one (or more) of these enzymes. Agents that are metabolized by CYP1A2 and CYP3A4 may have decreased plasma levels when administered concomitantly with carbamazepine. Thus, if a patient has been titrated to a stable dosage on one of the agents in these categories, and then begins a course of treatment with carbamazepine, it is reasonable to expect that a dose increase for the concomitant agent may be necessary).

No products indexed under this heading.

Trifluoperazine Hydrochloride (Because of its primary CNS effect, caution should be used when carbamazepine is taken with other centrally-acting drugs).

No products indexed under this heading.

Trimethaphan Camsylate (Carbamazepine is known to induce CYP1A2 and CYP3A4. Therefore, the potential exists for interaction between carbamazepine and any agent metabolized by one (or more) of these enzymes. Agents that are metabolized by CYP1A2 and CYP3A4 may have decreased plasma levels when administered concomitantly with carbamazepine. Thus, if a patient has been titrated to a stable dosage on one of the agents in these categories, and then begins a course of treatment with carbamazepine, it is reasonable to expect that a dose increase for the concomitant agent may be necessary).

No products indexed under this heading.

Trimipramine Maleate (Carbamazepine is known to induce CYP1A2 and CYP3A4. Therefore, the potential exists for interaction between carbamazepine and any agent metabolized by one (or more) of these enzymes. Agents that are metabolized by CYP1A2 and CYP3A4 may have decreased plasma levels when administered concomitantly with carbamazepine. Thus, if a patient has been titrated to a stable dosage on one of the agents in these categories, and then begins a course of treatment with carbamazepine, it is reasonable to expect that a dose increase for the concomitant agent may be necessary).

No products indexed under this heading.

Troglitazone (Carbamazepine is metabolized mainly by CYP3A4 the active carbamazepine 10,11-epoxide, which is futher metabolized to the trans-diol by epoxide hydrolase. Therefore, the potential exists for interaction between carbamazepine and any agent that inhibits CYP3A4 and/or epoxide hydrolase. Agents that are CYP3A4 inhibitors may increase the plasma levels of carbamazepine. Thus, if a patient has been titrated to a stable dosage of carbamazepine, and then begins a course of treatment with a CYP3A4 or epoxide hydrolase inhibitor, it is reasonable to expect that a dose reduction for carbamazepine may be necessary).

No products indexed under this heading.

Troleandomycin (Carbamazepine is metabolized mainly by CYP3A4 the active carbamazepine 10,11-epoxide, which is futher metabolized to the trans-diol by epoxide hydrolase. Therefore, the potential exists for interaction between carbamazepine and any agent that inhibits CYP3A4 and/or epoxide hydrolase. Agents that are CYP3A4 inhibitors may increase the plasma levels of carbamazepine. Thus, if a patient has been titrated to a stable dosage of carbamazepine, and then begins a course of treatment with a CYP3A4 or epoxide hydrolase inhibitor, it is reasonable to expect that a dose reduction for carbamazepine may be necessary).

No products indexed under this heading.

Trovafloxacin Mesylate (Carbamazepine is known to induce CYP1A2 and CYP3A4. Therefore, the potential exists for interaction between carbamazepine and any agent metabolized by one (or more) of these enzymes. Agents that are metabolized by CYP1A2 and CYP3A4 may have decreased plasma levels when administered concomitantly with carbamazepine. Thus, if a patient has been titrated to a stable dosage on one of the agents in these categories, and then begins a course of treatment with carbamazepine, it is reasonable to expect that a dose increase for the concomitant agent may be necessary).

No products indexed under this heading.

Valproate Sodium (Carbamazepine is metabolized mainly by CYP3A4 the active carbamazepine 10,11-epoxide, which is futher metabolized to the trans-diol by epoxide hydrolase. Therefore, the potential exists for interaction between carbamazepine and any agent that inhibits CYP3A4 and/or epoxide hydrolase. Agents that are CYP3A4 inhibitors may increase the plasma levels of carbamazepine. Thus, if a patient has been titrated to a stable dosage of carbamazepine, and then begins a course of treatment with a CYP3A4 or epoxide hydrolase inhibitor, it is reasonable to expect that a dose reduction for carbamazepine may be necessary). Products include:

Depacon Injection 412

Verapamil Hydrochloride (Carbamazepine is metabolized mainly by CYP3A4 the active carbamazepine 10,11-epoxide, which is futher metabolized to the trans-diol by epoxide hydrolase. Therefore, the potential exists for interaction between carbamazepine and any agent that inhibits CYP3A4 and/or epoxide hydrolase. Agents that are CYP3A4 inhibitors may increase the plasma levels of carbamazepine. Thus, if a patient has been titrated to a stable dosage of carbamazepine, and then begins a course of treatment with a CYP3A4 or epoxide hydrolase inhibitor, it is reasonable to expect that a dose reduction for carbamazepine may be necessary). Products include:

Covera-HS Tablets 3139
Tarka Tablets 524
Verelan PM Extended-Release Capsules, Controlled-Onset 3106

Vinblastine Sulfate (Carbamazepine is known to induce CYP1A2 and CYP3A4. Therefore, the potential exists for interaction between carbamazepine and any agent metabolized by one (or more) of these enzymes. Agents that are metabolized by CYP1A2 and CYP3A4 may have decreased plasma levels when administered concomitantly with carbamazepine. Thus, if a patient has been titrated to a stable dosage on one of the agents in these categories, and then begins a course of treatment with carbamazepine, it is reasonable to expect that a dose increase for the concomitant agent may be necessary).

No products indexed under this heading.

Vincristine Sulfate (Carbamazepine is known to induce CYP1A2 and CYP3A4. Therefore, the potential exists for interaction between carbamazepine and any agent metabolized by one (or more) of these enzymes. Agents that are metabolized by CYP1A2 and CYP3A4 may have decreased plasma levels when administered concomitantly with carbamazepine. Thus, if a patient has been titrated to a stable dosage on one of the agents in these categories, and then begins a course of treatment with carbamazepine, it is reasonable to expect that a dose increase for the concomitant agent may be necessary).

No products indexed under this heading.

Voriconazole (Carbamazepine is metabolized mainly by CYP3A4 the active carbamazepine 10,11-epoxide, which is futher metabolized to the trans-diol by epoxide hydrolase. Therefore, the potential exists for interaction between carbamazepine and any agent that inhibits CYP3A4 and/or epoxide hydrolase. Agents that are CYP3A4 inhibitors may increase the plasma levels of carbamazepine. Thus, if a patient has been titrated to a stable dosage of carbamazepine, and then begins a course of treatment with a CYP3A4 or epoxide hydrolase inhibitor, it is reasonable to expect that a dose reduction for carbamazepine may be necessary). Products include:

VFEND I.V. 2564
VFEND Oral Suspension 2564
VFEND Tablets 2564

Warfarin Sodium (Carbamazepine is known to induce CYP1A2 and CYP3A4. Therefore, the potential exists for interaction between carbamazepine and any agent metabolized by one (or more) of these enzymes. Agents that are metabolized by CYP1A2 or CYP3A4 may have decreased plasma levels when administered concomitantly with carbamazepine. Thus, if a patient has been titrated to a stable dosage on one of the agents in these categories, and then begins a course of treatment with carbamazepine, it is reasonable to expect that a dose increase for the concomitant agent may be necessary. Therefore, warfarin's anticoagulant effect may be reduced in the presence of carbamazepine and dosage adjustment may be necessary). Products include:

Coumadin for Injection 898
Coumadin Tablets 898

Zafirlukast (Carbamazepine is metabolized mainly by CYP3A4 the active carbamazepine 10,11-epoxide, which is futher metabolized to the trans-diol by epoxide hydrolase. Therefore, the potential exists for interaction between carbamazepine and any agent that inhibits CYP3A4 and/or epoxide hydrolase. Agents that are CYP3A4 inhibitors may increase the plasma levels of carbamazepine. Thus, if a patient has been titrated to a stable dosage of carbamazepine, and then begins a course of treatment with a CYP3A4 or epoxide hydrolase inhibitor, it is reasonable

to expect that a dose reduction for carbamazepine may be necessary). Products include:
Accolate Tablets **671**

Zaleplon (Because of its primary CNS effect, caution should be used when carbamazepine is taken with other centrally-acting drugs). Products include:
Sonata Capsules **1717**

Zileuton (Carbamazepine is metabolized mainly by CYP3A4 the active carbamazepine 10,11-epoxide, which is futher metabolized to the trans-diol by epoxide hydrolase. Therefore, the potential exists for interaction between carbamazepine and any agent that inhibits CYP3A4 and/or epoxide hydrolase. Agents that are CYP3A4 inhibitors may increase the plasma levels of carbamazepine. Thus, if a patient has been titrated to a stable dosage of carbamazepine, and then begins a course of treatment with a CYP3A4 or epoxide hydrolase inhibitor, it is reasonable to expect that a dose reduction for carbamazepine may be necessary). Products include:
Zyflo Tablets **1023**

Ziprasidone Hydrochloride (Because of its primary CNS effect, caution should be used when carbamazepine is taken with other centrally-acting drugs). Products include:
Geodon Capsules **2529**

Zolmitriptan (Carbamazepine is known to induce CYP1A2 and CYP3A4. Therefore, the potential exists for interaction between carbamazepine and any agent metabolized by one (or more) of these enzymes. Agents that are metabolized by CYP1A2 and CYP3A4 may have decreased plasma levels when administered concomitantly with carbamazepine. Thus, if a patient has been titrated to a stable dosage on one of the agents in these categories, and then begins a course of treatment with carbamazepine, it is reasonable to expect that a dose increase for the concomitant agent may be necessary). Products include:
Zomig Tablets **3519**
Zomig Nasal Spray **3523**
Zomig-ZMT Tablets **3519**

Zolpidem Tartrate (Because of its primary CNS effect, caution should be used when carbamazepine is taken with other centrally-acting drugs). Products include:
Ambien Tablets **2851**
Ambien CR Tablets **2855**

Food Interactions

Alcohol (Because of its primary CNS effect, caution should be used when carbamazepine is taken with alcohol).

Grapefruit (Carbamazepine is metabolized mainly by CYP3A4 the active carbamazepine 10,11-epoxide, which is futher metabolized to the trans-diol by epoxide hydrolase. Therefore, the potential exists for interaction between carbamazepine and any agent that inhibits CYP3A4 and/or epoxide hydrolase. Agents that are CYP3A4 inhibitors may increase the plasma levels of carbamazepine. Thus, if a patient has been titrated to a stable dosage of carbamazepine, and then begins a course of treatment with a CYP3A4 or epoxide hydrolase inhibitor, it is reasonable to expect that a dose reduction for carbamazepine may be necessary).

Grapefruit Juice (Carbamazepine is metabolized mainly by CYP3A4 the active carbamazepine 10,11-epoxide, which is futher metabolized to the trans-diol by epoxide hydrolase. Therefore, the potential exists for interaction between carbamazepine and any agent that inhibits CYP3A4 and/or epoxide hydrolase. Agents that are CYP3A4 inhibitors may increase the plasma levels of carbamazepine. Thus, if a patient has been titrated to a stable dosage of carbamazepine, and then begins a course of treatment with a CYP3A4 or epoxide hydrolase inhibitor, it is reasonable to expect that a dose reduction for carbamazepine may be necessary).

ERAXIS FOR INJECTION
(Anidulafungin) **2521**
None cited in PDR database.

ERBITUX
(Cetuximab) **910**
None cited in PDR database.

ERYPED 200 & ERYPED 400 ORAL SUSPENSION
(Erythromycin Ethylsuccinate) **447**
See EryPed Drops

ERYPED DROPS
(Erythromycin Ethylsuccinate) **447**
May interact with oral anticoagulants, HMG-CoA reductase inhibitors, phenytoin, triazolobenzodiazepines, valproate, xanthines, and certain other agents. Compounds in these categories include:

Alfentanil Hydrochloride (Concurrent use of erythromycin in patients receiving drugs metabolized by the cytochrome P450 system may be associated with elevation in serum levels of alfentanil).
No products indexed under this heading.

Alprazolam (Erythromycin has been reported to decrease the clearance of triazolam and midazolam; may increase the pharmacologic effect of these benzodiazepines). Products include:
Niravam Orally Disintegrating Tablets **3092**

Aminophylline (Co-administration in patients who are receiving high doses of theophylline may be associated with an increase in serum theophylline levels and potential theophylline toxicity).
No products indexed under this heading.

Anisindione (Co-administration has resulted in increased anticoagulant effects). Products include:
Miradon Tablets **3042**

Astemizole (Concurrent use of erythromycin in patients receiving drugs metabolized by the cytochrome P450 system may be associated with elevation in serum levels of astemizole; co-administration is contraindicated).
No products indexed under this heading.

Atorvastatin Calcium (Erythromycin has been reported to increase concentrations of HMG-CoA reductase inhibitors (e.g. lovastatin and simvastatin); rare reports of rhabdomyolysis have been reported in patients taking these drugs concomitantly). Products include:
Caduet Tablets **2508**
Lipitor Tablets **2483**

Bromocriptine Mesylate (Concurrent use of erythromycin in patients receiving drugs metabolized by the cytochrome P450 system may be associated with elevation in serum levels of bromocriptine).
No products indexed under this heading.

Carbamazepine (Concurrent use of erythromycin in patients receiving drugs metabolized by the cytochrome P450 system may be associated with elevation in serum levels of carbamazepine). Products include:
Carbatrol Capsules **3171**
Equetro Extended-Release Capsules **3180**
Tegretol/Tegretol-XR **2295**

Cerivastatin Sodium (Erythromycin has been reported to increase concentrations of HMG-CoA reductase inhibitors (e.g. lovastatin and simvastatin); rare reports of rhabdomyolysis have been reported in patients taking these drugs concomitantly).
No products indexed under this heading.

Cisapride (Post-marketing reports have shown concurrent use of erythromycin and cisapride may result in QT prolongation, cardiac arrhythmias, ventricular tachycardia, ventricular fibrillation, and torsade de pointes; most likely due to the inhibition of hepatic metabolism of cisapride by erythromycin; co-administration is contraindicated).
No products indexed under this heading.

Cyclosporine (Concurrent use of erythromycin in patients receiving drugs metabolized by the cytochrome P450 system may be associated with elevation in serum levels of cyclosporine). Products include:
Gengraf Capsules **459**
Neoral Oral Solution **2259**
Neoral Soft Gelatin Capsules **2259**
Restasis Ophthalmic Emulsion **575**
Sandimmune **2275**

Dicumarol (Co-administration has resulted in increased anticoagulant effects).
No products indexed under this heading.

Digoxin (Co-administration has been reported to result in elevated digoxin serum levels). Products include:
Lanoxicaps Capsules **1490**
Lanoxin Injection **1494**
Lanoxin Injection Pediatric **1497**
Lanoxin Tablets **1500**

Dihydroergotamine Mesylate (Co-administration has been associated in some patients with acute ergot toxicity characterized by severe peripheral vasospasm and dysesthesia). Products include:
Migranal Nasal Spray **3348**

Disopyramide Phosphate (Concurrent use of erythromycin in patients receiving drugs metabolized by the cytochrome P450 system may be associated with elevation in serum levels of disopyramide).
No products indexed under this heading.

Divalproex Sodium (There have been reports of interactions of erythromycin with drugs not thought to be metabolized by CYP3A, including valproate). Products include:
Depakote Sprinkle Capsules **422**
Depakote Tablets **427**
Depakote ER Tablets **434**

Dyphylline (Co-administration in patients who are receiving high doses of theophylline may be associated with an increase in serum theophylline levels and potential theophylline toxicity).
No products indexed under this heading.

Ergotamine Tartrate (Co-administration has been associated in some patients with acute ergot toxicity characterized by severe peripheral vasospasm and dysesthesia).
No products indexed under this heading.

Fluvastatin Sodium (Erythromycin has been reported to increase concentrations of HMG-CoA reductase inhibitors (e.g. lovastatin and simvastatin); rare reports of rhabdomyolysis have been reported in patients taking these drugs concomitantly). Products include:
Lescol Capsules **2233**
Lescol XL Tablets **2233**

Fosphenytoin Sodium (There have been reports of interactions of erythromycin with drugs not thought to be metabolized by CYP3A, including phenytoin).
No products indexed under this heading.

Hexobarbital (There have been reports of interactions of erythromycin with drugs not thought to be metabolized by CYP3A, including hexobarbital).
No products indexed under this heading.

Lovastatin (Erythromycin has been reported to increase concentrations of HMG-CoA reductase inhibitors (e.g. lovastatin and simvastatin); rare reports of rhabdomyolysis have been reported in patients taking these drugs concomitantly). Products include:
Advicor Tablets **1722**
Altoprev Extended-Release Tablets **3109**
Mevacor Tablets **2021**

Midazolam Hydrochloride (Erythromycin has been reported to decrease the clearance of triazolam and midazolam; may increase the pharmacologic effect of these benzodiazepines).
No products indexed under this heading.

Phenytoin (There have been reports of interactions of erythromycin with drugs not thought to be metabolized by CYP3A, including phenytoin).
No products indexed under this heading.

Phenytoin Sodium (There have been reports of interactions of erythromycin with drugs not thought to be metabolized by CYP3A, including phenytoin). Products include:
Phenytek Capsules **2160**

Pimozide (Concurrent use of erythromycin in patients receiving drugs metabolized by the cytochrome P450 system may be associated with elevation in serum levels of pimozide; co-administration is contraindicated).
No products indexed under this heading.

Pravastatin Sodium (Erythromycin has been reported to increase concentrations of HMG-CoA reductase inhibitors (e.g. lovastatin and simvastatin); rare reports of rhabdomyolysis have been reported in patients taking these drugs concomitantly).
No products indexed under this heading.

Sildenafil Citrate (Erythromycin has been reported to increase the systemic exposure (AUC) of sildenafil). Products include:
Revatio Tablets 2557
Viagra Tablets 2573

Simvastatin (Erythromycin has been reported to increase concentrations of HMG-CoA reductase inhibitors (e.g. lovastatin and simvastatin); rare reports of rhabdomyolysis have been reported in patients taking these drugs concomitantly). Products include:
Vytorin 10/10 Tablets 2114
Vytorin 10/10 Tablets 3077
Vytorin 10/20 Tablets 2114
Vytorin 10/20 Tablets 3077
Vytorin 10/40 Tablets 2114
Vytorin 10/40 Tablets 3077
Vytorin 10/80 Tablets 2114
Vytorin 10/80 Tablets 3077
Zocor Tablets 2105

Tacrolimus (Concurrent use of erythromycin in patients receiving drugs metabolized by the cytochrome P450 system may be associated with elevation in serum levels of tacrolimus). Products include:
Prograf Capsules and Injection 632
Protopic Ointment 638

Terfenadine (Erythromycin has been reported to significantly alter the metabolism of the nonsedating antihistamine terfenadine when taken concomitantly; rare cases of electrocardiographic QT/QTc interval prolongation, cardiac arrest, torsade de pointes, and other ventricular arrhythmias have been observed; co-administration is contraindicated).
No products indexed under this heading.

Theophylline (Co-administration in patients who are receiving high doses of theophylline may be associated with an increase in serum theophylline levels and potential theophylline toxicity).
No products indexed under this heading.

Theophylline Anhydrous (Co-administration in patients who are receiving high doses of theophylline may be associated with an increase in serum theophylline levels and potential theophylline toxicity). Products include:
Uniphyl Tablets 2710

Theophylline Calcium Salicylate (Co-administration in patients who are receiving high doses of theophylline may be associated with an increase in serum theophylline levels and potential theophylline toxicity).
No products indexed under this heading.

Theophylline Dihydroxypropyl (Glyceryl) (Co-administration in patients who are receiving high doses of theophylline may be associated with an increase in serum theophylline levels and potential theophylline toxicity).
No products indexed under this heading.

Theophylline Ethylenediamine (Co-administration in patients who are receiving high doses of theophylline may be associated with an increase in serum theophylline levels and potential theophylline toxicity).
No products indexed under this heading.

Theophylline Sodium Glycinate (Co-administration in patients who are receiving high doses of theophylline may be associated with an increase in serum theophylline levels and potential theophylline toxicity).
No products indexed under this heading.

Triazolam (Erythromycin has been reported to decrease the clearance of triazolam and midazolam; may increase the pharmacologic effect of these benzodiazepines).
No products indexed under this heading.

Valproate Sodium (There have been reports of interactions of erythromycin with drugs not thought to be metabolized by CYP3A, including valproate). Products include:
Depacon Injection 412

Valproic Acid (There have been reports of interactions of erythromycin with drugs not thought to be metabolized by CYP3A, including valproate). Products include:
Depakene 417

Warfarin Sodium (Co-administration has resulted in increased anticoagulant effects). Products include:
Coumadin for Injection 898
Coumadin Tablets 898

ERYPED CHEWABLE TABLETS

(Erythromycin Ethylsuccinate) 447
See EryPed Drops

ERY-TAB TABLETS

(Erythromycin) 449
May interact with oral anticoagulants, phenytoin, valproate, xanthines, and certain other agents. Compounds in these categories include:

Alfentanil Hydrochloride (Concurrent use of erythromycin in patients receiving drugs metabolized by the cytochrome P450 system may be associated with elevation in serum levels of alfentanil).
No products indexed under this heading.

Aminophylline (Co-administration in patients who are receiving high doses of theophylline may be associated with an increase in serum theophylline levels and potential theophylline toxicity).
No products indexed under this heading.

Anisindione (Co-administration has resulted in increased anticoagulant effects; these effects may be pronounced in the elderly). Products include:
Miradon Tablets 3042

Astemizole (Concurrent use of erythromycin in patients receiving astemizole has been reported to significantly alter the metabolism of astemizole; rare cases of cardiovascular adverse events, including prolonged QT interval, cardiac arrest, torsade de pointes, and other ventricular arrhythmias have been reported; co-administration is contraindicated).
No products indexed under this heading.

Bromocriptine Mesylate (Concurrent use of erythromycin in patients receiving drugs metabolized by the cytochrome P450 system may be associated with elevation in serum levels of bromocriptine).
No products indexed under this heading.

Carbamazepine (Concurrent use of erythromycin in patients receiving drugs metabolized by the cytochrome P450 system may be associated with elevation in serum levels of carbamazepine). Products include:
Carbatrol Capsules 3171
Equetro Extended-Release Capsules 3180
Tegretol/Tegretol-XR 2295

Cisapride (Concurrent use of erythromycin in patients receiving cisapride has been reported to inhibit the metabolism of cisapride; cases of cardiovascular adverse events, including prolonged QT interval, cardiac arrest, torsade de pointes, ventricular tachycardia,ventricular fibrillation and fatalities have been reported; co-administration is contraindicated).
No products indexed under this heading.

Cyclosporine (Concurrent use of erythromycin in patients receiving drugs metabolized by the cytochrome P450 system may be associated with elevation in serum levels of cyclosporine). Products include:
Gengraf Capsules 459
Neoral Oral Solution 2259
Neoral Soft Gelatin Capsules 2259
Restasis Ophthalmic Emulsion 575
Sandimmune 2275

Dicumarol (Co-administration has resulted in increased anticoagulant effects; these effects may be pronounced in the elderly).
No products indexed under this heading.

Digoxin (Co-administration has been reported to result in elevated digoxin serum levels). Products include:
Lanoxicaps Capsules 1490
Lanoxin Injection 1494
Lanoxin Injection Pediatric 1497
Lanoxin Tablets 1500

Dihydroergotamine Mesylate (Co-administration has been associated in some patients with acute ergot toxicity characterized by severe peripheral vasospasm and dysethesia). Products include:
Migranal Nasal Spray 3348

Disopyramide Phosphate (Concurrent use of erythromycin in patients receiving drugs metabolized by the cytochrome P450 system may be associated with elevation in serum levels of disopyramide).
No products indexed under this heading.

Divalproex Sodium (Concurrent use of erythromycin in patients receiving drugs metabolized by the cytochrome P450 system may be associated with elevation in serum levels of valproate). Products include:
Depakote Sprinkle Capsules 422
Depakote Tablets 427
Depakote ER Tablets 434

Dyphylline (Co-administration in patients who are receiving high doses of theophylline may be associated with an increase in serum theophylline levels and potential theophylline toxicity).
No products indexed under this heading.

Ergotamine Tartrate (Co-administration has been associated in some patients with acute ergot toxicity characterized by severe peripheral vasospasm and dysethesia).
No products indexed under this heading.

Fosphenytoin Sodium (Concurrent use of erythromycin in patients receiving drugs metabolized by the cytochrome P450 system may be associated with elevation in serum levels of phenytoin).
No products indexed under this heading.

Hexobarbital (Concurrent use of erythromycin in patients receiving drugs metabolized by the cytochrome P450 system may be associated with elevation in serum levels of hexobarbital).
No products indexed under this heading.

Lovastatin (Concurrent use of erythromycin in patients receiving drugs metabolized by the cytochrome P450 system may be associated with elevation in serum levels of lovastatin). Products include:
Advicor Tablets 1722
Altoprev Extended-Release Tablets 3109
Mevacor Tablets 2021

Midazolam Hydrochloride (Erythromycin has been reported to decrease clearance of midazolam and, thus, may increase the pharmacologic effect of the benzodiazepines).
No products indexed under this heading.

Phenytoin (Concurrent use of erythromycin in patients receiving drugs metabolized by the cytochrome P450 system may be associated with elevation in serum levels of phenytoin).
No products indexed under this heading.

Phenytoin Sodium (Concurrent use of erythromycin in patients receiving drugs metabolized by the cytochrome P450 system may be associated with elevation in serum levels of phenytoin). Products include:
Phenytek Capsules 2160

Tacrolimus (Concurrent use of erythromycin in patients receiving drugs metabolized by the cytochrome P450 system may be associated with elevation in serum levels of tacrolimus). Products include:
Prograf Capsules and Injection 632
Protopic Ointment 638

Terfenadine (Concurrent use of erythromycin in patients receiving terfenadine has been reported to significantly alter the metabolism of terfenadine; rare cases of cardiovascular adverse events, including prolonged QT interval, cardiac arrest, torsade de pointes, other ventricular arrhythmias, and death have been reported; co-administration is contraindicated).
> No products indexed under this heading.

Theophylline (Co-administration in patients who are receiving high doses of theophylline may be associated with an increase in serum theophylline levels and potential theophylline toxicity).
> No products indexed under this heading.

Theophylline Anhydrous (Co-administration in patients who are receiving high doses of theophylline may be associated with an increase in serum theophylline levels and potential theophylline toxicity). Products include:
> Uniphyl Tablets 2710

Theophylline Calcium Salicylate (Co-administration in patients who are receiving high doses of theophylline may be associated with an increase in serum theophylline levels and potential theophylline toxicity).
> No products indexed under this heading.

Theophylline Dihydroxypropyl (Glyceryl) (Co-administration in patients who are receiving high doses of theophylline may be associated with an increase in serum theophylline levels and potential theophylline toxicity).
> No products indexed under this heading.

Theophylline Ethylenediamine (Co-administration in patients who are receiving high doses of theophylline may be associated with an increase in serum theophylline levels and potential theophylline toxicity).
> No products indexed under this heading.

Theophylline Sodium Glycinate (Co-administration in patients who are receiving high doses of theophylline may be associated with an increase in serum theophylline levels and potential theophylline toxicity).
> No products indexed under this heading.

Triazolam (Erythromycin has been reported to decrease clearance of triazolam and, thus, may increase the pharmacologic effect of the benzodiazepines).
> No products indexed under this heading.

Valproate Sodium (Concurrent use of erythromycin in patients receiving drugs metabolized by the cytochrome P450 system may be associated with elevation in serum levels of valproate). Products include:
> Depacon Injection 412

Valproic Acid (Concurrent use of erythromycin in patients receiving drugs metabolized by the cytochrome P450 system may be associated with elevation in serum levels of valproate). Products include:
> Depakene 417

Warfarin Sodium (Co-administration has resulted in increased anticoagulant effects; these effects may be pronounced in the elderly). Products include:
> Coumadin for Injection 898
> Coumadin Tablets 898

ERYTHROCIN STEARATE FILMTAB TABLETS

(Erythromycin Stearate) 453
May interact with oral anticoagulants, HMG-CoA reductase inhibitors, phenytoin, valproate, xanthines, and certain other agents. Compounds in these categories include:

Alfentanil Hydrochloride (Potential for elevated serum alfentanil levels).
> No products indexed under this heading.

Aminophylline (Co-administration in patients who are receiving high doses of theophylline may be associated with an increase in serum theophylline levels and potential theophylline toxicity).
> No products indexed under this heading.

Anisindione (Co-administration has been reported to result in increased anticoagulant effects). Products include:
> Miradon Tablets 3042

Astemizole (Co-administration has produced a significant alteration in astemizole metabolism resulting in rare cases of serious cardiovascular adverse events, including QT prolongation, cardiac arrest, torsade de pointes and death; concurrent use is contraindicated).
> No products indexed under this heading.

Atorvastatin Calcium (Co-administration has been reported to increase concentrations of HMG-CoA reductase inhibitors. Rare reports of rhabdomyolysis have also been reported during concurrent therapy). Products include:
> Caduet Tablets 2508
> Lipitor Tablets 2483

Bromocriptine Mesylate (Potential for elevated serum bromocriptine levels).
> No products indexed under this heading.

Carbamazepine (Potential for elevated serum carbamazepine levels). Products include:
> Carbatrol Capsules 3171
> Equetro Extended-Release Capsules 3180
> Tegretol/Tegretol-XR 2295

Cerivastatin Sodium (Co-administration has been reported to increase concentrations of HMG-CoA reductase inhibitors. Rare reports of rhabdomyolysis have also been reported during concurrent therapy).
> No products indexed under this heading.

Cilostazol (Potential for elevated serum cilostazol levels). Products include:
> Pletal Tablets 2455

Cisapride (Co-administration has produced an inhibition of hepatic metabolism of cisapride metabolism resulting in QT prolongation, cardiac arrhythmias, ventricular tachycardia, ventricular fibrillation, and torsade de pointes; concurrent use is contraindicated).
> No products indexed under this heading.

Cyclosporine (Potential for elevated serum cyclosporine levels). Products include:
> Gengraf Capsules 459
> Neoral Oral Solution 2259
> Neoral Soft Gelatin Capsules 2259
> Restasis Ophthalmic Emulsion 575
> Sandimmune 2275

Dicumarol (Co-administration has been reported to result in increased anticoagulant effects).
> No products indexed under this heading.

Digoxin (Co-administration has been reported to result in elevated digoxin serum levels). Products include:
> Lanoxicaps Capsules 1490
> Lanoxin Injection 1494
> Lanoxin Injection Pediatric 1497
> Lanoxin Tablets 1500

Dihydroergotamine Mesylate (Co-administration has been reported to result in acute ergot toxicity characterized by severe peripheral vasospasm and dysesthesia). Products include:
> Migranal Nasal Spray 3348

Disopyramide Phosphate (Potential for elevated serum disopyramide levels).
> No products indexed under this heading.

Divalproex Sodium (Potential for elevated serum valproate levels). Products include:
> Depakote Sprinkle Capsules 422
> Depakote Tablets 427
> Depakote ER Tablets 434

Dyphylline (Co-administration in patients who are receiving high doses of theophylline may be associated with an increase in serum theophylline levels and potential theophylline toxicity).
> No products indexed under this heading.

Ergotamine Tartrate (Co-administration has been reported to result in acute ergot toxicity characterized by severe peripheral vasospasm and dysesthesia).
> No products indexed under this heading.

Fluvastatin Sodium (Co-administration has been reported to increase concentrations of HMG-CoA reductase inhibitors. Rare reports of rhabdomyolysis have also been reported during concurrent therapy). Products include:
> Lescol Capsules 2233
> Lescol XL Tablets 2233

Fosphenytoin Sodium (Potential for elevated serum phenytoin levels).
> No products indexed under this heading.

Hexobarbital (Potential for elevated serum hexobarbital levels).
> No products indexed under this heading.

Lovastatin (Co-administration has been reported to increase concentrations of HMG-CoA reductase inhibitors. Rare reports of rhabdomyolysis have also been reported during concurrent therapy). Products include:
> Advicor Tablets 1722
> Altoprev Extended-Release Tablets 3109
> Mevacor Tablets 2021

Methylprednisolone (Potential for elevated serum methylprednisolone levels).
> No products indexed under this heading.

Methylprednisolone Acetate (Potential for elevated serum methylprednisolone levels). Products include:
> Depo-Medrol Injectable Suspension 2617
> Depo-Medrol Single-Dose Vial 2619

Methylprednisolone Sodium Succinate (Potential for elevated serum methylprednisolone levels).
> No products indexed under this heading.

Midazolam Hydrochloride (Erythromycin has been reported to decrease the clearance of midazolam and may increase the pharmacologic effect of the benzodiazepine).
> No products indexed under this heading.

Phenytoin (Potential for elevated serum phenytoin levels).
> No products indexed under this heading.

Phenytoin Sodium (Potential for elevated serum phenytoin levels). Products include:
> Phenytek Capsules 2160

Pimozide (Concurrent use is contraindicated).
> No products indexed under this heading.

Pravastatin Sodium (Co-administration has been reported to increase concentrations of HMG-CoA reductase inhibitors. Rare reports of rhabdomyolysis have also been reported during concurrent therapy).
> No products indexed under this heading.

Quinidine (Potential for elevated serum quinidine levels).
> No products indexed under this heading.

Quinidine Gluconate (Potential for elevated serum quinidine levels).
> No products indexed under this heading.

Quinidine Hydrochloride (Potential for elevated serum quinidine levels).
> No products indexed under this heading.

Quinidine Polygalacturonate (Potential for elevated serum quinidine levels).
> No products indexed under this heading.

Quinidine Sulfate (Potential for elevated serum quinidine levels).
> No products indexed under this heading.

Rifabutin (Potential for elevated serum rifabutin levels).
> No products indexed under this heading.

Sildenafil Citrate (Co-administration has been reported to increase the systemic exposure (AUC) of sildenafil; reduction of sildenafil dosage should be considered). Products include:
> Revatio Tablets 2557
> Viagra Tablets 2573

Simvastatin (Co-administration has been reported to increase concentrations of HMG-CoA reductase inhibitors. Rare reports of rhabdomyolysis have also been reported during concurrent therapy). Products include:
> Vytorin 10/10 Tablets 2114
> Vytorin 10/10 Tablets 3077
> Vytorin 10/20 Tablets 2114
> Vytorin 10/20 Tablets 3077
> Vytorin 10/40 Tablets 2114

IMPORTANT NOTE: Always consult each drug listing in the patient's regimen for possible interactions.

Vytorin 10/40 Tablets **3077**
Vytorin 10/80 Tablets **2114**
Vytorin 10/80 Tablets **3077**
Zocor Tablets **2105**

Tacrolimus (Potential for elevated serum tacrolimus levels). Products include:
Prograf Capsules and Injection **632**
Protopic Ointment **638**

Terfenadine (Co-administration has produced a significant alteration in terfenadine metabolism resulting in rare cases of serious cardiovascular adverse events, including QT prolongation, cardiac arrest, torsade de pointes and death; concurrent use is contraindicated).
No products indexed under this heading.

Theophylline (Co-administration in patients who are receiving high doses of theophylline may be associated with an increase in serum theophylline levels and potential theophylline toxicity).
No products indexed under this heading.

Theophylline Anhydrous (Co-administration in patients who are receiving high doses of theophylline may be associated with an increase in serum theophylline levels and potential theophylline toxicity). Products include:
Uniphyl Tablets **2710**

Theophylline Calcium Salicylate (Co-administration in patients who are receiving high doses of theophylline may be associated with an increase in serum theophylline levels and potential theophylline toxicity).
No products indexed under this heading.

Theophylline Dihydroxypropyl (Glyceryl) (Co-administration in patients who are receiving high doses of theophylline may be associated with an increase in serum theophylline levels and potential theophylline toxicity).
No products indexed under this heading.

Theophylline Ethylenediamine (Co-administration in patients who are receiving high doses of theophylline may be associated with an increase in serum theophylline levels and potential theophylline toxicity).
No products indexed under this heading.

Theophylline Sodium Glycinate (Co-administration in patients who are receiving high doses of theophylline may be associated with an increase in serum theophylline levels and potential theophylline toxicity).
No products indexed under this heading.

Triazolam (Erythromycin has been reported to decrease the clearance of triazolam and may increase the pharmacologic effect of the benzodiazepine).
No products indexed under this heading.

Valproate Sodium (Potential for elevated serum valproate levels). Products include:
Depacon Injection **412**

Valproic Acid (Potential for elevated serum valproate levels). Products include:
Depakene **417**

Vinblastine Sulfate (Potential for elevated serum vinblastine levels).
No products indexed under this heading.

Warfarin Sodium (Co-administration has been reported to result in increased anticoagulant effects). Products include:
Coumadin for Injection **898**
Coumadin Tablets **898**

ERYTHROMYCIN BASE FILMTAB TABLETS

(Erythromycin) **455**
May interact with oral anticoagulants, phenytoin, valproate, xanthines, and certain other agents. Compounds in these categories include:

Alfentanil Hydrochloride (Potential for elevated serum alfentanil levels).
No products indexed under this heading.

Aminophylline (Co-administration in patients who are receiving high doses of theophylline may be associated with an increase in serum theophylline levels and potential theophylline toxicity).
No products indexed under this heading.

Anisindione (Co-administration has been reported to result in increased anticoagulant effects). Products include:
Miradon Tablets **3042**

Astemizole (Co-administration has produced a significant alteration in astemizole metabolism resulting in rare cases of serious cardiovascular adverse events, including QT prolongation, cardiac arrest, torsade de pointes and death; concurrent use is contraindicated).
No products indexed under this heading.

Bromocriptine Mesylate (Potential for elevated serum bromocriptine levels).
No products indexed under this heading.

Carbamazepine (Potential for elevated serum carbamazepine levels). Products include:
Carbatrol Capsules **3171**
Equetro Extended-Release Capsules **3180**
Tegretol/Tegretol-XR **2295**

Cisapride (Co-administration has produced an inhibition of hepatic metabolism of cisapride metabolism resulting in QT prolongation, cardiac arrhythmias, ventricular fibrillation, and torsade de pointes; concurrent use is contraindicated).
No products indexed under this heading.

Cyclosporine (Potential for elevated serum cyclosporine levels). Products include:
Gengraf Capsules **459**
Neoral Oral Solution **2259**
Neoral Soft Gelatin Capsules **2259**
Restasis Ophthalmic Emulsion **575**
Sandimmune **2275**

Dicumarol (Co-administration has been reported to result in increased anticoagulant effects).
No products indexed under this heading.

Digoxin (Co-administration has been reported to result in elevated digoxin serum levels). Products include:
Lanoxicaps Capsules **1490**
Lanoxin Injection **1494**
Lanoxin Injection Pediatric **1497**
Lanoxin Tablets **1500**

Dihydroergotamine Mesylate (Co-administration has been reported to result in acute ergot toxicity characterized by severe peripheral vasospasm and dysesthesia). Products include:
Migranal Nasal Spray **3348**

Disopyramide Phosphate (Potential for elevated serum disopyramide levels).
No products indexed under this heading.

Divalproex Sodium (Potential for elevated serum valproate levels). Products include:
Depakote Sprinkle Capsules **422**
Depakote Tablets **427**
Depakote ER Tablets **434**

Dyphylline (Co-administration in patients who are receiving high doses of theophylline may be associated with an increase in serum theophylline levels and potential theophylline toxicity).
No products indexed under this heading.

Ergotamine Tartrate (Co-administration has been reported to result in acute ergot toxicity characterized by severe peripheral vasospasm and dysesthesia).
No products indexed under this heading.

Fosphenytoin Sodium (Potential for elevated serum phenytoin levels).
No products indexed under this heading.

Hexobarbital (Potential for elevated serum hexobarbital levels).
No products indexed under this heading.

Lovastatin (Potential for elevated serum lovastatin levels). Products include:
Advicor Tablets **1722**
Altoprev Extended-Release Tablets **3109**
Mevacor Tablets **2021**

Midazolam Hydrochloride (Erythromycin has been reported to decrease the clearance of midazolam and may increase the pharmacologic effect of benzodiazepine).
No products indexed under this heading.

Phenytoin (Potential for elevated serum phenytoin levels).
No products indexed under this heading.

Phenytoin Sodium (Potential for elevated serum phenytoin levels). Products include:
Phenytek Capsules **2160**

Tacrolimus (Potential for elevated serum tacrolimus levels). Products include:
Prograf Capsules and Injection **632**
Protopic Ointment **638**

Terfenadine (Co-administration has produced a significant alteration in terfenadine metabolism resulting in rare cases of serious cardiovascular events, including QT prolongation, cardiac arrest, torsade de pointes and death; concurrent use is contraindicated).
No products indexed under this heading.

Theophylline (Co-administration in patients who are receiving high doses of theophylline may be associated with an increase in serum theophylline levels and potential theophylline toxicity).
No products indexed under this heading.

Theophylline Anhydrous (Co-administration in patients who are receiving high doses of theophylline may be associated with an increase in serum theophylline levels and potential theophylline toxicity). Products include:
Uniphyl Tablets **2710**

Theophylline Calcium Salicylate (Co-administration in patients who are receiving high doses of theophylline may be associated with an increase in serum theophylline levels and potential theophylline toxicity).
No products indexed under this heading.

Theophylline Dihydroxypropyl (Glyceryl) (Co-administration in patients who are receiving high doses of theophylline may be associated with an increase in serum theophylline levels and potential theophylline toxicity).
No products indexed under this heading.

Theophylline Ethylenediamine (Co-administration in patients who are receiving high doses of theophylline may be associated with an increase in serum theophylline levels and potential theophylline toxicity).
No products indexed under this heading.

Theophylline Sodium Glycinate (Co-administration in patients who are receiving high doses of theophylline may be associated with an increase in serum theophylline levels and potential theophylline toxicity).
No products indexed under this heading.

Triazolam (Erythromycin has been reported to decrease the clearance of triazolam and may increase the pharmacologic effect of the benzodiazepine).
No products indexed under this heading.

Valproate Sodium (Potential for elevated serum valproate levels). Products include:
Depacon Injection **412**

Valproic Acid (Potential for elevated serum valproate levels). Products include:
Depakene **417**

Warfarin Sodium (Co-administration has been reported to result in increased anticoagulant effects). Products include:
Coumadin for Injection **898**
Coumadin Tablets **898**

ERYTHROMYCIN DELAYED-RELEASE CAPSULES, USP

(Erythromycin) **457**
May interact with oral anticoagulants, cytochrome p450 3a substrates (selected), HMG-CoA reductase inhibitors, xanthines, and certain other agents. Compounds in these categories include:

Alfentanil Hydrochloride (Co-administration of erythromycin and a drug primarily matabolized by CYP3A, like alfentanil, may be associated with elevation in drug concentrations that could increase or prolong both the therapeutic and adverse effects of alfentanil).
No products indexed under this heading.

Alprazolam (Erythromycin is a substrate and inhibitor of the 3A isoform subfamily of the cytochrome p450 enzyme system (CYP3A). Co-administration of erythromycin and a drug primarily metabolized by CYP3A may be associated with elevations in drug concentrations

that could increase or prolong both the therapeutic and adverse effects of the concomitant drug). Products include:
- Niravam Orally Disintegrating Tablets 3092

Aminophylline (Concomitant administration with high doses of theophylline may be associated with increased theophylline levels and potential toxicity).
- No products indexed under this heading.

Amitriptyline Hydrochloride (Erythromycin is a substrate and inhibitor of the 3A isoform subfamily of the cytochrome p450 enzyme system (CYP3A). Co-administration of erythromycin and a drug primarily metabolized by CYP3A may be associated with elevations in drug concentrations that could increase or prolong both the therapeutic and adverse effects of the concomitant drug).
- No products indexed under this heading.

Amlodipine Besylate (Erythromycin is a substrate and inhibitor of the 3A isoform subfamily of the cytochrome p450 enzyme system (CYP3A). Co-administration of erythromycin and a drug primarily metabolized by CYP3A may be associated with elevations in drug concentrations that could increase or prolong both the therapeutic and adverse effects of the concomitant drug). Products include:
- Caduet Tablets 2508
- Lotrel Capsules 2249
- Norvasc Tablets 2545

Anisindione (Increased anticoagulant effects). Products include:
- Miradon Tablets 3042

Aprepitant (Erythromycin is a substrate and inhibitor of the 3A isoform subfamily of the cytochrome p450 enzyme system (CYP3A). Co-administration of erythromycin and a drug primarily metabolized by CYP3A may be associated with elevations in drug concentrations that could increase or prolong both the therapeutic and adverse effects of the concomitant drug). Products include:
- Emend Capsules 1963

Astemizole (Co-administration is contraindicated).
- No products indexed under this heading.

Atorvastatin Calcium (Erythromycin is a substrate and inhibitor of the 3A isoform subfamily of the cytochrome p450 enzyme system (CYP3A). Co-administration of erythromycin and a drug primarily metabolized by CYP3A may be associated with elevations in drug concentrations that could increase or prolong both the therapeutic and adverse effects of the concomitant drug). Products include:
- Caduet Tablets 2508
- Lipitor Tablets 2483

Bromocriptine Mesylate (Co-administration of erythromycin and a drug primarily matabolized by CYP3A, like bromocriptine, may be associated with elevation in drug concentrations that could increase or prolong both the therapeutic and adverse effects of bromocriptine).
- No products indexed under this heading.

Buspirone Hydrochloride (Erythromycin is a substrate and inhibitor of the 3A isoform subfamily of the cytochrome p450 enzyme system (CYP3A). Co-administration of erythromycin and a drug primarily metabolized by CYP3A may be associated with elevations in drug concentrations that could increase or prolong both the therapeutic and adverse effects of the concomitant drug).
- No products indexed under this heading.

Busulfan (Erythromycin is a substrate and inhibitor of the 3A isoform subfamily of the cytochrome p450 enzyme system (CYP3A). Co-administration of erythromycin and a drug primarily metabolized by CYP3A may be associated with elevations in drug concentrations that could increase or prolong both the therapeutic and adverse effects of the concomitant drug). Products include:
- I.V. Busulfex 2493
- Myleran Tablets 1525

Carbamazepine (Elevations in serum erythromycin and carbamazepine concentration). Products include:
- Carbatrol Capsules 3171
- Equetro Extended-Release Capsules 3180
- Tegretol/Tegretol-XR 2295

Cerivastatin Sodium (Erythromycin is a substrate and inhibitor of the 3A isoform subfamily of the cytochrome p450 enzyme system (CYP3A). Co-administration of erythromycin and a drug primarily metabolized by CYP3A may be associated with elevations in drug concentrations that could increase or prolong both the therapeutic and adverse effects of the concomitant drug).
- No products indexed under this heading.

Chlorpheniramine (Erythromycin is a substrate and inhibitor of the 3A isoform subfamily of the cytochrome p450 enzyme system (CYP3A). Co-administration of erythromycin and a drug primarily metabolized by CYP3A may be associated with elevations in drug concentrations that could increase or prolong both the therapeutic and adverse effects of the concomitant drug).
- No products indexed under this heading.

Chlorpheniramine Maleate (Erythromycin is a substrate and inhibitor of the 3A isoform subfamily of the cytochrome p450 enzyme system (CYP3A). Co-administration of erythromycin and a drug primarily metabolized by CYP3A may be associated with elevations in drug concentrations that could increase or prolong both the therapeutic and adverse effects of the concomitant drug). Products include:
- Advil Allergy Sinus Caplets 770
- Advil Multi-Symptom Cold Caplets 770
- BC Allergy Sinus Cold Powder 677
- Comtrex Maximum Strength Cold & Cough Day/Night Caplets - Night Formulation 726
- Comtrex Maximum Strength Day/Night Severe Cold & Sinus Caplets - Night Formulation 725
- Contac Cold and Flu Maximum Strength Caplets 728
- Contac Cold and Flu Day and Night Caplets (Night Formulation Only) 727
- Children's Dimetapp Long Acting Cough Plus Cold Syrup 731
- Robitussin Cough & Cold Long-Acting Liquid 735
- Robitussin Cough & Allergy Syrup .. 736
- Robitussin Cough & Cold Nighttime Liquid 736
- Robitussin Cough, Cold & Flu Nighttime Liquid 738
- Robitussin Pediatric Cough & Cold Long-Acting Liquid 735
- Robitussin Pediatric Cough & Cold Nighttime Liquid 736
- Triaminic Cold & Allergy Liquid 746
- Triaminic Cough & Runny Nose Softchews 748
- Children's Tylenol Plus Flu Oral Suspension 749
- Tylenol Allergy Multi-Symptom Caplets with Cool Burst and Gelcaps 1872
- Children's Tylenol Plus Cold Suspension Liquid 1879
- Children's Tylenol Plus Cough & Runny Nose Suspension Liquid 1879
- Children's Tylenol Plus Flu Suspension Liquid 1881
- Children's Tylenol Plus Multi-Symptom Cold Suspension Liquid 1879
- Tylenol Cold Head Congestion Nighttime Caplets with Cool Burst 1873
- Tylenol Cold Multi-Symptom Nighttime Caplets with Cool Burst 1874
- Tylenol Sinus Congestion & Pain Nighttime Caplets with Cool Burst 1876
- Vicks 44M Cough, Cold & Flu Relief Liquid 2680
- Pediatric Vicks 44m Cough & Cold Relief Liquid 2676
- Children's Vicks NyQuil Cold/Cough Relief 756
- Children's Vicks NyQuil Cold/Cough Relief Liquid 2680
- Zicam Maximum Strength Flu Daytime 768

Chlorpheniramine Polistirex (Erythromycin is a substrate and inhibitor of the 3A isoform subfamily of the cytochrome p450 enzyme system (CYP3A). Co-administration of erythromycin and a drug primarily metabolized by CYP3A may be associated with elevations in drug concentrations that could increase or prolong both the therapeutic and adverse effects of the concomitant drug). Products include:
- Tussionex Pennkinetic Extended-Release Suspension 3327

Chlorpheniramine Tannate (Erythromycin is a substrate and inhibitor of the 3A isoform subfamily of the cytochrome p450 enzyme system (CYP3A). Co-administration of erythromycin and a drug primarily metabolized by CYP3A may be associated with elevations in drug concentrations that could increase or prolong both the therapeutic and adverse effects of the concomitant drug).
- No products indexed under this heading.

Cilostazol (Co-administration of erythromycin and a drug primarily matabolized by CYP3A, like cilostazol, may be associated with elevation in drug concentrations that could increase or prolong both the therapeutic and adverse effects of cilostazol). Products include:
- Pletal Tablets 2455

Cisapride (Co-administration is contraindicated).
- No products indexed under this heading.

Clarithromycin (Erythromycin is a substrate and inhibitor of the 3A isoform subfamily of the cytochrome p450 enzyme system (CYP3A). Co-administration of erythromycin and a drug primarily metabolized by CYP3A may be associated with elevations in drug concentrations that could increase or prolong both the therapeutic and adverse effects of the concomitant drug). Products include:
- Biaxin/Biaxin XL 402
- PREVPAC 3284

Cyclosporine (Elevations in serum erythromycin and cyclosporine concentration). Products include:
- Gengraf Capsules 459
- Neoral Oral Solution 2259
- Neoral Soft Gelatin Capsules 2259
- Restasis Ophthalmic Emulsion 575
- Sandimmune 2275

Desogestrel (Erythromycin is a substrate and inhibitor of the 3A isoform subfamily of the cytochrome p450 enzyme system (CYP3A). Co-administration of erythromycin and a drug primarily metabolized by CYP3A may be associated with elevations in drug concentrations that could increase or prolong both the therapeutic and adverse effects of the concomitant drug). Products include:
- Mircette Tablets 1066

Dexamethasone (Erythromycin is a substrate and inhibitor of the 3A isoform subfamily of the cytochrome p450 enzyme system (CYP3A). Co-administration of erythromycin and a drug primarily metabolized by CYP3A may be associated with elevations in drug concentrations that could increase or prolong both the therapeutic and adverse effects of the concomitant drug). Products include:
- Ciprodex Otic Suspension 559
- Decadron Tablets 1951
- TobraDex Ophthalmic Ointment 562
- TobraDex Ophthalmic Suspension ... 563

Dexamethasone Acetate (Erythromycin is a substrate and inhibitor of the 3A isoform subfamily of the cytochrome p450 enzyme system (CYP3A). Co-administration of erythromycin and a drug primarily metabolized by CYP3A may be associated with elevations in drug concentrations that could increase or prolong both the therapeutic and adverse effects of the concomitant drug).
- No products indexed under this heading.

Dexamethasone Phosphate (Erythromycin is a substrate and inhibitor of the 3A isoform subfamily of the cytochrome p450 enzyme system (CYP3A). Co-administration of erythromycin and a drug primarily metabolized by CYP3A may be associated with elevations in drug concentrations that could increase or prolong both the therapeutic and adverse effects of the concomitant drug).
- No products indexed under this heading.

Dexamethasone Sodium (Erythromycin is a substrate and inhibitor of the 3A isoform subfamily of the cytochrome p450 enzyme system (CYP3A). Co-administration of erythromycin and a drug primarily metabolized by CYP3A may be associated with elevations in drug concentrations that could increase or prolong both the therapeutic and adverse effects of the concomitant drug).
- No products indexed under this heading.

Dexamethasone Sodium Phosphate (Erythromycin is a substrate and inhibitor of the 3A isoform subfamily of the cytochrome p450 enzyme system (CYP3A). Co-administration of erythromycin and a drug primarily metabolized by CYP3A may be associated with elevations in drug concentrations that could increase or prolong both the therapeutic and adverse effects of the concomitant drug).
No products indexed under this heading.

Diazepam (Erythromycin is a substrate and inhibitor of the 3A isoform subfamily of the cytochrome p450 enzyme system (CYP3A). Co-administration of erythromycin and a drug primarily metabolized by CYP3A may be associated with elevations in drug concentrations that could increase or prolong both the therapeutic and adverse effects of the concomitant drug). Products include:

Diastat Rectal Delivery System	3343
Valium Tablets	2819

Dicumarol (Increased anticoagulant effects).
No products indexed under this heading.

Digoxin (Elevated digoxin serum levels). Products include:

Lanoxicaps Capsules	1490
Lanoxin Injection	1494
Lanoxin Injection Pediatric	1497
Lanoxin Tablets	1500

Dihydroergotamine Mesylate (Potential for acute ergot toxicity characterized by severe peripheral vasospasm and dysesthesia). Products include:

Migranal Nasal Spray	3348

Diltiazem Hydrochloride (Erythromycin is a substrate and inhibitor of the 3A isoform subfamily of the cytochrome p450 enzyme system (CYP3A). Co-administration of erythromycin and a drug primarily metabolized by CYP3A may be associated with elevations in drug concentrations that could increase or prolong both the therapeutic and adverse effects of the concomitant drug). Products include:

Cardizem LA Extended Release Tablets	1728
Tiazac Capsules	1201

Diltiazem Maleate (Erythromycin is a substrate and inhibitor of the 3A isoform subfamily of the cytochrome p450 enzyme system (CYP3A). Co-administration of erythromycin and a drug primarily metabolized by CYP3A may be associated with elevations in drug concentrations that could increase or prolong both the therapeutic and adverse effects of the concomitant drug).
No products indexed under this heading.

Disopyramide (Co-administration of erythromycin and a drug primarily matabolized by CYP3A, like disopyramide, may be associated with elevation in drug concentrations that could increase or prolong both the therapeutic and adverse effects of disopyramide).
No products indexed under this heading.

Disopyramide Phosphate (Co-administration of erythromycin and a drug primarily matabolized by CYP3A, like disopyramide, may be associated with elevation in drug concentrations that could increase or prolong both the therapeutic and adverse effects of disopyramide).
No products indexed under this heading.

Doxorubicin Hydrochloride (Erythromycin is a substrate and inhibitor of the 3A isoform subfamily of the cytochrome p450 enzyme system (CYP3A). Co-administration of erythromycin and a drug primarily metabolized by CYP3A may be associated with elevations in drug concentrations that could increase or prolong both the therapeutic and adverse effects of the concomitant drug).
No products indexed under this heading.

Dronabinol (Erythromycin is a substrate and inhibitor of the 3A isoform subfamily of the cytochrome p450 enzyme system (CYP3A). Co-administration of erythromycin and a drug primarily metabolized by CYP3A may be associated with elevations in drug concentrations that could increase or prolong both the therapeutic and adverse effects of the concomitant drug). Products include:

Marinol Capsules	3333

Dyphylline (Concomitant administration with high doses of theophylline may be associated with increased theophylline levels and potential toxicity).
No products indexed under this heading.

Ergotamine Tartrate (Potential for acute ergot toxicity characterized by severe peripheral vasospasm and dysesthesia).
No products indexed under this heading.

Erythromycin Estolate (Erythromycin is a substrate and inhibitor of the 3A isoform subfamily of the cytochrome p450 enzyme system (CYP3A). Co-administration of erythromycin and a drug primarily metabolized by CYP3A may be associated with elevations in drug concentrations that could increase or prolong both the therapeutic and adverse effects of the concomitant drug).
No products indexed under this heading.

Erythromycin Ethylsuccinate (Erythromycin is a substrate and inhibitor of the 3A isoform subfamily of the cytochrome p450 enzyme system (CYP3A). Co-administration of erythromycin and a drug primarily metabolized by CYP3A may be associated with elevations in drug concentrations that could increase or prolong both the therapeutic and adverse effects of the concomitant drug). Products include:

E.E.S.	451
EryPed	447

Erythromycin Gluceptate (Erythromycin is a substrate and inhibitor of the 3A isoform subfamily of the cytochrome p450 enzyme system (CYP3A). Co-administration of erythromycin and a drug primarily metabolized by CYP3A may be associated with elevations in drug concentrations that could increase or prolong both the therapeutic and adverse effects of the concomitant drug).
No products indexed under this heading.

Erythromycin Lactobionate (Erythromycin is a substrate and inhibitor of the 3A isoform subfamily of the cytochrome p450 enzyme system (CYP3A). Co-administration of erythromycin and a drug primarily metabolized by CYP3A may be associated with elevations in drug concentrations that could increase or prolong both the therapeutic and adverse effects of the concomitant drug).
No products indexed under this heading.

Erythromycin Stearate (Erythromycin is a substrate and inhibitor of the 3A isoform subfamily of the cytochrome p450 enzyme system (CYP3A). Co-administration of erythromycin and a drug primarily metabolized by CYP3A may be associated with elevations in drug concentrations that could increase or prolong both the therapeutic and adverse effects of the concomitant drug). Products include:

Erythrocin Stearate Filmtab Tablets	453

Estrogen (Erythromycin is a substrate and inhibitor of the 3A isoform subfamily of the cytochrome p450 enzyme system (CYP3A). Co-administration of erythromycin and a drug primarily metabolized by CYP3A may be associated with elevations in drug concentrations that could increase or prolong both the therapeutic and adverse effects of the concomitant drug).
No products indexed under this heading.

Estrogens, Conjugated (Erythromycin is a substrate and inhibitor of the 3A isoform subfamily of the cytochrome p450 enzyme system (CYP3A). Co-administration of erythromycin and a drug primarily metabolized by CYP3A may be associated with elevations in drug concentrations that could increase or prolong both the therapeutic and adverse effects of the concomitant drug). Products include:

Premarin Intravenous	3442
Premarin Tablets	3446
Premarin Vaginal Cream	3452
Premphase Tablets	3456
Prempro Tablets	3456

Estrogens, Conjugated, Synthetic A (Erythromycin is a substrate and inhibitor of the 3A isoform subfamily of the cytochrome p450 enzyme system (CYP3A). Co-administration of erythromycin and a drug primarily metabolized by CYP3A may be associated with elevations in drug concentrations that could increase or prolong both the therapeutic and adverse effects of the concomitant drug).
No products indexed under this heading.

Estrogens, Esterified (Erythromycin is a substrate and inhibitor of the 3A isoform subfamily of the cyto-chrome p450 enzyme system (CYP3A). Co-administration of erythromycin and a drug primarily metabolized by CYP3A may be associated with elevations in drug concentrations that could increase or prolong both the therapeutic and adverse effects of the concomitant drug). Products include:

Estratest Tablets	3199
Estratest H.S. Tablets	3199

Ethinyl Estradiol (Erythromycin is a substrate and inhibitor of the 3A isoform subfamily of the cytochrome p450 enzyme system (CYP3A). Co-administration of erythromycin and a drug primarily metabolized by CYP3A may be associated with elevations in drug concentrations that could increase or prolong both the therapeutic and adverse effects of the concomitant drug). Products include:

Mircette Tablets	1066
NuvaRing	2340
Ortho-Cyclen/Ortho Tri-Cyclen	2429
Ortho Evra Transdermal System	2417
Ortho Tri-Cyclen Lo Tablets	2436
Seasonique Tablets	1077
Yasmin 28 Tablets	796
Yaz Tablets	803

Ethosuximide (Erythromycin is a substrate and inhibitor of the 3A isoform subfamily of the cytochrome p450 enzyme system (CYP3A). Co-administration of erythromycin and a drug primarily metabolized by CYP3A may be associated with elevations in drug concentrations that could increase or prolong both the therapeutic and adverse effects of the concomitant drug).
No products indexed under this heading.

Ethynodiol Diacetate (Erythromycin is a substrate and inhibitor of the 3A isoform subfamily of the cytochrome p450 enzyme system (CYP3A). Co-administration of erythromycin and a drug primarily metabolized by CYP3A may be associated with elevations in drug concentrations that could increase or prolong both the therapeutic and adverse effects of the concomitant drug).
No products indexed under this heading.

Etoposide (Erythromycin is a substrate and inhibitor of the 3A isoform subfamily of the cytochrome p450 enzyme system (CYP3A). Co-administration of erythromycin and a drug primarily metabolized by CYP3A may be associated with elevations in drug concentrations that could increase or prolong both the therapeutic and adverse effects of the concomitant drug).
No products indexed under this heading.

Etoposide Phosphate (Erythromycin is a substrate and inhibitor of the 3A isoform subfamily of the cytochrome p450 enzyme system (CYP3A). Co-administration of erythromycin and a drug primarily metabolized by CYP3A may be associated with elevations in drug concentrations that could increase or prolong both the therapeutic and adverse effects of the concomitant drug).
No products indexed under this heading.

Felodipine (Erythromycin is a substrate and inhibitor of the 3A isoform subfamily of the cytochrome p450 enzyme system (CYP3A). Co-administration of erythromycin and a drug primarily metabolized by CYP3A may be associated with elevations in drug concentrations that could increase or prolong both the therapeutic and adverse effects of the concomitant drug).
No products indexed under this heading.

Fentanyl (Erythromycin is a substrate and inhibitor of the 3A isoform subfamily of the cytochrome p450 enzyme system (CYP3A). Co-administration of erythromycin and a drug primarily metabolized by CYP3A may be associated with elevations in drug concentrations that could increase or prolong both the therapeutic and adverse effects of the concomitant drug). Products include:
Duragesic Transdermal System 2373
Ionsys Transdermal System 2379

Fentanyl Citrate (Erythromycin is a substrate and inhibitor of the 3A isoform subfamily of the cytochrome p450 enzyme system (CYP3A). Co-administration of erythromycin and a drug primarily metabolized by CYP3A may be associated with elevations in drug concentrations that could increase or prolong both the therapeutic and adverse effects of the concomitant drug). Products include:
Actiq 979

Fluvastatin Sodium (Erythromycin has been reported to increase concentrations of HMG-CoA reductase inhibitors (e.g., lovastatin and simvastatin); rare reports of rhabdomyolysis have been reported in patients taking these drugs concomitantly). Products include:
Lescol Capsules 2233
Lescol XL Tablets 2233

Glyburide (Erythromycin is a substrate and inhibitor of the 3A isoform subfamily of the cytochrome p450 enzyme system (CYP3A). Co-administration of erythromycin and a drug primarily metabolized by CYP3A may be associated with elevations in drug concentrations that could increase or prolong both the therapeutic and adverse effects of the concomitant drug).
No products indexed under this heading.

Haloperidol (Erythromycin is a substrate and inhibitor of the 3A isoform subfamily of the cytochrome p450 enzyme system (CYP3A). Co-administration of erythromycin and a drug primarily metabolized by CYP3A may be associated with elevations in drug concentrations that could increase or prolong both the therapeutic and adverse effects of the concomitant drug).
No products indexed under this heading.

Haloperidol Decanoate (Erythromycin is a substrate and inhibitor of the 3A isoform subfamily of the cytochrome p450 enzyme system (CYP3A). Co-administration of erythromycin and a drug primarily metabolized by CYP3A may be associated with elevations in drug concentrations that could increase or prolong both the therapeutic and adverse effects of the concomitant drug).
No products indexed under this heading.

Hexobarbital (There have been reportd of interactions of erythromyin with drugs not thought to be metaboilzed by CYP3A, including hexobarbital).
No products indexed under this heading.

Imipramine Hydrochloride (Erythromycin is a substrate and inhibitor of the 3A isoform subfamily of the cytochrome p450 enzyme system (CYP3A). Co-administration of erythromycin and a drug primarily metabolized by CYP3A may be associated with elevations in drug concentrations that could increase or prolong both the therapeutic and adverse effects of the concomitant drug).
No products indexed under this heading.

Imipramine Pamoate (Erythromycin is a substrate and inhibitor of the 3A isoform subfamily of the cytochrome p450 enzyme system (CYP3A). Co-administration of erythromycin and a drug primarily metabolized by CYP3A may be associated with elevations in drug concentrations that could increase or prolong both the therapeutic and adverse effects of the concomitant drug).
No products indexed under this heading.

Indinavir Sulfate (Erythromycin is a substrate and inhibitor of the 3A isoform subfamily of the cytochrome p450 enzyme system (CYP3A). Co-administration of erythromycin and a drug primarily metabolized by CYP3A may be associated with elevations in drug concentrations that could increase or prolong both the therapeutic and adverse effects of the concomitant drug). Products include:
Crixivan Capsules 1940

Isradipine (Erythromycin is a substrate and inhibitor of the 3A isoform subfamily of the cytochrome p450 enzyme system (CYP3A). Co-administration of erythromycin and a drug primarily metabolized by CYP3A may be associated with elevations in drug concentrations that could increase or prolong both the therapeutic and adverse effects of the concomitant drug). Products include:
DynaCirc CR Tablets 2721

Itraconazole (Erythromycin is a substrate and inhibitor of the 3A isoform subfamily of the cytochrome p450 enzyme system (CYP3A). Co-administration of erythromycin and a drug primarily metabolized by CYP3A may be associated with elevations in drug concentrations that could increase or prolong both the therapeutic and adverse effects of the concomitant drug).
No products indexed under this heading.

Ketoconazole (Erythromycin is a substrate and inhibitor of the 3A isoform subfamily of the cytochrome p450 enzyme system (CYP3A). Co-administration of erythromycin and a drug primarily metabolized by CYP3A may be associated with elevations in drug concentrations that could increase or prolong both the therapeutic and adverse effects of the concomitant drug). Products include:
Nizoral A-D Shampoo, 1% 1868

Levonorgestrel (Erythromycin is a substrate and inhibitor of the 3A isoform subfamily of the cytochrome p450 enzyme system (CYP3A). Co-administration of erythromycin and a drug primarily metabolized by CYP3A may be associated with elevations in drug concentrations that could increase or prolong both the therapeutic and adverse effects of the concomitant drug). Products include:
Climara Pro Transdermal System 776
Mirena Intrauterine System 787
Plan B Tablets 1076
Seasonique Tablets 1077

Lidocaine (Erythromycin is a substrate and inhibitor of the 3A isoform subfamily of the cytochrome p450 enzyme system (CYP3A). Co-administration of erythromycin and a drug primarily metabolized by CYP3A may be associated with elevations in drug concentrations that could increase or prolong both the therapeutic and adverse effects of the concomitant drug). Products include:
Lidoderm Patch 1118
Synera Topical Patch 1137

Lidocaine Hydrochloride (Erythromycin is a substrate and inhibitor of the 3A isoform subfamily of the cytochrome p450 enzyme system (CYP3A). Co-administration of erythromycin and a drug primarily metabolized by CYP3A may be associated with elevations in drug concentrations that could increase or prolong both the therapeutic and adverse effects of the concomitant drug).
No products indexed under this heading.

Lovastatin (Erythromycin has been reported to increase concentrations of HMG-CoA reductase inhibitors. Rare reports of rhabdomyolysis have been reported in patients taking these drugs concomitantly). Products include:
Advicor Tablets 1722
Altoprev Extended-Release Tablets 3109
Mevacor Tablets 2021

Mestranol (Erythromycin is a substrate and inhibitor of the 3A isoform subfamily of the cytochrome p450 enzyme system (CYP3A). Co-administration of erythromycin and a drug primarily metabolized by CYP3A may be associated with elevations in drug concentrations that could increase or prolong both the therapeutic and adverse effects of the concomitant drug).
No products indexed under this heading.

Methadone Hydrochloride (Erythromycin is a substrate and inhibitor of the 3A isoform subfamily of the cytochrome p450 enzyme system (CYP3A). Co-administration of erythromycin and a drug primarily metabolized by CYP3A may be associated with elevations in drug concentrations that could increase or prolong both the therapeutic and adverse effects of the concomitant drug).
No products indexed under this heading.

Methylprednisolone (Co-administration of erythromycin and a drug primarily matabolized by CYP3A, like methylprednisolone, may be associated with elevation in drug concentrations that could increase or prolong both the therapeutic and adverse effects of methylprednisolone).
No products indexed under this heading.

Methylprednisolone Acetate (Co-administration of erythromycin and a drug primarily matabolized by CYP3A, like methylprednisolone, may be associated with elevation in drug concentrations that could increase or prolong both the therapeutic and adverse effects of methylprednisolone). Products include:
Depo-Medrol Injectable Suspension 2617
Depo-Medrol Single-Dose Vial 2619

Methylprednisolone Sodium Succinate (Co-administration of erythromycin and a drug primarily matabolized by CYP3A, like methylprednisolone, may be associated with elevation in drug concentrations that could increase or prolong both the therapeutic and adverse effects of methylprednisolone).
No products indexed under this heading.

Midazolam Hydrochloride (Decreased clearance of midazolam, and thus, may increase the pharmacologic effect of midazolam).
No products indexed under this heading.

Nefazodone Hydrochloride (Erythromycin is a substrate and inhibitor of the 3A isoform subfamily of the cytochrome p450 enzyme system (CYP3A). Co-administration of erythromycin and a drug primarily metabolized by CYP3A may be associated with elevations in drug concentrations that could increase or prolong both the therapeutic and adverse effects of the concomitant drug).
No products indexed under this heading.

Nelfinavir Mesylate (Erythromycin is a substrate and inhibitor of the 3A isoform subfamily of the cytochrome p450 enzyme system (CYP3A). Co-administration of erythromycin and a drug primarily metabolized by CYP3A may be associated with elevations in drug concentrations that could increase or prolong both the therapeutic and adverse effects of the concomitant drug). Products include:
Viracept 2577

Nicardipine (Erythromycin is a substrate and inhibitor of the 3A isoform subfamily of the cytochrome p450 enzyme system (CYP3A). Co-administration of erythromycin and a drug primarily metabolized by CYP3A may be associated with elevations in drug concentrations that could increase or prolong both the therapeutic and adverse effects of the concomitant drug).
No products indexed under this heading.

Nicardipine Hydrochloride (Erythromycin is a substrate and inhibitor of the 3A isoform subfamily of the cytochrome p450 enzyme system (CYP3A). Co-administration of erythromycin and a drug primarily metabolized by CYP3A may be associated with elevations in drug concentrations that could increase or prolong both the therapeutic and adverse effects of the concomitant drug). Products include:
Cardene I.V. 2497

Nifedipine (Erythromycin is a substrate and inhibitor of the 3A isoform subfamily of the cytochrome p450 enzyme system (CYP3A). Co-administration of erythromycin and a drug primarily metabolized by

CYP3A may be associated with elevations in drug concentrations that could increase or prolong both the therapeutic and adverse effects of the concomitant drug). Products include:

Adalat CC Tablets 2964

Nimodipine (Erythromycin is a substrate and inhibitor of the 3A isoform subfamily of the cytochrome p450 enzyme system (CYP3A). Co-administration of erythromycin and a drug primarily metabolized by CYP3A may be associated with elevations in drug concentrations that could increase or prolong both the therapeutic and adverse effects of the concomitant drug). Products include:

Nimotop Capsules 749

Nisoldipine (Erythromycin is a substrate and inhibitor of the 3A isoform subfamily of the cytochrome p450 enzyme system (CYP3A). Co-administration of erythromycin and a drug primarily metabolized by CYP3A may be associated with elevations in drug concentrations that could increase or prolong both the therapeutic and adverse effects of the concomitant drug). Products include:

Sular Tablets 3122

Norethindrone (Erythromycin is a substrate and inhibitor of the 3A isoform subfamily of the cytochrome p450 enzyme system (CYP3A). Co-administration of erythromycin and a drug primarily metabolized by CYP3A may be associated with elevations in drug concentrations that could increase or prolong both the therapeutic and adverse effects of the concomitant drug). Products include:

Ortho Micronor Tablets 2426

Norgestrel (Erythromycin is a substrate and inhibitor of the 3A isoform subfamily of the cytochrome p450 enzyme system (CYP3A). Co-administration of erythromycin and a drug primarily metabolized by CYP3A may be associated with elevations in drug concentrations that could increase or prolong both the therapeutic and adverse effects of the concomitant drug).

No products indexed under this heading.

Ondansetron Hydrochloride (Erythromycin is a substrate and inhibitor of the 3A isoform subfamily of the cytochrome p450 enzyme system (CYP3A). Co-administration of erythromycin and a drug primarily metabolized by CYP3A may be associated with elevations in drug concentrations that could increase or prolong both the therapeutic and adverse effects of the concomitant drug). Products include:

Zofran Injection 1634
Zofran 1639

Paclitaxel (Erythromycin is a substrate and inhibitor of the 3A isoform subfamily of the cytochrome p450 enzyme system (CYP3A). Co-administration of erythromycin and a drug primarily metabolized by CYP3A may be associated with elevations in drug concentrations that could increase or prolong both the therapeutic and adverse effects of the concomitant drug).

No products indexed under this heading.

Phenytoin (There have been reports of interaction of erythromycin with drugs not thought to be metabolized by CYP3A, including phenytoin).

No products indexed under this heading.

Phenytoin Sodium (There have been reports of interaction of erythromycin with drugs not thought to be metabolized by CYP3A, including phenytoin). Products include:

Phenytek Capsules 2160

Pimozide (Co-administration is contraindicated).

No products indexed under this heading.

Pravastatin Sodium (Erythromycin has been reported to increase concentrations of HMG-CoA reductase inhibitors (e.g., lovastatin and simvastatin); rare reports of rhabdomyolysis have been reported in patients taking these drugs concomitantly).

No products indexed under this heading.

Quinidine (Co-administration of erythromycin and a drug primarily matabolized by CYP3A, like quinidine, may be associated with elevation in drug concentrations that could increase or prolong both the therapeutic and adverse effects of quinidine).

No products indexed under this heading.

Quinidine Gluconate (Co-administration of erythromycin and a drug primarily matabolized by CYP3A, like quinidine, may be associated with elevation in drug concentrations that could increase or prolong both the therapeutic and adverse effects of quinidine).

No products indexed under this heading.

Quinidine Hydrochloride (Co-administration of erythromycin and a drug primarily matabolized by CYP3A, like quinidine, may be associated with elevation in drug concentrations that could increase or prolong both the therapeutic and adverse effects of quinidine).

No products indexed under this heading.

Quinidine Polygalacturonate (Co-administration of erythromycin and a drug primarily matabolized by CYP3A, like quinidine, may be associated with elevation in drug concentrations that could increase or prolong both the therapeutic and adverse effects of quinidine).

No products indexed under this heading.

Quinidine Sulfate (Co-administration of erythromycin and a drug primarily matabolized by CYP3A, like quinidine, may be associated with elevation in drug concentrations that could increase or prolong both the therapeutic and adverse effects of quinidine).

No products indexed under this heading.

Quinine (Erythromycin is a substrate and inhibitor of the 3A isoform subfamily of the cytochrome p450 enzyme system (CYP3A). Co-administration of erythromycin and a drug primarily metabolized by CYP3A may be associated with elevations in drug concentrations that could increase or prolong both the therapeutic and adverse effects of the concomitant drug).

No products indexed under this heading.

Quinine Sulfate (Erythromycin is a substrate and inhibitor of the 3A isoform subfamily of the cytochrome p450 enzyme system (CYP3A). Co-administration of erythromycin and a drug primarily metabolized by CYP3A may be associated with elevations in drug concentrations that could increase or prolong both the therapeutic and adverse effects of the concomitant drug).

No products indexed under this heading.

Rifabutin (Co-administration of erythromycin and a drug primarily matabolized by CYP3A, like rifabutin, may be associated with elevation in drug concentrations that could increase or prolong both the therapeutic and adverse effects of rifabutin).

No products indexed under this heading.

Ritonavir (Erythromycin is a substrate and inhibitor of the 3A isoform subfamily of the cytochrome p450 enzyme system (CYP3A). Co-administration of erythromycin and a drug primarily metabolized by CYP3A may be associated with elevations in drug concentrations that could increase or prolong both the therapeutic and adverse effects of the concomitant drug). Products include:

Kaletra 476
Norvir 503

Saquinavir (Erythromycin is a substrate and inhibitor of the 3A isoform subfamily of the cytochrome p450 enzyme system (CYP3A). Co-administration of erythromycin and a drug primarily metabolized by CYP3A may be associated with elevations in drug concentrations that could increase or prolong both the therapeutic and adverse effects of the concomitant drug).

No products indexed under this heading.

Saquinavir Mesylate (Erythromycin is a substrate and inhibitor of the 3A isoform subfamily of the cytochrome p450 enzyme system (CYP3A). Co-administration of erythromycin and a drug primarily metabolized by CYP3A may be associated with elevations in drug concentrations that could increase or prolong both the therapeutic and adverse effects of the concomitant drug). Products include:

Invirase 2772

Sertraline Hydrochloride (Erythromycin is a substrate and inhibitor of the 3A isoform subfamily of the cytochrome p450 enzyme system (CYP3A). Co-administration of erythromycin and a drug primarily metabolized by CYP3A may be associated with elevations in drug concentrations that could increase or prolong both the therapeutic and adverse effects of the concomitant drug). Products include:

Zoloft 2586

Sildenafil Citrate (Erythromycin has been reported to increase the systemic exposure (AUC) of sildenafil; should consider reduction of sildenafil dosage). Products include:

Revatio Tablets 2557
Viagra Tablets 2573

Simvastatin (Erythromycin has been reported to increase concentrations of HMG-CoA reductase inhibitors. Rare reports of rhabdomyolysis have been reported in patients taking these drugs concomitantly). Products include:

Vytorin 10/10 Tablets 2114
Vytorin 10/10 Tablets 3077
Vytorin 10/20 Tablets 2114
Vytorin 10/20 Tablets 3077
Vytorin 10/40 Tablets 2114
Vytorin 10/40 Tablets 3077
Vytorin 10/80 Tablets 2114
Vytorin 10/80 Tablets 3077
Zocor Tablets 2105

Sirolimus (Erythromycin is a substrate and inhibitor of the 3A isoform subfamily of the cytochrome p450 enzyme system (CYP3A). Co-administration of erythromycin and a drug primarily metabolized by CYP3A may be associated with elevations in drug concentrations that could increase or prolong both the therapeutic and adverse effects of the concomitant drug). Products include:

Rapamune Oral Solution and Tablets 3475

Tacrolimus (Co-administration of erythromycin and a drug primarily matabolized by CYP3A, like tacrolimus, may be associated with elevation in drug concentrations that could increase or prolong both the therapeutic and adverse effects of tacrolimus). Products include:

Prograf Capsules and Injection 632
Protopic Ointment 638

Tamoxifen Citrate (Erythromycin is a substrate and inhibitor of the 3A isoform subfamily of the cytochrome p450 enzyme system (CYP3A). Co-administration of erythromycin and a drug primarily metabolized by CYP3A may be associated with elevations in drug concentrations that could increase or prolong both the therapeutic and adverse effects of the concomitant drug). Products include:

Soltamox Oral Solution 3527

Terfenadine (Potential for altered terfenadine metabolism. Co-administration is contraindicated).

No products indexed under this heading.

Testosterone (Erythromycin is a substrate and inhibitor of the 3A isoform subfamily of the cytochrome p450 enzyme system (CYP3A). Co-administration of erythromycin and a drug primarily metabolized by CYP3A may be associated with elevations in drug concentrations that could increase or prolong both the therapeutic and adverse effects of the concomitant drug). Products include:

AndroGel 3329
Striant Mucoadhesive 1007
Testim 1% Gel 695

Testosterone Cypionate (Erythromycin is a substrate and inhibitor of the 3A isoform subfamily of the cytochrome p450 enzyme system (CYP3A). Co-administration of erythromycin and a drug primarily metabolized by CYP3A may be associated with elevations in drug concentrations that could increase or prolong both the therapeutic and adverse effects of the concomitant drug).
No products indexed under this heading.

Testosterone Enanthate (Erythromycin is a substrate and inhibitor of the 3A isoform subfamily of the cytochrome p450 enzyme system (CYP3A). Co-administration of erythromycin and a drug primarily metabolized by CYP3A may be associated with elevations in drug concentrations that could increase or prolong both the therapeutic and adverse effects of the concomitant drug).
No products indexed under this heading.

Testosterone Propionate (Erythromycin is a substrate and inhibitor of the 3A isoform subfamily of the cytochrome p450 enzyme system (CYP3A). Co-administration of erythromycin and a drug primarily metabolized by CYP3A may be associated with elevations in drug concentrations that could increase or prolong both the therapeutic and adverse effects of the concomitant drug).
No products indexed under this heading.

Theophylline (Concomitant administration with high doses of theophylline may be associated with increased theophylline levels and potential toxicity).
No products indexed under this heading.

Theophylline Anhydrous (Concomitant administration with high doses of theophylline may be associated with increased theophylline levels and potential toxicity). Products include:
Uniphyl Tablets 2710

Theophylline Calcium Salicylate (Concomitant administration with high doses of theophylline may be associated with increased theophylline levels and potential toxicity).
No products indexed under this heading.

Theophylline Dihydroxypropyl (Glyceryl) (Concomitant administration with high doses of theophylline may be associated with increased theophylline levels and potential toxicity).
No products indexed under this heading.

Theophylline Ethylenediamine (Concomitant administration with high doses of theophylline may be associated with increased theophylline levels and potential toxicity).
No products indexed under this heading.

Theophylline Sodium Glycinate (Concomitant administration with high doses of theophylline may be associated with increased theophylline levels and potential toxicity).
No products indexed under this heading.

Tiagabine Hydrochloride (Erythromycin is a substrate and inhibitor of the 3A isoform subfamily of the cytochrome p450 enzyme system (CYP3A). Co-administration of erythromycin and a drug primarily metabolized by CYP3A may be associated with elevations in drug concentrations that could increase or prolong both the therapeutic and adverse effects of the concomitant drug). Products include:
Gabitril Tablets 984

Tolterodine Tartrate (Erythromycin is a substrate and inhibitor of the 3A isoform subfamily of the cytochrome p450 enzyme system (CYP3A). Co-administration of erythromycin and a drug primarily metabolized by CYP3A may be associated with elevations in drug concentrations that could increase or prolong both the therapeutic and adverse effects of the concomitant drug). Products include:
Detrol Tablets 2628
Detrol LA Capsules 2631

Trazodone Hydrochloride (Erythromycin is a substrate and inhibitor of the 3A isoform subfamily of the cytochrome p450 enzyme system (CYP3A). Co-administration of erythromycin and a drug primarily metabolized by CYP3A may be associated with elevations in drug concentrations that could increase or prolong both the therapeutic and adverse effects of the concomitant drug).
No products indexed under this heading.

Triazolam (Decreased clearance of triazolam, and thus, may increase the pharmacologic effect of triazolam).
No products indexed under this heading.

Valproate Sodium (There have been reports of interaction of erythromycin with drugs not thought to be metabolized by CYP3A, including valproate). Products include:
Depacon Injection 412

Venlafaxine Hydrochloride (Erythromycin is a substrate and inhibitor of the 3A isoform subfamily of the cytochrome p450 enzyme system (CYP3A). Co-administration of erythromycin and a drug primarily metabolized by CYP3A may be associated with elevations in drug concentrations that could increase or prolong both the therapeutic and adverse effects of the concomitant drug). Products include:
Effexor Tablets 3411
Effexor XR Capsules 3417

Verapamil Hydrochloride (Erythromycin is a substrate and inhibitor of the 3A isoform subfamily of the cytochrome p450 enzyme system (CYP3A). Co-administration of erythromycin and a drug primarily metabolized by CYP3A may be associated with elevations in drug concentrations that could increase or prolong both the therapeutic and adverse effects of the concomitant drug). Products include:
Covera-HS Tablets 3139
Tarka Tablets 524
Verelan PM Extended-Release Capsules, Controlled-Onset 3106

Vinblastine Sulfate (Co-administration of erythromycin and a drug primarily matabolized by CYP3A, like vinblastine, may be associated with elevation in drug concentrations that could increase or prolong both the therapeutic and adverse effects of vinblastine).
No products indexed under this heading.

Vincristine Sulfate (Erythromycin is a substrate and inhibitor of the 3A isoform subfamily of the cytochrome p450 enzyme system (CYP3A). Co-administration of erythromycin and a drug primarily metabolized by CYP3A may be associated with elevations in drug concentrations that could increase or prolong both the therapeutic and adverse effects of the concomitant drug).
No products indexed under this heading.

Warfarin Sodium (Erythromycin is a substrate and inhibitor of the 3A isoform subfamily of the cytochrome p450 enzyme system (CYP3A). Co-administration of erythromycin and a drug primarily metabolized by CYP3A may be associated with elevations in drug concentrations that could increase or prolong both the therapeutic and adverse effects of the concomitant drug). Products include:
Coumadin for Injection 898
Coumadin Tablets 898

Food Interactions

Food, unspecified (Lowers the blood levels of systemically available erythromycin).

ESTRASORB TOPICAL EMULSION

(Estradiol) 1147

May interact with cytochrome p450 3a4 inducers (selected), cytochrome p450 3a4 inhibitors (selected), thyroid preparations, and certain other agents. Compounds in these categories include:

Acetazolamide (Inhibitors of CYP3A4 may increase plasma concentrations of estrogens and may result in side effects).
No products indexed under this heading.

Allium sativum (Inducers of CYP3A4 may reduce plasma concentrations of estrogens, possibly resulting in a decrease in therapeutic effects and/or changes in the uterine bleeding profile).
No products indexed under this heading.

Amiodarone Hydrochloride (Inhibitors of CYP3A4 may increase plasma concentrations of estrogens and may result in side effects).
No products indexed under this heading.

Amprenavir (Inhibitors of CYP3A4 may increase plasma concentrations of estrogens and may result in side effects). Products include:
Agenerase Capsules 1327
Agenerase Oral Solution 1332

Anastrozole (Inhibitors of CYP3A4 may increase plasma concentrations of estrogens and may result in side effects). Products include:
Arimidex Tablets 673

Aprepitant (Inducers of CYP3A4 may reduce plasma concentrations of estrogens, possibly resulting in a decrease in therapeutic effects and/or changes in the uterine bleeding profile). Products include:
Emend Capsules 1963

Betamethasone Acetate (Inducers of CYP3A4 may reduce plasma concentrations of estrogens, possibly resulting in a decrease in therapeutic effects and/or changes in the uterine bleeding profile).
No products indexed under this heading.

Betamethasone Sodium Phosphate (Inducers of CYP3A4 may reduce plasma concentrations of estrogens, possibly resulting in a decrease in therapeutic effects and/or changes in the uterine bleeding profile).
No products indexed under this heading.

Carbamazepine (Inducers of CYP3A4 may reduce plasma concentrations of estrogens, possibly resulting in a decrease in therapeutic effects and/or changes in the uterine bleeding profile). Products include:
Carbatrol Capsules 3171
Equetro Extended-Release Capsules 3180
Tegretol/Tegretol-XR 2295

Cimetidine (Inhibitors of CYP3A4 may increase plasma concentrations of estrogens and may result in side effects). Products include:
Tagamet HB 200 Tablets ..... ▣664

Cimetidine Hydrochloride (Inhibitors of CYP3A4 may increase plasma concentrations of estrogens and may result in side effects).
No products indexed under this heading.

Ciprofloxacin (Inhibitors of CYP3A4 may increase plasma concentrations of estrogens and may result in side effects). Products include:
Cipro Oral Suspension 2977
Cipro I.V. 2984
Cipro XR Tablets 2990
Ciprodex Otic Suspension 559

Ciprofloxacin Hydrochloride (Inducers of CYP3A4 may reduce plasma concentrations of estrogens, possibly resulting in a decrease in therapeutic effects and/or changes in the uterine bleeding profile). Products include:
Ciloxan Ophthalmic Ointment 559
Ciloxan Ophthalmic Solution ..... ⊙206
Cipro Tablets 2977
Proquin XR Tablets 1153

Cisplatin (Inducers of CYP3A4 may reduce plasma concentrations of estrogens, possibly resulting in a decrease in therapeutic effects and/or changes in the uterine bleeding profile).
No products indexed under this heading.

Clarithromycin (Inhibitors of CYP3A4 may increase plasma concentrations of estrogens and may result in side effects). Products include:
Biaxin/Biaxin XL 402
PREVPAC 3284

Clotrimazole (Inhibitors of CYP3A4 may increase plasma concentrations of estrogens and may result in side effects). Products include:
Desenex Athlete's Foot Cream ..... ▣635
Lotrimin 3039
Lotrisone 3040

Cortisone Acetate (Inducers of CYP3A4 may reduce plasma concentrations of estrogens, possibly resulting in a decrease in therapeutic effects and/or changes in the uterine bleeding profile).
No products indexed under this heading.

Cyclosporine (Inhibitors of CYP3A4 may increase plasma concentrations of estrogens and may result in side effects). Products include:
Gengraf Capsules 459
Neoral Oral Solution 2259
Neoral Soft Gelatin Capsules 2259

Restasis Ophthalmic Emulsion 575
Sandimmune 2275

Dalfopristin (Inhibitors of CYP3A4 may increase plasma concentrations of estrogens and may result in side effects).
No products indexed under this heading.

Danazol (Inhibitors of CYP3A4 may increase plasma concentrations of estrogens and may result in side effects).
No products indexed under this heading.

Delavirdine Mesylate (Inhibitors of CYP3A4 may increase plasma concentrations of estrogens and may result in side effects). Products include:
Rescriptor Tablets 2551

Dexamethasone (Inducers of CYP3A4 may reduce plasma concentrations of estrogens, possibly resulting in a decrease in therapeutic effects and/or changes in the uterine bleeding profile). Products include:
Ciprodex Otic Suspension 559
Decadron Tablets 1951
TobraDex Ophthalmic Ointment 562
TobraDex Ophthalmic Suspension ... 563

Dexamethasone Acetate (Inducers of CYP3A4 may reduce plasma concentrations of estrogens, possibly resulting in a decrease in therapeutic effects and/or changes in the uterine bleeding profile).
No products indexed under this heading.

Dexamethasone Sodium Phosphate (Inducers of CYP3A4 may reduce plasma concentrations of estrogens, possibly resulting in a decrease in therapeutic effects and/or changes in the uterine bleeding profile).
No products indexed under this heading.

Diltiazem Hydrochloride (Inhibitors of CYP3A4 may increase plasma concentrations of estrogens and may result in side effects). Products include:
Cardizem LA Extended Release Tablets 1728
Tiazac Capsules 1201

Diltiazem Maleate (Inhibitors of CYP3A4 may increase plasma concentrations of estrogens and may result in side effects).
No products indexed under this heading.

Doxorubicin Hydrochloride (Inducers of CYP3A4 may reduce plasma concentrations of estrogens, possibly resulting in a decrease in therapeutic effects and/or changes in the uterine bleeding profile).
No products indexed under this heading.

Efavirenz (Inducers of CYP3A4 may reduce plasma concentrations of estrogens, possibly resulting in a decrease in therapeutic effects and/or changes in the uterine bleeding profile). Products include:
Atripla Tablets 945
Sustiva Capsules 930
Sustiva Tablets 930

Erythromycin (Inhibitors of CYP3A4 may increase plasma concentrations of estrogens and may result in side effects). Products include:
Ery-Tab Tablets 449
Erythromycin Base Filmtab Tablets 455
Erythromycin Delayed-Release Capsules, USP.............................. 457
PCE Dispertab Tablets 515

Erythromycin Estolate (Inhibitors of CYP3A4 may increase plasma concentrations of estrogens and may result in side effects).
No products indexed under this heading.

Erythromycin Ethylsuccinate (Inhibitors of CYP3A4 may increase plasma concentrations of estrogens and may result in side effects). Products include:
E.E.S. 451
EryPed 447

Erythromycin Gluceptate (Inhibitors of CYP3A4 may increase plasma concentrations of estrogens and may result in side effects).
No products indexed under this heading.

Erythromycin Lactobionate (Inhibitors of CYP3A4 may increase plasma concentrations of estrogens and may result in side effects).
No products indexed under this heading.

Erythromycin Stearate (Inhibitors of CYP3A4 may increase plasma concentrations of estrogens and may result in side effects). Products include:
Erythrocin Stearate Filmtab Tablets 453

Esomeprazole Magnesium (Inhibitors of CYP3A4 may increase plasma concentrations of estrogens and may result in side effects). Products include:
Nexium Delayed-Release Capsules...................................... 655

Ethosuximide (Inducers of CYP3A4 may reduce plasma concentrations of estrogens, possibly resulting in a decrease in therapeutic effects and/or changes in the uterine bleeding profile).
No products indexed under this heading.

Felbamate (Inducers of CYP3A4 may reduce plasma concentrations of estrogens, possibly resulting in a decrease in therapeutic effects and/or changes in the uterine bleeding profile).
No products indexed under this heading.

Fluconazole (Inhibitors of CYP3A4 may increase plasma concentrations of estrogens and may result in side effects).
No products indexed under this heading.

Fludrocortisone Acetate (Inducers of CYP3A4 may reduce plasma concentrations of estrogens, possibly resulting in a decrease in therapeutic effects and/or changes in the uterine bleeding profile).
No products indexed under this heading.

Fluoxetine Hydrochloride (Inhibitors of CYP3A4 may increase plasma concentrations of estrogens and may result in side effects). Products include:
Prozac Pulvules and Liquid 1801
Symbyax Capsules 1819

Fluvoxamine Maleate (Inhibitors of CYP3A4 may increase plasma concentrations of estrogens and may result in side effects).
No products indexed under this heading.

Fosamprenavir Calcium (Inhibitors of CYP3A4 may increase plasma concentrations of estrogens and may result in side effects). Products include:
Lexiva Tablets 1505

Fosphenytoin Sodium (Inducers of CYP3A4 may reduce plasma concentrations of estrogens, possibly resulting in a decrease in therapeutic effects and/or changes in the uterine bleeding profile).
No products indexed under this heading.

Garlic Extract (Inducers of CYP3A4 may reduce plasma concentrations of estrogens, possibly resulting in a decrease in therapeutic effects and/or changes in the uterine bleeding profile).
No products indexed under this heading.

Garlic Oil (Inducers of CYP3A4 may reduce plasma concentrations of estrogens, possibly resulting in a decrease in therapeutic effects and/or changes in the uterine bleeding profile).
No products indexed under this heading.

Hydrocortisone (Inducers of CYP3A4 may reduce plasma concentrations of estrogens, possibly resulting in a decrease in therapeutic effects and/or changes in the uterine bleeding profile). Products include:
Colocort Rectal Suspension, USP (Retention) 100 mg/60 mL........... 2476
Hydrocortone Tablets 1989
Preparation H Hydrocortisone Cream.. ▣646

Hydrocortisone Acetate (Inducers of CYP3A4 may reduce plasma concentrations of estrogens, possibly resulting in a decrease in therapeutic effects and/or changes in the uterine bleeding profile). Products include:
Analpram-HC 1159
Pramosone 1161
ProctoFoam-HC 3099

Hydrocortisone Butyrate (Inducers of CYP3A4 may reduce plasma concentrations of estrogens, possibly resulting in a decrease in therapeutic effects and/or changes in the uterine bleeding profile). Products include:
Locoid Lipocream Cream 1160

Hydrocortisone Cypionate (Inducers of CYP3A4 may reduce plasma concentrations of estrogens, possibly resulting in a decrease in therapeutic effects and/or changes in the uterine bleeding profile).
No products indexed under this heading.

Hydrocortisone Hemisuccinate (Inducers of CYP3A4 may reduce plasma concentrations of estrogens, possibly resulting in a decrease in therapeutic effects and/or changes in the uterine bleeding profile).
No products indexed under this heading.

Hydrocortisone Probutate (Inducers of CYP3A4 may reduce plasma concentrations of estrogens, possibly resulting in a decrease in therapeutic effects and/or changes in the uterine bleeding profile).
No products indexed under this heading.

Hydrocortisone Sodium Phosphate (Inducers of CYP3A4 may reduce plasma concentrations of estrogens, possibly resulting in a decrease in therapeutic effects and/or changes in the uterine bleeding profile).
No products indexed under this heading.

Hydrocortisone Sodium Succinate (Inducers of CYP3A4 may reduce plasma concentrations of estrogens, possibly resulting in a decrease in therapeutic effects and/or changes in the uterine bleeding profile).
No products indexed under this heading.

Hydrocortisone Valerate (Inducers of CYP3A4 may reduce plasma concentrations of estrogens, possibly resulting in a decrease in therapeutic effects and/or changes in the uterine bleeding profile).
No products indexed under this heading.

Hypericum (Inducers of CYP3A4 may reduce plasma concentrations of estrogens, possibly resulting in a decrease in therapeutic effects and/or changes in the uterine bleeding profile). Products include:
Satiete Tablets .... ▣832

Hypericum Perforatum (Inducers of CYP3A4 may reduce plasma concentrations of estrogens, possibly resulting in a decrease in therapeutic effects and/or changes in the uterine bleeding profile).
No products indexed under this heading.

Indinavir Sulfate (Inhibitors of CYP3A4 may increase plasma concentrations of estrogens and may result in side effects). Products include:
Crixivan Capsules 1940

Isoniazid (Inhibitors of CYP3A4 may increase plasma concentrations of estrogens and may result in side effects).
No products indexed under this heading.

Itraconazole (Inhibitors of CYP3A4 may increase plasma concentrations of estrogens and may result in side effects).
No products indexed under this heading.

Ketoconazole (Inhibitors of CYP3A4 may increase plasma concentrations of estrogens and may result in side effects). Products include:
Nizoral A-D Shampoo, 1% 1868

Levothyroxine Sodium (Estrogen administration leads to increased thyroid-binding globulin (TBG) levels. Patients dependent on thyroid hormone replacement therapy who are also receiving estrogens may require increased doses of their thyroid replacement therapy). Products include:
Levothroid Tablets 1186
Levoxyl Tablets 1712
Synthroid Tablets 520
Westhroid Tablets 3403

Liothyronine Sodium (Estrogen administration leads to increased thyroid-binding globulin (TBG) levels. Patients dependent on thyroid hormone replacement therapy who are also receiving estrogens may require increased doses of their thyroid replacement therapy). Products include:

Liotrix (Estrogen administration leads to increased thyroid-binding globulin (TBG) levels. Patients dependent on thyroid hormone replacement therapy who are also receiving estrogens may require increased doses of their thyroid replacement therapy). Products include:

Lopinavir (Inhibitors of CYP3A4 may increase plasma concentrations of estrogens and may result in side effects). Products include:

Loratadine (Inhibitors of CYP3A4 may increase plasma concentrations of estrogens and may result in side effects). Products include:

Mephenytoin (Inducers of CYP3A4 may reduce plasma concentrations of estrogens, possibly resulting in a decrease in therapeutic effects and/or changes in the uterine bleeding profile).
No products indexed under this heading.

Methsuximide (Inducers of CYP3A4 may reduce plasma concentrations of estrogens, possibly resulting in a decrease in therapeutic effects and/or changes in the uterine bleeding profile).
No products indexed under this heading.

Methylprednisolone (Inducers of CYP3A4 may reduce plasma concentrations of estrogens, possibly resulting in a decrease in therapeutic effects and/or changes in the uterine bleeding profile).
No products indexed under this heading.

Methylprednisolone Acetate (Inducers of CYP3A4 may reduce plasma concentrations of estrogens, possibly resulting in a decrease in therapeutic effects and/or changes in the uterine bleeding profile). Products include:

Methylprednisolone Sodium Succinate (Inducers of CYP3A4 may reduce plasma concentrations of estrogens, possibly resulting in a decrease in therapeutic effects and/or changes in the uterine bleeding profile).
No products indexed under this heading.

Metronidazole (Inhibitors of CYP3A4 may increase plasma concentrations of estrogens and may result in side effects). Products include:

Metronidazole Benzoate (Inhibitors of CYP3A4 may increase plasma concentrations of estrogens and may result in side effects).
No products indexed under this heading.

Metronidazole Hydrochloride (Inhibitors of CYP3A4 may increase plasma concentrations of estrogens and may result in side effects).
No products indexed under this heading.

Miconazole (Inhibitors of CYP3A4 may increase plasma concentrations of estrogens and may result in side effects).
No products indexed under this heading.

Miconazole Nitrate (Inhibitors of CYP3A4 may increase plasma concentrations of estrogens and may result in side effects). Products include:

Modafinil (Inducers of CYP3A4 may reduce plasma concentrations of estrogens, possibly resulting in a decrease in therapeutic effects and/or changes in the uterine bleeding profile). Products include:

Nefazodone Hydrochloride (Inhibitors of CYP3A4 may increase plasma concentrations of estrogens and may result in side effects).
No products indexed under this heading.

Nelfinavir Mesylate (Inhibitors of CYP3A4 may increase plasma concentrations of estrogens and may result in side effects). Products include:

Nevirapine (Inducers of CYP3A4 may reduce plasma concentrations of estrogens, possibly resulting in a decrease in therapeutic effects and/or changes in the uterine bleeding profile). Products include:

Niacinamide (Inhibitors of CYP3A4 may increase plasma concentrations of estrogens and may result in side effects).
No products indexed under this heading.

Nicotinamide (Inhibitors of CYP3A4 may increase plasma concentrations of estrogens and may result in side effects). Products include:

Nifedipine (Inhibitors of CYP3A4 may increase plasma concentrations of estrogens and may result in side effects). Products include:

Norfloxacin (Inhibitors of CYP3A4 may increase plasma concentrations of estrogens and may result in side effects). Products include:

Omeprazole (Inhibitors of CYP3A4 may increase plasma concentrations of estrogens and may result in side effects). Products include:

Oxcarbazepine (Inducers of CYP3A4 may reduce plasma concentrations of estrogens, possibly resulting in a decrease in therapeutic effects and/or changes in the uterine bleeding profile). Products include:

Paroxetine Hydrochloride (Inhibitors of CYP3A4 may increase plasma concentrations of estrogens and may result in side effects). Products include:

Phenobarbital (Inducers of CYP3A4 may reduce plasma concentrations of estrogens, possibly resulting in a decrease in therapeutic effects and/or changes in the uterine bleeding profile). Products include:

Phenobarbital Sodium (Inducers of CYP3A4 may reduce plasma concentrations of estrogens, possibly resulting in a decrease in therapeutic effects and/or changes in the uterine bleeding profile).
No products indexed under this heading.

Phenytoin (Inducers of CYP3A4 may reduce plasma concentrations of estrogens, possibly resulting in a decrease in therapeutic effects and/or changes in the uterine bleeding profile).
No products indexed under this heading.

Phenytoin Sodium (Inducers of CYP3A4 may reduce plasma concentrations of estrogens, possibly resulting in a decrease in therapeutic effects and/or changes in the uterine bleeding profile). Products include:

Prednisolone Acetate (Inducers of CYP3A4 may reduce plasma concentrations of estrogens, possibly resulting in a decrease in therapeutic effects and/or changes in the uterine bleeding profile). Products include:

Prednisolone Sodium Phosphate (Inducers of CYP3A4 may reduce plasma concentrations of estrogens, possibly resulting in a decrease in therapeutic effects and/or changes in the uterine bleeding profile).
No products indexed under this heading.

Prednisolone Tebutate (Inducers of CYP3A4 may reduce plasma concentrations of estrogens, possibly resulting in a decrease in therapeutic effects and/or changes in the uterine bleeding profile).
No products indexed under this heading.

Prednisone (Inducers of CYP3A4 may reduce plasma concentrations of estrogens, possibly resulting in a decrease in therapeutic effects and/or changes in the uterine bleeding profile).
No products indexed under this heading.

Primidone (Inducers of CYP3A4 may reduce plasma concentrations of estrogens, possibly resulting in a decrease in therapeutic effects and/or changes in the uterine bleeding profile).
No products indexed under this heading.

Propoxyphene Hydrochloride (Inhibitors of CYP3A4 may increase plasma concentrations of estrogens and may result in side effects).
No products indexed under this heading.

Propoxyphene Napsylate (Inhibitors of CYP3A4 may increase plasma concentrations of estrogens and may result in side effects).
No products indexed under this heading.

Quinidine (Inhibitors of CYP3A4 may increase plasma concentrations of estrogens and may result in side effects).
No products indexed under this heading.

Quinidine Hydrochloride (Inhibitors of CYP3A4 may increase plasma concentrations of estrogens and may result in side effects).
No products indexed under this heading.

Quinidine Polygalacturonate (Inhibitors of CYP3A4 may increase plasma concentrations of estrogens and may result in side effects).
No products indexed under this heading.

Quinidine Sulfate (Inhibitors of CYP3A4 may increase plasma concentrations of estrogens and may result in side effects).
No products indexed under this heading.

Quinine (Inhibitors of CYP3A4 may increase plasma concentrations of estrogens and may result in side effects).
No products indexed under this heading.

Quinine Sulfate (Inhibitors of CYP3A4 may increase plasma concentrations of estrogens and may result in side effects).
No products indexed under this heading.

Quinupristin (Inhibitors of CYP3A4 may increase plasma concentrations of estrogens and may result in side effects).
No products indexed under this heading.

Ranitidine Bismuth Citrate (Inhibitors of CYP3A4 may increase plasma concentrations of estrogens and may result in side effects).
No products indexed under this heading.

Ranitidine Hydrochloride (Inhibitors of CYP3A4 may increase plasma concentrations of estrogens and may result in side effects). Products include:

Rifabutin (Inducers of CYP3A4 may reduce plasma concentrations of estrogens, possibly resulting in a decrease in therapeutic effects and/or changes in the uterine bleeding profile).
No products indexed under this heading.

Rifampicin (Inducers of CYP3A4 may reduce plasma concentrations of estrogens, possibly resulting in a decrease in therapeutic effects and/or changes in the uterine bleeding profile).
No products indexed under this heading.

Rifampin (Inducers of CYP3A4 may reduce plasma concentrations of estrogens, possibly resulting in a decrease in therapeutic effects and/or changes in the uterine bleeding profile).
No products indexed under this heading.

Rifapentine (Inducers of CYP3A4 may reduce plasma concentrations of estrogens, possibly resulting in a decrease in therapeutic effects and/or changes in the uterine bleeding profile).
No products indexed under this heading.

Ritonavir (Inhibitors of CYP3A4 may increase plasma concentrations of estrogens and may result in side effects). Products include:
Kaletra 476
Norvir 503

Saquinavir (Inhibitors of CYP3A4 may increase plasma concentrations of estrogens and may result in side effects).
No products indexed under this heading.

Saquinavir Mesylate (Inhibitors of CYP3A4 may increase plasma concentrations of estrogens and may result in side effects). Products include:
Invirase 2772

Sertraline Hydrochloride (Inhibitors of CYP3A4 may increase plasma concentrations of estrogens and may result in side effects). Products include:
Zoloft 2586

Sulfinpyrazone (Inducers of CYP3A4 may reduce plasma concentrations of estrogens, possibly resulting in a decrease in therapeutic effects and/or changes in the uterine bleeding profile).
No products indexed under this heading.

Telithromycin (Inhibitors of CYP3A4 may increase plasma concentrations of estrogens and may result in side effects). Products include:
Ketek Tablets 2903

Theophylline (Inducers of CYP3A4 may reduce plasma concentrations of estrogens, possibly resulting in a decrease in therapeutic effects and/or changes in the uterine bleeding profile).
No products indexed under this heading.

Thyroglobulin (Estrogen administration leads to increased thyroid-binding globulin (TBG) levels. Patients dependent on thyroid hormone replacement therapy who are also receiving estrogens may require increased doses of their thyroid replacement therapy).
No products indexed under this heading.

Thyroid (Estrogen administration leads to increased thyroid-binding globulin (TBG) levels. Patients dependent on thyroid hormone replacement therapy who are also receiving estrogens may require increased doses of their thyroid replacement therapy).
No products indexed under this heading.

Thyroxine (Estrogen administration leads to increased thyroid-binding globulin (TBG) levels. Patients dependent on thyroid hormone replacement therapy who are also receiving estrogens may require increased doses of their thyroid replacement therapy).
No products indexed under this heading.

Thyroxine Sodium (Estrogen administration leads to increased thyroid-binding globulin (TBG) levels. Patients dependent on thyroid hormone replacement therapy who are also receiving estrogens may require increased doses of their thyroid replacement therapy).
No products indexed under this heading.

Triamcinolone (Inducers of CYP3A4 may reduce plasma concentrations of estrogens, possibly resulting in a decrease in therapeutic effects and/or changes in the uterine bleeding profile).
No products indexed under this heading.

Triamcinolone Acetonide (Inducers of CYP3A4 may reduce plasma concentrations of estrogens, possibly resulting in a decrease in therapeutic effects and/or changes in the uterine bleeding profile). Products include:
Azmacort Inhalation Aerosol 1726
Nasacort AQ Nasal Spray 2922

Triamcinolone Diacetate (Inducers of CYP3A4 may reduce plasma concentrations of estrogens, possibly resulting in a decrease in therapeutic effects and/or changes in the uterine bleeding profile).
No products indexed under this heading.

Triamcinolone Hexacetonide (Inducers of CYP3A4 may reduce plasma concentrations of estrogens, possibly resulting in a decrease in therapeutic effects and/or changes in the uterine bleeding profile).
No products indexed under this heading.

Troglitazone (Inducers of CYP3A4 may reduce plasma concentrations of estrogens, possibly resulting in a decrease in therapeutic effects and/or changes in the uterine bleeding profile).
No products indexed under this heading.

Troleandomycin (Inhibitors of CYP3A4 may increase plasma concentrations of estrogens and may result in side effects).
No products indexed under this heading.

Valproate Sodium (Inhibitors of CYP3A4 may increase plasma concentrations of estrogens and may result in side effects). Products include:
Depacon Injection 412

Verapamil Hydrochloride (Inhibitors of CYP3A4 may increase plasma concentrations of estrogens and may result in side effects). Products include:
Covera-HS Tablets 3139
Tarka Tablets 524
Verelan PM Extended-Release Capsules, Controlled-Onset 3106

Voriconazole (Inhibitors of CYP3A4 may increase plasma concentrations of estrogens and may result in side effects). Products include:
VFEND I.V. 2564
VFEND Oral Suspension 2564
VFEND Tablets 2564

Zafirlukast (Inhibitors of CYP3A4 may increase plasma concentrations of estrogens and may result in side effects). Products include:
Accolate Tablets 671

Zileuton (Inhibitors of CYP3A4 may increase plasma concentrations of estrogens and may result in side effects). Products include:
Zyflo Tablets 1023

Food Interactions

Grapefruit (Inhibitors of CYP3A4 may increase plasma concentrations of estrogens and may result in side effects).

Grapefruit Juice (Inhibitors of CYP3A4 may increase plasma concentrations of estrogens and may result in side effects).

ESTRATEST TABLETS

(Estrogens, Esterified, Methyltestosterone).......... 3199
See Estratest H.S. Tablets

ESTRATEST H.S. TABLETS

(Estrogens, Esterified, Methyltestosterone).......... 3199
May interact with oral anticoagulants, cytochrome p450 3a4 inducers (selected), cytochrome p450 3a4 inhibitors (selected), insulin, and certain other agents. Compounds in these categories include:

Acetazolamide (Co-administration with inhibitors of CYP3A4 may increase plasma concentrations of estrogens and may result in side effects).
No products indexed under this heading.

Allium sativum (Co-administration with inducers of CYP3A4 may reduce plasma concentrations of estrogens, possibly resulting in a decrease in therapeutic effects and/or changes in uterine bleeding profile).
No products indexed under this heading.

Amiodarone Hydrochloride (Co-administration with inhibitors of CYP3A4 may increase plasma concentrations of estrogens and may result in side effects).
No products indexed under this heading.

Amprenavir (Co-administration with inhibitors of CYP3A4 may increase plasma concentrations of estrogens and may result in side effects). Products include:
Agenerase Capsules 1327
Agenerase Oral Solution 1332

Anastrozole (Co-administration with inhibitors of CYP3A4 may increase plasma concentrations of estrogens and may result in side effects). Products include:
Arimidex Tablets 673

Anisindione (Decreased anticoagulant requirements). Products include:
Miradon Tablets 3042

Aprepitant (Co-administration with inducers of CYP3A4 may reduce plasma concentrations of estrogens, possibly resulting in a decrease in therapeutic effects and/or changes in uterine bleeding profile). Products include:
Emend Capsules 1963

Betamethasone Acetate (Co-administration with inducers of CYP3A4 may reduce plasma concentrations of estrogens, possibly resulting in a decrease in therapeutic effects and/or changes in uterine bleeding profile).
No products indexed under this heading.

Betamethasone Sodium Phosphate (Co-administration with inducers of CYP3A4 may reduce plasma concentrations of estrogens, possibly resulting in a decrease in therapeutic effects and/or changes in uterine bleeding profile).
No products indexed under this heading.

Carbamazepine (Co-administration with inducers of CYP3A4 may reduce plasma concentrations of estrogens, possibly resulting in a decrease in therapeutic effects and/or changes in uterine bleeding profile). Products include:
Carbatrol Capsules 3171
Equetro Extended-Release Capsules 3180
Tegretol/Tegretol-XR 2295

Cimetidine (Co-administration with inhibitors of CYP3A4 may increase plasma concentrations of estrogens and may result in side effects). Products include:
Tagamet HB 200 Tablets .... ▣664

Cimetidine Hydrochloride (Co-administration with inhibitors of CYP3A4 may increase plasma concentrations of estrogens and may result in side effects).
No products indexed under this heading.

Ciprofloxacin (Co-administration with inhibitors of CYP3A4 may increase plasma concentrations of estrogens and may result in side effects). Products include:
Cipro Oral Suspension 2977
Cipro I.V. 2984
Cipro XR Tablets 2990
Ciprodex Otic Suspension 559

Ciprofloxacin Hydrochloride (Co-administration with inducers of CYP3A4 may reduce plasma concentrations of estrogens, possibly resulting in a decrease in therapeutic effects and/or changes in uterine bleeding profile). Products include:
Ciloxan Ophthalmic Ointment 559
Ciloxan Ophthalmic Solution .... ⊙206
Cipro Tablets 2977
Proquin XR Tablets 1153

Cisplatin (Co-administration with inducers of CYP3A4 may reduce plasma concentrations of estrogens, possibly resulting in a decrease in therapeutic effects and/or changes in uterine bleeding profile).
No products indexed under this heading.

Clarithromycin (Co-administration with inhibitors of CYP3A4 may increase plasma concentrations of estrogens and may result in side effects). Products include:
Biaxin/Biaxin XL 402
PREVPAC 3284

Clotrimazole (Co-administration with inhibitors of CYP3A4 may increase plasma concentrations of estrogens and may result in side effects). Products include:

- Desenex Athlete's Foot Cream .... ■ **635**
- Lotrimin **3039**
- Lotrisone **3040**

Cortisone Acetate (Co-administration with inducers of CYP3A4 may reduce plasma concentrations of estrogens, possibly resulting in a decrease in therapeutic effects and/or changes in uterine bleeding profile).

No products indexed under this heading.

Cyclosporine (Co-administration with inhibitors of CYP3A4 may increase plasma concentrations of estrogens and may result in side effects). Products include:

- Gengraf Capsules **459**
- Neoral Oral Solution **2259**
- Neoral Soft Gelatin Capsules **2259**
- Restasis Ophthalmic Emulsion **575**
- Sandimmune **2275**

Dalfopristin (Co-administration with inhibitors of CYP3A4 may increase plasma concentrations of estrogens and may result in side effects).

No products indexed under this heading.

Danazol (Co-administration with inhibitors of CYP3A4 may increase plasma concentrations of estrogens and may result in side effects).

No products indexed under this heading.

Delavirdine Mesylate (Co-administration with inhibitors of CYP3A4 may increase plasma concentrations of estrogens and may result in side effects). Products include:

- Rescriptor Tablets **2551**

Dexamethasone (Co-administration with inducers of CYP3A4 may reduce plasma concentrations of estrogens, possibly resulting in a decrease in therapeutic effects and/or changes in uterine bleeding profile). Products include:

- Ciprodex Otic Suspension **559**
- Decadron Tablets **1951**
- TobraDex Ophthalmic Ointment **562**
- TobraDex Ophthalmic Suspension ... **563**

Dexamethasone Acetate (Co-administration with inducers of CYP3A4 may reduce plasma concentrations of estrogens, possibly resulting in a decrease in therapeutic effects and/or changes in uterine bleeding profile).

No products indexed under this heading.

Dexamethasone Sodium Phosphate (Co-administration with inducers of CYP3A4 may reduce plasma concentrations of estrogens, possibly resulting in a decrease in therapeutic effects and/or changes in uterine bleeding profile).

No products indexed under this heading.

Dicumarol (Decreased anticoagulant requirements).

No products indexed under this heading.

Diltiazem Hydrochloride (Co-administration with inhibitors of CYP3A4 may increase plasma concentrations of estrogens and may result in side effects). Products include:

- Cardizem LA Extended Release Tablets **1728**
- Tiazac Capsules **1201**

Diltiazem Maleate (Co-administration with inhibitors of CYP3A4 may increase plasma concentrations of estrogens and may result in side effects).

No products indexed under this heading.

Doxorubicin Hydrochloride (Co-administration with inducers of CYP3A4 may reduce plasma concentrations of estrogens, possibly resulting in a decrease in therapeutic effects and/or changes in uterine bleeding profile).

No products indexed under this heading.

Efavirenz (Co-administration with inducers of CYP3A4 may reduce plasma concentrations of estrogens, possibly resulting in a decrease in therapeutic effects and/or changes in uterine bleeding profile). Products include:

- Atripla Tablets **945**
- Sustiva Capsules **930**
- Sustiva Tablets **930**

Erythromycin (Co-administration with inhibitors of CYP3A4 may increase plasma concentrations of estrogens and may result in side effects). Products include:

- Ery-Tab Tablets **449**
- Erythromycin Base Filmtab Tablets **455**
- Erythromycin Delayed-Release Capsules, USP **457**
- PCE Dispertab Tablets **515**

Erythromycin Estolate (Co-administration with inhibitors of CYP3A4 may increase plasma concentrations of estrogens and may result in side effects).

No products indexed under this heading.

Erythromycin Ethylsuccinate (Co-administration with inhibitors of CYP3A4 may increase plasma concentrations of estrogens and may result in side effects). Products include:

- E.E.S. **451**
- EryPed **447**

Erythromycin Gluceptate (Co-administration with inhibitors of CYP3A4 may increase plasma concentrations of estrogens and may result in side effects).

No products indexed under this heading.

Erythromycin Lactobionate (Co-administration with inhibitors of CYP3A4 may increase plasma concentrations of estrogens and may result in side effects).

No products indexed under this heading.

Erythromycin Stearate (Co-administration with inhibitors of CYP3A4 may increase plasma concentrations of estrogens and may result in side effects). Products include:

- Erythrocin Stearate Filmtab Tablets **453**

Esomeprazole Magnesium (Co-administration with inhibitors of CYP3A4 may increase plasma concentrations of estrogens and may result in side effects). Products include:

- Nexium Delayed-Release Capsules **655**

Ethosuximide (Co-administration with inducers of CYP3A4 may reduce plasma concentrations of estrogens, possibly resulting in a decrease in therapeutic effects and/or changes in uterine bleeding profile).

No products indexed under this heading.

Felbamate (Co-administration with inducers of CYP3A4 may reduce plasma concentrations of estrogens, possibly resulting in a decrease in therapeutic effects and/or changes in uterine bleeding profile).

No products indexed under this heading.

Fluconazole (Co-administration with inhibitors of CYP3A4 may increase plasma concentrations of estrogens and may result in side effects).

No products indexed under this heading.

Fludrocortisone Acetate (Co-administration with inducers of CYP3A4 may reduce plasma concentrations of estrogens, possibly resulting in a decrease in therapeutic effects and/or changes in uterine bleeding profile).

No products indexed under this heading.

Fluoxetine Hydrochloride (Co-administration with inhibitors of CYP3A4 may increase plasma concentrations of estrogens and may result in side effects). Products include:

- Prozac Pulvules and Liquid **1801**
- Symbyax Capsules **1819**

Fluvoxamine Maleate (Co-administration with inhibitors of CYP3A4 may increase plasma concentrations of estrogens and may result in side effects).

No products indexed under this heading.

Fosamprenavir Calcium (Co-administration with inhibitors of CYP3A4 may increase plasma concentrations of estrogens and may result in side effects). Products include:

- Lexiva Tablets **1505**

Fosphenytoin Sodium (Co-administration with inducers of CYP3A4 may reduce plasma concentrations of estrogens, possibly resulting in a decrease in therapeutic effects and/or changes in uterine bleeding profile).

No products indexed under this heading.

Garlic Extract (Co-administration with inducers of CYP3A4 may reduce plasma concentrations of estrogens, possibly resulting in a decrease in therapeutic effects and/or changes in uterine bleeding profile).

No products indexed under this heading.

Garlic Oil (Co-administration with inducers of CYP3A4 may reduce plasma concentrations of estrogens, possibly resulting in a decrease in therapeutic effects and/or changes in uterine bleeding profile).

No products indexed under this heading.

Hydrocortisone (Co-administration with inducers of CYP3A4 may reduce plasma concentrations of estrogens, possibly resulting in a decrease in therapeutic effects and/or changes in uterine bleeding profile). Products include:

- Colocort Rectal Suspension, USP (Retention) 100 mg/60 mL **2476**
- Hydrocortone Tablets **1989**
- Preparation H Hydrocortisone Cream .... ■ **646**

Hydrocortisone Acetate (Co-administration with inducers of CYP3A4 may reduce plasma concentrations of estrogens, possibly resulting in a decrease in therapeutic effects and/or changes in uterine bleeding profile). Products include:

- Analpram-HC **1159**
- Pramosone **1161**
- ProctoFoam-HC **3099**

Hydrocortisone Butyrate (Co-administration with inducers of CYP3A4 may reduce plasma concentrations of estrogens, possibly resulting in a decrease in therapeutic effects and/or changes in uterine bleeding profile). Products include:

- Locoid Lipocream Cream **1160**

Hydrocortisone Cypionate (Co-administration with inducers of CYP3A4 may reduce plasma concentrations of estrogens, possibly resulting in a decrease in therapeutic effects and/or changes in uterine bleeding profile).

No products indexed under this heading.

Hydrocortisone Hemisuccinate (Co-administration with inducers of CYP3A4 may reduce plasma concentrations of estrogens, possibly resulting in a decrease in therapeutic effects and/or changes in uterine bleeding profile).

No products indexed under this heading.

Hydrocortisone Probutate (Co-administration with inducers of CYP3A4 may reduce plasma concentrations of estrogens, possibly resulting in a decrease in therapeutic effects and/or changes in uterine bleeding profile).

No products indexed under this heading.

Hydrocortisone Sodium Phosphate (Co-administration with inducers of CYP3A4 may reduce plasma concentrations of estrogens, possibly resulting in a decrease in therapeutic effects and/or changes in uterine bleeding profile).

No products indexed under this heading.

Hydrocortisone Sodium Succinate (Co-administration with inducers of CYP3A4 may reduce plasma concentrations of estrogens, possibly resulting in a decrease in therapeutic effects and/or changes in uterine bleeding profile).

No products indexed under this heading.

Hydrocortisone Valerate (Co-administration with inducers of CYP3A4 may reduce plasma concentrations of estrogens, possibly resulting in a decrease in therapeutic effects and/or changes in uterine bleeding profile).

No products indexed under this heading.

Hypericum (Co-administration with inducers of CYP3A4 may reduce plasma concentrations of estrogens, possibly resulting in a decrease in therapeutic effects and/or changes in uterine bleeding profile). Products include:

Satiete Tablets ...... ■832

Hypericum Perforatum (Co-administration with inducers of CYP3A4 may reduce plasma concentrations of estrogens, possibly resulting in a decrease in therapeutic effects and/or changes in uterine bleeding profile).
No products indexed under this heading.

Indinavir Sulfate (Co-administration with inhibitors of CYP3A4 may increase plasma concentrations of estrogens and may result in side effects). Products include:
Crixivan Capsules 1940

Insulin, Human, Zinc Suspension (Decreased blood glucose and insulin requirements). Products include:
Humulin L, 100 Units 1794
Humulin U, 100 Units 1800

Insulin, Human NPH (Decreased blood glucose and insulin requirements). Products include:
Humulin N, 100 Units 1795
Humulin N Pen 1797

Insulin, Human Regular (Decreased blood glucose and insulin requirements). Products include:
Humulin R, 100 Units 1798

Insulin, Human Regular and Human NPH Mixture (Decreased blood glucose and insulin requirements). Products include:
Humulin 50/50, 100 Units 1791
Humulin 70/30 Pen 1793

Insulin, NPH (Decreased blood glucose and insulin requirements).
No products indexed under this heading.

Insulin, Regular (Decreased blood glucose and insulin requirements).
No products indexed under this heading.

Insulin, Zinc Crystals (Decreased blood glucose and insulin requirements).
No products indexed under this heading.

Insulin, Zinc Suspension (Decreased blood glucose and insulin requirements).
No products indexed under this heading.

Insulin Aspart, Human Regular (Decreased blood glucose and insulin requirements). Products include:
NovoLog Injection 2326

Insulin glargine (Decreased blood glucose and insulin requirements). Products include:
Lantus Injection 2909

Insulin Lispro, Human (Decreased blood glucose and insulin requirements). Products include:
Humalog-Pen 1781
Humalog Mix 50/50-Pen 1783
Humalog Mix 75/25-Pen 1785

Insulin Lispro Protamine, Human (Decreased blood glucose and insulin requirements). Products include:
Humalog Mix 50/50-Pen 1783
Humalog Mix 75/25-Pen 1785

Isoniazid (Co-administration with inhibitors of CYP3A4 may increase plasma concentrations of estrogens and may result in side effects).
No products indexed under this heading.

Itraconazole (Co-administration with inhibitors of CYP3A4 may increase plasma concentrations of estrogens and may result in side effects).
No products indexed under this heading.

Ketoconazole (Co-administration with inhibitors of CYP3A4 may increase plasma concentrations of estrogens and may result in side effects). Products include:
Nizoral A-D Shampoo, 1% 1868

Lopinavir (Co-administration with inhibitors of CYP3A4 may increase plasma concentrations of estrogens and may result in side effects). Products include:
Kaletra 476

Loratadine (Co-administration with inhibitors of CYP3A4 may increase plasma concentrations of estrogens and may result in side effects). Products include:
Alavert Allergy & Sinus D-12 Hour Tablets ...... ■771
Alavert ...... ■771
Children's Claritin Allergy Oral Solution ...... ■771
Claritin Non-Drowsy 24 Hour Tablets ...... ■772
Claritin Reditabs 24 Hour Non-Drowsy Tablets ...... ■772
Claritin-D Non-Drowsy 12 Hour Tablets ...... ■772
Claritin-D Non-Drowsy 24 Hour Tablets ...... ■772

Mephenytoin (Co-administration with inducers of CYP3A4 may reduce plasma concentrations of estrogens, possibly resulting in a decrease in therapeutic effects and/or changes in uterine bleeding profile).
No products indexed under this heading.

Methsuximide (Co-administration with inducers of CYP3A4 may reduce plasma concentrations of estrogens, possibly resulting in a decrease in therapeutic effects and/or changes in uterine bleeding profile).
No products indexed under this heading.

Methylprednisolone (Co-administration with inducers of CYP3A4 may reduce plasma concentrations of estrogens, possibly resulting in a decrease in therapeutic effects and/or changes in uterine bleeding profile).
No products indexed under this heading.

Methylprednisolone Acetate (Co-administration with inducers of CYP3A4 may reduce plasma concentrations of estrogens, possibly resulting in a decrease in therapeutic effects and/or changes in uterine bleeding profile). Products include:
Depo-Medrol Injectable Suspension 2617
Depo-Medrol Single-Dose Vial 2619

Methylprednisolone Sodium Succinate (Co-administration with inducers of CYP3A4 may reduce plasma concentrations of estrogens, possibly resulting in a decrease in therapeutic effects and/or changes in uterine bleeding profile).
No products indexed under this heading.

Metronidazole (Co-administration with inhibitors of CYP3A4 may increase plasma concentrations of estrogens and may result in side effects). Products include:
Metrogel 1% 1211
MetroGel-Vaginal Gel 1855
Vandazole Vaginal Gel 3338

Metronidazole Benzoate (Co-administration with inhibitors of CYP3A4 may increase plasma concentrations of estrogens and may result in side effects).
No products indexed under this heading.

Metronidazole Hydrochloride (Co-administration with inhibitors of CYP3A4 may increase plasma concentrations of estrogens and may result in side effects).
No products indexed under this heading.

Miconazole (Co-administration with inhibitors of CYP3A4 may increase plasma concentrations of estrogens and may result in side effects).
No products indexed under this heading.

Miconazole Nitrate (Co-administration with inhibitors of CYP3A4 may increase plasma concentrations of estrogens and may result in side effects). Products include:
Desenex ...... ■635
Desenex Jock Itch Spray Powder ...... ■635

Modafinil (Co-administration with inducers of CYP3A4 may reduce plasma concentrations of estrogens, possibly resulting in a decrease in therapeutic effects and/or changes in uterine bleeding profile). Products include:
Provigil Tablets 988

Nefazodone Hydrochloride (Co-administration with inhibitors of CYP3A4 may increase plasma concentrations of estrogens and may result in side effects).
No products indexed under this heading.

Nelfinavir Mesylate (Co-administration with inhibitors of CYP3A4 may increase plasma concentrations of estrogens and may result in side effects). Products include:
Viracept 2577

Nevirapine (Co-administration with inducers of CYP3A4 may reduce plasma concentrations of estrogens, possibly resulting in a decrease in therapeutic effects and/or changes in uterine bleeding profile). Products include:
Viramune Oral Suspension 873
Viramune Tablets 873

Niacinamide (Co-administration with inhibitors of CYP3A4 may increase plasma concentrations of estrogens and may result in side effects).
No products indexed under this heading.

Nicotinamide (Co-administration with inhibitors of CYP3A4 may increase plasma concentrations of estrogens and may result in side effects). Products include:
Nicomide Tablets 1088

Nifedipine (Co-administration with inhibitors of CYP3A4 may increase plasma concentrations of estrogens and may result in side effects). Products include:
Adalat CC Tablets 2964

Norfloxacin (Co-administration with inhibitors of CYP3A4 may increase plasma concentrations of estrogens and may result in side effects). Products include:
Noroxin Tablets 2032

Omeprazole (Co-administration with inhibitors of CYP3A4 may increase plasma concentrations of estrogens and may result in side effects). Products include:
Zegerid Capsules 2958
Zegerid Powder for Oral Solution 2958

Oxcarbazepine (Co-administration with inducers of CYP3A4 may reduce plasma concentrations of estrogens, possibly resulting in a decrease in therapeutic effects and/or changes in uterine bleeding profile). Products include:
Trileptal Tablets 2300
Trileptal Oral Suspension 2300

Oxyphenbutazone (Concurrent use may result in elevated serum levels of oxyphenbutazone).
No products indexed under this heading.

Paroxetine Hydrochloride (Co-administration with inhibitors of CYP3A4 may increase plasma concentrations of estrogens and may result in side effects). Products include:
Paxil CR Controlled-Release Tablets 1538
Paxil 1530

Phenobarbital (Co-administration with inducers of CYP3A4 may reduce plasma concentrations of estrogens, possibly resulting in a decrease in therapeutic effects and/or changes in uterine bleeding profile). Products include:
Donnatal Extentabs 2493

Phenobarbital Sodium (Co-administration with inducers of CYP3A4 may reduce plasma concentrations of estrogens, possibly resulting in a decrease in therapeutic effects and/or changes in uterine bleeding profile).
No products indexed under this heading.

Phenytoin (Co-administration with inducers of CYP3A4 may reduce plasma concentrations of estrogens, possibly resulting in a decrease in therapeutic effects and/or changes in uterine bleeding profile).
No products indexed under this heading.

Phenytoin Sodium (Co-administration with inducers of CYP3A4 may reduce plasma concentrations of estrogens, possibly resulting in a decrease in therapeutic effects and/or changes in uterine bleeding profile). Products include:
Phenytek Capsules 2160

Prednisolone Acetate (Co-administration with inducers of CYP3A4 may reduce plasma concentrations of estrogens, possibly resulting in a decrease in therapeutic effects and/or changes in uterine bleeding profile). Products include:
Blephamide Ophthalmic Ointment 568
Blephamide Ophthalmic Suspension 569
Poly-Pred Ophthalmic Suspension ...... ⊙233
Pred Forte Ophthalmic Suspension ...... ⊙235
Pred Mild Ophthalmic Suspension ...... ⊙238
Pred-G Ophthalmic Ointment ...... ⊙237
Pred-G Ophthalmic Suspension ...... ⊙236

Prednisolone Sodium Phosphate (Co-administration with inducers of CYP3A4 may reduce plasma concentrations of estrogens, possibly resulting in a decrease in therapeutic effects and/or changes in uterine bleeding profile).
No products indexed under this heading.

Prednisolone Tebutate (Co-administration with inducers of CYP3A4 may reduce plasma concentrations of estrogens, possibly resulting in a decrease in therapeutic effects and/or changes in uterine bleeding profile).
No products indexed under this heading.

Prednisone (Co-administration with inducers of CYP3A4 may reduce plasma concentrations of estrogens, possibly resulting in a decrease in therapeutic effects and/or changes in uterine bleeding profile).
No products indexed under this heading.

Primidone (Co-administration with inducers of CYP3A4 may reduce plasma concentrations of estrogens, possibly resulting in a decrease in therapeutic effects and/or changes in uterine bleeding profile).
No products indexed under this heading.

Propoxyphene Hydrochloride (Co-administration with inhibitors of CYP3A4 may increase plasma concentrations of estrogens and may result in side effects).
No products indexed under this heading.

Propoxyphene Napsylate (Co-administration with inhibitors of CYP3A4 may increase plasma concentrations of estrogens and may result in side effects).
No products indexed under this heading.

Quinidine (Co-administration with inhibitors of CYP3A4 may increase plasma concentrations of estrogens and may result in side effects).
No products indexed under this heading.

Quinidine Hydrochloride (Co-administration with inhibitors of CYP3A4 may increase plasma concentrations of estrogens and may result in side effects).
No products indexed under this heading.

Quinidine Polygalacturonate (Co-administration with inhibitors of CYP3A4 may increase plasma concentrations of estrogens and may result in side effects).
No products indexed under this heading.

Quinidine Sulfate (Co-administration with inhibitors of CYP3A4 may increase plasma concentrations of estrogens and may result in side effects).
No products indexed under this heading.

Quinine (Co-administration with inhibitors of CYP3A4 may increase plasma concentrations of estrogens and may result in side effects).
No products indexed under this heading.

Quinine Sulfate (Co-administration with inhibitors of CYP3A4 may increase plasma concentrations of estrogens and may result in side effects).
No products indexed under this heading.

Quinupristin (Co-administration with inhibitors of CYP3A4 may increase plasma concentrations of estrogens and may result in side effects).
No products indexed under this heading.

Ranitidine Bismuth Citrate (Co-administration with inhibitors of CYP3A4 may increase plasma concentrations of estrogens and may result in side effects).
No products indexed under this heading.

Ranitidine Hydrochloride (Co-administration with inhibitors of CYP3A4 may increase plasma concentrations of estrogens and may result in side effects). Products include:

Rifabutin (Co-administration with inducers of CYP3A4 may reduce plasma concentrations of estrogens, possibly resulting in a decrease in therapeutic effects and/or changes in uterine bleeding profile).
No products indexed under this heading.

Rifampicin (Co-administration with inducers of CYP3A4 may reduce plasma concentrations of estrogens, possibly resulting in a decrease in therapeutic effects and/or changes in uterine bleeding profile).
No products indexed under this heading.

Rifampin (Co-administration with inducers of CYP3A4 may reduce plasma concentrations of estrogens, possibly resulting in a decrease in therapeutic effects and/or changes in uterine bleeding profile).
No products indexed under this heading.

Rifapentine (Co-administration with inducers of CYP3A4 may reduce plasma concentrations of estrogens, possibly resulting in a decrease in therapeutic effects and/or changes in uterine bleeding profile).
No products indexed under this heading.

Ritonavir (Co-administration with inhibitors of CYP3A4 may increase plasma concentrations of estrogens and may result in side effects). Products include:

Saquinavir (Co-administration with inhibitors of CYP3A4 may increase plasma concentrations of estrogens and may result in side effects).
No products indexed under this heading.

Saquinavir Mesylate (Co-administration with inhibitors of CYP3A4 may increase plasma concentrations of estrogens and may result in side effects). Products include:

Sertraline Hydrochloride (Co-administration with inhibitors of CYP3A4 may increase plasma con-

centrations of estrogens and may result in side effects). Products include:

Sulfinpyrazone (Co-administration with inducers of CYP3A4 may reduce plasma concentrations of estrogens, possibly resulting in a decrease in therapeutic effects and/or changes in uterine bleeding profile).
No products indexed under this heading.

Telithromycin (Co-administration with inhibitors of CYP3A4 may increase plasma concentrations of estrogens and may result in side effects). Products include:

Theophylline (Co-administration with inducers of CYP3A4 may reduce plasma concentrations of estrogens, possibly resulting in a decrease in therapeutic effects and/or changes in uterine bleeding profile).
No products indexed under this heading.

Triamcinolone (Co-administration with inducers of CYP3A4 may reduce plasma concentrations of estrogens, possibly resulting in a decrease in therapeutic effects and/or changes in uterine bleeding profile).
No products indexed under this heading.

Triamcinolone Acetonide (Co-administration with inducers of CYP3A4 may reduce plasma concentrations of estrogens, possibly resulting in a decrease in therapeutic effects and/or changes in uterine bleeding profile). Products include:

Triamcinolone Diacetate (Co-administration with inducers of CYP3A4 may reduce plasma concentrations of estrogens, possibly resulting in a decrease in therapeutic effects and/or changes in uterine bleeding profile).
No products indexed under this heading.

Triamcinolone Hexacetonide (Co-administration with inducers of CYP3A4 may reduce plasma concentrations of estrogens, possibly resulting in a decrease in therapeutic effects and/or changes in uterine bleeding profile).
No products indexed under this heading.

Troglitazone (Co-administration with inducers of CYP3A4 may reduce plasma concentrations of estrogens, possibly resulting in a decrease in therapeutic effects and/or changes in uterine bleeding profile).
No products indexed under this heading.

Troleandomycin (Co-administration with inhibitors of CYP3A4 may increase plasma concentrations of estrogens and may result in side effects).
No products indexed under this heading.

Valproate Sodium (Co-administration with inhibitors of CYP3A4 may increase plasma concentrations of estrogens and may result in side effects). Products include:

Verapamil Hydrochloride (Co-administration with inhibitors of CYP3A4 may increase plasma concentrations of estrogens and may result in side effects). Products include:

Voriconazole (Co-administration with inhibitors of CYP3A4 may increase plasma concentrations of estrogens and may result in side effects). Products include:

Warfarin Sodium (Decreased anti-coagulant requirements). Products include:

Zafirlukast (Co-administration with inhibitors of CYP3A4 may increase plasma concentrations of estrogens and may result in side effects). Products include:

Zileuton (Co-administration with inhibitors of CYP3A4 may increase plasma concentrations of estrogens and may result in side effects). Products include:

Food Interactions

Grapefruit (Co-administration with inhibitors of CYP3A4 may increase plasma concentrations of estrogens and may result in side effects).

Grapefruit Juice (Co-administration with inhibitors of CYP3A4 may increase plasma concentrations of estrogens and may result in side effects).

ESTRING VAGINAL RING
May interact with:

Vaginally administered preparations, unspecified (It is recommended that Estring be removed during treatment with other vaginally administered preparations).
No products indexed under this heading.

ETHYOL FOR INJECTION
May interact with antihypertensives. Compounds in these categories include:

Acebutolol Hydrochloride (Amifostine produces transient hypotension; caution is advised if it is used with other antihypertensive agents).
No products indexed under this heading.

Amlodipine Besylate (Amifostine produces transient hypotension; caution is advised if it is used with other antihypertensive agents). Products include:

Atenolol (Amifostine produces transient hypotension; caution is advised if it is used with other antihypertensive agents).
No products indexed under this heading.

Benazepril Hydrochloride (Amifostine produces transient hypoten-

IMPORTANT NOTE: Always consult each drug listing in the patient's regimen for possible interactions.

sion; caution is advised if it is used with other antihypertensive agents). Products include:
- Lotensin Tablets **2243**
- Lotensin HCT Tablets **2246**
- Lotrel Capsules **2249**

Bendroflumethiazide (Amifostine produces transient hypotension; caution is advised if it is used with other antihypertensive agents).
No products indexed under this heading.

Betaxolol Hydrochloride (Amifostine produces transient hypotension; caution is advised if it is used with other antihypertensive agents). Products include:
- Betoptic S Ophthalmic Suspension........ **558**

Bisoprolol Fumarate (Amifostine produces transient hypotension; caution is advised if it is used with other antihypertensive agents).
No products indexed under this heading.

Candesartan Cilexetil (Amifostine produces transient hypotension; caution is advised if it is used with other antihypertensive agents). Products include:
- Atacand Tablets **649**
- Atacand HCT **651**

Captopril (Amifostine produces transient hypotension; caution is advised if it is used with other antihypertensive agents). Products include:
- Captopril Tablets **2149**

Carteolol Hydrochloride (Amifostine produces transient hypotension; caution is advised if it is used with other antihypertensive agents). Products include:
- Carteolol Hydrochloride Ophthalmic Solution USP, 1%........ ⊙**249**

Chlorothiazide (Amifostine produces transient hypotension; caution is advised if it is used with other antihypertensive agents). Products include:
- Diuril Oral Suspension **1954**

Chlorothiazide Sodium (Amifostine produces transient hypotension; caution is advised if it is used with other antihypertensive agents). Products include:
- Diuril Sodium Intravenous **2467**

Chlorthalidone (Amifostine produces transient hypotension; caution is advised if it is used with other antihypertensive agents). Products include:
- Clorpres Tablets **2153**

Clonidine (Amifostine produces transient hypotension; caution is advised if it is used with other antihypertensive agents). Products include:
- Catapres-TTS **844**

Clonidine Hydrochloride (Amifostine produces transient hypotension; caution is advised if it is used with other antihypertensive agents). Products include:
- Catapres Tablets **843**
- Clorpres Tablets **2153**

Deserpidine (Amifostine produces transient hypotension; caution is advised if it is used with other antihypertensive agents).
No products indexed under this heading.

Diazoxide (Amifostine produces transient hypotension; caution is advised if it is used with other antihypertensive agents). Products include:
- Hyperstat I.V. **3017**

Diltiazem Hydrochloride (Amifostine produces transient hypotension; caution is advised if it is used with other antihypertensive agents). Products include:
- Cardizem LA Extended Release Tablets........ **1728**
- Tiazac Capsules **1201**

Doxazosin Mesylate (Amifostine produces transient hypotension; caution is advised if it is used with other antihypertensive agents). Products include:
- Cardura XL Tablets **2515**

Enalapril Maleate (Amifostine produces transient hypotension; caution is advised if it is used with other antihypertensive agents). Products include:
- Vasotec I.V. Injection **2103**

Enalaprilat (Amifostine produces transient hypotension; caution is advised if it is used with other antihypertensive agents).
No products indexed under this heading.

Eprosartan Mesylate (Amifostine produces transient hypotension; caution is advised if it is used with other antihypertensive agents). Products include:
- Teveten Tablets **1735**
- Teveten HCT Tablets **1737**

Esmolol Hydrochloride (Amifostine produces transient hypotension; caution is advised if it is used with other antihypertensive agents).
No products indexed under this heading.

Felodipine (Amifostine produces transient hypotension; caution is advised if it is used with other antihypertensive agents).
No products indexed under this heading.

Fosinopril Sodium (Amifostine produces transient hypotension; caution is advised if it is used with other antihypertensive agents).
No products indexed under this heading.

Furosemide (Amifostine produces transient hypotension; caution is advised if it is used with other antihypertensive agents). Products include:
- Furosemide Tablets **2154**

Guanabenz Acetate (Amifostine produces transient hypotension; caution is advised if it is used with other antihypertensive agents).
No products indexed under this heading.

Guanethidine Monosulfate (Amifostine produces transient hypotension; caution is advised if it is used with other antihypertensive agents).
No products indexed under this heading.

Hydralazine Hydrochloride (Amifostine produces transient hypotension; caution is advised if it is used with other antihypertensive agents). Products include:
- BiDil Tablets **2171**

Hydrochlorothiazide (Amifostine produces transient hypotension; caution is advised if it is used with other antihypertensive agents). Products include:
- Aldoril Tablets **1910**
- Atacand HCT **651**
- Avalide Tablets **888**
- Avalide Tablets **2874**
- Benicar HCT Tablets **1044**
- Diovan HCT Tablets **2196**
- Dyazide Capsules **1423**
- Hyzaar 50-12.5 Tablets **1990**
- Hyzaar 100-12.5 Tablets **1990**
- Hyzaar 100-25 Tablets **1990**
- Lopressor HCT 50/25 Tablets **2241**
- Lopressor HCT 100/25 Tablets **2241**
- Lopressor HCT 100/50 Tablets **2241**
- Lotensin HCT Tablets **2246**
- Micardis HCT Tablets **856**
- Moduretic Tablets **2028**
- Prinzide Tablets **2056**
- Teveten HCT Tablets **1737**
- Timolide Tablets **2086**
- Uniretic Tablets **3100**

Hydroflumethiazide (Amifostine produces transient hypotension; caution is advised if it is used with other antihypertensive agents).
No products indexed under this heading.

Indapamide (Amifostine produces transient hypotension; caution is advised if it is used with other antihypertensive agents). Products include:
- Indapamide Tablets **2156**

Irbesartan (Amifostine produces transient hypotension; caution is advised if it is used with other antihypertensive agents). Products include:
- Avalide Tablets **888**
- Avalide Tablets **2874**
- Avapro Tablets **891**
- Avapro Tablets **2871**

Isradipine (Amifostine produces transient hypotension; caution is advised if it is used with other antihypertensive agents). Products include:
- DynaCirc CR Tablets **2721**

Labetalol Hydrochloride (Amifostine produces transient hypotension; caution is advised if it is used with other antihypertensive agents).
No products indexed under this heading.

Lisinopril (Amifostine produces transient hypotension; caution is advised if it is used with other antihypertensive agents). Products include:
- Prinivil Tablets **2052**
- Prinzide Tablets **2056**

Losartan Potassium (Amifostine produces transient hypotension; caution is advised if it is used with other antihypertensive agents). Products include:
- Cozaar Tablets **1935**
- Hyzaar 50-12.5 Tablets **1990**
- Hyzaar 100-12.5 Tablets **1990**
- Hyzaar 100-25 Tablets **1990**

Mecamylamine Hydrochloride (Amifostine produces transient hypotension; caution is advised if it is used with other antihypertensive agents).
No products indexed under this heading.

Methyclothiazide (Amifostine produces transient hypotension; caution is advised if it is used with other antihypertensive agents).
No products indexed under this heading.

Methyldopa (Amifostine produces transient hypotension; caution is advised if it is used with other antihypertensive agents). Products include:
- Aldoril Tablets **1910**

Methyldopate Hydrochloride (Amifostine produces transient hypotension; caution is advised if it is used with other antihypertensive agents).
No products indexed under this heading.

Metolazone (Amifostine produces transient hypotension; caution is advised if it is used with other antihypertensive agents).
No products indexed under this heading.

Metoprolol Succinate (Amifostine produces transient hypotension; caution is advised if it is used with other antihypertensive agents). Products include:
- Toprol-XL Tablets **668**

Metoprolol Tartrate (Amifostine produces transient hypotension; caution is advised if it is used with other antihypertensive agents). Products include:
- Lopressor Injection **2238**
- Lopressor Tablets **2238**
- Lopressor HCT 50/25 Tablets **2241**
- Lopressor HCT 100/25 Tablets **2241**
- Lopressor HCT 100/50 Tablets **2241**

Metyrosine (Amifostine produces transient hypotension; caution is advised if it is used with other antihypertensive agents). Products include:
- Demser Capsules **1953**

Mibefradil Dihydrochloride (Amifostine produces transient hypotension; caution is advised if it is used with other antihypertensive agents).
No products indexed under this heading.

Minoxidil (Amifostine produces transient hypotension; caution is advised if it is used with other antihypertensive agents). Products include:
- Men's Rogaine Extra Strength Hair Regrowth Treatment Topical Solution, Ocean Rush Scent and Original Unscented........ ▣**633**
- Men's Rogaine Foam Hair Regrowth Treatment........ ▣**633**
- Women's Rogaine Hair Regrowth Treatment Topical Solution, Spring Bloom Scent and Original Unscented........ ▣**634**

Moexipril Hydrochloride (Amifostine produces transient hypotension; caution is advised if it is used with other antihypertensive agents). Products include:
- Uniretic Tablets **3100**
- Univasc Tablets **3104**

Nadolol (Amifostine produces transient hypotension; caution is advised if it is used with other antihypertensive agents). Products include:
- Nadolol Tablets **2159**

Nicardipine Hydrochloride (Amifostine produces transient hypotension; caution is advised if it is used with other antihypertensive agents). Products include:
- Cardene I.V. **2497**

Nifedipine (Amifostine produces transient hypotension; caution is advised if it is used with other antihypertensive agents). Products include:
- Adalat CC Tablets **2964**

Nisoldipine (Amifostine produces transient hypotension; caution is advised if it is used with other antihypertensive agents). Products include:
- Sular Tablets **3122**

Nitroglycerin (Amifostine produces transient hypotension; caution is

(▣ Described in PDR For Nonprescription Drugs) (⊙ Described in PDR For Ophthalmic Medicines™)

advised if it is used with other antihypertensive agents). Products include:
Nitro-Dur Transdermal Infusion System 3046
Nitrolingual Pumpspray 3120

Penbutolol Sulfate (Amifostine produces transient hypotension; caution is advised if it is used with other antihypertensive agents).
No products indexed under this heading.

Perindopril Erbumine (Amifostine produces transient hypotension; caution is advised if it is used with other antihypertensive agents). Products include:
Aceon Tablets (2 mg, 4 mg, 8 mg) 3194

Phenoxybenzamine Hydrochloride (Amifostine produces transient hypotension; caution is advised if it is used with other antihypertensive agents). Products include:
Dibenzyline Capsules 3399

Phentolamine Mesylate (Amifostine produces transient hypotension; caution is advised if it is used with other antihypertensive agents).
No products indexed under this heading.

Pindolol (Amifostine produces transient hypotension; caution is advised if it is used with other antihypertensive agents).
No products indexed under this heading.

Polythiazide (Amifostine produces transient hypotension; caution is advised if it is used with other antihypertensive agents).
No products indexed under this heading.

Prazosin Hydrochloride (Amifostine produces transient hypotension; caution is advised if it is used with other antihypertensive agents).
No products indexed under this heading.

Propranolol Hydrochloride (Amifostine produces transient hypotension; caution is advised if it is used with other antihypertensive agents). Products include:
Inderal LA Long-Acting Capsules 3429
InnoPran XL Capsules 2723

Quinapril Hydrochloride (Amifostine produces transient hypotension; caution is advised if it is used with other antihypertensive agents).
No products indexed under this heading.

Ramipril (Amifostine produces transient hypotension; caution is advised if it is used with other antihypertensive agents). Products include:
Altace Capsules 1702

Rauwolfia Serpentina (Amifostine produces transient hypotension; caution is advised if it is used with other antihypertensive agents).
No products indexed under this heading.

Rescinnamine (Amifostine produces transient hypotension; caution is advised if it is used with other antihypertensive agents).
No products indexed under this heading.

Reserpine (Amifostine produces transient hypotension; caution is advised if it is used with other antihypertensive agents).
No products indexed under this heading.

Sodium Nitroprusside (Amifostine produces transient hypotension; caution is advised if it is used with other antihypertensive agents).
No products indexed under this heading.

Sotalol Hydrochloride (Amifostine produces transient hypotension; caution is advised if it is used with other antihypertensive agents).
No products indexed under this heading.

Spirapril Hydrochloride (Amifostine produces transient hypotension; caution is advised if it is used with other antihypertensive agents).
No products indexed under this heading.

Telmisartan (Amifostine produces transient hypotension; caution is advised if it is used with other antihypertensive agents). Products include:
Micardis Tablets 854
Micardis HCT Tablets 856

Terazosin Hydrochloride (Amifostine produces transient hypotension; caution is advised if it is used with other antihypertensive agents). Products include:
Hytrin Capsules 471

Timolol Maleate (Amifostine produces transient hypotension; caution is advised if it is used with other antihypertensive agents). Products include:
Blocadren Tablets 1916
Cosopt Sterile Ophthalmic Solution 1931
Timolide Tablets 2086
Timoptic Sterile Ophthalmic Solution 2088
Timoptic in Ocudose 2091
Timoptic-XE Sterile Ophthalmic Gel Forming Solution 2092

Torsemide (Amifostine produces transient hypotension; caution is advised if it is used with other antihypertensive agents). Products include:
Demadex Injection 2759
Demadex Tablets 2759

Trandolapril (Amifostine produces transient hypotension; caution is advised if it is used with other antihypertensive agents). Products include:
Mavik Tablets 486
Tarka Tablets 524

Trimethaphan Camsylate (Amifostine produces transient hypotension; caution is advised if it is used with other antihypertensive agents).
No products indexed under this heading.

Valsartan (Amifostine produces transient hypotension; caution is advised if it is used with other antihypertensive agents). Products include:
Diovan Tablets 2193
Diovan HCT Tablets 2196

Verapamil Hydrochloride (Amifostine produces transient hypotension; caution is advised if it is used with other antihypertensive agents). Products include:
Covera-HS Tablets 3139
Tarka Tablets 524
Verelan PM Extended-Release Capsules, Controlled-Onset 3106

EUFLEXXA
(Sodium Hyaluronate) 1162
None cited in PDR database.

EULEXIN CAPSULES
(Flutamide) 3009
May interact with:

Warfarin Sodium (Increases in prothrombin time have been noted in patients receiving long-term warfarin therapy after flutamide was initiated). Products include:
Coumadin for Injection 898
Coumadin Tablets 898

EVISTA TABLETS
(Raloxifene Hydrochloride) 1763
May interact with:

Cholestyramine (Co-administration causes a 60% reduction in the absorption and enterohepatic cycling of raloxifene; concurrent use should be avoided).
No products indexed under this heading.

Diazepam (Raloxifene might affect the protein binding of other highly protein-bound drugs such as diazepam; caution should be exercised). Products include:
Diastat Rectal Delivery System 3343
Valium Tablets 2819

Diazoxide (Raloxifene might affect the protein binding of other highly protein-bound drugs such as diazoxide; caution should be exercised). Products include:
Hyperstat I.V. 3017

Lidocaine Hydrochloride (Raloxifene might affect the protein binding of other highly protein-bound drugs such as lidocaine; caution should be exercised).
No products indexed under this heading.

Warfarin Sodium (Co-administration has resulted in a 10% decrease in prothrombin time in single-dose studies; if used concurrently, prothrombin time should be monitored). Products include:
Coumadin for Injection 898
Coumadin Tablets 898

Food Interactions

Food, unspecified (Administration of raloxifene with a standardized, high fat meal increases the absorption of raloxifene, but does not lead to clinically meaningful changes in systemic exposure; Evista can be administered without regard to meals).

EVOCLIN FOAM, 1%
(Clindamycin Phosphate) 1009
May interact with neuromuscular blocking agents and certain other agents. Compounds in these categories include:

Atracurium Besylate (Clindamycin has been shown to have neuromuscular blocking properties that may enhance the action of other neuromuscular blocking agents; therefore, it should be used with caution in patients receiving such agents).
No products indexed under this heading.

Cisatracurium Besylate (Clindamycin has been shown to have neuromuscular blocking properties that may enhance the action of other neuromuscular blocking agents; therefore, it should be used with caution in patients receiving such agents). Products include:
Nimbex Injection 498

Doxacurium Chloride (Clindamycin has been shown to have neuromuscular blocking properties that may enhance the action of other neuromuscular blocking agents; therefore, it should be used with caution in patients receiving such agents).
No products indexed under this heading.

Metocurine Iodide (Clindamycin has been shown to have neuromuscular blocking properties that may enhance the action of other neuromuscular blocking agents; therefore, it should be used with caution in patients receiving such agents).
No products indexed under this heading.

Mivacurium Chloride (Clindamycin has been shown to have neuromuscular blocking properties that may enhance the action of other neuromuscular blocking agents; therefore, it should be used with caution in patients receiving such agents). Products include:
Mivacron Injection 493

Pancuronium Bromide (Clindamycin has been shown to have neuromuscular blocking properties that may enhance the action of other neuromuscular blocking agents; therefore, it should be used with caution in patients receiving such agents).
No products indexed under this heading.

Rapacuronium Bromide (Clindamycin has been shown to have neuromuscular blocking properties that may enhance the action of other neuromuscular blocking agents; therefore, it should be used with caution in patients receiving such agents).
No products indexed under this heading.

Rocuronium Bromide (Clindamycin has been shown to have neuromuscular blocking properties that may enhance the action of other neuromuscular blocking agents; therefore, it should be used with caution in patients receiving such agents). Products include:
Zemuron Injection 2346

Succinylcholine Chloride (Clindamycin has been shown to have neuromuscular blocking properties that may enhance the action of other neuromuscular blocking agents; therefore, it should be used with caution in patients receiving such agents).
No products indexed under this heading.

Vecuronium Bromide (Clindamycin has been shown to have neuromuscular blocking properties that may enhance the action of other neuromuscular blocking agents; therefore, it should be used with caution in patients receiving such agents).
No products indexed under this heading.

EVOXAC CAPSULES
(Cevimeline Hydrochloride) 1047
May interact with antimuscarinic drugs, beta blockers, cytochrome p450 2d6 inhibitors (selected), cytochrome p450 3a4 inhibitors (selected), parasympathomimetics, and certain other agents. Compounds in these categories include:

Acebutolol Hydrochloride (Possibility of conduction disturbances; co-administration with beta adrenergic antagonists requires caution).
No products indexed under this heading.

Acetazolamide (Drugs which inhibit CYP3A3/4 also inhibit the metabolism of cevimeline).
No products indexed under this heading.

Amiodarone Hydrochloride (Co-administration with drugs which inhibit CYP2D6, such as amiodarone, may inhibit the metabolism of cevimeline resulting in a higher risk of adverse events).
No products indexed under this heading.

Amitriptyline Hydrochloride (Drugs which inhibit CYP2D6 also inhibit the metabolism of cevimeline. Cevimeline should be used with caution in individuals known or suspected to be deficient in CYP2D6 activity, as they may be at a higher risk of adverse events).
No products indexed under this heading.

Amoxapine (Drugs which inhibit CYP2D6 also inhibit the metabolism of cevimeline. Cevimeline should be used with caution in individuals known or suspected to be deficient in CYP2D6 activity, as they may be at a higher risk of adverse events).
No products indexed under this heading.

Amprenavir (Drugs which inhibit CYP3A3/4 also inhibit the metabolism of cevimeline). Products include:
Agenerase Capsules 1327
Agenerase Oral Solution 1332

Anastrozole (Drugs which inhibit CYP3A3/4 also inhibit the metabolism of cevimeline). Products include:
Arimidex Tablets 673

Aprepitant (Drugs which inhibit CYP3A3/4 also inhibit the metabolism of cevimeline). Products include:
Emend Capsules 1963

Atenolol (Possibility of conduction disturbances; co-administration with beta adrenergic antagonists requires caution).
No products indexed under this heading.

Atropine Sulfate (Cevimeline might interfere with the desirable antimuscarinic effects of drugs used concomitantly). Products include:
Donnatal Extentabs 2493

Belladonna Alkaloids (Cevimeline might interfere with the desirable antimuscarinic effects of drugs used concomitantly). Products include:
Hyland's Teething Tablets .... ▣ 830

Betaxolol Hydrochloride (Possibility of conduction disturbances; co-administration with beta adrenergic antagonists requires caution). Products include:
Betoptic S Ophthalmic Suspension.................................. 558

Bisoprolol Fumarate (Possibility of conduction disturbances; co-administration with beta adrenergic antagonists requires caution).
No products indexed under this heading.

Bupropion Hydrochloride (Drugs which inhibit CYP2D6 also inhibit the metabolism of cevimeline. Cevimeline should be used with caution in individuals known or suspected to be deficient in CYP2D6 activity, as they may be at a higher risk of adverse events). Products include:
Wellbutrin Tablets 1603
Wellbutrin SR Sustained-Release Tablets 1607
Wellbutrin XL Extended-Release Tablets 1613
Zyban Sustained-Release Tablets 1644

Carteolol Hydrochloride (Possibility of conduction disturbances; co-administration with beta adrenergic antagonists requires caution). Products include:
Carteolol Hydrochloride Ophthalmic Solution USP, 1%....... ⊙ 249

Celecoxib (Drugs which inhibit CYP2D6 also inhibit the metabolism of cevimeline. Cevimeline should be used with caution in individuals known or suspected to be deficient in CYP2D6 activity, as they may be at a higher risk of adverse events). Products include:
Celebrex Capsules 3134

Chloroquine Hydrochloride (Drugs which inhibit CYP2D6 also inhibit the metabolism of cevimeline. Cevimeline should be used with caution in individuals known or suspected to be deficient in CYP2D6 activity, as they may be at a higher risk of adverse events).
No products indexed under this heading.

Chloroquine Phosphate (Drugs which inhibit CYP2D6 also inhibit the metabolism of cevimeline. Cevimeline should be used with caution in individuals known or suspected to be deficient in CYP2D6 activity, as they may be at a higher risk of adverse events).
No products indexed under this heading.

Chlorpheniramine (Drugs which inhibit CYP2D6 also inhibit the metabolism of cevimeline. Cevimeline should be used with caution in individuals known or suspected to be deficient in CYP2D6 activity, as they may be at a higher risk of adverse events).
No products indexed under this heading.

Chlorpheniramine Maleate (Drugs which inhibit CYP2D6 also inhibit the metabolism of cevimeline. Cevimeline should be used with caution in individuals known or suspected to be deficient in CYP2D6 activity, as they may be at a higher risk of adverse events). Products include:
Advil Allergy Sinus Caplets .... ▣ 770
Advil Multi-Symptom Cold Caplets.. ▣ 770
BC Allergy Sinus Cold Powder .... ▣ 677
Comtrex Maximum Strength Cold & Cough Day/Night Caplets - Night Formulation .... ▣ 726
Comtrex Maximum Strength Day/Night Severe Cold & Sinus Caplets - Night Formulation .... ▣ 725
Contac Cold and Flu Maximum Strength Caplets........................ ▣ 728
Contac Cold and Flu Day and Night Caplets (Night Formulation Only)....................... ▣ 727
Children's Dimetapp Long Acting Cough Plus Cold Syrup................ ▣ 731
Robitussin Cough & Cold Long-Acting Liquid .... ▣ 735
Robitussin Cough & Allergy Syrup .. ▣ 736
Robitussin Cough & Cold Nighttime Liquid............................ ▣ 736
Robitussin Cough, Cold & Flu Nighttime Liquid........................... ▣ 738
Robitussin Pediatric Cough & Cold Long-Acting Liquid............... ▣ 735
Robitussin Pediatric Cough & Cold Nighttime Liquid.................. ▣ 736
Triaminic Cold & Allergy Liquid .... ▣ 746
Triaminic Cough & Runny Nose Softchews .... ▣ 748
Children's Tylenol Plus Flu Oral Suspension...................................... ▣ 749
Tylenol Allergy Multi-Symptom Caplets with Cool Burst and Gelcaps.. 1872
Children's Tylenol Plus Cold Suspension Liquid 1879
Children's Tylenol Plus Cough & Runny Nose Suspension Liquid..... 1879
Children's Tylenol Plus Flu Suspension Liquid 1881
Children's Tylenol Plus Multi-Symptom Cold Suspension Liquid 1879
Tylenol Cold Head Congestion Nighttime Caplets with Cool Burst.. 1873
Tylenol Cold Multi-Symptom Nighttime Caplets with Cool Burst.. 1874
Tylenol Sinus Congestion & Pain Nighttime Caplets with Cool Burst.. 1876
Vicks 44M Cough, Cold & Flu Relief Liquid.................................. 2680
Pediatric Vicks 44m Cough & Cold Relief Liquid.......................... 2676
Children's Vicks NyQuil Cold/Cough Relief....................... ▣ 756
Children's Vicks NyQuil Cold/Cough Relief Liquid 2680
Zicam Maximum Strength Flu Daytime.................................... ▣ 768

Chlorpheniramine Polistirex (Drugs which inhibit CYP2D6 also inhibit the metabolism of cevimeline. Cevimeline should be used with caution in individuals known or suspected to be deficient in CYP2D6 activity, as they may be at a higher risk of adverse events). Products include:
Tussionex Pennkinetic Extended-Release Suspension...... 3327

Chlorpheniramine Tannate (Drugs which inhibit CYP2D6 also inhibit the metabolism of cevimeline. Cevimeline should be used with caution in individuals known or suspected to be deficient in CYP2D6 activity, as they may be at a higher risk of adverse events).
No products indexed under this heading.

Cimetidine (Co-administration with drugs which inhibit CYP2D6, such as cimetidine, may inhibit the metabolism of cevimeline resulting in a higher risk of adverse events). Products include:
Tagamet HB 200 Tablets .... ▣ 664

Cimetidine Hydrochloride (Co-administration with drugs which inhibit CYP2D6, such as cimetidine, may inhibit the metabolism of cevimeline resulting in a higher risk of adverse events).
No products indexed under this heading.

Ciprofloxacin (Drugs which inhibit CYP3A3/4 also inhibit the metabolism of cevimeline). Products include:
Cipro Oral Suspension 2977
Cipro I.V. 2984
Cipro XR Tablets 2990
Ciprodex Otic Suspension 559

Citalopram Hydrobromide (Drugs which inhibit CYP2D6 also inhibit the metabolism of cevimeline. Cevimeline should be used with caution in individuals known or suspected to be deficient in CYP2D6 activity, as they may be at a higher risk of adverse events). Products include:
Celexa 1176

Clarithromycin (Co-administration with drugs which inhibit CYP3A3/4, such as clarithromycin, may inhibit the metabolism of cevimeline resulting in a higher risk of adverse events). Products include:
Biaxin/Biaxin XL 402
PREVPAC 3284

Clidinium Bromide (Cevimeline might interfere with the desirable antimuscarinic effects of drugs used concomitantly).
No products indexed under this heading.

Clomipramine Hydrochloride (Drugs which inhibit CYP2D6 also inhibit the metabolism of cevimeline. Cevimeline should be used with caution in individuals known or suspected to be deficient in CYP2D6 activity, as they may be at a higher risk of adverse events).
No products indexed under this heading.

Clotrimazole (Drugs which inhibit CYP3A3/4 also inhibit the metabolism of cevimeline). Products include:
Desenex Athlete's Foot Cream .... ▣ 635
Lotrimin 3039
Lotrisone 3040

Cocaine Hydrochloride (Drugs which inhibit CYP2D6 also inhibit the metabolism of cevimeline. Cevimeline should be used with caution in individuals known or suspected to be deficient in CYP2D6 activity, as they may be at a higher risk of adverse events).
No products indexed under this heading.

Cyclosporine (Drugs which inhibit CYP3A3/4 also inhibit the metabolism of cevimeline). Products include:
Gengraf Capsules 459
Neoral Oral Solution 2259
Neoral Soft Gelatin Capsules 2259
Restasis Ophthalmic Emulsion 575
Sandimmune 2275

Dalfopristin (Drugs which inhibit CYP3A3/4 also inhibit the metabolism of cevimeline).
No products indexed under this heading.

Danazol (Drugs which inhibit CYP3A3/4 also inhibit the metabolism of cevimeline).
No products indexed under this heading.

Delavirdine Mesylate (Drugs which inhibit CYP3A3/4 also inhibit the metabolism of cevimeline). Products include:
Rescriptor Tablets 2551

Desipramine Hydrochloride (Drugs which inhibit CYP2D6 also inhibit the metabolism of cevimeline. Cevimeline should be used with caution in individuals known or suspected to be deficient in CYP2D6 activity, as they may be at a higher risk of adverse events).
No products indexed under this heading.

Dicyclomine Hydrochloride (Cevimeline might interfere with the desirable antimuscarinic effects of drugs used concomitantly). Products include:

- Bentyl Capsules 697
- Bentyl Injection 697
- Bentyl Syrup 697
- Bentyl Tablets 697

Diltiazem Hydrochloride (Co-administration with drugs which inhibit CYP3A3/4, such as diltiazem, may inhibit the metabolism of cevimeline resulting in a higher risk of adverse events). Products include:

- Cardizem LA Extended Release Tablets 1728
- Tiazac Capsules 1201

Diltiazem Maleate (Drugs which inhibit CYP3A3/4 also inhibit the metabolism of cevimeline).

No products indexed under this heading.

Diphenhydramine (Drugs which inhibit CYP2D6 also inhibit the metabolism of cevimeline. Cevimeline should be used with caution in individuals known or suspected to be deficient in CYP2D6 activity, as they may be at a higher risk of adverse events). Products include:

- Tylenol Sore Throat Nighttime Liquid with Cool Burst 1877

Diphenhydramine Hydrochloride (Drugs which inhibit CYP2D6 also inhibit the metabolism of cevimeline. Cevimeline should be used with caution in individuals known or suspected to be deficient in CYP2D6 activity, as they may be at a higher risk of adverse events). Products include:

- Nytol QuickCaps Caplets 615
- Nytol QuickGels Softgels Maximum Strength 616
- Simply Sleep Caplets 1868
- Sominex Original Formula Tablets .. 616
- TheraFlu Warming Relief Nighttime Severe Cold 743
- TheraFlu Thin Strips Multi Symptom 744
- Triaminic Nighttime Cold & Cough Liquid 746
- Triaminic Thin Strips Cough & Runny Nose 749
- Extra Strength Tylenol PM Caplets, Vanilla Caplets, Geltabs, Gelcaps and Liquid 1875
- Tylenol Sore Throat Nighttime Liquid with Cool Burst 790
- Tylenol Allergy Multi-Symptom Nighttime Caplets with Cool Burst 1872
- Tylenol Severe Allergy Caplets 1872
- Children's Tylenol Plus Cold & Allergy Suspension Liquid 1878

Doxepin Hydrochloride (Drugs which inhibit CYP2D6 also inhibit the metabolism of cevimeline. Cevimeline should be used with caution in individuals known or suspected to be deficient in CYP2D6 activity, as they may be at a higher risk of adverse events).

No products indexed under this heading.

Edrophonium Chloride (Co-administration with parasympathomimetic drugs can be expected to have additive effects).

No products indexed under this heading.

Efavirenz (Drugs which inhibit CYP3A3/4 also inhibit the metabolism of cevimeline). Products include:

- Atripla Tablets 945
- Sustiva Capsules 930
- Sustiva Tablets 930

Erythromycin (Drugs which inhibit CYP3A3/4 also inhibit the metabolism of cevimeline). Products include:

- Ery-Tab Tablets 449
- Erythromycin Base Filmtab Tablets 455
- Erythromycin Delayed-Release Capsules, USP 457
- PCE Dispertab Tablets 515

Erythromycin Estolate (Drugs which inhibit CYP3A3/4 also inhibit the metabolism of cevimeline).

No products indexed under this heading.

Erythromycin Ethylsuccinate (Drugs which inhibit CYP3A3/4 also inhibit the metabolism of cevimeline). Products include:

- E.E.S. 451
- EryPed 447

Erythromycin Gluceptate (Drugs which inhibit CYP3A3/4 also inhibit the metabolism of cevimeline).

No products indexed under this heading.

Erythromycin Lactobionate (Drugs which inhibit CYP3A3/4 also inhibit the metabolism of cevimeline).

No products indexed under this heading.

Erythromycin Stearate (Drugs which inhibit CYP3A3/4 also inhibit the metabolism of cevimeline). Products include:

- Erythrocin Stearate Filmtab Tablets 453

Escitalopram Oxalate (Drugs which inhibit CYP2D6 also inhibit the metabolism of cevimeline. Cevimeline should be used with caution in individuals known or suspected to be deficient in CYP2D6 activity, as they may be at a higher risk of adverse events). Products include:

- Lexapro Oral Solution 1190
- Lexapro Tablets 1190

Esmolol Hydrochloride (Possibility of conduction disturbances; co-administration with beta adrenergic antagonists requires caution).

No products indexed under this heading.

Esomeprazole Magnesium (Drugs which inhibit CYP3A3/4 also inhibit the metabolism of cevimeline). Products include:

- Nexium Delayed-Release Capsules 655

Fluconazole (Drugs which inhibit CYP3A3/4 also inhibit the metabolism of cevimeline).

No products indexed under this heading.

Fluoxetine (Drugs which inhibit CYP2D6 also inhibit the metabolism of cevimeline. Cevimeline should be used with caution in individuals known or suspected to be deficient in CYP2D6 activity, as they may be at a higher risk of adverse events).

No products indexed under this heading.

Fluoxetine Hydrochloride (Co-administration with drugs which inhibit CYP2D6, such as fluoxetine, may inhibit the metabolism of cevimeline resulting in a higher risk of adverse events). Products include:

- Prozac Pulvules and Liquid 1801
- Symbyax Capsules 1819

Fluphenazine Decanoate (Drugs which inhibit CYP2D6 also inhibit the metabolism of cevimeline. Cevimeline should be used with caution in individuals known or suspected to be deficient in CYP2D6 activity, as they may be at a higher risk of adverse events).

No products indexed under this heading.

Fluphenazine Enanthate (Drugs which inhibit CYP2D6 also inhibit the metabolism of cevimeline. Cevimeline should be used with caution in individuals known or suspected to be deficient in CYP2D6 activity, as they may be at a higher risk of adverse events).

No products indexed under this heading.

Fluphenazine Hydrochloride (Drugs which inhibit CYP2D6 also inhibit the metabolism of cevimeline. Cevimeline should be used with caution in individuals known or suspected to be deficient in CYP2D6 activity, as they may be at a higher risk of adverse events).

No products indexed under this heading.

Fluvoxamine Maleate (Drugs which inhibit CYP2D6 also inhibit the metabolism of cevimeline. Cevimeline should be used with caution in individuals known or suspected to be deficient in CYP2D6 activity, as they may be at a higher risk of adverse events).

No products indexed under this heading.

Fosamprenavir Calcium (Drugs which inhibit CYP3A3/4 also inhibit the metabolism of cevimeline). Products include:

- Lexiva Tablets 1505

Glycopyrrolate (Cevimeline might interfere with the desirable antimuscarinic effects of drugs used concomitantly).

No products indexed under this heading.

Halofantrine Hydrochloride (Drugs which inhibit CYP2D6 also inhibit the metabolism of cevimeline. Cevimeline should be used with caution in individuals known or suspected to be deficient in CYP2D6 activity, as they may be at a higher risk of adverse events).

No products indexed under this heading.

Haloperidol (Drugs which inhibit CYP2D6 also inhibit the metabolism of cevimeline. Cevimeline should be used with caution in individuals known or suspected to be deficient in CYP2D6 activity, as they may be at a higher risk of adverse events).

No products indexed under this heading.

Haloperidol Decanoate (Drugs which inhibit CYP2D6 also inhibit the metabolism of cevimeline. Cevimeline should be used with caution in individuals known or suspected to be deficient in CYP2D6 activity, as they may be at a higher risk of adverse events).

No products indexed under this heading.

Hydroxychloroquine Sulfate (Drugs which inhibit CYP2D6 also inhibit the metabolism of cevimeline. Cevimeline should be used with caution in individuals known or suspected to be deficient in CYP2D6 activity, as they may be at a higher risk of adverse events).

No products indexed under this heading.

Hyoscyamine (Cevimeline might interfere with the desirable antimuscarinic effects of drugs used concomitantly).

No products indexed under this heading.

Hyoscyamine Sulfate (Cevimeline might interfere with the desirable antimuscarinic effects of drugs used concomitantly). Products include:

- Donnatal Extentabs 2493
- Prosed/DS Tablets 1157

Imatinib Mesylate (Drugs which inhibit CYP2D6 also inhibit the metabolism of cevimeline. Cevimeline should be used with caution in individuals known or suspected to be deficient in CYP2D6 activity, as they may be at a higher risk of adverse events). Products include:

- Gleevec Tablets 2227

Imipramine Hydrochloride (Drugs which inhibit CYP2D6 also inhibit the metabolism of cevimeline. Cevimeline should be used with caution in individuals known or suspected to be deficient in CYP2D6 activity, as they may be at a higher risk of adverse events).

No products indexed under this heading.

Imipramine Pamoate (Drugs which inhibit CYP2D6 also inhibit the metabolism of cevimeline. Cevimeline should be used with caution in individuals known or suspected to be deficient in CYP2D6 activity, as they may be at a higher risk of adverse events).

No products indexed under this heading.

Indinavir Sulfate (Co-administration with drugs which inhibit CYP3A3/4, such as indinavir, may inhibit the metabolism of cevimeline resulting in a higher risk of adverse events). Products include:

- Crixivan Capsules 1940

Ipratropium Bromide (Cevimeline might interfere with the desirable antimuscarinic effects of drugs used concomitantly). Products include:

- Atrovent Inhalation Solution 835
- Atrovent HFA Inhalation Aerosol 841
- Atrovent Nasal Spray 0.03% 837
- Atrovent Nasal Spray 0.06% 839
- Combivent Inhalation Aerosol 847
- DuoNeb Inhalation Solution 1058

Isoniazid (Drugs which inhibit CYP3A3/4 also inhibit the metabolism of cevimeline).

No products indexed under this heading.

Itraconazole (Co-administration with drugs which inhibit CYP3A3/4, such as itraconazole, may inhibit the metabolism of cevimeline resulting in a higher risk of adverse events).

No products indexed under this heading.

Ketoconazole (Co-administration with drugs which inhibit CYP3A3/4, such as ketoconazole, may inhibit the metabolism of cevimeline resulting in a higher risk of adverse events). Products include:

IMPORTANT NOTE: Always consult each drug listing in the patient's regimen for possible interactions.

Nizoral A-D Shampoo, 1% 1868

Labetalol Hydrochloride (Possibility of conduction disturbances; co-administration with beta adrenergic antagonists requires caution).
No products indexed under this heading.

Levobunolol Hydrochloride (Possibility of conduction disturbances; co-administration with beta adrenergic antagonists requires caution). Products include:
Betagan Ophthalmic Solution, USP .... ⊙ 220

Lopinavir (Drugs which inhibit CYP3A3/4 also inhibit the metabolism of cevimeline). Products include:
Kaletra 476

Loratadine (Drugs which inhibit CYP3A3/4 also inhibit the metabolism of cevimeline). Products include:
Alavert Allergy & Sinus D-12 Hour Tablets .... ▣ 771
Alavert .... ▣ 771
Children's Claritin Allergy Oral Solution .... ▣ 771
Claritin Non-Drowsy 24 Hour Tablets .... ▣ 772
Claritin Reditabs 24 Hour Non-Drowsy Tablets .... ▣ 772
Claritin-D Non-Drowsy 12 Hour Tablets .... ▣ 772
Claritin-D Non-Drowsy 24 Hour Tablets .... ▣ 772

Maprotiline Hydrochloride (Drugs which inhibit CYP2D6 also inhibit the metabolism of cevimeline. Cevimeline should be used with caution in individuals known or suspected to be deficient in CYP2D6 activity, as they may be at a higher risk of adverse events).
No products indexed under this heading.

Mepenzolate Bromide (Cevimeline might interfere with the desirable antimuscarinic effects of drugs used concomitantly).
No products indexed under this heading.

Methadone Hydrochloride (Drugs which inhibit CYP2D6 also inhibit the metabolism of cevimeline. Cevimeline should be used with caution in individuals known or suspected to be deficient in CYP2D6 activity, as they may be at a higher risk of adverse events).
No products indexed under this heading.

Metipranolol Hydrochloride (Possibility of conduction disturbances; co-administration with beta adrenergic antagonists requires caution).
No products indexed under this heading.

Metoprolol Succinate (Possibility of conduction disturbances; co-administration with beta adrenergic antagonists requires caution). Products include:
Toprol-XL Tablets 668

Metoprolol Tartrate (Possibility of conduction disturbances; co-administration with beta adrenergic antagonists requires caution). Products include:
Lopressor Injection 2238
Lopressor Tablets 2238
Lopressor HCT 50/25 Tablets 2241
Lopressor HCT 100/25 Tablets 2241
Lopressor HCT 100/50 Tablets 2241

Metronidazole (Drugs which inhibit CYP3A3/4 also inhibit the metabolism of cevimeline). Products include:
Metrogel 1% 1211
MetroGel-Vaginal Gel 1855
Vandazole Vaginal Gel 3338

Metronidazole Benzoate (Drugs which inhibit CYP3A3/4 also inhibit the metabolism of cevimeline).
No products indexed under this heading.

Metronidazole Hydrochloride (Drugs which inhibit CYP3A3/4 also inhibit the metabolism of cevimeline).
No products indexed under this heading.

Mibefradil Dihydrochloride (Drugs which inhibit CYP2D6 also inhibit the metabolism of cevimeline. Cevimeline should be used with caution in individuals known or suspected to be deficient in CYP2D6 activity, as they may be at a higher risk of adverse events).
No products indexed under this heading.

Miconazole (Drugs which inhibit CYP3A3/4 also inhibit the metabolism of cevimeline).
No products indexed under this heading.

Miconazole Nitrate (Drugs which inhibit CYP3A3/4 also inhibit the metabolism of cevimeline). Products include:
Desenex .... ▣ 635
Desenex Jock Itch Spray Powder ... ▣ 635

Moclobemide (Drugs which inhibit CYP2D6 also inhibit the metabolism of cevimeline. Cevimeline should be used with caution in individuals known or suspected to be deficient in CYP2D6 activity, as they may be at a higher risk of adverse events).
No products indexed under this heading.

Nadolol (Possibility of conduction disturbances; co-administration with beta adrenergic antagonists requires caution). Products include:
Nadolol Tablets 2159

Nefazodone Hydrochloride (Co-administration with drugs which inhibit CYP3A3/4, such as nefazodone, may inhibit the metabolism of cevimeline resulting in a higher risk of adverse events).
No products indexed under this heading.

Nelfinavir Mesylate (Co-administration with drugs which inhibit CYP3A3/4, such as nelfinavir, may inhibit the metabolism of cevimeline resulting in a higher risk of adverse events). Products include:
Viracept 2577

Neostigmine Bromide (Co-administration with parasympathomimetic drugs can be expected to have additive effects).
No products indexed under this heading.

Neostigmine Methylsulfate (Co-administration with parasympathomimetic drugs can be expected to have additive effects).
No products indexed under this heading.

Nevirapine (Drugs which inhibit CYP3A3/4 also inhibit the metabolism of cevimeline). Products include:
Viramune Oral Suspension 873
Viramune Tablets 873

Niacinamide (Drugs which inhibit CYP3A3/4 also inhibit the metabolism of cevimeline).
No products indexed under this heading.

Nicotinamide (Drugs which inhibit CYP3A3/4 also inhibit the metabolism of cevimeline). Products include:
Nicomide Tablets 1088

Nifedipine (Drugs which inhibit CYP3A3/4 also inhibit the metabolism of cevimeline). Products include:
Adalat CC Tablets 2964

Norfloxacin (Drugs which inhibit CYP3A3/4 also inhibit the metabolism of cevimeline). Products include:
Noroxin Tablets 2032

Nortriptyline Hydrochloride (Drugs which inhibit CYP2D6 also inhibit the metabolism of cevimeline. Cevimeline should be used with caution in individuals known or suspected to be deficient in CYP2D6 activity, as they may be at a higher risk of adverse events).
No products indexed under this heading.

Omeprazole (Drugs which inhibit CYP3A3/4 also inhibit the metabolism of cevimeline). Products include:
Zegerid Capsules 2958
Zegerid Powder for Oral Solution 2958

Oxyphenonium Bromide (Cevimeline might interfere with the desirable antimuscarinic effects of drugs used concomitantly).
No products indexed under this heading.

Paroxetine Hydrochloride (Co-administration with drugs which inhibit CYP2D6, such as paroxetine, may inhibit the metabolism of cevimeline resulting in a higher risk of adverse events). Products include:
Paxil CR Controlled-Release Tablets 1538
Paxil 1530

Penbutolol Sulfate (Possibility of conduction disturbances; co-administration with beta adrenergic antagonists requires caution).
No products indexed under this heading.

Perphenazine (Drugs which inhibit CYP2D6 also inhibit the metabolism of cevimeline. Cevimeline should be used with caution in individuals known or suspected to be deficient in CYP2D6 activity, as they may be at a higher risk of adverse events).
No products indexed under this heading.

Pindolol (Possibility of conduction disturbances; co-administration with beta adrenergic antagonists requires caution).
No products indexed under this heading.

Propafenone Hydrochloride (Drugs which inhibit CYP2D6 also inhibit the metabolism of cevimeline. Cevimeline should be used with caution in individuals known or suspected to be deficient in CYP2D6 activity, as they may be at a higher risk of adverse events). Products include:
Rythmol SR Capsules 2727

Propantheline Bromide (Cevimeline might interfere with the desirable antimuscarinic effects of drugs used concomitantly).
No products indexed under this heading.

Propoxyphene Hydrochloride (Drugs which inhibit CYP2D6 also inhibit the metabolism of cevimeline. Cevimeline should be used with caution in individuals known or suspected to be deficient in CYP2D6 activity, as they may be at a higher risk of adverse events).
No products indexed under this heading.

Propoxyphene Napsylate (Drugs which inhibit CYP2D6 also inhibit the metabolism of cevimeline. Cevimeline should be used with caution in individuals known or suspected to be deficient in CYP2D6 activity, as they may be at a higher risk of adverse events).
No products indexed under this heading.

Propranolol Hydrochloride (Possibility of conduction disturbances; co-administration with beta adrenergic antagonists requires caution). Products include:
Inderal LA Long-Acting Capsules 3429
InnoPran XL Capsules 2723

Protriptyline Hydrochloride (Drugs which inhibit CYP2D6 also inhibit the metabolism of cevimeline. Cevimeline should be used with caution in individuals known or suspected to be deficient in CYP2D6 activity, as they may be at a higher risk of adverse events).
No products indexed under this heading.

Pyridostigmine Bromide (Co-administration with parasympathomimetic drugs can be expected to have additive effects).
No products indexed under this heading.

Quinacrine Hydrochloride (Drugs which inhibit CYP2D6 also inhibit the metabolism of cevimeline. Cevimeline should be used with caution in individuals known or suspected to be deficient in CYP2D6 activity, as they may be at a higher risk of adverse events).
No products indexed under this heading.

Quinidine (Drugs which inhibit CYP3A3/4 also inhibit the metabolism of cevimeline).
No products indexed under this heading.

Quinidine Gluconate (Drugs which inhibit CYP2D6 also inhibit the metabolism of cevimeline. Cevimeline should be used with caution in individuals known or suspected to be deficient in CYP2D6 activity, as they may be at a higher risk of adverse events).
No products indexed under this heading.

Quinidine Hydrochloride (Drugs which inhibit CYP2D6 also inhibit the metabolism of cevimeline. Cevimeline should be used with caution in individuals known or suspected to be deficient in CYP2D6 activity, as they may be at a higher risk of adverse events).
No products indexed under this heading.

Quinidine Polygalacturonate (Drugs which inhibit CYP2D6 also inhibit the metabolism of cevimeline. Cevimeline should be used with caution in individuals known or suspected to be deficient in CYP2D6 activity, as they may be at a higher risk of adverse events).
No products indexed under this heading.

Quinidine Sulfate (Drugs which inhibit CYP2D6 also inhibit the metabolism of cevimeline. Cevimeline should be used with caution in individuals known or suspected to be deficient in CYP2D6 activity, as they may be at a higher risk of adverse events).
No products indexed under this heading.

Quinine (Drugs which inhibit CYP3A3/4 also inhibit the metabolism of cevimeline).
No products indexed under this heading.

Quinine Sulfate (Drugs which inhibit CYP3A3/4 also inhibit the metabolism of cevimeline).
No products indexed under this heading.

Quinupristin (Drugs which inhibit CYP3A3/4 also inhibit the metabolism of cevimeline).
No products indexed under this heading.

Ranitidine Bismuth Citrate (Drugs which inhibit CYP2D6 also inhibit the metabolism of cevimeline. Cevimeline should be used with caution in individuals known or suspected to be deficient in CYP2D6 activity, as they may be at a higher risk of adverse events).
No products indexed under this heading.

Ranitidine Hydrochloride (Drugs which inhibit CYP2D6 also inhibit the metabolism of cevimeline. Cevimeline should be used with caution in individuals known or suspected to be deficient in CYP2D6 activity, as they may be at a higher risk of adverse events). Products include:
Zantac 1624
Zantac Injection 1619
Zantac Injection Pharmacy Bulk Package 1622

Ritonavir (Co-administration with drugs which inhibit CYP2D6 and/or CYP3A3/4, such as ritonavir, may inhibit the metabolism of cevimeline resulting in a higher risk of adverse events). Products include:
Kaletra 476
Norvir 503

Saquinavir (Drugs which inhibit CYP3A3/4 also inhibit the metabolism of cevimeline).
No products indexed under this heading.

Saquinavir Mesylate (Drugs which inhibit CYP3A3/4 also inhibit the metabolism of cevimeline). Products include:
Invirase 2772

Scopolamine (Cevimeline might interfere with the desirable antimuscarinic effects of drugs used concomitantly). Products include:
Transderm Scōp Transdermal Therapeutic System 2177

Scopolamine Hydrobromide (Cevimeline might interfere with the desirable antimuscarinic effects of drugs used concomitantly). Products include:
Donnatal Extentabs 2493

Sertraline Hydrochloride (Co-administration with drugs which inhibit CYP2D6, such as sertraline, may inhibit the metabolism of cevimeline resulting in a higher risk of adverse events). Products include:
Zoloft 2586

Sotalol Hydrochloride (Possibility of conduction disturbances; co-administration with beta adrenergic antagonists requires caution).
No products indexed under this heading.

Telithromycin (Drugs which inhibit CYP3A3/4 also inhibit the metabolism of cevimeline). Products include:
Ketek Tablets 2903

Terbinafine Hydrochloride (Drugs which inhibit CYP2D6 also inhibit the metabolism of cevimeline. Cevimeline should be used with caution in individuals known or suspected to be deficient in CYP2D6 activity, as they may be at a higher risk of adverse events). Products include:
Lamisil Tablets 2232
Lamisil AT Creams (Athlete's Foot & Jock Itch) .... ⊡636

Thioridazine Hydrochloride (Drugs which inhibit CYP2D6 also inhibit the metabolism of cevimeline. Cevimeline should be used with caution in individuals known or suspected to be deficient in CYP2D6 activity, as they may be at a higher risk of adverse events). Products include:
Thioridazine Hydrochloride Tablets 2163

Timolol Hemihydrate (Possibility of conduction disturbances; co-administration with beta adrenergic antagonists requires caution). Products include:
Betimol Ophthalmic Solution 3382
Betimol Ophthalmic Solution .... ⊙295

Timolol Maleate (Possibility of conduction disturbances; co-administration with beta adrenergic antagonists requires caution). Products include:
Blocadren Tablets 1916
Cosopt Sterile Ophthalmic Solution 1931
Timolide Tablets 2086
Timoptic Sterile Ophthalmic Solution 2088
Timoptic in Ocudose 2091
Timoptic-XE Sterile Ophthalmic Gel Forming Solution 2092

Tolterodine Tartrate (Cevimeline might interfere with the desirable antimuscarinic effects of drugs used concomitantly). Products include:
Detrol Tablets 2628
Detrol LA Capsules 2631

Tridihexethyl Chloride (Cevimeline might interfere with the desirable antimuscarinic effects of drugs used concomitantly).
No products indexed under this heading.

Trimipramine Maleate (Drugs which inhibit CYP2D6 also inhibit the metabolism of cevimeline. Cevimeline should be used with caution in individuals known or suspected to be deficient in CYP2D6 activity, as they may be at a higher risk of adverse events).
No products indexed under this heading.

Troglitazone (Drugs which inhibit CYP3A3/4 also inhibit the metabolism of cevimeline).
No products indexed under this heading.

Troleandomycin (Drugs which inhibit CYP3A3/4 also inhibit the metabolism of cevimeline).
No products indexed under this heading.

Valproate Sodium (Drugs which inhibit CYP3A3/4 also inhibit the metabolism of cevimeline). Products include:
Depacon Injection 412

Verapamil Hydrochloride (Co-administration with drugs which inhibit CYP3A3/4, such as verapamil, may inhibit the metabolism of cevimeline resulting in a higher risk of adverse events). Products include:
Covera-HS Tablets 3139
Tarka Tablets 524
Verelan PM Extended-Release Capsules, Controlled-Onset 3106

Voriconazole (Drugs which inhibit CYP3A3/4 also inhibit the metabolism of cevimeline). Products include:
VFEND I.V. 2564
VFEND Oral Suspension 2564
VFEND Tablets 2564

Zafirlukast (Drugs which inhibit CYP3A3/4 also inhibit the metabolism of cevimeline). Products include:
Accolate Tablets 671

Zileuton (Drugs which inhibit CYP3A3/4 also inhibit the metabolism of cevimeline). Products include:
Zyflo Tablets 1023

Food Interactions

Food, unspecified (Co-administration with food decreases the rate of absorption, with a fasting Tmax of 1.53 hours and a Tmax of 2.86 hours after a meal; the peak concentration is reduced by 17.3%).

Grapefruit (Drugs which inhibit CYP3A3/4 also inhibit the metabolism of cevimeline).

Grapefruit Juice (Co-administration with drugs which inhibit CYP3A3/4, such as grapefruit juice, may inhibit the metabolism of cevimeline resulting in a higher risk of adverse events).

EXCEDRIN EXTRA STRENGTH CAPLETS/ TABLETS/GELTABS

(Acetaminophen, Aspirin, Caffeine) .... ⊡684

Food Interactions

Alcohol (Concomitant consumption of alcohol may cause liver damage).

EXCEDRIN MIGRAINE CAPLETS/TABLETS/ GELTABS

(Acetaminophen, Aspirin, Caffeine) .... ⊡609

Food Interactions

Alcohol (Concomitant consumption of alcohol may cause liver damage).

EXCEDRIN PM CAPLETS/ TABLETS/GELTABS

(Acetaminophen, Diphenhydramine Citrate) .... ⊡610

Food Interactions

Alcohol (Concomitant consumption of alcohol may cause liver damage).

EXCEDRIN SINUS HEADACHE CAPLETS/ TABLETS

(Acetaminophen, Phenylephrine Hydrochloride) .... ⊡610
May interact with monoamine oxidase inhibitors and certain other agents. Compounds in these categories include:

Isocarboxazid (Concurrent or sequential use of MAO inhibitors is not recommended).
No products indexed under this heading.

Moclobemide (Concurrent or sequential use of MAO inhibitors is not recommended).
No products indexed under this heading.

Pargyline Hydrochloride (Concurrent or sequential use of MAO inhibitors is not recommended).
No products indexed under this heading.

Phenelzine Sulfate (Concurrent or sequential use of MAO inhibitors is not recommended).
No products indexed under this heading.

Procarbazine Hydrochloride (Concurrent or sequential use of MAO inhibitors is not recommended). Products include:
Matulane Capsules 3191

Selegiline Hydrochloride (Concurrent or sequential use of MAO inhibitors is not recommended). Products include:
Eldepryl Capsules 3208
Zelapar Tablets 3372

Tranylcypromine Sulfate (Concurrent or sequential use of MAO inhibitors is not recommended). Products include:
Parnate Tablets 1527

Food Interactions

Alcohol (Having 3 or more alcoholic beverages may cause liver damage).

EXCEDRIN TENSION HEADACHE CAPLETS/ TABLETS/GELTABS

(Acetaminophen, Caffeine) .... ⊡611

Food Interactions

Alcohol (Concomitant consumption of alcohol may cause liver damage).

EXELON CAPSULES

(Rivastigmine Tartrate) 2206
May interact with anticholinergics and certain other agents. Compounds in these categories include:

Atropine Sulfate (Rivastigmine, a cholinesterase inhibitor, has the potential to interfere with the activity of anticholinergic medications). Products include:
Donnatal Extentabs 2493

Belladonna Alkaloids (Rivastigmine, a cholinesterase inhibitor, has the potential to interfere with the activity of anticholinergic medications). Products include:
Hyland's Teething Tablets .... ⊡830

Benztropine Mesylate (Rivastigmine, a cholinesterase inhibitor, has the potential to interfere with the activity of anticholinergic medications).
No products indexed under this heading.

Bethanechol Chloride (Co-administration with cholinergic agonist, such as bethanechol, can be expected to result in a synergistic effect).
No products indexed under this heading.

Biperiden Hydrochloride (Rivastigmine, a cholinesterase inhibitor, has the potential to interfere with the activity of anticholinergic medications).
No products indexed under this heading.

Clidinium Bromide (Rivastigmine, a cholinesterase inhibitor, has the potential to interfere with the activity of anticholinergic medications).
No products indexed under this heading.

Dicyclomine Hydrochloride (Rivastigmine, a cholinesterase inhibitor, has the potential to interfere with the activity of anticholinergic medications). Products include:
Bentyl Capsules 697
Bentyl Injection 697
Bentyl Syrup 697
Bentyl Tablets 697

Glycopyrrolate (Rivastigmine, a cholinesterase inhibitor, has the potential to interfere with the activity of anticholinergic medications).
No products indexed under this heading.

Hyoscyamine (Rivastigmine, a cholinesterase inhibitor, has the potential to interfere with the activity of anticholinergic medications).
No products indexed under this heading.

Hyoscyamine Sulfate (Rivastigmine, a cholinesterase inhibitor, has the potential to interfere with the activity of anticholinergic medications). Products include:
Donnatal Extentabs 2493
Prosed/DS Tablets 1157

Ipratropium Bromide (Rivastigmine, a cholinesterase inhibitor, has the potential to interfere with the activity of anticholinergic medications). Products include:
Atrovent Inhalation Solution 835
Atrovent HFA Inhalation Aerosol 841
Atrovent Nasal Spray 0.03% 837
Atrovent Nasal Spray 0.06% 839
Combivent Inhalation Aerosol 847
DuoNeb Inhalation Solution 1058

Mepenzolate Bromide (Rivastigmine, a cholinesterase inhibitor, has the potential to interfere with the activity of anticholinergic medications).
No products indexed under this heading.

Oxybutynin Chloride (Rivastigmine, a cholinesterase inhibitor, has the potential to interfere with the activity of anticholinergic medications). Products include:
Ditropan XL Extended-Release Tablets 2413

Procyclidine Hydrochloride (Rivastigmine, a cholinesterase inhibitor, has the potential to interfere with the activity of anticholinergic medications).
No products indexed under this heading.

Propantheline Bromide (Rivastigmine, a cholinesterase inhibitor, has the potential to interfere with the activity of anticholinergic medications).
No products indexed under this heading.

Scopolamine (Rivastigmine, a cholinesterase inhibitor, has the potential to interfere with the activity of anticholinergic medications). Products include:
Transderm Scōp Transdermal Therapeutic System 2177

Scopolamine Hydrobromide (Rivastigmine, a cholinesterase inhibitor, has the potential to interfere with the activity of anticholinergic medications). Products include:
Donnatal Extentabs 2493

Succinylcholine Chloride (Co-administration with succinylcholine can be expected to result in a synergistic effect).
No products indexed under this heading.

Tolterodine Tartrate (Rivastigmine, a cholinesterase inhibitor, has the potential to interfere with the activity of anticholinergic medications). Products include:
Detrol Tablets 2628
Detrol LA Capsules 2631

Tridihexethyl Chloride (Rivastigmine, a cholinesterase inhibitor, has the potential to interfere with the activity of anticholinergic medications).
No products indexed under this heading.

Trihexyphenidyl Hydrochloride (Rivastigmine, a cholinesterase inhibitor, has the potential to interfere with the activity of anticholinergic medications).
No products indexed under this heading.

Food Interactions

Food, unspecified (Co-administration with food delays absorption (Tmax) by 90 minutes, lowers Cmax by approximately 30% and increases AUC by approximately 30%).

EXELON ORAL SOLUTION

(Rivastigmine Tartrate) 2206
See Exelon Capsules

EX•LAX CHOCOLATED LAXATIVE PIECES

(Sennosides) .... ▣649
None cited in PDR database.

EX•LAX REGULAR STRENGTH PILLS

(Sennosides) .... ▣649
None cited in PDR database.

EX•LAX MAXIMUM STRENGTH PILLS

(Sennosides) .... ▣649
None cited in PDR database.

EXPERIENCE CAPSULES

(Herbals, Multiple, Psyllium Preparations) .... ▣828
None cited in PDR database.

EXUBERA INHALATION POWDER

(Insulin, Human (rDNA origin)) 2524
May interact with ACE inhibitors, beta blockers, corticosteroids, diuretics, estrogens, fibrates, oral hypoglycemic agents, lithium preparations, monoamine oxidase inhibitors, oral contraceptives, phenothiazines, progestins, protease inhibitors, salicylates, sympathomimetic bronchodilators, sympathomimetics, sympathomimetic aerosol bronchodilators, thyroid preparations, and certain other agents. Compounds in these categories include:

Acarbose (Oral antidiabetic products may increase the blood glucose-lowering effect of insulin and susceptibility to hypoglycemia. Co-administration may require insulin dose adjustment and particularly close monitoring). Products include:
Precose Tablets 751

Acebutolol Hydrochloride (Beta-blockers may either increase or reduce the blood glucose-lowering effect of insulin. In addition, under the influence of sympatholytic medicinal products such as beta-blockers, the signs and symptoms of hypoglycemia may be reduced or absent. Co-administration may require insulin dose adjustment and particularly close monitoring).
No products indexed under this heading.

Albuterol (Sympathomimetics may reduce the blood glucose-lowering effect of insulin, which may result in hyperglycemia. Co-administration may require insulin dose adjustment and particularly close monitoring). Products include:
Proventil Inhalation Aerosol 3053

Albuterol Sulfate (Sympathomimetics may reduce the blood glucose-lowering effect of insulin, which may result in hyperglycemia. Co-administration may require insulin dose adjustment and particularly close monitoring). Products include:
AccuNeb Inhalation Solution 1055
Combivent Inhalation Aerosol 847
DuoNeb Inhalation Solution 1058
ProAir HFA Inhalation Aerosol 3300
Proventil Inhalation Solution 0.083% 3055
Proventil HFA Inhalation Aerosol 3056
Ventolin HFA Inhalation Aerosol 1600
VoSpire ER Tablets 1052

Amiloride Hydrochloride (Diuretics may reduce the blood glucose-lowering effect of insulin, which may result in hyperglycemia. Co-administration may require insulin dose adjustment and particularly close monitoring). Products include:
Midamor Tablets 2026
Moduretic Tablets 2028

Amprenavir (Protease inhibitors may reduce the blood glucose-lowering effect of insulin, which may result in hyperglycemia. Co-administration may require insulin dose adjustment and particularly close monitoring). Products include:
Agenerase Capsules 1327
Agenerase Oral Solution 1332

Aspirin (Salicylates may increase the blood glucose-lowering effect of insulin and susceptibility to hypoglycemia. Co-administration may require insulin dose adjustment and particularly close monitoring). Products include:
Aggrenox Capsules 822
Bayer Aspirin 744
BC Allergy Sinus Cold Powder .... ▣677
BC Headache Powder .... ▣677
Arthritis Strength BC Powder .... ▣677
BC Sinus Cold Powder .... ▣677
Excedrin Extra Strength Caplets/Tablets/Geltabs .... ▣684
Excedrin Migraine Caplets/Tablets/Geltabs .... ▣609
Goody's Body Pain Formula Powder .... ▣684
Goody's Extra Strength Headache Powders .... ▣611
Goody's Extra Strength Pain Relief Tablets .... ▣685
Percodan Tablets 1132
St. Joseph 81 mg Aspirin Chewable and Enteric Coated Tablets 1869

Aspirin, Enteric Coated (Salicylates may increase the blood glucose-lowering effect of insulin and susceptibility to hypoglycemia. Co-administration may require insulin dose adjustment and particularly close monitoring).
No products indexed under this heading.

Aspirin Buffered (Salicylates may increase the blood glucose lowering effect of insulin and susceptibility to hypoglycemia. Co-administration may require insulin dose adjustment and particularly close monitoring). Products include:
Bufferin Extra Strength Tablets .... ▣678
Bufferin Regular Strength Tablets .... ▣678

Atenolol (Beta-blockers may either increase or reduce the blood glucose-lowering effect of insulin. In addition, under the influence of sympatholytic medicinal products such as beta-blockers, the signs and symptoms of hypoglycemia may be reduced or absent. Co-administration may require insulin dose adjustment and particularly close monitoring).
No products indexed under this heading.

Benazepril Hydrochloride (ACE inhibitors may increase the blood glucose-lowering effect of insulin and susceptibility to hypoglycemia. Co-administration may require insulin dose adjustment and particularly close monitoring). Products include:
Lotensin Tablets 2243
Lotensin HCT Tablets 2246
Lotrel Capsules 2249

Bendroflumethiazide (Diuretics may reduce the blood glucose-lowering effect of insulin, which may result in hyperglycemia. Co-administration may require insulin dose adjustment and particularly close monitoring).
No products indexed under this heading.

Betamethasone Acetate (Corticosteroids may reduce the blood glucose-lowering effect of insulin, which may result in hyperglycemia. Co-administration may require insulin dose adjustment and particularly close monitoring).
No products indexed under this heading.

Betamethasone Sodium Phosphate (Corticosteroids may reduce the blood glucose-lowering effect of insulin, which may result in hyperglycemia. Co-administration may require insulin dose adjustment and particularly close monitoring).
No products indexed under this heading.

Betaxolol Hydrochloride (Beta-blockers may either increase or reduce the blood glucose-lowering effect of insulin. In addition, under the influence of sympatholytic medicinal products such as beta-blockers, the signs and symptoms of hypoglycemia may be reduced or absent. Co-administration may require insulin dose adjustment and particularly close monitoring). Products include:
Betoptic S Ophthalmic Suspension 558

Bisoprolol Fumarate (Beta-blockers may either increase or reduce the blood glucose-lowering effect of insulin. In addition, under the influence of sympatholytic medicinal products such as beta-blockers, the signs and symptoms of hypoglycemia may be reduced or absent. Co-administration may require insulin dose adjustment and particularly close monitoring).
 No products indexed under this heading.

Bitolterol Mesylate (Bronchodilators and other inhaled products may alter the absorption of inhaled human insulin. Consistent timing of dosing of bronchodilators relative to Exubera administration, close monitoring of blood glucose concentrations, and dose titration as appropriate are recommended. Co-administration may require insulin dose adjustment and particularly close monitoring).
 No products indexed under this heading.

Bumetanide (Diuretics may reduce the blood glucose-lowering effect of insulin, which may result in hyperglycemia. Co-administration may require insulin dose adjustment and particularly close monitoring). Products include:
 Bumex Tablets **2746**

Captopril (ACE inhibitors may increase the blood glucose-lowering effect of insulin and susceptibility to hypoglycemia. Co-administration may require insulin dose adjustment and particularly close monitoring). Products include:
 Captopril Tablets **2149**

Carteolol Hydrochloride (Beta-blockers may either increase or reduce the blood glucose-lowering effect of insulin. In addition, under the influence of sympatholytic medicinal products such as beta-blockers, the signs and symptoms of hypoglycemia may be reduced or absent. Co-administration may require insulin dose adjustment and particularly close monitoring). Products include:
 Carteolol Hydrochloride
 Ophthalmic Solution USP, 1%....... ⊙ **249**

Chlorothiazide (Diuretics may reduce the blood glucose-lowering effect of insulin, which may result in hyperglycemia. Co-administration may require insulin dose adjustment and particularly close monitoring). Products include:
 Diuril Oral Suspension **1954**

Chlorothiazide Sodium (Diuretics may reduce the blood glucose-lowering effect of insulin, which may result in hyperglycemia. Co-administration may require insulin dose adjustment and particularly close monitoring). Products include:
 Diuril Sodium Intravenous **2467**

Chlorotrianisene (Estrogens may reduce the blood glucose-lowering effect of insulin, which may result in hyperglycemia. Co-administration may require insulin dose adjustment and particularly close monitoring).
 No products indexed under this heading.

Chlorpromazine (Phenothiazine derivatives may reduce the blood glucose-lowering effect of insulin, which may result in hyperglycemia. Co-administration may require insulin dose adjustment and particularly close monitoring).
 No products indexed under this heading.

Chlorpromazine Hydrochloride (Phenothiazine derivatives may reduce the blood glucose-lowering effect of insulin, which may result in hyperglycemia. Co-administration may require insulin dose adjustment and particularly close monitoring).
 No products indexed under this heading.

Chlorpropamide (Oral antidiabetic products may increase the blood glucose-lowering effect of insulin and susceptibility to hypoglycemia. Co-administration may require insulin dose adjustment and particularly close monitoring).
 No products indexed under this heading.

Chlorthalidone (Diuretics may reduce the blood glucose-lowering effect of insulin, which may result in hyperglycemia. Co-administration may require insulin dose adjustment and particularly close monitoring). Products include:
 Clorpres Tablets **2153**

Choline Magnesium Trisalicylate (Salicylates may increase the blood glucose-lowering effect of insulin and susceptibility to hypoglycemia. Co-administration may require insulin dose adjustment and particularly close monitoring).
 No products indexed under this heading.

Clofibrate (Fibrates may increase the blood glucose-lowering effect of insulin and susceptibility to hypoglycemia. Co-administration may require insulin dose adjustment and particularly close monitoring).
 No products indexed under this heading.

Clonidine (Clonidine may either increase or reduce the blood glucose-lowering effect of insulin. In addition, under the influence of sympatholytic medicinal products such as clonidine, the signs and symptoms of hypoglycemia may be reduced or absent. In addition, under the influence of clonidine, the signs and symptoms of hypoglycemia may be reduced or absent. Co-administration may require insulin dose adjustment and particularly close monitoring). Products include:
 Catapres-TTS **844**

Clonidine Hydrochloride (Clonidine may either increase or reduce the blood glucose-lowering effect of insulin. In addition, under the influence of sympatholytic medicinal products such as clonidine, the signs and symptoms of hypoglycemia may be reduced or absent. In addition, under the influence of clonidine, the signs and symptoms of hypoglycemia may be reduced or absent. Co-administration may require insulin dose adjustment and particularly close monitoring). Products include:
 Catapres Tablets **843**
 Clorpres Tablets **2153**

Clozapine (Atypical antipsychotics, such as clozapine, may reduce the blood glucose-lowering effect of insulin, which may result in hyperglycemia. Co-administration may require insulin dose adjustment and particularly close monitoring). Products include:
 Clozaril Tablets **2184**
 FazaClo Orally Disintegrating
 Tablets .. **551**

Cortisone Acetate (Corticosteroids may reduce the blood glucose-lowering effect of insulin, which may result in hyperglycemia. Co-administration may require insulin dose adjustment and particularly close monitoring).
 No products indexed under this heading.

Danazol (Danazol may reduce the blood glucose-lowering effect of insulin, which may result in hyperglycemia. Co-administration may require insulin dose adjustment and particularly close monitoring).
 No products indexed under this heading.

Desogestrel (Oral contraceptives may reduce the blood glucose-lowering effect of insulin, which may result in hyperglycemia. Co-administration may require insulin dose adjustment and particularly close monitoring). Products include:
 Mircette Tablets **1066**

Dexamethasone (Corticosteroids may reduce the blood glucose-lowering effect of insulin, which may result in hyperglycemia. Co-administration may require insulin dose adjustment and particularly close monitoring). Products include:
 Ciprodex Otic Suspension **559**
 Decadron Tablets **1951**
 TobraDex Ophthalmic Ointment **562**
 TobraDex Ophthalmic Suspension ... **563**

Dexamethasone Acetate (Corticosteroids may reduce the blood glucose-lowering effect of insulin, which may result in hyperglycemia. Co-administration may require insulin dose adjustment and particularly close monitoring).
 No products indexed under this heading.

Dexamethasone Sodium Phosphate (Corticosteroids may reduce the blood glucose-lowering effect of insulin, which may result in hyperglycemia. Co-administration may require insulin dose adjustment and particularly close monitoring).
 No products indexed under this heading.

Diazoxide (Diazoxide may reduce the blood glucose-lowering effect of insulin, which may result in hyperglycemia. Co-administration may require insulin dose adjustment and particularly close monitoring). Products include:
 Hyperstat I.V. **3017**

Dienestrol (Estrogens may reduce the blood glucose-lowering effect of insulin, which may result in hyperglycemia. Co-administration may require insulin dose adjustment and particularly close monitoring).
 No products indexed under this heading.

Diethylstilbestrol (Estrogens may reduce the blood glucose-lowering effect of insulin, which may result in hyperglycemia. Co-administration may require insulin dose adjustment and particularly close monitoring).
 No products indexed under this heading.

Diflunisal (Salicylates may increase the blood glucose-lowering effect of insulin and susceptibility to hypoglycemia. Co-administration may require insulin dose adjustment and particularly close monitoring). Products include:
 Dolobid Tablets **1955**

Disopyramide (Disopyramide may increase the blood glucose-lowering effect of insulin and susceptibility to hypoglycemia. Co-administration may require insulin dose adjustment and particularly close monitoring).
 No products indexed under this heading.

Disopyramide Phosphate (Disopyramide may increase the blood glucose-lowering effect of insulin and susceptibility to hypoglycemia. Co-administration may require insulin dose adjustment and particularly close monitoring).
 No products indexed under this heading.

Dobutamine Hydrochloride (Sympathomimetics may reduce the blood glucose-lowering effect of insulin, which may result in hyperglycemia. Co-administration may require insulin dose adjustment and particularly close monitoring).
 No products indexed under this heading.

Dopamine Hydrochloride (Sympathomimetics may reduce the blood glucose-lowering effect of insulin, which may result in hyperglycemia. Co-administration may require insulin dose adjustment and particularly close monitoring).
 No products indexed under this heading.

Enalapril Maleate (ACE inhibitors may increase the blood glucose-lowering effect of insulin and susceptibility to hypoglycemia. Co-administration may require insulin dose adjustment and particularly close monitoring). Products include:
 Vasotec I.V. Injection **2103**

Enalaprilat (ACE inhibitors may increase the blood glucose-lowering effect of insulin and susceptibility to hypoglycemia. Co-administration may require insulin dose adjustment and particularly close monitoring).
 No products indexed under this heading.

Ephedrine Hydrochloride (Sympathomimetics may reduce the blood glucose-lowering effect of insulin, which may result in hyperglycemia. Co-administration may require insulin dose adjustment and particularly close monitoring).
 No products indexed under this heading.

Ephedrine Sulfate (Sympathomimetics may reduce the blood glucose-lowering effect of insulin, which may result in hyperglycemia. Co-administration may require insulin dose adjustment and particularly close monitoring).
 No products indexed under this heading.

Ephedrine Tannate (Sympathomimetics may reduce the blood glucose-lowering effect of insulin, which may result in hyperglycemia. Co-administration may require insulin dose adjustment and particularly close monitoring).
 No products indexed under this heading.

Epinephrine (Sympathomimetics may reduce the blood glucose-lowering effect of insulin, which may result in hyperglycemia. Co-administration may require insulin dose adjustment and particularly close monitoring). Products include:
 EpiPen .. **1061**

IMPORTANT NOTE: Always consult each drug listing in the patient's regimen for possible interactions.

Primatene Mist .... ▣719
Twinject 0.15 3379
Twinject 0.3 3378

Epinephrine Bitartrate (Sympathomimetics may reduce the blood glucose-lowering effect of insulin, which may result in hyperglycemia. Co-administration may require insulin dose adjustment and particularly close monitoring).
No products indexed under this heading.

Epinephrine Hydrochloride (Sympathomimetics may reduce the blood glucose-lowering effect of insulin, which may result in hyperglycemia. Co-administration may require insulin dose adjustment and particularly close monitoring).
No products indexed under this heading.

Esmolol Hydrochloride (Beta-blockers may either increase or reduce the blood glucose-lowering effect of insulin. In addition, under the influence of sympatholytic medicinal products such as beta-blockers, the signs and symptoms of hypoglycemia may be reduced or absent. Co-administration may require insulin dose adjustment and particularly close monitoring).
No products indexed under this heading.

Estradiol (Estrogents may reduce the blood glucose-lowering effect of insulin, which may result in hyperglycemia. Co-administration may require insulin dose adjustment and particularly close monitoring). Products include:
Angeliq Tablets 762
Climara Transdermal System 771
Climara Pro Transdermal System 776
Estrasorb Topical Emulsion 1147
Estring Vaginal Ring 2635
Menostar Transdermal System 782
Vagifem Tablets 2334

Estrogens, Conjugated (Estrogents may reduce the blood glucose-lowering effect of insulin, which may result in hyperglycemia. Co-administration may require insulin dose adjustment and particularly close monitoring). Products include:
Premarin Intravenous 3442
Premarin Tablets 3446
Premarin Vaginal Cream 3452
Premphase Tablets 3456
Prempro Tablets 3456

Estrogens, Esterified (Estrogents may reduce the blood glucose-lowering effect of insulin, which may result in hyperglycemia. Co-administration may require insulin dose adjustment and particularly close monitoring). Products include:
Estratest Tablets 3199
Estratest H.S. Tablets 3199

Estropipate (Estrogents may reduce the blood glucose-lowering effect of insulin, which may result in hyperglycemia. Co-administration may require insulin dose adjustment and particularly close monitoring).
No products indexed under this heading.

Ethacrynic Acid (Diuretics may reduce the blood glucose-lowering effect of insulin, which may result in hyperglycemia. Co-administration may require insulin dose adjustment and particularly close monitoring). Products include:
Edecrin Tablets 1959

Ethanol (Alcohol may either increase or reduce the blood glucose-lowering effect of insulin. Co-administration may require insulin dose adjustment and particularly close monitoring).
No products indexed under this heading.

Ethinyl Estradiol (Oral contraceptives may reduce the blood glucose-lowering effect of insulin, which may result in hyperglycemia. Co-administration may require insulin dose adjustment and particularly close monitoring). Products include:
Mircette Tablets 1066
NuvaRing 2340
Ortho-Cyclen/Ortho Tri-Cyclen 2429
Ortho Evra Transdermal System 2417
Ortho Tri-Cyclen Lo Tablets 2436
Seasonique Tablets 1077
Yasmin 28 Tablets 796
Yaz Tablets 803

Ethynodiol Diacetate (Oral contraceptives may reduce the blood glucose-lowering effect of insulin, which may result in hyperglycemia. Co-administration may require insulin dose adjustment and particularly close monitoring).
No products indexed under this heading.

Fenofibrate (Fibrates may increase the blood glucose-lowering effect of insulin and susceptibility to hypoglycemia. Co-administration may require insulin dose adjustment and particularly close monitoring). Products include:
Lofibra Tablets 1219
Lofibra Capsules 1216
Tricor Tablets 527
Triglide Tablets 3123

Fludrocortisone Acetate (Corticosteroids may reduce the blood glucose-lowering effect of insulin, which may result in hyperglycemia. Co-administration may require insulin dose adjustment and particularly close monitoring).
No products indexed under this heading.

Fluoxetine (Fluoxetine may increase the blood glucose-lowering effect of insulin and susceptibility to hypoglycemia. Co-administration may require insulin dose adjustment and particularly close monitoring).
No products indexed under this heading.

Fluoxetine Hydrochloride (Fluoxetine may increase the blood glucose-lowering effect of insulin and susceptibility to hypoglycemia. Co-administration may require insulin dose adjustment and particularly close monitoring). Products include:
Prozac Pulvules and Liquid 1801
Symbyax Capsules 1819

Fluphenazine Decanoate (Phenothiazine derivatives may reduce the blood glucose-lowering effect of insulin, which may result in hyperglycemia. Co-administration may require insulin dose adjustment and particularly close monitoring).
No products indexed under this heading.

Fluphenazine Enanthate (Phenothiazine derivatives may reduce the blood glucose-lowering effect of insulin, which may result in hyperglycemia. Co-administration may require insulin dose adjustment and particularly close monitoring).
No products indexed under this heading.

Fluphenazine Hydrochloride (Phenothiazine derivatives may reduce the blood glucose-lowering effect of insulin, which may result in hyperglycemia. Co-administration may require insulin dose adjustment and particularly close monitoring).
No products indexed under this heading.

Fosinopril Sodium (ACE inhibitors may increase the blood glucose-lowering effect of insulin and susceptibility to hypoglycemia. Co-administration may require insulin dose adjustment and particularly close monitoring).
No products indexed under this heading.

Furosemide (Diuretics may reduce the blood glucose-lowering effect of insulin, which may result in hyperglycemia. Co-administration may require insulin dose adjustment and particularly close monitoring). Products include:
Furosemide Tablets 2154

Gemfibrozil (Fibrates may increase the blood glucose-lowering effect of insulin and susceptibility to hypoglycemia. Co-administration may require insulin dose adjustment and particularly close monitoring).
No products indexed under this heading.

Glimepiride (Oral antidiabetic products may increase the blood glucose-lowering effect of insulin and susceptibility to hypoglycemia. Co-administration may require insulin dose adjustment and particularly close monitoring). Products include:
Avandaryl Tablets 1379
Duetact Tablets 3226

Glipizide (Oral antidiabetic products may increase the blood glucose-lowering effect of insulin and susceptibility to hypoglycemia. Co-administration may require insulin dose adjustment and particularly close monitoring).
No products indexed under this heading.

Glucagon (Glucagon may reduce the blood glucose-lowering effect of insulin, which may result in hyperglycemia. Co-administration may require insulin dose adjustment and particularly close monitoring). Products include:
GlucaGen 761
Glucagon for Injection Vials and Emergency Kit 1778

Glyburide (Oral antidiabetic products may increase the blood glucose-lowering effect of insulin and susceptibility to hypoglycemia. Co-administration may require insulin dose adjustment and particularly close monitoring).
No products indexed under this heading.

Guanethidine (Under the influence of sympatholytic medicinal products, such as guanethidine, the signs and symptoms of hypoglycemia may be reduced or absent. Co-administration may require insulin dose adjustment and particularly close monitoring).
No products indexed under this heading.

Guanethidine Monosulfate (Under the influence of sympatholytic medicinal products, such as guanethidine, the signs and symptoms of hypoglycemia may be reduced or absent. Co-administration may require insulin dose adjustment and particularly close monitoring).
No products indexed under this heading.

Guanethidine Sulfate (Under the influence of sympatholytic medicinal products, such as guanethidine, the signs and symptoms of hypoglycemia may be reduced or absent. Co-administration may require insulin dose adjustment and particularly close monitoring).
No products indexed under this heading.

Hydrochlorothiazide (Diuretics may reduce the blood glucose-lowering effect of insulin, which may result in hyperglycemia. Co-administration may require insulin dose adjustment and particularly close monitoring). Products include:
Aldoril Tablets 1910
Atacand HCT 651
Avalide Tablets 888
Avalide Tablets 2874
Benicar HCT Tablets 1044
Diovan HCT Tablets 2196
Dyazide Capsules 1423
Hyzaar 50-12.5 Tablets 1990
Hyzaar 100-12.5 Tablets 1990
Hyzaar 100-25 Tablets 1990
Lopressor HCT 50/25 Tablets 2241
Lopressor HCT 100/25 Tablets 2241
Lopressor HCT 100/50 Tablets 2241
Lotensin HCT Tablets 2246
Micardis HCT Tablets 856
Moduretic Tablets 2028
Prinzide Tablets 2056
Teveten HCT Tablets 1737
Timolide Tablets 2086
Uniretic Tablets 3100

Hydrocortisone (Corticosteroids may reduce the blood glucose-lowering effect of insulin, which may result in hyperglycemia. Co-administration may require insulin dose adjustment and particularly close monitoring). Products include:
Colocort Rectal Suspension, USP (Retention) 100 mg/60 mL 2476
Hydrocortone Tablets 1989
Preparation H Hydrocortisone Cream .... ▣646

Hydrocortisone Acetate (Corticosteroids may reduce the blood glucose-lowering effect of insulin, which may result in hyperglycemia. Co-administration may require insulin dose adjustment and particularly close monitoring). Products include:
Analpram-HC 1159
Pramosone 1161
ProctoFoam-HC 3099

Hydrocortisone Sodium Phosphate (Corticosteroids may reduce the blood glucose-lowering effect of insulin, which may result in hyperglycemia. Co-administration may require insulin dose adjustment and particularly close monitoring).
No products indexed under this heading.

Hydrocortisone Sodium Succinate (Corticosteroids may reduce the blood glucose-lowering effect of insulin, which may result in hyperglycemia. Co-administration may require insulin dose adjustment and particularly close monitoring).
No products indexed under this heading.

Hydroflumethiazide (Diuretics may reduce the blood glucose-lowering effect of insulin, which may result in hyperglycemia. Co-administration may require insulin dose adjustment and particularly close monitoring).

No products indexed under this heading.

Indapamide (Diuretics may reduce the blood glucose-lowering effect of insulin, which may result in hyperglycemia. Co-administration may require insulin dose adjustment and particularly close monitoring). Products include:

Indapamide Tablets 2156

Indinavir Sulfate (Protease inhibitors may reduce the blood glucose-lowering effect of insulin, which may result in hyperglycemia. Co-administration may require insulin dose adjustment and particularly close monitoring). Products include:

Crixivan Capsules 1940

Isocarboxazid (MAO inhibitors may increase the blood glucose-lowering effect of insulin and susceptibility to hypoglycemia. Co-administration may require insulin dose adjustment and particularly close monitoring).

No products indexed under this heading.

Isoetharine (Bronchodilators and other inhaled products may alter the absorption of inhaled human insulin. Consistent timing of dosing of bronchodilators relative to Exubera administration, close monitoring of blood glucose concentrations, and dose titration as appropriate are recommended. Co-administration may require insulin dose adjustment and particularly close monitoring).

No products indexed under this heading.

Isoniazid (Isoniazid may reduce the blood glucose-lowering effect of insulin, which may result in hyperglycemia. Co-administration may require insulin dose adjustment and particularly close monitoring).

No products indexed under this heading.

Isoproterenol Hydrochloride (Sympathomimetics may reduce the blood glucose-lowering effect of insulin, which may result in hyperglycemia. Co-administration may require insulin dose adjustment and particularly close monitoring).

No products indexed under this heading.

Isoproterenol Sulfate (Sympathomimetics may reduce the blood glucose-lowering effect of insulin, which may result in hyperglycemia. Co-administration may require insulin dose adjustment and particularly close monitoring).

No products indexed under this heading.

Labetalol Hydrochloride (Beta-blockers may either increase or reduce the blood glucose-lowering effect of insulin. In addition, under the influence of sympatholytic medicinal products such as beta-blockers, the signs and symptoms of hypoglycemia may be reduced or absent. Co-administration may require insulin dose adjustment and particularly close monitoring).

No products indexed under this heading.

Levalbuterol Hydrochloride (Sympathomimetics may reduce the

blood glucose-lowering effect of insulin, which may result in hyperglycemia. Co-administration may require insulin dose adjustment and particularly close monitoring). Products include:

Xopenex Inhalation Solution 3146
Xopenex Inhalation Solution
 Concentrate 3150

Levobunolol Hydrochloride (Beta-blockers may either increase or reduce the blood glucose-lowering effect of insulin. In addition, under the influence of sympatholytic medicinal products such as beta-blockers, the signs and symptoms of hypoglycemia may be reduced or absent. Co-administration may require insulin dose adjustment and particularly close monitoring). Products include:

Betagan Ophthalmic Solution,
 USP ... ⊙ 220

Levonorgestrel (Oral contraceptives may reduce the blood glucose-lowering effect of insulin, which may result in hyperglycemia. Co-administration may require insulin dose adjustment and particularly close monitoring). Products include:

Climara Pro Transdermal System 776
Mirena Intrauterine System 787
Plan B Tablets 1076
Seasonique Tablets 1077

Levothyroxine Sodium (Thyroid hormones may reduce the blood glucose-lowering effect of insulin, which may result in hyperglycemia. Co-administration may require insulin dose adjustment and particularly close monitoring). Products include:

Levothroid Tablets 1186
Levoxyl Tablets 1712
Synthroid Tablets 520
Westhroid Tablets 3403

Liothyronine Sodium (Thyroid hormones may reduce the blood glucose-lowering effect of insulin, which may result in hyperglycemia. Co-administration may require insulin dose adjustment and particularly close monitoring). Products include:

Cytomel Tablets 1710
Westhroid Tablets 3403

Liotrix (Thyroid hormones may reduce the blood glucose-lowering effect of insulin, which may result in hyperglycemia. Co-administration may require insulin dose adjustment and particularly close monitoring). Products include:

Thyrolar Tablets 1199

Lisinopril (ACE inhibitors may increase the blood glucose-lowering effect of insulin and susceptibility to hypoglycemia. Co-administration may require insulin dose adjustment and particularly close monitoring). Products include:

Prinivil Tablets 2052
Prinzide Tablets 2056

Lithium (Lithium salts may either increase or reduce the blood glucose-lowering effect of insulin. Co-administration may require insulin dose adjustment and particularly close monitoring).

No products indexed under this heading.

Lithium Carbonate (Lithium salts may either increase or reduce the blood glucose-lowering effect of insulin. Co-administration may require insulin dose adjustment and particularly close monitoring). Products include:

Lithobid Tablets 1692

Lithium Citrate (Lithium salts may either increase or reduce the blood glucose-lowering effect of insulin. Co-administration may require insulin dose adjustment and particularly close monitoring).

No products indexed under this heading.

Lopinavir (Protease inhibitors may reduce the blood glucose-lowering effect of insulin, which may result in hyperglycemia. Co-administration may require insulin dose adjustment and particularly close monitoring). Products include:

Kaletra .. 476

Magnesium Salicylate (Salicylates may increase the blood glucose-lowering effect of insulin and susceptibility to hypoglycemia. Co-administration may require insulin dose adjustment and particularly close monitoring).

No products indexed under this heading.

Medroxyprogesterone Acetate (Progestogens may reduce the blood glucose-lowering effect of insulin, which may result in hyperglycemia. Co-administration may require insulin dose adjustment and particularly close monitoring). Products include:

Depo-Provera Contraceptive
 Injection 2622
depo-subQ provera 104
 Injectable Suspension.................. 2624
Premphase Tablets 3456
Prempro Tablets 3456

Megestrol Acetate (Progestogens may reduce the blood glucose-lowering effect of insulin, which may result in hyperglycemia. Co-administration may require insulin dose adjustment and particularly close monitoring). Products include:

Megace ES Oral Suspension 2481

Mesoridazine Besylate (Phenothiazine derivatives may reduce the blood glucose-lowering effect of insulin, which may result in hyperglycemia. Co-administration may require insulin dose adjustment and particularly close monitoring).

No products indexed under this heading.

Mestranol (Oral contraceptives may reduce the blood glucose-lowering effect of insulin, which may result in hyperglycemia. Co-administration may require insulin dose adjustment and particularly close monitoring).

No products indexed under this heading.

Metaproterenol Sulfate (Sympathomimetics may reduce the blood glucose-lowering effect of insulin, which may result in hyperglycemia. Co-administration may require insulin dose adjustment and particularly close monitoring). Products include:

Alupent Inhalation Aerosol 826

Metaraminol Bitartrate (Sympathomimetics may reduce the blood glucose-lowering effect of insulin, which may result in hyperglycemia. Co-administration may require insulin dose adjustment and particularly close monitoring).

No products indexed under this heading.

Metformin Hydrochloride (Oral antidiabetic products may increase the blood glucose-lowering effect of insulin and susceptibility to hypoglycemia. Co-administration may

require insulin dose adjustment and particularly close monitoring). Products include:

ActoPlus Met Tablets 3214
Avandamet Tablets 1373
Fortamet Extended-Release
 Tablets 3115

Methotrimeprazine (Phenothiazine derivatives may reduce the blood glucose-lowering effect of insulin, which may result in hyperglycemia. Co-administration may require insulin dose adjustment and particularly close monitoring).

No products indexed under this heading.

Methoxamine Hydrochloride (Sympathomimetics may reduce the blood glucose-lowering effect of insulin, which may result in hyperglycemia. Co-administration may require insulin dose adjustment and particularly close monitoring).

No products indexed under this heading.

Methyclothiazide (Diuretics may reduce the blood glucose-lowering effect of insulin, which may result in hyperglycemia. Co-administration may require insulin dose adjustment and particularly close monitoring).

No products indexed under this heading.

Methylprednisolone Acetate (Corticosteroids may reduce the blood glucose-lowering effect of insulin, which may result in hyperglycemia. Co-administration may require insulin dose adjustment and particularly close monitoring). Products include:

Depo-Medrol Injectable
 Suspension 2617
Depo-Medrol Single-Dose Vial 2619

Methylprednisolone Sodium Succinate (Corticosteroids may reduce the blood glucose-lowering effect of insulin, which may result in hyperglycemia. Co-administration may require insulin dose adjustment and particularly close monitoring).

No products indexed under this heading.

Metipranolol Hydrochloride (Beta-blockers may either increase or reduce the blood glucose-lowering effect of insulin. In addition, under the influence of sympatholytic medicinal products such as beta-blockers, the signs and symptoms of hypoglycemia may be reduced or absent. Co-administration may require insulin dose adjustment and particularly close monitoring).

No products indexed under this heading.

Metolazone (Diuretics may reduce the blood glucose-lowering effect of insulin, which may result in hyperglycemia. Co-administration may require insulin dose adjustment and particularly close monitoring).

No products indexed under this heading.

Metoprolol Succinate (Beta-blockers may either increase or reduce the blood glucose-lowering effect of insulin. In addition, under the influence of sympatholytic medicinal products such as beta-blockers, the signs and symptoms of hypoglycemia may be reduced or absent. Co-administration may require insulin dose adjustment and particularly close monitoring). Products include:

Toprol-XL Tablets 668

Metoprolol Tartrate (Beta-blockers may either increase or reduce the

IMPORTANT NOTE: Always consult each drug listing in the patient's regimen for possible interactions.

blood glucose-lowering effect of insulin. In addition, under the influence of sympatholytic medicinal products such as beta-blockers, the signs and symptoms of hypoglycemia may be reduced or absent. Co-administration may require insulin dose adjustment and particularly close monitoring). Products include:

- Lopressor Injection 2238
- Lopressor Tablets 2238
- Lopressor HCT 50/25 Tablets 2241
- Lopressor HCT 100/25 Tablets 2241
- Lopressor HCT 100/50 Tablets 2241

Miglitol (Oral antidiabetic products may increase the blood glucose-lowering effect of insulin and susceptibility to hypoglycemia. Co-administration may require insulin dose adjustment and particularly close monitoring).

No products indexed under this heading.

Moclobemide (MAO inhibitors may increase the blood glucose-lowering effect of insulin and susceptibility to hypoglycemia. Co-administration may require insulin dose adjustment and particularly close monitoring).

No products indexed under this heading.

Moexipril Hydrochloride (ACE inhibitors may increase the blood glucose-lowering effect of insulin and susceptibility to hypoglycemia. Co-administration may require insulin dose adjustment and particularly close monitoring). Products include:

- Uniretic Tablets 3100
- Univasc Tablets 3104

Nadolol (Beta-blockers may either increase or reduce the blood glucose-lowering effect of insulin. In addition, under the influence of sympatholytic medicinal products such as beta-blockers, the signs and symptoms of hypoglycemia may be reduced or absent. Co-administration may require insulin dose adjustment and particularly close monitoring). Products include:

- Nadolol Tablets 2159

Nelfinavir Mesylate (Protease inhibitors may reduce the blood glucose-lowering effect of insulin, which may result in hyperglycemia. Co-administration may require insulin dose adjustment and particularly close monitoring). Products include:

- Viracept 2577

Norepinephrine Bitartrate (Sympathomimetics may reduce the blood glucose-lowering effect of insulin, which may result in hyperglycemia. Co-administration may require insulin dose adjustment and particularly close monitoring).

No products indexed under this heading.

Norethindrone (Oral contraceptives may reduce the blood glucose-lowering effect of insulin, which may result in hyperglycemia. Co-administration may require insulin dose adjustment and particularly close monitoring). Products include:

- Ortho Micronor Tablets 2426

Norethynodrel (Oral contraceptives may reduce the blood glucose-lowering effect of insulin, which may result in hyperglycemia. Co-administration may require insulin dose adjustment and particularly close monitoring).

No products indexed under this heading.

Norgestimate (Oral contraceptives may reduce the blood glucose-lowering effect of insulin, which may result in hyperglycemia. Co-administration may require insulin dose adjustment and particularly close monitoring). Products include:

- Ortho-Cyclen/Ortho Tri-Cyclen 2429
- Ortho Tri-Cyclen Lo Tablets 2436

Norgestrel (Oral contraceptives may reduce the blood glucose-lowering effect of insulin, which may result in hyperglycemia. Co-administration may require insulin dose adjustment and particularly close monitoring).

No products indexed under this heading.

Olanzapine (Atypical antipsychotics, such as olanzapine, may reduce the blood glucose-lowering effect of insulin, which may result in hyperglycemia. Co-administration may require insulin dose adjustment and particularly close monitoring). Products include:

- Symbyax Capsules 1819
- Zyprexa Tablets 1830
- Zyprexa IntraMuscular 1830
- Zyprexa ZYDIS Orally Disintegrating Tablets 1830

Pargyline Hydrochloride (MAO inhibitors may increase the blood glucose-lowering effect of insulin and susceptibility to hypoglycemia. Co-administration may require insulin dose adjustment and particularly close monitoring).

No products indexed under this heading.

Penbutolol Sulfate (Beta-blockers may either increase or reduce the blood glucose-lowering effect of insulin. In addition, under the influence of sympatholytic medicinal products such as beta-blockers, the signs and symptoms of hypoglycemia may be reduced or absent. Co-administration may require insulin dose adjustment and particularly close monitoring).

No products indexed under this heading.

Pentamidine Isethionate (Pentamidine may cause hypoglycemia, which may sometimes be followed by hyperglycemia. Co-administration may require insulin dose adjustment and particularly close monitoring).

No products indexed under this heading.

Pentoxifylline (Pentoxifylline may increase the blood glucose-lowering effect of insulin and susceptibility to hypoglycemia. Co-administration may require insulin dose adjustment and particularly close monitoring).

No products indexed under this heading.

Perindopril Erbumine (ACE inhibitors may increase the blood glucose-lowering effect of insulin and susceptibility to hypoglycemia. Co-administration may require insulin dose adjustment and particularly close monitoring). Products include:

- Aceon Tablets (2 mg, 4 mg, 8 mg) 3194

Perphenazine (Phenothiazine derivatives may reduce the blood glucose-lowering effect of insulin, which may result in hyperglycemia. Co-administration may require insulin dose adjustment and particularly close monitoring).

No products indexed under this heading.

Phenelzine Sulfate (MAO inhibitors may increase the blood glucose-lowering effect of insulin and susceptibility to hypoglycemia. Co-administration may require insulin dose adjustment and particularly close monitoring).

No products indexed under this heading.

Phenylephrine Bitartrate (Sympathomimetics may reduce the blood glucose-lowering effect of insulin, which may result in hyperglycemia. Co-administration may require insulin dose adjustment and particularly close monitoring).

No products indexed under this heading.

Phenylephrine Hydrochloride (Sympathomimetics may reduce the blood glucose-lowering effect of insulin, which may result in hyperglycemia. Co-administration may require insulin dose adjustment and particularly close monitoring). Products include:

- Comtrex Maximum Strength Non-Drowsy Cold & Cough Caplets .... ▣ 725
- Comtrex Maximum Strength Day/Night Severe Cold & Sinus Caplets - Day Formulation .... ▣ 725
- Comtrex Maximum Strength Day/Night Severe Cold & Sinus Caplets - Night Formulation .... ▣ 725
- Contac Cold and Flu Maximum Strength Caplets .... ▣ 728
- Contac Cold and Flu Day and Night Caplets (Day Formulation Only) .... ▣ 727
- Contac Cold and Flu Day and Night Caplets (Night Formulation Only) .... ▣ 727
- Contac Cold and Flu Non-Drowsy Caplets .... ▣ 728
- Contac-D Cold Non-Drowsy Tablets .... ▣ 729
- Children's Dimetapp Cold & Allergy Elixir .... ▣ 730
- Children's Dimetapp Cold & Allergy Chewable Tablets .... ▣ 730
- Children's Dimetapp DM Cold & Cough Elixir .... ▣ 731
- Toddler's Dimetapp Cold and Cough Drops .... ▣ 732
- Excedrin Sinus Headache Caplets/Tablets .... ▣ 610
- 4-Way Fast Acting Nasal Spray .... ▣ 775
- 4-Way Menthol Nasal Spray .... ▣ 775
- Preparation H Maximum Strength Cream .... ▣ 666
- Preparation H Cooling Gel .... ▣ 666
- Preparation H .... ▣ 666
- Refenesen PE Caplets .... ▣ 721
- Robitussin Cough & Allergy Syrup .. ▣ 736
- Robitussin Cough & Cold Nighttime Liquid .... ▣ 736
- Robitussin Cough, Cold & Flu Nighttime Liquid .... ▣ 738
- Robitussin Head & Chest Congestion PE Syrup .... ▣ 739
- Robitussin Pediatric Cough & Cold Nighttime Liquid .... ▣ 736
- TheraFlu Cold & Cough Hot Liquid .... ▣ 740
- TheraFlu Cold & Sore Throat Hot Liquid .... ▣ 741
- TheraFlu Flu & Sore Throat Hot Liquid .... ▣ 742
- TheraFlu Daytime Severe Cold Hot Liquid .... ▣ 742
- TheraFlu Nighttime Severe Cold Hot Liquid .... ▣ 740
- TheraFlu Warming Relief Daytime Severe Cold .... ▣ 743
- TheraFlu Warming Relief Nighttime Severe Cold .... ▣ 743
- Triaminic Chest & Nasal Congestion Liquid .... ▣ 746
- Triaminic Cold & Allergy Liquid .... ▣ 746
- Triaminic Daytime Cold & Cough Liquid .... ▣ 745
- Triaminic Nighttime Cold & Cough Liquid .... ▣ 746
- Triaminic Thin Strips Cold .... ▣ 748
- Triaminic Thin Strips Cold & Cough .... ▣ 778
- Triaminic Infant Thin Strips Decongestant .... ▣ 747
- Triaminic Infant Thin Strips Decongestant Plus Cough .... ▣ 747
- Children's Tylenol Plus Flu Oral Suspension .... ▣ 749
- Tylenol Cold Head Congestion Daytime Caplets with Cool Burst and Gelcaps .... ▣ 750
- Tylenol Cold Multi-Symptom Daytime Liquid .... ▣ 752
- Tylenol Cold Multi-Symptom Severe Daytime Liquid .... ▣ 752
- Concentrated Tylenol Infants' Drops Plus Cold & Cough .... ▣ 754
- Tylenol Allergy Multi-Symptom Caplets with Cool Burst and Gelcaps 1872
- Tylenol Allergy Multi-Symptom Nighttime Caplets with Cool Burst 1872
- Children's Tylenol Plus Cold Suspension Liquid 1879
- Children's Tylenol Plus Cold & Allergy Suspension Liquid 1878
- Children's Tylenol Plus Flu Suspension Liquid 1881
- Children's Tylenol Plus Multi-Symptom Cold Suspension Liquid 1879
- Tylenol Cold Head Congestion Daytime Caplets with Cool Burst 1873
- Tylenol Cold Head Congestion Nighttime Caplets with Cool Burst 1873
- Tylenol Cold Head Congestion Severe Caplets with Cool Burst..... 1873
- Tylenol Cold Multi-Symptom Daytime Caplets with Cool Burst and Gelcaps 1874
- Tylenol Cold Multi-Symptom Daytime Liquid with Citrus Burst... 1874
- Tylenol Cold Multi-Symptom Nighttime Caplets with Cool Burst 1874
- Tylenol Cold Multi-Symptom Nighttime Liquid with Cool Burst... 1874
- Tylenol Cold Multi-Symptom Severe Caplets with Cool Burst..... 1874
- Tylenol Cold Multi-Symptom Severe Daytime Liquid with Citrus Burst 1874
- Tylenol Sinus Congestion & Pain Daytime Caplets with Cool Burst and Gelcaps 1876
- Tylenol Sinus Congestion & Pain Nighttime Caplets with Cool Burst 1876
- Tylenol Sinus Congestion & Pain Severe Caplets with Cool Burst..... 1876
- Vicks 44D Cough & Head Congestion Relief Liquid .... ▣ 760
- Vicks DayQuil LiquiCaps/Liquid Multi-Symptom Cold/Flu Relief..... ▣ 761
- Zicam Cough Plus D Cough Spray .... ▣ 767

Phenylephrine Tannate (Sympathomimetics may reduce the blood glucose-lowering effect of insulin, which may result in hyperglycemia. Co-administration may require insulin dose adjustment and particularly close monitoring).

No products indexed under this heading.

Phenylpropanolamine Hydrochloride (Sympathomimetics may reduce the blood glucose-lowering effect of insulin, which may result in hyperglycemia. Co-administration may require insulin dose adjustment and particularly close monitoring).

No products indexed under this heading.

Pindolol (Beta-blockers may either increase or reduce the blood glucose-lowering effect of insulin. In addition, under the influence of sympatholytic medicinal products such as beta-blockers, the signs and symptoms of hypoglycemia may be reduced or absent. Co-administration may require insulin dose adjustment and particularly close monitoring).

No products indexed under this heading.

Pioglitazone Hydrochloride (Oral antidiabetic products may increase the blood glucose-lowering effect of insulin and susceptibility to hypoglycemia. Co-administration may require insulin dose adjustment and particularly close monitoring). Products include:

ActoPlus Met Tablets 3214
Actos Tablets 3219
Duetact Tablets 3226

Pirbuterol Acetate (Sympathomimetics may reduce the blood glucose-lowering effect of insulin, which may result in hyperglycemia. Co-administration may require insulin dose adjustment and particularly close monitoring). Products include:

Maxair Autohaler 1852

Polyestradiol Phosphate (Estrogents may reduce the blood glucose-lowering effect of insulin, which may result in hyperglycemia. Co-administration may require insulin dose adjustment and particularly close monitoring).

No products indexed under this heading.

Polythiazide (Diuretics may reduce the blood glucose-lowering effect of insulin, which may result in hyperglycemia. Co-administration may require insulin dose adjustment and particularly close monitoring).

No products indexed under this heading.

Prednisolone Acetate (Corticosteroids may reduce the blood glucose-lowering effect of insulin, which may result in hyperglycemia. Co-administration may require insulin dose adjustment and particularly close monitoring). Products include:

Blephamide Ophthalmic Ointment 568
Blephamide Ophthalmic Suspension................................ 569
Poly-Pred Ophthalmic Suspension .... ⊙233
Pred Forte Ophthalmic Suspension .... ⊙235
Pred Mild Ophthalmic Suspension .... ⊙238
Pred-G Ophthalmic Ointment .... ⊙237
Pred-G Ophthalmic Suspension ...... ⊙236

Prednisolone Sodium Phosphate (Corticosteroids may reduce the blood glucose-lowering effect of insulin, which may result in hyperglycemia. Co-administration may require insulin dose adjustment and particularly close monitoring).

No products indexed under this heading.

Prednisolone Tebutate (Corticosteroids may reduce the blood glucose-lowering effect of insulin, which may result in hyperglycemia. Co-administration may require insulin dose adjustment and particularly close monitoring).

No products indexed under this heading.

Prednisone (Corticosteroids may reduce the blood glucose-lowering effect of insulin, which may result in hyperglycemia. Co-administration may require insulin dose adjustment and particularly close monitoring).

No products indexed under this heading.

Procarbazine Hydrochloride (MAO inhibitors may increase the blood glucose-lowering effect of insulin and susceptibility to hypoglycemia. Co-administration may require insulin dose adjustment and particularly close monitoring). Products include:

Matulane Capsules 3191

Prochlorperazine (Phenothiazine derivatives may reduce the blood glucose-lowering effect of insulin, which may result in hyperglycemia. Co-administration may require insulin dose adjustment and particularly close monitoring).

No products indexed under this heading.

Promethazine Hydrochloride (Phenothiazine derivatives may reduce the blood glucose-lowering effect of insulin, which may result in hyperglycemia. Co-administration may require insulin dose adjustment and particularly close monitoring). Products include:

Phenergan Tablets and Suppositories................................ 3440

Propoxyphene Hydrochloride (Propoxyphene may increase the blood glucose-lowering effect of insulin and susceptibility to hypoglycemia.Co-administration may require insulin dose adjustment and particularly close monitoring).

No products indexed under this heading.

Propoxyphene Napsylate (Propoxyphene may increase the blood glucose-lowering effect of insulin and susceptibility to hypoglycemia. Co-administration may require insulin dose adjustment and particularly close monitoring).

No products indexed under this heading.

Propranolol Hydrochloride (Beta-blockers may either increase or reduce the blood glucose-lowering effect of insulin. In addition, under the influence of sympatholytic medicinal products such as beta-blockers, the signs and symptoms of hypoglycemia may be reduced or absent. Co-administration may require insulin dose adjustment and particularly close monitoring). Products include:

Inderal LA Long-Acting Capsules 3429
InnoPran XL Capsules 2723

Pseudoephedrine Hydrochloride (Sympathomimetics may reduce the blood glucose-lowering effect of insulin, which may result in hyperglycemia. Co-administration may require insulin dose adjustment and particularly close monitoring). Products include:

Advil Allergy Sinus Caplets 770
Advil Cold & Sinus 723
Advil Multi-Symptom Cold Caplets.................................... 770
Aleve Cold & Sinus Caplets 744
Allegra-D 12 Hour Extended-Release Tablets............ 2846
Allegra-D 24 Hour Extended-Release Tablets............ 2849
BC Cold Powder 677
Comtrex Maximum Strength Cold & Cough Day/Night Caplets - Day Formulation........................ 726
Comtrex Maximum Strength Cold & Cough Day/Night Caplets - Night Formulation 726
Children's Motrin Cold Oral Suspension 1867
Mucinex D Extended-Release Bi-Layer Tablets 776
Robitussin Cough & Cold CF Liquid 735
Robitussin Cough & Cold Pediatric Drops.......................... 735
Tylenol Sinus Congestion & Pain Nighttime Caplets with Cool Burst.. 778
Tylenol Cold Severe Congestion Non-Drowsy Caplets with Cool Burst.. 1874
Tylenol Sinus Severe Congestion Caplets with Cool Burst............... 1876
Vicks 44D Cough & Head Congestion Relief Liquid............. 2679
Vicks 44M Cough, Cold & Flu Relief Liquid................................ 2680
Vicks DayQuil Multi-Symptom Cold/Flu Relief LiquiCaps............. 2678
Vicks DayQuil Multi-Symptom Cold/Flu Relief Liquid.................. 2678
Vicks NyQuil Multi-Symptom Cold/Flu Relief Liquid.................. 2681
Vicks NyQuil Multi-Symptom Cold/Flu Relief LiquiCaps............. 2681
Children's Vicks NyQuil Cold/Cough Relief Liquid............... 2680
Zyrtec-D 12 Hour Extended Release Tablets......................... 2597

Pseudoephedrine Sulfate (Sympathomimetics may reduce the blood glucose-lowering effect of insulin, which may result in hyperglycemia. Co-administration may require insulin dose adjustment and particularly close monitoring). Products include:

Alavert Allergy & Sinus D-12 Hour Tablets.. 771
Clarinex-D 24-Hour Extended-Release Tablets............ 2998
Claritin-D Non-Drowsy 12 Hour Tablets.. 772
Claritin-D Non-Drowsy 24 Hour Tablets.. 772

Quinapril Hydrochloride (ACE inhibitors may increase the blood glucose-lowering effect of insulin and susceptibility to hypoglycemia. Co-administration may require insulin dose adjustment and particularly close monitoring).

No products indexed under this heading.

Quinestrol (Estrogents may reduce the blood glucose-lowering effect of insulin, which may result in hyperglycemia. Co-administration may require insulin dose adjustment and particularly close monitoring).

No products indexed under this heading.

Ramipril (ACE inhibitors may increase the blood glucose-lowering effect of insulin and susceptibility to hypoglycemia. Co-administration may require insulin dose adjustment and particularly close monitoring). Products include:

Altace Capsules 1702

Repaglinide (Oral antidiabetic products may increase the blood glucose-lowering effect of insulin and susceptibility to hypoglycemia. Co-administration may require insulin dose adjustment and particularly close monitoring).

No products indexed under this heading.

Reserpine (Under the influence of sympatholytic medicinal products, such as reserpine, the signs and symptoms of hypoglycemia may be reduced or absent. Co-administration may require insulin dose adjustment and particularly close monitoring).

No products indexed under this heading.

Ritonavir (Protease inhibitors may reduce the blood glucose-lowering effect of insulin, which may result in hyperglycemia. Co-administration may require insulin dose adjustment and particularly close monitoring). Products include:

Kaletra 476
Norvir 503

Rosiglitazone Maleate (Oral antidiabetic products may increase the blood glucose-lowering effect of insulin and susceptibility to hypoglycemia. Co-administration may require insulin dose adjustment and particularly close monitoring). Products include:

Avandamet Tablets 1373
Avandaryl Tablets 1379
Avandia Tablets 1384

Salmeterol Xinafoate (Sympathomimetics may reduce the blood glucose-lowering effect of insulin, which may result in hyperglycemia. Co-administration may require insulin dose adjustment and particularly close monitoring). Products include:

Advair Diskus 100/50 1308
Advair Diskus 250/50 1308
Advair Diskus 500/50 1308
Advair HFA Inhalation Aerosol 1318
Serevent Diskus 1568

Salsalate (Salicylates may increase the blood glucose-lowering effect of insulin and susceptibility to hypoglycemia. Co-administration may require insulin dose adjustment and particularly close monitoring).

No products indexed under this heading.

Saquinavir (Protease inhibitors may reduce the blood glucose-lowering effect of insulin, which may result in hyperglycemia. Co-administration may require insulin dose adjustment and particularly close monitoring).

No products indexed under this heading.

Saquinavir Mesylate (Protease inhibitors may reduce the blood glucose-lowering effect of insulin, which may result in hyperglycemia. Co-administration may require insulin dose adjustment and particularly close monitoring). Products include:

Invirase 2772

Selegiline Hydrochloride (MAO inhibitors may increase the blood glucose-lowering effect of insulin and susceptibility to hypoglycemia. Co-administration may require insulin dose adjustment and particularly close monitoring). Products include:

Eldepryl Capsules 3208
Zelapar Tablets 3372

Silver Sulfadiazine (Sulfonamide antibiotics may increase the blood glucose-lowering effect of insulin and susceptibility to hypoglycemia. Co-administration may require insulin dose adjustment and particularly close monitoring).

No products indexed under this heading.

Somatropin (Somatropin may reduce the blood glucose-lowering effect of insulin, which may result in hyperglycemia. Co-administration may require insulin dose adjustment and particularly close monitoring). Products include:

Somatropin (rDNA Origin) (Somatropin may reduce the blood glucose-lowering effect of insulin, which may result in hyperglycemia. Co-administration may require insulin dose adjustment and particularly close monitoring). Products include:

Sotalol Hydrochloride (Beta-blockers may either increase or reduce the blood glucose-lowering effect of insulin. In addition, under the influence of sympatholytic medicinal products such as beta-blockers, the signs and symptoms of hypoglycemia may be reduced or absent. Co-administration may require insulin dose adjustment and particularly close monitoring).
 No products indexed under this heading.

Spirapril Hydrochloride (ACE inhibitors may increase the blood glucose-lowering effect of insulin and susceptibility to hypoglycemia. Co-administration may require insulin dose adjustment and particularly close monitoring).
 No products indexed under this heading.

Spironolactone (Diuretics may reduce the blood glucose-lowering effect of insulin, which may result in hyperglycemia. Co-administration may require insulin dose adjustment and particularly close monitoring).
 No products indexed under this heading.

Sulfadiazine (Sulfonamide antibiotics may increase the blood glucose-lowering effect of insulin and susceptibility to hypoglycemia. Co-administration may require insulin dose adjustment and particularly close monitoring).
 No products indexed under this heading.

Sulfamethizole (Sulfonamide antibiotics may increase the blood glucose-lowering effect of insulin and susceptibility to hypoglycemia. Co-administration may require insulin dose adjustment and particularly close monitoring).
 No products indexed under this heading.

Sulfamethoprim (Sulfonamide antibiotics may increase the blood glucose-lowering effect of insulin and susceptibility to hypoglycemia. Co-administration may require insulin dose adjustment and particularly close monitoring).
 No products indexed under this heading.

Sulfamethoxazole (Sulfonamide antibiotics may increase the blood glucose-lowering effect of insulin and susceptibility to hypoglycemia. Co-administration may require insulin dose adjustment and particularly close monitoring).
 No products indexed under this heading.

Sulfisoxazole Acetyl (Sulfonamide antibiotics may increase the blood glucose-lowering effect of insulin and susceptibility to hypoglycemia. Co-administration may require insulin dose adjustment and particularly close monitoring).
 No products indexed under this heading.

Sulfisoxazole Diolamine (Sulfonamide antibiotics may increase the blood glucose-lowering effect of insulin and susceptibility to hypoglycemia. Co-administration may require insulin dose adjustment and particularly close monitoring).
 No products indexed under this heading.

Terbutaline Sulfate (Sympathomimetics may reduce the blood glucose-lowering effect of insulin, which may result in hyperglycemia. Co-administration may require insulin dose adjustment and particularly close monitoring).
 No products indexed under this heading.

Thioridazine Hydrochloride (Phenothiazine derivatives may reduce the blood glucose-lowering effect of insulin, which may result in hyperglycemia. Co-administration may require insulin dose adjustment and particularly close monitoring). Products include:

Thyroglobulin (Thyroid hormones may reduce the blood glucose-lowering effect of insulin, which may result in hyperglycemia. Co-administration may require insulin dose adjustment and particularly close monitoring).
 No products indexed under this heading.

Thyroid (Thyroid hormones may reduce the blood glucose-lowering effect of insulin, which may result in hyperglycemia. Co-administration may require insulin dose adjustment and particularly close monitoring).
 No products indexed under this heading.

Thyroxine (Thyroid hormones may reduce the blood glucose-lowering effect of insulin, which may result in hyperglycemia. Co-administration may require insulin dose adjustment and particularly close monitoring).
 No products indexed under this heading.

Thyroxine Sodium (Thyroid hormones may reduce the blood glucose-lowering effect of insulin, which may result in hyperglycemia. Co-administration may require insulin dose adjustment and particularly close monitoring).
 No products indexed under this heading.

Timolol Hemihydrate (Beta-blockers may either increase or reduce the blood glucose-lowering effect of insulin. In addition, under the influence of sympatholytic medicinal products such as beta-blockers, the signs and symptoms of hypoglycemia may be reduced or absent. Co-administration may require insulin dose adjustment and particularly close monitoring). Products include:

Timolol Maleate (Beta-blockers may either increase or reduce the blood glucose-lowering effect of

insulin. In addition, under the influence of sympatholytic medicinal products such as beta-blockers, the signs and symptoms of hypoglycemia may be reduced or absent. Co-administration may require insulin dose adjustment and particularly close monitoring). Products include:

Tolazamide (Oral antidiabetic products may increase the blood glucose-lowering effect of insulin and susceptibility to hypoglycemia. Co-administration may require insulin dose adjustment and particularly close monitoring).
 No products indexed under this heading.

Tolbutamide (Oral antidiabetic products may increase the blood glucose-lowering effect of insulin and susceptibility to hypoglycemia. Co-administration may require insulin dose adjustment and particularly close monitoring).
 No products indexed under this heading.

Torsemide (Diuretics may reduce the blood glucose-lowering effect of insulin, which may result in hyperglycemia. Co-administration may require insulin dose adjustment and particularly close monitoring). Products include:

Trandolapril (ACE inhibitors may increase the blood glucose-lowering effect of insulin and susceptibility to hypoglycemia. Co-administration may require insulin dose adjustment and particularly close monitoring). Products include:

Tranylcypromine Sulfate (MAO inhibitors may increase the blood glucose-lowering effect of insulin and susceptibility to hypoglycemia. Co-administration may require insulin dose adjustment and particularly close monitoring). Products include:

Triamcinolone (Corticosteroids may reduce the blood glucose-lowering effect of insulin, which may result in hyperglycemia. Co-administration may require insulin dose adjustment and particularly close monitoring).
 No products indexed under this heading.

Triamcinolone Acetonide (Corticosteroids may reduce the blood glucose-lowering effect of insulin, which may result in hyperglycemia. Co-administration may require insulin dose adjustment and particularly close monitoring). Products include:

Triamcinolone Diacetate (Corticosteroids may reduce the blood glucose-lowering effect of insulin, which may result in hyperglycemia. Co-administration may require insulin dose adjustment and particularly close monitoring).
 No products indexed under this heading.

Triamcinolone Hexacetonide (Corticosteroids may reduce the blood glucose-lowering effect of insulin, which may result in hyperglycemia. Co-administration may require insulin dose adjustment and particularly close monitoring).
 No products indexed under this heading.

Triamterene (Diuretics may reduce the blood glucose-lowering effect of insulin, which may result in hyperglycemia. Co-administration may require insulin dose adjustment and particularly close monitoring). Products include:

Trifluoperazine Hydrochloride (Phenothiazine derivatives may reduce the blood glucose-lowering effect of insulin, which may result in hyperglycemia. Co-administration may require insulin dose adjustment and particularly close monitoring).
 No products indexed under this heading.

Troglitazone (Oral antidiabetic products may increase the blood glucose-lowering effect of insulin and susceptibility to hypoglycemia. Co-administration may require insulin dose adjustment and particularly close monitoring).
 No products indexed under this heading.

Food Interactions

Alcohol (Alcohol may either increase or reduce the blood glucose-lowering effect of insulin. Co-administration may require insulin dose adjustment and particularly close monitoring).

FABRAZYME FOR INTRAVENOUS INFUSION
(Agalsidase beta) 1274
None cited in PDR database.

FAMVIR TABLETS
(Famciclovir) 2211
May interact with:

Probenecid (Concurrent use may result in increased plasma concentration of penciclovir).
 No products indexed under this heading.

Food Interactions

Meal, unspecified (Penciclovir Cmax decreased approximately 50% and Tmax was delayed by 1.5 hours when a capsule formulation of famciclovir was administered with food; there is no effect on the extent of availability (AUC) of penciclovir).

FANSIDAR TABLETS
(Pyrimethamine, Sulfadoxine) 2765
May interact with sulfonamides and certain other agents. Compounds in these categories include:

Bendroflumethiazide (Antifolic drugs such as sulfonamides or trimethoprim-sulfamethoxazole should not be used while the patient is receiving Fansidar for antimalarial prophylaxis).
 No products indexed under this heading.

Chloroquine (Reports may indicate an increase in incidence and severity of adverse reactions when chloroquine is used with Fansidar as compared to the use of Fansidar alone).
 No products indexed under this heading.

Chloroquine Hydrochloride (Reports may indicate an increase in incidence and severity of adverse reactions when chloroquine is used with Fansidar as compared to the use of Fansidar alone).
No products indexed under this heading.

Chloroquine Phosphate (Reports may indicate an increase in incidence and severity of adverse reactions when chloroquine is used with Fansidar as compared to the use of Fansidar alone).
No products indexed under this heading.

Chlorothiazide (Antifolic drugs such as sulfonamides or trimethoprim-sulfamethoxazole should not be used while the patient is receiving Fansidar for antimalarial prophylaxis). Products include:
Diuril Oral Suspension 1954

Chlorothiazide Sodium (Antifolic drugs such as sulfonamides or trimethoprim-sulfamethoxazole should not be used while the patient is receiving Fansidar for antimalarial prophylaxis). Products include:
Diuril Sodium Intravenous 2467

Chlorpropamide (Antifolic drugs such as sulfonamides or trimethoprim-sulfamethoxazole should not be used while the patient is receiving Fansidar for antimalarial prophylaxis).
No products indexed under this heading.

Glipizide (Antifolic drugs such as sulfonamides or trimethoprim-sulfamethoxazole should not be used while the patient is receiving Fansidar for antimalarial prophylaxis).
No products indexed under this heading.

Glyburide (Antifolic drugs such as sulfonamides or trimethoprim-sulfamethoxazole should not be used while the patient is receiving Fansidar for antimalarial prophylaxis).
No products indexed under this heading.

Hydrochlorothiazide (Antifolic drugs such as sulfonamides or trimethoprim-sulfamethoxazole should not be used while the patient is receiving Fansidar for antimalarial prophylaxis). Products include:
Aldoril Tablets 1910
Atacand HCT 651
Avalide Tablets 888
Avalide Tablets 2874
Benicar HCT Tablets 1044
Diovan HCT Tablets 2196
Dyazide Capsules 1423
Hyzaar 50-12.5 Tablets 1990
Hyzaar 100-12.5 Tablets 1990
Hyzaar 100-25 Tablets 1990
Lopressor HCT 50/25 Tablets 2241
Lopressor HCT 100/25 Tablets 2241
Lopressor HCT 100/50 Tablets 2241
Lotensin HCT Tablets 2246
Micardis HCT Tablets 856
Moduretic Tablets 2028
Prinzide Tablets 2056
Teveten HCT Tablets 1737
Timolide Tablets 2086
Uniretic Tablets 3100

Hydroflumethiazide (Antifolic drugs such as sulfonamides or trimethoprim-sulfamethoxazole should not be used while the patient is receiving Fansidar for antimalarial prophylaxis).
No products indexed under this heading.

Methyclothiazide (Antifolic drugs such as sulfonamides or trimethoprim-sulfamethoxazole should not be used while the patient is receiving Fansidar for antimalarial prophylaxis).
No products indexed under this heading.

Polythiazide (Antifolic drugs such as sulfonamides or trimethoprim-sulfamethoxazole should not be used while the patient is receiving Fansidar for antimalarial prophylaxis).
No products indexed under this heading.

Sulfacytine (Antifolic drugs such as sulfonamides or trimethoprim-sulfamethoxazole should not be used while the patient is receiving Fansidar for antimalarial prophylaxis).
No products indexed under this heading.

Sulfamethizole (Antifolic drugs such as sulfonamides or trimethoprim-sulfamethoxazole should not be used while the patient is receiving Fansidar for antimalarial prophylaxis).
No products indexed under this heading.

Sulfamethoxazole (Antifolic drugs such as sulfonamides or trimethoprim-sulfamethoxazole should not be used while the patient is receiving Fansidar for antimalarial prophylaxis).
No products indexed under this heading.

Sulfasalazine (Antifolic drugs such as sulfonamides or trimethoprim-sulfamethoxazole should not be used while the patient is receiving Fansidar for antimalarial prophylaxis).
No products indexed under this heading.

Sulfinpyrazone (Antifolic drugs such as sulfonamides or trimethoprim-sulfamethoxazole should not be used while the patient is receiving Fansidar for antimalarial prophylaxis).
No products indexed under this heading.

Sulfisoxazole Acetyl (Antifolic drugs such as sulfonamides or trimethoprim-sulfamethoxazole should not be used while the patient is receiving Fansidar for antimalarial prophylaxis).
No products indexed under this heading.

Sulfisoxazole Diolamine (Antifolic drugs such as sulfonamides or trimethoprim-sulfamethoxazole should not be used while the patient is receiving Fansidar for antimalarial prophylaxis).
No products indexed under this heading.

Tolazamide (Antifolic drugs such as sulfonamides or trimethoprim-sulfamethoxazole should not be used while the patient is receiving Fansidar for antimalarial prophylaxis).
No products indexed under this heading.

Tolbutamide (Antifolic drugs such as sulfonamides or trimethoprim-sulfamethoxazole should not be used while the patient is receiving Fansidar for antimalarial prophylaxis).
No products indexed under this heading.

Trimethoprim (Antifolic drugs such as sulfonamides or trimethoprim-sulfamethoxazole should not be used while the patient is receiving Fansidar for antimalarial prophylaxis).
No products indexed under this heading.

Trimethoprim Hydrochloride (Antifolic drugs such as sulfonamides or trimethoprim-sulfamethoxazole should not be used while the patient is receiving Fansidar for antimalarial prophylaxis).
No products indexed under this heading.

Trimethoprim Sulfate (Antifolic drugs such as sulfonamides or trimethoprim-sulfamethoxazole should not be used while the patient is receiving Fansidar for antimalarial prophylaxis). Products include:
Polytrim Ophthalmic Solution 574

FASLODEX INJECTION

(Fulvestrant) 681
None cited in PDR database.

FAZACLO ORALLY DISINTEGRATING TABLETS

(Clozapine) 551
May interact with anticholinergics, antihypertensives, benzodiazepines, central nervous system depressants, antidepressant drugs, erythromycin, general anesthetics, phenothiazines, phenytoin, psychotropics, quinidine, and certain other agents. Compounds in these categories include:

Acebutolol Hydrochloride (Clozapine may potentiate the hypotensive effects of antihypertensive drugs).
No products indexed under this heading.

Alfentanil Hydrochloride (Given the primary CNS effect of clozapine, caution is advised in using it concomitantly with CNS-active drugs).
No products indexed under this heading.

Alprazolam (Co-administration with benzodiazepines or other psychotropic agents may be accompanied by orthostatic hypotension leading to profound collapse and respiratory and/or cardiac arrest; caution is advised if used concurrently). Products include:
Niravam Orally Disintegrating Tablets 3092

Amitriptyline Hydrochloride (Concomitant use of clozapine with other drugs metabolized by CYP4502D6 may require lower than usual doses for either drug).
No products indexed under this heading.

Amlodipine Besylate (Clozapine may potentiate the hypotensive effects of antihypertensive drugs). Products include:
Caduet Tablets 2508
Lotrel Capsules 2249
Norvasc Tablets 2545

Amoxapine (Concomitant use of clozapine with other drugs metabolized by CYP4502D6 may require lower than usual doses for either drug).
No products indexed under this heading.

Aprobarbital (Given the primary CNS effect of clozapine, caution is advised in using it concomitantly with CNS-active drugs).
No products indexed under this heading.

Atenolol (Clozapine may potentiate the hypotensive effects of antihypertensive drugs).
No products indexed under this heading.

Atropine Sulfate (Clozapine may potentiate anticholinergic effects). Products include:
Donnatal Extentabs 2493

Belladonna Alkaloids (Clozapine may potentiate anticholinergic effects). Products include:
Hyland's Teething Tablets 830

Benazepril Hydrochloride (Clozapine may potentiate the hypotensive effects of antihypertensive drugs). Products include:
Lotensin Tablets 2243
Lotensin HCT Tablets 2246
Lotrel Capsules 2249

Bendroflumethiazide (Clozapine may potentiate the hypotensive effects of antihypertensive drugs).
No products indexed under this heading.

Benztropine Mesylate (Clozapine may potentiate anticholinergic effects).
No products indexed under this heading.

Betaxolol Hydrochloride (Clozapine may potentiate the hypotensive effects of antihypertensive drugs). Products include:
Betoptic S Ophthalmic Suspension.................................. 558

Biperiden Hydrochloride (Clozapine may potentiate anticholinergic effects).
No products indexed under this heading.

Bisoprolol Fumarate (Clozapine may potentiate the hypotensive effects of antihypertensive drugs).
No products indexed under this heading.

Bone Marrow Depressants, unspecified (Clozapine should not be used with agents having a well-known potential to suppress bone-marrow function. Co-administration may increase the risk and/or severity of bone marrow suppression).
No products indexed under this heading.

Buprenorphine Hydrochloride (Given the primary CNS effect of clozapine, caution is advised in using it concomitantly with CNS-active drugs). Products include:
Buprenex Injectable 2716
Suboxone Tablets 2717
Subutex Tablets 2717

Bupropion Hydrochloride (Concomitant use of clozapine with other drugs metabolized by CYP4502D6 may require lower than usual doses for either drug). Products include:
Wellbutrin Tablets 1603
Wellbutrin SR Sustained-Release Tablets 1607
Wellbutrin XL Extended-Release Tablets 1613

Zyban Sustained-Release Tablets 1644

Buspirone Hydrochloride (Co-administration with benzodiazepines or other psychotropic agents may be accompanied by orthostatic hypotension leading to profound collapse and respiratory and/or cardiac arrest; caution is advised if used concurrently).
No products indexed under this heading.

Butabarbital (Given the primary CNS effect of clozapine, caution is advised in using it concomitantly with CNS-active drugs).
No products indexed under this heading.

Butalbital (Given the primary CNS effect of clozapine, caution is advised in using it concomitantly with CNS-active drugs).
No products indexed under this heading.

Caffeine (May increase plasma levels of clozapine, potentially resulting in adverse effects). Products include:
BC Headache Powder .... ■ 677
Arthritis Strength BC Powder .... ■ 677
Excedrin Extra Strength Caplets/Tablets/Geltabs .... ■ 684
Excedrin Migraine Caplets/Tablets/Geltabs .... ■ 609
Excedrin Tension Headache Caplets/Tablets/Geltabs .... ■ 611
Goody's Extra Strength Headache Powders .... ■ 611
Goody's Extra Strength Pain Relief Tablets .... ■ 685
Vivarin .... ■ 602
Winrgy Dietary Supplement .... ■ 823

Caffeine Citrate (May increase plasma levels of clozapine, potentially resulting in adverse effects). Products include:
Cafcit 1886

Candesartan Cilexetil (Clozapine may potentiate the hypotensive effects of antihypertensive drugs). Products include:
Atacand Tablets 649
Atacand HCT 651

Captopril (Clozapine may potentiate the hypotensive effects of antihypertensive drugs). Products include:
Captopril Tablets 2149

Carbamazepine (Concomitant use is not recommended; discontinuation of concomitant carbamazepine administration may result in increase in clozapine levels). Products include:
Carbatrol Capsules 3171
Equetro Extended-Release Capsules 3180
Tegretol/Tegretol-XR 2295

Carteolol Hydrochloride (Clozapine may potentiate the hypotensive effects of antihypertensive drugs). Products include:
Carteolol Hydrochloride Ophthalmic Solution USP, 1%....... ⊙ 249

Chlordiazepoxide (Co-administration with benzodiazepines or other psychotropic agents may be accompanied by orthostatic hypotension leading to profound collapse and respiratory and/or cardiac arrest; caution is advised if used concurrently).
No products indexed under this heading.

Chlordiazepoxide Hydrochloride (Co-administration with benzodiazepines or other psychotropic agents may be accompanied by orthostatic hypotension leading to profound collapse and respiratory and/or cardiac arrest; caution is advised if used concurrently). Products include:
Librium Capsules 3347

Chlorothiazide (Clozapine may potentiate the hypotensive effects of antihypertensive drugs). Products include:
Diuril Oral Suspension 1954

Chlorothiazide Sodium (Clozapine may potentiate the hypotensive effects of antihypertensive drugs). Products include:
Diuril Sodium Intravenous 2467

Chlorpromazine (Co-administration with benzodiazepines or other psychotropic agents may be accompanied by orthostatic hypotension leading to profound collapse and respiratory and/or cardiac arrest; caution is advised if used concurrently).
No products indexed under this heading.

Chlorpromazine Hydrochloride (Co-administration with benzodiazepines or other psychotropic agents may be accompanied by orthostatic hypotension leading to profound collapse and respiratory and/or cardiac arrest; caution is advised if used concurrently).
No products indexed under this heading.

Chlorprothixene (Co-administration with benzodiazepines or other psychotropic agents may be accompanied by orthostatic hypotension leading to profound collapse and respiratory and/or cardiac arrest; caution is advised if used concurrently).
No products indexed under this heading.

Chlorprothixene Hydrochloride (Co-administration with benzodiazepines or other psychotropic agents may be accompanied by orthostatic hypotension leading to profound collapse and respiratory and/or cardiac arrest; caution is advised if used concurrently).
No products indexed under this heading.

Chlorprothixene Lactate (Given the primary CNS effect of clozapine, caution is advised in using it concomitantly with CNS-active drugs).
No products indexed under this heading.

Chlorthalidone (Clozapine may potentiate the hypotensive effects of antihypertensive drugs). Products include:
Clorpres Tablets 2153

Cimetidine (May increase plasma levels of clozapine, potentially resulting in adverse effects). Products include:
Tagamet HB 200 Tablets .... ■ 664

Cimetidine Hydrochloride (May increase plasma levels of clozapine, potentially resulting in adverse effects).
No products indexed under this heading.

Citalopram Hydrobromide (Concomitant use of clozapine with other drugs metabolized by CYP4502D6 may require lower than usual doses for either drug). Products include:
Celexa 1176

Clidinium Bromide (Clozapine may potentiate anticholinergic effects).
No products indexed under this heading.

Clonidine (Clozapine may potentiate the hypotensive effects of antihypertensive drugs). Products include:
Catapres-TTS 844

Clonidine Hydrochloride (Clozapine may potentiate the hypotensive effects of antihypertensive drugs). Products include:
Catapres Tablets 843
Clorpres Tablets 2153

Clorazepate Dipotassium (Co-administration with benzodiazepines or other psychotropic agents may be accompanied by orthostatic hypotension leading to profound collapse and respiratory and/or cardiac arrest; caution is advised if used concurrently). Products include:
Tranxene 2474

Codeine Phosphate (Given the primary CNS effect of clozapine, caution is advised in using it concomitantly with CNS-active drugs). Products include:
Tylenol with Codeine Tablets 2391

Deserpidine (Clozapine may potentiate the hypotensive effects of antihypertensive drugs).
No products indexed under this heading.

Desflurane (Given the primary CNS effect of clozapine, caution is advised in using it concomitantly with CNS-active drugs).
No products indexed under this heading.

Desipramine Hydrochloride (Concomitant use of clozapine with other drugs metabolized by CYP4502D6 may require lower than usual doses for either drug).
No products indexed under this heading.

Dezocine (Given the primary CNS effect of clozapine, caution is advised in using it concomitantly with CNS-active drugs).
No products indexed under this heading.

Diazepam (Co-administration with benzodiazepines or other psychotropic agents may be accompanied by orthostatic hypotension leading to profound collapse and respiratory and/or cardiac arrest; caution is advised if used concurrently). Products include:
Diastat Rectal Delivery System 3343
Valium Tablets 2819

Diazoxide (Clozapine may potentiate the hypotensive effects of antihypertensive drugs). Products include:
Hyperstat I.V. 3017

Dicyclomine Hydrochloride (Clozapine may potentiate anticholinergic effects). Products include:
Bentyl Capsules 697
Bentyl Injection 697
Bentyl Syrup 697
Bentyl Tablets 697

Diltiazem Hydrochloride (Clozapine may potentiate the hypotensive effects of antihypertensive drugs). Products include:
Cardizem LA Extended Release Tablets 1728
Tiazac Capsules 1201

Doxazosin Mesylate (Clozapine may potentiate the hypotensive effects of antihypertensive drugs). Products include:
Cardura XL Tablets 2515

Doxepin Hydrochloride (Concomitant use of clozapine with other drugs metabolized by CYP4502D6 may require lower than usual doses for either drug).
No products indexed under this heading.

Droperidol (Co-administration with benzodiazepines or other psychotropic agents may be accompanied by orthostatic hypotension leading to profound collapse and respiratory and/or cardiac arrest; caution is advised if used concurrently).
No products indexed under this heading.

Enalapril Maleate (Clozapine may potentiate the hypotensive effects of antihypertensive drugs). Products include:
Vasotec I.V. Injection 2103

Enalaprilat (Clozapine may potentiate the hypotensive effects of antihypertensive drugs).
No products indexed under this heading.

Encainide Hydrochloride (Concomitant use of clozapine with other drugs metabolized by CYP4502D6 may require lower than usual doses for either drug).
No products indexed under this heading.

Enflurane (Given the primary CNS effect of clozapine, caution is advised in using it concomitantly with CNS-active drugs).
No products indexed under this heading.

Epinephrine (The administration of epinephrine should be avoided in the treatment of clozapine-induced hypotension because of a possible reverse epinephrine effect). Products include:
EpiPen 1061
Primatene Mist .... ■ 719
Twinject 0.15 3379
Twinject 0.3 3378

Epinephrine Hydrochloride (The administration of epinephrine should be avoided in the treatment of clozapine-induced hypotension because of a possible reverse epinephrine effect).
No products indexed under this heading.

Eprosartan Mesylate (Clozapine may potentiate the hypotensive effects of antihypertensive drugs). Products include:
Teveten Tablets 1735
Teveten HCT Tablets 1737

Erythromycin (May increase plasma levels of clozapine, potentially resulting in adverse effects). Products include:
Ery-Tab Tablets 449
Erythromycin Base Filmtab Tablets 455
Erythromycin Delayed-Release Capsules, USP 457
PCE Dispertab Tablets 515

Erythromycin Estolate (May increase plasma levels of clozapine, potentially resulting in adverse effects).
No products indexed under this heading.

Erythromycin Ethylsuccinate (May increase plasma levels of clozapine, potentially resulting in adverse effects). Products include:
E.E.S. 451
EryPed 447

Isoflurane (Given the primary CNS effect of clozapine, caution is advised in using it concomitantly with CNS-active drugs).
No products indexed under this heading.

Isradipine (Clozapine may potentiate the hypotensive effects of antihypertensive drugs). Products include:
DynaCirc CR Tablets 2721

Ketamine Hydrochloride (Given the primary CNS effect of clozapine, caution is advised in using it concomitantly with CNS-active drugs).
No products indexed under this heading.

Labetalol Hydrochloride (Clozapine may potentiate the hypotensive effects of antihypertensive drugs).
No products indexed under this heading.

Levomethadyl Acetate Hydrochloride (Given the primary CNS effect of clozapine, caution is advised in using it concomitantly with CNS-active drugs).
No products indexed under this heading.

Levorphanol Tartrate (Given the primary CNS effect of clozapine, caution is advised in using it concomitantly with CNS-active drugs).
No products indexed under this heading.

Lisinopril (Clozapine may potentiate the hypotensive effects of antihypertensive drugs). Products include:
Prinivil Tablets 2052
Prinzide Tablets 2056

Lithium Carbonate (Co-administration with benzodiazepines or other psychotropic agents may be accompanied by orthostatic hypotension leading to profound collapse and respiratory and/or cardiac arrest; caution is advised if used concurrently). Products include:
Lithobid Tablets 1692

Lithium Citrate (Co-administration with benzodiazepines or other psychotropic agents may be accompanied by orthostatic hypotension leading to profound collapse and respiratory and/or cardiac arrest; caution is advised if used concurrently).
No products indexed under this heading.

Lorazepam (Co-administration with benzodiazepines or other psychotropic agents may be accompanied by orthostatic hypotension leading to profound collapse and respiratory and/or cardiac arrest; caution is advised if used concurrently).
No products indexed under this heading.

Losartan Potassium (Clozapine may potentiate the hypotensive effects of antihypertensive drugs). Products include:
Cozaar Tablets 1935
Hyzaar 50-12.5 Tablets 1990
Hyzaar 100-12.5 Tablets 1990
Hyzaar 100-25 Tablets 1990

Loxapine Hydrochloride (Co-administration with benzodiazepines or other psychotropic agents may be accompanied by orthostatic hypotension leading to profound collapse and respiratory and/or cardiac arrest; caution is advised if used concurrently).
No products indexed under this heading.

Loxapine Succinate (Co-administration with benzodiazepines or other psychotropic agents may be accompanied by orthostatic hypotension leading to profound collapse and respiratory and/or cardiac arrest; caution is advised if used concurrently).
No products indexed under this heading.

Maprotiline Hydrochloride (Concomitant use of clozapine with other drugs metabolized by CYP4502D6 may require lower than usual doses for either drug).
No products indexed under this heading.

Mecamylamine Hydrochloride (Clozapine may potentiate the hypotensive effects of antihypertensive drugs).
No products indexed under this heading.

Mepenzolate Bromide (Clozapine may potentiate anticholinergic effects).
No products indexed under this heading.

Meperidine Hydrochloride (Given the primary CNS effect of clozapine, caution is advised in using it concomitantly with CNS-active drugs).
No products indexed under this heading.

Mephobarbital (Given the primary CNS effect of clozapine, caution is advised in using it concomitantly with CNS-active drugs).
No products indexed under this heading.

Meprobamate (Co-administration with benzodiazepines or other psychotropic agents may be accompanied by orthostatic hypotension leading to profound collapse and respiratory and/or cardiac arrest; caution is advised if used concurrently).
No products indexed under this heading.

Mesoridazine Besylate (Co-administration with benzodiazepines or other psychotropic agents may be accompanied by orthostatic hypotension leading to profound collapse and respiratory and/or cardiac arrest; caution is advised if used concurrently).
No products indexed under this heading.

Methadone Hydrochloride (Given the primary CNS effect of clozapine, caution is advised in using it concomitantly with CNS-active drugs).
No products indexed under this heading.

Methohexital Sodium (Given the primary CNS effect of clozapine, caution is advised in using it concomitantly with CNS-active drugs).
No products indexed under this heading.

Methotrimeprazine (Given the primary CNS effect of clozapine, caution is advised in using it concomitantly with CNS-active drugs).
No products indexed under this heading.

Methoxyflurane (Given the primary CNS effect of clozapine, caution is advised in using it concomitantly with CNS-active drugs).
No products indexed under this heading.

Methyclothiazide (Clozapine may potentiate the hypotensive effects of antihypertensive drugs).
No products indexed under this heading.

Methyldopa (Clozapine may potentiate the hypotensive effects of antihypertensive drugs). Products include:
Aldoril Tablets 1910

Methyldopate Hydrochloride (Clozapine may potentiate the hypotensive effects of antihypertensive drugs).
No products indexed under this heading.

Metolazone (Clozapine may potentiate the hypotensive effects of antihypertensive drugs).
No products indexed under this heading.

Metoprolol Succinate (Clozapine may potentiate the hypotensive effects of antihypertensive drugs). Products include:
Toprol-XL Tablets 668

Metoprolol Tartrate (Clozapine may potentiate the hypotensive effects of antihypertensive drugs). Products include:
Lopressor Injection 2238
Lopressor Tablets 2238
Lopressor HCT 50/25 Tablets 2241
Lopressor HCT 100/25 Tablets 2241
Lopressor HCT 100/50 Tablets 2241

Metyrosine (Clozapine may potentiate the hypotensive effects of antihypertensive drugs). Products include:
Demser Capsules 1953

Mibefradil Dihydrochloride (Clozapine may potentiate the hypotensive effects of antihypertensive drugs).
No products indexed under this heading.

Midazolam Hydrochloride (Co-administration with benzodiazepines or other psychotropic agents may be accompanied by orthostatic hypotension leading to profound collapse and respiratory and/or cardiac arrest; caution is advised if used concurrently).
No products indexed under this heading.

Minoxidil (Clozapine may potentiate the hypotensive effects of antihypertensive drugs). Products include:
Men's Rogaine Extra Strength Hair Regrowth Treatment Topical Solution, Ocean Rush Scent and Original Unscented .... ◙633
Men's Rogaine Foam Hair Regrowth Treatment .... ◙633
Women's Rogaine Hair Regrowth Treatment Topical Solution, Spring Bloom Scent and Original Unscented .... ◙634

Mirtazapine (Concomitant use of clozapine with other drugs metabolized by CYP4502D6 may require lower than usual doses for either drug).
No products indexed under this heading.

Moexipril Hydrochloride (Clozapine may potentiate the hypotensive effects of antihypertensive drugs). Products include:
Uniretic Tablets 3100
Univasc Tablets 3104

Molindone Hydrochloride (Co-administration with benzodiazepines or other psychotropic agents may be accompanied by orthostatic hypotension leading to profound collapse and respiratory and/or cardiac arrest; caution is advised if used concurrently). Products include:
Moban Tablets 1119

Morphine Sulfate (Given the primary CNS effect of clozapine, caution is advised in using it concomitantly with CNS-active drugs). Products include:
Avinza Capsules 1741
Kadian Capsules 577
MS Contin Tablets 2701

Nadolol (Clozapine may potentiate the hypotensive effects of antihypertensive drugs). Products include:
Nadolol Tablets 2159

Nefazodone Hydrochloride (Concomitant use of clozapine with other drugs metabolized by CYP4502D6 may require lower than usual doses for either drug).
No products indexed under this heading.

Nicardipine Hydrochloride (Clozapine may potentiate the hypotensive effects of antihypertensive drugs). Products include:
Cardene I.V. 2497

Nicotine (May decrease clozapine plasma levels resulting in a decrease in effectiveness of a previously effective clozapine dose). Products include:
NicoDerm CQ Clear Patch .... ◙622

Nicotine Polacrilex (May decrease clozapine plasma levels resulting in a decrease in effectiveness of a previously effective clozapine dose).
No products indexed under this heading.

Nifedipine (Clozapine may potentiate the hypotensive effects of antihypertensive drugs). Products include:
Adalat CC Tablets 2964

Nisoldipine (Clozapine may potentiate the hypotensive effects of antihypertensive drugs). Products include:
Sular Tablets 3122

Nitroglycerin (Clozapine may potentiate the hypotensive effects of antihypertensive drugs). Products include:
Nitro-Dur Transdermal Infusion System 3046
Nitrolingual Pumpspray 3120

Nortriptyline Hydrochloride (Concomitant use of clozapine with other drugs metabolized by CYP4502D6 may require lower than usual doses for either drug).
No products indexed under this heading.

Olanzapine (Co-administration with benzodiazepines or other psychotropic agents may be accompanied by orthostatic hypotension leading to profound collapse and respiratory and/or cardiac arrest; caution is advised if used concurrently). Products include:
Symbyax Capsules 1819
Zyprexa Tablets 1830
Zyprexa IntraMuscular 1830
Zyprexa ZYDIS Orally Disintegrating Tablets 1830

Oxazepam (Co-administration with benzodiazepines or other psychotropic agents may be accompanied by orthostatic hypotension leading to profound collapse and respiratory and/or cardiac arrest; caution is advised if used concurrently).
No products indexed under this heading.

Oxybutynin Chloride (Clozapine may potentiate anticholinergic effects). Products include:

ing to profound collapse and respiratory and/or cardiac arrest; caution is advised if used concurrently). Products include:
Restoril Capsules **1860**

Terazosin Hydrochloride (Clozapine may potentiate the hypotensive effects of antihypertensive drugs). Products include:
Hytrin Capsules **471**

Thiamylal Sodium (Given the primary CNS effect of clozapine, caution is advised in using it concomitantly with CNS-active drugs).
No products indexed under this heading.

Thioridazine Hydrochloride (Co-administration with benzodiazepines or other psychotropic agents may be accompanied by orthostatic hypotension leading to profound collapse and respiratory and/or cardiac arrest; caution is advised if used concurrently). Products include:
Thioridazine Hydrochloride Tablets **2163**

Thiothixene (Co-administration with benzodiazepines or other psychotropic agents may be accompanied by orthostatic hypotension leading to profound collapse and respiratory and/or cardiac arrest; caution is advised if used concurrently). Products include:
Thiothixene Capsules **2165**

Timolol Maleate (Clozapine may potentiate the hypotensive effects of antihypertensive drugs). Products include:
Blocadren Tablets **1916**
Cosopt Sterile Ophthalmic Solution.. **1931**
Timolide Tablets **2086**
Timoptic Sterile Ophthalmic Solution.. **2088**
Timoptic in Ocudose **2091**
Timoptic-XE Sterile Ophthalmic Gel Forming Solution **2092**

Tolterodine Tartrate (Clozapine may potentiate anticholinergic effects). Products include:
Detrol Tablets **2628**
Detrol LA Capsules **2631**

Torsemide (Clozapine may potentiate the hypotensive effects of antihypertensive drugs). Products include:
Demadex Injection **2759**
Demadex Tablets **2759**

Trandolapril (Clozapine may potentiate the hypotensive effects of antihypertensive drugs). Products include:
Mavik Tablets **486**
Tarka Tablets **524**

Tranylcypromine Sulfate (Concomitant use of clozapine with other drugs metabolized by CYP4502D6 may require lower than usual doses for either drug). Products include:
Parnate Tablets **1527**

Trazodone Hydrochloride (Concomitant use of clozapine with other drugs metabolized by CYP4502D6 may require lower than usual doses for either drug).
No products indexed under this heading.

Triazolam (Co-administration with benzodiazepines or other psychotropic agents may be accompanied by orthostatic hypotension leading to profound collapse and respiratory and/or cardiac arrest; caution is advised if used concurrently).
No products indexed under this heading.

Tridihexethyl Chloride (Clozapine may potentiate anticholinergic effects).
No products indexed under this heading.

Trifluoperazine Hydrochloride (Co-administration with benzodiazepines or other psychotropic agents may be accompanied by orthostatic hypotension leading to profound collapse and respiratory and/or cardiac arrest; caution is advised if used concurrently).
No products indexed under this heading.

Trihexyphenidyl Hydrochloride (Clozapine may potentiate anticholinergic effects).
No products indexed under this heading.

Trimethaphan Camsylate (Clozapine may potentiate the hypotensive effects of antihypertensive drugs).
No products indexed under this heading.

Trimipramine Maleate (Concomitant use of clozapine with other drugs metabolized by CYP4502D6 may require lower than usual doses for either drug).
No products indexed under this heading.

Valsartan (Clozapine may potentiate the hypotensive effects of antihypertensive drugs). Products include:
Diovan Tablets **2193**
Diovan HCT Tablets **2196**

Venlafaxine Hydrochloride (Concomitant use of clozapine with other drugs metabolized by CYP4502D6 may require lower than usual doses for either drug). Products include:
Effexor Tablets **3411**
Effexor XR Capsules **3417**

Verapamil Hydrochloride (Clozapine may potentiate the hypotensive effects of antihypertensive drugs). Products include:
Covera-HS Tablets **3139**
Tarka Tablets **524**
Verelan PM Extended-Release Capsules, Controlled-Onset........... **3106**

Zaleplon (Given the primary CNS effect of clozapine, caution is advised in using it concomitantly with CNS-active drugs). Products include:
Sonata Capsules **1717**

Ziprasidone Hydrochloride (Co-administration with benzodiazepines or other psychotropic agents may be accompanied by orthostatic hypotension leading to profound collapse and respiratory and/or cardiac arrest; caution is advised if used concurrently). Products include:
Geodon Capsules **2529**

Zolpidem Tartrate (Given the primary CNS effect of clozapine, caution is advised in using it concomitantly with CNS-active drugs). Products include:
Ambien Tablets **2851**
Ambien CR Tablets **2855**

Food Interactions

Alcohol (Given the primary CNS effect of clozapine, caution is advised in using it concomitantly with alcohol).

FEIBA VH

(Anti-Inhibitor Coagulant Complex) **718**
None cited in PDR database.

FEMARA TABLETS

(Letrozole) **2214**
May interact with:

Tamoxifen Citrate (Co-administration of Femara and tamoxifen 20 mg daily resulted in a reduction of letrozole plasma levels of 38% on average. Clinical experience in the second-line breast cancer pivotal trials indicates that the therapeutic effect of Femara therapy is not impaired if Femara is administered immediately after tamoxifen). Products include:
Soltamox Oral Solution **3527**

FERRLECIT INJECTION

(Sodium Ferric Gluconate) **3388**
May interact with ACE inhibitors and iron containing oral preparations. Compounds in these categories include:

Benazepril Hydrochloride (Co-administration with ACE inhibitors has resulted in increased incidence of both drug intolerance or suspected allergic events). Products include:
Lotensin Tablets **2243**
Lotensin HCT Tablets **2246**
Lotrel Capsules **2249**

Captopril (Co-administration with ACE inhibitors has resulted in increased incidence of both drug intolerance or suspected allergic events). Products include:
Captopril Tablets **2149**

Enalapril Maleate (Co-administration with ACE inhibitors has resulted in increased incidence of both drug intolerance or suspected allergic events). Products include:
Vasotec I.V. Injection **2103**

Enalaprilat (Co-administration with ACE inhibitors has resulted in increased incidence of both drug intolerance or suspected allergic events).
No products indexed under this heading.

Ferrous Fumarate (Like other parenteral iron preparations, sodium ferric gluconate complex may be expected to reduce the absorption of concomitantly administered oral iron preparations).
No products indexed under this heading.

Ferrous Gluconate (Like other parenteral iron preparations, sodium ferric gluconate complex may be expected to reduce the absorption of concomitantly administered oral iron preparations).
No products indexed under this heading.

Ferrous Sulfate (Like other parenteral iron preparations, sodium ferric gluconate complex may be expected to reduce the absorption of concomitantly administered oral iron preparations). Products include:
Slow Fe Iron Tablets .... ⊡ **818**
Slow Fe with Folic Acid Tablets .... ⊡ **819**

Fosinopril Sodium (Co-administration with ACE inhibitors has resulted in increased incidence of both drug intolerance or suspected allergic events).
No products indexed under this heading.

Iron (Like other parenteral iron preparations, sodium ferric gluconate complex may be expected to reduce the absorption of concomitantly administered oral iron preparations).
No products indexed under this heading.

Lisinopril (Co-administration with ACE inhibitors has resulted in increased incidence of both drug intolerance or suspected allergic events). Products include:
Prinivil Tablets **2052**
Prinzide Tablets **2056**

Moexipril Hydrochloride (Co-administration with ACE inhibitors has resulted in increased incidence of both drug intolerance or suspected allergic events). Products include:
Uniretic Tablets **3100**
Univasc Tablets **3104**

Perindopril Erbumine (Co-administration with ACE inhibitors has resulted in increased incidence of both drug intolerance or suspected allergic events). Products include:
Aceon Tablets (2 mg, 4 mg, 8 mg).. **3194**

Polysaccharide Iron Complex (Like other parenteral iron preparations, sodium ferric gluconate complex may be expected to reduce the absorption of concomitantly administered oral iron preparations). Products include:
Nu-Iron 150 Capsules **2127**

Quinapril Hydrochloride (Co-administration with ACE inhibitors has resulted in increased incidence of both drug intolerance or suspected allergic events).
No products indexed under this heading.

Ramipril (Co-administration with ACE inhibitors has resulted in increased incidence of both drug intolerance or suspected allergic events). Products include:
Altace Capsules **1702**

Spirapril Hydrochloride (Co-administration with ACE inhibitors has resulted in increased incidence of both drug intolerance or suspected allergic events).
No products indexed under this heading.

Trandolapril (Co-administration with ACE inhibitors has resulted in increased incidence of both drug intolerance or suspected allergic events). Products include:
Mavik Tablets **486**
Tarka Tablets **524**

FIBERCON CAPLETS

(Calcium Polycarbophil) .... ⊡ **650**
May interact with tetracyclines. Compounds in these categories include:

Demeclocycline Hydrochloride (Fibercon should be taken at least one hour before or two hours after you have taken any form of tetracycline).
No products indexed under this heading.

Doxycycline Calcium (Fibercon should be taken at least one hour before or two hours after you have taken any form of tetracycline).
No products indexed under this heading.

Doxycycline Hyclate (Fibercon should be taken at least one hour before or two hours after you have taken any form of tetracycline).
No products indexed under this heading.

Doxycycline Monohydrate (Fibercon should be taken at least one hour before or two hours after you have taken any form of tetracycline). Products include:
Oracea Capsules **1000**

Methacycline Hydrochloride
(Fibercon should be taken at least one hour before or two hours after you have taken any form of tetracycline).
No products indexed under this heading.

Minocycline Hydrochloride
(Fibercon should be taken at least one hour before or two hours after you have taken any form of tetracycline). Products include:
Solodyn Extended Release Tablets 1890

Oxytetracycline Hydrochloride
(Fibercon should be taken at least one hour before or two hours after you have taken any form of tetracycline).
No products indexed under this heading.

Tetracycline Hydrochloride
(Fibercon should be taken at least one hour before or two hours after you have taken any form of tetracycline).
No products indexed under this heading.

FINACEA GEL
(Azelaic Acid) 1669
None cited in PDR database.

FLEBOGAMMA 5%, IMMUNE GLOBULIN INTRAVENOUS (HUMAN)
(Globulin, Immune (Human)) 1658
May interact with vaccines, live. Compounds in these categories include:

BCG Vaccine (Antibodies in immune globulin intravenous (Human) may interfere with the responses to live viral vaccines, such as measles, mumps, and rubella. Physicians should be informed of recent therapy with immune globulin intravenous (Human) so that administration of live viral vaccines, if indicated, can be appropriately delayed 3 or more months from the time of IGIV administration).
No products indexed under this heading.

Measles, Mumps, Rubella and Varicella Virus Vaccine Live (Antibodies in immune globulin intravenous (Human) may interfere with the responses to live viral vaccines, such as measles, mumps, and rubella. Physicians should be informed of recent therapy with immune globulin intravenous (Human) so that administration of live viral vaccines, if indicated, can be appropriately delayed 3 or more months from the time of IGIV administration). Products include:
ProQuad 2064

Measles, Mumps & Rubella Virus Vaccine, Live (Antibodies in immune globulin intravenous (Human) may interfere with the responses to live viral vaccines, such as measles, mumps, and rubella. Physicians should be informed of recent therapy with immune globulin intravenous (Human) so that administration of live viral vaccines, if indicated, can be appropriately delayed 3 or more months from the time of IGIV administration). Products include:
M-M-R II 2006

Measles & Rubella Virus Vaccine Live (Antibodies in immune globulin intravenous (Human) may interfere with the responses to live viral vaccines, such as measles, mumps, and rubella. Physicians should be informed of recent therapy with immune globulin intravenous (Human) so that administration of live viral vaccines, if indicated, can be appropriately delayed 3 or more months from the time of IGIV administration).
No products indexed under this heading.

Measles Virus Vaccine Live (Antibodies in immune globulin intravenous (Human) may interfere with the responses to live viral vaccines, such as measles, mumps, and rubella. Physicians should be informed of recent therapy with immune globulin intravenous (Human) so that administration of live viral vaccines, if indicated, can be appropriately delayed 3 or more months from the time of IGIV administration). Products include:
Attenuvax 1914

Mumps Virus Vaccine, Live (Antibodies in immune globulin intravenous (Human) may interfere with the responses to live viral vaccines, such as measles, mumps, and rubella. Physicians should be informed of recent therapy with immune globulin intravenous (Human) so that administration of live viral vaccines, if indicated, can be appropriately delayed 3 or more months from the time of IGIV administration). Products include:
Mumpsvax 2031

Poliovirus Vaccine, Live, Oral, Trivalent, Types 1,2,3 (Sabin) (Antibodies in immune globulin intravenous (Human) may interfere with the responses to live viral vaccines, such as measles, mumps, and rubella. Physicians should be informed of recent therapy with immune globulin intravenous (Human) so that administration of live viral vaccines, if indicated, can be appropriately delayed 3 or more months from the time of IGIV administration).
No products indexed under this heading.

Rotavirus Vaccine, Live, Oral, Tetravalent (Antibodies in immune globulin intravenous (Human) may interfere with the responses to live viral vaccines, such as measles, mumps, and rubella. Physicians should be informed of recent therapy with immune globulin intravenous (Human) so that administration of live viral vaccines, if indicated, can be appropriately delayed 3 or more months from the time of IGIV administration).
No products indexed under this heading.

Rubella & Mumps Virus Vaccine Live (Antibodies in immune globulin intravenous (Human) may interfere with the responses to live viral vaccines, such as measles, mumps, and rubella. Physicians should be informed of recent therapy with immune globulin intravenous (Human) so that administration of live viral vaccines, if indicated, can be appropriately delayed 3 or more months from the time of IGIV administration).
No products indexed under this heading.

Rubella Virus Vaccine Live (Antibodies in immune globulin intravenous (Human) may interfere with the responses to live viral vaccines, such as measles, mumps, and rubella. Physicians should be informed of recent therapy with immune globulin intravenous (Human) so that administration of live viral vaccines, if indicated, can be appropriately delayed 3 or more months from the time of IGIV administration). Products include:
Meruvax II 2019

Smallpox Vaccine (Antibodies in immune globulin intravenous (Human) may interfere with the responses to live viral vaccines, such as measles, mumps, and rubella. Physicians should be informed of recent therapy with immune globulin intravenous (Human) so that administration of live viral vaccines, if indicated, can be appropriately delayed 3 or more months from the time of IGIV administration).
No products indexed under this heading.

Typhoid Vaccine (Antibodies in immune globulin intravenous (Human) may interfere with the responses to live viral vaccines, such as measles, mumps, and rubella. Physicians should be informed of recent therapy with immune globulin intravenous (Human) so that administration of live viral vaccines, if indicated, can be appropriately delayed 3 or more months from the time of IGIV administration).
No products indexed under this heading.

Varicella Virus Vaccine Live (Antibodies in immune globulin intravenous (Human) may interfere with the responses to live viral vaccines, such as measles, mumps, and rubella. Physicians should be informed of recent therapy with immune globulin intravenous (Human) so that administration of live viral vaccines, if indicated, can be appropriately delayed 3 or more months from the time of IGIV administration). Products include:
Varivax 2100

Yellow Fever Vaccine (Antibodies in immune globulin intravenous (Human) may interfere with the responses to live viral vaccines, such as measles, mumps, and rubella. Physicians should be informed of recent therapy with immune globulin intravenous (Human) so that administration of live viral vaccines, if indicated, can be appropriately delayed 3 or more months from the time of IGIV administration).
No products indexed under this heading.

FLEET BISACODYL LAXATIVES
(Bisacodyl) 1165
None cited in PDR database.

FLEET ENEMA
(Sodium Phosphate) 1165
None cited in PDR database.

FLEET ENEMA FOR CHILDREN
(Sodium Phosphate) 1165
See Fleet Enema

FLEET GLYCERIN LAXATIVES
(Glycerin) 1165
None cited in PDR database.

FLEET GLYCERIN SUPPOSITORIES
(Glycerin) 1165
None cited in PDR database.

FLEET MINERAL OIL ENEMA
(Mineral Oil) 1166
None cited in PDR database.

FLEET PHOSPHO-SODA
(Sodium Phosphate) 1166
See Fleet Prep Kits

FLEET PHOSPHO-SODA ACCU-PREP
(Glycerin, Pramoxine Hydrochloride, Sodium Phosphate)..... 1168
May interact with antacids, diuretics, drugs that prolong the QT interval, and certain other agents. Compounds in these categories include:

Aluminum Carbonate (Concurrent use within one hour should be avoided).
No products indexed under this heading.

Aluminum Hydroxide (Concurrent use within one hour should be avoided). Products include:
Gaviscon Regular Strength Liquid .. 658
Gaviscon Regular Strength Tablets 658
Gaviscon Extra Strength Liquid 658
Gaviscon Extra Strength Tablets 658
Maalox Regular Strength Antacid/Antigas Liquid 2175
Maalox Max Maximum Strength Antacid/Anti-Gas Liquid 2176

Amiloride Hydrochloride (Electrolyte disturbances are a risk associated with this product; concurrent use in patients taking agents known to disturb electrolyte balance requires caution). Products include:
Midamor Tablets 2026
Moduretic Tablets 2028

Amiodarone Hydrochloride (Electrolyte disturbances are a risk associated with this product; concurrent use in patients taking agents known to disturb electrolyte balance requires caution).
No products indexed under this heading.

Amitriptyline Hydrochloride (Electrolyte disturbances are a risk associated with this product; concurrent use in patients taking agents known to disturb electrolyte balance requires caution).
No products indexed under this heading.

Amoxapine (Electrolyte disturbances are a risk associated with this product; concurrent use in patients taking agents known to disturb electrolyte balance requires caution).
No products indexed under this heading.

Astemizole (Electrolyte disturbances are a risk associated with this product; concurrent use in patients taking agents known to disturb electrolyte balance requires caution).
No products indexed under this heading.

Bendroflumethiazide (Electrolyte disturbances are a risk associated with this product; concurrent use in patients taking agents known to disturb electrolyte balance requires caution).
No products indexed under this heading.

Bretylium Tosylate (Electrolyte disturbances are a risk associated with this product; concurrent use in patients taking agents known to disturb electrolyte balance requires caution).
No products indexed under this heading.

Bumetanide (Electrolyte disturbances are a risk associated with this product; concurrent use in patients taking agents known to disturb electrolyte balance requires caution). Products include:
Bumex Tablets 2746

Chlorothiazide (Electrolyte disturbances are a risk associated with this product; concurrent use in patients taking agents known to disturb electrolyte balance requires caution). Products include:
Diuril Oral Suspension 1954

Chlorothiazide Sodium (Electrolyte disturbances are a risk associated with this product; concurrent use in patients taking agents known to disturb electrolyte balance requires caution). Products include:
Diuril Sodium Intravenous 2467

Chlorpromazine (Electrolyte disturbances are a risk associated with this product; concurrent use in patients taking agents known to disturb electrolyte balance requires caution).
No products indexed under this heading.

Chlorpromazine Hydrochloride (Electrolyte disturbances are a risk associated with this product; concurrent use in patients taking agents known to disturb electrolyte balance requires caution).
No products indexed under this heading.

Chlorthalidone (Electrolyte disturbances are a risk associated with this product; concurrent use in patients taking agents known to disturb electrolyte balance requires caution). Products include:
Clorpres Tablets 2153

Clomipramine Hydrochloride (Electrolyte disturbances are a risk associated with this product; concurrent use in patients taking agents known to disturb electrolyte balance requires caution).
No products indexed under this heading.

Desipramine Hydrochloride (Electrolyte disturbances are a risk associated with this product; concurrent use in patients taking agents known to disturb electrolyte balance requires caution).
No products indexed under this heading.

Disopyramide Phosphate (Electrolyte disturbances are a risk associated with this product; concurrent use in patients taking agents known to disturb electrolyte balance requires caution).
No products indexed under this heading.

Dofetilide (Electrolyte disturbances are a risk associated with this product; concurrent use in patients taking agents known to disturb electrolyte balance requires caution).
No products indexed under this heading.

Doxepin Hydrochloride (Electrolyte disturbances are a risk associated with this product; concurrent use in patients taking agents known to disturb electrolyte balance requires caution).
No products indexed under this heading.

Ethacrynic Acid (Electrolyte disturbances are a risk associated with this product; concurrent use in patients taking agents known to disturb electrolyte balance requires caution). Products include:
Edecrin Tablets 1959

Flecainide Acetate (Electrolyte disturbances are a risk associated with this product; concurrent use in patients taking agents known to disturb electrolyte balance requires caution). Products include:
Tambocor Tablets 1856

Fluphenazine Decanoate (Electrolyte disturbances are a risk associated with this product; concurrent use in patients taking agents known to disturb electrolyte balance requires caution).
No products indexed under this heading.

Fluphenazine Enanthate (Electrolyte disturbances are a risk associated with this product; concurrent use in patients taking agents known to disturb electrolyte balance requires caution).
No products indexed under this heading.

Fluphenazine Hydrochloride (Electrolyte disturbances are a risk associated with this product; concurrent use in patients taking agents known to disturb electrolyte balance requires caution).
No products indexed under this heading.

Furosemide (Electrolyte disturbances are a risk associated with this product; concurrent use in patients taking agents known to disturb electrolyte balance requires caution). Products include:
Furosemide Tablets 2154

Hydrochlorothiazide (Electrolyte disturbances are a risk associated with this product; concurrent use in patients taking agents known to disturb electrolyte balance requires caution). Products include:
Aldoril Tablets 1910
Atacand HCT 651
Avalide Tablets 888
Avalide Tablets 2874
Benicar HCT Tablets 1044
Diovan HCT Tablets 2196
Dyazide Capsules 1423
Hyzaar 50-12.5 Tablets 1990
Hyzaar 100-12.5 Tablets 1990
Hyzaar 100-25 Tablets 1990
Lopressor HCT 50/25 Tablets 2241
Lopressor HCT 100/25 Tablets 2241
Lopressor HCT 100/50 Tablets 2241
Lotensin HCT Tablets 2246
Micardis HCT Tablets 856
Moduretic Tablets 2028
Prinzide Tablets 2056
Teveten HCT Tablets 1737
Timolide Tablets 2086
Uniretic Tablets 3100

Hydroflumethiazide (Electrolyte disturbances are a risk associated with this product; concurrent use in patients taking agents known to disturb electrolyte balance requires caution).
No products indexed under this heading.

Imipramine Hydrochloride (Electrolyte disturbances are a risk associated with this product; concurrent use in patients taking agents known to disturb electrolyte balance requires caution).
No products indexed under this heading.

Imipramine Pamoate (Electrolyte disturbances are a risk associated with this product; concurrent use in patients taking agents known to disturb electrolyte balance requires caution).
No products indexed under this heading.

Indapamide (Electrolyte disturbances are a risk associated with this product; concurrent use in patients taking agents known to disturb electrolyte balance requires caution). Products include:
Indapamide Tablets 2156

Lidocaine Hydrochloride (Electrolyte disturbances are a risk associated with this product; concurrent use in patients taking agents known to disturb electrolyte balance requires caution).
No products indexed under this heading.

Magaldrate (Concurrent use within one hour should be avoided).
No products indexed under this heading.

Magnesium Hydroxide (Concurrent use within one hour should be avoided). Products include:
Maalox Regular Strength Antacid/Antigas Liquid 2175
Maalox Max Maximum Strength Antacid/Anti-Gas Liquid 2176
Pepcid Complete Chewable Tablets 1701

Magnesium Oxide (Concurrent use within one hour should be avoided). Products include:
Beelith Tablets 759
PremCal Light, Regular, and Extra Strength Tablets .... ▣818

Maprotiline Hydrochloride (Electrolyte disturbances are a risk associated with this product; concurrent use in patients taking agents known to disturb electrolyte balance requires caution).
No products indexed under this heading.

Mesoridazine Besylate (Electrolyte disturbances are a risk associated with this product; concurrent use in patients taking agents known to disturb electrolyte balance requires caution).
No products indexed under this heading.

Methyclothiazide (Electrolyte disturbances are a risk associated with this product; concurrent use in patients taking agents known to disturb electrolyte balance requires caution).
No products indexed under this heading.

Metolazone (Electrolyte disturbances are a risk associated with this product; concurrent use in patients taking agents known to disturb electrolyte balance requires caution).
No products indexed under this heading.

Mexiletine Hydrochloride (Electrolyte disturbances are a risk associated with this product; concurrent use in patients taking agents known to disturb electrolyte balance requires caution).
No products indexed under this heading.

Nortriptyline Hydrochloride (Electrolyte disturbances are a risk associated with this product; concurrent use in patients taking agents known to disturb electrolyte balance requires caution).
No products indexed under this heading.

Perphenazine (Electrolyte disturbances are a risk associated with this product; concurrent use in patients taking agents known to disturb electrolyte balance requires caution).
No products indexed under this heading.

Polythiazide (Electrolyte disturbances are a risk associated with this product; concurrent use in patients taking agents known to disturb electrolyte balance requires caution).
No products indexed under this heading.

Procainamide Hydrochloride (Electrolyte disturbances are a risk associated with this product; concurrent use in patients taking agents known to disturb electrolyte balance requires caution).
No products indexed under this heading.

Prochlorperazine (Electrolyte disturbances are a risk associated with this product; concurrent use in patients taking agents known to disturb electrolyte balance requires caution).
No products indexed under this heading.

Promethazine Hydrochloride (Electrolyte disturbances are a risk associated with this product; concurrent use in patients taking agents known to disturb electrolyte balance requires caution). Products include:
Phenergan Tablets and Suppositories 3440

Propafenone Hydrochloride (Electrolyte disturbances are a risk associated with this product; concurrent use in patients taking agents known to disturb electrolyte balance requires caution). Products include:
Rythmol SR Capsules 2727

Protriptyline Hydrochloride (Electrolyte disturbances are a risk associated with this product; concurrent use in patients taking agents known to disturb electrolyte balance requires caution).
No products indexed under this heading.

Quinidine Gluconate (Electrolyte disturbances are a risk associated with this product; concurrent use in patients taking agents known to disturb electrolyte balance requires caution).
No products indexed under this heading.

Quinidine Polygalacturonate (Electrolyte disturbances are a risk associated with this product; concurrent use in patients taking agents known to disturb electrolyte balance requires caution).
No products indexed under this heading.

Quinidine Sulfate (Electrolyte disturbances are a risk associated with this product; concurrent use in patients taking agents known to disturb electrolyte balance requires caution).

No products indexed under this heading.

Sodium Bicarbonate (Concurrent use within one hour should be avoided). Products include:

Colyte with Flavor Packs for Oral Solution.................................... 3088
HalfLytely and Bisacodyl Tablets Bowel Prep Kit with Flavors Packs .. 881
TriLyte with Flavor Packs for Oral Solution.................................... 3100

Spironolactone (Electrolyte disturbances are a risk associated with this product; concurrent use in patients taking agents known to disturb electrolyte balance requires caution).

No products indexed under this heading.

Thioridazine Hydrochloride (Electrolyte disturbances are a risk associated with this product; concurrent use in patients taking agents known to disturb electrolyte balance requires caution). Products include:

Thioridazine Hydrochloride Tablets.................................... 2163

Tocainide Hydrochloride (Electrolyte disturbances are a risk associated with this product; concurrent use in patients taking agents known to disturb electrolyte balance requires caution).

No products indexed under this heading.

Torsemide (Electrolyte disturbances are a risk associated with this product; concurrent use in patients taking agents known to disturb electrolyte balance requires caution). Products include:

Demadex Injection 2759
Demadex Tablets 2759

Triamterene (Electrolyte disturbances are a risk associated with this product; concurrent use in patients taking agents known to disturb electrolyte balance requires caution). Products include:

Dyazide Capsules 1423
Dyrenium Capsules 3400

Trifluoperazine Hydrochloride (Electrolyte disturbances are a risk associated with this product; concurrent use in patients taking agents known to disturb electrolyte balance requires caution).

No products indexed under this heading.

Trimipramine Maleate (Electrolyte disturbances are a risk associated with this product; concurrent use in patients taking agents known to disturb electrolyte balance requires caution).

No products indexed under this heading.

Ziprasidone Hydrochloride (Electrolyte disturbances are a risk associated with this product; concurrent use in patients taking agents known to disturb electrolyte balance requires caution). Products include:

Geodon Capsules 2529

Food Interactions

Dairy products (Concurrent use within one hour should be avoided).

FLEET PHOSPHO-SODA EZ-PREP

(Glycerin, Pramoxine Hydrochloride, Sodium Phosphate)..... 1169
See Fleet Phospho-soda ACCU-PREP

FLEET PREP KITS

(Bisacodyl, Sodium Phosphate) 1170
May interact with ACE inhibitors, angiotensin-II receptor antagonists, antacids, diuretics, lithium preparations, non-steroidal anti-inflammatory agents, drugs that prolong the QT interval, and certain other agents. Compounds in these categories include:

Aluminum Carbonate (Concurrent use within one hour should be avoided).

No products indexed under this heading.

Aluminum Hydroxide (Concurrent use within one hour should be avoided). Products include:

Gaviscon Regular Strength Liquid .. ☒658
Gaviscon Regular Strength Tablets................................... ☒658
Gaviscon Extra Strength Liquid ☒658
Gaviscon Extra Strength Tablets ☒658
Maalox Regular Strength Antacid/Antigas Liquid 2175
Maalox Max Maximum Strength Antacid/Anti-Gas Liquid................ 2176

Amiloride Hydrochloride (Electrolyte disturbances are a risk associated with this product; concurrent use in patients taking agents known to disturb electrolyte balance requires caution). Products include:

Midamor Tablets 2026
Moduretic Tablets 2028

Amiodarone Hydrochloride (Electrolyte disturbances are a risk associated with this product; concurrent use in patients taking agents known to prolong QT interval requires caution).

No products indexed under this heading.

Amitriptyline Hydrochloride (Electrolyte disturbances are a risk associated with this product; concurrent use in patients taking agents known to prolong QT interval requires caution).

No products indexed under this heading.

Amoxapine (Electrolyte disturbances are a risk associated with this product; concurrent use in patients taking agents known to prolong QT interval requires caution).

No products indexed under this heading.

Astemizole (Electrolyte disturbances are a risk associated with this product; concurrent use in patients taking agents known to prolong QT interval requires caution).

No products indexed under this heading.

Benazepril Hydrochloride (Electrolyte disturbances are a risk associated with this product; concurrent use in patients taking agents known to disturb electrolyte balance requires caution). Products include:

Lotensin Tablets 2243
Lotensin HCT Tablets 2246
Lotrel Capsules 2249

Bendroflumethiazide (Electrolyte disturbances are a risk associated with this product; concurrent use in patients taking agents known to disturb electrolyte balance requires caution).

No products indexed under this heading.

Bretylium Tosylate (Electrolyte disturbances are a risk associated with this product; concurrent use in patients taking agents known to prolong QT interval requires caution).

No products indexed under this heading.

Bumetanide (Electrolyte disturbances are a risk associated with this product; concurrent use in patients taking agents known to disturb electrolyte balance requires caution). Products include:

Bumex Tablets 2746

Candesartan Cilexetil (Electrolyte disturbances are a risk associated with this product; concurrent use in patients taking agents known to disturb electrolyte balance requires caution). Products include:

Atacand Tablets 649
Atacand HCT 651

Captopril (Electrolyte disturbances are a risk associated with this product; concurrent use in patients taking agents known to disturb electrolyte balance requires caution). Products include:

Captopril Tablets 2149

Celecoxib (Electrolyte disturbances are a risk associated with this product; concurrent use in patients taking agents known to disturb electrolyte balance requires caution). Products include:

Celebrex Capsules 3134

Chlorothiazide (Electrolyte disturbances are a risk associated with this product; concurrent use in patients taking agents known to disturb electrolyte balance requires caution). Products include:

Diuril Oral Suspension 1954

Chlorothiazide Sodium (Electrolyte disturbances are a risk associated with this product; concurrent use in patients taking agents known to disturb electrolyte balance requires caution). Products include:

Diuril Sodium Intravenous 2467

Chlorpromazine (Electrolyte disturbances are a risk associated with this product; concurrent use in patients taking agents known to prolong QT interval requires caution).

No products indexed under this heading.

Chlorpromazine Hydrochloride (Electrolyte disturbances are a risk associated with this product; concurrent use in patients taking agents known to prolong QT interval requires caution).

No products indexed under this heading.

Chlorthalidone (Electrolyte disturbances are a risk associated with this product; concurrent use in patients taking agents known to disturb electrolyte balance requires caution). Products include:

Clorpres Tablets 2153

Clomipramine Hydrochloride (Electrolyte disturbances are a risk associated with this product; concurrent use in patients taking agents known to prolong QT interval requires caution).

No products indexed under this heading.

Desipramine Hydrochloride (Electrolyte disturbances are a risk associated with this product; concurrent use in patients taking agents known to prolong QT interval requires caution).

No products indexed under this heading.

Diclofenac Potassium (Electrolyte disturbances are a risk associated with this product; concurrent use in patients taking agents known to disturb electrolyte balance requires caution).

No products indexed under this heading.

Diclofenac Sodium (Electrolyte disturbances are a risk associated with this product; concurrent use in patients taking agents known to disturb electrolyte balance requires caution). Products include:

Arthrotec Tablets 3129
Voltaren Ophthalmic Solution 2309
Voltaren Tablets 2307
Voltaren-XR Tablets 2310

Disopyramide Phosphate (Electrolyte disturbances are a risk associated with this product; concurrent use in patients taking agents known to prolong QT interval requires caution).

No products indexed under this heading.

Dofetilide (Electrolyte disturbances are a risk associated with this product; concurrent use in patients taking agents known to prolong QT interval requires caution).

No products indexed under this heading.

Doxepin Hydrochloride (Electrolyte disturbances are a risk associated with this product; concurrent use in patients taking agents known to prolong QT interval requires caution).

No products indexed under this heading.

Enalapril Maleate (Electrolyte disturbances are a risk associated with this product; concurrent use in patients taking agents known to disturb electrolyte balance requires caution). Products include:

Vasotec I.V. Injection 2103

Enalaprilat (Electrolyte disturbances are a risk associated with this product; concurrent use in patients taking agents known to disturb electrolyte balance requires caution).

No products indexed under this heading.

Eprosartan Mesylate (Electrolyte disturbances are a risk associated with this product; concurrent use in patients taking agents known to disturb electrolyte balance requires caution). Products include:

Teveten Tablets 1735
Teveten HCT Tablets 1737

Ethacrynic Acid (Electrolyte disturbances are a risk associated with this product; concurrent use in patients taking agents known to disturb electrolyte balance requires caution). Products include:

Edecrin Tablets 1959

Etodolac (Electrolyte disturbances are a risk associated with this product; concurrent use in patients taking agents known to disturb electrolyte balance requires caution).

No products indexed under this heading.

Fenoprofen Calcium (Electrolyte disturbances are a risk associated with this product; concurrent use in patients taking agents known to disturb electrolyte balance requires caution). Products include:

Nalfon Capsules 2502

Flecainide Acetate (Electrolyte disturbances are a risk associated with this product; concurrent use in patients taking agents known to prolong QT interval requires caution). Products include:

Tambocor Tablets 1856

Fluphenazine Decanoate (Electrolyte disturbances are a risk associated with this product; concurrent use in patients taking agents known to prolong QT interval requires caution).

No products indexed under this heading.

Fluphenazine Enanthate (Electrolyte disturbances are a risk associated with this product; concurrent use in patients taking agents known to prolong QT interval requires caution).

No products indexed under this heading.

Fluphenazine Hydrochloride (Electrolyte disturbances are a risk associated with this product; concurrent use in patients taking agents known to prolong QT interval requires caution).

No products indexed under this heading.

Flurbiprofen (Electrolyte disturbances are a risk associated with this product; concurrent use in patients taking agents known to disturb electrolyte balance requires caution).

No products indexed under this heading.

Fosinopril Sodium (Electrolyte disturbances are a risk associated with this product; concurrent use in patients taking agents known to disturb electrolyte balance requires caution).

No products indexed under this heading.

Furosemide (Electrolyte disturbances are a risk associated with this product; concurrent use in patients taking agents known to disturb electrolyte balance requires caution). Products include:

Furosemide Tablets 2154

Hydrochlorothiazide (Electrolyte disturbances are a risk associated with this product; concurrent use in patients taking agents known to disturb electrolyte balance requires caution). Products include:

Aldoril Tablets	1910
Atacand HCT	651
Avalide Tablets	888
Avalide Tablets	2874
Benicar HCT Tablets	1044
Diovan HCT Tablets	2196
Dyazide Capsules	1423
Hyzaar 50-12.5 Tablets	1990
Hyzaar 100-12.5 Tablets	1990
Hyzaar 100-25 Tablets	1990
Lopressor HCT 50/25 Tablets	2241
Lopressor HCT 100/25 Tablets	2241
Lopressor HCT 100/50 Tablets	2241
Lotensin HCT Tablets	2246
Micardis HCT Tablets	856
Moduretic Tablets	2028
Prinzide Tablets	2056
Teveten HCT Tablets	1737
Timolide Tablets	2086
Uniretic Tablets	3100

Hydroflumethiazide (Electrolyte disturbances are a risk associated with this product; concurrent use in patients taking agents known to disturb electrolyte balance requires caution).

No products indexed under this heading.

Ibuprofen (Electrolyte disturbances are a risk associated with this product; concurrent use in patients taking agents known to disturb electrolyte balance requires caution). Products include:

Advil Allergy Sinus Caplets	▣770
Advil ...	▣674
Children's Advil Oral Suspension	▣603
Children's Advil Chewable Tablets ..	▣603
Advil Cold & Sinus	▣723
Infants' Advil Concentrated Drops ..	▣604
Infants' Advil Concentrated Drops - White Grape (Dye-Free)...........	▣604
Junior Strength Advil Swallow Tablets.....................................	▣605
Advil Migraine Liquigels	▣608
Advil Multi-Symptom Cold Caplets.....................................	▣770
Advil PM Caplets	▣615
Motrin IB Tablets and Caplets	1866
Children's Motrin Oral Suspension ...	1867
Children's Motrin Non-Staining Dye-Free Oral Suspension.........	1867
Children's Motrin Cold Oral Suspension	1867
Infants' Motrin Concentrated Drops......................................	1867
Infants' Motrin Non-Staining Dye-Free Concentrated Drops.......	1867
Junior Strength Motrin Caplets and Chewable Tablets..................	1867
Vicoprofen Tablets	539

Imipramine Hydrochloride (Electrolyte disturbances are a risk associated with this product; concurrent use in patients taking agents known to prolong QT interval requires caution).

No products indexed under this heading.

Imipramine Pamoate (Electrolyte disturbances are a risk associated with this product; concurrent use in patients taking agents known to prolong QT interval requires caution).

No products indexed under this heading.

Indapamide (Electrolyte disturbances are a risk associated with this product; concurrent use in patients taking agents known to disturb electrolyte balance requires caution). Products include:

Indapamide Tablets 2156

Indomethacin (Electrolyte disturbances are a risk associated with this product; concurrent use in patients taking agents known to disturb electrolyte balance requires caution). Products include:

Indocin .. 1995

Indomethacin Sodium Trihydrate (Electrolyte disturbances are a risk associated with this product; concurrent use in patients taking agents known to disturb electrolyte balance requires caution). Products include:

Indocin I.V. 2465

Irbesartan (Electrolyte disturbances are a risk associated with this product; concurrent use in patients taking agents known to disturb electrolyte balance requires caution). Products include:

Avalide Tablets	888
Avalide Tablets	2874
Avapro Tablets	891
Avapro Tablets	2871

Ketoprofen (Electrolyte disturbances are a risk associated with this product; concurrent use in patients taking agents known to disturb electrolyte balance requires caution).

No products indexed under this heading.

Ketorolac Tromethamine (Electrolyte disturbances are a risk associated with this product; concurrent use in patients taking agents known to disturb electrolyte balance requires caution). Products include:

Acular Ophthalmic Solution	565
Acular LS Ophthalmic Solution	566

Lidocaine Hydrochloride (Electrolyte disturbances are a risk associated with this product; concurrent use in patients taking agents known to prolong QT interval requires caution).

No products indexed under this heading.

Lisinopril (Electrolyte disturbances are a risk associated with this product; concurrent use in patients taking agents known to disturb electrolyte balance requires caution). Products include:

Prinivil Tablets	2052
Prinzide Tablets	2056

Lithium (Electrolyte disturbances are a risk associated with this product; concurrent use in patients taking agents known to disturb electrolyte balance requires caution).

No products indexed under this heading.

Lithium Carbonate (Electrolyte disturbances are a risk associated with this product; concurrent use in patients taking agents known to disturb electrolyte balance requires caution). Products include:

Lithobid Tablets 1692

Lithium Citrate (Electrolyte disturbances are a risk associated with this product; concurrent use in patients taking agents known to disturb electrolyte balance requires caution).

No products indexed under this heading.

Losartan Potassium (Electrolyte disturbances are a risk associated with this product; concurrent use in patients taking agents known to disturb electrolyte balance requires caution). Products include:

Cozaar Tablets	1935
Hyzaar 50-12.5 Tablets	1990
Hyzaar 100-12.5 Tablets	1990
Hyzaar 100-25 Tablets	1990

Magaldrate (Concurrent use within one hour should be avoided).

No products indexed under this heading.

Magnesium Hydroxide (Concurrent use within one hour should be avoided). Products include:

Maalox Regular Strength Antacid/Antigas Liquid.................	2175
Maalox Max Maximum Strength Antacid/Anti-Gas Liquid...............	2176
Pepcid Complete Chewable Tablets.....................................	1701

Magnesium Oxide (Concurrent use within one hour should be avoided). Products include:

Beelith Tablets	759
PremCal Light, Regular, and Extra Strength Tablets................	▣818

Maprotiline Hydrochloride (Electrolyte disturbances are a risk associated with this product; concurrent use in patients taking agents known to prolong QT interval requires caution).

No products indexed under this heading.

Meclofenamate Sodium (Electrolyte disturbances are a risk associated with this product; concurrent use in patients taking agents known to disturb electrolyte balance requires caution).

No products indexed under this heading.

Mefenamic Acid (Electrolyte disturbances are a risk associated with this product; concurrent use in patients taking agents known to disturb electrolyte balance requires caution).

No products indexed under this heading.

Meloxicam (Electrolyte disturbances are a risk associated with this product; concurrent use in patients taking agents known to disturb electrolyte balance requires caution). Products include:

Mobic Oral Suspension	863
Mobic Tablets	863

Mesoridazine Besylate (Electrolyte disturbances are a risk associated with this product; concurrent use in patients taking agents known to prolong QT interval requires caution).

No products indexed under this heading.

Methyclothiazide (Electrolyte disturbances are a risk associated with this product; concurrent use in patients taking agents known to disturb electrolyte balance requires caution).

No products indexed under this heading.

Metolazone (Electrolyte disturbances are a risk associated with this product; concurrent use in patients taking agents known to disturb electrolyte balance requires caution).

No products indexed under this heading.

Mexiletine Hydrochloride (Electrolyte disturbances are a risk associated with this product; concurrent use in patients taking agents known to prolong QT interval requires caution).

No products indexed under this heading.

Moexipril Hydrochloride (Electrolyte disturbances are a risk associated with this product; concurrent use in patients taking agents known to disturb electrolyte balance requires caution). Products include:

Uniretic Tablets	3100
Univasc Tablets	3104

Nabumetone (Electrolyte disturbances are a risk associated with this product; concurrent use in patients taking agents known to disturb electrolyte balance requires caution).

No products indexed under this heading.

Naproxen (Electrolyte disturbances are a risk associated with this product; concurrent use in patients taking agents known to disturb electrolyte balance requires caution). Products include:

EC-Naprosyn Delayed-Release Tablets.....................................	2761
Naprosyn Suspension	2761
Naprosyn Tablets	2761

Prevacid NapraPAC 3280

Naproxen Sodium (Electrolyte disturbances are a risk associated with this product; concurrent use in patients taking agents known to disturb electrolyte balance requires caution). Products include:

Aleve Caplets 742
Aleve Gelcaps 743
Aleve Tablets 743
Aleve Cold & Sinus Caplets 744
Anaprox Tablets 2761
Anaprox DS Tablets 2761

Nortriptyline Hydrochloride (Electrolyte disturbances are a risk associated with this product; concurrent use in patients taking agents known to prolong QT interval requires caution).

No products indexed under this heading.

Oral Medications, unspecified (During the intake of sodium phosphate, the absorption of drugs from the gastrointestinal tract may be delayed or even completely prevented).

No products indexed under this heading.

Oxaprozin (Electrolyte disturbances are a risk associated with this product; concurrent use in patients taking agents known to disturb electrolyte balance requires caution).

No products indexed under this heading.

Perindopril Erbumine (Electrolyte disturbances are a risk associated with this product; concurrent use in patients taking agents known to disturb electrolyte balance requires caution). Products include:

Aceon Tablets (2 mg, 4 mg, 8 mg) 3194

Perphenazine (Electrolyte disturbances are a risk associated with this product; concurrent use in patients taking agents known to prolong QT interval requires caution).

No products indexed under this heading.

Phenylbutazone (Electrolyte disturbances are a risk associated with this product; concurrent use in patients taking agents known to disturb electrolyte balance requires caution).

No products indexed under this heading.

Piroxicam (Electrolyte disturbances are a risk associated with this product; concurrent use in patients taking agents known to disturb electrolyte balance requires caution).

No products indexed under this heading.

Polythiazide (Electrolyte disturbances are a risk associated with this product; concurrent use in patients taking agents known to disturb electrolyte balance requires caution).

No products indexed under this heading.

Procainamide Hydrochloride (Electrolyte disturbances are a risk associated with this product; concurrent use in patients taking agents known to prolong QT interval requires caution).

No products indexed under this heading.

Prochlorperazine (Electrolyte disturbances are a risk associated with this product; concurrent use in patients taking agents known to prolong QT interval requires caution).

No products indexed under this heading.

Promethazine Hydrochloride (Electrolyte disturbances are a risk associated with this product; concurrent use in patients taking agents known to prolong QT interval requires caution). Products include:

Phenergan Tablets and Suppositories 3440

Propafenone Hydrochloride (Electrolyte disturbances are a risk associated with this product; concurrent use in patients taking agents known to prolong QT interval requires caution). Products include:

Rythmol SR Capsules 2727

Protriptyline Hydrochloride (Electrolyte disturbances are a risk associated with this product; concurrent use in patients taking agents known to prolong QT interval requires caution).

No products indexed under this heading.

Quinapril Hydrochloride (Electrolyte disturbances are a risk associated with this product; concurrent use in patients taking agents known to disturb electrolyte balance requires caution).

No products indexed under this heading.

Quinidine Gluconate (Electrolyte disturbances are a risk associated with this product; concurrent use in patients taking agents known to prolong QT interval requires caution).

No products indexed under this heading.

Quinidine Polygalacturonate (Electrolyte disturbances are a risk associated with this product; concurrent use in patients taking agents known to prolong QT interval requires caution).

No products indexed under this heading.

Quinidine Sulfate (Electrolyte disturbances are a risk associated with this product; concurrent use in patients taking agents known to prolong QT interval requires caution).

No products indexed under this heading.

Ramipril (Electrolyte disturbances are a risk associated with this product; concurrent use in patients taking agents known to disturb electrolyte balance requires caution). Products include:

Altace Capsules 1702

Rofecoxib (Electrolyte disturbances are a risk associated with this product; concurrent use in patients taking agents known to disturb electrolyte balance requires caution).

No products indexed under this heading.

Sodium Bicarbonate (Concurrent use within one hour should be avoided). Products include:

Colyte with Flavor Packs for Oral Solution 3088
HalfLytely and Bisacodyl Tablets Bowel Prep Kit with Flavors Packs 881
TriLyte with Flavor Packs for Oral Solution 3100

Spirapril Hydrochloride (Electrolyte disturbances are a risk associated with this product; concurrent use in patients taking agents known to disturb electrolyte balance requires caution).

No products indexed under this heading.

Spironolactone (Electrolyte disturbances are a risk associated with this product; concurrent use in patients taking agents known to disturb electrolyte balance requires caution).

No products indexed under this heading.

Sulindac (Electrolyte disturbances are a risk associated with this product; concurrent use in patients taking agents known to disturb electrolyte balance requires caution). Products include:

Clinoril Tablets 1924

Telmisartan (Electrolyte disturbances are a risk associated with this product; concurrent use in patients taking agents known to disturb electrolyte balance requires caution). Products include:

Micardis Tablets 854
Micardis HCT Tablets 856

Thioridazine Hydrochloride (Electrolyte disturbances are a risk associated with this product; concurrent use in patients taking agents known to prolong QT interval requires caution). Products include:

Thioridazine Hydrochloride Tablets 2163

Tocainide Hydrochloride (Electrolyte disturbances are a risk associated with this product; concurrent use in patients taking agents known to prolong QT interval requires caution).

No products indexed under this heading.

Tolmetin Sodium (Electrolyte disturbances are a risk associated with this product; concurrent use in patients taking agents known to disturb electrolyte balance requires caution).

No products indexed under this heading.

Torsemide (Electrolyte disturbances are a risk associated with this product; concurrent use in patients taking agents known to disturb electrolyte balance requires caution). Products include:

Demadex Injection 2759
Demadex Tablets 2759

Trandolapril (Electrolyte disturbances are a risk associated with this product; concurrent use in patients taking agents known to disturb electrolyte balance requires caution). Products include:

Mavik Tablets 486
Tarka Tablets 524

Triamterene (Electrolyte disturbances are a risk associated with this product; concurrent use in patients taking agents known to disturb electrolyte balance requires caution). Products include:

Dyazide Capsules 1423
Dyrenium Capsules 3400

Trifluoperazine Hydrochloride (Electrolyte disturbances are a risk associated with this product; concurrent use in patients taking agents known to prolong QT interval requires caution).

No products indexed under this heading.

Trimipramine Maleate (Electrolyte disturbances are a risk associated with this product; concurrent use in patients taking agents known to prolong QT interval requires caution).

No products indexed under this heading.

Valdecoxib (Electrolyte disturbances are a risk associated with this product; concurrent use in patients taking agents known to disturb electrolyte balance requires caution).

No products indexed under this heading.

Valsartan (Electrolyte disturbances are a risk associated with this product; concurrent use in patients taking agents known to disturb electrolyte balance requires caution). Products include:

Diovan Tablets 2193
Diovan HCT Tablets 2196

Ziprasidone Hydrochloride (Electrolyte disturbances are a risk associated with this product; concurrent use in patients taking agents known to prolong QT interval requires caution). Products include:

Geodon Capsules 2529

Food Interactions

Dairy products (Concurrent use within one hour should be avoided).

FLEXBUMIN I.V.

(Albumin (human)) 720
None cited in PDR database.

FLINTSTONES COMPLETE WITH CHOLINE TABLETS

(Vitamins with Minerals) 813
None cited in PDR database.

FLINTSTONES GUMMIES

(Vitamins, Multiple) 813
None cited in PDR database.

FLOMAX CAPSULES

(Tamsulosin Hydrochloride) 850
May interact with alpha adrenergic blockers and certain other agents. Compounds in these categories include:

Cimetidine (Co-administration with highest recommended dose of cimetidine has resulted in a significant decrease (26%) in the clearance of tamsulosin which resulted in a moderate increase in tamsulosin AUC (44%)). Products include:

Tagamet HB 200 Tablets 664

Cimetidine Hydrochloride (Co-administration with highest recommended dose of cimetidine has resulted in a significant decrease (26%) in the clearance of tamsulosin which resulted in a moderate increase in tamsulosin AUC (44%)).

No products indexed under this heading.

Doxazosin Mesylate (The pharmacokinetic and pharmacodynamic interactions between tamsulosin and other alpha-adrenergic blockers have not been determined, however, interactions may be expected and co-administration should be avoided). Products include:

Cardura XL Tablets 2515

Furosemide (Co-administration produces an 11% to 12% reduction in tamsulosin Cmax and AUC; these changes are expected to be clinically insignificant). Products include:

Furosemide Tablets 2154

Prazosin Hydrochloride (The pharmacokinetic and pharmacodynamic interactions between tamsulosin and other alpha-adrenergic blockers have not been determined, however, interactions may be expected and co-administration should be avoided).

No products indexed under this heading.

Terazosin Hydrochloride (The pharmacokinetic and pharmacodynamic interactions between tamsulosin and other alpha-adrenergic blockers have not been determined, however, interactions may be expected and co-administration should be avoided). Products include:

Hytrin Capsules 471

Warfarin Sodium (Results from *in vitro* and *in vivo* interaction studies are inconclusive, therefore, caution should be exercised with concomitant use). Products include:

Coumadin for Injection 898
Coumadin Tablets 898

Food Interactions

Food, unspecified (Tmax is reached by 4 to 5 hours under fasting conditions and by 6 to 7 hours when tamsulosin is administered with food; taking tamsulosin under fasted conditions results in a 30% increase in AUC and 40% to 70% increase in Cmax compared to fed conditions; Flomax should be taken approximately 30 minutes following the meal).

FLONASE NASAL SPRAY

(Fluticasone Propionate) 1440

May interact with cytochrome p450 3a4 inhibitors (selected) and certain other agents. Compounds in these categories include:

Acetazolamide (Caution should be exercised when potent cytochrome P450 3A4 inhibitors are co-administered with fluticasone propionate).

No products indexed under this heading.

Amiodarone Hydrochloride (Caution should be exercised when potent cytochrome P450 3A4 inhibitors are co-administered with fluticasone propionate).

No products indexed under this heading.

Amprenavir (Caution should be exercised when potent cytochrome P450 3A4 inhibitors are co-administered with fluticasone propionate). Products include:

Agenerase Capsules 1327
Agenerase Oral Solution 1332

Anastrozole (Caution should be exercised when potent cytochrome P450 3A4 inhibitors are co-administered with fluticasone propionate). Products include:

Arimidex Tablets 673

Aprepitant (Caution should be exercised when potent cytochrome P450 3A4 inhibitors are co-administered with fluticasone propionate). Products include:

Emend Capsules 1963

Cimetidine (Caution should be exercised when potent cytochrome P450 3A4 inhibitors are co-administered with fluticasone propionate). Products include:

Tagamet HB 200 Tablets .... ■664

Cimetidine Hydrochloride (Caution should be exercised when potent cytochrome P450 3A4 inhibitors are co-administered with fluticasone propionate).

No products indexed under this heading.

Ciprofloxacin (Caution should be exercised when potent cytochrome P450 3A4 inhibitors are co-administered with fluticasone propionate). Products include:

Cipro Oral Suspension 2977
Cipro I.V. 2984
Cipro XR Tablets 2990
Ciprodex Otic Suspension 559

Clarithromycin (Caution should be exercised when potent cytochrome P450 3A4 inhibitors are co-administered with fluticasone propionate). Products include:

Biaxin/Biaxin XL 402
PREVPAC 3284

Clotrimazole (Caution should be exercised when potent cytochrome P450 3A4 inhibitors are co-administered with fluticasone propionate). Products include:

Desenex Athlete's Foot Cream .... ■635
Lotrimin 3039
Lotrisone 3040

Cyclosporine (Caution should be exercised when potent cytochrome P450 3A4 inhibitors are co-administered with fluticasone propionate). Products include:

Gengraf Capsules 459
Neoral Oral Solution 2259
Neoral Soft Gelatin Capsules 2259
Restasis Ophthalmic Emulsion 575
Sandimmune 2275

Dalfopristin (Caution should be exercised when potent cytochrome P450 3A4 inhibitors are co-administered with fluticasone propionate).

No products indexed under this heading.

Danazol (Caution should be exercised when potent cytochrome P450 3A4 inhibitors are co-administered with fluticasone propionate).

No products indexed under this heading.

Delavirdine Mesylate (Caution should be exercised when potent cytochrome P450 3A4 inhibitors are co-administered with fluticasone propionate). Products include:

Rescriptor Tablets 2551

Diltiazem Hydrochloride (Caution should be exercised when potent cytochrome P450 3A4 inhibitors are co-administered with fluticasone propionate). Products include:

Cardizem LA Extended Release Tablets 1728
Tiazac Capsules 1201

Diltiazem Maleate (Caution should be exercised when potent cytochrome P450 3A4 inhibitors are co-administered with fluticasone propionate).

No products indexed under this heading.

Efavirenz (Caution should be exercised when potent cytochrome P450 3A4 inhibitors are co-administered with fluticasone propionate). Products include:

Atripla Tablets 945
Sustiva Capsules 930
Sustiva Tablets 930

Erythromycin (Caution should be exercised when potent cytochrome P450 3A4 inhibitors are co-administered with fluticasone propionate). Products include:

Ery-Tab Tablets 449
Erythromycin Base Filmtab Tablets 455
Erythromycin Delayed-Release Capsules, USP 457
PCE Dispertab Tablets 515

Erythromycin Estolate (Caution should be exercised when potent cytochrome P450 3A4 inhibitors are co-administered with fluticasone propionate).

No products indexed under this heading.

Erythromycin Ethylsuccinate (Caution should be exercised when potent cytochrome P450 3A4 inhibitors are co-administered with fluticasone propionate). Products include:

E.E.S. 451
EryPed 447

Erythromycin Gluceptate (Caution should be exercised when potent cytochrome P450 3A4 inhibitors are co-administered with fluticasone propionate).

No products indexed under this heading.

Erythromycin Lactobionate (Caution should be exercised when potent cytochrome P450 3A4 inhibitors are co-administered with fluticasone propionate).

No products indexed under this heading.

Erythromycin Stearate (Caution should be exercised when potent cytochrome P450 3A4 inhibitors are co-administered with fluticasone propionate). Products include:

Erythrocin Stearate Filmtab Tablets 453

Esomeprazole Magnesium (Caution should be exercised when potent cytochrome P450 3A4 inhibitors are co-administered with fluticasone propionate). Products include:

Nexium Delayed-Release Capsules 655

Fluconazole (Caution should be exercised when potent cytochrome P450 3A4 inhibitors are co-administered with fluticasone propionate).

No products indexed under this heading.

Fluoxetine Hydrochloride (Caution should be exercised when potent cytochrome P450 3A4 inhibitors are co-administered with fluticasone propionate). Products include:

Prozac Pulvules and Liquid 1801
Symbyax Capsules 1819

Fluvoxamine Maleate (Caution should be exercised when potent cytochrome P450 3A4 inhibitors are co-administered with fluticasone propionate).

No products indexed under this heading.

Fosamprenavir Calcium (Caution should be exercised when potent cytochrome P450 3A4 inhibitors are co-administered with fluticasone propionate). Products include:

Lexiva Tablets 1505

Indinavir Sulfate (Caution should be exercised when potent cytochrome P450 3A4 inhibitors are co-administered with fluticasone propionate). Products include:

Crixivan Capsules 1940

Isoniazid (Caution should be exercised when potent cytochrome P450 3A4 inhibitors are co-administered with fluticasone propionate).

No products indexed under this heading.

Itraconazole (Caution should be exercised when potent cytochrome P450 3A4 inhibitors are co-administered with fluticasone propionate).

No products indexed under this heading.

Ketoconazole (Fluticasone propionate is a substrate of cytochrome P450 3A4. Co-administration with ketoconazole resulted in increased plasma fluticasone propionate exposure, a reduction in plasma cortisol AUC, and no effect on urinary excretion of cortisol. Caution should be exercised when potent cytochrome P450 3A inhibitors are co-administered with fluticasone propionate). Products include:

Nizoral A-D Shampoo, 1% 1868

Lopinavir (Caution should be exercised when potent cytochrome P450 3A4 inhibitors are co-administered with fluticasone propionate). Products include:

Kaletra 476

Loratadine (Caution should be exercised when potent cytochrome P450 3A4 inhibitors are co-administered with fluticasone propionate). Products include:

Alavert Allergy & Sinus D-12 Hour Tablets .... ■771
Alavert .... ■771
Children's Claritin Allergy Oral Solution .... ■771
Claritin Non-Drowsy 24 Hour Tablets .... ■772
Claritin Reditabs 24 Hour Non-Drowsy Tablets .... ■772
Claritin-D Non-Drowsy 12 Hour Tablets .... ■772
Claritin-D Non-Drowsy 24 Hour Tablets .... ■772

Metronidazole (Caution should be exercised when potent cytochrome P450 3A4 inhibitors are co-administered with fluticasone propionate). Products include:

Metrogel 1% 1211
MetroGel-Vaginal Gel 1855
Vandazole Vaginal Gel 3338

Metronidazole Benzoate (Caution should be exercised when potent cytochrome P450 3A4 inhibitors are co-administered with fluticasone propionate).

No products indexed under this heading.

Metronidazole Hydrochloride (Caution should be exercised when potent cytochrome P450 3A4 inhibitors are co-administered with fluticasone propionate).

No products indexed under this heading.

Miconazole (Caution should be exercised when potent cytochrome P450 3A4 inhibitors are co-administered with fluticasone propionate).

No products indexed under this heading.

Miconazole Nitrate (Caution should be exercised when potent cytochrome P450 3A4 inhibitors are co-administered with fluticasone propionate). Products include:

Desenex .... ■635
Desenex Jock Itch Spray Powder .... ■635

Nefazodone Hydrochloride (Caution should be exercised when potent cytochrome P450 3A4 inhibitors are co-administered with fluticasone propionate).

No products indexed under this heading.

Nelfinavir Mesylate (Caution should be exercised when potent cytochrome P450 3A4 inhibitors are co-administered with fluticasone propionate). Products include:

Viracept **2577**

Nevirapine (Caution should be exercised when potent cytochrome P450 3A4 inhibitors are co-administered with fluticasone propionate). Products include:

Viramune Oral Suspension **873**
Viramune Tablets **873**

Niacinamide (Caution should be exercised when potent cytochrome P450 3A4 inhibitors are co-administered with fluticasone propionate).

No products indexed under this heading.

Nicotinamide (Caution should be exercised when potent cytochrome P450 3A4 inhibitors are co-administered with fluticasone propionate). Products include:

Nicomide Tablets **1088**

Nifedipine (Caution should be exercised when potent cytochrome P450 3A4 inhibitors are co-administered with fluticasone propionate). Products include:

Adalat CC Tablets **2964**

Norfloxacin (Caution should be exercised when potent cytochrome P450 3A4 inhibitors are co-administered with fluticasone propionate). Products include:

Noroxin Tablets **2032**

Omeprazole (Caution should be exercised when potent cytochrome P450 3A4 inhibitors are co-administered with fluticasone propionate). Products include:

Zegerid Capsules **2958**
Zegerid Powder for Oral Solution **2958**

Paroxetine Hydrochloride (Caution should be exercised when potent cytochrome P450 3A4 inhibitors are co-administered with fluticasone propionate). Products include:

Paxil CR Controlled-Release Tablets **1538**
Paxil **1530**

Propoxyphene Hydrochloride (Caution should be exercised when potent cytochrome P450 3A4 inhibitors are co-administered with fluticasone propionate).

No products indexed under this heading.

Propoxyphene Napsylate (Caution should be exercised when potent cytochrome P450 3A4 inhibitors are co-administered with fluticasone propionate).

No products indexed under this heading.

Quinidine (Caution should be exercised when potent cytochrome P450 3A4 inhibitors are co-administered with fluticasone propionate).

No products indexed under this heading.

Quinidine Hydrochloride (Caution should be exercised when potent cytochrome P450 3A4 inhibitors are co-administered with fluticasone propionate).

No products indexed under this heading.

Quinidine Polygalacturonate (Caution should be exercised when potent cytochrome P450 3A4 inhibitors are co-administered with fluticasone propionate).

No products indexed under this heading.

Quinidine Sulfate (Caution should be exercised when potent cytochrome P450 3A4 inhibitors are co-administered with fluticasone propionate).

No products indexed under this heading.

Quinine (Caution should be exercised when potent cytochrome P450 3A4 inhibitors are co-administered with fluticasone propionate).

No products indexed under this heading.

Quinine Sulfate (Caution should be exercised when potent cytochrome P450 3A4 inhibitors are co-administered with fluticasone propionate).

No products indexed under this heading.

Quinupristin (Caution should be exercised when potent cytochrome P450 3A4 inhibitors are co-administered with fluticasone propionate).

No products indexed under this heading.

Ranitidine Bismuth Citrate (Caution should be exercised when potent cytochrome P450 3A4 inhibitors are co-administered with fluticasone propionate).

No products indexed under this heading.

Ranitidine Hydrochloride (Caution should be exercised when potent cytochrome P450 3A4 inhibitors are co-administered with fluticasone propionate). Products include:

Zantac **1624**
Zantac Injection **1619**
Zantac Injection Pharmacy Bulk Package **1622**

Ritonavir (Fluticasone propionate is a substrate of cytochrome P450 3A4. A drug interaction study has shown that ritonavir (a highly potent cytochrome P450 3A4 inhibitor) can significantly increase plasma fluticasone propionate exposure, resulting in significantly reduced serum cortisol concentrations. Therefore, co-administration of fluticasone propionate and ritonavir is not recommended unless the potential benefit to the patient outweighs the risk of systemic corticosteroid side effects). Products include:

Kaletra **476**
Norvir **503**

Saquinavir (Caution should be exercised when potent cytochrome P450 3A4 inhibitors are co-administered with fluticasone propionate).

No products indexed under this heading.

Saquinavir Mesylate (Caution should be exercised when potent cytochrome P450 3A4 inhibitors are co-administered with fluticasone propionate). Products include:

Invirase **2772**

Sertraline Hydrochloride (Caution should be exercised when potent cytochrome P450 3A4 inhibitors are co-administered with fluticasone propionate). Products include:

Zoloft **2586**

Telithromycin (Caution should be exercised when potent cytochrome P450 3A4 inhibitors are co-administered with fluticasone propionate). Products include:

Ketek Tablets **2903**

Troglitazone (Caution should be exercised when potent cytochrome P450 3A4 inhibitors are co-administered with fluticasone propionate).

No products indexed under this heading.

Troleandomycin (Caution should be exercised when potent cytochrome P450 3A4 inhibitors are co-administered with fluticasone propionate).

No products indexed under this heading.

Valproate Sodium (Caution should be exercised when potent cytochrome P450 3A4 inhibitors are co-administered with fluticasone propionate). Products include:

Depacon Injection **412**

Verapamil Hydrochloride (Caution should be exercised when potent cytochrome P450 3A4 inhibitors are co-administered with fluticasone propionate). Products include:

Covera-HS Tablets **3139**
Tarka Tablets **524**
Verelan PM Extended-Release Capsules, Controlled-Onset **3106**

Voriconazole (Caution should be exercised when potent cytochrome P450 3A4 inhibitors are co-administered with fluticasone propionate). Products include:

VFEND I.V. **2564**
VFEND Oral Suspension **2564**
VFEND Tablets **2564**

Zafirlukast (Caution should be exercised when potent cytochrome P450 3A4 inhibitors are co-administered with fluticasone propionate). Products include:

Accolate Tablets **671**

Zileuton (Caution should be exercised when potent cytochrome P450 3A4 inhibitors are co-administered with fluticasone propionate). Products include:

Zyflo Tablets **1023**

Food Interactions

Grapefruit (Caution should be exercised when potent cytochrome P450 3A4 inhibitors are co-administered with fluticasone propionate).

Grapefruit Juice (Caution should be exercised when potent cytochrome P450 3A4 inhibitors are co-administered with fluticasone propionate).

FLOVENT DISKUS 50 MCG

(Fluticasone Propionate) **1443**

May interact with cytochrome p450 3a4 inhibitors, potent and certain other agents. Compounds in these categories include:

Amprenavir (Caution should be exercised when potent cytochrome P450 3A4 inhibitors are co-administered with fluticasone. Interactions with ritonavir and ketoconazole, both potent CYP3A4 inhibitors, have resulted in increased fluticasone exposure). Products include:

Agenerase Capsules **1327**
Agenerase Oral Solution **1332**

Atazanavir (Caution should be exercised when potent cytochrome P450 3A4 inhibitors are co-administered with fluticasone. Interactions with ritonavir and ketoconazole, both potent CYP3A4 inhibitors, have resulted in increased fluticasone exposure).

No products indexed under this heading.

Atazanavir sulfate (Caution should be exercised when potent cytochrome P450 3A4 inhibitors are co-administered with fluticasone. Interactions with ritonavir and ketoconazole, both potent CYP3A4 inhibitors, have resulted in increased fluticasone exposure). Products include:

Reyataz Capsules **921**

Clarithromycin (Caution should be exercised when potent cytochrome P450 3A4 inhibitors are co-administered with fluticasone. Interactions with ritonavir and ketoconazole, both potent CYP3A4 inhibitors, have resulted in increased fluticasone exposure). Products include:

Biaxin/Biaxin XL **402**
PREVPAC **3284**

Fosamprenavir Calcium (Caution should be exercised when potent cytochrome P450 3A4 inhibitors are co-administered with fluticasone. Interactions with ritonavir and ketoconazole, both potent CYP3A4 inhibitors, have resulted in increased fluticasone exposure). Products include:

Lexiva Tablets **1505**

Indinavir Sulfate (Caution should be exercised when potent cytochrome P450 3A4 inhibitors are co-administered with fluticasone. Interactions with ritonavir and ketoconazole, both potent CYP3A4 inhibitors, have resulted in increased fluticasone exposure). Products include:

Crixivan Capsules **1940**

Itraconazole (Caution should be exercised when potent cytochrome P450 3A4 inhibitors are co-administered with fluticasone. Interactions with ritonavir and ketoconazole, both potent CYP3A4 inhibitors, have resulted in increased fluticasone exposure).

No products indexed under this heading.

Ketoconazole (Co-administration of a single dose of fluticasone (1000 mcg) with multiple doses of ketoconazole (200 mg) to steady state has resulted in increased mean fluticasone concentrations, a reduction in plasma cortisol AUC, and no effect on urinary excretion ofcortisol). Products include:

Nizoral A-D Shampoo, 1% **1868**

Lopinavir (Caution should be exercised when potent cytochrome P450 3A4 inhibitors are co-administered with fluticasone. Interactions with ritonavir and ketoconazole, both potent CYP3A4 inhibitors, have resulted in increased fluticasone exposure). Products include:

Kaletra **476**

Nefazodone Hydrochloride (Caution should be exercised when potent cytochrome P450 3A4 inhibitors are co-administered with fluticasone. Interactions with ritonavir and ketoconazole, both potent CYP3A4 inhibitors, have resulted in increased fluticasone exposure).

No products indexed under this heading.

Nelfinavir Mesylate (Caution should be exercised when potent cytochrome P450 3A4 inhibitors are co-administered with fluticasone. Interactions with ritonavir and ketoconazole, both potent CYP3A4 inhibitors, have resulted in increased fluticasone exposure). Products include:

Viracept **2577**

Ritonavir (Ritonavir can significantly increase plasma fluticasone expo-

IMPORTANT NOTE: Always consult each drug listing in the patient's regimen for possible interactions.

sure, resulting in significantly reduced serum cortisol concentrations. Cushing syndrome and adrenal suppression have been reported; therefore, co-administration is not recommended unless the potential benefit outweighs the risks).
Products include:
Kaletra **476**
Norvir **503**

Saquinavir (Caution should be exercised when potent cytochrome P450 3A4 inhibitors are co-administered with fluticasone. Interactions with ritonavir and ketoconazole, both potent CYP3A4 inhibitors, have resulted in increased fluticasone exposure).
No products indexed under this heading.

Saquinavir Mesylate (Caution should be exercised when potent cytochrome P450 3A4 inhibitors are co-administered with fluticasone. Interactions with ritonavir and ketoconazole, both potent CYP3A4 inhibitors, have resulted in increased fluticasone exposure). Products include:
Invirase **2772**

Telithromycin (Caution should be exercised when potent cytochrome P450 3A4 inhibitors are co-administered with fluticasone. Interactions with ritonavir and ketoconazole, both potent CYP3A4 inhibitors, have resulted in increased fluticasone exposure). Products include:
Ketek Tablets **2903**

Troleandomycin (Caution should be exercised when potent cytochrome P450 3A4 inhibitors are co-administered with fluticasone. Interactions with ritonavir and ketoconazole, both potent CYP3A4 inhibitors, have resulted in increased fluticasone exposure).
No products indexed under this heading.

Voriconazole (Caution should be exercised when potent cytochrome P450 3A4 inhibitors are co-administered with fluticasone. Interactions with ritonavir and ketoconazole, both potent CYP3A4 inhibitors, have resulted in increased fluticasone exposure). Products include:
VFEND I.V. **2564**
VFEND Oral Suspension **2564**
VFEND Tablets **2564**

FLOVENT DISKUS 100 MCG

(Fluticasone Propionate) **1443**
See Flovent Diskus 50 mcg

FLOVENT DISKUS 250 MCG

(Fluticasone Propionate) **1443**
See Flovent Diskus 50 mcg

FLOVENT HFA 44 MCG INHALATION AEROSOL

(Fluticasone Propionate HFA) **1447**
May interact with:

Ketoconazole (Co-administration of a single dose of fluticasone (1000 mcg) with multiple doses of ketoconazole (200 mg) to steady state has resulted in increased mean plasma fluticasone exposure, a reduction in plasma cortisol AUC, and no effect on urinary excretion of cortisol). Products include:
Nizoral A-D Shampoo, 1% **1868**

Ritonavir (Ritonavir can significantly increase plasma fluticasone exposure, resulting in significantly reduced serum cortisol concentrations. Cushing syndrome and adrenal suppression have been reported; therefore, co-administration is not recommended unless the potential benefit outweighs the risks).
Products include:
Kaletra **476**
Norvir **503**

FLOVENT HFA 110 MCG INHALATION AEROSOL

(Fluticasone Propionate HFA) **1447**
See Flovent HFA 44 mcg Inhalation Aerosol

FLOVENT HFA 220 MCG INHALATION AEROSOL

(Fluticasone Propionate HFA) **1447**
See Flovent HFA 44 mcg Inhalation Aerosol

FLOXIN OTIC SOLUTION

(Ofloxacin) **1049**
None cited in PDR database.

FLUARIX

(Influenza Virus Vaccine) **1451**
May interact with alkylating agents, antimetabolites, corticosteroids, cytotoxic drugs, phenytoin, theophyllines, and certain other agents. Compounds in these categories include:

Betamethasone Acetate (Immunosuppressive therapies, corticosteroids (used in greater than physiologic doses), may reduce the immune response to vaccines).
No products indexed under this heading.

Betamethasone Sodium Phosphate (Immunosuppressive therapies, corticosteroids (used in greater than physiologic doses), may reduce the immune response to vaccines).
No products indexed under this heading.

Bleomycin Sulfate (Immunosuppressive therapies, cytotoxic drugs, may reduce the immune response to vaccines).
No products indexed under this heading.

Busulfan (Immunosuppressive therapies, alkylating agents, may reduce the immune response to vaccines).
Products include:
I.V. Busulfex **2493**
Myleran Tablets **1525**

Capecitabine (Immunosuppressive therapies, antimetabolites, may reduce the immune response to vaccines). Products include:
Xeloda Tablets **2822**

Carmustine (BCNU) (Immunosuppressive therapies, alkylating agents, may reduce the immune response to vaccines).
No products indexed under this heading.

Chlorambucil (Immunosuppressive therapies, alkylating agents, may reduce the immune response to vaccines). Products include:
Leukeran Tablets **1504**

Cladribine (Immunosuppressive therapies, antimetabolites, may reduce the immune response to vaccines). Products include:
Leustatin Injection **2357**

Cortisone Acetate (Immunosuppressive therapies, corticosteroids (used in greater than physiologic doses), may reduce the immune response to vaccines).
No products indexed under this heading.

Cyclophosphamide (Immunosuppressive therapies, alkylating agents, may reduce the immune response to vaccines).
No products indexed under this heading.

Cytarabine (Immunosuppressive therapies, antimetabolites, may reduce the immune response to vaccines).
No products indexed under this heading.

Dacarbazine (Immunosuppressive therapies, alkylating agents, may reduce the immune response to vaccines).
No products indexed under this heading.

Daunorubicin Hydrochloride (Immunosuppressive therapies, cytotoxic drugs, may reduce the immune response to vaccines).
No products indexed under this heading.

Dexamethasone (Immunosuppressive therapies, corticosteroids (used in greater than physiologic doses), may reduce the immune response to vaccines). Products include:
Ciprodex Otic Suspension **559**
Decadron Tablets **1951**
TobraDex Ophthalmic Ointment **562**
TobraDex Ophthalmic Suspension **563**

Dexamethasone Acetate (Immunosuppressive therapies, corticosteroids (used in greater than physiologic doses), may reduce the immune response to vaccines).
No products indexed under this heading.

Dexamethasone Sodium Phosphate (Immunosuppressive therapies, corticosteroids (used in greater than physiologic doses), may reduce the immune response to vaccines).
No products indexed under this heading.

Doxorubicin Hydrochloride (Immunosuppressive therapies, cytotoxic drugs, may reduce the immune response to vaccines).
No products indexed under this heading.

Epirubicin Hydrochloride (Immunosuppressive therapies, cytotoxic drugs, may reduce the immune response to vaccines).
No products indexed under this heading.

Floxuridine (Immunosuppressive therapies, antimetabolites, may reduce the immune response to vaccines).
No products indexed under this heading.

Fludarabine Phosphate (Immunosuppressive therapies, antimetabolites, may reduce the immune response to vaccines).
No products indexed under this heading.

Fludrocortisone Acetate (Immunosuppressive therapies, corticosteroids (used in greater than physiologic doses), may reduce the immune response to vaccines).
No products indexed under this heading.

Fluorouracil (Immunosuppressive therapies, antimetabolites, may reduce the immune response to vaccines). Products include:
Carac Cream, 0.5% **2879**
Efudex **3363**

Fosphenytoin Sodium (Although it has been reported that influenza vaccination may inhibit the clearance of phenytoin, controlled studies have yielded inconsistent results regarding pharmacokinetic interactions between influenza vaccine and phenytoin. Nevertheless, clinicians should consider the potential for an interaction when influenza vaccine is administered to persons receiving phenytoin).
No products indexed under this heading.

Gemcitabine Hydrochloride (Immunosuppressive therapies, antimetabolites, may reduce the immune response to vaccines).
Products include:
Gemzar for Injection **1771**

Hydrocortisone (Immunosuppressive therapies, corticosteroids (used in greater than physiologic doses), may reduce the immune response to vaccines). Products include:
Colocort Rectal Suspension, USP (Retention) 100 mg/60 mL **2476**
Hydrocortone Tablets **1989**
Preparation H Hydrocortisone Cream .... ▣ **646**

Hydrocortisone Acetate (Immunosuppressive therapies, corticosteroids (used in greater than physiologic doses), may reduce the immune response to vaccines). Products include:
Analpram-HC **1159**
Pramosone **1161**
ProctoFoam-HC **3099**

Hydrocortisone Sodium Phosphate (Immunosuppressive therapies, corticosteroids (used in greater than physiologic doses), may reduce the immune response to vaccines).
No products indexed under this heading.

Hydrocortisone Sodium Succinate (Immunosuppressive therapies, corticosteroids (used in greater than physiologic doses), may reduce the immune response to vaccines).
No products indexed under this heading.

Hydroxyurea (Immunosuppressive therapies, cytotoxic drugs, may reduce the immune response to vaccines).
No products indexed under this heading.

Lomustine (CCNU) (Immunosuppressive therapies, alkylating agents, may reduce the immune response to vaccines).
No products indexed under this heading.

Mechlorethamine Hydrochloride (Immunosuppressive therapies, alkylating agents, may reduce the immune response to vaccines).
Products include:
Mustargen for Injection **2468**

Melphalan (Immunosuppressive therapies, alkylating agents, may reduce the immune response to vaccines). Products include:
Alkeran Tablets **956**

Mercaptopurine (Immunosuppressive therapies, antimetabolites, may reduce the immune response to vaccines).
No products indexed under this heading.

Methotrexate (Immunosuppressive therapies, antimetabolites, may reduce the immune response to vaccines).
No products indexed under this heading.

Methotrexate Sodium (Immunosuppressive therapies, cytotoxic drugs, may reduce the immune response to vaccines).
No products indexed under this heading.

Methylprednisolone Acetate (Immunosuppressive therapies, corticosteroids (used in greater than physiologic doses), may reduce the immune response to vaccines). Products include:
Depo-Medrol Injectable Suspension 2617
Depo-Medrol Single-Dose Vial 2619

Methylprednisolone Sodium Succinate (Immunosuppressive therapies, corticosteroids (used in greater than physiologic doses), may reduce the immune response to vaccines).
No products indexed under this heading.

Mitotane (Immunosuppressive therapies, cytotoxic drugs, may reduce the immune response to vaccines).
No products indexed under this heading.

Mitoxantrone Hydrochloride (Immunosuppressive therapies, cytotoxic drugs, may reduce the immune response to vaccines).
No products indexed under this heading.

Pentostatin (Immunosuppressive therapies, antimetabolites, may reduce the immune response to vaccines). Products include:
Nipent for Injection 1863

Phenytoin (Although it has been reported that influenza vaccination may inhibit the clearance of phenytoin, controlled studies have yielded inconsistent results regarding pharmacokinetic interactions between influenza vaccine and phenytoin. Nevertheless, clinicians should consider the potential for an interaction when influenza vaccine is administered to persons receiving phenytoin).
No products indexed under this heading.

Phenytoin Sodium (Although it has been reported that influenza vaccination may inhibit the clearance of phenytoin, controlled studies have yielded inconsistent results regarding pharmacokinetic interactions between influenza vaccine and phenytoin. Nevertheless, clinicians should consider the potential for an interaction when influenza vaccine is administered to persons receiving phenytoin). Products include:
Phenytek Capsules 2160

Prednisolone Acetate (Immunosuppressive therapies, corticosteroids (used in greater than physiologic doses), may reduce the immune response to vaccines). Products include:
Blephamide Ophthalmic Ointment 568
Blephamide Ophthalmic Suspension................................. 569
Poly-Pred Ophthalmic Suspension.............................. ⊘ 233
Pred Forte Ophthalmic Suspension ⊘ 235
Pred Mild Ophthalmic Suspension ⊘ 238
Pred-G Ophthalmic Ointment ⊘ 237
Pred-G Ophthalmic Suspension ⊘ 236

Prednisolone Sodium Phosphate (Immunosuppressive therapies, corticosteroids (used in greater than physiologic doses), may reduce the immune response to vaccines).
No products indexed under this heading.

Prednisolone Tebutate (Immunosuppressive therapies, corticosteroids (used in greater than physiologic doses), may reduce the immune response to vaccines).
No products indexed under this heading.

Prednisone (Immunosuppressive therapies, corticosteroids (used in greater than physiologic doses), may reduce the immune response to vaccines).
No products indexed under this heading.

Procarbazine Hydrochloride (Immunosuppressive therapies, cytotoxic drugs, may reduce the immune response to vaccines). Products include:
Matulane Capsules 3191

Tamoxifen Citrate (Immunosuppressive therapies, cytotoxic drugs, may reduce the immune response to vaccines). Products include:
Soltamox Oral Solution 3527

Theophylline (Although it has been reported that influenza vaccination may inhibit the clearance of theophylline, controlled studies have yielded inconsistent results regarding pharmacokinetic interactions between influenza vaccine and theophylline. Nevertheless, clinicians should consider the potential for an interaction when influenza vaccine is administered to persons receiving theophylline).
No products indexed under this heading.

Theophylline Anhydrous (Although it has been reported that influenza vaccination may inhibit the clearance of theophylline, controlled studies have yielded inconsistent results regarding pharmacokinetic interactions between influenza vaccine and theophylline. Nevertheless, clinicians should consider the potential for an interaction when influenza vaccine is administered to persons receiving theophylline). Products include:
Uniphyl Tablets 2710

Theophylline Calcium Salicylate (Although it has been reported that influenza vaccination may inhibit the clearance of theophylline, controlled studies have yielded inconsistent results regarding pharmacokinetic interactions between influenza vaccine and theophylline. Nevertheless, clinicians should consider the potential for an interaction when influenza vaccine is administered to persons receiving theophylline).
No products indexed under this heading.

Theophylline Dihydroxypropyl (Glyceryl) (Although it has been reported that influenza vaccination may inhibit the clearance of theophylline, controlled studies have yielded inconsistent results regarding pharmacokinetic interactions between influenza vaccine and theophylline. Nevertheless, clinicians should consider the potential for an interaction when influenza vaccine is administered to persons receiving theophylline).
No products indexed under this heading.

Theophylline Ethylenediamine (Although it has been reported that influenza vaccination may inhibit the clearance of theophylline, controlled studies have yielded inconsistent results regarding pharmacokinetic interactions between influenza vaccine and theophylline. Nevertheless, clinicians should consider the potential for an interaction when influenza vaccine is administered to persons receiving theophylline).
No products indexed under this heading.

Theophylline Sodium Glycinate (Although it has been reported that influenza vaccination may inhibit the clearance of theophylline, controlled studies have yielded inconsistent results regarding pharmacokinetic interactions between influenza vaccine and theophylline. Nevertheless, clinicians should consider the potential for an interaction when influenza vaccine is administered to persons receiving theophylline).
No products indexed under this heading.

Thioguanine (Immunosuppressive therapies, antimetabolites, may reduce the immune response to vaccines). Products include:
Tabloid Tablets 1575

Thiotepa (Immunosuppressive therapies, alkylating agents, may reduce the immune response to vaccines).
No products indexed under this heading.

Triamcinolone (Immunosuppressive therapies, corticosteroids (used in greater than physiologic doses), may reduce the immune response to vaccines).
No products indexed under this heading.

Triamcinolone Acetonide (Immunosuppressive therapies, corticosteroids (used in greater than physiologic doses), may reduce the immune response to vaccines). Products include:
Azmacort Inhalation Aerosol 1726
Nasacort AQ Nasal Spray 2922

Triamcinolone Diacetate (Immunosuppressive therapies, corticosteroids (used in greater than physiologic doses), may reduce the immune response to vaccines).
No products indexed under this heading.

Triamcinolone Hexacetonide (Immunosuppressive therapies, corticosteroids (used in greater than physiologic doses), may reduce the immune response to vaccines).
No products indexed under this heading.

Vincristine Sulfate (Immunosuppressive therapies, cytotoxic drugs, may reduce the immune response to vaccines).
No products indexed under this heading.

Warfarin Sodium (Although it has been reported that influenza vaccination may inhibit the clearance of warfarin, controlled studies have yielded inconsistent results regarding pharmacokinetic interactions between influenza vaccine and warfarin. Nevertheless, clinicians should consider the potential for an interaction when influenza vaccine is administered to persons receiving warfarin). Products include:
Coumadin for Injection 898
Coumadin Tablets 898

FLUMADINE SYRUP
(Rimantadine Hydrochloride) 1183
See Flumadine Tablets

FLUMADINE TABLETS
(Rimantadine Hydrochloride) 1183
May interact with:

Acetaminophen (Coadministration reduces the peak concentration and AUC values for rimantadine). Products include:
Comtrex Maximum Strength Cold & Cough Day/Night Caplets - Day Formulation.................... ▣726
Comtrex Maximum Strength Cold & Cough Day/Night Caplets - Night Formulation................... ▣726
Comtrex Maximum Strength Non-Drowsy Cold & Cough Caplets ▣725
Comtrex Maximum Strength Day/Night Severe Cold & Sinus Caplets - Day Formulation ▣725
Comtrex Maximum Strength Day/Night Severe Cold & Sinus Caplets - Night Formulation........ ▣725
Contac Cold and Flu Maximum Strength Caplets................... ▣728
Contac Cold and Flu Day and Night Caplets (Day Formulation Only).................................. ▣727
Contac Cold and Flu Day and Night Caplets (Night Formulation Only)........................ ▣727
Contac Cold and Flu Non-Drowsy Caplets............................... ▣728
Excedrin Extra Strength Caplets/Tablets/Geltabs............. ▣684
Excedrin Migraine Caplets/Tablets/Geltabs............. ▣609
Excedrin PM Caplets/Tablets/Geltabs............. ▣610
Excedrin Sinus Headache Caplets/Tablets...................... ▣610
Excedrin Tension Headache Caplets/Tablets/Geltabs............. ▣611
Goody's Body Pain Formula Powder.............................. ▣684
Goody's Extra Strength Headache Powders................... ▣611
Goody's Extra Strength Pain Relief Tablets...................... ▣685
Goody's PM Powder for Pain with Sleeplessness...................... ▣612
Percocet Tablets 1131
Robitussin Cough, Cold & Flu Nighttime Liquid.................... ▣738
TheraFlu Cold & Sore Throat Hot Liquid............................... ▣741
TheraFlu Flu & Chest Congestion Hot Liquid........................ ▣741
TheraFlu Flu & Sore Throat Hot Liquid............................... ▣742
TheraFlu Daytime Severe Cold Hot Liquid........................ ▣742
TheraFlu Nighttime Severe Cold Hot Liquid........................ ▣740
TheraFlu Warming Relief Daytime Severe Cold....................... ▣743
TheraFlu Warming Relief Nighttime Severe Cold............... ▣743
Triaminic Cough & Sore Throat Liquid............................... ▣747
Regular Strength Tylenol Tablets 1870
Children's Tylenol with Flavor Creator.............................. ▣679
Children's Tylenol Plus Flu Oral Suspension........................ ▣749
Tylenol Cold Head Congestion Daytime Caplets with Cool Burst and Gelcaps............... ▣750
Tylenol Cold Multi-Symptom Daytime Liquid................... ▣752
Tylenol Cold Multi-Symptom Severe Daytime Liquid ▣752
Tylenol 8 Hour Extended Release Caplets............................... 1870
Tylenol .. 1870

Extra Strength Tylenol PM Caplets, Vanilla Caplets, Geltabs, Gelcaps and Liquid.......... 1875
Extra Strength Tylenol Rapid Release Gels.............................. 1870
Concentrated Tylenol Infants' Drops Plus Cold & Cough............ ▣ 754
Tylenol with Codeine Tablets............ 2391
Tylenol Allergy Multi-Symptom Caplets with Cool Burst and Gelcaps.............................. 1872
Tylenol Allergy Multi-Symptom Nighttime Caplets with Cool Burst.............................. 1872
Tylenol Severe Allergy Caplets......... 1872
Tylenol Arthritis Pain Extended Release Caplets and Geltabs........ 1870
Tylenol Chest Congestion Caplets with Cool Burst.............................. 1872
Tylenol Chest Congestion Liquid with Cool Burst.............................. 1872
Children's Tylenol Suspension Liquid and Meltaways.................. 1878
Children's Tylenol Plus Cold Suspension Liquid.................. 1879
Children's Tylenol Plus Cold & Allergy Suspension Liquid............ 1878
Children's Tylenol Plus Cough & Runny Nose Suspension Liquid..... 1879
Children's Tylenol Plus Cough & Sore Throat Suspension Liquid..... 1879
Children's Tylenol Suspension with Flavor Creator...................... 1878
Children's Tylenol Plus Flu Suspension Liquid...................... 1881
Children's Tylenol Plus Multi-Symptom Cold Suspension Liquid...................... 1879
Tylenol Cold Severe Congestion Non-Drowsy Caplets with Cool Burst.............................. 1874
Tylenol Cold Head Congestion Daytime Caplets with Cool Burst.............................. 1873
Tylenol Cold Head Congestion Nighttime Caplets with Cool Burst.............................. 1873
Tylenol Cold Head Congestion Severe Caplets with Cool Burst..... 1873
Tylenol Cold Multi-Symptom Daytime Caplets with Cool Burst and Gelcaps...................... 1874
Tylenol Cold Multi-Symptom Daytime Liquid with Citrus Burst... 1874
Tylenol Cold Multi-Symptom Nighttime Caplets with Cool Burst.............................. 1874
Tylenol Cold Multi-Symptom Nighttime Liquid with Cool Burst... 1874
Tylenol Cold Multi-Symptom Severe Caplets with Cool Burst..... 1874
Tylenol Cold Multi-Symptom Severe Daytime Liquid with Citrus Burst.............................. 1874
Tylenol Cough & Sore Throat Daytime Liquid with Cool Burst...... 1877
Tylenol Cough & Sore Throat Nighttime Liquid with Cool Burst... 1877
Concentrated Tylenol Infants' Drops.............................. 1878
Concentrated Tylenol Infants' Drops Plus Cold.......................... 1879
Concentrated Tylenol Infants' Drops Plus Cold and Cough.......... 1879
Jr. Tylenol Meltaways...................... 1878
Tylenol Sinus Severe Congestion Caplets with Cool Burst............... 1876
Tylenol Sinus Congestion & Pain Daytime Caplets with Cool Burst and Gelcaps...................... 1876
Tylenol Sinus Congestion & Pain Nighttime Caplets with Cool Burst.............................. 1876
Tylenol Sinus Congestion & Pain Severe Caplets with Cool Burst..... 1876
Tylenol Sore Throat Daytime Liquid with Cool Burst.................. 1877
Tylenol Sore Throat Nighttime Liquid with Cool Burst.................. 1877
Women's Tylenol Menstrual Relief Caplets.............................. 1877
Vicks 44M Cough, Cold & Flu Relief Liquid.............................. 2680
Vicks DayQuil LiquiCaps/Liquid Multi-Symptom Cold/Flu Relief..... ▣ 761
Vicks DayQuil Multi-Symptom Cold/Flu Relief LiquiCaps............. 2678
Vicks DayQuil Multi-Symptom Cold/Flu Relief Liquid.................. 2678
Vicks NyQuil Multi-Symptom Cold/Flu Relief Liquid.................. 2681
Vicks NyQuil Multi-Symptom Cold/Flu Relief LiquiCaps............. 2681
Vicks NyQuil LiquiCaps/Liquid Multi-Symptom Cold/Flu Relief..... ▣ 763
Vicodin Tablets.............................. 535
Vicodin ES Tablets.......................... 536
Vicodin HP Tablets.......................... 538
Zicam Maximum Strength Flu Daytime.............................. ▣ 768
Zicam Maximum Strength Flu Nighttime.............................. ▣ 768
Zydone Tablets.............................. 1139

Aspirin (Coadministration reduces the peak concentration and AUC values for rimantadine). Products include:
Aggrenox Capsules.......................... 822
Bayer Aspirin.............................. 744
BC Allergy Sinus Cold Powder........ ▣ 677
BC Headache Powder...................... ▣ 677
Arthritis Strength BC Powder......... ▣ 677
BC Sinus Cold Powder.................... ▣ 677
Excedrin Extra Strength Caplets/Tablets/Geltabs............ ▣ 684
Excedrin Migraine Caplets/Tablets/Geltabs............ ▣ 609
Goody's Body Pain Formula Powder.............................. ▣ 684
Goody's Extra Strength Headache Powders...................... ▣ 611
Goody's Extra Strength Pain Relief Tablets............................ ▣ 685
Percodan Tablets.......................... 1132
St. Joseph 81 mg Aspirin Chewable and Enteric Coated Tablets.............................. 1869

Cimetidine (Potential for reduced clearance of total rimantadine). Products include:
Tagamet HB 200 Tablets.................. ▣ 664

Cimetidine Hydrochloride (Potential for reduced clearance of total rimantadine).
No products indexed under this heading.

Influenza Virus Vaccine Live, Intranasal (It is advisable that Influenza Virus Vaccine Live, Intranasal not be administered until 48 hours after cessation of rimantadine and that rimantadine not be administered until two weeks after the administration of Influenza Virus Vaccine Live, Intranasal unless medically indicated).
No products indexed under this heading.

FLUMIST VACCINE

(Influenza Virus Vaccine).................. 1901
May interact with alkylating agents, antivirals active against influenza, antimetabolites, corticosteroids, immunosuppressive agents, killed/inactivated vaccines, vaccines, live, and certain other agents. Compounds in these categories include:

Amantadine Hydrochloride (Based upon the potential for interference between Influenza Virus Vaccine Live, Intranasal and antiviral compounds that are active against influenza A and/or B viruses, it is advisable not to administer Influenza Virus Vaccine Live, Intranasal until 48 hours after the cessation of antiviral therapy. Antiviral agents should not be administered until two weeks after administration of Influenza Virus Vaccine Live, Intranasal unless medically indicated). Products include:
Symmetrel Tablets.......................... 1135

Aspirin (Influenza Virus Vaccine Live, Intranasal is contraindicated in children and adolescents receiving aspirin therapy or aspirin-containing therapy, because of the association of Reye syndrome with aspirin and wild-type influenza infection). Products include:
Aggrenox Capsules.......................... 822
Bayer Aspirin.............................. 744
BC Allergy Sinus Cold Powder........ ▣ 677
BC Headache Powder...................... ▣ 677
Arthritis Strength BC Powder......... ▣ 677
BC Sinus Cold Powder.................... ▣ 677
Excedrin Extra Strength Caplets/Tablets/Geltabs............ ▣ 684
Excedrin Migraine Caplets/Tablets/Geltabs............ ▣ 609
Goody's Body Pain Formula Powder.............................. ▣ 684
Goody's Extra Strength Headache Powders...................... ▣ 611
Goody's Extra Strength Pain Relief Tablets............................ ▣ 685
Percodan Tablets.......................... 1132
St. Joseph 81 mg Aspirin Chewable and Enteric Coated Tablets.............................. 1869

Azathioprine (Influenza Virus Vaccine Live, Intranasal is contraindicated in patients who have altered or compressed immune status as a consequence of immunosuppressive therapies).
No products indexed under this heading.

Basiliximab (Influenza Virus Vaccine Live, Intranasal is contraindicated in patients who have altered or compressed immune status as a consequence of immunosuppressive therapies). Products include:
Simulect for Injection...................... 2284

BCG Vaccine (The safety and immunogenicity of FluMist, when administered concurrently with other vaccines, have not been determined. Studies of FluMist in healthy individuals excluded subjects who received any live virus vaccine within one month of enrollment and anyinactivated or subunit vaccine within two weeks of enrollment. Therefore, healthcare providers should consider the risks and benefits of concurrent administration of FluMist with other vaccines).
No products indexed under this heading.

Betamethasone Acetate (Influenza Virus Vaccine Live, Intranasal is contraindicated in patients who may be immunosuppressed or have altered or compromised immune status as a consequence of treatment with systemic corticosteroids).
No products indexed under this heading.

Betamethasone Sodium Phosphate (Influenza Virus Vaccine Live, Intranasal is contraindicated in patients who may be immunosuppressed or have altered or compromised immune status as a consequence of treatment with systemic corticosteroids).
No products indexed under this heading.

Busulfan (Influenza Virus Vaccine Live, Intranasal is contraindicated in patients who may be immunosuppressed or have altered or compromised immune status as a consequence of treatment with alkylating drugs). Products include:
I.V. Busulfex.............................. 2493
Myleran Tablets.......................... 1525

Capecitabine (Influenza Virus Vaccine Live, Intranasal is contraindicated in patients who may be immunosuppressed or have altered or compromised immune status as a consequence of treatment with antimetabolites). Products include:
Xeloda Tablets.............................. 2822

Carmustine (BCNU) (Influenza Virus Vaccine Live, Intranasal is contraindicated in patients who may be immunosuppressed or have altered or compromised immune status as a consequence of treatment with alkylating drugs).
No products indexed under this heading.

Chlorambucil (Influenza Virus Vaccine Live, Intranasal is contraindicated in patients who may be immunosuppressed or have altered or compromised immune status as a consequence of treatment with alkylating drugs). Products include:
Leukeran Tablets.......................... 1504

Cladribine (Influenza Virus Vaccine Live, Intranasal is contraindicated in patients who may be immunosuppressed or have altered or compromised immune status as a consequence of treatment with antimetabolites). Products include:
Leustatin Injection.......................... 2357

Cortisone Acetate (Influenza Virus Vaccine Live, Intranasal is contraindicated in patients who may be immunosuppressed or have altered or compromised immune status as a consequence of treatment with systemic corticosteroids).
No products indexed under this heading.

Cyclophosphamide (Influenza Virus Vaccine Live, Intranasal is contraindicated in patients who may be immunosuppressed or have altered or compromised immune status as a consequence of treatment with alkylating drugs).
No products indexed under this heading.

Cyclosporine (Influenza Virus Vaccine Live, Intranasal is contraindicated in patients who have altered or compressed immune status as a consequence of immunosuppressive therapies). Products include:
Gengraf Capsules.......................... 459
Neoral Oral Solution...................... 2259
Neoral Soft Gelatin Capsules........... 2259
Restasis Ophthalmic Emulsion......... 575
Sandimmune.............................. 2275

Cytarabine (Influenza Virus Vaccine Live, Intranasal is contraindicated in patients who may be immunosuppressed or have altered or compromised immune status as a consequence of treatment with antimetabolites).
No products indexed under this heading.

Dacarbazine (Influenza Virus Vaccine Live, Intranasal is contraindicated in patients who may be immunosuppressed or have altered or compromised immune status as a consequence of treatment with alkylating drugs).
No products indexed under this heading.

Dexamethasone (Influenza Virus Vaccine Live, Intranasal is contraindicated in patients who may be immunosuppressed or have altered or compromised immune status as a consequence of treatment with systemic corticosteroids). Products include:
Ciprodex Otic Suspension............... 559
Decadron Tablets.......................... 1951
TobraDex Ophthalmic Ointment....... 562

TobraDex Ophthalmic Suspension ... **563**

Dexamethasone Acetate (Influenza Virus Vaccine Live, Intranasal is contraindicated in patients who may be immunosuppressed or have altered or compromised immune status as a consequence of treatment with systemic corticosteroids).
No products indexed under this heading.

Dexamethasone Sodium Phosphate (Influenza Virus Vaccine Live, Intranasal is contraindicated in patients who may be immunosuppressed or have altered or compromised immune status as a consequence of treatment with systemic corticosteroids).
No products indexed under this heading.

Diphtheria & Tetanus Toxoids and Acellular Pertussis Vaccine Adsorbed, Hepatitis B (recombinant) and Inactivated Poliovirus Vaccine Combined (The safety and immunogenicity of FluMist, when administered concurrently with other vaccines, have not been determined. Studies of FluMist in healthy individuals excluded subjects who received any live virus vaccine within one month of enrollment and anyinactivated or subunit vaccine within two weeks of enrollment. Therefore, healthcare providers should consider the risks and benefits of concurrent administration of FluMist with other vaccines).
No products indexed under this heading.

Estramustine Phosphate Sodium (Influenza Virus Vaccine Live, Intranasal is contraindicated in patients who may be immunosuppressed or have altered or compromised immune status as a consequence of treatment with alkylating drugs). Products include:
Emcyt Capsules ... **2634**

Floxuridine (Influenza Virus Vaccine Live, Intranasal is contraindicated in patients who may be immunosuppressed or have altered or compromised immune status as a consequence of treatment with antimetabolites).
No products indexed under this heading.

Fludarabine Phosphate (Influenza Virus Vaccine Live, Intranasal is contraindicated in patients who may be immunosuppressed or have altered or compromised immune status as a consequence of treatment with antimetabolites).
No products indexed under this heading.

Fludrocortisone Acetate (Influenza Virus Vaccine Live, Intranasal is contraindicated in patients who may be immunosuppressed or have altered or compromised immune status as a consequence of treatment with systemic corticosteroids).
No products indexed under this heading.

Fluorouracil (Influenza Virus Vaccine Live, Intranasal is contraindicated in patients who may be immunosuppressed or have altered or compromised immune status as a consequence of treatment with antimetabolites). Products include:
Carac Cream, 0.5% ... **2879**
Efudex ... **3363**

Gemcitabine Hydrochloride (Influenza Virus Vaccine Live, Intranasal is contraindicated in patients who may be immunosuppressed or have altered or compromised immune status as a consequence of treatment with antimetabolites). Products include:
Gemzar for Injection ... **1771**

Hepatitis A Vaccine, Inactivated (The safety and immunogenicity of FluMist, when administered concurrently with other vaccines, have not been determined. Studies of FluMist in healthy individuals excluded subjects who received any live virus vaccine within one month of enrollment and anyinactivated or subunit vaccine within two weeks of enrollment. Therefore, healthcare providers should consider the risks and benefits of concurrent administration of FluMist with other vaccines).
Products include:
Havrix Vaccine ... **1456**
Twinrix Vaccine ... **1595**
Vaqta ... **2097**

Hydrocortisone (Influenza Virus Vaccine Live, Intranasal is contraindicated in patients who may be immunosuppressed or have altered or compromised immune status as a consequence of treatment with systemic corticosteroids). Products include:
Colocort Rectal Suspension, USP (Retention) 100 mg/60 mL ... **2476**
Hydrocortone Tablets ... **1989**
Preparation H Hydrocortisone Cream ... **646**

Hydrocortisone Acetate (Influenza Virus Vaccine Live, Intranasal is contraindicated in patients who may be immunosuppressed or have altered or compromised immune status as a consequence of treatment with systemic corticosteroids). Products include:
Analpram-HC ... **1159**
Pramosone ... **1161**
ProctoFoam-HC ... **3099**

Hydrocortisone Sodium Phosphate (Influenza Virus Vaccine Live, Intranasal is contraindicated in patients who may be immunosuppressed or have altered or compromised immune status as a consequence of treatment with systemic corticosteroids).
No products indexed under this heading.

Hydrocortisone Sodium Succinate (Influenza Virus Vaccine Live, Intranasal is contraindicated in patients who may be immunosuppressed or have altered or compromised immune status as a consequence of treatment with systemic corticosteroids).
No products indexed under this heading.

Japanese Encephalitis Vaccine Inactivated (The safety and immunogenicity of FluMist, when administered concurrently with other vaccines, have not been determined. Studies of FluMist in healthy individuals excluded subjects who received any live virus vaccine within one month of enrollment and anyinactivated or subunit vaccine within two weeks of enrollment. Therefore, healthcare providers should consider the risks and benefits of concurrent administration of FluMist with other vaccines).
No products indexed under this heading.

Lomustine (CCNU) (Influenza Virus Vaccine Live, Intranasal is contraindicated in patients who may be immunosuppressed or have altered or compromised immune status as a consequence of treatment with alkylating drugs).
No products indexed under this heading.

Measles, Mumps, Rubella and Varicella Virus Vaccine Live (The safety and immunogenicity of FluMist, when administered concurrently with other vaccines, have not been determined. Studies of FluMist in healthy individuals excluded subjects who received any live virus vaccine within one month of enrollment and anyinactivated or subunit vaccine within two weeks of enrollment. Therefore, healthcare providers should consider the risks and benefits of concurrent administration of FluMist with other vaccines).
Products include:
ProQuad ... **2064**

Measles, Mumps & Rubella Virus Vaccine, Live (The safety and immunogenicity of FluMist, when administered concurrently with other vaccines, have not been determined. Studies of FluMist in healthy individuals excluded subjects who received any live virus vaccine within one month of enrollment and anyinactivated or subunit vaccine within two weeks of enrollment. Therefore, healthcare providers should consider the risks and benefits of concurrent administration of FluMist with other vaccines). Products include:
M-M-R II ... **2006**

Measles & Rubella Virus Vaccine Live (The safety and immunogenicity of FluMist, when administered concurrently with other vaccines, have not been determined. Studies of FluMist in healthy individuals excluded subjects who received any live virus vaccine within one month of enrollment and anyinactivated or subunit vaccine within two weeks of enrollment. Therefore, healthcare providers should consider the risks and benefits of concurrent administration of FluMist with other vaccines).
No products indexed under this heading.

Measles Virus Vaccine Live (The safety and immunogenicity of FluMist, when administered concurrently with other vaccines, have not been determined. Studies of FluMist in healthy individuals excluded subjects who received any live virus vaccine within one month of enrollment and anyinactivated or subunit vaccine within two weeks of enrollment. Therefore, healthcare providers should consider the risks and benefits of concurrent administration of FluMist with other vaccines).
Products include:
Attenuvax ... **1914**

Mechlorethamine Hydrochloride (Influenza Virus Vaccine Live, Intranasal is contraindicated in patients who may be immunosuppressed or have altered or compromised immune status as a consequence of treatment with alkylating drugs). Products include:
Mustargen for Injection ... **2468**

Melphalan (Influenza Virus Vaccine Live, Intranasal is contraindicated in patients who may be immunosuppressed or have altered or compromised immune status as a consequence of treatment with alkylating drugs). Products include:
Alkeran Tablets ... **956**

Mercaptopurine (Influenza Virus Vaccine Live, Intranasal is contraindicated in patients who may be immunosuppressed or have altered or compromised immune status as a consequence of treatment with antimetabolites).
No products indexed under this heading.

Methotrexate (Influenza Virus Vaccine Live, Intranasal is contraindicated in patients who may be immunosuppressed or have altered or compromised immune status as a consequence of treatment with antimetabolites).
No products indexed under this heading.

Methylprednisolone Acetate (Influenza Virus Vaccine Live, Intranasal is contraindicated in patients who may be immunosuppressed or have altered or compromised immune status as a consequence of treatment with systemic corticosteroids). Products include:
Depo-Medrol Injectable Suspension ... **2617**
Depo-Medrol Single-Dose Vial ... **2619**

Methylprednisolone Sodium Succinate (Influenza Virus Vaccine Live, Intranasal is contraindicated in patients who may be immunosuppressed or have altered or compromised immune status as a consequence of treatment with systemic corticosteroids).
No products indexed under this heading.

Mumps Virus Vaccine, Live (The safety and immunogenicity of FluMist, when administered concurrently with other vaccines, have not been determined. Studies of FluMist in healthy individuals excluded subjects who received any live virus vaccine within one month of enrollment and anyinactivated or subunit vaccine within two weeks of enrollment. Therefore, healthcare providers should consider the risks and benefits of concurrent administration of FluMist with other vaccines).
Products include:
Mumpsvax ... **2031**

Muromonab-CD3 (Influenza Virus Vaccine Live, Intranasal is contraindicated in patients who have altered or compressed immune status as a consequence of immunosuppressive therapies). Products include:
Orthoclone OKT3 Sterile Solution ... **2360**

Mycophenolate Mofetil (Influenza Virus Vaccine Live, Intranasal is contraindicated in patients who have altered or compressed immune status as a consequence of immunosuppressive therapies). Products include:
CellCept Capsules ... **2747**
CellCept Oral Suspension ... **2747**
CellCept Tablets ... **2747**

Oseltamivir Phosphate (Based upon the potential for interference between Influenza Virus Vaccine Live, Intranasal and antiviral compounds that are active against influenza A and/or B viruses, it is advisable not to administer Influenza Virus Vaccine Live, Intranasal until 48 hours after the cessation of antiviral therapy. Antiviral agents should not be administered until two weeks after administration of Influenza Virus Vaccine Live, Intranasal unless medically indicated). Products include:

Tamiflu Capsules 2807
Tamiflu Oral Suspension 2807

Pentostatin (Influenza Virus Vaccine Live, Intranasal is contraindicated in patients who may be immunosuppressed or have altered or compromised immune status as a consequence of treatment with antimetabolites). Products include:

Nipent for Injection 1863

Poliovirus Vaccine, Live, Oral, Trivalent, Types 1,2,3 (Sabin) (The safety and immunogenicity of FluMist, when administered concurrently with other vaccines, have not been determined. Studies of FluMist in healthy individuals excluded subjects who received any live virus vaccine within one month of enrollment and anyinactivated or subunit vaccine within two weeks of enrollment. Therefore, healthcare providers should consider the risks and benefits of concurrent administration of FluMist with other vaccines).

No products indexed under this heading.

Poliovirus Vaccine Inactivated, Trivalent Types 1,2,3 (The safety and immunogenicity of FluMist, when administered concurrently with other vaccines, have not been determined. Studies of FluMist in healthy individuals excluded subjects who received any live virus vaccine within one month of enrollment and anyinactivated or subunit vaccine within two weeks of enrollment. Therefore, healthcare providers should consider the risks and benefits of concurrent administration of FluMist with other vaccines). Products include:

Pediarix Vaccine 1548

Prednisolone Acetate (Influenza Virus Vaccine Live, Intranasal is contraindicated in patients who may be immunosuppressed or have altered or compromised immune status as a consequence of treatment with systemic corticosteroids). Products include:

Blephamide Ophthalmic Ointment 568
Blephamide Ophthalmic Suspension.................................. 569
Poly-Pred Ophthalmic Suspension .... ⊙233
Pred Forte Ophthalmic Suspension .... ⊙235
Pred Mild Ophthalmic Suspension .... ⊙238
Pred-G Ophthalmic Ointment .... ⊙237
Pred-G Ophthalmic Suspension ...... ⊙236

Prednisolone Sodium Phosphate (Influenza Virus Vaccine Live, Intranasal is contraindicated in patients who may be immunosuppressed or have altered or compromised immune status as a consequence of treatment with systemic corticosteroids).

No products indexed under this heading.

Prednisolone Tebutate (Influenza Virus Vaccine Live, Intranasal is contraindicated in patients who may be immunosuppressed or have altered or compromised immune status as a consequence of treatment with systemic corticosteroids).

No products indexed under this heading.

Prednisone (Influenza Virus Vaccine Live, Intranasal is contraindicated in patients who may be immunosuppressed or have altered or compromised immune status as a consequence of treatment with systemic corticosteroids).

No products indexed under this heading.

Rimantadine Hydrochloride (Based upon the potential for interference between Influenza Virus Vaccine Live, Intranasal and antiviral compounds that are active against influenza A and/or B viruses, it is advisable not to administer Influenza Virus Vaccine Live, Intranasal until 48 hours after the cessation of antiviral therapy. Antiviral agents should not be administered until two weeks after administration of Influenza Virus Vaccine Live, Intranasal unless medically indicated). Products include:

Flumadine 1183

Rotavirus Vaccine, Live, Oral, Tetravalent (The safety and immunogenicity of FluMist, when administered concurrently with other vaccines, have not been determined. Studies of FluMist in healthy individuals excluded subjects who received any live virus vaccine within one month of enrollment and anyinactivated or subunit vaccine within two weeks of enrollment. Therefore, healthcare providers should consider the risks and benefits of concurrent administration of FluMist with other vaccines).

No products indexed under this heading.

Rubella & Mumps Virus Vaccine Live (The safety and immunogenicity of FluMist, when administered concurrently with other vaccines, have not been determined. Studies of FluMist in healthy individuals excluded subjects who received any live virus vaccine within one month of enrollment and anyinactivated or subunit vaccine within two weeks of enrollment. Therefore, healthcare providers should consider the risks and benefits of concurrent administration of FluMist with other vaccines).

No products indexed under this heading.

Rubella Virus Vaccine Live (The safety and immunogenicity of FluMist, when administered concurrently with other vaccines, have not been determined. Studies of FluMist in healthy individuals excluded subjects who received any live virus vaccine within one month of enrollment and anyinactivated or subunit vaccine within two weeks of enrollment. Therefore, healthcare providers should consider the risks and benefits of concurrent administration of FluMist with other vaccines). Products include:

Meruvax II 2019

Sirolimus (Influenza Virus Vaccine Live, Intranasal is contraindicated in patients who have altered or compressed immune status as a consequence of immunosuppressive therapies). Products include:

Rapamune Oral Solution and Tablets 3475

Smallpox Vaccine (The safety and immunogenicity of FluMist, when administered concurrently with other vaccines, have not been determined. Studies of FluMist in healthy individuals excluded subjects who received any live virus vaccine within one month of enrollment and anyinactivated or subunit vaccine within two weeks of enrollment. Therefore, healthcare providers should consider the risks and benefits of concurrent administration of FluMist with other vaccines).

No products indexed under this heading.

Tacrolimus (Influenza Virus Vaccine Live, Intranasal is contraindicated in patients who have altered or compressed immune status as a consequence of immunosuppressive therapies). Products include:

Prograf Capsules and Injection 632
Protopic Ointment 638

Thioguanine (Influenza Virus Vaccine Live, Intranasal is contraindicated in patients who may be immunosuppressed or have altered or compromised immune status as a consequence of treatment with antimetabolites). Products include:

Tabloid Tablets 1575

Thiotepa (Influenza Virus Vaccine Live, Intranasal is contraindicated in patients who may be immunosuppressed or have altered or compromised immune status as a consequence of treatment with alkylating drugs).

No products indexed under this heading.

Triamcinolone (Influenza Virus Vaccine Live, Intranasal is contraindicated in patients who may be immunosuppressed or have altered or compromised immune status as a consequence of treatment with systemic corticosteroids).

No products indexed under this heading.

Triamcinolone Acetonide (Influenza Virus Vaccine Live, Intranasal is contraindicated in patients who may be immunosuppressed or have altered or compromised immune status as a consequence of treatment with systemic corticosteroids). Products include:

Azmacort Inhalation Aerosol 1726
Nasacort AQ Nasal Spray 2922

Triamcinolone Diacetate (Influenza Virus Vaccine Live, Intranasal is contraindicated in patients who may be immunosuppressed or have altered or compromised immune status as a consequence of treatment with systemic corticosteroids).

No products indexed under this heading.

Triamcinolone Hexacetonide (Influenza Virus Vaccine Live, Intranasal is contraindicated in patients who may be immunosuppressed or have altered or compromised immune status as a consequence of treatment with systemic corticosteroids).

No products indexed under this heading.

Typhoid Vaccine (The safety and immunogenicity of FluMist, when administered concurrently with other vaccines, have not been determined. Studies of FluMist in healthy individuals excluded subjects who received any live virus vaccine within one month of enrollment and anyinactivated or subunit vaccine within two weeks of enrollment. Therefore, healthcare providers should consider the risks and benefits of concurrent administration of FluMist with other vaccines).

No products indexed under this heading.

Varicella Virus Vaccine Live (The safety and immunogenicity of FluMist, when administered concurrently with other vaccines, have not been determined. Studies of FluMist in healthy individuals excluded subjects who received any live virus vaccine within one month of enrollment and anyinactivated or subunit vaccine within two weeks of enrollment. Therefore, healthcare providers should consider the risks and benefits of concurrent administration of FluMist with other vaccines). Products include:

Varivax 2100

Yellow Fever Vaccine (The safety and immunogenicity of FluMist, when administered concurrently with other vaccines, have not been determined. Studies of FluMist in healthy individuals excluded subjects who received any live virus vaccine within one month of enrollment and anyinactivated or subunit vaccine within two weeks of enrollment. Therefore, healthcare providers should consider the risks and benefits of concurrent administration of FluMist with other vaccines).

No products indexed under this heading.

Zanamivir (Based upon the potential for interference between Influenza Virus Vaccine Live, Intranasal and antiviral compounds that are active against influenza A and/or B viruses, it is advisable not to administer Influenza Virus Vaccine Live, Intranasal until 48 hours after the cessation of antiviral therapy. Antiviral agents should not be administered until two weeks after administration of Influenza Virus Vaccine Live, Intranasal unless medically indicated). Products include:

Relenza Rotadisk 1552

FLUORESCITE INJECTION

(Fluorescein Sodium) .... ⊙207
None cited in PDR database.

FLUOR-I-STRIP A.T. OPHTHALMIC STRIPS 1 MG

(Fluorescein Sodium) .... ⊙250
None cited in PDR database.

FML OPHTHALMIC OINTMENT

(Fluorometholone) .... ⊙228
None cited in PDR database.

FML OPHTHALMIC SUSPENSION

(Fluorometholone) .... ⊙227
None cited in PDR database.

FML FORTE OPHTHALMIC SUSPENSION

(Fluorometholone) .... ⊙226
None cited in PDR database.

FML-S OPHTHALMIC SUSPENSION

(Fluorometholone, Sulfacetamide Sodium).. ⊙229
May interact with silver preparations. Compounds in these categories include:

Silver Acetate (Sulfacetamide preparations are incompatible with silver preparations).

No products indexed under this heading.

Silver Nitrate (Sulfacetamide preparations are incompatible with silver preparations).
No products indexed under this heading.

Silver Sulfadiazine (Sulfacetamide preparations are incompatible with silver preparations).
No products indexed under this heading.

FOCALIN TABLETS

(Dexmethylphenidate Hydrochloride) ... 2220

May interact with antihypertensives, oral anticoagulants, monoamine oxidase inhibitors, phenytoin, selective serotonin reuptake inhibitors, tricyclic antidepressants, vasopressors, and certain other agents. Compounds in these categories include:

Acebutolol Hydrochloride (Methylphenidate may decrease the effectiveness of antihypertensive drugs).
No products indexed under this heading.

Amitriptyline Hydrochloride (Racemic methylphenidate may inhibit the metabolism of tricyclic antidepressants).
No products indexed under this heading.

Amlodipine Besylate (Methylphenidate may decrease the effectiveness of antihypertensive drugs). Products include:
- Caduet Tablets ... 2508
- Lotrel Capsules ... 2249
- Norvasc Tablets ... 2545

Amoxapine (Racemic methylphenidate may inhibit the metabolism of tricyclic antidepressants).
No products indexed under this heading.

Anisindione (Racemic methylphenidate may inhibit the metabolism of coumarin anticoagulants). Products include:
- Miradon Tablets ... 3042

Atenolol (Methylphenidate may decrease the effectiveness of antihypertensive drugs).
No products indexed under this heading.

Benazepril Hydrochloride (Methylphenidate may decrease the effectiveness of antihypertensive drugs). Products include:
- Lotensin Tablets ... 2243
- Lotensin HCT Tablets ... 2246
- Lotrel Capsules ... 2249

Bendroflumethiazide (Methylphenidate may decrease the effectiveness of antihypertensive drugs).
No products indexed under this heading.

Betaxolol Hydrochloride (Methylphenidate may decrease the effectiveness of antihypertensive drugs). Products include:
- Betoptic S Ophthalmic Suspension ... 558

Bisoprolol Fumarate (Methylphenidate may decrease the effectiveness of antihypertensive drugs).
No products indexed under this heading.

Candesartan Cilexetil (Methylphenidate may decrease the effectiveness of antihypertensive drugs). Products include:
- Atacand Tablets ... 649
- Atacand HCT ... 651

Captopril (Methylphenidate may decrease the effectiveness of antihypertensive drugs). Products include:
- Captopril Tablets ... 2149

Carteolol Hydrochloride (Methylphenidate may decrease the effectiveness of antihypertensive drugs). Products include:
- Carteolol Hydrochloride Ophthalmic Solution USP, 1% ... ⊙ 249

Chlorothiazide (Methylphenidate may decrease the effectiveness of antihypertensive drugs). Products include:
- Diuril Oral Suspension ... 1954

Chlorothiazide Sodium (Methylphenidate may decrease the effectiveness of antihypertensive drugs). Products include:
- Diuril Sodium Intravenous ... 2467

Chlorthalidone (Methylphenidate may decrease the effectiveness of antihypertensive drugs). Products include:
- Clorpres Tablets ... 2153

Citalopram Hydrobromide (Racemic methylphenidate may inhibit the metabolism of selective serotonin reuptake inhibitors). Products include:
- Celexa ... 1176

Clomipramine Hydrochloride (Racemic methylphenidate may inhibit the metabolism of tricyclic antidepressants).
No products indexed under this heading.

Clonidine (Co-administration has resulted in serious adverse events). Products include:
- Catapres-TTS ... 844

Clonidine Hydrochloride (Co-administration has resulted in serious adverse events). Products include:
- Catapres Tablets ... 843
- Clorpres Tablets ... 2153

Deserpidine (Methylphenidate may decrease the effectiveness of antihypertensive drugs).
No products indexed under this heading.

Desipramine Hydrochloride (Racemic methylphenidate may inhibit the metabolism of tricyclic antidepressants).
No products indexed under this heading.

Diazoxide (Methylphenidate may decrease the effectiveness of antihypertensive drugs). Products include:
- Hyperstat I.V. ... 3017

Dicumarol (Racemic methylphenidate may inhibit the metabolism of coumarin anticoagulants).
No products indexed under this heading.

Diltiazem Hydrochloride (Methylphenidate may decrease the effectiveness of antihypertensive drugs). Products include:
- Cardizem LA Extended Release Tablets ... 1728
- Tiazac Capsules ... 1201

Dobutamine (Methylphenidate has potential to increase blood pressure; concurrent use with pressor agents requires caution).
No products indexed under this heading.

Dobutamine Hydrochloride (Methylphenidate has potential to increase blood pressure; concurrent use with pressor agents requires caution).
No products indexed under this heading.

Dopamine Hydrochloride (Methylphenidate has potential to increase blood pressure; concurrent use with pressor agents requires caution).
No products indexed under this heading.

Doxazosin Mesylate (Methylphenidate may decrease the effectiveness of antihypertensive drugs). Products include:
- Cardura XL Tablets ... 2515

Doxepin Hydrochloride (Racemic methylphenidate may inhibit the metabolism of tricyclic antidepressants).
No products indexed under this heading.

Enalapril Maleate (Methylphenidate may decrease the effectiveness of antihypertensive drugs). Products include:
- Vasotec I.V. Injection ... 2103

Enalaprilat (Methylphenidate may decrease the effectiveness of antihypertensive drugs).
No products indexed under this heading.

Ephedrine Sulfate (Methylphenidate has potential to increase blood pressure; concurrent use with pressor agents requires caution).
No products indexed under this heading.

Epinephrine Bitartrate (Methylphenidate has potential to increase blood pressure; concurrent use with pressor agents requires caution).
No products indexed under this heading.

Epinephrine Hydrochloride (Methylphenidate has potential to increase blood pressure; concurrent use with pressor agents requires caution).
No products indexed under this heading.

Eprosartan Mesylate (Methylphenidate may decrease the effectiveness of antihypertensive drugs). Products include:
- Teveten Tablets ... 1735
- Teveten HCT Tablets ... 1737

Escitalopram Oxalate (Racemic methylphenidate may inhibit the metabolism of selective serotonin reuptake inhibitors). Products include:
- Lexapro Oral Solution ... 1190
- Lexapro Tablets ... 1190

Esmolol Hydrochloride (Methylphenidate may decrease the effectiveness of antihypertensive drugs).
No products indexed under this heading.

Felodipine (Methylphenidate may decrease the effectiveness of antihypertensive drugs).
No products indexed under this heading.

Fluoxetine Hydrochloride (Racemic methylphenidate may inhibit the metabolism of selective serotonin reuptake inhibitors). Products include:
- Prozac Pulvules and Liquid ... 1801
- Symbyax Capsules ... 1819

Fluvoxamine Maleate (Racemic methylphenidate may inhibit the metabolism of selective serotonin reuptake inhibitors).
No products indexed under this heading.

Fosinopril Sodium (Methylphenidate may decrease the effectiveness of antihypertensive drugs).
No products indexed under this heading.

Fosphenytoin Sodium (Racemic methylphenidate may inhibit the metabolism of phenytoin).
No products indexed under this heading.

Furosemide (Methylphenidate may decrease the effectiveness of antihypertensive drugs). Products include:
- Furosemide Tablets ... 2154

Guanabenz Acetate (Methylphenidate may decrease the effectiveness of antihypertensive drugs).
No products indexed under this heading.

Guanethidine Monosulfate (Methylphenidate may decrease the effectiveness of antihypertensive drugs).
No products indexed under this heading.

Hydralazine Hydrochloride (Methylphenidate may decrease the effectiveness of antihypertensive drugs). Products include:
- BiDil Tablets ... 2171

Hydrochlorothiazide (Methylphenidate may decrease the effectiveness of antihypertensive drugs). Products include:
- Aldoril Tablets ... 1910
- Atacand HCT ... 651
- Avalide Tablets ... 888
- Avalide Tablets ... 2874
- Benicar HCT Tablets ... 1044
- Diovan HCT Tablets ... 2196
- Dyazide Capsules ... 1423
- Hyzaar 50-12.5 Tablets ... 1990
- Hyzaar 100-12.5 Tablets ... 1990
- Hyzaar 100-25 Tablets ... 1990
- Lopressor HCT 50/25 Tablets ... 2241
- Lopressor HCT 100/25 Tablets ... 2241
- Lopressor HCT 100/50 Tablets ... 2241
- Lotensin HCT Tablets ... 2246
- Micardis HCT Tablets ... 856
- Moduretic Tablets ... 2028
- Prinzide Tablets ... 2056
- Teveten HCT Tablets ... 1737
- Timolide Tablets ... 2086
- Uniretic Tablets ... 3100

Hydroflumethiazide (Methylphenidate may decrease the effectiveness of antihypertensive drugs).
No products indexed under this heading.

Imipramine Hydrochloride (Racemic methylphenidate may inhibit the metabolism of tricyclic antidepressants).
No products indexed under this heading.

Imipramine Pamoate (Racemic methylphenidate may inhibit the metabolism of tricyclic antidepressants).
No products indexed under this heading.

Indapamide (Methylphenidate may decrease the effectiveness of antihypertensive drugs). Products include:
- Indapamide Tablets ... 2156

Irbesartan (Methylphenidate may decrease the effectiveness of antihypertensive drugs). Products include:
- Avalide Tablets ... 888
- Avalide Tablets ... 2874
- Avapro Tablets ... 891
- Avapro Tablets ... 2871

Isocarboxazid (Co-administration with MAO inhibitor may result in hypertensive crises; concurrent and/or sequential use is contraindicated).
No products indexed under this heading.

Isoproterenol Hydrochloride (Methylphenidate has potential to increase blood pressure; concurrent use with pressor agents requires caution).
No products indexed under this heading.

Isoproterenol Sulfate (Methylphenidate has potential to increase blood pressure; concurrent use with pressor agents requires caution).
No products indexed under this heading.

Isradipine (Methylphenidate may decrease the effectiveness of antihypertensive drugs). Products include:
DynaCirc CR Tablets 2721

Labetalol Hydrochloride (Methylphenidate may decrease the effectiveness of antihypertensive drugs).
No products indexed under this heading.

Lisinopril (Methylphenidate may decrease the effectiveness of antihypertensive drugs). Products include:
Prinivil Tablets 2052
Prinzide Tablets 2056

Losartan Potassium (Methylphenidate may decrease the effectiveness of antihypertensive drugs). Products include:
Cozaar Tablets 1935
Hyzaar 50-12.5 Tablets 1990
Hyzaar 100-12.5 Tablets 1990
Hyzaar 100-25 Tablets 1990

Maprotiline Hydrochloride (Racemic methylphenidate may inhibit the metabolism of tricyclic antidepressants).
No products indexed under this heading.

Mecamylamine Hydrochloride (Methylphenidate may decrease the effectiveness of antihypertensive drugs).
No products indexed under this heading.

Mephentermine Sulfate (Methylphenidate has potential to increase blood pressure; concurrent use with pressor agents requires caution).
No products indexed under this heading.

Metaraminol Bitartrate (Methylphenidate has potential to increase blood pressure; concurrent use with pressor agents requires caution).
No products indexed under this heading.

Methoxamine Hydrochloride (Methylphenidate has potential to increase blood pressure; concurrent use with pressor agents requires caution).
No products indexed under this heading.

Methyclothiazide (Methylphenidate may decrease the effectiveness of antihypertensive drugs).
No products indexed under this heading.

Methyldopa (Methylphenidate may decrease the effectiveness of antihypertensive drugs). Products include:
Aldoril Tablets 1910

Methyldopate Hydrochloride (Methylphenidate may decrease the effectiveness of antihypertensive drugs).
No products indexed under this heading.

Metolazone (Methylphenidate may decrease the effectiveness of antihypertensive drugs).
No products indexed under this heading.

Metoprolol Succinate (Methylphenidate may decrease the effectiveness of antihypertensive drugs). Products include:
Toprol-XL Tablets 668

Metoprolol Tartrate (Methylphenidate may decrease the effectiveness of antihypertensive drugs). Products include:
Lopressor Injection 2238
Lopressor Tablets 2238
Lopressor HCT 50/25 Tablets 2241
Lopressor HCT 100/25 Tablets 2241
Lopressor HCT 100/50 Tablets 2241

Metyrosine (Methylphenidate may decrease the effectiveness of antihypertensive drugs). Products include:
Demser Capsules 1953

Mibefradil Dihydrochloride (Methylphenidate may decrease the effectiveness of antihypertensive drugs).
No products indexed under this heading.

Minoxidil (Methylphenidate may decrease the effectiveness of antihypertensive drugs). Products include:
Men's Rogaine Extra Strength Hair Regrowth Treatment Topical Solution, Ocean Rush Scent and Original Unscented ■ 633
Men's Rogaine Foam Hair Regrowth Treatment ■ 633
Women's Rogaine Hair Regrowth Treatment Topical Solution, Spring Bloom Scent and Original Unscented ■ 634

Moclobemide (Co-administration with MAO inhibitor may result in hypertensive crises; concurrent and/or sequential use is contraindicated).
No products indexed under this heading.

Moexipril Hydrochloride (Methylphenidate may decrease the effectiveness of antihypertensive drugs). Products include:
Uniretic Tablets 3100
Univasc Tablets 3104

Nadolol (Methylphenidate may decrease the effectiveness of antihypertensive drugs). Products include:
Nadolol Tablets 2159

Nicardipine Hydrochloride (Methylphenidate may decrease the effectiveness of antihypertensive drugs). Products include:
Cardene I.V. 2497

Nifedipine (Methylphenidate may decrease the effectiveness of antihypertensive drugs). Products include:
Adalat CC Tablets 2964

Nisoldipine (Methylphenidate may decrease the effectiveness of antihypertensive drugs). Products include:
Sular Tablets 3122

Nitroglycerin (Methylphenidate may decrease the effectiveness of antihypertensive drugs). Products include:
Nitro-Dur Transdermal Infusion System 3046
Nitrolingual Pumpspray 3120

Norepinephrine Bitartrate (Methylphenidate has potential to increase blood pressure; concurrent use with pressor agents requires caution).
No products indexed under this heading.

Nortriptyline Hydrochloride (Racemic methylphenidate may inhibit the metabolism of tricyclic antidepressants).
No products indexed under this heading.

Pargyline Hydrochloride (Co-administration with MAO inhibitor may result in hypertensive crises; concurrent and/or sequential use is contraindicated).
No products indexed under this heading.

Paroxetine Hydrochloride (Racemic methylphenidate may inhibit the metabolism of selective serotonin reuptake inhibitors). Products include:
Paxil CR Controlled-Release Tablets 1538
Paxil 1530

Penbutolol Sulfate (Methylphenidate may decrease the effectiveness of antihypertensive drugs).
No products indexed under this heading.

Perindopril Erbumine (Methylphenidate may decrease the effectiveness of antihypertensive drugs). Products include:
Aceon Tablets (2 mg, 4 mg, 8 mg) 3194

Phenelzine Sulfate (Co-administration with MAO inhibitor may result in hypertensive crises; concurrent and/or sequential use is contraindicated).
No products indexed under this heading.

Phenobarbital (Racemic methylphenidate may inhibit the metabolism of phenobarbital). Products include:
Donnatal Extentabs 2493

Phenoxybenzamine Hydrochloride (Methylphenidate may decrease the effectiveness of antihypertensive drugs). Products include:
Dibenzyline Capsules 3399

Phentolamine Mesylate (Methylphenidate may decrease the effectiveness of antihypertensive drugs).
No products indexed under this heading.

Phenylephrine Hydrochloride (Methylphenidate has potential to increase blood pressure; concurrent use with pressor agents requires caution). Products include:
Comtrex Maximum Strength Non-Drowsy Cold & Cough Caplets ■ 725
Comtrex Maximum Strength Day/Night Severe Cold & Sinus Caplets - Day Formulation ■ 725
Comtrex Maximum Strength Day/Night Severe Cold & Sinus Caplets - Night Formulation ■ 725
Contac Cold and Flu Maximum Strength Caplets ■ 728
Contac Cold and Flu Day and Night Caplets (Day Formulation Only) ■ 727
Contac Cold and Flu Day and Night Caplets (Night Formulation Only) ■ 727
Contac Cold and Flu Non-Drowsy Caplets ■ 728
Contac-D Cold Non-Drowsy Tablets ■ 729
Children's Dimetapp Cold & Allergy Elixir ■ 730
Children's Dimetapp Cold & Allergy Chewable Tablets ■ 730
Children's Dimetapp DM Cold & Cough Elixir ■ 731
Toddler's Dimetapp Cold and Cough Drops ■ 732
Excedrin Sinus Headache Caplets/Tablets ■ 610
4-Way Fast Acting Nasal Spray ■ 775
4-Way Menthol Nasal Spray ■ 775
Preparation H Maximum Strength Cream ■ 666
Preparation H Cooling Gel ■ 666
Preparation H ■ 666
Refenesen PE Caplets ■ 721
Robitussin Cough & Allergy Syrup ■ 736
Robitussin Cough & Cold Nighttime Liquid ■ 736
Robitussin Cough, Cold & Flu Nighttime Liquid ■ 738
Robitussin Head & Chest Congestion PE Syrup ■ 739
Robitussin Pediatric Cough & Cold Nighttime Liquid ■ 736
TheraFlu Cold & Cough Hot Liquid ■ 740
TheraFlu Cold & Sore Throat Hot Liquid ■ 741
TheraFlu Flu & Sore Throat Hot Liquid ■ 742
TheraFlu Daytime Severe Cold Hot Liquid ■ 742
TheraFlu Nighttime Severe Cold Hot Liquid ■ 740
TheraFlu Warming Relief Daytime Severe Cold ■ 743
TheraFlu Warming Relief Nighttime Severe Cold ■ 743
Triaminic Chest & Nasal Congestion Liquid ■ 746
Triaminic Cold & Allergy Liquid ■ 746
Triaminic Daytime Cold & Cough Liquid ■ 745
Triaminic Nighttime Cold & Cough Liquid ■ 746
Triaminic Thin Strips Cold ■ 748
Triaminic Thin Strips Cold & Cough ■ 778
Triaminic Infant Thin Strips Decongestant ■ 747
Triaminic Infant Thin Strips Decongestant Plus Cough ■ 747
Children's Tylenol Plus Flu Oral Suspension ■ 749
Tylenol Cold Head Congestion Daytime Caplets with Cool Burst and Gelcaps ■ 750
Tylenol Cold Multi-Symptom Daytime Liquid ■ 752
Tylenol Cold Multi-Symptom Severe Daytime Liquid ■ 752
Concentrated Tylenol Infants' Drops Plus Cold & Cough ■ 754
Tylenol Allergy Multi-Symptom Caplets with Cool Burst and Gelcaps 1872
Tylenol Allergy Multi-Symptom Nighttime Caplets with Cool Burst 1872
Children's Tylenol Plus Cold Suspension Liquid 1879
Children's Tylenol Plus Cold & Allergy Suspension Liquid 1878
Children's Tylenol Plus Flu Suspension Liquid 1881
Children's Tylenol Plus Multi-Symptom Cold Suspension Liquid 1879
Tylenol Cold Head Congestion Daytime Caplets with Cool Burst 1873
Tylenol Cold Head Congestion Nighttime Caplets with Cool Burst 1873
Tylenol Cold Head Congestion Severe Caplets with Cool Burst 1873
Tylenol Cold Multi-Symptom Daytime Caplets with Cool Burst and Gelcaps 1874
Tylenol Cold Multi-Symptom Daytime Liquid with Citrus Burst 1874
Tylenol Cold Multi-Symptom Nighttime Caplets with Cool Burst 1874
Tylenol Cold Multi-Symptom Nighttime Liquid with Cool Burst 1874
Tylenol Cold Multi-Symptom Severe Caplets with Cool Burst 1874
Tylenol Cold Multi-Symptom Severe Daytime Liquid with Citrus Burst 1874
Tylenol Sinus Congestion & Pain Daytime Caplets with Cool Burst and Gelcaps 1876
Tylenol Sinus Congestion & Pain Nighttime Caplets with Cool Burst 1876
Tylenol Sinus Congestion & Pain Severe Caplets with Cool Burst 1876
Vicks 44D Cough & Head Congestion Relief Liquid ■ 760
Vicks DayQuil LiquiCaps/Liquid Multi-Symptom Cold/Flu Relief ■ 761

Zicam Cough Plus D Cough Spray 767

Phenytoin (Racemic methylphenidate may inhibit the metabolism of phenytoin).
No products indexed under this heading.

Phenytoin Sodium (Racemic methylphenidate may inhibit the metabolism of phenytoin). Products include:
Phenytek Capsules 2160

Pindolol (Methylphenidate may decrease the effectiveness of antihypertensive drugs).
No products indexed under this heading.

Polythiazide (Methylphenidate may decrease the effectiveness of antihypertensive drugs).
No products indexed under this heading.

Prazosin Hydrochloride (Methylphenidate may decrease the effectiveness of antihypertensive drugs).
No products indexed under this heading.

Primidone (Racemic methylphenidate may inhibit the metabolism of primidone).
No products indexed under this heading.

Procarbazine Hydrochloride (Co-administration with MAO inhibitor may result in hypertensive crises; concurrent and/or sequential use is contraindicated). Products include:
Matulane Capsules 3191

Propranolol Hydrochloride (Methylphenidate may decrease the effectiveness of antihypertensive drugs). Products include:
Inderal LA Long-Acting Capsules 3429
InnoPran XL Capsules 2723

Protriptyline Hydrochloride (Racemic methylphenidate may inhibit the metabolism of tricyclic antidepressants).
No products indexed under this heading.

Quinapril Hydrochloride (Methylphenidate may decrease the effectiveness of antihypertensive drugs).
No products indexed under this heading.

Ramipril (Methylphenidate may decrease the effectiveness of antihypertensive drugs). Products include:
Altace Capsules 1702

Rauwolfia Serpentina (Methylphenidate may decrease the effectiveness of antihypertensive drugs).
No products indexed under this heading.

Rescinnamine (Methylphenidate may decrease the effectiveness of antihypertensive drugs).
No products indexed under this heading.

Reserpine (Methylphenidate may decrease the effectiveness of antihypertensive drugs).
No products indexed under this heading.

Selegiline Hydrochloride (Co-administration with MAO inhibitor may result in hypertensive crises; concurrent and/or sequential use is contraindicated). Products include:
Eldepryl Capsules 3208
Zelapar Tablets 3372

Sertraline Hydrochloride (Racemic methylphenidate may inhibit the metabolism of selective serotonin reuptake inhibitors). Products include:
Zoloft 2586

Sodium Nitroprusside (Methylphenidate may decrease the effectiveness of antihypertensive drugs).
No products indexed under this heading.

Sotalol Hydrochloride (Methylphenidate may decrease the effectiveness of antihypertensive drugs).
No products indexed under this heading.

Spirapril Hydrochloride (Methylphenidate may decrease the effectiveness of antihypertensive drugs).
No products indexed under this heading.

Telmisartan (Methylphenidate may decrease the effectiveness of antihypertensive drugs). Products include:
Micardis Tablets 854
Micardis HCT Tablets 856

Terazosin Hydrochloride (Methylphenidate may decrease the effectiveness of antihypertensive drugs). Products include:
Hytrin Capsules 471

Timolol Maleate (Methylphenidate may decrease the effectiveness of antihypertensive drugs). Products include:
Blocadren Tablets 1916
Cosopt Sterile Ophthalmic Solution 1931
Timolide Tablets 2086
Timoptic Sterile Ophthalmic Solution 2088
Timoptic in Ocudose 2091
Timoptic-XE Sterile Ophthalmic Gel Forming Solution 2092

Torsemide (Methylphenidate may decrease the effectiveness of antihypertensive drugs). Products include:
Demadex Injection 2759
Demadex Tablets 2759

Trandolapril (Methylphenidate may decrease the effectiveness of antihypertensive drugs). Products include:
Mavik Tablets 486
Tarka Tablets 524

Tranylcypromine Sulfate (Co-administration with MAO inhibitor may result in hypertensive crises; concurrent and/or sequential use is contraindicated). Products include:
Parnate Tablets 1527

Trimethaphan Camsylate (Methylphenidate may decrease the effectiveness of antihypertensive drugs).
No products indexed under this heading.

Trimipramine Maleate (Racemic methylphenidate may inhibit the metabolism of tricyclic antidepressants).
No products indexed under this heading.

Valsartan (Methylphenidate may decrease the effectiveness of antihypertensive drugs). Products include:
Diovan Tablets 2193
Diovan HCT Tablets 2196

Verapamil Hydrochloride (Methylphenidate may decrease the effectiveness of antihypertensive drugs). Products include:
Covera-HS Tablets 3139
Tarka Tablets 524
Verelan PM Extended-Release Capsules, Controlled-Onset 3106

Warfarin Sodium (Racemic methylphenidate may inhibit the metabolism of coumarin anticoagulants). Products include:
Coumadin for Injection 898
Coumadin Tablets 898

FOCALIN XR CAPSULES

(Dexmethylphenidate Hydrochloride) 2223
May interact with antacids, antihypertensives, oral anticoagulants, histamine H2-receptor antagonists, monoamine oxidase inhibitors, phenytoin, proton pump inhibitor, tricyclic antidepressants, vasopressors, and certain other agents. Compounds in these categories include:

Acebutolol Hydrochloride (Methylphenidate may decrease the effectiveness of antihypertensive drugs).
No products indexed under this heading.

Aluminum Carbonate (The effects of gastrointestinal pH alterations on the absorption of dexmethylphenidate from Focalin XR have not been studied. Since the modified release characteristics of Focalin XR are pH dependent, the co-administration of antacids or acid suppressants could alter the release of dexmethylphenidate).
No products indexed under this heading.

Aluminum Hydroxide (The effects of gastrointestinal pH alterations on the absorption of dexmethylphenidate from Focalin XR have not been studied. Since the modified release characteristics of Focalin XR are pH dependent, the co-administration of antacids or acid suppressants could alter the release of dexmethylphenidate). Products include:
Gaviscon Regular Strength Liquid .. 658
Gaviscon Regular Strength Tablets 658
Gaviscon Extra Strength Liquid 658
Gaviscon Extra Strength Tablets 658
Maalox Regular Strength Antacid/Antigas Liquid 2175
Maalox Max Maximum Strength Antacid/Anti-Gas Liquid 2176

Amitriptyline Hydrochloride (Racemic methylphenidate may inhibit the metabolism of tricyclic antidepressants).
No products indexed under this heading.

Amlodipine Besylate (Methylphenidate may decrease the effectiveness of antihypertensive drugs). Products include:
Caduet Tablets 2508
Lotrel Capsules 2249
Norvasc Tablets 2545

Amoxapine (Racemic methylphenidate may inhibit the metabolism of tricyclic antidepressants).
No products indexed under this heading.

Anisindione (Racemic methylphenidate may inhibit the metabolism of coumarin anticoagulants). Products include:
Miradon Tablets 3042

Atenolol (Methylphenidate may decrease the effectiveness of antihypertensive drugs).
No products indexed under this heading.

Benazepril Hydrochloride (Methylphenidate may decrease the effectiveness of antihypertensive drugs). Products include:
Lotensin Tablets 2243
Lotensin HCT Tablets 2246
Lotrel Capsules 2249

Bendroflumethiazide (Methylphenidate may decrease the effectiveness of antihypertensive drugs).
No products indexed under this heading.

Betaxolol Hydrochloride (Methylphenidate may decrease the effectiveness of antihypertensive drugs). Products include:
Betoptic S Ophthalmic Suspension 558

Bisoprolol Fumarate (Methylphenidate may decrease the effectiveness of antihypertensive drugs).
No products indexed under this heading.

Candesartan Cilexetil (Methylphenidate may decrease the effectiveness of antihypertensive drugs). Products include:
Atacand Tablets 649
Atacand HCT 651

Captopril (Methylphenidate may decrease the effectiveness of antihypertensive drugs). Products include:
Captopril Tablets 2149

Carteolol Hydrochloride (Methylphenidate may decrease the effectiveness of antihypertensive drugs). Products include:
Carteolol Hydrochloride Ophthalmic Solution USP, 1% .... ⊙ 249

Chlorothiazide (Methylphenidate may decrease the effectiveness of antihypertensive drugs). Products include:
Diuril Oral Suspension 1954

Chlorothiazide Sodium (Methylphenidate may decrease the effectiveness of antihypertensive drugs). Products include:
Diuril Sodium Intravenous 2467

Chlorthalidone (Methylphenidate may decrease the effectiveness of antihypertensive drugs). Products include:
Clorpres Tablets 2153

Cimetidine (The effects of gastrointestinal pH alterations on the absorption of dexmethylphenidate from Focalin XR have not been studied. Since the modified release characteristics of Focalin XR are pH dependent, the co-administration of antacids or acid suppressants could alter the release of dexmethylphenidate). Products include:
Tagamet HB 200 Tablets 664

Cimetidine Hydrochloride (The effects of gastrointestinal pH alterations on the absorption of dexmethylphenidate from Focalin XR have not been studied. Since the modified release characteristics of Focalin XR are pH dependent, the co-administration of antacids or acid suppressants could alter the release of dexmethylphenidate).
No products indexed under this heading.

Clomipramine Hydrochloride (Racemic methylphenidate may inhibit the metabolism of tricyclic antidepressants).
No products indexed under this heading.

Clonidine (Co-administration has resulted in serious adverse events). Products include:
Catapres-TTS 844

Clonidine Hydrochloride (Co-administration has resulted in serious adverse events). Products include:
Catapres Tablets 843
Clorpres Tablets 2153

Deserpidine (Methylphenidate may decrease the effectiveness of antihypertensive drugs).
No products indexed under this heading.

Desipramine Hydrochloride (Racemic methylphenidate may inhibit the metabolism of tricyclic antidepressants).
No products indexed under this heading.

Diazoxide (Methylphenidate may decrease the effectiveness of antihypertensive drugs). Products include:
Hyperstat I.V. 3017

Dicumarol (Racemic methylphenidate may inhibit the metabolism of coumarin anticoagulants).
No products indexed under this heading.

Diltiazem Hydrochloride (Methylphenidate may decrease the effectiveness of antihypertensive drugs). Products include:
Cardizem LA Extended Release Tablets 1728
Tiazac Capsules 1201

Dobutamine (Methylphenidate has potential to increase blood pressure; concurrent use with pressor agents requires caution).
No products indexed under this heading.

Dobutamine Hydrochloride (Methylphenidate has potential to increase blood pressure; concurrent use with pressor agents requires caution).
No products indexed under this heading.

Dopamine Hydrochloride (Methylphenidate has potential to increase blood pressure; concurrent use with pressor agents requires caution).
No products indexed under this heading.

Doxazosin Mesylate (Methylphenidate may decrease the effectiveness of antihypertensive drugs). Products include:
Cardura XL Tablets 2515

Doxepin Hydrochloride (Racemic methylphenidate may inhibit the metabolism of tricyclic antidepressants).
No products indexed under this heading.

Enalapril Maleate (Methylphenidate may decrease the effectiveness of antihypertensive drugs). Products include:
Vasotec I.V. Injection 2103

Enalaprilat (Methylphenidate may decrease the effectiveness of antihypertensive drugs).
No products indexed under this heading.

Ephedrine Sulfate (Methylphenidate has potential to increase blood pressure; concurrent use with pressor agents requires caution).
No products indexed under this heading.

Epinephrine Bitartrate (Methylphenidate has potential to increase blood pressure; concurrent use with pressor agents requires caution).
No products indexed under this heading.

Epinephrine Hydrochloride (Methylphenidate has potential to increase blood pressure; concurrent use with pressor agents requires caution).
No products indexed under this heading.

Eprosartan Mesylate (Methylphenidate may decrease the effectiveness of antihypertensive drugs). Products include:
Teveten Tablets 1735
Teveten HCT Tablets 1737

Esmolol Hydrochloride (Methylphenidate may decrease the effectiveness of antihypertensive drugs).
No products indexed under this heading.

Esomeprazole Magnesium (The effects of gastrointestinal pH alterations on the absorption of dexmethylphenidate from Focalin XR have not been studied. Since the modified release characteristics of Focalin XR are pH dependent, the co-administration of antacids or acid suppressants could alter the release of dexmethylphenidate). Products include:
Nexium Delayed-Release Capsules 655

Famotidine (The effects of gastrointestinal pH alterations on the absorption of dexmethylphenidate from Focalin XR have not been studied. Since the modified release characteristics of Focalin XR are pH dependent, the co-administration of antacids or acid suppressants could alter the release of dexmethylphenidate). Products include:
Pepcid Injection 2040
Pepcid 2038
Pepcid AC Gelcaps 1701
Pepcid AC Tablets 1701
Maximum Strength Pepcid AC Tablets 1701
Pepcid Complete Chewable Tablets 1701

Felodipine (Methylphenidate may decrease the effectiveness of antihypertensive drugs).
No products indexed under this heading.

Fosinopril Sodium (Methylphenidate may decrease the effectiveness of antihypertensive drugs).
No products indexed under this heading.

Fosphenytoin Sodium (Racemic methylphenidate may inhibit the metabolism of phenytoin).
No products indexed under this heading.

Furosemide (Methylphenidate may decrease the effectiveness of antihypertensive drugs). Products include:
Furosemide Tablets 2154

Guanabenz Acetate (Methylphenidate may decrease the effectiveness of antihypertensive drugs).
No products indexed under this heading.

Guanethidine Monosulfate (Methylphenidate may decrease the effectiveness of antihypertensive drugs).
No products indexed under this heading.

Hydralazine Hydrochloride (Methylphenidate may decrease the effectiveness of antihypertensive drugs). Products include:
BiDil Tablets 2171

Hydrochlorothiazide (Methylphenidate may decrease the effectiveness of antihypertensive drugs). Products include:
Aldoril Tablets 1910
Atacand HCT 651
Avalide Tablets 888
Avalide Tablets 2874
Benicar HCT Tablets 1044
Diovan HCT Tablets 2196
Dyazide Capsules 1423
Hyzaar 50-12.5 Tablets 1990
Hyzaar 100-12.5 Tablets 1990
Hyzaar 100-25 Tablets 1990
Lopressor HCT 50/25 Tablets 2241
Lopressor HCT 100/25 Tablets 2241
Lopressor HCT 100/50 Tablets 2241
Lotensin HCT Tablets 2246
Micardis HCT Tablets 856
Moduretic Tablets 2028
Prinzide Tablets 2056
Teveten HCT Tablets 1737
Timolide Tablets 2086
Uniretic Tablets 3100

Hydroflumethiazide (Methylphenidate may decrease the effectiveness of antihypertensive drugs).
No products indexed under this heading.

Imipramine Hydrochloride (Racemic methylphenidate may inhibit the metabolism of tricyclic antidepressants).
No products indexed under this heading.

Imipramine Pamoate (Racemic methylphenidate may inhibit the metabolism of tricyclic antidepressants).
No products indexed under this heading.

Indapamide (Methylphenidate may decrease the effectiveness of antihypertensive drugs). Products include:
Indapamide Tablets 2156

Irbesartan (Methylphenidate may decrease the effectiveness of antihypertensive drugs). Products include:
Avalide Tablets 888
Avalide Tablets 2874
Avapro Tablets 891
Avapro Tablets 2871

Isocarboxazid (Co-administration with MAO inhibitor may result in hypertensive crises; concurrent and/or sequential use is contraindicated).
No products indexed under this heading.

Isoproterenol Hydrochloride (Methylphenidate has potential to increase blood pressure; concurrent use with pressor agents requires caution).
No products indexed under this heading.

Isoproterenol Sulfate (Methylphenidate has potential to increase blood pressure; concurrent use with pressor agents requires caution).
No products indexed under this heading.

Isradipine (Methylphenidate may decrease the effectiveness of antihypertensive drugs). Products include:
DynaCirc CR Tablets 2721

Labetalol Hydrochloride (Methylphenidate may decrease the effectiveness of antihypertensive drugs).
No products indexed under this heading.

Lansoprazole (The effects of gastrointestinal pH alterations on the absorption of dexmethylphenidate from Focalin XR have not been studied. Since the modified release characteristics of Focalin XR are pH dependent, the co-administration of antacids or acid suppressants could alter the release of dexmethylphenidate). Products include:
Prevacid Delayed-Release Capsules 3271
Prevacid for Delayed-Release Oral Suspension 3271
Prevacid SoluTab Delayed-Release Orally Disintegrating Tablets 3271
Prevacid I.V. for Injection 3277
Prevacid NapraPAC 3280
PREVPAC 3284

Lisinopril (Methylphenidate may decrease the effectiveness of antihypertensive drugs). Products include:
Prinivil Tablets 2052
Prinzide Tablets 2056

Losartan Potassium (Methylphenidate may decrease the effectiveness of antihypertensive drugs). Products include:
Cozaar Tablets 1935
Hyzaar 50-12.5 Tablets 1990
Hyzaar 100-12.5 Tablets 1990
Hyzaar 100-25 Tablets 1990

Magaldrate (The effects of gastrointestinal pH alterations on the absorption of dexmethylphenidate from Focalin XR have not been studied. Since the modified release characteristics of Focalin XR are pH dependent, the co-administration of antacids or acid suppressants could alter the release of dexmethylphenidate).
No products indexed under this heading.

Magnesium Hydroxide (The effects of gastrointestinal pH alterations on the absorption of dexmethylphenidate from Focalin XR have not been studied. Since the modified release characteristics of Focalin XR are pH dependent, the co-administration of antacids or acid suppressants could alter the release of dexmethylphenidate). Products include:
Maalox Regular Strength Antacid/Antigas Liquid 2175
Maalox Max Maximum Strength Antacid/Anti-Gas Liquid 2176
Pepcid Complete Chewable Tablets 1701

Magnesium Oxide (The effects of gastrointestinal pH alterations on the absorption of dexmethylphenidate from Focalin XR have not been studied. Since the modified release characteristics of Focalin XR are pH dependent, the co-administration of antacids or acid suppressants could alter the release of dexmethylphenidate). Products include:
Beelith Tablets 759
PremCal Light, Regular, and Extra Strength Tablets .... ▣ 818

Maprotiline Hydrochloride (Racemic methylphenidate may inhibit the metabolism of tricyclic antidepressants).
No products indexed under this heading.

Mecamylamine Hydrochloride (Methylphenidate may decrease the effectiveness of antihypertensive drugs).
No products indexed under this heading.

Mephentermine Sulfate (Methylphenidate has potential to increase blood pressure; concurrent use with pressor agents requires caution).
No products indexed under this heading.

Metaraminol Bitartrate (Methylphenidate has potential to increase blood pressure; concurrent use with pressor agents requires caution).
No products indexed under this heading.

Methoxamine Hydrochloride (Methylphenidate has potential to increase blood pressure; concurrent use with pressor agents requires caution).
No products indexed under this heading.

Methyclothiazide (Methylphenidate may decrease the effectiveness of antihypertensive drugs).
No products indexed under this heading.

Methyldopa (Methylphenidate may decrease the effectiveness of antihypertensive drugs). Products include:
Aldoril Tablets **1910**

Methyldopate Hydrochloride (Methylphenidate may decrease the effectiveness of antihypertensive drugs).
No products indexed under this heading.

Metolazone (Methylphenidate may decrease the effectiveness of antihypertensive drugs).
No products indexed under this heading.

Metoprolol Succinate (Methylphenidate may decrease the effectiveness of antihypertensive drugs). Products include:
Toprol-XL Tablets **668**

Metoprolol Tartrate (Methylphenidate may decrease the effectiveness of antihypertensive drugs). Products include:
Lopressor Injection **2238**
Lopressor Tablets **2238**
Lopressor HCT 50/25 Tablets **2241**
Lopressor HCT 100/25 Tablets **2241**
Lopressor HCT 100/50 Tablets **2241**

Metyrosine (Methylphenidate may decrease the effectiveness of antihypertensive drugs). Products include:
Demser Capsules **1953**

Mibefradil Dihydrochloride (Methylphenidate may decrease the effectiveness of antihypertensive drugs).
No products indexed under this heading.

Minoxidil (Methylphenidate may decrease the effectiveness of antihypertensive drugs). Products include:
Men's Rogaine Extra Strength Hair Regrowth Treatment Topical Solution, Ocean Rush Scent and Original Unscented ▣□**633**
Men's Rogaine Foam Hair Regrowth Treatment................... ▣□**633**
Women's Rogaine Hair Regrowth Treatment Topical Solution, Spring Bloom Scent and Original Unscented................... ▣□**634**

Moclobemide (Co-administration with MAO inhibitor may result in hypertensive crises; concurrent and/or sequential use is contraindicated).
No products indexed under this heading.

Moexipril Hydrochloride (Methylphenidate may decrease the effectiveness of antihypertensive drugs). Products include:
Uniretic Tablets **3100**
Univasc Tablets **3104**

Nadolol (Methylphenidate may decrease the effectiveness of antihypertensive drugs). Products include:
Nadolol Tablets **2159**

Nicardipine Hydrochloride (Methylphenidate may decrease the effectiveness of antihypertensive drugs). Products include:
Cardene I.V. **2497**

Nifedipine (Methylphenidate may decrease the effectiveness of antihypertensive drugs). Products include:
Adalat CC Tablets **2964**

Nisoldipine (Methylphenidate may decrease the effectiveness of antihypertensive drugs). Products include:
Sular Tablets **3122**

Nitroglycerin (Methylphenidate may decrease the effectiveness of antihypertensive drugs). Products include:
Nitro-Dur Transdermal Infusion System........................... **3046**

Nitrolingual Pumpspray **3120**

Nizatidine (The effects of gastrointestinal pH alterations on the absorption of dexmethylphenidate from Focalin XR have not been studied. Since the modified release characteristics of Focalin XR are pH dependent, the co-administration of antacids or acid suppressants could alter the release of dexmethylphenidate). Products include:
Axid Oral Solution **879**

Norepinephrine Bitartrate (Methylphenidate has potential to increase blood pressure; concurrent use with pressor agents requires caution).
No products indexed under this heading.

Nortriptyline Hydrochloride (Racemic methylphenidate may inhibit the metabolism of tricyclic antidepressants).
No products indexed under this heading.

Omeprazole (The effects of gastrointestinal pH alterations on the absorption of dexmethylphenidate from Focalin XR have not been studied. Since the modified release characteristics of Focalin XR are pH dependent, the co-administration of antacids or acid suppressants could alter the release of dexmethylphenidate). Products include:
Zegerid Capsules **2958**
Zegerid Powder for Oral Solution **2958**

Pantoprazole Sodium (The effects of gastrointestinal pH alterations on the absorption of dexmethylphenidate from Focalin XR have not been studied. Since the modified release characteristics of Focalin XR are pH dependent, the co-administration of antacids or acid suppressants could alter the release of dexmethylphenidate). Products include:
Protonix I.V. **3472**
Protonix Tablets **3469**

Pargyline Hydrochloride (Co-administration with MAO inhibitor may result in hypertensive crises; concurrent and/or sequential use is contraindicated).
No products indexed under this heading.

Penbutolol Sulfate (Methylphenidate may decrease the effectiveness of antihypertensive drugs).
No products indexed under this heading.

Perindopril Erbumine (Methylphenidate may decrease the effectiveness of antihypertensive drugs). Products include:
Aceon Tablets (2 mg, 4 mg, 8 mg)... **3194**

Phenelzine Sulfate (Co-administration with MAO inhibitor may result in hypertensive crises; concurrent and/or sequential use is contraindicated).
No products indexed under this heading.

Phenobarbital (Racemic methylphenidate may inhibit the metabolism of phenobarbital). Products include:
Donnatal Extentabs **2493**

Phenoxybenzamine Hydrochloride (Methylphenidate may decrease the effectiveness of antihypertensive drugs). Products include:
Dibenzyline Capsules **3399**

Phentolamine Mesylate (Methylphenidate may decrease the effectiveness of antihypertensive drugs).
No products indexed under this heading.

Phenylephrine Hydrochloride (Methylphenidate has potential to increase blood pressure; concurrent use with pressor agents requires caution). Products include:
Comtrex Maximum Strength Non-Drowsy Cold & Cough Caplets............................... ▣□**725**
Comtrex Maximum Strength Day/Night Severe Cold & Sinus Caplets - Day Formulation ▣□**725**
Comtrex Maximum Strength Day/Night Severe Cold & Sinus Caplets - Night Formulation........ ▣□**725**
Contac Cold and Flu Maximum Strength Caplets..................... ▣□**728**
Contac Cold and Flu Day and Night Caplets (Day Formulation Only)................................. ▣□**727**
Contac Cold and Flu Day and Night Caplets (Night Formulation Only)..................... ▣□**727**
Contac Cold and Flu Non-Drowsy Caplets............................... ▣□**728**
Contac-D Cold Non-Drowsy Tablets............................... ▣□**729**
Children's Dimetapp Cold & Allergy Elixir............................. ▣□**730**
Children's Dimetapp Cold & Allergy Chewable Tablets............. ▣□**730**
Children's Dimetapp DM Cold & Cough Elixir............................ ▣□**731**
Toddler's Dimetapp Cold and Cough Drops ▣□**732**
Excedrin Sinus Headache Caplets/Tablets..................... ▣□**610**
4-Way Fast Acting Nasal Spray ▣□**775**
4-Way Menthol Nasal Spray ▣□**775**
Preparation H Maximum Strength Cream ▣□**666**
Preparation H Cooling Gel ▣□**666**
Preparation H ▣□**666**
Refenesen PE Caplets ▣□**721**
Robitussin Cough & Allergy Syrup .. ▣□**736**
Robitussin Cough & Cold Nighttime Liquid...................... ▣□**736**
Robitussin Cough, Cold & Flu Nighttime Liquid...................... ▣□**738**
Robitussin Head & Chest Congestion PE Syrup ▣□**739**
Robitussin Pediatric Cough & Cold Nighttime Liquid................. ▣□**736**
TheraFlu Cold & Cough Hot Liquid ▣□**740**
TheraFlu Cold & Sore Throat Hot Liquid ▣□**741**
TheraFlu Flu & Sore Throat Hot Liquid ▣□**742**
TheraFlu Daytime Severe Cold Hot Liquid ▣□**742**
TheraFlu Nighttime Severe Cold Hot Liquid ▣□**740**
TheraFlu Warming Relief Daytime Severe Cold................................ ▣□**743**
TheraFlu Warming Relief Nighttime Severe Cold ▣□**743**
Triaminic Chest & Nasal Congestion Liquid................... ▣□**746**
Triaminic Cold & Allergy Liquid ▣□**746**
Triaminic Daytime Cold & Cough Liquid ▣□**745**
Triaminic Nighttime Cold & Cough Liquid............................. ▣□**746**
Triaminic Thin Strips Cold ▣□**748**
Triaminic Thin Strips Cold & Cough... ▣□**778**
Triaminic Infant Thin Strips Decongestant ▣□**747**
Triaminic Infant Thin Strips Decongestant Plus Cough........... ▣□**747**
Children's Tylenol Plus Flu Oral Suspension.......................... ▣□**749**
Tylenol Cold Head Congestion Daytime Caplets with Cool Burst and Gelcaps ▣□**750**
Tylenol Cold Multi-Symptom Daytime Liquid...................... ▣□**752**
Tylenol Cold Multi-Symptom Severe Daytime Liquid ▣□**752**
Concentrated Tylenol Infants' Drops Plus Cold & Cough........... ▣□**754**

Tylenol Allergy Multi-Symptom Caplets with Cool Burst and Gelcaps.................................... **1872**
Tylenol Allergy Multi-Symptom Nighttime Caplets with Cool Burst... **1872**
Children's Tylenol Plus Cold Suspension Liquid..................... **1879**
Children's Tylenol Plus Cold & Allergy Suspension Liquid **1878**
Children's Tylenol Plus Flu Suspension Liquid..................... **1881**
Children's Tylenol Plus Multi-Symptom Cold Suspension Liquid..................... **1879**
Tylenol Cold Head Congestion Daytime Caplets with Cool Burst... **1873**
Tylenol Cold Head Congestion Nighttime Caplets with Cool Burst... **1873**
Tylenol Cold Head Congestion Severe Caplets with Cool Burst..... **1873**
Tylenol Cold Multi-Symptom Daytime Caplets with Cool Burst and Gelcaps........................ **1874**
Tylenol Cold Multi-Symptom Daytime Liquid with Citrus Burst ... **1874**
Tylenol Cold Multi-Symptom Nighttime Caplets with Cool Burst... **1874**
Tylenol Cold Multi-Symptom Nighttime Liquid with Cool Burst... **1874**
Tylenol Cold Multi-Symptom Severe Caplets with Cool Burst..... **1874**
Tylenol Cold Multi-Symptom Severe Daytime Liquid with Citrus Burst............................. **1874**
Tylenol Sinus Congestion & Pain Daytime Caplets with Cool Burst and Gelcaps........................ **1876**
Tylenol Sinus Congestion & Pain Nighttime Caplets with Cool Burst... **1876**
Tylenol Sinus Congestion & Pain Severe Caplets with Cool Burst..... **1876**
Vicks 44D Cough & Head Congestion Relief Liquid............. ▣□**760**
Vicks DayQuil LiquiCaps/Liquid Multi-Symptom Cold/Flu Relief.... ▣□**761**
Zicam Cough Plus D Cough Spray.................................... ▣□**767**

Phenytoin (Racemic methylphenidate may inhibit the metabolism of phenytoin).
No products indexed under this heading.

Phenytoin Sodium (Racemic methylphenidate may inhibit the metabolism of phenytoin). Products include:
Phenytek Capsules **2160**

Pindolol (Methylphenidate may decrease the effectiveness of antihypertensive drugs).
No products indexed under this heading.

Polythiazide (Methylphenidate may decrease the effectiveness of antihypertensive drugs).
No products indexed under this heading.

Prazosin Hydrochloride (Methylphenidate may decrease the effectiveness of antihypertensive drugs).
No products indexed under this heading.

Primidone (Racemic methylphenidate may inhibit the metabolism of primidone).
No products indexed under this heading.

Procarbazine Hydrochloride (Co-administration with MAO inhibitor may result in hypertensive crises; concurrent and/or sequential use is contraindicated). Products include:
Matulane Capsules **3191**

Propranolol Hydrochloride (Methylphenidate may decrease the effectiveness of antihypertensive drugs). Products include:
Inderal LA Long-Acting Capsules **3429**

IMPORTANT NOTE: Always consult each drug listing in the patient's regimen for possible interactions.

InnoPran XL Capsules 2723

Protriptyline Hydrochloride (Racemic methylphenidate may inhibit the metabolism of tricyclic antidepressants).
No products indexed under this heading.

Quinapril Hydrochloride (Methylphenidate may decrease the effectiveness of antihypertensive drugs).
No products indexed under this heading.

Rabeprazole Sodium (The effects of gastrointestinal pH alterations on the absorption of dexmethylphenidate from Focalin XR have not been studied. Since the modified release characteristics of Focalin XR are pH dependent, the co-administration of antacids or acid suppressants could alter the release of dexmethylphenidate). Products include:
Aciphex Tablets 1090

Ramipril (Methylphenidate may decrease the effectiveness of antihypertensive drugs). Products include:
Altace Capsules 1702

Ranitidine Bismuth Citrate (The effects of gastrointestinal pH alterations on the absorption of dexmethylphenidate from Focalin XR have not been studied. Since the modified release characteristics of Focalin XR are pH dependent, the co-administration of antacids or acid suppressants could alter the release of dexmethylphenidate).
No products indexed under this heading.

Ranitidine Hydrochloride (The effects of gastrointestinal pH alterations on the absorption of dexmethylphenidate from Focalin XR have not been studied. Since the modified release characteristics of Focalin XR are pH dependent, the co-administration of antacids or acid suppressants could alter the release of dexmethylphenidate). Products include:
Zantac 1624
Zantac Injection 1619
Zantac Injection Pharmacy Bulk Package 1622

Rauwolfia Serpentina (Methylphenidate may decrease the effectiveness of antihypertensive drugs).
No products indexed under this heading.

Rescinnamine (Methylphenidate may decrease the effectiveness of antihypertensive drugs).
No products indexed under this heading.

Reserpine (Methylphenidate may decrease the effectiveness of antihypertensive drugs).
No products indexed under this heading.

Selegiline Hydrochloride (Co-administration with MAO inhibitor may result in hypertensive crises; concurrent and/or sequential use is contraindicated). Products include:
Eldepryl Capsules 3208
Zelapar Tablets 3372

Sodium Bicarbonate (The effects of gastrointestinal pH alterations on the absorption of dexmethylphenidate from Focalin XR have not been studied. Since the modified release characteristics of Focalin XR are pH dependent, the co-administration of antacids or acid suppressants could alter the release of dexmethylphenidate). Products include:
Colyte with Flavor Packs for Oral Solution 3088
HalfLytely and Bisacodyl Tablets Bowel Prep Kit with Flavors Packs 881
TriLyte with Flavor Packs for Oral Solution 3100

Sodium Nitroprusside (Methylphenidate may decrease the effectiveness of antihypertensive drugs).
No products indexed under this heading.

Sotalol Hydrochloride (Methylphenidate may decrease the effectiveness of antihypertensive drugs).
No products indexed under this heading.

Spirapril Hydrochloride (Methylphenidate may decrease the effectiveness of antihypertensive drugs).
No products indexed under this heading.

Telmisartan (Methylphenidate may decrease the effectiveness of antihypertensive drugs). Products include:
Micardis Tablets 854
Micardis HCT Tablets 856

Terazosin Hydrochloride (Methylphenidate may decrease the effectiveness of antihypertensive drugs). Products include:
Hytrin Capsules 471

Timolol Maleate (Methylphenidate may decrease the effectiveness of antihypertensive drugs). Products include:
Blocadren Tablets 1916
Cosopt Sterile Ophthalmic Solution 1931
Timolide Tablets 2086
Timoptic Sterile Ophthalmic Solution 2088
Timoptic in Ocudose 2091
Timoptic-XE Sterile Ophthalmic Gel Forming Solution 2092

Torsemide (Methylphenidate may decrease the effectiveness of antihypertensive drugs). Products include:
Demadex Injection 2759
Demadex Tablets 2759

Trandolapril (Methylphenidate may decrease the effectiveness of antihypertensive drugs). Products include:
Mavik Tablets 486
Tarka Tablets 524

Tranylcypromine Sulfate (Co-administration with MAO inhibitor may result in hypertensive crises; concurrent and/or sequential use is contraindicated). Products include:
Parnate Tablets 1527

Trimethaphan Camsylate (Methylphenidate may decrease the effectiveness of antihypertensive drugs).
No products indexed under this heading.

Trimipramine Maleate (Racemic methylphenidate may inhibit the metabolism of tricyclic antidepressants).
No products indexed under this heading.

Valsartan (Methylphenidate may decrease the effectiveness of antihypertensive drugs). Products include:
Diovan Tablets 2193
Diovan HCT Tablets 2196

Verapamil Hydrochloride (Methylphenidate may decrease the effectiveness of antihypertensive drugs). Products include:
Covera-HS Tablets 3139
Tarka Tablets 524
Verelan PM Extended-Release Capsules, Controlled-Onset 3106

Warfarin Sodium (Racemic methylphenidate may inhibit the metabolism of coumarin anticoagulants). Products include:
Coumadin for Injection 898
Coumadin Tablets 898

FOLGARD RX TABLETS

(Folic Acid, Vitamin B_{12}, Vitamin B_6) ... 3337
None cited in PDR database.

FOLLISTIM AQ CARTRIDGE

(Follitropin Beta) 2338
None cited in PDR database.

FOOD FOR THOUGHT DIETARY SUPPLEMENT

(Amino Acid Preparations, Vitamins with Minerals) .... ▣814
May interact with:

Aluminum Carbonate (Concomitant use with aluminum-containing antacids should be avoided).
No products indexed under this heading.

Aluminum Hydroxide (Concomitant use with aluminum-containing antacids should be avoided). Products include:
Gaviscon Regular Strength Liquid .. ▣658
Gaviscon Regular Strength Tablets .... ▣658
Gaviscon Extra Strength Liquid ...... ▣658
Gaviscon Extra Strength Tablets .... ▣658
Maalox Regular Strength Antacid/Antigas Liquid 2175
Maalox Max Maximum Strength Antacid/Anti-Gas Liquid 2176

FORADIL AEROLIZER

(Formoterol Fumarate) 3010
May interact with beta blockers, diuretics, glucocorticoids, monoamine oxidase inhibitors, potassium-depleting diuretics, drugs that prolong the QT interval, sympathomimetics, tricyclic antidepressants, and xanthines. Compounds in these categories include:

Acebutolol Hydrochloride (Co-administration with beta-blockers may inhibit the effect of each other. Beta-blockers not only block the therapeutic effect of beta-agonists, such as formoterol, but may produce severe bronchospasm in patients with asthma).
No products indexed under this heading.

Albuterol (Co-administration with additional adrenergic drugs may potentiate the sympathetic effects of formoterol). Products include:
Proventil Inhalation Aerosol 3053

Albuterol Sulfate (Co-administration with additional adrenergic drugs may potentiate the sympathetic effects of formoterol). Products include:
AccuNeb Inhalation Solution 1055
Combivent Inhalation Aerosol 847
DuoNeb Inhalation Solution 1058
ProAir HFA Inhalation Aerosol 3300
Proventil Inhalation Solution 0.083% 3055
Proventil HFA Inhalation Aerosol 3056
Ventolin HFA Inhalation Aerosol 1600
VoSpire ER Tablets 1052

Amiloride Hydrochloride (Concomitant treatment with diuretics may potentiate any hypokalemic effect of adrenergic agonists). Products include:
Midamor Tablets 2026
Moduretic Tablets 2028

Aminophylline (Co-administration with xanthine derivatives may potentiate hypokalemic effect of adrenergic agonists).
No products indexed under this heading.

Amiodarone Hydrochloride (Co-administration with drugs known to prolong the QTc interval may lead to an increased risk of ventricular arrhythmias; co-administer with extreme caution).
No products indexed under this heading.

Amitriptyline Hydrochloride (Concurrent and/or sequential administration with tricyclic antidepressants may potentiate the action of adrenergic agonists on the cardiovascular system; co-administer with extreme caution).
No products indexed under this heading.

Amoxapine (Concurrent and/or sequential administration with tricyclic antidepressants may potentiate the action of adrenergic agonists on the cardiovascular system; co-administer with extreme caution).
No products indexed under this heading.

Astemizole (Co-administration with drugs known to prolong the QTc interval may lead to an increased risk of ventricular arrhythmias; co-administer with extreme caution).
No products indexed under this heading.

Atenolol (Co-administration with beta-blockers may inhibit the effect of each other. Beta-blockers not only block the therapeutic effect of beta-agonists, such as formoterol, but may produce severe bronchospasm in patients with asthma).
No products indexed under this heading.

Bendroflumethiazide (The ECG changes and/or hypokalemia that may result from the administration of non-potassium sparing diuretics can be acutely worsened by beta-agonists, especially when the recommended dose of beta-agonist is exceeded).
No products indexed under this heading.

Betamethasone Acetate (Co-administration with glucocorticosteroids may potentiate hypokalemic effect of adrenergic agonists).
No products indexed under this heading.

Betamethasone Sodium Phosphate (Co-administration with glucocorticosteroids may potentiate hypokalemic effect of adrenergic agonists).
No products indexed under this heading.

Betaxolol Hydrochloride (Co-administration with beta-blockers may inhibit the effect of each other. Beta-blockers not only block the therapeutic effect of beta-agonists, such as formoterol, but may produce severe bronchospasm in patients with asthma). Products include:
Betoptic S Ophthalmic Suspension 558

Bisoprolol Fumarate (Co-administration with beta-blockers may inhibit the effect of each other. Beta-blockers not only block the therapeutic effect of beta-agonists, such as formoterol, but may produce severe bronchospasm in patients with asthma).
No products indexed under this heading.

Bretylium Tosylate (Co-administration with drugs known to prolong the QTc interval may lead to an increased risk of ventricular arrhythmias; co-administer with extreme caution).
No products indexed under this heading.

Bumetanide (The ECG changes and/or hypokalemia that may result from the administration of non-potassium sparing diuretics can be acutely worsened by beta-agonists, especially when the recommended dose of beta-agonist is exceeded). Products include:
Bumex Tablets 2746

Carteolol Hydrochloride (Co-administration with beta-blockers may inhibit the effect of each other. Beta-blockers not only block the therapeutic effect of beta-agonists, such as formoterol, but may produce severe bronchospasm in patients with asthma). Products include:
Carteolol Hydrochloride Ophthalmic Solution USP, 1%....... ⊙249

Chlorothiazide (The ECG changes and/or hypokalemia that may result from the administration of non-potassium sparing diuretics can be acutely worsened by beta-agonists, especially when the recommended dose of beta-agonist is exceeded). Products include:
Diuril Oral Suspension 1954

Chlorothiazide Sodium (The ECG changes and/or hypokalemia that may result from the administration of non-potassium sparing diuretics can be acutely worsened by beta-agonists, especially when the recommended dose of beta-agonist is exceeded). Products include:
Diuril Sodium Intravenous 2467

Chlorpromazine (Co-administration with drugs known to prolong the QTc interval may lead to an increased risk of ventricular arrhythmias; co-administer with extreme caution).
No products indexed under this heading.

Chlorpromazine Hydrochloride (Co-administration with drugs known to prolong the QTc interval may lead to an increased risk of ventricular arrhythmias; co-administer with extreme caution).
No products indexed under this heading.

Chlorthalidone (Concomitant treatment with diuretics may potentiate any hypokalemic effect of adrenergic agonists). Products include:
Clorpres Tablets 2153

Clomipramine Hydrochloride (Concurrent and/or sequential administration with tricyclic antidepressants may potentiate the action of adrenergic agonists on the cardiovascular system; co-administer with extreme caution).
No products indexed under this heading.

Cortisone Acetate (Co-administration with glucocorticosteroids may potentiate hypokalemic effect of adrenergic agonists).
No products indexed under this heading.

Desipramine Hydrochloride (Concurrent and/or sequential administration with tricyclic antidepressants may potentiate the action of adrenergic agonists on the cardiovascular system; co-administer with extreme caution).
No products indexed under this heading.

Dexamethasone (Co-administration with glucocorticosteroids may potentiate hypokalemic effect of adrenergic agonists). Products include:
Ciprodex Otic Suspension 559
Decadron Tablets 1951
TobraDex Ophthalmic Ointment 562
TobraDex Ophthalmic Suspension ... 563

Dexamethasone Acetate (Co-administration with glucocorticosteroids may potentiate hypokalemic effect of adrenergic agonists).
No products indexed under this heading.

Dexamethasone Sodium Phosphate (Co-administration with glucocorticosteroids may potentiate hypokalemic effect of adrenergic agonists).
No products indexed under this heading.

Disopyramide Phosphate (Co-administration with drugs known to prolong the QTc interval may lead to an increased risk of ventricular arrhythmias; co-administer with extreme caution).
No products indexed under this heading.

Dobutamine Hydrochloride (Co-administration with additional adrenergic drugs may potentiate the sympathetic effects of formoterol).
No products indexed under this heading.

Dofetilide (Co-administration with drugs known to prolong the QTc interval may lead to an increased risk of ventricular arrhythmias; co-administer with extreme caution).
No products indexed under this heading.

Dopamine Hydrochloride (Co-administration with additional adrenergic drugs may potentiate the sympathetic effects of formoterol).
No products indexed under this heading.

Doxepin Hydrochloride (Concurrent and/or sequential administration with tricyclic antidepressants may potentiate the action of adrenergic agonists on the cardiovascular system; co-administer with extreme caution).
No products indexed under this heading.

Dyphylline (Co-administration with xanthine derivatives may potentiate hypokalemic effect of adrenergic agonists).
No products indexed under this heading.

Ephedrine Hydrochloride (Co-administration with additional adrenergic drugs may potentiate the sympathetic effects of formoterol).
No products indexed under this heading.

Ephedrine Sulfate (Co-administration with additional adrenergic drugs may potentiate the sympathetic effects of formoterol).
No products indexed under this heading.

Ephedrine Tannate (Co-administration with additional adrenergic drugs may potentiate the sympathetic effects of formoterol).
No products indexed under this heading.

Epinephrine (Co-administration with additional adrenergic drugs may potentiate the sympathetic effects of formoterol). Products include:
EpiPen 1061
Primatene Mist .... ▣719
Twinject 0.15 3379
Twinject 0.3 3378

Epinephrine Bitartrate (Co-administration with additional adrenergic drugs may potentiate the sympathetic effects of formoterol).
No products indexed under this heading.

Epinephrine Hydrochloride (Co-administration with additional adrenergic drugs may potentiate the sympathetic effects of formoterol).
No products indexed under this heading.

Esmolol Hydrochloride (Co-administration with beta-blockers may inhibit the effect of each other. Beta-blockers not only block the therapeutic effect of beta-agonists, such as formoterol, but may produce severe bronchospasm in patients with asthma).
No products indexed under this heading.

Ethacrynic Acid (The ECG changes and/or hypokalemia that may result from the administration of non-potassium sparing diuretics can be acutely worsened by beta-agonists, especially when the recommended dose of beta-agonist is exceeded). Products include:
Edecrin Tablets 1959

Flecainide Acetate (Co-administration with drugs known to prolong the QTc interval may lead to an increased risk of ventricular arrhythmias; co-administer with extreme caution). Products include:
Tambocor Tablets 1856

Fludrocortisone Acetate (Co-administration with glucocorticosteroids may potentiate hypokalemic effect of adrenergic agonists).
No products indexed under this heading.

Fluphenazine Decanoate (Co-administration with drugs known to prolong the QTc interval may lead to an increased risk of ventricular arrhythmias; co-administer with extreme caution).
No products indexed under this heading.

Fluphenazine Enanthate (Co-administration with drugs known to prolong the QTc interval may lead to an increased risk of ventricular arrhythmias; co-administer with extreme caution).
No products indexed under this heading.

Fluphenazine Hydrochloride (Co-administration with drugs known to prolong the QTc interval may lead to an increased risk of ventricular arrhythmias; co-administer with extreme caution).
No products indexed under this heading.

Furosemide (The ECG changes and/or hypokalemia that may result from the administration of non-potassium sparing diuretics can be acutely worsened by beta-agonists, especially when the recommended dose of beta-agonist is exceeded). Products include:
Furosemide Tablets 2154

Hydrochlorothiazide (The ECG changes and/or hypokalemia that may result from the administration of non-potassium sparing diuretics can be acutely worsened by beta-agonists, especially when the recommended dose of beta-agonist is exceeded). Products include:
Aldoril Tablets 1910
Atacand HCT 651
Avalide Tablets 888
Avalide Tablets 2874
Benicar HCT Tablets 1044
Diovan HCT Tablets 2196
Dyazide Capsules 1423
Hyzaar 50-12.5 Tablets 1990
Hyzaar 100-12.5 Tablets 1990
Hyzaar 100-25 Tablets 1990
Lopressor HCT 50/25 Tablets 2241
Lopressor HCT 100/25 Tablets 2241
Lopressor HCT 100/50 Tablets 2241
Lotensin HCT Tablets 2246
Micardis HCT Tablets 856
Moduretic Tablets 2028
Prinzide Tablets 2056
Teveten HCT Tablets 1737
Timolide Tablets 2086
Uniretic Tablets 3100

Hydrocortisone (Co-administration with glucocorticosteroids may potentiate hypokalemic effect of adrenergic agonists). Products include:
Colocort Rectal Suspension, USP (Retention) 100 mg/60 mL.......... 2476
Hydrocortone Tablets 1989
Preparation H Hydrocortisone Cream .... ▣646

Hydrocortisone Acetate (Co-administration with glucocorticosteroids may potentiate hypokalemic effect of adrenergic agonists). Products include:
Analpram-HC 1159
Pramosone 1161
ProctoFoam-HC 3099

Hydrocortisone Sodium Phosphate (Co-administration with glucocorticosteroids may potentiate hypokalemic effect of adrenergic agonists).
No products indexed under this heading.

Hydrocortisone Sodium Succinate (Co-administration with glucocorticosteroids may potentiate hypokalemic effect of adrenergic agonists).
No products indexed under this heading.

Hydroflumethiazide (The ECG changes and/or hypokalemia that may result from the administration of non-potassium sparing diuretics can be acutely worsened by beta-agonists, especially when the recommended dose of beta-agonist is exceeded).
No products indexed under this heading.

Imipramine Hydrochloride (Concurrent and/or sequential administration with tricyclic antidepressants may potentiate the action of adrenergic agonists on the cardiovascular system; co-administer with extreme caution).
No products indexed under this heading.

Imipramine Pamoate (Concurrent and/or sequential administration with tricyclic antidepressants may potentiate the action of adrenergic agonists on the cardiovascular system; co-administer with extreme caution).
No products indexed under this heading.

Indapamide (Concomitant treatment with diuretics may potentiate any hypokalemic effect of adrenergic agonists). Products include:
Indapamide Tablets 2156

Isocarboxazid (Concurrent and/or sequential administration with MAO inhibitors may potentiate the action of adrenergic agonists on the cardiovascular system; co-administer with extreme caution).
No products indexed under this heading.

Isoproterenol Hydrochloride (Co-administration with additional adrenergic drugs may potentiate the sympathetic effects of formoterol).
No products indexed under this heading.

Isoproterenol Sulfate (Co-administration with additional adrenergic drugs may potentiate the sympathetic effects of formoterol).
No products indexed under this heading.

Labetalol Hydrochloride (Co-administration with beta-blockers may inhibit the effect of each other. Beta-blockers not only block the therapeutic effect of beta-agonists, such as formoterol, but may produce severe bronchospasm in patients with asthma).
No products indexed under this heading.

Levalbuterol Hydrochloride (Co-administration with additional adrenergic drugs may potentiate the sympathetic effects of formoterol). Products include:
Xopenex Inhalation Solution 3146
Xopenex Inhalation Solution Concentrate 3150

Levobunolol Hydrochloride (Co-administration with beta-blockers may inhibit the effect of each other. Beta-blockers not only block the therapeutic effect of beta-agonists, such as formoterol, but may produce severe bronchospasm in patients with asthma). Products include:
Betagan Ophthalmic Solution, USP.. ⊙ 220

Lidocaine Hydrochloride (Co-administration with drugs known to prolong the QTc interval may lead to an increased risk of ventricular arrhythmias; co-administer with extreme caution).
No products indexed under this heading.

Maprotiline Hydrochloride (Concurrent and/or sequential administration with tricyclic antidepressants may potentiate the action of adrenergic agonists on the cardiovascular system; co-administer with extreme caution).
No products indexed under this heading.

Mesoridazine Besylate (Co-administration with drugs known to prolong the QTc interval may lead to an increased risk of ventricular arrhythmias; co-administer with extreme caution).
No products indexed under this heading.

Metaproterenol Sulfate (Co-administration with additional adrenergic drugs may potentiate the sympathetic effects of formoterol). Products include:
Alupent Inhalation Aerosol 826

Metaraminol Bitartrate (Co-administration with additional adrenergic drugs may potentiate the sympathetic effects of formoterol).
No products indexed under this heading.

Methoxamine Hydrochloride (Co-administration with additional adrenergic drugs may potentiate the sympathetic effects of formoterol).
No products indexed under this heading.

Methyclothiazide (The ECG changes and/or hypokalemia that may result from the administration of non-potassium sparing diuretics can be acutely worsened by beta-agonists, especially when the recommended dose of beta-agonist is exceeded).
No products indexed under this heading.

Methylprednisolone Acetate (Co-administration with glucocorticosteroids may potentiate hypokalemic effect of adrenergic agonists). Products include:
Depo-Medrol Injectable Suspension 2617
Depo-Medrol Single-Dose Vial 2619

Methylprednisolone Sodium Succinate (Co-administration with glucocorticosteroids may potentiate hypokalemic effect of adrenergic agonists).
No products indexed under this heading.

Metipranolol Hydrochloride (Co-administration with beta-blockers may inhibit the effect of each other. Beta-blockers not only block the therapeutic effect of beta-agonists, such as formoterol, but may produce severe bronchospasm in patients with asthma).
No products indexed under this heading.

Metolazone (Concomitant treatment with diuretics may potentiate any hypokalemic effect of adrenergic agonists).
No products indexed under this heading.

Metoprolol Succinate (Co-administration with beta-blockers may inhibit the effect of each other. Beta-blockers not only block the therapeutic effect of beta-agonists, such as formoterol, but may produce severe bronchospasm in patients with asthma). Products include:
Toprol-XL Tablets 668

Metoprolol Tartrate (Co-administration with beta-blockers may inhibit the effect of each other. Beta-blockers not only block the therapeutic effect of beta-agonists, such as formoterol, but may produce severe bronchospasm in patients with asthma). Products include:
Lopressor Injection 2238
Lopressor Tablets 2238
Lopressor HCT 50/25 Tablets 2241
Lopressor HCT 100/25 Tablets 2241
Lopressor HCT 100/50 Tablets 2241

Mexiletine Hydrochloride (Co-administration with drugs known to prolong the QTc interval may lead to an increased risk of ventricular arrhythmias; co-administer with extreme caution).
No products indexed under this heading.

Moclobemide (Concurrent and/or sequential administration with MAO inhibitors may potentiate the action of adrenergic agonists on the cardiovascular system; co-administer with extreme caution).
No products indexed under this heading.

Nadolol (Co-administration with beta-blockers may inhibit the effect of each other. Beta-blockers not only block the therapeutic effect of beta-agonists, such as formoterol, but may produce severe bronchospasm in patients with asthma). Products include:
Nadolol Tablets 2159

Norepinephrine Bitartrate (Co-administration with additional adrenergic drugs may potentiate the sympathetic effects of formoterol).
No products indexed under this heading.

Nortriptyline Hydrochloride (Concurrent and/or sequential administration with tricyclic antidepressants may potentiate the action of adrenergic agonists on the cardiovascular system; co-administer with extreme caution).
No products indexed under this heading.

Pargyline Hydrochloride (Concurrent and/or sequential administration with MAO inhibitors may potentiate the action of adrenergic agonists on the cardiovascular system; co-administer with extreme caution).
No products indexed under this heading.

Penbutolol Sulfate (Co-administration with beta-blockers may inhibit the effect of each other. Beta-blockers not only block the therapeutic effect of beta-agonists, such as formoterol, but may produce severe bronchospasm in patients with asthma).
No products indexed under this heading.

Perphenazine (Co-administration with drugs known to prolong the QTc interval may lead to an increased risk of ventricular arrhythmias; co-administer with extreme caution).
No products indexed under this heading.

Phenelzine Sulfate (Concurrent and/or sequential administration with MAO inhibitors may potentiate the action of adrenergic agonists on the cardiovascular system; co-administer with extreme caution).
No products indexed under this heading.

Phenylephrine Bitartrate (Co-administration with additional adrenergic drugs may potentiate the sympathetic effects of formoterol).
No products indexed under this heading.

Phenylephrine Hydrochloride (Co-administration with additional adrenergic drugs may potentiate the sympathetic effects of formoterol). Products include:
Comtrex Maximum Strength Non-Drowsy Cold & Cough Caplets .... ▣ 725
Comtrex Maximum Strength Day/Night Severe Cold & Sinus Caplets - Day Formulation .... ▣ 725
Comtrex Maximum Strength Day/Night Severe Cold & Sinus Caplets - Night Formulation .... ▣ 725
Contac Cold and Flu Maximum Strength Caplets .... ▣ 728
Contac Cold and Flu Day and Night Caplets (Day Formulation Only).. ▣ 727
Contac Cold and Flu Day and Night Caplets (Night Formulation Only)......................... ▣ 727
Contac Cold and Flu Non-Drowsy Caplets.. ▣ 728
Contac-D Cold Non-Drowsy Tablets.. ▣ 729
Children's Dimetapp Cold & Allergy Elixir .... ▣ 730
Children's Dimetapp Cold & Allergy Chewable Tablets............... ▣ 730
Children's Dimetapp DM Cold & Cough Elixir .... ▣ 731
Toddler's Dimetapp Cold and Cough Drops .... ▣ 732
Excedrin Sinus Headache Caplets/Tablets .... ▣ 610
4-Way Fast Acting Nasal Spray ...... ▣ 775
4-Way Menthol Nasal Spray .... ▣ 775
Preparation H Maximum Strength Cream .... ▣ 666
Preparation H Cooling Gel .... ▣ 666
Preparation H .... ▣ 666
Refenesen PE Caplets .... ▣ 721
Robitussin Cough & Allergy Syrup .. ▣ 736
Robitussin Cough & Cold Nighttime Liquid............................. ▣ 736
Robitussin Cough, Cold & Flu Nighttime Liquid........................... ▣ 738
Robitussin Head & Chest Congestion PE Syrup .... ▣ 739
Robitussin Pediatric Cough & Cold Nighttime Liquid................... ▣ 736
TheraFlu Cold & Cough Hot Liquid .... ▣ 740
TheraFlu Cold & Sore Throat Hot Liquid .... ▣ 741
TheraFlu Flu & Sore Throat Hot Liquid .... ▣ 742
TheraFlu Daytime Severe Cold Hot Liquid.................................... ▣ 742
TheraFlu Nighttime Severe Cold Hot Liquid .... ▣ 740
TheraFlu Warming Relief Daytime Severe Cold................................... ▣ 743
TheraFlu Warming Relief Nighttime Severe Cold.................. ▣ 743
Triaminic Chest & Nasal Congestion Liquid .... ▣ 746
Triaminic Cold & Allergy Liquid .... ▣ 746
Triaminic Daytime Cold & Cough Liquid .... ▣ 745
Triaminic Nighttime Cold & Cough Liquid.................................. ▣ 746
Triaminic Thin Strips Cold .... ▣ 748
Triaminic Thin Strips Cold & Cough.. ▣ 778
Triaminic Infant Thin Strips Decongestant.................................. ▣ 747
Triaminic Infant Thin Strips Decongestant Plus Cough........... ▣ 747
Children's Tylenol Plus Flu Oral Suspension.................................... ▣ 749
Tylenol Cold Head Congestion Daytime Caplets with Cool Burst and Gelcaps .... ▣ 750
Tylenol Cold Multi-Symptom Daytime Liquid.............................. ▣ 752
Tylenol Cold Multi-Symptom Severe Daytime Liquid................ ▣ 752

Phenylephrine Tannate (Co-administration with additional adrenergic drugs may potentiate the sympathetic effects of formoterol).
 No products indexed under this heading.

Phenylpropanolamine Hydrochloride (Co-administration with additional adrenergic drugs may potentiate the sympathetic effects of formoterol).
 No products indexed under this heading.

Pindolol (Co-administration with beta-blockers may inhibit the effect of each other. Beta-blockers not only block the therapeutic effect of beta-agonists, such as formoterol, but may produce severe bronchospasm in patients with asthma).
 No products indexed under this heading.

Pirbuterol Acetate (Co-administration with additional adrenergic drugs may potentiate the sympathetic effects of formoterol).
 Products include:

Polythiazide (The ECG changes and/or hypokalemia that may result from the administration of non-potassium sparing diuretics can be acutely worsened by beta-agonists, especially when the recommended dose of beta-agonist is exceeded).
 No products indexed under this heading.

Prednisolone Acetate (Co-administration with glucocorticoster-

oids may potentiate hypokalemic effect of adrenergic agonists).
Products include:

Prednisolone Sodium Phosphate (Co-administration with glucocorticosteroids may potentiate hypokalemic effect of adrenergic agonists).
 No products indexed under this heading.

Prednisolone Tebutate (Co-administration with glucocorticosteroids may potentiate hypokalemic effect of adrenergic agonists).
 No products indexed under this heading.

Prednisone (Co-administration with glucocorticosteroids may potentiate hypokalemic effect of adrenergic agonists).
 No products indexed under this heading.

Procainamide Hydrochloride (Co-administration with drugs known to prolong the QTc interval may lead to an increased risk of ventricular arrhythmias; co-administer with extreme caution).
 No products indexed under this heading.

Procarbazine Hydrochloride (Concurrent and/or sequential administration with MAO inhibitors may potentiate the action of adrenergic agonists on the cardiovascular system; co-administer with extreme caution). Products include:

Prochlorperazine (Co-administration with drugs known to prolong the QTc interval may lead to an increased risk of ventricular arrhythmias; co-administer with extreme caution).
 No products indexed under this heading.

Promethazine Hydrochloride (Co-administration with drugs known to prolong the QTc interval may lead to an increased risk of ventricular arrhythmias; co-administer with extreme caution). Products include:
 Phenergan Tablets and

Propafenone Hydrochloride (Co-administration with drugs known to prolong the QTc interval may lead to an increased risk of ventricular arrhythmias; co-administer with extreme caution). Products include:

Propranolol Hydrochloride (Co-administration with beta-blockers may inhibit the effect of each other. Beta-blockers not only block the therapeutic effect of beta-agonists, such as formoterol, but may produce severe bronchospasm in patients with asthma). Products include:

Protriptyline Hydrochloride (Concurrent and/or sequential administration with tricyclic antidepressants may potentiate the action of adrenergic agonists on the cardiovascular system; co-administer with extreme caution).
 No products indexed under this heading.

Pseudoephedrine Hydrochloride (Co-administration with additional adrenergic drugs may potentiate the sympathetic effects of formoterol).
 Products include:

Pseudoephedrine Sulfate (Co-administration with additional adrenergic drugs may potentiate the sympathetic effects of formoterol).
 Products include:

Quinidine Gluconate (Co-administration with drugs known to prolong the QTc interval may lead to an increased risk of ventricular arrhythmias; co-administer with extreme caution).
 No products indexed under this heading.

Quinidine Polygalacturonate (Co-administration with drugs known to prolong the QTc interval may lead to an increased risk of ventricular arrhythmias; co-administer with extreme caution).
 No products indexed under this heading.

Quinidine Sulfate (Co-administration with drugs known to prolong the QTc interval may lead to an increased risk of ventricular arrhythmias; co-administer with extreme caution).
 No products indexed under this heading.

Salmeterol Xinafoate (Co-administration with additional adrenergic drugs may potentiate the sympathetic effects of formoterol).
 Products include:

Selegiline Hydrochloride (Concurrent and/or sequential administration with MAO inhibitors may potentiate the action of adrenergic agonists on the cardiovascular system; co-administer with extreme caution).
 Products include:

Sotalol Hydrochloride (Co-administration with beta-blockers may inhibit the effect of each other. Beta-blockers not only block the therapeutic effect of beta-agonists, such as formoterol, but may produce severe bronchospasm in patients with asthma).
 No products indexed under this heading.

Spironolactone (Concomitant treatment with diuretics may potentiate any hypokalemic effect of adrenergic agonists).
 No products indexed under this heading.

Terbutaline Sulfate (Co-administration with additional adrenergic drugs may potentiate the sympathetic effects of formoterol).
 No products indexed under this heading.

Theophylline (Co-administration with xanthine derivatives may potentiate hypokalemic effect of adrenergic agonists).
 No products indexed under this heading.

Theophylline Anhydrous (Co-administration with xanthine derivatives may potentiate hypokalemic effect of adrenergic agonists).
 Products include:

Theophylline Calcium Salicylate (Co-administration with xanthine derivatives may potentiate hypokalemic effect of adrenergic agonists).
 No products indexed under this heading.

Theophylline Dihydroxypropyl (Glyceryl) (Co-administration with xanthine derivatives may potentiate hypokalemic effect of adrenergic agonists).
 No products indexed under this heading.

Theophylline Ethylenediamine (Co-administration with xanthine derivatives may potentiate hypokalemic effect of adrenergic agonists).
 No products indexed under this heading.

Theophylline Sodium Glycinate (Co-administration with xanthine derivatives may potentiate hypokalemic effect of adrenergic agonists).
 No products indexed under this heading.

Thioridazine Hydrochloride (Co-administration with drugs known to prolong the QTc interval may lead to an increased risk of ventricular arrhythmias; co-administer with extreme caution). Products include:
Thioridazine Hydrochloride Tablets 2163

Timolol Hemihydrate (Co-administration with beta-blockers may inhibit the effect of each other. Beta-blockers not only block the therapeutic effect of beta-agonists, such as formoterol, but may produce severe bronchospasm in patients with asthma). Products include:
Betimol Ophthalmic Solution 3382
Betimol Ophthalmic Solution .... ⊙295

Timolol Maleate (Co-administration with beta-blockers may inhibit the effect of each other. Beta-blockers not only block the therapeutic effect of beta-agonists, such as formoterol, but may produce severe bronchospasm in patients with asthma). Products include:
Blocadren Tablets 1916
Cosopt Sterile Ophthalmic Solution 1931
Timolide Tablets 2086
Timoptic Sterile Ophthalmic Solution 2088
Timoptic in Ocudose 2091
Timoptic-XE Sterile Ophthalmic Gel Forming Solution 2092

Tocainide Hydrochloride (Co-administration with drugs known to prolong the QTc interval may lead to an increased risk of ventricular arrhythmias; co-administer with extreme caution).
No products indexed under this heading.

Torsemide (The ECG changes and/or hypokalemia that may result from the administration of non-potassium sparing diuretics can be acutely worsened by beta-agonists, especially when the recommended dose of beta-agonist is exceeded). Products include:
Demadex Injection 2759
Demadex Tablets 2759

Tranylcypromine Sulfate (Concurrent and/or sequential administration with MAO inhibitors may potentiate the action of adrenergic agonists on the cardiovascular system; co-administer with extreme caution). Products include:
Parnate Tablets 1527

Triamcinolone (Co-administration with glucocorticosteroids may potentiate hypokalemic effect of adrenergic agonists).
No products indexed under this heading.

Triamcinolone Acetonide (Co-administration with glucocorticosteroids may potentiate hypokalemic effect of adrenergic agonists). Products include:
Azmacort Inhalation Aerosol 1726
Nasacort AQ Nasal Spray 2922

Triamcinolone Diacetate (Co-administration with glucocorticosteroids may potentiate hypokalemic effect of adrenergic agonists).
No products indexed under this heading.

Triamcinolone Hexacetonide (Co-administration with glucocorticosteroids may potentiate hypokalemic effect of adrenergic agonists).
No products indexed under this heading.

Triamterene (Concomitant treatment with diuretics may potentiate any hypokalemic effect of adrenergic agonists). Products include:
Dyazide Capsules 1423
Dyrenium Capsules 3400

Trifluoperazine Hydrochloride (Co-administration with drugs known to prolong the QTc interval may lead to an increased risk of ventricular arrhythmias; co-administer with extreme caution).
No products indexed under this heading.

Trimipramine Maleate (Concurrent and/or sequential administration with tricyclic antidepressants may potentiate the action of adrenergic agonists on the cardiovascular system; co-administer with extreme caution).
No products indexed under this heading.

Ziprasidone Hydrochloride (Co-administration with drugs known to prolong the QTc interval may lead to an increased risk of ventricular arrhythmias; co-administer with extreme caution). Products include:
Geodon Capsules 2529

FORTAMET EXTENDED-RELEASE TABLETS

(Metformin Hydrochloride) 3115
May interact with cationic drugs that are eliminated by renal tubular, calcium channel blockers, corticosteroids, diuretics, estrogens, oral contraceptives, phenothiazines, phenytoin, radiographic iodinated contrast media, sympathomimetics, thiazides, thyroid preparations, and certain other agents. Compounds in these categories include:

Albuterol (Sympathomimetics tend to produce hyperglycemia and may lead to loss of glycemic control). Products include:
Proventil Inhalation Aerosol 3053

Albuterol Sulfate (Sympathomimetics tend to produce hyperglycemia and may lead to loss of glycemic control). Products include:
AccuNeb Inhalation Solution 1055
Combivent Inhalation Aerosol 847
DuoNeb Inhalation Solution 1058
ProAir HFA Inhalation Aerosol 3300
Proventil Inhalation Solution 0.083% 3055
Proventil HFA Inhalation Aerosol 3056
Ventolin HFA Inhalation Aerosol 1600
VoSpire ER Tablets 1052

Amiloride Hydrochloride (Diuretics tend to produce hyperglycemia and may lead to loss of glycemic control). Products include:
Midamor Tablets 2026
Moduretic Tablets 2028

Amlodipine Besylate (Calcium channel blocking drugs tend to produce hyperglycemia and may lead to loss of glycemic control). Products include:
Caduet Tablets 2508
Lotrel Capsules 2249
Norvasc Tablets 2545

Bendroflumethiazide (Thiazides tend to produce hyperglycemia and may lead to loss of glycemic control).
No products indexed under this heading.

Bepridil Hydrochloride (Calcium channel blocking drugs tend to produce hyperglycemia and may lead to loss of glycemic control).
No products indexed under this heading.

Betamethasone Acetate (Corticosteroids tend to produce hyperglycemia and may lead to loss of glycemic control).
No products indexed under this heading.

Betamethasone Sodium Phosphate (Corticosteroids tend to produce hyperglycemia and may lead to loss of glycemic control).
No products indexed under this heading.

Bumetanide (Diuretics tend to produce hyperglycemia and may lead to loss of glycemic control). Products include:
Bumex Tablets 2746

Chlorothiazide (Thiazides tend to produce hyperglycemia and may lead to loss of glycemic control). Products include:
Diuril Oral Suspension 1954

Chlorothiazide Sodium (Thiazides tend to produce hyperglycemia and may lead to loss of glycemic control). Products include:
Diuril Sodium Intravenous 2467

Chlorotrianisene (Estrogens tend to produce hyperglycemia and may lead to loss of glycemic control).
No products indexed under this heading.

Chlorpromazine (Phenothiazines tend to produce hyperglycemia and may lead to loss of glycemic control).
No products indexed under this heading.

Chlorpromazine Hydrochloride (Phenothiazines tend to produce hyperglycemia and may lead to loss of glycemic control).
No products indexed under this heading.

Chlorthalidone (Diuretics tend to produce hyperglycemia and may lead to loss of glycemic control). Products include:
Clorpres Tablets 2153

Cimetidine (Co-administration of cimetidine increased peak plasma metformin and whole blood concentrations by 60% and plasma and whole blood metformin AUC by 40%). Products include:
Tagamet HB 200 Tablets .... ▣664

Cimetidine Hydrochloride (Co-administration of cimetidine increased peak plasma metformin and whole blood concentrations by 60% and plasma and whole blood metformin AUC by 40%).
No products indexed under this heading.

Cortisone Acetate (Corticosteroids tend to produce hyperglycemia and may lead to loss of glycemic control).
No products indexed under this heading.

Desogestrel (Oral contraceptives tend to produce hyperglycemia and may lead to loss of glycemic control). Products include:
Mircette Tablets 1066

Dexamethasone (Corticosteroids tend to produce hyperglycemia and may lead to loss of glycemic control). Products include:
Ciprodex Otic Suspension 559
Decadron Tablets 1951
TobraDex Ophthalmic Ointment 562
TobraDex Ophthalmic Suspension 563

Dexamethasone Acetate (Corticosteroids tend to produce hyperglycemia and may lead to loss of glycemic control).
No products indexed under this heading.

Dexamethasone Sodium Phosphate (Corticosteroids tend to produce hyperglycemia and may lead to loss of glycemic control).
No products indexed under this heading.

Diatrizoate Meglumine (Intravascular contrast studies with iodinated materials can lead to acute alteration of renal function and have been associated with lactic acidosis in patients receiving metformin. Therefore, discontinue metformin at the time of or prior to the procedure, and for 48 hours subsequent to the procedure until renal function is normal).
No products indexed under this heading.

Diatrizoate Sodium (Intravascular contrast studies with iodinated materials can lead to acute alteration of renal function and have been associated with lactic acidosis in patients receiving metformin. Therefore, discontinue metformin at the time of or prior to the procedure, and for 48 hours subsequent to the procedure until renal function is normal).
No products indexed under this heading.

Dienestrol (Estrogens tend to produce hyperglycemia and may lead to loss of glycemic control).
No products indexed under this heading.

Diethylstilbestrol (Estrogens tend to produce hyperglycemia and may lead to loss of glycemic control).
No products indexed under this heading.

Digoxin (Cationic drugs that are eliminated by renal tubular secretion theoretically have the potential for interaction with metformin by competing for common renal tubular transport system). Products include:
Lanoxicaps Capsules 1490
Lanoxin Injection 1494
Lanoxin Injection Pediatric 1497
Lanoxin Tablets 1500

Diltiazem Hydrochloride (Calcium channel blocking drugs tend to produce hyperglycemia and may lead to loss of glycemic control). Products include:
Cardizem LA Extended Release Tablets 1728
Tiazac Capsules 1201

Dobutamine Hydrochloride (Sympathomimetics tend to produce hyperglycemia and may lead to loss of glycemic control).
No products indexed under this heading.

Dopamine Hydrochloride (Sympathomimetics tend to produce hyperglycemia and may lead to loss of glycemic control).
No products indexed under this heading.

Ephedrine Hydrochloride (Sympathomimetics tend to produce hyperglycemia and may lead to loss of glycemic control).
No products indexed under this heading.

Ephedrine Sulfate (Sympathomimetics tend to produce hyperglycemia and may lead to loss of glycemic control).
No products indexed under this heading.

Ephedrine Tannate (Sympathomimetics tend to produce hyperglycemia and may lead to loss of glycemic control).
No products indexed under this heading.

Epinephrine (Sympathomimetics tend to produce hyperglycemia and may lead to loss of glycemic control). Products include:
EpiPen **1061**
Primatene Mist **719**
Twinject 0.15 .... **3379**
Twinject 0.3 .... **3378**

Epinephrine Bitartrate (Sympathomimetics tend to produce hyperglycemia and may lead to loss of glycemic control).
No products indexed under this heading.

Epinephrine Hydrochloride (Sympathomimetics tend to produce hyperglycemia and may lead to loss of glycemic control).
No products indexed under this heading.

Estradiol (Estrogens tend to produce hyperglycemia and may lead to loss of glycemic control). Products include:
Angeliq Tablets **762**
Climara Transdermal System **771**
Climara Pro Transdermal System **776**
Estrasorb Topical Emulsion **1147**
Estring Vaginal Ring **2635**
Menostar Transdermal System **782**
Vagifem Tablets **2334**

Estrogens, Conjugated (Estrogens tend to produce hyperglycemia and may lead to loss of glycemic control). Products include:
Premarin Intravenous **3442**
Premarin Tablets **3446**
Premarin Vaginal Cream **3452**
Premphase Tablets **3456**
Prempro Tablets **3456**

Estrogens, Esterified (Estrogens tend to produce hyperglycemia and may lead to loss of glycemic control). Products include:
Estratest Tablets **3199**
Estratest H.S. Tablets **3199**

Estropipate (Estrogens tend to produce hyperglycemia and may lead to loss of glycemic control).
No products indexed under this heading.

Ethacrynic Acid (Diuretics tend to produce hyperglycemia and may lead to loss of glycemic control). Products include:
Edecrin Tablets **1959**

Ethinyl Estradiol (Estrogens tend to produce hyperglycemia and may lead to loss of glycemic control). Products include:
Mircette Tablets **1066**
NuvaRing **2340**
Ortho-Cyclen/Ortho Tri-Cyclen **2429**
Ortho Evra Transdermal System **2417**
Ortho Tri-Cyclen Lo Tablets **2436**
Seasonique Tablets **1077**
Yasmin 28 Tablets **796**
Yaz Tablets **803**

Ethiodized Oil (Intravascular contrast studies with iodinated materials can lead to acute alteration of renal function and have been associated with lactic acidosis in patients receiving metformin. Therefore, discontinue metformin at the time of or prior to the procedure, and for 48 hours subsequent to the procedure until renal function is normal).
No products indexed under this heading.

Ethynodiol Diacetate (Oral contraceptives tend to produce hyperglycemia and may lead to loss of glycemic control).
No products indexed under this heading.

Felodipine (Calcium channel blocking drugs tend to produce hyperglycemia and may lead to loss of glycemic control).
No products indexed under this heading.

Fludrocortisone Acetate (Corticosteroids tend to produce hyperglycemia and may lead to loss of glycemic control).
No products indexed under this heading.

Fluphenazine Decanoate (Phenothiazines tend to produce hyperglycemia and may lead to loss of glycemic control).
No products indexed under this heading.

Fluphenazine Enanthate (Phenothiazines tend to produce hyperglycemia and may lead to loss of glycemic control).
No products indexed under this heading.

Fluphenazine Hydrochloride (Phenothiazines tend to produce hyperglycemia and may lead to loss of glycemic control).
No products indexed under this heading.

Fosphenytoin Sodium (Phenytoin tends to produce hyperglycemia and may lead to loss of glycemic control).
No products indexed under this heading.

Furosemide (Furosemide increased the metformin plasma and blood Cmax by 22% and blood AUC by 15%, without any significant change in metformin renal clearance. When administered with metformin, the Cmax and AUC of furosemide were 31% and 12% smaller, respectively, and the terminal half-life was decreased by 32%, without any significant change in furosemide renal clearance). Products include:
Furosemide Tablets **2154**

Gadopentetate Dimeglumine (Intravascular contrast studies with iodinated materials can lead to acute alteration of renal function and have been associated with lactic acidosis in patients receiving metformin. Therefore, discontinue metformin at the time of or prior to the procedure, and for 48 hours subsequent to the procedure until renal function is normal).
No products indexed under this heading.

Hydrochlorothiazide (Thiazides tend to produce hyperglycemia and may lead to loss of glycemic control). Products include:
Aldoril Tablets **1910**
Atacand HCT **651**
Avalide Tablets **888**
Avalide Tablets **2874**
Benicar HCT Tablets **1044**
Diovan HCT Tablets **2196**
Dyazide Capsules **1423**
Hyzaar 50-12.5 Tablets **1990**
Hyzaar 100-12.5 Tablets **1990**
Hyzaar 100-25 Tablets **1990**
Lopressor HCT 50/25 Tablets **2241**
Lopressor HCT 100/25 Tablets **2241**
Lopressor HCT 100/50 Tablets **2241**
Lotensin HCT Tablets **2246**
Micardis HCT Tablets **856**
Moduretic Tablets **2028**
Prinzide Tablets **2056**
Teveten HCT Tablets **1737**
Timolide Tablets **2086**
Uniretic Tablets **3100**

Hydrocortisone (Corticosteroids tend to produce hyperglycemia and may lead to loss of glycemic control). Products include:
Colocort Rectal Suspension, USP (Retention) 100 mg/60 mL **2476**
Hydrocortone Tablets **1989**
Preparation H Hydrocortisone Cream **646**

Hydrocortisone Acetate (Corticosteroids tend to produce hyperglycemia and may lead to loss of glycemic control). Products include:
Analpram-HC **1159**
Pramosone **1161**
ProctoFoam-HC **3099**

Hydrocortisone Sodium Phosphate (Corticosteroids tend to produce hyperglycemia and may lead to loss of glycemic control).
No products indexed under this heading.

Hydrocortisone Sodium Succinate (Corticosteroids tend to produce hyperglycemia and may lead to loss of glycemic control).
No products indexed under this heading.

Hydroflumethiazide (Thiazides tend to produce hyperglycemia and may lead to loss of glycemic control).
No products indexed under this heading.

Indapamide (Diuretics tend to produce hyperglycemia and may lead to loss of glycemic control). Products include:
Indapamide Tablets **2156**

Iodamide Meglumine (Intravascular contrast studies with iodinated materials can lead to acute alteration of renal function and have been associated with lactic acidosis in patients receiving metformin. Therefore, discontinue metformin at the time of or prior to the procedure, and for 48 hours subsequent to the procedure until renal function is normal).
No products indexed under this heading.

Iohexol (Intravascular contrast studies with iodinated materials can lead to acute alteration of renal function and have been associated with lactic acidosis in patients receiving metformin. Therefore, discontinue metformin at the time of or prior to the procedure, and for 48 hours subsequent to the procedure until renal function is normal).
No products indexed under this heading.

Iopamidol (Intravascular contrast studies with iodinated materials can lead to acute alteration of renal function and have been associated with lactic acidosis in patients receiving metformin. Therefore, discontinue metformin at the time of or prior to the procedure, and for 48 hours subsequent to the procedure until renal function is normal).
No products indexed under this heading.

Iopanoic Acid (Intravascular contrast studies with iodinated materials can lead to acute alteration of renal function and have been associated with lactic acidosis in patients receiving metformin. Therefore, discontinue metformin at the time of or prior to the procedure, and for 48 hours subsequent to the procedure until renal function is normal).
No products indexed under this heading.

Iothalamate Meglumine (Intravascular contrast studies with iodinated materials can lead to acute alteration of renal function and have been associated with lactic acidosis in patients receiving metformin. Therefore, discontinue metformin at the time of or prior to the procedure, and for 48 hours subsequent to the procedure until renal function is normal).
No products indexed under this heading.

Ioxaglate Meglumine (Intravascular contrast studies with iodinated materials can lead to acute alteration of renal function and have been associated with lactic acidosis in patients receiving metformin. Therefore, discontinue metformin at the time of or prior to the procedure, and for 48 hours subsequent to the procedure until renal function is normal).
No products indexed under this heading.

Ioxaglate Sodium (Intravascular contrast studies with iodinated materials can lead to acute alteration of renal function and have been associated with lactic acidosis in patients receiving metformin. Therefore, discontinue metformin at the time of or prior to the procedure, and for 48 hours subsequent to the procedure until renal function is normal).
No products indexed under this heading.

Isoniazid (Isoniazid tends to produce hyperglycemia and may lead to loss of glycemic control).
No products indexed under this heading.

Isoproterenol Hydrochloride (Sympathomimetics tend to produce hyperglycemia and may lead to loss of glycemic control).
No products indexed under this heading.

Isoproterenol Sulfate (Sympathomimetics tend to produce hyperglycemia and may lead to loss of glycemic control).
No products indexed under this heading.

Isradipine (Calcium channel blocking drugs tend to produce hyperglycemia and may lead to loss of glycemic control). Products include:
DynaCirc CR Tablets **2721**

Levalbuterol Hydrochloride (Sympathomimetics tend to produce

hyperglycemia and may lead to loss of glycemic control). Products include:
- Xopenex Inhalation Solution 3146
- Xopenex Inhalation Solution Concentrate 3150

Levonorgestrel (Oral contraceptives tend to produce hyperglycemia and may lead to loss of glycemic control). Products include:
- Climara Pro Transdermal System 776
- Mirena Intrauterine System 787
- Plan B Tablets 1076
- Seasonique Tablets 1077

Levothyroxine Sodium (Thyroid products tend to produce hyperglycemia and may lead to loss of glycemic control). Products include:
- Levothroid Tablets 1186
- Levoxyl Tablets 1712
- Synthroid Tablets 520
- Westhroid Tablets 3403

Liothyronine Sodium (Thyroid products tend to produce hyperglycemia and may lead to loss of glycemic control). Products include:
- Cytomel Tablets 1710
- Westhroid Tablets 3403

Liotrix (Thyroid products tend to produce hyperglycemia and may lead to loss of glycemic control). Products include:
- Thyrolar Tablets 1199

Mesoridazine Besylate (Phenothiazines tend to produce hyperglycemia and may lead to loss of glycemic control).
No products indexed under this heading.

Mestranol (Oral contraceptives tend to produce hyperglycemia and may lead to loss of glycemic control).
No products indexed under this heading.

Metaproterenol Sulfate (Sympathomimetics tend to produce hyperglycemia and may lead to loss of glycemic control). Products include:
- Alupent Inhalation Aerosol 826

Metaraminol Bitartrate (Sympathomimetics tend to produce hyperglycemia and may lead to loss of glycemic control).
No products indexed under this heading.

Methotrimeprazine (Phenothiazines tend to produce hyperglycemia and may lead to loss of glycemic control).
No products indexed under this heading.

Methoxamine Hydrochloride (Sympathomimetics tend to produce hyperglycemia and may lead to loss of glycemic control).
No products indexed under this heading.

Methyclothiazide (Thiazides tend to produce hyperglycemia and may lead to loss of glycemic control).
No products indexed under this heading.

Methylprednisolone Acetate (Corticosteroids tend to produce hyperglycemia and may lead to loss of glycemic control). Products include:
- Depo-Medrol Injectable Suspension 2617
- Depo-Medrol Single-Dose Vial 2619

Methylprednisolone Sodium Succinate (Corticosteroids tend to produce hyperglycemia and may lead to loss of glycemic control).
No products indexed under this heading.

Metolazone (Diuretics tend to produce hyperglycemia and may lead to loss of glycemic control).
No products indexed under this heading.

Mibefradil Dihydrochloride (Calcium channel blocking drugs tend to produce hyperglycemia and may lead to loss of glycemic control).
No products indexed under this heading.

Morphine Sulfate (Cationic drugs that are eliminated by renal tubular secretion theoretically have the potential for interaction with metformin by competing for common renal tubular transport system). Products include:
- Avinza Capsules 1741
- Kadian Capsules 577
- MS Contin Tablets 2701

Nicardipine Hydrochloride (Calcium channel blocking drugs tend to produce hyperglycemia and may lead to loss of glycemic control). Products include:
- Cardene I.V. 2497

Nicotinic Acid (Nicotinic acid tends to produce hyperglycemia and may lead to loss of glycemic control).
No products indexed under this heading.

Nifedipine (Co-administration of nifedipine increased plasma metformin Cmax and AUC by 20% and 9%, respectively, and increased the amount excreted in the urine. Nifedipine appears to enhance the absorption of metformin). Products include:
- Adalat CC Tablets 2964

Nimodipine (Calcium channel blocking drugs tend to produce hyperglycemia and may lead to loss of glycemic control). Products include:
- Nimotop Capsules 749

Nisoldipine (Calcium channel blocking drugs tend to produce hyperglycemia and may lead to loss of glycemic control). Products include:
- Sular Tablets 3122

Norepinephrine Bitartrate (Sympathomimetics tend to produce hyperglycemia and may lead to loss of glycemic control).
No products indexed under this heading.

Norethindrone (Oral contraceptives tend to produce hyperglycemia and may lead to loss of glycemic control). Products include:
- Ortho Micronor Tablets 2426

Norethynodrel (Oral contraceptives tend to produce hyperglycemia and may lead to loss of glycemic control).
No products indexed under this heading.

Norgestimate (Oral contraceptives tend to produce hyperglycemia and may lead to loss of glycemic control). Products include:
- Ortho-Cyclen/Ortho Tri-Cyclen 2429
- Ortho Tri-Cyclen Lo Tablets 2436

Norgestrel (Oral contraceptives tend to produce hyperglycemia and may lead to loss of glycemic control).
No products indexed under this heading.

Perphenazine (Phenothiazines tend to produce hyperglycemia and may lead to loss of glycemic control).
No products indexed under this heading.

Phenylephrine Bitartrate (Sympathomimetics tend to produce hyperglycemia and may lead to loss of glycemic control).
No products indexed under this heading.

Phenylephrine Hydrochloride (Sympathomimetics tend to produce hyperglycemia and may lead to loss of glycemic control). Products include:
- Comtrex Maximum Strength Non-Drowsy Cold & Cough Caplets .... ■ 725
- Comtrex Maximum Strength Day/Night Severe Cold & Sinus Caplets - Day Formulation .... ■ 725
- Comtrex Maximum Strength Day/Night Severe Cold & Sinus Caplets - Night Formulation .... ■ 725
- Contac Cold and Flu Maximum Strength Caplets .... ■ 728
- Contac Cold and Flu Day and Night Caplets (Day Formulation Only) .... ■ 727
- Contac Cold and Flu Day and Night Caplets (Night Formulation Only) .... ■ 727
- Contac Cold and Flu Non-Drowsy Caplets .... ■ 728
- Contac-D Cold Non-Drowsy Tablets .... ■ 729
- Children's Dimetapp Cold & Allergy Elixir .... ■ 730
- Children's Dimetapp Cold & Allergy Chewable Tablets .... ■ 730
- Children's Dimetapp DM Cold & Cough Elixir .... ■ 731
- Toddler's Dimetapp Cold and Cough Drops .... ■ 732
- Excedrin Sinus Headache Caplets/Tablets .... ■ 610
- 4-Way Fast Acting Nasal Spray .... ■ 775
- 4-Way Menthol Nasal Spray .... ■ 775
- Preparation H Maximum Strength Cream .... ■ 666
- Preparation H Cooling Gel .... ■ 666
- Preparation H .... ■ 666
- Refenesen PE Caplets .... ■ 721
- Robitussin Cough & Allergy Syrup .. ■ 736
- Robitussin Cough & Cold Nighttime Liquid .... ■ 736
- Robitussin Cough, Cold & Flu Nighttime Liquid .... ■ 738
- Robitussin Head & Chest Congestion PE Syrup .... ■ 739
- Robitussin Pediatric Cough & Cold Nighttime Liquid .... ■ 736
- TheraFlu Cold & Cough Hot Liquid .... ■ 740
- TheraFlu Cold & Sore Throat Hot Liquid .... ■ 741
- TheraFlu Flu & Sore Throat Hot Liquid .... ■ 742
- TheraFlu Daytime Severe Cold Hot Liquid .... ■ 742
- TheraFlu Nighttime Severe Cold Hot Liquid .... ■ 740
- TheraFlu Warming Relief Daytime Severe Cold .... ■ 743
- TheraFlu Warming Relief Nighttime Severe Cold .... ■ 743
- Triaminic Chest & Nasal Congestion Liquid .... ■ 746
- Triaminic Cold & Allergy Liquid .... ■ 746
- Triaminic Daytime Cold & Cough Liquid .... ■ 745
- Triaminic Nighttime Cold & Cough Liquid .... ■ 746
- Triaminic Thin Strips Cold .... ■ 748
- Triaminic Thin Strips Cold & Cough .... ■ 778
- Triaminic Infant Thin Strips Decongestant .... ■ 747
- Triaminic Infant Thin Strips Decongestant Plus Cough .... ■ 747
- Children's Tylenol Plus Flu Oral Suspension .... ■ 749
- Tylenol Cold Head Congestion Daytime Caplets with Cool Burst and Gelcaps .... ■ 750
- Tylenol Cold Multi-Symptom Daytime Liquid .... ■ 752
- Tylenol Cold Multi-Symptom Severe Daytime Liquid .... ■ 752
- Concentrated Tylenol Infants' Drops Plus Cold & Cough .... ■ 754
- Tylenol Allergy Multi-Symptom Caplets with Cool Burst and Gelcaps 1872
- Tylenol Allergy Multi-Symptom Nighttime Caplets with Cool Burst 1872
- Children's Tylenol Plus Cold Suspension Liquid 1879
- Children's Tylenol Plus Cold & Allergy Suspension Liquid 1878
- Children's Tylenol Plus Flu Suspension Liquid 1881
- Children's Tylenol Plus Multi-Symptom Cold Suspension Liquid 1879
- Tylenol Cold Head Congestion Daytime Caplets with Cool Burst 1873
- Tylenol Cold Head Congestion Nighttime Caplets with Cool Burst 1873
- Tylenol Cold Head Congestion Severe Caplets with Cool Burst 1873
- Tylenol Cold Multi-Symptom Daytime Caplets with Cool Burst and Gelcaps 1874
- Tylenol Cold Multi-Symptom Daytime Liquid with Citrus Burst ... 1874
- Tylenol Cold Multi-Symptom Nighttime Caplets with Cool Burst 1874
- Tylenol Cold Multi-Symptom Nighttime Liquid with Cool Burst ... 1874
- Tylenol Cold Multi-Symptom Severe Caplets with Cool Burst 1874
- Tylenol Cold Multi-Symptom Severe Daytime Liquid with Citrus Burst 1874
- Tylenol Sinus Congestion & Pain Daytime Caplets with Cool Burst and Gelcaps 1876
- Tylenol Sinus Congestion & Pain Nighttime Caplets with Cool Burst 1876
- Tylenol Sinus Congestion & Pain Severe Caplets with Cool Burst 1876
- Vicks 44D Cough & Head Congestion Relief Liquid .... ■ 760
- Vicks DayQuil LiquiCaps/Liquid Multi-Symptom Cold/Flu Relief .... ■ 761
- Zicam Cough Plus D Cough Spray .... ■ 767

Phenylephrine Tannate (Sympathomimetics tend to produce hyperglycemia and may lead to loss of glycemic control).
No products indexed under this heading.

Phenylpropanolamine Hydrochloride (Sympathomimetics tend to produce hyperglycemia and may lead to loss of glycemic control).
No products indexed under this heading.

Phenytoin (Phenytoin tends to produce hyperglycemia and may lead to loss of glycemic control).
No products indexed under this heading.

Phenytoin Sodium (Phenytoin tends to produce hyperglycemia and may lead to loss of glycemic control). Products include:
- Phenytek Capsules 2160

Pirbuterol Acetate (Sympathomimetics tend to produce hyperglycemia and may lead to loss of glycemic control). Products include:
- Maxair Autohaler 1852

Food Interactions

Alcohol (Alcohol is known to potentiate the effect of metformin on lactate metabolism; therefore, patients should be warned against excessive acute or chronic intake).

FORTAZ INJECTION

(Ceftazidime) 1453
See Fortaz for Injection

FORTAZ FOR INJECTION

(Ceftazidime) 1453
May interact with aminoglycosides and certain other agents. Compounds in these categories include:

Amikacin Sulfate (Potential for nephrotoxicity following concomitant administration).

No products indexed under this heading.

Chloramphenicol (Possibility of antagonism *in vivo*, particularly when bactericidal activity is desired; avoid this combination).

No products indexed under this heading.

Chloramphenicol Palmitate (Possibility of antagonism *in vivo*, particularly when bactericidal activity is desired; avoid this combination).

No products indexed under this heading.

Chloramphenicol Sodium Succinate (Possibility of antagonism *in vivo*, particularly when bactericidal activity is desired; avoid this combination).
No products indexed under this heading.

Furosemide (Potential for nephrotoxicity following concomitant administration). Products include:
Furosemide Tablets 2154

Gentamicin Sulfate (Potential for nephrotoxicity following concomitant administration). Products include:
Garamycin Injectable 3014
Pred-G Ophthalmic Ointment .... ⊙237
Pred-G Ophthalmic Suspension ...... ⊙236

Kanamycin Sulfate (Potential for nephrotoxicity following concomitant administration).
No products indexed under this heading.

Streptomycin Sulfate (Potential for nephrotoxicity following concomitant administration).
No products indexed under this heading.

Tobramycin (Potential for nephrotoxicity following concomitant administration). Products include:
TOBI Solution for Inhalation 2298
TobraDex Ophthalmic Ointment 562
TobraDex Ophthalmic Suspension ... 563
Zylet Ophthalmic Suspension .... ⊙259

Tobramycin Sulfate (Potential for nephrotoxicity following concomitant administration).
No products indexed under this heading.

FORTEO FOR INJECTION

(Teriparatide) 1767
May interact with cardiac glycosides. Compounds in these categories include:

Deslanoside (Hypercalcemia may pre-dispose patients to digitalis toxicity. Because teriparatide transiently increases serum calcium, teriparatide should be used with caution in patients taking digitalis).
No products indexed under this heading.

Digitalis Glycoside Preparations (Hypercalcemia may pre-dispose patients to digitalis toxicity. Because teriparatide transiently increases serum calcium, teriparatide should be used with caution in patients taking digitalis).
No products indexed under this heading.

Digitoxin (Hypercalcemia may pre-dispose patients to digitalis toxicity. Because teriparatide transiently increases serum calcium, teriparatide should be used with caution in patients taking digitalis).
No products indexed under this heading.

Digoxin (Hypercalcemia may pre-dispose patients to digitalis toxicity. Because teriparatide transiently increases serum calcium, teriparatide should be used with caution in patients taking digitalis). Products include:
Lanoxicaps Capsules 1490
Lanoxin Injection 1494
Lanoxin Injection Pediatric 1497
Lanoxin Tablets 1500

FORTICAL NASAL SPRAY

(Calcitonin-Salmon) 3337
None cited in PDR database.

FOSAMAX ORAL SOLUTION

(Alendronate Sodium) 1969
See Fosamax Tablets

FOSAMAX TABLETS

(Alendronate Sodium) 1969
May interact with antacids containing aluminum, calcium and magnesium, calcium preparations, non-steroidal anti-inflammatory agents, and certain other agents. Compounds in these categories include:

Aluminum Carbonate (May interfere with the absorption of alendronate; patient must wait at least one-half hour after taking alendronate before taking any drug).
No products indexed under this heading.

Aluminum Hydroxide (May interfere with the absorption of alendronate; patient must wait at least one-half hour after taking alendronate before taking any drug). Products include:
Gaviscon Regular Strength Liquid .. ▣658
Gaviscon Regular Strength Tablets....................................... ▣658
Gaviscon Extra Strength Liquid ...... ▣658
Gaviscon Extra Strength Tablets .... ▣658
Maalox Regular Strength Antacid/Antigas Liquid................. 2175
Maalox Max Maximum Strength Antacid/Anti-Gas Liquid............. 2176

Aspirin (Co-administration with doses of alendronate greater than 10 mg/day and aspirin-containing compounds can increase the incidence of gastrointestinal adverse events; one case of anastomotic ulcer with mild hemorrhage has been reported in a patient with history of peptic ulcer disease and gastrectomy on alendronate 10 mg/day plus aspirin). Products include:
Aggrenox Capsules 822
Bayer Aspirin 744
BC Allergy Sinus Cold Powder .... ▣677
BC Headache Powder .... ▣677
Arthritis Strength BC Powder .... ▣677
BC Sinus Cold Powder .... ▣677
Excedrin Extra Strength Caplets/Tablets/Geltabs............. ▣684
Excedrin Migraine Caplets/Tablets/Geltabs............. ▣609
Goody's Body Pain Formula Powder.. ▣684
Goody's Extra Strength Headache Powders.................... ▣611
Goody's Extra Strength Pain Relief Tablets................................ ▣685
Percodan Tablets 1132
St. Joseph 81 mg Aspirin Chewable and Enteric Coated Tablets 1869

Aspirin, Enteric Coated (Co-administration with doses of alendronate greater than 10 mg/day and aspirin-containing compounds can increase the incidence of gastrointestinal adverse events; one case of anastomotic ulcer with mild hemorrhage has been reported in a patient with history of peptic ulcer disease and gastrectomy on alendronate 10 mg/day plus aspirin).
No products indexed under this heading.

Aspirin Buffered (Co-administration with doses of alendronate greater than 10 mg/day and aspirin-containing compounds can increase the incidence of gastrointestinal adverse events; one case of anastomotic ulcer with mild hemorrhage has been reported in a patient with history of peptic ulcer disease and gastrectomy on alendronate 10 mg/day plus aspirin). Products include:
Bufferin Extra Strength Tablets ...... ▣678
Bufferin Regular Strength Tablets ... ▣678

Calcium Carbonate (May interfere with the absorption of alendronate; patient must wait at least one-half hour after taking alendronate before taking any drug). Products include:
Actonel with Calcium Tablets 2688
Calcet Tablets 2138
Caltrate 600 PLUS .... ▣809
Caltrate 600 + D Tablets .... ▣809
D-Cal Chewable Caplets .... ▣812
Gas-X with Maalox .... ▣656
Maalox Regular Strength Antacid Chewable Tablets 2177
Maalox Max Maximum Strength Antacid/Antigas Chewable Tablets.. 2176
Maalox Max Maximum Strength Chewable Tablets........................ ▣660
Os-Cal Chewable Tablets .... ▣818
Pepcid Complete Chewable Tablets.. 1701
Children's Pepto 2674
PremCal Light, Regular, and Extra Strength Tablets................ ▣818
Tums .... ▣664

Calcium Chloride (May interfere with the absorption of alendronate; patient must wait at least one-half hour after taking alendronate before taking any drug).
No products indexed under this heading.

Calcium Citrate (May interfere with the absorption of alendronate; patient must wait at least one-half hour after taking alendronate before taking any drug). Products include:
Active Calcium Tablets 3339
Citracal Caplets .... ▣703
Citracal Lemon Cream Creamy Bites... 2139
Citracal Prenatal + DHA Tablets and Capsules............................. 2139

Calcium Glubionate (May interfere with the absorption of alendronate; patient must wait at least one-half hour after taking alendronate before taking any drug).
No products indexed under this heading.

Celecoxib (Since NSAID use is associated with gastrointestinal irritation, caution should be used during concomitant use; no increase in the incidence of gastrointestinal irritation was reported in clinical trials). Products include:
Celebrex Capsules 3134

Diclofenac Potassium (Since NSAID use is associated with gastrointestinal irritation, caution should be used during concomitant use; no increase in the incidence of gastrointestinal irritation was reported in clinical trials).
No products indexed under this heading.

Diclofenac Sodium (Since NSAID use is associated with gastrointestinal irritation, caution should be used during concomitant use; no increase in the incidence of gastrointestinal irritation was reported in clinical trials). Products include:
Arthrotec Tablets 3129
Voltaren Ophthalmic Solution 2309
Voltaren Tablets 2307
Voltaren-XR Tablets 2310

Etodolac (Since NSAID use is associated with gastrointestinal irritation, caution should be used during concomitant use; no increase in the incidence of gastrointestinal irritation was reported in clinical trials).
No products indexed under this heading.

Fenoprofen Calcium (Since NSAID use is associated with gastrointestinal irritation, caution should be used during concomitant use; no increase in the incidence of gastrointestinal irritation was reported in clinical trials). Products include:
Nalfon Capsules 2502

Flurbiprofen (Since NSAID use is associated with gastrointestinal irritation, caution should be used during concomitant use; no increase in the incidence of gastrointestinal irritation was reported in clinical trials).
No products indexed under this heading.

Ibuprofen (Since NSAID use is associated with gastrointestinal irritation, caution should be used during concomitant use; no increase in the incidence of gastrointestinal irritation was reported in clinical trials). Products include:
Advil Allergy Sinus Caplets .... ▣770
Advil .... ▣674
Children's Advil Oral Suspension .... ▣603
Children's Advil Chewable Tablets .. ▣603
Advil Cold & Sinus .... ▣723
Infants' Advil Concentrated Drops .. ▣604
Infants' Advil Concentrated Drops - White Grape (Dye-Free)............. ▣604
Junior Strength Advil Swallow Tablets.. ▣605
Advil Migraine Liquigels .... ▣608
Advil Multi-Symptom Cold Caplets... ▣770
Advil PM Caplets .... ▣615
Motrin IB Tablets and Caplets 1866
Children's Motrin Oral Suspension ... 1867
Children's Motrin Non-Staining Dye-Free Oral Suspension............ 1867
Children's Motrin Cold Oral Suspension.................................. 1867
Infants' Motrin Concentrated Drops... 1867
Infants' Motrin Non-Staining Dye-Free Concentrated Drops....... 1867
Junior Strength Motrin Caplets and Chewable Tablets................. 1867
Vicoprofen Tablets 539

Indomethacin (Since NSAID use is associated with gastrointestinal irritation, caution should be used during concomitant use; no increase in the incidence of gastrointestinal irritation was reported in clinical trials). Products include:
Indocin 1995

Indomethacin Sodium Trihydrate (Since NSAID use is associated with gastrointestinal irritation, caution should be used during concomitant use; no increase in the incidence of gastrointestinal irritation was reported in clinical trials). Products include:
Indocin I.V. 2465

Ketoprofen (Since NSAID use is associated with gastrointestinal irritation, caution should be used during concomitant use; no increase in the incidence of gastrointestinal irritation was reported in clinical trials).
No products indexed under this heading.

Ketorolac Tromethamine (Since NSAID use is associated with gastrointestinal irritation, caution should be used during concomitant use; no increase in the incidence of gastrointestinal irritation was reported in clinical trials). Products include:

Acular Ophthalmic Solution 565
Acular LS Ophthalmic Solution 566

Magaldrate (May interfere with the absorption of alendronate; patient must wait at least one-half hour after taking alendronate before taking any drug).
No products indexed under this heading.

Magnesium Hydroxide (May interfere with the absorption of alendronate; patient must wait at least one-half hour after taking alendronate before taking any drug). Products include:
Maalox Regular Strength Antacid/Antigas Liquid 2175
Maalox Max Maximum Strength Antacid/Anti-Gas Liquid 2176
Pepcid Complete Chewable Tablets 1701

Magnesium Oxide (May interfere with the absorption of alendronate; patient must wait at least one-half hour after taking alendronate before taking any drug). Products include:
Beelith Tablets 759
PremCal Light, Regular, and Extra Strength Tablets 818

Meclofenamate Sodium (Since NSAID use is associated with gastrointestinal irritation, caution should be used during concomitant use; no increase in the incidence of gastrointestinal irritation was reported in clinical trials).
No products indexed under this heading.

Mefenamic Acid (Since NSAID use is associated with gastrointestinal irritation, caution should be used during concomitant use; no increase in the incidence of gastrointestinal irritation was reported in clinical trials).
No products indexed under this heading.

Meloxicam (Since NSAID use is associated with gastrointestinal irritation, caution should be used during concomitant use; no increase in the incidence of gastrointestinal irritation was reported in clinical trials). Products include:
Mobic Oral Suspension 863
Mobic Tablets 863

Nabumetone (Since NSAID use is associated with gastrointestinal irritation, caution should be used during concomitant use; no increase in the incidence of gastrointestinal irritation was reported in clinical trials).
No products indexed under this heading.

Naproxen (Since NSAID use is associated with gastrointestinal irritation, caution should be used during concomitant use; no increase in the incidence of gastrointestinal irritation was reported in clinical trials). Products include:
EC-Naprosyn Delayed-Release Tablets 2761
Naprosyn Suspension 2761
Naprosyn Tablets 2761
Prevacid NapraPAC 3280

Naproxen Sodium (Since NSAID use is associated with gastrointestinal irritation, caution should be used during concomitant use; no increase in the incidence of gastrointestinal irritation was reported in clinical trials). Products include:
Aleve Caplets 742
Aleve Gelcaps 743
Aleve Tablets 743
Aleve Cold & Sinus Caplets 744
Anaprox Tablets 2761
Anaprox DS Tablets 2761

Oxaprozin (Since NSAID use is associated with gastrointestinal irritation, caution should be used during concomitant use; no increase in the incidence of gastrointestinal irritation was reported in clinical trials).
No products indexed under this heading.

Phenylbutazone (Since NSAID use is associated with gastrointestinal irritation, caution should be used during concomitant use; no increase in the incidence of gastrointestinal irritation was reported in clinical trials).
No products indexed under this heading.

Piroxicam (Since NSAID use is associated with gastrointestinal irritation, caution should be used during concomitant use; no increase in the incidence of gastrointestinal irritation was reported in clinical trials).
No products indexed under this heading.

Ranitidine Hydrochloride (Intravenous ranitidine has shown to double the bioavailability of oral alendronate; clinical significance of this increased bioavailability and whether similar increases will occur with oral ranitidine are unknown). Products include:
Zantac 1624
Zantac Injection 1619
Zantac Injection Pharmacy Bulk Package 1622

Rofecoxib (Since NSAID use is associated with gastrointestinal irritation, caution should be used during concomitant use; no increase in the incidence of gastrointestinal irritation was reported in clinical trials).
No products indexed under this heading.

Sulindac (Since NSAID use is associated with gastrointestinal irritation, caution should be used during concomitant use; no increase in the incidence of gastrointestinal irritation was reported in clinical trials). Products include:
Clinoril Tablets 1924

Tolmetin Sodium (Since NSAID use is associated with gastrointestinal irritation, caution should be used during concomitant use; no increase in the incidence of gastrointestinal irritation was reported in clinical trials).
No products indexed under this heading.

Valdecoxib (Since NSAID use is associated with gastrointestinal irritation, caution should be used during concomitant use; no increase in the incidence of gastrointestinal irritation was reported in clinical trials).
No products indexed under this heading.

Food Interactions

Beverages, caffeine-containing (Concomitant administration of alendronate with coffee reduces bioavailability by approximately 60%).

Meal, unspecified (Standardized breakfast decreases bioavailability by approximately 40% when alendronate is administered either one-half or 1 hour before breakfast).

Orange Juice (Concomitant administration of alendronate with orange juice reduces bioavailability by approximately 60%).

FOSAMAX PLUS D TABLETS

(Alendronate Sodium, Cholecalciferol) 1977

May interact with antacids containing aluminum, calcium and magnesium, aspirin-acetylsalicylic acid, calcium preparations, non-steroidal anti-inflammatory agents, and certain other agents. Compounds in these categories include:

Aluminum Carbonate (Antacids may interfere with the absorption of aledronate. Therefore, patients must wait at least one-half hour after taking aledronate sodium/cholecalciferol before taking any other oral medications).
No products indexed under this heading.

Aluminum Hydroxide (Antacids may interfere with the absorption of aledronate. Therefore, patients must wait at least one-half hour after taking aledronate sodium/cholecalciferol before taking any other oral medications). Products include:
Gaviscon Regular Strength Liquid .. 658
Gaviscon Regular Strength Tablets 658
Gaviscon Extra Strength Liquid 658
Gaviscon Extra Strength Tablets 658
Maalox Regular Strength Antacid/Antigas Liquid 2175
Maalox Max Maximum Strength Antacid/Anti-Gas Liquid 2176

Aspirin (Studies have shown an increased incidence of upper gastrointestinal adverse events in patients receiving concomitant therapy with daily doses of aledronate greater than 10 mg and aspirin-containing products). Products include:
Aggrenox Capsules 822
Bayer Aspirin 744
BC Allergy Sinus Cold Powder 677
BC Headache Powder 677
Arthritis Strength BC Powder 677
BC Sinus Cold Powder 677
Excedrin Extra Strength Caplets/Tablets/Geltabs 684
Excedrin Migraine Caplets/Tablets/Geltabs 609
Goody's Body Pain Formula Powder 684
Goody's Extra Strength Headache Powders 611
Goody's Extra Strength Pain Relief Tablets 685
Percodan Tablets 1132
St. Joseph 81 mg Aspirin Chewable and Enteric Coated Tablets 1869

Aspirin, Enteric Coated (Studies have shown an increased incidence of upper gastrointestinal adverse events in patients receiving concomitant therapy with daily doses of aledronate greater than 10 mg and aspirin-containing products).
No products indexed under this heading.

Aspirin Buffered (Studies have shown an increased incidence of upper gastrointestinal adverse events in patients receiving concomitant therapy with daily doses of aledronate greater than 10 mg and aspirin-containing products). Products include:
Bufferin Extra Strength Tablets 678
Bufferin Regular Strength Tablets ... 678

Calcium Carbonate (Calcium supplements may interfere with the absorption of aledronate. Therefore, patients must wait at least one-half hour after taking aledronate sodium/cholecalciferol before taking any other oral medications). Products include:
Actonel with Calcium Tablets 2688
Calcet Tablets 2138
Caltrate 600 PLUS 809
Caltrate 600 + D Tablets 809
D-Cal Chewable Caplets 812
Gas-X with Maalox 656
Maalox Regular Strength Antacid Chewable Tablets 2177
Maalox Max Maximum Strength Antacid/Antigas Chewable Tablets 2176
Maalox Max Maximum Strength Chewable Tablets 660
Os-Cal Chewable Tablets 818
Pepcid Complete Chewable Tablets 1701
Children's Pepto 2674
PremCal Light, Regular, and Extra Strength Tablets 818
Tums 664

Calcium Chloride (Calcium supplements may interfere with the absorption of aledronate. Therefore, patients must wait at least one-half hour after taking aledronate sodium/cholecalciferol before taking any other oral medications).
No products indexed under this heading.

Calcium Citrate (Calcium supplements may interfere with the absorption of aledronate. Therefore, patients must wait at least one-half hour after taking aledronate sodium/cholecalciferol before taking any other oral medications). Products include:
Active Calcium Tablets 3339
Citracal Caplets 703
Citracal Lemon Cream Creamy Bites 2139
Citracal Prenatal + DHA Tablets and Capsules 2139

Calcium Glubionate (Calcium supplements may interfere with the absorption of aledronate. Therefore, patients must wait at least one-half hour after taking aledronate sodium/cholecalciferol before taking any other oral medications).
No products indexed under this heading.

Celecoxib (Since NSAID use is associated with gastrointestinal irritation, caution should be used during concomitant use with aledronate sodium/cholecalciferol. No increase in the incidence of gastrointestinal irritation was reported in clinical trials). Products include:
Celebrex Capsules 3134

Cholestyramine (Concomitant use with bile acid sequestrants may impair the absorption of vitamin D).
No products indexed under this heading.

Colestipol (Concomitant use with bile acid sequestrants may impair the absorption of vitamin D).
No products indexed under this heading.

Diclofenac Potassium (Since NSAID use is associated with gastrointestinal irritation, caution should be used during concomitant use with aledronate sodium/cholecalciferol. No increase in the incidence of gastrointestinal irritation was reported in clinical trials).
No products indexed under this heading.

Diclofenac Sodium (Since NSAID use is associated with gastrointestinal irritation, caution should be used during concomitant use with aledronate sodium/cholecalciferol. No

increase in the incidence of gastrointestinal irritation was reported in clinical trials). Products include:
Arthrotec Tablets ... 3129
Voltaren Ophthalmic Solution ... 2309
Voltaren Tablets ... 2307
Voltaren-XR Tablets ... 2310

Etodolac (Since NSAID use is associated with gastrointestinal irritation, caution should be used during concomitant use with aledronate sodium/cholecalciferol. No increase in the incidence of gastrointestinal irritation was reported in clinical trials).
No products indexed under this heading.

Fenoprofen Calcium (Since NSAID use is associated with gastrointestinal irritation, caution should be used during concomitant use with aledronate sodium/cholecalciferol. No increase in the incidence of gastrointestinal irritation was reported in clinical trials). Products include:
Nalfon Capsules ... 2502

Flurbiprofen (Since NSAID use is associated with gastrointestinal irritation, caution should be used during concomitant use with aledronate sodium/cholecalciferol. No increase in the incidence of gastrointestinal irritation was reported in clinical trials).
No products indexed under this heading.

Ibuprofen (Since NSAID use is associated with gastrointestinal irritation, caution should be used during concomitant use with aledronate sodium/cholecalciferol. No increase in the incidence of gastrointestinal irritation was reported in clinical trials). Products include:
Advil Allergy Sinus Caplets ... ■ 770
Advil ... ■ 674
Children's Advil Oral Suspension ... ■ 603
Children's Advil Chewable Tablets ... ■ 603
Advil Cold & Sinus ... ■ 723
Infants' Advil Concentrated Drops ... ■ 604
Infants' Advil Concentrated Drops - White Grape (Dye-Free) ... ■ 604
Junior Strength Advil Swallow Tablets ... ■ 605
Advil Migraine Liquigels ... ■ 608
Advil Multi-Symptom Cold Caplets ... ■ 770
Advil PM Caplets ... ■ 615
Motrin IB Tablets and Caplets ... 1866
Children's Motrin Oral Suspension ... 1867
Children's Motrin Non-Staining Dye-Free Oral Suspension ... 1867
Children's Motrin Cold Oral Suspension ... 1867
Infants' Motrin Concentrated Drops ... 1867
Infants' Motrin Non-Staining Dye-Free Concentrated Drops ... 1867
Junior Strength Motrin Caplets and Chewable Tablets ... 1867
Vicoprofen Tablets ... 539

Indomethacin (Since NSAID use is associated with gastrointestinal irritation, caution should be used during concomitant use with aledronate sodium/cholecalciferol. No increase in the incidence of gastrointestinal irritation was reported in clinical trials). Products include:
Indocin ... 1995

Indomethacin Sodium Trihydrate (Since NSAID use is associated with gastrointestinal irritation, caution should be used during concomitant use with aledronate sodium/cholecalciferol. No increase in the incidence of gastrointestinal irritation was reported in clinical trials). Products include:
Indocin I.V. ... 2465

Ketoprofen (Since NSAID use is associated with gastrointestinal irritation, caution should be used during concomitant use with aledronate sodium/cholecalciferol. No increase in the incidence of gastrointestinal irritation was reported in clinical trials).
No products indexed under this heading.

Ketorolac Tromethamine (Since NSAID use is associated with gastrointestinal irritation, caution should be used during concomitant use with aledronate sodium/cholecalciferol. No increase in the incidence of gastrointestinal irritation was reported in clinical trials). Products include:
Acular Ophthalmic Solution ... 565
Acular LS Ophthalmic Solution ... 566

Magaldrate (Antacids may interfere with the absorption of aledronate. Therefore, patients must wait at least one-half hour after taking aledronate sodium/cholecalciferol before taking any other oral medications).
No products indexed under this heading.

Magnesium Hydroxide (Antacids may interfere with the absorption of aledronate. Therefore, patients must wait at least one-half hour after taking aledronate sodium/cholecalciferol before taking any other oral medications). Products include:
Maalox Regular Strength Antacid/Antigas Liquid ... 2175
Maalox Max Maximum Strength Antacid/Anti-Gas Liquid ... 2176
Pepcid Complete Chewable Tablets ... 1701

Magnesium Oxide (Antacids may interfere with the absorption of aledronate. Therefore, patients must wait at least one-half hour after taking aledronate sodium/cholecalciferol before taking any other oral medications). Products include:
Beelith Tablets ... 759
PremCal Light, Regular, and Extra Strength Tablets ... ■ 818

Meclofenamate Sodium (Since NSAID use is associated with gastrointestinal irritation, caution should be used during concomitant use with aledronate sodium/cholecalciferol. No increase in the incidence of gastrointestinal irritation was reported in clinical trials).
No products indexed under this heading.

Mefenamic Acid (Since NSAID use is associated with gastrointestinal irritation, caution should be used during concomitant use with aledronate sodium/cholecalciferol. No increase in the incidence of gastrointestinal irritation was reported in clinical trials).
No products indexed under this heading.

Meloxicam (Since NSAID use is associated with gastrointestinal irritation, caution should be used during concomitant use with aledronate sodium/cholecalciferol. No increase in the incidence of gastrointestinal irritation was reported in clinical trials). Products include:
Mobic Oral Suspension ... 863
Mobic Tablets ... 863

Nabumetone (Since NSAID use is associated with gastrointestinal irritation, caution should be used during concomitant use with aledronate sodium/cholecalciferol. No increase in the incidence of gastrointestinal irritation was reported in clinical trials).
No products indexed under this heading.

Naproxen (Since NSAID use is associated with gastrointestinal irritation, caution should be used during concomitant use with aledronate sodium/cholecalciferol. No increase in the incidence of gastrointestinal irritation was reported in clinical trials). Products include:
EC-Naprosyn Delayed-Release Tablets ... 2761
Naprosyn Suspension ... 2761
Naprosyn Tablets ... 2761
Prevacid NapraPAC ... 3280

Naproxen Sodium (Since NSAID use is associated with gastrointestinal irritation, caution should be used during concomitant use with aledronate sodium/cholecalciferol. No increase in the incidence of gastrointestinal irritation was reported in clinical trials). Products include:
Aleve Caplets ... 742
Aleve Gelcaps ... 743
Aleve Tablets ... 743
Aleve Cold & Sinus Caplets ... 744
Anaprox Tablets ... 2761
Anaprox DS Tablets ... 2761

Orlistat (Concomitant use with orlistat may impair the absorption of vitamin D). Products include:
Xenical Capsules ... 2831

Oxaprozin (Since NSAID use is associated with gastrointestinal irritation, caution should be used during concomitant use with aledronate sodium/cholecalciferol. No increase in the incidence of gastrointestinal irritation was reported in clinical trials).
No products indexed under this heading.

Phenylbutazone (Since NSAID use is associated with gastrointestinal irritation, caution should be used during concomitant use with aledronate sodium/cholecalciferol. No increase in the incidence of gastrointestinal irritation was reported in clinical trials).
No products indexed under this heading.

Piroxicam (Since NSAID use is associated with gastrointestinal irritation, caution should be used during concomitant use with aledronate sodium/cholecalciferol. No increase in the incidence of gastrointestinal irritation was reported in clinical trials).
No products indexed under this heading.

Ranitidine Hydrochloride (Intravenous ranitidine was shown to double the bioavailability of oral aledronate. The clinical significance of this increased bioavailability and whether similar increases will occur in patients given oral H2-antagonists is unknown). Products include:
Zantac ... 1624
Zantac Injection ... 1619
Zantac Injection Pharmacy Bulk Package ... 1622

Rofecoxib (Since NSAID use is associated with gastrointestinal irritation, caution should be used during concomitant use with aledronate sodium/cholecalciferol. No increase in the incidence of gastrointestinal irritation was reported in clinical trials).
No products indexed under this heading.

Sulindac (Since NSAID use is associated with gastrointestinal irritation, caution should be used during concomitant use with aledronate sodium/cholecalciferol. No increase in the incidence of gastrointestinal irritation was reported in clinical trials). Products include:
Clinoril Tablets ... 1924

Tolmetin Sodium (Since NSAID use is associated with gastrointestinal irritation, caution should be used during concomitant use with aledronate sodium/cholecalciferol. No increase in the incidence of gastrointestinal irritation was reported in clinical trials).
No products indexed under this heading.

Valdecoxib (Since NSAID use is associated with gastrointestinal irritation, caution should be used during concomitant use with aledronate sodium/cholecalciferol. No increase in the incidence of gastrointestinal irritation was reported in clinical trials).
No products indexed under this heading.

Food Interactions

Beverages, caffeine-containing (Concomitant administration of alendronate with coffee reduces bioavailability by approximately 60%).

Meal, unspecified (Bioavailability was decreased (by approximately 40%) when 10 mg alendronate was administered either 0.5 or 1 hour before a standardized breakfast, when compared to dosing 2 hours before eating).

Orange Juice (Concomitant administration of alendronate with orange juice reduces bioavailability by approximately 60%).

FOSRENOL CHEWABLE TABLETS

(Lanthanum Carbonate) ... 3183
May interact with antacids. Compounds in these categories include:

Aluminum Carbonate (Avoid administering within 2 hours of antacids).
No products indexed under this heading.

Aluminum Hydroxide (Avoid administering within 2 hours of antacids). Products include:
Gaviscon Regular Strength Liquid ... ■ 658
Gaviscon Regular Strength Tablets ... ■ 658
Gaviscon Extra Strength Liquid ... ■ 658
Gaviscon Extra Strength Tablets ... ■ 658
Maalox Regular Strength Antacid/Antigas Liquid ... 2175
Maalox Max Maximum Strength Antacid/Anti-Gas Liquid ... 2176

Magaldrate (Avoid administering within 2 hours of antacids).
No products indexed under this heading.

Magnesium Hydroxide (Avoid administering within 2 hours of antacids). Products include:

Maalox Regular Strength Antacid/Antigas Liquid 2175
Maalox Max Maximum Strength Antacid/Anti-Gas Liquid 2176
Pepcid Complete Chewable Tablets 1701

Magnesium Oxide (Avoid administering within 2 hours of antacids). Products include:
Beelith Tablets 759
PremCal Light, Regular, and Extra Strength Tablets 818

Sodium Bicarbonate (Avoid administering within 2 hours of antacids). Products include:
Colyte with Flavor Packs for Oral Solution 3088
HalfLytely and Bisacodyl Tablets Bowel Prep Kit with Flavors Packs 881
TriLyte with Flavor Packs for Oral Solution 3100

4-WAY FAST ACTING NASAL SPRAY

(Phenylephrine Hydrochloride) 775
None cited in PDR database.

4-WAY MENTHOL NASAL SPRAY

(Phenylephrine Hydrochloride) 775

4-WAY SALINE NASAL SPRAY

(Dietary Supplement) 775
None cited in PDR database.

FRAGMIN INJECTION

(Dalteparin Sodium) 1097
May interact with anesthetics, oral anticoagulants, platelet inhibitors, and thrombolytics. Compounds in these categories include:

Alfentanil Hydrochloride (Patients undergoing regional anesthesia should not receive dalteparin sodium for unstable angina or non-Q-wave myocardial infarction due to an increased risk of bleeding associated with the dosage of dalteparin sodium recommended for unstable angina and non-Q-wave myocardial infarction).
No products indexed under this heading.

Alteplase (Dalteparin sodium should be used with care in patients receiving oral anticoagulants, platelet inhibitors, and thrombolytic agents because of an increased risk of bleeding). Products include:
Activase I.V. 1223
Cathflo Activase 1231

Anisindione (Dalteparin sodium should be used with care in patients receiving oral anticoagulants, platelet inhibitors, and thrombolytic agents because of an increased risk of bleeding). Products include:
Miradon Tablets 3042

Anistreplase (Dalteparin sodium should be used with care in patients receiving oral anticoagulants, platelet inhibitors, and thrombolytic agents because of an increased risk of bleeding).
No products indexed under this heading.

Aspirin (Dalteparin sodium should be used with care in patients receiving oral anticoagulants, platelet inhibitors, and thrombolytic agents because of an increased risk of bleeding). Products include:
Aggrenox Capsules 822
Bayer Aspirin 744
BC Allergy Sinus Cold Powder 677
BC Headache Powder 677
Arthritis Strength BC Powder 677
BC Sinus Cold Powder 677
Excedrin Extra Strength Caplets/Tablets/Geltabs 684
Excedrin Migraine Caplets/Tablets/Geltabs 609
Goody's Body Pain Formula Powder 684
Goody's Extra Strength Headache Powders 611
Goody's Extra Strength Pain Relief Tablets 685
Percodan Tablets 1132
St. Joseph 81 mg Aspirin Chewable and Enteric Coated Tablets 1869

Aspirin, Enteric Coated (Dalteparin sodium should be used with care in patients receiving oral anticoagulants, platelet inhibitors, and thrombolytic agents because of an increased risk of bleeding).
No products indexed under this heading.

Aspirin Buffered (Dalteparin sodium should be used with care in patients receiving oral anticoagulants, platelet inhibitors, and thrombolytic agents because of an increased risk of bleeding). Products include:
Bufferin Extra Strength Tablets 678
Bufferin Regular Strength Tablets 678

Azlocillin Sodium (Dalteparin sodium should be used with care in patients receiving oral anticoagulants, platelet inhibitors, and thrombolytic agents because of an increased risk of bleeding).
No products indexed under this heading.

Carbenicillin Indanyl Sodium (Dalteparin sodium should be used with care in patients receiving oral anticoagulants, platelet inhibitors, and thrombolytic agents because of an increased risk of bleeding).
No products indexed under this heading.

Choline Magnesium Trisalicylate (Dalteparin sodium should be used with care in patients receiving oral anticoagulants, platelet inhibitors, and thrombolytic agents because of an increased risk of bleeding).
No products indexed under this heading.

Clopidogrel Bisulfate (Dalteparin sodium should be used with care in patients receiving oral anticoagulants, platelet inhibitors, and thrombolytic agents because of an increased risk of bleeding). Products include:
Plavix Tablets 917
Plavix Tablets 2926

Diclofenac Potassium (Dalteparin sodium should be used with care in patients receiving oral anticoagulants, platelet inhibitors, and thrombolytic agents because of an increased risk of bleeding).
No products indexed under this heading.

Diclofenac Sodium (Dalteparin sodium should be used with care in patients receiving oral anticoagulants, platelet inhibitors, and thrombolytic agents because of an increased risk of bleeding). Products include:
Arthrotec Tablets 3129
Voltaren Ophthalmic Solution 2309
Voltaren Tablets 2307
Voltaren-XR Tablets 2310

Dicumarol (Dalteparin sodium should be used with care in patients receiving oral anticoagulants, platelet inhibitors, and thrombolytic agents because of an increased risk of bleeding).
No products indexed under this heading.

Diflunisal (Dalteparin sodium should be used with care in patients receiving oral anticoagulants, platelet inhibitors, and thrombolytic agents because of an increased risk of bleeding). Products include:
Dolobid Tablets 1955

Dipyridamole (Dalteparin sodium should be used with care in patients receiving oral anticoagulants, platelet inhibitors, and thrombolytic agents because of an increased risk of bleeding). Products include:
Aggrenox Capsules 822
Persantine Tablets 868

Enflurane (Patients undergoing regional anesthesia should not receive dalteparin sodium for unstable angina or non-Q-wave myocardial infarction due to an increased risk of bleeding associated with the dosage of dalteparin sodium recommended for unstable angina and non-Q-wave myocardial infarction).
No products indexed under this heading.

Fenoprofen Calcium (Dalteparin sodium should be used with care in patients receiving oral anticoagulants, platelet inhibitors, and thrombolytic agents because of an increased risk of bleeding). Products include:
Nalfon Capsules 2502

Fentanyl Citrate (Patients undergoing regional anesthesia should not receive dalteparin sodium for unstable angina or non-Q-wave myocardial infarction due to an increased risk of bleeding associated with the dosage of dalteparin sodium recommended for unstable angina and non-Q-wave myocardial infarction). Products include:
Actiq 979

Flurbiprofen (Dalteparin sodium should be used with care in patients receiving oral anticoagulants, platelet inhibitors, and thrombolytic agents because of an increased risk of bleeding).
No products indexed under this heading.

Halothane (Patients undergoing regional anesthesia should not receive dalteparin sodium for unstable angina or non-Q-wave myocardial infarction due to an increased risk of bleeding associated with the dosage of dalteparin sodium recommended for unstable angina and non-Q-wave myocardial infarction).
No products indexed under this heading.

Ibuprofen (Dalteparin sodium should be used with care in patients receiving oral anticoagulants, platelet inhibitors, and thrombolytic agents because of an increased risk of bleeding). Products include:
Advil Allergy Sinus Caplets 770
Advil 674
Children's Advil Oral Suspension 603
Children's Advil Chewable Tablets 603
Advil Cold & Sinus 723
Infants' Advil Concentrated Drops 604
Infants' Advil Concentrated Drops - White Grape (Dye-Free) 604
Junior Strength Advil Swallow Tablets 605
Advil Migraine Liquigels 608
Advil Multi-Symptom Cold Caplets 770
Advil PM Caplets 615
Motrin IB Tablets and Caplets 1866
Children's Motrin Oral Suspension 1867
Children's Motrin Non-Staining Dye-Free Oral Suspension 1867
Children's Motrin Cold Oral Suspension 1867
Infants' Motrin Concentrated Drops 1867
Infants' Motrin Non-Staining Dye-Free Concentrated Drops 1867
Junior Strength Motrin Caplets and Chewable Tablets 1867
Vicoprofen Tablets 539

Indomethacin (Dalteparin sodium should be used with care in patients receiving oral anticoagulants, platelet inhibitors, and thrombolytic agents because of an increased risk of bleeding). Products include:
Indocin 1995

Indomethacin Sodium Trihydrate (Dalteparin sodium should be used with care in patients receiving oral anticoagulants, platelet inhibitors, and thrombolytic agents because of an increased risk of bleeding). Products include:
Indocin I.V. 2465

Isoflurane (Patients undergoing regional anesthesia should not receive dalteparin sodium for unstable angina or non-Q-wave myocardial infarction due to an increased risk of bleeding associated with the dosage of dalteparin sodium recommended for unstable angina and non-Q-wave myocardial infarction).
No products indexed under this heading.

Ketamine Hydrochloride (Patients undergoing regional anesthesia should not receive dalteparin sodium for unstable angina or non-Q-wave myocardial infarction due to an increased risk of bleeding associated with the dosage of dalteparin sodium recommended for unstable angina and non-Q-wave myocardial infarction).
No products indexed under this heading.

Ketoprofen (Dalteparin sodium should be used with care in patients receiving oral anticoagulants, platelet inhibitors, and thrombolytic agents because of an increased risk of bleeding).
No products indexed under this heading.

Magnesium Salicylate (Dalteparin sodium should be used with care in patients receiving oral anticoagulants, platelet inhibitors, and thrombolytic agents because of an increased risk of bleeding).
No products indexed under this heading.

Meclofenamate Sodium (Dalteparin sodium should be used with care in patients receiving oral anticoagulants, platelet inhibitors, and thrombolytic agents because of an increased risk of bleeding).
No products indexed under this heading.

Mefenamic Acid (Dalteparin sodium should be used with care in patients receiving oral anticoagulants, platelet inhibitors, and thrombolytic agents because of an increased risk of bleeding).
No products indexed under this heading.

Methohexital Sodium (Patients undergoing regional anesthesia should not receive dalteparin sodium for unstable angina or non-Q-wave myocardial infarction due to an increased risk of bleeding associated with the dosage of dalteparin sodium recommended for unstable angina and non-Q-wave myocardial infarction).
No products indexed under this heading.

Mezlocillin Sodium (Dalteparin sodium should be used with care in patients receiving oral anticoagulants, platelet inhibitors, and thrombolytic agents because of an increased risk of bleeding).
No products indexed under this heading.

Midazolam Hydrochloride (Patients undergoing regional anesthesia should not receive dalteparin sodium for unstable angina or non-Q-wave myocardial infarction due to an increased risk of bleeding associated with the dosage of dalteparin sodium recommended for unstable angina and non-Q-wave myocardial infarction).
No products indexed under this heading.

Nafcillin Sodium (Dalteparin sodium should be used with care in patients receiving oral anticoagulants, platelet inhibitors, and thrombolytic agents because of an increased risk of bleeding).
No products indexed under this heading.

Naproxen (Dalteparin sodium should be used with care in patients receiving oral anticoagulants, platelet inhibitors, and thrombolytic agents because of an increased risk of bleeding). Products include:

Naproxen Sodium (Dalteparin sodium should be used with care in patients receiving oral anticoagulants, platelet inhibitors, and thrombolytic agents because of an increased risk of bleeding). Products include:

Penicillin G Benzathine (Dalteparin sodium should be used with care in patients receiving oral anticoagulants, platelet inhibitors, and thrombolytic agents because of an increased risk of bleeding). Products include:

Penicillin G Procaine (Dalteparin sodium should be used with care in patients receiving oral anticoagulants, platelet inhibitors, and thrombolytic agents because of an increased risk of bleeding). Products include:

Phenylbutazone (Dalteparin sodium should be used with care in patients receiving oral anticoagulants, platelet inhibitors, and thrombolytic agents because of an increased risk of bleeding).
No products indexed under this heading.

Piroxicam (Dalteparin sodium should be used with care in patients receiving oral anticoagulants, platelet inhibitors, and thrombolytic agents because of an increased risk of bleeding).
No products indexed under this heading.

Propofol (Patients undergoing regional anesthesia should not receive dalteparin sodium for unstable angina or non-Q-wave myocardial infarction due to an increased risk of bleeding associated with the dosage of dalteparin sodium recommended for unstable angina and non-Q-wave myocardial infarction).
No products indexed under this heading.

Remifentanil Hydrochloride (Patients undergoing regional anesthesia should not receive dalteparin sodium for unstable angina or non-Q-wave myocardial infarction due to an increased risk of bleeding associated with the dosage of dalteparin sodium recommended for unstable angina and non-Q-wave myocardial infarction).
No products indexed under this heading.

Reteplase (Dalteparin sodium should be used with care in patients receiving oral anticoagulants, platelet inhibitors, and thrombolytic agents because of an increased risk of bleeding). Products include:

Salsalate (Dalteparin sodium should be used with care in patients receiving oral anticoagulants, platelet inhibitors, and thrombolytic agents because of an increased risk of bleeding).
No products indexed under this heading.

Streptokinase (Dalteparin sodium should be used with care in patients receiving oral anticoagulants, platelet inhibitors, and thrombolytic agents because of an increased risk of bleeding).
No products indexed under this heading.

Sufentanil Citrate (Patients undergoing regional anesthesia should not receive dalteparin sodium for unstable angina or non-Q-wave myocardial infarction due to an increased risk of bleeding associated with the dosage of dalteparin sodium recommended for unstable angina and non-Q-wave myocardial infarction).
No products indexed under this heading.

Sulindac (Dalteparin sodium should be used with care in patients receiving oral anticoagulants, platelet inhibitors, and thrombolytic agents because of an increased risk of bleeding). Products include:

Thiamylal Sodium (Patients undergoing regional anesthesia should not receive dalteparin sodium for unstable angina or non-Q-wave myocardial infarction due to an increased risk of bleeding associated with the dosage of dalteparin sodium recommended for unstable angina and non-Q-wave myocardial infarction).
No products indexed under this heading.

Ticarcillin Disodium (Dalteparin sodium should be used with care in patients receiving oral anticoagulants, platelet inhibitors, and throm-

bolytic agents because of an increased risk of bleeding). Products include:

Ticlopidine Hydrochloride (Dalteparin sodium should be used with care in patients receiving oral anticoagulants, platelet inhibitors, and thrombolytic agents because of an increased risk of bleeding). Products include:

Tolmetin Sodium (Dalteparin sodium should be used with care in patients receiving oral anticoagulants, platelet inhibitors, and thrombolytic agents because of an increased risk of bleeding).
No products indexed under this heading.

Urokinase (Dalteparin sodium should be used with care in patients receiving oral anticoagulants, platelet inhibitors, and thrombolytic agents because of an increased risk of bleeding).
No products indexed under this heading.

Warfarin Sodium (Dalteparin sodium should be used with care in patients receiving oral anticoagulants, platelet inhibitors, and thrombolytic agents because of an increased risk of bleeding). Products include:

FROVA TABLETS

(Frovatriptan Succinate) 1113
May interact with 5HT1-receptor agonists, ergot-containing drugs, oral contraceptives, selective serotonin reuptake inhibitors, and certain other agents. Compounds in these categories include:

Citalopram Hydrobromide (Co-administration of 5-HT$_1$ agonists with selective serotonin reuptake inhibitors (SSRIs) has resulted, rarely, in hyperreflexia, weakness and incoordination). Products include:

Desogestrel (Retrospective analysis of pharmacokinetic data indicates that mean C_{max} and AUC of frovatriptan are 30% higher in females taking oral contraceptives). Products include:

Dihydroergotamine Mesylate (Ergot-containing drugs have been reported to cause prolonged vasospastic reactions; because there is a theoretical basis that these effects may be additive, use of ergot-type agents and frovatriptan within 24 hours is contraindicated). Products include:

3-Diphenylacrylate (Co-administration with other 5-HT$_1$ agonists within 24 hours of each other is contraindicated).
No products indexed under this heading.

Ergonovine Maleate (Ergot-containing drugs have been reported to cause prolonged vasospastic reactions; because there is a theoretical basis that these effects may be additive, use of ergot-type agents and frovatriptan within 24 hours is contraindicated).
No products indexed under this heading.

Ergotamine Tartrate (Ergot-containing drugs have been reported to cause prolonged vasospastic reactions; because there is a theoretical basis that these effects may be additive, use of ergot-type agents and frovatriptan within 24 hours is contraindicated).
No products indexed under this heading.

Escitalopram Oxalate (Co-administration of 5-HT$_1$ agonists with selective serotonin reuptake inhibitors (SSRIs) has resulted, rarely, in hyperreflexia, weakness and incoordination). Products include:

Ethinyl Estradiol (Retrospective analysis of pharmacokinetic data indicates that mean C_{max} and AUC of frovatriptan are 30% higher in females taking oral contraceptives). Products include:

Ethynodiol Diacetate (Retrospective analysis of pharmacokinetic data indicates that mean C_{max} and AUC of frovatriptan are 30% higher in females taking oral contraceptives).
No products indexed under this heading.

Fluoxetine Hydrochloride (Co-administration of 5-HT$_1$ agonists with selective serotonin reuptake inhibitors (SSRIs) has resulted, rarely, in hyperreflexia, weakness and incoordination). Products include:

Fluvoxamine Maleate (Co-administration of 5-HT$_1$ agonists with selective serotonin reuptake inhibitors (SSRIs) has resulted, rarely, in hyperreflexia, weakness and incoordination).
No products indexed under this heading.

Levonorgestrel (Retrospective analysis of pharmacokinetic data indicates that mean C_{max} and AUC of frovatriptan are 30% higher in females taking oral contraceptives). Products include:

Mestranol (Retrospective analysis of pharmacokinetic data indicates that mean C_{max} and AUC of frovatriptan are 30% higher in females taking oral contraceptives).
No products indexed under this heading.

Methylergonovine Maleate (Ergot-containing drugs have been reported to cause prolonged vasospastic reactions; because there is a theoretical basis that these effects may be additive, use of ergot-type agents and frovatriptan within 24 hours is contraindicated).
No products indexed under this heading.

Methysergide Maleate (Ergot-containing drugs have been reported to cause prolonged vasospastic reactions; because there is a theoretical basis that these effects may be additive, use of ergot-type agents and frovatriptan within 24 hours is contraindicated).
No products indexed under this heading.

Naratriptan Hydrochloride (Co-administration with other 5-HT_1 agonists within 24 hours of each other is contraindicated). Products include:
Amerge Tablets **1339**

Norethindrone (Retrospective analysis of pharmacokinetic data indicates that mean C_{max} and AUC of frovatriptan are 30% higher in females taking oral contraceptives). Products include:
Ortho Micronor Tablets **2426**

Norethynodrel (Retrospective analysis of pharmacokinetic data indicates that mean C_{max} and AUC of frovatriptan are 30% higher in females taking oral contraceptives).
No products indexed under this heading.

Norgestimate (Retrospective analysis of pharmacokinetic data indicates that mean C_{max} and AUC of frovatriptan are 30% higher in females taking oral contraceptives). Products include:
Ortho-Cyclen/Ortho Tri-Cyclen **2429**
Ortho Tri-Cyclen Lo Tablets **2436**

Norgestrel (Retrospective analysis of pharmacokinetic data indicates that mean C_{max} and AUC of frovatriptan are 30% higher in females taking oral contraceptives).
No products indexed under this heading.

Paroxetine Hydrochloride (Co-administration of 5-HT_1 agonists with selective serotonin reuptake inhibitors (SSRIs) has resulted, rarely, in hyperreflexia, weakness and incoordination). Products include:
Paxil CR Controlled-Release Tablets **1538**
Paxil **1530**

Propranolol Hydrochloride (Increases AUC of frovatriptan in males by 60% and in females by 29%; Cmax was increased by 23% in males and 16% in females). Products include:
Inderal LA Long-Acting Capsules **3429**
InnoPran XL Capsules **2723**

Rizatriptan Benzoate (Co-administration with other 5-HT_1 agonists within 24 hours of each other is contraindicated). Products include:
Maxalt Tablets **2008**
Maxalt-MLT Orally Disintegrating Tablets **2008**

Sertraline Hydrochloride (Co-administration of 5-HT_1 agonists with selective serotonin reuptake inhibitors (SSRIs) has resulted, rarely, in hyperreflexia, weakness and incoordination). Products include:
Zoloft **2586**

Sumatriptan (Co-administration with other 5-HT_1 agonists within 24 hours of each other is contraindicated). Products include:
Imitrex Nasal Spray **1467**

Sumatriptan Succinate (Co-administration with other 5-HT_1 agonists within 24 hours of each other is contraindicated). Products include:
Imitrex Injection **1463**
Imitrex Tablets **1471**

Zolmitriptan (Co-administration with other 5-HT_1 agonists within 24 hours of each other is contraindicated). Products include:
Zomig Tablets **3519**
Zomig Nasal Spray **3523**
Zomig-ZMT Tablets **3519**

FUROSEMIDE TABLETS

(Furosemide) **2154**

May interact with aminoglycosides, antihypertensives, barbiturates, corticosteroids, cardiac glycosides, lithium preparations, narcotic analgesics, non-steroidal anti-inflammatory agents, salicylates, and certain other agents. Compounds in these categories include:

Acebutolol Hydrochloride (Furosemide may add to or potentiate the therapeutic effect of other antihypertensive drugs).
No products indexed under this heading.

ACTH (Co-administration with ACTH may increase the risk of hypokalemia).
No products indexed under this heading.

Alfentanil Hydrochloride (Aggravates orthostatic hypotension).
No products indexed under this heading.

Amikacin Sulfate (Potential for increased risk of ototoxicity with concomitant therapy, especially in the presence of impaired renal function; avoid concurrent use except in presence of life threatening situations).
No products indexed under this heading.

Amlodipine Besylate (Furosemide may add to or potentiate the therapeutic effect of other antihypertensive drugs). Products include:
Caduet Tablets **2508**
Lotrel Capsules **2249**
Norvasc Tablets **2545**

Aprobarbital (Aggravates orthostatic hypotension).
No products indexed under this heading.

Aspirin (Combination of furosemide and aspirin temporarily reduced creatinine clearance in patients with chronic renal insufficiency; co-administration in patients receiving high doses of salicylates may experience salicylate toxicity). Products include:
Aggrenox Capsules **822**
Bayer Aspirin **744**
BC Allergy Sinus Cold Powder .... ▣**677**
BC Headache Powder .... ▣**677**
Arthritis Strength BC Powder .... ▣**677**
BC Sinus Cold Powder .... ▣**677**
Excedrin Extra Strength Caplets/Tablets/Geltabs .... ▣**684**
Excedrin Migraine Caplets/Tablets/Geltabs .... ▣**609**
Goody's Body Pain Formula Powder .... ▣**684**
Goody's Extra Strength Headache Powders .... ▣**611**
Goody's Extra Strength Pain Relief Tablets .... ▣**685**
Percodan Tablets **1132**
St. Joseph 81 mg Aspirin Chewable and Enteric Coated Tablets **1869**

Aspirin, Enteric Coated (Co-administration in patients receiving high doses of salicylates may experience salicylate toxicity).
No products indexed under this heading.

Aspirin Buffered (Co-administration in patients receiving high doses of salicylates may experience salicylate toxicity). Products include:
Bufferin Extra Strength Tablets .... ▣**678**
Bufferin Regular Strength Tablets .... ▣**678**

Atenolol (Furosemide may add to or potentiate the therapeutic effect of other antihypertensive drugs).
No products indexed under this heading.

Benazepril Hydrochloride (Furosemide may add to or potentiate the therapeutic effect of other antihypertensive drugs). Products include:
Lotensin Tablets **2243**
Lotensin HCT Tablets **2246**
Lotrel Capsules **2249**

Bendroflumethiazide (Furosemide may add to or potentiate the therapeutic effect of other antihypertensive drugs).
No products indexed under this heading.

Betamethasone Acetate (Co-administration with corticosteroids may increase the risk of hypokalemia).
No products indexed under this heading.

Betamethasone Sodium Phosphate (Co-administration with corticosteroids may increase the risk of hypokalemia).
No products indexed under this heading.

Betaxolol Hydrochloride (Furosemide may add to or potentiate the therapeutic effect of other antihypertensive drugs). Products include:
Betoptic S Ophthalmic Suspension **558**

Bisoprolol Fumarate (Furosemide may add to or potentiate the therapeutic effect of other antihypertensive drugs).
No products indexed under this heading.

Buprenorphine Hydrochloride (Aggravates orthostatic hypotension). Products include:
Buprenex Injectable **2716**
Suboxone Tablets **2717**
Subutex Tablets **2717**

Butabarbital (Aggravates orthostatic hypotension).
No products indexed under this heading.

Butalbital (Aggravates orthostatic hypotension).
No products indexed under this heading.

Candesartan Cilexetil (Furosemide may add to or potentiate the therapeutic effect of other antihypertensive drugs). Products include:
Atacand Tablets **649**
Atacand HCT **651**

Captopril (Furosemide may add to or potentiate the therapeutic effect of other antihypertensive drugs). Products include:
Captopril Tablets **2149**

Carteolol Hydrochloride (Furosemide may add to or potentiate the therapeutic effect of other antihypertensive drugs). Products include:
Carteolol Hydrochloride Ophthalmic Solution USP, 1% .... ⊙**249**

Celecoxib (Co-administration with NSAIDs has resulted in increased BUN, serum creatinine and serum potassium levels, and weight gain). Products include:
Celebrex Capsules **3134**

Chlorothiazide (Furosemide may add to or potentiate the therapeutic effect of other antihypertensive drugs). Products include:
Diuril Oral Suspension **1954**

Chlorothiazide Sodium (Furosemide may add to or potentiate the therapeutic effect of other antihypertensive drugs). Products include:
Diuril Sodium Intravenous **2467**

Chlorthalidone (Furosemide may add to or potentiate the therapeutic effect of other antihypertensive drugs). Products include:
Clorpres Tablets **2153**

Choline Magnesium Trisalicylate (Co-administration in patients receiving high doses of salicylates may experience salicylate toxicity).
No products indexed under this heading.

Clonidine (Furosemide may add to or potentiate the therapeutic effect of other antihypertensive drugs). Products include:
Catapres-TTS **844**

Clonidine Hydrochloride (Furosemide may add to or potentiate the therapeutic effect of other antihypertensive drugs). Products include:
Catapres Tablets **843**
Clorpres Tablets **2153**

Codeine Phosphate (Aggravates orthostatic hypotension). Products include:
Tylenol with Codeine Tablets **2391**

Cortisone Acetate (Co-administration with corticosteroids may increase the risk of hypokalemia).
No products indexed under this heading.

Deserpidine (Furosemide may add to or potentiate the therapeutic effect of other antihypertensive drugs).
No products indexed under this heading.

Deslanoside (Concurrent digitalis therapy may exaggerate metabolic effects of hypokalemia, especially myocardial effects).
No products indexed under this heading.

Dexamethasone (Co-administration with corticosteroids may increase the risk of hypokalemia). Products include:
Ciprodex Otic Suspension **559**
Decadron Tablets **1951**
TobraDex Ophthalmic Ointment **562**
TobraDex Ophthalmic Suspension **563**

Dexamethasone Acetate (Co-administration with corticosteroids may increase the risk of hypokalemia).
No products indexed under this heading.

Dexamethasone Sodium Phosphate (Co-administration with corticosteroids may increase the risk of hypokalemia).
No products indexed under this heading.

Dezocine (Aggravates orthostatic hypotension).
No products indexed under this heading.

Diazoxide (Furosemide may add to or potentiate the therapeutic effect of other antihypertensive drugs). Products include:
Hyperstat I.V. 3017

Diclofenac Potassium (Co-administration with NSAIDs has resulted in increased BUN, serum creatinine and serum potassium levels, and weight gain).
No products indexed under this heading.

Diclofenac Sodium (Co-administration with NSAIDs has resulted in increased BUN, serum creatinine and serum potassium levels, and weight gain). Products include:
Arthrotec Tablets 3129
Voltaren Ophthalmic Solution 2309
Voltaren Tablets 2307
Voltaren-XR Tablets 2310

Diflunisal (Co-administration in patients receiving high doses of salicylates may experience salicylate toxicity). Products include:
Dolobid Tablets 1955

Digitalis Glycoside Preparations (Concurrent digitalis therapy may exaggerate metabolic effects of hypokalemia, especially myocardial effects).
No products indexed under this heading.

Digitoxin (Concurrent digitalis therapy may exaggerate metabolic effects of hypokalemia, especially myocardial effects).
No products indexed under this heading.

Digoxin (Concurrent digitalis therapy may exaggerate metabolic effects of hypokalemia, especially myocardial effects). Products include:
Lanoxicaps Capsules 1490
Lanoxin Injection 1494
Lanoxin Injection Pediatric 1497
Lanoxin Tablets 1500

Diltiazem Hydrochloride (Furosemide may add to or potentiate the therapeutic effect of other antihypertensive drugs). Products include:
Cardizem LA Extended Release Tablets 1728
Tiazac Capsules 1201

Doxazosin Mesylate (Furosemide may add to or potentiate the therapeutic effect of other antihypertensive drugs). Products include:
Cardura XL Tablets 2515

Enalapril Maleate (Furosemide may add to or potentiate the therapeutic effect of other antihypertensive drugs). Products include:
Vasotec I.V. Injection 2103

Enalaprilat (Furosemide may add to or potentiate the therapeutic effect of other antihypertensive drugs).
No products indexed under this heading.

Eprosartan Mesylate (Furosemide may add to or potentiate the therapeutic effect of other antihypertensive drugs). Products include:
Teveten Tablets 1735
Teveten HCT Tablets 1737

Esmolol Hydrochloride (Furosemide may add to or potentiate the therapeutic effect of other antihypertensive drugs).
No products indexed under this heading.

Ethacrynic Acid (Potential for increased risk of ototoxicity with concomitant therapy; concurrent use should be avoided). Products include:
Edecrin Tablets 1959

Etodolac (Co-administration with NSAIDs has resulted in increased BUN, serum creatinine and serum potassium levels, and weight gain).
No products indexed under this heading.

Felodipine (Furosemide may add to or potentiate the therapeutic effect of other antihypertensive drugs).
No products indexed under this heading.

Fenoprofen Calcium (Co-administration with NSAIDs has resulted in increased BUN, serum creatinine and serum potassium levels, and weight gain). Products include:
Nalfon Capsules 2502

Fentanyl (Aggravates orthostatic hypotension). Products include:
Duragesic Transdermal System 2373
Ionsys Transdermal System 2379

Fentanyl Citrate (Aggravates orthostatic hypotension). Products include:
Actiq 979

Fludrocortisone Acetate (Co-administration with corticosteroids may increase the risk of hypokalemia).
No products indexed under this heading.

Flurbiprofen (Co-administration with NSAIDs has resulted in increased BUN, serum creatinine and serum potassium levels, and weight gain).
No products indexed under this heading.

Fosinopril Sodium (Furosemide may add to or potentiate the therapeutic effect of other antihypertensive drugs).
No products indexed under this heading.

Gentamicin Sulfate (Potential for increased risk of ototoxicity with concomitant therapy, especially in the presence of impaired renal function; avoid concurrent use except in presence of life threatening situations). Products include:
Garamycin Injectable 3014
Pred-G Ophthalmic Ointment .... ⊙237
Pred-G Ophthalmic Suspension .... ⊙236

Guanabenz Acetate (Furosemide may add to or potentiate the therapeutic effect of other antihypertensive drugs).
No products indexed under this heading.

Guanethidine Monosulfate (Furosemide may add to or potentiate the therapeutic effect of other antihypertensive drugs).
No products indexed under this heading.

Hydralazine Hydrochloride (Furosemide may add to or potentiate the therapeutic effect of other antihypertensive drugs). Products include:
BiDil Tablets 2171

Hydrochlorothiazide (Furosemide may add to or potentiate the therapeutic effect of other antihypertensive drugs). Products include:
Aldoril Tablets 1910
Atacand HCT 651
Avalide Tablets 888
Avalide Tablets 2874
Benicar HCT Tablets 1044
Diovan HCT Tablets 2196
Dyazide Capsules 1423
Hyzaar 50-12.5 Tablets 1990
Hyzaar 100-12.5 Tablets 1990
Hyzaar 100-25 Tablets 1990
Lopressor HCT 50/25 Tablets 2241
Lopressor HCT 100/25 Tablets 2241
Lopressor HCT 100/50 Tablets 2241
Lotensin HCT Tablets 2246
Micardis HCT Tablets 856
Moduretic Tablets 2028
Prinzide Tablets 2056
Teveten HCT Tablets 1737
Timolide Tablets 2086
Uniretic Tablets 3100

Hydrocodone Bitartrate (Aggravates orthostatic hypotension). Products include:
Hycodan 1116
Hycotuss Expectorant Syrup 1117
Vicodin Tablets 535
Vicodin ES Tablets 536
Vicodin HP Tablets 538
Vicoprofen Tablets 539
Zydone Tablets 1139

Hydrocodone Polistirex (Aggravates orthostatic hypotension). Products include:
Tussionex Pennkinetic Extended-Release Suspension 3327

Hydrocortisone (Co-administration with corticosteroids may increase the risk of hypokalemia). Products include:
Colocort Rectal Suspension, USP (Retention) 100 mg/60 mL 2476
Hydrocortone Tablets 1989
Preparation H Hydrocortisone Cream .... ▣646

Hydrocortisone Acetate (Co-administration with corticosteroids may increase the risk of hypokalemia). Products include:
Analpram-HC 1159
Pramosone 1161
ProctoFoam-HC 3099

Hydrocortisone Sodium Phosphate (Co-administration with corticosteroids may increase the risk of hypokalemia).
No products indexed under this heading.

Hydrocortisone Sodium Succinate (Co-administration with corticosteroids may increase the risk of hypokalemia).
No products indexed under this heading.

Hydroflumethiazide (Furosemide may add to or potentiate the therapeutic effect of other antihypertensive drugs).
No products indexed under this heading.

Hydromorphone Hydrochloride (Aggravates orthostatic hypotension). Products include:
Dilaudid 440
Dilaudid Non-Sterile Powder 440
Dilaudid Oral Liquid 445
Dilaudid Rectal Suppositories 440
Dilaudid Tablets 440
Dilaudid Tablets - 8 mg 445
Dilaudid-HP 442

Ibuprofen (Co-administration with NSAIDs has resulted in increased BUN, serum creatinine and serum potassium levels, and weight gain). Products include:
Advil Allergy Sinus Caplets .... ▣770
Advil .... ▣674
Children's Advil Oral Suspension .... ▣603
Children's Advil Chewable Tablets .... ▣603
Advil Cold & Sinus .... ▣723
Infants' Advil Concentrated Drops .... ▣604
Infants' Advil Concentrated Drops - White Grape (Dye-Free) .... ▣604
Junior Strength Advil Swallow Tablets .... ▣605
Advil Migraine Liquigels .... ▣608
Advil Multi-Symptom Cold Caplets .... ▣770
Advil PM Caplets .... ▣615
Motrin IB Tablets and Caplets 1866
Children's Motrin Oral Suspension 1867
Children's Motrin Non-Staining Dye-Free Oral Suspension 1867
Children's Motrin Cold Oral Suspension 1867
Infants' Motrin Concentrated Drops 1867
Infants' Motrin Non-Staining Dye-Free Concentrated Drops 1867
Junior Strength Motrin Caplets and Chewable Tablets 1867
Vicoprofen Tablets 539

Indapamide (Furosemide may add to or potentiate the therapeutic effect of other antihypertensive drugs). Products include:
Indapamide Tablets 2156

Indomethacin (Co-administration may educe the natriuretic and antihypertensive effects of furosemide in some patients by inhibiting prostaglandin synthesis). Products include:
Indocin 1995

Indomethacin Sodium Trihydrate (Co-administration with NSAIDs has resulted in increased BUN, serum creatinine and serum potassium levels, and weight gain). Products include:
Indocin I.V. 2465

Irbesartan (Furosemide may add to or potentiate the therapeutic effect of other antihypertensive drugs). Products include:
Avalide Tablets 888
Avalide Tablets 2874
Avapro Tablets 891
Avapro Tablets 2871

Isradipine (Furosemide may add to or potentiate the therapeutic effect of other antihypertensive drugs). Products include:
DynaCirc CR Tablets 2721

Kanamycin Sulfate (Potential for increased risk of ototoxicity with concomitant therapy, especially in the presence of impaired renal function; avoid concurrent use except in presence of life threatening situations).
No products indexed under this heading.

Ketoprofen (Co-administration with NSAIDs has resulted in increased BUN, serum creatinine and serum potassium levels, and weight gain).
No products indexed under this heading.

Ketorolac Tromethamine (Co-administration with NSAIDs has resulted in increased BUN, serum creatinine and serum potassium levels, and weight gain). Products include:
Acular Ophthalmic Solution 565
Acular LS Ophthalmic Solution 566

Labetalol Hydrochloride (Furosemide may add to or potentiate the therapeutic effect of other antihypertensive drugs).
No products indexed under this heading.

Levorphanol Tartrate (Aggravates orthostatic hypotension).
No products indexed under this heading.

Lisinopril (Furosemide may add to or potentiate the therapeutic effect of other antihypertensive drugs). Products include:
Prinivil Tablets 2052
Prinzide Tablets 2056

Lithium (Diuretics reduce lithium's renal clearance and add a high risk of lithium toxicity).
No products indexed under this heading.

Lithium Carbonate (Diuretics reduce lithium's renal clearance and add a high risk of lithium toxicity). Products include:
Lithobid Tablets 1692

Lithium Citrate (Diuretics reduce lithium's renal clearance and add a high risk of lithium toxicity).
No products indexed under this heading.

Losartan Potassium (Furosemide may add to or potentiate the therapeutic effect of other antihypertensive drugs). Products include:
Cozaar Tablets 1935
Hyzaar 50-12.5 Tablets 1990
Hyzaar 100-12.5 Tablets 1990
Hyzaar 100-25 Tablets 1990

Magnesium Salicylate (Co-administration in patients receiving high doses of salicylates may experience salicylate toxicity).
No products indexed under this heading.

Mecamylamine Hydrochloride (Furosemide may add to or potentiate the therapeutic effect of other antihypertensive drugs).
No products indexed under this heading.

Meclofenamate Sodium (Co-administration with NSAIDs has resulted in increased BUN, serum creatinine and serum potassium levels, and weight gain).
No products indexed under this heading.

Mefenamic Acid (Co-administration with NSAIDs has resulted in increased BUN, serum creatinine and serum potassium levels, and weight gain).
No products indexed under this heading.

Meloxicam (Co-administration with NSAIDs has resulted in increased BUN, serum creatinine and serum potassium levels, and weight gain). Products include:
Mobic Oral Suspension 863
Mobic Tablets 863

Meperidine Hydrochloride (Aggravates orthostatic hypotension).
No products indexed under this heading.

Mephobarbital (Aggravates orthostatic hypotension).
No products indexed under this heading.

Methadone Hydrochloride (Aggravates orthostatic hypotension).
No products indexed under this heading.

Methyclothiazide (Furosemide may add to or potentiate the therapeutic effect of other antihypertensive drugs).
No products indexed under this heading.

Methyldopa (Furosemide may add to or potentiate the therapeutic effect of other antihypertensive drugs). Products include:
Aldoril Tablets 1910

Methyldopate Hydrochloride (Furosemide may add to or potentiate the therapeutic effect of other antihypertensive drugs).
No products indexed under this heading.

Methylprednisolone Acetate (Co-administration with corticosteroids may increase the risk of hypokalemia). Products include:
Depo-Medrol Injectable Suspension 2617
Depo-Medrol Single-Dose Vial 2619

Methylprednisolone Sodium Succinate (Co-administration with corticosteroids may increase the risk of hypokalemia).
No products indexed under this heading.

Metolazone (Furosemide may add to or potentiate the therapeutic effect of other antihypertensive drugs).
No products indexed under this heading.

Metoprolol Succinate (Furosemide may add to or potentiate the therapeutic effect of other antihypertensive drugs). Products include:
Toprol-XL Tablets 668

Metoprolol Tartrate (Furosemide may add to or potentiate the therapeutic effect of other antihypertensive drugs). Products include:
Lopressor Injection 2238
Lopressor Tablets 2238
Lopressor HCT 50/25 Tablets 2241
Lopressor HCT 100/25 Tablets 2241
Lopressor HCT 100/50 Tablets 2241

Metyrosine (Furosemide may add to or potentiate the therapeutic effect of other antihypertensive drugs). Products include:
Demser Capsules 1953

Mibefradil Dihydrochloride (Furosemide may add to or potentiate the therapeutic effect of other antihypertensive drugs).
No products indexed under this heading.

Minoxidil (Furosemide may add to or potentiate the therapeutic effect of other antihypertensive drugs). Products include:
Men's Rogaine Extra Strength Hair Regrowth Treatment Topical Solution, Ocean Rush Scent and Original Unscented 633
Men's Rogaine Foam Hair Regrowth Treatment 633
Women's Rogaine Hair Regrowth Treatment Topical Solution, Spring Bloom Scent and Original Unscented 634

Moexipril Hydrochloride (Furosemide may add to or potentiate the therapeutic effect of other antihypertensive drugs). Products include:
Uniretic Tablets 3100
Univasc Tablets 3104

Morphine Sulfate (Aggravates orthostatic hypotension). Products include:
Avinza Capsules 1741
Kadian Capsules 577
MS Contin Tablets 2701

Nabumetone (Co-administration with NSAIDs has resulted in increased BUN, serum creatinine and serum potassium levels, and weight gain).
No products indexed under this heading.

Nadolol (Furosemide may add to or potentiate the therapeutic effect of other antihypertensive drugs). Products include:
Nadolol Tablets 2159

Naproxen (Co-administration with NSAIDs has resulted in increased BUN, serum creatinine and serum potassium levels, and weight gain). Products include:
EC-Naprosyn Delayed-Release Tablets 2761
Naprosyn Suspension 2761
Naprosyn Tablets 2761
Prevacid NapraPAC 3280

Naproxen Sodium (Co-administration with NSAIDs has resulted in increased BUN, serum creatinine and serum potassium levels, and weight gain). Products include:
Aleve Caplets 742
Aleve Gelcaps 743
Aleve Tablets 743
Aleve Cold & Sinus Caplets 744
Anaprox Tablets 2761
Anaprox DS Tablets 2761

Nicardipine Hydrochloride (Furosemide may add to or potentiate the therapeutic effect of other antihypertensive drugs). Products include:
Cardene I.V. 2497

Nifedipine (Furosemide may add to or potentiate the therapeutic effect of other antihypertensive drugs). Products include:
Adalat CC Tablets 2964

Nisoldipine (Furosemide may add to or potentiate the therapeutic effect of other antihypertensive drugs). Products include:
Sular Tablets 3122

Nitroglycerin (Furosemide may add to or potentiate the therapeutic effect of other antihypertensive drugs). Products include:
Nitro-Dur Transdermal Infusion System 3046
Nitrolingual Pumpspray 3120

Norepinephrine Bitartrate (Furosemide may decrease arterial responsiveness to norepinephrine).
No products indexed under this heading.

Oxaprozin (Co-administration with NSAIDs has resulted in increased BUN, serum creatinine and serum potassium levels, and weight gain).
No products indexed under this heading.

Oxycodone Hydrochloride (Aggravates orthostatic hypotension). Products include:
OxyContin Tablets 2703
OxyFast Oral Concentrate Solution 2708
OxyIR Capsules 2708
Percocet Tablets 1131
Percodan Tablets 1132

Penbutolol Sulfate (Furosemide may add to or potentiate the therapeutic effect of other antihypertensive drugs).
No products indexed under this heading.

Pentobarbital Sodium (Aggravates orthostatic hypotension). Products include:
Nembutal Sodium Solution, USP 2470

Perindopril Erbumine (Furosemide may add to or potentiate the therapeutic effect of other antihypertensive drugs). Products include:
Aceon Tablets (2 mg, 4 mg, 8 mg) 3194

Phenobarbital (Aggravates orthostatic hypotension). Products include:
Donnatal Extentabs 2493

Phenoxybenzamine Hydrochloride (Furosemide may add to or potentiate the therapeutic effect of other antihypertensive drugs). Products include:
Dibenzyline Capsules 3399

Phentolamine Mesylate (Furosemide may add to or potentiate the therapeutic effect of other antihypertensive drugs).
No products indexed under this heading.

Phenylbutazone (Co-administration with NSAIDs has resulted in increased BUN, serum creatinine and serum potassium levels, and weight gain).
No products indexed under this heading.

Pindolol (Furosemide may add to or potentiate the therapeutic effect of other antihypertensive drugs).
No products indexed under this heading.

Piroxicam (Co-administration with NSAIDs has resulted in increased BUN, serum creatinine and serum potassium levels, and weight gain).
No products indexed under this heading.

Polythiazide (Furosemide may add to or potentiate the therapeutic effect of other antihypertensive drugs).
No products indexed under this heading.

Prazosin Hydrochloride (Furosemide may add to or potentiate the therapeutic effect of other antihypertensive drugs).
No products indexed under this heading.

Prednisolone Acetate (Co-administration with corticosteroids may increase the risk of hypokalemia). Products include:
Blephamide Ophthalmic Ointment 568
Blephamide Ophthalmic Suspension 569
Poly-Pred Ophthalmic Suspension .... ⊙ 233
Pred Forte Ophthalmic Suspension .... ⊙ 235
Pred Mild Ophthalmic Suspension .... ⊙ 238
Pred-G Ophthalmic Ointment .... ⊙ 237
Pred-G Ophthalmic Suspension .... ⊙ 236

Prednisolone Sodium Phosphate (Co-administration with corticosteroids may increase the risk of hypokalemia).
No products indexed under this heading.

Prednisolone Tebutate (Co-administration with corticosteroids may increase the risk of hypokalemia).
No products indexed under this heading.

Prednisone (Co-administration with corticosteroids may increase the risk of hypokalemia).
No products indexed under this heading.

Propoxyphene Hydrochloride (Aggravates orthostatic hypotension).
No products indexed under this heading.

Propoxyphene Napsylate (Aggravates orthostatic hypotension).
No products indexed under this heading.

Propranolol Hydrochloride (Furosemide may add to or potentiate the therapeutic effect of other antihypertensive drugs). Products include:
Inderal LA Long-Acting Capsules 3429
InnoPran XL Capsules 2723

Quinapril Hydrochloride (Furosemide may add to or potentiate the therapeutic effect of other antihypertensive drugs).
No products indexed under this heading.

Ramipril (Furosemide may add to or potentiate the therapeutic effect of other antihypertensive drugs). Products include:
Altace Capsules 1702

Rauwolfia Serpentina (Furosemide may add to or potentiate the therapeutic effect of other antihypertensive drugs).
No products indexed under this heading.

Remifentanil Hydrochloride (Aggravates orthostatic hypotension).
No products indexed under this heading.

Rescinnamine (Furosemide may add to or potentiate the therapeutic effect of other antihypertensive drugs).
No products indexed under this heading.

Reserpine (Furosemide may add to or potentiate the therapeutic effect of other antihypertensive drugs).
No products indexed under this heading.

Rofecoxib (Co-administration with NSAIDs has resulted in increased BUN, serum creatinine and serum potassium levels, and weight gain).
No products indexed under this heading.

Salsalate (Co-administration in patients receiving high doses of salicylates may experience salicylate toxicity).
No products indexed under this heading.

Secobarbital Sodium (Aggravates orthostatic hypotension).
No products indexed under this heading.

Sodium Nitroprusside (Furosemide may add to or potentiate the therapeutic effect of other antihypertensive drugs).
No products indexed under this heading.

Sotalol Hydrochloride (Furosemide may add to or potentiate the therapeutic effect of other antihypertensive drugs).
No products indexed under this heading.

Spirapril Hydrochloride (Furosemide may add to or potentiate the therapeutic effect of other antihypertensive drugs).
No products indexed under this heading.

Streptomycin Sulfate (Potential for increased risk of ototoxicity with concomitant therapy, especially in the presence of impaired renal function; avoid concurrent use except in presence of life threatening situations).
No products indexed under this heading.

Succinylcholine Chloride (Furosemide has a tendency to potentiate the action of succinylcholine).
No products indexed under this heading.

Sucralfate (Simultaneous administration of sucralfate and furosemide may reduce the natriuretic and antihypertensive effects of furosemide; the intake of these two drugs should be separated by at least two hours). Products include:
Carafate Suspension 701
Carafate Tablets 701

Sufentanil Citrate (Aggravates orthostatic hypotension).
No products indexed under this heading.

Sulindac (Co-administration with NSAIDs has resulted in increased BUN, serum creatinine and serum potassium levels, and weight gain). Products include:
Clinoril Tablets 1924

Telmisartan (Furosemide may add to or potentiate the therapeutic effect of other antihypertensive drugs). Products include:
Micardis Tablets 854
Micardis HCT Tablets 856

Terazosin Hydrochloride (Furosemide may add to or potentiate the therapeutic effect of other antihypertensive drugs). Products include:
Hytrin Capsules 471

Thiamylal Sodium (Aggravates orthostatic hypotension).
No products indexed under this heading.

Timolol Maleate (Furosemide may add to or potentiate the therapeutic effect of other antihypertensive drugs). Products include:
Blocadren Tablets 1916
Cosopt Sterile Ophthalmic Solution....................................... 1931
Timolide Tablets 2086
Timoptic Sterile Ophthalmic Solution....................................... 2088
Timoptic in Ocudose 2091
Timoptic-XE Sterile Ophthalmic Gel Forming Solution 2092

Tobramycin (Potential for increased risk of ototoxicity with concomitant therapy, especially in the presence of impaired renal function; avoid concurrent use except in presence of life threatening situations). Products include:
TOBI Solution for Inhalation 2298
TobraDex Ophthalmic Ointment 562
TobraDex Ophthalmic Suspension ... 563
Zylet Ophthalmic Suspension .... ⊙ 259

Tobramycin Sulfate (Potential for increased risk of ototoxicity with concomitant therapy, especially in the presence of impaired renal function; avoid concurrent use except in presence of life threatening situations).
No products indexed under this heading.

Tolmetin Sodium (Co-administration with NSAIDs has resulted in increased BUN, serum creatinine and serum potassium levels, and weight gain).
No products indexed under this heading.

Torsemide (Furosemide may add to or potentiate the therapeutic effect of other antihypertensive drugs). Products include:
Demadex Injection 2759
Demadex Tablets 2759

Trandolapril (Furosemide may add to or potentiate the therapeutic effect of other antihypertensive drugs). Products include:
Mavik Tablets 486
Tarka Tablets 524

Triamcinolone (Co-administration with corticosteroids may increase the risk of hypokalemia).
No products indexed under this heading.

Triamcinolone Acetonide (Co-administration with corticosteroids may increase the risk of hypokalemia). Products include:
Azmacort Inhalation Aerosol 1726
Nasacort AQ Nasal Spray 2922

Triamcinolone Diacetate (Co-administration with corticosteroids may increase the risk of hypokalemia).
No products indexed under this heading.

Triamcinolone Hexacetonide (Co-administration with corticosteroids may increase the risk of hypokalemia).
No products indexed under this heading.

Trimethaphan Camsylate (Furosemide may add to or potentiate the therapeutic effect of other antihypertensive drugs).
No products indexed under this heading.

Tubocurarine Chloride (Furosemide has a tendency to antagonize the skeletal muscle relaxing effects of tubocurarine).
No products indexed under this heading.

Valdecoxib (Co-administration with NSAIDs has resulted in increased BUN, serum creatinine and serum potassium levels, and weight gain).
No products indexed under this heading.

Valsartan (Furosemide may add to or potentiate the therapeutic effect of other antihypertensive drugs). Products include:
Diovan Tablets 2193
Diovan HCT Tablets 2196

Verapamil Hydrochloride (Furosemide may add to or potentiate the therapeutic effect of other antihypertensive drugs). Products include:
Covera-HS Tablets 3139
Tarka Tablets 524
Verelan PM Extended-Release Capsules, Controlled-Onset........... 3106

Food Interactions

Alcohol (Aggravates orthostatic hypotension).

FUZEON INJECTION

(Enfuvirtide) 2767
None cited in PDR database.

GABITRIL TABLETS

(Tiagabine Hydrochloride) 984
May interact with central nervous system depressants, phenytoin, highly protein bound drugs (selected), valproate, and certain other agents. Compounds in these categories include:

Alfentanil Hydrochloride (Possible additive depressive effects).
No products indexed under this heading.

Alprazolam (Possible additive depressive effects). Products include:
Niravam Orally Disintegrating Tablets.. 3092

Amiodarone Hydrochloride (Tiagabine is 96% bound to human plasma protein and therefore has the potential to interact with other highly protein bound compounds. Such an interaction can potentially lead to higher free fractions of either tiagabine or the competing drug).
No products indexed under this heading.

Amitriptyline Hydrochloride (Tiagabine is 96% bound to human plasma protein and therefore has the potential to interact with other highly protein bound compounds. Such an interaction can potentially lead to higher free fractions of either tiagabine or the competing drug).
No products indexed under this heading.

Aprobarbital (Possible additive depressive effects).
No products indexed under this heading.

Atovaquone (Tiagabine is 96% bound to human plasma protein and therefore has the potential to interact with other highly protein bound compounds. Such an interaction can potentially lead to higher free fractions of either tiagabine or the competing drug). Products include:
Malarone Pediatric Tablets 1517
Malarone Tablets 1517
Mepron Suspension 1521

Buprenorphine Hydrochloride (Possible additive depressive effects). Products include:
Buprenex Injectable 2716
Suboxone Tablets 2717
Subutex Tablets 2717

Buspirone Hydrochloride (Possible additive depressive effects).
No products indexed under this heading.

Butabarbital (Possible additive depressive effects).
No products indexed under this heading.

Butalbital (Possible additive depressive effects).
No products indexed under this heading.

Carbamazepine (Population pharmacokinetic analyses indicate that tiagabine clearance is 60% greater in patients taking carbamazepine with or without other enzyme-inducing antiepileptic drugs; tiagabine had no effect on the steady-state plasma concentrations of carbamazepine or its epoxide metabolite in patients with epilepsy). Products include:
Carbatrol Capsules 3171
Equetro Extended-Release Capsules..................................... 3180
Tegretol/Tegretol-XR 2295

Cefonicid Sodium (Tiagabine is 96% bound to human plasma protein and therefore has the potential to interact with other highly protein bound compounds. Such an interaction can potentially lead to higher free fractions of either tiagabine or the competing drug).
No products indexed under this heading.

Celecoxib (Tiagabine is 96% bound to human plasma protein and therefore has the potential to interact with other highly protein bound compounds. Such an interaction can potentially lead to higher free fractions of either tiagabine or the competing drug). Products include:
Celebrex Capsules 3134

Chlordiazepoxide (Possible additive depressive effects).
No products indexed under this heading.

Chlordiazepoxide Hydrochloride (Possible additive depressive effects). Products include:
Librium Capsules ... **3347**

Chlorpromazine (Possible additive depressive effects).
No products indexed under this heading.

Chlorpromazine Hydrochloride (Possible additive depressive effects).
No products indexed under this heading.

Chlorprothixene (Possible additive depressive effects).
No products indexed under this heading.

Chlorprothixene Hydrochloride (Possible additive depressive effects).
No products indexed under this heading.

Chlorprothixene Lactate (Possible additive depressive effects).
No products indexed under this heading.

Clomipramine Hydrochloride (Tiagabine is 96% bound to human plasma protein and therefore has the potential to interact with other highly protein bound compounds. Such an interaction can potentially lead to higher free fractions of either tiagabine or the competing drug).
No products indexed under this heading.

Clorazepate Dipotassium (Possible additive depressive effects). Products include:
Tranxene ... **2474**

Clozapine (Possible additive depressive effects). Products include:
Clozaril Tablets ... **2184**
FazaClo Orally Disintegrating Tablets ... **551**

Codeine Phosphate (Possible additive depressive effects). Products include:
Tylenol with Codeine Tablets ... **2391**

Cyclosporine (Tiagabine is 96% bound to human plasma protein and therefore has the potential to interact with other highly protein bound compounds. Such an interaction can potentially lead to higher free fractions of either tiagabine or the competing drug). Products include:
Gengraf Capsules ... **459**
Neoral Oral Solution ... **2259**
Neoral Soft Gelatin Capsules ... **2259**
Restasis Ophthalmic Emulsion ... **575**
Sandimmune ... **2275**

Desflurane (Possible additive depressive effects).
No products indexed under this heading.

Dezocine (Possible additive depressive effects).
No products indexed under this heading.

Diazepam (Possible additive depressive effects). Products include:
Diastat Rectal Delivery System ... **3343**
Valium Tablets ... **2819**

Diclofenac Potassium (Tiagabine is 96% bound to human plasma protein and therefore has the potential to interact with other highly protein bound compounds. Such an interaction can potentially lead to higher free fractions of either tiagabine or the competing drug).
No products indexed under this heading.

Diclofenac Sodium (Tiagabine is 96% bound to human plasma protein and therefore has the potential to interact with other highly protein bound compounds. Such an interaction can potentially lead to higher free fractions of either tiagabine or the competing drug). Products include:
Arthrotec Tablets ... **3129**
Voltaren Ophthalmic Solution ... **2309**
Voltaren Tablets ... **2307**
Voltaren-XR Tablets ... **2310**

Dipyridamole (Tiagabine is 96% bound to human plasma protein and therefore has the potential to interact with other highly protein bound compounds. Such an interaction can potentially lead to higher free fractions of either tiagabine or the competing drug). Products include:
Aggrenox Capsules ... **822**
Persantine Tablets ... **868**

Divalproex Sodium (Co-administration of tiagabine in patients taking valproate chronically had no effect on tiagabine pharmacokinetics, but valproate significantly decreased tiagabine binding in vitro from 96.3% to 94.8% which resulted in an increase of approximately 40% in the tiagabine concentrations; the clinical relevance of this in vitro finding is unknown). Products include:
Depakote Sprinkle Capsules ... **422**
Depakote Tablets ... **427**
Depakote ER Tablets ... **434**

Droperidol (Possible additive depressive effects).
No products indexed under this heading.

Enflurane (Possible additive depressive effects).
No products indexed under this heading.

Estazolam (Possible additive depressive effects). Products include:
ProSom Tablets ... **517**

Ethanol (Possible additive depressive effects).
No products indexed under this heading.

Ethchlorvynol (Possible additive depressive effects).
No products indexed under this heading.

Ethinamate (Possible additive depressive effects).
No products indexed under this heading.

Ethyl Alcohol (Possible additive depressive effects).
No products indexed under this heading.

Fenoprofen Calcium (Tiagabine is 96% bound to human plasma protein and therefore has the potential to interact with other highly protein bound compounds. Such an interaction can potentially lead to higher free fractions of either tiagabine or the competing drug). Products include:
Nalfon Capsules ... **2502**

Fentanyl (Possible additive depressive effects). Products include:
Duragesic Transdermal System ... **2373**
Ionsys Transdermal System ... **2379**

Fentanyl Citrate (Possible additive depressive effects). Products include:
Actiq ... **979**

Fluphenazine Decanoate (Possible additive depressive effects).
No products indexed under this heading.

Fluphenazine Enanthate (Possible additive depressive effects).
No products indexed under this heading.

Fluphenazine Hydrochloride (Possible additive depressive effects).
No products indexed under this heading.

Flurazepam Hydrochloride (Possible additive depressive effects). Products include:
Dalmane Capsules ... **3342**

Flurbiprofen (Tiagabine is 96% bound to human plasma protein and therefore has the potential to interact with other highly protein bound compounds. Such an interaction can potentially lead to higher free fractions of either tiagabine or the competing drug).
No products indexed under this heading.

Fosphenytoin Sodium (Population pharmacokinetic analyses indicate that tiagabine clearance is 60% greater in patients taking phenytoin with or without other enzyme-inducing antiepileptic drugs; tiagabine had no effect on the steady-state plasma concentrations of phenytoin in patients with epilepsy).
No products indexed under this heading.

Glipizide (Tiagabine is 96% bound to human plasma protein and therefore has the potential to interact with other highly protein bound compounds. Such an interaction can potentially lead to higher free fractions of either tiagabine or the competing drug).
No products indexed under this heading.

Glutethimide (Possible additive depressive effects).
No products indexed under this heading.

Haloperidol (Possible additive depressive effects).
No products indexed under this heading.

Haloperidol Decanoate (Possible additive depressive effects).
No products indexed under this heading.

Hydrocodone Bitartrate (Possible additive depressive effects). Products include:
Hycodan ... **1116**
Hycotuss Expectorant Syrup ... **1117**
Vicodin Tablets ... **535**
Vicodin ES Tablets ... **536**
Vicodin HP Tablets ... **538**
Vicoprofen Tablets ... **539**
Zydone Tablets ... **1139**

Hydrocodone Polistirex (Possible additive depressive effects). Products include:
Tussionex Pennkinetic Extended-Release Suspension ... **3327**

Hydromorphone Hydrochloride (Possible additive depressive effects). Products include:
Dilaudid ... **440**
Dilaudid Non-Sterile Powder ... **440**
Dilaudid Oral Liquid ... **445**
Dilaudid Rectal Suppositories ... **440**
Dilaudid Tablets ... **440**
Dilaudid Tablets - 8 mg ... **445**
Dilaudid-HP ... **442**

Hydroxyzine Hydrochloride (Possible additive depressive effects).
No products indexed under this heading.

Ibuprofen (Tiagabine is 96% bound to human plasma protein and therefore has the potential to interact with other highly protein bound compounds. Such an interaction can potentially lead to higher free fractions of either tiagabine or the competing drug). Products include:
Advil Allergy Sinus Caplets ... ▣**770**
Advil ... ▣**674**
Children's Advil Oral Suspension ... ▣**603**
Children's Advil Chewable Tablets ... ▣**603**
Advil Cold & Sinus ... ▣**723**
Infants' Advil Concentrated Drops ... ▣**604**
Infants' Advil Concentrated Drops - White Grape (Dye-Free) ... ▣**604**
Junior Strength Advil Swallow Tablets ... ▣**605**
Advil Migraine Liquigels ... ▣**608**
Advil Multi-Symptom Cold Caplets ... ▣**770**
Advil PM Caplets ... ▣**615**
Motrin IB Tablets and Caplets ... **1866**
Children's Motrin Oral Suspension ... **1867**
Children's Motrin Non-Staining Dye-Free Oral Suspension ... **1867**
Children's Motrin Cold Oral Suspension ... **1867**
Infants' Motrin Concentrated Drops ... **1867**
Infants' Motrin Non-Staining Dye-Free Concentrated Drops ... **1867**
Junior Strength Motrin Caplets and Chewable Tablets ... **1867**
Vicoprofen Tablets ... **539**

Imipramine Hydrochloride (Tiagabine is 96% bound to human plasma protein and therefore has the potential to interact with other highly protein bound compounds. Such an interaction can potentially lead to higher free fractions of either tiagabine or the competing drug).
No products indexed under this heading.

Imipramine Pamoate (Tiagabine is 96% bound to human plasma protein and therefore has the potential to interact with other highly protein bound compounds. Such an interaction can potentially lead to higher free fractions of either tiagabine or the competing drug).
No products indexed under this heading.

Indomethacin (Tiagabine is 96% bound to human plasma protein and therefore has the potential to interact with other highly protein bound compounds. Such an interaction can potentially lead to higher free fractions of either tiagabine or the competing drug). Products include:
Indocin ... **1995**

Indomethacin Sodium Trihydrate (Tiagabine is 96% bound to human plasma protein and therefore has the potential to interact with other highly protein bound compounds. Such an interaction can potentially lead to higher free fractions of either tiagabine or the competing drug). Products include:
Indocin I.V. ... **2465**

Isoflurane (Possible additive depressive effects).
No products indexed under this heading.

IMPORTANT NOTE: Always consult each drug listing in the patient's regimen for possible interactions.

Ketamine Hydrochloride (Possible additive depressive effects).
No products indexed under this heading.

Ketoprofen (Tiagabine is 96% bound to human plasma protein and therefore has the potential to interact with other highly protein bound compounds. Such an interaction can potentially lead to higher free fractions of either tiagabine or the competing drug).
No products indexed under this heading.

Ketorolac Tromethamine (Tiagabine is 96% bound to human plasma protein and therefore has the potential to interact with other highly protein bound compounds. Such an interaction can potentially lead to higher free fractions of either tiagabine or the competing drug). Products include:
Acular Ophthalmic Solution 565
Acular LS Ophthalmic Solution 566

Levomethadyl Acetate Hydrochloride (Possible additive depressive effects).
No products indexed under this heading.

Levorphanol Tartrate (Possible additive depressive effects).
No products indexed under this heading.

Lorazepam (Possible additive depressive effects).
No products indexed under this heading.

Loxapine Hydrochloride (Possible additive depressive effects).
No products indexed under this heading.

Loxapine Succinate (Possible additive depressive effects).
No products indexed under this heading.

Meclofenamate Sodium (Tiagabine is 96% bound to human plasma protein and therefore has the potential to interact with other highly protein bound compounds. Such an interaction can potentially lead to higher free fractions of either tiagabine or the competing drug).
No products indexed under this heading.

Mefenamic Acid (Tiagabine is 96% bound to human plasma protein and therefore has the potential to interact with other highly protein bound compounds. Such an interaction can potentially lead to higher free fractions of either tiagabine or the competing drug).
No products indexed under this heading.

Meperidine Hydrochloride (Possible additive depressive effects).
No products indexed under this heading.

Mephobarbital (Possible additive depressive effects).
No products indexed under this heading.

Meprobamate (Possible additive depressive effects).
No products indexed under this heading.

Mesoridazine Besylate (Possible additive depressive effects).
No products indexed under this heading.

Methadone Hydrochloride (Possible additive depressive effects).
No products indexed under this heading.

Methohexital Sodium (Possible additive depressive effects).
No products indexed under this heading.

Methotrimeprazine (Possible additive depressive effects).
No products indexed under this heading.

Methoxyflurane (Possible additive depressive effects).
No products indexed under this heading.

Midazolam Hydrochloride (Possible additive depressive effects).
No products indexed under this heading.

Molindone Hydrochloride (Possible additive depressive effects). Products include:
Moban Tablets 1119

Morphine Sulfate (Possible additive depressive effects). Products include:
Avinza Capsules 1741
Kadian Capsules 577
MS Contin Tablets 2701

Naproxen (Tiagabine is 96% bound to human plasma protein and therefore has the potential to interact with other highly protein bound compounds. Such an interaction can potentially lead to higher free fractions of either tiagabine or the competing drug). Products include:
EC-Naprosyn Delayed-Release Tablets 2761
Naprosyn Suspension 2761
Naprosyn Tablets 2761
Prevacid NapraPAC 3280

Naproxen Sodium (Tiagabine is 96% bound to human plasma protein and therefore has the potential to interact with other highly protein bound compounds. Such an interaction can potentially lead to higher free fractions of either tiagabine or the competing drug). Products include:
Aleve Caplets 742
Aleve Gelcaps 743
Aleve Tablets 743
Aleve Cold & Sinus Caplets 744
Anaprox Tablets 2761
Anaprox DS Tablets 2761

Nortriptyline Hydrochloride (Tiagabine is 96% bound to human plasma protein and therefore has the potential to interact with other highly protein bound compounds. Such an interaction can potentially lead to higher free fractions of either tiagabine or the competing drug).
No products indexed under this heading.

Olanzapine (Possible additive depressive effects). Products include:
Symbyax Capsules 1819
Zyprexa Tablets 1830
Zyprexa IntraMuscular 1830
Zyprexa ZYDIS Orally Disintegrating Tablets.................. 1830

Oxaprozin (Tiagabine is 96% bound to human plasma protein and therefore has the potential to interact with other highly protein bound compounds. Such an interaction can potentially lead to higher free fractions of either tiagabine or the competing drug).
No products indexed under this heading.

Oxazepam (Possible additive depressive effects).
No products indexed under this heading.

Oxycodone Hydrochloride (Possible additive depressive effects). Products include:
OxyContin Tablets 2703
OxyFast Oral Concentrate Solution.. 2708
OxyIR Capsules 2708
Percocet Tablets 1131
Percodan Tablets 1132

Pentobarbital Sodium (Possible additive depressive effects). Products include:
Nembutal Sodium Solution, USP 2470

Perphenazine (Possible additive depressive effects).
No products indexed under this heading.

Phenobarbital (Population pharmacokinetic analyses indicate that tiagabine clearance is 60% greater in patients taking phenobarbital with or without other enzyme-inducing antiepileptic drugs; possible additive depressive effects). Products include:
Donnatal Extentabs 2493

Phenylbutazone (Tiagabine is 96% bound to human plasma protein and therefore has the potential to interact with other highly protein bound compounds. Such an interaction can potentially lead to higher free fractions of either tiagabine or the competing drug).
No products indexed under this heading.

Phenytoin (Population pharmacokinetic analyses indicate that tiagabine clearance is 60% greater in patients taking phenytoin with or without other enzyme-inducing antiepileptic drugs; tiagabine had no effect on the steady-state plasma concentrations of phenytoin in patients with epilepsy).
No products indexed under this heading.

Phenytoin Sodium (Population pharmacokinetic analyses indicate that tiagabine clearance is 60% greater in patients taking phenytoin with or without other enzyme-inducing antiepileptic drugs; tiagabine had no effect on the steady-state plasma concentrations of phenytoin in patients with epilepsy). Products include:
Phenytek Capsules 2160

Piroxicam (Tiagabine is 96% bound to human plasma protein and therefore has the potential to interact with other highly protein bound compounds. Such an interaction can potentially lead to higher free fractions of either tiagabine or the competing drug).
No products indexed under this heading.

Prazepam (Possible additive depressive effects).
No products indexed under this heading.

Prochlorperazine (Possible additive depressive effects).
No products indexed under this heading.

Promethazine Hydrochloride (Possible additive depressive effects). Products include:
Phenergan Tablets and Suppositories.............................. 3440

Propofol (Possible additive depressive effects).
No products indexed under this heading.

Propoxyphene Hydrochloride (Possible additive depressive effects).
No products indexed under this heading.

Propoxyphene Napsylate (Possible additive depressive effects).
No products indexed under this heading.

Propranolol Hydrochloride (Tiagabine is 96% bound to human plasma protein and therefore has the potential to interact with other highly protein bound compounds. Such an interaction can potentially lead to higher free fractions of either tiagabine or the competing drug). Products include:
Inderal LA Long-Acting Capsules 3429
InnoPran XL Capsules 2723

Quazepam (Possible additive depressive effects).
No products indexed under this heading.

Quetiapine Fumarate (Possible additive depressive effects). Products include:
Seroquel Tablets 690

Remifentanil Hydrochloride (Possible additive depressive effects).
No products indexed under this heading.

Risperidone (Possible additive depressive effects). Products include:
Risperdal 1676
Risperdal Consta Long-Acting Injection 1682
Risperdal M-Tab Orally Disintegrating Tablets.................. 1676

Secobarbital Sodium (Possible additive depressive effects).
No products indexed under this heading.

Sevoflurane (Possible additive depressive effects). Products include:
Ultane Liquid for Inhalation 531

Sodium Oxybate (Possible additive depressive effects). Products include:
Xyrem Oral Solution 1688

Sufentanil Citrate (Possible additive depressive effects).
No products indexed under this heading.

Sulindac (Tiagabine is 96% bound to human plasma protein and therefore has the potential to interact with other highly protein bound compounds. Such an interaction can potentially lead to higher free fractions of either tiagabine or the competing drug). Products include:
Clinoril Tablets 1924

Temazepam (Possible additive depressive effects). Products include:
Restoril Capsules 1860

Thiamylal Sodium (Possible additive depressive effects).
No products indexed under this heading.

Thioridazine Hydrochloride (Possible additive depressive effects). Products include:
Thioridazine Hydrochloride Tablets 2163

Thiothixene (Possible additive depressive effects). Products include:
Thiothixene Capsules 2165

Tolbutamide (Tiagabine is 96% bound to human plasma protein and therefore has the potential to interact with other highly protein bound compounds. Such an interaction can potentially lead to higher free fractions of either tiagabine or the competing drug).
No products indexed under this heading.

Tolmetin Sodium (Tiagabine is 96% bound to human plasma protein and therefore has the potential to interact with other highly protein bound compounds. Such an interaction can potentially lead to higher free fractions of either tiagabine or the competing drug).
No products indexed under this heading.

Triazolam (Possible additive depressive effects).
No products indexed under this heading.

Trifluoperazine Hydrochloride (Possible additive depressive effects).
No products indexed under this heading.

Trimipramine Maleate (Tiagabine is 96% bound to human plasma protein and therefore has the potential to interact with other highly protein bound compounds. Such an interaction can potentially lead to higher free fractions of either tiagabine or the competing drug).
No products indexed under this heading.

Valproate Sodium (Co-administration of tiagabine in patients taking valproate chronically had no effect on tiagabine pharmacokinetics, but valproate significantly decreased tiagabine binding in vitro from 96.3% to 94.8% which resulted in an increase of approximately 40% in the tiagabine concentrations; the clinical relevance of this in vitro finding is unknown). Products include:
Depacon Injection 412

Valproic Acid (Co-administration of tiagabine in patients taking valproate chronically had no effect on tiagabine pharmacokinetics, but valproate significantly decreased tiagabine binding in vitro from 96.3% to 94.8% which resulted in an increase of approximately 40% in the tiagabine concentrations; the clinical relevance of this in vitro finding is unknown). Products include:
Depakene 417

Warfarin Sodium (Tiagabine is 96% bound to human plasma protein and therefore has the potential to interact with other highly protein bound compounds. Such an interaction can potentially lead to higher free fractions of either tiagabine or the competing drug). Products include:
Coumadin for Injection 898
Coumadin Tablets 898

Zaleplon (Possible additive depressive effects). Products include:
Sonata Capsules 1717

Ziprasidone Hydrochloride (Possible additive depressive effects). Products include:
Geodon Capsules 2529

Zolpidem Tartrate (Possible additive depressive effects). Products include:
Ambien Tablets 2851
Ambien CR Tablets 2855

Food Interactions

Alcohol (Possible additive depressive effects).

Food, unspecified (A high fat meal decreases the rate (mean Tmax was prolonged to 2.5 hours, and Cmax was reduced by about 40%) but not the extent (AUC) of tiagabine).

GAMASTAN

(Globulin, Immune (Human)) 3234
None cited in PDR database.

GAMMAGARD LIQUID

(Immune Globulin Intravenous (Human)) 721
May interact with vaccines, live. Compounds in these categories include:

BCG Vaccine (Antibodies in immune globulin intravenous products may interfere with patient responses to live vaccines, such as those for measles, mumps and rubella).
No products indexed under this heading.

Measles, Mumps, Rubella and Varicella Virus Vaccine Live (Antibodies in immune globulin intravenous products may interfere with patient responses to live vaccines, such as those for measles, mumps and rubella). Products include:
ProQuad 2064

Measles, Mumps & Rubella Virus Vaccine, Live (Antibodies in immune globulin intravenous products may interfere with patient responses to live vaccines, such as those for measles, mumps and rubella). Products include:
M-M-R II 2006

Measles & Rubella Virus Vaccine Live (Antibodies in immune globulin intravenous products may interfere with patient responses to live vaccines, such as those for measles, mumps and rubella).
No products indexed under this heading.

Measles Virus Vaccine Live (Antibodies in immune globulin intravenous products may interfere with patient responses to live vaccines, such as those for measles, mumps and rubella). Products include:
Attenuvax 1914

Mumps Virus Vaccine, Live (Antibodies in immune globulin intravenous products may interfere with patient responses to live vaccines, such as those for measles, mumps and rubella). Products include:
Mumpsvax 2031

Poliovirus Vaccine, Live, Oral, Trivalent, Types 1,2,3 (Sabin) (Antibodies in immune globulin intravenous products may interfere with patient responses to live vaccines, such as those for measles, mumps and rubella).
No products indexed under this heading.

Rotavirus Vaccine, Live, Oral, Tetravalent (Antibodies in immune globulin intravenous products may interfere with patient responses to live vaccines, such as those for measles, mumps and rubella).
No products indexed under this heading.

Rubella & Mumps Virus Vaccine Live (Antibodies in immune globulin intravenous products may interfere with patient responses to live vaccines, such as those for measles, mumps and rubella).
No products indexed under this heading.

Rubella Virus Vaccine Live (Antibodies in immune globulin intravenous products may interfere with patient responses to live vaccines, such as those for measles, mumps and rubella). Products include:
Meruvax II 2019

Smallpox Vaccine (Antibodies in immune globulin intravenous products may interfere with patient responses to live vaccines, such as those for measles, mumps and rubella).
No products indexed under this heading.

Typhoid Vaccine (Antibodies in immune globulin intravenous products may interfere with patient responses to live vaccines, such as those for measles, mumps and rubella).
No products indexed under this heading.

Varicella Virus Vaccine Live (Antibodies in immune globulin intravenous products may interfere with patient responses to live vaccines, such as those for measles, mumps and rubella). Products include:
Varivax 2100

Yellow Fever Vaccine (Antibodies in immune globulin intravenous products may interfere with patient responses to live vaccines, such as those for measles, mumps and rubella).
No products indexed under this heading.

GAMMAGARD S/D

(Immune Globulin Intravenous (Human)) 724
May interact with vaccines, live and certain other agents. Compounds in these categories include:

BCG Vaccine (Antibodies in immune globulin intravenous products may interfere with patient responses to live vaccines, such as those for measles, mumps and rubella).
No products indexed under this heading.

Measles, Mumps, Rubella and Varicella Virus Vaccine Live (Antibodies in immune globulin intravenous products may interfere with patient responses to live vaccines, such as those for measles, mumps and rubella). Products include:
ProQuad 2064

Measles, Mumps & Rubella Virus Vaccine, Live (Antibodies in immune globulin intravenous products may interfere with patient responses to live vaccines, such as those for measles, mumps and rubella). Products include:
M-M-R II 2006

Measles & Rubella Virus Vaccine Live (Antibodies in immune globulin intravenous products may interfere with patient responses to live vaccines, such as those for measles, mumps and rubella).
No products indexed under this heading.

Measles Virus Vaccine Live (Antibodies in immune globulin intravenous products may interfere with patient responses to live vaccines, such as those for measles, mumps and rubella). Products include:
Attenuvax 1914

Mumps Virus Vaccine, Live (Antibodies in immune globulin intravenous products may interfere with patient responses to live vaccines, such as those for measles, mumps and rubella). Products include:
Mumpsvax 2031

Poliovirus Vaccine, Live, Oral, Trivalent, Types 1,2,3 (Sabin) (Antibodies in immune globulin intravenous products may interfere with patient responses to live vaccines, such as those for measles, mumps and rubella).
No products indexed under this heading.

Rotavirus Vaccine, Live, Oral, Tetravalent (Antibodies in immune globulin intravenous products may interfere with patient responses to live vaccines, such as those for measles, mumps and rubella).
No products indexed under this heading.

Rubella & Mumps Virus Vaccine Live (Antibodies in immune globulin intravenous products may interfere with patient responses to live vaccines, such as those for measles, mumps and rubella).
No products indexed under this heading.

Rubella Virus Vaccine Live (Antibodies in immune globulin intravenous products may interfere with patient responses to live vaccines, such as those for measles, mumps and rubella). Products include:
Meruvax II 2019

Smallpox Vaccine (Antibodies in immune globulin intravenous products may interfere with patient responses to live vaccines, such as those for measles, mumps and rubella).
No products indexed under this heading.

Typhoid Vaccine (Antibodies in immune globulin intravenous products may interfere with patient responses to live vaccines, such as those for measles, mumps and rubella).
No products indexed under this heading.

Varicella Virus Vaccine Live (Antibodies in immune globulin intravenous products may interfere with patient responses to live vaccines, such as those for measles, mumps and rubella). Products include:
Varivax 2100

Yellow Fever Vaccine (Antibodies in immune globulin intravenous products may interfere with patient responses to live vaccines, such as those for measles, mumps and rubella).
No products indexed under this heading.

GAMUNEX IMMUNE GLOBULIN I.V., 10%

(Immune Globulin Intravenous (Human)) 3235
May interact with:

Measles, Mumps & Rubella Virus Vaccine, Live (Co-administration may interfere with the response to live viral vaccines such as measles. Therefore, use of such vaccines should be deferred until approximately 6 months after Immune Globulin Intravenous (Human) administration). Products include:

M-M-R II 2006

Measles & Rubella Virus Vaccine Live (Co-administration may interfere with the response to live viral vaccines such as measles. Therefore, use of such vaccines should be deferred until approximately 6 months after Immune Globulin Intravenous (Human) administration).

No products indexed under this heading.

Measles Virus Vaccine Live (Co-administration may interfere with the response to live viral vaccines such as measles. Therefore, use of such vaccines should be deferred until approximately 6 months after Immune Globulin Intravenous (Human) administration). Products include:

Attenuvax 1914

Mumps Skin Test Antigen (Co-administration may interfere with the response to live viral vaccines such as mumps. Therefore, use of such vaccines should be deferred until approximately 6 months after Immune Globulin Intravenous (Human) administration).

No products indexed under this heading.

Mumps Virus Vaccine, Live (Co-administration may interfere with the response to live viral vaccines such as mumps. Therefore, use of such vaccines should be deferred until approximately 6 months after Immune Globulin Intravenous (Human) administration). Products include:

Mumpsvax 2031

Rubella & Mumps Virus Vaccine Live (Co-administration may interfere with the response to live viral vaccines such as rubella. Therefore, use of such vaccines should be deferred until approximately 6 months after Immune Globulin Intravenous (Human) administration).

No products indexed under this heading.

Rubella Virus Vaccine Live (Co-administration may interfere with the response to live viral vaccines such as rubella. Therefore, use of such vaccines should be deferred until approximately 6 months after Immune Globulin Intravenous (Human) administration). Products include:

Meruvax II 2019

GANTRISIN PEDIATRIC SUSPENSION

(Acetyl Sulfisoxazole) 2770

May interact with anticoagulants, sulfonylureas, and certain other agents. Compounds in these categories include:

Anisindione (Sulfisoxazole may prolong the prothrombin time in patients who are receiving anticoagulants, including warfarin; monitor coagulation tests closely). Products include:

Miradon Tablets 3042

Ardeparin Sodium (Sulfisoxazole may prolong the prothrombin time in patients who are receiving anticoagulants, including warfarin; monitor coagulation tests closely).

No products indexed under this heading.

Chlorpropamide (Sulfisoxazole may potentiate the hypoglycemic activity of sulfonylureas, as well as cause hypoglycemia by itself).

No products indexed under this heading.

Dalteparin Sodium (Sulfisoxazole may prolong the prothrombin time in patients who are receiving anticoagulants, including warfarin; monitor coagulation tests closely). Products include:

Fragmin Injection 1097

Danaparoid Sodium (Sulfisoxazole may prolong the prothrombin time in patients who are receiving anticoagulants, including warfarin; monitor coagulation tests closely).

No products indexed under this heading.

Dicumarol (Sulfisoxazole may prolong the prothrombin time in patients who are receiving anticoagulants, including warfarin; monitor coagulation tests closely).

No products indexed under this heading.

Enoxaparin Sodium (Sulfisoxazole may prolong the prothrombin time in patients who are receiving anticoagulants, including warfarin; monitor coagulation tests closely). Products include:

Lovenox Injection 2915

Fondaparinux Sodium (Sulfisoxazole may prolong the prothrombin time in patients who are receiving anticoagulants, including warfarin; monitor coagulation tests closely). Products include:

Arixtra Injection 1351

Glimepiride (Sulfisoxazole may potentiate the hypoglycemic activity of sulfonylureas, as well as cause hypoglycemia by itself). Products include:

Avandaryl Tablets 1379

Duetact Tablets 3226

Glipizide (Sulfisoxazole may potentiate the hypoglycemic activity of sulfonylureas, as well as cause hypoglycemia by itself).

No products indexed under this heading.

Glyburide (Sulfisoxazole may potentiate the hypoglycemic activity of sulfonylureas, as well as cause hypoglycemia by itself).

No products indexed under this heading.

Heparin Calcium (Sulfisoxazole may prolong the prothrombin time in patients who are receiving anticoagulants, including warfarin; monitor coagulation tests closely).

No products indexed under this heading.

Heparin Sodium (Sulfisoxazole may prolong the prothrombin time in patients who are receiving anticoagulants, including warfarin; monitor coagulation tests closely).

No products indexed under this heading.

Low Molecular Weight Heparins (Sulfisoxazole may prolong the prothrombin time in patients who are receiving anticoagulants, including warfarin; monitor coagulation tests closely).

No products indexed under this heading.

Methotrexate (Sulfonamides can displace methotrexate from plasma protein-binding sites, thus increasing free methotrexate concentrations. Studies have shown sulfisoxazole infusions to decrease plasma protein-bound methotrexate by one-fourth.).

No products indexed under this heading.

Methotrexate Sodium (Sulfonamides can displace methotrexate from plasma protein-binding sites, thus increasing free methotrexate concentrations. Studies have shown sulfisoxazole infusions to decrease plasma protein-bound methotrexate by one-fourth.).

No products indexed under this heading.

Sodium Thiopental (Patients receiving sulfisoxazole may require less thiopental for anesthesia since sulfisoxazole may compete with thiopental for plasma protein-binding).

No products indexed under this heading.

Tinzaparin Sodium (Sulfisoxazole may prolong the prothrombin time in patients who are receiving anticoagulants, including warfarin; monitor coagulation tests closely).

No products indexed under this heading.

Tolazamide (Sulfisoxazole may potentiate the hypoglycemic activity of sulfonylureas, as well as cause hypoglycemia by itself).

No products indexed under this heading.

Tolbutamide (Sulfisoxazole may potentiate the hypoglycemic activity of sulfonylureas, as well as cause hypoglycemia by itself).

No products indexed under this heading.

Warfarin Sodium (Sulfisoxazole may prolong the prothrombin time in patients who are receiving anticoagulants, including warfarin; monitor coagulation tests closely). Products include:

Coumadin for Injection 898

Coumadin Tablets 898

GARAMYCIN INJECTABLE

(Gentamicin Sulfate) 3014

May interact with aminoglycosides, anesthetics, cephalosporins, neuromuscular blocking agents, and certain other agents. Compounds in these categories include:

Alfentanil Hydrochloride (Increased potential for neuromuscular blockade and respiratory paralysis).

No products indexed under this heading.

Amikacin Sulfate (Concurrent and/or sequential use increases the risk of neurotoxicity and/or nephrotoxicity).

No products indexed under this heading.

Atracurium Besylate (Increased potential for neuromuscular blockade and respiratory paralysis).

No products indexed under this heading.

Carbenicillin Indanyl Sodium (Potential for reduction in gentamicin serum half-life in patients with severe renal impairment receiving concomitant carbenicillin and gentamicin).

No products indexed under this heading.

Cefaclor (Potential for increased nephrotoxicity).

No products indexed under this heading.

Cefadroxil (Potential for increased nephrotoxicity).

No products indexed under this heading.

Cefamandole Nafate (Potential for increased nephrotoxicity).

No products indexed under this heading.

Cefazolin Sodium (Potential for increased nephrotoxicity).

No products indexed under this heading.

Cefdinir (Potential for increased nephrotoxicity). Products include:

Omnicef Capsules 511

Omnicef for Oral Suspension 511

Cefepime Hydrochloride (Potential for increased nephrotoxicity). Products include:

Maxipime for Injection 1105

Cefixime (Potential for increased nephrotoxicity). Products include:

Suprax 1843

Cefmetazole Sodium (Potential for increased nephrotoxicity).

No products indexed under this heading.

Cefonicid Sodium (Potential for increased nephrotoxicity).

No products indexed under this heading.

Cefoperazone Sodium (Potential for increased nephrotoxicity).

No products indexed under this heading.

Ceforanide (Potential for increased nephrotoxicity).

No products indexed under this heading.

Cefotaxime Sodium (Potential for increased nephrotoxicity).

No products indexed under this heading.

Cefotetan (Potential for increased nephrotoxicity).

No products indexed under this heading.

Cefoxitin Sodium (Potential for increased nephrotoxicity). Products include:

Mefoxin for Injection 2012

Mefoxin Premixed Intravenous Solution 2016

Cefpodoxime Proxetil (Potential for increased nephrotoxicity). Products include:

Vantin Tablets and Oral Suspension 2645

Cefprozil (Potential for increased nephrotoxicity).

No products indexed under this heading.

Ceftazidime (Potential for increased nephrotoxicity). Products include:

Fortaz 1453

Ceftizoxime Sodium (Potential for increased nephrotoxicity).

No products indexed under this heading.

Ceftriaxone Sodium (Potential for increased nephrotoxicity). Products include:

Rocephin Injectable Vials, ADD-Vantage, Galaxy, Bulk 2800

Cefuroxime Axetil (Potential for increased nephrotoxicity). Products include:
Ceftin 1407

Cefuroxime Sodium (Potential for increased nephrotoxicity).
No products indexed under this heading.

Cephalexin (Potential for increased nephrotoxicity). Products include:
Keflex Capsules 549

Cephaloridine (Concurrent and/or sequential use increases the risk of neurotoxicity and/or nephrotoxicity).
No products indexed under this heading.

Cephalothin Sodium (Potential for increased nephrotoxicity).
No products indexed under this heading.

Cephapirin Sodium (Potential for increased nephrotoxicity).
No products indexed under this heading.

Cephradine (Potential for increased nephrotoxicity).
No products indexed under this heading.

Cisatracurium Besylate (Increased potential for neuromuscular blockade and respiratory paralysis). Products include:
Nimbex Injection 498

Cisplatin (Concurrent and/or sequential use increases the risk of neurotoxicity and/or nephrotoxicity).
No products indexed under this heading.

Colistin Sulfate (Concurrent and/or sequential use increases the risk of neurotoxicity and/or nephrotoxicity).
No products indexed under this heading.

Doxacurium Chloride (Increased potential for neuromuscular blockade and respiratory paralysis).
No products indexed under this heading.

Enflurane (Increased potential for neuromuscular blockade and respiratory paralysis).
No products indexed under this heading.

Ethacrynic Acid (Potential for increased ototoxicity; concurrent use should be avoided). Products include:
Edecrin Tablets 1959

Fentanyl Citrate (Increased potential for neuromuscular blockade and respiratory paralysis). Products include:
Actiq 979

Furosemide (Potential for increased ototoxicity; concurrent use should be avoided). Products include:
Furosemide Tablets 2154

Halothane (Increased potential for neuromuscular blockade and respiratory paralysis).
No products indexed under this heading.

Isoflurane (Increased potential for neuromuscular blockade and respiratory paralysis).
No products indexed under this heading.

Kanamycin Sulfate (Concurrent and/or sequential use increases the risk of neurotoxicity and/or nephrotoxicity).
No products indexed under this heading.

Ketamine Hydrochloride (Increased potential for neuromuscular blockade and respiratory paralysis).
No products indexed under this heading.

Lithium Carbonate (Increased potential for neuromuscular blockade and respiratory paralysis). Products include:
Lithobid Tablets 1692

Lithium Citrate (Increased potential for neuromuscular blockade and respiratory paralysis).
No products indexed under this heading.

Loracarbef (Potential for increased nephrotoxicity).
No products indexed under this heading.

Methohexital Sodium (Increased potential for neuromuscular blockade and respiratory paralysis).
No products indexed under this heading.

Metocurine Iodide (Increased potential for neuromuscular blockade and respiratory paralysis).
No products indexed under this heading.

Midazolam Hydrochloride (Increased potential for neuromuscular blockade and respiratory paralysis).
No products indexed under this heading.

Mivacurium Chloride (Increased potential for neuromuscular blockade and respiratory paralysis). Products include:
Mivacron Injection 493

Neomycin, oral (Concurrent and/or sequential use increases the risk of neurotoxicity and/or nephrotoxicity).
No products indexed under this heading.

Neomycin Sulfate (Concurrent and/or sequential use increases the risk of neurotoxicity and/or nephrotoxicity). Products include:
Neosporin Ophthalmic Solution Sterile .... ⊙265
Poly-Pred Ophthalmic Suspension .... ⊙233

Pancuronium Bromide (Increased potential for neuromuscular blockade and respiratory paralysis).
No products indexed under this heading.

Paromomycin Sulfate (Concurrent and/or sequential use increases the risk of neurotoxicity and/or nephrotoxicity).
No products indexed under this heading.

Polymyxin B Sulfate (Concurrent and/or sequential use increases the risk of neurotoxicity and/or nephrotoxicity). Products include:
Neosporin Antibiotic Ointment .... ▣643
Neosporin Ophthalmic Solution Sterile .... ⊙265
Neosporin + Pain Relief Antibiotic Cream and Ointment (Maximum Strength)................... ▣643
Poly-Pred Ophthalmic Suspension .... ⊙233
Polysporin First Aid Antibiotic Ointment................................... ▣643
Polytrim Ophthalmic Solution 574

Propofol (Increased potential for neuromuscular blockade and respiratory paralysis).
No products indexed under this heading.

Rapacuronium Bromide (Increased potential for neuromuscular blockade and respiratory paralysis).
No products indexed under this heading.

Remifentanil Hydrochloride (Increased potential for neuromuscular blockade and respiratory paralysis).
No products indexed under this heading.

Rocuronium Bromide (Increased potential for neuromuscular blockade and respiratory paralysis). Products include:
Zemuron Injection 2346

Streptomycin Sulfate (Concurrent and/or sequential use increases the risk of neurotoxicity and/or nephrotoxicity).
No products indexed under this heading.

Succinylcholine Chloride (Increased potential for neuromuscular blockade and respiratory paralysis).
No products indexed under this heading.

Sufentanil Citrate (Increased potential for neuromuscular blockade and respiratory paralysis).
No products indexed under this heading.

Thiamylal Sodium (Increased potential for neuromuscular blockade and respiratory paralysis).
No products indexed under this heading.

Tobramycin (Concurrent and/or sequential use increases the risk of neurotoxicity and/or nephrotoxicity). Products include:
TOBI Solution for Inhalation 2298
TobraDex Ophthalmic Ointment 562
TobraDex Ophthalmic Suspension ... 563
Zylet Ophthalmic Suspension .... ⊙259

Tobramycin Sulfate (Concurrent and/or sequential use increases the risk of neurotoxicity and/or nephrotoxicity).
No products indexed under this heading.

Tubocurarine Chloride (Increased potential for neuromuscular blockade and respiratory paralysis).
No products indexed under this heading.

Vancomycin Hydrochloride (Concurrent and/or sequential use increases the risk of neurotoxicity and/or nephrotoxicity). Products include:
Vancocin HCl Capsules, USP 3380

Vecuronium Bromide (Increased potential for neuromuscular blockade and respiratory paralysis).
No products indexed under this heading.

Viomycin (Concurrent and/or sequential use increases the risk of neurotoxicity and/or nephrotoxicity).
No products indexed under this heading.

GARDASIL INJECTION

(Quadrivalent Human Papillomavirus (Types 6, 11, 16, 18) Recombinant Vaccine)................. 1984
May interact with alkylating agents, antimetabolites, corticosteroids, cytotoxic drugs, and immunosuppressive agents. Compounds in these categories include:

Azathioprine (Immunosuppressive agents may reduce the immune responses to vaccines).
No products indexed under this heading.

Basiliximab (Immunosuppressive agents may reduce the immune responses to vaccines). Products include:
Simulect for Injection 2284

Betamethasone Acetate (Corticosteroids may reduce the immune responses to vaccines).
No products indexed under this heading.

Betamethasone Sodium Phosphate (Corticosteroids may reduce the immune responses to vaccines).
No products indexed under this heading.

Bleomycin Sulfate (Cytotoxic drugs may reduce the immune responses to vaccines).
No products indexed under this heading.

Busulfan (Alkylating agents may reduce the immune responses to vaccines). Products include:
I.V. Busulfex 2493
Myleran Tablets 1525

Capecitabine (Antimetabolites may reduce the immune responses to vaccines). Products include:
Xeloda Tablets 2822

Carmustine (BCNU) (Alkylating agents may reduce the immune responses to vaccines).
No products indexed under this heading.

Chlorambucil (Alkylating agents may reduce the immune responses to vaccines). Products include:
Leukeran Tablets 1504

Cladribine (Antimetabolites may reduce the immune responses to vaccines). Products include:
Leustatin Injection 2357

Cortisone Acetate (Corticosteroids may reduce the immune responses to vaccines).
No products indexed under this heading.

Cyclophosphamide (Alkylating agents may reduce the immune responses to vaccines).
No products indexed under this heading.

Cyclosporine (Immunosuppressive agents may reduce the immune responses to vaccines). Products include:
Gengraf Capsules 459
Neoral Oral Solution 2259
Neoral Soft Gelatin Capsules 2259
Restasis Ophthalmic Emulsion 575
Sandimmune 2275

Cytarabine (Antimetabolites may reduce the immune responses to vaccines).
No products indexed under this heading.

Dacarbazine (Alkylating agents may reduce the immune responses to vaccines).
No products indexed under this heading.

Daunorubicin Hydrochloride (Cytotoxic drugs may reduce the immune responses to vaccines).
No products indexed under this heading.

Dexamethasone (Corticosteroids may reduce the immune responses to vaccines). Products include:
Ciprodex Otic Suspension 559
Decadron Tablets 1951
TobraDex Ophthalmic Ointment 562
TobraDex Ophthalmic Suspension ... 563

Dexamethasone Acetate (Corticosteroids may reduce the immune responses to vaccines).
No products indexed under this heading.

Dexamethasone Sodium Phosphate (Corticosteroids may reduce the immune responses to vaccines).
No products indexed under this heading.

Doxorubicin Hydrochloride (Cytotoxic drugs may reduce the immune responses to vaccines).
No products indexed under this heading.

Epirubicin Hydrochloride (Cytotoxic drugs may reduce the immune responses to vaccines).
No products indexed under this heading.

Floxuridine (Antimetabolites may reduce the immune responses to vaccines).
No products indexed under this heading.

Fludarabine Phosphate (Antimetabolites may reduce the immune responses to vaccines).
No products indexed under this heading.

Fludrocortisone Acetate (Corticosteroids may reduce the immune responses to vaccines).
No products indexed under this heading.

Fluorouracil (Antimetabolites may reduce the immune responses to vaccines). Products include:
Carac Cream, 0.5% 2879
Efudex 3363

Gemcitabine Hydrochloride (Antimetabolites may reduce the immune responses to vaccines). Products include:
Gemzar for Injection 1771

Hydrocortisone (Corticosteroids may reduce the immune responses to vaccines). Products include:
Colocort Rectal Suspension, USP (Retention) 100 mg/60 mL 2476
Hydrocortone Tablets 1989
Preparation H Hydrocortisone Cream .... ▣646

Hydrocortisone Acetate (Corticosteroids may reduce the immune responses to vaccines). Products include:
Analpram-HC 1159
Pramosone 1161
ProctoFoam-HC 3099

Hydrocortisone Sodium Phosphate (Corticosteroids may reduce the immune responses to vaccines).
No products indexed under this heading.

Hydrocortisone Sodium Succinate (Corticosteroids may reduce the immune responses to vaccines).
No products indexed under this heading.

Hydroxyurea (Cytotoxic drugs may reduce the immune responses to vaccines).
No products indexed under this heading.

Lomustine (CCNU) (Alkylating agents may reduce the immune responses to vaccines).
No products indexed under this heading.

Mechlorethamine Hydrochloride (Alkylating agents may reduce the immune responses to vaccines). Products include:
Mustargen for Injection 2468

Melphalan (Alkylating agents may reduce the immune responses to vaccines). Products include:
Alkeran Tablets 956

Mercaptopurine (Antimetabolites may reduce the immune responses to vaccines).
No products indexed under this heading.

Methotrexate (Antimetabolites may reduce the immune responses to vaccines).
No products indexed under this heading.

Methotrexate Sodium (Cytotoxic drugs may reduce the immune responses to vaccines).
No products indexed under this heading.

Methylprednisolone Acetate (Corticosteroids may reduce the immune responses to vaccines). Products include:
Depo-Medrol Injectable Suspension 2617
Depo-Medrol Single-Dose Vial 2619

Methylprednisolone Sodium Succinate (Corticosteroids may reduce the immune responses to vaccines).
No products indexed under this heading.

Mitotane (Cytotoxic drugs may reduce the immune responses to vaccines).
No products indexed under this heading.

Mitoxantrone Hydrochloride (Cytotoxic drugs may reduce the immune responses to vaccines).
No products indexed under this heading.

Muromonab-CD3 (Immunosuppressive agents may reduce the immune responses to vaccines). Products include:
Orthoclone OKT3 Sterile Solution 2360

Mycophenolate Mofetil (Immunosuppressive agents may reduce the immune responses to vaccines). Products include:
CellCept Capsules 2747
CellCept Oral Suspension 2747
CellCept Tablets 2747

Pentostatin (Antimetabolites may reduce the immune responses to vaccines). Products include:
Nipent for Injection 1863

Prednisolone Acetate (Corticosteroids may reduce the immune responses to vaccines). Products include:
Blephamide Ophthalmic Ointment 568
Blephamide Ophthalmic Suspension 569
Poly-Pred Ophthalmic Suspension .... ⊙233
Pred Forte Ophthalmic Suspension .... ⊙235
Pred Mild Ophthalmic Suspension .... ⊙238
Pred-G Ophthalmic Ointment .... ⊙237
Pred-G Ophthalmic Suspension ...... ⊙236

Prednisolone Sodium Phosphate (Corticosteroids may reduce the immune responses to vaccines).
No products indexed under this heading.

Prednisolone Tebutate (Corticosteroids may reduce the immune responses to vaccines).
No products indexed under this heading.

Prednisone (Corticosteroids may reduce the immune responses to vaccines).
No products indexed under this heading.

Procarbazine Hydrochloride (Cytotoxic drugs may reduce the immune responses to vaccines). Products include:
Matulane Capsules 3191

Sirolimus (Immunosuppressive agents may reduce the immune responses to vaccines). Products include:
Rapamune Oral Solution and Tablets 3475

Tacrolimus (Immunosuppressive agents may reduce the immune responses to vaccines). Products include:
Prograf Capsules and Injection 632
Protopic Ointment 638

Tamoxifen Citrate (Cytotoxic drugs may reduce the immune responses to vaccines). Products include:
Soltamox Oral Solution 3527

Thioguanine (Antimetabolites may reduce the immune responses to vaccines). Products include:
Tabloid Tablets 1575

Thiotepa (Alkylating agents may reduce the immune responses to vaccines).
No products indexed under this heading.

Triamcinolone (Corticosteroids may reduce the immune responses to vaccines).
No products indexed under this heading.

Triamcinolone Acetonide (Corticosteroids may reduce the immune responses to vaccines). Products include:
Azmacort Inhalation Aerosol 1726
Nasacort AQ Nasal Spray 2922

Triamcinolone Diacetate (Corticosteroids may reduce the immune responses to vaccines).
No products indexed under this heading.

Triamcinolone Hexacetonide (Corticosteroids may reduce the immune responses to vaccines).
No products indexed under this heading.

Vincristine Sulfate (Cytotoxic drugs may reduce the immune responses to vaccines).
No products indexed under this heading.

GAS-X EXTRA STRENGTH CHEWABLE TABLETS
(Simethicone) .... ▣656
None cited in PDR database.

GAS-X EXTRA STRENGTH SOFTGELS
(Simethicone) .... ▣656
None cited in PDR database.

GAS-X MAXIMUM STRENGTH SOFTGELS
(Simethicone) .... ▣656
None cited in PDR database.

GAS-X WITH MAALOX EXTRA STRENGTH CHEWABLE TABLETS
(Calcium Carbonate, Simethicone) ... ▣656
May interact with:

Prescription Drugs, unspecified (Antacids may interact with certain unspecified prescription drugs).
No products indexed under this heading.

GAS-X WITH MAALOX EXTRA STRENGTH SOFTGELS
(Calcium Carbonate, Simethicone) ... ▣656
See Gas-X with Maalox Extra Strength Chewable Tablets

GAS-X REGULAR STRENGTH CHEWABLE TABLETS
(Simethicone) .... ▣656
None cited in PDR database.

GAS-X EXTRA STRENGTH THIN STRIPS
(Simethicone) .... ▣657
None cited in PDR database.

GAVISCON REGULAR STRENGTH LIQUID
(Aluminum Hydroxide, Magnesium Carbonate) .... ▣658
May interact with:

Prescription Drugs, unspecified (Concurrent use with certain unspecified drugs is not recommended; consult your physicians).
No products indexed under this heading.

GAVISCON REGULAR STRENGTH TABLETS
(Aluminum Hydroxide, Magnesium Trisilicate) .... ▣658
May interact with:

Prescription Drugs, unspecified (Concurrent use with certain unspecified drugs is not recommended; consult your physicians).
No products indexed under this heading.

GAVISCON EXTRA STRENGTH LIQUID
(Aluminum Hydroxide, Magnesium Carbonate) .... ▣658
May interact with:

Prescription Drugs, unspecified (Concurrent use with certain unspecified drugs is not recommended; consult your physicians).
No products indexed under this heading.

GAVISCON EXTRA STRENGTH TABLETS
(Aluminum Hydroxide, Magnesium Carbonate) .... ▣658
May interact with:

Prescription Drugs, unspecified (Concurrent use with certain unspecified drugs is not recommended; consult your physicians).
No products indexed under this heading.

GEMZAR FOR INJECTION
(Gemcitabine Hydrochloride) 1771
None cited in PDR database.

GENGRAF CAPSULES
(Cyclosporine) 459
May interact with erythromycin, HMG-CoA reductase inhibitors, immunosuppressive agents, methylprednisolone, non-steroidal anti-inflammatory agents, phenytoin, prednisolone, potassium sparing diuretics, and certain other agents. Compounds in these categories include:

Allopurinol (Cyclosporine is extensively metabolized by CYP450 3A. Substances that inhibit this enzyme could decrease the metabolism and increase cyclosporine concentrations.).
No products indexed under this heading.

Amiloride Hydrochloride (Cyclosporine causes hyperkalemia; concurrent use with potassium-sparing diuretics can result in increased risk of hyperkalemia; co-administration should be avoided). Products include:
Midamor Tablets 2026
Moduretic Tablets 2028

Amiodarone Hydrochloride (Cyclosporine is extensively metabolized by CYP450 3A. Substances that inhibit this enzyme could decrease the metabolism and increase cyclosporine concentrations.).
No products indexed under this heading.

Amphotericin B (May potentiate renal dysfunction).
No products indexed under this heading.

Atorvastatin Calcium (Cyclosporine may reduce the clearance of HMG-CoA reductase inhibitors. Myotoxicity, including muscle pain and weakness, myositis, and rhabdomyolysis, have been reported with concomitant administration of cyclosporine with lovastatin, simvastatin, atorvastatin, pravastatin, and, rarely, fluvastatin. Dosage of these statins should be reduced). Products include:
Caduet Tablets 2508
Lipitor Tablets 2483

Azapropazon (May potentiate renal dysfunction).
No products indexed under this heading.

Azathioprine (Psoriasis patients who are treated with cyclosporine capsules should not receive concomitant immunosuppressive agents. Co-administration with other immunosuppressive agents increases the possibility of excessive immunosuppression).
No products indexed under this heading.

Basiliximab (Psoriasis patients who are treated with cyclosporine capsules should not receive concomitant immunosuppressive agents. Co-administration with other immunosuppressive agents increases the possibility of excessive immunosuppression). Products include:
Simulect for Injection 2284

Bromocriptine Mesylate (Cyclosporine is extensively metabolized by CYP450 3A. Substances that inhibit this enzyme could decrease the metabolism and increase cyclosporine concentrations.).
No products indexed under this heading.

Carbamazepine (Co-administration with drugs that are inducers of CYP450 3A, such as carbamazepine, could increase metabolism of cyclosporine and decrease its concentrations). Products include:
Carbatrol Capsules 3171
Equetro Extended-Release Capsules 3180
Tegretol/Tegretol-XR 2295

Celecoxib (Cyclosporine can cause nephrotoxicity; clinical status and serum creatinine should be closely monitored when cyclosporine is used with NSAIDs in rheumatoid arthritis patients). Products include:
Celebrex Capsules 3134

Cerivastatin Sodium (Cyclosporine may reduce the clearance of HMG-CoA reductase inhibitors. Myotoxicity, including muscle pain and weakness, myositis, and rhabdomyolysis, have been reported with concomitant administration of cyclosporine with lovastatin, simvastatin, atorvastatin, pravastatin, and, rarely, fluvastatin. Dosage of these statins should be reduced).
No products indexed under this heading.

Cimetidine (May potentiate renal dysfunction). Products include:
Tagamet HB 200 Tablets 664

Cimetidine Hydrochloride (May potentiate renal dysfunction).
No products indexed under this heading.

Clarithromycin (Cyclosporine is extensively metabolized by CYP450 3A. Substances that inhibit this enzyme could decrease the metabolism and increase cyclosporine concentrations). Products include:
Biaxin/Biaxin XL 402
PREVPAC 3284

Coal Tar (Psoriasis patients who are treated with cyclosporine capsules should not receive concomitant coal tar).
No products indexed under this heading.

Colchicine (Cyclosporine may reduce the clearance of colchicine and enhance its toxic effects, such as myopathy and neuropathy, especially in patients with renal dysfunction. Close clinical observation is required during concomitant administration).
No products indexed under this heading.

Dalfopristin (Cyclosporine is extensively metabolized by CYP450 3A. Substances that inhibit this enzyme could decrease the metabolism and increase cyclosporine concentrations.).
No products indexed under this heading.

Danazol (Cyclosporine is extensively metabolized by CYP450 3A. Substances that inhibit this enzyme could decrease the metabolism and increase cyclosporine concentrations.).
No products indexed under this heading.

Diclofenac Potassium (May potentiate renal dysfunction; potential for doubling of diclofenac blood levels and occasional reports of reversible decreases in renal function have been reported with concurrent use).
No products indexed under this heading.

Diclofenac Sodium (May potentiate renal dysfunction; potential for doubling of diclofenac blood levels and occasional reports of reversible decreases in renal function have been reported with concurrent use). Products include:
Arthrotec Tablets 3129
Voltaren Ophthalmic Solution 2309
Voltaren Tablets 2307
Voltaren-XR Tablets 2310

Digoxin (Cyclosporine may reduce the clearance of digoxin. Severe digitalis toxicity has been seen within days of starting cyclosporine. Close clinical observation is required during concomitant administration). Products include:
Lanoxicaps Capsules 1490
Lanoxin Injection 1494
Lanoxin Injection Pediatric 1497
Lanoxin Tablets 1500

Diltiazem Hydrochloride (Cyclosporine is extensively metabolized by CYP450 3A. Substances that inhibit this enzyme could decrease the metabolism and increase cyclosporine concentrations). Products include:
Cardizem LA Extended Release Tablets 1728
Tiazac Capsules 1201

Diltiazem Maleate (Cyclosporine is extensively metabolized by CYP450 3A. Substances that inhibit this enzyme could decrease the metabolism and increase cyclosporine concentrations.).
No products indexed under this heading.

Erythromycin (Cyclosporine is extensively metabolized by CYP450 3A. Substances that inhibit this enzyme could decrease the metabolism and increase cyclosporine concentrations). Products include:
Ery-Tab Tablets 449
Erythromycin Base Filmtab Tablets 455
Erythromycin Delayed-Release Capsules, USP 457
PCE Dispertab Tablets 515

Erythromycin Estolate (Cyclosporine is extensively metabolized by CYP450 3A. Substances that inhibit this enzyme could decrease the metabolism and increase cyclosporine concentrations.).
No products indexed under this heading.

Erythromycin Ethylsuccinate (Cyclosporine is extensively metabolized by CYP450 3A. Substances that inhibit this enzyme could decrease the metabolism and increase cyclosporine concentrations). Products include:
E.E.S. 451
EryPed 447

Erythromycin Gluceptate (Cyclosporine is extensively metabolized by CYP450 3A. Substances that inhibit this enzyme could decrease the metabolism and increase cyclosporine concentrations.).
No products indexed under this heading.

Erythromycin Lactobionate (Cyclosporine is extensively metabolized by CYP450 3A. Substances that inhibit this enzyme could decrease the metabolism and increase cyclosporine concentrations.).
No products indexed under this heading.

Erythromycin Stearate (Cyclosporine is extensively metabolized by CYP450 3A. Substances that inhibit this enzyme could decrease the metabolism and increase cyclosporine concentrations). Products include:
Erythrocin Stearate Filmtab Tablets 453

Etodolac (Cyclosporine can cause nephrotoxicity; clinical status and serum creatinine should be closely monitored when cyclosporine is used with NSAIDs in rheumatoid arthritis patients).
No products indexed under this heading.

Fenoprofen Calcium (Cyclosporine can cause nephrotoxicity; clinical status and serum creatinine should be closely monitored when cyclosporine is used with NSAIDs in rheumatoid arthritis patients). Products include:
Nalfon Capsules 2502

Fluconazole (Co-administration with drugs that inhibit CYP450 3A, such as fluconazole, could decrease metabolism of cyclosporine and increase its concentrations).
No products indexed under this heading.

Flurbiprofen (Cyclosporine can cause nephrotoxicity; clinical status and serum creatinine should be closely monitored when cyclosporine is used with NSAIDs in rheumatoid arthritis patients).
No products indexed under this heading.

Fluvastatin Sodium (Cyclosporine may reduce the clearance of HMG-CoA reductase inhibitors. Myotoxicity, including muscle pain and weakness, myositis, and rhabdomyolysis, have been reported with concomitant administration of cyclosporine with lovastatin, simvastatin, atorvastatin, pravastatin, and, rarely, fluvastatin. Dosage of these statins should be reduced). Products include:
Lescol Capsules 2233
Lescol XL Tablets 2233

Fosphenytoin Sodium (Co-administration with drugs that are inducers of CYP450 3A, such as phenytoin, could increase metabolism of cyclosporine and decrease its concentrations).
No products indexed under this heading.

Gentamicin Sulfate (May potentiate renal dysfunction). Products include:
Garamycin Injectable 3014
Pred-G Ophthalmic Ointment .... ⊙237
Pred-G Ophthalmic Suspension ...... ⊙236

Hypericum (Co-administration with drugs that are inducers of CYP450 3A could increase metabolism of cyclosporine and decrease its concentrations. This interaction has been reported to produce a marked reduction in the blood concentrations of cyclosporine, resultingin subtherapeutic levels, rejection of transplant organs, and graft loss). Products include:
Satiete Tablets 832

Ibuprofen (Cyclosporine can cause nephrotoxicity; clinical status and serum creatinine should be closely monitored when cyclosporine is used with NSAIDs in rheumatoid arthritis patients). Products include:
Advil Allergy Sinus Caplets 770
Advil 674
Children's Advil Oral Suspension 603
Children's Advil Chewable Tablets .. 603
Advil Cold & Sinus 723

Infants' Advil Concentrated Drops .. ■ 604
Infants' Advil Concentrated Drops - White Grape (Dye-Free) .... ■ 604
Junior Strength Advil Swallow Tablets .... ■ 605
Advil Migraine Liquigels .... ■ 608
Advil Multi-Symptom Cold Caplets .... ■ 770
Advil PM Caplets .... ■ 615
Motrin IB Tablets and Caplets 1866
Children's Motrin Oral Suspension ... 1867
Children's Motrin Non-Staining Dye-Free Oral Suspension 1867
Children's Motrin Cold Oral Suspension 1867
Infants' Motrin Concentrated Drops 1867
Infants' Motrin Non-Staining Dye-Free Concentrated Drops 1867
Junior Strength Motrin Caplets and Chewable Tablets 1867
Vicoprofen Tablets 539

Indomethacin (Cyclosporine can cause nephrotoxicity; clinical status and serum creatinine should be closely monitored when cyclosporine is used with NSAIDs in rheumatoid arthritis patients). Products include:
Indocin 1995

Indomethacin Sodium Trihydrate (Cyclosporine can cause nephrotoxicity; clinical status and serum creatinine should be closely monitored when cyclosporine is used with NSAIDs in rheumatoid arthritis patients). Products include:
Indocin I.V. 2465

Itraconazole (Co-administration with drugs that inhibit CYP450 3A, such as itraconazole, could decrease metabolism of cyclosporine and increase its concentrations).
No products indexed under this heading.

Ketoconazole (May potentiate renal dysfunction; co-administration with drugs that inhibit CYP4503A, such as ketoconazole, could decrease metabolism of cyclosporine and increase its concentrations). Products include:
Nizoral A-D Shampoo, 1% 1868

Ketoprofen (Cyclosporine can cause nephrotoxicity; clinical status and serum creatinine should be closely monitored when cyclosporine is used with NSAIDs in rheumatoid arthritis patients).
No products indexed under this heading.

Ketorolac Tromethamine (Cyclosporine can cause nephrotoxicity; clinical status and serum creatinine should be closely monitored when cyclosporine is used with NSAIDs in rheumatoid arthritis patients). Products include:
Acular Ophthalmic Solution 565
Acular LS Ophthalmic Solution 566

Lovastatin (Co-administration results in reduced clearance of lovastatin; myositis has been reported with concurrent use). Products include:
Advicor Tablets 1722
Altoprev Extended-Release Tablets 3109
Mevacor Tablets 2021

Meclofenamate Sodium (Cyclosporine can cause nephrotoxicity; clinical status and serum creatinine should be closely monitored when cyclosporine is used with NSAIDs in rheumatoid arthritis patients).
No products indexed under this heading.

Mefenamic Acid (Cyclosporine can cause nephrotoxicity; clinical status and serum creatinine should be closely monitored when cyclosporine is used with NSAIDs in rheumatoid arthritis patients).
No products indexed under this heading.

Meloxicam (Cyclosporine can cause nephrotoxicity; clinical status and serum creatinine should be closely monitored when cyclosporine is used with NSAIDs in rheumatoid arthritis patients). Products include:
Mobic Oral Suspension 863
Mobic Tablets 863

Melphalan (May potentiate renal dysfunction). Products include:
Alkeran Tablets 956

Methotrexate Sodium (Psoriasis patients who are treated with cyclosporine capsules should not receive concomitant methotrexate. Co-administration in rheumatoid arthritis patients has resulted in increased concentrations (AUC) of methotrexate by approximately 30% and the concentrations of its metabolite, 7-hydromethotrexate, were decreased by approximately 80%; the clinical significance of this otucome is nto know).
No products indexed under this heading.

Methylprednisolone (Co-administration with drugs that inhibit CYP450 3A such as methylprednisolone, could decrease metabolism of cyclosporine and increase its concentrations; convulsions have been reported with concurrent high dose methylprednisolone).
No products indexed under this heading.

Methylprednisolone Acetate (Co-administration with drugs that inhibit CYP450 3A such as methylprednisolone, could decrease metabolism of cyclosporine and increase its concentrations; convulsions have been reported with concurrent high dose methylprednisolone). Products include:
Depo-Medrol Injectable Suspension 2617
Depo-Medrol Single-Dose Vial 2619

Methylprednisolone Sodium Succinate (Co-administration with drugs that inhibit CYP450 3A such as methylprednisolone, could decrease metabolism of cyclosporine and increase its concentrations; convulsions have been reported with concurrent high dose methylprednisolone).
No products indexed under this heading.

Metoclopramide Hydrochloride (Cyclosporine is extensively metabolized by CYP450 3A. Substances that inhibit this enzyme could decrease the metabolism and increase cyclosporine concentrations.).
No products indexed under this heading.

Muromonab-CD3 (Psoriasis patients who are treated with cyclosporine capsules should not receive concomitant immunosuppressive agents. Co-administration with other immunosuppressive agents increases the possibility of excessive immunosuppression). Products include:
Orthoclone OKT3 Sterile Solution 2360

Mycophenolate Mofetil (Psoriasis patients who are treated with cyclosporine capsules should not receive concomitant immunosuppressive agents. Co-administration with other immunosuppressive agents increases the possibility of excessive immunosuppression). Products include:
CellCept Capsules 2747
CellCept Oral Suspension 2747
CellCept Tablets 2747

Nabumetone (Cyclosporine can cause nephrotoxicity; clinical status and serum creatinine should be closely monitored when cyclosporine is used with NSAIDs in rheumatoid arthritis patients).
No products indexed under this heading.

Nafcillin Sodium (Co-administration with drugs that are inducers of CYP450 3A, such as nafcillin, could increase metabolism of cyclosporine and decrease its concentrations).
No products indexed under this heading.

Naproxen (May potentiate renal dysfunction; co-administration is associated with additive decreases in renal function). Products include:
EC-Naprosyn Delayed-Release Tablets 2761
Naprosyn Suspension 2761
Naprosyn Tablets 2761
Prevacid NapraPAC 3280

Naproxen Sodium (May potentiate renal dysfunction; co-administration is associated with additive decreases in renal function). Products include:
Aleve Caplets 742
Aleve Gelcaps 743
Aleve Tablets 743
Aleve Cold & Sinus Caplets 744
Anaprox Tablets 2761
Anaprox DS Tablets 2761

Nicardipine Hydrochloride (Cyclosporine is extensively metabolized by CYP450 3A. Substances that inhibit this enzyme could decrease the metabolism and increase cyclosporine concentrations). Products include:
Cardene I.V. 2497

Nifedipine (Co-administration results in frequent episodes of gingival hyperplasia). Products include:
Adalat CC Tablets 2964

Octreotide Acetate (Co-administration with drugs that are inducers of CYP450 3A, such as octreotide, could increase metabolism of cyclosporine and decrease its concentrations). Products include:
Sandostatin Injection 2278
Sandostatin LAR Depot 2280

Orlistat (Co-administration with drugs that are inducers of CYP450 3A could increase metabolism of cyclosporine and decrease its concentrations). Products include:
Xenical Capsules 2831

Oxaprozin (Cyclosporine can cause nephrotoxicity; clinical status and serum creatinine should be closely monitored when cyclosporine is used with NSAIDs in rheumatoid arthritis patients).
No products indexed under this heading.

Phenobarbital (Co-administration with drugs that are inducers of CYP450 3A, such as phenobarbital, could increase metabolism of cyclosporine and decrease its concentrations). Products include:
Donnatal Extentabs 2493

Phenylbutazone (Cyclosporine can cause nephrotoxicity; clinical status and serum creatinine should be closely monitored when cyclosporine is used with NSAIDs in rheumatoid arthritis patients).
No products indexed under this heading.

Phenytoin (Co-administration with drugs that are inducers of CYP450 3A, such as phenytoin, could increase metabolism of cyclosporine and decrease its concentrations).
No products indexed under this heading.

Phenytoin Sodium (Co-administration with drugs that are inducers of CYP450 3A, such as phenytoin, could increase metabolism of cyclosporine and decrease its concentrations). Products include:
Phenytek Capsules 2160

Piroxicam (Cyclosporine can cause nephrotoxicity; clinical status and serum creatinine should be closely monitored when cyclosporine is used with NSAIDs in rheumatoid arthritis patients).
No products indexed under this heading.

Pravastatin Sodium (Cyclosporine may reduce the clearance of HMG-CoA reductase inhibitors. Myotoxicity, including muscle pain and weakness, myositis, and rhabdomyolysis, have been reported with concomitant administration of cyclosporine with lovastatin, simvastatin, atorvastatin, pravastatin, and, rarely, fluvastatin. Dosage of these statins should be reduced).
No products indexed under this heading.

Prednisolone (Co-administration results in reduced clearance of prednisolone).
No products indexed under this heading.

Prednisolone Acetate (Co-administration results in reduced clearance of prednisolone). Products include:
Blephamide Ophthalmic Ointment 568
Blephamide Ophthalmic Suspension 569
Poly-Pred Ophthalmic Suspension .... ⊙ 233
Pred Forte Ophthalmic Suspension .... ⊙ 235
Pred Mild Ophthalmic Suspension .... ⊙ 238
Pred-G Ophthalmic Ointment .... ⊙ 237
Pred-G Ophthalmic Suspension .... ⊙ 236

Prednisolone Sodium Phosphate (Co-administration results in reduced clearance of prednisolone).
No products indexed under this heading.

Prednisolone Tebutate (Co-administration results in reduced clearance of prednisolone).
No products indexed under this heading.

Quinupristin (Cyclosporine is extensively metabolized by CYP450 3A. Substances that inhibit this enzyme could decrease the metabolism and increase cyclosporine concentrations.).
No products indexed under this heading.

Ranitidine Hydrochloride (May potentiate renal dysfunction). Products include:
- Zantac 1624
- Zantac Injection 1619
- Zantac Injection Pharmacy Bulk Package 1622

Rifabutin (Rifabutin is known to increase the metabolism of other drugs metabolized by CYP450 system; cyclosporine is extensively metabolized by CYP450 3A system, therefore, caution should be exercised).
No products indexed under this heading.

Rifampin (Co-administration with drugs that are inducers of CYP450 3A, such as rifampin, could increase metabolism of cyclosporine and decrease its concentrations).
No products indexed under this heading.

Rofecoxib (Cyclosporine can cause nephrotoxicity; clinical status and serum creatinine should be closely monitored when cyclosporine is used with NSAIDs in rheumatoid arthritis patients).
No products indexed under this heading.

Simvastatin (Cyclosporine may reduce the clearance of HMG-CoA reductase inhibitors. Myotoxicity, including muscle pain and weakness, myositis, and rhabdomyolysis, have been reported with concomitant administration of cyclosporine with lovastatin, simvastatin, atorvastatin, pravastatin, and, rarely, fluvastatin. Dosage of these statins should be reduced). Products include:
- Vytorin 10/10 Tablets 2114
- Vytorin 10/10 Tablets 3077
- Vytorin 10/20 Tablets 2114
- Vytorin 10/20 Tablets 3077
- Vytorin 10/40 Tablets 2114
- Vytorin 10/40 Tablets 3077
- Vytorin 10/80 Tablets 2114
- Vytorin 10/80 Tablets 3077
- Zocor Tablets 2105

Sirolimus (Psoriasis patients who are treated with cyclosporine capsules should not receive concomitant immunosuppressive agents. Co-administration with other immunosuppressive agents increases the possibility of excessive immunosuppression). Products include:
- Rapamune Oral Solution and Tablets 3475

Spironolactone (Cyclosporine causes hyperkalemia; concurrent use with potassium-sparing diuretics can result in increased risk of hyperkalemia; co-administration should be avoided).
No products indexed under this heading.

Sulfamethoxazole (May potentiate renal dysfunction).
No products indexed under this heading.

Sulindac (May potentiate renal dysfunction; co-administration is associated with additive decreases in renal function). Products include:
- Clinoril Tablets 1924

Tacrolimus (May potentiate renal dysfunction; co-administration with other immunosuppressive agents increases the possibility of excessive immunosuppression). Products include:
- Prograf Capsules and Injection 632
- Protopic Ointment 638

Ticlopidine Hydrochloride (Co-administration with drugs that are inducers of CYP450 3A, such as ticlopidine, could increase metabolism of cyclosporine and decrease its concentrations). Products include:
- Ticlid Tablets 2810

Tobramycin (May potentiate renal dysfunction). Products include:
- TOBI Solution for Inhalation 2298
- TobraDex Ophthalmic Ointment 562
- TobraDex Ophthalmic Suspension 563
- Zylet Ophthalmic Suspension .... ⊙259

Tobramycin Sulfate (May potentiate renal dysfunction).
No products indexed under this heading.

Tolmetin Sodium (Cyclosporine can cause nephrotoxicity; clinical status and serum creatinine should be closely monitored when cyclosporine is used with NSAIDs in rheumatoid arthritis patients).
No products indexed under this heading.

Triamterene (Cyclosporine causes hyperkalemia; concurrent use with potassium-sparing diuretics can result in increased risk of hyperkalemia; co-administration should be avoided). Products include:
- Dyazide Capsules 1423
- Dyrenium Capsules 3400

Trimethoprim (May potentiate renal dysfunction).
No products indexed under this heading.

Ultraviolet radiation (Psoriasis patients who are treated with cyclosporine capsules should not receive concomitant PUVA or UVB therapy).
No products indexed under this heading.

Vaccines (Live) (During treatment with cyclosporine, vaccination may be less effective and the use of live attenuated vaccines should be avoided).
No products indexed under this heading.

Valdecoxib (Cyclosporine can cause nephrotoxicity; clinical status and serum creatinine should be closely monitored when cyclosporine is used with NSAIDs in rheumatoid arthritis patients).
No products indexed under this heading.

Vancomycin Hydrochloride (May potentiate renal dysfunction). Products include:
- Vancocin HCl Capsules, USP 3380

Verapamil Hydrochloride (Cyclosporine is extensively metabolized by CYP450 3A. Substances that inhibit this enzyme could decrease the metabolism and increase cyclosporine concentrations). Products include:
- Covera-HS Tablets 3139
- Tarka Tablets 524
- Verelan PM Extended-Release Capsules, Controlled-Onset 3106

Food Interactions

Diet, high-lipid (A high fat meal within one-half hour before cyclosporine administration decreases the AUC by 13% and Cmax by 33%).

Food, unspecified (The administration of food with Gengraf decreases the cyclosporine AUC and Cmax).

Grapefruit (Affects the metabolism of cyclosporine by increasing blood concentration of cyclosporine; concurrent use should be avoided).

Grapefruit Juice (Affects the metabolism of cyclosporine by increasing blood concentration of cyclosporine; concurrent use should be avoided).

GENOTROPIN LYOPHILIZED POWDER

(Somatropin) 2638

May interact with glucocorticoids and drugs which undergo biotransformation by cytochrome p-450 mixed function oxidase. Compounds in these categories include:

Acarbose (Growth hormone administration may alter the clearance of compounds known to be metabolized by CYP 450 liver enzymes; careful monitoring is advisable). Products include:
- Precose Tablets 751

Acetaminophen (Growth hormone administration may alter the clearance of compounds known to be metabolized by CYP 450 liver enzymes; careful monitoring is advisable). Products include:
- Comtrex Maximum Strength Cold & Cough Day/Night Caplets - Day Formulation 726
- Comtrex Maximum Strength Cold & Cough Day/Night Caplets - Night Formulation 726
- Comtrex Maximum Strength Non-Drowsy Cold & Cough Caplets 725
- Comtrex Maximum Strength Day/Night Severe Cold & Sinus Caplets - Day Formulation 725
- Comtrex Maximum Strength Day/Night Severe Cold & Sinus Caplets - Night Formulation 725
- Contac Cold and Flu Maximum Strength Caplets 728
- Contac Cold and Flu Day and Night Caplets (Day Formulation Only) 727
- Contac Cold and Flu Day and Night Caplets (Night Formulation Only) 727
- Contac Cold and Flu Non-Drowsy Caplets 728
- Excedrin Extra Strength Caplets/Tablets/Geltabs 684
- Excedrin Migraine Caplets/Tablets/Geltabs 609
- Excedrin PM Caplets/Tablets/Geltabs 610
- Excedrin Sinus Headache Caplets/Tablets 610
- Excedrin Tension Headache Caplets/Tablets/Geltabs 611
- Goody's Body Pain Formula Powder 684
- Goody's Extra Strength Headache Powders 611
- Goody's Extra Strength Pain Relief Tablets 685
- Goody's PM Powder for Pain with Sleeplessness 612
- Percocet Tablets 1131
- Robitussin Cough, Cold & Flu Nighttime Liquid 738
- TheraFlu Cold & Sore Throat Hot Liquid 741
- TheraFlu Flu & Chest Congestion Hot Liquid 741
- TheraFlu Flu & Sore Throat Hot Liquid 742
- TheraFlu Daytime Severe Cold Hot Liquid 742
- TheraFlu Nighttime Severe Cold Hot Liquid 740
- TheraFlu Warming Relief Daytime Severe Cold 743
- TheraFlu Warming Relief Nighttime Severe Cold 743
- Triaminic Cough & Sore Throat Liquid 747
- Regular Strength Tylenol Tablets 1870
- Children's Tylenol with Flavor Creator 679
- Children's Tylenol Plus Flu Oral Suspension 749
- Tylenol Cold Head Congestion Daytime Caplets with Cool Burst and Gelcaps 750
- Tylenol Cold Multi-Symptom Daytime Liquid 752
- Tylenol Cold Multi-Symptom Severe Daytime Liquid 752
- Tylenol 8 Hour Extended Release Caplets 1870
- Tylenol 1870
- Extra Strength Tylenol PM Caplets, Vanilla Caplets, Geltabs, Gelcaps and Liquid 1875
- Extra Strength Tylenol Rapid Release Gels 1870
- Concentrated Tylenol Infants' Drops Plus Cold & Cough 754
- Tylenol with Codeine Tablets 2391
- Tylenol Allergy Multi-Symptom Caplets with Cool Burst and Gelcaps 1872
- Tylenol Allergy Multi-Symptom Nighttime Caplets with Cool Burst 1872
- Tylenol Severe Allergy Caplets 1872
- Tylenol Arthritis Pain Extended Release Caplets and Geltabs 1870
- Tylenol Chest Congestion Caplets with Cool Burst 1872
- Tylenol Chest Congestion Liquid with Cool Burst 1872
- Children's Tylenol Suspension Liquid and Meltaways 1878
- Children's Tylenol Plus Cold Suspension Liquid 1879
- Children's Tylenol Plus Cold & Allergy Suspension Liquid 1878
- Children's Tylenol Plus Cough & Runny Nose Suspension Liquid 1879
- Children's Tylenol Plus Cough & Sore Throat Suspension Liquid 1879
- Children's Tylenol Suspension with Flavor Creator 1878
- Children's Tylenol Plus Flu Suspension Liquid 1881
- Children's Tylenol Plus Multi-Symptom Cold Suspension Liquid 1879
- Tylenol Cold Severe Congestion Non-Drowsy Caplets with Cool Burst 1874
- Tylenol Cold Head Congestion Daytime Caplets with Cool Burst 1873
- Tylenol Cold Head Congestion Nighttime Caplets with Cool Burst 1873
- Tylenol Cold Head Congestion Severe Caplets with Cool Burst 1873
- Tylenol Cold Multi-Symptom Daytime Caplets with Cool Burst and Gelcaps 1874
- Tylenol Cold Multi-Symptom Daytime Liquid with Citrus Burst 1874
- Tylenol Cold Multi-Symptom Nighttime Caplets with Cool Burst 1874
- Tylenol Cold Multi-Symptom Nighttime Liquid with Cool Burst 1874
- Tylenol Cold Multi-Symptom Severe Caplets with Cool Burst 1874
- Tylenol Cold Multi-Symptom Severe Daytime Liquid with Citrus Burst 1874
- Tylenol Cough & Sore Throat Daytime Liquid with Cool Burst 1877
- Tylenol Cough & Sore Throat Nighttime Liquid with Cool Burst 1877
- Concentrated Tylenol Infants' Drops 1878
- Concentrated Tylenol Infants' Drops Plus Cold 1879
- Concentrated Tylenol Infants' Drops Plus Cold and Cough 1879
- Jr. Tylenol Meltaways 1878
- Tylenol Sinus Severe Congestion Caplets with Cool Burst 1876
- Tylenol Sinus Congestion & Pain Daytime Caplets with Cool Burst and Gelcaps 1876
- Tylenol Sinus Congestion & Pain Nighttime Caplets with Cool Burst 1876
- Tylenol Sinus Congestion & Pain Severe Caplets with Cool Burst 1876
- Tylenol Sore Throat Daytime Liquid with Cool Burst 1877

Tylenol Sore Throat Nighttime Liquid with Cool Burst 1877
Women's Tylenol Menstrual Relief Caplets 1877
Vicks 44M Cough, Cold & Flu Relief Liquid 2680
Vicks DayQuil LiquiCaps/Liquid Multi-Symptom Cold/Flu Relief .... ■ 761
Vicks DayQuil Multi-Symptom Cold/Flu Relief LiquiCaps 2678
Vicks DayQuil Multi-Symptom Cold/Flu Relief Liquid 2678
Vicks NyQuil Multi-Symptom Cold/Flu Relief Liquid 2681
Vicks NyQuil Multi-Symptom Cold/Flu Relief LiquiCaps 2681
Vicks NyQuil LiquiCaps/Liquid Multi-Symptom Cold/Flu Relief .... ■ 763
Vicodin Tablets 535
Vicodin ES Tablets 536
Vicodin HP Tablets 538
Zicam Maximum Strength Flu Daytime .... ■ 768
Zicam Maximum Strength Flu Nighttime .... ■ 768
Zydone Tablets 1139

Alatrofloxacin Mesylate (Growth hormone administration may alter the clearance of compounds known to be metabolized by CYP 450 liver enzymes; careful monitoring is advisable).
No products indexed under this heading.

Alfentanil Hydrochloride (Growth hormone administration may alter the clearance of compounds known to be metabolized by CYP 450 liver enzymes; careful monitoring is advisable).
No products indexed under this heading.

Alprazolam (Growth hormone administration may alter the clearance of compounds known to be metabolized by CYP 450 liver enzymes; careful monitoring is advisable). Products include:
Niravam Orally Disintegrating Tablets 3092

Aminophylline (Growth hormone administration may alter the clearance of compounds known to be metabolized by CYP 450 liver enzymes; careful monitoring is advisable).
No products indexed under this heading.

Amiodarone Hydrochloride (Growth hormone administration may alter the clearance of compounds known to be metabolized by CYP 450 liver enzymes; careful monitoring is advisable).
No products indexed under this heading.

Amitriptyline Hydrochloride (Growth hormone administration may alter the clearance of compounds known to be metabolized by CYP 450 liver enzymes; careful monitoring is advisable).
No products indexed under this heading.

Amlodipine Besylate (Growth hormone administration may alter the clearance of compounds known to be metabolized by CYP 450 liver enzymes; careful monitoring is advisable). Products include:
Caduet Tablets 2508
Lotrel Capsules 2249
Norvasc Tablets 2545

Amoxapine (Growth hormone administration may alter the clearance of compounds known to be metabolized by CYP 450 liver enzymes; careful monitoring is advisable).
No products indexed under this heading.

Amphetamine Aspartate (Growth hormone administration may alter the clearance of compounds known to be metabolized by CYP 450 liver enzymes; careful monitoring is advisable). Products include:
Adderall Tablets 3164
Adderall XR Capsules 3166

Amphetamine Aspartate Monohydrate (Growth hormone administration may alter the clearance of compounds known to be metabolized by CYP 450 liver enzymes; careful monitoring is advisable).
No products indexed under this heading.

Amphetamine Sulfate (Growth hormone administration may alter the clearance of compounds known to be metabolized by CYP 450 liver enzymes; careful monitoring is advisable). Products include:
Adderall Tablets 3164
Adderall XR Capsules 3166

Aprepitant (Growth hormone administration may alter the clearance of compounds known to be metabolized by CYP 450 liver enzymes; careful monitoring is advisable). Products include:
Emend Capsules 1963

Astemizole (Growth hormone administration may alter the clearance of compounds known to be metabolized by CYP 450 liver enzymes; careful monitoring is advisable).
No products indexed under this heading.

Atomoxetine Hydrochloride (Growth hormone administration may alter the clearance of compounds known to be metabolized by CYP 450 liver enzymes; careful monitoring is advisable). Products include:
Strattera Capsules 1814

Atorvastatin Calcium (Growth hormone administration may alter the clearance of compounds known to be metabolized by CYP 450 liver enzymes; careful monitoring is advisable). Products include:
Caduet Tablets 2508
Lipitor Tablets 2483

Belladonna Ergotamine (Growth hormone administration may alter the clearance of compounds known to be metabolized by CYP 450 liver enzymes; careful monitoring is advisable).
No products indexed under this heading.

Benzphetamine Hydrochloride (Growth hormone administration may alter the clearance of compounds known to be metabolized by CYP 450 liver enzymes; careful monitoring is advisable).
No products indexed under this heading.

Betamethasone Acetate (Concomitant glucocorticoid therapy may inhibit human growth promoting effect).
No products indexed under this heading.

Betamethasone Sodium Phosphate (Concomitant glucocorticoid therapy may inhibit human growth promoting effect).
No products indexed under this heading.

Bisoprolol Fumarate (Growth hormone administration may alter the clearance of compounds known to be metabolized by CYP 450 liver enzymes; careful monitoring is advisable).
No products indexed under this heading.

Buspirone Hydrochloride (Growth hormone administration may alter the clearance of compounds known to be metabolized by CYP 450 liver enzymes; careful monitoring is advisable).
No products indexed under this heading.

Busulfan (Growth hormone administration may alter the clearance of compounds known to be metabolized by CYP 450 liver enzymes; careful monitoring is advisable). Products include:
I.V. Busulfex 2493
Myleran Tablets 1525

Caffeine (Growth hormone administration may alter the clearance of compounds known to be metabolized by CYP 450 liver enzymes; careful monitoring is advisable). Products include:
BC Headache Powder .... ■ 677
Arthritis Strength BC Powder .... ■ 677
Excedrin Extra Strength Caplets/Tablets/Geltabs .... ■ 684
Excedrin Migraine Caplets/Tablets/Geltabs .... ■ 609
Excedrin Tension Headache Caplets/Tablets/Geltabs .... ■ 611
Goody's Extra Strength Headache Powders .... ■ 611
Goody's Extra Strength Pain Relief Tablets .... ■ 685
Vivarin .... ■ 602
Winrgy Dietary Supplement .... ■ 823

Caffeine Anhydrous (Growth hormone administration may alter the clearance of compounds known to be metabolized by CYP 450 liver enzymes; careful monitoring is advisable).
No products indexed under this heading.

Caffeine Citrate (Growth hormone administration may alter the clearance of compounds known to be metabolized by CYP 450 liver enzymes; careful monitoring is advisable). Products include:
Cafcit 1886

Candesartan Cilexetil (Growth hormone administration may alter the clearance of compounds known to be metabolized by CYP 450 liver enzymes; careful monitoring is advisable). Products include:
Atacand Tablets 649
Atacand HCT 651

Captopril (Growth hormone administration may alter the clearance of compounds known to be metabolized by CYP 450 liver enzymes; careful monitoring is advisable). Products include:
Captopril Tablets 2149

Carbamazepine (Growth hormone administration may alter the clearance of compounds known to be metabolized by CYP 450 liver enzymes; careful monitoring is advisable). Products include:
Carbatrol Capsules 3171
Equetro Extended-Release Capsules 3180
Tegretol/Tegretol-XR 2295

Carisoprodol (Growth hormone administration may alter the clearance of compounds known to be metabolized by CYP 450 liver enzymes; careful monitoring is advisable).
No products indexed under this heading.

Carvedilol (Growth hormone administration may alter the clearance of compounds known to be metabolized by CYP 450 liver enzymes; careful monitoring is advisable). Products include:
Coreg Tablets 1414

Celecoxib (Growth hormone administration may alter the clearance of compounds known to be metabolized by CYP 450 liver enzymes; careful monitoring is advisable). Products include:
Celebrex Capsules 3134

Cerivastatin Sodium (Growth hormone administration may alter the clearance of compounds known to be metabolized by CYP 450 liver enzymes; careful monitoring is advisable).
No products indexed under this heading.

Cevimeline Hydrochloride (Growth hormone administration may alter the clearance of compounds known to be metabolized by CYP 450 liver enzymes; careful monitoring is advisable). Products include:
Evoxac Capsules 1047

Chlordiazepoxide (Growth hormone administration may alter the clearance of compounds known to be metabolized by CYP 450 liver enzymes; careful monitoring is advisable).
No products indexed under this heading.

Chlordiazepoxide Hydrochloride (Growth hormone administration may alter the clearance of compounds known to be metabolized by CYP 450 liver enzymes; careful monitoring is advisable). Products include:
Librium Capsules 3347

Chlorpheniramine (Growth hormone administration may alter the clearance of compounds known to be metabolized by CYP 450 liver enzymes; careful monitoring is advisable).
No products indexed under this heading.

Chlorpheniramine Maleate (Growth hormone administration may alter the clearance of compounds known to be metabolized by CYP 450 liver enzymes; careful monitoring is advisable). Products include:
Advil Allergy Sinus Caplets .... ■ 770
Advil Multi-Symptom Cold Caplets .... ■ 770
BC Allergy Sinus Cold Powder .... ■ 677
Comtrex Maximum Strength Cold & Cough Day/Night Caplets - Night Formulation .... ■ 726
Comtrex Maximum Strength Day/Night Severe Cold & Sinus Caplets - Night Formulation .... ■ 725
Contac Cold and Flu Maximum Strength Caplets .... ■ 728
Contac Cold and Flu Day and Night Caplets (Night Formulation Only) .... ■ 727
Children's Dimetapp Long Acting Cough Plus Cold Syrup .... ■ 731
Robitussin Cough & Cold Long-Acting Liquid .... ■ 735
Robitussin Cough & Allergy Syrup .... ■ 736

Chlorpheniramine Polistirex
(Growth hormone administration may
alter the clearance of compounds
known to be metabolized by CYP
450 liver enzymes; careful monitoring is advisable). Products include:

Chlorpheniramine Tannate
(Growth hormone administration may
alter the clearance of compounds
known to be metabolized by CYP
450 liver enzymes; careful monitoring is advisable).
No products indexed under this
heading.

Chlorpromazine (Growth hormone
administration may alter the clearance of compounds known to be
metabolized by CYP 450 liver
enzymes; careful monitoring is
advisable).
No products indexed under this
heading.

Chlorpromazine Hydrochloride
(Growth hormone administration may
alter the clearance of compounds
known to be metabolized by CYP
450 liver enzymes; careful monitoring is advisable).
No products indexed under this
heading.

Chlorpropamide (Growth hormone
administration may alter the clearance of compounds known to be
metabolized by CYP 450 liver
enzymes; careful monitoring is
advisable).
No products indexed under this
heading.

Cilostazol (Growth hormone administration may alter the clearance of
compounds known to be metabolized by CYP 450 liver enzymes;
careful monitoring is advisable).
Products include:

Cimetidine Hydrochloride
(Growth hormone administration may
alter the clearance of compounds
known to be metabolized by CYP
450 liver enzymes; careful monitoring is advisable).
No products indexed under this
heading.

Ciprofloxacin (Growth hormone
administration may alter the clearance of compounds known to be
metabolized by CYP 450 liver
enzymes; careful monitoring is advisable). Products include:

Ciprofloxacin Hydrochloride
(Growth hormone administration may
alter the clearance of compounds
known to be metabolized by CYP
450 liver enzymes; careful monitoring is advisable). Products include:

Cisapride (Growth hormone administration may alter the clearance of
compounds known to be metabolized by CYP 450 liver enzymes;
careful monitoring is advisable).
No products indexed under this
heading.

Citalopram Hydrobromide
(Growth hormone administration may
alter the clearance of compounds
known to be metabolized by CYP
450 liver enzymes; careful monitoring is advisable). Products include:

Clarithromycin (Growth hormone
administration may alter the clearance of compounds known to be
metabolized by CYP 450 liver
enzymes; careful monitoring is advisable). Products include:

Clomipramine Hydrochloride
(Growth hormone administration may
alter the clearance of compounds
known to be metabolized by CYP
450 liver enzymes; careful monitoring is advisable).
No products indexed under this
heading.

Clopidogrel Hydrogen Sulfate
(Growth hormone administration may
alter the clearance of compounds
known to be metabolized by CYP
450 liver enzymes; careful monitoring is advisable).
No products indexed under this
heading.

Clozapine (Growth hormone administration may alter the clearance of
compounds known to be metabolized by CYP 450 liver enzymes;
careful monitoring is advisable).
Products include:

Codeine Phosphate (Growth hormone administration may alter the
clearance of compounds known to
be metabolized by CYP 450 liver
enzymes; careful monitoring is advisable). Products include:

Codeine Sulfate (Growth hormone
administration may alter the clearance of compounds known to be
metabolized by CYP 450 liver
enzymes; careful monitoring is
advisable).
No products indexed under this
heading.

Cortisone Acetate (Concomitant
glucocorticoid therapy may inhibit
human growth promoting effect).
No products indexed under this
heading.

Cyclobenzaprine (Growth hormone administration may alter the
clearance of compounds known to
be metabolized by CYP 450 liver
enzymes; careful monitoring is
advisable).
No products indexed under this
heading.

Cyclobenzaprine Hydrochloride
(Growth hormone administration may
alter the clearance of compounds
known to be metabolized by CYP
450 liver enzymes; careful monitoring is advisable).
No products indexed under this
heading.

Cyclophosphamide (Growth hormone administration may alter the
clearance of compounds known to
be metabolized by CYP 450 liver
enzymes; careful monitoring is
advisable).
No products indexed under this
heading.

Cyclosporine (Growth hormone
administration may alter the clearance of compounds known to be
metabolized by CYP 450 liver
enzymes; careful monitoring is advisable). Products include:

Desipramine Hydrochloride
(Growth hormone administration may
alter the clearance of compounds
known to be metabolized by CYP
450 liver enzymes; careful monitoring is advisable).
No products indexed under this
heading.

Desogestrel (Growth hormone
administration may alter the clearance of compounds known to be
metabolized by CYP 450 liver
enzymes; careful monitoring is advisable). Products include:

Dexamethasone (Concomitant
glucocorticoid therapy may inhibit
human growth promoting effect).
Products include:

Dexamethasone Acetate (Concomitant glucocorticoid therapy may
inhibit human growth promoting
effect).
No products indexed under this
heading.

Dexamethasone Phosphate
(Growth hormone administration may
alter the clearance of compounds
known to be metabolized by CYP
450 liver enzymes; careful monitoring is advisable).
No products indexed under this
heading.

Dexamethasone Sodium (Growth
hormone administration may alter
the clearance of compounds known
to be metabolized by CYP 450 liver
enzymes; careful monitoring is
advisable).
No products indexed under this
heading.

**Dexamethasone Sodium Phos-
phate** (Concomitant glucocorticoid
therapy may inhibit human growth
promoting effect).
No products indexed under this
heading.

Dexfenfluramine Hydrochloride
(Growth hormone administration may
alter the clearance of compounds
known to be metabolized by CYP
450 liver enzymes; careful monitoring is advisable).
No products indexed under this
heading.

Dextromethorphan (Growth hormone administration may alter the
clearance of compounds known to
be metabolized by CYP 450 liver
enzymes; careful monitoring is
advisable).
No products indexed under this
heading.

**Dextromethorphan Hydrobro-
mide** (Growth hormone administration may alter the clearance of compounds known to be metabolized by
CYP 450 liver enzymes; careful monitoring is advisable). Products
include:

IMPORTANT NOTE: Always consult each drug listing in the patient's regimen for possible interactions.

Triaminic Cough & Runny Nose Softchews ▣748
Triaminic Thin Strips Cold & Cough ▣778
Triaminic Infant Thin Strips Decongestant Plus Cough ▣747
Children's Tylenol Plus Flu Oral Suspension ▣749
Tylenol Cold Head Congestion Daytime Caplets with Cool Burst and Gelcaps ▣750
Tylenol Cold Multi-Symptom Daytime Liquid ▣752
Tylenol Cold Multi-Symptom Severe Daytime Liquid ▣752
Concentrated Tylenol Infants' Drops Plus Cold & Cough ▣754
Children's Tylenol Plus Cough & Runny Nose Suspension Liquid 1879
Children's Tylenol Plus Cough & Sore Throat Suspension Liquid 1879
Children's Tylenol Plus Flu Suspension Liquid 1881
Children's Tylenol Plus Multi-Symptom Cold Suspension Liquid 1879
Tylenol Cold Severe Congestion Non-Drowsy Caplets with Cool Burst 1874
Tylenol Cold Head Congestion Daytime Caplets with Cool Burst 1873
Tylenol Cold Head Congestion Nighttime Caplets with Cool Burst 1873
Tylenol Cold Head Congestion Severe Caplets with Cool Burst 1873
Tylenol Cold Multi-Symptom Daytime Caplets with Cool Burst and Gelcaps 1874
Tylenol Cold Multi-Symptom Daytime Liquid with Citrus Burst 1874
Tylenol Cold Multi-Symptom Nighttime Caplets with Cool Burst 1874
Tylenol Cold Multi-Symptom Nighttime Liquid with Cool Burst 1874
Tylenol Cold Multi-Symptom Severe Caplets with Cool Burst 1874
Tylenol Cold Multi-Symptom Severe Daytime Liquid with Citrus Burst 1874
Tylenol Cough & Sore Throat Daytime Liquid with Cool Burst 1877
Tylenol Cough & Sore Throat Nighttime Liquid with Cool Burst 1877
Concentrated Tylenol Infants' Drops Plus Cold and Cough 1879
Vicks 44 Cough Relief Liquid 2679
Vicks 44D Cough & Head Congestion Relief Liquid 2679
Vicks 44E Cough & Chest Congestion Relief Liquid 2679
Pediatric Vicks 44e Cough & Chest Congestion Relief Liquid 2676
Vicks 44M Cough, Cold & Flu Relief Liquid 2680
Pediatric Vicks 44m Cough & Cold Relief Liquid 2676
Vicks DayQuil LiquiCaps/Liquid Multi-Symptom Cold/Flu Relief ▣761
Vicks DayQuil Multi-Symptom Cold/Flu Relief LiquiCaps 2678
Vicks DayQuil Multi-Symptom Cold/Flu Relief Liquid 2678
Vicks NyQuil Multi-Symptom Cold/Flu Relief Liquid 2681
Children's Vicks NyQuil Cold/Cough Relief ▣756
Vicks NyQuil Multi-Symptom Cold/Flu Relief LiquiCaps 2681
Vicks NyQuil LiquiCaps/Liquid Multi-Symptom Cold/Flu Relief ▣763
Vicks NyQuil Cough Liquid 2680
Children's Vicks NyQuil Cold/Cough Relief Liquid 2680
Zicam Cough Max Nighttime Cough Spray ▣767
Zicam Cough Max Cough Spray ▣767
Zicam Cough Max Cough Melts ▣767
Zicam Cough Plus D Cough Spray ▣767
Zicam Cough Relief Cough Spray ▣767
Zicam Maximum Strength Flu Daytime ▣768
Zicam Maximum Strength Flu Nighttime ▣768

Dextromethorphan Polistirex (Growth hormone administration may alter the clearance of compounds known to be metabolized by CYP 450 liver enzymes; careful monitoring is advisable). Products include:
Delsym Extended-Release Suspension 12 Hour Cough Suppressant ▣611

Diazepam (Growth hormone administration may alter the clearance of compounds known to be metabolized by CYP 450 liver enzymes; careful monitoring is advisable). Products include:
Diastat Rectal Delivery System 3343
Valium Tablets 2819

Diclofenac Potassium (Growth hormone administration may alter the clearance of compounds known to be metabolized by CYP 450 liver enzymes; careful monitoring is advisable).
No products indexed under this heading.

Diclofenac Sodium (Growth hormone administration may alter the clearance of compounds known to be metabolized by CYP 450 liver enzymes; careful monitoring is advisable). Products include:
Arthrotec Tablets 3129
Voltaren Ophthalmic Solution 2309
Voltaren Tablets 2307
Voltaren-XR Tablets 2310

Dihydroergotamine Mesylate (Growth hormone administration may alter the clearance of compounds known to be metabolized by CYP 450 liver enzymes; careful monitoring is advisable). Products include:
Migranal Nasal Spray 3348

Diltiazem Hydrochloride (Growth hormone administration may alter the clearance of compounds known to be metabolized by CYP 450 liver enzymes; careful monitoring is advisable). Products include:
Cardizem LA Extended Release Tablets 1728
Tiazac Capsules 1201

Diltiazem Maleate (Growth hormone administration may alter the clearance of compounds known to be metabolized by CYP 450 liver enzymes; careful monitoring is advisable).
No products indexed under this heading.

Disopyramide (Growth hormone administration may alter the clearance of compounds known to be metabolized by CYP 450 liver enzymes; careful monitoring is advisable).
No products indexed under this heading.

Disopyramide Phosphate (Growth hormone administration may alter the clearance of compounds known to be metabolized by CYP 450 liver enzymes; careful monitoring is advisable).
No products indexed under this heading.

Divalproex Sodium (Growth hormone administration may alter the clearance of compounds known to be metabolized by CYP 450 liver enzymes; careful monitoring is advisable). Products include:
Depakote Sprinkle Capsules 422
Depakote Tablets 427
Depakote ER Tablets 434

Docetaxel (Growth hormone administration may alter the clearance of compounds known to be metabolized by CYP 450 liver enzymes; careful monitoring is advisable). Products include:
Taxotere Injection Concentrate 2932

Dolasetron Mesylate (Growth hormone administration may alter the clearance of compounds known to be metabolized by CYP 450 liver enzymes; careful monitoring is advisable). Products include:
Anzemet Injection 2859
Anzemet Tablets 2862

Donepezil Hydrochloride (Growth hormone administration may alter the clearance of compounds known to be metabolized by CYP 450 liver enzymes; careful monitoring is advisable). Products include:
Aricept Tablets 1094
Aricept ODT Tablets 1094

Doxepin Hydrochloride (Growth hormone administration may alter the clearance of compounds known to be metabolized by CYP 450 liver enzymes; careful monitoring is advisable).
No products indexed under this heading.

Doxorubicin Hydrochloride (Growth hormone administration may alter the clearance of compounds known to be metabolized by CYP 450 liver enzymes; careful monitoring is advisable).
No products indexed under this heading.

Dronabinol (Growth hormone administration may alter the clearance of compounds known to be metabolized by CYP 450 liver enzymes; careful monitoring is advisable). Products include:
Marinol Capsules 3333

Drugs that Undergo Biotransformation by Cytochrome P-450 Mixed Function Oxidase (Growth hormone administration may alter the clearance of compounds known to be metabolized by CYP 450 liver enzymes; careful monitoring is advisable).
No products indexed under this heading.

Dyphylline (Growth hormone administration may alter the clearance of compounds known to be metabolized by CYP 450 liver enzymes; careful monitoring is advisable).
No products indexed under this heading.

Encainide Hydrochloride (Growth hormone administration may alter the clearance of compounds known to be metabolized by CYP 450 liver enzymes; careful monitoring is advisable).
No products indexed under this heading.

Enoxacin (Growth hormone administration may alter the clearance of compounds known to be metabolized by CYP 450 liver enzymes; careful monitoring is advisable).
No products indexed under this heading.

Eprosartan Mesylate (Growth hormone administration may alter the clearance of compounds known to be metabolized by CYP 450 liver enzymes; careful monitoring is advisable). Products include:
Teveten Tablets 1735
Teveten HCT Tablets 1737

Ergotamine Tartrate (Growth hormone administration may alter the clearance of compounds known to be metabolized by CYP 450 liver enzymes; careful monitoring is advisable).
No products indexed under this heading.

Erythromycin (Growth hormone administration may alter the clearance of compounds known to be metabolized by CYP 450 liver enzymes; careful monitoring is advisable). Products include:
Ery-Tab Tablets 449
Erythromycin Base Filmtab Tablets 455
Erythromycin Delayed-Release Capsules, USP 457
PCE Dispertab Tablets 515

Erythromycin Estolate (Growth hormone administration may alter the clearance of compounds known to be metabolized by CYP 450 liver enzymes; careful monitoring is advisable).
No products indexed under this heading.

Erythromycin Ethylsuccinate (Growth hormone administration may alter the clearance of compounds known to be metabolized by CYP 450 liver enzymes; careful monitoring is advisable). Products include:
E.E.S. 451
EryPed 447

Erythromycin Gluceptate (Growth hormone administration may alter the clearance of compounds known to be metabolized by CYP 450 liver enzymes; careful monitoring is advisable).
No products indexed under this heading.

Erythromycin Lactobionate (Growth hormone administration may alter the clearance of compounds known to be metabolized by CYP 450 liver enzymes; careful monitoring is advisable).
No products indexed under this heading.

Erythromycin Stearate (Growth hormone administration may alter the clearance of compounds known to be metabolized by CYP 450 liver enzymes; careful monitoring is advisable). Products include:
Erythrocin Stearate Filmtab Tablets 453

Esomeprazole Magnesium (Growth hormone administration may alter the clearance of compounds known to be metabolized by CYP 450 liver enzymes; careful monitoring is advisable). Products include:
Nexium Delayed-Release Capsules 655

Estradiol (Growth hormone administration may alter the clearance of compounds known to be metabolized by CYP 450 liver enzymes; careful monitoring is advisable). Products include:
Angeliq Tablets 762
Climara Transdermal System 771
Climara Pro Transdermal System 776
Estrasorb Topical Emulsion 1147
Estring Vaginal Ring 2635
Menostar Transdermal System 782
Vagifem Tablets 2334

Estradiol Benzoate (Growth hormone administration may alter the clearance of compounds known to be metabolized by CYP 450 liver enzymes; careful monitoring is advisable).
No products indexed under this heading.

Estradiol Cypionate (Growth hormone administration may alter the clearance of compounds known to be metabolized by CYP 450 liver enzymes; careful monitoring is advisable).
No products indexed under this heading.

Estradiol Valerate (Growth hormone administration may alter the clearance of compounds known to be metabolized by CYP 450 liver enzymes; careful monitoring is advisable).
No products indexed under this heading.

Estrogen (Growth hormone administration may alter the clearance of compounds known to be metabolized by CYP 450 liver enzymes; careful monitoring is advisable).
No products indexed under this heading.

Estrogens, Conjugated (Growth hormone administration may alter the clearance of compounds known to be metabolized by CYP 450 liver enzymes; careful monitoring is advisable). Products include:

Estrogens, Conjugated, Synthetic A (Growth hormone administration may alter the clearance of compounds known to be metabolized by CYP 450 liver enzymes; careful monitoring is advisable).
No products indexed under this heading.

Estrogens, Esterified (Growth hormone administration may alter the clearance of compounds known to be metabolized by CYP 450 liver enzymes; careful monitoring is advisable). Products include:

Ethinyl Estradiol (Growth hormone administration may alter the clearance of compounds known to be metabolized by CYP 450 liver enzymes; careful monitoring is advisable). Products include:

Ethosuximide (Growth hormone administration may alter the clearance of compounds known to be metabolized by CYP 450 liver enzymes; careful monitoring is advisable).
No products indexed under this heading.

Ethotoin (Growth hormone administration may alter the clearance of compounds known to be metabolized by CYP 450 liver enzymes; careful monitoring is advisable).
No products indexed under this heading.

Ethynodiol Diacetate (Growth hormone administration may alter the clearance of compounds known to be metabolized by CYP 450 liver enzymes; careful monitoring is advisable).
No products indexed under this heading.

Etodolac (Growth hormone administration may alter the clearance of compounds known to be metabolized by CYP 450 liver enzymes; careful monitoring is advisable).
No products indexed under this heading.

Etoposide (Growth hormone administration may alter the clearance of compounds known to be metabolized by CYP 450 liver enzymes; careful monitoring is advisable).
No products indexed under this heading.

Etoposide Phosphate (Growth hormone administration may alter the clearance of compounds known to be metabolized by CYP 450 liver enzymes; careful monitoring is advisable).
No products indexed under this heading.

Felbamate (Growth hormone administration may alter the clearance of compounds known to be metabolized by CYP 450 liver enzymes; careful monitoring is advisable).
No products indexed under this heading.

Felodipine (Growth hormone administration may alter the clearance of compounds known to be metabolized by CYP 450 liver enzymes; careful monitoring is advisable).
No products indexed under this heading.

Fenoprofen Calcium (Growth hormone administration may alter the clearance of compounds known to be metabolized by CYP 450 liver enzymes; careful monitoring is advisable). Products include:

Fentanyl (Growth hormone administration may alter the clearance of compounds known to be metabolized by CYP 450 liver enzymes; careful monitoring is advisable). Products include:

Fentanyl Citrate (Growth hormone administration may alter the clearance of compounds known to be metabolized by CYP 450 liver enzymes; careful monitoring is advisable). Products include:

Flecainide Acetate (Growth hormone administration may alter the clearance of compounds known to be metabolized by CYP 450 liver enzymes; careful monitoring is advisable). Products include:

Fludrocortisone Acetate (Concomitant glucocorticoid therapy may inhibit human growth promoting effect).
No products indexed under this heading.

Fluoxetine (Growth hormone administration may alter the clearance of compounds known to be metabolized by CYP 450 liver enzymes; careful monitoring is advisable).
No products indexed under this heading.

Fluoxetine Hydrochloride (Growth hormone administration may alter the clearance of compounds known to be metabolized by CYP 450 liver enzymes; careful monitoring is advisable). Products include:

Fluphenazine Decanoate (Growth hormone administration may alter the clearance of compounds known to be metabolized by CYP 450 liver enzymes; careful monitoring is advisable).
No products indexed under this heading.

Fluphenazine Enanthate (Growth hormone administration may alter the clearance of compounds known to be metabolized by CYP 450 liver enzymes; careful monitoring is advisable).
No products indexed under this heading.

Fluphenazine Hydrochloride (Growth hormone administration may alter the clearance of compounds known to be metabolized by CYP 450 liver enzymes; careful monitoring is advisable).
No products indexed under this heading.

Flurbiprofen (Growth hormone administration may alter the clearance of compounds known to be metabolized by CYP 450 liver enzymes; careful monitoring is advisable).
No products indexed under this heading.

Flurbiprofen Sodium (Growth hormone administration may alter the clearance of compounds known to be metabolized by CYP 450 liver enzymes; careful monitoring is advisable). Products include:

Flutamide (Growth hormone administration may alter the clearance of compounds known to be metabolized by CYP 450 liver enzymes; careful monitoring is advisable). Products include:

Fluticasone Propionate (Growth hormone administration may alter the clearance of compounds known to be metabolized by CYP 450 liver enzymes; careful monitoring is advisable). Products include:

Fluvastatin Sodium (Growth hormone administration may alter the clearance of compounds known to be metabolized by CYP 450 liver enzymes; careful monitoring is advisable). Products include:

Fluvoxamine Maleate (Growth hormone administration may alter the clearance of compounds known to be metabolized by CYP 450 liver enzymes; careful monitoring is advisable).
No products indexed under this heading.

Formoterol Fumarate (Growth hormone administration may alter

the clearance of compounds known to be metabolized by CYP 450 liver enzymes; careful monitoring is advisable). Products include:

Fosphenytoin (Growth hormone administration may alter the clearance of compounds known to be metabolized by CYP 450 liver enzymes; careful monitoring is advisable).
No products indexed under this heading.

Fosphenytoin Sodium (Growth hormone administration may alter the clearance of compounds known to be metabolized by CYP 450 liver enzymes; careful monitoring is advisable).
No products indexed under this heading.

Gabapentin (Growth hormone administration may alter the clearance of compounds known to be metabolized by CYP 450 liver enzymes; careful monitoring is advisable). Products include:

Galantamine Hydrobromide (Growth hormone administration may alter the clearance of compounds known to be metabolized by CYP 450 liver enzymes; careful monitoring is advisable). Products include:

Glimepiride (Growth hormone administration may alter the clearance of compounds known to be metabolized by CYP 450 liver enzymes; careful monitoring is advisable). Products include:

Glipizide (Growth hormone administration may alter the clearance of compounds known to be metabolized by CYP 450 liver enzymes; careful monitoring is advisable).
No products indexed under this heading.

Glyburide (Growth hormone administration may alter the clearance of compounds known to be metabolized by CYP 450 liver enzymes; careful monitoring is advisable).
No products indexed under this heading.

Grepafloxacin Hydrochloride (Growth hormone administration may alter the clearance of compounds known to be metabolized by CYP 450 liver enzymes; careful monitoring is advisable).
No products indexed under this heading.

Haloperidol (Growth hormone administration may alter the clearance of compounds known to be metabolized by CYP 450 liver enzymes; careful monitoring is advisable).
No products indexed under this heading.

Haloperidol Decanoate (Growth hormone administration may alter the clearance of compounds known to be metabolized by CYP 450 liver enzymes; careful monitoring is advisable).
No products indexed under this heading.

IMPORTANT NOTE: Always consult each drug listing in the patient's regimen for possible interactions.

Haloperidol Lactate (Growth hormone administration may alter the clearance of compounds known to be metabolized by CYP 450 liver enzymes; careful monitoring is advisable).
No products indexed under this heading.

Hydrocodone Bitartrate (Growth hormone administration may alter the clearance of compounds known to be metabolized by CYP 450 liver enzymes; careful monitoring is advisable). Products include:
Hycodan ... 1116
Hycotuss Expectorant Syrup ... 1117
Vicodin Tablets ... 535
Vicodin ES Tablets ... 536
Vicodin HP Tablets ... 538
Vicoprofen Tablets ... 539
Zydone Tablets ... 1139

Hydrocortisone (Concomitant glucocorticoid therapy may inhibit human growth promoting effect). Products include:
Colocort Rectal Suspension, USP (Retention) 100 mg/60 mL ... 2476
Hydrocortone Tablets ... 1989
Preparation H Hydrocortisone Cream ... ▣646

Hydrocortisone Acetate (Concomitant glucocorticoid therapy may inhibit human growth promoting effect). Products include:
Analpram-HC ... 1159
Pramosone ... 1161
ProctoFoam-HC ... 3099

Hydrocortisone Sodium Phosphate (Concomitant glucocorticoid therapy may inhibit human growth promoting effect).
No products indexed under this heading.

Hydrocortisone Sodium Succinate (Concomitant glucocorticoid therapy may inhibit human growth promoting effect).
No products indexed under this heading.

Ibuprofen (Growth hormone administration may alter the clearance of compounds known to be metabolized by CYP 450 liver enzymes; careful monitoring is advisable). Products include:
Advil Allergy Sinus Caplets ... ▣770
Advil ... ▣674
Children's Advil Oral Suspension ... ▣603
Children's Advil Chewable Tablets ... ▣603
Advil Cold & Sinus ... ▣723
Infants' Advil Concentrated Drops ... ▣604
Infants' Advil Concentrated Drops - White Grape (Dye-Free) ... ▣604
Junior Strength Advil Swallow Tablets ... ▣605
Advil Migraine Liquigels ... ▣608
Advil Multi-Symptom Cold Caplets ... ▣770
Advil PM Caplets ... ▣615
Motrin IB Tablets and Caplets ... 1866
Children's Motrin Oral Suspension ... 1867
Children's Motrin Non-Staining Dye-Free Oral Suspension ... 1867
Children's Motrin Cold Oral Suspension ... 1867
Infants' Motrin Concentrated Drops ... 1867
Infants' Motrin Non-Staining Dye-Free Concentrated Drops ... 1867
Junior Strength Motrin Caplets and Chewable Tablets ... 1867
Vicoprofen Tablets ... 539

Imipramine Hydrochloride (Growth hormone administration may alter the clearance of compounds known to be metabolized by CYP 450 liver enzymes; careful monitoring is advisable).
No products indexed under this heading.

Imipramine Pamoate (Growth hormone administration may alter the clearance of compounds known to be metabolized by CYP 450 liver enzymes; careful monitoring is advisable).
No products indexed under this heading.

Indinavir Sulfate (Growth hormone administration may alter the clearance of compounds known to be metabolized by CYP 450 liver enzymes; careful monitoring is advisable). Products include:
Crixivan Capsules ... 1940

Indomethacin (Growth hormone administration may alter the clearance of compounds known to be metabolized by CYP 450 liver enzymes; careful monitoring is advisable). Products include:
Indocin ... 1995

Indomethacin Sodium Trihydrate (Growth hormone administration may alter the clearance of compounds known to be metabolized by CYP 450 liver enzymes; careful monitoring is advisable). Products include:
Indocin I.V. ... 2465

Indoramin Hydrochloride (Growth hormone administration may alter the clearance of compounds known to be metabolized by CYP 450 liver enzymes; careful monitoring is advisable).
No products indexed under this heading.

Irbesartan (Growth hormone administration may alter the clearance of compounds known to be metabolized by CYP 450 liver enzymes; careful monitoring is advisable). Products include:
Avalide Tablets ... 888
Avalide Tablets ... 2874
Avapro Tablets ... 891
Avapro Tablets ... 2871

Isotretinoin (Growth hormone administration may alter the clearance of compounds known to be metabolized by CYP 450 liver enzymes; careful monitoring is advisable). Products include:
Accutane Capsules ... 2731

Isradipine (Growth hormone administration may alter the clearance of compounds known to be metabolized by CYP 450 liver enzymes; careful monitoring is advisable). Products include:
DynaCirc CR Tablets ... 2721

Itraconazole (Growth hormone administration may alter the clearance of compounds known to be metabolized by CYP 450 liver enzymes; careful monitoring is advisable).
No products indexed under this heading.

Ketoconazole (Growth hormone administration may alter the clearance of compounds known to be metabolized by CYP 450 liver enzymes; careful monitoring is advisable). Products include:
Nizoral A-D Shampoo, 1% ... 1868

Ketoprofen (Growth hormone administration may alter the clearance of compounds known to be metabolized by CYP 450 liver enzymes; careful monitoring is advisable).
No products indexed under this heading.

Ketorolac Tromethamine (Growth hormone administration may alter the clearance of compounds known to be metabolized by CYP 450 liver enzymes; careful monitoring is advisable). Products include:
Acular Ophthalmic Solution ... 565
Acular LS Ophthalmic Solution ... 566

Labetalol Hydrochloride (Growth hormone administration may alter the clearance of compounds known to be metabolized by CYP 450 liver enzymes; careful monitoring is advisable).
No products indexed under this heading.

Lamotrigine (Growth hormone administration may alter the clearance of compounds known to be metabolized by CYP 450 liver enzymes; careful monitoring is advisable). Products include:
Lamictal ... 1481

Lansoprazole (Growth hormone administration may alter the clearance of compounds known to be metabolized by CYP 450 liver enzymes; careful monitoring is advisable). Products include:
Prevacid Delayed-Release Capsules ... 3271
Prevacid for Delayed-Release Oral Suspension ... 3271
Prevacid SoluTab Delayed-Release Orally Disintegrating Tablets ... 3271
Prevacid I.V. for Injection ... 3277
Prevacid NapraPAC ... 3280
PREVPAC ... 3284

Levetiracetam (Growth hormone administration may alter the clearance of compounds known to be metabolized by CYP 450 liver enzymes; careful monitoring is advisable). Products include:
Keppra Injection ... 3320
Keppra Oral Solution ... 3314
Keppra Tablets ... 3314

Levobupivacaine Hydrochloride (Growth hormone administration may alter the clearance of compounds known to be metabolized by CYP 450 liver enzymes; careful monitoring is advisable).
No products indexed under this heading.

Levonorgestrel (Growth hormone administration may alter the clearance of compounds known to be metabolized by CYP 450 liver enzymes; careful monitoring is advisable). Products include:
Climara Pro Transdermal System ... 776
Mirena Intrauterine System ... 787
Plan B Tablets ... 1076
Seasonique Tablets ... 1077

Lidocaine (Growth hormone administration may alter the clearance of compounds known to be metabolized by CYP 450 liver enzymes; careful monitoring is advisable). Products include:
Lidoderm Patch ... 1118
Synera Topical Patch ... 1137

Lidocaine Base (Growth hormone administration may alter the clearance of compounds known to be metabolized by CYP 450 liver enzymes; careful monitoring is advisable).
No products indexed under this heading.

Lidocaine Hydrochloride (Growth hormone administration may alter the clearance of compounds known to be metabolized by CYP 450 liver enzymes; careful monitoring is advisable).
No products indexed under this heading.

Lomefloxacin Hydrochloride (Growth hormone administration may alter the clearance of compounds known to be metabolized by CYP 450 liver enzymes; careful monitoring is advisable).
No products indexed under this heading.

Losartan Potassium (Growth hormone administration may alter the clearance of compounds known to be metabolized by CYP 450 liver enzymes; careful monitoring is advisable). Products include:
Cozaar Tablets ... 1935
Hyzaar 50-12.5 Tablets ... 1990
Hyzaar 100-12.5 Tablets ... 1990
Hyzaar 100-25 Tablets ... 1990

Lovastatin (Growth hormone administration may alter the clearance of compounds known to be metabolized by CYP 450 liver enzymes; careful monitoring is advisable). Products include:
Advicor Tablets ... 1722
Altoprev Extended-Release Tablets ... 3109
Mevacor Tablets ... 2021

Maprotiline Hydrochloride (Growth hormone administration may alter the clearance of compounds known to be metabolized by CYP 450 liver enzymes; careful monitoring is advisable).
No products indexed under this heading.

Meclofenamate Sodium (Growth hormone administration may alter the clearance of compounds known to be metabolized by CYP 450 liver enzymes; careful monitoring is advisable).
No products indexed under this heading.

Mefenamic Acid (Growth hormone administration may alter the clearance of compounds known to be metabolized by CYP 450 liver enzymes; careful monitoring is advisable).
No products indexed under this heading.

Meloxicam (Growth hormone administration may alter the clearance of compounds known to be metabolized by CYP 450 liver enzymes; careful monitoring is advisable). Products include:
Mobic Oral Suspension ... 863
Mobic Tablets ... 863

Meperidine Hydrochloride (Growth hormone administration may alter the clearance of compounds known to be metabolized by CYP 450 liver enzymes; careful monitoring is advisable).
No products indexed under this heading.

Mephenytoin (Growth hormone administration may alter the clearance of compounds known to be metabolized by CYP 450 liver enzymes; careful monitoring is advisable).
No products indexed under this heading.

Mephobarbital (Growth hormone administration may alter the clearance of compounds known to be metabolized by CYP 450 liver enzymes; careful monitoring is advisable).
No products indexed under this heading.

Meprobamate (Growth hormone administration may alter the clearance of compounds known to be metabolized by CYP 450 liver enzymes; careful monitoring is advisable).

No products indexed under this heading.

Mestranol (Growth hormone administration may alter the clearance of compounds known to be metabolized by CYP 450 liver enzymes; careful monitoring is advisable).

No products indexed under this heading.

Metformin Hydrochloride (Growth hormone administration may alter the clearance of compounds known to be metabolized by CYP 450 liver enzymes; careful monitoring is advisable). Products include:

Methadone Hydrochloride (Growth hormone administration may alter the clearance of compounds known to be metabolized by CYP 450 liver enzymes; careful monitoring is advisable).

No products indexed under this heading.

Methamphetamine Hydrochloride (Growth hormone administration may alter the clearance of compounds known to be metabolized by CYP 450 liver enzymes; careful monitoring is advisable). Products include:

Methsuximide (Growth hormone administration may alter the clearance of compounds known to be metabolized by CYP 450 liver enzymes; careful monitoring is advisable).

No products indexed under this heading.

Methylprednisolone Acetate (Concomitant glucocorticoid therapy may inhibit human growth promoting effect). Products include:

Methylprednisolone Sodium Succinate (Concomitant glucocorticoid therapy may inhibit human growth promoting effect).

No products indexed under this heading.

Metoprolol Succinate (Growth hormone administration may alter the clearance of compounds known to be metabolized by CYP 450 liver enzymes; careful monitoring is advisable). Products include:

Metoprolol Tartrate (Growth hormone administration may alter the clearance of compounds known to be metabolized by CYP 450 liver enzymes; careful monitoring is advisable). Products include:

Mexiletine Hydrochloride (Growth hormone administration may alter the clearance of compounds known to be metabolized by CYP 450 liver enzymes; careful monitoring is advisable).

No products indexed under this heading.

Midazolam Hydrochloride (Growth hormone administration may alter the clearance of compounds known to be metabolized by CYP 450 liver enzymes; careful monitoring is advisable).

No products indexed under this heading.

Miglitol (Growth hormone administration may alter the clearance of compounds known to be metabolized by CYP 450 liver enzymes; careful monitoring is advisable).

No products indexed under this heading.

Mirtazapine (Growth hormone administration may alter the clearance of compounds known to be metabolized by CYP 450 liver enzymes; careful monitoring is advisable).

No products indexed under this heading.

Montelukast Sodium (Growth hormone administration may alter the clearance of compounds known to be metabolized by CYP 450 liver enzymes; careful monitoring is advisable). Products include:

Morphine Sulfate (Growth hormone administration may alter the clearance of compounds known to be metabolized by CYP 450 liver enzymes; careful monitoring is advisable). Products include:

Moxifloxacin Hydrochloride (Growth hormone administration may alter the clearance of compounds known to be metabolized by CYP 450 liver enzymes; careful monitoring is advisable). Products include:

Nabumetone (Growth hormone administration may alter the clearance of compounds known to be metabolized by CYP 450 liver enzymes; careful monitoring is advisable).

No products indexed under this heading.

Nafcillin Sodium (Growth hormone administration may alter the clearance of compounds known to be metabolized by CYP 450 liver enzymes; careful monitoring is advisable).

No products indexed under this heading.

Naproxen (Growth hormone administration may alter the clearance of compounds known to be metabolized by CYP 450 liver enzymes; careful monitoring is advisable). Products include:

Naproxen Sodium (Growth hormone administration may alter the clearance of compounds known to

be metabolized by CYP 450 liver enzymes; careful monitoring is advisable). Products include:

Nateglinide (Growth hormone administration may alter the clearance of compounds known to be metabolized by CYP 450 liver enzymes; careful monitoring is advisable). Products include:

Nefazodone Hydrochloride (Growth hormone administration may alter the clearance of compounds known to be metabolized by CYP 450 liver enzymes; careful monitoring is advisable).

No products indexed under this heading.

Nelfinavir Mesylate (Growth hormone administration may alter the clearance of compounds known to be metabolized by CYP 450 liver enzymes; careful monitoring is advisable). Products include:

Nicardipine (Growth hormone administration may alter the clearance of compounds known to be metabolized by CYP 450 liver enzymes; careful monitoring is advisable).

No products indexed under this heading.

Nicardipine Hydrochloride (Growth hormone administration may alter the clearance of compounds known to be metabolized by CYP 450 liver enzymes; careful monitoring is advisable). Products include:

Nicotine Polacrilex (Growth hormone administration may alter the clearance of compounds known to be metabolized by CYP 450 liver enzymes; careful monitoring is advisable).

No products indexed under this heading.

Nicotine Salicylate (Growth hormone administration may alter the clearance of compounds known to be metabolized by CYP 450 liver enzymes; careful monitoring is advisable).

No products indexed under this heading.

Nicotine Sulfate (Growth hormone administration may alter the clearance of compounds known to be metabolized by CYP 450 liver enzymes; careful monitoring is advisable).

No products indexed under this heading.

Nifedipine (Growth hormone administration may alter the clearance of compounds known to be metabolized by CYP 450 liver enzymes; careful monitoring is advisable). Products include:

Nilutamide (Growth hormone administration may alter the clearance of compounds known to be metabolized by CYP 450 liver enzymes; careful monitoring is advisable).

No products indexed under this heading.

Nimodipine (Growth hormone administration may alter the clear-

ance of compounds known to be metabolized by CYP 450 liver enzymes; careful monitoring is advisable). Products include:

Nisoldipine (Growth hormone administration may alter the clearance of compounds known to be metabolized by CYP 450 liver enzymes; careful monitoring is advisable). Products include:

Nitrendipine (Growth hormone administration may alter the clearance of compounds known to be metabolized by CYP 450 liver enzymes; careful monitoring is advisable).

No products indexed under this heading.

Norethindrone (Growth hormone administration may alter the clearance of compounds known to be metabolized by CYP 450 liver enzymes; careful monitoring is advisable). Products include:

Norethindrone Acetate (Growth hormone administration may alter the clearance of compounds known to be metabolized by CYP 450 liver enzymes; careful monitoring is advisable).

No products indexed under this heading.

Norfloxacin (Growth hormone administration may alter the clearance of compounds known to be metabolized by CYP 450 liver enzymes; careful monitoring is advisable). Products include:

Norgestrel (Growth hormone administration may alter the clearance of compounds known to be metabolized by CYP 450 liver enzymes; careful monitoring is advisable).

No products indexed under this heading.

Nortriptyline Hydrochloride (Growth hormone administration may alter the clearance of compounds known to be metabolized by CYP 450 liver enzymes; careful monitoring is advisable).

No products indexed under this heading.

Ofloxacin (Growth hormone administration may alter the clearance of compounds known to be metabolized by CYP 450 liver enzymes; careful monitoring is advisable). Products include:

Olanzapine (Growth hormone administration may alter the clearance of compounds known to be metabolized by CYP 450 liver enzymes; careful monitoring is advisable). Products include:

Omeprazole (Growth hormone administration may alter the clearance of compounds known to be metabolized by CYP 450 liver enzymes; careful monitoring is advisable). Products include:

Ondansetron (Growth hormone administration may alter the clearance of compounds known to be metabolized by CYP 450 liver enzymes; careful monitoring is advisable). Products include:

Ondansetron Hydrochloride (Growth hormone administration may alter the clearance of compounds known to be metabolized by CYP 450 liver enzymes; careful monitoring is advisable). Products include:

Oxaprozin (Growth hormone administration may alter the clearance of compounds known to be metabolized by CYP 450 liver enzymes; careful monitoring is advisable).
No products indexed under this heading.

Oxcarbazepine (Growth hormone administration may alter the clearance of compounds known to be metabolized by CYP 450 liver enzymes; careful monitoring is advisable). Products include:

Oxycodone Hydrochloride (Growth hormone administration may alter the clearance of compounds known to be metabolized by CYP 450 liver enzymes; careful monitoring is advisable). Products include:

Paclitaxel (Growth hormone administration may alter the clearance of compounds known to be metabolized by CYP 450 liver enzymes; careful monitoring is advisable).
No products indexed under this heading.

Pantoprazole Sodium (Growth hormone administration may alter the clearance of compounds known to be metabolized by CYP 450 liver enzymes; careful monitoring is advisable). Products include:

Paramethadione (Growth hormone administration may alter the clearance of compounds known to be metabolized by CYP 450 liver enzymes; careful monitoring is advisable).
No products indexed under this heading.

Paroxetine Hydrochloride (Growth hormone administration may alter the clearance of compounds known to be metabolized by CYP 450 liver enzymes; careful monitoring is advisable). Products include:

Pentamidine Isethionate (Growth hormone administration may alter the clearance of compounds known to be metabolized by CYP 450 liver enzymes; careful monitoring is advisable).
No products indexed under this heading.

Phenacemide (Growth hormone administration may alter the clearance of compounds known to be metabolized by CYP 450 liver enzymes; careful monitoring is advisable).
No products indexed under this heading.

Phenobarbital (Growth hormone administration may alter the clearance of compounds known to be metabolized by CYP 450 liver enzymes; careful monitoring is advisable). Products include:

Phenobarbital Sodium (Growth hormone administration may alter the clearance of compounds known to be metabolized by CYP 450 liver enzymes; careful monitoring is advisable).
No products indexed under this heading.

Phensuximide (Growth hormone administration may alter the clearance of compounds known to be metabolized by CYP 450 liver enzymes; careful monitoring is advisable).
No products indexed under this heading.

Phenylbutazone (Growth hormone administration may alter the clearance of compounds known to be metabolized by CYP 450 liver enzymes; careful monitoring is advisable).
No products indexed under this heading.

Phenytoin (Growth hormone administration may alter the clearance of compounds known to be metabolized by CYP 450 liver enzymes; careful monitoring is advisable).
No products indexed under this heading.

Phenytoin Sodium (Growth hormone administration may alter the clearance of compounds known to be metabolized by CYP 450 liver enzymes; careful monitoring is advisable). Products include:

Pimozide (Growth hormone administration may alter the clearance of compounds known to be metabolized by CYP 450 liver enzymes; careful monitoring is advisable).
No products indexed under this heading.

Pindolol (Growth hormone administration may alter the clearance of compounds known to be metabolized by CYP 450 liver enzymes; careful monitoring is advisable).
No products indexed under this heading.

Pioglitazone Hydrochloride (Growth hormone administration may alter the clearance of compounds known to be metabolized by CYP 450 liver enzymes; careful monitoring is advisable). Products include:

Piroxicam (Growth hormone administration may alter the clearance of compounds known to be metabolized by CYP 450 liver enzymes; careful monitoring is advisable).
No products indexed under this heading.

Polyestradiol Phosphate (Growth hormone administration may alter the clearance of compounds known to be metabolized by CYP 450 liver enzymes; careful monitoring is advisable).
No products indexed under this heading.

Prednisolone Acetate (Concomitant glucocorticoid therapy may inhibit human growth promoting effect). Products include:

Prednisolone Sodium Phosphate (Concomitant glucocorticoid therapy may inhibit human growth promoting effect).
No products indexed under this heading.

Prednisolone Tebutate (Concomitant glucocorticoid therapy may inhibit human growth promoting effect).
No products indexed under this heading.

Prednisone (Concomitant glucocorticoid therapy may inhibit human growth promoting effect).
No products indexed under this heading.

Primidone (Growth hormone administration may alter the clearance of compounds known to be metabolized by CYP 450 liver enzymes; careful monitoring is advisable).
No products indexed under this heading.

Progesterone (Growth hormone administration may alter the clearance of compounds known to be metabolized by CYP 450 liver enzymes; careful monitoring is advisable). Products include:

Proguanil Hydrochloride (Growth hormone administration may alter the clearance of compounds known to be metabolized by CYP 450 liver enzymes; careful monitoring is advisable). Products include:

Propafenone Hydrochloride (Growth hormone administration may alter the clearance of compounds known to be metabolized by CYP 450 liver enzymes; careful monitoring is advisable). Products include:

Propoxyphene Hydrochloride (Growth hormone administration may alter the clearance of compounds known to be metabolized by CYP 450 liver enzymes; careful monitoring is advisable).
No products indexed under this heading.

Propoxyphene Napsylate (Growth hormone administration may alter the clearance of compounds known to be metabolized by CYP 450 liver enzymes; careful monitoring is advisable).
No products indexed under this heading.

Propranolol Hydrochloride (Growth hormone administration may alter the clearance of compounds known to be metabolized by CYP 450 liver enzymes; careful monitoring is advisable). Products include:

Protriptyline Hydrochloride (Growth hormone administration may alter the clearance of compounds known to be metabolized by CYP 450 liver enzymes; careful monitoring is advisable).
No products indexed under this heading.

Quetiapine Fumarate (Growth hormone administration may alter the clearance of compounds known to be metabolized by CYP 450 liver enzymes; careful monitoring is advisable). Products include:

Quinidine Gluconate (Growth hormone administration may alter the clearance of compounds known to be metabolized by CYP 450 liver enzymes; careful monitoring is advisable).
No products indexed under this heading.

Quinidine Hydrochloride (Growth hormone administration may alter the clearance of compounds known to be metabolized by CYP 450 liver enzymes; careful monitoring is advisable).
No products indexed under this heading.

Quinidine Polygalacturonate (Growth hormone administration may alter the clearance of compounds known to be metabolized by CYP 450 liver enzymes; careful monitoring is advisable).
No products indexed under this heading.

Quinidine Sulfate (Growth hormone administration may alter the clearance of compounds known to be metabolized by CYP 450 liver enzymes; careful monitoring is advisable).
No products indexed under this heading.

Quinine (Growth hormone administration may alter the clearance of compounds known to be metabolized by CYP 450 liver enzymes; careful monitoring is advisable).
No products indexed under this heading.

Quinine Sulfate (Growth hormone administration may alter the clearance of compounds known to be metabolized by CYP 450 liver enzymes; careful monitoring is advisable).
No products indexed under this heading.

Rabeprazole Sodium (Growth hormone administration may alter the clearance of compounds known to be metabolized by CYP 450 liver enzymes; careful monitoring is advisable). Products include:

Repaglinide (Growth hormone administration may alter the clearance of compounds known to be metabolized by CYP 450 liver enzymes; careful monitoring is advisable).
No products indexed under this heading.

Rifabutin (Growth hormone administration may alter the clearance of compounds known to be metabolized by CYP 450 liver enzymes; careful monitoring is advisable).
No products indexed under this heading.

Riluzole (Growth hormone administration may alter the clearance of compounds known to be metabolized by CYP 450 liver enzymes; careful monitoring is advisable). Products include:

Risperidone (Growth hormone administration may alter the clearance of compounds known to be metabolized by CYP 450 liver enzymes; careful monitoring is advisable). Products include:

Ritonavir (Growth hormone administration may alter the clearance of compounds known to be metabolized by CYP 450 liver enzymes; careful monitoring is advisable). Products include:

Rofecoxib (Growth hormone administration may alter the clearance of compounds known to be metabolized by CYP 450 liver enzymes; careful monitoring is advisable).
No products indexed under this heading.

Ropinirole Hydrochloride (Growth hormone administration may alter the clearance of compounds known to be metabolized by CYP 450 liver enzymes; careful monitoring is advisable). Products include:

Ropivacaine Hydrochloride (Growth hormone administration may alter the clearance of compounds known to be metabolized by CYP 450 liver enzymes; careful monitoring is advisable).
No products indexed under this heading.

Rosiglitazone Maleate (Growth hormone administration may alter the clearance of compounds known to be metabolized by CYP 450 liver enzymes; careful monitoring is advisable). Products include:

Saquinavir (Growth hormone administration may alter the clearance of compounds known to be metabolized by CYP 450 liver enzymes; careful monitoring is advisable).
No products indexed under this heading.

Saquinavir Mesylate (Growth hormone administration may alter the clearance of compounds known to be metabolized by CYP 450 liver enzymes; careful monitoring is advisable). Products include:

Sertraline Hydrochloride (Growth hormone administration may alter the clearance of compounds known to be metabolized by CYP 450 liver enzymes; careful monitoring is advisable). Products include:

Sildenafil Citrate (Growth hormone administration may alter the clearance of compounds known to be metabolized by CYP 450 liver enzymes; careful monitoring is advisable). Products include:

Simvastatin (Growth hormone administration may alter the clearance of compounds known to be

metabolized by CYP 450 liver enzymes; careful monitoring is advisable). Products include:

Sirolimus (Growth hormone administration may alter the clearance of compounds known to be metabolized by CYP 450 liver enzymes; careful monitoring is advisable). Products include:

Sulfamethoxazole (Growth hormone administration may alter the clearance of compounds known to be metabolized by CYP 450 liver enzymes; careful monitoring is advisable).
No products indexed under this heading.

Sulindac (Growth hormone administration may alter the clearance of compounds known to be metabolized by CYP 450 liver enzymes; careful monitoring is advisable). Products include:

Suprofen (Growth hormone administration may alter the clearance of compounds known to be metabolized by CYP 450 liver enzymes; careful monitoring is advisable).
No products indexed under this heading.

Tacrine Hydrochloride (Growth hormone administration may alter the clearance of compounds known to be metabolized by CYP 450 liver enzymes; careful monitoring is advisable).
No products indexed under this heading.

Tacrolimus (Growth hormone administration may alter the clearance of compounds known to be metabolized by CYP 450 liver enzymes; careful monitoring is advisable). Products include:

Tamoxifen Citrate (Growth hormone administration may alter the clearance of compounds known to be metabolized by CYP 450 liver enzymes; careful monitoring is advisable). Products include:

Telmisartan (Growth hormone administration may alter the clearance of compounds known to be metabolized by CYP 450 liver enzymes; careful monitoring is advisable). Products include:

Teniposide (Growth hormone administration may alter the clearance of compounds known to be metabolized by CYP 450 liver enzymes; careful monitoring is advisable).
No products indexed under this heading.

Terfenadine (Growth hormone administration may alter the clearance of compounds known to be metabolized by CYP 450 liver enzymes; careful monitoring is advisable).
No products indexed under this heading.

Testosterone (Growth hormone administration may alter the clearance of compounds known to be metabolized by CYP 450 liver enzymes; careful monitoring is advisable). Products include:

Testosterone Cypionate (Growth hormone administration may alter the clearance of compounds known to be metabolized by CYP 450 liver enzymes; careful monitoring is advisable).
No products indexed under this heading.

Testosterone Enanthate (Growth hormone administration may alter the clearance of compounds known to be metabolized by CYP 450 liver enzymes; careful monitoring is advisable).
No products indexed under this heading.

Testosterone Propionate (Growth hormone administration may alter the clearance of compounds known to be metabolized by CYP 450 liver enzymes; careful monitoring is advisable).
No products indexed under this heading.

Theophylline (Growth hormone administration may alter the clearance of compounds known to be metabolized by CYP 450 liver enzymes; careful monitoring is advisable).
No products indexed under this heading.

Theophylline Anhydrous (Growth hormone administration may alter the clearance of compounds known to be metabolized by CYP 450 liver enzymes; careful monitoring is advisable). Products include:

Theophylline Sodium Glycinate (Growth hormone administration may alter the clearance of compounds known to be metabolized by CYP 450 liver enzymes; careful monitoring is advisable).
No products indexed under this heading.

Thioridazine (Growth hormone administration may alter the clearance of compounds known to be metabolized by CYP 450 liver enzymes; careful monitoring is advisable).
No products indexed under this heading.

Thioridazine Hydrochloride (Growth hormone administration may alter the clearance of compounds known to be metabolized by CYP 450 liver enzymes; careful monitoring is advisable). Products include:

Tiagabine Hydrochloride (Growth hormone administration may alter the clearance of compounds known to be metabolized by CYP 450 liver enzymes; careful monitoring is advisable). Products include:

Timolol Maleate (Growth hormone administration may alter the clearance of compounds known to be metabolized by CYP 450 liver enzymes; careful monitoring is advisable). Products include:

Tolazamide (Growth hormone administration may alter the clearance of compounds known to be metabolized by CYP 450 liver enzymes; careful monitoring is advisable).
No products indexed under this heading.

Tolbutamide (Growth hormone administration may alter the clearance of compounds known to be metabolized by CYP 450 liver enzymes; careful monitoring is advisable).
No products indexed under this heading.

Tolbutamide Sodium (Growth hormone administration may alter the clearance of compounds known to be metabolized by CYP 450 liver enzymes; careful monitoring is advisable).
No products indexed under this heading.

Tolmetin Sodium (Growth hormone administration may alter the clearance of compounds known to be metabolized by CYP 450 liver enzymes; careful monitoring is advisable).
No products indexed under this heading.

Tolterodine Tartrate (Growth hormone administration may alter the clearance of compounds known to be metabolized by CYP 450 liver enzymes; careful monitoring is advisable). Products include:

Topiramate (Growth hormone administration may alter the clearance of compounds known to be metabolized by CYP 450 liver enzymes; careful monitoring is advisable). Products include:

Torsemide (Growth hormone administration may alter the clearance of compounds known to be metabolized by CYP 450 liver enzymes; careful monitoring is advisable). Products include:

Tramadol Hydrochloride (Growth hormone administration may alter the clearance of compounds known to be metabolized by CYP 450 liver enzymes; careful monitoring is advisable). Products include:

Trazodone Hydrochloride (Growth hormone administration may alter the clearance of compounds known to be metabolized by CYP 450 liver enzymes; careful monitoring is advisable).
No products indexed under this heading.

Tretinoin (Growth hormone administration may alter the clearance of

compounds known to be metabolized by CYP 450 liver enzymes; careful monitoring is advisable). Products include:
Tri-Luma Cream 1213
Vesanoid Capsules 2820

Triamcinolone (Concomitant glucocorticoid therapy may inhibit human growth promoting effect).
No products indexed under this heading.

Triamcinolone Acetonide (Concomitant glucocorticoid therapy may inhibit human growth promoting effect). Products include:
Azmacort Inhalation Aerosol 1726
Nasacort AQ Nasal Spray 2922

Triamcinolone Diacetate (Concomitant glucocorticoid therapy may inhibit human growth promoting effect).
No products indexed under this heading.

Triamcinolone Hexacetonide (Concomitant glucocorticoid therapy may inhibit human growth promoting effect).
No products indexed under this heading.

Triazolam (Growth hormone administration may alter the clearance of compounds known to be metabolized by CYP 450 liver enzymes; careful monitoring is advisable).
No products indexed under this heading.

Trimethadione (Growth hormone administration may alter the clearance of compounds known to be metabolized by CYP 450 liver enzymes; careful monitoring is advisable).
No products indexed under this heading.

Trimethaphan Camsylate (Growth hormone administration may alter the clearance of compounds known to be metabolized by CYP 450 liver enzymes; careful monitoring is advisable).
No products indexed under this heading.

Trimipramine Maleate (Growth hormone administration may alter the clearance of compounds known to be metabolized by CYP 450 liver enzymes; careful monitoring is advisable).
No products indexed under this heading.

Troglitazone (Growth hormone administration may alter the clearance of compounds known to be metabolized by CYP 450 liver enzymes; careful monitoring is advisable).
No products indexed under this heading.

Trovafloxacin Mesylate (Growth hormone administration may alter the clearance of compounds known to be metabolized by CYP 450 liver enzymes; careful monitoring is advisable).
No products indexed under this heading.

Valdecoxib (Growth hormone administration may alter the clearance of compounds known to be metabolized by CYP 450 liver enzymes; careful monitoring is advisable).
No products indexed under this heading.

Valproate Sodium (Growth hormone administration may alter the clearance of compounds known to be metabolized by CYP 450 liver enzymes; careful monitoring is advisable). Products include:
Depacon Injection 412

Valproic Acid (Growth hormone administration may alter the clearance of compounds known to be metabolized by CYP 450 liver enzymes; careful monitoring is advisable). Products include:
Depakene 417

Valsartan (Growth hormone administration may alter the clearance of compounds known to be metabolized by CYP 450 liver enzymes; careful monitoring is advisable). Products include:
Diovan Tablets 2193
Diovan HCT Tablets 2196

Venlafaxine Hydrochloride (Growth hormone administration may alter the clearance of compounds known to be metabolized by CYP 450 liver enzymes; careful monitoring is advisable). Products include:
Effexor Tablets 3411
Effexor XR Capsules 3417

Verapamil Hydrochloride (Growth hormone administration may alter the clearance of compounds known to be metabolized by CYP 450 liver enzymes; careful monitoring is advisable). Products include:
Covera-HS Tablets 3139
Tarka Tablets 524
Verelan PM Extended-Release Capsules, Controlled-Onset 3106

Vinblastine Sulfate (Growth hormone administration may alter the clearance of compounds known to be metabolized by CYP 450 liver enzymes; careful monitoring is advisable).
No products indexed under this heading.

Vincristine Sulfate (Growth hormone administration may alter the clearance of compounds known to be metabolized by CYP 450 liver enzymes; careful monitoring is advisable).
No products indexed under this heading.

Vitamin A (Growth hormone administration may alter the clearance of compounds known to be metabolized by CYP 450 liver enzymes; careful monitoring is advisable). Products include:
Visutein Capsules 3329

Vitamin A Acetate (Growth hormone administration may alter the clearance of compounds known to be metabolized by CYP 450 liver enzymes; careful monitoring is advisable).
No products indexed under this heading.

Voriconazole (Growth hormone administration may alter the clearance of compounds known to be metabolized by CYP 450 liver enzymes; careful monitoring is advisable). Products include:
VFEND I.V. 2564
VFEND Oral Suspension 2564
VFEND Tablets 2564

Warfarin Sodium (Growth hormone administration may alter the clearance of compounds known to be metabolized by CYP 450 liver enzymes; careful monitoring is advisable). Products include:
Coumadin for Injection 898
Coumadin Tablets 898

Zafirlukast (Growth hormone administration may alter the clearance of compounds known to be metabolized by CYP 450 liver enzymes; careful monitoring is advisable). Products include:
Accolate Tablets 671

Zileuton (Growth hormone administration may alter the clearance of compounds known to be metabolized by CYP 450 liver enzymes; careful monitoring is advisable). Products include:
Zyflo Tablets 1023

Zolmitriptan (Growth hormone administration may alter the clearance of compounds known to be metabolized by CYP 450 liver enzymes; careful monitoring is advisable). Products include:
Zomig Tablets 3519
Zomig Nasal Spray 3523
Zomig-ZMT Tablets 3519

Zonisamide (Growth hormone administration may alter the clearance of compounds known to be metabolized by CYP 450 liver enzymes; careful monitoring is advisable). Products include:
Zonegran Capsules 1101

Zopiclone (Growth hormone administration may alter the clearance of compounds known to be metabolized by CYP 450 liver enzymes; careful monitoring is advisable).
No products indexed under this heading.

GEODON CAPSULES

(Ziprasidone Hydrochloride) 2529

May interact with antihypertensives, central nervous system depressants, dopamine agonists, erythromycin, potassium-depleting diuretics, quinidine, and certain other agents. Compounds in these categories include:

Acebutolol Hydrochloride (Ziprasidone may induce orthostatic hypotension; co-administration with certain antihypertensive drugs may enhance the hypotensive effects).
No products indexed under this heading.

Alfentanil Hydrochloride (Somnolence was a commonly reported adverse event in patients treated with ziprasidone; concurrent use with other CNS active drugs, such as depressants, should be undertaken with caution).
No products indexed under this heading.

Alprazolam (Somnolence was a commonly reported adverse event in patients treated with ziprasidone; concurrent use with other CNS active drugs, such as depressants, should be undertaken with caution). Products include:
Niravam Orally Disintegrating Tablets 3092

Amiodarone Hydrochloride (Ziprasidone produces dose-related prolongation of the QT interval; an additive effect of ziprasidone and other drugs that prolong cannot be excluded; concurrent use is not recommended).
No products indexed under this heading.

Amlodipine Besylate (Ziprasidone may induce orthostatic hypotension; co-administration with certain antihypertensive drugs may enhance the hypotensive effects). Products include:
Caduet Tablets 2508
Lotrel Capsules 2249
Norvasc Tablets 2545

Aprobarbital (Somnolence was a commonly reported adverse event in patients treated with ziprasidone; concurrent use with other CNS active drugs, such as depressants, should be undertaken with caution).
No products indexed under this heading.

Arsenic Trioxide (Ziprasidone produces dose-related prolongation of the QT interval; an additive effect of ziprasidone and other drugs that prolong cannot be excluded; concurrent use is not recommended). Products include:
Trisenox Injection 993

Atenolol (Ziprasidone may induce orthostatic hypotension; co-administration with certain antihypertensive drugs may enhance the hypotensive effects).
No products indexed under this heading.

Benazepril Hydrochloride (Ziprasidone may induce orthostatic hypotension; co-administration with certain antihypertensive drugs may enhance the hypotensive effects). Products include:
Lotensin Tablets 2243
Lotensin HCT Tablets 2246
Lotrel Capsules 2249

Bendroflumethiazide (Ziprasidone produces dose-related prolongation of the QT interval; hypokalemia may result from diuretic therapy and this may increase the risk of QT prolongation and arrhythmias; potential for enhanced hypotensive effect if used concurrently).
No products indexed under this heading.

Bepridil Hydrochloride (Ziprasidone produces dose-related prolongation of the QT interval; an additive effect of ziprasidone and other drugs that prolong cannot be excluded; concurrent use is not recommended).
No products indexed under this heading.

Betaxolol Hydrochloride (Ziprasidone may induce orthostatic hypotension; co-administration with certain antihypertensive drugs may enhance the hypotensive effects). Products include:
Betoptic S Ophthalmic Suspension 558

Bisoprolol Fumarate (Ziprasidone may induce orthostatic hypotension; co-administration with certain antihypertensive drugs may enhance the hypotensive effects).
No products indexed under this heading.

Bromocriptine Mesylate (Ziprasidone may antagonize the effects of dopamine agonists).
No products indexed under this heading.

Bumetanide (Ziprasidone produces dose-related prolongation of the QT interval; hypokalemia may result from diuretic therapy and this may increase the risk of QT prolongation and arrhythmias; potential for enhanced hypotensive effect if used concurrently). Products include:
Bumex Tablets 2746

Buprenorphine Hydrochloride (Somnolence was a commonly reported adverse event in patients treated with ziprasidone; concurrent use with other CNS active drugs, such as depressants, should be undertaken with caution). Products include:

Buprenex Injectable 2716
Suboxone Tablets 2717
Subutex Tablets 2717

Buspirone Hydrochloride (Somnolence was a commonly reported adverse event in patients treated with ziprasidone; concurrent use with other CNS active drugs, such as depressants, should be undertaken with caution).

No products indexed under this heading.

Butabarbital (Somnolence was a commonly reported adverse event in patients treated with ziprasidone; concurrent use with other CNS active drugs, such as depressants, should be undertaken with caution).

No products indexed under this heading.

Butalbital (Somnolence was a commonly reported adverse event in patients treated with ziprasidone; concurrent use with other CNS active drugs, such as depressants, should be undertaken with caution).

No products indexed under this heading.

Candesartan Cilexetil (Ziprasidone may induce orthostatic hypotension; co-administration with certain antihypertensive drugs may enhance the hypotensive effects). Products include:

Atacand Tablets 649
Atacand HCT 651

Captopril (Ziprasidone may induce orthostatic hypotension; co-administration with certain antihypertensive drugs may enhance the hypotensive effects). Products include:

Captopril Tablets 2149

Carbamazepine (Co-administration with carbamazepine, an inducer of CYP3A4, has resulted in a decrease of approximately 35% in AUC of ziprasidone; this effect may be greater when higher doses of carbamazepine are administered). Products include:

Carbatrol Capsules 3171
Equetro Extended-Release Capsules 3180
Tegretol/Tegretol-XR 2295

Carteolol Hydrochloride (Ziprasidone may induce orthostatic hypotension; co-administration with certain antihypertensive drugs may enhance the hypotensive effects). Products include:

Carteolol Hydrochloride Ophthalmic Solution USP, 1% .... ⊙ 249

Chlordiazepoxide (Somnolence was a commonly reported adverse event in patients treated with ziprasidone; concurrent use with other CNS active drugs, such as depressants, should be undertaken with caution).

No products indexed under this heading.

Chlordiazepoxide Hydrochloride (Somnolence was a commonly reported adverse event in patients treated with ziprasidone; concurrent use with other CNS active drugs, such as depressants, should be undertaken with caution). Products include:

Librium Capsules 3347

Chlorothiazide (Ziprasidone produces dose-related prolongation of the QT interval; hypokalemia may result from diuretic therapy and this may increase the risk of QT prolongation and arrhythmias; potential for enhanced hypotensive effect if used concurrently). Products include:

Diuril Oral Suspension 1954

Chlorothiazide Sodium (Ziprasidone produces dose-related prolongation of the QT interval; hypokalemia may result from diuretic therapy and this may increase the risk of QT prolongation and arrhythmias; potential for enhanced hypotensive effect if used concurrently). Products include:

Diuril Sodium Intravenous 2467

Chlorpromazine (Ziprasidone produces dose-related prolongation of the QT interval; an additive effect of ziprasidone and other drugs that prolong cannot be excluded; concurrent use is not recommended).

No products indexed under this heading.

Chlorpromazine Hydrochloride (Ziprasidone produces dose-related prolongation of the QT interval; an additive effect of ziprasidone and other drugs that prolong cannot be excluded; concurrent use is not recommended).

No products indexed under this heading.

Chlorprothixene (Somnolence was a commonly reported adverse event in patients treated with ziprasidone; concurrent use with other CNS active drugs, such as depressants, should be undertaken with caution).

No products indexed under this heading.

Chlorprothixene Hydrochloride (Ziprasidone produces dose-related prolongation of the QT interval; an additive effect of ziprasidone and other drugs that prolong cannot be excluded; concurrent use is not recommended).

No products indexed under this heading.

Chlorprothixene Lactate (Somnolence was a commonly reported adverse event in patients treated with ziprasidone; concurrent use with other CNS active drugs, such as depressants, should be undertaken with caution).

No products indexed under this heading.

Chlorthalidone (Ziprasidone may induce orthostatic hypotension; co-administration with certain antihypertensive drugs may enhance the hypotensive effects). Products include:

Clorpres Tablets 2153

Clonidine (Ziprasidone may induce orthostatic hypotension; co-administration with certain antihypertensive drugs may enhance the hypotensive effects). Products include:

Catapres-TTS 844

Clonidine Hydrochloride (Ziprasidone may induce orthostatic hypotension; co-administration with certain antihypertensive drugs may enhance the hypotensive effects). Products include:

Catapres Tablets 843
Clorpres Tablets 2153

Clorazepate Dipotassium (Somnolence was a commonly reported adverse event in patients treated with ziprasidone; concurrent use with other CNS active drugs, such as depressants, should be undertaken with caution). Products include:

Tranxene 2474

Clozapine (Somnolence was a commonly reported adverse event in patients treated with ziprasidone; concurrent use with other CNS active drugs, such as depressants, should be undertaken with caution). Products include:

Clozaril Tablets 2184
FazaClo Orally Disintegrating Tablets 551

Codeine Phosphate (Somnolence was a commonly reported adverse event in patients treated with ziprasidone; concurrent use with other CNS active drugs, such as depressants, should be undertaken with caution). Products include:

Tylenol with Codeine Tablets 2391

Deserpidine (Ziprasidone may induce orthostatic hypotension; co-administration with certain antihypertensive drugs may enhance the hypotensive effects).

No products indexed under this heading.

Desflurane (Somnolence was a commonly reported adverse event in patients treated with ziprasidone; concurrent use with other CNS active drugs, such as depressants, should be undertaken with caution).

No products indexed under this heading.

Desipramine Hydrochloride (Ziprasidone produces dose-related prolongation of the QT interval; an additive effect of ziprasidone and other drugs that prolong cannot be excluded; concurrent use is not recommended).

No products indexed under this heading.

Dezocine (Somnolence was a commonly reported adverse event in patients treated with ziprasidone; concurrent use with other CNS active drugs, such as depressants, should be undertaken with caution).

No products indexed under this heading.

Diazepam (Somnolence was a commonly reported adverse event in patients treated with ziprasidone; concurrent use with other CNS active drugs, such as depressants, should be undertaken with caution). Products include:

Diastat Rectal Delivery System 3343
Valium Tablets 2819

Diazoxide (Ziprasidone may induce orthostatic hypotension; co-administration with certain antihypertensive drugs may enhance the hypotensive effects). Products include:

Hyperstat I.V. 3017

Diltiazem Hydrochloride (Ziprasidone may induce orthostatic hypotension; co-administration with certain antihypertensive drugs may enhance the hypotensive effects). Products include:

Cardizem LA Extended Release Tablets 1728
Tiazac Capsules 1201

Disopyramide Phosphate (Ziprasidone produces dose-related prolongation of the QT interval; an additive effect of ziprasidone and other drugs that prolong cannot be excluded; concurrent use is not recommended).

No products indexed under this heading.

Dofetilide (Ziprasidone produces dose-related prolongation of the QT interval; an additive effect of ziprasidone and other drugs that prolong cannot be excluded; concurrent use is not recommended).

No products indexed under this heading.

Dolasetron Mesylate (Ziprasidone produces dose-related prolongation of the QT interval; an additive effect of ziprasidone and other drugs that prolong cannot be excluded; concurrent use is not recommended). Products include:

Anzemet Injection 2859
Anzemet Tablets 2862

Dopamine Hydrochloride (Ziprasidone may antagonize the effects of dopamine agonists).

No products indexed under this heading.

Doxazosin Mesylate (Ziprasidone may induce orthostatic hypotension; co-administration with certain antihypertensive drugs may enhance the hypotensive effects). Products include:

Cardura XL Tablets 2515

Droperidol (Ziprasidone produces dose-related prolongation of the QT interval; an additive effect of ziprasidone and other drugs that prolong cannot be excluded; concurrent use is not recommended).

No products indexed under this heading.

Enalapril Maleate (Ziprasidone may induce orthostatic hypotension; co-administration with certain antihypertensive drugs may enhance the hypotensive effects). Products include:

Vasotec I.V. Injection 2103

Enalaprilat (Ziprasidone may induce orthostatic hypotension; co-administration with certain antihypertensive drugs may enhance the hypotensive effects).

No products indexed under this heading.

Enflurane (Somnolence was a commonly reported adverse event in patients treated with ziprasidone; concurrent use with other CNS active drugs, such as depressants, should be undertaken with caution).

No products indexed under this heading.

Eprosartan Mesylate (Ziprasidone may induce orthostatic hypotension; co-administration with certain antihypertensive drugs may enhance the hypotensive effects). Products include:

Teveten Tablets 1735
Teveten HCT Tablets 1737

Erythromycin (Ziprasidone produces dose-related prolongation of the QT interval; an additive effect of ziprasidone and other drugs that prolong cannot be excluded; concurrent use is not recommended). Products include:

Ery-Tab Tablets 449
Erythromycin Base Filmtab Tablets 455

Erythromycin Delayed-Release Capsules, USP 457
PCE Dispertab Tablets 515

Erythromycin Estolate (Ziprasidone produces dose-related prolongation of the QT interval; an additive effect of ziprasidone and other drugs that prolong cannot be excluded; concurrent use is not recommended).
No products indexed under this heading.

Erythromycin Ethylsuccinate (Ziprasidone produces dose-related prolongation of the QT interval; an additive effect of ziprasidone and other drugs that prolong cannot be excluded; concurrent use is not recommended). Products include:
E.E.S. 451
EryPed 447

Erythromycin Gluceptate (Ziprasidone produces dose-related prolongation of the QT interval; an additive effect of ziprasidone and other drugs that prolong cannot be excluded; concurrent use is not recommended).
No products indexed under this heading.

Erythromycin Lactobionate (Ziprasidone produces dose-related prolongation of the QT interval; an additive effect of ziprasidone and other drugs that prolong cannot be excluded; concurrent use is not recommended).
No products indexed under this heading.

Erythromycin Stearate (Ziprasidone produces dose-related prolongation of the QT interval; an additive effect of ziprasidone and other drugs that prolong cannot be excluded; concurrent use is not recommended). Products include:
Erythrocin Stearate Filmtab Tablets 453

Esmolol Hydrochloride (Ziprasidone may induce orthostatic hypotension; co-administration with certain antihypertensive drugs may enhance the hypotensive effects).
No products indexed under this heading.

Estazolam (Somnolence was a commonly reported adverse event in patients treated with ziprasidone; concurrent use with other CNS active drugs, such as depressants, should be undertaken with caution). Products include:
ProSom Tablets 517

Ethacrynic Acid (Ziprasidone produces dose-related prolongation of the QT interval; hypokalemia may result from diuretic therapy and this may increase the risk of QT prolongation and arrhythmias; potential for enhanced hypotensive effect if used concurrently). Products include:
Edecrin Tablets 1959

Ethanol (Somnolence was a commonly reported adverse event in patients treated with ziprasidone; concurrent use with other CNS active drugs, such as depressants, should be undertaken with caution).
No products indexed under this heading.

Ethchlorvynol (Somnolence was a commonly reported adverse event in patients treated with ziprasidone; concurrent use with other CNS active drugs, such as depressants, should be undertaken with caution).
No products indexed under this heading.

Ethinamate (Somnolence was a commonly reported adverse event in patients treated with ziprasidone; concurrent use with other CNS active drugs, such as depressants, should be undertaken with caution).
No products indexed under this heading.

Ethyl Alcohol (Somnolence was a commonly reported adverse event in patients treated with ziprasidone; concurrent use with other CNS active drugs, such as depressants, should be undertaken with caution).
No products indexed under this heading.

Felodipine (Ziprasidone may induce orthostatic hypotension; co-administration with certain antihypertensive drugs may enhance the hypotensive effects).
No products indexed under this heading.

Fentanyl (Somnolence was a commonly reported adverse event in patients treated with ziprasidone; concurrent use with other CNS active drugs, such as depressants, should be undertaken with caution). Products include:
Duragesic Transdermal System 2373
Ionsys Transdermal System 2379

Fentanyl Citrate (Somnolence was a commonly reported adverse event in patients treated with ziprasidone; concurrent use with other CNS active drugs, such as depressants, should be undertaken with caution). Products include:
Actiq 979

Flecainide Acetate (Ziprasidone produces dose-related prolongation of the QT interval; an additive effect of ziprasidone and other drugs that prolong cannot be excluded; concurrent use is not recommended). Products include:
Tambocor Tablets 1856

Fluphenazine Decanoate (Somnolence was a commonly reported adverse event in patients treated with ziprasidone; concurrent use with other CNS active drugs, such as depressants, should be undertaken with caution).
No products indexed under this heading.

Fluphenazine Enanthate (Somnolence was a commonly reported adverse event in patients treated with ziprasidone; concurrent use with other CNS active drugs, such as depressants, should be undertaken with caution).
No products indexed under this heading.

Fluphenazine Hydrochloride (Somnolence was a commonly reported adverse event in patients treated with ziprasidone; concurrent use with other CNS active drugs, such as depressants, should be undertaken with caution).
No products indexed under this heading.

Flurazepam Hydrochloride (Somnolence was a commonly reported adverse event in patients treated with ziprasidone; concurrent use with other CNS active drugs, such as depressants, should be undertaken with caution). Products include:
Dalmane Capsules 3342

Fosinopril Sodium (Ziprasidone may induce orthostatic hypotension; co-administration with certain antihypertensive drugs may enhance the hypotensive effects).
No products indexed under this heading.

Furosemide (Ziprasidone produces dose-related prolongation of the QT interval; hypokalemia may result from diuretic therapy and this may increase the risk of QT prolongation and arrhythmias; potential for enhanced hypotensive effect if used concurrently). Products include:
Furosemide Tablets 2154

Gatifloxacin (Ziprasidone produces dose-related prolongation of the QT interval; an additive effect of ziprasidone and other drugs that prolong cannot be excluded; concurrent use is not recommended). Products include:
Tequin Injection 938
Tequin Injection in 5% Dextrose 938
Tequin Tablets 938
Zymar Ophthalmic Solution 575

Glutethimide (Somnolence was a commonly reported adverse event in patients treated with ziprasidone; concurrent use with other CNS active drugs, such as depressants, should be undertaken with caution).
No products indexed under this heading.

Guanabenz Acetate (Ziprasidone may induce orthostatic hypotension; co-administration with certain antihypertensive drugs may enhance the hypotensive effects).
No products indexed under this heading.

Guanethidine Monosulfate (Ziprasidone may induce orthostatic hypotension; co-administration with certain antihypertensive drugs may enhance the hypotensive effects).
No products indexed under this heading.

Halofantrine (Ziprasidone produces dose-related prolongation of the QT interval; an additive effect of ziprasidone and other drugs that prolong cannot be excluded; concurrent use is not recommended).
No products indexed under this heading.

Haloperidol (Somnolence was a commonly reported adverse event in patients treated with ziprasidone; concurrent use with other CNS active drugs, such as depressants, should be undertaken with caution).
No products indexed under this heading.

Haloperidol Decanoate (Somnolence was a commonly reported adverse event in patients treated with ziprasidone; concurrent use with other CNS active drugs, such as depressants, should be undertaken with caution).
No products indexed under this heading.

Hydralazine Hydrochloride (Ziprasidone may induce orthostatic hypotension; co-administration with certain antihypertensive drugs may enhance the hypotensive effects). Products include:
BiDil Tablets 2171

Hydrochlorothiazide (Ziprasidone produces dose-related prolongation of the QT interval; hypokalemia may result from diuretic therapy and this may increase the risk of QT prolongation and arrhythmias; potential for enhanced hypotensive effect if used concurrently). Products include:
Aldoril Tablets 1910
Atacand HCT 651
Avalide Tablets 888
Avalide Tablets 2874
Benicar HCT Tablets 1044
Diovan HCT Tablets 2196
Dyazide Capsules 1423
Hyzaar 50-12.5 Tablets 1990
Hyzaar 100-12.5 Tablets 1990
Hyzaar 100-25 Tablets 1990
Lopressor HCT 50/25 Tablets 2241
Lopressor HCT 100/25 Tablets 2241
Lopressor HCT 100/50 Tablets 2241
Lotensin HCT Tablets 2246
Micardis HCT Tablets 856
Moduretic Tablets 2028
Prinzide Tablets 2056
Teveten HCT Tablets 1737
Timolide Tablets 2086
Uniretic Tablets 3100

Hydrocodone Bitartrate (Somnolence was a commonly reported adverse event in patients treated with ziprasidone; concurrent use with other CNS active drugs, such as depressants, should be undertaken with caution). Products include:
Hycodan 1116
Hycotuss Expectorant Syrup 1117
Vicodin Tablets 535
Vicodin ES Tablets 536
Vicodin HP Tablets 538
Vicoprofen Tablets 539
Zydone Tablets 1139

Hydrocodone Polistirex (Somnolence was a commonly reported adverse event in patients treated with ziprasidone; concurrent use with other CNS active drugs, such as depressants, should be undertaken with caution). Products include:
Tussionex Pennkinetic Extended-Release Suspension 3327

Hydroflumethiazide (Ziprasidone produces dose-related prolongation of the QT interval; hypokalemia may result from diuretic therapy and this may increase the risk of QT prolongation and arrhythmias; potential for enhanced hypotensive effect if used concurrently).
No products indexed under this heading.

Hydromorphone Hydrochloride (Somnolence was a commonly reported adverse event in patients treated with ziprasidone; concurrent use with other CNS active drugs, such as depressants, should be undertaken with caution). Products include:
Dilaudid 440
Dilaudid Non-Sterile Powder 440
Dilaudid Oral Liquid 445
Dilaudid Rectal Suppositories 440
Dilaudid Tablets 440
Dilaudid Tablets - 8 mg 445
Dilaudid-HP 442

Hydroxyzine Hydrochloride (Somnolence was a commonly reported adverse event in patients treated with ziprasidone; concurrent use with other CNS active drugs, such as depressants, should be undertaken with caution).
No products indexed under this heading.

Ibutilide Fumarate (Ziprasidone produces dose-related prolongation of the QT interval; an additive effect of ziprasidone and other drugs that prolong cannot be excluded; concurrent use is not recommended).
No products indexed under this heading.

Indapamide (Ziprasidone may induce orthostatic hypotension; co-administration with certain antihypertensive drugs may enhance the hypotensive effects). Products include:

Irbesartan (Ziprasidone may induce orthostatic hypotension; co-administration with certain antihypertensive drugs may enhance the hypotensive effects). Products include:

Isoflurane (Somnolence was a commonly reported adverse event in patients treated with ziprasidone; concurrent use with other CNS active drugs, such as depressants, should be undertaken with caution).

No products indexed under this heading.

Isradipine (Ziprasidone may induce orthostatic hypotension; co-administration with certain antihypertensive drugs may enhance the hypotensive effects). Products include:

Itraconazole (Co-administration with inhibitors of CYP3A4, such as itraconazole, may result in increased AUC and Cmax of ziprasidone).

No products indexed under this heading.

Ketamine Hydrochloride (Somnolence was a commonly reported adverse event in patients treated with ziprasidone; concurrent use with other CNS active drugs, such as depressants, should be undertaken with caution).

No products indexed under this heading.

Ketoconazole (Co-administration with ketoconazole, a potent inhibitor of CYP3A4, has resulted in increased AUC and Cmax of ziprasidone by about 35-40%). Products include:

Labetalol Hydrochloride (Ziprasidone may induce orthostatic hypotension; co-administration with certain antihypertensive drugs may enhance the hypotensive effects).

No products indexed under this heading.

Levodopa (Ziprasidone may antagonize the effects of levodopa). Products include:

Levomethadyl Acetate Hydrochloride (Ziprasidone produces dose-related prolongation of the QT interval; an additive effect of ziprasidone and other drugs that prolong cannot be excluded; concurrent use is not recommended).

No products indexed under this heading.

Levorphanol Tartrate (Somnolence was a commonly reported adverse event in patients treated with ziprasidone; concurrent use with other CNS active drugs, such as depressants, should be undertaken with caution).

No products indexed under this heading.

Lisinopril (Ziprasidone may induce orthostatic hypotension; co-administration with certain antihyper-

tensive drugs may enhance the hypotensive effects). Products include:

Lorazepam (Somnolence was a commonly reported adverse event in patients treated with ziprasidone; concurrent use with other CNS active drugs, such as depressants, should be undertaken with caution).

No products indexed under this heading.

Losartan Potassium (Ziprasidone may induce orthostatic hypotension; co-administration with certain antihypertensive drugs may enhance the hypotensive effects). Products include:

Loxapine Hydrochloride (Somnolence was a commonly reported adverse event in patients treated with ziprasidone; concurrent use with other CNS active drugs, such as depressants, should be undertaken with caution).

No products indexed under this heading.

Loxapine Succinate (Somnolence was a commonly reported adverse event in patients treated with ziprasidone; concurrent use with other CNS active drugs, such as depressants, should be undertaken with caution).

No products indexed under this heading.

Mecamylamine Hydrochloride (Ziprasidone may induce orthostatic hypotension; co-administration with certain antihypertensive drugs may enhance the hypotensive effects).

No products indexed under this heading.

Mefloquine Hydrochloride (Ziprasidone produces dose-related prolongation of the QT interval; an additive effect of ziprasidone and other drugs that prolong cannot be excluded; concurrent use is not recommended). Products include:

Meperidine Hydrochloride (Somnolence was a commonly reported adverse event in patients treated with ziprasidone; concurrent use with other CNS active drugs, such as depressants, should be undertaken with caution).

No products indexed under this heading.

Mephobarbital (Somnolence was a commonly reported adverse event in patients treated with ziprasidone; concurrent use with other CNS active drugs, such as depressants, should be undertaken with caution).

No products indexed under this heading.

Meprobamate (Somnolence was a commonly reported adverse event in patients treated with ziprasidone; concurrent use with other CNS active drugs, such as depressants, should be undertaken with caution).

No products indexed under this heading.

Mesoridazine Besylate (Ziprasidone produces dose-related prolongation of the QT interval; an additive effect of ziprasidone and other drugs that prolong cannot be excluded; concurrent use is not recommended).

No products indexed under this heading.

Methadone Hydrochloride (Somnolence was a commonly reported adverse event in patients treated with ziprasidone; concurrent use with other CNS active drugs, such as depressants, should be undertaken with caution).

No products indexed under this heading.

Methohexital Sodium (Somnolence was a commonly reported adverse event in patients treated with ziprasidone; concurrent use with other CNS active drugs, such as depressants, should be undertaken with caution).

No products indexed under this heading.

Methotrimeprazine (Somnolence was a commonly reported adverse event in patients treated with ziprasidone; concurrent use with other CNS active drugs, such as depressants, should be undertaken with caution).

No products indexed under this heading.

Methoxyflurane (Somnolence was a commonly reported adverse event in patients treated with ziprasidone; concurrent use with other CNS active drugs, such as depressants, should be undertaken with caution).

No products indexed under this heading.

Methyclothiazide (Ziprasidone produces dose-related prolongation of the QT interval; hypokalemia may result from diuretic therapy and this may increase the risk of QT prolongation and arrhythmias; potential for enhanced hypotensive effect if used concurrently).

No products indexed under this heading.

Methyldopa (Ziprasidone may induce orthostatic hypotension; co-administration with certain antihypertensive drugs may enhance the hypotensive effects). Products include:

Methyldopate Hydrochloride (Ziprasidone may induce orthostatic hypotension; co-administration with certain antihypertensive drugs may enhance the hypotensive effects).

No products indexed under this heading.

Metolazone (Ziprasidone may induce orthostatic hypotension; co-administration with certain antihypertensive drugs may enhance the hypotensive effects).

No products indexed under this heading.

Metoprolol Succinate (Ziprasidone may induce orthostatic hypotension; co-administration with certain antihypertensive drugs may enhance the hypotensive effects). Products include:

Metoprolol Tartrate (Ziprasidone may induce orthostatic hypotension; co-administration with certain antihypertensive drugs may enhance the hypotensive effects). Products include:

Metyrosine (Ziprasidone may induce orthostatic hypotension; co-administration with certain antihypertensive drugs may enhance the hypotensive effects). Products include:

Mibefradil Dihydrochloride (Ziprasidone may induce orthostatic hypotension; co-administration with certain antihypertensive drugs may enhance the hypotensive effects).

No products indexed under this heading.

Midazolam Hydrochloride (Somnolence was a commonly reported adverse event in patients treated with ziprasidone; concurrent use with other CNS active drugs, such as depressants, should be undertaken with caution).

No products indexed under this heading.

Minoxidil (Ziprasidone may induce orthostatic hypotension; co-administration with certain antihypertensive drugs may enhance the hypotensive effects). Products include:

Moexipril Hydrochloride (Ziprasidone may induce orthostatic hypotension; co-administration with certain antihypertensive drugs may enhance the hypotensive effects). Products include:

Molindone Hydrochloride (Somnolence was a commonly reported adverse event in patients treated with ziprasidone; concurrent use with other CNS active drugs, such as depressants, should be undertaken with caution). Products include:

Morphine Sulfate (Somnolence was a commonly reported adverse event in patients treated with ziprasidone; concurrent use with other CNS active drugs, such as depressants, should be undertaken with caution). Products include:

Moxifloxacin Hydrochloride (Ziprasidone produces dose-related prolongation of the QT interval; an additive effect of ziprasidone and other drugs that prolong cannot be excluded; concurrent use is not recommended). Products include:

Nadolol (Ziprasidone may induce orthostatic hypotension; co-administration with certain antihypertensive drugs may enhance the hypotensive effects). Products include:

Nicardipine Hydrochloride (Ziprasidone may induce orthostatic

IMPORTANT NOTE: Always consult each drug listing in the patient's regimen for possible interactions.

hypotension; co-administration with certain antihypertensive drugs may enhance the hypotensive effects). Products include:

Nifedipine (Ziprasidone may induce orthostatic hypotension; co-administration with certain antihypertensive drugs may enhance the hypotensive effects). Products include:

Nisoldipine (Ziprasidone may induce orthostatic hypotension; co-administration with certain antihypertensive drugs may enhance the hypotensive effects). Products include:

Nitroglycerin (Ziprasidone may induce orthostatic hypotension; co-administration with certain antihypertensive drugs may enhance the hypotensive effects). Products include:

Olanzapine (Somnolence was a commonly reported adverse event in patients treated with ziprasidone; concurrent use with other CNS active drugs, such as depressants, should be undertaken with caution). Products include:

Oxazepam (Somnolence was a commonly reported adverse event in patients treated with ziprasidone; concurrent use with other CNS active drugs, such as depressants, should be undertaken with caution).

No products indexed under this heading.

Oxycodone Hydrochloride (Somnolence was a commonly reported adverse event in patients treated with ziprasidone; concurrent use with other CNS active drugs, such as depressants, should be undertaken with caution). Products include:

Penbutolol Sulfate (Ziprasidone may induce orthostatic hypotension; co-administration with certain antihypertensive drugs may enhance the hypotensive effects).

No products indexed under this heading.

Pentamidine Isethionate (Ziprasidone produces dose-related prolongation of the QT interval; an additive effect of ziprasidone and other drugs that prolong cannot be excluded; concurrent use is not recommended).

No products indexed under this heading.

Pentobarbital Sodium (Somnolence was a commonly reported adverse event in patients treated with ziprasidone; concurrent use with other CNS active drugs, such as depressants, should be undertaken with caution). Products include:

Pergolide Mesylate (Ziprasidone may antagonize the effects of dopamine agonists). Products include:

Perindopril Erbumine (Ziprasidone may induce orthostatic hypotension; co-administration with certain antihypertensive drugs may enhance the hypotensive effects). Products include:

Perphenazine (Somnolence was a commonly reported adverse event in patients treated with ziprasidone; concurrent use with other CNS active drugs, such as depressants, should be undertaken with caution).

No products indexed under this heading.

Phenobarbital (Somnolence was a commonly reported adverse event in patients treated with ziprasidone; concurrent use with other CNS active drugs, such as depressants, should be undertaken with caution). Products include:

Phenoxybenzamine Hydrochloride (Ziprasidone may induce orthostatic hypotension; co-administration with certain antihypertensive drugs may enhance the hypotensive effects). Products include:

Phentolamine Mesylate (Ziprasidone may induce orthostatic hypotension; co-administration with certain antihypertensive drugs may enhance the hypotensive effects).

No products indexed under this heading.

Pimozide (Ziprasidone produces dose-related prolongation of the QT interval; an additive effect of ziprasidone and other drugs that prolong cannot be excluded; concurrent use is not recommended).

No products indexed under this heading.

Pindolol (Ziprasidone may induce orthostatic hypotension; co-administration with certain antihypertensive drugs may enhance the hypotensive effects).

No products indexed under this heading.

Polythiazide (Ziprasidone produces dose-related prolongation of the QT interval; hypokalemia may result from diuretic therapy and this may increase the risk of QT prolongation and arrhythmias; potential for enhanced hypotensive effect if used concurrently).

No products indexed under this heading.

Pramipexole Dihydrochloride (Ziprasidone may antagonize the effects of dopamine agonists). Products include:

Prazepam (Somnolence was a commonly reported adverse event in patients treated with ziprasidone; concurrent use with other CNS active drugs, such as depressants, should be undertaken with caution).

No products indexed under this heading.

Prazosin Hydrochloride (Ziprasidone may induce orthostatic hypotension; co-administration with certain antihypertensive drugs may enhance the hypotensive effects).

No products indexed under this heading.

Probucol (Ziprasidone produces dose-related prolongation of the QT interval; an additive effect of ziprasidone and other drugs that prolong cannot be excluded; concurrent use is not recommended).

No products indexed under this heading.

Procainamide Hydrochloride (Ziprasidone produces dose-related prolongation of the QT interval; an additive effect of ziprasidone and other drugs that prolong cannot be excluded; concurrent use is not recommended).

No products indexed under this heading.

Prochlorperazine (Somnolence was a commonly reported adverse event in patients treated with ziprasidone; concurrent use with other CNS active drugs, such as depressants, should be undertaken with caution).

No products indexed under this heading.

Promethazine Hydrochloride (Somnolence was a commonly reported adverse event in patients treated with ziprasidone; concurrent use with other CNS active drugs, such as depressants, should be undertaken with caution). Products include:

Propofol (Somnolence was a commonly reported adverse event in patients treated with ziprasidone; concurrent use with other CNS active drugs, such as depressants, should be undertaken with caution).

No products indexed under this heading.

Propoxyphene Hydrochloride (Somnolence was a commonly reported adverse event in patients treated with ziprasidone; concurrent use with other CNS active drugs, such as depressants, should be undertaken with caution).

No products indexed under this heading.

Propoxyphene Napsylate (Somnolence was a commonly reported adverse event in patients treated with ziprasidone; concurrent use with other CNS active drugs, such as depressants, should be undertaken with caution).

No products indexed under this heading.

Propranolol Hydrochloride (Ziprasidone may induce orthostatic hypotension; co-administration with certain antihypertensive drugs may enhance the hypotensive effects). Products include:

Quazepam (Somnolence was a commonly reported adverse event in patients treated with ziprasidone; concurrent use with other CNS active drugs, such as depressants, should be undertaken with caution).

No products indexed under this heading.

Quetiapine Fumarate (Somnolence was a commonly reported adverse event in patients treated with ziprasidone; concurrent use with other CNS active drugs, such as depressants, should be undertaken with caution). Products include:

Quinapril Hydrochloride (Ziprasidone may induce orthostatic hypotension; co-administration with certain antihypertensive drugs may enhance the hypotensive effects).

No products indexed under this heading.

Quinidine (Ziprasidone produces dose-related prolongation of the QT interval; an additive effect of ziprasidone and other drugs that prolong cannot be excluded; concurrent use is not recommended).

No products indexed under this heading.

Quinidine Gluconate (Ziprasidone produces dose-related prolongation of the QT interval; an additive effect of ziprasidone and other drugs that prolong cannot be excluded; concurrent use is not recommended).

No products indexed under this heading.

Quinidine Hydrochloride (Ziprasidone produces dose-related prolongation of the QT interval; an additive effect of ziprasidone and other drugs that prolong cannot be excluded; concurrent use is not recommended).

No products indexed under this heading.

Quinidine Polygalacturonate (Ziprasidone produces dose-related prolongation of the QT interval; an additive effect of ziprasidone and other drugs that prolong cannot be excluded; concurrent use is not recommended).

No products indexed under this heading.

Quinidine Sulfate (Ziprasidone produces dose-related prolongation of the QT interval; an additive effect of ziprasidone and other drugs that prolong cannot be excluded; concurrent use is not recommended).

No products indexed under this heading.

Ramipril (Ziprasidone may induce orthostatic hypotension; co-administration with certain antihypertensive drugs may enhance the hypotensive effects). Products include:

Rauwolfia Serpentina (Ziprasidone may induce orthostatic hypotension; co-administration with certain antihypertensive drugs may enhance the hypotensive effects).

No products indexed under this heading.

Remifentanil Hydrochloride (Somnolence was a commonly reported adverse event in patients treated with ziprasidone; concurrent use with other CNS active drugs, such as depressants, should be undertaken with caution).

No products indexed under this heading.

Rescinnamine (Ziprasidone may induce orthostatic hypotension; co-administration with certain antihypertensive drugs may enhance the hypotensive effects).

No products indexed under this heading.

Reserpine (Ziprasidone may induce orthostatic hypotension; co-administration with certain antihypertensive drugs may enhance the hypotensive effects).

No products indexed under this heading.

Risperidone (Somnolence was a commonly reported adverse event in patients treated with ziprasidone; concurrent use with other CNS active drugs, such as depressants, should be undertaken with caution). Products include:

Risperdal **1676**
Risperdal Consta Long-Acting Injection **1682**
Risperdal M-Tab Orally Disintegrating Tablets.................. **1676**

Ropinirole Hydrochloride (Ziprasidone may antagonize the effects of dopamine agonists). Products include:

Requip Tablets **1555**

Secobarbital Sodium (Somnolence was a commonly reported adverse event in patients treated with ziprasidone; concurrent use with other CNS active drugs, such as depressants, should be undertaken with caution).

No products indexed under this heading.

Sevoflurane (Somnolence was a commonly reported adverse event in patients treated with ziprasidone; concurrent use with other CNS active drugs, such as depressants, should be undertaken with caution). Products include:

Ultane Liquid for Inhalation **531**

Sodium Nitroprusside (Ziprasidone may induce orthostatic hypotension; co-administration with certain antihypertensive drugs may enhance the hypotensive effects).

No products indexed under this heading.

Sodium Oxybate (Somnolence was a commonly reported adverse event in patients treated with ziprasidone; concurrent use with other CNS active drugs, such as depressants, should be undertaken with caution). Products include:

Xyrem Oral Solution **1688**

Sotalol Hydrochloride (Ziprasidone produces dose-related prolongation of the QT interval; an additive effect of ziprasidone and other drugs that prolong cannot be excluded; concurrent use is not recommended).

No products indexed under this heading.

Sparfloxacin (Ziprasidone produces dose-related prolongation of the QT interval; an additive effect of ziprasidone and other drugs that prolong cannot be excluded; concurrent use is not recommended).

No products indexed under this heading.

Spirapril Hydrochloride (Ziprasidone may induce orthostatic hypotension; co-administration with certain antihypertensive drugs may enhance the hypotensive effects).

No products indexed under this heading.

Sufentanil Citrate (Somnolence was a commonly reported adverse event in patients treated with ziprasidone; concurrent use with other CNS active drugs, such as depressants, should be undertaken with caution).

No products indexed under this heading.

Tacrolimus (Ziprasidone produces dose-related prolongation of the QT interval; an additive effect of ziprasidone and other drugs that prolong cannot be excluded; concurrent use is not recommended). Products include:

Prograf Capsules and Injection **632**
Protopic Ointment **638**

Telmisartan (Ziprasidone may induce orthostatic hypotension; co-administration with certain antihypertensive drugs may enhance the hypotensive effects). Products include:

Micardis Tablets **854**
Micardis HCT Tablets **856**

Temazepam (Somnolence was a commonly reported adverse event in patients treated with ziprasidone; concurrent use with other CNS active drugs, such as depressants, should be undertaken with caution). Products include:

Restoril Capsules **1860**

Terazosin Hydrochloride (Ziprasidone may induce orthostatic hypotension; co-administration with certain antihypertensive drugs may enhance the hypotensive effects). Products include:

Hytrin Capsules **471**

Thiamylal Sodium (Somnolence was a commonly reported adverse event in patients treated with ziprasidone; concurrent use with other CNS active drugs, such as depressants, should be undertaken with caution).

No products indexed under this heading.

Thioridazine Hydrochloride (Ziprasidone produces dose-related prolongation of the QT interval; an additive effect of ziprasidone and other drugs that prolong cannot be excluded; concurrent use is not recommended). Products include:

Thioridazine Hydrochloride Tablets ... **2163**

Thiothixene (Somnolence was a commonly reported adverse event in patients treated with ziprasidone; concurrent use with other CNS active drugs, such as depressants, should be undertaken with caution). Products include:

Thiothixene Capsules **2165**

Timolol Maleate (Ziprasidone may induce orthostatic hypotension; co-administration with certain antihypertensive drugs may enhance the hypotensive effects). Products include:

Blocadren Tablets **1916**
Cosopt Sterile Ophthalmic Solution................................... **1931**
Timolide Tablets **2086**
Timoptic Sterile Ophthalmic Solution **2088**
Timoptic in Ocudose **2091**
Timoptic-XE Sterile Ophthalmic Gel Forming Solution.................. **2092**

Torsemide (Ziprasidone produces dose-related prolongation of the QT interval; hypokalemia may result from diuretic therapy and this may increase the risk of QT prolongation and arrhythmias; potential for enhanced hypotensive effect if used concurrently). Products include:

Demadex Injection **2759**
Demadex Tablets **2759**

Trandolapril (Ziprasidone may induce orthostatic hypotension; co-administration with certain antihypertensive drugs may enhance the hypotensive effects). Products include:

Mavik Tablets **486**
Tarka Tablets **524**

Triazolam (Somnolence was a commonly reported adverse event in patients treated with ziprasidone; concurrent use with other CNS active drugs, such as depressants, should be undertaken with caution).

No products indexed under this heading.

Trifluoperazine Hydrochloride (Somnolence was a commonly reported adverse event in patients treated with ziprasidone; concurrent use with other CNS active drugs, such as depressants, should be undertaken with caution).

No products indexed under this heading.

Trimethaphan Camsylate (Ziprasidone may induce orthostatic hypotension; co-administration with certain antihypertensive drugs may enhance the hypotensive effects).

No products indexed under this heading.

Valsartan (Ziprasidone may induce orthostatic hypotension; co-administration with certain antihypertensive drugs may enhance the hypotensive effects). Products include:

Diovan Tablets **2193**
Diovan HCT Tablets **2196**

Verapamil Hydrochloride (Ziprasidone may induce orthostatic hypotension; co-administration with certain antihypertensive drugs may enhance the hypotensive effects). Products include:

Covera-HS Tablets **3139**
Tarka Tablets **524**
Verelan PM Extended-Release Capsules, Controlled-Onset.......... **3106**

Zaleplon (Somnolence was a commonly reported adverse event in patients treated with ziprasidone; concurrent use with other CNS active drugs, such as depressants, should be undertaken with caution). Products include:

Sonata Capsules **1717**

Zolpidem Tartrate (Somnolence was a commonly reported adverse event in patients treated with ziprasidone; concurrent use with other CNS active drugs, such as depressants, should be undertaken with caution). Products include:

Ambien Tablets **2851**
Ambien CR Tablets **2855**

Food Interactions

Alcohol (Somnolence was a commonly reported adverse event in patients treated with ziprasidone; concurrent use with alcohol or other CNS active drugs, such as depressants, should be undertaken with caution).

GEODON FOR INJECTION

(Ziprasidone Mesylate) **2529**
See Geodon Capsules

GLEEVEC TABLETS

(Imatinib Mesylate) **2227**
May interact with calcium channel blockers that are metabolized by CYP3A4, cytochrome p450 2c9 substrates (selected), cytochrome p450 2d6 substrates (selected), cytochrome p450 3a4 inducers (selected), cytochrome p450 3a4 inhibitors (selected), dexamethasone, erythromycin, phenytoin, triazolobenzodiazepines, and certain other agents. Compounds in these categories include:

Acarbose (Imatinib is a potent competitive inhibitor of CYP2C9; therefore, imatinib is likely to increase the blood levels of drugs that are substrates of this enzyme). Products include:

Precose Tablets **751**

Acetazolamide (Caution is recommended when administering Gleevec with inhibitors of the CYP3A4 family. Substances that inhibit CYP3A4 activity may decrease metabolism and increase imatinib concentrations. There is a significant increase in exposure to imatinib when Gleevec is co-administered with ketoconazole).

No products indexed under this heading.

Allium sativum (Substances that are inducers of CYP3A4 activity may increase metabolism and decrease imatinib plasma concentrations. Co-medications that induce CYP3A4 may significantly reduce exposure to Gleevec. Dosage of imatinib should be increased by at least 50% and clinical response should be carefully monitored in patients receiving imatinib with potent CYP3A4 inducers).

No products indexed under this heading.

Alprazolam (Imatinib will increase the plasma concentrations of triazolobenzodiazepines by inhibiting CYP3A4). Products include:

Niravam Orally Disintegrating Tablets .. **3092**

Amiodarone Hydrochloride (Caution is recommended when administering Gleevec with inhibitors of the CYP3A4 family. Substances that inhibit CYP3A4 activity may decrease metabolism and increase imatinib concentrations. There is a significant increase in exposure to imatinib when Gleevec is co-administered with ketoconazole).

No products indexed under this heading.

Amitriptyline Hydrochloride (Imatinib is a potent competitive inhibitor of CYP2D6; therefore, imatinib is likely to increase the blood levels of drugs that are substrates of this enzyme).

No products indexed under this heading.

Amlodipine Besylate (Imatinib will increase plasma concentration of CYP3A4 metabolized drugs. (e.g., dihydropyridine calcium channel blockers)). Products include:

Caduet Tablets **2508**
Lotrel Capsules **2249**
Norvasc Tablets **2545**

Amphetamine Aspartate (Imatinib is a potent competitive inhibitor of CYP2D6; therefore, imatinib is likely to increase the blood levels of drugs that are substrates of this enzyme). Products include:

Adderall Tablets **3164**
Adderall XR Capsules **3166**

Amphetamine Aspartate Monohydrate (Imatinib is a potent competitive inhibitor of CYP2D6; therefore, imatinib is likely to increase the blood levels of drugs that are substrates of this enzyme).

No products indexed under this heading.

Amphetamine Sulfate (Imatinib is a potent competitive inhibitor of CYP2D6; therefore, imatinib is likely to increase the blood levels of drugs that are substrates of this enzyme). Products include:

Adderall Tablets **3164**
Adderall XR Capsules **3166**

IMPORTANT NOTE: Always consult each drug listing in the patient's regimen for possible interactions.

Amprenavir (Caution is recommended when administering Gleevec with inhibitors of the CYP3A4 family. Substances that inhibit CYP3A4 activity may decrease metabolism and increase imatinib concentrations. There is a significant increase in exposure to imatinib when Gleevec is co-administered with ketoconazole). Products include:
- Agenerase Capsules **1327**
- Agenerase Oral Solution **1332**

Anastrozole (Caution is recommended when administering Gleevec with inhibitors of the CYP3A4 family. Substances that inhibit CYP3A4 activity may decrease metabolism and increase imatinib concentrations. There is a significant increase in exposure to imatinib when Gleevec is co-administered with ketoconazole). Products include:
- Arimidex Tablets **673**

Aprepitant (Caution is recommended when administering Gleevec with inhibitors of the CYP3A4 family. Substances that inhibit CYP3A4 activity may decrease metabolism and increase imatinib concentrations. There is a significant increase in exposure to imatinib when Gleevec is co-administered with ketoconazole). Products include:
- Emend Capsules **1963**

Atomoxetine Hydrochloride (Imatinib is a potent competitive inhibitor of CYP2D6; therefore, imatinib is likely to increase the blood levels of drugs that are substrates of this enzyme). Products include:
- Strattera Capsules **1814**

Atorvastatin Calcium (Imatinib will increase the plasma concentrations of certain HMG-CoA reductase inhibitors by inhibiting CYP3A4). Products include:
- Caduet Tablets **2508**
- Lipitor Tablets **2483**

Betamethasone Acetate (Substances that are inducers of CYP3A4 activity may increase metabolism and decrease imatinib plasma concentrations. Co-medications that induce CYP3A4 may significantly reduce exposure to Gleevec. Dosage of imatinib should be increased by at least 50% and clinical response should be carefully monitored in patients receiving imatinib with potent CYP3A4 inducers).

No products indexed under this heading.

Betamethasone Sodium Phosphate (Substances that are inducers of CYP3A4 activity may increase metabolism and decrease imatinib plasma concentrations. Co-medications that induce CYP3A4 may significantly reduce exposure to Gleevec. Dosage of imatinib should be increased by at least 50% and clinical response should be carefully monitored in patients receiving imatinib with potent CYP3A4 inducers).

No products indexed under this heading.

Bisoprolol Fumarate (Imatinib is a potent competitive inhibitor of CYP2D6; therefore, imatinib is likely to increase the blood levels of drugs that are substrates of this enzyme).

No products indexed under this heading.

Candesartan Cilexetil (Imatinib is a potent competitive inhibitor of CYP2C9; therefore, imatinib is likely to increase the blood levels of drugs that are substrates of this enzyme). Products include:
- Atacand Tablets **649**
- Atacand HCT **651**

Captopril (Imatinib is a potent competitive inhibitor of CYP2D6; therefore, imatinib is likely to increase the blood levels of drugs that are substrates of this enzyme). Products include:
- Captopril Tablets **2149**

Carbamazepine (Co-administration with inducers of CYP3A4, such as carbamazepine, may increase the metabolism and decrease imatinib concentrations). Products include:
- Carbatrol Capsules **3171**
- Equetro Extended-Release Capsules **3180**
- Tegretol/Tegretol-XR **2295**

Carvedilol (Imatinib is a potent competitive inhibitor of CYP2D6; therefore, imatinib is likely to increase the blood levels of drugs that are substrates of this enzyme). Products include:
- Coreg Tablets **1414**

Celecoxib (Imatinib is a potent competitive inhibitor of CYP2C9; therefore, imatinib is likely to increase the blood levels of drugs that are substrates of this enzyme). Products include:
- Celebrex Capsules **3134**

Cerivastatin Sodium (Imatinib will increase the plasma concentrations of certain HMG-CoA reductase inhibitors by inhibiting CYP3A4).

No products indexed under this heading.

Cevimeline Hydrochloride (Imatinib is a potent competitive inhibitor of CYP2D6; therefore, imatinib is likely to increase the blood levels of drugs that are substrates of this enzyme). Products include:
- Evoxac Capsules **1047**

Chlorpromazine (Imatinib is a potent competitive inhibitor of CYP2D6; therefore, imatinib is likely to increase the blood levels of drugs that are substrates of this enzyme).

No products indexed under this heading.

Chlorpromazine Hydrochloride (Imatinib is a potent competitive inhibitor of CYP2D6; therefore, imatinib is likely to increase the blood levels of drugs that are substrates of this enzyme).

No products indexed under this heading.

Chlorpropamide (Imatinib is a potent competitive inhibitor of CYP2D6; therefore, imatinib is likely to increase the blood levels of drugs that are substrates of this enzyme).

No products indexed under this heading.

Cimetidine (Caution is recommended when administering Gleevec with inhibitors of the CYP3A4 family. Substances that inhibit CYP3A4 activity may decrease metabolism and increase imatinib concentrations. There is a significant increase in exposure to imatinib when Gleevec is co-administered with ketoconazole). Products include:
- Tagamet HB 200 Tablets .... ▣**664**

Cimetidine Hydrochloride (Caution is recommended when administering Gleevec with inhibitors of the CYP3A4 family. Substances that inhibit CYP3A4 activity may decrease metabolism and increase imatinib concentrations. There is a significant increase in exposure to imatinib when Gleevec is co-administered with ketoconazole).

No products indexed under this heading.

Ciprofloxacin (Caution is recommended when administering Gleevec with inhibitors of the CYP3A4 family. Substances that inhibit CYP3A4 activity may decrease metabolism and increase imatinib concentrations. There is a significant increase in exposure to imatinib when Gleevec is co-administered with ketoconazole). Products include:
- Cipro Oral Suspension **2977**
- Cipro I.V. **2984**
- Cipro XR Tablets **2990**
- Ciprodex Otic Suspension **559**

Ciprofloxacin Hydrochloride (Substances that are inducers of CYP3A4 activity may increase metabolism and decrease imatinib plasma concentrations. Co-medications that induce CYP3A4 may significantly reduce exposure to Gleevec. Dosage of imatinib should be increased by at least 50% and clinical response should be carefully monitored in patients receiving imatinib with potent CYP3A4 inducers). Products include:
- Ciloxan Ophthalmic Ointment **559**
- Ciloxan Ophthalmic Solution .... ⊙**206**
- Cipro Tablets **2977**
- Proquin XR Tablets **1153**

Cisplatin (Substances that are inducers of CYP3A4 activity may increase metabolism and decrease imatinib plasma concentrations. Co-medications that induce CYP3A4 may significantly reduce exposure to Gleevec. Dosage of imatinib should be increased by at least 50% and clinical response should be carefully monitored in patients receiving imatinib with potent CYP3A4 inducers).

No products indexed under this heading.

Clarithromycin (Co-administration with CYP3A4 inhibitors, such as clarithromycin, may decrease the metabolism and increase imatinib concentrations). Products include:
- Biaxin/Biaxin XL **402**
- PREVPAC **3284**

Clomipramine Hydrochloride (Imatinib is a potent competitive inhibitor of CYP2D6; therefore, imatinib is likely to increase the blood levels of drugs that are substrates of this enzyme).

No products indexed under this heading.

Clotrimazole (Caution is recommended when administering Gleevec with inhibitors of the CYP3A4 family. Substances that inhibit CYP3A4 activity may decrease metabolism and increase imatinib concentrations. There is a significant increase in exposure to imatinib when Gleevec is co-administered with ketoconazole). Products include:
- Desenex Athlete's Foot Cream .... ▣**635**
- Lotrimin **3039**
- Lotrisone **3040**

Clozapine (Imatinib is a potent competitive inhibitor of CYP2D6; therefore, imatinib is likely to increase the blood levels of drugs that are substrates of this enzyme). Products include:
- Clozaril Tablets **2184**
- FazaClo Orally Disintegrating Tablets **551**

Codeine Phosphate (Imatinib is a potent competitive inhibitor of CYP2D6; therefore, imatinib is likely to increase the blood levels of drugs that are substrates of this enzyme). Products include:
- Tylenol with Codeine Tablets **2391**

Codeine Sulfate (Imatinib is a potent competitive inhibitor of CYP2D6; therefore, imatinib is likely to increase the blood levels of drugs that are substrates of this enzyme).

No products indexed under this heading.

Cortisone Acetate (Substances that are inducers of CYP3A4 activity may increase metabolism and decrease imatinib plasma concentrations. Co-medications that induce CYP3A4 may significantly reduce exposure to Gleevec. Dosage of imatinib should be increased by at least 50% and clinical response should be carefully monitored in patients receiving imatinib with potent CYP3A4 inducers).

No products indexed under this heading.

Cyclobenzaprine Hydrochloride (Imatinib is a potent competitive inhibitor of CYP2D6; therefore, imatinib is likely to increase the blood levels of drugs that are substrates of this enzyme).

No products indexed under this heading.

Cyclosporine (Particular caution is recommended when administering imatinib with CYP3A4 substrates that have a narrow therapeutic window). Products include:
- Gengraf Capsules **459**
- Neoral Oral Solution **2259**
- Neoral Soft Gelatin Capsules **2259**
- Restasis Ophthalmic Emulsion **575**
- Sandimmune **2275**

Dalfopristin (Caution is recommended when administering Gleevec with inhibitors of the CYP3A4 family. Substances that inhibit CYP3A4 activity may decrease metabolism and increase imatinib concentrations. There is a significant increase in exposure to imatinib when Gleevec is co-administered with ketoconazole).

No products indexed under this heading.

Danazol (Caution is recommended when administering Gleevec with inhibitors of the CYP3A4 family. Substances that inhibit CYP3A4 activity may decrease metabolism and increase imatinib concentrations. There is a significant increase in exposure to imatinib when Gleevec is co-administered with ketoconazole).

No products indexed under this heading.

Delavirdine Mesylate (Caution is recommended when administering Gleevec with inhibitors of the CYP3A4 family. Substances that inhibit CYP3A4 activity may decrease metabolism and increase imatinib concentrations. There is a significant increase in exposure to imatinib when Gleevec is co-administered with ketoconazole). Products include:
- Rescriptor Tablets **2551**

Desipramine Hydrochloride (Imatinib is a potent competitive inhibitor of CYP2D6; therefore, imatinib is likely to increase the blood levels of drugs that are substrates of this enzyme).
No products indexed under this heading.

Desogestrel (Imatinib is a potent competitive inhibitor of CYP2C9; therefore, imatinib is likely to increase the blood levels of drugs that are substrates of this enzyme). Products include:
Mircette Tablets 1066

Dexamethasone (Co-administration with inducers of CYP3A4, such as dexamethasone, may increase the metabolism and decrease imatinib concentrations). Products include:
Ciprodex Otic Suspension 559
Decadron Tablets 1951
TobraDex Ophthalmic Ointment 562
TobraDex Ophthalmic Suspension 563

Dexamethasone Acetate (Co-administration with inducers of CYP3A4, such as dexamethasone, may increase the metabolism and decrease imatinib concentrations).
No products indexed under this heading.

Dexamethasone Sodium Phosphate (Co-administration with inducers of CYP3A4, such as dexamethasone, may increase the metabolism and decrease imatinib concentrations).
No products indexed under this heading.

Dexfenfluramine Hydrochloride (Imatinib is a potent competitive inhibitor of CYP2D6; therefore, imatinib is likely to increase the blood levels of drugs that are substrates of this enzyme).
No products indexed under this heading.

Dextromethorphan (Imatinib is a potent competitive inhibitor of CYP2C9; therefore, imatinib is likely to increase the blood levels of drugs that are substrates of this enzyme).
No products indexed under this heading.

Dextromethorphan Hydrobromide (Imatinib is a potent competitive inhibitor of CYP2D6; therefore, imatinib is likely to increase the blood levels of drugs that are substrates of this enzyme). Products include:
Comtrex Maximum Strength Cold & Cough Day/Night Caplets - Day Formulation 726
Comtrex Maximum Strength Cold & Cough Day/Night Caplets - Night Formulation 726
Comtrex Maximum Strength Non-Drowsy Cold & Cough Caplets 725
Children's Dimetapp DM Cold & Cough Elixir 731
Children's Dimetapp Long Acting Cough Plus Cold Syrup 731
Toddler's Dimetapp Cold and Cough Drops 732
Mucinex DM Extended-Release Bi-Layer Tablets 720
Refenesen DM Caplets 721
Robitussin Cough & Cold CF Liquid 735
Robitussin Cough & Cold Long-Acting Liquid 735
Robitussin Cough & Allergy Syrup .. 736
Robitussin Cough & Cold Nighttime Liquid 736
Robitussin Cough & Cold Pediatric Drops 735
Robitussin Cough, Cold & Flu Nighttime Liquid 738
Robitussin Cough & Congestion Liquid 738
Robitussin Cough Gels Long-Acting 737
Robitussin Cough Long Acting Liquid 739
Robitussin Cough DM Syrup 738
Robitussin Cough DM Infant Drops 738
Robitussin Pediatric Cough Long Acting Liquid 739
Robitussin Pediatric Cough & Cold Long-Acting Liquid 735
Robitussin Pediatric Cough & Cold Nighttime Liquid 736
Robitussin Sugar Free Cough 738
TheraFlu Cold & Cough Hot Liquid 740
TheraFlu Warming Relief Daytime Severe Cold 743
TheraFlu Thin Strips Long Acting Cough 744
Triaminic Daytime Cold & Cough Liquid 745
Triaminic Cough & Sore Throat Liquid 747
Triaminic Cough & Runny Nose Softchews 748
Triaminic Thin Strips Cold & Cough 778
Triaminic Infant Thin Strips Decongestant Plus Cough 747
Children's Tylenol Plus Flu Oral Suspension 749
Tylenol Cold Head Congestion Daytime Caplets with Cool Burst and Gelcaps 750
Tylenol Cold Multi-Symptom Daytime Liquid 752
Tylenol Cold Multi-Symptom Severe Daytime Liquid 752
Concentrated Tylenol Infants' Drops Plus Cold & Cough 754
Children's Tylenol Plus Cough & Runny Nose Suspension Liquid 1879
Children's Tylenol Plus Cough & Sore Throat Suspension Liquid 1879
Children's Tylenol Plus Flu Suspension Liquid 1881
Children's Tylenol Plus Multi-Symptom Cold Suspension Liquid 1879
Tylenol Cold Severe Congestion Non-Drowsy Caplets with Cool Burst 1874
Tylenol Cold Head Congestion Daytime Caplets with Cool Burst 1873
Tylenol Cold Head Congestion Nighttime Caplets with Cool Burst 1873
Tylenol Cold Head Congestion Severe Caplets with Cool Burst 1873
Tylenol Cold Multi-Symptom Daytime Caplets with Cool Burst and Gelcaps 1874
Tylenol Cold Multi-Symptom Daytime Liquid with Citrus Burst 1874
Tylenol Cold Multi-Symptom Nighttime Caplets with Cool Burst 1874
Tylenol Cold Multi-Symptom Nighttime Liquid with Cool Burst 1874
Tylenol Cold Multi-Symptom Severe Caplets with Cool Burst 1874
Tylenol Cold Multi-Symptom Severe Daytime Liquid with Citrus Burst 1874
Tylenol Cough & Sore Throat Daytime Liquid with Cool Burst 1877
Tylenol Cough & Sore Throat Nighttime Liquid with Cool Burst 1877
Concentrated Tylenol Infants' Drops Plus Cold and Cough 1879
Vicks 44 Cough Relief Liquid 2679
Vicks 44D Cough & Head Congestion Relief Liquid 2679
Vicks 44E Cough & Chest Congestion Relief Liquid 2679
Pediatric Vicks 44e Cough & Chest Congestion Relief Liquid 2676
Vicks 44M Cough, Cold & Flu Relief Liquid 2680
Pediatric Vicks 44m Cough & Cold Relief Liquid 2676
Vicks DayQuil LiquiCaps/Liquid Multi-Symptom Cold/Flu Relief 761
Vicks DayQuil Multi-Symptom Cold/Flu Relief LiquiCaps 2678
Vicks DayQuil Multi-Symptom Cold/Flu Relief Liquid 2678
Vicks NyQuil Multi-Symptom Cold/Flu Relief Liquid 2681
Children's Vicks NyQuil Cold/Cough Relief 756
Vicks NyQuil Multi-Symptom Cold/Flu Relief LiquiCaps 2681
Vicks NyQuil LiquiCaps/Liquid Multi-Symptom Cold/Flu Relief 763
Vicks NyQuil Cough Liquid 2680
Children's Vicks NyQuil Cold/Cough Relief Liquid 2680
Zicam Cough Max Nighttime Cough Spray 767
Zicam Cough Max Cough Spray 767
Zicam Cough Max Cough Melts 767
Zicam Cough Plus D Cough Spray 767
Zicam Cough Relief Cough Spray 767
Zicam Maximum Strength Flu Daytime 768
Zicam Maximum Strength Flu Nighttime 768

Dextromethorphan Polistirex (Imatinib is a potent competitive inhibitor of CYP2D6; therefore, imatinib is likely to increase the blood levels of drugs that are substrates of this enzyme). Products include:
Delsym Extended-Release Suspension 12 Hour Cough Suppressant 611

Diazepam (Imatinib is a potent competitive inhibitor of CYP2C9; therefore, imatinib is likely to increase the blood levels of drugs that are substrates of this enzyme). Products include:
Diastat Rectal Delivery System 3343
Valium Tablets 2819

Diclofenac Potassium (Imatinib is a potent competitive inhibitor of CYP2C9; therefore, imatinib is likely to increase the blood levels of drugs that are substrates of this enzyme).
No products indexed under this heading.

Diclofenac Sodium (Imatinib is a potent competitive inhibitor of CYP2C9; therefore, imatinib is likely to increase the blood levels of drugs that are substrates of this enzyme). Products include:
Arthrotec Tablets 3129
Voltaren Ophthalmic Solution 2309
Voltaren Tablets 2307
Voltaren-XR Tablets 2310

Diltiazem Hydrochloride (Caution is recommended when administering Gleevec with inhibitors of the CYP3A4 family. Substances that inhibit CYP3A4 activity may decrease metabolism and increase imatinib concentrations. There is a significant increase in exposure to imatinib when Gleevec is co-administered with ketoconazole). Products include:
Cardizem LA Extended Release Tablets 1728
Tiazac Capsules 1201

Diltiazem Maleate (Caution is recommended when administering Gleevec with inhibitors of the CYP3A4 family. Substances that inhibit CYP3A4 activity may decrease metabolism and increase imatinib concentrations. There is a significant increase in exposure to imatinib when Gleevec is co-administered with ketoconazole).
No products indexed under this heading.

Dolasetron Mesylate (Imatinib is a potent competitive inhibitor of CYP2D6; therefore, imatinib is likely to increase the blood levels of drugs that are substrates of this enzyme). Products include:
Anzemet Injection 2859
Anzemet Tablets 2862

Donepezil Hydrochloride (Imatinib is a potent competitive inhibitor of CYP2D6; therefore, imatinib is likely to increase the blood levels of drugs that are substrates of this enzyme). Products include:
Aricept Tablets 1094
Aricept ODT Tablets 1094

Doxepin Hydrochloride (Imatinib is a potent competitive inhibitor of CYP2D6; therefore, imatinib is likely to increase the blood levels of drugs that are substrates of this enzyme).
No products indexed under this heading.

Doxorubicin Hydrochloride (Substances that are inducers of CYP3A4 activity may increase metabolism and decrease imatinib plasma concentrations. Co-medications that induce CYP3A4 may significantly reduce exposure to Gleevec. Dosage of imatinib should be increased by at least 50% and clinical response should be carefully monitored in patients receiving imatinib with potent CYP3A4 inducers).
No products indexed under this heading.

Dronabinol (Imatinib is a potent competitive inhibitor of CYP2C9; therefore, imatinib is likely to increase the blood levels of drugs that are substrates of this enzyme). Products include:
Marinol Capsules 3333

Efavirenz (Caution is recommended when administering Gleevec with inhibitors of the CYP3A4 family. Substances that inhibit CYP3A4 activity may decrease metabolism and increase imatinib concentrations. There is a significant increase in exposure to imatinib when Gleevec is co-administered with ketoconazole). Products include:
Atripla Tablets 945
Sustiva Capsules 930
Sustiva Tablets 930

Encainide Hydrochloride (Imatinib is a potent competitive inhibitor of CYP2D6; therefore, imatinib is likely to increase the blood levels of drugs that are substrates of this enzyme).
No products indexed under this heading.

Eprosartan Mesylate (Imatinib is a potent competitive inhibitor of CYP2C9; therefore, imatinib is likely to increase the blood levels of drugs that are substrates of this enzyme). Products include:
Teveten Tablets 1735
Teveten HCT Tablets 1737

Erythromycin (Co-administration with CYP3A4 inhibitors, such as erythromycin, may decrease the metabolism and increase imatinib concentrations). Products include:
Ery-Tab Tablets 449
Erythromycin Base Filmtab Tablets 455
Erythromycin Delayed-Release Capsules, USP 457
PCE Dispertab Tablets 515

Erythromycin Estolate (Co-administration with CYP3A4 inhibitors, such as erythromycin, may decrease the metabolism and increase imatinib concentrations).
No products indexed under this heading.

Erythromycin Ethylsuccinate (Co-administration with CYP3A4 inhibitors, such as erythromycin, may decrease the metabolism and increase imatinib concentrations). Products include:

Erythromycin Gluceptate (Co-administration with CYP3A4 inhibitors, such as erythromycin, may decrease the metabolism and increase imatinib concentrations).

No products indexed under this heading.

Erythromycin Lactobionate (Co-administration with CYP3A4 inhibitors, such as erythromycin, may decrease the metabolism and increase imatinib concentrations).

No products indexed under this heading.

Erythromycin Stearate (Co-administration with CYP3A4 inhibitors, such as erythromycin, may decrease the metabolism and increase imatinib concentrations). Products include:

Esomeprazole Magnesium (Caution is recommended when administering Gleevec with inhibitors of the CYP3A4 family. Substances that inhibit CYP3A4 activity may decrease metabolism and increase imatinib concentrations. There is a significant increase in exposure to imatinib when Gleevec is co-administered with ketoconazole). Products include:

Ethosuximide (Substances that are inducers of CYP3A4 activity may increase metabolism and decrease imatinib plasma concentrations. Co-medications that induce CYP3A4 may significantly reduce exposure to Gleevec. Dosage of imatinib should be increased by at least 50% and clinical response should be carefully monitored in patients receiving imatinib with potent CYP3A4 inducers).

No products indexed under this heading.

Etodolac (Imatinib is a potent competitive inhibitor of CYP2C9; therefore, imatinib is likely to increase the blood levels of drugs that are substrates of this enzyme).

No products indexed under this heading.

Felbamate (Substances that are inducers of CYP3A4 activity may increase metabolism and decrease imatinib plasma concentrations. Co-medications that induce CYP3A4 may significantly reduce exposure to Gleevec. Dosage of imatinib should be increased by at least 50% and clinical response should be carefully monitored in patients receiving imatinib with potent CYP3A4 inducers).

No products indexed under this heading.

Felodipine (Imatinib will increase plasma concentration of CYP3A4 metabolized drugs. (e.g., dihydropyridine calcium channel blockers)).

No products indexed under this heading.

Fenoprofen Calcium (Imatinib is a potent competitive inhibitor of CYP2C9; therefore, imatinib is likely to increase the blood levels of drugs that are substrates of this enzyme). Products include:

Fentanyl (Imatinib is a potent competitive inhibitor of CYP2D6; therefore, imatinib is likely to increase the blood levels of drugs that are substrates of this enzyme). Products include:

Fentanyl Citrate (Imatinib is a potent competitive inhibitor of CYP2D6; therefore, imatinib is likely to increase the blood levels of drugs that are substrates of this enzyme). Products include:

Flecainide Acetate (Imatinib is a potent competitive inhibitor of CYP2D6; therefore, imatinib is likely to increase the blood levels of drugs that are substrates of this enzyme). Products include:

Fluconazole (Caution is recommended when administering Gleevec with inhibitors of the CYP3A4 family. Substances that inhibit CYP3A4 activity may decrease metabolism and increase imatinib concentrations. There is a significant increase in exposure to imatinib when Gleevec is co-administered with ketoconazole).

No products indexed under this heading.

Fludrocortisone Acetate (Substances that are inducers of CYP3A4 activity may increase metabolism and decrease imatinib plasma concentrations. Co-medications that induce CYP3A4 may significantly reduce exposure to Gleevec. Dosage of imatinib should be increased by at least 50% and clinical response should be carefully monitored in patients receiving imatinib with potent CYP3A4 inducers).

No products indexed under this heading.

Fluoxetine (Imatinib is a potent competitive inhibitor of CYP2D6; therefore, imatinib is likely to increase the blood levels of drugs that are substrates of this enzyme).

No products indexed under this heading.

Fluoxetine Hydrochloride (Caution is recommended when administering Gleevec with inhibitors of the CYP3A4 family. Substances that inhibit CYP3A4 activity may decrease metabolism and increase imatinib concentrations. There is a significant increase in exposure to imatinib when Gleevec is co-administered with ketoconazole). Products include:

Fluphenazine Decanoate (Imatinib is a potent competitive inhibitor of CYP2D6; therefore, imatinib is likely to increase the blood levels of drugs that are substrates of this enzyme).

No products indexed under this heading.

Fluphenazine Enanthate (Imatinib is a potent competitive inhibitor of CYP2D6; therefore, imatinib is likely to increase the blood levels of drugs that are substrates of this enzyme).

No products indexed under this heading.

Fluphenazine Hydrochloride (Imatinib is a potent competitive inhibitor of CYP2D6; therefore, imatinib is likely to increase the blood levels of drugs that are substrates of this enzyme).

No products indexed under this heading.

Flurbiprofen (Imatinib is a potent competitive inhibitor of CYP2C9; therefore, imatinib is likely to increase the blood levels of drugs that are substrates of this enzyme).

No products indexed under this heading.

Flurbiprofen Sodium (Imatinib is a potent competitive inhibitor of CYP2C9; therefore, imatinib is likely to increase the blood levels of drugs that are substrates of this enzyme). Products include:

Fluvastatin Sodium (Imatinib is a potent competitive inhibitor of CYP2C9; therefore, imatinib is likely to increase the blood levels of drugs that are substrates of this enzyme). Products include:

Fluvoxamine Maleate (Caution is recommended when administering Gleevec with inhibitors of the CYP3A4 family. Substances that inhibit CYP3A4 activity may decrease metabolism and increase imatinib concentrations. There is a significant increase in exposure to imatinib when Gleevec is co-administered with ketoconazole).

No products indexed under this heading.

Formoterol Fumarate (Imatinib is a potent competitive inhibitor of CYP2D6; therefore, imatinib is likely to increase the blood levels of drugs that are substrates of this enzyme). Products include:

Fosamprenavir Calcium (Caution is recommended when administering Gleevec with inhibitors of the CYP3A4 family. Substances that inhibit CYP3A4 activity may decrease metabolism and increase imatinib concentrations. There is a significant increase in exposure to imatinib when Gleevec is co-administered with ketoconazole). Products include:

Fosphenytoin Sodium (Co-administration with inducers of CYP3A4, such as phenytoin, may increase the metabolism and decrease imatinib concentrations. Dosage of imatinib should be increased by at least 50% and clinical response should be carefully monitored in patients receiving imatinib with a potent CYP3A4 inducer such as phenytoin).

No products indexed under this heading.

Galantamine Hydrobromide (Imatinib is a potent competitive inhibitor of CYP2D6; therefore, imatinib is likely to increase the blood levels of drugs that are substrates of this enzyme). Products include:

Garlic Extract (Substances that are inducers of CYP3A4 activity may increase metabolism and decrease imatinib plasma concentrations. Co-medications that induce CYP3A4 may significantly reduce exposure to Gleevec. Dosage of imatinib should be increased by at least 50% and clinical response should be carefully monitored in patients receiving imatinib with potent CYP3A4 inducers).

No products indexed under this heading.

Garlic Oil (Substances that are inducers of CYP3A4 activity may increase metabolism and decrease imatinib plasma concentrations. Co-medications that induce CYP3A4 may significantly reduce exposure to Gleevec. Dosage of imatinib should be increased by at least 50% and clinical response should be carefully monitored in patients receiving imatinib with potent CYP3A4 inducers).

No products indexed under this heading.

Glimepiride (Imatinib is a potent competitive inhibitor of CYP2C9; therefore, imatinib is likely to increase the blood levels of drugs that are substrates of this enzyme). Products include:

Glipizide (Imatinib is a potent competitive inhibitor of CYP2C9; therefore, imatinib is likely to increase the blood levels of drugs that are substrates of this enzyme).

No products indexed under this heading.

Haloperidol (Imatinib is a potent competitive inhibitor of CYP2D6; therefore, imatinib is likely to increase the blood levels of drugs that are substrates of this enzyme).

No products indexed under this heading.

Haloperidol Decanoate (Imatinib is a potent competitive inhibitor of CYP2D6; therefore, imatinib is likely to increase the blood levels of drugs that are substrates of this enzyme).

No products indexed under this heading.

Hydrocodone Bitartrate (Imatinib is a potent competitive inhibitor of CYP2D6; therefore, imatinib is likely to increase the blood levels of drugs that are substrates of this enzyme). Products include:

Hydrocortisone (Substances that are inducers of CYP3A4 activity may increase metabolism and decrease imatinib plasma concentrations. Co-medications that induce CYP3A4 may significantly reduce exposure to Gleevec. Dosage of imatinib should be increased by at least 50% and clinical response should be carefully monitored in patients receiving imatinib with potent CYP3A4 inducers). Products include:

Hydrocortisone Acetate (Substances that are inducers of CYP3A4 activity may increase metabolism and decrease imatinib plasma concentrations. Co-medications that induce CYP3A4 may significantly reduce exposure to Gleevec. Dosage of imatinib should be increased by at least 50% and clinical response should be carefully monitored in patients receiving imatinib with potent CYP3A4 inducers). Products include:

Hydrocortisone Butyrate (Substances that are inducers of CYP3A4 activity may increase metabolism and decrease imatinib plasma concentrations. Co-medications that induce CYP3A4 may significantly reduce exposure to Gleevec. Dosage of imatinib should be increased by at least 50% and clinical response should be carefully monitored in patients receiving imatinib with potent CYP3A4 inducers). Products include:

Hydrocortisone Cypionate (Substances that are inducers of CYP3A4 activity may increase metabolism and decrease imatinib plasma concentrations. Co-medications that induce CYP3A4 may significantly reduce exposure to Gleevec. Dosage of imatinib should be increased by at least 50% and clinical response should be carefully monitored in patients receiving imatinib with potent CYP3A4 inducers).
No products indexed under this heading.

Hydrocortisone Hemisuccinate (Substances that are inducers of CYP3A4 activity may increase metabolism and decrease imatinib plasma concentrations. Co-medications that induce CYP3A4 may significantly reduce exposure to Gleevec. Dosage of imatinib should be increased by at least 50% and clinical response should be carefully monitored in patients receiving imatinib with potent CYP3A4 inducers).
No products indexed under this heading.

Hydrocortisone Probutate (Substances that are inducers of CYP3A4 activity may increase metabolism and decrease imatinib plasma concentrations. Co-medications that induce CYP3A4 may significantly reduce exposure to Gleevec. Dosage of imatinib should be increased by at least 50% and clinical response should be carefully monitored in patients receiving imatinib with potent CYP3A4 inducers).
No products indexed under this heading.

Hydrocortisone Sodium Phosphate (Substances that are inducers of CYP3A4 activity may increase metabolism and decrease imatinib plasma concentrations. Co-medications that induce CYP3A4 may significantly reduce exposure to Gleevec. Dosage of imatinib should be increased by at least 50% and clinical response should be carefully monitored in patients receiving imatinib with potent CYP3A4 inducers).
No products indexed under this heading.

Hydrocortisone Sodium Succinate (Substances that are inducers of CYP3A4 activity may increase metabolism and decrease imatinib plasma concentrations. Co-

medications that induce CYP3A4 may significantly reduce exposure to Gleevec. Dosage of imatinib should be increased by at least 50% and clinical response should be carefully monitored in patients receiving imatinib with potent CYP3A4 inducers).
No products indexed under this heading.

Hydrocortisone Valerate (Substances that are inducers of CYP3A4 activity may increase metabolism and decrease imatinib plasma concentrations. Co-medications that induce CYP3A4 may significantly reduce exposure to Gleevec. Dosage of imatinib should be increased by at least 50% and clinical response should be carefully monitored in patients receiving imatinib with potent CYP3A4 inducers).
No products indexed under this heading.

Hypericum (Co-administration with inducers of CYP3A4, such as St. John's Wort, may increase the metabolism and decrease imatinib concentrations). Products include:

Hypericum Perforatum (Substances that are inducers of CYP3A4 activity may increase metabolism and decrease imatinib plasma concentrations. Co-medications that induce CYP3A4 may significantly reduce exposure to Gleevec. Dosage of imatinib should be increased by at least 50% and clinical response should be carefully monitored in patients receiving imatinib with potent CYP3A4 inducers).
No products indexed under this heading.

Ibuprofen (Imatinib is a potent competitive inhibitor of CYP2C9; therefore, imatinib is likely to increase the blood levels of drugs that are substrates of this enzyme). Products include:

Imipramine Hydrochloride (Imatinib is a potent competitive inhibitor of CYP2D6; therefore, imatinib is likely to increase the blood levels of drugs that are substrates of this enzyme).
No products indexed under this heading.

Imipramine Pamoate (Imatinib is a potent competitive inhibitor of CYP2D6; therefore, imatinib is likely to increase the blood levels of drugs that are substrates of this enzyme).
No products indexed under this heading.

Indinavir Sulfate (Caution is recommended when administering Gleevec with inhibitors of the CYP3A4 family. Substances that inhibit CYP3A4 activity may decrease metabolism and increase imatinib concentrations. There is a significant increase in exposure to imatinib when Gleevec is co-administered with ketoconazole). Products include:

Indomethacin (Imatinib is a potent competitive inhibitor of CYP2C9; therefore, imatinib is likely to increase the blood levels of drugs that are substrates of this enzyme). Products include:

Indomethacin Sodium Trihydrate (Imatinib is a potent competitive inhibitor of CYP2C9; therefore, imatinib is likely to increase the blood levels of drugs that are substrates of this enzyme). Products include:

Indoramin Hydrochloride (Imatinib is a potent competitive inhibitor of CYP2D6; therefore, imatinib is likely to increase the blood levels of drugs that are substrates of this enzyme).
No products indexed under this heading.

Irbesartan (Imatinib is a potent competitive inhibitor of CYP2C9; therefore, imatinib is likely to increase the blood levels of drugs that are substrates of this enzyme). Products include:

Isoniazid (Caution is recommended when administering Gleevec with inhibitors of the CYP3A4 family. Substances that inhibit CYP3A4 activity may decrease metabolism and increase imatinib concentrations. There is a significant increase in exposure to imatinib when Gleevec is co-administered with ketoconazole).
No products indexed under this heading.

Itraconazole (Co-administration with CYP3A4 inhibitors, such as itraconazole, may decrease the metabolism and increase imatinib concentrations).
No products indexed under this heading.

Ketoconazole (Co-administration with inhibitors of CYP3A4, such as ketoconazole, may decrease the metabolism and increase imatinib concentrations; there is a significant increase in exposure to imatinib when co-administered with ketoconazole). Products include:

Ketoprofen (Imatinib is a potent competitive inhibitor of CYP2C9; therefore, imatinib is likely to increase the blood levels of drugs that are substrates of this enzyme).
No products indexed under this heading.

Ketorolac Tromethamine (Imatinib is a potent competitive inhibitor of CYP2C9; therefore, imatinib is likely to increase the blood levels of drugs that are substrates of this enzyme). Products include:

Labetalol Hydrochloride (Imatinib is a potent competitive inhibitor of CYP2D6; therefore, imatinib is likely to increase the blood levels of drugs that are substrates of this enzyme).
No products indexed under this heading.

Lansoprazole (Imatinib is a potent competitive inhibitor of CYP2C9; therefore, imatinib is likely to increase the blood levels of drugs that are substrates of this enzyme). Products include:

Lidocaine (Imatinib is a potent competitive inhibitor of CYP2D6; therefore, imatinib is likely to increase the blood levels of drugs that are substrates of this enzyme). Products include:

Lidocaine Hydrochloride (Imatinib is a potent competitive inhibitor of CYP2D6; therefore, imatinib is likely to increase the blood levels of drugs that are substrates of this enzyme).
No products indexed under this heading.

Lopinavir (Caution is recommended when administering Gleevec with inhibitors of the CYP3A4 family. Substances that inhibit CYP3A4 activity may decrease metabolism and increase imatinib concentrations. There is a significant increase in exposure to imatinib when Gleevec is co-administered with ketoconazole). Products include:

Loratadine (Caution is recommended when administering Gleevec with inhibitors of the CYP3A4 family. Substances that inhibit CYP3A4 activity may decrease metabolism and increase imatinib concentrations. There is a significant increase in exposure to imatinib when Gleevec is co-administered with ketoconazole). Products include:

Losartan Potassium (Imatinib is a potent competitive inhibitor of CYP2C9; therefore, imatinib is likely to increase the blood levels of drugs that are substrates of this enzyme). Products include:

Hyzaar 100-25 Tablets **1990**

Lovastatin (Imatinib will increase the plasma concentrations of certain HMG-CoA reductase inhibitors by inhibiting CYP3A4). Products include:

Advicor Tablets **1722**
Altoprev Extended-Release Tablets **3109**
Mevacor Tablets **2021**

Maprotiline Hydrochloride (Imatinib is a potent competitive inhibitor of CYP2D6; therefore, imatinib is likely to increase the blood levels of drugs that are substrates of this enzyme).

No products indexed under this heading.

Meclofenamate Sodium (Imatinib is a potent competitive inhibitor of CYP2C9; therefore, imatinib is likely to increase the blood levels of drugs that are substrates of this enzyme).

No products indexed under this heading.

Mefenamic Acid (Imatinib is a potent competitive inhibitor of CYP2C9; therefore, imatinib is likely to increase the blood levels of drugs that are substrates of this enzyme).

No products indexed under this heading.

Meloxicam (Imatinib is a potent competitive inhibitor of CYP2C9; therefore, imatinib is likely to increase the blood levels of drugs that are substrates of this enzyme). Products include:

Mobic Oral Suspension **863**
Mobic Tablets **863**

Meperidine Hydrochloride (Imatinib is a potent competitive inhibitor of CYP2D6; therefore, imatinib is likely to increase the blood levels of drugs that are substrates of this enzyme).

No products indexed under this heading.

Mephenytoin (Substances that are inducers of CYP3A4 activity may increase metabolism and decrease imatinib plasma concentrations. Co-medications that induce CYP3A4 may significantly reduce exposure to Gleevec. Dosage of imatinib should be increased by at least 50% and clinical response should be carefully monitored in patients receiving imatinib with potent CYP3A4 inducers).

No products indexed under this heading.

Metformin Hydrochloride (Imatinib is a potent competitive inhibitor of CYP2C9; therefore, imatinib is likely to increase the blood levels of drugs that are substrates of this enzyme). Products include:

ActoPlus Met Tablets **3214**
Avandamet Tablets **1373**
Fortamet Extended-Release Tablets **3115**

Methadone Hydrochloride (Imatinib is a potent competitive inhibitor of CYP2D6; therefore, imatinib is likely to increase the blood levels of drugs that are substrates of this enzyme).

No products indexed under this heading.

Methamphetamine Hydrochloride (Imatinib is a potent competitive inhibitor of CYP2D6; therefore, imatinib is likely to increase the blood levels of drugs that are substrates of this enzyme). Products include:

Desoxyn Tablets, USP **2462**

Methsuximide (Substances that are inducers of CYP3A4 activity may increase metabolism and decrease imatinib plasma concentrations. Co-medications that induce CYP3A4 may significantly reduce exposure to Gleevec. Dosage of imatinib should be increased by at least 50% and clinical response should be carefully monitored in patients receiving imatinib with potent CYP3A4 inducers).

No products indexed under this heading.

Methylprednisolone (Substances that are inducers of CYP3A4 activity may increase metabolism and decrease imatinib plasma concentrations. Co-medications that induce CYP3A4 may significantly reduce exposure to Gleevec. Dosage of imatinib should be increased by at least 50% and clinical response should be carefully monitored in patients receiving imatinib with potent CYP3A4 inducers).

No products indexed under this heading.

Methylprednisolone Acetate (Substances that are inducers of CYP3A4 activity may increase metabolism and decrease imatinib plasma concentrations. Co-medications that induce CYP3A4 may significantly reduce exposure to Gleevec. Dosage of imatinib should be increased by at least 50% and clinical response should be carefully monitored in patients receiving imatinib with potent CYP3A4 inducers). Products include:

Depo-Medrol Injectable Suspension **2617**
Depo-Medrol Single-Dose Vial **2619**

Methylprednisolone Sodium Succinate (Substances that are inducers of CYP3A4 activity may increase metabolism and decrease imatinib plasma concentrations. Co-medications that induce CYP3A4 may significantly reduce exposure to Gleevec. Dosage of imatinib should be increased by at least 50% and clinical response should be carefully monitored in patients receiving imatinib with potent CYP3A4 inducers).

No products indexed under this heading.

Metoprolol Succinate (Imatinib is a potent competitive inhibitor of CYP2D6; therefore, imatinib is likely to increase the blood levels of drugs that are substrates of this enzyme). Products include:

Toprol-XL Tablets **668**

Metoprolol Tartrate (Imatinib is a potent competitive inhibitor of CYP2D6; therefore, imatinib is likely to increase the blood levels of drugs that are substrates of this enzyme). Products include:

Lopressor Injection **2238**
Lopressor Tablets **2238**
Lopressor HCT 50/25 Tablets **2241**
Lopressor HCT 100/25 Tablets **2241**
Lopressor HCT 100/50 Tablets **2241**

Metronidazole (Caution is recommended when administering Gleevec with inhibitors of the CYP3A4 family. Substances that inhibit CYP3A4 activity may decrease metabolism and increase imatinib concentrations. There is a significant increase in exposure to imatinib when Gleevec is co-administered with ketoconazole). Products include:

Metrogel 1% **1211**
MetroGel-Vaginal Gel **1855**
Vandazole Vaginal Gel **3338**

Metronidazole Benzoate (Caution is recommended when administering Gleevec with inhibitors of the CYP3A4 family. Substances that inhibit CYP3A4 activity may decrease metabolism and increase imatinib concentrations. There is a significant increase in exposure to imatinib when Gleevec is co-administered with ketoconazole).

No products indexed under this heading.

Metronidazole Hydrochloride (Caution is recommended when administering Gleevec with inhibitors of the CYP3A4 family. Substances that inhibit CYP3A4 activity may decrease metabolism and increase imatinib concentrations. There is a significant increase in exposure to imatinib when Gleevec is co-administered with ketoconazole).

No products indexed under this heading.

Mexiletine Hydrochloride (Imatinib is a potent competitive inhibitor of CYP2D6; therefore, imatinib is likely to increase the blood levels of drugs that are substrates of this enzyme).

No products indexed under this heading.

Miconazole (Caution is recommended when administering Gleevec with inhibitors of the CYP3A4 family. Substances that inhibit CYP3A4 activity may decrease metabolism and increase imatinib concentrations. There is a significant increase in exposure to imatinib when Gleevec is co-administered with ketoconazole).

No products indexed under this heading.

Miconazole Nitrate (Caution is recommended when administering Gleevec with inhibitors of the CYP3A4 family. Substances that inhibit CYP3A4 activity may decrease metabolism and increase imatinib concentrations. There is a significant increase in exposure to imatinib when Gleevec is co-administered with ketoconazole). Products include:

Desenex .... ▣ **635**
Desenex Jock Itch Spray Powder ... ▣ **635**

Midazolam Hydrochloride (Imatinib will increase the plasma concentrations of triazolobenzodiazepines by inhibiting CYP3A4).

No products indexed under this heading.

Miglitol (Imatinib is a potent competitive inhibitor of CYP2C9; therefore, imatinib is likely to increase the blood levels of drugs that are substrates of this enzyme).

No products indexed under this heading.

Mirtazapine (Imatinib is a potent competitive inhibitor of CYP2D6; therefore, imatinib is likely to increase the blood levels of drugs that are substrates of this enzyme).

No products indexed under this heading.

Modafinil (Substances that are inducers of CYP3A4 activity may increase metabolism and decrease imatinib plasma concentrations. Co-medications that induce CYP3A4 may significantly reduce exposure to Gleevec. Dosage of imatinib should be increased by at least 50% and clinical response should be carefully monitored in patients receiving imatinib with potent CYP3A4 inducers). Products include:

Provigil Tablets **988**

Montelukast Sodium (Imatinib is a potent competitive inhibitor of CYP2C9; therefore, imatinib is likely to increase the blood levels of drugs that are substrates of this enzyme). Products include:

Singulair **2077**

Morphine Sulfate (Imatinib is a potent competitive inhibitor of CYP2D6; therefore, imatinib is likely to increase the blood levels of drugs that are substrates of this enzyme). Products include:

Avinza Capsules **1741**
Kadian Capsules **577**
MS Contin Tablets **2701**

Nabumetone (Imatinib is a potent competitive inhibitor of CYP2C9; therefore, imatinib is likely to increase the blood levels of drugs that are substrates of this enzyme).

No products indexed under this heading.

Naproxen (Imatinib is a potent competitive inhibitor of CYP2C9; therefore, imatinib is likely to increase the blood levels of drugs that are substrates of this enzyme). Products include:

EC-Naprosyn Delayed-Release Tablets **2761**
Naprosyn Suspension **2761**
Naprosyn Tablets **2761**
Prevacid NapraPAC **3280**

Naproxen Sodium (Imatinib is a potent competitive inhibitor of CYP2C9; therefore, imatinib is likely to increase the blood levels of drugs that are substrates of this enzyme). Products include:

Aleve Caplets **742**
Aleve Gelcaps **743**
Aleve Tablets **743**
Aleve Cold & Sinus Caplets **744**
Anaprox Tablets **2761**
Anaprox DS Tablets **2761**

Nateglinide (Imatinib is a potent competitive inhibitor of CYP2C9; therefore, imatinib is likely to increase the blood levels of drugs that are substrates of this enzyme). Products include:

Starlix Tablets **2292**

Nefazodone Hydrochloride (Caution is recommended when administering Gleevec with inhibitors of the CYP3A4 family. Substances that inhibit CYP3A4 activity may decrease metabolism and increase imatinib concentrations. There is a significant increase in exposure to imatinib when Gleevec is co-administered with ketoconazole).

No products indexed under this heading.

Nelfinavir Mesylate (Caution is recommended when administering Gleevec with inhibitors of the CYP3A4 family. Substances that inhibit CYP3A4 activity may decrease metabolism and increase imatinib concentrations. There is a significant increase in exposure to imatinib when Gleevec is co-administered with ketoconazole). Products include:

Viracept **2577**

Nevirapine (Caution is recommended when administering Gleevec with inhibitors of the CYP3A4 family. Substances that inhibit CYP3A4 activity may decrease metabolism and increase imatinib concentrations. There is a significant increase in exposure to imatinib when Gleevec is co-administered with ketoconazole). Products include:

Viramune Oral Suspension 873
Viramune Tablets 873

Niacinamide (Caution is recommended when administering Gleevec with inhibitors of the CYP3A4 family. Substances that inhibit CYP3A4 activity may decrease metabolism and increase imatinib concentrations. There is a significant increase in exposure to imatinib when Gleevec is co-administered with ketoconazole).

No products indexed under this heading.

Nicotinamide (Caution is recommended when administering Gleevec with inhibitors of the CYP3A4 family. Substances that inhibit CYP3A4 activity may decrease metabolism and increase imatinib concentrations. There is a significant increase in exposure to imatinib when Gleevec is co-administered with ketoconazole). Products include:

Nicomide Tablets 1088

Nifedipine (Caution is recommended when administering Gleevec with inhibitors of the CYP3A4 family. Substances that inhibit CYP3A4 activity may decrease metabolism and increase imatinib concentrations. There is a significant increase in exposure to imatinib when Gleevec is co-administered with ketoconazole). Products include:

Adalat CC Tablets 2964

Nisoldipine (Imatinib will increase plasma concentration of CYP3A4 metabolized drugs. (e.g., dihydropyridine calcium channel blockers)). Products include:

Sular Tablets 3122

Norfloxacin (Caution is recommended when administering Gleevec with inhibitors of the CYP3A4 family. Substances that inhibit CYP3A4 activity may decrease metabolism and increase imatinib concentrations. There is a significant increase in exposure to imatinib when Gleevec is co-administered with ketoconazole). Products include:

Noroxin Tablets 2032

Nortriptyline Hydrochloride (Imatinib is a potent competitive inhibitor of CYP2D6; therefore, imatinib is likely to increase the blood levels of drugs that are substrates of this enzyme).

No products indexed under this heading.

Olanzapine (Imatinib is a potent competitive inhibitor of CYP2D6; therefore, imatinib is likely to increase the blood levels of drugs that are substrates of this enzyme). Products include:

Symbyax Capsules 1819
Zyprexa Tablets 1830
Zyprexa IntraMuscular 1830
Zyprexa ZYDIS Orally Disintegrating Tablets 1830

Omeprazole (Caution is recommended when administering Gleevec with inhibitors of the CYP3A4 family. Substances that inhibit CYP3A4 activity may decrease metabolism and increase imatinib concentrations. There is a significant increase in exposure to imatinib when Gleevec is co-administered with ketoconazole). Products include:

Zegerid Capsules 2958
Zegerid Powder for Oral Solution 2958

Ondansetron (Imatinib is a potent competitive inhibitor of CYP2D6; therefore, imatinib is likely to increase the blood levels of drugs that are substrates of this enzyme). Products include:

Zofran ODT Orally Disintegrating Tablets 1639

Ondansetron Hydrochloride (Imatinib is a potent competitive inhibitor of CYP2D6; therefore, imatinib is likely to increase the blood levels of drugs that are substrates of this enzyme). Products include:

Zofran Injection 1634
Zofran 1639

Oxaprozin (Imatinib is a potent competitive inhibitor of CYP2C9; therefore, imatinib is likely to increase the blood levels of drugs that are substrates of this enzyme).

No products indexed under this heading.

Oxcarbazepine (Substances that are inducers of CYP3A4 activity may increase metabolism and decrease imatinib plasma concentrations. Co-medications that induce CYP3A4 may significantly reduce exposure to Gleevec. Dosage of imatinib should be increased by at least 50% and clinical response should be carefully monitored in patients receiving imatinib with potent CYP3A4 inducers). Products include:

Trileptal Tablets 2300
Trileptal Oral Suspension 2300

Oxycodone Hydrochloride (Imatinib is a potent competitive inhibitor of CYP2D6; therefore, imatinib is likely to increase the blood levels of drugs that are substrates of this enzyme). Products include:

OxyContin Tablets 2703
OxyFast Oral Concentrate Solution 2708
OxyIR Capsules 2708
Percocet Tablets 1131
Percodan Tablets 1132

Paclitaxel (Imatinib is a potent competitive inhibitor of CYP2D6; therefore, imatinib is likely to increase the blood levels of drugs that are substrates of this enzyme).

No products indexed under this heading.

Paroxetine Hydrochloride (Caution is recommended when administering Gleevec with inhibitors of the CYP3A4 family. Substances that inhibit CYP3A4 activity may decrease metabolism and increase imatinib concentrations. There is a significant increase in exposure to imatinib when Gleevec is co-administered with ketoconazole). Products include:

Paxil CR Controlled-Release Tablets 1538
Paxil 1530

Phenobarbital (Co-administration with inducers of CYP3A4, such as phenobarbital, may increase the metabolism and decrease imatinib concentrations). Products include:

Donnatal Extentabs 2493

Phenobarbital Sodium (Substances that are inducers of CYP3A4 activity may increase metabolism and decrease imatinib plasma concentrations. Co-medications that induce CYP3A4 may significantly reduce exposure to Gleevec. Dosage of imatinib should be increased by at least 50% and clinical response should be carefully monitored in patients receiving imatinib with potent CYP3A4 inducers).

No products indexed under this heading.

Phenylbutazone (Imatinib is a potent competitive inhibitor of CYP2C9; therefore, imatinib is likely to increase the blood levels of drugs that are substrates of this enzyme).

No products indexed under this heading.

Phenytoin (Co-administration with inducers of CYP3A4, such as phenytoin, may increase the metabolism and decrease imatinib concentrations. Dosage of imatinib should be increased by at least 50% and clinical response should be carefully monitored in patients receiving imatinib with a potent CYP3A4 inducer such as phenytoin).

No products indexed under this heading.

Phenytoin Sodium (Co-administration with inducers of CYP3A4, such as phenytoin, may increase the metabolism and decrease imatinib concentrations. Dosage of imatinib should be increased by at least 50% and clinical response should be carefully monitored in patients receiving imatinib with a potent CYP3A4 inducer such as phenytoin). Products include:

Phenytek Capsules 2160

Pimozide (Particular caution is recommended when administering imatinib with CYP3A4 substrates that have a narrow therapeutic window).

No products indexed under this heading.

Pindolol (Imatinib is a potent competitive inhibitor of CYP2D6; therefore, imatinib is likely to increase the blood levels of drugs that are substrates of this enzyme).

No products indexed under this heading.

Pioglitazone Hydrochloride (Imatinib is a potent competitive inhibitor of CYP2C9; therefore, imatinib is likely to increase the blood levels of drugs that are substrates of this enzyme). Products include:

ActoPlus Met Tablets 3214
Actos Tablets 3219
Duetact Tablets 3226

Piroxicam (Imatinib is a potent competitive inhibitor of CYP2C9; therefore, imatinib is likely to increase the blood levels of drugs that are substrates of this enzyme).

No products indexed under this heading.

Prednisolone Acetate (Substances that are inducers of CYP3A4 activity may increase metabolism and decrease imatinib plasma concentrations. Co-medications that induce CYP3A4 may significantly reduce exposure to Gleevec. Dosage of imatinib should be increased by at least 50% and clinical response should be carefully monitored in patients receiving imatinib with potent CYP3A4 inducers). Products include:

Blephamide Ophthalmic Ointment 568
Blephamide Ophthalmic Suspension 569
Poly-Pred Ophthalmic Suspension .... ⊙ 233
Pred Forte Ophthalmic Suspension .... ⊙ 235
Pred Mild Ophthalmic Suspension .... ⊙ 238
Pred-G Ophthalmic Ointment .... ⊙ 237
Pred-G Ophthalmic Suspension ...... ⊙ 236

Prednisolone Sodium Phosphate (Substances that are inducers of CYP3A4 activity may increase metabolism and decrease imatinib plasma concentrations. Co-medications that induce CYP3A4 may significantly reduce exposure to Gleevec. Dosage of imatinib should be increased by at least 50% and clinical response should be carefully monitored in patients receiving imatinib with potent CYP3A4 inducers).

No products indexed under this heading.

Prednisolone Tebutate (Substances that are inducers of CYP3A4 activity may increase metabolism and decrease imatinib plasma concentrations. Co-medications that induce CYP3A4 may significantly reduce exposure to Gleevec. Dosage of imatinib should be increased by at least 50% and clinical response should be carefully monitored in patients receiving imatinib with potent CYP3A4 inducers).

No products indexed under this heading.

Prednisone (Substances that are inducers of CYP3A4 activity may increase metabolism and decrease imatinib plasma concentrations. Co-medications that induce CYP3A4 may significantly reduce exposure to Gleevec. Dosage of imatinib should be increased by at least 50% and clinical response should be carefully monitored in patients receiving imatinib with potent CYP3A4 inducers).

No products indexed under this heading.

Primidone (Substances that are inducers of CYP3A4 activity may increase metabolism and decrease imatinib plasma concentrations. Co-medications that induce CYP3A4 may significantly reduce exposure to Gleevec. Dosage of imatinib should be increased by at least 50% and clinical response should be carefully monitored in patients receiving imatinib with potent CYP3A4 inducers).

No products indexed under this heading.

Propafenone Hydrochloride (Imatinib is a potent competitive inhibitor of CYP2D6; therefore, imatinib is likely to increase the blood levels of drugs that are substrates of this enzyme). Products include:

Rythmol SR Capsules 2727

Propoxyphene Hydrochloride (Caution is recommended when administering Gleevec with inhibitors of the CYP3A4 family. Substances that inhibit CYP3A4 activity may decrease metabolism and increase imatinib concentrations. There is a significant increase in exposure to imatinib when Gleevec is co-administered with ketoconazole).

No products indexed under this heading.

Propoxyphene Napsylate (Caution is recommended when administering Gleevec with inhibitors of the CYP3A4 family. Substances that inhibit CYP3A4 activity may decrease metabolism and increase imatinib concentrations. There is a significant increase in exposure to imatinib when Gleevec is co-administered with ketoconazole).

No products indexed under this heading.

Propranolol Hydrochloride (Imatinib is a potent competitive inhibitor of CYP2D6; therefore, imatinib is likely to increase the blood levels of drugs that are substrates of this enzyme). Products include:

Inderal LA Long-Acting Capsules 3429
InnoPran XL Capsules 2723

Quetiapine Fumarate (Imatinib is a potent competitive inhibitor of CYP2D6; therefore, imatinib is likely to increase the blood levels of drugs that are substrates of this enzyme). Products include:

Seroquel Tablets 690

Quinidine (Caution is recommended when administering Gleevec with inhibitors of the CYP3A4 family. Substances that inhibit CYP3A4 activity may decrease metabolism and increase imatinib concentrations. There is a significant increase in exposure to imatinib when Gleevec is co-administered with ketoconazole).

No products indexed under this heading.

Quinidine Gluconate (Imatinib is a potent competitive inhibitor of CYP2D6; therefore, imatinib is likely to increase the blood levels of drugs that are substrates of this enzyme).

No products indexed under this heading.

Quinidine Hydrochloride (Caution is recommended when administering Gleevec with inhibitors of the CYP3A4 family. Substances that inhibit CYP3A4 activity may decrease metabolism and increase imatinib concentrations. There is a significant increase in exposure to imatinib when Gleevec is co-administered with ketoconazole).

No products indexed under this heading.

Quinidine Polygalacturonate (Caution is recommended when administering Gleevec with inhibitors of the CYP3A4 family. Substances that inhibit CYP3A4 activity may decrease metabolism and increase imatinib concentrations. There is a significant increase in exposure to imatinib when Gleevec is co-administered with ketoconazole).

No products indexed under this heading.

Quinidine Sulfate (Caution is recommended when administering Gleevec with inhibitors of the CYP3A4 family. Substances that inhibit CYP3A4 activity may decrease metabolism and increase imatinib concentrations. There is a significant increase in exposure to imatinib when Gleevec is co-administered with ketoconazole).

No products indexed under this heading.

Quinine (Caution is recommended when administering Gleevec with inhibitors of the CYP3A4 family. Substances that inhibit CYP3A4 activity may decrease metabolism and increase imatinib concentrations. There is a significant increase in exposure to imatinib when Gleevec is co-administered with ketoconazole).

No products indexed under this heading.

Quinine Sulfate (Caution is recommended when administering Gleevec with inhibitors of the CYP3A4 family. Substances that inhibit CYP3A4 activity may decrease metabolism and increase imatinib concentrations. There is a significant increase in exposure to imatinib when Gleevec is co-administered with ketoconazole).

No products indexed under this heading.

Quinupristin (Caution is recommended when administering Gleevec with inhibitors of the CYP3A4 family. Substances that inhibit CYP3A4 activity may decrease metabolism and increase imatinib concentrations. There is a significant increase in exposure to imatinib when Gleevec is co-administered with ketoconazole).

No products indexed under this heading.

Ranitidine Bismuth Citrate (Caution is recommended when administering Gleevec with inhibitors of the CYP3A4 family. Substances that inhibit CYP3A4 activity may decrease metabolism and increase imatinib concentrations. There is a significant increase in exposure to imatinib when Gleevec is co-administered with ketoconazole).

No products indexed under this heading.

Ranitidine Hydrochloride (Caution is recommended when administering Gleevec with inhibitors of the CYP3A4 family. Substances that inhibit CYP3A4 activity may decrease metabolism and increase imatinib concentrations. There is a significant increase in exposure to imatinib when Gleevec is co-administered with ketoconazole). Products include:

Zantac .. 1624
Zantac Injection 1619
Zantac Injection Pharmacy Bulk Package .. 1622

Repaglinide (Imatinib is a potent competitive inhibitor of CYP2C9; therefore, imatinib is likely to increase the blood levels of drugs that are substrates of this enzyme).

No products indexed under this heading.

Rifabutin (Substances that are inducers of CYP3A4 activity may increase metabolism and decrease imatinib plasma concentrations. Co-medications that induce CYP3A4 may significantly reduce exposure to Gleevec. Dosage of imatinib should be increased by at least 50% and clinical response should be carefully monitored in patients receiving imatinib with potent CYP3A4 inducers).

No products indexed under this heading.

Rifampicin (Substances that are inducers of CYP3A4 activity may increase metabolism and decrease imatinib plasma concentrations. Co-medications that induce CYP3A4 may significantly reduce exposure to Gleevec. Dosage of imatinib should be increased by at least 50% and clinical response should be carefully monitored in patients receiving imatinib with potent CYP3A4 inducers).

No products indexed under this heading.

Rifampin (Co-administration with inducers of CYP3A4, such as rifampin, may increase the metabolism and decrease imatinib concentrations. Dosage of imatinib should be increased by at least 50% and clinical response should be carefully monitored in patients receiving imatinib with a potent CYP3A4 inducer, such as rifampin).

No products indexed under this heading.

Rifapentine (Substances that are inducers of CYP3A4 activity may increase metabolism and decrease imatinib plasma concentrations. Co-medications that induce CYP3A4 may significantly reduce exposure to Gleevec. Dosage of imatinib should be increased by at least 50% and clinical response should be carefully monitored in patients receiving imatinib with potent CYP3A4 inducers).

No products indexed under this heading.

Risperidone (Imatinib is a potent competitive inhibitor of CYP2D6; therefore, imatinib is likely to increase the blood levels of drugs that are substrates of this enzyme). Products include:

Risperdal .. 1676
Risperdal Consta Long-Acting Injection 1682
Risperdal M-Tab Orally Disintegrating Tablets 1676

Ritonavir (Caution is recommended when administering Gleevec with inhibitors of the CYP3A4 family. Substances that inhibit CYP3A4 activity may decrease metabolism and increase imatinib concentrations. There is a significant increase in exposure to imatinib when Gleevec is co-administered with ketoconazole). Products include:

Kaletra .. 476
Norvir .. 503

Rofecoxib (Imatinib is a potent competitive inhibitor of CYP2C9; therefore, imatinib is likely to increase the blood levels of drugs that are substrates of this enzyme).

No products indexed under this heading.

Rosiglitazone Maleate (Imatinib is a potent competitive inhibitor of CYP2C9; therefore, imatinib is likely to increase the blood levels of drugs that are substrates of this enzyme). Products include:

Avandamet Tablets 1373
Avandaryl Tablets 1379
Avandia Tablets 1384

Saquinavir (Caution is recommended when administering Gleevec with inhibitors of the CYP3A4 family. Substances that inhibit CYP3A4 activity may decrease metabolism and increase imatinib concentrations. There is a significant increase in exposure to imatinib when Gleevec is co-administered with ketoconazole).

No products indexed under this heading.

Saquinavir Mesylate (Caution is recommended when administering Gleevec with inhibitors of the CYP3A4 family. Substances that inhibit CYP3A4 activity may decrease metabolism and increase imatinib concentrations. There is a significant increase in exposure to imatinib when Gleevec is co-administered with ketoconazole). Products include:

Invirase ... 2772

Sertraline Hydrochloride (Caution is recommended when administering Gleevec with inhibitors of the CYP3A4 family. Substances that inhibit CYP3A4 activity may decrease metabolism and increase imatinib concentrations. There is a significant increase in exposure to imatinib when Gleevec is co-administered with ketoconazole). Products include:

Zoloft .. 2586

Sildenafil Citrate (Imatinib is a potent competitive inhibitor of CYP2C9; therefore, imatinib is likely to increase the blood levels of drugs that are substrates of this enzyme). Products include:

Revatio Tablets 2557
Viagra Tablets 2573

Simvastatin (Imatinib increases the mean Cmax and AUC of simvastatin 2- and 3.5-fold, respectively by inhibiting CYP3A4). Products include:

Vytorin 10/10 Tablets 2114
Vytorin 10/10 Tablets 3077
Vytorin 10/20 Tablets 2114
Vytorin 10/20 Tablets 3077
Vytorin 10/40 Tablets 2114
Vytorin 10/40 Tablets 3077
Vytorin 10/80 Tablets 2114
Vytorin 10/80 Tablets 3077
Zocor Tablets 2105

Sulfamethoxazole (Imatinib is a potent competitive inhibitor of CYP2C9; therefore, imatinib is likely to increase the blood levels of drugs that are substrates of this enzyme).

No products indexed under this heading.

Sulfinpyrazone (Substances that are inducers of CYP3A4 activity may increase metabolism and decrease imatinib plasma concentrations. Co-medications that induce CYP3A4 may significantly reduce exposure to Gleevec. Dosage of imatinib should be increased by at least 50% and clinical response should be carefully monitored in patients receiving imatinib with potent CYP3A4 inducers).

No products indexed under this heading.

Sulindac (Imatinib is a potent competitive inhibitor of CYP2C9; therefore, imatinib is likely to increase the blood levels of drugs that are substrates of this enzyme). Products include:

Clinoril Tablets 1924

Suprofen (Imatinib is a potent competitive inhibitor of CYP2C9; therefore, imatinib is likely to increase the blood levels of drugs that are substrates of this enzyme).

No products indexed under this heading.

Tamoxifen Citrate (Imatinib is a potent competitive inhibitor of CYP2D6; therefore, imatinib is likely to increase the blood levels of drugs that are substrates of this enzyme). Products include:

Soltamox Oral Solution 3527

Telithromycin (Caution is recommended when administering Gleevec with inhibitors of the CYP3A4 family. Substances that inhibit CYP3A4 activity may decrease metabolism and increase imatinib concentrations. There is a significant increase in exposure to imatinib when Gleevec is co-administered with ketoconazole). Products include:

Ketek Tablets 2903

Telmisartan (Imatinib is a potent competitive inhibitor of CYP2C9; therefore, imatinib is likely to increase the blood levels of drugs that are substrates of this enzyme). Products include:

Micardis Tablets 854
Micardis HCT Tablets 856

Teniposide (Imatinib is a potent competitive inhibitor of CYP2D6; therefore, imatinib is likely to increase the blood levels of drugs that are substrates of this enzyme).

No products indexed under this heading.

Testosterone (Imatinib is a potent competitive inhibitor of CYP2D6; therefore, imatinib is likely to increase the blood levels of drugs that are substrates of this enzyme). Products include:

- AndroGel ... 3329
- Striant Mucoadhesive ... 1007
- Testim 1% Gel ... 695

Testosterone Cypionate (Imatinib is a potent competitive inhibitor of CYP2D6; therefore, imatinib is likely to increase the blood levels of drugs that are substrates of this enzyme).
No products indexed under this heading.

Testosterone Enanthate (Imatinib is a potent competitive inhibitor of CYP2D6; therefore, imatinib is likely to increase the blood levels of drugs that are substrates of this enzyme).
No products indexed under this heading.

Testosterone Propionate (Imatinib is a potent competitive inhibitor of CYP2D6; therefore, imatinib is likely to increase the blood levels of drugs that are substrates of this enzyme).
No products indexed under this heading.

Theophylline (Substances that are inducers of CYP3A4 activity may increase metabolism and decrease imatinib plasma concentrations. Co-medications that induce CYP3A4 may significantly reduce exposure to Gleevec. Dosage of imatinib should be increased by at least 50% and clinical response should be carefully monitored in patients receiving imatinib with potent CYP3A4 inducers).
No products indexed under this heading.

Thioridazine (Imatinib is a potent competitive inhibitor of CYP2D6; therefore, imatinib is likely to increase the blood levels of drugs that are substrates of this enzyme).
No products indexed under this heading.

Thioridazine Hydrochloride (Imatinib is a potent competitive inhibitor of CYP2D6; therefore, imatinib is likely to increase the blood levels of drugs that are substrates of this enzyme). Products include:

- Thioridazine Hydrochloride Tablets ... 2163

Timolol Maleate (Imatinib is a potent competitive inhibitor of CYP2D6; therefore, imatinib is likely to increase the blood levels of drugs that are substrates of this enzyme). Products include:

- Blocadren Tablets ... 1916
- Cosopt Sterile Ophthalmic Solution ... 1931
- Timolide Tablets ... 2086
- Timoptic Sterile Ophthalmic Solution ... 2088
- Timoptic in Ocudose ... 2091
- Timoptic-XE Sterile Ophthalmic Gel Forming Solution ... 2092

Tolazamide (Imatinib is a potent competitive inhibitor of CYP2C9; therefore, imatinib is likely to increase the blood levels of drugs that are substrates of this enzyme).
No products indexed under this heading.

Tolbutamide (Imatinib is a potent competitive inhibitor of CYP2C9; therefore, imatinib is likely to increase the blood levels of drugs that are substrates of this enzyme).
No products indexed under this heading.

Tolbutamide Sodium (Imatinib is a potent competitive inhibitor of CYP2C9; therefore, imatinib is likely to increase the blood levels of drugs that are substrates of this enzyme).
No products indexed under this heading.

Tolmetin Sodium (Imatinib is a potent competitive inhibitor of CYP2C9; therefore, imatinib is likely to increase the blood levels of drugs that are substrates of this enzyme).
No products indexed under this heading.

Tolterodine Tartrate (Imatinib is a potent competitive inhibitor of CYP2D6; therefore, imatinib is likely to increase the blood levels of drugs that are substrates of this enzyme). Products include:

- Detrol Tablets ... 2628
- Detrol LA Capsules ... 2631

Torsemide (Imatinib is a potent competitive inhibitor of CYP2C9; therefore, imatinib is likely to increase the blood levels of drugs that are substrates of this enzyme). Products include:

- Demadex Injection ... 2759
- Demadex Tablets ... 2759

Tramadol Hydrochloride (Imatinib is a potent competitive inhibitor of CYP2D6; therefore, imatinib is likely to increase the blood levels of drugs that are substrates of this enzyme). Products include:

- Ultram ER Tablets ... 2392

Trazodone Hydrochloride (Imatinib is a potent competitive inhibitor of CYP2D6; therefore, imatinib is likely to increase the blood levels of drugs that are substrates of this enzyme).
No products indexed under this heading.

Triamcinolone (Substances that are inducers of CYP3A4 activity may increase metabolism and decrease imatinib plasma concentrations. Co-medications that induce CYP3A4 may significantly reduce exposure to Gleevec. Dosage of imatinib should be increased by at least 50% and clinical response should be carefully monitored in patients receiving imatinib with potent CYP3A4 inducers).
No products indexed under this heading.

Triamcinolone Acetonide (Substances that are inducers of CYP3A4 activity may increase metabolism and decrease imatinib plasma concentrations. Co-medications that induce CYP3A4 may significantly reduce exposure to Gleevec. Dosage of imatinib should be increased by at least 50% and clinical response should be carefully monitored in patients receiving imatinib with potent CYP3A4 inducers). Products include:

- Azmacort Inhalation Aerosol ... 1726
- Nasacort AQ Nasal Spray ... 2922

Triamcinolone Diacetate (Substances that are inducers of CYP3A4 activity may increase metabolism and decrease imatinib plasma concentrations. Co-medications that induce CYP3A4 may significantly reduce exposure to Gleevec. Dosage of imatinib should be increased by at least 50% and clinical response should be carefully monitored in patients receiving imatinib with potent CYP3A4 inducers).
No products indexed under this heading.

Triamcinolone Hexacetonide (Substances that are inducers of CYP3A4 activity may increase metabolism and decrease imatinib plasma concentrations. Co-medications that induce CYP3A4 may significantly reduce exposure to Gleevec. Dosage of imatinib should be increased by at least 50% and clinical response should be carefully monitored in patients receiving imatinib with potent CYP3A4 inducers).
No products indexed under this heading.

Triazolam (Imatinib is a potent competitive inhibitor of CYP2D6; therefore, imatinib is likely to increase the blood levels of drugs that are substrates of this enzyme).
No products indexed under this heading.

Trimipramine Maleate (Imatinib is a potent competitive inhibitor of CYP2D6; therefore, imatinib is likely to increase the blood levels of drugs that are substrates of this enzyme).
No products indexed under this heading.

Troglitazone (Caution is recommended when administering Gleevec with inhibitors of the CYP3A4 family. Substances that inhibit CYP3A4 activity may decrease metabolism and increase imatinib concentrations. There is a significant increase in exposure to imatinib when Gleevec is co-administered with ketoconazole).
No products indexed under this heading.

Troleandomycin (Caution is recommended when administering Gleevec with inhibitors of the CYP3A4 family. Substances that inhibit CYP3A4 activity may decrease metabolism and increase imatinib concentrations. There is a significant increase in exposure to imatinib when Gleevec is co-administered with ketoconazole).
No products indexed under this heading.

Valdecoxib (Imatinib is a potent competitive inhibitor of CYP2C9; therefore, imatinib is likely to increase the blood levels of drugs that are substrates of this enzyme).
No products indexed under this heading.

Valproate Sodium (Caution is recommended when administering Gleevec with inhibitors of the CYP3A4 family. Substances that inhibit CYP3A4 activity may decrease metabolism and increase imatinib concentrations. There is a significant increase in exposure to imatinib when Gleevec is co-administered with ketoconazole). Products include:

- Depacon Injection ... 412

Valsartan (Imatinib is a potent competitive inhibitor of CYP2C9; therefore, imatinib is likely to increase the blood levels of drugs that are substrates of this enzyme). Products include:

- Diovan Tablets ... 2193
- Diovan HCT Tablets ... 2196

Venlafaxine Hydrochloride (Imatinib is a potent competitive inhibitor of CYP2D6; therefore, imatinib is likely to increase the blood levels of drugs that are substrates of this enzyme). Products include:

- Effexor Tablets ... 3411
- Effexor XR Capsules ... 3417

Verapamil Hydrochloride (Caution is recommended when administering Gleevec with inhibitors of the CYP3A4 family. Substances that inhibit CYP3A4 activity may decrease metabolism and increase imatinib concentrations. There is a significant increase in exposure to imatinib when Gleevec is co-administered with ketoconazole). Products include:

- Covera-HS Tablets ... 3139
- Tarka Tablets ... 524
- Verelan PM Extended-Release Capsules, Controlled-Onset ... 3106

Vinblastine Sulfate (Imatinib is a potent competitive inhibitor of CYP2D6; therefore, imatinib is likely to increase the blood levels of drugs that are substrates of this enzyme).
No products indexed under this heading.

Voriconazole (Caution is recommended when administering Gleevec with inhibitors of the CYP3A4 family. Substances that inhibit CYP3A4 activity may decrease metabolism and increase imatinib concentrations. There is a significant increase in exposure to imatinib when Gleevec is co-administered with ketoconazole). Products include:

- VFEND I.V. ... 2564
- VFEND Oral Suspension ... 2564
- VFEND Tablets ... 2564

Warfarin Sodium (Imatinib is a potent competitive inhibitor of CYP2C9; warfarin is metabolized by CYP2C9; therefore, patients who require anticoagulation should receive low-molecular weight or standard heparin). Products include:

- Coumadin for Injection ... 898
- Coumadin Tablets ... 898

Zafirlukast (Caution is recommended when administering Gleevec with inhibitors of the CYP3A4 family. Substances that inhibit CYP3A4 activity may decrease metabolism and increase imatinib concentrations. There is a significant increase in exposure to imatinib when Gleevec is co-administered with ketoconazole). Products include:

- Accolate Tablets ... 671

Zileuton (Caution is recommended when administering Gleevec with inhibitors of the CYP3A4 family. Substances that inhibit CYP3A4 activity may decrease metabolism and increase imatinib concentrations. There is a significant increase in exposure to imatinib when Gleevec is co-administered with ketoconazole). Products include:

- Zyflo Tablets ... 1023

Zonisamide (Imatinib is a potent competitive inhibitor of CYP2D6; therefore, imatinib is likely to increase the blood levels of drugs that are substrates of this enzyme). Products include:

- Zonegran Capsules ... 1101

Food Interactions

Grapefruit (Caution is recommended when administering Gleevec with inhibitors of the CYP3A4 family. Substances that inhibit CYP3A4 activity may decrease metabolism and increase imatinib concentrations. There is a significant increase in exposure to imatinib when Gleevec is co-administered with ketoconazole).

Grapefruit Juice (Caution is recommended when administering Gleevec with inhibitors of the CYP3A4 family. Substances that inhibit CYP3A4 activity

may decrease metabolism and increase imatinib concentrations. There is a significant increase in exposure to imatinib when Gleevec is co-administered with ketoconazole).

GLUCAGEN
(Glucagon) 761
May interact with beta blockers. Compounds in these categories include:

Acebutolol Hydrochloride (Patients taking beta blockers might be expected to have a greater increase in both pulse and blood pressure).
No products indexed under this heading.

Atenolol (Patients taking beta blockers might be expected to have a greater increase in both pulse and blood pressure).
No products indexed under this heading.

Betaxolol Hydrochloride (Patients taking beta blockers might be expected to have a greater increase in both pulse and blood pressure). Products include:
Betoptic S Ophthalmic Suspension 558

Bisoprolol Fumarate (Patients taking beta blockers might be expected to have a greater increase in both pulse and blood pressure).
No products indexed under this heading.

Carteolol Hydrochloride (Patients taking beta blockers might be expected to have a greater increase in both pulse and blood pressure). Products include:
Carteolol Hydrochloride Ophthalmic Solution USP, 1%...... ⊙249

Esmolol Hydrochloride (Patients taking beta blockers might be expected to have a greater increase in both pulse and blood pressure).
No products indexed under this heading.

Labetalol Hydrochloride (Patients taking beta blockers might be expected to have a greater increase in both pulse and blood pressure).
No products indexed under this heading.

Levobunolol Hydrochloride (Patients taking beta blockers might be expected to have a greater increase in both pulse and blood pressure). Products include:
Betagan Ophthalmic Solution, USP .... ⊙220

Metipranolol Hydrochloride (Patients taking beta blockers might be expected to have a greater increase in both pulse and blood pressure).
No products indexed under this heading.

Metoprolol Succinate (Patients taking beta blockers might be expected to have a greater increase in both pulse and blood pressure). Products include:
Toprol-XL Tablets 668

Metoprolol Tartrate (Patients taking beta blockers might be expected to have a greater increase in both pulse and blood pressure). Products include:
Lopressor Injection 2238
Lopressor Tablets 2238
Lopressor HCT 50/25 Tablets 2241
Lopressor HCT 100/25 Tablets 2241
Lopressor HCT 100/50 Tablets 2241

Nadolol (Patients taking beta blockers might be expected to have a greater increase in both pulse and blood pressure). Products include:
Nadolol Tablets 2159

Penbutolol Sulfate (Patients taking beta blockers might be expected to have a greater increase in both pulse and blood pressure).
No products indexed under this heading.

Pindolol (Patients taking beta blockers might be expected to have a greater increase in both pulse and blood pressure).
No products indexed under this heading.

Propranolol Hydrochloride (Patients taking beta blockers might be expected to have a greater increase in both pulse and blood pressure). Products include:
Inderal LA Long-Acting Capsules 3429
InnoPran XL Capsules 2723

Sotalol Hydrochloride (Patients taking beta blockers might be expected to have a greater increase in both pulse and blood pressure).
No products indexed under this heading.

Timolol Hemihydrate (Patients taking beta blockers might be expected to have a greater increase in both pulse and blood pressure). Products include:
Betimol Ophthalmic Solution 3382
Betimol Ophthalmic Solution .... ⊙295

Timolol Maleate (Patients taking beta blockers might be expected to have a greater increase in both pulse and blood pressure). Products include:
Blocadren Tablets 1916
Cosopt Sterile Ophthalmic Solution.. 1931
Timolide Tablets 2086
Timoptic Sterile Ophthalmic Solution.. 2088
Timoptic in Ocudose 2091
Timoptic-XE Sterile Ophthalmic Gel Forming Solution.................. 2092

GLUCAGON FOR INJECTION VIALS AND EMERGENCY KIT
(Glucagon) 1778
None cited in PDR database.

GLY-OXIDE LIQUID
(Carbamide Peroxide) .... ▣709
None cited in PDR database.

GOODY'S BODY PAIN FORMULA POWDER
(Acetaminophen, Aspirin) .... ▣684
See Goody's Extra Strength Pain Relief Tablets

GOODY'S EXTRA STRENGTH HEADACHE POWDERS
(Acetaminophen, Aspirin, Caffeine)... ▣611
See Goody's Extra Strength Pain Relief Tablets

GOODY'S EXTRA STRENGTH PAIN RELIEF TABLETS
(Acetaminophen, Aspirin, Caffeine)... ▣685
May interact with oral anticoagulants, oral hypoglycemic agents, and certain other agents. Compounds in these categories include:

Acarbose (Concurrent use should be avoided unless directed by a physician). Products include:
Precose Tablets 751

Anisindione (Concurrent use should be avoided unless directed by a physician). Products include:
Miradon Tablets 3042

Chlorpropamide (Concurrent use should be avoided unless directed by a physician).
No products indexed under this heading.

Dicumarol (Concurrent use should be avoided unless directed by a physician).
No products indexed under this heading.

Glimepiride (Concurrent use should be avoided unless directed by a physician). Products include:
Avandaryl Tablets 1379
Duetact Tablets 3226

Glipizide (Concurrent use should be avoided unless directed by a physician).
No products indexed under this heading.

Glyburide (Concurrent use should be avoided unless directed by a physician).
No products indexed under this heading.

Metformin Hydrochloride (Concurrent use should be avoided unless directed by a physician). Products include:
ActoPlus Met Tablets 3214
Avandamet Tablets 1373
Fortamet Extended-Release Tablets 3115

Miglitol (Concurrent use should be avoided unless directed by a physician).
No products indexed under this heading.

Pioglitazone Hydrochloride (Concurrent use should be avoided unless directed by a physician). Products include:
ActoPlus Met Tablets 3214
Actos Tablets 3219
Duetact Tablets 3226

Repaglinide (Concurrent use should be avoided unless directed by a physician).
No products indexed under this heading.

Rosiglitazone Maleate (Concurrent use should be avoided unless directed by a physician). Products include:
Avandamet Tablets 1373
Avandaryl Tablets 1379
Avandia Tablets 1384

Tolazamide (Concurrent use should be avoided unless directed by a physician).
No products indexed under this heading.

Tolbutamide (Concurrent use should be avoided unless directed by a physician).
No products indexed under this heading.

Troglitazone (Concurrent use should be avoided unless directed by a physician).
No products indexed under this heading.

Warfarin Sodium (Concurrent use should be avoided unless directed by a physician). Products include:
Coumadin for Injection 898
Coumadin Tablets 898

Food Interactions

Alcohol (Individuals consuming 3 or more alcohol-containing drinks per day should consult their physicians for advice on when and how they should take this product).

GOODY'S PM POWDER FOR PAIN WITH SLEEPLESSNESS
(Acetaminophen, Diphenhydramine Citrate)................. ▣612
May interact with hypnotics and sedatives, tranquilizers, and certain other agents. Compounds in these categories include:

Alprazolam (Concurrent use is not recommended). Products include:
Niravam Orally Disintegrating Tablets 3092

Buspirone Hydrochloride (Concurrent use is not recommended).
No products indexed under this heading.

Chlordiazepoxide (Concurrent use is not recommended).
No products indexed under this heading.

Chlordiazepoxide Hydrochloride (Concurrent use is not recommended). Products include:
Librium Capsules 3347

Chlorpromazine (Concurrent use is not recommended).
No products indexed under this heading.

Chlorpromazine Hydrochloride (Concurrent use is not recommended).
No products indexed under this heading.

Chlorprothixene (Concurrent use is not recommended).
No products indexed under this heading.

Chlorprothixene Hydrochloride (Concurrent use is not recommended).
No products indexed under this heading.

Clorazepate Dipotassium (Concurrent use is not recommended). Products include:
Tranxene 2474

Diazepam (Concurrent use is not recommended). Products include:
Diastat Rectal Delivery System 3343
Valium Tablets 2819

Diphenhydramine (Concurrent use with other diphenhydramine-containing products is not recommended). Products include:
Tylenol Sore Throat Nighttime Liquid with Cool Burst.................. 1877

Diphenhydramine Hydrochloride (Concurrent use with any other product containing diphenhydramine, including topical preparations, should be avoided). Products include:
Nytol QuickCaps Caplets .... ▣615
Nytol QuickGels Softgels Maximum Strength........................ ▣616
Simply Sleep Caplets 1868
Sominex Original Formula Tablets .. ▣616
TheraFlu Warming Relief Nighttime Severe Cold .... ▣743
TheraFlu Thin Strips Multi Symptom... ▣744
Triaminic Nighttime Cold & Cough Liquid.............................. ▣746
Triaminic Thin Strips Cough & Runny Nose .... ▣749
Extra Strength Tylenol PM Caplets, Vanilla Caplets, Geltabs, Gelcaps and Liquid........... 1875

Tylenol Sore Throat Nighttime Liquid with Cool Burst 790
Tylenol Allergy Multi-Symptom Nighttime Caplets with Cool Burst 1872
Tylenol Severe Allergy Caplets 1872
Children's Tylenol Plus Cold & Allergy Suspension Liquid 1878

Droperidol (Concurrent use is not recommended).
No products indexed under this heading.

Estazolam (Concurrent use is not recommended). Products include:
ProSom Tablets 517

Ethchlorvynol (Concurrent use is not recommended).
No products indexed under this heading.

Ethinamate (Concurrent use is not recommended).
No products indexed under this heading.

Fluphenazine Decanoate (Concurrent use is not recommended).
No products indexed under this heading.

Fluphenazine Enanthate (Concurrent use is not recommended).
No products indexed under this heading.

Fluphenazine Hydrochloride (Concurrent use is not recommended).
No products indexed under this heading.

Flurazepam Hydrochloride (Concurrent use is not recommended). Products include:
Dalmane Capsules 3342

Glutethimide (Concurrent use is not recommended).
No products indexed under this heading.

Haloperidol (Concurrent use is not recommended).
No products indexed under this heading.

Haloperidol Decanoate (Concurrent use is not recommended).
No products indexed under this heading.

Hydroxyzine Hydrochloride (Concurrent use is not recommended).
No products indexed under this heading.

Lorazepam (Concurrent use is not recommended).
No products indexed under this heading.

Loxapine Hydrochloride (Concurrent use is not recommended).
No products indexed under this heading.

Loxapine Succinate (Concurrent use is not recommended).
No products indexed under this heading.

Meprobamate (Concurrent use is not recommended).
No products indexed under this heading.

Mesoridazine Besylate (Concurrent use is not recommended).
No products indexed under this heading.

Midazolam Hydrochloride (Concurrent use is not recommended).
No products indexed under this heading.

Molindone Hydrochloride (Concurrent use is not recommended). Products include:
Moban Tablets 1119

Oxazepam (Concurrent use is not recommended).
No products indexed under this heading.

Perphenazine (Concurrent use is not recommended).
No products indexed under this heading.

Prazepam (Concurrent use is not recommended).
No products indexed under this heading.

Prochlorperazine (Concurrent use is not recommended).
No products indexed under this heading.

Promethazine Hydrochloride (Concurrent use is not recommended). Products include:
Phenergan Tablets and Suppositories 3440

Propofol (Concurrent use is not recommended).
No products indexed under this heading.

Quazepam (Concurrent use is not recommended).
No products indexed under this heading.

Ramelteon (Concurrent use is not recommended). Products include:
Rozerem Tablets 3231

Secobarbital Sodium (Concurrent use is not recommended).
No products indexed under this heading.

Temazepam (Concurrent use is not recommended). Products include:
Restoril Capsules 1860

Thioridazine Hydrochloride (Concurrent use is not recommended). Products include:
Thioridazine Hydrochloride Tablets 2163

Thiothixene (Concurrent use is not recommended). Products include:
Thiothixene Capsules 2165

Triazolam (Concurrent use is not recommended).
No products indexed under this heading.

Trifluoperazine Hydrochloride (Concurrent use is not recommended).
No products indexed under this heading.

Zaleplon (Concurrent use is not recommended). Products include:
Sonata Capsules 1717

Zolpidem Tartrate (Concurrent use is not recommended). Products include:
Ambien Tablets 2851
Ambien CR Tablets 2855

Food Interactions

Alcohol (Individuals consuming 3 or more alcohol-containing drinks per day should consult their physicians for advice on when and how they should take this product; avoid alcoholic beverages since diphenhydramine causes drowsiness).

GORDOCHOM SOLUTION

(Chloroxylenol, Undecylenic Acid) 1650
None cited in PDR database.

GRIS-PEG TABLETS

(Griseofulvin) 2502
May interact with barbiturates, oral contraceptives, and certain other agents. Compounds in these categories include:

Aprobarbital (Barbiturates usually depress griseofulvin activity and co-administration requires a dosage adjustment of the antifungal agent).
No products indexed under this heading.

Butabarbital (Barbiturates usually depress griseofulvin activity and co-administration requires a dosage adjustment of the antifungal agent).
No products indexed under this heading.

Butalbital (Barbiturates usually depress griseofulvin activity and co-administration requires a dosage adjustment of the antifungal agent).
No products indexed under this heading.

Desogestrel (There have been reports in the literature of possible interactions between griseofulvin and oral contraceptives). Products include:
Mircette Tablets 1066

Ethinyl Estradiol (There have been reports in the literature of possible interactions between griseofulvin and oral contraceptives). Products include:
Mircette Tablets 1066
NuvaRing 2340
Ortho-Cyclen/Ortho Tri-Cyclen 2429
Ortho Evra Transdermal System 2417
Ortho Tri-Cyclen Lo Tablets 2436
Seasonique Tablets 1077
Yasmin 28 Tablets 796
Yaz Tablets 803

Ethynodiol Diacetate (There have been reports in the literature of possible interactions between griseofulvin and oral contraceptives).
No products indexed under this heading.

Levonorgestrel (There have been reports in the literature of possible interactions between griseofulvin and oral contraceptives). Products include:
Climara Pro Transdermal System 776
Mirena Intrauterine System 787
Plan B Tablets 1076
Seasonique Tablets 1077

Mephobarbital (Barbiturates usually depress griseofulvin activity and co-administration requires a dosage adjustment of the antifungal agent).
No products indexed under this heading.

Mestranol (There have been reports in the literature of possible interactions between griseofulvin and oral contraceptives).
No products indexed under this heading.

Norethindrone (There have been reports in the literature of possible interactions between griseofulvin and oral contraceptives). Products include:
Ortho Micronor Tablets 2426

Norethynodrel (There have been reports in the literature of possible interactions between griseofulvin and oral contraceptives).
No products indexed under this heading.

Norgestimate (There have been reports in the literature of possible interactions between griseofulvin and oral contraceptives). Products include:
Ortho-Cyclen/Ortho Tri-Cyclen 2429
Ortho Tri-Cyclen Lo Tablets 2436

Norgestrel (There have been reports in the literature of possible interactions between griseofulvin and oral contraceptives).
No products indexed under this heading.

Pentobarbital Sodium (Barbiturates usually depress griseofulvin activity and co-administration requires a dosage adjustment of the antifungal agent). Products include:
Nembutal Sodium Solution, USP 2470

Phenobarbital (Barbiturates usually depress griseofulvin activity and co-administration requires a dosage adjustment of the antifungal agent). Products include:
Donnatal Extentabs 2493

Secobarbital Sodium (Barbiturates usually depress griseofulvin activity and co-administration requires a dosage adjustment of the antifungal agent).
No products indexed under this heading.

Thiamylal Sodium (Barbiturates usually depress griseofulvin activity and co-administration requires a dosage adjustment of the antifungal agent).
No products indexed under this heading.

Warfarin Sodium (Griseofulvin decreases the activity of warfarin-type anticoagulants). Products include:
Coumadin for Injection 898
Coumadin Tablets 898

Food Interactions

Alcohol (The effects of alcohol may be potentiated by griseofulvin, producing such effects as tachycardia and flushing).

GUANIDINE HYDROCHLORIDE TABLETS

(Guanidine Hydrochloride) 3016
None cited in PDR database.

HALFLYTELY AND BISACODYL TABLETS BOWEL PREP KIT WITH FLAVORS PACKS

(Bisacodyl, Polyethylene Glycol, Potassium Chloride, Sodium Bicarbonate, Sodium Chloride)............ 881
May interact with antacids and certain other agents. Compounds in these categories include:

Aluminum Carbonate (Bisacodyl tablets should not be taken within one hour of taking an antacid).
No products indexed under this heading.

Aluminum Hydroxide (Bisacodyl tablets should not be taken within one hour of taking an antacid). Products include:
Gaviscon Regular Strength Liquid .. 658
Gaviscon Regular Strength Tablets.. 658
Gaviscon Extra Strength Liquid 658
Gaviscon Extra Strength Tablets 658
Maalox Regular Strength Antacid/Antigas Liquid................. 2175
Maalox Max Maximum Strength Antacid/Anti-Gas Liquid................ 2176

Magaldrate (Bisacodyl tablets should not be taken within one hour of taking an antacid).
No products indexed under this heading.

Magnesium Hydroxide (Bisacodyl tablets should not be taken within one hour of taking an antacid). Products include:
- Maalox Regular Strength Antacid/Antigas Liquid 2175
- Maalox Max Maximum Strength Antacid/Anti-Gas Liquid 2176
- Pepcid Complete Chewable Tablets 1701

Magnesium Oxide (Bisacodyl tablets should not be taken within one hour of taking an antacid). Products include:
- Beelith Tablets 759
- PremCal Light, Regular, and Extra Strength Tablets .... ▣818

Oral Medications, unspecified (Oral medication administered within one hour of the start of administration of the solution may be flushed from the gastrointestinal tract and not absorbed).
No products indexed under this heading.

HAVRIX VACCINE

(Hepatitis A Vaccine, Inactivated) 1456
May interact with anticoagulants. Compounds in these categories include:

Anisindione (Havrix should be given with caution to individuals on anticoagulant therapy). Products include:
- Miradon Tablets 3042

Ardeparin Sodium (Havrix should be given with caution to individuals on anticoagulant therapy).
No products indexed under this heading.

Dalteparin Sodium (Havrix should be given with caution to individuals on anticoagulant therapy). Products include:
- Fragmin Injection 1097

Danaparoid Sodium (Havrix should be given with caution to individuals on anticoagulant therapy).
No products indexed under this heading.

Dicumarol (Havrix should be given with caution to individuals on anticoagulant therapy).
No products indexed under this heading.

Enoxaparin Sodium (Havrix should be given with caution to individuals on anticoagulant therapy). Products include:
- Lovenox Injection 2915

Fondaparinux Sodium (Havrix should be given with caution to individuals on anticoagulant therapy). Products include:
- Arixtra Injection 1351

Heparin Calcium (Havrix should be given with caution to individuals on anticoagulant therapy).
No products indexed under this heading.

Heparin Sodium (Havrix should be given with caution to individuals on anticoagulant therapy).
No products indexed under this heading.

Low Molecular Weight Heparins (Havrix should be given with caution to individuals on anticoagulant therapy).
No products indexed under this heading.

Tinzaparin Sodium (Havrix should be given with caution to individuals on anticoagulant therapy).
No products indexed under this heading.

Warfarin Sodium (Havrix should be given with caution to individuals on anticoagulant therapy). Products include:
- Coumadin for Injection 898
- Coumadin Tablets 898

HEAD & SHOULDERS INTENSIVE SOLUTIONS DANDRUFF SHAMPOO

(Pyrithione Zinc) 2674
None cited in PDR database.

HECTOROL CAPSULES

(Doxercalciferol) 1275
May interact with cytochrome p450 3a4 inhibitors (selected), phenytoin, and certain other agents. Compounds in these categories include:

Acetazolamide (Cytochrome P450 inhibitors may inhibit the 25-hydroxylation of doxercalciferol. Hence, formation of the active doxercalciferol moiety may be hindered).
No products indexed under this heading.

Amiodarone Hydrochloride (Cytochrome P450 inhibitors may inhibit the 25-hydroxylation of doxercalciferol. Hence, formation of the active doxercalciferol moiety may be hindered).
No products indexed under this heading.

Amprenavir (Cytochrome P450 inhibitors may inhibit the 25-hydroxylation of doxercalciferol. Hence, formation of the active doxercalciferol moiety may be hindered). Products include:
- Agenerase Capsules 1327
- Agenerase Oral Solution 1332

Anastrozole (Cytochrome P450 inhibitors may inhibit the 25-hydroxylation of doxercalciferol. Hence, formation of the active doxercalciferol moiety may be hindered). Products include:
- Arimidex Tablets 673

Aprepitant (Cytochrome P450 inhibitors may inhibit the 25-hydroxylation of doxercalciferol. Hence, formation of the active doxercalciferol moiety may be hindered). Products include:
- Emend Capsules 1963

Cholestyramine (Reduces the intestinal absorption of fat-soluble vitamins; therefore, it may impair absorption of doxercalciferol).
No products indexed under this heading.

Cimetidine (Cytochrome P450 inhibitors may inhibit the 25-hydroxylation of doxercalciferol. Hence, formation of the active doxercalciferol moiety may be hindered). Products include:
- Tagamet HB 200 Tablets .... ▣664

Cimetidine Hydrochloride (Cytochrome P450 inhibitors may inhibit the 25-hydroxylation of doxercalciferol. Hence, formation of the active doxercalciferol moiety may be hindered).
No products indexed under this heading.

Ciprofloxacin (Cytochrome P450 inhibitors may inhibit the 25-hydroxylation of doxercalciferol. Hence, formation of the active doxercalciferol moiety may be hindered). Products include:
- Cipro Oral Suspension 2977
- Cipro I.V. 2984
- Cipro XR Tablets 2990
- Ciprodex Otic Suspension 559

Clarithromycin (Cytochrome P450 inhibitors may inhibit the 25-hydroxylation of doxercalciferol. Hence, formation of the active doxercalciferol moiety may be hindered). Products include:
- Biaxin/Biaxin XL 402
- PREVPAC 3284

Clotrimazole (Cytochrome P450 inhibitors may inhibit the 25-hydroxylation of doxercalciferol. Hence, formation of the active doxercalciferol moiety may be hindered). Products include:
- Desenex Athlete's Foot Cream .... ▣635
- Lotrimin 3039
- Lotrisone 3040

Cyclosporine (Cytochrome P450 inhibitors may inhibit the 25-hydroxylation of doxercalciferol. Hence, formation of the active doxercalciferol moiety may be hindered). Products include:
- Gengraf Capsules 459
- Neoral Oral Solution 2259
- Neoral Soft Gelatin Capsules 2259
- Restasis Ophthalmic Emulsion 575
- Sandimmune 2275

Dalfopristin (Cytochrome P450 inhibitors may inhibit the 25-hydroxylation of doxercalciferol. Hence, formation of the active doxercalciferol moiety may be hindered).
No products indexed under this heading.

Danazol (Cytochrome P450 inhibitors may inhibit the 25-hydroxylation of doxercalciferol. Hence, formation of the active doxercalciferol moiety may be hindered).
No products indexed under this heading.

Delavirdine Mesylate (Cytochrome P450 inhibitors may inhibit the 25-hydroxylation of doxercalciferol. Hence, formation of the active doxercalciferol moiety may be hindered). Products include:
- Rescriptor Tablets 2551

Diltiazem Hydrochloride (Cytochrome P450 inhibitors may inhibit the 25-hydroxylation of doxercalciferol. Hence, formation of the active doxercalciferol moiety may be hindered). Products include:
- Cardizem LA Extended Release Tablets 1728
- Tiazac Capsules 1201

Diltiazem Maleate (Cytochrome P450 inhibitors may inhibit the 25-hydroxylation of doxercalciferol. Hence, formation of the active doxercalciferol moiety may be hindered).
No products indexed under this heading.

Efavirenz (Cytochrome P450 inhibitors may inhibit the 25-hydroxylation of doxercalciferol. Hence, formation of the active doxercalciferol moiety may be hindered). Products include:
- Atripla Tablets 945
- Sustiva Capsules 930
- Sustiva Tablets 930

Erythromycin (Cytochrome P450 inhibitors may inhibit the 25-hydroxylation of doxercalciferol. Hence, formation of the active doxercalciferol moiety may be hindered). Products include:
- Ery-Tab Tablets 449
- Erythromycin Base Filmtab Tablets 455
- Erythromycin Delayed-Release Capsules, USP 457
- PCE Dispertab Tablets 515

Erythromycin Estolate (Cytochrome P450 inhibitors may inhibit the 25-hydroxylation of doxercalciferol. Hence, formation of the active doxercalciferol moiety may be hindered).
No products indexed under this heading.

Erythromycin Ethylsuccinate (Cytochrome P450 inhibitors may inhibit the 25-hydroxylation of doxercalciferol. Hence, formation of the active doxercalciferol moiety may be hindered). Products include:
- E.E.S. 451
- EryPed 447

Erythromycin Gluceptate (Cytochrome P450 inhibitors may inhibit the 25-hydroxylation of doxercalciferol. Hence, formation of the active doxercalciferol moiety may be hindered).
No products indexed under this heading.

Erythromycin Lactobionate (Cytochrome P450 inhibitors may inhibit the 25-hydroxylation of doxercalciferol. Hence, formation of the active doxercalciferol moiety may be hindered).
No products indexed under this heading.

Erythromycin Stearate (Cytochrome P450 inhibitors may inhibit the 25-hydroxylation of doxercalciferol. Hence, formation of the active doxercalciferol moiety may be hindered). Products include:
- Erythrocin Stearate Filmtab Tablets 453

Esomeprazole Magnesium (Cytochrome P450 inhibitors may inhibit the 25-hydroxylation of doxercalciferol. Hence, formation of the active doxercalciferol moiety may be hindered). Products include:
- Nexium Delayed-Release Capsules 655

Fluconazole (Cytochrome P450 inhibitors may inhibit the 25-hydroxylation of doxercalciferol. Hence, formation of the active doxercalciferol moiety may be hindered).
No products indexed under this heading.

Fluoxetine Hydrochloride (Cytochrome P450 inhibitors may inhibit the 25-hydroxylation of doxercalciferol. Hence, formation of the active doxercalciferol moiety may be hindered). Products include:
- Prozac Pulvules and Liquid 1801
- Symbyax Capsules 1819

Fluvoxamine Maleate (Cytochrome P450 inhibitors may inhibit the 25-hydroxylation of doxercalciferol. Hence, formation of the active doxercalciferol moiety may be hindered).
No products indexed under this heading.

Fosamprenavir Calcium (Cytochrome P450 inhibitors may inhibit the 25-hydroxylation of doxercalciferol. Hence, formation of the active doxercalciferol moiety may be hindered). Products include:
- Lexiva Tablets 1505

Fosphenytoin Sodium (Coadministration with enzyme inhibitors, such as phenytoin, may affect the 25-hydroxylation of Hectorol and may necessitate dosage adjustment).
No products indexed under this heading.

Glutethimide (Co-administration with enzyme inducers, such as glutethimide, may affect the 25-hydroxylation of Hectorol and may necessitate dosage adjustment).
No products indexed under this heading.

Indinavir Sulfate (Cytochrome P450 inhibitors may inhibit the 25-hydroxylation of doxercalciferol. Hence, formation of the active doxercalciferol moiety may be hindered). Products include:
Crixivan Capsules 1940

Isoniazid (Cytochrome P450 inhibitors may inhibit the 25-hydroxylation of doxercalciferol. Hence, formation of the active doxercalciferol moiety may be hindered).
No products indexed under this heading.

Itraconazole (Cytochrome P450 inhibitors may inhibit the 25-hydroxylation of doxercalciferol. Hence, formation of the active doxercalciferol moiety may be hindered).
No products indexed under this heading.

Ketoconazole (Cytochrome P450 inhibitors may inhibit the 25-hydroxylation of doxercalciferol. Hence, formation of the active doxercalciferol moiety may be hindered). Products include:
Nizoral A-D Shampoo, 1% 1868

Lopinavir (Cytochrome P450 inhibitors may inhibit the 25-hydroxylation of doxercalciferol. Hence, formation of the active doxercalciferol moiety may be hindered). Products include:
Kaletra 476

Loratadine (Cytochrome P450 inhibitors may inhibit the 25-hydroxylation of doxercalciferol. Hence, formation of the active doxercalciferol moiety may be hindered). Products include:
Alavert Allergy & Sinus D-12 Hour Tablets .... ◘771
Alavert .... ◘771
Children's Claritin Allergy Oral Solution .... ◘771
Claritin Non-Drowsy 24 Hour Tablets .... ◘772
Claritin Reditabs 24 Hour Non-Drowsy Tablets .... ◘772
Claritin-D Non-Drowsy 12 Hour Tablets .... ◘772
Claritin-D Non-Drowsy 24 Hour Tablets .... ◘772

Magnesium Hydroxide (Co-administration with magnesium-containing antacids and Hectorol may lead to the development of hypermagnesemia; concurrent use should be avoided). Products include:
Maalox Regular Strength Antacid/Antigas Liquid 2175
Maalox Max Maximum Strength Antacid/Anti-Gas Liquid 2176
Pepcid Complete Chewable Tablets 1701

Magnesium Oxide (Co-administration with magnesium-containing antacids and Hectorol may lead to the development of hypermagnesemia; concurrent use should be avoided). Products include:
Beelith Tablets 759
PremCal Light, Regular, and Extra Strength Tablets .... ◘818

Metronidazole (Cytochrome P450 inhibitors may inhibit the 25-hydroxylation of doxercalciferol. Hence, formation of the active doxercalciferol moiety may be hindered). Products include:
Metrogel 1% 1211
MetroGel-Vaginal Gel 1855
Vandazole Vaginal Gel 3338

Metronidazole Benzoate (Cytochrome P450 inhibitors may inhibit the 25-hydroxylation of doxercalciferol. Hence, formation of the active doxercalciferol moiety may be hindered).
No products indexed under this heading.

Metronidazole Hydrochloride (Cytochrome P450 inhibitors may inhibit the 25-hydroxylation of doxercalciferol. Hence, formation of the active doxercalciferol moiety may be hindered).
No products indexed under this heading.

Miconazole (Cytochrome P450 inhibitors may inhibit the 25-hydroxylation of doxercalciferol. Hence, formation of the active doxercalciferol moiety may be hindered).
No products indexed under this heading.

Miconazole Nitrate (Cytochrome P450 inhibitors may inhibit the 25-hydroxylation of doxercalciferol. Hence, formation of the active doxercalciferol moiety may be hindered). Products include:
Desenex .... ◘635
Desenex Jock Itch Spray Powder .... ◘635

Mineral Oil (The use of mineral oil or other substances that affect absorption of the fat may influence the absorption and availability of Hectorol). Products include:
Fleet Mineral Oil Enema 1166
Preparation H Ointment .... ◘666
Refresh P.M. Lubricant Eye Ointment .... ⊙241

Nefazodone Hydrochloride (Cytochrome P450 inhibitors may inhibit the 25-hydroxylation of doxercalciferol. Hence, formation of the active doxercalciferol moiety may be hindered).
No products indexed under this heading.

Nelfinavir Mesylate (Cytochrome P450 inhibitors may inhibit the 25-hydroxylation of doxercalciferol. Hence, formation of the active doxercalciferol moiety may be hindered). Products include:
Viracept 2577

Nevirapine (Cytochrome P450 inhibitors may inhibit the 25-hydroxylation of doxercalciferol. Hence, formation of the active doxercalciferol moiety may be hindered). Products include:
Viramune Oral Suspension 873
Viramune Tablets 873

Niacinamide (Cytochrome P450 inhibitors may inhibit the 25-hydroxylation of doxercalciferol. Hence, formation of the active doxercalciferol moiety may be hindered).
No products indexed under this heading.

Nicotinamide (Cytochrome P450 inhibitors may inhibit the 25-hydroxylation of doxercalciferol. Hence, formation of the active doxercalciferol moiety may be hindered). Products include:
Nicomide Tablets 1088

Nifedipine (Cytochrome P450 inhibitors may inhibit the 25-hydroxylation of doxercalciferol. Hence, formation of the active doxercalciferol moiety may be hindered). Products include:
Adalat CC Tablets 2964

Norfloxacin (Cytochrome P450 inhibitors may inhibit the 25-hydroxylation of doxercalciferol. Hence, formation of the active doxercalciferol moiety may be hindered). Products include:
Noroxin Tablets 2032

Omeprazole (Cytochrome P450 inhibitors may inhibit the 25-hydroxylation of doxercalciferol. Hence, formation of the active doxercalciferol moiety may be hindered). Products include:
Zegerid Capsules 2958
Zegerid Powder for Oral Solution 2958

Paroxetine Hydrochloride (Cytochrome P450 inhibitors may inhibit the 25-hydroxylation of doxercalciferol. Hence, formation of the active doxercalciferol moiety may be hindered). Products include:
Paxil CR Controlled-Release Tablets 1538
Paxil 1530

Phenobarbital (Co-administration with enzyme inducers, such as phenobarbital, may affect the 25-hydroxylation of Hectorol and may necessitate dosage adjustment). Products include:
Donnatal Extentabs 2493

Phenytoin (Co-administration with enzyme inhibitors, such as phenytoin, may affect the 25-hydroxylation of Hectorol and may necessitate dosage adjustment).
No products indexed under this heading.

Phenytoin Sodium (Co-administration with enzyme inhibitors, such as phenytoin, may affect the 25-hydroxylation of Hectorol and may necessitate dosage adjustment). Products include:
Phenytek Capsules 2160

Propoxyphene Hydrochloride (Cytochrome P450 inhibitors may inhibit the 25-hydroxylation of doxercalciferol. Hence, formation of the active doxercalciferol moiety may be hindered).
No products indexed under this heading.

Propoxyphene Napsylate (Cytochrome P450 inhibitors may inhibit the 25-hydroxylation of doxercalciferol. Hence, formation of the active doxercalciferol moiety may be hindered).
No products indexed under this heading.

Quinidine (Cytochrome P450 inhibitors may inhibit the 25-hydroxylation of doxercalciferol. Hence, formation of the active doxercalciferol moiety may be hindered).
No products indexed under this heading.

Quinidine Hydrochloride (Cytochrome P450 inhibitors may inhibit the 25-hydroxylation of doxercalciferol. Hence, formation of the active doxercalciferol moiety may be hindered).
No products indexed under this heading.

Quinidine Polygalacturonate (Cytochrome P450 inhibitors may inhibit the 25-hydroxylation of doxercalciferol. Hence, formation of the active doxercalciferol moiety may be hindered).
No products indexed under this heading.

Quinidine Sulfate (Cytochrome P450 inhibitors may inhibit the 25-hydroxylation of doxercalciferol. Hence, formation of the active doxercalciferol moiety may be hindered).
No products indexed under this heading.

Quinine (Cytochrome P450 inhibitors may inhibit the 25-hydroxylation of doxercalciferol. Hence, formation of the active doxercalciferol moiety may be hindered).
No products indexed under this heading.

Quinine Sulfate (Cytochrome P450 inhibitors may inhibit the 25-hydroxylation of doxercalciferol. Hence, formation of the active doxercalciferol moiety may be hindered).
No products indexed under this heading.

Quinupristin (Cytochrome P450 inhibitors may inhibit the 25-hydroxylation of doxercalciferol. Hence, formation of the active doxercalciferol moiety may be hindered).
No products indexed under this heading.

Ranitidine Bismuth Citrate (Cytochrome P450 inhibitors may inhibit the 25-hydroxylation of doxercalciferol. Hence, formation of the active doxercalciferol moiety may be hindered).
No products indexed under this heading.

Ranitidine Hydrochloride (Cytochrome P450 inhibitors may inhibit the 25-hydroxylation of doxercalciferol. Hence, formation of the active doxercalciferol moiety may be hindered). Products include:
Zantac 1624
Zantac Injection 1619
Zantac Injection Pharmacy Bulk Package 1622

Ritonavir (Cytochrome P450 inhibitors may inhibit the 25-hydroxylation of doxercalciferol. Hence, formation of the active doxercalciferol moiety may be hindered). Products include:
Kaletra 476
Norvir 503

Saquinavir (Cytochrome P450 inhibitors may inhibit the 25-hydroxylation of doxercalciferol. Hence, formation of the active doxercalciferol moiety may be hindered).
No products indexed under this heading.

Saquinavir Mesylate (Cytochrome P450 inhibitors may inhibit the 25-hydroxylation of doxercalciferol. Hence, formation of the active doxercalciferol moiety may be hindered). Products include:
Invirase 2772

Sertraline Hydrochloride (Cytochrome P450 inhibitors may inhibit the 25-hydroxylation of doxercalciferol. Hence, formation of the active doxercalciferol moiety may be hindered). Products include:
Zoloft 2586

Telithromycin (Cytochrome P450 inhibitors may inhibit the 25-hydroxylation of doxercalciferol.

Hence, formation of the active doxercalciferol moiety may be hindered). Products include:
Ketek Tablets 2903

Troglitazone (Cytochrome P450 inhibitors may inhibit the 25-hydroxylation of doxercalciferol. Hence, formation of the active doxercalciferol moiety may be hindered).
No products indexed under this heading.

Troleandomycin (Cytochrome P450 inhibitors may inhibit the 25-hydroxylation of doxercalciferol. Hence, formation of the active doxercalciferol moiety may be hindered).
No products indexed under this heading.

Valproate Sodium (Cytochrome P450 inhibitors may inhibit the 25-hydroxylation of doxercalciferol. Hence, formation of the active doxercalciferol moiety may be hindered). Products include:
Depacon Injection 412

Verapamil Hydrochloride (Cytochrome P450 inhibitors may inhibit the 25-hydroxylation of doxercalciferol. Hence, formation of the active doxercalciferol moiety may be hindered). Products include:
Covera-HS Tablets 3139
Tarka Tablets 524
Verelan PM Extended-Release Capsules, Controlled-Onset........... 3106

Vitamin D (Pharmacologic doses of Vitamin D and its derivatives should be withheld during doxercalciferol treatment to avoid possible additive effects and hypercalcemia). Products include:
Active Calcium Tablets 3339
Caltrate 600 PLUS .... ▣809
Caltrate 600 + D Tablets .... ▣809
D-Cal Chewable Caplets .... ▣812
Os-Cal 250 + D Tablets .... ▣817
Os-Cal 500 + D Tablets .... ▣817

Vitamin D_2 (Pharmacologic doses of Vitamin D and its derivatives should be withheld during doxercalciferol treatment to avoid possible additive effects and hypercalcemia).
No products indexed under this heading.

Voriconazole (Cytochrome P450 inhibitors may inhibit the 25-hydroxylation of doxercalciferol. Hence, formation of the active doxercalciferol moiety may be hindered). Products include:
VFEND I.V. 2564
VFEND Oral Suspension 2564
VFEND Tablets 2564

Zafirlukast (Cytochrome P450 inhibitors may inhibit the 25-hydroxylation of doxercalciferol. Hence, formation of the active doxercalciferol moiety may be hindered). Products include:
Accolate Tablets 671

Zileuton (Cytochrome P450 inhibitors may inhibit the 25-hydroxylation of doxercalciferol. Hence, formation of the active doxercalciferol moiety may be hindered). Products include:
Zyflo Tablets 1023

Food Interactions

Grapefruit (Cytochrome P450 inhibitors may inhibit the 25-hydroxylation of doxercalciferol. Hence, formation of the active doxercalciferol moiety may be hindered).

Grapefruit Juice (Cytochrome P450 inhibitors may inhibit the 25-hydroxylation of doxercalciferol. Hence, formation of the active doxercalciferol moiety may be hindered).

HECTOROL INJECTION
(Doxercalciferol) 1278
May interact with:

See (Hectorol Capsules).
No products indexed under this heading.

HEMOFIL M
(Antihemophilic Factor (Human)) 728
None cited in PDR database.

HEP-FORTE CAPSULES
(Vitamins with Minerals) 1862
None cited in PDR database.

HEPSERA TABLETS
(Adefovir dipivoxil) 1292
May interact with inhibitors of renal tubular secretion or resorption and certain other agents. Compounds in these categories include:

Ibuprofen (When adefovir was co-administered with ibuprofen, increases in adefovir Cmax (33%), AUC (23%) and urinary recovery were observed. These increases appear to be due to higher oral bioavailability, not a reduction in renal clearance of adefovir). Products include:
Advil Allergy Sinus Caplets .... ▣770
Advil .... ▣674
Children's Advil Oral Suspension .... ▣603
Children's Advil Chewable Tablets .. ▣603
Advil Cold & Sinus .... ▣723
Infants' Advil Concentrated Drops .. ▣604
Infants' Advil Concentrated Drops - White Grape (Dye-Free)............. ▣604
Junior Strength Advil Swallow Tablets .... ▣605
Advil Migraine Liquigels .... ▣608
Advil Multi-Symptom Cold Caplets .... ▣770
Advil PM Caplets .... ▣615
Motrin IB Tablets and Caplets 1866
Children's Motrin Oral Suspension ... 1867
Children's Motrin Non-Staining Dye-Free Oral Suspension............ 1867
Children's Motrin Cold Oral Suspension 1867
Infants' Motrin Concentrated Drops 1867
Infants' Motrin Non-Staining Dye-Free Concentrated Drops....... 1867
Junior Strength Motrin Caplets and Chewable Tablets.................. 1867
Vicoprofen Tablets 539

Probenecid (Since adefovir is eliminated by the kidney, co-administration of adefovir with drugs that compete for active tubular secretion may increase serum concentrations of either adefovir and/or these co-administered drugs).
No products indexed under this heading.

Sulfinpyrazone (Since adefovir is eliminated by the kidney, co-administration of adefovir with drugs that compete for active tubular secretion may increase serum concentrations of either adefovir and/or these co-administered drugs).
No products indexed under this heading.

HERCEPTIN I.V.
(Trastuzumab) 1233
May interact with anthracycline antibiotics and their derivatives and certain other agents. Compounds in these categories include:

Cyclophosphamide (The increase and severity of cardiac dysfunction is particularly high in patients who receive trastuzumab in combination with cyclophosphamide).
No products indexed under this heading.

Daunorubicin Hydrochloride (The increase and severity of cardiac dysfunction is particularly high in patients who receive trastuzumab in combination with anthracyclines).
No products indexed under this heading.

Doxorubicin Hydrochloride (The increase and severity of cardiac dysfunction is particularly high in patients who receive trastuzumab in combination with anthracyclines).
No products indexed under this heading.

Epirubicin Hydrochloride (The increase and severity of cardiac dysfunction is particularly high in patients who receive trastuzumab in combination with anthracyclines).
No products indexed under this heading.

Idarubicin Hydrochloride (The increase and severity of cardiac dysfunction is particularly high in patients who receive trastuzumab in combination with anthracyclines).
No products indexed under this heading.

Paclitaxel (Co-administration has resulted in a two-fold decrease in trastuzumab clearance in a non-human primate study and in a 1.5-fold increase in trastuzumab serum levels in clinical studies).
No products indexed under this heading.

HIBTITER
(Haemophilus B Conjugate Vaccine).. 3426
May interact with alkylating agents, antimetabolites, anticoagulants, corticosteroids, cytotoxic drugs, immunosuppressive agents, and certain other agents. Compounds in these categories include:

Anisindione (HibTITER should be given with caution to children on anticoagulant therapy). Products include:
Miradon Tablets 3042

Ardeparin Sodium (HibTITER should be given with caution to children on anticoagulant therapy).
No products indexed under this heading.

Azathioprine (Reduces antibody response to active immunization procedures).
No products indexed under this heading.

Basiliximab (Reduces antibody response to active immunization procedures). Products include:
Simulect for Injection 2284

Betamethasone Acetate (Reduces antibody response to active immunization procedures).
No products indexed under this heading.

Betamethasone Sodium Phosphate (Reduces antibody response to active immunization procedures).
No products indexed under this heading.

Bleomycin Sulfate (Reduces antibody response to active immunization procedures).
No products indexed under this heading.

Busulfan (Reduces antibody response to active immunization procedures). Products include:
I.V. Busulfex 2493
Myleran Tablets 1525

Capecitabine (Children with impaired immune responsiveness may have reduced antibody response to active immunization procedures. Deferral of administration of vaccine may be considered in individuals receiving immunosuppressive therapy). Products include:
Xeloda Tablets 2822

Carmustine (BCNU) (Reduces antibody response to active immunization procedures).
No products indexed under this heading.

Chlorambucil (Reduces antibody response to active immunization procedures). Products include:
Leukeran Tablets 1504

Cladribine (Children with impaired immune responsiveness may have reduced antibody response to active immunization procedures. Deferral of administration of vaccine may be considered in individuals receiving immunosuppressive therapy). Products include:
Leustatin Injection 2357

Cortisone Acetate (Reduces antibody response to active immunization procedures).
No products indexed under this heading.

Cyclophosphamide (Reduces antibody response to active immunization procedures).
No products indexed under this heading.

Cyclosporine (Reduces antibody response to active immunization procedures). Products include:
Gengraf Capsules 459
Neoral Oral Solution 2259
Neoral Soft Gelatin Capsules 2259
Restasis Ophthalmic Emulsion 575
Sandimmune 2275

Cytarabine (Children with impaired immune responsiveness may have reduced antibody response to active immunization procedures. Deferral of administration of vaccine may be considered in individuals receiving immunosuppressive therapy).
No products indexed under this heading.

Dacarbazine (Reduces antibody response to active immunization procedures).
No products indexed under this heading.

Dalteparin Sodium (HibTITER should be given with caution to children on anticoagulant therapy). Products include:
Fragmin Injection 1097

Danaparoid Sodium (HibTITER should be given with caution to children on anticoagulant therapy).
No products indexed under this heading.

Daunorubicin Hydrochloride (Reduces antibody response to active immunization procedures).
No products indexed under this heading.

Dexamethasone (Reduces antibody response to active immunization procedures). Products include:
Ciprodex Otic Suspension 559
Decadron Tablets 1951
TobraDex Ophthalmic Ointment 562
TobraDex Ophthalmic Suspension ... 563

Dexamethasone Acetate (Reduces antibody response to active immunization procedures).
No products indexed under this heading.

Dexamethasone Sodium Phosphate (Reduces antibody response to active immunization procedures).
No products indexed under this heading.

Dicumarol (HibTITER should be given with caution to children on anticoagulant therapy).
No products indexed under this heading.

Doxorubicin Hydrochloride (Reduces antibody response to active immunization procedures).
No products indexed under this heading.

Enoxaparin Sodium (HibTITER should be given with caution to children on anticoagulant therapy). Products include:
Lovenox Injection 2915

Epirubicin Hydrochloride (Reduces antibody response to active immunization procedures).
No products indexed under this heading.

Floxuridine (Children with impaired immune responsiveness may have reduced antibody response to active immunization procedures. Deferral of administration of vaccine may be considered in individuals receiving immunosuppressive therapy).
No products indexed under this heading.

Fludarabine Phosphate (Children with impaired immune responsiveness may have reduced antibody response to active immunization procedures. Deferral of administration of vaccine may be considered in individuals receiving immunosuppressive therapy).
No products indexed under this heading.

Fludrocortisone Acetate (Reduces antibody response to active immunization procedures).
No products indexed under this heading.

Fluorouracil (Reduces antibody response to active immunization procedures). Products include:
Carac Cream, 0.5% 2879
Efudex 3363

Fondaparinux Sodium (HibTITER should be given with caution to children on anticoagulant therapy). Products include:
Arixtra Injection 1351

Gemcitabine Hydrochloride (Children with impaired immune responsiveness may have reduced antibody response to active immunization procedures. Deferral of administration of vaccine may be considered in individuals receiving immunosuppressive therapy). Products include:
Gemzar for Injection 1771

Heparin Calcium (HibTITER should be given with caution to children on anticoagulant therapy).
No products indexed under this heading.

Heparin Sodium (HibTITER should be given with caution to children on anticoagulant therapy).
No products indexed under this heading.

Hydrocortisone (Reduces antibody response to active immunization procedures). Products include:
Colocort Rectal Suspension, USP (Retention) 100 mg/60 mL 2476
Hydrocortone Tablets 1989
Preparation H Hydrocortisone Cream .... ▣646

Hydrocortisone Acetate (Reduces antibody response to active immunization procedures). Products include:
Analpram-HC 1159
Pramosone 1161
ProctoFoam-HC 3099

Hydrocortisone Sodium Phosphate (Reduces antibody response to active immunization procedures).
No products indexed under this heading.

Hydrocortisone Sodium Succinate (Reduces antibody response to active immunization procedures).
No products indexed under this heading.

Hydroxyurea (Reduces antibody response to active immunization procedures).
No products indexed under this heading.

Immune Globulin Intravenous (Human) (Reduces antibody response to active immunization procedures). Products include:
Carimune NF 3499
Gammagard Liquid 721
Gammagard S/D 724
Gamunex Immune Globulin I.V., 10% 3235

Lomustine (CCNU) (Reduces antibody response to active immunization procedures).
No products indexed under this heading.

Low Molecular Weight Heparins (HibTITER should be given with caution to children on anticoagulant therapy).
No products indexed under this heading.

Mechlorethamine Hydrochloride (Reduces antibody response to active immunization procedures). Products include:
Mustargen for Injection 2468

Melphalan (Reduces antibody response to active immunization procedures). Products include:
Alkeran Tablets 956

Mercaptopurine (Children with impaired immune responsiveness may have reduced antibody response to active immunization procedures. Deferral of administration of vaccine may be considered in individuals receiving immunosuppressive therapy).
No products indexed under this heading.

Methotrexate (Children with impaired immune responsiveness may have reduced antibody response to active immunization procedures. Deferral of administration of vaccine may be considered in individuals receiving immunosuppressive therapy).
No products indexed under this heading.

Methotrexate Sodium (Reduces antibody response to active immunization procedures).
No products indexed under this heading.

Methylprednisolone Acetate (Reduces antibody response to active immunization procedures). Products include:
Depo-Medrol Injectable Suspension 2617
Depo-Medrol Single-Dose Vial 2619

Methylprednisolone Sodium Succinate (Reduces antibody response to active immunization procedures).
No products indexed under this heading.

Mitotane (Reduces antibody response to active immunization procedures).
No products indexed under this heading.

Mitoxantrone Hydrochloride (Reduces antibody response to active immunization procedures).
No products indexed under this heading.

Muromonab-CD3 (Reduces antibody response to active immunization procedures). Products include:
Orthoclone OKT3 Sterile Solution 2360

Mycophenolate Mofetil (Reduces antibody response to active immunization procedures). Products include:
CellCept Capsules 2747
CellCept Oral Suspension 2747
CellCept Tablets 2747

Pentostatin (Children with impaired immune responsiveness may have reduced antibody response to active immunization procedures. Deferral of administration of vaccine may be considered in individuals receiving immunosuppressive therapy). Products include:
Nipent for Injection 1863

Prednisolone Acetate (Reduces antibody response to active immunization procedures). Products include:
Blephamide Ophthalmic Ointment 568
Blephamide Ophthalmic Suspension 569
Poly-Pred Ophthalmic Suspension .... ⊙233
Pred Forte Ophthalmic Suspension .... ⊙235
Pred Mild Ophthalmic Suspension .... ⊙238
Pred-G Ophthalmic Ointment .... ⊙237
Pred-G Ophthalmic Suspension .... ⊙236

Prednisolone Sodium Phosphate (Reduces antibody response to active immunization procedures).
No products indexed under this heading.

Prednisolone Tebutate (Reduces antibody response to active immunization procedures).
No products indexed under this heading.

Prednisone (Reduces antibody response to active immunization procedures).
No products indexed under this heading.

Procarbazine Hydrochloride (Reduces antibody response to active immunization procedures). Products include:
Matulane Capsules 3191

Sirolimus (Reduces antibody response to active immunization procedures). Products include:
Rapamune Oral Solution and Tablets 3475

Tacrolimus (Reduces antibody response to active immunization procedures). Products include:
Prograf Capsules and Injection 632
Protopic Ointment 638

Tamoxifen Citrate (Reduces antibody response to active immunization procedures). Products include:
Soltamox Oral Solution 3527

Thioguanine (Children with impaired immune responsiveness may have reduced antibody response to active immunization procedures. Deferral of administration of vaccine may be considered in individuals receiving immunosuppressive therapy). Products include:
Tabloid Tablets 1575

Thiotepa (Reduces antibody response to active immunization procedures).
No products indexed under this heading.

Tinzaparin Sodium (HibTITER should be given with caution to children on anticoagulant therapy).
No products indexed under this heading.

Triamcinolone (Reduces antibody response to active immunization procedures).
No products indexed under this heading.

Triamcinolone Acetonide (Reduces antibody response to active immunization procedures). Products include:
Azmacort Inhalation Aerosol 1726
Nasacort AQ Nasal Spray 2922

Triamcinolone Diacetate (Reduces antibody response to active immunization procedures).
No products indexed under this heading.

Triamcinolone Hexacetonide (Reduces antibody response to active immunization procedures).
No products indexed under this heading.

Vincristine Sulfate (Reduces antibody response to active immunization procedures).
No products indexed under this heading.

Warfarin Sodium (HibTITER should be given with caution to children on anticoagulant therapy). Products include:
Coumadin for Injection 898
Coumadin Tablets 898

HUMALOG-PEN

(Insulin Lispro, Human) 1781
May interact with ACE inhibitors, beta blockers, corticosteroids, estrogens, oral hypoglycemic agents, oral contraceptives, phenothiazines, salicylates, thyroid preparations, and certain other agents. Compounds in these categories include:

Acarbose (Co-administration with drugs with hypoglycemic activity, such as oral hypoglycemic agents, may result in decreased insulin requirements). Products include:
Precose Tablets 751

Acebutolol Hydrochloride (Co-administration with drugs with hypoglycemic activity, such as beta blockers, may result in decreased insulin requirements; beta blockers may mask the symptoms of hypoglycemia in some patients).
No products indexed under this heading.

Aspirin (Co-administration with drugs with hypoglycemic activity, such as salicylates, may result in decreased insulin requirements). Products include:
Aggrenox Capsules 822
Bayer Aspirin 744
BC Allergy Sinus Cold Powder .... ▣677
BC Headache Powder .... ▣677
Arthritis Strength BC Powder .... ▣677
BC Sinus Cold Powder .... ▣677
Excedrin Extra Strength Caplets/Tablets/Geltabs .... ▣684

Excedrin Migraine Caplets/Tablets/Geltabs .... ▣609
Goody's Body Pain Formula Powder .... ▣684
Goody's Extra Strength Headache Powders .... ▣611
Goody's Extra Strength Pain Relief Tablets .... ▣685
Percodan Tablets 1132
St. Joseph 81 mg Aspirin Chewable and Enteric Coated Tablets 1869

Aspirin, Enteric Coated (Co-administration with drugs with hypoglycemic activity, such as salicylates, may result in decreased insulin requirements).
No products indexed under this heading.

Aspirin Buffered (Co-administration with drugs with hypoglycemic activity, such as salicylates, may result in decreased insulin requirements). Products include:
Bufferin Extra Strength Tablets ...... ▣678
Bufferin Regular Strength Tablets ... ▣678

Atenolol (Co-administration with drugs with hypoglycemic activity, such as beta blockers, may result in decreased insulin requirements; beta blockers may mask the symptoms of hypoglycemia in some patients).
No products indexed under this heading.

Benazepril Hydrochloride (Co-administration with drugs with hypoglycemic activity, such as certain ACE inhibitors, may result in decreased insulin requirements). Products include:
Lotensin Tablets 2243
Lotensin HCT Tablets 2246
Lotrel Capsules 2249

Betamethasone Acetate (Co-administration may result in increased insulin requirements).
No products indexed under this heading.

Betamethasone Sodium Phosphate (Co-administration may result in increased insulin requirements).
No products indexed under this heading.

Betaxolol Hydrochloride (Co-administration with drugs with hypoglycemic activity, such as beta blockers, may result in decreased insulin requirements; beta blockers may mask the symptoms of hypoglycemia in some patients). Products include:
Betoptic S Ophthalmic Suspension 558

Bisoprolol Fumarate (Co-administration with drugs with hypoglycemic activity, such as beta blockers, may result in decreased insulin requirements; beta blockers may mask the symptoms of hypoglycemia in some patients).
No products indexed under this heading.

Captopril (Co-administration with drugs with hypoglycemic activity, such as certain ACE inhibitors, may result in decreased insulin requirements). Products include:
Captopril Tablets 2149

Carteolol Hydrochloride (Co-administration with drugs with hypoglycemic activity, such as beta blockers, may result in decreased insulin requirements; beta blockers may mask the symptoms of hypoglycemia in some patients). Products include:
Carteolol Hydrochloride Ophthalmic Solution USP, 1%...... ⊙249

Chlorotrianisene (Co-administration may result in increased insulin requirements).
No products indexed under this heading.

Chlorpromazine (Co-administration with phenothiazines may result in increased insulin requirements).
No products indexed under this heading.

Chlorpromazine Hydrochloride (Co-administration with phenothiazines may result in increased insulin requirements).
No products indexed under this heading.

Chlorpropamide (Co-administration with drugs with hypoglycemic activity, such as oral hypoglycemic agents, may result in decreased insulin requirements).
No products indexed under this heading.

Choline Magnesium Trisalicylate (Co-administration with drugs with hypoglycemic activity, such as salicylates, may result in decreased insulin requirements).
No products indexed under this heading.

Cortisone Acetate (Co-administration may result in increased insulin requirements).
No products indexed under this heading.

Desogestrel (Co-admininstration with oral contraceptives may result in increased insulin requirements). Products include:
Mircette Tablets 1066

Dexamethasone (Co-administration may result in increased insulin requirements). Products include:
Ciprodex Otic Suspension 559
Decadron Tablets 1951
TobraDex Ophthalmic Ointment 562
TobraDex Ophthalmic Suspension ... 563

Dexamethasone Acetate (Co-administration may result in increased insulin requirements).
No products indexed under this heading.

Dexamethasone Sodium Phosphate (Co-administration may result in increased insulin requirements).
No products indexed under this heading.

Dienestrol (Co-administration may result in increased insulin requirements).
No products indexed under this heading.

Diethylstilbestrol (Co-administration may result in increased insulin requirements).
No products indexed under this heading.

Diflunisal (Co-administration with drugs with hypoglycemic activity, such as salicylates, may result in decreased insulin requirements). Products include:
Dolobid Tablets 1955

Enalapril Maleate (Co-administration with drugs with hypoglycemic activity, such as certain ACE inhibitors, may result in decreased insulin requirements). Products include:
Vasotec I.V. Injection 2103

Enalaprilat (Co-administration with drugs with hypoglycemic activity, such as certain ACE inhibitors, may result in decreased insulin requirements).
No products indexed under this heading.

Esmolol Hydrochloride (Co-administration with drugs with hypoglycemic activity, such as beta blockers, may result in decreased insulin requirements; beta blockers may mask the symptoms of hypoglycemia in some patients).
No products indexed under this heading.

Estradiol (Co-administration may result in increased insulin requirements). Products include:
Angeliq Tablets 762
Climara Transdermal System 771
Climara Pro Transdermal System 776
Estrasorb Topical Emulsion 1147
Estring Vaginal Ring 2635
Menostar Transdermal System 782
Vagifem Tablets 2334

Estrogens, Conjugated (Co-administration may result in increased insulin requirements). Products include:
Premarin Intravenous 3442
Premarin Tablets 3446
Premarin Vaginal Cream 3452
Premphase Tablets 3456
Prempro Tablets 3456

Estrogens, Esterified (Co-administration may result in increased insulin requirements). Products include:
Estratest Tablets 3199
Estratest H.S. Tablets 3199

Estropipate (Co-administration may result in increased insulin requirements).
No products indexed under this heading.

Ethinyl Estradiol (Co-administration may result in increased insulin requirements). Products include:
Mircette Tablets 1066
NuvaRing 2340
Ortho-Cyclen/Ortho Tri-Cyclen 2429
Ortho Evra Transdermal System 2417
Ortho Tri-Cyclen Lo Tablets 2436
Seasonique Tablets 1077
Yasmin 28 Tablets 796
Yaz Tablets 803

Ethynodiol Diacetate (Co-admininstration with oral contraceptives may result in increased insulin requirements).
No products indexed under this heading.

Fludrocortisone Acetate (Co-administration may result in increased insulin requirements).
No products indexed under this heading.

Fluphenazine Decanoate (Co-administration with phenothiazines may result in increased insulin requirements).
No products indexed under this heading.

Fluphenazine Enanthate (Co-administration with phenothiazines may result in increased insulin requirements).
No products indexed under this heading.

Fluphenazine Hydrochloride (Co-administration with phenothiazines may result in increased insulin requirements).
No products indexed under this heading.

Fosinopril Sodium (Co-administration with drugs with hypoglycemic activity, such as certain ACE inhibitors, may result in decreased insulin requirements).
No products indexed under this heading.

Glimepiride (Co-administration with drugs with hypoglycemic activity, such as oral hypoglycemic agents, may result in decreased insulin requirements). Products include:
Avandaryl Tablets 1379
Duetact Tablets 3226

Glipizide (Co-administration with drugs with hypoglycemic activity, such as oral hypoglycemic agents, may result in decreased insulin requirements).
No products indexed under this heading.

Glyburide (Co-administration with drugs with hypoglycemic activity, such as oral hypoglycemic agents, may result in decreased insulin requirements).
No products indexed under this heading.

Hydrocortisone (Co-administration may result in increased insulin requirements). Products include:
Colocort Rectal Suspension, USP (Retention) 100 mg/60 mL........... 2476
Hydrocortone Tablets 1989
Preparation H Hydrocortisone Cream .... ▣646

Hydrocortisone Acetate (Co-administration may result in increased insulin requirements). Products include:
Analpram-HC 1159
Pramosone 1161
ProctoFoam-HC 3099

Hydrocortisone Sodium Phosphate (Co-administration may result in increased insulin requirements).
No products indexed under this heading.

Hydrocortisone Sodium Succinate (Co-administration may result in increased insulin requirements).
No products indexed under this heading.

Isoniazid (Co-administration may result in increased insulin requirements).
No products indexed under this heading.

Labetalol Hydrochloride (Co-administration with drugs with hypoglycemic activity, such as beta blockers, may result in decreased insulin requirements; beta blockers may mask the symptoms of hypoglycemia in some patients).
No products indexed under this heading.

Levobunolol Hydrochloride (Co-administration with drugs with hypoglycemic activity, such as beta blockers, may result in decreased insulin requirements; beta blockers may mask the symptoms of hypoglycemia in some patients). Products include:
Betagan Ophthalmic Solution, USP .... ⊙220

Levonorgestrel (Co-admininstration with oral contraceptives may result in increased insulin requirements). Products include:
Climara Pro Transdermal System 776
Mirena Intrauterine System 787
Plan B Tablets 1076
Seasonique Tablets 1077

Levothyroxine Sodium (Co-administration with thyroid replace-

ment therapy may result in increased insulin requirements). Products include:
- Levothroid Tablets 1186
- Levoxyl Tablets 1712
- Synthroid Tablets 520
- Westhroid Tablets 3403

Liothyronine Sodium (Co-administration with thyroid replacement therapy may result in increased insulin requirements). Products include:
- Cytomel Tablets 1710
- Westhroid Tablets 3403

Liotrix (Co-administration with thyroid replacement therapy may result in increased insulin requirements). Products include:
- Thyrolar Tablets 1199

Lisinopril (Co-administration with drugs with hypoglycemic activity, such as certain ACE inhibitors, may result in decreased insulin requirements). Products include:
- Prinivil Tablets 2052
- Prinzide Tablets 2056

Magnesium Salicylate (Co-administration with drugs with hypoglycemic activity, such as salicylates, may result in decreased insulin requirements).
No products indexed under this heading.

Mesoridazine Besylate (Co-administration with phenothiazines may result in increased insulin requirements).
No products indexed under this heading.

Mestranol (Co-admininstration with oral contraceptives may result in increased insulin requirements).
No products indexed under this heading.

Metformin Hydrochloride (Co-administration with drugs with hypoglycemic activity, such as oral hypoglycemic agents, may result in decreased insulin requirements). Products include:
- ActoPlus Met Tablets 3214
- Avandamet Tablets 1373
- Fortamet Extended-Release Tablets 3115

Methotrimeprazine (Co-administration with phenothiazines may result in increased insulin requirements).
No products indexed under this heading.

Methylprednisolone Acetate (Co-administration may result in increased insulin requirements). Products include:
- Depo-Medrol Injectable Suspension 2617
- Depo-Medrol Single-Dose Vial 2619

Methylprednisolone Sodium Succinate (Co-administration may result in increased insulin requirements).
No products indexed under this heading.

Metipranolol Hydrochloride (Co-administration with drugs with hypoglycemic activity, such as beta blockers, may result in decreased insulin requirements; beta blockers may mask the symptoms of hypoglycemia in some patients).
No products indexed under this heading.

Metoprolol Succinate (Co-administration with drugs with hypoglycemic activity, such as beta blockers, may result in decreased insulin requirements; beta blockers may mask the symptoms of hypoglycemia in some patients). Products include:
- Toprol-XL Tablets 668

Metoprolol Tartrate (Co-administration with drugs with hypoglycemic activity, such as beta blockers, may result in decreased insulin requirements; beta blockers may mask the symptoms of hypoglycemia in some patients). Products include:
- Lopressor Injection 2238
- Lopressor Tablets 2238
- Lopressor HCT 50/25 Tablets 2241
- Lopressor HCT 100/25 Tablets 2241
- Lopressor HCT 100/50 Tablets 2241

Miglitol (Co-administration with drugs with hypoglycemic activity, such as oral hypoglycemic agents, may result in decreased insulin requirements).
No products indexed under this heading.

Moexipril Hydrochloride (Co-administration with drugs with hypoglycemic activity, such as certain ACE inhibitors, may result in decreased insulin requirements). Products include:
- Uniretic Tablets 3100
- Univasc Tablets 3104

Nadolol (Co-administration with drugs with hypoglycemic activity, such as beta blockers, may result in decreased insulin requirements; beta blockers may mask the symptoms of hypoglycemia in some patients). Products include:
- Nadolol Tablets 2159

Niacin (Co-administration may result in increased insulin requirements). Products include:
- Advicor Tablets 1722
- Niaspan Extended-Release Tablets 1730

Norethindrone (Co-admininstration with oral contraceptives may result in increased insulin requirements). Products include:
- Ortho Micronor Tablets 2426

Norethynodrel (Co-admininstration with oral contraceptives may result in increased insulin requirements).
No products indexed under this heading.

Norgestimate (Co-admininstration with oral contraceptives may result in increased insulin requirements). Products include:
- Ortho-Cyclen/Ortho Tri-Cyclen 2429
- Ortho Tri-Cyclen Lo Tablets 2436

Norgestrel (Co-admininstration with oral contraceptives may result in increased insulin requirements).
No products indexed under this heading.

Octreotide Acetate (Co-administration with drugs with hypoglycemic activity, such as inhibitors of pancreatic function, may result in decreased insulin requirements). Products include:
- Sandostatin Injection 2278
- Sandostatin LAR Depot 2280

Penbutolol Sulfate (Co-administration with drugs with hypoglycemic activity, such as beta blockers, may result in decreased insulin requirements; beta blockers may mask the symptoms of hypoglycemia in some patients).
No products indexed under this heading.

Perindopril Erbumine (Co-administration with drugs with hypoglycemic activity, such as certain ACE inhibitors, may result in decreased insulin requirements). Products include:
- Aceon Tablets (2 mg, 4 mg, 8 mg) 3194

Perphenazine (Co-administration with phenothiazines may result in increased insulin requirements).
No products indexed under this heading.

Phenelzine Sulfate (Co-administration with drugs with hypoglycemic activity, such as certain MAO inhibitor antidepressants, may result in decreased insulin requirements).
No products indexed under this heading.

Pindolol (Co-administration with drugs with hypoglycemic activity, such as beta blockers, may result in decreased insulin requirements; beta blockers may mask the symptoms of hypoglycemia in some patients).
No products indexed under this heading.

Pioglitazone Hydrochloride (Co-administration with drugs with hypoglycemic activity, such as oral hypoglycemic agents, may result in decreased insulin requirements). Products include:
- ActoPlus Met Tablets 3214
- Actos Tablets 3219
- Duetact Tablets 3226

Polyestradiol Phosphate (Co-administration may result in increased insulin requirements).
No products indexed under this heading.

Prednisolone Acetate (Co-administration may result in increased insulin requirements). Products include:
- Blephamide Ophthalmic Ointment 568
- Blephamide Ophthalmic Suspension 569
- Poly-Pred Ophthalmic Suspension .... ⊙ 233
- Pred Forte Ophthalmic Suspension .... ⊙ 235
- Pred Mild Ophthalmic Suspension .... ⊙ 238
- Pred-G Ophthalmic Ointment .... ⊙ 237
- Pred-G Ophthalmic Suspension .... ⊙ 236

Prednisolone Sodium Phosphate (Co-administration may result in increased insulin requirements).
No products indexed under this heading.

Prednisolone Tebutate (Co-administration may result in increased insulin requirements).
No products indexed under this heading.

Prednisone (Co-administration may result in increased insulin requirements).
No products indexed under this heading.

Prochlorperazine (Co-administration with phenothiazines may result in increased insulin requirements).
No products indexed under this heading.

Promethazine Hydrochloride (Co-administration with phenothiazines may result in increased insulin requirements). Products include:
- Phenergan Tablets and Suppositories 3440

Propranolol Hydrochloride (Co-administration with drugs with hypoglycemic activity, such as beta blockers, may result in decreased insulin requirements; beta blockers may mask the symptoms of hypoglycemia in some patients). Products include:
- Inderal LA Long-Acting Capsules 3429
- InnoPran XL Capsules 2723

Quinapril Hydrochloride (Co-administration with drugs with hypoglycemic activity, such as certain ACE inhibitors, may result in decreased insulin requirements).
No products indexed under this heading.

Quinestrol (Co-administration may result in increased insulin requirements).
No products indexed under this heading.

Ramipril (Co-administration with drugs with hypoglycemic activity, such as certain ACE inhibitors, may result in decreased insulin requirements). Products include:
- Altace Capsules 1702

Repaglinide (Co-administration with drugs with hypoglycemic activity, such as oral hypoglycemic agents, may result in decreased insulin requirements).
No products indexed under this heading.

Rosiglitazone Maleate (Co-administration with drugs with hypoglycemic activity, such as oral hypoglycemic agents, may result in decreased insulin requirements). Products include:
- Avandamet Tablets 1373
- Avandaryl Tablets 1379
- Avandia Tablets 1384

Salsalate (Co-administration with drugs with hypoglycemic activity, such as salicylates, may result in decreased insulin requirements).
No products indexed under this heading.

Sotalol Hydrochloride (Co-administration with drugs with hypoglycemic activity, such as beta blockers, may result in decreased insulin requirements; beta blockers may mask the symptoms of hypoglycemia in some patients).
No products indexed under this heading.

Spirapril Hydrochloride (Co-administration with drugs with hypoglycemic activity, such as certain ACE inhibitors, may result in decreased insulin requirements).
No products indexed under this heading.

Sulfacytine (Co-administration with drugs with hypoglycemic activity, such as sulfa antibiotics, may result in decreased insulin requirements).
No products indexed under this heading.

Sulfamethizole (Co-administration with drugs with hypoglycemic activity, such as sulfa antibiotics, may result in decreased insulin requirements).
No products indexed under this heading.

Sulfamethoxazole (Co-administration with drugs with hypoglycemic activity, such as sulfa antibiotics, may result in decreased insulin requirements).
No products indexed under this heading.

Sulfasalazine (Co-administration with drugs with hypoglycemic activity, such as sulfa antibiotics, may result in decreased insulin requirements).
No products indexed under this heading.

Thioridazine Hydrochloride (Co-administration with phenothiazines may result in increased insulin requirements). Products include:
Thioridazine Hydrochloride Tablets 2163

Thyroglobulin (Co-administration with thyroid replacement therapy may result in increased insulin requirements).
No products indexed under this heading.

Thyroid (Co-administration with thyroid replacement therapy may result in increased insulin requirements).
No products indexed under this heading.

Thyroxine (Co-administration with thyroid replacement therapy may result in increased insulin requirements).
No products indexed under this heading.

Thyroxine Sodium (Co-administration with thyroid replacement therapy may result in increased insulin requirements).
No products indexed under this heading.

Timolol Hemihydrate (Co-administration with drugs with hypoglycemic activity, such as beta blockers, may result in decreased insulin requirements; beta blockers may mask the symptoms of hypoglycemia in some patients). Products include:
Betimol Ophthalmic Solution 3382
Betimol Ophthalmic Solution .... ⊙295

Timolol Maleate (Co-administration with drugs with hypoglycemic activity, such as beta blockers, may result in decreased insulin requirements; beta blockers may mask the symptoms of hypoglycemia in some patients). Products include:
Blocadren Tablets 1916
Cosopt Sterile Ophthalmic Solution 1931
Timolide Tablets 2086
Timoptic Sterile Ophthalmic Solution 2088
Timoptic in Ocudose 2091
Timoptic-XE Sterile Ophthalmic Gel Forming Solution 2092

Tolazamide (Co-administration with drugs with hypoglycemic activity, such as oral hypoglycemic agents, may result in decreased insulin requirements).
No products indexed under this heading.

Tolbutamide (Co-administration with drugs with hypoglycemic activity, such as oral hypoglycemic agents, may result in decreased insulin requirements).
No products indexed under this heading.

Trandolapril (Co-administration with drugs with hypoglycemic activity, such as certain ACE inhibitors, may result in decreased insulin requirements). Products include:
Mavik Tablets 486
Tarka Tablets 524

Tranylcypromine Sulfate (Co-administration with drugs with hypoglycemic activity, such as certain MAO inhibitor antidepressants, may result in decreased insulin requirements). Products include:
Parnate Tablets 1527

Triamcinolone (Co-administration may result in increased insulin requirements).
No products indexed under this heading.

Triamcinolone Acetonide (Co-administration may result in increased insulin requirements). Products include:
Azmacort Inhalation Aerosol 1726
Nasacort AQ Nasal Spray 2922

Triamcinolone Diacetate (Co-administration may result in increased insulin requirements).
No products indexed under this heading.

Triamcinolone Hexacetonide (Co-administration may result in increased insulin requirements).
No products indexed under this heading.

Trifluoperazine Hydrochloride (Co-administration with phenothiazines may result in increased insulin requirements).
No products indexed under this heading.

Troglitazone (Co-administration with drugs with hypoglycemic activity, such as oral hypoglycemic agents, may result in decreased insulin requirements).
No products indexed under this heading.

Food Interactions

Alcohol (Co-administration with drugs with hypoglycemic activity may result in decreased insulin requirements).

HUMALOG MIX 50/50-PEN

(Insulin Lispro, Human, Insulin Lispro Protamine, Human) 1783
May interact with ACE inhibitors, beta blockers, corticosteroids, estrogens, oral hypoglycemic agents, monoamine oxidase inhibitors, oral contraceptives, phenothiazines, salicylates, thyroid preparations, and certain other agents. Compounds in these categories include:

Acarbose (Insulin requirements may be decreased in the presence of drugs with with hypoglycemic activity, such as oral antidiabetic agents). Products include:
Precose Tablets 751

Acebutolol Hydrochloride (Beta-adrenergic blockers may mask the symptoms of hypoglycemia in some patients).
No products indexed under this heading.

Aspirin (Insulin requirements may be decreased in the presence of drugs with hypoglycemic activity, such as salicylates). Products include:
Aggrenox Capsules 822
Bayer Aspirin 744
BC Allergy Sinus Cold Powder .... ▣677
BC Headache Powder .... ▣677
Arthritis Strength BC Powder .... ▣677
BC Sinus Cold Powder .... ▣677
Excedrin Extra Strength Caplets/Tablets/Geltabs .... ▣684
Excedrin Migraine Caplets/Tablets/Geltabs .... ▣609
Goody's Body Pain Formula Powder .... ▣684
Goody's Extra Strength Headache Powders .... ▣611
Goody's Extra Strength Pain Relief Tablets .... ▣685
Percodan Tablets 1132
St. Joseph 81 mg Aspirin Chewable and Enteric Coated Tablets 1869

Aspirin, Enteric Coated (Insulin requirements may be decreased in the presence of drugs with hypoglycemic activity, such as salicylates).
No products indexed under this heading.

Aspirin Buffered (Insulin requirements may be decreased in the presence of drugs with hypoglycemic activity, such as salicylates). Products include:
Bufferin Extra Strength Tablets .... ▣678
Bufferin Regular Strength Tablets .... ▣678

Atenolol (Beta-adrenergic blockers may mask the symptoms of hypoglycemia in some patients).
No products indexed under this heading.

Benazepril Hydrochloride (Insulin requirements may be decreased in the presence of drugs with hypoglycemic activity, such as certain angiotensin converting enzyme inhibitors). Products include:
Lotensin Tablets 2243
Lotensin HCT Tablets 2246
Lotrel Capsules 2249

Betamethasone Acetate (Insulin requirements may be increased by medications with hypoglycemic activity, such as corticosteroids).
No products indexed under this heading.

Betamethasone Sodium Phosphate (Insulin requirements may be increased by medications with hypoglycemic activity, such as corticosteroids).
No products indexed under this heading.

Betaxolol Hydrochloride (Beta-adrenergic blockers may mask the symptoms of hypoglycemia in some patients). Products include:
Betoptic S Ophthalmic Suspension 558

Bisoprolol Fumarate (Beta-adrenergic blockers may mask the symptoms of hypoglycemia in some patients).
No products indexed under this heading.

Captopril (Insulin requirements may be decreased in the presence of drugs with hypoglycemic activity, such as certain angiotensin converting enzyme inhibitors). Products include:
Captopril Tablets 2149

Carteolol Hydrochloride (Beta-adrenergic blockers may mask the symptoms of hypoglycemia in some patients). Products include:
Carteolol Hydrochloride Ophthalmic Solution USP, 1% .... ⊙249

Chlorotrianisene (Insulin requirements may be increased by medications with hypoglycemic activity, such as estrogens).
No products indexed under this heading.

Chlorpromazine (Insulin requirements may be increased by medications with hypoglycemic activity, such as phenothiazines).
No products indexed under this heading.

Chlorpromazine Hydrochloride (Insulin requirements may be increased by medications with hypoglycemic activity, such as phenothiazines).
No products indexed under this heading.

Chlorpropamide (Insulin requirements may be decreased in the presence of drugs with with hypoglycemic activity, such as oral antidiabetic agents).
No products indexed under this heading.

Choline Magnesium Trisalicylate (Insulin requirements may be decreased in the presence of drugs with hypoglycemic activity, such as salicylates).
No products indexed under this heading.

Cortisone Acetate (Insulin requirements may be increased by medications with hypoglycemic activity, such as corticosteroids).
No products indexed under this heading.

Desogestrel (Insulin requirements may be increased by medications with hypoglycemic activity, such as oral contraceptives). Products include:
Mircette Tablets 1066

Dexamethasone (Insulin requirements may be increased by medications with hypoglycemic activity, such as corticosteroids). Products include:
Ciprodex Otic Suspension 559
Decadron Tablets 1951
TobraDex Ophthalmic Ointment 562
TobraDex Ophthalmic Suspension 563

Dexamethasone Acetate (Insulin requirements may be increased by medications with hypoglycemic activity, such as corticosteroids).
No products indexed under this heading.

Dexamethasone Sodium Phosphate (Insulin requirements may be increased by medications with hypoglycemic activity, such as corticosteroids).
No products indexed under this heading.

Dienestrol (Insulin requirements may be increased by medications with hypoglycemic activity, such as estrogens).
No products indexed under this heading.

Diethylstilbestrol (Insulin requirements may be increased by medications with hypoglycemic activity, such as estrogens).
No products indexed under this heading.

Diflunisal (Insulin requirements may be decreased in the presence of drugs with hypoglycemic activity, such as salicylates). Products include:
Dolobid Tablets 1955

Enalapril Maleate (Insulin requirements may be decreased in the presence of drugs with hypoglycemic activity, such as certain angiotensin converting enzyme inhibitors). Products include:
Vasotec I.V. Injection 2103

Enalaprilat (Insulin requirements may be decreased in the presence of drugs with hypoglycemic activity, such as certain angiotensin converting enzyme inhibitors).

No products indexed under this heading.

Esmolol Hydrochloride (Beta-adrenergic blockers may mask the symptoms of hypoglycemia in some patients).

No products indexed under this heading.

Estradiol (Insulin requirements may be increased by medications with hypoglycemic activity, such as estrogens). Products include:

Angeliq Tablets	762
Climara Transdermal System	771
Climara Pro Transdermal System	776
Estrasorb Topical Emulsion	1147
Estring Vaginal Ring	2635
Menostar Transdermal System	782
Vagifem Tablets	2334

Estrogens, Conjugated (Insulin requirements may be increased by medications with hypoglycemic activity, such as estrogens). Products include:

Premarin Intravenous	3442
Premarin Tablets	3446
Premarin Vaginal Cream	3452
Premphase Tablets	3456
Prempro Tablets	3456

Estrogens, Esterified (Insulin requirements may be increased by medications with hypoglycemic activity, such as estrogens). Products include:

Estratest Tablets	3199
Estratest H.S. Tablets	3199

Estropipate (Insulin requirements may be increased by medications with hypoglycemic activity, such as estrogens).

No products indexed under this heading.

Ethanol (Insulin requirements may be decreased in the presence of drugs with hypoglycemic activity, such as ethanol).

No products indexed under this heading.

Ethinyl Estradiol (Insulin requirements may be increased by medications with hypoglycemic activity, such as oral contraceptives). Products include:

Mircette Tablets	1066
NuvaRing	2340
Ortho-Cyclen/Ortho Tri-Cyclen	2429
Ortho Evra Transdermal System	2417
Ortho Tri-Cyclen Lo Tablets	2436
Seasonique Tablets	1077
Yasmin 28 Tablets	796
Yaz Tablets	803

Ethyl Alcohol (Insulin requirements may be decreased in the presence of drugs with hypoglycemic activity, such as alcohol).

No products indexed under this heading.

Ethynodiol Diacetate (Insulin requirements may be increased by medications with hypoglycemic activity, such as oral contraceptives).

No products indexed under this heading.

Fludrocortisone Acetate (Insulin requirements may be increased by medications with hypoglycemic activity, such as corticosteroids).

No products indexed under this heading.

Fluphenazine Decanoate (Insulin requirements may be increased by medications with hypoglycemic activity, such as phenothiazines).

No products indexed under this heading.

Fluphenazine Enanthate (Insulin requirements may be increased by medications with hypoglycemic activity, such as phenothiazines).

No products indexed under this heading.

Fluphenazine Hydrochloride (Insulin requirements may be increased by medications with hypoglycemic activity, such as phenothiazines).

No products indexed under this heading.

Fosinopril Sodium (Insulin requirements may be decreased in the presence of drugs with hypoglycemic activity, such as certain angiotensin converting enzyme inhibitors).

No products indexed under this heading.

Glimepiride (Insulin requirements may be decreased in the presence of drugs with with hypoglycemic activity, such as oral antidiabetic agents). Products include:

Avandaryl Tablets	1379
Duetact Tablets	3226

Glipizide (Insulin requirements may be decreased in the presence of drugs with with hypoglycemic activity, such as oral antidiabetic agents).

No products indexed under this heading.

Glyburide (Insulin requirements may be decreased in the presence of drugs with with hypoglycemic activity, such as oral antidiabetic agents).

No products indexed under this heading.

Hydrocortisone (Insulin requirements may be increased by medications with hypoglycemic activity, such as corticosteroids). Products include:

Colocort Rectal Suspension, USP (Retention) 100 mg/60 mL	2476
Hydrocortone Tablets	1989
Preparation H Hydrocortisone Cream	▣▣646

Hydrocortisone Acetate (Insulin requirements may be increased by medications with hypoglycemic activity, such as corticosteroids). Products include:

Analpram-HC	1159
Pramosone	1161
ProctoFoam-HC	3099

Hydrocortisone Sodium Phosphate (Insulin requirements may be increased by medications with hypoglycemic activity, such as corticosteroids).

No products indexed under this heading.

Hydrocortisone Sodium Succinate (Insulin requirements may be increased by medications with hypoglycemic activity, such as corticosteroids).

No products indexed under this heading.

Isocarboxazid (Insulin requirements may be decreased in the presence of drugs with hypoglycemic activity, such as monoamine oxidase inhibitors).

No products indexed under this heading.

Isoniazid (Insulin requirements may be increased by medications with hypoglycemic activity, such as isoniazid).

No products indexed under this heading.

Labetalol Hydrochloride (Beta-adrenergic blockers may mask the symptoms of hypoglycemia in some patients).

No products indexed under this heading.

Levobunolol Hydrochloride (Beta-adrenergic blockers may mask the symptoms of hypoglycemia in some patients). Products include:

Betagan Ophthalmic Solution, USP	⊙220

Levonorgestrel (Insulin requirements may be increased by medications with hypoglycemic activity, such as oral contraceptives). Products include:

Climara Pro Transdermal System	776
Mirena Intrauterine System	787
Plan B Tablets	1076
Seasonique Tablets	1077

Levothyroxine Sodium (Insulin requirements may be increased by medications with hypoglycemic activity, such as thyroid replacement therapy). Products include:

Levothroid Tablets	1186
Levoxyl Tablets	1712
Synthroid Tablets	520
Westhroid Tablets	3403

Liothyronine Sodium (Insulin requirements may be increased by medications with hypoglycemic activity, such as thyroid replacement therapy). Products include:

Cytomel Tablets	1710
Westhroid Tablets	3403

Liotrix (Insulin requirements may be increased by medications with hypoglycemic activity, such as thyroid replacement therapy). Products include:

Thyrolar Tablets	1199

Lisinopril (Insulin requirements may be decreased in the presence of drugs with hypoglycemic activity, such as certain angiotensin converting enzyme inhibitors). Products include:

Prinivil Tablets	2052
Prinzide Tablets	2056

Magnesium Salicylate (Insulin requirements may be decreased in the presence of drugs with hypoglycemic activity, such as salicylates).

No products indexed under this heading.

Mesoridazine Besylate (Insulin requirements may be increased by medications with hypoglycemic activity, such as phenothiazines).

No products indexed under this heading.

Mestranol (Insulin requirements may be increased by medications with hypoglycemic activity, such as oral contraceptives).

No products indexed under this heading.

Metformin Hydrochloride (Insulin requirements may be decreased in the presence of drugs with with hypoglycemic activity, such as oral antidiabetic agents). Products include:

ActoPlus Met Tablets	3214
Avandamet Tablets	1373
Fortamet Extended-Release Tablets	3115

Methotrimeprazine (Insulin requirements may be increased by medications with hypoglycemic activity, such as phenothiazines).

No products indexed under this heading.

Methylprednisolone Acetate (Insulin requirements may be increased by medications with hypoglycemic activity, such as corticosteroids). Products include:

Depo-Medrol Injectable Suspension	2617
Depo-Medrol Single-Dose Vial	2619

Methylprednisolone Sodium Succinate (Insulin requirements may be increased by medications with hypoglycemic activity, such as corticosteroids).

No products indexed under this heading.

Metipranolol Hydrochloride (Beta-adrenergic blockers may mask the symptoms of hypoglycemia in some patients).

No products indexed under this heading.

Metoprolol Succinate (Beta-adrenergic blockers may mask the symptoms of hypoglycemia in some patients). Products include:

Toprol-XL Tablets	668

Metoprolol Tartrate (Beta-adrenergic blockers may mask the symptoms of hypoglycemia in some patients). Products include:

Lopressor Injection	2238
Lopressor Tablets	2238
Lopressor HCT 50/25 Tablets	2241
Lopressor HCT 100/25 Tablets	2241
Lopressor HCT 100/50 Tablets	2241

Miglitol (Insulin requirements may be decreased in the presence of drugs with with hypoglycemic activity, such as oral antidiabetic agents).

No products indexed under this heading.

Moclobemide (Insulin requirements may be decreased in the presence of drugs with hypoglycemic activity, such as monoamine oxidase inhibitors).

No products indexed under this heading.

Moexipril Hydrochloride (Insulin requirements may be decreased in the presence of drugs with hypoglycemic activity, such as certain angiotensin converting enzyme inhibitors). Products include:

Uniretic Tablets	3100
Univasc Tablets	3104

Nadolol (Beta-adrenergic blockers may mask the symptoms of hypoglycemia in some patients). Products include:

Nadolol Tablets	2159

Niacin (Insulin requirements may be increased by medications with hypoglycemic activity such as certain lipid-lowering drugs (niacin)). Products include:

Advicor Tablets	1722
Niaspan Extended-Release Tablets	1730

Niacinamide (Insulin requirements may be increased by medications with hypoglycemic activity such as certain lipid-lowering drugs (niacin)).

No products indexed under this heading.

Norethindrone (Insulin requirements may be increased by medications with hypoglycemic activity, such as oral contraceptives). Products include:

Ortho Micronor Tablets	2426

IMPORTANT NOTE: Always consult each drug listing in the patient's regimen for possible interactions.

Norethynodrel (Insulin requirements may be increased by medications with hypoglycemic activity, such as oral contraceptives).
No products indexed under this heading.

Norgestimate (Insulin requirements may be increased by medications with hypoglycemic activity, such as oral contraceptives). Products include:
Ortho-Cyclen/Ortho Tri-Cyclen 2429
Ortho Tri-Cyclen Lo Tablets 2436

Norgestrel (Insulin requirements may be increased by medications with hypoglycemic activity, such as oral contraceptives).
No products indexed under this heading.

Octreotide Acetate (Insulin requirements may be decreased in the presence of drugs with hypoglycemic activity, such as inhibitors of pancreatic function (octreotide)). Products include:
Sandostatin Injection 2278
Sandostatin LAR Depot 2280

Pargyline Hydrochloride (Insulin requirements may be decreased in the presence of drugs with hypoglycemic activity, such as monoamine oxidase inhibitors).
No products indexed under this heading.

Penbutolol Sulfate (Beta-adrenergic blockers may mask the symptoms of hypoglycemia in some patients).
No products indexed under this heading.

Perindopril Erbumine (Insulin requirements may be decreased in the presence of drugs with hypoglycemic activity, such as certain angiotensin converting enzyme inhibitors). Products include:
Aceon Tablets (2 mg, 4 mg, 8 mg) 3194

Perphenazine (Insulin requirements may be increased by medications with hypoglycemic activity, such as phenothiazines).
No products indexed under this heading.

Phenelzine Sulfate (Insulin requirements may be decreased in the presence of drugs with hypoglycemic activity, such as monoamine oxidase inhibitors).
No products indexed under this heading.

Pindolol (Beta-adrenergic blockers may mask the symptoms of hypoglycemia in some patients).
No products indexed under this heading.

Pioglitazone Hydrochloride (Insulin requirements may be decreased in the presence of drugs with with hypoglycemic activity, such as oral antidiabetic agents). Products include:
ActoPlus Met Tablets 3214
Actos Tablets 3219
Duetact Tablets 3226

Polyestradiol Phosphate (Insulin requirements may be increased by medications with hypoglycemic activity, such as estrogens).
No products indexed under this heading.

Prednisolone Acetate (Insulin requirements may be increased by medications with hypoglycemic activity, such as corticosteroids). Products include:
Blephamide Ophthalmic Ointment 568
Blephamide Ophthalmic Suspension................................. 569
Poly-Pred Ophthalmic Suspension .... ⊙233
Pred Forte Ophthalmic Suspension .... ⊙235
Pred Mild Ophthalmic Suspension .... ⊙238
Pred-G Ophthalmic Ointment .... ⊙237
Pred-G Ophthalmic Suspension ...... ⊙236

Prednisolone Sodium Phosphate (Insulin requirements may be increased by medications with hypoglycemic activity, such as corticosteroids).
No products indexed under this heading.

Prednisolone Tebutate (Insulin requirements may be increased by medications with hypoglycemic activity, such as corticosteroids).
No products indexed under this heading.

Prednisone (Insulin requirements may be increased by medications with hypoglycemic activity, such as corticosteroids).
No products indexed under this heading.

Procarbazine Hydrochloride (Insulin requirements may be decreased in the presence of drugs with hypoglycemic activity, such as monoamine oxidase inhibitors). Products include:
Matulane Capsules 3191

Prochlorperazine (Insulin requirements may be increased by medications with hypoglycemic activity, such as phenothiazines).
No products indexed under this heading.

Promethazine Hydrochloride (Insulin requirements may be increased by medications with hypoglycemic activity, such as phenothiazines). Products include:
Phenergan Tablets and Suppositories.............................. 3440

Propranolol Hydrochloride (Beta-adrenergic blockers may mask the symptoms of hypoglycemia in some patients). Products include:
Inderal LA Long-Acting Capsules 3429
InnoPran XL Capsules 2723

Quinapril Hydrochloride (Insulin requirements may be decreased in the presence of drugs with hypoglycemic activity, such as certain angiotensin converting enzyme inhibitors).
No products indexed under this heading.

Quinestrol (Insulin requirements may be increased by medications with hypoglycemic activity, such as estrogens).
No products indexed under this heading.

Ramipril (Insulin requirements may be decreased in the presence of drugs with hypoglycemic activity, such as certain angiotensin converting enzyme inhibitors). Products include:
Altace Capsules 1702

Repaglinide (Insulin requirements may be decreased in the presence of drugs with with hypoglycemic activity, such as oral antidiabetic agents).
No products indexed under this heading.

Rosiglitazone Maleate (Insulin requirements may be decreased in the presence of drugs with with hypoglycemic activity, such as oral antidiabetic agents). Products include:
Avandamet Tablets 1373
Avandaryl Tablets 1379
Avandia Tablets 1384

Salsalate (Insulin requirements may be decreased in the presence of drugs with hypoglycemic activity, such as salicylates).
No products indexed under this heading.

Selegiline Hydrochloride (Insulin requirements may be decreased in the presence of drugs with hypoglycemic activity, such as monoamine oxidase inhibitors). Products include:
Eldepryl Capsules 3208
Zelapar Tablets 3372

Sotalol Hydrochloride (Beta-adrenergic blockers may mask the symptoms of hypoglycemia in some patients).
No products indexed under this heading.

Spirapril Hydrochloride (Insulin requirements may be decreased in the presence of drugs with hypoglycemic activity, such as certain angiotensin converting enzyme inhibitors).
No products indexed under this heading.

Thioridazine Hydrochloride (Insulin requirements may be increased by medications with hypoglycemic activity, such as phenothiazines). Products include:
Thioridazine Hydrochloride Tablets 2163

Thyroglobulin (Insulin requirements may be increased by medications with hypoglycemic activity, such as thyroid replacement therapy).
No products indexed under this heading.

Thyroid (Insulin requirements may be increased by medications with hypoglycemic activity, such as thyroid replacement therapy).
No products indexed under this heading.

Thyroxine (Insulin requirements may be increased by medications with hypoglycemic activity, such as thyroid replacement therapy).
No products indexed under this heading.

Thyroxine Sodium (Insulin requirements may be increased by medications with hypoglycemic activity, such as thyroid replacement therapy).
No products indexed under this heading.

Timolol Hemihydrate (Beta-adrenergic blockers may mask the symptoms of hypoglycemia in some patients). Products include:
Betimol Ophthalmic Solution 3382
Betimol Ophthalmic Solution .... ⊙295

Timolol Maleate (Beta-adrenergic blockers may mask the symptoms of hypoglycemia in some patients). Products include:
Blocadren Tablets 1916
Cosopt Sterile Ophthalmic Solution.. 1931
Timolide Tablets 2086
Timoptic Sterile Ophthalmic Solution.. 2088
Timoptic in Ocudose 2091
Timoptic-XE Sterile Ophthalmic Gel Forming Solution 2092

Tolazamide (Insulin requirements may be decreased in the presence of drugs with with hypoglycemic activity, such as oral antidiabetic agents).
No products indexed under this heading.

Tolbutamide (Insulin requirements may be decreased in the presence of drugs with with hypoglycemic activity, such as oral antidiabetic agents).
No products indexed under this heading.

Trandolapril (Insulin requirements may be decreased in the presence of drugs with hypoglycemic activity, such as certain angiotensin converting enzyme inhibitors). Products include:
Mavik Tablets 486
Tarka Tablets 524

Tranylcypromine Sulfate (Insulin requirements may be decreased in the presence of drugs with hypoglycemic activity, such as monoamine oxidase inhibitors). Products include:
Parnate Tablets 1527

Triamcinolone (Insulin requirements may be increased by medications with hypoglycemic activity, such as corticosteroids).
No products indexed under this heading.

Triamcinolone Acetonide (Insulin requirements may be increased by medications with hypoglycemic activity, such as corticosteroids). Products include:
Azmacort Inhalation Aerosol 1726
Nasacort AQ Nasal Spray 2922

Triamcinolone Diacetate (Insulin requirements may be increased by medications with hypoglycemic activity, such as corticosteroids).
No products indexed under this heading.

Triamcinolone Hexacetonide (Insulin requirements may be increased by medications with hypoglycemic activity, such as corticosteroids).
No products indexed under this heading.

Trifluoperazine Hydrochloride (Insulin requirements may be increased by medications with hypoglycemic activity, such as phenothiazines).
No products indexed under this heading.

Troglitazone (Insulin requirements may be decreased in the presence of drugs with with hypoglycemic activity, such as oral antidiabetic agents).
No products indexed under this heading.

Food Interactions

Alcohol (Insulin requirements may be decreased in the presence of drugs with hypoglycemic activity, such as alcohol).

HUMALOG MIX 75/25-PEN

(Insulin Lispro, Human, Insulin Lispro Protamine, Human)................. 1785
See Humalog-Pen

HUMAN ALBUMIN GRIFOLS 20%, ALBUMIN (HUMAN)

(Albumin (human)) 1651
None cited in PDR database.

HUMAN ALBUMIN GRIFOLS 25%, ALBUMIN (HUMAN)
(Albumin (human)) 1652
None cited in PDR database.

HUMATE-P
(Antihemophilic Factor (Human), von Willebrand Factor (Human))........... 3502
None cited in PDR database.

HUMATROPE VIALS AND CARTRIDGES
(Somatropin) 1787
May interact with corticosteroids, glucocorticoids, insulin, phenytoin, sex steroids, and certain other agents. Compounds in these categories include:

ACTH (Excessive glucocorticoid therapy will inhibit the growth promoting effect of somatropin; growth hormone administration may alter the clearance of compounds known to be metabolized by cytochrome P450 liver enzymes; such as corticosteroids).
No products indexed under this heading.

Betamethasone Acetate (Excessive glucocorticoid therapy will inhibit the growth promoting effect of somatropin; growth hormone administration may alter the clearance of compounds known to be metabolized by cytochrome P450 liver enzymes; such as corticosteroids).
No products indexed under this heading.

Betamethasone Sodium Phosphate (Excessive glucocorticoid therapy will inhibit the growth promoting effect of somatropin; growth hormone administration may alter the clearance of compounds known to be metabolized by cytochrome P450 liver enzymes; such as corticosteroids).
No products indexed under this heading.

Cortisone Acetate (Excessive glucocorticoid therapy will inhibit the growth promoting effect of somatropin; growth hormone administration may alter the clearance of compounds known to be metabolized by cytochrome P450 liver enzymes; such as corticosteroids).
No products indexed under this heading.

Cyclosporine (Growth hormone administration may alter the clearance of compounds known to be metabolized by cytochrome P450 liver enzymes, such as cyclosporine). Products include:
Gengraf Capsules 459
Neoral Oral Solution 2259
Neoral Soft Gelatin Capsules 2259
Restasis Ophthalmic Emulsion 575
Sandimmune 2275

Desogestrel (Growth hormone administration may alter the clearance of compounds known to be metabolized by cytochrome P450 liver enzymes, such as sex steroids). Products include:
Mircette Tablets 1066

Dexamethasone (Excessive glucocorticoid therapy will inhibit the growth promoting effect of somatropin; growth hormone administration may alter the clearance of compounds known to be metabolized by cytochrome P450 liver enzymes; such as corticosteroids). Products include:
Ciprodex Otic Suspension 559
Decadron Tablets 1951
TobraDex Ophthalmic Ointment 562
TobraDex Ophthalmic Suspension ... 563

Dexamethasone Acetate (Excessive glucocorticoid therapy will inhibit the growth promoting effect of somatropin; growth hormone administration may alter the clearance of compounds known to be metabolized by cytochrome P450 liver enzymes; such as corticosteroids).
No products indexed under this heading.

Dexamethasone Sodium Phosphate (Excessive glucocorticoid therapy will inhibit the growth promoting effect of somatropin; growth hormone administration may alter the clearance of compounds known to be metabolized by cytochrome P450 liver enzymes; such as corticosteroids).
No products indexed under this heading.

Estradiol (Growth hormone administration may alter the clearance of compounds known to be metabolized by cytochrome P450 liver enzymes, such as sex steroids). Products include:
Angeliq Tablets 762
Climara Transdermal System 771
Climara Pro Transdermal System 776
Estrasorb Topical Emulsion 1147
Estring Vaginal Ring 2635
Menostar Transdermal System 782
Vagifem Tablets 2334

Estrogens, Conjugated (Growth hormone administration may alter the clearance of compounds known to be metabolized by cytochrome P450 liver enzymes, such as sex steroids). Products include:
Premarin Intravenous 3442
Premarin Tablets 3446
Premarin Vaginal Cream 3452
Premphase Tablets 3456
Prempro Tablets 3456

Ethinyl Estradiol (Growth hormone administration may alter the clearance of compounds known to be metabolized by cytochrome P450 liver enzymes, such as sex steroids). Products include:
Mircette Tablets 1066
NuvaRing 2340
Ortho-Cyclen/Ortho Tri-Cyclen 2429
Ortho Evra Transdermal System 2417
Ortho Tri-Cyclen Lo Tablets 2436
Seasonique Tablets 1077
Yasmin 28 Tablets 796
Yaz Tablets 803

Ethynodiol Diacetate (Growth hormone administration may alter the clearance of compounds known to be metabolized by cytochrome P450 liver enzymes, such as sex steroids).
No products indexed under this heading.

Fludrocortisone Acetate (Excessive glucocorticoid therapy will inhibit the growth promoting effect of somatropin; growth hormone administration may alter the clearance of compounds known to be metabolized by cytochrome P450 liver enzymes; such as corticosteroids).
No products indexed under this heading.

Fluoxymesterone (Growth hormone administration may alter the clearance of compounds known to be metabolized by cytochrome P450 liver enzymes, such as sex steroids). Products include:
Androxy Tablets 3335

Fosphenytoin Sodium (Growth hormone administration may alter the clearance of compounds known to be metabolized by CYP450 liver enzymes, such as anticonvulsants).
No products indexed under this heading.

Hydrocortisone (Excessive glucocorticoid therapy will inhibit the growth promoting effect of somatropin; growth hormone administration may alter the clearance of compounds known to be metabolized by cytochrome P450 liver enzymes; such as corticosteroids). Products include:
Colocort Rectal Suspension, USP (Retention) 100 mg/60 mL 2476
Hydrocortone Tablets 1989
Preparation H Hydrocortisone Cream 646

Hydrocortisone Acetate (Excessive glucocorticoid therapy will inhibit the growth promoting effect of somatropin; growth hormone administration may alter the clearance of compounds known to be metabolized by cytochrome P450 liver enzymes; such as corticosteroids). Products include:
Analpram-HC 1159
Pramosone 1161
ProctoFoam-HC 3099

Hydrocortisone Sodium Phosphate (Excessive glucocorticoid therapy will inhibit the growth promoting effect of somatropin; growth hormone administration may alter the clearance of compounds known to be metabolized by cytochrome P450 liver enzymes; such as corticosteroids).
No products indexed under this heading.

Hydrocortisone Sodium Succinate (Excessive glucocorticoid therapy will inhibit the growth promoting effect of somatropin; growth hormone administration may alter the clearance of compounds known to be metabolized by cytochrome P450 liver enzymes; such as corticosteroids).
No products indexed under this heading.

Insulin, Human, Zinc Suspension (For diabetics, the insulin dose may require adjustment when somatropin therapy is instituted; growth hormone may induce a state of insulin resistance; patients should be observed for evidence of glucose intolerance). Products include:
Humulin L, 100 Units 1794
Humulin U, 100 Units 1800

Insulin, Human NPH (For diabetics, the insulin dose may require adjustment when somatropin therapy is instituted; growth hormone may induce a state of insulin resistance; patients should be observed for evidence of glucose intolerance). Products include:
Humulin N, 100 Units 1795
Humulin N Pen 1797

Insulin, Human Regular (For diabetics, the insulin dose may require adjustment when somatropin therapy is instituted; growth hormone may induce a state of insulin resistance; patients should be observed for evidence of glucose intolerance). Products include:
Humulin R, 100 Units 1798

Insulin, Human Regular and Human NPH Mixture (For diabetics, the insulin dose may require adjustment when somatropin therapy is instituted; growth hormone may induce a state of insulin resistance; patients should be observed for evidence of glucose intolerance). Products include:
Humulin 50/50, 100 Units 1791
Humulin 70/30 Pen 1793

Insulin, NPH (For diabetics, the insulin dose may require adjustment when somatropin therapy is instituted; growth hormone may induce a state of insulin resistance; patients should be observed for evidence of glucose intolerance).
No products indexed under this heading.

Insulin, Regular (For diabetics, the insulin dose may require adjustment when somatropin therapy is instituted; growth hormone may induce a state of insulin resistance; patients should be observed for evidence of glucose intolerance).
No products indexed under this heading.

Insulin, Zinc Crystals (For diabetics, the insulin dose may require adjustment when somatropin therapy is instituted; growth hormone may induce a state of insulin resistance; patients should be observed for evidence of glucose intolerance).
No products indexed under this heading.

Insulin, Zinc Suspension (For diabetics, the insulin dose may require adjustment when somatropin therapy is instituted; growth hormone may induce a state of insulin resistance; patients should be observed for evidence of glucose intolerance).
No products indexed under this heading.

Insulin Aspart, Human Regular (For diabetics, the insulin dose may require adjustment when somatropin therapy is instituted; growth hormone may induce a state of insulin resistance; patients should be observed for evidence of glucose intolerance). Products include:
NovoLog Injection 2326

Insulin glargine (For diabetics, the insulin dose may require adjustment when somatropin therapy is instituted; growth hormone may induce a state of insulin resistance; patients should be observed for evidence of glucose intolerance). Products include:
Lantus Injection 2909

Insulin Lispro, Human (For diabetics, the insulin dose may require adjustment when somatropin therapy is instituted; growth hormone may induce a state of insulin resistance; patients should be observed for evidence of glucose intolerance). Products include:
Humalog-Pen 1781
Humalog Mix 50/50-Pen 1783
Humalog Mix 75/25-Pen 1785

Insulin Lispro Protamine, Human (For diabetics, the insulin dose may require adjustment when somatropin therapy is instituted; growth hormone may induce a state of insulin resistance; patients should be observed for evidence of glucose intolerance). Products include:
Humalog Mix 50/50-Pen 1783
Humalog Mix 75/25-Pen 1785

Levonorgestrel (Growth hormone administration may alter the clearance of compounds known to be metabolized by cytochrome P450 liver enzymes, such as sex steroids). Products include:

- Climara Pro Transdermal System 776
- Mirena Intrauterine System 787
- Plan B Tablets 1076
- Seasonique Tablets 1077

Mestranol (Growth hormone administration may alter the clearance of compounds known to be metabolized by cytochrome P450 liver enzymes, such as sex steroids).

No products indexed under this heading.

Methylprednisolone Acetate (Excessive glucocorticoid therapy will inhibit the growth promoting effect of somatropin; growth hormone administration may alter the clearance of compounds known to be metabolized by cytochrome P450 liver enzymes; such as corticosteroids). Products include:

- Depo-Medrol Injectable Suspension 2617
- Depo-Medrol Single-Dose Vial 2619

Methylprednisolone Sodium Succinate (Excessive glucocorticoid therapy will inhibit the growth promoting effect of somatropin; growth hormone administration may alter the clearance of compounds known to be metabolized by cytochrome P450 liver enzymes; such as corticosteroids).

No products indexed under this heading.

Methyltestosterone (Growth hormone administration may alter the clearance of compounds known to be metabolized by cytochrome P450 liver enzymes, such as sex steroids). Products include:

- Estratest Tablets 3199
- Estratest H.S. Tablets 3199

Norethindrone (Growth hormone administration may alter the clearance of compounds known to be metabolized by cytochrome P450 liver enzymes, such as sex steroids). Products include:

- Ortho Micronor Tablets 2426

Norethindrone Acetate (Growth hormone administration may alter the clearance of compounds known to be metabolized by cytochrome P450 liver enzymes, such as sex steroids).

No products indexed under this heading.

Norgestimate (Growth hormone administration may alter the clearance of compounds known to be metabolized by cytochrome P450 liver enzymes, such as sex steroids). Products include:

- Ortho-Cyclen/Ortho Tri-Cyclen 2429
- Ortho Tri-Cyclen Lo Tablets 2436

Phenobarbital (Growth hormone administration may alter the clearance of compounds known to be metabolized by CYP450 liver enzymes, such as anticonvulsants). Products include:

- Donnatal Extentabs 2493

Phenytoin (Growth hormone administration may alter the clearance of compounds known to be metabolized by CYP450 liver enzymes, such as anticonvulsants).

No products indexed under this heading.

Phenytoin Sodium (Growth hormone administration may alter the clearance of compounds known to be metabolized by CYP450 liver enzymes, such as anticonvulsants). Products include:

- Phenytek Capsules 2160

Prednisolone Acetate (Excessive glucocorticoid therapy will inhibit the growth promoting effect of somatropin; growth hormone administration may alter the clearance of compounds known to be metabolized by cytochrome P450 liver enzymes; such as corticosteroids). Products include:

- Blephamide Ophthalmic Ointment 568
- Blephamide Ophthalmic Suspension................................ 569
- Poly-Pred Ophthalmic Suspension .... ⊙233
- Pred Forte Ophthalmic Suspension .... ⊙235
- Pred Mild Ophthalmic Suspension .... ⊙238
- Pred-G Ophthalmic Ointment .... ⊙237
- Pred-G Ophthalmic Suspension ...... ⊙236

Prednisolone Sodium Phosphate (Excessive glucocorticoid therapy will inhibit the growth promoting effect of somatropin; growth hormone administration may alter the clearance of compounds known to be metabolized by cytochrome P450 liver enzymes; such as corticosteroids).

No products indexed under this heading.

Prednisolone Tebutate (Excessive glucocorticoid therapy will inhibit the growth promoting effect of somatropin; growth hormone administration may alter the clearance of compounds known to be metabolized by cytochrome P450 liver enzymes; such as corticosteroids).

No products indexed under this heading.

Prednisone (Excessive glucocorticoid therapy will inhibit the growth promoting effect of somatropin; growth hormone administration may alter the clearance of compounds known to be metabolized by cytochrome P450 liver enzymes; such as corticosteroids).

No products indexed under this heading.

Testosterone (Growth hormone administration may alter the clearance of compounds known to be metabolized by cytochrome P450 liver enzymes, such as sex steroids). Products include:

- AndroGel 3329
- Striant Mucoadhesive 1007
- Testim 1% Gel 695

Triamcinolone (Excessive glucocorticoid therapy will inhibit the growth promoting effect of somatropin; growth hormone administration may alter the clearance of compounds known to be metabolized by cytochrome P450 liver enzymes; such as corticosteroids).

No products indexed under this heading.

Triamcinolone Acetonide (Excessive glucocorticoid therapy will inhibit the growth promoting effect of somatropin; growth hormone administration may alter the clearance of compounds known to be metabolized by cytochrome P450 liver enzymes; such as corticosteroids). Products include:

- Azmacort Inhalation Aerosol 1726
- Nasacort AQ Nasal Spray 2922

Triamcinolone Diacetate (Excessive glucocorticoid therapy will inhibit the growth promoting effect of somatropin; growth hormone administration may alter the clearance of compounds known to be metabolized by cytochrome P450 liver enzymes; such as corticosteroids).

No products indexed under this heading.

Triamcinolone Hexacetonide (Excessive glucocorticoid therapy will inhibit the growth promoting effect of somatropin; growth hormone administration may alter the clearance of compounds known to be metabolized by cytochrome P450 liver enzymes; such as corticosteroids).

No products indexed under this heading.

HUMIBID EXTENDED-RELEASE BI-LAYER TABLETS

(Guaifenesin) .... ▣720
None cited in PDR database.

HUMIRA INJECTION

(Adalimumab) 466
May interact with:

Anakinra (Concurrent administration of anakinra (an interleukin-1 antagonist) and another TNF-blocking agent has been associated with an increased risk of serious infections, an increased risk of neutropenia and no additional benefit compared to these medicinal agents alone. Therefore, the combination of anakinra with other TNF-blocking agents, including adalimumab, may also result in similar toxicities). Products include:

- Kineret Injection 599

Methotrexate (Methotrexate reduced adalimumab apparent clearance after single and multiple dosing by 29% and 44% respectively).

No products indexed under this heading.

Vaccines (Live) (Live vaccines should not be given concurrently with Humira).

No products indexed under this heading.

HUMULIN 50/50, 100 UNITS

(Insulin, Human Regular and Human NPH Mixture)........................... 1791
See Humulin N Pen

HUMULIN 70/30 PEN

(Insulin, Human Regular and Human NPH Mixture)........................... 1793
See Humulin N Pen

HUMULIN L, 100 UNITS

(Insulin, Human, Zinc Suspension) 1794
See Humulin N Pen

HUMULIN N, 100 UNITS

(Insulin, Human NPH) 1795
See Humulin N Pen

HUMULIN N PEN

(Insulin, Human NPH) 1797
May interact with corticosteroids, oral hypoglycemic agents, oral contraceptives, salicylates, thyroid preparations, and certain other agents. Compounds in these categories include:

Acarbose (Co-administration with drugs with hypoglycemic activity, such as oral hypoglycemic agents, may result in decreased insulin requirements). Products include:

- Precose Tablets 751

Aspirin (Co-administration with drugs with hypoglycemic activity, such as salicylates, may result in decreased insulin requirements). Products include:

- Aggrenox Capsules 822
- Bayer Aspirin 744
- BC Allergy Sinus Cold Powder .... ▣677
- BC Headache Powder .... ▣677
- Arthritis Strength BC Powder .... ▣677
- BC Sinus Cold Powder .... ▣677
- Excedrin Extra Strength Caplets/Tablets/Geltabs............ ▣684
- Excedrin Migraine Caplets/Tablets/Geltabs............ ▣609
- Goody's Body Pain Formula Powder.. ▣684
- Goody's Extra Strength Headache Powders.......................... ▣611
- Goody's Extra Strength Pain Relief Tablets .... ▣685
- Percodan Tablets 1132
- St. Joseph 81 mg Aspirin Chewable and Enteric Coated Tablets 1869

Aspirin, Enteric Coated (Co-administration with drugs with hypoglycemic activity, such as salicylates, may result in decreased insulin requirements).

No products indexed under this heading.

Aspirin Buffered (Co-administration with drugs with hypoglycemic activity, such as salicylates, may result in decreased insulin requirements). Products include:

- Bufferin Extra Strength Tablets ...... ▣678
- Bufferin Regular Strength Tablets ... ▣678

Betamethasone Acetate (Co-administration may result in increased insulin requirements).

No products indexed under this heading.

Betamethasone Sodium Phosphate (Co-administration may result in increased insulin requirements).

No products indexed under this heading.

Chlorpropamide (Co-administration with drugs with hypoglycemic activity, such as oral hypoglycemic agents, may result in decreased insulin requirements).

No products indexed under this heading.

Choline Magnesium Trisalicylate (Co-administration with drugs with hypoglycemic activity, such as salicylates, may result in decreased insulin requirements).

No products indexed under this heading.

Cortisone Acetate (Co-administration may result in increased insulin requirements).

No products indexed under this heading.

Desogestrel (Co-administration with oral contraceptives may result in increased insulin requirements). Products include:

- Mircette Tablets 1066

Dexamethasone (Co-administration may result in increased insulin requirements). Products include:

- Ciprodex Otic Suspension 559
- Decadron Tablets 1951
- TobraDex Ophthalmic Ointment 562
- TobraDex Ophthalmic Suspension ... 563

Dexamethasone Acetate (Co-administration may result in increased insulin requirements).

No products indexed under this heading.

Dexamethasone Sodium Phosphate (Co-administration may result in increased insulin requirements).

No products indexed under this heading.

Diflunisal (Co-administration with drugs with hypoglycemic activity, such as salicylates, may result in decreased insulin requirements). Products include:

Dolobid Tablets 1955

Ethinyl Estradiol (Co-administration with oral contraceptives may result in increased insulin requirements). Products include:

Mircette Tablets 1066
NuvaRing 2340
Ortho-Cyclen/Ortho Tri-Cyclen 2429
Ortho Evra Transdermal System 2417
Ortho Tri-Cyclen Lo Tablets 2436
Seasonique Tablets 1077
Yasmin 28 Tablets 796
Yaz Tablets 803

Ethynodiol Diacetate (Co-administration with oral contraceptives may result in increased insulin requirements).

No products indexed under this heading.

Fludrocortisone Acetate (Co-administration may result in increased insulin requirements).

No products indexed under this heading.

Glimepiride (Co-administration with drugs with hypoglycemic activity, such as oral hypoglycemic agents, may result in decreased insulin requirements). Products include:

Avandaryl Tablets 1379
Duetact Tablets 3226

Glipizide (Co-administration with drugs with hypoglycemic activity, such as oral hypoglycemic agents, may result in decreased insulin requirements).

No products indexed under this heading.

Glyburide (Co-administration with drugs with hypoglycemic activity, such as oral hypoglycemic agents, may result in decreased insulin requirements).

No products indexed under this heading.

Hydrocortisone (Co-administration may result in increased insulin requirements). Products include:

Colocort Rectal Suspension, USP (Retention) 100 mg/60 mL 2476
Hydrocortone Tablets 1989
Preparation H Hydrocortisone Cream ▣646

Hydrocortisone Acetate (Co-administration may result in increased insulin requirements). Products include:

Analpram-HC 1159
Pramosone 1161
ProctoFoam-HC 3099

Hydrocortisone Sodium Phosphate (Co-administration may result in increased insulin requirements).

No products indexed under this heading.

Hydrocortisone Sodium Succinate (Co-administration may result in increased insulin requirements).

No products indexed under this heading.

Levonorgestrel (Co-administration with oral contraceptives may result in increased insulin requirements). Products include:

Climara Pro Transdermal System 776
Mirena Intrauterine System.............. 787
Plan B Tablets 1076
Seasonique Tablets 1077

Levothyroxine Sodium (Co-administration with thyroid replacement therapy may result in increased insulin requirements). Products include:

Levothroid Tablets 1186
Levoxyl Tablets 1712
Synthroid Tablets 520
Westhroid Tablets 3403

Liothyronine Sodium (Co-administration with thyroid replacement therapy may result in increased insulin requirements). Products include:

Cytomel Tablets 1710
Westhroid Tablets 3403

Liotrix (Co-administration with thyroid replacement therapy may result in increased insulin requirements). Products include:

Thyrolar Tablets 1199

Magnesium Salicylate (Co-administration with drugs with hypoglycemic activity, such as salicylates, may result in decreased insulin requirements).

No products indexed under this heading.

Mestranol (Co-administration with oral contraceptives may result in increased insulin requirements).

No products indexed under this heading.

Metformin Hydrochloride (Co-administration with drugs with hypoglycemic activity, such as oral hypoglycemic agents, may result in decreased insulin requirements). Products include:

ActoPlus Met Tablets 3214
Avandamet Tablets 1373
Fortamet Extended-Release Tablets 3115

Methylprednisolone Acetate (Co-administration may result in increased insulin requirements). Products include:

Depo-Medrol Injectable Suspension 2617
Depo-Medrol Single-Dose Vial 2619

Methylprednisolone Sodium Succinate (Co-administration may result in increased insulin requirements).

No products indexed under this heading.

Miglitol (Co-administration with drugs with hypoglycemic activity, such as oral hypoglycemic agents, may result in decreased insulin requirements).

No products indexed under this heading.

Norethindrone (Co-administration with oral contraceptives may result in increased insulin requirements). Products include:

Ortho Micronor Tablets 2426

Norethynodrel (Co-administration with oral contraceptives may result in increased insulin requirements).

No products indexed under this heading.

Norgestimate (Co-administration with oral contraceptives may result in increased insulin requirements). Products include:

Ortho-Cyclen/Ortho Tri-Cyclen 2429
Ortho Tri-Cyclen Lo Tablets 2436

Norgestrel (Co-administration with oral contraceptives may result in increased insulin requirements).

No products indexed under this heading.

Phenelzine Sulfate (Co-administration with drugs with hypoglycemic activity, such as certain MAO inhibitor antidepressants, may result in decreased insulin requirements).

No products indexed under this heading.

Pioglitazone Hydrochloride (Co-administration with drugs with hypoglycemic activity, such as oral hypoglycemic agents, may result in decreased insulin requirements). Products include:

ActoPlus Met Tablets 3214
Actos Tablets 3219
Duetact Tablets 3226

Prednisolone Acetate (Co-administration may result in increased insulin requirements). Products include:

Blephamide Ophthalmic Ointment 568
Blephamide Ophthalmic Suspension................................. 569
Poly-Pred Ophthalmic Suspension............................ ⊙233
Pred Forte Ophthalmic Suspension............................ ⊙235
Pred Mild Ophthalmic Suspension............................ ⊙238
Pred-G Ophthalmic Ointment ⊙237
Pred-G Ophthalmic Suspension ⊙236

Prednisolone Sodium Phosphate (Co-administration may result in increased insulin requirements).

No products indexed under this heading.

Prednisolone Tebutate (Co-administration may result in increased insulin requirements).

No products indexed under this heading.

Prednisone (Co-administration may result in increased insulin requirements).

No products indexed under this heading.

Repaglinide (Co-administration with drugs with hypoglycemic activity, such as oral hypoglycemic agents, may result in decreased insulin requirements).

No products indexed under this heading.

Rosiglitazone Maleate (Co-administration with drugs with hypoglycemic activity, such as oral hypoglycemic agents, may result in decreased insulin requirements). Products include:

Avandamet Tablets 1373
Avandaryl Tablets 1379
Avandia Tablets 1384

Salsalate (Co-administration with drugs with hypoglycemic activity, such as salicylates, may result in decreased insulin requirements).

No products indexed under this heading.

Sulfacytine (Co-administration with drugs with hypoglycemic activity, such as sulfa antibiotics, may result in decreased insulin requirements).

No products indexed under this heading.

Sulfamethizole (Co-administration with drugs with hypoglycemic activity, such as sulfa antibiotics, may result in decreased insulin requirements).

No products indexed under this heading.

Sulfamethoxazole (Co-administration with drugs with hypoglycemic activity, such as sulfa antibiotics, may result in decreased insulin requirements).

No products indexed under this heading.

Sulfasalazine (Co-administration with drugs with hypoglycemic activity, such as sulfa antibiotics, may result in decreased insulin requirements).

No products indexed under this heading.

Thyroglobulin (Co-administration with thyroid replacement therapy may result in increased insulin requirements).

No products indexed under this heading.

Thyroid (Co-administration with thyroid replacement therapy may result in increased insulin requirements).

No products indexed under this heading.

Thyroxine (Co-administration with thyroid replacement therapy may result in increased insulin requirements).

No products indexed under this heading.

Thyroxine Sodium (Co-administration with thyroid replacement therapy may result in increased insulin requirements).

No products indexed under this heading.

Tolazamide (Co-administration with drugs with hypoglycemic activity, such as oral hypoglycemic agents, may result in decreased insulin requirements).

No products indexed under this heading.

Tolbutamide (Co-administration with drugs with hypoglycemic activity, such as oral hypoglycemic agents, may result in decreased insulin requirements).

No products indexed under this heading.

Tranylcypromine Sulfate (Co-administration with drugs with hypoglycemic activity, such as certain MAO inhibitor antidepressants, may result in decreased insulin requirements). Products include:

Parnate Tablets 1527

Triamcinolone (Co-administration may result in increased insulin requirements).

No products indexed under this heading.

Triamcinolone Acetonide (Co-administration may result in increased insulin requirements). Products include:

Azmacort Inhalation Aerosol 1726
Nasacort AQ Nasal Spray 2922

Triamcinolone Diacetate (Co-administration may result in increased insulin requirements).

No products indexed under this heading.

Triamcinolone Hexacetonide (Co-administration may result in increased insulin requirements).

No products indexed under this heading.

Troglitazone (Co-administration with drugs with hypoglycemic activity, such as oral hypoglycemic agents, may result in decreased insulin requirements).

No products indexed under this heading.

IMPORTANT NOTE: Always consult each drug listing in the patient's regimen for possible interactions.

HUMULIN R, 100 UNITS

(Insulin, Human Regular) 1798

May interact with oral hypoglycemic agents. Compounds in these categories include:

Acarbose (The concurrent use of oral hypoglycemic agents with regular human insulin is not recommended). Products include:

Precose Tablets 751

Chlorpropamide (The concurrent use of oral hypoglycemic agents with regular human insulin is not recommended).

No products indexed under this heading.

Glimepiride (The concurrent use of oral hypoglycemic agents with regular human insulin is not recommended). Products include:

Avandaryl Tablets 1379
Duetact Tablets 3226

Glipizide (The concurrent use of oral hypoglycemic agents with regular human insulin is not recommended).

No products indexed under this heading.

Glyburide (The concurrent use of oral hypoglycemic agents with regular human insulin is not recommended).

No products indexed under this heading.

Metformin Hydrochloride (The concurrent use of oral hypoglycemic agents with regular human insulin is not recommended). Products include:

ActoPlus Met Tablets 3214
Avandamet Tablets 1373
Fortamet Extended-Release Tablets 3115

Miglitol (The concurrent use of oral hypoglycemic agents with regular human insulin is not recommended).

No products indexed under this heading.

Pioglitazone Hydrochloride (The concurrent use of oral hypoglycemic agents with regular human insulin is not recommended). Products include:

ActoPlus Met Tablets 3214
Actos Tablets 3219
Duetact Tablets 3226

Repaglinide (The concurrent use of oral hypoglycemic agents with regular human insulin is not recommended).

No products indexed under this heading.

Rosiglitazone Maleate (The concurrent use of oral hypoglycemic agents with regular human insulin is not recommended). Products include:

Avandamet Tablets 1373
Avandaryl Tablets 1379
Avandia Tablets 1384

Tolazamide (The concurrent use of oral hypoglycemic agents with regular human insulin is not recommended).

No products indexed under this heading.

Tolbutamide (The concurrent use of oral hypoglycemic agents with regular human insulin is not recommended).

No products indexed under this heading.

Troglitazone (The concurrent use of oral hypoglycemic agents with regular human insulin is not recommended).

No products indexed under this heading.

HUMULIN U, 100 UNITS

(Insulin, Human, Zinc Suspension) 1800
See Humulin N Pen

HURRICAINE TOPICAL ANESTHETIC GEL, 1 OZ. WILD CHERRY, PINA COLADA, WATERMELON, AND FRESH MINT, 5.25 G. WILD CHERRY

(Benzocaine) .... ▣712
None cited in PDR database.

HURRICAINE TOPICAL ANESTHETIC LIQUID, 1 OZ. WILD CHERRY, PINA COLADA, 0.005 FL. OZ. SNAP-N-GO SWABS WILD CHERRY

(Benzocaine) .... ▣712
None cited in PDR database.

HURRICAINE TOPICAL ANESTHETIC SPRAY EXTENSION TUBES (200)

(Benzocaine) .... ▣712
None cited in PDR database.

HURRICAINE TOPICAL ANESTHETIC SPRAY KIT, 2 OZ. WILD CHERRY WITH DISPOSABLE EXTENSION TUBES (200)

(Benzocaine) .... ▣712
None cited in PDR database.

HURRICAINE TOPICAL ANESTHETIC SPRAY, 2 OZ. WILD CHERRY

(Benzocaine) .... ▣712
None cited in PDR database.

HYALGAN SOLUTION

(Sodium Hyaluronate) 2901
None cited in PDR database.

HYCAMTIN FOR INJECTION

(Topotecan Hydrochloride) 1458

May interact with cytotoxic drugs and certain other agents. Compounds in these categories include:

Bleomycin Sulfate (Greater myelosuppression is also likely to be seen when Hycamtin is used in combination with other cytotoxic agents, thereby necessitating a dose reduction).

No products indexed under this heading.

Carboplatin (Greater myelosuppression is likely to be seen when topotecan hydrochloride is used in combination with other cytotoxic agents, thereby necessitating a dose reduction. However, when combining topotecan hydrochloride with platinum agents (eg, carboplatin),a distinct sequence dependent interaction on myelosuppression has been reported).

No products indexed under this heading.

Cisplatin (Co-administration has resulted in severe myelosuppression; a case of neutropenia and fatal neutropenic sepsis has been reported).

No products indexed under this heading.

Cyclophosphamide (Greater myelosuppression is also likely to be seen when Hycamtin is used in combination with other cytotoxic agents, thereby necessitating a dose reduction).

No products indexed under this heading.

Daunorubicin Hydrochloride (Greater myelosuppression is also likely to be seen when Hycamtin is used in combination with other cytotoxic agents, thereby necessitating a dose reduction).

No products indexed under this heading.

Doxorubicin Hydrochloride (Greater myelosuppression is also likely to be seen when Hycamtin is used in combination with other cytotoxic agents, thereby necessitating a dose reduction).

No products indexed under this heading.

Epirubicin Hydrochloride (Greater myelosuppression is also likely to be seen when Hycamtin is used in combination with other cytotoxic agents, thereby necessitating a dose reduction).

No products indexed under this heading.

Filgrastim (Concomitant administration of granulocyte colony stimulating factor (G-CSF) can prolong the duration of neutropenia, so if G-CSF is to be used, it should not be initiated until day 6 of the course of therapy, 24 hours after completion of treatment with topotecan hydrochloride). Products include:

Neupogen for Injection 603

Fluorouracil (Greater myelosuppression is also likely to be seen when Hycamtin is used in combination with other cytotoxic agents, thereby necessitating a dose reduction). Products include:

Carac Cream, 0.5% 2879
Efudex 3363

Hydroxyurea (Greater myelosuppression is also likely to be seen when Hycamtin is used in combination with other cytotoxic agents, thereby necessitating a dose reduction).

No products indexed under this heading.

Methotrexate Sodium (Greater myelosuppression is also likely to be seen when Hycamtin is used in combination with other cytotoxic agents, thereby necessitating a dose reduction).

No products indexed under this heading.

Mitotane (Greater myelosuppression is also likely to be seen when Hycamtin is used in combination with other cytotoxic agents, thereby necessitating a dose reduction).

No products indexed under this heading.

Mitoxantrone Hydrochloride (Greater myelosuppression is also likely to be seen when Hycamtin is used in combination with other cytotoxic agents, thereby necessitating a dose reduction).

No products indexed under this heading.

Procarbazine Hydrochloride (Greater myelosuppression is also likely to be seen when Hycamtin is used in combination with other cytotoxic agents, thereby necessitating a dose reduction). Products include:

Matulane Capsules 3191

Tamoxifen Citrate (Greater myelosuppression is also likely to be seen when Hycamtin is used in combination with other cytotoxic agents, thereby necessitating a dose reduction). Products include:

Soltamox Oral Solution 3527

Vincristine Sulfate (Greater myelosuppression is also likely to be seen when Hycamtin is used in combination with other cytotoxic agents, thereby necessitating a dose reduction).

No products indexed under this heading.

HYCODAN SYRUP

(Homatropine Methylbromide, Hydrocodone Bitartrate).................... 1116
See Hycodan Tablets

HYCODAN TABLETS

(Homatropine Methylbromide, Hydrocodone Bitartrate).................... 1116

May interact with antihistamines, central nervous system depressants, monoamine oxidase inhibitors, narcotic analgesics, antipsychotic agents, tranquilizers, tricyclic antidepressants, and certain other agents. Compounds in these categories include:

Acrivastine (Exhibits an additive CNS depression).

No products indexed under this heading.

Alfentanil Hydrochloride (Exhibits an additive CNS depression).

No products indexed under this heading.

Alprazolam (Exhibits an additive CNS depression). Products include:

Niravam Orally Disintegrating Tablets 3092

Amitriptyline Hydrochloride (Increased effect of either the antidepressant or hydrocodone).

No products indexed under this heading.

Amoxapine (Increased effect of either the antidepressant or hydrocodone).

No products indexed under this heading.

Aprobarbital (Exhibits an additive CNS depression).

No products indexed under this heading.

Aripiprazole (Exhibits an additive CNS depression). Products include:

Abilify Oral Solution 882
Abilify Oral Solution 2450
Abilify Discmelt Orally Disintegrating Tablets.................. 882
Abilify Discmelt Orally Disintegrating Tablets.................. 2450
Abilify Tablets 882
Abilify Tablets 2450

Astemizole (Exhibits an additive CNS depression).

No products indexed under this heading.

Azatadine Maleate (Exhibits an additive CNS depression).
No products indexed under this heading.

Bromodiphenhydramine Hydrochloride (Exhibits an additive CNS depression).
No products indexed under this heading.

Brompheniramine Maleate (Exhibits an additive CNS depression). Products include:
Children's Dimetapp Cold & Allergy Elixir 730
Children's Dimetapp Cold & Allergy Chewable Tablets 730
Children's Dimetapp DM Cold & Cough Elixir 731

Buprenorphine Hydrochloride (Exhibits an additive CNS depression). Products include:
Buprenex Injectable 2716
Suboxone Tablets 2717
Subutex Tablets 2717

Buspirone Hydrochloride (Exhibits an additive CNS depression).
No products indexed under this heading.

Butabarbital (Exhibits an additive CNS depression).
No products indexed under this heading.

Butalbital (Exhibits an additive CNS depression).
No products indexed under this heading.

Cetirizine Hydrochloride (Exhibits an additive CNS depression). Products include:
Zyrtec Chewable Tablets 2594
Zyrtec 2594
Zyrtec-D 12 Hour Extended Release Tablets 2597

Chlordiazepoxide (Exhibits an additive CNS depression).
No products indexed under this heading.

Chlordiazepoxide Hydrochloride (Exhibits an additive CNS depression). Products include:
Librium Capsules 3347

Chlorpheniramine Maleate (Exhibits an additive CNS depression). Products include:
Advil Allergy Sinus Caplets 770
Advil Multi-Symptom Cold Caplets 770
BC Allergy Sinus Cold Powder 677
Comtrex Maximum Strength Cold & Cough Day/Night Caplets - Night Formulation 726
Comtrex Maximum Strength Day/Night Severe Cold & Sinus Caplets - Night Formulation 725
Contac Cold and Flu Maximum Strength Caplets 728
Contac Cold and Flu Day and Night Caplets (Night Formulation Only) 727
Children's Dimetapp Long Acting Cough Plus Cold Syrup 731
Robitussin Cough & Cold Long-Acting Liquid 735
Robitussin Cough & Allergy Syrup .. 736
Robitussin Cough & Cold Nighttime Liquid 736
Robitussin Cough, Cold & Flu Nighttime Liquid 738
Robitussin Pediatric Cough & Cold Long-Acting Liquid 735
Robitussin Pediatric Cough & Cold Nighttime Liquid 736
Triaminic Cold & Allergy Liquid 746
Triaminic Cough & Runny Nose Softchews 748
Children's Tylenol Plus Flu Oral Suspension 749
Tylenol Allergy Multi-Symptom Caplets with Cool Burst and Gelcaps 1872
Children's Tylenol Plus Cold Suspension Liquid 1879
Children's Tylenol Plus Cough & Runny Nose Suspension Liquid 1879
Children's Tylenol Plus Flu Suspension Liquid 1881
Children's Tylenol Plus Multi-Symptom Cold Suspension Liquid 1879
Tylenol Cold Head Congestion Nighttime Caplets with Cool Burst 1873
Tylenol Cold Multi-Symptom Nighttime Caplets with Cool Burst 1874
Tylenol Sinus Congestion & Pain Nighttime Caplets with Cool Burst 1876
Vicks 44M Cough, Cold & Flu Relief Liquid 2680
Pediatric Vicks 44m Cough & Cold Relief Liquid 2676
Children's Vicks NyQuil Cold/Cough Relief 756
Children's Vicks NyQuil Cold/Cough Relief Liquid 2680
Zicam Maximum Strength Flu Daytime 768

Chlorpheniramine Polistirex (Exhibits an additive CNS depression). Products include:
Tussionex Pennkinetic Extended-Release Suspension 3327

Chlorpheniramine Tannate (Exhibits an additive CNS depression).
No products indexed under this heading.

Chlorpromazine (Exhibits an additive CNS depression).
No products indexed under this heading.

Chlorpromazine Hydrochloride (Exhibits an additive CNS depression).
No products indexed under this heading.

Chlorprothixene (Exhibits an additive CNS depression).
No products indexed under this heading.

Chlorprothixene Hydrochloride (Exhibits an additive CNS depression).
No products indexed under this heading.

Chlorprothixene Lactate (Exhibits an additive CNS depression).
No products indexed under this heading.

Clemastine Fumarate (Exhibits an additive CNS depression).
No products indexed under this heading.

Clomipramine Hydrochloride (Increased effect of either the antidepressant or hydrocodone).
No products indexed under this heading.

Clorazepate Dipotassium (Exhibits an additive CNS depression). Products include:
Tranxene 2474

Clozapine (Exhibits an additive CNS depression). Products include:
Clozaril Tablets 2184
FazaClo Orally Disintegrating Tablets 551

Codeine Phosphate (Exhibits an additive CNS depression). Products include:
Tylenol with Codeine Tablets 2391

Cyproheptadine Hydrochloride (Exhibits an additive CNS depression).
No products indexed under this heading.

Desflurane (Exhibits an additive CNS depression).
No products indexed under this heading.

Desipramine Hydrochloride (Increased effect of either the antidepressant or hydrocodone).
No products indexed under this heading.

Dexchlorpheniramine Maleate (Exhibits an additive CNS depression).
No products indexed under this heading.

Dezocine (Exhibits an additive CNS depression).
No products indexed under this heading.

Diazepam (Exhibits an additive CNS depression). Products include:
Diastat Rectal Delivery System 3343
Valium Tablets 2819

Diphenhydramine Citrate (Exhibits an additive CNS depression). Products include:
Advil PM Caplets 615
Excedrin PM Caplets/Tablets/Geltabs 610
Goody's PM Powder for Pain with Sleeplessness 612

Diphenhydramine Hydrochloride (Exhibits an additive CNS depression). Products include:
Nytol QuickCaps Caplets 615
Nytol QuickGels Softgels Maximum Strength 616
Simply Sleep Caplets 1868
Sominex Original Formula Tablets .. 616
TheraFlu Warming Relief Nighttime Severe Cold 743
TheraFlu Thin Strips Multi Symptom 744
Triaminic Nighttime Cold & Cough Liquid 746
Triaminic Thin Strips Cough & Runny Nose 749
Extra Strength Tylenol PM Caplets, Vanilla Caplets, Geltabs, Gelcaps and Liquid 1875
Tylenol Sore Throat Nighttime Liquid with Cool Burst 790
Tylenol Allergy Multi-Symptom Nighttime Caplets with Cool Burst 1872
Tylenol Severe Allergy Caplets 1872
Children's Tylenol Plus Cold & Allergy Suspension Liquid 1878

Diphenylpyraline Hydrochloride (Exhibits an additive CNS depression).
No products indexed under this heading.

Doxepin Hydrochloride (Increased effect of either the antidepressant or hydrocodone).
No products indexed under this heading.

Droperidol (Exhibits an additive CNS depression).
No products indexed under this heading.

Enflurane (Exhibits an additive CNS depression).
No products indexed under this heading.

Estazolam (Exhibits an additive CNS depression). Products include:
ProSom Tablets 517

Ethanol (Exhibits an additive CNS depression).
No products indexed under this heading.

Ethchlorvynol (Exhibits an additive CNS depression).
No products indexed under this heading.

Ethinamate (Exhibits an additive CNS depression).
No products indexed under this heading.

Ethyl Alcohol (Exhibits an additive CNS depression).
No products indexed under this heading.

Fentanyl (Exhibits an additive CNS depression). Products include:
Duragesic Transdermal System 2373
Ionsys Transdermal System 2379

Fentanyl Citrate (Exhibits an additive CNS depression). Products include:
Actiq 979

Fexofenadine Hydrochloride (Exhibits an additive CNS depression). Products include:
Allegra 2844
Allegra-D 12 Hour Extended-Release Tablets 2846
Allegra-D 24 Hour Extended-Release Tablets 2849

Fluphenazine Decanoate (Exhibits an additive CNS depression).
No products indexed under this heading.

Fluphenazine Enanthate (Exhibits an additive CNS depression).
No products indexed under this heading.

Fluphenazine Hydrochloride (Exhibits an additive CNS depression).
No products indexed under this heading.

Flurazepam Hydrochloride (Exhibits an additive CNS depression). Products include:
Dalmane Capsules 3342

Glutethimide (Exhibits an additive CNS depression).
No products indexed under this heading.

Haloperidol (Exhibits an additive CNS depression).
No products indexed under this heading.

Haloperidol Decanoate (Exhibits an additive CNS depression).
No products indexed under this heading.

Hydrocodone Polistirex (Exhibits an additive CNS depression). Products include:
Tussionex Pennkinetic Extended-Release Suspension 3327

Hydromorphone Hydrochloride (Exhibits an additive CNS depression). Products include:
Dilaudid 440
Dilaudid Non-Sterile Powder 440
Dilaudid Oral Liquid 445
Dilaudid Rectal Suppositories 440
Dilaudid Tablets 440
Dilaudid Tablets - 8 mg 445
Dilaudid-HP 442

Hydroxyzine Hydrochloride (Exhibits an additive CNS depression).
No products indexed under this heading.

Imipramine Hydrochloride (Increased effect of either the antidepressant or hydrocodone).
No products indexed under this heading.

Imipramine Pamoate (Increased effect of either the antidepressant or hydrocodone).
No products indexed under this heading.

Isocarboxazid (May increase the effect of either MAO inhibitor or hydrocodone).
No products indexed under this heading.

Isoflurane (Exhibits an additive CNS depression).
No products indexed under this heading.

Ketamine Hydrochloride (Exhibits an additive CNS depression).
No products indexed under this heading.

Levomethadyl Acetate Hydrochloride (Exhibits an additive CNS depression).
No products indexed under this heading.

Levorphanol Tartrate (Exhibits an additive CNS depression).
No products indexed under this heading.

Lithium Carbonate (Exhibits an additive CNS depression). Products include:
Lithobid Tablets 1692

Lithium Citrate (Exhibits an additive CNS depression).
No products indexed under this heading.

Loratadine (Exhibits an additive CNS depression). Products include:
Alavert Allergy & Sinus D-12 Hour Tablets............................... ▣771
Alavert ▣771
Children's Claritin Allergy Oral Solution ▣771
Claritin Non-Drowsy 24 Hour Tablets............................... ▣772
Claritin Reditabs 24 Hour Non-Drowsy Tablets ▣772
Claritin-D Non-Drowsy 12 Hour Tablets............................... ▣772
Claritin-D Non-Drowsy 24 Hour Tablets............................... ▣772

Lorazepam (Exhibits an additive CNS depression).
No products indexed under this heading.

Loxapine Hydrochloride (Exhibits an additive CNS depression).
No products indexed under this heading.

Loxapine Succinate (Exhibits an additive CNS depression).
No products indexed under this heading.

Maprotiline Hydrochloride (Increased effect of either the antidepressant or hydrocodone).
No products indexed under this heading.

Meperidine Hydrochloride (Exhibits an additive CNS depression).
No products indexed under this heading.

Mephobarbital (Exhibits an additive CNS depression).
No products indexed under this heading.

Meprobamate (Exhibits an additive CNS depression).
No products indexed under this heading.

Mesoridazine Besylate (Exhibits an additive CNS depression).
No products indexed under this heading.

Methadone Hydrochloride (Exhibits an additive CNS depression).
No products indexed under this heading.

Methdilazine Hydrochloride (Exhibits an additive CNS depression).
No products indexed under this heading.

Methohexital Sodium (Exhibits an additive CNS depression).
No products indexed under this heading.

Methotrimeprazine (Exhibits an additive CNS depression).
No products indexed under this heading.

Methoxyflurane (Exhibits an additive CNS depression).
No products indexed under this heading.

Midazolam Hydrochloride (Exhibits an additive CNS depression).
No products indexed under this heading.

Moclobemide (May increase the effect of either MAO inhibitor or hydrocodone).
No products indexed under this heading.

Molindone Hydrochloride (Exhibits an additive CNS depression). Products include:
Moban Tablets 1119

Morphine Sulfate (Exhibits an additive CNS depression). Products include:
Avinza Capsules 1741
Kadian Capsules 577
MS Contin Tablets 2701

Nortriptyline Hydrochloride (Increased effect of either the antidepressant or hydrocodone).
No products indexed under this heading.

Olanzapine (Exhibits an additive CNS depression). Products include:
Symbyax Capsules 1819
Zyprexa Tablets 1830
Zyprexa IntraMuscular 1830
Zyprexa ZYDIS Orally Disintegrating Tablets 1830

Oxazepam (Exhibits an additive CNS depression).
No products indexed under this heading.

Oxycodone Hydrochloride (Exhibits an additive CNS depression). Products include:
OxyContin Tablets 2703
OxyFast Oral Concentrate Solution 2708
OxyIR Capsules 2708
Percocet Tablets 1131
Percodan Tablets 1132

Pargyline Hydrochloride (May increase the effect of either MAO inhibitor or hydrocodone).
No products indexed under this heading.

Pentobarbital Sodium (Exhibits an additive CNS depression). Products include:
Nembutal Sodium Solution, USP 2470

Perphenazine (Exhibits an additive CNS depression).
No products indexed under this heading.

Phenelzine Sulfate (May increase the effect of either MAO inhibitor or hydrocodone).
No products indexed under this heading.

Phenobarbital (Exhibits an additive CNS depression). Products include:
Donnatal Extentabs 2493

Pimozide (Exhibits an additive CNS depression).
No products indexed under this heading.

Prazepam (Exhibits an additive CNS depression).
No products indexed under this heading.

Procarbazine Hydrochloride (May increase the effect of either MAO inhibitor or hydrocodone). Products include:
Matulane Capsules 3191

Prochlorperazine (Exhibits an additive CNS depression).
No products indexed under this heading.

Promethazine Hydrochloride (Exhibits an additive CNS depression). Products include:
Phenergan Tablets and Suppositories.............................. 3440

Propofol (Exhibits an additive CNS depression).
No products indexed under this heading.

Propoxyphene Hydrochloride (Exhibits an additive CNS depression).
No products indexed under this heading.

Propoxyphene Napsylate (Exhibits an additive CNS depression).
No products indexed under this heading.

Protriptyline Hydrochloride (Increased effect of either the antidepressant or hydrocodone).
No products indexed under this heading.

Pyrilamine Maleate (Exhibits an additive CNS depression).
No products indexed under this heading.

Pyrilamine Tannate (Exhibits an additive CNS depression).
No products indexed under this heading.

Quazepam (Exhibits an additive CNS depression).
No products indexed under this heading.

Quetiapine Fumarate (Exhibits an additive CNS depression). Products include:
Seroquel Tablets 690

Remifentanil Hydrochloride (Exhibits an additive CNS depression).
No products indexed under this heading.

Risperidone (Exhibits an additive CNS depression). Products include:
Risperdal 1676
Risperdal Consta Long-Acting Injection 1682
Risperdal M-Tab Orally Disintegrating Tablets................... 1676

Secobarbital Sodium (Exhibits an additive CNS depression).
No products indexed under this heading.

Selegiline Hydrochloride (May increase the effect of either MAO inhibitor or hydrocodone). Products include:
Eldepryl Capsules 3208
Zelapar Tablets 3372

Sevoflurane (Exhibits an additive CNS depression). Products include:
Ultane Liquid for Inhalation 531

Sodium Oxybate (Exhibits an additive CNS depression). Products include:
Xyrem Oral Solution 1688

Sufentanil Citrate (Exhibits an additive CNS depression).
No products indexed under this heading.

Temazepam (Exhibits an additive CNS depression). Products include:
Restoril Capsules 1860

Terfenadine (Exhibits an additive CNS depression).
No products indexed under this heading.

Thiamylal Sodium (Exhibits an additive CNS depression).
No products indexed under this heading.

Thioridazine Hydrochloride (Exhibits an additive CNS depression). Products include:
Thioridazine Hydrochloride Tablets...................................... 2163

Thiothixene (Exhibits an additive CNS depression). Products include:
Thiothixene Capsules 2165

Tranylcypromine Sulfate (May increase the effect of either MAO inhibitor or hydrocodone). Products include:
Parnate Tablets 1527

Triazolam (Exhibits an additive CNS depression).
No products indexed under this heading.

Trifluoperazine Hydrochloride (Exhibits an additive CNS depression).
No products indexed under this heading.

Trimeprazine Tartrate (Exhibits an additive CNS depression).
No products indexed under this heading.

Trimipramine Maleate (Increased effect of either the antidepressant or hydrocodone).
No products indexed under this heading.

Tripelennamine Hydrochloride (Exhibits an additive CNS depression).
No products indexed under this heading.

Triprolidine Hydrochloride (Exhibits an additive CNS depression).
No products indexed under this heading.

Zaleplon (Exhibits an additive CNS depression). Products include:
Sonata Capsules 1717

Ziprasidone Hydrochloride (Exhibits an additive CNS depression). Products include:
Geodon Capsules 2529

Zolpidem Tartrate (Exhibits an additive CNS depression). Products include:
Ambien Tablets 2851
Ambien CR Tablets 2855

Food Interactions

Alcohol (Exhibits an additive CNS depression).

HYCOTUSS EXPECTORANT SYRUP
(Guaifenesin, Hydrocodone Bitartrate).. 1117
May interact with central nervous system depressants, narcotic analgesics, antipsychotic agents, tranquilizers, and certain other agents. Compounds in these categories include:

Alfentanil Hydrochloride (Exhibits an additive CNS depression).
No products indexed under this heading.

Alprazolam (Exhibits an additive CNS depression). Products include:
Niravam Orally Disintegrating Tablets..................................... 3092

Aprobarbital (Exhibits an additive CNS depression).
No products indexed under this heading.

Aripiprazole (Exhibits an additive CNS depression). Products include:
Abilify Oral Solution ... 882
Abilify Oral Solution ... 2450
Abilify Discmelt Orally Disintegrating Tablets ... 882
Abilify Discmelt Orally Disintegrating Tablets ... 2450
Abilify Tablets ... 882
Abilify Tablets ... 2450

Buprenorphine Hydrochloride (Exhibits an additive CNS depression). Products include:
Buprenex Injectable ... 2716
Suboxone Tablets ... 2717
Subutex Tablets ... 2717

Buspirone Hydrochloride (Exhibits an additive CNS depression).
No products indexed under this heading.

Butabarbital (Exhibits an additive CNS depression).
No products indexed under this heading.

Butalbital (Exhibits an additive CNS depression).
No products indexed under this heading.

Chlordiazepoxide (Exhibits an additive CNS depression).
No products indexed under this heading.

Chlordiazepoxide Hydrochloride (Exhibits an additive CNS depression). Products include:
Librium Capsules ... 3347

Chlorpromazine (Exhibits an additive CNS depression).
No products indexed under this heading.

Chlorpromazine Hydrochloride (Exhibits an additive CNS depression).
No products indexed under this heading.

Chlorprothixene (Exhibits an additive CNS depression).
No products indexed under this heading.

Chlorprothixene Hydrochloride (Exhibits an additive CNS depression).
No products indexed under this heading.

Chlorprothixene Lactate (Exhibits an additive CNS depression).
No products indexed under this heading.

Clorazepate Dipotassium (Exhibits an additive CNS depression). Products include:
Tranxene ... 2474

Clozapine (Exhibits an additive CNS depression). Products include:
Clozaril Tablets ... 2184
FazaClo Orally Disintegrating Tablets ... 551

Codeine Phosphate (Exhibits an additive CNS depression). Products include:
Tylenol with Codeine Tablets ... 2391

Desflurane (Exhibits an additive CNS depression).
No products indexed under this heading.

Dezocine (Exhibits an additive CNS depression).
No products indexed under this heading.

Diazepam (Exhibits an additive CNS depression). Products include:
Diastat Rectal Delivery System ... 3343
Valium Tablets ... 2819

Droperidol (Exhibits an additive CNS depression).
No products indexed under this heading.

Enflurane (Exhibits an additive CNS depression).
No products indexed under this heading.

Estazolam (Exhibits an additive CNS depression). Products include:
ProSom Tablets ... 517

Ethanol (Exhibits an additive CNS depression).
No products indexed under this heading.

Ethchlorvynol (Exhibits an additive CNS depression).
No products indexed under this heading.

Ethinamate (Exhibits an additive CNS depression).
No products indexed under this heading.

Ethyl Alcohol (Exhibits an additive CNS depression).
No products indexed under this heading.

Fentanyl (Exhibits an additive CNS depression). Products include:
Duragesic Transdermal System ... 2373
Ionsys Transdermal System ... 2379

Fentanyl Citrate (Exhibits an additive CNS depression). Products include:
Actiq ... 979

Fluphenazine Decanoate (Exhibits an additive CNS depression).
No products indexed under this heading.

Fluphenazine Enanthate (Exhibits an additive CNS depression).
No products indexed under this heading.

Fluphenazine Hydrochloride (Exhibits an additive CNS depression).
No products indexed under this heading.

Flurazepam Hydrochloride (Exhibits an additive CNS depression). Products include:
Dalmane Capsules ... 3342

Glutethimide (Exhibits an additive CNS depression).
No products indexed under this heading.

Haloperidol (Exhibits an additive CNS depression).
No products indexed under this heading.

Haloperidol Decanoate (Exhibits an additive CNS depression).
No products indexed under this heading.

Hydrocodone Polistirex (Exhibits an additive CNS depression). Products include:
Tussionex Pennkinetic Extended-Release Suspension ... 3327

Hydromorphone Hydrochloride (Exhibits an additive CNS depression). Products include:
Dilaudid ... 440
Dilaudid Non-Sterile Powder ... 440
Dilaudid Oral Liquid ... 445
Dilaudid Rectal Suppositories ... 440
Dilaudid Tablets ... 440
Dilaudid Tablets - 8 mg ... 445
Dilaudid-HP ... 442

Hydroxyzine Hydrochloride (Exhibits an additive CNS depression).
No products indexed under this heading.

Isoflurane (Exhibits an additive CNS depression).
No products indexed under this heading.

Ketamine Hydrochloride (Exhibits an additive CNS depression).
No products indexed under this heading.

Levomethadyl Acetate Hydrochloride (Exhibits an additive CNS depression).
No products indexed under this heading.

Levorphanol Tartrate (Exhibits an additive CNS depression).
No products indexed under this heading.

Lithium Carbonate (Exhibits an additive CNS depression). Products include:
Lithobid Tablets ... 1692

Lithium Citrate (Exhibits an additive CNS depression).
No products indexed under this heading.

Lorazepam (Exhibits an additive CNS depression).
No products indexed under this heading.

Loxapine Hydrochloride (Exhibits an additive CNS depression).
No products indexed under this heading.

Loxapine Succinate (Exhibits an additive CNS depression).
No products indexed under this heading.

Meperidine Hydrochloride (Exhibits an additive CNS depression).
No products indexed under this heading.

Mephobarbital (Exhibits an additive CNS depression).
No products indexed under this heading.

Meprobamate (Exhibits an additive CNS depression).
No products indexed under this heading.

Mesoridazine Besylate (Exhibits an additive CNS depression).
No products indexed under this heading.

Methadone Hydrochloride (Exhibits an additive CNS depression).
No products indexed under this heading.

Methohexital Sodium (Exhibits an additive CNS depression).
No products indexed under this heading.

Methotrimeprazine (Exhibits an additive CNS depression).
No products indexed under this heading.

Methoxyflurane (Exhibits an additive CNS depression).
No products indexed under this heading.

Midazolam Hydrochloride (Exhibits an additive CNS depression).
No products indexed under this heading.

Molindone Hydrochloride (Exhibits an additive CNS depression). Products include:
Moban Tablets ... 1119

Morphine Sulfate (Exhibits an additive CNS depression). Products include:
Avinza Capsules ... 1741
Kadian Capsules ... 577
MS Contin Tablets ... 2701

Olanzapine (Exhibits an additive CNS depression). Products include:
Symbyax Capsules ... 1819
Zyprexa Tablets ... 1830
Zyprexa IntraMuscular ... 1830
Zyprexa ZYDIS Orally Disintegrating Tablets ... 1830

Oxazepam (Exhibits an additive CNS depression).
No products indexed under this heading.

Oxycodone Hydrochloride (Exhibits an additive CNS depression). Products include:
OxyContin Tablets ... 2703
OxyFast Oral Concentrate Solution ... 2708
OxyIR Capsules ... 2708
Percocet Tablets ... 1131
Percodan Tablets ... 1132

Pentobarbital Sodium (Exhibits an additive CNS depression). Products include:
Nembutal Sodium Solution, USP ... 2470

Perphenazine (Exhibits an additive CNS depression).
No products indexed under this heading.

Phenobarbital (Exhibits an additive CNS depression). Products include:
Donnatal Extentabs ... 2493

Pimozide (Exhibits an additive CNS depression).
No products indexed under this heading.

Prazepam (Exhibits an additive CNS depression).
No products indexed under this heading.

Prochlorperazine (Exhibits an additive CNS depression).
No products indexed under this heading.

Promethazine Hydrochloride (Exhibits an additive CNS depression). Products include:
Phenergan Tablets and Suppositories ... 3440

Propofol (Exhibits an additive CNS depression).
No products indexed under this heading.

Propoxyphene Hydrochloride (Exhibits an additive CNS depression).
No products indexed under this heading.

Propoxyphene Napsylate (Exhibits an additive CNS depression).
No products indexed under this heading.

Quazepam (Exhibits an additive CNS depression).
No products indexed under this heading.

Quetiapine Fumarate (Exhibits an additive CNS depression). Products include:
Seroquel Tablets ... 690

Remifentanil Hydrochloride (Exhibits an additive CNS depression).
No products indexed under this heading.

Risperidone (Exhibits an additive CNS depression). Products include:
Risperdal ... 1676
Risperdal Consta Long-Acting Injection ... 1682
Risperdal M-Tab Orally Disintegrating Tablets ... 1676

Secobarbital Sodium (Exhibits an additive CNS depression).
No products indexed under this heading.

Sevoflurane (Exhibits an additive CNS depression). Products include:
Ultane Liquid for Inhalation ... 531

Sodium Oxybate (Exhibits an additive CNS depression). Products include:
Xyrem Oral Solution 1688

Sufentanil Citrate (Exhibits an additive CNS depression).
No products indexed under this heading.

Temazepam (Exhibits an additive CNS depression). Products include:
Restoril Capsules 1860

Thiamylal Sodium (Exhibits an additive CNS depression).
No products indexed under this heading.

Thioridazine Hydrochloride (Exhibits an additive CNS depression). Products include:
Thioridazine Hydrochloride Tablets 2163

Thiothixene (Exhibits an additive CNS depression). Products include:
Thiothixene Capsules 2165

Triazolam (Exhibits an additive CNS depression).
No products indexed under this heading.

Trifluoperazine Hydrochloride (Exhibits an additive CNS depression).
No products indexed under this heading.

Zaleplon (Exhibits an additive CNS depression). Products include:
Sonata Capsules 1717

Ziprasidone Hydrochloride (Exhibits an additive CNS depression). Products include:
Geodon Capsules 2529

Zolpidem Tartrate (Exhibits an additive CNS depression). Products include:
Ambien Tablets 2851
Ambien CR Tablets 2855

Food Interactions

Alcohol (Exhibits an additive CNS depression).

HYDROCORTONE TABLETS

(Hydrocortisone) 1989

May interact with oral anticoagulants, oral hypoglycemic agents, insulin, potassium-depleting diuretics, killed/inactivated vaccines, vaccines, live, and certain other agents. Compounds in these categories include:

Acarbose (Potential for increased requirements of oral hypoglycemic agents). Products include:
Precose Tablets 751

Anisindione (Potential for altered response to coumarin anticoagulants). Products include:
Miradon Tablets 3042

Aspirin (Aspirin should be used cautiously in conjunction with corticosteroids in hypoprothrombinemia). Products include:
Aggrenox Capsules 822
Bayer Aspirin 744
BC Allergy Sinus Cold Powder .... ▣677
BC Headache Powder .... ▣677
Arthritis Strength BC Powder .... ▣677
BC Sinus Cold Powder .... ▣677
Excedrin Extra Strength Caplets/Tablets/Geltabs .... ▣684
Excedrin Migraine Caplets/Tablets/Geltabs .... ▣609
Goody's Body Pain Formula Powder .... ▣684
Goody's Extra Strength Headache Powders .... ▣611
Goody's Extra Strength Pain Relief Tablets .... ▣685
Percodan Tablets 1132
St. Joseph 81 mg Aspirin Chewable and Enteric Coated Tablets 1869

BCG Vaccine (Administration of live virus vaccines, including smallpox, is contraindicated in patients receiving immunosuppressive doses of corticosteroids).
No products indexed under this heading.

Bendroflumethiazide (Co-administration may result in hypokalemia).
No products indexed under this heading.

Bumetanide (Co-administration may result in hypokalemia). Products include:
Bumex Tablets 2746

Chlorothiazide (Co-administration may result in hypokalemia). Products include:
Diuril Oral Suspension 1954

Chlorothiazide Sodium (Co-administration may result in hypokalemia). Products include:
Diuril Sodium Intravenous 2467

Chlorpropamide (Potential for increased requirements of oral hypoglycemic agents).
No products indexed under this heading.

Dicumarol (Potential for altered response to coumarin anticoagulants).
No products indexed under this heading.

Diphtheria & Tetanus Toxoids and Acellular Pertussis Vaccine Adsorbed, Hepatitis B (recombinant) and Inactivated Poliovirus Vaccine Combined (If inactivated viral or bacterial vaccines are administered to individuals receiving immunosuppressive doses of corticosteroids, the expected serum antibody response may not be obtained. However, immunization procedures may be undertaken in patients whoare receiving corticosteroids as replacement therapy, e.g., for Addison's disease).
No products indexed under this heading.

Ephedrine Hydrochloride (Enhances metabolic clearance of corticosteroids resulting in decreased blood levels and lessened physiologic activity).
No products indexed under this heading.

Ephedrine Sulfate (Enhances metabolic clearance of corticosteroids resulting in decreased blood levels and lessened physiologic activity).
No products indexed under this heading.

Ephedrine Tannate (Enhances metabolic clearance of corticosteroids resulting in decreased blood levels and lessened physiologic activity).
No products indexed under this heading.

Ethacrynic Acid (Co-administration may result in hypokalemia). Products include:
Edecrin Tablets 1959

Fosphenytoin Sodium (Enhances metabolic clearance of corticosteroids resulting in decreased blood levels and lessened physiologic activity).
No products indexed under this heading.

Furosemide (Co-administration may result in hypokalemia). Products include:
Furosemide Tablets 2154

Glimepiride (Potential for increased requirements of oral hypoglycemic agents). Products include:
Avandaryl Tablets 1379
Duetact Tablets 3226

Glipizide (Potential for increased requirements of oral hypoglycemic agents).
No products indexed under this heading.

Glyburide (Potential for increased requirements of oral hypoglycemic agents).
No products indexed under this heading.

Hepatitis A Vaccine, Inactivated (If inactivated viral or bacterial vaccines are administered to individuals receiving immunosuppressive doses of corticosteroids, the expected serum antibody response may not be obtained. However, immunization procedures may be undertaken in patients whoare receiving corticosteroids as replacement therapy, e.g., for Addison's disease). Products include:
Havrix Vaccine 1456
Twinrix Vaccine 1595
Vaqta 2097

Hydrochlorothiazide (Co-administration may result in hypokalemia). Products include:
Aldoril Tablets 1910
Atacand HCT 651
Avalide Tablets 888
Avalide Tablets 2874
Benicar HCT Tablets 1044
Diovan HCT Tablets 2196
Dyazide Capsules 1423
Hyzaar 50-12.5 Tablets 1990
Hyzaar 100-12.5 Tablets 1990
Hyzaar 100-25 Tablets 1990
Lopressor HCT 50/25 Tablets 2241
Lopressor HCT 100/25 Tablets 2241
Lopressor HCT 100/50 Tablets 2241
Lotensin HCT Tablets 2246
Micardis HCT Tablets 856
Moduretic Tablets 2028
Prinzide Tablets 2056
Teveten HCT Tablets 1737
Timolide Tablets 2086
Uniretic Tablets 3100

Hydroflumethiazide (Co-administration may result in hypokalemia).
No products indexed under this heading.

Influenza Virus Vaccine (If inactivated viral or bacterial vaccines are administered to individuals receiving immunosuppressive doses of corticosteroids, the expected serum antibody response may not be obtained. However, immunization procedures may be undertaken in patients whoare receiving corticosteroids as replacement therapy, e.g., for Addison's disease). Products include:
Fluarix 1451
Flumist Vaccine 1901

Insulin, Human, Zinc Suspension (Potential for increased requirements of insulin). Products include:
Humulin L, 100 Units 1794
Humulin U, 100 Units 1800

Insulin, Human NPH (Potential for increased requirements of insulin). Products include:
Humulin N, 100 Units 1795
Humulin N Pen 1797

Insulin, Human Regular (Potential for increased requirements of insulin). Products include:
Humulin R, 100 Units 1798

Insulin, Human Regular and Human NPH Mixture (Potential for increased requirements of insulin). Products include:
Humulin 50/50, 100 Units 1791
Humulin 70/30 Pen 1793

Insulin, NPH (Potential for increased requirements of insulin).
No products indexed under this heading.

Insulin, Regular (Potential for increased requirements of insulin).
No products indexed under this heading.

Insulin, Zinc Crystals (Potential for increased requirements of insulin).
No products indexed under this heading.

Insulin, Zinc Suspension (Potential for increased requirements of insulin).
No products indexed under this heading.

Insulin Aspart, Human Regular (Potential for increased requirements of insulin). Products include:
NovoLog Injection 2326

Insulin glargine (Potential for increased requirements of insulin). Products include:
Lantus Injection 2909

Insulin Lispro, Human (Potential for increased requirements of insulin). Products include:
Humalog-Pen 1781
Humalog Mix 50/50-Pen 1783
Humalog Mix 75/25-Pen 1785

Insulin Lispro Protamine, Human (Potential for increased requirements of insulin). Products include:
Humalog Mix 50/50-Pen 1783
Humalog Mix 75/25-Pen 1785

Japanese Encephalitis Vaccine Inactivated (If inactivated viral or bacterial vaccines are administered to individuals receiving immunosuppressive doses of corticosteroids, the expected serum antibody response may not be obtained. However, immunization procedures may be undertaken in patients whoare receiving corticosteroids as replacement therapy, e.g., for Addison's disease).
No products indexed under this heading.

Ketoconazole (Inhibits adrenal corticosteroid synthesis and may cause cortical insufficiency during corticosteroid withdrawal). Products include:
Nizoral A-D Shampoo, 1% 1868

Live Virus Vaccines (Co-administration is contraindicated in patients receiving immunosuppressive doses of corticosteroids).
No products indexed under this heading.

Measles, Mumps, Rubella and Varicella Virus Vaccine Live (Administration of live virus vaccines, including smallpox, is contraindicated in patients receiving immunosuppressive doses of corticosteroids). Products include:
ProQuad 2064

Measles, Mumps & Rubella Virus Vaccine, Live (Administration of live virus vaccines, including smallpox, is contraindicated in patients receiving immunosuppressive doses of corticosteroids). Products include:
M-M-R II 2006

Measles & Rubella Virus Vaccine Live (Administration of live virus vaccines, including smallpox, is contraindicated in patients receiving immunosuppressive doses of corticosteroids).
No products indexed under this heading.

Measles Virus Vaccine Live (Administration of live virus vaccines, including smallpox, is contraindicated in patients receiving immunosuppressive doses of corticosteroids). Products include:
Attenuvax 1914

Metformin Hydrochloride (Potential for increased requirements of oral hypoglycemic agents). Products include:
ActoPlus Met Tablets 3214
Avandamet Tablets 1373
Fortamet Extended-Release Tablets 3115

Methyclothiazide (Co-administration may result in hypokalemia).
No products indexed under this heading.

Miglitol (Potential for increased requirements of oral hypoglycemic agents).
No products indexed under this heading.

Mumps Virus Vaccine, Live (Administration of live virus vaccines, including smallpox, is contraindicated in patients receiving immunosuppressive doses of corticosteroids). Products include:
Mumpsvax 2031

Phenobarbital (Enhances metabolic clearance of corticosteroids resulting in decreased blood levels and lessened physiologic activity). Products include:
Donnatal Extentabs 2493

Phenytoin (Enhances metabolic clearance of corticosteroids resulting in decreased blood levels and lessened physiologic activity).
No products indexed under this heading.

Phenytoin Sodium (Enhances metabolic clearance of corticosteroids resulting in decreased blood levels and lessened physiologic activity). Products include:
Phenytek Capsules 2160

Pioglitazone Hydrochloride (Potential for increased requirements of oral hypoglycemic agents). Products include:
ActoPlus Met Tablets 3214
Actos Tablets 3219
Duetact Tablets 3226

Poliovirus Vaccine, Live, Oral, Trivalent, Types 1,2,3 (Sabin) (Administration of live virus vaccines, including smallpox, is contraindicated in patients receiving immunosuppressive doses of corticosteroids).
No products indexed under this heading.

Poliovirus Vaccine Inactivated, Trivalent Types 1,2,3 (If inactivated viral or bacterial vaccines are administered to individuals receiving immunosuppressive doses of corticosteroids, the expected serum antibody response may not be obtained. However, immunization procedures may be undertaken in patients whoare receiving corticosteroids as replacement therapy, e.g., for Addison's disease). Products include:
Pediarix Vaccine 1548

Polythiazide (Co-administration may result in hypokalemia).
No products indexed under this heading.

Repaglinide (Potential for increased requirements of oral hypoglycemic agents).
No products indexed under this heading.

Rifampin (Enhances metabolic clearance of corticosteroids resulting in decreased blood levels and lessened physiologic activity).
No products indexed under this heading.

Rosiglitazone Maleate (Potential for increased requirements of oral hypoglycemic agents). Products include:
Avandamet Tablets 1373
Avandaryl Tablets 1379
Avandia Tablets 1384

Rotavirus Vaccine, Live, Oral, Tetravalent (Administration of live virus vaccines, including smallpox, is contraindicated in patients receiving immunosuppressive doses of corticosteroids).
No products indexed under this heading.

Rubella & Mumps Virus Vaccine Live (Administration of live virus vaccines, including smallpox, is contraindicated in patients receiving immunosuppressive doses of corticosteroids).
No products indexed under this heading.

Rubella Virus Vaccine Live (Administration of live virus vaccines, including smallpox, is contraindicated in patients receiving immunosuppressive doses of corticosteroids). Products include:
Meruvax II 2019

Smallpox Vaccine (Administration of live virus vaccines, including smallpox, is contraindicated in patients receiving immunosuppressive doses of corticosteroids).
No products indexed under this heading.

Tolazamide (Potential for increased requirements of oral hypoglycemic agents).
No products indexed under this heading.

Tolbutamide (Potential for increased requirements of oral hypoglycemic agents).
No products indexed under this heading.

Torsemide (Co-administration may result in hypokalemia). Products include:
Demadex Injection 2759
Demadex Tablets 2759

Troglitazone (Potential for increased requirements of oral hypoglycemic agents).
No products indexed under this heading.

Typhoid Vaccine (Administration of live virus vaccines, including smallpox, is contraindicated in patients receiving immunosuppressive doses of corticosteroids).
No products indexed under this heading.

Varicella Virus Vaccine Live (Administration of live virus vaccines, including smallpox, is contraindicated in patients receiving immunosuppressive doses of corticosteroids). Products include:
Varivax 2100

Warfarin Sodium (Potential for altered response to coumarin anticoagulants). Products include:
Coumadin for Injection 898
Coumadin Tablets 898

Yellow Fever Vaccine (Administration of live virus vaccines, including smallpox, is contraindicated in patients receiving immunosuppressive doses of corticosteroids).
No products indexed under this heading.

HYLAND'S BACKACHE WITH ARNICA CAPLETS
(Homeopathic Formulations) 828
None cited in PDR database.

HYLAND'S CALM FORTE 4 KIDS TABLETS
(Homeopathic Formulations, Sulfur) 828
None cited in PDR database.

HYLAND'S CALMS FORTE TABLETS AND CAPLETS
(Homeopathic Formulations) 828
None cited in PDR database.

HYLAND'S COMPLETE FLU CARE TABLETS
(Herbals, Multiple) 828
None cited in PDR database.

HYLAND'S COMPLETE FLU CARE 4 KIDS TABLETS
(Dietary Supplement) 732
None cited in PDR database.

HYLAND'S EARACHE DROPS
(Herbals, Multiple) 828
None cited in PDR database.

HYLAND'S EARACHE TABLETS
(Homeopathic Formulations) 829
None cited in PDR database.

HYLAND'S LEG CRAMPS WITH QUININE TABLETS AND CAPLETS
(Homeopathic Formulations) 829
None cited in PDR database.

HYLAND'S NERVE TONIC TABLETS AND CAPLETS
(Homeopathic Formulations) 829
None cited in PDR database.

HYLAND'S RESTFUL LEGS TABLETS
(Dietary Supplement) 829
None cited in PDR database.

HYLAND'S SNIFFLES 'N SNEEZES 4 KIDS TABLETS
(Dietary Supplement) 732
None cited in PDR database.

HYLAND'S TEETHING GEL
(Homeopathic Formulations) 830
None cited in PDR database.

HYLAND'S TEETHING TABLETS
(Belladonna Alkaloids, Homeopathic Formulations)................ 830
None cited in PDR database.

HYPERHEP B S/D
(Hepatitis B Immune Globulin (Human)).. 3240
May interact with:

Vaccines (Live) (May interfere with response. Use should be deferred for 3 months after administration of HyperHep).
No products indexed under this heading.

HYPERRAB
(Rabies Immune Globulin (Human)) 3242
May interact with:

Measles, Mumps & Rubella Virus Vaccine, Live (Interference with the response to live viral vaccines). Products include:
M-M-R II 2006

Measles & Rubella Virus Vaccine Live (Interference with the response to live viral vaccines).
No products indexed under this heading.

Measles Virus Vaccine Live (Interference with the response to live viral vaccines). Products include:
Attenuvax 1914

Mumps Virus Vaccine, Live (Interference with the response to live viral vaccines). Products include:
Mumpsvax 2031

Poliovirus Vaccine, Live, Oral, Trivalent, Types 1,2,3 (Sabin) (Interference with the response to live viral vaccines).
No products indexed under this heading.

Rubella & Mumps Virus Vaccine Live (Interference with the response to live viral vaccines).
No products indexed under this heading.

Rubella Virus Vaccine Live (Interference with the response to live viral vaccines). Products include:
Meruvax II 2019

HYPERRHO S/D MINI-DOSE
(Rh_o (D) Immune Globulin (Human)) 3244
See HyperRho S/D Full Dose

HYPERRHO S/D FULL DOSE
(Rh_o (D) Immune Globulin (Human)) 3246
May interact with:

Measles, Mumps & Rubella Virus Vaccine, Live (Interference with response to live vaccines). Products include:
M-M-R II 2006

Measles & Rubella Virus Vaccine Live (Interference with response to live vaccines).
No products indexed under this heading.

Measles Virus Vaccine Live (Interference with response to live vaccines). Products include:
Attenuvax 1914

Rubella & Mumps Virus Vaccine Live (Interference with response to live vaccines).
No products indexed under this heading.

Rubella Virus Vaccine Live (Interference with response to live vaccines). Products include:
Meruvax II 2019

HYPERSTAT I.V.
(Diazoxide) ... 3017
May interact with antihypertensives, beta blockers, oral anticoagulants, diuretics, and certain other agents. Compounds in these categories include:

Acebutolol Hydrochloride (An undesirable hypotension may result when diazoxide is administered to patients who have received other antihypertensive agents within six hours; do not administer within six hours).
No products indexed under this heading.

Amiloride Hydrochloride (Potentiates the hyperuricemic and antihypertensive effects of diazoxide). Products include:
Midamor Tablets ... 2026
Moduretic Tablets ... 2028

Amlodipine Besylate (An undesirable hypotension may result when diazoxide is administered to patients who have received other antihypertensive agents within six hours). Products include:
Caduet Tablets ... 2508
Lotrel Capsules ... 2249
Norvasc Tablets ... 2545

Anisindione (Increased blood levels of coumarin derivatives due to displacement from protein binding sites). Products include:
Miradon Tablets ... 3042

Atenolol (An undesirable hypotension may result when diazoxide is administered to patients who have received other antihypertensive agents within six hours; do not administer within six hours).
No products indexed under this heading.

Benazepril Hydrochloride (An undesirable hypotension may result when diazoxide is administered to patients who have received other antihypertensive agents within six hours). Products include:
Lotensin Tablets ... 2243
Lotensin HCT Tablets ... 2246
Lotrel Capsules ... 2249

Bendroflumethiazide (Potentiates the hyperuricemic and antihypertensive effects of diazoxide).
No products indexed under this heading.

Betaxolol Hydrochloride (An undesirable hypotension may result when diazoxide is administered to patients who have received other antihypertensive agents within six hours; do not administer within six hours). Products include:
Betoptic S Ophthalmic Suspension ... 558

Bisoprolol Fumarate (An undesirable hypotension may result when diazoxide is administered to patients who have received other antihypertensive agents within six hours; do not administer within six hours).
No products indexed under this heading.

Bumetanide (Potentiates the hyperuricemic and antihypertensive effects of diazoxide). Products include:
Bumex Tablets ... 2746

Candesartan Cilexetil (An undesirable hypotension may result when diazoxide is administered to patients who have received other antihypertensive agents within six hours). Products include:
Atacand Tablets ... 649
Atacand HCT ... 651

Captopril (An undesirable hypotension may result when diazoxide is administered to patients who have received other antihypertensive agents within six hours). Products include:
Captopril Tablets ... 2149

Carteolol Hydrochloride (An undesirable hypotension may result when diazoxide is administered to patients who have received other antihypertensive agents within six hours; do not administer within six hours). Products include:
Carteolol Hydrochloride Ophthalmic Solution USP, 1% ... ⊙249

Chlorothiazide (Potentiates the hyperuricemic and antihypertensive effects of diazoxide). Products include:
Diuril Oral Suspension ... 1954

Chlorothiazide Sodium (Potentiates the hyperuricemic and antihypertensive effects of diazoxide). Products include:
Diuril Sodium Intravenous ... 2467

Chlorthalidone (Potentiates the hyperuricemic and antihypertensive effects of diazoxide). Products include:
Clorpres Tablets ... 2153

Clonidine (An undesirable hypotension may result when diazoxide is administered to patients who have received other antihypertensive agents within six hours). Products include:
Catapres-TTS ... 844

Clonidine Hydrochloride (An undesirable hypotension may result when diazoxide is administered to patients who have received other antihypertensive agents within six hours). Products include:
Catapres Tablets ... 843
Clorpres Tablets ... 2153

Deserpidine (An undesirable hypotension may result when diazoxide is administered to patients who have received other antihypertensive agents within six hours).
No products indexed under this heading.

Dicumarol (Increased blood levels of coumarin derivatives due to displacement from protein binding sites).
No products indexed under this heading.

Diltiazem Hydrochloride (An undesirable hypotension may result when diazoxide is administered to patients who have received other antihypertensive agents within six hours). Products include:
Cardizem LA Extended Release Tablets ... 1728
Tiazac Capsules ... 1201

Doxazosin Mesylate (An undesirable hypotension may result when diazoxide is administered to patients who have received other antihypertensive agents within six hours). Products include:
Cardura XL Tablets ... 2515

Enalapril Maleate (An undesirable hypotension may result when diazoxide is administered to patients who have received other antihypertensive agents within six hours). Products include:
Vasotec I.V. Injection ... 2103

Enalaprilat (An undesirable hypotension may result when diazoxide is administered to patients who have received other antihypertensive agents within six hours).
No products indexed under this heading.

Eprosartan Mesylate (An undesirable hypotension may result when diazoxide is administered to patients who have received other antihypertensive agents within six hours). Products include:
Teveten Tablets ... 1735
Teveten HCT Tablets ... 1737

Esmolol Hydrochloride (An undesirable hypotension may result when diazoxide is administered to patients who have received other antihypertensive agents within six hours; do not administer within six hours).
No products indexed under this heading.

Ethacrynic Acid (Potentiates the hyperuricemic and antihypertensive effects of diazoxide). Products include:
Edecrin Tablets ... 1959

Felodipine (An undesirable hypotension may result when diazoxide is administered to patients who have received other antihypertensive agents within six hours).
No products indexed under this heading.

Fosinopril Sodium (An undesirable hypotension may result when diazoxide is administered to patients who have received other antihypertensive agents within six hours).
No products indexed under this heading.

Furosemide (Potentiates the hyperuricemic and antihypertensive effects of diazoxide). Products include:
Furosemide Tablets ... 2154

Guanabenz Acetate (An undesirable hypotension may result when diazoxide is administered to patients who have received other antihypertensive agents within six hours).
No products indexed under this heading.

Guanethidine Monosulfate (An undesirable hypotension may result when diazoxide is administered to patients who have received other antihypertensive agents within six hours).
No products indexed under this heading.

Hydralazine Hydrochloride (Co-administration with methyldopa and hydralazine has produced excessive hypotension; do not administer within six hours). Products include:
BiDil Tablets ... 2171

Hydrochlorothiazide (Potentiates the hyperuricemic and antihypertensive effects of diazoxide). Products include:
Aldoril Tablets ... 1910
Atacand HCT ... 651
Avalide Tablets ... 888
Avalide Tablets ... 2874
Benicar HCT Tablets ... 1044
Diovan HCT Tablets ... 2196
Dyazide Capsules ... 1423
Hyzaar 50-12.5 Tablets ... 1990
Hyzaar 100-12.5 Tablets ... 1990
Hyzaar 100-25 Tablets ... 1990
Lopressor HCT 50/25 Tablets ... 2241
Lopressor HCT 100/25 Tablets ... 2241
Lopressor HCT 100/50 Tablets ... 2241
Lotensin HCT Tablets ... 2246
Micardis HCT Tablets ... 856
Moduretic Tablets ... 2028
Prinzide Tablets ... 2056
Teveten HCT Tablets ... 1737
Timolide Tablets ... 2086
Uniretic Tablets ... 3100

Hydroflumethiazide (Potentiates the hyperuricemic and antihypertensive effects of diazoxide).
No products indexed under this heading.

Indapamide (Potentiates the hyperuricemic and antihypertensive effects of diazoxide). Products include:
Indapamide Tablets ... 2156

Irbesartan (An undesirable hypotension may result when diazoxide is administered to patients who have received other antihypertensive agents within six hours). Products include:
Avalide Tablets ... 888
Avalide Tablets ... 2874
Avapro Tablets ... 891
Avapro Tablets ... 2871

Isradipine (An undesirable hypotension may result when diazoxide is administered to patients who have received other antihypertensive agents within six hours). Products include:
DynaCirc CR Tablets ... 2721

Labetalol Hydrochloride (An undesirable hypotension may result when diazoxide is administered to patients who have received other antihypertensive agents within six hours; do not administer within six hours).
No products indexed under this heading.

Levobunolol Hydrochloride (An undesirable hypotension may result when diazoxide is administered to patients who have received other antihypertensive agents within six hours; do not administer within six hours). Products include:
Betagan Ophthalmic Solution, USP ... ⊙220

Lisinopril (An undesirable hypotension may result when diazoxide is administered to patients who have received other antihypertensive agents within six hours). Products include:
Prinivil Tablets ... 2052
Prinzide Tablets ... 2056

Losartan Potassium (An undesirable hypotension may result when diazoxide is administered to patients who have received other antihypertensive agents within six hours). Products include:
Cozaar Tablets ... 1935
Hyzaar 50-12.5 Tablets ... 1990
Hyzaar 100-12.5 Tablets ... 1990
Hyzaar 100-25 Tablets ... 1990

Mecamylamine Hydrochloride (An undesirable hypotension may result when diazoxide is administered to patients who have received other antihypertensive agents within six hours).
No products indexed under this heading.

Methyclothiazide (Potentiates the hyperuricemic and antihypertensive effects of diazoxide).
No products indexed under this heading.

Methyldopa (Co-administration with methyldopa and hydralazine has produced excessive hypotension; do not administer within six hours). Products include:
Aldoril Tablets ... 1910

Methyldopate Hydrochloride (Co-administration with methyldopa and hydralazine has produced excessive hypotension; do not administer within six hours).
No products indexed under this heading.

Metipranolol Hydrochloride (An undesirable hypotension may result when diazoxide is administered to patients who have received other antihypertensive agents within six hours; do not administer within six hours).
No products indexed under this heading.

Metolazone (Potentiates the hyperuricemic and antihypertensive effects of diazoxide).
No products indexed under this heading.

Metoprolol Succinate (An undesirable hypotension may result when diazoxide is administered to patients who have received other antihypertensive agents within six hours; do not administer within six hours). Products include:
Toprol-XL Tablets 668

Metoprolol Tartrate (An undesirable hypotension may result when diazoxide is administered to patients who have received other antihypertensive agents within six hours; do not administer within six hours). Products include:
Lopressor Injection 2238
Lopressor Tablets 2238
Lopressor HCT 50/25 Tablets 2241
Lopressor HCT 100/25 Tablets 2241
Lopressor HCT 100/50 Tablets 2241

Metyrosine (An undesirable hypotension may result when diazoxide is administered to patients who have received other antihypertensive agents within six hours). Products include:
Demser Capsules 1953

Mibefradil Dihydrochloride (An undesirable hypotension may result when diazoxide is administered to patients who have received other antihypertensive agents within six hours).
No products indexed under this heading.

Minoxidil (An undesirable hypotension may result when diazoxide is administered to patients who have received other antihypertensive agents within six hours; do not administer within six hours). Products include:
Men's Rogaine Extra Strength Hair Regrowth Treatment Topical Solution, Ocean Rush Scent and Original Unscented..... ▣◧633
Men's Rogaine Foam Hair Regrowth Treatment.................... ▣◧633
Women's Rogaine Hair Regrowth Treatment Topical Solution, Spring Bloom Scent and Original Unscented..................... ▣◧634

Moexipril Hydrochloride (An undesirable hypotension may result when diazoxide is administered to patients who have received other antihypertensive agents within six hours). Products include:
Uniretic Tablets 3100
Univasc Tablets 3104

Nadolol (An undesirable hypotension may result when diazoxide is administered to patients who have received other antihypertensive agents within six hours; do not administer within six hours). Products include:

Nadolol Tablets 2159

Nicardipine Hydrochloride (An undesirable hypotension may result when diazoxide is administered to patients who have received other antihypertensive agents within six hours). Products include:
Cardene I.V. 2497

Nifedipine (An undesirable hypotension may result when diazoxide is administered to patients who have received other antihypertensive agents within six hours). Products include:
Adalat CC Tablets 2964

Nisoldipine (An undesirable hypotension may result when diazoxide is administered to patients who have received other antihypertensive agents within six hours). Products include:
Sular Tablets 3122

Nitroglycerin (An undesirable hypotension may result when diazoxide is administered to patients who have received other antihypertensive agents within six hours; do not administer within six hours). Products include:
Nitro-Dur Transdermal Infusion System 3046
Nitrolingual Pumpspray 3120

Papaverine Hydrochloride (An undesirable hypotension may result when diazoxide is administered to patients who have received other antihypertensive agents within six hours; do not administer within six hours).
No products indexed under this heading.

Penbutolol Sulfate (An undesirable hypotension may result when diazoxide is administered to patients who have received other antihypertensive agents within six hours; do not administer within six hours).
No products indexed under this heading.

Perindopril Erbumine (An undesirable hypotension may result when diazoxide is administered to patients who have received other antihypertensive agents within six hours). Products include:
Aceon Tablets (2 mg, 4 mg, 8 mg)...................................... 3194

Phenoxybenzamine Hydrochloride (An undesirable hypotension may result when diazoxide is administered to patients who have received other antihypertensive agents within six hours). Products include:
Dibenzyline Capsules 3399

Phentolamine Mesylate (An undesirable hypotension may result when diazoxide is administered to patients who have received other antihypertensive agents within six hours).
No products indexed under this heading.

Pindolol (An undesirable hypotension may result when diazoxide is administered to patients who have received other antihypertensive agents within six hours; do not administer within six hours).
No products indexed under this heading.

Polythiazide (Potentiates the hyperuricemic and antihypertensive effects of diazoxide).
No products indexed under this heading.

Prazosin Hydrochloride (An undesirable hypotension may result when diazoxide is administered to patients who have received other antihypertensive agents within six hours; do not administer within six hours).
No products indexed under this heading.

Propranolol Hydrochloride (An undesirable hypotension may result when diazoxide is administered to patients who have received other antihypertensive agents within six hours; do not administer within six hours). Products include:
Inderal LA Long-Acting Capsules 3429
InnoPran XL Capsules 2723

Quinapril Hydrochloride (An undesirable hypotension may result when diazoxide is administered to patients who have received other antihypertensive agents within six hours).
No products indexed under this heading.

Ramipril (An undesirable hypotension may result when diazoxide is administered to patients who have received other antihypertensive agents within six hours). Products include:
Altace Capsules 1702

Rauwolfia Serpentina (An undesirable hypotension may result when diazoxide is administered to patients who have received other antihypertensive agents within six hours).
No products indexed under this heading.

Rescinnamine (An undesirable hypotension may result when diazoxide is administered to patients who have received other antihypertensive agents within six hours).
No products indexed under this heading.

Reserpine (Co-administration with reserpine and hydralazine has produced maternal hypotension and fetal bradycardia in a patient in labor; do not administer within six hours).
No products indexed under this heading.

Sodium Nitroprusside (An undesirable hypotension may result when diazoxide is administered to patients who have received other antihypertensive agents within six hours).
No products indexed under this heading.

Sotalol Hydrochloride (An undesirable hypotension may result when diazoxide is administered to patients who have received other antihypertensive agents within six hours; do not administer within six hours).
No products indexed under this heading.

Spirapril Hydrochloride (An undesirable hypotension may result when diazoxide is administered to patients who have received other antihypertensive agents within six hours).
No products indexed under this heading.

Spironolactone (Potentiates the hyperuricemic and antihypertensive effects of diazoxide).
No products indexed under this heading.

Telmisartan (An undesirable hypotension may result when diazoxide is administered to patients who have received other antihypertensive agents within six hours). Products include:

Micardis Tablets 854
Micardis HCT Tablets 856

Terazosin Hydrochloride (An undesirable hypotension may result when diazoxide is administered to patients who have received other antihypertensive agents within six hours). Products include:
Hytrin Capsules 471

Timolol Hemihydrate (An undesirable hypotension may result when diazoxide is administered to patients who have received other antihypertensive agents within six hours; do not administer within six hours). Products include:
Betimol Ophthalmic Solution 3382
Betimol Ophthalmic Solution ⊙295

Timolol Maleate (An undesirable hypotension may result when diazoxide is administered to patients who have received other antihypertensive agents within six hours; do not administer within six hours). Products include:
Blocadren Tablets 1916
Cosopt Sterile Ophthalmic Solution....................................... 1931
Timolide Tablets 2086
Timoptic Sterile Ophthalmic Solution....................................... 2088
Timoptic in Ocudose 2091
Timoptic-XE Sterile Ophthalmic Gel Forming Solution 2092

Torsemide (Potentiates the hyperuricemic and antihypertensive effects of diazoxide). Products include:
Demadex Injection 2759
Demadex Tablets 2759

Trandolapril (An undesirable hypotension may result when diazoxide is administered to patients who have received other antihypertensive agents within six hours). Products include:
Mavik Tablets 486
Tarka Tablets 524

Triamterene (Potentiates the hyperuricemic and antihypertensive effects of diazoxide). Products include:
Dyazide Capsules 1423
Dyrenium Capsules 3400

Trimethaphan Camsylate (An undesirable hypotension may result when diazoxide is administered to patients who have received other antihypertensive agents within six hours).
No products indexed under this heading.

Valsartan (An undesirable hypotension may result when diazoxide is administered to patients who have received other antihypertensive agents within six hours). Products include:
Diovan Tablets 2193
Diovan HCT Tablets 2196

Verapamil Hydrochloride (An undesirable hypotension may result when diazoxide is administered to patients who have received other antihypertensive agents within six hours). Products include:
Covera-HS Tablets 3139
Tarka Tablets 524
Verelan PM Extended-Release Capsules, Controlled-Onset......... 3106

Warfarin Sodium (Increased blood levels of coumarin derivatives due to displacement from protein binding sites). Products include:
Coumadin for Injection 898
Coumadin Tablets 898

IMPORTANT NOTE: Always consult each drug listing in the patient's regimen for possible interactions.

HYPERTET

(Tetanus Immune Globulin (Human)) ... 3248
May interact with:

Vaccines (Live) (May interfere with response. Use should be deferred for 3 months).
No products indexed under this heading.

HYTRIN CAPSULES

(Terazosin Hydrochloride) 471
May interact with antihypertensives and certain other agents. Compounds in these categories include:

Acebutolol Hydrochloride (Possibility of significant hypotension; dosage adjustment may be necessary).
No products indexed under this heading.

Amlodipine Besylate (Possibility of significant hypotension; dosage adjustment may be necessary). Products include:
- Caduet Tablets 2508
- Lotrel Capsules 2249
- Norvasc Tablets 2545

Atenolol (Possibility of significant hypotension; dosage adjustment may be necessary).
No products indexed under this heading.

Benazepril Hydrochloride (Possibility of significant hypotension; dosage adjustment may be necessary). Products include:
- Lotensin Tablets 2243
- Lotensin HCT Tablets 2246
- Lotrel Capsules 2249

Bendroflumethiazide (Possibility of significant hypotension; dosage adjustment may be necessary).
No products indexed under this heading.

Betaxolol Hydrochloride (Possibility of significant hypotension; dosage adjustment may be necessary). Products include:
- Betoptic S Ophthalmic Suspension.................................. 558

Bisoprolol Fumarate (Possibility of significant hypotension; dosage adjustment may be necessary).
No products indexed under this heading.

Candesartan Cilexetil (Possibility of significant hypotension; dosage adjustment may be necessary). Products include:
- Atacand Tablets 649
- Atacand HCT 651

Captopril (Co-administration increases terazosin's maximum plasma concentrations linearly with dose at steady-state after administration of terazosin plus captopril). Products include:
- Captopril Tablets 2149

Carteolol Hydrochloride (Possibility of significant hypotension; dosage adjustment may be necessary). Products include:
- Carteolol Hydrochloride Ophthalmic Solution USP, 1%....... ⊙249

Chlorothiazide (Possibility of significant hypotension; dosage adjustment may be necessary). Products include:
- Diuril Oral Suspension 1954

Chlorothiazide Sodium (Possibility of significant hypotension; dosage adjustment may be necessary). Products include:
- Diuril Sodium Intravenous 2467

Chlorthalidone (Possibility of significant hypotension; dosage adjustment may be necessary). Products include:
- Clorpres Tablets 2153

Clonidine (Possibility of significant hypotension; dosage adjustment may be necessary). Products include:
- Catapres-TTS 844

Clonidine Hydrochloride (Possibility of significant hypotension; dosage adjustment may be necessary). Products include:
- Catapres Tablets 843
- Clorpres Tablets 2153

Deserpidine (Possibility of significant hypotension; dosage adjustment may be necessary).
No products indexed under this heading.

Diazoxide (Possibility of significant hypotension; dosage adjustment may be necessary). Products include:
- Hyperstat I.V. 3017

Diltiazem Hydrochloride (Possibility of significant hypotension; dosage adjustment may be necessary). Products include:
- Cardizem LA Extended Release Tablets 1728
- Tiazac Capsules 1201

Doxazosin Mesylate (Possibility of significant hypotension; dosage adjustment may be necessary). Products include:
- Cardura XL Tablets 2515

Enalapril Maleate (Possibility of significant hypotension; dosage adjustment may be necessary). Products include:
- Vasotec I.V. Injection....................... 2103

Enalaprilat (Possibility of significant hypotension; dosage adjustment may be necessary).
No products indexed under this heading.

Eprosartan Mesylate (Possibility of significant hypotension; dosage adjustment may be necessary). Products include:
- Teveten Tablets 1735
- Teveten HCT Tablets 1737

Esmolol Hydrochloride (Possibility of significant hypotension; dosage adjustment may be necessary).
No products indexed under this heading.

Felodipine (Possibility of significant hypotension; dosage adjustment may be necessary).
No products indexed under this heading.

Fosinopril Sodium (Possibility of significant hypotension; dosage adjustment may be necessary).
No products indexed under this heading.

Furosemide (Possibility of significant hypotension; dosage adjustment may be necessary). Products include:
- Furosemide Tablets 2154

Guanabenz Acetate (Possibility of significant hypotension; dosage adjustment may be necessary).
No products indexed under this heading.

Guanethidine Monosulfate (Possibility of significant hypotension; dosage adjustment may be necessary).
No products indexed under this heading.

Hydralazine Hydrochloride (Possibility of significant hypotension; dosage adjustment may be necessary). Products include:
- BiDil Tablets 2171

Hydrochlorothiazide (Possibility of significant hypotension; dosage adjustment may be necessary). Products include:
- Aldoril Tablets 1910
- Atacand HCT 651
- Avalide Tablets 888
- Avalide Tablets 2874
- Benicar HCT Tablets 1044
- Diovan HCT Tablets 2196
- Dyazide Capsules 1423
- Hyzaar 50-12.5 Tablets 1990
- Hyzaar 100-12.5 Tablets 1990
- Hyzaar 100-25 Tablets 1990
- Lopressor HCT 50/25 Tablets 2241
- Lopressor HCT 100/25 Tablets 2241
- Lopressor HCT 100/50 Tablets 2241
- Lotensin HCT Tablets 2246
- Micardis HCT Tablets 856
- Moduretic Tablets 2028
- Prinzide Tablets 2056
- Teveten HCT Tablets 1737
- Timolide Tablets 2086
- Uniretic Tablets 3100

Hydroflumethiazide (Possibility of significant hypotension; dosage adjustment may be necessary).
No products indexed under this heading.

Indapamide (Possibility of significant hypotension; dosage adjustment may be necessary). Products include:
- Indapamide Tablets 2156

Irbesartan (Possibility of significant hypotension; dosage adjustment may be necessary). Products include:
- Avalide Tablets 888
- Avalide Tablets 2874
- Avapro Tablets 891
- Avapro Tablets 2871

Isradipine (Possibility of significant hypotension; dosage adjustment may be necessary). Products include:
- DynaCirc CR Tablets 2721

Labetalol Hydrochloride (Possibility of significant hypotension; dosage adjustment may be necessary).
No products indexed under this heading.

Lisinopril (Possibility of significant hypotension; dosage adjustment may be necessary). Products include:
- Prinivil Tablets 2052
- Prinzide Tablets 2056

Losartan Potassium (Possibility of significant hypotension; dosage adjustment may be necessary). Products include:
- Cozaar Tablets 1935
- Hyzaar 50-12.5 Tablets 1990
- Hyzaar 100-12.5 Tablets 1990
- Hyzaar 100-25 Tablets 1990

Mecamylamine Hydrochloride (Possibility of significant hypotension; dosage adjustment may be necessary).
No products indexed under this heading.

Methyclothiazide (Possibility of significant hypotension; dosage adjustment may be necessary).
No products indexed under this heading.

Methyldopa (Possibility of significant hypotension; dosage adjustment may be necessary). Products include:
- Aldoril Tablets 1910

Methyldopate Hydrochloride (Possibility of significant hypotension; dosage adjustment may be necessary).
No products indexed under this heading.

Metipranolol Hydrochloride (Possibility of significant hypotension; dosage adjustment may be necessary).
No products indexed under this heading.

Metolazone (Possibility of significant hypotension; dosage adjustment may be necessary).
No products indexed under this heading.

Metoprolol Succinate (Possibility of significant hypotension; dosage adjustment may be necessary). Products include:
- Toprol-XL Tablets 668

Metoprolol Tartrate (Possibility of significant hypotension; dosage adjustment may be necessary). Products include:
- Lopressor Injection 2238
- Lopressor Tablets 2238
- Lopressor HCT 50/25 Tablets 2241
- Lopressor HCT 100/25 Tablets 2241
- Lopressor HCT 100/50 Tablets 2241

Metyrosine (Possibility of significant hypotension; dosage adjustment may be necessary). Products include:
- Demser Capsules 1953

Mibefradil Dihydrochloride (Possibility of significant hypotension; dosage adjustment may be necessary).
No products indexed under this heading.

Minoxidil (Possibility of significant hypotension; dosage adjustment may be necessary). Products include:
- Men's Rogaine Extra Strength Hair Regrowth Treatment Topical Solution, Ocean Rush Scent and Original Unscented..... ▣633
- Men's Rogaine Foam Hair Regrowth Treatment.................... ▣633
- Women's Rogaine Hair Regrowth Treatment Topical Solution, Spring Bloom Scent and Original Unscented........................ ▣634

Moexipril Hydrochloride (Possibility of significant hypotension; dosage adjustment may be necessary). Products include:
- Uniretic Tablets 3100
- Univasc Tablets 3104

Nadolol (Possibility of significant hypotension; dosage adjustment may be necessary). Products include:
- Nadolol Tablets 2159

Nicardipine Hydrochloride (Possibility of significant hypotension; dosage adjustment may be necessary). Products include:
- Cardene I.V. 2497

Nifedipine (Possibility of significant hypotension; dosage adjustment may be necessary). Products include:
- Adalat CC Tablets 2964

Nisoldipine (Possibility of significant hypotension; dosage adjustment may be necessary). Products include:
- Sular Tablets 3122

Nitroglycerin (Possibility of significant hypotension; dosage adjustment may be necessary). Products include:

Nitro-Dur Transdermal Infusion System.. 3046
Nitrolingual Pumpspray 3120

Penbutolol Sulfate (Possibility of significant hypotension; dosage adjustment may be necessary).
No products indexed under this heading.

Perindopril Erbumine (Possibility of significant hypotension; dosage adjustment may be necessary). Products include:
Aceon Tablets (2 mg, 4 mg, 8 mg).. 3194

Phenoxybenzamine Hydrochloride (Possibility of significant hypotension; dosage adjustment may be necessary). Products include:
Dibenzyline Capsules 3399

Phentolamine Mesylate (Possibility of significant hypotension; dosage adjustment may be necessary).
No products indexed under this heading.

Pindolol (Possibility of significant hypotension; dosage adjustment may be necessary).
No products indexed under this heading.

Polythiazide (Possibility of significant hypotension; dosage adjustment may be necessary).
No products indexed under this heading.

Prazosin Hydrochloride (Possibility of significant hypotension; dosage adjustment may be necessary).
No products indexed under this heading.

Propranolol Hydrochloride (Possibility of significant hypotension; dosage adjustment may be necessary). Products include:
Inderal LA Long-Acting Capsules 3429
InnoPran XL Capsules 2723

Quinapril Hydrochloride (Possibility of significant hypotension; dosage adjustment may be necessary).
No products indexed under this heading.

Ramipril (Possibility of significant hypotension; dosage adjustment may be necessary). Products include:
Altace Capsules 1702

Rauwolfia Serpentina (Possibility of significant hypotension; dosage adjustment may be necessary).
No products indexed under this heading.

Rescinnamine (Possibility of significant hypotension; dosage adjustment may be necessary).
No products indexed under this heading.

Reserpine (Possibility of significant hypotension; dosage adjustment may be necessary).
No products indexed under this heading.

Sodium Nitroprusside (Possibility of significant hypotension; dosage adjustment may be necessary).
No products indexed under this heading.

Sotalol Hydrochloride (Possibility of significant hypotension; dosage adjustment may be necessary).
No products indexed under this heading.

Spirapril Hydrochloride (Possibility of significant hypotension; dosage adjustment may be necessary).
No products indexed under this heading.

Telmisartan (Possibility of significant hypotension; dosage adjustment may be necessary). Products include:
Micardis Tablets 854
Micardis HCT Tablets 856

Timolol Maleate (Possibility of significant hypotension; dosage adjustment may be necessary). Products include:
Blocadren Tablets 1916
Cosopt Sterile Ophthalmic Solution.. 1931
Timolide Tablets 2086
Timoptic Sterile Ophthalmic Solution.. 2088
Timoptic in Ocudose 2091
Timoptic-XE Sterile Ophthalmic Gel Forming Solution 2092

Torsemide (Possibility of significant hypotension; dosage adjustment may be necessary). Products include:
Demadex Injection.......................... 2759
Demadex Tablets 2759

Trandolapril (Possibility of significant hypotension; dosage adjustment may be necessary). Products include:
Mavik Tablets 486
Tarka Tablets 524

Trimethaphan Camsylate (Possibility of significant hypotension; dosage adjustment may be necessary).
No products indexed under this heading.

Valsartan (Possibility of significant hypotension; dosage adjustment may be necessary). Products include:
Diovan Tablets 2193
Diovan HCT Tablets 2196

Verapamil Hydrochloride (Co-administration increases terazosin's mean AUC0-24 by 11% to 24% with associated increase in Cmax (25%) and Cmin (32%)). Products include:
Covera-HS Tablets 3139
Tarka Tablets 524
Verelan PM Extended-Release Capsules, Controlled-Onset........... 3106

Food Interactions

Food, unspecified (Delays the time to peak concentration by about 40 minutes; minimal effect on the extent of absorption).

HYZAAR 50-12.5 TABLETS

(Hydrochlorothiazide, Losartan Potassium).. 1990

May interact with antihypertensives, barbiturates, corticosteroids, erythromycin, oral hypoglycemic agents, insulin, lithium preparations, narcotic analgesics, nondepolarizing neuromuscular blocking agents, non-steroidal anti-inflammatory agents, potassium preparations, potassium sparing diuretics, and certain other agents. Compounds in these categories include:

Acarbose (Hyperglycemia may occur with thiazide diuretics; dosage adjustment of the antidiabetic drug may be required). Products include:
Precose Tablets 751

Acebutolol Hydrochloride (Additive effect or potentiation of other antihypertensives).
No products indexed under this heading.

ACTH (Potential for intensified electrolyte depletion, particularly hypokalemia).
No products indexed under this heading.

Alfentanil Hydrochloride (Potentiation of orthostatic hypotension).
No products indexed under this heading.

Amiloride Hydrochloride (Concomitant use with potassium-sparing diuretics may lead to hyperkalemia). Products include:
Midamor Tablets 2026
Moduretic Tablets 2028

Amlodipine Besylate (Additive effect or potentiation of other antihypertensives). Products include:
Caduet Tablets 2508
Lotrel Capsules 2249
Norvasc Tablets 2545

Aprobarbital (Potentiation of orthostatic hypotension).
No products indexed under this heading.

Atenolol (Additive effect or potentiation of other antihypertensives).
No products indexed under this heading.

Atracurium Besylate (Possible increased responsiveness to the muscle relaxant).
No products indexed under this heading.

Benazepril Hydrochloride (Additive effect or potentiation of other antihypertensives). Products include:
Lotensin Tablets.............................. 2243
Lotensin HCT Tablets 2246
Lotrel Capsules 2249

Bendroflumethiazide (Additive effect or potentiation of other antihypertensives).
No products indexed under this heading.

Betamethasone Acetate (Potential for intensified electrolyte depletion, particularly hypokalemia).
No products indexed under this heading.

Betamethasone Sodium Phosphate (Potential for intensified electrolyte depletion, particularly hypokalemia).
No products indexed under this heading.

Betaxolol Hydrochloride (Additive effect or potentiation of other antihypertensives). Products include:
Betoptic S Ophthalmic Suspension.. 558

Bisoprolol Fumarate (Additive effect or potentiation of other antihypertensives).
No products indexed under this heading.

Buprenorphine Hydrochloride (Potentiation of orthostatic hypotension). Products include:
Buprenex Injectable........................ 2716
Suboxone Tablets 2717
Subutex Tablets 2717

Butabarbital (Potentiation of orthostatic hypotension).
No products indexed under this heading.

Butalbital (Potentiation of orthostatic hypotension).
No products indexed under this heading.

Candesartan Cilexetil (Additive effect or potentiation of other antihypertensives). Products include:
Atacand Tablets 649
Atacand HCT 651

Captopril (Additive effect or potentiation of other antihypertensives). Products include:
Captopril Tablets 2149

Carteolol Hydrochloride (Additive effect or potentiation of other antihypertensives). Products include:
Carteolol Hydrochloride Ophthalmic Solution USP, 1%....... ⊙249

Celecoxib (In some patients with compromised renal function who are being treated with non-steroidal anti-inflammatory drugs (NSAIDs), including those that selectively inhibit cyclooxygenase-2 inhibitors (COX-2 inhibitors), the co-administration of angiotensin II receptor antagonists including losartan may result in a further deterioration of renal function. These effects are usually reversible. Reports suggest that NSAIDs, including selective COX-2 inhibitors, may diminish the antihypertensive effect of angiotensin II receptor antagonists, including losartan. This interaction should be given consideration in patients taking NSAIDs, including selective COX-2 inhibitors, concomitantly with angiotensin II receptor antagonists). Products include:
Celebrex Capsules 3134

Chlorothiazide (Additive effect or potentiation of other antihypertensives). Products include:
Diuril Oral Suspension 1954

Chlorothiazide Sodium (Additive effect or potentiation of other antihypertensives). Products include:
Diuril Sodium Intravenous 2467

Chlorpropamide (Hyperglycemia may occur with thiazide diuretics; dosage adjustment of the antidiabetic drug may be required).
No products indexed under this heading.

Chlorthalidone (Additive effect or potentiation of other antihypertensives). Products include:
Clorpres Tablets 2153

Cholestyramine (Absorption of hydrochlorothiazide is impaired in the presence of anionic exchange resins; cholestyramine binds hydrochlorothiazide and reduces its absorption from GI tract by up to 85%).
No products indexed under this heading.

Cimetidine (Co-administration led to an increase of about 18% in AUC of losartan but did not affect the pharmacokinetics of its active metabolite). Products include:
Tagamet HB 200 Tablets .... ▣664

Cimetidine Hydrochloride (Co-administration led to an increase of about 18% in AUC of losartan but did not affect the pharmacokinetics of its active metabolite).
No products indexed under this heading.

Cisatracurium Besylate (Possible increased responsiveness to the muscle relaxant). Products include:
Nimbex Injection............................. 498

Clonidine (Additive effect or potentiation of other antihypertensives). Products include:
Catapres-TTS 844

Clonidine Hydrochloride (Additive effect or potentiation of other antihypertensives). Products include:
Catapres Tablets 843
Clorpres Tablets 2153

Codeine Phosphate (Potentiation of orthostatic hypotension). Products include:
Tylenol with Codeine Tablets 2391

IMPORTANT NOTE: Always consult each drug listing in the patient's regimen for possible interactions.

Colestipol Hydrochloride (Absorption of hydrochlorothiazide is impaired in the presence of anionic exchange resins; cholestyramine binds hydrochlorothiazide and reduces its absorption from GI tract by up to 85%).
No products indexed under this heading.

Cortisone Acetate (Potential for intensified electrolyte depletion, particularly hypokalemia).
No products indexed under this heading.

Deserpidine (Additive effect or potentiation of other antihypertensives).
No products indexed under this heading.

Dexamethasone (Potential for intensified electrolyte depletion, particularly hypokalemia). Products include:
Ciprodex Otic Suspension 559
Decadron Tablets 1951
TobraDex Ophthalmic Ointment 562
TobraDex Ophthalmic Suspension ... 563

Dexamethasone Acetate (Potential for intensified electrolyte depletion, particularly hypokalemia).
No products indexed under this heading.

Dexamethasone Sodium Phosphate (Potential for intensified electrolyte depletion, particularly hypokalemia).
No products indexed under this heading.

Dezocine (Potentiation of orthostatic hypotension).
No products indexed under this heading.

Diazoxide (Additive effect or potentiation of other antihypertensives). Products include:
Hyperstat I.V. 3017

Diclofenac Potassium (In some patients with compromised renal function who are being treated with non-steroidal anti-inflammatory drugs (NSAIDs), including those that selectively inhibit cyclooxygenase-2 inhibitors (COX-2 inhibitors), the co-administration of angiotensin II receptor antagonists including losartan may result in a further deterioration of renal function. These effects are usually reversible. Reports suggest that NSAIDs, including selective COX-2 inhibitors, may diminish the antihypertensive effect of angiotensin II receptor antagonists, including losartan. This interaction should be given consideration in patients taking NSAIDs, including selective COX-2 inhibitors, concomitantly with angiotensin II receptor antagonists).
No products indexed under this heading.

Diclofenac Sodium (In some patients with compromised renal function who are being treated with non-steroidal anti-inflammatory drugs (NSAIDs), including those that selectively inhibit cyclooxygenase-2 inhibitors (COX-2 inhibitors), the co-administration of angiotensin II receptor antagonists including losartan may result in a further deterioration of renal function. These effects are usually reversible. Reports suggest that NSAIDs, including selective COX-2 inhibitors, may diminish the antihypertensive effect of angiotensin II receptor antagonists, including losartan. This interaction should be given consideration in patients taking NSAIDs, including selective COX-2 inhibitors, concomitantly with angiotensin II receptor antagonists). Products include:
Arthrotec Tablets 3129
Voltaren Ophthalmic Solution 2309
Voltaren Tablets 2307
Voltaren-XR Tablets 2310

Diltiazem Hydrochloride (Additive effect or potentiation of other antihypertensives). Products include:
Cardizem LA Extended Release Tablets 1728
Tiazac Capsules 1201

Doxazosin Mesylate (Additive effect or potentiation of other antihypertensives). Products include:
Cardura XL Tablets 2515

Enalapril Maleate (Additive effect or potentiation of other antihypertensives). Products include:
Vasotec I.V. Injection 2103

Enalaprilat (Additive effect or potentiation of other antihypertensives).
No products indexed under this heading.

Eprosartan Mesylate (Additive effect or potentiation of other antihypertensives). Products include:
Teveten Tablets 1735
Teveten HCT Tablets 1737

Erythromycin (Erythromycin increased the AUC of losartan by 30%). Products include:
Ery-Tab Tablets 449
Erythromycin Base Filmtab Tablets 455
Erythromycin Delayed-Release Capsules, USP.............................. 457
PCE Dispertab Tablets 515

Erythromycin Estolate (Erythromycin increased the AUC of losartan by 30%).
No products indexed under this heading.

Erythromycin Ethylsuccinate (Erythromycin increased the AUC of losartan by 30%). Products include:
E.E.S. 451
EryPed 447

Erythromycin Gluceptate (Erythromycin increased the AUC of losartan by 30%).
No products indexed under this heading.

Erythromycin Lactobionate (Erythromycin increased the AUC of losartan by 30%).
No products indexed under this heading.

Erythromycin Stearate (Erythromycin increased the AUC of losartan by 30%). Products include:
Erythrocin Stearate Filmtab Tablets 453

Esmolol Hydrochloride (Additive effect or potentiation of other antihypertensives).
No products indexed under this heading.

Etodolac (In some patients with compromised renal function who are being treated with non-steroidal anti-inflammatory drugs (NSAIDs), including those that selectively inhibit cyclooxygenase-2 inhibitors (COX-2 inhibitors), the co-administration of angiotensin II receptor antagonists including losartan may result in a further deterioration of renal function. These effects are usually reversible. Reports suggest that NSAIDs, including selective COX-2 inhibitors, may diminish the antihypertensive effect of angiotensin II receptor antagonists, including losartan. This interaction should be given consideration in patients taking NSAIDs, including selective COX-2 inhibitors, concomitantly with angiotensin II receptor antagonists).
No products indexed under this heading.

Felodipine (Additive effect or potentiation of other antihypertensives).
No products indexed under this heading.

Fenoprofen Calcium (In some patients with compromised renal function who are being treated with non-steroidal anti-inflammatory drugs (NSAIDs), including those that selectively inhibit cyclooxygenase-2 inhibitors (COX-2 inhibitors), the co-administration of angiotensin II receptor antagonists including losartan may result in a further deterioration of renal function. These effects are usually reversible. Reports suggest that NSAIDs, including selective COX-2 inhibitors, may diminish the antihypertensive effect of angiotensin II receptor antagonists, including losartan. This interaction should be given consideration in patients taking NSAIDs, including selective COX-2 inhibitors, concomitantly with angiotensin II receptor antagonists). Products include:
Nalfon Capsules 2502

Fentanyl (Potentiation of orthostatic hypotension). Products include:
Duragesic Transdermal System 2373
Ionsys Transdermal System 2379

Fentanyl Citrate (Potentiation of orthostatic hypotension). Products include:
Actiq 979

Fluconazole (Fluconazole decreased the AUC of the active metabolite of losartan by approximately 40%, but increased the AUC of losartan by 70%).
No products indexed under this heading.

Fludrocortisone Acetate (Potential for intensified electrolyte depletion, particularly hypokalemia).
No products indexed under this heading.

Flurbiprofen (In some patients with compromised renal function who are being treated with non-steroidal anti-inflammatory drugs (NSAIDs), including those that selectively inhibit cyclooxygenase-2 inhibitors (COX-2 inhibitors), the co-administration of angiotensin II receptor antagonists including losartan may result in a further deterioration of renal function. These effects are usually reversible. Reports suggest that NSAIDs, including selective COX-2 inhibitors, may diminish the antihypertensive effect of angiotensin II receptor antagonists, including losartan. This interaction should be given consideration in patients taking NSAIDs, including selective COX-2 inhibitors, concomitantly with angiotensin II receptor antagonists).
No products indexed under this heading.

Fosinopril Sodium (Additive effect or potentiation of other antihypertensives).
No products indexed under this heading.

Furosemide (Additive effect or potentiation of other antihypertensives). Products include:
Furosemide Tablets 2154

Gestodene (In vitro studies show significant inhibition of the formation of the active metabolite by inhibitors of CYP4503A4, such as gestodene; pharmacodynamic consequences of concomitant use are undefined).
No products indexed under this heading.

Glimepiride (Hyperglycemia may occur with thiazide diuretics; dosage adjustment of the antidiabetic drug may be required). Products include:
Avandaryl Tablets 1379
Duetact Tablets 3226

Glipizide (Hyperglycemia may occur with thiazide diuretics; dosage adjustment of the antidiabetic drug may be required).
No products indexed under this heading.

Glyburide (Hyperglycemia may occur with thiazide diuretics; dosage adjustment of the antidiabetic drug may be required).
No products indexed under this heading.

Guanabenz Acetate (Additive effect or potentiation of other antihypertensives).
No products indexed under this heading.

Guanethidine Monosulfate (Additive effect or potentiation of other antihypertensives).
No products indexed under this heading.

Hydralazine Hydrochloride (Additive effect or potentiation of other antihypertensives). Products include:
BiDil Tablets 2171

Hydrocodone Bitartrate (Potentiation of orthostatic hypotension). Products include:
Hycodan 1116
Hycotuss Expectorant Syrup 1117
Vicodin Tablets 535
Vicodin ES Tablets 536
Vicodin HP Tablets 538
Vicoprofen Tablets 539
Zydone Tablets 1139

Hydrocodone Polistirex (Potentiation of orthostatic hypotension). Products include:
Tussionex Pennkinetic Extended-Release Suspension...... 3327

Hydrocortisone (Potential for intensified electrolyte depletion, particularly hypokalemia). Products include:
Colocort Rectal Suspension, USP (Retention) 100 mg/60 mL........... 2476
Hydrocortone Tablets 1989
Preparation H Hydrocortisone Cream .... ▣646

Hydrocortisone Acetate (Potential for intensified electrolyte depletion, particularly hypokalemia). Products include:
Analpram-HC 1159
Pramosone 1161
ProctoFoam-HC 3099

Hydrocortisone Sodium Phosphate (Potential for intensified electrolyte depletion, particularly hypokalemia).
No products indexed under this heading.

Hydrocortisone Sodium Succinate (Potential for intensified electrolyte depletion, particularly hypokalemia).
No products indexed under this heading.

Hydroflumethiazide (Additive effect or potentiation of other antihypertensives).
No products indexed under this heading.

Hydromorphone Hydrochloride (Potentiation of orthostatic hypotension). Products include:

- Dilaudid ... 440
- Dilaudid Non-Sterile Powder ... 440
- Dilaudid Oral Liquid ... 445
- Dilaudid Rectal Suppositories ... 440
- Dilaudid Tablets ... 440
- Dilaudid Tablets - 8 mg ... 445
- Dilaudid-HP ... 442

Ibuprofen (In some patients with compromised renal function who are being treated with non-steroidal anti-inflammatory drugs (NSAIDs), including those that selectively inhibit cyclooxygenase-2 inhibitors (COX-2 inhibitors), the co-administration of angiotensin II receptor antagonists including losartan may result in a further deterioration of renal function. These effects are usually reversible. Reports suggest that NSAIDs, including selective COX-2 inhibitors, may diminish the antihypertensive effect of angiotensin II receptor antagonists, including losartan. This interaction should be given consideration in patients taking NSAIDs, including selective COX-2 inhibitors, concomitantly with angiotensin II receptor antagonists). Products include:

- Advil Allergy Sinus Caplets ... 770
- Advil ... 674
- Children's Advil Oral Suspension ... 603
- Children's Advil Chewable Tablets ... 603
- Advil Cold & Sinus ... 723
- Infants' Advil Concentrated Drops ... 604
- Infants' Advil Concentrated Drops - White Grape (Dye-Free) ... 604
- Junior Strength Advil Swallow Tablets ... 605
- Advil Migraine Liquigels ... 608
- Advil Multi-Symptom Cold Caplets ... 770
- Advil PM Caplets ... 615
- Motrin IB Tablets and Caplets ... 1866
- Children's Motrin Oral Suspension ... 1867
- Children's Motrin Non-Staining Dye-Free Oral Suspension ... 1867
- Children's Motrin Cold Oral Suspension ... 1867
- Infants' Motrin Concentrated Drops ... 1867
- Infants' Motrin Non-Staining Dye-Free Concentrated Drops ... 1867
- Junior Strength Motrin Caplets and Chewable Tablets ... 1867
- Vicoprofen Tablets ... 539

Indapamide (Additive effect or potentiation of other antihypertensives). Products include:

- Indapamide Tablets ... 2156

Indomethacin (Antihypertensive effect of losartan may be blunted by indomethacin). Products include:

- Indocin ... 1995

Indomethacin Sodium Trihydrate (Antihypertensive effect of losartan may be blunted by indomethacin). Products include:

- Indocin I.V. ... 2465

Insulin, Human, Zinc Suspension (Hyperglycemia may occur with thiazide diuretics; dosage adjustment of the antidiabetic drug may be required). Products include:

- Humulin L, 100 Units ... 1794
- Humulin U, 100 Units ... 1800

Insulin, Human NPH (Hyperglycemia may occur with thiazide diuretics; dosage adjustment of the antidiabetic drug may be required). Products include:

- Humulin N, 100 Units ... 1795
- Humulin N Pen ... 1797

Insulin, Human Regular (Hyperglycemia may occur with thiazide diuretics; dosage adjustment of the antidiabetic drug may be required). Products include:

- Humulin R, 100 Units ... 1798

Insulin, Human Regular and Human NPH Mixture (Hyperglycemia may occur with thiazide diuretics; dosage adjustment of the antidiabetic drug may be required). Products include:

- Humulin 50/50, 100 Units ... 1791
- Humulin 70/30 Pen ... 1793

Insulin, NPH (Hyperglycemia may occur with thiazide diuretics; dosage adjustment of the antidiabetic drug may be required).

No products indexed under this heading.

Insulin, Regular (Hyperglycemia may occur with thiazide diuretics; dosage adjustment of the antidiabetic drug may be required).

No products indexed under this heading.

Insulin, Zinc Crystals (Hyperglycemia may occur with thiazide diuretics; dosage adjustment of the antidiabetic drug may be required).

No products indexed under this heading.

Insulin, Zinc Suspension (Hyperglycemia may occur with thiazide diuretics; dosage adjustment of the antidiabetic drug may be required).

No products indexed under this heading.

Insulin Aspart, Human Regular (Hyperglycemia may occur with thiazide diuretics; dosage adjustment of the antidiabetic drug may be required). Products include:

- NovoLog Injection ... 2326

Insulin glargine (Hyperglycemia may occur with thiazide diuretics; dosage adjustment of the antidiabetic drug may be required). Products include:

- Lantus Injection ... 2909

Insulin Lispro, Human (Hyperglycemia may occur with thiazide diuretics; dosage adjustment of the antidiabetic drug may be required). Products include:

- Humalog-Pen ... 1781
- Humalog Mix 50/50-Pen ... 1783
- Humalog Mix 75/25-Pen ... 1785

Insulin Lispro Protamine, Human (Hyperglycemia may occur with thiazide diuretics; dosage adjustment of the antidiabetic drug may be required). Products include:

- Humalog Mix 50/50-Pen ... 1783
- Humalog Mix 75/25-Pen ... 1785

Irbesartan (Additive effect or potentiation of other antihypertensives). Products include:

- Avalide Tablets ... 888
- Avalide Tablets ... 2874
- Avapro Tablets ... 891
- Avapro Tablets ... 2871

Isradipine (Additive effect or potentiation of other antihypertensives). Products include:

- DynaCirc CR Tablets ... 2721

Ketoconazole (In vitro studies show significant inhibition of the formation of the active metabolite by inhibitors of CYP4503A4, such as ketoconazole or complete inhibition by the combination of ketoconazole and sulfaphenazole; pharmacodynamic consequences of concomitant use are undefined). Products include:

- Nizoral A-D Shampoo, 1% ... 1868

Ketoprofen (In some patients with compromised renal function who are being treated with non-steroidal anti-inflammatory drugs (NSAIDs), including those that selectively inhibit cyclooxygenase-2 inhibitors (COX-2 inhibitors), the co-administration of angiotensin II receptor antagonists including losartan may result in a further deterioration of renal function. These effects are usually reversible. Reports suggest that NSAIDs, including selective COX-2 inhibitors, may diminish the antihypertensive effect of angiotensin II receptor antagonists, including losartan. This interaction should be given consideration in patients taking NSAIDs, including selective COX-2 inhibitors, concomitantly with angiotensin II receptor antagonists).

No products indexed under this heading.

Ketorolac Tromethamine (In some patients with compromised renal function who are being treated with non-steroidal anti-inflammatory drugs (NSAIDs), including those that selectively inhibit cyclooxygenase-2 inhibitors (COX-2 inhibitors), the co-administration of angiotensin II receptor antagonists including losartan may result in a further deterioration of renal function. These effects are usually reversible. Reports suggest that NSAIDs, including selective COX-2 inhibitors, may diminish the antihypertensive effect of angiotensin II receptor antagonists, including losartan. This interaction should be given consideration in patients taking NSAIDs, including selective COX-2 inhibitors, concomitantly with angiotensin II receptor antagonists). Products include:

- Acular Ophthalmic Solution ... 565
- Acular LS Ophthalmic Solution ... 566

Labetalol Hydrochloride (Additive effect or potentiation of other antihypertensives).

No products indexed under this heading.

Levobunolol Hydrochloride (Additive effect or potentiation of other antihypertensives). Products include:

- Betagan Ophthalmic Solution, USP ... ⊙220

Levorphanol Tartrate (Potentiation of orthostatic hypotension).

No products indexed under this heading.

Lisinopril (Additive effect or potentiation of other antihypertensives). Products include:

- Prinivil Tablets ... 2052
- Prinzide Tablets ... 2056

Lithium (Diuretics reduce the renal clearance of lithium and add a high risk of lithium toxicity; concurrent use should be avoided).

No products indexed under this heading.

Lithium Carbonate (Diuretics reduce the renal clearance of lithium and add a high risk of lithium toxicity; concurrent use should be avoided). Products include:

- Lithobid Tablets ... 1692

Lithium Citrate (Diuretics reduce the renal clearance of lithium and add a high risk of lithium toxicity; concurrent use should be avoided).

No products indexed under this heading.

Mecamylamine Hydrochloride (Additive effect or potentiation of other antihypertensives).

No products indexed under this heading.

Meclofenamate Sodium (In some patients with compromised renal function who are being treated with non-steroidal anti-inflammatory drugs (NSAIDs), including those that selectively inhibit cyclooxygenase-2 inhibitors (COX-2 inhibitors), the co-administration of angiotensin II receptor antagonists including losartan may result in a further deterioration of renal function. These effects are usually reversible. Reports suggest that NSAIDs, including selective COX-2 inhibitors, may diminish the antihypertensive effect of angiotensin II receptor antagonists, including losartan. This interaction should be given consideration in patients taking NSAIDs, including selective COX-2 inhibitors, concomitantly with angiotensin II receptor antagonists).

No products indexed under this heading.

Mefenamic Acid (In some patients with compromised renal function who are being treated with non-steroidal anti-inflammatory drugs (NSAIDs), including those that selectively inhibit cyclooxygenase-2 inhibitors (COX-2 inhibitors), the co-administration of angiotensin II receptor antagonists including losartan may result in a further deterioration of renal function. These effects are usually reversible. Reports suggest that NSAIDs, including selective COX-2 inhibitors, may diminish the antihypertensive effect of angiotensin II receptor antagonists, including losartan. This interaction should be given consideration in patients taking NSAIDs, including selective COX-2 inhibitors, concomitantly with angiotensin II receptor antagonists).

No products indexed under this heading.

Meloxicam (In some patients with compromised renal function who are being treated with non-steroidal anti-inflammatory drugs (NSAIDs), including those that selectively inhibit cyclooxygenase-2 inhibitors (COX-2 inhibitors), the co-administration of angiotensin II receptor antagonists including losartan may result in a further deterioration of renal function. These effects are usually reversible. Reports suggest that NSAIDs, including selective COX-2 inhibitors, may diminish the antihypertensive effect of angiotensin II receptor antagonists, including losartan. This interaction should be given consideration in patients taking NSAIDs, including selective COX-2 inhibitors, concomitantly with angiotensin II receptor antagonists). Products include:

- Mobic Oral Suspension ... 863
- Mobic Tablets ... 863

Meperidine Hydrochloride (Potentiation of orthostatic hypotension).

No products indexed under this heading.

Mephobarbital (Potentiation of orthostatic hypotension).

No products indexed under this heading.

Metformin Hydrochloride (Hyperglycemia may occur with thiazide diuretics; dosage adjustment of the antidiabetic drug may be required). Products include:

- ActoPlus Met Tablets ... 3214
- Avandamet Tablets ... 1373
- Fortamet Extended-Release Tablets ... 3115

Methadone Hydrochloride
(Potentiation of orthostatic
hypotension).
 No products indexed under this
 heading.

Methyclothiazide (Additive effect
or potentiation of other
antihypertensives).
 No products indexed under this
 heading.

Methyldopa (Additive effect or
potentiation of other antihypertensives). Products include:
 Aldoril Tablets **1910**

Methyldopate Hydrochloride
(Additive effect or potentiation of
other antihypertensives).
 No products indexed under this
 heading.

Methylprednisolone Acetate
(Potential for intensified electrolyte
depletion, particularly hypokalemia).
Products include:
 Depo-Medrol Injectable
 Suspension **2617**
 Depo-Medrol Single-Dose Vial **2619**

**Methylprednisolone Sodium
Succinate** (Potential for intensified
electrolyte depletion, particularly
hypokalemia).
 No products indexed under this
 heading.

Metipranolol Hydrochloride
(Additive effect or potentiation of
other antihypertensives).
 No products indexed under this
 heading.

Metocurine Iodide (Possible
increased responsiveness to the
muscle relaxant).
 No products indexed under this
 heading.

Metolazone (Additive effect or
potentiation of other antihypertensives).
 No products indexed under this
 heading.

Metoprolol Succinate (Additive
effect or potentiation of other antihypertensives). Products include:
 Toprol-XL Tablets **668**

Metoprolol Tartrate (Additive
effect or potentiation of other antihy-
pertensives). Products include:
 Lopressor Injection **2238**
 Lopressor Tablets **2238**
 Lopressor HCT 50/25 Tablets **2241**
 Lopressor HCT 100/25 Tablets **2241**
 Lopressor HCT 100/50 Tablets **2241**

Metyrosine (Additive effect or
potentiation of other antihypertensives). Products include:
 Demser Capsules **1953**

Mibefradil Dihydrochloride (Additive effect or potentiation of other
antihypertensives).
 No products indexed under this
 heading.

Miglitol (Hyperglycemia may occur
with thiazide diuretics; dosage
adjustment of the antidiabetic drug
may be required).
 No products indexed under this
 heading.

Minoxidil (Additive effect or potenti-
ation of other antihypertensives).
Products include:
 Men's Rogaine Extra Strength
 Hair Regrowth Treatment
 Topical Solution, Ocean Rush
 Scent and Original Unscented ▣**633**
 Men's Rogaine Foam Hair
 Regrowth Treatment.................... ▣**633**
 Women's Rogaine Hair Regrowth
 Treatment Topical Solution,
 Spring Bloom Scent and
 Original Unscented...................... ▣**634**

Mivacurium Chloride (Possible
increased responsiveness to the
muscle relaxant). Products include:
 Mivacron Injection **493**

Moexipril Hydrochloride (Additive
effect or potentiation of other antihypertensives). Products include:
 Uniretic Tablets **3100**
 Univasc Tablets **3104**

Morphine Sulfate (Potentiation of
orthostatic hypotension). Products
include:
 Avinza Capsules **1741**
 Kadian Capsules **577**
 MS Contin Tablets **2701**

Nabumetone (In some patients
with compromised renal function
who are being treated with non-
steroidal anti-inflammatory drugs
(NSAIDs), including those that selectively inhibit cyclooxygenase-2 inhibitors (COX-2 inhibitors), the co-
administration of angiotensin II
receptor antagonists including losartan may result in a further deterioration of renal function. These effects
are usually reversible. Reports suggest that NSAIDs, including selective
COX-2 inhibitors, may diminish the
antihypertensive effect of angiotensin II receptor antagonists, including
losartan. This interaction should be
given consideration in patients taking NSAIDs, including selective
COX-2 inhibitors, concomitantly with
angiotensin II receptor antagonists).
 No products indexed under this
 heading.

Nadolol (Additive effect or potentia-
tion of other antihypertensives).
Products include:
 Nadolol Tablets **2159**

Naproxen (In some patients with
compromised renal function who are
being treated with non-steroidal
anti-inflammatory drugs (NSAIDs),
including those that selectively inhibit
cyclooxygenase-2 inhibitors (COX-2
inhibitors), the co-administration of
angiotensin II receptor antagonists
including losartan may result in a
further deterioration of renal function. These effects are usually
reversible. Reports suggest that
NSAIDs, including selective COX-2
inhibitors, may diminish the antihypertensive effect of angiotensin II
receptor antagonists, including losartan. This interaction should be given
consideration in patients taking
NSAIDs, including selective COX-2
inhibitors, concomitantly with angiotensin II receptor antagonists).
Products include:
 EC-Naprosyn Delayed-Release
 Tablets **2761**
 Naprosyn Suspension **2761**
 Naprosyn Tablets **2761**
 Prevacid NapraPAC **3280**

Naproxen Sodium (In some
patients with compromised renal
function who are being treated with
non-steroidal anti-inflammatory drugs
(NSAIDs), including those that selectively inhibit cyclooxygenase-2 inhibitors (COX-2 inhibitors), the co-
administration of angiotensin II
receptor antagonists including losartan may result in a further deterioration of renal function. These effects
are usually reversible. Reports suggest that NSAIDs, including selective
COX-2 inhibitors, may diminish the
antihypertensive effect of angiotensin II receptor antagonists, including
losartan. This interaction should be
given consideration in patients taking NSAIDs, including selective

COX-2 inhibitors, concomitantly with
angiotensin II receptor antagonists).
Products include:
 Aleve Caplets **742**
 Aleve Gelcaps **743**
 Aleve Tablets **743**
 Aleve Cold & Sinus Caplets **744**
 Anaprox Tablets **2761**
 Anaprox DS Tablets **2761**

Nicardipine Hydrochloride (Additive effect or potentiation of other
antihypertensives). Products include:
 Cardene I.V. **2497**

Nifedipine (Additive effect or poten-
tiation of other antihypertensives).
Products include:
 Adalat CC Tablets **2964**

Nisoldipine (Additive effect or
potentiation of other antihypertensives). Products include:
 Sular Tablets **3122**

Nitroglycerin (Additive effect or
potentiation of other antihyperten-
sives). Products include:
 Nitro-Dur Transdermal Infusion
 System **3046**
 Nitrolingual Pumpspray **3120**

Oxaprozin (In some patients with
compromised renal function who are
being treated with non-steroidal
anti-inflammatory drugs (NSAIDs),
including those that selectively inhibit
cyclooxygenase-2 inhibitors (COX-2
inhibitors), the co-administration of
angiotensin II receptor antagonists
including losartan may result in a
further deterioration of renal function. These effects are usually
reversible. Reports suggest that
NSAIDs, including selective COX-2
inhibitors, may diminish the antihypertensive effect of angiotensin II
receptor antagonists, including losartan. This interaction should be given
consideration in patients taking
NSAIDs, including selective COX-2
inhibitors, concomitantly with angiotensin II receptor antagonists).
 No products indexed under this
 heading.

Oxycodone Hydrochloride
(Potentiation of orthostatic hypoten-
sion). Products include:
 OxyContin Tablets **2703**
 OxyFast Oral Concentrate
 Solution **2708**
 OxyIR Capsules **2708**
 Percocet Tablets **1131**
 Percodan Tablets **1132**

Pancuronium Bromide (Possible
increased responsiveness to the
muscle relaxant).
 No products indexed under this
 heading.

Penbutolol Sulfate (Additive effect
or potentiation of other
antihypertensives).
 No products indexed under this
 heading.

Pentobarbital Sodium (Potentia-
tion of orthostatic hypotension).
Products include:
 Nembutal Sodium Solution, USP **2470**

Perindopril Erbumine (Additive
effect or potentiation of other antihypertensives). Products include:
 Aceon Tablets (2 mg, 4 mg,
 8 mg)...................................... **3194**

Phenobarbital (Co-administration
may lead to a reduction of about
20% in AUC of losartan and its active
metabolite; potentiation of orthostatic hypotension). Products
include:
 Donnatal Extentabs **2493**

**Phenoxybenzamine Hydrochlo-
ride** (Additive effect or potentiation
of other antihypertensives). Products
include:
 Dibenzyline Capsules **3399**

Phentolamine Mesylate (Additive
effect or potentiation of other
antihypertensives).
 No products indexed under this
 heading.

Phenylbutazone (In some patients
with compromised renal function
who are being treated with non-
steroidal anti-inflammatory drugs
(NSAIDs), including those that selectively inhibit cyclooxygenase-2 inhibitors (COX-2 inhibitors), the co-
administration of angiotensin II
receptor antagonists including losartan may result in a further deterioration of renal function. These effects
are usually reversible. Reports suggest that NSAIDs, including selective
COX-2 inhibitors, may diminish the
antihypertensive effect of angiotensin II receptor antagonists, including
losartan. This interaction should be
given consideration in patients taking NSAIDs, including selective
COX-2 inhibitors, concomitantly with
angiotensin II receptor antagonists).
 No products indexed under this
 heading.

Pindolol (Additive effect or potentiation of other antihypertensives).
 No products indexed under this
 heading.

Pioglitazone Hydrochloride
(Hyperglycemia may occur with thia-
zide diuretics; dosage adjustment of
the antidiabetic drug may be
required). Products include:
 ActoPlus Met Tablets **3214**
 Actos Tablets **3219**
 Duetact Tablets **3226**

Piroxicam (In some patients with
compromised renal function who are
being treated with non-steroidal
anti-inflammatory drugs (NSAIDs),
including those that selectively inhibit
cyclooxygenase-2 inhibitors (COX-2
inhibitors), the co-administration of
angiotensin II receptor antagonists
including losartan may result in a
further deterioration of renal function. These effects are usually
reversible. Reports suggest that
NSAIDs, including selective COX-2
inhibitors, may diminish the antihypertensive effect of angiotensin II
receptor antagonists, including losartan. This interaction should be given
consideration in patients taking
NSAIDs, including selective COX-2
inhibitors, concomitantly with angiotensin II receptor antagonists).
 No products indexed under this
 heading.

Polythiazide (Additive effect or
potentiation of other
antihypertensives).
 No products indexed under this
 heading.

Potassium Acid Phosphate (Con-
comitant use with potassium supple-
ments may lead to hyperkalemia).
Products include:
 K-Phos Original (Sodium Free)
 Tablets **760**

Potassium Bicarbonate (Concomitant use with potassium supplements may lead to hyperkalemia).
 No products indexed under this
 heading.

Potassium Chloride (Concomitant use with potassium supplements may lead to hyperkalemia). Products include:
- Colyte with Flavor Packs for Oral Solution 3088
- HalfLytely and Bisacodyl Tablets Bowel Prep Kit with Flavors Packs 881
- K-Dur Extended-Relase Tablets 3033
- K-Lor Oral Solution 474
- K-Tab Tablets 475
- MoviPrep Oral Solution 2839
- TriLyte with Flavor Packs for Oral Solution 3100

Potassium Citrate (Concomitant use with potassium supplements may lead to hyperkalemia). Products include:
- Urocit-K Tablets 2144

Potassium Gluconate (Concomitant use with potassium supplements may lead to hyperkalemia).
No products indexed under this heading.

Potassium Phosphate (Concomitant use with potassium supplements may lead to hyperkalemia). Products include:
- K-Phos Neutral Tablets 760

Prazosin Hydrochloride (Additive effect or potentiation of other antihypertensives).
No products indexed under this heading.

Prednisolone Acetate (Potential for intensified electrolyte depletion, particularly hypokalemia). Products include:
- Blephamide Ophthalmic Ointment 568
- Blephamide Ophthalmic Suspension 569
- Poly-Pred Ophthalmic Suspension .... ⊙233
- Pred Forte Ophthalmic Suspension .... ⊙235
- Pred Mild Ophthalmic Suspension .... ⊙238
- Pred-G Ophthalmic Ointment .... ⊙237
- Pred-G Ophthalmic Suspension .... ⊙236

Prednisolone Sodium Phosphate (Potential for intensified electrolyte depletion, particularly hypokalemia).
No products indexed under this heading.

Prednisolone Tebutate (Potential for intensified electrolyte depletion, particularly hypokalemia).
No products indexed under this heading.

Prednisone (Potential for intensified electrolyte depletion, particularly hypokalemia).
No products indexed under this heading.

Propoxyphene Hydrochloride (Potentiation of orthostatic hypotension).
No products indexed under this heading.

Propoxyphene Napsylate (Potentiation of orthostatic hypotension).
No products indexed under this heading.

Propranolol Hydrochloride (Additive effect or potentiation of other antihypertensives). Products include:
- Inderal LA Long-Acting Capsules 3429
- InnoPran XL Capsules 2723

Quinapril Hydrochloride (Additive effect or potentiation of other antihypertensives).
No products indexed under this heading.

Ramipril (Additive effect or potentiation of other antihypertensives). Products include:
- Altace Capsules 1702

Rapacuronium Bromide (Possible increased responsiveness to the muscle relaxant).
No products indexed under this heading.

Rauwolfia Serpentina (Additive effect or potentiation of other antihypertensives).
No products indexed under this heading.

Remifentanil Hydrochloride (Potentiation of orthostatic hypotension).
No products indexed under this heading.

Repaglinide (Hyperglycemia may occur with thiazide diuretics; dosage adjustment of the antidiabetic drug may be required).
No products indexed under this heading.

Rescinnamine (Additive effect or potentiation of other antihypertensives).
No products indexed under this heading.

Reserpine (Additive effect or potentiation of other antihypertensives).
No products indexed under this heading.

Rifampin (Rifampin decreased the concentrations of losartan and its active metabolite).
No products indexed under this heading.

Rocuronium Bromide (Possible increased responsiveness to the muscle relaxant). Products include:
- Zemuron Injection 2346

Rofecoxib (In some patients with compromised renal function who are being treated with non-steroidal anti-inflammatory drugs (NSAIDs), including those that selectively inhibit cyclooxygenase-2 inhibitors (COX-2 inhibitors), the co-administration of angiotensin II receptor antagonists including losartan may result in a further deterioration of renal function. These effects are usually reversible. Reports suggest that NSAIDs, including selective COX-2 inhibitors, may diminish the antihypertensive effect of angiotensin II receptor antagonists, including losartan. This interaction should be given consideration in patients taking NSAIDs, including selective COX-2 inhibitors, concomitantly with angiotensin II receptor antagonists).
No products indexed under this heading.

Rosiglitazone Maleate (Hyperglycemia may occur with thiazide diuretics; dosage adjustment of the antidiabetic drug may be required). Products include:
- Avandamet Tablets 1373
- Avandaryl Tablets 1379
- Avandia Tablets 1384

Salt Substitutes (Concomitant use with salt substitutes may lead to hyperkalemia).
No products indexed under this heading.

Secobarbital Sodium (Potentiation of orthostatic hypotension).
No products indexed under this heading.

Sodium Nitroprusside (Additive effect or potentiation of other antihypertensives).
No products indexed under this heading.

Sotalol Hydrochloride (Additive effect or potentiation of other antihypertensives).
No products indexed under this heading.

Spirapril Hydrochloride (Additive effect or potentiation of other antihypertensives).
No products indexed under this heading.

Spironolactone (Concomitant use with potassium-sparing diuretics may lead to hyperkalemia).
No products indexed under this heading.

Sufentanil Citrate (Potentiation of orthostatic hypotension).
No products indexed under this heading.

Sulfaphenazole (In vitro studies show significant inhibition of the formation of the active metabolite by inhibitors of CYP4503A4, such as sulfaphenazole; pharmacodynamic consequences of concomitant use are undefined).
No products indexed under this heading.

Sulindac (In some patients with compromised renal function who are being treated with non-steroidal anti-inflammatory drugs (NSAIDs), including those that selectively inhibit cyclooxygenase-2 inhibitors (COX-2 inhibitors), the co-administration of angiotensin II receptor antagonists including losartan may result in a further deterioration of renal function. These effects are usually reversible. Reports suggest that NSAIDs, including selective COX-2 inhibitors, may diminish the antihypertensive effect of angiotensin II receptor antagonists, including losartan. This interaction should be given consideration in patients taking NSAIDs, including selective COX-2 inhibitors, concomitantly with angiotensin II receptor antagonists). Products include:
- Clinoril Tablets 1924

Telmisartan (Additive effect or potentiation of other antihypertensives). Products include:
- Micardis Tablets 854
- Micardis HCT Tablets 856

Terazosin Hydrochloride (Additive effect or potentiation of other antihypertensives). Products include:
- Hytrin Capsules 471

Thiamylal Sodium (Potentiation of orthostatic hypotension).
No products indexed under this heading.

Timolol Maleate (Additive effect or potentiation of other antihypertensives). Products include:
- Blocadren Tablets 1916
- Cosopt Sterile Ophthalmic Solution 1931
- Timolide Tablets 2086
- Timoptic Sterile Ophthalmic Solution 2088
- Timoptic in Ocudose 2091
- Timoptic-XE Sterile Ophthalmic Gel Forming Solution 2092

Tolazamide (Hyperglycemia may occur with thiazide diuretics; dosage adjustment of the antidiabetic drug may be required).
No products indexed under this heading.

Tolbutamide (Hyperglycemia may occur with thiazide diuretics; dosage adjustment of the antidiabetic drug may be required).
No products indexed under this heading.

Tolmetin Sodium (In some patients with compromised renal function who are being treated with non-steroidal anti-inflammatory drugs (NSAIDs), including those that selectively inhibit cyclooxygenase-2 inhibitors (COX-2 inhibitors), the co-administration of angiotensin II receptor antagonists including losartan may result in a further deterioration of renal function. These effects are usually reversible. Reports suggest that NSAIDs, including selective COX-2 inhibitors, may diminish the antihypertensive effect of angiotensin II receptor antagonists, including losartan. This interaction should be given consideration in patients taking NSAIDs, including selective COX-2 inhibitors, concomitantly with angiotensin II receptor antagonists).
No products indexed under this heading.

Torsemide (Additive effect or potentiation of other antihypertensives). Products include:
- Demadex Injection 2759
- Demadex Tablets 2759

Trandolapril (Additive effect or potentiation of other antihypertensives). Products include:
- Mavik Tablets 486
- Tarka Tablets 524

Triamcinolone (Potential for intensified electrolyte depletion, particularly hypokalemia).
No products indexed under this heading.

Triamcinolone Acetonide (Potential for intensified electrolyte depletion, particularly hypokalemia). Products include:
- Azmacort Inhalation Aerosol 1726
- Nasacort AQ Nasal Spray 2922

Triamcinolone Diacetate (Potential for intensified electrolyte depletion, particularly hypokalemia).
No products indexed under this heading.

Triamcinolone Hexacetonide (Potential for intensified electrolyte depletion, particularly hypokalemia).
No products indexed under this heading.

Triamterene (Concomitant use with potassium-sparing diuretics may lead to hyperkalemia). Products include:
- Dyazide Capsules 1423
- Dyrenium Capsules 3400

Trimethaphan Camsylate (Additive effect or potentiation of other antihypertensives).
No products indexed under this heading.

Troglitazone (Hyperglycemia may occur with thiazide diuretics; dosage adjustment of the antidiabetic drug may be required).
No products indexed under this heading.

Troleandomycin (In vitro studies show significant inhibition of the formation of the active metabolite by inhibitors of CYP4503A4, such as troleandomycin; pharmacodynamic consequences of concomitant use are undefined).
No products indexed under this heading.

Valdecoxib (In some patients with compromised renal function who are being treated with non-steroidal anti-inflammatory drugs (NSAIDs), including those that selectively inhibit cyclooxygenase-2 inhibitors (COX-2 inhibitors), the co-administration of angiotensin II receptor antagonists including losartan may result in a further deterioration of renal function. These effects are usually reversible. Reports suggest that NSAIDs, including selective COX-2 inhibitors, may diminish the antihypertensive effect of angiotensin II receptor antagonists, including losartan. This interaction should be given consideration in patients taking NSAIDs, including selective COX-2 inhibitors, concomitantly with angiotensin II receptor antagonists).
No products indexed under this heading.

Valsartan (Additive effect or potentiation of other antihypertensives). Products include:
Diovan Tablets **2193**
Diovan HCT Tablets **2196**

Vecuronium Bromide (Possible increased responsiveness to the muscle relaxant).
No products indexed under this heading.

Verapamil Hydrochloride (Additive effect or potentiation of other antihypertensives). Products include:
Covera-HS Tablets **3139**
Tarka Tablets **524**
Verelan PM Extended-Release Capsules, Controlled-Onset **3106**

Food Interactions

Alcohol (Potentiation of orthostatic hypotension).

Meal, unspecified (Meal slows absorption and decreases Cmax but has minor effects on losartan AUC or on the AUC of the metabolite).

HYZAAR 100-12.5 TABLETS

(Hydrochlorothiazide, Losartan Potassium) **1990**
See Hyzaar 50-12.5 Tablets

HYZAAR 100-25 TABLETS

(Hydrochlorothiazide, Losartan Potassium) **1990**
See Hyzaar 50-12.5 Tablets

IMDUR TABLETS

(Isosorbide Mononitrate) **3018**
May interact with calcium channel blockers, vasodilators, and certain other agents. Compounds in these categories include:

Amlodipine Besylate (Marked symptomatic orthostatic hypotension has been reported when calcium channel blockers and organic nitrates were used in combination). Products include:
Caduet Tablets **2508**
Lotrel Capsules **2249**
Norvasc Tablets **2545**

Amyl Nitrite (Additive vasodilating effects).
No products indexed under this heading.

Bepridil Hydrochloride (Marked symptomatic orthostatic hypotension has been reported when calcium channel blockers and organic nitrates were used in combination).
No products indexed under this heading.

Diazoxide (Additive vasodilating effects). Products include:
Hyperstat I.V. **3017**

Diltiazem Hydrochloride (Marked symptomatic orthostatic hypotension has been reported when calcium channel blockers and organic nitrates were used in combination). Products include:
Cardizem LA Extended Release Tablets **1728**
Tiazac Capsules **1201**

Epoprostenol Sodium (Additive vasodilating effects).
No products indexed under this heading.

Ethaverine Hydrochloride (Additive vasodilating effects).
No products indexed under this heading.

Felodipine (Marked symptomatic orthostatic hypotension has been reported when calcium channel blockers and organic nitrates were used in combination).
No products indexed under this heading.

Hydralazine Hydrochloride (Additive vasodilating effects). Products include:
BiDil Tablets **2171**

Isosorbide Dinitrate (Additive vasodilating effects). Products include:
BiDil Tablets **2171**

Isoxsuprine Hydrochloride (Additive vasodilating effects).
No products indexed under this heading.

Isradipine (Marked symptomatic orthostatic hypotension has been reported when calcium channel blockers and organic nitrates were used in combination). Products include:
DynaCirc CR Tablets **2721**

Mibefradil Dihydrochloride (Marked symptomatic orthostatic hypotension has been reported when calcium channel blockers and organic nitrates were used in combination).
No products indexed under this heading.

Minoxidil (Additive vasodilating effects). Products include:
Men's Rogaine Extra Strength Hair Regrowth Treatment Topical Solution, Ocean Rush Scent and Original Unscented .... ◘ **633**
Men's Rogaine Foam Hair Regrowth Treatment .... ◘ **633**
Women's Rogaine Hair Regrowth Treatment Topical Solution, Spring Bloom Scent and Original Unscented .... ◘ **634**

Nicardipine Hydrochloride (Marked symptomatic orthostatic hypotension has been reported when calcium channel blockers and organic nitrates were used in combination). Products include:
Cardene I.V. **2497**

Nifedipine (Marked symptomatic orthostatic hypotension has been reported when calcium channel blockers and organic nitrates were used in combination). Products include:
Adalat CC Tablets **2964**

Nimodipine (Marked symptomatic orthostatic hypotension has been reported when calcium channel blockers and organic nitrates were used in combination). Products include:
Nimotop Capsules **749**

Nisoldipine (Marked symptomatic orthostatic hypotension has been reported when calcium channel blockers and organic nitrates were used in combination). Products include:
Sular Tablets **3122**

Nitroglycerin (Additive vasodilating effects). Products include:
Nitro-Dur Transdermal Infusion System **3046**
Nitrolingual Pumpspray **3120**

Nitroglycerin, long-acting formulations (Additive vasodilating effects).
No products indexed under this heading.

Nitroglycerin Intravenous (Additive vasodilating effects).
No products indexed under this heading.

Papaverine (Additive vasodilating effects).
No products indexed under this heading.

Papaverine Hydrochloride (Additive vasodilating effects).
No products indexed under this heading.

Sildenafil Citrate (Amplification of the vasodilatory effects of Imdur by sildenafil can result in severe hypotension). Products include:
Revatio Tablets **2557**
Viagra Tablets **2573**

Tolazoline Hydrochloride (Additive vasodilating effects).
No products indexed under this heading.

Verapamil Hydrochloride (Marked symptomatic orthostatic hypotension has been reported when calcium channel blockers and organic nitrates were used in combination). Products include:
Covera-HS Tablets **3139**
Tarka Tablets **524**
Verelan PM Extended-Release Capsules, Controlled-Onset **3106**

Food Interactions

Alcohol (Additive vasodilating effects).

Food, unspecified (May decrease the rate (increase in Tmax) but not the extent (AUC) of absorption).

IMITREX INJECTION

(Sumatriptan Succinate) **1463**
See Imitrex Tablets

IMITREX NASAL SPRAY

(Sumatriptan) **1467**
See Imitrex Tablets

IMITREX TABLETS

(Sumatriptan Succinate) **1471**
May interact with 5HT1-receptor agonists, ergot-containing drugs, nonselective MAO inhibitors, selective serotonin reuptake inhibitors, and certain other agents. Compounds in these categories include:

Citalopram Hydrobromide (Cases of life-threatening serotonin syndrome have been reported during combined use of selective serotonin reuptake inhibitors (SSRIs) and triptans. If concomitant treatment with sumatriptan succinate is clinically warranted, careful observation of the patient is advised, particularly during treatment initiation and dose increases. Serotonin syndrome symptoms may include mental status changes, autonomic instability, neuromuscular aberrations and/or gastrointestinal symptoms). Products include:
Celexa **1176**

Dihydroergotamine Mesylate (Ergot-containing drugs have been reported to cause prolonged vasospastic reactions; because there is a theoretical basis that these effects may be additive, use of ergot-type agents and sumatriptan within 24 hours is contraindicated). Products include:
Migranal Nasal Spray **3348**

3-Diphenylacrylate (Co-administration with other 5-HT_1 agonists within 24 hours of each other is contraindicated because the vasospastic effects may be additive).
No products indexed under this heading.

Duloxetine Hydrochloride (Cases of life-threatening serotonin syndrome have been reported during combined use of serotonin and norepinephrine reuptake inhibitors (SNRIs) and triptans. If concomitant treatment with sumatriptan succinate is clinically warranted, careful observation of the patient is advised, particularly during treatment initiation and dose increases. Serotonin syndrome symptoms may include mental status changes, autonomic instability, neuromuscular aberrations and/or gastrointestinal symptoms). Products include:
Cymbalta Delayed-Release Capsules **1757**

Ergonovine Maleate (Ergot-containing drugs have been reported to cause prolonged vasospastic reactions; because there is a theoretical basis that these effects may be additive, use of ergot-type agents and sumatriptan within 24 hours is contraindicated).
No products indexed under this heading.

Ergotamine Tartrate (Ergot-containing drugs have been reported to cause prolonged vasospastic reactions; because there is a theoretical basis that these effects may be additive, use of ergot-type agents and sumatriptan within 24 hours is contraindicated).
No products indexed under this heading.

Escitalopram Oxalate (Cases of life-threatening serotonin syndrome have been reported during combined use of selective serotonin reuptake inhibitors (SSRIs) and triptans. If concomitant treatment with sumatriptan succinate is clinically warranted, careful observation of the patient is advised, particularly during treatment initiation and dose increases. Serotonin syndrome symptoms may include mental status changes, autonomic instability, neuromuscular aberrations and/or gastrointestinal symptoms). Products include:
Lexapro Oral Solution **1190**
Lexapro Tablets **1190**

Fluoxetine Hydrochloride (Cases of life-threatening serotonin syndrome have been reported during combined use of selective serotonin reuptake inhibitors (SSRIs) and triptans. If concomitant treatment with sumatriptan succinate is clinically warranted, careful observation of the patient is advised, particularly during treatment initiation and dose increases. Serotonin syndrome symptoms may include mental status changes, autonomic instability, neuromuscular aberrations and/or gastrointestinal symptoms). Products include:

Prozac Pulvules and Liquid 1801
Symbyax Capsules 1819

Fluvoxamine Maleate (Cases of life-threatening serotonin syndrome have been reported during combined use of selective serotonin reuptake inhibitors (SSRIs) and triptans. If concomitant treatment with sumatriptan succinate is clinically warranted, careful observation of the patient is advised, particularly during treatment initiation and dose increases. Serotonin syndrome symptoms may include mental status changes, autonomic instability, neuromuscular aberrations and/or gastrointestinal symptoms).

No products indexed under this heading.

Isocarboxazid (MAO-A inhibitors reduce sumatriptan clearance and significantly increasing systemic exposure; concurrent and/or sequential use is contraindicated).

No products indexed under this heading.

Methylergonovine Maleate (Ergot-containing drugs have been reported to cause prolonged vasospastic reactions; because there is a theoretical basis that these effects may be additive, use of ergot-type agents and sumatriptan within 24 hours is contraindicated).

No products indexed under this heading.

Methysergide Maleate (Ergot-containing drugs have been reported to cause prolonged vasospastic reactions; because there is a theoretical basis that these effects may be additive, use of ergot-type agents and sumatriptan within 24 hours is contraindicated).

No products indexed under this heading.

Naratriptan Hydrochloride (Co-administration with other 5-HT_1 agonists within 24 hours of each other is contraindicated because the vasospastic effects may be additive). Products include:

Amerge Tablets 1339

Nefazodone Hydrochloride (Cases of life-threatening serotonin syndrome have been reported during combined use of serotonin and norepinephrine reuptake inhibitors (SNRIs) and triptans. If concomitant treatment with sumatriptan succinate is clinically warranted, careful observation of the patient is advised, particularly during treatment initiation and dose increases. Serotonin syndrome symptoms may include mental status changes, autonomic instability, neuromuscular aberrations and/or gastrointestinal symptoms).

No products indexed under this heading.

Pargyline Hydrochloride (MAO-A inhibitors reduce sumatriptan clearance and significantly increasing systemic exposure; concurrent and/or sequential use is contraindicated).

No products indexed under this heading.

Paroxetine Hydrochloride (Cases of life-threatening serotonin syndrome have been reported during combined use of selective serotonin reuptake inhibitors (SSRIs) and triptans. If concomitant treatment with sumatriptan succinate is clinically warranted, careful observation of the patient is advised, particularly during treatment initiation and dose increases. Serotonin syndrome symptoms may include mental status changes, autonomic instability, neuromuscular aberrations and/or gastrointestinal symptoms). Products include:

Paxil CR Controlled-Release Tablets 1538
Paxil 1530

Phenelzine Sulfate (MAO-A inhibitors reduce sumatriptan clearance and significantly increasing systemic exposure; concurrent and/or sequential use is contraindicated).

No products indexed under this heading.

Procarbazine Hydrochloride (MAO-A inhibitors reduce sumatriptan clearance and significantly increasing systemic exposure; concurrent and/or sequential use is contraindicated). Products include:

Matulane Capsules 3191

Rizatriptan Benzoate (Co-administration with other 5-HT_1 agonists within 24 hours of each other is contraindicated because the vasospastic effects may be additive). Products include:

Maxalt Tablets 2008
Maxalt-MLT Orally Disintegrating Tablets 2008

Sertraline Hydrochloride (Cases of life-threatening serotonin syndrome have been reported during combined use of selective serotonin reuptake inhibitors (SSRIs) and triptans. If concomitant treatment with sumatriptan succinate is clinically warranted, careful observation of the patient is advised, particularly during treatment initiation and dose increases. Serotonin syndrome symptoms may include mental status changes, autonomic instability, neuromuscular aberrations and/or gastrointestinal symptoms). Products include:

Zoloft 2586

Sumatriptan (Co-administration with other 5-HT_1 agonists within 24 hours of each other is contraindicated because the vasospastic effects may be additive). Products include:

Imitrex Nasal Spray 1467

Tranylcypromine Sulfate (MAO-A inhibitors reduce sumatriptan clearance and significantly increasing systemic exposure; concurrent and/or sequential use is contraindicated). Products include:

Parnate Tablets 1527

Venlafaxine Hydrochloride (Cases of life-threatening serotonin syndrome have been reported during combined use of serotonin and norepinephrine reuptake inhibitors (SNRIs) and triptans. If concomitant treatment with sumatriptan succinate is clinically warranted, careful observation of the patient is advised, particularly during treatment initiation and dose increases. Serotonin syndrome symptoms may include mental status changes, autonomic instability, neuromuscular aberrations and/or gastrointestinal symptoms). Products include:

Effexor Tablets 3411
Effexor XR Capsules 3417

Zolmitriptan (Co-administration with other 5-HT_1 agonists within 24 hours of each other is contraindicated because the vasospastic effects may be additive). Products include:

Zomig Tablets 3519
Zomig Nasal Spray 3523
Zomig-ZMT Tablets 3519

Food Interactions

Food, unspecified (Delays the Tmax slightly by about 0.5 hour with no significant effect on the bioavailability).

IMMUNE[26] BALANCE POWDER SHAKE MIX

(Egg product, hyperimmune) 815
None cited in PDR database.

IMMUNE[26] COMPLETE SUPPORT POWDER SHAKE MIX

(Egg product, hyperimmune) 815
None cited in PDR database.

IMMUNE[26] POWDER, CAPSULES AND CHEWABLE TABLETS

(Egg product, hyperimmune) 815
None cited in PDR database.

IMMUNE[26] POWER CHEWS CHILDREN'S CHEWABLE TABLETS

(Egg product, hyperimmune) 815
None cited in PDR database.

IMMUNOCAL POWDER SACHETS

(Whey Protein Isolate) 1668
None cited in PDR database.

IMODIUM A-D LIQUID AND CAPLETS

(Loperamide Hydrochloride) 1865
None cited in PDR database.

IMODIUM ADVANCED CAPLETS AND CHEWABLE TABLETS

(Loperamide Hydrochloride, Simethicone) 1866
None cited in PDR database.

INCRELEX INJECTION

(Mecasermin [rDNA origin]) 3291
None cited in PDR database.

INDAPAMIDE TABLETS

(Indapamide) 2156
May interact with antihypertensives, barbiturates, corticosteroids, cardiac glycosides, insulin, lithium preparations, narcotic analgesics, and certain other agents. Compounds in these categories include:

Acebutolol Hydrochloride (Indapamide may add to or potentiate the therapeutic effect of other antihypertensive drugs).

No products indexed under this heading.

ACTH (Co-administration with ACTH may increase the risk of hypokalemia).

No products indexed under this heading.

Alfentanil Hydrochloride (Aggravates orthostatic hypotension).

No products indexed under this heading.

Amlodipine Besylate (Indapamide may add to or potentiate the therapeutic effect of other antihypertensive drugs). Products include:

Caduet Tablets 2508
Lotrel Capsules 2249
Norvasc Tablets 2545

Aprobarbital (Aggravates orthostatic hypotension).

No products indexed under this heading.

Atenolol (Indapamide may add to or potentiate the therapeutic effect of other antihypertensive drugs).

No products indexed under this heading.

Benazepril Hydrochloride (Indapamide may add to or potentiate the therapeutic effect of other antihypertensive drugs). Products include:

Lotensin Tablets 2243
Lotensin HCT Tablets 2246
Lotrel Capsules 2249

Bendroflumethiazide (Indapamide may add to or potentiate the therapeutic effect of other antihypertensive drugs).

No products indexed under this heading.

Betamethasone Acetate (Co-administration with corticosteroids may increase the risk of hypokalemia).

No products indexed under this heading.

Betamethasone Sodium Phosphate (Co-administration with corticosteroids may increase the risk of hypokalemia).

No products indexed under this heading.

Betaxolol Hydrochloride (Indapamide may add to or potentiate the therapeutic effect of other antihypertensive drugs). Products include:

Betoptic S Ophthalmic Suspension..................................... 558

Bisoprolol Fumarate (Indapamide may add to or potentiate the therapeutic effect of other antihypertensive drugs).

No products indexed under this heading.

Buprenorphine Hydrochloride (Aggravates orthostatic hypotension). Products include:

Buprenex Injectable 2716
Suboxone Tablets 2717
Subutex Tablets 2717

Butabarbital (Aggravates orthostatic hypotension).

No products indexed under this heading.

Butalbital (Aggravates orthostatic hypotension).

No products indexed under this heading.

Candesartan Cilexetil (Indapamide may add to or potentiate the therapeutic effect of other antihypertensive drugs). Products include:

Atacand Tablets 649
Atacand HCT 651

Captopril (Indapamide may add to or potentiate the therapeutic effect of other antihypertensive drugs). Products include:

Captopril Tablets 2149

Carteolol Hydrochloride (Indapamide may add to or potentiate the therapeutic effect of other antihypertensive drugs). Products include:

Carteolol Hydrochloride Ophthalmic Solution USP, 1%....... ⊙249

Chlorothiazide (Indapamide may add to or potentiate the therapeutic effect of other antihypertensive drugs). Products include:

Diuril Oral Suspension 1954

Chlorothiazide Sodium (Indapamide may add to or potentiate the therapeutic effect of other antihypertensive drugs). Products include:
- Diuril Sodium Intravenous **2467**

Chlorthalidone (Indapamide may add to or potentiate the therapeutic effect of other antihypertensive drugs). Products include:
- Clorpres Tablets **2153**

Clonidine (Indapamide may add to or potentiate the therapeutic effect of other antihypertensive drugs). Products include:
- Catapres-TTS **844**

Clonidine Hydrochloride (Indapamide may add to or potentiate the therapeutic effect of other antihypertensive drugs). Products include:
- Catapres Tablets **843**
- Clorpres Tablets **2153**

Codeine Phosphate (Aggravates orthostatic hypotension). Products include:
- Tylenol with Codeine Tablets **2391**

Cortisone Acetate (Co-administration with corticosteroids may increase the risk of hypokalemia).
No products indexed under this heading.

Deserpidine (Indapamide may add to or potentiate the therapeutic effect of other antihypertensive drugs).
No products indexed under this heading.

Deslanoside (Concurrent digitalis therapy may exaggerate metabolic effects of hypokalemia; especially myocardial effects such as increase ventricular irritability).
No products indexed under this heading.

Dexamethasone (Co-administration with corticosteroids may increase the risk of hypokalemia). Products include:
- Ciprodex Otic Suspension **559**
- Decadron Tablets **1951**
- TobraDex Ophthalmic Ointment **562**
- TobraDex Ophthalmic Suspension ... **563**

Dexamethasone Acetate (Co-administration with corticosteroids may increase the risk of hypokalemia).
No products indexed under this heading.

Dexamethasone Sodium Phosphate (Co-administration with corticosteroids may increase the risk of hypokalemia).
No products indexed under this heading.

Dezocine (Aggravates orthostatic hypotension).
No products indexed under this heading.

Diazoxide (Indapamide may add to or potentiate the therapeutic effect of other antihypertensive drugs). Products include:
- Hyperstat I.V. **3017**

Digitalis Glycoside Preparations (Concurrent digitalis therapy may exaggerate metabolic effects of hypokalemia; especially myocardial effects such as increase ventricular irritability).
No products indexed under this heading.

Digitoxin (Concurrent digitalis therapy may exaggerate metabolic effects of hypokalemia; especially myocardial effects such as increase ventricular irritability).
No products indexed under this heading.

Digoxin (Concurrent digitalis therapy may exaggerate metabolic effects of hypokalemia; especially myocardial effects such as increase ventricular irritability). Products include:
- Lanoxicaps Capsules **1490**
- Lanoxin Injection **1494**
- Lanoxin Injection Pediatric **1497**
- Lanoxin Tablets **1500**

Diltiazem Hydrochloride (Indapamide may add to or potentiate the therapeutic effect of other antihypertensive drugs). Products include:
- Cardizem LA Extended Release Tablets **1728**
- Tiazac Capsules **1201**

Doxazosin Mesylate (Indapamide may add to or potentiate the therapeutic effect of other antihypertensive drugs). Products include:
- Cardura XL Tablets **2515**

Enalapril Maleate (Indapamide may add to or potentiate the therapeutic effect of other antihypertensive drugs). Products include:
- Vasotec I.V. Injection **2103**

Enalaprilat (Indapamide may add to or potentiate the therapeutic effect of other antihypertensive drugs).
No products indexed under this heading.

Eprosartan Mesylate (Indapamide may add to or potentiate the therapeutic effect of other antihypertensive drugs). Products include:
- Teveten Tablets **1735**
- Teveten HCT Tablets **1737**

Esmolol Hydrochloride (Indapamide may add to or potentiate the therapeutic effect of other antihypertensive drugs).
No products indexed under this heading.

Felodipine (Indapamide may add to or potentiate the therapeutic effect of other antihypertensive drugs).
No products indexed under this heading.

Fentanyl (Aggravates orthostatic hypotension). Products include:
- Duragesic Transdermal System **2373**
- Ionsys Transdermal System **2379**

Fentanyl Citrate (Aggravates orthostatic hypotension). Products include:
- Actiq **979**

Fludrocortisone Acetate (Co-administration with corticosteroids may increase the risk of hypokalemia).
No products indexed under this heading.

Fosinopril Sodium (Indapamide may add to or potentiate the therapeutic effect of other antihypertensive drugs).
No products indexed under this heading.

Furosemide (Indapamide may add to or potentiate the therapeutic effect of other antihypertensive drugs). Products include:
- Furosemide Tablets **2154**

Guanabenz Acetate (Indapamide may add to or potentiate the therapeutic effect of other antihypertensive drugs).
No products indexed under this heading.

Guanethidine Monosulfate (Indapamide may add to or potentiate the therapeutic effect of other antihypertensive drugs).
No products indexed under this heading.

Hydralazine Hydrochloride (Indapamide may add to or potentiate the therapeutic effect of other antihypertensive drugs). Products include:
- BiDil Tablets **2171**

Hydrochlorothiazide (Indapamide may add to or potentiate the therapeutic effect of other antihypertensive drugs). Products include:
- Aldoril Tablets **1910**
- Atacand HCT **651**
- Avalide Tablets **888**
- Avalide Tablets **2874**
- Benicar HCT Tablets **1044**
- Diovan HCT Tablets **2196**
- Dyazide Capsules **1423**
- Hyzaar 50-12.5 Tablets **1990**
- Hyzaar 100-12.5 Tablets **1990**
- Hyzaar 100-25 Tablets **1990**
- Lopressor HCT 50/25 Tablets **2241**
- Lopressor HCT 100/25 Tablets **2241**
- Lopressor HCT 100/50 Tablets **2241**
- Lotensin HCT Tablets **2246**
- Micardis HCT Tablets **856**
- Moduretic Tablets **2028**
- Prinzide Tablets **2056**
- Teveten HCT Tablets **1737**
- Timolide Tablets **2086**
- Uniretic Tablets **3100**

Hydrocodone Bitartrate (Aggravates orthostatic hypotension). Products include:
- Hycodan **1116**
- Hycotuss Expectorant Syrup **1117**
- Vicodin Tablets **535**
- Vicodin ES Tablets **536**
- Vicodin HP Tablets **538**
- Vicoprofen Tablets **539**
- Zydone Tablets **1139**

Hydrocodone Polistirex (Aggravates orthostatic hypotension). Products include:
- Tussionex Pennkinetic Extended-Release Suspension **3327**

Hydrocortisone (Co-administration with corticosteroids may increase the risk of hypokalemia). Products include:
- Colocort Rectal Suspension, USP (Retention) 100 mg/60 mL **2476**
- Hydrocortone Tablets **1989**
- Preparation H Hydrocortisone Cream .... ▣ **646**

Hydrocortisone Acetate (Co-administration with corticosteroids may increase the risk of hypokalemia). Products include:
- Analpram-HC **1159**
- Pramosone **1161**
- ProctoFoam-HC **3099**

Hydrocortisone Sodium Phosphate (Co-administration with corticosteroids may increase the risk of hypokalemia).
No products indexed under this heading.

Hydrocortisone Sodium Succinate (Co-administration with corticosteroids may increase the risk of hypokalemia).
No products indexed under this heading.

Hydroflumethiazide (Indapamide may add to or potentiate the therapeutic effect of other antihypertensive drugs).
No products indexed under this heading.

Hydromorphone Hydrochloride (Aggravates orthostatic hypotension). Products include:
- Dilaudid **440**
- Dilaudid Non-Sterile Powder **440**
- Dilaudid Oral Liquid **445**
- Dilaudid Rectal Suppositories **440**
- Dilaudid Tablets **440**
- Dilaudid Tablets - 8 mg **445**
- Dilaudid-HP **442**

Insulin, Human, Zinc Suspension (Hyperglycemia has been reported with the use of indapamide; co-administration may require adjustment in insulin dosage in diabetic patients). Products include:
- Humulin L, 100 Units **1794**
- Humulin U, 100 Units **1800**

Insulin, Human NPH (Hyperglycemia has been reported with the use of indapamide; co-administration may require adjustment in insulin dosage in diabetic patients). Products include:
- Humulin N, 100 Units **1795**
- Humulin N Pen **1797**

Insulin, Human Regular (Hyperglycemia has been reported with the use of indapamide; co-administration may require adjustment in insulin dosage in diabetic patients). Products include:
- Humulin R, 100 Units **1798**

Insulin, Human Regular and Human NPH Mixture (Hyperglycemia has been reported with the use of indapamide; co-administration may require adjustment in insulin dosage in diabetic patients). Products include:
- Humulin 50/50, 100 Units **1791**
- Humulin 70/30 Pen **1793**

Insulin, NPH (Hyperglycemia has been reported with the use of indapamide; co-administration may require adjustment in insulin dosage in diabetic patients).
No products indexed under this heading.

Insulin, Regular (Hyperglycemia has been reported with the use of indapamide; co-administration may require adjustment in insulin dosage in diabetic patients).
No products indexed under this heading.

Insulin, Zinc Crystals (Hyperglycemia has been reported with the use of indapamide; co-administration may require adjustment in insulin dosage in diabetic patients).
No products indexed under this heading.

Insulin, Zinc Suspension (Hyperglycemia has been reported with the use of indapamide; co-administration may require adjustment in insulin dosage in diabetic patients).
No products indexed under this heading.

Insulin Aspart, Human Regular (Hyperglycemia has been reported with the use of indapamide; co-administration may require adjustment in insulin dosage in diabetic patients). Products include:
- NovoLog Injection **2326**

Insulin glargine (Hyperglycemia has been reported with the use of indapamide; co-administration may require adjustment in insulin dosage in diabetic patients). Products include:
- Lantus Injection **2909**

Insulin Lispro, Human (Hyperglycemia has been reported with the use of indapamide; co-administration may require adjustment in insulin dosage in diabetic patients). Products include:
- Humalog-Pen **1781**
- Humalog Mix 50/50-Pen **1783**

Humalog Mix 75/25-Pen 1785

Insulin Lispro Protamine, Human
(Hyperglycemia has been reported with the use of indapamide; co-administration may require adjustment in insulin dosage in diabetic patients). Products include:
Humalog Mix 50/50-Pen 1783
Humalog Mix 75/25-Pen 1785

Irbesartan (Indapamide may add to or potentiate the therapeutic effect of other antihypertensive drugs). Products include:
Avalide Tablets 888
Avalide Tablets 2874
Avapro Tablets 891
Avapro Tablets 2871

Isradipine (Indapamide may add to or potentiate the therapeutic effect of other antihypertensive drugs). Products include:
DynaCirc CR Tablets 2721

Labetalol Hydrochloride (Indapamide may add to or potentiate the therapeutic effect of other antihypertensive drugs).
No products indexed under this heading.

Levorphanol Tartrate (Aggravates orthostatic hypotension).
No products indexed under this heading.

Lisinopril (Indapamide may add to or potentiate the therapeutic effect of other antihypertensive drugs). Products include:
Prinivil Tablets 2052
Prinzide Tablets 2056

Lithium (Diuretics reduce lithium's renal clearance and add a high risk of lithium toxicity).
No products indexed under this heading.

Lithium Carbonate (Diuretics reduce lithium's renal clearance and add a high risk of lithium toxicity). Products include:
Lithobid Tablets 1692

Lithium Citrate (Diuretics reduce lithium's renal clearance and add a high risk of lithium toxicity).
No products indexed under this heading.

Losartan Potassium (Indapamide may add to or potentiate the therapeutic effect of other antihypertensive drugs). Products include:
Cozaar Tablets 1935
Hyzaar 50-12.5 Tablets 1990
Hyzaar 100-12.5 Tablets 1990
Hyzaar 100-25 Tablets 1990

Mecamylamine Hydrochloride
(Indapamide may add to or potentiate the therapeutic effect of other antihypertensive drugs).
No products indexed under this heading.

Meperidine Hydrochloride
(Aggravates orthostatic hypotension).
No products indexed under this heading.

Mephobarbital (Aggravates orthostatic hypotension).
No products indexed under this heading.

Methadone Hydrochloride
(Aggravates orthostatic hypotension).
No products indexed under this heading.

Methyclothiazide (Indapamide may add to or potentiate the therapeutic effect of other antihypertensive drugs).
No products indexed under this heading.

Methyldopa (Indapamide may add to or potentiate the therapeutic effect of other antihypertensive drugs). Products include:
Aldoril Tablets 1910

Methyldopate Hydrochloride
(Indapamide may add to or potentiate the therapeutic effect of other antihypertensive drugs).
No products indexed under this heading.

Methylprednisolone Acetate (Co-administration with corticosteroids may increase the risk of hypokalemia). Products include:
Depo-Medrol Injectable Suspension 2617
Depo-Medrol Single-Dose Vial 2619

Methylprednisolone Sodium Succinate (Co-administration with corticosteroids may increase the risk of hypokalemia).
No products indexed under this heading.

Metolazone (Indapamide may add to or potentiate the therapeutic effect of other antihypertensive drugs).
No products indexed under this heading.

Metoprolol Succinate (Indapamide may add to or potentiate the therapeutic effect of other antihypertensive drugs). Products include:
Toprol-XL Tablets 668

Metoprolol Tartrate (Indapamide may add to or potentiate the therapeutic effect of other antihypertensive drugs). Products include:
Lopressor Injection 2238
Lopressor Tablets 2238
Lopressor HCT 50/25 Tablets 2241
Lopressor HCT 100/25 Tablets 2241
Lopressor HCT 100/50 Tablets 2241

Metyrosine (Indapamide may add to or potentiate the therapeutic effect of other antihypertensive drugs). Products include:
Demser Capsules 1953

Mibefradil Dihydrochloride (Indapamide may add to or potentiate the therapeutic effect of other antihypertensive drugs).
No products indexed under this heading.

Minoxidil (Indapamide may add to or potentiate the therapeutic effect of other antihypertensive drugs). Products include:
Men's Rogaine Extra Strength Hair Regrowth Treatment Topical Solution, Ocean Rush Scent and Original Unscented ▣▣633
Men's Rogaine Foam Hair Regrowth Treatment.................... ▣▣633
Women's Rogaine Hair Regrowth Treatment Topical Solution, Spring Bloom Scent and Original Unscented.................... ▣▣634

Moexipril Hydrochloride (Indapamide may add to or potentiate the therapeutic effect of other antihypertensive drugs). Products include:
Uniretic Tablets 3100
Univasc Tablets 3104

Morphine Sulfate (Aggravates orthostatic hypotension). Products include:
Avinza Capsules 1741
Kadian Capsules 577
MS Contin Tablets 2701

Nadolol (Indapamide may add to or potentiate the therapeutic effect of other antihypertensive drugs). Products include:
Nadolol Tablets 2159

Nicardipine Hydrochloride (Indapamide may add to or potentiate the therapeutic effect of other antihypertensive drugs). Products include:
Cardene I.V. 2497

Nifedipine (Indapamide may add to or potentiate the therapeutic effect of other antihypertensive drugs). Products include:
Adalat CC Tablets 2964

Nisoldipine (Indapamide may add to or potentiate the therapeutic effect of other antihypertensive drugs). Products include:
Sular Tablets 3122

Nitroglycerin (Indapamide may add to or potentiate the therapeutic effect of other antihypertensive drugs). Products include:
Nitro-Dur Transdermal Infusion System.. 3046
Nitrolingual Pumpspray 3120

Norepinephrine Bitartrate (Indapamide may decrease arterial responsiveness to norepinephrine).
No products indexed under this heading.

Oxycodone Hydrochloride
(Aggravates orthostatic hypotension). Products include:
OxyContin Tablets 2703
OxyFast Oral Concentrate Solution..................................... 2708
OxyIR Capsules 2708
Percocet Tablets 1131
Percodan Tablets 1132

Penbutolol Sulfate (Indapamide may add to or potentiate the therapeutic effect of other antihypertensive drugs).
No products indexed under this heading.

Pentobarbital Sodium (Aggravates orthostatic hypotension). Products include:
Nembutal Sodium Solution, USP 2470

Perindopril Erbumine (Indapamide may add to or potentiate the therapeutic effect of other antihypertensive drugs). Products include:
Aceon Tablets (2 mg, 4 mg, 8 mg) 3194

Phenobarbital (Aggravates orthostatic hypotension). Products include:
Donnatal Extentabs 2493

Phenoxybenzamine Hydrochloride (Indapamide may add to or potentiate the therapeutic effect of other antihypertensive drugs). Products include:
Dibenzyline Capsules 3399

Phentolamine Mesylate (Indapamide may add to or potentiate the therapeutic effect of other antihypertensive drugs).
No products indexed under this heading.

Pindolol (Indapamide may add to or potentiate the therapeutic effect of other antihypertensive drugs).
No products indexed under this heading.

Polythiazide (Indapamide may add to or potentiate the therapeutic effect of other antihypertensive drugs).
No products indexed under this heading.

Prazosin Hydrochloride (Indapamide may add to or potentiate the therapeutic effect of other antihypertensive drugs).
No products indexed under this heading.

Prednisolone Acetate (Co-administration with corticosteroids may increase the risk of hypokalemia). Products include:
Blephamide Ophthalmic Ointment 568
Blephamide Ophthalmic Suspension 569
Poly-Pred Ophthalmic Suspension ⊙233
Pred Forte Ophthalmic Suspension ⊙235
Pred Mild Ophthalmic Suspension ⊙238
Pred-G Ophthalmic Ointment ⊙237
Pred-G Ophthalmic Suspension ⊙236

Prednisolone Sodium Phosphate
(Co-administration with corticosteroids may increase the risk of hypokalemia).
No products indexed under this heading.

Prednisolone Tebutate (Co-administration with corticosteroids may increase the risk of hypokalemia).
No products indexed under this heading.

Prednisone (Co-administration with corticosteroids may increase the risk of hypokalemia).
No products indexed under this heading.

Propoxyphene Hydrochloride
(Aggravates orthostatic hypotension).
No products indexed under this heading.

Propoxyphene Napsylate (Aggravates orthostatic hypotension).
No products indexed under this heading.

Propranolol Hydrochloride (Indapamide may add to or potentiate the therapeutic effect of other antihypertensive drugs). Products include:
Inderal LA Long-Acting Capsules 3429
InnoPran XL Capsules 2723

Quinapril Hydrochloride (Indapamide may add to or potentiate the therapeutic effect of other antihypertensive drugs).
No products indexed under this heading.

Ramipril (Indapamide may add to or potentiate the therapeutic effect of other antihypertensive drugs). Products include:
Altace Capsules 1702

Rauwolfia Serpentina (Indapamide may add to or potentiate the therapeutic effect of other antihypertensive drugs).
No products indexed under this heading.

Remifentanil Hydrochloride
(Aggravates orthostatic hypotension).
No products indexed under this heading.

Rescinnamine (Indapamide may add to or potentiate the therapeutic effect of other antihypertensive drugs).
No products indexed under this heading.

Reserpine (Indapamide may add to or potentiate the therapeutic effect of other antihypertensive drugs).
No products indexed under this heading.

Secobarbital Sodium (Aggravates orthostatic hypotension).
No products indexed under this heading.

IMPORTANT NOTE: Always consult each drug listing in the patient's regimen for possible interactions.

Sodium Nitroprusside (Indapamide may add to or potentiate the therapeutic effect of other antihypertensive drugs).
No products indexed under this heading.

Sotalol Hydrochloride (Indapamide may add to or potentiate the therapeutic effect of other antihypertensive drugs).
No products indexed under this heading.

Spirapril Hydrochloride (Indapamide may add to or potentiate the therapeutic effect of other antihypertensive drugs).
No products indexed under this heading.

Sufentanil Citrate (Aggravates orthostatic hypotension).
No products indexed under this heading.

Telmisartan (Indapamide may add to or potentiate the therapeutic effect of other antihypertensive drugs). Products include:
Micardis Tablets ... 854
Micardis HCT Tablets ... 856

Terazosin Hydrochloride (Indapamide may add to or potentiate the therapeutic effect of other antihypertensive drugs). Products include:
Hytrin Capsules ... 471

Thiamylal Sodium (Aggravates orthostatic hypotension).
No products indexed under this heading.

Timolol Maleate (Indapamide may add to or potentiate the therapeutic effect of other antihypertensive drugs). Products include:
Blocadren Tablets ... 1916
Cosopt Sterile Ophthalmic Solution ... 1931
Timolide Tablets ... 2086
Timoptic Sterile Ophthalmic Solution ... 2088
Timoptic in Ocudose ... 2091
Timoptic-XE Sterile Ophthalmic Gel Forming Solution ... 2092

Torsemide (Indapamide may add to or potentiate the therapeutic effect of other antihypertensive drugs). Products include:
Demadex Injection ... 2759
Demadex Tablets ... 2759

Trandolapril (Indapamide may add to or potentiate the therapeutic effect of other antihypertensive drugs). Products include:
Mavik Tablets ... 486
Tarka Tablets ... 524

Triamcinolone (Co-administration with corticosteroids may increase the risk of hypokalemia).
No products indexed under this heading.

Triamcinolone Acetonide (Co-administration with corticosteroids may increase the risk of hypokalemia). Products include:
Azmacort Inhalation Aerosol ... 1726
Nasacort AQ Nasal Spray ... 2922

Triamcinolone Diacetate (Co-administration with corticosteroids may increase the risk of hypokalemia).
No products indexed under this heading.

Triamcinolone Hexacetonide (Co-administration with corticosteroids may increase the risk of hypokalemia).
No products indexed under this heading.

Trimethaphan Camsylate (Indapamide may add to or potentiate the therapeutic effect of other antihypertensive drugs).
No products indexed under this heading.

Valsartan (Indapamide may add to or potentiate the therapeutic effect of other antihypertensive drugs). Products include:
Diovan Tablets ... 2193
Diovan HCT Tablets ... 2196

Verapamil Hydrochloride (Indapamide may add to or potentiate the therapeutic effect of other antihypertensive drugs). Products include:
Covera-HS Tablets ... 3139
Tarka Tablets ... 524
Verelan PM Extended-Release Capsules, Controlled-Onset ... 3106

Food Interactions

Alcohol (Aggravates orthostatic hypotension).

INDERAL LA LONG-ACTING CAPSULES

(Propranolol Hydrochloride) ... 3429

May interact with beta-adrenergic stimulating agents, calcium channel blockers, oral hypoglycemic agents, insulin, non-steroidal anti-inflammatory agents, phenytoin, xanthines, and certain other agents. Compounds in these categories include:

Acarbose (Beta-adrenergic blockade may prevent the appearance of certain premonitory signs and symptoms of acute hypoglycemia in labile insulin-dependent diabetes). Products include:
Precose Tablets ... 751

Albuterol (Propranolol may block bronchodilation produced by exogenous catecholamine stimulation of beta receptors). Products include:
Proventil Inhalation Aerosol ... 3053

Albuterol Sulfate (Propranolol may block bronchodilation produced by exogenous catecholamine stimulation of beta receptors). Products include:
AccuNeb Inhalation Solution ... 1055
Combivent Inhalation Aerosol ... 847
DuoNeb Inhalation Solution ... 1058
ProAir HFA Inhalation Aerosol ... 3300
Proventil Inhalation Solution 0.083% ... 3055
Proventil HFA Inhalation Aerosol ... 3056
Ventolin HFA Inhalation Aerosol ... 1600
VoSpire ER Tablets ... 1052

Aluminum Hydroxide (Greatly reduces intestinal absorption of propranolol). Products include:
Gaviscon Regular Strength Liquid ... ▣ 658
Gaviscon Regular Strength Tablets ... ▣ 658
Gaviscon Extra Strength Liquid ... ▣ 658
Gaviscon Extra Strength Tablets ... ▣ 658
Maalox Regular Strength Antacid/Antigas Liquid ... 2175
Maalox Max Maximum Strength Antacid/Anti-Gas Liquid ... 2176

Aminophylline (Co-administration of theophylline with propranolol results in reduced theophylline clearance).
No products indexed under this heading.

Amlodipine Besylate (Both agents may depress myocardial contractility or AV conduction resulting in increased adverse reactions). Products include:
Caduet Tablets ... 2508
Lotrel Capsules ... 2249
Norvasc Tablets ... 2545

Antipyrine (Reduced clearance of antipyrine).
No products indexed under this heading.

Bepridil Hydrochloride (Both agents may depress myocardial contractility or AV conduction resulting in increased adverse reactions).
No products indexed under this heading.

Bitolterol Mesylate (Propranolol may block bronchodilation produced by exogenous catecholamine stimulation of beta receptors).
No products indexed under this heading.

Celecoxib (Blunts antihypertensive effect of beta-blocker). Products include:
Celebrex Capsules ... 3134

Chlorpromazine (Increased plasma levels of both drugs).
No products indexed under this heading.

Chlorpromazine Hydrochloride (Increased plasma levels of both drugs).
No products indexed under this heading.

Chlorpropamide (Beta-adrenergic blockade may prevent the appearance of certain premonitory signs and symptoms of acute hypoglycemia in labile insulin-dependent diabetes).
No products indexed under this heading.

Cimetidine (Decreases hepatic metabolism of propranolol resulting in increased blood levels). Products include:
Tagamet HB 200 Tablets ... ▣ 664

Cimetidine Hydrochloride (Decreases hepatic metabolism of propranolol resulting in increased blood levels).
No products indexed under this heading.

Diclofenac Potassium (Blunts antihypertensive effect of beta-blocker).
No products indexed under this heading.

Diclofenac Sodium (Blunts antihypertensive effect of beta-blocker). Products include:
Arthrotec Tablets ... 3129
Voltaren Ophthalmic Solution ... 2309
Voltaren Tablets ... 2307
Voltaren-XR Tablets ... 2310

Diltiazem Hydrochloride (Both agents may depress myocardial contractility or AV conduction resulting in increased adverse reactions). Products include:
Cardizem LA Extended Release Tablets ... 1728
Tiazac Capsules ... 1201

Dobutamine (Propranolol may block bronchodilation produced by exogenous catecholamine stimulation of beta receptors).
No products indexed under this heading.

Dobutamine Hydrochloride (Reversed effects of propranolol).
No products indexed under this heading.

Dyphylline (Co-administration of theophylline with propranolol results in reduced theophylline clearance).
No products indexed under this heading.

Ephedrine Hydrochloride (Propranolol may block bronchodilation produced by exogenous catecholamine stimulation of beta receptors).
No products indexed under this heading.

Ephedrine Sulfate (Propranolol may block bronchodilation produced by exogenous catecholamine stimulation of beta receptors).
No products indexed under this heading.

Ephedrine Tannate (Propranolol may block bronchodilation produced by exogenous catecholamine stimulation of beta receptors).
No products indexed under this heading.

Epinephrine (Potential for unresponsiveness to the usual dose of epinephrine to treat allergic reaction). Products include:
EpiPen ... 1061
Primatene Mist ... ▣ 719
Twinject 0.15 ... 3379
Twinject 0.3 ... 3378

Epinephrine Hydrochloride (Potential for unresponsiveness to the usual dose of epinephrine to treat allergic reaction).
No products indexed under this heading.

Etodolac (Blunts antihypertensive effect of beta-blocker).
No products indexed under this heading.

Felodipine (Both agents may depress myocardial contractility or AV conduction resulting in increased adverse reactions).
No products indexed under this heading.

Fenoprofen Calcium (Blunts antihypertensive effect of beta-blocker). Products include:
Nalfon Capsules ... 2502

Flurbiprofen (Blunts antihypertensive effect of beta-blocker).
No products indexed under this heading.

Fosphenytoin Sodium (Accelerates propranolol clearance).
No products indexed under this heading.

Glimepiride (Beta-adrenergic blockade may prevent the appearance of certain premonitory signs and symptoms of acute hypoglycemia in labile insulin-dependent diabetes). Products include:
Avandaryl Tablets ... 1379
Duetact Tablets ... 3226

Glipizide (Beta-adrenergic blockade may prevent the appearance of certain premonitory signs and symptoms of acute hypoglycemia in labile insulin-dependent diabetes).
No products indexed under this heading.

Glyburide (Beta-adrenergic blockade may prevent the appearance of certain premonitory signs and symptoms of acute hypoglycemia in labile insulin-dependent diabetes).
No products indexed under this heading.

Haloperidol (Hypotension and cardiac arrest have been reported with the concomitant use of propranolol and haloperidol).
No products indexed under this heading.

Haloperidol Decanoate (Hypotension and cardiac arrest have been reported with the concomitant use of propranolol and haloperidol).
No products indexed under this heading.

Ibuprofen (Blunts antihypertensive effect of beta-blocker). Products include:
Advil Allergy Sinus Caplets ... 770
Advil ... 674
Children's Advil Oral Suspension ... 603
Children's Advil Chewable Tablets ... 603
Advil Cold & Sinus ... 723
Infants' Advil Concentrated Drops ... 604
Infants' Advil Concentrated Drops - White Grape (Dye-Free) ... 604
Junior Strength Advil Swallow Tablets ... 605
Advil Migraine Liquigels ... 608
Advil Multi-Symptom Cold Caplets ... 770
Advil PM Caplets ... 615
Motrin IB Tablets and Caplets ... 1866
Children's Motrin Oral Suspension ... 1867
Children's Motrin Non-Staining Dye-Free Oral Suspension ... 1867
Children's Motrin Cold Oral Suspension ... 1867
Infants' Motrin Concentrated Drops ... 1867
Infants' Motrin Non-Staining Dye-Free Concentrated Drops ... 1867
Junior Strength Motrin Caplets and Chewable Tablets ... 1867
Vicoprofen Tablets ... 539

Indomethacin (Blunts antihypertensive effect of beta-blocker). Products include:
Indocin ... 1995

Indomethacin Sodium Trihydrate (Blunts antihypertensive effect of beta-blocker). Products include:
Indocin I.V. ... 2465

Insulin, Human, Zinc Suspension (Beta-adrenergic blockade may prevent the appearance of certain premonitory signs and symptoms of acute hypoglycemia in labile insulin-dependent diabetes; acute increases in blood pressure occurred after insulin-induced hypoglycemia in patients on propranolol). Products include:
Humulin L, 100 Units ... 1794
Humulin U, 100 Units ... 1800

Insulin, Human NPH (Beta-adrenergic blockade may prevent the appearance of certain premonitory signs and symptoms of acute hypoglycemia in labile insulin-dependent diabetes; acute increases in blood pressure occurred after insulin-induced hypoglycemia in patients on propranolol). Products include:
Humulin N, 100 Units ... 1795
Humulin N Pen ... 1797

Insulin, Human Regular (Beta-adrenergic blockade may prevent the appearance of certain premonitory signs and symptoms of acute hypoglycemia in labile insulin-dependent diabetes; acute increases in blood pressure occurred after insulin-induced hypoglycemia in patients on propranolol). Products include:
Humulin R, 100 Units ... 1798

Insulin, Human Regular and Human NPH Mixture (Beta-adrenergic blockade may prevent the appearance of certain premonitory signs and symptoms of acute hypoglycemia in labile insulin-dependent diabetes; acute increases in blood pressure occurred after insulin-induced hypoglycemia in patients on propranolol). Products include:
Humulin 50/50, 100 Units ... 1791
Humulin 70/30 Pen ... 1793

Insulin, NPH (Beta-adrenergic blockade may prevent the appearance of certain premonitory signs and symptoms of acute hypoglycemia in labile insulin-dependent diabetes; acute increases in blood pressure occurred after insulin-induced hypoglycemia in patients on propranolol).
No products indexed under this heading.

Insulin, Regular (Beta-adrenergic blockade may prevent the appearance of certain premonitory signs and symptoms of acute hypoglycemia in labile insulin-dependent diabetes; acute increases in blood pressure occurred after insulin-induced hypoglycemia in patients on propranolol).
No products indexed under this heading.

Insulin, Zinc Crystals (Beta-adrenergic blockade may prevent the appearance of certain premonitory signs and symptoms of acute hypoglycemia in labile insulin-dependent diabetes; acute increases in blood pressure occurred after insulin-induced hypoglycemia in patients on propranolol).
No products indexed under this heading.

Insulin, Zinc Suspension (Beta-adrenergic blockade may prevent the appearance of certain premonitory signs and symptoms of acute hypoglycemia in labile insulin-dependent diabetes; acute increases in blood pressure occurred after insulin-induced hypoglycemia in patients on propranolol).
No products indexed under this heading.

Insulin Aspart, Human Regular (Beta-adrenergic blockade may prevent the appearance of certain premonitory signs and symptoms of acute hypoglycemia in labile insulin-dependent diabetes; acute increases in blood pressure occurred after insulin-induced hypoglycemia in patients on propranolol). Products include:
NovoLog Injection ... 2326

Insulin glargine (Beta-adrenergic blockade may prevent the appearance of certain premonitory signs and symptoms of acute hypoglycemia in labile insulin-dependent diabetes; acute increases in blood pressure occurred after insulin-induced hypoglycemia in patients on propranolol). Products include:
Lantus Injection ... 2909

Insulin Lispro, Human (Beta-adrenergic blockade may prevent the appearance of certain premonitory signs and symptoms of acute hypoglycemia in labile insulin-dependent diabetes; acute increases in blood pressure occurred after insulin-induced hypoglycemia in patients on propranolol). Products include:
Humalog-Pen ... 1781
Humalog Mix 50/50-Pen ... 1783
Humalog Mix 75/25-Pen ... 1785

Insulin Lispro Protamine, Human (Beta-adrenergic blockade may prevent the appearance of certain premonitory signs and symptoms of acute hypoglycemia in labile insulin-dependent diabetes; acute increases in blood pressure occurred after insulin-induced hypoglycemia in patients on propranolol). Products include:
Humalog Mix 50/50-Pen ... 1783
Humalog Mix 75/25-Pen ... 1785

Isoetharine (Propranolol may block bronchodilation produced by exogenous catecholamine stimulation of beta receptors).
No products indexed under this heading.

Isoproterenol Hydrochloride (Propranolol may block bronchodilation produced by exogenous catecholamine stimulation of beta receptors).
No products indexed under this heading.

Isoproterenol Sulfate (Propranolol may block bronchodilation produced by exogenous catecholamine stimulation of beta receptors).
No products indexed under this heading.

Isradipine (Both agents may depress myocardial contractility or AV conduction resulting in increased adverse reactions). Products include:
DynaCirc CR Tablets ... 2721

Ketoprofen (Blunts antihypertensive effect of beta-blocker).
No products indexed under this heading.

Ketorolac Tromethamine (Blunts antihypertensive effect of beta-blocker). Products include:
Acular Ophthalmic Solution ... 565
Acular LS Ophthalmic Solution ... 566

Levalbuterol Hydrochloride (Propranolol may block bronchodilation produced by exogenous catecholamine stimulation of beta receptors). Products include:
Xopenex Inhalation Solution ... 3146
Xopenex Inhalation Solution Concentrate ... 3150

Levothyroxine Sodium (Concurrent use may result in lower than expected T_3 concentration). Products include:
Levothroid Tablets ... 1186
Levoxyl Tablets ... 1712
Synthroid Tablets ... 520
Westhroid Tablets ... 3403

Lidocaine Hydrochloride (Reduced clearance of lidocaine).
No products indexed under this heading.

Meclofenamate Sodium (Blunts antihypertensive effect of beta-blocker).
No products indexed under this heading.

Mefenamic Acid (Blunts antihypertensive effect of beta-blocker).
No products indexed under this heading.

Meloxicam (Blunts antihypertensive effect of beta-blocker). Products include:
Mobic Oral Suspension ... 863
Mobic Tablets ... 863

Metaproterenol Sulfate (Propranolol may block bronchodilation produced by exogenous catecholamine stimulation of beta receptors). Products include:
Alupent Inhalation Aerosol ... 826

Metformin Hydrochloride (Beta-adrenergic blockade may prevent the appearance of certain premonitory signs and symptoms of acute hypoglycemia in labile insulin-dependent diabetes). Products include:
ActoPlus Met Tablets ... 3214
Avandamet Tablets ... 1373
Fortamet Extended-Release Tablets ... 3115

Mibefradil Dihydrochloride (Both agents may depress myocardial contractility or AV conduction resulting in increased adverse reactions).
No products indexed under this heading.

Miglitol (Beta-adrenergic blockade may prevent the appearance of certain premonitory signs and symptoms of acute hypoglycemia in labile insulin-dependent diabetes).
No products indexed under this heading.

Nabumetone (Blunts antihypertensive effect of beta-blocker).
No products indexed under this heading.

Naproxen (Blunts antihypertensive effect of beta-blocker). Products include:
EC-Naprosyn Delayed-Release Tablets ... 2761
Naprosyn Suspension ... 2761
Naprosyn Tablets ... 2761
Prevacid NapraPAC ... 3280

Naproxen Sodium (Blunts antihypertensive effect of beta-blocker). Products include:
Aleve Caplets ... 742
Aleve Gelcaps ... 743
Aleve Tablets ... 743
Aleve Cold & Sinus Caplets ... 744
Anaprox Tablets ... 2761
Anaprox DS Tablets ... 2761

Nicardipine Hydrochloride (Both agents may depress myocardial contractility or AV conduction resulting in increased adverse reactions). Products include:
Cardene I.V. ... 2497

Nifedipine (Both agents may depress myocardial contractility or AV conduction resulting in increased adverse reactions). Products include:
Adalat CC Tablets ... 2964

Nimodipine (Both agents may depress myocardial contractility or AV conduction resulting in increased adverse reactions). Products include:
Nimotop Capsules ... 749

Nisoldipine (Both agents may depress myocardial contractility or AV conduction resulting in increased adverse reactions). Products include:
Sular Tablets ... 3122

Oxaprozin (Blunts antihypertensive effect of beta-blocker).
No products indexed under this heading.

Phenobarbital (Accelerates propranolol clearance). Products include:
Donnatal Extentabs ... 2493

Phenylbutazone (Blunts antihypertensive effect of beta-blocker).
No products indexed under this heading.

Phenytoin (Accelerates propranolol clearance).
No products indexed under this heading.

Phenytoin Sodium (Accelerates propranolol clearance). Products include:
Phenytek Capsules ... 2160

Pioglitazone Hydrochloride (Beta-adrenergic blockade may prevent the appearance of certain premonitory signs and symptoms of acute hypoglycemia in labile insulin-dependent diabetes). Products include:

ActoPlus Met Tablets 3214
Actos Tablets 3219
Duetact Tablets 3226

Pirbuterol Acetate (Propranolol may block bronchodilation produced by exogenous catecholamine stimulation of beta receptors). Products include:
Maxair Autohaler 1852

Piroxicam (Blunts antihypertensive effect of beta-blocker).
No products indexed under this heading.

Repaglinide (Beta-adrenergic blockade may prevent the appearance of certain premonitory signs and symptoms of acute hypoglycemia in labile insulin-dependent diabetes).
No products indexed under this heading.

Reserpine (Co-administration of catecholamine-depleting drugs, such as reserpine, may produce an excessive reduction of resting sympathetic nervous activity, which may result in hypotension, vertigo, marked bradycardia, syncopal attacks or orthostatic hypotension).
No products indexed under this heading.

Rifampin (Accelerates propranolol clearance).
No products indexed under this heading.

Rofecoxib (Blunts antihypertensive effect of beta-blocker).
No products indexed under this heading.

Rosiglitazone Maleate (Beta-adrenergic blockade may prevent the appearance of certain premonitory signs and symptoms of acute hypoglycemia in labile insulin-dependent diabetes). Products include:
Avandamet Tablets 1373
Avandaryl Tablets 1379
Avandia Tablets 1384

Salmeterol Xinafoate (Propranolol may block bronchodilation produced by exogenous catecholamine stimulation of beta receptors). Products include:
Advair Diskus 100/50 1308
Advair Diskus 250/50 1308
Advair Diskus 500/50 1308
Advair HFA Inhalation Aerosol 1318
Serevent Diskus 1568

Sulindac (Blunts antihypertensive effect of beta-blocker). Products include:
Clinoril Tablets 1924

Terbutaline Sulfate (Propranolol may block bronchodilation produced by exogenous catecholamine stimulation of beta receptors).
No products indexed under this heading.

Theophylline (Co-administration of theophylline with propranolol results in reduced theophylline clearance).
No products indexed under this heading.

Theophylline Anhydrous (Co-administration of theophylline with propranolol results in reduced theophylline clearance). Products include:
Uniphyl Tablets 2710

Theophylline Calcium Salicylate (Co-administration of theophylline with propranolol results in reduced theophylline clearance).
No products indexed under this heading.

Theophylline Dihydroxypropyl (Glyceryl) (Co-administration of theophylline with propranolol results in reduced theophylline clearance).
No products indexed under this heading.

Theophylline Ethylenediamine (Co-administration of theophylline with propranolol results in reduced theophylline clearance).
No products indexed under this heading.

Theophylline Sodium Glycinate (Co-administration of theophylline with propranolol results in reduced theophylline clearance).
No products indexed under this heading.

Thyroxine (Thyroxine may result in a lower than expected T3 concentration when used concomitantly with propranolol).
No products indexed under this heading.

Thyroxine Sodium (Thyroxine may result in a lower than expected T3 concentration when used concomitantly with propranolol).
No products indexed under this heading.

Tolazamide (Beta-adrenergic blockade may prevent the appearance of certain premonitory signs and symptoms of acute hypoglycemia in labile insulin-dependent diabetes).
No products indexed under this heading.

Tolbutamide (Beta-adrenergic blockade may prevent the appearance of certain premonitory signs and symptoms of acute hypoglycemia in labile insulin-dependent diabetes).
No products indexed under this heading.

Tolmetin Sodium (Blunts antihypertensive effect of beta-blocker).
No products indexed under this heading.

Troglitazone (Beta-adrenergic blockade may prevent the appearance of certain premonitory signs and symptoms of acute hypoglycemia in labile insulin-dependent diabetes).
No products indexed under this heading.

Valdecoxib (Blunts antihypertensive effect of beta-blocker).
No products indexed under this heading.

Verapamil Hydrochloride (On rare occasion, co-administration of intravenous beta-blocker and verapamil, has resulted in serious adverse reactions, especially in patients with severe cardiomyopathy, congestive heart failure or recent myocardial infarction; calcium channel blockers and beta-blockers may depress myocardial contractility or AV conduction). Products include:
Covera-HS Tablets 3139
Tarka Tablets 524
Verelan PM Extended-Release Capsules, Controlled-Onset........... 3106

Food Interactions

Alcohol (Slows the rate of absorption of propranolol).

INDOCIN CAPSULES

(Indomethacin) 1995
May interact with ACE inhibitors, angiotensin-II receptor antagonists, beta blockers, anticoagulants, lithium preparations, loop diuretics, non-steroidal anti-inflammatory agents, potassium sparing diuretics, thiazides, and certain other agents. Compounds in these categories include:

Acebutolol Hydrochloride (Blunting of antihypertensive effect of beta blockers).
No products indexed under this heading.

Amiloride Hydrochloride (Reduced diuretic, natriuretic and antihypertensive effects of increased serum potassium levels). Products include:
Midamor Tablets 2026
Moduretic Tablets 2028

Anisindione (Bleeding has been reported in patients on concomitant treatment with anticoagulants and indomethacin. Caution should be exercised when indomethacin and anticoagulants are administered concomitantly). Products include:
Miradon Tablets 3042

Ardeparin Sodium (Bleeding has been reported in patients on concomitant treatment with anticoagulants and indomethacin. Caution should be exercised when indomethacin and anticoagulants are administered concomitantly).
No products indexed under this heading.

Aspirin (When indomethacin is administered with aspirin, its protein binding is reduced, although the clearance of free indomethacin is not altered. The clinical significance of this interaction is not known; however, as with other NSAIDs, concomitant administration of indomethacin and aspirin is not generally recommended because of the potential of increased adverse effects). Products include:
Aggrenox Capsules 822
Bayer Aspirin 744
BC Allergy Sinus Cold Powder .... ■677
BC Headache Powder .... ■677
Arthritis Strength BC Powder .... ■677
BC Sinus Cold Powder .... ■677
Excedrin Extra Strength Caplets/Tablets/Geltabs............ ■684
Excedrin Migraine Caplets/Tablets/Geltabs............ ■609
Goody's Body Pain Formula Powder....................................... ■684
Goody's Extra Strength Headache Powders.......................... ■611
Goody's Extra Strength Pain Relief Tablets.............................. ■685
Percodan Tablets 1132
St. Joseph 81 mg Aspirin Chewable and Enteric Coated Tablets... 1869

Atenolol (Blunting of antihypertensive effect of beta blockers).
No products indexed under this heading.

Benazepril Hydrochloride (Reports suggest that NSAIDs may diminish the antihypertensive effect of ACE-inhibitors and angiotensin II antagonists. These interactions should be given consideration in patients taking NSAIDs concomitantly with ACE-inhibitors or angiotensin II antagonists. In some patients with compromised renal function, the co-administration of an NSAID and an ACE-inhibitor or an angiotensin II antagonist may result in further deterioration of renal funchtion, including possible acute renal failure, which is usually reversible). Products include:
Lotensin Tablets 2243
Lotensin HCT Tablets 2246
Lotrel Capsules 2249

Bendroflumethiazide (Reduced diuretic, natriuretic, and antihypertensive effects of thiazide diuretics).
No products indexed under this heading.

Betaxolol Hydrochloride (Blunting of antihypertensive effect of beta blockers). Products include:
Betoptic S Ophthalmic Suspension.................................. 558

Bisoprolol Fumarate (Blunting of antihypertensive effect of beta blockers).
No products indexed under this heading.

Bumetanide (Reduced diuretic, natriuretic, and antihypertensive effects of loop diuretics). Products include:
Bumex Tablets 2746

Candesartan Cilexetil (Reports suggest that NSAIDs may diminish the antihypertensive effect of ACE-inhibitors and angiotensin II antagonists. These interactions should be given consideration in patients taking NSAIDs concomitantly with ACE-inhibitors or angiotensin II antagonists. In some patients with compromised renal function, the co-administration of an NSAID and an ACE-inhibitor or an angiotensin II antagonist may result in further deterioration of renal funchtion, including possible acute renal failure, which is usually reversible). Products include:
Atacand Tablets 649
Atacand HCT 651

Captopril (Reduced antihypertensive effect of captopril). Products include:
Captopril Tablets 2149

Carteolol Hydrochloride (Blunting of antihypertensive effect of beta blockers). Products include:
Carteolol Hydrochloride Ophthalmic Solution USP, 1%....... ⊙249

Celecoxib (Concomitant use is not recommended due to the increased possibility of gastrointestinal toxicity, with little or no increase in efficacy). Products include:
Celebrex Capsules 3134

Chlorothiazide (Reduced diuretic, natriuretic, and antihypertensive effects of thiazide diuretics). Products include:
Diuril Oral Suspension 1954

Chlorothiazide Sodium (Reduced diuretic, natriuretic, and antihypertensive effects of thiazide diuretics). Products include:
Diuril Sodium Intravenous 2467

Cyclosporine (Increase in cyclosporine-induced toxicity). Products include:
Gengraf Capsules 459
Neoral Oral Solution 2259
Neoral Soft Gelatin Capsules 2259
Restasis Ophthalmic Emulsion 575
Sandimmune 2275

Dalteparin Sodium (Bleeding has been reported in patients on concomitant treatment with anticoagulants and indomethacin. Caution should be exercised when indomethacin and anticoagulants are administered concomitantly). Products include:
Fragmin Injection 1097

Danaparoid Sodium (Bleeding has been reported in patients on concomitant treatment with anticoagulants and indomethacin. Caution should be exercised when indomethacin and anticoagulants are administered concomitantly).
No products indexed under this heading.

Dexamethasone (False-negative results in dexamethasone suppression test). Products include:
Ciprodex Otic Suspension 559
Decadron Tablets 1951
TobraDex Ophthalmic Ointment 562
TobraDex Ophthalmic Suspension ... 563

Dexamethasone Acetate (False-negative results in dexamethasone suppression test).
No products indexed under this heading.

Dexamethasone Sodium Phosphate (False-negative results in dexamethasone suppression test).
No products indexed under this heading.

Diclofenac Potassium (Concomitant use is not recommended due to the increased possibility of gastrointestinal toxicity, with little or no increase in efficacy).
No products indexed under this heading.

Diclofenac Sodium (Concomitant use is not recommended due to the increased possibility of gastrointestinal toxicity, with little or no increase in efficacy). Products include:
Arthrotec Tablets 3129
Voltaren Ophthalmic Solution 2309
Voltaren Tablets 2307
Voltaren-XR Tablets 2310

Dicumarol (Bleeding has been reported in patients on concomitant treatment with anticoagulants and indomethacin. Caution should be exercised when indomethacin and anticoagulants are administered concomitantly).
No products indexed under this heading.

Diflunisal (Co-administration results in decreased renal clearance and significant increase in the plasma levels of indomethacin; in some patients combined therapy has been associated with fatal gastrointestinal hemorrhage; concurrent use is not recommended). Products include:
Dolobid Tablets 1955

Digoxin (Increased serum digoxin concentration and prolonged half-life). Products include:
Lanoxicaps Capsules 1490
Lanoxin Injection 1494
Lanoxin Injection Pediatric 1497
Lanoxin Tablets 1500

Enalapril Maleate (Reports suggest that NSAIDs may diminish the antihypertensive effect of ACE-inhibitors and angiotensin II antagonists. These interactions should be given consideration in patients taking NSAIDs concomitantly with ACE-inhibitors or angiotensin II antagonists. In some patients with compromised renal function, the co-administration of an NSAID and an ACE-inhibitor or an angiotensin II antagonist may result in further deterioration of renal funchtion, including possible acute renal failure, which is usually reversible). Products include:
Vasotec I.V. Injection 2103

Enalaprilat (Reports suggest that NSAIDs may diminish the antihypertensive effect of ACE-inhibitors and angiotensin II antagonists. These interactions should be given consideration in patients taking NSAIDs concomitantly with ACE-inhibitors or angiotensin II antagonists. In some patients with compromised renal function, the co-administration of an NSAID and an ACE-inhibitor or an angiotensin II antagonist may result in further deterioration of renal funchtion, including possible acute renal failure, which is usually reversible).
No products indexed under this heading.

Enoxaparin Sodium (Bleeding has been reported in patients on concomitant treatment with anticoagulants and indomethacin. Caution should be exercised when indomethacin and anticoagulants are administered concomitantly). Products include:
Lovenox Injection 2915

Eprosartan Mesylate (Reports suggest that NSAIDs may diminish the antihypertensive effect of ACE-inhibitors and angiotensin II antagonists. These interactions should be given consideration in patients taking NSAIDs concomitantly with ACE-inhibitors or angiotensin II antagonists. In some patients with compromised renal function, the co-administration of an NSAID and an ACE-inhibitor or an angiotensin II antagonist may result in further deterioration of renal funchtion, including possible acute renal failure, which is usually reversible). Products include:
Teveten Tablets 1735
Teveten HCT Tablets 1737

Esmolol Hydrochloride (Blunting of antihypertensive effect of beta blockers).
No products indexed under this heading.

Ethacrynic Acid (Reduced diuretic, natriuretic, and antihypertensive effects of loop diuretics). Products include:
Edecrin Tablets 1959

Etodolac (Concomitant use is not recommended due to the increased possibility of gastrointestinal toxicity, with little or no increase in efficacy).
No products indexed under this heading.

Fenoprofen Calcium (Concomitant use is not recommended due to the increased possibility of gastrointestinal toxicity, with little or no increase in efficacy). Products include:
Nalfon Capsules 2502

Flurbiprofen (Concomitant use is not recommended due to the increased possibility of gastrointestinal toxicity, with little or no increase in efficacy).
No products indexed under this heading.

Fondaparinux Sodium (Bleeding has been reported in patients on concomitant treatment with anticoagulants and indomethacin. Caution should be exercised when indomethacin and anticoagulants are administered concomitantly). Products include:
Arixtra Injection 1351

Fosinopril Sodium (Reports suggest that NSAIDs may diminish the antihypertensive effect of ACE-inhibitors and angiotensin II antagonists. These interactions should be given consideration in patients taking NSAIDs concomitantly with ACE-inhibitors or angiotensin II antagonists. In some patients with compromised renal function, the co-administration of an NSAID and an ACE-inhibitor or an angiotensin II antagonist may result in further deterioration of renal funchtion, including possible acute renal failure, which is usually reversible).
No products indexed under this heading.

Furosemide (Indomethacin reduces basal plasma renin activity (PRA) induced by furosemide; reduced diuretic, natriuretic, and antihypertensive effects of loop diuretics). Products include:
Furosemide Tablets 2154

Heparin Calcium (Bleeding has been reported in patients on concomitant treatment with anticoagulants and indomethacin. Caution should be exercised when indomethacin and anticoagulants are administered concomitantly).
No products indexed under this heading.

Heparin Sodium (Bleeding has been reported in patients on concomitant treatment with anticoagulants and indomethacin. Caution should be exercised when indomethacin and anticoagulants are administered concomitantly).
No products indexed under this heading.

Hydrochlorothiazide (Reduced diuretic, natriuretic, and antihypertensive effects of thiazide diuretics). Products include:
Aldoril Tablets 1910
Atacand HCT 651
Avalide Tablets 888
Avalide Tablets 2874
Benicar HCT Tablets 1044
Diovan HCT Tablets 2196
Dyazide Capsules 1423
Hyzaar 50-12.5 Tablets 1990
Hyzaar 100-12.5 Tablets 1990
Hyzaar 100-25 Tablets 1990
Lopressor HCT 50/25 Tablets 2241
Lopressor HCT 100/25 Tablets 2241
Lopressor HCT 100/50 Tablets 2241
Lotensin HCT Tablets 2246
Micardis HCT Tablets 856
Moduretic Tablets 2028
Prinzide Tablets 2056
Teveten HCT Tablets 1737
Timolide Tablets 2086
Uniretic Tablets 3100

Hydroflumethiazide (Reduced diuretic, natriuretic, and antihypertensive effects of thiazide diuretics).
No products indexed under this heading.

Ibuprofen (Concomitant use is not recommended due to the increased possibility of gastrointestinal toxicity, with little or no increase in efficacy). Products include:
Advil Allergy Sinus Caplets 770
Advil 674
Children's Advil Oral Suspension 603
Children's Advil Chewable Tablets .. 603
Advil Cold & Sinus 723
Infants' Advil Concentrated Drops .. 604
Infants' Advil Concentrated Drops - White Grape (Dye-Free) 604
Junior Strength Advil Swallow Tablets 605
Advil Migraine Liquigels 608
Advil Multi-Symptom Cold Caplets 770
Advil PM Caplets 615
Motrin IB Tablets and Caplets 1866
Children's Motrin Oral Suspension ... 1867
Children's Motrin Non-Staining Dye-Free Oral Suspension 1867
Children's Motrin Cold Oral Suspension 1867
Infants' Motrin Concentrated Drops 1867
Infants' Motrin Non-Staining Dye-Free Concentrated Drops 1867
Junior Strength Motrin Caplets and Chewable Tablets 1867
Vicoprofen Tablets 539

Indomethacin Sodium Trihydrate (Concomitant use is not recommended due to the increased possibility of gastrointestinal toxicity, with little or no increase in efficacy). Products include:
Indocin I.V. 2465

Irbesartan (Reports suggest that NSAIDs may diminish the antihypertensive effect of ACE-inhibitors and angiotensin II antagonists. These interactions should be given consideration in patients taking NSAIDs concomitantly with ACE-inhibitors or angiotensin II antagonists. In some patients with compromised renal function, the co-administration of an NSAID and an ACE-inhibitor or an angiotensin II antagonist may result in further deterioration of renal funchtion, including possible acute renal failure, which is usually reversible). Products include:
Avalide Tablets 888
Avalide Tablets 2874
Avapro Tablets 891
Avapro Tablets 2871

Ketoprofen (Concomitant use is not recommended due to the increased possibility of gastrointestinal toxicity, with little or no increase in efficacy).
No products indexed under this heading.

Ketorolac Tromethamine (Concomitant use is not recommended due to the increased possibility of gastrointestinal toxicity, with little or no increase in efficacy). Products include:
Acular Ophthalmic Solution 565
Acular LS Ophthalmic Solution 566

Labetalol Hydrochloride (Blunting of antihypertensive effect of beta blockers).
No products indexed under this heading.

Levobunolol Hydrochloride (Blunting of antihypertensive effect of beta blockers). Products include:
Betagan Ophthalmic Solution, USP .... ⊙220

Lisinopril (Reports suggest that NSAIDs may diminish the antihypertensive effect of ACE-inhibitors and angiotensin II antagonists. These interactions should be given consideration in patients taking NSAIDs concomitantly with ACE-inhibitors or angiotensin II antagonists. In some patients with compromised renal function, the co-administration of an NSAID and an ACE-inhibitor or an angiotensin II antagonist may result in further deterioration of renal funchtion, including possible acute renal failure, which is usually reversible). Products include:
Prinivil Tablets 2052
Prinzide Tablets 2056

Lithium (Co-administration produces a clinically relevant elevation of plasma lithium and reduction in renal lithium clearance with a potential for lithium toxicity).
No products indexed under this heading.

Lithium Carbonate (Co-administration produces a clinically relevant elevation of plasma lithium

and reduction in renal lithium clearance with a potential for lithium toxicity). Products include:

Lithobid Tablets 1692

Lithium Citrate (Co-administration produces a clinically relevant elevation of plasma lithium and reduction in renal lithium clearance with a potential for lithium toxicity).

No products indexed under this heading.

Losartan Potassium (Reports suggest that NSAIDs may diminish the antihypertensive effect of ACE-inhibitors and angiotensin II antagonists. These interactions should be given consideration in patients taking NSAIDs concomitantly with ACE-inhibitors or angiotensin II antagonists. In some patients with compromised renal function, the co-administration of an NSAID and an ACE-inhibitor or an angiotensin II antagonist may result in further deterioration of renal funchtion, including possible acute renal failure, which is usually reversible). Products include:

Cozaar Tablets 1935
Hyzaar 50-12.5 Tablets 1990
Hyzaar 100-12.5 Tablets 1990
Hyzaar 100-25 Tablets 1990

Low Molecular Weight Heparins (Bleeding has been reported in patients on concomitant treatment with anticoagulants and indomethacin. Caution should be exercised when indomethacin and anticoagulants are administered concomitantly).

No products indexed under this heading.

Meclofenamate Sodium (Concomitant use is not recommended due to the increased possibility of gastrointestinal toxicity, with little or no increase in efficacy).

No products indexed under this heading.

Mefenamic Acid (Concomitant use is not recommended due to the increased possibility of gastrointestinal toxicity, with little or no increase in efficacy).

No products indexed under this heading.

Meloxicam (Concomitant use is not recommended due to the increased possibility of gastrointestinal toxicity, with little or no increase in efficacy). Products include:

Mobic Oral Suspension 863
Mobic Tablets 863

Methotrexate Sodium (Potentiation of methotrexate toxicity).

No products indexed under this heading.

Methyclothiazide (Reduced diuretic, natriuretic, and antihypertensive effects of thiazide diuretics).

No products indexed under this heading.

Metipranolol Hydrochloride (Blunting of antihypertensive effect of beta blockers).

No products indexed under this heading.

Metoprolol Succinate (Blunting of antihypertensive effect of beta blockers). Products include:

Toprol-XL Tablets 668

Metoprolol Tartrate (Blunting of antihypertensive effect of beta blockers). Products include:

Lopressor Injection 2238
Lopressor Tablets 2238
Lopressor HCT 50/25 Tablets 2241
Lopressor HCT 100/25 Tablets 2241

Lopressor HCT 100/50 Tablets 2241

Moexipril Hydrochloride (Reports suggest that NSAIDs may diminish the antihypertensive effect of ACE-inhibitors and angiotensin II antagonists. These interactions should be given consideration in patients taking NSAIDs concomitantly with ACE-inhibitors or angiotensin II antagonists. In some patients with compromised renal function, the co-administration of an NSAID and an ACE-inhibitor or an angiotensin II antagonist may result in further deterioration of renal funchtion, including possible acute renal failure, which is usually reversible). Products include:

Uniretic Tablets 3100
Univasc Tablets 3104

Nabumetone (Concomitant use is not recommended due to the increased possibility of gastrointestinal toxicity, with little or no increase in efficacy).

No products indexed under this heading.

Nadolol (Blunting of antihypertensive effect of beta blockers). Products include:

Nadolol Tablets 2159

Naproxen (Concomitant use is not recommended due to the increased possibility of gastrointestinal toxicity, with little or no increase in efficacy). Products include:

EC-Naprosyn Delayed-Release Tablets 2761
Naprosyn Suspension 2761
Naprosyn Tablets 2761
Prevacid NapraPAC 3280

Naproxen Sodium (Concomitant use is not recommended due to the increased possibility of gastrointestinal toxicity, with little or no increase in efficacy). Products include:

Aleve Caplets 742
Aleve Gelcaps 743
Aleve Tablets 743
Aleve Cold & Sinus Caplets 744
Anaprox Tablets 2761
Anaprox DS Tablets 2761

Nephrotoxic Drugs (Overt renal decompensation).

No products indexed under this heading.

Oxaprozin (Concomitant use is not recommended due to the increased possibility of gastrointestinal toxicity, with little or no increase in efficacy).

No products indexed under this heading.

Penbutolol Sulfate (Blunting of antihypertensive effect of beta blockers).

No products indexed under this heading.

Perindopril Erbumine (Reports suggest that NSAIDs may diminish the antihypertensive effect of ACE-inhibitors and angiotensin II antagonists. These interactions should be given consideration in patients taking NSAIDs concomitantly with ACE-inhibitors or angiotensin II antagonists. In some patients with compromised renal function, the co-administration of an NSAID and an ACE-inhibitor or an angiotensin II antagonist may result in further deterioration of renal funchtion, including possible acute renal failure, which is usually reversible). Products include:

Aceon Tablets (2 mg, 4 mg, 8 mg) 3194

Phenylbutazone (Concomitant use is not recommended due to the increased possibility of gastrointestinal toxicity, with little or no increase in efficacy).

No products indexed under this heading.

Pindolol (Blunting of antihypertensive effect of beta blockers).

No products indexed under this heading.

Piroxicam (Concomitant use is not recommended due to the increased possibility of gastrointestinal toxicity, with little or no increase in efficacy).

No products indexed under this heading.

Polythiazide (Reduced diuretic, natriuretic, and antihypertensive effects of thiazide diuretics).

No products indexed under this heading.

Probenecid (Increased plasma levels of indomethacin).

No products indexed under this heading.

Propranolol Hydrochloride (Blunting of antihypertensive effect of beta blockers). Products include:

Inderal LA Long-Acting Capsules 3429
InnoPran XL Capsules 2723

Quinapril Hydrochloride (Reports suggest that NSAIDs may diminish the antihypertensive effect of ACE-inhibitors and angiotensin II antagonists. These interactions should be given consideration in patients taking NSAIDs concomitantly with ACE-inhibitors or angiotensin II antagonists. In some patients with compromised renal function, the co-administration of an NSAID and an ACE-inhibitor or an angiotensin II antagonist may result in further deterioration of renal funchtion, including possible acute renal failure, which is usually reversible).

No products indexed under this heading.

Ramipril (Reports suggest that NSAIDs may diminish the antihypertensive effect of ACE-inhibitors and angiotensin II antagonists. These interactions should be given consideration in patients taking NSAIDs concomitantly with ACE-inhibitors or angiotensin II antagonists. In some patients with compromised renal function, the co-administration of an NSAID and an ACE-inhibitor or an angiotensin II antagonist may result in further deterioration of renal funchtion, including possible acute renal failure, which is usually reversible). Products include:

Altace Capsules 1702

Rofecoxib (Concomitant use is not recommended due to the increased possibility of gastrointestinal toxicity, with little or no increase in efficacy).

No products indexed under this heading.

Sotalol Hydrochloride (Blunting of antihypertensive effect of beta blockers).

No products indexed under this heading.

Spirapril Hydrochloride (Reports suggest that NSAIDs may diminish the antihypertensive effect of ACE-inhibitors and angiotensin II antagonists. These interactions should be given consideration in patients taking NSAIDs concomitantly with ACE-inhibitors or angiotensin II antagonists. In some patients with compromised renal function, the

co-administration of an NSAID and an ACE-inhibitor or an angiotensin II antagonist may result in further deterioration of renal funchtion, including possible acute renal failure, which is usually reversible).

No products indexed under this heading.

Spironolactone (Reduced diuretic, natriuretic and antihypertensive effects of increased serum potassium levels).

No products indexed under this heading.

Sulindac (Concomitant use is not recommended due to the increased possibility of gastrointestinal toxicity, with little or no increase in efficacy). Products include:

Clinoril Tablets 1924

Telmisartan (Reports suggest that NSAIDs may diminish the antihypertensive effect of ACE-inhibitors and angiotensin II antagonists. These interactions should be given consideration in patients taking NSAIDs concomitantly with ACE-inhibitors or angiotensin II antagonists. In some patients with compromised renal function, the co-administration of an NSAID and an ACE-inhibitor or an angiotensin II antagonist may result in further deterioration of renal funchtion, including possible acute renal failure, which is usually reversible). Products include:

Micardis Tablets 854
Micardis HCT Tablets 856

Timolol Hemihydrate (Blunting of antihypertensive effect of beta blockers). Products include:

Betimol Ophthalmic Solution 3382
Betimol Ophthalmic Solution ⊙295

Timolol Maleate (Blunting of antihypertensive effect of beta blockers). Products include:

Blocadren Tablets 1916
Cosopt Sterile Ophthalmic Solution 1931
Timolide Tablets 2086
Timoptic Sterile Ophthalmic Solution 2088
Timoptic in Ocudose 2091
Timoptic-XE Sterile Ophthalmic Gel Forming Solution 2092

Tinzaparin Sodium (Bleeding has been reported in patients on concomitant treatment with anticoagulants and indomethacin. Caution should be exercised when indomethacin and anticoagulants are administered concomitantly).

No products indexed under this heading.

Tolmetin Sodium (Concomitant use is not recommended due to the increased possibility of gastrointestinal toxicity, with little or no increase in efficacy).

No products indexed under this heading.

Torsemide (Reduced diuretic, natriuretic, and antihypertensive effects of loop diuretics). Products include:

Demadex Injection 2759
Demadex Tablets 2759

Trandolapril (Reports suggest that NSAIDs may diminish the antihypertensive effect of ACE-inhibitors and angiotensin II antagonists. These interactions should be given consideration in patients taking NSAIDs concomitantly with ACE-inhibitors or angiotensin II antagonists. In some patients with compromised renal function, the co-administration of an NSAID and an ACE-inhibitor or an angiotensin II antagonist may result in further deterioration of renal funchtion, including possible acute renal failure, which is usually reversible). Products include:

- Mavik Tablets ... 486
- Tarka Tablets ... 524

Triamterene (The addition of triamterene to maintenance schedule of indomethacin has resulted in reversible acute renal failure; potential for increased hyperkalemia; concurrent therapy should be avoided). Products include:

- Dyazide Capsules ... 1423
- Dyrenium Capsules ... 3400

Valdecoxib (Concomitant use is not recommended due to the increased possibility of gastrointestinal toxicity, with little or no increase in efficacy).

No products indexed under this heading.

Valsartan (Reports suggest that NSAIDs may diminish the antihypertensive effect of ACE-inhibitors and angiotensin II antagonists. These interactions should be given consideration in patients taking NSAIDs concomitantly with ACE-inhibitors or angiotensin II antagonists. In some patients with compromised renal function, the co-administration of an NSAID and an ACE-inhibitor or an angiotensin II antagonist may result in further deterioration of renal funchtion, including possible acute renal failure, which is usually reversible). Products include:

- Diovan Tablets ... 2193
- Diovan HCT Tablets ... 2196

Warfarin Sodium (Bleeding has been reported in patients on concomitant treatment with anticoagulants and indomethacin. Caution should be exercised when indomethacin and anticoagulants are administered concomitantly). Products include:

- Coumadin for Injection ... 898
- Coumadin Tablets ... 898

INDOCIN I.V.

(Indomethacin Sodium Trihydrate) ... 2465

May interact with cardiac glycosides and certain other agents. Compounds in these categories include:

Amikacin Sulfate (Serum levels of amikacin significantly elevated).

No products indexed under this heading.

Deslanoside (Half-life of digitalis may be prolonged when given concomitantly).

No products indexed under this heading.

Digitalis Glycoside Preparations (Half-life of digitalis may be prolonged when given concomitantly).

No products indexed under this heading.

Digitoxin (Half-life of digitalis may be prolonged when given concomitantly).

No products indexed under this heading.

Digoxin (Half-life of digitalis may be prolonged when given concomitantly). Products include:

- Lanoxicaps Capsules ... 1490
- Lanoxin Injection ... 1494
- Lanoxin Injection Pediatric ... 1497
- Lanoxin Tablets ... 1500

Furosemide (Blunted natriuretic effect of furosemide). Products include:

- Furosemide Tablets ... 2154

Gentamicin Sulfate (Serum levels of gentamicin significantly elevated). Products include:

- Garamycin Injectable ... 3014
- Pred-G Ophthalmic Ointment ... ⊙237
- Pred-G Ophthalmic Suspension ... ⊙236

INDOCIN ORAL SUSPENSION

(Indomethacin) ... 1995

See Indocin Capsules

INDOCIN SUPPOSITORIES

(Indomethacin) ... 1995

See Indocin Capsules

INFANRIX VACCINE

(Diphtheria & Tetanus Toxoids and Acellular Pertussis Vaccine Adsorbed) ... 1476

May interact with alkylating agents, antimetabolites, corticosteroids, cytotoxic drugs, and immunosuppressive agents. Compounds in these categories include:

Azathioprine (Concurrent immunosuppressive therapy may reduce the immune response to vaccine).

No products indexed under this heading.

Basiliximab (Concurrent immunosuppressive therapy may reduce the immune response to vaccine). Products include:

- Simulect for Injection ... 2284

Betamethasone Acetate (Concurrent immunosuppressive therapy with greater than physiologic doses of corticosteroids may reduce the immune response to vaccine).

No products indexed under this heading.

Betamethasone Sodium Phosphate (Concurrent immunosuppressive therapy with greater than physiologic doses of corticosteroids may reduce the immune response to vaccine).

No products indexed under this heading.

Bleomycin Sulfate (Cytotoxic drugs may reduce the immune response to vaccine).

No products indexed under this heading.

Busulfan (Alkylating drugs may reduce the immune response to vaccine). Products include:

- I.V. Busulfex ... 2493
- Myleran Tablets ... 1525

Capecitabine (Immunosuppressive therapies may reduce the immune response to vaccines). Products include:

- Xeloda Tablets ... 2822

Carmustine (BCNU) (Alkylating drugs may reduce the immune response to vaccine).

No products indexed under this heading.

Chlorambucil (Alkylating drugs may reduce the immune response to vaccine). Products include:

- Leukeran Tablets ... 1504

Cladribine (Immunosuppressive therapies may reduce the immune response to vaccines). Products include:

- Leustatin Injection ... 2357

Cortisone Acetate (Concurrent immunosuppressive therapy with greater than physiologic doses of corticosteroids may reduce the immune response to vaccine).

No products indexed under this heading.

Cyclophosphamide (Alkylating drugs may reduce the immune response to vaccine).

No products indexed under this heading.

Cyclosporine (Concurrent immunosuppressive therapy may reduce the immune response to vaccine). Products include:

- Gengraf Capsules ... 459
- Neoral Oral Solution ... 2259
- Neoral Soft Gelatin Capsules ... 2259
- Restasis Ophthalmic Emulsion ... 575
- Sandimmune ... 2275

Cytarabine (Immunosuppressive therapies may reduce the immune response to vaccines).

No products indexed under this heading.

Dacarbazine (Alkylating drugs may reduce the immune response to vaccine).

No products indexed under this heading.

Daunorubicin Hydrochloride (Cytotoxic drugs may reduce the immune response to vaccine).

No products indexed under this heading.

Dexamethasone (Concurrent immunosuppressive therapy with greater than physiologic doses of corticosteroids may reduce the immune response to vaccine). Products include:

- Ciprodex Otic Suspension ... 559
- Decadron Tablets ... 1951
- TobraDex Ophthalmic Ointment ... 562
- TobraDex Ophthalmic Suspension ... 563

Dexamethasone Acetate (Concurrent immunosuppressive therapy with greater than physiologic doses of corticosteroids may reduce the immune response to vaccine).

No products indexed under this heading.

Dexamethasone Sodium Phosphate (Concurrent immunosuppressive therapy with greater than physiologic doses of corticosteroids may reduce the immune response to vaccine).

No products indexed under this heading.

Doxorubicin Hydrochloride (Cytotoxic drugs may reduce the immune response to vaccine).

No products indexed under this heading.

Epirubicin Hydrochloride (Cytotoxic drugs may reduce the immune response to vaccine).

No products indexed under this heading.

Floxuridine (Immunosuppressive therapies may reduce the immune response to vaccines).

No products indexed under this heading.

Fludarabine Phosphate (Immunosuppressive therapies may reduce the immune response to vaccines).

No products indexed under this heading.

Fludrocortisone Acetate (Concurrent immunosuppressive therapy with greater than physiologic doses of corticosteroids may reduce the immune response to vaccine).

No products indexed under this heading.

Fluorouracil (Immunosuppressive therapies may reduce the immune response to vaccines). Products include:

- Carac Cream, 0.5% ... 2879
- Efudex ... 3363

Gemcitabine Hydrochloride (Immunosuppressive therapies may reduce the immune response to vaccines). Products include:

- Gemzar for Injection ... 1771

Hydrocortisone (Concurrent immunosuppressive therapy with greater than physiologic doses of corticosteroids may reduce the immune response to vaccine). Products include:

- Colocort Rectal Suspension, USP (Retention) 100 mg/60 mL ... 2476
- Hydrocortone Tablets ... 1989
- Preparation H Hydrocortisone Cream ... 646

Hydrocortisone Acetate (Concurrent immunosuppressive therapy with greater than physiologic doses of corticosteroids may reduce the immune response to vaccine). Products include:

- Analpram-HC ... 1159
- Pramosone ... 1161
- ProctoFoam-HC ... 3099

Hydrocortisone Sodium Phosphate (Concurrent immunosuppressive therapy with greater than physiologic doses of corticosteroids may reduce the immune response to vaccine).

No products indexed under this heading.

Hydrocortisone Sodium Succinate (Concurrent immunosuppressive therapy with greater than physiologic doses of corticosteroids may reduce the immune response to vaccine).

No products indexed under this heading.

Hydroxyurea (Cytotoxic drugs may reduce the immune response to vaccine).

No products indexed under this heading.

Lomustine (CCNU) (Alkylating drugs may reduce the immune response to vaccine).

No products indexed under this heading.

Mechlorethamine Hydrochloride (Alkylating drugs may reduce the immune response to vaccine). Products include:

- Mustargen for Injection ... 2468

Melphalan (Alkylating drugs may reduce the immune response to vaccine). Products include:

- Alkeran Tablets ... 956

Mercaptopurine (Immunosuppressive therapies may reduce the immune response to vaccines).

No products indexed under this heading.

Methotrexate (Immunosuppressive therapies may reduce the immune response to vaccines).

No products indexed under this heading.

Methotrexate Sodium (Cytotoxic drugs may reduce the immune response to vaccine).

No products indexed under this heading.

Methylprednisolone Acetate (Concurrent immunosuppressive therapy with greater than physiologic doses of corticosteroids may reduce the immune response to vaccine). Products include:

- Depo-Medrol Injectable Suspension ... 2617
- Depo-Medrol Single-Dose Vial ... 2619

Methylprednisolone Sodium Succinate (Concurrent immunosuppressive therapy with greater than physiologic doses of corticosteroids may reduce the immune response to vaccine).
No products indexed under this heading.

Mitotane (Cytotoxic drugs may reduce the immune response to vaccine).
No products indexed under this heading.

Mitoxantrone Hydrochloride (Cytotoxic drugs may reduce the immune response to vaccine).
No products indexed under this heading.

Muromonab-CD3 (Concurrent immunosuppressive therapy may reduce the immune response to vaccine). Products include:
Orthoclone OKT3 Sterile Solution 2360

Mycophenolate Mofetil (Concurrent immunosuppressive therapy may reduce the immune response to vaccine). Products include:
CellCept Capsules 2747
CellCept Oral Suspension 2747
CellCept Tablets 2747

Pentostatin (Immunosuppressive therapies may reduce the immune response to vaccines). Products include:
Nipent for Injection 1863

Prednisolone Acetate (Concurrent immunosuppressive therapy with greater than physiologic doses of corticosteroids may reduce the immune response to vaccine). Products include:
Blephamide Ophthalmic Ointment 568
Blephamide Ophthalmic Suspension 569
Poly-Pred Ophthalmic Suspension .... ⊙233
Pred Forte Ophthalmic Suspension .... ⊙235
Pred Mild Ophthalmic Suspension .... ⊙238
Pred-G Ophthalmic Ointment .... ⊙237
Pred-G Ophthalmic Suspension .... ⊙236

Prednisolone Sodium Phosphate (Concurrent immunosuppressive therapy with greater than physiologic doses of corticosteroids may reduce the immune response to vaccine).
No products indexed under this heading.

Prednisolone Tebutate (Concurrent immunosuppressive therapy with greater than physiologic doses of corticosteroids may reduce the immune response to vaccine).
No products indexed under this heading.

Prednisone (Concurrent immunosuppressive therapy with greater than physiologic doses of corticosteroids may reduce the immune response to vaccine).
No products indexed under this heading.

Procarbazine Hydrochloride (Cytotoxic drugs may reduce the immune response to vaccine). Products include:
Matulane Capsules 3191

Sirolimus (Concurrent immunosuppressive therapy may reduce the immune response to vaccine). Products include:
Rapamune Oral Solution and Tablets 3475

Tacrolimus (Concurrent immunosuppressive therapy may reduce the immune response to vaccine). Products include:
Prograf Capsules and Injection 632
Protopic Ointment 638

Tamoxifen Citrate (Cytotoxic drugs may reduce the immune response to vaccine). Products include:
Soltamox Oral Solution 3527

Thioguanine (Immunosuppressive therapies may reduce the immune response to vaccines). Products include:
Tabloid Tablets 1575

Thiotepa (Alkylating drugs may reduce the immune response to vaccine).
No products indexed under this heading.

Triamcinolone (Concurrent immunosuppressive therapy with greater than physiologic doses of corticosteroids may reduce the immune response to vaccine).
No products indexed under this heading.

Triamcinolone Acetonide (Concurrent immunosuppressive therapy with greater than physiologic doses of corticosteroids may reduce the immune response to vaccine). Products include:
Azmacort Inhalation Aerosol 1726
Nasacort AQ Nasal Spray 2922

Triamcinolone Diacetate (Concurrent immunosuppressive therapy with greater than physiologic doses of corticosteroids may reduce the immune response to vaccine).
No products indexed under this heading.

Triamcinolone Hexacetonide (Concurrent immunosuppressive therapy with greater than physiologic doses of corticosteroids may reduce the immune response to vaccine).
No products indexed under this heading.

Vincristine Sulfate (Cytotoxic drugs may reduce the immune response to vaccine).
No products indexed under this heading.

INFASURF INTRATRACHEAL SUSPENSION

(Calfactant) 1184
None cited in PDR database.

INFED INJECTION

(Iron Dextran) 3390
None cited in PDR database.

INFERGEN

(Interferon Alfacon-1) 3364
May interact with drugs which undergo biotransformation by cytochrome p-450 mixed function oxidase and certain other agents. Compounds in these categories include:

Acarbose (Concurrent use with agents known to be metabolized via cytochrome P450 pathway requires caution). Products include:
Precose Tablets 751

Acetaminophen (Concurrent use with agents known to be metabolized via cytochrome P450 pathway requires caution). Products include:
Comtrex Maximum Strength Cold & Cough Day/Night Caplets - Day Formulation .... ▣726
Comtrex Maximum Strength Cold & Cough Day/Night Caplets - Night Formulation .... ▣726
Comtrex Maximum Strength Non-Drowsy Cold & Cough Caplets .... ▣725
Comtrex Maximum Strength Day/Night Severe Cold & Sinus Caplets - Day Formulation .... ▣725
Comtrex Maximum Strength Day/Night Severe Cold & Sinus Caplets - Night Formulation .... ▣725
Contac Cold and Flu Maximum Strength Caplets .... ▣728
Contac Cold and Flu Day and Night Caplets (Day Formulation Only) .... ▣727
Contac Cold and Flu Day and Night Caplets (Night Formulation Only) .... ▣727
Contac Cold and Flu Non-Drowsy Caplets .... ▣728
Excedrin Extra Strength Caplets/Tablets/Geltabs .... ▣684
Excedrin Migraine Caplets/Tablets/Geltabs .... ▣609
Excedrin PM Caplets/Tablets/Geltabs .... ▣610
Excedrin Sinus Headache Caplets/Tablets .... ▣610
Excedrin Tension Headache Caplets/Tablets/Geltabs .... ▣611
Goody's Body Pain Formula Powder .... ▣684
Goody's Extra Strength Headache Powders .... ▣611
Goody's Extra Strength Pain Relief Tablets .... ▣685
Goody's PM Powder for Pain with Sleeplessness .... ▣612
Percocet Tablets 1131
Robitussin Cough, Cold & Flu Nighttime Liquid .... ▣738
TheraFlu Cold & Sore Throat Hot Liquid .... ▣741
TheraFlu Flu & Chest Congestion Hot Liquid .... ▣741
TheraFlu Flu & Sore Throat Hot Liquid .... ▣742
TheraFlu Daytime Severe Cold Hot Liquid .... ▣742
TheraFlu Nighttime Severe Cold Hot Liquid .... ▣740
TheraFlu Warming Relief Daytime Severe Cold .... ▣743
TheraFlu Warming Relief Nighttime Severe Cold .... ▣743
Triaminic Cough & Sore Throat Liquid .... ▣747
Regular Strength Tylenol Tablets 1870
Children's Tylenol with Flavor Creator .... ▣679
Children's Tylenol Plus Flu Oral Suspension .... ▣749
Tylenol Cold Head Congestion Daytime Caplets with Cool Burst and Gelcaps .... ▣750
Tylenol Cold Multi-Symptom Daytime Liquid .... ▣752
Tylenol Cold Multi-Symptom Severe Daytime Liquid .... ▣752
Tylenol 8 Hour Extended Release Caplets 1870
Tylenol 1870
Extra Strength Tylenol PM Caplets, Vanilla Caplets, Geltabs, Gelcaps and Liquid 1875
Extra Strength Tylenol Rapid Release Gels 1870
Concentrated Tylenol Infants' Drops Plus Cold & Cough .... ▣754
Tylenol with Codeine Tablets 2391
Tylenol Allergy Multi-Symptom Caplets with Cool Burst and Gelcaps 1872
Tylenol Allergy Multi-Symptom Nighttime Caplets with Cool Burst 1872
Tylenol Severe Allergy Caplets 1872
Tylenol Arthritis Pain Extended Release Caplets and Geltabs 1870
Tylenol Chest Congestion Caplets with Cool Burst 1872
Tylenol Chest Congestion Liquid with Cool Burst 1872
Children's Tylenol Suspension Liquid and Meltaways 1878
Children's Tylenol Plus Cold Suspension Liquid 1879
Children's Tylenol Plus Cold & Allergy Suspension Liquid 1878
Children's Tylenol Plus Cough & Runny Nose Suspension Liquid 1879
Children's Tylenol Plus Cough & Sore Throat Suspension Liquid 1879
Children's Tylenol Suspension with Flavor Creator 1878
Children's Tylenol Plus Flu Suspension Liquid 1881
Children's Tylenol Plus Multi-Symptom Cold Suspension Liquid 1879
Tylenol Cold Severe Congestion Non-Drowsy Caplets with Cool Burst 1874
Tylenol Cold Head Congestion Daytime Caplets with Cool Burst 1873
Tylenol Cold Head Congestion Nighttime Caplets with Cool Burst 1873
Tylenol Cold Head Congestion Severe Caplets with Cool Burst 1873
Tylenol Cold Multi-Symptom Daytime Caplets with Cool Burst and Gelcaps 1874
Tylenol Cold Multi-Symptom Daytime Liquid with Citrus Burst 1874
Tylenol Cold Multi-Symptom Nighttime Caplets with Cool Burst 1874
Tylenol Cold Multi-Symptom Nighttime Liquid with Cool Burst 1874
Tylenol Cold Multi-Symptom Severe Caplets with Cool Burst 1874
Tylenol Cold Multi-Symptom Severe Daytime Liquid with Citrus Burst 1874
Tylenol Cough & Sore Throat Daytime Liquid with Cool Burst 1877
Tylenol Cough & Sore Throat Nighttime Liquid with Cool Burst 1877
Concentrated Tylenol Infants' Drops 1878
Concentrated Tylenol Infants' Drops Plus Cold 1879
Concentrated Tylenol Infants' Drops Plus Cold and Cough 1879
Jr. Tylenol Meltaways 1878
Tylenol Sinus Severe Congestion Caplets with Cool Burst 1876
Tylenol Sinus Congestion & Pain Daytime Caplets with Cool Burst and Gelcaps 1876
Tylenol Sinus Congestion & Pain Nighttime Caplets with Cool Burst 1876
Tylenol Sinus Congestion & Pain Severe Caplets with Cool Burst 1876
Tylenol Sore Throat Daytime Liquid with Cool Burst 1877
Tylenol Sore Throat Nighttime Liquid with Cool Burst 1877
Women's Tylenol Menstrual Relief Caplets 1877
Vicks 44M Cough, Cold & Flu Relief Liquid 2680
Vicks DayQuil LiquiCaps/Liquid Multi-Symptom Cold/Flu Relief .... ▣761
Vicks DayQuil Multi-Symptom Cold/Flu Relief LiquiCaps 2678
Vicks DayQuil Multi-Symptom Cold/Flu Relief Liquid 2678
Vicks NyQuil Multi-Symptom Cold/Flu Relief Liquid 2681
Vicks NyQuil Multi-Symptom Cold/Flu Relief LiquiCaps 2681
Vicks NyQuil LiquiCaps/Liquid Multi-Symptom Cold/Flu Relief .... ▣763
Vicodin Tablets 535
Vicodin ES Tablets 536
Vicodin HP Tablets 538
Zicam Maximum Strength Flu Daytime .... ▣768
Zicam Maximum Strength Flu Nighttime .... ▣768
Zydone Tablets 1139

Alatrofloxacin Mesylate (Concurrent use with agents known to be metabolized via cytochrome P450 pathway requires caution).
No products indexed under this heading.

Alfentanil Hydrochloride (Concurrent use with agents known to be metabolized via cytochrome P450 pathway requires caution).
No products indexed under this heading.

Alprazolam (Concurrent use with agents known to be metabolized via cytochrome P450 pathway requires caution). Products include:
Niravam Orally Disintegrating Tablets ... 3092

Aminophylline (Concurrent use with agents known to be metabolized via cytochrome P450 pathway requires caution).
No products indexed under this heading.

Amiodarone Hydrochloride (Concurrent use with agents known to be metabolized via cytochrome P450 pathway requires caution).
No products indexed under this heading.

Amitriptyline Hydrochloride (Concurrent use with agents known to be metabolized via cytochrome P450 pathway requires caution).
No products indexed under this heading.

Amlodipine Besylate (Concurrent use with agents known to be metabolized via cytochrome P450 pathway requires caution). Products include:
Caduet Tablets ... 2508
Lotrel Capsules ... 2249
Norvasc Tablets ... 2545

Amoxapine (Concurrent use with agents known to be metabolized via cytochrome P450 pathway requires caution).
No products indexed under this heading.

Amphetamine Aspartate (Concurrent use with agents known to be metabolized via cytochrome P450 pathway requires caution). Products include:
Adderall Tablets ... 3164
Adderall XR Capsules ... 3166

Amphetamine Aspartate Monohydrate (Concurrent use with agents known to be metabolized via cytochrome P450 pathway requires caution).
No products indexed under this heading.

Amphetamine Sulfate (Concurrent use with agents known to be metabolized via cytochrome P450 pathway requires caution). Products include:
Adderall Tablets ... 3164
Adderall XR Capsules ... 3166

Aprepitant (Concurrent use with agents known to be metabolized via cytochrome P450 pathway requires caution). Products include:
Emend Capsules ... 1963

Astemizole (Concurrent use with agents known to be metabolized via cytochrome P450 pathway requires caution).
No products indexed under this heading.

Atomoxetine Hydrochloride (Concurrent use with agents known to be metabolized via cytochrome P450 pathway requires caution). Products include:
Strattera Capsules ... 1814

Atorvastatin Calcium (Concurrent use with agents known to be metabolized via cytochrome P450 pathway requires caution). Products include:
Caduet Tablets ... 2508
Lipitor Tablets ... 2483

Belladonna Ergotamine (Concurrent use with agents known to be metabolized via cytochrome P450 pathway requires caution).
No products indexed under this heading.

Benzphetamine Hydrochloride (Concurrent use with agents known to be metabolized via cytochrome P450 pathway requires caution).
No products indexed under this heading.

Bisoprolol Fumarate (Concurrent use with agents known to be metabolized via cytochrome P450 pathway requires caution).
No products indexed under this heading.

Bone Marrow Depressants, unspecified (Concurrent use with agents known to cause myelosuppression requires caution).
No products indexed under this heading.

Buspirone Hydrochloride (Concurrent use with agents known to be metabolized via cytochrome P450 pathway requires caution).
No products indexed under this heading.

Busulfan (Concurrent use with agents known to be metabolized via cytochrome P450 pathway requires caution). Products include:
I.V. Busulfex ... 2493
Myleran Tablets ... 1525

Caffeine (Concurrent use with agents known to be metabolized via cytochrome P450 pathway requires caution). Products include:
BC Headache Powder ... 677
Arthritis Strength BC Powder ... 677
Excedrin Extra Strength Caplets/Tablets/Geltabs ... 684
Excedrin Migraine Caplets/Tablets/Geltabs ... 609
Excedrin Tension Headache Caplets/Tablets/Geltabs ... 611
Goody's Extra Strength Headache Powders ... 611
Goody's Extra Strength Pain Relief Tablets ... 685
Vivarin ... 602
Winrgy Dietary Supplement ... 823

Caffeine Anhydrous (Concurrent use with agents known to be metabolized via cytochrome P450 pathway requires caution).
No products indexed under this heading.

Caffeine Citrate (Concurrent use with agents known to be metabolized via cytochrome P450 pathway requires caution). Products include:
Cafcit ... 1886

Candesartan Cilexetil (Concurrent use with agents known to be metabolized via cytochrome P450 pathway requires caution). Products include:
Atacand Tablets ... 649
Atacand HCT ... 651

Captopril (Concurrent use with agents known to be metabolized via cytochrome P450 pathway requires caution). Products include:
Captopril Tablets ... 2149

Carbamazepine (Concurrent use with agents known to be metabolized via cytochrome P450 pathway requires caution). Products include:
Carbatrol Capsules ... 3171
Equetro Extended-Release Capsules ... 3180
Tegretol/Tegretol-XR ... 2295

Carisoprodol (Concurrent use with agents known to be metabolized via cytochrome P450 pathway requires caution).
No products indexed under this heading.

Carvedilol (Concurrent use with agents known to be metabolized via cytochrome P450 pathway requires caution). Products include:
Coreg Tablets ... 1414

Celecoxib (Concurrent use with agents known to be metabolized via cytochrome P450 pathway requires caution). Products include:
Celebrex Capsules ... 3134

Cerivastatin Sodium (Concurrent use with agents known to be metabolized via cytochrome P450 pathway requires caution).
No products indexed under this heading.

Cevimeline Hydrochloride (Concurrent use with agents known to be metabolized via cytochrome P450 pathway requires caution). Products include:
Evoxac Capsules ... 1047

Chlordiazepoxide (Concurrent use with agents known to be metabolized via cytochrome P450 pathway requires caution).
No products indexed under this heading.

Chlordiazepoxide Hydrochloride (Concurrent use with agents known to be metabolized via cytochrome P450 pathway requires caution). Products include:
Librium Capsules ... 3347

Chlorpheniramine (Concurrent use with agents known to be metabolized via cytochrome P450 pathway requires caution).
No products indexed under this heading.

Chlorpheniramine Maleate (Concurrent use with agents known to be metabolized via cytochrome P450 pathway requires caution). Products include:
Advil Allergy Sinus Caplets ... 770
Advil Multi-Symptom Cold Caplets ... 770
BC Allergy Sinus Cold Powder ... 677
Comtrex Maximum Strength Cold & Cough Day/Night Caplets - Night Formulation ... 726
Comtrex Maximum Strength Day/Night Severe Cold & Sinus Caplets - Night Formulation ... 725
Contac Cold and Flu Maximum Strength Caplets ... 728
Contac Cold and Flu Day and Night Caplets (Night Formulation Only) ... 727
Children's Dimetapp Long Acting Cough Plus Cold Syrup ... 731
Robitussin Cough & Cold Long-Acting Liquid ... 735
Robitussin Cough & Allergy Syrup ... 736
Robitussin Cough & Cold Nighttime Liquid ... 736
Robitussin Cough, Cold & Flu Nighttime Liquid ... 738
Robitussin Pediatric Cough & Cold Long-Acting Liquid ... 735
Robitussin Pediatric Cough & Cold Nighttime Liquid ... 736
Triaminic Cold & Allergy Liquid ... 746
Triaminic Cough & Runny Nose Softchews ... 748
Children's Tylenol Plus Flu Oral Suspension ... 749
Tylenol Allergy Multi-Symptom Caplets with Cool Burst and Gelcaps ... 1872
Children's Tylenol Plus Cold Suspension Liquid ... 1879
Children's Tylenol Plus Cough & Runny Nose Suspension Liquid ... 1879
Children's Tylenol Plus Flu Suspension Liquid ... 1881
Children's Tylenol Plus Multi-Symptom Cold Suspension Liquid ... 1879
Tylenol Cold Head Congestion Nighttime Caplets with Cool Burst ... 1873
Tylenol Cold Multi-Symptom Nighttime Caplets with Cool Burst ... 1874
Tylenol Sinus Congestion & Pain Nighttime Caplets with Cool Burst ... 1876
Vicks 44M Cough, Cold & Flu Relief Liquid ... 2680
Pediatric Vicks 44m Cough & Cold Relief Liquid ... 2676
Children's Vicks NyQuil Cold/Cough Relief ... 756
Children's Vicks NyQuil Cold/Cough Relief Liquid ... 2680
Zicam Maximum Strength Flu Daytime ... 768

Chlorpheniramine Polistirex (Concurrent use with agents known to be metabolized via cytochrome P450 pathway requires caution). Products include:
Tussionex Pennkinetic Extended-Release Suspension ... 3327

Chlorpheniramine Tannate (Concurrent use with agents known to be metabolized via cytochrome P450 pathway requires caution).
No products indexed under this heading.

Chlorpromazine (Concurrent use with agents known to be metabolized via cytochrome P450 pathway requires caution).
No products indexed under this heading.

Chlorpromazine Hydrochloride (Concurrent use with agents known to be metabolized via cytochrome P450 pathway requires caution).
No products indexed under this heading.

Chlorpropamide (Concurrent use with agents known to be metabolized via cytochrome P450 pathway requires caution).
No products indexed under this heading.

Cilostazol (Concurrent use with agents known to be metabolized via cytochrome P450 pathway requires caution). Products include:
Pletal Tablets ... 2455

Cimetidine Hydrochloride (Concurrent use with agents known to be metabolized via cytochrome P450 pathway requires caution).
No products indexed under this heading.

Ciprofloxacin (Concurrent use with agents known to be metabolized via cytochrome P450 pathway requires caution). Products include:
Cipro Oral Suspension ... 2977
Cipro I.V. ... 2984
Cipro XR Tablets ... 2990
Ciprodex Otic Suspension ... 559

Ciprofloxacin Hydrochloride (Concurrent use with agents known to be metabolized via cytochrome P450 pathway requires caution). Products include:
Ciloxan Ophthalmic Ointment ... 559
Ciloxan Ophthalmic Solution ... ⊙206
Cipro Tablets ... 2977
Proquin XR Tablets ... 1153

Cisapride (Concurrent use with agents known to be metabolized via cytochrome P450 pathway requires caution).
No products indexed under this heading.

Citalopram Hydrobromide (Concurrent use with agents known to be metabolized via cytochrome P450 pathway requires caution). Products include:
Celexa ... 1176

Clarithromycin (Concurrent use with agents known to be metabolized via cytochrome P450 pathway requires caution). Products include:
Biaxin/Biaxin XL ... 402
PREVPAC ... 3284

Clomipramine Hydrochloride (Concurrent use with agents known to be metabolized via cytochrome P450 pathway requires caution).
No products indexed under this heading.

Clopidogrel Hydrogen Sulfate (Concurrent use with agents known to be metabolized via cytochrome P450 pathway requires caution).
No products indexed under this heading.

Clozapine (Concurrent use with agents known to be metabolized via cytochrome P450 pathway requires caution). Products include:
Clozaril Tablets ... 2184
FazaClo Orally Disintegrating Tablets ... 551

Codeine Phosphate (Concurrent use with agents known to be metabolized via cytochrome P450 pathway requires caution). Products include:
Tylenol with Codeine Tablets ... 2391

Codeine Sulfate (Concurrent use with agents known to be metabolized via cytochrome P450 pathway requires caution).
No products indexed under this heading.

Cyclobenzaprine (Concurrent use with agents known to be metabolized via cytochrome P450 pathway requires caution).
No products indexed under this heading.

Cyclobenzaprine Hydrochloride (Concurrent use with agents known to be metabolized via cytochrome P450 pathway requires caution).
No products indexed under this heading.

Cyclophosphamide (Concurrent use with agents known to be metabolized via cytochrome P450 pathway requires caution).
No products indexed under this heading.

Cyclosporine (Concurrent use with agents known to be metabolized via cytochrome P450 pathway requires caution). Products include:
Gengraf Capsules ... 459
Neoral Oral Solution ... 2259
Neoral Soft Gelatin Capsules ... 2259
Restasis Ophthalmic Emulsion ... 575
Sandimmune ... 2275

Desipramine Hydrochloride (Concurrent use with agents known to be metabolized via cytochrome P450 pathway requires caution).
No products indexed under this heading.

Desogestrel (Concurrent use with agents known to be metabolized via cytochrome P450 pathway requires caution). Products include:
Mircette Tablets ... 1066

Dexamethasone (Concurrent use with agents known to be metabolized via cytochrome P450 pathway requires caution). Products include:
Ciprodex Otic Suspension ... 559
Decadron Tablets ... 1951
TobraDex Ophthalmic Ointment ... 562
TobraDex Ophthalmic Suspension ... 563

Dexamethasone Acetate (Concurrent use with agents known to be metabolized via cytochrome P450 pathway requires caution).
No products indexed under this heading.

Dexamethasone Phosphate (Concurrent use with agents known to be metabolized via cytochrome P450 pathway requires caution).
No products indexed under this heading.

Dexamethasone Sodium (Concurrent use with agents known to be metabolized via cytochrome P450 pathway requires caution).
No products indexed under this heading.

Dexamethasone Sodium Phosphate (Concurrent use with agents known to be metabolized via cytochrome P450 pathway requires caution).
No products indexed under this heading.

Dexfenfluramine Hydrochloride (Concurrent use with agents known to be metabolized via cytochrome P450 pathway requires caution).
No products indexed under this heading.

Dextromethorphan (Concurrent use with agents known to be metabolized via cytochrome P450 pathway requires caution).
No products indexed under this heading.

Dextromethorphan Hydrobromide (Concurrent use with agents known to be metabolized via cytochrome P450 pathway requires caution). Products include:
Comtrex Maximum Strength Cold & Cough Day/Night Caplets - Day Formulation ... ■ 726
Comtrex Maximum Strength Cold & Cough Day/Night Caplets - Night Formulation ... ■ 726
Comtrex Maximum Strength Non-Drowsy Cold & Cough Caplets ... ■ 725
Children's Dimetapp DM Cold & Cough Elixir ... ■ 731
Children's Dimetapp Long Acting Cough Plus Cold Syrup ... ■ 731
Toddler's Dimetapp Cold and Cough Drops ... ■ 732
Mucinex DM Extended-Release Bi-Layer Tablets ... ■ 720
Refenesen DM Caplets ... ■ 721
Robitussin Cough & Cold CF Liquid ... ■ 735
Robitussin Cough & Cold Long-Acting Liquid ... ■ 735
Robitussin Cough & Allergy Syrup ... ■ 736
Robitussin Cough & Cold Nighttime Liquid ... ■ 736
Robitussin Cough & Cold Pediatric Drops ... ■ 735
Robitussin Cough, Cold & Flu Nighttime Liquid ... ■ 738
Robitussin Cough & Congestion Liquid ... ■ 738
Robitussin Cough Gels Long-Acting ... ■ 737
Robitussin Cough Long Acting Liquid ... ■ 739
Robitussin Cough DM Syrup ... ■ 738
Robitussin Cough DM Infant Drops ... ■ 738
Robitussin Pediatric Cough Long Acting Liquid ... ■ 739
Robitussin Pediatric Cough & Cold Long-Acting Liquid ... ■ 735
Robitussin Pediatric Cough & Cold Nighttime Liquid ... ■ 736
Robitussin Sugar Free Cough ... ■ 738
TheraFlu Cold & Cough Hot Liquid ... ■ 740
TheraFlu Warming Relief Daytime Severe Cold ... ■ 743
TheraFlu Thin Strips Long Acting Cough ... ■ 744
Triaminic Daytime Cold & Cough Liquid ... ■ 745
Triaminic Cough & Sore Throat Liquid ... ■ 747
Triaminic Cough & Runny Nose Softchews ... ■ 748
Triaminic Thin Strips Cold & Cough ... ■ 778
Triaminic Infant Thin Strips Decongestant Plus Cough ... ■ 747
Children's Tylenol Plus Flu Oral Suspension ... ■ 749
Tylenol Cold Head Congestion Daytime Caplets with Cool Burst and Gelcaps ... ■ 750
Tylenol Cold Multi-Symptom Daytime Liquid ... ■ 752
Tylenol Cold Multi-Symptom Severe Daytime Liquid ... ■ 752
Concentrated Tylenol Infants' Drops Plus Cold & Cough ... ■ 754
Children's Tylenol Plus Cough & Runny Nose Suspension Liquid ... 1879
Children's Tylenol Plus Cough & Sore Throat Suspension Liquid ... 1879
Children's Tylenol Plus Flu Suspension Liquid ... 1881
Children's Tylenol Plus Multi-Symptom Cold Suspension Liquid ... 1879
Tylenol Cold Severe Congestion Non-Drowsy Caplets with Cool Burst ... 1874
Tylenol Cold Head Congestion Daytime Caplets with Cool Burst ... 1873
Tylenol Cold Head Congestion Nighttime Caplets with Cool Burst ... 1873
Tylenol Cold Head Congestion Severe Caplets with Cool Burst ... 1873
Tylenol Cold Multi-Symptom Daytime Caplets with Cool Burst and Gelcaps ... 1874
Tylenol Cold Multi-Symptom Daytime Liquid with Citrus Burst ... 1874
Tylenol Cold Multi-Symptom Nighttime Caplets with Cool Burst ... 1874
Tylenol Cold Multi-Symptom Nighttime Liquid with Cool Burst ... 1874
Tylenol Cold Multi-Symptom Severe Caplets with Cool Burst ... 1874
Tylenol Cold Multi-Symptom Severe Daytime Liquid with Citrus Burst ... 1874
Tylenol Cough & Sore Throat Daytime Liquid with Cool Burst ... 1877
Tylenol Cough & Sore Throat Nighttime Liquid with Cool Burst ... 1877
Concentrated Tylenol Infants' Drops Plus Cold and Cough ... 1879
Vicks 44 Cough Relief Liquid ... 2679
Vicks 44D Cough & Head Congestion Relief Liquid ... 2679
Vicks 44E Cough & Chest Congestion Relief Liquid ... 2679
Pediatric Vicks 44e Cough & Chest Congestion Relief Liquid ... 2676
Vicks 44M Cough, Cold & Flu Relief Liquid ... 2680
Pediatric Vicks 44m Cough & Cold Relief Liquid ... 2676
Vicks DayQuil LiquiCaps/Liquid Multi-Symptom Cold/Flu Relief ... ■ 761
Vicks DayQuil Multi-Symptom Cold/Flu Relief LiquiCaps ... 2678
Vicks DayQuil Multi-Symptom Cold/Flu Relief Liquid ... 2678
Vicks NyQuil Multi-Symptom Cold/Flu Relief Liquid ... 2681
Children's Vicks NyQuil Cold/Cough Relief ... ■ 756
Vicks NyQuil Multi-Symptom Cold/Flu Relief LiquiCaps ... 2681
Vicks NyQuil LiquiCaps/Liquid Multi-Symptom Cold/Flu Relief ... ■ 763
Vicks NyQuil Cough Liquid ... 2680
Children's Vicks NyQuil Cold/Cough Relief Liquid ... 2680
Zicam Cough Max Nighttime Cough Spray ... ■ 767
Zicam Cough Max Cough Spray ... ■ 767
Zicam Cough Max Cough Melts ... ■ 767
Zicam Cough Plus D Cough Spray ... ■ 767
Zicam Cough Relief Cough Spray ... ■ 767
Zicam Maximum Strength Flu Daytime ... ■ 768
Zicam Maximum Strength Flu Nighttime ... ■ 768

Dextromethorphan Polistirex (Concurrent use with agents known to be metabolized via cytochrome P450 pathway requires caution). Products include:
Delsym Extended-Release Suspension 12 Hour Cough Suppressant ... ■ 611

Diazepam (Concurrent use with agents known to be metabolized via cytochrome P450 pathway requires caution). Products include:
Diastat Rectal Delivery System ... 3343
Valium Tablets ... 2819

Diclofenac Potassium (Concurrent use with agents known to be metabolized via cytochrome P450 pathway requires caution).
No products indexed under this heading.

Diclofenac Sodium (Concurrent use with agents known to be metabolized via cytochrome P450 pathway requires caution). Products include:
Arthrotec Tablets ... 3129
Voltaren Ophthalmic Solution ... 2309
Voltaren Tablets ... 2307
Voltaren-XR Tablets ... 2310

Dihydroergotamine Mesylate (Concurrent use with agents known to be metabolized via cytochrome P450 pathway requires caution). Products include:
Migranal Nasal Spray ... 3348

Diltiazem Hydrochloride (Concurrent use with agents known to be metabolized via cytochrome P450 pathway requires caution). Products include:
Cardizem LA Extended Release Tablets ... 1728
Tiazac Capsules ... 1201

Diltiazem Maleate (Concurrent use with agents known to be metabolized via cytochrome P450 pathway requires caution).
No products indexed under this heading.

Disopyramide (Concurrent use with agents known to be metabolized via cytochrome P450 pathway requires caution).
No products indexed under this heading.

Disopyramide Phosphate (Concurrent use with agents known to be metabolized via cytochrome P450 pathway requires caution).
No products indexed under this heading.

Divalproex Sodium (Concurrent use with agents known to be metabolized via cytochrome P450 pathway requires caution). Products include:
Depakote Sprinkle Capsules ... 422
Depakote Tablets ... 427
Depakote ER Tablets ... 434

Docetaxel (Concurrent use with agents known to be metabolized via cytochrome P450 pathway requires caution). Products include:
Taxotere Injection Concentrate ... 2932

Dolasetron Mesylate (Concurrent use with agents known to be metabolized via cytochrome P450 pathway requires caution). Products include:
Anzemet Injection ... 2859
Anzemet Tablets ... 2862

Donepezil Hydrochloride (Concurrent use with agents known to be

metabolized via cytochrome P450 pathway requires caution). Products include:
Aricept Tablets ... 1094
Aricept ODT Tablets ... 1094

Doxepin Hydrochloride (Concurrent use with agents known to be metabolized via cytochrome P450 pathway requires caution).
No products indexed under this heading.

Doxorubicin Hydrochloride (Concurrent use with agents known to be metabolized via cytochrome P450 pathway requires caution).
No products indexed under this heading.

Dronabinol (Concurrent use with agents known to be metabolized via cytochrome P450 pathway requires caution). Products include:
Marinol Capsules ... 3333

Drugs that Undergo Biotransformation by Cytochrome P-450 Mixed Function Oxidase (Concurrent use with agents known to be metabolized via cytochrome P450 pathway requires caution).
No products indexed under this heading.

Dyphylline (Concurrent use with agents known to be metabolized via cytochrome P450 pathway requires caution).
No products indexed under this heading.

Encainide Hydrochloride (Concurrent use with agents known to be metabolized via cytochrome P450 pathway requires caution).
No products indexed under this heading.

Enoxacin (Concurrent use with agents known to be metabolized via cytochrome P450 pathway requires caution).
No products indexed under this heading.

Eprosartan Mesylate (Concurrent use with agents known to be metabolized via cytochrome P450 pathway requires caution). Products include:
Teveten Tablets ... 1735
Teveten HCT Tablets ... 1737

Ergotamine Tartrate (Concurrent use with agents known to be metabolized via cytochrome P450 pathway requires caution).
No products indexed under this heading.

Erythromycin (Concurrent use with agents known to be metabolized via cytochrome P450 pathway requires caution). Products include:
Ery-Tab Tablets ... 449
Erythromycin Base Filmtab Tablets ... 455
Erythromycin Delayed-Release Capsules, USP ... 457
PCE Dispertab Tablets ... 515

Erythromycin Estolate (Concurrent use with agents known to be metabolized via cytochrome P450 pathway requires caution).
No products indexed under this heading.

Erythromycin Ethylsuccinate (Concurrent use with agents known to be metabolized via cytochrome P450 pathway requires caution). Products include:
E.E.S. ... 451
EryPed ... 447

Erythromycin Gluceptate (Concurrent use with agents known to be metabolized via cytochrome P450 pathway requires caution).
No products indexed under this heading.

Erythromycin Lactobionate (Concurrent use with agents known to be metabolized via cytochrome P450 pathway requires caution).
No products indexed under this heading.

Erythromycin Stearate (Concurrent use with agents known to be metabolized via cytochrome P450 pathway requires caution). Products include:
Erythrocin Stearate Filmtab Tablets ... 453

Esomeprazole Magnesium (Concurrent use with agents known to be metabolized via cytochrome P450 pathway requires caution). Products include:
Nexium Delayed-Release Capsules ... 655

Estradiol (Concurrent use with agents known to be metabolized via cytochrome P450 pathway requires caution). Products include:
Angeliq Tablets ... 762
Climara Transdermal System ... 771
Climara Pro Transdermal System ... 776
Estrasorb Topical Emulsion ... 1147
Estring Vaginal Ring ... 2635
Menostar Transdermal System ... 782
Vagifem Tablets ... 2334

Estradiol Benzoate (Concurrent use with agents known to be metabolized via cytochrome P450 pathway requires caution).
No products indexed under this heading.

Estradiol Cypionate (Concurrent use with agents known to be metabolized via cytochrome P450 pathway requires caution).
No products indexed under this heading.

Estradiol Valerate (Concurrent use with agents known to be metabolized via cytochrome P450 pathway requires caution).
No products indexed under this heading.

Estrogen (Concurrent use with agents known to be metabolized via cytochrome P450 pathway requires caution).
No products indexed under this heading.

Estrogens, Conjugated (Concurrent use with agents known to be metabolized via cytochrome P450 pathway requires caution). Products include:
Premarin Intravenous ... 3442
Premarin Tablets ... 3446
Premarin Vaginal Cream ... 3452
Premphase Tablets ... 3456
Prempro Tablets ... 3456

Estrogens, Conjugated, Synthetic A (Concurrent use with agents known to be metabolized via cytochrome P450 pathway requires caution).
No products indexed under this heading.

Estrogens, Esterified (Concurrent use with agents known to be metabolized via cytochrome P450 pathway requires caution). Products include:
Estratest Tablets ... 3199
Estratest H.S. Tablets ... 3199

Ethinyl Estradiol (Concurrent use with agents known to be metabolized via cytochrome P450 pathway requires caution). Products include:
Mircette Tablets ... 1066
NuvaRing ... 2340
Ortho-Cyclen/Ortho Tri-Cyclen ... 2429
Ortho Evra Transdermal System ... 2417
Ortho Tri-Cyclen Lo Tablets ... 2436
Seasonique Tablets ... 1077
Yasmin 28 Tablets ... 796
Yaz Tablets ... 803

Ethosuximide (Concurrent use with agents known to be metabolized via cytochrome P450 pathway requires caution).
No products indexed under this heading.

Ethotoin (Concurrent use with agents known to be metabolized via cytochrome P450 pathway requires caution).
No products indexed under this heading.

Ethynodiol Diacetate (Concurrent use with agents known to be metabolized via cytochrome P450 pathway requires caution).
No products indexed under this heading.

Etodolac (Concurrent use with agents known to be metabolized via cytochrome P450 pathway requires caution).
No products indexed under this heading.

Etoposide (Concurrent use with agents known to be metabolized via cytochrome P450 pathway requires caution).
No products indexed under this heading.

Etoposide Phosphate (Concurrent use with agents known to be metabolized via cytochrome P450 pathway requires caution).
No products indexed under this heading.

Felbamate (Concurrent use with agents known to be metabolized via cytochrome P450 pathway requires caution).
No products indexed under this heading.

Felodipine (Concurrent use with agents known to be metabolized via cytochrome P450 pathway requires caution).
No products indexed under this heading.

Fenoprofen Calcium (Concurrent use with agents known to be metabolized via cytochrome P450 pathway requires caution). Products include:
Nalfon Capsules ... 2502

Fentanyl (Concurrent use with agents known to be metabolized via cytochrome P450 pathway requires caution). Products include:
Duragesic Transdermal System ... 2373
Ionsys Transdermal System ... 2379

Fentanyl Citrate (Concurrent use with agents known to be metabolized via cytochrome P450 pathway requires caution). Products include:
Actiq ... 979

Flecainide Acetate (Concurrent use with agents known to be metabolized via cytochrome P450 pathway requires caution). Products include:
Tambocor Tablets ... 1856

Fluoxetine (Concurrent use with agents known to be metabolized via cytochrome P450 pathway requires caution).
No products indexed under this heading.

Fluoxetine Hydrochloride (Concurrent use with agents known to be metabolized via cytochrome P450 pathway requires caution). Products include:
Prozac Pulvules and Liquid ... 1801
Symbyax Capsules ... 1819

Fluphenazine Decanoate (Concurrent use with agents known to be metabolized via cytochrome P450 pathway requires caution).
No products indexed under this heading.

Fluphenazine Enanthate (Concurrent use with agents known to be metabolized via cytochrome P450 pathway requires caution).
No products indexed under this heading.

Fluphenazine Hydrochloride (Concurrent use with agents known to be metabolized via cytochrome P450 pathway requires caution).
No products indexed under this heading.

Flurbiprofen (Concurrent use with agents known to be metabolized via cytochrome P450 pathway requires caution).
No products indexed under this heading.

Flurbiprofen Sodium (Concurrent use with agents known to be metabolized via cytochrome P450 pathway requires caution). Products include:
Ocufen Ophthalmic Solution ... ⊙232

Flutamide (Concurrent use with agents known to be metabolized via cytochrome P450 pathway requires caution). Products include:
Eulexin Capsules ... 3009

Fluticasone Propionate (Concurrent use with agents known to be metabolized via cytochrome P450 pathway requires caution). Products include:
Advair Diskus 100/50 ... 1308
Advair Diskus 250/50 ... 1308
Advair Diskus 500/50 ... 1308
Advair HFA Inhalation Aerosol ... 1318
Cutivate Cream ... 2662
Cutivate Lotion 0.05% ... 2664
Cutivate Ointment ... 2665
Flonase Nasal Spray ... 1440
Flovent Diskus ... 1443

Fluvastatin Sodium (Concurrent use with agents known to be metabolized via cytochrome P450 pathway requires caution). Products include:
Lescol Capsules ... 2233
Lescol XL Tablets ... 2233

Fluvoxamine Maleate (Concurrent use with agents known to be metabolized via cytochrome P450 pathway requires caution).
No products indexed under this heading.

Formoterol Fumarate (Concurrent use with agents known to be metabolized via cytochrome P450 pathway requires caution). Products include:
Foradil Aerolizer ... 3010

Fosphenytoin (Concurrent use with agents known to be metabolized via cytochrome P450 pathway requires caution).
No products indexed under this heading.

Fosphenytoin Sodium (Concurrent use with agents known to be metabolized via cytochrome P450 pathway requires caution).
No products indexed under this heading.

Gabapentin (Concurrent use with agents known to be metabolized via cytochrome P450 pathway requires caution). Products include:

Neurontin Capsules 2487
Neurontin Oral Solution 2487
Neurontin Tablets 2487

Galantamine Hydrobromide (Concurrent use with agents known to be metabolized via cytochrome P450 pathway requires caution). Products include:
Razadyne 2399
Razadyne ER Extended-Release Capsules 2399

Glimepiride (Concurrent use with agents known to be metabolized via cytochrome P450 pathway requires caution). Products include:
Avandaryl Tablets 1379
Duetact Tablets 3226

Glipizide (Concurrent use with agents known to be metabolized via cytochrome P450 pathway requires caution).
No products indexed under this heading.

Glyburide (Concurrent use with agents known to be metabolized via cytochrome P450 pathway requires caution).
No products indexed under this heading.

Grepafloxacin Hydrochloride (Concurrent use with agents known to be metabolized via cytochrome P450 pathway requires caution).
No products indexed under this heading.

Haloperidol (Concurrent use with agents known to be metabolized via cytochrome P450 pathway requires caution).
No products indexed under this heading.

Haloperidol Decanoate (Concurrent use with agents known to be metabolized via cytochrome P450 pathway requires caution).
No products indexed under this heading.

Haloperidol Lactate (Concurrent use with agents known to be metabolized via cytochrome P450 pathway requires caution).
No products indexed under this heading.

Hydrocodone Bitartrate (Concurrent use with agents known to be metabolized via cytochrome P450 pathway requires caution). Products include:
Hycodan 1116
Hycotuss Expectorant Syrup 1117
Vicodin Tablets 535
Vicodin ES Tablets 536
Vicodin HP Tablets 538
Vicoprofen Tablets 539
Zydone Tablets 1139

Ibuprofen (Concurrent use with agents known to be metabolized via cytochrome P450 pathway requires caution). Products include:
Advil Allergy Sinus Caplets .... ■ 770
Advil .... ■ 674
Children's Advil Oral Suspension .... ■ 603
Children's Advil Chewable Tablets .. ■ 603
Advil Cold & Sinus .... ■ 723
Infants' Advil Concentrated Drops .. ■ 604
Infants' Advil Concentrated Drops - White Grape (Dye-Free)............. ■ 604
Junior Strength Advil Swallow Tablets.. ■ 605
Advil Migraine Liquigels .... ■ 608
Advil Multi-Symptom Cold Caplets.. ■ 770
Advil PM Caplets .... ■ 615
Motrin IB Tablets and Caplets 1866
Children's Motrin Oral Suspension ... 1867
Children's Motrin Non-Staining Dye-Free Oral Suspension............. 1867
Children's Motrin Cold Oral Suspension 1867
Infants' Motrin Concentrated Drops.. 1867
Infants' Motrin Non-Staining Dye-Free Concentrated Drops....... 1867
Junior Strength Motrin Caplets and Chewable Tablets.................. 1867
Vicoprofen Tablets 539

Imipramine Hydrochloride (Concurrent use with agents known to be metabolized via cytochrome P450 pathway requires caution).
No products indexed under this heading.

Imipramine Pamoate (Concurrent use with agents known to be metabolized via cytochrome P450 pathway requires caution).
No products indexed under this heading.

Indinavir Sulfate (Concurrent use with agents known to be metabolized via cytochrome P450 pathway requires caution). Products include:
Crixivan Capsules 1940

Indomethacin (Concurrent use with agents known to be metabolized via cytochrome P450 pathway requires caution). Products include:
Indocin 1995

Indomethacin Sodium Trihydrate (Concurrent use with agents known to be metabolized via cytochrome P450 pathway requires caution). Products include:
Indocin I.V. 2465

Indoramin Hydrochloride (Concurrent use with agents known to be metabolized via cytochrome P450 pathway requires caution).
No products indexed under this heading.

Irbesartan (Concurrent use with agents known to be metabolized via cytochrome P450 pathway requires caution). Products include:
Avalide Tablets 888
Avalide Tablets 2874
Avapro Tablets 891
Avapro Tablets 2871

Isotretinoin (Concurrent use with agents known to be metabolized via cytochrome P450 pathway requires caution). Products include:
Accutane Capsules 2731

Isradipine (Concurrent use with agents known to be metabolized via cytochrome P450 pathway requires caution). Products include:
DynaCirc CR Tablets 2721

Itraconazole (Concurrent use with agents known to be metabolized via cytochrome P450 pathway requires caution).
No products indexed under this heading.

Ketoconazole (Concurrent use with agents known to be metabolized via cytochrome P450 pathway requires caution). Products include:
Nizoral A-D Shampoo, 1%................ 1868

Ketoprofen (Concurrent use with agents known to be metabolized via cytochrome P450 pathway requires caution).
No products indexed under this heading.

Ketorolac Tromethamine (Concurrent use with agents known to be metabolized via cytochrome P450 pathway requires caution). Products include:
Acular Ophthalmic Solution 565
Acular LS Ophthalmic Solution 566

Labetalol Hydrochloride (Concurrent use with agents known to be metabolized via cytochrome P450 pathway requires caution).
No products indexed under this heading.

Lamotrigine (Concurrent use with agents known to be metabolized via cytochrome P450 pathway requires caution). Products include:
Lamictal 1481

Lansoprazole (Concurrent use with agents known to be metabolized via cytochrome P450 pathway requires caution). Products include:
Prevacid Delayed-Release Capsules.. 3271
Prevacid for Delayed-Release Oral Suspension 3271
Prevacid SoluTab Delayed-Release Orally Disintegrating Tablets................. 3271
Prevacid I.V. for Injection 3277
Prevacid NapraPAC 3280
PREVPAC 3284

Levetiracetam (Concurrent use with agents known to be metabolized via cytochrome P450 pathway requires caution). Products include:
Keppra Injection 3320
Keppra Oral Solution 3314
Keppra Tablets 3314

Levobupivacaine Hydrochloride (Concurrent use with agents known to be metabolized via cytochrome P450 pathway requires caution).
No products indexed under this heading.

Levonorgestrel (Concurrent use with agents known to be metabolized via cytochrome P450 pathway requires caution). Products include:
Climara Pro Transdermal System 776
Mirena Intrauterine System 787
Plan B Tablets 1076
Seasonique Tablets 1077

Lidocaine (Concurrent use with agents known to be metabolized via cytochrome P450 pathway requires caution). Products include:
Lidoderm Patch 1118
Synera Topical Patch 1137

Lidocaine Base (Concurrent use with agents known to be metabolized via cytochrome P450 pathway requires caution).
No products indexed under this heading.

Lidocaine Hydrochloride (Concurrent use with agents known to be metabolized via cytochrome P450 pathway requires caution).
No products indexed under this heading.

Lomefloxacin Hydrochloride (Concurrent use with agents known to be metabolized via cytochrome P450 pathway requires caution).
No products indexed under this heading.

Losartan Potassium (Concurrent use with agents known to be metabolized via cytochrome P450 pathway requires caution). Products include:
Cozaar Tablets 1935
Hyzaar 50-12.5 Tablets 1990
Hyzaar 100-12.5 Tablets 1990
Hyzaar 100-25 Tablets 1990

Lovastatin (Concurrent use with agents known to be metabolized via cytochrome P450 pathway requires caution). Products include:
Advicor Tablets 1722
Altoprev Extended-Release Tablets.. 3109
Mevacor Tablets 2021

Maprotiline Hydrochloride (Concurrent use with agents known to be metabolized via cytochrome P450 pathway requires caution).
No products indexed under this heading.

Meclofenamate Sodium (Concurrent use with agents known to be metabolized via cytochrome P450 pathway requires caution).
No products indexed under this heading.

Mefenamic Acid (Concurrent use with agents known to be metabolized via cytochrome P450 pathway requires caution).
No products indexed under this heading.

Meloxicam (Concurrent use with agents known to be metabolized via cytochrome P450 pathway requires caution). Products include:
Mobic Oral Suspension 863
Mobic Tablets 863

Meperidine Hydrochloride (Concurrent use with agents known to be metabolized via cytochrome P450 pathway requires caution).
No products indexed under this heading.

Mephenytoin (Concurrent use with agents known to be metabolized via cytochrome P450 pathway requires caution).
No products indexed under this heading.

Mephobarbital (Concurrent use with agents known to be metabolized via cytochrome P450 pathway requires caution).
No products indexed under this heading.

Meprobamate (Concurrent use with agents known to be metabolized via cytochrome P450 pathway requires caution).
No products indexed under this heading.

Mestranol (Concurrent use with agents known to be metabolized via cytochrome P450 pathway requires caution).
No products indexed under this heading.

Metformin Hydrochloride (Concurrent use with agents known to be metabolized via cytochrome P450 pathway requires caution). Products include:
ActoPlus Met Tablets 3214
Avandamet Tablets 1373
Fortamet Extended-Release Tablets.. 3115

Methadone Hydrochloride (Concurrent use with agents known to be metabolized via cytochrome P450 pathway requires caution).
No products indexed under this heading.

Methamphetamine Hydrochloride (Concurrent use with agents known to be metabolized via cytochrome P450 pathway requires caution). Products include:
Desoxyn Tablets, USP 2462

Methsuximide (Concurrent use with agents known to be metabolized via cytochrome P450 pathway requires caution).
No products indexed under this heading.

Metoprolol Succinate (Concurrent use with agents known to be metabolized via cytochrome P450 pathway requires caution). Products include:
Toprol-XL Tablets 668

Metoprolol Tartrate (Concurrent use with agents known to be metabolized via cytochrome P450 pathway requires caution). Products include:

Lopressor Injection 2238
Lopressor Tablets 2238
Lopressor HCT 50/25 Tablets 2241
Lopressor HCT 100/25 Tablets 2241
Lopressor HCT 100/50 Tablets 2241

Mexiletine Hydrochloride (Concurrent use with agents known to be metabolized via cytochrome P450 pathway requires caution).

No products indexed under this heading.

Midazolam Hydrochloride (Concurrent use with agents known to be metabolized via cytochrome P450 pathway requires caution).

No products indexed under this heading.

Miglitol (Concurrent use with agents known to be metabolized via cytochrome P450 pathway requires caution).

No products indexed under this heading.

Mirtazapine (Concurrent use with agents known to be metabolized via cytochrome P450 pathway requires caution).

No products indexed under this heading.

Montelukast Sodium (Concurrent use with agents known to be metabolized via cytochrome P450 pathway requires caution). Products include:

Singulair 2077

Morphine Sulfate (Concurrent use with agents known to be metabolized via cytochrome P450 pathway requires caution). Products include:

Avinza Capsules 1741
Kadian Capsules 577
MS Contin Tablets 2701

Moxifloxacin Hydrochloride (Concurrent use with agents known to be metabolized via cytochrome P450 pathway requires caution). Products include:

Avelox ... 2970
Vigamox Ophthalmic Solution 564

Nabumetone (Concurrent use with agents known to be metabolized via cytochrome P450 pathway requires caution).

No products indexed under this heading.

Nafcillin Sodium (Concurrent use with agents known to be metabolized via cytochrome P450 pathway requires caution).

No products indexed under this heading.

Naproxen (Concurrent use with agents known to be metabolized via cytochrome P450 pathway requires caution). Products include:

EC-Naprosyn Delayed-Release
Tablets 2761
Naprosyn Suspension 2761
Naprosyn Tablets 2761
Prevacid NapraPAC 3280

Naproxen Sodium (Concurrent use with agents known to be metabolized via cytochrome P450 pathway requires caution). Products include:

Aleve Caplets 742
Aleve Gelcaps 743
Aleve Tablets 743
Aleve Cold & Sinus Caplets 744
Anaprox Tablets 2761
Anaprox DS Tablets 2761

Nateglinide (Concurrent use with agents known to be metabolized via cytochrome P450 pathway requires caution). Products include:

Starlix Tablets 2292

Nefazodone Hydrochloride (Concurrent use with agents known to be metabolized via cytochrome P450 pathway requires caution).

No products indexed under this heading.

Nelfinavir Mesylate (Concurrent use with agents known to be metabolized via cytochrome P450 pathway requires caution). Products include:

Viracept .. 2577

Nicardipine (Concurrent use with agents known to be metabolized via cytochrome P450 pathway requires caution).

No products indexed under this heading.

Nicardipine Hydrochloride (Concurrent use with agents known to be metabolized via cytochrome P450 pathway requires caution). Products include:

Cardene I.V. 2497

Nicotine Polacrilex (Concurrent use with agents known to be metabolized via cytochrome P450 pathway requires caution).

No products indexed under this heading.

Nicotine Salicylate (Concurrent use with agents known to be metabolized via cytochrome P450 pathway requires caution).

No products indexed under this heading.

Nicotine Sulfate (Concurrent use with agents known to be metabolized via cytochrome P450 pathway requires caution).

No products indexed under this heading.

Nifedipine (Concurrent use with agents known to be metabolized via cytochrome P450 pathway requires caution). Products include:

Adalat CC Tablets 2964

Nilutamide (Concurrent use with agents known to be metabolized via cytochrome P450 pathway requires caution).

No products indexed under this heading.

Nimodipine (Concurrent use with agents known to be metabolized via cytochrome P450 pathway requires caution). Products include:

Nimotop Capsules 749

Nisoldipine (Concurrent use with agents known to be metabolized via cytochrome P450 pathway requires caution). Products include:

Sular Tablets 3122

Nitrendipine (Concurrent use with agents known to be metabolized via cytochrome P450 pathway requires caution).

No products indexed under this heading.

Norethindrone (Concurrent use with agents known to be metabolized via cytochrome P450 pathway requires caution). Products include:

Ortho Micronor Tablets 2426

Norethindrone Acetate (Concurrent use with agents known to be metabolized via cytochrome P450 pathway requires caution).

No products indexed under this heading.

Norfloxacin (Concurrent use with agents known to be metabolized via cytochrome P450 pathway requires caution). Products include:

Noroxin Tablets 2032

Norgestrel (Concurrent use with agents known to be metabolized via cytochrome P450 pathway requires caution).

No products indexed under this heading.

Nortriptyline Hydrochloride (Concurrent use with agents known to be metabolized via cytochrome P450 pathway requires caution).

No products indexed under this heading.

Ofloxacin (Concurrent use with agents known to be metabolized via cytochrome P450 pathway requires caution). Products include:

Floxin Otic Solution 1049

Olanzapine (Concurrent use with agents known to be metabolized via cytochrome P450 pathway requires caution). Products include:

Symbyax Capsules 1819
Zyprexa Tablets 1830
Zyprexa IntraMuscular 1830
Zyprexa ZYDIS Orally
Disintegrating Tablets 1830

Omeprazole (Concurrent use with agents known to be metabolized via cytochrome P450 pathway requires caution). Products include:

Zegerid Capsules 2958
Zegerid Powder for Oral Solution 2958

Ondansetron (Concurrent use with agents known to be metabolized via cytochrome P450 pathway requires caution). Products include:

Zofran ODT Orally Disintegrating
Tablets 1639

Ondansetron Hydrochloride (Concurrent use with agents known to be metabolized via cytochrome P450 pathway requires caution). Products include:

Zofran Injection 1634
Zofran ... 1639

Oxaprozin (Concurrent use with agents known to be metabolized via cytochrome P450 pathway requires caution).

No products indexed under this heading.

Oxcarbazepine (Concurrent use with agents known to be metabolized via cytochrome P450 pathway requires caution). Products include:

Trileptal Tablets 2300
Trileptal Oral Suspension 2300

Oxycodone Hydrochloride (Concurrent use with agents known to be metabolized via cytochrome P450 pathway requires caution). Products include:

OxyContin Tablets 2703
OxyFast Oral Concentrate
Solution 2708
OxyIR Capsules 2708
Percocet Tablets 1131
Percodan Tablets 1132

Paclitaxel (Concurrent use with agents known to be metabolized via cytochrome P450 pathway requires caution).

No products indexed under this heading.

Pantoprazole Sodium (Concurrent use with agents known to be metabolized via cytochrome P450 pathway requires caution). Products include:

Protonix I.V. 3472
Protonix Tablets 3469

Paramethadione (Concurrent use with agents known to be metabolized via cytochrome P450 pathway requires caution).

No products indexed under this heading.

Paroxetine Hydrochloride (Concurrent use with agents known to be metabolized via cytochrome P450 pathway requires caution). Products include:

Paxil CR Controlled-Release
Tablets 1538
Paxil ... 1530

Pentamidine Isethionate (Concurrent use with agents known to be metabolized via cytochrome P450 pathway requires caution).

No products indexed under this heading.

Phenacemide (Concurrent use with agents known to be metabolized via cytochrome P450 pathway requires caution).

No products indexed under this heading.

Phenobarbital (Concurrent use with agents known to be metabolized via cytochrome P450 pathway requires caution). Products include:

Donnatal Extentabs 2493

Phenobarbital Sodium (Concurrent use with agents known to be metabolized via cytochrome P450 pathway requires caution).

No products indexed under this heading.

Phensuximide (Concurrent use with agents known to be metabolized via cytochrome P450 pathway requires caution).

No products indexed under this heading.

Phenylbutazone (Concurrent use with agents known to be metabolized via cytochrome P450 pathway requires caution).

No products indexed under this heading.

Phenytoin (Concurrent use with agents known to be metabolized via cytochrome P450 pathway requires caution).

No products indexed under this heading.

Phenytoin Sodium (Concurrent use with agents known to be metabolized via cytochrome P450 pathway requires caution). Products include:

Phenytek Capsules 2160

Pimozide (Concurrent use with agents known to be metabolized via cytochrome P450 pathway requires caution).

No products indexed under this heading.

Pindolol (Concurrent use with agents known to be metabolized via cytochrome P450 pathway requires caution).

No products indexed under this heading.

Pioglitazone Hydrochloride (Concurrent use with agents known to be metabolized via cytochrome P450 pathway requires caution). Products include:

ActoPlus Met Tablets 3214
Actos Tablets 3219
Duetact Tablets 3226

Piroxicam (Concurrent use with agents known to be metabolized via cytochrome P450 pathway requires caution).

No products indexed under this heading.

Polyestradiol Phosphate (Concurrent use with agents known to be metabolized via cytochrome P450 pathway requires caution).

No products indexed under this heading.

IMPORTANT NOTE: Always consult each drug listing in the patient's regimen for possible interactions.

Primidone (Concurrent use with agents known to be metabolized via cytochrome P450 pathway requires caution).

No products indexed under this heading.

Progesterone (Concurrent use with agents known to be metabolized via cytochrome P450 pathway requires caution). Products include:

Proguanil Hydrochloride (Concurrent use with agents known to be metabolized via cytochrome P450 pathway requires caution). Products include:

Propafenone Hydrochloride (Concurrent use with agents known to be metabolized via cytochrome P450 pathway requires caution). Products include:

Propoxyphene Hydrochloride (Concurrent use with agents known to be metabolized via cytochrome P450 pathway requires caution).

No products indexed under this heading.

Propoxyphene Napsylate (Concurrent use with agents known to be metabolized via cytochrome P450 pathway requires caution).

No products indexed under this heading.

Propranolol Hydrochloride (Concurrent use with agents known to be metabolized via cytochrome P450 pathway requires caution). Products include:

Protriptyline Hydrochloride (Concurrent use with agents known to be metabolized via cytochrome P450 pathway requires caution).

No products indexed under this heading.

Quetiapine Fumarate (Concurrent use with agents known to be metabolized via cytochrome P450 pathway requires caution). Products include:

Quinidine Gluconate (Concurrent use with agents known to be metabolized via cytochrome P450 pathway requires caution).

No products indexed under this heading.

Quinidine Hydrochloride (Concurrent use with agents known to be metabolized via cytochrome P450 pathway requires caution).

No products indexed under this heading.

Quinidine Polygalacturonate (Concurrent use with agents known to be metabolized via cytochrome P450 pathway requires caution).

No products indexed under this heading.

Quinidine Sulfate (Concurrent use with agents known to be metabolized via cytochrome P450 pathway requires caution).

No products indexed under this heading.

Quinine (Concurrent use with agents known to be metabolized via cytochrome P450 pathway requires caution).

No products indexed under this heading.

Quinine Sulfate (Concurrent use with agents known to be metabolized via cytochrome P450 pathway requires caution).

No products indexed under this heading.

Rabeprazole Sodium (Concurrent use with agents known to be metabolized via cytochrome P450 pathway requires caution). Products include:

Repaglinide (Concurrent use with agents known to be metabolized via cytochrome P450 pathway requires caution).

No products indexed under this heading.

Rifabutin (Concurrent use with agents known to be metabolized via cytochrome P450 pathway requires caution).

No products indexed under this heading.

Riluzole (Concurrent use with agents known to be metabolized via cytochrome P450 pathway requires caution). Products include:

Risperidone (Concurrent use with agents known to be metabolized via cytochrome P450 pathway requires caution). Products include:

Ritonavir (Concurrent use with agents known to be metabolized via cytochrome P450 pathway requires caution). Products include:

Rofecoxib (Concurrent use with agents known to be metabolized via cytochrome P450 pathway requires caution).

No products indexed under this heading.

Ropinirole Hydrochloride (Concurrent use with agents known to be metabolized via cytochrome P450 pathway requires caution). Products include:

Ropivacaine Hydrochloride (Concurrent use with agents known to be metabolized via cytochrome P450 pathway requires caution).

No products indexed under this heading.

Rosiglitazone Maleate (Concurrent use with agents known to be metabolized via cytochrome P450 pathway requires caution). Products include:

Saquinavir (Concurrent use with agents known to be metabolized via cytochrome P450 pathway requires caution).

No products indexed under this heading.

Saquinavir Mesylate (Concurrent use with agents known to be metabolized via cytochrome P450 pathway requires caution). Products include:

Sertraline Hydrochloride (Concurrent use with agents known to be metabolized via cytochrome P450 pathway requires caution). Products include:

Sildenafil Citrate (Concurrent use with agents known to be metabolized via cytochrome P450 pathway requires caution). Products include:

Simvastatin (Concurrent use with agents known to be metabolized via cytochrome P450 pathway requires caution). Products include:

Sirolimus (Concurrent use with agents known to be metabolized via cytochrome P450 pathway requires caution). Products include:

Sulfamethoxazole (Concurrent use with agents known to be metabolized via cytochrome P450 pathway requires caution).

No products indexed under this heading.

Sulindac (Concurrent use with agents known to be metabolized via cytochrome P450 pathway requires caution). Products include:

Suprofen (Concurrent use with agents known to be metabolized via cytochrome P450 pathway requires caution).

No products indexed under this heading.

Tacrine Hydrochloride (Concurrent use with agents known to be metabolized via cytochrome P450 pathway requires caution).

No products indexed under this heading.

Tacrolimus (Concurrent use with agents known to be metabolized via cytochrome P450 pathway requires caution). Products include:

Tamoxifen Citrate (Concurrent use with agents known to be metabolized via cytochrome P450 pathway requires caution). Products include:

Telmisartan (Concurrent use with agents known to be metabolized via cytochrome P450 pathway requires caution). Products include:

Teniposide (Concurrent use with agents known to be metabolized via cytochrome P450 pathway requires caution).

No products indexed under this heading.

Terfenadine (Concurrent use with agents known to be metabolized via cytochrome P450 pathway requires caution).

No products indexed under this heading.

Testosterone (Concurrent use with agents known to be metabolized via cytochrome P450 pathway requires caution). Products include:

Testosterone Cypionate (Concurrent use with agents known to be metabolized via cytochrome P450 pathway requires caution).

No products indexed under this heading.

Testosterone Enanthate (Concurrent use with agents known to be metabolized via cytochrome P450 pathway requires caution).

No products indexed under this heading.

Testosterone Propionate (Concurrent use with agents known to be metabolized via cytochrome P450 pathway requires caution).

No products indexed under this heading.

Theophylline (Concurrent use with agents known to be metabolized via cytochrome P450 pathway requires caution).

No products indexed under this heading.

Theophylline Anhydrous (Concurrent use with agents known to be metabolized via cytochrome P450 pathway requires caution). Products include:

Theophylline Sodium Glycinate (Concurrent use with agents known to be metabolized via cytochrome P450 pathway requires caution).

No products indexed under this heading.

Thioridazine (Concurrent use with agents known to be metabolized via cytochrome P450 pathway requires caution).

No products indexed under this heading.

Thioridazine Hydrochloride (Concurrent use with agents known to be metabolized via cytochrome P450 pathway requires caution). Products include:

Tiagabine Hydrochloride (Concurrent use with agents known to be metabolized via cytochrome P450 pathway requires caution). Products include:

Timolol Maleate (Concurrent use with agents known to be metabolized via cytochrome P450 pathway requires caution). Products include:

Tolazamide (Concurrent use with agents known to be metabolized via cytochrome P450 pathway requires caution).

No products indexed under this heading.

Tolbutamide (Concurrent use with agents known to be metabolized via cytochrome P450 pathway requires caution).

No products indexed under this heading.

Tolbutamide Sodium (Concurrent use with agents known to be metabolized via cytochrome P450 pathway requires caution).

No products indexed under this heading.

Tylenol Sinus Congestion & Pain Severe Caplets with Cool Burst..... 1876
Tylenol Sore Throat Daytime Liquid with Cool Burst.................. 1877
Tylenol Sore Throat Nighttime Liquid with Cool Burst.................. 1877
Women's Tylenol Menstrual Relief Caplets.................................... 1877
Vicks 44M Cough, Cold & Flu Relief Liquid................................ 2680
Vicks DayQuil LiquiCaps/Liquid Multi-Symptom Cold/Flu Relief..... ▣761
Vicks DayQuil Multi-Symptom Cold/Flu Relief LiquiCaps............. 2678
Vicks DayQuil Multi-Symptom Cold/Flu Relief Liquid.................. 2678
Vicks NyQuil Multi-Symptom Cold/Flu Relief Liquid.................. 2681
Vicks NyQuil Multi-Symptom Cold/Flu Relief LiquiCaps............. 2681
Vicks NyQuil LiquiCaps/Liquid Multi-Symptom Cold/Flu Relief..... ▣763
Vicodin Tablets 535
Vicodin ES Tablets 536
Vicodin HP Tablets 538
Zicam Maximum Strength Flu Daytime.................................... ▣768
Zicam Maximum Strength Flu Nighttime.................................. ▣768
Zydone Tablets 1139

Alatrofloxacin Mesylate (Blood levels and/or toxicity of propranolol may be increased by administration of propranolol hydrochloride extended-release capsules with substrates of CYP1A2).
No products indexed under this heading.

Albuterol (Propranolol is a competitive inhibitor of beta-receptor agonists and its effects can be reversed by administration of such agents (e.g., isoproterenol)). Products include:
Proventil Inhalation Aerosol 3053

Albuterol Sulfate (Propranolol is a competitive inhibitor of beta-receptor agonists and its effects can be reversed by administration of such agents (e.g., isoproterenol)). Products include:
AccuNeb Inhalation Solution 1055
Combivent Inhalation Aerosol 847
DuoNeb Inhalation Solution 1058
ProAir HFA Inhalation Aerosol 3300
Proventil Inhalation Solution 0.083%...................................... 3055
Proventil HFA Inhalation Aerosol....... 3056
Ventolin HFA Inhalation Aerosol 1600
VoSpire ER Tablets 1052

Aluminum Hydroxide (Co-administration of propranolol with aluminum hydroxide gel (1200 mg) resulted in a 50% decrease in propranolol concentrations). Products include:
Gaviscon Regular Strength Liquid .. ▣658
Gaviscon Regular Strength Tablets.................................... ▣658
Gaviscon Extra Strength Liquid ..... ▣658
Gaviscon Extra Strength Tablets .... ▣658
Maalox Regular Strength Antacid/Antigas Liquid................. 2175
Maalox Max Maximum Strength Antacid/Anti-Gas Liquid................ 2176

Aluminum Hydroxide Preparations (Co-administration of propranolol with aluminum hydroxide gel (1200 mg) resulted in a 50% decrease in propranolol concentrations).
No products indexed under this heading.

Amiodarone Hydrochloride (Amiodarone is an antiarrhythmic agent with negative chronotropic properties that may be additive to those seen with propranolol).
No products indexed under this heading.

Amitriptyline Hydrochloride (Blood levels and/or toxicity of propranolol may be increased by administration of propranolol hydrochloride extended-release capsules with substrates of CYP2D6).
No products indexed under this heading.

Amlodipine Besylate (Caution should be exercised when patients receiving a beta-blocker are administered a calcium channel blocking drug with negative inotropic and/or chronotropic effects. Both agents may depress cardiac contractility or atrioventricular conduction). Products include:
Caduet Tablets 2508
Lotrel Capsules 2249
Norvasc Tablets 2545

Amoxapine (Blood levels and/or toxicity of propranolol may be increased by administration of propranolol hydrochloride extended-release capsules with inhibitors of CYP2D6).
No products indexed under this heading.

Amphetamine Aspartate (Blood levels and/or toxicity of propranolol may be increased by administration of propranolol hydrochloride extended-release capsules with substrates of CYP2D6). Products include:
Adderall Tablets 3164
Adderall XR Capsules 3166

Amphetamine Aspartate Monohydrate (Blood levels and/or toxicity of propranolol may be increased by administration of propranolol hydrochloride extended-release capsules with substrates of CYP2D6).
No products indexed under this heading.

Amphetamine Sulfate (Blood levels and/or toxicity of propranolol may be increased by administration of propranolol hydrochloride extended-release capsules with substrates of CYP2D6). Products include:
Adderall Tablets 3164
Adderall XR Capsules 3166

Anagrelide Hydrochloride (Blood levels and/or toxicity of propranolol may be increased by administration of propranolol hydrochloride extended-release capsules with substrates of CYP1A2). Products include:
Agrylin Capsules 3169

Anastrozole (Blood levels and/or toxicity of propranolol may be increased by administration of propranolol hydrochloride extended-release capsules with inhibitors of CYP1A2). Products include:
Arimidex Tablets 673

Atomoxetine Hydrochloride (Blood levels and/or toxicity of propranolol may be increased by administration of propranolol hydrochloride extended-release capsules with substrates of CYP2D6). Products include:
Strattera Capsules 1814

Benazepril Hydrochloride (When combined with beta-blockers, ACE inhibitors can cause hypotension, particularly in the setting of acute myocardial infarction. Certain ACE inhibitors have been reported to increase bronchial hyper-reactivity when administered with propranolol). Products include:
Lotensin Tablets 2243
Lotensin HCT Tablets 2246
Lotrel Capsules 2249

Bepridil Hydrochloride (Caution should be exercised when patients receiving a beta-blocker are administered a calcium channel blocking drug with negative inotropic and/or chronotropic effects. Both agents may depress cardiac contractility or atrioventricular conduction).
No products indexed under this heading.

Bisoprolol Fumarate (Blood levels and/or toxicity of propranolol may be increased by administration of propranolol hydrochloride extended-release capsules with substrates of CYP2D6).
No products indexed under this heading.

Bitolterol Mesylate (Propranolol is a competitive inhibitor of beta-receptor agonists and its effects can be reversed by administration of such agents (e.g., isoproterenol)).
No products indexed under this heading.

Bupropion Hydrochloride (Blood levels and/or toxicity of propranolol may be increased by administration of propranolol hydrochloride extended-release capsules with inhibitors of CYP2D6). Products include:
Wellbutrin Tablets 1603
Wellbutrin SR Sustained-Release Tablets.. 1607
Wellbutrin XL Extended-Release Tablets.. 1613
Zyban Sustained-Release Tablets..... 1644

Caffeine (Blood levels and/or toxicity of propranolol may be increased by administration of propranolol hydrochloride extended-release capsules with substrates of CYP1A2). Products include:
BC Headache Powder .... ▣677
Arthritis Strength BC Powder .... ▣677
Excedrin Extra Strength Caplets/Tablets/Geltabs............ ▣684
Excedrin Migraine Caplets/Tablets/Geltabs............ ▣609
Excedrin Tension Headache Caplets/Tablets/Geltabs............ ▣611
Goody's Extra Strength Headache Powders.................... ▣611
Goody's Extra Strength Pain Relief Tablets............................ ▣685
Vivarin .... ▣602
Winrgy Dietary Supplement .... ▣823

Caffeine Anhydrous (Blood levels and/or toxicity of propranolol may be increased by administration of propranolol hydrochloride extended-release capsules with substrates of CYP1A2).
No products indexed under this heading.

Captopril (Blood levels and/or toxicity of propranolol may be increased by administration of propranolol hydrochloride extended-release capsules with substrates of CYP2D6). Products include:
Captopril Tablets 2149

Carbamazepine (Blood levels of propranolol may be decreased by co-administration of propranolol hydrochloride extended-release capsules with inducers of hepatic drug metabolism). Products include:
Carbatrol Capsules 3171
Equetro Extended-Release Capsules...................................... 3180
Tegretol/Tegretol-XR 2295

Carisoprodol (Blood levels and/or toxicity of propranolol may be increased by administration of propranolol hydrochloride extended-release capsules with substrates of CYP2C19).
No products indexed under this heading.

Carvedilol (Blood levels and/or toxicity of propranolol may be increased by administration of propranolol hydrochloride extended-release capsules with substrates of CYP2D6). Products include:
Coreg Tablets 1414

Celecoxib (Blood levels and/or toxicity of propranolol may be increased by administration of propranolol hydrochloride extended-release capsules with inhibitors of CYP2D6). Products include:
Celebrex Capsules 3134

Cevimeline Hydrochloride (Blood levels and/or toxicity of propranolol may be increased by administration of propranolol hydrochloride extended-release capsules with substrates of CYP2D6). Products include:
Evoxac Capsules 1047

Chlordiazepoxide (Blood levels and/or toxicity of propranolol may be increased by administration of propranolol hydrochloride extended-release capsules with substrates of CYP1A2).
No products indexed under this heading.

Chlordiazepoxide Hydrochloride (Blood levels and/or toxicity of propranolol may be increased by administration of propranolol hydrochloride extended-release capsules with substrates of CYP1A2). Products include:
Librium Capsules 3347

Chloroquine Hydrochloride (Blood levels and/or toxicity of propranolol may be increased by administration of propranolol hydrochloride extended-release capsules with inhibitors of CYP2D6).
No products indexed under this heading.

Chloroquine Phosphate (Blood levels and/or toxicity of propranolol may be increased by administration of propranolol hydrochloride extended-release capsules with inhibitors of CYP2D6).
No products indexed under this heading.

Chlorpheniramine (Blood levels and/or toxicity of propranolol may be increased by administration of propranolol hydrochloride extended-release capsules with inhibitors of CYP2D6).
No products indexed under this heading.

Chlorpheniramine Maleate (Blood levels and/or toxicity of propranolol may be increased by administration of propranolol hydrochloride extended-release capsules with inhibitors of CYP2D6). Products include:
Advil Allergy Sinus Caplets .... ▣770
Advil Multi-Symptom Cold Caplets...................................... ▣770
BC Allergy Sinus Cold Powder .... ▣677
Comtrex Maximum Strength Cold & Cough Day/Night Caplets - Night Formulation .... ▣726
Comtrex Maximum Strength Day/Night Severe Cold & Sinus Caplets - Night Formulation .... ▣725

Contac Cold and Flu Maximum Strength Caplets 728
Contac Cold and Flu Day and Night Caplets (Night Formulation Only) 727
Children's Dimetapp Long Acting Cough Plus Cold Syrup 731
Robitussin Cough & Cold Long-Acting Liquid 735
Robitussin Cough & Allergy Syrup .. 736
Robitussin Cough & Cold Nighttime Liquid 736
Robitussin Cough, Cold & Flu Nighttime Liquid 738
Robitussin Pediatric Cough & Cold Long-Acting Liquid 735
Robitussin Pediatric Cough & Cold Nighttime Liquid 736
Triaminic Cold & Allergy Liquid 746
Triaminic Cough & Runny Nose Softchews 748
Children's Tylenol Plus Flu Oral Suspension 749
Tylenol Allergy Multi-Symptom Caplets with Cool Burst and Gelcaps 1872
Children's Tylenol Plus Cold Suspension Liquid 1879
Children's Tylenol Plus Cough & Runny Nose Suspension Liquid 1879
Children's Tylenol Plus Flu Suspension Liquid 1881
Children's Tylenol Plus Multi-Symptom Cold Suspension Liquid 1879
Tylenol Cold Head Congestion Nighttime Caplets with Cool Burst 1873
Tylenol Cold Multi-Symptom Nighttime Caplets with Cool Burst 1874
Tylenol Sinus Congestion & Pain Nighttime Caplets with Cool Burst 1876
Vicks 44M Cough, Cold & Flu Relief Liquid 2680
Pediatric Vicks 44m Cough & Cold Relief Liquid 2676
Children's Vicks NyQuil Cold/Cough Relief 756
Children's Vicks NyQuil Cold/Cough Relief Liquid 2680
Zicam Maximum Strength Flu Daytime 768

Chlorpheniramine Polistirex (Blood levels and/or toxicity of propranolol may be increased by administration of propranolol hydrochloride extended-release capsules with inhibitors of CYP2D6). Products include:
Tussionex Pennkinetic Extended-Release Suspension 3327

Chlorpheniramine Tannate (Blood levels and/or toxicity of propranolol may be increased by administration of propranolol hydrochloride extended-release capsules with inhibitors of CYP2D6).
No products indexed under this heading.

Chlorpromazine (Co-administration of chlorpromazine with propranolol resulted in increased plasma levels of both drugs (70% increase in propranolol concentrations)).
No products indexed under this heading.

Chlorpromazine Hydrochloride (Co-administration of chlorpromazine with propranolol resulted in increased plasma levels of both drugs (70% increase in propranolol concentrations)).
No products indexed under this heading.

Chlorpropamide (Blood levels and/or toxicity of propranolol may be increased by administration of propranolol hydrochloride extended-release capsules with substrates of CYP2D6).
No products indexed under this heading.

Cholestyramine (Co-administration of cholestyramine with propranolol decreased propranolol concentrations by up to 50%).
No products indexed under this heading.

Cilostazol (Blood levels and/or toxicity of propranolol may be increased by administration of propranolol hydrochloride extended-release capsules with substrates of CYP2C19). Products include:
Pletal Tablets 2455

Cimetidine (Co-administration of propranolol with cimetidine, a non-specific CYP450 inhibitor, increased propranolol concentrations by about 40%). Products include:
Tagamet HB 200 Tablets 664

Cimetidine Hydrochloride (Co-administration of propranolol with cimetidine, a non-specific CYP450 inhibitor, increased propranolol concentrations by about 40%).
No products indexed under this heading.

Ciprofloxacin (Blood levels and/or toxicity of propranolol may be increased by administration of propranolol hydrochloride extended-release capsules with substrates of CYP1A2). Products include:
Cipro Oral Suspension 2977
Cipro I.V. 2984
Cipro XR Tablets 2990
Ciprodex Otic Suspension 559

Ciprofloxacin Hydrochloride (Blood levels and/or toxicity of propranolol may be increased by administration of propranolol hydrochloride extended-release capsules with substrates of CYP1A2). Products include:
Ciloxan Ophthalmic Ointment 559
Ciloxan Ophthalmic Solution .... ⊙206
Cipro Tablets 2977
Proquin XR Tablets 1153

Citalopram Hydrobromide (Blood levels and/or toxicity of propranolol may be increased by administration of propranolol hydrochloride extended-release capsules with inhibitors of CYP2D6). Products include:
Celexa 1176

Clarithromycin (Blood levels and/or toxicity of propranolol may be increased by administration of propranolol hydrochloride extended-release capsules with inhibitors of CYP1A2). Products include:
Biaxin/Biaxin XL 402
PREVPAC 3284

Clomipramine Hydrochloride (Blood levels and/or toxicity of propranolol may be increased by administration of propranolol hydrochloride extended-release capsules with substrates of CYP2D6).
No products indexed under this heading.

Clonidine (The antihypertensive effects of clonidine may be antagonized by beta-blockers. Propranolol extended-release capsules should be administered cautiously to patients withdrawing from clonidine). Products include:
Catapres-TTS 844

Clonidine Hydrochloride (The antihypertensive effects of clonidine may be antagonized by beta-blockers. Propranolol extended-release capsules should be administered cautiously to patients withdrawing from clonidine). Products include:
Catapres Tablets 843
Clorpres Tablets 2153

Clopidogrel Bisulfate (Blood levels and/or toxicity of propranolol may be increased by administration of propranolol hydrochloride extended-release capsules with substrates of CYP1A2). Products include:
Plavix Tablets 917
Plavix Tablets 2926

Clozapine (Blood levels and/or toxicity of propranolol may be increased by administration of propranolol hydrochloride extended-release capsules with substrates of CYP2D6). Products include:
Clozaril Tablets 2184
FazaClo Orally Disintegrating Tablets 551

Cocaine Hydrochloride (Blood levels and/or toxicity of propranolol may be increased by administration of propranolol hydrochloride extended-release capsules with inhibitors of CYP2D6).
No products indexed under this heading.

Codeine Phosphate (Blood levels and/or toxicity of propranolol may be increased by administration of propranolol hydrochloride extended-release capsules with substrates of CYP2D6). Products include:
Tylenol with Codeine Tablets 2391

Codeine Sulfate (Blood levels and/or toxicity of propranolol may be increased by administration of propranolol hydrochloride extended-release capsules with substrates of CYP2D6).
No products indexed under this heading.

Colestipol (Co-administration of colestipol with propranolol decreased propranolol concentrations by up to 50%).
No products indexed under this heading.

Colestipol Hydrochloride (Co-administration of colestipol with propranolol decreased propranolol concentrations by up to 50%).
No products indexed under this heading.

Cyclobenzaprine (Blood levels and/or toxicity of propranolol may be increased by administration of propranolol hydrochloride extended-release capsules with substrates of CYP1A2).
No products indexed under this heading.

Cyclobenzaprine Hydrochloride (Blood levels and/or toxicity of propranolol may be increased by administration of propranolol hydrochloride extended-release capsules with substrates of CYP2D6).
No products indexed under this heading.

Cyclophosphamide (Blood levels and/or toxicity of propranolol may be increased by administration of propranolol hydrochloride extended-release capsules with substrates of CYP2C19).
No products indexed under this heading.

Delavirdine Mesylate (Blood levels and/or toxicity of propranolol may be increased by administration of propranolol hydrochloride extended-release capsules with inhibitors of CYP2C19). Products include:
Rescriptor Tablets 2551

Deserpidine (Patients receiving catecholamine-depleting drugs (e.g., reserpine) and propranolol hydrochloride extended-release capsules should be observed closely for excessive reduction of resting sympathetic nervous activity, which may result in hypotension, marked bradycardia, vertigo, syncopal attacks, or orthostatic hypotension).
No products indexed under this heading.

Desipramine Hydrochloride (Blood levels and/or toxicity of propranolol may be increased by administration of propranolol hydrochloride extended-release capsules with substrates of CYP2D6).
No products indexed under this heading.

Deslanoside (Use caution when administering propranolol hydrochloride extended-release tablets with drugs that slow AV nodal conduction (e.g., digitalis)).
No products indexed under this heading.

Desogestrel (Blood levels and/or toxicity of propranolol may be increased by administration of propranolol hydrochloride extended-release capsules with inhibitors of CYP1A2). Products include:
Mircette Tablets 1066

Dexfenfluramine Hydrochloride (Blood levels and/or toxicity of propranolol may be increased by administration of propranolol hydrochloride extended-release capsules with substrates of CYP2D6).
No products indexed under this heading.

Dextromethorphan (Blood levels and/or toxicity of propranolol may be increased by administration of propranolol hydrochloride extended-release capsules with substrates of CYP2C19).
No products indexed under this heading.

Dextromethorphan Hydrobromide (Blood levels and/or toxicity of propranolol may be increased by administration of propranolol hydrochloride extended-release capsules with substrates of CYP2D6). Products include:
Comtrex Maximum Strength Cold & Cough Day/Night Caplets - Day Formulation 726
Comtrex Maximum Strength Cold & Cough Day/Night Caplets - Night Formulation 726
Comtrex Maximum Strength Non-Drowsy Cold & Cough Caplets 725
Children's Dimetapp DM Cold & Cough Elixir 731
Children's Dimetapp Long Acting Cough Plus Cold Syrup 731
Toddler's Dimetapp Cold and Cough Drops 732
Mucinex DM Extended-Release Bi-Layer Tablets 720
Refenesen DM Caplets 721
Robitussin Cough & Cold CF Liquid 735
Robitussin Cough & Cold Long-Acting Liquid 735
Robitussin Cough & Allergy Syrup .. 736
Robitussin Cough & Cold Nighttime Liquid 736
Robitussin Cough & Cold Pediatric Drops 735
Robitussin Cough, Cold & Flu Nighttime Liquid 738
Robitussin Cough & Congestion Liquid 738

Robitussin Cough Gels Long-Acting .... ■ 737
Robitussin Cough Long Acting Liquid .... ■ 739
Robitussin Cough DM Syrup .... ■ 738
Robitussin Cough DM Infant Drops .... ■ 738
Robitussin Pediatric Cough Long Acting Liquid .... ■ 739
Robitussin Pediatric Cough & Cold Long-Acting Liquid .... ■ 735
Robitussin Pediatric Cough & Cold Nighttime Liquid .... ■ 736
Robitussin Sugar Free Cough .... ■ 738
TheraFlu Cold & Cough Hot Liquid .... ■ 740
TheraFlu Warming Relief Daytime Severe Cold .... ■ 743
TheraFlu Thin Strips Long Acting Cough .... ■ 744
Triaminic Daytime Cold & Cough Liquid .... ■ 745
Triaminic Cough & Sore Throat Liquid .... ■ 747
Triaminic Cough & Runny Nose Softchews .... ■ 748
Triaminic Thin Strips Cold & Cough .... ■ 778
Triaminic Infant Thin Strips Decongestant Plus Cough .... ■ 747
Children's Tylenol Plus Flu Oral Suspension .... ■ 749
Tylenol Cold Head Congestion Daytime Caplets with Cool Burst and Gelcaps .... ■ 750
Tylenol Cold Multi-Symptom Daytime Liquid .... ■ 752
Tylenol Cold Multi-Symptom Severe Daytime Liquid .... ■ 752
Concentrated Tylenol Infants' Drops Plus Cold & Cough .... ■ 754
Children's Tylenol Plus Cough & Runny Nose Suspension Liquid 1879
Children's Tylenol Plus Cough & Sore Throat Suspension Liquid 1879
Children's Tylenol Plus Flu Suspension Liquid 1881
Children's Tylenol Plus Multi-Symptom Cold Suspension Liquid 1879
Tylenol Cold Severe Congestion Non-Drowsy Caplets with Cool Burst 1874
Tylenol Cold Head Congestion Daytime Caplets with Cool Burst 1873
Tylenol Cold Head Congestion Nighttime Caplets with Cool Burst 1873
Tylenol Cold Head Congestion Severe Caplets with Cool Burst 1873
Tylenol Cold Multi-Symptom Daytime Caplets with Cool Burst and Gelcaps 1874
Tylenol Cold Multi-Symptom Daytime Liquid with Citrus Burst 1874
Tylenol Cold Multi-Symptom Nighttime Caplets with Cool Burst 1874
Tylenol Cold Multi-Symptom Nighttime Liquid with Cool Burst 1874
Tylenol Cold Multi-Symptom Severe Caplets with Cool Burst 1874
Tylenol Cold Multi-Symptom Severe Daytime Liquid with Citrus Burst 1874
Tylenol Cough & Sore Throat Daytime Liquid with Cool Burst 1877
Tylenol Cough & Sore Throat Nighttime Liquid with Cool Burst 1877
Concentrated Tylenol Infants' Drops Plus Cold and Cough 1879
Vicks 44 Cough Relief Liquid 2679
Vicks 44D Cough & Head Congestion Relief Liquid 2679
Vicks 44E Cough & Chest Congestion Relief Liquid 2679
Pediatric Vicks 44e Cough & Chest Congestion Relief Liquid 2676
Vicks 44M Cough, Cold & Flu Relief Liquid 2680
Pediatric Vicks 44m Cough & Cold Relief Liquid 2676
Vicks DayQuil LiquiCaps/Liquid Multi-Symptom Cold/Flu Relief .... ■ 761
Vicks DayQuil Multi-Symptom Cold/Flu Relief LiquiCaps 2678
Vicks DayQuil Multi-Symptom Cold/Flu Relief Liquid 2678
Vicks NyQuil Multi-Symptom Cold/Flu Relief Liquid 2681
Children's Vicks NyQuil Cold/Cough Relief .... ■ 756
Vicks NyQuil Multi-Symptom Cold/Flu Relief LiquiCaps 2681
Vicks NyQuil LiquiCaps/Liquid Multi Symptom Cold/Flu Relief .... ■ 763
Vicks NyQuil Cough Liquid 2680
Children's Vicks NyQuil Cold/Cough Relief Liquid 2680
Zicam Cough Max Nighttime Cough Spray .... ■ 767
Zicam Cough Max Cough Spray .... ■ 767
Zicam Cough Max Cough Melts .... ■ 767
Zicam Cough Plus D Cough Spray .... ■ 767
Zicam Cough Relief Cough Spray .... ■ 767
Zicam Maximum Strength Flu Daytime .... ■ 768
Zicam Maximum Strength Flu Nighttime .... ■ 768

Dextromethorphan Polistirex (Blood levels and/or toxicity of propranolol may be increased by administration of propranolol hydrochloride extended-release capsules with substrates of CYP2D6). Products include:

Delsym Extended-Release Suspension 12 Hour Cough Suppressant .... ■ 611

Diazepam (Propranolol can inhibit the metabolism of diazepam, resulting in increased concentrations of diazepam and its metabolites. Diazepam does not alter the pharmacokinetics of propranolol). Products include:

Diastat Rectal Delivery System 3343
Valium Tablets 2819

Diclofenac Potassium (Non-steroidal anti-inflammatory drugs have been reported to blunt the antihypertensive effects of beta-adrenoreceptor blocking agents).

No products indexed under this heading.

Diclofenac Sodium (Non-steroidal anti-inflammatory drugs have been reported to blunt the antihypertensive effects of beta-adrenoreceptor blocking agents). Products include:

Arthrotec Tablets 3129
Voltaren Ophthalmic Solution 2309
Voltaren Tablets 2307
Voltaren-XR Tablets 2310

Digitalis Glycoside Preparations (Use caution when administering propranolol hydrochloride extended-release tablets with drugs that slow AV nodal conduction (e.g., digitalis)).

No products indexed under this heading.

Digitoxin (Use caution when administering propranolol hydrochloride extended-release tablets with drugs that slow AV nodal conduction (e.g., digitalis)).

No products indexed under this heading.

Digoxin (Use caution when administering propranolol hydrochloride extended-release tablets with drugs that slow AV nodal conduction (e.g., digitalis)). Products include:

Lanoxicaps Capsules 1490
Lanoxin Injection 1494
Lanoxin Injection Pediatric 1497
Lanoxin Tablets 1500

Diltiazem Hydrochloride (Co-administration of propranolol and diltiazem in patients with cardiac disease has been associated with bradycardia, hypotension, high degree heart block, and heart failure). Products include:

Cardizem LA Extended Release Tablets 1728
Tiazac Capsules 1201

Diltiazem Maleate (Co-administration of propranolol and diltiazem in patients with cardiac disease has been associated with bradycardia, hypotension, high degree heart block, and heart failure).

No products indexed under this heading.

Diphenhydramine (Blood levels and/or toxicity of propranolol may be increased by administration of propranolol hydrochloride extended-release capsules with inhibitors of CYP2D6). Products include:

Tylenol Sore Throat Nighttime Liquid with Cool Burst 1877

Diphenhydramine Hydrochloride (Blood levels and/or toxicity of propranolol may be increased by administration of propranolol hydrochloride extended-release capsules with inhibitors of CYP2D6). Products include:

Nytol QuickCaps Caplets .... ■ 615
Nytol QuickGels Softgels Maximum Strength .... ■ 616
Simply Sleep Caplets 1868
Sominex Original Formula Tablets .... ■ 616
TheraFlu Warming Relief Nighttime Severe Cold .... ■ 743
TheraFlu Thin Strips Multi Symptom .... ■ 744
Triaminic Nighttime Cold & Cough Liquid .... ■ 746
Triaminic Thin Strips Cough & Runny Nose .... ■ 749
Extra Strength Tylenol PM Caplets, Vanilla Caplets, Geltabs, Gelcaps and Liquid 1875
Tylenol Sore Throat Nighttime Liquid with Cool Burst .... ■ 790
Tylenol Allergy Multi-Symptom Nighttime Caplets with Cool Burst 1872
Tylenol Severe Allergy Caplets 1872
Children's Tylenol Plus Cold & Allergy Suspension Liquid 1878

Disopyramide (Disopyramide, a Type I antiarrhythmic drug with potent negative inotropic and chronotropic effects, has been associated with severe bradycardia, asystole, and heart failure when administered with propranolol).

No products indexed under this heading.

Disopyramide Phosphate (Disopyramide, a Type I antiarrhythmic drug with potent negative inotropic and chronotropic effects, has been associated with severe bradycardia, asystole, and heart failure when administered with propranolol).

No products indexed under this heading.

Divalproex Sodium (Blood levels and/or toxicity of propranolol may be increased by administration of propranolol hydrochloride extended-release capsules with substrates of CYP2C19). Products include:

Depakote Sprinkle Capsules 422
Depakote Tablets 427
Depakote ER Tablets 434

Dobutamine (Propranolol is a competitive inhibitor of beta-receptor agonists and its effects can be reversed by administration of such agents (e.g., dobutamine)).

No products indexed under this heading.

Dobutamine Hydrochloride (Propranolol is a competitive inhibitor of beta-receptor agonists and its effects can be reversed by administration of such agents (e.g., dobutamine)).

No products indexed under this heading.

Dolasetron Mesylate (Blood levels and/or toxicity of propranolol may be increased by administration of propranolol hydrochloride extended-release capsules with substrates of CYP2D6). Products include:

Anzemet Injection 2859
Anzemet Tablets 2862

Donepezil Hydrochloride (Blood levels and/or toxicity of propranolol may be increased by administration of propranolol hydrochloride extended-release capsules with substrates of CYP2D6). Products include:

Aricept Tablets 1094
Aricept ODT Tablets 1094

Doxazosin Mesylate (Postural hypotension has been reported in patients taking both beta-blockers and doxazosin). Products include:

Cardura XL Tablets 2515

Doxepin Hydrochloride (Blood levels and/or toxicity of propranolol may be increased by administration of propranolol hydrochloride extended-release capsules with substrates of CYP2D6).

No products indexed under this heading.

Efavirenz (Blood levels and/or toxicity of propranolol may be increased by administration of propranolol hydrochloride extended-release capsules with inhibitors of CYP2C19). Products include:

Atripla Tablets 945
Sustiva Capsules 930
Sustiva Tablets 930

Enalapril Maleate (When combined with beta-blockers, ACE inhibitors can cause hypotension, particularly in the setting of acute myocardial infarction. Certain ACE inhibitors have been reported to increase bronchial hyper-reactivity when administered with propranolol). Products include:

Vasotec I.V. Injection 2103

Enalaprilat (When combined with beta-blockers, ACE inhibitors can cause hypotension, particularly in the setting of acute myocardial infarction. Certain ACE inhibitors have been reported to increase bronchial hyper-reactivity when administered with propranolol).

No products indexed under this heading.

Encainide Hydrochloride (Blood levels and/or toxicity of propranolol may be increased by administration of propranolol hydrochloride extended-release capsules with substrates of CYP2D6).

No products indexed under this heading.

Enoxacin (Blood levels and/or toxicity of propranolol may be increased by administration of propranolol hydrochloride extended-release capsules with substrates of CYP1A2).

No products indexed under this heading.

Ephedrine Hydrochloride (Propranolol is a competitive inhibitor of beta-receptor agonists and its effects can be reversed by administration of such agents (e.g., isoproterenol)).
No products indexed under this heading.

Ephedrine Sulfate (Propranolol is a competitive inhibitor of beta-receptor agonists and its effects can be reversed by administration of such agents (e.g., isoproterenol)).
No products indexed under this heading.

Ephedrine Tannate (Propranolol is a competitive inhibitor of beta-receptor agonists and its effects can be reversed by administration of such agents (e.g., isoproterenol)).
No products indexed under this heading.

Epinephrine (Patients on long-term therapy with propranolol may experience uncontrolled hypertension if they are administered epinephrine as a consequence of unopposed alpha-receptor stimulation. Epinephrine is, therefore, not indicated in the treatment of propranolol overdose). Products include:

Epinephrine, Racemic (Patients on long-term therapy with propranolol may experience uncontrolled hypertension if they are administered epinephrine as a consequence of unopposed alpha-receptor stimulation. Epinephrine is, therefore, not indicated in the treatment of propranolol overdose).
No products indexed under this heading.

Epinephrine Bitartrate (Patients on long-term therapy with propranolol may experience uncontrolled hypertension if they are administered epinephrine as a consequence of unopposed alpha-receptor stimulation. Epinephrine is, therefore, not indicated in the treatment of propranolol overdose).
No products indexed under this heading.

Epinephrine Hydrochloride (Patients on long-term therapy with propranolol may experience uncontrolled hypertension if they are administered epinephrine as a consequence of unopposed alpha-receptor stimulation. Epinephrine is, therefore, not indicated in the treatment of propranolol overdose).
No products indexed under this heading.

Erythromycin (Blood levels and/or toxicity of propranolol may be increased by administration of propranolol hydrochloride extended-release capsules with substrates of CYP1A2). Products include:

Erythromycin Estolate (Blood levels and/or toxicity of propranolol may be increased by administration of propranolol hydrochloride extended-release capsules with substrates of CYP1A2).
No products indexed under this heading.

Erythromycin Ethylsuccinate (Blood levels and/or toxicity of propranolol may be increased by administration of propranolol hydrochloride extended-release capsules with substrates of CYP1A2). Products include:

Erythromycin Gluceptate (Blood levels and/or toxicity of propranolol may be increased by administration of propranolol hydrochloride extended-release capsules with substrates of CYP1A2).
No products indexed under this heading.

Erythromycin Lactobionate (Blood levels and/or toxicity of propranolol may be increased by administration of propranolol hydrochloride extended-release capsules with substrates of CYP1A2).
No products indexed under this heading.

Erythromycin Stearate (Blood levels and/or toxicity of propranolol may be increased by administration of propranolol hydrochloride extended-release capsules with substrates of CYP1A2). Products include:

Escitalopram Oxalate (Blood levels and/or toxicity of propranolol may be increased by administration of propranolol hydrochloride extended-release capsules with inhibitors of CYP2D6). Products include:

Esomeprazole Magnesium (Blood levels and/or toxicity of propranolol may be increased by administration of propranolol hydrochloride extended-release capsules with substrates of CYP2C19). Products include:

Estradiol (Blood levels and/or toxicity of propranolol may be increased by administration of propranolol hydrochloride extended-release capsules with substrates of CYP1A2). Products include:

Estradiol Benzoate (Blood levels and/or toxicity of propranolol may be increased by administration of propranolol hydrochloride extended-release capsules with substrates of CYP1A2).
No products indexed under this heading.

Estradiol Cypionate (Blood levels and/or toxicity of propranolol may be increased by administration of propranolol hydrochloride extended-release capsules with substrates of CYP1A2).
No products indexed under this heading.

Ethanol (Blood levels of propranolol may be decreased by co-administration of propranolol hydrochloride extended-release capsules with inducers of hepatic drug metabolism (e.g., ethanol)).
No products indexed under this heading.

Ethinyl Estradiol (Blood levels and/or toxicity of propranolol may be increased by administration of propranolol hydrochloride extended-release capsules with inhibitors of CYP1A2). Products include:

Ethosuximide (Blood levels and/or toxicity of propranolol may be increased by administration of propranolol hydrochloride extended-release capsules with substrates of CYP2C19).
No products indexed under this heading.

Ethotoin (Blood levels and/or toxicity of propranolol may be increased by administration of propranolol hydrochloride extended-release capsules with substrates of CYP2C19).
No products indexed under this heading.

Ethynodiol Diacetate (Blood levels and/or toxicity of propranolol may be increased by administration of propranolol hydrochloride extended-release capsules with inhibitors of CYP2C19).
No products indexed under this heading.

Etodolac (Non-steroidal anti-inflammatory drugs have been reported to blunt the antihypertensive effects of beta-adrenoreceptor blocking agents).
No products indexed under this heading.

Felbamate (Blood levels and/or toxicity of propranolol may be increased by administration of propranolol hydrochloride extended-release capsules with inhibitors of CYP2C19).
No products indexed under this heading.

Felodipine (Caution should be exercised when patients receiving a beta-blocker are administered a calcium channel blocking drug with negative inotropic and/or chronotropic effects. Both agents may depress cardiac contractility or atrioventricular conduction).
No products indexed under this heading.

Fenoprofen Calcium (Non-steroidal anti-inflammatory drugs have been reported to blunt the antihypertensive effects of beta-adrenoreceptor blocking agents). Products include:

Fentanyl (Blood levels and/or toxicity of propranolol may be increased by administration of propranolol hydrochloride extended-release capsules with substrates of CYP2D6). Products include:

Fentanyl Citrate (Blood levels and/or toxicity of propranolol may be increased by administration of propranolol hydrochloride extended-release capsules with substrates of CYP2D6). Products include:

Flecainide Acetate (Blood levels and/or toxicity of propranolol may be increased by administration of propranolol hydrochloride extended-release capsules with substrates of CYP2D6). Products include:

Fluoxetine (Blood levels and/or toxicity of propranolol may be increased by administration of propranolol hydrochloride extended-release capsules with substrates of CYP2D6).
No products indexed under this heading.

Fluoxetine Hydrochloride (Blood levels and/or toxicity of propranolol may be increased by administration of propranolol hydrochloride extended-release capsules with substrates of CYP2D6). Products include:

Fluphenazine Decanoate (Blood levels and/or toxicity of propranolol may be increased by administration of propranolol hydrochloride extended-release capsules with substrates of CYP2D6).
No products indexed under this heading.

Fluphenazine Enanthate (Blood levels and/or toxicity of propranolol may be increased by administration of propranolol hydrochloride extended-release capsules with substrates of CYP2D6).
No products indexed under this heading.

Fluphenazine Hydrochloride (Blood levels and/or toxicity of propranolol may be increased by administration of propranolol hydrochloride extended-release capsules with substrates of CYP2D6).
No products indexed under this heading.

Flurbiprofen (Non-steroidal anti-inflammatory drugs have been reported to blunt the antihypertensive effects of beta-adrenoreceptor blocking agents).
No products indexed under this heading.

Flutamide (Blood levels and/or toxicity of propranolol may be increased by administration of propranolol hydrochloride extended-release capsules with substrates of CYP1A2). Products include:

Fluticasone Propionate (Blood levels and/or toxicity of propranolol may be increased by administration of propranolol hydrochloride extended-release capsules with substrates of CYP1A2). Products include:

Fluvastatin Sodium (Blood levels and/or toxicity of propranolol may be increased by administration of

IMPORTANT NOTE: Always consult each drug listing in the patient's regimen for possible interactions.

propranolol hydrochloride extended-release capsules with inhibitors of CYP2C19). Products include:

Lescol Capsules 2233
Lescol XL Tablets 2233

Fluvoxamine (Blood levels and/or toxicity of propranolol may be increased by administration of propranolol hydrochloride extended-release capsules with inhibitors of CYP1A2).

No products indexed under this heading.

Fluvoxamine Maleate (Blood levels and/or toxicity of propranolol may be increased by administration of propranolol hydrochloride extended-release capsules with substrates of CYP2D6).

No products indexed under this heading.

Formoterol Fumarate (Blood levels and/or toxicity of propranolol may be increased by administration of propranolol hydrochloride extended-release capsules with substrates of CYP2D6). Products include:

Foradil Aerolizer 3010

Fosinopril Sodium (When combined with beta-blockers, ACE inhibitors can cause hypotension, particularly in the setting of acute myocardial infarction. Certain ACE inhibitors have been reported to increase bronchial hyper-reactivity when administered with propranolol).

No products indexed under this heading.

Fosphenytoin (Blood levels and/or toxicity of propranolol may be increased by administration of propranolol hydrochloride extended-release capsules with substrates of CYP2C19).

No products indexed under this heading.

Fosphenytoin Sodium (Blood levels and/or toxicity of propranolol may be increased by administration of propranolol hydrochloride extended-release capsules with substrates of CYP2C19).

No products indexed under this heading.

Gabapentin (Blood levels and/or toxicity of propranolol may be increased by administration of propranolol hydrochloride extended-release capsules with substrates of CYP2C19). Products include:

Neurontin Capsules 2487
Neurontin Oral Solution 2487
Neurontin Tablets 2487

Galantamine Hydrobromide (Blood levels and/or toxicity of propranolol may be increased by administration of propranolol hydrochloride extended-release capsules with substrates of CYP2D6). Products include:

Razadyne 2399
Razadyne ER Extended-Release Capsules 2399

Gatifloxacin (Blood levels and/or toxicity of propranolol may be increased by administration of propranolol hydrochloride extended-release capsules with inhibitors of CYP1A2). Products include:

Tequin Injection 938
Tequin Injection in 5% Dextrose 938
Tequin Tablets 938
Zymar Ophthalmic Solution 575

Gemifloxacin Mesylate (Blood levels and/or toxicity of propranolol may be increased by administration of propranolol hydrochloride extended-release capsules with inhibitors of CYP1A2).

No products indexed under this heading.

Glipizide (Blood levels of propranolol may be decreased by co-administration of propranolol hydrochloride extended-release capsules with inducers of hepatic drug metabolism).

No products indexed under this heading.

Glyburide (Blood levels of propranolol may be decreased by co-administration of propranolol hydrochloride extended-release capsules with inducers of hepatic drug metabolism).

No products indexed under this heading.

Grepafloxacin Hydrochloride (Blood levels and/or toxicity of propranolol may be increased by administration of propranolol hydrochloride extended-release capsules with substrates of CYP1A2).

No products indexed under this heading.

Guanethidine Monosulfate (Patients receiving catecholamine-depleting drugs (e.g., reserpine) and propranolol hydrochloride extended-release capsules should be observed closely for excessive reduction of resting sympathetic nervous activity, which may result in hypotension, marked bradycardia, vertigo, syncopal attacks, or orthostatic hypotension).

No products indexed under this heading.

Halofantrine Hydrochloride (Blood levels and/or toxicity of propranolol may be increased by administration of propranolol hydrochloride extended-release capsules with inhibitors of CYP2D6).

No products indexed under this heading.

Haloperidol (Hypotension and cardiac arrest have been reported with the concomitant use of propranolol and haloperidol).

No products indexed under this heading.

Haloperidol Decanoate (Hypotension and cardiac arrest have been reported with the concomitant use of propranolol and haloperidol).

No products indexed under this heading.

Haloperidol Lactate (Hypotension and cardiac arrest have been reported with the concomitant use of propranolol and haloperidol).

No products indexed under this heading.

Hydrocodone Bitartrate (Blood levels and/or toxicity of propranolol may be increased by administration of propranolol hydrochloride extended-release capsules with substrates of CYP2D6). Products include:

Hycodan 1116
Hycotuss Expectorant Syrup 1117
Vicodin Tablets 535
Vicodin ES Tablets 536
Vicodin HP Tablets 538
Vicoprofen Tablets 539
Zydone Tablets 1139

Hydroxychloroquine Sulfate (Blood levels and/or toxicity of propranolol may be increased by administration of propranolol hydrochloride extended-release capsules with inhibitors of CYP2D6).

No products indexed under this heading.

Ibuprofen (Non-steroidal anti-inflammatory drugs have been reported to blunt the antihypertensive effects of beta-adrenoreceptor blocking agents). Products include:

Advil Allergy Sinus Caplets .... ▣770
Advil .... ▣674
Children's Advil Oral Suspension .... ▣603
Children's Advil Chewable Tablets .. ▣603
Advil Cold & Sinus .... ▣723
Infants' Advil Concentrated Drops .. ▣604
Infants' Advil Concentrated Drops - White Grape (Dye-Free) .... ▣604
Junior Strength Advil Swallow Tablets .... ▣605
Advil Migraine Liquigels .... ▣608
Advil Multi-Symptom Cold Caplets .... ▣770
Advil PM Caplets .... ▣615
Motrin IB Tablets and Caplets 1866
Children's Motrin Oral Suspension ... 1867
Children's Motrin Non-Staining Dye-Free Oral Suspension 1867
Children's Motrin Cold Oral Suspension 1867
Infants' Motrin Concentrated Drops 1867
Infants' Motrin Non-Staining Dye-Free Concentrated Drops 1867
Junior Strength Motrin Caplets and Chewable Tablets 1867
Vicoprofen Tablets 539

Imatinib Mesylate (Blood levels and/or toxicity of propranolol may be increased by administration of propranolol hydrochloride extended-release capsules with inhibitors of CYP2D6). Products include:

Gleevec Tablets 2227

Imipramine Hydrochloride (Blood levels and/or toxicity of propranolol may be increased by administration of propranolol hydrochloride extended-release capsules with substrates of CYP2D6).

No products indexed under this heading.

Imipramine Pamoate (Blood levels and/or toxicity of propranolol may be increased by administration of propranolol hydrochloride extended-release capsules with substrates of CYP2D6).

No products indexed under this heading.

Indomethacin (Administration of indomethacin with propranolol may reduce the efficacy of propranolol in reducing blood pressure and heart rate). Products include:

Indocin 1995

Indomethacin Sodium Trihydrate (Administration of indomethacin with propranolol may reduce the efficacy of propranolol in reducing blood pressure and heart rate). Products include:

Indocin I.V. 2465

Indoramin Hydrochloride (Blood levels and/or toxicity of propranolol may be increased by administration of propranolol hydrochloride extended-release capsules with substrates of CYP2D6).

No products indexed under this heading.

Isocarboxazid (The hypotensive effects of MAO inhibitors may be exacerbated when administered with beta-blockers by interfering with the beta-blocking activity of propranolol).

No products indexed under this heading.

Isoetharine (Propranolol is a competitive inhibitor of beta-receptor agonists and its effects can be reversed by administration of such agents (e.g., isoproterenol)).

No products indexed under this heading.

Isoniazid (Blood levels and/or toxicity of propranolol may be increased by administration of propranolol hydrochloride extended-release capsules with inhibitors of CYP1A2).

No products indexed under this heading.

Isoproterenol Hydrochloride (Propranolol is a competitive inhibitor of beta-receptor agonists and its effects can be reversed by administration of such agents (e.g., isoproterenol)).

No products indexed under this heading.

Isoproterenol Sulfate (Propranolol is a competitive inhibitor of beta-receptor agonists and its effects can be reversed by administration of such agents (e.g., isoproterenol)).

No products indexed under this heading.

Isradipine (Caution should be exercised when patients receiving a beta-blocker are administered a calcium channel blocking drug with negative inotropic and/or chronotropic effects. Both agents may depress cardiac contractility or atrioventricular conduction). Products include:

DynaCirc CR Tablets 2721

Ketoconazole (Blood levels and/or toxicity of propranolol may be increased by administration of propranolol hydrochloride extended-release capsules with inhibitors of CYP1A2). Products include:

Nizoral A-D Shampoo, 1% 1868

Ketoprofen (Non-steroidal anti-inflammatory drugs have been reported to blunt the antihypertensive effects of beta-adrenoreceptor blocking agents).

No products indexed under this heading.

Ketorolac Tromethamine (Non-steroidal anti-inflammatory drugs have been reported to blunt the anti-hypertensive effects of beta-adrenoreceptor blocking agents). Products include:

Acular Ophthalmic Solution 565
Acular LS Ophthalmic Solution 566

Labetalol Hydrochloride (Blood levels and/or toxicity of propranolol may be increased by administration of propranolol hydrochloride extended-release capsules with substrates of CYP2D6).

No products indexed under this heading.

Lamotrigine (Blood levels and/or toxicity of propranolol may be increased by administration of propranolol hydrochloride extended-release capsules with substrates of CYP2C19). Products include:

Lamictal 1481

Lansoprazole (Although blood levels and/or toxicity of propranolol may be increased by administration of propranolol hydrochloride extended-release capsules with sub-

strates or inhibitors of CYP2D6, no interaction was observed with lansoprazole). Products include:
Prevacid Delayed-Release Capsules 3271
Prevacid for Delayed-Release Oral Suspension 3271
Prevacid SoluTab Delayed-Release Orally Disintegrating Tablets 3271
Prevacid I.V. for Injection 3277
Prevacid NapraPAC 3280
PREVPAC 3284

Letrozole (Blood levels and/or toxicity of propranolol may be increased by administration of propranolol hydrochloride extended-release capsules with inhibitors of CYP2C19). Products include:
Femara Tablets 2214

Levalbuterol Hydrochloride (Propranolol is a competitive inhibitor of beta-receptor agonists and its effects can be reversed by administration of such agents (e.g., isoproterenol)). Products include:
Xopenex Inhalation Solution 3146
Xopenex Inhalation Solution Concentrate 3150

Levetiracetam (Blood levels and/or toxicity of propranolol may be increased by administration of propranolol hydrochloride extended-release capsules with substrates of CYP2C19). Products include:
Keppra Injection 3320
Keppra Oral Solution 3314
Keppra Tablets 3314

Levobupivacaine Hydrochloride (Blood levels and/or toxicity of propranolol may be increased by administration of propranolol hydrochloride extended-release capsules with substrates of CYP1A2).
No products indexed under this heading.

Levofloxacin (Blood levels and/or toxicity of propranolol may be increased by administration of propranolol hydrochloride extended-release capsules with inhibitors of CYP1A2). Products include:
Levaquin 2384
Levaquin in 5% Dextrose Injection 2384
Quixin Ophthalmic Solution 3383

Levonorgestrel (Blood levels and/or toxicity of propranolol may be increased by administration of propranolol hydrochloride extended-release capsules with inhibitors of CYP1A2). Products include:
Climara Pro Transdermal System 776
Mirena Intrauterine System 787
Plan B Tablets 1076
Seasonique Tablets 1077

Lidocaine (The clearance of lidocaine is reduced with administration of propranolol. Lidocaine toxicity has been reported following co-administration with propranolol. Use caution when administering propranolol hydrochloride extended-release capsules with drugs that slow AV nodal conduction (e.g., lidocaine)). Products include:
Lidoderm Patch 1118
Synera Topical Patch 1137

Lidocaine Base (The clearance of lidocaine is reduced with administration of propranolol. Lidocaine toxicity has been reported following co-administration with propranolol. Use caution when administering propranolol hydrochloride extended-release capsules with drugs that slow AV nodal conduction (e.g., lidocaine)).
No products indexed under this heading.

Lidocaine Hydrochloride (The clearance of lidocaine is reduced with administration of propranolol. Lidocaine toxicity has been reported following co-administration with propranolol. Use caution when administering propranolol hydrochloride extended-release capsules with drugs that slow AV nodal conduction (e.g., lidocaine)).
No products indexed under this heading.

Lisinopril (When combined with beta-blockers, ACE inhibitors can cause hypotension, particularly in the setting of acute myocardial infarction. Certain ACE inhibitors have been reported to increase bronchial hyper-reactivity when administered with propranolol). Products include:
Prinivil Tablets 2052
Prinzide Tablets 2056

Lomefloxacin Hydrochloride (Blood levels and/or toxicity of propranolol may be increased by administration of propranolol hydrochloride extended-release capsules with substrates of CYP1A2).
No products indexed under this heading.

Lovastatin (Co-administration of propranolol with lovastatin decreased the AUC of lovastatin but did not alter its pharmacodynamics). Products include:
Advicor Tablets 1722
Altoprev Extended-Release Tablets 3109
Mevacor Tablets 2021

Maprotiline Hydrochloride (Blood levels and/or toxicity of propranolol may be increased by administration of propranolol hydrochloride extended-release capsules with substrates of CYP2D6).
No products indexed under this heading.

Meclofenamate Sodium (Non-steroidal anti-inflammatory drugs have been reported to blunt the antihypertensive effects of beta-adrenoreceptor blocking agents).
No products indexed under this heading.

Mefenamic Acid (Non-steroidal anti-inflammatory drugs have been reported to blunt the antihypertensive effects of beta-adrenoreceptor blocking agents).
No products indexed under this heading.

Meloxicam (Non-steroidal anti-inflammatory drugs have been reported to blunt the antihypertensive effects of beta-adrenoreceptor blocking agents). Products include:
Mobic Oral Suspension 863
Mobic Tablets 863

Meperidine Hydrochloride (Blood levels and/or toxicity of propranolol may be increased by administration of propranolol hydrochloride extended-release capsules with substrates of CYP2D6).
No products indexed under this heading.

Mephenytoin (Blood levels and/or toxicity of propranolol may be increased by administration of propranolol hydrochloride extended-release capsules with substrates of CYP2C19).
No products indexed under this heading.

Mephobarbital (Blood levels and/or toxicity of propranolol may be increased by administration of propranolol hydrochloride extended-release capsules with substrates of CYP2C19).
No products indexed under this heading.

Meprobamate (Blood levels and/or toxicity of propranolol may be increased by administration of propranolol hydrochloride extended-release capsules with substrates of CYP2C19).
No products indexed under this heading.

Mestranol (Blood levels and/or toxicity of propranolol may be increased by administration of propranolol hydrochloride extended-release capsules with inhibitors of CYP1A2).
No products indexed under this heading.

Metaproterenol Sulfate (Propranolol is a competitive inhibitor of beta-receptor agonists and its effects can be reversed by administration of such agents (e.g., isoproterenol)). Products include:
Alupent Inhalation Aerosol 826

Methadone Hydrochloride (Blood levels and/or toxicity of propranolol may be increased by administration of propranolol hydrochloride extended-release capsules with substrates of CYP2D6).
No products indexed under this heading.

Methamphetamine Hydrochloride (Blood levels and/or toxicity of propranolol may be increased by administration of propranolol hydrochloride extended-release capsules with substrates of CYP2D6). Products include:
Desoxyn Tablets, USP 2462

Methoxsalen (Blood levels and/or toxicity of propranolol may be increased by administration of propranolol hydrochloride extended-release capsules with inhibitors of CYP1A2). Products include:
Oxsoralen Lotion 1% 3352
Oxsoralen-Ultra Capsules 3353

Methoxyflurane (May depress myocardial contractility when administered with propranolol).
No products indexed under this heading.

Methsuximide (Blood levels and/or toxicity of propranolol may be increased by administration of propranolol hydrochloride extended-release capsules with substrates of CYP2C19).
No products indexed under this heading.

Metoprolol Succinate (Blood levels and/or toxicity of propranolol may be increased by administration of propranolol hydrochloride extended-release capsules with substrates of CYP2D6). Products include:
Toprol-XL Tablets 668

Metoprolol Tartrate (Blood levels and/or toxicity of propranolol may be increased by administration of propranolol hydrochloride extended-release capsules with substrates of CYP2D6). Products include:
Lopressor Injection 2238
Lopressor Tablets 2238
Lopressor HCT 50/25 Tablets 2241
Lopressor HCT 100/25 Tablets 2241
Lopressor HCT 100/50 Tablets 2241

Mexiletine Hydrochloride (Blood levels and/or toxicity of propranolol may be increased by administration of propranolol hydrochloride extended-release capsules with substrates of CYP2D6).
No products indexed under this heading.

Mibefradil Dihydrochloride (Blood levels and/or toxicity of propranolol may be increased by administration of propranolol hydrochloride extended-release capsules with inhibitors of CYP2D6).
No products indexed under this heading.

Midazolam Hydrochloride (Blood levels and/or toxicity of propranolol may be increased by administration of propranolol hydrochloride extended-release capsules with substrates of CYP2C19).
No products indexed under this heading.

Mirtazapine (Blood levels and/or toxicity of propranolol may be increased by administration of propranolol hydrochloride extended-release capsules with substrates of CYP2D6).
No products indexed under this heading.

Moclobemide (Blood levels and/or toxicity of propranolol may be increased by administration of propranolol hydrochloride extended-release capsules with inhibitors of CYP2D6).
No products indexed under this heading.

Modafinil (Blood levels and/or toxicity of propranolol may be increased by administration of propranolol hydrochloride extended-release capsules with inhibitors of CYP2C19). Products include:
Provigil Tablets 988

Moexipril Hydrochloride (When combined with beta-blockers, ACE inhibitors can cause hypotension, particularly in the setting of acute myocardial infarction. Certain ACE inhibitors have been reported to increase bronchial hyper-reactivity when administered with propranolol). Products include:
Uniretic Tablets 3100
Univasc Tablets 3104

Morphine Sulfate (Blood levels and/or toxicity of propranolol may be increased by administration of propranolol hydrochloride extended-release capsules with substrates of CYP2D6). Products include:
Avinza Capsules 1741
Kadian Capsules 577
MS Contin Tablets 2701

Moxifloxacin Hydrochloride (Blood levels and/or toxicity of propranolol may be increased by administration of propranolol hydrochloride extended-release capsules with substrates of CYP1A2). Products include:
Avelox 2970
Vigamox Ophthalmic Solution 564

Nabumetone (Non-steroidal anti-inflammatory drugs have been reported to blunt the antihypertensive effects of beta-adrenoreceptor blocking agents).
No products indexed under this heading.

Nafcillin Sodium (Blood levels and/or toxicity of propranolol may be increased by administration of propranolol hydrochloride extended-release capsules with substrates of CYP1A2).
No products indexed under this heading.

Nalidixic Acid (Blood levels and/or toxicity of propranolol may be increased by administration of propranolol hydrochloride extended-release capsules with inhibitors of CYP1A2).
No products indexed under this heading.

Naproxen (Blood levels and/or toxicity of propranolol may be increased by administration of propranolol hydrochloride extended-release capsules with substrates of CYP1A2). Products include:
EC-Naprosyn Delayed-Release Tablets **2761**
Naprosyn Suspension **2761**
Naprosyn Tablets **2761**
Prevacid NapraPAC **3280**

Naproxen Sodium (Blood levels and/or toxicity of propranolol may be increased by administration of propranolol hydrochloride extended-release capsules with substrates of CYP1A2). Products include:
Aleve Caplets **742**
Aleve Gelcaps **743**
Aleve Tablets **743**
Aleve Cold & Sinus Caplets **744**
Anaprox Tablets **2761**
Anaprox DS Tablets **2761**

Nelfinavir Mesylate (Blood levels and/or toxicity of propranolol may be increased by administration of propranolol hydrochloride extended-release capsules with substrates of CYP2D6). Products include:
Viracept **2577**

Nicardipine (The mean Cmax and AUC of propranolol are increased by 80% and 47%, respectively, by co-administration with nicardipine).
No products indexed under this heading.

Nicardipine Hydrochloride (The mean Cmax and AUC of propranolol are increased by 80% and 47%, respectively, by co-administration with nicardipine). Products include:
Cardene I.V. **2497**

Nicotine Polacrilex (Blood levels and/or toxicity of propranolol may be increased by administration of propranolol hydrochloride extended-release capsules with substrates of CYP1A2).
No products indexed under this heading.

Nicotine Salicylate (Blood levels and/or toxicity of propranolol may be increased by administration of propranolol hydrochloride extended-release capsules with substrates of CYP1A2).
No products indexed under this heading.

Nicotine Sulfate (Blood levels and/or toxicity of propranolol may be increased by administration of propranolol hydrochloride extended-release capsules with substrates of CYP1A2).
No products indexed under this heading.

Nifedipine (The mean Cmax and AUC of nifedipine are increased by 64% and 79%, respectively, by co-administration with propranolol). Products include:
Adalat CC Tablets **2964**

Nilutamide (Blood levels and/or toxicity of propranolol may be increased by administration of propranolol hydrochloride extended-release capsules with substrates of CYP2C19).
No products indexed under this heading.

Nimodipine (Caution should be exercised when patients receiving a beta-blocker are administered a calcium channel blocking drug with negative inotropic and/or chronotropic effects. Both agents may depress cardiac contractility or atrioventricular conduction). Products include:
Nimotop Capsules **749**

Nisoldipine (The mean Cmax and AUC of propranolol are increased by 50% and 30%, respectively, by co-administration with nisoldipine). Products include:
Sular Tablets **3122**

Norethindrone (Blood levels and/or toxicity of propranolol may be increased by administration of propranolol hydrochloride extended-release capsules with inhibitors of CYP1A2). Products include:
Ortho Micronor Tablets **2426**

Norethindrone Acetate (Blood levels and/or toxicity of propranolol may be increased by administration of propranolol hydrochloride extended-release capsules with substrates of CYP1A2).
No products indexed under this heading.

Norethynodrel (Blood levels and/or toxicity of propranolol may be increased by administration of propranolol hydrochloride extended-release capsules with inhibitors of CYP2C19).
No products indexed under this heading.

Norfloxacin (Blood levels and/or toxicity of propranolol may be increased by administration of propranolol hydrochloride extended-release capsules with substrates of CYP1A2). Products include:
Noroxin Tablets **2032**

Norgestimate (Blood levels and/or toxicity of propranolol may be increased by administration of propranolol hydrochloride extended-release capsules with inhibitors of CYP2C19). Products include:
Ortho-Cyclen/Ortho Tri-Cyclen **2429**
Ortho Tri-Cyclen Lo Tablets **2436**

Norgestrel (Blood levels and/or toxicity of propranolol may be increased by administration of propranolol hydrochloride extended-release capsules with inhibitors of CYP1A2).
No products indexed under this heading.

Nortriptyline Hydrochloride (Blood levels and/or toxicity of propranolol may be increased by administration of propranolol hydrochloride extended-release capsules with substrates of CYP2D6).
No products indexed under this heading.

Ofloxacin (Blood levels and/or toxicity of propranolol may be increased by administration of propranolol hydrochloride extended-release capsules with substrates of CYP1A2). Products include:
Floxin Otic Solution **1049**

Olanzapine (Blood levels and/or toxicity of propranolol may be increased by administration of propranolol hydrochloride extended-release capsules with substrates of CYP2D6). Products include:
Symbyax Capsules **1819**
Zyprexa Tablets **1830**
Zyprexa IntraMuscular **1830**
Zyprexa ZYDIS Orally Disintegrating Tablets **1830**

Omeprazole (Although blood levels and/or toxicity of propranolol may be increased by administration of propranolol hydrochloride extended-release capsules with substrates or inhibitors of CYP2C19, no interaction was observed with omeprazole). Products include:
Zegerid Capsules **2958**
Zegerid Powder for Oral Solution **2958**

Omeprazole magnesium (Although blood levels and/or toxicity of propranolol may be increased by administration of propranolol hydrochloride extended-release capsules with substrates or inhibitors of CYP2C19, no interaction was observed with omeprazole). Products include:
Prilosec OTC Delayed-Release Tablets **2677**

Ondansetron (Blood levels and/or toxicity of propranolol may be increased by administration of propranolol hydrochloride extended-release capsules with substrates of CYP2D6). Products include:
Zofran ODT Orally Disintegrating Tablets **1639**

Ondansetron Hydrochloride (Blood levels and/or toxicity of propranolol may be increased by administration of propranolol hydrochloride extended-release capsules with substrates of CYP2D6). Products include:
Zofran Injection **1634**
Zofran **1639**

Oxaprozin (Non-steroidal anti-inflammatory drugs have been reported to blunt the antihypertensive effects of beta-adrenoreceptor blocking agents).
No products indexed under this heading.

Oxcarbazepine (Blood levels and/or toxicity of propranolol may be increased by administration of propranolol hydrochloride extended-release capsules with inhibitors of CYP2C19). Products include:
Trileptal Tablets **2300**
Trileptal Oral Suspension **2300**

Oxycodone Hydrochloride (Blood levels and/or toxicity of propranolol may be increased by administration of propranolol hydrochloride extended-release capsules with substrates of CYP2D6). Products include:
OxyContin Tablets **2703**
OxyFast Oral Concentrate Solution **2708**
OxyIR Capsules **2708**
Percocet Tablets **1131**
Percodan Tablets **1132**

Paclitaxel (Blood levels and/or toxicity of propranolol may be increased by administration of propranolol hydrochloride extended-release capsules with substrates of CYP2D6).
No products indexed under this heading.

Pantoprazole Sodium (Blood levels and/or toxicity of propranolol may be increased by administration of propranolol hydrochloride extended-release capsules with substrates of CYP2C19). Products include:
Protonix I.V. **3472**
Protonix Tablets **3469**

Paramethadione (Blood levels and/or toxicity of propranolol may be increased by administration of propranolol hydrochloride extended-release capsules with substrates of CYP2C19).
No products indexed under this heading.

Pargyline Hydrochloride (The hypotensive effects of MAO inhibitors may be exacerbated when administered with beta-blockers by interfering with the beta-blocking activity of propranolol).
No products indexed under this heading.

Paroxetine Hydrochloride (Blood levels and/or toxicity of propranolol may be increased by administration of propranolol hydrochloride extended-release capsules with substrates of CYP2D6). Products include:
Paxil CR Controlled-Release Tablets **1538**
Paxil **1530**

Pentamidine Isethionate (Blood levels and/or toxicity of propranolol may be increased by administration of propranolol hydrochloride extended-release capsules with substrates of CYP2C19).
No products indexed under this heading.

Perindopril Erbumine (When combined with beta-blockers, ACE inhibitors can cause hypotension, particularly in the setting of acute myocardial infarction. Certain ACE inhibitors have been reported to increase bronchial hyper-reactivity when administered with propranolol). Products include:
Aceon Tablets (2 mg, 4 mg, 8 mg) **3194**

Perphenazine (Blood levels and/or toxicity of propranolol may be increased by administration of propranolol hydrochloride extended-release capsules with inhibitors of CYP2D6).
No products indexed under this heading.

Phenacemide (Blood levels and/or toxicity of propranolol may be increased by administration of propranolol hydrochloride extended-release capsules with substrates of CYP2C19).
No products indexed under this heading.

Phenelzine Sulfate (The hypotensive effects of MAO inhibitors may be exacerbated when administered with beta-blockers by interfering with the beta-blocking activity of propranolol).
No products indexed under this heading.

Phenobarbital (Blood levels and/or toxicity of propranolol may be increased by administration of propranolol hydrochloride extended-release capsules with substrates of CYP2C19). Products include:
Donnatal Extentabs **2493**

Phenobarbital Sodium (Blood levels and/or toxicity of propranolol may be increased by administration of propranolol hydrochloride extended-release capsules with substrates of CYP1A2).

No products indexed under this heading.

Phensuximide (Blood levels and/or toxicity of propranolol may be increased by administration of propranolol hydrochloride extended-release capsules with substrates of CYP2C19).

No products indexed under this heading.

Phenylbutazone (Non-steroidal anti-inflammatory drugs have been reported to blunt the antihypertensive effects of beta-adrenoreceptor blocking agents).

No products indexed under this heading.

Phenytoin (Blood levels and/or toxicity of propranolol may be increased by administration of propranolol hydrochloride extended-release capsules with substrates of CYP2C19).

No products indexed under this heading.

Phenytoin Sodium (Blood levels and/or toxicity of propranolol may be increased by administration of propranolol hydrochloride extended-release capsules with substrates of CYP1A2). Products include:

Phenytek Capsules 2160

Pindolol (Blood levels and/or toxicity of propranolol may be increased by administration of propranolol hydrochloride extended-release capsules with substrates of CYP2D6).

No products indexed under this heading.

Pirbuterol Acetate (Propranolol is a competitive inhibitor of beta-receptor agonists and its effects can be reversed by administration of such agents (e.g., isoproterenol)). Products include:

Maxair Autohaler 1852

Piroxicam (Non-steroidal anti-inflammatory drugs have been reported to blunt the antihypertensive effects of beta-adrenoreceptor blocking agents).

No products indexed under this heading.

Pravastatin Sodium (Co-administration of propranolol with pravastatin decreased the AUC of pravastatin but did not alter its pharmacodynamics).

No products indexed under this heading.

Prazosin Hydrochloride (Prazosin has been associated with prolongation of first dose hypotension in the presence of beta-blockers).

No products indexed under this heading.

Primidone (Blood levels and/or toxicity of propranolol may be increased by administration of propranolol hydrochloride extended-release capsules with substrates of CYP2C19).

No products indexed under this heading.

Procarbazine Hydrochloride (The hypotensive effects of MAO inhibitors may be exacerbated when administered with beta-blockers by interfering with the beta-blocking activity of propranolol). Products include:

Matulane Capsules 3191

Progesterone (Blood levels and/or toxicity of propranolol may be increased by administration of propranolol hydrochloride extended-release capsules with substrates of CYP2C19). Products include:

Prochieve 4% Gel 1003
Prochieve 8% Gel 1003
Prometrium Capsules (100 mg, 200 mg)......................... 3203

Proguanil Hydrochloride (Blood levels and/or toxicity of propranolol may be increased by administration of propranolol hydrochloride extended-release capsules with substrates of CYP2C19). Products include:

Malarone Pediatric Tablets 1517
Malarone Tablets 1517

Propafenone Hydrochloride (Propafenone has negative inotropic and beta-blocking properties that can be additive to those of propranolol. The AUC of propafenone is increased by more than 200% by co-administration with propranolol). Products include:

Rythmol SR Capsules 2727

Propoxyphene Hydrochloride (Blood levels and/or toxicity of propranolol may be increased by administration of propranolol hydrochloride extended-release capsules with substrates of CYP2D6).

No products indexed under this heading.

Propoxyphene Napsylate (Blood levels and/or toxicity of propranolol may be increased by administration of propranolol hydrochloride extended-release capsules with substrates of CYP2D6).

No products indexed under this heading.

Protriptyline Hydrochloride (Blood levels and/or toxicity of propranolol may be increased by administration of propranolol hydrochloride extended-release capsules with inhibitors of CYP2D6).

No products indexed under this heading.

Quetiapine Fumarate (Blood levels and/or toxicity of propranolol may be increased by administration of propranolol hydrochloride extended-release capsules with substrates of CYP2D6). Products include:

Seroquel Tablets 690

Quinacrine Hydrochloride (Blood levels and/or toxicity of propranolol may be increased by administration of propranolol hydrochloride extended-release capsules with inhibitors of CYP2D6).

No products indexed under this heading.

Quinapril Hydrochloride (When combined with beta-blockers, ACE inhibitors can cause hypotension, particularly in the setting of acute myocardial infarction. Certain ACE inhibitors have been reported to increase bronchial hyper-reactivity when administered with propranolol).

No products indexed under this heading.

Quinidine (Quinidine increases the concentration of propranolol and produces greater degrees of clinical beta-blockade and may cause postural hypotension).

No products indexed under this heading.

Quinidine Gluconate (Quinidine increases the concentration of propranolol and produces greater degrees of clinical beta-blockade and may cause postural hypotension).

No products indexed under this heading.

Quinidine Hydrochloride (Quinidine increases the concentration of propranolol and produces greater degrees of clinical beta-blockade and may cause postural hypotension).

No products indexed under this heading.

Quinidine Polygalacturonate (Quinidine increases the concentration of propranolol and produces greater degrees of clinical beta-blockade and may cause postural hypotension).

No products indexed under this heading.

Quinidine Sulfate (Quinidine increases the concentration of propranolol and produces greater degrees of clinical beta-blockade and may cause postural hypotension).

No products indexed under this heading.

Rabeprazole Sodium (Blood levels and/or toxicity of propranolol may be increased by administration of propranolol hydrochloride extended-release capsules with substrates of CYP2C19). Products include:

Aciphex Tablets 1090

Ramipril (When combined with beta-blockers, ACE inhibitors can cause hypotension, particularly in the setting of acute myocardial infarction. Certain ACE inhibitors have been reported to increase bronchial hyper-reactivity when administered with propranolol). Products include:

Altace Capsules 1702

Ranitidine Bismuth Citrate (Although blood levels and/or toxicity of propranolol may be increased by administration of propranolol hydrochloride extended-release capsules with substrates or inhibitors of CYP2D6, no interaction was observed with ranitidine).

No products indexed under this heading.

Ranitidine Hydrochloride (Although blood levels and/or toxicity of propranolol may be increased by administration of propranolol hydrochloride extended-release capsules with substrates or inhibitors of CYP2D6, no interaction was observed with ranitidine). Products include:

Zantac 1624
Zantac Injection 1619
Zantac Injection Pharmacy Bulk Package......................... 1622

Rauwolfia Serpentina (Patients receiving catecholamine-depleting drugs (e.g., reserpine) and propranolol hydrochloride extended-release capsules should be observed closely for excessive reduction of resting sympathetic nervous activity, which may result in hypotension, marked bradycardia, vertigo, syncopal attacks, or orthostatic hypotension).

No products indexed under this heading.

Rescinnamine (Patients receiving catecholamine-depleting drugs (e.g., reserpine) and propranolol hydrochloride extended-release capsules should be observed closely for excessive reduction of resting sympathetic nervous activity, which may result in hypotension, marked bradycardia, vertigo, syncopal attacks, or orthostatic hypotension).

No products indexed under this heading.

Reserpine (Patients receiving catecholamine-depleting drugs (e.g., reserpine) and propranolol hydrochloride extended-release capsules should be observed closely for excessive reduction of resting sympathetic nervous activity, which may result in hypotension, marked bradycardia, vertigo, syncopal attacks, or orthostatic hypotension. Administration of reserpine with propranolol may also potentiate depression).

No products indexed under this heading.

Rifampin (Blood levels of propranolol may be decreased by administration of propranolol hydrochloride extended-release capsules with inducers of hepatic drug metabolism, such as rifampin).

No products indexed under this heading.

Rifapentine (Blood levels of propranolol may be decreased by co-administration of propranolol hydrochloride extended-release capsules with inducers of hepatic drug metabolism).

No products indexed under this heading.

Riluzole (Blood levels and/or toxicity of propranolol may be increased by administration of propranolol hydrochloride extended-release capsules with substrates of CYP1A2). Products include:

Rilutek Tablets 2930

Risperidone (Blood levels and/or toxicity of propranolol may be increased by administration of propranolol hydrochloride extended-release capsules with substrates of CYP2D6). Products include:

Risperdal 1676
Risperdal Consta Long-Acting Injection 1682
Risperdal M-Tab Orally Disintegrating Tablets.................. 1676

Ritonavir (Blood levels and/or toxicity of propranolol may be increased by administration of propranolol hydrochloride extended-release capsules with substrates of CYP2D6). Products include:

Kaletra 476
Norvir 503

Rizatriptan Benzoate (Co-administration of rizatriptan with propranolol resulted in increased concentrations of rizatriptan (AUC increased by 67% and Cmax by 75%)). Products include:

Maxalt Tablets 2008
Maxalt-MLT Orally Disintegrating Tablets 2008

Rofecoxib (Non-steroidal anti-inflammatory drugs have been reported to blunt the antihypertensive effects of beta-adrenoreceptor blocking agents).

No products indexed under this heading.

Ropinirole Hydrochloride (Blood levels and/or toxicity of propranolol may be increased by administration of propranolol hydrochloride

IMPORTANT NOTE: Always consult each drug listing in the patient's regimen for possible interactions.

extended-release capsules with substrates of CYP1A2). Products include:

Ropivacaine Hydrochloride (Blood levels and/or toxicity of propranolol may be increased by administration of propranolol hydrochloride extended-release capsules with substrates of CYP1A2).

No products indexed under this heading.

Salmeterol Xinafoate (Propranolol is a competitive inhibitor of beta-receptor agonists and its effects can be reversed by administration of such agents (e.g., isoproterenol)). Products include:

Selegiline Hydrochloride (The hypotensive effects of MAO inhibitors may be exacerbated when administered with beta-blockers by interfering with the beta-blocking activity of propranolol). Products include:

Sertraline Hydrochloride (Blood levels and/or toxicity of propranolol may be increased by administration of propranolol hydrochloride extended-release capsules with inhibitors of CYP2D6). Products include:

Sparfloxacin (Blood levels and/or toxicity of propranolol may be increased by administration of propranolol hydrochloride extended-release capsules with inhibitors of CYP1A2).

No products indexed under this heading.

Spirapril Hydrochloride (When combined with beta-blockers, ACE inhibitors can cause hypotension, particularly in the setting of acute myocardial infarction. Certain ACE inhibitors have been reported to increase bronchial hyper-reactivity when administered with propranolol).

No products indexed under this heading.

Sulfaphenazole (Blood levels and/or toxicity of propranolol may be increased by administration of propranolol hydrochloride extended-release capsules with inhibitors of CYP2C19).

No products indexed under this heading.

Sulindac (Non-steroidal anti-inflammatory drugs have been reported to blunt the antihypertensive effects of beta-adrenoreceptor blocking agents). Products include:

Tacrine Hydrochloride (Blood levels and/or toxicity of propranolol may be increased by administration of propranolol hydrochloride extended-release capsules with substrates of CYP1A2).

No products indexed under this heading.

Tamoxifen Citrate (Blood levels and/or toxicity of propranolol may be increased by administration of propranolol hydrochloride extended-release capsules with substrates of CYP2D6). Products include:

Telmisartan (Blood levels and/or toxicity of propranolol may be increased by administration of propranolol hydrochloride extended-release capsules with inhibitors of CYP2C19). Products include:

Teniposide (Blood levels and/or toxicity of propranolol may be increased by administration of propranolol hydrochloride extended-release capsules with substrates of CYP2D6).

No products indexed under this heading.

Terazosin Hydrochloride (Postural hypotension has been reported in patients taking both beta-blockers and terazosin). Products include:

Terbinafine Hydrochloride (Blood levels and/or toxicity of propranolol may be increased by administration of propranolol hydrochloride extended-release capsules with inhibitors of CYP2D6). Products include:

Terbutaline Sulfate (Propranolol is a competitive inhibitor of beta-receptor agonists and its effects can be reversed by administration of such agents (e.g., isoproterenol)).

No products indexed under this heading.

Testosterone (Blood levels and/or toxicity of propranolol may be increased by administration of propranolol hydrochloride extended-release capsules with substrates of CYP2D6). Products include:

Testosterone Cypionate (Blood levels and/or toxicity of propranolol may be increased by administration of propranolol hydrochloride extended-release capsules with substrates of CYP2D6).

No products indexed under this heading.

Testosterone Enanthate (Blood levels and/or toxicity of propranolol may be increased by administration of propranolol hydrochloride extended-release capsules with substrates of CYP2D6).

No products indexed under this heading.

Testosterone Propionate (Blood levels and/or toxicity of propranolol may be increased by administration of propranolol hydrochloride extended-release capsules with substrates of CYP2D6).

No products indexed under this heading.

Theophylline (Co-administration of theophylline with propranolol decreases theophylline oral clearance by 33% to 52%).

No products indexed under this heading.

Theophylline Anhydrous (Co-administration of theophylline with propranolol decreases theophylline oral clearance by 33% to 52%). Products include:

Theophylline Calcium Salicylate (Co-administration of theophylline with propranolol decreases theophylline oral clearance by 33% to 52%).

No products indexed under this heading.

Theophylline Dihydroxypropyl (Glyceryl) (Co-administration of theophylline with propranolol decreases theophylline oral clearance by 33% to 52%).

No products indexed under this heading.

Theophylline Ethylenediamine (Co-administration of theophylline with propranolol decreases theophylline oral clearance by 33% to 52%).

No products indexed under this heading.

Theophylline Sodium Glycinate (Co-administration of theophylline with propranolol decreases theophylline oral clearance by 33% to 52%).

No products indexed under this heading.

Thioridazine (Co-administration of propranolol at doses greater than or equal to 160 mg/day resulted in increased thioridazine plasma concentrations, ranging from 50% to 370%, and increased thioridazine metabolites concentrations, ranging from 33% to 210%).

No products indexed under this heading.

Thioridazine Hydrochloride (Co-administration of propranolol at doses greater than or equal to 160 mg/day resulted in increased thioridazine plasma concentrations, ranging from 50% to 370%, and increased thioridazine metabolites concentrations, ranging from 33% to 210%). Products include:

Thyroxine (Thyroxine may result in a lower than expected T3 concentration when used concomitantly with propranolol).

No products indexed under this heading.

Thyroxine Sodium (Thyroxine may result in a lower than expected T3 concentration when used concomitantly with propranolol).

No products indexed under this heading.

Tiagabine Hydrochloride (Blood levels and/or toxicity of propranolol may be increased by administration of propranolol hydrochloride extended-release capsules with substrates of CYP2C19). Products include:

Ticlopidine Hydrochloride (Blood levels and/or toxicity of propranolol may be increased by administration of propranolol hydrochloride extended-release capsules with inhibitors of CYP1A2). Products include:

Timolol Maleate (Blood levels and/or toxicity of propranolol may be increased by administration of propranolol hydrochloride extended-release capsules with substrates of CYP2D6). Products include:

Tolazamide (Blood levels of propranolol may be decreased by co-administration of propranolol hydrochloride extended-release capsules with inducers of hepatic drug metabolism).

No products indexed under this heading.

Tolbutamide (Blood levels and/or toxicity of propranolol may be increased by administration of propranolol hydrochloride extended-release capsules with inhibitors of CYP2C19).

No products indexed under this heading.

Tolbutamide Sodium (Blood levels and/or toxicity of propranolol may be increased by administration of propranolol hydrochloride extended-release capsules with inhibitors of CYP2C19).

No products indexed under this heading.

Tolmetin Sodium (Non-steroidal anti-inflammatory drugs have been reported to blunt the antihypertensive effects of beta-adrenoreceptor blocking agents).

No products indexed under this heading.

Tolterodine Tartrate (Blood levels and/or toxicity of propranolol may be increased by administration of propranolol hydrochloride extended-release capsules with substrates of CYP2D6). Products include:

Topiramate (Blood levels and/or toxicity of propranolol may be increased by administration of propranolol hydrochloride extended-release capsules with inhibitors of CYP2C19). Products include:

Tramadol Hydrochloride (Blood levels and/or toxicity of propranolol may be increased by administration of propranolol hydrochloride extended-release capsules with substrates of CYP2D6). Products include:

Trandolapril (When combined with beta-blockers, ACE inhibitors can cause hypotension, particularly in the setting of acute myocardial infarction. Certain ACE inhibitors have been reported to increase bronchial hyper-reactivity when administered with propranolol). Products include:

Tranylcypromine Sulfate (The hypotensive effects of MAO inhibitors may be exacerbated when administered with beta-blockers by interfering with the beta-blocking activity of propranolol). Products include:

Trazodone Hydrochloride (Blood levels and/or toxicity of propranolol may be increased by administration of propranolol hydrochloride extended-release capsules with substrates of CYP2D6).

No products indexed under this heading.

Triazolam (Blood levels and/or toxicity of propranolol may be increased by administration of propranolol hydrochloride extended-release capsules with substrates of CYP2D6).
No products indexed under this heading.

Trichloroethylene (May depress myocardial contractility when administered with propranolol).
No products indexed under this heading.

Trimethadione (Blood levels and/or toxicity of propranolol may be increased by administration of propranolol hydrochloride extended-release capsules with substrates of CYP2C19).
No products indexed under this heading.

Trimethaphan Camsylate (Blood levels and/or toxicity of propranolol may be increased by administration of propranolol hydrochloride extended-release capsules with substrates of CYP1A2).
No products indexed under this heading.

Trimipramine Maleate (Blood levels and/or toxicity of propranolol may be increased by administration of propranolol hydrochloride extended-release capsules with substrates of CYP2D6).
No products indexed under this heading.

Troleandomycin (Blood levels and/or toxicity of propranolol may be increased by administration of propranolol hydrochloride extended-release capsules with inhibitors of CYP1A2).
No products indexed under this heading.

Trovafloxacin Mesylate (Blood levels and/or toxicity of propranolol may be increased by administration of propranolol hydrochloride extended-release capsules with substrates of CYP1A2).
No products indexed under this heading.

Valdecoxib (Non-steroidal anti-inflammatory drugs have been reported to blunt the antihypertensive effects of beta-adrenoreceptor blocking agents).
No products indexed under this heading.

Valproate Sodium (Blood levels and/or toxicity of propranolol may be increased by administration of propranolol hydrochloride extended-release capsules with substrates of CYP2C19). Products include:
Depacon Injection **412**

Valproic Acid (Blood levels and/or toxicity of propranolol may be increased by administration of propranolol hydrochloride extended-release capsules with substrates of CYP2C19). Products include:
Depakene **417**

Venlafaxine Hydrochloride (Blood levels and/or toxicity of propranolol may be increased by administration of propranolol hydrochloride extended-release capsules with substrates of CYP2D6). Products include:
Effexor Tablets **3411**
Effexor XR Capsules **3417**

Verapamil Hydrochloride (There have been reports of significant bradycardia, heart failure, and cardiovascular collapse with concurrent use of verapamil and beta-blockers). Products include:
Covera-HS Tablets **3139**
Tarka Tablets **524**
Verelan PM Extended-Release Capsules, Controlled-Onset........... **3106**

Vinblastine Sulfate (Blood levels and/or toxicity of propranolol may be increased by administration of propranolol hydrochloride extended-release capsules with substrates of CYP2D6).
No products indexed under this heading.

Voriconazole (Blood levels and/or toxicity of propranolol may be increased by administration of propranolol hydrochloride extended-release capsules with inhibitors of CYP2C19). Products include:
VFEND I.V. **2564**
VFEND Oral Suspension **2564**
VFEND Tablets **2564**

Warfarin Sodium (Concomitant administration of propranolol and warfarin has been shown to increase warfarin bioavailability and concentration, as well as increasing prothrombin time; therefore, prothrombin time should be monitored). Products include:
Coumadin for Injection **898**
Coumadin Tablets **898**

Zileuton (Blood levels and/or toxicity of propranolol may be increased by administration of propranolol hydrochloride extended-release capsules with substrates of CYP1A2). Products include:
Zyflo Tablets **1023**

Zolmitriptan (Co-administration of zolmitriptan with propranolol resulted in increased concentrations of zolmitriptan (AUC increased by 56% and Cmax by 37%)). Products include:
Zomig Tablets **3519**
Zomig Nasal Spray **3523**
Zomig-ZMT Tablets **3519**

Zonisamide (Blood levels and/or toxicity of propranolol may be increased by administration of propranolol hydrochloride extended-release capsules with substrates of CYP2D6). Products include:
Zonegran Capsules **1101**

Food Interactions

Grapefruit Juice (Blood levels and/or toxicity of propranolol may be increased by administration of propranolol hydrochloride extended-release capsules with inhibitors of CYP1A2).

INSPRA TABLETS

(Eplerenone) **2536**
May interact with ACE inhibitors, angiotensin-II receptor antagonists, cytochrome p450 3a4 inhibitors (selected), non-steroidal anti-inflammatory agents, potassium preparations, potassium sparing diuretics, and certain other agents. Compounds in these categories include:

Acetazolamide (Eplerenone should not be used with strong inhibitors of CYP450 3A4. Potent inhibitors of CYP3A4 caused increased exposure of about 5-fold, while less potent CYP3A4 inhibitors (e.g., erythromycin, saquinavir, verapamil, fluconazole) gave approximately 2-fold increases in exposure. Grapefruit juice caused only a small increase (about 25%) in exposure).
No products indexed under this heading.

Amiloride Hydrochloride (Eplerenone is contraindicated in patients treated concomitantly with potassium-sparing diuretics). Products include:
Midamor Tablets **2026**
Moduretic Tablets **2028**

Amiodarone Hydrochloride (Eplerenone should not be used with strong inhibitors of CYP450 3A4. Potent inhibitors of CYP3A4 caused increased exposure of about 5-fold, while less potent CYP3A4 inhibitors (e.g., erythromycin, saquinavir, verapamil, fluconazole) gave approximately 2-fold increases in exposure. Grapefruit juice caused only a small increase (about 25%) in exposure).
No products indexed under this heading.

Amprenavir (Eplerenone should not be used with strong inhibitors of CYP450 3A4. Potent inhibitors of CYP3A4 caused increased exposure of about 5-fold, while less potent CYP3A4 inhibitors (e.g., erythromycin, saquinavir, verapamil, fluconazole) gave approximately 2-fold increases in exposure. Grapefruit juice caused only a small increase (about 25%) in exposure). Products include:
Agenerase Capsules **1327**
Agenerase Oral Solution **1332**

Anastrozole (Eplerenone should not be used with strong inhibitors of CYP450 3A4. Potent inhibitors of CYP3A4 caused increased exposure of about 5-fold, while less potent CYP3A4 inhibitors (e.g., erythromycin, saquinavir, verapamil, fluconazole) gave approximately 2-fold increases in exposure. Grapefruit juice caused only a small increase (about 25%) in exposure). Products include:
Arimidex Tablets **673**

Aprepitant (Eplerenone should not be used with strong inhibitors of CYP450 3A4. Potent inhibitors of CYP3A4 caused increased exposure of about 5-fold, while less potent CYP3A4 inhibitors (e.g., erythromycin, saquinavir, verapamil, fluconazole) gave approximately 2-fold increases in exposure. Grapefruit juice caused only a small increase (about 25%) in exposure). Products include:
Emend Capsules **1963**

Benazepril Hydrochloride (Because the concomitant use of another mineralocorticoid receptor blocker and ACE inhibitors has led to clinically relevant hyperkalemia; caution should be used). Products include:
Lotensin Tablets **2243**
Lotensin HCT Tablets **2246**
Lotrel Capsules **2249**

Candesartan Cilexetil (Because the concomitant use of another mineralocorticoid receptor blocker and angiotensin II receptor antagonists has led to clinically relevant hyperkalemia; caution should be used). Products include:
Atacand Tablets **649**
Atacand HCT **651**

Captopril (Because the concomitant use of another mineralocorticoid receptor blocker and ACE inhibitors has led to clinically relevant hyperkalemia; caution should be used). Products include:
Captopril Tablets **2149**

Celecoxib (When eplerenone and NSAIDs are used concomitantly, patients should be observed to determine whether the desired effect on blood pressure is obtained). Products include:
Celebrex Capsules **3134**

Cimetidine (Eplerenone should not be used with strong inhibitors of CYP450 3A4. Potent inhibitors of CYP3A4 caused increased exposure of about 5-fold, while less potent CYP3A4 inhibitors (e.g., erythromycin, saquinavir, verapamil, fluconazole) gave approximately 2-fold increases in exposure. Grapefruit juice caused only a small increase (about 25%) in exposure). Products include:
Tagamet HB 200 Tablets **664**

Cimetidine Hydrochloride (Eplerenone should not be used with strong inhibitors of CYP450 3A4. Potent inhibitors of CYP3A4 caused increased exposure of about 5-fold, while less potent CYP3A4 inhibitors (e.g., erythromycin, saquinavir, verapamil, fluconazole) gave approximately 2-fold increases in exposure. Grapefruit juice caused only a small increase (about 25%) in exposure).
No products indexed under this heading.

Ciprofloxacin (Eplerenone should not be used with strong inhibitors of CYP450 3A4. Potent inhibitors of CYP3A4 caused increased exposure of about 5-fold, while less potent CYP3A4 inhibitors (e.g., erythromycin, saquinavir, verapamil, fluconazole) gave approximately 2-fold increases in exposure. Grapefruit juice caused only a small increase (about 25%) in exposure). Products include:
Cipro Oral Suspension **2977**
Cipro I.V. **2984**
Cipro XR Tablets **2990**
Ciprodex Otic Suspension **559**

Clarithromycin (Concomitant use with the potent CYP3A4 inhibitor clarithromycin is contraindicated). Products include:
Biaxin/Biaxin XL **402**
PREVPAC **3284**

Clotrimazole (Eplerenone should not be used with strong inhibitors of CYP450 3A4. Potent inhibitors of CYP3A4 caused increased exposure of about 5-fold, while less potent CYP3A4 inhibitors (e.g., erythromycin, saquinavir, verapamil, fluconazole) gave approximately 2-fold increases in exposure. Grapefruit juice caused only a small increase (about 25%) in exposure). Products include:
Desenex Athlete's Foot Cream **635**
Lotrimin **3039**
Lotrisone **3040**

Cyclosporine (Eplerenone should not be used with strong inhibitors of CYP450 3A4. Potent inhibitors of CYP3A4 caused increased exposure of about 5-fold, while less potent CYP3A4 inhibitors (e.g., erythromycin, saquinavir, verapamil, fluconazole) gave approximately 2-fold increases in exposure. Grapefruit juice caused only a small increase (about 25%) in exposure). Products include:
Gengraf Capsules **459**
Neoral Oral Solution **2259**
Neoral Soft Gelatin Capsules **2259**
Restasis Ophthalmic Emulsion **575**
Sandimmune **2275**

Dalfopristin (Eplerenone should not be used with strong inhibitors of CYP450 3A4. Potent inhibitors of CYP3A4 caused increased exposure of about 5-fold, while less potent CYP3A4 inhibitors (e.g., erythromycin, saquinavir, verapamil, fluconazole) gave approximately 2-fold increases in exposure. Grapefruit juice caused only a small increase (about 25%) in exposure).

No products indexed under this heading.

Danazol (Eplerenone should not be used with strong inhibitors of CYP450 3A4. Potent inhibitors of CYP3A4 caused increased exposure of about 5-fold, while less potent CYP3A4 inhibitors (e.g., erythromycin, saquinavir, verapamil, fluconazole) gave approximately 2-fold increases in exposure. Grapefruit juice caused only a small increase (about 25%) in exposure).

No products indexed under this heading.

Delavirdine Mesylate (Eplerenone should not be used with strong inhibitors of CYP450 3A4. Potent inhibitors of CYP3A4 caused increased exposure of about 5-fold, while less potent CYP3A4 inhibitors (e.g., erythromycin, saquinavir, verapamil, fluconazole) gave approximately 2-fold increases in exposure. Grapefruit juice caused only a small increase (about 25%) in exposure). Products include:

Rescriptor Tablets 2551

Diclofenac Potassium (When eplerenone and NSAIDs are used concomitantly, patients should be observed to determine whether the desired effect on blood pressure is obtained).

No products indexed under this heading.

Diclofenac Sodium (When eplerenone and NSAIDs are used concomitantly, patients should be observed to determine whether the desired effect on blood pressure is obtained). Products include:

Arthrotec Tablets 3129
Voltaren Ophthalmic Solution 2309
Voltaren Tablets 2307
Voltaren-XR Tablets 2310

Diltiazem Hydrochloride (Eplerenone should not be used with strong inhibitors of CYP450 3A4. Potent inhibitors of CYP3A4 caused increased exposure of about 5-fold, while less potent CYP3A4 inhibitors (e.g., erythromycin, saquinavir, verapamil, fluconazole) gave approximately 2-fold increases in exposure. Grapefruit juice caused only a small increase (about 25%) in exposure). Products include:

Cardizem LA Extended Release Tablets 1728
Tiazac Capsules 1201

Diltiazem Maleate (Eplerenone should not be used with strong inhibitors of CYP450 3A4. Potent inhibitors of CYP3A4 caused increased exposure of about 5-fold, while less potent CYP3A4 inhibitors (e.g., erythromycin, saquinavir, verapamil, fluconazole) gave approximately 2-fold increases in exposure. Grapefruit juice caused only a small increase (about 25%) in exposure).

No products indexed under this heading.

Efavirenz (Eplerenone should not be used with strong inhibitors of CYP450 3A4. Potent inhibitors of CYP3A4 caused increased exposure of about 5-fold, while less potent CYP3A4 inhibitors (e.g., erythromycin, saquinavir, verapamil, fluconazole) gave approximately 2-fold increases in exposure. Grapefruit juice caused only a small increase (about 25%) in exposure). Products include:

Atripla Tablets 945
Sustiva Capsules 930
Sustiva Tablets 930

Enalapril Maleate (Because the concomitant use of another mineralocorticoid receptor blocker and ACE inhibitors has led to clinically relevant hyperkalemia; caution should be used). Products include:

Vasotec I.V. Injection 2103

Enalaprilat (Because the concomitant use of another mineralocorticoid receptor blocker and ACE inhibitors has led to clinically relevant hyperkalemia; caution should be used).

No products indexed under this heading.

Eprosartan Mesylate (Because the concomitant use of another mineralocorticoid receptor blocker and angiotensin II receptor antagonists has led to clinically relevant hyperkalemia; caution should be used). Products include:

Teveten Tablets 1735
Teveten HCT Tablets 1737

Erythromycin (Eplerenone should not be used with strong inhibitors of CYP450 3A4. Potent inhibitors of CYP3A4 caused increased exposure of about 5-fold, while less potent CYP3A4 inhibitors (e.g., erythromycin, saquinavir, verapamil, fluconazole) gave approximately 2-fold increases in exposure. Grapefruit juice caused only a small increase (about 25%) in exposure). Products include:

Ery-Tab Tablets 449
Erythromycin Base Filmtab Tablets 455
Erythromycin Delayed-Release Capsules, USP 457
PCE Dispertab Tablets 515

Erythromycin Estolate (Eplerenone should not be used with strong inhibitors of CYP450 3A4. Potent inhibitors of CYP3A4 caused increased exposure of about 5-fold, while less potent CYP3A4 inhibitors (e.g., erythromycin, saquinavir, verapamil, fluconazole) gave approximately 2-fold increases in exposure. Grapefruit juice caused only a small increase (about 25%) in exposure).

No products indexed under this heading.

Erythromycin Ethylsuccinate (Eplerenone should not be used with strong inhibitors of CYP450 3A4. Potent inhibitors of CYP3A4 caused increased exposure of about 5-fold, while less potent CYP3A4 inhibitors (e.g., erythromycin, saquinavir, verapamil, fluconazole) gave approximately 2-fold increases in exposure. Grapefruit juice caused only a small increase (about 25%) in exposure). Products include:

E.E.S. 451
EryPed 447

Erythromycin Gluceptate (Eplerenone should not be used with strong inhibitors of CYP450 3A4. Potent inhibitors of CYP3A4 caused increased exposure of about 5-fold, while less potent CYP3A4 inhibitors (e.g., erythromycin, saquinavir, verapamil, fluconazole) gave approximately 2-fold increases in exposure. Grapefruit juice caused only a small increase (about 25%) in exposure).

No products indexed under this heading.

Erythromycin Lactobionate (Eplerenone should not be used with strong inhibitors of CYP450 3A4. Potent inhibitors of CYP3A4 caused increased exposure of about 5-fold, while less potent CYP3A4 inhibitors (e.g., erythromycin, saquinavir, verapamil, fluconazole) gave approximately 2-fold increases in exposure. Grapefruit juice caused only a small increase (about 25%) in exposure).

No products indexed under this heading.

Erythromycin Stearate (Eplerenone should not be used with strong inhibitors of CYP450 3A4. Potent inhibitors of CYP3A4 caused increased exposure of about 5-fold, while less potent CYP3A4 inhibitors (e.g., erythromycin, saquinavir, verapamil, fluconazole) gave approximately 2-fold increases in exposure. Grapefruit juice caused only a small increase (about 25%) in exposure). Products include:

Erythrocin Stearate Filmtab Tablets 453

Esomeprazole Magnesium (Eplerenone should not be used with strong inhibitors of CYP450 3A4. Potent inhibitors of CYP3A4 caused increased exposure of about 5-fold, while less potent CYP3A4 inhibitors (e.g., erythromycin, saquinavir, verapamil, fluconazole) gave approximately 2-fold increases in exposure. Grapefruit juice caused only a small increase (about 25%) in exposure). Products include:

Nexium Delayed-Release Capsules 655

Etodolac (When eplerenone and NSAIDs are used concomitantly, patients should be observed to determine whether the desired effect on blood pressure is obtained).

No products indexed under this heading.

Fenoprofen Calcium (When eplerenone and NSAIDs are used concomitantly, patients should be observed to determine whether the desired effect on blood pressure is obtained). Products include:

Nalfon Capsules 2502

Fluconazole (Eplerenone should not be used with strong inhibitors of CYP450 3A4. Potent inhibitors of CYP3A4 caused increased exposure of about 5-fold, while less potent CYP3A4 inhibitors (e.g., erythromycin, saquinavir, verapamil, fluconazole) gave approximately 2-fold increases in exposure. Grapefruit juice caused only a small increase (about 25%) in exposure).

No products indexed under this heading.

Fluoxetine Hydrochloride (Eplerenone should not be used with strong inhibitors of CYP450 3A4. Potent inhibitors of CYP3A4 caused increased exposure of about 5-fold, while less potent CYP3A4 inhibitors (e.g., erythromycin, saquinavir, verapamil, fluconazole) gave approximately 2-fold increases in exposure. Grapefruit juice caused only a small increase (about 25%) in exposure). Products include:

Prozac Pulvules and Liquid 1801
Symbyax Capsules 1819

Flurbiprofen (When eplerenone and NSAIDs are used concomitantly, patients should be observed to determine whether the desired effect on blood pressure is obtained).

No products indexed under this heading.

Fluvoxamine Maleate (Eplerenone should not be used with strong inhibitors of CYP450 3A4. Potent inhibitors of CYP3A4 caused increased exposure of about 5-fold, while less potent CYP3A4 inhibitors (e.g., erythromycin, saquinavir, verapamil, fluconazole) gave approximately 2-fold increases in exposure. Grapefruit juice caused only a small increase (about 25%) in exposure).

No products indexed under this heading.

Fosamprenavir Calcium (Eplerenone should not be used with strong inhibitors of CYP450 3A4. Potent inhibitors of CYP3A4 caused increased exposure of about 5-fold, while less potent CYP3A4 inhibitors (e.g., erythromycin, saquinavir, verapamil, fluconazole) gave approximately 2-fold increases in exposure. Grapefruit juice caused only a small increase (about 25%) in exposure). Products include:

Lexiva Tablets 1505

Fosinopril Sodium (Because the concomitant use of another mineralocorticoid receptor blocker and ACE inhibitors has led to clinically relevant hyperkalemia; caution should be used).

No products indexed under this heading.

Ibuprofen (When eplerenone and NSAIDs are used concomitantly, patients should be observed to determine whether the desired effect on blood pressure is obtained). Products include:

Advil Allergy Sinus Caplets .... ▣770
Advil .... ▣674
Children's Advil Oral Suspension .... ▣603
Children's Advil Chewable Tablets .... ▣603
Advil Cold & Sinus .... ▣723
Infants' Advil Concentrated Drops .... ▣604
Infants' Advil Concentrated Drops - White Grape (Dye-Free) .... ▣604
Junior Strength Advil Swallow Tablets .... ▣605
Advil Migraine Liquigels .... ▣608
Advil Multi-Symptom Cold Caplets .... ▣770
Advil PM Caplets .... ▣615
Motrin IB Tablets and Caplets 1866
Children's Motrin Oral Suspension 1867
Children's Motrin Non-Staining Dye-Free Oral Suspension 1867
Children's Motrin Cold Oral Suspension 1867
Infants' Motrin Concentrated Drops 1867
Infants' Motrin Non-Staining Dye-Free Concentrated Drops 1867
Junior Strength Motrin Caplets and Chewable Tablets 1867
Vicoprofen Tablets 539

Indinavir Sulfate (Eplerenone should not be used with strong inhibitors of CYP450 3A4. Potent inhibitors of CYP3A4 caused increased exposure of about 5-fold, while less potent CYP3A4 inhibitors (e.g., erythromycin, saquinavir, verapamil,

fluconazole) gave approximately 2-fold increases in exposure. Grapefruit juice caused only a small increase (about 25%) in exposure). Products include:
Crixivan Capsules 1940

Indomethacin (When eplerenone and NSAIDs are used concomitantly, patients should be observed to determine whether the desired effect on blood pressure is obtained). Products include:
Indocin 1995

Indomethacin Sodium Trihydrate (When eplerenone and NSAIDs are used concomitantly, patients should be observed to determine whether the desired effect on blood pressure is obtained). Products include:
Indocin I.V. 2465

Irbesartan (Because the concomitant use of another mineralocorticoid receptor blocker and angiotensin II receptor antagonists has led to clinically relevant hyperkalemia; caution should be used). Products include:
Avalide Tablets 888
Avalide Tablets 2874
Avapro Tablets 891
Avapro Tablets 2871

Isoniazid (Eplerenone should not be used with strong inhibitors of CYP450 3A4. Potent inhibitors of CYP3A4 caused increased exposure of about 5-fold, while less potent CYP3A4 inhibitors (e.g., erythromycin, saquinavir, verapamil, fluconazole) gave approximately 2-fold increases in exposure. Grapefruit juice caused only a small increase (about 25%) in exposure).
No products indexed under this heading.

Itraconazole (Concomitant use with the potent CYP3A4 inhibitor itraconazole is contraindicated).
No products indexed under this heading.

Ketoconazole (Concomitant use with the potent CYP3A4 inhibitor ketoconazole is contraindicated). Products include:
Nizoral A-D Shampoo, 1% 1868

Ketoprofen (When eplerenone and NSAIDs are used concomitantly, patients should be observed to determine whether the desired effect on blood pressure is obtained).
No products indexed under this heading.

Ketorolac Tromethamine (When eplerenone and NSAIDs are used concomitantly, patients should be observed to determine whether the desired effect on blood pressure is obtained). Products include:
Acular Ophthalmic Solution 565
Acular LS Ophthalmic Solution 566

Lisinopril (Because the concomitant use of another mineralocorticoid receptor blocker and ACE inhibitors has led to clinically relevant hyperkalemia; caution should be used). Products include:
Prinivil Tablets 2052
Prinzide Tablets 2056

Lithium (Serum lithium levels should be monitored frequently if eplerenone is administered concomitantly with lithium).
No products indexed under this heading.

Lithium Carbonate (Serum lithium levels should be monitored frequently if eplerenone is administered concomitantly with lithium). Products include:
Lithobid Tablets 1692

Lithium Citrate (Serum lithium levels should be monitored frequently if eplerenone is administered concomitantly with lithium).
No products indexed under this heading.

Lopinavir (Eplerenone should not be used with strong inhibitors of CYP450 3A4. Potent inhibitors of CYP3A4 caused increased exposure of about 5-fold, while less potent CYP3A4 inhibitors (e.g., erythromycin, saquinavir, verapamil, fluconazole) gave approximately 2-fold increases in exposure. Grapefruit juice caused only a small increase (about 25%) in exposure). Products include:
Kaletra 476

Loratadine (Eplerenone should not be used with strong inhibitors of CYP450 3A4. Potent inhibitors of CYP3A4 caused increased exposure of about 5-fold, while less potent CYP3A4 inhibitors (e.g., erythromycin, saquinavir, verapamil, fluconazole) gave approximately 2-fold increases in exposure. Grapefruit juice caused only a small increase (about 25%) in exposure). Products include:
Alavert Allergy & Sinus D-12 Hour Tablets 771
Alavert 771
Children's Claritin Allergy Oral Solution 771
Claritin Non-Drowsy 24 Hour Tablets 772
Claritin Reditabs 24 Hour Non-Drowsy Tablets 772
Claritin-D Non-Drowsy 12 Hour Tablets 772
Claritin-D Non-Drowsy 24 Hour Tablets 772

Losartan Potassium (Because the concomitant use of another mineralocorticoid receptor blocker and angiotensin II receptor antagonists has led to clinically relevant hyperkalemia; caution should be used). Products include:
Cozaar Tablets 1935
Hyzaar 50-12.5 Tablets 1990
Hyzaar 100-12.5 Tablets 1990
Hyzaar 100-25 Tablets 1990

Meclofenamate Sodium (When eplerenone and NSAIDs are used concomitantly, patients should be observed to determine whether the desired effect on blood pressure is obtained).
No products indexed under this heading.

Mefenamic Acid (When eplerenone and NSAIDs are used concomitantly, patients should be observed to determine whether the desired effect on blood pressure is obtained).
No products indexed under this heading.

Meloxicam (When eplerenone and NSAIDs are used concomitantly, patients should be observed to determine whether the desired effect on blood pressure is obtained). Products include:
Mobic Oral Suspension 863
Mobic Tablets 863

Metronidazole (Eplerenone should not be used with strong inhibitors of CYP450 3A4. Potent inhibitors of CYP3A4 caused increased exposure of about 5-fold, while less potent CYP3A4 inhibitors (e.g., erythromycin, saquinavir, verapamil, fluconazole) gave approximately 2-fold increases in exposure. Grapefruit juice caused only a small increase (about 25%) in exposure). Products include:
Metrogel 1% 1211
MetroGel-Vaginal Gel 1855
Vandazole Vaginal Gel 3338

Metronidazole Benzoate (Eplerenone should not be used with strong inhibitors of CYP450 3A4. Potent inhibitors of CYP3A4 caused increased exposure of about 5-fold, while less potent CYP3A4 inhibitors (e.g., erythromycin, saquinavir, verapamil, fluconazole) gave approximately 2-fold increases in exposure. Grapefruit juice caused only a small increase (about 25%) in exposure).
No products indexed under this heading.

Metronidazole Hydrochloride (Eplerenone should not be used with strong inhibitors of CYP450 3A4. Potent inhibitors of CYP3A4 caused increased exposure of about 5-fold, while less potent CYP3A4 inhibitors (e.g., erythromycin, saquinavir, verapamil, fluconazole) gave approximately 2-fold increases in exposure. Grapefruit juice caused only a small increase (about 25%) in exposure).
No products indexed under this heading.

Miconazole (Eplerenone should not be used with strong inhibitors of CYP450 3A4. Potent inhibitors of CYP3A4 caused increased exposure of about 5-fold, while less potent CYP3A4 inhibitors (e.g., erythromycin, saquinavir, verapamil, fluconazole) gave approximately 2-fold increases in exposure. Grapefruit juice caused only a small increase (about 25%) in exposure).
No products indexed under this heading.

Miconazole Nitrate (Eplerenone should not be used with strong inhibitors of CYP450 3A4. Potent inhibitors of CYP3A4 caused increased exposure of about 5-fold, while less potent CYP3A4 inhibitors (e.g., erythromycin, saquinavir, verapamil, fluconazole) gave approximately 2-fold increases in exposure. Grapefruit juice caused only a small increase (about 25%) in exposure). Products include:
Desenex 635
Desenex Jock Itch Spray Powder 635

Moexipril Hydrochloride (Because the concomitant use of another mineralocorticoid receptor blocker and ACE inhibitors has led to clinically relevant hyperkalemia; caution should be used). Products include:
Uniretic Tablets 3100
Univasc Tablets 3104

Nabumetone (When eplerenone and NSAIDs are used concomitantly, patients should be observed to determine whether the desired effect on blood pressure is obtained).
No products indexed under this heading.

Naproxen (When eplerenone and NSAIDs are used concomitantly, patients should be observed to determine whether the desired effect on blood pressure is obtained). Products include:
EC-Naprosyn Delayed-Release Tablets 2761
Naprosyn Suspension 2761
Naprosyn Tablets 2761
Prevacid NapraPAC 3280

Naproxen Sodium (When eplerenone and NSAIDs are used concomitantly, patients should be observed to determine whether the desired effect on blood pressure is obtained). Products include:
Aleve Caplets 742
Aleve Gelcaps 743
Aleve Tablets 743
Aleve Cold & Sinus Caplets 744
Anaprox Tablets 2761
Anaprox DS Tablets 2761

Nefazodone Hydrochloride (Concomitant use with the potent CYP3A4 inhibitor nefazodone is contraindicated).
No products indexed under this heading.

Nelfinavir Mesylate (Concomitant use with the potent CYP3A4 inhibitor nelfinavir is contraindicated). Products include:
Viracept 2577

Nevirapine (Eplerenone should not be used with strong inhibitors of CYP450 3A4. Potent inhibitors of CYP3A4 caused increased exposure of about 5-fold, while less potent CYP3A4 inhibitors (e.g., erythromycin, saquinavir, verapamil, fluconazole) gave approximately 2-fold increases in exposure. Grapefruit juice caused only a small increase (about 25%) in exposure). Products include:
Viramune Oral Suspension 873
Viramune Tablets 873

Niacinamide (Eplerenone should not be used with strong inhibitors of CYP450 3A4. Potent inhibitors of CYP3A4 caused increased exposure of about 5-fold, while less potent CYP3A4 inhibitors (e.g., erythromycin, saquinavir, verapamil, fluconazole) gave approximately 2-fold increases in exposure. Grapefruit juice caused only a small increase (about 25%) in exposure).
No products indexed under this heading.

Nicotinamide (Eplerenone should not be used with strong inhibitors of CYP450 3A4. Potent inhibitors of CYP3A4 caused increased exposure of about 5-fold, while less potent CYP3A4 inhibitors (e.g., erythromycin, saquinavir, verapamil, fluconazole) gave approximately 2-fold increases in exposure. Grapefruit juice caused only a small increase (about 25%) in exposure). Products include:
Nicomide Tablets 1088

Nifedipine (Eplerenone should not be used with strong inhibitors of CYP450 3A4. Potent inhibitors of CYP3A4 caused increased exposure of about 5-fold, while less potent CYP3A4 inhibitors (e.g., erythromycin, saquinavir, verapamil, fluconazole) gave approximately 2-fold increases in exposure. Grapefruit juice caused only a small increase (about 25%) in exposure). Products include:
Adalat CC Tablets 2964

Norfloxacin (Eplerenone should not be used with strong inhibitors of CYP450 3A4. Potent inhibitors of CYP3A4 caused increased exposure of about 5-fold, while less potent CYP3A4 inhibitors (e.g., erythromycin, saquinavir, verapamil, fluconazole) gave approximately 2-fold increases in exposure. Grapefruit juice caused only a small increase (about 25%) in exposure). Products include:

Telmisartan (Because the concomitant use of another mineralocorticoid receptor blocker and angiotensin II receptor antagonists has led to clinically relevant hyperkalemia; caution should be used). Products include:
- Micardis Tablets ... 854
- Micardis HCT Tablets ... 856

Tolmetin Sodium (When eplerenone and NSAIDs are used concomitantly, patients should be observed to determine whether the desired effect on blood pressure is obtained).
No products indexed under this heading.

Trandolapril (Because the concomitant use of another mineralocorticoid receptor blocker and ACE inhibitors has led to clinically relevant hyperkalemia; caution should be used). Products include:
- Mavik Tablets ... 486
- Tarka Tablets ... 524

Triamterene (Eplerenone is contraindicated in patients treated concomitantly with potassium-sparing diuretics). Products include:
- Dyazide Capsules ... 1423
- Dyrenium Capsules ... 3400

Troglitazone (Eplerenone should not be used with strong inhibitors of CYP450 3A4. Potent inhibitors of CYP3A4 caused increased exposure of about 5-fold, while less potent CYP3A4 inhibitors (e.g., erythromycin, saquinavir, verapamil, fluconazole) gave approximately 2-fold increases in exposure. Grapefruit juice caused only a small increase (about 25%) in exposure).
No products indexed under this heading.

Troleandomycin (Concomitant use with the potent CYP3A4 inhibitor troleandomycin is contraindicated).
No products indexed under this heading.

Valdecoxib (When eplerenone and NSAIDs are used concomitantly, patients should be observed to determine whether the desired effect on blood pressure is obtained).
No products indexed under this heading.

Valproate Sodium (Eplerenone should not be used with strong inhibitors of CYP450 3A4. Potent inhibitors of CYP3A4 caused increased exposure of about 5-fold, while less potent CYP3A4 inhibitors (e.g., erythromycin, saquinavir, verapamil, fluconazole) gave approximately 2-fold increases in exposure. Grapefruit juice caused only a small increase (about 25%) in exposure). Products include:
- Depacon Injection ... 412

Valsartan (Because the concomitant use of another mineralocorticoid receptor blocker and angiotensin II receptor antagonists has led to clinically relevant hyperkalemia; caution should be used). Products include:
- Diovan Tablets ... 2193
- Diovan HCT Tablets ... 2196

Verapamil Hydrochloride (Eplerenone should not be used with strong inhibitors of CYP450 3A4. Potent inhibitors of CYP3A4 caused increased exposure of about 5-fold, while less potent CYP3A4 inhibitors (e.g., erythromycin, saquinavir, verapamil, fluconazole) gave approximately 2-fold increases in exposure. Grapefruit juice caused only a small increase (about 25%) in exposure). Products include:
- Covera-HS Tablets ... 3139
- Tarka Tablets ... 524
- Verelan PM Extended-Release Capsules, Controlled-Onset ... 3106

Voriconazole (Eplerenone should not be used with strong inhibitors of CYP450 3A4. Potent inhibitors of CYP3A4 caused increased exposure of about 5-fold, while less potent CYP3A4 inhibitors (e.g., erythromycin, saquinavir, verapamil, fluconazole) gave approximately 2-fold increases in exposure. Grapefruit juice caused only a small increase (about 25%) in exposure). Products include:
- VFEND I.V. ... 2564
- VFEND Oral Suspension ... 2564
- VFEND Tablets ... 2564

Zafirlukast (Eplerenone should not be used with strong inhibitors of CYP450 3A4. Potent inhibitors of CYP3A4 caused increased exposure of about 5-fold, while less potent CYP3A4 inhibitors (e.g., erythromycin, saquinavir, verapamil, fluconazole) gave approximately 2-fold increases in exposure. Grapefruit juice caused only a small increase (about 25%) in exposure). Products include:
- Accolate Tablets ... 671

Zileuton (Eplerenone should not be used with strong inhibitors of CYP450 3A4. Potent inhibitors of CYP3A4 caused increased exposure of about 5-fold, while less potent CYP3A4 inhibitors (e.g., erythromycin, saquinavir, verapamil, fluconazole) gave approximately 2-fold increases in exposure. Grapefruit juice caused only a small increase (about 25%) in exposure). Products include:
- Zyflo Tablets ... 1023

Food Interactions

Grapefruit (Eplerenone should not be used with strong inhibitors of CYP450 3A4. Potent inhibitors of CYP3A4 caused increased exposure of about 5-fold, while less potent CYP3A4 inhibitors (e.g., erythromycin, saquinavir, verapamil, fluconazole) gave approximately 2-fold increases in exposure. Grapefruit juice caused only a small increase (about 25%) in exposure).

Grapefruit Juice (Eplerenone should not be used with strong inhibitors of CYP450 3A4. Potent inhibitors of CYP3A4 caused increased exposure of about 5-fold, while less potent CYP3A4 inhibitors (e.g., erythromycin, saquinavir, verapamil, fluconazole) gave approximately 2-fold increases in exposure. Grapefruit juice caused only a small increase (about 25%) in exposure).

Salt Substitutes, Potassium-Containing (Eplerenone is contraindicated in patients treated concomitantly with salt substitutes containing potassium).

INTEGRILIN INJECTION

(Eptifibatide) ... 3020

May interact with oral anticoagulants, glycoprotein (GP) IIb/IIIa inhibitors, non-steroidal anti-inflammatory agents, and certain other agents. Compounds in these categories include:

Abciximab (Current or planned administration of another parenteral GP IIb/IIIa inhibitor is contraindicated). Products include:
- ReoPro Vials ... 1809

Anisindione (Potential for additive pharmacologic effects because eptifibatide inhibits platelet aggregation; concurrent use requires caution). Products include:
- Miradon Tablets ... 3042

Aspirin (Co-administration of eptifibatide with heparin and aspirin has resulted in cerebral, GI and pulmonary hemorrhage). Products include:
- Aggrenox Capsules ... 822
- Bayer Aspirin ... 744
- BC Allergy Sinus Cold Powder ... 677
- BC Headache Powder ... 677
- Arthritis Strength BC Powder ... 677
- BC Sinus Cold Powder ... 677
- Excedrin Extra Strength Caplets/Tablets/Geltabs ... 684
- Excedrin Migraine Caplets/Tablets/Geltabs ... 609
- Goody's Body Pain Formula Powder ... 684
- Goody's Extra Strength Headache Powders ... 611
- Goody's Extra Strength Pain Relief Tablets ... 685
- Percodan Tablets ... 1132
- St. Joseph 81 mg Aspirin Chewable and Enteric Coated Tablets ... 1869

Celecoxib (Potential for additive pharmacologic effects because eptifibatide inhibits platelet aggregation; concurrent use requires caution). Products include:
- Celebrex Capsules ... 3134

Clopidogrel Bisulfate (Potential for additive pharmacologic effects because eptifibatide inhibits platelet aggregation; concurrent use requires caution). Products include:
- Plavix Tablets ... 917
- Plavix Tablets ... 2926

Diclofenac Potassium (Potential for additive pharmacologic effects because eptifibatide inhibits platelet aggregation; concurrent use requires caution).
No products indexed under this heading.

Diclofenac Sodium (Potential for additive pharmacologic effects because eptifibatide inhibits platelet aggregation; concurrent use requires caution). Products include:
- Arthrotec Tablets ... 3129
- Voltaren Ophthalmic Solution ... 2309
- Voltaren Tablets ... 2307
- Voltaren-XR Tablets ... 2310

Dicumarol (Potential for additive pharmacologic effects because eptifibatide inhibits platelet aggregation; concurrent use requires caution).
No products indexed under this heading.

Dipyridamole (Potential for additive pharmacologic effects because eptifibatide inhibits platelet aggregation; concurrent use requires caution). Products include:
- Aggrenox Capsules ... 822
- Persantine Tablets ... 868

Etodolac (Potential for additive pharmacologic effects because eptifibatide inhibits platelet aggregation; concurrent use requires caution).
No products indexed under this heading.

Fenoprofen Calcium (Potential for additive pharmacologic effects because eptifibatide inhibits platelet aggregation; concurrent use requires caution). Products include:
- Nalfon Capsules ... 2502

Flurbiprofen (Potential for additive pharmacologic effects because eptifibatide inhibits platelet aggregation; concurrent use requires caution).
No products indexed under this heading.

Heparin Sodium (Co-administration of eptifibatide with heparin and aspirin has resulted in cerebral, GI and pulmonary hemorrhage).
No products indexed under this heading.

Ibuprofen (Potential for additive pharmacologic effects because eptifibatide inhibits platelet aggregation; concurrent use requires caution). Products include:
- Advil Allergy Sinus Caplets ... 770
- Advil ... 674
- Children's Advil Oral Suspension ... 603
- Children's Advil Chewable Tablets ... 603
- Advil Cold & Sinus ... 723
- Infants' Advil Concentrated Drops ... 604
- Infants' Advil Concentrated Drops - White Grape (Dye-Free) ... 604
- Junior Strength Advil Swallow Tablets ... 605
- Advil Migraine Liquigels ... 608
- Advil Multi-Symptom Cold Caplets ... 770
- Advil PM Caplets ... 615
- Motrin IB Tablets and Caplets ... 1866
- Children's Motrin Oral Suspension ... 1867
- Children's Motrin Non-Staining Dye-Free Oral Suspension ... 1867
- Children's Motrin Cold Oral Suspension ... 1867
- Infants' Motrin Concentrated Drops ... 1867
- Infants' Motrin Non-Staining Dye-Free Concentrated Drops ... 1867
- Junior Strength Motrin Caplets and Chewable Tablets ... 1867
- Vicoprofen Tablets ... 539

Indomethacin (Potential for additive pharmacologic effects because eptifibatide inhibits platelet aggregation; concurrent use requires caution). Products include:
- Indocin ... 1995

Indomethacin Sodium Trihydrate (Potential for additive pharmacologic effects because eptifibatide inhibits platelet aggregation; concurrent use requires caution). Products include:
- Indocin I.V. ... 2465

Ketoprofen (Potential for additive pharmacologic effects because eptifibatide inhibits platelet aggregation; concurrent use requires caution).
No products indexed under this heading.

Ketorolac Tromethamine (Potential for additive pharmacologic effects because eptifibatide inhibits platelet aggregation; concurrent use requires caution). Products include:
- Acular Ophthalmic Solution ... 565
- Acular LS Ophthalmic Solution ... 566

Meclofenamate Sodium (Potential for additive pharmacologic effects because eptifibatide inhibits platelet aggregation; concurrent use requires caution).
No products indexed under this heading.

Mefenamic Acid (Potential for additive pharmacologic effects because eptifibatide inhibits platelet aggregation; concurrent use requires caution).
No products indexed under this heading.

Meloxicam (Potential for additive pharmacologic effects because eptifibatide inhibits platelet aggregation; concurrent use requires caution). Products include:

Mobic Oral Suspension 863
Mobic Tablets 863

Nabumetone (Potential for additive pharmacologic effects because eptifibatide inhibits platelet aggregation; concurrent use requires caution).
No products indexed under this heading.

Naproxen (Potential for additive pharmacologic effects because eptifibatide inhibits platelet aggregation; concurrent use requires caution). Products include:
EC-Naprosyn Delayed-Release Tablets 2761
Naprosyn Suspension 2761
Naprosyn Tablets 2761
Prevacid NapraPAC 3280

Naproxen Sodium (Potential for additive pharmacologic effects because eptifibatide inhibits platelet aggregation; concurrent use requires caution). Products include:
Aleve Caplets 742
Aleve Gelcaps 743
Aleve Tablets 743
Aleve Cold & Sinus Caplets 744
Anaprox Tablets 2761
Anaprox DS Tablets 2761

Oxaprozin (Potential for additive pharmacologic effects because eptifibatide inhibits platelet aggregation; concurrent use requires caution).
No products indexed under this heading.

Phenylbutazone (Potential for additive pharmacologic effects because eptifibatide inhibits platelet aggregation; concurrent use requires caution).
No products indexed under this heading.

Piroxicam (Potential for additive pharmacologic effects because eptifibatide inhibits platelet aggregation; concurrent use requires caution).
No products indexed under this heading.

Rofecoxib (Potential for additive pharmacologic effects because eptifibatide inhibits platelet aggregation; concurrent use requires caution).
No products indexed under this heading.

Sulindac (Potential for additive pharmacologic effects because eptifibatide inhibits platelet aggregation; concurrent use requires caution). Products include:
Clinoril Tablets 1924

Ticlopidine Hydrochloride (Potential for additive pharmacologic effects because eptifibatide inhibits platelet aggregation; concurrent use requires caution). Products include:
Ticlid Tablets 2810

Tirofiban Hydrochloride (Current or planned administration of another parenteral GP IIb/IIIa inhibitor is contraindicated). Products include:
Aggrastat 1907

Tolmetin Sodium (Potential for additive pharmacologic effects because eptifibatide inhibits platelet aggregation; concurrent use requires caution).
No products indexed under this heading.

Valdecoxib (Potential for additive pharmacologic effects because eptifibatide inhibits platelet aggregation; concurrent use requires caution).
No products indexed under this heading.

Warfarin Sodium (Potential for additive pharmacologic effects because eptifibatide inhibits platelet aggregation; concurrent use requires caution). Products include:
Coumadin for Injection 898
Coumadin Tablets 898

INTELECTOL TABLETS

(Vinpocetine) .... ▣830
None cited in PDR database.

INTRON A FOR INJECTION

(Interferon alfa-2b, Recombinant) 3024
May interact with xanthines and certain other agents. Compounds in these categories include:

Aminophylline (Co-administration results in decreased theophylline clearance resulting in a 100% increase in serum theophylline levels).
No products indexed under this heading.

Bone Marrow Depressants, unspecified (Careful monitoring of the WBC count is indicated).
No products indexed under this heading.

Dyphylline (Co-administration results in decreased theophylline clearance resulting in a 100% increase in serum theophylline levels).
No products indexed under this heading.

Theophylline (Co-administration results in decreased theophylline clearance resulting in a 100% increase in serum theophylline levels).
No products indexed under this heading.

Theophylline Anhydrous (Co-administration results in decreased theophylline clearance resulting in a 100% increase in serum theophylline levels). Products include:
Uniphyl Tablets 2710

Theophylline Calcium Salicylate (Co-administration results in decreased theophylline clearance resulting in a 100% increase in serum theophylline levels).
No products indexed under this heading.

Theophylline Dihydroxypropyl (Glyceryl) (Co-administration results in decreased theophylline clearance resulting in a 100% increase in serum theophylline levels).
No products indexed under this heading.

Theophylline Ethylenediamine (Co-administration results in decreased theophylline clearance resulting in a 100% increase in serum theophylline levels).
No products indexed under this heading.

Theophylline Sodium Glycinate (Co-administration results in decreased theophylline clearance resulting in a 100% increase in serum theophylline levels).
No products indexed under this heading.

Zidovudine (Concomitant administration may result in a higher incidence of neutropenia). Products include:
Combivir Tablets 1411
Retrovir 1560
Retrovir IV Infusion 1564
Trizivir Tablets 1589

INVANZ FOR INJECTION

(Ertapenem) 1999
May interact with:

Probenecid (Competes for active tubular secretion and reduces the renal clearance of ertapenem).
No products indexed under this heading.

INVIRASE CAPSULES

(Saquinavir Mesylate) 2772
May interact with calcium channel blockers, cytochrome p450 3a4 inducers (selected), cytochrome p450 3a4 substrates (selected), dexamethasone, ergot-containing drugs, oral contraceptives, phenytoin, and certain other agents. Compounds in these categories include:

Alfentanil Hydrochloride (Co-administration with drugs that are mainly metabolized by CYP3A4 may have elevated plasma concentrations when co-administered with saquinavir; these combinations should be used with caution).
No products indexed under this heading.

Allium sativum (Co-administration with compounds that are potent inducers of CYP3A4 may result in decreased plasma levels of saquinavir).
No products indexed under this heading.

Alprazolam (Concomitant administration with saquinavir may lead to increased alprazolam levels; a decrease in alprazolam dose may be needed). Products include:
Niravam Orally Disintegrating Tablets 3092

Amiodarone Hydrochloride (Inhibition of CYP3A4 by saquinavir could result in elevated plasma concentrations of amiodarone, potentially causing serious or life-threatening reactions; concurrent use is contraindicated).
No products indexed under this heading.

Amitriptyline Hydrochloride (Concomitant administration with saquinavir may cause increased levels of amitriptyline; therapeutic concentration monitoring is recommended for tricyclic antidepressants when co-administered with saquinavir).
No products indexed under this heading.

Amlodipine Besylate (Concomitant administration with saquinavir may lead to increased amlodipine levels; caution is warranted and clinical monitoring of patient is recommended). Products include:
Caduet Tablets 2508
Lotrel Capsules 2249
Norvasc Tablets 2545

Aprepitant (Co-administration with drugs that are mainly metabolized by CYP3A4 may have elevated plasma concentrations when co-administered with saquinavir; these combinations should be used with caution). Products include:
Emend Capsules 1963

Astemizole (Inhibition of CYP3A4 by saquinavir could result in increased astemizole plasma levels and create the potential for serious and/or life-threatening reactions, such as rare cases of serious cardiovascular adverse events; concurrent use is contraindicated).
No products indexed under this heading.

Atazanavir (Concomitant administration with saquinavir may cause increased plasma concentrations of atazanavir).
No products indexed under this heading.

Atazanavir sulfate (Concomitant administration with saquinavir may cause increased plasma concentrations of atazanavir). Products include:
Reyataz Capsules 921

Atorvastatin Calcium (Concomitant administration with saquinavir may cause increased atorvastatin levels. Use lowest possible dose of atorvastatin and with careful monitoring or consider other HMG-CoA reductase inhibitors, such as pravastatin, fluvastatin, and rosuvastatin). Products include:
Caduet Tablets 2508
Lipitor Tablets 2483

Belladonna Ergotamine (Co-administration with drugs that are mainly metabolized by CYP3A4 may have elevated plasma concentrations when co-administered with saquinavir; these combinations should be used with caution).
No products indexed under this heading.

Bepridil Hydrochloride (Inhibition of CYP3A4 by saquinavir could result in elevated plasma concentrations of bepridil, potentially causing serious or life-threatening reactions; concurrent use is contraindicated).
No products indexed under this heading.

Betamethasone Acetate (Co-administration with compounds that are potent inducers of CYP3A4 may result in decreased plasma levels of saquinavir).
No products indexed under this heading.

Betamethasone Sodium Phosphate (Co-administration with compounds that are potent inducers of CYP3A4 may result in decreased plasma levels of saquinavir).
No products indexed under this heading.

Buspirone Hydrochloride (Co-administration with drugs that are mainly metabolized by CYP3A4 may have elevated plasma concentrations when co-administered with saquinavir; these combinations should be used with caution).
No products indexed under this heading.

Busulfan (Co-administration with drugs that are mainly metabolized by CYP3A4 may have elevated plasma concentrations when co-administered with saquinavir; these combinations should be used with caution). Products include:
I.V. Busulfex 2493
Myleran Tablets 1525

Carbamazepine (Concomitant administration with saquinavir may decrease saquinavir levels. Use with caution since saquinavir may be less effective due to decreased saquinavir plasma concentrations). Products include:

Carbatrol Capsules ... 3171
Equetro Extended-Release Capsules ... 3180
Tegretol/Tegretol-XR ... 2295

Cerivastatin Sodium (Co-administration of Invirase and other HMG-CoA reductase inhibitors that are metabolized by the CYP3A4 pathway, such as cerivastatin, may result in increased concentrations of statins; potential for, in rare cases, severe adverse events, such as myopathy, including rhabdomyolysis).

No products indexed under this heading.

Chlorpheniramine (Co-administration with drugs that are mainly metabolized by CYP3A4 may have elevated plasma concentrations when co-administered with saquinavir; these combinations should be used with caution).

No products indexed under this heading.

Chlorpheniramine Maleate (Co-administration with drugs that are mainly metabolized by CYP3A4 may have elevated plasma concentrations when co-administered with saquinavir; these combinations should be used with caution). Products include:

Advil Allergy Sinus Caplets ... ▪770
Advil Multi-Symptom Cold Caplets ... ▪770
BC Allergy Sinus Cold Powder ... ▪677
Comtrex Maximum Strength Cold & Cough Day/Night Caplets - Night Formulation ... ▪726
Comtrex Maximum Strength Day/Night Severe Cold & Sinus Caplets - Night Formulation ... ▪725
Contac Cold and Flu Maximum Strength Caplets ... ▪728
Contac Cold and Flu Day and Night Caplets (Night Formulation Only) ... ▪727
Children's Dimetapp Long Acting Cough Plus Cold Syrup ... ▪731
Robitussin Cough & Cold Long-Acting Liquid ... ▪735
Robitussin Cough & Allergy Syrup ... ▪736
Robitussin Cough & Cold Nighttime Liquid ... ▪736
Robitussin Cough, Cold & Flu Nighttime Liquid ... ▪738
Robitussin Pediatric Cough & Cold Long-Acting Liquid ... ▪735
Robitussin Pediatric Cough & Cold Nighttime Liquid ... ▪736
Triaminic Cold & Allergy Liquid ... ▪746
Triaminic Cough & Runny Nose Softchews ... ▪748
Children's Tylenol Plus Flu Oral Suspension ... ▪749
Tylenol Allergy Multi-Symptom Caplets with Cool Burst and Gelcaps ... 1872
Children's Tylenol Plus Cold Suspension Liquid ... 1879
Children's Tylenol Plus Cough & Runny Nose Suspension Liquid ... 1879
Children's Tylenol Plus Flu Suspension Liquid ... 1881
Children's Tylenol Plus Multi-Symptom Cold Suspension Liquid ... 1879
Tylenol Cold Head Congestion Nighttime Caplets with Cool Burst ... 1873
Tylenol Cold Multi-Symptom Nighttime Caplets with Cool Burst ... 1874
Tylenol Sinus Congestion & Pain Nighttime Caplets with Cool Burst ... 1876
Vicks 44M Cough, Cold & Flu Relief Liquid ... 2680
Pediatric Vicks 44m Cough & Cold Relief Liquid ... 2676
Children's Vicks NyQuil Cold/Cough Relief ... ▪756
Children's Vicks NyQuil Cold/Cough Relief Liquid ... 2680
Zicam Maximum Strength Flu Daytime ... ▪768

Chlorpheniramine Polistirex (Co-administration with drugs that are mainly metabolized by CYP3A4 may have elevated plasma concentrations when co-administered with saquinavir; these combinations should be used with caution). Products include:

Tussionex Pennkinetic Extended-Release Suspension ... 3327

Chlorpheniramine Tannate (Co-administration with drugs that are mainly metabolized by CYP3A4 may have elevated plasma concentrations when co-administered with saquinavir; these combinations should be used with caution).

No products indexed under this heading.

Ciprofloxacin Hydrochloride (Co-administration with compounds that are potent inducers of CYP3A4 may result in decreased plasma levels of saquinavir). Products include:

Ciloxan Ophthalmic Ointment ... 559
Ciloxan Ophthalmic Solution ... ⊙206
Cipro Tablets ... 2977
Proquin XR Tablets ... 1153

Cisapride (Inhibition of CYP3A4 by saquinavir could result in increased cisapride plasma levels and create the potential for serious and/or life-threatening reactions, such as rare cases of serious cardiovascular adverse events; concurrent use is contraindicated).

No products indexed under this heading.

Cisplatin (Co-administration with compounds that are potent inducers of CYP3A4 may result in decreased plasma levels of saquinavir).

No products indexed under this heading.

Clarithromycin (Concomitant administration with saquinavir may cause increased levels of clarithromycin and/or saquinavir). Products include:

Biaxin/Biaxin XL ... 402
PREVPAC ... 3284

Clindamycin Hydrochloride (Potential for elevated plasma concentrations of compounds that are substrate of CYP3A4, such as clindamycin). Products include:

Cleocin Vaginal Ovules ... 2616

Clindamycin Palmitate Hydrochloride (Potential for elevated plasma concentrations of compounds that are substrate of CYP3A4, such as clindamycin).

No products indexed under this heading.

Clindamycin Phosphate (Potential for elevated plasma concentrations of compounds that are substrate of CYP3A4, such as clindamycin). Products include:

Benzaclin Topical Gel ... 2877
Clindagel ... 1203
Evoclin Foam, 1% ... 1009

Clorazepate Dipotassium (Concomitant administration with saquinavir may lead to increased clorazepate levels; a decrease in clorazepate dose may be needed). Products include:

Tranxene ... 2474

Cortisone Acetate (Co-administration with compounds that are potent inducers of CYP3A4 may result in decreased plasma levels of saquinavir).

No products indexed under this heading.

Cyclosporine (Concomitant administration with saquinavir may lead to increased levels of cyclosporine. Therapeutic concentration monitoring is recommended for all immunosuppressant agents when co-administered with saquinavir). Products include:

Gengraf Capsules ... 459
Neoral Oral Solution ... 2259
Neoral Soft Gelatin Capsules ... 2259
Restasis Ophthalmic Emulsion ... 575
Sandimmune ... 2275

Dapsone (Potential for elevated plasma concentrations of compounds that are substrate of CYP3A4, such as dapsone). Products include:

Dapsone Tablets USP ... 1673

Delavirdine Mesylate (Co-administration has resulted in a 5-fold increase in saquinavir plasma AUC; currently, there are no safety and efficacy data available from use of this combination; hepatocellular enzyme elevations have occurred in some patients). Products include:

Rescriptor Tablets ... 2551

Desogestrel (Concomitant administration with saquinavir/ritonavir may lead to decreased ethinyl estradiol levels. Alternative or additional contraceptive measures should be used when estrogen-based oral contraceptives and saquinavir/ritonavir are co-administered). Products include:

Mircette Tablets ... 1066

Dexamethasone (Concomitant administration with saquinavir may cause decreased saquinavir levels. Use with caution since saquinavir may be less effective due to decreased saquinavir plasma concentrations). Products include:

Ciprodex Otic Suspension ... 559
Decadron Tablets ... 1951
TobraDex Ophthalmic Ointment ... 562
TobraDex Ophthalmic Suspension ... 563

Dexamethasone Acetate (Concomitant administration with saquinavir may cause decreased saquinavir levels. Use with caution since saquinavir may be less effective due to decreased saquinavir plasma concentrations).

No products indexed under this heading.

Dexamethasone Sodium Phosphate (Concomitant administration with saquinavir may cause decreased saquinavir levels. Use with caution since saquinavir may be less effective due to decreased saquinavir plasma concentrations).

No products indexed under this heading.

Diazepam (Concomitant administration with saquinavir may lead to increased diazepam levels; a decrease in diazepam dose may be needed). Products include:

Diastat Rectal Delivery System ... 3343
Valium Tablets ... 2819

Dihydroergotamine Mesylate (Inhibition of CYP3A4 by saquinavir could result in increased ergot derivatives plasma levels and create the potential for serious and/or life-threatening reactions; concurrent use is contraindicated). Products include:

Migranal Nasal Spray ... 3348

Diltiazem Hydrochloride (Concomitant administration with saquinavir may lead to increased diltiazem levels; caution is warranted and clinical monitoring of patient is recommended). Products include:

Cardizem LA Extended Release Tablets ... 1728
Tiazac Capsules ... 1201

Diltiazem Maleate (Concomitant administration with saquinavir may lead to increased diltiazem levels; caution is warranted and clinical monitoring of patient is recommended).

No products indexed under this heading.

Disopyramide (Co-administration with drugs that are mainly metabolized by CYP3A4 may have elevated plasma concentrations when co-administered with saquinavir; these combinations should be used with caution).

No products indexed under this heading.

Disopyramide Phosphate (Co-administration with drugs that are mainly metabolized by CYP3A4 may have elevated plasma concentrations when co-administered with saquinavir; these combinations should be used with caution).

No products indexed under this heading.

Disulfiram (Co-administration with drugs that are mainly metabolized by CYP3A4 may have elevated plasma concentrations when co-administered with saquinavir; these combinations should be used with caution).

No products indexed under this heading.

Doxorubicin Hydrochloride (Co-administration with drugs that are mainly metabolized by CYP3A4 may have elevated plasma concentrations when co-administered with saquinavir; these combinations should be used with caution).

No products indexed under this heading.

Dronabinol (Co-administration with drugs that are mainly metabolized by CYP3A4 may have elevated plasma concentrations when co-administered with saquinavir; these combinations should be used with caution). Products include:

Marinol Capsules ... 3333

Efavirenz (Concomitant administration with saquinavir may lead to decreased levels of saquinavir and efavirenz. Saquinavir should not be given as the sole protease inhibitor to patients taking efavirenz). Products include:

Atripla Tablets ... 945
Sustiva Capsules ... 930
Sustiva Tablets ... 930

Ergonovine Maleate (Inhibition of CYP3A4 by saquinavir could result in increased ergot derivatives plasma levels and create the potential for serious and/or life-threatening reactions; concurrent use is contraindicated).

No products indexed under this heading.

Ergotamine Tartrate (Inhibition of CYP3A4 by saquinavir could result in increased ergot derivatives plasma levels and create the potential for serious and/or life-threatening reactions; concurrent use is contraindicated).
No products indexed under this heading.

Erythromycin (Co-administration with drugs that are mainly metabolized by CYP3A4 may have elevated plasma concentrations when co-administered with saquinavir; these combinations should be used with caution). Products include:
Ery-Tab Tablets 449
Erythromycin Base Filmtab Tablets 455
Erythromycin Delayed-Release Capsules, USP 457
PCE Dispertab Tablets 515

Erythromycin Estolate (Co-administration with drugs that are mainly metabolized by CYP3A4 may have elevated plasma concentrations when co-administered with saquinavir; these combinations should be used with caution).
No products indexed under this heading.

Erythromycin Ethylsuccinate (Co-administration with drugs that are mainly metabolized by CYP3A4 may have elevated plasma concentrations when co-administered with saquinavir; these combinations should be used with caution). Products include:
E.E.S. 451
EryPed 447

Erythromycin Gluceptate (Co-administration with drugs that are mainly metabolized by CYP3A4 may have elevated plasma concentrations when co-administered with saquinavir; these combinations should be used with caution).
No products indexed under this heading.

Erythromycin Lactobionate (Co-administration with drugs that are mainly metabolized by CYP3A4 may have elevated plasma concentrations when co-administered with saquinavir; these combinations should be used with caution).
No products indexed under this heading.

Erythromycin Stearate (Co-administration with drugs that are mainly metabolized by CYP3A4 may have elevated plasma concentrations when co-administered with saquinavir; these combinations should be used with caution). Products include:
Erythrocin Stearate Filmtab Tablets 453

Estradiol (Co-administration with drugs that are mainly metabolized by CYP3A4 may have elevated plasma concentrations when co-administered with saquinavir; these combinations should be used with caution). Products include:
Angeliq Tablets 762
Climara Transdermal System 771
Climara Pro Transdermal System 776
Estrasorb Topical Emulsion 1147
Estring Vaginal Ring 2635
Menostar Transdermal System 782
Vagifem Tablets 2334

Estradiol Benzoate (Co-administration with drugs that are mainly metabolized by CYP3A4 may have elevated plasma concentrations when co-administered with saquinavir; these combinations should be used with caution).
No products indexed under this heading.

Estradiol Cypionate (Co-administration with drugs that are mainly metabolized by CYP3A4 may have elevated plasma concentrations when co-administered with saquinavir; these combinations should be used with caution).
No products indexed under this heading.

Estradiol Valerate (Co-administration with drugs that are mainly metabolized by CYP3A4 may have elevated plasma concentrations when co-administered with saquinavir; these combinations should be used with caution).
No products indexed under this heading.

Ethinyl Estradiol (Concomitant administration with saquinavir/ritonavir may lead to decreased ethinyl estradiol levels. Alternative or additional contraceptive measures should be used when estrogen-based oral contraceptives and saquinavir/ritonavir are co-administered). Products include:
Mircette Tablets 1066
NuvaRing 2340
Ortho-Cyclen/Ortho Tri-Cyclen 2429
Ortho Evra Transdermal System 2417
Ortho Tri-Cyclen Lo Tablets 2436
Seasonique Tablets 1077
Yasmin 28 Tablets 796
Yaz Tablets 803

Ethosuximide (Co-administration with drugs that are mainly metabolized by CYP3A4 may have elevated plasma concentrations when co-administered with saquinavir; these combinations should be used with caution).
No products indexed under this heading.

Ethynodiol Diacetate (Concomitant administration with saquinavir/ritonavir may lead to decreased ethinyl estradiol levels. Alternative or additional contraceptive measures should be used when estrogen-based oral contraceptives and saquinavir/ritonavir are co-administered).
No products indexed under this heading.

Etoposide (Co-administration with drugs that are mainly metabolized by CYP3A4 may have elevated plasma concentrations when co-administered with saquinavir; these combinations should be used with caution).
No products indexed under this heading.

Etoposide Phosphate (Co-administration with drugs that are mainly metabolized by CYP3A4 may have elevated plasma concentrations when co-administered with saquinavir; these combinations should be used with caution).
No products indexed under this heading.

Felbamate (Co-administration with compounds that are potent inducers of CYP3A4 may result in decreased plasma levels of saquinavir).
No products indexed under this heading.

Felodipine (Concomitant administration with saquinavir may lead to increased felodipine levels; caution is warranted and clinical monitoring of patient is recommended).
No products indexed under this heading.

Fentanyl (Co-administration with drugs that are mainly metabolized by CYP3A4 may have elevated plasma concentrations when co-administered with saquinavir; these combinations should be used with caution). Products include:
Duragesic Transdermal System 2373
Ionsys Transdermal System 2379

Fentanyl Citrate (Co-administration with drugs that are mainly metabolized by CYP3A4 may have elevated plasma concentrations when co-administered with saquinavir; these combinations should be used with caution). Products include:
Actiq 979

Flecainide Acetate (Inhibition of CYP3A4 by saquinavir could result in elevated plasma concentrations of flecainide, potentially causing serious or life-threatening reactions; concurrent use is contraindicated). Products include:
Tambocor Tablets 1856

Fludrocortisone Acetate (Co-administration with compounds that are potent inducers of CYP3A4 may result in decreased plasma levels of saquinavir).
No products indexed under this heading.

Flurazepam Hydrochloride (Concomitant administration with saquinavir may lead to increased flurazepam levels; a decrease in flurazepam dose may be needed). Products include:
Dalmane Capsules 3342

Fluticasone Propionate (Concomitant use of ritonavir with saquinavir may significantly increase plasma fluticasone proprionate exposures, resulting in significantly decreased serum cortisol concentrations. Systemic corticosteroid effects including Cushing's syndrome and adrenal suppression have been reported. Therefore, co-administration of fluticasone proprionate and saquinavir with ritonavir is not recommended unless the potential benefit to the patient outweighs the risk of systemic corticosteroid side effects). Products include:
Advair Diskus 100/50 1308
Advair Diskus 250/50 1308
Advair Diskus 500/50 1308
Advair HFA Inhalation Aerosol 1318
Cutivate Cream 2662
Cutivate Lotion 0.05% 2664
Cutivate Ointment 2665
Flonase Nasal Spray 1440
Flovent Diskus 1443

Fosamprenavir Calcium (Concomitant administration with saquinavir may cause decreased plasma concentrations of fosamprenavir). Products include:
Lexiva Tablets 1505

Fosphenytoin Sodium (Concomitant administration with saquinavir may decrease saquinavir levels. Use with caution since saquinavir may be less effective due to decreased saquinavir plasma concentrations).
No products indexed under this heading.

Garlic Extract (Garlic capsules should not be used while taking saquinavir as the sole protease inhibitor due to the increased risk of decreased saquinavir plasma concentrations).
No products indexed under this heading.

Garlic Oil (Garlic capsules should not be used while taking saquinavir as the sole protease inhibitor due to the increased risk of decreased saquinavir plasma concentrations).
No products indexed under this heading.

Haloperidol (Co-administration with drugs that are mainly metabolized by CYP3A4 may have elevated plasma concentrations when co-administered with saquinavir; these combinations should be used with caution).
No products indexed under this heading.

Haloperidol Decanoate (Co-administration with drugs that are mainly metabolized by CYP3A4 may have elevated plasma concentrations when co-administered with saquinavir; these combinations should be used with caution).
No products indexed under this heading.

Haloperidol Lactate (Co-administration with drugs that are mainly metabolized by CYP3A4 may have elevated plasma concentrations when co-administered with saquinavir; these combinations should be used with caution).
No products indexed under this heading.

Hydrocortisone (Co-administration with compounds that are potent inducers of CYP3A4 may result in decreased plasma levels of saquinavir). Products include:
Colocort Rectal Suspension, USP (Retention) 100 mg/60 mL 2476
Hydrocortone Tablets 1989
Preparation H Hydrocortisone Cream .... ▣ 646

Hydrocortisone Acetate (Co-administration with compounds that are potent inducers of CYP3A4 may result in decreased plasma levels of saquinavir). Products include:
Analpram-HC 1159
Pramosone 1161
ProctoFoam-HC 3099

Hydrocortisone Butyrate (Co-administration with compounds that are potent inducers of CYP3A4 may result in decreased plasma levels of saquinavir). Products include:
Locoid Lipocream Cream 1160

Hydrocortisone Cypionate (Co-administration with compounds that are potent inducers of CYP3A4 may result in decreased plasma levels of saquinavir).
No products indexed under this heading.

Hydrocortisone Hemisuccinate (Co-administration with compounds that are potent inducers of CYP3A4 may result in decreased plasma levels of saquinavir).
No products indexed under this heading.

Hydrocortisone Probutate (Co-administration with compounds that are potent inducers of CYP3A4 may result in decreased plasma levels of saquinavir).
No products indexed under this heading.

Hydrocortisone Sodium Phosphate (Co-administration with compounds that are potent inducers of CYP3A4 may result in decreased plasma levels of saquinavir).

No products indexed under this heading.

Hydrocortisone Sodium Succinate (Co-administration with compounds that are potent inducers of CYP3A4 may result in decreased plasma levels of saquinavir).

No products indexed under this heading.

Hydrocortisone Valerate (Co-administration with compounds that are potent inducers of CYP3A4 may result in decreased plasma levels of saquinavir).

No products indexed under this heading.

Hypericum (Co-administration of protease inhibitors with St. John's Wort is expected to substantially decrease protease inhibitor concentrations and may result in suboptimal levels of protease inhibitor and loss of virologic response and possible resistance to protease inhibitors; concurrent use is not recommended). Products include:

Hypericum Perforatum (Co-administration with compounds that are potent inducers of CYP3A4 may result in decreased plasma levels of saquinavir).

No products indexed under this heading.

Imipramine Hydrochloride (Concomitant administration with saquinavir may cause increased levels of imipramine; therapeutic concentration monitoring is recommended for tricyclic antidepressants when co-administered with saquinavir).

No products indexed under this heading.

Imipramine Pamoate (Concomitant administration with saquinavir may cause increased levels of imipramine; therapeutic concentration monitoring is recommended for tricyclic antidepressants when co-administered with saquinavir).

No products indexed under this heading.

Indinavir Sulfate (Co-administration with drugs that are mainly metabolized by CYP3A4 may have elevated plasma concentrations when co-administered with saquinavir; these combinations should be used with caution). Products include:

Isradipine (Concomitant administration with saquinavir may lead to increased isradipine levels; caution is warranted and clinical monitoring of patient is recommended). Products include:

Itraconazole (Concomitant administration with saquinavir may lead to increased saquinavir levels).

No products indexed under this heading.

Ketoconazole (Concomitant administration with saquinavir may lead to increased saquinavir levels). Products include:

Levonorgestrel (Concomitant administration with saquinavir/ritonavir may lead to decreased ethi-

nyl estradiol levels. Alternative or additional contraceptive measures should be used when estrogen-based oral contraceptives and saquinavir/ritonavir are co-administered). Products include:

Lidocaine (Caution is warranted and therapeutic concentration monitoring is recommended for antiarrhythmics given with saquinavir). Products include:

Lidocaine Hydrochloride (Caution is warranted and therapeutic concentration monitoring is recommended for antiarrhythmics given with saquinavir).

No products indexed under this heading.

Lovastatin (Co-administration of Invirase and lovastatin may result in increased concentrations of statins; potential for, in rare cases, severe adverse events, such as myopathy including rhabdomyolysis; concomitant use is not recommended). Products include:

Mephenytoin (Co-administration with compounds that are potent inducers of CYP3A4 may result in decreased plasma levels of saquinavir).

No products indexed under this heading.

Mestranol (Concomitant administration with saquinavir/ritonavir may lead to decreased ethinyl estradiol levels. Alternative or additional contraceptive measures should be used when estrogen-based oral contraceptives and saquinavir/ritonavir are co-administered).

No products indexed under this heading.

Methadone Hydrochloride (Concomitant administration with saquinavir/ritonavir may lead to decreased methadone levels. Dosage of methadone may need to be increased when co-administered with saquinavir/ritonavir).

No products indexed under this heading.

Methsuximide (Co-administration with compounds that are potent inducers of CYP3A4 may result in decreased plasma levels of saquinavir).

No products indexed under this heading.

Methylergonovine Maleate (Inhibition of CYP3A4 by saquinavir could result in increased ergot derivatives plasma levels and create the potential for serious and/or life-threatening reactions; concurrent use is contraindicated).

No products indexed under this heading.

Methylprednisolone (Co-administration with compounds that are potent inducers of CYP3A4 may result in decreased plasma levels of saquinavir).

No products indexed under this heading.

Methylprednisolone Acetate (Co-administration with compounds that

are potent inducers of CYP3A4 may result in decreased plasma levels of saquinavir). Products include:

Methylprednisolone Sodium Succinate (Co-administration with compounds that are potent inducers of CYP3A4 may result in decreased plasma levels of saquinavir).

No products indexed under this heading.

Methysergide Maleate (Inhibition of CYP3A4 by saquinavir could result in increased ergot derivatives plasma levels and create the potential for serious and/or life-threatening reactions; concurrent use is contraindicated).

No products indexed under this heading.

Mibefradil Dihydrochloride (Potential for elevated plasma concentrations of compounds that are substrate of CYP3A4, such as calcium channel blockers).

No products indexed under this heading.

Midazolam Hydrochloride (Inhibition of CYP3A4 by saquinavir could result in increased midazolam plasma levels and create the potential for serious and/or life-threatening reactions; concurrent use is contraindicated).

No products indexed under this heading.

Modafinil (Co-administration with compounds that are potent inducers of CYP3A4 may result in decreased plasma levels of saquinavir). Products include:

Nefazodone Hydrochloride (Co-administration with drugs that are mainly metabolized by CYP3A4 may have elevated plasma concentrations when co-administered with saquinavir; these combinations should be used with caution).

No products indexed under this heading.

Nelfinavir Mesylate (Co-administration has resulted in an 18% increase in nelfinavir plasma AUC and a 392% increase in saquinavir plasma AUC; currently, there are no safety and efficacy data available from use of this combination). Products include:

Nevirapine (Co-administration has resulted in a 24% decrease in saquinavir plasma AUC; currently, there are no safety and efficacy data available from use of this combination). Products include:

Nicardipine (Concomitant administration with saquinavir may lead to increased nicardipine levels; caution is warranted and clinical monitoring of patient is recommended).

No products indexed under this heading.

Nicardipine Hydrochloride (Concomitant administration with saquinavir may lead to increased nicardipine levels; caution is warranted and clinical monitoring of patient is recommended). Products include:

Nifedipine (Concomitant administration with saquinavir may lead to

increased nifedipine levels; caution is warranted and clinical monitoring of patient is recommended). Products include:

Nimodipine (Concomitant administration with saquinavir may lead to increased nimodipine levels; caution is warranted and clinical monitoring of patient is recommended). Products include:

Nisoldipine (Concomitant administration with saquinavir may lead to increased nisoldipine levels; caution is warranted and clinical monitoring of patient is recommended). Products include:

Nitrendipine (Co-administration with drugs that are mainly metabolized by CYP3A4 may have elevated plasma concentrations when co-administered with saquinavir; these combinations should be used with caution).

No products indexed under this heading.

Norethindrone (Concomitant administration with saquinavir/ ritonavir may lead to decreased ethinyl estradiol levels. Alternative or additional contraceptive measures should be used when estrogen-based oral contraceptives and saquinavir/ritonavir are co-administered). Products include:

Norethindrone Acetate (Co-administration with drugs that are mainly metabolized by CYP3A4 may have elevated plasma concentrations when co-administered with saquinavir; these combinations should be used with caution).

No products indexed under this heading.

Norethynodrel (Concomitant administration with saquinavir/ ritonavir may lead to decreased ethinyl estradiol levels. Alternative or additional contraceptive measures should be used when estrogen-based oral contraceptives and saquinavir/ritonavir are co-administered).

No products indexed under this heading.

Norgestimate (Concomitant administration with saquinavir/ritonavir may lead to decreased ethinyl estradiol levels. Alternative or additional contraceptive measures should be used when estrogen-based oral contraceptives and saquinavir/ritonavir are co-administered). Products include:

Norgestrel (Concomitant administration with saquinavir/ritonavir may lead to decreased ethinyl estradiol levels. Alternative or additional contraceptive measures should be used when estrogen-based oral contraceptives and saquinavir/ritonavir are co-administered).

No products indexed under this heading.

Ondansetron (Co-administration with drugs that are mainly metabolized by CYP3A4 may have elevated plasma concentrations when co-administered with saquinavir; these combinations should be used with caution). Products include:

Zofran ODT Orally Disintegrating Tablets ... 1639

Ondansetron Hydrochloride (Co-administration with drugs that are mainly metabolized by CYP3A4 may have elevated plasma concentrations when co-administered with saquinavir; these combinations should be used with caution). Products include:

Zofran Injection ... 1634
Zofran ... 1639

Oxcarbazepine (Co-administration with compounds that are potent inducers of CYP3A4 may result in decreased plasma levels of saquinavir). Products include:

Trileptal Tablets ... 2300
Trileptal Oral Suspension ... 2300

Paclitaxel (Co-administration with drugs that are mainly metabolized by CYP3A4 may have elevated plasma concentrations when co-administered with saquinavir; these combinations should be used with caution).

No products indexed under this heading.

Phenobarbital (Anticonvulsants, such as phenobarbital, may decrease saquinavir plasma concentrations). Products include:

Donnatal Extentabs ... 2493

Phenobarbital Sodium (Co-administration with compounds that are potent inducers of CYP3A4 may result in decreased plasma levels of saquinavir).

No products indexed under this heading.

Phenytoin (Concomitant administration with saquinavir may decrease saquinavir levels. Use with caution since saquinavir may be less effective due to decreased saquinavir plasma concentrations).

No products indexed under this heading.

Phenytoin Sodium (Concomitant administration with saquinavir may decrease saquinavir levels. Use with caution since saquinavir may be less effective due to decreased saquinavir plasma concentrations). Products include:

Phenytek Capsules ... 2160

Pimozide (Inhibition of CYP3A4 by saquinavir could result in elevated plasma concentrations of pimozide, potentially causing serious or life-threatening reactions; concurrent use is contraindicated).

No products indexed under this heading.

Polyestradiol Phosphate (Co-administration with drugs that are mainly metabolized by CYP3A4 may have elevated plasma concentrations when co-administered with saquinavir; these combinations should be used with caution).

No products indexed under this heading.

Prednisolone Acetate (Co-administration with compounds that are potent inducers of CYP3A4 may result in decreased plasma levels of saquinavir). Products include:

Blephamide Ophthalmic Ointment ... 568
Blephamide Ophthalmic Suspension ... 569
Poly-Pred Ophthalmic Suspension ... ⊙233
Pred Forte Ophthalmic Suspension ... ⊙235
Pred Mild Ophthalmic Suspension ... ⊙238
Pred-G Ophthalmic Ointment ... ⊙237
Pred-G Ophthalmic Suspension ... ⊙236

Prednisolone Sodium Phosphate (Co-administration with compounds that are potent inducers of CYP3A4 may result in decreased plasma levels of saquinavir).

No products indexed under this heading.

Prednisolone Tebutate (Co-administration with compounds that are potent inducers of CYP3A4 may result in decreased plasma levels of saquinavir).

No products indexed under this heading.

Prednisone (Co-administration with compounds that are potent inducers of CYP3A4 may result in decreased plasma levels of saquinavir).

No products indexed under this heading.

Primidone (Co-administration with compounds that are potent inducers of CYP3A4 may result in decreased plasma levels of saquinavir).

No products indexed under this heading.

Propafenone Hydrochloride (Inhibition of CYP3A4 by saquinavir could result in elevated plasma concentrations of propafenone, potentially causing serious or life-threatening reactions; concurrent use is contraindicated). Products include:

Rythmol SR Capsules ... 2727

Quinidine (Inhibition of CYP3A4 by saquinavir could result in elevated plasma concentrations of quinidine, potentially causing serious or life-threatening reactions; concurrent use is contraindicated).

No products indexed under this heading.

Quinidine Gluconate (Inhibition of CYP3A4 by saquinavir could result in elevated plasma concentrations of quinidine, potentially causing serious or life-threatening reactions; concurrent use is contraindicated).

No products indexed under this heading.

Quinidine Hydrochloride (Inhibition of CYP3A4 by saquinavir could result in elevated plasma concentrations of quinidine, potentially causing serious or life-threatening reactions; concurrent use is contraindicated).

No products indexed under this heading.

Quinidine Polygalacturonate (Inhibition of CYP3A4 by saquinavir could result in elevated plasma concentrations of quinidine, potentially causing serious or life-threatening reactions; concurrent use is contraindicated).

No products indexed under this heading.

Quinidine Sulfate (Inhibition of CYP3A4 by saquinavir could result in elevated plasma concentrations of quinidine, potentially causing serious or life-threatening reactions; concurrent use is contraindicated).

No products indexed under this heading.

Ranitidine Hydrochloride (Concomitant administration may cause increased saquinavir levels; no dosage adjustment of saquinavir is recommended). Products include:

Zantac ... 1624
Zantac Injection ... 1619
Zantac Injection Pharmacy Bulk Package ... 1622

Rapamycin (Concomitant administration with saquinavir may lead to increased levels of rapamycin. Therapeutic concentration monitoring is recommended for all immunosuppressant agents when co-administered with saquinavir).

No products indexed under this heading.

Rifabutin (Concomitant administration with saquinavir may lead to decreased saquinavir and/or increased rifabutin levels. Saquinavir should not be given as the sole protease inhibitor to patients taking rifabutin).

No products indexed under this heading.

Rifampicin (Co-administration with compounds that are potent inducers of CYP3A4 may result in decreased plasma levels of saquinavir).

No products indexed under this heading.

Rifampin (Inhibition of CYP3A4 by saquinavir could result in elevated plasma concentrations of rifampin, potentially causing severe hepatocellular toxicity or serious, life-threatening reactions).

No products indexed under this heading.

Rifapentine (Co-administration with compounds that are potent inducers of CYP3A4 may result in decreased plasma levels of saquinavir).

No products indexed under this heading.

Ritonavir (Combination therapy in HIV-infected patients has resulted in AUC values which were at least 17-fold greater than historical AUC values from patients who received saquinavir without ritonavir). Products include:

Kaletra ... 476
Norvir ... 503

Saquinavir (Co-administration with drugs that are mainly metabolized by CYP3A4 may have elevated plasma concentrations when co-administered with saquinavir; these combinations should be used with caution).

No products indexed under this heading.

Sertraline Hydrochloride (Co-administration with drugs that are mainly metabolized by CYP3A4 may have elevated plasma concentrations when co-administered with saquinavir; these combinations should be used with caution). Products include:

Zoloft ... 2586

Sildenafil Citrate (Concomitant administration may lead to increased sildenafil levels; use sildenafil with caution at reduced doses of 25mg every 48 hours with increased monitoring of adverse events when co-administered with saquinavir). Products include:

Revatio Tablets ... 2557
Viagra Tablets ... 2573

Simvastatin (Co-administration of Invirase and simvastatin may result in increased concentrations of statins; potential for, in rare cases, severe adverse events, such as myopathy including rhabdomyolysis; concomitant use is not recommended). Products include:

Vytorin 10/10 Tablets ... 2114
Vytorin 10/10 Tablets ... 3077
Vytorin 10/20 Tablets ... 2114
Vytorin 10/20 Tablets ... 3077
Vytorin 10/40 Tablets ... 2114
Vytorin 10/40 Tablets ... 3077
Vytorin 10/80 Tablets ... 2114
Vytorin 10/80 Tablets ... 3077
Zocor Tablets ... 2105

Sirolimus (Co-administration with drugs that are mainly metabolized by CYP3A4 may have elevated plasma concentrations when co-administered with saquinavir; these combinations should be used with caution). Products include:

Rapamune Oral Solution and Tablets ... 3475

Sulfinpyrazone (Co-administration with compounds that are potent inducers of CYP3A4 may result in decreased plasma levels of saquinavir).

No products indexed under this heading.

Tacrolimus (Concomitant administration with saquinavir may lead to increased levels of tacrolimus. Therapeutic concentration monitoring is recommended for all immunosuppressant agents when co-administered with saquinavir). Products include:

Prograf Capsules and Injection ... 632
Protopic Ointment ... 638

Tadalafil (Concomitant administration may lead to increased tadalafil levels; use tadalafil with caution at reduced doses of no more than 10mg every 72 hours with increased monitoring of adverse events when co-administered with saquinavir). Products include:

Cialis Tablets ... 1838

Tamoxifen Citrate (Co-administration with drugs that are mainly metabolized by CYP3A4 may have elevated plasma concentrations when co-administered with saquinavir; these combinations should be used with caution). Products include:

Soltamox Oral Solution ... 3527

Terfenadine (Inhibition of CYP3A4 by saquinavir could result in increased terfenadine plasma levels and create the potential for serious and/or life-threatening reactions, such as rare cases of serious cardiovascular adverse events; concurrent use is contraindicated).

No products indexed under this heading.

Theophylline (Co-administration with compounds that are potent inducers of CYP3A4 may result in decreased plasma levels of saquinavir).

No products indexed under this heading.

Tiagabine Hydrochloride (Co-administration with drugs that are mainly metabolized by CYP3A4 may have elevated plasma concentrations when co-administered with saquinavir; these combinations should be used with caution). Products include:

Gabitril Tablets ... 984

Tolterodine Tartrate (Co-administration with drugs that are mainly metabolized by CYP3A4 may have elevated plasma concentrations when co-administered with saquinavir; these combinations should be used with caution). Products include:

Detrol Tablets ... 2628
Detrol LA Capsules ... 2631

Trazodone Hydrochloride (Concomitant use of trazadone and

saquinavir with ritonaivir may increase plasma concentrations of trazadone. Adverse events of nausea, dizziness, hypotension, and syncope have been observed following co-administration of trazadone and ritonavir. If trazadone is used with CYP3A4 inhibitors such as saquinavir with ritonavir, the combination should be used with caution and lower doses of trazadone should be considered).
No products indexed under this heading.

Triamcinolone (Co-administration with compounds that are potent inducers of CYP3A4 may result in decreased plasma levels of saquinavir).
No products indexed under this heading.

Triamcinolone Acetonide (Co-administration with compounds that are potent inducers of CYP3A4 may result in decreased plasma levels of saquinavir). Products include:
Azmacort Inhalation Aerosol 1726
Nasacort AQ Nasal Spray 2922

Triamcinolone Diacetate (Co-administration with compounds that are potent inducers of CYP3A4 may result in decreased plasma levels of saquinavir).
No products indexed under this heading.

Triamcinolone Hexacetonide (Co-administration with compounds that are potent inducers of CYP3A4 may result in decreased plasma levels of saquinavir).
No products indexed under this heading.

Triazolam (Inhibition of CYP3A4 by saquinavir could result in increased triazolam plasma levels and create the potential for serious and/or life-threatening reactions; concurrent use is contraindicated).
No products indexed under this heading.

Troglitazone (Co-administration with compounds that are potent inducers of CYP3A4 may result in decreased plasma levels of saquinavir).
No products indexed under this heading.

Vardenafil Hydrochloride (Concomitant administration may lead to increased vardenafil levels; use vardenafil with caution at reduced doses of no more than 2.5mg every 72 hours with increased monitoring of adverse events when co-administered with saquinavir). Products include:
Levitra Tablets 3034

Verapamil Hydrochloride (Concomitant administration with saquinavir may lead to increased verapamil levels; caution is warranted and clinical monitoring of patient is recommended). Products include:
Covera-HS Tablets 3139
Tarka Tablets 524
Verelan PM Extended-Release Capsules, Controlled-Onset........... 3106

Vinblastine Sulfate (Co-administration with drugs that are mainly metabolized by CYP3A4 may have elevated plasma concentrations when co-administered with saquinavir; these combinations should be used with caution).
No products indexed under this heading.

Vincristine Sulfate (Co-administration with drugs that are mainly metabolized by CYP3A4 may have elevated plasma concentrations when co-administered with saquinavir; these combinations should be used with caution).
No products indexed under this heading.

Warfarin Sodium (Concentrations of warfarin may be affected. It is recommended that INR be monitored). Products include:
Coumadin for Injection 898
Coumadin Tablets 898

Food Interactions

Food, unspecified (Saquinavir 24-hour AUC and Cmax following the administration of a high calorie meal were an average two times higher than after a lower calorie, lower fat meal; the effect of food has been shown to persist for up to 2 hours).

INVIRASE TABLETS
(Saquinavir Mesylate) 2772
See Invirase Capsules

IONSYS TRANSDERMAL SYSTEM
(Fentanyl) 2379
May interact with anesthetics, cytochrome p450 3a4 inducers (selected), cytochrome p450 3a4 inhibitors (selected), hypnotics and sedatives, narcotic analgesics, phenothiazines, sedating antihistamines, skeletal muscle relaxants, tranquilizers, and certain other agents. Compounds in these categories include:

Acetazolamide (The concomitant use of fentanyl with CYP3A4 inhibitors may result in a decreases in fentanyl clearance, which could increase or prolong adverse drug effects including serious respiratory depression. In this situation, special patient care and observation is appropriate).
No products indexed under this heading.

Acrivastine (The concomitant use of other central nervous system depressants, such as sedating antihistamines, may produce additive depressant effects. Hypoventilation, hypotension, profound sedation, and coma may occur. Therefore, use of concomitant CNS depressants requires individual adjustment of dosage of the concomitant medication and observation of a given patient).
No products indexed under this heading.

Alfentanil Hydrochloride (The concomitant use of other central nervous system depressants, such as opiods, may produce additive depressant effects. Hypoventilation, hypotension, profound sedation, and coma may occur. Therefore, use of concomitant CNS depressants requires individual adjustment of dosage of the concomitant medication and observation of a given patient).
No products indexed under this heading.

Allium sativum (Co-administration with agents that induce CYP3A4 activity may cause increased clearance of fentanyl and reduce its efficacy).
No products indexed under this heading.

Alprazolam (The concomitant use of other central nervous system depressants, such as tranquilizers, may produce additive depressant effects. Hypoventilation, hypotension, profound sedation, and coma may occur. Therefore, use of concomitant CNS depressants requires individual adjustment of dosage of the concomitant medication and observation of a given patient). Products include:
Niravam Orally Disintegrating Tablets 3092

Amiodarone Hydrochloride (The concomitant use of fentanyl with CYP3A4 inhibitors may result in a decreases in fentanyl clearance, which could increase or prolong adverse drug effects including serious respiratory depression. In this situation, special patient care and observation is appropriate).
No products indexed under this heading.

Amprenavir (The concomitant use of fentanyl with CYP3A4 inhibitors may result in a decreases in fentanyl clearance, which could increase or prolong adverse drug effects including serious respiratory depression. In this situation, special patient care and observation is appropriate). Products include:
Agenerase Capsules 1327
Agenerase Oral Solution 1332

Anastrozole (The concomitant use of fentanyl with CYP3A4 inhibitors may result in a decreases in fentanyl clearance, which could increase or prolong adverse drug effects including serious respiratory depression. In this situation, special patient care and observation is appropriate). Products include:
Arimidex Tablets 673

Aprepitant (The concomitant use of fentanyl with CYP3A4 inhibitors may result in a decreases in fentanyl clearance, which could increase or prolong adverse drug effects including serious respiratory depression. In this situation, special patient care and observation is appropriate). Products include:
Emend Capsules 1963

Azatadine Maleate (The concomitant use of other central nervous system depressants, such as sedating antihistamines, may produce additive depressant effects. Hypoventilation, hypotension, profound sedation, and coma may occur. Therefore, use of concomitant CNS depressants requires individual adjustment of dosage of the concomitant medication and observation of a given patient).
No products indexed under this heading.

Baclofen (The concomitant use of other central nervous system depressants, such as skeletal muscle relaxants, may produce additive depressant effects. Hypoventilation, hypotension, profound sedation, and coma may occur. Therefore, use of concomitant CNS depressants requires individual adjustment of dosage of the concomitant medication and observation of a given patient).
No products indexed under this heading.

Betamethasone Acetate (Co-administration with agents that induce CYP3A4 activity may cause increased clearance of fentanyl and reduce its efficacy).
No products indexed under this heading.

Betamethasone Sodium Phosphate (Co-administration with agents that induce CYP3A4 activity may cause increased clearance of fentanyl and reduce its efficacy).
No products indexed under this heading.

Bromodiphenhydramine Hydrochloride (The concomitant use of other central nervous system depressants, such as sedating antihistamines, may produce additive depressant effects. Hypoventilation, hypotension, profound sedation, and coma may occur. Therefore, use of concomitant CNS depressants requires individual adjustment of dosage of the concomitant medication and observation of a given patient).
No products indexed under this heading.

Brompheniramine Maleate (The concomitant use of other central nervous system depressants, such as sedating antihistamines, may produce additive depressant effects. Hypoventilation, hypotension, profound sedation, and coma may occur. Therefore, use of concomitant CNS depressants requires individual adjustment of dosage of the concomitant medication and observation of a given patient). Products include:
Children's Dimetapp Cold & Allergy Elixir 730
Children's Dimetapp Cold & Allergy Chewable Tablets............. 730
Children's Dimetapp DM Cold & Cough Elixir 731

Buprenorphine Hydrochloride (The concomitant use of other central nervous system depressants, such as opiods, may produce additive depressant effects. Hypoventilation, hypotension, profound sedation, and coma may occur. Therefore, use of concomitant CNS depressants requires individual adjustment of dosage of the concomitant medication and observation of a given patient). Products include:
Buprenex Injectable 2716
Suboxone Tablets 2717
Subutex Tablets 2717

Buspirone Hydrochloride (The concomitant use of other central nervous system depressants, such as tranquilizers, may produce additive depressant effects. Hypoventilation, hypotension, profound sedation, and coma may occur. Therefore, use of concomitant CNS depressants requires individual adjustment of dosage of the concomitant medication and observation of a given patient).
No products indexed under this heading.

Carbamazepine (Co-administration with agents that induce CYP3A4 activity may cause increased clearance of fentanyl and reduce its efficacy). Products include:
Carbatrol Capsules 3171
Equetro Extended-Release Capsules.................................... 3180
Tegretol/Tegretol-XR 2295

Carisoprodol (The concomitant use of other central nervous system depressants, such as skeletal muscle relaxants, may produce additive depressant effects. Hypoventilation, hypotension, profound sedation, and coma may occur. Therefore, use of concomitant CNS depressants requires individual adjustment of dosage of the concomitant medication and observation of a given patient).
No products indexed under this heading.

Chlordiazepoxide (The concomitant use of other central nervous system depressants, such as tranquilizers, may produce additive depressant effects. Hypoventilation, hypotension, profound sedation, and coma may occur. Therefore, use of concomitant CNS depressants requires individual adjustment of dosage of the concomitant medication and observation of a given patient).
No products indexed under this heading.

Chlordiazepoxide Hydrochloride (The concomitant use of other central nervous system depressants, such as tranquilizers, may produce additive depressant effects. Hypoventilation, hypotension, profound sedation, and coma may occur. Therefore, use of concomitant CNS depressants requires individual adjustment of dosage of the concomitant medication and observation of a given patient). Products include:
Librium Capsules **3347**

Chlorpheniramine Maleate (The concomitant use of other central nervous system depressants, such as sedating antihistamines, may produce additive depressant effects. Hypoventilation, hypotension, profound sedation, and coma may occur. Therefore, use of concomitant CNS depressants requires individual adjustment of dosage of the concomitant medication and observation of a given patient). Products include:
Advil Allergy Sinus Caplets .... ■**770**
Advil Multi-Symptom Cold Caplets..................................... ■**770**
BC Allergy Sinus Cold Powder .... ■**677**
Comtrex Maximum Strength Cold & Cough Day/Night Caplets - Night Formulation........................ ■**726**
Comtrex Maximum Strength Day/Night Severe Cold & Sinus Caplets - Night Formulation......... ■**725**
Contac Cold and Flu Maximum Strength Caplets........................ ■**728**
Contac Cold and Flu Day and Night Caplets (Night Formulation Only)....................... ■**727**
Children's Dimetapp Long Acting Cough Plus Cold Syrup.............. ■**731**
Robitussin Cough & Cold Long-Acting Liquid..................... ■**735**
Robitussin Cough & Allergy Syrup .. ■**736**
Robitussin Cough & Cold Nighttime Liquid......................... ■**736**
Robitussin Cough, Cold & Flu Nighttime Liquid........................ ■**738**
Robitussin Pediatric Cough & Cold Long-Acting Liquid.............. ■**735**
Robitussin Pediatric Cough & Cold Nighttime Liquid................. ■**736**
Triaminic Cold & Allergy Liquid .... ■**746**
Triaminic Cough & Runny Nose Softchews.................................. ■**748**
Children's Tylenol Plus Flu Oral Suspension................................ ■**749**
Tylenol Allergy Multi-Symptom Caplets with Cool Burst and Gelcaps...................................... **1872**
Children's Tylenol Plus Cold Suspension Liquid........................ **1879**
Children's Tylenol Plus Cough & Runny Nose Suspension Liquid..... **1879**
Children's Tylenol Plus Flu Suspension Liquid........................ **1881**
Children's Tylenol Plus Multi-Symptom Cold Suspension Liquid........................ **1879**
Tylenol Cold Head Congestion Nighttime Caplets with Cool Burst.. **1873**
Tylenol Cold Multi-Symptom Nighttime Caplets with Cool Burst.. **1874**
Tylenol Sinus Congestion & Pain Nighttime Caplets with Cool Burst.. **1876**
Vicks 44M Cough, Cold & Flu Relief Liquid................................ **2680**
Pediatric Vicks 44m Cough & Cold Relief Liquid......................... **2676**
Children's Vicks NyQuil Cold/Cough Relief...................... ■**756**
Children's Vicks NyQuil Cold/Cough Relief Liquid............ **2680**
Zicam Maximum Strength Flu Daytime.................................... ■**768**

Chlorpheniramine Polistirex (The concomitant use of other central nervous system depressants, such as sedating antihistamines, may produce additive depressant effects. Hypoventilation, hypotension, profound sedation, and coma may occur. Therefore, use of concomitant CNS depressants requires individual adjustment of dosage of the concomitant medication and observation of a given patient). Products include:
Tussionex Pennkinetic Extended-Release Suspension...... **3327**

Chlorpheniramine Tannate (The concomitant use of other central nervous system depressants, such as sedating antihistamines, may produce additive depressant effects. Hypoventilation, hypotension, profound sedation, and coma may occur. Therefore, use of concomitant CNS depressants requires individual adjustment of dosage of the concomitant medication and observation of a given patient).
No products indexed under this heading.

Chlorpromazine (The concomitant use of other central nervous system depressants, such as phenothiazines, may produce additive depressant effects. Hypoventilation, hypotension, profound sedation, and coma may occur. Therefore, use of concomitant CNS depressants requires individual adjustment of dosage of the concomitant medication and observation of a given patient).
No products indexed under this heading.

Chlorpromazine Hydrochloride (The concomitant use of other central nervous system depressants, such as phenothiazines, may produce additive depressant effects. Hypoventilation, hypotension, profound sedation, and coma may occur. Therefore, use of concomitant CNS depressants requires individual adjustment of dosage of the concomitant medication and observation of a given patient).
No products indexed under this heading.

Chlorprothixene (The concomitant use of other central nervous system depressants, such as tranquilizers, may produce additive depressant effects. Hypoventilation, hypotension, profound sedation, and coma may occur. Therefore, use of concomitant CNS depressants requires individual adjustment of dosage of the concomitant medication and observation of a given patient).
No products indexed under this heading.

Chlorprothixene Hydrochloride (The concomitant use of other central nervous system depressants, such as tranquilizers, may produce additive depressant effects. Hypoventilation, hypotension, profound sedation, and coma may occur. Therefore, use of concomitant CNS depressants requires individual adjustment of dosage of the concomitant medication and observation of a given patient).
No products indexed under this heading.

Chlorzoxazone (The concomitant use of other central nervous system depressants, such as skeletal muscle relaxants, may produce additive depressant effects. Hypoventilation, hypotension, profound sedation, and coma may occur. Therefore, use of concomitant CNS depressants requires individual adjustment of dosage of the concomitant medication and observation of a given patient).
No products indexed under this heading.

Cimetidine (The concomitant use of fentanyl with CYP3A4 inhibitors may result in a decreases in fentanyl clearance, which could increase or prolong adverse drug effects including serious respiratory depression. In this situation, special patient care and observation is appropriate). Products include:
Tagamet HB 200 Tablets .... ■**664**

Cimetidine Hydrochloride (The concomitant use of fentanyl with CYP3A4 inhibitors may result in a decreases in fentanyl clearance, which could increase or prolong adverse drug effects including serious respiratory depression. In this situation, special patient care and observation is appropriate).
No products indexed under this heading.

Ciprofloxacin (The concomitant use of fentanyl with CYP3A4 inhibitors may result in a decreases in fentanyl clearance, which could increase or prolong adverse drug effects including serious respiratory depression. In this situation, special patient care and observation is appropriate). Products include:
Cipro Oral Suspension **2977**
Cipro I.V. **2984**
Cipro XR Tablets **2990**
Ciprodex Otic Suspension **559**

Ciprofloxacin Hydrochloride (Co-administration with agents that induce CYP3A4 activity may cause increased clearance of fentanyl and reduce its efficacy). Products include:
Ciloxan Ophthalmic Ointment........... **559**
Ciloxan Ophthalmic Solution .... ⊙**206**
Cipro Tablets **2977**
Proquin XR Tablets **1153**

Cisplatin (Co-administration with agents that induce CYP3A4 activity may cause increased clearance of fentanyl and reduce its efficacy).
No products indexed under this heading.

Clarithromycin (The concomitant use of fentanyl with CYP3A4 inhibitors may result in a decreases in fentanyl clearance, which could increase or prolong adverse drug effects including serious respiratory depression. In this situation, special patient care and observation is appropriate). Products include:
Biaxin/Biaxin XL **402**
PREVPAC **3284**

Clemastine Fumarate (The concomitant use of other central nervous system depressants, such as sedating antihistamines, may produce additive depressant effects. Hypoventilation, hypotension, profound sedation, and coma may occur. Therefore, use of concomitant CNS depressants requires individual adjustment of dosage of the concomitant medication and observation of a given patient).
No products indexed under this heading.

Clorazepate Dipotassium (The concomitant use of other central nervous system depressants, such as tranquilizers, may produce additive depressant effects. Hypoventilation, hypotension, profound sedation, and coma may occur. Therefore, use of concomitant CNS depressants requires individual adjustment of dosage of the concomitant medication and observation of a given patient). Products include:
Tranxene **2474**

Clotrimazole (The concomitant use of fentanyl with CYP3A4 inhibitors may result in a decreases in fentanyl clearance, which could increase or prolong adverse drug effects including serious respiratory depression. In this situation, special patient care and observation is appropriate). Products include:
Desenex Athlete's Foot Cream .... ■**635**
Lotrimin **3039**
Lotrisone **3040**

Codeine Phosphate (The concomitant use of other central nervous system depressants, such as opiods, may produce additive depressant effects. Hypoventilation, hypotension, profound sedation, and coma may occur. Therefore, use of concomitant CNS depressants requires individual adjustment of dosage of the concomitant medication and observation of a given patient). Products include:
Tylenol with Codeine Tablets **2391**

Cortisone Acetate (Co-administration with agents that induce CYP3A4 activity may cause increased clearance of fentanyl and reduce its efficacy).
No products indexed under this heading.

Cyclobenzaprine Hydrochloride (The concomitant use of other central nervous system depressants, such as skeletal muscle relaxants, may produce additive depressant effects. Hypoventilation, hypotension, profound sedation, and coma may occur. Therefore, use of concomitant CNS depressants requires individual adjustment of dosage of the concomitant medication and observation of a given patient).
No products indexed under this heading.

Cyclosporine (The concomitant use of fentanyl with CYP3A4 inhibitors may result in a decreases in fentanyl clearance, which could increase or prolong adverse drug effects including serious respiratory depression. In this situation, special patient care and observation is appropriate). Products include:
Gengraf Capsules **459**
Neoral Oral Solution **2259**
Neoral Soft Gelatin Capsules **2259**
Restasis Ophthalmic Emulsion **575**
Sandimmune **2275**

Cyproheptadine Hydrochloride (The concomitant use of other central nervous system depressants, such as sedating antihistamines, may produce additive depressant effects. Hypoventilation, hypotension, profound sedation, and coma may occur. Therefore, use of concomitant CNS depressants requires individual adjustment of dosage of the concomitant medication and observation of a given patient).
No products indexed under this heading.

Dalfopristin (The concomitant use of fentanyl with CYP3A4 inhibitors may result in a decreases in fentanyl clearance, which could increase or prolong adverse drug effects including serious respiratory depression. In this situation, special patient care and observation is appropriate).
No products indexed under this heading.

Danazol (The concomitant use of fentanyl with CYP3A4 inhibitors may result in a decreases in fentanyl clearance, which could increase or prolong adverse drug effects including serious respiratory depression. In this situation, special patient care and observation is appropriate).
No products indexed under this heading.

Dantrolene Sodium (The concomitant use of other central nervous system depressants, such as skeletal muscle relaxants, may produce additive depressant effects. Hypoventilation, hypotension, profound sedation, and coma may occur. Therefore, use of concomitant CNS depressants requires individual adjustment of dosage of the concomitant medication and observation of a given patient). Products include:
- Dantrium Capsules **2694**
- Dantrium Intravenous **2695**

Delavirdine Mesylate (The concomitant use of fentanyl with CYP3A4 inhibitors may result in a decreases in fentanyl clearance, which could increase or prolong adverse drug effects including serious respiratory depression. In this situation, special patient care and observation is appropriate).
Products include:
- Rescriptor Tablets **2551**

Dexamethasone (Co-administration with agents that induce CYP3A4 activity may cause increased clearance of fentanyl and reduce its efficacy). Products include:
- Ciprodex Otic Suspension **559**
- Decadron Tablets **1951**
- TobraDex Ophthalmic Ointment **562**
- TobraDex Ophthalmic Suspension ... **563**

Dexamethasone Acetate (Co-administration with agents that induce CYP3A4 activity may cause increased clearance of fentanyl and reduce its efficacy).
No products indexed under this heading.

Dexamethasone Sodium Phosphate (Co-administration with agents that induce CYP3A4 activity may cause increased clearance of fentanyl and reduce its efficacy).
No products indexed under this heading.

Dexchlorpheniramine Maleate (The concomitant use of other central nervous system depressants, such as sedating antihistamines, may produce additive depressant effects. Hypoventilation, hypotension, profound sedation, and coma may occur. Therefore, use of concomitant CNS depressants requires individual adjustment of dosage of the concomitant medication and observation of a given patient).
No products indexed under this heading.

Dezocine (The concomitant use of other central nervous system depressants, such as opiods, may produce additive depressant effects. Hypoventilation, hypotension, profound sedation, and coma may occur. Therefore, use of concomitant CNS depressants requires individual adjustment of dosage of the concomitant medication and observation of a given patient).
No products indexed under this heading.

Diazepam (The concomitant use of other central nervous system depressants, such as tranquilizers, may produce additive depressant effects. Hypoventilation, hypotension, profound sedation, and coma may occur. Therefore, use of concomitant CNS depressants requires individual adjustment of dosage of the concomitant medication and observation of a given patient).
Products include:
- Diastat Rectal Delivery System **3343**
- Valium Tablets **2819**

Diltiazem Hydrochloride (The concomitant use of fentanyl with CYP3A4 inhibitors may result in a decreases in fentanyl clearance, which could increase or prolong adverse drug effects including serious respiratory depression. In this situation, special patient care and observation is appropriate).
Products include:
- Cardizem LA Extended Release Tablets **1728**
- Tiazac Capsules **1201**

Diltiazem Maleate (The concomitant use of fentanyl with CYP3A4 inhibitors may result in a decreases in fentanyl clearance, which could increase or prolong adverse drug effects including serious respiratory depression. In this situation, special patient care and observation is appropriate).
No products indexed under this heading.

Diphenhydramine Citrate (The concomitant use of other central nervous system depressants, such as sedating antihistamines, may produce additive depressant effects. Hypoventilation, hypotension, profound sedation, and coma may occur. Therefore, use of concomitant CNS depressants requires individual adjustment of dosage of the concomitant medication and observation of a given patient). Products include:
- Advil PM Caplets **615**
- Excedrin PM Caplets/Tablets/Geltabs **610**
- Goody's PM Powder for Pain with Sleeplessness **612**

Diphenhydramine Hydrochloride (The concomitant use of other central nervous system depressants, such as sedating antihistamines, may produce additive depressant effects. Hypoventilation, hypotension, profound sedation, and coma may occur. Therefore, use of concomitant CNS depressants requires individual adjustment of dosage of the concomitant medication and observation of a given patient).
Products include:
- Nytol QuickCaps Caplets **615**
- Nytol QuickGels Softgels Maximum Strength **616**
- Simply Sleep Caplets **1868**
- Sominex Original Formula Tablets .. **616**
- TheraFlu Warming Relief Nighttime Severe Cold **743**
- TheraFlu Thin Strips Multi Symptom **744**
- Triaminic Nighttime Cold & Cough Liquid **746**
- Triaminic Thin Strips Cough & Runny Nose **749**
- Extra Strength Tylenol PM Caplets, Vanilla Caplets, Geltabs, Gelcaps and Liquid **1875**
- Tylenol Sore Throat Nighttime Liquid with Cool Burst **790**
- Tylenol Allergy Multi-Symptom Nighttime Caplets with Cool Burst **1872**
- Tylenol Severe Allergy Caplets **1872**
- Children's Tylenol Plus Cold & Allergy Suspension Liquid **1878**

Diphenylpyraline Hydrochloride (The concomitant use of other central nervous system depressants, such as sedating antihistamines, may produce additive depressant effects. Hypoventilation, hypotension, profound sedation, and coma may occur. Therefore, use of concomitant CNS depressants requires individual adjustment of dosage of the concomitant medication and observation of a given patient).
No products indexed under this heading.

Doxorubicin Hydrochloride (Co-administration with agents that induce CYP3A4 activity may cause increased clearance of fentanyl and reduce its efficacy).
No products indexed under this heading.

Droperidol (The concomitant use of other central nervous system depressants, such as tranquilizers, may produce additive depressant effects. Hypoventilation, hypotension, profound sedation, and coma may occur. Therefore, use of concomitant CNS depressants requires individual adjustment of dosage of the concomitant medication and observation of a given patient).
No products indexed under this heading.

Efavirenz (The concomitant use of fentanyl with CYP3A4 inhibitors may result in a decreases in fentanyl clearance, which could increase or prolong adverse drug effects including serious respiratory depression. In this situation, special patient care and observation is appropriate).
Products include:
- Atripla Tablets **945**
- Sustiva Capsules **930**
- Sustiva Tablets **930**

Enflurane (The concomitant use of other central nervous system depressants, such as general anesthetics, may produce additive depressant effects. Hypoventilation, hypotension, profound sedation, and coma may occur. Therefore, use of concomitant CNS depressants requires individual adjustment of dosage of the concomitant medication and observation of a given patient).
No products indexed under this heading.

Erythromycin (The concomitant use of fentanyl with CYP3A4 inhibitors may result in a decreases in fentanyl clearance, which could increase or prolong adverse drug effects including serious respiratory depression. In this situation, special patient care and observation is appropriate). Products include:
- Ery-Tab Tablets **449**
- Erythromycin Base Filmtab Tablets **455**
- Erythromycin Delayed-Release Capsules, USP **457**
- PCE Dispertab Tablets **515**

Erythromycin Estolate (The concomitant use of fentanyl with CYP3A4 inhibitors may result in a decreases in fentanyl clearance, which could increase or prolong adverse drug effects including serious respiratory depression. In this situation, special patient care and observation is appropriate).
No products indexed under this heading.

Erythromycin Ethylsuccinate (The concomitant use of fentanyl with CYP3A4 inhibitors may result in a decreases in fentanyl clearance, which could increase or prolong adverse drug effects including serious respiratory depression. In this situation, special patient care and observation is appropriate).
Products include:
- E.E.S. **451**
- EryPed **447**

Erythromycin Gluceptate (The concomitant use of fentanyl with CYP3A4 inhibitors may result in a decreases in fentanyl clearance, which could increase or prolong adverse drug effects including serious respiratory depression. In this situation, special patient care and observation is appropriate).
No products indexed under this heading.

Erythromycin Lactobionate (The concomitant use of fentanyl with CYP3A4 inhibitors may result in a decreases in fentanyl clearance, which could increase or prolong adverse drug effects including serious respiratory depression. In this situation, special patient care and observation is appropriate).
No products indexed under this heading.

Erythromycin Stearate (The concomitant use of fentanyl with CYP3A4 inhibitors may result in a decreases in fentanyl clearance, which could increase or prolong adverse drug effects including serious respiratory depression. In this situation, special patient care and observation is appropriate).
Products include:
- Erythrocin Stearate Filmtab Tablets **453**

Esomeprazole Magnesium (The concomitant use of fentanyl with CYP3A4 inhibitors may result in a decreases in fentanyl clearance, which could increase or prolong adverse drug effects including serious respiratory depression. In this situation, special patient care and observation is appropriate).
Products include:
- Nexium Delayed-Release Capsules **655**

Estazolam (The concomitant use of other central nervous system depressants, such as sedatives and hypnotics, may produce additive depressant effects. Hypoventilation, hypotension, profound sedation, and coma may occur. Therefore, use of concomitant CNS depressants

requires individual adjustment of dosage of the concomitant medication and observation of a given patient). Products include:
ProSom Tablets 517

Ethchlorvynol (The concomitant use of other central nervous system depressants, such as sedatives and hypnotics, may produce additive depressant effects. Hypoventilation, hypotension, profound sedation, and coma may occur. Therefore, use of concomitant CNS depressants requires individual adjustment of dosage of the concomitant medication and observation of a given patient).
No products indexed under this heading.

Ethinamate (The concomitant use of other central nervous system depressants, such as sedatives and hypnotics, may produce additive depressant effects. Hypoventilation, hypotension, profound sedation, and coma may occur. Therefore, use of concomitant CNS depressants requires individual adjustment of dosage of the concomitant medication and observation of a given patient).
No products indexed under this heading.

Ethosuximide (Co-administration with agents that induce CYP3A4 activity may cause increased clearance of fentanyl and reduce its efficacy).
No products indexed under this heading.

Felbamate (Co-administration with agents that induce CYP3A4 activity may cause increased clearance of fentanyl and reduce its efficacy).
No products indexed under this heading.

Fentanyl Citrate (The concomitant use of other central nervous system depressants, such as opiods, may produce additive depressant effects. Hypoventilation, hypotension, profound sedation, and coma may occur. Therefore, use of concomitant CNS depressants requires individual adjustment of dosage of the concomitant medication and observation of a given patient). Products include:
Actiq 979

Fluconazole (The concomitant use of fentanyl with CYP3A4 inhibitors may result in a decreases in fentanyl clearance, which could increase or prolong adverse drug effects including serious respiratory depression. In this situation, special patient care and observation is appropriate).
No products indexed under this heading.

Fludrocortisone Acetate (Co-administration with agents that induce CYP3A4 activity may cause increased clearance of fentanyl and reduce its efficacy).
No products indexed under this heading.

Fluoxetine Hydrochloride (The concomitant use of fentanyl with CYP3A4 inhibitors may result in a decreases in fentanyl clearance, which could increase or prolong adverse drug effects including serious respiratory depression. In this situation, special patient care and observation is appropriate).
Products include:
Prozac Pulvules and Liquid 1801
Symbyax Capsules 1819

Fluphenazine Decanoate (The concomitant use of other central nervous system depressants, such as phenothiazines, may produce additive depressant effects. Hypoventilation, hypotension, profound sedation, and coma may occur. Therefore, use of concomitant CNS depressants requires individual adjustment of dosage of the concomitant medication and observation of a given patient).
No products indexed under this heading.

Fluphenazine Enanthate (The concomitant use of other central nervous system depressants, such as phenothiazines, may produce additive depressant effects. Hypoventilation, hypotension, profound sedation, and coma may occur. Therefore, use of concomitant CNS depressants requires individual adjustment of dosage of the concomitant medication and observation of a given patient).
No products indexed under this heading.

Fluphenazine Hydrochloride (The concomitant use of other central nervous system depressants, such as phenothiazines, may produce additive depressant effects. Hypoventilation, hypotension, profound sedation, and coma may occur. Therefore, use of concomitant CNS depressants requires individual adjustment of dosage of the concomitant medication and observation of a given patient).
No products indexed under this heading.

Flurazepam Hydrochloride (The concomitant use of other central nervous system depressants, such as sedatives and hypnotics, may produce additive depressant effects. Hypoventilation, hypotension, profound sedation, and coma may occur. Therefore, use of concomitant CNS depressants requires individual adjustment of dosage of the concomitant medication and observation of a given patient). Products include:
Dalmane Capsules 3342

Fluvoxamine Maleate (The concomitant use of fentanyl with CYP3A4 inhibitors may result in a decreases in fentanyl clearance, which could increase or prolong adverse drug effects including serious respiratory depression. In this situation, special patient care and observation is appropriate).
No products indexed under this heading.

Fosamprenavir Calcium (The concomitant use of fentanyl with CYP3A4 inhibitors may result in a decreases in fentanyl clearance, which could increase or prolong adverse drug effects including serious respiratory depression. In this situation, special patient care and observation is appropriate).
Products include:
Lexiva Tablets 1505

Fosphenytoin Sodium (Co-administration with agents that induce CYP3A4 activity may cause increased clearance of fentanyl and reduce its efficacy).
No products indexed under this heading.

Garlic Extract (Co-administration with agents that induce CYP3A4 activity may cause increased clearance of fentanyl and reduce its efficacy).
No products indexed under this heading.

Garlic Oil (Co-administration with agents that induce CYP3A4 activity may cause increased clearance of fentanyl and reduce its efficacy).
No products indexed under this heading.

Glutethimide (The concomitant use of other central nervous system depressants, such as sedatives and hypnotics, may produce additive depressant effects. Hypoventilation, hypotension, profound sedation, and coma may occur. Therefore, use of concomitant CNS depressants requires individual adjustment of dosage of the concomitant medication and observation of a given patient).
No products indexed under this heading.

Haloperidol (The concomitant use of other central nervous system depressants, such as tranquilizers, may produce additive depressant effects. Hypoventilation, hypotension, profound sedation, and coma may occur. Therefore, use of concomitant CNS depressants requires individual adjustment of dosage of the concomitant medication and observation of a given patient).
No products indexed under this heading.

Haloperidol Decanoate (The concomitant use of other central nervous system depressants, such as tranquilizers, may produce additive depressant effects. Hypoventilation, hypotension, profound sedation, and coma may occur. Therefore, use of concomitant CNS depressants requires individual adjustment of dosage of the concomitant medication and observation of a given patient).
No products indexed under this heading.

Halothane (The concomitant use of other central nervous system depressants, such as general anesthetics, may produce additive depressant effects. Hypoventilation, hypotension, profound sedation, and coma may occur. Therefore, use of concomitant CNS depressants requires individual adjustment of dosage of the concomitant medication and observation of a given patient).
No products indexed under this heading.

Hydrocodone Bitartrate (The concomitant use of other central nervous system depressants, such as opiods, may produce additive depressant effects. Hypoventilation, hypotension, profound sedation, and coma may occur. Therefore, use of concomitant CNS depressants requires individual adjustment of dosage of the concomitant medication and observation of a given patient).
Products include:
Hycodan 1116
Hycotuss Expectorant Syrup 1117
Vicodin Tablets 535
Vicodin ES Tablets 536
Vicodin HP Tablets 538
Vicoprofen Tablets 539
Zydone Tablets 1139

Hydrocodone Polistirex (The concomitant use of other central nervous system depressants, such as opiods, may produce additive depressant effects. Hypoventilation, hypotension, profound sedation, and coma may occur. Therefore, use of concomitant CNS depressants requires individual adjustment of dosage of the concomitant medication and observation of a given patient). Products include:
Tussionex Pennkinetic Extended-Release Suspension 3327

Hydrocortisone (Co-administration with agents that induce CYP3A4 activity may cause increased clearance of fentanyl and reduce its efficacy). Products include:
Colocort Rectal Suspension, USP (Retention) 100 mg/60 mL 2476
Hydrocortone Tablets 1989
Preparation H Hydrocortisone Cream .... ▣646

Hydrocortisone Acetate (Co-administration with agents that induce CYP3A4 activity may cause increased clearance of fentanyl and reduce its efficacy). Products include:
Analpram-HC 1159
Pramosone 1161
ProctoFoam-HC 3099

Hydrocortisone Butyrate (Co-administration with agents that induce CYP3A4 activity may cause increased clearance of fentanyl and reduce its efficacy). Products include:
Locoid Lipocream Cream 1160

Hydrocortisone Cypionate (Co-administration with agents that induce CYP3A4 activity may cause increased clearance of fentanyl and reduce its efficacy).
No products indexed under this heading.

Hydrocortisone Hemisuccinate (Co-administration with agents that induce CYP3A4 activity may cause increased clearance of fentanyl and reduce its efficacy).
No products indexed under this heading.

Hydrocortisone Probutate (Co-administration with agents that induce CYP3A4 activity may cause increased clearance of fentanyl and reduce its efficacy).
No products indexed under this heading.

Hydrocortisone Sodium Phosphate (Co-administration with agents that induce CYP3A4 activity may cause increased clearance of fentanyl and reduce its efficacy).
No products indexed under this heading.

Hydrocortisone Sodium Succinate (Co-administration with agents that induce CYP3A4 activity may cause increased clearance of fentanyl and reduce its efficacy).
No products indexed under this heading.

Hydrocortisone Valerate (Co-administration with agents that induce CYP3A4 activity may cause increased clearance of fentanyl and reduce its efficacy).
No products indexed under this heading.

Hydromorphone Hydrochloride (The concomitant use of other central nervous system depressants, such as opiods, may produce additive depressant effects. Hypoventilation, hypotension, profound sedation, and coma may occur. Therefore, use of concomitant CNS depressants requires individual adjustment of dosage of the concomitant medication and observation of a given patient). Products include:

Dilaudid 440
Dilaudid Non-Sterile Powder 440
Dilaudid Oral Liquid 445
Dilaudid Rectal Suppositories 440
Dilaudid Tablets 440
Dilaudid Tablets - 8 mg 445
Dilaudid-HP 442

Hydroxyzine Hydrochloride (The concomitant use of other central nervous system depressants, such as tranquilizers, may produce additive depressant effects. Hypoventilation, hypotension, profound sedation, and coma may occur. Therefore, use of concomitant CNS depressants requires individual adjustment of dosage of the concomitant medication and observation of a given patient).
No products indexed under this heading.

Hypericum (Co-administration with agents that induce CYP3A4 activity may cause increased clearance of fentanyl and reduce its efficacy). Products include:

Satiete Tablets 832

Hypericum Perforatum (Co-administration with agents that induce CYP3A4 activity may cause increased clearance of fentanyl and reduce its efficacy).
No products indexed under this heading.

Indinavir Sulfate (The concomitant use of fentanyl with CYP3A4 inhibitors may result in a decreases in fentanyl clearance, which could increase or prolong adverse drug effects including serious respiratory depression. In this situation, special patient care and observation is appropriate). Products include:

Crixivan Capsules 1940

Isoflurane (The concomitant use of other central nervous system depressants, such as general anesthetics, may produce additive depressant effects. Hypoventilation, hypotension, profound sedation, and coma may occur. Therefore, use of concomitant CNS depressants requires individual adjustment of dosage of the concomitant medication and observation of a given patient).
No products indexed under this heading.

Isoniazid (The concomitant use of fentanyl with CYP3A4 inhibitors may result in a decreases in fentanyl clearance, which could increase or prolong adverse drug effects including serious respiratory depression. In this situation, special patient care and observation is appropriate).
No products indexed under this heading.

Itraconazole (The concomitant use of fentanyl with CYP3A4 inhibitors may result in a decreases in fentanyl clearance, which could increase or prolong adverse drug effects including serious respiratory depression. In this situation, special patient care and observation is appropriate).
No products indexed under this heading.

Ketamine Hydrochloride (The concomitant use of other central nervous system depressants, such as general anesthetics, may produce additive depressant effects. Hypoventilation, hypotension, profound sedation, and coma may occur. Therefore, use of concomitant CNS depressants requires individual adjustment of dosage of the concomitant medication and observation of a given patient).
No products indexed under this heading.

Ketoconazole (The concomitant use of fentanyl with CYP3A4 inhibitors may result in a decreases in fentanyl clearance, which could increase or prolong adverse drug effects including serious respiratory depression. In this situation, special patient care and observation is appropriate). Products include:

Nizoral A-D Shampoo, 1% 1868

Levorphanol Tartrate (The concomitant use of other central nervous system depressants, such as opiods, may produce additive depressant effects. Hypoventilation, hypotension, profound sedation, and coma may occur. Therefore, use of concomitant CNS depressants requires individual adjustment of dosage of the concomitant medication and observation of a given patient).
No products indexed under this heading.

Lopinavir (The concomitant use of fentanyl with CYP3A4 inhibitors may result in a decreases in fentanyl clearance, which could increase or prolong adverse drug effects including serious respiratory depression. In this situation, special patient care and observation is appropriate). Products include:

Kaletra 476

Loratadine (The concomitant use of fentanyl with CYP3A4 inhibitors may result in a decreases in fentanyl clearance, which could increase or prolong adverse drug effects including serious respiratory depression. In this situation, special patient care and observation is appropriate). Products include:

Alavert Allergy & Sinus D-12 Hour Tablets 771
Alavert 771
Children's Claritin Allergy Oral Solution 771
Claritin Non-Drowsy 24 Hour Tablets 772
Claritin Reditabs 24 Hour Non-Drowsy Tablets 772
Claritin-D Non-Drowsy 12 Hour Tablets 772
Claritin-D Non-Drowsy 24 Hour Tablets 772

Lorazepam (The concomitant use of other central nervous system depressants, such as sedatives and hypnotics, may produce additive depressant effects. Hypoventilation, hypotension, profound sedation, and coma may occur. Therefore, use of concomitant CNS depressants requires individual adjustment of dosage of the concomitant medication and observation of a given patient).
No products indexed under this heading.

Loxapine Hydrochloride (The concomitant use of other central nervous system depressants, such as tranquilizers, may produce additive depressant effects. Hypoventilation, hypotension, profound sedation, and coma may occur. Therefore, use of concomitant CNS depressants requires individual adjustment of dosage of the concomitant medication and observation of a given patient).
No products indexed under this heading.

Loxapine Succinate (The concomitant use of other central nervous system depressants, such as tranquilizers, may produce additive depressant effects. Hypoventilation, hypotension, profound sedation, and coma may occur. Therefore, use of concomitant CNS depressants requires individual adjustment of dosage of the concomitant medication and observation of a given patient).
No products indexed under this heading.

Meperidine Hydrochloride (The concomitant use of other central nervous system depressants, such as opiods, may produce additive depressant effects. Hypoventilation, hypotension, profound sedation, and coma may occur. Therefore, use of concomitant CNS depressants requires individual adjustment of dosage of the concomitant medication and observation of a given patient).
No products indexed under this heading.

Mephenytoin (Co-administration with agents that induce CYP3A4 activity may cause increased clearance of fentanyl and reduce its efficacy).
No products indexed under this heading.

Meprobamate (The concomitant use of other central nervous system depressants, such as tranquilizers, may produce additive depressant effects. Hypoventilation, hypotension, profound sedation, and coma may occur. Therefore, use of concomitant CNS depressants requires individual adjustment of dosage of the concomitant medication and observation of a given patient).
No products indexed under this heading.

Mesoridazine Besylate (The concomitant use of other central nervous system depressants, such as phenothiazines, may produce additive depressant effects. Hypoventilation, hypotension, profound sedation, and coma may occur. Therefore, use of concomitant CNS depressants requires individual adjustment of dosage of the concomitant medication and observation of a given patient).
No products indexed under this heading.

Metaxalone (The concomitant use of other central nervous system depressants, such as skeletal muscle relaxants, may produce additive depressant effects. Hypoventilation, hypotension, profound sedation, and coma may occur. Therefore, use of concomitant CNS depressants requires individual adjustment of dosage of the concomitant medication and observation of a given patient). Products include:

Skelaxin Tablets 1716

Methadone Hydrochloride (The concomitant use of other central nervous system depressants, such as opiods, may produce additive depressant effects. Hypoventilation, hypotension, profound sedation, and coma may occur. Therefore, use of concomitant CNS depressants requires individual adjustment of dosage of the concomitant medication and observation of a given patient).
No products indexed under this heading.

Methdilazine Hydrochloride (The concomitant use of other central nervous system depressants, such as sedating antihistamines, may produce additive depressant effects. Hypoventilation, hypotension, profound sedation, and coma may occur. Therefore, use of concomitant CNS depressants requires individual adjustment of dosage of the concomitant medication and observation of a given patient).
No products indexed under this heading.

Methocarbamol (The concomitant use of other central nervous system depressants, such as skeletal muscle relaxants, may produce additive depressant effects. Hypoventilation, hypotension, profound sedation, and coma may occur. Therefore, use of concomitant CNS depressants requires individual adjustment of dosage of the concomitant medication and observation of a given patient).
No products indexed under this heading.

Methohexital Sodium (The concomitant use of other central nervous system depressants, such as general anesthetics, may produce additive depressant effects. Hypoventilation, hypotension, profound sedation, and coma may occur. Therefore, use of concomitant CNS depressants requires individual adjustment of dosage of the concomitant medication and observation of a given patient).
No products indexed under this heading.

Methotrimeprazine (The concomitant use of other central nervous system depressants, such as phenothiazines, may produce additive depressant effects. Hypoventilation, hypotension, profound sedation, and coma may occur. Therefore, use of concomitant CNS depressants requires individual adjustment of dosage of the concomitant medication and observation of a given patient).
No products indexed under this heading.

Methsuximide (Co-administration with agents that induce CYP3A4 activity may cause increased clearance of fentanyl and reduce its efficacy).
No products indexed under this heading.

Methylprednisolone (Co-administration with agents that induce CYP3A4 activity may cause increased clearance of fentanyl and reduce its efficacy).
No products indexed under this heading.

Methylprednisolone Acetate (Co-administration with agents that induce CYP3A4 activity may cause increased clearance of fentanyl and reduce its efficacy). Products include:

Depo-Medrol Injectable Suspension 2617
Depo-Medrol Single-Dose Vial 2619

Methylprednisolone Sodium Succinate (Co-administration with agents that induce CYP3A4 activity may cause increased clearance of fentanyl and reduce its efficacy).
No products indexed under this heading.

Metronidazole (The concomitant use of fentanyl with CYP3A4 inhibitors may result in a decreases in fentanyl clearance, which could increase or prolong adverse drug effects including serious respiratory depression. In this situation, special patient care and observation is appropriate). Products include:
Metrogel 1% 1211
MetroGel-Vaginal Gel 1855
Vandazole Vaginal Gel 3338

Metronidazole Benzoate (The concomitant use of fentanyl with CYP3A4 inhibitors may result in a decreases in fentanyl clearance, which could increase or prolong adverse drug effects including serious respiratory depression. In this situation, special patient care and observation is appropriate).
No products indexed under this heading.

Metronidazole Hydrochloride (The concomitant use of fentanyl with CYP3A4 inhibitors may result in a decreases in fentanyl clearance, which could increase or prolong adverse drug effects including serious respiratory depression. In this situation, special patient care and observation is appropriate).
No products indexed under this heading.

Miconazole (The concomitant use of fentanyl with CYP3A4 inhibitors may result in a decreases in fentanyl clearance, which could increase or prolong adverse drug effects including serious respiratory depression. In this situation, special patient care and observation is appropriate).
No products indexed under this heading.

Miconazole Nitrate (The concomitant use of fentanyl with CYP3A4 inhibitors may result in a decreases in fentanyl clearance, which could increase or prolong adverse drug effects including serious respiratory depression. In this situation, special patient care and observation is appropriate). Products include:
Desenex .... ▣635
Desenex Jock Itch Spray Powder ... ▣635

Midazolam Hydrochloride (The concomitant use of other central nervous system depressants, such as sedatives and hypnotics, may produce additive depressant effects. Hypoventilation, hypotension, profound sedation, and coma may occur. Therefore, use of concomitant CNS depressants requires individual adjustment of dosage of the concomitant medication and observation of a given patient).
No products indexed under this heading.

Modafinil (Co-administration with agents that induce CYP3A4 activity may cause increased clearance of fentanyl and reduce its efficacy). Products include:
Provigil Tablets 988

Molindone Hydrochloride (The concomitant use of other central nervous system depressants, such as tranquilizers, may produce additive depressant effects. Hypoventilation, hypotension, profound sedation, and coma may occur. Therefore, use of concomitant CNS depressants requires individual adjustment of dosage of the concomitant medication and observation of a given patient). Products include:
Moban Tablets 1119

Morphine Sulfate (The concomitant use of other central nervous system depressants, such as opioids, may produce additive depressant effects. Hypoventilation, hypotension, profound sedation, and coma may occur. Therefore, use of concomitant CNS depressants requires individual adjustment of dosage of the concomitant medication and observation of a given patient). Products include:
Avinza Capsules 1741
Kadian Capsules 577
MS Contin Tablets 2701

Nefazodone Hydrochloride (The concomitant use of fentanyl with CYP3A4 inhibitors may result in a decreases in fentanyl clearance, which could increase or prolong adverse drug effects including serious respiratory depression. In this situation, special patient care and observation is appropriate).
No products indexed under this heading.

Nelfinavir Mesylate (The concomitant use of fentanyl with CYP3A4 inhibitors may result in a decreases in fentanyl clearance, which could increase or prolong adverse drug effects including serious respiratory depression. In this situation, special patient care and observation is appropriate). Products include:
Viracept 2577

Nevirapine (The concomitant use of fentanyl with CYP3A4 inhibitors may result in a decreases in fentanyl clearance, which could increase or prolong adverse drug effects including serious respiratory depression. In this situation, special patient care and observation is appropriate). Products include:
Viramune Oral Suspension 873
Viramune Tablets 873

Niacinamide (The concomitant use of fentanyl with CYP3A4 inhibitors may result in a decreases in fentanyl clearance, which could increase or prolong adverse drug effects including serious respiratory depression. In this situation, special patient care and observation is appropriate).
No products indexed under this heading.

Nicotinamide (The concomitant use of fentanyl with CYP3A4 inhibitors may result in a decreases in fentanyl clearance, which could increase or prolong adverse drug effects including serious respiratory depression. In this situation, special patient care and observation is appropriate). Products include:
Nicomide Tablets 1088

Nifedipine (The concomitant use of fentanyl with CYP3A4 inhibitors may result in a decreases in fentanyl clearance, which could increase or prolong adverse drug effects including serious respiratory depression. In this situation, special patient care and observation is appropriate). Products include:
Adalat CC Tablets 2964

Norfloxacin (The concomitant use of fentanyl with CYP3A4 inhibitors may result in a decreases in fentanyl clearance, which could increase or prolong adverse drug effects including serious respiratory depression. In this situation, special patient care and observation is appropriate). Products include:
Noroxin Tablets 2032

Omeprazole (The concomitant use of fentanyl with CYP3A4 inhibitors may result in a decreases in fentanyl clearance, which could increase or prolong adverse drug effects including serious respiratory depression. In this situation, special patient care and observation is appropriate). Products include:
Zegerid Capsules 2958
Zegerid Powder for Oral Solution 2958

Orphenadrine Citrate (The concomitant use of other central nervous system depressants, such as skeletal muscle relaxants, may produce additive depressant effects. Hypoventilation, hypotension, profound sedation, and coma may occur. Therefore, use of concomitant CNS depressants requires individual adjustment of dosage of the concomitant medication and observation of a given patient). Products include:
Norflex Injection 1856

Oxazepam (The concomitant use of other central nervous system depressants, such as tranquilizers, may produce additive depressant effects. Hypoventilation, hypotension, profound sedation, and coma may occur. Therefore, use of concomitant CNS depressants requires individual adjustment of dosage of the concomitant medication and observation of a given patient).
No products indexed under this heading.

Oxcarbazepine (Co-administration with agents that induce CYP3A4 activity may cause increased clearance of fentanyl and reduce its efficacy). Products include:
Trileptal Tablets 2300
Trileptal Oral Suspension 2300

Oxycodone Hydrochloride (The concomitant use of other central nervous system depressants, such as opioids, may produce additive depressant effects. Hypoventilation, hypotension, profound sedation, and coma may occur. Therefore, use of concomitant CNS depressants requires individual adjustment of dosage of the concomitant medication and observation of a given patient). Products include:
OxyContin Tablets 2703
OxyFast Oral Concentrate Solution 2708
OxyIR Capsules 2708
Percocet Tablets 1131
Percodan Tablets 1132

Paroxetine Hydrochloride (The concomitant use of fentanyl with CYP3A4 inhibitors may result in a decreases in fentanyl clearance, which could increase or prolong adverse drug effects including serious respiratory depression. In this situation, special patient care and observation is appropriate). Products include:
Paxil CR Controlled-Release Tablets 1538
Paxil 1530

Perphenazine (The concomitant use of other central nervous system depressants, such as phenothiazines, may produce additive depressant effects. Hypoventilation, hypotension, profound sedation, and coma may occur. Therefore, use of concomitant CNS depressants requires individual adjustment of dosage of the concomitant medication and observation of a given patient).
No products indexed under this heading.

Phenobarbital (Co-administration with agents that induce CYP3A4 activity may cause increased clearance of fentanyl and reduce its efficacy). Products include:
Donnatal Extentabs 2493

Phenobarbital Sodium (Co-administration with agents that induce CYP3A4 activity may cause increased clearance of fentanyl and reduce its efficacy).
No products indexed under this heading.

Phenytoin (Co-administration with agents that induce CYP3A4 activity may cause increased clearance of fentanyl and reduce its efficacy).
No products indexed under this heading.

Phenytoin Sodium (Co-administration with agents that induce CYP3A4 activity may cause increased clearance of fentanyl and reduce its efficacy). Products include:
Phenytek Capsules 2160

Prazepam (The concomitant use of other central nervous system depressants, such as tranquilizers, may produce additive depressant effects. Hypoventilation, hypotension, profound sedation, and coma may occur. Therefore, use of concomitant CNS depressants requires individual adjustment of dosage of the concomitant medication and observation of a given patient).
No products indexed under this heading.

Prednisolone Acetate (Co-administration with agents that induce CYP3A4 activity may cause increased clearance of fentanyl and reduce its efficacy). Products include:
Blephamide Ophthalmic Ointment 568
Blephamide Ophthalmic Suspension 569
Poly-Pred Ophthalmic Suspension .... ⊙233
Pred Forte Ophthalmic Suspension .... ⊙235
Pred Mild Ophthalmic Suspension .... ⊙238
Pred-G Ophthalmic Ointment .... ⊙237
Pred-G Ophthalmic Suspension ...... ⊙236

Prednisolone Sodium Phosphate (Co-administration with agents that induce CYP3A4 activity may cause increased clearance of fentanyl and reduce its efficacy).
No products indexed under this heading.

Prednisolone Tebutate (Co-administration with agents that induce CYP3A4 activity may cause increased clearance of fentanyl and reduce its efficacy).
No products indexed under this heading.

Prednisone (Co-administration with agents that induce CYP3A4 activity may cause increased clearance of fentanyl and reduce its efficacy).

No products indexed under this heading.

Primidone (Co-administration with agents that induce CYP3A4 activity may cause increased clearance of fentanyl and reduce its efficacy).

No products indexed under this heading.

Prochlorperazine (The concomitant use of other central nervous system depressants, such as phenothiazines, may produce additive depressant effects. Hypoventilation, hypotension, profound sedation, and coma may occur. Therefore, use of concomitant CNS depressants requires individual adjustment of dosage of the concomitant medication and observation of a given patient).

No products indexed under this heading.

Promethazine Hydrochloride (The concomitant use of other central nervous system depressants, such as phenothiazines, may produce additive depressant effects. Hypoventilation, hypotension, profound sedation, and coma may occur. Therefore, use of concomitant CNS depressants requires individual adjustment of dosage of the concomitant medication and observation of a given patient). Products include:

Phenergan Tablets and
Suppositories 3440

Propofol (The concomitant use of other central nervous system depressants, such as sedatives and hypnotics, may produce additive depressant effects. Hypoventilation, hypotension, profound sedation, and coma may occur. Therefore, use of concomitant CNS depressants requires individual adjustment of dosage of the concomitant medication and observation of a given patient).

No products indexed under this heading.

Propoxyphene Hydrochloride (The concomitant use of other central nervous system depressants, such as opiods, may produce additive depressant effects. Hypoventilation, hypotension, profound sedation, and coma may occur. Therefore, use of concomitant CNS depressants requires individual adjustment of dosage of the concomitant medication and observation of a given patient).

No products indexed under this heading.

Propoxyphene Napsylate (The concomitant use of other central nervous system depressants, such as opiods, may produce additive depressant effects. Hypoventilation, hypotension, profound sedation, and coma may occur. Therefore, use of concomitant CNS depressants requires individual adjustment of dosage of the concomitant medication and observation of a given patient).

No products indexed under this heading.

Pyrilamine Maleate (The concomitant use of other central nervous system depressants, such as sedating antihistamines, may produce additive depressant effects. Hypoventilation, hypotension, profound sedation, and coma may occur. Therefore, use of concomitant CNS depressants requires individual adjustment of dosage of the concomitant medication and observation of a given patient).

No products indexed under this heading.

Pyrilamine Tannate (The concomitant use of other central nervous system depressants, such as sedating antihistamines, may produce additive depressant effects. Hypoventilation, hypotension, profound sedation, and coma may occur. Therefore, use of concomitant CNS depressants requires individual adjustment of dosage of the concomitant medication and observation of a given patient).

No products indexed under this heading.

Quazepam (The concomitant use of other central nervous system depressants, such as sedatives and hypnotics, may produce additive depressant effects. Hypoventilation, hypotension, profound sedation, and coma may occur. Therefore, use of concomitant CNS depressants requires individual adjustment of dosage of the concomitant medication and observation of a given patient).

No products indexed under this heading.

Quinidine (The concomitant use of fentanyl with CYP3A4 inhibitors may result in a decreases in fentanyl clearance, which could increase or prolong adverse drug effects including serious respiratory depression. In this situation, special patient care and observation is appropriate).

No products indexed under this heading.

Quinidine Hydrochloride (The concomitant use of fentanyl with CYP3A4 inhibitors may result in a decreases in fentanyl clearance, which could increase or prolong adverse drug effects including serious respiratory depression. In this situation, special patient care and observation is appropriate).

No products indexed under this heading.

Quinidine Polygalacturonate (The concomitant use of fentanyl with CYP3A4 inhibitors may result in a decreases in fentanyl clearance, which could increase or prolong adverse drug effects including serious respiratory depression. In this situation, special patient care and observation is appropriate).

No products indexed under this heading.

Quinidine Sulfate (The concomitant use of fentanyl with CYP3A4 inhibitors may result in a decreases in fentanyl clearance, which could increase or prolong adverse drug effects including serious respiratory depression. In this situation, special patient care and observation is appropriate).

No products indexed under this heading.

Quinine (The concomitant use of fentanyl with CYP3A4 inhibitors may result in a decreases in fentanyl clearance, which could increase or prolong adverse drug effects including serious respiratory depression. In this situation, special patient care and observation is appropriate).

No products indexed under this heading.

Quinine Sulfate (The concomitant use of fentanyl with CYP3A4 inhibitors may result in a decreases in fentanyl clearance, which could increase or prolong adverse drug effects including serious respiratory depression. In this situation, special patient care and observation is appropriate).

No products indexed under this heading.

Quinupristin (The concomitant use of fentanyl with CYP3A4 inhibitors may result in a decreases in fentanyl clearance, which could increase or prolong adverse drug effects including serious respiratory depression. In this situation, special patient care and observation is appropriate).

No products indexed under this heading.

Ramelteon (The concomitant use of other central nervous system depressants, such as sedatives and hypnotics, may produce additive depressant effects. Hypoventilation, hypotension, profound sedation, and coma may occur. Therefore, use of concomitant CNS depressants requires individual adjustment of dosage of the concomitant medication and observation of a given patient). Products include:

Rozerem Tablets 3231

Ranitidine Bismuth Citrate (The concomitant use of fentanyl with CYP3A4 inhibitors may result in a decreases in fentanyl clearance, which could increase or prolong adverse drug effects including serious respiratory depression. In this situation, special patient care and observation is appropriate).

No products indexed under this heading.

Ranitidine Hydrochloride (The concomitant use of fentanyl with CYP3A4 inhibitors may result in a decreases in fentanyl clearance, which could increase or prolong adverse drug effects including serious respiratory depression. In this situation, special patient care and observation is appropriate). Products include:

Zantac ... 1624
Zantac Injection 1619
Zantac Injection Pharmacy Bulk
Package 1622

Remifentanil Hydrochloride (The concomitant use of other central nervous system depressants, such as opiods, may produce additive depressant effects. Hypoventilation, hypotension, profound sedation, and coma may occur. Therefore, use of concomitant CNS depressants requires individual adjustment of dosage of the concomitant medication and observation of a given patient).

No products indexed under this heading.

Rifabutin (Co-administration with agents that induce CYP3A4 activity may cause increased clearance of fentanyl and reduce its efficacy).

No products indexed under this heading.

Rifampicin (Co-administration with agents that induce CYP3A4 activity may cause increased clearance of fentanyl and reduce its efficacy).

No products indexed under this heading.

Rifampin (Co-administration with agents that induce CYP3A4 activity may cause increased clearance of fentanyl and reduce its efficacy).

No products indexed under this heading.

Rifapentine (Co-administration with agents that induce CYP3A4 activity may cause increased clearance of fentanyl and reduce its efficacy).

No products indexed under this heading.

Ritonavir (The concomitant use of fentanyl with CYP3A4 inhibitors may result in a decreases in fentanyl clearance, which could increase or prolong adverse drug effects including serious respiratory depression. In this situation, special patient care and observation is appropriate). Products include:

Kaletra ... 476
Norvir ... 503

Saquinavir (The concomitant use of fentanyl with CYP3A4 inhibitors may result in a decreases in fentanyl clearance, which could increase or prolong adverse drug effects including serious respiratory depression. In this situation, special patient care and observation is appropriate).

No products indexed under this heading.

Saquinavir Mesylate (The concomitant use of fentanyl with CYP3A4 inhibitors may result in a decreases in fentanyl clearance, which could increase or prolong adverse drug effects including serious respiratory depression. In this situation, special patient care and observation is appropriate). Products include:

Invirase ... 2772

Secobarbital Sodium (The concomitant use of other central nervous system depressants, such as sedatives and hypnotics, may produce additive depressant effects. Hypoventilation, hypotension, profound sedation, and coma may occur. Therefore, use of concomitant CNS depressants requires individual adjustment of dosage of the concomitant medication and observation of a given patient).

No products indexed under this heading.

Sertraline Hydrochloride (The concomitant use of fentanyl with CYP3A4 inhibitors may result in a decreases in fentanyl clearance, which could increase or prolong adverse drug effects including serious respiratory depression. In this situation, special patient care and observation is appropriate). Products include:

Zoloft ... 2586

Sufentanil Citrate (The concomitant use of other central nervous system depressants, such as opiods, may produce additive depressant effects. Hypoventilation, hypotension, profound sedation, and coma may occur. Therefore, use of concomitant CNS depressants requires individual adjustment of dosage of the concomitant medication and observation of a given patient).

No products indexed under this heading.

IMPORTANT NOTE: Always consult each drug listing in the patient's regimen for possible interactions.

Sulfinpyrazone (Co-administration with agents that induce CYP3A4 activity may cause increased clearance of fentanyl and reduce its efficacy).
No products indexed under this heading.

Telithromycin (The concomitant use of fentanyl with CYP3A4 inhibitors may result in a decreases in fentanyl clearance, which could increase or prolong adverse drug effects including serious respiratory depression. In this situation, special patient care and observation is appropriate). Products include:
Ketek Tablets 2903

Temazepam (The concomitant use of other central nervous system depressants, such as sedatives and hypnotics, may produce additive depressant effects. Hypoventilation, hypotension, profound sedation, and coma may occur. Therefore, use of concomitant CNS depressants requires individual adjustment of dosage of the concomitant medication and observation of a given patient). Products include:
Restoril Capsules 1860

Theophylline (Co-administration with agents that induce CYP3A4 activity may cause increased clearance of fentanyl and reduce its efficacy).
No products indexed under this heading.

Thiamylal Sodium (The concomitant use of other central nervous system depressants, such as general anesthetics, may produce additive depressant effects. Hypoventilation, hypotension, profound sedation, and coma may occur. Therefore, use of concomitant CNS depressants requires individual adjustment of dosage of the concomitant medication and observation of a given patient).
No products indexed under this heading.

Thioridazine Hydrochloride (The concomitant use of other central nervous system depressants, such as phenothiazines, may produce additive depressant effects. Hypoventilation, hypotension, profound sedation, and coma may occur. Therefore, use of concomitant CNS depressants requires individual adjustment of dosage of the concomitant medication and observation of a given patient). Products include:
Thioridazine Hydrochloride Tablets 2163

Thiothixene (The concomitant use of other central nervous system depressants, such as tranquilizers, may produce additive depressant effects. Hypoventilation, hypotension, profound sedation, and coma may occur. Therefore, use of concomitant CNS depressants requires individual adjustment of dosage of the concomitant medication and observation of a given patient). Products include:
Thiothixene Capsules 2165

Triamcinolone (Co-administration with agents that induce CYP3A4 activity may cause increased clearance of fentanyl and reduce its efficacy).
No products indexed under this heading.

Triamcinolone Acetonide (Co-administration with agents that induce CYP3A4 activity may cause increased clearance of fentanyl and reduce its efficacy). Products include:
Azmacort Inhalation Aerosol 1726
Nasacort AQ Nasal Spray 2922

Triamcinolone Diacetate (Co-administration with agents that induce CYP3A4 activity may cause increased clearance of fentanyl and reduce its efficacy).
No products indexed under this heading.

Triamcinolone Hexacetonide (Co-administration with agents that induce CYP3A4 activity may cause increased clearance of fentanyl and reduce its efficacy).
No products indexed under this heading.

Triazolam (The concomitant use of other central nervous system depressants, such as sedatives and hypnotics, may produce additive depressant effects. Hypoventilation, hypotension, profound sedation, and coma may occur. Therefore, use of concomitant CNS depressants requires individual adjustment of dosage of the concomitant medication and observation of a given patient).
No products indexed under this heading.

Trifluoperazine Hydrochloride (The concomitant use of other central nervous system depressants, such as phenothiazines, may produce additive depressant effects. Hypoventilation, hypotension, profound sedation, and coma may occur. Therefore, use of concomitant CNS depressants requires individual adjustment of dosage of the concomitant medication and observation of a given patient).
No products indexed under this heading.

Trimeprazine Tartrate (The concomitant use of other central nervous system depressants, such as sedating antihistamines, may produce additive depressant effects. Hypoventilation, hypotension, profound sedation, and coma may occur. Therefore, use of concomitant CNS depressants requires individual adjustment of dosage of the concomitant medication and observation of a given patient).
No products indexed under this heading.

Tripelennamine Hydrochloride (The concomitant use of other central nervous system depressants, such as sedating antihistamines, may produce additive depressant effects. Hypoventilation, hypotension, profound sedation, and coma may occur. Therefore, use of concomitant CNS depressants requires individual adjustment of dosage of the concomitant medication and observation of a given patient).
No products indexed under this heading.

Triprolidine Hydrochloride (The concomitant use of other central nervous system depressants, such as sedating antihistamines, may produce additive depressant effects. Hypoventilation, hypotension, profound sedation, and coma may occur. Therefore, use of concomitant CNS depressants requires individual adjustment of dosage of the concomitant medication and observation of a given patient).
No products indexed under this heading.

Troglitazone (The concomitant use of fentanyl with CYP3A4 inhibitors may result in a decreases in fentanyl clearance, which could increase or prolong adverse drug effects including serious respiratory depression. In this situation, special patient care and observation is appropriate).
No products indexed under this heading.

Troleandomycin (The concomitant use of fentanyl with CYP3A4 inhibitors may result in a decreases in fentanyl clearance, which could increase or prolong adverse drug effects including serious respiratory depression. In this situation, special patient care and observation is appropriate).
No products indexed under this heading.

Valproate Sodium (The concomitant use of fentanyl with CYP3A4 inhibitors may result in a decreases in fentanyl clearance, which could increase or prolong adverse drug effects including serious respiratory depression. In this situation, special patient care and observation is appropriate). Products include:
Depacon Injection 412

Verapamil Hydrochloride (The concomitant use of fentanyl with CYP3A4 inhibitors may result in a decreases in fentanyl clearance, which could increase or prolong adverse drug effects including serious respiratory depression. In this situation, special patient care and observation is appropriate). Products include:
Covera-HS Tablets 3139
Tarka Tablets 524
Verelan PM Extended-Release Capsules, Controlled-Onset........... 3106

Voriconazole (The concomitant use of fentanyl with CYP3A4 inhibitors may result in a decreases in fentanyl clearance, which could increase or prolong adverse drug effects including serious respiratory depression. In this situation, special patient care and observation is appropriate). Products include:
VFEND I.V. 2564
VFEND Oral Suspension 2564
VFEND Tablets 2564

Zafirlukast (The concomitant use of fentanyl with CYP3A4 inhibitors may result in a decreases in fentanyl clearance, which could increase or prolong adverse drug effects including serious respiratory depression. In this situation, special patient care and observation is appropriate). Products include:
Accolate Tablets 671

Zaleplon (The concomitant use of other central nervous system depressants, such as sedatives and hypnotics, may produce additive depressant effects. Hypoventilation, hypotension, profound sedation, and coma may occur. Therefore, use of concomitant CNS depressants requires individual adjustment of dosage of the concomitant medication and observation of a given patient). Products include:
Sonata Capsules 1717

Zileuton (The concomitant use of fentanyl with CYP3A4 inhibitors may result in a decreases in fentanyl clearance, which could increase or prolong adverse drug effects including serious respiratory depression. In this situation, special patient care and observation is appropriate). Products include:
Zyflo Tablets 1023

Zolpidem Tartrate (The concomitant use of other central nervous system depressants, such as sedatives and hypnotics, may produce additive depressant effects. Hypoventilation, hypotension, profound sedation, and coma may occur. Therefore, use of concomitant CNS depressants requires individual adjustment of dosage of the concomitant medication and observation of a given patient). Products include:
Ambien Tablets 2851
Ambien CR Tablets 2855

Food Interactions

Alcohol (The concomitant use of other central nervous system depressants, such as alcoholic beverages, may produce additive depressant effects. Hypoventilation, hypotension, profound sedation, and coma may occur. Therefore, use of concomitant CNS depressants requires individual adjustment of dosage of the concomitant medication and observation of a given patient).

Grapefruit (The concomitant use of fentanyl with CYP3A4 inhibitors may result in a decreases in fentanyl clearance, which could increase or prolong adverse drug effects including serious respiratory depression. In this situation, special patient care and observation is appropriate).

Grapefruit Juice (The concomitant use of fentanyl with CYP3A4 inhibitors may result in a decreases in fentanyl clearance, which could increase or prolong adverse drug effects including serious respiratory depression. In this situation, special patient care and observation is appropriate).

IRESSA TABLETS

(Gefitinib) 684

May interact with cytochrome p450 2c19 substrates (selected), cytochrome p450 2d6 substrates (selected), cytochrome p450 3a4 inducers (selected), cytochrome p450 3a4 inhibitors (selected), histamine H2-receptor antagonists, phenytoin, and certain other agents. Compounds in these categories include:

Acetazolamide (Substances that are potent inhibitors of CYP3A4 (e.g., ketoconazole and itraconazole) decrease gefitinib metabolism and increase gefitinib plasma concentrations).
No products indexed under this heading.

Allium sativum (Substances that are inducers of CYP3A4 activity increase the metabolism of gefitinib and decrease its plasma concentrations).
No products indexed under this heading.

Amiodarone Hydrochloride (Substances that are potent inhibitors of CYP3A4 (e.g., ketoconazole and itraconazole) decrease gefitinib metabolism and increase gefitinib plasma concentrations).
No products indexed under this heading.

Amitriptyline Hydrochloride (In the highest concentration studied (5000ng/ml), gefitinib inhibited CYP2D6 by 43%).
No products indexed under this heading.

Amoxapine (In the highest concentration studied (5000ng/ml), gefitinib inhibited CYP2D6 by 24%).
No products indexed under this heading.

Amphetamine Aspartate (In the highest concentration studied (5000ng/ml), gefitinib inhibited CYP2D6 by 43%). Products include:
Adderall Tablets 3164
Adderall XR Capsules 3166

Amphetamine Aspartate Monohydrate (In the highest concentration studied (5000ng/ml), gefitinib inhibited CYP2D6 by 43%).
No products indexed under this heading.

Amphetamine Sulfate (In the highest concentration studied (5000ng/ml), gefitinib inhibited CYP2D6 by 43%). Products include:
Adderall Tablets 3164
Adderall XR Capsules 3166

Amprenavir (Substances that are potent inhibitors of CYP3A4 (e.g., ketoconazole and itraconazole) decrease gefitinib metabolism and increase gefitinib plasma concentrations). Products include:
Agenerase Capsules 1327
Agenerase Oral Solution 1332

Anastrozole (Substances that are potent inhibitors of CYP3A4 (e.g., ketoconazole and itraconazole) decrease gefitinib metabolism and increase gefitinib plasma concentrations). Products include:
Arimidex Tablets 673

Aprepitant (Substances that are inducers of CYP3A4 activity increase the metabolism of gefitinib and decrease its plasma concentrations). Products include:
Emend Capsules 1963

Atomoxetine Hydrochloride (In the highest concentration studied (5000ng/ml), gefitinib inhibited CYP2D6 by 43%). Products include:
Strattera Capsules 1814

Betamethasone Acetate (Substances that are inducers of CYP3A4 activity increase the metabolism of gefitinib and decrease its plasma concentrations).
No products indexed under this heading.

Betamethasone Sodium Phosphate (Substances that are inducers of CYP3A4 activity increase the metabolism of gefitinib and decrease its plasma concentrations).
No products indexed under this heading.

Bisoprolol Fumarate (In the highest concentration studied (5000ng/ml), gefitinib inhibited CYP2D6 by 43%).
No products indexed under this heading.

Captopril (In the highest concentration studied (5000ng/ml), gefitinib inhibited CYP2D6 by 43%). Products include:
Captopril Tablets 2149

Carbamazepine (Substances that are inducers of CYP3A4 activity increase the metabolism of gefitinib and decrease its plasma concentrations). Products include:
Carbatrol Capsules 3171
Equetro Extended-Release Capsules 3180
Tegretol/Tegretol-XR 2295

Carisoprodol (In the highest concentration studied (5000ng/ml), gefitinib inhibited CYP2D6 by 24%).
No products indexed under this heading.

Carvedilol (In the highest concentration studied (5000ng/ml), gefitinib inhibited CYP2D6 by 43%). Products include:
Coreg Tablets 1414

Cevimeline Hydrochloride (In the highest concentration studied (5000ng/ml), gefitinib inhibited CYP2D6 by 43%). Products include:
Evoxac Capsules 1047

Chlorpromazine (In the highest concentration studied (5000ng/ml), gefitinib inhibited CYP2D6 by 43%).
No products indexed under this heading.

Chlorpromazine Hydrochloride (In the highest concentration studied (5000ng/ml), gefitinib inhibited CYP2D6 by 43%).
No products indexed under this heading.

Chlorpropamide (In the highest concentration studied (5000ng/ml), gefitinib inhibited CYP2D6 by 43%).
No products indexed under this heading.

Cilostazol (In the highest concentration studied (5000ng/ml), gefitinib inhibited CYP2D6 by 24%). Products include:
Pletal Tablets 2455

Cimetidine (Drugs that cause significant sustained elevation in gastric pH may reduce plasma concentrations of gefitinib and therefore potentially may reduce efficacy). Products include:
Tagamet HB 200 Tablets .... ■664

Cimetidine Hydrochloride (Drugs that cause significant sustained elevation in gastric pH may reduce plasma concentrations of gefitinib and therefore potentially may reduce efficacy).
No products indexed under this heading.

Ciprofloxacin (Substances that are potent inhibitors of CYP3A4 (e.g., ketoconazole and itraconazole) decrease gefitinib metabolism and increase gefitinib plasma concentrations). Products include:
Cipro Oral Suspension 2977
Cipro I.V. 2984
Cipro XR Tablets 2990
Ciprodex Otic Suspension 559

Ciprofloxacin Hydrochloride (Substances that are inducers of CYP3A4 activity increase the metabolism of gefitinib and decrease its plasma concentrations). Products include:
Ciloxan Ophthalmic Ointment 559
Ciloxan Ophthalmic Solution .... ⊙206
Cipro Tablets 2977
Proquin XR Tablets 1153

Cisplatin (Substances that are inducers of CYP3A4 activity increase the metabolism of gefitinib and decrease its plasma concentrations).
No products indexed under this heading.

Citalopram Hydrobromide (In the highest concentration studied (5000ng/ml), gefitinib inhibited CYP2D6 by 24%). Products include:
Celexa 1176

Clarithromycin (Substances that are potent inhibitors of CYP3A4 (e.g., ketoconazole and itraconazole) decrease gefitinib metabolism and increase gefitinib plasma concentrations). Products include:
Biaxin/Biaxin XL 402
PREVPAC 3284

Clomipramine Hydrochloride (In the highest concentration studied (5000ng/ml), gefitinib inhibited CYP2D6 by 43%).
No products indexed under this heading.

Clotrimazole (Substances that are potent inhibitors of CYP3A4 (e.g., ketoconazole and itraconazole) decrease gefitinib metabolism and increase gefitinib plasma concentrations). Products include:
Desenex Athlete's Foot Cream .... ■635
Lotrimin 3039
Lotrisone 3040

Clozapine (In the highest concentration studied (5000ng/ml), gefitinib inhibited CYP2D6 by 43%). Products include:
Clozaril Tablets 2184
FazaClo Orally Disintegrating Tablets 551

Codeine Phosphate (In the highest concentration studied (5000ng/ml), gefitinib inhibited CYP2D6 by 43%). Products include:
Tylenol with Codeine Tablets 2391

Codeine Sulfate (In the highest concentration studied (5000ng/ml), gefitinib inhibited CYP2D6 by 43%).
No products indexed under this heading.

Cortisone Acetate (Substances that are inducers of CYP3A4 activity increase the metabolism of gefitinib and decrease its plasma concentrations).
No products indexed under this heading.

Cyclobenzaprine Hydrochloride (In the highest concentration studied (5000ng/ml), gefitinib inhibited CYP2D6 by 43%).
No products indexed under this heading.

Cyclophosphamide (In the highest concentration studied (5000ng/ml), gefitinib inhibited CYP2D6 by 24%).
No products indexed under this heading.

Cyclosporine (Substances that are potent inhibitors of CYP3A4 (e.g., ketoconazole and itraconazole) decrease gefitinib metabolism and increase gefitinib plasma concentrations). Products include:
Gengraf Capsules 459
Neoral Oral Solution 2259
Neoral Soft Gelatin Capsules 2259
Restasis Ophthalmic Emulsion 575
Sandimmune 2275

Dalfopristin (Substances that are potent inhibitors of CYP3A4 (e.g., ketoconazole and itraconazole) decrease gefitinib metabolism and increase gefitinib plasma concentrations).
No products indexed under this heading.

Danazol (Substances that are potent inhibitors of CYP3A4 (e.g., ketoconazole and itraconazole) decrease gefitinib metabolism and increase gefitinib plasma concentrations).
No products indexed under this heading.

Delavirdine Mesylate (Substances that are potent inhibitors of CYP3A4 (e.g., ketoconazole and itraconazole) decrease gefitinib metabolism and increase gefitinib plasma concentrations). Products include:
Rescriptor Tablets 2551

Desipramine Hydrochloride (In the highest concentration studied (5000ng/ml), gefitinib inhibited CYP2D6 by 43%).
No products indexed under this heading.

Dexamethasone (Substances that are inducers of CYP3A4 activity increase the metabolism of gefitinib and decrease its plasma concentrations). Products include:
Ciprodex Otic Suspension 559
Decadron Tablets 1951
TobraDex Ophthalmic Ointment 562
TobraDex Ophthalmic Suspension 563

Dexamethasone Acetate (Substances that are inducers of CYP3A4 activity increase the metabolism of gefitinib and decrease its plasma concentrations).
No products indexed under this heading.

Dexamethasone Sodium Phosphate (Substances that are inducers of CYP3A4 activity increase the metabolism of gefitinib and decrease its plasma concentrations).
No products indexed under this heading.

Dexfenfluramine Hydrochloride (In the highest concentration studied (5000ng/ml), gefitinib inhibited CYP2D6 by 43%).
No products indexed under this heading.

Dextromethorphan (In the highest concentration studied (5000ng/ml), gefitinib inhibited CYP2D6 by 24%).
No products indexed under this heading.

Dextromethorphan Hydrobromide (In the highest concentration studied (5000ng/ml), gefitinib inhibited CYP2D6 by 43%). Products include:
Comtrex Maximum Strength Cold & Cough Day/Night Caplets - Day Formulation .... ■726
Comtrex Maximum Strength Cold & Cough Day/Night Caplets - Night Formulation .... ■726
Comtrex Maximum Strength Non-Drowsy Cold & Cough Caplets .... ■725
Children's Dimetapp DM Cold & Cough Elixir .... ■731
Children's Dimetapp Long Acting Cough Plus Cold Syrup .... ■731
Toddler's Dimetapp Cold and Cough Drops .... ■732
Mucinex DM Extended-Release Bi-Layer Tablets .... ■720
Refenesen DM Caplets .... ■721
Robitussin Cough & Cold CF Liquid .... ■735
Robitussin Cough & Cold Long-Acting Liquid .... ■735
Robitussin Cough & Allergy Syrup .. ■736
Robitussin Cough & Cold Nighttime Liquid .... ■736
Robitussin Cough & Cold Pediatric Drops .... ■735
Robitussin Cough, Cold & Flu Nighttime Liquid .... ■738
Robitussin Cough & Congestion Liquid .... ■738
Robitussin Cough Gels Long-Acting .... ■737
Robitussin Cough Long Acting Liquid .... ■739
Robitussin Cough DM Syrup .... ■738
Robitussin Cough DM Infant Drops .... ■738
Robitussin Pediatric Cough Long Acting Liquid .... ■739
Robitussin Pediatric Cough & Cold Long-Acting Liquid .... ■735

Dextromethorphan Polistirex (In the highest concentration studied (5000ng/ml), gefitinib inhibited CYP2D6 by 43%). Products include:

Diazepam (In the highest concentration studied (5000ng/ml), gefitinib inhibited CYP2D6 by 24%). Products include:

Diltiazem Hydrochloride (Substances that are potent inhibitors of CYP3A4 (e.g., ketoconazole and itraconazole) decrease gefitinib metabolism and increase gefitinib plasma concentrations). Products include:

Diltiazem Maleate (Substances that are potent inhibitors of CYP3A4 (e.g., ketoconazole and itraconazole) decrease gefitinib metabolism and increase gefitinib plasma concentrations).
 No products indexed under this heading.

Divalproex Sodium (In the highest concentration studied (5000ng/ml), gefitinib inhibited CYP2D6 by 24%). Products include:

Dolasetron Mesylate (In the highest concentration studied (5000ng/ml), gefitinib inhibited CYP2D6 by 43%). Products include:

Donepezil Hydrochloride (In the highest concentration studied (5000ng/ml), gefitinib inhibited CYP2D6 by 43%). Products include:

Doxepin Hydrochloride (In the highest concentration studied (5000ng/ml), gefitinib inhibited CYP2D6 by 43%).
 No products indexed under this heading.

Doxorubicin Hydrochloride (Substances that are inducers of CYP3A4 activity increase the metabolism of gefitinib and decrease its plasma concentrations).
 No products indexed under this heading.

Efavirenz (Substances that are inducers of CYP3A4 activity increase the metabolism of gefitinib and decrease its plasma concentrations). Products include:

Encainide Hydrochloride (In the highest concentration studied (5000ng/ml), gefitinib inhibited CYP2D6 by 43%).
 No products indexed under this heading.

Erythromycin (Substances that are potent inhibitors of CYP3A4 (e.g., ketoconazole and itraconazole) decrease gefitinib metabolism and increase gefitinib plasma concentrations). Products include:

Erythromycin Estolate (Substances that are potent inhibitors of CYP3A4 (e.g., ketoconazole and itraconazole) decrease gefitinib metabolism and increase gefitinib plasma concentrations).
 No products indexed under this heading.

Erythromycin Ethylsuccinate (Substances that are potent inhibitors of CYP3A4 (e.g., ketoconazole and itraconazole) decrease gefitinib metabolism and increase gefitinib plasma concentrations). Products include:

Erythromycin Gluceptate (Substances that are potent inhibitors of CYP3A4 (e.g., ketoconazole and itraconazole) decrease gefitinib metabolism and increase gefitinib plasma concentrations).
 No products indexed under this heading.

Erythromycin Lactobionate (Substances that are potent inhibitors of CYP3A4 (e.g., ketoconazole and itraconazole) decrease gefitinib metabolism and increase gefitinib plasma concentrations).
 No products indexed under this heading.

Erythromycin Stearate (Substances that are potent inhibitors of CYP3A4 (e.g., ketoconazole and itraconazole) decrease gefitinib metabolism and increase gefitinib plasma concentrations). Products include:

Esomeprazole Magnesium (Substances that are potent inhibitors of CYP3A4 (e.g., ketoconazole and itraconazole) decrease gefitinib metabolism and increase gefitinib plasma concentrations). Products include:

Ethosuximide (Substances that are inducers of CYP3A4 activity increase the metabolism of gefitinib and decrease its plasma concentrations).
 No products indexed under this heading.

Ethotoin (In the highest concentration studied (5000ng/ml), gefitinib inhibited CYP2D6 by 24%).
 No products indexed under this heading.

Famotidine (Drugs that cause significant sustained elevation in gastric pH may reduce plasma concentrations of gefitinib and therefore potentially may reduce efficacy). Products include:

Felbamate (Substances that are inducers of CYP3A4 activity increase the metabolism of gefitinib and decrease its plasma concentrations).
 No products indexed under this heading.

Fentanyl (In the highest concentration studied (5000ng/ml), gefitinib inhibited CYP2D6 by 43%). Products include:

Fentanyl Citrate (In the highest concentration studied (5000ng/ml), gefitinib inhibited CYP2D6 by 43%). Products include:

Flecainide Acetate (In the highest concentration studied (5000ng/ml), gefitinib inhibited CYP2D6 by 43%). Products include:

Fluconazole (Substances that are potent inhibitors of CYP3A4 (e.g., ketoconazole and itraconazole) decrease gefitinib metabolism and increase gefitinib plasma concentrations).
 No products indexed under this heading.

Fludrocortisone Acetate (Substances that are inducers of CYP3A4 activity increase the metabolism of gefitinib and decrease its plasma concentrations).
 No products indexed under this heading.

Fluoxetine (In the highest concentration studied (5000ng/ml), gefitinib inhibited CYP2D6 by 43%).
 No products indexed under this heading.

Fluoxetine Hydrochloride (Substances that are potent inhibitors of CYP3A4 (e.g., ketoconazole and itraconazole) decrease gefitinib metabolism and increase gefitinib plasma concentrations). Products include:

Fluphenazine Decanoate (In the highest concentration studied (5000ng/ml), gefitinib inhibited CYP2D6 by 43%).
 No products indexed under this heading.

Fluphenazine Enanthate (In the highest concentration studied (5000ng/ml), gefitinib inhibited CYP2D6 by 43%).
 No products indexed under this heading.

Fluphenazine Hydrochloride (In the highest concentration studied (5000ng/ml), gefitinib inhibited CYP2D6 by 43%).
 No products indexed under this heading.

Fluvoxamine Maleate (Substances that are potent inhibitors of CYP3A4 (e.g., ketoconazole and itraconazole) decrease gefitinib metabolism and increase gefitinib plasma concentrations).
 No products indexed under this heading.

Formoterol Fumarate (In the highest concentration studied (5000ng/ml), gefitinib inhibited CYP2D6 by 43%). Products include:
Foradil Aerolizer 3010

Fosamprenavir Calcium (Substances that are potent inhibitors of CYP3A4 (e.g., ketoconazole and itraconazole) decrease gefitinib metabolism and increase gefitinib plasma concentrations). Products include:
Lexiva Tablets 1505

Fosphenytoin (In the highest concentration studied (5000ng/ml), gefitinib inhibited CYP2D6 by 24%).
No products indexed under this heading.

Fosphenytoin Sodium (Substances that are inducers of CYP3A4 increase the metabolism of gefitinib and decrease its plasma concentrations. In patients receiving a potent CYP3A4 inducer such as phenytoin, a dose increase to 500mg daily should be considered in the absence of severe adverse drug reaction, and clinical response and adverse events should be carefully monitored).
No products indexed under this heading.

Gabapentin (In the highest concentration studied (5000ng/ml), gefitinib inhibited CYP2D6 by 24%). Products include:
Neurontin Capsules 2487
Neurontin Oral Solution 2487
Neurontin Tablets 2487

Galantamine Hydrobromide (In the highest concentration studied (5000ng/ml), gefitinib inhibited CYP2D6 by 43%). Products include:
Razadyne 2399
Razadyne ER Extended-Release Capsules 2399

Garlic Extract (Substances that are inducers of CYP3A4 activity increase the metabolism of gefitinib and decrease its plasma concentrations).
No products indexed under this heading.

Garlic Oil (Substances that are inducers of CYP3A4 activity increase the metabolism of gefitinib and decrease its plasma concentrations).
No products indexed under this heading.

Haloperidol (In the highest concentration studied (5000ng/ml), gefitinib inhibited CYP2D6 by 43%).
No products indexed under this heading.

Haloperidol Decanoate (In the highest concentration studied (5000ng/ml), gefitinib inhibited CYP2D6 by 43%).
No products indexed under this heading.

Hydrocodone Bitartrate (In the highest concentration studied (5000ng/ml), gefitinib inhibited CYP2D6 by 43%). Products include:
Hycodan 1116
Hycotuss Expectorant Syrup 1117
Vicodin Tablets 535
Vicodin ES Tablets 536
Vicodin HP Tablets 538
Vicoprofen Tablets 539
Zydone Tablets 1139

Hydrocortisone (Substances that are inducers of CYP3A4 activity increase the metabolism of gefitinib and decrease its plasma concentrations). Products include:
Colocort Rectal Suspension, USP (Retention) 100 mg/60 mL 2476
Hydrocortone Tablets 1989
Preparation H Hydrocortisone Cream 646

Hydrocortisone Acetate (Substances that are inducers of CYP3A4 activity increase the metabolism of gefitinib and decrease its plasma concentrations). Products include:
Analpram-HC 1159
Pramosone 1161
ProctoFoam-HC 3099

Hydrocortisone Butyrate (Substances that are inducers of CYP3A4 activity increase the metabolism of gefitinib and decrease its plasma concentrations). Products include:
Locoid Lipocream Cream 1160

Hydrocortisone Cypionate (Substances that are inducers of CYP3A4 activity increase the metabolism of gefitinib and decrease its plasma concentrations).
No products indexed under this heading.

Hydrocortisone Hemisuccinate (Substances that are inducers of CYP3A4 activity increase the metabolism of gefitinib and decrease its plasma concentrations).
No products indexed under this heading.

Hydrocortisone Probutate (Substances that are inducers of CYP3A4 activity increase the metabolism of gefitinib and decrease its plasma concentrations).
No products indexed under this heading.

Hydrocortisone Sodium Phosphate (Substances that are inducers of CYP3A4 activity increase the metabolism of gefitinib and decrease its plasma concentrations).
No products indexed under this heading.

Hydrocortisone Sodium Succinate (Substances that are inducers of CYP3A4 activity increase the metabolism of gefitinib and decrease its plasma concentrations).
No products indexed under this heading.

Hydrocortisone Valerate (Substances that are inducers of CYP3A4 activity increase the metabolism of gefitinib and decrease its plasma concentrations).
No products indexed under this heading.

Hypericum (Substances that are inducers of CYP3A4 activity increase the metabolism of gefitinib and decrease its plasma concentrations). Products include:
Satiete Tablets 832

Hypericum Perforatum (Substances that are inducers of CYP3A4 activity increase the metabolism of gefitinib and decrease its plasma concentrations).
No products indexed under this heading.

Imipramine Hydrochloride (In the highest concentration studied (5000ng/ml), gefitinib inhibited CYP2D6 by 43%).
No products indexed under this heading.

Imipramine Pamoate (In the highest concentration studied (5000ng/ml), gefitinib inhibited CYP2D6 by 43%).
No products indexed under this heading.

Indinavir Sulfate (Substances that are potent inhibitors of CYP3A4 (e.g., ketoconazole and itraconazole) decrease gefitinib metabolism and increase gefitinib plasma concentrations). Products include:
Crixivan Capsules 1940

Indomethacin (In the highest concentration studied (5000ng/ml), gefitinib inhibited CYP2D6 by 24%). Products include:
Indocin 1995

Indomethacin Sodium Trihydrate (In the highest concentration studied (5000ng/ml), gefitinib inhibited CYP2D6 by 24%). Products include:
Indocin I.V. 2465

Indoramin Hydrochloride (In the highest concentration studied (5000ng/ml), gefitinib inhibited CYP2D6 by 43%).
No products indexed under this heading.

Isoniazid (Substances that are potent inhibitors of CYP3A4 (e.g., ketoconazole and itraconazole) decrease gefitinib metabolism and increase gefitinib plasma concentrations).
No products indexed under this heading.

Itraconazole (Substances that are potent inhibitors of CYP3A4 activity decrease gefitinib metabolism and increase gefitinib plasma concentrations. Co-administration of itraconazole, an inhibitor of CYP3A4, with gefitinib to healthy male volunteers, increased mean gefitinib AUC by 88%).
No products indexed under this heading.

Ketoconazole (Substances that are potent inhibitors of CYP3A4 (e.g., ketoconazole and itraconazole) decrease gefitinib metabolism and increase gefitinib plasma concentrations). Products include:
Nizoral A-D Shampoo, 1% 1868

Labetalol Hydrochloride (In the highest concentration studied (5000ng/ml), gefitinib inhibited CYP2D6 by 43%).
No products indexed under this heading.

Lamotrigine (In the highest concentration studied (5000ng/ml), gefitinib inhibited CYP2D6 by 24%). Products include:
Lamictal 1481

Lansoprazole (In the highest concentration studied (5000ng/ml), gefitinib inhibited CYP2D6 by 24%). Products include:
Prevacid Delayed-Release Capsules 3271
Prevacid for Delayed-Release Oral Suspension 3271
Prevacid SoluTab Delayed-Release Orally Disintegrating Tablets 3271
Prevacid I.V. for Injection 3277
Prevacid NapraPAC 3280
PREVPAC 3284

Levetiracetam (In the highest concentration studied (5000ng/ml), gefitinib inhibited CYP2D6 by 24%). Products include:
Keppra Injection 3320
Keppra Oral Solution 3314
Keppra Tablets 3314

Lidocaine (In the highest concentration studied (5000ng/ml), gefitinib inhibited CYP2D6 by 43%). Products include:
Lidoderm Patch 1118
Synera Topical Patch 1137

Lidocaine Hydrochloride (In the highest concentration studied (5000ng/ml), gefitinib inhibited CYP2D6 by 43%).
No products indexed under this heading.

Lopinavir (Substances that are potent inhibitors of CYP3A4 (e.g., ketoconazole and itraconazole) decrease gefitinib metabolism and increase gefitinib plasma concentrations). Products include:
Kaletra 476

Loratadine (Substances that are potent inhibitors of CYP3A4 (e.g., ketoconazole and itraconazole) decrease gefitinib metabolism and increase gefitinib plasma concentrations). Products include:
Alavert Allergy & Sinus D-12 Hour Tablets 771
Alavert 771
Children's Claritin Allergy Oral Solution 771
Claritin Non-Drowsy 24 Hour Tablets 772
Claritin Reditabs 24 Hour Non-Drowsy Tablets 772
Claritin-D Non-Drowsy 12 Hour Tablets 772
Claritin-D Non-Drowsy 24 Hour Tablets 772

Maprotiline Hydrochloride (In the highest concentration studied (5000ng/ml), gefitinib inhibited CYP2D6 by 43%).
No products indexed under this heading.

Meperidine Hydrochloride (In the highest concentration studied (5000ng/ml), gefitinib inhibited CYP2D6 by 43%).
No products indexed under this heading.

Mephenytoin (Substances that are inducers of CYP3A4 activity increase the metabolism of gefitinib and decrease its plasma concentrations).
No products indexed under this heading.

Mephobarbital (In the highest concentration studied (5000ng/ml), gefitinib inhibited CYP2D6 by 24%).
No products indexed under this heading.

Meprobamate (In the highest concentration studied (5000ng/ml), gefitinib inhibited CYP2D6 by 24%).
No products indexed under this heading.

Methadone Hydrochloride (In the highest concentration studied (5000ng/ml), gefitinib inhibited CYP2D6 by 43%).
No products indexed under this heading.

Methamphetamine Hydrochloride (In the highest concentration studied (5000ng/ml), gefitinib inhibited CYP2D6 by 43%). Products include:
Desoxyn Tablets, USP 2462

Methsuximide (Substances that are inducers of CYP3A4 activity increase the metabolism of gefitinib and decrease its plasma concentrations).
No products indexed under this heading.

Methylprednisolone (Substances that are inducers of CYP3A4 activity increase the metabolism of gefitinib and decrease its plasma concentrations).
No products indexed under this heading.

Methylprednisolone Acetate (Substances that are inducers of

CYP3A4 activity increase the metabolism of gefitinib and decrease its plasma concentrations). Products include:
Depo-Medrol Injectable Suspension 2617
Depo-Medrol Single-Dose Vial 2619

Methylprednisolone Sodium Succinate (Substances that are inducers of CYP3A4 activity increase the metabolism of gefitinib and decrease its plasma concentrations).
No products indexed under this heading.

Metoprolol Succinate (Exposure to metoprolol, a substrate of CYP2D6, was increased by 30% when it was given in combination with gefitinib in patients with solid tumors). Products include:
Toprol-XL Tablets 668

Metoprolol Tartrate (Exposure to metoprolol, a substrate of CYP2D6, was increased by 30% when it was given in combination with gefitinib in patients with solid tumors). Products include:
Lopressor Injection 2238
Lopressor Tablets 2238
Lopressor HCT 50/25 Tablets 2241
Lopressor HCT 100/25 Tablets 2241
Lopressor HCT 100/50 Tablets 2241

Metronidazole (Substances that are potent inhibitors of CYP3A4 (e.g., ketoconazole and itraconazole) decrease gefitinib metabolism and increase gefitinib plasma concentrations). Products include:
Metrogel 1% 1211
MetroGel-Vaginal Gel 1855
Vandazole Vaginal Gel 3338

Metronidazole Benzoate (Substances that are potent inhibitors of CYP3A4 (e.g., ketoconazole and itraconazole) decrease gefitinib metabolism and increase gefitinib plasma concentrations).
No products indexed under this heading.

Metronidazole Hydrochloride (Substances that are potent inhibitors of CYP3A4 (e.g., ketoconazole and itraconazole) decrease gefitinib metabolism and increase gefitinib plasma concentrations).
No products indexed under this heading.

Mexiletine Hydrochloride (In the highest concentration studied (5000ng/ml), gefitinib inhibited CYP2D6 by 43%).
No products indexed under this heading.

Miconazole (Substances that are potent inhibitors of CYP3A4 (e.g., ketoconazole and itraconazole) decrease gefitinib metabolism and increase gefitinib plasma concentrations).
No products indexed under this heading.

Miconazole Nitrate (Substances that are potent inhibitors of CYP3A4 (e.g., ketoconazole and itraconazole) decrease gefitinib metabolism and increase gefitinib plasma concentrations). Products include:
Desenex .... ▣635
Desenex Jock Itch Spray Powder ... ▣635

Midazolam Hydrochloride (In the highest concentration studied (5000ng/ml), gefitinib inhibited CYP2D6 by 24%).
No products indexed under this heading.

Mirtazapine (In the highest concentration studied (5000ng/ml), gefitinib inhibited CYP2D6 by 43%).
No products indexed under this heading.

Modafinil (Substances that are inducers of CYP3A4 activity increase the metabolism of gefitinib and decrease its plasma concentrations). Products include:
Provigil Tablets 988

Morphine Sulfate (In the highest concentration studied (5000ng/ml), gefitinib inhibited CYP2D6 by 43%). Products include:
Avinza Capsules 1741
Kadian Capsules 577
MS Contin Tablets 2701

Nefazodone Hydrochloride (Substances that are potent inhibitors of CYP3A4 (e.g., ketoconazole and itraconazole) decrease gefitinib metabolism and increase gefitinib plasma concentrations).
No products indexed under this heading.

Nelfinavir Mesylate (Substances that are potent inhibitors of CYP3A4 (e.g., ketoconazole and itraconazole) decrease gefitinib metabolism and increase gefitinib plasma concentrations). Products include:
Viracept 2577

Nevirapine (Substances that are inducers of CYP3A4 activity increase the metabolism of gefitinib and decrease its plasma concentrations). Products include:
Viramune Oral Suspension 873
Viramune Tablets 873

Niacinamide (Substances that are potent inhibitors of CYP3A4 (e.g., ketoconazole and itraconazole) decrease gefitinib metabolism and increase gefitinib plasma concentrations).
No products indexed under this heading.

Nicotinamide (Substances that are potent inhibitors of CYP3A4 (e.g., ketoconazole and itraconazole) decrease gefitinib metabolism and increase gefitinib plasma concentrations). Products include:
Nicomide Tablets 1088

Nifedipine (Substances that are potent inhibitors of CYP3A4 (e.g., ketoconazole and itraconazole) decrease gefitinib metabolism and increase gefitinib plasma concentrations). Products include:
Adalat CC Tablets 2964

Nilutamide (In the highest concentration studied (5000ng/ml), gefitinib inhibited CYP2D6 by 24%).
No products indexed under this heading.

Nizatidine (Drugs that cause significant sustained elevation in gastric pH may reduce plasma concentrations of gefitinib and therefore potentially may reduce efficacy). Products include:
Axid Oral Solution 879

Norfloxacin (Substances that are potent inhibitors of CYP3A4 (e.g., ketoconazole and itraconazole) decrease gefitinib metabolism and increase gefitinib plasma concentrations). Products include:
Noroxin Tablets 2032

Nortriptyline Hydrochloride (In the highest concentration studied (5000ng/ml), gefitinib inhibited CYP2D6 by 43%).
No products indexed under this heading.

Olanzapine (In the highest concentration studied (5000ng/ml), gefitinib inhibited CYP2D6 by 43%). Products include:
Symbyax Capsules 1819
Zyprexa Tablets 1830
Zyprexa IntraMuscular 1830
Zyprexa ZYDIS Orally Disintegrating Tablets 1830

Omeprazole (Substances that are potent inhibitors of CYP3A4 (e.g., ketoconazole and itraconazole) decrease gefitinib metabolism and increase gefitinib plasma concentrations). Products include:
Zegerid Capsules 2958
Zegerid Powder for Oral Solution 2958

Ondansetron (In the highest concentration studied (5000ng/ml), gefitinib inhibited CYP2D6 by 43%). Products include:
Zofran ODT Orally Disintegrating Tablets 1639

Ondansetron Hydrochloride (In the highest concentration studied (5000ng/ml), gefitinib inhibited CYP2D6 by 43%). Products include:
Zofran Injection 1634
Zofran 1639

Oxcarbazepine (Substances that are inducers of CYP3A4 activity increase the metabolism of gefitinib and decrease its plasma concentrations). Products include:
Trileptal Tablets 2300
Trileptal Oral Suspension 2300

Oxycodone Hydrochloride (In the highest concentration studied (5000ng/ml), gefitinib inhibited CYP2D6 by 43%). Products include:
OxyContin Tablets 2703
OxyFast Oral Concentrate Solution 2708
OxyIR Capsules 2708
Percocet Tablets 1131
Percodan Tablets 1132

Paclitaxel (In the highest concentration studied (5000ng/ml), gefitinib inhibited CYP2D6 by 43%).
No products indexed under this heading.

Pantoprazole Sodium (In the highest concentration studied (5000ng/ml), gefitinib inhibited CYP2D6 by 24%). Products include:
Protonix I.V. 3472
Protonix Tablets 3469

Paramethadione (In the highest concentration studied (5000ng/ml), gefitinib inhibited CYP2D6 by 24%).
No products indexed under this heading.

Paroxetine Hydrochloride (Substances that are potent inhibitors of CYP3A4 (e.g., ketoconazole and itraconazole) decrease gefitinib metabolism and increase gefitinib plasma concentrations). Products include:
Paxil CR Controlled-Release Tablets 1538
Paxil 1530

Pentamidine Isethionate (In the highest concentration studied (5000ng/ml), gefitinib inhibited CYP2D6 by 24%).
No products indexed under this heading.

Phenacemide (In the highest concentration studied (5000ng/ml), gefitinib inhibited CYP2D6 by 24%).
No products indexed under this heading.

Phenobarbital (Substances that are inducers of CYP3A4 activity increase the metabolism of gefitinib and decrease its plasma concentrations). Products include:
Donnatal Extentabs 2493

Phenobarbital Sodium (Substances that are inducers of CYP3A4 activity increase the metabolism of gefitinib and decrease its plasma concentrations).
No products indexed under this heading.

Phensuximide (In the highest concentration studied (5000ng/ml), gefitinib inhibited CYP2D6 by 24%).
No products indexed under this heading.

Phenytoin (Substances that are inducers of CYP3A4 increase the metabolism of gefitinib and decrease its plasma concentrations. In patients receiving a potent CYP3A4 inducer such as phenytoin, a dose increase to 500mg daily should be considered in the absence of severe adverse drug reaction, and clinical response and adverse events should be carefully monitored).
No products indexed under this heading.

Phenytoin Sodium (Substances that are inducers of CYP3A4 increase the metabolism of gefitinib and decrease its plasma concentrations. In patients receiving a potent CYP3A4 inducer such as phenytoin, a dose increase to 500mg daily should be considered in the absence of severe adverse drug reaction, and clinical response and adverse events should be carefully monitored). Products include:
Phenytek Capsules 2160

Pindolol (In the highest concentration studied (5000ng/ml), gefitinib inhibited CYP2D6 by 43%).
No products indexed under this heading.

Prednisolone Acetate (Substances that are inducers of CYP3A4 activity increase the metabolism of gefitinib and decrease its plasma concentrations). Products include:
Blephamide Ophthalmic Ointment 568
Blephamide Ophthalmic Suspension 569
Poly-Pred Ophthalmic Suspension .... ⊙233
Pred Forte Ophthalmic Suspension .... ⊙235
Pred Mild Ophthalmic Suspension .... ⊙238
Pred-G Ophthalmic Ointment .... ⊙237
Pred-G Ophthalmic Suspension ...... ⊙236

Prednisolone Sodium Phosphate (Substances that are inducers of CYP3A4 activity increase the metabolism of gefitinib and decrease its plasma concentrations).
No products indexed under this heading.

Prednisolone Tebutate (Substances that are inducers of CYP3A4 activity increase the metabolism of gefitinib and decrease its plasma concentrations).
No products indexed under this heading.

Prednisone (Substances that are inducers of CYP3A4 activity increase the metabolism of gefitinib and decrease its plasma concentrations).
No products indexed under this heading.

Primidone (Substances that are inducers of CYP3A4 activity increase the metabolism of gefitinib and decrease its plasma concentrations).
No products indexed under this heading.

Progesterone (In the highest concentration studied (5000ng/ml), gefitinib inhibited CYP2D6 by 24%). Products include:
Prochieve 4% Gel 1003
Prochieve 8% Gel 1003
Prometrium Capsules (100 mg, 200 mg) 3203

Proguanil Hydrochloride (In the highest concentration studied (5000ng/ml), gefitinib inhibited CYP2D6 by 24%). Products include:
Malarone Pediatric Tablets 1517
Malarone Tablets 1517

Propafenone Hydrochloride (In the highest concentration studied (5000ng/ml), gefitinib inhibited CYP2D6 by 43%). Products include:
Rythmol SR Capsules 2727

Propoxyphene Hydrochloride (Substances that are potent inhibitors of CYP3A4 (e.g., ketoconazole and itraconazole) decrease gefitinib metabolism and increase gefitinib plasma concentrations).
No products indexed under this heading.

Propoxyphene Napsylate (Substances that are potent inhibitors of CYP3A4 (e.g., ketoconazole and itraconazole) decrease gefitinib metabolism and increase gefitinib plasma concentrations).
No products indexed under this heading.

Propranolol Hydrochloride (In the highest concentration studied (5000ng/ml), gefitinib inhibited CYP2D6 by 43%). Products include:
Inderal LA Long-Acting Capsules 3429
InnoPran XL Capsules 2723

Protriptyline Hydrochloride (In the highest concentration studied (5000ng/ml), gefitinib inhibited CYP2D6 by 24%).
No products indexed under this heading.

Quetiapine Fumarate (In the highest concentration studied (5000ng/ml), gefitinib inhibited CYP2D6 by 43%). Products include:
Seroquel Tablets 690

Quinidine (Substances that are potent inhibitors of CYP3A4 (e.g., ketoconazole and itraconazole) decrease gefitinib metabolism and increase gefitinib plasma concentrations).
No products indexed under this heading.

Quinidine Gluconate (In the highest concentration studied (5000ng/ml), gefitinib inhibited CYP2D6 by 43%).
No products indexed under this heading.

Quinidine Hydrochloride (Substances that are potent inhibitors of CYP3A4 (e.g., ketoconazole and itraconazole) decrease gefitinib metabolism and increase gefitinib plasma concentrations).
No products indexed under this heading.

Quinidine Polygalacturonate (Substances that are potent inhibitors of CYP3A4 (e.g., ketoconazole and itraconazole) decrease gefitinib metabolism and increase gefitinib plasma concentrations).
No products indexed under this heading.

Quinidine Sulfate (Substances that are potent inhibitors of CYP3A4 (e.g., ketoconazole and itraconazole) decrease gefitinib metabolism and increase gefitinib plasma concentrations).
No products indexed under this heading.

Quinine (Substances that are potent inhibitors of CYP3A4 (e.g., ketoconazole and itraconazole) decrease gefitinib metabolism and increase gefitinib plasma concentrations).
No products indexed under this heading.

Quinine Sulfate (Substances that are potent inhibitors of CYP3A4 (e.g., ketoconazole and itraconazole) decrease gefitinib metabolism and increase gefitinib plasma concentrations).
No products indexed under this heading.

Quinupristin (Substances that are potent inhibitors of CYP3A4 (e.g., ketoconazole and itraconazole) decrease gefitinib metabolism and increase gefitinib plasma concentrations).
No products indexed under this heading.

Rabeprazole Sodium (In the highest concentration studied (5000ng/ml), gefitinib inhibited CYP2D6 by 24%). Products include:
Aciphex Tablets 1090

Ranitidine Bismuth Citrate (Drugs that cause significant sustained elevation in gastric pH may reduce plasma concentrations of gefitinib and therefore potentially may reduce efficacy. Co-administration of high doses of ranitidine with sodium bicarbonate (to maintain the gastric pH above pH 5.0) reduced mean gefitinib AUC by 44%).
No products indexed under this heading.

Ranitidine Hydrochloride (Drugs that cause significant sustained elevation in gastric pH may reduce plasma concentrations of gefitinib and therefore potentially may reduce efficacy. Co-administration of high doses of ranitidine with sodium bicarbonate (to maintain the gastric pH above pH 5.0) reduced mean gefitinib AUV by 44%). Products include:
Zantac 1624
Zantac Injection 1619
Zantac Injection Pharmacy Bulk Package 1622

Rifabutin (Substances that are inducers of CYP3A4 activity increase the metabolism of gefitinib and decrease its plasma concentrations).
No products indexed under this heading.

Rifampicin (Substances that are inducers of CYP3A4 activity increase the metabolism of gefitinib and decrease its plasma concentrations. Rifampicin reduced mean AUC of gefitinib by 85% in healthy male volunteers. In patients receiving a potent CYP3A4 inducer such as rifampicin, a dose increase to 500mg daily should be considered in the absence of severe adverse drug reaction, and clinical response and adverse events should be carefully monitored).
No products indexed under this heading.

Rifampin (Substances that are inducers of CYP3A4 activity increase the metabolism of gefitinib and decrease its plasma concentrations).
No products indexed under this heading.

Rifapentine (Substances that are inducers of CYP3A4 activity increase the metabolism of gefitinib and decrease its plasma concentrations).
No products indexed under this heading.

Risperidone (In the highest concentration studied (5000ng/ml), gefitinib inhibited CYP2D6 by 43%). Products include:
Risperdal 1676
Risperdal Consta Long-Acting Injection 1682
Risperdal M-Tab Orally Disintegrating Tablets 1676

Ritonavir (Substances that are potent inhibitors of CYP3A4 (e.g., ketoconazole and itraconazole) decrease gefitinib metabolism and increase gefitinib plasma concentrations). Products include:
Kaletra 476
Norvir 503

Saquinavir (Substances that are potent inhibitors of CYP3A4 (e.g., ketoconazole and itraconazole) decrease gefitinib metabolism and increase gefitinib plasma concentrations).
No products indexed under this heading.

Saquinavir Mesylate (Substances that are potent inhibitors of CYP3A4 (e.g., ketoconazole and itraconazole) decrease gefitinib metabolism and increase gefitinib plasma concentrations). Products include:
Invirase 2772

Sertraline Hydrochloride (Substances that are potent inhibitors of CYP3A4 (e.g., ketoconazole and itraconazole) decrease gefitinib metabolism and increase gefitinib plasma concentrations). Products include:
Zoloft 2586

Sodium Bicarbonate (Co-administration of high doses of ranitidine with sodium bicarbonate (to maintain the gastric pH above pH 5.0) reduced mean gefitinib AUC by 44%). Products include:
Colyte with Flavor Packs for Oral Solution 3088
HalfLytely and Bisacodyl Tablets Bowel Prep Kit with Flavors Packs 881
TriLyte with Flavor Packs for Oral Solution 3100

Sulfinpyrazone (Substances that are inducers of CYP3A4 activity increase the metabolism of gefitinib and decrease its plasma concentrations).
No products indexed under this heading.

Tamoxifen Citrate (In the highest concentration studied (5000ng/ml), gefitinib inhibited CYP2D6 by 43%). Products include:
Soltamox Oral Solution 3527

Telithromycin (Substances that are potent inhibitors of CYP3A4 (e.g., ketoconazole and itraconazole) decrease gefitinib metabolism and increase gefitinib plasma concentrations). Products include:
Ketek Tablets 2903

Teniposide (In the highest concentration studied (5000ng/ml), gefitinib inhibited CYP2D6 by 43%).
No products indexed under this heading.

Testosterone (In the highest concentration studied (5000ng/ml), gefitinib inhibited CYP2D6 by 43%). Products include:
AndroGel 3329
Striant Mucoadhesive 1007
Testim 1% Gel 695

Testosterone Cypionate (In the highest concentration studied (5000ng/ml), gefitinib inhibited CYP2D6 by 43%).
No products indexed under this heading.

Testosterone Enanthate (In the highest concentration studied (5000ng/ml), gefitinib inhibited CYP2D6 by 43%).
No products indexed under this heading.

Testosterone Propionate (In the highest concentration studied (5000ng/ml), gefitinib inhibited CYP2D6 by 43%).
No products indexed under this heading.

Theophylline (Substances that are inducers of CYP3A4 activity increase the metabolism of gefitinib and decrease its plasma concentrations).
No products indexed under this heading.

Thioridazine (In the highest concentration studied (5000ng/ml), gefitinib inhibited CYP2D6 by 43%).
No products indexed under this heading.

Thioridazine Hydrochloride (In the highest concentration studied (5000ng/ml), gefitinib inhibited CYP2D6 by 43%). Products include:
Thioridazine Hydrochloride Tablets 2163

Tiagabine Hydrochloride (In the highest concentration studied (5000ng/ml), gefitinib inhibited CYP2D6 by 24%). Products include:
Gabitril Tablets 984

Timolol Maleate (In the highest concentration studied (5000ng/ml), gefitinib inhibited CYP2D6 by 43%). Products include:
Blocadren Tablets 1916
Cosopt Sterile Ophthalmic Solution 1931
Timolide Tablets 2086
Timoptic Sterile Ophthalmic Solution 2088
Timoptic in Ocudose 2091
Timoptic-XE Sterile Ophthalmic Gel Forming Solution 2092

Tolbutamide (In the highest concentration studied (5000ng/ml), gefitinib inhibited CYP2D6 by 24%).
No products indexed under this heading.

Tolbutamide Sodium (In the highest concentration studied (5000ng/ml), gefitinib inhibited CYP2D6 by 24%).
No products indexed under this heading.

Tolterodine Tartrate (In the highest concentration studied (5000ng/ml), gefitinib inhibited CYP2D6 by 43%). Products include:
Detrol Tablets 2628
Detrol LA Capsules 2631

Topiramate (In the highest concentration studied (5000ng/ml), gefitinib inhibited CYP2D6 by 24%). Products include:
Topamax Sprinkle Capsules 2404

Topamax Tablets **2404**

Tramadol Hydrochloride (In the highest concentration studied (5000ng/ml), gefitinib inhibited CYP2D6 by 43%). Products include:

Ultram ER Tablets **2392**

Trazodone Hydrochloride (In the highest concentration studied (5000ng/ml), gefitinib inhibited CYP2D6 by 43%).

No products indexed under this heading.

Triamcinolone (Substances that are inducers of CYP3A4 activity increase the metabolism of gefitinib and decrease its plasma concentrations).

No products indexed under this heading.

Triamcinolone Acetonide (Substances that are inducers of CYP3A4 activity increase the metabolism of gefitinib and decrease its plasma concentrations). Products include:

Azmacort Inhalation Aerosol **1726**
Nasacort AQ Nasal Spray **2922**

Triamcinolone Diacetate (Substances that are inducers of CYP3A4 activity increase the metabolism of gefitinib and decrease its plasma concentrations).

No products indexed under this heading.

Triamcinolone Hexacetonide (Substances that are inducers of CYP3A4 activity increase the metabolism of gefitinib and decrease its plasma concentrations).

No products indexed under this heading.

Triazolam (In the highest concentration studied (5000ng/ml), gefitinib inhibited CYP2D6 by 43%).

No products indexed under this heading.

Trimethadione (In the highest concentration studied (5000ng/ml), gefitinib inhibited CYP2D6 by 24%).

No products indexed under this heading.

Trimipramine Maleate (In the highest concentration studied (5000ng/ml), gefitinib inhibited CYP2D6 by 43%).

No products indexed under this heading.

Troglitazone (Substances that are inducers of CYP3A4 activity increase the metabolism of gefitinib and decrease its plasma concentrations).

No products indexed under this heading.

Troleandomycin (Substances that are potent inhibitors of CYP3A4 (e.g., ketoconazole and itraconazole) decrease gefitinib metabolism and increase gefitinib plasma concentrations).

No products indexed under this heading.

Valproate Sodium (Substances that are potent inhibitors of CYP3A4 (e.g., ketoconazole and itraconazole) decrease gefitinib metabolism and increase gefitinib plasma concentrations). Products include:

Depacon Injection **412**

Valproic Acid (In the highest concentration studied (5000ng/ml), gefitinib inhibited CYP2D6 by 24%). Products include:

Depakene **417**

Venlafaxine Hydrochloride (In the highest concentration studied (5000ng/ml), gefitinib inhibited CYP2D6 by 43%). Products include:

Effexor Tablets **3411**
Effexor XR Capsules **3417**

Verapamil Hydrochloride (Substances that are potent inhibitors of CYP3A4 (e.g., ketoconazole and itraconazole) decrease gefitinib metabolism and increase gefitinib plasma concentrations). Products include:

Covera-HS Tablets **3139**
Tarka Tablets **524**
Verelan PM Extended-Release Capsules, Controlled-Onset **3106**

Vinblastine Sulfate (In the highest concentration studied (5000ng/ml), gefitinib inhibited CYP2D6 by 43%).

No products indexed under this heading.

Vinorelbine Tartrate (Phase II clinical trial data, where gefitinib and vinorelbine have been used concomitantly, indicates that gefitinib may exacerbate the neutropenic effect of vinorelbine).

No products indexed under this heading.

Voriconazole (Substances that are potent inhibitors of CYP3A4 (e.g., ketoconazole and itraconazole) decrease gefitinib metabolism and increase gefitinib plasma concentrations). Products include:

VFEND I.V. **2564**
VFEND Oral Suspension **2564**
VFEND Tablets **2564**

Warfarin Sodium (International Normalized Ratio (INR) elevations and/or bleeding events have been reported in some patients taking warfarin while on gefitinib. Patients taking warfarin should be monitored regularly for changes in prothrombin time or INR). Products include:

Coumadin for Injection **898**
Coumadin Tablets **898**

Zafirlukast (Substances that are potent inhibitors of CYP3A4 (e.g., ketoconazole and itraconazole) decrease gefitinib metabolism and increase gefitinib plasma concentrations). Products include:

Accolate Tablets **671**

Zileuton (Substances that are potent inhibitors of CYP3A4 (e.g., ketoconazole and itraconazole) decrease gefitinib metabolism and increase gefitinib plasma concentrations). Products include:

Zyflo Tablets **1023**

Zonisamide (In the highest concentration studied (5000ng/ml), gefitinib inhibited CYP2D6 by 43%). Products include:

Zonegran Capsules **1101**

Food Interactions

Grapefruit (Substances that are potent inhibitors of CYP3A4 (e.g., ketoconazole and itraconazole) decrease gefitinib metabolism and increase gefitinib plasma concentrations).

Grapefruit Juice (Substances that are potent inhibitors of CYP3A4 (e.g., ketoconazole and itraconazole) decrease gefitinib metabolism and increase gefitinib plasma concentrations).

I.V. BUSULFEX

(Busulfan) **2493**

May interact with phenytoin and certain other agents. Compounds in these categories include:

Acetaminophen (Use of acetaminophen prior to (less than 72 hours) or concurrent with Busulfex may result in reduced busulfan clearance since acetaminophen decreases glutathione levels in the blood and tissues). Products include:

Comtrex Maximum Strength Cold & Cough Day/Night Caplets - Day Formulation .... ▣ **726**
Comtrex Maximum Strength Cold & Cough Day/Night Caplets - Night Formulation .... ▣ **726**
Comtrex Maximum Strength Non-Drowsy Cold & Cough Caplets .... ▣ **725**
Comtrex Maximum Strength Day/Night Severe Cold & Sinus Caplets - Day Formulation .... ▣ **725**
Comtrex Maximum Strength Day/Night Severe Cold & Sinus Caplets - Night Formulation .... ▣ **725**
Contac Cold and Flu Maximum Strength Caplets .... ▣ **728**
Contac Cold and Flu Day and Night Caplets (Day Formulation Only) .... ▣ **727**
Contac Cold and Flu Day and Night Caplets (Night Formulation Only) .... ▣ **727**
Contac Cold and Flu Non-Drowsy Caplets .... ▣ **728**
Excedrin Extra Strength Caplets/Tablets/Geltabs .... ▣ **684**
Excedrin Migraine Caplets/Tablets/Geltabs .... ▣ **609**
Excedrin PM Caplets/Tablets/Geltabs .... ▣ **610**
Excedrin Sinus Headache Caplets/Tablets .... ▣ **610**
Excedrin Tension Headache Caplets/Tablets/Geltabs .... ▣ **611**
Goody's Body Pain Formula Powder .... ▣ **684**
Goody's Extra Strength Headache Powders .... ▣ **611**
Goody's Extra Strength Pain Relief Tablets .... ▣ **685**
Goody's PM Powder for Pain with Sleeplessness .... ▣ **612**
Percocet Tablets **1131**
Robitussin Cough, Cold & Flu Nighttime Liquid .... ▣ **738**
TheraFlu Cold & Sore Throat Hot Liquid .... ▣ **741**
TheraFlu Flu & Chest Congestion Hot Liquid .... ▣ **741**
TheraFlu Flu & Sore Throat Hot Liquid .... ▣ **742**
TheraFlu Daytime Severe Cold Hot Liquid .... ▣ **742**
TheraFlu Nighttime Severe Cold Hot Liquid .... ▣ **740**
TheraFlu Warming Relief Daytime Severe Cold .... ▣ **743**
TheraFlu Warming Relief Nighttime Severe Cold .... ▣ **743**
Triaminic Cough & Sore Throat Liquid .... ▣ **747**
Regular Strength Tylenol Tablets **1870**
Children's Tylenol with Flavor Creator .... ▣ **679**
Children's Tylenol Plus Flu Oral Suspension .... ▣ **749**
Tylenol Cold Head Congestion Daytime Caplets with Cool Burst and Gelcaps .... ▣ **750**
Tylenol Cold Multi-Symptom Daytime Liquid .... ▣ **752**
Tylenol Cold Multi-Symptom Severe Daytime Liquid .... ▣ **752**
Tylenol 8 Hour Extended Release Caplets **1870**
Tylenol **1870**
Extra Strength Tylenol PM Caplets, Vanilla Caplets, Geltabs, Gelcaps and Liquid **1875**
Extra Strength Tylenol Rapid Release Gels **1870**
Concentrated Tylenol Infants' Drops Plus Cold & Cough .... ▣ **754**
Tylenol with Codeine Tablets **2391**
Tylenol Allergy Multi-Symptom Caplets with Cool Burst and Gelcaps **1872**
Tylenol Allergy Multi-Symptom Nighttime Caplets with Cool Burst **1872**
Tylenol Severe Allergy Caplets **1872**
Tylenol Arthritis Pain Extended Release Caplets and Geltabs **1870**
Tylenol Chest Congestion Caplets with Cool Burst **1872**
Tylenol Chest Congestion Liquid with Cool Burst **1872**
Children's Tylenol Suspension Liquid and Meltaways **1878**
Children's Tylenol Plus Cold Suspension Liquid **1879**
Children's Tylenol Plus Cold & Allergy Suspension Liquid **1878**
Children's Tylenol Plus Cough & Runny Nose Suspension Liquid **1879**
Children's Tylenol Plus Cough & Sore Throat Suspension Liquid **1879**
Children's Tylenol Suspension with Flavor Creator **1878**
Children's Tylenol Plus Flu Suspension Liquid **1881**
Children's Tylenol Plus Multi-Symptom Cold Suspension Liquid **1879**
Tylenol Cold Severe Congestion Non-Drowsy Caplets with Cool Burst **1874**
Tylenol Cold Head Congestion Daytime Caplets with Cool Burst **1873**
Tylenol Cold Head Congestion Nighttime Caplets with Cool Burst **1873**
Tylenol Cold Head Congestion Severe Caplets with Cool Burst **1873**
Tylenol Cold Multi-Symptom Daytime Caplets with Cool Burst and Gelcaps **1874**
Tylenol Cold Multi-Symptom Daytime Liquid with Citrus Burst **1874**
Tylenol Cold Multi-Symptom Nighttime Caplets with Cool Burst **1874**
Tylenol Cold Multi-Symptom Nighttime Liquid with Cool Burst **1874**
Tylenol Cold Multi-Symptom Severe Caplets with Cool Burst **1874**
Tylenol Cold Multi-Symptom Severe Daytime Liquid with Citrus Burst **1874**
Tylenol Cough & Sore Throat Daytime Liquid with Cool Burst **1877**
Tylenol Cough & Sore Throat Nighttime Liquid with Cool Burst **1877**
Concentrated Tylenol Infants' Drops **1878**
Concentrated Tylenol Infants' Drops Plus Cold **1879**
Concentrated Tylenol Infants' Drops Plus Cold and Cough **1879**
Jr. Tylenol Meltaways **1878**
Tylenol Sinus Severe Congestion Caplets with Cool Burst **1876**
Tylenol Sinus Congestion & Pain Daytime Caplets with Cool Burst and Gelcaps **1876**
Tylenol Sinus Congestion & Pain Nighttime Caplets with Cool Burst **1876**
Tylenol Sinus Congestion & Pain Severe Caplets with Cool Burst **1876**
Tylenol Sore Throat Daytime Liquid with Cool Burst **1877**
Tylenol Sore Throat Nighttime Liquid with Cool Burst **1877**
Women's Tylenol Menstrual Relief Caplets **1877**
Vicks 44M Cough, Cold & Flu Relief Liquid **2680**
Vicks DayQuil LiquiCaps/Liquid Multi-Symptom Cold/Flu Relief .... ▣ **761**
Vicks DayQuil Multi-Symptom Cold/Flu Relief LiquiCaps **2678**
Vicks DayQuil Multi-Symptom Cold/Flu Relief Liquid **2678**
Vicks NyQuil Multi-Symptom Cold/Flu Relief Liquid **2681**
Vicks NyQuil Multi-Symptom Cold/Flu Relief LiquiCaps **2681**
Vicks NyQuil LiquiCaps/Liquid Multi-Symptom Cold/Flu Relief .... ▣ **763**
Vicodin Tablets **535**
Vicodin ES Tablets **536**
Vicodin HP Tablets **538**
Zicam Maximum Strength Flu Daytime .... ▣ **768**
Zicam Maximum Strength Flu Nighttime .... ▣ **768**
Zydone Tablets **1139**

Fosphenytoin Sodium (Phenytoin increases the clearance of busulfan by 15% or more, possibly due to the induction of glutathione-S-transferase).

No products indexed under this heading.

Itraconazole (Itraconazole decreases busulfan clearance by up to 25%).
No products indexed under this heading.

Phenytoin (Phenytoin increases the clearance of busulfan by 15% or more, possibly due to the induction of glutathione-S-transferase).
No products indexed under this heading.

Phenytoin Sodium (Phenytoin increases the clearance of busulfan by 15% or more, possibly due to the induction of glutathione-S-transferase). Products include:
Phenytek Capsules 2160

KADIAN CAPSULES

(Morphine Sulfate) 577

May interact with central nervous system depressants, diuretics, general anesthetics, hypnotics and sedatives, monoamine oxidase inhibitors, mixed agonist/antagonist opioid analgesics, neuromuscular blocking agents, phenothiazines, and tranquilizers. Compounds in these categories include:

Alfentanil Hydrochloride (Co-administration may increase the risk of respiratory depression, hypotension and profound sedation and coma; when such combined therapy is contemplated, the initial dose of one or both agents should be reduced by at least 50%).
No products indexed under this heading.

Alprazolam (Co-administration may increase the risk of respiratory depression, hypotension and profound sedation and coma; when such combined therapy is contemplated, the initial dose of one or both agents should be reduced by at least 50%). Products include:
Niravam Orally Disintegrating Tablets 3092

Amiloride Hydrochloride (Morphine can reduce the efficacy of diuretics by inducing the release of antidiuretic hormone and by causing spasm of the sphincter of the bladder leading to acute retention of urine). Products include:
Midamor Tablets 2026
Moduretic Tablets 2028

Aprobarbital (Co-administration may increase the risk of respiratory depression, hypotension and profound sedation and coma; when such combined therapy is contemplated, the initial dose of one or both agents should be reduced by at least 50%).
No products indexed under this heading.

Atracurium Besylate (Morphine may enhance the neuromuscular blocking action of skeletal relaxants and produce an increased degree of respiratory depression).
No products indexed under this heading.

Bendroflumethiazide (Morphine can reduce the efficacy of diuretics by inducing the release of antidiuretic hormone and by causing spasm of the sphincter of the bladder leading to acute retention of urine).
No products indexed under this heading.

Bumetanide (Morphine can reduce the efficacy of diuretics by inducing the release of antidiuretic hormone and by causing spasm of the sphincter of the bladder leading to acute retention of urine). Products include:
Bumex Tablets 2746

Buprenorphine Hydrochloride (May reduce the analgesic effect and/or precipitate withdrawal symptoms). Products include:
Buprenex Injectable 2716
Suboxone Tablets 2717
Subutex Tablets 2717

Buspirone Hydrochloride (Co-administration may increase the risk of respiratory depression, hypotension and profound sedation and coma; when such combined therapy is contemplated, the initial dose of one or both agents should be reduced by at least 50%).
No products indexed under this heading.

Butabarbital (Co-administration may increase the risk of respiratory depression, hypotension and profound sedation and coma; when such combined therapy is contemplated, the initial dose of one or both agents should be reduced by at least 50%).
No products indexed under this heading.

Butalbital (Co-administration may increase the risk of respiratory depression, hypotension and profound sedation and coma; when such combined therapy is contemplated, the initial dose of one or both agents should be reduced by at least 50%).
No products indexed under this heading.

Butorphanol Tartrate (May reduce the analgesic effect and/or precipitate withdrawal symptoms).
No products indexed under this heading.

Chlordiazepoxide (Co-administration may increase the risk of respiratory depression, hypotension and profound sedation and coma; when such combined therapy is contemplated, the initial dose of one or both agents should be reduced by at least 50%).
No products indexed under this heading.

Chlordiazepoxide Hydrochloride (Co-administration may increase the risk of respiratory depression, hypotension and profound sedation and coma; when such combined therapy is contemplated, the initial dose of one or both agents should be reduced by at least 50%). Products include:
Librium Capsules 3347

Chlorothiazide (Morphine can reduce the efficacy of diuretics by inducing the release of antidiuretic hormone and by causing spasm of the sphincter of the bladder leading to acute retention of urine). Products include:
Diuril Oral Suspension 1954

Chlorothiazide Sodium (Morphine can reduce the efficacy of diuretics by inducing the release of antidiuretic hormone and by causing spasm of the sphincter of the bladder leading to acute retention of urine). Products include:
Diuril Sodium Intravenous 2467

Chlorpromazine (Co-administration may increase the risk of respiratory depression, hypotension and profound sedation and coma; when such combined therapy is contemplated, the initial dose of one or both agents should be reduced by at least 50%).
No products indexed under this heading.

Chlorpromazine Hydrochloride (Co-administration may increase the risk of respiratory depression, hypotension and profound sedation and coma; when such combined therapy is contemplated, the initial dose of one or both agents should be reduced by at least 50%).
No products indexed under this heading.

Chlorprothixene (Co-administration may increase the risk of respiratory depression, hypotension and profound sedation and coma; when such combined therapy is contemplated, the initial dose of one or both agents should be reduced by at least 50%).
No products indexed under this heading.

Chlorprothixene Hydrochloride (Co-administration may increase the risk of respiratory depression, hypotension and profound sedation and coma; when such combined therapy is contemplated, the initial dose of one or both agents should be reduced by at least 50%).
No products indexed under this heading.

Chlorprothixene Lactate (Co-administration may increase the risk of respiratory depression, hypotension and profound sedation and coma; when such combined therapy is contemplated, the initial dose of one or both agents should be reduced by at least 50%).
No products indexed under this heading.

Chlorthalidone (Morphine can reduce the efficacy of diuretics by inducing the release of antidiuretic hormone and by causing spasm of the sphincter of the bladder leading to acute retention of urine). Products include:
Clorpres Tablets 2153

Cimetidine (Co-administration has resulted in an isolated report of confusion and severe respiratory depression). Products include:
Tagamet HB 200 Tablets 664

Cimetidine Hydrochloride (Co-administration has resulted in an isolated report of confusion and severe respiratory depression).
No products indexed under this heading.

Cisatracurium Besylate (Morphine may enhance the neuromuscular blocking action of skeletal relaxants and produce an increased degree of respiratory depression). Products include:
Nimbex Injection 498

Clorazepate Dipotassium (Co-administration may increase the risk of respiratory depression, hypotension and profound sedation and coma; when such combined therapy is contemplated, the initial dose of one or both agents should be reduced by at least 50%). Products include:
Tranxene 2474

Clozapine (Co-administration may increase the risk of respiratory depression, hypotension and profound sedation and coma; when such combined therapy is contemplated, the initial dose of one or both agents should be reduced by at least 50%). Products include:
Clozaril Tablets 2184
FazaClo Orally Disintegrating Tablets 551

Codeine Phosphate (Co-administration may increase the risk of respiratory depression, hypotension and profound sedation and coma; when such combined therapy is contemplated, the initial dose of one or both agents should be reduced by at least 50%). Products include:
Tylenol with Codeine Tablets 2391

Desflurane (Co-administration may increase the risk of respiratory depression, hypotension and profound sedation and coma; when such combined therapy is contemplated, the initial dose of one or both agents should be reduced by at least 50%).
No products indexed under this heading.

Dezocine (Co-administration may increase the risk of respiratory depression, hypotension and profound sedation and coma; when such combined therapy is contemplated, the initial dose of one or both agents should be reduced by at least 50%).
No products indexed under this heading.

Diazepam (Co-administration may increase the risk of respiratory depression, hypotension and profound sedation and coma; when such combined therapy is contemplated, the initial dose of one or both agents should be reduced by at least 50%). Products include:
Diastat Rectal Delivery System 3343
Valium Tablets 2819

Doxacurium Chloride (Morphine may enhance the neuromuscular blocking action of skeletal relaxants and produce an increased degree of respiratory depression).
No products indexed under this heading.

Droperidol (Co-administration may increase the risk of respiratory depression, hypotension and profound sedation and coma; when such combined therapy is contemplated, the initial dose of one or both agents should be reduced by at least 50%).
No products indexed under this heading.

Enflurane (Co-administration may increase the risk of respiratory depression, hypotension and profound sedation and coma; when such combined therapy is contemplated, the initial dose of one or both agents should be reduced by at least 50%).
No products indexed under this heading.

Estazolam (Co-administration may increase the risk of respiratory depression, hypotension and profound sedation and coma; when such combined therapy is contemplated, the initial dose of one or both agents should be reduced by at least 50%). Products include:
ProSom Tablets 517

Ethacrynic Acid (Morphine can reduce the efficacy of diuretics by inducing the release of antidiuretic hormone and by causing spasm of the sphincter of the bladder leading to acute retention of urine). Products include:
Edecrin Tablets 1959

Ethanol (Co-administration may increase the risk of respiratory depression, hypotension and profound sedation and coma; when such combined therapy is contemplated, the initial dose of one or both agents should be reduced by at least 50%).
No products indexed under this heading.

Ethchlorvynol (Co-administration may increase the risk of respiratory depression, hypotension and profound sedation and coma; when such combined therapy is contemplated, the initial dose of one or both agents should be reduced by at least 50%).
No products indexed under this heading.

Ethinamate (Co-administration may increase the risk of respiratory depression, hypotension and profound sedation and coma; when such combined therapy is contemplated, the initial dose of one or both agents should be reduced by at least 50%).
No products indexed under this heading.

Ethyl Alcohol (Co-administration may increase the risk of respiratory depression, hypotension and profound sedation and coma; when such combined therapy is contemplated, the initial dose of one or both agents should be reduced by at least 50%).
No products indexed under this heading.

Fentanyl (Co-administration may increase the risk of respiratory depression, hypotension and profound sedation and coma; when such combined therapy is contemplated, the initial dose of one or both agents should be reduced by at least 50%). Products include:
Duragesic Transdermal System 2373
Ionsys Transdermal System 2379

Fentanyl Citrate (Co-administration may increase the risk of respiratory depression, hypotension and profound sedation and coma; when such combined therapy is contemplated, the initial dose of one or both agents should be reduced by at least 50%). Products include:
Actiq ... 979

Fluphenazine Decanoate (Co-administration may increase the risk of respiratory depression, hypotension and profound sedation and coma; when such combined therapy is contemplated, the initial dose of one or both agents should be reduced by at least 50%).
No products indexed under this heading.

Fluphenazine Enanthate (Co-administration may increase the risk of respiratory depression, hypotension and profound sedation and coma; when such combined therapy is contemplated, the initial dose of one or both agents should be reduced by at least 50%).
No products indexed under this heading.

Fluphenazine Hydrochloride (Co-administration may increase the risk of respiratory depression, hypotension and profound sedation and coma; when such combined therapy is contemplated, the initial dose of one or both agents should be reduced by at least 50%).
No products indexed under this heading.

Flurazepam Hydrochloride (Co-administration may increase the risk of respiratory depression, hypotension and profound sedation and coma; when such combined therapy is contemplated, the initial dose of one or both agents should be reduced by at least 50%). Products include:
Dalmane Capsules 3342

Furosemide (Morphine can reduce the efficacy of diuretics by inducing the release of antidiuretic hormone and by causing spasm of the sphincter of the bladder leading to acute retention of urine). Products include:
Furosemide Tablets 2154

Glutethimide (Co-administration may increase the risk of respiratory depression, hypotension and profound sedation and coma; when such combined therapy is contemplated, the initial dose of one or both agents should be reduced by at least 50%).
No products indexed under this heading.

Haloperidol (Co-administration may increase the risk of respiratory depression, hypotension and profound sedation and coma; when such combined therapy is contemplated, the initial dose of one or both agents should be reduced by at least 50%).
No products indexed under this heading.

Haloperidol Decanoate (Co-administration may increase the risk of respiratory depression, hypotension and profound sedation and coma; when such combined therapy is contemplated, the initial dose of one or both agents should be reduced by at least 50%).
No products indexed under this heading.

Hydrochlorothiazide (Morphine can reduce the efficacy of diuretics by inducing the release of antidiuretic hormone and by causing spasm of the sphincter of the bladder leading to acute retention of urine). Products include:
Aldoril Tablets 1910
Atacand HCT 651
Avalide Tablets 888
Avalide Tablets 2874
Benicar HCT Tablets 1044
Diovan HCT Tablets 2196
Dyazide Capsules 1423
Hyzaar 50-12.5 Tablets 1990
Hyzaar 100-12.5 Tablets 1990
Hyzaar 100-25 Tablets 1990
Lopressor HCT 50/25 Tablets 2241
Lopressor HCT 100/25 Tablets 2241
Lopressor HCT 100/50 Tablets 2241
Lotensin HCT Tablets 2246
Micardis HCT Tablets 856
Moduretic Tablets 2028
Prinzide Tablets 2056
Teveten HCT Tablets 1737
Timolide Tablets 2086
Uniretic Tablets 3100

Hydrocodone Bitartrate (Co-administration may increase the risk of respiratory depression, hypotension and profound sedation and coma; when such combined therapy is contemplated, the initial dose of one or both agents should be reduced by at least 50%). Products include:
Hycodan ... 1116
Hycotuss Expectorant Syrup 1117
Vicodin Tablets 535
Vicodin ES Tablets 536
Vicodin HP Tablets 538
Vicoprofen Tablets 539
Zydone Tablets 1139

Hydrocodone Polistirex (Co-administration may increase the risk of respiratory depression, hypotension and profound sedation and coma; when such combined therapy is contemplated, the initial dose of one or both agents should be reduced by at least 50%). Products include:
Tussionex Pennkinetic
Extended-Release Suspension 3327

Hydroflumethiazide (Morphine can reduce the efficacy of diuretics by inducing the release of antidiuretic hormone and by causing spasm of the sphincter of the bladder leading to acute retention of urine).
No products indexed under this heading.

Hydromorphone Hydrochloride (Co-administration may increase the risk of respiratory depression, hypotension and profound sedation and coma; when such combined therapy is contemplated, the initial dose of one or both agents should be reduced by at least 50%). Products include:
Dilaudid ... 440
Dilaudid Non-Sterile Powder 440
Dilaudid Oral Liquid 445
Dilaudid Rectal Suppositories 440
Dilaudid Tablets 440
Dilaudid Tablets - 8 mg 445
Dilaudid-HP 442

Hydroxyzine Hydrochloride (Co-administration may increase the risk of respiratory depression, hypotension and profound sedation and coma; when such combined therapy is contemplated, the initial dose of one or both agents should be reduced by at least 50%).
No products indexed under this heading.

Indapamide (Morphine can reduce the efficacy of diuretics by inducing the release of antidiuretic hormone and by causing spasm of the sphincter of the bladder leading to acute retention of urine). Products include:
Indapamide Tablets 2156

Isocarboxazid (MAO inhibitors have been reported to intensify the effects of opioids causing anxiety, confusion and significant depression of respiration or coma; concurrent and/or sequential use is not recommended).
No products indexed under this heading.

Isoflurane (Co-administration may increase the risk of respiratory depression, hypotension and profound sedation and coma; when such combined therapy is contemplated, the initial dose of one or both agents should be reduced by at least 50%).
No products indexed under this heading.

Ketamine Hydrochloride (Co-administration may increase the risk of respiratory depression, hypotension and profound sedation and coma; when such combined therapy is contemplated, the initial dose of one or both agents should be reduced by at least 50%).
No products indexed under this heading.

Levomethadyl Acetate Hydrochloride (Co-administration may increase the risk of respiratory depression, hypotension and profound sedation and coma; when such combined therapy is contemplated, the initial dose of one or both agents should be reduced by at least 50%).
No products indexed under this heading.

Levorphanol Tartrate (Co-administration may increase the risk of respiratory depression, hypotension and profound sedation and coma; when such combined therapy is contemplated, the initial dose of one or both agents should be reduced by at least 50%).
No products indexed under this heading.

Lorazepam (Co-administration may increase the risk of respiratory depression, hypotension and profound sedation and coma; when such combined therapy is contemplated, the initial dose of one or both agents should be reduced by at least 50%).
No products indexed under this heading.

Loxapine Hydrochloride (Co-administration may increase the risk of respiratory depression, hypotension and profound sedation and coma; when such combined therapy is contemplated, the initial dose of one or both agents should be reduced by at least 50%).
No products indexed under this heading.

Loxapine Succinate (Co-administration may increase the risk of respiratory depression, hypotension and profound sedation and coma; when such combined therapy is contemplated, the initial dose of one or both agents should be reduced by at least 50%).
No products indexed under this heading.

Meperidine Hydrochloride (Co-administration may increase the risk of respiratory depression, hypotension and profound sedation and coma; when such combined therapy is contemplated, the initial dose of one or both agents should be reduced by at least 50%).
No products indexed under this heading.

Mephobarbital (Co-administration may increase the risk of respiratory depression, hypotension and profound sedation and coma; when such combined therapy is contemplated, the initial dose of one or both agents should be reduced by at least 50%).
No products indexed under this heading.

Meprobamate (Co-administration may increase the risk of respiratory depression, hypotension and profound sedation and coma; when such combined therapy is contemplated, the initial dose of one or both agents should be reduced by at least 50%).

No products indexed under this heading.

Mesoridazine Besylate (Co-administration may increase the risk of respiratory depression, hypotension and profound sedation and coma; when such combined therapy is contemplated, the initial dose of one or both agents should be reduced by at least 50%).

No products indexed under this heading.

Methadone Hydrochloride (Co-administration may increase the risk of respiratory depression, hypotension and profound sedation and coma; when such combined therapy is contemplated, the initial dose of one or both agents should be reduced by at least 50%).

No products indexed under this heading.

Methohexital Sodium (Co-administration may increase the risk of respiratory depression, hypotension and profound sedation and coma; when such combined therapy is contemplated, the initial dose of one or both agents should be reduced by at least 50%).

No products indexed under this heading.

Methotrimeprazine (Co-administration may increase the risk of respiratory depression, hypotension and profound sedation and coma; when such combined therapy is contemplated, the initial dose of one or both agents should be reduced by at least 50%).

No products indexed under this heading.

Methoxyflurane (Co-administration may increase the risk of respiratory depression, hypotension and profound sedation and coma; when such combined therapy is contemplated, the initial dose of one or both agents should be reduced by at least 50%).

No products indexed under this heading.

Methyclothiazide (Morphine can reduce the efficacy of diuretics by inducing the release of antidiuretic hormone and by causing spasm of the sphincter of the bladder leading to acute retention of urine).

No products indexed under this heading.

Metocurine Iodide (Morphine may enhance the neuromuscular blocking action of skeletal relaxants and produce an increased degree of respiratory depression).

No products indexed under this heading.

Metolazone (Morphine can reduce the efficacy of diuretics by inducing the release of antidiuretic hormone and by causing spasm of the sphincter of the bladder leading to acute retention of urine).

No products indexed under this heading.

Midazolam Hydrochloride (Co-administration may increase the risk of respiratory depression, hypotension and profound sedation and coma; when such combined therapy is contemplated, the initial dose of one or both agents should be reduced by at least 50%).

No products indexed under this heading.

Mivacurium Chloride (Morphine may enhance the neuromuscular blocking action of skeletal relaxants and produce an increased degree of respiratory depression). Products include:

Mivacron Injection **493**

Moclobemide (MAO inhibitors have been reported to intensify the effects of opioids causing anxiety, confusion and significant depression of respiration or coma; concurrent and/or sequential use is not recommended).

No products indexed under this heading.

Molindone Hydrochloride (Co-administration may increase the risk of respiratory depression, hypotension and profound sedation and coma; when such combined therapy is contemplated, the initial dose of one or both agents should be reduced by at least 50%). Products include:

Moban Tablets **1119**

Nalbuphine Hydrochloride (May reduce the analgesic effect and/or precipitate withdrawal symptoms).

No products indexed under this heading.

Olanzapine (Co-administration may increase the risk of respiratory depression, hypotension and profound sedation and coma; when such combined therapy is contemplated, the initial dose of one or both agents should be reduced by at least 50%). Products include:

Symbyax Capsules **1819**
Zyprexa Tablets **1830**
Zyprexa IntraMuscular **1830**
Zyprexa ZYDIS Orally
 Disintegrating Tablets **1830**

Oxazepam (Co-administration may increase the risk of respiratory depression, hypotension and profound sedation and coma; when such combined therapy is contemplated, the initial dose of one or both agents should be reduced by at least 50%).

No products indexed under this heading.

Oxycodone Hydrochloride (Co-administration may increase the risk of respiratory depression, hypotension and profound sedation and coma; when such combined therapy is contemplated, the initial dose of one or both agents should be reduced by at least 50%). Products include:

OxyContin Tablets **2703**
OxyFast Oral Concentrate
 Solution...................................... **2708**
OxyIR Capsules **2708**
Percocet Tablets **1131**
Percodan Tablets **1132**

Pancuronium Bromide (Morphine may enhance the neuromuscular blocking action of skeletal relaxants and produce an increased degree of respiratory depression).

No products indexed under this heading.

Pargyline Hydrochloride (MAO inhibitors have been reported to intensify the effects of opioids causing anxiety, confusion and significant depression of respiration or coma; concurrent and/or sequential use is not recommended).

No products indexed under this heading.

Pentazocine Hydrochloride (May reduce the analgesic effect and/or precipitate withdrawal symptoms).

No products indexed under this heading.

Pentazocine Lactate (May reduce the analgesic effect and/or precipitate withdrawal symptoms).

No products indexed under this heading.

Pentobarbital Sodium (Co-administration may increase the risk of respiratory depression, hypotension and profound sedation and coma; when such combined therapy is contemplated, the initial dose of one or both agents should be reduced by at least 50%). Products include:

Nembutal Sodium Solution, USP **2470**

Perphenazine (Co-administration may increase the risk of respiratory depression, hypotension and profound sedation and coma; when such combined therapy is contemplated, the initial dose of one or both agents should be reduced by at least 50%).

No products indexed under this heading.

Phenelzine Sulfate (MAO inhibitors have been reported to intensify the effects of opioids causing anxiety, confusion and significant depression of respiration or coma; concurrent and/or sequential use is not recommended).

No products indexed under this heading.

Phenobarbital (Co-administration may increase the risk of respiratory depression, hypotension and profound sedation and coma; when such combined therapy is contemplated, the initial dose of one or both agents should be reduced by at least 50%). Products include:

Donnatal Extentabs **2493**

Polythiazide (Morphine can reduce the efficacy of diuretics by inducing the release of antidiuretic hormone and by causing spasm of the sphincter of the bladder leading to acute retention of urine).

No products indexed under this heading.

Prazepam (Co-administration may increase the risk of respiratory depression, hypotension and profound sedation and coma; when such combined therapy is contemplated, the initial dose of one or both agents should be reduced by at least 50%).

No products indexed under this heading.

Procarbazine Hydrochloride (MAO inhibitors have been reported to intensify the effects of opioids causing anxiety, confusion and significant depression of respiration or coma; concurrent and/or sequential use is not recommended). Products include:

Matulane Capsules **3191**

Prochlorperazine (Co-administration may increase the risk of respiratory depression, hypotension and profound sedation and coma; when such combined therapy is contemplated, the initial dose of one or both agents should be reduced by at least 50%).

No products indexed under this heading.

Promethazine Hydrochloride (Co-administration may increase the risk of respiratory depression, hypotension and profound sedation and coma; when such combined therapy is contemplated, the initial dose of one or both agents should be reduced by at least 50%). Products include:

Phenergan Tablets and
 Suppositories.............................. **3440**

Propofol (Co-administration may increase the risk of respiratory depression, hypotension and coma; when such combined therapy is contemplated, the initial dose of one or both agents should be reduced by at least 50%).

No products indexed under this heading.

Propoxyphene Hydrochloride (Co-administration may increase the risk of respiratory depression, hypotension and profound sedation and coma; when such combined therapy is contemplated, the initial dose of one or both agents should be reduced by at least 50%).

No products indexed under this heading.

Propoxyphene Napsylate (Co-administration may increase the risk of respiratory depression, hypotension and profound sedation and coma; when such combined therapy is contemplated, the initial dose of one or both agents should be reduced by at least 50%).

No products indexed under this heading.

Quazepam (Co-administration may increase the risk of respiratory depression, hypotension and profound sedation and coma; when such combined therapy is contemplated, the initial dose of one or both agents should be reduced by at least 50%).

No products indexed under this heading.

Quetiapine Fumarate (Co-administration may increase the risk of respiratory depression, hypotension and profound sedation and coma; when such combined therapy is contemplated, the initial dose of one or both agents should be reduced by at least 50%). Products include:

Seroquel Tablets **690**

Ramelteon (Co-administration may increase the risk of respiratory depression, hypotension and profound sedation and coma; when such combined therapy is contemplated, the initial dose of one or both agents should be reduced by at least 50%). Products include:

Rozerem Tablets **3231**

Rapacuronium Bromide (Morphine may enhance the neuromuscular blocking action of skeletal relaxants and produce an increased degree of respiratory depression).

No products indexed under this heading.

IMPORTANT NOTE: Always consult each drug listing in the patient's regimen for possible interactions.

Remifentanil Hydrochloride (Co-administration may increase the risk of respiratory depression, hypotension and profound sedation and coma; when such combined therapy is contemplated, the initial dose of one or both agents should be reduced by at least 50%).
No products indexed under this heading.

Risperidone (Co-administration may increase the risk of respiratory depression, hypotension and profound sedation and coma; when such combined therapy is contemplated, the initial dose of one or both agents should be reduced by at least 50%). Products include:
Risperdal 1676
Risperdal Consta Long-Acting Injection 1682
Risperdal M-Tab Orally Disintegrating Tablets 1676

Rocuronium Bromide (Morphine may enhance the neuromuscular blocking action of skeletal relaxants and produce an increased degree of respiratory depression). Products include:
Zemuron Injection 2346

Secobarbital Sodium (Co-administration may increase the risk of respiratory depression, hypotension and profound sedation and coma; when such combined therapy is contemplated, the initial dose of one or both agents should be reduced by at least 50%).
No products indexed under this heading.

Selegiline Hydrochloride (MAO inhibitors have been reported to intensify the effects of opioids causing anxiety, confusion and significant depression of respiration or coma; concurrent and/or sequential use is not recommended). Products include:
Eldepryl Capsules 3208
Zelapar Tablets 3372

Sevoflurane (Co-administration may increase the risk of respiratory depression, hypotension and profound sedation and coma; when such combined therapy is contemplated, the initial dose of one or both agents should be reduced by at least 50%). Products include:
Ultane Liquid for Inhalation 531

Spironolactone (Morphine can reduce the efficacy of diuretics by inducing the release of antidiuretic hormone and by causing spasm of the sphincter of the bladder leading to acute retention of urine).
No products indexed under this heading.

Succinylcholine Chloride (Morphine may enhance the neuromuscular blocking action of skeletal relaxants and produce an increased degree of respiratory depression).
No products indexed under this heading.

Sufentanil Citrate (Co-administration may increase the risk of respiratory depression, hypotension and profound sedation and coma; when such combined therapy is contemplated, the initial dose of one or both agents should be reduced by at least 50%).
No products indexed under this heading.

Temazepam (Co-administration may increase the risk of respiratory depression, hypotension and profound sedation and coma; when such combined therapy is contemplated, the initial dose of one or both agents should be reduced by at least 50%). Products include:
Restoril Capsules 1860

Thiamylal Sodium (Co-administration may increase the risk of respiratory depression, hypotension and profound sedation and coma; when such combined therapy is contemplated, the initial dose of one or both agents should be reduced by at least 50%).
No products indexed under this heading.

Thioridazine Hydrochloride (Co-administration may increase the risk of respiratory depression, hypotension and profound sedation and coma; when such combined therapy is contemplated, the initial dose of one or both agents should be reduced by at least 50%). Products include:
Thioridazine Hydrochloride Tablets 2163

Thiothixene (Co-administration may increase the risk of respiratory depression, hypotension and profound sedation and coma; when such combined therapy is contemplated, the initial dose of one or both agents should be reduced by at least 50%). Products include:
Thiothixene Capsules 2165

Torsemide (Morphine can reduce the efficacy of diuretics by inducing the release of antidiuretic hormone and by causing spasm of the sphincter of the bladder leading to acute retention of urine). Products include:
Demadex Injection 2759
Demadex Tablets 2759

Tranylcypromine Sulfate (MAO inhibitors have been reported to intensify the effects of opioids causing anxiety, confusion and significant depression of respiration or coma; concurrent and/or sequential use is not recommended). Products include:
Parnate Tablets 1527

Triamterene (Morphine can reduce the efficacy of diuretics by inducing the release of antidiuretic hormone and by causing spasm of the sphincter of the bladder leading to acute retention of urine). Products include:
Dyazide Capsules 1423
Dyrenium Capsules 3400

Triazolam (Co-administration may increase the risk of respiratory depression, hypotension and profound sedation and coma; when such combined therapy is contemplated, the initial dose of one or both agents should be reduced by at least 50%).
No products indexed under this heading.

Trifluoperazine Hydrochloride (Co-administration may increase the risk of respiratory depression, hypotension and profound sedation and coma; when such combined therapy is contemplated, the initial dose of one or both agents should be reduced by at least 50%).
No products indexed under this heading.

Vecuronium Bromide (Morphine may enhance the neuromuscular blocking action of skeletal relaxants and produce an increased degree of respiratory depression).
No products indexed under this heading.

Zaleplon (Co-administration may increase the risk of respiratory depression, hypotension and profound sedation and coma; when such combined therapy is contemplated, the initial dose of one or both agents should be reduced by at least 50%). Products include:
Sonata Capsules 1717

Ziprasidone Hydrochloride (Co-administration may increase the risk of respiratory depression, hypotension and profound sedation and coma; when such combined therapy is contemplated, the initial dose of one or both agents should be reduced by at least 50%). Products include:
Geodon Capsules 2529

Zolpidem Tartrate (Co-administration may increase the risk of respiratory depression, hypotension and profound sedation and coma; when such combined therapy is contemplated, the initial dose of one or both agents should be reduced by at least 50%). Products include:
Ambien Tablets 2851
Ambien CR Tablets 2855

Food Interactions

Alcohol (Co-administration may increase the risk of respiratory depression, hypotension and profound sedation and coma).

Food, unspecified (Slows the rate of absorption of Kadian, the extent of absorption is not affected and Kadian can be administered without regard to meals; the pellets in Kadian should not be dissolved).

KALETRA ORAL SOLUTION

(Lopinavir, Ritonavir) 476
See Kaletra Tablets

KALETRA TABLETS

(Lopinavir, Ritonavir) 476
May interact with dexamethasone, dihydropyridine calcium channel blockers, ergot-containing drugs, phenytoin, quinidine, and certain other agents. Compounds in these categories include:

Abacavir Sulfate (Kaletra induces glucuronidation; therefore, Kaletra has the potential to reduce abacavir plasma concentrations; the clinical significance is unknown). Products include:
Epzicom Tablets 1436
Trizivir Tablets 1589
Ziagen 1626

Amiodarone Hydrochloride (Co-administration can result in increased amiodarone plasma concentrations; caution and monitoring is recommended).
No products indexed under this heading.

Amlodipine Besylate (Increased plasma concentrations of dihydropyridine calcium channel blockers; caution is warranted and clinical monitoring of patients is recommended). Products include:
Caduet Tablets 2508
Lotrel Capsules 2249
Norvasc Tablets 2545

Amprenavir (Co-administration results in increased amprenavir plasma concentrations and may increase AUC and Cmin; dosage adjustments may be needed). Products include:
Agenerase Capsules 1327
Agenerase Oral Solution 1332

Astemizole (Kaletra is an inhibitor of the CYP450 3A. Co-administration with drugs that are highly dependent on CYP450 3A for clearance and for which elevated plasma concentrations are associated with serious and/or life threatening events, such as astemizole, is contraindicated).
No products indexed under this heading.

Atorvastatin Calcium (Co-administration with HMG-CoA reductase inhibitors that are metabolized by the CYP3A pathway, such as atorvastatin, increases the risk of myopathy including rhabdomyolysis; caution is recommended). Products include:
Caduet Tablets 2508
Lipitor Tablets 2483

Atovaquone (Co-administration can result in decreased atovaquone plasma concentrations; clinical significance is unknown; however, increase in atovaquone doses may be needed). Products include:
Malarone Pediatric Tablets 1517
Malarone Tablets 1517
Mepron Suspension 1521

Bepridil Hydrochloride (Co-administration can result in increased bepridil plasma concentrations; caution and monitoring is recommended).
No products indexed under this heading.

Carbamazepine (Co-administration can result in decreased lopinavir plasma concentrations; Kaletra may be less effective due to decreased lopinavir plasma concentrations; use with caution). Products include:
Carbatrol Capsules 3171
Equetro Extended-Release Capsules 3180
Tegretol/Tegretol-XR 2295

Cisapride (Kaletra is an inhibitor of the CYP450 3A. Co-administration with drugs that are highly dependent on CYP450 3A for clearance and for which elevated plasma concentrations are associated with serious and/or life threatening events, such as cisapride, is contraindicated).
No products indexed under this heading.

Clarithromycin (Co-administration can result in increased clarithromycin plasma concentrations; for patients with renal impairment, the dosage may need to be adjusted). Products include:
Biaxin/Biaxin XL 402
PREVPAC 3284

Cyclosporine (Co-administration results in increased plasma concentrations of immunosuppressants; monitoring is recommended). Products include:
Gengraf Capsules 459
Neoral Oral Solution 2259
Neoral Soft Gelatin Capsules 2259
Restasis Ophthalmic Emulsion 575
Sandimmune 2275

Delavirdine Mesylate (Co-administration has a potential to increase lopinavir plasma concentrations). Products include:
Rescriptor Tablets 2551

Dexamethasone (Co-administration can result in decreased lopinavir plasma concentrations; Kaletra may be less effective due to decreased lopinavir plasma concentrations in patients taking

these agents concomitantly. Co-administer with caution). Products include:
- Ciprodex Otic Suspension 559
- Decadron Tablets 1951
- TobraDex Ophthalmic Ointment 562
- TobraDex Ophthalmic Suspension ... 563

Dexamethasone Acetate (Co-administration can result in decreased lopinavir plasma concentrations; Kaletra may be less effective due to decreased lopinavir plasma concentrations in patients taking these agents concomitantly. Co-administer with caution).
- No products indexed under this heading.

Dexamethasone Sodium Phosphate (Co-administration can result in decreased lopinavir plasma concentrations; Kaletra may be less effective due to decreased lopinavir plasma concentrations in patients taking these agents concomitantly. Co-administer with caution).
- No products indexed under this heading.

Didanosine (Kaletra tablets can be administered simultaneously with didanosine without food. For Kaletra oral solution, it is recommended that didanosine be administered on an empty stomach, therefore, didanosine should be given one hour before or two hours after Kaletra oral solution (given with food)).
- No products indexed under this heading.

Dihydroergotamine Mesylate (Kaletra is an inhibitor of CYP450 3A. Co-administration is contraindicated due to potential for serious and/or life threatening reactions such as acute ergot toxicity). Products include:
- Migranal Nasal Spray 3348

Disulfiram (Kaletra oral solution contains alcohol which can produce disulfiram-like reactions when co-administered with disulfiram).
- No products indexed under this heading.

Efavirenz (Efavirenz may decrease concentration of lopinavir. Kaletra should not be administered once-daily in combination with enfavirenz). Products include:
- Atripla Tablets 945
- Sustiva Capsules 930
- Sustiva Tablets 930

Ergonovine Maleate (Kaletra is an inhibitor of CYP450 3A. Co-administration is contraindicated due to potential for serious and/or life threatening reactions such as acute ergot toxicity).
- No products indexed under this heading.

Ergotamine Tartrate (Kaletra is an inhibitor of CYP450 3A. Co-administration is contraindicated due to potential for serious and/or life threatening reactions such as acute ergot toxicity).
- No products indexed under this heading.

Ethinyl Estradiol (Co-administration results in decreased plasma concentrations of ethinyl estradiol; alternative methods of non-hormonal contraception should be used when estrogen-based oral contraceptives and Kaletra are co-administered). Products include:
- Mircette Tablets 1066
- NuvaRing 2340
- Ortho-Cyclen/Ortho Tri-Cyclen 2429
- Ortho Evra Transdermal System 2417
- Ortho Tri-Cyclen Lo Tablets 2436
- Seasonique Tablets 1077
- Yasmin 28 Tablets 796
- Yaz Tablets 803

Felodipine (Increased plasma concentrations of dihydropyridine calcium channel blockers; caution is warranted and clinical monitoring of patients is recommended).
- No products indexed under this heading.

Flecainide Acetate (Kaletra is an in vitro inhibitor of the CYP450 3A and inhibits CYP2D6 to a lesser extent; co-administration with drugs that are highly dependent on these isoforms for clearance and for which elevated plasma concentrations are associated with serious and/or life threatening events, such as flecainide, is contraindicated). Products include:
- Tambocor Tablets 1856

Fluticasone Propionate (Concomitant use of fluticasone propionate and Kaletra may increase plasma concentrations of fluticasone propionate, resulting in significantly reduced serum cortisol concentrations. Co-administration of fluticasone propionate and Kaletra is not recommended unless the potential benefit to the patient outweighs the risk of system corticosteroid side effect). Products include:
- Advair Diskus 100/50 1308
- Advair Diskus 250/50 1308
- Advair Diskus 500/50 1308
- Advair HFA Inhalation Aerosol 1318
- Cutivate Cream 2662
- Cutivate Lotion 0.05% 2664
- Cutivate Ointment 2665
- Flonase Nasal Spray 1440
- Flovent Diskus 1443

Fluticasone Propionate HFA (Concomitant use of fluticasone propionate and Kaletra may increase plasma concentrations of fluticasone propionate, resulting in significantly reduced serum cortisol concentrations. Co-administration of fluticasone propionate and Kaletra is not recommended unless the potential benefit to the patient outweighs the risk of system corticosteroid side effect). Products include:
- Flovent HFA 1447

Fosamprenavir Calcium (Co-administration may result in decreased levels of amprenavir and/or lopinavir. An increased rate of adverse effects has also been observed with co-administration of these medications). Products include:
- Lexiva Tablets 1505

Fosphenytoin Sodium (Co-administration can result in decreased lopinavir plasma concentrations; Kaletra may be less effective due to decreased lopinavir plasma concentrations. Co-administer with caution).
- No products indexed under this heading.

Hypericum (Co-administration is expected to substantially decrease protease inhibitor concentrations and may result in sub-optimal levels of lopinavir and lead to loss of virologic response and possible resistance to lopinavir or to the class of protease inhibitors; concomitant use is not recommended). Products include:
- Satiete Tablets 832

Indinavir Sulfate (Co-administration may result in increased indinavir concentrations, decreased Cmax and increased Cmin. Decreased indinavir dose to 600mg BID, when co-administered with Kaletra 400/100mg BID. Kaletra once-daily has not been studied in combination with indinavir). Products include:
- Crixivan Capsules 1940

Isradipine (Increased plasma concentrations of dihydropyridine calcium channel blockers; caution is warranted and clinical monitoring of patients is recommended). Products include:
- DynaCirc CR Tablets 2721

Itraconazole (Co-administration can result in increased itraconazole plasma concentrations; high doses of itraconazole (>200 mg/day) are not recommended).
- No products indexed under this heading.

Ketoconazole (Co-administration can result in increased ketoconazole plasma concentrations; high doses of ketoconazole (>200 mg/day) are not recommended). Products include:
- Nizoral A-D Shampoo, 1% 1868

Lidocaine Hydrochloride (Co-administration with systemic lidocaine can result in increased lidocaine plasma concentrations; caution and monitoring is recommended).
- No products indexed under this heading.

Lovastatin (Co-administration of Kaletra and lovastatin may increase the risk of myopathy, including rhabdomyolysis; concomitant use is not recommended). Products include:
- Advicor Tablets 1722
- Altoprev Extended-Release Tablets 3109
- Mevacor Tablets 2021

Methadone Hydrochloride (Co-administration results in decreased plasma concentrations of methadone; dosage of methadone may need to be increased when co-administered).
- No products indexed under this heading.

Methylergonovine Maleate (Kaletra is an inhibitor of CYP450 3A. Co-administration is contraindicated due to potential for serious and/or life threatening reactions such as acute ergot toxicity).
- No products indexed under this heading.

Methysergide Maleate (Kaletra is an inhibitor of CYP450 3A. Co-administration is contraindicated due to potential for serious and/or life threatening reactions such as acute ergot toxicity).
- No products indexed under this heading.

Metronidazole (Kaletra oral solution contains alcohol, which can produce disulfiram-like reactions when co-administered with disulfiram or other drugs that produce this reaction, such as metronidazole). Products include:
- Metrogel 1% 1211
- MetroGel-Vaginal Gel 1855
- Vandazole Vaginal Gel 3338

Metronidazole Hydrochloride (Kaletra oral solution contains alcohol, which can produce disulfiram-like reactions when co-administered with disulfiram or other drugs that produce this reaction, such as metronidazole).
- No products indexed under this heading.

Midazolam Hydrochloride (Kaletra is an in vitro inhibitor of the CYP450 3A and inhibits CYP2D6 to a lesser extent; co-administration with drugs that are highly dependent on these isoforms for clearance and for which elevated plasma concentrations are associated with serious and/or life threatening events, such as midazolam, is contraindicated).
- No products indexed under this heading.

Nelfinavir Mesylate (Co-administration may require dosage adjustment). Products include:
- Viracept 2577

Nevirapine (Nevirapine may decrease concentration of lopinavir. Kaletra should not be administered once-daily in combination with nevirapine). Products include:
- Viramune Oral Suspension 873
- Viramune Tablets 873

Nicardipine Hydrochloride (Increased plasma concentrations of dihydropyridine calcium channel blockers; caution is warranted and clinical monitoring of patients is recommended). Products include:
- Cardene I.V. 2497

Nifedipine (Increased plasma concentrations of dihydropyridine calcium channel blockers; caution is warranted and clinical monitoring of patients is recommended). Products include:
- Adalat CC Tablets 2964

Nimodipine (Increased plasma concentrations of dihydropyridine calcium channel blockers; caution is warranted and clinical monitoring of patients is recommended). Products include:
- Nimotop Capsules 749

Phenobarbital (Co-administration can result in decreased lopinavir plasma concentrations; Kaletra may be less effective due to decreased lopinavir plasma concentrations. Co-administer with caution). Products include:
- Donnatal Extentabs 2493

Phenytoin (Co-administration can result in decreased lopinavir plasma concentrations; Kaletra may be less effective due to decreased lopinavir plasma concentrations. Co-administer with caution).
- No products indexed under this heading.

Phenytoin Sodium (Co-administration can result in decreased lopinavir plasma concentrations; Kaletra may be less effective due to decreased lopinavir plasma concentrations. Co-administer with caution). Products include:
- Phenytek Capsules 2160

Pimozide (Kaletra is an inhibitor of CYP450 3A. Co-administration with drugs that are highly dependent on CYP450 3A for clearance and for which elevated plasma concentrations are associated with serious and/or life threatening events, such as pimozide, is contraindicated).
- No products indexed under this heading.

Propafenone Hydrochloride (Kaletra is an inhibitor of CYP450 3A. Co-administration with drugs that are highly dependent on CYP450 3A for clearance and for which elevated plasma concentrations are associated with serious and/or life threatening events, such as propafenone, is contraindicated). Products include:
Rythmol SR Capsules 2727

Quinidine (Co-administration can result in increased quinidine plasma concentrations; caution and monitoring is recommended).
No products indexed under this heading.

Quinidine Gluconate (Co-administration can result in increased quinidine plasma concentrations; caution and monitoring is recommended).
No products indexed under this heading.

Quinidine Hydrochloride (Co-administration can result in increased quinidine plasma concentrations; caution and monitoring is recommended).
No products indexed under this heading.

Quinidine Polygalacturonate (Co-administration can result in increased quinidine plasma concentrations; caution and monitoring is recommended).
No products indexed under this heading.

Quinidine Sulfate (Co-administration can result in increased quinidine plasma concentrations; caution and monitoring is recommended).
No products indexed under this heading.

Rapamycin (Co-administration results in increased plasma concentrations of immunosuppressants; monitoring is recommended).
No products indexed under this heading.

Rifabutin (Co-administration can result in increased rifabutin and rifabutin metabolite plasma concentrations; dosage reduction of rifabutin by at least 75% of the usual dose of 300 mg/day is recommended; increased monitoring for adverse reactions is warranted).
No products indexed under this heading.

Rifampin (Co-administration may lead to loss of virologic response and possible resistance to Kaletra; concomitant use should be avoided).
No products indexed under this heading.

Saquinavir (Co-administration may increase saquinavir concentrations. The saquinavir dose is 1000mg BID, when co-administered with Kaletra 400/100mg. Kaletra once-daily has not been studied in combination with saquinavir).
No products indexed under this heading.

Saquinavir Mesylate (Co-administration may increase saquinavir concentrations. The saquinavir dose is 1000mg BID, when co-administered with Kaletra 400/100mg. Kaletra once-daily has not been studied in combination with saquinavir). Products include:
Invirase 2772

Sildenafil Citrate (Co-administration is expected to substantially increase sildenafil concentrations and may result in an increase in sildenafil-associated adverse events including hypotension, syncope, visual changes and prolonged erection; Dosage reductions of 25 mg every 48 hours with increased monitoring for adverse events). Products include:
Revatio Tablets 2557
Viagra Tablets 2573

Simvastatin (Co-administration of Kaletra and simvastatin may increase the risk of myopathy, including rhabdomyolysis; concomitant use is not recommended). Products include:
Vytorin 10/10 Tablets 2114
Vytorin 10/10 Tablets 3077
Vytorin 10/20 Tablets 2114
Vytorin 10/20 Tablets 3077
Vytorin 10/40 Tablets 2114
Vytorin 10/40 Tablets 3077
Vytorin 10/80 Tablets 2114
Vytorin 10/80 Tablets 3077
Zocor Tablets 2105

Tacrolimus (Co-administration results in increased plasma concentrations of immunosuppressants; monitoring is recommended). Products include:
Prograf Capsules and Injection 632
Protopic Ointment 638

Tadalafil (Co-administration is expected to substantially increase tadalafil concentrations and may result in an increase in tadalafil associated adverse drug events including hypotension, syncope, visual changes and prolonged erection; Dosage reduction recommended10 mg every 72 hours with increased monitoring for adverse events). Products include:
Cialis Tablets 1838

Tenofovir Disoproxil Fumarate (Co-administration results in increased plasma concentrations of nucleoside reverse transcriptase inhibitors; Co-administer with caution). Products include:
Atripla Tablets 945
Truvada Tablets 1296
Viread Tablets 1301

Terfenadine (Kaletra is an inhibitor of CYP450 3A. Co-administration with drugs that are highly dependent on CYP450 3A for clearance and for which elevated plasma concentrations are associated with serious and/or life threatening events, such as terfenadine, is contraindicated).
No products indexed under this heading.

Trazodone Hydrochloride (Concomitant use of trazodone and Kaletra may increase concentrations of trazodone. Adverse events of nausea, dizziness, hypotension and syncope have been observed following co-administration of trazodone and ritonavir. If trazodone is used with a CYP3A4 inhibitor such as ritonavir, the combination should be used with caution and a lower dose of trazodone should be considered).
No products indexed under this heading.

Triazolam (Kaletra is an inhibitor of CYP450 3A. Co-administration with drugs that are highly dependent on CYP450 3A for clearance and for which elevated plasma concentrations are associated with serious and/or life threatening events, such as triazolam, is contraindicated).
No products indexed under this heading.

Vardenafil Hydrochloride (Co-administration is expected to substantially increase vardenafil concentrations and may result in an increase in vardenafil associated adverse drug events including hypotension, syncope, visual changes and prolonged erection; Dosage reduction of 2.5 mg every 72 hours with increased monitoring for adverse effects). Products include:
Levitra Tablets 3034

Voriconazole (Co-administration of voriconazole with Kaletra has not been studied. However, administration of voriconazole with ritonavir 400 mg every 12 hours decreased voriconazole steady-state AUC by an average of 82%. The effect of lower ritonavir doses on voriconazole is not known at this time. Until data is available, voriconazole should not be administered to patients receiving Kaletra). Products include:
VFEND I.V. 2564
VFEND Oral Suspension 2564
VFEND Tablets 2564

Warfarin Sodium (Co-administration can affect concentrations of warfarin; it is recommended that INR be monitored). Products include:
Coumadin for Injection 898
Coumadin Tablets 898

Zidovudine (Kaletra induces glucuronidation; therefore, Kaletra has the potential to reduce zidovudine plasma concentrations; the clinical significance is unknown). Products include:
Combivir Tablets 1411
Retrovir 1560
Retrovir IV Infusion 1564
Trizivir Tablets 1589

Food Interactions

Food, unspecified (Co-administration with moderate fat meal was associated with a mean increase in AUC and Cmax; to enhance bioavailability Kaletra should be taken with food).

K-DUR EXTENDED-RELASE TABLETS

(Potassium Chloride) 3033
May interact with ACE inhibitors, potassium sparing diuretics, and certain other agents. Compounds in these categories include:

Amiloride Hydrochloride (Co-administration of these agents can produce severe hyperkalemia; concurrent use is not recommended). Products include:
Midamor Tablets 2026
Moduretic Tablets 2028

Benazepril Hydrochloride (Potential for increased potassium retention). Products include:
Lotensin Tablets 2243
Lotensin HCT Tablets 2246
Lotrel Capsules 2249

Captopril (Potential for increased potassium retention). Products include:
Captopril Tablets 2149

Enalapril Maleate (Potential for increased potassium retention). Products include:
Vasotec I.V. Injection 2103

Enalaprilat (Potential for increased potassium retention).
No products indexed under this heading.

Fosinopril Sodium (Potential for increased potassium retention).
No products indexed under this heading.

Lisinopril (Potential for increased potassium retention). Products include:
Prinivil Tablets 2052
Prinzide Tablets 2056

Moexipril Hydrochloride (Potential for increased potassium retention). Products include:
Uniretic Tablets 3100
Univasc Tablets 3104

Perindopril Erbumine (Potential for increased potassium retention). Products include:
Aceon Tablets (2 mg, 4 mg, 8 mg) 3194

Quinapril Hydrochloride (Potential for increased potassium retention).
No products indexed under this heading.

Ramipril (Potential for increased potassium retention). Products include:
Altace Capsules 1702

Spirapril Hydrochloride (Potential for increased potassium retention).
No products indexed under this heading.

Spironolactone (Co-administration of these agents can produce severe hyperkalemia; concurrent use is not recommended).
No products indexed under this heading.

Trandolapril (Potential for increased potassium retention). Products include:
Mavik Tablets 486
Tarka Tablets 524

Triamterene (Co-administration of these agents can produce severe hyperkalemia; concurrent use is not recommended). Products include:
Dyazide Capsules 1423
Dyrenium Capsules 3400

KEFLEX CAPSULES

(Cephalexin) 549
May interact with:

Metformin (Co-administration increased plasma metformin Cmax and AUC by 34% and 24%, respectively, and decreased metformin renal clearance by 14%).
No products indexed under this heading.

Metformin Hydrochloride (Co-administration increased plasma metformin Cmax and AUC by 34% and 24%, respectively, and decreased metformin renal clearance by 14%). Products include:
ActoPlus Met Tablets 3214
Avandamet Tablets 1373
Fortamet Extended-Release Tablets 3115

Probenecid (The renal excretion of cephalexin is inhibited by probenecid).
No products indexed under this heading.

KEPIVANCE

(Palifermin) 597
May interact with:

Heparin Calcium (Palifermin has been shown to bind to heparin in vitro. Therefore, if heparin is used to maintain an IV line, saline should be used to rinse the line prior to and after palifermin administration).
No products indexed under this heading.

Heparin Sodium (Palifermin has been shown to bind to heparin in vitro. Therefore, if heparin is used to maintain an IV line, saline should be used to rinse the line prior to and after palifermin administration).
No products indexed under this heading.

KEPPRA INJECTION

(Levetiracetam) 3320
May interact with:

Probenecid (Co-administration has resulted in double Cmax of the metabolite, ucb L057, while the fraction of the drug excreted remained unchanged in the urine; renal clearance of ucb L057 in the presence decreased 60%).
No products indexed under this heading.

KEPPRA ORAL SOLUTION

(Levetiracetam) 3314
See Keppra Tablets

KEPPRA TABLETS

(Levetiracetam) 3314
May interact with:

Probenecid (Co-administration has resulted in double Cmax of the metabolite, ucb L057, while the fraction of the drug excreted remained unchanged in the urine; renal clearance of ucb L057 in the presence of probenecid decreased 60%).
No products indexed under this heading.

Food Interactions

Food, unspecified (Decreases Cmax by 20% and delays Tmax by 1.5 hours; does not affect the extent of absorption).

KETEK TABLETS

(Telithromycin) 2903
May interact with benzodiazepine that are metabolized by CYP3A4, cytochrome p450 3a4 inducers (selected), cytochrome p450 3a4 substrates (selected), ergot-containing drugs, and drugs which undergo biotransformation by cytochrome p-450 mixed function oxidase. Compounds in these categories include:

Acarbose (Elevated levels of drugs metabolized by the CYP450 system may be observed when co-administered with telithromycin; therefore, increases or prolongation of the therapeutic and/or adverse effects of the concomitant drug may be observed). Products include:
Precose Tablets 751

Acetaminophen (Elevated levels of drugs metabolized by the CYP450 system may be observed when co-administered with telithromycin; therefore, increases or prolongation of the therapeutic and/or adverse effects of the concomitant drug may be observed). Products include:
Comtrex Maximum Strength Cold & Cough Day/Night Caplets - Day Formulation .... ■726
Comtrex Maximum Strength Cold & Cough Day/Night Caplets - Night Formulation .... ■726
Comtrex Maximum Strength Non-Drowsy Cold & Cough Caplets .... ■725
Comtrex Maximum Strength Day/Night Severe Cold & Sinus Caplets - Day Formulation .... ■725
Comtrex Maximum Strength Day/Night Severe Cold & Sinus Caplets - Night Formulation .... ■725
Contac Cold and Flu Maximum Strength Caplets .... ■728
Contac Cold and Flu Day and Night Caplets (Day Formulation Only) .... ■727
Contac Cold and Flu Day and Night Caplets (Night Formulation Only) .... ■727
Contac Cold and Flu Non-Drowsy Caplets .... ■728
Excedrin Extra Strength Caplets/Tablets/Geltabs .... ■684
Excedrin Migraine Caplets/Tablets/Geltabs .... ■609
Excedrin PM Caplets/Tablets/Geltabs .... ■610
Excedrin Sinus Headache Caplets/Tablets .... ■610
Excedrin Tension Headache Caplets/Tablets/Geltabs .... ■611
Goody's Body Pain Formula Powder .... ■684
Goody's Extra Strength Headache Powders .... ■611
Goody's Extra Strength Pain Relief Tablets .... ■685
Goody's PM Powder for Pain with Sleeplessness .... ■612
Percocet Tablets 1131
Robitussin Cough, Cold & Flu Nighttime Liquid .... ■738
TheraFlu Cold & Sore Throat Hot Liquid .... ■741
TheraFlu Flu & Chest Congestion Hot Liquid .... ■741
TheraFlu Flu & Sore Throat Hot Liquid .... ■742
TheraFlu Daytime Severe Cold Hot Liquid .... ■742
TheraFlu Nighttime Severe Cold Hot Liquid .... ■740
TheraFlu Warming Relief Daytime Severe Cold .... ■743
TheraFlu Warming Relief Nighttime Severe Cold .... ■743
Triaminic Cough & Sore Throat Liquid .... ■747
Regular Strength Tylenol Tablets 1870
Children's Tylenol with Flavor Creator .... ■679
Children's Tylenol Plus Flu Oral Suspension .... ■749
Tylenol Cold Head Congestion Daytime Caplets with Cool Burst and Gelcaps .... ■750
Tylenol Cold Multi-Symptom Daytime Liquid .... ■752
Tylenol Cold Multi-Symptom Severe Daytime Liquid .... ■752
Tylenol 8 Hour Extended Release Caplets 1870
Tylenol 1870
Extra Strength Tylenol PM Caplets, Vanilla Caplets, Geltabs, Gelcaps and Liquid 1875
Extra Strength Tylenol Rapid Release Gels 1870
Concentrated Tylenol Infants' Drops Plus Cold & Cough .... ■754
Tylenol with Codeine Tablets 2391
Tylenol Allergy Multi-Symptom Caplets with Cool Burst and Gelcaps 1872
Tylenol Allergy Multi-Symptom Nighttime Caplets with Cool Burst 1872
Tylenol Severe Allergy Caplets 1872
Tylenol Arthritis Pain Extended Release Caplets and Geltabs 1870
Tylenol Chest Congestion Caplets with Cool Burst 1872
Tylenol Chest Congestion Liquid with Cool Burst 1872
Children's Tylenol Suspension Liquid and Meltaways 1878
Children's Tylenol Plus Cold Suspension Liquid 1879
Children's Tylenol Plus Cold & Allergy Suspension Liquid 1878
Children's Tylenol Plus Cough & Runny Nose Suspension Liquid 1879
Children's Tylenol Plus Cough & Sore Throat Suspension Liquid 1879
Children's Tylenol Suspension with Flavor Creator 1878
Children's Tylenol Plus Flu Suspension Liquid 1881
Children's Tylenol Plus Multi-Symptom Cold Suspension Liquid 1879
Tylenol Cold Severe Congestion Non-Drowsy Caplets with Cool Burst 1874
Tylenol Cold Head Congestion Daytime Caplets with Cool Burst 1873
Tylenol Cold Head Congestion Nighttime Caplets with Cool Burst 1873
Tylenol Cold Head Congestion Severe Caplets with Cool Burst 1873
Tylenol Cold Multi-Symptom Daytime Caplets with Cool Burst and Gelcaps 1874
Tylenol Cold Multi-Symptom Daytime Liquid with Citrus Burst 1874
Tylenol Cold Multi-Symptom Nighttime Caplets with Cool Burst 1874
Tylenol Cold Multi-Symptom Nighttime Liquid with Cool Burst 1874
Tylenol Cold Multi-Symptom Severe Caplets with Cool Burst 1874
Tylenol Cold Multi-Symptom Severe Daytime Liquid with Citrus Burst 1874
Tylenol Cough & Sore Throat Daytime Liquid with Cool Burst 1877
Tylenol Cough & Sore Throat Nighttime Liquid with Cool Burst 1877
Concentrated Tylenol Infants' Drops 1878
Concentrated Tylenol Infants' Drops Plus Cold 1879
Concentrated Tylenol Infants' Drops Plus Cold and Cough 1879
Jr. Tylenol Meltaways 1878
Tylenol Sinus Severe Congestion Caplets with Cool Burst 1876
Tylenol Sinus Congestion & Pain Daytime Caplets with Cool Burst and Gelcaps 1876
Tylenol Sinus Congestion & Pain Nighttime Caplets with Cool Burst 1876
Tylenol Sinus Congestion & Pain Severe Caplets with Cool Burst 1876
Tylenol Sore Throat Daytime Liquid with Cool Burst 1877
Tylenol Sore Throat Nighttime Liquid with Cool Burst 1877
Women's Tylenol Menstrual Relief Caplets 1877
Vicks 44M Cough, Cold & Flu Relief Liquid 2680
Vicks DayQuil LiquiCaps/Liquid Multi-Symptom Cold/Flu Relief .... ■761
Vicks DayQuil Multi-Symptom Cold/Flu Relief LiquiCaps 2678
Vicks DayQuil Multi-Symptom Cold/Flu Relief Liquid 2678
Vicks NyQuil Multi-Symptom Cold/Flu Relief Liquid 2681
Vicks NyQuil Multi-Symptom Cold/Flu Relief LiquiCaps 2681
Vicks NyQuil LiquiCaps/Liquid Multi-Symptom Cold/Flu Relief .... ■763
Vicodin Tablets 535
Vicodin ES Tablets 536
Vicodin HP Tablets 538
Zicam Maximum Strength Flu Daytime .... ■768
Zicam Maximum Strength Flu Nighttime .... ■768
Zydone Tablets 1139

Alatrofloxacin Mesylate (Elevated levels of drugs metabolized by the CYP450 system may be observed when co-administered with telithromycin; therefore, increases or prolongation of the therapeutic and/or adverse effects of the concomitant drug may be observed).
No products indexed under this heading.

Alfentanil Hydrochloride (Co-administration of telithromycin with a drug primarily metabolized by the CYP 3A4 enzyme system may result in increased plasma concentrations of the drug co-administered with telithromycin that could increase or prolong both the therapeutic and adverse effects).
No products indexed under this heading.

Allium sativum (Concomitant administration of CYP 3A4 inducers is likely to result in subtherapeutic levels of telithromycin and loss of effect).
No products indexed under this heading.

Alprazolam (Co-administration of telithromycin with a drug primarily metabolized by the CYP 3A4 enzyme system may result in increased plasma concentrations of the drug co-administered with telithromycin that could increase or prolong both the therapeutic and adverse effects). Products include:
Niravam Orally Disintegrating Tablets 3092

Aminophylline (Elevated levels of drugs metabolized by the CYP450 system may be observed when co-administered with telithromycin; therefore, increases or prolongation of the therapeutic and/or adverse effects of the concomitant drug may be observed).
No products indexed under this heading.

Amiodarone Hydrochloride (Elevated levels of drugs metabolized by the CYP450 system may be observed when co-administered with telithromycin; therefore, increases or prolongation of the therapeutic and/or adverse effects of the concomitant drug may be observed).
No products indexed under this heading.

Amitriptyline Hydrochloride (Co-administration of telithromycin with a drug primarily metabolized by the CYP 3A4 enzyme system may result in increased plasma concentrations of the drug co-administered with telithromycin that could increase or prolong both the therapeutic and adverse effects).
No products indexed under this heading.

Amlodipine Besylate (Co-administration of telithromycin with a drug primarily metabolized by the CYP 3A4 enzyme system may result in increased plasma concentrations of the drug co-administered with telithromycin that could increase or prolong both the therapeutic and adverse effects). Products include:
Caduet Tablets 2508
Lotrel Capsules 2249
Norvasc Tablets 2545

Amoxapine (Elevated levels of drugs metabolized by the CYP450 system may be observed when co-administered with telithromycin; therefore, increases or prolongation of the therapeutic and/or adverse effects of the concomitant drug may be observed).

No products indexed under this heading.

Amphetamine Aspartate (Elevated levels of drugs metabolized by the CYP450 system may be observed when co-administered with telithromycin; therefore, increases or prolongation of the therapeutic and/or adverse effects of the concomitant drug may be observed).
Products include:

Amphetamine Aspartate Monohydrate (Elevated levels of drugs metabolized by the CYP450 system may be observed when co-administered with telithromycin; therefore, increases or prolongation of the therapeutic and/or adverse effects of the concomitant drug may be observed).

No products indexed under this heading.

Amphetamine Sulfate (Elevated levels of drugs metabolized by the CYP450 system may be observed when co-administered with telithromycin; therefore, increases or prolongation of the therapeutic and/or adverse effects of the concomitant drug may be observed). Products include:

Aprepitant (Co-administration of telithromycin with a drug primarily metabolized by the CYP 3A4 enzyme system may result in increased plasma concentrations of the drug co-administered with telithromycin that could increase or prolong both the therapeutic and adverse effects). Products include:

Astemizole (Co-administration of telithromycin with a drug primarily metabolized by the CYP 3A4 enzyme system may result in increased plasma concentrations of the drug co-administered with telithromycin that could increase or prolong both the therapeutic and adverse effects).

No products indexed under this heading.

Atomoxetine Hydrochloride (Elevated levels of drugs metabolized by the CYP450 system may be observed when co-administered with telithromycin; therefore, increases or prolongation of the therapeutic and/or adverse effects of the concomitant drug may be observed). Products include:

Atorvastatin Calcium (Atorvastatin levels were increased due to CYP 3A4 inhibition by telithromycin, thereby increasing the risk of myopathy. Co-administration should be avoided). Products include:

Belladonna Ergotamine (Co-administration of telithromycin with a drug primarily metabolized by the CYP 3A4 enzyme system may result in increased plasma concentrations of the drug co-administered with telithromycin that could increase or prolong both the therapeutic and adverse effects).

No products indexed under this heading.

Benzphetamine Hydrochloride (Elevated levels of drugs metabolized by the CYP450 system may be observed when co-administered with telithromycin; therefore, increases or prolongation of the therapeutic and/or adverse effects of the concomitant drug may be observed).

No products indexed under this heading.

Betamethasone Acetate (Concomitant administration of CYP 3A4 inducers is likely to result in subtherapeutic levels of telithromycin and loss of effect).

No products indexed under this heading.

Betamethasone Sodium Phosphate (Concomitant administration of CYP 3A4 inducers is likely to result in subtherapeutic levels of telithromycin and loss of effect).

No products indexed under this heading.

Bisoprolol Fumarate (Elevated levels of drugs metabolized by the CYP450 system may be observed when co-administered with telithromycin; therefore, increases or prolongation of the therapeutic and/or adverse effects of the concomitant drug may be observed).

No products indexed under this heading.

Buspirone Hydrochloride (Co-administration of telithromycin with a drug primarily metabolized by the CYP 3A4 enzyme system may result in increased plasma concentrations of the drug co-administered with telithromycin that could increase or prolong both the therapeutic and adverse effects).

No products indexed under this heading.

Busulfan (Co-administration of telithromycin with a drug primarily metabolized by the CYP 3A4 enzyme system may result in increased plasma concentrations of the drug co-administered with telithromycin that could increase or prolong both the therapeutic and adverse effects). Products include:

Caffeine (Elevated levels of drugs metabolized by the CYP450 system may be observed when co-administered with telithromycin; therefore, increases or prolongation of the therapeutic and/or adverse effects of the concomitant drug may be observed). Products include:

Caffeine Anhydrous (Elevated levels of drugs metabolized by the CYP450 system may be observed when co-administered with telithromycin; therefore, increases or prolongation of the therapeutic and/or adverse effects of the concomitant drug may be observed).

No products indexed under this heading.

Caffeine Citrate (Elevated levels of drugs metabolized by the CYP450 system may be observed when co-administered with telithromycin; therefore, increases or prolongation of the therapeutic and/or adverse effects of the concomitant drug may be observed). Products include:

Candesartan Cilexetil (Elevated levels of drugs metabolized by the CYP450 system may be observed when co-administered with telithromycin; therefore, increases or prolongation of the therapeutic and/or adverse effects of the concomitant drug may be observed). Products include:

Captopril (Elevated levels of drugs metabolized by the CYP450 system may be observed when co-administered with telithromycin; therefore, increases or prolongation of the therapeutic and/or adverse effects of the concomitant drug may be observed). Products include:

Carbamazepine (Co-administration of telithromycin with a drug primarily metabolized by the CYP 3A4 enzyme system may result in increased plasma concentrations of the drug co-administered with telithromycin that could increase or prolong both the therapeutic and adverse effects). Products include:

Carisoprodol (Elevated levels of drugs metabolized by the CYP450 system may be observed when co-administered with telithromycin; therefore, increases or prolongation of the therapeutic and/or adverse effects of the concomitant drug may be observed).

No products indexed under this heading.

Carvedilol (Elevated levels of drugs metabolized by the CYP450 system may be observed when co-administered with telithromycin; therefore, increases or prolongation of the therapeutic and/or adverse effects of the concomitant drug may be observed). Products include:

Celecoxib (Elevated levels of drugs metabolized by the CYP450 system may be observed when co-administered with telithromycin; therefore, increases or prolongation of the therapeutic and/or adverse effects of the concomitant drug may be observed). Products include:

Cerivastatin Sodium (Co-administration of telithromycin with a drug primarily metabolized by the CYP 3A4 enzyme system may result in increased plasma concentrations of the drug co-administered with telithromycin that could increase or prolong both the therapeutic and adverse effects).

No products indexed under this heading.

Cevimeline Hydrochloride (Elevated levels of drugs metabolized by the CYP450 system may be observed when co-administered with telithromycin; therefore, increases or prolongation of the therapeutic and/or adverse effects of the concomitant drug may be observed). Products include:

Chlordiazepoxide (Elevated levels of drugs metabolized by the CYP450 system may be observed when co-administered with telithromycin; therefore, increases or prolongation of the therapeutic and/or adverse effects of the concomitant drug may be observed).

No products indexed under this heading.

Chlordiazepoxide Hydrochloride (Elevated levels of drugs metabolized by the CYP450 system may be observed when co-administered with telithromycin; therefore, increases or prolongation of the therapeutic and/or adverse effects of the concomitant drug may be observed). Products include:

Chlorpheniramine (Co-administration of telithromycin with a drug primarily metabolized by the CYP 3A4 enzyme system may result in increased plasma concentrations of the drug co-administered with telithromycin that could increase or prolong both the therapeutic and adverse effects).

No products indexed under this heading.

Chlorpheniramine Maleate (Co-administration of telithromycin with a drug primarily metabolized by the CYP 3A4 enzyme system may result in increased plasma concentrations of the drug co-administered with telithromycin that could increase or prolong both the therapeutic and adverse effects). Products include:

Triaminic Cough & Runny Nose Softchews 748
Children's Tylenol Plus Flu Oral Suspension 749
Tylenol Allergy Multi-Symptom Caplets with Cool Burst and Gelcaps 1872
Children's Tylenol Plus Cold Suspension Liquid 1879
Children's Tylenol Plus Cough & Runny Nose Suspension Liquid 1879
Children's Tylenol Plus Flu Suspension Liquid 1881
Children's Tylenol Plus Multi-Symptom Cold Suspension Liquid 1879
Tylenol Cold Head Congestion Nighttime Caplets with Cool Burst 1873
Tylenol Cold Multi-Symptom Nighttime Caplets with Cool Burst 1874
Tylenol Sinus Congestion & Pain Nighttime Caplets with Cool Burst 1876
Vicks 44M Cough, Cold & Flu Relief Liquid 2680
Pediatric Vicks 44m Cough & Cold Relief Liquid 2676
Children's Vicks NyQuil Cold/Cough Relief 756
Children's Vicks NyQuil Cold/Cough Relief Liquid 2680
Zicam Maximum Strength Flu Daytime 768

Chlorpheniramine Polistirex (Co-administration of telithromycin with a drug primarily metabolized by the CYP 3A4 enzyme system may result in increased plasma concentrations of the drug co-administered with telithromycin that could increase or prolong both the therapeutic and adverse effects). Products include:
Tussionex Pennkinetic Extended-Release Suspension 3327

Chlorpheniramine Tannate (Co-administration of telithromycin with a drug primarily metabolized by the CYP 3A4 enzyme system may result in increased plasma concentrations of the drug co-administered with telithromycin that could increase or prolong both the therapeutic and adverse effects).
No products indexed under this heading.

Chlorpromazine (Elevated levels of drugs metabolized by the CYP450 system may be observed when co-administered with telithromycin; therefore, increases or prolongation of the therapeutic and/or adverse effects of the concomitant drug may be observed).
No products indexed under this heading.

Chlorpromazine Hydrochloride (Elevated levels of drugs metabolized by the CYP450 system may be observed when co-administered with telithromycin; therefore, increases or prolongation of the therapeutic and/or adverse effects of the concomitant drug may be observed).
No products indexed under this heading.

Chlorpropamide (Elevated levels of drugs metabolized by the CYP450 system may be observed when co-administered with telithromycin; therefore, increases or prolongation of the therapeutic and/or adverse effects of the concomitant drug may be observed).
No products indexed under this heading.

Cilostazol (Elevated levels of drugs metabolized by the CYP450 system may be observed when co-administered with telithromycin; therefore, increases or prolongation of the therapeutic and/or adverse effects of the concomitant drug may be observed). Products include:
Pletal Tablets 2455

Cimetidine Hydrochloride (Elevated levels of drugs metabolized by the CYP450 system may be observed when co-administered with telithromycin; therefore, increases or prolongation of the therapeutic and/or adverse effects of the concomitant drug may be observed).
No products indexed under this heading.

Ciprofloxacin (Elevated levels of drugs metabolized by the CYP450 system may be observed when co-administered with telithromycin; therefore, increases or prolongation of the therapeutic and/or adverse effects of the concomitant drug may be observed). Products include:
Cipro Oral Suspension 2977
Cipro I.V. 2984
Cipro XR Tablets 2990
Ciprodex Otic Suspension 559

Ciprofloxacin Hydrochloride (Concomitant administration of CYP 3A4 inducers is likely to result in subtherapeutic levels of telithromycin and loss of effect). Products include:
Ciloxan Ophthalmic Ointment 559
Ciloxan Ophthalmic Solution .... ⊙206
Cipro Tablets 2977
Proquin XR Tablets 1153

Cisapride (Steady-state peak plasma concentrations of cisapride were increased when co-administered with repeated doses of telithromycin, resulting in significant increases in QTc. Co-administration is contraindicated).
No products indexed under this heading.

Cisplatin (Concomitant administration of CYP 3A4 inducers is likely to result in subtherapeutic levels of telithromycin and loss of effect).
No products indexed under this heading.

Citalopram Hydrobromide (Elevated levels of drugs metabolized by the CYP450 system may be observed when co-administered with telithromycin; therefore, increases or prolongation of the therapeutic and/or adverse effects of the concomitant drug may be observed). Products include:
Celexa 1176

Clarithromycin (Co-administration of telithromycin with a drug primarily metabolized by the CYP 3A4 enzyme system may result in increased plasma concentrations of the drug co-administered with telithromycin that could increase or prolong both the therapeutic and adverse effects). Products include:
Biaxin/Biaxin XL 402
PREVPAC 3284

Clomipramine Hydrochloride (Elevated levels of drugs metabolized by the CYP450 system may be observed when co-administered with telithromycin; therefore, increases or prolongation of the therapeutic and/or adverse effects of the concomitant drug may be observed).
No products indexed under this heading.

Clopidogrel Hydrogen Sulfate (Elevated levels of drugs metabolized by the CYP450 system may be observed when co-administered with telithromycin; therefore, increases or prolongation of the therapeutic and/or adverse effects of the concomitant drug may be observed).
No products indexed under this heading.

Clozapine (Elevated levels of drugs metabolized by the CYP450 system may be observed when co-administered with telithromycin; therefore, increases or prolongation of the therapeutic and/or adverse effects of the concomitant drug may be observed). Products include:
Clozaril Tablets 2184
FazaClo Orally Disintegrating Tablets 551

Codeine Phosphate (Elevated levels of drugs metabolized by the CYP450 system may be observed when co-administered with telithromycin; therefore, increases or prolongation of the therapeutic and/or adverse effects of the concomitant drug may be observed). Products include:
Tylenol with Codeine Tablets 2391

Codeine Sulfate (Elevated levels of drugs metabolized by the CYP450 system may be observed when co-administered with telithromycin; therefore, increases or prolongation of the therapeutic and/or adverse effects of the concomitant drug may be observed).
No products indexed under this heading.

Cortisone Acetate (Concomitant administration of CYP 3A4 inducers is likely to result in subtherapeutic levels of telithromycin and loss of effect).
No products indexed under this heading.

Cyclobenzaprine (Elevated levels of drugs metabolized by the CYP450 system may be observed when co-administered with telithromycin; therefore, increases or prolongation of the therapeutic and/or adverse effects of the concomitant drug may be observed).
No products indexed under this heading.

Cyclobenzaprine Hydrochloride (Elevated levels of drugs metabolized by the CYP450 system may be observed when co-administered with telithromycin; therefore, increases or prolongation of the therapeutic and/or adverse effects of the concomitant drug may be observed).
No products indexed under this heading.

Cyclophosphamide (Elevated levels of drugs metabolized by the CYP450 system may be observed when co-administered with telithromycin; therefore, increases or prolongation of the therapeutic and/or adverse effects of the concomitant drug may be observed).
No products indexed under this heading.

Cyclosporine (Co-administration of telithromycin with a drug primarily metabolized by the CYP 3A4 enzyme system may result in increased plasma concentrations of the drug co-administered with telithromycin that could increase or prolong both the therapeutic and adverse effects). Products include:
Gengraf Capsules 459
Neoral Oral Solution 2259
Neoral Soft Gelatin Capsules 2259
Restasis Ophthalmic Emulsion 575
Sandimmune 2275

Desipramine Hydrochloride (Elevated levels of drugs metabolized by the CYP450 system may be observed when co-administered with telithromycin; therefore, increases or prolongation of the therapeutic and/or adverse effects of the concomitant drug may be observed).
No products indexed under this heading.

Desogestrel (Co-administration of telithromycin with a drug primarily metabolized by the CYP 3A4 enzyme system may result in increased plasma concentrations of the drug co-administered with telithromycin that could increase or prolong both the therapeutic and adverse effects). Products include:
Mircette Tablets 1066

Dexamethasone (Concomitant administration of CYP 3A4 inducers is likely to result in subtherapeutic levels of telithromycin and loss of effect). Products include:
Ciprodex Otic Suspension 559
Decadron Tablets 1951
TobraDex Ophthalmic Ointment 562
TobraDex Ophthalmic Suspension 563

Dexamethasone Acetate (Concomitant administration of CYP 3A4 inducers is likely to result in subtherapeutic levels of telithromycin and loss of effect).
No products indexed under this heading.

Dexamethasone Phosphate (Elevated levels of drugs metabolized by the CYP450 system may be observed when co-administered with telithromycin; therefore, increases or prolongation of the therapeutic and/or adverse effects of the concomitant drug may be observed).
No products indexed under this heading.

Dexamethasone Sodium (Elevated levels of drugs metabolized by the CYP450 system may be observed when co-administered with telithromycin; therefore, increases or prolongation of the therapeutic and/or adverse effects of the concomitant drug may be observed).
No products indexed under this heading.

Dexamethasone Sodium Phosphate (Concomitant administration of CYP 3A4 inducers is likely to result in subtherapeutic levels of telithromycin and loss of effect).
No products indexed under this heading.

Dexfenfluramine Hydrochloride (Elevated levels of drugs metabolized by the CYP450 system may be observed when co-administered with telithromycin; therefore, increases or prolongation of the therapeutic and/or adverse effects of the concomitant drug may be observed).
No products indexed under this heading.

Dextromethorphan (Elevated levels of drugs metabolized by the CYP450 system may be observed when co-administered with telithromycin; therefore, increases or prolongation of the therapeutic and/or adverse effects of the concomitant drug may be observed).
No products indexed under this heading.

Dextromethorphan Hydrobromide (Elevated levels of drugs metabolized by the CYP450 system may be observed when co-administered with telithromycin; therefore, increases or prolongation of the therapeutic and/or adverse effects of the concomitant drug may be observed). Products include:

- Comtrex Maximum Strength Cold & Cough Day/Night Caplets - Day Formulation ▣ 726
- Comtrex Maximum Strength Cold & Cough Day/Night Caplets - Night Formulation ▣ 726
- Comtrex Maximum Strength Non-Drowsy Cold & Cough Caplets ▣ 725
- Children's Dimetapp DM Cold & Cough Elixir ▣ 731
- Children's Dimetapp Long Acting Cough Plus Cold Syrup ▣ 731
- Toddler's Dimetapp Cold and Cough Drops ▣ 732
- Mucinex DM Extended-Release Bi-Layer Tablets ▣ 720
- Refenesen DM Caplets ▣ 721
- Robitussin Cough & Cold CF Liquid ▣ 735
- Robitussin Cough & Cold Long-Acting Liquid ▣ 735
- Robitussin Cough & Allergy Syrup ▣ 736
- Robitussin Cough & Cold Nighttime Liquid ▣ 736
- Robitussin Cough & Cold Pediatric Drops ▣ 735
- Robitussin Cough, Cold & Flu Nighttime Liquid ▣ 738
- Robitussin Cough & Congestion Liquid ▣ 738
- Robitussin Cough Gels Long-Acting ▣ 737
- Robitussin Cough Long Acting Liquid ▣ 739
- Robitussin Cough DM Syrup ▣ 738
- Robitussin Cough DM Infant Drops ▣ 738
- Robitussin Pediatric Cough Long Acting Liquid ▣ 739
- Robitussin Pediatric Cough & Cold Long-Acting Liquid ▣ 735
- Robitussin Pediatric Cough & Cold Nighttime Liquid ▣ 736
- Robitussin Sugar Free Cough ▣ 738
- TheraFlu Cold & Cough Hot Liquid ▣ 740
- TheraFlu Warming Relief Daytime Severe Cold ▣ 743
- TheraFlu Thin Strips Long Acting Cough ▣ 744
- Triaminic Daytime Cold & Cough Liquid ▣ 745
- Triaminic Cough & Sore Throat Liquid ▣ 747
- Triaminic Cough & Runny Nose Softchews ▣ 748
- Triaminic Thin Strips Cold & Cough ▣ 778
- Triaminic Infant Thin Strips Decongestant Plus Cough ▣ 747
- Children's Tylenol Plus Flu Oral Suspension ▣ 749
- Tylenol Cold Head Congestion Daytime Caplets with Cool Burst and Gelcaps ▣ 750
- Tylenol Cold Multi-Symptom Daytime Liquid ▣ 752
- Tylenol Cold Multi-Symptom Severe Daytime Liquid ▣ 752
- Concentrated Tylenol Infants' Drops Plus Cold & Cough ▣ 754
- Children's Tylenol Plus Cough & Runny Nose Suspension Liquid 1879
- Children's Tylenol Plus Cough & Sore Throat Suspension Liquid 1879
- Children's Tylenol Plus Flu Suspension Liquid 1881
- Children's Tylenol Plus Multi-Symptom Cold Suspension Liquid 1879
- Tylenol Cold Severe Congestion Non-Drowsy Caplets with Cool Burst 1874
- Tylenol Cold Head Congestion Daytime Caplets with Cool Burst 1873
- Tylenol Cold Head Congestion Nighttime Caplets with Cool Burst 1873
- Tylenol Cold Head Congestion Severe Caplets with Cool Burst 1873
- Tylenol Cold Multi-Symptom Daytime Caplets with Cool Burst and Gelcaps 1874
- Tylenol Cold Multi-Symptom Daytime Liquid with Citrus Burst 1874
- Tylenol Cold Multi-Symptom Nighttime Caplets with Cool Burst 1874
- Tylenol Cold Multi-Symptom Nighttime Liquid with Cool Burst 1874
- Tylenol Cold Multi-Symptom Severe Caplets with Cool Burst 1874
- Tylenol Cold Multi-Symptom Severe Daytime Liquid with Citrus Burst 1874
- Tylenol Cough & Sore Throat Daytime Liquid with Cool Burst 1877
- Tylenol Cough & Sore Throat Nighttime Liquid with Cool Burst 1877
- Concentrated Tylenol Infants' Drops Plus Cold and Cough 1879
- Vicks 44 Cough Relief Liquid 2679
- Vicks 44D Cough & Head Congestion Relief Liquid 2679
- Vicks 44E Cough & Chest Congestion Relief Liquid 2679
- Pediatric Vicks 44e Cough & Chest Congestion Relief Liquid 2676
- Vicks 44M Cough, Cold & Flu Relief Liquid 2680
- Pediatric Vicks 44m Cough & Cold Relief Liquid 2676
- Vicks DayQuil LiquiCaps/Liquid Multi-Symptom Cold/Flu Relief ▣ 761
- Vicks DayQuil Multi-Symptom Cold/Flu Relief LiquiCaps 2678
- Vicks DayQuil Multi-Symptom Cold/Flu Relief Liquid 2678
- Vicks NyQuil Multi-Symptom Cold/Flu Relief Liquid 2681
- Children's Vicks NyQuil Cold/Cough Relief ▣ 756
- Vicks NyQuil Multi-Symptom Cold/Flu Relief LiquiCaps 2681
- Vicks NyQuil LiquiCaps/Liquid Multi-Symptom Cold/Flu Relief ▣ 763
- Vicks NyQuil Cough Liquid 2680
- Children's Vicks NyQuil Cold/Cough Relief Liquid 2680
- Zicam Cough Max Nighttime Cough Spray ▣ 767
- Zicam Cough Max Cough Spray ▣ 767
- Zicam Cough Max Cough Melts ▣ 767
- Zicam Cough Plus D Cough Spray ▣ 767
- Zicam Cough Relief Cough Spray ▣ 767
- Zicam Maximum Strength Flu Daytime ▣ 768
- Zicam Maximum Strength Flu Nighttime ▣ 768

Dextromethorphan Polistirex (Elevated levels of drugs metabolized by the CYP450 system may be observed when co-administered with telithromycin; therefore, increases or prolongation of the therapeutic and/or adverse effects of the concomitant drug may be observed). Products include:

- Delsym Extended-Release Suspension 12 Hour Cough Suppressant ▣ 611

Diazepam (Co-administration of telithromycin with a drug primarily metabolized by the CYP 3A4 enzyme system may result in increased plasma concentrations of the drug co-administered with telithromycin that could increase or prolong both the therapeutic and adverse effects). Products include:

- Diastat Rectal Delivery System 3343
- Valium Tablets 2819

Diclofenac Potassium (Elevated levels of drugs metabolized by the CYP450 system may be observed when co-administered with telithromycin; therefore, increases or prolongation of the therapeutic and/or adverse effects of the concomitant drug may be observed).

No products indexed under this heading.

Diclofenac Sodium (Elevated levels of drugs metabolized by the CYP450 system may be observed when co-administered with telithromycin; therefore, increases or prolongation of the therapeutic and/or adverse effects of the concomitant drug may be observed). Products include:

- Arthrotec Tablets 3129
- Voltaren Ophthalmic Solution 2309
- Voltaren Tablets 2307
- Voltaren-XR Tablets 2310

Digoxin (Plasma peak and trough levels of digoxin were increased when co-adminstered with telithromycin; however, trough concentrations of digoxin ranged from 0.74 to 2.17 ng/mL). Products include:

- Lanoxicaps Capsules 1490
- Lanoxin Injection 1494
- Lanoxin Injection Pediatric 1497
- Lanoxin Tablets 1500

Dihydroergotamine Mesylate (Co-administration is not recommended because acute ergot toxicity characterized by severe peripheral vasospasm and dyesthesia have been reported with macrolide antibiotics). Products include:

- Migranal Nasal Spray 3348

Diltiazem Hydrochloride (Co-administration of telithromycin with a drug primarily metabolized by the CYP 3A4 enzyme system may result in increased plasma concentrations of the drug co-administered with telithromycin that could increase or prolong both the therapeutic and adverse effects). Products include:

- Cardizem LA Extended Release Tablets 1728
- Tiazac Capsules 1201

Diltiazem Maleate (Co-administration of telithromycin with a drug primarily metabolized by the CYP 3A4 enzyme system may result in increased plasma concentrations of the drug co-administered with telithromycin that could increase or prolong both the therapeutic and adverse effects).

No products indexed under this heading.

Disopyramide (Co-administration of telithromycin with a drug primarily metabolized by the CYP 3A4 enzyme system may result in increased plasma concentrations of the drug co-administered with telithromycin that could increase or prolong both the therapeutic and adverse effects).

No products indexed under this heading.

Disopyramide Phosphate (Co-administration of telithromycin with a drug primarily metabolized by the CYP 3A4 enzyme system may result in increased plasma concentrations of the drug co-administered with telithromycin that could increase or prolong both the therapeutic and adverse effects).

No products indexed under this heading.

Disulfiram (Co-administration of telithromycin with a drug primarily metabolized by the CYP 3A4 enzyme system may result in increased plasma concentrations of the drug co-administered with telithromycin that could increase or prolong both the therapeutic and adverse effects).

No products indexed under this heading.

Divalproex Sodium (Elevated levels of drugs metabolized by the CYP450 system may be observed when co-administered with telithromycin; therefore, increases or prolongation of the therapeutic and/or adverse effects of the concomitant drug may be observed). Products include:

- Depakote Sprinkle Capsules 422
- Depakote Tablets 427
- Depakote ER Tablets 434

Docetaxel (Elevated levels of drugs metabolized by the CYP450 system may be observed when co-administered with telithromycin; therefore, increases or prolongation of the therapeutic and/or adverse effects of the concomitant drug may be observed). Products include:

- Taxotere Injection Concentrate 2932

Dolasetron Mesylate (Elevated levels of drugs metabolized by the CYP450 system may be observed when co-administered with telithromycin; therefore, increases or prolongation of the therapeutic and/or adverse effects of the concomitant drug may be observed). Products include:

- Anzemet Injection 2859
- Anzemet Tablets 2862

Donepezil Hydrochloride (Elevated levels of drugs metabolized by the CYP450 system may be observed when co-administered with telithromycin; therefore, increases or prolongation of the therapeutic and/or adverse effects of the concomitant drug may be observed). Products include:

- Aricept Tablets 1094
- Aricept ODT Tablets 1094

Doxepin Hydrochloride (Elevated levels of drugs metabolized by the CYP450 system may be observed when co-administered with telithromycin; therefore, increases or prolongation of the therapeutic and/or adverse effects of the concomitant drug may be observed).

No products indexed under this heading.

Doxorubicin Hydrochloride (Co-administration of telithromycin with a drug primarily metabolized by the CYP 3A4 enzyme system may result in increased plasma concentrations of the drug co-administered with telithromycin that could increase or prolong both the therapeutic and adverse effects).

No products indexed under this heading.

Dronabinol (Co-administration of telithromycin with a drug primarily metabolized by the CYP 3A4 enzyme system may result in increased plasma concentrations of the drug co-administered with telithromycin that could increase or prolong both the therapeutic and adverse effects). Products include:

- Marinol Capsules 3333

Drugs that Undergo Biotransformation by Cytochrome P-450 Mixed Function Oxidase (Elevated levels of drugs metabolized by the CYP450 system may be observed when co-administered with telithromycin; therefore, increases or prolongation of the therapeutic and/or adverse effects of the concomitant drug may be observed).

No products indexed under this heading.

Dyphylline (Elevated levels of drugs metabolized by the CYP450 system may be observed when co-administered with telithromycin; therefore, increases or prolongation of the therapeutic and/or adverse effects of the concomitant drug may be observed).

No products indexed under this heading.

Efavirenz (Concomitant administration of CYP 3A4 inducers is likely to result in subtherapeutic levels of telithromycin and loss of effect). Products include:

Encainide Hydrochloride (Elevated levels of drugs metabolized by the CYP450 system may be observed when co-administered with telithromycin; therefore, increases or prolongation of the therapeutic and/or adverse effects of the concomitant drug may be observed).

No products indexed under this heading.

Enoxacin (Elevated levels of drugs metabolized by the CYP450 system may be observed when co-administered with telithromycin; therefore, increases or prolongation of the therapeutic and/or adverse effects of the concomitant drug may be observed).

No products indexed under this heading.

Eprosartan Mesylate (Elevated levels of drugs metabolized by the CYP450 system may be observed when co-administered with telithromycin; therefore, increases or prolongation of the therapeutic and/or adverse effects of the concomitant drug may be observed). Products include:

Ergonovine Maleate (Co-administration is not recommended because acute ergot toxicity characterized by severe peripheral vasospasm and dyesthesia have been reported with macrolide antibiotics).

No products indexed under this heading.

Ergotamine Tartrate (Co-administration is not recommended because acute ergot toxicity characterized by severe peripheral vasospasm and dyesthesia have been reported with macrolide antibiotics).

No products indexed under this heading.

Erythromycin (Co-administration of telithromycin with a drug primarily metabolized by the CYP 3A4 enzyme system may result in increased plasma concentrations of the drug co-administered with telithromycin that could increase or prolong both the therapeutic and adverse effects). Products include:

Erythromycin Estolate (Co-administration of telithromycin with a drug primarily metabolized by the CYP 3A4 enzyme system may result in increased plasma concentrations of the drug co-administered with telithromycin that could increase or prolong both the therapeutic and adverse effects).

No products indexed under this heading.

Erythromycin Ethylsuccinate (Co-administration of telithromycin with a drug primarily metabolized by the CYP 3A4 enzyme system may result in increased plasma concentrations of the drug co-administered with telithromycin that could increase or prolong both the therapeutic and adverse effects). Products include:

Erythromycin Gluceptate (Co-administration of telithromycin with a drug primarily metabolized by the CYP 3A4 enzyme system may result in increased plasma concentrations of the drug co-administered with telithromycin that could increase or prolong both the therapeutic and adverse effects).

No products indexed under this heading.

Erythromycin Lactobionate (Co-administration of telithromycin with a drug primarily metabolized by the CYP 3A4 enzyme system may result in increased plasma concentrations of the drug co-administered with telithromycin that could increase or prolong both the therapeutic and adverse effects).

No products indexed under this heading.

Erythromycin Stearate (Co-administration of telithromycin with a drug primarily metabolized by the CYP 3A4 enzyme system may result in increased plasma concentrations of the drug co-administered with telithromycin that could increase or prolong both the therapeutic and adverse effects). Products include:

Esomeprazole Magnesium (Elevated levels of drugs metabolized by the CYP450 system may be observed when co-administered with telithromycin; therefore, increases or prolongation of the therapeutic and/or adverse effects of the concomitant drug may be observed). Products include:

Estradiol (Co-administration of telithromycin with a drug primarily metabolized by the CYP 3A4 enzyme system may result in increased plasma concentrations of the drug co-administered with telithromycin that could increase or prolong both the therapeutic and adverse effects). Products include:

Estradiol Benzoate (Co-administration of telithromycin with a drug primarily metabolized by the CYP 3A4 enzyme system may result in increased plasma concentrations of the drug co-administered with telithromycin that could increase or prolong both the therapeutic and adverse effects).

No products indexed under this heading.

Estradiol Cypionate (Co-administration of telithromycin with a drug primarily metabolized by the CYP 3A4 enzyme system may result in increased plasma concentrations of the drug co-administered with telithromycin that could increase or prolong both the therapeutic and adverse effects).

No products indexed under this heading.

Estradiol Valerate (Co-administration of telithromycin with a drug primarily metabolized by the CYP 3A4 enzyme system may result in increased plasma concentrations of the drug co-administered with telithromycin that could increase or prolong both the therapeutic and adverse effects).

No products indexed under this heading.

Estrogen (Elevated levels of drugs metabolized by the CYP450 system may be observed when co-administered with telithromycin; therefore, increases or prolongation of the therapeutic and/or adverse effects of the concomitant drug may be observed).

No products indexed under this heading.

Estrogens, Conjugated (Elevated levels of drugs metabolized by the CYP450 system may be observed when co-administered with telithromycin; therefore, increases or prolongation of the therapeutic and/or adverse effects of the concomitant drug may be observed). Products include:

Estrogens, Conjugated, Synthetic A (Elevated levels of drugs metabolized by the CYP450 system may be observed when co-administered with telithromycin; therefore, increases or prolongation of the therapeutic and/or adverse effects of the concomitant drug may be observed).

No products indexed under this heading.

Estrogens, Esterified (Elevated levels of drugs metabolized by the CYP450 system may be observed when co-administered with telithromycin; therefore, increases or prolongation of the therapeutic and/or adverse effects of the concomitant drug may be observed). Products include:

Ethinyl Estradiol (Co-administration of telithromycin with a drug primarily metabolized by the CYP 3A4 enzyme system may result in increased plasma concentrations of the drug co-administered with telithromycin that could increase or prolong both the therapeutic and adverse effects). Products include:

Ethosuximide (Co-administration of telithromycin with a drug primarily metabolized by the CYP 3A4 enzyme system may result in increased plasma concentrations of the drug co-administered with telithromycin that could increase or prolong both the therapeutic and adverse effects).

No products indexed under this heading.

Ethotoin (Elevated levels of drugs metabolized by the CYP450 system may be observed when co-administered with telithromycin; therefore, increases or prolongation of the therapeutic and/or adverse effects of the concomitant drug may be observed).

No products indexed under this heading.

Ethynodiol Diacetate (Co-administration of telithromycin with a drug primarily metabolized by the CYP 3A4 enzyme system may result in increased plasma concentrations of the drug co-administered with telithromycin that could increase or prolong both the therapeutic and adverse effects).

No products indexed under this heading.

Etodolac (Elevated levels of drugs metabolized by the CYP450 system may be observed when co-administered with telithromycin; therefore, increases or prolongation of the therapeutic and/or adverse effects of the concomitant drug may be observed).

No products indexed under this heading.

Etoposide (Co-administration of telithromycin with a drug primarily metabolized by the CYP 3A4 enzyme system may result in increased plasma concentrations of the drug co-administered with telithromycin that could increase or prolong both the therapeutic and adverse effects).

No products indexed under this heading.

Etoposide Phosphate (Co-administration of telithromycin with a drug primarily metabolized by the CYP 3A4 enzyme system may result in increased plasma concentrations of the drug co-administered with telithromycin that could increase or prolong both the therapeutic and adverse effects).

No products indexed under this heading.

Felbamate (Concomitant administration of CYP 3A4 inducers is likely to result in subtherapeutic levels of telithromycin and loss of effect).

No products indexed under this heading.

Felodipine (Co-administration of telithromycin with a drug primarily metabolized by the CYP 3A4 enzyme system may result in increased plasma concentrations of the drug co-administered with telithromycin that could increase or prolong both the therapeutic and adverse effects).

No products indexed under this heading.

Fenoprofen Calcium (Elevated levels of drugs metabolized by the CYP450 system may be observed when co-administered with telithromycin; therefore, increases or prolongation of the therapeutic and/or adverse effects of the concomitant drug may be observed). Products include:

Nalfon Capsules 2502

Fentanyl (Co-administration of telithromycin with a drug primarily metabolized by the CYP 3A4 enzyme system may result in increased plasma concentrations of the drug co-administered with telithromycin that could increase or prolong both the therapeutic and adverse effects). Products include:

Duragesic Transdermal System 2373
Ionsys Transdermal System 2379

Fentanyl Citrate (Co-administration of telithromycin with a drug primarily metabolized by the CYP 3A4 enzyme system may result in increased plasma concentrations of the drug co-administered with telithromycin that could increase or prolong both the therapeutic and adverse effects). Products include:

Actiq ... 979

Flecainide Acetate (Elevated levels of drugs metabolized by the CYP450 system may be observed when co-administered with telithromycin; therefore, increases or prolongation of the therapeutic and/or adverse effects of the concomitant drug may be observed). Products include:

Tambocor Tablets 1856

Fludrocortisone Acetate (Concomitant administration of CYP 3A4 inducers is likely to result in subtherapeutic levels of telithromycin and loss of effect).

No products indexed under this heading.

Fluoxetine (Elevated levels of drugs metabolized by the CYP450 system may be observed when co-administered with telithromycin; therefore, increases or prolongation of the therapeutic and/or adverse effects of the concomitant drug may be observed).

No products indexed under this heading.

Fluoxetine Hydrochloride (Elevated levels of drugs metabolized by the CYP450 system may be observed when co-administered with telithromycin; therefore, increases or prolongation of the therapeutic and/or adverse effects of the concomitant drug may be observed). Products include:

Prozac Pulvules and Liquid 1801
Symbyax Capsules 1819

Fluphenazine Decanoate (Elevated levels of drugs metabolized by the CYP450 system may be observed when co-administered with telithromycin; therefore, increases or prolongation of the therapeutic and/or adverse effects of the concomitant drug may be observed).

No products indexed under this heading.

Fluphenazine Enanthate (Elevated levels of drugs metabolized by the CYP450 system may be observed when co-administered with telithromycin; therefore, increases or prolongation of the therapeutic and/or adverse effects of the concomitant drug may be observed).

No products indexed under this heading.

Fluphenazine Hydrochloride (Elevated levels of drugs metabolized by the CYP450 system may be observed when co-administered with telithromycin; therefore, increases or prolongation of the therapeutic and/or adverse effects of the concomitant drug may be observed).

No products indexed under this heading.

Flurbiprofen (Elevated levels of drugs metabolized by the CYP450 system may be observed when co-administered with telithromycin; therefore, increases or prolongation of the therapeutic and/or adverse effects of the concomitant drug may be observed).

No products indexed under this heading.

Flurbiprofen Sodium (Elevated levels of drugs metabolized by the CYP450 system may be observed when co-administered with telithromycin; therefore, increases or prolongation of the therapeutic and/or adverse effects of the concomitant drug may be observed). Products include:

Ocufen Ophthalmic Solution ☉232

Flutamide (Elevated levels of drugs metabolized by the CYP450 system may be observed when co-administered with telithromycin; therefore, increases or prolongation of the therapeutic and/or adverse effects of the concomitant drug may be observed). Products include:

Eulexin Capsules 3009

Fluticasone Propionate (Elevated levels of drugs metabolized by the CYP450 system may be observed when co-administered with telithromycin; therefore, increases or prolongation of the therapeutic and/or adverse effects of the concomitant drug may be observed). Products include:

Advair Diskus 100/50 1308
Advair Diskus 250/50 1308
Advair Diskus 500/50 1308
Advair HFA Inhalation Aerosol 1318
Cutivate Cream 2662
Cutivate Lotion 0.05% 2664
Cutivate Ointment 2665
Flonase Nasal Spray 1440
Flovent Diskus 1443

Fluvastatin Sodium (Elevated levels of drugs metabolized by the CYP450 system may be observed when co-administered with telithromycin; therefore, increases or prolongation of the therapeutic and/or adverse effects of the concomitant drug may be observed). Products include:

Lescol Capsules 2233
Lescol XL Tablets 2233

Fluvoxamine Maleate (Elevated levels of drugs metabolized by the CYP450 system may be observed when co-administered with telithromycin; therefore, increases or prolongation of the therapeutic and/or adverse effects of the concomitant drug may be observed).

No products indexed under this heading.

Formoterol Fumarate (Elevated levels of drugs metabolized by the CYP450 system may be observed when co-administered with telithromycin; therefore, increases or prolongation of the therapeutic and/or adverse effects of the concomitant drug may be observed). Products include:

Foradil Aerolizer 3010

Fosphenytoin (Elevated levels of drugs metabolized by the CYP450 system may be observed when co-administered with telithromycin; therefore, increases or prolongation of the therapeutic and/or adverse effects of the concomitant drug may be observed).

No products indexed under this heading.

Fosphenytoin Sodium (Concomitant administration of CYP 3A4 inducers is likely to result in subtherapeutic levels of telithromycin and loss of effect).

No products indexed under this heading.

Gabapentin (Elevated levels of drugs metabolized by the CYP450 system may be observed when co-administered with telithromycin; therefore, increases or prolongation of the therapeutic and/or adverse effects of the concomitant drug may be observed). Products include:

Neurontin Capsules 2487
Neurontin Oral Solution 2487
Neurontin Tablets 2487

Galantamine Hydrobromide (Elevated levels of drugs metabolized by the CYP450 system may be observed when co-administered with telithromycin; therefore, increases or prolongation of the therapeutic and/or adverse effects of the concomitant drug may be observed). Products include:

Razadyne 2399
Razadyne ER Extended-Release
Capsules 2399

Garlic Extract (Concomitant administration of CYP 3A4 inducers is likely to result in subtherapeutic levels of telithromycin and loss of effect).

No products indexed under this heading.

Garlic Oil (Concomitant administration of CYP 3A4 inducers is likely to result in subtherapeutic levels of telithromycin and loss of effect).

No products indexed under this heading.

Glimepiride (Elevated levels of drugs metabolized by the CYP450 system may be observed when co-administered with telithromycin; therefore, increases or prolongation of the therapeutic and/or adverse effects of the concomitant drug may be observed). Products include:

Avandaryl Tablets 1379
Duetact Tablets 3226

Glipizide (Elevated levels of drugs metabolized by the CYP450 system may be observed when co-administered with telithromycin; therefore, increases or prolongation of the therapeutic and/or adverse effects of the concomitant drug may be observed).

No products indexed under this heading.

Glyburide (Elevated levels of drugs metabolized by the CYP450 system may be observed when co-administered with telithromycin; therefore, increases or prolongation of the therapeutic and/or adverse effects of the concomitant drug may be observed).

No products indexed under this heading.

Grepafloxacin Hydrochloride (Elevated levels of drugs metabolized by the CYP450 system may be observed when co-administered with telithromycin; therefore, increases or prolongation of the therapeutic and/or adverse effects of the concomitant drug may be observed).

No products indexed under this heading.

Haloperidol (Co-administration of telithromycin with a drug primarily metabolized by the CYP 3A4 enzyme system may result in increased plasma concentrations of the drug co-administered with telithromycin that could increase or prolong both the therapeutic and adverse effects).

No products indexed under this heading.

Haloperidol Decanoate (Co-administration of telithromycin with a drug primarily metabolized by the CYP 3A4 enzyme system may result in increased plasma concentrations of the drug co-administered with telithromycin that could increase or prolong both the therapeutic and adverse effects).

No products indexed under this heading.

Haloperidol Lactate (Co-administration of telithromycin with a drug primarily metabolized by the CYP 3A4 enzyme system may result in increased plasma concentrations of the drug co-administered with telithromycin that could increase or prolong both the therapeutic and adverse effects).

No products indexed under this heading.

Hydrocodone Bitartrate (Elevated levels of drugs metabolized by the CYP450 system may be observed when co-administered with telithromycin; therefore, increases or prolongation of the therapeutic and/or adverse effects of the concomitant drug may be observed). Products include:

Hycodan 1116
Hycotuss Expectorant Syrup 1117
Vicodin Tablets 535
Vicodin ES Tablets 536
Vicodin HP Tablets 538
Vicoprofen Tablets 539
Zydone Tablets 1139

Hydrocortisone (Concomitant administration of CYP 3A4 inducers is likely to result in subtherapeutic levels of telithromycin and loss of effect). Products include:

Colocort Rectal Suspension, USP
(Retention) 100 mg/60 mL........... 2476
Hydrocortone Tablets 1989
Preparation H Hydrocortisone
Cream ▣646

Hydrocortisone Acetate (Concomitant administration of CYP 3A4 inducers is likely to result in subtherapeutic levels of telithromycin and loss of effect). Products include:

Analpram-HC 1159
Pramosone 1161
ProctoFoam-HC 3099

Hydrocortisone Butyrate (Concomitant administration of CYP 3A4 inducers is likely to result in subtherapeutic levels of telithromycin and loss of effect). Products include:

Locoid Lipocream Cream 1160

Hydrocortisone Cypionate (Concomitant administration of CYP 3A4 inducers is likely to result in subtherapeutic levels of telithromycin and loss of effect).
No products indexed under this heading.

Hydrocortisone Hemisuccinate (Concomitant administration of CYP 3A4 inducers is likely to result in subtherapeutic levels of telithromycin and loss of effect).
No products indexed under this heading.

Hydrocortisone Probutate (Concomitant administration of CYP 3A4 inducers is likely to result in subtherapeutic levels of telithromycin and loss of effect).
No products indexed under this heading.

Hydrocortisone Sodium Phosphate (Concomitant administration of CYP 3A4 inducers is likely to result in subtherapeutic levels of telithromycin and loss of effect).
No products indexed under this heading.

Hydrocortisone Sodium Succinate (Concomitant administration of CYP 3A4 inducers is likely to result in subtherapeutic levels of telithromycin and loss of effect).
No products indexed under this heading.

Hydrocortisone Valerate (Concomitant administration of CYP 3A4 inducers is likely to result in subtherapeutic levels of telithromycin and loss of effect).
No products indexed under this heading.

Hypericum (Concomitant administration of CYP 3A4 inducers is likely to result in subtherapeutic levels of telithromycin and loss of effect). Products include:
Satiete Tablets 832

Hypericum Perforatum (Concomitant administration of CYP 3A4 inducers is likely to result in subtherapeutic levels of telithromycin and loss of effect).
No products indexed under this heading.

Ibuprofen (Elevated levels of drugs metabolized by the CYP450 system may be observed when co-administered with telithromycin; therefore, increases or prolongation of the therapeutic and/or adverse effects of the concomitant drug may be observed). Products include:
Advil Allergy Sinus Caplets 770
Advil 674
Children's Advil Oral Suspension 603
Children's Advil Chewable Tablets 603
Advil Cold & Sinus 723
Infants' Advil Concentrated Drops 604
Infants' Advil Concentrated Drops - White Grape (Dye-Free) 604
Junior Strength Advil Swallow Tablets 605
Advil Migraine Liquigels 608
Advil Multi-Symptom Cold Caplets 770
Advil PM Caplets 615
Motrin IB Tablets and Caplets 1866
Children's Motrin Oral Suspension 1867
Children's Motrin Non-Staining Dye-Free Oral Suspension 1867
Children's Motrin Cold Oral Suspension 1867
Infants' Motrin Concentrated Drops 1867
Infants' Motrin Non-Staining Dye-Free Concentrated Drops 1867
Junior Strength Motrin Caplets and Chewable Tablets 1867
Vicoprofen Tablets 539

Imipramine Hydrochloride (Elevated levels of drugs metabolized by the CYP450 system may be observed when co-administered with telithromycin; therefore, increases or prolongation of the therapeutic and/or adverse effects of the concomitant drug may be observed).
No products indexed under this heading.

Imipramine Pamoate (Elevated levels of drugs metabolized by the CYP450 system may be observed when co-administered with telithromycin; therefore, increases or prolongation of the therapeutic and/or adverse effects of the concomitant drug may be observed).
No products indexed under this heading.

Indinavir Sulfate (Co-administration of telithromycin with a drug primarily metabolized by the CYP 3A4 enzyme system may result in increased plasma concentrations of the drug co-administered with telithromycin that could increase or prolong both the therapeutic and adverse effects). Products include:
Crixivan Capsules 1940

Indomethacin (Elevated levels of drugs metabolized by the CYP450 system may be observed when co-administered with telithromycin; therefore, increases or prolongation of the therapeutic and/or adverse effects of the concomitant drug may be observed). Products include:
Indocin 1995

Indomethacin Sodium Trihydrate (Elevated levels of drugs metabolized by the CYP450 system may be observed when co-administered with telithromycin; therefore, increases or prolongation of the therapeutic and/or adverse effects of the concomitant drug may be observed). Products include:
Indocin I.V. 2465

Indoramin Hydrochloride (Elevated levels of drugs metabolized by the CYP450 system may be observed when co-administered with telithromycin; therefore, increases or prolongation of the therapeutic and/or adverse effects of the concomitant drug may be observed).
No products indexed under this heading.

Irbesartan (Elevated levels of drugs metabolized by the CYP450 system may be observed when co-administered with telithromycin; therefore, increases or prolongation of the therapeutic and/or adverse effects of the concomitant drug may be observed). Products include:
Avalide Tablets 888
Avalide Tablets 2874
Avapro Tablets 891
Avapro Tablets 2871

Isotretinoin (Elevated levels of drugs metabolized by the CYP450 system may be observed when co-administered with telithromycin; therefore, increases or prolongation of the therapeutic and/or adverse effects of the concomitant drug may be observed). Products include:
Accutane Capsules 2731

Isradipine (Co-administration of telithromycin with a drug primarily metabolized by the CYP 3A4 enzyme system may result in increased plasma concentrations of the drug co-administered with telithromycin that could increase or prolong both the therapeutic and adverse effects). Products include:
DynaCirc CR Tablets 2721

Itraconazole (A study with itraconazole showed the Cmax and AUC of telithromycin were increased).
No products indexed under this heading.

Ketoconazole (A study with ketoconazole showed the Cmax and AUC of telithromycin were increased). Products include:
Nizoral A-D Shampoo, 1% 1868

Ketoprofen (Elevated levels of drugs metabolized by the CYP450 system may be observed when co-administered with telithromycin; therefore, increases or prolongation of the therapeutic and/or adverse effects of the concomitant drug may be observed).
No products indexed under this heading.

Ketorolac Tromethamine (Elevated levels of drugs metabolized by the CYP450 system may be observed when co-administered with telithromycin; therefore, increases or prolongation of the therapeutic and/or adverse effects of the concomitant drug may be observed). Products include:
Acular Ophthalmic Solution 565
Acular LS Ophthalmic Solution 566

Labetalol Hydrochloride (Elevated levels of drugs metabolized by the CYP450 system may be observed when co-administered with telithromycin; therefore, increases or prolongation of the therapeutic and/or adverse effects of the concomitant drug may be observed).
No products indexed under this heading.

Lamotrigine (Elevated levels of drugs metabolized by the CYP450 system may be observed when co-administered with telithromycin; therefore, increases or prolongation of the therapeutic and/or adverse effects of the concomitant drug may be observed). Products include:
Lamictal 1481

Lansoprazole (Elevated levels of drugs metabolized by the CYP450 system may be observed when co-administered with telithromycin; therefore, increases or prolongation of the therapeutic and/or adverse effects of the concomitant drug may be observed). Products include:
Prevacid Delayed-Release Capsules 3271
Prevacid for Delayed-Release Oral Suspension 3271
Prevacid SoluTab Delayed-Release Orally Disintegrating Tablets 3271
Prevacid I.V. for Injection 3277
Prevacid NapraPAC 3280
PREVPAC 3284

Levetiracetam (Elevated levels of drugs metabolized by the CYP450 system may be observed when co-administered with telithromycin; therefore, increases or prolongation of the therapeutic and/or adverse effects of the concomitant drug may be observed). Products include:
Keppra Injection 3320
Keppra Oral Solution 3314
Keppra Tablets 3314

Levobupivacaine Hydrochloride (Elevated levels of drugs metabolized by the CYP450 system may be observed when co-administered with telithromycin; therefore, increases or prolongation of the therapeutic and/or adverse effects of the concomitant drug may be observed).
No products indexed under this heading.

Levonorgestrel (When oral contraceptives containing ethinyl estradiol and levonorgestrel were co-administered with telithromycin, the steady-state AUC of ethinyl estradiol did not change but the AUC of levonorgestrel increased. However, telithromycin did not interfere with the antiovulatory effect of the oral contraceptives). Products include:
Climara Pro Transdermal System 776
Mirena Intrauterine System 787
Plan B Tablets 1076
Seasonique Tablets 1077

Lidocaine (Co-administration of telithromycin with a drug primarily metabolized by the CYP 3A4 enzyme system may result in increased plasma concentrations of the drug co-administered with telithromycin that could increase or prolong both the therapeutic and adverse effects). Products include:
Lidoderm Patch 1118
Synera Topical Patch 1137

Lidocaine Base (Elevated levels of drugs metabolized by the CYP450 system may be observed when co-administered with telithromycin; therefore, increases or prolongation of the therapeutic and/or adverse effects of the concomitant drug may be observed).
No products indexed under this heading.

Lidocaine Hydrochloride (Co-administration of telithromycin with a drug primarily metabolized by the CYP 3A4 enzyme system may result in increased plasma concentrations of the drug co-administered with telithromycin that could increase or prolong both the therapeutic and adverse effects).
No products indexed under this heading.

Lomefloxacin Hydrochloride (Elevated levels of drugs metabolized by the CYP450 system may be observed when co-administered with telithromycin; therefore, increases or prolongation of the therapeutic and/or adverse effects of the concomitant drug may be observed).
No products indexed under this heading.

Losartan Potassium (Elevated levels of drugs metabolized by the CYP450 system may be observed when co-administered with telithromycin; therefore, increases or prolongation of the therapeutic and/or adverse effects of the concomitant drug may be observed). Products include:
Cozaar Tablets 1935
Hyzaar 50-12.5 Tablets 1990
Hyzaar 100-12.5 Tablets 1990
Hyzaar 100-25 Tablets 1990

Lovastatin (Lovastatin levels were increased due to CYP 3A4 inhibition by telithromycin, thereby increasing the risk of myopathy. Co-administration should be avoided). Products include:
Advicor Tablets 1722
Altoprev Extended-Release Tablets 3109

Mevacor Tablets 2021

Maprotiline Hydrochloride (Elevated levels of drugs metabolized by the CYP450 system may be observed when co-administered with telithromycin; therefore, increases or prolongation of the therapeutic and/or adverse effects of the concomitant drug may be observed).
No products indexed under this heading.

Meclofenamate Sodium (Elevated levels of drugs metabolized by the CYP450 system may be observed when co-administered with telithromycin; therefore, increases or prolongation of the therapeutic and/or adverse effects of the concomitant drug may be observed).
No products indexed under this heading.

Mefenamic Acid (Elevated levels of drugs metabolized by the CYP450 system may be observed when co-administered with telithromycin; therefore, increases or prolongation of the therapeutic and/or adverse effects of the concomitant drug may be observed).
No products indexed under this heading.

Meloxicam (Elevated levels of drugs metabolized by the CYP450 system may be observed when co-administered with telithromycin; therefore, increases or prolongation of the therapeutic and/or adverse effects of the concomitant drug may be observed). Products include:
Mobic Oral Suspension 863
Mobic Tablets 863

Meperidine Hydrochloride (Elevated levels of drugs metabolized by the CYP450 system may be observed when co-administered with telithromycin; therefore, increases or prolongation of the therapeutic and/or adverse effects of the concomitant drug may be observed).
No products indexed under this heading.

Mephenytoin (Concomitant administration of CYP 3A4 inducers is likely to result in subtherapeutic levels of telithromycin and loss of effect).
No products indexed under this heading.

Mephobarbital (Elevated levels of drugs metabolized by the CYP450 system may be observed when co-administered with telithromycin; therefore, increases or prolongation of the therapeutic and/or adverse effects of the concomitant drug may be observed).
No products indexed under this heading.

Meprobamate (Elevated levels of drugs metabolized by the CYP450 system may be observed when co-administered with telithromycin; therefore, increases or prolongation of the therapeutic and/or adverse effects of the concomitant drug may be observed).
No products indexed under this heading.

Mestranol (Co-administration of telithromycin with a drug primarily metabolized by the CYP 3A4 enzyme system may result in increased plasma concentrations of the drug co-administered with telithromycin that could increase or prolong both the therapeutic and adverse effects).
No products indexed under this heading.

Metformin Hydrochloride (Elevated levels of drugs metabolized by the CYP450 system may be observed when co-administered with telithromycin; therefore, increases or prolongation of the therapeutic and/or adverse effects of the concomitant drug may be observed). Products include:
ActoPlus Met Tablets 3214
Avandamet Tablets 1373
Fortamet Extended-Release Tablets 3115

Methadone Hydrochloride (Co-administration of telithromycin with a drug primarily metabolized by the CYP 3A4 enzyme system may result in increased plasma concentrations of the drug co-administered with telithromycin that could increase or prolong both the therapeutic and adverse effects).
No products indexed under this heading.

Methamphetamine Hydrochloride (Elevated levels of drugs metabolized by the CYP450 system may be observed when co-administered with telithromycin; therefore, increases or prolongation of the therapeutic and/or adverse effects of the concomitant drug may be observed). Products include:
Desoxyn Tablets, USP 2462

Methsuximide (Concomitant administration of CYP 3A4 inducers is likely to result in subtherapeutic levels of telithromycin and loss of effect).
No products indexed under this heading.

Methylergonovine Maleate (Co-administration is not recommended because acute ergot toxicity characterized by severe peripheral vasospasm and dyesthesia have been reported with macrolide antibiotics).
No products indexed under this heading.

Methylprednisolone (Concomitant administration of CYP 3A4 inducers is likely to result in subtherapeutic levels of telithromycin and loss of effect).
No products indexed under this heading.

Methylprednisolone Acetate (Concomitant administration of CYP 3A4 inducers is likely to result in subtherapeutic levels of telithromycin and loss of effect). Products include:
Depo-Medrol Injectable Suspension 2617
Depo-Medrol Single-Dose Vial 2619

Methylprednisolone Sodium Succinate (Concomitant administration of CYP 3A4 inducers is likely to result in subtherapeutic levels of telithromycin and loss of effect).
No products indexed under this heading.

Methysergide Maleate (Co-administration is not recommended because acute ergot toxicity characterized by severe peripheral vasospasm and dyesthesia have been reported with macrolide antibiotics).
No products indexed under this heading.

Metoprolol Succinate (Co-administration increased the Cmax and AUC of metoprolol; however, there was no effect on the elimination half-life. The increased exposure to metoprolol may be of clinical importance). Products include:
Toprol-XL Tablets 668

Metoprolol Tartrate (Co-administration increased the Cmax and AUC of metoprolol; however, there was no effect on the elimination half-life. The increased exposure to metoprolol may be of clinical importance). Products include:
Lopressor Injection 2238
Lopressor Tablets 2238
Lopressor HCT 50/25 Tablets 2241
Lopressor HCT 100/25 Tablets 2241
Lopressor HCT 100/50 Tablets 2241

Mexiletine Hydrochloride (Elevated levels of drugs metabolized by the CYP450 system may be observed when co-administered with telithromycin; therefore, increases or prolongation of the therapeutic and/or adverse effects of the concomitant drug may be observed).
No products indexed under this heading.

Midazolam Hydrochloride (Concomitant administration of telithromycin with midazolam increased the AUC of midazolam. Dosage adjustment of midazolam should be considered if necessary).
No products indexed under this heading.

Miglitol (Elevated levels of drugs metabolized by the CYP450 system may be observed when co-administered with telithromycin; therefore, increases or prolongation of the therapeutic and/or adverse effects of the concomitant drug may be observed).
No products indexed under this heading.

Mirtazapine (Elevated levels of drugs metabolized by the CYP450 system may be observed when co-administered with telithromycin; therefore, increases or prolongation of the therapeutic and/or adverse effects of the concomitant drug may be observed).
No products indexed under this heading.

Modafinil (Concomitant administration of CYP 3A4 inducers is likely to result in subtherapeutic levels of telithromycin and loss of effect). Products include:
Provigil Tablets 988

Montelukast Sodium (Elevated levels of drugs metabolized by the CYP450 system may be observed when co-administered with telithromycin; therefore, increases or prolongation of the therapeutic and/or adverse effects of the concomitant drug may be observed). Products include:
Singulair 2077

Morphine Sulfate (Elevated levels of drugs metabolized by the CYP450 system may be observed when co-administered with telithromycin; therefore, increases or prolongation of the therapeutic and/or adverse effects of the concomitant drug may be observed). Products include:
Avinza Capsules 1741
Kadian Capsules 577
MS Contin Tablets 2701

Moxifloxacin Hydrochloride (Elevated levels of drugs metabolized by the CYP450 system may be observed when co-administered with telithromycin; therefore, increases or prolongation of the therapeutic and/or adverse effects of the concomitant drug may be observed). Products include:
Avelox 2970
Vigamox Ophthalmic Solution 564

Nabumetone (Elevated levels of drugs metabolized by the CYP450 system may be observed when co-administered with telithromycin; therefore, increases or prolongation of the therapeutic and/or adverse effects of the concomitant drug may be observed).
No products indexed under this heading.

Nafcillin Sodium (Elevated levels of drugs metabolized by the CYP450 system may be observed when co-administered with telithromycin; therefore, increases or prolongation of the therapeutic and/or adverse effects of the concomitant drug may be observed).
No products indexed under this heading.

Naproxen (Elevated levels of drugs metabolized by the CYP450 system may be observed when co-administered with telithromycin; therefore, increases or prolongation of the therapeutic and/or adverse effects of the concomitant drug may be observed). Products include:
EC-Naprosyn Delayed-Release Tablets 2761
Naprosyn Suspension 2761
Naprosyn Tablets 2761
Prevacid NapraPAC 3280

Naproxen Sodium (Elevated levels of drugs metabolized by the CYP450 system may be observed when co-administered with telithromycin; therefore, increases or prolongation of the therapeutic and/or adverse effects of the concomitant drug may be observed). Products include:
Aleve Caplets 742
Aleve Gelcaps 743
Aleve Tablets 743
Aleve Cold & Sinus Caplets 744
Anaprox Tablets 2761
Anaprox DS Tablets 2761

Nateglinide (Elevated levels of drugs metabolized by the CYP450 system may be observed when co-administered with telithromycin; therefore, increases or prolongation of the therapeutic and/or adverse effects of the concomitant drug may be observed). Products include:
Starlix Tablets 2292

Nefazodone Hydrochloride (Co-administration of telithromycin with a drug primarily metabolized by the CYP 3A4 enzyme system may result in increased plasma concentrations of the drug co-administered with telithromycin that could increase or prolong both the therapeutic and adverse effects).
No products indexed under this heading.

Nelfinavir Mesylate (Co-administration of telithromycin with a drug primarily metabolized by the CYP 3A4 enzyme system may result in increased plasma concentrations of the drug co-administered with telithromycin that could increase or prolong both the therapeutic and adverse effects). Products include:
Viracept 2577

Nevirapine (Concomitant administration of CYP 3A4 inducers is likely to result in subtherapeutic levels of telithromycin and loss of effect). Products include:
Viramune Oral Suspension 873
Viramune Tablets 873

Nicardipine (Elevated levels of drugs metabolized by the CYP450 system may be observed when co-administered with telithromycin; therefore, increases or prolongation of the therapeutic and/or adverse effects of the concomitant drug may be observed).

No products indexed under this heading.

Nicardipine Hydrochloride (Co-administration of telithromycin with a drug primarily metabolized by the CYP 3A4 enzyme system may result in increased plasma concentrations of the drug co-administered with telithromycin that could increase or prolong both the therapeutic and adverse effects). Products include:

Nicotine Polacrilex (Elevated levels of drugs metabolized by the CYP450 system may be observed when co-administered with telithromycin; therefore, increases or prolongation of the therapeutic and/or adverse effects of the concomitant drug may be observed).

No products indexed under this heading.

Nicotine Salicylate (Elevated levels of drugs metabolized by the CYP450 system may be observed when co-administered with telithromycin; therefore, increases or prolongation of the therapeutic and/or adverse effects of the concomitant drug may be observed).

No products indexed under this heading.

Nicotine Sulfate (Elevated levels of drugs metabolized by the CYP450 system may be observed when co-administered with telithromycin; therefore, increases or prolongation of the therapeutic and/or adverse effects of the concomitant drug may be observed).

No products indexed under this heading.

Nifedipine (Co-administration of telithromycin with a drug primarily metabolized by the CYP 3A4 enzyme system may result in increased plasma concentrations of the drug co-administered with telithromycin that could increase or prolong both the therapeutic and adverse effects). Products include:

Nilutamide (Elevated levels of drugs metabolized by the CYP450 system may be observed when co-administered with telithromycin; therefore, increases or prolongation of the therapeutic and/or adverse effects of the concomitant drug may be observed).

No products indexed under this heading.

Nimodipine (Co-administration of telithromycin with a drug primarily metabolized by the CYP 3A4 enzyme system may result in increased plasma concentrations of the drug co-administered with telithromycin that could increase or prolong both the therapeutic and adverse effects). Products include:

Nisoldipine (Co-administration of telithromycin with a drug primarily metabolized by the CYP 3A4 enzyme system may result in increased plasma concentrations of the drug co-administered with telithromycin that

could increase or prolong both the therapeutic and adverse effects). Products include:

Nitrendipine (Co-administration of telithromycin with a drug primarily metabolized by the CYP 3A4 enzyme system may result in increased plasma concentrations of the drug co-administered with telithromycin that could increase and prolong both the therapeutic and adverse effects).

No products indexed under this heading.

Norethindrone (Co-administration of telithromycin with a drug primarily metabolized by the CYP 3A4 enzyme system may result in increased plasma concentrations of the drug co-administered with telithromycin that could increase or prolong both the therapeutic and adverse effects). Products include:

Norethindrone Acetate (Co-administration of telithromycin with a drug primarily metabolized by the CYP 3A4 enzyme system may result in increased plasma concentrations of the drug co-administered with telithromycin that could increase or prolong both the therapeutic and adverse effects).

No products indexed under this heading.

Norfloxacin (Elevated levels of drugs metabolized by the CYP450 system may be observed when co-administered with telithromycin; therefore, increases or prolongation of the therapeutic and/or adverse effects of the concomitant drug may be observed). Products include:

Norgestrel (Co-administration of telithromycin with a drug primarily metabolized by the CYP 3A4 enzyme system may result in increased plasma concentrations of the drug co-administered with telithromycin that could increase or prolong both the therapeutic and adverse effects).

No products indexed under this heading.

Nortriptyline Hydrochloride (Elevated levels of drugs metabolized by the CYP450 system may be observed when co-administered with telithromycin; therefore, increases or prolongation of the therapeutic and/or adverse effects of the concomitant drug may be observed).

No products indexed under this heading.

Ofloxacin (Elevated levels of drugs metabolized by the CYP450 system may be observed when co-administered with telithromycin; therefore, increases or prolongation of the therapeutic and/or adverse effects of the concomitant drug may be observed). Products include:

Olanzapine (Elevated levels of drugs metabolized by the CYP450 system may be observed when co-administered with telithromycin; therefore, increases or prolongation of the therapeutic and/or adverse effects of the concomitant drug may be observed). Products include:

Omeprazole (Elevated levels of drugs metabolized by the CYP450 system may be observed when co-administered with telithromycin; therefore, increases or prolongation of the therapeutic and/or adverse effects of the concomitant drug may be observed). Products include:

Ondansetron (Co-administration of telithromycin with a drug primarily metabolized by the CYP 3A4 enzyme system may result in increased plasma concentrations of the drug co-administered with telithromycin that could increase or prolong both the therapeutic and adverse effects). Products include:

Ondansetron Hydrochloride (Co-administration of telithromycin with a drug primarily metabolized by the CYP 3A4 enzyme system may result in increased plasma concentrations of the drug co-administered with telithromycin that could increase or prolong both the therapeutic and adverse effects). Products include:

Oxaprozin (Elevated levels of drugs metabolized by the CYP450 system may be observed when co-administered with telithromycin; therefore, increases or prolongation of the therapeutic and/or adverse effects of the concomitant drug may be observed).

No products indexed under this heading.

Oxcarbazepine (Concomitant administration of CYP 3A4 inducers is likely to result in subtherapeutic levels of telithromycin and loss of effect). Products include:

Oxycodone Hydrochloride (Elevated levels of drugs metabolized by the CYP450 system may be observed when co-administered with telithromycin; therefore, increases or prolongation of the therapeutic and/or adverse effects of the concomitant drug may be observed). Products include:

Paclitaxel (Co-administration of telithromycin with a drug primarily metabolized by the CYP 3A4 enzyme system may result in increased plasma concentrations of the drug co-administered with telithromycin that could increase or prolong both the therapeutic and adverse effects).

No products indexed under this heading.

Pantoprazole Sodium (Elevated levels of drugs metabolized by the CYP450 system may be observed when co-administered with telithromycin; therefore, increases or prolongation of the therapeutic and/or adverse effects of the concomitant drug may be observed). Products include:

Paramethadione (Elevated levels of drugs metabolized by the CYP450 system may be observed when co-administered with telithromycin; therefore, increases or prolongation of the therapeutic and/or adverse effects of the concomitant drug may be observed).

No products indexed under this heading.

Paroxetine Hydrochloride (Elevated levels of drugs metabolized by the CYP450 system may be observed when co-administered with telithromycin; therefore, increases or prolongation of the therapeutic and/or adverse effects of the concomitant drug may be observed). Products include:

Pentamidine Isethionate (Elevated levels of drugs metabolized by the CYP450 system may be observed when co-administered with telithromycin; therefore, increases or prolongation of the therapeutic and/or adverse effects of the concomitant drug may be observed).

No products indexed under this heading.

Phenacemide (Elevated levels of drugs metabolized by the CYP450 system may be observed when co-administered with telithromycin; therefore, increases or prolongation of the therapeutic and/or adverse effects of the concomitant drug may be observed).

No products indexed under this heading.

Phenobarbital (Concomitant administration of CYP 3A4 inducers is likely to result in subtherapeutic levels of telithromycin and loss of effect). Products include:

Phenobarbital Sodium (Concomitant administration of CYP 3A4 inducers is likely to result in sub-therapeutic levels of telithromycin and loss of effect).

No products indexed under this heading.

Phensuximide (Elevated levels of drugs metabolized by the CYP450 system may be observed when co-administered with telithromycin; therefore, increases or prolongation of the therapeutic and/or adverse effects of the concomitant drug may be observed).

No products indexed under this heading.

Phenylbutazone (Elevated levels of drugs metabolized by the CYP450 system may be observed when co-administered with telithromycin; therefore, increases or prolongation of the therapeutic and/or adverse effects of the concomitant drug may be observed).

No products indexed under this heading.

Phenytoin (Concomitant administration of CYP 3A4 inducers is likely to result in subtherapeutic levels of telithromycin and loss of effect).

No products indexed under this heading.

Phenytoin Sodium (Concomitant administration of CYP 3A4 inducers is likely to result in subtherapeutic levels of telithromycin and loss of effect). Products include:

IMPORTANT NOTE: Always consult each drug listing in the patient's regimen for possible interactions.

Pimozide (There is a potential risk of increased pimozide plasma levels by inhibition of CYP 3A4 pathways by telithromycin. Coadministration is contraindicated).
No products indexed under this heading.

Pindolol (Elevated levels of drugs metabolized by the CYP450 system may be observed when co-administered with telithromycin; therefore, increases or prolongation of the therapeutic and/or adverse effects of the concomitant drug may be observed).
No products indexed under this heading.

Pioglitazone Hydrochloride (Elevated levels of drugs metabolized by the CYP450 system may be observed when co-administered with telithromycin; therefore, increases or prolongation of the therapeutic and/or adverse effects of the concomitant drug may be observed).
Products include:
ActoPlus Met Tablets 3214
Actos Tablets 3219
Duetact Tablets 3226

Piroxicam (Elevated levels of drugs metabolized by the CYP450 system may be observed when co-administered with telithromycin; therefore, increases or prolongation of the therapeutic and/or adverse effects of the concomitant drug may be observed).
No products indexed under this heading.

Polyestradiol Phosphate (Co-administration of telithromycin with a drug primarily metabolized by the CYP 3A4 enzyme system may result in increased plasma concentrations of the drug co-administered with telithromycin that could increase or prolong both the therapeutic and adverse effects).
No products indexed under this heading.

Prednisolone Acetate (Concomitant administration of CYP 3A4 inducers is likely to result in subtherapeutic levels of telithromycin and loss of effect). Products include:
Blephamide Ophthalmic Ointment 568
Blephamide Ophthalmic Suspension 569
Poly-Pred Ophthalmic Suspension .... ⊙233
Pred Forte Ophthalmic Suspension .... ⊙235
Pred Mild Ophthalmic Suspension .... ⊙238
Pred-G Ophthalmic Ointment .... ⊙237
Pred-G Ophthalmic Suspension ...... ⊙236

Prednisolone Sodium Phosphate (Concomitant administration of CYP 3A4 inducers is likely to result in subtherapeutic levels of telithromycin and loss of effect).
No products indexed under this heading.

Prednisolone Tebutate (Concomitant administration of CYP 3A4 inducers is likely to result in subtherapeutic levels of telithromycin and loss of effect).
No products indexed under this heading.

Prednisone (Concomitant administration of CYP 3A4 inducers is likely to result in subtherapeutic levels of telithromycin and loss of effect).
No products indexed under this heading.

Primidone (Concomitant administration of CYP 3A4 inducers is likely to result in subtherapeutic levels of telithromycin and loss of effect).
No products indexed under this heading.

Progesterone (Elevated levels of drugs metabolized by the CYP450 system may be observed when co-administered with telithromycin; therefore, increases or prolongation of the therapeutic and/or adverse effects of the concomitant drug may be observed). Products include:
Prochieve 4% Gel 1003
Prochieve 8% Gel 1003
Prometrium Capsules (100 mg, 200 mg) 3203

Proguanil Hydrochloride (Elevated levels of drugs metabolized by the CYP450 system may be observed when co-administered with telithromycin; therefore, increases or prolongation of the therapeutic and/or adverse effects of the concomitant drug may be observed).
Products include:
Malarone Pediatric Tablets 1517
Malarone Tablets 1517

Propafenone Hydrochloride (Elevated levels of drugs metabolized by the CYP450 system may be observed when co-administered with telithromycin; therefore, increases or prolongation of the therapeutic and/or adverse effects of the concomitant drug may be observed).
Products include:
Rythmol SR Capsules 2727

Propoxyphene Hydrochloride (Elevated levels of drugs metabolized by the CYP450 system may be observed when co-administered with telithromycin; therefore, increases or prolongation of the therapeutic and/or adverse effects of the concomitant drug may be observed).
No products indexed under this heading.

Propoxyphene Napsylate (Elevated levels of drugs metabolized by the CYP450 system may be observed when co-administered with telithromycin; therefore, increases or prolongation of the therapeutic and/or adverse effects of the concomitant drug may be observed).
No products indexed under this heading.

Propranolol Hydrochloride (Elevated levels of drugs metabolized by the CYP450 system may be observed when co-administered with telithromycin; therefore, increases or prolongation of the therapeutic and/or adverse effects of the concomitant drug may be observed).
Products include:
Inderal LA Long-Acting Capsules 3429
InnoPran XL Capsules 2723

Protriptyline Hydrochloride (Elevated levels of drugs metabolized by the CYP450 system may be observed when co-administered with telithromycin; therefore, increases or prolongation of the therapeutic and/or adverse effects of the concomitant drug may be observed).
No products indexed under this heading.

Quetiapine Fumarate (Elevated levels of drugs metabolized by the CYP450 system may be observed when co-administered with telithromycin; therefore, increases or prolongation of the therapeutic and/or adverse effects of the concomitant drug may be observed). Products include:
Seroquel Tablets 690

Quinidine Gluconate (Co-administration of telithromycin with a drug primarily metabolized by the CYP 3A4 enzyme system may result in increased plasma concentrations of the drug co-administered with telithromycin that could increase or prolong both the therapeutic and adverse effects).
No products indexed under this heading.

Quinidine Hydrochloride (Elevated levels of drugs metabolized by the CYP450 system may be observed when co-administered with telithromycin; therefore, increases or prolongation of the therapeutic and/or adverse effects of the concomitant drug may be observed).
No products indexed under this heading.

Quinidine Polygalacturonate (Co-administration of telithromycin with a drug primarily metabolized by the CYP 3A4 enzyme system may result in increased plasma concentrations of the drug co-administered with telithromycin that could increase or prolong both the therapeutic and adverse effects).
No products indexed under this heading.

Quinidine Sulfate (Co-administration of telithromycin with a drug primarily metabolized by the CYP 3A4 enzyme system may result in increased plasma concentrations of the drug co-administered with telithromycin that could increase or prolong both the therapeutic and adverse effects).
No products indexed under this heading.

Quinine (Elevated levels of drugs metabolized by the CYP450 system may be observed when co-administered with telithromycin; therefore, increases or prolongation of the therapeutic and/or adverse effects of the concomitant drug may be observed).
No products indexed under this heading.

Quinine Sulfate (Elevated levels of drugs metabolized by the CYP450 system may be observed when co-administered with telithromycin; therefore, increases or prolongation of the therapeutic and/or adverse effects of the concomitant drug may be observed).
No products indexed under this heading.

Rabeprazole Sodium (Elevated levels of drugs metabolized by the CYP450 system may be observed when co-administered with telithromycin; therefore, increases or prolongation of the therapeutic and/or adverse effects of the concomitant drug may be observed). Products include:
Aciphex Tablets 1090

Repaglinide (Elevated levels of drugs metabolized by the CYP450 system may be observed when co-administered with telithromycin; therefore, increases or prolongation of the therapeutic and/or adverse effects of the concomitant drug may be observed).
No products indexed under this heading.

Rifabutin (Co-administration of telithromycin with a drug primarily metabolized by the CYP 3A4 enzyme system may result in increased plasma concentrations of the drug co-administered with telithromycin that could increase or prolong both the therapeutic and adverse effects).
No products indexed under this heading.

Rifampicin (Concomitant administration of CYP 3A4 inducers is likely to result in subtherapeutic levels of telithromycin and loss of effect).
No products indexed under this heading.

Rifampin (Co-administration of rifampin, a CYP 3A4 inducer, with telithromycin in repeated doses decreased the Cmax and AUC of telithromycin. Avoid concomitant treatment).
No products indexed under this heading.

Rifapentine (Concomitant administration of CYP 3A4 inducers is likely to result in subtherapeutic levels of telithromycin and loss of effect).
No products indexed under this heading.

Riluzole (Elevated levels of drugs metabolized by the CYP450 system may be observed when co-administered with telithromycin; therefore, increases or prolongation of the therapeutic and/or adverse effects of the concomitant drug may be observed). Products include:
Rilutek Tablets 2930

Risperidone (Elevated levels of drugs metabolized by the CYP450 system may be observed when co-administered with telithromycin; therefore, increases or prolongation of the therapeutic and/or adverse effects of the concomitant drug may be observed). Products include:
Risperdal 1676
Risperdal Consta Long-Acting Injection 1682
Risperdal M-Tab Orally Disintegrating Tablets 1676

Ritonavir (Co-administration of telithromycin with a drug primarily metabolized by the CYP 3A4 enzyme system may result in increased plasma concentrations of the drug co-administered with telithromycin that could increase or prolong both the therapeutic and adverse effects).
Products include:
Kaletra 476
Norvir 503

Rofecoxib (Elevated levels of drugs metabolized by the CYP450 system may be observed when co-administered with telithromycin; therefore, increases or prolongation of the therapeutic and/or adverse effects of the concomitant drug may be observed).
No products indexed under this heading.

Ropinirole Hydrochloride (Elevated levels of drugs metabolized by the CYP450 system may be observed when co-administered with telithromycin; therefore, increases or prolongation of the therapeutic and/or adverse effects of the concomitant drug may be observed).
Products include:
Requip Tablets 1555

Ropivacaine Hydrochloride (Elevated levels of drugs metabolized by the CYP450 system may be observed when co-administered with telithromycin; therefore, increases or prolongation of the therapeutic and/or adverse effects of the concomitant drug may be observed).

No products indexed under this heading.

Rosiglitazone Maleate (Elevated levels of drugs metabolized by the CYP450 system may be observed when co-administered with telithromycin; therefore, increases or prolongation of the therapeutic and/or adverse effects of the concomitant drug may be observed). Products include:

Saquinavir (Co-administration of telithromycin with a drug primarily metabolized by the CYP 3A4 enzyme system may result in increased plasma concentrations of the drug co-administered with telithromycin that could increase or prolong both the therapeutic and adverse effects).

No products indexed under this heading.

Saquinavir Mesylate (Co-administration of telithromycin with a drug primarily metabolized by the CYP 3A4 enzyme system may result in increased plasma concentrations of the drug co-administered with telithromycin that could increase or prolong both the therapeutic and adverse effects). Products include:

Sertraline Hydrochloride (Co-administration of telithromycin with a drug primarily metabolized by the CYP 3A4 enzyme system may result in increased plasma concentrations of the drug co-administered with telithromycin that could increase or prolong both the therapeutic and adverse effects). Products include:

Sildenafil Citrate (Co-administration of telithromycin with a drug primarily metabolized by the CYP 3A4 enzyme system may result in increased plasma concentrations of the drug co-administered with telithromycin that could increase or prolong both the therapeutic and adverse effects). Products include:

Simvastatin (Simvastatin levels were increased due to CYP 3A4 inhibition by telithromycin, thereby increasing the risk of myopathy. Co-administration should be avoided). Products include:

Sirolimus (Co-administration of telithromycin with a drug primarily metabolized by the CYP 3A4 enzyme system may result in increased plasma concentrations of the drug co-administered with telithromycin that could increase or prolong both the therapeutic and adverse effects). Products include:

Rapamune Oral Solution and

Sotalol Hydrochloride (Telithromycin has been shown to decrease the Cmax and AUC of sotalol due to decreased absorption).

No products indexed under this heading.

Sulfamethoxazole (Elevated levels of drugs metabolized by the CYP450 system may be observed when co-administered with telithromycin; therefore, increases or prolongation of the therapeutic and/or adverse effects of the concomitant drug may be observed).

No products indexed under this heading.

Sulfinpyrazone (Concomitant administration of CYP 3A4 inducers is likely to result in subtherapeutic levels of telithromycin and loss of effect).

No products indexed under this heading.

Sulindac (Elevated levels of drugs metabolized by the CYP450 system may be observed when co-administered with telithromycin; therefore, increases or prolongation of the therapeutic and/or adverse effects of the concomitant drug may be observed). Products include:

Suprofen (Elevated levels of drugs metabolized by the CYP450 system may be observed when co-administered with telithromycin; therefore, increases or prolongation of the therapeutic and/or adverse effects of the concomitant drug may be observed).

No products indexed under this heading.

Tacrine Hydrochloride (Elevated levels of drugs metabolized by the CYP450 system may be observed when co-administered with telithromycin; therefore, increases or prolongation of the therapeutic and/or adverse effects of the concomitant drug may be observed).

No products indexed under this heading.

Tacrolimus (Co-administration of telithromycin with a drug primarily metabolized by the CYP 3A4 enzyme system may result in increased plasma concentrations of the drug co-administered with telithromycin that could increase or prolong both the therapeutic and adverse effects). Products include:

Tamoxifen Citrate (Co-administration of telithromycin with a drug primarily metabolized by the CYP 3A4 enzyme system may result in increased plasma concentrations of the drug co-administered with telithromycin that could increase or prolong both the therapeutic and adverse effects). Products include:

Telmisartan (Elevated levels of drugs metabolized by the CYP450 system may be observed when co-administered with telithromycin; therefore, increases or prolongation of the therapeutic and/or adverse effects of the concomitant drug may be observed). Products include:

Teniposide (Elevated levels of drugs metabolized by the CYP450 system may be observed when co-administered with telithromycin; therefore, increases or prolongation of the therapeutic and/or adverse effects of the concomitant drug may be observed).

No products indexed under this heading.

Terfenadine (Elevated levels of drugs metabolized by the CYP450 system may be observed when co-administered with telithromycin; therefore, increases or prolongation of the therapeutic and/or adverse effects of the concomitant drug may be observed).

No products indexed under this heading.

Testosterone (Elevated levels of drugs metabolized by the CYP450 system may be observed when co-administered with telithromycin; therefore, increases or prolongation of the therapeutic and/or adverse effects of the concomitant drug may be observed). Products include:

Testosterone Cypionate (Elevated levels of drugs metabolized by the CYP450 system may be observed when co-administered with telithromycin; therefore, increases or prolongation of the therapeutic and/or adverse effects of the concomitant drug may be observed).

No products indexed under this heading.

Testosterone Enanthate (Elevated levels of drugs metabolized by the CYP450 system may be observed when co-administered with telithromycin; therefore, increases or prolongation of the therapeutic and/or adverse effects of the concomitant drug may be observed).

No products indexed under this heading.

Testosterone Propionate (Elevated levels of drugs metabolized by the CYP450 system may be observed when co-administered with telithromycin; therefore, increases or prolongation of the therapeutic and/or adverse effects of the concomitant drug may be observed).

No products indexed under this heading.

Theophylline (Co-administration increased steady state Cmax and AUC of theophylline and may worsen GI side effects, especially in female patients. Theophylline and telithromycin should be taken 1 hour apart).

No products indexed under this heading.

Theophylline Anhydrous (Co-administration increased steady state Cmax and AUC of theophylline and may worsen GI side effects, especially in female patients. Theophylline and telithromycin should be taken 1 hour apart). Products include:

Theophylline Calcium Salicylate (Co-administration increased steady state Cmax and AUC of theophylline and may worsen GI side effects, especially in female patients. Theophylline and telithromycin should be taken 1 hour apart).

No products indexed under this heading.

Theophylline Dihydroxypropyl (Glyceryl) (Co-administration increased steady state Cmax and AUC of theophylline and may worsen GI side effects, especially in female patients. Theophylline and telithromycin should be taken 1 hour apart).

No products indexed under this heading.

Theophylline Ethylenediamine (Co-administration increased steady state Cmax and AUC of theophylline and may worsen GI side effects, especially in female patients. Theophylline and telithromycin should be taken 1 hour apart).

No products indexed under this heading.

Theophylline Sodium Glycinate (Co-administration increased steady state Cmax and AUC of theophylline and may worsen GI side effects, especially in female patients. Theophylline and telithromycin should be taken 1 hour apart).

No products indexed under this heading.

Thioridazine (Elevated levels of drugs metabolized by the CYP450 system may be observed when co-administered with telithromycin; therefore, increases or prolongation of the therapeutic and/or adverse effects of the concomitant drug may be observed).

No products indexed under this heading.

Thioridazine Hydrochloride (Elevated levels of drugs metabolized by the CYP450 system may be observed when co-administered with telithromycin; therefore, increases or prolongation of the therapeutic and/or adverse effects of the concomitant drug may be observed). Products include:

Tiagabine Hydrochloride (Co-administration of telithromycin with a drug primarily metabolized by the CYP 3A4 enzyme system may result in increased plasma concentrations of the drug co-administered with telithromycin that could increase or prolong both the therapeutic and adverse effects). Products include:

Timolol Maleate (Elevated levels of drugs metabolized by the CYP450 system may be observed when co-administered with telithromycin; therefore, increases or prolongation of the therapeutic and/or adverse effects of the concomitant drug may be observed). Products include:

Tolazamide (Elevated levels of drugs metabolized by the CYP450 system may be observed when co-administered with telithromycin; therefore, increases or prolongation of the therapeutic and/or adverse effects of the concomitant drug may be observed).

No products indexed under this heading.

IMPORTANT NOTE: Always consult each drug listing in the patient's regimen for possible interactions.

Tolbutamide (Elevated levels of drugs metabolized by the CYP450 system may be observed when co-administered with telithromycin; therefore, increases or prolongation of the therapeutic and/or adverse effects of the concomitant drug may be observed).
 No products indexed under this heading.

Tolbutamide Sodium (Elevated levels of drugs metabolized by the CYP450 system may be observed when co-administered with telithromycin; therefore, increases or prolongation of the therapeutic and/or adverse effects of the concomitant drug may be observed).
 No products indexed under this heading.

Tolmetin Sodium (Elevated levels of drugs metabolized by the CYP450 system may be observed when co-administered with telithromycin; therefore, increases or prolongation of the therapeutic and/or adverse effects of the concomitant drug may be observed).
 No products indexed under this heading.

Tolterodine Tartrate (Co-administration of telithromycin with a drug primarily metabolized by the CYP 3A4 enzyme system may result in increased plasma concentrations of the drug co-administered with telithromycin that could increase or prolong both the therapeutic and adverse effects). Products include:
Detrol Tablets 2628
Detrol LA Capsules 2631

Topiramate (Elevated levels of drugs metabolized by the CYP450 system may be observed when co-administered with telithromycin; therefore, increases or prolongation of the therapeutic and/or adverse effects of the concomitant drug may be observed). Products include:
Topamax Sprinkle Capsules 2404
Topamax Tablets 2404

Torsemide (Elevated levels of drugs metabolized by the CYP450 system may be observed when co-administered with telithromycin; therefore, increases or prolongation of the therapeutic and/or adverse effects of the concomitant drug may be observed). Products include:
Demadex Injection 2759
Demadex Tablets 2759

Tramadol Hydrochloride (Elevated levels of drugs metabolized by the CYP450 system may be observed when co-administered with telithromycin; therefore, increases or prolongation of the therapeutic and/or adverse effects of the concomitant drug may be observed). Products include:
Ultram ER Tablets 2392

Trazodone Hydrochloride (Co-administration of telithromycin with a drug primarily metabolized by the CYP 3A4 enzyme system may result in increased plasma concentrations of the drug co-administered with telithromycin that could increase or prolong both the therapeutic and adverse effects).
 No products indexed under this heading.

Tretinoin (Elevated levels of drugs metabolized by the CYP450 system may be observed when co-administered with telithromycin; therefore, increases or prolongation

of the therapeutic and/or adverse effects of the concomitant drug may be observed). Products include:
Tri-Luma Cream 1213
Vesanoid Capsules 2820

Triamcinolone (Concomitant administration of CYP 3A4 inducers is likely to result in subtherapeutic levels of telithromycin and loss of effect).
 No products indexed under this heading.

Triamcinolone Acetonide (Concomitant administration of CYP 3A4 inducers is likely to result in subtherapeutic levels of telithromycin and loss of effect). Products include:
Azmacort Inhalation Aerosol 1726
Nasacort AQ Nasal Spray 2922

Triamcinolone Diacetate (Concomitant administration of CYP 3A4 inducers is likely to result in subtherapeutic levels of telithromycin and loss of effect).
 No products indexed under this heading.

Triamcinolone Hexacetonide (Concomitant administration of CYP 3A4 inducers is likely to result in subtherapeutic levels of telithromycin and loss of effect).
 No products indexed under this heading.

Triazolam (Co-administration of telithromycin with a drug primarily metabolized by the CYP 3A4 enzyme system may result in increased plasma concentrations of the drug co-administered with telithromycin that could increase or prolong both the therapeutic and adverse effects).
 No products indexed under this heading.

Trimethadione (Elevated levels of drugs metabolized by the CYP450 system may be observed when co-administered with telithromycin; therefore, increases or prolongation of the therapeutic and/or adverse effects of the concomitant drug may be observed).
 No products indexed under this heading.

Trimethaphan Camsylate (Elevated levels of drugs metabolized by the CYP450 system may be observed when co-administered with telithromycin; therefore, increases or prolongation of the therapeutic and/or adverse effects of the concomitant drug may be observed).
 No products indexed under this heading.

Trimipramine Maleate (Elevated levels of drugs metabolized by the CYP450 system may be observed when co-administered with telithromycin; therefore, increases or prolongation of the therapeutic and/or adverse effects of the concomitant drug may be observed).
 No products indexed under this heading.

Troglitazone (Concomitant administration of CYP 3A4 inducers is likely to result in subtherapeutic levels of telithromycin and loss of effect).
 No products indexed under this heading.

Trovafloxacin Mesylate (Elevated levels of drugs metabolized by the CYP450 system may be observed when co-administered with telithromycin; therefore, increases or prolongation of the therapeutic and/or adverse effects of the concomitant drug may be observed).
 No products indexed under this heading.

Valdecoxib (Elevated levels of drugs metabolized by the CYP450 system may be observed when co-administered with telithromycin; therefore, increases or prolongation of the therapeutic and/or adverse effects of the concomitant drug may be observed).
 No products indexed under this heading.

Valproate Sodium (Elevated levels of drugs metabolized by the CYP450 system may be observed when co-administered with telithromycin; therefore, increases or prolongation of the therapeutic and/or adverse effects of the concomitant drug may be observed). Products include:
Depacon Injection 412

Valproic Acid (Elevated levels of drugs metabolized by the CYP450 system may be observed when co-administered with telithromycin; therefore, increases or prolongation of the therapeutic and/or adverse effects of the concomitant drug may be observed). Products include:
Depakene 417

Valsartan (Elevated levels of drugs metabolized by the CYP450 system may be observed when co-administered with telithromycin; therefore, increases or prolongation of the therapeutic and/or adverse effects of the concomitant drug may be observed). Products include:
Diovan Tablets 2193
Diovan HCT Tablets 2196

Venlafaxine Hydrochloride (Elevated levels of drugs metabolized by the CYP450 system may be observed when co-administered with telithromycin; therefore, increases or prolongation of the therapeutic and/or adverse effects of the concomitant drug may be observed). Products include:
Effexor Tablets 3411
Effexor XR Capsules 3417

Verapamil Hydrochloride (Co-administration of telithromycin with a drug primarily metabolized by the CYP 3A4 enzyme system may result in increased plasma concentrations of the drug co-administered with telithromycin that could increase or prolong both the therapeutic and adverse effects). Products include:
Covera-HS Tablets 3139
Tarka Tablets 524
Verelan PM Extended-Release Capsules, Controlled-Onset.......... 3106

Vinblastine Sulfate (Co-administration of telithromycin with a drug primarily metabolized by the CYP 3A4 enzyme system may result in increased plasma concentrations of the drug co-administered with telithromycin that could increase or prolong both the therapeutic and adverse effects).
 No products indexed under this heading.

Vincristine Sulfate (Co-administration of telithromycin with a drug primarily metabolized by the CYP 3A4 enzyme system may result in increased plasma concentrations of the drug co-administered with telithromycin that could increase or prolong both the therapeutic and adverse effects).
 No products indexed under this heading.

Vitamin A (Elevated levels of drugs metabolized by the CYP450 system may be observed when co-administered with telithromycin; therefore, increases or prolongation of the therapeutic and/or adverse effects of the concomitant drug may be observed). Products include:
Visutein Capsules 3329

Vitamin A Acetate (Elevated levels of drugs metabolized by the CYP450 system may be observed when co-administered with telithromycin; therefore, increases or prolongation of the therapeutic and/or adverse effects of the concomitant drug may be observed).
 No products indexed under this heading.

Voriconazole (Elevated levels of drugs metabolized by the CYP450 system may be observed when co-administered with telithromycin; therefore, increases or prolongation of the therapeutic and/or adverse effects of the concomitant drug may be observed). Products include:
VFEND I.V. 2564
VFEND Oral Suspension 2564
VFEND Tablets 2564

Warfarin Sodium (Co-administration of telithromycin with a drug primarily metabolized by the CYP 3A4 enzyme system may result in increased plasma concentrations of the drug co-administered with telithromycin that could increase or prolong both the therapeutic and adverse effects). Products include:
Coumadin for Injection 898
Coumadin Tablets 898

Zafirlukast (Elevated levels of drugs metabolized by the CYP450 system may be observed when co-administered with telithromycin; therefore, increases or prolongation of the therapeutic and/or adverse effects of the concomitant drug may be observed). Products include:
Accolate Tablets 671

Zileuton (Elevated levels of drugs metabolized by the CYP450 system may be observed when co-administered with telithromycin; therefore, increases or prolongation of the therapeutic and/or adverse effects of the concomitant drug may be observed). Products include:
Zyflo Tablets 1023

Zolmitriptan (Elevated levels of drugs metabolized by the CYP450 system may be observed when co-administered with telithromycin; therefore, increases or prolongation of the therapeutic and/or adverse effects of the concomitant drug may be observed). Products include:
Zomig Tablets 3519
Zomig Nasal Spray 3523
Zomig-ZMT Tablets 3519

Zonisamide (Elevated levels of drugs metabolized by the CYP450 system may be observed when co-administered with telithromycin; therefore, increases or prolongation of the therapeutic and/or adverse effects of the concomitant drug may be observed). Products include:

Zonegran Capsules 1101

Zopiclone (Elevated levels of drugs metabolized by the CYP450 system may be observed when co-administered with telithromycin; therefore, increases or prolongation of the therapeutic and/or adverse effects of the concomitant drug may be observed).

No products indexed under this heading.

KINERET INJECTION

(Anakinra) 599

May interact with killed/inactivated vaccines and certain other agents. Compounds in these categories include:

Adalimumab (Use of anakinra in combination with TNF-blocking agents is not recommended). Products include:

Humira Injection 466

Diphtheria & Tetanus Toxoids and Acellular Pertussis Vaccine Adsorbed, Hepatitis B (recombinant) and Inactivated Poliovirus Vaccine Combined (Vaccination may not be effective in patients receiving anakinra).

No products indexed under this heading.

Etanercept (In a study in which patients with active RA were treated for up to 24 weeks with concurrent anakinra and etanercept therapy, a 7% rate of serious infections was observed, which was higher than that observed with etanercept alone (0%). Two percent of patients treated concurrently with anakinra and etanercept developed neutropenia. Use of anakinra in combination with TNF-blocking agents is not recommended). Products include:

Enbrel for Injection 584

Hepatitis A Vaccine, Inactivated (Vaccination may not be effective in patients receiving anakinra). Products include:

Havrix Vaccine 1456
Twinrix Vaccine 1595
Vaqta 2097

Infliximab (Use of anakinra in combination with TNF-blocking agents is not recommended). Products include:

Remicade for IV Injection 971

Influenza Virus Vaccine (Vaccination may not be effective in patients receiving anakinra). Products include:

Fluarix 1451
Flumist Vaccine 1901

Japanese Encephalitis Vaccine Inactivated (Vaccination may not be effective in patients receiving anakinra).

No products indexed under this heading.

Poliovirus Vaccine Inactivated, Trivalent Types 1,2,3 (Vaccination may not be effective in patients receiving anakinra). Products include:

Pediarix Vaccine 1548

Vaccines (Live) (Vaccination may not be effective in patients receiving anakinra. Live vaccines should not be given concurrently with anakinra).

No products indexed under this heading.

KIONEX POWDER

(Sodium Polystyrene Sulfonate) 2477

May interact with antacids containing aluminum, calcium and magnesium, cardiac glycosides, and certain other agents. Compounds in these categories include:

Aluminum Carbonate (Simultaneous oral administration of Kionex with nonabsorbable cation-donating antacids may reduce the resin's potassium exchange capability; systemic alkalosis has been reported with concurrent use).

No products indexed under this heading.

Aluminum Hydroxide (Simultaneous oral administration of Kionex with nonabsorbable cation-donating antacids may reduce the resin's potassium exchange capability; systemic alkalosis has been reported with concurrent use; intestinal impaction due to concretions of aluminum hydroxide has been reported with concurrent use). Products include:

Gaviscon Regular Strength Liquid .. 658
Gaviscon Regular Strength Tablets 658
Gaviscon Extra Strength Liquid 658
Gaviscon Extra Strength Tablets 658
Maalox Regular Strength Antacid/Antigas Liquid 2176
Maalox Max Maximum Strength Antacid/Anti-Gas Liquid 2176

Deslanoside (The toxic effects of digitalis on the heart, especially various ventricular arrhythmias and A-V nodal dissociation, are likely to be exaggerated by hypokalemia).

No products indexed under this heading.

Digitoxin (The toxic effects of digitalis on the heart, especially various ventricular arrhythmias and A-V nodal dissociation, are likely to be exaggerated by hypokalemia).

No products indexed under this heading.

Digoxin (The toxic effects of digitalis on the heart, especially various ventricular arrhythmias and A-V nodal dissociation, are likely to be exaggerated by hypokalemia). Products include:

Lanoxicaps Capsules 1490
Lanoxin Injection 1494
Lanoxin Injection Pediatric 1497
Lanoxin Tablets 1500

Lithium (Kionex may decrease the absorption of lithium).

No products indexed under this heading.

Magnesium Hydroxide (Systemic alkalosis has been reported with concurrent use; one case of grand mal seizure has been reported in a patient with chronic hypocalcemia of renal failure with concurrent use; magnesium hydroxide should not be administered with Kionex). Products include:

Maalox Regular Strength Antacid/Antigas Liquid 2175
Maalox Max Maximum Strength Antacid/Anti-Gas Liquid 2176
Pepcid Complete Chewable Tablets 1701

Sorbitol (Concomitant use of sorbitol with Kionex has been implicated in cases of chronic necrosis).

No products indexed under this heading.

Thyroxine (Kionex may decrease the absorption of thyroxine).

No products indexed under this heading.

KLARON LOTION 10%

(Sulfacetamide Sodium) 2909

None cited in PDR database.

KLONOPIN TABLETS

(Clonazepam) 2778

May interact with central nervous system depressants, anticonvulsants, monoamine oxidase inhibitors, phenytoin, tricyclic antidepressants, and certain other agents. Compounds in these categories include:

Alfentanil Hydrochloride (Potentiates CNS-depressant action).

No products indexed under this heading.

Alprazolam (Potentiates CNS-depressant action). Products include:

Niravam Orally Disintegrating Tablets 3092

Amitriptyline Hydrochloride (Potentiates CNS-depressant action).

No products indexed under this heading.

Amoxapine (Potentiates CNS-depressant action).

No products indexed under this heading.

Aprobarbital (Potentiates CNS-depressant action).

No products indexed under this heading.

Buprenorphine Hydrochloride (Potentiates CNS-depressant action). Products include:

Buprenex Injectable 2716
Suboxone Tablets 2717
Subutex Tablets 2717

Buspirone Hydrochloride (Potentiates CNS-depressant action).

No products indexed under this heading.

Butabarbital (Potentiates CNS-depressant action).

No products indexed under this heading.

Butalbital (Potentiates CNS-depressant action).

No products indexed under this heading.

Carbamazepine (Induces clonazepam metabolism causing an approximately 30% decrease in plasma clonazepam levels). Products include:

Carbatrol Capsules 3171
Equetro Extended-Release Capsules 3180
Tegretol/Tegretol-XR 2295

Chlordiazepoxide (Potentiates CNS-depressant action).

No products indexed under this heading.

Chlordiazepoxide Hydrochloride (Potentiates CNS-depressant action). Products include:

Librium Capsules 3347

Chlorpromazine (Potentiates CNS-depressant action).

No products indexed under this heading.

Chlorpromazine Hydrochloride (Potentiates CNS-depressant action).

No products indexed under this heading.

Chlorprothixene (Potentiates CNS-depressant action).

No products indexed under this heading.

Chlorprothixene Hydrochloride (Potentiates CNS-depressant action).

No products indexed under this heading.

Chlorprothixene Lactate (Potentiates CNS-depressant action).

No products indexed under this heading.

Clomipramine Hydrochloride (Potentiates CNS-depressant action).

No products indexed under this heading.

Clorazepate Dipotassium (Potentiates CNS-depressant action). Products include:

Tranxene 2474

Clozapine (Potentiates CNS-depressant action). Products include:

Clozaril Tablets 2184
FazaClo Orally Disintegrating Tablets 551

Codeine Phosphate (Potentiates CNS-depressant action). Products include:

Tylenol with Codeine Tablets 2391

Desflurane (Potentiates CNS-depressant action).

No products indexed under this heading.

Desipramine Hydrochloride (Potentiates CNS-depressant action).

No products indexed under this heading.

Dezocine (Potentiates CNS-depressant action).

No products indexed under this heading.

Diazepam (Potentiates CNS-depressant action). Products include:

Diastat Rectal Delivery System 3343
Valium Tablets 2819

Divalproex Sodium (Potentiates CNS-depressant action). Products include:

Depakote Sprinkle Capsules 422
Depakote Tablets 427
Depakote ER Tablets 434

Doxepin Hydrochloride (Potentiates CNS-depressant action).

No products indexed under this heading.

Droperidol (Potentiates CNS-depressant action).

No products indexed under this heading.

Enflurane (Potentiates CNS-depressant action).

No products indexed under this heading.

Estazolam (Potentiates CNS-depressant action). Products include:

ProSom Tablets 517

Ethanol (Potentiates CNS-depressant action).

No products indexed under this heading.

Ethchlorvynol (Potentiates CNS-depressant action).

No products indexed under this heading.

Ethinamate (Potentiates CNS-depressant action).

No products indexed under this heading.

Ethosuximide (Potentiates CNS-depressant action).

No products indexed under this heading.

Ethotoin (Potentiates CNS-depressant action).

No products indexed under this heading.

Ethyl Alcohol (Potentiates CNS-depressant action).

No products indexed under this heading.

Felbamate (Potentiates CNS-depressant action).

No products indexed under this heading.

Fentanyl (Potentiates CNS-depressant action). Products include:
Duragesic Transdermal System 2373
Ionsys Transdermal System 2379

Fentanyl Citrate (Potentiates CNS-depressant action). Products include:
Actiq 979

Fluphenazine Decanoate (Potentiates CNS-depressant action).
No products indexed under this heading.

Fluphenazine Enanthate (Potentiates CNS-depressant action).
No products indexed under this heading.

Fluphenazine Hydrochloride (Potentiates CNS-depressant action).
No products indexed under this heading.

Flurazepam Hydrochloride (Potentiates CNS-depressant action). Products include:
Dalmane Capsules 3342

Fosphenytoin (Potentiates CNS-depressant action).
No products indexed under this heading.

Fosphenytoin Sodium (Induces clonazepam metabolism causing an approximately 30% decrease in plasma clonazepam levels).
No products indexed under this heading.

Gabapentin (Potentiates CNS-depressant action). Products include:
Neurontin Capsules 2487
Neurontin Oral Solution 2487
Neurontin Tablets 2487

Glutethimide (Potentiates CNS-depressant action).
No products indexed under this heading.

Haloperidol (Potentiates CNS-depressant action).
No products indexed under this heading.

Haloperidol Decanoate (Potentiates CNS-depressant action).
No products indexed under this heading.

Hydrocodone Bitartrate (Potentiates CNS-depressant action). Products include:
Hycodan 1116
Hycotuss Expectorant Syrup 1117
Vicodin Tablets 535
Vicodin ES Tablets 536
Vicodin HP Tablets 538
Vicoprofen Tablets 539
Zydone Tablets 1139

Hydrocodone Polistirex (Potentiates CNS-depressant action). Products include:
Tussionex Pennkinetic Extended-Release Suspension 3327

Hydromorphone Hydrochloride (Potentiates CNS-depressant action). Products include:
Dilaudid 440
Dilaudid Non-Sterile Powder 440
Dilaudid Oral Liquid 445
Dilaudid Rectal Suppositories 440
Dilaudid Tablets 440
Dilaudid Tablets - 8 mg 445
Dilaudid-HP 442

Hydroxyzine Hydrochloride (Potentiates CNS-depressant action).
No products indexed under this heading.

Imipramine Hydrochloride (Potentiates CNS-depressant action).
No products indexed under this heading.

Imipramine Pamoate (Potentiates CNS-depressant action).
No products indexed under this heading.

Isocarboxazid (Potentiates CNS-depressant action).
No products indexed under this heading.

Isoflurane (Potentiates CNS depressant action).
No products indexed under this heading.

Itraconazole (Co-administration with CYP450 3A inhibitors should be undertaken with caution).
No products indexed under this heading.

Ketamine Hydrochloride (Potentiates CNS-depressant action).
No products indexed under this heading.

Ketoconazole (Co-administration with CYP450 3A inhibitors should be undertaken with caution). Products include:
Nizoral A-D Shampoo, 1% 1868

Lamotrigine (Potentiates CNS-depressant action). Products include:
Lamictal 1481

Levetiracetam (Potentiates CNS-depressant action). Products include:
Keppra Injection 3320
Keppra Oral Solution 3314
Keppra Tablets 3314

Levomethadyl Acetate Hydrochloride (Potentiates CNS-depressant action).
No products indexed under this heading.

Levorphanol Tartrate (Potentiates CNS-depressant action).
No products indexed under this heading.

Lorazepam (Potentiates CNS-depressant action).
No products indexed under this heading.

Loxapine Hydrochloride (Potentiates CNS-depressant action).
No products indexed under this heading.

Loxapine Succinate (Potentiates CNS-depressant action).
No products indexed under this heading.

Maprotiline Hydrochloride (Potentiates CNS-depressant action).
No products indexed under this heading.

Meperidine Hydrochloride (Potentiates CNS-depressant action).
No products indexed under this heading.

Mephenytoin (Potentiates CNS-depressant action).
No products indexed under this heading.

Mephobarbital (Potentiates CNS-depressant action).
No products indexed under this heading.

Meprobamate (Potentiates CNS-depressant action).
No products indexed under this heading.

Mesoridazine Besylate (Potentiates CNS-depressant action).
No products indexed under this heading.

Methadone Hydrochloride (Potentiates CNS-depressant action).
No products indexed under this heading.

Methohexital Sodium (Potentiates CNS-depressant action).
No products indexed under this heading.

Methotrimeprazine (Potentiates CNS-depressant action).
No products indexed under this heading.

Methoxyflurane (Potentiates CNS-depressant action).
No products indexed under this heading.

Methsuximide (Potentiates CNS-depressant action).
No products indexed under this heading.

Midazolam Hydrochloride (Potentiates CNS-depressant action).
No products indexed under this heading.

Moclobemide (Potentiates CNS-depressant action).
No products indexed under this heading.

Molindone Hydrochloride (Potentiates CNS-depressant action). Products include:
Moban Tablets 1119

Morphine Sulfate (Potentiates CNS-depressant action). Products include:
Avinza Capsules 1741
Kadian Capsules 577
MS Contin Tablets 2701

Nortriptyline Hydrochloride (Potentiates CNS-depressant action).
No products indexed under this heading.

Olanzapine (Potentiates CNS-depressant action). Products include:
Symbyax Capsules 1819
Zyprexa Tablets 1830
Zyprexa IntraMuscular 1830
Zyprexa ZYDIS Orally Disintegrating Tablets 1830

Oxazepam (Potentiates CNS-depressant action).
No products indexed under this heading.

Oxcarbazepine (Potentiates CNS-depressant action). Products include:
Trileptal Tablets 2300
Trileptal Oral Suspension 2300

Oxycodone Hydrochloride (Potentiates CNS-depressant action). Products include:
OxyContin Tablets 2703
OxyFast Oral Concentrate Solution 2708
OxyIR Capsules 2708
Percocet Tablets 1131
Percodan Tablets 1132

Paramethadione (Potentiates CNS-depressant action).
No products indexed under this heading.

Pargyline Hydrochloride (Potentiates CNS-depressant action).
No products indexed under this heading.

Pentobarbital Sodium (Potentiates CNS-depressant action). Products include:
Nembutal Sodium Solution, USP 2470

Perphenazine (Potentiates CNS-depressant action).
No products indexed under this heading.

Phenacemide (Potentiates CNS-depressant action).
No products indexed under this heading.

Phenelzine Sulfate (Potentiates CNS-depressant action).
No products indexed under this heading.

Phenobarbital (Induces clonazepam metabolism causing an approximately 30% decrease in plasma clonazepam levels; CNS depressant action may be potentiated). Products include:
Donnatal Extentabs 2493

Phensuximide (Potentiates CNS-depressant action).
No products indexed under this heading.

Phenytoin (Induces clonazepam metabolism causing an approximately 30% decrease in plasma clonazepam levels).
No products indexed under this heading.

Phenytoin Sodium (Induces clonazepam metabolism causing an approximately 30% decrease in plasma clonazepam levels). Products include:
Phenytek Capsules 2160

Prazepam (Potentiates CNS-depressant action).
No products indexed under this heading.

Primidone (Potentiates CNS-depressant action).
No products indexed under this heading.

Procarbazine Hydrochloride (Potentiates CNS-depressant action). Products include:
Matulane Capsules 3191

Prochlorperazine (Potentiates CNS-depressant action).
No products indexed under this heading.

Promethazine Hydrochloride (Potentiates CNS-depressant action). Products include:
Phenergan Tablets and Suppositories 3440

Propofol (Potentiates CNS-depressant action).
No products indexed under this heading.

Propoxyphene Hydrochloride (Potentiates CNS-depressant action).
No products indexed under this heading.

Propoxyphene Napsylate (Potentiates CNS-depressant action).
No products indexed under this heading.

Protriptyline Hydrochloride (Potentiates CNS-depressant action).
No products indexed under this heading.

Quazepam (Potentiates CNS-depressant action).
No products indexed under this heading.

Quetiapine Fumarate (Potentiates CNS-depressant action). Products include:
Seroquel Tablets 690

Remifentanil Hydrochloride (Potentiates CNS-depressant action).
No products indexed under this heading.

Risperidone (Potentiates CNS-depressant action). Products include:
Risperdal 1676
Risperdal Consta Long-Acting Injection 1682
Risperdal M-Tab Orally Disintegrating Tablets 1676

Secobarbital Sodium (Potentiates CNS-depressant action).
No products indexed under this heading.

Selegiline Hydrochloride (Potentiates CNS-depressant action). Products include:
Eldepryl Capsules 3208
Zelapar Tablets 3372

Sevoflurane (Potentiates CNS-depressant action). Products include:
Ultane Liquid for Inhalation 531

Sufentanil Citrate (Potentiates CNS-depressant action).
No products indexed under this heading.

Temazepam (Potentiates CNS-depressant action). Products include:
Restoril Capsules 1860

Thiamylal Sodium (Potentiates CNS-depressant action).
No products indexed under this heading.

Thioridazine Hydrochloride (Potentiates CNS-depressant action). Products include:
Thioridazine Hydrochloride Tablets 2163

Thiothixene (Potentiates CNS-depressant action). Products include:
Thiothixene Capsules 2165

Tiagabine Hydrochloride (Potentiates CNS-depressant action). Products include:
Gabitril Tablets 984

Topiramate (Potentiates CNS-depressant action). Products include:
Topamax Sprinkle Capsules 2404
Topamax Tablets 2404

Tranylcypromine Sulfate (Potentiates CNS-depressant action). Products include:
Parnate Tablets 1527

Triazolam (Potentiates CNS-depressant action).
No products indexed under this heading.

Trifluoperazine Hydrochloride (Potentiates CNS-depressant action).
No products indexed under this heading.

Trimethadione (Potentiates CNS-depressant action).
No products indexed under this heading.

Trimipramine Maleate (Potentiates CNS-depressant action).
No products indexed under this heading.

Valproate Sodium (Potentiates CNS-depressant action). Products include:
Depacon Injection 412

Valproic Acid (Potentiates CNS-depressant action). Products include:
Depakene 417

Zaleplon (Potentiates CNS-depressant action). Products include:
Sonata Capsules 1717

Ziprasidone Hydrochloride (Potentiates CNS-depressant action). Products include:
Geodon Capsules 2529

Zolpidem Tartrate (Potentiates CNS-depressant action). Products include:
Ambien Tablets 2851
Ambien CR Tablets 2855

Zonisamide (Potentiates CNS-depressant action). Products include:
Zonegran Capsules 1101

Food Interactions

Alcohol (Potentiates CNS-depressant action).

KLONOPIN WAFERS
(Clonazepam) 2778
See Klonopin Tablets

K-LOR ORAL SOLUTION
(Potassium Chloride) 474
May interact with ACE inhibitors and potassium sparing diuretics. Compounds in these categories include:

Amiloride Hydrochloride (Co-administration of these agents can produce severe hyperkalemia; concurrent use is not recommended). Products include:
Midamor Tablets 2026
Moduretic Tablets 2028

Benazepril Hydrochloride (Potential for hyperkalemia). Products include:
Lotensin Tablets 2243
Lotensin HCT Tablets 2246
Lotrel Capsules 2249

Captopril (Potential for hyperkalemia). Products include:
Captopril Tablets 2149

Enalapril Maleate (Potential for hyperkalemia). Products include:
Vasotec I.V. Injection 2103

Enalaprilat (Potential for hyperkalemia).
No products indexed under this heading.

Fosinopril Sodium (Potential for hyperkalemia).
No products indexed under this heading.

Lisinopril (Potential for hyperkalemia). Products include:
Prinivil Tablets 2052
Prinzide Tablets 2056

Moexipril Hydrochloride (Potential for hyperkalemia). Products include:
Uniretic Tablets 3100
Univasc Tablets 3104

Perindopril Erbumine (Potential for hyperkalemia). Products include:
Aceon Tablets (2 mg, 4 mg, 8 mg) 3194

Quinapril Hydrochloride (Potential for hyperkalemia).
No products indexed under this heading.

Ramipril (Potential for hyperkalemia). Products include:
Altace Capsules 1702

Spirapril Hydrochloride (Potential for hyperkalemia).
No products indexed under this heading.

Spironolactone (Co-administration of these agents can produce severe hyperkalemia; concurrent use is not recommended).
No products indexed under this heading.

Trandolapril (Potential for hyperkalemia). Products include:
Mavik Tablets 486
Tarka Tablets 524

Triamterene (Co-administration of these agents can produce severe hyperkalemia; concurrent use is not recommended). Products include:
Dyazide Capsules 1423
Dyrenium Capsules 3400

KOĀTE-DVI
(Antihemophilic Factor (Human)) 3250
None cited in PDR database.

KOGENATE FS
(Antihemophilic Factor (Recombinant)) 738
None cited in PDR database.

KOGENATE FS WITH BIO-SET
(Antihemophilic Factor (Recombinant)) 740
None cited in PDR database.

K-PHOS ORIGINAL (SODIUM FREE) TABLETS
(Potassium Acid Phosphate) 760
May interact with antacids, potassium preparations, potassium sparing diuretics, salicylates, and certain other agents. Compounds in these categories include:

Aluminum Carbonate (May bind phosphate and prevent its absorption).
No products indexed under this heading.

Aluminum Hydroxide (May bind phosphate and prevent its absorption). Products include:
Gaviscon Regular Strength Liquid 658
Gaviscon Regular Strength Tablets 658
Gaviscon Extra Strength Liquid 658
Gaviscon Extra Strength Tablets 658
Maalox Regular Strength Antacid/Antigas Liquid 2175
Maalox Max Maximum Strength Antacid/Anti-Gas Liquid 2176

Amiloride Hydrochloride (Hyperkalemia). Products include:
Midamor Tablets 2026
Moduretic Tablets 2028

Aspirin (Increased serum salicylate levels; possible toxicity). Products include:
Aggrenox Capsules 822
Bayer Aspirin 744
BC Allergy Sinus Cold Powder 677
BC Headache Powder 677
Arthritis Strength BC Powder 677
BC Sinus Cold Powder 677
Excedrin Extra Strength Caplets/Tablets/Geltabs 684
Excedrin Migraine Caplets/Tablets/Geltabs 609
Goody's Body Pain Formula Powder 684
Goody's Extra Strength Headache Powders 611
Goody's Extra Strength Pain Relief Tablets 685
Percodan Tablets 1132
St. Joseph 81 mg Aspirin Chewable and Enteric Coated Tablets 1869

Aspirin, Enteric Coated (Increased serum salicylate levels; possible toxicity).
No products indexed under this heading.

Aspirin Buffered (Increased serum salicylate levels; possible toxicity). Products include:
Bufferin Extra Strength Tablets 678
Bufferin Regular Strength Tablets 678

Choline Magnesium Trisalicylate (Increased serum salicylate levels; possible toxicity).
No products indexed under this heading.

Diflunisal (Increased serum salicylate levels; possible toxicity). Products include:
Dolobid Tablets 1955

Magaldrate (May bind phosphate and prevent its absorption).
No products indexed under this heading.

Magnesium Hydroxide (May bind phosphate and prevent its absorption). Products include:
Maalox Regular Strength Antacid/Antigas Liquid 2175
Maalox Max Maximum Strength Antacid/Anti-Gas Liquid 2176
Pepcid Complete Chewable Tablets 1701

Magnesium Oxide (May bind phosphate and prevent its absorption). Products include:
Beelith Tablets 759
PremCal Light, Regular, and Extra Strength Tablets 818

Magnesium Salicylate (Increased serum salicylate levels; possible toxicity).
No products indexed under this heading.

Potassium Bicarbonate (Potential for hyperkalemia).
No products indexed under this heading.

Potassium Chloride (Potential for hyperkalemia). Products include:
Colyte with Flavor Packs for Oral Solution 3088
HalfLytely and Bisacodyl Tablets Bowel Prep Kit with Flavors Packs 881
K-Dur Extended-Relase Tablets 3033
K-Lor Oral Solution 474
K-Tab Tablets 475
MoviPrep Oral Solution 2839
TriLyte with Flavor Packs for Oral Solution 3100

Potassium Citrate (Potential for hyperkalemia). Products include:
Urocit-K Tablets 2144

Potassium Gluconate (Potential for hyperkalemia).
No products indexed under this heading.

Potassium Phosphate (Potential for hyperkalemia). Products include:
K-Phos Neutral Tablets 760

Salsalate (Increased serum salicylate levels; possible toxicity).
No products indexed under this heading.

Sodium Bicarbonate (May bind phosphate and prevent its absorption). Products include:
Colyte with Flavor Packs for Oral Solution 3088
HalfLytely and Bisacodyl Tablets Bowel Prep Kit with Flavors Packs 881
TriLyte with Flavor Packs for Oral Solution 3100

Spironolactone (Hyperkalemia).
No products indexed under this heading.

Triamterene (Hyperkalemia). Products include:
Dyazide Capsules 1423
Dyrenium Capsules 3400

K-PHOS NEUTRAL TABLETS
(Potassium Phosphate, Sodium Phosphate) 760
May interact with antacids containing aluminum, calcium and magnesium, calcium preparations, potassium preparations, potassium sparing diuretics, and certain other agents. Compounds in these categories include:

ACTH (Concurrent use with corticotropin may result in hypernatremia).
No products indexed under this heading.

Aluminum Carbonate (Co-administration with antacids may bind the phosphate and prevent its absorption).
No products indexed under this heading.

Aluminum Hydroxide (Co-administration with antacids may bind the phosphate and prevent its absorption). Products include:
Gaviscon Regular Strength Liquid .. ▣658
Gaviscon Regular Strength Tablets .... ▣658
Gaviscon Extra Strength Liquid ...... ▣658
Gaviscon Extra Strength Tablets .... ▣658
Maalox Regular Strength Antacid/Antigas Liquid 2175
Maalox Max Maximum Strength Antacid/Anti-Gas Liquid 2176

Amiloride Hydrochloride (Concurrent use with potassium-sparing diuretics may cause hyperkalemia). Products include:
Midamor Tablets 2026
Moduretic Tablets 2028

Calcium Carbonate (Concurrent use with calcium-containing preparations may antagonize the effects of phosphates in the treatment of hypercalcemia). Products include:
Actonel with Calcium Tablets 2688
Calcet Tablets 2138
Caltrate 600 PLUS .... ▣809
Caltrate 600 + D Tablets .... ▣809
D-Cal Chewable Caplets .... ▣812
Gas-X with Maalox .... ▣656
Maalox Regular Strength Antacid Chewable Tablets 2177
Maalox Max Maximum Strength Antacid/Antigas Chewable Tablets 2176
Maalox Max Maximum Strength Chewable Tablets .... ▣660
Os-Cal Chewable Tablets .... ▣818
Pepcid Complete Chewable Tablets 1701
Children's Pepto 2674
PremCal Light, Regular, and Extra Strength Tablets .... ▣818
Tums .... ▣664

Calcium Chloride (Concurrent use with calcium-containing preparations may antagonize the effects of phosphates in the treatment of hypercalcemia).
No products indexed under this heading.

Calcium Citrate (Concurrent use with calcium-containing preparations may antagonize the effects of phosphates in the treatment of hypercalcemia). Products include:
Active Calcium Tablets 3339
Citracal Caplets .... ▣703
Citracal Lemon Cream Creamy Bites 2139
Citracal Prenatal + DHA Tablets and Capsules 2139

Calcium Glubionate (Concurrent use with calcium-containing preparations may antagonize the effects of phosphates in the treatment of hypercalcemia).
No products indexed under this heading.

Deserpidine (Concurrent use with antihypertensives, such as rauwolfia alkaloids, may result in hypernatremia).
No products indexed under this heading.

Diazoxide (Concurrent use with antihypertensives, such as diazoxide, may result in hypernatremia). Products include:
Hyperstat I.V. 3017

Fludrocortisone Acetate (Concurrent use with mineralocorticoids may result in hypernatremia).
No products indexed under this heading.

Guanethidine Monosulfate (Concurrent use with antihypertensives, such as guanethidine, may result in hypernatremia).
No products indexed under this heading.

Hydralazine Hydrochloride (Concurrent use with antihypertensives, such as hydralazine, may result in hypernatremia). Products include:
BiDil Tablets 2171

Magaldrate (Co-administration with antacids may bind the phosphate and prevent its absorption).
No products indexed under this heading.

Magnesium Hydroxide (Co-administration with antacids may bind the phosphate and prevent its absorption). Products include:
Maalox Regular Strength Antacid/Antigas Liquid 2175
Maalox Max Maximum Strength Antacid/Anti-Gas Liquid 2176
Pepcid Complete Chewable Tablets 1701

Magnesium Oxide (Co-administration with antacids may bind the phosphate and prevent its absorption). Products include:
Beelith Tablets 759
PremCal Light, Regular, and Extra Strength Tablets .... ▣818

Methyldopa (Concurrent use with antihypertensives, such as methyldopa, may result in hypernatremia). Products include:
Aldoril Tablets 1910

Potassium Acid Phosphate (Concurrent use with potassium-containing medications may cause hyperkalemia). Products include:
K-Phos Original (Sodium Free) Tablets 760

Potassium Bicarbonate (Concurrent use with potassium-containing medications may cause hyperkalemia).
No products indexed under this heading.

Potassium Chloride (Concurrent use with potassium-containing medications may cause hyperkalemia). Products include:
Colyte with Flavor Packs for Oral Solution 3088
HalfLytely and Bisacodyl Tablets Bowel Prep Kit with Flavors Packs 881
K-Dur Extended-Relase Tablets 3033
K-Lor Oral Solution 474
K-Tab Tablets 475
MoviPrep Oral Solution 2839
TriLyte with Flavor Packs for Oral Solution 3100

Potassium Citrate (Concurrent use with potassium-containing medications may cause hyperkalemia). Products include:
Urocit-K Tablets 2144

Potassium Gluconate (Concurrent use with potassium-containing medications may cause hyperkalemia).
No products indexed under this heading.

Rauwolfia Serpentina (Concurrent use with antihypertensives, such as rauwolfia alkaloids, may result in hypernatremia).
No products indexed under this heading.

Rescinnamine (Concurrent use with antihypertensives, such as rauwolfia alkaloids, may result in hypernatremia).
No products indexed under this heading.

Reserpine (Concurrent use with antihypertensives, such as rauwolfia alkaloids, may result in hypernatremia).
No products indexed under this heading.

Spironolactone (Concurrent use with potassium-sparing diuretics may cause hyperkalemia).
No products indexed under this heading.

Triamterene (Concurrent use with potassium-sparing diuretics may cause hyperkalemia). Products include:
Dyazide Capsules 1423
Dyrenium Capsules 3400

Vitamin D (Concurrent use with vitamin D may antagonize the effects of phosphates in the treatment of hypercalcemia). Products include:
Active Calcium Tablets 3339
Caltrate 600 PLUS .... ▣809
Caltrate 600 + D Tablets .... ▣809
D-Cal Chewable Caplets .... ▣812
Os-Cal 250 + D Tablets .... ▣817
Os-Cal 500 + D Tablets .... ▣817

KRISTALOSE FOR ORAL SOLUTION

(Lactulose) 1034
May interact with nonabsorbable antacids. Compounds in these categories include:

Aluminum Carbonate (Results of preliminary studies suggests that nonabsorbable antacids given concurrently with lactulose may inhibit the desired lactulose-induced drop in colonic pH).
No products indexed under this heading.

Aluminum Hydroxide (Results of preliminary studies suggests that nonabsorbable antacids given concurrently with lactulose may inhibit the desired lactulose-induced drop in colonic pH). Products include:
Gaviscon Regular Strength Liquid .. ▣658
Gaviscon Regular Strength Tablets .... ▣658
Gaviscon Extra Strength Liquid ...... ▣658
Gaviscon Extra Strength Tablets .... ▣658
Maalox Regular Strength Antacid/Antigas Liquid 2175
Maalox Max Maximum Strength Antacid/Anti-Gas Liquid 2176

Calcium Carbonate (Results of preliminary studies suggests that nonabsorbable antacids given concurrently with lactulose may inhibit the desired lactulose-induced drop in colonic pH). Products include:
Actonel with Calcium Tablets 2688
Calcet Tablets 2138
Caltrate 600 PLUS .... ▣809
Caltrate 600 + D Tablets .... ▣809
D-Cal Chewable Caplets .... ▣812
Gas-X with Maalox .... ▣656
Maalox Regular Strength Antacid Chewable Tablets 2177
Maalox Max Maximum Strength Antacid/Antigas Chewable Tablets 2176
Maalox Max Maximum Strength Chewable Tablets .... ▣660
Os-Cal Chewable Tablets .... ▣818
Pepcid Complete Chewable Tablets 1701
Children's Pepto 2674
PremCal Light, Regular, and Extra Strength Tablets .... ▣818
Tums .... ▣664

Magnesium Carbonate (Results of preliminary studies suggests that nonabsorbable antacids given concurrently with lactulose may inhibit the desired lactulose-induced drop in colonic pH). Products include:
Gaviscon Regular Strength Liquid .. ▣658
Gaviscon Extra Strength Liquid ...... ▣658
Gaviscon Extra Strength Tablets .... ▣658

Magnesium Hydroxide (Results of preliminary studies suggests that nonabsorbable antacids given concurrently with lactulose may inhibit the desired lactulose-induced drop in colonic pH). Products include:
Maalox Regular Strength Antacid/Antigas Liquid 2175
Maalox Max Maximum Strength Antacid/Anti-Gas Liquid 2176
Pepcid Complete Chewable Tablets 1701

K-TAB TABLETS

(Potassium Chloride) 475
May interact with ACE inhibitors, anticholinergics, and potassium sparing diuretics. Compounds in these categories include:

Amiloride Hydrochloride (Potential for severe hyperkalemia). Products include:
Midamor Tablets 2026
Moduretic Tablets 2028

Atropine Sulfate (Anticholinergic drugs can be cause for delay or arrest in tablet passage through the gastrointestinal tract; concomitant administration of drugs capable of decreasing GI motility should be avoided). Products include:
Donnatal Extentabs 2493

Belladonna Alkaloids (Anticholinergic drugs can be cause for delay or arrest in tablet passage through the gastrointestinal tract; concomitant administration of drugs capable of decreasing GI motility should be avoided). Products include:
Hyland's Teething Tablets .... ▣830

Benazepril Hydrochloride (Concomitant therapy may result in hyperkalemia; close monitoring is advised). Products include:
Lotensin Tablets 2243
Lotensin HCT Tablets 2246
Lotrel Capsules 2249

Benztropine Mesylate (Anticholinergic drugs can be cause for delay or arrest in tablet passage through the gastrointestinal tract; concomitant administration of drugs capable of decreasing GI motility should be avoided).
No products indexed under this heading.

Biperiden Hydrochloride (Anticholinergic drugs can be cause for delay or arrest in tablet passage through the gastrointestinal tract; concomitant administration of drugs capable of decreasing GI motility should be avoided).
No products indexed under this heading.

Captopril (Concomitant therapy may result in hyperkalemia; close monitoring is advised). Products include:
Captopril Tablets 2149

Clidinium Bromide (Anticholinergic drugs can be cause for delay or arrest in tablet passage through the gastrointestinal tract; concomitant administration of drugs capable of decreasing GI motility should be avoided).
No products indexed under this heading.

Dicyclomine Hydrochloride (Anticholinergic drugs can be cause for delay or arrest in tablet passage through the gastrointestinal tract; concomitant administration of drugs capable of decreasing GI motility should be avoided). Products include:
- Bentyl Capsules 697
- Bentyl Injection 697
- Bentyl Syrup 697
- Bentyl Tablets 697

Enalapril Maleate (Concomitant therapy may result in hyperkalemia; close monitoring is advised). Products include:
- Vasotec I.V. Injection 2103

Enalaprilat (Concomitant therapy may result in hyperkalemia; close monitoring is advised).
No products indexed under this heading.

Fosinopril Sodium (Concomitant therapy may result in hyperkalemia; close monitoring is advised).
No products indexed under this heading.

Glycopyrrolate (Anticholinergic drugs can be cause for delay or arrest in tablet passage through the gastrointestinal tract; concomitant administration of drugs capable of decreasing GI motility should be avoided).
No products indexed under this heading.

Hyoscyamine (Anticholinergic drugs can be cause for delay or arrest in tablet passage through the gastrointestinal tract; concomitant administration of drugs capable of decreasing GI motility should be avoided).
No products indexed under this heading.

Hyoscyamine Sulfate (Anticholinergic drugs can be cause for delay or arrest in tablet passage through the gastrointestinal tract; concomitant administration of drugs capable of decreasing GI motility should be avoided). Products include:
- Donnatal Extentabs 2493
- Prosed/DS Tablets 1157

Ipratropium Bromide (Anticholinergic drugs can be cause for delay or arrest in tablet passage through the gastrointestinal tract; concomitant administration of drugs capable of decreasing GI motility should be avoided). Products include:
- Atrovent Inhalation Solution 835
- Atrovent HFA Inhalation Aerosol 841
- Atrovent Nasal Spray 0.03% 837
- Atrovent Nasal Spray 0.06% 839
- Combivent Inhalation Aerosol 847
- DuoNeb Inhalation Solution 1058

Lisinopril (Concomitant therapy may result in hyperkalemia; close monitoring is advised). Products include:
- Prinivil Tablets 2052
- Prinzide Tablets 2056

Mepenzolate Bromide (Anticholinergic drugs can be cause for delay or arrest in tablet passage through the gastrointestinal tract; concomitant administration of drugs capable of decreasing GI motility should be avoided).
No products indexed under this heading.

Moexipril Hydrochloride (Concomitant therapy may result in hyperkalemia; close monitoring is advised). Products include:
- Uniretic Tablets 3100
- Univasc Tablets 3104

Oxybutynin Chloride (Anticholinergic drugs can be cause for delay or arrest in tablet passage through the gastrointestinal tract; concomitant administration of drugs capable of decreasing GI motility should be avoided). Products include:
- Ditropan XL Extended-Release Tablets 2413

Perindopril Erbumine (Concomitant therapy may result in hyperkalemia; close monitoring is advised). Products include:
- Aceon Tablets (2 mg, 4 mg, 8 mg) 3194

Procyclidine Hydrochloride (Anticholinergic drugs can be cause for delay or arrest in tablet passage through the gastrointestinal tract; concomitant administration of drugs capable of decreasing GI motility should be avoided).
No products indexed under this heading.

Propantheline Bromide (Anticholinergic drugs can be cause for delay or arrest in tablet passage through the gastrointestinal tract; concomitant administration of drugs capable of decreasing GI motility should be avoided).
No products indexed under this heading.

Quinapril Hydrochloride (Concomitant therapy may result in hyperkalemia; close monitoring is advised).
No products indexed under this heading.

Ramipril (Concomitant therapy may result in hyperkalemia; close monitoring is advised). Products include:
- Altace Capsules 1702

Scopolamine (Anticholinergic drugs can be cause for delay or arrest in tablet passage through the gastrointestinal tract; concomitant administration of drugs capable of decreasing GI motility should be avoided). Products include:
- Transderm Scōp Transdermal Therapeutic System 2177

Scopolamine Hydrobromide (Anticholinergic drugs can be cause for delay or arrest in tablet passage through the gastrointestinal tract; concomitant administration of drugs capable of decreasing GI motility should be avoided). Products include:
- Donnatal Extentabs 2493

Spirapril Hydrochloride (Concomitant therapy may result in hyperkalemia; close monitoring is advised).
No products indexed under this heading.

Spironolactone (Potential for severe hyperkalemia).
No products indexed under this heading.

Tolterodine Tartrate (Anticholinergic drugs can be cause for delay or arrest in tablet passage through the gastrointestinal tract; concomitant administration of drugs capable of decreasing GI motility should be avoided). Products include:
- Detrol Tablets 2628
- Detrol LA Capsules 2631

Trandolapril (Concomitant therapy may result in hyperkalemia; close monitoring is advised). Products include:
- Mavik Tablets 486
- Tarka Tablets 524

Triamterene (Potential for severe hyperkalemia). Products include:
- Dyazide Capsules 1423
- Dyrenium Capsules 3400

Tridihexethyl Chloride (Anticholinergic drugs can be cause for delay or arrest in tablet passage through the gastrointestinal tract; concomitant administration of drugs capable of decreasing GI motility should be avoided).
No products indexed under this heading.

Trihexyphenidyl Hydrochloride (Anticholinergic drugs can be cause for delay or arrest in tablet passage through the gastrointestinal tract; concomitant administration of drugs capable of decreasing GI motility should be avoided).
No products indexed under this heading.

KYTRIL INJECTION
(Granisetron Hydrochloride) 2781
See Kytril Tablets

KYTRIL ORAL SOLUTION
(Granisetron Hydrochloride) 2784
See Kytril Tablets

KYTRIL TABLETS
(Granisetron Hydrochloride) 2784
May interact with drugs affecting hepatic drug metabolizing enzyme systems and certain other agents. Compounds in these categories include:

Carbamazepine (May change the clearance and, hence the half-life of granisetron). Products include:
- Carbatrol Capsules 3171
- Equetro Extended-Release Capsules 3180
- Tegretol/Tegretol-XR 2295

Cimetidine (May change the clearance and, hence the half-life of granisetron). Products include:
- Tagamet HB 200 Tablets 664

Cimetidine Hydrochloride (May change the clearance and, hence the half-life of granisetron).
No products indexed under this heading.

Fosphenytoin Sodium (May change the clearance and, hence the half-life of granisetron).
No products indexed under this heading.

Ketoconazole (During in vitro human microsomal studies, ketoconazole inhibited ring oxidation of granisetron hydrochloride). Products include:
- Nizoral A-D Shampoo, 1% 1868

Phenobarbital (May change the clearance and, hence the half-life of granisetron). Products include:
- Donnatal Extentabs 2493

Phenytoin (May change the clearance and, hence the half-life of granisetron).
No products indexed under this heading.

Phenytoin Sodium (May change the clearance and, hence the half-life of granisetron). Products include:
- Phenytek Capsules 2160

Food Interactions

Food, unspecified (When oral granisetron was administered with food, AUC was decreased by 5% and Cmax increased by 30% in non-fasted individuals).

LACRISERT STERILE OPHTHALMIC INSERT
(Hydroxypropyl Cellulose) 2005
None cited in PDR database.

LACTAID ORIGINAL STRENGTH CAPLETS
(Lactase (beta-d-Galactosidase)) 1881
None cited in PDR database.

LACTAID FAST ACT CAPLETS AND CHEWABLE TABLETS
(Lactase (beta-d-Galactosidase)) 1881
None cited in PDR database.

LAMICTAL CHEWABLE DISPERSIBLE TABLETS
(Lamotrigine) 1481
See Lamictal Tablets

LAMICTAL TABLETS
(Lamotrigine) 1481
May interact with dihydrofolate reductase inhibitors, oral contraceptives, phenytoin, valproate, and certain other agents. Compounds in these categories include:

Carbamazepine (Potential for higher incidence of dizziness, diplopia, ataxia, and blurred vision; decreases lamotrigine steady-state concentrations by approximately 40%; lamotrigine has no appreciable effect on steady-state carbamazepine plasma concentration). Products include:
- Carbatrol Capsules 3171
- Equetro Extended-Release Capsules 3180
- Tegretol/Tegretol-XR 2295

Desogestrel (Oral contraceptive have been shown to increase the apparent clearance of lamotrigine. There have been reports of decreased lamotrigine concentrations following introduction of oral contraceptives and reports of increased lamotrigine concentrations following withdrawal of oral contraceptives). Products include:
- Mircette Tablets 1066

Divalproex Sodium (Co-administration in healthy volunteers resulted in decreased trough steady-state VPA concentrations; the addition of VPA increases lamotrigine steady-state concentrations in normal volunteers by slightly more than two-fold). Products include:
- Depakote Sprinkle Capsules 422
- Depakote Tablets 427
- Depakote ER Tablets 434

Ethinyl Estradiol (Oral contraceptive have been shown to increase the apparent clearance of lamotrigine. There have been reports of decreased lamotrigine concentrations following introduction of oral contraceptives and reports of increased lamotrigine concentrations following withdrawal of oral contraceptives). Products include:
- Mircette Tablets 1066
- NuvaRing 2340
- Ortho-Cyclen/Ortho Tri-Cyclen 2429
- Ortho Evra Transdermal System 2417
- Ortho Tri-Cyclen Lo Tablets 2436
- Seasonique Tablets 1077
- Yasmin 28 Tablets 796
- Yaz Tablets 803

Ethynodiol Diacetate (Oral contraceptive have been shown to increase the apparent clearance of lamotrigine. There have been reports of decreased lamotrigine concentrations following introduction of oral contraceptives and reports of increased lamotrigine concentrations following withdrawal of oral contraceptives).
No products indexed under this heading.

Fosphenytoin Sodium (Decreases lamotrigine steady-state concentrations by approximately 40%).
No products indexed under this heading.

Levonorgestrel (Oral contraceptive have been shown to increase the apparent clearance of lamotrigine. There have been reports of decreased lamotrigine concentrations following introduction of oral contraceptives and reports of increased lamotrigine concentrations following withdrawal of oral contraceptives). Products include:
Climara Pro Transdermal System 776
Mirena Intrauterine System 787
Plan B Tablets 1076
Seasonique Tablets 1077

Mestranol (Oral contraceptive have been shown to increase the apparent clearance of lamotrigine. There have been reports of decreased lamotrigine concentrations following introduction of oral contraceptives and reports of increased lamotrigine concentrations following withdrawal of oral contraceptives).
No products indexed under this heading.

Methotrexate Sodium (Lamotrigine is an inhibitor of dihydrofolate reductase; use caution when prescribing other medications that inhibit folate metabolism).
No products indexed under this heading.

Norethindrone (Oral contraceptive have been shown to increase the apparent clearance of lamotrigine. There have been reports of decreased lamotrigine concentrations following introduction of oral contraceptives and reports of increased lamotrigine concentrations following withdrawal of oral contraceptives). Products include:
Ortho Micronor Tablets 2426

Norethynodrel (Oral contraceptive have been shown to increase the apparent clearance of lamotrigine. There have been reports of decreased lamotrigine concentrations following introduction of oral contraceptives and reports of increased lamotrigine concentrations following withdrawal of oral contraceptives).
No products indexed under this heading.

Norgestimate (Oral contraceptive have been shown to increase the apparent clearance of lamotrigine. There have been reports of decreased lamotrigine concentrations following introduction of oral contraceptives and reports of increased lamotrigine concentrations following withdrawal of oral contraceptives). Products include:
Ortho-Cyclen/Ortho Tri-Cyclen 2429
Ortho Tri-Cyclen Lo Tablets 2436

Norgestrel (Oral contraceptive have been shown to increase the apparent clearance of lamotrigine. There have been reports of decreased lamotrigine concentrations following introduction of oral contraceptives and reports of increased lamotrigine concentrations following withdrawal of oral contraceptives).
No products indexed under this heading.

Olanzapine (The AUC and Cmax of lamotrigine was reduced on average by 24% and 20%, respectively, following the addition of olanzapine (15 mg once daily) to lamotrigine (200 mg once daily) in healthy male volunteers (n=16) compared to healthy male volunteers receiving lamotrigine alone (n=12). This reduction in lamotrigine plasma concentration is not expected to be clinically relevant). Products include:
Symbyax Capsules 1819
Zyprexa Tablets 1830
Zyprexa IntraMuscular 1830
Zyprexa ZYDIS Orally Disintegrating Tablets.................. 1830

Oral Contraceptives (There have been reports of decreased lamotrigine concentrations following introduction of oral contraceptives and reports of increased lamotrigine concentrations following withdrawal of oral contraceptives).
No products indexed under this heading.

Phenobarbital (Decreases lamotrigine steady-state concentrations by approximately 40%). Products include:
Donnatal Extentabs 2493

Phenytoin (Decreases lamotrigine steady-state concentrations by approximately 40%).
No products indexed under this heading.

Phenytoin Sodium (Decreases lamotrigine steady-state concentrations by approximately 40%). Products include:
Phenytek Capsules 2160

Primidone (Decreases lamotrigine steady-state concentrations by approximately 40%).
No products indexed under this heading.

Rifampin (Co-administration of rifampin has been shown to increase the apparent clearance of lamotrigine).
No products indexed under this heading.

Trimethoprim (Lamotrigine is an inhibitor of dihydrofolate reductase; use caution when prescribing other medications that inhibit folate metabolism).
No products indexed under this heading.

Trimetrexate Glucuronate (Lamotrigine is an inhibitor of dihydrofolate reductase; use caution when prescribing other medications that inhibit folate metabolism).
No products indexed under this heading.

Valproate Sodium (Co-administration in healthy volunteers resulted in decreased trough steady-state VPA concentrations; the addition of VPA increases lamotrigine steady-state concentrations in normal volunteers by slightly more than two-fold). Products include:
Depacon Injection 412

Valproic Acid (Co-administration in healthy volunteers resulted in decreased trough steady-state VPA concentrations; the addition of VPA increases lamotrigine steady-state concentrations in normal volunteers by slightly more than two-fold). Products include:
Depakene 417

LAMISIL TABLETS

(Terbinafine Hydrochloride) 2232
May interact with beta blockers, cytochrome p450 2d6 substrates (selected), monoamine oxidase inhibitors, selective serotonin reuptake inhibitors, tricyclic antidepressants, and certain other agents. Compounds in these categories include:

Acebutolol Hydrochloride (Studies have shown that terbinafine is an inhibitor of the CYP450 2D6 isoenzyme. Co-administration of terbinafine with drugs predominantly metabolized by the CYP450 2D6 isoenzyme should be done with careful monitoring and may require a reduction in dose of the 2D6-metabolized drug).
No products indexed under this heading.

Amitriptyline Hydrochloride (Studies have shown that terbinafine is an inhibitor of the CYP450 2D6 isoenzyme. Co-administration of terbinafine with drugs predominantly metabolized by the CYP450 2D6 isoenzyme should be done with careful monitoring and may require a reduction in dose of the 2D6-metabolized drug).
No products indexed under this heading.

Amoxapine (Studies have shown that terbinafine is an inhibitor of the CYP450 2D6 isoenzyme. Co-administration of terbinafine with drugs predominantly metabolized by the CYP450 2D6 isoenzyme should be done with careful monitoring and may require a reduction in dose of the 2D6-metabolized drug).
No products indexed under this heading.

Amphetamine Aspartate (Studies have shown that terbinafine is an inhibitor of the CYP450 2D6 isoenzyme. Co-administration of terbinafine with drugs predominantly metabolized by the CYP450 2D6 isoenzyme should be done with careful monitoring and may require a reduction in dose of the 2D6-metabolized drug). Products include:
Adderall Tablets 3164
Adderall XR Capsules 3166

Amphetamine Aspartate Monohydrate (Studies have shown that terbinafine is an inhibitor of the CYP450 2D6 isoenzyme. Co-administration of terbinafine with drugs predominantly metabolized by the CYP450 2D6 isoenzyme should be done with careful monitoring and may require a reduction in dose of the 2D6-metabolized drug).
No products indexed under this heading.

Amphetamine Sulfate (Studies have shown that terbinafine is an inhibitor of the CYP450 2D6 isoenzyme. Co-administration of terbinafine with drugs predominantly metabolized by the CYP450 2D6 isoenzyme should be done with careful monitoring and may require a reduction in dose of the 2D6-metabolized drug). Products include:
Adderall Tablets 3164
Adderall XR Capsules 3166

Atenolol (Studies have shown that terbinafine is an inhibitor of the CYP450 2D6 isoenzyme. Co-administration of terbinafine with drugs predominantly metabolized by the CYP450 2D6 isoenzyme should be done with careful monitoring and may require a reduction in dose of the 2D6-metabolized drug).
No products indexed under this heading.

Atomoxetine Hydrochloride (Studies have shown that terbinafine is an inhibitor of the CYP450 2D6 isoenzyme. Co-administration of terbinafine with drugs predominantly metabolized by the CYP450 2D6 isoenzyme should be done with careful monitoring and may require a reduction in dose of the 2D6-metabolized drug). Products include:
Strattera Capsules 1814

Betaxolol Hydrochloride (Studies have shown that terbinafine is an inhibitor of the CYP450 2D6 isoenzyme. Co-administration of terbinafine with drugs predominantly metabolized by the CYP450 2D6 isoenzyme should be done with careful monitoring and may require a reduction in dose of the 2D6-metabolized drug). Products include:
Betoptic S Ophthalmic Suspension................................. ⊙ 558

Bisoprolol Fumarate (Studies have shown that terbinafine is an inhibitor of the CYP450 2D6 isoenzyme. Co-administration of terbinafine with drugs predominantly metabolized by the CYP450 2D6 isoenzyme should be done with careful monitoring and may require a reduction in dose of the 2D6-metabolized drug).
No products indexed under this heading.

Caffeine (Terbinafine decreases the clearance of intravenously administered caffeine by 19%). Products include:
BC Headache Powder .... ■ 677
Arthritis Strength BC Powder .... ■ 677
Excedrin Extra Strength Caplets/Tablets/Geltabs .... ■ 684
Excedrin Migraine Caplets/Tablets/Geltabs .... ■ 609
Excedrin Tension Headache Caplets/Tablets/Geltabs .... ■ 611
Goody's Extra Strength Headache Powders.................... ■ 611
Goody's Extra Strength Pain Relief Tablets .... ■ 685
Vivarin .... ■ 602
Winrgy Dietary Supplement .... ■ 823

Caffeine Citrate (Terbinafine decreases the clearance of intravenously administered caffeine by 19%). Products include:
Cafcit 1886

Captopril (Studies have shown that terbinafine is an inhibitor of the CYP450 2D6 isoenzyme. Co-administration of terbinafine with drugs predominantly metabolized by the CYP450 2D6 isoenzyme should be done with careful monitoring and may require a reduction in dose of the 2D6-metabolized drug). Products include:
Captopril Tablets 2149

Carteolol Hydrochloride (Studies have shown that terbinafine is an inhibitor of the CYP450 2D6 isoenzyme. Co-administration of terbinafine with drugs predominantly metabolized by the CYP450 2D6 isoenzyme should be done with careful monitoring and may require a reduction in dose of the 2D6-metabolized drug). Products include:

- Carteolol Hydrochloride Ophthalmic Solution USP, 1% ... ⊙249

Carvedilol (Studies have shown that terbinafine is an inhibitor of the CYP450 2D6 isoenzyme. Co-administration of terbinafine with drugs predominantly metabolized by the CYP450 2D6 isoenzyme should be done with careful monitoring and may require a reduction in dose of the 2D6-metabolized drug). Products include:

- Coreg Tablets ... 1414

Cevimeline Hydrochloride (Studies have shown that terbinafine is an inhibitor of the CYP450 2D6 isoenzyme. Co-administration of terbinafine with drugs predominantly metabolized by the CYP450 2D6 isoenzyme should be done with careful monitoring and may require a reduction in dose of the 2D6-metabolized drug). Products include:

- Evoxac Capsules ... 1047

Chlorpromazine (Studies have shown that terbinafine is an inhibitor of the CYP450 2D6 isoenzyme. Co-administration of terbinafine with drugs predominantly metabolized by the CYP450 2D6 isoenzyme should be done with careful monitoring and may require a reduction in dose of the 2D6-metabolized drug).

No products indexed under this heading.

Chlorpromazine Hydrochloride (Studies have shown that terbinafine is an inhibitor of the CYP450 2D6 isoenzyme. Co-administration of terbinafine with drugs predominantly metabolized by the CYP450 2D6 isoenzyme should be done with careful monitoring and may require a reduction in dose of the 2D6-metabolized drug).

No products indexed under this heading.

Chlorpropamide (Studies have shown that terbinafine is an inhibitor of the CYP450 2D6 isoenzyme. Co-administration of terbinafine with drugs predominantly metabolized by the CYP450 2D6 isoenzyme should be done with careful monitoring and may require a reduction in dose of the 2D6-metabolized drug).

No products indexed under this heading.

Cimetidine (Terbinafine clearance is decreased 33% by cimetidine, a CYP450 enzyme inhibitor). Products include:

- Tagamet HB 200 Tablets ... 664

Cimetidine Hydrochloride (Terbinafine clearance is decreased 33% by cimetidine, a CYP450 enzyme inhibitor).

No products indexed under this heading.

Citalopram Hydrobromide (Studies have shown that terbinafine is an inhibitor of the CYP450 2D6 isoenzyme. Co-administration of terbinafine with drugs predominantly metabolized by the CYP450 2D6 isoenzyme should be done with careful monitoring and may require a reduction in dose of the 2D6-metabolized drug). Products include:

- Celexa ... 1176

Clomipramine Hydrochloride (Studies have shown that terbinafine is an inhibitor of the CYP450 2D6 isoenzyme. Co-administration of terbinafine with drugs predominantly metabolized by the CYP450 2D6 isoenzyme should be done with careful monitoring and may require a reduction in dose of the 2D6-metabolized drug).

No products indexed under this heading.

Clozapine (Studies have shown that terbinafine is an inhibitor of the CYP450 2D6 isoenzyme. Co-administration of terbinafine with drugs predominantly metabolized by the CYP450 2D6 isoenzyme should be done with careful monitoring and may require a reduction in dose of the 2D6-metabolized drug). Products include:

- Clozaril Tablets ... 2184
- FazaClo Orally Disintegrating Tablets ... 551

Codeine Phosphate (Studies have shown that terbinafine is an inhibitor of the CYP450 2D6 isoenzyme. Co-administration of terbinafine with drugs predominantly metabolized by the CYP450 2D6 isoenzyme should be done with careful monitoring and may require a reduction in dose of the 2D6-metabolized drug). Products include:

- Tylenol with Codeine Tablets ... 2391

Codeine Sulfate (Studies have shown that terbinafine is an inhibitor of the CYP450 2D6 isoenzyme. Co-administration of terbinafine with drugs predominantly metabolized by the CYP450 2D6 isoenzyme should be done with careful monitoring and may require a reduction in dose of the 2D6-metabolized drug).

No products indexed under this heading.

Cyclobenzaprine Hydrochloride (Studies have shown that terbinafine is an inhibitor of the CYP450 2D6 isoenzyme. Co-administration of terbinafine with drugs predominantly metabolized by the CYP450 2D6 isoenzyme should be done with careful monitoring and may require a reduction in dose of the 2D6-metabolized drug).

No products indexed under this heading.

Cyclosporine (Terbinafine increases the clearance of cyclosporine by 15%; terbinafine clearance is unaffected by cyclosporine). Products include:

- Gengraf Capsules ... 459
- Neoral Oral Solution ... 2259
- Neoral Soft Gelatin Capsules ... 2259
- Restasis Ophthalmic Emulsion ... 575
- Sandimmune ... 2275

Desipramine Hydrochloride (Studies have shown that terbinafine is an inhibitor of the CYP450 2D6 isoenzyme. Co-administration of terbinafine with drugs predominantly metabolized by the CYP450 2D6 isoenzyme should be done with careful monitoring and may require a reduction in dose of the 2D6-metabolized drug).

No products indexed under this heading.

Dexfenfluramine Hydrochloride (Studies have shown that terbinafine is an inhibitor of the CYP450 2D6 isoenzyme. Co-administration of terbinafine with drugs predominantly metabolized by the CYP450 2D6 isoenzyme should be done with careful monitoring and may require a reduction in dose of the 2D6-metabolized drug).

No products indexed under this heading.

Dextromethorphan Hydrobromide (Studies have shown that terbinafine is an inhibitor of the CYP450 2D6 isoenzyme. Co-administration of terbinafine with drugs predominantly metabolized by the CYP450 2D6 isoenzyme should be done with careful monitoring and may require a reduction in dose of the 2D6-metabolized drug). Products include:

- Comtrex Maximum Strength Cold & Cough Day/Night Caplets - Day Formulation ... 726
- Comtrex Maximum Strength Cold & Cough Day/Night Caplets - Night Formulation ... 726
- Comtrex Maximum Strength Non-Drowsy Cold & Cough Caplets ... 725
- Children's Dimetapp DM Cold & Cough Elixir ... 731
- Children's Dimetapp Long Acting Cough Plus Cold Syrup ... 731
- Toddler's Dimetapp Cold and Cough Drops ... 732
- Mucinex DM Extended-Release Bi-Layer Tablets ... 720
- Refenesen DM Caplets ... 721
- Robitussin Cough & Cold CF Liquid ... 735
- Robitussin Cough & Cold Long-Acting Liquid ... 735
- Robitussin Cough & Allergy Syrup ... 736
- Robitussin Cough & Cold Nighttime Liquid ... 736
- Robitussin Cough & Cold Pediatric Drops ... 735
- Robitussin Cough, Cold & Flu Nighttime Liquid ... 738
- Robitussin Cough & Congestion Liquid ... 738
- Robitussin Cough Gels Long-Acting ... 737
- Robitussin Cough Long Acting Liquid ... 739
- Robitussin Cough DM Syrup ... 738
- Robitussin Cough DM Infant Drops ... 738
- Robitussin Pediatric Cough Long Acting Liquid ... 739
- Robitussin Pediatric Cough & Cold Long-Acting Liquid ... 735
- Robitussin Pediatric Cough & Cold Nighttime Liquid ... 736
- Robitussin Sugar Free Cough ... 738
- TheraFlu Cold & Cough Hot Liquid ... 740
- TheraFlu Warming Relief Daytime Severe Cold ... 743
- TheraFlu Thin Strips Long Acting Cough ... 744
- Triaminic Daytime Cold & Cough Liquid ... 745
- Triaminic Cough & Sore Throat Liquid ... 747
- Triaminic Cough & Runny Nose Softchews ... 748
- Triaminic Thin Strips Cold & Cough ... 778
- Triaminic Infant Thin Strips Decongestant Plus Cough ... 747
- Children's Tylenol Plus Flu Oral Suspension ... 749
- Tylenol Cold Head Congestion Daytime Caplets with Cool Burst and Gelcaps ... 750
- Tylenol Cold Multi-Symptom Daytime Liquid ... 752
- Tylenol Cold Multi-Symptom Severe Daytime Liquid ... 752
- Concentrated Tylenol Infants' Drops Plus Cold & Cough ... 754
- Children's Tylenol Plus Cough & Runny Nose Suspension Liquid ... 1879
- Children's Tylenol Plus Cough & Sore Throat Suspension Liquid ... 1879
- Children's Tylenol Plus Flu Suspension Liquid ... 1881
- Children's Tylenol Plus Multi-Symptom Cold Suspension Liquid ... 1879
- Tylenol Cold Severe Congestion Non-Drowsy Caplets with Cool Burst ... 1874
- Tylenol Cold Head Congestion Daytime Caplets with Cool Burst ... 1873
- Tylenol Cold Head Congestion Nighttime Caplets with Cool Burst ... 1873
- Tylenol Cold Head Congestion Severe Caplets with Cool Burst ... 1873
- Tylenol Cold Multi-Symptom Daytime Caplets with Cool Burst and Gelcaps ... 1874
- Tylenol Cold Multi-Symptom Daytime Liquid with Citrus Burst ... 1874
- Tylenol Cold Multi-Symptom Nighttime Caplets with Cool Burst ... 1874
- Tylenol Cold Multi-Symptom Nighttime Liquid with Cool Burst ... 1874
- Tylenol Cold Multi-Symptom Severe Caplets with Cool Burst ... 1874
- Tylenol Cold Multi-Symptom Severe Daytime Liquid with Citrus Burst ... 1874
- Tylenol Cough & Sore Throat Daytime Liquid with Cool Burst ... 1877
- Tylenol Cough & Sore Throat Nighttime Liquid with Cool Burst ... 1877
- Concentrated Tylenol Infants' Drops Plus Cold and Cough ... 1879
- Vicks 44 Cough Relief Liquid ... 2679
- Vicks 44D Cough & Head Congestion Relief Liquid ... 2679
- Vicks 44E Cough & Chest Congestion Relief Liquid ... 2679
- Pediatric Vicks 44e Cough & Chest Congestion Relief Liquid ... 2676
- Vicks 44M Cough, Cold & Flu Relief Liquid ... 2680
- Pediatric Vicks 44m Cough & Cold Relief Liquid ... 2676
- Vicks DayQuil LiquiCaps/Liquid Multi-Symptom Cold/Flu Relief ... 761
- Vicks DayQuil Multi-Symptom Cold/Flu Relief LiquiCaps ... 2678
- Vicks DayQuil Multi-Symptom Cold/Flu Relief Liquid ... 2678
- Vicks NyQuil Multi-Symptom Cold/Flu Relief Liquid ... 2681
- Children's Vicks NyQuil Cold/Cough Relief ... 756
- Vicks NyQuil Multi-Symptom Cold/Flu Relief LiquiCaps ... 2681
- Vicks NyQuil LiquiCaps/Liquid Multi-Symptom Cold/Flu Relief ... 763
- Vicks NyQuil Cough Liquid ... 2680
- Children's Vicks NyQuil Cold/Cough Relief Liquid ... 2680
- Zicam Cough Max Nighttime Cough Spray ... 767
- Zicam Cough Max Cough Spray ... 767
- Zicam Cough Max Cough Melts ... 767
- Zicam Cough Plus D Cough Spray ... 767
- Zicam Cough Relief Cough Spray ... 767
- Zicam Maximum Strength Flu Daytime ... 768
- Zicam Maximum Strength Flu Nighttime ... 768

Dextromethorphan Polistirex (Studies have shown that terbinafine is an inhibitor of the CYP450 2D6 isoenzyme. Co-administration of terbinafine with drugs predominantly metabolized by the CYP450 2D6 isoenzyme should be done with careful monitoring and may require a reduction in dose of the 2D6-metabolized drug). Products include:

- Delsym Extended-Release Suspension 12 Hour Cough Suppressant ... 611

Dolasetron Mesylate (Studies have shown that terbinafine is an inhibitor of the CYP450 2D6 isoenzyme. Co-administration of terbinafine with drugs predominantly metabolized by the CYP450 2D6 isoenzyme should be done with careful monitoring and may require a reduction in dose of the 2D6-metabolized drug). Products include:

Anzemet Injection 2859
Anzemet Tablets 2862

Donepezil Hydrochloride (Studies have shown that terbinafine is an inhibitor of the CYP450 2D6 isoenzyme. Co-administration of terbinafine with drugs predominantly metabolized by the CYP450 2D6 isoenzyme should be done with careful monitoring and may require a reduction in dose of the 2D6-metabolized drug). Products include:

Aricept Tablets 1094
Aricept ODT Tablets 1094

Doxepin Hydrochloride (Studies have shown that terbinafine is an inhibitor of the CYP450 2D6 isoenzyme. Co-administration of terbinafine with drugs predominantly metabolized by the CYP450 2D6 isoenzyme should be done with careful monitoring and may require a reduction in dose of the 2D6-metabolized drug).

No products indexed under this heading.

Encainide Hydrochloride (Studies have shown that terbinafine is an inhibitor of the CYP450 2D6 isoenzyme. Co-administration of terbinafine with drugs predominantly metabolized by the CYP450 2D6 isoenzyme should be done with careful monitoring and may require a reduction in dose of the 2D6-metabolized drug).

No products indexed under this heading.

Escitalopram Oxalate (Studies have shown that terbinafine is an inhibitor of the CYP450 2D6 isoenzyme. Co-administration of terbinafine with drugs predominantly metabolized by the CYP450 2D6 isoenzyme should be done with careful monitoring and may require a reduction in dose of the 2D6-metabolized drug). Products include:

Lexapro Oral Solution 1190
Lexapro Tablets 1190

Esmolol Hydrochloride (Studies have shown that terbinafine is an inhibitor of the CYP450 2D6 isoenzyme. Co-administration of terbinafine with drugs predominantly metabolized by the CYP450 2D6 isoenzyme should be done with careful monitoring and may require a reduction in dose of the 2D6-metabolized drug).

No products indexed under this heading.

Fentanyl (Studies have shown that terbinafine is an inhibitor of the CYP450 2D6 isoenzyme. Co-administration of terbinafine with drugs predominantly metabolized by the CYP450 2D6 isoenzyme should be done with careful monitoring and may require a reduction in dose of the 2D6-metabolized drug). Products include:

Duragesic Transdermal System 2373
Ionsys Transdermal System 2379

Fentanyl Citrate (Studies have shown that terbinafine is an inhibitor of the CYP450 2D6 isoenzyme. Co-administration of terbinafine with drugs predominantly metabolized by the CYP450 2D6 isoenzyme should be done with careful monitoring and may require a reduction in dose of the 2D6-metabolized drug). Products include:

Actiq 979

Flecainide Acetate (Studies have shown that terbinafine is an inhibitor of the CYP450 2D6 isoenzyme. Co-administration of terbinafine with drugs predominantly metabolized by the CYP450 2D6 isoenzyme should be done with careful monitoring and may require a reduction in dose of the 2D6-metabolized drug). Products include:

Tambocor Tablets 1856

Fluoxetine (Studies have shown that terbinafine is an inhibitor of the CYP450 2D6 isoenzyme. Co-administration of terbinafine with drugs predominantly metabolized by the CYP450 2D6 isoenzyme should be done with careful monitoring and may require a reduction in dose of the 2D6-metabolized drug).

No products indexed under this heading.

Fluoxetine Hydrochloride (Studies have shown that terbinafine is an inhibitor of the CYP450 2D6 isoenzyme. Co-administration of terbinafine with drugs predominantly metabolized by the CYP450 2D6 isoenzyme should be done with careful monitoring and may require a reduction in dose of the 2D6-metabolized drug). Products include:

Prozac Pulvules and Liquid 1801
Symbyax Capsules 1819

Fluphenazine Decanoate (Studies have shown that terbinafine is an inhibitor of the CYP450 2D6 isoenzyme. Co-administration of terbinafine with drugs predominantly metabolized by the CYP450 2D6 isoenzyme should be done with careful monitoring and may require a reduction in dose of the 2D6-metabolized drug).

No products indexed under this heading.

Fluphenazine Enanthate (Studies have shown that terbinafine is an inhibitor of the CYP450 2D6 isoenzyme. Co-administration of terbinafine with drugs predominantly metabolized by the CYP450 2D6 isoenzyme should be done with careful monitoring and may require a reduction in dose of the 2D6-metabolized drug).

No products indexed under this heading.

Fluphenazine Hydrochloride (Studies have shown that terbinafine is an inhibitor of the CYP450 2D6 isoenzyme. Co-administration of terbinafine with drugs predominantly metabolized by the CYP450 2D6 isoenzyme should be done with careful monitoring and may require a reduction in dose of the 2D6-metabolized drug).

No products indexed under this heading.

Fluvoxamine Maleate (Studies have shown that terbinafine is an inhibitor of the CYP450 2D6 isoenzyme. Co-administration of terbinafine with drugs predominantly metabolized by the CYP450 2D6 isoenzyme should be done with careful monitoring and may require a reduction in dose of the 2D6-metabolized drug).

No products indexed under this heading.

Formoterol Fumarate (Studies have shown that terbinafine is an inhibitor of the CYP450 2D6 isoenzyme. Co-administration of terbinafine with drugs predominantly metabolized by the CYP450 2D6 isoenzyme should be done with careful monitoring and may require a reduction in dose of the 2D6-metabolized drug). Products include:

Foradil Aerolizer 3010

Galantamine Hydrobromide (Studies have shown that terbinafine is an inhibitor of the CYP450 2D6 isoenzyme. Co-administration of terbinafine with drugs predominantly metabolized by the CYP450 2D6 isoenzyme should be done with careful monitoring and may require a reduction in dose of the 2D6-metabolized drug). Products include:

Razadyne 2399
Razadyne ER Extended-Release Capsules 2399

Haloperidol (Studies have shown that terbinafine is an inhibitor of the CYP450 2D6 isoenzyme. Co-administration of terbinafine with drugs predominantly metabolized by the CYP450 2D6 isoenzyme should be done with careful monitoring and may require a reduction in dose of the 2D6-metabolized drug).

No products indexed under this heading.

Haloperidol Decanoate (Studies have shown that terbinafine is an inhibitor of the CYP450 2D6 isoenzyme. Co-administration of terbinafine with drugs predominantly metabolized by the CYP450 2D6 isoenzyme should be done with careful monitoring and may require a reduction in dose of the 2D6-metabolized drug).

No products indexed under this heading.

Hydrocodone Bitartrate (Studies have shown that terbinafine is an inhibitor of the CYP450 2D6 isoenzyme. Co-administration of terbinafine with drugs predominantly metabolized by the CYP450 2D6 isoenzyme should be done with careful monitoring and may require a reduction in dose of the 2D6-metabolized drug). Products include:

Hycodan 1116
Hycotuss Expectorant Syrup 1117
Vicodin Tablets 535
Vicodin ES Tablets 536
Vicodin HP Tablets 538
Vicoprofen Tablets 539
Zydone Tablets 1139

Imipramine Hydrochloride (Studies have shown that terbinafine is an inhibitor of the CYP450 2D6 isoenzyme. Co-administration of terbinafine with drugs predominantly metabolized by the CYP450 2D6 isoenzyme should be done with careful monitoring and may require a reduction in dose of the 2D6-metabolized drug).

No products indexed under this heading.

Imipramine Pamoate (Studies have shown that terbinafine is an inhibitor of the CYP450 2D6 isoenzyme. Co-administration of terbinafine with drugs predominantly metabolized by the CYP450 2D6 isoenzyme should be done with careful monitoring and may require a reduction in dose of the 2D6-metabolized drug).

No products indexed under this heading.

Indoramin Hydrochloride (Studies have shown that terbinafine is an inhibitor of the CYP450 2D6 isoenzyme. Co-administration of terbinafine with drugs predominantly metabolized by the CYP450 2D6 isoenzyme should be done with careful monitoring and may require a reduction in dose of the 2D6-metabolized drug).

No products indexed under this heading.

Isocarboxazid (Studies have shown that terbinafine is an inhibitor of the CYP450 2D6 isoenzyme. Co-administration of terbinafine with drugs predominantly metabolized by the CYP450 2D6 isoenzyme should be done with careful monitoring and may require a reduction in dose of the 2D6-metabolized drug).

No products indexed under this heading.

Labetalol Hydrochloride (Studies have shown that terbinafine is an inhibitor of the CYP450 2D6 isoenzyme. Co-administration of terbinafine with drugs predominantly metabolized by the CYP450 2D6 isoenzyme should be done with careful monitoring and may require a reduction in dose of the 2D6-metabolized drug).

No products indexed under this heading.

Levobunolol Hydrochloride (Studies have shown that terbinafine is an inhibitor of the CYP450 2D6 isoenzyme. Co-administration of terbinafine with drugs predominantly metabolized by the CYP450 2D6 isoenzyme should be done with careful monitoring and may require a reduction in dose of the 2D6-metabolized drug). Products include:

Betagan Ophthalmic Solution, USP .... ⊙220

Lidocaine (Studies have shown that terbinafine is an inhibitor of the CYP450 2D6 isoenzyme. Co-administration of terbinafine with drugs predominantly metabolized by the CYP450 2D6 isoenzyme should be done with careful monitoring and may require a reduction in dose of the 2D6-metabolized drug). Products include:

Lidoderm Patch 1118
Synera Topical Patch 1137

Lidocaine Hydrochloride (Studies have shown that terbinafine is an inhibitor of the CYP450 2D6 isoenzyme. Co-administration of terbinafine with drugs predominantly metabolized by the CYP450 2D6 isoenzyme should be done with careful monitoring and may require a reduction in dose of the 2D6-metabolized drug).
No products indexed under this heading.

Maprotiline Hydrochloride (Studies have shown that terbinafine is an inhibitor of the CYP450 2D6 isoenzyme. Co-administration of terbinafine with drugs predominantly metabolized by the CYP450 2D6 isoenzyme should be done with careful monitoring and may require a reduction in dose of the 2D6-metabolized drug).
No products indexed under this heading.

Meperidine Hydrochloride (Studies have shown that terbinafine is an inhibitor of the CYP450 2D6 isoenzyme. Co-administration of terbinafine with drugs predominantly metabolized by the CYP450 2D6 isoenzyme should be done with careful monitoring and may require a reduction in dose of the 2D6-metabolized drug).
No products indexed under this heading.

Methadone Hydrochloride (Studies have shown that terbinafine is an inhibitor of the CYP450 2D6 isoenzyme. Co-administration of terbinafine with drugs predominantly metabolized by the CYP450 2D6 isoenzyme should be done with careful monitoring and may require a reduction in dose of the 2D6-metabolized drug).
No products indexed under this heading.

Methamphetamine Hydrochloride (Studies have shown that terbinafine is an inhibitor of the CYP450 2D6 isoenzyme. Co-administration of terbinafine with drugs predominantly metabolized by the CYP450 2D6 isoenzyme should be done with careful monitoring and may require a reduction in dose of the 2D6-metabolized drug). Products include:
Desoxyn Tablets, USP 2462

Metipranolol Hydrochloride (Studies have shown that terbinafine is an inhibitor of the CYP450 2D6 isoenzyme. Co-administration of terbinafine with drugs predominantly metabolized by the CYP450 2D6 isoenzyme should be done with careful monitoring and may require a reduction in dose of the 2D6-metabolized drug).
No products indexed under this heading.

Metoprolol Succinate (Studies have shown that terbinafine is an inhibitor of the CYP450 2D6 isoenzyme. Co-administration of terbinafine with drugs predominantly metabolized by the CYP450 2D6 isoenzyme should be done with careful monitoring and may require a reduction in dose of the 2D6-metabolized drug). Products include:
Toprol-XL Tablets 668

Metoprolol Tartrate (Studies have shown that terbinafine is an inhibitor of the CYP450 2D6 isoenzyme. Co-administration of terbinafine with drugs predominantly metabolized by the CYP450 2D6 isoenzyme should be done with careful monitoring and may require a reduction in dose of the 2D6-metabolized drug). Products include:
Lopressor Injection 2238
Lopressor Tablets 2238
Lopressor HCT 50/25 Tablets 2241
Lopressor HCT 100/25 Tablets 2241
Lopressor HCT 100/50 Tablets 2241

Mexiletine Hydrochloride (Studies have shown that terbinafine is an inhibitor of the CYP450 2D6 isoenzyme. Co-administration of terbinafine with drugs predominantly metabolized by the CYP450 2D6 isoenzyme should be done with careful monitoring and may require a reduction in dose of the 2D6-metabolized drug).
No products indexed under this heading.

Mirtazapine (Studies have shown that terbinafine is an inhibitor of the CYP450 2D6 isoenzyme. Co-administration of terbinafine with drugs predominantly metabolized by the CYP450 2D6 isoenzyme should be done with careful monitoring and may require a reduction in dose of the 2D6-metabolized drug).
No products indexed under this heading.

Moclobemide (Studies have shown that terbinafine is an inhibitor of the CYP450 2D6 isoenzyme. Co-administration of terbinafine with drugs predominantly metabolized by the CYP450 2D6 isoenzyme should be done with careful monitoring and may require a reduction in dose of the 2D6-metabolized drug).
No products indexed under this heading.

Morphine Sulfate (Studies have shown that terbinafine is an inhibitor of the CYP450 2D6 isoenzyme. Co-administration of terbinafine with drugs predominantly metabolized by the CYP450 2D6 isoenzyme should be done with careful monitoring and may require a reduction in dose of the 2D6-metabolized drug). Products include:
Avinza Capsules 1741
Kadian Capsules 577
MS Contin Tablets 2701

Nadolol (Studies have shown that terbinafine is an inhibitor of the CYP450 2D6 isoenzyme. Co-administration of terbinafine with drugs predominantly metabolized by the CYP450 2D6 isoenzyme should be done with careful monitoring and may require a reduction in dose of the 2D6-metabolized drug). Products include:
Nadolol Tablets 2159

Nelfinavir Mesylate (Studies have shown that terbinafine is an inhibitor of the CYP450 2D6 isoenzyme. Co-administration of terbinafine with drugs predominantly metabolized by the CYP450 2D6 isoenzyme should be done with careful monitoring and may require a reduction in dose of the 2D6-metabolized drug). Products include:
Viracept 2577

Nortriptyline Hydrochloride (Studies have shown that terbinafine is an inhibitor of the CYP450 2D6 isoenzyme. Co-administration of terbinafine with drugs predominantly metabolized by the CYP450 2D6 isoenzyme should be done with careful monitoring and may require a reduction in dose of the 2D6-metabolized drug).
No products indexed under this heading.

Olanzapine (Studies have shown that terbinafine is an inhibitor of the CYP450 2D6 isoenzyme. Co-administration of terbinafine with drugs predominantly metabolized by the CYP450 2D6 isoenzyme should be done with careful monitoring and may require a reduction in dose of the 2D6-metabolized drug). Products include:
Symbyax Capsules 1819
Zyprexa Tablets 1830
Zyprexa IntraMuscular 1830
Zyprexa ZYDIS Orally Disintegrating Tablets 1830

Omeprazole (Studies have shown that terbinafine is an inhibitor of the CYP450 2D6 isoenzyme. Co-administration of terbinafine with drugs predominantly metabolized by the CYP450 2D6 isoenzyme should be done with careful monitoring and may require a reduction in dose of the 2D6-metabolized drug). Products include:
Zegerid Capsules 2958
Zegerid Powder for Oral Solution 2958

Ondansetron (Studies have shown that terbinafine is an inhibitor of the CYP450 2D6 isoenzyme. Co-administration of terbinafine with drugs predominantly metabolized by the CYP450 2D6 isoenzyme should be done with careful monitoring and may require a reduction in dose of the 2D6-metabolized drug). Products include:
Zofran ODT Orally Disintegrating Tablets 1639

Ondansetron Hydrochloride (Studies have shown that terbinafine is an inhibitor of the CYP450 2D6 isoenzyme. Co-administration of terbinafine with drugs predominantly metabolized by the CYP450 2D6 isoenzyme should be done with careful monitoring and may require a reduction in dose of the 2D6-metabolized drug). Products include:
Zofran Injection 1634
Zofran 1639

Oxycodone Hydrochloride (Studies have shown that terbinafine is an inhibitor of the CYP450 2D6 isoenzyme. Co-administration of terbinafine with drugs predominantly metabolized by the CYP450 2D6 isoenzyme should be done with careful monitoring and may require a reduction in dose of the 2D6-metabolized drug). Products include:
OxyContin Tablets 2703
OxyFast Oral Concentrate Solution 2708
OxyIR Capsules 2708
Percocet Tablets 1131
Percodan Tablets 1132

Paclitaxel (Studies have shown that terbinafine is an inhibitor of the CYP450 2D6 isoenzyme. Co-administration of terbinafine with drugs predominantly metabolized by the CYP450 2D6 isoenzyme should be done with careful monitoring and may require a reduction in dose of the 2D6-metabolized drug).
No products indexed under this heading.

Pargyline Hydrochloride (Studies have shown that terbinafine is an inhibitor of the CYP450 2D6 isoenzyme. Co-administration of terbinafine with drugs predominantly metabolized by the CYP450 2D6 isoenzyme should be done with careful monitoring and may require a reduction in dose of the 2D6-metabolized drug).
No products indexed under this heading.

Paroxetine Hydrochloride (Studies have shown that terbinafine is an inhibitor of the CYP450 2D6 isoenzyme. Co-administration of terbinafine with drugs predominantly metabolized by the CYP450 2D6 isoenzyme should be done with careful monitoring and may require a reduction in dose of the 2D6-metabolized drug). Products include:
Paxil CR Controlled-Release Tablets 1538
Paxil 1530

Penbutolol Sulfate (Studies have shown that terbinafine is an inhibitor of the CYP450 2D6 isoenzyme. Co-administration of terbinafine with drugs predominantly metabolized by the CYP450 2D6 isoenzyme should be done with careful monitoring and may require a reduction in dose of the 2D6-metabolized drug).
No products indexed under this heading.

Phenelzine Sulfate (Studies have shown that terbinafine is an inhibitor of the CYP450 2D6 isoenzyme. Co-administration of terbinafine with drugs predominantly metabolized by the CYP450 2D6 isoenzyme should be done with careful monitoring and may require a reduction in dose of the 2D6-metabolized drug).
No products indexed under this heading.

Pindolol (Studies have shown that terbinafine is an inhibitor of the CYP450 2D6 isoenzyme. Co-administration of terbinafine with drugs predominantly metabolized by the CYP450 2D6 isoenzyme should be done with careful monitoring and may require a reduction in dose of the 2D6-metabolized drug).
No products indexed under this heading.

Procarbazine Hydrochloride (Studies have shown that terbinafine is an inhibitor of the CYP450 2D6 isoenzyme. Co-administration of terbinafine with drugs predominantly metabolized by the CYP450 2D6 isoenzyme should be done with careful monitoring and may require a reduction in dose of the 2D6-metabolized drug). Products include:
Matulane Capsules 3191

Propafenone Hydrochloride (Studies have shown that terbinafine is an inhibitor of the CYP450 2D6 isoenzyme. Co-administration of terbinafine with drugs predominantly

metabolized by the CYP450 2D6 isoenzyme should be done with careful monitoring and may require a reduction in dose of the 2D6-metabolized drug). Products include:

Propoxyphene Hydrochloride (Studies have shown that terbinafine is an inhibitor of the CYP450 2D6 isoenzyme. Co-administration of terbinafine with drugs predominantly metabolized by the CYP450 2D6 isoenzyme should be done with careful monitoring and may require a reduction in dose of the 2D6-metabolized drug).

 No products indexed under this heading.

Propoxyphene Napsylate (Studies have shown that terbinafine is an inhibitor of the CYP450 2D6 isoenzyme. Co-administration of terbinafine with drugs predominantly metabolized by the CYP450 2D6 isoenzyme should be done with careful monitoring and may require a reduction in dose of the 2D6-metabolized drug).

 No products indexed under this heading.

Propranolol Hydrochloride (Studies have shown that terbinafine is an inhibitor of the CYP450 2D6 isoenzyme. Co-administration of terbinafine with drugs predominantly metabolized by the CYP450 2D6 isoenzyme should be done with careful monitoring and may require a reduction in dose of the 2D6-metabolized drug). Products include:

Protriptyline Hydrochloride (Studies have shown that terbinafine is an inhibitor of the CYP450 2D6 isoenzyme. Co-administration of terbinafine with drugs predominantly metabolized by the CYP450 2D6 isoenzyme should be done with careful monitoring and may require a reduction in dose of the 2D6-metabolized drug).

 No products indexed under this heading.

Quetiapine Fumarate (Studies have shown that terbinafine is an inhibitor of the CYP450 2D6 isoenzyme. Co-administration of terbinafine with drugs predominantly metabolized by the CYP450 2D6 isoenzyme should be done with careful monitoring and may require a reduction in dose of the 2D6-metabolized drug). Products include:

Quinidine Gluconate (Studies have shown that terbinafine is an inhibitor of the CYP450 2D6 isoenzyme. Co-administration of terbinafine with drugs predominantly metabolized by the CYP450 2D6 isoenzyme should be done with careful monitoring and may require a reduction in dose of the 2D6-metabolized drug).

 No products indexed under this heading.

Quinidine Hydrochloride (Studies have shown that terbinafine is an inhibitor of the CYP450 2D6 isoenzyme. Co-administration of terbinafine with drugs predominantly metabolized by the CYP450 2D6 isoenzyme should be done with careful monitoring and may require a reduction in dose of the 2D6-metabolized drug).

 No products indexed under this heading.

Quinidine Polygalacturonate (Studies have shown that terbinafine is an inhibitor of the CYP450 2D6 isoenzyme. Co-administration of terbinafine with drugs predominantly metabolized by the CYP450 2D6 isoenzyme should be done with careful monitoring and may require a reduction in dose of the 2D6-metabolized drug).

 No products indexed under this heading.

Quinidine Sulfate (Studies have shown that terbinafine is an inhibitor of the CYP450 2D6 isoenzyme. Co-administration of terbinafine with drugs predominantly metabolized by the CYP450 2D6 isoenzyme should be done with careful monitoring and may require a reduction in dose of the 2D6-metabolized drug).

 No products indexed under this heading.

Rifampin (Terbinafine clearance is increased 100% by rifampin, a CYP450 enzyme inducer).

 No products indexed under this heading.

Risperidone (Studies have shown that terbinafine is an inhibitor of the CYP450 2D6 isoenzyme. Co-administration of terbinafine with drugs predominantly metabolized by the CYP450 2D6 isoenzyme should be done with careful monitoring and may require a reduction in dose of the 2D6-metabolized drug). Products include:

Ritonavir (Studies have shown that terbinafine is an inhibitor of the CYP450 2D6 isoenzyme. Co-administration of terbinafine with drugs predominantly metabolized by the CYP450 2D6 isoenzyme should be done with careful monitoring and may require a reduction in dose of the 2D6-metabolized drug). Products include:

Selegiline Hydrochloride (In vitro studies show that terbinafine inhibits CYP2D6 mediated metabolism; this may be of clinical relevance for compounds predominantly metabolized by this enzyme, such as type B MAO inhibitor, if they have a narrow therapeutic window). Products include:

Sertraline Hydrochloride (Studies have shown that terbinafine is an inhibitor of the CYP450 2D6 isoenzyme. Co-administration of terbinafine with drugs predominantly metabolized by the CYP450 2D6 isoenzyme should be done with careful monitoring and may require a

reduction in dose of the 2D6-metabolized drug). Products include:

Sotalol Hydrochloride (Studies have shown that terbinafine is an inhibitor of the CYP450 2D6 isoenzyme. Co-administration of terbinafine with drugs predominantly metabolized by the CYP450 2D6 isoenzyme should be done with careful monitoring and may require a reduction in dose of the 2D6-metabolized drug).

 No products indexed under this heading.

Tamoxifen Citrate (Studies have shown that terbinafine is an inhibitor of the CYP450 2D6 isoenzyme. Co-administration of terbinafine with drugs predominantly metabolized by the CYP450 2D6 isoenzyme should be done with careful monitoring and may require a reduction in dose of the 2D6-metabolized drug). Products include:

Teniposide (Studies have shown that terbinafine is an inhibitor of the CYP450 2D6 isoenzyme. Co-administration of terbinafine with drugs predominantly metabolized by the CYP450 2D6 isoenzyme should be done with careful monitoring and may require a reduction in dose of the 2D6-metabolized drug).

 No products indexed under this heading.

Terfenadine (Terbinafine clearance is decreased 16% by terfenadine).

 No products indexed under this heading.

Testosterone (Studies have shown that terbinafine is an inhibitor of the CYP450 2D6 isoenzyme. Co-administration of terbinafine with drugs predominantly metabolized by the CYP450 2D6 isoenzyme should be done with careful monitoring and may require a reduction in dose of the 2D6-metabolized drug). Products include:

Testosterone Cypionate (Studies have shown that terbinafine is an inhibitor of the CYP450 2D6 isoenzyme. Co-administration of terbinafine with drugs predominantly metabolized by the CYP450 2D6 isoenzyme should be done with careful monitoring and may require a reduction in dose of the 2D6-metabolized drug).

 No products indexed under this heading.

Testosterone Enanthate (Studies have shown that terbinafine is an inhibitor of the CYP450 2D6 isoenzyme. Co-administration of terbinafine with drugs predominantly metabolized by the CYP450 2D6 isoenzyme should be done with careful monitoring and may require a reduction in dose of the 2D6-metabolized drug).

 No products indexed under this heading.

Testosterone Propionate (Studies have shown that terbinafine is an inhibitor of the CYP450 2D6 isoenzyme. Co-administration of terbinafine with drugs predominantly metabolized by the CYP450 2D6 isoenzyme should be done with careful monitoring and may require a reduction in dose of the 2D6-metabolized drug).

 No products indexed under this heading.

Thioridazine (Studies have shown that terbinafine is an inhibitor of the CYP450 2D6 isoenzyme. Co-administration of terbinafine with drugs predominantly metabolized by the CYP450 2D6 isoenzyme should be done with careful monitoring and may require a reduction in dose of the 2D6-metabolized drug).

 No products indexed under this heading.

Thioridazine Hydrochloride (Studies have shown that terbinafine is an inhibitor of the CYP450 2D6 isoenzyme. Co-administration of terbinafine with drugs predominantly metabolized by the CYP450 2D6 isoenzyme should be done with careful monitoring and may require a reduction in dose of the 2D6-metabolized drug). Products include:

Timolol Hemihydrate (Studies have shown that terbinafine is an inhibitor of the CYP450 2D6 isoenzyme. Co-administration of terbinafine with drugs predominantly metabolized by the CYP450 2D6 isoenzyme should be done with careful monitoring and may require a reduction in dose of the 2D6-metabolized drug). Products include:

Timolol Maleate (Studies have shown that terbinafine is an inhibitor of the CYP450 2D6 isoenzyme. Co-administration of terbinafine with drugs predominantly metabolized by the CYP450 2D6 isoenzyme should be done with careful monitoring and may require a reduction in dose of the 2D6-metabolized drug). Products include:

Tolterodine Tartrate (Studies have shown that terbinafine is an inhibitor of the CYP450 2D6 isoenzyme. Co-administration of terbinafine with drugs predominantly metabolized by the CYP450 2D6 isoenzyme should be done with careful monitoring and may require a reduction in dose of the 2D6-metabolized drug). Products include:

Tramadol Hydrochloride (Studies have shown that terbinafine is an inhibitor of the CYP450 2D6 isoenzyme. Co-administration of terbinafine with drugs predominantly metabolized by the CYP450 2D6 isoenzyme should be done with careful monitoring and may require a reduction in dose of the 2D6-metabolized drug). Products include:

Ultram ER Tablets 2392

Tranylcypromine Sulfate (Studies have shown that terbinafine is an inhibitor of the CYP450 2D6 isoenzyme. Co-administration of terbinafine with drugs predominantly metabolized by the CYP450 2D6 isoenzyme should be done with careful monitoring and may require a reduction in dose of the 2D6-metabolized drug). Products include:

Parnate Tablets 1527

Trazodone Hydrochloride (Studies have shown that terbinafine is an inhibitor of the CYP450 2D6 isoenzyme. Co-administration of terbinafine with drugs predominantly metabolized by the CYP450 2D6 isoenzyme should be done with careful monitoring and may require a reduction in dose of the 2D6-metabolized drug).

No products indexed under this heading.

Triazolam (Studies have shown that terbinafine is an inhibitor of the CYP450 2D6 isoenzyme. Co-administration of terbinafine with drugs predominantly metabolized by the CYP450 2D6 isoenzyme should be done with careful monitoring and may require a reduction in dose of the 2D6-metabolized drug).

No products indexed under this heading.

Trimipramine Maleate (Studies have shown that terbinafine is an inhibitor of the CYP450 2D6 isoenzyme. Co-administration of terbinafine with drugs predominantly metabolized by the CYP450 2D6 isoenzyme should be done with careful monitoring and may require a reduction in dose of the 2D6-metabolized drug).

No products indexed under this heading.

Venlafaxine Hydrochloride (Studies have shown that terbinafine is an inhibitor of the CYP450 2D6 isoenzyme. Co-administration of terbinafine with drugs predominantly metabolized by the CYP450 2D6 isoenzyme should be done with careful monitoring and may require a reduction in dose of the 2D6-metabolized drug). Products include:

Effexor Tablets 3411
Effexor XR Capsules 3417

Vinblastine Sulfate (Studies have shown that terbinafine is an inhibitor of the CYP450 2D6 isoenzyme. Co-administration of terbinafine with drugs predominantly metabolized by the CYP450 2D6 isoenzyme should be done with careful monitoring and may require a reduction in dose of the 2D6-metabolized drug).

No products indexed under this heading.

Warfarin Sodium (Co-administration has resulted in altered prothrombin time (prolongation and reduction)). Products include:

Coumadin for Injection 898
Coumadin Tablets 898

Zonisamide (Studies have shown that terbinafine is an inhibitor of the CYP450 2D6 isoenzyme. Co-administration of terbinafine with drugs predominantly metabolized by the CYP450 2D6 isoenzyme should be done with careful monitoring and may require a reduction in dose of the 2D6-metabolized drug). Products include:

Zonegran Capsules 1101

Food Interactions

Food, unspecified (Co-administration has resulted in an increase in the AUC of terbinafine of less than 20%).

LAMISIL AT CREAMS (ATHLETE'S FOOT & JOCK ITCH)

(Terbinafine Hydrochloride) 636
None cited in PDR database.

LAMISIL AF DEFENSE POWDERS (SHAKE & SPRAY)

(Tolnaftate) 636
None cited in PDR database.

LANOXICAPS CAPSULES

(Digoxin) 1490
See Lanoxin Tablets

LANOXIN INJECTION

(Digoxin) 1494
See Lanoxin Tablets

LANOXIN INJECTION PEDIATRIC

(Digoxin) 1497
See Lanoxin Tablets

LANOXIN TABLETS

(Digoxin) 1500

May interact with antacids, beta blockers, calcium channel blockers, corticosteroids, erythromycin, macrolide antibiotics, potassium-depleting diuretics, quinidine, sympathomimetics, tetracyclines, thyroid preparations, and certain other agents. Compounds in these categories include:

Acebutolol Hydrochloride (Concomitant use of digoxin and beta-andrenergic blockers may result in the additive effects on AV node conduction).

No products indexed under this heading.

Albuterol (Concomitant use of digoxin and sympathomimetics increases the risk of cardiac arrhythmias). Products include:

Proventil Inhalation Aerosol 3053

Albuterol Sulfate (Concomitant use of digoxin and sympathomimetics increases the risk of cardiac arrhythmias). Products include:

AccuNeb Inhalation Solution 1055
Combivent Inhalation Aerosol 847
DuoNeb Inhalation Solution 1058
ProAir HFA Inhalation Aerosol 3300
Proventil Inhalation Solution 0.083%.. 3055
Proventil HFA Inhalation Aerosol 3056
Ventolin HFA Inhalation Aerosol 1600
VoSpire ER Tablets 1052

Alprazolam (Raises the serum digoxin concentration due to reduction in clearance and/or volume of distribution of the drug, with the implication that digitalis intoxication may result). Products include:

Niravam Orally Disintegrating Tablets 3092

Aluminum Carbonate (Antacids may interfere with intestinal digoxin absorption, resulting in unexpectedly low serum concentrations; antacids may cause hypokalemia or hypomagnesemia and co-administration can cause digitalis toxicity).

No products indexed under this heading.

Aluminum Hydroxide (Antacids may interfere with intestinal digoxin absorption, resulting in unexpectedly low serum concentrations; antacids may cause hypokalemia or hypomagnesemia and co-administration can cause digitalis toxicity). Products include:

Gaviscon Regular Strength Liquid .. 658
Gaviscon Regular Strength Tablets....................................... 658
Gaviscon Extra Strength Liquid 658
Gaviscon Extra Strength Tablets 658
Maalox Regular Strength Antacid/Antigas Liquid................. 2175
Maalox Max Maximum Strength Antacid/Anti-Gas Liquid................ 2176

Amiodarone Hydrochloride (Raises the serum digoxin concentration due to reduction in clearance and/or volume of distribution of the drug, with the implication that digitalis intoxication may result).

No products indexed under this heading.

Amlodipine Besylate (Concomitant use of digoxin and calcium channel blockers may result in the additive effects on AV node conduction). Products include:

Caduet Tablets 2508
Lotrel Capsules 2249
Norvasc Tablets 2545

Amphotericin B (Can cause hypokalemia or hypomagnesemia and potassium or magnesium depletion can sensitize the myocardium to digoxin resulting in digitails toxicity).

No products indexed under this heading.

Anticancer Drugs, unspecified (May interfere with intestinal digoxin absorption, resulting in unexpectedly low serum concentrations).

No products indexed under this heading.

Atenolol (Concomitant use of digoxin and beta-andrenergic blockers may result in the additive effects on AV node conduction).

No products indexed under this heading.

Azithromycin Dihydrate (Macrolide antibiotics may possibly increase digoxin absorption in patients who inactivate digoxin by bacterial metabolism in the lower intestine, so that digitalis intoxication may result).

No products indexed under this heading.

Bendroflumethiazide (Potassium-depleting diuretics can cause hypokalemia and co-administration can result in digitalis toxicity).

No products indexed under this heading.

Bepridil Hydrochloride (Concomitant use of digoxin and calcium channel blockers may result in the additive effects on AV node conduction).

No products indexed under this heading.

Betamethasone Acetate (Corticosteroids can cause hypokalemia or hypomagnesemia and potassium or magnesium depletion can sensitize the myocardium to digoxin resulting in digitalis toxicity).

No products indexed under this heading.

Betamethasone Sodium Phosphate (Corticosteroids can cause hypokalemia or hypomagnesemia and potassium or magnesium depletion can sensitize the myocardium to digoxin resulting in digitalis toxicity).

No products indexed under this heading.

Betaxolol Hydrochloride (Concomitant use of digoxin and beta-andrenergic blockers may result in the additive effects on AV node conduction). Products include:

Betoptic S Ophthalmic Suspension.................................. 558

Bisoprolol Fumarate (Concomitant use of digoxin and beta-andrenergic blockers may result in the additive effects on AV node conduction).

No products indexed under this heading.

Bumetanide (Potassium-depleting diuretics can cause hypokalemia and co-administration can result in digitalis toxicity). Products include:

Bumex Tablets 2746

Calcium, intravenous (Co-administration with calcium, particularly if administered rapidly by the intravenous route may produce serious arrhythmias in digitalized patients).

No products indexed under this heading.

Carteolol Hydrochloride (Concomitant use of digoxin and beta-andrenergic blockers may result in the additive effects on AV node conduction). Products include:

Carteolol Hydrochloride Ophthalmic Solution USP, 1%....... ⊙249

Chlorothiazide (Potassium-depleting diuretics can cause hypokalemia and co-administration can result in digitalis toxicity). Products include:

Diuril Oral Suspension 1954

Chlorothiazide Sodium (Potassium-depleting diuretics can cause hypokalemia and co-administration can result in digitalis toxicity). Products include:

Diuril Sodium Intravenous 2467

Cholestyramine (May interfere with intestinal digoxin absorption, resulting in unexpectedly low serum concentrations).

No products indexed under this heading.

Clarithromycin (May increase digoxin absorption in patients who inactivate digoxin by bacterial metabolism in the lower intestine, so that digitalis intoxication may result). Products include:

Biaxin/Biaxin XL 402
PREVPAC 3284

Cortisone Acetate (Corticosteroids can cause hypokalemia or hypomagnesemia and potassium or magnesium depletion can sensitize the myocardium to digoxin resulting in digitalis toxicity).

No products indexed under this heading.

Demeclocycline Hydrochloride (May increase digoxin absorption in patients who inactivate digoxin by bacterial metabolism in the lower intestine, so that digitalis intoxication may result).
No products indexed under this heading.

Dexamethasone (Corticosteroids can cause hypokalemia or hypomagnesemia and potassium or magnesium depletion can sensitize the myocardium to digoxin resulting in digitalis toxicity). Products include:
Ciprodex Otic Suspension 559
Decadron Tablets 1951
TobraDex Ophthalmic Ointment 562
TobraDex Ophthalmic Suspension 563

Dexamethasone Acetate (Corticosteroids can cause hypokalemia or hypomagnesemia and potassium or magnesium depletion can sensitize the myocardium to digoxin resulting in digitalis toxicity).
No products indexed under this heading.

Dexamethasone Sodium Phosphate (Corticosteroids can cause hypokalemia or hypomagnesemia and potassium or magnesium depletion can sensitize the myocardium to digoxin resulting in digitalis toxicity).
No products indexed under this heading.

Diltiazem Hydrochloride (Concomitant use of digoxin and calcium channel blockers may result in the additive effects on AV node conduction). Products include:
Cardizem LA Extended Release Tablets 1728
Tiazac Capsules 1201

Diphenoxylate Hydrochloride (Decreases gut motility and may increase digoxin absorption).
No products indexed under this heading.

Dirithromycin (Macrolide antibiotics may possibly increase digoxin absorption in patients who inactivate digoxin by bacterial metabolism in the lower intestine, so that digitalis intoxication may result).
No products indexed under this heading.

Dobutamine Hydrochloride (Concomitant use of digoxin and sympathomimetics increases the risk of cardiac arrhythmias).
No products indexed under this heading.

Dopamine Hydrochloride (Concomitant use of digoxin and sympathomimetics increases the risk of cardiac arrhythmias).
No products indexed under this heading.

Doxycycline Calcium (May increase digoxin absorption in patients who inactivate digoxin by bacterial metabolism in the lower intestine, so that digitalis intoxication may result).
No products indexed under this heading.

Doxycycline Hyclate (May increase digoxin absorption in patients who inactivate digoxin by bacterial metabolism in the lower intestine, so that digitalis intoxication may result).
No products indexed under this heading.

Doxycycline Monohydrate (May increase digoxin absorption in patients who inactivate digoxin by bacterial metabolism in the lower intestine, so that digitalis intoxication may result). Products include:
Oracea Capsules 1000

Ephedrine Hydrochloride (Concomitant use of digoxin and sympathomimetics increases the risk of cardiac arrhythmias).
No products indexed under this heading.

Ephedrine Sulfate (Concomitant use of digoxin and sympathomimetics increases the risk of cardiac arrhythmias).
No products indexed under this heading.

Ephedrine Tannate (Concomitant use of digoxin and sympathomimetics increases the risk of cardiac arrhythmias).
No products indexed under this heading.

Epinephrine (Concomitant use of digoxin and sympathomimetics increases the risk of cardiac arrhythmias). Products include:
EpiPen 1061
Primatene Mist .... ▣ 719
Twinject 0.15 3379
Twinject 0.3 3378

Epinephrine Bitartrate (Concomitant use of digoxin and sympathomimetics increases the risk of cardiac arrhythmias).
No products indexed under this heading.

Epinephrine Hydrochloride (Concomitant use of digoxin and sympathomimetics increases the risk of cardiac arrhythmias).
No products indexed under this heading.

Erythromycin (May increase digoxin absorption in patients who inactivate digoxin by bacterial metabolism in the lower intestine, so that digitalis intoxication may result). Products include:
Ery-Tab Tablets 449
Erythromycin Base Filmtab Tablets 455
Erythromycin Delayed-Release Capsules, USP 457
PCE Dispertab Tablets 515

Erythromycin Estolate (May increase digoxin absorption in patients who inactivate digoxin by bacterial metabolism in the lower intestine, so that digitalis intoxication may result).
No products indexed under this heading.

Erythromycin Ethylsuccinate (May increase digoxin absorption in patients who inactivate digoxin by bacterial metabolism in the lower intestine, so that digitalis intoxication may result). Products include:
E.E.S. 451
EryPed 447

Erythromycin Gluceptate (May increase digoxin absorption in patients who inactivate digoxin by bacterial metabolism in the lower intestine, so that digitalis intoxication may result).
No products indexed under this heading.

Erythromycin Lactobionate (May increase digoxin absorption in patients who inactivate digoxin by bacterial metabolism in the lower intestine, so that digitalis intoxication may result).
No products indexed under this heading.

Erythromycin Stearate (May increase digoxin absorption in patients who inactivate digoxin by bacterial metabolism in the lower intestine, so that digitalis intoxication may result). Products include:
Erythrocin Stearate Filmtab Tablets 453

Esmolol Hydrochloride (Concomitant use of digoxin and beta-andrenergic blockers may result in the additive effects on AV node conduction).
No products indexed under this heading.

Ethacrynic Acid (Potassium-depleting diuretics can cause hypokalemia and co-administration can result in digitalis toxicity). Products include:
Edecrin Tablets 1959

Felodipine (Concomitant use of digoxin and calcium channel blockers may result in the additive effects on AV node conduction).
No products indexed under this heading.

Fludrocortisone Acetate (Corticosteroids can cause hypokalemia or hypomagnesemia and potassium or magnesium depletion can sensitize the myocardium to digoxin resulting in digitalis toxicity).
No products indexed under this heading.

Furosemide (Potassium-depleting diuretics can cause hypokalemia and co-administration can result in digitalis toxicity). Products include:
Furosemide Tablets 2154

Hydrochlorothiazide (Potassium-depleting diuretics can cause hypokalemia and co-administration can result in digitalis toxicity). Products include:
Aldoril Tablets 1910
Atacand HCT 651
Avalide Tablets 888
Avalide Tablets 2874
Benicar HCT Tablets 1044
Diovan HCT Tablets 2196
Dyazide Capsules 1423
Hyzaar 50-12.5 Tablets 1990
Hyzaar 100-12.5 Tablets 1990
Hyzaar 100-25 Tablets 1990
Lopressor HCT 50/25 Tablets 2241
Lopressor HCT 100/25 Tablets 2241
Lopressor HCT 100/50 Tablets 2241
Lotensin HCT Tablets 2246
Micardis HCT Tablets 856
Moduretic Tablets 2028
Prinzide Tablets 2056
Teveten HCT Tablets 1737
Timolide Tablets 2086
Uniretic Tablets 3100

Hydrocortisone (Corticosteroids can cause hypokalemia or hypomagnesemia and potassium or magnesium depletion can sensitize the myocardium to digoxin resulting in digitalis toxicity). Products include:
Colocort Rectal Suspension, USP (Retention) 100 mg/60 mL.......... 2476
Hydrocortone Tablets 1989
Preparation H Hydrocortisone Cream .... ▣ 646

Hydrocortisone Acetate (Corticosteroids can cause hypokalemia or hypomagnesemia and potassium or magnesium depletion can sensitize the myocardium to digoxin resulting in digitalis toxicity). Products include:
Analpram-HC 1159
Pramosone 1161
ProctoFoam-HC 3099

Hydrocortisone Sodium Phosphate (Corticosteroids can cause hypokalemia or hypomagnesemia and potassium or magnesium depletion can sensitize the myocardium to digoxin resulting in digitalis toxicity).
No products indexed under this heading.

Hydrocortisone Sodium Succinate (Corticosteroids can cause hypokalemia or hypomagnesemia and potassium or magnesium depletion can sensitize the myocardium to digoxin resulting in digitalis toxicity).
No products indexed under this heading.

Hydroflumethiazide (Potassium-depleting diuretics can cause hypokalemia and co-administration can result in digitalis toxicity).
No products indexed under this heading.

Indomethacin (Raises the serum digoxin concentration due to reduction in clearance and/or volume of distribution of the drug, with the implication that digitalis intoxication may result). Products include:
Indocin 1995

Indomethacin Sodium Trihydrate (Raises the serum digoxin concentration due to reduction in clearance and/or volume of distribution of the drug, with the implication that digitalis intoxication may result). Products include:
Indocin I.V. 2465

Isoproterenol Hydrochloride (Concomitant use of digoxin and sympathomimetics increases the risk of cardiac arrhythmias).
No products indexed under this heading.

Isoproterenol Sulfate (Concomitant use of digoxin and sympathomimetics increases the risk of cardiac arrhythmias).
No products indexed under this heading.

Isradipine (Concomitant use of digoxin and calcium channel blockers may result in the additive effects on AV node conduction). Products include:
DynaCirc CR Tablets 2721

Itraconazole (Raises the serum digoxin concentration due to reduction in clearance and/or volume of distribution of the drug, with the implication that digitalis intoxication may result).
No products indexed under this heading.

Kaolin (May interfere with intestinal digoxin absorption, resulting in unexpectedly low serum concentrations).
No products indexed under this heading.

Labetalol Hydrochloride (Concomitant use of digoxin and beta-andrenergic blockers may result in the additive effects on AV node conduction).
No products indexed under this heading.

Levalbuterol Hydrochloride (Concomitant use of digoxin and sympathomimetics increases the risk of cardiac arrhythmias). Products include:
Xopenex Inhalation Solution 3146
Xopenex Inhalation Solution Concentrate 3150

Levobunolol Hydrochloride (Concomitant use of digoxin and beta-

andrenergic blockers may result in the additive effects on AV node conduction). Products include:
- Betagan Ophthalmic Solution, USP ... ⊙ 220

Levothyroxine Sodium (Thyroid administration to a digitalized, hypothyroid patient may increase the dose requirement of digoxin). Products include:
- Levothroid Tablets ... 1186
- Levoxyl Tablets ... 1712
- Synthroid Tablets ... 520
- Westhroid Tablets ... 3403

Liothyronine Sodium (Thyroid administration to a digitalized, hypothyroid patient may increase the dose requirement of digoxin). Products include:
- Cytomel Tablets ... 1710
- Westhroid Tablets ... 3403

Liotrix (Thyroid administration to a digitalized, hypothyroid patient may increase the dose requirement of digoxin). Products include:
- Thyrolar Tablets ... 1199

Magaldrate (Antacids may interfere with intestinal digoxin absorption, resulting in unexpectedly low serum concentrations; antacids may cause hypokalemia or hypomagnesemia and co-administration can cause digitalis toxicity).
No products indexed under this heading.

Magnesium Hydroxide (Antacids may interfere with intestinal digoxin absorption, resulting in unexpectedly low serum concentrations; antacids may cause hypokalemia or hypomagnesemia and co-administration can cause digitalis toxicity). Products include:
- Maalox Regular Strength Antacid/Antigas Liquid ... 2175
- Maalox Max Maximum Strength Antacid/Anti-Gas Liquid ... 2176
- Pepcid Complete Chewable Tablets ... 1701

Magnesium Oxide (Antacids may interfere with intestinal digoxin absorption, resulting in unexpectedly low serum concentrations; antacids may cause hypokalemia or hypomagnesemia and co-administration can cause digitalis toxicity). Products include:
- Beelith Tablets ... 759
- PremCal Light, Regular, and Extra Strength Tablets ... 818

Metaproterenol Sulfate (Concomitant use of digoxin and sympathomimetics increases the risk of cardiac arrhythmias). Products include:
- Alupent Inhalation Aerosol ... 826

Metaraminol Bitartrate (Concomitant use of digoxin and sympathomimetics increases the risk of cardiac arrhythmias).
No products indexed under this heading.

Methacycline Hydrochloride (May increase digoxin absorption in patients who inactivate digoxin by bacterial metabolism in the lower intestine, so that digitalis intoxication may result).
No products indexed under this heading.

Methoxamine Hydrochloride (Concomitant use of digoxin and sympathomimetics increases the risk of cardiac arrhythmias).
No products indexed under this heading.

Methyclothiazide (Potassium-depleting diuretics can cause hypokalemia and co-administration can result in digitalis toxicity).
No products indexed under this heading.

Methylprednisolone Acetate (Corticosteroids can cause hypokalemia or hypomagnesemia and potassium or magnesium depletion can sensitize the myocardium to digoxin resulting in digitalis toxicity). Products include:
- Depo-Medrol Injectable Suspension ... 2617
- Depo-Medrol Single-Dose Vial ... 2619

Methylprednisolone Sodium Succinate (Corticosteroids can cause hypokalemia or hypomagnesemia and potassium or magnesium depletion can sensitize the myocardium to digoxin resulting in digitalis toxicity).
No products indexed under this heading.

Metipranolol Hydrochloride (Concomitant use of digoxin and beta-andrenergic blockers may result in the additive effects on AV node conduction).
No products indexed under this heading.

Metoclopramide Hydrochloride (May interfere with intestinal digoxin absorption, resulting in unexpectedly low serum concentrations).
No products indexed under this heading.

Metoprolol Succinate (Concomitant use of digoxin and beta-andrenergic blockers may result in the additive effects on AV node conduction). Products include:
- Toprol-XL Tablets ... 668

Metoprolol Tartrate (Concomitant use of digoxin and beta-andrenergic blockers may result in the additive effects on AV node conduction). Products include:
- Lopressor Injection ... 2238
- Lopressor Tablets ... 2238
- Lopressor HCT 50/25 Tablets ... 2241
- Lopressor HCT 100/25 Tablets ... 2241
- Lopressor HCT 100/50 Tablets ... 2241

Mibefradil Dihydrochloride (Concomitant use of digoxin and calcium channel blockers may result in the additive effects on AV node conduction).
No products indexed under this heading.

Minocycline Hydrochloride (May increase digoxin absorption in patients who inactivate digoxin by bacterial metabolism in the lower intestine, so that digitalis intoxication may result). Products include:
- Solodyn Extended Release Tablets ... 1890

Nadolol (Concomitant use of digoxin and beta-andrenergic blockers may result in the additive effects on AV node conduction). Products include:
- Nadolol Tablets ... 2159

Neomycin, oral (May interfere with intestinal digoxin absorption, resulting in unexpectedly low serum concentrations).
No products indexed under this heading.

Nicardipine Hydrochloride (Concomitant use of digoxin and calcium channel blockers may result in the additive effects on AV node conduction). Products include:
- Cardene I.V. ... 2497

Nifedipine (Concomitant use of digoxin and calcium channel blockers may result in the additive effects on AV node conduction). Products include:
- Adalat CC Tablets ... 2964

Nimodipine (Concomitant use of digoxin and calcium channel blockers may result in the additive effects on AV node conduction). Products include:
- Nimotop Capsules ... 749

Nisoldipine (Concomitant use of digoxin and calcium channel blockers may result in the additive effects on AV node conduction). Products include:
- Sular Tablets ... 3122

Norepinephrine Bitartrate (Concomitant use of digoxin and sympathomimetics increases the risk of cardiac arrhythmias).
No products indexed under this heading.

Oxytetracycline Hydrochloride (May increase digoxin absorption in patients who inactivate digoxin by bacterial metabolism in the lower intestine, so that digitalis intoxication may result).
No products indexed under this heading.

Pectin (May interfere with intestinal digoxin absorption, resulting in unexpectedly low serum concentrations).
No products indexed under this heading.

Penbutolol Sulfate (Concomitant use of digoxin and beta-andrenergic blockers may result in the additive effects on AV node conduction).
No products indexed under this heading.

Penicillamine (Co-administration has resulted in inconsistent reports regarding the effects of penicillamine on serum digoxin concentration). Products include:
- Cuprimine Capsules ... 1947

Phenylephrine Bitartrate (Concomitant use of digoxin and sympathomimetics increases the risk of cardiac arrhythmias).
No products indexed under this heading.

Phenylephrine Hydrochloride (Concomitant use of digoxin and sympathomimetics increases the risk of cardiac arrhythmias). Products include:
- Comtrex Maximum Strength Non-Drowsy Cold & Cough Caplets ... 725
- Comtrex Maximum Strength Day/Night Severe Cold & Sinus Caplets - Day Formulation ... 725
- Comtrex Maximum Strength Day/Night Severe Cold & Sinus Caplets - Night Formulation ... 725
- Contac Cold and Flu Maximum Strength Caplets ... 728
- Contac Cold and Flu Day and Night Caplets (Day Formulation Only) ... 727
- Contac Cold and Flu Day and Night Caplets (Night Formulation Only) ... 727
- Contac Cold and Flu Non-Drowsy Caplets ... 728
- Contac-D Cold Non-Drowsy Tablets ... 729
- Children's Dimetapp Cold & Allergy Elixir ... 730
- Children's Dimetapp Cold & Allergy Chewable Tablets ... 730
- Children's Dimetapp DM Cold & Cough Elixir ... 731
- Toddler's Dimetapp Cold and Cough Drops ... 732
- Excedrin Sinus Headache Caplets/Tablets ... 610
- 4-Way Fast Acting Nasal Spray ... 775
- 4-Way Menthol Nasal Spray ... 775
- Preparation H Maximum Strength Cream ... 666
- Preparation H Cooling Gel ... 666
- Preparation H ... 666
- Refenesen PE Caplets ... 721
- Robitussin Cough & Allergy Syrup ... 736
- Robitussin Cough & Cold Nighttime Liquid ... 736
- Robitussin Cough, Cold & Flu Nighttime Liquid ... 738
- Robitussin Head & Chest Congestion PE Syrup ... 739
- Robitussin Pediatric Cough & Cold Nighttime Liquid ... 736
- TheraFlu Cold & Cough Hot Liquid ... 740
- TheraFlu Cold & Sore Throat Hot Liquid ... 741
- TheraFlu Flu & Sore Throat Hot Liquid ... 742
- TheraFlu Daytime Severe Cold Hot Liquid ... 742
- TheraFlu Nighttime Severe Cold Hot Liquid ... 740
- TheraFlu Warming Relief Daytime Severe Cold ... 743
- TheraFlu Warming Relief Nighttime Severe Cold ... 743
- Triaminic Chest & Nasal Congestion Liquid ... 746
- Triaminic Cold & Allergy Liquid ... 746
- Triaminic Daytime Cold & Cough Liquid ... 745
- Triaminic Nighttime Cold & Cough Liquid ... 746
- Triaminic Thin Strips Cold ... 748
- Triaminic Thin Strips Cold & Cough ... 778
- Triaminic Infant Thin Strips Decongestant ... 747
- Triaminic Infant Thin Strips Decongestant Plus Cough ... 747
- Children's Tylenol Plus Flu Oral Suspension ... 749
- Tylenol Cold Head Congestion Daytime Caplets with Cool Burst and Gelcaps ... 750
- Tylenol Cold Multi-Symptom Daytime Liquid ... 752
- Tylenol Cold Multi-Symptom Severe Daytime Liquid ... 752
- Concentrated Tylenol Infants' Drops Plus Cold & Cough ... 754
- Tylenol Allergy Multi-Symptom Caplets with Cool Burst and Gelcaps ... 1872
- Tylenol Allergy Multi-Symptom Nighttime Caplets with Cool Burst ... 1872
- Children's Tylenol Plus Cold Suspension Liquid ... 1879
- Children's Tylenol Plus Cold & Allergy Suspension Liquid ... 1878
- Children's Tylenol Plus Flu Suspension Liquid ... 1881
- Children's Tylenol Plus Multi-Symptom Cold Suspension Liquid ... 1879
- Tylenol Cold Head Congestion Daytime Caplets with Cool Burst ... 1873
- Tylenol Cold Head Congestion Nighttime Caplets with Cool Burst ... 1873
- Tylenol Cold Head Congestion Severe Caplets with Cool Burst ... 1873
- Tylenol Cold Multi-Symptom Daytime Caplets with Cool Burst and Gelcaps ... 1874
- Tylenol Cold Multi-Symptom Daytime Liquid with Citrus Burst ... 1874
- Tylenol Cold Multi-Symptom Nighttime Caplets with Cool Burst ... 1874
- Tylenol Cold Multi-Symptom Nighttime Liquid with Cool Burst ... 1874
- Tylenol Cold Multi-Symptom Severe Caplets with Cool Burst ... 1874
- Tylenol Cold Multi-Symptom Severe Daytime Liquid with Citrus Burst ... 1874
- Tylenol Sinus Congestion & Pain Daytime Caplets with Cool Burst and Gelcaps ... 1876

Tylenol Sinus Congestion & Pain Nighttime Caplets with Cool Burst 1876
Tylenol Sinus Congestion & Pain Severe Caplets with Cool Burst 1876
Vicks 44D Cough & Head Congestion Relief Liquid .... ■760
Vicks DayQuil LiquiCaps/Liquid Multi-Symptom Cold/Flu Relief ..... ■761
Zicam Cough Plus D Cough Spray .... ■767

Phenylephrine Tannate (Concomitant use of digoxin and sympathomimetics increases the risk of cardiac arrhythmias).
No products indexed under this heading.

Phenylpropanolamine Hydrochloride (Concomitant use of digoxin and sympathomimetics increases the risk of cardiac arrhythmias).
No products indexed under this heading.

Pindolol (Concomitant use of digoxin and beta-andrenergic blockers may result in the additive effects on AV node conduction).
No products indexed under this heading.

Pirbuterol Acetate (Concomitant use of digoxin and sympathomimetics increases the risk of cardiac arrhythmias). Products include:
Maxair Autohaler 1852

Polythiazide (Potassium-depleting diuretics can cause hypokalemia and co-administration can result in digitalis toxicity).
No products indexed under this heading.

Prednisolone Acetate (Corticosteroids can cause hypokalemia or hypomagnesemia and potassium or magnesium depletion can sensitize the myocardium to digoxin resulting in digitalis toxicity). Products include:
Blephamide Ophthalmic Ointment 568
Blephamide Ophthalmic Suspension 569
Poly-Pred Ophthalmic Suspension .... ⊙233
Pred Forte Ophthalmic Suspension .... ⊙235
Pred Mild Ophthalmic Suspension .... ⊙238
Pred-G Ophthalmic Ointment .... ⊙237
Pred-G Ophthalmic Suspension ...... ⊙236

Prednisolone Sodium Phosphate (Corticosteroids can cause hypokalemia or hypomagnesemia and potassium or magnesium depletion can sensitize the myocardium to digoxin resulting in digitalis toxicity).
No products indexed under this heading.

Prednisolone Tebutate (Corticosteroids can cause hypokalemia or hypomagnesemia and potassium or magnesium depletion can sensitize the myocardium to digoxin resulting in digitalis toxicity).
No products indexed under this heading.

Prednisone (Corticosteroids can cause hypokalemia or hypomagnesemia and potassium or magnesium depletion can sensitize the myocardium to digoxin resulting in digitalis toxicity).
No products indexed under this heading.

Propafenone Hydrochloride (Raises the serum digoxin concentration due to reduction in clearance and/or volume of distribution of the drug, with the implication that digitalis intoxication may result). Products include:
Rythmol SR Capsules 2727

Propantheline Bromide (Decreases gut motility and may increase digoxin absorption).
No products indexed under this heading.

Propranolol Hydrochloride (Concomitant use of digoxin and beta-andrenergic blockers may result in the additive effects on AV node conduction). Products include:
Inderal LA Long-Acting Capsules 3429
InnoPran XL Capsules 2723

Pseudoephedrine Hydrochloride (Concomitant use of digoxin and sympathomimetics increases the risk of cardiac arrhythmias). Products include:
Advil Allergy Sinus Caplets .... ■770
Advil Cold & Sinus .... ■723
Advil Multi-Symptom Cold Caplets .... ■770
Aleve Cold & Sinus Caplets 744
Allegra-D 12 Hour Extended-Release Tablets 2846
Allegra-D 24 Hour Extended-Release Tablets 2849
BC Cold Powder .... ■677
Comtrex Maximum Strength Cold & Cough Day/Night Caplets - Day Formulation .... ■726
Comtrex Maximum Strength Cold & Cough Day/Night Caplets - Night Formulation .... ■726
Children's Motrin Cold Oral Suspension 1867
Mucinex D Extended-Release Bi-Layer Tablets .... ■776
Robitussin Cough & Cold CF Liquid .... ■735
Robitussin Cough & Cold Pediatric Drops .... ■735
Tylenol Sinus Congestion & Pain Nighttime Caplets with Cool Burst .... ■778
Tylenol Cold Severe Congestion Non-Drowsy Caplets with Cool Burst 1874
Tylenol Sinus Severe Congestion Caplets with Cool Burst 1876
Vicks 44D Cough & Head Congestion Relief Liquid 2679
Vicks 44M Cough, Cold & Flu Relief Liquid 2680
Vicks DayQuil Multi-Symptom Cold/Flu Relief LiquiCaps 2678
Vicks DayQuil Multi-Symptom Cold/Flu Relief Liquid 2678
Vicks NyQuil Multi-Symptom Cold/Flu Relief Liquid 2681
Vicks NyQuil Multi-Symptom Cold/Flu Relief LiquiCaps 2681
Children's Vicks NyQuil Cold/Cough Relief Liquid 2680
Zyrtec-D 12 Hour Extended Release Tablets 2597

Pseudoephedrine Sulfate (Concomitant use of digoxin and sympathomimetics increases the risk of cardiac arrhythmias). Products include:
Alavert Allergy & Sinus D-12 Hour Tablets .... ■771
Clarinex-D 24-Hour Extended-Release Tablets 2998
Claritin-D Non-Drowsy 12 Hour Tablets .... ■772
Claritin-D Non-Drowsy 24 Hour Tablets .... ■772

Quinidine (Raises the serum digoxin concentration due to reduction in clearance and/or volume of distribution of the drug, with the implication that digitalis intoxication may result).
No products indexed under this heading.

Quinidine Gluconate (Raises the serum digoxin concentration due to reduction in clearance and/or volume of distribution of the drug, with the implication that digitalis intoxication may result).
No products indexed under this heading.

Quinidine Hydrochloride (Raises the serum digoxin concentration due to reduction in clearance and/or volume of distribution of the drug, with the implication that digitalis intoxication may result).
No products indexed under this heading.

Quinidine Polygalacturonate (Raises the serum digoxin concentration due to reduction in clearance and/or volume of distribution of the drug, with the implication that digitalis intoxication may result).
No products indexed under this heading.

Quinidine Sulfate (Raises the serum digoxin concentration due to reduction in clearance and/or volume of distribution of the drug, with the implication that digitalis intoxication may result).
No products indexed under this heading.

Quinine (Co-administration has resulted in inconsistent reports regarding the effects of quinine on serum digoxin concentration).
No products indexed under this heading.

Rifampin (May decrease serum digoxin concentration, especially in patients with renal dysfunction, by increasing the non-renal clearance of digoxin).
No products indexed under this heading.

Salmeterol Xinafoate (Concomitant use of digoxin and sympathomimetics increases the risk of cardiac arrhythmias). Products include:
Advair Diskus 100/50 1308
Advair Diskus 250/50 1308
Advair Diskus 500/50 1308
Advair HFA Inhalation Aerosol 1318
Serevent Diskus 1568

Sodium Bicarbonate (Antacids may interfere with intestinal digoxin absorption, resulting in unexpectedly low serum concentrations; antacids may cause hypokalemia or hypomagnesemia and co-administration can cause digitalis toxicity). Products include:
Colyte with Flavor Packs for Oral Solution 3088
HalfLytely and Bisacodyl Tablets Bowel Prep Kit with Flavors Packs 881
TriLyte with Flavor Packs for Oral Solution 3100

Sotalol Hydrochloride (Concomitant use of digoxin and beta-andrenergic blockers may result in the additive effects on AV node conduction).
No products indexed under this heading.

Spironolactone (Raises the serum digoxin concentration due to reduction in clearance and/or volume of distribution of the drug, with the implication that digitalis intoxication may result).
No products indexed under this heading.

Succinylcholine Chloride (May cause a sudden extrusion of potassium from muscle cells, and may thereby cause arrhythmias in digitalized patients).
No products indexed under this heading.

Sulfasalazine (May interfere with intestinal digoxin absorption, resulting in unexpectedly low serum concentrations).
No products indexed under this heading.

Terbutaline Sulfate (Concomitant use of digoxin and sympathomimetics increases the risk of cardiac arrhythmias).
No products indexed under this heading.

Tetracycline Hydrochloride (May increase digoxin absorption in patients who inactivate digoxin by bacterial metabolism in the lower intestine, so that digitalis intoxication may result).
No products indexed under this heading.

Thyroglobulin (Thyroid administration to a digitalized, hypothyroid patient may increase the dose requirement of digoxin).
No products indexed under this heading.

Thyroid (Thyroid administration to a digitalized, hypothyroid patient may increase the dose requirement of digoxin).
No products indexed under this heading.

Thyroxine (Thyroid administration to a digitalized, hypothyroid patient may increase the dose requirement of digoxin).
No products indexed under this heading.

Thyroxine Sodium (Thyroid administration to a digitalized, hypothyroid patient may increase the dose requirement of digoxin).
No products indexed under this heading.

Timolol Hemihydrate (Concomitant use of digoxin and beta-andrenergic blockers may result in the additive effects on AV node conduction). Products include:
Betimol Ophthalmic Solution 3382
Betimol Ophthalmic Solution .... ⊙295

Timolol Maleate (Concomitant use of digoxin and beta-andrenergic blockers may result in the additive effects on AV node conduction). Products include:
Blocadren Tablets 1916
Cosopt Sterile Ophthalmic Solution 1931
Timolide Tablets 2086
Timoptic Sterile Ophthalmic Solution 2088
Timoptic in Ocudose 2091
Timoptic-XE Sterile Ophthalmic Gel Forming Solution 2092

Torsemide (Potassium-depleting diuretics can cause hypokalemia and co-administration can result in digitalis toxicity). Products include:
Demadex Injection 2759
Demadex Tablets 2759

Triamcinolone (Corticosteroids can cause hypokalemia or hypomagnesemia and potassium or magnesium depletion can sensitize the myocardium to digoxin resulting in digitalis toxicity).
No products indexed under this heading.

Triamcinolone Acetonide (Corticosteroids can cause hypokalemia or hypomagnesemia and potassium or magnesium depletion can sensitize the myocardium to digoxin resulting in digitalis toxicity). Products include:
- Azmacort Inhalation Aerosol 1726
- Nasacort AQ Nasal Spray 2922

Triamcinolone Diacetate (Corticosteroids can cause hypokalemia or hypomagnesemia and potassium or magnesium depletion can sensitize the myocardium to digoxin resulting in digitalis toxicity).
No products indexed under this heading.

Triamcinolone Hexacetonide (Corticosteroids can cause hypokalemia or hypomagnesemia and potassium or magnesium depletion can sensitize the myocardium to digoxin resulting in digitalis toxicity).
No products indexed under this heading.

Troleandomycin (Macrolide antibiotics may possibly increase digoxin absorption in patients who inactivate digoxin by bacterial metabolism in the lower intestine, so that digitalis intoxication may result).
No products indexed under this heading.

Verapamil Hydrochloride (Raises the serum digoxin concentration due to reduction in clearance and/or volume of distribution of the drug, with the implication that digitalis intoxication may result). Products include:
- Covera-HS Tablets 3139
- Tarka Tablets 524
- Verelan PM Extended-Release Capsules, Controlled-Onset 3106

Food Interactions

Meal, high in bran fiber (The amount of digoxin from an oral dose may be reduced).

Meal, unspecified (Slows the rate of absorption).

LANTUS INJECTION

(Insulin glargine) 2909

May interact with ACE inhibitors, beta blockers, corticosteroids, diuretics, fibrates, oral hypoglycemic agents, lithium preparations, monoamine oxidase inhibitors, oral contraceptives, phenothiazines, salicylates, sympathomimetics, thyroid preparations, and certain other agents. Compounds in these categories include:

Acarbose (May increase the blood-glucose-lowering effect and susceptibility to hypoglycemia). Products include:
- Precose Tablets 751

Acebutolol Hydrochloride (Beta-blockers may either potentiate or weaken the blood-glucose-lowering effect of insulin; signs of hypoglycemia may be reduced or absent with co-administration).
No products indexed under this heading.

Albuterol (Sympathomimetic agents may reduce the blood-glucose-lowering effect of insulin). Products include:
- Proventil Inhalation Aerosol 3053

Albuterol Sulfate (Sympathomimetic agents may reduce the blood-glucose-lowering effect of insulin). Products include:
- AccuNeb Inhalation Solution 1055
- Combivent Inhalation Aerosol 847
- DuoNeb Inhalation Solution 1058
- ProAir HFA Inhalation Aerosol 3300
- Proventil Inhalation Solution 0.083% 3055
- Proventil HFA Inhalation Aerosol 3056
- Ventolin HFA Inhalation Aerosol 1600
- VoSpire ER Tablets 1052

Amiloride Hydrochloride (Diuretics may reduce the blood-glucose-lowering effect of insulin). Products include:
- Midamor Tablets 2026
- Moduretic Tablets 2028

Aspirin (May increase the blood-glucose-lowering effect and susceptibility to hypoglycemia). Products include:
- Aggrenox Capsules 822
- Bayer Aspirin 744
- BC Allergy Sinus Cold Powder .... ■677
- BC Headache Powder .... ■677
- Arthritis Strength BC Powder .... ■677
- BC Sinus Cold Powder .... ■677
- Excedrin Extra Strength Caplets/Tablets/Geltabs .... ■684
- Excedrin Migraine Caplets/Tablets/Geltabs .... ■609
- Goody's Body Pain Formula Powder .... ■684
- Goody's Extra Strength Headache Powders .... ■611
- Goody's Extra Strength Pain Relief Tablets .... ■685
- Percodan Tablets 1132
- St. Joseph 81 mg Aspirin Chewable and Enteric Coated Tablets 1869

Aspirin, Enteric Coated (May increase the blood-glucose-lowering effect and susceptibility to hypoglycemia).
No products indexed under this heading.

Aspirin Buffered (May increase the blood-glucose-lowering effect and susceptibility to hypoglycemia). Products include:
- Bufferin Extra Strength Tablets .... ■678
- Bufferin Regular Strength Tablets .... ■678

Atenolol (Beta-blockers may either potentiate or weaken the blood-glucose-lowering effect of insulin; signs of hypoglycemia may be reduced or absent with co-administration).
No products indexed under this heading.

Benazepril Hydrochloride (May increase the blood-glucose-lowering effect and susceptibility to hypoglycemia). Products include:
- Lotensin Tablets 2243
- Lotensin HCT Tablets 2246
- Lotrel Capsules 2249

Bendroflumethiazide (Diuretics may reduce the blood-glucose-lowering effect of insulin).
No products indexed under this heading.

Betamethasone Acetate (Co-administration with corticosteroids may reduce the blood-glucose-lowering effect of insulin).
No products indexed under this heading.

Betamethasone Sodium Phosphate (Co-administration with corticosteroids may reduce the blood-glucose-lowering effect of insulin).
No products indexed under this heading.

Betaxolol Hydrochloride (Beta-blockers may either potentiate or weaken the blood-glucose-lowering effect of insulin; signs of hypoglycemia may be reduced or absent with co-administration). Products include:
- Betoptic S Ophthalmic Suspension 558

Bisoprolol Fumarate (Beta-blockers may either potentiate or weaken the blood-glucose-lowering effect of insulin; signs of hypoglycemia may be reduced or absent with co-administration).
No products indexed under this heading.

Bumetanide (Diuretics may reduce the blood-glucose-lowering effect of insulin). Products include:
- Bumex Tablets 2746

Captopril (May increase the blood-glucose-lowering effect and susceptibility to hypoglycemia). Products include:
- Captopril Tablets 2149

Carteolol Hydrochloride (Beta-blockers may either potentiate or weaken the blood-glucose-lowering effect of insulin; signs of hypoglycemia may be reduced or absent with co-administration). Products include:
- Carteolol Hydrochloride Ophthalmic Solution USP, 1% .... ⊙249

Chlorothiazide (Diuretics may reduce the blood-glucose-lowering effect of insulin). Products include:
- Diuril Oral Suspension 1954

Chlorothiazide Sodium (Diuretics may reduce the blood-glucose-lowering effect of insulin). Products include:
- Diuril Sodium Intravenous 2467

Chlorpromazine (Phenothiazine derivatives may reduce the blood-glucose-lowering effect of insulin).
No products indexed under this heading.

Chlorpromazine Hydrochloride (Phenothiazine derivatives may reduce the blood-glucose-lowering effect of insulin).
No products indexed under this heading.

Chlorpropamide (May increase the blood-glucose-lowering effect and susceptibility to hypoglycemia).
No products indexed under this heading.

Chlorthalidone (Diuretics may reduce the blood-glucose-lowering effect of insulin). Products include:
- Clorpres Tablets 2153

Choline Magnesium Trisalicylate (May increase the blood-glucose-lowering effect and susceptibility to hypoglycemia).
No products indexed under this heading.

Clofibrate (May increase the blood-glucose-lowering effect and susceptibility to hypoglycemia).
No products indexed under this heading.

Clonidine (Signs of hypoglycemia may be reduced or absent with co-administration). Products include:
- Catapres-TTS 844

Clonidine Hydrochloride (Signs of hypoglycemia may be reduced or absent with co-administration). Products include:
- Catapres Tablets 843
- Clorpres Tablets 2153

Cortisone Acetate (Co-administration with corticosteroids may reduce the blood-glucose-lowering effect of insulin).
No products indexed under this heading.

Danazol (May reduce the blood-glucose-lowering effect of insulin).
No products indexed under this heading.

Desogestrel (Oral contraceptives may reduce the blood-glucose-lowering effect of insulin). Products include:
- Mircette Tablets 1066

Dexamethasone (Co-administration with corticosteroids may reduce the blood-glucose-lowering effect of insulin). Products include:
- Ciprodex Otic Suspension 559
- Decadron Tablets 1951
- TobraDex Ophthalmic Ointment 562
- TobraDex Ophthalmic Suspension 563

Dexamethasone Acetate (Co-administration with corticosteroids may reduce the blood-glucose-lowering effect of insulin).
No products indexed under this heading.

Dexamethasone Sodium Phosphate (Co-administration with corticosteroids may reduce the blood-glucose-lowering effect of insulin).
No products indexed under this heading.

Diflunisal (May increase the blood-glucose-lowering effect and susceptibility to hypoglycemia). Products include:
- Dolobid Tablets 1955

Disopyramide Phosphate (May increase the blood-glucose-lowering effect and susceptibility to hypoglycemia).
No products indexed under this heading.

Dobutamine Hydrochloride (Sympathomimetic agents may reduce the blood-glucose-lowering effect of insulin).
No products indexed under this heading.

Dopamine Hydrochloride (Sympathomimetic agents may reduce the blood-glucose-lowering effect of insulin).
No products indexed under this heading.

Enalapril Maleate (May increase the blood-glucose-lowering effect and susceptibility to hypoglycemia). Products include:
- Vasotec I.V. Injection 2103

Enalaprilat (May increase the blood-glucose-lowering effect and susceptibility to hypoglycemia).
No products indexed under this heading.

Ephedrine Hydrochloride (Sympathomimetic agents may reduce the blood-glucose-lowering effect of insulin).
No products indexed under this heading.

Ephedrine Sulfate (Sympathomimetic agents may reduce the blood-glucose-lowering effect of insulin).
No products indexed under this heading.

Ephedrine Tannate (Sympathomimetic agents may reduce the blood-glucose-lowering effect of insulin).
No products indexed under this heading.

Epinephrine (Sympathomimetic agents may reduce the blood-glucose-lowering effect of insulin). Products include:
- EpiPen 1061
- Primatene Mist .... ■719
- Twinject 0.15 3379
- Twinject 0.3 3378

Epinephrine Bitartrate (Sympathomimetic agents may reduce the blood-glucose-lowering effect of insulin).
> No products indexed under this heading.

Epinephrine Hydrochloride (Sympathomimetic agents may reduce the blood-glucose-lowering effect of insulin).
> No products indexed under this heading.

Esmolol Hydrochloride (Beta-blockers may either potentiate or weaken the blood-glucose-lowering effect of insulin; signs of hypoglycemia may be reduced or absent with co-administration).
> No products indexed under this heading.

Ethacrynic Acid (Diuretics may reduce the blood-glucose-lowering effect of insulin). Products include:

Ethinyl Estradiol (Oral contraceptives may reduce the blood-glucose-lowering effect of insulin). Products include:

Ethynodiol Diacetate (Oral contraceptives may reduce the blood-glucose-lowering effect of insulin).
> No products indexed under this heading.

Fenofibrate (May increase the blood-glucose-lowering effect and susceptibility to hypoglycemia). Products include:

Fludrocortisone Acetate (Co-administration with corticosteroids may reduce the blood-glucose-lowering effect of insulin).
> No products indexed under this heading.

Fluoxetine Hydrochloride (May increase the blood-glucose-lowering effect and susceptibility to hypoglycemia). Products include:

Fluphenazine Decanoate (Phenothiazine derivatives may reduce the blood-glucose-lowering effect of insulin).
> No products indexed under this heading.

Fluphenazine Enanthate (Phenothiazine derivatives may reduce the blood-glucose-lowering effect of insulin).
> No products indexed under this heading.

Fluphenazine Hydrochloride (Phenothiazine derivatives may reduce the blood-glucose-lowering effect of insulin).
> No products indexed under this heading.

Fosinopril Sodium (May increase the blood-glucose-lowering effect and susceptibility to hypoglycemia).
> No products indexed under this heading.

Furosemide (Diuretics may reduce the blood-glucose-lowering effect of insulin). Products include:

Gemfibrozil (May increase the blood-glucose-lowering effect and susceptibility to hypoglycemia).
> No products indexed under this heading.

Glimepiride (May increase the blood-glucose-lowering effect and susceptibility to hypoglycemia). Products include:

Glipizide (May increase the blood-glucose-lowering effect and susceptibility to hypoglycemia).
> No products indexed under this heading.

Glyburide (May increase the blood-glucose-lowering effect and susceptibility to hypoglycemia).
> No products indexed under this heading.

Guanethidine Monosulfate (Signs of hypoglycemia may be reduced or absent with co-administration).
> No products indexed under this heading.

Hydrochlorothiazide (Diuretics may reduce the blood-glucose-lowering effect of insulin). Products include:

Hydrocortisone (Co-administration with corticosteroids may reduce the blood-glucose-lowering effect of insulin). Products include:

Hydrocortisone Acetate (Co-administration with corticosteroids may reduce the blood-glucose-lowering effect of insulin). Products include:

Hydrocortisone Sodium Phosphate (Co-administration with corticosteroids may reduce the blood-glucose-lowering effect of insulin).
> No products indexed under this heading.

Hydrocortisone Sodium Succinate (Co-administration with corticosteroids may reduce the blood-glucose-lowering effect of insulin).
> No products indexed under this heading.

Hydroflumethiazide (Diuretics may reduce the blood-glucose-lowering effect of insulin).
> No products indexed under this heading.

Indapamide (Diuretics may reduce the blood-glucose-lowering effect of insulin). Products include:

Isocarboxazid (May increase the blood-glucose-lowering effect and susceptibility to hypoglycemia).
> No products indexed under this heading.

Isoniazid (May reduce the blood-glucose-lowering effect of insulin).
> No products indexed under this heading.

Isoproterenol Hydrochloride (Sympathomimetic agents may reduce the blood-glucose-lowering effect of insulin).
> No products indexed under this heading.

Isoproterenol Sulfate (Sympathomimetic agents may reduce the blood-glucose-lowering effect of insulin).
> No products indexed under this heading.

Labetalol Hydrochloride (Beta-blockers may either potentiate or weaken the blood-glucose-lowering effect of insulin; signs of hypoglycemia may be reduced or absent with co-administration).
> No products indexed under this heading.

Levalbuterol Hydrochloride (Sympathomimetic agents may reduce the blood-glucose-lowering effect of insulin). Products include:

Levobunolol Hydrochloride (Beta-blockers may either potentiate or weaken the blood-glucose-lowering effect of insulin; signs of hypoglycemia may be reduced or absent with co-administration). Products include:

Levonorgestrel (Oral contraceptives may reduce the blood-glucose-lowering effect of insulin). Products include:

Levothyroxine Sodium (May reduce the blood-glucose-lowering effect of insulin). Products include:

Liothyronine Sodium (May reduce the blood-glucose-lowering effect of insulin). Products include:

Liotrix (May reduce the blood-glucose-lowering effect of insulin). Products include:

Lisinopril (May increase the blood-glucose-lowering effect and susceptibility to hypoglycemia). Products include:

Lithium (May either potentiate or weaken the blood-glucose-lowering effect of insulin).
> No products indexed under this heading.

Lithium Carbonate (May either potentiate or weaken the blood-glucose-lowering effect of insulin). Products include:

Lithium Citrate (May either potentiate or weaken the blood-glucose-lowering effect of insulin).
> No products indexed under this heading.

Magnesium Salicylate (May increase the blood-glucose-lowering effect and susceptibility to hypoglycemia).
> No products indexed under this heading.

Mesoridazine Besylate (Phenothiazine derivatives may reduce the blood-glucose-lowering effect of insulin).
> No products indexed under this heading.

Mestranol (Oral contraceptives may reduce the blood-glucose-lowering effect of insulin).
> No products indexed under this heading.

Metaproterenol Sulfate (Sympathomimetic agents may reduce the blood-glucose-lowering effect of insulin). Products include:

Metaraminol Bitartrate (Sympathomimetic agents may reduce the blood-glucose-lowering effect of insulin).
> No products indexed under this heading.

Metformin Hydrochloride (May increase the blood-glucose-lowering effect and susceptibility to hypoglycemia). Products include:

Methotrimeprazine (Phenothiazine derivatives may reduce the blood-glucose-lowering effect of insulin).
> No products indexed under this heading.

Methoxamine Hydrochloride (Sympathomimetic agents may reduce the blood-glucose-lowering effect of insulin).
> No products indexed under this heading.

Methyclothiazide (Diuretics may reduce the blood-glucose-lowering effect of insulin).
> No products indexed under this heading.

Methylprednisolone Acetate (Co-administration with corticosteroids may reduce the blood-glucose-lowering effect of insulin). Products include:

Methylprednisolone Sodium Succinate (Co-administration with corticosteroids may reduce the blood-glucose-lowering effect of insulin).
> No products indexed under this heading.

Metipranolol Hydrochloride (Beta-blockers may either potentiate or weaken the blood-glucose-lowering effect of insulin; signs of hypoglycemia may be reduced or absent with co-administration).
> No products indexed under this heading.

Metolazone (Diuretics may reduce the blood-glucose-lowering effect of insulin).
> No products indexed under this heading.

Metoprolol Succinate (Beta-blockers may either potentiate or

weaken the blood-glucose-lowering effect of insulin; signs of hypoglycemia may be reduced or absent with co-administration). Products include:
Toprol-XL Tablets 668

Metoprolol Tartrate (Beta-blockers may either potentiate or weaken the blood-glucose-lowering effect of insulin; signs of hypoglycemia may be reduced or absent with co-administration). Products include:
Lopressor Injection 2238
Lopressor Tablets 2238
Lopressor HCT 50/25 Tablets 2241
Lopressor HCT 100/25 Tablets 2241
Lopressor HCT 100/50 Tablets 2241

Miglitol (May increase the blood-glucose-lowering effect and susceptibility to hypoglycemia).
No products indexed under this heading.

Moclobemide (May increase the blood-glucose-lowering effect and susceptibility to hypoglycemia).
No products indexed under this heading.

Moexipril Hydrochloride (May increase the blood-glucose-lowering effect and susceptibility to hypoglycemia). Products include:
Uniretic Tablets 3100
Univasc Tablets 3104

Nadolol (Beta-blockers may either potentiate or weaken the blood-glucose-lowering effect of insulin; signs of hypoglycemia may be reduced or absent with co-administration). Products include:
Nadolol Tablets 2159

Norepinephrine Bitartrate (Sympathomimetic agents may reduce the blood-glucose-lowering effect of insulin).
No products indexed under this heading.

Norethindrone (Oral contraceptives may reduce the blood-glucose-lowering effect of insulin). Products include:
Ortho Micronor Tablets 2426

Norethynodrel (Oral contraceptives may reduce the blood-glucose-lowering effect of insulin).
No products indexed under this heading.

Norgestimate (Oral contraceptives may reduce the blood-glucose-lowering effect of insulin). Products include:
Ortho-Cyclen/Ortho Tri-Cyclen 2429
Ortho Tri-Cyclen Lo Tablets 2436

Norgestrel (Oral contraceptives may reduce the blood-glucose-lowering effect of insulin).
No products indexed under this heading.

Octreotide Acetate (May increase the blood-glucose-lowering effect and susceptibility to hypoglycemia). Products include:
Sandostatin Injection 2278
Sandostatin LAR Depot 2280

Pargyline Hydrochloride (May increase the blood-glucose-lowering effect and susceptibility to hypoglycemia).
No products indexed under this heading.

Penbutolol Sulfate (Beta-blockers may either potentiate or weaken the blood-glucose-lowering effect of insulin; signs of hypoglycemia may be reduced or absent with co-administration).
No products indexed under this heading.

Pentamidine Isethionate (May cause hypoglycemia, which may sometimes be followed by hyperglycemia).
No products indexed under this heading.

Perindopril Erbumine (May increase the blood-glucose-lowering effect and susceptibility to hypoglycemia). Products include:
Aceon Tablets (2 mg, 4 mg, 8 mg) 3194

Perphenazine (Phenothiazine derivatives may reduce the blood-glucose-lowering effect of insulin).
No products indexed under this heading.

Phenelzine Sulfate (May increase the blood-glucose-lowering effect and susceptibility to hypoglycemia).
No products indexed under this heading.

Phenylephrine Bitartrate (Sympathomimetic agents may reduce the blood-glucose-lowering effect of insulin).
No products indexed under this heading.

Phenylephrine Hydrochloride (Sympathomimetic agents may reduce the blood-glucose-lowering effect of insulin). Products include:
Comtrex Maximum Strength Non-Drowsy Cold & Cough Caplets 725
Comtrex Maximum Strength Day/Night Severe Cold & Sinus Caplets - Day Formulation 725
Comtrex Maximum Strength Day/Night Severe Cold & Sinus Caplets - Night Formulation 725
Contac Cold and Flu Maximum Strength Caplets 728
Contac Cold and Flu Day and Night Caplets (Day Formulation Only) 727
Contac Cold and Flu Day and Night Caplets (Night Formulation Only) 727
Contac Cold and Flu Non-Drowsy Caplets 728
Contac-D Cold Non-Drowsy Tablets 729
Children's Dimetapp Cold & Allergy Elixir 730
Children's Dimetapp Cold & Allergy Chewable Tablets 730
Children's Dimetapp DM Cold & Cough Elixir 731
Toddler's Dimetapp Cold and Cough Drops 732
Excedrin Sinus Headache Caplets/Tablets 610
4-Way Fast Acting Nasal Spray 775
4-Way Menthol Nasal Spray 775
Preparation H Maximum Strength Cream 666
Preparation H Cooling Gel 666
Preparation H 666
Refenesen PE Caplets 721
Robitussin Cough & Allergy Syrup .. 736
Robitussin Cough & Cold Nighttime Liquid........................ 736
Robitussin Cough, Cold & Flu Nighttime Liquid 738
Robitussin Head & Chest Congestion PE Syrup 739
Robitussin Pediatric Cough & Cold Nighttime Liquid............... 736
TheraFlu Cold & Cough Hot Liquid 740
TheraFlu Cold & Sore Throat Hot Liquid 741
TheraFlu Flu & Sore Throat Hot Liquid 742
TheraFlu Daytime Severe Cold Hot Liquid 742
TheraFlu Nighttime Severe Cold Hot Liquid 740
TheraFlu Warming Relief Daytime Severe Cold....................... 743
TheraFlu Warming Relief Nighttime Severe Cold................ 743

Triaminic Chest & Nasal Congestion Liquid...................... 746
Triaminic Cold & Allergy Liquid 746
Triaminic Daytime Cold & Cough Liquid 745
Triaminic Nighttime Cold & Cough Liquid 746
Triaminic Thin Strips Cold 748
Triaminic Thin Strips Cold & Cough 778
Triaminic Infant Thin Strips Decongestant 747
Triaminic Infant Thin Strips Decongestant Plus Cough........... 747
Children's Tylenol Plus Flu Oral Suspension 749
Tylenol Cold Head Congestion Daytime Caplets with Cool Burst and Gelcaps..................... 750
Tylenol Cold Multi-Symptom Daytime Liquid....................... 752
Tylenol Cold Multi-Symptom Severe Daytime Liquid 752
Concentrated Tylenol Infants' Drops Plus Cold & Cough........... 754
Tylenol Allergy Multi-Symptom Caplets with Cool Burst and Gelcaps.................................. 1872
Tylenol Allergy Multi-Symptom Nighttime Caplets with Cool Burst...................................... 1872
Children's Tylenol Plus Cold Suspension Liquid 1879
Children's Tylenol Plus Cold & Allergy Suspension Liquid........... 1878
Children's Tylenol Plus Flu Suspension Liquid 1881
Children's Tylenol Plus Multi-Symptom Cold Suspension Liquid 1879
Tylenol Cold Head Congestion Daytime Caplets with Cool Burst...................................... 1873
Tylenol Cold Head Congestion Nighttime Caplets with Cool Burst...................................... 1873
Tylenol Cold Head Congestion Severe Caplets with Cool Burst..... 1873
Tylenol Cold Multi-Symptom Daytime Caplets with Cool Burst and Gelcaps..................... 1874
Tylenol Cold Multi-Symptom Daytime Liquid with Citrus Burst ... 1874
Tylenol Cold Multi-Symptom Nighttime Caplets with Cool Burst...................................... 1874
Tylenol Cold Multi-Symptom Nighttime Liquid with Cool Burst ... 1874
Tylenol Cold Multi-Symptom Severe Caplets with Cool Burst..... 1874
Tylenol Cold Multi-Symptom Severe Daytime Liquid with Citrus Burst............................ 1874
Tylenol Sinus Congestion & Pain Daytime Caplets with Cool Burst and Gelcaps..................... 1876
Tylenol Sinus Congestion & Pain Nighttime Caplets with Cool Burst...................................... 1876
Tylenol Sinus Congestion & Pain Severe Caplets with Cool Burst..... 1876
Vicks 44D Cough & Head Congestion Relief Liquid............. 760
Vicks DayQuil LiquiCaps/Liquid Multi-Symptom Cold/Flu Relief..... 761
Zicam Cough Plus D Cough Spray 767

Phenylephrine Tannate (Sympathomimetic agents may reduce the blood-glucose-lowering effect of insulin).
No products indexed under this heading.

Phenylpropanolamine Hydrochloride (Sympathomimetic agents may reduce the blood-glucose-lowering effect of insulin).
No products indexed under this heading.

Pindolol (Beta-blockers may either potentiate or weaken the blood-glucose-lowering effect of insulin; signs of hypoglycemia may be reduced or absent with co-administration).
No products indexed under this heading.

Pioglitazone Hydrochloride (May increase the blood-glucose-lowering effect and susceptibility to hypoglycemia). Products include:
ActoPlus Met Tablets 3214
Actos Tablets 3219
Duetact Tablets 3226

Pirbuterol Acetate (Sympathomimetic agents may reduce the blood-glucose-lowering effect of insulin). Products include:
Maxair Autohaler 1852

Polythiazide (Diuretics may reduce the blood-glucose-lowering effect of insulin).
No products indexed under this heading.

Prednisolone Acetate (Co-administration with corticosteroids may reduce the blood-glucose-lowering effect of insulin). Products include:
Blephamide Ophthalmic Ointment 568
Blephamide Ophthalmic Suspension............................. 569
Poly-Pred Ophthalmic Suspension............................. ⊙233
Pred Forte Ophthalmic Suspension............................. ⊙235
Pred Mild Ophthalmic Suspension............................. ⊙238
Pred-G Ophthalmic Ointment ⊙237
Pred-G Ophthalmic Suspension ⊙236

Prednisolone Sodium Phosphate (Co-administration with corticosteroids may reduce the blood-glucose-lowering effect of insulin).
No products indexed under this heading.

Prednisolone Tebutate (Co-administration with corticosteroids may reduce the blood-glucose-lowering effect of insulin).
No products indexed under this heading.

Prednisone (Co-administration with corticosteroids may reduce the blood-glucose-lowering effect of insulin).
No products indexed under this heading.

Procarbazine Hydrochloride (May increase the blood-glucose-lowering effect and susceptibility to hypoglycemia). Products include:
Matulane Capsules 3191

Prochlorperazine (Phenothiazine derivatives may reduce the blood-glucose-lowering effect of insulin).
No products indexed under this heading.

Promethazine Hydrochloride (Phenothiazine derivatives may reduce the blood-glucose-lowering effect of insulin). Products include:
Phenergan Tablets and Suppositories........................... 3440

Propoxyphene Hydrochloride (May increase the blood-glucose-lowering effect and susceptibility to hypoglycemia).
No products indexed under this heading.

Propoxyphene Napsylate (May increase the blood-glucose-lowering effect and susceptibility to hypoglycemia).
No products indexed under this heading.

Propranolol Hydrochloride (Beta-blockers may either potentiate or weaken the blood-glucose-lowering effect of insulin; signs of hypoglycemia may be reduced or absent with co-administration). Products include:
Inderal LA Long-Acting Capsules 3429
InnoPran XL Capsules 2723

Pseudoephedrine Hydrochloride (Sympathomimetic agents may reduce the blood-glucose-lowering effect of insulin). Products include:

- Advil Allergy Sinus Caplets .... ▣ 770
- Advil Cold & Sinus .... ▣ 723
- Advil Multi-Symptom Cold Caplets .... ▣ 770
- Aleve Cold & Sinus Caplets 744
- Allegra-D 12 Hour Extended-Release Tablets 2846
- Allegra-D 24 Hour Extended-Release Tablets 2849
- BC Cold Powder .... ▣ 677
- Comtrex Maximum Strength Cold & Cough Day/Night Caplets - Day Formulation .... ▣ 726
- Comtrex Maximum Strength Cold & Cough Day/Night Caplets - Night Formulation .... ▣ 726
- Children's Motrin Cold Oral Suspension 1867
- Mucinex D Extended-Release Bi-Layer Tablets .... ▣ 776
- Robitussin Cough & Cold CF Liquid .... ▣ 735
- Robitussin Cough & Cold Pediatric Drops .... ▣ 735
- Tylenol Sinus Congestion & Pain Nighttime Caplets with Cool Burst .... ▣ 778
- Tylenol Cold Severe Congestion Non-Drowsy Caplets with Cool Burst 1874
- Tylenol Sinus Severe Congestion Caplets with Cool Burst 1876
- Vicks 44D Cough & Head Congestion Relief Liquid 2679
- Vicks 44M Cough, Cold & Flu Relief Liquid 2680
- Vicks DayQuil Multi-Symptom Cold/Flu Relief LiquiCaps 2678
- Vicks DayQuil Multi-Symptom Cold/Flu Relief Liquid 2678
- Vicks NyQuil Multi-Symptom Cold/Flu Relief Liquid 2681
- Vicks NyQuil Multi-Symptom Cold/Flu Relief LiquiCaps 2681
- Children's Vicks NyQuil Cold/Cough Relief Liquid 2680
- Zyrtec-D 12 Hour Extended Release Tablets 2597

Pseudoephedrine Sulfate (Sympathomimetic agents may reduce the blood-glucose-lowering effect of insulin). Products include:

- Alavert Allergy & Sinus D-12 Hour Tablets .... ▣ 771
- Clarinex-D 24-Hour Extended-Release Tablets 2998
- Claritin-D Non-Drowsy 12 Hour Tablets .... ▣ 772
- Claritin-D Non-Drowsy 24 Hour Tablets .... ▣ 772

Quinapril Hydrochloride (May increase the blood-glucose-lowering effect and susceptibility to hypoglycemia).

No products indexed under this heading.

Ramipril (May increase the blood-glucose-lowering effect and susceptibility to hypoglycemia). Products include:

- Altace Capsules 1702

Repaglinide (May increase the blood-glucose-lowering effect and susceptibility to hypoglycemia).

No products indexed under this heading.

Reserpine (Signs of hypoglycemia may be reduced or absent with co-administration).

No products indexed under this heading.

Rosiglitazone Maleate (May increase the blood-glucose-lowering effect and susceptibility to hypoglycemia). Products include:

- Avandamet Tablets 1373
- Avandaryl Tablets 1379
- Avandia Tablets 1384

Salmeterol Xinafoate (Sympathomimetic agents may reduce the blood-glucose-lowering effect of insulin). Products include:

- Advair Diskus 100/50 1308
- Advair Diskus 250/50 1308
- Advair Diskus 500/50 1308
- Advair HFA Inhalation Aerosol 1318
- Serevent Diskus 1568

Salsalate (May increase the blood-glucose-lowering effect and susceptibility to hypoglycemia).

No products indexed under this heading.

Selegiline Hydrochloride (May increase the blood-glucose-lowering effect and susceptibility to hypoglycemia). Products include:

- Eldepryl Capsules 3208
- Zelapar Tablets 3372

Somatropin (May reduce the blood-glucose-lowering effect of insulin). Products include:

- Genotropin Lyophilized Powder 2638
- Humatrope Vials and Cartridges 1787
- Norditropin Cartridges 2323
- Nutropin for Injection 1239
- Nutropin AQ Injection 1243
- Nutropin AQ Pen 1243
- Nutropin AQ Pen Cartridge 1243

Sotalol Hydrochloride (Beta-blockers may either potentiate or weaken the blood-glucose-lowering effect of insulin; signs of hypoglycemia may be reduced or absent with co-administration).

No products indexed under this heading.

Spirapril Hydrochloride (May increase the blood-glucose-lowering effect and susceptibility to hypoglycemia).

No products indexed under this heading.

Spironolactone (Diuretics may reduce the blood-glucose-lowering effect of insulin).

No products indexed under this heading.

Sulfamethoxazole (Co-administration with sulfonamide antibiotics may increase the blood-glucose-lowering effect and susceptibility to hypoglycemia).

No products indexed under this heading.

Sulfisoxazole Acetyl (Co-administration with sulfonamide antibiotics may increase the blood-glucose-lowering effect and susceptibility to hypoglycemia).

No products indexed under this heading.

Terbutaline Sulfate (Sympathomimetic agents may reduce the blood-glucose-lowering effect of insulin).

No products indexed under this heading.

Thioridazine Hydrochloride (Phenothiazine derivatives may reduce the blood-glucose-lowering effect of insulin). Products include:

- Thioridazine Hydrochloride Tablets 2163

Thyroglobulin (May reduce the blood-glucose-lowering effect of insulin).

No products indexed under this heading.

Thyroid (May reduce the blood-glucose-lowering effect of insulin).

No products indexed under this heading.

Thyroxine (May reduce the blood-glucose-lowering effect of insulin).

No products indexed under this heading.

Thyroxine Sodium (May reduce the blood-glucose-lowering effect of insulin).

No products indexed under this heading.

Timolol Hemihydrate (Beta-blockers may either potentiate or weaken the blood-glucose-lowering effect of insulin; signs of hypoglycemia may be reduced or absent with co-administration). Products include:

- Betimol Ophthalmic Solution 3382
- Betimol Ophthalmic Solution .... ⊙ 295

Timolol Maleate (Beta-blockers may either potentiate or weaken the blood-glucose-lowering effect of insulin; signs of hypoglycemia may be reduced or absent with co-administration). Products include:

- Blocadren Tablets 1916
- Cosopt Sterile Ophthalmic Solution 1931
- Timolide Tablets 2086
- Timoptic Sterile Ophthalmic Solution 2088
- Timoptic in Ocudose 2091
- Timoptic-XE Sterile Ophthalmic Gel Forming Solution 2092

Tolazamide (May increase the blood-glucose-lowering effect and susceptibility to hypoglycemia).

No products indexed under this heading.

Tolbutamide (May increase the blood-glucose-lowering effect and susceptibility to hypoglycemia).

No products indexed under this heading.

Torsemide (Diuretics may reduce the blood-glucose-lowering effect of insulin). Products include:

- Demadex Injection 2759
- Demadex Tablets 2759

Trandolapril (May increase the blood-glucose-lowering effect and susceptibility to hypoglycemia). Products include:

- Mavik Tablets 486
- Tarka Tablets 524

Tranylcypromine Sulfate (May increase the blood-glucose-lowering effect and susceptibility to hypoglycemia). Products include:

- Parnate Tablets 1527

Triamcinolone (Co-administration with corticosteroids may reduce the blood-glucose-lowering effect of insulin).

No products indexed under this heading.

Triamcinolone Acetonide (Co-administration with corticosteroids may reduce the blood-glucose-lowering effect of insulin). Products include:

- Azmacort Inhalation Aerosol 1726
- Nasacort AQ Nasal Spray 2922

Triamcinolone Diacetate (Co-administration with corticosteroids may reduce the blood-glucose-lowering effect of insulin).

No products indexed under this heading.

Triamcinolone Hexacetonide (Co-administration with corticosteroids may reduce the blood-glucose-lowering effect of insulin).

No products indexed under this heading.

Triamterene (Diuretics may reduce the blood-glucose-lowering effect of insulin). Products include:

- Dyazide Capsules 1423
- Dyrenium Capsules 3400

Trifluoperazine Hydrochloride (Phenothiazine derivatives may reduce the blood-glucose-lowering effect of insulin).

No products indexed under this heading.

Troglitazone (May increase the blood-glucose-lowering effect and susceptibility to hypoglycemia).

No products indexed under this heading.

Food Interactions

Alcohol (May either potentiate or weaken the blood-glucose-lowering effect of insulin).

LARIAM TABLETS

(Mefloquine Hydrochloride) 2786

May interact with antiarrhythmics, beta blockers, calcium channel blockers, anticonvulsants, phenothiazines, quinidine, tricyclic antidepressants, and certain other agents. Compounds in these categories include:

Acebutolol Hydrochloride (There is a theoretical possibility that co-administration of other drugs known to alter cardiac conduction, such as beta blockers, might also contribute to a prolongation of the QTc interval).

No products indexed under this heading.

Adenosine (There is a theoretical possibility that co-administration of other drugs known to alter cardiac conduction, such as antiarrhythmic agents, might also contribute to a prolongation of the QTc interval). Products include:

- Adenocard Injection 617
- Adenoscan 619

Amiodarone Hydrochloride (There is a theoretical possibility that co-administration of other drugs known to alter cardiac conduction, such as antiarrhythmic agents, might also contribute to a prolongation of the QTc interval).

No products indexed under this heading.

Amitriptyline Hydrochloride (There is a theoretical possibility that co-administration of other drugs known to alter cardiac conduction, such as tricyclic antidepressants, might also contribute to a prolongation of the QTc interval).

No products indexed under this heading.

Amlodipine Besylate (There is a theoretical possibility that co-administration of other drugs known to alter cardiac conduction, such as calcium channel blockers, might also contribute to a prolongation of the QTc interval). Products include:

- Caduet Tablets 2508
- Lotrel Capsules 2249
- Norvasc Tablets 2545

Amoxapine (There is a theoretical possibility that co-administration of other drugs known to alter cardiac conduction, such as tricyclic antidepressants, might also contribute to a prolongation of the QTc interval).

No products indexed under this heading.

Astemizole (There is a theoretical possibility that co-administration of other drugs known to alter cardiac conduction, such as antihistamine astemizole, might also contribute to a prolongation of the QTc interval).

No products indexed under this heading.

Atenolol (There is a theoretical possibility that co-administration of other drugs known to alter cardiac conduction, such as beta blockers, might also contribute to a prolongation of the QTc interval).
No products indexed under this heading.

Bepridil Hydrochloride (There is a theoretical possibility that co-administration of other drugs known to alter cardiac conduction, such as calcium channel blockers, might also contribute to a prolongation of the QTc interval).
No products indexed under this heading.

Betaxolol Hydrochloride (There is a theoretical possibility that co-administration of other drugs known to alter cardiac conduction, such as beta blockers, might also contribute to a prolongation of the QTc interval). Products include:
Betoptic S Ophthalmic
Suspension................................... 558

Bisoprolol Fumarate (There is a theoretical possibility that co-administration of other drugs known to alter cardiac conduction, such as beta blockers, might also contribute to a prolongation of the QTc interval).
No products indexed under this heading.

Bretylium Tosylate (There is a theoretical possibility that co-administration of other drugs known to alter cardiac conduction, such as antiarrhythmic agents, might also contribute to a prolongation of the QTc interval).
No products indexed under this heading.

Carbamazepine (Co-administration may reduce seizure control by lowering the plasma levels of anticonvulsant; dosage of anticonvulsant may need to be adjusted). Products include:
Carbatrol Capsules 3171
Equetro Extended-Release
Capsules..................................... 3180
Tegretol/Tegretol-XR 2295

Carteolol Hydrochloride (There is a theoretical possibility that co-administration of other drugs known to alter cardiac conduction, such as beta blockers, might also contribute to a prolongation of the QTc interval). Products include:
Carteolol Hydrochloride
Ophthalmic Solution USP, 1%....... ⊙249

Chloroquine Hydrochloride (Co-administration may produce electrocardiographic abnormalities and increase the risk of convulsions; if these drugs are to be used in the initial treatment of severe malaria, mefloquine administration should be delayed at least 12 hours after the last dose).
No products indexed under this heading.

Chloroquine Phosphate (Co-administration may produce electrocardiographic abnormalities and increase the risk of convulsions; if these drugs are to be used in the initial treatment of severe malaria, mefloquine administration should be delayed at least 12 hours after the last dose).
No products indexed under this heading.

Chlorpromazine (There is a theoretical possibility that co-administration of other drugs known to alter cardiac conduction, such as phenothiazines, might also contribute to a prolongation of the QTc interval).
No products indexed under this heading.

Chlorpromazine Hydrochloride (There is a theoretical possibility that co-administration of other drugs known to alter cardiac conduction, such as phenothiazines, might also contribute to a prolongation of the QTc interval).
No products indexed under this heading.

Clomipramine Hydrochloride (There is a theoretical possibility that co-administration of other drugs known to alter cardiac conduction, such as tricyclic antidepressants, might also contribute to a prolongation of the QTc interval).
No products indexed under this heading.

Desipramine Hydrochloride (There is a theoretical possibility that co-administration of other drugs known to alter cardiac conduction, such as tricyclic antidepressants, might also contribute to a prolongation of the QTc interval).
No products indexed under this heading.

Diltiazem Hydrochloride (There is a theoretical possibility that co-administration of other drugs known to alter cardiac conduction, such as calcium channel blockers, might also contribute to a prolongation of the QTc interval). Products include:
Cardizem LA Extended Release
Tablets 1728
Tiazac Capsules 1201

Disopyramide Phosphate (There is a theoretical possibility that co-administration of other drugs known to alter cardiac conduction, such as antiarrhythmic agents, might also contribute to a prolongation of the QTc interval).
No products indexed under this heading.

Divalproex Sodium (Co-administration may reduce seizure control by lowering the plasma levels of anticonvulsant; dosage of anticonvulsant may need to be adjusted). Products include:
Depakote Sprinkle Capsules 422
Depakote Tablets 427
Depakote ER Tablets 434

Dofetilide (There is a theoretical possibility that co-administration of other drugs known to alter cardiac conduction, such as antiarrhythmic agents, might also contribute to a prolongation of the QTc interval).
No products indexed under this heading.

Doxepin Hydrochloride (There is a theoretical possibility that co-administration of other drugs known to alter cardiac conduction, such as tricyclic antidepressants, might also contribute to a prolongation of the QTc interval).
No products indexed under this heading.

Esmolol Hydrochloride (There is a theoretical possibility that co-administration of other drugs known to alter cardiac conduction, such as beta blockers, might also contribute to a prolongation of the QTc interval).
No products indexed under this heading.

Ethosuximide (Co-administration may reduce seizure control by lowering the plasma levels of anticonvulsant; dosage of anticonvulsant may need to be adjusted).
No products indexed under this heading.

Ethotoin (Co-administration may reduce seizure control by lowering the plasma levels of anticonvulsant; dosage of anticonvulsant may need to be adjusted).
No products indexed under this heading.

Felbamate (Co-administration may reduce seizure control by lowering the plasma levels of anticonvulsant; dosage of anticonvulsant may need to be adjusted).
No products indexed under this heading.

Felodipine (There is a theoretical possibility that co-administration of other drugs known to alter cardiac conduction, such as calcium channel blockers, might also contribute to a prolongation of the QTc interval).
No products indexed under this heading.

Flecainide Acetate (There is a theoretical possibility that co-administration of other drugs known to alter cardiac conduction, such as antiarrhythmic agents, might also contribute to a prolongation of the QTc interval). Products include:
Tambocor Tablets 1856

Fluphenazine Decanoate (There is a theoretical possibility that co-administration of other drugs known to alter cardiac conduction, such as phenothiazines, might also contribute to a prolongation of the QTc interval).
No products indexed under this heading.

Fluphenazine Enanthate (There is a theoretical possibility that co-administration of other drugs known to alter cardiac conduction, such as phenothiazines, might also contribute to a prolongation of the QTc interval).
No products indexed under this heading.

Fluphenazine Hydrochloride (There is a theoretical possibility that co-administration of other drugs known to alter cardiac conduction, such as phenothiazines, might also contribute to a prolongation of the QTc interval).
No products indexed under this heading.

Fosphenytoin (Co-administration may reduce seizure control by lowering the plasma levels of anticonvulsant; dosage of anticonvulsant may need to be adjusted).
No products indexed under this heading.

Fosphenytoin Sodium (Co-administration may reduce seizure control by lowering the plasma levels of anticonvulsant; dosage of anticonvulsant may need to be adjusted).
No products indexed under this heading.

Gabapentin (Co-administration may reduce seizure control by lowering the plasma levels of anticonvulsant; dosage of anticonvulsant may need to be adjusted). Products include:
Neurontin Capsules 2487
Neurontin Oral Solution 2487
Neurontin Tablets 2487

Halofantrine (Administration of halofantrine subsequent to mefloquine suggests a significant, potentially fatal, prolongation of the QTc interval of ECG; halofantrine must not be given simultaneously with or subsequent to mefloquine).
No products indexed under this heading.

Imipramine Hydrochloride (There is a theoretical possibility that co-administration of other drugs known to alter cardiac conduction, such as tricyclic antidepressants, might also contribute to a prolongation of the QTc interval).
No products indexed under this heading.

Imipramine Pamoate (There is a theoretical possibility that co-administration of other drugs known to alter cardiac conduction, such as tricyclic antidepressants, might also contribute to a prolongation of the QTc interval).
No products indexed under this heading.

Isradipine (There is a theoretical possibility that co-administration of other drugs known to alter cardiac conduction, such as calcium channel blockers, might also contribute to a prolongation of the QTc interval). Products include:
DynaCirc CR Tablets 2721

Labetalol Hydrochloride (There is a theoretical possibility that co-administration of other drugs known to alter cardiac conduction, such as beta blockers, might also contribute to a prolongation of the QTc interval).
No products indexed under this heading.

Lamotrigine (Co-administration may reduce seizure control by lowering the plasma levels of anticonvulsant; dosage of anticonvulsant may need to be adjusted). Products include:
Lamictal 1481

Levetiracetam (Co-administration may reduce seizure control by lowering the plasma levels of anticonvulsant; dosage of anticonvulsant may need to be adjusted). Products include:
Keppra Injection 3320
Keppra Oral Solution 3314
Keppra Tablets 3314

Levobunolol Hydrochloride (There is a theoretical possibility that co-administration of other drugs known to alter cardiac conduction, such as beta blockers, might also contribute to a prolongation of the QTc interval). Products include:
Betagan Ophthalmic Solution,
USP.. ⊙220

Lidocaine Hydrochloride (There is a theoretical possibility that co-administration of other drugs known to alter cardiac conduction, such as antiarrhythmic agents, might also contribute to a prolongation of the QTc interval).
No products indexed under this heading.

IMPORTANT NOTE: Always consult each drug listing in the patient's regimen for possible interactions.

Maprotiline Hydrochloride (There is a theoretical possibility that co-administration of other drugs known to alter cardiac conduction, such as tricyclic antidepressants, might also contribute to a prolongation of the QTc interval).

No products indexed under this heading.

Mephenytoin (Co-administration may reduce seizure control by lowering the plasma levels of anticonvulsant; dosage of anticonvulsant may need to be adjusted).

No products indexed under this heading.

Mesoridazine Besylate (There is a theoretical possibility that co-administration of other drugs known to alter cardiac conduction, such as phenothiazines, might also contribute to a prolongation of the QTc interval).

No products indexed under this heading.

Methotrimeprazine (There is a theoretical possibility that co-administration of other drugs known to alter cardiac conduction, such as phenothiazines, might also contribute to a prolongation of the QTc interval).

No products indexed under this heading.

Methsuximide (Co-administration may reduce seizure control by lowering the plasma levels of anticonvulsant; dosage of anticonvulsant may need to be adjusted).

No products indexed under this heading.

Metipranolol Hydrochloride (There is a theoretical possibility that co-administration of other drugs known to alter cardiac conduction, such as beta blockers, might also contribute to a prolongation of the QTc interval).

No products indexed under this heading.

Metoprolol Succinate (There is a theoretical possibility that co-administration of other drugs known to alter cardiac conduction, such as beta blockers, might also contribute to a prolongation of the QTc interval). Products include:

Toprol-XL Tablets 668

Metoprolol Tartrate (There is a theoretical possibility that co-administration of other drugs known to alter cardiac conduction, such as beta blockers, might also contribute to a prolongation of the QTc interval). Products include:

Lopressor Injection 2238
Lopressor Tablets 2238
Lopressor HCT 50/25 Tablets 2241
Lopressor HCT 100/25 Tablets 2241
Lopressor HCT 100/50 Tablets 2241

Mexiletine Hydrochloride (There is a theoretical possibility that co-administration of other drugs known to alter cardiac conduction, such as antiarrhythmic agents, might also contribute to a prolongation of the QTc interval).

No products indexed under this heading.

Mibefradil Dihydrochloride (There is a theoretical possibility that co-administration of other drugs known to alter cardiac conduction, such as calcium channel blockers, might also contribute to a prolongation of the QTc interval).

No products indexed under this heading.

Moricizine Hydrochloride (There is a theoretical possibility that co-administration of other drugs known to alter cardiac conduction, such as antiarrhythmic agents, might also contribute to a prolongation of the QTc interval).

No products indexed under this heading.

Nadolol (There is a theoretical possibility that co-administration of other drugs known to alter cardiac conduction, such as beta blockers, might also contribute to a prolongation of the QTc interval). Products include:

Nadolol Tablets 2159

Nicardipine Hydrochloride (There is a theoretical possibility that co-administration of other drugs known to alter cardiac conduction, such as calcium channel blockers, might also contribute to a prolongation of the QTc interval). Products include:

Cardene I.V. 2497

Nifedipine (There is a theoretical possibility that co-administration of other drugs known to alter cardiac conduction, such as calcium channel blockers, might also contribute to a prolongation of the QTc interval). Products include:

Adalat CC Tablets 2964

Nimodipine (There is a theoretical possibility that co-administration of other drugs known to alter cardiac conduction, such as calcium channel blockers, might also contribute to a prolongation of the QTc interval). Products include:

Nimotop Capsules 749

Nisoldipine (There is a theoretical possibility that co-administration of other drugs known to alter cardiac conduction, such as calcium channel blockers, might also contribute to a prolongation of the QTc interval). Products include:

Sular Tablets 3122

Nortriptyline Hydrochloride (There is a theoretical possibility that co-administration of other drugs known to alter cardiac conduction, such as tricyclic antidepressants, might also contribute to a prolongation of the QTc interval).

No products indexed under this heading.

Oxcarbazepine (Co-administration may reduce seizure control by lowering the plasma levels of anticonvulsant; dosage of anticonvulsant may need to be adjusted). Products include:

Trileptal Tablets 2300
Trileptal Oral Suspension 2300

Paramethadione (Co-administration may reduce seizure control by lowering the plasma levels of anticonvulsant; dosage of anticonvulsant may need to be adjusted).

No products indexed under this heading.

Penbutolol Sulfate (There is a theoretical possibility that co-administration of other drugs known to alter cardiac conduction, such as beta blockers, might also contribute to a prolongation of the QTc interval).

No products indexed under this heading.

Perphenazine (There is a theoretical possibility that co-administration of other drugs known to alter cardiac conduction, such as phenothiazines, might also contribute to a prolongation of the QTc interval).

No products indexed under this heading.

Phenacemide (Co-administration may reduce seizure control by lowering the plasma levels of anticonvulsant; dosage of anticonvulsant may need to be adjusted).

No products indexed under this heading.

Phenobarbital (Co-administration may reduce seizure control by lowering the plasma levels of anticonvulsant; dosage of anticonvulsant may need to be adjusted). Products include:

Donnatal Extentabs 2493

Phensuximide (Co-administration may reduce seizure control by lowering the plasma levels of anticonvulsant; dosage of anticonvulsant may need to be adjusted).

No products indexed under this heading.

Phenytoin (Co-administration may reduce seizure control by lowering the plasma levels of anticonvulsant; dosage of anticonvulsant may need to be adjusted).

No products indexed under this heading.

Phenytoin Sodium (Co-administration may reduce seizure control by lowering the plasma levels of anticonvulsant; dosage of anticonvulsant may need to be adjusted). Products include:

Phenytek Capsules 2160

Pindolol (There is a theoretical possibility that co-administration of other drugs known to alter cardiac conduction, such as beta blockers, might also contribute to a prolongation of the QTc interval).

No products indexed under this heading.

Primidone (Co-administration may reduce seizure control by lowering the plasma levels of anticonvulsant; dosage of anticonvulsant may need to be adjusted).

No products indexed under this heading.

Procainamide Hydrochloride (There is a theoretical possibility that co-administration of other drugs known to alter cardiac conduction, such as antiarrhythmic agents, might also contribute to a prolongation of the QTc interval).

No products indexed under this heading.

Prochlorperazine (There is a theoretical possibility that co-administration of other drugs known to alter cardiac conduction, such as phenothiazines, might also contribute to a prolongation of the QTc interval).

No products indexed under this heading.

Promethazine Hydrochloride (There is a theoretical possibility that co-administration of other drugs

known to alter cardiac conduction, such as phenothiazines, might also contribute to a prolongation of the QTc interval). Products include:

Phenergan Tablets and
Suppositories................................ 3440

Propafenone Hydrochloride (There is a theoretical possibility that co-administration of other drugs known to alter cardiac conduction, such as antiarrhythmic agents, might also contribute to a prolongation of the QTc interval). Products include:

Rythmol SR Capsules 2727

Propranolol Hydrochloride (Co-administration has resulted in one report of cardiopulmonary arrest, with full recovery, in a patient; there is a theoretical possibility that co-administration of other drugs known to alter cardiac conduction, such as beta blockers, might also contribute to a prolongation of the QTc interval). Products include:

Inderal LA Long-Acting Capsules 3429
InnoPran XL Capsules 2723

Protriptyline Hydrochloride (There is a theoretical possibility that co-administration of other drugs known to alter cardiac conduction, such as tricyclic antidepressants, might also contribute to a prolongation of the QTc interval).

No products indexed under this heading.

Quinidine (Co-administration may produce electrocardiographic abnormalities and increase the risk of convulsions; if these drugs are to be used in the initial treatment of severe malaria, mefloquine administration should be delayed at least 12 hours after the last dose).

No products indexed under this heading.

Quinidine Gluconate (Co-administration may produce electrocardiographic abnormalities and increase the risk of convulsions; if these drugs are to be used in the initial treatment of severe malaria, mefloquine administration should be delayed at least 12 hours after the last dose).

No products indexed under this heading.

Quinidine Hydrochloride (Co-administration may produce electrocardiographic abnormalities and increase the risk of convulsions; if these drugs are to be used in the initial treatment of severe malaria, mefloquine administration should be delayed at least 12 hours after the last dose).

No products indexed under this heading.

Quinidine Polygalacturonate (Co-administration may produce electrocardiographic abnormalities and increase the risk of convulsions; if these drugs are to be used in the initial treatment of severe malaria, mefloquine administration should be delayed at least 12 hours after the last dose).

No products indexed under this heading.

Quinidine Sulfate (Co-administration may produce electrocardiographic abnormalities and increase the risk of convulsions; if these drugs are to be used in the initial treatment of severe malaria, mefloquine administration should be delayed at least 12 hours after the last dose).

No products indexed under this heading.

Quinine Sulfate (Co-administration may produce electrocardiographic abnormalities and increase the risk of convulsions; if these drugs are to be used in the initial treatment of severe malaria, mefloquine administration should be delayed at least 12 hours after the last dose).
No products indexed under this heading.

Sotalol Hydrochloride (There is a theoretical possibility that co-administration of other drugs known to alter cardiac conduction, such as beta blockers, might also contribute to a prolongation of the QTc interval).
No products indexed under this heading.

Terfenadine (There is a theoretical possibility that the co-administration of other drugs known to alter cardiac conduction, such as antihistamine terfenadine, might also contribute to a prolongation of the QTc interval).
No products indexed under this heading.

Thioridazine Hydrochloride (There is a theoretical possibility that co-administration of other drugs known to alter cardiac conduction, such as phenothiazines, might also contribute to a prolongation of the QTc interval). Products include:
Thioridazine Hydrochloride Tablets **2163**

Tiagabine Hydrochloride (Co-administration may reduce seizure control by lowering the plasma levels of anticonvulsant; dosage of anticonvulsant may need to be adjusted). Products include:
Gabitril Tablets **984**

Timolol Hemihydrate (There is a theoretical possibility that co-administration of other drugs known to alter cardiac conduction, such as beta blockers, might also contribute to a prolongation of the QTc interval). Products include:
Betimol Ophthalmic Solution **3382**
Betimol Ophthalmic Solution .... **⊙295**

Timolol Maleate (There is a theoretical possibility that co-administration of other drugs known to alter cardiac conduction, such as beta blockers, might also contribute to a prolongation of the QTc interval). Products include:
Blocadren Tablets **1916**
Cosopt Sterile Ophthalmic Solution **1931**
Timolide Tablets **2086**
Timoptic Sterile Ophthalmic Solution **2088**
Timoptic in Ocudose **2091**
Timoptic-XE Sterile Ophthalmic Gel Forming Solution **2092**

Tocainide Hydrochloride (There is a theoretical possibility that co-administration of other drugs known to alter cardiac conduction, such as antiarrhythmic agents, might also contribute to a prolongation of the QTc interval).
No products indexed under this heading.

Topiramate (Co-administration may reduce seizure control by lowering the plasma levels of anticonvulsant; dosage of anticonvulsant may need to be adjusted). Products include:
Topamax Sprinkle Capsules **2404**
Topamax Tablets **2404**

Trifluoperazine Hydrochloride (There is a theoretical possibility that co-administration of other drugs known to alter cardiac conduction, such as phenothiazines, might also contribute to a prolongation of the QTc interval).
No products indexed under this heading.

Trimethadione (Co-administration may reduce seizure control by lowering the plasma levels of anticonvulsant; dosage of anticonvulsant may need to be adjusted).
No products indexed under this heading.

Trimipramine Maleate (There is a theoretical possibility that co-administration of other drugs known to alter cardiac conduction, such as tricyclic antidepressants, might also contribute to a prolongation of the QTc interval).
No products indexed under this heading.

Typhoid Vaccine Live Oral TY21a (Attenuation of immunization cannot be excluded when co-administered). Products include:
Vivotif **819**

Valproate Sodium (Co-administration may reduce seizure control by lowering the plasma levels of anticonvulsant; dosage of anticonvulsant may need to be adjusted). Products include:
Depacon Injection **412**

Valproic Acid (Co-administration may reduce seizure control by lowering the plasma levels of anticonvulsant; dosage of anticonvulsant may need to be adjusted). Products include:
Depakene **417**

Verapamil Hydrochloride (There is a theoretical possibility that co-administration of other drugs known to alter cardiac conduction, such as calcium channel blockers, might also contribute to a prolongation of the QTc interval). Products include:
Covera-HS Tablets **3139**
Tarka Tablets **524**
Verelan PM Extended-Release Capsules, Controlled-Onset **3106**

Zonisamide (Co-administration may reduce seizure control by lowering the plasma levels of anticonvulsant; dosage of anticonvulsant may need to be adjusted). Products include:
Zonegran Capsules **1101**

LESCOL CAPSULES

(Fluvastatin Sodium) **2233**
May interact with erythromycin, fibrates, and certain other agents. Compounds in these categories include:

Cholestyramine (Administration of fluvastatin with, or up to 4 hours after cholestyramine results in significant reductions in AUC and Cmax of fluvastatin; however, use of fluvastatin 4 hours after resin results in clinically significant additive effect).
No products indexed under this heading.

Cimetidine (Co-administration results in a significant increase in the fluvastatin Cmax and AUC and a decrease in plasma clearance). Products include:
Tagamet HB 200 Tablets .... **▣664**

Cimetidine Hydrochloride (Co-administration results in a significant increase in the fluvastatin Cmax and AUC and a decrease in plasma clearance).
No products indexed under this heading.

Clofibrate (Myopathy has occasionally been associated with fibrates; combined use should generally be avoided).
No products indexed under this heading.

Cyclosporine (The risk of myopathy and/or rhabdomyolysis during treatment with HMG-CoA reductase inhibitor has been reported to be increased with concurrent cyclosporine; caution should be exercised). Products include:
Gengraf Capsules **459**
Neoral Oral Solution **2259**
Neoral Soft Gelatin Capsules **2259**
Restasis Ophthalmic Emulsion **575**
Sandimmune **2275**

Diclofenac Potassium (Co-administration increases the mean Cmax and AUC of diclofenac by 60% and 25% respectively).
No products indexed under this heading.

Diclofenac Sodium (Co-administration increases the mean Cmax and AUC of diclofenac by 60% and 25% respectively). Products include:
Arthrotec Tablets **3129**
Voltaren Ophthalmic Solution **2309**
Voltaren Tablets **2307**
Voltaren-XR Tablets **2310**

Digoxin (Co-administration in patients on chronic digoxin may result in a small increase in digoxin Cmax (11%) and urinary clearance). Products include:
Lanoxicaps Capsules **1490**
Lanoxin Injection **1494**
Lanoxin Injection Pediatric **1497**
Lanoxin Tablets **1500**

Erythromycin (The risk of myopathy and/or rhabdomyolysis during treatment with HMG-CoA reductase inhibitor has been reported to be increased with concurrent erythromycin; caution should be exercised). Products include:
Ery-Tab Tablets **449**
Erythromycin Base Filmtab Tablets **455**
Erythromycin Delayed-Release Capsules, USP **457**
PCE Dispertab Tablets **515**

Erythromycin Estolate (The risk of myopathy and/or rhabdomyolysis during treatment with HMG-CoA reductase inhibitor has been reported to be increased with concurrent erythromycin; caution should be exercised).
No products indexed under this heading.

Erythromycin Ethylsuccinate (The risk of myopathy and/or rhabdomyolysis during treatment with HMG-CoA reductase inhibitor has been reported to be increased with concurrent erythromycin; caution should be exercised). Products include:
E.E.S. **451**
EryPed **447**

Erythromycin Gluceptate (The risk of myopathy and/or rhabdomyolysis during treatment with HMG-CoA reductase inhibitor has been reported to be increased with concurrent erythromycin; caution should be exercised).
No products indexed under this heading.

Erythromycin Lactobionate (The risk of myopathy and/or rhabdomyolysis during treatment with HMG-CoA reductase inhibitor has been reported to be increased with concurrent erythromycin; caution should be exercised).
No products indexed under this heading.

Erythromycin Stearate (The risk of myopathy and/or rhabdomyolysis during treatment with HMG-CoA reductase inhibitor has been reported to be increased with concurrent erythromycin; caution should be exercised). Products include:
Erythrocin Stearate Filmtab Tablets **453**

Fenofibrate (Myopathy has occasionally been associated with fibrates; combined use should generally be avoided). Products include:
Lofibra Tablets **1219**
Lofibra Capsules **1216**
Tricor Tablets **527**
Triglide Tablets **3123**

Fluconazole (Administration of fluvastatin to volunteers pre-treated with fluconazole for 4 days results in an increase of fluvastatin Cmax and AUC by 44% and 84% respectively; caution should be exercised when fluvastatin is co-administered with fluconazole).
No products indexed under this heading.

Gemfibrozil (The risk of myopathy and/or rhabdomyolysis during treatment with HMG-CoA reductase inhibitor has been reported to be increased with concurrent gemfibrozil; combined use should generally be avoided).
No products indexed under this heading.

Glyburide (Co-administration results in increased mean Cmax, AUC, and t1/2 of glyburide approximately 50%, 69% and 121% respectively; glyburide increased the mean Cmax and AUC of fluvastatin by 44% and 51% respectively).
No products indexed under this heading.

Ketoconazole (Caution should be exercised if used concurrently with drugs that may decrease the levels of endogenous steroid hormones; increased potential for endocrine dysfunction). Products include:
Nizoral A-D Shampoo, 1% **1868**

Nicotinic Acid (The risk of myopathy and/or rhabdomyolysis during treatment with HMG-CoA reductase inhibitor has been reported to be increased with concurrent niacin; caution should be exercised).
No products indexed under this heading.

Omeprazole (Co-administration results in a significant increase in the fluvastatin Cmax and AUC and a decrease in plasma clearance). Products include:
Zegerid Capsules **2958**
Zegerid Powder for Oral Solution **2958**

Ranitidine Hydrochloride (Co-administration results in a significant

IMPORTANT NOTE: Always consult each drug listing in the patient's regimen for possible interactions.

increase in the fluvastatin Cmax and AUC and a decrease in plasma clearance). Products include:

Zantac **1624**
Zantac Injection **1619**
Zantac Injection Pharmacy Bulk Package **1622**

Rifampicin (Co-administration in patients pretreated with rifampin results in significant reduction in Cmax (59%) and AUC (51%) with a large increase (95%) in plasma clearance).

No products indexed under this heading.

Spironolactone (Caution should be exercised if used concurrently with drugs that may decrease the levels of endogenous steroid hormones; increased potential for endocrine dysfunction).

No products indexed under this heading.

Warfarin Sodium (Bleeding and/or increased prothrombin time has been reported with other HMG-CoA reductase inhibitors when used concurrently; no interactions at therapeutic concentrations have been demonstrated with fluvastatin and warfarin). Products include:

Coumadin for Injection **898**
Coumadin Tablets **898**

Food Interactions

Food, unspecified (Administration of regular formulation of fluvastatin with food reduces the rate but not the extent of absorption; administration with evening meal results in a two-fold decrease in Cmax and more than a two-fold increase in tmax as compared to administration 4 hours after the evening meal; administration of Lescol XL with a high fat meal delayed the absorption and increased the bioavailability by 50%).

LESCOL XL TABLETS

(Fluvastatin Sodium) **2233**
See Lescol Capsules

LEUKERAN TABLETS

(Chlorambucil) **1504**
May interact with vaccines, live. Compounds in these categories include:

BCG Vaccine (Administration of live vaccines to immunocompromised patients should be avoided).

No products indexed under this heading.

Measles, Mumps, Rubella and Varicella Virus Vaccine Live (Administration of live vaccines to immunocompromised patients should be avoided). Products include:

ProQuad **2064**

Measles, Mumps & Rubella Virus Vaccine, Live (Administration of live vaccines to immunocompromised patients should be avoided). Products include:

M-M-R II **2006**

Measles & Rubella Virus Vaccine Live (Administration of live vaccines to immunocompromised patients should be avoided).

No products indexed under this heading.

Measles Virus Vaccine Live (Administration of live vaccines to immunocompromised patients should be avoided). Products include:

Attenuvax **1914**

Mumps Virus Vaccine, Live (Administration of live vaccines to immunocompromised patients should be avoided). Products include:

Mumpsvax **2031**

Poliovirus Vaccine, Live, Oral, Trivalent, Types 1,2,3 (Sabin) (Administration of live vaccines to immunocompromised patients should be avoided).

No products indexed under this heading.

Rotavirus Vaccine, Live, Oral, Tetravalent (Administration of live vaccines to immunocompromised patients should be avoided).

No products indexed under this heading.

Rubella & Mumps Virus Vaccine Live (Administration of live vaccines to immunocompromised patients should be avoided).

No products indexed under this heading.

Rubella Virus Vaccine Live (Administration of live vaccines to immunocompromised patients should be avoided). Products include:

Meruvax II **2019**

Smallpox Vaccine (Administration of live vaccines to immunocompromised patients should be avoided).

No products indexed under this heading.

Typhoid Vaccine (Administration of live vaccines to immunocompromised patients should be avoided).

No products indexed under this heading.

Varicella Virus Vaccine Live (Administration of live vaccines to immunocompromised patients should be avoided). Products include:

Varivax **2100**

Yellow Fever Vaccine (Administration of live vaccines to immunocompromised patients should be avoided).

No products indexed under this heading.

LEUKINE

(Sargramostim) **814**
May interact with antimetabolites, cytotoxic drugs, drugs with myeloproliferative effects, and certain other agents. Compounds in these categories include:

Betamethasone Acetate (May potentiate the myeloproliferative effect).

No products indexed under this heading.

Betamethasone Sodium Phosphate (May potentiate the myeloproliferative effect).

No products indexed under this heading.

Bleomycin Sulfate (Coadministration within 24 hours preceding or following chemotherapy is not recommended because of potential sensitivity of rapidly dividing hematopoietic progenitor cells to cytotoxic therapy).

No products indexed under this heading.

Capecitabine (In patients who have been exposed to multiple myelotoxic agents, the effect of Leukine on myeloid reconstitution may be limited). Products include:

Xeloda Tablets **2822**

Cladribine (In patients who have been exposed to multiple myelotoxic agents, the effect of Leukine on myeloid reconstitution may be limited). Products include:

Leustatin Injection **2357**

Cortisone Acetate (May potentiate the myeloproliferative effect).

No products indexed under this heading.

Cyclophosphamide (Coadministration within 24 hours preceding or following chemotherapy is not recommended because of potential sensitivity of rapidly dividing hematopoietic progenitor cells to cytotoxic therapy).

No products indexed under this heading.

Cytarabine (In patients who have been exposed to multiple myelotoxic agents, the effect of Leukine on myeloid reconstitution may be limited).

No products indexed under this heading.

Daunorubicin Hydrochloride (Coadministration within 24 hours preceding or following chemotherapy is not recommended because of potential sensitivity of rapidly dividing hematopoietic progenitor cells to cytotoxic therapy).

No products indexed under this heading.

Dexamethasone (May potentiate the myeloproliferative effect). Products include:

Ciprodex Otic Suspension **559**
Decadron Tablets **1951**
TobraDex Ophthalmic Ointment **562**
TobraDex Ophthalmic Suspension **563**

Dexamethasone Acetate (May potentiate the myeloproliferative effect).

No products indexed under this heading.

Dexamethasone Sodium Phosphate (May potentiate the myeloproliferative effect).

No products indexed under this heading.

Doxorubicin Hydrochloride (Coadministration within 24 hours preceding or following chemotherapy is not recommended because of potential sensitivity of rapidly dividing hematopoietic progenitor cells to cytotoxic therapy).

No products indexed under this heading.

Epirubicin Hydrochloride (Coadministration within 24 hours preceding or following chemotherapy is not recommended because of potential sensitivity of rapidly dividing hematopoietic progenitor cells to cytotoxic therapy).

No products indexed under this heading.

Floxuridine (In patients who have been exposed to multiple myelotoxic agents, the effect of Leukine on myeloid reconstitution may be limited).

No products indexed under this heading.

Fludarabine Phosphate (In patients who have been exposed to multiple myelotoxic agents, the effect of Leukine on myeloid reconstitution may be limited).

No products indexed under this heading.

Fluorouracil (Coadministration within 24 hours preceding or following chemotherapy is not recommended because of potential sensitivity of rapidly dividing hematopoietic progenitor cells to cytotoxic therapy). Products include:

Carac Cream, 0.5% **2879**
Efudex **3363**

Gemcitabine Hydrochloride (In patients who have been exposed to multiple myelotoxic agents, the effect of Leukine on myeloid reconstitution may be limited). Products include:

Gemzar for Injection **1771**

Hydrocortisone (May potentiate the myeloproliferative effect). Products include:

Colocort Rectal Suspension, USP (Retention) 100 mg/60 mL **2476**
Hydrocortone Tablets **1989**
Preparation H Hydrocortisone Cream .... ▣**646**

Hydrocortisone Acetate (May potentiate the myeloproliferative effect). Products include:

Analpram-HC **1159**
Pramosone **1161**
ProctoFoam-HC **3099**

Hydrocortisone Sodium Phosphate (May potentiate the myeloproliferative effect).

No products indexed under this heading.

Hydrocortisone Sodium Succinate (May potentiate the myeloproliferative effect).

No products indexed under this heading.

Hydroxyurea (Coadministration within 24 hours preceding or following chemotherapy is not recommended because of potential sensitivity of rapidly dividing hematopoietic progenitor cells to cytotoxic therapy).

No products indexed under this heading.

Lithium Carbonate (May potentiate the myeloproliferative effect). Products include:

Lithobid Tablets **1692**

Lithium Citrate (May potentiate the myeloproliferative effect).

No products indexed under this heading.

Mercaptopurine (In patients who have been exposed to multiple myelotoxic agents, the effect of Leukine on myeloid reconstitution may be limited).

No products indexed under this heading.

Methotrexate (In patients who have been exposed to multiple myelotoxic agents, the effect of Leukine on myeloid reconstitution may be limited).

No products indexed under this heading.

Methotrexate Sodium (Coadministration within 24 hours preceding or following chemotherapy is not recommended because of potential sensitivity of rapidly dividing hematopoietic progenitor cells to cytotoxic therapy).

No products indexed under this heading.

Methylprednisolone Acetate (May potentiate the myeloproliferative effect). Products include:

Depo-Medrol Injectable Suspension **2617**
Depo-Medrol Single-Dose Vial **2619**

Methylprednisolone Sodium Succinate (May potentiate the myeloproliferative effect).
No products indexed under this heading.

Mitotane (Coadministration within 24 hours preceding or following chemotherapy is not recommended because of potential sensitivity of rapidly dividing hematopoietic progenitor cells to cytotoxic therapy).
No products indexed under this heading.

Mitoxantrone Hydrochloride (Coadministration within 24 hours preceding or following chemotherapy is not recommended because of potential sensitivity of rapidly dividing hematopoietic progenitor cells to cytotoxic therapy).
No products indexed under this heading.

Pentostatin (In patients who have been exposed to multiple myelotoxic agents, the effect of Leukine on myeloid reconstitution may be limited). Products include:
Nipent for Injection 1863

Prednisolone Acetate (May potentiate the myeloproliferative effect). Products include:
Blephamide Ophthalmic Ointment 568
Blephamide Ophthalmic Suspension 569
Poly-Pred Ophthalmic Suspension .... ⊙233
Pred Forte Ophthalmic Suspension .... ⊙235
Pred Mild Ophthalmic Suspension .... ⊙238
Pred-G Ophthalmic Ointment .... ⊙237
Pred-G Ophthalmic Suspension .... ⊙236

Prednisolone Sodium Phosphate (May potentiate the myeloproliferative effect).
No products indexed under this heading.

Prednisolone Tebutate (May potentiate the myeloproliferative effect).
No products indexed under this heading.

Prednisone (May potentiate the myeloproliferative effect).
No products indexed under this heading.

Procarbazine Hydrochloride (Coadministration within 24 hours preceding or following chemotherapy is not recommended because of potential sensitivity of rapidly dividing hematopoietic progenitor cells to cytotoxic therapy). Products include:
Matulane Capsules 3191

Tamoxifen Citrate (Coadministration within 24 hours preceding or following chemotherapy is not recommended because of potential sensitivity of rapidly dividing hematopoietic progenitor cells to cytotoxic therapy). Products include:
Soltamox Oral Solution 3527

Thioguanine (In patients who have been exposed to multiple myelotoxic agents, the effect of Leukine on myeloid reconstitution may be limited). Products include:
Tabloid Tablets 1575

Triamcinolone (May potentiate the myeloproliferative effect).
No products indexed under this heading.

Triamcinolone Acetonide (May potentiate the myeloproliferative effect). Products include:
Azmacort Inhalation Aerosol 1726
Nasacort AQ Nasal Spray 2922

Triamcinolone Diacetate (May potentiate the myeloproliferative effect).
No products indexed under this heading.

Triamcinolone Hexacetonide (May potentiate the myeloproliferative effect).
No products indexed under this heading.

Vincristine Sulfate (Coadministration within 24 hours preceding or following chemotherapy is not recommended because of potential sensitivity of rapidly dividing hematopoietic progenitor cells to cytotoxic therapy).
No products indexed under this heading.

LEUSTATIN INJECTION

(Cladribine) 2357
May interact with immunosuppressive agents, agents associated with myelosuppression, and certain other agents. Compounds in these categories include:

Altretamine (Caution should be exercised if co-administered with other drugs known to cause immunosuppression).
No products indexed under this heading.

Azathioprine (Caution should be exercised if co-administered with other drugs known to cause immunosuppression).
No products indexed under this heading.

Basiliximab (Caution should be exercised if co-administered with other drugs known to cause immunosuppression). Products include:
Simulect for Injection 2284

Bone Marrow Depressants, unspecified (Caution should be exercised if co-administered with other drugs known to cause myelosuppression).
No products indexed under this heading.

Busulfan (Caution should be exercised if co-administered with other drugs known to cause immunosuppression). Products include:
I.V. Busulfex 2493
Myleran Tablets 1525

Chlorambucil (Caution should be exercised if co-administered with other drugs known to cause immunosuppression). Products include:
Leukeran Tablets 1504

Cyclosporine (Caution should be exercised if co-administered with other drugs known to cause immunosuppression). Products include:
Gengraf Capsules 459
Neoral Oral Solution 2259
Neoral Soft Gelatin Capsules 2259
Restasis Ophthalmic Emulsion 575
Sandimmune 2275

Daunorubicin Citrate Liposome (Caution should be exercised if co-administered with other drugs known to cause immunosuppression).
No products indexed under this heading.

Daunorubicin Hydrochloride (Caution should be exercised if co-administered with other drugs known to cause immunosuppression).
No products indexed under this heading.

Dexrazoxane (Caution should be exercised if co-administered with other drugs known to cause immunosuppression). Products include:
Zinecard for Injection 2650

Doxorubicin Hydrochloride (Caution should be exercised if co-administered with other drugs known to cause immunosuppression).
No products indexed under this heading.

Doxorubicin Hydrochloride Liposome (Caution should be exercised if co-administered with other drugs known to cause immunosuppression). Products include:
Doxil Injection 2351

Fludarabine Phosphate (Caution should be exercised if co-administered with other drugs known to cause immunosuppression).
No products indexed under this heading.

Gemcitabine Hydrochloride (Caution should be exercised if co-administered with other drugs known to cause immunosuppression). Products include:
Gemzar for Injection 1771

Gemtuzumab Ozogamicin (Caution should be exercised if co-administered with other drugs known to cause immunosuppression). Products include:
Mylotarg for Injection 3431

Idarubicin Hydrochloride (Caution should be exercised if co-administered with other drugs known to cause immunosuppression).
No products indexed under this heading.

Immunosuppressants (Caution should be exercised if co-administered with other drugs known to cause immunosuppression).
No products indexed under this heading.

Interferon alfa-2a, Recombinant (Caution should be exercised if co-administered with other drugs known to cause immunosuppression).
No products indexed under this heading.

Irinotecan Hydrochloride (Caution should be exercised if co-administered with other drugs known to cause immunosuppression). Products include:
Camptosar Injection 2604

Melphalan Hydrochloride (Caution should be exercised if co-administered with other drugs known to cause immunosuppression). Products include:
Alkeran for Injection 955

Mercaptopurine (Caution should be exercised if co-administered with other drugs known to cause immunosuppression).
No products indexed under this heading.

Mitoxantrone Hydrochloride (Caution should be exercised if co-administered with other drugs known to cause immunosuppression).
No products indexed under this heading.

Muromonab-CD3 (Caution should be exercised if co-administered with other drugs known to cause immunosuppression). Products include:
Orthoclone OKT3 Sterile Solution 2360

Mycophenolate Mofetil (Caution should be exercised if co-administered with other drugs known to cause immunosuppression). Products include:
CellCept Capsules 2747
CellCept Oral Suspension 2747
CellCept Tablets 2747

Sirolimus (Caution should be exercised if co-administered with other drugs known to cause immunosuppression). Products include:
Rapamune Oral Solution and Tablets 3475

Tacrolimus (Caution should be exercised if co-administered with other drugs known to cause immunosuppression). Products include:
Prograf Capsules and Injection 632
Protopic Ointment 638

Temozolomide (Caution should be exercised if co-administered with other drugs known to cause immunosuppression). Products include:
Temodar Capsules 3073

Thioguanine (Caution should be exercised if co-administered with other drugs known to cause immunosuppression). Products include:
Tabloid Tablets 1575

Vinorelbine Tartrate (Caution should be exercised if co-administered with other drugs known to cause immunosuppression).
No products indexed under this heading.

LEVAQUIN ORAL SOLUTION

(Levofloxacin) 2384
See Levaquin Tablets

LEVAQUIN INJECTION

(Levofloxacin) 2384
May interact with class 1A antiarrhythmics, class III antiarrhythmics, corticosteroids, erythromycin, oral hypoglycemic agents, non-steroidal anti-inflammatory agents, psychotropics, quinidine, tricyclic antidepressants, xanthines, and certain other agents. Compounds in these categories include:

Acarbose (Disturbances of blood glucose, including hyper- and hypoglycemia, have been reported in patients treated concomitantly with quinolones and an antidiabetic agent; careful monitoring of blood glucose levels is recommended). Products include:
Precose Tablets 751

Alprazolam (Levofloxacin has been associated with prolongation of the QTc interval; co-administration with drugs known to prolong QT interval should be avoided). Products include:
Niravam Orally Disintegrating Tablets 3092

Aminophylline (Co-administration of other quinolones with theophylline has resulted in prolonged elimination half-life, elevated serum theophylline levels, and increased risk of theophylline related toxicity; no significant effect of levofloxacin on theophylline pharmacokinetic parameters has been detected, however, caution should be exercised).
No products indexed under this heading.

Amiodarone Hydrochloride (Levofloxacin has been associated with prolongation of the QTc interval; co-administration with drugs known to prolong QT interval should be avoided).
No products indexed under this heading.

Amitriptyline Hydrochloride (Levofloxacin has been associated with prolongation of the QTc interval; co-administration with drugs known to prolong QT interval should be avoided).

No products indexed under this heading.

Amoxapine (Levofloxacin has been associated with prolongation of the QTc interval; co-administration with drugs known to prolong QT interval should be avoided).

No products indexed under this heading.

Arsenic Trioxide (Levofloxacin has been associated with prolongation of the QTc interval; co-administration with drugs known to prolong QT interval should be avoided). Products include:

Trisenox Injection 993

Betamethasone Acetate (Achilles and other tendon ruptures have been reported with quinolones, post-market surveillance reports indicate that the risk may be increased in patients on concomitant corticosteroids).

No products indexed under this heading.

Betamethasone Sodium Phosphate (Achilles and other tendon ruptures have been reported with quinolones, post-market surveillance reports indicate that the risk may be increased in patients on concomitant corticosteroids).

No products indexed under this heading.

Bretylium Tosylate (Levofloxacin has been associated with prolongation of the QT interval and infrequent cases of arrhythmia. Rare cases of torsades de pointes have been spontaneously reported during post-marketing surveillance in patients receiving levofloxacin. Levofloxacin should be avoided in patients receiving class III antiarrhythmic agents).

No products indexed under this heading.

Buspirone Hydrochloride (Levofloxacin has been associated with prolongation of the QTc interval; co-administration with drugs known to prolong QT interval should be avoided).

No products indexed under this heading.

Celecoxib (Co-administration may increase the risk of CNS stimulation and convulsive seizures). Products include:

Celebrex Capsules 3134

Chlordiazepoxide (Levofloxacin has been associated with prolongation of the QTc interval; co-administration with drugs known to prolong QT interval should be avoided).

No products indexed under this heading.

Chlordiazepoxide Hydrochloride (Levofloxacin has been associated with prolongation of the QTc interval; co-administration with drugs known to prolong QT interval should be avoided). Products include:

Librium Capsules 3347

Chlorpromazine (Levofloxacin has been associated with prolongation of the QTc interval; co-administration with drugs known to prolong QT interval should be avoided).

No products indexed under this heading.

Chlorpromazine Hydrochloride (Levofloxacin has been associated with prolongation of the QTc interval; co-administration with drugs known to prolong QT interval should be avoided).

No products indexed under this heading.

Chlorpropamide (Disturbances of blood glucose, including hyper- and hypoglycemia, have been reported in patients treated concomitantly with quinolones and an antidiabetic agent; careful monitoring of blood glucose levels is recommended).

No products indexed under this heading.

Chlorprothixene (Levofloxacin has been associated with prolongation of the QTc interval; co-administration with drugs known to prolong QT interval should be avoided).

No products indexed under this heading.

Chlorprothixene Hydrochloride (Levofloxacin has been associated with prolongation of the QTc interval; co-administration with drugs known to prolong QT interval should be avoided).

No products indexed under this heading.

Cimetidine (Co-administration has resulted in higher levofloxacin AUC and t1/2, while CL/F and CLr were lower during concomitant treatment with cimetidine). Products include:

Tagamet HB 200 Tablets ▣ 664

Cimetidine Hydrochloride (Co-administration has resulted in higher levofloxacin AUC and t1/2, while CL/F and CLr were lower during concomitant treatment with cimetidine).

No products indexed under this heading.

Cisapride (Levofloxacin has been associated with prolongation of the QTc interval; co-administration with drugs known to prolong QT interval should be avoided).

No products indexed under this heading.

Clomipramine Hydrochloride (Levofloxacin has been associated with prolongation of the QTc interval; co-administration with drugs known to prolong QT interval should be avoided).

No products indexed under this heading.

Clorazepate Dipotassium (Levofloxacin has been associated with prolongation of the QTc interval; co-administration with drugs known to prolong QT interval should be avoided). Products include:

Tranxene .. 2474

Clozapine (Levofloxacin has been associated with prolongation of the QTc interval; co-administration with drugs known to prolong QT interval should be avoided). Products include:

Clozaril Tablets 2184
FazaClo Orally Disintegrating Tablets .. 551

Cortisone Acetate (Achilles and other tendon ruptures have been reported with quinolones, post-market surveillance reports indicate that the risk may be increased in patients on concomitant corticosteroids).

No products indexed under this heading.

Cyclosporine (Levofloxacin Cmax and Ke were slightly lower while

Tmax and t1/2 were slightly longer in the presence of cyclosporine; these differences, however, are not clinically significant, therefore, no dosage adjustment is required).
Products include:

Gengraf Capsules 459
Neoral Oral Solution 2259
Neoral Soft Gelatin Capsules 2259
Restasis Ophthalmic Emulsion 575
Sandimmune 2275

Desipramine Hydrochloride (Levofloxacin has been associated with prolongation of the QTc interval; co-administration with drugs known to prolong QT interval should be avoided).

No products indexed under this heading.

Dexamethasone (Achilles and other tendon ruptures have been reported with quinolones, post-market surveillance reports indicate that the risk may be increased in patients on concomitant corticosteroids).
Products include:

Ciprodex Otic Suspension 559
Decadron Tablets 1951
TobraDex Ophthalmic Ointment 562
TobraDex Ophthalmic Suspension ... 563

Dexamethasone Acetate (Achilles and other tendon ruptures have been reported with quinolones, post-market surveillance reports indicate that the risk may be increased in patients on concomitant corticosteroids).

No products indexed under this heading.

Dexamethasone Sodium Phosphate (Achilles and other tendon ruptures have been reported with quinolones, post-market surveillance reports indicate that the risk may be increased in patients on concomitant corticosteroids).

No products indexed under this heading.

Diazepam (Levofloxacin has been associated with prolongation of the QTc interval; co-administration with drugs known to prolong QT interval should be avoided). Products include:

Diastat Rectal Delivery System 3343
Valium Tablets 2819

Diclofenac Potassium (Co-administration may increase the risk of CNS stimulation and convulsive seizures).

No products indexed under this heading.

Diclofenac Sodium (Co-administration may increase the risk of CNS stimulation and convulsive seizures). Products include:

Arthrotec Tablets 3129
Voltaren Ophthalmic Solution 2309
Voltaren Tablets 2307
Voltaren-XR Tablets 2310

Disopyramide (Levofloxacin has been associated with prolongation of the QT interval and infrequent cases of arrhythmia. Rare cases of torsades de pointes have been spontaneously reported during post-marketing surveillance in patients receiving levofloxacin. Levofloxacin should be avoided in patients receiving class IA antiarrhythmic agents).

No products indexed under this heading.

Doxepin Hydrochloride (Levofloxacin has been associated with prolongation of the QTc interval; co-administration with drugs known to prolong QT interval should be avoided).

No products indexed under this heading.

Droperidol (Levofloxacin has been associated with prolongation of the QTc interval; co-administration with drugs known to prolong QT interval should be avoided).

No products indexed under this heading.

Dyphylline (Co-administration of other quinolones with theophylline has resulted in prolonged elimination half-life, elevated serum theophylline levels, and increased risk of theophylline related toxicity; no significant effect of levofloxacin on theophylline pharmacokinetic parameters has been detected, however, caution should be exercised).

No products indexed under this heading.

Erythromycin (Levofloxacin has been associated with prolongation of the QTc interval; co-administration with drugs known to prolong QT interval should be avoided). Products include:

Ery-Tab Tablets 449
Erythromycin Base Filmtab Tablets .. 455
Erythromycin Delayed-Release Capsules, USP............................. 457
PCE Dispertab Tablets 515

Erythromycin Estolate (Levofloxacin has been associated with prolongation of the QTc interval; co-administration with drugs known to prolong QT interval should be avoided).

No products indexed under this heading.

Erythromycin Ethylsuccinate (Levofloxacin has been associated with prolongation of the QTc interval; co-administration with drugs known to prolong QT interval should be avoided). Products include:

E.E.S. ... 451
EryPed .. 447

Erythromycin Gluceptate (Levofloxacin has been associated with prolongation of the QTc interval; co-administration with drugs known to prolong QT interval should be avoided).

No products indexed under this heading.

Erythromycin Lactobionate (Levofloxacin has been associated with prolongation of the QTc interval; co-administration with drugs known to prolong QT interval should be avoided).

No products indexed under this heading.

Erythromycin Stearate (Levofloxacin has been associated with prolongation of the QTc interval; co-administration with drugs known to prolong QT interval should be avoided). Products include:

Erythrocin Stearate Filmtab Tablets .. 453

Etodolac (Co-administration may increase the risk of CNS stimulation and convulsive seizures).

No products indexed under this heading.

Fenoprofen Calcium (Co-administration may increase the risk of CNS stimulation and convulsive seizures). Products include:

Nalfon Capsules 2502

Fludrocortisone Acetate (Achilles and other tendon ruptures have been reported with quinolones, post-market surveillance reports indicate that the risk may be increased in patients on concomitant corticosteroids).
No products indexed under this heading.

Fluphenazine Decanoate (Levofloxacin has been associated with prolongation of the QTc interval; co-administration with drugs known to prolong QT interval should be avoided).
No products indexed under this heading.

Fluphenazine Enanthate (Levofloxacin has been associated with prolongation of the QTc interval; co-administration with drugs known to prolong QT interval should be avoided).
No products indexed under this heading.

Fluphenazine Hydrochloride (Levofloxacin has been associated with prolongation of the QTc interval; co-administration with drugs known to prolong QT interval should be avoided).
No products indexed under this heading.

Flurbiprofen (Co-administration may increase the risk of CNS stimulation and convulsive seizures).
No products indexed under this heading.

Glimepiride (Disturbances of blood glucose, including hyper- and hypoglycemia, have been reported in patients treated concomitantly with quinolones and an antidiabetic agent; careful monitoring of blood glucose levels is recommended). Products include:
Avandaryl Tablets 1379
Duetact Tablets 3226

Glipizide (Disturbances of blood glucose, including hyper- and hypoglycemia, have been reported in patients treated concomitantly with quinolones and an antidiabetic agent; careful monitoring of blood glucose levels is recommended).
No products indexed under this heading.

Glyburide (Disturbances of blood glucose, including hyper- and hypoglycemia, have been reported in patients treated concomitantly with quinolones and an antidiabetic agent; careful monitoring of blood glucose levels is recommended).
No products indexed under this heading.

Haloperidol (Levofloxacin has been associated with prolongation of the QTc interval; co-administration with drugs known to prolong QT interval should be avoided).
No products indexed under this heading.

Haloperidol Decanoate (Levofloxacin has been associated with prolongation of the QTc interval; co-administration with drugs known to prolong QT interval should be avoided).
No products indexed under this heading.

Hydrocortisone (Achilles and other tendon ruptures have been reported with quinolones, post-market surveillance reports indicate that the risk may be increased in patients on concomitant corticosteroids). Products include:
Colocort Rectal Suspension, USP (Retention) 100 mg/60 mL........... 2476
Hydrocortone Tablets 1989
Preparation H Hydrocortisone Cream 646

Hydrocortisone Acetate (Achilles and other tendon ruptures have been reported with quinolones, post-market surveillance reports indicate that the risk may be increased in patients on concomitant corticosteroids). Products include:
Analpram-HC 1159
Pramosone 1161
ProctoFoam-HC 3099

Hydrocortisone Sodium Phosphate (Achilles and other tendon ruptures have been reported with quinolones, post-market surveillance reports indicate that the risk may be increased in patients on concomitant corticosteroids).
No products indexed under this heading.

Hydrocortisone Sodium Succinate (Achilles and other tendon ruptures have been reported with quinolones, post-market surveillance reports indicate that the risk may be increased in patients on concomitant corticosteroids).
No products indexed under this heading.

Hydroxyzine Hydrochloride (Levofloxacin has been associated with prolongation of the QTc interval; co-administration with drugs known to prolong QT interval should be avoided).
No products indexed under this heading.

Ibuprofen (Co-administration may increase the risk of CNS stimulation and convulsive seizures). Products include:
Advil Allergy Sinus Caplets 770
Advil 674
Children's Advil Oral Suspension 603
Children's Advil Chewable Tablets .. 603
Advil Cold & Sinus 723
Infants' Advil Concentrated Drops .. 604
Infants' Advil Concentrated Drops - White Grape (Dye-Free)............. 604
Junior Strength Advil Swallow Tablets.. 605
Advil Migraine Liquigels 608
Advil Multi-Symptom Cold Caplets....................................... 770
Advil PM Caplets 615
Motrin IB Tablets and Caplets 1866
Children's Motrin Oral Suspension ... 1867
Children's Motrin Non-Staining Dye-Free Oral Suspension............ 1867
Children's Motrin Cold Oral Suspension 1867
Infants' Motrin Concentrated Drops.. 1867
Infants' Motrin Non-Staining Dye-Free Concentrated Drops....... 1867
Junior Strength Motrin Caplets and Chewable Tablets.................. 1867
Vicoprofen Tablets 539

Imipramine Hydrochloride (Levofloxacin has been associated with prolongation of the QTc interval; co-administration with drugs known to prolong QT interval should be avoided).
No products indexed under this heading.

Imipramine Pamoate (Levofloxacin has been associated with prolongation of the QTc interval; co-administration with drugs known to prolong QT interval should be avoided).
No products indexed under this heading.

Indomethacin (Co-administration may increase the risk of CNS stimulation and convulsive seizures). Products include:
Indocin 1995

Indomethacin Sodium Trihydrate (Co-administration may increase the risk of CNS stimulation and convulsive seizures). Products include:
Indocin I.V. 2465

Isocarboxazid (Levofloxacin has been associated with prolongation of the QTc interval; co-administration with drugs known to prolong QT interval should be avoided).
No products indexed under this heading.

Ketoprofen (Co-administration may increase the risk of CNS stimulation and convulsive seizures).
No products indexed under this heading.

Ketorolac Tromethamine (Co-administration may increase the risk of CNS stimulation and convulsive seizures). Products include:
Acular Ophthalmic Solution 565
Acular LS Ophthalmic Solution 566

Lithium Carbonate (Levofloxacin has been associated with prolongation of the QTc interval; co-administration with drugs known to prolong QT interval should be avoided). Products include:
Lithobid Tablets 1692

Lithium Citrate (Levofloxacin has been associated with prolongation of the QTc interval; co-administration with drugs known to prolong QT interval should be avoided).
No products indexed under this heading.

Lorazepam (Levofloxacin has been associated with prolongation of the QTc interval; co-administration with drugs known to prolong QT interval should be avoided).
No products indexed under this heading.

Loxapine Hydrochloride (Levofloxacin has been associated with prolongation of the QTc interval; co-administration with drugs known to prolong QT interval should be avoided).
No products indexed under this heading.

Loxapine Succinate (Levofloxacin has been associated with prolongation of the QTc interval; co-administration with drugs known to prolong QT interval should be avoided).
No products indexed under this heading.

Maprotiline Hydrochloride (Levofloxacin has been associated with prolongation of the QTc interval; co-administration with drugs known to prolong QT interval should be avoided).
No products indexed under this heading.

Meclofenamate Sodium (Co-administration may increase the risk of CNS stimulation and convulsive seizures).
No products indexed under this heading.

Mefenamic Acid (Co-administration may increase the risk of CNS stimulation and convulsive seizures).
No products indexed under this heading.

Meloxicam (Co-administration may increase the risk of CNS stimulation and convulsive seizures). Products include:
Mobic Oral Suspension 863
Mobic Tablets 863

Meprobamate (Levofloxacin has been associated with prolongation of the QTc interval; co-administration with drugs known to prolong QT interval should be avoided).
No products indexed under this heading.

Mesoridazine Besylate (Levofloxacin has been associated with prolongation of the QTc interval; co-administration with drugs known to prolong QT interval should be avoided).
No products indexed under this heading.

Metformin Hydrochloride (Disturbances of blood glucose, including hyper- and hypoglycemia, have been reported in patients treated concomitantly with quinolones and an antidiabetic agent; careful monitoring of blood glucose levels is recommended). Products include:
ActoPlus Met Tablets 3214
Avandamet Tablets 1373
Fortamet Extended-Release Tablets.. 3115

Methylprednisolone Acetate (Achilles and other tendon ruptures have been reported with quinolones, post-market surveillance reports indicate that the risk may be increased in patients on concomitant corticosteroids). Products include:
Depo-Medrol Injectable Suspension 2617
Depo-Medrol Single-Dose Vial 2619

Methylprednisolone Sodium Succinate (Achilles and other tendon ruptures have been reported with quinolones, post-market surveillance reports indicate that the risk may be increased in patients on concomitant corticosteroids).
No products indexed under this heading.

Midazolam Hydrochloride (Levofloxacin has been associated with prolongation of the QTc interval; co-administration with drugs known to prolong QT interval should be avoided).
No products indexed under this heading.

Miglitol (Disturbances of blood glucose, including hyper- and hypoglycemia, have been reported in patients treated concomitantly with quinolones and an antidiabetic agent; careful monitoring of blood glucose levels is recommended).
No products indexed under this heading.

Molindone Hydrochloride (Levofloxacin has been associated with prolongation of the QTc interval; co-administration with drugs known to prolong QT interval should be avoided). Products include:

Moricizine Hydrochloride (Levofloxacin has been associated with prolongation of the QT interval and infrequent cases of arrhythmia. Rare cases of torsades de pointes have been spontaneously reported during post-marketing surveillance in patients receiving levofloxacin. Levofloxacin should be avoided in patients receiving class IA antiarrhythmic agents).

 No products indexed under this heading.

Nabumetone (Co-administration may increase the risk of CNS stimulation and convulsive seizures).

 No products indexed under this heading.

Naproxen (Co-administration may increase the risk of CNS stimulation and convulsive seizures). Products include:

Naproxen Sodium (Co-administration may increase the risk of CNS stimulation and convulsive seizures). Products include:

Nortriptyline Hydrochloride (Levofloxacin has been associated with prolongation of the QTc interval; co-administration with drugs known to prolong QT interval should be avoided).

 No products indexed under this heading.

Olanzapine (Levofloxacin has been associated with prolongation of the QTc interval; co-administration with drugs known to prolong QT interval should be avoided). Products include:

Oxaprozin (Co-administration may increase the risk of CNS stimulation and convulsive seizures).

 No products indexed under this heading.

Oxazepam (Levofloxacin has been associated with prolongation of the QTc interval; co-administration with drugs known to prolong QT interval should be avoided).

 No products indexed under this heading.

Perphenazine (Levofloxacin has been associated with prolongation of the QTc interval; co-administration with drugs known to prolong QT interval should be avoided).

 No products indexed under this heading.

Phenelzine Sulfate (Levofloxacin has been associated with prolongation of the QTc interval; co-administration with drugs known to prolong QT interval should be avoided).

 No products indexed under this heading.

Phenylbutazone (Co-administration may increase the risk of CNS stimulation and convulsive seizures).

 No products indexed under this heading.

Pimozide (Levofloxacin has been associated with prolongation of the QTc interval; co-administration with drugs known to prolong QT interval should be avoided).

 No products indexed under this heading.

Pioglitazone Hydrochloride (Disturbances of blood glucose, including hyper- and hypoglycemia, have been reported in patients treated concomitantly with quinolones and an antidiabetic agent; careful monitoring of blood glucose levels is recommended). Products include:

Piroxicam (Co-administration may increase the risk of CNS stimulation and convulsive seizures).

 No products indexed under this heading.

Prazepam (Levofloxacin has been associated with prolongation of the QTc interval; co-administration with drugs known to prolong QT interval should be avoided).

 No products indexed under this heading.

Prednisolone Acetate (Achilles and other tendon ruptures have been reported with quinolones, post-market surveillance reports indicate that the risk may be increased in patients on concomitant corticosteroids). Products include:

Prednisolone Sodium Phosphate (Achilles and other tendon ruptures have been reported with quinolones, post-market surveillance reports indicate that the risk may be increased in patients on concomitant corticosteroids).

 No products indexed under this heading.

Prednisolone Tebutate (Achilles and other tendon ruptures have been reported with quinolones, post-market surveillance reports indicate that the risk may be increased in patients on concomitant corticosteroids).

 No products indexed under this heading.

Prednisone (Achilles and other tendon ruptures have been reported with quinolones, post-market surveillance reports indicate that the risk may be increased in patients on concomitant corticosteroids).

 No products indexed under this heading.

Probenecid (Co-administration has resulted in higher levofloxacin AUC and t1/2, while CL/F and CLr were lower during concomitant treatment with probenecid).

 No products indexed under this heading.

Procainamide (Levofloxacin has been associated with prolongation of the QT interval and infrequent cases of arrhythmia. Rare cases of torsades de pointes have been spontaneously reported during post-marketing surveillance in patients receiving levofloxacin. Levofloxacin should be avoided in patients receiving class IA antiarrhythmic agents).

 No products indexed under this heading.

Procainamide Hydrochloride (Levofloxacin has been associated with prolongation of the QTc interval; co-administration with drugs known to prolong QT interval should be avoided).

 No products indexed under this heading.

Prochlorperazine (Levofloxacin has been associated with prolongation of the QTc interval; co-administration with drugs known to prolong QT interval should be avoided).

 No products indexed under this heading.

Promethazine Hydrochloride (Levofloxacin has been associated with prolongation of the QTc interval; co-administration with drugs known to prolong QT interval should be avoided). Products include:

Protriptyline Hydrochloride (Levofloxacin has been associated with prolongation of the QTc interval; co-administration with drugs known to prolong QT interval should be avoided).

 No products indexed under this heading.

Quetiapine Fumarate (Levofloxacin has been associated with prolongation of the QTc interval; co-administration with drugs known to prolong QT interval should be avoided). Products include:

Quinidine (Levofloxacin has been associated with prolongation of the QTc interval; co-administration with drugs known to prolong QT interval should be avoided).

 No products indexed under this heading.

Quinidine Gluconate (Levofloxacin has been associated with prolongation of the QTc interval; co-administration with drugs known to prolong QT interval should be avoided).

 No products indexed under this heading.

Quinidine Hydrochloride (Levofloxacin has been associated with prolongation of the QTc interval; co-administration with drugs known to prolong QT interval should be avoided).

 No products indexed under this heading.

Quinidine Polygalacturonate (Levofloxacin has been associated with prolongation of the QTc interval; co-administration with drugs known to prolong QT interval should be avoided).

 No products indexed under this heading.

Quinidine Sulfate (Levofloxacin has been associated with prolongation of the QTc interval; co-administration with drugs known to prolong QT interval should be avoided).

 No products indexed under this heading.

Repaglinide (Disturbances of blood glucose, including hyper- and hypoglycemia, have been reported in patients treated concomitantly with quinolones and an antidiabetic agent; careful monitoring of blood glucose levels is recommended)

 No products indexed under this heading.

Risperidone (Levofloxacin has been associated with prolongation of the QTc interval; co-administration with drugs known to prolong QT interval should be avoided). Products include:

Rofecoxib (Co-administration may increase the risk of CNS stimulation and convulsive seizures).

 No products indexed under this heading.

Rosiglitazone Maleate (Disturbances of blood glucose, including hyper- and hypoglycemia, have been reported in patients treated concomitantly with quinolones and an antidiabetic agent; careful monitoring of blood glucose levels is recommended). Products include:

Sotalol Hydrochloride (Levofloxacin has been associated with prolongation of the QTc interval; co-administration with drugs known to prolong QT interval should be avoided).

 No products indexed under this heading.

Sucralfate (May interfere with the gastrointestinal absorption of levofloxacin resulting in systemic levels considerably lower than desired; sucralfate should be taken at least 2 hours before or after levofloxacin administration). Products include:

Sulindac (Co-administration may increase the risk of CNS stimulation and convulsive seizures). Products include:

Theophylline (Co-administration of other quinolones with theophylline has resulted in prolonged elimination half-life, elevated serum theophylline levels, and increased risk of theophylline related toxicity; no significant effect of levofloxacin on theophylline pharmacokinetic parameters has been detected, however, caution should be exercised).

 No products indexed under this heading.

Theophylline Anhydrous (Co-administration of other quinolones with theophylline has resulted in prolonged elimination half-life, elevated serum theophylline levels, and increased risk of theophylline related toxicity; no significant effect of levofloxacin on theophylline pharmacokinetic parameters has been detected, however, caution should be exercised). Products include:

Uniphyl Tablets 2710

Theophylline Calcium Salicylate (Co-administration of other quinolones with theophylline has resulted in prolonged elimination half-life, elevated serum theophylline levels, and increased risk of theophylline related toxicity; no significant effect of levofloxacin on theophylline pharmacokinetic parameters has been detected, however, caution should be exercised).

No products indexed under this heading.

Theophylline Dihydroxypropyl (Glyceryl) (Co-administration of other quinolones with theophylline has resulted in prolonged elimination half-life, elevated serum theophylline levels, and increased risk of theophylline related toxicity; no significant effect of levofloxacin on theophylline pharmacokinetic parameters has been detected, however, caution should be exercised).

No products indexed under this heading.

Theophylline Ethylenediamine (Co-administration of other quinolones with theophylline has resulted in prolonged elimination half-life, elevated serum theophylline levels, and increased risk of theophylline related toxicity; no significant effect of levofloxacin on theophylline pharmacokinetic parameters has been detected, however, caution should be exercised).

No products indexed under this heading.

Theophylline Sodium Glycinate (Co-administration of other quinolones with theophylline has resulted in prolonged elimination half-life, elevated serum theophylline levels, and increased risk of theophylline related toxicity; no significant effect of levofloxacin on theophylline pharmacokinetic parameters has been detected, however, caution should be exercised).

No products indexed under this heading.

Thioridazine Hydrochloride (Levofloxacin has been associated with prolongation of the QTc interval; co-administration with drugs known to prolong QT interval should be avoided). Products include:

Thioridazine Hydrochloride Tablets 2163

Thiothixene (Levofloxacin has been associated with prolongation of the QTc interval; co-administration with drugs known to prolong QT interval should be avoided). Products include:

Thiothixene Capsules 2165

Tolazamide (Disturbances of blood glucose, including hyper- and hypoglycemia, have been reported in patients treated concomitantly with quinolones and an antidiabetic agent; careful monitoring of blood glucose levels is recommended).

No products indexed under this heading.

Tolbutamide (Disturbances of blood glucose, including hyper- and hypoglycemia, have been reported in patients treated concomitantly with quinolones and an antidiabetic agent; careful monitoring of blood glucose levels is recommended).

No products indexed under this heading.

Tolmetin Sodium (Co-administration may increase the risk of CNS stimulation and convulsive seizures).

No products indexed under this heading.

Tranylcypromine Sulfate (Levofloxacin has been associated with prolongation of the QTc interval; co-administration with drugs known to prolong QT interval should be avoided). Products include:

Parnate Tablets 1527

Triamcinolone (Achilles and other tendon ruptures have been reported with quinolones, post-market surveillance reports indicate that the risk may be increased in patients on concomitant corticosteroids).

No products indexed under this heading.

Triamcinolone Acetonide (Achilles and other tendon ruptures have been reported with quinolones, post-market surveillance reports indicate that the risk may be increased in patients on concomitant corticosteroids). Products include:

Azmacort Inhalation Aerosol 1726
Nasacort AQ Nasal Spray 2922

Triamcinolone Diacetate (Achilles and other tendon ruptures have been reported with quinolones, post-market surveillance reports indicate that the risk may be increased in patients on concomitant corticosteroids).

No products indexed under this heading.

Triamcinolone Hexacetonide (Achilles and other tendon ruptures have been reported with quinolones, post-market surveillance reports indicate that the risk may be increased in patients on concomitant corticosteroids).

No products indexed under this heading.

Trifluoperazine Hydrochloride (Levofloxacin has been associated with prolongation of the QTc interval; co-administration with drugs known to prolong QT interval should be avoided).

No products indexed under this heading.

Trimipramine Maleate (Levofloxacin has been associated with prolongation of the QTc interval; co-administration with drugs known to prolong QT interval should be avoided).

No products indexed under this heading.

Troglitazone (Disturbances of blood glucose, including hyper- and hypoglycemia, have been reported in patients treated concomitantly with quinolones and an antidiabetic agent; careful monitoring of blood glucose levels is recommended).

No products indexed under this heading.

Valdecoxib (Co-administration may increase the risk of CNS stimulation and convulsive seizures).

No products indexed under this heading.

Warfarin Sodium (Co-administration of other quinolones with warfarin has resulted in enhanced effects of warfarin; no significant effect of levofloxacin on warfarin pharmacokinetic parameters has been detected in clinical studies, however, caution should be exercised and coagulation test should be closely monitored). Products include:

Coumadin for Injection 898
Coumadin Tablets 898

Ziprasidone Hydrochloride (Levofloxacin has been associated with prolongation of the QTc interval; co-administration with drugs known to prolong QT interval should be avoided). Products include:

Geodon Capsules 2529

Food Interactions

Food, unspecified (Co-administration slightly prolongs the time to peak concentration by approximately 1 hour and slightly decreases the peak concentration by approximately 14%; levofloxacin can be administered without regard to food).

LEVAQUIN TABLETS

(Levofloxacin) 2384

May interact with antacids containing aluminum, calcium and magnesium, class 1A antiarrhythmics, class III antiarrhythmics, cations, corticosteroids, erythromycin, oral hypoglycemic agents, iron containing oral preparations, non-steroidal anti-inflammatory agents, psychotropics, quinidine, tricyclic antidepressants, xanthines, and certain other agents. Compounds in these categories include:

Acarbose (Disturbances of blood glucose, including hyper- and hypoglycemia, have been reported in patients treated concomitantly with quinolones and an antidiabetic agent; careful monitoring of blood glucose levels is recommended). Products include:

Precose Tablets 751

Alprazolam (Levofloxacin has been associated with prolongation of the QTc interval; co-administration with drugs known to prolong QT interval should be avoided). Products include:

Niravam Orally Disintegrating Tablets 3092

Aluminum Carbonate (Antacids containing aluminum or magnesium may interfere with the gastrointestinal absorption of levofloxacin resulting in systemic levels considerably lower than desired; these agents should be taken at least 2 hours before or after levofloxacin administration).

No products indexed under this heading.

Aluminum-containing Compounds, unspecified (Concurrent administration of levofloxacin with metal cations may interfere with the GI absorption of levofloxacin, resulting in systemic levels considerably lower than desired; these agents containing metal cations should be taken at least 2 hours before or 2 hours after levofloxacin administration).

No products indexed under this heading.

Aluminum Hydroxide (Antacids containing aluminum or magnesium may interfere with the gastrointestinal absorption of levofloxacin resulting in systemic levels considerably lower than desired; these agents should be taken at least 2 hours before or after levofloxacin administration). Products include:

Gaviscon Regular Strength Liquid .. 658
Gaviscon Regular Strength Tablets 658
Gaviscon Extra Strength Liquid 658
Gaviscon Extra Strength Tablets 658
Maalox Regular Strength Antacid/Antigas Liquid................. 2175
Maalox Max Maximum Strength Antacid/Anti-Gas Liquid................ 2176

Aminophylline (Co-administration of other quinolones with theophylline has resulted in prolonged elimination half-life, elevated serum theophylline levels, and increased risk of theophylline related toxicity; no significant effect of levofloxacin on theophylline pharmacokinetic parameters has been detected, however, caution should be exercised).

No products indexed under this heading.

Amiodarone Hydrochloride (Levofloxacin has been associated with prolongation of the QTc interval; co-administration with drugs known to prolong QT interval should be avoided).

No products indexed under this heading.

Amitriptyline Hydrochloride (Levofloxacin has been associated with prolongation of the QTc interval; co-administration with drugs known to prolong QT interval should be avoided).

No products indexed under this heading.

Amoxapine (Levofloxacin has been associated with prolongation of the QTc interval; co-administration with drugs known to prolong QT interval should be avoided).

No products indexed under this heading.

Arsenic Trioxide (Levofloxacin has been associated with prolongation of the QTc interval; co-administration with drugs known to prolong QT interval should be avoided). Products include:

Trisenox Injection 993

Betamethasone Acetate (Achilles and other tendon ruptures have been reported with quinolones, post-market surveillance reports indicate that the risk may be increased in patients on concomitant corticosteroids).

No products indexed under this heading.

Betamethasone Sodium Phosphate (Achilles and other tendon ruptures have been reported with quinolones, post-market surveillance reports indicate that the risk may be increased in patients on concomitant corticosteroids).

No products indexed under this heading.

Bretylium Tosylate (Levofloxacin has been associated with prolongation of the QT interval and infrequent cases of arrhythmia. Rare cases of torsades de pointes have been spontaneously reported during post-marketing surveillance in patients receiving levofloxacin. Levofloxacin should be avoided in patients receiving class III antiarrhythmic agents).

No products indexed under this heading.

Buspirone Hydrochloride (Levofloxacin has been associated with prolongation of the QTc interval; co-administration with drugs known to prolong QT interval should be avoided).

No products indexed under this heading.

Calcium (Concurrent administration of levofloxacin with metal cations may interfere with the GI absorption of levofloxacin, resulting in systemic levels considerably lower than desired; these agents containing metal cations should be taken at least 2 hours before or 2 hours after levofloxacin administration). Products include:

Os-Cal 250 + D Tablets ▣□817
Os-Cal 500 Tablets ▣□817
Os-Cal 500 + D Tablets ▣□817

Celecoxib (Co-administration may increase the risk of CNS stimulation and convulsive seizures). Products include:

Celebrex Capsules 3134

Chlordiazepoxide (Levofloxacin has been associated with prolongation of the QTc interval; co-administration with drugs known to prolong QT interval should be avoided).

No products indexed under this heading.

Chlordiazepoxide Hydrochloride (Levofloxacin has been associated with prolongation of the QTc interval; co-administration with drugs known to prolong QT interval should be avoided). Products include:

Librium Capsules 3347

Chlorpromazine (Levofloxacin has been associated with prolongation of the QTc interval; co-administration with drugs known to prolong QT interval should be avoided).

No products indexed under this heading.

Chlorpromazine Hydrochloride (Levofloxacin has been associated with prolongation of the QTc interval; co-administration with drugs known to prolong QT interval should be avoided).

No products indexed under this heading.

Chlorpropamide (Disturbances of blood glucose, including hyper- and hypoglycemia, have been reported in patients treated concomitantly with quinolones and an antidiabetic agent; careful monitoring of blood glucose levels is recommended).

No products indexed under this heading.

Chlorprothixene (Levofloxacin has been associated with prolongation of the QTc interval; co-administration with drugs known to prolong QT interval should be avoided).

No products indexed under this heading.

Chlorprothixene Hydrochloride (Levofloxacin has been associated with prolongation of the QTc interval; co-administration with drugs known to prolong QT interval should be avoided).

No products indexed under this heading.

Cimetidine (Co-administration has resulted in higher levofloxacin AUC and t1/2, while CL/F and CLr were lower during concomitant treatment with cimetidine). Products include:

Tagamet HB 200 Tablets ▣□664

Cimetidine Hydrochloride (Co-administration has resulted in higher levofloxacin AUC and t1/2, while CL/F and CLr were lower during con-comitant treatment with cimetidine).

No products indexed under this heading.

Cisapride (Levofloxacin has been associated with prolongation of the QTc interval; co-administration with drugs known to prolong QT interval should be avoided).

No products indexed under this heading.

Clomipramine Hydrochloride (Levofloxacin has been associated with prolongation of the QTc interval; co-administration with drugs known to prolong QT interval should be avoided).

No products indexed under this heading.

Clorazepate Dipotassium (Levofloxacin has been associated with prolongation of the QTc interval; co-administration with drugs known to prolong QT interval should be avoided). Products include:

Tranxene .. 2474

Clozapine (Levofloxacin has been associated with prolongation of the QTc interval; co-administration with drugs known to prolong QT interval should be avoided). Products include:

Clozaril Tablets 2184
FazaClo Orally Disintegrating Tablets .. 551

Cortisone Acetate (Achilles and other tendon ruptures have been reported with quinolones, post-market surveillance reports indicate that the risk may be increased in patients on concomitant corticosteroids).

No products indexed under this heading.

Cyclosporine (Levofloxacin Cmax and Ke were slightly lower while Tmax and t1/2 were slightly longer in the presence of cyclosporine; these differences, however, are not clinically significant, therefore, no dosage adjustment is required). Products include:

Gengraf Capsules 459
Neoral Oral Solution 2259
Neoral Soft Gelatin Capsules 2259
Restasis Ophthalmic Emulsion 575
Sandimmune 2275

Desipramine Hydrochloride (Levofloxacin has been associated with prolongation of the QTc interval; co-administration with drugs known to prolong QT interval should be avoided).

No products indexed under this heading.

Dexamethasone (Achilles and other tendon ruptures have been reported with quinolones, post-market surveillance reports indicate that the risk may be increased in patients on concomitant corticosteroids). Products include:

Ciprodex Otic Suspension 559
Decadron Tablets 1951
TobraDex Ophthalmic Ointment 562
TobraDex Ophthalmic Suspension ... 563

Dexamethasone Acetate (Achilles and other tendon ruptures have been reported with quinolones, post-market surveillance reports indicate that the risk may be increased in patients on concomitant corticosteroids).

No products indexed under this heading.

Dexamethasone Sodium Phosphate (Achilles and other tendon ruptures have been reported with quinolones, post-market surveillance reports indicate that the risk may be increased in patients on concomitant corticosteroids).

No products indexed under this heading.

Diazepam (Levofloxacin has been associated with prolongation of the QTc interval; co-administration with drugs known to prolong QT interval should be avoided). Products include:

Diastat Rectal Delivery System 3343
Valium Tablets 2819

Diclofenac Potassium (Co-administration may increase the risk of CNS stimulation and convulsive seizures).

No products indexed under this heading.

Diclofenac Sodium (Co-administration may increase the risk of CNS stimulation and convulsive seizures). Products include:

Arthrotec Tablets 3129
Voltaren Ophthalmic Solution 2309
Voltaren Tablets 2307
Voltaren-XR Tablets 2310

Didanosine (Antacids contained in Videx chewable/buffered tablets or pediatric powder for oral solution may substantially interfere with the gastrointestinal absorption of levofloxacin, resulting in systemic levels considerably lower than desired).

No products indexed under this heading.

Disopyramide (Levofloxacin has been associated with prolongation of the QT interval and infrequent cases of arrhythmia. Rare cases of torsades de pointes have been spontaneously reported during post-marketing surveillance in patients receiving levofloxacin. Levofloxacin should be avoided in patients receiving class IA antiarrhythmic agents).

No products indexed under this heading.

Doxepin Hydrochloride (Levofloxacin has been associated with prolongation of the QTc interval; co-administration with drugs known to prolong QT interval should be avoided).

No products indexed under this heading.

Droperidol (Levofloxacin has been associated with prolongation of the QTc interval; co-administration with drugs known to prolong QT interval should be avoided).

No products indexed under this heading.

Dyphylline (Co-administration of other quinolones with theophylline has resulted in prolonged elimination half-life, elevated serum theophylline levels, and increased risk of theophylline related toxicity; no significant effect of levofloxacin on theophylline pharmacokinetic parameters has been detected, however, caution should be exercised).

No products indexed under this heading.

Erythromycin (Levofloxacin has been associated with prolongation of the QTc interval; co-administration with drugs known to prolong QT interval should be avoided). Products include:

Ery-Tab Tablets 449

Erythromycin Base Filmtab Tablets ... 455
Erythromycin Delayed-Release Capsules, USP 457
PCE Dispertab Tablets 515

Erythromycin Estolate (Levofloxacin has been associated with prolongation of the QTc interval; co-administration with drugs known to prolong QT interval should be avoided).

No products indexed under this heading.

Erythromycin Ethylsuccinate (Levofloxacin has been associated with prolongation of the QTc interval; co-administration with drugs known to prolong QT interval should be avoided). Products include:

E.E.S. ... 451
EryPed ... 447

Erythromycin Gluceptate (Levofloxacin has been associated with prolongation of the QTc interval; co-administration with drugs known to prolong QT interval should be avoided).

No products indexed under this heading.

Erythromycin Lactobionate (Levofloxacin has been associated with prolongation of the QTc interval; co-administration with drugs known to prolong QT interval should be avoided).

No products indexed under this heading.

Erythromycin Stearate (Levofloxacin has been associated with prolongation of the QTc interval; co-administration with drugs known to prolong QT interval should be avoided). Products include:

Erythrocin Stearate Filmtab Tablets .. 453

Etodolac (Co-administration may increase the risk of CNS stimulation and convulsive seizures).

No products indexed under this heading.

Fenoprofen Calcium (Co-administration may increase the risk of CNS stimulation and convulsive seizures). Products include:

Nalfon Capsules 2502

Ferrous Fumarate (Iron-containing preparations may interfere with the gastrointestinal absorption of levofloxacin resulting in systemic levels considerably lower than desired; these agents should be taken at least 2 hours before or after levofloxacin administration).

No products indexed under this heading.

Ferrous Gluconate (Iron-containing preparations may interfere with the gastrointestinal absorption of levofloxacin resulting in systemic levels considerably lower than desired; these agents should be taken at least 2 hours before or after levofloxacin administration).

No products indexed under this heading.

Ferrous Sulfate (Iron-containing preparations may interfere with the gastrointestinal absorption of levofloxacin resulting in systemic levels considerably lower than desired; these agents should be taken at least 2 hours before or after levofloxacin administration). Products include:

Slow Fe Iron Tablets ▣□818
Slow Fe with Folic Acid Tablets ▣□819

Fludrocortisone Acetate (Achilles and other tendon ruptures have been reported with quinolones, post-market surveillance reports indicate that the risk may be increased in patients on concomitant corticosteroids).
No products indexed under this heading.

Fluphenazine Decanoate (Levofloxacin has been associated with prolongation of the QTc interval; co-administration with drugs known to prolong QT interval should be avoided).
No products indexed under this heading.

Fluphenazine Enanthate (Levofloxacin has been associated with prolongation of the QTc interval; co-administration with drugs known to prolong QT interval should be avoided).
No products indexed under this heading.

Fluphenazine Hydrochloride (Levofloxacin has been associated with prolongation of the QTc interval; co-administration with drugs known to prolong QT interval should be avoided).
No products indexed under this heading.

Flurbiprofen (Co-administration may increase the risk of CNS stimulation and convulsive seizures).
No products indexed under this heading.

Glimepiride (Disturbances of blood glucose, including hyper- and hypoglycemia, have been reported in patients treated concomitantly with quinolones and an antidiabetic agent; careful monitoring of blood glucose levels is recommended). Products include:
Avandaryl Tablets 1379
Duetact Tablets 3226

Glipizide (Disturbances of blood glucose, including hyper- and hypoglycemia, have been reported in patients treated concomitantly with quinolones and an antidiabetic agent; careful monitoring of blood glucose levels is recommended).
No products indexed under this heading.

Glyburide (Disturbances of blood glucose, including hyper- and hypoglycemia, have been reported in patients treated concomitantly with quinolones and an antidiabetic agent; careful monitoring of blood glucose levels is recommended).
No products indexed under this heading.

Haloperidol (Levofloxacin has been associated with prolongation of the QTc interval; co-administration with drugs known to prolong QT interval should be avoided).
No products indexed under this heading.

Haloperidol Decanoate (Levofloxacin has been associated with prolongation of the QTc interval; co-administration with drugs known to prolong QT interval should be avoided).
No products indexed under this heading.

Hydrocortisone (Achilles and other tendon ruptures have been reported with quinolones, post-market surveillance reports indicate that the risk

may be increased in patients on concomitant corticosteroids). Products include:
Colocort Rectal Suspension, USP (Retention) 100 mg/60 mL 2476
Hydrocortone Tablets 1989
Preparation H Hydrocortisone Cream 646

Hydrocortisone Acetate (Achilles and other tendon ruptures have been reported with quinolones, post-market surveillance reports indicate that the risk may be increased in patients on concomitant corticosteroids). Products include:
Analpram-HC 1159
Pramosone 1161
ProctoFoam-HC 3099

Hydrocortisone Sodium Phosphate (Achilles and other tendon ruptures have been reported with quinolones, post-market surveillance reports indicate that the risk may be increased in patients on concomitant corticosteroids).
No products indexed under this heading.

Hydrocortisone Sodium Succinate (Achilles and other tendon ruptures have been reported with quinolones, post-market surveillance reports indicate that the risk may be increased in patients on concomitant corticosteroids).
No products indexed under this heading.

Hydroxyzine Hydrochloride (Levofloxacin has been associated with prolongation of the QTc interval; co-administration with drugs known to prolong QT interval should be avoided).
No products indexed under this heading.

Ibuprofen (Co-administration may increase the risk of CNS stimulation and convulsive seizures). Products include:
Advil Allergy Sinus Caplets 770
Advil ... 674
Children's Advil Oral Suspension 603
Children's Advil Chewable Tablets .. 603
Advil Cold & Sinus 723
Infants' Advil Concentrated Drops .. 604
Infants' Advil Concentrated Drops - White Grape (Dye-Free)............. 604
Junior Strength Advil Swallow Tablets..................................... 605
Advil Migraine Liquigels 608
Advil Multi-Symptom Cold Caplets.................................... 770
Advil PM Caplets 615
Motrin IB Tablets and Caplets 1866
Children's Motrin Oral Suspension ... 1867
Children's Motrin Non-Staining Dye-Free Oral Suspension............. 1867
Children's Motrin Cold Oral Suspension 1867
Infants' Motrin Concentrated Drops...................................... 1867
Infants' Motrin Non-Staining Dye-Free Concentrated Drops....... 1867
Junior Strength Motrin Caplets and Chewable Tablets.................. 1867
Vicoprofen Tablets 539

Imipramine Hydrochloride (Levofloxacin has been associated with prolongation of the QTc interval; co-administration with drugs known to prolong QT interval should be avoided).
No products indexed under this heading.

Imipramine Pamoate (Levofloxacin has been associated with prolongation of the QTc interval; co-administration with drugs known to prolong QT interval should be avoided).
No products indexed under this heading.

Indomethacin (Co-administration may increase the risk of CNS stimulation and convulsive seizures). Products include:
Indocin .. 1995

Indomethacin Sodium Trihydrate (Co-administration may increase the risk of CNS stimulation and convulsive seizures). Products include:
Indocin I.V. 2465

Iron (Iron-containing preparations may interfere with the gastrointestinal absorption of levofloxacin resulting in systemic levels considerably lower than desired; these agents should be taken at least 2 hours before or after levofloxacin administration).
No products indexed under this heading.

Isocarboxazid (Levofloxacin has been associated with prolongation of the QTc interval; co-administration with drugs known to prolong QT interval should be avoided).
No products indexed under this heading.

Ketoprofen (Co-administration may increase the risk of CNS stimulation and convulsive seizures).
No products indexed under this heading.

Ketorolac Tromethamine (Co-administration may increase the risk of CNS stimulation and convulsive seizures). Products include:
Acular Ophthalmic Solution 565
Acular LS Ophthalmic Solution 566

Lithium Carbonate (Levofloxacin has been associated with prolongation of the QTc interval; co-administration with drugs known to prolong QT interval should be avoided). Products include:
Lithobid Tablets 1692

Lithium Citrate (Levofloxacin has been associated with prolongation of the QTc interval; co-administration with drugs known to prolong QT interval should be avoided).
No products indexed under this heading.

Lorazepam (Levofloxacin has been associated with prolongation of the QTc interval; co-administration with drugs known to prolong QT interval should be avoided).
No products indexed under this heading.

Loxapine Hydrochloride (Levofloxacin has been associated with prolongation of the QTc interval; co-administration with drugs known to prolong QT interval should be avoided).
No products indexed under this heading.

Loxapine Succinate (Levofloxacin has been associated with prolongation of the QTc interval; co-administration with drugs known to prolong QT interval should be avoided).
No products indexed under this heading.

Magaldrate (Antacids containing aluminum or magnesium may interfere with the gastrointestinal absorption of levofloxacin resulting in systemic levels considerably lower than desired; these agents should be taken at least 2 hours before or after levofloxacin administration).
No products indexed under this heading.

Magnesium (Concurrent administration of levofloxacin with metal cations may interfere with the GI absorption of levofloxacin, resulting in systemic levels considerably lower than desired; these agents containing metal cations should be taken at least 2 hours before or 2 hours after levofloxacin administration).
No products indexed under this heading.

Magnesium Hydroxide (Antacids containing aluminum or magnesium may interfere with the gastrointestinal absorption of levofloxacin resulting in systemic levels considerably lower than desired; these agents should be taken at least 2 hours before or after levofloxacin administration). Products include:
Maalox Regular Strength Antacid/Antigas Liquid................. 2175
Maalox Max Maximum Strength Antacid/Anti-Gas Liquid................ 2176
Pepcid Complete Chewable Tablets.................................... 1701

Magnesium Oxide (Antacids containing aluminum or magnesium may interfere with the gastrointestinal absorption of levofloxacin resulting in systemic levels considerably lower than desired; these agents should be taken at least 2 hours before or after levofloxacin administration). Products include:
Beelith Tablets 759
PremCal Light, Regular, and Extra Strength Tablets................. 818

Maprotiline Hydrochloride (Levofloxacin has been associated with prolongation of the QTc interval; co-administration with drugs known to prolong QT interval should be avoided).
No products indexed under this heading.

Meclofenamate Sodium (Co-administration may increase the risk of CNS stimulation and convulsive seizures).
No products indexed under this heading.

Mefenamic Acid (Co-administration may increase the risk of CNS stimulation and convulsive seizures).
No products indexed under this heading.

Meloxicam (Co-administration may increase the risk of CNS stimulation and convulsive seizures). Products include:
Mobic Oral Suspension 863
Mobic Tablets 863

Meprobamate (Levofloxacin has been associated with prolongation of the QTc interval; co-administration with drugs known to prolong QT interval should be avoided).
No products indexed under this heading.

IMPORTANT NOTE: Always consult each drug listing in the patient's regimen for possible interactions.

Mesoridazine Besylate (Levofloxacin has been associated with prolongation of the QTc interval; co-administration with drugs known to prolong QT interval should be avoided).

No products indexed under this heading.

Metformin Hydrochloride (Disturbances of blood glucose, including hyper- and hypoglycemia, have been reported in patients treated concomitantly with quinolones and an antidiabetic agent; careful monitoring of blood glucose levels is recommended). Products include:

Methylprednisolone Acetate (Achilles and other tendon ruptures have been reported with quinolones, post-market surveillance reports indicate that the risk may be increased in patients on concomitant corticosteroids). Products include:

Methylprednisolone Sodium Succinate (Achilles and other tendon ruptures have been reported with quinolones, post-market surveillance reports indicate that the risk may be increased in patients on concomitant corticosteroids).

No products indexed under this heading.

Midazolam Hydrochloride (Levofloxacin has been associated with prolongation of the QTc interval; co-administration with drugs known to prolong QT interval should be avoided).

No products indexed under this heading.

Miglitol (Disturbances of blood glucose, including hyper- and hypoglycemia, have been reported in patients treated concomitantly with quinolones and an antidiabetic agent; careful monitoring of blood glucose levels is recommended).

No products indexed under this heading.

Molindone Hydrochloride (Levofloxacin has been associated with prolongation of the QTc interval; co-administration with drugs known to prolong QT interval should be avoided). Products include:

Moricizine Hydrochloride (Levofloxacin has been associated with prolongation of the QT interval and infrequent cases of arrhythmia. Rare cases of torsades de pointes have been spontaneously reported during post-marketing surveillance in patients receiving levofloxacin. Levofloxacin should be avoided in patients receiving class IA antiarrhythmic agents).

No products indexed under this heading.

Nabumetone (Co-administration may increase the risk of CNS stimulation and convulsive seizures).

No products indexed under this heading.

Naproxen (Co-administration may increase the risk of CNS stimulation and convulsive seizures). Products include:

Naproxen Sodium (Co-administration may increase the risk of CNS stimulation and convulsive seizures). Products include:

Nortriptyline Hydrochloride (Levofloxacin has been associated with prolongation of the QTc interval; co-administration with drugs known to prolong QT interval should be avoided).

No products indexed under this heading.

Olanzapine (Levofloxacin has been associated with prolongation of the QTc interval; co-administration with drugs known to prolong QT interval should be avoided). Products include:

Oxaprozin (Co-administration may increase the risk of CNS stimulation and convulsive seizures).

No products indexed under this heading.

Oxazepam (Levofloxacin has been associated with prolongation of the QTc interval; co-administration with drugs known to prolong QT interval should be avoided).

No products indexed under this heading.

Perphenazine (Levofloxacin has been associated with prolongation of the QTc interval; co-administration with drugs known to prolong QT interval should be avoided).

No products indexed under this heading.

Phenelzine Sulfate (Levofloxacin has been associated with prolongation of the QTc interval; co-administration with drugs known to prolong QT interval should be avoided).

No products indexed under this heading.

Phenylbutazone (Co-administration may increase the risk of CNS stimulation and convulsive seizures).

No products indexed under this heading.

Pimozide (Levofloxacin has been associated with prolongation of the QTc interval; co-administration with drugs known to prolong QT interval should be avoided).

No products indexed under this heading.

Pioglitazone Hydrochloride (Disturbances of blood glucose, including hyper- and hypoglycemia, have been reported in patients treated concomitantly with quinolones and an antidiabetic agent; careful monitoring of blood glucose levels is recommended). Products include:

Piroxicam (Co-administration may increase the risk of CNS stimulation and convulsive seizures).

No products indexed under this heading.

Polysaccharide Iron Complex (Iron-containing preparations may interfere with the gastrointestinal absorption of levofloxacin resulting in systemic levels considerably lower than desired; these agents should be taken at least 2 hours before or after levofloxacin administration). Products include:

Prazepam (Levofloxacin has been associated with prolongation of the QTc interval; co-administration with drugs known to prolong QT interval should be avoided).

No products indexed under this heading.

Prednisolone Acetate (Achilles and other tendon ruptures have been reported with quinolones, post-market surveillance reports indicate that the risk may be increased in patients on concomitant corticosteroids). Products include:

Prednisolone Sodium Phosphate (Achilles and other tendon ruptures have been reported with quinolones, post-market surveillance reports indicate that the risk may be increased in patients on concomitant corticosteroids).

No products indexed under this heading.

Prednisolone Tebutate (Achilles and other tendon ruptures have been reported with quinolones, post-market surveillance reports indicate that the risk may be increased in patients on concomitant corticosteroids).

No products indexed under this heading.

Prednisone (Achilles and other tendon ruptures have been reported with quinolones, post-market surveillance reports indicate that the risk may be increased in patients on concomitant corticosteroids).

No products indexed under this heading.

Probenecid (Co-administration has resulted in higher levofloxacin AUC and t1/2, while CL/F and CLr were lower during concomitant treatment with probenecid).

No products indexed under this heading.

Procainamide (Levofloxacin has been associated with prolongation of the QT interval and infrequent cases of arrhythmia. Rare cases of torsades de pointes have been spontaneously reported during post-marketing surveillance in patients receiving levofloxacin. Levofloxacin should be avoided in patients receiving class IA antiarrhythmic agents).

No products indexed under this heading.

Procainamide Hydrochloride (Levofloxacin has been associated with prolongation of the QTc interval; co-administration with drugs known to prolong QT interval should be avoided).

No products indexed under this heading.

Prochlorperazine (Levofloxacin has been associated with prolongation of the QTc interval; co-administration with drugs known to prolong QT interval should be avoided).

No products indexed under this heading.

Promethazine Hydrochloride (Levofloxacin has been associated with prolongation of the QTc interval; co-administration with drugs known to prolong QT interval should be avoided). Products include:

Protriptyline Hydrochloride (Levofloxacin has been associated with prolongation of the QTc interval; co-administration with drugs known to prolong QT interval should be avoided).

No products indexed under this heading.

Quetiapine Fumarate (Levofloxacin has been associated with prolongation of the QTc interval; co-administration with drugs known to prolong QT interval should be avoided). Products include:

Quinidine (Levofloxacin has been associated with prolongation of the QTc interval; co-administration with drugs known to prolong QT interval should be avoided).

No products indexed under this heading.

Quinidine Gluconate (Levofloxacin has been associated with prolongation of the QTc interval; co-administration with drugs known to prolong QT interval should be avoided).

No products indexed under this heading.

Quinidine Hydrochloride (Levofloxacin has been associated with prolongation of the QTc interval; co-administration with drugs known to prolong QT interval should be avoided).

No products indexed under this heading.

Quinidine Polygalacturonate (Levofloxacin has been associated with prolongation of the QTc interval; co-administration with drugs known to prolong QT interval should be avoided).

No products indexed under this heading.

Quinidine Sulfate (Levofloxacin has been associated with prolongation of the QTc interval; co-administration with drugs known to prolong QT interval should be avoided).

No products indexed under this heading.

Repaglinide (Disturbances of blood glucose, including hyper- and hypoglycemia, have been reported in patients treated concomitantly with quinolones and an antidiabetic agent; careful monitoring of blood glucose levels is recommended).

No products indexed under this heading.

Risperidone (Levofloxacin has been associated with prolongation of the QTc interval; co-administration with drugs known to prolong QT interval should be avoided). Products include:

Risperdal Consta Long-Acting Injection **1682**
Risperdal M-Tab Orally Disintegrating Tablets **1676**

Rofecoxib (Co-administration may increase the risk of CNS stimulation and convulsive seizures).
No products indexed under this heading.

Rosiglitazone Maleate (Disturbances of blood glucose, including hyper- and hypoglycemia, have been reported in patients treated concomitantly with quinolones and an antidiabetic agent; careful monitoring of blood glucose levels is recommended). Products include:
Avandamet Tablets **1373**
Avandaryl Tablets **1379**
Avandia Tablets **1384**

Sotalol Hydrochloride (Levofloxacin has been associated with prolongation of the QTc interval; co-administration with drugs known to prolong QT interval should be avoided).
No products indexed under this heading.

Sucralfate (May interfere with the gastrointestinal absorption of levofloxacin resulting in systemic levels considerably lower than desired; sucralfate should be taken at least 2 hours before or after levofloxacin administration). Products include:
Carafate Suspension **701**
Carafate Tablets **701**

Sulindac (Co-administration may increase the risk of CNS stimulation and convulsive seizures). Products include:
Clinoril Tablets **1924**

Theophylline (Co-administration of other quinolones with theophylline has resulted in prolonged elimination half-life, elevated serum theophylline levels, and increased risk of theophylline related toxicity; no significant effect of levofloxacin on theophylline pharmacokinetic parameters has been detected, however, caution should be exercised).
No products indexed under this heading.

Theophylline Anhydrous (Co-administration of other quinolones with theophylline has resulted in prolonged elimination half-life, elevated serum theophylline levels, and increased risk of theophylline related toxicity; no significant effect of levofloxacin on theophylline pharmacokinetic parameters has been detected, however, caution should be exercised). Products include:
Uniphyl Tablets **2710**

Theophylline Calcium Salicylate (Co-administration of other quinolones with theophylline has resulted in prolonged elimination half-life, elevated serum theophylline levels, and increased risk of theophylline related toxicity; no significant effect of levofloxacin on theophylline pharmacokinetic parameters has been detected, however, caution should be exercised).
No products indexed under this heading.

Theophylline Dihydroxypropyl (Glyceryl) (Co-administration of other quinolones with theophylline has resulted in prolonged elimination half-life, elevated serum theophylline levels, and increased risk of theophylline related toxicity; no significant effect of levofloxacin on theophylline pharmacokinetic parameters has been detected, however, caution should be exercised).
No products indexed under this heading.

Theophylline Ethylenediamine (Co-administration of other quinolones with theophylline has resulted in prolonged elimination half-life, elevated serum theophylline levels, and increased risk of theophylline related toxicity; no significant effect of levofloxacin on theophylline pharmacokinetic parameters has been detected, however, caution should be exercised).
No products indexed under this heading.

Theophylline Sodium Glycinate (Co-administration of other quinolones with theophylline has resulted in prolonged elimination half-life, elevated serum theophylline levels, and increased risk of theophylline related toxicity; no significant effect of levofloxacin on theophylline pharmacokinetic parameters has been detected, however, caution should be exercised).
No products indexed under this heading.

Thioridazine Hydrochloride (Levofloxacin has been associated with prolongation of the QTc interval; co-administration with drugs known to prolong QT interval should be avoided). Products include:
Thioridazine Hydrochloride Tablets **2163**

Thiothixene (Levofloxacin has been associated with prolongation of the QTc interval; co-administration with drugs known to prolong QT interval should be avoided). Products include:
Thiothixene Capsules **2165**

Tolazamide (Disturbances of blood glucose, including hyper- and hypoglycemia, have been reported in patients treated concomitantly with quinolones and an antidiabetic agent; careful monitoring of blood glucose levels is recommended).
No products indexed under this heading.

Tolbutamide (Disturbances of blood glucose, including hyper- and hypoglycemia, have been reported in patients treated concomitantly with quinolones and an antidiabetic agent; careful monitoring of blood glucose levels is recommended).
No products indexed under this heading.

Tolmetin Sodium (Co-administration may increase the risk of CNS stimulation and convulsive seizures).
No products indexed under this heading.

Tranylcypromine Sulfate (Levofloxacin has been associated with prolongation of the QTc interval; co-administration with drugs known to prolong QT interval should be avoided). Products include:
Parnate Tablets **1527**

Triamcinolone (Achilles and other tendon ruptures have been reported with quinolones, post-market surveillance reports indicate that the risk may be increased in patients on concomitant corticosteroids).
No products indexed under this heading.

Triamcinolone Acetonide (Achilles and other tendon ruptures have been reported with quinolones, post-market surveillance reports indicate that the risk may be increased in patients on concomitant corticosteroids). Products include:
Azmacort Inhalation Aerosol **1726**
Nasacort AQ Nasal Spray **2922**

Triamcinolone Diacetate (Achilles and other tendon ruptures have been reported with quinolones, post-market surveillance reports indicate that the risk may be increased in patients on concomitant corticosteroids).
No products indexed under this heading.

Triamcinolone Hexacetonide (Achilles and other tendon ruptures have been reported with quinolones, post-market surveillance reports indicate that the risk may be increased in patients on concomitant corticosteroids).
No products indexed under this heading.

Trifluoperazine Hydrochloride (Levofloxacin has been associated with prolongation of the QTc interval; co-administration with drugs known to prolong QT interval should be avoided).
No products indexed under this heading.

Trimipramine Maleate (Levofloxacin has been associated with prolongation of the QTc interval; co-administration with drugs known to prolong QT interval should be avoided).
No products indexed under this heading.

Troglitazone (Disturbances of blood glucose, including hyper- and hypoglycemia, have been reported in patients treated concomitantly with quinolones and an antidiabetic agent; careful monitoring of blood glucose levels is recommended).
No products indexed under this heading.

Valdecoxib (Co-administration may increase the risk of CNS stimulation and convulsive seizures).
No products indexed under this heading.

Warfarin Sodium (Co-administration of other quinolones with warfarin has resulted in enhanced effects of warfarin; no significant effect of levofloxacin on warfarin pharmacokinetic parameters has been detected in clinical studies, however, caution should be exercised and coagulation test should be closely monitored). Products include:
Coumadin for Injection **898**
Coumadin Tablets **898**

Zinc (Concurrent administration of levofloxacin with metal cations may interfere with the GI absorption of levofloxacin, resulting in systemic levels considerably lower than desired; these agents containing metal cations should be taken at least 2 hours before or 2 hours after levofloxacin administration). Products include:
Visutein Capsules **3329**

Ziprasidone Hydrochloride (Levofloxacin has been associated with prolongation of the QTc interval; co-administration with drugs known to prolong QT interval should be avoided). Products include:
Geodon Capsules **2529**

Food Interactions

Food, unspecified (Co-administration slightly prolongs the time to peak concentration by approximately 1 hour and slightly decreases the peak concentration by approximately 14%; levofloxacin can be administered without regard to food).

LEVAQUIN IN 5% DEXTROSE INJECTION

(Levofloxacin) **2384**
See Levaquin Injection

LEVEMIR INJECTION

(Insulin Detemir (rDNA Origin)) **2320**
May interact with ACE inhibitors, beta blockers, corticosteroids, diuretics, estrogens, fibrates, oral hypoglycemic agents, lithium preparations, monoamine oxidase inhibitors, phenothiazines, progestins, salicylates, sulfonamides, sympathomimetics, thyroid preparations, and certain other agents. Compounds in these categories include:

Acarbose (Co-administration may reduce the blood-glucose-lowering effect of insulin and susceptibility to hypoglycemia). Products include:
Precose Tablets **751**

Acebutolol Hydrochloride (Co-administration may either potentiate or weaken the blood-glucose-lowering effect of insulin. Signs of hypoglycemia may be reduced or absent).
No products indexed under this heading.

Albuterol (Co-administration may reduce the blood-glucose-lowering effect of insulin). Products include:
Proventil Inhalation Aerosol **3053**

Albuterol Sulfate (Co-administration may reduce the blood-glucose-lowering effect of insulin). Products include:
AccuNeb Inhalation Solution **1055**
Combivent Inhalation Aerosol **847**
DuoNeb Inhalation Solution **1058**
ProAir HFA Inhalation Aerosol **3300**
Proventil Inhalation Solution 0.083% **3055**
Proventil HFA Inhalation Aerosol **3056**
Ventolin HFA Inhalation Aerosol **1600**
VoSpire ER Tablets **1052**

Amiloride Hydrochloride (Co-administration may reduce the blood-glucose-lowering effect of insulin). Products include:
Midamor Tablets **2026**
Moduretic Tablets **2028**

Aspirin (Co-administration may reduce the blood-glucose-lowering effect of insulin and susceptibility to hypoglycemia). Products include:
Aggrenox Capsules **822**
Bayer Aspirin **744**
BC Allergy Sinus Cold Powder **677**
BC Headache Powder **677**
Arthritis Strength BC Powder **677**
BC Sinus Cold Powder **677**
Excedrin Extra Strength Caplets/Tablets/Geltabs **684**
Excedrin Migraine Caplets/Tablets/Geltabs **609**

Goody's Body Pain Formula Powder .... ▣ 684
Goody's Extra Strength Headache Powders .... ▣ 611
Goody's Extra Strength Pain Relief Tablets .... ▣ 685
Percodan Tablets 1132
St. Joseph 81 mg Aspirin Chewable and Enteric Coated Tablets 1869

Aspirin, Enteric Coated (Co-administration may reduce the blood-glucose-lowering effect of insulin and susceptibility to hypoglycemia).
No products indexed under this heading.

Aspirin Buffered (Co-administration may reduce the blood-glucose-lowering effect of insulin and susceptibility to hypoglycemia). Products include:
Bufferin Extra Strength Tablets .... ▣ 678
Bufferin Regular Strength Tablets .... ▣ 678

Atenolol (Co-administration may either potentiate or weaken the blood-glucose-lowering effect of insulin. Signs of hypoglycemia may be reduced or absent).
No products indexed under this heading.

Benazepril Hydrochloride (Co-administration may reduce the blood-glucose-lowering effect of insulin and susceptibility to hypoglycemia). Products include:
Lotensin Tablets 2243
Lotensin HCT Tablets 2246
Lotrel Capsules 2249

Bendroflumethiazide (Co-administration may reduce the blood-glucose-lowering effect of insulin).
No products indexed under this heading.

Betamethasone Acetate (Co-administration may reduce the blood-glucose-lowering effect of insulin).
No products indexed under this heading.

Betamethasone Sodium Phosphate (Co-administration may reduce the blood-glucose-lowering effect of insulin).
No products indexed under this heading.

Betaxolol Hydrochloride (Co-administration may either potentiate or weaken the blood-glucose-lowering effect of insulin. Signs of hypoglycemia may be reduced or absent). Products include:
Betoptic S Ophthalmic Suspension 558

Bisoprolol Fumarate (Co-administration may either potentiate or weaken the blood-glucose-lowering effect of insulin. Signs of hypoglycemia may be reduced or absent).
No products indexed under this heading.

Bumetanide (Co-administration may reduce the blood-glucose-lowering effect of insulin). Products include:
Bumex Tablets 2746

Captopril (Co-administration may reduce the blood-glucose-lowering effect of insulin and susceptibility to hypoglycemia). Products include:
Captopril Tablets 2149

Carteolol Hydrochloride (Co-administration may either potentiate or weaken the blood-glucose-lowering effect of insulin. Signs of hypoglycemia may be reduced or absent). Products include:
Carteolol Hydrochloride Ophthalmic Solution USP, 1% .... ⊙ 249

Chlorothiazide (Co-administration may reduce the blood-glucose-lowering effect of insulin). Products include:
Diuril Oral Suspension 1954

Chlorothiazide Sodium (Co-administration may reduce the blood-glucose-lowering effect of insulin). Products include:
Diuril Sodium Intravenous 2467

Chlorotrianisene (Co-administration may reduce the blood-glucose-lowering effect of insulin).
No products indexed under this heading.

Chlorpromazine (Co-administration may reduce the blood-glucose-lowering effect of insulin).
No products indexed under this heading.

Chlorpromazine Hydrochloride (Co-administration may reduce the blood-glucose-lowering effect of insulin).
No products indexed under this heading.

Chlorpropamide (Co-administration may reduce the blood-glucose-lowering effect of insulin and susceptibility to hypoglycemia).
No products indexed under this heading.

Chlorthalidone (Co-administration may reduce the blood-glucose-lowering effect of insulin). Products include:
Clorpres Tablets 2153

Choline Magnesium Trisalicylate (Co-administration may reduce the blood-glucose-lowering effect of insulin and susceptibility to hypoglycemia).
No products indexed under this heading.

Clofibrate (Co-administration may reduce the blood-glucose-lowering effect of insulin and susceptibility to hypoglycemia).
No products indexed under this heading.

Clonidine (Co-administration may either potentiate or weaken the blood-glucose lowering effect of insulin. Signs of hypoglycemia may be reduced or absent). Products include:
Catapres-TTS 844

Cortisone Acetate (Co-administration may reduce the blood-glucose-lowering effect of insulin).
No products indexed under this heading.

Danazol (Co-administration may reduce the blood-glucose-lowering effect of insulin).
No products indexed under this heading.

Desogestrel (Co-administration may reduce the blood-glucose-lowering effect of insulin). Products include:
Mircette Tablets 1066

Dexamethasone (Co-administration may reduce the blood-glucose-lowering effect of insulin). Products include:
Ciprodex Otic Suspension 559
Decadron Tablets 1951
TobraDex Ophthalmic Ointment 562
TobraDex Ophthalmic Suspension 563

Dexamethasone Acetate (Co-administration may reduce the blood-glucose-lowering effect of insulin).
No products indexed under this heading.

Dexamethasone Sodium Phosphate (Co-administration may reduce the blood-glucose-lowering effect of insulin).
No products indexed under this heading.

Dienestrol (Co-administration may reduce the blood-glucose-lowering effect of insulin).
No products indexed under this heading.

Diethylstilbestrol (Co-administration may reduce the blood-glucose-lowering effect of insulin).
No products indexed under this heading.

Diflunisal (Co-administration may reduce the blood-glucose-lowering effect of insulin and susceptibility to hypoglycemia). Products include:
Dolobid Tablets 1955

Disopyramide (Co-administration may reduce the blood-glucose-lowering effect of insulin and susceptibility to hypoglycemia).
No products indexed under this heading.

Dobutamine Hydrochloride (Co-administration may reduce the blood-glucose-lowering effect of insulin).
No products indexed under this heading.

Dopamine Hydrochloride (Co-administration may reduce the blood-glucose-lowering effect of insulin).
No products indexed under this heading.

Enalapril Maleate (Co-administration may reduce the blood-glucose-lowering effect of insulin and susceptibility to hypoglycemia). Products include:
Vasotec I.V. Injection 2103

Enalaprilat (Co-administration may reduce the blood-glucose-lowering effect of insulin and susceptibility to hypoglycemia).
No products indexed under this heading.

Ephedrine Hydrochloride (Co-administration may reduce the blood-glucose-lowering effect of insulin).
No products indexed under this heading.

Ephedrine Sulfate (Co-administration may reduce the blood-glucose-lowering effect of insulin).
No products indexed under this heading.

Ephedrine Tannate (Co-administration may reduce the blood-glucose-lowering effect of insulin).
No products indexed under this heading.

Epinephrine (Co-administration may reduce the blood-glucose-lowering effect of insulin). Products include:
EpiPen 1061
Primatene Mist .... ▣ 719
Twinject 0.15 3379
Twinject 0.3 3378

Epinephrine Bitartrate (Co-administration may reduce the blood-glucose-lowering effect of insulin).
No products indexed under this heading.

Epinephrine Hydrochloride (Co-administration may reduce the blood-glucose-lowering effect of insulin).
No products indexed under this heading.

Esmolol Hydrochloride (Co-administration may either potentiate or weaken the blood-glucose-lowering effect of insulin. Signs of hypoglycemia may be reduced or absent).
No products indexed under this heading.

Estradiol (Co-administration may reduce the blood-glucose-lowering effect of insulin). Products include:
Angeliq Tablets 762
Climara Transdermal System 771
Climara Pro Transdermal System 776
Estrasorb Topical Emulsion 1147
Estring Vaginal Ring 2635
Menostar Transdermal System 782
Vagifem Tablets 2334

Estrogens, Conjugated (Co-administration may reduce the blood-glucose-lowering effect of insulin). Products include:
Premarin Intravenous 3442
Premarin Tablets 3446
Premarin Vaginal Cream 3452
Premphase Tablets 3456
Prempro Tablets 3456

Estrogens, Esterified (Co-administration may reduce the blood-glucose-lowering effect of insulin). Products include:
Estratest Tablets 3199
Estratest H.S. Tablets 3199

Estropipate (Co-administration may reduce the blood-glucose-lowering effect of insulin).
No products indexed under this heading.

Ethacrynic Acid (Co-administration may reduce the blood-glucose-lowering effect of insulin). Products include:
Edecrin Tablets 1959

Ethinyl Estradiol (Co-administration may reduce the blood-glucose-lowering effect of insulin). Products include:
Mircette Tablets 1066
NuvaRing 2340
Ortho-Cyclen/Ortho Tri-Cyclen 2429
Ortho Evra Transdermal System 2417
Ortho Tri-Cyclen Lo Tablets 2436
Seasonique Tablets 1077
Yasmin 28 Tablets 796
Yaz Tablets 803

Fenofibrate (Co-administration may reduce the blood-glucose-lowering effect of insulin and susceptibility to hypoglycemia). Products include:
Lofibra Tablets 1219
Lofibra Capsules 1216
Tricor Tablets 527
Triglide Tablets 3123

Fludrocortisone Acetate (Co-administration may reduce the blood-glucose-lowering effect of insulin).
No products indexed under this heading.

Fluoxetine (Co-administration may reduce the blood-glucose-lowering effect of insulin and susceptibility to hypoglycemia).
No products indexed under this heading.

Fluphenazine Decanoate (Co-administration may reduce the blood-glucose-lowering effect of insulin).
No products indexed under this heading.

Fluphenazine Enanthate (Co-administration may reduce the blood-glucose-lowering effect of insulin).

 No products indexed under this heading.

Fluphenazine Hydrochloride (Co-administration may reduce the blood-glucose-lowering effect of insulin).

 No products indexed under this heading.

Fosinopril Sodium (Co-administration may reduce the blood-glucose-lowering effect of insulin and susceptibility to hypoglycemia).

 No products indexed under this heading.

Furosemide (Co-administration may reduce the blood-glucose-lowering effect of insulin). Products include:

 Furosemide Tablets 2154

Gemfibrozil (Co-administration may reduce the blood-glucose-lowering effect of insulin and susceptibility to hypoglycemia).

 No products indexed under this heading.

Glimepiride (Co-administration may reduce the blood-glucose-lowering effect of insulin and susceptibility to hypoglycemia). Products include:

 Avandaryl Tablets 1379
 Duetact Tablets 3226

Glipizide (Co-administration may reduce the blood-glucose-lowering effect of insulin and susceptibility to hypoglycemia).

 No products indexed under this heading.

Glyburide (Co-administration may reduce the blood-glucose-lowering effect of insulin and susceptibility to hypoglycemia).

 No products indexed under this heading.

Guanethidine (Signs of hypoglycemia may be reduced or absent).

 No products indexed under this heading.

Hydrochlorothiazide (Co-administration may reduce the blood-glucose-lowering effect of insulin). Products include:

 Aldoril Tablets 1910
 Atacand HCT 651
 Avalide Tablets 888
 Avalide Tablets 2874
 Benicar HCT Tablets 1044
 Diovan HCT Tablets 2196
 Dyazide Capsules 1423
 Hyzaar 50-12.5 Tablets 1990
 Hyzaar 100-12.5 Tablets 1990
 Hyzaar 100-25 Tablets 1990
 Lopressor HCT 50/25 Tablets 2241
 Lopressor HCT 100/25 Tablets 2241
 Lopressor HCT 100/50 Tablets 2241
 Lotensin HCT Tablets 2246
 Micardis HCT Tablets 856
 Moduretic Tablets 2028
 Prinzide Tablets 2056
 Teveten HCT Tablets 1737
 Timolide Tablets 2086
 Uniretic Tablets 3100

Hydrocortisone (Co-administration may reduce the blood-glucose-lowering effect of insulin). Products include:

 Colocort Rectal Suspension, USP (Retention) 100 mg/60 mL.......... 2476
 Hydrocortone Tablets 1989
 Preparation H Hydrocortisone Cream 646

Hydrocortisone Acetate (Co-administration may reduce the blood-glucose-lowering effect of insulin). Products include:

 Analpram-HC 1159
 Pramosone 1161
 ProctoFoam-HC 3099

Hydrocortisone Sodium Phosphate (Co-administration may reduce the blood-glucose-lowering effect of insulin).

 No products indexed under this heading.

Hydrocortisone Sodium Succinate (Co-administration may reduce the blood-glucose-lowering effect of insulin).

 No products indexed under this heading.

Hydroflumethiazide (Co-administration may reduce the blood-glucose-lowering effect of insulin).

 No products indexed under this heading.

Indapamide (Co-administration may reduce the blood-glucose-lowering effect of insulin). Products include:

 Indapamide Tablets 2156

Isocarboxazid (Co-administration may reduce the blood-glucose-lowering effect of insulin and susceptibility to hypoglycemia).

 No products indexed under this heading.

Isoniazid (Co-administration may reduce the blood-glucose-lowering effect of insulin).

 No products indexed under this heading.

Isoproterenol Hydrochloride (Co-administration may reduce the blood-glucose-lowering effect of insulin).

 No products indexed under this heading.

Isoproterenol Sulfate (Co-administration may reduce the blood-glucose-lowering effect of insulin).

 No products indexed under this heading.

Labetalol Hydrochloride (Co-administration may either potentiate or weaken the blood-glucose-lowering effect of insulin. Signs of hypoglycemia may be reduced or absent).

 No products indexed under this heading.

Levalbuterol Hydrochloride (Co-administration may reduce the blood-glucose-lowering effect of insulin). Products include:

 Xopenex Inhalation Solution 3146
 Xopenex Inhalation Solution Concentrate 3150

Levobunolol Hydrochloride (Co-administration may either potentiate or weaken the blood-glucose-lowering effect of insulin. Signs of hypoglycemia may be reduced or absent). Products include:

 Betagan Ophthalmic Solution, USP ☉220

Levothyroxine Sodium (Co-administration may reduce the blood-glucose-lowering effect of insulin). Products include:

 Levothroid Tablets 1186
 Levoxyl Tablets 1712
 Synthroid Tablets 520
 Westhroid Tablets 3403

Liothyronine Sodium (Co-administration may reduce the blood-glucose-lowering effect of insulin). Products include:

 Cytomel Tablets 1710
 Westhroid Tablets 3403

Liotrix (Co-administration may reduce the blood-glucose-lowering effect of insulin). Products include:

 Thyrolar Tablets 1199

Lisinopril (Co-administration may reduce the blood-glucose-lowering effect of insulin and susceptibility to hypoglycemia). Products include:

 Prinivil Tablets 2052
 Prinzide Tablets 2056

Lithium (Co-administration may either potentiate or weaken the blood-glucose-lowering effect of insulin).

 No products indexed under this heading.

Lithium Carbonate (Co-administration may either potentiate or weaken the blood-glucose-lowering effect of insulin). Products include:

 Lithobid Tablets 1692

Lithium Citrate (Co-administration may either potentiate or weaken the blood-glucose-lowering effect of insulin).

 No products indexed under this heading.

Magnesium Salicylate (Co-administration may reduce the blood-glucose-lowering effect of insulin and susceptibility to hypoglycemia).

 No products indexed under this heading.

Medroxyprogesterone Acetate (Co-administration may reduce the blood-glucose-lowering effect of insulin). Products include:

 Depo-Provera Contraceptive Injection 2622
 depo-subQ provera 104 Injectable Suspension................... 2624
 Premphase Tablets 3456
 Prempro Tablets 3456

Megestrol Acetate (Co-administration may reduce the blood-glucose-lowering effect of insulin). Products include:

 Megace ES Oral Suspension 2481

Mesoridazine Besylate (Co-administration may reduce the blood-glucose-lowering effect of insulin).

 No products indexed under this heading.

Metaproterenol Sulfate (Co-administration may reduce the blood-glucose-lowering effect of insulin). Products include:

 Alupent Inhalation Aerosol 826

Metaraminol Bitartrate (Co-administration may reduce the blood-glucose-lowering effect of insulin).

 No products indexed under this heading.

Metformin Hydrochloride (Co-administration may reduce the blood-glucose-lowering effect of insulin and susceptibility to hypoglycemia). Products include:

 ActoPlus Met Tablets 3214
 Avandamet Tablets 1373
 Fortamet Extended-Release Tablets 3115

Methotrimeprazine (Co-administration may reduce the blood-glucose-lowering effect of insulin).

 No products indexed under this heading.

Methoxamine Hydrochloride (Co-administration may reduce the blood-glucose-lowering effect of insulin).

 No products indexed under this heading.

Methyclothiazide (Co-administration may reduce the blood-glucose-lowering effect of insulin).

 No products indexed under this heading.

Methylprednisolone Acetate (Co-administration may reduce the blood-glucose-lowering effect of insulin). Products include:

 Depo-Medrol Injectable Suspension.............................. 2617
 Depo-Medrol Single-Dose Vial 2619

Methylprednisolone Sodium Succinate (Co-administration may reduce the blood-glucose-lowering effect of insulin).

 No products indexed under this heading.

Metipranolol Hydrochloride (Co-administration may either potentiate or weaken the blood-glucose-lowering effect of insulin. Signs of hypoglycemia may be reduced or absent).

 No products indexed under this heading.

Metolazone (Co-administration may reduce the blood-glucose-lowering effect of insulin).

 No products indexed under this heading.

Metoprolol Succinate (Co-administration may either potentiate or weaken the blood-glucose-lowering effect of insulin. Signs of hypoglycemia may be reduced or absent). Products include:

 Toprol-XL Tablets 668

Metoprolol Tartrate (Co-administration may either potentiate or weaken the blood-glucose-lowering effect of insulin. Signs of hypoglycemia may be reduced or absent). Products include:

 Lopressor Injection 2238
 Lopressor Tablets 2238
 Lopressor HCT 50/25 Tablets 2241
 Lopressor HCT 100/25 Tablets 2241
 Lopressor HCT 100/50 Tablets 2241

Miglitol (Co-administration may reduce the blood-glucose-lowering effect of insulin and susceptibility to hypoglycemia).

 No products indexed under this heading.

Moclobemide (Co-administration may reduce the blood-glucose-lowering effect of insulin and susceptibility to hypoglycemia).

 No products indexed under this heading.

Moexipril Hydrochloride (Co-administration may reduce the blood-glucose-lowering effect of insulin and susceptibility to hypoglycemia). Products include:

 Uniretic Tablets 3100
 Univasc Tablets 3104

Nadolol (Co-administration may either potentiate or weaken the blood-glucose-lowering effect of insulin. Signs of hypoglycemia may be reduced or absent). Products include:

 Nadolol Tablets 2159

Norepinephrine Bitartrate (Co-administration may reduce the blood-glucose-lowering effect of insulin).

 No products indexed under this heading.

Norgestimate (Co-administration may reduce the blood-glucose-lowering effect of insulin). Products include:

 Ortho-Cyclen/Ortho Tri-Cyclen 2429
 Ortho Tri-Cyclen Lo Tablets 2436

Octreotide Acetate (Co-administration may increase the blood-glucose-lowering effect of insulin and susceptibility to hypoglycemia). Products include:

 Sandostatin Injection 2278

IMPORTANT NOTE: Always consult each drug listing in the patient's regimen for possible interactions.

Quinapril Hydrochloride (Co-administration may reduce the blood-glucose-lowering effect of insulin and susceptibility to hypoglycemia).
No products indexed under this heading.

Quinestrol (Co-administration may reduce the blood-glucose-lowering effect of insulin).
No products indexed under this heading.

Ramipril (Co-administration may reduce the blood-glucose-lowering effect of insulin and susceptibility to hypoglycemia). Products include:
Altace Capsules 1702

Repaglinide (Co-administration may reduce the blood-glucose-lowering effect of insulin and susceptibility to hypoglycemia).
No products indexed under this heading.

Reserpine (Signs of hypoglycemia may be reduced or absent).
No products indexed under this heading.

Rosiglitazone Maleate (Co-administration may reduce the blood-glucose-lowering effect of insulin and susceptibility to hypoglycemia).
Products include:
Avandamet Tablets 1373
Avandaryl Tablets 1379
Avandia Tablets 1384

Salmeterol Xinafoate (Co-administration may reduce the blood-glucose-lowering effect of insulin).
Products include:
Advair Diskus 100/50 1308
Advair Diskus 250/50 1308
Advair Diskus 500/50 1308
Advair HFA Inhalation Aerosol 1318
Serevent Diskus 1568

Salsalate (Co-administration may reduce the blood-glucose-lowering effect of insulin and susceptibility to hypoglycemia).
No products indexed under this heading.

Selegiline Hydrochloride (Co-administration may reduce the blood-glucose-lowering effect of insulin and susceptibility to hypoglycemia).
Products include:
Eldepryl Capsules 3208
Zelapar Tablets 3372

Somatropin (Co-administration may reduce the blood-glucose-lowering effect of insulin). Products include:
Genotropin Lyophilized Powder 2638
Humatrope Vials and Cartridges 1787
Norditropin Cartridges 2323
Nutropin for Injection 1239
Nutropin AQ Injection 1243
Nutropin AQ Pen 1243
Nutropin AQ Pen Cartridge 1243

Sotalol Hydrochloride (Co-administration may either potentiate or weaken the blood-glucose-lowering effect of insulin. Signs of hypoglycemia may be reduced or absent).
No products indexed under this heading.

Spirapril Hydrochloride (Co-administration may reduce the blood-glucose-lowering effect of insulin and susceptibility to hypoglycemia).
No products indexed under this heading.

Spironolactone (Co-administration may reduce the blood-glucose-lowering effect of insulin).
No products indexed under this heading.

Sulfacytine (Co-administration may reduce the blood-glucose-lowering effect of insulin and susceptibility to hypoglycemia).
No products indexed under this heading.

Sulfamethizole (Co-administration may reduce the blood-glucose-lowering effect of insulin and susceptibility to hypoglycemia).
No products indexed under this heading.

Sulfamethoxazole (Co-administration may reduce the blood-glucose-lowering effect of insulin and susceptibility to hypoglycemia).
No products indexed under this heading.

Sulfasalazine (Co-administration may reduce the blood-glucose-lowering effect of insulin and susceptibility to hypoglycemia).
No products indexed under this heading.

Sulfinpyrazone (Co-administration may reduce the blood-glucose-lowering effect of insulin and susceptibility to hypoglycemia).
No products indexed under this heading.

Sulfisoxazole Acetyl (Co-administration may reduce the blood-glucose-lowering effect of insulin and susceptibility to hypoglycemia).
No products indexed under this heading.

Sulfisoxazole Diolamine (Co-administration may reduce the blood-glucose-lowering effect of insulin and susceptibility to hypoglycemia).
No products indexed under this heading.

Terbutaline Sulfate (Co-administration may reduce the blood-glucose-lowering effect of insulin).
No products indexed under this heading.

Thioridazine Hydrochloride (Co-administration may reduce the blood-glucose-lowering effect of insulin).
Products include:
Thioridazine Hydrochloride Tablets 2163

Thyroglobulin (Co-administration may reduce the blood-glucose-lowering effect of insulin).
No products indexed under this heading.

Thyroid (Co-administration may reduce the blood-glucose-lowering effect of insulin).
No products indexed under this heading.

Thyroxine (Co-administration may reduce the blood-glucose-lowering effect of insulin).
No products indexed under this heading.

Thyroxine Sodium (Co-administration may reduce the blood-glucose-lowering effect of insulin).
No products indexed under this heading.

Timolol Hemihydrate (Co-administration may either potentiate or weaken the blood-glucose-lowering effect of insulin. Signs of hypoglycemia may be reduced or absent). Products include:
Betimol Ophthalmic Solution 3382
Betimol Ophthalmic Solution .... ⊙295

Timolol Maleate (Co-administration may either potentiate or weaken the blood-glucose-lowering effect of insulin. Signs of hypoglycemia may be reduced or absent). Products include:
Blocadren Tablets 1916
Cosopt Sterile Ophthalmic Solution....................................... 1931
Timolide Tablets 2086
Timoptic Sterile Ophthalmic Solution..................................... 2088
Timoptic in Ocudose 2091
Timoptic-XE Sterile Ophthalmic Gel Forming Solution 2092

Tolazamide (Co-administration may reduce the blood-glucose-lowering effect of insulin and susceptibility to hypoglycemia).
No products indexed under this heading.

Tolbutamide (Co-administration may reduce the blood-glucose-lowering effect of insulin and susceptibility to hypoglycemia).
No products indexed under this heading.

Torsemide (Co-administration may reduce the blood-glucose-lowering effect of insulin). Products include:
Demadex Injection 2759
Demadex Tablets 2759

Trandolapril (Co-administration may reduce the blood-glucose-lowering effect of insulin and susceptibility to hypoglycemia). Products include:
Mavik Tablets 486
Tarka Tablets 524

Tranylcypromine Sulfate (Co-administration may reduce the blood-glucose-lowering effect of insulin and susceptibility to hypoglycemia).
Products include:
Parnate Tablets 1527

Triamcinolone (Co-administration may reduce the blood-glucose-lowering effect of insulin).
No products indexed under this heading.

Triamcinolone Acetonide (Co-administration may reduce the blood-glucose-lowering effect of insulin).
Products include:
Azmacort Inhalation Aerosol 1726
Nasacort AQ Nasal Spray 2922

Triamcinolone Diacetate (Co-administration may reduce the blood-glucose-lowering effect of insulin).
No products indexed under this heading.

Triamcinolone Hexacetonide (Co-administration may reduce the blood-glucose-lowering effect of insulin).
No products indexed under this heading.

Triamterene (Co-administration may reduce the blood-glucose-lowering effect of insulin). Products include:
Dyazide Capsules 1423
Dyrenium Capsules 3400

Trifluoperazine Hydrochloride (Co-administration may reduce the blood-glucose-lowering effect of insulin).
No products indexed under this heading.

Troglitazone (Co-administration may reduce the blood-glucose-lowering effect of insulin and susceptibility to hypoglycemia).
No products indexed under this heading.

Food Interactions

Alcohol (Co-administration may either potentiate or weaken the blood-glucose lowering effect of insulin).

LEVITRA TABLETS

(Vardenafil Hydrochloride) 3034
May interact with alpha adrenergic blockers, class 1A antiarrhythmics, class III antiarrhythmics, cytochrome p450 3a4 inhibitors (selected), erythromycin, nitrates and nitrites, and certain other agents. Compounds in these categories include:

Acetazolamide (Concomitant use with moderate/strong CYP 3A4 inhibitors results in significant increases in plasma levels of vardenafil).
No products indexed under this heading.

Amiodarone Hydrochloride (Vardenafil hydrochloride may increase the QTc interval. Patients with congenital QT prolongation and those taking Class III antiarrhythmic medications should avoid using vardenafil hydrochloride).
No products indexed under this heading.

Amprenavir (Concomitant use with moderate/strong CYP 3A4 inhibitors results in significant increases in plasma levels of vardenafil).
Products include:
Agenerase Capsules 1327
Agenerase Oral Solution 1332

Amyl Nitrite (The blood pressure lowering effects of sublingual nitrates taken 1 and 4 hours after vardenafil and increases in heart rate when taken at 1, 4 and 8 hours, were potentiated by vardenafil hydrochloride. These effects were not observed when vardenafil hydrochloride was taken 24 hours before the nitroglycerin. Concomitant use of vardenafil and nitrates is contraindicated).
No products indexed under this heading.

Anastrozole (Concomitant use with moderate/strong CYP 3A4 inhibitors results in significant increases in plasma levels of vardenafil).
Products include:
Arimidex Tablets 673

Aprepitant (Concomitant use with moderate/strong CYP 3A4 inhibitors results in significant increases in plasma levels of vardenafil).
Products include:
Emend Capsules 1963

Bretylium Tosylate (Vardenafil hydrochloride may increase the QTc interval. Patients with congenital QT prolongation and those taking Class III antiarrhythmic medications should avoid using vardenafil hydrochloride).
No products indexed under this heading.

Cimetidine (Concomitant use with moderate/strong CYP 3A4 inhibitors results in significant increases in plasma levels of vardenafil).
Products include:
Tagamet HB 200 Tablets 664

Cimetidine Hydrochloride (Concomitant use with moderate/strong CYP 3A4 inhibitors results in significant increases in plasma levels of vardenafil).
No products indexed under this heading.

Ciprofloxacin (Concomitant use with moderate/strong CYP 3A4 inhibitors results in significant increases in plasma levels of vardenafil). Products include:
Cipro Oral Suspension 2977
Cipro I.V. 2984
Cipro XR Tablets 2990

Ciprodex Otic Suspension 559

Clarithromycin (Concomitant use with moderate/strong CYP 3A4 inhibitors results in significant increases in plasma levels of vardenafil). Products include:

Biaxin/Biaxin XL 402
PREVPAC 3284

Clotrimazole (Concomitant use with moderate/strong CYP 3A4 inhibitors results in significant increases in plasma levels of vardenafil). Products include:

Desenex Athlete's Foot Cream .... ▣635
Lotrimin 3039
Lotrisone 3040

Cyclosporine (Concomitant use with moderate/strong CYP 3A4 inhibitors results in significant increases in plasma levels of vardenafil). Products include:

Gengraf Capsules 459
Neoral Oral Solution 2259
Neoral Soft Gelatin Capsules 2259
Restasis Ophthalmic Emulsion 575
Sandimmune 2275

Dalfopristin (Concomitant use with moderate/strong CYP 3A4 inhibitors results in significant increases in plasma levels of vardenafil).

No products indexed under this heading.

Danazol (Concomitant use with moderate/strong CYP 3A4 inhibitors results in significant increases in plasma levels of vardenafil).

No products indexed under this heading.

Delavirdine Mesylate (Concomitant use with moderate/strong CYP 3A4 inhibitors results in significant increases in plasma levels of vardenafil). Products include:

Rescriptor Tablets 2551

Diltiazem Hydrochloride (Concomitant use with moderate/strong CYP 3A4 inhibitors results in significant increases in plasma levels of vardenafil). Products include:

Cardizem LA Extended Release Tablets 1728
Tiazac Capsules 1201

Diltiazem Maleate (Concomitant use with moderate/strong CYP 3A4 inhibitors results in significant increases in plasma levels of vardenafil).

No products indexed under this heading.

Disopyramide (Vardenafil hydrochloride may increase the QTc interval. Patients with congenital QT prolongation and those taking Class IA antiarrhythmic medications should avoid using vardenafil hydrochloride).

No products indexed under this heading.

Doxazosin Mesylate (Caution is advised when Phosphodiesterase Type 5 (PDE5) inhibitors are co-administered with alpha-blockers. Concomitant use of these two drug classes may lower blood pressure significantly leading to symptomatic hypotention. Patients should be stable on alpha-blocker therapy prior to initiating a PDE5 inhibitor. Patients who demonstrate hemodynamic instability on alpha-blocker therapy alone are at an increased risk of symptomatic hypotention with concomitant use of PDE5 inhibitors. In those patients who are stable on alpha-blocker therapy, PDE5 inhibitors should be initiated at the lowest recommended starting dose. In those patients already taking an optimized dose of PDE5 inhibitor, alpha-blocker therapy should be initiated at the lowest dose). Products include:

Cardura XL Tablets 2515

Efavirenz (Concomitant use with moderate/strong CYP 3A4 inhibitors results in significant increases in plasma levels of vardenafil). Products include:

Atripla Tablets 945
Sustiva Capsules 930
Sustiva Tablets 930

Erythrityl Tetranitrate (The blood pressure lowering effects of sublingual nitrates taken 1 and 4 hours after vardenafil and increases in heart rate when taken at 1, 4 and 8 hours, were potentiated by vardenafil hydrochloride. These effects were not observed when vardenafil hydrochloride was taken 24 hours before the nitroglycerin. Concomitant use of vardenafil and nitrates is contraindicated).

No products indexed under this heading.

Erythromycin (Erythromycin produced a 4-fold increase in vardenafil AUC and a 3-fold increase in Cmax when co-administered with vardenafil hydrochloride in healthy volunteers. It is not recommended to exceed a single 5mg dose of vardenafil hydrochloride in a 24-hour period when used in combination with erythromycin). Products include:

Ery-Tab Tablets 449
Erythromycin Base Filmtab Tablets 455
Erythromycin Delayed-Release Capsules, USP 457
PCE Dispertab Tablets 515

Erythromycin Estolate (Erythromycin produced a 4-fold increase in vardenafil AUC and a 3-fold increase in Cmax when co-administered with vardenafil hydrochloride in healthy volunteers. It is not recommended to exceed a single 5mg dose of vardenafil hydrochloride in a 24-hour period when used in combination with erythromycin).

No products indexed under this heading.

Erythromycin Ethylsuccinate (Erythromycin produced a 4-fold increase in vardenafil AUC and a 3-fold increase in Cmax when co-administered with vardenafil hydrochloride in healthy volunteers. It is not recommended to exceed a single 5mg dose of vardenafil hydrochloride in a 24-hour period when used in combination with erythromycin). Products include:

E.E.S. 451
EryPed 447

Erythromycin Gluceptate (Erythromycin produced a 4-fold increase in vardenafil AUC and a 3-fold increase in Cmax when co-administered with vardenafil hydrochloride in healthy volunteers. It is not recommended to exceed a single 5mg dose of vardenafil hydrochloride in a 24-hour period when used in combination with erythromycin).

No products indexed under this heading.

Erythromycin Lactobionate (Erythromycin produced a 4-fold increase in vardenafil AUC and a 3-fold increase in Cmax when co-administered with vardenafil hydrochloride in healthy volunteers. It is not recommended to exceed a single 5mg dose of vardenafil hydrochloride in a 24-hour period when used in combination with erythromycin).

No products indexed under this heading.

Erythromycin Stearate (Erythromycin produced a 4-fold increase in vardenafil AUC and a 3-fold increase in Cmax when co-administered with vardenafil hydrochloride in healthy volunteers. It is not recommended to exceed a single 5mg dose of vardenafil hydrochloride in a 24-hour period when used in combination with erythromycin). Products include:

Erythrocin Stearate Filmtab Tablets 453

Esomeprazole Magnesium (Concomitant use with moderate/strong CYP 3A4 inhibitors results in significant increases in plasma levels of vardenafil). Products include:

Nexium Delayed-Release Capsules 655

Fluconazole (Concomitant use with moderate/strong CYP 3A4 inhibitors results in significant increases in plasma levels of vardenafil).

No products indexed under this heading.

Fluoxetine Hydrochloride (Concomitant use with moderate/strong CYP 3A4 inhibitors results in significant increases in plasma levels of vardenafil). Products include:

Prozac Pulvules and Liquid 1801
Symbyax Capsules 1819

Fluvoxamine Maleate (Concomitant use with moderate/strong CYP 3A4 inhibitors results in significant increases in plasma levels of vardenafil).

No products indexed under this heading.

Fosamprenavir Calcium (Concomitant use with moderate/strong CYP 3A4 inhibitors results in significant increases in plasma levels of vardenafil). Products include:

Lexiva Tablets 1505

Indinavir Sulfate (Indinavir, co-administered with vardenafil hydrochloride, resulted in a 16-fold increase in vardenafil AUC, a 7-fold increase in vardenafil Cmax and a 2-fold increase in vardenafil half-life. It is recommended not to exceed a single 2.5mg vardenafil hydrochloride dose in a 24-hour period when used in combination with indinavir). Products include:

Crixivan Capsules 1940

Isoniazid (Concomitant use with moderate/strong CYP 3A4 inhibitors results in significant increases in plasma levels of vardenafil).

No products indexed under this heading.

Isosorbide Dinitrate (The blood pressure lowering effects of sublingual nitrates taken 1 and 4 hours after vardenafil and increases in heart rate when taken at 1, 4 and 8 hours, were potentiated by vardenafil hydrochloride. These effects were not observed when vardenafil hydrochloride was taken 24 hours before the nitroglycerin. Concomitant use of vardenafil and nitrates is contraindicated). Products include:

BiDil Tablets 2171

Isosorbide Mononitrate (The blood pressure lowering effects of sublingual nitrates taken 1 and 4 hours after vardenafil and increases in heart rate when taken at 1, 4 and 8 hours, were potentiated by vardenafil hydrochloride. These effects were not observed when vardenafil hydrochloride was taken 24 hours before the nitroglycerin. Concomitant use of vardenafil and nitrates is contraindicated). Products include:

Imdur Tablets 3018

Itraconazole (Patients taking itraconazole 400mg daily should not exceed vardenafil hydrochloride 2.5mg once daily. For patients taking itraconazole 200mg daily, a single dose of 5mg vardenafil hydrochloride should not be exceeded in a 24-hour period).

No products indexed under this heading.

Ketoconazole (Ketoconazole may produce an increase in vardenafil AUC and Cmax when co-administered. Patients taking ketoconazole 400mg daily should not exceed vardenafil hydrochloride 2.5mg once daily. For patients taking ketoconazole 200mg daily, a single dose of 5mg vardenafil hydrochloride should not be exceeded in a 24-hour period). Products include:

Nizoral A-D Shampoo, 1% 1868

Lopinavir (Concomitant use with moderate/strong CYP 3A4 inhibitors results in significant increases in plasma levels of vardenafil). Products include:

Kaletra 476

Loratadine (Concomitant use with moderate/strong CYP 3A4 inhibitors results in significant increases in plasma levels of vardenafil). Products include:

Alavert Allergy & Sinus D-12 Hour Tablets .... ▣771
Alavert .... ▣771
Children's Claritin Allergy Oral Solution .... ▣771
Claritin Non-Drowsy 24 Hour Tablets .... ▣772
Claritin Reditabs 24 Hour Non-Drowsy Tablets .... ▣772
Claritin-D Non-Drowsy 12 Hour Tablets .... ▣772
Claritin-D Non-Drowsy 24 Hour Tablets .... ▣772

Metronidazole (Concomitant use with moderate/strong CYP 3A4 inhibitors results in significant increases in plasma levels of vardenafil). Products include:

Metrogel 1% 1211
MetroGel-Vaginal Gel 1855
Vandazole Vaginal Gel 3338

Metronidazole Benzoate (Concomitant use with moderate/strong CYP 3A4 inhibitors results in significant increases in plasma levels of vardenafil).

No products indexed under this heading.

Metronidazole Hydrochloride (Concomitant use with moderate/strong CYP 3A4 inhibitors results in significant increases in plasma levels of vardenafil).

No products indexed under this heading.

Miconazole (Concomitant use with moderate/strong CYP 3A4 inhibitors results in significant increases in plasma levels of vardenafil).

No products indexed under this heading.

Miconazole Nitrate (Concomitant use with moderate/strong CYP 3A4 inhibitors results in significant increases in plasma levels of vardenafil). Products include:

Moricizine Hydrochloride (Vardenafil hydrochloride may increase the QTc interval. Patients with congenital QT prolongation and those taking Class IA antiarrhythmic medications should avoid using vardenafil hydrochloride).

No products indexed under this heading.

Nefazodone Hydrochloride (Concomitant use with moderate/strong CYP 3A4 inhibitors results in significant increases in plasma levels of vardenafil).

No products indexed under this heading.

Nelfinavir Mesylate (Concomitant use with moderate/strong CYP 3A4 inhibitors results in significant increases in plasma levels of vardenafil). Products include:

Nevirapine (Concomitant use with moderate/strong CYP 3A4 inhibitors results in significant increases in plasma levels of vardenafil). Products include:

Niacinamide (Concomitant use with moderate/strong CYP 3A4 inhibitors results in significant increases in plasma levels of vardenafil).

No products indexed under this heading.

Nicotinamide (Concomitant use with moderate/strong CYP 3A4 inhibitors results in significant increases in plasma levels of vardenafil). Products include:

Nifedipine (In patients whose hypertension was controlled with nifedipine, vardenafil hydrochloride produced mean additional supine systolic/diastolic blood pressure reductions of 6/5mm Hg compared to placebo). Products include:

Nitroglycerin (The blood pressure lowering effects of sublingual nitrates taken 1 and 4 hours after vardenafil and increases in heart rate when taken at 1, 4 and 8 hours, were potentiated by vardenafil hydrochloride. These effects were not observed when vardenafil hydrochloride was taken 24 hours before the nitroglycerin. Concomitant use of vardenafil and nitrates is contraindicated). Products include:

Norfloxacin (Concomitant use with moderate/strong CYP 3A4 inhibitors results in significant increases in plasma levels of vardenafil). Products include:

Omeprazole (Concomitant use with moderate/strong CYP 3A4 inhibitors

results in significant increases in plasma levels of vardenafil). Products include:

Paroxetine Hydrochloride (Concomitant use with moderate/strong CYP 3A4 inhibitors results in significant increases in plasma levels of vardenafil). Products include:

Pentaerythritol Tetranitrate (The blood pressure lowering effects of sublingual nitrates taken 1 and 4 hours after vardenafil and increases in heart rate when taken at 1, 4 and 8 hours, were potentiated by vardenafil hydrochloride. These effects were not observed when vardenafil hydrochloride was taken 24 hours before the nitroglycerin. Concomitant use of vardenafil and nitrates is contraindicated).

No products indexed under this heading.

Prazosin Hydrochloride (Caution is advised when Phosphodiesterase Type 5 (PDE5) inhibitors are co-administered with alpha-blockers. Concomitant use of these two drug classes may lower blood pressure significantly leading to symptomatic hypotention. Patients should be stable on alpha-blocker therapy prior to initiating a PDE5 inhibitor. Patients who demonstrate hemodynamic instability on alpha-blocker therapy alone are at an increased risk of symptomatic hypotention with concomitant use of PDE5 inhibitors. In those patients who are stable on alpha-blocker therapy, PDE5 inhibitors should be initiated at the lowest recommended starting dose. In those patients already taking an optimized dose of PDE5 inhibitor, alpha-blocker therapy should be initiated at the lowest dose).

No products indexed under this heading.

Procainamide (Vardenafil hydrochloride may increase the QTc interval. Patients with congenital QT prolongation and those taking Class IA antiarrhythmic medications should avoid using vardenafil hydrochloride).

No products indexed under this heading.

Propoxyphene Hydrochloride (Concomitant use with moderate/strong CYP 3A4 inhibitors results in significant increases in plasma levels of vardenafil).

No products indexed under this heading.

Propoxyphene Napsylate (Concomitant use with moderate/strong CYP 3A4 inhibitors results in significant increases in plasma levels of vardenafil).

No products indexed under this heading.

Quinidine (Vardenafil hydrochloride may increase the QTc interval. Patients with congenital QT prolongation and those taking Class IA antiarrhythmic medications should avoid using vardenafil hydrochloride).

No products indexed under this heading.

Quinidine Gluconate (Vardenafil hydrochloride may increase the QTc interval. Patients with congenital QT prolongation and those taking Class IA antiarrhythmic medications should avoid using vardenafil hydrochloride).

No products indexed under this heading.

Quinidine Hydrochloride (Concomitant use with moderate/strong CYP 3A4 inhibitors results in significant increases in plasma levels of vardenafil).

No products indexed under this heading.

Quinidine Polygalacturonate (Concomitant use with moderate/strong CYP 3A4 inhibitors results in significant increases in plasma levels of vardenafil).

No products indexed under this heading.

Quinidine Sulfate (Concomitant use with moderate/strong CYP 3A4 inhibitors results in significant increases in plasma levels of vardenafil).

No products indexed under this heading.

Quinine (Concomitant use with moderate/strong CYP 3A4 inhibitors results in significant increases in plasma levels of vardenafil).

No products indexed under this heading.

Quinine Sulfate (Concomitant use with moderate/strong CYP 3A4 inhibitors results in significant increases in plasma levels of vardenafil).

No products indexed under this heading.

Quinupristin (Concomitant use with moderate/strong CYP 3A4 inhibitors results in significant increases in plasma levels of vardenafil).

No products indexed under this heading.

Ranitidine Bismuth Citrate (Concomitant use with moderate/strong CYP 3A4 inhibitors results in significant increases in plasma levels of vardenafil).

No products indexed under this heading.

Ranitidine Hydrochloride (Concomitant use with moderate/strong CYP 3A4 inhibitors results in significant increases in plasma levels of vardenafil). Products include:

Ritonavir (Ritonavir co-administered with vardenafil hydrochloride resulted in a 49-fold increase in vardenafil AUC, a 13-fold increase in vardenafil Cmax, and significantly prolonged the half-life of vardenafil to 26 hours. The interaction is a consequence of blocking the hepatic metabolism of vardenafil by ritonavir, a highly potent CYP3A4 inhibitor. It is recommended not to exceed a single 2.5mg dose of vardenafil hydrochloride in a 72-hour period when used in combination with ritonavir). Products include:

Saquinavir (Concomitant use with moderate/strong CYP 3A4 inhibitors results in significant increases in plasma levels of vardenafil).

No products indexed under this heading.

Saquinavir Mesylate (Concomitant use with moderate/strong CYP 3A4 inhibitors results in significant increases in plasma levels of vardenafil). Products include:

Sertraline Hydrochloride (Concomitant use with moderate/strong CYP 3A4 inhibitors results in significant increases in plasma levels of vardenafil). Products include:

Sildenafil Citrate (The safety and efficacy of vardenafil hydrochloride used in combination with other treatments for erectile dysfunction have not been studied. Therefore, the use of such combinations is not recommended). Products include:

Sotalol Hydrochloride (Vardenafil hydrochloride may increase the QTc interval. Patients with congenital QT prolongation and those taking Class III antiarrhythmic medications should avoid using vardenafil hydrochloride).

No products indexed under this heading.

Tamsulosin Hydrochloride (Caution is advised when Phosphodiesterase Type 5 (PDE5) inhibitors are co-administered with alpha-blockers. Concomitant use of these two drug classes may lower blood pressure significantly leading to symptomatic hypotention. Patients should be stable on alpha-blocker therapy prior to initiating a PDE5 inhibitor. Patients who demonstrate hemodynamic instability on alpha-blocker therapy alone are at an increased risk of symptomatic hypotention with concomitant use of PDE5 inhibitors. In those patients who are stable on alpha-blocker therapy, PDE5 inhibitors should be initiated at the lowest recommended starting dose. In those patients already taking an optimized dose of PDE5 inhibitor, alpha-blocker therapy should be initiated at the lowest dose). Products include:

Telithromycin (Concomitant use with moderate/strong CYP 3A4 inhibitors results in significant increases in plasma levels of vardenafil). Products include:

Terazosin Hydrochloride (Caution is advised when Phosphodiesterase Type 5 (PDE5) inhibitors are co-administered with alpha-blockers. Concomitant use of these two drug classes may lower blood pressure significantly leading to symptomatic hypotention. Patients should be stable on alpha-blocker therapy prior to initiating a PDE5 inhibitor. Patients who demonstrate hemodynamic instability on alpha-blocker therapy alone are at an increased risk of symptomatic hypotention with concomitant use of PDE5 inhibitors. In those patients who are stable on alpha-blocker therapy, PDE5 inhibitors should be initiated at the lowest recommended starting dose. In those patients already taking an optimized dose of PDE5 inhibitor, alpha-blocker therapy should be initiated at the lowest dose). Products include:

Troglitazone (Concomitant use with moderate/strong CYP 3A4 inhibitors results in significant increases in plasma levels of vardenafil).
No products indexed under this heading.

Troleandomycin (Concomitant use with moderate/strong CYP 3A4 inhibitors results in significant increases in plasma levels of vardenafil).
No products indexed under this heading.

Valproate Sodium (Concomitant use with moderate/strong CYP 3A4 inhibitors results in significant increases in plasma levels of vardenafil). Products include:
Depacon Injection 412

Verapamil Hydrochloride (Concomitant use with moderate/strong CYP 3A4 inhibitors results in significant increases in plasma levels of vardenafil). Products include:
Covera-HS Tablets 3139
Tarka Tablets 524
Verelan PM Extended-Release Capsules, Controlled-Onset 3106

Voriconazole (Concomitant use with moderate/strong CYP 3A4 inhibitors results in significant increases in plasma levels of vardenafil). Products include:
VFEND I.V. 2564
VFEND Oral Suspension 2564
VFEND Tablets 2564

Zafirlukast (Concomitant use with moderate/strong CYP 3A4 inhibitors results in significant increases in plasma levels of vardenafil). Products include:
Accolate Tablets 671

Zileuton (Concomitant use with moderate/strong CYP 3A4 inhibitors results in significant increases in plasma levels of vardenafil). Products include:
Zyflo Tablets 1023

Food Interactions

Grapefruit (Concomitant use with moderate/strong CYP 3A4 inhibitors results in significant increases in plasma levels of vardenafil).

Grapefruit Juice (Concomitant use with moderate/strong CYP 3A4 inhibitors results in significant increases in plasma levels of vardenafil).

LEVOTHROID TABLETS

(Levothyroxine Sodium) 1186
May interact with androgens, antacids, beta blockers, oral anticoagulants, dopamine agonists, estrogens, glucocorticoids, cardiac glycosides, hydantoin anticonvulsants, oral hypoglycemic agents, insulin, oral contraceptives, radiographic iodinated contrast media, salicylates, sympathomimetics, thiazides, tricyclic antidepressants, xanthines, and certain other agents. Compounds in these categories include:

Acarbose (Addition of levothyroxine to antidiabetic therapy may result in increased antidiabetic agent requirements. Careful monitoring of diabetic control is recommended, especially when thyroid therapy is started, changed, or discontinued). Products include:
Precose Tablets 751

Acebutolol Hydrochloride (Actions of particular beta-adrenergic antagonists may be impaired when the hypothyroid patient is converted to the euthroid state).
No products indexed under this heading.

Albuterol (Concurrent use may increase the effects of sympathomimetics or thyroid hormone. Thyroid hormones may increase the risk of coronary insufficiency when sympathomimetic agents are administered to patients with coronary artery disease). Products include:
Proventil Inhalation Aerosol 3053

Albuterol Sulfate (Concurrent use may increase the effects of sympathomimetics or thyroid hormone. Thyroid hormones may increase the risk of coronary insufficiency when sympathomimetic agents are administered to patients with coronary artery disease). Products include:
AccuNeb Inhalation Solution 1055
Combivent Inhalation Aerosol 847
DuoNeb Inhalation Solution 1058
ProAir HFA Inhalation Aerosol 3300
Proventil Inhalation Solution 0.083% 3055
Proventil HFA Inhalation Aerosol 3056
Ventolin HFA Inhalation Aerosol 1600
VoSpire ER Tablets 1052

Aluminum Carbonate (Concurrent use with antacids may reduce the efficacy of levothyroxine by binding and delaying or preventing the absorption, potentially resulting in hypothyroidism. Administer levothyroxine at least four hours apart from these agents).
No products indexed under this heading.

Aluminum Hydroxide (Concurrent use with antacids may reduce the efficacy of levothyroxine by binding and delaying or preventing the absorption, potentially resulting in hypothyroidism. Administer levothyroxine at least four hours apart from these agents). Products include:
Gaviscon Regular Strength Liquid .... ▣ 658
Gaviscon Regular Strength Tablets .... ▣ 658
Gaviscon Extra Strength Liquid .... ▣ 658
Gaviscon Extra Strength Tablets .... ▣ 658
Maalox Regular Strength Antacid/Antigas Liquid 2175
Maalox Max Maximum Strength Antacid/Anti-Gas Liquid 2176

Aminoglutethimide (Long-term aminoglutethimide therapy may minimally decrease T4 and T3 levels and increase TSH, although all values remain within normal limits in most patients).
No products indexed under this heading.

Aminophylline (Decreased theophylline clearance may occur in hypothyroid patients; clearance returns to normal when the euthroid state is achieved).
No products indexed under this heading.

Amiodarone Hydrochloride (Administration may decrease the peripheral conversion of T4 to T3, leading to decreased T3 levels. However, serum T4 levels are usually normal but may occasionally be slightly increased. Amiodarone may also induce hyperthyroidism by causing thyroiditis).
No products indexed under this heading.

Amitriptyline Hydrochloride (Concurrent use of tricyclic antidepressants and levothyroxine may increase the therapeutic and toxic effects of both drugs, possibly due to increased receptor sensitivity to catecholamines. Onset of action of tricyclics may be accelerated).
No products indexed under this heading.

Amoxapine (Concurrent use of tricyclic antidepressants and levothyroxine may increase the therapeutic and toxic effects of both drugs, possibly due to increased receptor sensitivity to catecholamines. Onset of action of tricyclics may be accelerated).
No products indexed under this heading.

Anisindione (Thyroid hormones appear to increase the catabolism of vitamin-K dependent clotting factors, thereby increasing the anticoagulant activity of oral anticoagulants. Concomitant use of these agents impairs the compensatory increases in clotting factor synthesis. Prothrombin time should be carefully monitored in patients taking levothyroxine and oral anticoagulants and the dose of anticoagulant therapy adjusted accordingly). Products include:
Miradon Tablets 3042

Asparaginase (Asparaginase may decrease serum TBG concentration). Products include:
Elspar for Injection 2463
Elspar for Injection 1960

Aspirin (Salicylates inhibit binding of T4 and T3 to TBG and transthyretin. An initial increase in FT4 is followed by return of FT4 to normal levels with sustained therapeutic serum salicylate concentrations, although total T4 levels may decrease by as much as 30%). Products include:
Aggrenox Capsules 822
Bayer Aspirin 744
BC Allergy Sinus Cold Powder .... ▣ 677
BC Headache Powder .... ▣ 677
Arthritis Strength BC Powder .... ▣ 677
BC Sinus Cold Powder .... ▣ 677
Excedrin Extra Strength Caplets/Tablets/Geltabs .... ▣ 684
Excedrin Migraine Caplets/Tablets/Geltabs .... ▣ 609
Goody's Body Pain Formula Powder .... ▣ 684
Goody's Extra Strength Headache Powders .... ▣ 611
Goody's Extra Strength Pain Relief Tablets .... ▣ 685
Percodan Tablets 1132
St. Joseph 81 mg Aspirin Chewable and Enteric Coated Tablets 1869

Aspirin, Enteric Coated (Salicylates inhibit binding of T4 and T3 to TBG and transthyretin. An initial increase in FT4 is followed by return of FT4 to normal levels with sustained therapeutic serum salicylate concentrations, although total T4 levels may decrease by as much as 30%).
No products indexed under this heading.

Aspirin Buffered (Salicylates inhibit binding of T4 and T3 to TBG and transthyretin. An initial increase in FT4 is followed by return of FT4 to normal levels with sustained therapeutic serum salicylate concentrations, although total T4 levels may decrease by as much as 30%). Products include:
Bufferin Extra Strength Tablets .... ▣ 678
Bufferin Regular Strength Tablets .... ▣ 678

Atenolol (Actions of particular beta-adrenergic antagonists may be impaired when the hypothyroid patient is converted to the euthroid state).
No products indexed under this heading.

Bendroflumethiazide (Thiazide diuretics are associated with thyroid hormone and/or TSH level alterations).
No products indexed under this heading.

Betamethasone Acetate (Glucocorticoids may result in a transient reduction in TSH secretion when administered at doses greater than 100mg/day of hydrocortisone or equivalent. Short-term administration of large doses of glucocorticoids may decrease serum T3 concentrations by 30% with minimal change in serum T4 levels. However, long-term glucocorticoid therapy may result in slightly decreased T3 and T4 levels due to decreased TBG production).
No products indexed under this heading.

Betamethasone Sodium Phosphate (Glucocorticoids may result in a transient reduction in TSH secretion when administered at doses greater than 100mg/day of hydrocortisone or equivalent. Short-term administration of large doses of glucocorticoids may decrease serum T3 concentrations by 30% with minimal change in serum T4 levels. However, long-term glucocorticoid therapy may result in slightly decreased T3 and T4 levels due to decreased TBG production).
No products indexed under this heading.

Betaxolol Hydrochloride (Actions of particular beta-adrenergic antagonists may be impaired when the hypothyroid patient is converted to the euthroid state). Products include:
Betoptic S Ophthalmic Suspension 558

Bisoprolol Fumarate (Actions of particular beta-adrenergic antagonists may be impaired when the hypothyroid patient is converted to the euthroid state).
No products indexed under this heading.

Bromocriptine Mesylate (Dopamine and dopamine agonists may result in a transient reduction in TSH secretion when administered at dopamine doses greater than or equal to 1 mcg/kg/min).
No products indexed under this heading.

Calcium Carbonate (Calcium carbonate may form an insoluble chelate with levothyroxine. Concurrent use may reduce the efficacy of levothyroxine by binding and delaying or preventing the absorption, potentially resulting in hypothyroidism. Administer levothyroxine at least four hours apart from calcium carbonate-containing products). Products include:
Actonel with Calcium Tablets 2688
Calcet Tablets 2138
Caltrate 600 PLUS .... ▣ 809
Caltrate 600 + D Tablets .... ▣ 809
D-Cal Chewable Caplets .... ▣ 812
Gas-X with Maalox .... ▣ 656
Maalox Regular Strength Antacid Chewable Tablets 2177
Maalox Max Maximum Strength Antacid/Antigas Chewable Tablets 2176
Maalox Max Maximum Strength Chewable Tablets .... ▣ 660
Os-Cal Chewable Tablets .... ▣ 818
Pepcid Complete Chewable Tablets 1701
Children's Pepto 2674
PremCal Light, Regular, and Extra Strength Tablets .... ▣ 818

Tums .... ▣ 664

Carbamazepine (Stimulation of hepatic microsomal drug-metabolizing activity may cause increased hepatic degradation of levothyroxine, resulting in increased levothyroxine requirements). Products include:

Carbatrol Capsules 3171
Equetro Extended-Release Capsules 3180
Tegretol/Tegretol-XR 2295

Carteolol Hydrochloride (Actions of particular beta-adrenergic antagonists may be impaired when the hypothyroid patient is converted to the euthroid state). Products include:

Carteolol Hydrochloride Ophthalmic Solution USP, 1%....... ⊙ 249

Chloral Hydrate (Chloral Hydrate has been associated with thyroid hormone and/or TSH level alterations).

No products indexed under this heading.

Chlorothiazide (Thiazide diuretics are associated with thyroid hormone and/or TSH level alterations). Products include:

Diuril Oral Suspension 1954

Chlorothiazide Sodium (Thiazide diuretics are associated with thyroid hormone and/or TSH level alterations). Products include:

Diuril Sodium Intravenous 2467

Chlorotrianisene (Estrogen may increase serum TBG concentration).

No products indexed under this heading.

Chlorpropamide (Addition of levothyroxine to antidiabetic therapy may result in increased antidiabetic agent requirements. Careful monitoring of diabetic control is recommended, especially when thyroid therapy is started, changed, or discontinued).

No products indexed under this heading.

Cholestyramine (Concurrent use with cholestyramine may reduce the efficacy of levothyroxine by binding and delaying or preventing the absorption, potentially resulting in hypothyroidism. Administer levothyroxine at least four hours apart from cholestyramine).

No products indexed under this heading.

Choline Magnesium Trisalicylate (Salicylates inhibit binding of T4 and T3 to TBG and transthyretin. An initial increase in FT4 is followed by return of FT4 to normal levels with sustained therapeutic serum salicylate concentrations, although total T4 levels may decrease by as much as 30%).

No products indexed under this heading.

Clofibrate (Clofibrate may increase serum TBG concentration).

No products indexed under this heading.

Clomipramine Hydrochloride (Concurrent use of tricyclic antidepressants and levothyroxine may increase the therapeutic and toxic effects of both drugs, possibly due to increased receptor sensitivity to catecholamines. Onset of action of tricyclics may be accelerated).

No products indexed under this heading.

Colestipol (Concurrent use with colestipol may reduce the efficacy of levothyroxine by binding and delaying or preventing the absorption, potentially resulting in hypothyroidism. Administer levothyroxine at least four hours apart from colestipol).

No products indexed under this heading.

Colestipol Hydrochloride (Concurrent use with colestipol may reduce the efficacy of levothyroxine by binding and delaying or preventing the absorption, potentially resulting in hypothyroidism. Administer levothyroxine at least four hours apart from colestipol).

No products indexed under this heading.

Cortisone Acetate (Glucocorticoids may result in a transient reduction in TSH secretion when administered at doses greater than 100mg/day of hydrocortisone or equivalent. Short-term administration of large doses of glucocorticoids may decrease serum T3 concentrations by 30% with minimal change in serum T4 levels. However, long-term glucocorticoid therapy may result in slightly decreased T3 and T4 levels due to decreased TBG production).

No products indexed under this heading.

Desipramine Hydrochloride (Concurrent use of tricyclic antidepressants and levothyroxine may increase the therapeutic and toxic effects of both drugs, possibly due to increased receptor sensitivity to catecholamines. Onset of action of tricyclics may be accelerated).

No products indexed under this heading.

Deslanoside (Serum digitalis glycoside levels may be reduced in hyperthyroidism or when the hypothyroid patient is converted to the euthroid state. Therapeutic effect of digitalis glycosides may be reduced).

No products indexed under this heading.

Desogestrel (Estrogen-containing oral contraceptives may increase serum TBG concentration). Products include:

Mircette Tablets 1066

Dexamethasone (Glucocorticoids may result in a transient reduction in TSH secretion when administered at doses greater than 100mg/day of hydrocortisone or equivalent. Short-term administration of large doses of glucocorticoids may decrease serum T3 concentrations by 30% with minimal change in serum T4 levels. However, long-term glucocorticoid therapy may result in slightly decreased T3 and T4 levels due to decreased TBG production). Products include:

Ciprodex Otic Suspension 559
Decadron Tablets 1951
TobraDex Ophthalmic Ointment 562
TobraDex Ophthalmic Suspension ... 563

Dexamethasone Acetate (Glucocorticoids may result in a transient reduction in TSH secretion when administered at doses greater than 100mg/day of hydrocortisone or equivalent. Short-term administration of large doses of glucocorticoids may decrease serum T3 concentrations by 30% with minimal change in serum T4 levels. However, long-term glucocorticoid therapy may result in slightly decreased T3 and T4 levels due to decreased TBG production).

No products indexed under this heading.

Dexamethasone Sodium Phosphate (Glucocorticoids may result in a transient reduction in TSH secretion when administered at doses greater than 100mg/day of hydrocortisone or equivalent. Short-term administration of large doses of glucocorticoids may decrease serum T3 concentrations by 30% with minimal change in serum T4 levels. However, long-term glucocorticoid therapy may result in slightly decreased T3 and T4 levels due to decreased TBG production).

No products indexed under this heading.

Diatrizoate Meglumine (Iodide and drugs that contain pharmacologic amounts of iodide may cause hyperthyroidism in euthroid patients with Grave's disease previously treated with antithyroid drugs or in euthroid patients with thyroid autonomy. Hyperthyroidism may develop over several weeks and may persist for several months after therapy discontinuation. Thyroid hormones may also reduce the uptake of I-123 and I-131).

No products indexed under this heading.

Diatrizoate Sodium (Iodide and drugs that contain pharmacologic amounts of iodide may cause hyperthyroidism in euthroid patients with Grave's disease previously treated with antithyroid drugs or in euthroid patients with thyroid autonomy. Hyperthyroidism may develop over several weeks and may persist for several months after therapy discontinuation. Thyroid hormones may also reduce the uptake of I-123 and I-131).

No products indexed under this heading.

Diazepam (Diazepam is associated with thyroid hormone and/or TSH level alterations). Products include:

Diastat Rectal Delivery System 3343
Valium Tablets 2819

Dicumarol (Thyroid hormones appear to increase the catabolism of vitamin-K dependent clotting factors, thereby increasing the anticoagulant activity of oral anticoagulants. Concomitant use of these agents impairs the compensatory increases in clotting factor synthesis. Prothrombin time should be carefully monitored in patients taking levothyroxine and oral anticoagulants and the dose of anticoagulant therapy adjusted accordingly).

No products indexed under this heading.

Dienestrol (Estrogen may increase serum TBG concentration).

No products indexed under this heading.

Diethylstilbestrol (Estrogen may increase serum TBG concentration).

No products indexed under this heading.

Diflunisal (Salicylates inhibit binding of T4 and T3 to TBG and transthyretin. An initial increase in FT4 is followed by return of FT4 to normal levels with sustained therapeutic serum salicylate concentrations, although total T4 levels may decrease by as much as 30%). Products include:

Dolobid Tablets 1955

Digitalis Glycoside Preparations (Serum digitalis glycoside levels may be reduced in hyperthyroidism or when the hypothyroid patient is converted to the euthroid state. Therapeutic effect of digitalis glycosides may be reduced).

No products indexed under this heading.

Digitoxin (Serum digitalis glycoside levels may be reduced in hyperthyroidism or when the hypothyroid patient is converted to the euthroid state. Therapeutic effect of digitalis glycosides may be reduced).

No products indexed under this heading.

Digoxin (Serum digitalis glycoside levels may be reduced in hyperthyroidism or when the hypothyroid patient is converted to the euthroid state. Therapeutic effect of digitalis glycosides may be reduced). Products include:

Lanoxicaps Capsules 1490
Lanoxin Injection 1494
Lanoxin Injection Pediatric 1497
Lanoxin Tablets 1500

Dobutamine Hydrochloride (Concurrent use may increase the effects of sympathomimetics or thyroid hormone. Thyroid hormones may increase the risk of coronary insufficiency when sympathomimetic agents are administered to patients with coronary artery disease).

No products indexed under this heading.

Dopamine Hydrochloride (Concurrent use may increase the effects of sympathomimetics or thyroid hormone. Thyroid hormones may increase the risk of coronary insufficiency when sympathomimetic agents are administered to patients with coronary artery disease).

No products indexed under this heading.

Doxepin Hydrochloride (Concurrent use of tricyclic antidepressants and levothyroxine may increase the therapeutic and toxic effects of both drugs, possibly due to increased receptor sensitivity to catecholamines. Onset of action of tricyclics may be accelerated).

No products indexed under this heading.

Dyphylline (Decreased theophylline clearance may occur in hypothyroid patients; clearance returns to normal when the euthroid state is achieved).

No products indexed under this heading.

Ephedrine Hydrochloride (Concurrent use may increase the effects of sympathomimetics or thyroid hormone. Thyroid hormones may increase the risk of coronary insufficiency when sympathomimetic agents are administered to patients with coronary artery disease).

No products indexed under this heading.

Ephedrine Sulfate (Concurrent use may increase the effects of sympathomimetics or thyroid hormone. Thyroid hormones may increase the risk of coronary insufficiency when sympathomimetic agents are administered to patients with coronary artery disease).

No products indexed under this heading.

Ephedrine Tannate (Concurrent use may increase the effects of sympathomimetics or thyroid hormone. Thyroid hormones may increase the risk of coronary insufficiency when sympathomimetic agents are administered to patients with coronary artery disease).
No products indexed under this heading.

Epinephrine (Concurrent use may increase the effects of sympathomimetics or thyroid hormone. Thyroid hormones may increase the risk of coronary insufficiency when sympathomimetic agents are administered to patients with coronary artery disease). Products include:
- EpiPen **1061**
- Primatene Mist .... ◘ **719**
- Twinject 0.15 .... **3379**
- Twinject 0.3 .... **3378**

Epinephrine Bitartrate (Concurrent use may increase the effects of sympathomimetics or thyroid hormone. Thyroid hormones may increase the risk of coronary insufficiency when sympathomimetic agents are administered to patients with coronary artery disease).
No products indexed under this heading.

Epinephrine Hydrochloride (Concurrent use may increase the effects of sympathomimetics or thyroid hormone. Thyroid hormones may increase the risk of coronary insufficiency when sympathomimetic agents are administered to patients with coronary artery disease).
No products indexed under this heading.

Esmolol Hydrochloride (Actions of particular beta-adrenergic antagonists may be impaired when the hypothyroid patient is converted to the euthroid state).
No products indexed under this heading.

Estradiol (Estrogen may increase serum TBG concentration). Products include:
- Angeliq Tablets **762**
- Climara Transdermal System **771**
- Climara Pro Transdermal System **776**
- Estrasorb Topical Emulsion **1147**
- Estring Vaginal Ring **2635**
- Menostar Transdermal System **782**
- Vagifem Tablets **2334**

Estrogens, Conjugated (Estrogen may increase serum TBG concentration). Products include:
- Premarin Intravenous **3442**
- Premarin Tablets **3446**
- Premarin Vaginal Cream **3452**
- Premphase Tablets **3456**
- Prempro Tablets **3456**

Estrogens, Esterified (Estrogen may increase serum TBG concentration). Products include:
- Estratest Tablets **3199**
- Estratest H.S. Tablets **3199**

Estropipate (Estrogen may increase serum TBG concentration).
No products indexed under this heading.

Ethinyl Estradiol (Estrogen-containing oral contraceptives may increase serum TBG concentration). Products include:
- Mircette Tablets **1066**
- NuvaRing **2340**
- Ortho-Cyclen/Ortho Tri-Cyclen **2429**
- Ortho Evra Transdermal System **2417**
- Ortho Tri-Cyclen Lo Tablets **2436**
- Seasonique Tablets **1077**
- Yasmin 28 Tablets **796**
- Yaz Tablets **803**

Ethiodized Oil (Iodide and drugs that contain pharmacologic amounts of iodide may cause hyperthyroidism in euthroid patients with Grave's disease previously treated with antithyroid drugs or in euthroid patients with thyroid autonomy. Hyperthyroidism may develop over several weeks and may persist for several months after therapy discontinuation. Thyroid hormones may also reduce the uptake of I-123 and I-131).
No products indexed under this heading.

Ethionamide (Ethionamide is associated with thyroid hormone and/or TSH level alterations). Products include:
- Trecator Tablets **3487**

Ethotoin (Stimulation of hepatic microsomal drug-metabolizing activity may cause increased hepatic degradation of levothyroxine, resulting in increased levothyroxine requirements).
No products indexed under this heading.

Ethynodiol Diacetate (Estrogen-containing oral contraceptives may increase serum TBG concentration).
No products indexed under this heading.

Ferrous Sulfate (Ferrous sulfate likely forms a ferric-thyroxine complex. Concurrent use may reduce the efficacy of levothyroxine by binding and delaying or preventing the absorption, potentially resulting in hypothyroidism. Administer levothyroxine at least four hours apart from ferrous sulfate-containing products). Products include:
- Slow Fe Iron Tablets .... ◘ **818**
- Slow Fe with Folic Acid Tablets .... ◘ **819**

Fludrocortisone Acetate (Glucocorticoids may result in a transient reduction in TSH secretion when administered at doses greater than 100mg/day of hydrocortisone or equivalent. Short-term administration of large doses of glucocorticoids may decrease serum T3 concentrations by 30% with minimal change in serum T4 levels. However, long-term glucocorticoid therapy may result in slightly decreased T3 and T4 levels due to decreased TBG production).
No products indexed under this heading.

Fluorouracil (Fluorouracil may increase serum TBG concentration). Products include:
- Carac Cream, 0.5% **2879**
- Efudex **3363**

Fluoxymesterone (Androgens/anabolic steroids may decrease serum TBG concentration). Products include:
- Androxy Tablets **3335**

Fosphenytoin Sodium (Stimulation of hepatic microsomal drug-metabolizing activity may cause increased hepatic degradation of levothyroxine, resulting in increased levothyroxine requirements).
No products indexed under this heading.

Furosemide (Co-administration of furosemide (greater than 80mg IV) with levothyroxine results in an initial transient increase in FT4. Continued administration results in a decrease in serum T4 and normal FT4 and TSH concentrations and, therefore, patients are clinically euthroid). Products include:
- Furosemide Tablets **2154**

Gadopentetate Dimeglumine (Iodide and drugs that contain pharmacologic amounts of iodide may cause hyperthyroidism in euthroid patients with Grave's disease previously treated with antithyroid drugs or in euthroid patients with thyroid autonomy. Hyperthyroidism may develop over several weeks and may persist for several months after therapy discontinuation. Thyroid hormones may also reduce the uptake of I-123 and I-131).
No products indexed under this heading.

Glimepiride (Addition of levothyroxine to antidiabetic therapy may result in increased antidiabetic agent requirements. Careful monitoring of diabetic control is recommended, especially when thyroid therapy is started, changed, or discontinued). Products include:
- Avandaryl Tablets **1379**
- Duetact Tablets **3226**

Glipizide (Addition of levothyroxine to antidiabetic therapy may result in increased antidiabetic agent requirements. Careful monitoring of diabetic control is recommended, especially when thyroid therapy is started, changed, or discontinued).
No products indexed under this heading.

Glyburide (Addition of levothyroxine to antidiabetic therapy may result in increased antidiabetic agent requirements. Careful monitoring of diabetic control is recommended, especially when thyroid therapy is started, changed, or discontinued).
No products indexed under this heading.

Heparin Calcium (Co-administration of heparin with levothyroxine results in an initial transient increase in FT4. Continued administration results in a decrease in serum T4 and normal FT4 and TSH concentrations and, therefore, patients are clinically euthroid).
No products indexed under this heading.

Heparin Sodium (Co-administration of heparin with levothyroxine results in an initial transient increase in FT4. Continued administration results in a decrease in serum T4 and normal FT4 and TSH concentrations and, therefore, patients are clinically euthroid).
No products indexed under this heading.

Heroin (Heroin may increase serum TBG concentration).
No products indexed under this heading.

Hydrochlorothiazide (Thiazide diuretics are associated with thyroid hormone and/or TSH level alterations). Products include:
- Aldoril Tablets **1910**
- Atacand HCT **651**
- Avalide Tablets **888**
- Avalide Tablets **2874**
- Benicar HCT Tablets **1044**
- Diovan HCT Tablets **2196**
- Dyazide Capsules **1423**
- Hyzaar 50-12.5 Tablets **1990**
- Hyzaar 100-12.5 Tablets **1990**
- Hyzaar 100-25 Tablets **1990**
- Lopressor HCT 50/25 Tablets **2241**
- Lopressor HCT 100/25 Tablets **2241**
- Lopressor HCT 100/50 Tablets **2241**
- Lotensin HCT Tablets **2246**
- Micardis HCT Tablets **856**
- Moduretic Tablets **2028**
- Prinzide Tablets **2056**
- Teveten HCT Tablets **1737**
- Timolide Tablets **2086**
- Uniretic Tablets **3100**

Hydrocortisone (Glucocorticoids may result in a transient reduction in TSH secretion when administered at doses greater than 100mg/day of hydrocortisone or equivalent. Short-term administration of large doses of glucocorticoids may decrease serum T3 concentrations by 30% with minimal change in serum T4 levels. However, long-term glucocorticoid therapy may result in slightly decreased T3 and T4 levels due to decreased TBG production). Products include:
- Colocort Rectal Suspension, USP (Retention) 100 mg/60 mL **2476**
- Hydrocortone Tablets **1989**
- Preparation H Hydrocortisone Cream .... ◘ **646**

Hydrocortisone Acetate (Glucocorticoids may result in a transient reduction in TSH secretion when administered at doses greater than 100mg/day of hydrocortisone or equivalent. Short-term administration of large doses of glucocorticoids may decrease serum T3 concentrations by 30% with minimal change in serum T4 levels. However, long-term glucocorticoid therapy may result in slightly decreased T3 and T4 levels due to decreased TBG production). Products include:
- Analpram-HC **1159**
- Pramosone **1161**
- ProctoFoam-HC **3099**

Hydrocortisone Sodium Phosphate (Glucocorticoids may result in a transient reduction in TSH secretion when administered at doses greater than 100mg/day of hydrocortisone or equivalent. Short-term administration of large doses of glucocorticoids may decrease serum T3 concentrations by 30% with minimal change in serum T4 levels. However, long-term glucocorticoid therapy may result in slightly decreased T3 and T4 levels due to decreased TBG production).
No products indexed under this heading.

Hydrocortisone Sodium Succinate (Glucocorticoids may result in a transient reduction in TSH secretion when administered at doses greater than 100mg/day of hydrocortisone or equivalent. Short-term administration of large doses of glucocorticoids may decrease serum T3 concentrations by 30% with minimal change in serum T4 levels. However, long-term glucocorticoid therapy may result in slightly decreased T3 and T4 levels due to decreased TBG production).
No products indexed under this heading.

Hydroflumethiazide (Thiazide diuretics are associated with thyroid hormone and/or TSH level alterations).
No products indexed under this heading.

Imipramine Hydrochloride (Concurrent use of tricyclic antidepressants and levothyroxine may increase the therapeutic and toxic effects of both drugs, possibly due to increased receptor sensitivity to catecholamines. Onset of action of tricyclics may be accelerated).
No products indexed under this heading.

Imipramine Pamoate (Concurrent use of tricyclic antidepressants and levothyroxine may increase the therapeutic and toxic effects of both drugs, possibly due to increased receptor sensitivity to catecholamines. Onset of action of tricyclics may be accelerated).

No products indexed under this heading.

Insulin, Human, Zinc Suspension (Addition of levothyroxine to insulin therapy may result in increased insulin requirements. Careful monitoring of diabetic control is recommended, especially when thyroid therapy is started, changed, or discontinued). Products include:

Insulin, Human NPH (Addition of levothyroxine to insulin therapy may result in increased insulin requirements. Careful monitoring of diabetic control is recommended, especially when thyroid therapy is started, changed, or discontinued). Products include:

Insulin, Human Regular (Addition of levothyroxine to insulin therapy may result in increased insulin requirements. Careful monitoring of diabetic control is recommended, especially when thyroid therapy is started, changed, or discontinued). Products include:

Insulin, Human Regular and Human NPH Mixture (Addition of levothyroxine to insulin therapy may result in increased insulin requirements. Careful monitoring of diabetic control is recommended, especially when thyroid therapy is started, changed, or discontinued). Products include:

Insulin, NPH (Addition of levothyroxine to insulin therapy may result in increased insulin requirements. Careful monitoring of diabetic control is recommended, especially when thyroid therapy is started, changed, or discontinued).

No products indexed under this heading.

Insulin, Regular (Addition of levothyroxine to insulin therapy may result in increased insulin requirements. Careful monitoring of diabetic control is recommended, especially when thyroid therapy is started, changed, or discontinued).

No products indexed under this heading.

Insulin, Zinc Crystals (Addition of levothyroxine to insulin therapy may result in increased insulin requirements. Careful monitoring of diabetic control is recommended, especially when thyroid therapy is started, changed, or discontinued).

No products indexed under this heading.

Insulin, Zinc Suspension (Addition of levothyroxine to insulin therapy may result in increased insulin requirements. Careful monitoring of diabetic control is recommended, especially when thyroid therapy is started, changed, or discontinued).

No products indexed under this heading.

Insulin Aspart, Human Regular (Addition of levothyroxine to insulin therapy may result in increased insulin requirements. Careful monitoring of diabetic control is recommended, especially when thyroid therapy is started, changed, or discontinued). Products include:

Insulin glargine (Addition of levothyroxine to insulin therapy may result in increased insulin requirements. Careful monitoring of diabetic control is recommended, especially when thyroid therapy is started, changed, or discontinued). Products include:

Insulin Lispro, Human (Addition of levothyroxine to insulin therapy may result in increased insulin requirements. Careful monitoring of diabetic control is recommended, especially when thyroid therapy is started, changed, or discontinued). Products include:

Insulin Lispro Protamine, Human (Addition of levothyroxine to insulin therapy may result in increased insulin requirements. Careful monitoring of diabetic control is recommended, especially when thyroid therapy is started, changed, or discontinued). Products include:

Interferon alfa-2a, Recombinant (Therapy with interferon-alpha has been associated with the development of antithyroid microsomal antibodies in 20% of patients and some have transient hypothyroidism, hyperthyroidism, or both).

No products indexed under this heading.

Interferon alfa-2b, Recombinant (Therapy with interferon-alpha has been associated with the development of antithyroid microsomal antibodies in 20% of patients and some have transient hypothyroidism, hyperthyroidism, or both). Products include:

Iodamide Meglumine (Iodide and drugs that contain pharmacologic amounts of iodide may cause hyperthyroidism in euthroid patients with Grave's disease previously treated with antithyroid drugs or in euthroid patients with thyroid autonomy. Hyperthyroidism may develop over several weeks and may persist for several months after therapy discontinuation. Thyroid hormones may also reduce the uptake of I-123 and I-131).

No products indexed under this heading.

Iohexol (Iodide and drugs that contain pharmacologic amounts of iodide may cause hyperthyroidism in euthroid patients with Grave's disease previously treated with antithyroid drugs or in euthroid patients with thyroid autonomy. Hyperthyroidism may develop over several weeks and may persist for several months after therapy discontinuation. Thyroid hormones may also reduce the uptake of I-123 and I-131).

No products indexed under this heading.

Iopamidol (Iodide and drugs that contain pharmacologic amounts of iodide may cause hyperthyroidism in euthroid patients with Grave's disease previously treated with antithyroid drugs or in euthroid patients with thyroid autonomy. Hyperthyroidism may develop over several weeks and may persist for several months after therapy discontinuation. Thyroid hormones may also reduce the uptake of I-123 and I-131).

No products indexed under this heading.

Iopanoic Acid (Iodide and drugs that contain pharmacologic amounts of iodide may cause hyperthyroidism in euthroid patients with Grave's disease previously treated with antithyroid drugs or in euthroid patients with thyroid autonomy. Hyperthyroidism may develop over several weeks and may persist for several months after therapy discontinuation. Thyroid hormones may also reduce the uptake of I-123 and I-131).

No products indexed under this heading.

Iothalamate Meglumine (Iodide and drugs that contain pharmacologic amounts of iodide may cause hyperthyroidism in euthroid patients with Grave's disease previously treated with antithyroid drugs or in euthroid patients with thyroid autonomy. Hyperthyroidism may develop over several weeks and may persist for several months after therapy discontinuation. Thyroid hormones may also reduce the uptake of I-123 and I-131).

No products indexed under this heading.

Ioxaglate Meglumine (Iodide and drugs that contain pharmacologic amounts of iodide may cause hyperthyroidism in euthroid patients with Grave's disease previously treated with antithyroid drugs or in euthroid patients with thyroid autonomy. Hyperthyroidism may develop over several weeks and may persist for several months after therapy discontinuation. Thyroid hormones may also reduce the uptake of I-123 and I-131).

No products indexed under this heading.

Ioxaglate Sodium (Iodide and drugs that contain pharmacologic amounts of iodide may cause hyperthyroidism in euthroid patients with Grave's disease previously treated with antithyroid drugs or in euthroid patients with thyroid autonomy. Hyperthyroidism may develop over several weeks and may persist for several months after therapy discontinuation. Thyroid hormones may also reduce the uptake of I-123 and I-131).

No products indexed under this heading.

Isoproterenol Hydrochloride (Concurrent use may increase the effects of sympathomimetics or thyroid hormone. Thyroid hormones may increase the risk of coronary insufficiency when sympathomimetic agents are administered to patients with coronary artery disease).

No products indexed under this heading.

Isoproterenol Sulfate (Concurrent use may increase the effects of sympathomimetics or thyroid hormone. Thyroid hormones may increase the risk of coronary insufficiency when sympathomimetic agents are administered to patients with coronary artery disease).

No products indexed under this heading.

Ketamine (Concurrent use may produce marked hypertension and tachycardia; cautious administration to patients receiving thyroid therapy is recommended).

No products indexed under this heading.

Ketamine Hydrochloride (Concurrent use may produce marked hypertension and tachycardia; cautious administration to patients receiving thyroid therapy is recommended).

No products indexed under this heading.

Labetalol Hydrochloride (Actions of particular beta-adrenergic antagonists may be impaired when the hypothyroid patient is converted to the euthroid state).

No products indexed under this heading.

Levalbuterol Hydrochloride (Concurrent use may increase the effects of sympathomimetics or thyroid hormone. Thyroid hormones may increase the risk of coronary insufficiency when sympathomimetic agents are administered to patients with coronary artery disease). Products include:

Levobunolol Hydrochloride (Actions of particular beta-adrenergic antagonists may be impaired when the hypothyroid patient is converted to the euthroid state). Products include:

Levonorgestrel (Estrogen-containing oral contraceptives may increase serum TBG concentration). Products include:

Lithium (Long-term lithium therapy can result in goiter in up to 50% of patients, and either subclinical or overt hypothyroidism, each in up to 20% of patients).

No products indexed under this heading.

Lithium Carbonate (Long-term lithium therapy can result in goiter in up to 50% of patients, and either subclinical or overt hypothyroidism, each in up to 20% of patients). Products include:

Lithium Citrate (Long-term lithium therapy can result in goiter in up to 50% of patients, and either subclinical or overt hypothyroidism, each in up to 20% of patients).

No products indexed under this heading.

Lovastatin (Lovastatin is associated with thyroid hormone and/or TSH level alterations). Products include:

IMPORTANT NOTE: Always consult each drug listing in the patient's regimen for possible interactions.

Magaldrate (Concurrent use with antacids may reduce the efficacy of levothyroxine by binding and delaying or preventing the absorption, potentially resulting in hypothyroidism. Administer levothyroxine at least four hours apart from these agents).
No products indexed under this heading.

Magnesium Hydroxide (Concurrent use with antacids may reduce the efficacy of levothyroxine by binding and delaying or preventing the absorption, potentially resulting in hypothyroidism. Administer levothyroxine at least four hours apart from these agents). Products include:
Maalox Regular Strength Antacid/Antigas Liquid.................. 2175
Maalox Max Maximum Strength Antacid/Anti-Gas Liquid................ 2176
Pepcid Complete Chewable Tablets.. 1701

Magnesium Oxide (Concurrent use with antacids may reduce the efficacy of levothyroxine by binding and delaying or preventing the absorption, potentially resulting in hypothyroidism. Administer levothyroxine at least four hours apart from these agents). Products include:
Beelith Tablets.................................... 759
PremCal Light, Regular, and Extra Strength Tablets................ ▣818

Magnesium Salicylate (Salicylates inhibit binding of T4 and T3 to TBG and transthyretin. An initial increase in FT4 is followed by return of FT4 to normal levels with sustained therapeutic serum salicylate concentrations, although total T4 levels may decrease by as much as 30%).
No products indexed under this heading.

Maprotiline Hydrochloride (Concurrent use of tetracyclic antidepressants and levothyroxine may increase the therapeutic and toxic effects of both drugs, possibly due to increased receptor sensitivity to catecholamines).
No products indexed under this heading.

Meclofenamate Sodium (Co-administration of fenamates with levothyroxine results in an initial transient increase in FT4. Continued administration results in a decrease in serum T4 and normal FT4 and TSH concentrations and, therefore, patients are clinically euthroid).
No products indexed under this heading.

Mephenytoin (Stimulation of hepatic microsomal drug-metabolizing activity may cause increased hepatic degradation of levothyroxine, resulting in increased levothyroxine requirements).
No products indexed under this heading.

Mercaptopurine (Mercaptopurine is associated with thyroid hormone and/or TSH level alterations).
No products indexed under this heading.

Mestranol (Estrogen-containing oral contraceptives may increase serum TBG concentration).
No products indexed under this heading.

Metaproterenol Sulfate (Concurrent use may increase the effects of sympathomimetics or thyroid hormone. Thyroid hormones may increase the risk of coronary insufficiency when sympathomimetic agents are administered to patients with coronary artery disease). Products include:
Alupent Inhalation Aerosol 826

Metaraminol Bitartrate (Concurrent use may increase the effects of sympathomimetics or thyroid hormone. Thyroid hormones may increase the risk of coronary insufficiency when sympathomimetic agents are administered to patients with coronary artery disease).
No products indexed under this heading.

Metformin Hydrochloride (Addition of levothyroxine to antidiabetic therapy may result in increased antidiabetic agent requirements. Careful monitoring of diabetic control is recommended, especially when thyroid therapy is started, changed, or discontinued). Products include:
ActoPlus Met Tablets 3214
Avandamet Tablets 1373
Fortamet Extended-Release Tablets....................................... 3115

Methadone Hydrochloride (Methadone may increase serum TBG concentration).
No products indexed under this heading.

Methoxamine Hydrochloride (Concurrent use may increase the effects of sympathomimetics or thyroid hormone. Thyroid hormones may increase the risk of coronary insufficiency when sympathomimetic agents are administered to patients with coronary artery disease).
No products indexed under this heading.

Methyclothiazide (Thiazide diuretics are associated with thyroid hormone and/or TSH level alterations).
No products indexed under this heading.

Methylprednisolone Acetate (Glucocorticoids may result in a transient reduction in TSH secretion when administered at doses greater than 100mg/day of hydrocortisone or equivalent. Short-term administration of large doses of glucocorticoids may decrease serum T3 concentrations by 30% with minimal change in serum T4 levels. However, long-term glucocorticoid therapy may result in slightly decreased T3 and T4 levels due to decreased TBG production). Products include:
Depo-Medrol Injectable Suspension................................ 2617
Depo-Medrol Single-Dose Vial 2619

Methylprednisolone Sodium Succinate (Glucocorticoids may result in a transient reduction in TSH secretion when administered at doses greater than 100mg/day of hydrocortisone or equivalent. Short-term administration of large doses of glucocorticoids may decrease serum T3 concentrations by 30% with minimal change in serum T4 levels. However, long-term glucocorticoid therapy may result in slightly decreased T3 and T4 levels due to decreased TBG production).
No products indexed under this heading.

Methyltestosterone (Androgens/anabolic steroids may decrease serum TBG concentration). Products include:
Estratest Tablets 3199
Estratest H.S. Tablets 3199

Metipranolol Hydrochloride (Actions of particular beta-adrenergic antagonists may be impaired when the hypothyroid patient is converted to the euthroid state).
No products indexed under this heading.

Metoclopramide Hydrochloride (Metoclopramide is associated with thyroid hormone and/or TSH level alterations).
No products indexed under this heading.

Metoprolol Succinate (Actions of particular beta-adrenergic antagonists may be impaired when the hypothyroid patient is converted to the euthroid state). Products include:
Toprol-XL Tablets 668

Metoprolol Tartrate (Actions of particular beta-adrenergic antagonists may be impaired when the hypothyroid patient is converted to the euthroid state). Products include:
Lopressor Injection 2238
Lopressor Tablets 2238
Lopressor HCT 50/25 Tablets 2241
Lopressor HCT 100/25 Tablets 2241
Lopressor HCT 100/50 Tablets 2241

Miglitol (Addition of levothyroxine to antidiabetic therapy may result in increased antidiabetic agent requirements. Careful monitoring of diabetic control is recommended, especially when thyroid therapy is started, changed, or discontinued).
No products indexed under this heading.

Mirtazapine (Concurrent use of tetracyclic antidepressants and levothyroxine may increase the therapeutic and toxic effects of both drugs, possibly due to increased receptor sensitivity to catecholamines).
No products indexed under this heading.

Mitotane (Mitotane may increase serum TBG concentration).
No products indexed under this heading.

Nadolol (Actions of particular beta-adrenergic antagonists may be impaired when the hypothyroid patient is converted to the euthroid state). Products include:
Nadolol Tablets 2159

Nicotinic Acid (Slow-release nicotinic acid may decrease TBG concentration).
No products indexed under this heading.

Norepinephrine Bitartrate (Concurrent use may increase the effects of sympathomimetics or thyroid hormone. Thyroid hormones may increase the risk of coronary insufficiency when sympathomimetic agents are administered to patients with coronary artery disease).
No products indexed under this heading.

Norethindrone (Estrogen-containing oral contraceptives may increase serum TBG concentration). Products include:
Ortho Micronor Tablets 2426

Norethynodrel (Estrogen-containing oral contraceptives may increase serum TBG concentration).
No products indexed under this heading.

Norgestimate (Estrogen-containing oral contraceptives may increase serum TBG concentration). Products include:
Ortho-Cyclen/Ortho Tri-Cyclen 2429
Ortho Tri-Cyclen Lo Tablets 2436

Norgestrel (Estrogen-containing oral contraceptives may increase serum TBG concentration).
No products indexed under this heading.

Nortriptyline Hydrochloride (Concurrent use of tricyclic antidepressants and levothyroxine may increase the therapeutic and toxic effects of both drugs, possibly due to increased receptor sensitivity to catecholamines. Onset of action of tricyclics may be accelerated).
No products indexed under this heading.

Octreotide Acetate (Octreotide may result in a transient reduction in TSH secretion when administered at doses greater than 100 mcg/day). Products include:
Sandostatin Injection 2278
Sandostatin LAR Depot 2280

Oxandrolone (Androgens/anabolic steroids may decrease serum TBG concentration). Products include:
Oxandrin Tablets 2962

Oxymetholone (Androgens/anabolic steroids may decrease serum TBG concentration).
No products indexed under this heading.

Para-Aminosalicylate Sodium (Para-aminosalicylate sodium is associated with thyroid hormone and/or TSH level alterations).
No products indexed under this heading.

Penbutolol Sulfate (Actions of particular beta-adrenergic antagonists may be impaired when the hypothyroid patient is converted to the euthroid state).
No products indexed under this heading.

Pergolide Mesylate (Dopamine and dopamine agonists may result in a transient reduction in TSH secretion when administered at dopamine doses greater than or equal to 1 mcg/kg/min). Products include:
Permax Tablets 3356

Perphenazine (Perphenazine is associated with thyroid hormone and/or TSH level alterations).
No products indexed under this heading.

Phenobarbital (Stimulation of hepatic microsomal drug-metabolizing activity may cause increased hepatic degradation of levothyroxine, resulting in increased levothyroxine requirements). Products include:
Donnatal Extentabs 2493

Phenobarbital Sodium (Stimulation of hepatic microsomal drug-metabolizing activity may cause increased hepatic degradation of levothyroxine, resulting in increased levothyroxine requirements).
No products indexed under this heading.

Phenylbutazone (Co-administration of phenylbutazone with levothyroxine results in an initial transient increase in FT4. Continued administration results in a decrease in serum T4 and normal FT4 and TSH concentrations and, therefore, patients are clinically euthroid).
No products indexed under this heading.

Phenylephrine Bitartrate (Concurrent use may increase the effects of sympathomimetics or thyroid hormone. Thyroid hormones may increase the risk of coronary insufficiency when sympathomimetic agents are administered to patients with coronary artery disease).
No products indexed under this heading.

Phenylephrine Hydrochloride (Concurrent use may increase the effects of sympathomimetics or thyroid hormone. Thyroid hormones may increase the risk of coronary insufficiency when sympathomimetic agents are administered to patients with coronary artery disease).
Products include:
- Comtrex Maximum Strength Non-Drowsy Cold & Cough Caplets 725
- Comtrex Maximum Strength Day/Night Severe Cold & Sinus Caplets - Day Formulation 725
- Comtrex Maximum Strength Day/Night Severe Cold & Sinus Caplets - Night Formulation 725
- Contac Cold and Flu Maximum Strength Caplets 728
- Contac Cold and Flu Day and Night Caplets (Day Formulation Only) 727
- Contac Cold and Flu Day and Night Caplets (Night Formulation Only) 727
- Contac Cold and Flu Non-Drowsy Caplets 728
- Contac-D Cold Non-Drowsy Tablets 729
- Children's Dimetapp Cold & Allergy Elixir 730
- Children's Dimetapp Cold & Allergy Chewable Tablets 730
- Children's Dimetapp DM Cold & Cough Elixir 731
- Toddler's Dimetapp Cold and Cough Drops 732
- Excedrin Sinus Headache Caplets/Tablets 610
- 4-Way Fast Acting Nasal Spray 775
- 4-Way Menthol Nasal Spray 775
- Preparation H Maximum Strength Cream 666
- Preparation H Cooling Gel 666
- Preparation H 666
- Refenesen PE Caplets 721
- Robitussin Cough & Allergy Syrup 736
- Robitussin Cough & Cold Nighttime Liquid 736
- Robitussin Cough, Cold & Flu Nighttime Liquid 738
- Robitussin Head & Chest Congestion PE Syrup 739
- Robitussin Pediatric Cough & Cold Nighttime Liquid 736
- TheraFlu Cold & Cough Hot Liquid 740
- TheraFlu Cold & Sore Throat Hot Liquid 741
- TheraFlu Flu & Sore Throat Hot Liquid 742
- TheraFlu Daytime Severe Cold Hot Liquid 742
- TheraFlu Nighttime Severe Cold Hot Liquid 740
- TheraFlu Warming Relief Daytime Severe Cold 743
- TheraFlu Warming Relief Nighttime Severe Cold 743
- Triaminic Chest & Nasal Congestion Liquid 746
- Triaminic Cold & Allergy Liquid 746
- Triaminic Daytime Cold & Cough Liquid 745
- Triaminic Nighttime Cold & Cough Liquid 746
- Triaminic Thin Strips Cold 748
- Triaminic Thin Strips Cold & Cough 778
- Triaminic Infant Thin Strips Decongestant 747
- Triaminic Infant Thin Strips Decongestant Plus Cough 747
- Children's Tylenol Plus Flu Oral Suspension 749
- Tylenol Cold Head Congestion Daytime Caplets with Cool Burst and Gelcaps 750
- Tylenol Cold Multi-Symptom Daytime Liquid 752
- Tylenol Cold Multi-Symptom Severe Daytime Liquid 752
- Concentrated Tylenol Infants' Drops Plus Cold & Cough 754
- Tylenol Allergy Multi-Symptom Caplets with Cool Burst and Gelcaps 1872
- Tylenol Allergy Multi-Symptom Nighttime Caplets with Cool Burst 1872
- Children's Tylenol Plus Cold Suspension Liquid 1879
- Children's Tylenol Plus Cold & Allergy Suspension Liquid 1878
- Children's Tylenol Plus Flu Suspension Liquid 1881
- Children's Tylenol Plus Multi-Symptom Cold Suspension Liquid 1879
- Tylenol Cold Head Congestion Daytime Caplets with Cool Burst 1873
- Tylenol Cold Head Congestion Nighttime Caplets with Cool Burst 1873
- Tylenol Cold Head Congestion Severe Caplets with Cool Burst 1873
- Tylenol Cold Multi-Symptom Daytime Caplets with Cool Burst and Gelcaps 1874
- Tylenol Cold Multi-Symptom Daytime Liquid with Citrus Burst 1874
- Tylenol Cold Multi-Symptom Nighttime Caplets with Cool Burst 1874
- Tylenol Cold Multi-Symptom Nighttime Liquid with Cool Burst 1874
- Tylenol Cold Multi-Symptom Severe Caplets with Cool Burst 1874
- Tylenol Cold Multi-Symptom Severe Daytime Liquid with Citrus Burst 1874
- Tylenol Sinus Congestion & Pain Daytime Caplets with Cool Burst and Gelcaps 1876
- Tylenol Sinus Congestion & Pain Nighttime Caplets with Cool Burst 1876
- Tylenol Sinus Congestion & Pain Severe Caplets with Cool Burst 1876
- Vicks 44D Cough & Head Congestion Relief Liquid 760
- Vicks DayQuil LiquiCaps/Liquid Multi-Symptom Cold/Flu Relief 761
- Zicam Cough Plus D Cough Spray 767

Phenylephrine Tannate (Concurrent use may increase the effects of sympathomimetics or thyroid hormone. Thyroid hormones may increase the risk of coronary insufficiency when sympathomimetic agents are administered to patients with coronary artery disease).
No products indexed under this heading.

Phenylpropanolamine Hydrochloride (Concurrent use may increase the effects of sympathomimetics or thyroid hormone. Thyroid hormones may increase the risk of coronary insufficiency when sympathomimetic agents are administered to patients with coronary artery disease).
No products indexed under this heading.

Phenytoin (Stimulation of hepatic microsomal drug-metabolizing activity may cause increased hepatic degradation of levothyroxine, resulting in increased levothyroxine requirements).
No products indexed under this heading.

Phenytoin Sodium (Stimulation of hepatic microsomal drug-metabolizing activity may cause increased hepatic degradation of levothyroxine, resulting in increased levothyroxine requirements).
Products include:
- Phenytek Capsules 2160

Pindolol (Actions of particular beta-adrenergic antagonists may be impaired when the hypothyroid patient is converted to the euthroid state).
No products indexed under this heading.

Pioglitazone Hydrochloride (Addition of levothyroxine to antidiabetic therapy may result in increased antidiabetic agent requirements. Careful monitoring of diabetic control is recommended, especially when thyroid therapy is started, changed, or discontinued). Products include:
- ActoPlus Met Tablets 3214
- Actos Tablets 3219
- Duetact Tablets 3226

Pirbuterol Acetate (Concurrent use may increase the effects of sympathomimetics or thyroid hormone. Thyroid hormones may increase the risk of coronary insufficiency when sympathomimetic agents are administered to patients with coronary artery disease). Products include:
- Maxair Autohaler 1852

Polyestradiol Phosphate (Estrogen may increase serum TBG concentration).
No products indexed under this heading.

Polythiazide (Thiazide diuretics are associated with thyroid hormone and/or TSH level alterations).
No products indexed under this heading.

Pramipexole Dihydrochloride (Dopamine and dopamine agonists may result in a transient reduction in TSH secretion when administered at dopamine doses greater than or equal to 1 mcg/kg/min). Products include:
- Mirapex Tablets 859

Prednisolone Acetate (Glucocorticoids may result in a transient reduction in TSH secretion when administered at doses greater than 100mg/day of hydrocortisone or equivalent. Short-term administration of large doses of glucocorticoids may decrease serum T3 concentrations by 30% with minimal change in serum T4 levels. However, long-term glucocorticoid therapy may result in slightly decreased T3 and T4 levels due to decreased TBG production).
Products include:
- Blephamide Ophthalmic Ointment 568
- Blephamide Ophthalmic Suspension 569
- Poly-Pred Ophthalmic Suspension .... ⊙233
- Pred Forte Ophthalmic Suspension .... ⊙235
- Pred Mild Ophthalmic Suspension .... ⊙238
- Pred-G Ophthalmic Ointment .... ⊙237
- Pred-G Ophthalmic Suspension .... ⊙236

Prednisolone Sodium Phosphate (Glucocorticoids may result in a transient reduction in TSH secretion when administered at doses greater than 100mg/day of hydrocortisone or equivalent. Short-term administration of large doses of glucocorticoids may decrease serum T3 concentrations by 30% with minimal change in serum T4 levels. However, long-term glucocorticoid therapy may result in slightly decreased T3 and T4 levels due to decreased TBG production).
No products indexed under this heading.

Prednisolone Tebutate (Glucocorticoids may result in a transient reduction in TSH secretion when administered at doses greater than 100mg/day of hydrocortisone or equivalent. Short-term administration of large doses of glucocorticoids may decrease serum T3 concentrations by 30% with minimal change in serum T4 levels. However, long-term glucocorticoid therapy may result in slightly decreased T3 and T4 levels due to decreased TBG production).
No products indexed under this heading.

Prednisone (Glucocorticoids may result in a transient reduction in TSH secretion when administered at doses greater than 100mg/day of hydrocortisone or equivalent. Short-term administration of large doses of glucocorticoids may decrease serum T3 concentrations by 30% with minimal change in serum T4 levels. However, long-term glucocorticoid therapy may result in slightly decreased T3 and T4 levels due to decreased TBG production).
No products indexed under this heading.

Propranolol Hydrochloride (In patients treated with large doses of propranolol (greater than 160mg/day), T3 and T4 levels change slightly, TSH levels remain normal, and patients are clinically euthroid).
Products include:
- Inderal LA Long-Acting Capsules 3429
- InnoPran XL Capsules 2723

Protriptyline Hydrochloride (Concurrent use of tricyclic antidepressants and levothyroxine may increase the therapeutic and toxic effects of both drugs, possibly due to increased receptor sensitivity to catecholamines. Onset of action of tricyclics may be accelerated).
No products indexed under this heading.

Pseudoephedrine Hydrochloride (Concurrent use may increase the effects of sympathomimetics or thyroid hormone. Thyroid hormones may increase the risk of coronary insufficiency when sympathomimetic agents are administered to patients with coronary artery disease).
Products include:
- Advil Allergy Sinus Caplets 770
- Advil Cold & Sinus 723
- Advil Multi-Symptom Cold Caplets 770
- Aleve Cold & Sinus Caplets 744
- Allegra-D 12 Hour Extended-Release Tablets 2846
- Allegra-D 24 Hour Extended-Release Tablets 2849
- BC Cold Powder 677
- Comtrex Maximum Strength Cold & Cough Day/Night Caplets - Day Formulation 726
- Comtrex Maximum Strength Cold & Cough Day/Night Caplets - Night Formulation 726
- Children's Motrin Cold Oral Suspension 1867
- Mucinex D Extended-Release Bi-Layer Tablets 776
- Robitussin Cough & Cold CF Liquid 735
- Robitussin Cough & Cold Pediatric Drops 735
- Tylenol Sinus Congestion & Pain Nighttime Caplets with Cool Burst 778

Pseudoephedrine Sulfate (Concurrent use may increase the effects of sympathomimetics or thyroid hormone. Thyroid hormones may increase the risk of coronary insufficiency when sympathomimetic agents are administered to patients with coronary artery disease). Products include:

Quinestrol (Estrogen may increase serum TBG concentration).
No products indexed under this heading.

Repaglinide (Addition of levothyroxine to antidiabetic therapy may result in increased antidiabetic agent requirements. Careful monitoring of diabetic control is recommended, especially when thyroid therapy is started, changed, or discontinued).
No products indexed under this heading.

Resorcinol (Excessive topical use of resorcinol has been associated with thyroid hormone and/or TSH level alterations).
No products indexed under this heading.

Rifampin (Stimulation of hepatic microsomal drug-metabolizing activity may cause increased hepatic degradation of levothyroxine, resulting in increased levothyroxine requirements).
No products indexed under this heading.

Ropinirole Hydrochloride (Dopamine and dopamine agonists may result in a transient reduction in TSH secretion when administered at dopamine doses greater than or equal to 1 mcg/kg/min). Products include:

Rosiglitazone Maleate (Addition of levothyroxine to antidiabetic therapy may result in increased antidiabetic agent requirements. Careful monitoring of diabetic control is recommended, especially when thyroid therapy is started, changed, or discontinued). Products include:

Salmeterol Xinafoate (Concurrent use may increase the effects of sympathomimetics or thyroid hormone. Thyroid hormones may increase the risk of coronary insufficiency when sympathomimetic agents are administered to patients with coronary artery disease). Products include:

Salsalate (Salicylates inhibit binding of T4 and T3 to TBG and transthyretin. An initial increase in FT4 is followed by return of FT4 to normal levels with sustained therapeutic serum salicylate concentrations, although total T4 levels may decrease by as much as 30%).
No products indexed under this heading.

Sertraline Hydrochloride (Administration of sertraline in patients stabilized on levothyroxine may result in increased levothyroxine requirements). Products include:

Simethicone (Concurrent use with simethicone may reduce the efficacy of levothyroxine by binding and delaying or preventing the absorption, potentially resulting in hypothyroidism. Administer levothyroxine at least 4 hours apart from simethicone). Products include:

Sodium Bicarbonate (Concurrent use with antacids may reduce the efficacy of levothyroxine by binding and delaying or preventing the absorption, potentially resulting in hypothyroidism. Administer levothyroxine at least four hours apart from these agents). Products include:

Sodium Nitroprusside (Nitroprusside is associated with thyroid hormone and/or TSH level alterations).
No products indexed under this heading.

Sodium Polystyrene Sulfonate (Concurrent use with sodium polystyrene sulfonate may reduce the efficacy of levothyroxine by binding and delaying or preventing the absorption, potentially resulting in hypothyroidism. Administer levothyroxine at least 4 hours apart from sodium polystyrene sodium).
No products indexed under this heading.

Somatrem (Excessive use of thyroid hormones with growth hormones may accelerate epiphyseal closure. However, untreated hypothyroidism may interfere with growth response to growth hormone).
No products indexed under this heading.

Somatropin (Excessive use of thyroid hormones with growth hormones may accelerate epiphyseal closure. However, untreated hypothyroidism may interfere with growth response to growth hormone). Products include:

Sotalol Hydrochloride (Actions of particular beta-adrenergic antagonists may be impaired when the hypothyroid patient is converted to the euthroid state).
No products indexed under this heading.

Stanozolol (Androgens/anabolic steroids may decrease serum TBG concentration).
No products indexed under this heading.

Sucralfate (Concurrent use with sucralfate may reduce the efficacy of levothyroxine by binding and delaying or preventing the absorption, potentially resulting in hypothyroidism. Administer levothyroxine at least four hours apart from sucralfate). Products include:

Tamoxifen Citrate (Tamoxifen may increase serum TBG concentration). Products include:

Terbutaline Sulfate (Concurrent use may increase the effects of sympathomimetics or thyroid hormone. Thyroid hormones may increase the risk of coronary insufficiency when sympathomimetic agents are administered to patients with coronary artery disease).
No products indexed under this heading.

Theophylline (Decreased theophylline clearance may occur in hypothyroid patients; clearance returns to normal when the euthroid state is achieved).
No products indexed under this heading.

Theophylline Anhydrous (Decreased theophylline clearance may occur in hypothyroid patients; clearance returns to normal when the euthroid state is achieved). Products include:

Theophylline Calcium Salicylate (Decreased theophylline clearance may occur in hypothyroid patients; clearance returns to normal when the euthroid state is achieved).
No products indexed under this heading.

Theophylline Dihydroxypropyl (Glyceryl) (Decreased theophylline clearance may occur in hypothyroid patients; clearance returns to normal when the euthroid state is achieved).
No products indexed under this heading.

Theophylline Ethylenediamine (Decreased theophylline clearance may occur in hypothyroid patients; clearance returns to normal when the euthroid state is achieved).
No products indexed under this heading.

Theophylline Sodium Glycinate (Decreased theophylline clearance may occur in hypothyroid patients; clearance returns to normal when the euthroid state is achieved).
No products indexed under this heading.

Timolol Hemihydrate (Actions of particular beta-adrenergic antagonists may be impaired when the hypothyroid patient is converted to the euthroid state). Products include:

Timolol Maleate (Actions of particular beta-adrenergic antagonists may be impaired when the hypothyroid patient is converted to the euthroid state). Products include:

Tolazamide (Addition of levothyroxine to antidiabetic therapy may result in increased antidiabetic agent requirements. Careful monitoring of diabetic control is recommended, especially when thyroid therapy is started, changed, or discontinued).
No products indexed under this heading.

Tolbutamide (Addition of levothyroxine to antidiabetic therapy may result in increased antidiabetic agent requirements. Careful monitoring of diabetic control is recommended, especially when thyroid therapy is started, changed, or discontinued).
No products indexed under this heading.

Triamcinolone (Glucocorticoids may result in a transient reduction in TSH secretion when administered at doses greater than 100mg/day of hydrocortisone or equivalent. Short-term administration of large doses of glucocorticoids may decrease serum T3 concentrations by 30% with minimal change in serum T4 levels. However, long-term glucocorticoid therapy may result in slightly decreased T3 and T4 levels due to decreased TBG production).
No products indexed under this heading.

Triamcinolone Acetonide (Glucocorticoids may result in a transient reduction in TSH secretion when administered at doses greater than 100mg/day of hydrocortisone or equivalent. Short-term administration of large doses of glucocorticoids may decrease serum T3 concentrations by 30% with minimal change in serum T4 levels. However, long-term glucocorticoid therapy may result in slightly decreased T3 and T4 levels due to decreased TBG production). Products include:

Triamcinolone Diacetate (Glucocorticoids may result in a transient reduction in TSH secretion when administered at doses greater than 100mg/day of hydrocortisone or equivalent. Short-term administration of large doses of glucocorticoids may decrease serum T3 concentrations by 30% with minimal change in serum T4 levels. However, long-term glucocorticoid therapy may result in

slightly decreased T3 and T4 levels due to decreased TBG production).
No products indexed under this heading.

Triamcinolone Hexacetonide (Glucocorticoids may result in a transient reduction in TSH secretion when administered at doses greater than 100mg/day of hydrocortisone or equivalent. Short-term administration of large doses of glucocorticoids may decrease serum T3 concentrations by 30% with minimal change in serum T4 levels. However, long-term glucocorticoid therapy may result in slightly decreased T3 and T4 levels due to decreased TBG production).
No products indexed under this heading.

Trimipramine Maleate (Concurrent use of tricyclic antidepressants and levothyroxine may increase the therapeutic and toxic effects of both drugs, possibly due to increased receptor sensitivity to catecholamines. Onset of action of tricyclics may be accelerated).
No products indexed under this heading.

Troglitazone (Addition of levothyroxine to antidiabetic therapy may result in increased antidiabetic agent requirements. Careful monitoring of diabetic control is recommended, especially when thyroid therapy is started, changed, or discontinued).
No products indexed under this heading.

Tyropanoate Sodium (Iodide and drugs that contain pharmacologic amounts of iodide may cause hyperthyroidism in euthroid patients with Grave's disease previously treated with antithyroid drugs or in euthroid patients with thyroid autonomy. Hyperthyroidism may develop over several weeks and may persist for several months after therapy discontinuation. Thyroid hormones may also reduce the uptake of I-123 and I-131).
No products indexed under this heading.

Warfarin Sodium (Thyroid hormones appear to increase the catabolism of vitamin-K dependent clotting factors, thereby increasing the anticoagulant activity of oral anticoagulants. Concomitant use of these agents impairs the compensatory increases in clotting factor synthesis. Prothrombin time should be carefully monitored in patients taking levothyroxine and oral anticoagulants and the dose of anticoagulant therapy adjusted accordingly).
Products include:
Coumadin for Injection 898
Coumadin Tablets 898

LEVOXYL TABLETS

(Levothyroxine Sodium) 1712

May interact with androgens, antacids containing aluminum, calcium and magnesium, beta blockers, oral anticoagulants, dopamine agonists, estrogens, glucocorticoids, cardiac glycosides, hydantoin anticonvulsants, oral hypoglycemic agents, insulin, lithium preparations, phenytoin, radiographic iodinated contrast media, salicylates, sympathomimetics, thiazides, tricyclic antidepressants, and xanthines. Compounds in these categories include:

Acarbose (Addition of levothyroxine to antidiabetic therapy may result in increased antidiabetic agent requirements). Products include:
Precose Tablets 751

Acebutolol Hydrochloride (Co-administration with beta-blockers may decrease T_4 5'-deiodinase activity; action of beta-blocker may be impaired when the hypothyroid patient is converted to euthyroid).
No products indexed under this heading.

Albuterol (Co-administration of sympathomimetic agents may increase the effects of sympathomimetics or thyroid hormone; thyroid hormones may increase risk of coronary insufficiency when sympathomimetic agents are administered to patients with coronary disease). Products include:
Proventil Inhalation Aerosol 3053

Albuterol Sulfate (Co-administration of sympathomimetic agents may increase the effects of sympathomimetics or thyroid hormone; thyroid hormones may increase risk of coronary insufficiency when sympathomimetic agents are administered to patients with coronary disease). Products include:
AccuNeb Inhalation Solution 1055
Combivent Inhalation Aerosol 847
DuoNeb Inhalation Solution 1058
ProAir HFA Inhalation Aerosol 3300
Proventil Inhalation Solution 0.083%.. 3055
Proventil HFA Inhalation Aerosol 3056
Ventolin HFA Inhalation Aerosol 1600
VoSpire ER Tablets 1052

Aldesleukin (Co-administration has been associated with transient painless thyroiditis in 20% of patients). Products include:
Proleukin for Injection 2266

Aluminum Carbonate (Co-administration with antacids may reduce the efficacy of levothyroxine by binding and delaying or preventing absorption, potentially resulting in hypothyroidism; administer levothyroxine at least 4 hours apart from these agents).
No products indexed under this heading.

Aluminum Hydroxide (Co-administration with antacids may reduce the efficacy of levothyroxine by binding and delaying or preventing absorption, potentially resulting in hypothyroidism; administer levothyroxine at least 4 hours apart from these agents). Products include:
Gaviscon Regular Strength Liquid .. 658
Gaviscon Regular Strength Tablets... 658
Gaviscon Extra Strength Liquid 658
Gaviscon Extra Strength Tablets 658
Maalox Regular Strength Antacid/Antigas Liquid................. 2175
Maalox Max Maximum Strength Antacid/Anti-Gas Liquid................ 2176

Aminoglutethimide (May decrease thyroid hormone secretion, which may result in hypothyrodism).
No products indexed under this heading.

Aminophylline (Decreased theophylline clearance may occur in hypothyroid patients; clearance returns to normal when euthyroid state is achieved).
No products indexed under this heading.

p-Aminosalicylic Acid (Co-administration has been associated with thyroid hormone and/or TSH level alterations by various mechanisms).
No products indexed under this heading.

Amiodarone Hydrochloride (May decrease thyroid hormone secretion, which may result in hypothyrodism; amiodarone is slowly excreted, producing more prolonged hypothyroidism; amiodarone may induce hyperthyroidism by causing thyroiditis).
No products indexed under this heading.

Amitriptyline Hydrochloride (Co-administration may increase the therapeutic and toxic effects of both drugs possibly due to increased receptor sensitivity to catecholamines; toxic effects may include increased risk of arrhythmias and CNS stimulation; onset of tricyclics may be accelerated).
No products indexed under this heading.

Amoxapine (Co-administration may increase the therapeutic and toxic effects of both drugs possibly due to increased receptor sensitivity to catecholamines; toxic effects may include increased risk of arrhythmias and CNS stimulation; onset of tricyclics may be accelerated).
No products indexed under this heading.

Anisindione (Thyroid hormones appear to increase the catabolism of vitamin K-dependent clotting factors, thereby increasing the anticoagulant activity of oral anticoagulants). Products include:
Miradon Tablets 3042

Asparaginase (Co-administration may result in decreased serum TBG concentration). Products include:
Elspar for Injection 2463
Elspar for Injection 1960

Aspirin (Co-administration with salicylates at greater than 2 gm inhibit binding of T_4 and T_3 to TBG and transthyrelin; an initial increase in serum FT_4 is followed by return of FT_4 to normal levels with sustained therapeutic salicylate concentrations, although total T_4 levels may decrease by as much as 30%). Products include:
Aggrenox Capsules 822
Bayer Aspirin 744
BC Allergy Sinus Cold Powder 677
BC Headache Powder 677
Arthritis Strength BC Powder 677
BC Sinus Cold Powder 677
Excedrin Extra Strength Caplets/Tablets/Geltabs............ 684
Excedrin Migraine Caplets/Tablets/Geltabs............ 609
Goody's Body Pain Formula Powder.. 684
Goody's Extra Strength Headache Powders.................... 611
Goody's Extra Strength Pain Relief Tablets............................. 685
Percodan Tablets 1132
St. Joseph 81 mg Aspirin Chewable and Enteric Coated Tablets 1869

Aspirin, Enteric Coated (Co-administration with salicylates at greater than 2 gm inhibit binding of T_4 and T_3 to TBG and transthyrelin; an initial increase in serum FT_4 is followed by return of FT_4 to normal levels with sustained therapeutic salicylate concentrations, although total T_4 levels may decrease by as much as 30%).
No products indexed under this heading.

Aspirin Buffered (Co-administration with salicylates at greater than 2 gm inhibit binding of T_4 and T_3 to TBG and transthyrelin; an initial increase in serum FT_4 is followed by return of FT_4 to normal levels with sustained therapeutic salicylate concentrations, although total T_4 levels may decrease by as much as 30%). Products include:
Bufferin Extra Strength Tablets 678
Bufferin Regular Strength Tablets ... 678

Atenolol (Co-administration with beta-blockers may decrease T_4 5'-deiodinase activity; action of beta-blocker may be impaired when the hypothyroid patient is converted to euthyroid).
No products indexed under this heading.

Bendroflumethiazide (Co-administration has been associated with thyroid hormone and/or TSH level alterations by various mechanisms).
No products indexed under this heading.

Betamethasone Acetate (Co-administration with glucocorticoids may result in a transient reduction in TSH secretion; the reduction is not sustained, therefore, hypothyroidism does not occur; glucocorticoids may decrease serum TBG concentration).
No products indexed under this heading.

Betamethasone Sodium Phosphate (Co-administration with glucocorticoids may result in a transient reduction in TSH secretion; the reduction is not sustained, therefore, hypothyroidism does not occur; glucocorticoids may decrease serum TBG concentration).
No products indexed under this heading.

Betaxolol Hydrochloride (Co-administration with beta-blockers may decrease T_4 5'-deiodinase activity; action of beta-blocker may be impaired when the hypothyroid patient is converted to euthyroid). Products include:
Betoptic S Ophthalmic Suspension................................... 558

Bisoprolol Fumarate (Co-administration with beta-blockers may decrease T_4 5'-deiodinase activity; action of beta-blocker may be impaired when the hypothyroid patient is converted to euthyroid).
No products indexed under this heading.

Bromocriptine Mesylate (Co-administration with dopamine agonists may result in a transient reduction in TSH secretion; the reduction is not sustained, therefore, hypothyroidism does not occur).
No products indexed under this heading.

Calcium Carbonate (Co-administration with calcium carbonate may form insoluble chelate with levothyroxine, which may result in hypothyroidism; administer levothyroxine at least 4 hours apart from these agents). Products include:
Actonel with Calcium Tablets 2688
Calcet Tablets 2138
Caltrate 600 PLUS 809
Caltrate 600 + D Tablets 809
D-Cal Chewable Caplets 812
Gas-X with Maalox 656
Maalox Regular Strength Antacid Chewable Tablets 2177

Carbamazepine (Co-administration may increase hepatic metabolism, which may result in hypothyroidism, resulting in increased levothyroxine requirements; carbamazepine reduces serum protein binding of levothyroxine, and total- and free-T_4 may be reduced by 20% to 40%, but most patients have normal serum TSH levels and are clinically euthyroid). Products include:

Carteolol Hydrochloride (Co-administration with beta-blockers may decrease T_4 5'-deiodinase activity; action of beta-blocker may be impaired when the hypothyroid patient is converted to euthyroid). Products include:

Chloral Hydrate (Co-administration has been associated with thyroid hormone and/or TSH level alterations by various mechanisms).
No products indexed under this heading.

Chlorothiazide (Co-administration has been associated with thyroid hormone and/or TSH level alterations by various mechanisms). Products include:

Chlorothiazide Sodium (Co-administration has been associated with thyroid hormone and/or TSH level alterations by various mechanisms). Products include:

Chlorotrianisene (Co-administration with oral estrogens may result in increased serum TBG concentrations).
No products indexed under this heading.

Chlorpropamide (Addition of levothyroxine to antidiabetic therapy may result in increased antidiabetic agent requirements).
No products indexed under this heading.

Cholestyramine (Co-administration may result in decreased T_4 absorption, which may result in hypothyroidism; administer levothyroxine at least 4 hours apart from these agents).
No products indexed under this heading.

Choline Magnesium Trisalicylate (Co-administration with salicylates at greater than 2 gm inhibit binding of T_4 and T_3 to TBG and transthyrelin; an initial increase in serum FT_4 is followed by return of FT_4 to normal levels with sustained therapeutic salicylate concentrations, although total T_4 levels may decrease by as much as 30%).
No products indexed under this heading.

Clofibrate (Co-administration may result in increased serum TBG concentrations).
No products indexed under this heading.

Clomipramine Hydrochloride (Co-administration may increase the therapeutic and toxic effects of both drugs possibly due to increased receptor sensitivity to catecholamines; toxic effects may include increased risk of arrhythmias and CNS stimulation; onset of tricyclics may be accelerated).
No products indexed under this heading.

Colestipol Hydrochloride (Co-administration may result in decreased T_4 absorption, which may result in hypothyroidism; administer levothyroxine at least 4 hours apart from these agents).
No products indexed under this heading.

Cortisone Acetate (Co-administration with glucocorticoids may result in a transient reduction in TSH secretion; the reduction is not sustained, therefore, hypothyroidism does not occur; glucocorticoids may decrease serum TBG concentration).
No products indexed under this heading.

Desipramine Hydrochloride (Co-administration may increase the therapeutic and toxic effects of both drugs possibly due to increased receptor sensitivity to catecholamines; toxic effects may include increased risk of arrhythmias and CNS stimulation; onset of tricyclics may be accelerated).
No products indexed under this heading.

Deslanoside (Co-administration may result in reduced serum digitalis glycosides in hyperthyroidism or when the hypothyroid patient is converted to euthyroid state; therapeutic effect of digitalis glycoside may be reduced).
No products indexed under this heading.

Dexamethasone (Co-administration with glucocorticoids may result in a transient reduction in TSH secretion; the reduction is not sustained, therefore, hypothyroidism does not occur; glucocorticoids may decrease serum TBG concentration). Products include:

Dexamethasone Acetate (Co-administration with glucocorticoids may result in a transient reduction in TSH secretion; the reduction is not sustained, therefore, hypothyroidism does not occur; glucocorticoids may decrease serum TBG concentration).
No products indexed under this heading.

Dexamethasone Sodium Phosphate (Co-administration with glucocorticoids may result in a transient reduction in TSH secretion; the reduction is not sustained, therefore, hypothyroidism does not occur; glucocorticoids may decrease serum TBG concentration).
No products indexed under this heading.

Diatrizoate Meglumine (May decrease thyroid hormone secretion, which may result in hypothyrodism;

the fetus, elderly, and euthyroid patients with underlying thyroid disease are among those individuals who are susceptible to iodine-induced hypothyroidism; oral cholecytographic agents slowly excreted, producing more prolonged hypothyroidism; iodide drugs that contain pharmacologic amounts of iodide may cause hypothyroidism in euthyroid patients with Grave's disease previously treated with thyroid autonomy; hyperthyroidism may develop over several weeks and may persist for several months after therapy discontinuation).
No products indexed under this heading.

Diatrizoate Sodium (May decrease thyroid hormone secretion, which may result in hypothyroidism; the fetus, elderly, and euthyroid patients with underlying thyroid disease are among those individuals who are susceptible to iodine-induced hypothyroidism; oral cholecytographic agents slowly excreted, producing more prolonged hypothyroidism; iodide drugs that contain pharmacologic amounts of iodide may cause hypothyroidism in euthyroid patients with Grave's disease previously treated with thyroid autonomy; hyperthyroidism may develop over several weeks and may persist for several months after therapy discontinuation).
No products indexed under this heading.

Diazepam (Co-administration has been associated with thyroid hormone and/or TSH level alterations by various mechanisms). Products include:

Dicumarol (Thyroid hormones appear to increase the catabolism of vitamin K-dependent clotting factors, thereby increasing the anticoagulant activity of oral anticoagulants).
No products indexed under this heading.

Dienestrol (Co-administration with oral estrogens may result in increased serum TBG concentrations).
No products indexed under this heading.

Diethylstilbestrol (Co-administration with oral estrogens may result in increased serum TBG concentrations).
No products indexed under this heading.

Diflunisal (Co-administration with salicylates at greater than 2 gm inhibit binding of T_4 and T_3 to TBG and transthyrelin; an initial increase in serum FT_4 is followed by return of FT_4 to normal levels with sustained therapeutic salicylate concentrations, although total T_4 levels may decrease by as much as 30%). Products include:

Digitalis Glycoside Preparations (Co-administration may result in reduced serum digitalis glycosides in hyperthyroidism or when the hypothyroid patient is converted to euthyroid state; therapeutic effect of digitalis glycoside may be reduced).
No products indexed under this heading.

Digitoxin (Co-administration may result in reduced serum digitalis glycosides in hyperthyroidism or when the hypothyroid patient is converted to euthyroid state; therapeutic effect of digitalis glycoside may be reduced).
No products indexed under this heading.

Digoxin (Co-administration may result in reduced serum digitalis glycosides in hyperthyroidism or when the hypothyroid patient is converted to euthyroid state; therapeutic effect of digitalis glycoside may be reduced). Products include:

Dobutamine Hydrochloride (Co-administration of sympathomimetic agents may increase the effects of sympathomimetics or thyroid hormone; thyroid hormones may increase risk of coronary insufficiency when sympathomimetic agents are administered to patients with coronary disease).
No products indexed under this heading.

Dopamine Hydrochloride (Co-administration with dopamine may result in a transient reduction in TSH secretion; the reduction is not sustained, therefore, hypothyroidism does not occur).
No products indexed under this heading.

Doxepin Hydrochloride (Co-administration may increase the therapeutic and toxic effects of both drugs possibly due to increased receptor sensitivity to catecholamines; toxic effects may include increased risk of arrhythmias and CNS stimulation; onset of tricyclics may be accelerated).
No products indexed under this heading.

Dyphylline (Decreased theophylline clearance may occur in hypothyroid patients; clearance returns to normal when euthyroid state is achieved).
No products indexed under this heading.

Ephedrine Hydrochloride (Co-administration of sympathomimetic agents may increase the effects of sympathomimetics or thyroid hormone; thyroid hormones may increase risk of coronary insufficiency when sympathomimetic agents are administered to patients with coronary disease).
No products indexed under this heading.

Ephedrine Sulfate (Co-administration of sympathomimetic agents may increase the effects of sympathomimetics or thyroid hormone; thyroid hormones may increase risk of coronary insufficiency when sympathomimetic agents are administered to patients with coronary disease).
No products indexed under this heading.

Ephedrine Tannate (Co-administration of sympathomimetic agents may increase the effects of sympathomimetics or thyroid hormone; thyroid hormones may increase risk of coronary insufficiency when sympathomimetic agents are administered to patients with coronary disease).
No products indexed under this heading.

Epinephrine (Co-administration of sympathomimetic agents may increase the effects of sympathomimetics or thyroid hormone; thyroid hormones may increase risk of coronary insufficiency when sympathomimetic agents are administered to patients with coronary disease). Products include:

Epinephrine Bitartrate (Co-administration of sympathomimetic agents may increase the effects of sympathomimetics or thyroid hormone; thyroid hormones may increase risk of coronary insufficiency when sympathomimetic agents are administered to patients with coronary disease).

No products indexed under this heading.

Epinephrine Hydrochloride (Co-administration of sympathomimetic agents may increase the effects of sympathomimetic or thyroid hormone; thyroid hormones may increase risk of coronary insufficiency when sympathomimetic agents are administered to patients with coronary disease).

No products indexed under this heading.

Esmolol Hydrochloride (Co-administration with beta-blockers may decrease T_4 5'-deiodinase activity; action of beta-blocker may be impaired when the hypothyroid patient is converted to euthyroid).

No products indexed under this heading.

Estradiol (Co-administration with oral estrogens may result in increased serum TBG concentrations). Products include:

Estrogens, Conjugated (Co-administration with oral estrogens may result in increased serum TBG concentrations). Products include:

Estrogens, Esterified (Co-administration with oral estrogens may result in increased serum TBG concentrations). Products include:

Estropipate (Co-administration with oral estrogens may result in increased serum TBG concentrations).

No products indexed under this heading.

Ethinyl Estradiol (Co-administration with estrogen containing oral contraceptives may result in increased serum TBG concentrations). Products include:

Ethiodized Oil (May decrease thyroid hormone secretion, which may result in hypothyrodism; the fetus, elderly, and euthyroid patients with underlying thyroid disease are among those individuals who are susceptible to iodine-induced hypothyroidism; oral cholecytographic agents slowly excreted, producing more prolonged hypothyroidism; iodide drugs that contain pharmacologic amounts of iodide may cause hypothyroidism in euthyroid patients with Grave's disease previously treated with thyroid autonomy; hyperthyroidism may develop over several weeks and may persist for several months after therapy discontinuation).

No products indexed under this heading.

Ethionamide (Co-administration has been associated with thyroid hormone and/or TSH level alterations by various mechanisms). Products include:

Ethotoin (Hydantoins may cause protein-binding site displacement; co-administration results in an initial transient increase in FT_4; continued administration results in a decrease in serum T_4 and normal FT_4 and TSH concentrations and, therefore, patients are clinically euthyroid).

No products indexed under this heading.

Ferrous Sulfate (Co-administration may result in decreased T_4 absorption, which may result in hypothyroidism; ferrous sulfate may form a ferric-thyroxine complex; administer levothyroxine at least 4 hours apart from these agents). Products include:

Fiber Supplement (Concurrent use of dietary fiber may bind and decrease the absorption of levothyroxine sodium from GI tract).

No products indexed under this heading.

Fludrocortisone Acetate (Co-administration with glucocorticoids may result in a transient reduction in TSH secretion; the reduction is not sustained, therefore, hypothyroidism does not occur; glucocorticoids may decrease serum TBG concentration).

No products indexed under this heading.

Fluorouracil (Co-administration with 5-FU may result in increased serum TBG concentrations). Products include:

Fluoxymesterone (Co-administration with androgens/anabolic steroids may result in decreased serum TBG concentration). Products include:

Fosphenytoin Sodium (Hydantoins may cause protein-binding site displacement; co-administration results in an initial transient increase in FT_4; co-administration may increase hepatic metabolism, which may result in hypothyroidism, resulting in increased levothyroxine requirements; phenytoin reduces serum protein binding of levothyroxine, and total- and free-T_4 may be reduced by 20% to 40%, but most patients have normal serum TSH levels and are clinically euthyroid).

No products indexed under this heading.

Furosemide (May cause protein-binding site displacement at greater than 80 mg IV; co-administration results in an initial transient increase in FT_4; continued administration results in a decrease in serum T_4 and normal FT4 and TSH concentrations and, therefore, patients are clinically euthyroid). Products include:

Gadopentetate Dimeglumine (May decrease thyroid hormone secretion, which may result in hypothyrodism; the fetus, elderly, and euthyroid patients with underlying thyroid disease are among those individuals who are susceptible to iodine-induced hypothyroidism; oral cholecytographic agents slowly excreted, producing more prolonged hypothyroidism; iodide drugs that contain pharmacologic amounts of iodide may cause hypothyroidism in euthyroid patients with Grave's disease previously treated with thyroid autonomy; hyperthyroidism may develop over several weeks and may persist for several months after therapy discontinuation).

No products indexed under this heading.

Glimepiride (Addition of levothyroxine to antidiabetic therapy may result in increased antidiabetic agent requirements). Products include:

Glipizide (Addition of levothyroxine to antidiabetic therapy may result in increased antidiabetic agent requirements).

No products indexed under this heading.

Glyburide (Addition of levothyroxine to antidiabetic therapy may result in increased antidiabetic agent requirements).

No products indexed under this heading.

Heparin Sodium (May cause protein-binding site displacement; co-administration results in an initial transient increase in FT_4; continued administration results in a decrease in serum T_4 and normal FT4 and TSH concentrations and, therefore, patients are clinically euthyroid).

No products indexed under this heading.

Heroin (Co-administration may result in increased serum TBG concentrations).

No products indexed under this heading.

Hydrochlorothiazide (Co-administration has been associated with thyroid hormone and/or TSH level alterations by various mechanisms). Products include:

Hydrocortisone (Co-administration with glucocorticoids may result in a transient reduction in TSH secretion; the reduction is not sustained, therefore, hypothyroidism does not occur; glucocorticoids may decrease serum TBG concentration). Products include:

Hydrocortisone Acetate (Co-administration with glucocorticoids may result in a transient reduction in TSH secretion; the reduction is not sustained, therefore, hypothyroidism does not occur; glucocorticoids may decrease serum TBG concentration). Products include:

Hydrocortisone Sodium Phosphate (Co-administration with glucocorticoids may result in a transient reduction in TSH secretion; the reduction is not sustained, therefore, hypothyroidism does not occur; glucocorticoids may decrease serum TBG concentration).

No products indexed under this heading.

Hydrocortisone Sodium Succinate (Co-administration with glucocorticoids may result in a transient reduction in TSH secretion; the reduction is not sustained, therefore, hypothyroidism does not occur; glucocorticoids may decrease serum TBG concentration).

No products indexed under this heading.

Hydroflumethiazide (Co-administration has been associated with thyroid hormone and/or TSH level alterations by various mechanisms).

No products indexed under this heading.

Imipramine Hydrochloride (Co-administration may increase the therapeutic and toxic effects of both drugs possibly due to increased receptor sensitivity to catecholamines; toxic effects may include increased risk of arrhythmias and CNS stimulation; onset of tricyclics may be accelerated).

No products indexed under this heading.

Imipramine Pamoate (Co-administration may increase the therapeutic and toxic effects of both drugs possibly due to increased receptor sensitivity to catecholamines; toxic effects may include increased risk of arrhythmias and CNS stimulation; onset of tricyclics may be accelerated).

No products indexed under this heading.

Infant Formula (Concurrent use of soybean flour may bind and decrease the absorption of levothyroxine sodium from GI tract).

No products indexed under this heading.

Insulin, Human, Zinc Suspension (Addition of levothyroxine to insulin therapy may result in increased insulin requirements). Products include:

Humulin L, 100 Units 1794
Humulin U, 100 Units 1800

Insulin, Human NPH (Addition of levothyroxine to insulin therapy may result in increased insulin requirements). Products include:
Humulin N, 100 Units 1795
Humulin N Pen 1797

Insulin, Human Regular (Addition of levothyroxine to insulin therapy may result in increased insulin requirements). Products include:
Humulin R, 100 Units 1798

Insulin, Human Regular and Human NPH Mixture (Addition of levothyroxine to insulin therapy may result in increased insulin requirements). Products include:
Humulin 50/50, 100 Units 1791
Humulin 70/30 Pen 1793

Insulin, NPH (Addition of levothyroxine to insulin therapy may result in increased insulin requirements).
No products indexed under this heading.

Insulin, Regular (Addition of levothyroxine to insulin therapy may result in increased insulin requirements).
No products indexed under this heading.

Insulin, Zinc Crystals (Addition of levothyroxine to insulin therapy may result in increased insulin requirements).
No products indexed under this heading.

Insulin, Zinc Suspension (Addition of levothyroxine to insulin therapy may result in increased insulin requirements).
No products indexed under this heading.

Insulin Aspart, Human Regular (Addition of levothyroxine to insulin therapy may result in increased insulin requirements). Products include:
NovoLog Injection 2326

Insulin glargine (Addition of levothyroxine to insulin therapy may result in increased insulin requirements). Products include:
Lantus Injection 2909

Insulin Lispro, Human (Addition of levothyroxine to insulin therapy may result in increased insulin requirements). Products include:
Humalog-Pen 1781
Humalog Mix 50/50-Pen 1783
Humalog Mix 75/25-Pen 1785

Insulin Lispro Protamine, Human (Addition of levothyroxine to insulin therapy may result in increased insulin requirements). Products include:
Humalog Mix 50/50-Pen 1783
Humalog Mix 75/25-Pen 1785

Interferon alfa-2a, Recombinant (Co-administration with interferon alpha has been associated with the development of antithyroid microsomal antibodies in 20% of patients and some have transient hypothyroidism, hyperthyroidism, or both; patients who have antithyroid antibodies before treatment are at higher risk for thyroid dysfunction).
No products indexed under this heading.

Interferon alfa-2b, Recombinant (Co-administration with interferon alpha has been associated with the development of antithyroid microsomal antibodies in 20% of patients and some have transient hypothyroidism, hyperthyroidism, or both; patients who have antithyroid antibodies before treatment are at higher risk for thyroid dysfunction). Products include:
Intron A for Injection 3024
Rebetron Combination Therapy 3063

Interferon alfa-N3 (Human Leukocyte Derived) (Co-administration with interferon alpha has been associated with the development of antithyroid microsomal antibodies in 20% of patients and some have transient hypothyroidism, hyperthyroidism, or both; patients who have antithyroid antibodies before treatment are at higher risk for thyroid dysfunction). Products include:
Alferon N Injection 1665

Iodamide Meglumine (May decrease thyroid hormone secretion, which may result in hypothyrodism; the fetus, elderly, and euthyroid patients with underlying thyroid disease are among those individuals who are susceptible to iodine-induced hypothyroidism; oral cholecytographic agents slowly excreted, producing more prolonged hypothyroidism; iodide drugs that contain pharmacologic amounts of iodide may cause hypothyroidism in euthyroid patients with Grave's disease previously treated with thyroid autonomy; hyperthyroidism may develop over several weeks and may persist for several months after therapy discontinuation).
No products indexed under this heading.

Iohexol (May decrease thyroid hormone secretion, which may result in hypothyrodism; the fetus, elderly, and euthyroid patients with underlying thyroid disease are among those individuals who are susceptible to iodine-induced hypothyroidism; oral cholecytographic agents slowly excreted, producing more prolonged hypothyroidism; iodide drugs that contain pharmacologic amounts of iodide may cause hypothyroidism in euthyroid patients with Grave's disease previously treated with thyroid autonomy; hyperthyroidism may develop over several weeks and may persist for several months after therapy discontinuation).
No products indexed under this heading.

Iopamidol (May decrease thyroid hormone secretion, which may result in hypothyrodism; the fetus, elderly, and euthyroid patients with underlying thyroid disease are among those individuals who are susceptible to iodine-induced hypothyroidism; oral cholecytographic agents slowly excreted, producing more prolonged hypothyroidism; iodide drugs that contain pharmacologic amounts of iodide may cause hypothyroidism in euthyroid patients with Grave's disease previously treated with thyroid autonomy; hyperthyroidism may develop over several weeks and may persist for several months after therapy discontinuation).
No products indexed under this heading.

Iopanoic Acid (May decrease thyroid hormone secretion, which may result in hypothyrodism; the fetus, elderly, and euthyroid patients with underlying thyroid disease are among those individuals who are susceptible to iodine-induced hypothyroidism; oral cholecytographic agents slowly excreted, producing more prolonged hypothyroidism; iodide drugs that contain pharmacologic amounts of iodide may cause hypothyroidism in euthyroid patients with Grave's disease previously treated with thyroid autonomy; hyperthyroidism may develop over several weeks and may persist for several months after therapy discontinuation).
No products indexed under this heading.

Iothalamate Meglumine (May decrease thyroid hormone secretion, which may result in hypothyrodism; the fetus, elderly, and euthyroid patients with underlying thyroid disease are among those individuals who are susceptible to iodine-induced hypothyroidism; oral cholecytographic agents slowly excreted, producing more prolonged hypothyroidism; iodide drugs that contain pharmacologic amounts of iodide may cause hypothyroidism in euthyroid patients with Grave's disease previously treated with thyroid autonomy; hyperthyroidism may develop over several weeks and may persist for several months after therapy discontinuation).
No products indexed under this heading.

Ioxaglate Meglumine (May decrease thyroid hormone secretion, which may result in hypothyrodism; the fetus, elderly, and euthyroid patients with underlying thyroid disease are among those individuals who are susceptible to iodine-induced hypothyroidism; oral cholecytographic agents slowly excreted, producing more prolonged hypothyroidism; iodide drugs that contain pharmacologic amounts of iodide may cause hypothyroidism in euthyroid patients with Grave's disease previously treated with thyroid autonomy; hyperthyroidism may develop over several weeks and may persist for several months after therapy discontinuation).
No products indexed under this heading.

Ioxaglate Sodium (May decrease thyroid hormone secretion, which may result in hypothyrodism; the fetus, elderly, and euthyroid patients with underlying thyroid disease are among those individuals who are susceptible to iodine-induced hypothyroidism; oral cholecytographic agents slowly excreted, producing more prolonged hypothyroidism; iodide drugs that contain pharmacologic amounts of iodide may cause hypothyroidism in euthyroid patients with Grave's disease previously treated with thyroid autonomy; hyperthyroidism may develop over several weeks and may persist for several months after therapy discontinuation).
No products indexed under this heading.

Isoproterenol Hydrochloride (Co-administration of sympathomimetic agents may increase the effects of sympathomimetics or thyroid hormone; thyroid hormones may increase risk of coronary insufficiency when sympathomimetic agents are administered to patients with coronary disease).
No products indexed under this heading.

Isoproterenol Sulfate (Co-administration of sympathomimetic agents may increase the effects of sympathomimetics or thyroid hormone; thyroid hormones may increase risk of coronary insufficiency when sympathomimetic agents are administered to patients with coronary disease).
No products indexed under this heading.

Ketamine Hydrochloride (Co-administration may produce marked hypertension and tachycardia).
No products indexed under this heading.

Labetalol Hydrochloride (Co-administration with beta-blockers may decrease T_4 5'-deiodinase activity; action of beta-blocker may be impaired when the hypothyroid patient is converted to euthyroid).
No products indexed under this heading.

Levalbuterol Hydrochloride (Co-administration of sympathomimetic agents may increase the effects of sympathomimetics or thyroid hormone; thyroid hormones may increase risk of coronary insufficiency when sympathomimetic agents are administered to patients with coronary disease). Products include:
Xopenex Inhalation Solution 3146
Xopenex Inhalation Solution Concentrate 3150

Levobunolol Hydrochloride (Co-administration with beta-blockers may decrease T_4 5'-deiodinase activity; action of beta-blocker may be impaired when the hypothyroid patient is converted to euthyroid). Products include:
Betagan Ophthalmic Solution, USP .... ⊙220

Lithium (May decrease thyroid hormone secretion, which may result in hypothyrodism; long-term lithium therapy can result in goiter in up to 50% of patients, and either subclinical or overt hypothyroidism, each in up to 20% of patients).
No products indexed under this heading.

Lithium Carbonate (May decrease thyroid hormone secretion, which may result in hypothyrodism; long-term lithium therapy can result in goiter in up to 50% of patients, and either subclinical or overt hypothyroidism, each in up to 20% of patients). Products include:
Lithobid Tablets 1692

Lithium Citrate (May decrease thyroid hormone secretion, which may result in hypothyrodism; long-term lithium therapy can result in goiter in up to 50% of patients, and either subclinical or overt hypothyroidism, each in up to 20% of patients).
No products indexed under this heading.

Lovastatin (Co-administration has been associated with thyroid hormone and/or TSH level alterations by various mechanisms). Products include:
Advicor Tablets 1722
Altoprev Extended-Release Tablets 3109
Mevacor Tablets 2021

Magaldrate (Co-administration with antacids may reduce the efficacy of levothyroxine by binding and delaying or preventing absorption, potentially resulting in hypothyroidism; administer levothyroxine at least 4 hours apart from these agents).

 No products indexed under this heading.

Magnesium Hydroxide (Co-administration with antacids may reduce the efficacy of levothyroxine by binding and delaying or preventing absorption, potentially resulting in hypothyroidism; administer levothyroxine at least 4 hours apart from these agents). Products include:

Magnesium Oxide (Co-administration with antacids may reduce the efficacy of levothyroxine by binding and delaying or preventing absorption, potentially resulting in hypothyroidism; administer levothyroxine at least 4 hours apart from these agents). Products include:

Magnesium Salicylate (Co-administration with salicylates at greater than 2 gm inhibit binding of T_4 and T_3 to TBG and transthyrelin; an initial increase in serum FT_4 is followed by return of FT_4 to normal levels with sustained therapeutic salicylate concentrations, although total T_4 levels may decrease by as much as 30%).

 No products indexed under this heading.

Maprotiline Hydrochloride (Co-administration may increase the therapeutic and toxic effects of both drugs possibly due to increased receptor sensitivity to catecholamines; toxic effects may include increased risk of arrhythmias and CNS stimulation; onset of tricyclics may be accelerated).

 No products indexed under this heading.

Meclofenamate Sodium (Co-administration with fenamate NSAID may result in decreased serum TBG concentration).

 No products indexed under this heading.

Mefenamic Acid (Co-administration with fenamate NSAID may result in decreased serum TBG concentration).

 No products indexed under this heading.

Mephenytoin (Hydantoins may cause protein-binding site displacement; co-administration results in an initial transient increase in FT_4; continued administration results in a decrease in serum T_4 and normal FT_4 and TSH concentrations and, therefore, patients are clinically euthyroid).

 No products indexed under this heading.

Mercaptopurine (Co-administration has been associated with thyroid hormone and/or TSH level alterations by various mechanisms).

 No products indexed under this heading.

Mestranol (Co-administration with estrogen containing oral contraceptives may result in increased serum TBG concentrations).

 No products indexed under this heading.

Metaproterenol Sulfate (Co-administration of sympathomimetic agents may increase the effects of sympathomimetics or thyroid hormone; thyroid hormones may increase risk of coronary insufficiency when sympathomimetic agents are administered to patients with coronary disease). Products include:

Metaraminol Bitartrate (Co-administration of sympathomimetic agents may increase the effects of sympathomimetics or thyroid hormone; thyroid hormones may increase risk of coronary insufficiency when sympathomimetic agents are administered to patients with coronary disease).

 No products indexed under this heading.

Metformin Hydrochloride (Addition of levothyroxine to antidiabetic therapy may result in increased antidiabetic agent requirements). Products include:

Methadone Hydrochloride (Co-administration may result in increased serum TBG concentrations).

 No products indexed under this heading.

Methimazole (May decrease thyroid hormone secretion, which may result in hypothyrodism).

 No products indexed under this heading.

Methoxamine Hydrochloride (Co-administration of sympathomimetic agents may increase the effects of sympathomimetics or thyroid hormone; thyroid hormones may increase risk of coronary insufficiency when sympathomimetic agents are administered to patients with coronary disease).

 No products indexed under this heading.

Methyclothiazide (Co-administration has been associated with thyroid hormone and/or TSH level alterations by various mechanisms).

 No products indexed under this heading.

Methylprednisolone Acetate (Co-administration with glucocorticoids may result in a transient reduction in TSH secretion; the reduction is not sustained, therefore, hypothyroidism does not occur; glucocorticoids may decrease serum TBG concentration). Products include:

Methylprednisolone Sodium Succinate (Co-administration with glucocorticoids may result in a transient reduction in TSH secretion; the reduction is not sustained, therefore, hypothyroidism does not occur; glucocorticoids may decrease serum TBG concentration).

 No products indexed under this heading.

Methyltestosterone (Co-administration with androgens/anabolic steroids may result in decreased serum TBG concentration). Products include:

Metipranolol Hydrochloride (Co-administration with beta-blockers may decrease T_4 5'-deiodinase activity; action of beta-blocker may be impaired when the hypothyroid patient is converted to euthyroid).

 No products indexed under this heading.

Metoclopramide Hydrochloride (Co-administration has been associated with thyroid hormone and/or TSH level alterations by various mechanisms).

 No products indexed under this heading.

Metoprolol Succinate (Co-administration with beta-blockers may decrease T_4 5'-deiodinase activity; action of beta-blocker may be impaired when the hypothyroid patient is converted to euthyroid). Products include:

Metoprolol Tartrate (Co-administration with beta-blockers may decrease T_4 5'-deiodinase activity; action of beta-blocker may be impaired when the hypothyroid patient is converted to euthyroid). Products include:

Miglitol (Addition of levothyroxine to antidiabetic therapy may result in increased antidiabetic agent requirements).

 No products indexed under this heading.

Mitotane (Co-administration may result in increased serum TBG concentrations).

 No products indexed under this heading.

Nadolol (Co-administration with beta-blockers may decrease T_4 5'-deiodinase activity; action of beta-blocker may be impaired when the hypothyroid patient is converted to euthyroid). Products include:

Niacin (Co-administration with slow-release nicotinic acid may result in decreased serum TBG concentration). Products include:

Norepinephrine Bitartrate (Co-administration of sympathomimetic agents may increase the effects of sympathomimetics or thyroid hormone; thyroid hormones may increase risk of coronary insufficiency when sympathomimetic agents are administered to patients with coronary disease).

 No products indexed under this heading.

Nortriptyline Hydrochloride (Co-administration may increase the therapeutic and toxic effects of both drugs possibly due to increased receptor sensitivity to catecholamines; toxic effects may include increased risk of arrhythmias and CNS stimulation; onset of tricyclics may be accelerated).

 No products indexed under this heading.

Octreotide Acetate (Co-administration with octreotide may result in a transient reduction in TSH secretion; the reduction is not sustained, therefore, hypothyroidism does not occur). Products include:

Oxandrolone (Co-administration with androgens/anabolic steroids may result in decreased serum TBG concentration). Products include:

Oxymetholone (Co-administration with androgens/anabolic steroids may result in decreased serum TBG concentration).

 No products indexed under this heading.

Penbutolol Sulfate (Co-administration with beta-blockers may decrease T_4 5'-deiodinase activity; action of beta-blocker may be impaired when the hypothyroid patient is converted to euthyroid).

 No products indexed under this heading.

Pergolide Mesylate (Co-administration with dopamine agonists may result in a transient reduction in TSH secretion; the reduction is not sustained, therefore, hypothyroidism does not occur). Products include:

Perphenazine (Co-administration has been associated with thyroid hormone and/or TSH level alterations by various mechanisms).

 No products indexed under this heading.

Phenobarbital (Co-administration may increase hepatic metabolism, which may result in hypothyroidism, resulting in increased levothyroxine requirements). Products include:

Phenylbutazone (Co-administration may cause protein-binding site displacement).

 No products indexed under this heading.

Phenylephrine Bitartrate (Co-administration of sympathomimetic agents may increase the effects of sympathomimetics or thyroid hormone; thyroid hormones may increase risk of coronary insufficiency when sympathomimetic agents are administered to patients with coronary disease).

 No products indexed under this heading.

Phenylephrine Hydrochloride (Co-administration of sympathomimetic agents may increase the effects of sympathomimetics or thyroid hormone; thyroid hormones may increase risk of coronary insufficiency when sympathomimetic agents are administered to patients with coronary disease). Products include:

IMPORTANT NOTE: Always consult each drug listing in the patient's regimen for possible interactions.

Comtrex Maximum Strength Day/Night Severe Cold & Sinus Caplets - Day Formulation .... ▣ 725
Comtrex Maximum Strength Day/Night Severe Cold & Sinus Caplets - Night Formulation .... ▣ 725
Contac Cold and Flu Maximum Strength Caplets .... ▣ 728
Contac Cold and Flu Day and Night Caplets (Day Formulation Only) .... ▣ 727
Contac Cold and Flu Day and Night Caplets (Night Formulation Only) .... ▣ 727
Contac Cold and Flu Non-Drowsy Caplets .... ▣ 728
Contac-D Cold Non-Drowsy Tablets .... ▣ 729
Children's Dimetapp Cold & Allergy Elixir .... ▣ 730
Children's Dimetapp Cold & Allergy Chewable Tablets .... ▣ 730
Children's Dimetapp DM Cold & Cough Elixir .... ▣ 731
Toddler's Dimetapp Cold and Cough Drops .... ▣ 732
Excedrin Sinus Headache Caplets/Tablets .... ▣ 610
4-Way Fast Acting Nasal Spray ...... ▣ 775
4-Way Menthol Nasal Spray .... ▣ 775
Preparation H Maximum Strength Cream .... ▣ 666
Preparation H Cooling Gel .... ▣ 666
Preparation H .... ▣ 666
Refenesen PE Caplets .... ▣ 721
Robitussin Cough & Allergy Syrup .. ▣ 736
Robitussin Cough & Cold Nighttime Liquid .... ▣ 736
Robitussin Cough, Cold & Flu Nighttime Liquid .... ▣ 738
Robitussin Head & Chest Congestion PE Syrup .... ▣ 739
Robitussin Pediatric Cough & Cold Nighttime Liquid .... ▣ 736
TheraFlu Cold & Cough Hot Liquid .... ▣ 740
TheraFlu Cold & Sore Throat Hot Liquid .... ▣ 741
TheraFlu Flu & Sore Throat Hot Liquid .... ▣ 742
TheraFlu Daytime Severe Cold Hot Liquid .... ▣ 742
TheraFlu Nighttime Severe Cold Hot Liquid .... ▣ 740
TheraFlu Warming Relief Daytime Severe Cold .... ▣ 743
TheraFlu Warming Relief Nighttime Severe Cold .... ▣ 743
Triaminic Chest & Nasal Congestion Liquid .... ▣ 746
Triaminic Cold & Allergy Liquid .... ▣ 746
Triaminic Daytime Cold & Cough Liquid .... ▣ 745
Triaminic Nighttime Cold & Cough Liquid .... ▣ 746
Triaminic Thin Strips Cold .... ▣ 748
Triaminic Thin Strips Cold & Cough .... ▣ 778
Triaminic Infant Thin Strips Decongestant .... ▣ 747
Triaminic Infant Thin Strips Decongestant Plus Cough .... ▣ 747
Children's Tylenol Plus Flu Oral Suspension .... ▣ 749
Tylenol Cold Head Congestion Daytime Caplets with Cool Burst and Gelcaps .... ▣ 750
Tylenol Cold Multi-Symptom Daytime Liquid .... ▣ 752
Tylenol Cold Multi-Symptom Severe Daytime Liquid .... ▣ 752
Concentrated Tylenol Infants' Drops Plus Cold & Cough .... ▣ 754
Tylenol Allergy Multi-Symptom Caplets with Cool Burst and Gelcaps 1872
Tylenol Allergy Multi-Symptom Nighttime Caplets with Cool Burst 1872
Children's Tylenol Plus Cold Suspension Liquid 1879
Children's Tylenol Plus Cold & Allergy Suspension Liquid 1878
Children's Tylenol Plus Flu Suspension Liquid 1881
Children's Tylenol Plus Multi-Symptom Cold Suspension Liquid 1879
Tylenol Cold Head Congestion Daytime Caplets with Cool Burst 1873
Tylenol Cold Head Congestion Nighttime Caplets with Cool Burst 1873
Tylenol Cold Head Congestion Severe Caplets with Cool Burst..... 1873
Tylenol Cold Multi-Symptom Daytime Caplets with Cool Burst and Gelcaps 1874
Tylenol Cold Multi-Symptom Daytime Liquid with Citrus Burst ... 1874
Tylenol Cold Multi-Symptom Nighttime Caplets with Cool Burst 1874
Tylenol Cold Multi-Symptom Nighttime Liquid with Cool Burst ... 1874
Tylenol Cold Multi-Symptom Severe Caplets with Cool Burst..... 1874
Tylenol Cold Multi-Symptom Severe Daytime Liquid with Citrus Burst 1874
Tylenol Sinus Congestion & Pain Daytime Caplets with Cool Burst and Gelcaps 1876
Tylenol Sinus Congestion & Pain Nighttime Caplets with Cool Burst 1876
Tylenol Sinus Congestion & Pain Severe Caplets with Cool Burst..... 1876
Vicks 44D Cough & Head Congestion Relief Liquid............. ▣ 760
Vicks DayQuil LiquiCaps/Liquid Multi-Symptom Cold/Flu Relief..... ▣ 761
Zicam Cough Plus D Cough Spray .... ▣ 767

Phenylephrine Tannate (Co-administration of sympathomimetic agents may increase the effects of sympathomimetics or thyroid hormone; thyroid hormones may increase risk of coronary insufficiency when sympathomimetic agents are administered to patients with coronary disease).
No products indexed under this heading.

Phenylpropanolamine Hydrochloride (Co-administration of sympathomimetic agents may increase the effects of sympathomimetics or thyroid hormone; thyroid hormones may increase risk of coronary insufficiency when sympathomimetic agents are administered to patients with coronary disease).
No products indexed under this heading.

Phenytoin (Hydantoins may cause protein-binding site displacement; co-administration results in an initial transient increase in FT_4; co-administration may increase hepatic metabolism, which may result in hypothyroidism, resulting in increased levothyroxine requirements; phenytoin reduces serum protein binding of levothyroxine, and total- and free-T_4 may be reduced by 20% to 40%, but most patients have normal serum TSH levels and are clinicly euthyroid).
No products indexed under this heading.

Phenytoin Sodium (Hydantoins may cause protein-binding site displacement; co-administration results in an initial transient increase in FT_4; co-administration may increase hepatic metabolism, which may result in hypothyroidism, resulting in increased levothyroxine requirements; phenytoin reduces serum protein binding of levothyroxine, and total- and free-T_4 may be reduced by 20% to 40%, but most patients have normal serum TSH levels and are clinicly euthyroid). Products include:
Phenytek Capsules 2160

Pindolol (Co-administration with beta-blockers may decrease T_4 5'-deiodinase activity; action of beta-blocker may be impaired when the hypothyroid patient is converted to euthyroid).
No products indexed under this heading.

Pioglitazone Hydrochloride (Addition of levothyroxine to antidiabetic therapy may result in increased antidiabetic agent requirements). Products include:
ActoPlus Met Tablets 3214
Actos Tablets 3219
Duetact Tablets 3226

Pirbuterol Acetate (Co-administration of sympathomimetic agents may increase the effects of sympathomimetics or thyroid hormone; thyroid hormones may increase risk of coronary insufficiency when sympathomimetic agents are administered to patients with coronary disease). Products include:
Maxair Autohaler 1852

Polyestradiol Phosphate (Co-administration with oral estrogens may result in increased serum TBG concentrations).
No products indexed under this heading.

Polythiazide (Co-administration has been associated with thyroid hormone and/or TSH level alterations by various mechanisms).
No products indexed under this heading.

Potassium Iodide (May decrease thyroid hormone secretion, which may result in hypothyroidism; iodide drugs that contain pharmacologic amounts of iodide may cause hypothyroidism in euthyroid patients with Grave's disease previously treated with thyroid autonomy; hyperthyroidism may develop over several weeks and may persist for several months after therapy discontinuation).
No products indexed under this heading.

Pramipexole Dihydrochloride (Co-administration with dopamine agonists may result in a transient reduction in TSH secretion; the reduction is not sustained, therefore, hypothyroidism does not occur). Products include:
Mirapex Tablets 859

Prednisolone Acetate (Co-administration with glucocorticoids may result in a transient reduction in TSH secretion; the reduction is not sustained, therefore, hypothyroidism does not occur; glucocorticoids may decrease serum TBG concentration). Products include:
Blephamide Ophthalmic Ointment 568
Blephamide Ophthalmic Suspension.. 569
Poly-Pred Ophthalmic Suspension .... ⊙ 233
Pred Forte Ophthalmic Suspension .... ⊙ 235
Pred Mild Ophthalmic Suspension .... ⊙ 238
Pred-G Ophthalmic Ointment .... ⊙ 237
Pred-G Ophthalmic Suspension ...... ⊙ 236

Prednisolone Sodium Phosphate (Co-administration with glucocorticoids may result in a transient reduction in TSH secretion; the reduction is not sustained, therefore, hypothyroidism does not occur; glucocorticoids may decrease serum TBG concentration).
No products indexed under this heading.

Prednisolone Tebutate (Co-administration with glucocorticoids may result in a transient reduction in TSH secretion; the reduction is not sustained, therefore, hypothyroidism does not occur; glucocorticoids may decrease serum TBG concentration).
No products indexed under this heading.

Prednisone (Co-administration with glucocorticoids may result in a transient reduction in TSH secretion; the reduction is not sustained, therefore, hypothyroidism does not occur; glucocorticoids may decrease serum TBG concentration).
No products indexed under this heading.

Propranolol Hydrochloride (Co-administration with beta-blockers may decrease T_4 5'-deiodinase activity; in patients treated with large doses of propranolol, greater than 160 mg/day, T_3 and T_4 levels change slightly, TSH levels remain normal, and patients are clinically euthyroid; action of beta-blocker may be impaired when the hypothyroid patient is converted to euthyroid). Products include:
Inderal LA Long-Acting Capsules 3429
InnoPran XL Capsules 2723

Propylthiouracil (May decrease thyroid hormone secretion, which may result in hypothyrodism).
No products indexed under this heading.

Protriptyline Hydrochloride (Co-administration may increase the therapeutic and toxic effects of both drugs possibly due to increased receptor sensitivity to catecholamines; toxic effects may include increased risk of arrhythmias and CNS stimulation; onset of tricyclics may be accelerated).
No products indexed under this heading.

Pseudoephedrine Hydrochloride (Co-administration of sympathomimetic agents may increase the effects of sympathomimetics or thyroid hormone; thyroid hormones may increase risk of coronary insufficiency when sympathomimetic agents are administered to patients with coronary disease). Products include:
Advil Allergy Sinus Caplets .... ▣ 770
Advil Cold & Sinus .... ▣ 723
Advil Multi-Symptom Cold Caplets .... ▣ 770
Aleve Cold & Sinus Caplets 744
Allegra-D 12 Hour Extended-Release Tablets............ 2846
Allegra-D 24 Hour Extended-Release Tablets............ 2849
BC Cold Powder .... ▣ 677
Comtrex Maximum Strength Cold & Cough Day/Night Caplets - Day Formulation........................ ▣ 726
Comtrex Maximum Strength Cold & Cough Day/Night Caplets - Night Formulation .... ▣ 726
Children's Motrin Cold Oral Suspension 1867
Mucinex D Extended-Release Bi-Layer Tablets .... ▣ 776

Robitussin Cough & Cold CF Liquid 735
Robitussin Cough & Cold Pediatric Drops 735
Tylenol Sinus Congestion & Pain Nighttime Caplets with Cool Burst 778
Tylenol Cold Severe Congestion Non-Drowsy Caplets with Cool Burst 1874
Tylenol Sinus Severe Congestion Caplets with Cool Burst 1876
Vicks 44D Cough & Head Congestion Relief Liquid 2679
Vicks 44M Cough, Cold & Flu Relief Liquid 2680
Vicks DayQuil Multi-Symptom Cold/Flu Relief LiquiCaps 2678
Vicks DayQuil Multi-Symptom Cold/Flu Relief Liquid 2678
Vicks NyQuil Multi-Symptom Cold/Flu Relief Liquid 2681
Vicks NyQuil Multi-Symptom Cold/Flu Relief LiquiCaps 2681
Children's Vicks NyQuil Cold/Cough Relief Liquid 2680
Zyrtec-D 12 Hour Extended Release Tablets 2597

Pseudoephedrine Sulfate (Co-administration of sympathomimetic agents may increase the effects of sympathomimetics or thyroid hormone; thyroid hormones may increase risk of coronary insufficiency when sympathomimetic agents are administered to patients with coronary disease). Products include:
Alavert Allergy & Sinus D-12 Hour Tablets 771
Clarinex-D 24-Hour Extended-Release Tablets 2998
Claritin-D Non-Drowsy 12 Hour Tablets 772
Claritin-D Non-Drowsy 24 Hour Tablets 772

Quinestrol (Co-administration with oral estrogens may result in increased serum TBG concentrations).
No products indexed under this heading.

Repaglinide (Addition of levothyroxine to antidiabetic therapy may result in increased antidiabetic agent requirements).
No products indexed under this heading.

Resorcinol (Co-administration of excessive topical use of resorcinol has been associated with thyroid hormone and/or TSH level alterations by various mechanisms).
No products indexed under this heading.

Rifampin (Co-administration may increase hepatic metabolism, which may result in hypothyroidism, resulting in increased levothyroxine requirements).
No products indexed under this heading.

Ropinirole Hydrochloride (Co-administration with dopamine agonists may result in a transient reduction in TSH secretion; the reduction is not sustained, therefore, hypothyroidism does not occur). Products include:
Requip Tablets 1555

Rosiglitazone Maleate (Addition of levothyroxine to antidiabetic therapy may result in increased antidiabetic agent requirements). Products include:
Avandamet Tablets 1373
Avandaryl Tablets 1379
Avandia Tablets 1384

Salmeterol Xinafoate (Co-administration of sympathomimetic agents may increase the effects of sympathomimetics or thyroid hormone; thyroid hormones may increase risk of coronary insufficiency when sympathomimetic agents are administered to patients with coronary disease). Products include:
Advair Diskus 100/50 1308
Advair Diskus 250/50 1308
Advair Diskus 500/50 1308
Advair HFA Inhalation Aerosol 1318
Serevent Diskus 1568

Salsalate (Co-administration with salicylates at greater than 2 gm inhibit binding of T_4 and T_3 to TBG and transthyrelin; an initial increase in serum FT_4 is followed by return of FT_4 to normal levels with sustained therapeutic salicylate concentrations, although total T_4 levels may decrease by as much as 30%).
No products indexed under this heading.

Sertraline Hydrochloride (Co-administration of sertraline in patients stabilized on levothyroxine may result in increased levothyroxine requirements). Products include:
Zoloft 2586

Sodium Nitroprusside (Co-administration has been associated with thyroid hormone and/or TSH level alterations by various mechanisms).
No products indexed under this heading.

Sodium Polystyrene Sulfonate (Co-administration may result in decreased T_4 absorption, which may result in hypothyroidism; administer levothyroxine at least 4 hours apart from these agents).
No products indexed under this heading.

Somatrem (Excessive use of thyroid hormone with growth hormones may accelerate epiphyseal closure; however, untreated hypothyroidism may interfere with growth response to growth hormone).
No products indexed under this heading.

Somatropin (Excessive use of thyroid hormone with growth hormones may accelerate epiphyseal closure; however, untreated hypothyroidism may interfere with growth response to growth hormone). Products include:
Genotropin Lyophilized Powder 2638
Humatrope Vials and Cartridges 1787
Norditropin Cartridges 2323
Nutropin for Injection 1239
Nutropin AQ Injection 1243
Nutropin AQ Pen 1243
Nutropin AQ Pen Cartridge 1243

Sotalol Hydrochloride (Co-administration with beta-blockers may decrease T_4 5'-deiodinase activity; action of beta-blocker may be impaired when the hypothyroid patient is converted to euthyroid).
No products indexed under this heading.

Soybean Preparations (Concurrent use of soybean flour may bind and decrease the absorption of levothyroxine sodium from GI tract).
No products indexed under this heading.

Stanozolol (Co-administration with androgens/anabolic steroids may result in decreased serum TBG concentration).
No products indexed under this heading.

Sucralfate (Co-administration may result in decreased T_4 absorption, which may result in hypothyroidism; administer levothyroxine at least 4 hours apart from these agents). Products include:
Carafate Suspension 701
Carafate Tablets 701

Sulfamethoxazole (May decrease thyroid hormone secretion, which may result in hypothyrodism).
No products indexed under this heading.

Sulfisoxazole Acetyl (May decrease thyroid hormone secretion, which may result in hypothyrodism).
No products indexed under this heading.

Tamoxifen Citrate (Co-administration may result in increased serum TBG concentrations). Products include:
Soltamox Oral Solution 3527

Terbutaline Sulfate (Co-administration of sympathomimetic agents may increase the effects of sympathomimetics or thyroid hormone; thyroid hormones may increase risk of coronary insufficiency when sympathomimetic agents are administered to patients with coronary disease).
No products indexed under this heading.

Theophylline (Decreased theophylline clearance may occur in hypothyroid patients; clearance returns to normal when euthyroid state is achieved).
No products indexed under this heading.

Theophylline Anhydrous (Decreased theophylline clearance may occur in hypothyroid patients; clearance returns to normal when euthyroid state is achieved). Products include:
Uniphyl Tablets 2710

Theophylline Calcium Salicylate (Decreased theophylline clearance may occur in hypothyroid patients; clearance returns to normal when euthyroid state is achieved).
No products indexed under this heading.

Theophylline Dihydroxypropyl (Glyceryl) (Decreased theophylline clearance may occur in hypothyroid patients; clearance returns to normal when euthyroid state is achieved).
No products indexed under this heading.

Theophylline Ethylenediamine (Decreased theophylline clearance may occur in hypothyroid patients; clearance returns to normal when euthyroid state is achieved).
No products indexed under this heading.

Theophylline Sodium Glycinate (Decreased theophylline clearance may occur in hypothyroid patients; clearance returns to normal when euthyroid state is achieved).
No products indexed under this heading.

Timolol Hemihydrate (Co-administration with beta-blockers may decrease T_4 5'-deiodinase activity; action of beta-blocker may be impaired when the hypothyroid patient is converted to euthyroid). Products include:
Betimol Ophthalmic Solution 3382
Betimol Ophthalmic Solution .... ⊙ 295

Timolol Maleate (Co-administration with beta-blockers may decrease T_4 5'-deiodinase activity; action of beta-blocker may be impaired when the hypothyroid patient is converted to euthyroid). Products include:
Blocadren Tablets 1916
Cosopt Sterile Ophthalmic Solution 1931
Timolide Tablets 2086
Timoptic Sterile Ophthalmic Solution 2088
Timoptic in Ocudose 2091
Timoptic-XE Sterile Ophthalmic Gel Forming Solution 2092

Tolazamide (Addition of levothyroxine to antidiabetic therapy may result in increased antidiabetic agent requirements).
No products indexed under this heading.

Tolbutamide (May decrease thyroid hormone secretion, which may result in hypothyrodism).
No products indexed under this heading.

Triamcinolone (Co-administration with glucocorticoids may result in a transient reduction in TSH secretion; the reduction is not sustained, therefore, hypothyroidism does not occur; glucocorticoids may decrease serum TBG concentration).
No products indexed under this heading.

Triamcinolone Acetonide (Co-administration with glucocorticoids may result in a transient reduction in TSH secretion; the reduction is not sustained, therefore, hypothyroidism does not occur; glucocorticoids may decrease serum TBG concentration). Products include:
Azmacort Inhalation Aerosol 1726
Nasacort AQ Nasal Spray 2922

Triamcinolone Diacetate (Co-administration with glucocorticoids may result in a transient reduction in TSH secretion; the reduction is not sustained, therefore, hypothyroidism does not occur; glucocorticoids may decrease serum TBG concentration).
No products indexed under this heading.

Triamcinolone Hexacetonide (Co-administration with glucocorticoids may result in a transient reduction in TSH secretion; the reduction is not sustained, therefore, hypothyroidism does not occur; glucocorticoids may decrease serum TBG concentration).
No products indexed under this heading.

Trimipramine Maleate (Co-administration may increase the therapeutic and toxic effects of both drugs possibly due to increased receptor sensitivity to catecholamines; toxic effects may include increased risk of arrhythmias and CNS stimulation; onset of tricyclics may be accelerated).
No products indexed under this heading.

Troglitazone (Addition of levothyroxine to antidiabetic therapy may result in increased antidiabetic agent requirements).
No products indexed under this heading.

Tyropanoate Sodium (May decrease thyroid hormone secretion, which may result in hypothyrodism; the fetus, elderly, and euthyroid patients with underlying thyroid disease are among those individuals who are susceptible to iodine-induced hypothyroidism; oral cholecytographic agents slowly excreted, producing more prolonged hypothyroidism; iodide drugs that contain pharmacologic amounts of iodide may cause hypothyroidism in euthyroid patients with Grave's disease previously treated with thyroid autonomy; hyperthyroidism may develop over several weeks and may persist for several months after therapy discontinuation).

No products indexed under this heading.

Warfarin Sodium (Thyroid hormones appear to increase the catabolism of vitamin K-dependent clotting factors, thereby increasing the anticoagulant activity of oral anticoagulants). Products include:

Food Interactions

Cotton seed meal (Concurrent use of cotton seed meal may bind and decrease the absorption of levothyroxine sodium from GI tract).

Dietary Fiber (Concurrent use of dietary fiber may bind and decrease the absorption of levothyroxine sodium from GI tract).

Soybean Formula, Children's (Concurrent use of soybean flour may bind and decrease the absorption of levothyroxine sodium from GI tract).

Walnuts (Concurrent use of walnuts may bind and decrease the absorption of levothyroxine sodium from GI tract).

LEVULAN KERASTICK FOR TOPICAL SOLUTION, 20%

(Aminolevulinic Acid Hydrochloride) ... 1085
May interact with phenothiazines, sulfonamides, sulfonylureas, tetracyclines, thiazides, and certain other agents. Compounds in these categories include:

Bendroflumethiazide (Co-administration with other photosensitizing agents, such as thiazide diuretics, might increase photosensitivity reactions of actinic ketoses treated with aminolevulinic acid HCL).

No products indexed under this heading.

Chlorothiazide (Co-administration with other photosensitizing agents, such as thiazide diuretics, might increase photosensitivity reactions of actinic ketoses treated with aminolevulinic acid HCL). Products include:

Chlorothiazide Sodium (Co-administration with other photosensitizing agents, such as thiazide diuretics, might increase photosensitivity reactions of actinic ketoses treated with aminolevulinic acid HCL). Products include:

Chlorpromazine (Co-administration with other photosensitizing agents, such as phenothiazines, might increase photosensitivity reactions of actinic ketoses treated with aminolevulinic acid HCL).

No products indexed under this heading.

Chlorpromazine Hydrochloride (Co-administration with other photosensitizing agents, such as phenothiazines, might increase photosensitivity reactions of actinic ketoses treated with aminolevulinic acid HCL).

No products indexed under this heading.

Chlorpropamide (Co-administration with other photosensitizing agents, such as sulfonylureas, might increase photosensitivity reactions of actinic ketoses treated with aminolevulinic acid HCL).

No products indexed under this heading.

Demeclocycline Hydrochloride (Co-administration with other photosensitizing agents, such as tetracyclines, might increase photosensitivity reactions of actinic ketoses treated with aminolevulinic acid HCL).

No products indexed under this heading.

Doxycycline Calcium (Co-administration with other photosensitizing agents, such as tetracyclines, might increase photosensitivity reactions of actinic ketoses treated with aminolevulinic acid HCL).

No products indexed under this heading.

Doxycycline Hyclate (Co-administration with other photosensitizing agents, such as tetracyclines, might increase photosensitivity reactions of actinic ketoses treated with aminolevulinic acid HCL).

No products indexed under this heading.

Doxycycline Monohydrate (Co-administration with other photosensitizing agents, such as tetracyclines, might increase photosensitivity reactions of actinic ketoses treated with aminolevulinic acid HCL). Products include:

Fluphenazine Decanoate (Co-administration with other photosensitizing agents, such as phenothiazines, might increase photosensitivity reactions of actinic ketoses treated with aminolevulinic acid HCL).

No products indexed under this heading.

Fluphenazine Enanthate (Co-administration with other photosensitizing agents, such as phenothiazines, might increase photosensitivity reactions of actinic ketoses treated with aminolevulinic acid HCL).

No products indexed under this heading.

Fluphenazine Hydrochloride (Co-administration with other photosensitizing agents, such as phenothiazines, might increase photosensitivity reactions of actinic ketoses treated with aminolevulinic acid HCL).

No products indexed under this heading.

Glimepiride (Co-administration with other photosensitizing agents, such as sulfonylureas, might increase photosensitivity reactions of actinic ketoses treated with aminolevulinic acid HCL). Products include:

Glipizide (Co-administration with other photosensitizing agents, such as sulfonylureas, might increase photosensitivity reactions of actinic ketoses treated with aminolevulinic acid HCL).

No products indexed under this heading.

Glyburide (Co-administration with other photosensitizing agents, such as sulfonylureas, might increase photosensitivity reactions of actinic ketoses treated with aminolevulinic acid HCL).

No products indexed under this heading.

Griseofulvin (Co-administration with other photosensitizing agents, such as griseofulvin, might increase photosensitivity reactions of actinic ketoses treated with aminolevulinic acid HCL). Products include:

Hydrochlorothiazide (Co-administration with other photosensitizing agents, such as thiazide diuretics, might increase photosensitivity reactions of actinic ketoses treated with aminolevulinic acid HCL). Products include:

Hydroflumethiazide (Co-administration with other photosensitizing agents, such as thiazide diuretics, might increase photosensitivity reactions of actinic ketoses treated with aminolevulinic acid HCL).

No products indexed under this heading.

Mesoridazine Besylate (Co-administration with other photosensitizing agents, such as phenothiazines, might increase photosensitivity reactions of actinic ketoses treated with aminolevulinic acid HCL).

No products indexed under this heading.

Methacycline Hydrochloride (Co-administration with other photosensitizing agents, such as tetracyclines, might increase photosensitivity reactions of actinic ketoses treated with aminolevulinic acid HCL).

No products indexed under this heading.

Methotrimeprazine (Co-administration with other photosensitizing agents, such as phenothiazines, might increase photosensitivity reactions of actinic ketoses treated with aminolevulinic acid HCL).

No products indexed under this heading.

Methyclothiazide (Co-administration with other photosensitizing agents, such as thiazide diuretics, might increase photosensitivity reactions of actinic ketoses treated with aminolevulinic acid HCL).

No products indexed under this heading.

Minocycline Hydrochloride (Co-administration with other photosensitizing agents, such as tetracyclines, might increase photosensitivity reac-

tions of actinic ketoses treated with aminolevulinic acid HCL). Products include:

Oxytetracycline Hydrochloride (Co-administration with other photosensitizing agents, such as tetracyclines, might increase photosensitivity reactions of actinic ketoses treated with aminolevulinic acid HCL).

No products indexed under this heading.

Perphenazine (Co-administration with other photosensitizing agents, such as phenothiazines, might increase photosensitivity reactions of actinic ketoses treated with aminolevulinic acid HCL).

No products indexed under this heading.

Polythiazide (Co-administration with other photosensitizing agents, such as thiazide diuretics, might increase photosensitivity reactions of actinic ketoses treated with aminolevulinic acid HCL).

No products indexed under this heading.

Prochlorperazine (Co-administration with other photosensitizing agents, such as phenothiazines, might increase photosensitivity reactions of actinic ketoses treated with aminolevulinic acid HCL).

No products indexed under this heading.

Promethazine Hydrochloride (Co-administration with other photosensitizing agents, such as phenothiazines, might increase photosensitivity reactions of actinic ketoses treated with aminolevulinic acid HCL). Products include:

Sulfacytine (Co-administration with other photosensitizing agents, such as sulfonamides, might increase photosensitivity reactions of actinic ketoses treated with aminolevulinic acid HCL).

No products indexed under this heading.

Sulfamethizole (Co-administration with other photosensitizing agents, such as sulfonamides, might increase photosensitivity reactions of actinic ketoses treated with aminolevulinic acid HCL).

No products indexed under this heading.

Sulfamethoxazole (Co-administration with other photosensitizing agents, such as sulfonamides, might increase photosensitivity reactions of actinic ketoses treated with aminolevulinic acid HCL).

No products indexed under this heading.

Sulfasalazine (Co-administration with other photosensitizing agents, such as sulfonamides, might increase photosensitivity reactions of actinic ketoses treated with aminolevulinic acid HCL).

No products indexed under this heading.

Sulfinpyrazone (Co-administration with other photosensitizing agents, such as sulfonamides, might increase photosensitivity reactions of actinic ketoses treated with aminolevulinic acid HCL).
No products indexed under this heading.

Sulfisoxazole Acetyl (Co-administration with other photosensitizing agents, such as sulfonamides, might increase photosensitivity reactions of actinic ketoses treated with aminolevulinic acid HCL).
No products indexed under this heading.

Sulfisoxazole Diolamine (Co-administration with other photosensitizing agents, such as sulfonamides, might increase photosensitivity reactions of actinic ketoses treated with aminolevulinic acid HCL).
No products indexed under this heading.

Tetracycline Hydrochloride (Co-administration with other photosensitizing agents, such as tetracyclines, might increase photosensitivity reactions of actinic ketoses treated with aminolevulinic acid HCL).
No products indexed under this heading.

Thioridazine Hydrochloride (Co-administration with other photosensitizing agents, such as phenothiazines, might increase photosensitivity reactions of actinic ketoses treated with aminolevulinic acid HCL). Products include:
Thioridazine Hydrochloride Tablets ... 2163

Tolazamide (Co-administration with other photosensitizing agents, such as sulfonylureas, might increase photosensitivity reactions of actinic ketoses treated with aminolevulinic acid HCL).
No products indexed under this heading.

Tolbutamide (Co-administration with other photosensitizing agents, such as sulfonylureas, might increase photosensitivity reactions of actinic ketoses treated with aminolevulinic acid HCL).
No products indexed under this heading.

Trifluoperazine Hydrochloride (Co-administration with other photosensitizing agents, such as phenothiazines, might increase photosensitivity reactions of actinic ketoses treated with aminolevulinic acid HCL).
No products indexed under this heading.

LEXAPRO ORAL SOLUTION

(Escitalopram Oxalate) ... 1190
See Lexapro Tablets

LEXAPRO TABLETS

(Escitalopram Oxalate) ... 1190
May interact with anticoagulants, cytochrome p450 2d6 substrates (selected), lithium preparations, monoamine oxidase inhibitors, non-steroidal anti-inflammatory agents, and certain other agents. Compounds in these categories include:

Amitriptyline Hydrochloride (Caution is indicated in the co-administration of escitalopram and drugs metabolized by CYP2D6).
No products indexed under this heading.

Amphetamine Aspartate (Caution is indicated in the co-administration of escitalopram and drugs metabolized by CYP2D6). Products include:
Adderall Tablets ... 3164
Adderall XR Capsules ... 3166

Amphetamine Aspartate Monohydrate (Caution is indicated in the co-administration of escitalopram and drugs metabolized by CYP2D6).
No products indexed under this heading.

Amphetamine Sulfate (Caution is indicated in the co-administration of escitalopram and drugs metabolized by CYP2D6). Products include:
Adderall Tablets ... 3164
Adderall XR Capsules ... 3166

Anisindione (The combined use of psychotropic drugs that interfere with serotonin reuptake and drugs that affect coagulation has been associated with an increased risk of bleeding). Products include:
Miradon Tablets ... 3042

Ardeparin Sodium (The combined use of psychotropic drugs that interfere with serotonin reuptake and drugs that affect coagulation has been associated with an increased risk of bleeding).
No products indexed under this heading.

Aspirin (The combined use of psychotropic drugs that interfere with serotonin reuptake and drugs that affect coagulation has been associated with an increased risk of bleeding. Use caution when co-administering). Products include:
Aggrenox Capsules ... 822
Bayer Aspirin ... 744
BC Allergy Sinus Cold Powder ... 677
BC Headache Powder ... 677
Arthritis Strength BC Powder ... 677
BC Sinus Cold Powder ... 677
Excedrin Extra Strength Caplets/Tablets/Geltabs ... 684
Excedrin Migraine Caplets/Tablets/Geltabs ... 609
Goody's Body Pain Formula Powder ... 684
Goody's Extra Strength Headache Powders ... 611
Goody's Extra Strength Pain Relief Tablets ... 685
Percodan Tablets ... 1132
St. Joseph 81 mg Aspirin Chewable and Enteric Coated Tablets ... 1869

Aspirin, Enteric Coated (The combined use of psychotropic drugs that interfere with serotonin reuptake and drugs that affect coagulation has been associated with an increased risk of bleeding. Use caution when co-administering).
No products indexed under this heading.

Aspirin Buffered (The combined use of psychotropic drugs that interfere with serotonin reuptake and drugs that affect coagulation has been associated with an increased risk of bleeding. Use caution when co-administering). Products include:
Bufferin Extra Strength Tablets ... 678
Bufferin Regular Strength Tablets ... 678

Atomoxetine Hydrochloride (Caution is indicated in the co-administration of escitalopram and drugs metabolized by CYP2D6). Products include:
Strattera Capsules ... 1814

Bisoprolol Fumarate (Caution is indicated in the co-administration of escitalopram and drugs metabolized by CYP2D6).
No products indexed under this heading.

Captopril (Caution is indicated in the co-administration of escitalopram and drugs metabolized by CYP2D6). Products include:
Captopril Tablets ... 2149

Carbamazepine (Potential for increased clearance of escitalopram, although trough citalopram plasma levels were unaffected during co-administration. The possibility that carbamazepine might increase the clearance of escitalopram should be considered if the two drugs are co-administered). Products include:
Carbatrol Capsules ... 3171
Equetro Extended-Release Capsules ... 3180
Tegretol/Tegretol-XR ... 2295

Carvedilol (Caution is indicated in the co-administration of escitalopram and drugs metabolized by CYP2D6). Products include:
Coreg Tablets ... 1414

Celecoxib (The combined use of psychotropic drugs that interfere with serotonin reuptake and drugs that affect coagulation has been associated with an increased risk of bleeding; use caution when co-administering). Products include:
Celebrex Capsules ... 3134

Cevimeline Hydrochloride (Caution is indicated in the co-administration of escitalopram and drugs metabolized by CYP2D6). Products include:
Evoxac Capsules ... 1047

Chlorpromazine (Caution is indicated in the co-administration of escitalopram and drugs metabolized by CYP2D6).
No products indexed under this heading.

Chlorpromazine Hydrochloride (Caution is indicated in the co-administration of escitalopram and drugs metabolized by CYP2D6).
No products indexed under this heading.

Chlorpropamide (Caution is indicated in the co-administration of escitalopram and drugs metabolized by CYP2D6).
No products indexed under this heading.

Cimetidine (Co-administration of racemic citalopram with cimetidine has resulted in an increase in citalopram AUC and Cmax). Products include:
Tagamet HB 200 Tablets ... 664

Cimetidine Hydrochloride (Co-administration of racemic citalopram with cimetidine has resulted in an increase in citalopram AUC and Cmax).
No products indexed under this heading.

Citalopram Hydrobromide (Since escitalopram is the active isomer of racemic citalopram, the two agents should not be co-administered). Products include:
Celexa ... 1176

Clomipramine Hydrochloride (Caution is indicated in the co-administration of escitalopram and drugs metabolized by CYP2D6).
No products indexed under this heading.

Clozapine (Caution is indicated in the co-administration of escitalopram and drugs metabolized by CYP2D6). Products include:
Clozaril Tablets ... 2184
FazaClo Orally Disintegrating Tablets ... 551

Codeine Phosphate (Caution is indicated in the co-administration of escitalopram and drugs metabolized by CYP2D6). Products include:
Tylenol with Codeine Tablets ... 2391

Codeine Sulfate (Caution is indicated in the co-administration of escitalopram and drugs metabolized by CYP2D6).
No products indexed under this heading.

Cyclobenzaprine Hydrochloride (Caution is indicated in the co-administration of escitalopram and drugs metabolized by CYP2D6).
No products indexed under this heading.

Dalteparin Sodium (The combined use of psychotropic drugs that interfere with serotonin reuptake and drugs that affect coagulation has been associated with an increased risk of bleeding). Products include:
Fragmin Injection ... 1097

Danaparoid Sodium (The combined use of psychotropic drugs that interfere with serotonin reuptake and drugs that affect coagulation has been associated with an increased risk of bleeding).
No products indexed under this heading.

Desipramine Hydrochloride (Co-administration has resulted in an increase in Cmax and AUC of desipramine; the clinical significance of this finding is unknown).
No products indexed under this heading.

Dexfenfluramine Hydrochloride (Caution is indicated in the co-administration of escitalopram and drugs metabolized by CYP2D6).
No products indexed under this heading.

Dextromethorphan Hydrobromide (Caution is indicated in the co-administration of escitalopram and drugs metabolized by CYP2D6). Products include:
Comtrex Maximum Strength Cold & Cough Day/Night Caplets - Day Formulation ... 726
Comtrex Maximum Strength Cold & Cough Day/Night Caplets - Night Formulation ... 726
Comtrex Maximum Strength Non-Drowsy Cold & Cough Caplets ... 725
Children's Dimetapp DM Cold & Cough Elixir ... 731
Children's Dimetapp Long Acting Cough Plus Cold Syrup ... 731
Toddler's Dimetapp Cold and Cough Drops ... 732
Mucinex DM Extended-Release Bi-Layer Tablets ... 720
Refenesen DM Caplets ... 721
Robitussin Cough & Cold CF Liquid ... 735
Robitussin Cough & Cold Long-Acting Liquid ... 735
Robitussin Cough & Allergy Syrup ... 736
Robitussin Cough & Cold Nighttime Liquid ... 736
Robitussin Cough & Cold Pediatric Drops ... 735
Robitussin Cough, Cold & Flu Nighttime Liquid ... 738
Robitussin Cough & Congestion Liquid ... 738
Robitussin Cough Gels Long-Acting ... 737

Dextromethorphan Polistirex
(Caution is indicated in the co-administration of escitalopram and drugs metabolized by CYP2D6). Products include:

Diclofenac Potassium (The combined use of psychotropic drugs that interfere with serotonin reuptake and drugs that affect coagulation has been associated with an increased risk of bleeding; use caution when co-administering).
 No products indexed under this heading.

Diclofenac Sodium (The combined use of psychotropic drugs that interfere with serotonin reuptake and drugs that affect coagulation has been associated with an increased risk of bleeding; use caution when co-administering). Products include:

Dicumarol (The combined use of psychotropic drugs that interfere with serotonin reuptake and drugs that affect coagulation has been associated with an increased risk of bleeding).
 No products indexed under this heading.

Dolasetron Mesylate (Caution is indicated in the co-administration of escitalopram and drugs metabolized by CYP2D6). Products include:

Donepezil Hydrochloride (Caution is indicated in the co-administration of escitalopram and drugs metabolized by CYP2D6). Products include:

Doxepin Hydrochloride (Caution is indicated in the co-administration of escitalopram and drugs metabolized by CYP2D6).
 No products indexed under this heading.

Encainide Hydrochloride (Caution is indicated in the co-administration of escitalopram and drugs metabolized by CYP2D6).
 No products indexed under this heading.

Enoxaparin Sodium (The combined use of psychotropic drugs that interfere with serotonin reuptake and drugs that affect coagulation has been associated with an increased risk of bleeding). Products include:

Etodolac (The combined use of psychotropic drugs that interfere with serotonin reuptake and drugs that affect coagulation has been associated with an increased risk of bleeding; use caution when co-administering).
 No products indexed under this heading.

Fenoprofen Calcium (The combined use of psychotropic drugs that interfere with serotonin reuptake and drugs that affect coagulation has been associated with an increased risk of bleeding; use caution when co-administering). Products include:

Fentanyl (Caution is indicated in the co-administration of escitalopram and drugs metabolized by CYP2D6). Products include:

Fentanyl Citrate (Caution is indicated in the co-administration of escitalopram and drugs metabolized by CYP2D6). Products include:

Flecainide Acetate (Caution is indicated in the co-administration of escitalopram and drugs metabolized by CYP2D6). Products include:

Fluoxetine (Caution is indicated in the co-administration of escitalopram and drugs metabolized by CYP2D6).
 No products indexed under this heading.

Fluoxetine Hydrochloride (Caution is indicated in the co-administration of escitalopram and drugs metabolized by CYP2D6). Products include:

Fluphenazine Decanoate (Caution is indicated in the co-administration of escitalopram and drugs metabolized by CYP2D6).
 No products indexed under this heading.

Fluphenazine Enanthate (Caution is indicated in the co-administration of escitalopram and drugs metabolized by CYP2D6).
 No products indexed under this heading.

Fluphenazine Hydrochloride (Caution is indicated in the co-administration of escitalopram and drugs metabolized by CYP2D6).
 No products indexed under this heading.

Flurbiprofen (The combined use of psychotropic drugs that interfere with serotonin reuptake and drugs that affect coagulation has been associated with an increased risk of bleeding; use caution when co-administering).
 No products indexed under this heading.

Fluvoxamine Maleate (Caution is indicated in the co-administration of escitalopram and drugs metabolized by CYP2D6).
 No products indexed under this heading.

Fondaparinux Sodium (The combined use of psychotropic drugs that interfere with serotonin reuptake and drugs that affect coagulation has been associated with an increased risk of bleeding). Products include:

Formoterol Fumarate (Caution is indicated in the co-administration of escitalopram and drugs metabolized by CYP2D6). Products include:

Galantamine Hydrobromide (Caution is indicated in the co-administration of escitalopram and drugs metabolized by CYP2D6). Products include:

Haloperidol (Caution is indicated in the co-administration of escitalopram and drugs metabolized by CYP2D6).
 No products indexed under this heading.

Haloperidol Decanoate (Caution is indicated in the co-administration of escitalopram and drugs metabolized by CYP2D6).
 No products indexed under this heading.

Heparin Calcium (The combined use of psychotropic drugs that interfere with serotonin reuptake and drugs that affect coagulation has been associated with an increased risk of bleeding).
 No products indexed under this heading.

Heparin Sodium (The combined use of psychotropic drugs that interfere with serotonin reuptake and drugs that affect coagulation has been associated with an increased risk of bleeding).
 No products indexed under this heading.

Hydrocodone Bitartrate (Caution is indicated in the co-administration of escitalopram and drugs metabolized by CYP2D6). Products include:

Ibuprofen (The combined use of psychotropic drugs that interfere with serotonin reuptake and drugs that affect coagulation has been associated with an increased risk of bleeding; use caution when co-administering). Products include:

Imipramine Hydrochloride (Caution is indicated in the co-administration of escitalopram and drugs metabolized by CYP2D6).
No products indexed under this heading.

Imipramine Pamoate (Caution is indicated in the co-administration of escitalopram and drugs metabolized by CYP2D6).
No products indexed under this heading.

Indomethacin (The combined use of psychotropic drugs that interfere with serotonin reuptake and drugs that affect coagulation has been associated with an increased risk of bleeding; use caution when co-administering). Products include:
Indocin 1995

Indomethacin Sodium Trihydrate (The combined use of psychotropic drugs that interfere with serotonin reuptake and drugs that affect coagulation has been associated with an increased risk of bleeding; use caution when co-administering). Products include:
Indocin I.V. 2465

Indoramin Hydrochloride (Caution is indicated in the co-administration of escitalopram and drugs metabolized by CYP2D6).
No products indexed under this heading.

Isocarboxazid (Co-administration of SSRIs and MAO inhibitors has resulted in serious, sometimes fatal, reactions including hyperthermia, rigidity, myoclonus, autonomic instability, agitation progressing to delirium and coma; concurrent and/or sequential use is contraindicated).
No products indexed under this heading.

Ketoconazole (Co-administration of racemic citalopram and ketoconazole resulted in decrease in Cmax and AUC of ketoconazole). Products include:
Nizoral A-D Shampoo, 1% 1868

Ketoprofen (The combined use of psychotropic drugs that interfere with serotonin reuptake and drugs that affect coagulation has been associated with an increased risk of bleeding; use caution when co-administering).
No products indexed under this heading.

Ketorolac Tromethamine (The combined use of psychotropic drugs that interfere with serotonin reuptake and drugs that affect coagulation has been associated with an increased risk of bleeding; use caution when co-administering). Products include:
Acular Ophthalmic Solution 565
Acular LS Ophthalmic Solution 566

Labetalol Hydrochloride (Caution is indicated in the co-administration of escitalopram and drugs metabolized by CYP2D6).
No products indexed under this heading.

Lidocaine (Caution is indicated in the co-administration of escitalopram and drugs metabolized by CYP2D6). Products include:
Lidoderm Patch 1118
Synera Topical Patch 1137

Lidocaine Hydrochloride (Caution is indicated in the co-administration of escitalopram and drugs metabolized by CYP2D6).
No products indexed under this heading.

Lithium (Serotonergic effects of escitalopram may be enhanced by lithium; co-administration had no significant effect on the pharmacokinetics of citalopram or lithium. Use caution when co-administering).
No products indexed under this heading.

Lithium Carbonate (Serotonergic effects of escitalopram may be enhanced by lithium; co-administration had no significant effect on the pharmacokinetics of citalopram or lithium. Use caution when co-administering). Products include:
Lithobid Tablets 1692

Lithium Citrate (Serotonergic effects of escitalopram may be enhanced by lithium; co-administration had no significant effect on the pharmacokinetics of citalopram or lithium. Use caution when co-administering).
No products indexed under this heading.

Low Molecular Weight Heparins (The combined use of psychotropic drugs that interfere with serotonin reuptake and drugs that affect coagulation has been associated with an increased risk of bleeding).
No products indexed under this heading.

Maprotiline Hydrochloride (Caution is indicated in the co-administration of escitalopram and drugs metabolized by CYP2D6).
No products indexed under this heading.

Meclofenamate Sodium (The combined use of psychotropic drugs that interfere with serotonin reuptake and drugs that affect coagulation has been associated with an increased risk of bleeding; use caution when co-administering).
No products indexed under this heading.

Mefenamic Acid (The combined use of psychotropic drugs that interfere with serotonin reuptake and drugs that affect coagulation has been associated with an increased risk of bleeding; use caution when co-administering).
No products indexed under this heading.

Meloxicam (The combined use of psychotropic drugs that interfere with serotonin reuptake and drugs that affect coagulation has been associated with an increased risk of bleeding; use caution when co-administering). Products include:
Mobic Oral Suspension 863
Mobic Tablets 863

Meperidine Hydrochloride (Caution is indicated in the co-administration of escitalopram and drugs metabolized by CYP2D6).
No products indexed under this heading.

Methadone Hydrochloride (Caution is indicated in the co-administration of escitalopram and drugs metabolized by CYP2D6).
No products indexed under this heading.

Methamphetamine Hydrochloride (Caution is indicated in the co-administration of escitalopram and drugs metabolized by CYP2D6). Products include:
Desoxyn Tablets, USP 2462

Metoprolol Succinate (Co-administration has resulted in an increase in Cmax and AUC of metoprolol; increased metoprolol plasma levels have been associated with decreased cardioselectivity). Products include:
Toprol-XL Tablets 668

Metoprolol Tartrate (Co-administration has resulted in an increase in Cmax and AUC of metoprolol; increased metoprolol plasma levels have been associated with decreased cardioselectivity). Products include:
Lopressor Injection 2238
Lopressor Tablets 2238
Lopressor HCT 50/25 Tablets 2241
Lopressor HCT 100/25 Tablets 2241
Lopressor HCT 100/50 Tablets 2241

Mexiletine Hydrochloride (Caution is indicated in the co-administration of escitalopram and drugs metabolized by CYP2D6).
No products indexed under this heading.

Mirtazapine (Caution is indicated in the co-administration of escitalopram and drugs metabolized by CYP2D6).
No products indexed under this heading.

Moclobemide (Co-administration of SSRIs and MAO inhibitors has resulted in serious, sometimes fatal, reactions including hyperthermia, rigidity, myoclonus, autonomic instability, agitation progressing to delirium and coma; concurrent and/or sequential use is contraindicated).
No products indexed under this heading.

Morphine Sulfate (Caution is indicated in the co-administration of escitalopram and drugs metabolized by CYP2D6). Products include:
Avinza Capsules 1741
Kadian Capsules 577
MS Contin Tablets 2701

Nabumetone (The combined use of psychotropic drugs that interfere with serotonin reuptake and drugs that affect coagulation has been associated with an increased risk of bleeding; use caution when co-administering).
No products indexed under this heading.

Naproxen (The combined use of psychotropic drugs that interfere with serotonin reuptake and drugs that affect coagulation has been associated with an increased risk of bleeding; use caution when co-administering). Products include:
EC-Naprosyn Delayed-Release Tablets 2761
Naprosyn Suspension 2761
Naprosyn Tablets 2761
Prevacid NapraPAC 3280

Naproxen Sodium (The combined use of psychotropic drugs that interfere with serotonin reuptake and drugs that affect coagulation has been associated with an increased risk of bleeding; use caution when co-administering). Products include:
Aleve Caplets 742
Aleve Gelcaps 743
Aleve Tablets 743
Aleve Cold & Sinus Caplets 744
Anaprox Tablets 2761
Anaprox DS Tablets 2761

Nelfinavir Mesylate (Caution is indicated in the co-administration of escitalopram and drugs metabolized by CYP2D6). Products include:
Viracept 2577

Nortriptyline Hydrochloride (Caution is indicated in the co-administration of escitalopram and drugs metabolized by CYP2D6).
No products indexed under this heading.

Olanzapine (Caution is indicated in the co-administration of escitalopram and drugs metabolized by CYP2D6). Products include:
Symbyax Capsules 1819
Zyprexa Tablets 1830
Zyprexa IntraMuscular 1830
Zyprexa ZYDIS Orally Disintegrating Tablets 1830

Omeprazole (Caution is indicated in the co-administration of escitalopram and drugs metabolized by CYP2D6). Products include:
Zegerid Capsules 2958
Zegerid Powder for Oral Solution 2958

Ondansetron (Caution is indicated in the co-administration of escitalopram and drugs metabolized by CYP2D6). Products include:
Zofran ODT Orally Disintegrating Tablets 1639

Ondansetron Hydrochloride (Caution is indicated in the co-administration of escitalopram and drugs metabolized by CYP2D6). Products include:
Zofran Injection 1634
Zofran 1639

Oxaprozin (The combined use of psychotropic drugs that interfere with serotonin reuptake and drugs that affect coagulation has been associated with an increased risk of bleeding; use caution when co-administering).
No products indexed under this heading.

Oxycodone Hydrochloride (Caution is indicated in the co-administration of escitalopram and drugs metabolized by CYP2D6). Products include:
OxyContin Tablets 2703
OxyFast Oral Concentrate Solution 2708
OxyIR Capsules 2708
Percocet Tablets 1131
Percodan Tablets 1132

Paclitaxel (Caution is indicated in the co-administration of escitalopram and drugs metabolized by CYP2D6).
No products indexed under this heading.

Pargyline Hydrochloride (Co-administration of SSRIs and MAO inhibitors has resulted in serious, sometimes fatal, reactions including hyperthermia, rigidity, myoclonus, autonomic instability, agitation progressing to delirium and coma; concurrent and/or sequential use is contraindicated).
No products indexed under this heading.

Paroxetine Hydrochloride (Caution is indicated in the co-administration of escitalopram and drugs metabolized by CYP2D6). Products include:
Paxil CR Controlled-Release Tablets 1538
Paxil 1530

Phenelzine Sulfate (Co-administration of SSRIs and MAO inhibitors has resulted in serious, sometimes fatal, reactions including hyperthermia, rigidity, myoclonus, autonomic instability, agitation progressing to delirium and coma; concurrent and/or sequential use is contraindicated).
No products indexed under this heading.

Phenylbutazone (The combined use of psychotropic drugs that interfere with serotonin reuptake and drugs that affect coagulation has been associated with an increased risk of bleeding; use caution when co-administering).
No products indexed under this heading.

Pimozide (In a controlled study, a single dose of pimozide 2 mg co-administered with citalopram 40 mg given once daily for 11 days was associated with a mean increase in QTc values of approximately 10 msec. compared to pimozide given alone).
No products indexed under this heading.

Pindolol (Caution is indicated in the co-administration of escitalopram and drugs metabolized by CYP2D6).
No products indexed under this heading.

Piroxicam (The combined use of psychotropic drugs that interfere with serotonin reuptake and drugs that affect coagulation has been associated with an increased risk of bleeding; use caution when co-administering).
No products indexed under this heading.

Procarbazine Hydrochloride (Co-administration of SSRIs and MAO inhibitors has resulted in serious, sometimes fatal, reactions including hyperthermia, rigidity, myoclonus, autonomic instability, agitation progressing to delirium and coma; concurrent and/or sequential use is contraindicated). Products include:
Matulane Capsules 3191

Propafenone Hydrochloride (Caution is indicated in the co-administration of escitalopram and drugs metabolized by CYP2D6). Products include:
Rythmol SR Capsules 2727

Propoxyphene Hydrochloride (Caution is indicated in the co-administration of escitalopram and drugs metabolized by CYP2D6).
No products indexed under this heading.

Propoxyphene Napsylate (Caution is indicated in the co-administration of escitalopram and drugs metabolized by CYP2D6).
No products indexed under this heading.

Propranolol Hydrochloride (Caution is indicated in the co-administration of escitalopram and drugs metabolized by CYP2D6).
Products include:
Inderal LA Long-Acting Capsules 3429
InnoPran XL Capsules 2723

Quetiapine Fumarate (Caution is indicated in the co-administration of escitalopram and drugs metabolized by CYP2D6). Products include:
Seroquel Tablets 690

Quinidine Gluconate (Caution is indicated in the co-administration of escitalopram and drugs metabolized by CYP2D6).
No products indexed under this heading.

Quinidine Hydrochloride (Caution is indicated in the co-administration of escitalopram and drugs metabolized by CYP2D6).
No products indexed under this heading.

Quinidine Polygalacturonate (Caution is indicated in the co-administration of escitalopram and drugs metabolized by CYP2D6).
No products indexed under this heading.

Quinidine Sulfate (Caution is indicated in the co-administration of escitalopram and drugs metabolized by CYP2D6).
No products indexed under this heading.

Risperidone (Caution is indicated in the co-administration of escitalopram and drugs metabolized by CYP2D6). Products include:
Risperdal 1676
Risperdal Consta Long-Acting Injection 1682
Risperdal M-Tab Orally Disintegrating Tablets 1676

Ritonavir (Caution is indicated in the co-administration of escitalopram and drugs metabolized by CYP2D6). Products include:
Kaletra 476
Norvir .. 503

Rofecoxib (The combined use of psychotropic drugs that interfere with serotonin reuptake and drugs that affect coagulation has been associated with an increased risk of bleeding; use caution when co-administering).
No products indexed under this heading.

Selegiline Hydrochloride (Co-administration of SSRIs and MAO inhibitors has resulted in serious, sometimes fatal, reactions including hyperthermia, rigidity, myoclonus, autonomic instability, agitation progressing to delirium and coma; concurrent and/or sequential use is contraindicated). Products include:
Eldepryl Capsules 3208
Zelapar Tablets 3372

Sulindac (The combined use of psychotropic drugs that interfere with serotonin reuptake and drugs that affect coagulation has been associated with an increased risk of bleeding; use caution when co-administering). Products include:
Clinoril Tablets 1924

Sumatriptan (Co-administration of SSRIs and sumatriptan has resulted in weakness, hyperreflexia, and incoordination). Products include:
Imitrex Nasal Spray 1467

Sumatriptan Succinate (Co-administration of SSRIs and

sumatriptan has resulted in weakness, hyperreflexia, and incoordination). Products include:
Imitrex Injection 1463
Imitrex Tablets 1471

Tamoxifen Citrate (Caution is indicated in the co-administration of escitalopram and drugs metabolized by CYP2D6). Products include:
Soltamox Oral Solution 3527

Teniposide (Caution is indicated in the co-administration of escitalopram and drugs metabolized by CYP2D6).
No products indexed under this heading.

Testosterone (Caution is indicated in the co-administration of escitalopram and drugs metabolized by CYP2D6). Products include:
AndroGel 3329
Striant Mucoadhesive 1007
Testim 1% Gel 695

Testosterone Cypionate (Caution is indicated in the co-administration of escitalopram and drugs metabolized by CYP2D6).
No products indexed under this heading.

Testosterone Enanthate (Caution is indicated in the co-administration of escitalopram and drugs metabolized by CYP2D6).
No products indexed under this heading.

Testosterone Propionate (Caution is indicated in the co-administration of escitalopram and drugs metabolized by CYP2D6).
No products indexed under this heading.

Thioridazine (Caution is indicated in the co-administration of escitalopram and drugs metabolized by CYP2D6).
No products indexed under this heading.

Thioridazine Hydrochloride (Caution is indicated in the co-administration of escitalopram and drugs metabolized by CYP2D6). Products include:
Thioridazine Hydrochloride Tablets 2163

Timolol Maleate (Caution is indicated in the co-administration of escitalopram and drugs metabolized by CYP2D6). Products include:
Blocadren Tablets 1916
Cosopt Sterile Ophthalmic Solution 1931
Timolide Tablets 2086
Timoptic Sterile Ophthalmic Solution 2088
Timoptic in Ocudose 2091
Timoptic-XE Sterile Ophthalmic Gel Forming Solution 2092

Tinzaparin Sodium (The combined use of psychotropic drugs that interfere with serotonin reuptake and drugs that affect coagulation has been associated with an increased risk of bleeding).
No products indexed under this heading.

Tolmetin Sodium (The combined use of psychotropic drugs that interfere with serotonin reuptake and drugs that affect coagulation has been associated with an increased risk of bleeding; use caution when co-administering).
No products indexed under this heading.

Tolterodine Tartrate (Caution is indicated in the co-administration of escitalopram and drugs metabolized by CYP2D6). Products include:
Detrol Tablets 2628
Detrol LA Capsules 2631

Tramadol Hydrochloride (Caution is indicated in the co-administration of escitalopram and drugs metabolized by CYP2D6). Products include:
Ultram ER Tablets 2392

Tranylcypromine Sulfate (Co-administration of SSRIs and MAO inhibitors has resulted in serious, sometimes fatal, reactions including hyperthermia, rigidity, myoclonus, autonomic instability, agitation progressing to delirium and coma; concurrent and/or sequential use is contraindicated). Products include:
Parnate Tablets 1527

Trazodone Hydrochloride (Caution is indicated in the co-administration of escitalopram and drugs metabolized by CYP2D6).
No products indexed under this heading.

Triazolam (Caution is indicated in the co-administration of escitalopram and drugs metabolized by CYP2D6).
No products indexed under this heading.

Trimipramine Maleate (Caution is indicated in the co-administration of escitalopram and drugs metabolized by CYP2D6).
No products indexed under this heading.

Valdecoxib (The combined use of psychotropic drugs that interfere with serotonin reuptake and drugs that affect coagulation has been associated with an increased risk of bleeding; use caution when co-administering).
No products indexed under this heading.

Venlafaxine Hydrochloride (Caution is indicated in the co-administration of escitalopram and drugs metabolized by CYP2D6). Products include:
Effexor Tablets 3411
Effexor XR Capsules 3417

Vinblastine Sulfate (Caution is indicated in the co-administration of escitalopram and drugs metabolized by CYP2D6).
No products indexed under this heading.

Warfarin Sodium (The combined use of psychotropic drugs that interfere with serotonin reuptake and drugs that affect coagulation has been associated with an increased risk of bleeding). Products include:
Coumadin for Injection 898
Coumadin Tablets 898

Zonisamide (Caution is indicated in the co-administration of escitalopram and drugs metabolized by CYP2D6). Products include:
Zonegran Capsules 1101

Food Interactions

Alcohol (Given the primary CNS effects of escitalopram, concurrent use is not recommended).

LEXIVA TABLETS

(Fosamprenavir Calcium) 1505
May interact with cytochrome p450 3a4 inducers (selected), cytochrome p450 3a4 inhibitors (selected), cytochrome p450 3a4 substrates (selected), histamine H2-receptor antagonists, phenytoin, and certain other agents. Compounds in these categories include:

Acetazolamide (Amprenavir, the active metabolite of fosamprenavir, is metabolized in the liver by the cytochrome P450 enzyme system. Amprenavir may inhibit or induce CYP3A4. Caution should be used when co-administering medications that are substrates, inhibitors, or inducers of CYP3A4, or potentially toxic medications that are metabolized by CYP3A4).
No products indexed under this heading.

Alfentanil Hydrochloride (Amprenavir, the active metabolite of fosamprenavir, is metabolized in the liver by the cytochrome P450 enzyme system. Amprenavir may inhibit or induce CYP3A4. Caution should be used when co-administering medications that are substrates, inhibitors, or inducers of CYP3A4, or potentially toxic medications that are metabolized by CYP3A4).
No products indexed under this heading.

Allium sativum (Amprenavir, the active metabolite of fosamprenavir, is metabolized in the liver by the cytochrome P450 enzyme system. Amprenavir may inhibit or induce CYP3A4. Caution should be used when co-administering medications that are substrates, inhibitors, or inducers of CYP3A4, or potentially toxic medications that are metabolized by CYP3A4).
No products indexed under this heading.

Alprazolam (Co-administration may increase alprazolam levels; may need to decrease alprazolam dose). Products include:
Niravam Orally Disintegrating Tablets 3092

Amiodarone Hydrochloride (Co-administration may lead to increased levels of amiodarone. Caution is warranted and therapeutic concentration monitoring is recommended for antiarrhythmics when co-administered with fosamprenavir).
No products indexed under this heading.

Amitriptyline Hydrochloride (Co-administration may lead to increased levels of amitriptyline. Therapeutic concentration monitoring is recommended for tricyclic antidepressants when co-administered with fosamprenavir).
No products indexed under this heading.

Amlodipine Besylate (Co-administration may increase levels of amlodipine; caution is warranted and clinical monitoring is recommended). Products include:
Caduet Tablets 2508
Lotrel Capsules 2249
Norvasc Tablets 2545

Amprenavir (Amprenavir, the active metabolite of fosamprenavir, is metabolized in the liver by the cytochrome P450 enzyme system. Amprenavir may inhibit or induce CYP3A4. Caution should be used when co-administering medications that are substrates, inhibitors, or inducers of CYP3A4, or potentially toxic medications that are metabolized by CYP3A4). Products include:
Agenerase Capsules 1327
Agenerase Oral Solution 1332

Anastrozole (Amprenavir, the active metabolite of fosamprenavir, is metabolized in the liver by the cytochrome P450 enzyme system. Amprenavir may inhibit or induce CYP3A4. Caution should be used when co-administering medications that are substrates, inhibitors, or inducers of CYP3A4, or potentially toxic medications that are metabolized by CYP3A4). Products include:
Arimidex Tablets 673

Aprepitant (Amprenavir, the active metabolite of fosamprenavir, is metabolized in the liver by the cytochrome P450 enzyme system. Amprenavir may inhibit or induce CYP3A4. Caution should be used when co-administering medications that are substrates, inhibitors, or inducers of CYP3A4, or potentially toxic medications that are metabolized by CYP3A4). Products include:
Emend Capsules 1963

Astemizole (Amprenavir, the active metabolite of fosamprenavir, is metabolized in the liver by the cytochrome P450 enzyme system. Amprenavir may inhibit or induce CYP3A4. Caution should be used when co-administering medications that are substrates, inhibitors, or inducers of CYP3A4, or potentially toxic medications that are metabolized by CYP3A4).
No products indexed under this heading.

Atazanavir (Co-administration with fosamprenavir/ritonavir combination may lead to decreased levels of atazanavir).
No products indexed under this heading.

Atazanavir sulfate (Co-administration with fosamprenavir/ritonavir combination may lead to decreased levels of atazanavir). Products include:
Reyataz Capsules 921

Atorvastatin Calcium (Co-administration may lead to increased atorvastatin levels. Use ≤20mg/day of atorvastatin with careful monitoring or consider other HMG-CoA reductase inhibitors in combination with fosamprenavir). Products include:
Caduet Tablets 2508
Lipitor Tablets 2483

Belladonna Ergotamine (Amprenavir, the active metabolite of fosamprenavir, is metabolized in the liver by the cytochrome P450 enzyme system. Amprenavir may inhibit or induce CYP3A4. Caution should be used when co-administering medications that are substrates, inhibitors, or inducers of CYP3A4, or potentially toxic medications that are metabolized by CYP3A4).
No products indexed under this heading.

Bepridil Hydrochloride (Co-administration may lead to increased levels of bepridil. Use with caution; increased levels of bepridil may be associated with life-threatening reactions such as cardiac arrhythmias).
No products indexed under this heading.

Betamethasone Acetate (Amprenavir, the active metabolite of fosamprenavir, is metabolized in the liver by the cytochrome P450 enzyme system. Amprenavir may inhibit or induce CYP3A4. Caution should be used when co-administering medications that are substrates, inhibitors, or inducers of CYP3A4, or potentially toxic medications that are metabolized by CYP3A4).
No products indexed under this heading.

Betamethasone Sodium Phosphate (Amprenavir, the active metabolite of fosamprenavir, is metabolized in the liver by the cytochrome P450 enzyme system. Amprenavir may inhibit or induce CYP3A4. Caution should be used when co-administering medications that are substrates, inhibitors, or inducers of CYP3A4, or potentially toxic medications that are metabolized by CYP3A4).
No products indexed under this heading.

Buspirone Hydrochloride (Amprenavir, the active metabolite of fosamprenavir, is metabolized in the liver by the cytochrome P450 enzyme system. Amprenavir may inhibit or induce CYP3A4. Caution should be used when co-administering medications that are substrates, inhibitors, or inducers of CYP3A4, or potentially toxic medications that are metabolized by CYP3A4).
No products indexed under this heading.

Busulfan (Amprenavir, the active metabolite of fosamprenavir, is metabolized in the liver by the cytochrome P450 enzyme system. Amprenavir may inhibit or induce CYP3A4. Caution should be used when co-administering medications that are substrates, inhibitors, or inducers of CYP3A4, or potentially toxic medications that are metabolized by CYP3A4). Products include:
I.V. Busulfex 2493
Myleran Tablets 1525

Carbamazepine (Co-administration may lead to decreased amprenavir levels. Use with caution; fosamprenavir may be less effective due to decreased plasma concentrations in patients taking these agents concomitantly). Products include:
Carbatrol Capsules 3171
Equetro Extended-Release Capsules 3180
Tegretol/Tegretol-XR 2295

Cerivastatin Sodium (Amprenavir, the active metabolite of fosamprenavir, is metabolized in the liver by the cytochrome P450 enzyme system. Amprenavir may inhibit or induce CYP3A4. Caution should be used when co-administering medications that are substrates, inhibitors, or inducers of CYP3A4, or potentially toxic medications that are metabolized by CYP3A4).
No products indexed under this heading.

Chlorpheniramine (Amprenavir, the active metabolite of fosamprenavir, is metabolized in the liver by the cytochrome P450 enzyme system. Amprenavir may inhibit or induce CYP3A4. Caution should be used when co-administering medications that are substrates, inhibitors, or inducers of CYP3A4, or potentially toxic medications that are metabolized by CYP3A4).
No products indexed under this heading.

Chlorpheniramine Maleate (Amprenavir, the active metabolite of fosamprenavir, is metabolized in the liver by the cytochrome P450 enzyme system. Amprenavir may inhibit or induce CYP3A4. Caution should be used when co-administering medications that are substrates, inhibitors, or inducers of CYP3A4, or potentially toxic medications that are metabolized by CYP3A4). Products include:
Advil Allergy Sinus Caplets 770
Advil Multi-Symptom Cold Caplets 770
BC Allergy Sinus Cold Powder 677
Comtrex Maximum Strength Cold & Cough Day/Night Caplets - Night Formulation 726
Comtrex Maximum Strength Day/Night Severe Cold & Sinus Caplets - Night Formulation 725
Contac Cold and Flu Maximum Strength Caplets 728
Contac Cold and Flu Day and Night Caplets (Night Formulation Only) 727
Children's Dimetapp Long Acting Cough Plus Cold Syrup 731
Robitussin Cough & Cold Long-Acting Liquid 735
Robitussin Cough & Allergy Syrup .. 736
Robitussin Cough & Cold Nighttime Liquid 736
Robitussin Cough, Cold & Flu Nighttime Liquid 738
Robitussin Pediatric Cough & Cold Long-Acting Liquid 735
Robitussin Pediatric Cough & Cold Nighttime Liquid 736
Triaminic Cold & Allergy Liquid 746
Triaminic Cough & Runny Nose Softchews 748
Children's Tylenol Plus Flu Oral Suspension 749
Tylenol Allergy Multi-Symptom Caplets with Cool Burst and Gelcaps 1872
Children's Tylenol Plus Cold Suspension Liquid 1879
Children's Tylenol Plus Cough & Runny Nose Suspension Liquid 1879
Children's Tylenol Plus Flu Suspension Liquid 1881
Children's Tylenol Plus Multi-Symptom Cold Suspension Liquid 1879
Tylenol Cold Head Congestion Nighttime Caplets with Cool Burst 1873
Tylenol Cold Multi-Symptom Nighttime Caplets with Cool Burst 1874
Tylenol Sinus Congestion & Pain Nighttime Caplets with Cool Burst 1876

Vicks 44M Cough, Cold & Flu Relief Liquid.......... **2680**
Pediatric Vicks 44m Cough & Cold Relief Liquid.......... **2676**
Children's Vicks NyQuil Cold/Cough Relief.......... ▣**756**
Children's Vicks NyQuil Cold/Cough Relief Liquid.......... **2680**
Zicam Maximum Strength Flu Daytime.......... ▣**768**

Chlorpheniramine Polistirex (Amprenavir, the active metabolite of fosamprenavir, is metabolized in the liver by the cytochrome P450 enzyme system. Amprenavir may inhibit or induce CYP3A4. Caution should be used when co-administering medications that are substrates, inhibitors, or inducers of CYP3A4, or potentially toxic medications that are metabolized by CYP3A4). Products include:
Tussionex Pennkinetic Extended-Release Suspension.......... **3327**

Chlorpheniramine Tannate (Amprenavir, the active metabolite of fosamprenavir, is metabolized in the liver by the cytochrome P450 enzyme system. Amprenavir may inhibit or induce CYP3A4. Caution should be used when co-administering medications that are substrates, inhibitors, or inducers of CYP3A4, or potentially toxic medications that are metabolized by CYP3A4).
No products indexed under this heading.

Cimetidine (Co-administration of fosamprenavir alone and histamine H2-receptor antagonists may lead to decreased levels of fosamprenavir. Use with caution since fosamprenavir may be less effective due to decreased amprenavir plasma concentrations in patients taking these agents concomitantly). Products include:
Tagamet HB 200 Tablets.......... ▣**664**

Cimetidine Hydrochloride (Co-administration of fosamprenavir alone and histamine H2-receptor antagonists may lead to decreased levels of fosamprenavir. Use with caution since fosamprenavir may be less effective due to decreased amprenavir plasma concentrations in patients taking these agents concomitantly).
No products indexed under this heading.

Ciprofloxacin (Amprenavir, the active metabolite of fosamprenavir, is metabolized in the liver by the cytochrome P450 enzyme system. Amprenavir may inhibit or induce CYP3A4. Caution should be used when co-administering medications that are substrates, inhibitors, or inducers of CYP3A4, or potentially toxic medications that are metabolized by CYP3A4). Products include:
Cipro Oral Suspension.......... **2977**
Cipro I.V. **2984**
Cipro XR Tablets.......... **2990**
Ciprodex Otic Suspension.......... **559**

Ciprofloxacin Hydrochloride (Amprenavir, the active metabolite of fosamprenavir, is metabolized in the liver by the cytochrome P450 enzyme system. Amprenavir may inhibit or induce CYP3A4. Caution should be used when co-administering medications that are substrates, inhibitors, or inducers of CYP3A4, or potentially toxic medications that are metabolized by CYP3A4). Products include:
Ciloxan Ophthalmic Ointment.......... **559**
Ciloxan Ophthalmic Solution.......... ⊙**206**
Cipro Tablets.......... **2977**
Proquin XR Tablets.......... **1153**

Cisapride (Co-administration with cisapride is contraindicated due to the potential for serious and/or life-threatening reactions such as cardiac arrhythmias).
No products indexed under this heading.

Cisplatin (Amprenavir, the active metabolite of fosamprenavir, is metabolized in the liver by the cytochrome P450 enzyme system. Amprenavir may inhibit or induce CYP3A4. Caution should be used when co-administering medications that are substrates, inhibitors, or inducers of CYP3A4, or potentially toxic medications that are metabolized by CYP3A4).
No products indexed under this heading.

Clarithromycin (Amprenavir, the active metabolite of fosamprenavir, is metabolized in the liver by the cytochrome P450 enzyme system. Amprenavir may inhibit or induce CYP3A4. Caution should be used when co-administering medications that are substrates, inhibitors, or inducers of CYP3A4, or potentially toxic medications that are metabolized by CYP3A4). Products include:
Biaxin/Biaxin XL.......... **402**
PREVPAC.......... **3284**

Clorazepate Dipotassium (Co-administration may increase clorazepate levels; may need to decrease clorazepate dose). Products include:
Tranxene.......... **2474**

Clotrimazole (Amprenavir, the active metabolite of fosamprenavir, is metabolized in the liver by the cytochrome P450 enzyme system. Amprenavir may inhibit or induce CYP3A4. Caution should be used when co-administering medications that are substrates, inhibitors, or inducers of CYP3A4, or potentially toxic medications that are metabolized by CYP3A4). Products include:
Desenex Athlete's Foot Cream.......... ▣**635**
Lotrimin.......... **3039**
Lotrisone.......... **3040**

Cortisone Acetate (Amprenavir, the active metabolite of fosamprenavir, is metabolized in the liver by the cytochrome P450 enzyme system. Amprenavir may inhibit or induce CYP3A4. Caution should be used when co-administering medications that are substrates, inhibitors, or inducers of CYP3A4, or potentially toxic medications that are metabolized by CYP3A4).
No products indexed under this heading.

Cyclosporine (Co-administration may lead to increased levels of cyclosporine. Therapeutic concentration monitoring is recommended for immunosuppressant agents when co-administered with fosamprenavir). Products include:
Gengraf Capsules.......... **459**
Neoral Oral Solution.......... **2259**
Neoral Soft Gelatin Capsules.......... **2259**
Restasis Ophthalmic Emulsion.......... **575**
Sandimmune.......... **2275**

Dalfopristin (Amprenavir, the active metabolite of fosamprenavir, is metabolized in the liver by the cytochrome P450 enzyme system. Amprenavir may inhibit or induce CYP3A4. Caution should be used when co-administering medications that are substrates, inhibitors, or inducers of CYP3A4, or potentially toxic medications that are metabolized by CYP3A4).
No products indexed under this heading.

Danazol (Amprenavir, the active metabolite of fosamprenavir, is metabolized in the liver by the cytochrome P450 enzyme system. Amprenavir may inhibit or induce CYP3A4. Caution should be used when co-administering medications that are substrates, inhibitors, or inducers of CYP3A4, or potentially toxic medications that are metabolized by CYP3A4).
No products indexed under this heading.

Delavirdine Mesylate (Co-administration may lead to loss of virologic response and possible resistance to delavirdine). Products include:
Rescriptor Tablets.......... **2551**

Desogestrel (Amprenavir, the active metabolite of fosamprenavir, is metabolized in the liver by the cytochrome P450 enzyme system. Amprenavir may inhibit or induce CYP3A4. Caution should be used when co-administering medications that are substrates, inhibitors, or inducers of CYP3A4, or potentially toxic medications that are metabolized by CYP3A4). Products include:
Mircette Tablets.......... **1066**

Dexamethasone (Co-administration may decrease amprenavir levels. Use with caution since fosamprenavir may be less effective due to decreased amprenavir plasma concentrations in patients taking these agents concomitantly). Products include:
Ciprodex Otic Suspension.......... **559**
Decadron Tablets.......... **1951**
TobraDex Ophthalmic Ointment.......... **562**
TobraDex Ophthalmic Suspension.......... **563**

Dexamethasone Acetate (Co-administration may decrease amprenavir levels. Use with caution since fosamprenavir may be less effective due to decreased amprenavir plasma concentrations in patients taking these agents concomitantly).
No products indexed under this heading.

Dexamethasone Phosphate (Co-administration may decrease amprenavir levels. Use with caution since fosamprenavir may be less effective due to decreased amprenavir plasma concentrations in patients taking these agents concomitantly).
No products indexed under this heading.

Dexamethasone Sodium (Co-administration may decrease amprenavir levels. Use with caution since fosamprenavir may be less effective due to decreased amprenavir plasma concentrations in patients taking these agents concomitantly).
No products indexed under this heading.

Dexamethasone Sodium Phosphate (Co-administration may decrease amprenavir levels. Use with caution since fosamprenavir may be less effective due to decreased amprenavir plasma concentrations in patients taking these agents concomitantly).
No products indexed under this heading.

Dexamethasone Sodium Phosphate Injection (Co-administration may decrease amprenavir levels. Use with caution since fosamprenavir may be less effective due to decreased amprenavir plasma concentrations in patients taking these agents concomitantly).
No products indexed under this heading.

Diazepam (Co-administration may increase diazepam levels; may need to decrease diazepam dose). Products include:
Diastat Rectal Delivery System.......... **3343**
Valium Tablets.......... **2819**

Dihydroergotamine Mesylate (Co-administration with dihydroergotamine is contraindicated due to the potential for serious and/or life-threatening reactions such as acute ergot toxicity characterized by peripheral vasospasm and ischemia of the extremities and other tissues). Products include:
Migranal Nasal Spray.......... **3348**

Diltiazem Hydrochloride (Co-administration may increase levels of diltiazem; caution is warranted and clinical monitoring is recommended). Products include:
Cardizem LA Extended Release Tablets.......... **1728**
Tiazac Capsules.......... **1201**

Diltiazem Maleate (Co-administration may increase levels of diltiazem; caution is warranted and clinical monitoring is recommended).
No products indexed under this heading.

Disopyramide (Amprenavir, the active metabolite of fosamprenavir, is metabolized in the liver by the cytochrome P450 enzyme system. Amprenavir may inhibit or induce CYP3A4. Caution should be used when co-administering medications that are substrates, inhibitors, or inducers of CYP3A4, or potentially toxic medications that are metabolized by CYP3A4).
No products indexed under this heading.

Disopyramide Phosphate (Amprenavir, the active metabolite of fosamprenavir, is metabolized in the liver by the cytochrome P450 enzyme system. Amprenavir may inhibit or induce CYP3A4. Caution should be used when co-administering medications that are substrates, inhibitors, or inducers of CYP3A4, or potentially toxic medications that are metabolized by CYP3A4).
No products indexed under this heading.

Disulfiram (Amprenavir, the active metabolite of fosamprenavir, is metabolized in the liver by the cytochrome P450 enzyme system. Amprenavir may inhibit or induce CYP3A4. Caution should be used when co-administering medications that are substrates, inhibitors, or inducers of CYP3A4, or potentially toxic medications that are metabolized by CYP3A4).

No products indexed under this heading.

Doxorubicin Hydrochloride (Amprenavir, the active metabolite of fosamprenavir, is metabolized in the liver by the cytochrome P450 enzyme system. Amprenavir may inhibit or induce CYP3A4. Caution should be used when co-administering medications that are substrates, inhibitors, or inducers of CYP3A4, or potentially toxic medications that are metabolized by CYP3A4).

No products indexed under this heading.

Dronabinol (Amprenavir, the active metabolite of fosamprenavir, is metabolized in the liver by the cytochrome P450 enzyme system. Amprenavir may inhibit or induce CYP3A4. Caution should be used when co-administering medications that are substrates, inhibitors, or inducers of CYP3A4, or potentially toxic medications that are metabolized by CYP3A4). Products include:

Efavirenz (Co-administration may lead to decreased amprenavir levels. An additional 100mg/day (300mg total) of ritonavir is recommended when efavirenz is administered with fosamprenavir/ritonavir once daily. No change in the ritonavir dose is required when efavirenz is administered with fosamprenavir plus ritonavir twice daily). Products include:

Ergonovine Maleate (Co-administration with ergonovine is contraindicated due to the potential for serious and/or life-threatening reactions such as acute ergot toxicity characterized by peripheral vasospasm and ischemia of the extremities and other tissues).

No products indexed under this heading.

Ergotamine Tartrate (Co-administration with ergotamine is contraindicated due to the potential for serious and/or life-threatening reactions such as acute ergot toxicity characterized by peripheral vasospasm and ischemia of the extremities and other tissues).

No products indexed under this heading.

Erythromycin (Amprenavir, the active metabolite of fosamprenavir, is metabolized in the liver by the cytochrome P450 enzyme system. Amprenavir may inhibit or induce CYP3A4. Caution should be used when co-administering medications that are substrates, inhibitors, or inducers of CYP3A4, or potentially toxic medications that are metabolized by CYP3A4). Products include:

Erythromycin Estolate (Amprenavir, the active metabolite of fosamprenavir, is metabolized in the liver by the cytochrome P450 enzyme system. Amprenavir may inhibit or induce CYP3A4. Caution should be used when co-administering medications that are substrates, inhibitors, or inducers of CYP3A4, or potentially toxic medications that are metabolized by CYP3A4).

No products indexed under this heading.

Erythromycin Ethylsuccinate (Amprenavir, the active metabolite of fosamprenavir, is metabolized in the liver by the cytochrome P450 enzyme system. Amprenavir may inhibit or induce CYP3A4. Caution should be used when co-administering medications that are substrates, inhibitors, or inducers of CYP3A4, or potentially toxic medications that are metabolized by CYP3A4). Products include:

Erythromycin Gluceptate (Amprenavir, the active metabolite of fosamprenavir, is metabolized in the liver by the cytochrome P450 enzyme system. Amprenavir may inhibit or induce CYP3A4. Caution should be used when co-administering medications that are substrates, inhibitors, or inducers of CYP3A4, or potentially toxic medications that are metabolized by CYP3A4).

No products indexed under this heading.

Erythromycin Lactobionate (Amprenavir, the active metabolite of fosamprenavir, is metabolized in the liver by the cytochrome P450 enzyme system. Amprenavir may inhibit or induce CYP3A4. Caution should be used when co-administering medications that are substrates, inhibitors, or inducers of CYP3A4, or potentially toxic medications that are metabolized by CYP3A4).

No products indexed under this heading.

Erythromycin Stearate (Amprenavir, the active metabolite of fosamprenavir, is metabolized in the liver by the cytochrome P450 enzyme system. Amprenavir may inhibit or induce CYP3A4. Caution should be used when co-administering medications that are substrates, inhibitors, or inducers of CYP3A4, or potentially toxic medications that are metabolized by CYP3A4). Products include:

Esomeprazole Magnesium (Concurrent administration may lead to increased levels of esomeprazole). Products include:

Estradiol (Amprenavir, the active metabolite of fosamprenavir, is metabolized in the liver by the cytochrome P450 enzyme system. Amprenavir may inhibit or induce CYP3A4. Caution should be used when co-administering medications that are substrates, inhibitors, or inducers of CYP3A4, or potentially

toxic medications that are metabolized by CYP3A4). Products include:

Estradiol Benzoate (Amprenavir, the active metabolite of fosamprenavir, is metabolized in the liver by the cytochrome P450 enzyme system. Amprenavir may inhibit or induce CYP3A4. Caution should be used when co-administering medications that are substrates, inhibitors, or inducers of CYP3A4, or potentially toxic medications that are metabolized by CYP3A4).

No products indexed under this heading.

Estradiol Cypionate (Amprenavir, the active metabolite of fosamprenavir, is metabolized in the liver by the cytochrome P450 enzyme system. Amprenavir may inhibit or induce CYP3A4. Caution should be used when co-administering medications that are substrates, inhibitors, or inducers of CYP3A4, or potentially toxic medications that are metabolized by CYP3A4).

No products indexed under this heading.

Estradiol Valerate (Amprenavir, the active metabolite of fosamprenavir, is metabolized in the liver by the cytochrome P450 enzyme system. Amprenavir may inhibit or induce CYP3A4. Caution should be used when co-administering medications that are substrates, inhibitors, or inducers of CYP3A4, or potentially toxic medications that are metabolized by CYP3A4).

No products indexed under this heading.

Ethinyl Estradiol (Co-administration of fosamprenavir alone with oral contraceptives containing the combination ethinyl estradiol/norethindrone may lead to increased levels of ethinyl estradiol/norethindrone. Because these hormonal levels may be altered, alternative methods of non-hormonal contraception are recommended). Products include:

Ethosuximide (Amprenavir, the active metabolite of fosamprenavir, is metabolized in the liver by the cytochrome P450 enzyme system. Amprenavir may inhibit or induce CYP3A4. Caution should be used when co-administering medications that are substrates, inhibitors, or inducers of CYP3A4, or potentially toxic medications that are metabolized by CYP3A4).

No products indexed under this heading.

Ethynodiol Diacetate (Amprenavir, the active metabolite of fosamprenavir, is metabolized in the liver by the cytochrome P450 enzyme system. Amprenavir may inhibit or induce CYP3A4. Caution should be used when co-administering medications that are substrates, inhibitors, or inducers of CYP3A4, or potentially toxic medications that are metabolized by CYP3A4).

No products indexed under this heading.

Etoposide (Amprenavir, the active metabolite of fosamprenavir, is metabolized in the liver by the cytochrome P450 enzyme system. Amprenavir may inhibit or induce CYP3A4. Caution should be used when co-administering medications that are substrates, inhibitors, or inducers of CYP3A4, or potentially toxic medications that are metabolized by CYP3A4).

No products indexed under this heading.

Etoposide Phosphate (Amprenavir, the active metabolite of fosamprenavir, is metabolized in the liver by the cytochrome P450 enzyme system. Amprenavir may inhibit or induce CYP3A4. Caution should be used when co-administering medications that are substrates, inhibitors, or inducers of CYP3A4, or potentially toxic medications that are metabolized by CYP3A4).

No products indexed under this heading.

Famotidine (Co-administration of fosamprenavir alone and histamine H2-receptor antagonists may lead to decreased levels of fosamprenavir. Use with caution since fosamprenavir may be less effective due to decreased amprenavir plasma concentrations in patients taking these agents concomitantly). Products include:

Felbamate (Amprenavir, the active metabolite of fosamprenavir, is metabolized in the liver by the cytochrome P450 enzyme system. Amprenavir may inhibit or induce CYP3A4. Caution should be used when co-administering medications that are substrates, inhibitors, or inducers of CYP3A4, or potentially toxic medications that are metabolized by CYP3A4).

No products indexed under this heading.

Felodipine (Co-administration may increase levels of felodipine; caution is warranted and clinical monitoring is recommended).

No products indexed under this heading.

Fentanyl (Amprenavir, the active metabolite of fosamprenavir, is metabolized in the liver by the cytochrome P450 enzyme system. Amprenavir may inhibit or induce CYP3A4. Caution should be used when co-administering medications that are substrates, inhibitors, or inducers of CYP3A4, or potentially

toxic medications that are metabolized by CYP3A4). Products include:
Duragesic Transdermal System 2373
Ionsys Transdermal System 2379

Fentanyl Citrate (Amprenavir, the active metabolite of fosamprenavir, is metabolized in the liver by the cytochrome P450 enzyme system. Amprenavir may inhibit or induce CYP3A4. Caution should be used when co-administering medications that are substrates, inhibitors, or inducers of CYP3A4, or potentially toxic medications that are metabolized by CYP3A4). Products include:
Actiq 979

Flecainide Acetate (If fosamprenavir is co-administered with ritonavir, the antiarrhythmic agent flecainide is contraindicated due to the potential for serious and/or life-threatening reactions such as cardiac arrhythmias secondary to increases in plasma concentrations of flecainide). Products include:
Tambocor Tablets 1856

Fluconazole (Amprenavir, the active metabolite of fosamprenavir, is metabolized in the liver by the cytochrome P450 enzyme system. Amprenavir may inhibit or induce CYP3A4. Caution should be used when co-administering medications that are substrates, inhibitors, or inducers of CYP3A4, or potentially toxic medications that are metabolized by CYP3A4).
No products indexed under this heading.

Fludrocortisone Acetate (Amprenavir, the active metabolite of fosamprenavir, is metabolized in the liver by the cytochrome P450 enzyme system. Amprenavir may inhibit or induce CYP3A4. Caution should be used when co-administering medications that are substrates, inhibitors, or inducers of CYP3A4, or potentially toxic medications that are metabolized by CYP3A4).
No products indexed under this heading.

Fluoxetine Hydrochloride (Amprenavir, the active metabolite of fosamprenavir, is metabolized in the liver by the cytochrome P450 enzyme system. Amprenavir may inhibit or induce CYP3A4. Caution should be used when co-administering medications that are substrates, inhibitors, or inducers of CYP3A4, or potentially toxic medications that are metabolized by CYP3A4). Products include:
Prozac Pulvules and Liquid 1801
Symbyax Capsules 1819

Flurazepam Hydrochloride (Co-administration may increase flurazepam levels; may need to decrease flurazepam dose). Products include:
Dalmane Capsules 3342

Fluticasone Propionate (Co-administration may lead to increased fluticasone levels. Concomitant use of fluticasone propionate and fosamprenavir calcium (without ritonavir) may increase plasma concentrations of fluticasone propionate; use with caution and consider alternatives to fluticasone propionate, particularly for long-term use. Concomitant use of fluticasone propionate and fosamprenavir calcium/ritonavir may increase plasma concentrations of fluticasone propionate, resulting in significantly reduce serum cortisol concentrations. Co-administration of fluticasone propionate and fosamprenavir calcium/ritonavir is not recommended unless the potential benefit to the patient outweighs the risk of systemic corticosteroid side effects). Products include:
Advair Diskus 100/50 1308
Advair Diskus 250/50 1308
Advair Diskus 500/50 1308
Advair HFA Inhalation Aerosol 1318
Cutivate Cream 2662
Cutivate Lotion 0.05% 2664
Cutivate Ointment 2665
Flonase Nasal Spray 1440
Flovent Diskus 1443

Fluticasone Propionate HFA (Co-administration may lead to increased fluticasone levels. Concomitant use of fluticasone propionate and fosamprenavir calcium (without ritonavir) may increase plasma concentrations of fluticasone propionate; use with caution and consider alternatives to fluticasone propionate, particularly for long-term use. Concomitant use of fluticasone propionate and fosamprenavir calcium/ritonavir may increase plasma concentrations of fluticasone propionate, resulting in significantly reduce serum cortisol concentrations. Co-administration of fluticasone propionate and fosamprenavir calcium/ritonavir is not recommended unless the potential benefit to the patient outweighs the risk of systemic corticosteroid side effects Apr 5 2006 9:34:48:876AM). Products include:
Flovent HFA 1447

Fluvoxamine Maleate (Amprenavir, the active metabolite of fosamprenavir, is metabolized in the liver by the cytochrome P450 enzyme system. Amprenavir may inhibit or induce CYP3A4. Caution should be used when co-administering medications that are substrates, inhibitors, or inducers of CYP3A4, or potentially toxic medications that are metabolized by CYP3A4).
No products indexed under this heading.

Fosphenytoin Sodium (Co-administration may lead to decreased amprenavir levels. Use with caution; fosamprenavir may be less effective due to decreased plasma concentrations in patients taking these agents concomitantly).
No products indexed under this heading.

Garlic Extract (Amprenavir, the active metabolite of fosamprenavir, is metabolized in the liver by the cytochrome P450 enzyme system. Amprenavir may inhibit or induce CYP3A4. Caution should be used when co-administering medications that are substrates, inhibitors, or inducers of CYP3A4, or potentially toxic medications that are metabolized by CYP3A4).
No products indexed under this heading.

Garlic Oil (Amprenavir, the active metabolite of fosamprenavir, is metabolized in the liver by the cytochrome P450 enzyme system. Amprenavir may inhibit or induce CYP3A4. Caution should be used when co-administering medications that are substrates, inhibitors, or inducers of CYP3A4, or potentially toxic medications that are metabolized by CYP3A4).
No products indexed under this heading.

Haloperidol (Amprenavir, the active metabolite of fosamprenavir, is metabolized in the liver by the cytochrome P450 enzyme system. Amprenavir may inhibit or induce CYP3A4. Caution should be used when co-administering medications that are substrates, inhibitors, or inducers of CYP3A4, or potentially toxic medications that are metabolized by CYP3A4).
No products indexed under this heading.

Haloperidol Decanoate (Amprenavir, the active metabolite of fosamprenavir, is metabolized in the liver by the cytochrome P450 enzyme system. Amprenavir may inhibit or induce CYP3A4. Caution should be used when co-administering medications that are substrates, inhibitors, or inducers of CYP3A4, or potentially toxic medications that are metabolized by CYP3A4).
No products indexed under this heading.

Haloperidol Lactate (Amprenavir, the active metabolite of fosamprenavir, is metabolized in the liver by the cytochrome P450 enzyme system. Amprenavir may inhibit or induce CYP3A4. Caution should be used when co-administering medications that are substrates, inhibitors, or inducers of CYP3A4, or potentially toxic medications that are metabolized by CYP3A4).
No products indexed under this heading.

Hydrocortisone (Amprenavir, the active metabolite of fosamprenavir, is metabolized in the liver by the cytochrome P450 enzyme system. Amprenavir may inhibit or induce CYP3A4. Caution should be used when co-administering medications that are substrates, inhibitors, or inducers of CYP3A4, or potentially toxic medications that are metabolized by CYP3A4). Products include:
Colocort Rectal Suspension, USP (Retention) 100 mg/60 mL 2476
Hydrocortone Tablets 1989
Preparation H Hydrocortisone Cream .... ▣ 646

Hydrocortisone Acetate (Amprenavir, the active metabolite of fosamprenavir, is metabolized in the liver by the cytochrome P450 enzyme system. Amprenavir may inhibit or induce CYP3A4. Caution should be used when co-administering medications that are substrates, inhibitors, or inducers of CYP3A4, or potentially toxic medications that are metabolized by CYP3A4). Products include:
Analpram-HC 1159
Pramosone 1161
ProctoFoam-HC 3099

Hydrocortisone Butyrate (Amprenavir, the active metabolite of fosamprenavir, is metabolized in the liver by the cytochrome P450 enzyme system. Amprenavir may inhibit or induce CYP3A4. Caution should be used when co-administering medications that are substrates, inhibitors, or inducers of CYP3A4, or potentially toxic medications that are metabolized by CYP3A4). Products include:
Locoid Lipocream Cream 1160

Hydrocortisone Cypionate (Amprenavir, the active metabolite of fosamprenavir, is metabolized in the liver by the cytochrome P450 enzyme system. Amprenavir may inhibit or induce CYP3A4. Caution should be used when co-administering medications that are substrates, inhibitors, or inducers of CYP3A4, or potentially toxic medications that are metabolized by CYP3A4).
No products indexed under this heading.

Hydrocortisone Hemisuccinate (Amprenavir, the active metabolite of fosamprenavir, is metabolized in the liver by the cytochrome P450 enzyme system. Amprenavir may inhibit or induce CYP3A4. Caution should be used when co-administering medications that are substrates, inhibitors, or inducers of CYP3A4, or potentially toxic medications that are metabolized by CYP3A4).
No products indexed under this heading.

Hydrocortisone Probutate (Amprenavir, the active metabolite of fosamprenavir, is metabolized in the liver by the cytochrome P450 enzyme system. Amprenavir may inhibit or induce CYP3A4. Caution should be used when co-administering medications that are substrates, inhibitors, or inducers of CYP3A4, or potentially toxic medications that are metabolized by CYP3A4).
No products indexed under this heading.

Hydrocortisone Sodium Phosphate (Amprenavir, the active metabolite of fosamprenavir, is metabolized in the liver by the cytochrome P450 enzyme system. Amprenavir may inhibit or induce CYP3A4. Caution should be used when co-administering medications that are substrates, inhibitors, or inducers of CYP3A4, or potentially toxic medications that are metabolized by CYP3A4).
No products indexed under this heading.

Hydrocortisone Sodium Succinate (Amprenavir, the active metabolite of fosamprenavir, is metabolized in the liver by the cytochrome P450 enzyme system. Amprenavir may inhibit or induce CYP3A4. Caution should be used when co-administering medications that are substrates, inhibitors, or inducers of CYP3A4, or potentially toxic medications that are metabolized by CYP3A4).
No products indexed under this heading.

Hydrocortisone Valerate (Amprenavir, the active metabolite of fosamprenavir, is metabolized in the liver by the cytochrome P450 enzyme system. Amprenavir may inhibit or induce CYP3A4. Caution should be used when co-administering medications that are substrates, inhibitors, or inducers of CYP3A4, or potentially toxic medications that are metabolized by CYP3A4).
No products indexed under this heading.

Hypericum (Co-administration may lead to loss of virologic response and possible resistance to fosamprenavir or other protease inhibitors). Products include:

Satiete Tablets 832

Hypericum Perforatum (Co-administration may lead to loss of virologic response and possible resistance to fosamprenavir or other protease inhibitors).

No products indexed under this heading.

Imipramine Hydrochloride (Co-administration may lead to increased levels of imipramine. Therapeutic concentration monitoring is recommended for tricyclic antidepressants when co-administered with fosamprenavir).

No products indexed under this heading.

Imipramine Pamoate (Co-administration may lead to increased levels of imipramine. Therapeutic concentration monitoring is recommended for tricyclic antidepressants when co-administered with fosamprenavir).

No products indexed under this heading.

Indinavir Sulfate (Co-administration with fosamprenavir alone may lead to increased amprenavir levels). Products include:

Crixivan Capsules 1940

Isoniazid (Amprenavir, the active metabolite of fosamprenavir, is metabolized in the liver by the cytochrome P450 enzyme system. Amprenavir may inhibit or induce CYP3A4. Caution should be used when co-administering medications that are substrates, inhibitors, or inducers of CYP3A4, or potentially toxic medications that are metabolized by CYP3A4).

No products indexed under this heading.

Isradipine (Co-administration may increase levels of isradipine; caution is warranted and clinical monitoring is recommended). Products include:

DynaCirc CR Tablets 2721

Itraconazole (Co-administration may increase itraconazole levels; increase monitoring for adverse events due to itraconazole. When co-administered with fosamprenavir alone, itraconazole dose reduction may be needed for patients receiving more than 400mg of itraconazole per day. If patient is receiving fosamprenavir/ritonavir combination, co-administration of high doses of itraconazole (>200mg/day) are not recommended).

No products indexed under this heading.

Ketoconazole (Co-administration may increase ketoconazole levels; increase monitoring for adverse events due to ketoconazole. When co-administered with fosamprenavir alone, ketoconazole dose reduction may be needed for patients receiving more than 400mg of ketoconazole per day. If patient is receiving fosamprenavir/ritonavir combination, co-administration of high doses of ketoconazole (>200mg/day) are not recommended). Products include:

Nizoral A-D Shampoo, 1% 1868

Levonorgestrel (Amprenavir, the active metabolite of fosamprenavir, is metabolized in the liver by the cytochrome P450 enzyme system. Amprenavir may inhibit or induce CYP3A4. Caution should be used when co-administering medications that are substrates, inhibitors, or inducers of CYP3A4, or potentially toxic medications that are metabolized by CYP3A4). Products include:

Climara Pro Transdermal System 776
Mirena Intrauterine System 787
Plan B Tablets 1076
Seasonique Tablets 1077

Lidocaine (Co-administration may lead to increased levels of lidocaine. Caution is warranted and therapeutic concentration monitoring is recommended for antiarrhythmics when co-administered with fosamprenavir). Products include:

Lidoderm Patch 1118
Synera Topical Patch 1137

Lidocaine Hydrochloride (Co-administration may lead to increased levels of lidocaine. Caution is warranted and therapeutic concentration monitoring is recommended for antiarrhythmics when co-administered with fosamprenavir).

No products indexed under this heading.

Lopinavir (Co-administration of lopinavir/ritonavir and fosamprenavir may lead to decreased levels of amprenavir and lopinavir. An increased rate of adverse events has also been observed with co-administration of these medications). Products include:

Kaletra 476

Loratadine (Amprenavir, the active metabolite of fosamprenavir, is metabolized in the liver by the cytochrome P450 enzyme system. Amprenavir may inhibit or induce CYP3A4. Caution should be used when co-administering medications that are substrates, inhibitors, or inducers of CYP3A4, or potentially toxic medications that are metabolized by CYP3A4). Products include:

Alavert Allergy & Sinus D-12 Hour Tablets 771
Alavert 771
Children's Claritin Allergy Oral Solution 771
Claritin Non-Drowsy 24 Hour Tablets 772
Claritin Reditabs 24 Hour Non-Drowsy Tablets 772
Claritin-D Non-Drowsy 12 Hour Tablets 772
Claritin-D Non-Drowsy 24 Hour Tablets 772

Lovastatin (Co-administration may lead to the potential for serious reactions such as risk of myopathy including rhabdomyolysis). Products include:

Advicor Tablets 1722
Altoprev Extended-Release Tablets 3109
Mevacor Tablets 2021

Mephenytoin (Amprenavir, the active metabolite of fosamprenavir, is metabolized in the liver by the cytochrome P450 enzyme system. Amprenavir may inhibit or induce CYP3A4. Caution should be used when co-administering medications that are substrates, inhibitors, or inducers of CYP3A4, or potentially toxic medications that are metabolized by CYP3A4).

No products indexed under this heading.

Mestranol (Amprenavir, the active metabolite of fosamprenavir, is metabolized in the liver by the cytochrome P450 enzyme system. Amprenavir may inhibit or induce CYP3A4. Caution should be used when co-administering medications that are substrates, inhibitors, or inducers of CYP3A4, or potentially toxic medications that are metabolized by CYP3A4).

No products indexed under this heading.

Methadone Hydrochloride (Co-administration may lead to decreased levels of methadone; dosage of methadone may need to be increased when co-administered with fosamprenavir).

No products indexed under this heading.

Methsuximide (Amprenavir, the active metabolite of fosamprenavir, is metabolized in the liver by the cytochrome P450 enzyme system. Amprenavir may inhibit or induce CYP3A4. Caution should be used when co-administering medications that are substrates, inhibitors, or inducers of CYP3A4, or potentially toxic medications that are metabolized by CYP3A4).

No products indexed under this heading.

Methylergonovine Maleate (Co-administration with methylergonovine is contraindicated due to the potential for serious and/or life-threatening reactions such as acute ergot toxicity characterized by peripheral vasospasm and ischemia of the extremities and other tissues).

No products indexed under this heading.

Methylprednisolone (Amprenavir, the active metabolite of fosamprenavir, is metabolized in the liver by the cytochrome P450 enzyme system. Amprenavir may inhibit or induce CYP3A4. Caution should be used when co-administering medications that are substrates, inhibitors, or inducers of CYP3A4, or potentially toxic medications that are metabolized by CYP3A4).

No products indexed under this heading.

Methylprednisolone Acetate (Amprenavir, the active metabolite of fosamprenavir, is metabolized in the liver by the cytochrome P450 enzyme system. Amprenavir may inhibit or induce CYP3A4. Caution should be used when co-administering medications that are substrates, inhibitors, or inducers of CYP3A4, or potentially toxic medications that are metabolized by CYP3A4). Products include:

Depo-Medrol Injectable Suspension 2617
Depo-Medrol Single-Dose Vial 2619

Methylprednisolone Sodium Succinate (Amprenavir, the active metabolite of fosamprenavir, is metabolized in the liver by the cytochrome P450 enzyme system. Amprenavir may inhibit or induce CYP3A4. Caution should be used when co-administering medications that are substrates, inhibitors, or inducers of CYP3A4, or potentially toxic medications that are metabolized by CYP3A4).

No products indexed under this heading.

Metronidazole (Amprenavir, the active metabolite of fosamprenavir, is metabolized in the liver by the cytochrome P450 enzyme system. Amprenavir may inhibit or induce CYP3A4. Caution should be used when co-administering medications that are substrates, inhibitors, or inducers of CYP3A4, or potentially toxic medications that are metabolized by CYP3A4). Products include:

Metrogel 1% 1211
MetroGel-Vaginal Gel 1855
Vandazole Vaginal Gel 3338

Metronidazole Benzoate (Amprenavir, the active metabolite of fosamprenavir, is metabolized in the liver by the cytochrome P450 enzyme system. Amprenavir may inhibit or induce CYP3A4. Caution should be used when co-administering medications that are substrates, inhibitors, or inducers of CYP3A4, or potentially toxic medications that are metabolized by CYP3A4).

No products indexed under this heading.

Metronidazole Hydrochloride (Amprenavir, the active metabolite of fosamprenavir, is metabolized in the liver by the cytochrome P450 enzyme system. Amprenavir may inhibit or induce CYP3A4. Caution should be used when co-administering medications that are substrates, inhibitors, or inducers of CYP3A4, or potentially toxic medications that are metabolized by CYP3A4).

No products indexed under this heading.

Miconazole (Amprenavir, the active metabolite of fosamprenavir, is metabolized in the liver by the cytochrome P450 enzyme system. Amprenavir may inhibit or induce CYP3A4. Caution should be used when co-administering medications that are substrates, inhibitors, or inducers of CYP3A4, or potentially toxic medications that are metabolized by CYP3A4).

No products indexed under this heading.

Miconazole Nitrate (Amprenavir, the active metabolite of fosamprenavir, is metabolized in the liver by the cytochrome P450 enzyme system. Amprenavir may inhibit or induce CYP3A4. Caution should be used when co-administering medications that are substrates, inhibitors, or inducers of CYP3A4, or potentially toxic medications that are metabolized by CYP3A4). Products include:

Desenex 635
Desenex Jock Itch Spray Powder ... 635

Midazolam Hydrochloride (Co-administration with midazolam is contraindicated due to potential for serious and/or life-threatening reactions such as prolonged or increased sedation or respiratory depression).

No products indexed under this heading.

Modafinil (Amprenavir, the active metabolite of fosamprenavir, is metabolized in the liver by the cytochrome P450 enzyme system. Amprenavir may inhibit or induce CYP3A4. Caution should be used when co-administering medications that are substrates, inhibitors, or inducers of CYP3A4, or potentially toxic medications that are metabolized by CYP3A4). Products include:

Provivil Tablets 988

Nefazodone Hydrochloride
(Amprenavir, the active metabolite of fosamprenavir, is metabolized in the liver by the cytochrome P450 enzyme system. Amprenavir may inhibit or induce CYP3A4. Caution should be used when co-administering medications that are substrates, inhibitors, or inducers of CYP3A4, or potentially toxic medications that are metabolized by CYP3A4).
No products indexed under this heading.

Nelfinavir Mesylate
(Co-administration with fosamprenavir alone may lead to increased amprenavir levels). Products include:
Viracept .. 2577

Nevirapine
(Co-administration may lead to decreased amprenavir levels and increased nevirapine levels. Co-administration of nevirapine and fos-amprenavir calcium without ritonavir is not recommended). Products include:
Viramune Oral Suspension 873
Viramune Tablets 873

Niacinamide
(Amprenavir, the active metabolite of fosamprenavir, is metabolized in the liver by the cytochrome P450 enzyme system. Amprenavir may inhibit or induce CYP3A4. Caution should be used when co-administering medications that are substrates, inhibitors, or inducers of CYP3A4, or potentially toxic medications that are metabolized by CYP3A4).
No products indexed under this heading.

Nicardipine
(Co-administration may increase levels of nicardipine; caution is warranted and clinical monitoring is recommended).
No products indexed under this heading.

Nicardipine Hydrochloride
(Co-administration may increase levels of nicardipine; caution is warranted and clinical monitoring is recommended). Products include:
Cardene I.V. 2497

Nicotinamide
(Amprenavir, the active metabolite of fosamprenavir, is metabolized in the liver by the cytochrome P450 enzyme system. Amprenavir may inhibit or induce CYP3A4. Caution should be used when co-administering medications that are substrates, inhibitors, or inducers of CYP3A4, or potentially toxic medications that are metabolized by CYP3A4). Products include:
Nicomide Tablets 1088

Nifedipine
(Co-administration may increase levels of nifedipine, caution is warranted and clinical monitoring is recommended). Products include:
Adalat CC Tablets 2964

Nimodipine
(Co-administration may increase levels of nimodipine; caution is warranted and clinical monitoring is recommended). Products include:
Nimotop Capsules 749

Nisoldipine
(Co-administration may increase levels of nisoldipine; caution is warranted and clinical monitoring is recommended). Products include:
Sular Tablets 3122

Nitrendipine
(Amprenavir, the active metabolite of fosamprenavir, is metabolized in the liver by the cytochrome P450 enzyme system. Amprenavir may inhibit or induce CYP3A4. Caution should be used when co-administering medications that are substrates, inhibitors, or inducers of CYP3A4, or potentially toxic medications that are metabolized by CYP3A4).
No products indexed under this heading.

Nizatidine
(Co-administration of fosamprenavir alone and histamine H2-receptor antagonists may lead to decreased levels of fosamprenavir. Use with caution since fosam-prenavir may be less effective due to decreased amprenavir plasma concentrations in patients taking these agents concomitantly). Products include:
Axid Oral Solution 879

Norethindrone
(Co-administration of fosamprenavir alone with oral contraceptives containing the combination ethinyl estradiol/norethindrone may lead to increased levels of ethinyl estradiol/norethindrone. Because these hormonal levels may be altered, alternative methods of non-hormonal contraception are recommended). Products include:
Ortho Micronor Tablets 2426

Norethindrone Acetate
(Co-administration of fosamprenavir alone with oral contraceptives containing the combination ethinyl estradiol/norethindrone may lead to increased levels of ethinyl estradiol/norethindrone. Because these hormonal levels may be altered, alternative methods of non-hormonal contraception are recommended).
No products indexed under this heading.

Norfloxacin
(Amprenavir, the active metabolite of fosamprenavir, is metabolized in the liver by the cytochrome P450 enzyme system. Amprenavir may inhibit or induce CYP3A4. Caution should be used when co-administering medications that are substrates, inhibitors, or inducers of CYP3A4, or potentially toxic medications that are metabolized by CYP3A4). Products include:
Noroxin Tablets 2032

Norgestrel
(Amprenavir, the active metabolite of fosamprenavir, is metabolized in the liver by the cytochrome P450 enzyme system. Amprenavir may inhibit or induce CYP3A4. Caution should be used when co-administering medications that are substrates, inhibitors, or inducers of CYP3A4, or potentially toxic medications that are metabolized by CYP3A4).
No products indexed under this heading.

Omeprazole
(Amprenavir, the active metabolite of fosamprenavir, is metabolized in the liver by the cytochrome P450 enzyme system. Amprenavir may inhibit or induce CYP3A4. Caution should be used when co-administering medications that are substrates, inhibitors, or inducers of CYP3A4, or potentially toxic medications that are metabolized by CYP3A4). Products include:
Zegerid Capsules 2958
Zegerid Powder for Oral Solution 2958

Ondansetron
(Amprenavir, the active metabolite of fosamprenavir, is metabolized in the liver by the cytochrome P450 enzyme system. Amprenavir may inhibit or induce CYP3A4. Caution should be used when co-administering medications that are substrates, inhibitors, or inducers of CYP3A4, or potentially toxic medications that are metabolized by CYP3A4). Products include:
Zofran ODT Orally Disintegrating Tablets .. 1639

Ondansetron Hydrochloride
(Amprenavir, the active metabolite of fosamprenavir, is metabolized in the liver by the cytochrome P450 enzyme system. Amprenavir may inhibit or induce CYP3A4. Caution should be used when co-administering medications that are substrates, inhibitors, or inducers of CYP3A4, or potentially toxic medications that are metabolized by CYP3A4). Products include:
Zofran Injection 1634
Zofran ... 1639

Oxcarbazepine
(Amprenavir, the active metabolite of fosamprenavir, is metabolized in the liver by the cytochrome P450 enzyme system. Amprenavir may inhibit or induce CYP3A4. Caution should be used when co-administering medications that are substrates, inhibitors, or inducers of CYP3A4, or potentially toxic medications that are metabolized by CYP3A4). Products include:
Trileptal Tablets 2300
Trileptal Oral Suspension 2300

Paclitaxel
(Amprenavir, the active metabolite of fosamprenavir, is metabolized in the liver by the cytochrome P450 enzyme system. Amprenavir may inhibit or induce CYP3A4. Caution should be used when co-administering medications that are substrates, inhibitors, or inducers of CYP3A4, or potentially toxic medications that are metabolized by CYP3A4).
No products indexed under this heading.

Paroxetine Hydrochloride
(Amprenavir, the active metabolite of fosamprenavir, is metabolized in the liver by the cytochrome P450 enzyme system. Amprenavir may inhibit or induce CYP3A4. Caution should be used when co-administering medications that are substrates, inhibitors, or inducers of CYP3A4, or potentially toxic medications that are metabolized by CYP3A4). Products include:
Paxil CR Controlled-Release Tablets .. 1538
Paxil ... 1530

Phenobarbital
(Co-administration may lead to decreased amprenavir levels. Use with caution; fosam-prenavir may be less effective due to decreased plasma concentrations in patients taking these agents con-comitantly). Products include:
Donnatal Extentabs 2493

Phenobarbital Sodium
(Co-administration may lead to decreased amprenavir levels. Use with caution; fosamprenavir may be less effective due to decreased plas-ma concentrations in patients taking these agents concomitantly).
No products indexed under this heading.

Phenytoin
(Co-administration may lead to decreased amprenavir levels. Use with caution; fosamprenavir may be less effective due to decreased plasma concentrations in patients taking these agents concomitantly).
No products indexed under this heading.

Phenytoin Sodium
(Co-administration may lead to decreased amprenavir levels. Use with caution; fosamprenavir may be less effective due to decreased plas-ma concentrations in patients taking these agents concomitantly). Products include:
Phenytek Capsules 2160

Pimozide
(Co-administration with pimozide is contraindicated due to potential for serious and/or life-threatening reactions such as cardi-ac arrhythmias).
No products indexed under this heading.

Polyestradiol Phosphate
(Amprenavir, the active metabolite of fosamprenavir, is metabolized in the liver by the cytochrome P450 enzyme system. Amprenavir may inhibit or induce CYP3A4. Caution should be used when co-administering medications that are substrates, inhibitors, or inducers of CYP3A4, or potentially toxic medications that are metabolized by CYP3A4).
No products indexed under this heading.

Prednisolone Acetate
(Amprenavir, the active metabolite of fosamprenavir, is metabolized in the liver by the cytochrome P450 enzyme system. Amprenavir may inhibit or induce CYP3A4. Caution should be used when co-administering medications that are substrates, inhibitors, or inducers of CYP3A4, or potentially toxic medications that are metabolized by CYP3A4). Products include:
Blephamide Ophthalmic Ointment **568**
Blephamide Ophthalmic Suspension **569**
Poly-Pred Ophthalmic Suspension ☉**233**
Pred Forte Ophthalmic Suspension ☉**235**
Pred Mild Ophthalmic Suspension ☉**238**
Pred-G Ophthalmic Ointment ☉**237**
Pred-G Ophthalmic Suspension ☉**236**

Prednisolone Sodium Phosphate
(Amprenavir, the active metabolite of fosamprenavir, is metabolized in the liver by the cytochrome P450 enzyme system. Amprenavir may inhibit or induce CYP3A4. Caution should be used when co-administering medications that are substrates, inhibitors, or inducers of CYP3A4, or potentially toxic medica-tions that are metabolized by CYP3A4).
No products indexed under this heading.

Prednisolone Tebutate
(Amprenavir, the active metabolite of fosamprenavir, is metabolized in the liver by the cytochrome P450 enzyme system. Amprenavir may inhibit or induce CYP3A4. Caution should be used when co-administering medications that are substrates, inhibitors, or inducers of CYP3A4, or potentially toxic medica-tions that are metabolized by CYP3A4).
No products indexed under this heading.

Prednisone (Amprenavir, the active metabolite of fosamprenavir, is metabolized in the liver by the cytochrome P450 enzyme system. Amprenavir may inhibit or induce CYP3A4. Caution should be used when co-administering medications that are substrates, inhibitors, or inducers of CYP3A4, or potentially toxic medications that are metabolized by CYP3A4).

No products indexed under this heading.

Primidone (Amprenavir, the active metabolite of fosamprenavir, is metabolized in the liver by the cytochrome P450 enzyme system. Amprenavir may inhibit or induce CYP3A4. Caution should be used when co-administering medications that are substrates, inhibitors, or inducers of CYP3A4, or potentially toxic medications that are metabolized by CYP3A4).

No products indexed under this heading.

Propafenone Hydrochloride (If fosamprenavir is co-administered with ritonavir, the antiarrhythmic agent propafenone is contraindicated due to the potential for serious and/or life-threatening reactions such as cardiac arrhythmias secondary to increases in plasma concentrations of propafenone). Products include:

Rythmol SR Capsules **2727**

Propoxyphene Hydrochloride (Amprenavir, the active metabolite of fosamprenavir, is metabolized in the liver by the cytochrome P450 enzyme system. Amprenavir may inhibit or induce CYP3A4. Caution should be used when co-administering medications that are substrates, inhibitors, or inducers of CYP3A4, or potentially toxic medications that are metabolized by CYP3A4).

No products indexed under this heading.

Propoxyphene Napsylate (Amprenavir, the active metabolite of fosamprenavir, is metabolized in the liver by the cytochrome P450 enzyme system. Amprenavir may inhibit or induce CYP3A4. Caution should be used when co-administering medications that are substrates, inhibitors, or inducers of CYP3A4, or potentially toxic medications that are metabolized by CYP3A4).

No products indexed under this heading.

Quinidine (Co-administration may lead to increased levels of quinidine. Caution is warranted and therapeutic concentration monitoring is recommended for antiarrhythmics when co-administered with fosamprenavir).

No products indexed under this heading.

Quinidine Gluconate (Co-administration may lead to increased levels of quinidine. Caution is warranted and therapeutic concentration monitoring is recommended for antiarrhythmics when co-administered with fosamprenavir).

No products indexed under this heading.

Quinidine Hydrochloride (Co-administration may lead to increased levels of quinidine. Caution is warranted and therapeutic concentration monitoring is recommended for antiarrhythmics when co-administered with fosamprenavir).

No products indexed under this heading.

Quinidine Polygalacturonate (Co-administration may lead to increased levels of quinidine. Caution is warranted and therapeutic concentration monitoring is recommended for antiarrhythmics when co-administered with fosamprenavir).

No products indexed under this heading.

Quinidine Sulfate (Co-administration may lead to increased levels of quinidine. Caution is warranted and therapeutic concentration monitoring is recommended for antiarrhythmics when co-administered with fosamprenavir).

No products indexed under this heading.

Quinine (Amprenavir, the active metabolite of fosamprenavir, is metabolized in the liver by the cytochrome P450 enzyme system. Amprenavir may inhibit or induce CYP3A4. Caution should be used when co-administering medications that are substrates, inhibitors, or inducers of CYP3A4, or potentially toxic medications that are metabolized by CYP3A4).

No products indexed under this heading.

Quinine Sulfate (Amprenavir, the active metabolite of fosamprenavir, is metabolized in the liver by the cytochrome P450 enzyme system. Amprenavir may inhibit or induce CYP3A4. Caution should be used when co-administering medications that are substrates, inhibitors, or inducers of CYP3A4, or potentially toxic medications that are metabolized by CYP3A4).

No products indexed under this heading.

Quinupristin (Amprenavir, the active metabolite of fosamprenavir, is metabolized in the liver by the cytochrome P450 enzyme system. Amprenavir may inhibit or induce CYP3A4. Caution should be used when co-administering medications that are substrates, inhibitors, or inducers of CYP3A4, or potentially toxic medications that are metabolized by CYP3A4).

No products indexed under this heading.

Ranitidine Bismuth Citrate (Co-administration of fosamprenavir alone and histamine H2-receptor antagonists may lead to decreased levels of fosamprenavir. Use with caution since fosamprenavir may be less effective due to decreased amprenavir plasma concentrations in patients taking these agents concomitantly).

No products indexed under this heading.

Ranitidine Hydrochloride (Co-administration of fosamprenavir alone and histamine H2-receptor antagonists may lead to decreased levels of fosamprenavir. Use with caution since fosamprenavir may be less effective due to decreased amprenavir plasma concentrations in patients taking these agents concomitantly). Products include:

Zantac **1624**
Zantac Injection **1619**
Zantac Injection Pharmacy Bulk Package **1622**

Rapamycin (Co-administration may lead to increased levels of rapamycin. Therapeutic concentration monitoring is recommended for immunosuppressant agents when co-administered with fosamprenavir).

No products indexed under this heading.

Rifabutin (Co-administration may cause increased levels of rifabutin and its metabolite; perform CBC weekly and as clinically indicated in order to monitor for neutropenia in patients receiving concurrent administration. In patients receiving fosamprenavir alone, a dosage reduction of rifabutin by at least half the recommended dose is required. In patients receiving fosamprenavir/ritonavir combination, dosage reduction of rifabutin by at least 75% of the usual dose of 300mg/day is recommended (maximum dose of 150mg every other day or three times weekly)).

No products indexed under this heading.

Rifampicin (Amprenavir, the active metabolite of fosamprenavir, is metabolized in the liver by the cytochrome P450 enzyme system. Amprenavir may inhibit or induce CYP3A4. Caution should be used when co-administering medications that are substrates, inhibitors, or inducers of CYP3A4, or potentially toxic medications that are metabolized by CYP3A4).

No products indexed under this heading.

Rifampin (Co-administration may lead to loss of virologic response and possible resistance to fosamprenavir or other protease inhibitors).

No products indexed under this heading.

Rifapentine (Amprenavir, the active metabolite of fosamprenavir, is metabolized in the liver by the cytochrome P450 enzyme system. Amprenavir may inhibit or induce CYP3A4. Caution should be used when co-administering medications that are substrates, inhibitors, or inducers of CYP3A4, or potentially toxic medications that are metabolized by CYP3A4).

No products indexed under this heading.

Ritonavir (Co-administration of lopinavir/ritonavir and fosamprenavir may lead to decreased levels of amprenavir and lopinavir (when given in combination with ritonavir). An increased rate of adverse events has also been observed with co-administration of these medications). Products include:

Kaletra **476**
Norvir **503**

Saquinavir (Co-administration with fosamprenavir alone may lead to decreased levels of amprenavir).

No products indexed under this heading.

Saquinavir Mesylate (Amprenavir, the active metabolite of fosamprenavir, is metabolized in the liver by the cytochrome P450 enzyme system. Amprenavir may inhibit or induce CYP3A4. Caution should be used when co-administering medications that are substrates, inhibitors, or inducers of CYP3A4, or potentially toxic medications that are metabolized by CYP3A4). Products include:

Invirase **2772**

Sertraline Hydrochloride (Amprenavir, the active metabolite of fosamprenavir, is metabolized in the liver by the cytochrome P450 enzyme system. Amprenavir may inhibit or induce CYP3A4. Caution should be used when co-administering medications that are substrates, inhibitors, or inducers of CYP3A4, or potentially toxic medications that are metabolized by CYP3A4). Products include:

Zoloft **2586**

Sildenafil Citrate (Co-administration may lead to increased levels of sildenafil; use sildenafil with caution at reduced doses of 25mg every 48 hours with increased monitoring for adverse events). Products include:

Revatio Tablets **2557**
Viagra Tablets **2573**

Simvastatin (Co-administration may lead to the potential for serious reactions such as risk of myopathy including rhabdomyolysis). Products include:

Vytorin 10/10 Tablets **2114**
Vytorin 10/10 Tablets **3077**
Vytorin 10/20 Tablets **2114**
Vytorin 10/20 Tablets **3077**
Vytorin 10/40 Tablets **2114**
Vytorin 10/40 Tablets **3077**
Vytorin 10/80 Tablets **2114**
Vytorin 10/80 Tablets **3077**
Zocor Tablets **2105**

Sirolimus (Amprenavir, the active metabolite of fosamprenavir, is metabolized in the liver by the cytochrome P450 enzyme system. Amprenavir may inhibit or induce CYP3A4. Caution should be used when co-administering medications that are substrates, inhibitors, or inducers of CYP3A4, or potentially toxic medications that are metabolized by CYP3A4). Products include:

Rapamune Oral Solution and Tablets **3475**

Sulfinpyrazone (Amprenavir, the active metabolite of fosamprenavir, is metabolized in the liver by the cytochrome P450 enzyme system. Amprenavir may inhibit or induce CYP3A4. Caution should be used when co-administering medications that are substrates, inhibitors, or inducers of CYP3A4, or potentially toxic medications that are metabolized by CYP3A4).

No products indexed under this heading.

Tacrolimus (Co-administration may lead to increased levels of tacrolimus. Therapeutic concentration monitoring is recommended for immunosuppressant agents when co-administered with fosamprenavir). Products include:

Prograf Capsules and Injection **632**
Protopic Ointment **638**

Tamoxifen Citrate (Amprenavir, the active metabolite of fosamprenavir, is metabolized in the liver by the cytochrome P450 enzyme system. Amprenavir may inhibit or induce CYP3A4. Caution should be used when co-administering medications that are substrates, inhibitors, or inducers of CYP3A4, or potentially toxic medications that are metabolized by CYP3A4). Products include:

Soltamox Oral Solution **3527**

Telithromycin (Amprenavir, the active metabolite of fosamprenavir, is metabolized in the liver by the cytochrome P450 enzyme system. Amprenavir may inhibit or induce CYP3A4. Caution should be used when co-administering medications that are substrates, inhibitors, or inducers of CYP3A4, or potentially toxic medications that are metabolized by CYP3A4). Products include:
Ketek Tablets 2903

Theophylline (Amprenavir, the active metabolite of fosamprenavir, is metabolized in the liver by the cytochrome P450 enzyme system. Amprenavir may inhibit or induce CYP3A4. Caution should be used when co-administering medications that are substrates, inhibitors, or inducers of CYP3A4, or potentially toxic medications that are metabolized by CYP3A4).
No products indexed under this heading.

Tiagabine Hydrochloride (Amprenavir, the active metabolite of fosamprenavir, is metabolized in the liver by the cytochrome P450 enzyme system. Amprenavir may inhibit or induce CYP3A4. Caution should be used when co-administering medications that are substrates, inhibitors, or inducers of CYP3A4, or potentially toxic medications that are metabolized by CYP3A4). Products include:
Gabitril Tablets 984

Tolterodine Tartrate (Amprenavir, the active metabolite of fosamprenavir, is metabolized in the liver by the cytochrome P450 enzyme system. Amprenavir may inhibit or induce CYP3A4. Caution should be used when co-administering medications that are substrates, inhibitors, or inducers of CYP3A4, or potentially toxic medications that are metabolized by CYP3A4). Products include:
Detrol Tablets 2628
Detrol LA Capsules 2631

Trazodone Hydrochloride (Concomitant use of trazodone and fosamprenavir calcium with or without ritonavir may increase plasma concentrations of trazodone. Adverse events have been observed during co-administration. If trazodone is used with a CYP3A4 inhibitor such as fosamaprenavir calcium, the combination should be used with caution and a lower dose of trazodone should be considered).
No products indexed under this heading.

Triamcinolone (Amprenavir, the active metabolite of fosamprenavir, is metabolized in the liver by the cytochrome P450 enzyme system. Amprenavir may inhibit or induce CYP3A4. Caution should be used when co-administering medications that are substrates, inhibitors, or inducers of CYP3A4, or potentially toxic medications that are metabolized by CYP3A4).
No products indexed under this heading.

Triamcinolone Acetonide (Amprenavir, the active metabolite of fosamprenavir, is metabolized in the liver by the cytochrome P450 enzyme system. Amprenavir may inhibit or induce CYP3A4. Caution should be used when co-administering medications that are substrates, inhibitors, or inducers of

CYP3A4, or potentially toxic medications that are metabolized by CYP3A4). Products include:
Azmacort Inhalation Aerosol 1726
Nasacort AQ Nasal Spray 2922

Triamcinolone Diacetate (Amprenavir, the active metabolite of fosamprenavir, is metabolized in the liver by the cytochrome P450 enzyme system. Amprenavir may inhibit or induce CYP3A4. Caution should be used when co-administering medications that are substrates, inhibitors, or inducers of CYP3A4, or potentially toxic medications that are metabolized by CYP3A4).
No products indexed under this heading.

Triamcinolone Hexacetonide (Amprenavir, the active metabolite of fosamprenavir, is metabolized in the liver by the cytochrome P450 enzyme system. Amprenavir may inhibit or induce CYP3A4. Caution should be used when co-administering medications that are substrates, inhibitors, or inducers of CYP3A4, or potentially toxic medications that are metabolized by CYP3A4).
No products indexed under this heading.

Triazolam (Co-administration with triazolam is contraindicated due to potential for serious and/or life-threatening reactions such as prolonged or increased sedation or respiratory depression).
No products indexed under this heading.

Troglitazone (Amprenavir, the active metabolite of fosamprenavir, is metabolized in the liver by the cytochrome P450 enzyme system. Amprenavir may inhibit or induce CYP3A4. Caution should be used when co-administering medications that are substrates, inhibitors, or inducers of CYP3A4, or potentially toxic medications that are metabolized by CYP3A4).
No products indexed under this heading.

Troleandomycin (Amprenavir, the active metabolite of fosamprenavir, is metabolized in the liver by the cytochrome P450 enzyme system. Amprenavir may inhibit or induce CYP3A4. Caution should be used when co-administering medications that are substrates, inhibitors, or inducers of CYP3A4, or potentially toxic medications that are metabolized by CYP3A4).
No products indexed under this heading.

Valproate Sodium (Amprenavir, the active metabolite of fosamprenavir, is metabolized in the liver by the cytochrome P450 enzyme system. Amprenavir may inhibit or induce CYP3A4. Caution should be used when co-administering medications that are substrates, inhibitors, or inducers of CYP3A4, or potentially toxic medications that are metabolized by CYP3A4). Products include:
Depacon Injection 412

Vardenafil Hydrochloride (Co-administration may lead to increased levels of vardenafil. When co-administered with fosamprenavir alone, use vardenafil with caution at reduced doses of no more than 2.5mg every 24 hours with increased monitoring for adverse

events. When co-administered with fosamprenavir/ritonavir combination, use vardenafil with caution at reduced doses of no more than 2.5mg every 72 hours with increased monitoring for adverse events). Products include:
Levitra Tablets 3034

Verapamil Hydrochloride (Co-administration may increase levels of verapamil; caution is warranted and clinical monitoring is recommended). Products include:
Covera-HS Tablets 3139
Tarka Tablets 524
Verelan PM Extended-Release
Capsules, Controlled-Onset........... 3106

Vinblastine Sulfate (Amprenavir, the active metabolite of fosamprenavir, is metabolized in the liver by the cytochrome P450 enzyme system. Amprenavir may inhibit or induce CYP3A4. Caution should be used when co-administering medications that are substrates, inhibitors, or inducers of CYP3A4, or potentially toxic medications that are metabolized by CYP3A4).
No products indexed under this heading.

Vincristine Sulfate (Amprenavir, the active metabolite of fosamprenavir, is metabolized in the liver by the cytochrome P450 enzyme system. Amprenavir may inhibit or induce CYP3A4. Caution should be used when co-administering medications that are substrates, inhibitors, or inducers of CYP3A4, or potentially toxic medications that are metabolized by CYP3A4).
No products indexed under this heading.

Voriconazole (Amprenavir, the active metabolite of fosamprenavir, is metabolized in the liver by the cytochrome P450 enzyme system. Amprenavir may inhibit or induce CYP3A4. Caution should be used when co-administering medications that are substrates, inhibitors, or inducers of CYP3A4, or potentially toxic medications that are metabolized by CYP3A4). Products include:
VFEND I.V. 2564
VFEND Oral Suspension 2564
VFEND Tablets 2564

Warfarin Sodium (Concentrations of warfarin may be affected. It is recommended that INR be monitored). Products include:
Coumadin for Injection 898
Coumadin Tablets 898

Zafirlukast (Amprenavir, the active metabolite of fosamprenavir, is metabolized in the liver by the cytochrome P450 enzyme system. Amprenavir may inhibit or induce CYP3A4. Caution should be used when co-administering medications that are substrates, inhibitors, or inducers of CYP3A4, or potentially toxic medications that are metabolized by CYP3A4). Products include:
Accolate Tablets 671

Zileuton (Amprenavir, the active metabolite of fosamprenavir, is metabolized in the liver by the cytochrome P450 enzyme system. Amprenavir may inhibit or induce CYP3A4. Caution should be used when co-administering medications that are substrates, inhibitors, or inducers of CYP3A4, or potentially toxic medications that are metabolized by CYP3A4). Products include:
Zyflo Tablets 1023

Food Interactions

Grapefruit (Amprenavir, the active metabolite of fosamprenavir, is metabolized in the liver by the cytochrome P450 enzyme system. Amprenavir may inhibit or induce CYP3A4. Caution should be used when co-administering medications that are substrates, inhibitors, or inducers of CYP3A4, or potentially toxic medications that are metabolized by CYP3A4).

Grapefruit Juice (Amprenavir, the active metabolite of fosamprenavir, is metabolized in the liver by the cytochrome P450 enzyme system. Amprenavir may inhibit or induce CYP3A4. Caution should be used when co-administering medications that are substrates, inhibitors, or inducers of CYP3A4, or potentially toxic medications that are metabolized by CYP3A4).

LIBRIUM CAPSULES

(Chlordiazepoxide Hydrochloride) 3347
None cited in PDR database.

LIDODERM PATCH

(Lidocaine) 1118
May interact with class 1A antiarrhythmics, local anesthetics, and certain other agents. Compounds in these categories include:

Bupivacaine Hydrochloride (When used concomitantly with other products containing local anesthetic agents, the amount absorbed from all formulations must be considered).
No products indexed under this heading.

Chloroprocaine Hydrochloride (When used concomitantly with other products containing local anesthetic agents, the amount absorbed from all formulations must be considered).
No products indexed under this heading.

Disopyramide (Should be used with caution in patients receiving Class I antiarrhythmic drugs since the toxic effects are additive and potentially synergistic).
No products indexed under this heading.

Etidocaine Hydrochloride (When used concomitantly with other products containing local anesthetic agents, the amount absorbed from all formulations must be considered).
No products indexed under this heading.

Levobupivacaine Hydrochloride (When used concomitantly with other products containing local anesthetic agents, the amount absorbed from all formulations must be considered).
No products indexed under this heading.

Lidocaine Hydrochloride (When used concomitantly with other products containing local anesthetic agents, the amount absorbed from all formulations must be considered).
No products indexed under this heading.

Mepivacaine Hydrochloride (When used concomitantly with other products containing local anesthetic agents, the amount absorbed from all formulations must be considered).
No products indexed under this heading.

Mexiletine Hydrochloride (Co-administration in patients receiving Class-1 antiarrhythmic drugs, such as mexiletine, may result in additive toxic effects).
No products indexed under this heading.

Moricizine Hydrochloride (Should be used with caution in patients receiving Class I antiarrhythmic drugs since the toxic effects are additive and potentially synergistic).
No products indexed under this heading.

Procainamide (Should be used with caution in patients receiving Class I antiarrhythmic drugs since the toxic effects are additive and potentially synergistic).
No products indexed under this heading.

Procaine Hydrochloride (When used concomitantly with other products containing local anesthetic agents, the amount absorbed from all formulations must be considered).
No products indexed under this heading.

Quinidine (Should be used with caution in patients receiving Class I antiarrhythmic drugs since the toxic effects are additive and potentially synergistic).
No products indexed under this heading.

Quinidine Gluconate (Should be used with caution in patients receiving Class I antiarrhythmic drugs since the toxic effects are additive and potentially synergistic).
No products indexed under this heading.

Tetracaine Hydrochloride (When used concomitantly with other products containing local anesthetic agents, the amount absorbed from all formulations must be considered). Products include:
Cetacaine Topical Anesthetic 999

Tocainide Hydrochloride (Co-administration in patients receiving Class-1 antiarrhythmic drugs, such as tocainide, may result in additive toxic effects).
No products indexed under this heading.

LIFEPAK CAPSULES
(Vitamins with Minerals) 2672
None cited in PDR database.

LIMBREL CAPSULES
(Flavocoxid) 2672
None cited in PDR database.

LIPITOR TABLETS
(Atorvastatin Calcium) 2483
May interact with azole antifungals, erythromycin, fibrates, and certain other agents. Compounds in these categories include:

Aluminum Hydroxide (Co-administration with aluminum hydroxide/magnesium hydroxide antacid has resulted in decreased atorvastatin plasma concentrations by 35%; LDL-C reduction was unaltered). Products include:
Gaviscon Regular Strength Liquid .. 658
Gaviscon Regular Strength Tablets 658
Gaviscon Extra Strength Liquid 658
Gaviscon Extra Strength Tablets 658
Maalox Regular Strength Antacid/Antigas Liquid 2175
Maalox Max Maximum Strength Antacid/Anti-Gas Liquid 2176

Clofibrate (Co-administration with fibric acid derivatives increases the risk of myopathy).
No products indexed under this heading.

Clotrimazole (Co-administration with azole antifungals increases the risk of myopathy). Products include:
Desenex Athlete's Foot Cream 635
Lotrimin 3039
Lotrisone 3040

Colestipol Hydrochloride (Co-administration has resulted in decreased atorvastatin plasma concentrations by 25%; however, LDL-C reduction was greater when these drugs were given together than when either drug was given alone).
No products indexed under this heading.

Cyclosporine (Co-administration increases the risk of myopathy). Products include:
Gengraf Capsules 459
Neoral Oral Solution 2259
Neoral Soft Gelatin Capsules 2259
Restasis Ophthalmic Emulsion 575
Sandimmune 2275

Digoxin (Co-administration has resulted in increased steady-state digoxin plasma concentrations by 20%). Products include:
Lanoxicaps Capsules 1490
Lanoxin Injection 1494
Lanoxin Injection Pediatric 1497
Lanoxin Tablets 1500

Erythromycin (Co-administration increases the risk of myopathy; plasma concentrations of atorvastatin have increased by 40% when co-administered with erythromycin, a known inhibitor of cytochrome P4503A4). Products include:
Ery-Tab Tablets 449
Erythromycin Base Filmtab Tablets 455
Erythromycin Delayed-Release Capsules, USP 457
PCE Dispertab Tablets 515

Erythromycin Estolate (Co-administration increases the risk of myopathy; plasma concentrations of atorvastatin have increased by 40% when co-administered with erythromycin, a known inhibitor of cytochrome P4503A4).
No products indexed under this heading.

Erythromycin Ethylsuccinate (Co-administration increases the risk of myopathy; plasma concentrations of atorvastatin have increased by 40% when co-administered with erythromycin, a known inhibitor of cytochrome P4503A4). Products include:
E.E.S. 451
EryPed 447

Erythromycin Gluceptate (Co-administration increases the risk of myopathy; plasma concentrations of atorvastatin have increased by 40% when co-administered with erythromycin, a known inhibitor of cytochrome P4503A4).
No products indexed under this heading.

Erythromycin Lactobionate (Co-administration increases the risk of myopathy; plasma concentrations of atorvastatin have increased by 40% when co-administered with erythromycin, a known inhibitor of cytochrome P4503A4).
No products indexed under this heading.

Erythromycin Stearate (Co-administration increases the risk of myopathy; plasma concentrations of atorvastatin have increased by 40% when co-administered with erythromycin, a known inhibitor of cytochrome P4503A4). Products include:
Erythrocin Stearate Filmtab Tablets 453

Ethinyl Estradiol (Co-administration with an oral contraceptive has increased AUC values for norethindrone and ethinyl estradiol by 30% and 20%, respectively). Products include:
Mircette Tablets 1066
NuvaRing 2340
Ortho-Cyclen/Ortho Tri-Cyclen 2429
Ortho Evra Transdermal System 2417
Ortho Tri-Cyclen Lo Tablets 2436
Seasonique Tablets 1077
Yasmin 28 Tablets 796
Yaz Tablets 803

Fenofibrate (Co-administration with fibric acid derivatives increases the risk of myopathy). Products include:
Lofibra Tablets 1219
Lofibra Capsules 1216
Tricor Tablets 527
Triglide Tablets 3123

Fluconazole (Co-administration with azole antifungals increases the risk of myopathy).
No products indexed under this heading.

Gemfibrozil (Co-administration with fibric acid derivatives increases the risk of myopathy).
No products indexed under this heading.

Itraconazole (Co-administration with azole antifungals increases the risk of myopathy).
No products indexed under this heading.

Ketoconazole (Co-administration with azole antifungals increases the risk of myopathy). Products include:
Nizoral A-D Shampoo, 1% 1868

Miconazole (Co-administration with azole antifungals increases the risk of myopathy).
No products indexed under this heading.

Niacin (Co-administration increases the risk of myopathy). Products include:
Advicor Tablets 1722
Niaspan Extended-Release Tablets 1730

Norethindrone (Co-administration with an oral contraceptive has increased AUC values for norethindrone and ethinyl estradiol by 30% and 20%, respectively). Products include:
Ortho Micronor Tablets 2426

Oxiconazole Nitrate (Co-administration with azole antifungals increases the risk of myopathy). Products include:
Oxistat 2667

Terconazole (Co-administration with azole antifungals increases the risk of myopathy).
No products indexed under this heading.

LITHOBID TABLETS
(Lithium Carbonate) 1692
May interact with ACE inhibitors, calcium channel blockers, diuretics, nondepolarizing neuromuscular blocking agents, antipsychotic agents, non-steroidal anti-inflammatory agents, urinary alkalinizing agents, xanthines, and certain other agents. Compounds in these categories include:

Acetazolamide (Concurrent use of acetazolamide with lithium may lower serum lithium concentrations by increasing urinary lithium excretion).
No products indexed under this heading.

Acetazolamide Sodium (Concurrent use of acetazolamide with lithium may lower serum lithium concentrations by increasing urinary lithium excretion).
No products indexed under this heading.

Amiloride Hydrochloride (Concurrent use of lithium with diuretics is not recommended since the risk of lithium toxicity is very high. If psychiatric indication is life threatening, and if such a patient fails to respond to other measures, lithium treatment may be undertaken withextreme caution including daily serum lithium determinations and adjustment to the usually low doses ordinarily tolerated by these individuals. In such instances, hospitilization is a necessity). Products include:
Midamor Tablets 2026
Moduretic Tablets 2028

Aminophylline (Concurrent use of xanthine preparations with lithium may lower serum lithium concentrations by increasing urinary lithium excretion).
No products indexed under this heading.

Amlodipine Besylate (Concurrent use of calcium channel blocking agents with lithium may increase the risk of neurotoxicity in the form of ataxia, tremors, nausea, vomiting, diarrhea and/or tinnitus). Products include:
Caduet Tablets 2508
Lotrel Capsules 2249
Norvasc Tablets 2545

Aripiprazole (An encephalopathic syndrome (characterized by weakness, lethargy, fever, tremulousness and confusion, extrapyramidal symptoms, leukocytosis, elevated serum enzymes, BUN and FBS) has occurred in a few patients treated with lithium plus a neuroleptic, most notably haloperidol. In some instance, the syndrome was followed by irreversible brain damage. Monitor these patients closely for early evidence of neurologic toxicity and discontinue treatment promptly if such signs appear). Products include:
Abilify Oral Solution 882
Abilify Oral Solution 2450
Abilify Discmelt Orally Disintegrating Tablets 882
Abilify Discmelt Orally Disintegrating Tablets 2450
Abilify Tablets 882
Abilify Tablets 2450

Atracurium Besylate (Concurrent use of lithium with neuromuscular blocking agents may prolong the effect of neuromuscular blocking agents. Neuromuscular blocking agents should be given with caution to patients receiving lithium).

No products indexed under this heading.

Benazepril Hydrochloride (Concurrent use of lithium with ACE inhibitors is not recommended since the risk of lithium toxicity is very high. If psychiatric indication is life threatening, and if such a patient fails to respond to other measures, lithium treatment may be undertaken with extreme caution including daily serum lithium determinations and adjustment to the usually low doses ordinarily tolerated by these individuals. In such instances, hospitalization is a necessity). Products include:

Bendroflumethiazide (Concurrent use of lithium with diuretics is not recommended since the risk of lithium toxicity is very high. If psychiatric indication is life threatening, and if such a patient fails to respond to other measures, lithium treatment may be undertaken with extreme caution including daily serum lithium determinations and adjustment to the usually low doses ordinarily tolerated by these individuals. In such instances, hospitalization is a necessity).

No products indexed under this heading.

Bepridil Hydrochloride (Concurrent use of calcium channel blocking agents with lithium may increase the risk of neurotoxicity in the form of ataxia, tremors, nausea, vomiting, diarrhea and/or tinnitus).

No products indexed under this heading.

Bismuth Oxyiodide (Concomitant use of iodide preparations with lithium may produce hypothyroidism).

No products indexed under this heading.

Bumetanide (Concurrent use of lithium with diuretics is not recommended since the risk of lithium toxicity is very high. If psychiatric indication is life threatening, and if such a patient fails to respond to other measures, lithium treatment may be undertaken with extreme caution including daily serum lithium determinations and adjustment to the usually low doses ordinarily tolerated by these individuals. In such instances, hospitalization is a necessity). Products include:

Calcium Iodide (Concomitant use of iodide preparations with lithium may produce hypothyroidism).

No products indexed under this heading.

Captopril (Concurrent use of lithium with ACE inhibitors is not recommended since the risk of lithium toxicity is very high. If psychiatric indication is life threatening, and if such a patient fails to respond to other measures, lithium treatment may be undertaken with extreme caution including daily serum lithium determinations and adjustment to the usually low doses ordinarily tolerated by

these individuals. In such instances, hospitalization is a necessity). Products include:

Carbamazepine (Concomitant administration of carbamazepine and lithium may increase the risk of neurotoxic side effects). Products include:

Celecoxib (Lithium levels should be closely monitored when patients initiate or discontinue NSAID use. In some cases, lithium toxicity has resulted from interactions between an NSAID and lithium. Significantly increased steady-state plasma lithium concentrations are reported with concurrent use of lithium with NSAIDs and selective COX-2 inhibitors). Products include:

Chlorothiazide (Concurrent use of lithium with diuretics is not recommended since the risk of lithium toxicity is very high. If psychiatric indication is life threatening, and if such a patient fails to respond to other measures, lithium treatment may be undertaken with extreme caution including daily serum lithium determinations and adjustment to the usually low doses ordinarily tolerated by these individuals. In such instances, hospitalization is a necessity). Products include:

Chlorothiazide Sodium (Concurrent use of lithium with diuretics is not recommended since the risk of lithium toxicity is very high. If psychiatric indication is life threatening, and if such a patient fails to respond to other measures, lithium treatment may be undertaken with extreme caution including daily serum lithium determinations and adjustment to the usually low doses ordinarily tolerated by these individuals. In such instances, hospitalization is a necessity). Products include:

Chlorpromazine (An encephalopathic syndrome characterized by weakness, lethargy, fever, tremulousness and confusion, extrapyramidal symptoms, leukocytois, elevated serum enzymes, BUN and FBS) has occurred in a few patients treated with lithium plus a neuroleptic, most notably haloperidol. In some instance, the syndrome was followed by irreversible brain damage. Monitor these patients closely for early evidence of neurologic toxicity and discontinue treatment promptly if such signs appear).

No products indexed under this heading.

Chlorpromazine Hydrochloride (An encephalopathic syndrome characterized by weakness, lethargy, fever, tremulousness and confusion, extrapyramidal symptoms, leukocytois, elevated serum enzymes, BUN and FBS) has occurred in a few patients treated with lithium plus a neuroleptic, most notably haloperidol. In some instance, the syndrome was followed by irreversible brain damage. Monitor these patients closely for early evidence of neurologic toxicity and discontinue treat-

ment promptly if such signs appear).

No products indexed under this heading.

Chlorprothixene (An encephalopathic syndrome (characterized by weakness, lethargy, fever, tremulousness and confusion, extrapyramidal symptoms, leukocytois, elevated serum enzymes, BUN and FBS) has occurred in a few patients treated with lithium plus a neuroleptic, most notably haloperidol. In some instance, the syndrome was followed by irreversible brain damage. Monitor these patients closely for early evidence of neurologic toxicity and discontinue treatment promptly if such signs appear).

No products indexed under this heading.

Chlorprothixene Hydrochloride (An encephalopathic syndrome (characterized by weakness, lethargy, fever, tremulousness and confusion, extrapyramidal symptoms, leukocytois, elevated serum enzymes, BUN and FBS) has occurred in a few patients treated with lithium plus a neuroleptic, most notably haloperidol. In some instance, the syndrome was followed by irreversible brain damage. Monitor these patients closely for early evidence of neurologic toxicity and discontinue treatment promptly if such signs appear).

No products indexed under this heading.

Chlorthalidone (Concurrent use of lithium with diuretics is not recommended since the risk of lithium toxicity is very high. If psychiatric indication is life threatening, and if such a patient fails to respond to other measures, lithium treatment may be undertaken with extreme caution including daily serum lithium determinations and adjustment to the usually low doses ordinarily tolerated by these individuals. In such instances, hospitalization is a necessity). Products include:

Cisatracurium Besylate (Concurrent use of lithium with neuromuscular blocking agents may prolong the effect of neuromuscular blocking agents. Neuromuscular blocking agents should be given with caution to patients receiving lithium). Products include:

Clozapine (An encephalopathic syndrome (characterized by weakness, lethargy, fever, tremulousness and confusion, extrapyramidal symptoms, leukocytois, elevated serum enzymes, BUN and FBS) has occurred in a few patients treated with lithium plus a neuroleptic, most notably haloperidol. In some instance, the syndrome was followed by irreversible brain damage. Monitor these patients closely for early evidence of neurologic toxicity and discontinue treatment promptly if such signs appear). Products include:

Diclofenac Potassium (Lithium levels should be closely monitored when patients initiate or discontinue NSAID use. In some cases, lithium toxicity has resulted from interactions between an NSAID and lithium. Significantly increased steady-state plasma lithium concentrations are reported with concurrent use of lithium with NSAIDs and selective COX-2 inhibitors).

No products indexed under this heading.

Diclofenac Sodium (Lithium levels should be closely monitored when patients initiate or discontinue NSAID use. In some cases, lithium toxicity has resulted from interactions between an NSAID and lithium. Significantly increased steady-state plasma lithium concentrations are reported with concurrent use of lithium with NSAIDs and selective COX-2 inhibitors). Products include:

Diltiazem Hydrochloride (Concurrent use of calcium channel blocking agents with lithium may increase the risk of neurotoxicity in the form of ataxia, tremors, nausea, vomiting, diarrhea and/or tinnitus). Products include:

Dyphilline (Concurrent use of xanthine preparations with lithium may lower serum lithium concentrations by increasing urinary lithium excretion).

No products indexed under this heading.

Echothiophate Iodide (Concomitant use of iodide preparations with lithium may produce hypothyroidism).

No products indexed under this heading.

Enalapril Maleate (Concurrent use of lithium with ACE inhibitors is not recommended since the risk of lithium toxicity is very high. If psychiatric indication is life threatening, and if such a patient fails to respond to other measures, lithium treatment may be undertaken with extreme caution including daily serum lithium determinations and adjustment to the usually low doses ordinarily tolerated by these individuals. In such instances, hospitalization is a necessity). Products include:

Enalaprilat (Concurrent use of lithium with ACE inhibitors is not recommended since the risk of lithium toxicity is very high. If psychiatric indication is life threatening, and if such a patient fails to respond to other measures, lithium treatment may be undertaken with extreme caution including daily serum lithium determinations and adjustment to the usually low doses ordinarily tolerated by these individuals. In such instances, hospitilization is a necessity).

No products indexed under this heading.

Ethacrynic Acid (Concurrent use of lithium with diuretics is not recommended since the risk of lithium toxicity is very high. If psychiatric indication is life threatening, and if such a patient fails to respond to other measures, lithium treatment may be undertaken withextreme caution including daily serum lithium determinations and adjustment to the usually low doses ordinarily tolerated by these individuals. In such instances, hospitilization is a necessity). Products include:

Edecrin Tablets 1959

Etodolac (Lithium levels should be closely monitored when patients initiate or discontinue NSAID use. In some cases, lithium toxicity has resulted from interactions between an NSAID and lithium. Significantly increased steady-state plasma lithium concentrations are reported with concurrent use of lithium with NSAIDs and selective COX-2 inhibitors).

No products indexed under this heading.

Felodipine (Concurrent use of calcium channel blocking agents with lithium may increase the risk of neurotoxicity in the form of ataxia, tremors, nausea, vomiting, diarrhea and/or tinnitus).

No products indexed under this heading.

Fenoprofen Calcium (Lithium levels should be closely monitored when patients initiate or discontinue NSAID use. In some cases, lithium toxicity has resulted from interactions between an NSAID and lithium. Significantly increased steady-state plasma lithium concentrations are reported with concurrent use of lithium with NSAIDs and selective COX-2 inhibitors). Products include:

Nalfon Capsules 2502

Fluoxetine (Concurrent use of fluoxetine with lithium has resulted in both increased and decreased serum lithium concentration. Patients receiving such combined therapy should be monitored closely).

No products indexed under this heading.

Fluoxetine Hydrochloride (Concurrent use of fluoxetine with lithium has resulted in both increased and decreased serum lithium concentration. Patients receiving such combined therapy should be monitored closely). Products include:

Prozac Pulvules and Liquid 1801
Symbyax Capsules 1819

Fluphenazine Decanoate (An encephalopathic syndrome (characterized by weakness, lethargy, fever, tremulousness and confusion, extrapyramidal symptoms, leukocytois, elevated serum enzymes, BUN and FBS) has occurred in a few patients treated with lithium plus a neuroleptic, most notably haloperidol. In some instance, the syndrome was followed by irreversible brain damage. Monitor these patients closely for early evidence of neurologic toxicity and discontinue treatment promptly if such signs appear).

No products indexed under this heading.

Fluphenazine Enanthate (An encephalopathic syndrome (characterized by weakness, lethargy, fever, tremulousness and confusion, extrapyramidal symptoms, leukocytois, elevated serum enzymes, BUN and FBS) has occurred in a few patients treated with lithium plus a neuroleptic, most notably haloperidol. In some instance, the syndrome was followed by irreversible brain damage. Monitor these patients closely for early evidence of neurologic toxicity and discontinue treatment promptly if such signs appear).

No products indexed under this heading.

Fluphenazine Hydrochloride (An encephalopathic syndrome (characterized by weakness, lethargy, fever, tremulousness and confusion, extrapyramidal symptoms, leukocytois, elevated serum enzymes, BUN and FBS) has occurred in a few patients treated with lithium plus a neuroleptic, most notably haloperidol. In some instance, the syndrome was followed by irreversible brain damage. Monitor these patients closely for early evidence of neurologic toxicity and discontinue treatment promptly if such signs appear).

No products indexed under this heading.

Flurbiprofen (Lithium levels should be closely monitored when patients initiate or discontinue NSAID use. In some cases, lithium toxicity has resulted from interactions between an NSAID and lithium. Significantly increased steady-state plasma lithium concentrations are reported with concurrent use of lithium with NSAIDs and selective COX-2 inhibitors).

No products indexed under this heading.

Fosinopril Sodium (Concurrent use of lithium with ACE inhibitors is not recommended since the risk of lithium toxicity is very high. If psychiatric indication is life threatening, and if such a patient fails to respond to other measures, lithium treatment may be undertakenwith extreme caution including daily serum lithium determinations and adjustment to the usually low doses ordinarily tolerated by these individuals. In such instances, hospitilization is a necessity).

No products indexed under this heading.

Furosemide (Concurrent use of lithium with diuretics is not recommended since the risk of lithium toxicity is very high. If psychiatric indication is life threatening, and if such a patient fails to respond to other measures, lithium treatment may be undertaken withextreme caution including daily serum lithium determinations and adjustment to the usually low doses ordinarily tolerated by these individuals. In such instances, hospitilization is a necessity). Products include:

Furosemide Tablets 2154

Gallamine Triethiodide (Concomitant use of iodide preparations with lithium may produce hypothyroidism).

No products indexed under this heading.

Haloperidol (An encephalopathic syndrome (characterized by weakness, lethargy, fever, tremulousness and confusion, extrapyramidal symptoms, leukocytois, elevated serum enzymes, BUN and FBS) has occurred in a few patients treated with lithium plus a neuroleptic, most notably haloperidol. In some instance, the syndrome was followed by irreversible brain damage. Monitor these patients closely for early evidence of neurologic toxicity and discontinue treatment promptly if such signs appear).

No products indexed under this heading.

Haloperidol Decanoate (An encephalopathic syndrome (characterized by weakness, lethargy, fever, tremulousness and confusion, extrapyramidal symptoms, leukocytois, elevated serum enzymes, BUN and FBS) has occurred in a few patients treated with lithium plus a neuroleptic, most notably haloperidol. In some instance, the syndrome was followed by irreversible brain damage. Monitor these patients closely for early evidence of neurologic toxicity and discontinue treatment promptly if such signs appear).

No products indexed under this heading.

Hydrochlorothiazide (Concurrent use of lithium with diuretics is not recommended since the risk of lithium toxicity is very high. If psychiatric indication is life threatening, and if such a patient fails to respond to other measures, lithium treatment may be undertaken withextreme caution including daily serum lithium determinations and adjustment to the usually low doses ordinarily tolerated by these individuals. In such instances, hospitilization is a necessity). Products include:

Aldoril Tablets 1910
Atacand HCT 651
Avalide Tablets 888
Avalide Tablets 2874
Benicar HCT Tablets 1044
Diovan HCT Tablets 2196
Dyazide Capsules 1423
Hyzaar 50-12.5 Tablets 1990
Hyzaar 100-12.5 Tablets 1990
Hyzaar 100-25 Tablets 1990
Lopressor HCT 50/25 Tablets 2241
Lopressor HCT 100/25 Tablets 2241
Lopressor HCT 100/50 Tablets 2241
Lotensin HCT Tablets 2246
Micardis HCT Tablets 856
Moduretic Tablets 2028
Prinzide Tablets 2056
Teveten HCT Tablets 1737
Timolide Tablets 2086
Uniretic Tablets 3100

Hydroflumethiazide (Concurrent use of lithium with diuretics is not recommended since the risk of lithium toxicity is very high. If psychiatric indication is life threatening, and if such a patient fails to respond to other measures, lithium treatment may be undertaken withextreme caution including daily serum lithium determinations and adjustment to the usually low doses ordinarily tolerated by these individuals. In such instances, hospitilization is a necessity).

No products indexed under this heading.

Ibuprofen (Lithium levels should be closely monitored when patients initiate or discontinue NSAID use. In some cases, lithium toxicity has resulted from interactions between an NSAID and lithium. Significantly increased steady-state plasma lithium concentrations are reported with concurrent use of lithium with NSAIDs and selective COX-2 inhibitors). Products include:

Advil Allergy Sinus Caplets 770
Advil 674
Children's Advil Oral Suspension 603
Children's Advil Chewable Tablets .. 603
Advil Cold & Sinus 723
Infants' Advil Concentrated Drops .. 604
Infants' Advil Concentrated Drops - White Grape (Dye-Free) 604
Junior Strength Advil Swallow Tablets 605
Advil Migraine Liquigels 608
Advil Multi-Symptom Cold Caplets 770
Advil PM Caplets 615
Motrin IB Tablets and Caplets 1866
Children's Motrin Oral Suspension ... 1867
Children's Motrin Non-Staining Dye-Free Oral Suspension 1867
Children's Motrin Cold Oral Suspension 1867
Infants' Motrin Concentrated Drops 1867
Infants' Motrin Non-Staining Dye-Free Concentrated Drops 1867
Junior Strength Motrin Caplets and Chewable Tablets 1867
Vicoprofen Tablets 539

Indapamide (Concurrent use of lithium with diuretics is not recommended since the risk of lithium toxicity is very high. If psychiatric indication is life threatening, and if such a patient fails to respond to other measures, lithium treatment may be undertaken withextreme caution including daily serum lithium determinations and adjustment to the usually low doses ordinarily tolerated by these individuals. In such instances, hospitilization is a necessity). Products include:

Indapamide Tablets 2156

Indomethacin (Lithium levels should be closely monitored when patients initiate or discontinue NSAID use. In some cases, lithium toxicity has resulted from interactions between an NSAID and lithium. Significantly increased steady-state plasma lithium concentrations are reported with concurrent use of lithium with NSAIDs and selective COX-2 inhibitors). Products include:

Indocin 1995

Indomethacin Sodium Trihydrate (Lithium levels should be closely monitored when patients initiate or discontinue NSAID use. In some cases, lithium toxicity has resulted from interactions between an NSAID and lithium. Significantly increased steady-state plasma lithium concentrations are reported with concurrent use of lithium with NSAIDs and selective COX-2 inhibitors). Products include:

Indocin I.V. 2465

Isopropamide Iodide (Concomitant use of iodide preparations with lithium may produce hypothyroidism).

No products indexed under this heading.

Isradipine (Concurrent use of calcium channel blocking agents with lithium may increase the risk of neurotoxicity in the form of ataxia, tremors, nausea, vomiting, diarrhea and/or tinnitus). Products include:

DynaCirc CR Tablets 2721

Ketoprofen (Lithium levels should be closely monitored when patients initiate or discontinue NSAID use. In some cases, lithium toxicity has resulted from interactions between an NSAID and lithium. Significantly increased steady-state plasma lithium concentrations are reported with concurrent use of lithium with NSAIDs and selective COX-2 inhibitors).

No products indexed under this heading.

Ketorolac Tromethamine (Lithium levels should be closely monitored when patients initiate or discontinue NSAID use. In some cases, lithium toxicity has resulted from interactions between an NSAID and lithium. Significantly increased steady-state plasma lithium concentrations are reported with concurrent use of lithium with NSAIDs and selective COX-2 inhibitors). Products include:

Lisinopril (Concurrent use of lithium with ACE inhibitors is not recommended since the risk of lithium toxicity is very high. If psychiatric indication is life threatening, and if such a patient fails to respond to other measures, lithium treatment may be undertakenwith extreme caution including daily serum lithium determinations and adjustment to the usually low doses ordinarily tolerated by these individuals. In such instances, hospitilization is a necessity). Products include:

Lithium Citrate (An encephalopathic syndrome (characterized by weakness, lethargy, fever, tremulousness and confusion, extrapyramidal symptoms, leukocytois, elevated serum enzymes, BUN and FBS) has occurred in a few patients treated with lithium plus a neuroleptic, most notably haloperidol. In some instance, the syndrome was followed by irreversible brain damage. Monitor these patients closely for early evidence of neurologic toxicity and discontinue treatment promptly if such signs appear).
No products indexed under this heading.

Loxapine Hydrochloride (An encephalopathic syndrome (characterized by weakness, lethargy, fever, tremulousness and confusion, extrapyramidal symptoms, leukocytois, elevated serum enzymes, BUN and FBS) has occurred in a few patients treated with lithium plus a neuroleptic, most notably haloperidol. In some instance, the syndrome was followed by irreversible brain damage. Monitor these patients closely for early evidence of neurologic toxicity and discontinue treatment promptly if such signs appear).
No products indexed under this heading.

Loxapine Succinate (An encephalopathic syndrome (characterized by weakness, lethargy, fever, tremulousness and confusion, extrapyramidal symptoms, leukocytois, elevated serum enzymes, BUN and FBS) has occurred in a few patients treated with lithium plus a neuroleptic, most notably haloperidol. In some instance, the syndrome was followed by irreversible brain damage. Monitor these patients closely for early evidence of neurologic toxicity and discontinue treatment promptly if such signs appear).
No products indexed under this heading.

Meclofenamate Sodium (Lithium levels should be closely monitored when patients initiate or discontinue NSAID use. In some cases, lithium toxicity has resulted from interactions between an NSAID and lithium. Significantly increased steady-state plasma lithium concentrations are reported with concurrent use of lithium with NSAIDs and selective COX-2 inhibitors).
No products indexed under this heading.

Mefenamic Acid (Lithium levels should be closely monitored when patients initiate or discontinue NSAID use. In some cases, lithium toxicity has resulted from interactions between an NSAID and lithium. Significantly increased steady-state plasma lithium concentrations are reported with concurrent use of lithium with NSAIDs and selective COX-2 inhibitors).
No products indexed under this heading.

Meloxicam (Lithium levels should be closely monitored when patients initiate or discontinue NSAID use. In some cases, lithium toxicity has resulted from interactions between an NSAID and lithium. Significantly increased steady-state plasma lithium concentrations are reported with concurrent use of lithium with NSAIDs and selective COX-2 inhibitors). Products include:

Mesoridazine Besylate (An encephalopathic syndrome (characterized by weakness, lethargy, fever, tremulousness and confusion, extrapyramidal symptoms, leukocytois, elevated serum enzymes, BUN and FBS) has occurred in a few patients treated with lithium plus a neuroleptic, most notably haloperidol. In some instance, the syndrome was followed by irreversible brain damage. Monitor these patients closely for early evidence of neurologic toxicity and discontinue treatment promptly if such signs appear).
No products indexed under this heading.

Methotrimeprazine (An encephalopathic syndrome (characterized by weakness, lethargy, fever, tremulousness and confusion, extrapyramidal symptoms, leukocytois, elevated serum enzymes, BUN and FBS) has occurred in a few patients treated with lithium plus a neuroleptic, most notably haloperidol. In some instance, the syndrome was followed by irreversible brain damage. Monitor these patients closely for early evidence of neurologic toxicity and discontinue treatment promptly if such signs appear).
No products indexed under this heading.

Methyclothiazide (Concurrent use of lithium with diuretics is not recommended since the risk of lithium toxicity is very high. If psychiatric indication is life threatening, and if such a patient fails to respond to other measures, lithium treatment may be undertaken withextreme caution including daily serum lithium determinations and adjustment to the usually low doses ordinarily tolerated by these individuals. In such instances, hospitilization is a necessity).
No products indexed under this heading.

Metocurine Iodide (Concomitant use of iodide preparations with lithium may produce hypothyroidism).
No products indexed under this heading.

Metolazone (Concurrent use of lithium with diuretics is not recommended since the risk of lithium toxicity is very high. If psychiatric indication is life threatening, and if such a patient fails to respond to other measures, lithium treatment may be undertaken withextreme caution

including daily serum lithium determinations and adjustment to the usually low doses ordinarily tolerated by these individuals. In such instances, hospitilization is a necessity).
No products indexed under this heading.

Metronidazole (Concurrent use of metronidazole with lithium may provoke lithium toxicity due to reduced renal clearance. Patients receiving such combined therapy should be monitored closely). Products include:

Metronidazole Benzoate (Concurrent use of metronidazole with lithium may provoke lithium toxicity due to reduced renal clearance. Patients receiving such combined therapy should be monitored closely).
No products indexed under this heading.

Metronidazole Hydrochloride (Concurrent use of metronidazole with lithium may provoke lithium toxicity due to reduced renal clearance. Patients receiving such combined therapy should be monitored closely).
No products indexed under this heading.

Metronidazole Sodium (Concurrent use of metronidazole with lithium may provoke lithium toxicity due to reduced renal clearance. Patients receiving such combined therapy should be monitored closely).
No products indexed under this heading.

Mibefradil Dihydrochloride (Concurrent use of calcium channel blocking agents with lithium may increase the risk of neurotoxicity in the form of ataxia, tremors, nausea, vomiting, diarrhea and/or tinnitus).
No products indexed under this heading.

Mivacurium Chloride (Concurrent use of lithium with neuromuscular blocking agents may prolong the effect of neuromuscular blocking agents. Neuromuscular blocking agents should be given with caution to patients receiving lithium). Products include:

Moexipril Hydrochloride (Concurrent use of lithium with ACE inhibitors is not recommended since the risk of lithium toxicity is very high. If psychiatric indication is life threatening, and if such a patient fails to respond to other measures, lithium treatment may be undertakenwith extreme caution including daily serum lithium determinations and adjustment to the usually low doses ordinarily tolerated by these individuals. In such instances, hospitilization is a necessity). Products include:

Molindone Hydrochloride (An encephalopathic syndrome (characterized by weakness, lethargy, fever, tremulousness and confusion, extrapyramidal symptoms, leukocytois, elevated serum enzymes, BUN and FBS) has occurred in a few patients treated with lithium plus a neuroleptic, most notably haloperidol. In some instance, the syndrome was followed by irreversible brain damage. Monitor these patients closely for early evidence of neurologic tox-

icity and discontinue treatment promptly if such signs appear). Products include:

Nabumetone (Lithium levels should be closely monitored when patients initiate or discontinue NSAID use. In some cases, lithium toxicity has resulted from interactions between an NSAID and lithium. Significantly increased steady-state plasma lithium concentrations are reported with concurrent use of lithium with NSAIDs and selective COX-2 inhibitors).
No products indexed under this heading.

Naproxen (Lithium levels should be closely monitored when patients initiate or discontinue NSAID use. In some cases, lithium toxicity has resulted from interactions between an NSAID and lithium. Significantly increased steady-state plasma lithium concentrations are reported with concurrent use of lithium with NSAIDs and selective COX-2 inhibitors). Products include:

Naproxen Sodium (Lithium levels should be closely monitored when patients initiate or discontinue NSAID use. In some cases, lithium toxicity has resulted from interactions between an NSAID and lithium. Significantly increased steady-state plasma lithium concentrations are reported with concurrent use of lithium with NSAIDs and selective COX-2 inhibitors). Products include:

Niacinamide Hydroiodide (Concomitant use of iodide preparations with lithium may produce hypothyroidism).
No products indexed under this heading.

Nicardipine Hydrochloride (Concurrent use of calcium channel blocking agents with lithium may increase the risk of neurotoxicity in the form of ataxia, tremors, nausea, vomiting, diarrhea and/or tinnitus). Products include:

Nifedipine (Concurrent use of calcium channel blocking agents with lithium may increase the risk of neurotoxicity in the form of ataxia, tremors, nausea, vomiting, diarrhea and/or tinnitus). Products include:

Nimodipine (Concurrent use of calcium channel blocking agents with lithium may increase the risk of neurotoxicity in the form of ataxia, tremors, nausea, vomiting, diarrhea and/or tinnitus). Products include:

Nisoldipine (Concurrent use of calcium channel blocking agents with lithium may increase the risk of neurotoxicity in the form of ataxia, tremors, nausea, vomiting, diarrhea and/or tinnitus). Products include:

Olanzapine (An encephalopathic syndrome (characterized by weakness, lethargy, fever, tremulousness and confusion, extrapyramidal symptoms, leukocytois, elevated serum enzymes, BUN and FBS) has occurred in a few patients treated with lithium plus a neuroleptic, most notably haloperidol. In some instance, the syndrome was followed by irreversible brain damage. Monitor these patients closely for early evidence of neurologic toxicity and discontinue treatment promptly if such signs appear). Products include:

Oxaprozin (Lithium levels should be closely monitored when patients initiate or discontinue NSAID use. In some cases, lithium toxicity has resulted from interactions between an NSAID and lithium. Significantly increased steady-state plasma lithium concentrations are reported with concurrent use of lithium with NSAIDs and selective COX-2 inhibitors).
 No products indexed under this heading.

Pancuronium Bromide (Concurrent use of lithium with neuromuscular blocking agents may prolong the effect of neuromuscular blocking agents. Neuromuscular blocking agents should be given with caution to patients receiving lithium).
 No products indexed under this heading.

Perindopril Erbumine (Concurrent use of lithium with ACE inhibitors is not recommended since the risk of lithium toxicity is very high. If psychiatric indication is life threatening, and if such a patient fails to respond to other measures, lithium treatment may be undertaken with extreme caution including daily serum lithium determinations and adjustment to the usually low doses ordinarily tolerated by these individuals. In such instances, hospitilization is a necessity). Products include:

Perphenazine (An encephalopathic syndrome (characterized by weakness, lethargy, fever, tremulousness and confusion, extrapyramidal symptoms, leukocytois, elevated serum enzymes, BUN and FBS) has occurred in a few patients treated with lithium plus a neuroleptic, most notably haloperidol. In some instance, the syndrome was followed by irreversible brain damage. Monitor these patients closely for early evidence of neurologic toxicity and discontinue treatment promptly if such signs appear).
 No products indexed under this heading.

Phenylbutazone (Lithium levels should be closely monitored when patients initiate or discontinue NSAID use. In some cases, lithium toxicity has resulted from interactions between an NSAID and lithium. Significantly increased steady-state plasma lithium concentrations are reported with concurrent use of lithium with NSAIDs and selective COX-2 inhibitors).
 No products indexed under this heading.

Pimozide (An encephalopathic syndrome (characterized by weakness,

lethargy, fever, tremulousness and confusion, extrapyramidal symptoms, leukocytois, elevated serum enzymes, BUN and FBS) has occurred in a few patients treated with lithium plus a neuroleptic, most notably haloperidol. In some instance, the syndrome was followed by irreversible brain damage. Monitor these patients closely for early evidence of neurologic toxicity and discontinue treatment promptly if such signs appear).
 No products indexed under this heading.

Piroxicam (Lithium levels should be closely monitored when patients initiate or discontinue NSAID use. In some cases, lithium toxicity has resulted from interactions between an NSAID and lithium. Significantly increased steady-state plasma lithium concentrations are reported with concurrent use of lithium with NSAIDs and selective COX-2 inhibitors).
 No products indexed under this heading.

Polythiazide (Concurrent use of lithium with diuretics is not recommended since the risk of lithium toxicity is very high. If psychiatric indication is life threatening, and if such a patient fails to respond to other measures, lithium treatment may be undertaken with extreme caution including daily serum lithium determinations and adjustment to the usually low doses ordinarily tolerated by these individuals. In such instances, hospitilization is a necessity).
 No products indexed under this heading.

Potassium Citrate (Concurrent use of alkalinizing agents, such as sodium bicarbonate, with lithium may lower the serum lithium concentration by increasing urinary lithium excretion). Products include:

Potassium Iodide (Concomitant use of iodide preparations, especially potassium iodide, with lithium may produce hypothyroidism).
 No products indexed under this heading.

Prochlorperazine (An encephalopathic syndrome (characterized by weakness, lethargy, fever, tremulousness and confusion, extrapyramidal symptoms, leukocytois, elevated serum enzymes, BUN and FBS) has occurred in a few patients treated with lithium plus a neuroleptic, most notably haloperidol. In some instance, the syndrome was followed by irreversible brain damage. Monitor these patients closely for early evidence of neurologic toxicity and discontinue treatment promptly if such signs appear).
 No products indexed under this heading.

Promethazine Hydrochloride (An encephalopathic syndrome (characterized by weakness, lethargy, fever, tremulousness and confusion, extrapyramidal symptoms, leukocytois, elevated serum enzymes, BUN and FBS) has occurred in a few patients treated with lithium plus a neuroleptic, most notably haloperidol. In some instance, the syndrome was followed by irreversible brain damage. Monitor these patients closely for early evidence of neurologic tox-

icity and discontinue treatment promptly if such signs appear). Products include:

Quetiapine Fumarate (An encephalopathic syndrome (characterized by weakness, lethargy, fever, tremulousness and confusion, extrapyramidal symptoms, leukocytois, elevated serum enzymes, BUN and FBS) has occurred in a few patients treated with lithium plus a neuroleptic, most notably haloperidol. In some instance, the syndrome was followed by irreversible brain damage. Monitor these patients closely for early evidence of neurologic toxicity and discontinue treatment promptly if such signs appear). Products include:

Quinapril Hydrochloride (Concurrent use of lithium with ACE inhibitors is not recommended since the risk of lithium toxicity is very high. If psychiatric indication is life threatening, and if such a patient fails to respond to other measures, lithium treatment may be undertaken with extreme caution including daily serum lithium determinations and adjustment to the usually low doses ordinarily tolerated by these individuals. In such instances, hospitilization is a necessity.
 No products indexed under this heading.

Ramipril (Concurrent use of lithium with ACE inhibitors is not recommended since the risk of lithium toxicity is very high. If psychiatric indication is life threatening, and if such a patient fails to respond to other measures, lithium treatment may be undertaken with extreme caution including daily serum lithium determinations and adjustment to the usually low doses ordinarily tolerated by these individuals. In such instances, hospitilization is a necessity). Products include:

Rapacuronium Bromide (Concurrent use of lithium with neuromuscular blocking agents may prolong the effect of neuromuscular blocking agents. Neuromuscular blocking agents should be given with caution to patients receiving lithium).
 No products indexed under this heading.

Risperidone (An encephalopathic syndrome (characterized by weakness, lethargy, fever, tremulousness and confusion, extrapyramidal symptoms, leukocytois, elevated serum enzymes, BUN and FBS) has occurred in a few patients treated with lithium plus a neuroleptic, most notably haloperidol. In some instance, the syndrome was followed by irreversible brain damage. Monitor these patients closely for early evidence of neurologic toxicity and discontinue treatment promptly if such signs appear). Products include:

Rocuronium Bromide (Concurrent use of lithium with neuromuscular blocking agents may prolong the effect of neuromuscular blocking agents. Neuromuscular blocking

agents should be given with caution to patients receiving lithium). Products include:

Rofecoxib (Lithium levels should be closely monitored when patients initiate or discontinue NSAID use. In some cases, lithium toxicity has resulted from interactions between an NSAID and lithium. Significantly increased steady-state plasma lithium concentrations are reported with concurrent use of lithium with NSAIDs and selective COX-2 inhibitors).
 No products indexed under this heading.

Sodium Bicarbonate (Concurrent use of alkalinizing agents, such as sodium bicarbonate, with lithium may lower the serum lithium concentration by increasing urinary lithium excretion). Products include:

Sodium Citrate (Concurrent use of alkalinizing agents, such as sodium bicarbonate, with lithium may lower the serum lithium concentration by increasing urinary lithium excretion).
 No products indexed under this heading.

Sodium Iodide I 123 (Concomitant use of iodide preparations with lithium may produce hypothyroidism).
 No products indexed under this heading.

Sodium Iodide I 131 (Concomitant use of iodide preparations with lithium may produce hypothyroidism).
 No products indexed under this heading.

Spirapril Hydrochloride (Concurrent use of lithium with ACE inhibitors is not recommended since the risk of lithium toxicity is very high. If psychiatric indication is life threatening, and if such a patient fails to respond to other measures, lithium treatment may be undertaken with extreme caution including daily serum lithium determinations and adjustment to the usually low doses ordinarily tolerated by these individuals. In such instances, hospitilization is a necessity).
 No products indexed under this heading.

Spironolactone (Concurrent use of lithium with diuretics is not recommended since the risk of lithium toxicity is very high. If psychiatric indication is life threatening, and if such a patient fails to respond to other measures, lithium treatment may be undertaken with extreme caution including daily serum lithium determinations and adjustment to the usually low doses ordinarily tolerated by these individuals. In such instances, hospitilization is a necessity).
 No products indexed under this heading.

Sulindac (Lithium levels should be closely monitored when patients initiate or discontinue NSAID use. In some cases, lithium toxicity has resulted from interactions between an NSAID and lithium. Significantly increased steady-state plasma lithium concentrations are reported with concurrent use of lithium with NSAIDs and selective COX-2 inhibitors). Products include:

Clinoril Tablets 1924

Theophylline (Concurrent use of xanthine preparations with lithium may lower serum lithium concentrations by increasing urinary lithium excretion).

No products indexed under this heading.

Theophylline Anhydrous (Concurrent use of xanthine preparations with lithium may lower serum lithium concentrations by increasing urinary lithium excretion). Products include:

Uniphyl Tablets 2710

Theophylline Calcium Salicylate (Concurrent use of xanthine preparations with lithium may lower serum lithium concentrations by increasing urinary lithium excretion).

No products indexed under this heading.

Theophylline Dihydroxypropyl (Glyceryl) (Concurrent use of xanthine preparations with lithium may lower serum lithium concentrations by increasing urinary lithium excretion).

No products indexed under this heading.

Theophylline Ethylenediamine (Concurrent use of xanthine preparations with lithium may lower serum lithium concentrations by increasing urinary lithium excretion).

No products indexed under this heading.

Theophylline Sodium Glycinate (Concurrent use of xanthine preparations with lithium may lower serum lithium concentrations by increasing urinary lithium excretion).

No products indexed under this heading.

Thioridazine Hydrochloride (An encephalopathic syndrome (characterized by weakness, lethargy, fever, tremulousness and confusion, extrapyramidal symptoms, leukocytois, elevated serum enzymes, BUN and FBS) has occurred in a few patients treated with lithium plus a neuroleptic, most notably haloperidol. In some instance, the syndrome was followed by irreversible brain damage. Monitor these patients closely for early evidence of neurologic toxicity and discontinue treatment promptly if such signs appear). Products include:

Thioridazine Hydrochloride Tablets 2163

Thiothixene (An encephalopathic syndrome (characterized by weakness, lethargy, fever, tremulousness and confusion, extrapyramidal symptoms, leukocytois, elevated serum enzymes, BUN and FBS) has occurred in a few patients treated with lithium plus a neuroleptic, most notably haloperidol. In some instance, the syndrome was followed by irreversible brain damage. Monitor these patients closely for early evidence of neurologic toxicity and discontinue treatment promptly if such signs appear). Products include:

Thiothixene Capsules 2165

Tolmetin Sodium (Lithium levels should be closely monitored when patients initiate or discontinue NSAID use. In some cases, lithium toxicity has resulted from interactions between an NSAID and lithium. Significantly increased steady-state plasma lithium concentrations are reported with concurrent use of lithium with NSAIDs and selective COX 2 inhibitors).

No products indexed under this heading.

Torsemide (Concurrent use of lithium with diuretics is not recommended since the risk of lithium toxicity is very high. If psychiatric indication is life threatening, and if such a patient fails to respond to other measures, lithium treatment may be undertaken withextreme caution including daily serum lithium determinations and adjustment to the usually low doses ordinarily tolerated by these individuals. In such instances, hospitilization is a necessity). Products include:

Demadex Injection 2759
Demadex Tablets 2759

Trandolapril (Concurrent use of lithium with ACE inhibitors is not recommended since the risk of lithium toxicity is very high. If psychiatric indication is life threatening, and if such a patient fails to respond to other measures, lithium treatment may be undertakenwith extreme caution including daily serum lithium determinations and adjustment to the usually low doses ordinarily tolerated by these individuals. In such instances, hospitilization is a necessity). Products include:

Mavik Tablets 486
Tarka Tablets 524

Triamterene (Concurrent use of lithium with diuretics is not recommended since the risk of lithium toxicity is very high. If psychiatric indication is life threatening, and if such a patient fails to respond to other measures, lithium treatment may be undertaken withextreme caution including daily serum lithium determinations and adjustment to the usually low doses ordinarily tolerated by these individuals. In such instances, hospitilization is a necessity). Products include:

Dyazide Capsules 1423
Dyrenium Capsules 3400

Trifluoperazine Hydrochloride (An encephalopathic syndrome (characterized by weakness, lethargy, fever, tremulousness and confusion, extrapyramidal symptoms, leukocytois, elevated serum enzymes, BUN and FBS) has occurred in a few patients treated with lithium plus a neuroleptic, most notably haloperidol. In some instance, the syndrome was followed by irreversible brain damage. Monitor these patients closely for early evidence of neurologic toxicity and discontinue treatment promptly if such signs appear).

No products indexed under this heading.

Urea (Concurrent use of urea with lithium may lower serum lithium concentrations by increasing urinary lithium excretion). Products include:

Accuzyme Debriding Ointment 1662
Accuzyme SE Spray Emulsion 1662
Panafil Ointment 1663
Panafil SE Spray Emulsion 1663

Valdecoxib (Lithium levels should be closely monitored when patients initiate or discontinue NSAID use. In some cases, lithium toxicity has resulted from interactions between an NSAID and lithium. Significantly increased steady-state plasma lithium concentrations are reported with concurrent use of lithium with NSAIDs and selective COX-2 inhibitors).

No products indexed under this heading.

Vecuronium Bromide (Concurrent use of lithium with neuromuscular blocking agents may prolong the effect of neuromuscular blocking agents. Neuromuscular blocking agents should be given with caution to patients receiving lithium).

No products indexed under this heading.

Verapamil Hydrochloride (Concurrent use of calcium channel blocking agents with lithium may increase the risk of neurotoxicity in the form of ataxia, tremors, nausea, vomiting, diarrhea and/or tinnitus). Products include:

Covera-HS Tablets 3139
Tarka Tablets 524
Verelan PM Extended-Release Capsules, Controlled-Onset........... 3106

Ziprasidone Hydrochloride (An encephalopathic syndrome (characterized by weakness, lethargy, fever, tremulousness and confusion, extrapyramidal symptoms, leukocytois, elevated serum enzymes, BUN and FBS) has occurred in a few patients treated with lithium plus a neuroleptic, most notably haloperidol. In some instance, the syndrome was followed by irreversible brain damage. Monitor these patients closely for early evidence of neurologic toxicity and discontinue treatment promptly if such signs appear). Products include:

Geodon Capsules 2529

LITHOSTAT TABLETS

(Acetohydroxamic Acid) 2140
May interact with:

Iron (Acetohydroxamic acid chelates heavy metals - notably iron. The absorption of iron and acetohydroxamic acid from the intestinal lumen may be reduced when both drugs are taken concomitantly. When iron administration is indicated, intramuscular iron is probably the product of choice).

No products indexed under this heading.

Food Interactions

Alcohol (Acetohydroxamic acid taken in association with alcoholic beverages has resulted in rash).

LOCOID LIPOCREAM CREAM

(Hydrocortisone Butyrate) 1160
None cited in PDR database.

LOFIBRA TABLETS

(Fenofibrate) 1219
May interact with bile acid sequestering agents, oral anticoagulants, HMG-CoA reductase inhibitors, and certain other agents. Compounds in these categories include:

Anisindione (Caution should be exercised when coumarin anticoagulants are given in conjunction with fenofibrate. The dosage of the anticoagulants should be reduced to maintain the prothrombin time/INR at the desired level to prevent bleeding complications. Frequent prothrombin time/INR determinations are advisable until it has been definitely determined that the prothrombin time/INR has been stabilized). Products include:

Miradon Tablets 3042

Atorvastatin Calcium (Co-administration of fibric acid derivatives and HMG-CoA reductase inhibitors has been associated, in numerous case reports, with rhabdomyolysis, markedly elevated creatine kinase (CK) levels and myoglobulinuria, leading in a high proportion of cases to acute renal failure; the combined use should be avoided unless the benefit of further alterations in lipid levels is likely to outweigh the increased risk of this combination). Products include:

Caduet Tablets 2508
Lipitor Tablets 2483

Cerivastatin Sodium (Co-administration of fibric acid derivatives and HMG-CoA reductase inhibitors has been associated, in numerous case reports, with rhabdomyolysis, markedly elevated creatine kinase (CK) levels and myoglobulinuria, leading in a high proportion of cases to acute renal failure; the combined use should be avoided unless the benefit of further alterations in lipid levels is likely to outweigh the increased risk of this combination).

No products indexed under this heading.

Cholestyramine (Bile acid sequestrants may bind fenofibrate; Lofibra should be taken at least 1 hour before or 4-6 hours after a bile acid binding resin to avoid impeding its absorption).

No products indexed under this heading.

Colesevelam Hydrochloride (Bile acid sequestrants may bind fenofibrate; Lofibra should be taken at least 1 hour before or 4-6 hours after a bile acid binding resin to avoid impeding its absorption). Products include:

WelChol Tablets 1050

Colestipol Hydrochloride (Bile acid sequestrants may bind fenofibrate; Lofibra should be taken at least 1 hour before or 4-6 hours after a bile acid binding resin to avoid impeding its absorption).

No products indexed under this heading.

Cyclosporine (Renal excretion is the primary elimination route for fibrates and because cyclosporine can produce nephrotoxicity with decrease in creatinine clearance and rise in serum clearance, there is a risk that an interaction will lead to deterioration). Products include:

Gengraf Capsules 459
Neoral Oral Solution 2259
Neoral Soft Gelatin Capsules 2259
Restasis Ophthalmic Emulsion 575
Sandimmune 2275

Dicumarol (Caution should be exercised when coumarin anticoagulants are given in conjunction with fenofibrate. The dosage of the anticoagulants should be reduced to maintain the prothrombin time/INR at the desired level to prevent bleeding complications. Frequent prothrombin time/INR determinations are advisable until it has been definitely determined that the prothrombin time/INR has been stabilized).

No products indexed under this heading.

Fluvastatin Sodium (Co-administration of fibric acid derivatives and HMG-CoA reductase inhibitors has been associated, in numerous case reports, with rhabdomyolysis, markedly elevated creatine kinase (CK) levels and myoglobulinuria, leading in a high proportion of cases to acute renal failure; the combined use should be avoided unless the benefit of further alterations in lipid levels is likely to outweigh the increased risk of this combination). Products include:

Lescol Capsules 2233
Lescol XL Tablets 2233

Lovastatin (Co-administration of fibric acid derivatives and HMG-CoA reductase inhibitors has been associated, in numerous case reports, with rhabdomyolysis, markedly elevated creatine kinase (CK) levels and myoglobulinuria, leading in a high proportion of cases to acute renal failure; the combined use should be avoided unless the benefit of further alterations in lipid levels is likely to outweigh the increased risk of this combination). Products include:

Advicor Tablets 1722
Altoprev Extended-Release Tablets 3109
Mevacor Tablets 2021

Pravastatin Sodium (Co-administration of fibric acid derivatives and HMG-CoA reductase inhibitors has been associated, in numerous case reports, with rhabdomyolysis, markedly elevated creatine kinase (CK) levels and myoglobulinuria, leading in a high proportion of cases to acute renal failure; the combined use should be avoided unless the benefit of further alterations in lipid levels is likely to outweigh the increased risk of this combination).

No products indexed under this heading.

Simvastatin (Co-administration of fibric acid derivatives and HMG-CoA reductase inhibitors has been associated, in numerous case reports, with rhabdomyolysis, markedly elevated creatine kinase (CK) levels and myoglobulinuria, leading in a high proportion of cases to acute renal failure; the combined use should be avoided unless the benefit of further alterations in lipid levels is likely to outweigh the increased risk of this combination). Products include:

Vytorin 10/10 Tablets 2114
Vytorin 10/10 Tablets 3077
Vytorin 10/20 Tablets 2114
Vytorin 10/20 Tablets 3077
Vytorin 10/40 Tablets 2114
Vytorin 10/40 Tablets 3077
Vytorin 10/80 Tablets 2114
Vytorin 10/80 Tablets 3077
Zocor Tablets 2105

Warfarin Sodium (Caution should be exercised when coumarin anticoagulants are given in conjunction with fenofibrate. The dosage of the anticoagulants should be reduced to maintain the prothrombin time/INR at the desired level to prevent bleeding complications. Frequent prothrombin time/INR determinations are advisable until it has been definitely determined that the prothrombin time/INR has been stabilized). Products include:

Coumadin for Injection 898
Coumadin Tablets 898

Food Interactions

Food, unspecified (The absorption of fenofibrate is increased when administered with food; Lofibra should be given with meals).

LOFIBRA CAPSULES

(Fenofibrate) 1216
See Lofibra Tablets

LOPRESSOR INJECTION

(Metoprolol Tartrate) 2238

May interact with catecholamine depleting drugs, cytochrome p450 2d6 inhibitors (selected), general anesthetics, and certain other agents. Compounds in these categories include:

Amiodarone Hydrochloride (Potent inhibitors of the CYP2D6 enzyme may increase the plasma concentration of metoprolol tartrate. Strong inhibition of CYP2D6 would mimic the pharmacokintetics of CYP2D6 poor metabolizers. Caution should therefore be exercised when administering potent CYP2D6 inhibitors with metoprolol tartrate).

No products indexed under this heading.

Amitriptyline Hydrochloride (Potent inhibitors of the CYP2D6 enzyme may increase the plasma concentration of metoprolol tartrate. Strong inhibition of CYP2D6 would mimic the pharmacokintetics of CYP2D6 poor metabolizers. Caution should therefore be exercised when administering potent CYP2D6 inhibitors with metoprolol tartrate).

No products indexed under this heading.

Amoxapine (Potent inhibitors of the CYP2D6 enzyme may increase the plasma concentration of metoprolol tartrate. Strong inhibition of CYP2D6 would mimic the pharmacokintetics of CYP2D6 poor metabolizers. Caution should therefore be exercised when administering potent CYP2D6 inhibitors with metoprolol tartrate).

No products indexed under this heading.

Bupropion Hydrochloride (Potent inhibitors of the CYP2D6 enzyme may increase the plasma concentration of metoprolol tartrate. Strong inhibition of CYP2D6 would mimic the pharmacokintetics of CYP2D6 poor metabolizers. Caution should therefore be exercised when administering potent CYP2D6 inhibitors with metoprolol tartrate). Products include:

Wellbutrin Tablets 1603
Wellbutrin SR Sustained-Release Tablets 1607
Wellbutrin XL Extended-Release Tablets 1613
Zyban Sustained-Release Tablets 1644

Celecoxib (Potent inhibitors of the CYP2D6 enzyme may increase the plasma concentration of metoprolol tartrate. Strong inhibition of CYP2D6 would mimic the pharmacokintetics of CYP2D6 poor metabolizers. Caution should therefore be exercised when administering potent CYP2D6 inhibitors with metoprolol tartrate). Products include:

Celebrex Capsules 3134

Chloroquine Hydrochloride (Potent inhibitors of the CYP2D6 enzyme may increase the plasma concentration of metoprolol tartrate. Strong inhibition of CYP2D6 would mimic the pharmacokintetics of CYP2D6 poor metabolizers. Caution should therefore be exercised when administering potent CYP2D6 inhibitors with metoprolol tartrate).

No products indexed under this heading.

Chloroquine Phosphate (Potent inhibitors of the CYP2D6 enzyme may increase the plasma concentration of metoprolol tartrate. Strong inhibition of CYP2D6 would mimic the pharmacokintetics of CYP2D6 poor metabolizers. Caution should therefore be exercised when administering potent CYP2D6 inhibitors with metoprolol tartrate).

No products indexed under this heading.

Chlorpheniramine (Potent inhibitors of the CYP2D6 enzyme may increase the plasma concentration of metoprolol tartrate. Strong inhibition of CYP2D6 would mimic the pharmacokintetics of CYP2D6 poor metabolizers. Caution should therefore be exercised when administering potent CYP2D6 inhibitors with metoprolol tartrate).

No products indexed under this heading.

Chlorpheniramine Maleate (Potent inhibitors of the CYP2D6 enzyme may increase the plasma concentration of metoprolol tartrate. Strong inhibition of CYP2D6 would mimic the pharmacokintetics of CYP2D6 poor metabolizers. Caution should therefore be exercised when administering potent CYP2D6 inhibitors with metoprolol tartrate). Products include:

Advil Allergy Sinus Caplets ..... ■ 770
Advil Multi-Symptom Cold Caplets ..... ■ 770
BC Allergy Sinus Cold Powder ..... ■ 677
Comtrex Maximum Strength Cold & Cough Day/Night Caplets - Night Formulation ..... ■ 726
Comtrex Maximum Strength Day/Night Severe Cold & Sinus Caplets - Night Formulation ..... ■ 725
Contac Cold and Flu Maximum Strength Caplets ..... ■ 728
Contac Cold and Flu Day and Night Caplets (Night Formulation Only) ..... ■ 727
Children's Dimetapp Long Acting Cough Plus Cold Syrup ..... ■ 731
Robitussin Cough & Cold Long-Acting Liquid ..... ■ 735
Robitussin Cough & Allergy Syrup .. ■ 736
Robitussin Cough & Cold Nighttime Liquid ..... ■ 736
Robitussin Cough, Cold & Flu Nighttime Liquid ..... ■ 738
Robitussin Pediatric Cough & Cold Long-Acting Liquid ..... ■ 735
Robitussin Pediatric Cough & Cold Nighttime Liquid ..... ■ 736
Triaminic Cold & Allergy Liquid ..... ■ 746
Triaminic Cough & Runny Nose Softchews ..... ■ 748
Children's Tylenol Plus Flu Oral Suspension ..... ■ 749
Tylenol Allergy Multi-Symptom Caplets with Cool Burst and Gelcaps 1872
Children's Tylenol Plus Cold Suspension Liquid 1879
Children's Tylenol Plus Cough & Runny Nose Suspension Liquid 1879
Children's Tylenol Plus Flu Suspension Liquid 1881
Children's Tylenol Plus Multi-Symptom Cold Suspension Liquid 1879
Tylenol Cold Head Congestion Nighttime Caplets with Cool Burst 1873
Tylenol Cold Multi-Symptom Nighttime Caplets with Cool Burst 1874
Tylenol Sinus Congestion & Pain Nighttime Caplets with Cool Burst 1876
Vicks 44M Cough, Cold & Flu Relief Liquid 2680
Pediatric Vicks 44m Cough & Cold Relief Liquid 2676
Children's Vicks NyQuil Cold/Cough Relief ..... ■ 756
Children's Vicks NyQuil Cold/Cough Relief Liquid 2680
Zicam Maximum Strength Flu Daytime ..... ■ 768

Chlorpheniramine Polistirex (Potent inhibitors of the CYP2D6 enzyme may increase the plasma concentration of metoprolol tartrate. Strong inhibition of CYP2D6 would mimic the pharmacokintetics of CYP2D6 poor metabolizers. Caution should therefore be exercised when administering potent CYP2D6 inhibitors with metoprolol tartrate). Products include:

Tussionex Pennkinetic Extended-Release Suspension 3327

Chlorpheniramine Tannate (Potent inhibitors of the CYP2D6 enzyme may increase the plasma concentration of metoprolol tartrate. Strong inhibition of CYP2D6 would mimic the pharmacokintetics of CYP2D6 poor metabolizers. Caution should therefore be exercised when administering potent CYP2D6 inhibitors with metoprolol tartrate).

No products indexed under this heading.

Cimetidine (Potent inhibitors of the CYP2D6 enzyme may increase the plasma concentration of metoprolol tartrate. Strong inhibition of CYP2D6 would mimic the pharmacokintetics of CYP2D6 poor metabolizers. Caution should therefore be exercised when administering potent CYP2D6 inhibitors with metoprolol tartrate). Products include:

Tagamet HB 200 Tablets ..... ■ 664

Cimetidine Hydrochloride (Potent inhibitors of the CYP2D6 enzyme may increase the plasma concentration of metoprolol tartrate. Strong inhibition of CYP2D6 would mimic the pharmacokintetics of CYP2D6 poor metabolizers. Caution should therefore be exercised when administering potent CYP2D6 inhibitors with metoprolol tartrate).

No products indexed under this heading.

Citalopram Hydrobromide (Potent inhibitors of the CYP2D6 enzyme may increase the plasma concentration of metoprolol tartrate. Strong inhibition of CYP2D6 would mimic the pharmacokintetics of CYP2D6 poor metabolizers. Caution should therefore be exercised when administering potent CYP2D6 inhibitors with metoprolol tartrate). Products include:

Celexa 1176

Clomipramine Hydrochloride (Potent inhibitors of the CYP2D6 enzyme may increase the plasma concentration of metoprolol tartrate. Strong inhibition of CYP2D6 would mimic the pharmacokintetics of CYP2D6 poor metabolizers. Caution should therefore be exercised when administering potent CYP2D6 inhibitors with metoprolol tartrate).

No products indexed under this heading.

Clonidine (If a patient is treated with clonidine and metoprolol tartrate concurrently, and clonidine treatment is to be discontinued, metoprolol tartrate should be stopped several days before clonidine is withdrawn. Rebound hypertension that can follow withdrawalof clonidine may be increased in patients receiving concurrent beta-blocker treatment). Products include:

Catapres-TTS 844

Clonidine Hydrochloride (If a patient is treated with clonidine and metoprolol tartrate concurrently, and clonidine treatment is to be discontinued, metoprolol tartrate should be stopped several days before clonidine is withdrawn. Rebound hypertension that can follow withdrawalof clonidine may be increased in patients receiving concurrent beta-clocker treatment). Products include:

Catapres Tablets 843
Clorpres Tablets 2153

Cocaine Hydrochloride (Potent inhibitors of the CYP2D6 enzyme may increase the plasma concentration of metoprolol tartrate. Strong inhibition of CYP2D6 would mimic the pharmacokintetics of CYP2D6 poor metabolizers. Caution should therefore be exercised when administering potent CYP2D6 inhibitors with metoprolol tartrate).

No products indexed under this heading.

Deserpidine (Catecholamine-depleting drugs may have an additive effect when given with beta-blocking agents; observe closely for evidence of hypotension or marked bradycardia).

No products indexed under this heading.

Desipramine Hydrochloride (Potent inhibitors of the CYP2D6 enzyme may increase the plasma concentration of metoprolol tartrate. Strong inhibition of CYP2D6 would mimic the pharmacokintetics of CYP2D6 poor metabolizers. Caution should therefore be exercised when administering potent CYP2D6 inhibitors with metoprolol tartrate).

No products indexed under this heading.

Diphenhydramine (Potent inhibitors of the CYP2D6 enzyme may increase the plasma concentration of metoprolol tartrate. Strong inhibition of CYP2D6 would mimic the pharmacokintetics of CYP2D6 poor metabolizers. Caution should therefore be exercised when administering potent CYP2D6 inhibitors with metoprolol tartrate). Products include:

Tylenol Sore Throat Nighttime Liquid with Cool Burst 1877

Diphenhydramine Hydrochloride (Potent inhibitors of the CYP2D6 enzyme may increase the plasma concentration of metoprolol tartrate. Strong inhibition of CYP2D6 would mimic the pharmacokintetics of CYP2D6 poor metabolizers. Caution should therefore be exercised when administering potent CYP2D6 inhibitors with metoprolol tartrate). Products include:

Nytol QuickCaps Caplets .... ▣615
Nytol QuickGels Softgels Maximum Strength .... ▣616
Simply Sleep Caplets 1868
Sominex Original Formula Tablets .. ▣616
TheraFlu Warming Relief Nighttime Severe Cold .... ▣743
TheraFlu Thin Strips Multi Symptom .... ▣744
Triaminic Nighttime Cold & Cough Liquid .... ▣746
Triaminic Thin Strips Cough & Runny Nose .... ▣749
Extra Strength Tylenol PM Caplets, Vanilla Caplets, Geltabs, Gelcaps and Liquid 1875
Tylenol Sore Throat Nighttime Liquid with Cool Burst .... ▣790
Tylenol Allergy Multi-Symptom Nighttime Caplets with Cool Burst 1872
Tylenol Severe Allergy Caplets 1872
Children's Tylenol Plus Cold & Allergy Suspension Liquid 1878

Doxepin Hydrochloride (Potent inhibitors of the CYP2D6 enzyme may increase the plasma concentration of metoprolol tartrate. Strong inhibition of CYP2D6 would mimic the pharmacokintetics of CYP2D6 poor metabolizers. Caution should therefore be exercised when administering potent CYP2D6 inhibitors with metoprolol tartrate).

No products indexed under this heading.

Enflurane (Some inhalation anesthetics may enhance the cardiodepressant effect of beta-blockers).

No products indexed under this heading.

Epinephrine (Patients with a history of severe anaphylactic reaction may be unresponsive to the usual doses of epinephrine used to treat allergic reaction). Products include:

EpiPen 1061
Primatene Mist .... ▣719
Twinject 0.15 3379
Twinject 0.3 3378

Epinephrine Bitartrate (Patients with a history of severe anaphylactic reaction may be unresponsive to the usual doses of epinephrine used to treat allergic reaction).

No products indexed under this heading.

Epinephrine Hydrochloride (Patients with a history of severe anaphylactic reaction may be unresponsive to the usual doses of epinephrine used to treat allergic reaction).

No products indexed under this heading.

Escitalopram Oxalate (Potent inhibitors of the CYP2D6 enzyme may increase the plasma concentration of metoprolol tartrate. Strong inhibition of CYP2D6 would mimic the pharmacokintetics of CYP2D6 poor metabolizers. Caution should therefore be exercised when administering potent CYP2D6 inhibitors with metoprolol tartrate). Products include:

Lexapro Oral Solution 1190
Lexapro Tablets 1190

Fluoxetine (Potent inhibitors of the CYP2D6 enzyme may increase the plasma concentration of metoprolol tartrate. Strong inhibition of CYP2D6 would mimic the pharmacokintetics of CYP2D6 poor metabolizers. Caution should therefore be exercised when administering potent CYP2D6 inhibitors with metoprolol tartrate).

No products indexed under this heading.

Fluoxetine Hydrochloride (Potent inhibitors of the CYP2D6 enzyme may increase the plasma concentration of metoprolol tartrate. Strong inhibition of CYP2D6 would mimic the pharmacokintetics of CYP2D6 poor metabolizers. Caution should therefore be exercised when administering potent CYP2D6 inhibitors with metoprolol tartrate). Products include:

Prozac Pulvules and Liquid 1801
Symbyax Capsules 1819

Fluphenazine Decanoate (Potent inhibitors of the CYP2D6 enzyme may increase the plasma concentration of metoprolol tartrate. Strong inhibition of CYP2D6 would mimic the pharmacokintetics of CYP2D6 poor metabolizers. Caution should therefore be exercised when administering potent CYP2D6 inhibitors with metoprolol tartrate).

No products indexed under this heading.

Fluphenazine Enanthate (Potent inhibitors of the CYP2D6 enzyme may increase the plasma concentration of metoprolol tartrate. Strong inhibition of CYP2D6 would mimic the pharmacokintetics of CYP2D6 poor metabolizers. Caution should therefore be exercised when administering potent CYP2D6 inhibitors with metoprolol tartrate).

No products indexed under this heading.

Fluphenazine Hydrochloride (Potent inhibitors of the CYP2D6 enzyme may increase the plasma concentration of metoprolol tartrate. Strong inhibition of CYP2D6 would mimic the pharmacokintetics of CYP2D6 poor metabolizers. Caution should therefore be exercised when administering potent CYP2D6 inhibitors with metoprolol tartrate).

No products indexed under this heading.

Fluvoxamine Maleate (Potent inhibitors of the CYP2D6 enzyme may increase the plasma concentration of metoprolol tartrate. Strong inhibition of CYP2D6 would mimic the pharmacokintetics of CYP2D6 poor metabolizers. Caution should therefore be exercised when administering potent CYP2D6 inhibitors with metoprolol tartrate).

No products indexed under this heading.

Guanethidine Monosulfate (Catecholamine-depleting drugs may have an additive effect when given with beta-blocking agents; observe closely for evidence of hypotension or marked bradycardia).

No products indexed under this heading.

Halofantrine Hydrochloride (Potent inhibitors of the CYP2D6 enzyme may increase the plasma concentration of metoprolol tartrate. Strong inhibition of CYP2D6 would mimic the pharmacokintetics of CYP2D6 poor metabolizers. Caution should therefore be exercised when administering potent CYP2D6 inhibitors with metoprolol tartrate).

No products indexed under this heading.

Haloperidol (Potent inhibitors of the CYP2D6 enzyme may increase the plasma concentration of metoprolol tartrate. Strong inhibition of CYP2D6 would mimic the pharmacokintetics of CYP2D6 poor metabolizers. Caution should therefore be exercised when administering potent CYP2D6 inhibitors with metoprolol tartrate).

No products indexed under this heading.

Haloperidol Decanoate (Potent inhibitors of the CYP2D6 enzyme may increase the plasma concentration of metoprolol tartrate. Strong inhibition of CYP2D6 would mimic the pharmacokintetics of CYP2D6 poor metabolizers. Caution should therefore be exercised when administering potent CYP2D6 inhibitors with metoprolol tartrate).

No products indexed under this heading.

Hydroxychloroquine Sulfate (Potent inhibitors of the CYP2D6 enzyme may increase the plasma concentration of metoprolol tartrate. Strong inhibition of CYP2D6 would mimic the pharmacokintetics of CYP2D6 poor metabolizers. Caution should therefore be exercised when administering potent CYP2D6 inhibitors with metoprolol tartrate).

No products indexed under this heading.

Imatinib Mesylate (Potent inhibitors of the CYP2D6 enzyme may increase the plasma concentration of metoprolol tartrate. Strong inhibition of CYP2D6 would mimic the pharmacokintetics of CYP2D6 poor metabolizers. Caution should therefore be exercised when administering potent CYP2D6 inhibitors with metoprolol tartrate). Products include:

Gleevec Tablets 2227

Imipramine Hydrochloride (Potent inhibitors of the CYP2D6 enzyme may increase the plasma concentration of metoprolol tartrate. Strong inhibition of CYP2D6 would mimic the pharmacokintetics of CYP2D6 poor metabolizers. Caution should therefore be exercised when administering potent CYP2D6 inhibitors with metoprolol tartrate).

No products indexed under this heading.

Imipramine Pamoate (Potent inhibitors of the CYP2D6 enzyme may increase the plasma concentration of metoprolol tartrate. Strong inhibition of CYP2D6 would mimic the pharmacokintetics of CYP2D6 poor metabolizers. Caution should therefore be exercised when administering potent CYP2D6 inhibitors with metoprolol tartrate).

No products indexed under this heading.

Isoflurane (Some inhalation anesthetics may enhance the cardiodepressant effect of beta-blockers).

No products indexed under this heading.

Ketamine Hydrochloride (Some inhalation anesthetics may enhance the cardiodepressant effect of beta-blockers).

No products indexed under this heading.

Maprotiline Hydrochloride (Potent inhibitors of the CYP2D6 enzyme may increase the plasma concentration of metoprolol tartrate. Strong inhibition of CYP2D6 would mimic the pharmacokintetics of CYP2D6 poor metabolizers. Caution should therefore be exercised when administering potent CYP2D6 inhibitors with metoprolol tartrate).

No products indexed under this heading.

Methadone Hydrochloride (Potent inhibitors of the CYP2D6 enzyme may increase the plasma concentration of metoprolol tartrate. Strong inhibition of CYP2D6 would mimic the pharmacokintetics of CYP2D6 poor metabolizers. Caution should therefore be exercised when administering potent CYP2D6 inhibitors with metoprolol tartrate).

No products indexed under this heading.

Methohexital Sodium (Some inhalation anesthetics may enhance the cardiodepressant effect of beta-blockers).

No products indexed under this heading.

Methoxyflurane (Some inhalation anesthetics may enhance the cardiodepressant effect of beta-blockers).

No products indexed under this heading.

Mibefradil Dihydrochloride (Potent inhibitors of the CYP2D6 enzyme may increase the plasma concentration of metoprolol tartrate. Strong inhibition of CYP2D6 would mimic the pharmacokintetics of CYP2D6 poor metabolizers. Caution should therefore be exercised when administering potent CYP2D6 inhibitors with metoprolol tartrate).

No products indexed under this heading.

Moclobemide (Potent inhibitors of the CYP2D6 enzyme may increase the plasma concentration of metoprolol tartrate. Strong inhibition of CYP2D6 would mimic the pharmacokintetics of CYP2D6 poor metabolizers. Caution should therefore be exercised when administering potent CYP2D6 inhibitors with metoprolol tartrate).

No products indexed under this heading.

Nortriptyline Hydrochloride (Potent inhibitors of the CYP2D6 enzyme may increase the plasma concentration of metoprolol tartrate. Strong inhibition of CYP2D6 would mimic the pharmacokintetics of CYP2D6 poor metabolizers. Caution should therefore be exercised when administering potent CYP2D6 inhibitors with metoprolol tartrate).

No products indexed under this heading.

Paroxetine Hydrochloride (Potent inhibitors of the CYP2D6 enzyme may increase the plasma concentration of metoprolol tartrate. Strong inhibition of CYP2D6 would mimic the pharmacokintetics of CYP2D6 poor metabolizers. Caution should therefore be exercised when administering potent CYP2D6 inhibitors with metoprolol tartrate). Products include:

Paxil CR Controlled-Release Tablets 1538
Paxil 1530

Perphenazine (Potent inhibitors of the CYP2D6 enzyme may increase the plasma concentration of metoprolol tartrate. Strong inhibition of CYP2D6 would mimic the pharmacokintetics of CYP2D6 poor metabolizers. Caution should therefore be exercised when administering potent CYP2D6 inhibitors with metoprolol tartrate).

No products indexed under this heading.

Propafenone Hydrochloride (Potent inhibitors of the CYP2D6 enzyme may increase the plasma concentration of metoprolol tartrate. Strong inhibition of CYP2D6 would mimic the pharmacokintetics of CYP2D6 poor metabolizers. Caution should therefore be exercised when administering potent CYP2D6 inhibitors with metoprolol tartrate). Products include:

Rythmol SR Capsules 2727

Propofol (Some inhalation anesthetics may enhance the cardiodepressant effect of beta-blockers).

No products indexed under this heading.

Propoxyphene Hydrochloride (Potent inhibitors of the CYP2D6 enzyme may increase the plasma concentration of metoprolol tartrate. Strong inhibition of CYP2D6 would mimic the pharmacokintetics of CYP2D6 poor metabolizers. Caution should therefore be exercised when administering potent CYP2D6 inhibitors with metoprolol tartrate).

No products indexed under this heading.

Propoxyphene Napsylate (Potent inhibitors of the CYP2D6 enzyme may increase the plasma concentration of metoprolol tartrate. Strong inhibition of CYP2D6 would mimic the pharmacokintetics of CYP2D6 poor metabolizers. Caution should therefore be exercised when administering potent CYP2D6 inhibitors with metoprolol tartrate).

No products indexed under this heading.

Protriptyline Hydrochloride (Potent inhibitors of the CYP2D6 enzyme may increase the plasma concentration of metoprolol tartrate. Strong inhibition of CYP2D6 would mimic the pharmacokintetics of CYP2D6 poor metabolizers. Caution should therefore be exercised when administering potent CYP2D6 inhibitors with metoprolol tartrate).

No products indexed under this heading.

Quinacrine Hydrochloride (Potent inhibitors of the CYP2D6 enzyme may increase the plasma concentration of metoprolol tartrate. Strong inhibition of CYP2D6 would mimic the pharmacokintetics of CYP2D6 poor metabolizers. Caution should therefore be exercised when administering potent CYP2D6 inhibitors with metoprolol tartrate).

No products indexed under this heading.

Quinidine Gluconate (Potent inhibitors of the CYP2D6 enzyme may increase the plasma concentration of metoprolol tartrate. Strong inhibition of CYP2D6 would mimic the pharmacokintetics of CYP2D6 poor metabolizers. Caution should therefore be exercised when administering potent CYP2D6 inhibitors with metoprolol tartrate).

No products indexed under this heading.

Quinidine Hydrochloride (Potent inhibitors of the CYP2D6 enzyme may increase the plasma concentration of metoprolol tartrate. Strong inhibition of CYP2D6 would mimic the pharmacokintetics of CYP2D6 poor metabolizers. Caution should therefore be exercised when administering potent CYP2D6 inhibitors with metoprolol tartrate).

No products indexed under this heading.

Quinidine Polygalacturonate (Potent inhibitors of the CYP2D6 enzyme may increase the plasma concentration of metoprolol tartrate. Strong inhibition of CYP2D6 would mimic the pharmacokintetics of CYP2D6 poor metabolizers. Caution should therefore be exercised when administering potent CYP2D6 inhibitors with metoprolol tartrate).

No products indexed under this heading.

Quinidine Sulfate (Potent inhibitors of the CYP2D6 enzyme may increase the plasma concentration of metoprolol tartrate. Strong inhibition of CYP2D6 would mimic the pharmacokintetics of CYP2D6 poor metabolizers. Caution should therefore be exercised when administering potent CYP2D6 inhibitors with metoprolol tartrate).

No products indexed under this heading.

Ranitidine Bismuth Citrate (Potent inhibitors of the CYP2D6 enzyme may increase the plasma concentration of metoprolol tartrate. Strong inhibition of CYP2D6 would mimic the pharmacokintetics of CYP2D6 poor metabolizers. Caution should therefore be exercised when administering potent CYP2D6 inhibitors with metoprolol tartrate).

No products indexed under this heading.

Ranitidine Hydrochloride (Potent inhibitors of the CYP2D6 enzyme may increase the plasma concentration of metoprolol tartrate. Strong inhibition of CYP2D6 would mimic the pharmacokintetics of CYP2D6 poor metabolizers. Caution should therefore be exercised when administering potent CYP2D6 inhibitors with metoprolol tartrate). Products include:

Zantac 1624
Zantac Injection 1619
Zantac Injection Pharmacy Bulk Package 1622

Rauwolfia Serpentina (Catecholamine-depleting drugs may have an additive effect when given with beta-blocking agents; observe closely for evidence of hypotension or marked bradycardia).

No products indexed under this heading.

Rescinnamine (Catecholamine-depleting drugs may have an additive effect when given with beta-blocking agents; observe closely for evidence of hypotension or marked bradycardia).

No products indexed under this heading.

Reserpine (Catecholamine-depleting drugs may have an additive effect when given with beta-blocking agents; observe closely for evidence of hypotension or marked bradycardia).

No products indexed under this heading.

Ritonavir (Potent inhibitors of the CYP2D6 enzyme may increase the plasma concentration of metoprolol tartrate. Strong inhibition of CYP2D6 would mimic the pharmacokintetics of CYP2D6 poor metabolizers. Caution should therefore be exercised when administering potent CYP2D6 inhibitors with metoprolol tartrate). Products include:

Kaletra 476
Norvir 503

Sertraline Hydrochloride (Potent inhibitors of the CYP2D6 enzyme may increase the plasma concentration of metoprolol tartrate. Strong inhibition of CYP2D6 would mimic the pharmacokintetics of CYP2D6 poor metabolizers. Caution should therefore be exercised when administering potent CYP2D6 inhibitors with metoprolol tartrate). Products include:

Zoloft 2586

Sevoflurane (Some inhalation anesthetics may enhance the cardiodepressant effect of beta-blockers). Products include:

Ultane Liquid for Inhalation 531

Terbinafine Hydrochloride (Potent inhibitors of the CYP2D6 enzyme may increase the plasma concentration of metoprolol tartrate. Strong inhibition of CYP2D6 would mimic the pharmacokintetics of CYP2D6 poor metabolizers. Caution should therefore be exercised when administering potent CYP2D6 inhibitors with metoprolol tartrate). Products include:

Lamisil Tablets 2232
Lamisil AT Creams (Athlete's Foot & Jock Itch) 636

Thioridazine Hydrochloride (Potent inhibitors of the CYP2D6 enzyme may increase the plasma concentration of metoprolol tartrate. Strong inhibition of CYP2D6 would mimic the pharmacokintetics of CYP2D6 poor metabolizers. Caution should therefore be exercised when administering potent CYP2D6 inhibitors with metoprolol tartrate). Products include:

Thioridazine Hydrochloride Tablets 2163

Trimipramine Maleate (Potent inhibitors of the CYP2D6 enzyme may increase the plasma concentration of metoprolol tartrate. Strong inhibition of CYP2D6 would mimic the pharmacokintetics of CYP2D6 poor metabolizers. Caution should therefore be exercised when administering potent CYP2D6 inhibitors with metoprolol tartrate).

No products indexed under this heading.

LOPRESSOR TABLETS

(Metoprolol Tartrate) 2238

See Lopressor Injection

LOPRESSOR HCT 50/25 TABLETS

(Hydrochlorothiazide, Metoprolol Tartrate) 2241

May interact with catecholamine depleting drugs, corticosteroids, cytochrome p450 2d6 inhibitors (selected), general anesthetics, insulin, non-steroidal anti-inflammatory agents, sex steroids, and certain other agents. Compounds in these categories include:

ACTH (Hypokalemia may develop during concomitant use of ACTH).

No products indexed under this heading.

Amiodarone Hydrochloride (Potent inhibitors of the CYP2D6 enzyme may increase the plasma concentration of metoprolol tartrate. Strong inhibition of CYP2D6 would mimic the pharmacokine tics of CYP2D6 poor metabolizers. Caution should therefore be exercised when administering potent CYP2D6 inhibitors with metoprolol tartrate).

No products indexed under this heading.

Amitriptyline Hydrochloride (Potent inhibitors of the CYP2D6 enzyme may increase the plasma concentration of metoprolol tartrate. Strong inhibition of CYP2D6 would mimic the pharmacokine tics of CYP2D6 poor metabolizers. Caution should therefore be exercised when administering potent CYP2D6 inhibitors with metoprolol tartrate).
No products indexed under this heading.

Amoxapine (Potent inhibitors of the CYP2D6 enzyme may increase the plasma concentration of metoprolol tartrate. Strong inhibition of CYP2D6 would mimic the pharmacokine tics of CYP2D6 poor metabolizers. Caution should therefore be exercised when administering potent CYP2D6 inhibitors with metoprolol tartrate).
No products indexed under this heading.

Betamethasone Acetate (Hypokalemia may develop during concomitant use of steroids).
No products indexed under this heading.

Betamethasone Sodium Phosphate (Hypokalemia may develop during concomitant use of steroids).
No products indexed under this heading.

Bupropion Hydrochloride (Potent inhibitors of the CYP2D6 enzyme may increase the plasma concentration of metoprolol tartrate. Strong inhibition of CYP2D6 would mimic the pharmacokine tics of CYP2D6 poor metabolizers. Caution should therefore be exercised when administering potent CYP2D6 inhibitors with metoprolol tartrate). Products include:
Wellbutrin Tablets 1603
Wellbutrin SR Sustained-Release Tablets 1607
Wellbutrin XL Extended-Release Tablets 1613
Zyban Sustained-Release Tablets 1644

Celecoxib (Concurrent administration of some nonsteroidal anti-inflammatory agents may reduce the diuretic, natriuretic, and antihypertensive effects of thiazide diuretics). Products include:
Celebrex Capsules 3134

Chloroquine Hydrochloride (Potent inhibitors of the CYP2D6 enzyme may increase the plasma concentration of metoprolol tartrate. Strong inhibition of CYP2D6 would mimic the pharmacokine tics of CYP2D6 poor metabolizers. Caution should therefore be exercised when administering potent CYP2D6 inhibitors with metoprolol tartrate).
No products indexed under this heading.

Chloroquine Phosphate (Potent inhibitors of the CYP2D6 enzyme may increase the plasma concentration of metoprolol tartrate. Strong inhibition of CYP2D6 would mimic the pharmacokine tics of CYP2D6 poor metabolizers. Caution should therefore be exercised when administering potent CYP2D6 inhibitors with metoprolol tartrate).
No products indexed under this heading.

Chlorpheniramine (Potent inhibitors of the CYP2D6 enzyme may increase the plasma concentration of metoprolol tartrate. Strong inhibition of CYP2D6 would mimic the pharmacokine tics of CYP2D6 poor metabolizers. Caution should therefore be exercised when administering potent CYP2D6 inhibitors with metoprolol tartrate).
No products indexed under this heading.

Chlorpheniramine Maleate (Potent inhibitors of the CYP2D6 enzyme may increase the plasma concentration of metoprolol tartrate. Strong inhibition of CYP2D6 would mimic the pharmacokine tics of CYP2D6 poor metabolizers. Caution should therefore be exercised when administering potent CYP2D6 inhibitors with metoprolol tartrate). Products include:
Advil Allergy Sinus Caplets .... ▣ 770
Advil Multi-Symptom Cold Caplets .... ▣ 770
BC Allergy Sinus Cold Powder .... ▣ 677
Comtrex Maximum Strength Cold & Cough Day/Night Caplets - Night Formulation .... ▣ 726
Comtrex Maximum Strength Day/Night Severe Cold & Sinus Caplets - Night Formulation .... ▣ 725
Contac Cold and Flu Maximum Strength Caplets .... ▣ 728
Contac Cold and Flu Day and Night Caplets (Night Formulation Only) .... ▣ 727
Children's Dimetapp Long Acting Cough Plus Cold Syrup .... ▣ 731
Robitussin Cough & Cold Long-Acting Liquid .... ▣ 735
Robitussin Cough & Allergy Syrup .. ▣ 736
Robitussin Cough & Cold Nighttime Liquid .... ▣ 736
Robitussin Cough, Cold & Flu Nighttime Liquid .... ▣ 738
Robitussin Pediatric Cough & Cold Long-Acting Liquid .... ▣ 735
Robitussin Pediatric Cough & Cold Nighttime Liquid .... ▣ 736
Triaminic Cold & Allergy Liquid .... ▣ 746
Triaminic Cough & Runny Nose Softchews .... ▣ 748
Children's Tylenol Plus Flu Oral Suspension .... ▣ 749
Tylenol Allergy Multi-Symptom Caplets with Cool Burst and Gelcaps 1872
Children's Tylenol Plus Cold Suspension Liquid 1879
Children's Tylenol Plus Cough & Runny Nose Suspension Liquid 1879
Children's Tylenol Plus Flu Suspension Liquid 1881
Children's Tylenol Plus Multi-Symptom Cold Suspension Liquid 1879
Tylenol Cold Head Congestion Nighttime Caplets with Cool Burst 1873
Tylenol Cold Multi-Symptom Nighttime Caplets with Cool Burst 1874
Tylenol Sinus Congestion & Pain Nighttime Caplets with Cool Burst 1876
Vicks 44M Cough, Cold & Flu Relief Liquid 2680
Pediatric Vicks 44m Cough & Cold Relief Liquid 2676
Children's Vicks NyQuil Cold/Cough Relief .... ▣ 756
Children's Vicks NyQuil Cold/Cough Relief Liquid 2680
Zicam Maximum Strength Flu Daytime .... ▣ 768

Chlorpheniramine Polistirex (Potent inhibitors of the CYP2D6 enzyme may increase the plasma concentration of metoprolol tartrate. Strong inhibition of CYP2D6 would mimic the pharmacokine tics of CYP2D6 poor metabolizers. Caution should therefore be exercised when administering potent CYP2D6 inhibitors with metoprolol tartrate). Products include:
Tussionex Pennkinetic Extended-Release Suspension 3327

Chlorpheniramine Tannate (Potent inhibitors of the CYP2D6 enzyme may increase the plasma concentration of metoprolol tartrate. Strong inhibition of CYP2D6 would mimic the pharmacokine tics of CYP2D6 poor metabolizers. Caution should therefore be exercised when administering potent CYP2D6 inhibitors with metoprolol tartrate).
No products indexed under this heading.

Cholestyramine (Absorption of hydrochlorothiazide is impaired in the presence of anionic exchange resins. Single doses of cholestyramine may bind hydrochlorothiazide and reduce its absorption from the gastrointestinal tract by up to 85%.).
No products indexed under this heading.

Cimetidine (Potent inhibitors of the CYP2D6 enzyme may increase the plasma concentration of metoprolol tartrate. Strong inhibition of CYP2D6 would mimic the pharmacokine tics of CYP2D6 poor metabolizers. Caution should therefore be exercised when administering potent CYP2D6 inhibitors with metoprolol tartrate). Products include:
Tagamet HB 200 Tablets .... ▣ 664

Cimetidine Hydrochloride (Potent inhibitors of the CYP2D6 enzyme may increase the plasma concentration of metoprolol tartrate. Strong inhibition of CYP2D6 would mimic the pharmacokine tics of CYP2D6 poor metabolizers. Caution should therefore be exercised when administering potent CYP2D6 inhibitors with metoprolol tartrate).
No products indexed under this heading.

Citalopram Hydrobromide (Potent inhibitors of the CYP2D6 enzyme may increase the plasma concentration of metoprolol tartrate. Strong inhibition of CYP2D6 would mimic the pharmacokine tics of CYP2D6 poor metabolizers. Caution should therefore be exercised when administering potent CYP2D6 inhibitors with metoprolol tartrate). Products include:
Celexa 1176

Clomipramine Hydrochloride (Potent inhibitors of the CYP2D6 enzyme may increase the plasma concentration of metoprolol tartrate. Strong inhibition of CYP2D6 would mimic the pharmacokine tics of CYP2D6 poor metabolizers. Caution should therefore be exercised when administering potent CYP2D6 inhibitors with metoprolol tartrate).
No products indexed under this heading.

Clonidine (If a patient is treated with clonidine and metoprolol tartrate concurrently, and clonidine treatment is to be discontinued, metoprolol tartrate should be stopped several days before clonidine is withdrawn. Rebound hypertension that can follow withdrawalof clonidine may be increased in patients receiving concurrent betaclocker treatment). Products include:
Catapres-TTS 844

Clonidine Hydrochloride (If a patient is treated with clonidine and metoprolol tartrate concurrently, and clonidine treatment is to be discontinued, metoprolol tartrate should be stopped several days before clonidine is withdrawn. Rebound hypertension that can follow withdrawal of clonidine may be increased in patients receiving concurrent betablocker treatment). Products include:
Catapres Tablets 843
Clorpres Tablets 2153

Cocaine Hydrochloride (Potent inhibitors of the CYP2D6 enzyme may increase the plasma concentration of metoprolol tartrate. Strong inhibition of CYP2D6 would mimic the pharmacokine tics of CYP2D6 poor metabolizers. Caution should therefore be exercised when administering potent CYP2D6 inhibitors with metoprolol tartrate).
No products indexed under this heading.

Colestipol (Absorption of hydrochlorothiazide is impaired in the presence of anionic exchange resins. Single doses of colestipol may bind hydrochlorothiazide and reduce its absorption from the gastrointestinal tract by up to 43%).
No products indexed under this heading.

Colestipol Hydrochloride (Absorption of hydrochlorothiazide is impaired in the presence of anionic exchange resins. Single doses of colestipol may bind hydrochlorothiazide and reduce its absorption from the gastrointestinal tract by up to 43%.).
No products indexed under this heading.

Cortisone Acetate (Hypokalemia may develop during concomitant use of steroids).
No products indexed under this heading.

Deserpidine (Catecholamine-depleting drugs may have an additive effect when given with beta-blocking agents; observe closely for evidence of hypotension or marked bradycardia).
No products indexed under this heading.

Desipramine Hydrochloride (Potent inhibitors of the CYP2D6 enzyme may increase the plasma concentration of metoprolol tartrate. Strong inhibition of CYP2D6 would mimic the pharmacokine tics of CYP2D6 poor metabolizers. Caution should therefore be exercised when administering potent CYP2D6 inhibitors with metoprolol tartrate).
No products indexed under this heading.

Desogestrel (Hypokalemia may develop during concomitant use of steroids). Products include:
Mircette Tablets 1066

Dexamethasone (Hypokalemia may develop during concomitant use of steroids). Products include:
Ciprodex Otic Suspension 559
Decadron Tablets 1951
TobraDex Ophthalmic Ointment 562
TobraDex Ophthalmic Suspension ... 563

Dexamethasone Acetate (Hypokalemia may develop during concomitant use of steroids).
No products indexed under this heading.

Dexamethasone Sodium Phosphate (Hypokalemia may develop during concomitant use of steroids).
No products indexed under this heading.

Diclofenac Potassium (Concurrent administration of some nonsteroidal anti-inflammatory agents may reduce the diuretic, natriuretic, and antihypertensive effects of thiazide diuretics).
No products indexed under this heading.

Diclofenac Sodium (Concurrent administration of some nonsteroidal anti-inflammatory agents may reduce the diuretic, natriuretic, and antihypertensive effects of thiazide diuretics). Products include:
- Arthrotec Tablets **3129**
- Voltaren Ophthalmic Solution **2309**
- Voltaren Tablets **2307**
- Voltaren-XR Tablets **2310**

Digitalis Glycoside Preparations (Hypokalemia can sensitize or exaggerate the response of the heart to the toxic effects of digitalis (e.g., increased ventricular irritability)).
No products indexed under this heading.

Diphenhydramine (Potent inhibitors of the CYP2D6 enzyme may increase the plasma concentration of metoprolol tartrate. Strong inhibition of CYP2D6 would mimic the pharmacokine tics of CYP2D6 poor metabolizers. Caution should therefore be exercised when administering potent CYP2D6 inhibitors with metoprolol tartrate). Products include:
- Tylenol Sore Throat Nighttime Liquid with Cool Burst **1877**

Diphenhydramine Hydrochloride (Potent inhibitors of the CYP2D6 enzyme may increase the plasma concentration of metoprolol tartrate. Strong inhibition of CYP2D6 would mimic the pharmacokine tics of CYP2D6 poor metabolizers. Caution should therefore be exercised when administering potent CYP2D6 inhibitors with metoprolol tartrate). Products include:
- Nytol QuickCaps Caplets **615**
- Nytol QuickGels Softgels Maximum Strength **616**
- Simply Sleep Caplets **1868**
- Sominex Original Formula Tablets .. **616**
- TheraFlu Warming Relief Nighttime Severe Cold **743**
- TheraFlu Thin Strips Multi Symptom **744**
- Triaminic Nighttime Cold & Cough Liquid **746**
- Triaminic Thin Strips Cough & Runny Nose **749**
- Extra Strength Tylenol PM Caplets, Vanilla Caplets, Geltabs, Gelcaps and Liquid **1875**
- Tylenol Sore Throat Nighttime Liquid with Cool Burst **790**
- Tylenol Allergy Multi-Symptom Nighttime Caplets with Cool Burst **1872**
- Tylenol Severe Allergy Caplets **1872**
- Children's Tylenol Plus Cold & Allergy Suspension Liquid **1878**

Doxepin Hydrochloride (Potent inhibitors of the CYP2D6 enzyme may increase the plasma concentration of metoprolol tartrate. Strong inhibition of CYP2D6 would mimic the pharmacokine tics of CYP2D6 poor metabolizers. Caution should therefore be exercised when administering potent CYP2D6 inhibitors with metoprolol tartrate).
No products indexed under this heading.

Enflurane (Some inhalation anesthetics may enhance the cardiodepressant effect of beta-blockers).
No products indexed under this heading.

Epinephrine (Patients with a history of severe anaphylactic reaction may be unresponsive to the usual doses of epinephrine used to treat allergic reaction). Products include:
- EpiPen **1061**
- Primatene Mist **719**
- Twinject 0.15 .... **3379**
- Twinject 0.3 .... **3378**

Epinephrine Bitartrate (Patients with a history of severe anaphylactic reaction may be unresponsive to the usual doses of epinephrine used to treat allergic reaction).
No products indexed under this heading.

Epinephrine Hydrochloride (Patients with a history of severe anaphylactic reaction may be unresponsive to the usual doses of epinephrine used to treat allergic reaction).
No products indexed under this heading.

Escitalopram Oxalate (Potent inhibitors of the CYP2D6 enzyme may increase the plasma concentration of metoprolol tartrate. Strong inhibition of CYP2D6 would mimic the pharmacokine tics of CYP2D6 poor metabolizers. Caution should therefore be exercised when administering potent CYP2D6 inhibitors with metoprolol tartrate). Products include:
- Lexapro Oral Solution **1190**
- Lexapro Tablets **1190**

Estradiol (Hypokalemia may develop during concomitant use of steroids). Products include:
- Angeliq Tablets **762**
- Climara Transdermal System **771**
- Climara Pro Transdermal System **776**
- Estrasorb Topical Emulsion **1147**
- Estring Vaginal Ring **2635**
- Menostar Transdermal System **782**
- Vagifem Tablets **2334**

Estrogens, Conjugated (Hypokalemia may develop during concomitant use of steroids). Products include:
- Premarin Intravenous **3442**
- Premarin Tablets **3446**
- Premarin Vaginal Cream **3452**
- Premphase Tablets **3456**
- Prempro Tablets **3456**

Ethinyl Estradiol (Hypokalemia may develop during concomitant use of steroids). Products include:
- Mircette Tablets **1066**
- NuvaRing **2340**
- Ortho-Cyclen/Ortho Tri-Cyclen **2429**
- Ortho Evra Transdermal System **2417**
- Ortho Tri-Cyclen Lo Tablets **2436**
- Seasonique Tablets **1077**
- Yasmin 28 Tablets **796**
- Yaz Tablets **803**

Ethynodiol Diacetate (Hypokalemia may develop during concomitant use of steroids).
No products indexed under this heading.

Etodolac (Concurrent administration of some nonsteroidal anti-inflammatory agents may reduce the diuretic, natriuretic, and antihypertensive effects of thiazide diuretics).
No products indexed under this heading.

Fenoprofen Calcium (Concurrent administration of some nonsteroidal anti-inflammatory agents may reduce the diuretic, natriuretic, and antihypertensive effects of thiazide diuretics). Products include:
- Nalfon Capsules **2502**

Fludrocortisone Acetate (Hypokalemia may develop during concomitant use of steroids).
No products indexed under this heading.

Fluoxetine (Potent inhibitors of the CYP2D6 enzyme may increase the plasma concentration of metoprolol tartrate. Strong inhibition of CYP2D6 would mimic the pharmacokine tics of CYP2D6 poor metabolizers. Caution should therefore be exercised when administering potent CYP2D6 inhibitors with metoprolol tartrate).
No products indexed under this heading.

Fluoxetine Hydrochloride (Potent inhibitors of the CYP2D6 enzyme may increase the plasma concentration of metoprolol tartrate. Strong inhibition of CYP2D6 would mimic the pharmacokine tics of CYP2D6 poor metabolizers. Caution should therefore be exercised when administering potent CYP2D6 inhibitors with metoprolol tartrate). Products include:
- Prozac Pulvules and Liquid **1801**
- Symbyax Capsules **1819**

Fluoxymesterone (Hypokalemia may develop during concomitant use of steroids). Products include:
- Androxy Tablets **3335**

Fluphenazine Decanoate (Potent inhibitors of the CYP2D6 enzyme may increase the plasma concentration of metoprolol tartrate. Strong inhibition of CYP2D6 would mimic the pharmacokine tics of CYP2D6 poor metabolizers. Caution should therefore be exercised when administering potent CYP2D6 inhibitors with metoprolol tartrate).
No products indexed under this heading.

Fluphenazine Enanthate (Potent inhibitors of the CYP2D6 enzyme may increase the plasma concentration of metoprolol tartrate. Strong inhibition of CYP2D6 would mimic the pharmacokine tics of CYP2D6 poor metabolizers. Caution should therefore be exercised when administering potent CYP2D6 inhibitors with metoprolol tartrate).
No products indexed under this heading.

Fluphenazine Hydrochloride (Potent inhibitors of the CYP2D6 enzyme may increase the plasma concentration of metoprolol tartrate. Strong inhibition of CYP2D6 would mimic the pharmacokine tics of CYP2D6 poor metabolizers. Caution should therefore be exercised when administering potent CYP2D6 inhibitors with metoprolol tartrate).
No products indexed under this heading.

Flurbiprofen (Concurrent administration of some nonsteroidal anti-inflammatory agents may reduce the diuretic, natriuretic, and antihypertensive effects of thiazide diuretics).
No products indexed under this heading.

Fluvoxamine Maleate (Potent inhibitors of the CYP2D6 enzyme may increase the plasma concentration of metoprolol tartrate. Strong inhibition of CYP2D6 would mimic the pharmacokine tics of CYP2D6 poor metabolizers. Caution should therefore be exercised when administering potent CYP2D6 inhibitors with metoprolol tartrate).
No products indexed under this heading.

Guanethidine Monosulfate (Catecholamine-depleting drugs may have an additive effect when given with beta-blocking agents; observe closely for evidence of hypotension or marked bradycardia).
No products indexed under this heading.

Halofantrine Hydrochloride (Potent inhibitors of the CYP2D6 enzyme may increase the plasma concentration of metoprolol tartrate. Strong inhibition of CYP2D6 would mimic the pharmacokine tics of CYP2D6 poor metabolizers. Caution should therefore be exercised when administering potent CYP2D6 inhibitors with metoprolol tartrate).
No products indexed under this heading.

Haloperidol (Potent inhibitors of the CYP2D6 enzyme may increase the plasma concentration of metoprolol tartrate. Strong inhibition of CYP2D6 would mimic the pharmacokine tics of CYP2D6 poor metabolizers. Caution should therefore be exercised when administering potent CYP2D6 inhibitors with metoprolol tartrate).
No products indexed under this heading.

Haloperidol Decanoate (Potent inhibitors of the CYP2D6 enzyme may increase the plasma concentration of metoprolol tartrate. Strong inhibition of CYP2D6 would mimic the pharmacokine tics of CYP2D6 poor metabolizers. Caution should therefore be exercised when administering potent CYP2D6 inhibitors with metoprolol tartrate).
No products indexed under this heading.

Hydrocortisone (Hypokalemia may develop during concomitant use of steroids). Products include:
- Colocort Rectal Suspension, USP (Retention) 100 mg/60 mL **2476**
- Hydrocortone Tablets **1989**
- Preparation H Hydrocortisone Cream **646**

Hydrocortisone Acetate (Hypokalemia may develop during concomitant use of steroids). Products include:
- Analpram-HC **1159**
- Pramosone **1161**
- ProctoFoam-HC **3099**

Hydrocortisone Sodium Phosphate (Hypokalemia may develop during concomitant use of steroids).
No products indexed under this heading.

Hydrocortisone Sodium Succinate (Hypokalemia may develop during concomitant use of steroids).
No products indexed under this heading.

Hydroxychloroquine Sulfate (Potent inhibitors of the CYP2D6 enzyme may increase the plasma concentration of metoprolol tartrate. Strong inhibition of CYP2D6 would mimic the pharmacokine tics of CYP2D6 poor metabolizers. Caution should therefore be exercised when administering potent CYP2D6 inhibitors with metoprolol tartrate).
No products indexed under this heading.

Ibuprofen (Concurrent administration of some nonsteroidal anti-inflammatory agents may reduce the diuretic, natriuretic, and antihypertensive effects of thiazide diuretics). Products include:
- Advil Allergy Sinus Caplets .... ▣ 770
- Advil .... ▣ 674
- Children's Advil Oral Suspension .... ▣ 603
- Children's Advil Chewable Tablets .... ▣ 603
- Advil Cold & Sinus .... ▣ 723
- Infants' Advil Concentrated Drops .... ▣ 604
- Infants' Advil Concentrated Drops - White Grape (Dye-Free) .... ▣ 604
- Junior Strength Advil Swallow Tablets .... ▣ 605
- Advil Migraine Liquigels .... ▣ 608
- Advil Multi-Symptom Cold Caplets .... ▣ 770
- Advil PM Caplets .... ▣ 615
- Motrin IB Tablets and Caplets 1866
- Children's Motrin Oral Suspension 1867
- Children's Motrin Non-Staining Dye-Free Oral Suspension 1867
- Children's Motrin Cold Oral Suspension 1867
- Infants' Motrin Concentrated Drops 1867
- Infants' Motrin Non-Staining Dye-Free Concentrated Drops 1867
- Junior Strength Motrin Caplets and Chewable Tablets 1867
- Vicoprofen Tablets 539

Imatinib Mesylate (Potent inhibitors of the CYP2D6 enzyme may increase the plasma concentration of metoprolol tartrate. Strong inhibition of CYP2D6 would mimic the pharmacokine tics of CYP2D6 poor metabolizers. Caution should therefore be exercised when administering potent CYP2D6 inhibitors with metoprolol tartrate). Products include:
- Gleevec Tablets 2227

Imipramine Hydrochloride (Potent inhibitors of the CYP2D6 enzyme may increase the plasma concentration of metoprolol tartrate. Strong inhibition of CYP2D6 would mimic the pharmacokine tics of CYP2D6 poor metabolizers. Caution should therefore be exercised when administering potent CYP2D6 inhibitors with metoprolol tartrate).
No products indexed under this heading.

Imipramine Pamoate (Potent inhibitors of the CYP2D6 enzyme may increase the plasma concentration of metoprolol tartrate. Strong inhibition of CYP2D6 would mimic the pharmacokine tics of CYP2D6 poor metabolizers. Caution should therefore be exercised when administering potent CYP2D6 inhibitors with metoprolol tartrate).
No products indexed under this heading.

Indomethacin (Concurrent administration of some nonsteroidal anti-inflammatory agents may reduce the diuretic, natriuretic, and antihypertensive effects of thiazide diuretics). Products include:
- Indocin 1995

Indomethacin Sodium Trihydrate (Concurrent administration of some nonsteroidal anti-inflammatory agents may reduce the diuretic, natriuretic, and antihypertensive effects of thiazide diuretics). Products include:
- Indocin I.V. 2465

Insulin, Human, Zinc Suspension (Insulin requirements in diabetic patients may be increased, decreased, or unchanged). Products include:
- Humulin L, 100 Units 1794
- Humulin U, 100 Units 1800

Insulin, Human NPH (Insulin requirements in diabetic patients may be increased, decreased, or unchanged). Products include:
- Humulin N, 100 Units 1795
- Humulin N Pen 1797

Insulin, Human Regular (Insulin requirements in diabetic patients may be increased, decreased, or unchanged). Products include:
- Humulin R, 100 Units 1798

Insulin, Human Regular and Human NPH Mixture (Insulin requirements in diabetic patients may be increased, decreased, or unchanged). Products include:
- Humulin 50/50, 100 Units 1791
- Humulin 70/30 Pen 1793

Insulin, NPH (Insulin requirements in diabetic patients may be increased, decreased, or unchanged).
No products indexed under this heading.

Insulin, Regular (Insulin requirements in diabetic patients may be increased, decreased, or unchanged).
No products indexed under this heading.

Insulin, Zinc Crystals (Insulin requirements in diabetic patients may be increased, decreased, or unchanged).
No products indexed under this heading.

Insulin, Zinc Suspension (Insulin requirements in diabetic patients may be increased, decreased, or unchanged).
No products indexed under this heading.

Insulin Aspart, Human Regular (Insulin requirements in diabetic patients may be increased, decreased, or unchanged). Products include:
- NovoLog Injection 2326

Insulin glargine (Insulin requirements in diabetic patients may be increased, decreased, or unchanged). Products include:
- Lantus Injection 2909

Insulin Lispro, Human (Insulin requirements in diabetic patients may be increased, decreased, or unchanged). Products include:
- Humalog-Pen 1781
- Humalog Mix 50/50-Pen 1783
- Humalog Mix 75/25-Pen 1785

Insulin Lispro Protamine, Human (Insulin requirements in diabetic patients may be increased, decreased, or unchanged). Products include:
- Humalog Mix 50/50-Pen 1783
- Humalog Mix 75/25-Pen 1785

Isoflurane (Some inhalation anesthetics may enhance the cardiodepressant effect of beta-blockers).
No products indexed under this heading.

Ketamine Hydrochloride (Some inhalation anesthetics may enhance the cardiodepressant effect of beta-blockers).
No products indexed under this heading.

Ketoprofen (Concurrent administration of some nonsteroidal anti-inflammatory agents may reduce the diuretic, natriuretic, and antihypertensive effects of thiazide diuretics).
No products indexed under this heading.

Ketorolac Tromethamine (Concurrent administration of some nonsteroidal anti-inflammatory agents may reduce the diuretic, natriuretic, and antihypertensive effects of thiazide diuretics). Products include:
- Acular Ophthalmic Solution 565
- Acular LS Ophthalmic Solution 566

Levonorgestrel (Hypokalemia may develop during concomitant use of steroids). Products include:
- Climara Pro Transdermal System 776
- Mirena Intrauterine System 787
- Plan B Tablets 1076
- Seasonique Tablets 1077

Lithium (Lithium renal clearance is reduced by thiazides, increasing the risk of lithium toxicity).
No products indexed under this heading.

Lithium Carbonate (Lithium renal clearance is reduced by thiazides, increasing the risk of lithium toxicity). Products include:
- Lithobid Tablets 1692

Lithium Citrate (Lithium renal clearance is reduced by thiazides, increasing the risk of lithium toxicity).
No products indexed under this heading.

Maprotiline Hydrochloride (Potent inhibitors of the CYP2D6 enzyme may increase the plasma concentration of metoprolol tartrate. Strong inhibition of CYP2D6 would mimic the pharmacokine tics of CYP2D6 poor metabolizers. Caution should therefore be exercised when administering potent CYP2D6 inhibitors with metoprolol tartrate).
No products indexed under this heading.

Meclofenamate Sodium (Concurrent administration of some nonsteroidal anti-inflammatory agents may reduce the diuretic, natriuretic, and antihypertensive effects of thiazide diuretics).
No products indexed under this heading.

Mefenamic Acid (Concurrent administration of some nonsteroidal anti-inflammatory agents may reduce the diuretic, natriuretic, and antihypertensive effects of thiazide diuretics).
No products indexed under this heading.

Meloxicam (Concurrent administration of some nonsteroidal anti-inflammatory agents may reduce the diuretic, natriuretic, and antihypertensive effects of thiazide diuretics). Products include:
- Mobic Oral Suspension 863
- Mobic Tablets 863

Mestranol (Hypokalemia may develop during concomitant use of steroids).
No products indexed under this heading.

Methadone Hydrochloride (Potent inhibitors of the CYP2D6 enzyme may increase the plasma concentration of metoprolol tartrate. Strong inhibition of CYP2D6 would mimic the pharmacokine tics of CYP2D6 poor metabolizers. Caution should therefore be exercised when administering potent CYP2D6 inhibitors with metoprolol tartrate).
No products indexed under this heading.

Methohexital Sodium (Some inhalation anesthetics may enhance the cardiodepressant effect of beta-blockers).
No products indexed under this heading.

Methoxyflurane (Some inhalation anesthetics may enhance the cardiodepressant effect of beta-blockers).
No products indexed under this heading.

Methyldopa (There have been rare reports of hemolytic anemia occurring with the concomitant use of hydrochlorothiazide and methyldopa). Products include:
- Aldoril Tablets 1910

Methylprednisolone Acetate (Hypokalemia may develop during concomitant use of steroids). Products include:
- Depo-Medrol Injectable Suspension 2617
- Depo-Medrol Single-Dose Vial 2619

Methylprednisolone Sodium Succinate (Hypokalemia may develop during concomitant use of steroids).
No products indexed under this heading.

Methyltestosterone (Hypokalemia may develop during concomitant use of steroids). Products include:
- Estratest Tablets 3199
- Estratest H.S. Tablets 3199

Mibefradil Dihydrochloride (Potent inhibitors of the CYP2D6 enzyme may increase the plasma concentration of metoprolol tartrate. Strong inhibition of CYP2D6 would mimic the pharmacokine tics of CYP2D6 poor metabolizers. Caution should therefore be exercised when administering potent CYP2D6 inhibitors with metoprolol tartrate).
No products indexed under this heading.

Moclobemide (Potent inhibitors of the CYP2D6 enzyme may increase the plasma concentration of metoprolol tartrate. Strong inhibition of CYP2D6 would mimic the pharmacokine tics of CYP2D6 poor metabolizers. Caution should therefore be exercised when administering potent CYP2D6 inhibitors with metoprolol tartrate).
No products indexed under this heading.

Nabumetone (Concurrent administration of some nonsteroidal anti-inflammatory agents may reduce the diuretic, natriuretic, and antihypertensive effects of thiazide diuretics).
No products indexed under this heading.

Naproxen (Concurrent administration of some nonsteroidal anti-inflammatory agents may reduce the diuretic, natriuretic, and antihypertensive effects of thiazide diuretics). Products include:
- EC-Naprosyn Delayed-Release Tablets 2761

Naprosyn Suspension 2761
Naprosyn Tablets 2761
Prevacid NapraPAC 3280

Naproxen Sodium (Concurrent administration of some nonsteroidal anti-inflammatory agents may reduce the diuretic, natriuretic, and antihypertensive effects of thiazide diuretics). Products include:

Aleve Caplets 742
Aleve Gelcaps 743
Aleve Tablets 743
Aleve Cold & Sinus Caplets 744
Anaprox Tablets 2761
Anaprox DS Tablets 2761

Norepinephrine Bitartrate (Thiazides may decrease arterial responsiveness to norepinephrine, but not enough to preclude effectiveness of the pressor agent for therapeutic use).
No products indexed under this heading.

Norepinephrine Hydrochloride (Thiazides may decrease arterial responsiveness to norepinephrine, but not enough to preclude effectiveness of the pressor agent for therapeutic use).
No products indexed under this heading.

Norethindrone (Hypokalemia may develop during concomitant use of steroids). Products include:

Ortho Micronor Tablets 2426

Norethindrone Acetate (Hypokalemia may develop during concomitant use of steroids).
No products indexed under this heading.

Norgestimate (Hypokalemia may develop during concomitant use of steroids). Products include:

Ortho-Cyclen/Ortho Tri-Cyclen 2429
Ortho Tri-Cyclen Lo Tablets 2436

Nortriptyline Hydrochloride (Potent inhibitors of the CYP2D6 enzyme may increase the plasma concentration of metoprolol tartrate. Strong inhibition of CYP2D6 would mimic the pharmacokine tics of CYP2D6 poor metabolizers. Caution should therefore be exercised when administering potent CYP2D6 inhibitors with metoprolol tartrate).
No products indexed under this heading.

Oxaprozin (Concurrent administration of some nonsteroidal anti-inflammatory agents may reduce the diuretic, natriuretic, and antihypertensive effects of thiazide diuretics).
No products indexed under this heading.

Paroxetine Hydrochloride (Potent inhibitors of the CYP2D6 enzyme may increase the plasma concentration of metoprolol tartrate. Strong inhibition of CYP2D6 would mimic the pharmacokine tics of CYP2D6 poor metabolizers. Caution should therefore be exercised when administering potent CYP2D6 inhibitors with metoprolol tartrate). Products include:

Paxil CR Controlled-Release Tablets 1538
Paxil 1530

Perphenazine (Potent inhibitors of the CYP2D6 enzyme may increase the plasma concentration of metoprolol tartrate. Strong inhibition of CYP2D6 would mimic the pharmacokine tics of CYP2D6 poor metabolizers. Caution should therefore be exercised when administering potent CYP2D6 inhibitors with metoprolol tartrate).
No products indexed under this heading.

Phenylbutazone (Concurrent administration of some nonsteroidal anti-inflammatory agents may reduce the diuretic, natriuretic, and antihypertensive effects of thiazide diuretics).
No products indexed under this heading.

Piroxicam (Concurrent administration of some nonsteroidal anti-inflammatory agents may reduce the diuretic, natriuretic, and antihypertensive effects of thiazide diuretics).
No products indexed under this heading.

Prednisolone Acetate (Hypokalemia may develop during concomitant use of steroids). Products include:

Blephamide Ophthalmic Ointment 568
Blephamide Ophthalmic Suspension 569
Poly-Pred Ophthalmic Suspension .... ⊙233
Pred Forte Ophthalmic Suspension .... ⊙235
Pred Mild Ophthalmic Suspension .... ⊙238
Pred-G Ophthalmic Ointment .... ⊙237
Pred-G Ophthalmic Suspension ...... ⊙236

Prednisolone Sodium Phosphate (Hypokalemia may develop during concomitant use of steroids).
No products indexed under this heading.

Prednisolone Tebutate (Hypokalemia may develop during concomitant use of steroids).
No products indexed under this heading.

Prednisone (Hypokalemia may develop during concomitant use of steroids).
No products indexed under this heading.

Propafenone Hydrochloride (Potent inhibitors of the CYP2D6 enzyme may increase the plasma concentration of metoprolol tartrate. Strong inhibition of CYP2D6 would mimic the pharmacokine tics of CYP2D6 poor metabolizers. Caution should therefore be exercised when administering potent CYP2D6 inhibitors with metoprolol tartrate). Products include:

Rythmol SR Capsules 2727

Propofol (Some inhalation anesthetics may enhance the cardiodepressant effect of beta-blockers).
No products indexed under this heading.

Propoxyphene Hydrochloride (Potent inhibitors of the CYP2D6 enzyme may increase the plasma concentration of metoprolol tartrate. Strong inhibition of CYP2D6 would mimic the pharmacokine tics of CYP2D6 poor metabolizers. Caution should therefore be exercised when administering potent CYP2D6 inhibitors with metoprolol tartrate).
No products indexed under this heading.

Propoxyphene Napsylate (Potent inhibitors of the CYP2D6 enzyme may increase the plasma concentration of metoprolol tartrate. Strong inhibition of CYP2D6 would mimic the pharmacokine tics of CYP2D6 poor metabolizers. Caution should therefore be exercised when administering potent CYP2D6 inhibitors with metoprolol tartrate).
No products indexed under this heading.

Protriptyline Hydrochloride (Potent inhibitors of the CYP2D6 enzyme may increase the plasma concentration of metoprolol tartrate. Strong inhibition of CYP2D6 would mimic the pharmacokine tics of CYP2D6 poor metabolizers. Caution should therefore be exercised when administering potent CYP2D6 inhibitors with metoprolol tartrate).
No products indexed under this heading.

Quinacrine Hydrochloride (Potent inhibitors of the CYP2D6 enzyme may increase the plasma concentration of metoprolol tartrate. Strong inhibition of CYP2D6 would mimic the pharmacokine tics of CYP2D6 poor metabolizers. Caution should therefore be exercised when administering potent CYP2D6 inhibitors with metoprolol tartrate).
No products indexed under this heading.

Quinidine Gluconate (Potent inhibitors of the CYP2D6 enzyme may increase the plasma concentration of metoprolol tartrate. Strong inhibition of CYP2D6 would mimic the pharmacokine tics of CYP2D6 poor metabolizers. Caution should therefore be exercised when administering potent CYP2D6 inhibitors with metoprolol tartrate).
No products indexed under this heading.

Quinidine Hydrochloride (Potent inhibitors of the CYP2D6 enzyme may increase the plasma concentration of metoprolol tartrate. Strong inhibition of CYP2D6 would mimic the pharmacokine tics of CYP2D6 poor metabolizers. Caution should therefore be exercised when administering potent CYP2D6 inhibitors with metoprolol tartrate).
No products indexed under this heading.

Quinidine Polygalacturonate (Potent inhibitors of the CYP2D6 enzyme may increase the plasma concentration of metoprolol tartrate. Strong inhibition of CYP2D6 would mimic the pharmacokine tics of CYP2D6 poor metabolizers. Caution should therefore be exercised when administering potent CYP2D6 inhibitors with metoprolol tartrate).
No products indexed under this heading.

Quinidine Sulfate (Potent inhibitors of the CYP2D6 enzyme may increase the plasma concentration of metoprolol tartrate. Strong inhibition of CYP2D6 would mimic the pharmacokine tics of CYP2D6 poor metabolizers. Caution should therefore be exercised when administering potent CYP2D6 inhibitors with metoprolol tartrate).
No products indexed under this heading.

Ranitidine Bismuth Citrate (Potent inhibitors of the CYP2D6 enzyme may increase the plasma concentration of metoprolol tartrate. Strong inhibition of CYP2D6 would mimic the pharmacokine tics of CYP2D6 poor metabolizers. Caution should therefore be exercised when administering potent CYP2D6 inhibitors with metoprolol tartrate).
No products indexed under this heading.

Ranitidine Hydrochloride (Potent inhibitors of the CYP2D6 enzyme may increase the plasma concentration of metoprolol tartrate. Strong inhibition of CYP2D6 would mimic the pharmacokine tics of CYP2D6 poor metabolizers. Caution should therefore be exercised when administering potent CYP2D6 inhibitors with metoprolol tartrate). Products include:

Zantac 1624
Zantac Injection 1619
Zantac Injection Pharmacy Bulk Package 1622

Rauwolfia Serpentina (Catecholamine-depleting drugs may have an additive effect when given with beta-blocking agents; observe closely for evidence of hypotension or marked bradycardia).
No products indexed under this heading.

Rescinnamine (Catecholamine-depleting drugs may have an additive effect when given with beta-blocking agents; observe closely for evidence of hypotension or marked bradycardia).
No products indexed under this heading.

Reserpine (Catecholamine-depleting drugs may have an additive effect when given with beta-blocking agents; observe closely for evidence of hypotension or marked bradycardia).
No products indexed under this heading.

Rofecoxib (Concurrent administration of some nonsteroidal anti-inflammatory agents may reduce the diuretic, natriuretic, and antihypertensive effects of thiazide diuretics).
No products indexed under this heading.

Sevoflurane (Some inhalation anesthetics may enhance the cardiodepressant effect of beta-blockers). Products include:

Ultane Liquid for Inhalation 531

Sulindac (Concurrent administration of some nonsteroidal anti-inflammatory agents may reduce the diuretic, natriuretic, and antihypertensive effects of thiazide diuretics). Products include:

Clinoril Tablets 1924

Testosterone (Hypokalemia may develop during concomitant use of steroids). Products include:

AndroGel 3329
Striant Mucoadhesive 1007
Testim 1% Gel 695

Tolmetin Sodium (Concurrent administration of some nonsteroidal anti-inflammatory agents may reduce the diuretic, natriuretic, and antihypertensive effects of thiazide diuretics).
No products indexed under this heading.

Triamcinolone (Hypokalemia may develop during concomitant use of steroids).
No products indexed under this heading.

Triamcinolone Acetonide (Hypokalemia may develop during concomitant use of steroids). Products include:
Azmacort Inhalation Aerosol 1726
Nasacort AQ Nasal Spray 2922

Triamcinolone Diacetate (Hypokalemia may develop during concomitant use of steroids).
No products indexed under this heading.

Triamcinolone Hexacetonide (Hypokalemia may develop during concomitant use of steroids).
No products indexed under this heading.

Tubocurarine Chloride (Thiazides may increase the responsiveness to tubocurarine).
No products indexed under this heading.

Valdecoxib (Concurrent administration of some nonsteroidal anti-inflammatory agents may reduce the diuretic, natriuretic, and antihypertensive effects of thiazide diuretics).
No products indexed under this heading.

LOPRESSOR HCT 100/25 TABLETS
(Hydrochlorothiazide, Metoprolol Tartrate).. 2241
See Lopressor HCT 50/25 Tablets

LOPRESSOR HCT 100/50 TABLETS
(Hydrochlorothiazide, Metoprolol Tartrate).. 2241
See Lopressor HCT 50/25 Tablets

LOPROX SHAMPOO
(Ciclopirox) 1888
None cited in PDR database.

LOTEMAX OPHTHALMIC SUSPENSION 0.5%
(Loteprednol Etabonate) .... ⊙251
None cited in PDR database.

LOTENSIN TABLETS
(Benazepril Hydrochloride) 2243
May interact with diuretics, lithium preparations, potassium preparations, and potassium sparing diuretics. Compounds in these categories include:

Amiloride Hydrochloride (Co-administration with potassium-sparing diuretics can increase the risk of hyperkalemia). Products include:
Midamor Tablets 2026
Moduretic Tablets 2028

Bendroflumethiazide (Patients on diuretics, especially those in whom diuretic therapy was recently instituted, may occasionally experience an excessive reduction in blood pressure).
No products indexed under this heading.

Bumetanide (Patients on diuretics, especially those in whom diuretic therapy was recently instituted, may occasionally experience an excessive reduction in blood pressure). Products include:
Bumex Tablets 2746

Chlorothiazide (Patients on diuretics, especially those in whom diuretic therapy was recently instituted, may occasionally experience an excessive reduction in blood pressure). Products include:
Diuril Oral Suspension 1954

Chlorothiazide Sodium (Patients on diuretics, especially those in whom diuretic therapy was recently instituted, may occasionally experience an excessive reduction in blood pressure). Products include:
Diuril Sodium Intravenous 2467

Chlorthalidone (Patients on diuretics, especially those in whom diuretic therapy was recently instituted, may occasionally experience an excessive reduction in blood pressure). Products include:
Clorpres Tablets 2153

Ethacrynic Acid (Patients on diuretics, especially those in whom diuretic therapy was recently instituted, may occasionally experience an excessive reduction in blood pressure). Products include:
Edecrin Tablets 1959

Furosemide (Patients on diuretics, especially those in whom diuretic therapy was recently instituted, may occasionally experience an excessive reduction in blood pressure). Products include:
Furosemide Tablets 2154

Hydrochlorothiazide (Patients on diuretics, especially those in whom diuretic therapy was recently instituted, may occasionally experience an excessive reduction in blood pressure). Products include:
Aldoril Tablets 1910
Atacand HCT 651
Avalide Tablets 888
Avalide Tablets 2874
Benicar HCT Tablets 1044
Diovan HCT Tablets 2196
Dyazide Capsules 1423
Hyzaar 50-12.5 Tablets 1990
Hyzaar 100-12.5 Tablets 1990
Hyzaar 100-25 Tablets 1990
Lopressor HCT 50/25 Tablets 2241
Lopressor HCT 100/25 Tablets 2241
Lopressor HCT 100/50 Tablets 2241
Lotensin HCT Tablets 2246
Micardis HCT Tablets 856
Moduretic Tablets 2028
Prinzide Tablets 2056
Teveten HCT Tablets 1737
Timolide Tablets 2086
Uniretic Tablets 3100

Hydroflumethiazide (Patients on diuretics, especially those in whom diuretic therapy was recently instituted, may occasionally experience an excessive reduction in blood pressure).
No products indexed under this heading.

Indapamide (Patients on diuretics, especially those in whom diuretic therapy was recently instituted, may occasionally experience an excessive reduction in blood pressure). Products include:
Indapamide Tablets 2156

Lithium (Co-administration with lithium results in increased serum lithium levels and symptoms of lithium toxicity).
No products indexed under this heading.

Lithium Carbonate (Co-administration with lithium results in increased serum lithium levels and symptoms of lithium toxicity). Products include:
Lithobid Tablets 1692

Lithium Citrate (Co-administration with lithium results in increased serum lithium levels and symptoms of lithium toxicity).
No products indexed under this heading.

Methyclothiazide (Patients on diuretics, especially those in whom diuretic therapy was recently instituted, may occasionally experience an excessive reduction in blood pressure).
No products indexed under this heading.

Metolazone (Patients on diuretics, especially those in whom diuretic therapy was recently instituted, may occasionally experience an excessive reduction in blood pressure).
No products indexed under this heading.

Polythiazide (Patients on diuretics, especially those in whom diuretic therapy was recently instituted, may occasionally experience an excessive reduction in blood pressure).
No products indexed under this heading.

Potassium Acid Phosphate (Co-administration with potassium supplements can increase the risk of hyperkalemia). Products include:
K-Phos Original (Sodium Free) Tablets 760

Potassium Bicarbonate (Co-administration with potassium supplements can increase the risk of hyperkalemia).
No products indexed under this heading.

Potassium Chloride (Co-administration with potassium supplements can increase the risk of hyperkalemia). Products include:
Colyte with Flavor Packs for Oral Solution.. 3088
HalfLytely and Bisacodyl Tablets Bowel Prep Kit with Flavors Packs.. 881
K-Dur Extended-Relase Tablets 3033
K-Lor Oral Solution 474
K-Tab Tablets 475
MoviPrep Oral Solution 2839
TriLyte with Flavor Packs for Oral Solution.. 3100

Potassium Citrate (Co-administration with potassium supplements can increase the risk of hyperkalemia). Products include:
Urocit-K Tablets 2144

Potassium Gluconate (Co-administration with potassium supplements can increase the risk of hyperkalemia).
No products indexed under this heading.

Potassium Phosphate (Co-administration with potassium supplements can increase the risk of hyperkalemia). Products include:
K-Phos Neutral Tablets 760

Spironolactone (Co-administration with potassium-sparing diuretics can increase the risk of hyperkalemia).
No products indexed under this heading.

Torsemide (Patients on diuretics, especially those in whom diuretic therapy was recently instituted, may occasionally experience an excessive reduction in blood pressure). Products include:
Demadex Injection 2759
Demadex Tablets 2759

Triamterene (Co-administration with potassium-sparing diuretics can increase the risk of hyperkalemia). Products include:
Dyazide Capsules 1423
Dyrenium Capsules 3400

LOTENSIN HCT TABLETS
(Benazepril Hydrochloride, Hydrochlorothiazide)........................... 2246
May interact with barbiturates, insulin, lithium preparations, narcotic analgesics, non-steroidal anti-inflammatory agents, potassium preparations, potassium sparing diuretics, and certain other agents. Compounds in these categories include:

Alfentanil Hydrochloride (Orthostatic hypotension produced by thiazides may be potentiated by narcotics).
No products indexed under this heading.

Amiloride Hydrochloride (Co-administration with potassium-sparing diuretics can increase the risk of hyperkalemia). Products include:
Midamor Tablets 2026
Moduretic Tablets 2028

Aprobarbital (Orthostatic hypotension produced by thiazides may be potentiated by barbiturates).
No products indexed under this heading.

Buprenorphine Hydrochloride (Orthostatic hypotension produced by thiazides may be potentiated by narcotics). Products include:
Buprenex Injectable 2716
Suboxone Tablets 2717
Subutex Tablets 2717

Butabarbital (Orthostatic hypotension produced by thiazides may be potentiated by barbiturates).
No products indexed under this heading.

Butalbital (Orthostatic hypotension produced by thiazides may be potentiated by barbiturates).
No products indexed under this heading.

Celecoxib (The diuretic, natriuretic, and antihypertensive effects of thiazide diuretics may be reduced by concurrent administration of non-steroidal anti-inflammatory agents). Products include:
Celebrex Capsules 3134

Cholestyramine (Absorption of hydrochlorothiazide is impaired in the presence of anionic exchange resins; cholestyramine resins bind the hydrochlorothiazide and reduce its absorption from GI tract by up to 85%).
No products indexed under this heading.

Codeine Phosphate (Orthostatic hypotension produced by thiazides may be potentiated by narcotics). Products include:
Tylenol with Codeine Tablets 2391

Colestipol Hydrochloride (Absorption of hydrochlorothiazide is impaired in the presence of anionic exchange resins; colestipol resins bind the hydrochlorothiazide and reduce its absorption from GI tract by up to 43%).
No products indexed under this heading.

Dezocine (Orthostatic hypotension produced by thiazides may be potentiated by narcotics).
No products indexed under this heading.

Diclofenac Potassium (The diuretic, natriuretic, and antihypertensive effects of thiazide diuretics may be reduced by concurrent administration of non-steroidal anti-inflammatory agents).
No products indexed under this heading.

Diclofenac Sodium (The diuretic, natriuretic, and antihypertensive effects of thiazide diuretics may be reduced by concurrent administration of non-steroidal anti-inflammatory agents). Products include:
Arthrotec Tablets 3129
Voltaren Ophthalmic Solution 2309
Voltaren Tablets 2307
Voltaren-XR Tablets 2310

Etodolac (The diuretic, natriuretic, and antihypertensive effects of thiazide diuretics may be reduced by concurrent administration of non-steroidal anti-inflammatory agents).
No products indexed under this heading.

Fenoprofen Calcium (The diuretic, natriuretic, and antihypertensive effects of thiazide diuretics may be reduced by concurrent administration of non-steroidal anti-inflammatory agents). Products include:
Nalfon Capsules 2502

Fentanyl (Orthostatic hypotension produced by thiazides may be potentiated by narcotics). Products include:
Duragesic Transdermal System 2373
Ionsys Transdermal System 2379

Fentanyl Citrate (Orthostatic hypotension produced by thiazides may be potentiated by narcotics). Products include:
Actiq 979

Flurbiprofen (The diuretic, natriuretic, and antihypertensive effects of thiazide diuretics may be reduced by concurrent administration of non-steroidal anti-inflammatory agents).
No products indexed under this heading.

Hydrocodone Bitartrate (Orthostatic hypotension produced by thiazides may be potentiated by narcotics). Products include:
Hycodan 1116
Hycotuss Expectorant Syrup 1117
Vicodin Tablets 535
Vicodin ES Tablets 536
Vicodin HP Tablets 538
Vicoprofen Tablets 539
Zydone Tablets 1139

Hydrocodone Polistirex (Orthostatic hypotension produced by thiazides may be potentiated by narcotics). Products include:
Tussionex Pennkinetic Extended-Release Suspension 3327

Hydromorphone Hydrochloride (Orthostatic hypotension produced by thiazides may be potentiated by narcotics). Products include:
Dilaudid 440
Dilaudid Non-Sterile Powder 440
Dilaudid Oral Liquid 445
Dilaudid Rectal Suppositories 440
Dilaudid Tablets 440
Dilaudid Tablets - 8 mg 445
Dilaudid-HP 442

Ibuprofen (The diuretic, natriuretic, and antihypertensive effects of thiazide diuretics may be reduced by concurrent administration of non-steroidal anti-inflammatory agents). Products include:
Advil Allergy Sinus Caplets 770
Advil 674
Children's Advil Oral Suspension 603
Children's Advil Chewable Tablets 603
Advil Cold & Sinus 723
Infants' Advil Concentrated Drops 604
Infants' Advil Concentrated Drops - White Grape (Dye-Free) 604
Junior Strength Advil Swallow Tablets 605
Advil Migraine Liquigels 608
Advil Multi-Symptom Cold Caplets 770
Advil PM Caplets 615
Motrin IB Tablets and Caplets 1866
Children's Motrin Oral Suspension 1867
Children's Motrin Non-Staining Dye-Free Oral Suspension 1867
Children's Motrin Cold Oral Suspension 1867
Infants' Motrin Concentrated Drops 1867
Infants' Motrin Non-Staining Dye-Free Concentrated Drops 1867
Junior Strength Motrin Caplets and Chewable Tablets 1867
Vicoprofen Tablets 539

Indomethacin (The diuretic, natriuretic, and antihypertensive effects of thiazide diuretics may be reduced by concurrent administration of non-steroidal anti-inflammatory agents). Products include:
Indocin 1995

Indomethacin Sodium Trihydrate (The diuretic, natriuretic, and antihypertensive effects of thiazide diuretics may be reduced by concurrent administration of non-steroidal anti-inflammatory agents). Products include:
Indocin I.V. 2465

Insulin, Human, Zinc Suspension (Hydrochlorothiazide causes hyperglycemia and tends to reduce glucose tolerance; insulin requirements may be increased, decreased, or unchanged). Products include:
Humulin L, 100 Units 1794
Humulin U, 100 Units 1800

Insulin, Human NPH (Hydrochlorothiazide causes hyperglycemia and tends to reduce glucose tolerance; insulin requirements may be increased, decreased, or unchanged). Products include:
Humulin N, 100 Units 1795
Humulin N Pen 1797

Insulin, Human Regular (Hydrochlorothiazide causes hyperglycemia and tends to reduce glucose tolerance; insulin requirements may be increased, decreased, or unchanged). Products include:
Humulin R, 100 Units 1798

Insulin, Human Regular and Human NPH Mixture (Hydrochlorothiazide causes hyperglycemia and tends to reduce glucose tolerance; insulin requirements may be increased, decreased, or unchanged). Products include:
Humulin 50/50, 100 Units 1791
Humulin 70/30 Pen 1793

Insulin, NPH (Hydrochlorothiazide causes hyperglycemia and tends to reduce glucose tolerance; insulin requirements may be increased, decreased, or unchanged).
No products indexed under this heading.

Insulin, Regular (Hydrochlorothiazide causes hyperglycemia and tends to reduce glucose tolerance; insulin requirements may be increased, decreased, or unchanged).
No products indexed under this heading.

Insulin, Zinc Crystals (Hydrochlorothiazide causes hyperglycemia and tends to reduce glucose tolerance; insulin requirements may be increased, decreased, or unchanged).
No products indexed under this heading.

Insulin, Zinc Suspension (Hydrochlorothiazide causes hyperglycemia and tends to reduce glucose tolerance; insulin requirements may be increased, decreased, or unchanged).
No products indexed under this heading.

Insulin Aspart, Human Regular (Hydrochlorothiazide causes hyperglycemia and tends to reduce glucose tolerance; insulin requirements may be increased, decreased, or unchanged). Products include:
NovoLog Injection 2326

Insulin glargine (Hydrochlorothiazide causes hyperglycemia and tends to reduce glucose tolerance; insulin requirements may be increased, decreased, or unchanged). Products include:
Lantus Injection 2909

Insulin Lispro, Human (Hydrochlorothiazide causes hyperglycemia and tends to reduce glucose tolerance; insulin requirements may be increased, decreased, or unchanged). Products include:
Humalog-Pen 1781
Humalog Mix 50/50-Pen 1783
Humalog Mix 75/25-Pen 1785

Insulin Lispro Protamine, Human (Hydrochlorothiazide causes hyperglycemia and tends to reduce glucose tolerance; insulin requirements may be increased, decreased, or unchanged). Products include:
Humalog Mix 50/50-Pen 1783
Humalog Mix 75/25-Pen 1785

Ketoprofen (The diuretic, natriuretic, and antihypertensive effects of thiazide diuretics may be reduced by concurrent administration of non-steroidal anti-inflammatory agents).
No products indexed under this heading.

Ketorolac Tromethamine (The diuretic, natriuretic, and antihypertensive effects of thiazide diuretics may be reduced by concurrent administration of non-steroidal anti-inflammatory agents). Products include:
Acular Ophthalmic Solution 565
Acular LS Ophthalmic Solution 566

Levorphanol Tartrate (Orthostatic hypotension produced by thiazides may be potentiated by narcotics).
No products indexed under this heading.

Lithium (Co-administration with lithium results in increased serum lithium levels; renal clearance of lithium is reduced by thiazides; increased risk of lithium toxicity).
No products indexed under this heading.

Lithium Carbonate (Co-administration with lithium results in increased serum lithium levels; renal clearance of lithium is reduced by thiazides; increased risk of lithium toxicity). Products include:
Lithobid Tablets 1692

Lithium Citrate (Co-administration with lithium results in increased serum lithium levels; renal clearance of lithium is reduced by thiazides; increased risk of lithium toxicity).
No products indexed under this heading.

Meclofenamate Sodium (The diuretic, natriuretic, and antihypertensive effects of thiazide diuretics may be reduced by concurrent administration of non-steroidal anti-inflammatory agents).
No products indexed under this heading.

Mefenamic Acid (The diuretic, natriuretic, and antihypertensive effects of thiazide diuretics may be reduced by concurrent administration of non-steroidal anti-inflammatory agents).
No products indexed under this heading.

Meloxicam (The diuretic, natriuretic, and antihypertensive effects of thiazide diuretics may be reduced by concurrent administration of non-steroidal anti-inflammatory agents). Products include:
Mobic Oral Suspension 863
Mobic Tablets 863

Meperidine Hydrochloride (Orthostatic hypotension produced by thiazides may be potentiated by narcotics).
No products indexed under this heading.

Mephobarbital (Orthostatic hypotension produced by thiazides may be potentiated by barbiturates).
No products indexed under this heading.

Methadone Hydrochloride (Orthostatic hypotension produced by thiazides may be potentiated by narcotics).
No products indexed under this heading.

Morphine Sulfate (Orthostatic hypotension produced by thiazides may be potentiated by narcotics). Products include:
Avinza Capsules 1741
Kadian Capsules 577
MS Contin Tablets 2701

Nabumetone (The diuretic, natriuretic, and antihypertensive effects of thiazide diuretics may be reduced by concurrent administration of non-steroidal anti-inflammatory agents).
No products indexed under this heading.

Naproxen (The diuretic, natriuretic, and antihypertensive effects of thiazide diuretics may be reduced by concurrent administration of non-steroidal anti-inflammatory agents). Products include:
EC-Naprosyn Delayed-Release Tablets 2761
Naprosyn Suspension 2761
Naprosyn Tablets 2761
Prevacid NapraPAC 3280

Naproxen Sodium (The diuretic, natriuretic, and antihypertensive effects of thiazide diuretics may be reduced by concurrent administration of non-steroidal anti-inflammatory agents). Products include:
Aleve Caplets 742
Aleve Gelcaps 743
Aleve Tablets 743
Aleve Cold & Sinus Caplets 744
Anaprox Tablets 2761
Anaprox DS Tablets 2761

Norepinephrine Hydrochloride
(Thiazides may decrease arterial responsiveness to norepinephrine).
No products indexed under this heading.

Oxaprozin (The diuretic, natriuretic, and antihypertensive effects of thiazide diuretics may be reduced by concurrent administration of non-steroidal anti-inflammatory agents).
No products indexed under this heading.

Oxycodone Hydrochloride (Orthostatic hypotension produced by thiazides may be potentiated by narcotics). Products include:
OxyContin Tablets 2703
OxyFast Oral Concentrate
　Solution...................................... 2708
OxyIR Capsules 2708
Percocet Tablets 1131
Percodan Tablets 1132

Pentobarbital Sodium (Orthostatic hypotension produced by thiazides may be potentiated by barbiturates). Products include:
Nembutal Sodium Solution, USP 2470

Phenobarbital (Orthostatic hypotension produced by thiazides may be potentiated by barbiturates). Products include:
Donnatal Extentabs 2493

Phenylbutazone (The diuretic, natriuretic, and antihypertensive effects of thiazide diuretics may be reduced by concurrent administration of non-steroidal anti-inflammatory agents).
No products indexed under this heading.

Piroxicam (The diuretic, natriuretic, and antihypertensive effects of thiazide diuretics may be reduced by concurrent administration of non-steroidal anti-inflammatory agents).
No products indexed under this heading.

Potassium Acid Phosphate (Co-administration with potassium supplements can increase the risk of hyperkalemia). Products include:
K-Phos Original (Sodium Free)
　Tablets 760

Potassium Bicarbonate (Co-administration with potassium supplements can increase the risk of hyperkalemia).
No products indexed under this heading.

Potassium Chloride (Co-administration with potassium supplements can increase the risk of hyperkalemia). Products include:
Colyte with Flavor Packs for Oral
　Solution...................................... 3088
HalfLytely and Bisacodyl Tablets
　Bowel Prep Kit with Flavors
　Packs...................................... 881
K-Dur Extended-Relase Tablets 3033
K-Lor Oral Solution 474
K-Tab Tablets 475
MoviPrep Oral Solution 2839
TriLyte with Flavor Packs for Oral
　Solution...................................... 3100

Potassium Citrate (Co-administration with potassium supplements can increase the risk of hyperkalemia). Products include:
Urocit-K Tablets 2144

Potassium Gluconate (Co-administration with potassium supplements can increase the risk of hyperkalemia).
No products indexed under this heading.

Potassium Phosphate (Co-administration with potassium supplements can increase the risk of hyperkalemia). Products include:
K-Phos Neutral Tablets 760

Propoxyphene Hydrochloride (Orthostatic hypotension produced by thiazides may be potentiated by narcotics).
No products indexed under this heading.

Propoxyphene Napsylate (Orthostatic hypotension produced by thiazides may be potentiated by narcotics).
No products indexed under this heading.

Remifentanil Hydrochloride (Orthostatic hypotension produced by thiazides may be potentiated by narcotics).
No products indexed under this heading.

Rofecoxib (The diuretic, natriuretic, and antihypertensive effects of thiazide diuretics may be reduced by concurrent administration of non-steroidal anti-inflammatory agents).
No products indexed under this heading.

Secobarbital Sodium (Orthostatic hypotension produced by thiazides may be potentiated by barbiturates).
No products indexed under this heading.

Spironolactone (Co-administration with potassium-sparing diuretics can increase the risk of hyperkalemia).
No products indexed under this heading.

Sufentanil Citrate (Orthostatic hypotension produced by thiazides may be potentiated by narcotics).
No products indexed under this heading.

Sulindac (The diuretic, natriuretic, and antihypertensive effects of thiazide diuretics may be reduced by concurrent administration of non-steroidal anti-inflammatory agents). Products include:
Clinoril Tablets 1924

Thiamylal Sodium (Orthostatic hypotension produced by thiazides may be potentiated by barbiturates).
No products indexed under this heading.

Tolmetin Sodium (The diuretic, natriuretic, and antihypertensive effects of thiazide diuretics may be reduced by concurrent administration of non-steroidal anti-inflammatory agents).
No products indexed under this heading.

Triamterene (Co-administration with potassium-sparing diuretics can increase the risk of hyperkalemia). Products include:
Dyazide Capsules 1423
Dyrenium Capsules 3400

Tubocurarine Chloride (Thiazides may increase the responsiveness to tubocurarine).
No products indexed under this heading.

Valdecoxib (The diuretic, natriuretic, and antihypertensive effects of thiazide diuretics may be reduced by concurrent administration of non-steroidal anti-inflammatory agents).
No products indexed under this heading.

Food Interactions

Alcohol (Orthostatic hypotension produced by thiazides may be potentiated by alcohol).

LOTREL CAPSULES

(Amlodipine Besylate, Benazepril Hydrochloride)................................ 2249
May interact with diuretics, lithium preparations, potassium preparations, and potassium sparing diuretics. Compounds in these categories include:

Amiloride Hydrochloride (Potential for the increased risk of hyperkalemia; patients on diuretics, especially those in whom diuretic therapy was recently instituted, may experience an excessive reduction in blood pressure). Products include:
Midamor Tablets 2026
Moduretic Tablets 2028

Bendroflumethiazide (Patients on diuretics, especially those in whom diuretic therapy was recently instituted, may experience an excessive reduction in blood pressure).
No products indexed under this heading.

Bumetanide (Patients on diuretics, especially those in whom diuretic therapy was recently instituted, may experience an excessive reduction in blood pressure). Products include:
Bumex Tablets 2746

Chlorothiazide (Patients on diuretics, especially those in whom diuretic therapy was recently instituted, may experience an excessive reduction in blood pressure). Products include:
Diuril Oral Suspension 1954

Chlorothiazide Sodium (Patients on diuretics, especially those in whom diuretic therapy was recently instituted, may experience an excessive reduction in blood pressure). Products include:
Diuril Sodium Intravenous 2467

Chlorthalidone (Patients on diuretics, especially those in whom diuretic therapy was recently instituted, may experience an excessive reduction in blood pressure). Products include:
Clorpres Tablets 2153

Ethacrynic Acid (Patients on diuretics, especially those in whom diuretic therapy was recently instituted, may experience an excessive reduction in blood pressure). Products include:
Edecrin Tablets 1959

Furosemide (Patients on diuretics, especially those in whom diuretic therapy was recently instituted, may experience an excessive reduction in blood pressure). Products include:
Furosemide Tablets 2154

Hydrochlorothiazide (Patients on diuretics, especially those in whom diuretic therapy was recently instituted, may experience an excessive reduction in blood pressure). Products include:
Aldoril Tablets 1910
Atacand HCT 651
Avalide Tablets 888
Avalide Tablets 2874
Benicar HCT Tablets 1044
Diovan HCT Tablets 2196
Dyazide Capsules 1423
Hyzaar 12.5 Tablets 1990
Hyzaar 100-12.5 Tablets 1990
Hyzaar 100-25 Tablets 1990
Lopressor HCT 50/25 Tablets 2241
Lopressor HCT 100/25 Tablets 2241
Lopressor HCT 100/50 Tablets 2241
Lotensin HCT Tablets 2246
Micardis HCT Tablets 856
Moduretic Tablets 2028
Prinzide Tablets 2056
Teveten HCT Tablets 1737
Timolide Tablets 2086
Uniretic Tablets 3100

Hydroflumethiazide (Patients on diuretics, especially those in whom diuretic therapy was recently instituted, may experience an excessive reduction in blood pressure).
No products indexed under this heading.

Indapamide (Patients on diuretics, especially those in whom diuretic therapy was recently instituted, may experience an excessive reduction in blood pressure). Products include:
Indapamide Tablets 2156

Lithium (Potential for increased serum lithium levels and symptoms of lithium toxicity).
No products indexed under this heading.

Lithium Carbonate (Potential for increased serum lithium levels and symptoms of lithium toxicity). Products include:
Lithobid Tablets 1692

Lithium Citrate (Potential for increased serum lithium levels and symptoms of lithium toxicity).
No products indexed under this heading.

Methyclothiazide (Patients on diuretics, especially those in whom diuretic therapy was recently instituted, may experience an excessive reduction in blood pressure).
No products indexed under this heading.

Metolazone (Patients on diuretics, especially those in whom diuretic therapy was recently instituted, may experience an excessive reduction in blood pressure).
No products indexed under this heading.

Polythiazide (Patients on diuretics, especially those in whom diuretic therapy was recently instituted, may experience an excessive reduction in blood pressure).
No products indexed under this heading.

Potassium Acid Phosphate (Potential for the increased risk of hyperkalemia). Products include:
K-Phos Original (Sodium Free)
　Tablets 760

Potassium Bicarbonate (Potential for the increased risk of hyperkalemia).
No products indexed under this heading.

Potassium Chloride (Potential for the increased risk of hyperkalemia). Products include:
Colyte with Flavor Packs for Oral
　Solution...................................... 3088
HalfLytely and Bisacodyl Tablets
　Bowel Prep Kit with Flavors
　Packs...................................... 881
K-Dur Extended-Release Tablets 3033
K-Lor Oral Solution 474
K-Tab Tablets 475
MoviPrep Oral Solution 2839
TriLyte with Flavor Packs for Oral
　Solution...................................... 3100

Potassium Citrate (Potential for the increased risk of hyperkalemia). Products include:
Urocit-K Tablets 2144

Potassium Gluconate (Potential for the increased risk of hyperkalemia).
No products indexed under this heading.

Potassium Phosphate (Potential for the increased risk of hyperkalemia). Products include:
K-Phos Neutral Tablets 760

Spironolactone (Potential for the increased risk of hyperkalemia; patients on diuretics, especially those in whom diuretic therapy was recently instituted, may experience an excessive reduction in blood pressure).
No products indexed under this heading.

Torsemide (Patients on diuretics, especially those in whom diuretic therapy was recently instituted, may experience an excessive reduction in blood pressure). Products include:
Demadex Injection 2759
Demadex Tablets 2759

Triamterene (Potential for the increased risk of hyperkalemia; patients on diuretics, especially those in whom diuretic therapy was recently instituted, may experience an excessive reduction in blood pressure). Products include:
Dyazide Capsules 1423
Dyrenium Capsules 3400

LOTRIMIN CREAM
(Clotrimazole) 3039
None cited in PDR database.

LOTRIMIN LOTION 1%
(Clotrimazole) 3039
None cited in PDR database.

LOTRIMIN TOPICAL SOLUTION 1%
(Clotrimazole) 3039
None cited in PDR database.

LOTRISONE CREAM
(Betamethasone Dipropionate, Clotrimazole) 3040
None cited in PDR database.

LOTRISONE LOTION
(Betamethasone Dipropionate, Clotrimazole) 3040
None cited in PDR database.

LOTRONEX TABLETS
(Alosetron Hydrochloride) 1512
May interact with cytochrome p450 1a2 inhibitors (selected), cytochrome p450 3a4 inhibitors (selected), and certain other agents. Compounds in these categories include:

Acetazolamide (Co-administration of alosetron and strong CYP3A4 inhibitors has not been evaluated but should be undertaken with caution because of similar potential drug interactions).
No products indexed under this heading.

Alatrofloxacin Mesylate (Concomitant administration of alosetron and moderate CYP1A2 inhibitors, including quinolone antibiotics and cimetidine, has not been evaluated, but should be avoided unless clinically necessary because of potential drug interactions).
No products indexed under this heading.

Amiodarone Hydrochloride (Co-administration of alosetron and strong CYP3A4 inhibitors has not been evaluated but should be undertaken with caution because of similar potential drug interactions).
No products indexed under this heading.

Amprenavir (Co-administration of alosetron and strong CYP3A4 inhibitors has not been evaluated but should be undertaken with caution because of similar potential drug interactions). Products include:
Agenerase Capsules 1327
Agenerase Oral Solution 1332

Anastrozole (Co-administration of alosetron and strong CYP3A4 inhibitors has not been evaluated but should be undertaken with caution because of similar potential drug interactions). Products include:
Arimidex Tablets 673

Aprepitant (Co-administration of alosetron and strong CYP3A4 inhibitors has not been evaluated but should be undertaken with caution because of similar potential drug interactions). Products include:
Emend Capsules 1963

Cimetidine (Co-administration of alosetron and strong CYP3A4 inhibitors has not been evaluated but should be undertaken with caution because of similar potential drug interactions). Products include:
Tagamet HB 200 Tablets 664

Cimetidine Hydrochloride (Co-administration of alosetron and strong CYP3A4 inhibitors has not been evaluated but should be undertaken with caution because of similar potential drug interactions).
No products indexed under this heading.

Ciprofloxacin (Co-administration of alosetron and strong CYP3A4 inhibitors has not been evaluated but should be undertaken with caution because of similar potential drug interactions). Products include:
Cipro Oral Suspension 2977
Cipro I.V. 2984
Cipro XR Tablets 2990
Ciprodex Otic Suspension 559

Ciprofloxacin Hydrochloride (Concomitant administration of alosetron and moderate CYP1A2 inhibitors, including quinolone antibiotics and cimetidine, has not been evaluated, but should be avoided unless clinically necessary because of potential drug interactions).
Products include:
Ciloxan Ophthalmic Ointment 559
Ciloxan Ophthalmic Solution 206
Cipro Tablets 2977
Proquin XR Tablets 1153

Clarithromycin (Co-administration of alosetron and strong CYP3A4 inhibitors has not been evaluated but should be undertaken with caution because of similar potential drug interactions). Products include:
Biaxin/Biaxin XL 402
PREVPAC 3284

Clotrimazole (Co-administration of alosetron and strong CYP3A4 inhibitors has not been evaluated but should be undertaken with caution because of similar potential drug interactions). Products include:
Desenex Athlete's Foot Cream 635
Lotrimin 3039
Lotrisone 3040

Cyclosporine (Co-administration of alosetron and strong CYP3A4 inhibitors has not been evaluated but should be undertaken with caution because of similar potential drug interactions). Products include:
Gengraf Capsules 459
Neoral Oral Solution 2259
Neoral Soft Gelatin Capsules 2259
Restasis Ophthalmic Emulsion 575
Sandimmune 2275

Dalfopristin (Co-administration of alosetron and strong CYP3A4 inhibitors has not been evaluated but should be undertaken with caution because of similar potential drug interactions).
No products indexed under this heading.

Danazol (Co-administration of alosetron and strong CYP3A4 inhibitors has not been evaluated but should be undertaken with caution because of similar potential drug interactions).
No products indexed under this heading.

Delavirdine Mesylate (Co-administration of alosetron and strong CYP3A4 inhibitors has not been evaluated but should be undertaken with caution because of similar potential drug interactions).
Products include:
Rescriptor Tablets 2551

Desogestrel (Concomitant administration of alosetron and moderate CYP1A2 inhibitors, including quinolone antibiotics and cimetidine, has not been evaluated, but should be avoided unless clinically necessary because of potential drug interactions). Products include:
Mircette Tablets 1066

Diltiazem Hydrochloride (Co-administration of alosetron and strong CYP3A4 inhibitors has not been evaluated but should be undertaken with caution because of similar potential drug interactions).
Products include:
Cardizem LA Extended Release Tablets 1728
Tiazac Capsules 1201

Diltiazem Maleate (Co-administration of alosetron and strong CYP3A4 inhibitors has not been evaluated but should be undertaken with caution because of similar potential drug interactions).
No products indexed under this heading.

Efavirenz (Co-administration of alosetron and strong CYP3A4 inhibitors has not been evaluated but should be undertaken with caution because of similar potential drug interactions). Products include:
Atripla Tablets 945
Sustiva Capsules 930
Sustiva Tablets 930

Enoxacin (Concomitant administration of alosetron and moderate CYP1A2 inhibitors, including quinolone antibiotics and cimetidine, has not been evaluated, but should be avoided unless clinically necessary because of potential drug interactions).
No products indexed under this heading.

Erythromycin (Co-administration of alosetron and strong CYP3A4 inhibitors has not been evaluated but should be undertaken with caution because of similar potential drug interactions). Products include:
Ery-Tab Tablets 449
Erythromycin Base Filmtab Tablets 455
Erythromycin Delayed-Release Capsules, USP 457
PCE Dispertab Tablets 515

Erythromycin Estolate (Co-administration of alosetron and strong CYP3A4 inhibitors has not been evaluated but should be undertaken with caution because of similar potential drug interactions).
No products indexed under this heading.

Erythromycin Ethylsuccinate (Co-administration of alosetron and strong CYP3A4 inhibitors has not been evaluated but should be undertaken with caution because of similar potential drug interactions).
Products include:
E.E.S. 451
EryPed 447

Erythromycin Gluceptate (Co-administration of alosetron and strong CYP3A4 inhibitors has not been evaluated but should be undertaken with caution because of similar potential drug interactions).
No products indexed under this heading.

Erythromycin Lactobionate (Co-administration of alosetron and strong CYP3A4 inhibitors has not been evaluated but should be undertaken with caution because of similar potential drug interactions).
No products indexed under this heading.

Erythromycin Stearate (Co-administration of alosetron and strong CYP3A4 inhibitors has not been evaluated but should be undertaken with caution because of similar potential drug interactions).
Products include:
Erythrocin Stearate Filmtab Tablets 453

Esomeprazole Magnesium (Co-administration of alosetron and strong CYP3A4 inhibitors has not been evaluated but should be undertaken with caution because of similar potential drug interactions).
Products include:
Nexium Delayed-Release Capsules 655

Ethinyl Estradiol (Concomitant administration of alosetron and moderate CYP1A2 inhibitors, including quinolone antibiotics and cimetidine, has not been evaluated, but should be avoided unless clinically necessary because of potential drug interactions). Products include:
Mircette Tablets 1066
NuvaRing 2340
Ortho-Cyclen/Ortho Tri-Cyclen 2429
Ortho Evra Transdermal System 2417
Ortho Tri-Cyclen Lo Tablets 2436
Seasonique Tablets 1077
Yasmin 28 Tablets 796
Yaz Tablets 803

Fluconazole (Co-administration of alosetron and strong CYP3A4 inhibitors has not been evaluated but should be undertaken with caution because of similar potential drug interactions).
No products indexed under this heading.

Fluoxetine Hydrochloride (Co-administration of alosetron and strong CYP3A4 inhibitors has not been evaluated but should be undertaken with caution because of similar potential drug interactions).
Products include:
Prozac Pulvules and Liquid 1801

Symbyax Capsules 1819

Fluvoxamine (Concomitant administration of alosetron with fluvoxamine is contraindicated. Fluvoxamine, a known strong inhibitor of CYP1A2, has been shown to increase mean alosetron plasma concentrations (AUC) approximately 6 fold and prolong the half-life by approximately 3 fold).
 No products indexed under this heading.

Fluvoxamine Maleate (Concomitant administration of alosetron with fluvoxamine is contraindicated. Fluvoxamine, a known strong inhibitor of CYP1A2, has been shown to increase mean alosetron plasma concentrations (AUC) approximately 6 fold and prolong the half-life by approximately 3 fold).
 No products indexed under this heading.

Fosamprenavir Calcium (Co-administration of alosetron and strong CYP3A4 inhibitors has not been evaluated but should be undertaken with caution because of similar potential drug interactions). Products include:
 Lexiva Tablets 1505

Gatifloxacin (Concomitant administration of alosetron and moderate CYP1A2 inhibitors, including quinolone antibiotics and cimetidine, has not been evaluated, but should be avoided unless clinically necessary because of potential drug interactions). Products include:
 Tequin Injection 938
 Tequin Injection in 5% Dextrose 938
 Tequin Tablets 938
 Zymar Ophthalmic Solution 575

Gemifloxacin Mesylate (Concomitant administration of alosetron and moderate CYP1A2 inhibitors, including quinolone antibiotics and cimetidine, has not been evaluated, but should be avoided unless clinically necessary because of potential drug interactions).
 No products indexed under this heading.

Grepafloxacin Hydrochloride (Concomitant administration of alosetron and moderate CYP1A2 inhibitors, including quinolone antibiotics and cimetidine, has not been evaluated, but should be avoided unless clinically necessary because of potential drug interactions).
 No products indexed under this heading.

Hydralazine Hydrochloride (Although not studied with alosetron, inhibition of N-acetyltransferase may have clinically relevant consequences for drugs such as hydralazine). Products include:
 BiDil Tablets 2171

Indinavir Sulfate (Co-administration of alosetron and strong CYP3A4 inhibitors has not been evaluated but should be undertaken with caution because of similar potential drug interactions). Products include:
 Crixivan Capsules 1940

Isoniazid (Although not studied with alosetron, inhibition of N-acetyltransferase may have clinically relevant consequences for drugs such as isoniazid).
 No products indexed under this heading.

Itraconazole (Co-administration of alosetron and strong CYP3A4 inhibitors has not been evaluated but should be undertaken with caution because of similar potential drug interactions).
 No products indexed under this heading.

Ketoconazole (Ketoconazole is a known strong inhibitor of CYP3A4. In a pharmacokinetic study, 38 healthy female subjects recieved ketoconazole 200 mg twice daily for 7 days, with co-administration of alosetron 1 mg on the last day. Ketoconazole increased mean alosetron plasma concentrations (AUC) by 29%. Caution should be used when alosetron and ketoconazole are administered concomitantly). Products include:
 Nizoral A-D Shampoo, 1% 1868

Levofloxacin (Concomitant administration of alosetron and moderate CYP1A2 inhibitors, including quinolone antibiotics and cimetidine, has not been evaluated, but should be avoided unless clinically necessary because of potential drug interactions). Products include:
 Levaquin 2384
 Levaquin in 5% Dextrose Injection 2384
 Quixin Ophthalmic Solution 3383

Levonorgestrel (Concomitant administration of alosetron and moderate CYP1A2 inhibitors, including quinolone antibiotics and cimetidine, has not been evaluated, but should be avoided unless clinically necessary because of potential drug interactions). Products include:
 Climara Pro Transdermal System 776
 Mirena Intrauterine System 787
 Plan B Tablets 1076
 Seasonique Tablets 1077

Lomefloxacin Hydrochloride (Concomitant administration of alosetron and moderate CYP1A2 inhibitors, including quinolone antibiotics and cimetidine, has not been evaluated, but should be avoided unless clinically necessary because of potential drug interactions).
 No products indexed under this heading.

Lopinavir (Co-administration of alosetron and strong CYP3A4 inhibitors has not been evaluated but should be undertaken with caution because of similar potential drug interactions). Products include:
 Kaletra .. 476

Loratadine (Co-administration of alosetron and strong CYP3A4 inhibitors has not been evaluated but should be undertaken with caution because of similar potential drug interactions). Products include:
 Alavert Allergy & Sinus D-12 Hour Tablets.. ▣⊙771
 Alavert ... ▣⊙771
 Children's Claritin Allergy Oral Solution...................................... ▣⊙771
 Claritin Non-Drowsy 24 Hour Tablets.. ▣⊙772
 Claritin Reditabs 24 Hour Non-Drowsy Tablets.................... ▣⊙772
 Claritin-D Non-Drowsy 12 Hour Tablets.. ▣⊙772
 Claritin-D Non-Drowsy 24 Hour Tablets.. ▣⊙772

Mestranol (Concomitant administration of alosetron and moderate CYP1A2 inhibitors, including quinolone antibiotics and cimetidine, has not been evaluated, but should be avoided unless clinically necessary because of potential drug interactions).
 No products indexed under this heading.

Methoxsalen (Concomitant administration of alosetron and moderate CYP1A2 inhibitors, including quinolone antibiotics and cimetidine, has not been evaluated, but should be avoided unless clinically necessary because of potential drug interactions). Products include:
 Oxsoralen Lotion 1% 3352
 Oxsoralen-Ultra Capsules 3353

Metronidazole (Co-administration of alosetron and strong CYP3A4 inhibitors has not been evaluated but should be undertaken with caution because of similar potential drug interactions). Products include:
 Metrogel 1% 1211
 MetroGel-Vaginal Gel 1855
 Vandazole Vaginal Gel 3338

Metronidazole Benzoate (Co-administration of alosetron and strong CYP3A4 inhibitors has not been evaluated but should be undertaken with caution because of similar potential drug interactions).
 No products indexed under this heading.

Metronidazole Hydrochloride (Co-administration of alosetron and strong CYP3A4 inhibitors has not been evaluated but should be undertaken with caution because of similar potential drug interactions).
 No products indexed under this heading.

Mexiletine Hydrochloride (Concomitant administration of alosetron and moderate CYP1A2 inhibitors, including quinolone antibiotics and cimetidine, has not been evaluated, but should be avoided unless clinically necessary because of potential drug interactions).
 No products indexed under this heading.

Mibefradil Dihydrochloride (Concomitant administration of alosetron and moderate CYP1A2 inhibitors, including quinolone antibiotics and cimetidine, has not been evaluated, but should be avoided unless clinically necessary because of potential drug interactions).
 No products indexed under this heading.

Miconazole (Co-administration of alosetron and strong CYP3A4 inhibitors has not been evaluated but should be undertaken with caution because of similar potential drug interactions).
 No products indexed under this heading.

Miconazole Nitrate (Co-administration of alosetron and strong CYP3A4 inhibitors has not been evaluated but should be undertaken with caution because of similar potential drug interactions). Products include:
 Desenex ▣⊙635
 Desenex Jock Itch Spray Powder ... ▣⊙635

Moxifloxacin Hydrochloride (Concomitant administration of alosetron and moderate CYP1A2 inhibitors, including quinolone antibiotics and cimetidine, has not been evaluated, but should be avoided unless clinically necessary because of potential drug interactions). Products include:
 Avelox ... 2970
 Vigamox Ophthalmic Solution 564

Nalidixic Acid (Concomitant administration of alosetron and moderate CYP1A2 inhibitors, including quinolone antibiotics and cimetidine, has not been evaluated, but should be avoided unless clinically necessary because of potential drug interactions).
 No products indexed under this heading.

Nefazodone Hydrochloride (Co-administration of alosetron and strong CYP3A4 inhibitors has not been evaluated but should be undertaken with caution because of similar potential drug interactions).
 No products indexed under this heading.

Nelfinavir Mesylate (Co-administration of alosetron and strong CYP3A4 inhibitors has not been evaluated but should be undertaken with caution because of similar potential drug interactions). Products include:
 Viracept ... 2577

Nevirapine (Co-administration of alosetron and strong CYP3A4 inhibitors has not been evaluated but should be undertaken with caution because of similar potential drug interactions). Products include:
 Viramune Oral Suspension 873
 Viramune Tablets 873

Niacinamide (Co-administration of alosetron and strong CYP3A4 inhibitors has not been evaluated but should be undertaken with caution because of similar potential drug interactions).
 No products indexed under this heading.

Nicotinamide (Co-administration of alosetron and strong CYP3A4 inhibitors has not been evaluated but should be undertaken with caution because of similar potential drug interactions). Products include:
 Nicomide Tablets 1088

Nifedipine (Co-administration of alosetron and strong CYP3A4 inhibitors has not been evaluated but should be undertaken with caution because of similar potential drug interactions). Products include:
 Adalat CC Tablets 2964

Norethindrone (Concomitant administration of alosetron and moderate CYP1A2 inhibitors, including quinolone antibiotics and cimetidine, has not been evaluated, but should be avoided unless clinically necessary because of potential drug interactions). Products include:
 Ortho Micronor Tablets 2426

Norfloxacin (Co-administration of alosetron and strong CYP3A4 inhibitors has not been evaluated but should be undertaken with caution because of similar potential drug interactions). Products include:
 Noroxin Tablets 2032

Norgestrel (Concomitant administration of alosetron and moderate CYP1A2 inhibitors, including quinolone antibiotics and cimetidine, has not been evaluated, but should be avoided unless clinically necessary because of potential drug interactions).
 No products indexed under this heading.

Ofloxacin (Concomitant administration of alosetron and moderate CYP1A2 inhibitors, including quinolone antibiotics and cimetidine, has not been evaluated, but should be avoided unless clinically necessary because of potential drug interactions). Products include:

Floxin Otic Solution **1049**

Omeprazole (Co-administration of alosetron and strong CYP3A4 inhibitors has not been evaluated but should be undertaken with caution because of similar potential drug interactions). Products include:

Zegerid Capsules **2958**
Zegerid Powder for Oral Solution **2958**

Paroxetine Hydrochloride (Co-administration of alosetron and strong CYP3A4 inhibitors has not been evaluated but should be undertaken with caution because of similar potential drug interactions). Products include:

Paxil CR Controlled-Release Tablets **1538**
Paxil **1530**

Procainamide Hydrochloride (Although not studied with alosetron, inhibition of N-acetyltransferase may have clinically relevant consequences for drugs such as procainamide).

No products indexed under this heading.

Propoxyphene Hydrochloride (Co-administration of alosetron and strong CYP3A4 inhibitors has not been evaluated but should be undertaken with caution because of similar potential drug interactions).

No products indexed under this heading.

Propoxyphene Napsylate (Co-administration of alosetron and strong CYP3A4 inhibitors has not been evaluated but should be undertaken with caution because of similar potential drug interactions).

No products indexed under this heading.

Quinidine (Co-administration of alosetron and strong CYP3A4 inhibitors has not been evaluated but should be undertaken with caution because of similar potential drug interactions).

No products indexed under this heading.

Quinidine Hydrochloride (Co-administration of alosetron and strong CYP3A4 inhibitors has not been evaluated but should be undertaken with caution because of similar potential drug interactions).

No products indexed under this heading.

Quinidine Polygalacturonate (Co-administration of alosetron and strong CYP3A4 inhibitors has not been evaluated but should be undertaken with caution because of similar potential drug interactions).

No products indexed under this heading.

Quinidine Sulfate (Co-administration of alosetron and strong CYP3A4 inhibitors has not been evaluated but should be undertaken with caution because of similar potential drug interactions).

No products indexed under this heading.

Quinine (Co-administration of alosetron and strong CYP3A4 inhibitors has not been evaluated but should be undertaken with caution because of similar potential drug interactions).

No products indexed under this heading.

Quinine Sulfate (Co-administration of alosetron and strong CYP3A4 inhibitors has not been evaluated but should be undertaken with caution because of similar potential drug interactions).

No products indexed under this heading.

Quinupristin (Co-administration of alosetron and strong CYP3A4 inhibitors has not been evaluated but should be undertaken with caution because of similar potential drug interactions).

No products indexed under this heading.

Ranitidine Bismuth Citrate (Co-administration of alosetron and strong CYP3A4 inhibitors has not been evaluated but should be undertaken with caution because of similar potential drug interactions).

No products indexed under this heading.

Ranitidine Hydrochloride (Co-administration of alosetron and strong CYP3A4 inhibitors has not been evaluated but should be undertaken with caution because of similar potential drug interactions). Products include:

Zantac **1624**
Zantac Injection **1619**
Zantac Injection Pharmacy Bulk Package.. **1622**

Ritonavir (Co-administration of alosetron and strong CYP3A4 inhibitors has not been evaluated but should be undertaken with caution because of similar potential drug interactions). Products include:

Kaletra **476**
Norvir **503**

Saquinavir (Co-administration of alosetron and strong CYP3A4 inhibitors has not been evaluated but should be undertaken with caution because of similar potential drug interactions).

No products indexed under this heading.

Saquinavir Mesylate (Co-administration of alosetron and strong CYP3A4 inhibitors has not been evaluated but should be undertaken with caution because of similar potential drug interactions). Products include:

Invirase **2772**

Sertraline Hydrochloride (Co-administration of alosetron and strong CYP3A4 inhibitors has not been evaluated but should be undertaken with caution because of similar potential drug interactions). Products include:

Zoloft **2586**

Sparfloxacin (Concomitant administration of alosetron and moderate CYP1A2 inhibitors, including quinolone antibiotics and cimetidine, has not been evaluated, but should be avoided unless clinically necessary because of potential drug interactions).

No products indexed under this heading.

Tacrine Hydrochloride (Concomitant administration of alosetron and moderate CYP1A2 inhibitors, including quinolone antibiotics and cimetidine, has not been evaluated, but should be avoided unless clinically necessary because of potential drug interactions).

No products indexed under this heading.

Telithromycin (Co-administration of alosetron and strong CYP3A4 inhibitors has not been evaluated but should be undertaken with caution because of similar potential drug interactions). Products include:

Ketek Tablets **2903**

Ticlopidine Hydrochloride (Concomitant administration of alosetron and moderate CYP1A2 inhibitors, including quinolone antibiotics and cimetidine, has not been evaluated, but should be avoided unless clinically necessary because of potential drug interactions). Products include:

Ticlid Tablets **2810**

Troglitazone (Co-administration of alosetron and strong CYP3A4 inhibitors has not been evaluated but should be undertaken with caution because of similar potential drug interactions).

No products indexed under this heading.

Troleandomycin (Co-administration of alosetron and strong CYP3A4 inhibitors has not been evaluated but should be undertaken with caution because of similar potential drug interactions).

No products indexed under this heading.

Trovafloxacin Mesylate (Concomitant administration of alosetron and moderate CYP1A2 inhibitors, including quinolone antibiotics and cimetidine, has not been evaluated, but should be avoided unless clinically necessary because of potential drug interactions).

No products indexed under this heading.

Valproate Sodium (Co-administration of alosetron and strong CYP3A4 inhibitors has not been evaluated but should be undertaken with caution because of similar potential drug interactions). Products include:

Depacon Injection **412**

Verapamil Hydrochloride (Co-administration of alosetron and strong CYP3A4 inhibitors has not been evaluated but should be undertaken with caution because of similar potential drug interactions). Products include:

Covera-HS Tablets **3139**
Tarka Tablets **524**
Verelan PM Extended-Release Capsules, Controlled-Onset........... **3106**

Voriconazole (Co-administration of alosetron and strong CYP3A4 inhibitors has not been evaluated but should be undertaken with caution because of similar potential drug interactions). Products include:

VFEND I.V. **2564**
VFEND Oral Suspension **2564**
VFEND Tablets **2564**

Zafirlukast (Co-administration of alosetron and strong CYP3A4 inhibitors has not been evaluated but should be undertaken with caution because of similar potential drug interactions). Products include:

Accolate Tablets **671**

Zileuton (Co-administration of alosetron and strong CYP3A4 inhibitors has not been evaluated but should be undertaken with caution because of similar potential drug interactions). Products include:

Zyflo Tablets **1023**

Food Interactions

Food, unspecified (Alosetron absorption is decreased by approximately 25% by co-administration with food with a mean delay in time to peak concentration of 15 minutes; Lotronex can be taken with or without food).

Grapefruit (Co-administration of alosetron and strong CYP3A4 inhibitors has not been evaluated but should be undertaken with caution because of similar potential drug interactions).

Grapefruit Juice (Co-administration of alosetron and strong CYP3A4 inhibitors has not been evaluated but should be undertaken with caution because of similar potential drug interactions).

LOVENOX INJECTION

(Enoxaparin Sodium) **2915**

May interact with anticoagulants, non-steroidal anti-inflammatory agents, salicylates, and certain other agents. Compounds in these categories include:

Anisindione (Agents which may enhance the risk of hemorrhage, such as other anticoagulants, should be discontinued prior to initiation of Lovenox therapy; the risk of developing epidural or spinal hematoma which can result in long-term or permanent paralysis is increased by the concomitant use of drugs affecting hemostasis). Products include:

Miradon Tablets **3042**

Ardeparin Sodium (Agents which may enhance the risk of hemorrhage, such as other anticoagulants, should be discontinued prior to initiation of Lovenox therapy; the risk of developing epidural or spinal hematoma which can result in long-term or permanent paralysis is increased by the concomitant use of drugs affecting hemostasis).

No products indexed under this heading.

Aspirin (Agents which may enhance the risk of hemorrhage, such as platelet inhibitors, should be discontinued prior to initiation of Lovenox therapy; the risk of developing epidural or spinal hematoma which can result in long-term or permanent paralysis is increased by the concomitant use of drugs affecting hemostasis). Products include:

Aggrenox Capsules **822**
Bayer Aspirin **744**
BC Allergy Sinus Cold Powder **677**
BC Headache Powder **677**
Arthritis Strength BC Powder **677**
BC Sinus Cold Powder **677**
Excedrin Extra Strength Caplets/Tablets/Geltabs............. **684**
Excedrin Migraine Caplets/Tablets/Geltabs............. **609**
Goody's Body Pain Formula Powder.. **684**
Goody's Extra Strength Headache Powders...................... **611**
Goody's Extra Strength Pain Relief Tablets **685**
Percodan Tablets **1132**
St. Joseph 81 mg Aspirin Chewable and Enteric Coated Tablets... **1869**

Aspirin, Enteric Coated (Agents which may enhance the risk of hemorrhage, such as platelet inhibitors, should be discontinued prior to initiation of Lovenox therapy; the risk of developing epidural or spinal hematoma which can result in long-term or permanent paralysis is increased by the concomitant use of drugs affecting hemostasis).

No products indexed under this heading.

Aspirin Buffered (Agents which may enhance the risk of hemorrhage, such as platelet inhibitors, should be discontinued prior to initiation of Lovenox therapy; the risk of developing epidural or spinal hematoma which can result in long-term or permanent paralysis is increased by the concomitant use of drugs affecting hemostasis). Products include:

Bufferin Extra Strength Tablets ...... ▣678
Bufferin Regular Strength Tablets ... ▣678

Celecoxib (Agents which may enhance the risk of hemorrhage, such as platelet inhibitors, should be discontinued prior to initiation of Lovenox therapy; the risk of developing epidural or spinal hematoma which can result in long-term or permanent paralysis is increased by the concomitant use of drugs affecting hemostasis). Products include:

Celebrex Capsules 3134

Choline Magnesium Trisalicylate (Agents which may enhance the risk of hemorrhage, such as platelet inhibitors, should be discontinued prior to initiation of Lovenox therapy; the risk of developing epidural or spinal hematoma which can result in long-term or permanent paralysis is increased by the concomitant use of drugs affecting hemostasis).

No products indexed under this heading.

Clopidogrel Bisulfate (Agents which may enhance the risk of hemorrhage, such as platelet aggregation inhibitors, should be discontinued prior to initiation of Lovenox therapy; the risk of developing epidural or spinal hematoma which can result in long-term or permanent paralysis is increased by the concomitant use of drugs affecting hemostasis). Products include:

Plavix Tablets 917
Plavix Tablets 2926

Dalteparin Sodium (Agents which may enhance the risk of hemorrhage, such as other anticoagulants, should be discontinued prior to initiation of Lovenox therapy; the risk of developing epidural or spinal hematoma which can result in long-term or permanent paralysis is increased by the concomitant use of drugs affecting hemostasis). Products include:

Fragmin Injection 1097

Danaparoid Sodium (Agents which may enhance the risk of hemorrhage, such as other anticoagulants, should be discontinued prior to initiation of Lovenox therapy; the risk of developing epidural or spinal hematoma which can result in long-term or permanent paralysis is increased by the concomitant use of drugs affecting hemostasis).

No products indexed under this heading.

Diclofenac Potassium (Agents which may enhance the risk of hemorrhage, such as platelet inhibitors, should be discontinued prior to initiation of Lovenox therapy; the risk of developing epidural or spinal hematoma which can result in long-term or permanent paralysis is increased by the concomitant use of drugs affecting hemostasis).

No products indexed under this heading.

Diclofenac Sodium (Agents which may enhance the risk of hemorrhage, such as platelet inhibitors, should be discontinued prior to initiation of Lovenox therapy; the risk of developing epidural or spinal hematoma which can result in long-term or permanent paralysis is increased by the concomitant use of drugs affecting hemostasis). Products include:

Arthrotec Tablets 3129
Voltaren Ophthalmic Solution 2309
Voltaren Tablets 2307
Voltaren-XR Tablets 2310

Dicumarol (Agents which may enhance the risk of hemorrhage, such as other anticoagulants, should be discontinued prior to initiation of Lovenox therapy; the risk of developing epidural or spinal hematoma which can result in long-term or permanent paralysis is increased by the concomitant use of drugs affecting hemostasis).

No products indexed under this heading.

Diflunisal (Agents which may enhance the risk of hemorrhage, such as platelet inhibitors, should be discontinued prior to initiation of Lovenox therapy; the risk of developing epidural or spinal hematoma which can result in long-term or permanent paralysis is increased by the concomitant use of drugs affecting hemostasis). Products include:

Dolobid Tablets 1955

Dipyridamole (Agents which may enhance the risk of hemorrhage, such as dipyridamole, should be discontinued prior to initiation of Lovenox therapy). Products include:

Aggrenox Capsules 822
Persantine Tablets 868

Eptifibatide (Agents which may enhance the risk of hemorrhage, such as platelet aggregation inhibitors, should be discontinued prior to initiation of Lovenox therapy; the risk of developing epidural or spinal hematoma which can result in long-term or permanent paralysis is increased by the concomitant use of drugs affecting hemostasis). Products include:

Integrilin Injection 3020

Etodolac (Agents which may enhance the risk of hemorrhage, such as platelet inhibitors, should be discontinued prior to initiation of Lovenox therapy; the risk of developing epidural or spinal hematoma which can result in long-term or permanent paralysis is increased by the concomitant use of drugs affecting hemostasis).

No products indexed under this heading.

Fenoprofen Calcium (Agents which may enhance the risk of hemorrhage, such as platelet inhibitors, should be discontinued prior to initiation of Lovenox therapy; the risk of developing epidural or spinal hematoma which can result in long-term or permanent paralysis is increased by the concomitant use of drugs affecting hemostasis). Products include:

Nalfon Capsules 2502

Flurbiprofen (Agents which may enhance the risk of hemorrhage, such as platelet inhibitors, should be discontinued prior to initiation of Lovenox therapy; the risk of developing epidural or spinal hematoma which can result in long-term or permanent paralysis is increased by the concomitant use of drugs affecting hemostasis).

No products indexed under this heading.

Fondaparinux Sodium (Agents which may enhance the risk of hemorrhage, such as other anticoagulants, should be discontinued prior to initiation of Lovenox therapy; the risk of developing epidural or spinal hematoma which can result in long-term or permanent paralysis is increased by the concomitant use of drugs affecting hemostasis). Products include:

Arixtra Injection 1351

Heparin Calcium (Agents which may enhance the risk of hemorrhage, such as other anticoagulants, should be discontinued prior to initiation of Lovenox therapy; the risk of developing epidural or spinal hematoma which can result in long-term or permanent paralysis is increased by the concomitant use of drugs affecting hemostasis).

No products indexed under this heading.

Heparin Sodium (Agents which may enhance the risk of hemorrhage, such as other anticoagulants, should be discontinued prior to initiation of Lovenox therapy; the risk of developing epidural or spinal hematoma which can result in long-term or permanent paralysis is increased by the concomitant use of drugs affecting hemostasis).

No products indexed under this heading.

Ibuprofen (Agents which may enhance the risk of hemorrhage, such as platelet inhibitors, should be discontinued prior to initiation of Lovenox therapy; the risk of developing epidural or spinal hematoma which can result in long-term or permanent paralysis is increased by the concomitant use of drugs affecting hemostasis). Products include:

Advil Allergy Sinus Caplets .... ▣770
Advil .... ▣674
Children's Advil Oral Suspension .... ▣603
Children's Advil Chewable Tablets .. ▣603
Advil Cold & Sinus .... ▣723
Infants' Advil Concentrated Drops .. ▣604
Infants' Advil Concentrated Drops - White Grape (Dye-Free) .... ▣604
Junior Strength Advil Swallow Tablets .... ▣605
Advil Migraine Liquigels .... ▣608
Advil Multi-Symptom Cold Caplets .... ▣770
Advil PM Caplets .... ▣615
Motrin IB Tablets and Caplets 1866
Children's Motrin Oral Suspension ... 1867
Children's Motrin Non-Staining Dye-Free Oral Suspension 1867
Children's Motrin Cold Oral Suspension 1867
Infants' Motrin Concentrated Drops 1867
Infants' Motrin Non-Staining Dye-Free Concentrated Drops 1867
Junior Strength Motrin Caplets and Chewable Tablets 1867
Vicoprofen Tablets 539

Indomethacin (Agents which may enhance the risk of hemorrhage, such as platelet inhibitors, should be discontinued prior to initiation of Lovenox therapy; the risk of developing epidural or spinal hematoma which can result in long-term or permanent paralysis is increased by the concomitant use of drugs affecting hemostasis). Products include:

Indocin 1995

Indomethacin Sodium Trihydrate (Agents which may enhance the risk of hemorrhage, such as platelet inhibitors, should be discontinued prior to initiation of Lovenox therapy; the risk of developing epidural or spinal hematoma which can result in long-term or permanent paralysis is increased by the concomitant use of drugs affecting hemostasis). Products include:

Indocin I.V. 2465

Ketoprofen (Agents which may enhance the risk of hemorrhage, such as platelet inhibitors, should be discontinued prior to initiation of Lovenox therapy; the risk of developing epidural or spinal hematoma which can result in long-term or permanent paralysis is increased by the concomitant use of drugs affecting hemostasis).

No products indexed under this heading.

Ketorolac Tromethamine (Agents which may enhance the risk of hemorrhage, such as platelet inhibitors, should be discontinued prior to initiation of Lovenox therapy; the risk of developing epidural or spinal hematoma which can result in long-term or permanent paralysis is increased by the concomitant use of drugs affecting hemostasis). Products include:

Acular Ophthalmic Solution 565
Acular LS Ophthalmic Solution 566

Low Molecular Weight Heparins (Agents which may enhance the risk of hemorrhage, such as other anticoagulants, should be discontinued prior to initiation of Lovenox therapy; the risk of developing epidural or spinal hematoma which can result in long-term or permanent paralysis is increased by the concomitant use of drugs affecting hemostasis).

No products indexed under this heading.

Magnesium Salicylate (Agents which may enhance the risk of hemorrhage, such as platelet inhibitors, should be discontinued prior to initiation of Lovenox therapy; the risk of developing epidural or spinal hematoma which can result in long-term or permanent paralysis is increased by the concomitant use of drugs affecting hemostasis).

No products indexed under this heading.

Meclofenamate Sodium (Agents which may enhance the risk of hemorrhage, such as platelet inhibitors, should be discontinued prior to initiation of Lovenox therapy; the risk of developing epidural or spinal hematoma which can result in long-term or permanent paralysis is increased by the concomitant use of drugs affecting hemostasis).

No products indexed under this heading.

Mefenamic Acid (Agents which may enhance the risk of hemorrhage, such as platelet inhibitors, should be discontinued prior to initiation of Lovenox therapy; the risk of developing epidural or spinal hematoma which can result in long-term or permanent paralysis is increased by the concomitant use of drugs affecting hemostasis).

No products indexed under this heading.

Meloxicam (Agents which may enhance the risk of hemorrhage, such as platelet inhibitors, should be discontinued prior to initiation of Lovenox therapy; the risk of developing epidural or spinal hematoma which can result in long-term or permanent paralysis is increased by the concomitant use of drugs affecting hemostasis). Products include:

Mobic Oral Suspension 863
Mobic Tablets 863

Nabumetone (Agents which may enhance the risk of hemorrhage, such as platelet inhibitors, should be discontinued prior to initiation of Lovenox therapy; the risk of developing epidural or spinal hematoma which can result in long-term or permanent paralysis is increased by the concomitant use of drugs affecting hemostasis).

No products indexed under this heading.

Naproxen (Agents which may enhance the risk of hemorrhage, such as platelet inhibitors, should be discontinued prior to initiation of Lovenox therapy; the risk of developing epidural or spinal hematoma which can result in long-term or permanent paralysis is increased by the concomitant use of drugs affecting hemostasis). Products include:

EC-Naprosyn Delayed-Release Tablets 2761
Naprosyn Suspension 2761
Naprosyn Tablets 2761
Prevacid NapraPAC 3280

Naproxen Sodium (Agents which may enhance the risk of hemorrhage, such as platelet inhibitors, should be discontinued prior to initiation of Lovenox therapy; the risk of developing epidural or spinal hematoma which can result in long-term or permanent paralysis is increased by the concomitant use of drugs affecting hemostasis). Products include:

Aleve Caplets 742
Aleve Gelcaps 743
Aleve Tablets 743
Aleve Cold & Sinus Caplets 744
Anaprox Tablets 2761
Anaprox DS Tablets 2761

Oxaprozin (Agents which may enhance the risk of hemorrhage, such as platelet inhibitors, should be discontinued prior to initiation of Lovenox therapy; the risk of developing epidural or spinal hematoma which can result in long-term or permanent paralysis is increased by the concomitant use of drugs affecting hemostasis).

No products indexed under this heading.

Phenylbutazone (Agents which may enhance the risk of hemorrhage, such as platelet inhibitors, should be discontinued prior to initiation of Lovenox therapy; the risk of developing epidural or spinal hematoma which can result in long-term or permanent paralysis is increased by the concomitant use of drugs affecting hemostasis).

No products indexed under this heading.

Piroxicam (Agents which may enhance the risk of hemorrhage, such as platelet inhibitors, should be discontinued prior to initiation of Lovenox therapy; the risk of developing epidural or spinal hematoma which can result in long-term or permanent paralysis is increased by the concomitant use of drugs affecting hemostasis).

No products indexed under this heading.

Rofecoxib (Agents which may enhance the risk of hemorrhage, such as platelet inhibitors, should be discontinued prior to initiation of Lovenox therapy; the risk of developing epidural or spinal hematoma which can result in long-term or permanent paralysis is increased by the concomitant use of drugs affecting hemostasis).

No products indexed under this heading.

Salsalate (Agents which may enhance the risk of hemorrhage, such as platelet inhibitors, should be discontinued prior to initiation of Lovenox therapy; the risk of developing epidural or spinal hematoma which can result in long-term or permanent paralysis is increased by the concomitant use of drugs affecting hemostasis).

No products indexed under this heading.

Sulfinpyrazone (Agents which may enhance the risk of hemorrhage, such as sulfinpyrazone, should be discontinued prior to initiation of Lovenox therapy).

No products indexed under this heading.

Sulindac (Agents which may enhance the risk of hemorrhage, such as platelet inhibitors, should be discontinued prior to initiation of Lovenox therapy; the risk of developing epidural or spinal hematoma which can result in long-term or permanent paralysis is increased by the concomitant use of drugs affecting hemostasis). Products include:

Clinoril Tablets 1924

Tinzaparin Sodium (Agents which may enhance the risk of hemorrhage, such as other anticoagulants, should be discontinued prior to initiation of Lovenox therapy; the risk of developing epidural or spinal hematoma which can result in long-term or permanent paralysis is increased by the concomitant use of drugs affecting hemostasis).

No products indexed under this heading.

Tirofiban Hydrochloride (Agents which may enhance the risk of hemorrhage, such as platelet aggregation inhibitors, should be discontinued prior to initiation of Lovenox therapy; the risk of developing epidural or spinal hematoma which can result in long-term or permanent paralysis is increased by the concomitant use of drugs affecting hemostasis). Products include:

Aggrastat 1907

Tolmetin Sodium (Agents which may enhance the risk of hemorrhage, such as platelet inhibitors, should be discontinued prior to initiation of Lovenox therapy; the risk of developing epidural or spinal hematoma which can result in long-term or permanent paralysis is increased by the concomitant use of drugs affecting hemostasis).

No products indexed under this heading.

Valdecoxib (Agents which may enhance the risk of hemorrhage, such as platelet inhibitors, should be discontinued prior to initiation of Lovenox therapy; the risk of developing epidural or spinal hematoma which can result in long-term or permanent paralysis is increased by the concomitant use of drugs affecting hemostasis).

No products indexed under this heading.

Warfarin Sodium (Agents which may enhance the risk of hemorrhage, such as other anticoagulants, should be discontinued prior to initiation of Lovenox therapy; the risk of developing epidural or spinal hematoma which can result in long-term or permanent paralysis is increased by the concomitant use of drugs affecting hemostasis). Products include:

Coumadin for Injection 898
Coumadin Tablets 898

L-TRYPTOPHAN CAPSULES

(L-Tryptophan) 2145
None cited in PDR database.

LUCENTIS INJECTION

(Ranibizumab) 1237
May interact with:

Verteporfin (11% of patients developed serious intraocular inflammation when ranibizumab was used concomitantly with verteporfin). Products include:

Visudyne for Injection 2305

LUMIGAN OPHTHALMIC SOLUTION

(Bimatoprost) 573
None cited in PDR database.

LUNESTA TABLETS

(Eszopiclone) 3142
May interact with cytochrome p450 3a4 inhibitors, potent and certain other agents. Compounds in these categories include:

Amprenavir (CYP3A4 is a major metabolic pathway for elimination of eszopiclone. The AUC of eszopiclone was increased 2.2-fold by co-administration of ketoconazole, a potent inhibitor of CYP3A4, 400 mg daily for 5 days. Cmax and T1/2 were increased 1.4-fold and 1.3-fold, respectively. Other strong inhibitors of CYP3A4 (e.g., itraconazole, clarithromycin, nefazodone, troleandomycin, ritonavir, nelfinavir) would be expected to behave similarly). Products include:

Agenerase Capsules 1327
Agenerase Oral Solution 1332

Atazanavir (CYP3A4 is a major metabolic pathway for elimination of eszopiclone. The AUC of eszopiclone was increased 2.2-fold by co-administration of ketoconazole, a potent inhibitor of CYP3A4, 400 mg daily for 5 days. Cmax and T1/2 were increased 1.4-fold and 1.3-fold, respectively. Other strong inhibitors of CYP3A4 (e.g., itraconazole, clarithromycin, nefazodone, troleandomycin, ritonavir, nelfinavir) would be expected to behave similarly).

No products indexed under this heading.

Atazanavir sulfate (CYP3A4 is a major metabolic pathway for elimination of eszopiclone. The AUC of eszopiclone was increased 2.2-fold by co-administration of ketoconazole, a potent inhibitor of CYP3A4, 400 mg daily for 5 days. Cmax and T1/2 were increased 1.4-fold and 1.3-fold, respectively. Other strong inhibitors of CYP3A4 (e.g., itraconazole, clarithromycin, nefazodone, troleandomycin, ritonavir, nelfinavir) would be expected to behave similarly). Products include:

Reyataz Capsules 921

Clarithromycin (CYP3A4 is a major metabolic pathway for elimination of eszopiclone. The AUC of eszopiclone was increased 2.2-fold by co-administration of ketoconazole, a potent inhibitor of CYP3A4, 400 mg daily for 5 days. Cmax and T1/2 were increased 1.4-fold and 1.3-fold, respectively. Other strong inhibitors of CYP3A4 (e.g., itraconazole, clarithromycin, nefazodone, troleandomycin, ritonavir, nelfinavir) would be expected to behave similarly). Products include:

Biaxin/Biaxin XL 402
PREVPAC 3284

Ethanol (An additive effect on psychomotor performance was seen with co-administration of eszopiclone and ethanol 0.70 g/kg for up to 4 hours after ethanol administration).

No products indexed under this heading.

Fosamprenavir Calcium (CYP3A4 is a major metabolic pathway for elimination of eszopiclone. The AUC of eszopiclone was increased 2.2-fold by co-administration of ketoconazole, a potent inhibitor of CYP3A4, 400 mg daily for 5 days. Cmax and T1/2 were increased 1.4-fold and 1.3-fold, respectively. Other strong inhibitors of CYP3A4 (e.g., itraconazole, clarithromycin, nefazodone, troleandomycin, ritonavir, nelfinavir) would be expected to behave similarly). Products include:

Lexiva Tablets 1505

Indinavir Sulfate (CYP3A4 is a major metabolic pathway for elimination of eszopiclone. The AUC of eszopiclone was increased 2.2-fold by co-administration of ketoconazole, a potent inhibitor of CYP3A4, 400 mg daily for 5 days. Cmax and T1/2 were increased 1.4-fold and 1.3-fold, respectively. Other strong inhibitors of CYP3A4 (e.g., itraconazole, clarithromycin, nefazodone, troleandomycin, ritonavir, nelfinavir) would be expected to behave similarly). Products include:

Crixivan Capsules 1940

Itraconazole (CYP3A4 is a major metabolic pathway for elimination of eszopiclone. The AUC of eszopiclone was increased 2.2-fold by co-administration of ketoconazole, a potent inhibitor of CYP3A4, 400 mg daily for 5 days. Cmax and T1/2 were increased 1.4-fold and 1.3-fold, respectively. Other strong inhibitors of CYP3A4 (e.g., itraconazole, clarithromycin, nefazodone, troleandomycin, ritonavir, nelfinavir) would be expected to behave similarly).

No products indexed under this heading.

Ketoconazole (CYP3A4 is a major metabolic pathway for elimination of eszopiclone. The AUC of eszopiclone was increased 2.2-fold by co-administration of ketoconazole, a potent inhibitor of CYP3A4, 400 mg daily for 5 days. Cmax and T1/2 were increased 1.4-fold and 1.3-fold, respectively. Other strong inhibitors of CYP3A4 (e.g., itraconazole, clarithromycin, nefazodone, troleandomycin, ritonavir, nelfinavir) would be expected to behave similarly). Products include:

Nizoral A-D Shampoo, 1% 1868

Lopinavir (CYP3A4 is a major metabolic pathway for elimination of eszopiclone. The AUC of eszopiclone was increased 2.2-fold by co-administration of ketoconazole, a potent inhibitor of CYP3A4, 400 mg daily for 5 days. Cmax and T1/2 were increased 1.4-fold and 1.3-fold, respectively. Other strong inhibitors of CYP3A4 (e.g., itraconazole, clarithromycin, nefazodone, troleandomycin, ritonavir, nelfinavir) would be expected to behave similarly). Products include:

Kaletra 476

Lorazepam (Co-administration of Eszopiclone and lorazepam decreased the Cmax of both drugs by 22%).

No products indexed under this heading.

Nefazodone Hydrochloride (CYP3A4 is a major metabolic pathway for elimination of eszopiclone. The AUC of eszopiclone was increased 2.2-fold by co-administration of ketoconazole, a potent inhibitor of CYP3A4, 400 mg daily for 5 days. Cmax and T1/2 were increased 1.4-fold and 1.3-fold, respectively. Other strong inhibitors of CYP3A4 (e.g., itraconazole, clarithromycin, nefazodone, troleandomycin, ritonavir, nelfinavir) would be expected to behave similarly).

No products indexed under this heading.

Nelfinavir Mesylate (CYP3A4 is a major metabolic pathway for elimination of eszopiclone. The AUC of eszopiclone was increased 2.2-fold by co-administration of ketoconazole, a potent inhibitor of CYP3A4, 400 mg daily for 5 days. Cmax and T1/2 were increased 1.4-fold and 1.3-fold, respectively. Other strong inhibitors of CYP3A4 (e.g., itraconazole, clarithromycin, nefazodone, troleandomycin, ritonavir, nelfinavir) would be expected to behave similarly). Products include:

Viracept 2577

Olanzapine (Co-administration of eszopiclone 3 mg and olanzapine 10 mg produced a decrease in DSST scores. The interaction was pharmacodynamic; there was no alteration in the pharmacokinetics of either drug). Products include:

Symbyax Capsules 1819
Zyprexa Tablets 1830
Zyprexa IntraMuscular 1830
Zyprexa ZYDIS Orally Disintegrating Tablets 1830

Rifampicin (Racemic zopiclone exposure was decreased 80% by concomitant use of rifampicin, a potent inducer of CYP3A4. A similar effect would be expected with eszopiclone).

No products indexed under this heading.

Ritonavir (CYP3A4 is a major metabolic pathway for elimination of eszopiclone. The AUC of eszopiclone was increased 2.2-fold by co-administration of ketoconazole, a potent inhibitor of CYP3A4, 400 mg daily for 5 days. Cmax and T1/2 were increased 1.4-fold and 1.3-fold, respectively. Other strong inhibitors of CYP3A4 (e.g., itraconazole, clarithromycin, nefazodone, troleandomycin, ritonavir, nelfinavir) would be expected to behave similarly). Products include:

Kaletra 476
Norvir 503

Saquinavir (CYP3A4 is a major metabolic pathway for elimination of eszopiclone. The AUC of eszopiclone was increased 2.2-fold by co-administration of ketoconazole, a potent inhibitor of CYP3A4, 400 mg daily for 5 days. Cmax and T1/2 were increased 1.4-fold and 1.3-fold, respectively. Other strong inhibitors of CYP3A4 (e.g., itraconazole, clarithromycin, nefazodone, troleandomycin, ritonavir, nelfinavir) would be expected to behave similarly).

No products indexed under this heading.

Saquinavir Mesylate (CYP3A4 is a major metabolic pathway for elimination of eszopiclone. The AUC of eszopiclone was increased 2.2-fold by co-administration of ketoconazole, a potent inhibitor of CYP3A4, 400 mg daily for 5 days. Cmax and T1/2 were increased 1.4-fold and 1.3-fold, respectively. Other strong inhibitors of CYP3A4 (e.g., itraconazole, clarithromycin, nefazodone, troleandomycin, ritonavir, nelfinavir) would be expected to behave similarly). Products include:

Invirase 2772

Telithromycin (CYP3A4 is a major metabolic pathway for elimination of eszopiclone. The AUC of eszopiclone was increased 2.2-fold by co-administration of ketoconazole, a potent inhibitor of CYP3A4, 400 mg daily for 5 days. Cmax and T1/2 were increased 1.4-fold and 1.3-fold, respectively. Other strong inhibitors of CYP3A4 (e.g., itraconazole, clarithromycin, nefazodone, troleandomycin, ritonavir, nelfinavir) would be expected to behave similarly). Products include:

Ketek Tablets 2903

Troleandomycin (CYP3A4 is a major metabolic pathway for elimination of eszopiclone. The AUC of eszopiclone was increased 2.2-fold by co-administration of ketoconazole, a potent inhibitor of CYP3A4, 400 mg daily for 5 days. Cmax and T1/2 were increased 1.4-fold and 1.3-fold, respectively. Other strong inhibitors of CYP3A4 (e.g., itraconazole, clarithromycin, nefazodone, troleandomycin, ritonavir, nelfinavir) would be expected to behave similarly).

No products indexed under this heading.

Voriconazole (CYP3A4 is a major metabolic pathway for elimination of eszopiclone. The AUC of eszopiclone was increased 2.2-fold by co-administration of ketoconazole, a potent inhibitor of CYP3A4, 400 mg daily for 5 days. Cmax and T1/2 were increased 1.4-fold and 1.3-fold, respectively. Other strong inhibitors of CYP3A4 (e.g., itraconazole, clarithromycin, nefazodone, troleandomycin, ritonavir, nelfinavir) would be expected to behave similarly). Products include:

VFEND I.V. 2564
VFEND Oral Suspension 2564
VFEND Tablets 2564

Food Interactions

Alcohol (An additive effect on psychomotor performance was seen with co-administration of eszopiclone and alcohol 0.70 g/kg for up to 4 hours after alcohol consumption).

LUPRON DEPOT 3.75 MG
(Leuprolide Acetate) 3260
None cited in PDR database.

LUPRON DEPOT 7.5 MG
(Leuprolide Acetate) 3264
None cited in PDR database.

LUPRON DEPOT--3 MONTH 11.25 MG
(Leuprolide Acetate) 3265
None cited in PDR database.

LUPRON DEPOT-PED 7.5 MG, 11.25 MG AND 15 MG
(Leuprolide Acetate) 3269
None cited in PDR database.

LUPRON INJECTION PEDIATRIC
(Leuprolide Acetate) 3259
None cited in PDR database.

LUSTRA CREAM
(Hydroquinone) 3289
None cited in PDR database.

LUSTRA-AF CREAM
(Hydroquinone) 3289
None cited in PDR database.

LUSTRA-ULTRA CREAM
(Hydroquinone) 3289
None cited in PDR database.

LUXIQ FOAM
(Betamethasone Valerate) 1010
None cited in PDR database.

LYRICA CAPSULES
(Pregabalin) 2539
May interact with central nervous system depressants. Compounds in these categories include:

Alfentanil Hydrochloride (Patients who require concomitant treatment with CNS depressants (eg, opiates or benzodiazepines) should be informed that they may experience additive CNS side effects, such as somnolence).

No products indexed under this heading.

Alprazolam (Patients who require concomitant treatment with CNS depressants (eg, opiates or benzodiazepines) should be informed that they may experience additive CNS side effects, such as somnolence). Products include:

Niravam Orally Disintegrating Tablets 3092

Aprobarbital (Patients who require concomitant treatment with CNS depressants (eg, opiates or benzodiazepines) should be informed that they may experience additive CNS side effects, such as somnolence).

No products indexed under this heading.

Buprenorphine Hydrochloride (Patients who require concomitant treatment with CNS depressants (eg, opiates or benzodiazepines) should be informed that they may experience additive CNS side effects, such as somnolence). Products include:

Buprenex Injectable 2716
Suboxone Tablets 2717
Subutex Tablets 2717

Buspirone Hydrochloride (Patients who require concomitant treatment with CNS depressants (eg, opiates or benzodiazepines) should be informed that they may experience additive CNS side effects, such as somnolence).

No products indexed under this heading.

Butabarbital (Patients who require concomitant treatment with CNS depressants (eg, opiates or benzodiazepines) should be informed that they may experience additive CNS side effects, such as somnolence).

No products indexed under this heading.

Butalbital (Patients who require concomitant treatment with CNS depressants (eg, opiates or benzodiazepines) should be informed that they may experience additive CNS side effects, such as somnolence).

No products indexed under this heading.

Chlordiazepoxide (Patients who require concomitant treatment with CNS depressants (eg, opiates or benzodiazepines) should be informed that they may experience additive CNS side effects, such as somnolence).

No products indexed under this heading.

Chlordiazepoxide Hydrochloride (Patients who require concomitant treatment with CNS depressants (eg, opiates or benzodiazepines) should be informed that they may experience additive CNS side effects, such as somnolence). Products include:

Librium Capsules 3347

Chlorpromazine (Patients who require concomitant treatment with CNS depressants (eg, opiates or benzodiazepines) should be informed that they may experience additive CNS side effects, such as somnolence).

No products indexed under this heading.

Chlorpromazine Hydrochloride (Patients who require concomitant treatment with CNS depressants (eg, opiates or benzodiazepines) should be informed that they may experience additive CNS side effects, such as somnolence).

No products indexed under this heading.

Chlorprothixene (Patients who require concomitant treatment with CNS depressants (eg, opiates or benzodiazepines) should be informed that they may experience additive CNS side effects, such as somnolence).

No products indexed under this heading.

Chlorprothixene Hydrochloride (Patients who require concomitant treatment with CNS depressants (eg, opiates or benzodiazepines) should be informed that they may experience additive CNS side effects, such as somnolence).

No products indexed under this heading.

Chlorprothixene Lactate (Patients who require concomitant treatment with CNS depressants (eg, opiates or benzodiazepines) should be informed that they may experience additive CNS side effects, such as somnolence).
No products indexed under this heading.

Clorazepate Dipotassium (Patients who require concomitant treatment with CNS depressants (eg, opiates or benzodiazepines) should be informed that they may experience additive CNS side effects, such as somnolence). Products include:
Tranxene 2474

Clozapine (Patients who require concomitant treatment with CNS depressants (eg, opiates or benzodiazepines) should be informed that they may experience additive CNS side effects, such as somnolence). Products include:
Clozaril Tablets 2184
FazaClo Orally Disintegrating Tablets 551

Codeine Phosphate (Patients who require concomitant treatment with CNS depressants (eg, opiates or benzodiazepines) should be informed that they may experience additive CNS side effects, such as somnolence). Products include:
Tylenol with Codeine Tablets 2391

Desflurane (Patients who require concomitant treatment with CNS depressants (eg, opiates or benzodiazepines) should be informed that they may experience additive CNS side effects, such as somnolence).
No products indexed under this heading.

Dezocine (Patients who require concomitant treatment with CNS depressants (eg, opiates or benzodiazepines) should be informed that they may experience additive CNS side effects, such as somnolence).
No products indexed under this heading.

Diazepam (Patients who require concomitant treatment with CNS depressants (eg, opiates or benzodiazepines) should be informed that they may experience additive CNS side effects, such as somnolence). Products include:
Diastat Rectal Delivery System 3343
Valium Tablets 2819

Droperidol (Patients who require concomitant treatment with CNS depressants (eg, opiates or benzodiazepines) should be informed that they may experience additive CNS side effects, such as somnolence).
No products indexed under this heading.

Enflurane (Patients who require concomitant treatment with CNS depressants (eg, opiates or benzodiazepines) should be informed that they may experience additive CNS side effects, such as somnolence).
No products indexed under this heading!

Estazolam (Patients who require concomitant treatment with CNS depressants (eg, opiates or benzodiazepines) should be informed that they may experience additive CNS side effects, such as somnolence). Products include:
ProSom Tablets 517

Ethanol (Alcohol consumption should be avoided while taking pregabalin, as pregabalin may potentiate the impairment of motor skills and sedation of alcohol).
No products indexed under this heading.

Ethchlorvynol (Patients who require concomitant treatment with CNS depressants (eg, opiates or benzodiazepines) should be informed that they may experience additive CNS side effects, such as somnolence).
No products indexed under this heading.

Ethinamate (Patients who require concomitant treatment with CNS depressants (eg, opiates or benzodiazepines) should be informed that they may experience additive CNS side effects, such as somnolence).
No products indexed under this heading.

Ethyl Alcohol (Alcohol consumption should be avoided while taking pregabalin, as pregabalin may potentiate the impairment of motor skills and sedation of alcohol).
No products indexed under this heading.

Fentanyl (Patients who require concomitant treatment with CNS depressants (eg, opiates or benzodiazepines) should be informed that they may experience additive CNS side effects, such as somnolence). Products include:
Duragesic Transdermal System 2373
Ionsys Transdermal System 2379

Fentanyl Citrate (Patients who require concomitant treatment with CNS depressants (eg, opiates or benzodiazepines) should be informed that they may experience additive CNS side effects, such as somnolence). Products include:
Actiq ... 979

Fluphenazine Decanoate (Patients who require concomitant treatment with CNS depressants (eg, opiates or benzodiazepines) should be informed that they may experience additive CNS side effects, such as somnolence).
No products indexed under this heading.

Fluphenazine Enanthate (Patients who require concomitant treatment with CNS depressants (eg, opiates or benzodiazepines) should be informed that they may experience additive CNS side effects, such as somnolence).
No products indexed under this heading.

Fluphenazine Hydrochloride (Patients who require concomitant treatment with CNS depressants (eg, opiates or benzodiazepines) should be informed that they may experience additive CNS side effects, such as somnolence).
No products indexed under this heading.

Flurazepam Hydrochloride (Patients who require concomitant treatment with CNS depressants (eg, opiates or benzodiazepines) should be informed that they may experience additive CNS side effects, such as somnolence). Products include:
Dalmane Capsules 3342

Glutethimide (Patients who require concomitant treatment with CNS depressants (eg, opiates or benzodiazepines) should be informed that they may experience additive CNS side effects, such as somnolence).
No products indexed under this heading.

Haloperidol (Patients who require concomitant treatment with CNS depressants (eg, opiates or benzodiazepines) should be informed that they may experience additive CNS side effects, such as somnolence).
No products indexed under this heading.

Haloperidol Decanoate (Patients who require concomitant treatment with CNS depressants (eg, opiates or benzodiazepines) should be informed that they may experience additive CNS side effects, such as somnolence).
No products indexed under this heading.

Hydrocodone Bitartrate (Patients who require concomitant treatment with CNS depressants (eg, opiates or benzodiazepines) should be informed that they may experience additive CNS side effects, such as somnolence). Products include:
Hycodan ... 1116
Hycotuss Expectorant Syrup 1117
Vicodin Tablets 535
Vicodin ES Tablets 536
Vicodin HP Tablets 538
Vicoprofen Tablets 539
Zydone Tablets 1139

Hydrocodone Polistirex (Patients who require concomitant treatment with CNS depressants (eg, opiates or benzodiazepines) should be informed that they may experience additive CNS side effects, such as somnolence). Products include:
Tussionex Pennkinetic Extended-Release Suspension 3327

Hydromorphone Hydrochloride (Patients who require concomitant treatment with CNS depressants (eg, opiates or benzodiazepines) should be informed that they may experience additive CNS side effects, such as somnolence). Products include:
Dilaudid ... 440
Dilaudid Non-Sterile Powder 440
Dilaudid Oral Liquid 445
Dilaudid Rectal Suppositories 440
Dilaudid Tablets 440
Dilaudid Tablets - 8 mg 445
Dilaudid-HP 442

Hydroxyzine Hydrochloride (Patients who require concomitant treatment with CNS depressants (eg, opiates or benzodiazepines) should be informed that they may experience additive CNS side effects, such as somnolence).
No products indexed under this heading.

Isoflurane (Patients who require concomitant treatment with CNS depressants (eg, opiates or benzodiazepines) should be informed that they may experience additive CNS side effects, such as somnolence).
No products indexed under this heading.

Ketamine Hydrochloride (Patients who require concomitant treatment with CNS depressants (eg, opiates or benzodiazepines) should be informed that they may experience additive CNS side effects, such as somnolence).
No products indexed under this heading.

Levomethadyl Acetate Hydrochloride (Patients who require concomitant treatment with CNS depressants (eg, opiates or benzodiazepines) should be informed that they may experience additive CNS side effects, such as somnolence).
No products indexed under this heading.

Levorphanol Tartrate (Patients who require concomitant treatment with CNS depressants (eg, opiates or benzodiazepines) should be informed that they may experience additive CNS side effects, such as somnolence).
No products indexed under this heading.

Lorazepam (Patients who require concomitant treatment with CNS depressants (eg, opiates or benzodiazepines) should be informed that they may experience additive CNS side effects, such as somnolence).
No products indexed under this heading.

Loxapine Hydrochloride (Patients who require concomitant treatment with CNS depressants (eg, opiates or benzodiazepines) should be informed that they may experience additive CNS side effects, such as somnolence).
No products indexed under this heading.

Loxapine Succinate (Patients who require concomitant treatment with CNS depressants (eg, opiates or benzodiazepines) should be informed that they may experience additive CNS side effects, such as somnolence).
No products indexed under this heading.

Meperidine Hydrochloride (Patients who require concomitant treatment with CNS depressants (eg, opiates or benzodiazepines) should be informed that they may experience additive CNS side effects, such as somnolence).
No products indexed under this heading.

Mephobarbital (Patients who require concomitant treatment with CNS depressants (eg, opiates or benzodiazepines) should be informed that they may experience additive CNS side effects, such as somnolence).
No products indexed under this heading.

Meprobamate (Patients who require concomitant treatment with CNS depressants (eg, opiates or benzodiazepines) should be informed that they may experience additive CNS side effects, such as somnolence).
No products indexed under this heading.

Mesoridazine Besylate (Patients who require concomitant treatment with CNS depressants (eg, opiates or benzodiazepines) should be informed that they may experience additive CNS side effects, such as somnolence).
No products indexed under this heading.

IMPORTANT NOTE: Always consult each drug listing in the patient's regimen for possible interactions.

Methadone Hydrochloride
(Patients who require concomitant treatment with CNS depressants (eg, opiates or benzodiazepines) should be informed that they may experience additive CNS side effects, such as somnolence).

No products indexed under this heading.

Methohexital Sodium (Patients who require concomitant treatment with CNS depressants (eg, opiates or benzodiazepines) should be informed that they may experience additive CNS side effects, such as somnolence).

No products indexed under this heading.

Methotrimeprazine (Patients who require concomitant treatment with CNS depressants (eg, opiates or benzodiazepines) should be informed that they may experience additive CNS side effects, such as somnolence).

No products indexed under this heading.

Methoxyflurane (Patients who require concomitant treatment with CNS depressants (eg, opiates or benzodiazepines) should be informed that they may experience additive CNS side effects, such as somnolence).

No products indexed under this heading.

Midazolam Hydrochloride
(Patients who require concomitant treatment with CNS depressants (eg, opiates or benzodiazepines) should be informed that they may experience additive CNS side effects, such as somnolence).

No products indexed under this heading.

Molindone Hydrochloride
(Patients who require concomitant treatment with CNS depressants (eg, opiates or benzodiazepines) should be informed that they may experience additive CNS side effects, such as somnolence). Products include:

Morphine Sulfate (Patients who require concomitant treatment with CNS depressants (eg, opiates or benzodiazepines) should be informed that they may experience additive CNS side effects, such as somnolence). Products include:

Olanzapine (Patients who require concomitant treatment with CNS depressants (eg, opiates or benzodiazepines) should be informed that they may experience additive CNS side effects, such as somnolence). Products include:

Oxazepam (Patients who require concomitant treatment with CNS depressants (eg, opiates or benzodiazepines) should be informed that they may experience additive CNS side effects, such as somnolence).

No products indexed under this heading.

Oxycodone Hydrochloride
(Patients who require concomitant treatment with CNS depressants (eg, opiates or benzodiazepines) should

be informed that they may experience additive CNS side effects, such as somnolence). Products include:

Pentobarbital Sodium (Patients who require concomitant treatment with CNS depressants (eg, opiates or benzodiazepines) should be informed that they may experience additive CNS side effects, such as somnolence). Products include:

Perphenazine (Patients who require concomitant treatment with CNS depressants (eg, opiates or benzodiazepines) should be informed that they may experience additive CNS side effects, such as somnolence).

No products indexed under this heading.

Phenobarbital (Patients who require concomitant treatment with CNS depressants (eg, opiates or benzodiazepines) should be informed that they may experience additive CNS side effects, such as somnolence). Products include:

Prazepam (Patients who require concomitant treatment with CNS depressants (eg, opiates or benzodiazepines) should be informed that they may experience additive CNS side effects, such as somnolence).

No products indexed under this heading.

Prochlorperazine (Patients who require concomitant treatment with CNS depressants (eg, opiates or benzodiazepines) should be informed that they may experience additive CNS side effects, such as somnolence).

No products indexed under this heading.

Promethazine Hydrochloride
(Patients who require concomitant treatment with CNS depressants (eg, opiates or benzodiazepines) should be informed that they may experience additive CNS side effects, such as somnolence). Products include:

Propofol (Patients who require concomitant treatment with CNS depressants (eg, opiates or benzodiazepines) should be informed that they may experience additive CNS side effects, such as somnolence).

No products indexed under this heading.

Propoxyphene Hydrochloride
(Patients who require concomitant treatment with CNS depressants (eg, opiates or benzodiazepines) should be informed that they may experience additive CNS side effects, such as somnolence).

No products indexed under this heading.

Propoxyphene Napsylate
(Patients who require concomitant treatment with CNS depressants (eg, opiates or benzodiazepines) should be informed that they may experience additive CNS side effects, such as somnolence).

No products indexed under this heading.

Quazepam (Patients who require concomitant treatment with CNS depressants (eg, opiates or benzodiazepines) should be informed that they may experience additive CNS side effects, such as somnolence).

No products indexed under this heading.

Quetiapine Fumarate (Patients who require concomitant treatment with CNS depressants (eg, opiates or benzodiazepines) should be informed that they may experience additive CNS side effects, such as somnolence). Products include:

Remifentanil Hydrochloride
(Patients who require concomitant treatment with CNS depressants (eg, opiates or benzodiazepines) should be informed that they may experience additive CNS side effects, such as somnolence).

No products indexed under this heading.

Risperidone (Patients who require concomitant treatment with CNS depressants (eg, opiates or benzodiazepines) should be informed that they may experience additive CNS side effects, such as somnolence). Products include:

Secobarbital Sodium (Patients who require concomitant treatment with CNS depressants (eg, opiates or benzodiazepines) should be informed that they may experience additive CNS side effects, such as somnolence).

No products indexed under this heading.

Sevoflurane (Patients who require concomitant treatment with CNS depressants (eg, opiates or benzodiazepines) should be informed that they may experience additive CNS side effects, such as somnolence). Products include:

Sodium Oxybate (Patients who require concomitant treatment with CNS depressants (eg, opiates or benzodiazepines) should be informed that they may experience additive CNS side effects, such as somnolence). Products include:

Sufentanil Citrate (Patients who require concomitant treatment with CNS depressants (eg, opiates or benzodiazepines) should be informed that they may experience additive CNS side effects, such as somnolence).

No products indexed under this heading.

Temazepam (Patients who require concomitant treatment with CNS depressants (eg, opiates or benzodiazepines) should be informed that they may experience additive CNS side effects, such as somnolence). Products include:

Thiamylal Sodium (Patients who require concomitant treatment with CNS depressants (eg, opiates or benzodiazepines) should be informed that they may experience additive CNS side effects, such as somnolence).

No products indexed under this heading.

Thioridazine Hydrochloride
(Patients who require concomitant treatment with CNS depressants (eg, opiates or benzodiazepines) should be informed that they may experience additive CNS side effects, such as somnolence). Products include:

Thiothixene (Patients who require concomitant treatment with CNS depressants (eg, opiates or benzodiazepines) should be informed that they may experience additive CNS side effects, such as somnolence). Products include:

Triazolam (Patients who require concomitant treatment with CNS depressants (eg, opiates or benzodiazepines) should be informed that they may experience additive CNS side effects, such as somnolence).

No products indexed under this heading.

Trifluoperazine Hydrochloride
(Patients who require concomitant treatment with CNS depressants (eg, opiates or benzodiazepines) should be informed that they may experience additive CNS side effects, such as somnolence).

No products indexed under this heading.

Zaleplon (Patients who require concomitant treatment with CNS depressants (eg, opiates or benzodiazepines) should be informed that they may experience additive CNS side effects, such as somnolence). Products include:

Ziprasidone Hydrochloride
(Patients who require concomitant treatment with CNS depressants (eg, opiates or benzodiazepines) should be informed that they may experience additive CNS side effects, such as somnolence). Products include:

Zolpidem Tartrate (Patients who require concomitant treatment with CNS depressants (eg, opiates or benzodiazepines) should be informed that they may experience additive CNS side effects, such as somnolence). Products include:

Food Interactions

Alcohol (Alcohol consumption should be avoided while taking pregabalin, as pregabalin may potentiate the impairment of motor skills and sedation of alcohol).

MAALOX REGULAR STRENGTH ANTACID/ ANTI-GAS LIQUID
(Aluminum Hydroxide, Magnesium Hydroxide, Simethicone).................. ▣660
May interact with:

Prescription Drugs, unspecified
(Antacids may interact with certain unspecified prescription drugs).

No products indexed under this heading.

MAALOX REGULAR STRENGTH ANTACID/ ANTIGAS LIQUID
(Aluminum Hydroxide, Magnesium Hydroxide, Simethicone).................... 2175
May interact with:

Prescription Drugs, unspecified (Antacids may interact with certain unspecified prescription drugs).
No products indexed under this heading.

MAALOX REGULAR STRENGTH ANTACID CHEWABLE TABLETS
(Calcium Carbonate) 2177
May interact with:

Drugs, Oral, unspecified (Antacids may interact with certain unspecified prescription drugs).
No products indexed under this heading.

MAALOX MAX MAXIMUM STRENGTH ANTACID/ ANTI-GAS LIQUID
(Aluminum Hydroxide, Magnesium Hydroxide, Simethicone).................. ▣659
May interact with:

Prescription Drugs, unspecified (Antacids may interact with certain unspecified prescription drugs).
No products indexed under this heading.

MAALOX MAXIMUM STRENGTH TOTAL STOMACH RELIEF PEPPERMINT LIQUID
(Bismuth Subsalicylate) .... ▣660
None cited in PDR database.

MAALOX MAXIMUM STRENGTH TOTAL STOMACH RELIEF STRAWBERRY LIQUID
(Bismuth Subsalicylate) .... ▣672
None cited in PDR database.

MAALOX MAX MAXIMUM STRENGTH ANTACID/ ANTIGAS CHEWABLE TABLETS
(Calcium Carbonate) 2176
See Maalox Regular Strength Antacid Chewable Tablets

MAALOX MAX MAXIMUM STRENGTH CHEWABLE TABLETS
(Calcium Carbonate, Simethicone) ... ▣660
May interact with:

Prescription Drugs, unspecified (Antacids may interact with certain unspecified prescription drugs).
No products indexed under this heading.

MAALOX MAX MAXIMUM STRENGTH ANTACID/ ANTI-GAS LIQUID
(Aluminum Hydroxide, Magnesium Hydroxide, Simethicone).................... 2176
May interact with:

Prescription Drugs, unspecified (Antacids may interfere with certain unspecified prescription drugs; resulting effect not specified).
No products indexed under this heading.

MACUGEN INJECTION
(Pegaptanib sodium, Pegaptinab) ..... ⊙261
None cited in PDR database.

MALARONE PEDIATRIC TABLETS
(Atovaquone, Proguanil Hydrochloride).................................. 1517
See Malarone Tablets

MALARONE TABLETS
(Atovaquone, Proguanil Hydrochloride).................................. 1517
May interact with tetracyclines and certain other agents. Compounds in these categories include:

Demeclocycline Hydrochloride (Co-administration with tetracyclines has been associated with approximately a 40% reduction in plasma concentrations of atovaquone).
No products indexed under this heading.

Doxycycline Calcium (Co-administration with tetracyclines has been associated with approximately a 40% reduction in plasma concentrations of atovaquone).
No products indexed under this heading.

Doxycycline Hyclate (Co-administration with tetracyclines has been associated with approximately a 40% reduction in plasma concentrations of atovaquone).
No products indexed under this heading.

Doxycycline Monohydrate (Co-administration with tetracyclines has been associated with approximately a 40% reduction in plasma concentrations of atovaquone). Products include:
Oracea Capsules 1000

Methacycline Hydrochloride (Co-administration with tetracyclines has been associated with approximately a 40% reduction in plasma concentrations of atovaquone).
No products indexed under this heading.

Metoclopramide Hydrochloride (May reduce the bioavailability of atovaquone and should be used only if other antiemetics are not available).
No products indexed under this heading.

Minocycline Hydrochloride (Co-administration with tetracyclines has been associated with approximately a 40% reduction in plasma concentrations of atovaquone). Products include:
Solodyn Extended Release Tablets 1890

Oxytetracycline Hydrochloride (Co-administration with tetracyclines has been associated with approximately a 40% reduction in plasma concentrations of atovaquone).
No products indexed under this heading.

Rifabutin (Co-administration of rifabutin is known to reduce atovaquone levels by approximately 34%; concomitant therapy is not recommended).
No products indexed under this heading.

Rifampin (Co-administration of rifampin is known to reduce atovaquone levels by approximately 50%; concomitant therapy is not recommended).
No products indexed under this heading.

Tetracycline Hydrochloride (Co-administration with tetracyclines has been associated with approximately a 40% reduction in plasma concentrations of atovaquone).
No products indexed under this heading.

Food Interactions

Food, unspecified (Dietary fat intake with atovaquone increases the rate and extent of absorption; Malarone should be taken with food or milky drink).

MARINEOMEGA SOFTGEL CAPSULES
(Fatty Acids, Vitamin E) 2672
None cited in PDR database.

MARINOL CAPSULES
(Dronabinol) 3333
May interact with anticholinergics, antihistamines, barbiturates, benzodiazepines, central nervous system depressants, lithium preparations, muscle relaxants, narcotic analgesics, sympathomimetics, tricyclic antidepressants, xanthines, and certain other agents. Compounds in these categories include:

Acrivastine (Co-administration results in additive CNS depression or super-additive tachycardia and drowsiness).
No products indexed under this heading.

Albuterol (Co-administration with sympathomimetics may result in additive hypertension, tachycardia, and possibly cardiotoxicity).
Products include:
Proventil Inhalation Aerosol 3053

Albuterol Sulfate (Co-administration with sympathomimetics may result in additive hypertension, tachycardia, and possibly cardiotoxicity). Products include:
AccuNeb Inhalation Solution 1055
Combivent Inhalation Aerosol 847
DuoNeb Inhalation Solution 1058
ProAir HFA Inhalation Aerosol 3300
Proventil Inhalation Solution 0.083%... 3055
Proventil HFA Inhalation Aerosol 3056
Ventolin HFA Inhalation Aerosol 1600
VoSpire ER Tablets 1052

Alfentanil Hydrochloride (Co-administration results in additive drowsiness and CNS depression).
No products indexed under this heading.

Alprazolam (Co-administration results in additive drowsiness and CNS depression). Products include:
Niravam Orally Disintegrating Tablets 3092

Aminophylline (Increased theophylline metabolism has resulted with smoking marijuana).
No products indexed under this heading.

Amitriptyline Hydrochloride (Co-administration results in additive tachycardia, hypertension, and drowsiness).
No products indexed under this heading.

Amoxapine (Co-administration results in additive tachycardia, hypertension, and drowsiness).
No products indexed under this heading.

Amphetamine Sulfate (Co-administration with amphetamine may result in additive hypertension, tachycardia, and possibly cardiotoxicity). Products include:
Adderall Tablets 3164
Adderall XR Capsules 3166

Antipyrine (Co-administration results in decreased clearance of barbiturates via competitive inhibition of metabolism; additive drowsiness and CNS depression).
No products indexed under this heading.

Aprobarbital (Co-administration results in decreased clearance of barbiturates via competitive inhibition of metabolism; additive drowsiness and CNS depression).
No products indexed under this heading.

Astemizole (Co-administration results in additive CNS depression or super-additive tachycardia and drowsiness).
No products indexed under this heading.

Atracurium Besylate (Co-administration results in additive drowsiness and CNS depression).
No products indexed under this heading.

Atropine Sulfate (Co-administration with anticholinergic agents may result in additive or super-additive tachycardia and drowsiness).
Products include:
Donnatal Extentabs 2493

Azatadine Maleate (Co-administration results in additive CNS depression or super-additive tachycardia and drowsiness).
No products indexed under this heading.

Baclofen (Co-administration results in additive drowsiness and CNS depression).
No products indexed under this heading.

Belladonna Alkaloids (Co-administration with anticholinergic agents may result in additive or super-additive tachycardia and drowsiness). Products include:
Hyland's Teething Tablets .... ▣830

Benztropine Mesylate (Co-administration with anticholinergic agents may result in additive or super-additive tachycardia and drowsiness).
No products indexed under this heading.

Biperiden Hydrochloride (Co-administration with anticholinergic agents may result in additive or super-additive tachycardia and drowsiness).
No products indexed under this heading.

Bromodiphenhydramine Hydrochloride (Co-administration results in additive CNS depression or super-additive tachycardia and drowsiness).
No products indexed under this heading.

Brompheniramine Maleate (Co-administration results in additive CNS depression or super-additive tachycardia and drowsiness).
Products include:
Children's Dimetapp Cold & Allergy Elixir .... ▣730
Children's Dimetapp Cold & Allergy Chewable Tablets............ ▣730
Children's Dimetapp DM Cold & Cough Elixir .... ▣731

Buprenorphine Hydrochloride (Co-administration results in additive drowsiness and CNS depression).
Products include:

Buprenex Injectable 2716
Suboxone Tablets 2717
Subutex Tablets 2717

Buspirone Hydrochloride (Co-administration results in additive drowsiness and CNS depression).
No products indexed under this heading.

Butabarbital (Co-administration results in decreased clearance of barbiturates via competitive inhibition of metabolism; additive drowsiness and CNS depression).
No products indexed under this heading.

Butalbital (Co-administration results in decreased clearance of barbiturates via competitive inhibition of metabolism; additive drowsiness and CNS depression).
No products indexed under this heading.

Carisoprodol (Co-administration with muscle relaxants may result in additive drowsiness and CNS depression).
No products indexed under this heading.

Cetirizine Hydrochloride (Co-administration results in additive CNS depression or super-additive tachycardia and drowsiness).
Products include:
Zyrtec Chewable Tablets 2594
Zyrtec 2594
Zyrtec-D 12 Hour Extended Release Tablets 2597

Chlordiazepoxide (Co-administration results in additive drowsiness and CNS depression).
No products indexed under this heading.

Chlordiazepoxide Hydrochloride (Co-administration results in additive drowsiness and CNS depression).
Products include:
Librium Capsules 3347

Chlorpheniramine Maleate (Co-administration results in additive CNS depression or super-additive tachycardia and drowsiness).
Products include:
Advil Allergy Sinus Caplets .... ■770
Advil Multi-Symptom Cold Caplets .... ■770
BC Allergy Sinus Cold Powder .... ■677
Comtrex Maximum Strength Cold & Cough Day/Night Caplets - Night Formulation .... ■726
Comtrex Maximum Strength Day/Night Severe Cold & Sinus Caplets - Night Formulation .... ■725
Contac Cold and Flu Maximum Strength Caplets .... ■728
Contac Cold and Flu Day and Night Caplets (Night Formulation Only) .... ■727
Children's Dimetapp Long Acting Cough Plus Cold Syrup .... ■731
Robitussin Cough & Cold Long-Acting Liquid .... ■735
Robitussin Cough & Allergy Syrup .. ■736
Robitussin Cough & Cold Nighttime Liquid .... ■736
Robitussin Cough, Cold & Flu Nighttime Liquid .... ■738
Robitussin Pediatric Cough & Cold Long-Acting Liquid .... ■735
Robitussin Pediatric Cough & Cold Nighttime Liquid .... ■736
Triaminic Cold & Allergy Liquid .... ■746
Triaminic Cough & Runny Nose Softchews .... ■748
Children's Tylenol Plus Flu Oral Suspension .... ■749
Tylenol Allergy Multi-Symptom Caplets with Cool Burst and Gelcaps 1872
Children's Tylenol Plus Cold Suspension Liquid 1879
Children's Tylenol Plus Cough & Runny Nose Suspension Liquid 1879
Children's Tylenol Plus Flu Suspension Liquid 1881
Children's Tylenol Plus Multi-Symptom Cold Suspension Liquid 1879
Tylenol Cold Head Congestion Nighttime Caplets with Cool Burst 1873
Tylenol Cold Multi-Symptom Nighttime Caplets with Cool Burst 1874
Tylenol Sinus Congestion & Pain Nighttime Caplets with Cool Burst 1876
Vicks 44M Cough, Cold & Flu Relief Liquid 2680
Pediatric Vicks 44m Cough & Cold Relief Liquid 2676
Children's Vicks NyQuil Cold/Cough Relief .... ■756
Children's Vicks NyQuil Cold/Cough Relief Liquid 2680
Zicam Maximum Strength Flu Daytime .... ■768

Chlorpheniramine Polistirex (Co-administration results in additive CNS depression or super-additive tachycardia and drowsiness).
Products include:
Tussionex Pennkinetic Extended-Release Suspension 3327

Chlorpheniramine Tannate (Co-administration results in additive CNS depression or super-additive tachycardia and drowsiness).
No products indexed under this heading.

Chlorpromazine (Co-administration results in additive drowsiness and CNS depression).
No products indexed under this heading.

Chlorpromazine Hydrochloride (Co-administration results in additive drowsiness and CNS depression).
No products indexed under this heading.

Chlorprothixene (Co-administration results in additive drowsiness and CNS depression).
No products indexed under this heading.

Chlorprothixene Hydrochloride (Co-administration results in additive drowsiness and CNS depression).
No products indexed under this heading.

Chlorprothixene Lactate (Co-administration results in additive drowsiness and CNS depression).
No products indexed under this heading.

Chlorzoxazone (Co-administration with muscle relaxants may result in additive drowsiness and CNS depression).
No products indexed under this heading.

Cisatracurium Besylate (Co-administration results in additive drowsiness and CNS depression).
Products include:
Nimbex Injection 498

Clemastine Fumarate (Co-administration results in additive CNS depression or super-additive tachycardia and drowsiness).
No products indexed under this heading.

Clidinium Bromide (Co-administration with anticholinergic agents may result in additive or super-additive tachycardia and drowsiness).
No products indexed under this heading.

Clomipramine Hydrochloride (Co-administration results in additive tachycardia, hypertension, and drowsiness).
No products indexed under this heading.

Clorazepate Dipotassium (Co-administration results in additive drowsiness and CNS depression).
Products include:
Tranxene 2474

Clozapine (Co-administration results in additive drowsiness and CNS depression). Products include:
Clozaril Tablets 2184
FazaClo Orally Disintegrating Tablets 551

Cocaine Hydrochloride (Co-administration with cocaine may result in additive hypertension, tachycardia, and possibly cardiotoxicity).
No products indexed under this heading.

Codeine Phosphate (Co-administration results in additive drowsiness and CNS depression).
Products include:
Tylenol with Codeine Tablets 2391

Cyclobenzaprine Hydrochloride (Co-administration with muscle relaxants may result in additive drowsiness and CNS depression).
No products indexed under this heading.

Cyproheptadine Hydrochloride (Co-administration results in additive CNS depression or super-additive tachycardia and drowsiness).
No products indexed under this heading.

Dantrolene Sodium (Co-administration results in additive drowsiness and CNS depression).
Products include:
Dantrium Capsules 2694
Dantrium Intravenous 2695

Desflurane (Co-administration results in additive drowsiness and CNS depression).
No products indexed under this heading.

Desipramine Hydrochloride (Co-administration results in additive tachycardia, hypertension, and drowsiness).
No products indexed under this heading.

Dexchlorpheniramine Maleate (Co-administration results in additive CNS depression or super-additive tachycardia and drowsiness).
No products indexed under this heading.

Dextroamphetamine Sulfate (Co-administration with amphetamine may result in additive hypertension, tachycardia, and possibly cardiotoxicity). Products include:
Adderall Tablets 3164
Adderall XR Capsules 3166
Dexedrine 1420
DextroStat Tablets 3179

Dezocine (Co-administration results in additive drowsiness and CNS depression).
No products indexed under this heading.

Diazepam (Co-administration results in additive drowsiness and CNS depression). Products include:
Diastat Rectal Delivery System 3343
Valium Tablets 2819

Dicyclomine Hydrochloride (Co-administration with anticholinergic agents may result in additive or super-additive tachycardia and drowsiness). Products include:
Bentyl Capsules 697
Bentyl Injection 697
Bentyl Syrup 697
Bentyl Tablets 697

Diphenhydramine Citrate (Co-administration results in additive CNS depression or super-additive tachycardia and drowsiness).
Products include:
Advil PM Caplets .... ■615
Excedrin PM Caplets/Tablets/Geltabs .... ■610
Goody's PM Powder for Pain with Sleeplessness .... ■612

Diphenhydramine Hydrochloride (Co-administration results in additive CNS depression or super-additive tachycardia and drowsiness).
Products include:
Nytol QuickCaps Caplets .... ■615
Nytol QuickGels Softgels Maximum Strength .... ■616
Simply Sleep Caplets 1868
Sominex Original Formula Tablets .. ■616
TheraFlu Warming Relief Nighttime Severe Cold .... ■743
TheraFlu Thin Strips Multi Symptom .... ■744
Triaminic Nighttime Cold & Cough Liquid .... ■746
Triaminic Thin Strips Cough & Runny Nose .... ■749
Extra Strength Tylenol PM Caplets, Vanilla Caplets, Geltabs, Gelcaps and Liquid 1875
Tylenol Sore Throat Nighttime Liquid with Cool Burst .... ■790
Tylenol Allergy Multi-Symptom Nighttime Caplets with Cool Burst 1872
Tylenol Severe Allergy Caplets 1872
Children's Tylenol Plus Cold & Allergy Suspension Liquid 1878

Diphenylpyraline Hydrochloride (Co-administration results in additive CNS depression or super-additive tachycardia and drowsiness).
No products indexed under this heading.

Disulfiram (Co-administration of disulfiram in a patient who smoked marijuana has resulted in a reversible hypomanic reaction).
No products indexed under this heading.

Dobutamine Hydrochloride (Co-administration with sympathomimetics may result in additive hypertension, tachycardia, and possibly cardiotoxicity).
No products indexed under this heading.

Dopamine Hydrochloride (Co-administration with sympathomimetics may result in additive hypertension, tachycardia, and possibly cardiotoxicity).
No products indexed under this heading.

Doxacurium Chloride (Co-administration results in additive drowsiness and CNS depression).
No products indexed under this heading.

Doxepin Hydrochloride (Co-administration results in additive tachycardia, hypertension, and drowsiness).
No products indexed under this heading.

Droperidol (Co-administration results in additive drowsiness and CNS depression).
No products indexed under this heading.

Dyphylline (Increased theophylline metabolism has resulted with smoking marijuana).
No products indexed under this heading.

Enflurane (Co-administration results in additive drowsiness and CNS depression).
No products indexed under this heading.

Ephedrine Hydrochloride (Co-administration with sympathomimetics may result in additive hypertension, tachycardia, and possibly cardiotoxicity).
No products indexed under this heading.

Ephedrine Sulfate (Co-administration with sympathomimetics may result in additive hypertension, tachycardia, and possibly cardiotoxicity).
No products indexed under this heading.

Ephedrine Tannate (Co-administration with sympathomimetics may result in additive hypertension, tachycardia, and possibly cardiotoxicity).
No products indexed under this heading.

Epinephrine (Co-administration with sympathomimetics may result in additive hypertension, tachycardia, and possibly cardiotoxicity).
Products include:
EpiPen 1061
Primatene Mist 719
Twinject 0.15 3379
Twinject 0.3 3378

Epinephrine Bitartrate (Co-administration with sympathomimetics may result in additive hypertension, tachycardia, and possibly cardiotoxicity).
No products indexed under this heading.

Epinephrine Hydrochloride (Co-administration with sympathomimetics may result in additive hypertension, tachycardia, and possibly cardiotoxicity).
No products indexed under this heading.

Estazolam (Co-administration results in additive drowsiness and CNS depression). Products include:
ProSom Tablets 517

Ethanol (Co-administration results in additive drowsiness and CNS depression).
No products indexed under this heading.

Ethchlorvynol (Co-administration results in additive drowsiness and CNS depression).
No products indexed under this heading.

Ethinamate (Co-administration results in additive drowsiness and CNS depression).
No products indexed under this heading.

Ethyl Alcohol (Co-administration results in additive drowsiness and CNS depression).
No products indexed under this heading.

Fentanyl (Co-administration results in additive drowsiness and CNS depression). Products include:
Duragesic Transdermal System 2373
Ionsys Transdermal System 2379

Fentanyl Citrate (Co-administration results in additive drowsiness and CNS depression). Products include:
Actiq 979

Fexofenadine Hydrochloride (Co-administration results in additive CNS depression or super-additive tachycardia and drowsiness).
Products include:
Allegra 2844
Allegra-D 12 Hour Extended-Release Tablets 2846
Allegra-D 24 Hour Extended-Release Tablets 2849

Fluoxetine Hydrochloride (Co-administration of fluoxetine in a patient who smoked marijuana has resulted in a hypomanic reaction).
Products include:
Prozac Pulvules and Liquid 1801
Symbyax Capsules 1819

Fluphenazine Decanoate (Co-administration results in additive drowsiness and CNS depression).
No products indexed under this heading.

Fluphenazine Enanthate (Co-administration results in additive drowsiness and CNS depression).
No products indexed under this heading.

Fluphenazine Hydrochloride (Co-administration results in additive drowsiness and CNS depression).
No products indexed under this heading.

Flurazepam Hydrochloride (Co-administration results in additive drowsiness and CNS depression).
Products include:
Dalmane Capsules 3342

Glutethimide (Co-administration results in additive drowsiness and CNS depression).
No products indexed under this heading.

Glycopyrrolate (Co-administration with anticholinergic agents may result in additive or super-additive tachycardia and drowsiness).
No products indexed under this heading.

Halazepam (Co-administration results in additive drowsiness and CNS depression).
No products indexed under this heading.

Haloperidol (Co-administration results in additive drowsiness and CNS depression).
No products indexed under this heading.

Haloperidol Decanoate (Co-administration results in additive drowsiness and CNS depression).
No products indexed under this heading.

Hydrocodone Bitartrate (Co-administration results in additive drowsiness and CNS depression).
Products include:
Hycodan 1116
Hycotuss Expectorant Syrup 1117
Vicodin Tablets 535
Vicodin ES Tablets 536
Vicodin HP Tablets 538
Vicoprofen Tablets 539
Zydone Tablets 1139

Hydrocodone Polistirex (Co-administration results in additive drowsiness and CNS depression).
Products include:
Tussionex Pennkinetic Extended-Release Suspension 3327

Hydromorphone Hydrochloride (Co-administration results in additive drowsiness and CNS depression).
Products include:
Dilaudid 440
Dilaudid Non-Sterile Powder 440
Dilaudid Oral Liquid 445
Dilaudid Rectal Suppositories 440
Dilaudid Tablets 440
Dilaudid Tablets - 8 mg 445
Dilaudid-HP 442

Hydroxyzine Hydrochloride (Co-administration results in additive drowsiness and CNS depression).
No products indexed under this heading.

Hyoscyamine (Co-administration with anticholinergic agents may result in additive or super-additive tachycardia and drowsiness).
No products indexed under this heading.

Hyoscyamine Sulfate (Co-administration with anticholinergic agents may result in additive or super-additive tachycardia and drowsiness). Products include:
Donnatal Extentabs 2493
Prosed/DS Tablets 1157

Imipramine Hydrochloride (Co-administration results in additive tachycardia, hypertension, and drowsiness).
No products indexed under this heading.

Imipramine Pamoate (Co-administration results in additive tachycardia, hypertension, and drowsiness).
No products indexed under this heading.

Ipratropium Bromide (Co-administration with anticholinergic agents may result in additive or super-additive tachycardia and drowsiness). Products include:
Atrovent Inhalation Solution 835
Atrovent HFA Inhalation Aerosol 841
Atrovent Nasal Spray 0.03% 837
Atrovent Nasal Spray 0.06% 839
Combivent Inhalation Aerosol 847
DuoNeb Inhalation Solution 1058

Isoflurane (Co-administration results in additive drowsiness and CNS depression).
No products indexed under this heading.

Isoproterenol Hydrochloride (Co-administration with sympathomimetics may result in additive hypertension, tachycardia, and possibly cardiotoxicity).
No products indexed under this heading.

Isoproterenol Sulfate (Co-administration with sympathomimetics may result in additive hypertension, tachycardia, and possibly cardiotoxicity).
No products indexed under this heading.

Ketamine Hydrochloride (Co-administration results in additive drowsiness and CNS depression).
No products indexed under this heading.

Levalbuterol Hydrochloride (Co-administration with sympathomimetics may result in additive hypertension, tachycardia, and possibly cardiotoxicity). Products include:
Xopenex Inhalation Solution 3146
Xopenex Inhalation Solution Concentrate 3150

Levomethadyl Acetate Hydrochloride (Co-administration results in additive drowsiness and CNS depression).
No products indexed under this heading.

Levorphanol Tartrate (Co-administration results in additive drowsiness and CNS depression).
No products indexed under this heading.

Lithium (Co-administration results in additive drowsiness and CNS depression).
No products indexed under this heading.

Lithium Carbonate (Co-administration results in additive drowsiness and CNS depression).
Products include:
Lithobid Tablets 1692

Lithium Citrate (Co-administration results in additive drowsiness and CNS depression).
No products indexed under this heading.

Loratadine (Co-administration results in additive CNS depression or super-additive tachycardia and drowsiness). Products include:
Alavert Allergy & Sinus D-12 Hour Tablets 771
Alavert 771
Children's Claritin Allergy Oral Solution 771
Claritin Non-Drowsy 24 Hour Tablets 772
Claritin Reditabs 24 Hour Non-Drowsy Tablets 772
Claritin-D Non-Drowsy 12 Hour Tablets 772
Claritin-D Non-Drowsy 24 Hour Tablets 772

Lorazepam (Co-administration results in additive drowsiness and CNS depression).
No products indexed under this heading.

Loxapine Hydrochloride (Co-administration results in additive drowsiness and CNS depression).
No products indexed under this heading.

Loxapine Succinate (Co-administration results in additive drowsiness and CNS depression).
No products indexed under this heading.

Maprotiline Hydrochloride (Co-administration results in additive tachycardia, hypertension, and drowsiness).
No products indexed under this heading.

Mepenzolate Bromide (Co-administration with anticholinergic agents may result in additive or super-additive tachycardia and drowsiness).
No products indexed under this heading.

Meperidine Hydrochloride (Co-administration results in additive drowsiness and CNS depression).
No products indexed under this heading.

Mephobarbital (Co-administration results in decreased clearance of barbiturates via competitive inhibition of metabolism; additive drowsiness and CNS depression).
No products indexed under this heading.

Meprobamate (Co-administration results in additive drowsiness and CNS depression).
No products indexed under this heading.

Mesoridazine Besylate (Co-administration results in additive drowsiness and CNS depression).
No products indexed under this heading.

Metaproterenol Sulfate (Co-administration with sympathomimetics may result in additive hypertension, tachycardia, and possibly cardiotoxicity). Products include:
Alupent Inhalation Aerosol 826

Metaraminol Bitartrate (Co-administration with sympathomimetics may result in additive hypertension, tachycardia, and possibly cardiotoxicity).
No products indexed under this heading.

Metaxalone (Co-administration results in additive drowsiness and CNS depression). Products include:
Skelaxin Tablets 1716

Methadone Hydrochloride (Co-administration results in additive drowsiness and CNS depression).
No products indexed under this heading.

Methamphetamine Hydrochloride (Co-administration with amphetamine may result in additive hypertension, tachycardia, and possibly cardiotoxicity). Products include:
Desoxyn Tablets, USP 2462

Methdilazine Hydrochloride (Co-administration results in additive CNS depression or super-additive tachycardia and drowsiness).
No products indexed under this heading.

Methocarbamol (Co-administration with muscle relaxants may result in additive drowsiness and CNS depression).
No products indexed under this heading.

Methohexital Sodium (Co-administration results in additive drowsiness and CNS depression).
No products indexed under this heading.

Methotrimeprazine (Co-administration results in additive drowsiness and CNS depression).
No products indexed under this heading.

Methoxamine Hydrochloride (Co-administration with sympathomimetics may result in additive hypertension, tachycardia, and possibly cardiotoxicity).
No products indexed under this heading.

Methoxyflurane (Co-administration results in additive drowsiness and CNS depression).
No products indexed under this heading.

Metocurine Iodide (Co-administration results in additive drowsiness and CNS depression).
No products indexed under this heading.

Midazolam Hydrochloride (Co-administration results in additive drowsiness and CNS depression).
No products indexed under this heading.

Mivacurium Chloride (Co-administration results in additive drowsiness and CNS depression). Products include:
Mivacron Injection 493

Molindone Hydrochloride (Co-administration results in additive drowsiness and CNS depression). Products include:
Moban Tablets 1119

Morphine Sulfate (Co-administration results in additive drowsiness and CNS depression). Products include:

Avinza Capsules 1741
Kadian Capsules 577
MS Contin Tablets 2701

Norepinephrine Bitartrate (Co-administration with sympathomimetics may result in additive hypertension, tachycardia, and possibly cardiotoxicity).
No products indexed under this heading.

Nortriptyline Hydrochloride (Co-administration results in additive tachycardia, hypertension, and drowsiness).
No products indexed under this heading.

Olanzapine (Co-administration results in additive drowsiness and CNS depression). Products include:
Symbyax Capsules 1819
Zyprexa Tablets 1830
Zyprexa IntraMuscular 1830
Zyprexa ZYDIS Orally
Disintegrating Tablets 1830

Orphenadrine Citrate (Co-administration with muscle relaxants may result in additive drowsiness and CNS depression). Products include:
Norflex Injection 1856

Oxazepam (Co-administration results in additive drowsiness and CNS depression).
No products indexed under this heading.

Oxybutynin Chloride (Co-administration with anticholinergic agents may result in additive or super-additive tachycardia and drowsiness). Products include:
Ditropan XL Extended-Release
Tablets 2413

Oxycodone Hydrochloride (Co-administration results in additive drowsiness and CNS depression). Products include:
OxyContin Tablets 2703
OxyFast Oral Concentrate
Solution 2708
OxyIR Capsules 2708
Percocet Tablets 1131
Percodan Tablets 1132

Pancuronium Bromide (Co-administration results in additive drowsiness and CNS depression).
No products indexed under this heading.

Pentobarbital Sodium (Co-administration results in decreased clearance of barbiturates via competitive inhibition of metabolism; additive drowsiness and CNS depression). Products include:
Nembutal Sodium Solution, USP 2470

Perphenazine (Co-administration results in additive drowsiness and CNS depression).
No products indexed under this heading.

Phenobarbital (Co-administration results in decreased clearance of barbiturates via competitive inhibition of metabolism; additive drowsiness and CNS depression). Products include:
Donnatal Extentabs 2493

Phenylephrine Bitartrate (Co-administration with sympathomimetics may result in additive hypertension, tachycardia, and possibly cardiotoxicity).
No products indexed under this heading.

Phenylephrine Hydrochloride (Co-administration with sympathomi-

metics may result in additive hypertension, tachycardia, and possibly cardiotoxicity). Products include:
Comtrex Maximum Strength
Non-Drowsy Cold & Cough
Caplets ⊞725
Comtrex Maximum Strength
Day/Night Severe Cold & Sinus
Caplets - Day Formulation ⊞725
Comtrex Maximum Strength
Day/Night Severe Cold & Sinus
Caplets - Night Formulation ⊞725
Contac Cold and Flu Maximum
Strength Caplets ⊞728
Contac Cold and Flu Day and
Night Caplets (Day Formulation
Only) ⊞727
Contac Cold and Flu Day and
Night Caplets (Night
Formulation Only) ⊞727
Contac Cold and Flu Non-Drowsy
Caplets ⊞728
Contac-D Cold Non-Drowsy
Tablets ⊞729
Children's Dimetapp Cold &
Allergy Elixir ⊞730
Children's Dimetapp Cold &
Allergy Chewable Tablets ⊞730
Children's Dimetapp DM Cold &
Cough Elixir ⊞731
Toddler's Dimetapp Cold and
Cough Drops ⊞732
Excedrin Sinus Headache
Caplets/Tablets ⊞610
4-Way Fast Acting Nasal Spray ⊞775
4-Way Menthol Nasal Spray ⊞775
Preparation H Maximum Strength
Cream ⊞666
Preparation H Cooling Gel ⊞666
Preparation H ⊞666
Refenesen PE Caplets ⊞721
Robitussin Cough & Allergy Syrup .. ⊞736
Robitussin Cough & Cold
Nighttime Liquid ⊞736
Robitussin Cough, Cold & Flu
Nighttime Liquid ⊞738
Robitussin Head & Chest
Congestion PE Syrup ⊞739
Robitussin Pediatric Cough &
Cold Nighttime Liquid ⊞736
TheraFlu Cold & Cough Hot
Liquid ⊞740
TheraFlu Cold & Sore Throat Hot
Liquid ⊞741
TheraFlu Flu & Sore Throat Hot
Liquid ⊞742
TheraFlu Daytime Severe Cold
Hot Liquid ⊞742
TheraFlu Nighttime Severe Cold
Hot Liquid ⊞740
TheraFlu Warming Relief Daytime
Severe Cold ⊞743
TheraFlu Warming Relief
Nighttime Severe Cold ⊞743
Triaminic Chest & Nasal
Congestion Liquid ⊞746
Triaminic Cold & Allergy Liquid ⊞746
Triaminic Daytime Cold & Cough
Liquid ⊞745
Triaminic Nighttime Cold &
Cough Liquid ⊞746
Triaminic Thin Strips Cold ⊞748
Triaminic Thin Strips Cold &
Cough ⊞778
Triaminic Infant Thin Strips
Decongestant ⊞747
Triaminic Infant Thin Strips
Decongestant Plus Cough ⊞747
Children's Tylenol Plus Flu Oral
Suspension ⊞749
Tylenol Cold Head Congestion
Daytime Caplets with Cool
Burst and Gelcaps ⊞750
Tylenol Cold Multi-Symptom
Daytime Liquid ⊞752
Tylenol Cold Multi-Symptom
Severe Daytime Liquid ⊞752
Concentrated Tylenol Infants'
Drops Plus Cold & Cough ⊞754
Tylenol Allergy Multi-Symptom
Caplets with Cool Burst and
Gelcaps 1872
Tylenol Allergy Multi-Symptom
Nighttime Caplets with Cool
Burst 1872
Children's Tylenol Plus Cold
Suspension Liquid 1879

Children's Tylenol Plus Cold &
Allergy Suspension Liquid 1878
Children's Tylenol Plus Flu
Suspension Liquid 1881
Children's Tylenol Plus
Multi-Symptom Cold
Suspension Liquid 1879
Tylenol Cold Head Congestion
Daytime Caplets with Cool
Burst 1873
Tylenol Cold Head Congestion
Nighttime Caplets with Cool
Burst 1873
Tylenol Cold Head Congestion
Severe Caplets with Cool Burst..... 1873
Tylenol Cold Multi-Symptom
Daytime Caplets with Cool
Burst and Gelcaps 1874
Tylenol Cold Multi-Symptom
Daytime Liquid with Citrus Burst ... 1874
Tylenol Cold Multi-Symptom
Nighttime Caplets with Cool
Burst 1874
Tylenol Cold Multi-Symptom
Nighttime Liquid with Cool Burst ... 1874
Tylenol Cold Multi-Symptom
Severe Caplets with Cool Burst..... 1874
Tylenol Cold Multi-Symptom
Severe Daytime Liquid with
Citrus Burst, 1874
Tylenol Sinus Congestion & Pain
Daytime Caplets with Cool
Burst and Gelcaps 1876
Tylenol Sinus Congestion & Pain
Nighttime Caplets with Cool
Burst 1876
Tylenol Sinus Congestion & Pain
Severe Caplets with Cool Burst..... 1876
Vicks 44D Cough & Head
Congestion Relief Liquid.............. ⊞760
Vicks DayQuil LiquiCaps/Liquid
Multi-Symptom Cold/Flu Relief..... ⊞761
Zicam Cough Plus D Cough
Spray...................................... ⊞767

Phenylephrine Tannate (Co-administration with sympathomimetics may result in additive hypertension, tachycardia, and possibly cardiotoxicity).
No products indexed under this heading.

Phenylpropanolamine Hydrochloride (Co-administration with sympathomimetics may result in additive hypertension, tachycardia, and possibly cardiotoxicity).
No products indexed under this heading.

Pirbuterol Acetate (Co-administration with sympathomimetics may result in additive hypertension, tachycardia, and possibly cardiotoxicity). Products include:
Maxair Autohaler 1852

Prazepam (Co-administration results in additive drowsiness and CNS depression).
No products indexed under this heading.

Prochlorperazine (Co-administration results in additive drowsiness and CNS depression).
No products indexed under this heading.

Procyclidine Hydrochloride (Co-administration with anticholinergic agents may result in additive or super-additive tachycardia and drowsiness).
No products indexed under this heading.

Promethazine Hydrochloride (Co-administration results in additive drowsiness and CNS depression). Products include:
Phenergan Tablets and
Suppositories............................ 3440

Propantheline Bromide (Co-administration with anticholinergic agents may result in additive or super-additive tachycardia and drowsiness).
No products indexed under this heading.

Propofol (Co-administration results in additive drowsiness and CNS depression).
No products indexed under this heading.

Propoxyphene Hydrochloride (Co-administration results in additive drowsiness and CNS depression).
No products indexed under this heading.

Propoxyphene Napsylate (Co-administration results in additive drowsiness and CNS depression).
No products indexed under this heading.

Protriptyline Hydrochloride (Co-administration results in additive tachycardia, hypertension, and drowsiness).
No products indexed under this heading.

Pseudoephedrine Hydrochloride (Co-administration with sympathomimetics may result in additive hypertension, tachycardia, and possibly cardiotoxicity). Products include:
- Advil Allergy Sinus Caplets 770
- Advil Cold & Sinus 723
- Advil Multi-Symptom Cold Caplets 770
- Aleve Cold & Sinus Caplets 744
- Allegra-D 12 Hour Extended-Release Tablets 2846
- Allegra-D 24 Hour Extended-Release Tablets 2849
- BC Cold Powder 677
- Comtrex Maximum Strength Cold & Cough Day/Night Caplets - Day Formulation 726
- Comtrex Maximum Strength Cold & Cough Day/Night Caplets - Night Formulation 726
- Children's Motrin Cold Oral Suspension 1867
- Mucinex D Extended-Release Bi-Layer Tablets 776
- Robitussin Cough & Cold CF Liquid 735
- Robitussin Cough & Cold Pediatric Drops 735
- Tylenol Sinus Congestion & Pain Nighttime Caplets with Cool Burst 778
- Tylenol Cold Severe Congestion Non-Drowsy Caplets with Cool Burst 1874
- Tylenol Sinus Severe Congestion Caplets with Cool Burst 1876
- Vicks 44D Cough & Head Congestion Relief Liquid 2679
- Vicks 44M Cough, Cold & Flu Relief Liquid 2680
- Vicks DayQuil Multi-Symptom Cold/Flu Relief LiquiCaps 2678
- Vicks DayQuil Multi-Symptom Cold/Flu Relief Liquid 2678
- Vicks NyQuil Multi-Symptom Cold/Flu Relief Liquid 2681
- Vicks NyQuil Multi-Symptom Cold/Flu Relief LiquiCaps 2681
- Children's Vicks NyQuil Cold/Cough Relief Liquid 2680
- Zyrtec-D 12 Hour Extended Release Tablets 2597

Pseudoephedrine Sulfate (Co-administration with sympathomimetics may result in additive hypertension, tachycardia, and possibly cardiotoxicity). Products include:
- Alavert Allergy & Sinus D-12 Hour Tablets 771
- Clarinex-D 24-Hour Extended-Release Tablets 2998
- Claritin-D Non-Drowsy 12 Hour Tablets 772
- Claritin-D Non-Drowsy 24 Hour Tablets 772

Pyrilamine Maleate (Co-administration results in additive CNS depression or super-additive tachycardia and drowsiness).
No products indexed under this heading.

Pyrilamine Tannate (Co-administration results in additive CNS depression or super-additive tachycardia and drowsiness).
No products indexed under this heading.

Quazepam (Co-administration results in additive drowsiness and CNS depression).
No products indexed under this heading.

Quetiapine Fumarate (Co-administration results in additive drowsiness and CNS depression). Products include:
- Seroquel Tablets 690

Rapacuronium Bromide (Co-administration results in additive drowsiness and CNS depression).
No products indexed under this heading.

Remifentanil Hydrochloride (Co-administration results in additive drowsiness and CNS depression).
No products indexed under this heading.

Risperidone (Co-administration results in additive drowsiness and CNS depression). Products include:
- Risperdal 1676
- Risperdal Consta Long-Acting Injection 1682
- Risperdal M-Tab Orally Disintegrating Tablets 1676

Rocuronium Bromide (Co-administration results in additive drowsiness and CNS depression). Products include:
- Zemuron Injection 2346

Salmeterol Xinafoate (Co-administration with sympathomimetics may result in additive hypertension, tachycardia, and possibly cardiotoxicity). Products include:
- Advair Diskus 100/50 1308
- Advair Diskus 250/50 1308
- Advair Diskus 500/50 1308
- Advair HFA Inhalation Aerosol 1318
- Serevent Diskus 1568

Scopolamine (Co-administration with anticholinergic agents may result in additive or super-additive tachycardia and drowsiness). Products include:
- Transderm Scōp Transdermal Therapeutic System 2177

Scopolamine Hydrobromide (Co-administration with anticholinergic agents may result in additive or super-additive tachycardia and drowsiness). Products include:
- Donnatal Extentabs 2493

Secobarbital Sodium (Co-administration results in decreased clearance of barbiturates via competitive inhibition of metabolism; additive drowsiness and CNS depression).
No products indexed under this heading.

Sevoflurane (Co-administration results in additive drowsiness and CNS depression). Products include:
- Ultane Liquid for Inhalation 531

Sodium Oxybate (Co-administration results in additive drowsiness and CNS depression). Products include:
- Xyrem Oral Solution 1688

Succinylcholine Chloride (Co-administration results in additive drowsiness and CNS depression).
No products indexed under this heading.

Sufentanil Citrate (Co-administration results in additive drowsiness and CNS depression).
No products indexed under this heading.

Temazepam (Co-administration results in additive drowsiness and CNS depression). Products include:
- Restoril Capsules 1860

Terbutaline Sulfate (Co-administration with sympathomimetics may result in additive hypertension, tachycardia, and possibly cardiotoxicity).
No products indexed under this heading.

Terfenadine (Co-administration results in additive CNS depression or super-additive tachycardia and drowsiness).
No products indexed under this heading.

Theophylline (Increased theophylline metabolism has resulted with smoking marijuana).
No products indexed under this heading.

Theophylline Anhydrous (Increased theophylline metabolism has resulted with smoking marijuana). Products include:
- Uniphyl Tablets 2710

Theophylline Calcium Salicylate (Increased theophylline metabolism has resulted with smoking marijuana).
No products indexed under this heading.

Theophylline Dihydroxypropyl (Glyceryl) (Increased theophylline metabolism has resulted with smoking marijuana).
No products indexed under this heading.

Theophylline Ethylenediamine (Increased theophylline metabolism has resulted with smoking marijuana).
No products indexed under this heading.

Theophylline Sodium Glycinate (Increased theophylline metabolism has resulted with smoking marijuana).
No products indexed under this heading.

Thiamylal Sodium (Co-administration results in decreased clearance of barbiturates via competitive inhibition of metabolism; additive drowsiness and CNS depression).
No products indexed under this heading.

Thioridazine Hydrochloride (Co-administration results in additive drowsiness and CNS depression). Products include:
- Thioridazine Hydrochloride Tablets 2163

Thiothixene (Co-administration results in additive drowsiness and CNS depression). Products include:
- Thiothixene Capsules 2165

Tolterodine Tartrate (Co-administration with anticholinergic agents may result in additive or super-additive tachycardia and drowsiness). Products include:
- Detrol Tablets 2628
- Detrol LA Capsules 2631

Triazolam (Co-administration results in additive drowsiness and CNS depression).
No products indexed under this heading.

Tridihexethyl Chloride (Co-administration with anticholinergic agents may result in additive or super-additive tachycardia and drowsiness).
No products indexed under this heading.

Trifluoperazine Hydrochloride (Co-administration results in additive drowsiness and CNS depression).
No products indexed under this heading.

Trihexyphenidyl Hydrochloride (Co-administration with anticholinergic agents may result in additive or super-additive tachycardia and drowsiness).
No products indexed under this heading.

Trimeprazine Tartrate (Co-administration results in additive CNS depression or super-additive tachycardia and drowsiness).
No products indexed under this heading.

Trimipramine Maleate (Co-administration results in additive tachycardia, hypertension, and drowsiness).
No products indexed under this heading.

Tripelennamine Hydrochloride (Co-administration results in additive CNS depression or super-additive tachycardia and drowsiness).
No products indexed under this heading.

Triprolidine Hydrochloride (Co-administration results in additive CNS depression or super-additive tachycardia and drowsiness).
No products indexed under this heading.

Vecuronium Bromide (Co-administration results in additive drowsiness and CNS depression).
No products indexed under this heading.

Zaleplon (Co-administration results in additive drowsiness and CNS depression). Products include:
- Sonata Capsules 1717

Ziprasidone Hydrochloride (Co-administration results in additive drowsiness and CNS depression). Products include:
- Geodon Capsules 2529

Zolpidem Tartrate (Co-administration results in additive drowsiness and CNS depression). Products include:
- Ambien Tablets 2851
- Ambien CR Tablets 2855

Food Interactions

Alcohol (Co-administration results in additive drowsiness and CNS depression).

MARLYN FORMULA 50 CAPSULES

(Amino Acid Preparations, Vitamin B_6) 1862
None cited in PDR database.

MASS APPEAL TABLETS

(Amino Acid Preparations, Minerals) 830
None cited in PDR database.

MASSENGILL FEMININE CLEANSING WASH
(Cleanser) .... ▣801
None cited in PDR database.

MASSENGILL BABY POWDER SCENT SOFT CLOTH TOWELETTE
(Lactic Acid, Potassium Sorbate, Sodium Lactate)............................... ▣801
None cited in PDR database.

MATULANE CAPSULES
(Procarbazine Hydrochloride) 3191
May interact with antihistamines, antihypertensives, barbiturates, narcotic analgesics, phenothiazines, sympathomimetics, tricyclic antidepressants, and certain other agents. Compounds in these categories include:

Acebutolol Hydrochloride (To minimize CNS depression and possible potentiation, hypotensive agents should be used with caution).
No products indexed under this heading.

Acrivastine (Potential for increased CNS depression and possible potentiation).
No products indexed under this heading.

Albuterol (Procarbazine exhibits some MAO inhibitory activity; concurrent use should be avoided).
Products include:
Proventil Inhalation Aerosol 3053

Albuterol Sulfate (Procarbazine exhibits some MAO inhibitory activity; concurrent use should be avoided). Products include:
AccuNeb Inhalation Solution 1055
Combivent Inhalation Aerosol 847
DuoNeb Inhalation Solution 1058
ProAir HFA Inhalation Aerosol 3300
Proventil Inhalation Solution 0.083%.. 3055
Proventil HFA Inhalation Aerosol 3056
Ventolin HFA Inhalation Aerosol 1600
VoSpire ER Tablets 1052

Alfentanil Hydrochloride (Potential for increased CNS depression and possible potentiation).
No products indexed under this heading.

Amitriptyline Hydrochloride (Procarbazine exhibits some MAO inhibitory activity; concurrent use should be avoided).
No products indexed under this heading.

Amlodipine Besylate (To minimize CNS depression and possible potentiation, hypotensive agents should be used with caution). Products include:
Caduet Tablets 2508
Lotrel Capsules 2249
Norvasc Tablets 2545

Amoxapine (Procarbazine exhibits some MAO inhibitory activity; concurrent use should be avoided).
No products indexed under this heading.

Aprobarbital (Potential for increased CNS depression and possible potentiation).
No products indexed under this heading.

Astemizole (Potential for increased CNS depression and possible potentiation).
No products indexed under this heading.

Atenolol (To minimize CNS depression and possible potentiation, hypotensive agents should be used with caution).
No products indexed under this heading.

Azatadine Maleate (Potential for increased CNS depression and possible potentiation).
No products indexed under this heading.

Benazepril Hydrochloride (To minimize CNS depression and possible potentiation, hypotensive agents should be used with caution).
Products include:
Lotensin Tablets 2243
Lotensin HCT Tablets 2246
Lotrel Capsules 2249

Bendroflumethiazide (To minimize CNS depression and possible potentiation, hypotensive agents should be used with caution).
No products indexed under this heading.

Betaxolol Hydrochloride (To minimize CNS depression and possible potentiation, hypotensive agents should be used with caution).
Products include:
Betoptic S Ophthalmic Suspension.. 558

Bisoprolol Fumarate (To minimize CNS depression and possible potentiation, hypotensive agents should be used with caution).
No products indexed under this heading.

Bromodiphenhydramine Hydrochloride (Potential for increased CNS depression and possible potentiation).
No products indexed under this heading.

Brompheniramine Maleate (Potential for increased CNS depression and possible potentiation).
Products include:
Children's Dimetapp Cold & Allergy Elixir .... ▣730
Children's Dimetapp Cold & Allergy Chewable Tablets............ ▣730
Children's Dimetapp DM Cold & Cough Elixir .... ▣731

Buprenorphine Hydrochloride (Potential for increased CNS depression and possible potentiation).
Products include:
Buprenex Injectable 2716
Suboxone Tablets 2717
Subutex Tablets 2717

Butabarbital (Potential for increased CNS depression and possible potentiation).
No products indexed under this heading.

Butalbital (Potential for increased CNS depression and possible potentiation).
No products indexed under this heading.

Candesartan Cilexetil (To minimize CNS depression and possible potentiation, hypotensive agents should be used with caution).
Products include:
Atacand Tablets 649
Atacand HCT 651

Captopril (To minimize CNS depression and possible potentiation, hypotensive agents should be used with caution). Products include:
Captopril Tablets 2149

Carteolol Hydrochloride (To minimize CNS depression and possible potentiation, hypotensive agents should be used with caution).
Products include:
Carteolol Hydrochloride Ophthalmic Solution USP, 1%....... ⊙249

Cetirizine Hydrochloride (Potential for increased CNS depression and possible potentiation). Products include:
Zyrtec Chewable Tablets 2594
Zyrtec 2594
Zyrtec-D 12 Hour Extended Release Tablets 2597

Chlorothiazide (To minimize CNS depression and possible potentiation, hypotensive agents should be used with caution). Products include:
Diuril Oral Suspension 1954

Chlorothiazide Sodium (To minimize CNS depression and possible potentiation, hypotensive agents should be used with caution).
Products include:
Diuril Sodium Intravenous 2467

Chlorpheniramine Maleate (Potential for increased CNS depression and possible potentiation).
Products include:
Advil Allergy Sinus Caplets .... ▣770
Advil Multi-Symptom Cold Caplets....................................... ▣770
BC Allergy Sinus Cold Powder .... ▣677
Comtrex Maximum Strength Cold & Cough Day/Night Caplets - Night Formulation .... ▣726
Comtrex Maximum Strength Day/Night Severe Cold & Sinus Caplets - Night Formulation .... ▣725
Contac Cold and Flu Maximum Strength Caplets.......................... ▣728
Contac Cold and Flu Day and Night Caplets (Night Formulation Only)........................ ▣727
Children's Dimetapp Long Acting Cough Plus Cold Syrup............... ▣731
Robitussin Cough & Cold Long-Acting Liquid .... ▣735
Robitussin Cough & Allergy Syrup .. ▣736
Robitussin Cough & Cold Nighttime Liquid.......................... ▣736
Robitussin Cough, Cold & Flu Nighttime Liquid.......................... ▣738
Robitussin Pediatric Cough & Cold Long-Acting Liquid............... ▣735
Robitussin Pediatric Cough & Cold Nighttime Liquid................. ▣736
Triaminic Cold & Allergy Liquid .... ▣746
Triaminic Cough & Runny Nose Softchews .... ▣748
Children's Tylenol Plus Flu Oral Suspension.................................. ▣749
Tylenol Allergy Multi-Symptom Caplets with Cool Burst and Gelcaps.. 1872
Children's Tylenol Plus Cold Suspension Liquid 1879
Children's Tylenol Plus Cough & Runny Nose Suspension Liquid..... 1879
Children's Tylenol Plus Flu Suspension Liquid 1881
Children's Tylenol Plus Multi-Symptom Cold Suspension Liquid 1879
Tylenol Cold Head Congestion Nighttime Caplets with Cool Burst... 1873
Tylenol Cold Multi-Symptom Nighttime Caplets with Cool Burst... 1874
Tylenol Sinus Congestion & Pain Nighttime Caplets with Cool Burst... 1876
Vicks 44M Cough, Cold & Flu Relief Liquid................................. 2680
Pediatric Vicks 44m Cough & Cold Relief Liquid......................... 2676
Children's Vicks NyQuil Cold/Cough Relief........................ ▣756
Children's Vicks NyQuil Cold/Cough Relief Liquid............. 2680
Zicam Maximum Strength Flu Daytime.. ▣768

Chlorpheniramine Polistirex (Potential for increased CNS depression and possible potentiation).
Products include:
Tussionex Pennkinetic Extended-Release Suspension 3327

Chlorpheniramine Tannate (Potential for increased CNS depression and possible potentiation).
No products indexed under this heading.

Chlorpromazine (Potential for increased CNS depression and possible potentiation).
No products indexed under this heading.

Chlorpromazine Hydrochloride (Potential for increased CNS depression and possible potentiation).
No products indexed under this heading.

Chlorthalidone (To minimize CNS depression and possible potentiation, hypotensive agents should be used with caution). Products include:
Clorpres Tablets 2153

Clemastine Fumarate (Potential for increased CNS depression and possible potentiation).
No products indexed under this heading.

Clomipramine Hydrochloride (Procarbazine exhibits some MAO inhibitory activity; concurrent use should be avoided).
No products indexed under this heading.

Clonidine (To minimize CNS depression and possible potentiation, hypotensive agents should be used with caution). Products include:
Catapres-TTS 844

Clonidine Hydrochloride (To minimize CNS depression and possible potentiation, hypotensive agents should be used with caution).
Products include:
Catapres Tablets 843
Clorpres Tablets 2153

Codeine Phosphate (Potential for increased CNS depression and possible potentiation). Products include:
Tylenol with Codeine Tablets 2391

Cyproheptadine Hydrochloride (Potential for increased CNS depression and possible potentiation).
No products indexed under this heading.

Deserpidine (To minimize CNS depression and possible potentiation, hypotensive agents should be used with caution).
No products indexed under this heading.

Desipramine Hydrochloride (Procarbazine exhibits some MAO inhibitory activity; concurrent use should be avoided).
No products indexed under this heading.

Dexchlorpheniramine Maleate (Potential for increased CNS depression and possible potentiation).
No products indexed under this heading.

Dezocine (Potential for increased CNS depression and possible potentiation).
No products indexed under this heading.

Diazoxide (To minimize CNS depression and possible potentiation, hypotensive agents should be used with caution). Products include:
Hyperstat I.V. 3017

Diltiazem Hydrochloride (To minimize CNS depression and possible potentiation, hypotensive agents should be used with caution). Products include:

Diphenhydramine Citrate (Potential for increased CNS depression and possible potentiation). Products include:

Diphenhydramine Hydrochloride (Potential for increased CNS depression and possible potentiation). Products include:

Diphenylpyraline Hydrochloride (Potential for increased CNS depression and possible potentiation). No products indexed under this heading.

Dobutamine Hydrochloride (Procarbazine exhibits some MAO inhibitory activity; concurrent use should be avoided). No products indexed under this heading.

Dopamine Hydrochloride (Procarbazine exhibits some MAO inhibitory activity; concurrent use should be avoided). No products indexed under this heading.

Doxazosin Mesylate (To minimize CNS depression and possible potentiation, hypotensive agents should be used with caution). Products include:

Doxepin Hydrochloride (Procarbazine exhibits some MAO inhibitory activity; concurrent use should be avoided). No products indexed under this heading.

Enalapril Maleate (To minimize CNS depression and possible potentiation, hypotensive agents should be used with caution). Products include:

Enalaprilat (To minimize CNS depression and possible potentiation, hypotensive agents should be used with caution). No products indexed under this heading.

Ephedrine Hydrochloride (Procarbazine exhibits some MAO inhibitory activity; concurrent use should be avoided). No products indexed under this heading.

Ephedrine Sulfate (Procarbazine exhibits some MAO inhibitory activity; concurrent use should be avoided). No products indexed under this heading.

Ephedrine Tannate (Procarbazine exhibits some MAO inhibitory activity; concurrent use should be avoided). No products indexed under this heading.

Epinephrine (Procarbazine exhibits some MAO inhibitory activity; concurrent use should be avoided). Products include:

Epinephrine Bitartrate (Procarbazine exhibits some MAO inhibitory activity; concurrent use should be avoided). No products indexed under this heading.

Epinephrine Hydrochloride (Procarbazine exhibits some MAO inhibitory activity; concurrent use should be avoided). No products indexed under this heading.

Eprosartan Mesylate (To minimize CNS depression and possible potentiation, hypotensive agents should be used with caution). Products include:

Esmolol Hydrochloride (To minimize CNS depression and possible potentiation, hypotensive agents should be used with caution). No products indexed under this heading.

Felodipine (To minimize CNS depression and possible potentiation, hypotensive agents should be used with caution). No products indexed under this heading.

Fentanyl (Potential for increased CNS depression and possible potentiation). Products include:

Fentanyl Citrate (Potential for increased CNS depression and possible potentiation). Products include:

Fexofenadine Hydrochloride (Potential for increased CNS depression and possible potentiation). Products include:

Fluphenazine Decanoate (Potential for increased CNS depression and possible potentiation). No products indexed under this heading.

Fluphenazine Enanthate (Potential for increased CNS depression and possible potentiation). No products indexed under this heading.

Fluphenazine Hydrochloride (Potential for increased CNS depression and possible potentiation). No products indexed under this heading.

Fosinopril Sodium (To minimize CNS depression and possible potentiation, hypotensive agents should be used with caution). No products indexed under this heading.

Furosemide (To minimize CNS depression and possible potentiation, hypotensive agents should be used with caution). Products include:

Guanabenz Acetate (To minimize CNS depression and possible potentiation, hypotensive agents should be used with caution). No products indexed under this heading.

Guanethidine Monosulfate (To minimize CNS depression and possible potentiation, hypotensive agents should be used with caution). No products indexed under this heading.

Hydralazine Hydrochloride (To minimize CNS depression and possible potentiation, hypotensive agents should be used with caution). Products include:

Hydrochlorothiazide (To minimize CNS depression and possible potentiation, hypotensive agents should be used with caution). Products include:

Hydrocodone Bitartrate (Potential for increased CNS depression and possible potentiation). Products include:

Hydrocodone Polistirex (Potential for increased CNS depression and possible potentiation). Products include:

Hydroflumethiazide (To minimize CNS depression and possible potentiation, hypotensive agents should be used with caution). No products indexed under this heading.

Hydromorphone Hydrochloride (Potential for increased CNS depression and possible potentiation). Products include:

Imipramine Hydrochloride (Procarbazine exhibits some MAO inhibitory activity; concurrent use should be avoided). No products indexed under this heading.

Imipramine Pamoate (Procarbazine exhibits some MAO inhibitory activity; concurrent use should be avoided). No products indexed under this heading.

Indapamide (To minimize CNS depression and possible potentiation, hypotensive agents should be used with caution). Products include:

Irbesartan (To minimize CNS depression and possible potentiation, hypotensive agents should be used with caution). Products include:

Isoproterenol Hydrochloride (Procarbazine exhibits some MAO inhibitory activity; concurrent use should be avoided). No products indexed under this heading.

Isoproterenol Sulfate (Procarbazine exhibits some MAO inhibitory activity; concurrent use should be avoided). No products indexed under this heading.

Isradipine (To minimize CNS depression and possible potentiation, hypotensive agents should be used with caution). Products include:

Labetalol Hydrochloride (To minimize CNS depression and possible potentiation, hypotensive agents should be used with caution). No products indexed under this heading.

Levalbuterol Hydrochloride (Procarbazine exhibits some MAO inhibitory activity; concurrent use should be avoided). Products include:

Levorphanol Tartrate (Potential for increased CNS depression and possible potentiation). No products indexed under this heading.

Lisinopril (To minimize CNS depression and possible potentiation, hypotensive agents should be used with caution). Products include:

Loratadine (Potential for increased CNS depression and possible potentiation). Products include:

Losartan Potassium (To minimize CNS depression and possible potentiation, hypotensive agents should be used with caution). Products include:
- Cozaar Tablets 1935
- Hyzaar 50-12.5 Tablets 1990
- Hyzaar 100-12.5 Tablets 1990
- Hyzaar 100-25 Tablets 1990

Maprotiline Hydrochloride (Procarbazine exhibits some MAO inhibitory activity; concurrent use should be avoided).
- No products indexed under this heading.

Mecamylamine Hydrochloride (To minimize CNS depression and possible potentiation, hypotensive agents should be used with caution).
- No products indexed under this heading.

Meperidine Hydrochloride (Potential for increased CNS depression and possible potentiation).
- No products indexed under this heading.

Mephobarbital (Potential for increased CNS depression and possible potentiation).
- No products indexed under this heading.

Mesoridazine Besylate (Potential for increased CNS depression and possible potentiation).
- No products indexed under this heading.

Metaproterenol Sulfate (Procarbazine exhibits some MAO inhibitory activity; concurrent use should be avoided). Products include:
- Alupent Inhalation Aerosol 826

Metaraminol Bitartrate (Procarbazine exhibits some MAO inhibitory activity; concurrent use should be avoided).
- No products indexed under this heading.

Methadone Hydrochloride (Potential for increased CNS depression and possible potentiation).
- No products indexed under this heading.

Methdilazine Hydrochloride (Potential for increased CNS depression and possible potentiation).
- No products indexed under this heading.

Methotrimeprazine (Potential for increased CNS depression and possible potentiation).
- No products indexed under this heading.

Methoxamine Hydrochloride (Procarbazine exhibits some MAO inhibitory activity; concurrent use should be avoided).
- No products indexed under this heading.

Methyclothiazide (To minimize CNS depression and possible potentiation, hypotensive agents should be used with caution).
- No products indexed under this heading.

Methyldopa (To minimize CNS depression and possible potentiation, hypotensive agents should be used with caution). Products include:
- Aldoril Tablets 1910

Methyldopate Hydrochloride (To minimize CNS depression and possible potentiation, hypotensive agents should be used with caution).
- No products indexed under this heading.

Metolazone (To minimize CNS depression and possible potentiation, hypotensive agents should be used with caution).
- No products indexed under this heading.

Metoprolol Succinate (To minimize CNS depression and possible potentiation, hypotensive agents should be used with caution). Products include:
- Toprol-XL Tablets 668

Metoprolol Tartrate (To minimize CNS depression and possible potentiation, hypotensive agents should be used with caution). Products include:
- Lopressor Injection 2238
- Lopressor Tablets 2238
- Lopressor HCT 50/25 Tablets 2241
- Lopressor HCT 100/25 Tablets 2241
- Lopressor HCT 100/50 Tablets 2241

Metyrosine (To minimize CNS depression and possible potentiation, hypotensive agents should be used with caution). Products include:
- Demser Capsules 1953

Mibefradil Dihydrochloride (To minimize CNS depression and possible potentiation, hypotensive agents should be used with caution).
- No products indexed under this heading.

Minoxidil (To minimize CNS depression and possible potentiation, hypotensive agents should be used with caution). Products include:
- Men's Rogaine Extra Strength Hair Regrowth Treatment Topical Solution, Ocean Rush Scent and Original Unscented ..... ▣633
- Men's Rogaine Foam Hair Regrowth Treatment ..... ▣633
- Women's Rogaine Hair Regrowth Treatment Topical Solution, Spring Bloom Scent and Original Unscented ..... ▣634

Moexipril Hydrochloride (To minimize CNS depression and possible potentiation, hypotensive agents should be used with caution). Products include:
- Uniretic Tablets 3100
- Univasc Tablets 3104

Morphine Sulfate (Potential for increased CNS depression and possible potentiation). Products include:
- Avinza Capsules 1741
- Kadian Capsules 577
- MS Contin Tablets 2701

Nadolol (To minimize CNS depression and possible potentiation, hypotensive agents should be used with caution). Products include:
- Nadolol Tablets 2159

Nicardipine Hydrochloride (To minimize CNS depression and possible potentiation, hypotensive agents should be used with caution). Products include:
- Cardene I.V. 2497

Nifedipine (To minimize CNS depression and possible potentiation, hypotensive agents should be used with caution). Products include:
- Adalat CC Tablets 2964

Nisoldipine (To minimize CNS depression and possible potentiation, hypotensive agents should be used with caution). Products include:
- Sular Tablets 3122

Nitroglycerin (To minimize CNS depression and possible potentiation, hypotensive agents should be used with caution). Products include:
- Nitro-Dur Transdermal Infusion System 3046
- Nitrolingual Pumpspray 3120

Norepinephrine Bitartrate (Procarbazine exhibits some MAO inhibitory activity; concurrent use should be avoided).
- No products indexed under this heading.

Nortriptyline Hydrochloride (Procarbazine exhibits some MAO inhibitory activity; concurrent use should be avoided).
- No products indexed under this heading.

Oxycodone Hydrochloride (Potential for increased CNS depression and possible potentiation). Products include:
- OxyContin Tablets 2703
- OxyFast Oral Concentrate Solution 2708
- OxyIR Capsules 2708
- Percocet Tablets 1131
- Percodan Tablets 1132

Penbutolol Sulfate (To minimize CNS depression and possible potentiation, hypotensive agents should be used with caution).
- No products indexed under this heading.

Pentobarbital Sodium (Potential for increased CNS depression and possible potentiation). Products include:
- Nembutal Sodium Solution, USP 2470

Perindopril Erbumine (To minimize CNS depression and possible potentiation, hypotensive agents should be used with caution). Products include:
- Aceon Tablets (2 mg, 4 mg, 8 mg) 3194

Perphenazine (Potential for increased CNS depression and possible potentiation).
- No products indexed under this heading.

Phenobarbital (Potential for increased CNS depression and possible potentiation). Products include:
- Donnatal Extentabs 2493

Phenoxybenzamine Hydrochloride (To minimize CNS depression and possible potentiation, hypotensive agents should be used with caution). Products include:
- Dibenzyline Capsules 3399

Phentolamine Mesylate (To minimize CNS depression and possible potentiation, hypotensive agents should be used with caution).
- No products indexed under this heading.

Phenylephrine Bitartrate (Procarbazine exhibits some MAO inhibitory activity; concurrent use should be avoided).
- No products indexed under this heading.

Phenylephrine Hydrochloride (Procarbazine exhibits some MAO inhibitory activity; concurrent use should be avoided). Products include:
- Comtrex Maximum Strength Non-Drowsy Cold & Cough Caplets ..... ▣725
- Comtrex Maximum Strength Day/Night Severe Cold & Sinus Caplets - Day Formulation ..... ▣725
- Comtrex Maximum Strength Day/Night Severe Cold & Sinus Caplets - Night Formulation ..... ▣725
- Contac Cold and Flu Maximum Strength Caplets ..... ▣728
- Contac Cold and Flu Day and Night Caplets (Day Formulation Only) ..... ▣727
- Contac Cold and Flu Day and Night Caplets (Night Formulation Only) ..... ▣727
- Contac Cold and Flu Non-Drowsy Caplets ..... ▣728
- Contac-D Cold Non-Drowsy Tablets ..... ▣729
- Children's Dimetapp Cold & Allergy Elixir ..... ▣730
- Children's Dimetapp Cold & Allergy Chewable Tablets ..... ▣730
- Children's Dimetapp DM Cold & Cough Elixir ..... ▣731
- Toddler's Dimetapp Cold and Cough Drops ..... ▣732
- Excedrin Sinus Headache Caplets/Tablets ..... ▣610
- 4-Way Fast Acting Nasal Spray ..... ▣775
- 4-Way Menthol Nasal Spray ..... ▣775
- Preparation H Maximum Strength Cream ..... ▣666
- Preparation H Cooling Gel ..... ▣666
- Preparation H ..... ▣666
- Refenesen PE Caplets ..... ▣721
- Robitussin Cough & Allergy Syrup ..... ▣736
- Robitussin Cough & Cold Nighttime Liquid ..... ▣736
- Robitussin Cough, Cold & Flu Nighttime Liquid ..... ▣738
- Robitussin Head & Chest Congestion PE Syrup ..... ▣739
- Robitussin Pediatric Cough & Cold Nighttime Liquid ..... ▣736
- TheraFlu Cold & Cough Hot Liquid ..... ▣740
- TheraFlu Cold & Sore Throat Hot Liquid ..... ▣741
- TheraFlu Flu & Sore Throat Hot Liquid ..... ▣742
- TheraFlu Daytime Severe Cold Hot Liquid ..... ▣742
- TheraFlu Nighttime Severe Cold Hot Liquid ..... ▣740
- TheraFlu Warming Relief Daytime Severe Cold ..... ▣743
- TheraFlu Warming Relief Nighttime Severe Cold ..... ▣743
- Triaminic Chest & Nasal Congestion Liquid ..... ▣746
- Triaminic Cold & Allergy Liquid ..... ▣746
- Triaminic Daytime Cold & Cough Liquid ..... ▣745
- Triaminic Nighttime Cold & Cough Liquid ..... ▣746
- Triaminic Thin Strips Cold ..... ▣748
- Triaminic Thin Strips Cold & Cough ..... ▣778
- Triaminic Infant Thin Strips Decongestant ..... ▣747
- Triaminic Infant Thin Strips Decongestant Plus Cough ..... ▣747
- Children's Tylenol Plus Flu Oral Suspension ..... ▣749
- Tylenol Cold Head Congestion Daytime Caplets with Cool Burst and Gelcaps ..... ▣750
- Tylenol Cold Multi-Symptom Daytime Liquid ..... ▣752
- Tylenol Cold Multi-Symptom Severe Daytime Liquid ..... ▣752
- Concentrated Tylenol Infants' Drops Plus Cold & Cough ..... ▣754
- Tylenol Allergy Multi-Symptom Caplets with Cool Burst and Gelcaps 1872
- Tylenol Allergy Multi-Symptom Nighttime Caplets with Cool Burst 1872
- Children's Tylenol Plus Cold Suspension Liquid 1879
- Children's Tylenol Plus Cold & Allergy Suspension Liquid 1878
- Children's Tylenol Plus Flu Suspension Liquid 1881
- Children's Tylenol Plus Multi-Symptom Cold Suspension Liquid 1879
- Tylenol Cold Head Congestion Daytime Caplets with Cool Burst 1873
- Tylenol Cold Head Congestion Nighttime Caplets with Cool Burst 1873
- Tylenol Cold Head Congestion Severe Caplets with Cool Burst 1873
- Tylenol Cold Multi-Symptom Daytime Caplets with Cool Burst and Gelcaps 1874

Tylenol Cold Multi-Symptom Daytime Liquid with Citrus Burst ... 1874
Tylenol Cold Multi-Symptom Nighttime Caplets with Cool Burst ... 1874
Tylenol Cold Multi-Symptom Nighttime Liquid with Cool Burst ... 1874
Tylenol Cold Multi-Symptom Severe Caplets with Cool Burst ... 1874
Tylenol Cold Multi-Symptom Severe Daytime Liquid with Citrus Burst ... 1874
Tylenol Sinus Congestion & Pain Daytime Caplets with Cool Burst and Gelcaps ... 1876
Tylenol Sinus Congestion & Pain Nighttime Caplets with Cool Burst ... 1876
Tylenol Sinus Congestion & Pain Severe Caplets with Cool Burst ... 1876
Vicks 44D Cough & Head Congestion Relief Liquid ... 760
Vicks DayQuil LiquiCaps/Liquid Multi-Symptom Cold/Flu Relief ... 761
Zicam Cough Plus D Cough Spray ... 767

Phenylephrine Tannate (Procarbazine exhibits some MAO inhibitory activity; concurrent use should be avoided).
No products indexed under this heading.

Phenylpropanolamine Hydrochloride (Procarbazine exhibits some MAO inhibitory activity; concurrent use should be avoided).
No products indexed under this heading.

Pindolol (To minimize CNS depression and possible potentiation, hypotensive agents should be used with caution).
No products indexed under this heading.

Pirbuterol Acetate (Procarbazine exhibits some MAO inhibitory activity; concurrent use should be avoided). Products include:
Maxair Autohaler ... 1852

Polythiazide (To minimize CNS depression and possible potentiation, hypotensive agents should be used with caution).
No products indexed under this heading.

Prazosin Hydrochloride (To minimize CNS depression and possible potentiation, hypotensive agents should be used with caution).
No products indexed under this heading.

Prochlorperazine (Potential for increased CNS depression and possible potentiation).
No products indexed under this heading.

Promethazine Hydrochloride (Potential for increased CNS depression and possible potentiation). Products include:
Phenergan Tablets and Suppositories ... 3440

Propoxyphene Hydrochloride (Potential for increased CNS depression and possible potentiation).
No products indexed under this heading.

Propoxyphene Napsylate (Potential for increased CNS depression and possible potentiation).
No products indexed under this heading.

Propranolol Hydrochloride (To minimize CNS depression and possible potentiation, hypotensive agents should be used with caution). Products include:
Inderal LA Long-Acting Capsules ... 3429
InnoPran XL Capsules ... 2723

Protriptyline Hydrochloride (Procarbazine exhibits some MAO inhibitory activity; concurrent use should be avoided).
No products indexed under this heading.

Pseudoephedrine Hydrochloride (Procarbazine exhibits some MAO inhibitory activity; concurrent use should be avoided). Products include:
Advil Allergy Sinus Caplets ... 770
Advil Cold & Sinus ... 723
Advil Multi-Symptom Cold Caplets ... 770
Aleve Cold & Sinus Caplets ... 744
Allegra-D 12 Hour Extended-Release Tablets ... 2846
Allegra-D 24 Hour Extended-Release Tablets ... 2849
BC Cold Powder ... 677
Comtrex Maximum Strength Cold & Cough Day/Night Caplets - Day Formulation ... 726
Comtrex Maximum Strength Cold & Cough Day/Night Caplets - Night Formulation ... 726
Children's Motrin Cold Oral Suspension ... 1867
Mucinex D Extended-Release Bi-Layer Tablets ... 776
Robitussin Cough & Cold CF Liquid ... 735
Robitussin Cough & Cold Pediatric Drops ... 735
Tylenol Sinus Congestion & Pain Nighttime Caplets with Cool Burst ... 778
Tylenol Cold Severe Congestion Non-Drowsy Caplets with Cool Burst ... 1874
Tylenol Sinus Severe Congestion Caplets with Cool Burst ... 1876
Vicks 44D Cough & Head Congestion Relief Liquid ... 2679
Vicks 44M Cough, Cold & Flu Relief Liquid ... 2680
Vicks DayQuil Multi-Symptom Cold/Flu Relief LiquiCaps ... 2678
Vicks DayQuil Multi-Symptom Cold/Flu Relief Liquid ... 2678
Vicks NyQuil Multi-Symptom Cold/Flu Relief Liquid ... 2681
Vicks NyQuil Multi-Symptom Cold/Flu Relief LiquiCaps ... 2681
Children's Vicks NyQuil Cold/Cough Relief Liquid ... 2680
Zyrtec-D 12 Hour Extended Release Tablets ... 2597

Pseudoephedrine Sulfate (Procarbazine exhibits some MAO inhibitory activity; concurrent use should be avoided). Products include:
Alavert Allergy & Sinus D-12 Hour Tablets ... 771
Clarinex-D 24-Hour Extended-Release Tablets ... 2998
Claritin-D Non-Drowsy 12 Hour Tablets ... 772
Claritin-D Non-Drowsy 24 Hour Tablets ... 772

Pyrilamine Maleate (Potential for increased CNS depression and possible potentiation).
No products indexed under this heading.

Pyrilamine Tannate (Potential for increased CNS depression and possible potentiation).
No products indexed under this heading.

Quinapril Hydrochloride (To minimize CNS depression and possible potentiation, hypotensive agents should be used with caution).
No products indexed under this heading.

Ramipril (To minimize CNS depression and possible potentiation, hypotensive agents should be used with caution). Products include:
Altace Capsules ... 1702

Rauwolfia Serpentina (To minimize CNS depression and possible potentiation, hypotensive agents should be used with caution).
No products indexed under this heading.

Remifentanil Hydrochloride (Potential for increased CNS depression and possible potentiation).
No products indexed under this heading.

Rescinnamine (To minimize CNS depression and possible potentiation, hypotensive agents should be used with caution).
No products indexed under this heading.

Reserpine (To minimize CNS depression and possible potentiation, hypotensive agents should be used with caution).
No products indexed under this heading.

Salmeterol Xinafoate (Procarbazine exhibits some MAO inhibitory activity; concurrent use should be avoided). Products include:
Advair Diskus 100/50 ... 1308
Advair Diskus 250/50 ... 1308
Advair Diskus 500/50 ... 1308
Advair HFA Inhalation Aerosol ... 1318
Serevent Diskus ... 1568

Secobarbital Sodium (Potential for increased CNS depression and possible potentiation).
No products indexed under this heading.

Sodium Nitroprusside (To minimize CNS depression and possible potentiation, hypotensive agents should be used with caution).
No products indexed under this heading.

Sotalol Hydrochloride (To minimize CNS depression and possible potentiation, hypotensive agents should be used with caution).
No products indexed under this heading.

Spirapril Hydrochloride (To minimize CNS depression and possible potentiation, hypotensive agents should be used with caution).
No products indexed under this heading.

Sufentanil Citrate (Potential for increased CNS depression and possible potentiation).
No products indexed under this heading.

Telmisartan (To minimize CNS depression and possible potentiation, hypotensive agents should be used with caution). Products include:
Micardis Tablets ... 854
Micardis HCT Tablets ... 856

Terazosin Hydrochloride (To minimize CNS depression and possible potentiation, hypotensive agents should be used with caution). Products include:
Hytrin Capsules ... 471

Terbutaline Sulfate (Procarbazine exhibits some MAO inhibitory activity; concurrent use should be avoided).
No products indexed under this heading.

Terfenadine (Potential for increased CNS depression and possible potentiation).
No products indexed under this heading.

Thiamylal Sodium (Potential for increased CNS depression and possible potentiation).
No products indexed under this heading.

Thioridazine Hydrochloride (Potential for increased CNS depression and possible potentiation). Products include:
Thioridazine Hydrochloride Tablets ... 2163

Timolol Maleate (To minimize CNS depression and possible potentiation, hypotensive agents should be used with caution). Products include:
Blocadren Tablets ... 1916
Cosopt Sterile Ophthalmic Solution ... 1931
Timolide Tablets ... 2086
Timoptic Sterile Ophthalmic Solution ... 2088
Timoptic in Ocudose ... 2091
Timoptic-XE Sterile Ophthalmic Gel Forming Solution ... 2092

Torsemide (To minimize CNS depression and possible potentiation, hypotensive agents should be used with caution). Products include:
Demadex Injection ... 2759
Demadex Tablets ... 2759

Trandolapril (To minimize CNS depression and possible potentiation, hypotensive agents should be used with caution). Products include:
Mavik Tablets ... 486
Tarka Tablets ... 524

Trifluoperazine Hydrochloride (Potential for increased CNS depression and possible potentiation).
No products indexed under this heading.

Trimeprazine Tartrate (Potential for increased CNS depression and possible potentiation).
No products indexed under this heading.

Trimethaphan Camsylate (To minimize CNS depression and possible potentiation, hypotensive agents should be used with caution).
No products indexed under this heading.

Trimipramine Maleate (Procarbazine exhibits some MAO inhibitory activity; concurrent use should be avoided).
No products indexed under this heading.

Tripelennamine Hydrochloride (Potential for increased CNS depression and possible potentiation).
No products indexed under this heading.

Triprolidine Hydrochloride (Potential for increased CNS depression and possible potentiation).
No products indexed under this heading.

Valsartan (To minimize CNS depression and possible potentiation, hypotensive agents should be used with caution). Products include:
Diovan Tablets ... 2193
Diovan HCT Tablets ... 2196

Verapamil Hydrochloride (To minimize CNS depression and possible potentiation, hypotensive agents should be used with caution). Products include:
Covera-HS Tablets ... 3139
Tarka Tablets ... 524
Verelan PM Extended-Release Capsules, Controlled-Onset ... 3106

Food Interactions

Alcohol (Concurrent use may produce an Antabuse-like reaction; concomitant use should be avoided).

Bananas (Procarbazine exhibits some MAO inhibitory activity: concurrent use should be avoided).

Cheese, aged (Procarbazine exhibits some MAO inhibitory activity: concurrent use should be avoided).

Food with high concentration of tyramine (Procarbazine exhibits some MAO inhibitory activity: concurrent use should be avoided).

Wine, unspecified (Procarbazine exhibits some MAO inhibitory activity: concurrent use should be avoided).

Yogurt (Procarbazine exhibits some MAO inhibitory activity: concurrent use should be avoided).

MAVIK TABLETS

(Trandolapril) 486

May interact with diuretics, lithium preparations, potassium preparations, potassium sparing diuretics, and certain other agents. Compounds in these categories include:

Amiloride Hydrochloride (Co-administration increases the risk of hyperkalemia; patients on diuretics, especially those on recently instituted diuretic therapy, may experience an excessive reduction in blood pressure after initiation of therapy with trandolapril). Products include:
- Midamor Tablets 2026
- Moduretic Tablets 2028

Bendroflumethiazide (Patients on diuretics, especially those on recently instituted diuretic therapy, may experience an excessive reduction in blood pressure after initiation of therapy with trandolapril).
- No products indexed under this heading.

Bumetanide (Patients on diuretics, especially those on recently instituted diuretic therapy, may experience an excessive reduction in blood pressure after initiation of therapy with trandolapril). Products include:
- Bumex Tablets 2746

Chlorothiazide (Patients on diuretics, especially those on recently instituted diuretic therapy, may experience an excessive reduction in blood pressure after initiation of therapy with trandolapril). Products include:
- Diuril Oral Suspension 1954

Chlorothiazide Sodium (Patients on diuretics, especially those on recently instituted diuretic therapy, may experience an excessive reduction in blood pressure after initiation of therapy with trandolapril). Products include:
- Diuril Sodium Intravenous 2467

Chlorthalidone (Patients on diuretics, especially those on recently instituted diuretic therapy, may experience an excessive reduction in blood pressure after initiation of therapy with trandolapril). Products include:
- Clorpres Tablets 2153

Cimetidine (Co-administration has led to an increase of about 44% in Cmax for trandolapril with no effect on ACE inhibition). Products include:
- Tagamet HB 200 Tablets .... ▣664

Cimetidine Hydrochloride (Co-administration has led to an increase of about 44% in Cmax for trandolapril with no effect on ACE inhibition).
- No products indexed under this heading.

Ethacrynic Acid (Patients on diuretics, especially those on recently instituted diuretic therapy, may experience an excessive reduction in blood pressure after initiation of therapy with trandolapril). Products include:
- Edecrin Tablets 1959

Furosemide (Co-administration has led to an increase of about 25% in the renal clearance of trandolapril with no effect on ACE inhibition; patients on diuretics, especially those on recently instituted diuretic therapy, may experience an excessive reduction in blood pressure after initiation of therapy with trandolapril). Products include:
- Furosemide Tablets 2154

Hydrochlorothiazide (Patients on diuretics, especially those on recently instituted diuretic therapy, may experience an excessive reduction in blood pressure after initiation of therapy with trandolapril). Products include:
- Aldoril Tablets 1910
- Atacand HCT 651
- Avalide Tablets 888
- Avalide Tablets 2874
- Benicar HCT Tablets 1044
- Diovan HCT Tablets 2196
- Dyazide Capsules 1423
- Hyzaar 50-12.5 Tablets 1990
- Hyzaar 100-12.5 Tablets 1990
- Hyzaar 100-25 Tablets 1990
- Lopressor HCT 50/25 Tablets 2241
- Lopressor HCT 100/25 Tablets 2241
- Lopressor HCT 100/50 Tablets 2241
- Lotensin HCT Tablets 2246
- Micardis HCT Tablets 856
- Moduretic Tablets 2028
- Prinzide Tablets 2056
- Teveten HCT Tablets 1737
- Timolide Tablets 2086
- Uniretic Tablets 3100

Hydroflumethiazide (Patients on diuretics, especially those on recently instituted diuretic therapy, may experience an excessive reduction in blood pressure after initiation of therapy with trandolapril).
- No products indexed under this heading.

Indapamide (Patients on diuretics, especially those on recently instituted diuretic therapy, may experience an excessive reduction in blood pressure after initiation of therapy with trandolapril). Products include:
- Indapamide Tablets 2156

Lithium (Co-administration of ACE inhibitors and lithium has resulted in increased serum lithium levels and symptoms of lithium toxicity).
- No products indexed under this heading.

Lithium Carbonate (Co-administration of ACE inhibitors and lithium has resulted in increased serum lithium levels and symptoms of lithium toxicity). Products include:
- Lithobid Tablets 1692

Lithium Citrate (Co-administration of ACE inhibitors and lithium has resulted in increased serum lithium levels and symptoms of lithium toxicity).
- No products indexed under this heading.

Methyclothiazide (Patients on diuretics, especially those on recently instituted diuretic therapy, may experience an excessive reduction in blood pressure after initiation of therapy with trandolapril).
- No products indexed under this heading.

Metolazone (Patients on diuretics, especially those on recently instituted diuretic therapy, may experience an excessive reduction in blood pressure after initiation of therapy with trandolapril).
- No products indexed under this heading.

Polythiazide (Patients on diuretics, especially those on recently instituted diuretic therapy, may experience an excessive reduction in blood pressure after initiation of therapy with trandolapril).
- No products indexed under this heading.

Potassium Acid Phosphate (Co-administration increases the risk of hyperkalemia). Products include:
- K-Phos Original (Sodium Free) Tablets 760

Potassium Bicarbonate (Co-administration increases the risk of hyperkalemia).
- No products indexed under this heading.

Potassium Chloride (Co-administration increases the risk of hyperkalemia). Products include:
- Colyte with Flavor Packs for Oral Solution 3088
- HalfLytely and Bisacodyl Tablets Bowel Prep Kit with Flavors Packs 881
- K-Dur Extended-Relase Tablets 3033
- K-Lor Oral Solution 474
- K-Tab Tablets 475
- MoviPrep Oral Solution 2839
- TriLyte with Flavor Packs for Oral Solution 3100

Potassium Citrate (Co-administration increases the risk of hyperkalemia). Products include:
- Urocit-K Tablets 2144

Potassium Gluconate (Co-administration increases the risk of hyperkalemia).
- No products indexed under this heading.

Potassium Phosphate (Co-administration increases the risk of hyperkalemia). Products include:
- K-Phos Neutral Tablets 760

Spironolactone (Co-administration increases the risk of hyperkalemia; patients on diuretics, especially those on recently instituted diuretic therapy, may experience an excessive reduction in blood pressure after initiation of therapy with trandolapril).
- No products indexed under this heading.

Torsemide (Patients on diuretics, especially those on recently instituted diuretic therapy, may experience an excessive reduction in blood pressure after initiation of therapy with trandolapril). Products include:
- Demadex Injection 2759
- Demadex Tablets 2759

Triamterene (Co-administration increases the risk of hyperkalemia; patients on diuretics, especially those on recently instituted diuretic therapy, may experience an excessive reduction in blood pressure after initiation of therapy with trandolapril). Products include:
- Dyazide Capsules 1423
- Dyrenium Capsules 3400

Food Interactions

Food, unspecified (Slows absorption of trandolapril but does not affect AUC or Cmax).

MAXAIR AUTOHALER

(Pirbuterol Acetate) 1852

May interact with beta blockers, monoamine oxidase inhibitors, potassium-depleting diuretics, sympathomimetic aerosol bronchodilators, and tricyclic antidepressants. Compounds in these categories include:

Acebutolol Hydrochloride (Co-administration with beta adrenergic receptor blocking agents blocks the pulmonary effect of pirbuterol and may produce severe bronchospasm in asthmatic patients).
- No products indexed under this heading.

Albuterol (Potential for additive effects). Products include:
- Proventil Inhalation Aerosol 3053

Amitriptyline Hydrochloride (Concurrent and/or sequential use with tricyclic antidepressants can result in the potentiation of pirbuterol's action on the vascular system).
- No products indexed under this heading.

Amoxapine (Concurrent and/or sequential use with tricyclic antidepressants can result in the potentiation of pirbuterol's action on the vascular system).
- No products indexed under this heading.

Atenolol (Co-administration with beta adrenergic receptor blocking agents blocks the pulmonary effect of pirbuterol and may produce severe bronchospasm in asthmatic patients).
- No products indexed under this heading.

Bendroflumethiazide (The ECG changes and/or hypokalemia that may result from administration of non-potassium sparing diuretics can be acutely worsened by beta-agonists; clinical significance is not known).
- No products indexed under this heading.

Betaxolol Hydrochloride (Co-administration with beta adrenergic receptor blocking agents blocks the pulmonary effect of pirbuterol and may produce severe bronchospasm in asthmatic patients). Products include:
- Betoptic S Ophthalmic Suspension.................................. 558

Bisoprolol Fumarate (Co-administration with beta adrenergic receptor blocking agents blocks the pulmonary effect of pirbuterol and may produce severe bronchospasm in asthmatic patients).
- No products indexed under this heading.

Bitolterol Mesylate (Potential for additive effects).
- No products indexed under this heading.

Bumetanide (The ECG changes and/or hypokalemia that may result from administration of non-potassium sparing diuretics can be acutely worsened by beta-agonists; clinical significance is not known). Products include:
- Bumex Tablets 2746

Carteolol Hydrochloride (Co-administration with beta adrenergic receptor blocking agents blocks the pulmonary effect of pirbuterol and may produce severe bronchospasm in asthmatic patients). Products include:

Carteolol Hydrochloride Ophthalmic Solution USP, 1%....... ⊙249

Chlorothiazide (The ECG changes and/or hypokalemia that may result from administration of non-potassium sparing diuretics can be acutely worsened by beta-agonists; clinical significance is not known). Products include:

Diuril Oral Suspension **1954**

Chlorothiazide Sodium (The ECG changes and/or hypokalemia that may result from administration of non-potassium sparing diuretics can be acutely worsened by beta-agonists; clinical significance is not known). Products include:

Diuril Sodium Intravenous **2467**

Clomipramine Hydrochloride (Concurrent and/or sequential use with tricyclic antidepressants can result in the potentiation of pirbuterol's action on the vascular system).

No products indexed under this heading.

Desipramine Hydrochloride (Concurrent and/or sequential use with tricyclic antidepressants can result in the potentiation of pirbuterol's action on the vascular system).

No products indexed under this heading.

Doxepin Hydrochloride (Concurrent and/or sequential use with tricyclic antidepressants can result in the potentiation of pirbuterol's action on the vascular system).

No products indexed under this heading.

Esmolol Hydrochloride (Co-administration with beta adrenergic receptor blocking agents blocks the pulmonary effect of pirbuterol and may produce severe bronchospasm in asthmatic patients).

No products indexed under this heading.

Ethacrynic Acid (The ECG changes and/or hypokalemia that may result from administration of non-potassium sparing diuretics can be acutely worsened by beta-agonists; clinical significance is not known). Products include:

Edecrin Tablets **1959**

Furosemide (The ECG changes and/or hypokalemia that may result from administration of non-potassium sparing diuretics can be acutely worsened by beta-agonists; clinical significance is not known). Products include:

Furosemide Tablets **2154**

Hydrochlorothiazide (The ECG changes and/or hypokalemia that may result from administration of non-potassium sparing diuretics can be acutely worsened by beta-agonists; clinical significance is not known). Products include:

Aldoril Tablets **1910**
Atacand HCT **651**
Avalide Tablets **888**
Avalide Tablets **2874**
Benicar HCT Tablets **1044**
Diovan HCT Tablets **2196**
Dyazide Capsules **1423**
Hyzaar 50-12.5 Tablets **1990**
Hyzaar 100-12.5 Tablets **1990**
Hyzaar 100-25 Tablets **1990**
Lopressor HCT 50/25 Tablets **2241**
Lopressor HCT 100/25 Tablets **2241**
Lopressor HCT 100/50 Tablets **2241**
Lotensin HCT Tablets **2246**
Micardis HCT Tablets **856**
Moduretic Tablets **2028**
Prinzide Tablets **2056**
Teveten HCT Tablets **1737**
Timolide Tablets **2086**
Uniretic Tablets **3100**

Hydroflumethiazide (The ECG changes and/or hypokalemia that may result from administration of non-potassium sparing diuretics can be acutely worsened by beta-agonists; clinical significance is not known).

No products indexed under this heading.

Imipramine Hydrochloride (Concurrent and/or sequential use with tricyclic antidepressants can result in the potentiation of pirbuterol's action on the vascular system).

No products indexed under this heading.

Imipramine Pamoate (Concurrent and/or sequential use with tricyclic antidepressants can result in the potentiation of pirbuterol's action on the vascular system).

No products indexed under this heading.

Isocarboxazid (Concurrent and/or sequential use with MAO inhibitors can result in the potentiation of pirbuterol's action on the vascular system).

No products indexed under this heading.

Isoetharine (Potential for additive effects).

No products indexed under this heading.

Isoproterenol Hydrochloride (Potential for additive effects).

No products indexed under this heading.

Labetalol Hydrochloride (Co-administration with beta adrenergic receptor blocking agents blocks the pulmonary effect of pirbuterol and may produce severe bronchospasm in asthmatic patients).

No products indexed under this heading.

Levalbuterol Hydrochloride (Potential for additive effects). Products include:

Xopenex Inhalation Solution **3146**
Xopenex Inhalation Solution Concentrate **3150**

Levobunolol Hydrochloride (Co-administration with beta adrenergic receptor blocking agents blocks the pulmonary effect of pirbuterol and may produce severe bronchospasm in asthmatic patients). Products include:

Betagan Ophthalmic Solution, USP.. ⊙220

Maprotiline Hydrochloride (Concurrent and/or sequential use with tricyclic antidepressants can result in the potentiation of pirbuterol's action on the vascular system).

No products indexed under this heading.

Metaproterenol Sulfate (Potential for additive effects). Products include:

Alupent Inhalation Aerosol **826**

Methyclothiazide (The ECG changes and/or hypokalemia that may result from administration of non-potassium sparing diuretics can be acutely worsened by beta-agonists; clinical significance is not known).

No products indexed under this heading.

Metipranolol Hydrochloride (Co-administration with beta adrenergic receptor blocking agents blocks the pulmonary effect of pirbuterol and may produce severe bronchospasm in asthmatic patients).

No products indexed under this heading.

Metoprolol Succinate (Co-administration with beta adrenergic receptor blocking agents blocks the pulmonary effect of pirbuterol and may produce severe bronchospasm in asthmatic patients). Products include:

Toprol-XL Tablets **668**

Metoprolol Tartrate (Co-administration with beta adrenergic receptor blocking agents blocks the pulmonary effect of pirbuterol and may produce severe bronchospasm in asthmatic patients). Products include:

Lopressor Injection **2238**
Lopressor Tablets **2238**
Lopressor HCT 50/25 Tablets **2241**
Lopressor HCT 100/25 Tablets **2241**
Lopressor HCT 100/50 Tablets **2241**

Moclobemide (Concurrent and/or sequential use with MAO inhibitors can result in the potentiation of pirbuterol's action on the vascular system).

No products indexed under this heading.

Nadolol (Co-administration with beta adrenergic receptor blocking agents blocks the pulmonary effect of pirbuterol and may produce severe bronchospasm in asthmatic patients). Products include:

Nadolol Tablets **2159**

Nortriptyline Hydrochloride (Concurrent and/or sequential use with tricyclic antidepressants can result in the potentiation of pirbuterol's action on the vascular system).

No products indexed under this heading.

Pargyline Hydrochloride (Concurrent and/or sequential use with MAO inhibitors can result in the potentiation of pirbuterol's action on the vascular system).

No products indexed under this heading.

Penbutolol Sulfate (Co-administration with beta adrenergic receptor blocking agents blocks the pulmonary effect of pirbuterol and may produce severe bronchospasm in asthmatic patients).

No products indexed under this heading.

Phenelzine Sulfate (Concurrent and/or sequential use with MAO inhibitors can result in the potentiation of pirbuterol's action on the vascular system).

No products indexed under this heading.

Pindolol (Co-administration with beta adrenergic receptor blocking agents blocks the pulmonary effect of pirbuterol and may produce severe bronchospasm in asthmatic patients).

No products indexed under this heading.

Polythiazide (The ECG changes and/or hypokalemia that may result from administration of non-potassium sparing diuretics can be acutely worsened by beta-agonists; clinical significance is not known).

No products indexed under this heading.

Procarbazine Hydrochloride (Concurrent and/or sequential use with MAO inhibitors can result in the potentiation of pirbuterol's action on the vascular system). Products include:

Matulane Capsules **3191**

Propranolol Hydrochloride (Co-administration with beta adrenergic receptor blocking agents blocks the pulmonary effect of pirbuterol and may produce severe bronchospasm in asthmatic patients). Products include:

Inderal LA Long-Acting Capsules **3429**
InnoPran XL Capsules **2723**

Protriptyline Hydrochloride (Concurrent and/or sequential use with tricyclic antidepressants can result in the potentiation of pirbuterol's action on the vascular system).

No products indexed under this heading.

Salmeterol Xinafoate (Potential for additive effects). Products include:

Advair Diskus 100/50 .... **1308**
Advair Diskus 250/50 .... **1308**
Advair Diskus 500/50 .... **1308**
Advair HFA Inhalation Aerosol **1318**
Serevent Diskus **1568**

Selegiline Hydrochloride (Concurrent and/or sequential use with MAO inhibitors can result in the potentiation of pirbuterol's action on the vascular system). Products include:

Eldepryl Capsules **3208**
Zelapar Tablets **3372**

Sotalol Hydrochloride (Co-administration with beta adrenergic receptor blocking agents blocks the pulmonary effect of pirbuterol and may produce severe bronchospasm in asthmatic patients).

No products indexed under this heading.

Terbutaline Sulfate (Potential for additive effects).

No products indexed under this heading.

Timolol Hemihydrate (Co-administration with beta adrenergic receptor blocking agents blocks the pulmonary effect of pirbuterol and may produce severe bronchospasm in asthmatic patients). Products include:

Betimol Ophthalmic Solution **3382**
Betimol Ophthalmic Solution .... ⊙295

Timolol Maleate (Co-administration with beta adrenergic receptor blocking agents blocks the pulmonary effect of pirbuterol and may produce severe bronchospasm in asthmatic patients). Products include:

Blocadren Tablets **1916**
Cosopt Sterile Ophthalmic Solution.. **1931**
Timolide Tablets **2086**
Timoptic Sterile Ophthalmic Solution.. **2088**
Timoptic in Ocudose **2091**
Timoptic-XE Sterile Ophthalmic Gel Forming Solution **2092**

Torsemide (The ECG changes and/or hypokalemia that may result from administration of non-potassium sparing diuretics can be acutely worsened by beta-agonists; clinical significance is not known). Products include:

Demadex Injection **2759**
Demadex Tablets **2759**

Tranylcypromine Sulfate (Concurrent and/or sequential use with MAO inhibitors can result in the potentiation of pirbuterol's action on the vascular system). Products include:

Parnate Tablets 1527

Trimipramine Maleate (Concurrent and/or sequential use with tricyclic antidepressants can result in the potentiation of pirbuterol's action on the vascular system).

No products indexed under this heading.

MAXALT TABLETS

(Rizatriptan Benzoate) 2008

May interact with 5HT1-receptor agonists, ergot-containing drugs, monoamine oxidase inhibitors, selective serotonin reuptake inhibitors, and certain other agents. Compounds in these categories include:

Citalopram Hydrobromide (Co-administration of 5-HT1 agonists with selective serotonin reuptake inhibitors (SSRIs) has resulted, rarely, in hyperreflexia, weakness, and incoordination). Products include:

Celexa 1176

Desipramine Hydrochloride (Cases of life-threatening serotonin syndrome have been reported during combined use of serotonin-norepinephrine reuptake inhibitors).

No products indexed under this heading.

Dihydroergotamine Mesylate (Ergot-containing drugs have been reported to cause prolonged vasospastic reactions; because there is a theoretical basis that these effects may be additive, use of ergot-type agents and rizatriptan within 24 hours is contraindicated). Products include:

Migranal Nasal Spray 3348

3-Diphenylacrylate (Co-administration with other 5-HT1 agonists within 24 hours of each other is contraindicated because the vasospastic effects may be additive).

No products indexed under this heading.

Duloxetine Hydrochloride (Cases of life-threatening serotonin syndrome have been reported during combined use of serotonin-norepinephrine reuptake inhibitors). Products include:

Cymbalta Delayed-Release Capsules 1757

Ergonovine Maleate (Ergot-containing drugs have been reported to cause prolonged vasospastic reactions; because there is a theoretical basis that these effects may be additive, use of ergot-type agents and rizatriptan within 24 hours is contraindicated).

No products indexed under this heading.

Ergotamine Tartrate (Ergot-containing drugs have been reported to cause prolonged vasospastic reactions; because there is a theoretical basis that these effects may be additive, use of ergot-type agents and rizatriptan within 24 hours is contraindicated).

No products indexed under this heading.

Escitalopram Oxalate (Co-administration of 5-HT1 agonists with selective serotonin reuptake inhibitors (SSRIs) has resulted, rarely, in hyperreflexia, weakness, and incoordination). Products include:

Lexapro Oral Solution 1190
Lexapro Tablets 1190

Fluoxetine Hydrochloride (Co-administration of 5-HT1 agonists with selective serotonin reuptake inhibitors (SSRIs) has resulted, rarely, in hyperreflexia, weakness, and incoordination). Products include:

Prozac Pulvules and Liquid 1801
Symbyax Capsules 1819

Fluvoxamine Maleate (Co-administration of 5-HT1 agonists with selective serotonin reuptake inhibitors (SSRIs) has resulted, rarely, in hyperreflexia, weakness, and incoordination).

No products indexed under this heading.

Isocarboxazid (Plasma concentrations of rizatriptan may be increased by MAO inhibitors; concurrent and/or sequential use is contraindicated).

No products indexed under this heading.

Methylergonovine Maleate (Ergot-containing drugs have been reported to cause prolonged vasospastic reactions; because there is a theoretical basis that these effects may be additive, use of ergot-type agents and rizatriptan within 24 hours is contraindicated).

No products indexed under this heading.

Methysergide Maleate (Ergot-containing drugs have been reported to cause prolonged vasospastic reactions; because there is a theoretical basis that these effects may be additive, use of ergot-type agents and rizatriptan within 24 hours is contraindicated).

No products indexed under this heading.

Moclobemide (Concomitant therapy with the selective, reversible MAO-A inhibitor, moclobemide, has resulted in increased systemic exposure of rizatriptan and its metabolite; concurrent and/or sequential use is contraindicated).

No products indexed under this heading.

Naratriptan Hydrochloride (Co-administration with other 5-HT1 agonists within 24 hours of each other is contraindicated because the vasospastic effects may be additive). Products include:

Amerge Tablets 1339

Nefazodone Hydrochloride (Cases of life-threatening serotonin syndrome have been reported during combined use of serotonin-norepinephrine reuptake inhibitors).

No products indexed under this heading.

Pargyline Hydrochloride (Plasma concentrations of rizatriptan may be increased by MAO inhibitors; concurrent and/or sequential use is contraindicated).

No products indexed under this heading.

Paroxetine Hydrochloride (Co-administration of 5-HT1 agonists with selective serotonin reuptake inhibitors (SSRIs) has resulted, rarely, in hyperreflexia, weakness, and incoordination; no pharmacokinetic interaction was observed with a single dose study). Products include:

Paxil CR Controlled-Release Tablets 1538
Paxil 1530

Phenelzine Sulfate (Plasma concentrations of rizatriptan may be increased by MAO inhibitors; concurrent and/or sequential use is contraindicated).

No products indexed under this heading.

Procarbazine Hydrochloride (Plasma concentrations of rizatriptan may be increased by MAO inhibitors; concurrent and/or sequential use is contraindicated). Products include:

Matulane Capsules 3191

Propranolol Hydrochloride (Co-administration has resulted in an increase in mean plasma AUC for rizatriptan by 70%). Products include:

Inderal LA Long-Acting Capsules 3429
InnoPran XL Capsules 2723

Selegiline Hydrochloride (Plasma concentrations of rizatriptan may be increased by MAO inhibitors; concurrent and/or sequential use is contraindicated). Products include:

Eldepryl Capsules 3208
Zelapar Tablets 3372

Sertraline Hydrochloride (Co-administration of 5-HT1 agonists with selective serotonin reuptake inhibitors (SSRIs) has resulted, rarely, in hyperreflexia, weakness, and incoordination). Products include:

Zoloft 2586

Sumatriptan (Co-administration with other 5-HT1 agonists within 24 hours of each other is contraindicated because the vasospastic effects may be additive). Products include:

Imitrex Nasal Spray 1467

Sumatriptan Succinate (Co-administration with other 5-HT1 agonists within 24 hours of each other is contraindicated because the vasospastic effects may be additive). Products include:

Imitrex Injection 1463
Imitrex Tablets 1471

Tranylcypromine Sulfate (Plasma concentrations of rizatriptan may be increased by MAO inhibitors; concurrent and/or sequential use is contraindicated). Products include:

Parnate Tablets 1527

Venlafaxine Hydrochloride (Cases of life-threatening serotonin syndrome have been reported during combined use of serotonin-norepinephrine reuptake inhibitors). Products include:

Effexor Tablets 3411
Effexor XR Capsules 3417

Zolmitriptan (Co-administration with other 5-HT1 agonists within 24 hours of each other is contraindicated because the vasospastic effects may be additive). Products include:

Zomig Tablets 3519
Zomig Nasal Spray 3523
Zomig-ZMT Tablets 3519

Food Interactions

Food, unspecified (Delays the time to reach peak concentration by an hour; no significant effect on the bioavailability).

MAXALT-MLT ORALLY DISINTEGRATING TABLETS

(Rizatriptan Benzoate) 2008

See Maxalt Tablets

MAXIPIME FOR INJECTION

(Cefepime Hydrochloride) 1105

May interact with aminoglycosides and certain other agents. Compounds in these categories include:

Amikacin Sulfate (Co-administration increases the potential for nephrotoxicity and ototoxicity of aminoglycoside antibiotics).

No products indexed under this heading.

Furosemide (Co-administration with furosemide and other cephalosporins has resulted in nephrotoxicity). Products include:

Furosemide Tablets 2154

Gentamicin Sulfate (Co-administration increases the potential for nephrotoxicity and ototoxicity of aminoglycoside antibiotics). Products include:

Garamycin Injectable 3014
Pred-G Ophthalmic Ointment .... ⊙237
Pred-G Ophthalmic Suspension ...... ⊙236

Kanamycin Sulfate (Co-administration increases the potential for nephrotoxicity and ototoxicity of aminoglycoside antibiotics).

No products indexed under this heading.

Streptomycin Sulfate (Co-administration increases the potential for nephrotoxicity and ototoxicity of aminoglycoside antibiotics).

No products indexed under this heading.

Tobramycin (Co-administration increases the potential for nephrotoxicity and ototoxicity of aminoglycoside antibiotics). Products include:

TOBI Solution for Inhalation 2298
TobraDex Ophthalmic Ointment 562
TobraDex Ophthalmic Suspension ... 563
Zylet Ophthalmic Suspension .... ⊙259

Tobramycin Sulfate (Co-administration increases the potential for nephrotoxicity and ototoxicity of aminoglycoside antibiotics).

No products indexed under this heading.

MDR FITNESS TABS FOR MEN AND WOMEN

(Vitamins with Minerals) 1886

None cited in PDR database.

MDR VITAL FACTORS

(Vitamins with Minerals) 1886

None cited in PDR database.

MEDERMA TOPICAL GEL

(Allantoin, Allium cepa) 2126

None cited in PDR database.

MEDERMA FOR KIDS TOPICAL GEL

(Allantoin, Allium cepa) 2126

None cited in PDR database.

MEFOXIN FOR INJECTION

(Cefoxitin Sodium) 2012

May interact with aminoglycosides and certain other agents. Compounds in these categories include:

Amikacin Sulfate (Increased nephrotoxicity).

No products indexed under this heading.

Gentamicin Sulfate (Increased nephrotoxicity). Products include:

Garamycin Injectable 3014
Pred-G Ophthalmic Ointment .... ⊙237
Pred-G Ophthalmic Suspension ...... ⊙236

Kanamycin Sulfate (Increased nephrotoxicity).
No products indexed under this heading.

Probenecid (Higher serum levels of cefoxitin).
No products indexed under this heading.

Streptomycin Sulfate (Increased nephrotoxicity).
No products indexed under this heading.

Tobramycin (Increased nephrotoxicity). Products include:
TOBI Solution for Inhalation **2298**
TobraDex Ophthalmic Ointment **562**
TobraDex Ophthalmic Suspension ... **563**
Zylet Ophthalmic Suspension .... ⊙**259**

Tobramycin Sulfate (Increased nephrotoxicity).
No products indexed under this heading.

MEFOXIN PREMIXED INTRAVENOUS SOLUTION

(Cefoxitin Sodium) **2016**
May interact with aminoglycosides and certain other agents. Compounds in these categories include:

Amikacin Sulfate (Increased nephrotoxicity).
No products indexed under this heading.

Gentamicin Sulfate (Increased nephrotoxicity). Products include:
Garamycin Injectable **3014**
Pred-G Ophthalmic Ointment .... ⊙**237**
Pred-G Ophthalmic Suspension ...... ⊙**236**

Kanamycin Sulfate (Increased nephrotoxicity).
No products indexed under this heading.

Probenecid (Higher serum levels of cefoxitin).
No products indexed under this heading.

Streptomycin Sulfate (Increased nephrotoxicity).
No products indexed under this heading.

Tobramycin (Increased nephrotoxicity). Products include:
TOBI Solution for Inhalation **2298**
TobraDex Ophthalmic Ointment **562**
TobraDex Ophthalmic Suspension ... **563**
Zylet Ophthalmic Suspension .... ⊙**259**

Tobramycin Sulfate (Increased nephrotoxicity).
No products indexed under this heading.

MEGA ANTIOXIDANT TABLETS

(Vitamins, Multiple) **3339**
None cited in PDR database.

MEGACE ES ORAL SUSPENSION

(Megestrol Acetate) **2481**
May interact with insulin and certain other agents. Compounds in these categories include:

Indinavir Sulfate (A pharmacokinetic study demonstrated that co-administration of megestrol acetate and indinavir results in a significant decrease in the pharmacokinetic parameters (approximately 36% for Cmax and approximately 28% for AUC) of indinavir. Administration of a higher dose of indinavir should be considered when co-administering with megestrol acetate). Products include:
Crixivan Capsules **1940**

Insulin, Human, Zinc Suspension (Exacerbation of pre-existing diabetes with increased insulin requirements has been reported in association with concomitant use of megestrol acetate). Products include:
Humulin L, 100 Units **1794**
Humulin U, 100 Units **1800**

Insulin, Human NPH (Exacerbation of pre-existing diabetes with increased insulin requirements has been reported in association with concomitant use of megestrol acetate). Products include:
Humulin N, 100 Units **1795**
Humulin N Pen **1797**

Insulin, Human Regular (Exacerbation of pre-existing diabetes with increased insulin requirements has been reported in association with concomitant use of megestrol acetate). Products include:
Humulin R, 100 Units **1798**

Insulin, Human Regular and Human NPH Mixture (Exacerbation of pre-existing diabetes with increased insulin requirements has been reported in association with concomitant use of megestrol acetate). Products include:
Humulin 50/50, 100 Units **1791**
Humulin 70/30 Pen **1793**

Insulin, NPH (Exacerbation of pre-existing diabetes with increased insulin requirements has been reported in association with concomitant use of megestrol acetate).
No products indexed under this heading.

Insulin, Regular (Exacerbation of pre-existing diabetes with increased insulin requirements has been reported in association with concomitant use of megestrol acetate).
No products indexed under this heading.

Insulin, Zinc Crystals (Exacerbation of pre-existing diabetes with increased insulin requirements has been reported in association with concomitant use of megestrol acetate).
No products indexed under this heading.

Insulin, Zinc Suspension (Exacerbation of pre-existing diabetes with increased insulin requirements has been reported in association with concomitant use of megestrol acetate).
No products indexed under this heading.

Insulin Aspart, Human Regular (Exacerbation of pre-existing diabetes with increased insulin requirements has been reported in association with concomitant use of megestrol acetate). Products include:
NovoLog Injection **2326**

Insulin glargine (Exacerbation of pre-existing diabetes with increased insulin requirements has been reported in association with concomitant use of megestrol acetate). Products include:
Lantus Injection **2909**

Insulin Lispro, Human (Exacerbation of pre-existing diabetes with increased insulin requirements has been reported in association with concomitant use of megestrol acetate). Products include:
Humalog-Pen **1781**
Humalog Mix 50/50-Pen **1783**
Humalog Mix 75/25-Pen **1785**

Insulin Lispro Protamine, Human (Exacerbation of pre-existing diabetes with increased insulin requirements has been reported in association with concomitant use of megestrol acetate). Products include:
Humalog Mix 50/50-Pen **1783**
Humalog Mix 75/25-Pen **1785**

MENACTRA VACCINE

(Meningoccal Polysaccharide Diphtheria Toxoid Conjugate Vaccine) **2954**
May interact with alkylating agents, antimetabolites, anticoagulants, corticosteroids, oral anticoagulants, cytotoxic drugs, immunosuppressive agents, and nitrogen-mustard-type alkylating agents. Compounds in these categories include:

Anisindione (Because of the risk of hemorrhage, avoid use with concomitant anticoagulant therapy unless the potential benefit clearly outweighs the risk of administration). Products include:
Miradon Tablets **3042**

Ardeparin Sodium (Because of the risk of hemorrhage, avoid use with concomitant anticoagulant therapy unless the potential benefit clearly outweighs the risk of administration).
No products indexed under this heading.

Azathioprine (Immunosuppressive therapies, including irradiation, antimetabolites, alkylating agents, cytotoxic drugs, and corticosteroids (used in greater than physiologic doses) may reduce the immune response to vaccines).
No products indexed under this heading.

Basiliximab (Immunosuppressive therapies, including irradiation, antimetabolites, alkylating agents, cytotoxic drugs, and corticosteroids (used in greater than physiologic doses) may reduce the immune response to vaccines). Products include:
Simulect for Injection **2284**

Betamethasone Acetate (Immunosuppressive therapies, including irradiation, antimetabolites, alkylating agents, cytotoxic drugs, and corticosteroids (used in greater than physiologic doses) may reduce the immune response to vaccines).
No products indexed under this heading.

Betamethasone Sodium Phosphate (Immunosuppressive therapies, including irradiation, antimetabolites, alkylating agents, cytotoxic drugs, and corticosteroids (used in greater than physiologic doses) may reduce the immune response to vaccines).
No products indexed under this heading.

Bleomycin Sulfate (Immunosuppressive therapies, including irradiation, antimetabolites, alkylating agents, cytotoxic drugs, and corticosteroids (used in greater than physiologic doses) may reduce the immune response to vaccines).
No products indexed under this heading.

Busulfan (Immunosuppressive therapies, including irradiation, antimetabolites, alkylating agents, cytotoxic drugs, and corticosteroids (used in greater than physiologic doses) may reduce the immune response to vaccines). Products include:
I.V. Busulfex **2493**
Myleran Tablets **1525**

Capecitabine (Immunosuppressive therapies, including irradiation, antimetabolites, alkylating agents, cytotoxic drugs, and corticosteroids (used in greater than physiologic doses) may reduce the immune response to vaccines). Products include:
Xeloda Tablets **2822**

Carmustine (BCNU) (Immunosuppressive therapies, including irradiation, antimetabolites, alkylating agents, cytotoxic drugs, and corticosteroids (used in greater than physiologic doses) may reduce the immune response to vaccines).
No products indexed under this heading.

Chlorambucil (Immunosuppressive therapies, including irradiation, antimetabolites, alkylating agents, cytotoxic drugs, and corticosteroids (used in greater than physiologic doses) may reduce the immune response to vaccines). Products include:
Leukeran Tablets **1504**

Cladribine (Immunosuppressive therapies, including irradiation, antimetabolites, alkylating agents, cytotoxic drugs, and corticosteroids (used in greater than physiologic doses) may reduce the immune response to vaccines). Products include:
Leustatin Injection **2357**

Cortisone Acetate (Immunosuppressive therapies, including irradiation, antimetabolites, alkylating agents, cytotoxic drugs, and corticosteroids (used in greater than physiologic doses) may reduce the immune response to vaccines).
No products indexed under this heading.

Cyclophosphamide (Immunosuppressive therapies, including irradiation, antimetabolites, alkylating agents, cytotoxic drugs, and corticosteroids (used in greater than physiologic doses) may reduce the immune response to vaccines).
No products indexed under this heading.

Cyclosporine (Immunosuppressive therapies, including irradiation, antimetabolites, alkylating agents, cytotoxic drugs, and corticosteroids (used in greater than physiologic doses) may reduce the immune response to vaccines). Products include:
Gengraf Capsules **459**
Neoral Oral Solution **2259**
Neoral Soft Gelatin Capsules **2259**
Restasis Ophthalmic Emulsion **575**
Sandimmune **2275**

Cytarabine (Immunosuppressive therapies, including irradiation, antimetabolites, alkylating agents, cytotoxic drugs, and corticosteroids (used in greater than physiologic doses) may reduce the immune response to vaccines).
No products indexed under this heading.

Dacarbazine (Immunosuppressive therapies, including irradiation, antimetabolites, alkylating agents, cytotoxic drugs, and corticosteroids (used in greater than physiologic doses) may reduce the immune response to vaccines).

No products indexed under this heading.

Dalteparin Sodium (Because of the risk of hemorrhage, avoid use with concomitant anticoagulant therapy unless the potential benefit clearly outweighs the risk of administration). Products include:

Fragmin Injection 1097

Danaparoid Sodium (Because of the risk of hemorrhage, avoid use with concomitant anticoagulant therapy unless the potential benefit clearly outweighs the risk of administration).

No products indexed under this heading.

Daunorubicin Hydrochloride (Immunosuppressive therapies, including irradiation, antimetabolites, alkylating agents, cytotoxic drugs, and corticosteroids (used in greater than physiologic doses) may reduce the immune response to vaccines).

No products indexed under this heading.

Dexamethasone (Immunosuppressive therapies, including irradiation, antimetabolites, alkylating agents, cytotoxic drugs, and corticosteroids (used in greater than physiologic doses) may reduce the immune response to vaccines). Products include:

Ciprodex Otic Suspension	559
Decadron Tablets	1951
TobraDex Ophthalmic Ointment	562
TobraDex Ophthalmic Suspension	563

Dexamethasone Acetate (Immunosuppressive therapies, including irradiation, antimetabolites, alkylating agents, cytotoxic drugs, and corticosteroids (used in greater than physiologic doses) may reduce the immune response to vaccines).

No products indexed under this heading.

Dexamethasone Sodium Phosphate (Immunosuppressive therapies, including irradiation, antimetabolites, alkylating agents, cytotoxic drugs, and corticosteroids (used in greater than physiologic doses) may reduce the immune response to vaccines).

No products indexed under this heading.

Dicumarol (Because of the risk of hemorrhage, avoid use with concomitant anticoagulant therapy unless the potential benefit clearly outweighs the risk of administration).

No products indexed under this heading.

Doxorubicin Hydrochloride (Immunosuppressive therapies, including irradiation, antimetabolites, alkylating agents, cytotoxic drugs, and corticosteroids (used in greater than physiologic doses) may reduce the immune response to vaccines).

No products indexed under this heading.

Enoxaparin Sodium (Because of the risk of hemorrhage, avoid use with concomitant anticoagulant therapy unless the potential benefit clearly outweighs the risk of administration). Products include:

Lovenox Injection 2915

Epirubicin Hydrochloride (Immunosuppressive therapies, including irradiation, antimetabolites, alkylating agents, cytotoxic drugs, and corticosteroids (used in greater than physiologic doses) may reduce the immune response to vaccines).

No products indexed under this heading.

Estramustine Phosphate Sodium (Immunosuppressive therapies, including irradiation, antimetabolites, alkylating agents, cytotoxic drugs, and corticosteroids (used in greater than physiologic doses) may reduce the immune response to vaccines). Products include:

Emcyt Capsules 2634

Floxuridine (Immunosuppressive therapies, including irradiation, antimetabolites, alkylating agents, cytotoxic drugs, and corticosteroids (used in greater than physiologic doses) may reduce the immune response to vaccines).

No products indexed under this heading.

Fludarabine Phosphate (Immunosuppressive therapies, including irradiation, antimetabolites, alkylating agents, cytotoxic drugs, and corticosteroids (used in greater than physiologic doses) may reduce the immune response to vaccines).

No products indexed under this heading.

Fludrocortisone Acetate (Immunosuppressive therapies, including irradiation, antimetabolites, alkylating agents, cytotoxic drugs, and corticosteroids (used in greater than physiologic doses) may reduce the immune response to vaccines).

No products indexed under this heading.

Fluorouracil (Immunosuppressive therapies, including irradiation, antimetabolites, alkylating agents, cytotoxic drugs, and corticosteroids (used in greater than physiologic doses) may reduce the immune response to vaccines). Products include:

| Carac Cream, 0.5% | 2879 |
| Efudex | 3363 |

Fondaparinux Sodium (Because of the risk of hemorrhage, avoid use with concomitant anticoagulant therapy unless the potential benefit clearly outweighs the risk of administration). Products include:

Arixtra Injection 1351

Gemcitabine Hydrochloride (Immunosuppressive therapies, including irradiation, antimetabolites, alkylating agents, cytotoxic drugs, and corticosteroids (used in greater than physiologic doses) may reduce the immune response to vaccines). Products include:

Gemzar for Injection 1771

Heparin Calcium (Because of the risk of hemorrhage, avoid use with concomitant anticoagulant therapy unless the potential benefit clearly outweighs the risk of administration).

No products indexed under this heading.

Heparin Sodium (Because of the risk of hemorrhage, avoid use with concomitant anticoagulant therapy unless the potential benefit clearly outweighs the risk of administration).

No products indexed under this heading.

Hydrocortisone (Immunosuppressive therapies, including irradiation,

antimetabolites, alkylating agents, cytotoxic drugs, and corticosteroids (used in greater than physiologic doses) may reduce the immune response to vaccines). Products include:

Colocort Rectal Suspension, USP (Retention) 100 mg/60 mL	2476
Hydrocortone Tablets	1989
Preparation H Hydrocortisone Cream	⬛646

Hydrocortisone Acetate (Immunosuppressive therapies, including irradiation, antimetabolites, alkylating agents, cytotoxic drugs, and corticosteroids (used in greater than physiologic doses) may reduce the immune response to vaccines). Products include:

Analpram-HC	1159
Pramosone	1161
ProctoFoam-HC	3099

Hydrocortisone Sodium Phosphate (Immunosuppressive therapies, including irradiation, antimetabolites, alkylating agents, cytotoxic drugs, and corticosteroids (used in greater than physiologic doses) may reduce the immune response to vaccines).

No products indexed under this heading.

Hydrocortisone Sodium Succinate (Immunosuppressive therapies, including irradiation, antimetabolites, alkylating agents, cytotoxic drugs, and corticosteroids (used in greater than physiologic doses) may reduce the immune response to vaccines).

No products indexed under this heading.

Hydroxyurea (Immunosuppressive therapies, including irradiation, antimetabolites, alkylating agents, cytotoxic drugs, and corticosteroids (used in greater than physiologic doses) may reduce the immune response to vaccines).

No products indexed under this heading.

Lomustine (CCNU) (Immunosuppressive therapies, including irradiation, antimetabolites, alkylating agents, cytotoxic drugs, and corticosteroids (used in greater than physiologic doses) may reduce the immune response to vaccines).

No products indexed under this heading.

Low Molecular Weight Heparins (Because of the risk of hemorrhage, avoid use with concomitant anticoagulant therapy unless the potential benefit clearly outweighs the risk of administration).

No products indexed under this heading.

Mechlorethamine Hydrochloride (Immunosuppressive therapies, including irradiation, antimetabolites, alkylating agents, cytotoxic drugs, and corticosteroids (used in greater than physiologic doses) may reduce the immune response to vaccines). Products include:

Mustargen for Injection 2468

Melphalan (Immunosuppressive therapies, including irradiation, antimetabolites, alkylating agents, cytotoxic drugs, and corticosteroids (used in greater than physiologic doses) may reduce the immune response to vaccines). Products include:

Alkeran Tablets 956

Mercaptopurine (Immunosuppressive therapies, including irradiation, antimetabolites, alkylating agents, cytotoxic drugs, and corticosteroids (used in greater than physiologic doses) may reduce the immune response to vaccines).

No products indexed under this heading.

Methotrexate (Immunosuppressive therapies, including irradiation, antimetabolites, alkylating agents, cytotoxic drugs, and corticosteroids (used in greater than physiologic doses) may reduce the immune response to vaccines).

No products indexed under this heading.

Methotrexate Sodium (Immunosuppressive therapies, including irradiation, antimetabolites, alkylating agents, cytotoxic drugs, and corticosteroids (used in greater than physiologic doses) may reduce the immune response to vaccines).

No products indexed under this heading.

Methylprednisolone Acetate (Immunosuppressive therapies, including irradiation, antimetabolites, alkylating agents, cytotoxic drugs, and corticosteroids (used in greater than physiologic doses) may reduce the immune response to vaccines). Products include:

| Depo-Medrol Injectable Suspension | 2617 |
| Depo-Medrol Single-Dose Vial | 2619 |

Methylprednisolone Sodium Succinate (Immunosuppressive therapies, including irradiation, antimetabolites, alkylating agents, cytotoxic drugs, and corticosteroids (used in greater than physiologic doses) may reduce the immune response to vaccines).

No products indexed under this heading.

Mitotane (Immunosuppressive therapies, including irradiation, antimetabolites, alkylating agents, cytotoxic drugs, and corticosteroids (used in greater than physiologic doses) may reduce the immune response to vaccines).

No products indexed under this heading.

Mitoxantrone Hydrochloride (Immunosuppressive therapies, including irradiation, antimetabolites, alkylating agents, cytotoxic drugs, and corticosteroids (used in greater than physiologic doses) may reduce the immune response to vaccines).

No products indexed under this heading.

Muromonab-CD3 (Immunosuppressive therapies, including irradiation, antimetabolites, alkylating agents, cytotoxic drugs, and corticosteroids (used in greater than physiologic doses) may reduce the immune response to vaccines). Products include:

Orthoclone OKT3 Sterile Solution 2360

Mycophenolate Mofetil (Immunosuppressive therapies, including irradiation, antimetabolites, alkylating agents, cytotoxic drugs, and corticosteroids (used in greater than physiologic doses) may reduce the immune response to vaccines). Products include:

CellCept Capsules	2747
CellCept Oral Suspension	2747
CellCept Tablets	2747

(⬛ Described in PDR For Nonprescription Drugs) (⊙ Described in PDR For Ophthalmic Medicines™)

Pentostatin (Immunosuppressive therapies, including irradiation, antimetabolites, alkylating agents, cytotoxic drugs, and corticosteroids (used in greater than physiologic doses) may reduce the immune response to vaccines). Products include:
- Nipent for Injection 1863

Prednisolone Acetate (Immunosuppressive therapies, including irradiation, antimetabolites, alkylating agents, cytotoxic drugs, and corticosteroids (used in greater than physiologic doses) may reduce the immune response to vaccines). Products include:
- Blephamide Ophthalmic Ointment 568
- Blephamide Ophthalmic Suspension.................................. 569
- Poly-Pred Ophthalmic Suspension .... ⊙233
- Pred Forte Ophthalmic Suspension .... ⊙235
- Pred Mild Ophthalmic Suspension .... ⊙238
- Pred-G Ophthalmic Ointment .... ⊙237
- Pred-G Ophthalmic Suspension ...... ⊙236

Prednisolone Sodium Phosphate (Immunosuppressive therapies, including irradiation, antimetabolites, alkylating agents, cytotoxic drugs, and corticosteroids (used in greater than physiologic doses) may reduce the immune response to vaccines).
No products indexed under this heading.

Prednisolone Tebutate (Immunosuppressive therapies, including irradiation, antimetabolites, alkylating agents, cytotoxic drugs, and corticosteroids (used in greater than physiologic doses) may reduce the immune response to vaccines).
No products indexed under this heading.

Prednisone (Immunosuppressive therapies, including irradiation, antimetabolites, alkylating agents, cytotoxic drugs, and corticosteroids (used in greater than physiologic doses) may reduce the immune response to vaccines).
No products indexed under this heading.

Procarbazine Hydrochloride (Immunosuppressive therapies, including irradiation, antimetabolites, alkylating agents, cytotoxic drugs, and corticosteroids (used in greater than physiologic doses) may reduce the immune response to vaccines). Products include:
- Matulane Capsules 3191

Sirolimus (Immunosuppressive therapies, including irradiation, antimetabolites, alkylating agents, cytotoxic drugs, and corticosteroids (used in greater than physiologic doses) may reduce the immune response to vaccines). Products include:
- Rapamune Oral Solution and Tablets.. 3475

Tacrolimus (Immunosuppressive therapies, including irradiation, antimetabolites, alkylating agents, cytotoxic drugs, and corticosteroids (used in greater than physiologic doses) may reduce the immune response to vaccines). Products include:
- Prograf Capsules and Injection 632
- Protopic Ointment 638

Tamoxifen Citrate (Immunosuppressive therapies, including irradiation, antimetabolites, alkylating agents, cytotoxic drugs, and corticosteroids (used in greater than physiologic doses) may reduce the immune response to vaccines). Products include:
- Soltamox Oral Solution 3527

Thioguanine (Immunosuppressive therapies, including irradiation, antimetabolites, alkylating agents, cytotoxic drugs, and corticosteroids (used in greater than physiologic doses) may reduce the immune response to vaccines). Products include:
- Tabloid Tablets 1575

Thiotepa (Immunosuppressive therapies, including irradiation, antimetabolites, alkylating agents, cytotoxic drugs, and corticosteroids (used in greater than physiologic doses) may reduce the immune response to vaccines).
No products indexed under this heading.

Tinzaparin Sodium (Because of the risk of hemorrhage, avoid use with concomitant anticoagulant therapy unless the potential benefit clearly outweighs the risk of administration).
No products indexed under this heading.

Triamcinolone (Immunosuppressive therapies, including irradiation, antimetabolites, alkylating agents, cytotoxic drugs, and corticosteroids (used in greater than physiologic doses) may reduce the immune response to vaccines).
No products indexed under this heading.

Triamcinolone Acetonide (Immunosuppressive therapies, including irradiation, antimetabolites, alkylating agents, cytotoxic drugs, and corticosteroids (used in greater than physiologic doses) may reduce the immune response to vaccines). Products include:
- Azmacort Inhalation Aerosol 1726
- Nasacort AQ Nasal Spray 2922

Triamcinolone Diacetate (Immunosuppressive therapies, including irradiation, antimetabolites, alkylating agents, cytotoxic drugs, and corticosteroids (used in greater than physiologic doses) may reduce the immune response to vaccines).
No products indexed under this heading.

Triamcinolone Hexacetonide (Immunosuppressive therapies, including irradiation, antimetabolites, alkylating agents, cytotoxic drugs, and corticosteroids (used in greater than physiologic doses) may reduce the immune response to vaccines).
No products indexed under this heading.

Vincristine Sulfate (Immunosuppressive therapies, including irradiation, antimetabolites, alkylating agents, cytotoxic drugs, and corticosteroids (used in greater than physiologic doses) may reduce the immune response to vaccines).
No products indexed under this heading.

Warfarin Sodium (Because of the risk of hemorrhage, avoid use with concomitant anticoagulant therapy unless the potential benefit clearly outweighs the risk of administration). Products include:
- Coumadin for Injection 898
- Coumadin Tablets 898

MENOSTAR TRANSDERMAL SYSTEM

(Estradiol) 782

May interact with cytochrome p450 3a4 inducers (selected), cytochrome p450 3a4 inhibitors (selected), and certain other agents. Compounds in these categories include:

Acetazolamide (Inhibitors of CYP3A4 may increase plasma concentrations of estrogens and may result in side effects).
No products indexed under this heading.

Allium sativum (Inducers of CYP3A4 may reduce plasma concentrations of estrogens, possibly resulting in a decrease in therapeutic effects and/or changes in the uterine bleeding profile).
No products indexed under this heading.

Amiodarone Hydrochloride (Inhibitors of CYP3A4 may increase plasma concentrations of estrogens and may result in side effects).
No products indexed under this heading.

Amprenavir (Inhibitors of CYP3A4 may increase plasma concentrations of estrogens and may result in side effects). Products include:
- Agenerase Capsules 1327
- Agenerase Oral Solution 1332

Anastrozole (Inhibitors of CYP3A4 may increase plasma concentrations of estrogens and may result in side effects). Products include:
- Arimidex Tablets 673

Aprepitant (Inducers of CYP3A4 may reduce plasma concentrations of estrogens, possibly resulting in a decrease in therapeutic effects and/or changes in the uterine bleeding profile). Products include:
- Emend Capsules 1963

Betamethasone Acetate (Inducers of CYP3A4 may reduce plasma concentrations of estrogens, possibly resulting in a decrease in therapeutic effects and/or changes in the uterine bleeding profile).
No products indexed under this heading.

Betamethasone Sodium Phosphate (Inducers of CYP3A4 may reduce plasma concentrations of estrogens, possibly resulting in a decrease in therapeutic effects and/or changes in the uterine bleeding profile).
No products indexed under this heading.

Carbamazepine (Inducers of CYP3A4 may reduce plasma concentrations of estrogens, possibly resulting in a decrease in therapeutic effects and/or changes in the uterine bleeding profile). Products include:
- Carbatrol Capsules 3171
- Equetro Extended-Release Capsules.................................... 3180
- Tegretol/Tegretol-XR 2295

Cimetidine (Inhibitors of CYP3A4 may increase plasma concentrations of estrogens and may result in side effects). Products include:
- Tagamet HB 200 Tablets 664

Cimetidine Hydrochloride (Inhibitors of CYP3A4 may increase plasma concentrations of estrogens and may result in side effects).
No products indexed under this heading.

Ciprofloxacin (Inhibitors of CYP3A4 may increase plasma concentrations of estrogens and may result in side effects). Products include:
- Cipro Oral Suspension 2977
- Cipro I.V. 2984
- Cipro XR Tablets 2990
- Ciprodex Otic Suspension 559

Ciprofloxacin Hydrochloride (Inducers of CYP3A4 may reduce plasma concentrations of estrogens, possibly resulting in a decrease in therapeutic effects and/or changes in the uterine bleeding profile). Products include:
- Ciloxan Ophthalmic Ointment 559
- Ciloxan Ophthalmic Solution .... ⊙206
- Cipro Tablets 2977
- Proquin XR Tablets 1153

Cisplatin (Inducers of CYP3A4 may reduce plasma concentrations of estrogens, possibly resulting in a decrease in therapeutic effects and/or changes in the uterine bleeding profile).
No products indexed under this heading.

Clarithromycin (Inhibitors of CYP3A4, such as clarithromycin, may increase plasma concentrations of estrogens and may result in side effects). Products include:
- Biaxin/Biaxin XL 402
- PREVPAC 3284

Clotrimazole (Inhibitors of CYP3A4 may increase plasma concentrations of estrogens and may result in side effects). Products include:
- Desenex Athlete's Foot Cream 635
- Lotrimin 3039
- Lotrisone 3040

Cortisone Acetate (Inducers of CYP3A4 may reduce plasma concentrations of estrogens, possibly resulting in a decrease in therapeutic effects and/or changes in the uterine bleeding profile).
No products indexed under this heading.

Cyclosporine (Inhibitors of CYP3A4 may increase plasma concentrations of estrogens and may result in side effects). Products include:
- Gengraf Capsules 459
- Neoral Oral Solution 2259
- Neoral Soft Gelatin Capsules 2259
- Restasis Ophthalmic Emulsion 575
- Sandimmune 2275

Dalfopristin (Inhibitors of CYP3A4 may increase plasma concentrations of estrogens and may result in side effects).
No products indexed under this heading.

Danazol (Inhibitors of CYP3A4 may increase plasma concentrations of estrogens and may result in side effects).
No products indexed under this heading.

Delavirdine Mesylate (Inhibitors of CYP3A4 may increase plasma concentrations of estrogens and may result in side effects). Products include:
- Rescriptor Tablets 2551

Dexamethasone (Inducers of CYP3A4 may reduce plasma concentrations of estrogens, possibly resulting in a decrease in therapeutic effects and/or changes in the uterine bleeding profile). Products include:
- Ciprodex Otic Suspension 559
- Decadron Tablets 1951
- TobraDex Ophthalmic Ointment 562
- TobraDex Ophthalmic Suspension ... 563

Dexamethasone Acetate (Inducers of CYP3A4 may reduce plasma concentrations of estrogens, possibly resulting in a decrease in therapeutic effects and/or changes in the uterine bleeding profile).
No products indexed under this heading.

Dexamethasone Sodium Phosphate (Inducers of CYP3A4 may reduce plasma concentrations of estrogens, possibly resulting in a decrease in therapeutic effects and/or changes in the uterine bleeding profile).
No products indexed under this heading.

Diltiazem Hydrochloride (Inhibitors of CYP3A4 may increase plasma concentrations of estrogens and may result in side effects). Products include:
Cardizem LA Extended Release Tablets .. 1728
Tiazac Capsules 1201

Diltiazem Maleate (Inhibitors of CYP3A4 may increase plasma concentrations of estrogens and may result in side effects).
No products indexed under this heading.

Doxorubicin Hydrochloride (Inducers of CYP3A4 may reduce plasma concentrations of estrogens, possibly resulting in a decrease in therapeutic effects and/or changes in the uterine bleeding profile).
No products indexed under this heading.

Efavirenz (Inducers of CYP3A4 may reduce plasma concentrations of estrogens, possibly resulting in a decrease in therapeutic effects and/or changes in the uterine bleeding profile). Products include:
Atripla Tablets 945
Sustiva Capsules 930
Sustiva Tablets 930

Erythromycin (Inhibitors of CYP3A4 may increase plasma concentrations of estrogens and may result in side effects). Products include:
Ery-Tab Tablets 449
Erythromycin Base Filmtab Tablets .. 455
Erythromycin Delayed-Release Capsules, USP 457
PCE Dispertab Tablets 515

Erythromycin Estolate (Inhibitors of CYP3A4 may increase plasma concentrations of estrogens and may result in side effects).
No products indexed under this heading.

Erythromycin Ethylsuccinate (Inhibitors of CYP3A4 may increase plasma concentrations of estrogens and may result in side effects). Products include:
E.E.S. ... 451
EryPed .. 447

Erythromycin Gluceptate (Inhibitors of CYP3A4 may increase plasma concentrations of estrogens and may result in side effects).
No products indexed under this heading.

Erythromycin Lactobionate (Inhibitors of CYP3A4 may increase plasma concentrations of estrogens and may result in side effects).
No products indexed under this heading.

Erythromycin Stearate (Inhibitors of CYP3A4 may increase plasma

concentrations of estrogens and may result in side effects). Products include:
Erythrocin Stearate Filmtab Tablets .. 453

Esomeprazole Magnesium (Inhibitors of CYP3A4 may increase plasma concentrations of estrogens and may result in side effects). Products include:
Nexium Delayed-Release Capsules 655

Ethosuximide (Inducers of CYP3A4 may reduce plasma concentrations of estrogens, possibly resulting in a decrease in therapeutic effects and/or changes in the uterine bleeding profile).
No products indexed under this heading.

Felbamate (Inducers of CYP3A4 may reduce plasma concentrations of estrogens, possibly resulting in a decrease in therapeutic effects and/or changes in the uterine bleeding profile).
No products indexed under this heading.

Fluconazole (Inhibitors of CYP3A4 may increase plasma concentrations of estrogens and may result in side effects).
No products indexed under this heading.

Fludrocortisone Acetate (Inducers of CYP3A4 may reduce plasma concentrations of estrogens, possibly resulting in a decrease in therapeutic effects and/or changes in the uterine bleeding profile).
No products indexed under this heading.

Fluoxetine Hydrochloride (Inhibitors of CYP3A4 may increase plasma concentrations of estrogens and may result in side effects). Products include:
Prozac Pulvules and Liquid 1801
Symbyax Capsules 1819

Fluvoxamine Maleate (Inhibitors of CYP3A4 may increase plasma concentrations of estrogens and may result in side effects).
No products indexed under this heading.

Fosamprenavir Calcium (Inhibitors of CYP3A4 may increase plasma concentrations of estrogens and may result in side effects). Products include:
Lexiva Tablets 1505

Fosphenytoin Sodium (Inducers of CYP3A4 may reduce plasma concentrations of estrogens, possibly resulting in a decrease in therapeutic effects and/or changes in the uterine bleeding profile).
No products indexed under this heading.

Garlic Extract (Inducers of CYP3A4 may reduce plasma concentrations of estrogens, possibly resulting in a decrease in therapeutic effects and/or changes in the uterine bleeding profile).
No products indexed under this heading.

Garlic Oil (Inducers of CYP3A4 may reduce plasma concentrations of estrogens, possibly resulting in a decrease in therapeutic effects and/or changes in the uterine bleeding profile).
No products indexed under this heading.

Hydrocortisone (Inducers of CYP3A4 may reduce plasma concen-

trations of estrogens, possibly resulting in a decrease in therapeutic effects and/or changes in the uterine bleeding profile). Products include:
Colocort Rectal Suspension, USP (Retention) 100 mg/60 mL 2476
Hydrocortone Tablets 1989
Preparation H Hydrocortisone Cream ▣646

Hydrocortisone Acetate (Inducers of CYP3A4 may reduce plasma concentrations of estrogens, possibly resulting in a decrease in therapeutic effects and/or changes in the uterine bleeding profile). Products include:
Analpram-HC 1159
Pramosone 1161
ProctoFoam-HC 3099

Hydrocortisone Butyrate (Inducers of CYP3A4 may reduce plasma concentrations of estrogens, possibly resulting in a decrease in therapeutic effects and/or changes in the uterine bleeding profile). Products include:
Locoid Lipocream Cream 1160

Hydrocortisone Cypionate (Inducers of CYP3A4 may reduce plasma concentrations of estrogens, possibly resulting in a decrease in therapeutic effects and/or changes in the uterine bleeding profile).
No products indexed under this heading.

Hydrocortisone Hemisuccinate (Inducers of CYP3A4 may reduce plasma concentrations of estrogens, possibly resulting in a decrease in therapeutic effects and/or changes in the uterine bleeding profile).
No products indexed under this heading.

Hydrocortisone Probutate (Inducers of CYP3A4 may reduce plasma concentrations of estrogens, possibly resulting in a decrease in therapeutic effects and/or changes in the uterine bleeding profile).
No products indexed under this heading.

Hydrocortisone Sodium Phosphate (Inducers of CYP3A4 may reduce plasma concentrations of estrogens, possibly resulting in a decrease in therapeutic effects and/or changes in the uterine bleeding profile).
No products indexed under this heading.

Hydrocortisone Sodium Succinate (Inducers of CYP3A4 may reduce plasma concentrations of estrogens, possibly resulting in a decrease in therapeutic effects and/or changes in the uterine bleeding profile).
No products indexed under this heading.

Hydrocortisone Valerate (Inducers of CYP3A4 may reduce plasma concentrations of estrogens, possibly resulting in a decrease in therapeutic effects and/or changes in the uterine bleeding profile).
No products indexed under this heading.

Hypericum (Inducers of CYP3A4 may reduce plasma concentrations of estrogens, possibly resulting in a decrease in therapeutic effects and/or changes in the uterine bleeding profile). Products include:
Satiete Tablets ▣832

Hypericum Perforatum (Inducers of CYP3A4 may reduce plasma concentrations of estrogens, possibly resulting in a decrease in therapeutic effects and/or changes in the uterine bleeding profile).
No products indexed under this heading.

Indinavir Sulfate (Inhibitors of CYP3A4 may increase plasma concentrations of estrogens and may result in side effects). Products include:
Crixivan Capsules 1940

Isoniazid (Inhibitors of CYP3A4 may increase plasma concentrations of estrogens and may result in side effects).
No products indexed under this heading.

Itraconazole (Inhibitors of CYP3A4 may increase plasma concentrations of estrogens and may result in side effects).
No products indexed under this heading.

Ketoconazole (Inhibitors of CYP3A4 may increase plasma concentrations of estrogens and may result in side effects). Products include:
Nizoral A-D Shampoo, 1% 1868

Lopinavir (Inhibitors of CYP3A4 may increase plasma concentrations of estrogens and may result in side effects). Products include:
Kaletra ... 476

Loratadine (Inhibitors of CYP3A4 may increase plasma concentrations of estrogens and may result in side effects). Products include:
Alavert Allergy & Sinus D-12 Hour Tablets ▣771
Alavert ... ▣771
Children's Claritin Allergy Oral Solution ▣771
Claritin Non-Drowsy 24 Hour Tablets ▣772
Claritin Reditabs 24 Hour Non-Drowsy Tablets ▣772
Claritin-D Non-Drowsy 12 Hour Tablets ▣772
Claritin-D Non-Drowsy 24 Hour Tablets ▣772

Mephenytoin (Inducers of CYP3A4 may reduce plasma concentrations of estrogens, possibly resulting in a decrease in therapeutic effects and/or changes in the uterine bleeding profile).
No products indexed under this heading.

Methsuximide (Inducers of CYP3A4 may reduce plasma concentrations of estrogens, possibly resulting in a decrease in therapeutic effects and/or changes in the uterine bleeding profile).
No products indexed under this heading.

Methylprednisolone (Inducers of CYP3A4 may reduce plasma concentrations of estrogens, possibly resulting in a decrease in therapeutic effects and/or changes in the uterine bleeding profile).
No products indexed under this heading.

Methylprednisolone Acetate (Inducers of CYP3A4 may reduce plasma concentrations of estrogens, possibly resulting in a decrease in therapeutic effects and/or changes in the uterine bleeding profile). Products include:
Depo-Medrol Injectable Suspension 2617
Depo-Medrol Single-Dose Vial 2619

Methylprednisolone Sodium Succinate (Inducers of CYP3A4 may reduce plasma concentrations of estrogens, possibly resulting in a decrease in therapeutic effects and/or changes in the uterine bleeding profile).
No products indexed under this heading.

Metronidazole (Inhibitors of CYP3A4 may increase plasma concentrations of estrogens and may result in side effects). Products include:
Metrogel 1% 1211
MetroGel-Vaginal Gel 1855
Vandazole Vaginal Gel 3338

Metronidazole Benzoate (Inhibitors of CYP3A4 may increase plasma concentrations of estrogens and may result in side effects).
No products indexed under this heading.

Metronidazole Hydrochloride (Inhibitors of CYP3A4 may increase plasma concentrations of estrogens and may result in side effects).
No products indexed under this heading.

Miconazole (Inhibitors of CYP3A4 may increase plasma concentrations of estrogens and may result in side effects).
No products indexed under this heading.

Miconazole Nitrate (Inhibitors of CYP3A4 may increase plasma concentrations of estrogens and may result in side effects). Products include:
Desenex ▣635
Desenex Jock Itch Spray Powder ... ▣635

Modafinil (Inducers of CYP3A4 may reduce plasma concentrations of estrogens, possibly resulting in a decrease in therapeutic effects and/or changes in the uterine bleeding profile). Products include:
Provigil Tablets 988

Nefazodone Hydrochloride (Inhibitors of CYP3A4 may increase plasma concentrations of estrogens and may result in side effects).
No products indexed under this heading.

Nelfinavir Mesylate (Inhibitors of CYP3A4 may increase plasma concentrations of estrogens and may result in side effects). Products include:
Viracept 2577

Nevirapine (Inducers of CYP3A4 may reduce plasma concentrations of estrogens, possibly resulting in a decrease in therapeutic effects and/or changes in the uterine bleeding profile). Products include:
Viramune Oral Suspension 873
Viramune Tablets 873

Niacinamide (Inhibitors of CYP3A4 may increase plasma concentrations of estrogens and may result in side effects).
No products indexed under this heading.

Nicotinamide (Inhibitors of CYP3A4 may increase plasma concentrations of estrogens and may result in side effects). Products include:
Nicomide Tablets 1088

Nifedipine (Inhibitors of CYP3A4 may increase plasma concentrations of estrogens and may result in side effects). Products include:
Adalat CC Tablets 2964

Norfloxacin (Inhibitors of CYP3A4 may increase plasma concentrations of estrogens and may result in side effects). Products include:
Noroxin Tablets 2032

Omeprazole (Inhibitors of CYP3A4 may increase plasma concentrations of estrogens and may result in side effects). Products include:
Zegerid Capsules 2958
Zegerid Powder for Oral Solution 2958

Oxcarbazepine (Inducers of CYP3A4 may reduce plasma concentrations of estrogens, possibly resulting in a decrease in therapeutic effects and/or changes in the uterine bleeding profile). Products include:
Trileptal Tablets 2300
Trileptal Oral Suspension 2300

Paroxetine Hydrochloride (Inhibitors of CYP3A4 may increase plasma concentrations of estrogens and may result in side effects). Products include:
Paxil CR Controlled-Release Tablets 1538
Paxil ... 1530

Phenobarbital (Inducers of CYP3A4 may reduce plasma concentrations of estrogens, possibly resulting in a decrease in therapeutic effects and/or changes in the uterine bleeding profile). Products include:
Donnatal Extentabs 2493

Phenobarbital Sodium (Inducers of CYP3A4 may reduce plasma concentrations of estrogens, possibly resulting in a decrease in therapeutic effects and/or changes in the uterine bleeding profile).
No products indexed under this heading.

Phenytoin (Inducers of CYP3A4 may reduce plasma concentrations of estrogens, possibly resulting in a decrease in therapeutic effects and/or changes in the uterine bleeding profile).
No products indexed under this heading.

Phenytoin Sodium (Inducers of CYP3A4 may reduce plasma concentrations of estrogens, possibly resulting in a decrease in therapeutic effects and/or changes in the uterine bleeding profile). Products include:
Phenytek Capsules 2160

Prednisolone Acetate (Inducers of CYP3A4 may reduce plasma concentrations of estrogens, possibly resulting in a decrease in therapeutic effects and/or changes in the uterine bleeding profile). Products include:
Blephamide Ophthalmic Ointment 568
Blephamide Ophthalmic Suspension.............................. 569
Poly-Pred Ophthalmic Suspension ⊙233
Pred Forte Ophthalmic Suspension ⊙235
Pred Mild Ophthalmic Suspension ⊙238
Pred-G Ophthalmic Ointment ⊙237
Pred-G Ophthalmic Suspension ⊙236

Prednisolone Sodium Phosphate (Inducers of CYP3A4 may reduce plasma concentrations of estrogens, possibly resulting in a decrease in therapeutic effects and/or changes in the uterine bleeding profile).
No products indexed under this heading.

Prednisolone Tebutate (Inducers of CYP3A4 may reduce plasma concentrations of estrogens, possibly resulting in a decrease in therapeutic effects and/or changes in the uterine bleeding profile).
No products indexed under this heading.

Prednisone (Inducers of CYP3A4 may reduce plasma concentrations of estrogens, possibly resulting in a decrease in therapeutic effects and/or changes in the uterine bleeding profile).
No products indexed under this heading.

Primidone (Inducers of CYP3A4 may reduce plasma concentrations of estrogens, possibly resulting in a decrease in therapeutic effects and/or changes in the uterine bleeding profile).
No products indexed under this heading.

Propoxyphene Hydrochloride (Inhibitors of CYP3A4 may increase plasma concentrations of estrogens and may result in side effects).
No products indexed under this heading.

Propoxyphene Napsylate (Inhibitors of CYP3A4 may increase plasma concentrations of estrogens and may result in side effects).
No products indexed under this heading.

Quinidine (Inhibitors of CYP3A4 may increase plasma concentrations of estrogens and may result in side effects).
No products indexed under this heading.

Quinidine Hydrochloride (Inhibitors of CYP3A4 may increase plasma concentrations of estrogens and may result in side effects).
No products indexed under this heading.

Quinidine Polygalacturonate (Inhibitors of CYP3A4 may increase plasma concentrations of estrogens and may result in side effects).
No products indexed under this heading.

Quinidine Sulfate (Inhibitors of CYP3A4 may increase plasma concentrations of estrogens and may result in side effects).
No products indexed under this heading.

Quinine (Inhibitors of CYP3A4 may increase plasma concentrations of estrogens and may result in side effects).
No products indexed under this heading.

Quinine Sulfate (Inhibitors of CYP3A4 may increase plasma concentrations of estrogens and may result in side effects).
No products indexed under this heading.

Quinupristin (Inhibitors of CYP3A4 may increase plasma concentrations of estrogens and may result in side effects).
No products indexed under this heading.

Ranitidine Bismuth Citrate (Inhibitors of CYP3A4 may increase plasma concentrations of estrogens and may result in side effects).
No products indexed under this heading.

Ranitidine Hydrochloride (Inhibitors of CYP3A4 may increase plas-

ma concentrations of estrogens and may result in side effects). Products include:
Zantac .. 1624
Zantac Injection 1619
Zantac Injection Pharmacy Bulk Package.................................... 1622

Rifabutin (Inducers of CYP3A4 may reduce plasma concentrations of estrogens, possibly resulting in a decrease in therapeutic effects and/or changes in the uterine bleeding profile).
No products indexed under this heading.

Rifampicin (Inducers of CYP3A4 may reduce plasma concentrations of estrogens, possibly resulting in a decrease in therapeutic effects and/or changes in the uterine bleeding profile).
No products indexed under this heading.

Rifampin (Inducers of CYP3A4 may reduce plasma concentrations of estrogens, possibly resulting in a decrease in therapeutic effects and/or changes in the uterine bleeding profile).
No products indexed under this heading.

Rifapentine (Inducers of CYP3A4 may reduce plasma concentrations of estrogens, possibly resulting in a decrease in therapeutic effects and/or changes in the uterine bleeding profile).
No products indexed under this heading.

Ritonavir (Inhibitors of CYP3A4 may increase plasma concentrations of estrogens and may result in side effects). Products include:
Kaletra 476
Norvir .. 503

Saquinavir (Inhibitors of CYP3A4 may increase plasma concentrations of estrogens and may result in side effects).
No products indexed under this heading.

Saquinavir Mesylate (Inhibitors of CYP3A4 may increase plasma concentrations of estrogens and may result in side effects). Products include:
Invirase 2772

Sertraline Hydrochloride (Inhibitors of CYP3A4 may increase plasma concentrations of estrogens and may result in side effects). Products include:
Zoloft .. 2586

Sulfinpyrazone (Inducers of CYP3A4 may reduce plasma concentrations of estrogens, possibly resulting in a decrease in therapeutic effects and/or changes in the uterine bleeding profile).
No products indexed under this heading.

Telithromycin (Inhibitors of CYP3A4 may increase plasma concentrations of estrogens and may result in side effects). Products include:
Ketek Tablets 2903

Theophylline (Inducers of CYP3A4 may reduce plasma concentrations of estrogens, possibly resulting in a decrease in therapeutic effects and/or changes in the uterine bleeding profile).
No products indexed under this heading.

IMPORTANT NOTE: Always consult each drug listing in the patient's regimen for possible interactions.

Triamcinolone (Inducers of CYP3A4 may reduce plasma concentrations of estrogens, possibly resulting in a decrease in therapeutic effects and/or changes in the uterine bleeding profile).
No products indexed under this heading.

Triamcinolone Acetonide (Inducers of CYP3A4 may reduce plasma concentrations of estrogens, possibly resulting in a decrease in therapeutic effects and/or changes in the uterine bleeding profile). Products include:
Azmacort Inhalation Aerosol **1726**
Nasacort AQ Nasal Spray **2922**

Triamcinolone Diacetate (Inducers of CYP3A4 may reduce plasma concentrations of estrogens, possibly resulting in a decrease in therapeutic effects and/or changes in the uterine bleeding profile).
No products indexed under this heading.

Triamcinolone Hexacetonide (Inducers of CYP3A4 may reduce plasma concentrations of estrogens, possibly resulting in a decrease in therapeutic effects and/or changes in the uterine bleeding profile).
No products indexed under this heading.

Troglitazone (Inducers of CYP3A4 may reduce plasma concentrations of estrogens, possibly resulting in a decrease in therapeutic effects and/or changes in the uterine bleeding profile).
No products indexed under this heading.

Troleandomycin (Inhibitors of CYP3A4 may increase plasma concentrations of estrogens and may result in side effects).
No products indexed under this heading.

Valproate Sodium (Inhibitors of CYP3A4 may increase plasma concentrations of estrogens and may result in side effects). Products include:
Depacon Injection **412**

Verapamil Hydrochloride (Inhibitors of CYP3A4 may increase plasma concentrations of estrogens and may result in side effects). Products include:
Covera-HS Tablets **3139**
Tarka Tablets **524**
Verelan PM Extended-Release Capsules, Controlled-Onset........... **3106**

Voriconazole (Inhibitors of CYP3A4 may increase plasma concentrations of estrogens and may result in side effects). Products include:
VFEND I.V. **2564**
VFEND Oral Suspension **2564**
VFEND Tablets **2564**

Zafirlukast (Inhibitors of CYP3A4 may increase plasma concentrations of estrogens and may result in side effects). Products include:
Accolate Tablets **671**

Zileuton (Inhibitors of CYP3A4 may increase plasma concentrations of estrogens and may result in side effects). Products include:
Zyflo Tablets **1023**

Food Interactions

Grapefruit (Inhibitors of CYP3A4 may increase plasma concentrations of estrogens and may result in side effects).

Grapefruit Juice (Inhibitors of CYP3A4 may increase plasma concentrations of estrogens and may result in side effects).

MENTAX CREAM

(Butenafine Hydrochloride) **2158**
None cited in PDR database.

MEPHYTON TABLETS

(Vitamin K_1) **2018**
None cited in PDR database.

MEPRON SUSPENSION

(Atovaquone) **1521**
May interact with highly protein bound drugs (selected) and certain other agents. Compounds in these categories include:

Amiodarone Hydrochloride (Atovaquone is highly bound to plasma protein (greater than 99.9%); caution is advised when co-administered with other highly protein bound drugs with narrow therapeutic indices).
No products indexed under this heading.

Amitriptyline Hydrochloride (Atovaquone is highly bound to plasma protein (greater than 99.9%); caution is advised when co-administered with other highly protein bound drugs with narrow therapeutic indices).
No products indexed under this heading.

Cefonicid Sodium (Atovaquone is highly bound to plasma protein (greater than 99.9%); caution is advised when co-administered with other highly protein bound drugs with narrow therapeutic indices).
No products indexed under this heading.

Celecoxib (Atovaquone is highly bound to plasma protein (greater than 99.9%); caution is advised when co-administered with other highly protein bound drugs with narrow therapeutic indices). Products include:
Celebrex Capsules **3134**

Chlordiazepoxide (Atovaquone is highly bound to plasma protein (greater than 99.9%); caution is advised when co-administered with other highly protein bound drugs with narrow therapeutic indices).
No products indexed under this heading.

Chlordiazepoxide Hydrochloride (Atovaquone is highly bound to plasma protein (greater than 99.9%); caution is advised when co-administered with other highly protein bound drugs with narrow therapeutic indices). Products include:
Librium Capsules **3347**

Chlorpromazine (Atovaquone is highly bound to plasma protein (greater than 99.9%); caution is advised when co-administered with other highly protein bound drugs with narrow therapeutic indices).
No products indexed under this heading.

Chlorpromazine Hydrochloride (Atovaquone is highly bound to plasma protein (greater than 99.9%); caution is advised when co-administered with other highly protein bound drugs with narrow therapeutic indices).
No products indexed under this heading.

Clomipramine Hydrochloride (Atovaquone is highly bound to plasma protein (greater than 99.9%); caution is advised when co-administered with other highly protein bound drugs with narrow therapeutic indices).
No products indexed under this heading.

Clozapine (Atovaquone is highly bound to plasma protein (greater than 99.9%); caution is advised when co-administered with other highly protein bound drugs with narrow therapeutic indices). Products include:
Clozaril Tablets **2184**
FazaClo Orally Disintegrating Tablets **551**

Cyclosporine (Atovaquone is highly bound to plasma protein (greater than 99.9%); caution is advised when co-administered with other highly protein bound drugs with narrow therapeutic indices). Products include:
Gengraf Capsules **459**
Neoral Oral Solution **2259**
Neoral Soft Gelatin Capsules **2259**
Restasis Ophthalmic Emulsion **575**
Sandimmune **2275**

Diazepam (Atovaquone is highly bound to plasma protein (greater than 99.9%); caution is advised when co-administered with other highly protein bound drugs with narrow therapeutic indices). Products include:
Diastat Rectal Delivery System **3343**
Valium Tablets **2819**

Diclofenac Potassium (Atovaquone is highly bound to plasma protein (greater than 99.9%); caution is advised when co-administered with other highly protein bound drugs with narrow therapeutic indices).
No products indexed under this heading.

Diclofenac Sodium (Atovaquone is highly bound to plasma protein (greater than 99.9%); caution is advised when co-administered with other highly protein bound drugs with narrow therapeutic indices). Products include:
Arthrotec Tablets **3129**
Voltaren Ophthalmic Solution **2309**
Voltaren Tablets **2307**
Voltaren-XR Tablets **2310**

Dipyridamole (Atovaquone is highly bound to plasma protein (greater than 99.9%); caution is advised when co-administered with other highly protein bound drugs with narrow therapeutic indices). Products include:
Aggrenox Capsules **822**
Persantine Tablets **868**

Fenoprofen Calcium (Atovaquone is highly bound to plasma protein (greater than 99.9%); caution is advised when co-administered with other highly protein bound drugs with narrow therapeutic indices). Products include:
Nalfon Capsules **2502**

Flurazepam Hydrochloride (Atovaquone is highly bound to plasma protein (greater than 99.9%); caution is advised when co-administered with other highly protein bound drugs with narrow therapeutic indices). Products include:
Dalmane Capsules **3342**

Flurbiprofen (Atovaquone is highly bound to plasma protein (greater than 99.9%); caution is advised when co-administered with other highly protein bound drugs with narrow therapeutic indices).
No products indexed under this heading.

Glipizide (Atovaquone is highly bound to plasma protein (greater than 99.9%); caution is advised when co-administered with other highly protein bound drugs with narrow therapeutic indices).
No products indexed under this heading.

Ibuprofen (Atovaquone is highly bound to plasma protein (greater than 99.9%); caution is advised when co-administered with other highly protein bound drugs with narrow therapeutic indices). Products include:
Advil Allergy Sinus Caplets .... ▣ **770**
Advil .... ▣ **674**
Children's Advil Oral Suspension .... ▣ **603**
Children's Advil Chewable Tablets .. ▣ **603**
Advil Cold & Sinus .... ▣ **723**
Infants' Advil Concentrated Drops .. ▣ **604**
Infants' Advil Concentrated Drops - White Grape (Dye-Free)............. ▣ **604**
Junior Strength Advil Swallow Tablets.. ▣ **605**
Advil Migraine Liquigels .... ▣ **608**
Advil Multi-Symptom Cold Caplets....................................... ▣ **770**
Advil PM Caplets .... ▣ **615**
Motrin IB Tablets and Caplets **1866**
Children's Motrin Oral Suspension ... **1867**
Children's Motrin Non-Staining Dye-Free Oral Suspension............ **1867**
Children's Motrin Cold Oral Suspension **1867**
Infants' Motrin Concentrated Drops **1867**
Infants' Motrin Non-Staining Dye-Free Concentrated Drops....... **1867**
Junior Strength Motrin Caplets and Chewable Tablets.................. **1867**
Vicoprofen Tablets **539**

Imipramine Hydrochloride (Atovaquone is highly bound to plasma protein (greater than 99.9%); caution is advised when co-administered with other highly protein bound drugs with narrow therapeutic indices).
No products indexed under this heading.

Imipramine Pamoate (Atovaquone is highly bound to plasma protein (greater than 99.9%); caution is advised when co-administered with other highly protein bound drugs with narrow therapeutic indices).
No products indexed under this heading.

Indomethacin (Atovaquone is highly bound to plasma protein (greater than 99.9%); caution is advised when co-administered with other highly protein bound drugs with narrow therapeutic indices). Products include:
Indocin **1995**

Indomethacin Sodium Trihydrate (Atovaquone is highly bound to plasma protein (greater than 99.9%); caution is advised when co-administered with other highly protein bound drugs with narrow therapeutic indices). Products include:
Indocin I.V. **2465**

Ketoprofen (Atovaquone is highly bound to plasma protein (greater than 99.9%); caution is advised when co-administered with other highly protein bound drugs with narrow therapeutic indices).
No products indexed under this heading.

Ketorolac Tromethamine (Atovaquone is highly bound to plasma protein (greater than 99.9%); caution is advised when co-administered with other highly protein bound drugs with narrow therapeutic indices). Products include:
- Acular Ophthalmic Solution 565
- Acular LS Ophthalmic Solution 566

Meclofenamate Sodium (Atovaquone is highly bound to plasma protein (greater than 99.9%); caution is advised when co-administered with other highly protein bound drugs with narrow therapeutic indices).
No products indexed under this heading.

Mefenamic Acid (Atovaquone is highly bound to plasma protein (greater than 99.9%); caution is advised when co-administered with other highly protein bound drugs with narrow therapeutic indices).
No products indexed under this heading.

Midazolam Hydrochloride (Atovaquone is highly bound to plasma protein (greater than 99.9%); caution is advised when co-administered with other highly protein bound drugs with narrow therapeutic indices).
No products indexed under this heading.

Naproxen (Atovaquone is highly bound to plasma protein (greater than 99.9%); caution is advised when co-administered with other highly protein bound drugs with narrow therapeutic indices). Products include:
- EC-Naprosyn Delayed-Release Tablets 2761
- Naprosyn Suspension 2761
- Naprosyn Tablets 2761
- Prevacid NapraPAC 3280

Naproxen Sodium (Atovaquone is highly bound to plasma protein (greater than 99.9%); caution is advised when co-administered with other highly protein bound drugs with narrow therapeutic indices). Products include:
- Aleve Caplets 742
- Aleve Gelcaps 743
- Aleve Tablets 743
- Aleve Cold & Sinus Caplets 744
- Anaprox Tablets 2761
- Anaprox DS Tablets 2761

Nortriptyline Hydrochloride (Atovaquone is highly bound to plasma protein (greater than 99.9%); caution is advised when co-administered with other highly protein bound drugs with narrow therapeutic indices).
No products indexed under this heading.

Oxaprozin (Atovaquone is highly bound to plasma protein (greater than 99.9%); caution is advised when co-administered with other highly protein bound drugs with narrow therapeutic indices).
No products indexed under this heading.

Oxazepam (Atovaquone is highly bound to plasma protein (greater than 99.9%); caution is advised when co-administered with other highly protein bound drugs with narrow therapeutic indices).
No products indexed under this heading.

Phenylbutazone (Atovaquone is highly bound to plasma protein (greater than 99.9%); caution is advised when co-administered with other highly protein bound drugs with narrow therapeutic indices).
No products indexed under this heading.

Piroxicam (Atovaquone is highly bound to plasma protein (greater than 99.9%); caution is advised when co-administered with other highly protein bound drugs with narrow therapeutic indices).
No products indexed under this heading.

Propranolol Hydrochloride (Atovaquone is highly bound to plasma protein (greater than 99.9%); caution is advised when co-administered with other highly protein bound drugs with narrow therapeutic indices). Products include:
- Inderal LA Long-Acting Capsules 3429
- InnoPran XL Capsules 2723

Rifabutin (Due to structural similarity to rifampin, rifabutin may decrease average steady-state plasma atovaquone concentration).
No products indexed under this heading.

Rifampin (Co-administration with oral rifampin in HIV-infected individuals may result in a 52% ± 13% decrease in the average steady-state plasma atovaquone concentration and a 37% +/- 42% increase in the average steady-state plasma rifampin concentration).
No products indexed under this heading.

Sulfamethoxazole (Co-administration with TMP-SMX may result in slight decrease in average steady-state concentrations of TMP-SMX; this effect is minor and would not expect to produce clinically significant events).
No products indexed under this heading.

Sulindac (Atovaquone is highly bound to plasma protein (greater than 99.9%); caution is advised when co-administered with other highly protein bound drugs with narrow therapeutic indices). Products include:
- Clinoril Tablets 1924

Temazepam (Atovaquone is highly bound to plasma protein (greater than 99.9%); caution is advised when co-administered with other highly protein bound drugs with narrow therapeutic indices). Products include:
- Restoril Capsules 1860

Tolbutamide (Atovaquone is highly bound to plasma protein (greater than 99.9%); caution is advised when co-administered with other highly protein bound drugs with narrow therapeutic indices).
No products indexed under this heading.

Tolmetin Sodium (Atovaquone is highly bound to plasma protein (greater than 99.9%); caution is advised when co-administered with other highly protein bound drugs with narrow therapeutic indices).
No products indexed under this heading.

Trimethoprim (Co-administration with TMP-SMX may result in slight decrease in average steady-state concentrations of TMP-SMX; this effect is minor and would not expect to produce clinically significant events).
No products indexed under this heading.

Trimipramine Maleate (Atovaquone is highly bound to plasma protein (greater than 99.9%); caution is advised when co-administered with other highly protein bound drugs with narrow therapeutic indices).
No products indexed under this heading.

Warfarin Sodium (Atovaquone is highly bound to plasma protein (greater than 99.9%); caution is advised when co-administered with other highly protein bound drugs with narrow therapeutic indices). Products include:
- Coumadin for Injection 898
- Coumadin Tablets 898

Zidovudine (Atovaquone tablets have shown to decrease zidovudine apparent oral clearance leading to an increase in plasma zidovudine AUC; this effect is minor and would not expect to produce clinically significant events). Products include:
- Combivir Tablets 1411
- Retrovir 1560
- Retrovir IV Infusion 1564
- Trizivir Tablets 1589

Food Interactions

Food, unspecified (Food enhances absorption by approximately two-fold).

MERIDIA CAPSULES

(Sibutramine Hydrochloride Monohydrate) 489

May interact with anorexiants, erythromycin, lithium preparations, monoamine oxidase inhibitors, serotoninergic agents, and certain other agents. Compounds in these categories include:

Amphetamine Resins (Concurrent use with other centrally acting appetite suppressant drugs is contraindicated).
No products indexed under this heading.

Benzphetamine Hydrochloride (Concurrent use with other centrally acting appetite suppressant drugs is contraindicated).
No products indexed under this heading.

Cimetidine (Co-administration has resulted in small increases in combined (M1 and M2 metabolites) plasma Cmax and AUC; these differences are unlikely to be of clinical significance). Products include:
- Tagamet HB 200 Tablets 664

Cimetidine Hydrochloride (Co-administration has resulted in small increases in combined (M1 and M2 metabolites) plasma Cmax and AUC; these differences are unlikely to be of clinical significance).
No products indexed under this heading.

Citalopram Hydrobromide (Sibutramine inhibits serotonin reuptake and serotonin syndrome, a rare, but serious constellation of symptoms, has been reported with the concomitant use of two SSRIs; concurrent use should be avoided). Products include:
- Celexa 1176

Dexfenfluramine Hydrochloride (Concurrent use with other centrally acting appetite suppressant drugs is contraindicated).
No products indexed under this heading.

Dextroamphetamine Sulfate (Concurrent use with other centrally acting appetite suppressant drugs is contraindicated). Products include:
- Adderall Tablets 3164
- Adderall XR Capsules 3166
- Dexedrine 1420
- DextroStat Tablets 3179

Dextromethorphan Hydrobromide (Sibutramine inhibits serotonin reuptake and combination of SSRIs and dextromethorphan has resulted in serious, sometimes fatal, reactions, serotonin syndrome). Products include:
- Comtrex Maximum Strength Cold & Cough Day/Night Caplets - Day Formulation 726
- Comtrex Maximum Strength Cold & Cough Day/Night Caplets - Night Formulation 726
- Comtrex Maximum Strength Non-Drowsy Cold & Cough Caplets 725
- Children's Dimetapp DM Cold & Cough Elixir 731
- Children's Dimetapp Long Acting Cough Plus Cold Syrup 731
- Toddler's Dimetapp Cold and Cough Drops 732
- Mucinex DM Extended-Release Bi-Layer Tablets 720
- Refenesen DM Caplets 721
- Robitussin Cough & Cold CF Liquid 735
- Robitussin Cough & Cold Long-Acting Liquid 735
- Robitussin Cough & Allergy Syrup 736
- Robitussin Cough & Cold Nighttime Liquid 736
- Robitussin Cough & Cold Pediatric Drops 735
- Robitussin Cough, Cold & Flu Nighttime Liquid 738
- Robitussin Cough & Congestion Liquid 738
- Robitussin Cough Gels Long-Acting 737
- Robitussin Cough Long Acting Liquid 739
- Robitussin Cough DM Syrup 738
- Robitussin Cough DM Infant Drops 738
- Robitussin Pediatric Cough Long Acting Liquid 739
- Robitussin Pediatric Cough & Cold Long-Acting Liquid 735
- Robitussin Pediatric Cough & Cold Nighttime Liquid 736
- Robitussin Sugar Free Cough 738
- TheraFlu Cold & Cough Hot Liquid 740
- TheraFlu Warming Relief Daytime Severe Cold 743
- TheraFlu Thin Strips Long Acting Cough 744
- Triaminic Daytime Cold & Cough Liquid 745
- Triaminic Cough & Sore Throat Liquid 747
- Triaminic Cough & Runny Nose Softchews 748
- Triaminic Thin Strips Cold & Cough 778
- Triaminic Infant Thin Strips Decongestant Plus Cough 747
- Children's Tylenol Plus Flu Oral Suspension 749
- Tylenol Cold Head Congestion Daytime Caplets with Cool Burst and Gelcaps 750

Tylenol Cold Multi-Symptom Daytime Liquid .... ▣752
Tylenol Cold Multi-Symptom Severe Daytime Liquid .... ▣752
Concentrated Tylenol Infants' Drops Plus Cold & Cough .... ▣754
Children's Tylenol Plus Cough & Runny Nose Suspension Liquid 1879
Children's Tylenol Plus Cough & Sore Throat Suspension Liquid 1879
Children's Tylenol Plus Flu Suspension Liquid 1881
Children's Tylenol Plus Multi-Symptom Cold Suspension Liquid 1879
Tylenol Cold Severe Congestion Non-Drowsy Caplets with Cool Burst 1874
Tylenol Cold Head Congestion Daytime Caplets with Cool Burst 1873
Tylenol Cold Head Congestion Nighttime Caplets with Cool Burst 1873
Tylenol Cold Head Congestion Severe Caplets with Cool Burst..... 1873
Tylenol Cold Multi-Symptom Daytime Caplets with Cool Burst and Gelcaps 1874
Tylenol Cold Multi-Symptom Daytime Liquid with Citrus Burst ... 1874
Tylenol Cold Multi-Symptom Nighttime Caplets with Cool Burst 1874
Tylenol Cold Multi-Symptom Nighttime Liquid with Cool Burst ... 1874
Tylenol Cold Multi-Symptom Severe Caplets with Cool Burst..... 1874
Tylenol Cold Multi-Symptom Severe Daytime Liquid with Citrus Burst 1874
Tylenol Cough & Sore Throat Daytime Liquid with Cool Burst...... 1877
Tylenol Cough & Sore Throat Nighttime Liquid with Cool Burst ... 1877
Concentrated Tylenol Infants' Drops Plus Cold and Cough 1879
Vicks 44 Cough Relief Liquid 2679
Vicks 44D Cough & Head Congestion Relief Liquid 2679
Vicks 44E Cough & Chest Congestion Relief Liquid 2679
Pediatric Vicks 44e Cough & Chest Congestion Relief Liquid...... 2676
Vicks 44M Cough, Cold & Flu Relief Liquid 2680
Pediatric Vicks 44m Cough & Cold Relief Liquid 2676
Vicks DayQuil LiquiCaps/Liquid Multi-Symptom Cold/Flu Relief..... ▣761
Vicks DayQuil Multi-Symptom Cold/Flu Relief LiquiCaps 2678
Vicks DayQuil Multi-Symptom Cold/Flu Relief Liquid 2678
Vicks NyQuil Multi-Symptom Cold/Flu Relief Liquid 2681
Children's Vicks NyQuil Cold/Cough Relief .... ▣756
Vicks NyQuil Multi-Symptom Cold/Flu Relief LiquiCaps 2681
Vicks NyQuil LiquiCaps/Liquid Multi-Symptom Cold/Flu Relief..... ▣763
Vicks NyQuil Cough Liquid 2680
Children's Vicks NyQuil Cold/Cough Relief Liquid 2680
Zicam Cough Max Nighttime Cough Spray .... ▣767
Zicam Cough Max Cough Spray ..... ▣767
Zicam Cough Max Cough Melts ...... ▣767
Zicam Cough Plus D Cough Spray .... ▣767
Zicam Cough Relief Cough Spray ... ▣767
Zicam Maximum Strength Flu Daytime .... ▣768
Zicam Maximum Strength Flu Nighttime .... ▣768

Dextromethorphan Polistirex (Sibutramine inhibits serotonin reuptake and combination of SSRIs and dextromethorphan has resulted in serious, sometimes fatal, reactions, serotonin syndrome). Products include:
Delsym Extended-Release Suspension 12 Hour Cough Suppressant .... ▣611

Diethylpropion Hydrochloride (Concurrent use with other centrally acting appetite suppressant drugs is contraindicated).
No products indexed under this heading.

Dihydroergotamine Mesylate (Sibutramine inhibits serotonin reuptake and combination of SSRIs and agents for migraine, such as dihydroergotamine, has resulted in serious, sometimes fatal, reactions, serotonin syndrome). Products include:
Migranal Nasal Spray 3348

Erythromycin (Co-administration has resulted in a small increase in the AUC and a small reduction in Cmax of sibutramine metabolites). Products include:
Ery-Tab Tablets 449
Erythromycin Base Filmtab Tablets 455
Erythromycin Delayed-Release Capsules, USP 457
PCE Dispertab Tablets 515

Erythromycin Estolate (Co-administration has resulted in a small increase in the AUC and a small reduction in Cmax of sibutramine metabolites).
No products indexed under this heading.

Erythromycin Ethylsuccinate (Co-administration has resulted in a small increase in the AUC and a small reduction in Cmax of sibutramine metabolites). Products include:
E.E.S. 451
EryPed 447

Erythromycin Gluceptate (Co-administration has resulted in a small increase in the AUC and a small reduction in Cmax of sibutramine metabolites).
No products indexed under this heading.

Erythromycin Lactobionate (Co-administration has resulted in a small increase in the AUC and a small reduction in Cmax of sibutramine metabolites).
No products indexed under this heading.

Erythromycin Stearate (Co-administration has resulted in a small increase in the AUC and a small reduction in Cmax of sibutramine metabolites). Products include:
Erythrocin Stearate Filmtab Tablets 453

Escitalopram Oxalate (Sibutramine inhibits serotonin reuptake and serotonin syndrome, a rare, but serious constellation of symptoms, has been reported with the concomitant use of two SSRIs; concurrent use should be avoided). Products include:
Lexapro Oral Solution 1190
Lexapro Tablets 1190

Fenfluramine Hydrochloride (Concurrent use with other centrally acting appetite suppressant drugs is contraindicated).
No products indexed under this heading.

Fentanyl (Sibutramine inhibits serotonin reuptake and combination of SSRIs and certain opioids, such as fentanyl, has resulted in serious, sometimes fatal, reactions, serotonin syndrome). Products include:
Duragesic Transdermal System 2373
Ionsys Transdermal System 2379

Fentanyl Citrate (Sibutramine inhibits serotonin reuptake and combination of SSRIs and certain opioids, such as fentanyl, has resulted in serious, sometimes fatal, reactions, serotonin syndrome). Products include:
Actiq 979

Fluoxetine Hydrochloride (Sibutramine inhibits serotonin reuptake and serotonin syndrome, a rare, but serious constellation of symptoms, has been reported with the concomitant use of two SSRIs; concurrent use should be avoided). Products include:
Prozac Pulvules and Liquid 1801
Symbyax Capsules 1819

Fluvoxamine Maleate (Sibutramine inhibits serotonin reuptake and serotonin syndrome, a rare, but serious constellation of symptoms, has been reported with the concomitant use of two SSRIs; concurrent use should be avoided).
No products indexed under this heading.

Isocarboxazid (Concurrent and/or sequential use with MAO inhibitors is contraindicated; sibutramine inhibits serotonin reuptake and combination of MAO inhibitor and serotonergic agents has resulted in serious, sometimes fatal, reactions, serotonin syndrome).
No products indexed under this heading.

Ketoconazole (Co-administration has resulted in a moderate increase in AUC and Cmax of sibutramine). Products include:
Nizoral A-D Shampoo, 1% 1868

Lithium (Sibutramine inhibits serotonin reuptake and combination of SSRIs and lithium has resulted in serious, sometimes fatal, reactions, serotonin syndrome).
No products indexed under this heading.

Lithium Carbonate (Sibutramine inhibits serotonin reuptake and combination of SSRIs and lithium has resulted in serious, sometimes fatal, reactions, serotonin syndrome). Products include:
Lithobid Tablets 1692

Lithium Citrate (Sibutramine inhibits serotonin reuptake and combination of SSRIs and lithium has resulted in serious, sometimes fatal, reactions, serotonin syndrome).
No products indexed under this heading.

Mazindol (Concurrent use with other centrally acting appetite suppressant drugs is contraindicated).
No products indexed under this heading.

Meperidine Hydrochloride (Sibutramine inhibits serotonin reuptake and combination of SSRIs and certain opioids, such as meperidine, has resulted in serious, sometimes fatal, reactions, serotonin syndrome).
No products indexed under this heading.

Methamphetamine Hydrochloride (Concurrent use with other centrally acting appetite suppressant drugs is contraindicated). Products include:
Desoxyn Tablets, USP 2462

Moclobemide (Concurrent and/or sequential use with MAO inhibitors is contraindicated; sibutramine inhibits serotonin reuptake and combination of MAO inhibitor and serotonergic agents has resulted in serious, sometimes fatal, reactions, serotonin syndrome).
No products indexed under this heading.

Pargyline Hydrochloride (Concurrent and/or sequential use with MAO inhibitors is contraindicated; sibutramine inhibits serotonin reuptake and combination of MAO inhibitor and serotonergic agents has resulted in serious, sometimes fatal, reactions, serotonin syndrome).
No products indexed under this heading.

Paroxetine Hydrochloride (Sibutramine inhibits serotonin reuptake and serotonin syndrome, a rare, but serious constellation of symptoms, has been reported with the concomitant use of two SSRIs; concurrent use should be avoided). Products include:
Paxil CR Controlled-Release Tablets 1538
Paxil 1530

Pentazocine Hydrochloride (Sibutramine inhibits serotonin reuptake and combination of SSRIs and pentazocine has resulted in serious, sometimes fatal, reactions, serotonin syndrome).
No products indexed under this heading.

Phendimetrazine Tartrate (Concurrent use with other centrally acting appetite suppressant drugs is contraindicated).
No products indexed under this heading.

Phenelzine Sulfate (Concurrent and/or sequential use with MAO inhibitors is contraindicated; sibutramine inhibits serotonin reuptake and combination of MAO inhibitor and serotonergic agents has resulted in serious, sometimes fatal, reactions, serotonin syndrome).
No products indexed under this heading.

Phenmetrazine Hydrochloride (Concurrent use with other centrally acting appetite suppressant drugs is contraindicated).
No products indexed under this heading.

Phentermine Hydrochloride (Concurrent use with other centrally acting appetite suppressant drugs is contraindicated). Products include:
Adipex-P 1215

Phentermine Resin (Concurrent use with other centrally acting appetite suppressant drugs is contraindicated).
No products indexed under this heading.

Phenylephrine Hydrochloride (Sibutramine substantially raises blood in some patients and concomitant use of sibutramine and drugs that raise blood pressure and/or heart rate, such as decongestants, requires caution). Products include:
Comtrex Maximum Strength Non-Drowsy Cold & Cough Caplets .... ▣725
Comtrex Maximum Strength Day/Night Severe Cold & Sinus Caplets - Day Formulation .... ▣725
Comtrex Maximum Strength Day/Night Severe Cold & Sinus Caplets - Night Formulation .... ▣725

Contac Cold and Flu Maximum Strength Caplets 728
Contac Cold and Flu Day and Night Caplets (Day Formulation Only) 727
Contac Cold and Flu Day and Night Caplets (Night Formulation Only) 727
Contac Cold and Flu Non-Drowsy Caplets 728
Contac-D Cold Non-Drowsy Tablets 729
Children's Dimetapp Cold & Allergy Elixir 730
Children's Dimetapp Cold & Allergy Chewable Tablets 730
Children's Dimetapp DM Cold & Cough Elixir 731
Toddler's Dimetapp Cold and Cough Drops 732
Excedrin Sinus Headache Caplets/Tablets 610
4-Way Fast Acting Nasal Spray 775
4-Way Menthol Nasal Spray 775
Preparation H Maximum Strength Cream 666
Preparation H Cooling Gel 666
Preparation H 666
Refenesen PE Caplets 721
Robitussin Cough & Allergy Syrup 736
Robitussin Cough & Cold Nighttime Liquid 736
Robitussin Cough, Cold & Flu Nighttime Liquid 738
Robitussin Head & Chest Congestion PE Syrup 739
Robitussin Pediatric Cough & Cold Nighttime Liquid 736
TheraFlu Cold & Cough Hot Liquid 740
TheraFlu Cold & Sore Throat Hot Liquid 741
TheraFlu Flu & Sore Throat Hot Liquid 742
TheraFlu Daytime Severe Cold Hot Liquid 742
TheraFlu Nighttime Severe Cold Hot Liquid 740
TheraFlu Warming Relief Daytime Severe Cold 743
TheraFlu Warming Relief Nighttime Severe Cold 743
Triaminic Chest & Nasal Congestion Liquid 746
Triaminic Cold & Allergy Liquid 746
Triaminic Daytime Cold & Cough Liquid 745
Triaminic Nighttime Cold & Cough Liquid 746
Triaminic Thin Strips Cold 748
Triaminic Thin Strips Cold & Cough 778
Triaminic Infant Thin Strips Decongestant 747
Triaminic Infant Thin Strips Decongestant Plus Cough 747
Children's Tylenol Plus Flu Oral Suspension 749
Tylenol Cold Head Congestion Daytime Caplets with Cool Burst and Gelcaps 750
Tylenol Cold Multi-Symptom Daytime Liquid 752
Tylenol Cold Multi-Symptom Severe Daytime Liquid 752
Concentrated Tylenol Infants' Drops Plus Cold & Cough 754
Tylenol Allergy Multi-Symptom Caplets with Cool Burst and Gelcaps 1872
Tylenol Allergy Multi-Symptom Nighttime Caplets with Cool Burst 1872
Children's Tylenol Plus Cold Suspension Liquid 1879
Children's Tylenol Plus Cold & Allergy Suspension Liquid 1878
Children's Tylenol Plus Flu Suspension Liquid 1881
Children's Tylenol Plus Multi-Symptom Cold Suspension Liquid 1879
Tylenol Cold Head Congestion Daytime Caplets with Cool Burst 1873
Tylenol Cold Head Congestion Nighttime Caplets with Cool Burst 1873
Tylenol Cold Head Congestion Severe Caplets with Cool Burst 1873
Tylenol Cold Multi-Symptom Daytime Caplets with Cool Burst and Gelcaps 1874
Tylenol Cold Multi-Symptom Daytime Liquid with Citrus Burst 1874
Tylenol Cold Multi-Symptom Nighttime Caplets with Cool Burst 1874
Tylenol Cold Multi-Symptom Nighttime Liquid with Cool Burst 1874
Tylenol Cold Multi-Symptom Severe Caplets with Cool Burst 1874
Tylenol Cold Multi-Symptom Severe Daytime Liquid with Citrus Burst 1874
Tylenol Sinus Congestion & Pain Daytime Caplets with Cool Burst and Gelcaps 1876
Tylenol Sinus Congestion & Pain Nighttime Caplets with Cool Burst 1876
Tylenol Sinus Congestion & Pain Severe Caplets with Cool Burst 1876
Vicks 44D Cough & Head Congestion Relief Liquid 760
Vicks DayQuil LiquiCaps/Liquid Multi-Symptom Cold/Flu Relief 761
Zicam Cough Plus D Cough Spray 767

Phenylephrine Tannate (Sibutramine substantially raises blood in some patients and concomitant use of sibutramine and drugs that raise blood pressure and/or heart rate, such as decongestants, requires caution).
No products indexed under this heading.

Phenylpropanolamine Hydrochloride (Sibutramine substantially raises blood in some patients and concomitant use of sibutramine and drugs that raise blood pressure and/or heart rate, such as decongestants, requires caution).
No products indexed under this heading.

Procarbazine Hydrochloride (Concurrent and/or sequential use with MAO inhibitors is contraindicated; sibutramine inhibits serotonin reuptake and combination of MAO inhibitor and serotonergic agents has resulted in serious, sometimes fatal, reactions, serotonin syndrome). Products include:
Matulane Capsules 3191

Pseudoephedrine Hydrochloride (Sibutramine substantially raises blood in some patients and concomitant use of sibutramine and drugs that raise blood pressure and/or heart rate, such as decongestants, requires caution). Products include:
Advil Allergy Sinus Caplets 770
Advil Cold & Sinus 723
Advil Multi-Symptom Cold Caplets 770
Aleve Cold & Sinus Caplets 744
Allegra-D 12 Hour Extended-Release Tablets 2846
Allegra-D 24 Hour Extended-Release Tablets 2849
BC Cold Powder 677
Comtrex Maximum Strength Cold & Cough Day/Night Caplets - Day Formulation 726
Comtrex Maximum Strength Cold & Cough Day/Night Caplets - Night Formulation 726
Children's Motrin Cold Oral Suspension 1867
Mucinex D Extended-Release Bi-Layer Tablets 776
Robitussin Cough & Cold CF Liquid 735
Robitussin Cough & Cold Pediatric Drops 735
Tylenol Sinus Congestion & Pain Nighttime Caplets with Cool Burst 778
Tylenol Cold Severe Congestion Non-Drowsy Caplets with Cool Burst 1874
Tylenol Sinus Severe Congestion Caplets with Cool Burst 1876
Vicks 44D Cough & Head Congestion Relief Liquid 2679
Vicks 44M Cough, Cold & Flu Relief Liquid 2680
Vicks DayQuil Multi-Symptom Cold/Flu Relief LiquiCaps 2678
Vicks DayQuil Multi-Symptom Cold/Flu Relief Liquid 2678
Vicks NyQuil Multi-Symptom Cold/Flu Relief Liquid 2681
Vicks NyQuil Multi-Symptom Cold/Flu Relief LiquiCaps 2681
Children's Vicks NyQuil Cold/Cough Relief Liquid 2680
Zyrtec-D 12 Hour Extended Release Tablets 2597

Pseudoephedrine Sulfate (Sibutramine substantially raises blood in some patients and concomitant use of sibutramine and drugs that raise blood pressure and/or heart rate, such as decongestants, requires caution). Products include:
Alavert Allergy & Sinus D-12 Hour Tablets 771
Clarinex-D 24-Hour Extended-Release Tablets 2998
Claritin-D Non-Drowsy 12 Hour Tablets 772
Claritin-D Non-Drowsy 24 Hour Tablets 772

Selegiline Hydrochloride (Concurrent and/or sequential use with MAO inhibitors is contraindicated; sibutramine inhibits serotonin reuptake and combination of MAO inhibitor and serotonergic agents has resulted in serious, sometimes fatal, reactions, serotonin syndrome). Products include:
Eldepryl Capsules 3208
Zelapar Tablets 3372

Sertraline Hydrochloride (Sibutramine inhibits serotonin reuptake and serotonin syndrome, a rare, but serious constellation of symptoms, has been reported with the concomitant use of two SSRIs; concurrent use should be avoided). Products include:
Zoloft 2586

Sumatriptan (Sibutramine inhibits serotonin reuptake and combination of SSRIs and agents for migraine, such as sumatriptan, has resulted in serious, sometimes fatal, reactions, serotonin syndrome). Products include:
Imitrex Nasal Spray 1467

Sumatriptan Succinate (Sibutramine inhibits serotonin reuptake and combination of SSRIs and agents for migraine, such as sumatriptan, has resulted in serious, sometimes fatal, reactions, serotonin syndrome). Products include:
Imitrex Injection 1463
Imitrex Tablets 1471

Tranylcypromine Sulfate (Concurrent and/or sequential use with MAO inhibitors is contraindicated; sibutramine inhibits serotonin reuptake and combination of MAO inhibitor and serotonergic agents has resulted in serious, sometimes fatal, reactions, serotonin syndrome). Products include:
Parnate Tablets 1527

L-Tryptophan (Sibutramine inhibits serotonin reuptake and combination of SSRIs and tryptophan has resulted in serious, sometimes fatal, reactions, serotonin syndrome). Products include:
L-Tryptophan Capsules 2145

Venlafaxine Hydrochloride (Sibutramine inhibits serotonin reuptake and serotonin syndrome, a rare, but serious constellation of symptoms, has been reported with the concomitant use of two SSRIs; concurrent use should be avoided). Products include:
Effexor Tablets 3411
Effexor XR Capsules 3417

Food Interactions

Alcohol (Concurrent use has not resulted in psychomotor reactions of clinical significance, however, concomitant use with excessive alcohol is not recommended).

Food, unspecified (Co-administration with a standard breakfast has resulted in reduced peak M1 and M2 amine concentrations and delayed the time to peak by approximately three hours; the AUCs of M1 and M2 were not significantly altered).

MERREM I.V.
(Meropenem) 686
May interact with:

Probenecid (Competes with meropenem for active tubular secretion and, thus, inhibits the renal excretion of meropenem. Statistically significant increases in the elimination half-life and the extent of systemic exposure have been reported; co-administration is not recommended).
No products indexed under this heading.

MERUVAX II
(Rubella Virus Vaccine Live) 2019
May interact with immunosuppressive agents. Compounds in these categories include:

Azathioprine (Concurrent immunosuppressive therapy is contraindicated).
No products indexed under this heading.

Basiliximab (Concurrent immunosuppressive therapy is contraindicated). Products include:
Simulect for Injection 2284

Cyclosporine (Concurrent immunosuppressive therapy is contraindicated). Products include:
Gengraf Capsules 459
Neoral Oral Solution 2259
Neoral Soft Gelatin Capsules 2259
Restasis Ophthalmic Emulsion 575
Sandimmune 2275

Muromonab-CD3 (Concurrent immunosuppressive therapy is contraindicated). Products include:
Orthoclone OKT3 Sterile Solution 2360

Mycophenolate Mofetil (Concurrent immunosuppressive therapy is contraindicated). Products include:
CellCept Capsules 2747
CellCept Oral Suspension 2747
CellCept Tablets 2747

Sirolimus (Concurrent immunosuppressive therapy is contraindicated). Products include:
Rapamune Oral Solution and Tablets 3475

Tacrolimus (Concurrent immunosuppressive therapy is contraindicated). Products include:
Prograf Capsules and Injection 632
Protopic Ointment 638

METADATE CD CAPSULES

(Methylphenidate Hydrochloride) 3323
May interact with oral anticoagulants, monoamine oxidase inhibitors, phenytoin, selective serotonin reuptake inhibitors, tricyclic antidepressants, vasopressors, and certain other agents. Compounds in these categories include:

Amitriptyline Hydrochloride
(Methylphenidate may inhibit the metabolism of tricyclic antidepressants; downward dosage adjustment of tricyclic antidepressants may be required).
 No products indexed under this heading.

Amoxapine (Methylphenidate may inhibit the metabolism of tricyclic antidepressants; downward dosage adjustment of tricyclic antidepressants may be required).
 No products indexed under this heading.

Anisindione (Methylphenidate may inhibit the metabolism of coumarin anticoagulants; downward dosage adjustment of anticoagulants may be required). Products include:
 Miradon Tablets 3042

Citalopram Hydrobromide (Methylphenidate may inhibit the metabolism of selective serotonin reuptake inhibitors; downward dosage adjustment of SSRI may be required). Products include:
 Celexa .. 1176

Clomipramine Hydrochloride
(Methylphenidate may inhibit the metabolism of tricyclic antidepressants; downward dosage adjustment of tricyclic antidepressants may be required).
 No products indexed under this heading.

Clonidine (Co-administration has resulted in serious adverse events; the safety of this combination has not been systemically established). Products include:
 Catapres-TTS 844

Clonidine Hydrochloride (Co-administration has resulted in serious adverse events; the safety of this combination has not been systemically established). Products include:
 Catapres Tablets 843
 Clorpres Tablets 2153

Desipramine Hydrochloride
(Methylphenidate may inhibit the metabolism of tricyclic antidepressants; downward dosage adjustment of tricyclic antidepressants may be required).
 No products indexed under this heading.

Dicumarol (Methylphenidate may inhibit the metabolism of coumarin anticoagulants; downward dosage adjustment of anticoagulants may be required).
 No products indexed under this heading.

Dobutamine (Methylphenidate causes rise in blood pressure; co-administration with other pressor agents should be undertaken with caution).
 No products indexed under this heading.

Dobutamine Hydrochloride
(Methylphenidate causes rise in blood pressure; co-administration with other pressor agents should be undertaken with caution).
 No products indexed under this heading.

Dopamine Hydrochloride (Methylphenidate causes rise in blood pressure; co-administration with other pressor agents should be undertaken with caution).
 No products indexed under this heading.

Doxepin Hydrochloride (Methylphenidate may inhibit the metabolism of tricyclic antidepressants; downward dosage adjustment of tricyclic antidepressants may be required).
 No products indexed under this heading.

Ephedrine Sulfate (Methylphenidate causes rise in blood pressure; co-administration with other pressor agents should be undertaken with caution).
 No products indexed under this heading.

Epinephrine Bitartrate (Methylphenidate causes rise in blood pressure; co-administration with other pressor agents should be undertaken with caution).
 No products indexed under this heading.

Epinephrine Hydrochloride
(Methylphenidate causes rise in blood pressure; co-administration with other pressor agents should be undertaken with caution).
 No products indexed under this heading.

Escitalopram Oxalate (Methylphenidate may inhibit the metabolism of selective serotonin reuptake inhibitors; downward dosage adjustment of SSRI may be required). Products include:
 Lexapro Oral Solution 1190
 Lexapro Tablets 1190

Fluoxetine Hydrochloride (Methylphenidate may inhibit the metabolism of selective serotonin reuptake inhibitors; downward dosage adjustment of SSRI may be required). Products include:
 Prozac Pulvules and Liquid 1801
 Symbyax Capsules 1819

Fluvoxamine Maleate (Methylphenidate may inhibit the metabolism of selective serotonin reuptake inhibitors; downward dosage adjustment of SSRI may be required).
 No products indexed under this heading.

Fosphenytoin Sodium (Methylphenidate may inhibit the metabolism of anticonvulsants, such as phenytoin; additionally methylphenidate may lower the convulsive threshold in patients with prior history of seizures).
 No products indexed under this heading.

Guanethidine Monosulfate (Methylphenidate may decrease the hypotensive effect of guanethidine).
 No products indexed under this heading.

Imipramine Hydrochloride (Methylphenidate may inhibit the metabolism of tricyclic antidepressants; downward dosage adjustment of tricyclic antidepressants may be required).
 No products indexed under this heading.

Imipramine Pamoate (Methylphenidate may inhibit the metabolism of tricyclic antidepressants; downward dosage adjustment of tricyclic antidepressants may be required).
 No products indexed under this heading.

Isocarboxazid (Co-administration is contraindicated during treatment with monoamine oxidase inhibitors, and also within a minimum of 14 days following discontinuation of a monoamine oxidase inhibitor (hypertensive crises may result).).
 No products indexed under this heading.

Isoproterenol Hydrochloride (Methylphenidate causes rise in blood pressure; co-administration with other pressor agents should be undertaken with caution).
 No products indexed under this heading.

Isoproterenol Sulfate (Methylphenidate causes rise in blood pressure; co-administration with other pressor agents should be undertaken with caution).
 No products indexed under this heading.

Maprotiline Hydrochloride (Methylphenidate may inhibit the metabolism of tricyclic antidepressants; downward dosage adjustment of tricyclic antidepressants may be required).
 No products indexed under this heading.

Mephentermine Sulfate (Methylphenidate causes rise in blood pressure; co-administration with other pressor agents should be undertaken with caution).
 No products indexed under this heading.

Metaraminol Bitartrate (Methylphenidate causes rise in blood pressure; co-administration with other pressor agents should be undertaken with caution).
 No products indexed under this heading.

Methoxamine Hydrochloride
(Methylphenidate causes rise in blood pressure; co-administration with other pressor agents should be undertaken with caution).
 No products indexed under this heading.

Moclobemide (Co-administration is contraindicated during treatment with monoamine oxidase inhibitors, and also within a minimum of 14 days following discontinuation of a monoamine oxidase inhibitor (hypertensive crises may result).).
 No products indexed under this heading.

Norepinephrine Bitartrate (Methylphenidate causes rise in blood pressure; co-administration with other pressor agents should be undertaken with caution).
 No products indexed under this heading.

Nortriptyline Hydrochloride
(Methylphenidate may inhibit the metabolism of tricyclic antidepressants; downward dosage adjustment of tricyclic antidepressants may be required).
 No products indexed under this heading.

Pargyline Hydrochloride (Co-administration is contraindicated during treatment with monoamine oxidase inhibitors, and also within a minimum of 14 days following discontinuation of a monoamine oxidase inhibitor (hypertensive crises may result).).
 No products indexed under this heading.

Paroxetine Hydrochloride (Methylphenidate may inhibit the metabolism of selective serotonin reuptake inhibitors; downward dosage adjustment of SSRI may be required). Products include:
 Paxil CR Controlled-Release Tablets ... 1538
 Paxil ... 1530

Phenelzine Sulfate (Co-administration is contraindicated during treatment with monoamine oxidase inhibitors, and also within a minimum of 14 days following discontinuation of a monoamine oxidase inhibitor (hypertensive crises may result).).
 No products indexed under this heading.

Phenobarbital (Methylphenidate may inhibit the metabolism of anticonvulsants, such as phenobarbital; additionally methylphenidate may lower the convulsive threshold in patients with prior history of seizures). Products include:
 Donnatal Extentabs 2493

Phenylephrine Hydrochloride
(Methylphenidate causes rise in blood pressure; co-administration with other pressor agents should be undertaken with caution). Products include:
 Comtrex Maximum Strength Non-Drowsy Cold & Cough Caplets.. ▣ 725
 Comtrex Maximum Strength Day/Night Severe Cold & Sinus Caplets - Day Formulation ▣ 725
 Comtrex Maximum Strength Day/Night Severe Cold & Sinus Caplets - Night Formulation ▣ 725
 Contac Cold and Flu Maximum Strength Caplets ▣ 728
 Contac Cold and Flu Day and Night Caplets (Day Formulation Only) ▣ 727
 Contac Cold and Flu Day and Night Caplets (Night Formulation Only) ▣ 727
 Contac Cold and Flu Non-Drowsy Caplets.................................... ▣ 728
 Contac-D Cold Non-Drowsy Tablets....................................... ▣ 729
 Children's Dimetapp Cold & Allergy Elixir................................ ▣ 730
 Children's Dimetapp Cold & Allergy Chewable Tablets............ ▣ 730
 Children's Dimetapp DM Cold & Cough Elixir ▣ 731
 Toddler's Dimetapp Cold and Cough Drops ▣ 732
 Excedrin Sinus Headache Caplets/Tablets......................... ▣ 610
 4-Way Fast Acting Nasal Spray ▣ 775
 4-Way Menthol Nasal Spray ▣ 775
 Preparation H Maximum Strength Cream ... ▣ 666
 Preparation H Cooling Gel ▣ 666
 Preparation H ▣ 666
 Refenesen PE Caplets ▣ 721
 Robitussin Cough & Allergy Syrup .. ▣ 736

Robitussin Cough & Cold Nighttime Liquid 736
Robitussin Cough, Cold & Flu Nighttime Liquid 738
Robitussin Head & Chest Congestion PE Syrup 739
Robitussin Pediatric Cough & Cold Nighttime Liquid 736
TheraFlu Cold & Cough Hot Liquid 740
TheraFlu Cold & Sore Throat Hot Liquid 741
TheraFlu Flu & Sore Throat Hot Liquid 742
TheraFlu Daytime Severe Cold Hot Liquid 742
TheraFlu Nighttime Severe Cold Hot Liquid 740
TheraFlu Warming Relief Daytime Severe Cold 743
TheraFlu Warming Relief Nighttime Severe Cold 743
Triaminic Chest & Nasal Congestion Liquid 746
Triaminic Cold & Allergy Liquid 746
Triaminic Daytime Cold & Cough Liquid 745
Triaminic Nighttime Cold & Cough Liquid 746
Triaminic Thin Strips Cold 748
Triaminic Thin Strips Cold & Cough 778
Triaminic Infant Thin Strips Decongestant 747
Triaminic Infant Thin Strips Decongestant Plus Cough 747
Children's Tylenol Plus Flu Oral Suspension 749
Tylenol Cold Head Congestion Daytime Caplets with Cool Burst and Gelcaps 750
Tylenol Cold Multi-Symptom Daytime Liquid 752
Tylenol Cold Multi-Symptom Severe Daytime Liquid 752
Concentrated Tylenol Infants' Drops Plus Cold & Cough 754
Tylenol Allergy Multi-Symptom Caplets with Cool Burst and Gelcaps 1872
Tylenol Allergy Multi-Symptom Nighttime Caplets with Cool Burst 1872
Children's Tylenol Plus Cold Suspension Liquid 1879
Children's Tylenol Plus Cold & Allergy Suspension Liquid 1878
Children's Tylenol Plus Flu Suspension Liquid 1881
Children's Tylenol Plus Multi-Symptom Cold Suspension Liquid 1879
Tylenol Cold Head Congestion Daytime Caplets with Cool Burst 1873
Tylenol Cold Head Congestion Nighttime Caplets with Cool Burst 1873
Tylenol Cold Head Congestion Severe Caplets with Cool Burst 1873
Tylenol Cold Multi-Symptom Daytime Caplets with Cool Burst and Gelcaps 1874
Tylenol Cold Multi-Symptom Daytime Liquid with Citrus Burst 1874
Tylenol Cold Multi-Symptom Nighttime Caplets with Cool Burst 1874
Tylenol Cold Multi-Symptom Nighttime Liquid with Cool Burst 1874
Tylenol Cold Multi-Symptom Severe Caplets with Cool Burst 1874
Tylenol Cold Multi-Symptom Severe Daytime Liquid with Citrus Burst 1874
Tylenol Sinus Congestion & Pain Daytime Caplets with Cool Burst and Gelcaps 1876
Tylenol Sinus Congestion & Pain Nighttime Caplets with Cool Burst 1876
Tylenol Sinus Congestion & Pain Severe Caplets with Cool Burst 1876
Vicks 44D Cough & Head Congestion Relief Liquid 760
Vicks DayQuil LiquiCaps/Liquid Multi-Symptom Cold/Flu Relief 761
Zicam Cough Plus D Cough Spray 767

Phenytoin (Methylphenidate may inhibit the metabolism of anticonvulsants, such as phenytoin; additionally methylphenidate may lower the convulsive threshold in patients with prior history of seizures).
No products indexed under this heading.

Phenytoin Sodium (Methylphenidate may inhibit the metabolism of anticonvulsants, such as phenytoin; additionally methylphenidate may lower the convulsive threshold in patients with prior history of seizures). Products include:
Phenytek Capsules 2160

Primidone (Methylphenidate may inhibit the metabolism of anticonvulsants, such as primidone; additionally methylphenidate may lower the convulsive threshold in patients with prior history of seizures).
No products indexed under this heading.

Procarbazine Hydrochloride (Co-administration is contraindicated during treatment with monoamine oxidase inhibitors, and also within a minimum of 14 days following discontinuation of a monoamine oxidase inhibitor (hypertensive crises may result)). Products include:
Matulane Capsules 3191

Protriptyline Hydrochloride (Methylphenidate may inhibit the metabolism of tricyclic antidepressants; downward dosage adjustment of tricyclic antidepressants may be required).
No products indexed under this heading.

Selegiline Hydrochloride (Co-administration is contraindicated during treatment with monoamine oxidase inhibitors, and also within a minimum of 14 days following discontinuation of a monoamine oxidase inhibitor (hypertensive crises may result)). Products include:
Eldepryl Capsules 3208
Zelapar Tablets 3372

Sertraline Hydrochloride (Methylphenidate may inhibit the metabolism of selective serotonin reuptake inhibitors; downward dosage adjustment of SSRI may be required). Products include:
Zoloft 2586

Tranylcypromine Sulfate (Co-administration is contraindicated during treatment with monoamine oxidase inhibitors, and also within a minimum of 14 days following discontinuation of a monoamine oxidase inhibitor (hypertensive crises may result)). Products include:
Parnate Tablets 1527

Trimipramine Maleate (Methylphenidate may inhibit the metabolism of tricyclic antidepressants; downward dosage adjustment of tricyclic antidepressants may be required).
No products indexed under this heading.

Venlafaxine Hydrochloride (Co-administration in a patient on methylphenidate for 18 months has resulted in neuroleptic malignant syndrome within 45 minutes of ingesting his first dose of venlafaxine). Products include:
Effexor Tablets 3411
Effexor XR Capsules 3417

Warfarin Sodium (Methylphenidate may inhibit the metabolism of coumarin anticoagulants; downward dosage adjustment of anticoagulants may be required). Products include:
Coumadin for Injection 898
Coumadin Tablets 898

METAMUCIL CAPSULES
(Psyllium Preparations) 2675
None cited in PDR database.

METAMUCIL COARSE MILLED UNFLAVORED POWDER
(Psyllium Preparations) 2675
None cited in PDR database.

METAMUCIL COARSE MILLED ORANGE FLAVOR POWDER
(Psyllium Preparations) 2675
None cited in PDR database.

METAMUCIL DIETARY FIBER SUPPLEMENT
(Psyllium Preparations) 650
None cited in PDR database.

METAMUCIL SMOOTH TEXTURE ORANGE FLAVOR POWDER
(Psyllium Preparations) 2675
None cited in PDR database.

METAMUCIL SMOOTH TEXTURE SUGAR-FREE UNFLAVORED POWDER
(Psyllium Preparations) 2675
None cited in PDR database.

METAMUCIL SMOOTH TEXTURE SUGAR-FREE ORANGE FLAVOR POWDER
(Psyllium Preparations) 2675
None cited in PDR database.

METAMUCIL WAFERS, APPLE AND CINNAMON FLAVORS
(Psyllium Preparations) 2675
None cited in PDR database.

METROGEL 1%
(Metronidazole) 1211
May interact with oral anticoagulants. Compounds in these categories include:

Anisindione (Prolonged prothrombin time and potentiation of oral anticoagulant with oral metronidazole; the effect of topical metronidazole on prothrombin time is unknown). Products include:
Miradon Tablets 3042

Dicumarol (Prolonged prothrombin time and potentiation of oral anticoagulant with oral metronidazole; the effect of topical metronidazole on prothrombin time is unknown).
No products indexed under this heading.

Warfarin Sodium (Prolonged prothrombin time and potentiation of oral anticoagulant with oral metronidazole; the effect of topical metronidazole on prothrombin time is unknown). Products include:
Coumadin for Injection 898
Coumadin Tablets 898

METROGEL-VAGINAL GEL
(Metronidazole) 1855
May interact with oral anticoagulants and certain other agents. Compounds in these categories include:

Anisindione (Oral metronidazole potentiates the anticoagulant effect of warfarin). Products include:
Miradon Tablets 3042

Dicumarol (Oral metronidazole potentiates the anticoagulant effect of warfarin).
No products indexed under this heading.

Disulfiram (Psychotic reactions to oral metronidazole have been reported in alcoholics who are using metronidazole and disulfiram concurrently).
No products indexed under this heading.

Warfarin Sodium (Oral metronidazole potentiates the anticoagulant effect of warfarin). Products include:
Coumadin for Injection 898
Coumadin Tablets 898

Food Interactions

Alcohol (Possibility of a disulfiram-like reaction).

MEVACOR TABLETS
(Lovastatin) 2021
May interact with azole antifungals, oral anticoagulants, cytochrome p450 3a4 inhibitors (selected), erythromycin, fibrates, protease inhibitors, and certain other agents. Compounds in these categories include:

Acetazolamide (The risk of myopathy/rhabdomyolysis is increased by concomitant use of lovastatin with potent inhibitors of CYP3A4, particularly with higher doses of lovastatin; concomitant use should be avoided unless the benefits of combined therapy outweigh the increased risk).
No products indexed under this heading.

Amiodarone Hydrochloride (The combined use of lovastatin at doses higher than 40 mg daily with amiodarone should be avoided unless the clinical benefit is likely to outweigh the increased risk of myopathy).
No products indexed under this heading.

Amprenavir (The risk of myopathy/rhabdomyolysis is increased by concomitant use of lovastatin with potent inhibitors of CYP3A4, particularly with higher doses of lovastatin; concomitant use should be avoided unless the benefits of combined therapy outweigh the increased risk). Products include:
Agenerase Capsules 1327
Agenerase Oral Solution 1332

Anastrozole (The risk of myopathy/rhabdomyolysis is increased by concomitant use of lovastatin with potent inhibitors of CYP3A4, particularly with higher doses of lovastatin; concomitant use should be avoided unless the benefits of combined therapy outweigh the increased risk). Products include:
Arimidex Tablets 673

Anisindione (Co-administration has resulted in bleeding and/or increased prothrombin time in few patients). Products include:
Miradon Tablets 3042

Aprepitant (The risk of myopathy/rhabdomyolysis is increased by concomitant use of lovastatin with potent inhibitors of CYP3A4, particularly with higher doses of lovastatin; concomitant use should be avoided unless the benefits of combined therapy outweigh the increased risk). Products include:
Emend Capsules 1963

Cimetidine (The risk of myopathy/rhabdomyolysis is increased by concomitant use of lovastatin with potent inhibitors of CYP3A4, particularly with higher doses of lovastatin; concomitant use should be avoided unless the benefits of combined therapy outweigh the increased risk). Products include:
- Tagamet HB 200 Tablets .... ▣ 664

Cimetidine Hydrochloride (The risk of myopathy/rhabdomyolysis is increased by concomitant use of lovastatin with potent inhibitors of CYP3A4, particularly with higher doses of lovastatin; concomitant use should be avoided unless the benefits of combined therapy outweigh the increased risk).
No products indexed under this heading.

Ciprofloxacin (The risk of myopathy/rhabdomyolysis is increased by concomitant use of lovastatin with potent inhibitors of CYP3A4, particularly with higher doses of lovastatin; concomitant use should be avoided unless the benefits of combined therapy outweigh the increased risk). Products include:
- Cipro Oral Suspension 2977
- Cipro I.V. 2984
- Cipro XR Tablets 2990
- Ciprodex Otic Suspension 559

Clarithromycin (The risk of myopathy appears to be increased by high levels of HMG-CoA reductase inhibitory activity in plasma; lovastatin is metabolized by CYP3A4 isoenzyme, certain agents, such as macrolide antibiotics clarithromycin, share this metabolic pathway and can raise the plasma levels of lovastatin and may increase the risk of myopathy). Products include:
- Biaxin/Biaxin XL 402
- PREVPAC 3284

Clofibrate (The incidence and severity of myopathy are increased by co-administration of HMG-CoA reductase inhibitors with drugs that cause myopathy when given alone, such as fibrates; combined use should be avoided; if used concurrently, the dose of lovastatin should generally not exceed 20 mg).
No products indexed under this heading.

Clotrimazole (The risk of myopathy appears to be increased by high levels of HMG-CoA reductase inhibitory activity in plasma; lovastatin is metabolized by CYP3A4 isoenzyme, certain agents, such as azole antifungals, share this metabolic pathway and can raise the plasma levels of lovastatin and may increase the risk of myopathy). Products include:
- Desenex Athlete's Foot Cream .... ▣ 635
- Lotrimin 3039
- Lotrisone 3040

Cyclosporine (The risk of myopathy appears to be increased by high levels of HMG-CoA reductase inhibitory activity in plasma; lovastatin is metabolized by CYP3A4 isoenzyme, certain agents, such as cyclosporine, share this metabolic pathway and can raise the plasma levels of lovastatin and may increase the risk of myopathy; the dose of lovastatin should generally not exceed 20 mg if used concomitantly). Products include:
- Gengraf Capsules 459
- Neoral Oral Solution 2259
- Neoral Soft Gelatin Capsules 2259
- Restasis Ophthalmic Emulsion 575
- Sandimmune 2275

Dalfopristin (The risk of myopathy/rhabdomyolysis is increased by concomitant use of lovastatin with potent inhibitors of CYP3A4, particularly with higher doses of lovastatin; concomitant use should be avoided unless the benefits of combined therapy outweigh the increased risk).
No products indexed under this heading.

Danazol (The risk of rhabdomyolysis/myopathy is increased by concomitant administration of danazol, particularly with higher doses of lovastatin. The dose of lovastatin should not exceed 20 mg daily in patients receiving concomitant medication with danazol).
No products indexed under this heading.

Delavirdine Mesylate (The risk of myopathy/rhabdomyolysis is increased by concomitant use of lovastatin with potent inhibitors of CYP3A4, particularly with higher doses of lovastatin; concomitant use should be avoided unless the benefits of combined therapy outweigh the increased risk). Products include:
- Rescriptor Tablets 2551

Dicumarol (Co-administration has resulted in bleeding and/or increased prothrombin time in few patients).
No products indexed under this heading.

Diltiazem Hydrochloride (The risk of myopathy/rhabdomyolysis is increased by concomitant use of lovastatin with potent inhibitors of CYP3A4, particularly with higher doses of lovastatin; concomitant use should be avoided unless the benefits of combined therapy outweigh the increased risk). Products include:
- Cardizem LA Extended Release Tablets 1728
- Tiazac Capsules 1201

Diltiazem Maleate (The risk of myopathy/rhabdomyolysis is increased by concomitant use of lovastatin with potent inhibitors of CYP3A4, particularly with higher doses of lovastatin; concomitant use should be avoided unless the benefits of combined therapy outweigh the increased risk).
No products indexed under this heading.

Efavirenz (The risk of myopathy/rhabdomyolysis is increased by concomitant use of lovastatin with potent inhibitors of CYP3A4, particularly with higher doses of lovastatin; concomitant use should be avoided unless the benefits of combined therapy outweigh the increased risk). Products include:
- Atripla Tablets 945
- Sustiva Capsules 930
- Sustiva Tablets 930

Erythromycin (The risk of myopathy/rhabdomyolysis is increased by concomitant use of lovastatin with potent inhibitors of CYP3A4, particularly with higher doses of lovastatin; concomitant use should be avoided unless the benefits of combined therapy outweigh the increased risk). Products include:
- Ery-Tab Tablets 449
- Erythromycin Base Filmtab Tablets 455
- Erythromycin Delayed-Release Capsules, USP 457
- PCE Dispertab Tablets 515

Erythromycin Estolate (The risk of myopathy/rhabdomyolysis is increased by concomitant use of lovastatin with potent inhibitors of CYP3A4, particularly with higher doses of lovastatin; concomitant use should be avoided unless the benefits of combined therapy outweigh the increased risk).
No products indexed under this heading.

Erythromycin Ethylsuccinate (The risk of myopathy/rhabdomyolysis is increased by concomitant use of lovastatin with potent inhibitors of CYP3A4, particularly with higher doses of lovastatin; concomitant use should be avoided unless the benefits of combined therapy outweigh the increased risk). Products include:
- E.E.S. 451
- EryPed 447

Erythromycin Gluceptate (The risk of myopathy/rhabdomyolysis is increased by concomitant use of lovastatin with potent inhibitors of CYP3A4, particularly with higher doses of lovastatin; concomitant use should be avoided unless the benefits of combined therapy outweigh the increased risk).
No products indexed under this heading.

Erythromycin Lactobionate (The risk of myopathy/rhabdomyolysis is increased by concomitant use of lovastatin with potent inhibitors of CYP3A4, particularly with higher doses of lovastatin; concomitant use should be avoided unless the benefits of combined therapy outweigh the increased risk).
No products indexed under this heading.

Erythromycin Stearate (The risk of myopathy/rhabdomyolysis is increased by concomitant use of lovastatin with potent inhibitors of CYP3A4, particularly with higher doses of lovastatin; concomitant use should be avoided unless the benefits of combined therapy outweigh the increased risk). Products include:
- Erythrocin Stearate Filmtab Tablets 453

Esomeprazole Magnesium (The risk of myopathy/rhabdomyolysis is increased by concomitant use of lovastatin with potent inhibitors of CYP3A4, particularly with higher doses of lovastatin; concomitant use should be avoided unless the benefits of combined therapy outweigh the increased risk). Products include:
- Nexium Delayed-Release Capsules 655

Fenofibrate (The incidence and severity of myopathy are increased by co-administration of HMG-CoA reductase inhibitors with drugs that cause myopathy when given alone, such as fibrates; combined use should be avoided; if used concurrently, the dose of lovastatin should generally not exceed 20 mg). Products include:
- Lofibra Tablets 1219
- Lofibra Capsules 1216
- Tricor Tablets 527
- Triglide Tablets 3123

Fluconazole (The risk of myopathy appears to be increased by high levels of HMG-CoA reductase inhibitory activity in plasma; lovastatin is metabolized by CYP3A4 isoenzyme, certain agents, such as azole antifungals, share this metabolic pathway and can raise the plasma levels of lovastatin and may increase the risk of myopathy).
No products indexed under this heading.

Fluoxetine Hydrochloride (The risk of myopathy/rhabdomyolysis is increased by concomitant use of lovastatin with potent inhibitors of CYP3A4, particularly with higher doses of lovastatin; concomitant use should be avoided unless the benefits of combined therapy outweigh the increased risk). Products include:
- Prozac Pulvules and Liquid 1801
- Symbyax Capsules 1819

Fluvoxamine Maleate (The risk of myopathy/rhabdomyolysis is increased by concomitant use of lovastatin with potent inhibitors of CYP3A4, particularly with higher doses of lovastatin; concomitant use should be avoided unless the benefits of combined therapy outweigh the increased risk).
No products indexed under this heading.

Fosamprenavir Calcium (The risk of myopathy/rhabdomyolysis is increased by concomitant use of lovastatin with potent inhibitors of CYP3A4, particularly with higher doses of lovastatin; concomitant use should be avoided unless the benefits of combined therapy outweigh the increased risk). Products include:
- Lexiva Tablets 1505

Gemfibrozil (The incidence and severity of myopathy are increased by co-administration of HMG-CoA reductase inhibitors with drugs that cause myopathy when given alone, such as fibrates; combined use should be avoided; if used concurrently, the dose of lovastatin should generally not exceed 20 mg).
No products indexed under this heading.

Indinavir Sulfate (The risk of myopathy/rhabdomyolysis is increased by concomitant use of lovastatin with potent inhibitors of CYP3A4, particularly with higher doses of lovastatin; concomitant use should be avoided unless the benefits of combined therapy outweigh the increased risk). Products include:
- Crixivan Capsules 1940

Isoniazid (The risk of myopathy/rhabdomyolysis is increased by concomitant use of lovastatin with potent inhibitors of CYP3A4, particularly with higher doses of lovastatin; concomitant use should be avoided unless the benefits of combined therapy outweigh the increased risk).
No products indexed under this heading.

Itraconazole (The risk of myopathy appears to be increased by high levels of HMG-CoA reductase inhibitory activity in plasma; lovastatin is metabolized by CYP3A4 isoenzyme, certain agents, such as itraconazole, share this metabolic pathway and can raise the plasma levels of lovastatin and may increase the risk of myopathy).
No products indexed under this heading.

Ketoconazole (The risk of myopathy appears to be increased by high levels of HMG-CoA reductase inhibitory activity in plasma; lovastatin is metabolized by CYP3A4 isoenzyme, certain agents, such as ketoconazole, share this metabolic pathway and can raise the plasma levels of lovastatin and may increase the risk of myopathy). Products include:
Nizoral A-D Shampoo, 1% 1868

Lopinavir (The risk of myopathy/rhabdomyolysis is increased by concomitant use of lovastatin with potent inhibitors of CYP3A4, particularly with higher doses of lovastatin; concomitant use should be avoided unless the benefits of combined therapy outweigh the increased risk). Products include:
Kaletra 476

Loratadine (The risk of myopathy/rhabdomyolysis is increased by concomitant use of lovastatin with potent inhibitors of CYP3A4, particularly with higher doses of lovastatin; concomitant use should be avoided unless the benefits of combined therapy outweigh the increased risk). Products include:
Alavert Allergy & Sinus D-12 Hour Tablets.. 771
Alavert 771
Children's Claritin Allergy Oral Solution...................................... 771
Claritin Non-Drowsy 24 Hour Tablets.. 772
Claritin Reditabs 24 Hour Non-Drowsy Tablets.................... 772
Claritin-D Non-Drowsy 12 Hour Tablets.. 772
Claritin-D Non-Drowsy 24 Hour Tablets.. 772

Metronidazole (The risk of myopathy/rhabdomyolysis is increased by concomitant use of lovastatin with potent inhibitors of CYP3A4, particularly with higher doses of lovastatin; concomitant use should be avoided unless the benefits of combined therapy outweigh the increased risk). Products include:
Metrogel 1% 1211
MetroGel-Vaginal Gel 1855
Vandazole Vaginal Gel 3338

Metronidazole Benzoate (The risk of myopathy/rhabdomyolysis is increased by concomitant use of lovastatin with potent inhibitors of CYP3A4, particularly with higher doses of lovastatin; concomitant use should be avoided unless the benefits of combined therapy outweigh the increased risk).
No products indexed under this heading.

Metronidazole Hydrochloride (The risk of myopathy/rhabdomyolysis is increased by concomitant use of lovastatin with potent inhibitors of CYP3A4, particularly with higher doses of lovastatin; concomitant use should be avoided unless the benefits of combined therapy outweigh the increased risk).
No products indexed under this heading.

Miconazole (The risk of myopathy appears to be increased by high levels of HMG-CoA reductase inhibitory activity in plasma; lovastatin is metabolized by CYP3A4 isoenzyme, certain agents, such as azole antifungals, share this metabolic pathway and can raise the plasma levels of lovastatin and may increase the risk of myopathy).
No products indexed under this heading.

Miconazole Nitrate (The risk of myopathy/rhabdomyolysis is increased by concomitant use of lovastatin with potent inhibitors of CYP3A4, particularly with higher doses of lovastatin; concomitant use should be avoided unless the benefits of combined therapy outweigh the increased risk). Products include:
Desenex 635
Desenex Jock Itch Spray Powder ... 635

Nefazodone Hydrochloride (The risk of myopathy appears to be increased by high levels of HMG-CoA reductase inhibitory activity in plasma; lovastatin is metabolized by CYP3A4 isoenzyme, certain agents, such as antidepressant nefazodone, share this metabolic pathway and can raise the plasma levels of lovastatin and may increase the risk of myopathy).
No products indexed under this heading.

Nelfinavir Mesylate (The risk of myopathy/rhabdomyolysis is increased by concomitant use of lovastatin with potent inhibitors of CYP3A4, particularly with higher doses of lovastatin; concomitant use should be avoided unless the benefits of combined therapy outweigh the increased risk). Products include:
Viracept 2577

Nevirapine (The risk of myopathy/rhabdomyolysis is increased by concomitant use of lovastatin with potent inhibitors of CYP3A4, particularly with higher doses of lovastatin; concomitant use should be avoided unless the benefits of combined therapy outweigh the increased risk). Products include:
Viramune Oral Suspension 873
Viramune Tablets 873

Niacin (The incidence and severity of myopathy are increased by coadministration of HMG-CoA reductase inhibitors with drugs that cause myopathy when given alone, such as lipid-lowering doses of niacin; combined use should be avoided; if used concurrently, the dose of lovastatin should generally not exceed 20 mg). Products include:
Advicor Tablets 1722
Niaspan Extended-Release Tablets... 1730

Niacinamide (The risk of myopathy/rhabdomyolysis is increased by concomitant use of lovastatin with potent inhibitors of CYP3A4, particularly with higher doses of lovastatin; concomitant use should be avoided unless the benefits of combined therapy outweigh the increased risk).
No products indexed under this heading.

Nicotinamide (The risk of myopathy/rhabdomyolysis is increased by concomitant use of lovastatin with potent inhibitors of CYP3A4, particularly with higher doses of lovastatin; concomitant use should be avoided unless the benefits of combined therapy outweigh the increased risk). Products include:
Nicomide Tablets 1088

Nifedipine (The risk of myopathy/rhabdomyolysis is increased by concomitant use of lovastatin with potent inhibitors of CYP3A4, particularly with higher doses of lovastatin; concomitant use should be avoided unless the benefits of combined therapy outweigh the increased risk). Products include:
Adalat CC Tablets 2964

Norfloxacin (The risk of myopathy/rhabdomyolysis is increased by concomitant use of lovastatin with potent inhibitors of CYP3A4, particularly with higher doses of lovastatin; concomitant use should be avoided unless the benefits of combined therapy outweigh the increased risk). Products include:
Noroxin Tablets 2032

Omeprazole (The risk of myopathy/rhabdomyolysis is increased by concomitant use of lovastatin with potent inhibitors of CYP3A4, particularly with higher doses of lovastatin; concomitant use should be avoided unless the benefits of combined therapy outweigh the increased risk). Products include:
Zegerid Capsules 2958
Zegerid Powder for Oral Solution 2958

Oxiconazole Nitrate (The risk of myopathy appears to be increased by high levels of HMG-CoA reductase inhibitory activity in plasma; lovastatin is metabolized by CYP3A4 isoenzyme, certain agents, such as azole antifungals, share this metabolic pathway and can raise the plasma levels of lovastatin and may increase the risk of myopathy). Products include:
Oxistat 2667

Paroxetine Hydrochloride (The risk of myopathy/rhabdomyolysis is increased by concomitant use of lovastatin with potent inhibitors of CYP3A4, particularly with higher doses of lovastatin; concomitant use should be avoided unless the benefits of combined therapy outweigh the increased risk). Products include:
Paxil CR Controlled-Release Tablets.. 1538
Paxil 1530

Propoxyphene Hydrochloride (The risk of myopathy/rhabdomyolysis is increased by concomitant use of lovastatin with potent inhibitors of CYP3A4, particularly with higher doses of lovastatin; concomitant use should be avoided unless the benefits of combined therapy outweigh the increased risk).
No products indexed under this heading.

Propoxyphene Napsylate (The risk of myopathy/rhabdomyolysis is increased by concomitant use of lovastatin with potent inhibitors of CYP3A4, particularly with higher doses of lovastatin; concomitant use should be avoided unless the benefits of combined therapy outweigh the increased risk).
No products indexed under this heading.

Quinidine (The risk of myopathy/rhabdomyolysis is increased by concomitant use of lovastatin with potent inhibitors of CYP3A4, particularly with higher doses of lovastatin; concomitant use should be avoided unless the benefits of combined therapy outweigh the increased risk).
No products indexed under this heading.

Quinidine Hydrochloride (The risk of myopathy/rhabdomyolysis is increased by concomitant use of lovastatin with potent inhibitors of CYP3A4, particularly with higher doses of lovastatin; concomitant use should be avoided unless the benefits of combined therapy outweigh the increased risk).
No products indexed under this heading.

Quinidine Polygalacturonate (The risk of myopathy/rhabdomyolysis is increased by concomitant use of lovastatin with potent inhibitors of CYP3A4, particularly with higher doses of lovastatin; concomitant use should be avoided unless the benefits of combined therapy outweigh the increased risk).
No products indexed under this heading.

Quinidine Sulfate (The risk of myopathy/rhabdomyolysis is increased by concomitant use of lovastatin with potent inhibitors of CYP3A4, particularly with higher doses of lovastatin; concomitant use should be avoided unless the benefits of combined therapy outweigh the increased risk).
No products indexed under this heading.

Quinine (The risk of myopathy/rhabdomyolysis is increased by concomitant use of lovastatin with potent inhibitors of CYP3A4, particularly with higher doses of lovastatin; concomitant use should be avoided unless the benefits of combined therapy outweigh the increased risk).
No products indexed under this heading.

Quinine Sulfate (The risk of myopathy/rhabdomyolysis is increased by concomitant use of lovastatin with potent inhibitors of CYP3A4, particularly with higher doses of lovastatin; concomitant use should be avoided unless the benefits of combined therapy outweigh the increased risk).
No products indexed under this heading.

Quinupristin (The risk of myopathy/rhabdomyolysis is increased by concomitant use of lovastatin with potent inhibitors of CYP3A4, particularly with higher doses of lovastatin; concomitant use should be avoided unless the benefits of combined therapy outweigh the increased risk).
No products indexed under this heading.

Ranitidine Bismuth Citrate (The risk of myopathy/rhabdomyolysis is increased by concomitant use of lovastatin with potent inhibitors of CYP3A4, particularly with higher doses of lovastatin; concomitant use should be avoided unless the benefits of combined therapy outweigh the increased risk).
No products indexed under this heading.

Ranitidine Hydrochloride (The risk of myopathy/rhabdomyolysis is increased by concomitant use of lovastatin with potent inhibitors of CYP3A4, particularly with higher doses of lovastatin; concomitant use should be avoided unless the benefits of combined therapy outweigh the increased risk). Products include:

Zantac ... **1624**
Zantac Injection ... **1619**
Zantac Injection Pharmacy Bulk Package ... **1622**

Ritonavir (The risk of myopathy/rhabdomyolysis is increased by concomitant use of lovastatin with potent inhibitors of CYP3A4, particularly with higher doses of lovastatin; concomitant use should be avoided unless the benefits of combined therapy outweigh the increased risk). Products include:

Kaletra ... **476**
Norvir ... **503**

Saquinavir (The risk of myopathy/rhabdomyolysis is increased by concomitant use of lovastatin with potent inhibitors of CYP3A4, particularly with higher doses of lovastatin; concomitant use should be avoided unless the benefits of combined therapy outweigh the increased risk).

No products indexed under this heading.

Saquinavir Mesylate (The risk of myopathy/rhabdomyolysis is increased by concomitant use of lovastatin with potent inhibitors of CYP3A4, particularly with higher doses of lovastatin; concomitant use should be avoided unless the benefits of combined therapy outweigh the increased risk). Products include:

Invirase ... **2772**

Sertraline Hydrochloride (The risk of myopathy/rhabdomyolysis is increased by concomitant use of lovastatin with potent inhibitors of CYP3A4, particularly with higher doses of lovastatin; concomitant use should be avoided unless the benefits of combined therapy outweigh the increased risk). Products include:

Zoloft ... **2586**

Telithromycin (The risk of myopathy appears to be increased by high levels of HMG-CoA reductase inhibitory activity in plasma; lovastatin is metabolized by CYP3A4 isoenzyme, certain agents, such as macrolide antibiotics telithromycin, share this metabolic pathway and can raise the plasma levels of lovastatin and may increase the risk of myopathy). Products include:

Ketek Tablets ... **2903**

Terconazole (The risk of myopathy appears to be increased by high levels of HMG-CoA reductase inhibitory activity in plasma; lovastatin is metabolized by CYP3A4 isoenzyme, certain agents, such as azole antifungals, share this metabolic pathway and can raise the plasma levels of lovastatin and may increase the risk of myopathy).

No products indexed under this heading.

Troglitazone (The risk of myopathy/rhabdomyolysis is increased by concomitant use of lovastatin with potent inhibitors of CYP3A4, particularly with higher doses of lovastatin; concomitant use should be avoided unless the benefits of combined therapy outweigh the increased risk).

No products indexed under this heading.

Troleandomycin (The risk of myopathy/rhabdomyolysis is increased by concomitant use of lovastatin with potent inhibitors of CYP3A4, particularly with higher doses of lovastatin; concomitant use should be avoided unless the benefits of combined therapy outweigh the increased risk).

No products indexed under this heading.

Valproate Sodium (The risk of myopathy/rhabdomyolysis is increased by concomitant use of lovastatin with potent inhibitors of CYP3A4, particularly with higher doses of lovastatin; concomitant use should be avoided unless the benefits of combined therapy outweigh the increased risk). Products include:

Depacon Injection ... **412**

Verapamil Hydrochloride (The combined use of lovastatin at doses higher than 40 mg daily with verapamil should be avoided unless the clinical benefit is likely to outweigh the increased risk of myopathy). Products include:

Covera-HS Tablets ... **3139**
Tarka Tablets ... **524**
Verelan PM Extended-Release Capsules, Controlled-Onset ... **3106**

Voriconazole (The risk of myopathy/rhabdomyolysis is increased by concomitant use of lovastatin with potent inhibitors of CYP3A4, particularly with higher doses of lovastatin; concomitant use should be avoided unless the benefits of combined therapy outweigh the increased risk). Products include:

VFEND I.V. ... **2564**
VFEND Oral Suspension ... **2564**
VFEND Tablets ... **2564**

Warfarin Sodium (Co-administration has resulted in bleeding and/or increased prothrombin time in few patients). Products include:

Coumadin for Injection ... **898**
Coumadin Tablets ... **898**

Zafirlukast (The risk of myopathy/rhabdomyolysis is increased by concomitant use of lovastatin with potent inhibitors of CYP3A4, particularly with higher doses of lovastatin; concomitant use should be avoided unless the benefits of combined therapy outweigh the increased risk). Products include:

Accolate Tablets ... **671**

Zileuton (The risk of myopathy/rhabdomyolysis is increased by concomitant use of lovastatin with potent inhibitors of CYP3A4, particularly with higher doses of lovastatin; concomitant use should be avoided unless the benefits of combined therapy outweigh the increased risk). Products include:

Zyflo Tablets ... **1023**

Food Interactions

Alcohol (Lovastatin should be used with caution in patients who have consumed substantial quantity of alcohol and have a past history of liver disease; active liver disease and unexplained elevation in transaminase are contraindications to the use of lovastatin).

Grapefruit (The risk of myopathy/rhabdomyolysis is increased by concomitant use of lovastatin with potent inhibitors of CYP3A4, particularly with higher doses of lovastatin; concomitant use should be avoided unless the benefits of combined therapy outweigh the increased risk).

Grapefruit Juice (The risk of myopathy/rhabdomyolysis is increased by concomitant use of lovastatin with potent inhibitors of CYP3A4, particularly with higher doses of lovastatin; concomitant use should be avoided unless the benefits of combined therapy outweigh the increased risk).

Meal, unspecified (When lovastatin was given under fasting conditions, plasma concentrations of total inhibitors were on average about two-thirds those found when lovastatin was administered immediately after a standard meal).

MIACALCIN INJECTION

(Calcitonin-Salmon) ... **2252**
None cited in PDR database.

MIACALCIN NASAL SPRAY

(Calcitonin-Salmon) ... **2253**
May interact with:

Etidronate Disodium (Diphosphonate) (Prior diphosphonate use may reduce the anti-resorptive response to calcitonin-salmon nasal spray).

No products indexed under this heading.

Pamidronate Disodium (Prior diphosphonate use may reduce the anti-resorptive response to calcitonin-salmon nasal spray). Products include:

Aredia for Injection ... **2179**

MICARDIS TABLETS

(Telmisartan) ... **854**
May interact with cytochrome p450 2c19 substrates (selected) and certain other agents. Compounds in these categories include:

Amitriptyline Hydrochloride (Possible inhibition of the metabolism of drugs metabolized by CYP2C19).

No products indexed under this heading.

Amoxapine (Possible inhibition of the metabolism of drugs metabolized by CYP2C19).

No products indexed under this heading.

Carisoprodol (Possible inhibition of the metabolism of drugs metabolized by CYP2C19).

No products indexed under this heading.

Cilostazol (Possible inhibition of the metabolism of drugs metabolized by CYP2C19). Products include:

Pletal Tablets ... **2455**

Citalopram Hydrobromide (Possible inhibition of the metabolism of drugs metabolized by CYP2C19). Products include:

Celexa ... **1176**

Clomipramine Hydrochloride (Possible inhibition of the metabolism of drugs metabolized by CYP2C19).

No products indexed under this heading.

Cyclophosphamide (Possible inhibition of the metabolism of drugs metabolized by CYP2C19).

No products indexed under this heading.

Desipramine Hydrochloride (Possible inhibition of the metabolism of drugs metabolized by CYP2C19).

No products indexed under this heading.

Dextromethorphan (Possible inhibition of the metabolism of drugs metabolized by CYP2C19).

No products indexed under this heading.

Dextromethorphan Hydrobromide (Possible inhibition of the metabolism of drugs metabolized by CYP2C19). Products include:

Comtrex Maximum Strength Cold & Cough Day/Night Caplets - Day Formulation ... ■ **726**
Comtrex Maximum Strength Cold & Cough Day/Night Caplets - Night Formulation ... ■ **726**
Comtrex Maximum Strength Non-Drowsy Cold & Cough Caplets ... ■ **725**
Children's Dimetapp DM Cold & Cough Elixir ... ■ **731**
Children's Dimetapp Long Acting Cough Plus Cold Syrup ... ■ **731**
Toddler's Dimetapp Cold and Cough Drops ... ■ **732**
Mucinex DM Extended-Release Bi-Layer Tablets ... ■ **720**
Refenesen DM Caplets ... ■ **721**
Robitussin Cough & Cold CF Liquid ... ■ **735**
Robitussin Cough & Cold Long-Acting Liquid ... ■ **735**
Robitussin Cough & Allergy Syrup ... ■ **736**
Robitussin Cough & Cold Nighttime Liquid ... ■ **736**
Robitussin Cough & Cold Pediatric Drops ... ■ **735**
Robitussin Cough, Cold & Flu Nighttime Liquid ... ■ **738**
Robitussin Cough & Congestion Liquid ... ■ **738**
Robitussin Cough Gels Long-Acting ... ■ **737**
Robitussin Cough Long Acting Liquid ... ■ **739**
Robitussin Cough DM Syrup ... ■ **738**
Robitussin Cough DM Infant Drops ... ■ **738**
Robitussin Pediatric Cough Long Acting Liquid ... ■ **739**
Robitussin Pediatric Cough & Cold Long-Acting Liquid ... ■ **735**
Robitussin Pediatric Cough & Cold Nighttime Liquid ... ■ **736**
Robitussin Sugar Free Cough ... ■ **738**
TheraFlu Cold & Cough Hot Liquid ... ■ **740**
TheraFlu Warming Relief Daytime Severe Cold ... ■ **743**
TheraFlu Thin Strips Long Acting Cough ... ■ **744**
Triaminic Daytime Cold & Cough Liquid ... ■ **745**
Triaminic Cough & Sore Throat Liquid ... ■ **747**
Triaminic Cough & Runny Nose Softchews ... ■ **748**
Triaminic Thin Strips Cold & Cough ... ■ **778**
Triaminic Infant Thin Strips Decongestant Plus Cough ... ■ **747**
Children's Tylenol Plus Flu Oral Suspension ... ■ **749**
Tylenol Cold Head Congestion Daytime Caplets with Cool Burst and Gelcaps ... ■ **750**
Tylenol Cold Multi-Symptom Daytime Liquid ... ■ **752**

Tylenol Cold Multi-Symptom Severe Daytime Liquid 752
Concentrated Tylenol Infants' Drops Plus Cold & Cough 754
Children's Tylenol Plus Cough & Runny Nose Suspension Liquid 1879
Children's Tylenol Plus Cough & Sore Throat Suspension Liquid 1879
Children's Tylenol Plus Flu Suspension Liquid 1881
Children's Tylenol Plus Multi-Symptom Cold Suspension Liquid 1879
Tylenol Cold Severe Congestion Non-Drowsy Caplets with Cool Burst 1874
Tylenol Cold Head Congestion Daytime Caplets with Cool Burst 1873
Tylenol Cold Head Congestion Nighttime Caplets with Cool Burst 1873
Tylenol Cold Head Congestion Severe Caplets with Cool Burst 1873
Tylenol Cold Multi-Symptom Daytime Caplets with Cool Burst and Gelcaps 1874
Tylenol Cold Multi-Symptom Daytime Liquid with Citrus Burst ... 1874
Tylenol Cold Multi-Symptom Nighttime Caplets with Cool Burst 1874
Tylenol Cold Multi-Symptom Nighttime Liquid with Cool Burst ... 1874
Tylenol Cold Multi-Symptom Severe Caplets with Cool Burst 1874
Tylenol Cold Multi-Symptom Severe Daytime Liquid with Citrus Burst 1874
Tylenol Cough & Sore Throat Daytime Liquid with Cool Burst 1877
Tylenol Cough & Sore Throat Nighttime Liquid with Cool Burst ... 1877
Concentrated Tylenol Infants' Drops Plus Cold and Cough 1879
Vicks 44 Cough Relief Liquid 2679
Vicks 44D Cough & Head Congestion Relief Liquid 2679
Vicks 44E Cough & Chest Congestion Relief Liquid 2679
Pediatric Vicks 44e Cough & Chest Congestion Relief Liquid 2676
Vicks 44M Cough, Cold & Flu Relief Liquid 2680
Pediatric Vicks 44m Cough & Cold Relief Liquid 2676
Vicks DayQuil LiquiCaps/Liquid Multi-Symptom Cold/Flu Relief 761
Vicks DayQuil Multi-Symptom Cold/Flu Relief LiquiCaps 2678
Vicks DayQuil Multi-Symptom Cold/Flu Relief Liquid 2678
Vicks NyQuil Multi-Symptom Cold/Flu Relief Liquid 2681
Children's Vicks NyQuil Cold/Cough Relief 756
Vicks NyQuil Multi-Symptom Cold/Flu Relief LiquiCaps 2681
Vicks NyQuil LiquiCaps/Liquid Multi-Symptom Cold/Flu Relief 763
Vicks NyQuil Cough Liquid 2680
Children's Vicks NyQuil Cold/Cough Relief Liquid 2680
Zicam Cough Max Nighttime Cough Spray 767
Zicam Cough Max Cough Spray 767
Zicam Cough Max Cough Melts 767
Zicam Cough Plus D Cough Spray 767
Zicam Cough Relief Cough Spray ... 767
Zicam Maximum Strength Flu Daytime 768
Zicam Maximum Strength Flu Nighttime 768

Diazepam (Possible inhibition of the metabolism of drugs metabolized by CYP2C19). Products include:
Diastat Rectal Delivery System 3343
Valium Tablets 2819

Digoxin (Co-administration has resulted in median increases in digoxin peak plasma concentration (49%) and in trough concentration (20%); digoxin levels should be monitored when initiating, adjusting, and discontinuing telmisartan to avoid possible over- or under- digitalization). Products include:
Lanoxicaps Capsules 1490
Lanoxin Injection 1494
Lanoxin Injection Pediatric 1497
Lanoxin Tablets 1500

Divalproex Sodium (Possible inhibition of the metabolism of drugs metabolized by CYP2C19). Products include:
Depakote Sprinkle Capsules 422
Depakote Tablets 427
Depakote ER Tablets 434

Doxepin Hydrochloride (Possible inhibition of the metabolism of drugs metabolized by CYP2C19).
No products indexed under this heading.

Esomeprazole Magnesium (Possible inhibition of the metabolism of drugs metabolized by CYP2C19). Products include:
Nexium Delayed-Release Capsules 655

Ethosuximide (Possible inhibition of the metabolism of drugs metabolized by CYP2C19).
No products indexed under this heading.

Ethotoin (Possible inhibition of the metabolism of drugs metabolized by CYP2C19).
No products indexed under this heading.

Felbamate (Possible inhibition of the metabolism of drugs metabolized by CYP2C19).
No products indexed under this heading.

Formoterol Fumarate (Possible inhibition of the metabolism of drugs metabolized by CYP2C19). Products include:
Foradil Aerolizer 3010

Fosphenytoin (Possible inhibition of the metabolism of drugs metabolized by CYP2C19).
No products indexed under this heading.

Fosphenytoin Sodium (Possible inhibition of the metabolism of drugs metabolized by CYP2C19).
No products indexed under this heading.

Gabapentin (Possible inhibition of the metabolism of drugs metabolized by CYP2C19). Products include:
Neurontin Capsules 2487
Neurontin Oral Solution 2487
Neurontin Tablets 2487

Imipramine Hydrochloride (Possible inhibition of the metabolism of drugs metabolized by CYP2C19).
No products indexed under this heading.

Imipramine Pamoate (Possible inhibition of the metabolism of drugs metabolized by CYP2C19).
No products indexed under this heading.

Indomethacin (Possible inhibition of the metabolism of drugs metabolized by CYP2C19). Products include:
Indocin 1995

Indomethacin Sodium Trihydrate (Possible inhibition of the metabolism of drugs metabolized by CYP2C19). Products include:
Indocin I.V. 2465

Lamotrigine (Possible inhibition of the metabolism of drugs metabolized by CYP2C19). Products include:
Lamictal 1481

Lansoprazole (Possible inhibition of the metabolism of drugs metabolized by CYP2C19). Products include:
Prevacid Delayed-Release Capsules 3271
Prevacid for Delayed-Release Oral Suspension 3271
Prevacid SoluTab Delayed-Release Orally Disintegrating Tablets 3271
Prevacid I.V. for Injection 3277
Prevacid NapraPAC 3280
PREVPAC 3284

Levetiracetam (Possible inhibition of the metabolism of drugs metabolized by CYP2C19). Products include:
Keppra Injection 3320
Keppra Oral Solution 3314
Keppra Tablets 3314

Maprotiline Hydrochloride (Possible inhibition of the metabolism of drugs metabolized by CYP2C19).
No products indexed under this heading.

Mephenytoin (Possible inhibition of the metabolism of drugs metabolized by CYP2C19).
No products indexed under this heading.

Mephobarbital (Possible inhibition of the metabolism of drugs metabolized by CYP2C19).
No products indexed under this heading.

Meprobamate (Possible inhibition of the metabolism of drugs metabolized by CYP2C19).
No products indexed under this heading.

Methsuximide (Possible inhibition of the metabolism of drugs metabolized by CYP2C19).
No products indexed under this heading.

Midazolam Hydrochloride (Possible inhibition of the metabolism of drugs metabolized by CYP2C19).
No products indexed under this heading.

Nelfinavir Mesylate (Possible inhibition of the metabolism of drugs metabolized by CYP2C19). Products include:
Viracept 2577

Nilutamide (Possible inhibition of the metabolism of drugs metabolized by CYP2C19).
No products indexed under this heading.

Nortriptyline Hydrochloride (Possible inhibition of the metabolism of drugs metabolized by CYP2C19).
No products indexed under this heading.

Omeprazole (Possible inhibition of the metabolism of drugs metabolized by CYP2C19). Products include:
Zegerid Capsules 2958
Zegerid Powder for Oral Solution 2958

Oxcarbazepine (Possible inhibition of the metabolism of drugs metabolized by CYP2C19). Products include:
Trileptal Tablets 2300
Trileptal Oral Suspension 2300

Pantoprazole Sodium (Possible inhibition of the metabolism of drugs metabolized by CYP2C19). Products include:
Protonix I.V. 3472
Protonix Tablets 3469

Paramethadione (Possible inhibition of the metabolism of drugs metabolized by CYP2C19).
No products indexed under this heading.

Pentamidine Isethionate (Possible inhibition of the metabolism of drugs metabolized by CYP2C19).
No products indexed under this heading.

Phenacemide (Possible inhibition of the metabolism of drugs metabolized by CYP2C19).
No products indexed under this heading.

Phenobarbital (Possible inhibition of the metabolism of drugs metabolized by CYP2C19). Products include:
Donnatal Extentabs 2493

Phenobarbital Sodium (Possible inhibition of the metabolism of drugs metabolized by CYP2C19).
No products indexed under this heading.

Phensuximide (Possible inhibition of the metabolism of drugs metabolized by CYP2C19).
No products indexed under this heading.

Phenytoin (Possible inhibition of the metabolism of drugs metabolized by CYP2C19).
No products indexed under this heading.

Phenytoin Sodium (Possible inhibition of the metabolism of drugs metabolized by CYP2C19). Products include:
Phenytek Capsules 2160

Primidone (Possible inhibition of the metabolism of drugs metabolized by CYP2C19).
No products indexed under this heading.

Progesterone (Possible inhibition of the metabolism of drugs metabolized by CYP2C19). Products include:
Prochieve 4% Gel 1003
Prochieve 8% Gel 1003
Prometrium Capsules (100 mg, 200 mg) 3203

Proguanil Hydrochloride (Possible inhibition of the metabolism of drugs metabolized by CYP2C19). Products include:
Malarone Pediatric Tablets 1517
Malarone Tablets 1517

Propranolol Hydrochloride (Possible inhibition of the metabolism of drugs metabolized by CYP2C19). Products include:
Inderal LA Long-Acting Capsules 3429
InnoPran XL Capsules 2723

Protriptyline Hydrochloride (Possible inhibition of the metabolism of drugs metabolized by CYP2C19).
No products indexed under this heading.

Rabeprazole Sodium (Possible inhibition of the metabolism of drugs metabolized by CYP2C19). Products include:
Aciphex Tablets 1090

Sertraline Hydrochloride (Possible inhibition of the metabolism of drugs metabolized by CYP2C19). Products include:
Zoloft 2586

Teniposide (Possible inhibition of the metabolism of drugs metabolized by CYP2C19).
No products indexed under this heading.

Thioridazine (Possible inhibition of the metabolism of drugs metabolized by CYP2C19).

No products indexed under this heading.

Thioridazine Hydrochloride (Possible inhibition of the metabolism of drugs metabolized by CYP2C19). Products include:

Thioridazine Hydrochloride Tablets 2163

Tiagabine Hydrochloride (Possible inhibition of the metabolism of drugs metabolized by CYP2C19). Products include:

Gabitril Tablets 984

Tolbutamide (Possible inhibition of the metabolism of drugs metabolized by CYP2C19).

No products indexed under this heading.

Tolbutamide Sodium (Possible inhibition of the metabolism of drugs metabolized by CYP2C19).

No products indexed under this heading.

Topiramate (Possible inhibition of the metabolism of drugs metabolized by CYP2C19). Products include:

Topamax Sprinkle Capsules 2404
Topamax Tablets 2404

Trimethadione (Possible inhibition of the metabolism of drugs metabolized by CYP2C19).

No products indexed under this heading.

Trimipramine Maleate (Possible inhibition of the metabolism of drugs metabolized by CYP2C19).

No products indexed under this heading.

Valproate Sodium (Possible inhibition of the metabolism of drugs metabolized by CYP2C19). Products include:

Depacon Injection 412

Valproic Acid (Possible inhibition of the metabolism of drugs metabolized by CYP2C19). Products include:

Depakene 417

Voriconazole (Possible inhibition of the metabolism of drugs metabolized by CYP2C19). Products include:

VFEND I.V. 2564
VFEND Oral Suspension 2564
VFEND Tablets 2564

Warfarin Sodium (Co-administration has resulted in slight decrease in the mean warfarin trough plasma concentration; this decrease did not result in a change in INR). Products include:

Coumadin for Injection 898
Coumadin Tablets 898

Zonisamide (Possible inhibition of the metabolism of drugs metabolized by CYP2C19). Products include:

Zonegran Capsules 1101

Food Interactions

Food, unspecified (Slightly reduces the bioavailability of telmisartan; Micardis tablets may be administered with or without food).

MICARDIS HCT TABLETS

(Hydrochlorothiazide, Telmisartan) 856
May interact with antihypertensives, barbiturates, corticosteroids, cytochrome p450 2c19 substrates (selected), oral hypoglycemic agents, insulin, lithium preparations, narcotic analgesics, nondepolarizing neuromuscular blocking agents, non-steroidal anti-inflammatory agents, potassium preparations, and certain other agents. Compounds in these categories include:

Acarbose (Thiazide diuretics may cause hyperglycemia; dosage adjustment of oral hypoglycemia agents may be required). Products include:

Precose Tablets 751

Acebutolol Hydrochloride (Co-administration with other antihypertensive agents may result in additive effect or potentiation).

No products indexed under this heading.

ACTH (Intensifies electrolyte depletion, particularly hypokalemia).

No products indexed under this heading.

Alfentanil Hydrochloride (Potentiation of orthostatic hypotension).

No products indexed under this heading.

Amitriptyline Hydrochloride (Possible inhibition of the metabolism of drugs metabolized by CYP2C19).

No products indexed under this heading.

Amlodipine Besylate (Co-administration with other antihypertensive agents may result in additive effect or potentiation). Products include:

Caduet Tablets 2508
Lotrel Capsules 2249
Norvasc Tablets 2545

Amoxapine (Possible inhibition of the metabolism of drugs metabolized by CYP2C19).

No products indexed under this heading.

Aprobarbital (Potentiation of orthostatic hypotension).

No products indexed under this heading.

Atenolol (Co-administration with other antihypertensive agents may result in additive effect or potentiation).

No products indexed under this heading.

Atracurium Besylate (Possible increased responsiveness to the muscle relaxants).

No products indexed under this heading.

Benazepril Hydrochloride (Co-administration with other antihypertensive agents may result in additive effect or potentiation). Products include:

Lotensin Tablets 2243
Lotensin HCT Tablets 2246
Lotrel Capsules 2249

Bendroflumethiazide (Co-administration with other antihypertensive agents may result in additive effect or potentiation).

No products indexed under this heading.

Betamethasone Acetate (Corticosteroids intensify electrolyte depletion, particularly hypokalemia).

No products indexed under this heading.

Betamethasone Sodium Phosphate (Corticosteroids intensify electrolyte depletion, particularly hypokalemia).

No products indexed under this heading.

Betaxolol Hydrochloride (Co-administration with other antihypertensive agents may result in additive effect or potentiation). Products include:

Betoptic S Ophthalmic Suspension ⊙ 558

Bisoprolol Fumarate (Co-administration with other antihypertensive agents may result in additive effect or potentiation).

No products indexed under this heading.

Buprenorphine Hydrochloride (Potentiation of orthostatic hypotension). Products include:

Buprenex Injectable 2716
Suboxone Tablets 2717
Subutex Tablets 2717

Butabarbital (Potentiation of orthostatic hypotension).

No products indexed under this heading.

Butalbital (Potentiation of orthostatic hypotension).

No products indexed under this heading.

Candesartan Cilexetil (Co-administration with other antihypertensive agents may result in additive effect or potentiation). Products include:

Atacand Tablets 649
Atacand HCT 651

Captopril (Co-administration with other antihypertensive agents may result in additive effect or potentiation). Products include:

Captopril Tablets 2149

Carisoprodol (Possible inhibition of the metabolism of drugs metabolized by CYP2C19).

No products indexed under this heading.

Carteolol Hydrochloride (Co-administration with other antihypertensive agents may result in additive effect or potentiation). Products include:

Carteolol Hydrochloride Ophthalmic Solution USP, 1%....... ⊙ 249

Celecoxib (Co-administration in some patients can result in reduced diuretic, natriuretic, and antihypertensive effects). Products include:

Celebrex Capsules 3134

Chlorothiazide (Co-administration with other antihypertensive agents may result in additive effect or potentiation). Products include:

Diuril Oral Suspension 1954

Chlorothiazide Sodium (Co-administration with other antihypertensive agents may result in additive effect or potentiation). Products include:

Diuril Sodium Intravenous 2467

Chlorpropamide (Thiazide diuretics may cause hyperglycemia; dosage adjustment of oral hypoglycemia agents may be required).

No products indexed under this heading.

Chlorthalidone (Co-administration with other antihypertensive agents may result in additive effect or potentiation). Products include:

Clorpres Tablets 2153

Cholestyramine (Absorption of hydrochlorothiazide is impaired in the presence of anionic exchange resins; cholestyramine binds the hydrochlorothiazide from the GI tract by up to 85%).

No products indexed under this heading.

Cilostazol (Possible inhibition of the metabolism of drugs metabolized by CYP2C19). Products include:

Pletal Tablets 2455

Cisatracurium Besylate (Possible increased responsiveness to the muscle relaxants). Products include:

Nimbex Injection 498

Citalopram Hydrobromide (Possible inhibition of the metabolism of drugs metabolized by CYP2C19). Products include:

Celexa 1176

Clomipramine Hydrochloride (Possible inhibition of the metabolism of drugs metabolized by CYP2C19).

No products indexed under this heading.

Clonidine (Co-administration with other antihypertensive agents may result in additive effect or potentiation). Products include:

Catapres-TTS 844

Clonidine Hydrochloride (Co-administration with other antihypertensive agents may result in additive effect or potentiation). Products include:

Catapres Tablets 843
Clorpres Tablets 2153

Codeine Phosphate (Potentiation of orthostatic hypotension). Products include:

Tylenol with Codeine Tablets 2391

Colestipol Hydrochloride (Absorption of hydrochlorothiazide is impaired in the presence of anionic exchange resins; colestipol binds the hydroclorothiazide from the GI tract by up to 43%).

No products indexed under this heading.

Cortisone Acetate (Corticosteroids intensify electrolyte depletion, particularly hypokalemia).

No products indexed under this heading.

Cyclophosphamide (Possible inhibition of the metabolism of drugs metabolized by CYP2C19).

No products indexed under this heading.

Deserpidine (Co-administration with other antihypertensive agents may result in additive effect or potentiation).

No products indexed under this heading.

Desipramine Hydrochloride (Possible inhibition of the metabolism of drugs metabolized by CYP2C19).

No products indexed under this heading.

Dexamethasone (Corticosteroids intensify electrolyte depletion, particularly hypokalemia). Products include:

Ciprodex Otic Suspension 559
Decadron Tablets 1951
TobraDex Ophthalmic Ointment ⊙ 562
TobraDex Ophthalmic Suspension ... ⊙ 563

Dexamethasone Acetate (Corticosteroids intensify electrolyte depletion, particularly hypokalemia).

No products indexed under this heading.

Dexamethasone Sodium Phosphate (Corticosteroids intensify electrolyte depletion, particularly hypokalemia).
No products indexed under this heading.

Dextromethorphan (Possible inhibition of the metabolism of drugs metabolized by CYP2C19).
No products indexed under this heading.

Dextromethorphan Hydrobromide (Possible inhibition of the metabolism of drugs metabolized by CYP2C19). Products include:
- Comtrex Maximum Strength Cold & Cough Day/Night Caplets - Day Formulation 726
- Comtrex Maximum Strength Cold & Cough Day/Night Caplets - Night Formulation 726
- Comtrex Maximum Strength Non-Drowsy Cold & Cough Caplets 725
- Children's Dimetapp DM Cold & Cough Elixir 731
- Children's Dimetapp Long Acting Cough Plus Cold Syrup 731
- Toddler's Dimetapp Cold and Cough Drops 732
- Mucinex DM Extended-Release Bi-Layer Tablets 720
- Refenesen DM Caplets 721
- Robitussin Cough & Cold CF Liquid 735
- Robitussin Cough & Cold Long-Acting Liquid 735
- Robitussin Cough & Allergy Syrup 736
- Robitussin Cough & Cold Nighttime Liquid 736
- Robitussin Cough & Cold Pediatric Drops 735
- Robitussin Cough, Cold & Flu Nighttime Liquid 738
- Robitussin Cough & Congestion Liquid 738
- Robitussin Cough Gels Long-Acting 737
- Robitussin Cough Long Acting Liquid 739
- Robitussin Cough DM Syrup 738
- Robitussin Cough DM Infant Drops 738
- Robitussin Pediatric Cough Long Acting Liquid 739
- Robitussin Pediatric Cough & Cold Long-Acting Liquid 735
- Robitussin Pediatric Cough & Cold Nighttime Liquid 736
- Robitussin Sugar Free Cough 738
- TheraFlu Cold & Cough Hot Liquid 740
- TheraFlu Warming Relief Daytime Severe Cold 743
- TheraFlu Thin Strips Long Acting Cough 744
- Triaminic Daytime Cold & Cough Liquid 745
- Triaminic Cough & Sore Throat Liquid 747
- Triaminic Cough & Runny Nose Softchews 748
- Triaminic Thin Strips Cold & Cough 778
- Triaminic Infant Thin Strips Decongestant Plus Cough 747
- Children's Tylenol Plus Flu Oral Suspension 749
- Tylenol Cold Head Congestion Daytime Caplets with Cool Burst and Gelcaps 750
- Tylenol Cold Multi-Symptom Daytime Liquid 752
- Tylenol Cold Multi-Symptom Severe Daytime Liquid 752
- Concentrated Tylenol Infants' Drops Plus Cold & Cough 754
- Children's Tylenol Plus Cough & Runny Nose Suspension Liquid 1879
- Children's Tylenol Plus Cough & Sore Throat Suspension Liquid 1879
- Children's Tylenol Plus Flu Suspension Liquid 1881
- Children's Tylenol Plus Multi-Symptom Cold Suspension Liquid 1879
- Tylenol Cold Severe Congestion Non-Drowsy Caplets with Cool Burst 1874
- Tylenol Cold Head Congestion Daytime Caplets with Cool Burst 1873
- Tylenol Cold Head Congestion Nighttime Caplets with Cool Burst 1873
- Tylenol Cold Head Congestion Severe Caplets with Cool Burst 1873
- Tylenol Cold Multi-Symptom Daytime Caplets with Cool Burst and Gelcaps 1874
- Tylenol Cold Multi-Symptom Daytime Liquid with Citrus Burst 1874
- Tylenol Cold Multi-Symptom Nighttime Caplets with Cool Burst 1874
- Tylenol Cold Multi-Symptom Nighttime Liquid with Cool Burst 1874
- Tylenol Cold Multi-Symptom Severe Caplets with Cool Burst 1874
- Tylenol Cold Multi-Symptom Severe Daytime Liquid with Citrus Burst 1874
- Tylenol Cough & Sore Throat Daytime Liquid with Cool Burst 1877
- Tylenol Cough & Sore Throat Nighttime Liquid with Cool Burst 1877
- Concentrated Tylenol Infants' Drops Plus Cold and Cough 1879
- Vicks 44 Cough Relief Liquid 2679
- Vicks 44D Cough & Head Congestion Relief Liquid 2679
- Vicks 44E Cough & Chest Congestion Relief Liquid 2679
- Pediatric Vicks 44e Cough & Chest Congestion Relief Liquid 2676
- Vicks 44M Cough, Cold & Flu Relief Liquid 2680
- Pediatric Vicks 44m Cough & Cold Relief Liquid 2676
- Vicks DayQuil LiquiCaps/Liquid Multi-Symptom Cold/Flu Relief 761
- Vicks DayQuil Multi-Symptom Cold/Flu Relief LiquiCaps 2678
- Vicks DayQuil Multi-Symptom Cold/Flu Relief Liquid 2678
- Vicks NyQuil Multi-Symptom Cold/Flu Relief Liquid 2681
- Children's Vicks NyQuil Cold/Cough Relief 756
- Vicks NyQuil Multi-Symptom Cold/Flu Relief LiquiCaps 2681
- Vicks NyQuil LiquiCaps/Liquid Multi-Symptom Cold/Flu Relief 763
- Vicks NyQuil Cough Liquid 2680
- Children's Vicks NyQuil Cold/Cough Relief Liquid 2680
- Zicam Cough Max Nighttime Cough Spray 767
- Zicam Cough Max Cough Spray 767
- Zicam Cough Max Cough Melts 767
- Zicam Cough Plus D Cough Spray 767
- Zicam Cough Relief Cough Spray 767
- Zicam Maximum Strength Flu Daytime 768
- Zicam Maximum Strength Flu Nighttime 768

Dezocine (Potentiation of orthostatic hypotension).
No products indexed under this heading.

Diazepam (Possible inhibition of the metabolism of drugs metabolized by CYP2C19). Products include:
- Diastat Rectal Delivery System 3343
- Valium Tablets 2819

Diazoxide (Co-administration with other antihypertensive agents may result in additive effect or potentiation). Products include:
- Hyperstat I.V. 3017

Diclofenac Potassium (Co-administration in some patients can result in reduced diuretic, natriuretic, and antihypertensive effects).
No products indexed under this heading.

Diclofenac Sodium (Co-administration in some patients can result in reduced diuretic, natriuretic, and antihypertensive effects). Products include:
- Arthrotec Tablets 3129
- Voltaren Ophthalmic Solution 2309
- Voltaren Tablets 2307
- Voltaren-XR Tablets 2310

Digoxin (Co-administration has resulted in median increases in digoxin peak plasma concentration (49%) and in trough concentration (20%); digoxin levels should be monitored when initiating, adjusting, and discontinuing telmisartan to avoid possible over- or under-digitalization; thiazide-induced hypokalemia exaggerates or sensitizes the response of the heart to the toxic effects of digitalis, i.e., increased ventricular irritability). Products include:
- Lanoxicaps Capsules 1490
- Lanoxin Injection 1494
- Lanoxin Injection Pediatric 1497
- Lanoxin Tablets 1500

Diltiazem Hydrochloride (Co-administration with other antihypertensive agents may result in additive effect or potentiation). Products include:
- Cardizem LA Extended Release Tablets 1728
- Tiazac Capsules 1201

Divalproex Sodium (Possible inhibition of the metabolism of drugs metabolized by CYP2C19). Products include:
- Depakote Sprinkle Capsules 422
- Depakote Tablets 427
- Depakote ER Tablets 434

Doxazosin Mesylate (Co-administration with other antihypertensive agents may result in additive effect or potentiation). Products include:
- Cardura XL Tablets 2515

Doxepin Hydrochloride (Possible inhibition of the metabolism of drugs metabolized by CYP2C19).
No products indexed under this heading.

Enalapril Maleate (Co-administration with other antihypertensive agents may result in additive effect or potentiation). Products include:
- Vasotec I.V. Injection 2103

Enalaprilat (Co-administration with other antihypertensive agents may result in additive effect or potentiation).
No products indexed under this heading.

Eprosartan Mesylate (Co-administration with other antihypertensive agents may result in additive effect or potentiation). Products include:
- Teveten Tablets 1735
- Teveten HCT Tablets 1737

Esmolol Hydrochloride (Co-administration with other antihypertensive agents may result in additive effect or potentiation).
No products indexed under this heading.

Esomeprazole Magnesium (Possible inhibition of the metabolism of drugs metabolized by CYP2C19). Products include:
- Nexium Delayed-Release Capsules 655

Ethosuximide (Possible inhibition of the metabolism of drugs metabolized by CYP2C19).
No products indexed under this heading.

Ethotoin (Possible inhibition of the metabolism of drugs metabolized by CYP2C19).
No products indexed under this heading.

Etodolac (Co-administration in some patients can result in reduced diuretic, natriuretic, and antihypertensive effects).
No products indexed under this heading.

Felbamate (Possible inhibition of the metabolism of drugs metabolized by CYP2C19).
No products indexed under this heading.

Felodipine (Co-administration with other antihypertensive agents may result in additive effect or potentiation).
No products indexed under this heading.

Fenoprofen Calcium (Co-administration in some patients can result in reduced diuretic, natriuretic, and antihypertensive effects). Products include:
- Nalfon Capsules 2502

Fentanyl (Potentiation of orthostatic hypotension). Products include:
- Duragesic Transdermal System 2373
- Ionsys Transdermal System 2379

Fentanyl Citrate (Potentiation of orthostatic hypotension). Products include:
- Actiq 979

Fludrocortisone Acetate (Corticosteroids intensify electrolyte depletion, particularly hypokalemia).
No products indexed under this heading.

Flurbiprofen (Co-administration in some patients can result in reduced diuretic, natriuretic, and antihypertensive effects).
No products indexed under this heading.

Formoterol Fumarate (Possible inhibition of the metabolism of drugs metabolized by CYP2C19). Products include:
- Foradil Aerolizer 3010

Fosinopril Sodium (Co-administration with other antihypertensive agents may result in additive effect or potentiation).
No products indexed under this heading.

Fosphenytoin (Possible inhibition of the metabolism of drugs metabolized by CYP2C19).
No products indexed under this heading.

Fosphenytoin Sodium (Possible inhibition of the metabolism of drugs metabolized by CYP2C19).
No products indexed under this heading.

Furosemide (Co-administration with other antihypertensive agents may result in additive effect or potentiation). Products include:
- Furosemide Tablets 2154

Gabapentin (Possible inhibition of the metabolism of drugs metabolized by CYP2C19). Products include:
- Neurontin Capsules 2487
- Neurontin Oral Solution 2487
- Neurontin Tablets 2487

Glimepiride (Thiazide diuretics may cause hyperglycemia; dosage adjustment of oral hypoglycemia agents may be required). Products include:
- Avandaryl Tablets 1379

Duetact Tablets 3226

Glipizide (Thiazide diuretics may cause hyperglycemia; dosage adjustment of oral hypoglycemia agents may be required).
No products indexed under this heading.

Glyburide (Thiazide diuretics may cause hyperglycemia; dosage adjustment of oral hypoglycemia agents may be required).
No products indexed under this heading.

Guanabenz Acetate (Co-administration with other antihypertensive agents may result in additive effect or potentiation).
No products indexed under this heading.

Guanethidine Monosulfate (Co-administration with other antihypertensive agents may result in additive effect or potentiation).
No products indexed under this heading.

Hydralazine Hydrochloride (Co-administration with other antihypertensive agents may result in additive effect or potentiation). Products include:
BiDil Tablets 2171

Hydrocodone Bitartrate (Potentiation of orthostatic hypotension). Products include:
Hycodan 1116
Hycotuss Expectorant Syrup 1117
Vicodin Tablets 535
Vicodin ES Tablets 536
Vicodin HP Tablets 538
Vicoprofen Tablets 539
Zydone Tablets 1139

Hydrocodone Polistirex (Potentiation of orthostatic hypotension). Products include:
Tussionex Pennkinetic Extended-Release Suspension 3327

Hydrocortisone (Corticosteroids intensify electrolyte depletion, particularly hypokalemia). Products include:
Colocort Rectal Suspension, USP (Retention) 100 mg/60 mL 2476
Hydrocortone Tablets 1989
Preparation H Hydrocortisone Cream .... ▣646

Hydrocortisone Acetate (Corticosteroids intensify electrolyte depletion, particularly hypokalemia). Products include:
Analpram-HC 1159
Pramosone 1161
ProctoFoam-HC 3099

Hydrocortisone Sodium Phosphate (Corticosteroids intensify electrolyte depletion, particularly hypokalemia).
No products indexed under this heading.

Hydrocortisone Sodium Succinate (Corticosteroids intensify electrolyte depletion, particularly hypokalemia).
No products indexed under this heading.

Hydroflumethiazide (Co-administration with other antihypertensive agents may result in additive effect or potentiation).
No products indexed under this heading.

Hydromorphone Hydrochloride (Potentiation of orthostatic hypotension). Products include:
Dilaudid 440
Dilaudid Non-Sterile Powder 440
Dilaudid Oral Liquid 445
Dilaudid Rectal Suppositories 440
Dilaudid Tablets 440
Dilaudid Tablets - 8 mg 445
Dilaudid-HP 442

Ibuprofen (Co-administration in some patients can result in reduced diuretic, natriuretic, and antihypertensive effects). Products include:
Advil Allergy Sinus Caplets .... ▣770
Advil .... ▣674
Children's Advil Oral Suspension .... ▣603
Children's Advil Chewable Tablets .... ▣603
Advil Cold & Sinus .... ▣723
Infants' Advil Concentrated Drops .... ▣604
Infants' Advil Concentrated Drops - White Grape (Dye-Free) .... ▣604
Junior Strength Advil Swallow Tablets .... ▣605
Advil Migraine Liquigels .... ▣608
Advil Multi-Symptom Cold Caplets .... ▣770
Advil PM Caplets .... ▣615
Motrin IB Tablets and Caplets 1866
Children's Motrin Oral Suspension 1867
Children's Motrin Non-Staining Dye-Free Oral Suspension 1867
Children's Motrin Cold Oral Suspension 1867
Infants' Motrin Concentrated Drops 1867
Infants' Motrin Non-Staining Dye-Free Concentrated Drops 1867
Junior Strength Motrin Caplets and Chewable Tablets 1867
Vicoprofen Tablets 539

Imipramine Hydrochloride (Possible inhibition of the metabolism of drugs metabolized by CYP2C19).
No products indexed under this heading.

Imipramine Pamoate (Possible inhibition of the metabolism of drugs metabolized by CYP2C19).
No products indexed under this heading.

Indapamide (Co-administration with other antihypertensive agents may result in additive effect or potentiation). Products include:
Indapamide Tablets 2156

Indomethacin (Possible inhibition of the metabolism of drugs metabolized by CYP2C19). Products include:
Indocin 1995

Indomethacin Sodium Trihydrate (Possible inhibition of the metabolism of drugs metabolized by CYP2C19). Products include:
Indocin I.V. 2465

Insulin, Human, Zinc Suspension (Thiazide diuretics may cause hyperglycemia; dosage adjustment of insulin may be required). Products include:
Humulin L, 100 Units 1794
Humulin U, 100 Units 1800

Insulin, Human NPH (Thiazide diuretics may cause hyperglycemia; dosage adjustment of insulin may be required). Products include:
Humulin N, 100 Units 1795
Humulin N Pen 1797

Insulin, Human Regular (Thiazide diuretics may cause hyperglycemia; dosage adjustment of insulin may be required). Products include:
Humulin R, 100 Units 1798

Insulin, Human Regular and Human NPH Mixture (Thiazide diuretics may cause hyperglycemia; dosage adjustment of insulin may be required). Products include:
Humulin 50/50, 100 Units 1791
Humulin 70/30 Pen 1793

Insulin, NPH (Thiazide diuretics may cause hyperglycemia; dosage adjustment of insulin may be required).
No products indexed under this heading.

Insulin, Regular (Thiazide diuretics may cause hyperglycemia; dosage adjustment of insulin may be required).
No products indexed under this heading.

Insulin, Zinc Crystals (Thiazide diuretics may cause hyperglycemia; dosage adjustment of insulin may be required).
No products indexed under this heading.

Insulin, Zinc Suspension (Thiazide diuretics may cause hyperglycemia; dosage adjustment of insulin may be required).
No products indexed under this heading.

Insulin Aspart, Human Regular (Thiazide diuretics may cause hyperglycemia; dosage adjustment of insulin may be required). Products include:
NovoLog Injection 2326

Insulin glargine (Thiazide diuretics may cause hyperglycemia; dosage adjustment of insulin may be required). Products include:
Lantus Injection 2909

Insulin Lispro, Human (Thiazide diuretics may cause hyperglycemia; dosage adjustment of insulin may be required). Products include:
Humalog-Pen 1781
Humalog Mix 50/50-Pen 1783
Humalog Mix 75/25-Pen 1785

Insulin Lispro Protamine, Human (Thiazide diuretics may cause hyperglycemia; dosage adjustment of insulin may be required). Products include:
Humalog Mix 50/50-Pen 1783
Humalog Mix 75/25-Pen 1785

Irbesartan (Co-administration with other antihypertensive agents may result in additive effect or potentiation). Products include:
Avalide Tablets 888
Avalide Tablets 2874
Avapro Tablets 891
Avapro Tablets 2871

Isradipine (Co-administration with other antihypertensive agents may result in additive effect or potentiation). Products include:
DynaCirc CR Tablets 2721

Ketoprofen (Co-administration in some patients can result in reduced diuretic, natriuretic, and antihypertensive effects).
No products indexed under this heading.

Ketorolac Tromethamine (Co-administration in some patients can result in reduced diuretic, natriuretic, and antihypertensive effects). Products include:
Acular Ophthalmic Solution 565
Acular LS Ophthalmic Solution 566

Labetalol Hydrochloride (Co-administration with other antihypertensive agents may result in additive effect or potentiation).
No products indexed under this heading.

Lamotrigine (Possible inhibition of the metabolism of drugs metabolized by CYP2C19). Products include:
Lamictal 1481

Lansoprazole (Possible inhibition of the metabolism of drugs metabolized by CYP2C19). Products include:
Prevacid Delayed-Release Capsules 3271
Prevacid for Delayed-Release Oral Suspension 3271
Prevacid SoluTab Delayed-Release Orally Disintegrating Tablets 3271
Prevacid I.V. for Injection 3277
Prevacid NapraPAC 3280
PREVPAC 3284

Levetiracetam (Possible inhibition of the metabolism of drugs metabolized by CYP2C19). Products include:
Keppra Injection 3320
Keppra Oral Solution 3314
Keppra Tablets 3314

Levorphanol Tartrate (Potentiation of orthostatic hypotension).
No products indexed under this heading.

Lisinopril (Co-administration with other antihypertensive agents may result in additive effect or potentiation). Products include:
Prinivil Tablets 2052
Prinzide Tablets 2056

Lithium (Diuretics reduce the renal clearance of lithium and add a high risk of lithium toxicity; concurrent use should be avoided).
No products indexed under this heading.

Lithium Carbonate (Diuretics reduce the renal clearance of lithium and add a high risk of lithium toxicity; concurrent use should be avoided). Products include:
Lithobid Tablets 1692

Lithium Citrate (Diuretics reduce the renal clearance of lithium and add a high risk of lithium toxicity; concurrent use should be avoided).
No products indexed under this heading.

Losartan Potassium (Co-administration with other antihypertensive agents may result in additive effect or potentiation). Products include:
Cozaar Tablets 1935
Hyzaar 50-12.5 Tablets 1990
Hyzaar 100-12.5 Tablets 1990
Hyzaar 100-25 Tablets 1990

Maprotiline Hydrochloride (Possible inhibition of the metabolism of drugs metabolized by CYP2C19).
No products indexed under this heading.

Mecamylamine Hydrochloride (Co-administration with other antihypertensive agents may result in additive effect or potentiation).
No products indexed under this heading.

Meclofenamate Sodium (Co-administration in some patients can result in reduced diuretic, natriuretic, and antihypertensive effects).
No products indexed under this heading.

Mefenamic Acid (Co-administration in some patients can result in reduced diuretic, natriuretic, and antihypertensive effects).
No products indexed under this heading.

Meloxicam (Co-administration in some patients can result in reduced diuretic, natriuretic, and antihypertensive effects). Products include:
Mobic Oral Suspension 863
Mobic Tablets 863

Meperidine Hydrochloride (Potentiation of orthostatic hypotension).
No products indexed under this heading.

Mephenytoin (Possible inhibition of the metabolism of drugs metabolized by CYP2C19).
No products indexed under this heading.

Mephobarbital (Potentiation of orthostatic hypotension).
No products indexed under this heading.

Meprobamate (Possible inhibition of the metabolism of drugs metabolized by CYP2C19).
No products indexed under this heading.

Metformin Hydrochloride (Thiazide diuretics may cause hyperglycemia; dosage adjustment of oral hypoglycemia agents may be required). Products include:
ActoPlus Met Tablets 3214
Avandamet Tablets 1373
Fortamet Extended-Release Tablets 3115

Methadone Hydrochloride (Potentiation of orthostatic hypotension).
No products indexed under this heading.

Methsuximide (Possible inhibition of the metabolism of drugs metabolized by CYP2C19).
No products indexed under this heading.

Methyclothiazide (Co-administration with other antihypertensive agents may result in additive effect or potentiation).
No products indexed under this heading.

Methyldopa (Co-administration with other antihypertensive agents may result in additive effect or potentiation). Products include:
Aldoril Tablets 1910

Methyldopate Hydrochloride (Co-administration with other antihypertensive agents may result in additive effect or potentiation).
No products indexed under this heading.

Methylprednisolone Acetate (Corticosteroids intensify electrolyte depletion, particularly hypokalemia). Products include:
Depo-Medrol Injectable Suspension 2617
Depo-Medrol Single-Dose Vial 2619

Methylprednisolone Sodium Succinate (Corticosteroids intensify electrolyte depletion, particularly hypokalemia).
No products indexed under this heading.

Metocurine Iodide (Possible increased responsiveness to the muscle relaxants).
No products indexed under this heading.

Metolazone (Co-administration with other antihypertensive agents may result in additive effect or potentiation).
No products indexed under this heading.

Metoprolol Succinate (Co-administration with other antihypertensive agents may result in additive effect or potentiation). Products include:
Toprol-XL Tablets 668

Metoprolol Tartrate (Co-administration with other antihypertensive agents may result in additive effect or potentiation). Products include:
Lopressor Injection 2238
Lopressor Tablets 2238
Lopressor HCT 50/25 Tablets 2241
Lopressor HCT 100/25 Tablets 2241
Lopressor HCT 100/50 Tablets 2241

Metyrosine (Co-administration with other antihypertensive agents may result in additive effect or potentiation). Products include:
Demser Capsules 1953

Mibefradil Dihydrochloride (Co-administration with other antihypertensive agents may result in additive effect or potentiation).
No products indexed under this heading.

Midazolam Hydrochloride (Possible inhibition of the metabolism of drugs metabolized by CYP2C19).
No products indexed under this heading.

Miglitol (Thiazide diuretics may cause hyperglycemia; dosage adjustment of oral hypoglycemia agents may be required).
No products indexed under this heading.

Minoxidil (Co-administration with other antihypertensive agents may result in additive effect or potentiation). Products include:
Men's Rogaine Extra Strength Hair Regrowth Treatment Topical Solution, Ocean Rush Scent and Original Unscented 633
Men's Rogaine Foam Hair Regrowth Treatment.................. 633
Women's Rogaine Hair Regrowth Treatment Topical Solution, Spring Bloom Scent and Original Unscented..................... 634

Mivacurium Chloride (Possible increased responsiveness to the muscle relaxants). Products include:
Mivacron Injection 493

Moexipril Hydrochloride (Co-administration with other antihypertensive agents may result in additive effect or potentiation). Products include:
Uniretic Tablets 3100
Univasc Tablets 3104

Morphine Sulfate (Potentiation of orthostatic hypotension). Products include:
Avinza Capsules 1741
Kadian Capsules 577
MS Contin Tablets 2701

Nabumetone (Co-administration in some patients can result in reduced diuretic, natriuretic, and antihypertensive effects).
No products indexed under this heading.

Nadolol (Co-administration with other antihypertensive agents may result in additive effect or potentiation). Products include:
Nadolol Tablets 2159

Naproxen (Co-administration in some patients can result in reduced diuretic, natriuretic, and antihypertensive effects). Products include:
EC-Naprosyn Delayed-Release Tablets 2761
Naprosyn Suspension 2761
Naprosyn Tablets 2761
Prevacid NapraPAC 3280

Naproxen Sodium (Co-administration in some patients can result in reduced diuretic, natriuretic, and antihypertensive effects). Products include:
Aleve Caplets 742
Aleve Gelcaps 743
Aleve Tablets 743
Aleve Cold & Sinus Caplets 744
Anaprox Tablets 2761
Anaprox DS Tablets 2761

Nelfinavir Mesylate (Possible inhibition of the metabolism of drugs metabolized by CYP2C19). Products include:
Viracept 2577

Nicardipine Hydrochloride (Co-administration with other antihypertensive agents may result in additive effect or potentiation). Products include:
Cardene I.V. 2497

Nifedipine (Co-administration with other antihypertensive agents may result in additive effect or potentiation). Products include:
Adalat CC Tablets 2964

Nilutamide (Possible inhibition of the metabolism of drugs metabolized by CYP2C19).
No products indexed under this heading.

Nisoldipine (Co-administration with other antihypertensive agents may result in additive effect or potentiation). Products include:
Sular Tablets 3122

Nitroglycerin (Co-administration with other antihypertensive agents may result in additive effect or potentiation). Products include:
Nitro-Dur Transdermal Infusion System.. 3046
Nitrolingual Pumpspray 3120

Norepinephrine Bitartrate (Possible decreased response to pressor amines).
No products indexed under this heading.

Nortriptyline Hydrochloride (Possible inhibition of the metabolism of drugs metabolized by CYP2C19).
No products indexed under this heading.

Omeprazole (Possible inhibition of the metabolism of drugs metabolized by CYP2C19). Products include:
Zegerid Capsules 2958
Zegerid Powder for Oral Solution 2958

Oxaprozin (Co-administration in some patients can result in reduced diuretic, natriuretic, and antihypertensive effects).
No products indexed under this heading.

Oxcarbazepine (Possible inhibition of the metabolism of drugs metabolized by CYP2C19). Products include:
Trileptal Tablets 2300
Trileptal Oral Suspension 2300

Oxycodone Hydrochloride (Potentiation of orthostatic hypotension). Products include:
OxyContin Tablets 2703
OxyFast Oral Concentrate Solution.. 2708
OxyIR Capsules 2708
Percocet Tablets 1131
Percodan Tablets 1132

Pancuronium Bromide (Possible increased responsiveness to the muscle relaxants).
No products indexed under this heading.

Pantoprazole Sodium (Possible inhibition of the metabolism of drugs metabolized by CYP2C19). Products include:
Protonix I.V. 3472
Protonix Tablets 3469

Paramethadione (Possible inhibition of the metabolism of drugs metabolized by CYP2C19).
No products indexed under this heading.

Penbutolol Sulfate (Co-administration with other antihypertensive agents may result in additive effect or potentiation).
No products indexed under this heading.

Pentamidine Isethionate (Possible inhibition of the metabolism of drugs metabolized by CYP2C19).
No products indexed under this heading.

Pentobarbital Sodium (Potentiation of orthostatic hypotension). Products include:
Nembutal Sodium Solution, USP 2470

Perindopril Erbumine (Co-administration with other antihypertensive agents may result in additive effect or potentiation). Products include:
Aceon Tablets (2 mg, 4 mg, 8 mg).. 3194

Phenacemide (Possible inhibition of the metabolism of drugs metabolized by CYP2C19).
No products indexed under this heading.

Phenobarbital (Potentiation of orthostatic hypotension). Products include:
Donnatal Extentabs 2493

Phenobarbital Sodium (Possible inhibition of the metabolism of drugs metabolized by CYP2C19).
No products indexed under this heading.

Phenoxybenzamine Hydrochloride (Co-administration with other antihypertensive agents may result in additive effect or potentiation). Products include:
Dibenzyline Capsules 3399

Phensuximide (Possible inhibition of the metabolism of drugs metabolized by CYP2C19).
No products indexed under this heading.

Phentolamine Mesylate (Co-administration with other antihypertensive agents may result in additive effect or potentiation).
No products indexed under this heading.

Phenylbutazone (Co-administration in some patients can result in reduced diuretic, natriuretic, and antihypertensive effects).
No products indexed under this heading.

Phenytoin (Possible inhibition of the metabolism of drugs metabolized by CYP2C19).
No products indexed under this heading.

Phenytoin Sodium (Possible inhibition of the metabolism of drugs metabolized by CYP2C19). Products include:
Phenytek Capsules 2160

Pindolol (Co-administration with other antihypertensive agents may result in additive effect or potentiation).
No products indexed under this heading.

Pioglitazone Hydrochloride (Thiazide diuretics may cause hyperglycemia; dosage adjustment of oral hypoglycemia agents may be required). Products include:

ActoPlus Met Tablets 3214
Actos Tablets 3219
Duetact Tablets 3226

Piroxicam (Co-administration in some patients can result in reduced diuretic, natriuretic, and antihypertensive effects).
No products indexed under this heading.

Polythiazide (Co-administration with other antihypertensive agents may result in additive effect or potentiation).
No products indexed under this heading.

Potassium Acid Phosphate (Concurrent use of potassium supplements or salt substitute is not recommended). Products include:
K-Phos Original (Sodium Free) Tablets 760

Potassium Bicarbonate (Concurrent use of potassium supplements or salt substitute is not recommended).
No products indexed under this heading.

Potassium Chloride (Concurrent use of potassium supplements or salt substitute is not recommended). Products include:
Colyte with Flavor Packs for Oral Solution 3088
HalfLytely and Bisacodyl Tablets Bowel Prep Kit with Flavors Packs 881
K-Dur Extended-Relase Tablets 3033
K-Lor Oral Solution 474
K-Tab Tablets 475
MoviPrep Oral Solution 2839
TriLyte with Flavor Packs for Oral Solution 3100

Potassium Citrate (Concurrent use of potassium supplements or salt substitute is not recommended). Products include:
Urocit-K Tablets 2144

Potassium Gluconate (Concurrent use of potassium supplements or salt substitute is not recommended).
No products indexed under this heading.

Potassium Phosphate (Concurrent use of potassium supplements or salt substitute is not recommended). Products include:
K-Phos Neutral Tablets 760

Prazosin Hydrochloride (Co-administration with other antihypertensive agents may result in additive effect or potentiation).
No products indexed under this heading.

Prednisolone Acetate (Corticosteroids intensify electrolyte depletion, particularly hypokalemia). Products include:
Blephamide Ophthalmic Ointment 568
Blephamide Ophthalmic Suspension 569
Poly-Pred Ophthalmic Suspension .... ⊙233
Pred Forte Ophthalmic Suspension .... ⊙235
Pred Mild Ophthalmic Suspension .... ⊙238
Pred-G Ophthalmic Ointment .... ⊙237
Pred-G Ophthalmic Suspension .... ⊙236

Prednisolone Sodium Phosphate (Corticosteroids intensify electrolyte depletion, particularly hypokalemia).
No products indexed under this heading.

Prednisolone Tebutate (Corticosteroids intensify electrolyte depletion, particularly hypokalemia).
No products indexed under this heading.

Prednisone (Corticosteroids intensify electrolyte depletion, particularly hypokalemia).
No products indexed under this heading.

Primidone (Possible inhibition of the metabolism of drugs metabolized by CYP2C19).
No products indexed under this heading.

Progesterone (Possible inhibition of the metabolism of drugs metabolized by CYP2C19). Products include:
Prochieve 4% Gel 1003
Prochieve 8% Gel 1003
Prometrium Capsules (100 mg, 200 mg) 3203

Proguanil Hydrochloride (Possible inhibition of the metabolism of drugs metabolized by CYP2C19). Products include:
Malarone Pediatric Tablets 1517
Malarone Tablets 1517

Propoxyphene Hydrochloride (Potentiation of orthostatic hypotension).
No products indexed under this heading.

Propoxyphene Napsylate (Potentiation of orthostatic hypotension).
No products indexed under this heading.

Propranolol Hydrochloride (Possible inhibition of the metabolism of drugs metabolized by CYP2C19). Products include:
Inderal LA Long-Acting Capsules 3429
InnoPran XL Capsules 2723

Protriptyline Hydrochloride (Possible inhibition of the metabolism of drugs metabolized by CYP2C19).
No products indexed under this heading.

Quinapril Hydrochloride (Co-administration with other antihypertensive agents may result in additive effect or potentiation).
No products indexed under this heading.

Rabeprazole Sodium (Possible inhibition of the metabolism of drugs metabolized by CYP2C19). Products include:
Aciphex Tablets 1090

Ramipril (Co-administration with other antihypertensive agents may result in additive effect or potentiation). Products include:
Altace Capsules 1702

Rapacuronium Bromide (Possible increased responsiveness to the muscle relaxants).
No products indexed under this heading.

Rauwolfia Serpentina (Co-administration with other antihypertensive agents may result in additive effect or potentiation).
No products indexed under this heading.

Remifentanil Hydrochloride (Potentiation of orthostatic hypotension).
No products indexed under this heading.

Repaglinide (Thiazide diuretics may cause hyperglycemia; dosage adjustment of oral hypoglycemia agents may be required).
No products indexed under this heading.

Rescinnamine (Co-administration with other antihypertensive agents may result in additive effect or potentiation).
No products indexed under this heading.

Reserpine (Co-administration with other antihypertensive agents may result in additive effect or potentiation).
No products indexed under this heading.

Rocuronium Bromide (Possible increased responsiveness to the muscle relaxants). Products include:
Zemuron Injection 2346

Rofecoxib (Co-administration in some patients can result in reduced diuretic, natriuretic, and antihypertensive effects).
No products indexed under this heading.

Rosiglitazone Maleate (Thiazide diuretics may cause hyperglycemia; dosage adjustment of oral hypoglycemia agents may be required). Products include:
Avandamet Tablets 1373
Avandaryl Tablets 1379
Avandia Tablets 1384

Secobarbital Sodium (Potentiation of orthostatic hypotension).
No products indexed under this heading.

Sertraline Hydrochloride (Possible inhibition of the metabolism of drugs metabolized by CYP2C19). Products include:
Zoloft 2586

Sodium Nitroprusside (Co-administration with other antihypertensive agents may result in additive effect or potentiation).
No products indexed under this heading.

Sotalol Hydrochloride (Co-administration with other antihypertensive agents may result in additive effect or potentiation).
No products indexed under this heading.

Spirapril Hydrochloride (Co-administration with other antihypertensive agents may result in additive effect or potentiation).
No products indexed under this heading.

Sufentanil Citrate (Potentiation of orthostatic hypotension).
No products indexed under this heading.

Sulindac (Co-administration in some patients can result in reduced diuretic, natriuretic, and antihypertensive effects). Products include:
Clinoril Tablets 1924

Teniposide (Possible inhibition of the metabolism of drugs metabolized by CYP2C19).
No products indexed under this heading.

Terazosin Hydrochloride (Co-administration with other antihypertensive agents may result in additive effect or potentiation). Products include:
Hytrin Capsules 471

Thiamylal Sodium (Potentiation of orthostatic hypotension).
No products indexed under this heading.

Thioridazine (Possible inhibition of the metabolism of drugs metabolized by CYP2C19).
No products indexed under this heading.

Thioridazine Hydrochloride (Possible inhibition of the metabolism of drugs metabolized by CYP2C19). Products include:
Thioridazine Hydrochloride Tablets 2163

Tiagabine Hydrochloride (Possible inhibition of the metabolism of drugs metabolized by CYP2C19). Products include:
Gabitril Tablets 984

Timolol Maleate (Co-administration with other antihypertensive agents may result in additive effect or potentiation). Products include:
Blocadren Tablets 1916
Cosopt Sterile Ophthalmic Solution 1931
Timolide Tablets 2086
Timoptic Sterile Ophthalmic Solution 2088
Timoptic in Ocudose 2091
Timoptic-XE Sterile Ophthalmic Gel Forming Solution 2092

Tolazamide (Thiazide diuretics may cause hyperglycemia; dosage adjustment of oral hypoglycemia agents may be required).
No products indexed under this heading.

Tolbutamide (Possible inhibition of the metabolism of drugs metabolized by CYP2C19).
No products indexed under this heading.

Tolbutamide Sodium (Possible inhibition of the metabolism of drugs metabolized by CYP2C19).
No products indexed under this heading.

Tolmetin Sodium (Co-administration in some patients can result in reduced diuretic, natriuretic, and antihypertensive effects).
No products indexed under this heading.

Topiramate (Possible inhibition of the metabolism of drugs metabolized by CYP2C19). Products include:
Topamax Sprinkle Capsules 2404
Topamax Tablets 2404

Torsemide (Co-administration with other antihypertensive agents may result in additive effect or potentiation). Products include:
Demadex Injection 2759
Demadex Tablets 2759

Trandolapril (Co-administration with other antihypertensive agents may result in additive effect or potentiation). Products include:
Mavik Tablets 486
Tarka Tablets 524

Triamcinolone (Corticosteroids intensify electrolyte depletion, particularly hypokalemia).
No products indexed under this heading.

Triamcinolone Acetonide (Corticosteroids intensify electrolyte depletion, particularly hypokalemia). Products include:
Azmacort Inhalation Aerosol 1726
Nasacort AQ Nasal Spray 2922

Triamcinolone Diacetate (Corticosteroids intensify electrolyte depletion, particularly hypokalemia).
No products indexed under this heading.

Triamcinolone Hexacetonide (Corticosteroids intensify electrolyte depletion, particularly hypokalemia).
No products indexed under this heading.

Trimethadione (Possible inhibition of the metabolism of drugs metabolized by CYP2C19).
 No products indexed under this heading.

Trimethaphan Camsylate (Co-administration with other antihypertensive agents may result in additive effect or potentiation).
 No products indexed under this heading.

Trimipramine Maleate (Possible inhibition of the metabolism of drugs metabolized by CYP2C19).
 No products indexed under this heading.

Troglitazone (Thiazide diuretics may cause hyperglycemia; dosage adjustment of oral hypoglycemia agents may be required).
 No products indexed under this heading.

Valdecoxib (Co-administration in some patients can result in reduced diuretic, natriuretic, and antihypertensive effects).
 No products indexed under this heading.

Valproate Sodium (Possible inhibition of the metabolism of drugs metabolized by CYP2C19). Products include:
 Depacon Injection **412**

Valproic Acid (Possible inhibition of the metabolism of drugs metabolized by CYP2C19). Products include:
 Depakene **417**

Valsartan (Co-administration with other antihypertensive agents may result in additive effect or potentiation). Products include:
 Diovan Tablets **2193**
 Diovan HCT Tablets **2196**

Vecuronium Bromide (Possible increased responsiveness to the muscle relaxants).
 No products indexed under this heading.

Verapamil Hydrochloride (Co-administration with other antihypertensive agents may result in additive effect or potentiation). Products include:
 Covera-HS Tablets **3139**
 Tarka Tablets **524**
 Verelan PM Extended-Release Capsules, Controlled-Onset **3106**

Voriconazole (Possible inhibition of the metabolism of drugs metabolized by CYP2C19). Products include:
 VFEND I.V. **2564**
 VFEND Oral Suspension **2564**
 VFEND Tablets **2564**

Warfarin Sodium (Co-administration has resulted in slight decrease in the mean warfarin trough plasma concentration; this decrease did not result in a change in INR). Products include:
 Coumadin for Injection **898**
 Coumadin Tablets **898**

Zonisamide (Possible inhibition of the metabolism of drugs metabolized by CYP2C19). Products include:
 Zonegran Capsules **1101**

Food Interactions

Alcohol (Potentiation of orthostatic hypotension).

Food, unspecified (Slightly reduces the bioavailability of telmisartan with reduction in AUC of about 6%).

MICRHOGAM ULTRA-FILTERED

(Rh_o (D) Immune Globulin (Human)) **2371**
None cited in PDR database.

MIDAMOR TABLETS

(Amiloride Hydrochloride) **2026**
May interact with ACE inhibitors, angiotensin-II receptor antagonists, diuretics, lithium preparations, nonsteroidal anti-inflammatory agents, potassium preparations, potassium sparing diuretics, and certain other agents. Compounds in these categories include:

Benazepril Hydrochloride (Co-administration increases the risk of hyperkalemia). Products include:
 Lotensin Tablets **2243**
 Lotensin HCT Tablets **2246**
 Lotrel Capsules **2249**

Bendroflumethiazide (Co-administration with other diuretics may result in hypochloremia, hyponatremia, and increases in BUN).
 No products indexed under this heading.

Bumetanide (Co-administration with other diuretics may result in hypochloremia, hyponatremia, and increases in BUN). Products include:
 Bumex Tablets **2746**

Candesartan Cilexetil (Co-administration increases the risk of hyperkalemia). Products include:
 Atacand Tablets **649**
 Atacand HCT **651**

Captopril (Co-administration increases the risk of hyperkalemia). Products include:
 Captopril Tablets **2149**

Celecoxib (Co-administration of non-steroidal anti-inflammatory agents can reduce the diuretic, natriuretic, and antihypertensive effects). Products include:
 Celebrex Capsules **3134**

Chlorothiazide (Co-administration with other diuretics may result in hypochloremia, hyponatremia, and increases in BUN). Products include:
 Diuril Oral Suspension **1954**

Chlorothiazide Sodium (Co-administration with other diuretics may result in hypochloremia, hyponatremia, and increases in BUN). Products include:
 Diuril Sodium Intravenous **2467**

Chlorthalidone (Co-administration with other diuretics may result in hypochloremia, hyponatremia, and increases in BUN). Products include:
 Clorpres Tablets **2153**

Cyclosporine (Co-administration increases the risk of hyperkalemia). Products include:
 Gengraf Capsules **459**
 Neoral Oral Solution **2259**
 Neoral Soft Gelatin Capsules **2259**
 Restasis Ophthalmic Emulsion **575**
 Sandimmune **2275**

Diclofenac Potassium (Co-administration of non-steroidal anti-inflammatory agents can reduce the diuretic, natriuretic, and antihypertensive effects).
 No products indexed under this heading.

Diclofenac Sodium (Co-administration of non-steroidal anti-inflammatory agents can reduce the diuretic, natriuretic, and antihypertensive effects). Products include:
 Arthrotec Tablets **3129**
 Voltaren Ophthalmic Solution **2309**
 Voltaren Tablets **2307**
 Voltaren-XR Tablets **2310**

Enalapril Maleate (Co-administration increases the risk of hyperkalemia). Products include:
 Vasotec I.V. Injection **2103**

Enalaprilat (Co-administration increases the risk of hyperkalemia).
 No products indexed under this heading.

Eprosartan Mesylate (Co-administration increases the risk of hyperkalemia). Products include:
 Teveten Tablets **1735**
 Teveten HCT Tablets **1737**

Ethacrynic Acid (Co-administration with other diuretics may result in hypochloremia, hyponatremia, and increases in BUN). Products include:
 Edecrin Tablets **1959**

Etodolac (Co-administration of non-steroidal anti-inflammatory agents can reduce the diuretic, natriuretic, and antihypertensive effects).
 No products indexed under this heading.

Fenoprofen Calcium (Co-administration of non-steroidal anti-inflammatory agents can reduce the diuretic, natriuretic, and antihypertensive effects). Products include:
 Nalfon Capsules **2502**

Flurbiprofen (Co-administration of non-steroidal anti-inflammatory agents can reduce the diuretic, natriuretic, and antihypertensive effects).
 No products indexed under this heading.

Fosinopril Sodium (Co-administration increases the risk of hyperkalemia).
 No products indexed under this heading.

Furosemide (Co-administration with other diuretics may result in hypochloremia, hyponatremia, and increases in BUN). Products include:
 Furosemide Tablets **2154**

Hydrochlorothiazide (Co-administration with other diuretics may result in hypochloremia, hyponatremia, and increases in BUN). Products include:
 Aldoril Tablets **1910**
 Atacand HCT **651**
 Avalide Tablets **888**
 Avalide Tablets **2874**
 Benicar HCT Tablets **1044**
 Diovan HCT Tablets **2196**
 Dyazide Capsules **1423**
 Hyzaar 50-12.5 Tablets **1990**
 Hyzaar 100-12.5 Tablets **1990**
 Hyzaar 100-25 Tablets **1990**
 Lopressor HCT 50/25 Tablets **2241**
 Lopressor HCT 100/25 Tablets **2241**
 Lopressor HCT 100/50 Tablets **2241**
 Lotensin HCT Tablets **2246**
 Micardis HCT Tablets **856**
 Moduretic Tablets **2028**
 Prinzide Tablets **2056**
 Teveten HCT Tablets **1737**
 Timolide Tablets **2086**
 Uniretic Tablets **3100**

Hydroflumethiazide (Co-administration with other diuretics may result in hypochloremia, hyponatremia, and increases in BUN).
 No products indexed under this heading.

Ibuprofen (Co-administration of non-steroidal anti-inflammatory agents can reduce the diuretic, natriuretic, and antihypertensive effects). Products include:
 Advil Allergy Sinus Caplets .... ▣ **770**
 Advil .... ▣ **674**
 Children's Advil Oral Suspension .... ▣ **603**
 Children's Advil Chewable Tablets .... ▣ **603**
 Advil Cold & Sinus .... ▣ **723**
 Infants' Advil Concentrated Drops .... ▣ **604**
 Infants' Advil Concentrated Drops - White Grape (Dye-Free) .... ▣ **604**
 Junior Strength Advil Swallow Tablets .... ▣ **605**
 Advil Migraine Liquigels .... ▣ **608**
 Advil Multi-Symptom Cold Caplets .... ▣ **770**
 Advil PM Caplets .... ▣ **615**
 Motrin IB Tablets and Caplets **1866**
 Children's Motrin Oral Suspension **1867**
 Children's Motrin Non-Staining Dye-Free Oral Suspension **1867**
 Children's Motrin Cold Oral Suspension **1867**
 Infants' Motrin Concentrated Drops **1867**
 Infants' Motrin Non-Staining Dye-Free Concentrated Drops **1867**
 Junior Strength Motrin Caplets and Chewable Tablets **1867**
 Vicoprofen Tablets **539**

Indapamide (Co-administration with other diuretics may result in hypochloremia, hyponatremia, and increases in BUN). Products include:
 Indapamide Tablets **2156**

Indomethacin (Co-administration of non-steroidal anti-inflammatory agents can reduce the diuretic, natriuretic, and antihypertensive effects; both indomethacin and amiloride are associated with hyperkalemia, the potential effect on potassium kinetic and renal function should be considered if used concurrently). Products include:
 Indocin **1995**

Indomethacin Sodium Trihydrate (Co-administration of non-steroidal anti-inflammatory agents can reduce the diuretic, natriuretic, and antihypertensive effects; both indomethacin and amiloride are associated with hyperkalemia, the potential effect on potassium kinetic and renal function should be considered if used concurrently). Products include:
 Indocin I.V. **2465**

Irbesartan (Co-administration increases the risk of hyperkalemia). Products include:
 Avalide Tablets **888**
 Avalide Tablets **2874**
 Avapro Tablets **891**
 Avapro Tablets **2871**

Ketoprofen (Co-administration of non-steroidal anti-inflammatory agents can reduce the diuretic, natriuretic, and antihypertensive effects).
 No products indexed under this heading.

Ketorolac Tromethamine (Co-administration of non-steroidal anti-inflammatory agents can reduce the diuretic, natriuretic, and antihypertensive effects). Products include:
 Acular Ophthalmic Solution **565**
 Acular LS Ophthalmic Solution **566**

Lisinopril (Co-administration increases the risk of hyperkalemia). Products include:
 Prinivil Tablets **2052**
 Prinzide Tablets **2056**

Lithium (Diuretics reduce the renal clearance and add a high risk of lithium toxicity).
 No products indexed under this heading.

Lithium Carbonate (Diuretics reduce the renal clearance and add a high risk of lithium toxicity). Products include:
 Lithobid Tablets **1692**

Lithium Citrate (Diuretics reduce the renal clearance and add a high risk of lithium toxicity).
 No products indexed under this heading.

Losartan Potassium (Co-administration increases the risk of hyperkalemia). Products include:
- Cozaar Tablets 1935
- Hyzaar 50-12.5 Tablets 1990
- Hyzaar 100-12.5 Tablets 1990
- Hyzaar 100-25 Tablets 1990

Meclofenamate Sodium (Co-administration of non-steroidal anti-inflammatory agents can reduce the diuretic, natriuretic, and antihypertensive effects).
No products indexed under this heading.

Mefenamic Acid (Co-administration of non-steroidal anti-inflammatory agents can reduce the diuretic, natriuretic, and antihypertensive effects).
No products indexed under this heading.

Meloxicam (Co-administration of non-steroidal anti-inflammatory agents can reduce the diuretic, natriuretic, and antihypertensive effects). Products include:
- Mobic Oral Suspension 863
- Mobic Tablets 863

Methyclothiazide (Co-administration with other diuretics may result in hypochloremia, hyponatremia, and increases in BUN).
No products indexed under this heading.

Metolazone (Co-administration with other diuretics may result in hypochloremia, hyponatremia, and increases in BUN).
No products indexed under this heading.

Moexipril Hydrochloride (Co-administration increases the risk of hyperkalemia). Products include:
- Uniretic Tablets 3100
- Univasc Tablets 3104

Nabumetone (Co-administration of non-steroidal anti-inflammatory agents can reduce the diuretic, natriuretic, and antihypertensive effects).
No products indexed under this heading.

Naproxen (Co-administration of non-steroidal anti-inflammatory agents can reduce the diuretic, natriuretic, and antihypertensive effects). Products include:
- EC-Naprosyn Delayed-Release Tablets 2761
- Naprosyn Suspension 2761
- Naprosyn Tablets 2761
- Prevacid NapraPAC 3280

Naproxen Sodium (Co-administration of non-steroidal anti-inflammatory agents can reduce the diuretic, natriuretic, and antihypertensive effects). Products include:
- Aleve Caplets 742
- Aleve Gelcaps 743
- Aleve Tablets 743
- Aleve Cold & Sinus Caplets 744
- Anaprox Tablets 2761
- Anaprox DS Tablets 2761

Oxaprozin (Co-administration of non-steroidal anti-inflammatory agents can reduce the diuretic, natriuretic, and antihypertensive effects).
No products indexed under this heading.

Perindopril Erbumine (Co-administration increases the risk of hyperkalemia). Products include:
- Aceon Tablets (2 mg, 4 mg, 8 mg) 3194

Phenylbutazone (Co-administration of non-steroidal anti-inflammatory agents can reduce the diuretic, natriuretic, and antihypertensive effects).
No products indexed under this heading.

Piroxicam (Co-administration of non-steroidal anti-inflammatory agents can reduce the diuretic, natriuretic, and antihypertensive effects).
No products indexed under this heading.

Polythiazide (Co-administration with other diuretics may result in hypochloremia, hyponatremia, and increases in BUN).
No products indexed under this heading.

Potassium Acid Phosphate (Amiloride is associated with hyperkalemia; concurrent use with potassium supplements is contraindicated). Products include:
- K-Phos Original (Sodium Free) Tablets 760

Potassium Bicarbonate (Amiloride is associated with hyperkalemia; concurrent use with potassium supplements is contraindicated).
No products indexed under this heading.

Potassium Chloride (Amiloride is associated with hyperkalemia; concurrent use with potassium supplements is contraindicated). Products include:
- Colyte with Flavor Packs for Oral Solution 3088
- HalfLytely and Bisacodyl Tablets Bowel Prep Kit with Flavors Packs 881
- K-Dur Extended-Relase Tablets 3033
- K-Lor Oral Solution 474
- K-Tab Tablets 475
- MoviPrep Oral Solution 2839
- TriLyte with Flavor Packs for Oral Solution 3100

Potassium Citrate (Amiloride is associated with hyperkalemia; concurrent use with potassium supplements is contraindicated). Products include:
- Urocit-K Tablets 2144

Potassium Gluconate (Amiloride is associated with hyperkalemia; concurrent use with potassium supplements is contraindicated).
No products indexed under this heading.

Potassium Phosphate (Amiloride is associated with hyperkalemia; concurrent use with potassium supplements is contraindicated). Products include:
- K-Phos Neutral Tablets 760

Quinapril Hydrochloride (Co-administration increases the risk of hyperkalemia).
No products indexed under this heading.

Ramipril (Co-administration increases the risk of hyperkalemia). Products include:
- Altace Capsules 1702

Rofecoxib (Co-administration of non-steroidal anti-inflammatory agents can reduce the diuretic, natriuretic, and antihypertensive effects).
No products indexed under this heading.

Spirapril Hydrochloride (Co-administration increases the risk of hyperkalemia).
No products indexed under this heading.

Spironolactone (Amiloride is associated with hyperkalemia; concurrent use with potassium sparing diuretics is contraindicated).
No products indexed under this heading.

Sulindac (Co-administration of non-steroidal anti-inflammatory agents can reduce the diuretic, natriuretic, and antihypertensive effects). Products include:
- Clinoril Tablets 1924

Tacrolimus (Co-administration increases the risk of hyperkalemia). Products include:
- Prograf Capsules and Injection 632
- Protopic Ointment 638

Telmisartan (Co-administration increases the risk of hyperkalemia). Products include:
- Micardis Tablets 854
- Micardis HCT Tablets 856

Tolmetin Sodium (Co-administration of non-steroidal anti-inflammatory agents can reduce the diuretic, natriuretic, and antihypertensive effects).
No products indexed under this heading.

Torsemide (Co-administration with other diuretics may result in hypochloremia, hyponatremia, and increases in BUN). Products include:
- Demadex Injection 2759
- Demadex Tablets 2759

Trandolapril (Co-administration increases the risk of hyperkalemia). Products include:
- Mavik Tablets 486
- Tarka Tablets 524

Triamterene (Amiloride is associated with hyperkalemia; concurrent use with potassium sparing diuretics is contraindicated). Products include:
- Dyazide Capsules 1423
- Dyrenium Capsules 3400

Valdecoxib (Co-administration of non-steroidal anti-inflammatory agents can reduce the diuretic, natriuretic, and antihypertensive effects).
No products indexed under this heading.

Valsartan (Co-administration increases the risk of hyperkalemia). Products include:
- Diovan Tablets 2193
- Diovan HCT Tablets 2196

Food Interactions

Diet, potassium-rich (Potential for rapid increases in serum potassium levels).

MIGRANAL NASAL SPRAY

(Dihydroergotamine Mesylate) 3348

May interact with 5HT1-receptor agonists, cytochrome p450 3a4 inhibitors (selected), cytochrome p450 3a4 inhibitors, potent, macrolide antibiotics, vasopressors, and certain other agents. Compounds in these categories include:

Acetazolamide (Co-administration of dihydroergotamin with potent CYP3A4 inhibitors results in vasospasm that can lead to cerebral ischemia and/or ischemia of the extremities, therefore it is contraindicated).
No products indexed under this heading.

Amiodarone Hydrochloride (Co-administration of dihydroergotamin with potent CYP3A4 inhibitors results in vasospasm that can lead to cerebral ischemia and/or ischemia of the extremities, therefore it is contraindicated).
No products indexed under this heading.

Amprenavir (Co-administration of dihydroergotamin and potent CYP3A4 inhibitors results in vasospasm that can lead to cerebral ischemia and/or ischemia of the extremities, therefore it is contraindicated). Products include:
- Agenerase Capsules 1327
- Agenerase Oral Solution 1332

Anastrozole (Co-administration of dihydroergotamin with potent CYP3A4 inhibitors results in vasospasm that can lead to cerebral ischemia and/or ischemia of the extremities, therefore it is contraindicated). Products include:
- Arimidex Tablets 673

Aprepitant (Co-administration of dihydroergotamin with potent CYP3A4 inhibitors results in vasospasm that can lead to cerebral ischemia and/or ischemia of the extremities, therefore it is contraindicated). Products include:
- Emend Capsules 1963

Atazanavir (Co-administration of dihydroergotamin and potent CYP3A4 inhibitors results in vasospasm that can lead to cerebral ischemia and/or ischemia of the extremities, therefore it is contraindicated).
No products indexed under this heading.

Atazanavir sulfate (Co-administration of dihydroergotamin and potent CYP3A4 inhibitors results in vasospasm that can lead to cerebral ischemia and/or ischemia of the extremities, therefore it is contraindicated). Products include:
- Reyataz Capsules 921

Azithromycin Dihydrate (Co-administration of ergot alkaloids with macrolide antibiotics has resulted in increased plasma levels of unchanged alkaloids and peripheral vasoconstriction; vasospastic reactions have been reported with concurrent use at therapeutic doses).
No products indexed under this heading.

Cimetidine (Co-administration of dihydroergotamin with potent CYP3A4 inhibitors results in vasospasm that can lead to cerebral ischemia and/or ischemia of the extremities, therefore it is contraindicated). Products include:
- Tagamet HB 200 Tablets .... ◘664

Cimetidine Hydrochloride (Co-administration of dihydroergotamin with potent CYP3A4 inhibitors results in vasospasm that can lead to cerebral ischemia and/or ischemia of the extremities, therefore it is contraindicated).
No products indexed under this heading.

Ciprofloxacin (Co-administration of dihydroergotamin with potent CYP3A4 inhibitors results in vasospasm that can lead to cerebral ischemia and/or ischemia of the extremities, therefore it is contraindicated). Products include:
- Cipro Oral Suspension 2977
- Cipro I.V. 2984

Cipro XR Tablets 2990
Ciprodex Otic Suspension 559

Clarithromycin (Co-administration of dihydroergotamin and potent CYP3A4 inhibitors results in vasospasm that can lead to cerebral ischemia and/or ischemia of the extremities, therefore it is contraindicated). Products include:
Biaxin/Biaxin XL 402
PREVPAC 3284

Clotrimazole (Co-administration of dihydroergotamin with potent CYP3A4 inhibitors results in vasospasm that can lead to cerebral ischemia and/or ischemia of the extremities, therefore it is contraindicated). Products include:
Desenex Athlete's Foot Cream 635
Lotrimin 3039
Lotrisone 3040

Cyclosporine (Co-administration of dihydroergotamin with potent CYP3A4 inhibitors results in vasospasm that can lead to cerebral ischemia and/or ischemia of the extremities, therefore it is contraindicated). Products include:
Gengraf Capsules 459
Neoral Oral Solution 2259
Neoral Soft Gelatin Capsules 2259
Restasis Ophthalmic Emulsion 575
Sandimmune 2275

Dalfopristin (Co-administration of dihydroergotamin with potent CYP3A4 inhibitors results in vasospasm that can lead to cerebral ischemia and/or ischemia of the extremities, therefore it is contraindicated).
No products indexed under this heading.

Danazol (Co-administration of dihydroergotamin with potent CYP3A4 inhibitors results in vasospasm that can lead to cerebral ischemia and/or ischemia of the extremities, therefore it is contraindicated).
No products indexed under this heading.

Delavirdine Mesylate (Co-administration of dihydroergotamin with potent CYP3A4 inhibitors results in vasospasm that can lead to cerebral ischemia and/or ischemia of the extremities, therefore it is contraindicated). Products include:
Rescriptor Tablets 2551

Diltiazem Hydrochloride (Co-administration of dihydroergotamin with potent CYP3A4 inhibitors results in vasospasm that can lead to cerebral ischemia and/or ischemia of the extremities, therefore it is contraindicated). Products include:
Cardizem LA Extended Release Tablets 1728
Tiazac Capsules 1201

Diltiazem Maleate (Co-administration of dihydroergotamin with potent CYP3A4 inhibitors results in vasospasm that can lead to cerebral ischemia and/or ischemia of the extremities, therefore it is contraindicated).
No products indexed under this heading.

3-Diphenylacrylate (Concurrent use of 5-HT1 agonists and ergot-containing or ergot-type medications should not be undertaken within 24 hours of each other).
No products indexed under this heading.

Dirithromycin (Co-administration of ergot alkaloids with macrolide antibiotics has resulted in increased plasma levels of unchanged alkaloids and peripheral vasoconstriction; vasospastic reactions have been reported with concurrent use at therapeutic doses).
No products indexed under this heading.

Dobutamine (Concurrent use with peripheral and central vasoconstrictors is not recommended because the combination may result in additive or synergistic elevation of blood pressure).
No products indexed under this heading.

Dobutamine Hydrochloride (Concurrent use with peripheral and central vasoconstrictors is not recommended because the combination may result in additive or synergistic elevation of blood pressure).
No products indexed under this heading.

Dopamine Hydrochloride (Concurrent use with peripheral and central vasoconstrictors is not recommended because the combination may result in additive or synergistic elevation of blood pressure).
No products indexed under this heading.

Efavirenz (Co-administration of dihydroergotamin with potent CYP3A4 inhibitors results in vasospasm that can lead to cerebral ischemia and/or ischemia of the extremities, therefore it is contraindicated). Products include:
Atripla Tablets 945
Sustiva Capsules 930
Sustiva Tablets 930

Ephedrine Sulfate (Concurrent use with peripheral and central vasoconstrictors is not recommended because the combination may result in additive or synergistic elevation of blood pressure).
No products indexed under this heading.

Epinephrine Bitartrate (Concurrent use with peripheral and central vasoconstrictors is not recommended because the combination may result in additive or synergistic elevation of blood pressure).
No products indexed under this heading.

Epinephrine Hydrochloride (Concurrent use with peripheral and central vasoconstrictors is not recommended because the combination may result in additive or synergistic elevation of blood pressure).
No products indexed under this heading.

Erythromycin (Co-administration of dihydroergotamin with potent CYP3A4 inhibitors results in vasospasm that can lead to cerebral ischemia and/or ischemia of the extremities, therefore it is contraindicated). Products include:
Ery-Tab Tablets 449
Erythromycin Base Filmtab Tablets 455
Erythromycin Delayed-Release Capsules, USP 457
PCE Dispertab Tablets 515

Erythromycin Estolate (Co-administration of dihydroergotamin with potent CYP3A4 inhibitors results in vasospasm that can lead to cerebral ischemia and/or ischemia of the extremities, therefore it is contraindicated).
No products indexed under this heading.

Erythromycin Ethylsuccinate (Co-administration of dihydroergotamin with potent CYP3A4 inhibitors results in vasospasm that can lead to cerebral ischemia and/or ischemia of the extremities, therefore it is contraindicated). Products include:
E.E.S. 451
EryPed 447

Erythromycin Gluceptate (Co-administration of dihydroergotamin with potent CYP3A4 inhibitors results in vasospasm that can lead to cerebral ischemia and/or ischemia of the extremities, therefore it is contraindicated).
No products indexed under this heading.

Erythromycin Lactobionate (Co-administration of dihydroergotamin with potent CYP3A4 inhibitors results in vasospasm that can lead to cerebral ischemia and/or ischemia of the extremities, therefore it is contraindicated).
No products indexed under this heading.

Erythromycin Stearate (Co-administration of dihydroergotamin with potent CYP3A4 inhibitors results in vasospasm that can lead to cerebral ischemia and/or ischemia of the extremities, therefore it is contraindicated). Products include:
Erythrocin Stearate Filmtab Tablets 453

Esomeprazole Magnesium (Co-administration of dihydroergotamin with potent CYP3A4 inhibitors results in vasospasm that can lead to cerebral ischemia and/or ischemia of the extremities, therefore it is contraindicated). Products include:
Nexium Delayed-Release Capsules 655

Fluconazole (Co-administration of dihydroergotamin with potent CYP3A4 inhibitors results in vasospasm that can lead to cerebral ischemia and/or ischemia of the extremities, therefore it is contraindicated).
No products indexed under this heading.

Fluoxetine Hydrochloride (Co-administration of dihydroergotamin with potent CYP3A4 inhibitors results in vasospasm that can lead to cerebral ischemia and/or ischemia of the extremities, therefore it is contraindicated). Products include:
Prozac Pulvules and Liquid 1801
Symbyax Capsules 1819

Fluvoxamine Maleate (Co-administration of dihydroergotamin with potent CYP3A4 inhibitors results in vasospasm that can lead to cerebral ischemia and/or ischemia of the extremities, therefore it is contraindicated).
No products indexed under this heading.

Fosamprenavir Calcium (Co-administration of dihydroergotamin and potent CYP3A4 inhibitors results in vasospasm that can lead to cerebral ischemia and/or ischemia of the extremities, therefore it is contraindicated). Products include:
Lexiva Tablets 1505

Indinavir Sulfate (Co-administration of dihydroergotamin and potent CYP3A4 inhibitors results in vasospasm that can lead to cerebral ischemia and/or ischemia of the extremities, therefore it is contraindicated). Products include:
Crixivan Capsules 1940

Isoniazid (Co-administration of dihydroergotamin with potent CYP3A4 inhibitors results in vasospasm that can lead to cerebral ischemia and/or ischemia of the extremities, therefore it is contraindicated).
No products indexed under this heading.

Isoproterenol Hydrochloride (Concurrent use with peripheral and central vasoconstrictors is not recommended because the combination may result in additive or synergistic elevation of blood pressure).
No products indexed under this heading.

Isoproterenol Sulfate (Concurrent use with peripheral and central vasoconstrictors is not recommended because the combination may result in additive or synergistic elevation of blood pressure).
No products indexed under this heading.

Itraconazole (Co-administration of dihydroergotamin and potent CYP3A4 inhibitors results in vasospasm that can lead to cerebral ischemia and/or ischemia of the extremities, therefore it is contraindicated).
No products indexed under this heading.

Ketoconazole (Co-administration of dihydroergotamin and potent CYP3A4 inhibitors results in vasospasm that can lead to cerebral ischemia and/or ischemia of the extremities, therefore it is contraindicated). Products include:
Nizoral A-D Shampoo, 1% 1868

Lopinavir (Co-administration of dihydroergotamin and potent CYP3A4 inhibitors results in vasospasm that can lead to cerebral ischemia and/or ischemia of the extremities, therefore it is contraindicated). Products include:
Kaletra 476

Loratadine (Co-administration of dihydroergotamin with potent CYP3A4 inhibitors results in vasospasm that can lead to cerebral ischemia and/or ischemia of the extremities, therefore it is contraindicated). Products include:
Alavert Allergy & Sinus D-12 Hour Tablets 771
Alavert 771
Children's Claritin Allergy Oral Solution 771
Claritin Non-Drowsy 24 Hour Tablets 772
Claritin Reditabs 24 Hour Non-Drowsy Tablets 772
Claritin-D Non-Drowsy 12 Hour Tablets 772
Claritin-D Non-Drowsy 24 Hour Tablets 772

Mephentermine Sulfate (Concurrent use with peripheral and central vasoconstrictors is not recommended because the combination may result in additive or synergistic elevation of blood pressure).
No products indexed under this heading.

Metaraminol Bitartrate (Concurrent use with peripheral and central vasoconstrictors is not recommended because the combination may result in additive or synergistic elevation of blood pressure).
No products indexed under this heading.

Methoxamine Hydrochloride (Concurrent use with peripheral and central vasoconstrictors is not recommended because the combination may result in additive or synergistic elevation of blood pressure).
No products indexed under this heading.

Metronidazole (Co-administration of dihydroergotamin with potent CYP3A4 inhibitors results in vasospasm that can lead to cerebral ischemia and/or ischemia of the extremities, therefore it is contraindicated). Products include:
Metrogel 1% 1211
MetroGel-Vaginal Gel 1855
Vandazole Vaginal Gel 3338

Metronidazole Benzoate (Co-administration of dihydroergotamin with potent CYP3A4 inhibitors results in vasospasm that can lead to cerebral ischemia and/or ischemia of the extremities, therefore it is contraindicated).
No products indexed under this heading.

Metronidazole Hydrochloride (Co-administration of dihydroergotamin with potent CYP3A4 inhibitors results in vasospasm that can lead to cerebral ischemia and/or ischemia of the extremities, therefore it is contraindicated).
No products indexed under this heading.

Miconazole (Co-administration of dihydroergotamin with potent CYP3A4 inhibitors results in vasospasm that can lead to cerebral ischemia and/or ischemia of the extremities, therefore it is contraindicated).
No products indexed under this heading.

Miconazole Nitrate (Co-administration of dihydroergotamin with potent CYP3A4 inhibitors results in vasospasm that can lead to cerebral ischemia and/or ischemia of the extremities, therefore it is contraindicated). Products include:
Desenex .... ■635
Desenex Jock Itch Spray Powder ... ■635

Naratriptan Hydrochloride (Concurrent use of 5-HT1 agonists and ergot-containing or ergot-type medications should not be undertaken within 24 hours of each other). Products include:
Amerge Tablets 1339

Nefazodone Hydrochloride (Co-administration of dihydroergotamin and potent CYP3A4 inhibitors results in vasospasm that can lead to cerebral ischemia and/or ischemia of the extremities, therefore it is contraindicated).
No products indexed under this heading.

Nelfinavir Mesylate (Co-administration of dihydroergotamin and potent CYP3A4 inhibitors results in vasospasm that can lead to cerebral ischemia and/or ischemia of the extremities, therefore it is contraindicated). Products include:
Viracept 2577

Nevirapine (Co-administration of dihydroergotamin with potent CYP3A4 inhibitors results in vasospasm that can lead to cerebral ischemia and/or ischemia of the extremities, therefore it is contraindicated). Products include:
Viramune Oral Suspension 873
Viramune Tablets 873

Niacinamide (Co-administration of dihydroergotamin with potent CYP3A4 inhibitors results in vasospasm that can lead to cerebral ischemia and/or ischemia of the extremities, therefore it is contraindicated).
No products indexed under this heading.

Nicotinamide (Co-administration of dihydroergotamin with potent CYP3A4 inhibitors results in vasospasm that can lead to cerebral ischemia and/or ischemia of the extremities, therefore it is contraindicated). Products include:
Nicomide Tablets 1088

Nicotine (May provoke vasoconstriction in some patients, predisposing to a greater ischemic response to ergot). Products include:
NicoDerm CQ Clear Patch .... ■622

Nicotine Polacrilex (May provoke vasoconstriction in some patients, predisposing to a greater ischemic response to ergot).
No products indexed under this heading.

Nifedipine (Co-administration of dihydroergotamin with potent CYP3A4 inhibitors results in vasospasm that can lead to cerebral ischemia and/or ischemia of the extremities, therefore it is contraindicated). Products include:
Adalat CC Tablets 2964

Norepinephrine Bitartrate (Concurrent use with peripheral and central vasoconstrictors is not recommended because the combination may result in additive or synergistic elevation of blood pressure).
No products indexed under this heading.

Norfloxacin (Co-administration of dihydroergotamin with potent CYP3A4 inhibitors results in vasospasm that can lead to cerebral ischemia and/or ischemia of the extremities, therefore it is contraindicated). Products include:
Noroxin Tablets 2032

Omeprazole (Co-administration of dihydroergotamin with potent CYP3A4 inhibitors results in vasospasm that can lead to cerebral ischemia and/or ischemia of the extremities, therefore it is contraindicated). Products include:
Zegerid Capsules 2958
Zegerid Powder for Oral Solution 2958

Paroxetine Hydrochloride (Co-administration of dihydroergotamin with potent CYP3A4 inhibitors results in vasospasm that can lead to cerebral ischemia and/or ischemia of the extremities, therefore it is contraindicated). Products include:
Paxil CR Controlled-Release Tablets 1538
Paxil 1530

Phenylephrine Hydrochloride (Concurrent use with peripheral and central vasoconstrictors is not recommended because the combination may result in additive or synergistic elevation of blood pressure). Products include:
Comtrex Maximum Strength Non-Drowsy Cold & Cough Caplets .... ■725
Comtrex Maximum Strength Day/Night Severe Cold & Sinus Caplets - Day Formulation .... ■725
Comtrex Maximum Strength Day/Night Severe Cold & Sinus Caplets - Night Formulation .... ■725
Contac Cold and Flu Maximum Strength Caplets .... ■728
Contac Cold and Flu Day and Night Caplets (Day Formulation Only) .... ■727
Contac Cold and Flu Day and Night Caplets (Night Formulation Only) .... ■727
Contac Cold and Flu Non-Drowsy Caplets .... ■728
Contac-D Cold Non-Drowsy Tablets .... ■729
Children's Dimetapp Cold & Allergy Elixir .... ■730
Children's Dimetapp Cold & Allergy Chewable Tablets .... ■730
Children's Dimetapp DM Cold & Cough Elixir .... ■731
Toddler's Dimetapp Cold and Cough Drops .... ■732
Excedrin Sinus Headache Caplets/Tablets .... ■610
4-Way Fast Acting Nasal Spray ...... ■775
4-Way Menthol Nasal Spray .... ■775
Preparation H Maximum Strength Cream .... ■666
Preparation H Cooling Gel .... ■666
Preparation H .... ■666
Refenesen PE Caplets .... ■721
Robitussin Cough & Allergy Syrup .. ■736
Robitussin Cough & Cold Nighttime Liquid .... ■736
Robitussin Cough, Cold & Flu Nighttime Liquid .... ■738
Robitussin Head & Chest Congestion PE Syrup .... ■739
Robitussin Pediatric Cough & Cold Nighttime Liquid .... ■736
TheraFlu Cold & Cough Hot Liquid .... ■740
TheraFlu Cold & Sore Throat Hot Liquid .... ■741
TheraFlu Flu & Sore Throat Hot Liquid .... ■742
TheraFlu Daytime Severe Cold Hot Liquid .... ■742
TheraFlu Nighttime Severe Cold Hot Liquid .... ■740
TheraFlu Warming Relief Daytime Severe Cold .... ■743
TheraFlu Warming Relief Nighttime Severe Cold .... ■743
Triaminic Chest & Nasal Congestion Liquid .... ■746
Triaminic Cold & Allergy Liquid .... ■746
Triaminic Daytime Cold & Cough Liquid .... ■745
Triaminic Nighttime Cold & Cough Liquid .... ■746
Triaminic Thin Strips Cold .... ■748
Triaminic Thin Strips Cold & Cough .... ■778
Triaminic Infant Thin Strips Decongestant .... ■747
Triaminic Infant Thin Strips Decongestant Plus Cough .... ■747
Children's Tylenol Plus Flu Oral Suspension .... ■749
Tylenol Cold Head Congestion Daytime Caplets with Cool Burst and Gelcaps .... ■750
Tylenol Cold Multi-Symptom Daytime Liquid .... ■752
Tylenol Cold Multi-Symptom Severe Daytime Liquid .... ■752
Concentrated Tylenol Infants' Drops Plus Cold & Cough .... ■754
Tylenol Allergy Multi-Symptom Caplets with Cool Burst and Gelcaps 1872
Tylenol Allergy Multi-Symptom Nighttime Caplets with Cool Burst 1872
Children's Tylenol Plus Cold Suspension Liquid 1879
Children's Tylenol Plus Cold & Allergy Suspension Liquid 1878
Children's Tylenol Plus Flu Suspension Liquid 1881
Children's Tylenol Plus Multi-Symptom Cold Suspension Liquid 1879
Tylenol Cold Head Congestion Daytime Caplets with Cool Burst 1873
Tylenol Cold Head Congestion Nighttime Caplets with Cool Burst 1873
Tylenol Cold Head Congestion Severe Caplets with Cool Burst..... 1873
Tylenol Cold Multi-Symptom Daytime Caplets with Cool Burst and Gelcaps 1874
Tylenol Cold Multi-Symptom Daytime Liquid with Citrus Burst... 1874
Tylenol Cold Multi-Symptom Nighttime Caplets with Cool Burst 1874
Tylenol Cold Multi-Symptom Nighttime Liquid with Cool Burst... 1874
Tylenol Cold Multi-Symptom Severe Caplets with Cool Burst..... 1874
Tylenol Cold Multi-Symptom Severe Daytime Liquid with Citrus Burst 1874
Tylenol Sinus Congestion & Pain Daytime Caplets with Cool Burst and Gelcaps 1876
Tylenol Sinus Congestion & Pain Nighttime Caplets with Cool Burst 1876
Tylenol Sinus Congestion & Pain Severe Caplets with Cool Burst..... 1876
Vicks 44D Cough & Head Congestion Relief Liquid .... ■760
Vicks DayQuil LiquiCaps/Liquid Multi-Symptom Cold/Flu Relief..... ■761
Zicam Cough Plus D Cough Spray .... ■767

Propoxyphene Hydrochloride (Co-administration of dihydroergotamin with potent CYP3A4 inhibitors results in vasospasm that can lead to cerebral ischemia and/or ischemia of the extremities, therefore it is contraindicated).
No products indexed under this heading.

Propoxyphene Napsylate (Co-administration of dihydroergotamin with potent CYP3A4 inhibitors results in vasospasm that can lead to cerebral ischemia and/or ischemia of the extremities, therefore it is contraindicated).
No products indexed under this heading.

Propranolol Hydrochloride (May potentiate the vasoconstrictive action of ergotamine by blocking the vasodilating property of epinephrine). Products include:
Inderal LA Long-Acting Capsules 3429
InnoPran XL Capsules 2723

Quinidine (Co-administration of dihydroergotamin with potent CYP3A4 inhibitors results in vasospasm that can lead to cerebral ischemia and/or ischemia of the extremities, therefore it is contraindicated).
No products indexed under this heading.

Quinidine Hydrochloride (Co-administration of dihydroergotamin with potent CYP3A4 inhibitors results in vasospasm that can lead to cerebral ischemia and/or ischemia of the extremities, therefore it is contraindicated).
No products indexed under this heading.

Quinidine Polygalacturonate (Co-administration of dihydroergotamin with potent CYP3A4 inhibitors results in vasospasm that can lead to cerebral ischemia and/or ischemia of the extremities, therefore it is contraindicated).
No products indexed under this heading.

Quinidine Sulfate (Co-administration of dihydroergotamin with potent CYP3A4 inhibitors results in vasospasm that can lead to cerebral ischemia and/or ischemia of the extremities, therefore it is contraindicated).
No products indexed under this heading.

Quinine (Co-administration of dihydroergotamin with potent CYP3A4 inhibitors results in vasospasm that can lead to cerebral ischemia and/or ischemia of the extremities, therefore it is contraindicated).
No products indexed under this heading.

Quinine Sulfate (Co-administration of dihydroergotamin with potent CYP3A4 inhibitors results in vasospasm that can lead to cerebral ischemia and/or ischemia of the extremities, therefore it is contraindicated).
No products indexed under this heading.

Quinupristin (Co-administration of dihydroergotamin with potent CYP3A4 inhibitors results in vasospasm that can lead to cerebral ischemia and/or ischemia of the extremities, therefore it is contraindicated).
No products indexed under this heading.

Ranitidine Bismuth Citrate (Co-administration of dihydroergotamin with potent CYP3A4 inhibitors results in vasospasm that can lead to cerebral ischemia and/or ischemia of the extremities, therefore it is contraindicated).
No products indexed under this heading.

Ranitidine Hydrochloride (Co-administration of dihydroergotamin with potent CYP3A4 inhibitors results in vasospasm that can lead to cerebral ischemia and/or ischemia of the extremities, therefore it is contraindicated). Products include:
Zantac 1624
Zantac Injection 1619
Zantac Injection Pharmacy Bulk Package 1622

Ritonavir (Co-administration of dihydroergotamin and potent CYP3A4 inhibitors results in vasospasm that can lead to cerebral ischemia and/or ischemia of the extremities, therefore it is contraindicated). Products include:
Kaletra 476
Norvir 503

Rizatriptan Benzoate (Concurrent use of 5-HT1 agonists and ergot-containing or ergot-type medications should not be undertaken within 24 hours of each other). Products include:
Maxalt Tablets 2008
Maxalt-MLT Orally Disintegrating Tablets 2008

Saquinavir (Co-administration of dihydroergotamin and potent CYP3A4 inhibitors results in vasospasm that can lead to cerebral ischemia and/or ischemia of the extremities, therefore it is contraindicated).
No products indexed under this heading.

Saquinavir Mesylate (Co-administration of dihydroergotamin and potent CYP3A4 inhibitors results in vasospasm that can lead to cerebral ischemia and/or ischemia of the extremities, therefore it is contraindicated). Products include:
Invirase 2772

Sertraline Hydrochloride (Co-administration of dihydroergotamin with potent CYP3A4 inhibitors results in vasospasm that can lead to cerebral ischemia and/or ischemia of the extremities, therefore it is contraindicated). Products include:
Zoloft 2586

Sumatriptan (Co-administration could lead to additive coronary artery vasospasm effect; concurrent use should not be undertaken within 24 hours of each other). Products include:
Imitrex Nasal Spray 1467

Sumatriptan Succinate (Co-administration could lead to additive coronary artery vasospasm effect; concurrent use should not be undertaken within 24 hours of each other). Products include:
Imitrex Injection 1463
Imitrex Tablets 1471

Telithromycin (Co-administration of dihydroergotamin and potent CYP3A4 inhibitors results in vasospasm that can lead to cerebral ischemia and/or ischemia of the extremities, therefore it is contraindicated). Products include:
Ketek Tablets 2903

Troglitazone (Co-administration of dihydroergotamin with potent CYP3A4 inhibitors results in vasospasm that can lead to cerebral ischemia and/or ischemia of the extremities, therefore it is contraindicated).
No products indexed under this heading.

Troleandomycin (Co-administration of dihydroergotamin and potent CYP3A4 inhibitors results in vasospasm that can lead to cerebral ischemia and/or ischemia of the extremities, therefore it is contraindicated).
No products indexed under this heading.

Valproate Sodium (Co-administration of dihydroergotamin with potent CYP3A4 inhibitors results in vasospasm that can lead to cerebral ischemia and/or ischemia of the extremities, therefore it is contraindicated). Products include:
Depacon Injection 412

Verapamil Hydrochloride (Co-administration of dihydroergotamin with potent CYP3A4 inhibitors results in vasospasm that can lead to cerebral ischemia and/or ischemia of the extremities, therefore it is contraindicated). Products include:
Covera-HS Tablets 3139
Tarka Tablets 524
Verelan PM Extended-Release Capsules, Controlled-Onset 3106

Voriconazole (Co-administration of dihydroergotamin and potent CYP3A4 inhibitors results in vasospasm that can lead to cerebral ischemia and/or ischemia of the extremities, therefore it is contraindicated). Products include:
VFEND I.V. 2564
VFEND Oral Suspension 2564
VFEND Tablets 2564

Zafirlukast (Co-administration of dihydroergotamin with potent CYP3A4 inhibitors results in vasospasm that can lead to cerebral ischemia and/or ischemia of the extremities, therefore it is contraindicated). Products include:
Accolate Tablets 671

Zileuton (Co-administration of dihydroergotamin with potent CYP3A4 inhibitors results in vasospasm that can lead to cerebral ischemia and/or ischemia of the extremities, therefore it is contraindicated). Products include:
Zyflo Tablets 1023

Zolmitriptan (Concurrent use of 5-HT1 agonists and ergot-containing or ergot-type medications should not be undertaken within 24 hours of each other). Products include:
Zomig Tablets 3519
Zomig Nasal Spray 3523
Zomig-ZMT Tablets 3519

Food Interactions

Grapefruit (Co-administration of dihydroergotamin with potent CYP3A4 inhibitors results in vasospasm that can lead to cerebral ischemia and/or ischemia of the extremities, therefore it is contraindicated).

Grapefruit Juice (Co-administration of dihydroergotamin with potent CYP3A4 inhibitors results in vasospasm that can lead to cerebral ischemia and/or ischemia of the extremities, therefore it is contraindicated).

MIMYX CREAM

(Glycerin) 3213
None cited in PDR database.

MINERAL ICE

(Menthol) .... ▣685
May interact with topical nonsteroidal anti-inflammatory agents. Compounds in these categories include:

Diclofenac Sodium (Do not use with other topical pain relievers). Products include:
Arthrotec Tablets 3129
Voltaren Ophthalmic Solution 2309
Voltaren Tablets 2307
Voltaren-XR Tablets 2310

Flurbiprofen Sodium (Do not use with other topical pain relievers). Products include:
Ocufen Ophthalmic Solution .... ⊙232

Suprofen (Do not use with other topical pain relievers).
No products indexed under this heading.

MINTEZOL SUSPENSION

(Thiabendazole) 2027
See Mintezol Chewable Tablets

MINTEZOL CHEWABLE TABLETS

(Thiabendazole) 2027
May interact with xanthines. Compounds in these categories include:

Aminophylline (Thiabendazole may compete with theophylline for sites of metabolism in the liver, thus elevating the serum levels of theophylline to toxic levels; monitor theophylline blood levels).
No products indexed under this heading.

Dyphylline (Thiabendazole may compete with theophylline for sites of metabolism in the liver, thus elevating the serum levels of theophylline to toxic levels; monitor theophylline blood levels).
No products indexed under this heading.

Theophylline (Thiabendazole may compete with theophylline for sites of metabolism in the liver, thus elevating the serum levels of theophylline to toxic levels; monitor theophylline blood levels).
No products indexed under this heading.

Theophylline Anhydrous (Thiabendazole may compete with theophylline for sites of metabolism in the liver, thus elevating the serum levels of theophylline to toxic levels; monitor theophylline blood levels). Products include:
Uniphyl Tablets 2710

Theophylline Calcium Salicylate (Thiabendazole may compete with theophylline for sites of metabolism in the liver, thus elevating the serum levels of theophylline to toxic levels; monitor theophylline blood levels).
No products indexed under this heading.

Theophylline Dihydroxypropyl (Glyceryl) (Thiabendazole may compete with theophylline for sites of metabolism in the liver, thus elevating the serum levels of theophylline to toxic levels; monitor theophylline blood levels).
No products indexed under this heading.

Theophylline Ethylenediamine (Thiabendazole may compete with theophylline for sites of metabolism in the liver, thus elevating the serum levels of theophylline to toxic levels; monitor theophylline blood levels).
No products indexed under this heading.

Theophylline Sodium Glycinate (Thiabendazole may compete with theophylline for sites of metabolism in the liver, thus elevating the serum levels of theophylline to toxic levels; monitor theophylline blood levels).
No products indexed under this heading.

MIRADON TABLETS

(Anisindione) 3042
May interact with androgens, antacids, antihistamines, barbiturates, corticosteroids, diuretics, inhalant anesthetics, monoamine oxidase inhibitors, narcotic analgesics, nonsteroidal anti-inflammatory agents, oral contraceptives, phenytoin, pyrazolon derivatives, quinidine, salicylates, thrombolytics, thyroid preparations, and certain other agents. Compounds in these categories include:

Acrivastine (Antihistamines have been reported to diminish oral anticoagulant response, i.e., decreased prothrombin time response significantly).
No products indexed under this heading.

Alfentanil Hydrochloride (Prolonged use of narcotics may increase oral anticoagulant response, i.e., increased prothrombin time response).
No products indexed under this heading.

Allopurinol (May increase oral anticoagulant response, i.e., increased prothrombin time response).
No products indexed under this heading.

Alteplase (Co-administration with thrombolytics is not recommended and may be hazardous). Products include:

Activase I.V. 1223
Cathflo Activase 1231

Aluminum Carbonate (Antacids have been reported to diminish oral anticoagulant response, i.e., decreased prothrombin time response significantly).
No products indexed under this heading.

Aluminum Hydroxide (Antacids have been reported to diminish oral anticoagulant response, i.e., decreased prothrombin time response significantly). Products include:
Gaviscon Regular Strength Liquid .. ▣ 658
Gaviscon Regular Strength Tablets........ ▣ 658
Gaviscon Extra Strength Liquid ...... ▣ 658
Gaviscon Extra Strength Tablets .... ▣ 658
Maalox Regular Strength Antacid/Antigas Liquid........ 2175
Maalox Max Maximum Strength Antacid/Anti-Gas Liquid........ 2176

Amiloride Hydrochloride (Diuretics have been reported to diminish or increase oral anticoagulant response, i.e., decreased or increased prothrombin time response significantly). Products include:
Midamor Tablets 2026
Moduretic Tablets 2028

p-Aminosalicylic Acid (May increase oral anticoagulant response, i.e., increased prothrombin time response).
No products indexed under this heading.

Amiodarone Hydrochloride (May increase oral anticoagulant response, i.e., increased prothrombin time response).
No products indexed under this heading.

Anistreplase (Co-administration with thrombolytics is not recommended and may be hazardous).
No products indexed under this heading.

Antipyrine (May increase oral anticoagulant response, i.e., increased prothrombin time response).
No products indexed under this heading.

Aprobarbital (Barbiturates have been reported to diminish oral anticoagulant response, i.e., decreased prothrombin time response significantly).
No products indexed under this heading.

Aspirin (May increase oral anticoagulant response, i.e., increased prothrombin time response; aspirin may increase the bleeding tendency produced by anticoagulants without altering prothrombin time determination). Products include:
Aggrenox Capsules 822
Bayer Aspirin 744
BC Allergy Sinus Cold Powder .... ▣ 677
BC Headache Powder .... ▣ 677
Arthritis Strength BC Powder .... ▣ 677
BC Sinus Cold Powder .... ▣ 677
Excedrin Extra Strength Caplets/Tablets/Geltabs........ ▣ 684
Excedrin Migraine Caplets/Tablets/Geltabs........ ▣ 609
Goody's Body Pain Formula Powder........ ▣ 684
Goody's Extra Strength Headache Powders........ ▣ 611
Goody's Extra Strength Pain Relief Tablets........ ▣ 685
Percodan Tablets 1132
St. Joseph 81 mg Aspirin Chewable and Enteric Coated Tablets........ 1869

Astemizole (Antihistamines have been reported to diminish oral anticoagulant response, i.e., decreased prothrombin time response significantly).
No products indexed under this heading.

Azatadine Maleate (Antihistamines have been reported to diminish oral anticoagulant response, i.e., decreased prothrombin time response significantly).
No products indexed under this heading.

Bendroflumethiazide (Diuretics have been reported to diminish or increase oral anticoagulant response, i.e., decreased or increased prothrombin time response significantly).
No products indexed under this heading.

Betamethasone Acetate (Adrenocorticosteroids have been reported to diminish oral anticoagulant response, i.e., decreased prothrombin time response significantly).
No products indexed under this heading.

Betamethasone Sodium Phosphate (Adrenocorticosteroids have been reported to diminish oral anticoagulant response, i.e., decreased prothrombin time response significantly).
No products indexed under this heading.

Bromelains (May increase oral anticoagulant response, i.e., increased prothrombin time response).
No products indexed under this heading.

Bromodiphenhydramine Hydrochloride (Antihistamines have been reported to diminish oral anticoagulant response, i.e., decreased prothrombin time response significantly).
No products indexed under this heading.

Brompheniramine Maleate (Antihistamines have been reported to diminish oral anticoagulant response, i.e., decreased prothrombin time response significantly). Products include:
Children's Dimetapp Cold & Allergy Elixir........ ▣ 730
Children's Dimetapp Cold & Allergy Chewable Tablets........ ▣ 730
Children's Dimetapp DM Cold & Cough Elixir .... ▣ 731

Bumetanide (Diuretics have been reported to diminish or increase oral anticoagulant response, i.e., decreased or increased prothrombin time response significantly). Products include:
Bumex Tablets 2746

Buprenorphine Hydrochloride (Prolonged use of narcotics may increase oral anticoagulant response, i.e., increased prothrombin time response). Products include:
Buprenex Injectable 2716
Suboxone Tablets 2717
Subutex Tablets 2717

Butabarbital (Barbiturates have been reported to diminish oral anticoagulant response, i.e., decreased prothrombin time response significantly).
No products indexed under this heading.

Butalbital (Barbiturates have been reported to diminish oral anticoagulant response, i.e., decreased prothrombin time response significantly).
No products indexed under this heading.

Carbamazepine (Has been reported to diminish oral anticoagulant response, i.e., decreased prothrombin time response significantly). Products include:
Carbatrol Capsules 3171
Equetro Extended-Release Capsules........ 3180
Tegretol/Tegretol-XR 2295

Celecoxib (Drugs that reduce the number of blood platelets by causing bone marrow depression, such as non-steroidal anti-inflammatory agents, may increase the bleeding tendency produced by anticoagulants without altering prothrombin time determination). Products include:
Celebrex Capsules 3134

Cetirizine Hydrochloride (Antihistamines have been reported to diminish oral anticoagulant response, i.e., decreased prothrombin time response significantly). Products include:
Zyrtec Chewable Tablets 2594
Zyrtec 2594
Zyrtec-D 12 Hour Extended Release Tablets........ 2597

Chloral Hydrate (May cause an increased prothrombin response by displacing the anticoagulant from protein binding sites or an increased metabolism of the unbound drug by hepatic enzyme induction).
No products indexed under this heading.

Chlorothiazide (Diuretics have been reported to diminish or increase oral anticoagulant response, i.e., decreased or increased prothrombin time response significantly). Products include:
Diuril Oral Suspension 1954

Chlorothiazide Sodium (Diuretics have been reported to diminish or increase oral anticoagulant response, i.e., decreased or increased prothrombin time response significantly). Products include:
Diuril Sodium Intravenous 2467

Chlorpheniramine Maleate (Antihistamines have been reported to diminish oral anticoagulant response, i.e., decreased prothrombin time response significantly). Products include:
Advil Allergy Sinus Caplets .... ▣ 770
Advil Multi-Symptom Cold Caplets........ ▣ 770
BC Allergy Sinus Cold Powder .... ▣ 677
Comtrex Maximum Strength Cold & Cough Day/Night Caplets - Night Formulation........ ▣ 726
Comtrex Maximum Strength Day/Night Severe Cold & Sinus Caplets - Night Formulation........ ▣ 725
Contac Cold and Flu Maximum Strength Caplets........ ▣ 728
Contac Cold and Flu Day and Night Caplets (Night Formulation Only)........ ▣ 727
Children's Dimetapp Long Acting Cough Plus Cold Syrup........ ▣ 731
Robitussin Cough & Cold Long-Acting Liquid........ ▣ 735
Robitussin Cough & Allergy Syrup .. ▣ 736
Robitussin Cough & Cold Nighttime Liquid........ ▣ 736
Robitussin Cough, Cold & Flu Nighttime Liquid........ ▣ 738
Robitussin Pediatric Cough & Cold Long-Acting Liquid........ ▣ 735
Robitussin Pediatric Cough & Cold Nighttime Liquid........ ▣ 736
Triaminic Cold & Allergy Liquid .... ▣ 746
Triaminic Cough & Runny Nose Softchews .... ▣ 748
Children's Tylenol Plus Flu Oral Suspension........ ▣ 749
Tylenol Allergy Multi-Symptom Caplets with Cool Burst and Gelcaps........ 1872
Children's Tylenol Plus Cold Suspension Liquid........ 1879
Children's Tylenol Plus Cough & Runny Nose Suspension Liquid........ 1879
Children's Tylenol Plus Flu Suspension Liquid........ 1881
Children's Tylenol Plus Multi-Symptom Cold Suspension Liquid........ 1879
Tylenol Cold Head Congestion Nighttime Caplets with Cool Burst........ 1873
Tylenol Cold Multi-Symptom Nighttime Caplets with Cool Burst........ 1874
Tylenol Sinus Congestion & Pain Nighttime Caplets with Cool Burst........ 1876
Vicks 44M Cough, Cold & Flu Relief Liquid........ 2680
Pediatric Vicks 44m Cough & Cold Relief Liquid........ 2676
Children's Vicks NyQuil Cold/Cough Relief........ ▣ 756
Children's Vicks NyQuil Cold/Cough Relief Liquid........ 2680
Zicam Maximum Strength Flu Daytime........ ▣ 768

Chlorpheniramine Polistirex (Antihistamines have been reported to diminish oral anticoagulant response, i.e., decreased prothrombin time response significantly). Products include:
Tussionex Pennkinetic Extended-Release Suspension........ 3327

Chlorpheniramine Tannate (Antihistamines have been reported to diminish oral anticoagulant response, i.e., decreased prothrombin time response significantly).
No products indexed under this heading.

Chlorpropamide (May increase oral anticoagulant response, i.e., increased prothrombin time response; oral anticoagulants may potentiate the hypoglycemic agents; such as chlorpropamide by inhibiting their metabolism in the liver).
No products indexed under this heading.

Chlorthalidone (Diuretics have been reported to diminish or increase oral anticoagulant response, i.e., decreased or increased prothrombin time response significantly). Products include:
Clorpres Tablets 2153

Cholestyramine (May reduce the gastrointestinal absorption of both the anticoagulants and Vitamin K; net effect is unpredictable).
No products indexed under this heading.

Choline Magnesium Trisalicylate (May increase oral anticoagulant response, i.e., increased prothrombin time response).
No products indexed under this heading.

Chymotrypsin (May increase oral anticoagulant response, i.e., increased prothrombin time response).
No products indexed under this heading.

Cimetidine (May increase oral anti-coagulant response, i.e., increased prothrombin time response). Products include:
Tagamet HB 200 Tablets ▣▫664

Cimetidine Hydrochloride (May increase oral anticoagulant response, i.e., increased prothrombin time response).
No products indexed under this heading.

Cinchophen (May increase oral anticoagulant response, i.e., increased prothrombin time response).
No products indexed under this heading.

Clemastine Fumarate (Antihistamines have been reported to diminish oral anticoagulant response, i.e., decreased prothrombin time response significantly).
No products indexed under this heading.

Clofibrate (Drugs that reduce the number of blood platelets by causing bone marrow depression, such as clofibrate, may increase the bleeding tendency produced by anticoagulants without altering prothrombin time determination; may increase oral anticoagulant response, i.e. increased prothrombin time response).
No products indexed under this heading.

Clopidogrel Bisulfate (Drugs that reduce the number of blood platelets by causing bone marrow depression, such as clopidogrel, may increase the bleeding tendency produced by anticoagulants without altering prothrombin time determination). Products include:
Plavix Tablets 917
Plavix Tablets 2926

Codeine Phosphate (Prolonged use of narcotics may increase oral anticoagulant response, i.e., increased prothrombin time response). Products include:
Tylenol with Codeine Tablets 2391

Cortisone Acetate (Adrenocorticosteroids have been reported to diminish oral anticoagulant response, i.e., decreased prothrombin time response significantly).
No products indexed under this heading.

Cyproheptadine Hydrochloride (Antihistamines have been reported to diminish oral anticoagulant response, i.e., decreased prothrombin time response significantly).
No products indexed under this heading.

Desflurane (May increase oral anticoagulant response, i.e., increased prothrombin time response).
No products indexed under this heading.

Desogestrel (Oral contraceptives have been reported to diminish oral anticoagulant response, i.e., decreased prothrombin time response significantly). Products include:
Mircette Tablets 1066

Dexamethasone (Adrenocorticosteroids have been reported to diminish oral anticoagulant response, i.e., decreased prothrombin time response significantly). Products include:
Ciprodex Otic Suspension 559
Decadron Tablets 1951

TobraDex Ophthalmic Ointment 562
TobraDex Ophthalmic Suspension ... 563

Dexamethasone Acetate (Adrenocorticosteroids have been reported to diminish oral anticoagulant response, i.e., decreased prothrombin time response significantly).
No products indexed under this heading.

Dexamethasone Sodium Phosphate (Adrenocorticosteroids have been reported to diminish oral anticoagulant response, i.e., decreased prothrombin time response significantly).
No products indexed under this heading.

Dexchlorpheniramine Maleate (Antihistamines have been reported to diminish oral anticoagulant response, i.e., decreased prothrombin time response significantly).
No products indexed under this heading.

Dextrans (Low Molecular Weight) (May increase oral anticoagulant response, i.e., increased prothrombin time response; drugs that reduce the number of blood platelets by causing bone marrow depression, such as dextran, may increase the bleeding tendency produced by anticoagulants without altering prothrombin time determination).
No products indexed under this heading.

Dextrothyroxine Sodium (May increase oral anticoagulant response, i.e., increased prothrombin time response).
No products indexed under this heading.

Dezocine (Prolonged use of narcotics may increase oral anticoagulant response, i.e., increased prothrombin time response).
No products indexed under this heading.

Diazoxide (May increase oral anticoagulant response, i.e., increased prothrombin time response). Products include:
Hyperstat I.V. 3017

Diclofenac Potassium (Drugs that reduce the number of blood platelets by causing bone marrow depression, such as non-steroidal anti-inflammatory agents, may increase the bleeding tendency produced by anticoagulants without altering prothrombin time determination).
No products indexed under this heading.

Diclofenac Sodium (Drugs that reduce the number of blood platelets by causing bone marrow depression, such as non-steroidal anti-inflammatory agents, may increase the bleeding tendency produced by anticoagulants without altering prothrombin time determination). Products include:
Arthrotec Tablets 3129
Voltaren Ophthalmic Solution 2309
Voltaren Tablets 2307
Voltaren-XR Tablets 2310

Diflunisal (May increase oral anticoagulant response, i.e., increased prothrombin time response; drugs that reduce the number of platelets by causing bone marrow depression, such as non-steroidal anti-inflammatory agents, may increase the bleeding tendency produced by anticoagu-

lants without altering prothrombin time determination). Products include:
Dolobid Tablets 1955

Diphenhydramine Citrate (Antihistamines have been reported to diminish oral anticoagulant response, i.e., decreased prothrombin time response significantly). Products include:
Advil PM Caplets ▣▫615
Excedrin PM
Caplets/Tablets/Geltabs ▣▫610
Goody's PM Powder for Pain with
Sleeplessness ▣▫612

Diphenhydramine Hydrochloride (Antihistamines have been reported to diminish oral anticoagulant response, i.e., decreased prothrombin time response significantly). Products include:
Nytol QuickCaps Caplets ▣▫615
Nytol QuickGels Softgels
Maximum Strength..................... ▣▫616
Simply Sleep Caplets 1868
Sominex Original Formula Tablets .. ▣▫616
TheraFlu Warming Relief
Nighttime Severe Cold............... ▣▫743
TheraFlu Thin Strips Multi
Symptom.............................. ▣▫744
Triaminic Nighttime Cold &
Cough Liquid........................ ▣▫746
Triaminic Thin Strips Cough &
Runny Nose ▣▫749
Extra Strength Tylenol PM
Caplets, Vanilla Caplets,
Geltabs, Gelcaps and Liquid......... 1875
Tylenol Sore Throat Nighttime
Liquid with Cool Burst ▣▫790
Tylenol Allergy Multi-Symptom
Nighttime Caplets with Cool
Burst 1872
Tylenol Severe Allergy Caplets 1872
Children's Tylenol Plus Cold &
Allergy Suspension Liquid........... 1878

Diphenylpyraline Hydrochloride (Antihistamines have been reported to diminish oral anticoagulant response, i.e., decreased prothrombin time response significantly).
No products indexed under this heading.

Dipyridamole (Drugs that reduce the number of blood platelets by causing bone marrow depression, such as dipyridamole, may increase the bleeding tendency produced by anticoagulants without altering prothrombin time determination). Products include:
Aggrenox Capsules 822
Persantine Tablets 868

Disulfiram (May increase oral anticoagulant response, i.e., increased prothrombin time response).
No products indexed under this heading.

Enflurane (May increase oral anticoagulant response, i.e., increased prothrombin time response).
No products indexed under this heading.

Ethacrynic Acid (Diuretics have been reported to diminish or increase oral anticoagulant response, i.e., decreased or increased prothrombin time response significantly). Products include:
Edecrin Tablets 1959

Ethchlorvynol (Has been reported to diminish oral anticoagulant response, i.e., decreased prothrombin time response significantly).
No products indexed under this heading.

Ethinyl Estradiol (Oral contraceptives have been reported to diminish oral anticoagulant response, i.e.,

decreased prothrombin time response significantly). Products include:
Mircette Tablets 1066
NuvaRing 2340
Ortho-Cyclen/Ortho Tri-Cyclen 2429
Ortho Evra Transdermal System 2417
Ortho Tri-Cyclen Lo Tablets 2436
Seasonique Tablets 1077
Yasmin 28 Tablets 796
Yaz Tablets 803

Ethynodiol Diacetate (Oral contraceptives have been reported to diminish oral anticoagulant response, i.e., decreased prothrombin time response significantly).
No products indexed under this heading.

Etodolac (Drugs that reduce the number of blood platelets by causing bone marrow depression, such as non-steroidal anti-inflammatory agents, may increase the bleeding tendency produced by anticoagulants without altering prothrombin time determination).
No products indexed under this heading.

Fenoprofen Calcium (May increase oral anticoagulant response, i.e., increased prothrombin time response; drugs that reduce the number of blood platelets by causing bone marrow depression, such as non-steroidal anti-inflammatory agents, may increase the bleeding tendency produced by anticoagulants without altering prothrombin time determination). Products include:
Nalfon Capsules 2502

Fentanyl (Prolonged use of narcotics may increase oral anticoagulant response, i.e., increased prothrombin time response). Products include:
Duragesic Transdermal System 2373
Ionsys Transdermal System 2379

Fentanyl Citrate (Prolonged use of narcotics may increase oral anticoagulant response, i.e., increased prothrombin time response). Products include:
Actiq 979

Fexofenadine Hydrochloride (Antihistamines have been reported to diminish oral anticoagulant response, i.e., decreased prothrombin time response significantly). Products include:
Allegra 2844
Allegra-D 12 Hour
Extended-Release Tablets............ 2846
Allegra-D 24 Hour
Extended-Release Tablets............ 2849

Fludrocortisone Acetate (Adrenocorticosteroids have been reported to diminish oral anticoagulant response, i.e., decreased prothrombin time response significantly).
No products indexed under this heading.

Fluoxymesterone (Anabolic steroids may increase oral anticoagulant response, i.e., increased prothrombin time response). Products include:
Androxy Tablets 3335

Flurbiprofen (Drugs that reduce the number of blood platelets by causing bone marrow depression, such as non-steroidal anti-inflammatory agents, may increase the bleeding tendency produced by anticoagulants without altering prothrombin time determination).
No products indexed under this heading.

IMPORTANT NOTE: Always consult each drug listing in the patient's regimen for possible interactions.

Fosphenytoin Sodium (May increase oral anticoagulant response, i.e., increased prothrombin time response; oral anticoagulants may interfere with the hepatic metabolism of phenytoin, toxic levels of phenytoin may occur).
No products indexed under this heading.

Furosemide (Diuretics have been reported to diminish or increase oral anticoagulant response, i.e., decreased or increased prothrombin time response significantly).
Products include:
Furosemide Tablets 2154

Glucagon (May increase oral anticoagulant response, i.e., increased prothrombin time response).
Products include:
GlucaGen 761
Glucagon for Injection Vials and Emergency Kit 1778

Glutethimide (Has been reported to diminish oral anticoagulant response, i.e., decreased prothrombin time response significantly).
No products indexed under this heading.

Griseofulvin (Has been reported to diminish oral anticoagulant response, i.e., decreased prothrombin time response significantly).
Products include:
Gris-PEG Tablets 2502

Haloperidol (Has been reported to diminish oral anticoagulant response, i.e., decreased prothrombin time response significantly).
No products indexed under this heading.

Haloperidol Decanoate (Has been reported to diminish oral anticoagulant response, i.e., decreased prothrombin time response significantly).
No products indexed under this heading.

Halothane (May increase oral anticoagulant response, i.e., increased prothrombin time response).
No products indexed under this heading.

Hepatotoxic Drugs, unspecified (May increase oral anticoagulant response, i.e., increased prothrombin time response).
No products indexed under this heading.

Hydrochloroquine (Drugs that reduce the number of blood platelets by causing bone marrow depression, such as hydrochloroquine, may increase the bleeding tendency produced by anticoagulants without altering prothrombin time determination).
No products indexed under this heading.

Hydrochlorothiazide (Diuretics have been reported to diminish or increase oral anticoagulant response, i.e., decreased or increased prothrombin time response significantly). Products include:
Aldoril Tablets 1910
Atacand HCT 651
Avalide Tablets 888
Avalide Tablets 2874
Benicar HCT Tablets 1044
Diovan HCT Tablets 2196
Dyazide Capsules 1423
Hyzaar 50-12.5 Tablets 1990
Hyzaar 100-12.5 Tablets 1990
Hyzaar 100-25 Tablets 1990
Lopressor HCT 50/25 Tablets 2241
Lopressor HCT 100/25 Tablets 2241
Lopressor HCT 100/50 Tablets 2241
Lotensin HCT Tablets 2246
Micardis HCT Tablets 856
Moduretic Tablets 2028
Prinzide Tablets 2056
Teveten HCT Tablets 1737
Timolide Tablets 2086
Uniretic Tablets 3100

Hydrocodone Bitartrate (Prolonged use of narcotics may increase oral anticoagulant response, i.e., increased prothrombin time response). Products include:
Hycodan 1116
Hycotuss Expectorant Syrup 1117
Vicodin Tablets 535
Vicodin ES Tablets 536
Vicodin HP Tablets 538
Vicoprofen Tablets 539
Zydone Tablets 1139

Hydrocodone Polistirex (Prolonged use of narcotics may increase oral anticoagulant response, i.e., increased prothrombin time response). Products include:
Tussionex Pennkinetic Extended-Release Suspension 3327

Hydrocortisone (Adrenocorticosteroids have been reported to diminish oral anticoagulant response, i.e., decreased prothrombin time response significantly). Products include:
Colocort Rectal Suspension, USP (Retention) 100 mg/60 mL 2476
Hydrocortone Tablets 1989
Preparation H Hydrocortisone Cream .... ▣646

Hydrocortisone Acetate (Adrenocorticosteroids have been reported to diminish oral anticoagulant response, i.e., decreased prothrombin time response significantly).
Products include:
Analpram-HC 1159
Pramosone 1161
ProctoFoam-HC 3099

Hydrocortisone Sodium Phosphate (Adrenocorticosteroids have been reported to diminish oral anticoagulant response, i.e., decreased prothrombin time response significantly).
No products indexed under this heading.

Hydrocortisone Sodium Succinate (Adrenocorticosteroids have been reported to diminish oral anticoagulant response, i.e., decreased prothrombin time response significantly).
No products indexed under this heading.

Hydroflumethiazide (Diuretics have been reported to diminish or increase oral anticoagulant response, i.e., decreased or increased prothrombin time response significantly).
No products indexed under this heading.

Hydromorphone Hydrochloride (Prolonged use of narcotics may increase oral anticoagulant response, i.e., increased prothrombin time response). Products include:
Dilaudid 440
Dilaudid Non-Sterile Powder 440
Dilaudid Oral Liquid 445
Dilaudid Rectal Suppositories 440
Dilaudid Tablets 440
Dilaudid Tablets - 8 mg 445
Dilaudid-HP 442

Ibuprofen (May increase oral anticoagulant response, i.e., increased prothrombin time response; drugs that reduce the number of blood platelets by causing bone marrow depression, such as non-steroidal anti-inflammatory agents, may increase the bleeding tendency produced by anticoagulants without altering prothrombin time determination). Products include:
Advil Allergy Sinus Caplets .... ▣770
Advil .... ▣674
Children's Advil Oral Suspension .... ▣603
Children's Advil Chewable Tablets .... ▣603
Advil Cold & Sinus .... ▣723
Infants' Advil Concentrated Drops .... ▣604
Infants' Advil Concentrated Drops - White Grape (Dye-Free) .... ▣604
Junior Strength Advil Swallow Tablets .... ▣605
Advil Migraine Liquigels .... ▣608
Advil Multi-Symptom Cold Caplets .... ▣770
Advil PM Caplets .... ▣615
Motrin IB Tablets and Caplets 1866
Children's Motrin Oral Suspension 1867
Children's Motrin Non-Staining Dye-Free Oral Suspension 1867
Children's Motrin Cold Oral Suspension 1867
Infants' Motrin Concentrated Drops 1867
Infants' Motrin Non-Staining Dye-Free Concentrated Drops 1867
Junior Strength Motrin Caplets and Chewable Tablets 1867
Vicoprofen Tablets 539

Indapamide (Diuretics have been reported to diminish or increase oral anticoagulant response, i.e., decreased or increased prothrombin time response significantly).
Products include:
Indapamide Tablets 2156

Indomethacin (May increase oral anticoagulant response, i.e., increased prothrombin time response; drugs that reduce the number of blood platelets by causing bone marrow depression, such as non-steroidal anti-inflammatory agents, may increase the bleeding tendency produced by anticoagulants without altering prothrombin time determination). Products include:
Indocin 1995

Indomethacin Sodium Trihydrate (Drugs that reduce the number of blood platelets by causing bone marrow depression, such as non-steroidal anti-inflammatory agents, may increase the bleeding tendency produced by anticoagulants without altering prothrombin time determination). Products include:
Indocin I.V. 2465

Influenza Virus Vaccine (May increase oral anticoagulant response, i.e., increased prothrombin time response). Products include:
Fluarix 1451
Flumist Vaccine 1901

Isocarboxazid (May increase oral anticoagulant response, i.e., increased prothrombin time response).
No products indexed under this heading.

Isoflurane (May increase oral anticoagulant response, i.e., increased prothrombin time response).
No products indexed under this heading.

Ketoprofen (Drugs that reduce the number of blood platelets by causing bone marrow depression, such as non-steroidal anti-inflammatory agents, may increase the bleeding tendency produced by anticoagulants without altering prothrombin time determination).
No products indexed under this heading.

Ketorolac Tromethamine (Drugs that reduce the number of blood platelets by causing bone marrow depression, such as non-steroidal anti-inflammatory agents, may increase the bleeding tendency produced by anticoagulants without altering prothrombin time determination). Products include:
Acular Ophthalmic Solution 565
Acular LS Ophthalmic Solution 566

Levonorgestrel (Oral contraceptives have been reported to diminish oral anticoagulant response, i.e., decreased prothrombin time response significantly). Products include:
Climara Pro Transdermal System 776
Mirena Intrauterine System 787
Plan B Tablets 1076
Seasonique Tablets 1077

Levorphanol Tartrate (Prolonged use of narcotics may increase oral anticoagulant response, i.e., increased prothrombin time response).
No products indexed under this heading.

Levothyroxine Sodium (May increase oral anticoagulant response, i.e., increased prothrombin time response). Products include:
Levothroid Tablets 1186
Levoxyl Tablets 1712
Synthroid Tablets 520
Westhroid Tablets 3403

Liothyronine Sodium (May increase oral anticoagulant response, i.e., increased prothrombin time response). Products include:
Cytomel Tablets 1710
Westhroid Tablets 3403

Liotrix (May increase oral anticoagulant response, i.e., increased prothrombin time response). Products include:
Thyrolar Tablets 1199

Loratadine (Antihistamines have been reported to diminish oral anticoagulant response, i.e., decreased prothrombin time response significantly). Products include:
Alavert Allergy & Sinus D-12 Hour Tablets .... ▣771
Alavert .... ▣771
Children's Claritin Allergy Oral Solution .... ▣771
Claritin Non-Drowsy 24 Hour Tablets .... ▣772
Claritin Reditabs 24 Hour Non-Drowsy Tablets .... ▣772
Claritin-D Non-Drowsy 12 Hour Tablets .... ▣772
Claritin-D Non-Drowsy 24 Hour Tablets .... ▣772

Magaldrate (Antacids have been reported to diminish oral anticoagulant response, i.e., decreased prothrombin time response significantly).
No products indexed under this heading.

Magnesium Hydroxide (Antacids have been reported to diminish oral anticoagulant response, i.e.,

decreased prothrombin time response significantly). Products include:
- Maalox Regular Strength Antacid/Antigas Liquid 2175
- Maalox Max Maximum Strength Antacid/Anti-Gas Liquid 2176
- Pepcid Complete Chewable Tablets 1701

Magnesium Oxide (Antacids have been reported to diminish oral anticoagulant response, i.e., decreased prothrombin time response significantly). Products include:
- Beelith Tablets 759
- PremCal Light, Regular, and Extra Strength Tablets 818

Magnesium Salicylate (May increase oral anticoagulant response, i.e., increased prothrombin time response).
No products indexed under this heading.

Meclofenamate Sodium (Drugs that reduce the number of blood platelets by causing bone marrow depression, such as non-steroidal anti-inflammatory agents, may increase the bleeding tendency produced by anticoagulants without altering prothrombin time determination).
No products indexed under this heading.

Mefenamic Acid (May increase oral anticoagulant response, i.e., increased prothrombin time response; drugs that reduce the number of blood platelets by causing bone marrow depression, such as non-steroidal anti-inflammatory agents, may increase the bleeding tendency produced by anticoagulants without altering prothrombin time determination).
No products indexed under this heading.

Meloxicam (Drugs that reduce the number of blood platelets by causing bone marrow depression, such as non-steroidal anti-inflammatory agents, may increase the bleeding tendency produced by anticoagulants without altering prothrombin time determination). Products include:
- Mobic Oral Suspension 863
- Mobic Tablets 863

Meperidine Hydrochloride (Prolonged use of narcotics may increase oral anticoagulant response, i.e., increased prothrombin time response).
No products indexed under this heading.

Mephobarbital (Barbiturates have been reported to diminish oral anticoagulant response, i.e., decreased prothrombin time response significantly).
No products indexed under this heading.

Meprobamate (Has been reported to diminish oral anticoagulant response, i.e., decreased prothrombin time response significantly).
No products indexed under this heading.

Mestranol (Oral contraceptives have been reported to diminish oral anticoagulant response, i.e., decreased prothrombin time response significantly).
No products indexed under this heading.

Methadone Hydrochloride (Prolonged use of narcotics may increase oral anticoagulant response, i.e., increased prothrombin time response).
No products indexed under this heading.

Methdilazine Hydrochloride (Antihistamines have been reported to diminish oral anticoagulant response, i.e., decreased prothrombin time response significantly).
No products indexed under this heading.

Methoxyflurane (May increase oral anticoagulant response, i.e., increased prothrombin time response).
No products indexed under this heading.

Methyclothiazide (Diuretics have been reported to diminish or increase oral anticoagulant response, i.e., decreased or increased prothrombin time response significantly).
No products indexed under this heading.

Methyldopa (May increase oral anticoagulant response, i.e., increased prothrombin time response). Products include:
- Aldoril Tablets 1910

Methylphenidate Hydrochloride (May increase oral anticoagulant response, i.e., increased prothrombin time response). Products include:
- Concerta Extended-Release Tablets 1881
- Metadate CD Capsules 3323
- Ritalin Hydrochloride Tablets 2269
- Ritalin LA Capsules 2271
- Ritalin-SR Tablets 2269

Methylprednisolone Acetate (Adrenocorticosteroids have been reported to diminish oral anticoagulant response, i.e., decreased prothrombin time response significantly). Products include:
- Depo-Medrol Injectable Suspension 2617
- Depo-Medrol Single-Dose Vial 2619

Methylprednisolone Sodium Succinate (Adrenocorticosteroids have been reported to diminish oral anticoagulant response, i.e., decreased prothrombin time response significantly).
No products indexed under this heading.

Methyltestosterone (Anabolic steroids may increase oral anticoagulant response, i.e., increased prothrombin time response). Products include:
- Estratest Tablets 3199
- Estratest H.S. Tablets 3199

Metolazone (Diuretics have been reported to diminish or increase oral anticoagulant response, i.e., decreased or increased prothrombin time response significantly).
No products indexed under this heading.

Metronidazole (May increase oral anticoagulant response, i.e., increased prothrombin time response). Products include:
- Metrogel 1% 1211
- MetroGel-Vaginal Gel 1855
- Vandazole Vaginal Gel 3338

Metronidazole Hydrochloride (May increase oral anticoagulant response, i.e., increased prothrombin time response).
No products indexed under this heading.

Miconazole (May increase oral anticoagulant response, i.e., increased prothrombin time response).
No products indexed under this heading.

Moclobemide (May increase oral anticoagulant response, i.e., increased prothrombin time response).
No products indexed under this heading.

Morphine Sulfate (Prolonged use of narcotics may increase oral anticoagulant response, i.e., increased prothrombin time response). Products include:
- Avinza Capsules 1741
- Kadian Capsules 577
- MS Contin Tablets 2701

Nabumetone (Drugs that reduce the number of blood platelets by causing bone marrow depression, such as non-steroidal anti-inflammatory agents, may increase the bleeding tendency produced by anticoagulants without altering prothrombin time determination).
No products indexed under this heading.

Nalidixic Acid (May increase oral anticoagulant response, i.e., increased prothrombin time response).
No products indexed under this heading.

Naproxen (May increase oral anticoagulant response, i.e., increased prothrombin time response; drugs that reduce the number of blood platelets by causing bone marrow depression, such as non-steroidal anti-inflammatory agents, may increase the bleeding tendency produced by anticoagulants without altering prothrombin time determination). Products include:
- EC-Naprosyn Delayed-Release Tablets 2761
- Naprosyn Suspension 2761
- Naprosyn Tablets 2761
- Prevacid NapraPAC 3280

Naproxen Sodium (May increase oral anticoagulant response, i.e., increased prothrombin time response; drugs that reduce the number of blood platelets by causing bone marrow depression, such as non-steroidal anti-inflammatory agents, may increase the bleeding tendency produced by anticoagulants without altering prothrombin time determination). Products include:
- Aleve Caplets 742
- Aleve Gelcaps 743
- Aleve Tablets 743
- Aleve Cold & Sinus Caplets 744
- Anaprox Tablets 2761
- Anaprox DS Tablets 2761

Norethindrone (Oral contraceptives have been reported to diminish oral anticoagulant response, i.e., decreased prothrombin time response significantly). Products include:
- Ortho Micronor Tablets 2426

Norethynodrel (Oral contraceptives have been reported to diminish oral anticoagulant response, i.e., decreased prothrombin time response significantly).
No products indexed under this heading.

Norgestimate (Oral contraceptives have been reported to diminish oral anticoagulant response, i.e., decreased prothrombin time response significantly). Products include:
- Ortho-Cyclen/Ortho Tri-Cyclen 2429
- Ortho Tri-Cyclen Lo Tablets 2436

Norgestrel (Oral contraceptives have been reported to diminish oral anticoagulant response, i.e., decreased prothrombin time response significantly).
No products indexed under this heading.

Oxandrolone (Anabolic steroids may increase oral anticoagulant response, i.e., increased prothrombin time response). Products include:
- Oxandrin Tablets 2962

Oxaprozin (Drugs that reduce the number of blood platelets by causing bone marrow depression, such as non-steroidal anti-inflammatory agents, may increase the bleeding tendency produced by anticoagulants without altering prothrombin time determination).
No products indexed under this heading.

Oxolinic Acid (May increase oral anticoagulant response, i.e., increased prothrombin time response).
No products indexed under this heading.

Oxycodone Hydrochloride (Prolonged use of narcotics may increase oral anticoagulant response, i.e., increased prothrombin time response). Products include:
- OxyContin Tablets 2703
- OxyFast Oral Concentrate Solution 2708
- OxyIR Capsules 2708
- Percocet Tablets 1131
- Percodan Tablets 1132

Oxymetholone (Anabolic steroids may increase oral anticoagulant response, i.e., increased prothrombin time response).
No products indexed under this heading.

Oxyphenbutazone (May increase oral anticoagulant response, i.e., increased prothrombin time response).
No products indexed under this heading.

Paraldehyde (Has been reported to diminish oral anticoagulant response, i.e., decreased prothrombin time response significantly).
No products indexed under this heading.

Pargyline Hydrochloride (May increase oral anticoagulant response, i.e., increased prothrombin time response).
No products indexed under this heading.

Pentobarbital Sodium (Barbiturates have been reported to diminish oral anticoagulant response, i.e., decreased prothrombin time response significantly). Products include:

Nembutal Sodium Solution, USP 2470

Phenelzine Sulfate (May increase oral anticoagulant response, i.e., increased prothrombin time response).
No products indexed under this heading.

Phenobarbital (Barbiturates have been reported to diminish oral anticoagulant response, i.e., decreased prothrombin time response significantly). Products include:
Donnatal Extentabs 2493

Phenylbutazone (May increase oral anticoagulant response, i.e., increased prothrombin time response).
No products indexed under this heading.

Phenyramidol (May increase oral anticoagulant response, i.e., increased prothrombin time response).
No products indexed under this heading.

Phenytoin (May increase oral anticoagulant response, i.e., increased prothrombin time response; oral anticoagulants may interfere with the hepatic metabolism of phenytoin, toxic levels of phenytoin may occur).
No products indexed under this heading.

Phenytoin Sodium (May increase oral anticoagulant response, i.e., increased prothrombin time response; oral anticoagulants may interfere with the hepatic metabolism of phenytoin, toxic levels of phenytoin may occur). Products include:
Phenytek Capsules 2160

Piroxicam (Drugs that reduce the number of blood platelets by causing bone marrow depression, such as non-steroidal anti-inflammatory agents, may increase the bleeding tendency produced by anticoagulants without altering prothrombin time determination).
No products indexed under this heading.

Polythiazide (Diuretics have been reported to diminish or increase oral anticoagulant response, i.e., decreased or increased prothrombin time response significantly).
No products indexed under this heading.

Prednisolone Acetate (Adrenocorticosteroids have been reported to diminish oral anticoagulant response, i.e., decreased prothrombin time response significantly). Products include:
Blephamide Ophthalmic Ointment 568
Blephamide Ophthalmic
Suspension................................. 569
Poly-Pred Ophthalmic
Suspension................................. ⊙233
Pred Forte Ophthalmic
Suspension................................. ⊙235
Pred Mild Ophthalmic
Suspension ⊙238
Pred-G Ophthalmic Ointment ⊙237
Pred-G Ophthalmic Suspension ⊙236

Prednisolone Sodium Phosphate (Adrenocorticosteroids have been reported to diminish oral anticoagulant response, i.e., decreased prothrombin time response significantly).
No products indexed under this heading.

Prednisolone Tebutate (Adrenocorticosteroids have been reported to diminish oral anticoagulant response, i.e., decreased prothrombin time response significantly).
No products indexed under this heading.

Prednisone (Adrenocorticosteroids have been reported to diminish oral anticoagulant response, i.e., decreased prothrombin time response significantly).
No products indexed under this heading.

Primidone (Has been reported to diminish oral anticoagulant response, i.e., decreased prothrombin time response significantly).
No products indexed under this heading.

Procarbazine Hydrochloride (May increase oral anticoagulant response, i.e., increased prothrombin time response). Products include:
Matulane Capsules 3191

Promethazine Hydrochloride (Antihistamines have been reported to diminish oral anticoagulant response, i.e., decreased prothrombin time response significantly). Products include:
Phenergan Tablets and
Suppositories.............................. 3440

Propoxyphene Hydrochloride (Prolonged use of narcotics may increase oral anticoagulant response, i.e., increased prothrombin time response).
No products indexed under this heading.

Propoxyphene Napsylate (Prolonged use of narcotics may increase oral anticoagulant response, i.e., increased prothrombin time response).
No products indexed under this heading.

Pyrilamine Maleate (Antihistamines have been reported to diminish oral anticoagulant response, i.e., decreased prothrombin time response significantly).
No products indexed under this heading.

Pyrilamine Tannate (Antihistamines have been reported to diminish oral anticoagulant response, i.e., decreased prothrombin time response significantly).
No products indexed under this heading.

Quinidine Gluconate (May increase oral anticoagulant response, i.e., increased prothrombin time response).
No products indexed under this heading.

Quinidine Polygalacturonate (May increase oral anticoagulant response, i.e., increased prothrombin time response).
No products indexed under this heading.

Quinidine Sulfate (May increase oral anticoagulant response, i.e., increased prothrombin time response).
No products indexed under this heading.

Quinine Sulfate (May increase oral anticoagulant response, i.e., increased prothrombin time response).
No products indexed under this heading.

Ranitidine Hydrochloride (Has been reported to diminish or increase oral anticoagulant response, i.e., decreased or increased prothrombin time response significantly). Products include:
Zantac ... 1624
Zantac Injection 1619
Zantac Injection Pharmacy Bulk
Package.................................... 1622

Remifentanil Hydrochloride (Prolonged use of narcotics may increase oral anticoagulant response, i.e., increased prothrombin time response).
No products indexed under this heading.

Reteplase (Co-administration with thrombolytics is not recommended and may be hazardous). Products include:
Retavase 2499

Rifampin (Has been reported to diminish oral anticoagulant response, i.e., decreased prothrombin time response significantly).
No products indexed under this heading.

Rofecoxib (Drugs that reduce the number of blood platelets by causing bone marrow depression, such as non-steroidal anti-inflammatory agents, may increase the bleeding tendency produced by anticoagulants without altering prothrombin time determination).
No products indexed under this heading.

Salsalate (May increase oral anticoagulant response, i.e., increased prothrombin time response).
No products indexed under this heading.

Secobarbital Sodium (Barbiturates have been reported to diminish oral anticoagulant response, i.e., decreased prothrombin time response significantly).
No products indexed under this heading.

Selegiline Hydrochloride (May increase oral anticoagulant response, i.e., increased prothrombin time response). Products include:
Eldepryl Capsules 3208
Zelapar Tablets 3372

Sodium Bicarbonate (Antacids have been reported to diminish oral anticoagulant response, i.e., decreased prothrombin time response significantly). Products include:
Colyte with Flavor Packs for Oral
Solution 3088
HalfLytely and Bisacodyl Tablets
Bowel Prep Kit with Flavors
Packs 881
TriLyte with Flavor Packs for Oral
Solution.................................... 3100

Spironolactone (Diuretics have been reported to diminish or increase oral anticoagulant response, i.e., decreased or increased prothrombin time response significantly).
No products indexed under this heading.

Stanozolol (Anabolic steroids may increase oral anticoagulant response, i.e., increased prothrombin time response).
No products indexed under this heading.

Streptokinase (Co-administration with thrombolytics is not recommended and may be hazardous).
No products indexed under this heading.

Sufentanil Citrate (Prolonged use of narcotics may increase oral anticoagulant response, i.e., increased prothrombin time response).
No products indexed under this heading.

Sulfamethizole (May increase oral anticoagulant response, i.e., increased prothrombin time response).
No products indexed under this heading.

Sulfamethoxazole (May increase oral anticoagulant response, i.e., increased prothrombin time response).
No products indexed under this heading.

Sulfinpyrazone (May increase oral anticoagulant response, i.e., increased prothrombin time response).
No products indexed under this heading.

Sulfisoxazole Acetyl (May increase oral anticoagulant response, i.e., increased prothrombin time response).
No products indexed under this heading.

Sulindac (Long acting sulindac may increase oral anticoagulant response, i.e., increased prothrombin time response; drugs that reduce the number of blood platelets by causing bone marrow depression, such as non-steroidal anti-inflammatory agents, may increase the bleeding tendency produced by anticoagulants without altering prothrombin time determination). Products include:
Clinoril Tablets 1924

Terfenadine (Antihistamines have been reported to diminish oral anticoagulant response, i.e., decreased prothrombin time response significantly).
No products indexed under this heading.

Thiamylal Sodium (Barbiturates have been reported to diminish oral anticoagulant response, i.e., decreased prothrombin time response significantly).
No products indexed under this heading.

Thyroglobulin (May increase oral anticoagulant response, i.e., increased prothrombin time response).
No products indexed under this heading.

Thyroid (May increase oral anticoagulant response, i.e., increased prothrombin time response).
No products indexed under this heading.

Thyroxine (May increase oral anticoagulant response, i.e., increased prothrombin time response).
No products indexed under this heading.

Thyroxine Sodium (May increase oral anticoagulant response, i.e., increased prothrombin time response).
No products indexed under this heading.

Tolbutamide (May increase oral anticoagulant response, i.e., increased prothrombin time response; oral anticoagulants may potentiate the hypoglycemic agents; such as tolbutamide by inhibiting their metabolism in the liver).
No products indexed under this heading.

Tolmetin Sodium (Drugs that reduce the number of blood platelets by causing bone marrow depression, such as non-steroidal anti-inflammatory agents, may increase the bleeding tendency produced by anticoagulants without altering prothrombin time determination).
No products indexed under this heading.

Torsemide (Diuretics have been reported to diminish or increase oral anticoagulant response, i.e., decreased or increased prothrombin time response significantly). Products include:
Demadex Injection 2759
Demadex Tablets 2759

Tranylcypromine Sulfate (May increase oral anticoagulant response, i.e., increased prothrombin time response). Products include:
Parnate Tablets 1527

Triamcinolone (Adrenocorticosteroids have been reported to diminish oral anticoagulant response, i.e., decreased prothrombin time response significantly).
No products indexed under this heading.

Triamcinolone Acetonide (Adrenocorticosteroids have been reported to diminish oral anticoagulant response, i.e., decreased prothrombin time response significantly). Products include:
Azmacort Inhalation Aerosol 1726
Nasacort AQ Nasal Spray 2922

Triamcinolone Diacetate (Adrenocorticosteroids have been reported to diminish oral anticoagulant response, i.e., decreased prothrombin time response significantly).
No products indexed under this heading.

Triamcinolone Hexacetonide (Adrenocorticosteroids have been reported to diminish oral anticoagulant response, i.e., decreased prothrombin time response significantly).
No products indexed under this heading.

Triamterene (Diuretics have been reported to diminish or increase oral anticoagulant response, i.e., decreased or increased prothrombin time response significantly). Products include:
Dyazide Capsules 1423
Dyrenium Capsules 3400

Trimeprazine Tartrate (Antihistamines have been reported to diminish oral anticoagulant response, i.e., decreased prothrombin time response significantly).
No products indexed under this heading.

Trimethoprim (Sulfamethoxazole/trimethoprim may increase oral anticoagulant response, i.e., increased prothrombin time response).
No products indexed under this heading.

Tripelennamine Hydrochloride (Antihistamines have been reported to diminish oral anticoagulant response, i.e., decreased prothrombin time response significantly).
No products indexed under this heading.

Triprolidine Hydrochloride (Antihistamines have been reported to diminish oral anticoagulant response, i.e., decreased prothrombin time response significantly).
No products indexed under this heading.

Urokinase (Co-administration with thrombolytics is not recommended and may be hazardous).
No products indexed under this heading.

Valdecoxib (Drugs that reduce the number of blood platelets by causing bone marrow depression, such as non-steroidal anti-inflammatory agents, may increase the bleeding tendency produced by anticoagulants without altering prothrombin time determination).
No products indexed under this heading.

Vitamin C (Has been reported to diminish oral anticoagulant response, i.e., decreased prothrombin time response significantly). Products include:
Bausch & Lomb Ocuvite Adult Eye Vitamin and Mineral Supplement Soft Gels 706
Bausch & Lomb Ocuvite Adult 50+ Eye Vitamin and Mineral Supplement Soft Gels 706
Ocuvite Adult Vitamin and Mineral Supplement .... ⊙253
Ocuvite Adult 50+ Vitamin and Mineral Supplement .... ⊙253
Peridin-C Vitamin C Supplement 818

Warfarin Sodium (Under dosage of warfarin sodium has been reported to diminish oral anticoagulant response, i.e., decreased prothrombin time response significantly; overdosage of warfarin may increase oral anticoagulant response, i.e., increased prothrombin time response). Products include:
Coumadin for Injection 898
Coumadin Tablets 898

Food Interactions

Alcohol (Has been reported to diminish and/or increase oral anticoagulant response, i.e., decreased prothrombin time response significantly).

Diet high in vitamin K (Has been reported to diminish oral anticoagulant response, i.e., decreased prothrombin time response significantly).

MIRAPEX TABLETS

(Pramipexole Dihydrochloride) 859
May interact with dopamine D2 antagonists, quinidine, and certain other agents. Compounds in these categories include:

Amantadine Hydrochloride (Population pharmacokinetic analyses suggest that amantadine may slightly decrease the oral clearance of pramipexole). Products include:
Symmetrel Tablets 1135

Chlorpromazine (Co-administration with dopamine antagonists may diminish the effectiveness of pramipexole).
No products indexed under this heading.

Chlorpromazine Hydrochloride (Co-administration with dopamine antagonists may diminish the effectiveness of pramipexole).
No products indexed under this heading.

Chlorprothixene (Co-administration with dopamine antagonists may diminish the effectiveness of pramipexole).
No products indexed under this heading.

Chlorprothixene Hydrochloride (Co-administration with dopamine antagonists may diminish the effectiveness of pramipexole).
No products indexed under this heading.

Cimetidine (Co-administration with cimetidine, a known inhibitor of renal tubular secretion of organic acids via anionic transport, has caused a 50% increase in pramipexole AUC and a 40% increase in half-life). Products include:
Tagamet HB 200 Tablets 664

Cimetidine Hydrochloride (Co-administration with cimetidine, a known inhibitor of renal tubular secretion of organic acids via anionic transport, has caused a 50% increase in pramipexole AUC and a 40% increase in half-life).
No products indexed under this heading.

Diltiazem Hydrochloride (Co-administration of drugs that are secreted by the cationic transport system, e.g., diltiazem, decrease the oral clearance of pramipexole by about 20%). Products include:
Cardizem LA Extended Release Tablets 1728
Tiazac Capsules 1201

Fluphenazine Decanoate (Co-administration with dopamine antagonists may diminish the effectiveness of pramipexole).
No products indexed under this heading.

Fluphenazine Enanthate (Co-administration with dopamine antagonists may diminish the effectiveness of pramipexole).
No products indexed under this heading.

Fluphenazine Hydrochloride (Co-administration with dopamine antagonists may diminish the effectiveness of pramipexole).
No products indexed under this heading.

Haloperidol (Co-administration with dopamine antagonists may diminish the effectiveness of pramipexole).
No products indexed under this heading.

Haloperidol Decanoate (Co-administration with dopamine antagonists may diminish the effectiveness of pramipexole).
No products indexed under this heading.

Levodopa (Pramipexole may potentiate the dopaminergic side effects of levodopa and may cause or exacerbate pre-existing dyskinesia; pramipexole may cause an increase in levodopa Cmax by about 40% and a decrease in Tmax from 2.5 to 0.6 hours). Products include:
Parcopa Orally Disintegrating Tablets 3097
Stalevo Tablets 2287

Loxapine Hydrochloride (Co-administration with dopamine antagonists may diminish the effectiveness of pramipexole).
No products indexed under this heading.

Loxapine Succinate (Co-administration with dopamine antagonists may diminish the effectiveness of pramipexole).
No products indexed under this heading.

Mesoridazine Besylate (Co-administration with dopamine antagonists may diminish the effectiveness of pramipexole).
No products indexed under this heading.

Methotrimeprazine (Co-administration with dopamine antagonists may diminish the effectiveness of pramipexole).
No products indexed under this heading.

Metoclopramide Hydrochloride (Co-administration with dopamine antagonists may diminish the effectiveness of pramipexole).
No products indexed under this heading.

Molindone Hydrochloride (Co-administration with dopamine antagonists may diminish the effectiveness of pramipexole). Products include:
Moban Tablets 1119

Perphenazine (Co-administration with dopamine antagonists may diminish the effectiveness of pramipexole).
No products indexed under this heading.

Prochlorperazine (Co-administration with dopamine antagonists may diminish the effectiveness of pramipexole).
No products indexed under this heading.

Promethazine Hydrochloride (Co-administration with dopamine antagonists may diminish the effectiveness of pramipexole). Products include:
Phenergan Tablets and Suppositories 3440

Quetiapine Fumarate (Co-administration with dopamine antagonists may diminish the effectiveness of pramipexole). Products include:
Seroquel Tablets 690

Quinidine (Co-administration of drugs that are secreted by the cationic transport system, e.g., quinidine, decrease the oral clearance of pramipexole by about 20%).
No products indexed under this heading.

Quinidine Gluconate (Co-administration of drugs that are secreted by the cationic transport system, e.g., quinidine, decrease the oral clearance of pramipexole by about 20%).
No products indexed under this heading.

Quinidine Hydrochloride (Co-administration of drugs that are secreted by the cationic transport system, e.g., quinidine, decrease the oral clearance of pramipexole by about 20%).
No products indexed under this heading.

Quinidine Polygalacturonate (Co-administration of drugs that are secreted by the cationic transport system, e.g., quinidine, decrease the oral clearance of pramipexole by about 20%).
No products indexed under this heading.

Quinidine Sulfate (Co-administration of drugs that are secreted by the cationic transport system, e.g., quinidine, decrease the oral clearance of pramipexole by about 20%).
No products indexed under this heading.

Quinine Sulfate (Co-administration of drugs that are secreted by the cationic transport system, e.g., quinine, decrease the oral clearance of pramipexole by about 20%).
No products indexed under this heading.

Ranitidine Hydrochloride (Co-administration of drugs that are secreted by the cationic transport system, e.g., ranitidine, decrease the oral clearance of pramipexole by about 20%). Products include:
Zantac 1624
Zantac Injection 1619
Zantac Injection Pharmacy Bulk Package 1622

Risperidone (Co-administration with dopamine antagonists may diminish the effectiveness of pramipexole). Products include:
Risperdal 1676
Risperdal Consta Long-Acting Injection 1682
Risperdal M-Tab Orally Disintegrating Tablets 1676

Thioridazine Hydrochloride (Co-administration with dopamine antagonists may diminish the effectiveness of pramipexole). Products include:
Thioridazine Hydrochloride Tablets 2163

Thiothixene (Co-administration with dopamine antagonists may diminish the effectiveness of pramipexole). Products include:
Thiothixene Capsules 2165

Triamterene (Co-administration of drugs that are secreted by the cationic transport system, e.g., triamterene, decrease the oral clearance of pramipexole by about 20%). Products include:
Dyazide Capsules 1423
Dyrenium Capsules 3400

Trifluoperazine Hydrochloride (Co-administration with dopamine antagonists may diminish the effectiveness of pramipexole).
No products indexed under this heading.

Verapamil Hydrochloride (Co-administration of drugs that are secreted by the cationic transport system, e.g., verapamil, decrease the oral clearance of pramipexole by about 20%). Products include:
Covera-HS Tablets 3139
Tarka Tablets 524
Verelan PM Extended-Release Capsules, Controlled-Onset 3106

Food Interactions

Food, unspecified (Food does not affect the extent of pramipexole absorption, although the time of maximum plasma concentration is increased by about 1 hour when the drug is taken with a meal).

MIRCETTE TABLETS

(Desogestrel, Ethinyl Estradiol) 1066
May interact with barbiturates, tetracyclines, and certain other agents. Compounds in these categories include:

Ampicillin (Potential for reduced efficacy and increased incidence of breakthrough bleeding and menstrual irregularities with concomitant use).
No products indexed under this heading.

Ampicillin Sodium (Potential for reduced efficacy and increased incidence of breakthrough bleeding and menstrual irregularities with concomitant use).
No products indexed under this heading.

Ampicillin Trihydrate (Potential for reduced efficacy and increased incidence of breakthrough bleeding and menstrual irregularities with concomitant use).
No products indexed under this heading.

Aprobarbital (Potential for reduced efficacy and increased incidence of breakthrough bleeding and menstrual irregularities with concomitant use).
No products indexed under this heading.

Butabarbital (Potential for reduced efficacy and increased incidence of breakthrough bleeding and menstrual irregularities with concomitant use).
No products indexed under this heading.

Butalbital (Potential for reduced efficacy and increased incidence of breakthrough bleeding and menstrual irregularities with concomitant use).
No products indexed under this heading.

Carbamazepine (Potential for reduced efficacy and increased incidence of breakthrough bleeding and menstrual irregularities with concomitant use). Products include:
Carbatrol Capsules 3171
Equetro Extended-Release Capsules 3180
Tegretol/Tegretol-XR 2295

Demeclocycline Hydrochloride (Potential for reduced efficacy and increased incidence of breakthrough bleeding and menstrual irregularities with concomitant use).
No products indexed under this heading.

Doxycycline Calcium (Potential for reduced efficacy and increased incidence of breakthrough bleeding and menstrual irregularities with concomitant use).
No products indexed under this heading.

Doxycycline Hyclate (Potential for reduced efficacy and increased incidence of breakthrough bleeding and menstrual irregularities with concomitant use).
No products indexed under this heading.

Doxycycline Monohydrate (Potential for reduced efficacy and increased incidence of breakthrough bleeding and menstrual irregularities with concomitant use). Products include:
Oracea Capsules 1000

Griseofulvin (Potential for reduced efficacy and increased incidence of breakthrough bleeding and menstrual irregularities with concomitant use). Products include:
Gris-PEG Tablets 2502

Mephobarbital (Potential for reduced efficacy and increased incidence of breakthrough bleeding and menstrual irregularities with concomitant use).
No products indexed under this heading.

Methacycline Hydrochloride (Potential for reduced efficacy and increased incidence of breakthrough bleeding and menstrual irregularities with concomitant use).
No products indexed under this heading.

Minocycline Hydrochloride (Potential for reduced efficacy and increased incidence of breakthrough bleeding and menstrual irregularities with concomitant use). Products include:
Solodyn Extended Release Tablets 1890

Oxytetracycline Hydrochloride (Potential for reduced efficacy and increased incidence of breakthrough bleeding and menstrual irregularities with concomitant use).
No products indexed under this heading.

Pentobarbital Sodium (Potential for reduced efficacy and increased incidence of breakthrough bleeding and menstrual irregularities with concomitant use). Products include:
Nembutal Sodium Solution, USP 2470

Phenobarbital (Potential for reduced efficacy and increased incidence of breakthrough bleeding and menstrual irregularities with concomitant use). Products include:
Donnatal Extentabs 2493

Phenylbutazone (Potential for reduced efficacy and increased incidence of breakthrough bleeding and menstrual irregularities with concomitant use).
No products indexed under this heading.

Phenytoin (Potential for reduced efficacy and increased incidence of breakthrough bleeding and menstrual irregularities with concomitant use).
No products indexed under this heading.

Rifampin (Co-administration with rifampin has been associated with reduced efficacy and increased incidence of breakthrough bleeding and menstrual irregularities).
No products indexed under this heading.

Secobarbital Sodium (Potential for reduced efficacy and increased incidence of breakthrough bleeding and menstrual irregularities with concomitant use).
No products indexed under this heading.

Tetracycline Hydrochloride (Potential for reduced efficacy and increased incidence of breakthrough bleeding and menstrual irregularities with concomitant use).
No products indexed under this heading.

Thiamylal Sodium (Potential for reduced efficacy and increased incidence of breakthrough bleeding and menstrual irregularities with concomitant use).
No products indexed under this heading.

MIRENA INTRAUTERINE SYSTEM

(Levonorgestrel) 787
May interact with phenytoin and certain other agents. Compounds in these categories include:

Carbamazepine (Co-administration with drugs that induce liver enzymes may impair the effect of hormonal contraceptives). Products include:
Carbatrol Capsules 3171
Equetro Extended-Release Capsules 3180
Tegretol/Tegretol-XR 2295

Fosphenytoin Sodium (Co-administration with drugs that induce liver enzymes may impair the effect of hormonal contraceptives).
No products indexed under this heading.

Phenytoin (Co-administration with drugs that induce liver enzymes may impair the effect of hormonal contraceptives).
No products indexed under this heading.

Phenytoin Sodium (Co-administration with drugs that induce liver enzymes may impair the effect of hormonal contraceptives). Products include:
Phenytek Capsules 2160

Rifampin (Co-administration with drugs that induce liver enzymes may impair the effect of hormonal contraceptives).
No products indexed under this heading.

MIVACRON INJECTION

(Mivacurium Chloride) 493
May interact with aminoglycosides, antineoplastics, glucocorticoids, lithium preparations, local anesthetics, monoamine oxidase inhibitors, oral contraceptives, phenytoin, quinidine, tetracyclines, and certain other agents. Compounds in these categories include:

Altretamine (Irreversible inhibition of plasma cholinesterase by certain unspecified antineoplastic drugs resulting in possible prolonged neuromuscular block).
No products indexed under this heading.

Amikacin Sulfate (Enhances the neuromuscular blocking action).
No products indexed under this heading.

Anastrozole (Irreversible inhibition of plasma cholinesterase by certain unspecified antineoplastic drugs resulting in possible prolonged neuromuscular block). Products include:
Arimidex Tablets 673

Asparaginase (Irreversible inhibition of plasma cholinesterase by certain unspecified antineoplastic drugs resulting in possible prolonged neuromuscular block). Products include:
Elspar for Injection 2463
Elspar for Injection 1960

Bacitracin (Enhances neuromuscular blocking action). Products include:
Neosporin Antibiotic Ointment .... ▣643
Polysporin First Aid Antibiotic Ointment .... ▣643

Betamethasone Acetate
(Enhances the neuromuscular blocking effects by a reduction in plasma cholinesterase activity induced by chronic administration of glucocorticoids).
 No products indexed under this heading.

Betamethasone Sodium Phosphate (Enhances the neuromuscular blocking effects by a reduction in plasma cholinesterase activity induced by chronic administration of glucocorticoids).
 No products indexed under this heading.

Bicalutamide (Irreversible inhibition of plasma cholinesterase by certain unspecified antineoplastic drugs resulting in possible prolonged neuromuscular block).
 No products indexed under this heading.

Bleomycin Sulfate (Irreversible inhibition of plasma cholinesterase by certain unspecified antineoplastic drugs resulting in possible prolonged neuromuscular block).
 No products indexed under this heading.

Bupivacaine Hydrochloride (Enhances neuromuscular blocking action).
 No products indexed under this heading.

Busulfan (Irreversible inhibition of plasma cholinesterase by certain unspecified antineoplastic drugs resulting in possible prolonged neuromuscular block). Products include:
 I.V. Busulfex 2493
 Myleran Tablets 1525

Carbamazepine (Potential for resistance to the neuromuscular blocking action in patients on chronic carbamazepine therapy). Products include:
 Carbatrol Capsules 3171
 Equetro Extended-Release
 Capsules 3180
 Tegretol/Tegretol-XR 2295

Carboplatin (Irreversible inhibition of plasma cholinesterase by certain unspecified antineoplastic drugs resulting in possible prolonged neuromuscular block).
 No products indexed under this heading.

Carmustine (BCNU) (Irreversible inhibition of plasma cholinesterase by certain unspecified antineoplastic drugs resulting in possible prolonged neuromuscular block).
 No products indexed under this heading.

Chlorambucil (Irreversible inhibition of plasma cholinesterase by certain unspecified antineoplastic drugs resulting in possible prolonged neuromuscular block). Products include:
 Leukeran Tablets 1504

Chloroprocaine Hydrochloride (Enhances neuromuscular blocking action).
 No products indexed under this heading.

Cisplatin (Irreversible inhibition of plasma cholinesterase by certain unspecified antineoplastic drugs resulting in possible prolonged neuromuscular block).
 No products indexed under this heading.

Clindamycin Hydrochloride (Enhances neuromuscular blocking action). Products include:

Cleocin Vaginal Ovules 2616

Clindamycin Palmitate Hydrochloride (Enhances neuromuscular blocking action).
 No products indexed under this heading.

Clindamycin Phosphate (Enhances neuromuscular blocking action). Products include:
 Benzaclin Topical Gel 2877
 Clindagel .. 1203
 Evoclin Foam, 1% 1009

Colistimethate Sodium (Enhances neuromuscular blocking action).
 No products indexed under this heading.

Colistin Sulfate (Enhances neuromuscular blocking action).
 No products indexed under this heading.

Cortisone Acetate (Enhances the neuromuscular blocking effects by a reduction in plasma cholinesterase activity induced by chronic administration of glucocorticoids).
 No products indexed under this heading.

Cyclophosphamide (Irreversible inhibition of plasma cholinesterase by certain unspecified antineoplastic drugs resulting in possible prolonged neuromuscular block).
 No products indexed under this heading.

Dacarbazine (Irreversible inhibition of plasma cholinesterase by certain unspecified antineoplastic drugs resulting in possible prolonged neuromuscular block).
 No products indexed under this heading.

Daunorubicin Citrate (Irreversible inhibition of plasma cholinesterase by certain unspecified antineoplastic drugs resulting in possible prolonged neuromuscular block).
 No products indexed under this heading.

Daunorubicin Hydrochloride (Irreversible inhibition of plasma cholinesterase by certain unspecified antineoplastic drugs resulting in possible prolonged neuromuscular block).
 No products indexed under this heading.

Demeclocycline Hydrochloride (Enhances neuromuscular blocking action).
 No products indexed under this heading.

Denileukin Diftitox (Irreversible inhibition of plasma cholinesterase by certain unspecified antineoplastic drugs resulting in possible prolonged neuromuscular block). Products include:
 Ontak Vials 1745

Desogestrel (Enhances the neuromuscular blocking effects by a reduction in plasma cholinesterase activity induced by chronic administration of oral contraceptives). Products include:
 Mircette Tablets 1066

Dexamethasone (Enhances the neuromuscular blocking effects by a reduction in plasma cholinesterase activity induced by chronic administration of glucocorticoids). Products include:
 Ciprodex Otic Suspension 559
 Decadron Tablets 1951
 TobraDex Ophthalmic Ointment 562
 TobraDex Ophthalmic Suspension ... 563

Dexamethasone Acetate (Enhances the neuromuscular blocking effects by a reduction in plasma cholinesterase activity induced by chronic administration of glucocorticoids).
 No products indexed under this heading.

Dexamethasone Sodium Phosphate (Enhances the neuromuscular blocking effects by a reduction in plasma cholinesterase activity induced by chronic administration of glucocorticoids).
 No products indexed under this heading.

Docetaxel (Irreversible inhibition of plasma cholinesterase by certain unspecified antineoplastic drugs resulting in possible prolonged neuromuscular block). Products include:
 Taxotere Injection Concentrate 2932

Doxorubicin Hydrochloride (Irreversible inhibition of plasma cholinesterase by certain unspecified antineoplastic drugs resulting in possible prolonged neuromuscular block).
 No products indexed under this heading.

Doxycycline Calcium (Enhances neuromuscular blocking action).
 No products indexed under this heading.

Doxycycline Hyclate (Enhances neuromuscular blocking action).
 No products indexed under this heading.

Doxycycline Monohydrate (Enhances neuromuscular blocking action). Products include:
 Oracea Capsules 1000

Echothiophate Iodide (Irreversible inhibition of plasma cholinesterase by echothiophate resulting in possible prolonged neuromuscular block).
 No products indexed under this heading.

Enflurane (Decreases ED_{50} of Mivacron by as much as 35% to 40%; prolongs the clinically effective duration of action).
 No products indexed under this heading.

Epirubicin Hydrochloride (Irreversible inhibition of plasma cholinesterase by certain unspecified antineoplastic drugs resulting in possible prolonged neuromuscular block).
 No products indexed under this heading.

Estramustine Phosphate Sodium (Irreversible inhibition of plasma cholinesterase by certain unspecified antineoplastic drugs resulting in possible prolonged neuromuscular block). Products include:
 Emcyt Capsules 2634

Ethinyl Estradiol (Enhances the neuromuscular blocking effects by a reduction in plasma cholinesterase activity induced by chronic administration of oral contraceptives). Products include:
 Mircette Tablets 1066
 NuvaRing 2340
 Ortho-Cyclen/Ortho Tri-Cyclen 2429
 Ortho Evra Transdermal System 2417
 Ortho Tri-Cyclen Lo Tablets 2436
 Seasonique Tablets 1077
 Yasmin 28 Tablets 796
 Yaz Tablets 803

Ethynodiol Diacetate (Enhances the neuromuscular blocking effects by a reduction in plasma cholinesterase activity induced by chronic administration of oral contraceptives).
 No products indexed under this heading.

Etidocaine Hydrochloride (Enhances neuromuscular blocking action).
 No products indexed under this heading.

Etoposide (Irreversible inhibition of plasma cholinesterase by certain unspecified antineoplastic drugs resulting in possible prolonged neuromuscular block).
 No products indexed under this heading.

Exemestane (Irreversible inhibition of plasma cholinesterase by certain unspecified antineoplastic drugs resulting in possible prolonged neuromuscular block). Products include:
 Aromasin Tablets 2600

Floxuridine (Irreversible inhibition of plasma cholinesterase by certain unspecified antineoplastic drugs resulting in possible prolonged neuromuscular block).
 No products indexed under this heading.

Fludrocortisone Acetate (Enhances the neuromuscular blocking effects by a reduction in plasma cholinesterase activity induced by chronic administration of glucocorticoids).
 No products indexed under this heading.

Fluorouracil (Irreversible inhibition of plasma cholinesterase by certain unspecified antineoplastic drugs resulting in possible prolonged neuromuscular block). Products include:
 Carac Cream, 0.5% 2879
 Efudex ... 3363

Flutamide (Irreversible inhibition of plasma cholinesterase by certain unspecified antineoplastic drugs resulting in possible prolonged neuromuscular block). Products include:
 Eulexin Capsules 3009

Fosphenytoin Sodium (Potential for resistance to the neuromuscular blocking action in patients on chronic phenytoin therapy).
 No products indexed under this heading.

Gemcitabine Hydrochloride (Irreversible inhibition of plasma cholinesterase by certain unspecified antineoplastic drugs resulting in possible prolonged neuromuscular block). Products include:
 Gemzar for Injection 1771

Gentamicin Sulfate (Enhances the neuromuscular blocking action). Products include:
 Garamycin Injectable 3014
 Pred-G Ophthalmic Ointment ⊙237
 Pred-G Ophthalmic Suspension ⊙236

Halothane (Prolongs the duration of action).
 No products indexed under this heading.

Hydrocortisone (Enhances the neuromuscular blocking effects by a reduction in plasma cholinesterase activity induced by chronic administration of glucocorticoids). Products include:
 Colocort Rectal Suspension, USP
 (Retention) 100 mg/60 mL........... 2476
 Hydrocortone Tablets 1989

IMPORTANT NOTE: Always consult each drug listing in the patient's regimen for possible interactions.

Preparation H Hydrocortisone
Cream .. ▣646

Hydrocortisone Acetate
(Enhances the neuromuscular blocking effects by a reduction in plasma
cholinesterase activity induced by
chronic administration of glucocorticoids). Products include:
Analpram-HC 1159
Pramosone 1161
ProctoFoam-HC 3099

Hydrocortisone Sodium Phos-phate
(Enhances the neuromuscular
blocking effects by a reduction in
plasma cholinesterase activity
induced by chronic administration of
glucocorticoids).
No products indexed under this
heading.

Hydrocortisone Sodium Succin-ate
(Enhances the neuromuscular
blocking effects by a reduction in
plasma cholinesterase activity
induced by chronic administration of
glucocorticoids).
No products indexed under this
heading.

Hydroxyurea (Irreversible inhibition
of plasma cholinesterase by certain
unspecified antineoplastic drugs
resulting in possible prolonged neuromuscular block).
No products indexed under this
heading.

Idarubicin Hydrochloride (Irreversible inhibition of plasma cholinesterase by certain unspecified antineoplastic drugs resulting in possible
prolonged neuromuscular block).
No products indexed under this
heading.

Ifosfamide (Irreversible inhibition of
plasma cholinesterase by certain
unspecified antineoplastic drugs
resulting in possible prolonged neuromuscular block).
No products indexed under this
heading.

Interferon alfa-2a, Recombinant
(Irreversible inhibition of plasma cholinesterase by certain unspecified
antineoplastic drugs resulting in possible prolonged neuromuscular
block).
No products indexed under this
heading.

Interferon alfa-2b, Recombinant
(Irreversible inhibition of plasma cholinesterase by certain unspecified
antineoplastic drugs resulting in possible prolonged neuromuscular
block). Products include:
Intron A for Injection 3024
Rebetron Combination Therapy 3063

Irinotecan Hydrochloride (Irreversible inhibition of plasma cholinesterase by certain unspecified antineoplastic drugs resulting in possible
prolonged neuromuscular block).
Products include:
Camptosar Injection 2604

Isocarboxazid (Enhances the neuromuscular blocking effects by a
reduction in plasma cholinesterase
activity induced by chronic administration of certain unspecified monoamine oxidase inhibitors).
No products indexed under this
heading.

Isoflurane (Decreases ED$_{50}$ of
Mivacron by as much as 35% to
40%; prolongs the clinically effective
duration of action).
No products indexed under this
heading.

Kanamycin Sulfate (Enhances the
neuromuscular blocking action).
No products indexed under this
heading.

Levamisole Hydrochloride (Irreversible inhibition of plasma cholinesterase by certain unspecified antineoplastic drugs resulting in
possible prolonged neuromuscular
block).
No products indexed under this
heading.

Levobupivacaine Hydrochloride
(Enhances neuromuscular blocking
action).
No products indexed under this
heading.

Levonorgestrel (Enhances the neu-
romuscular blocking effects by a
reduction in plasma cholinesterase
activity induced by chronic adminis-
tration of oral contraceptives).
Products include:
Climara Pro Transdermal System 776
Mirena Intrauterine System 787
Plan B Tablets 1076
Seasonique Tablets 1077

Lidocaine Hydrochloride
(Enhances neuromuscular blocking
action).
No products indexed under this
heading.

Lincomycin Hydrochloride
(Enhances neuromuscular blocking
action).
No products indexed under this
heading.

Lithium (Enhances neuromuscular
blocking action).
No products indexed under this
heading.

Lithium Carbonate (Enhances neu-
romuscular blocking action).
Products include:
Lithobid Tablets 1692

Lithium Citrate (Enhances neuromuscular blocking action).
No products indexed under this
heading.

Lomustine (CCNU) (Irreversible
inhibition of plasma cholinesterase
by certain unspecified antineoplastic
drugs resulting in possible prolonged
neuromuscular block).
No products indexed under this
heading.

Magnesium Salts (Enhances neuromuscular blocking action).
No products indexed under this
heading.

Mechlorethamine Hydrochloride
(Irreversible inhibition of plasma cholinesterase by certain unspecified
antineoplastic drugs resulting in possible prolonged neuromuscular
block). Products include:
Mustargen for Injection 2468

Megestrol Acetate (Irreversible
inhibition of plasma cholinesterase
by certain unspecified antineoplastic
drugs resulting in possible prolonged
neuromuscular block). Products
include:
Megace ES Oral Suspension 2481

Melphalan (Irreversible inhibition of
plasma cholinesterase by certain
unspecified antineoplastic drugs
resulting in possible prolonged neuromuscular block). Products include:
Alkeran Tablets 956

Mepivacaine Hydrochloride
(Enhances neuromuscular blocking
action).
No products indexed under this
heading.

Mercaptopurine (Irreversible inhibition of plasma cholinesterase by
certain unspecified antineoplastic
drugs resulting in possible prolonged
neuromuscular block).
No products indexed under this
heading.

Mestranol (Enhances the neuromuscular blocking effects by a
reduction in plasma cholinesterase
activity induced by chronic administration of oral contraceptives).
No products indexed under this
heading.

Methacycline Hydrochloride
(Enhances neuromuscular blocking
action).
No products indexed under this
heading.

Methotrexate Sodium (Irreversible
inhibition of plasma cholinesterase
by certain unspecified antineoplastic
drugs resulting in possible prolonged
neuromuscular block).
No products indexed under this
heading.

Methylprednisolone Acetate
(Enhances the neuromuscular blocking effects by a reduction in plasma
cholinesterase activity induced by
chronic administration of glucocorticoids). Products include:
Depo-Medrol Injectable
Suspension 2617
Depo-Medrol Single-Dose Vial 2619

Methylprednisolone Sodium Succinate
(Enhances the neuro-
muscular blocking effects by a
reduction in plasma cholinesterase
activity induced by chronic administration of glucocorticoids).
No products indexed under this
heading.

Minocycline Hydrochloride
(Enhances neuromuscular blocking
action). Products include:
Solodyn Extended Release
Tablets ... 1890

Mitomycin (Mitomycin-C) (Irreversible inhibition of plasma cholinesterase by certain unspecified antineoplastic drugs resulting in possible
prolonged neuromuscular block).
No products indexed under this
heading.

Mitotane (Irreversible inhibition of
plasma cholinesterase by certain
unspecified antineoplastic drugs
resulting in possible prolonged neuromuscular block).
No products indexed under this
heading.

Mitoxantrone Hydrochloride (Irreversible inhibition of plasma cholinesterase by certain unspecified antineoplastic drugs resulting in
possible prolonged neuromuscular
block).
No products indexed under this
heading.

Moclobemide (Enhances the neuromuscular blocking effects by a
reduction in plasma cholinesterase
activity induced by chronic administration of certain unspecified monoamine oxidase inhibitors).
No products indexed under this
heading.

Norethindrone (Enhances the neuromuscular blocking effects by a
reduction in plasma cholinesterase
activity induced by chronic administration of oral contraceptives).
Products include:
Ortho Micronor Tablets 2426

Norethynodrel (Enhances the neuromuscular blocking effects by a
reduction in plasma cholinesterase
activity induced by chronic administration of oral contraceptives).
No products indexed under this
heading.

Norgestimate (Enhances the neuromuscular blocking effects by a
reduction in plasma cholinesterase
activity induced by chronic administration of oral contraceptives).
Products include:
Ortho-Cyclen/Ortho Tri-Cyclen 2429
Ortho Tri-Cyclen Lo Tablets 2436

Norgestrel (Enhances the neuromuscular blocking effects by a
reduction in plasma cholinesterase
activity induced by chronic administration of oral contraceptives).
No products indexed under this
heading.

Oxaliplatin (Irreversible inhibition of
plasma cholinesterase by certain
unspecified antineoplastic drugs
resulting in possible prolonged neuromuscular block). Products include:
Eloxatin for Injection 2892

Oxytetracycline Hydrochloride
(Enhances neuromuscular blocking
action).
No products indexed under this
heading.

Paclitaxel (Irreversible inhibition of
plasma cholinesterase by certain
unspecified antineoplastic drugs
resulting in possible prolonged neuromuscular block).
No products indexed under this
heading.

Pargyline Hydrochloride
(Enhances the neuromuscular blocking effects by a reduction in plasma
cholinesterase activity induced by
chronic administration of certain
unspecified monoamine oxidase
inhibitors).
No products indexed under this
heading.

Phenelzine Sulfate (Enhances the
neuromuscular blocking effects by a
reduction in plasma cholinesterase
activity induced by chronic administration of certain unspecified monoamine oxidase inhibitors).
No products indexed under this
heading.

Phenytoin (Potential for resistance
to the neuromuscular blocking action
in patients on chronic phenytoin
therapy).
No products indexed under this
heading.

Phenytoin Sodium (Potential for
resistance to the neuromuscular
blocking action in patients on chronic phenytoin therapy). Products
include:
Phenytek Capsules 2160

Polymyxin Preparations
(Enhances neuromuscular blocking
action).
No products indexed under this
heading.

Prednisolone Acetate (Enhances
the neuromuscular blocking effects
by a reduction in plasma cholinester-
ase activity induced by chronic
administration of glucocorticoids).
Products include:
Blephamide Ophthalmic Ointment 568
Blephamide Ophthalmic
Suspension 569
Poly-Pred Ophthalmic
Suspension ☉233
Pred Forte Ophthalmic
Suspension ☉235

Pred Mild Ophthalmic Suspension ⊙238
Pred-G Ophthalmic Ointment ⊙237
Pred-G Ophthalmic Suspension ⊙236

Prednisolone Sodium Phosphate (Enhances the neuromuscular blocking effects by a reduction in plasma cholinesterase activity induced by chronic administration of glucocorticoids).
No products indexed under this heading.

Prednisolone Tebutate (Enhances the neuromuscular blocking effects by a reduction in plasma cholinesterase activity induced by chronic administration of glucocorticoids).
No products indexed under this heading.

Prednisone (Enhances the neuromuscular blocking effects by a reduction in plasma cholinesterase activity induced by chronic administration of glucocorticoids).
No products indexed under this heading.

Procainamide Hydrochloride (Enhances neuromuscular blocking action).
No products indexed under this heading.

Procaine Hydrochloride (Enhances neuromuscular blocking action).
No products indexed under this heading.

Procarbazine Hydrochloride (Irreversible inhibition of plasma cholinesterase by certain unspecified antineoplastic drugs resulting in possible prolonged neuromuscular block). Products include:
Matulane Capsules 3191

Quinidine (Enhances neuromuscular blocking action).
No products indexed under this heading.

Quinidine Gluconate (Enhances neuromuscular blocking action).
No products indexed under this heading.

Quinidine Hydrochloride (Enhances neuromuscular blocking action).
No products indexed under this heading.

Quinidine Polygalacturonate (Enhances neuromuscular blocking action).
No products indexed under this heading.

Quinidine Sulfate (Enhances neuromuscular blocking action).
No products indexed under this heading.

Selegiline Hydrochloride (Enhances the neuromuscular blocking effects by a reduction in plasma cholinesterase activity induced by chronic administration of certain unspecified monoamine oxidase inhibitors). Products include:
Eldepryl Capsules 3208
Zelapar Tablets 3372

Streptomycin Sulfate (Enhances the neuromuscular blocking action).
No products indexed under this heading.

Streptozocin (Irreversible inhibition of plasma cholinesterase by certain unspecified antineoplastic drugs resulting in possible prolonged neuromuscular block).
No products indexed under this heading.

Succinylcholine Chloride (Prior administration of succinylcholine can potentiate neuromuscular blockade).
No products indexed under this heading.

Tamoxifen Citrate (Irreversible inhibition of plasma cholinesterase by certain unspecified antineoplastic drugs resulting in possible prolonged neuromuscular block). Products include:
Soltamox Oral Solution 3527

Teniposide (Irreversible inhibition of plasma cholinesterase by certain unspecified antineoplastic drugs resulting in possible prolonged neuromuscular block).
No products indexed under this heading.

Tetracaine Hydrochloride (Enhances neuromuscular blocking action). Products include:
Cetacaine Topical Anesthetic 999

Tetracycline Hydrochloride (Enhances neuromuscular blocking action).
No products indexed under this heading.

Thioguanine (Irreversible inhibition of plasma cholinesterase by certain unspecified antineoplastic drugs resulting in possible prolonged neuromuscular block). Products include:
Tabloid Tablets 1575

Thiotepa (Irreversible inhibition of plasma cholinesterase by certain unspecified antineoplastic drugs resulting in possible prolonged neuromuscular block).
No products indexed under this heading.

Tobramycin (Enhances the neuromuscular blocking action). Products include:
TOBI Solution for Inhalation 2298
TobraDex Ophthalmic Ointment 562
TobraDex Ophthalmic Suspension 563
Zylet Ophthalmic Suspension ⊙259

Tobramycin Sulfate (Enhances the neuromuscular blocking action).
No products indexed under this heading.

Topotecan Hydrochloride (Irreversible inhibition of plasma cholinesterase by certain unspecified antineoplastic drugs resulting in possible prolonged neuromuscular block). Products include:
Hycamtin for Injection 1458

Toremifene Citrate (Irreversible inhibition of plasma cholinesterase by certain unspecified antineoplastic drugs resulting in possible prolonged neuromuscular block).
No products indexed under this heading.

Tranylcypromine Sulfate (Enhances the neuromuscular blocking effects by a reduction in plasma cholinesterase activity induced by chronic administration of certain unspecified monoamine oxidase inhibitors). Products include:
Parnate Tablets 1527

Triamcinolone (Enhances the neuromuscular blocking effects by a reduction in plasma cholinesterase activity induced by chronic administration of glucocorticoids).
No products indexed under this heading.

Triamcinolone Acetonide (Enhances the neuromuscular blocking effects by a reduction in plasma cholinesterase activity induced by chronic administration of glucocorticoids). Products include:
Azmacort Inhalation Aerosol 1726
Nasacort AQ Nasal Spray 2922

Triamcinolone Diacetate (Enhances the neuromuscular blocking effects by a reduction in plasma cholinesterase activity induced by chronic administration of glucocorticoids).
No products indexed under this heading.

Triamcinolone Hexacetonide (Enhances the neuromuscular blocking effects by a reduction in plasma cholinesterase activity induced by chronic administration of glucocorticoids).
No products indexed under this heading.

Valrubicin (Irreversible inhibition of plasma cholinesterase by certain unspecified antineoplastic drugs resulting in possible prolonged neuromuscular block).
No products indexed under this heading.

Vincristine Sulfate (Irreversible inhibition of plasma cholinesterase by certain unspecified antineoplastic drugs resulting in possible prolonged neuromuscular block).
No products indexed under this heading.

Vinorelbine Tartrate (Irreversible inhibition of plasma cholinesterase by certain unspecified antineoplastic drugs resulting in possible prolonged neuromuscular block).
No products indexed under this heading.

M-M-R II

(Measles, Mumps & Rubella Virus Vaccine, Live) 2006
May interact with immunosuppressive agents. Compounds in these categories include:

Azathioprine (Concurrent administration with immunosuppressant is contraindicated).
No products indexed under this heading.

Basiliximab (Concurrent administration with immunosuppressant is contraindicated). Products include:
Simulect for Injection 2284

Cyclosporine (Concurrent administration with immunosuppressant is contraindicated). Products include:
Gengraf Capsules 459
Neoral Oral Solution 2259
Neoral Soft Gelatin Capsules 2259
Restasis Ophthalmic Emulsion 575
Sandimmune 2275

Muromonab-CD3 (Concurrent administration with immunosuppressant is contraindicated). Products include:
Orthoclone OKT3 Sterile Solution 2360

Mycophenolate Mofetil (Concurrent administration with immunosuppressant is contraindicated). Products include:
CellCept Capsules 2747
CellCept Oral Suspension 2747
CellCept Tablets 2747

Sirolimus (Concurrent administration with immunosuppressant is contraindicated). Products include:
Rapamune Oral Solution and Tablets 3475

Tacrolimus (Concurrent administration with immunosuppressant is contraindicated). Products include:
Prograf Capsules and Injection 632
Protopic Ointment 638

MOBAN TABLETS

(Molindone Hydrochloride) 1119
May interact with tetracyclines and certain other agents. Compounds in these categories include:

Demeclocycline Hydrochloride (Calcium sulfate present as an excipient may interfere with the absorption of oral tetracyclines).
No products indexed under this heading.

Doxycycline Calcium (Calcium sulfate present as an excipient may interfere with the absorption of oral tetracyclines).
No products indexed under this heading.

Doxycycline Hyclate (Calcium sulfate present as an excipient may interfere with the absorption of oral tetracyclines).
No products indexed under this heading.

Doxycycline Monohydrate (Calcium sulfate present as an excipient may interfere with the absorption of oral tetracyclines). Products include:
Oracea Capsules 1000

Methacycline Hydrochloride (Calcium sulfate present as an excipient may interfere with the absorption of oral tetracyclines).
No products indexed under this heading.

Minocycline Hydrochloride (Calcium sulfate present as an excipient may interfere with the absorption of oral tetracyclines). Products include:
Solodyn Extended Release Tablets 1890

Oxytetracycline Hydrochloride (Calcium sulfate present as an excipient may interfere with the absorption of oral tetracyclines).
No products indexed under this heading.

Phenytoin Sodium (Calcium sulfate present as an excipient may interfere with the absorption of oral phenytoin sodium). Products include:
Phenytek Capsules 2160

Tetracycline Hydrochloride (Calcium sulfate present as an excipient may interfere with the absorption of oral tetracyclines).
No products indexed under this heading.

MOBIC ORAL SUSPENSION

(Meloxicam) 863
See Mobic Tablets

MOBIC TABLETS

(Meloxicam) 863
May interact with ACE inhibitors, lithium preparations, loop diuretics, thiazides, and certain other agents. Compounds in these categories include:

Aspirin (Co-administration of aspirin to healthy volunteers tended to increase the AUC and Cmax of meloxicam; the clinical significance of this interaction is not known; concurrent use may result in an increased rate of GI ulceration or other complications). Products include:
Aggrenox Capsules 822
Bayer Aspirin 744
BC Allergy Sinus Cold Powder ▣677
BC Headache Powder ▣677
Arthritis Strength BC Powder ▣677
BC Sinus Cold Powder ▣677

IMPORTANT NOTE: Always consult each drug listing in the patient's regimen for possible interactions.

Excedrin Extra Strength Caplets/Tablets/Geltabs .... ▣684
Excedrin Migraine Caplets/Tablets/Geltabs .... ▣609
Goody's Body Pain Formula Powder .... ▣684
Goody's Extra Strength Headache Powders .... ▣611
Goody's Extra Strength Pain Relief Tablets .... ▣685
Percodan Tablets 1132
St. Joseph 81 mg Aspirin Chewable and Enteric Coated Tablets 1869

Benazepril Hydrochloride (Co-administration of NSAIDs with ACE inhibitors may diminish the antihypertensive effects of ACE inhibitors). Products include:
Lotensin Tablets 2243
Lotensin HCT Tablets 2246
Lotrel Capsules 2249

Bendroflumethiazide (NSAIDs can reduce the natriuretic effect of thiazide diuretics in some patients. Patients taking thiazides may have impaired response when taking NSAIDs).
No products indexed under this heading.

Bumetanide (Patients taking loop diuretics may have impaired response when taking NSAIDs). Products include:
Bumex Tablets 2746

Captopril (Co-administration of NSAIDs with ACE inhibitors may diminish the antihypertensive effects of ACE inhibitors). Products include:
Captopril Tablets 2149

Chlorothiazide (NSAIDs can reduce the natriuretic effect of thiazide diuretics in some patients. Patients taking thiazides may have impaired response when taking NSAIDs). Products include:
Diuril Oral Suspension 1954

Chlorothiazide Sodium (NSAIDs can reduce the natriuretic effect of thiazide diuretics in some patients. Patients taking thiazides may have impaired response when taking NSAIDs). Products include:
Diuril Sodium Intravenous 2467

Cholestyramine (Pretreatment for four days with cholestyramine significantly increased clearance of meloxicam by 50% resulting in a decrease in t1/2 from 19.2 hours to 12.5 hours and a 35% reduction in AUC; the clinical significance of this interaction is not known).
No products indexed under this heading.

Enalapril Maleate (Co-administration of NSAIDs with ACE inhibitors may diminish the antihypertensive effects of ACE inhibitors). Products include:
Vasotec I.V. Injection 2103

Enalaprilat (Co-administration of NSAIDs with ACE inhibitors may diminish the antihypertensive effects of ACE inhibitors).
No products indexed under this heading.

Ethacrynic Acid (Patients taking loop diuretics may have impaired response when taking NSAIDs). Products include:
Edecrin Tablets 1959

Fosinopril Sodium (Co-administration of NSAIDs with ACE inhibitors may diminish the antihypertensive effects of ACE inhibitors).
No products indexed under this heading.

Furosemide (NSAIDs can reduce the natriuretic effect of furosemide in some patients; in clinical studies, pharmacokinetics and pharmacodynamics of furosemide were not affected by multiple doses of meloxicam). Products include:
Furosemide Tablets 2154

Hydrochlorothiazide (NSAIDs can reduce the natriuretic effect of thiazide diuretics in some patients. Patients taking thiazides may have impaired response when taking NSAIDs). Products include:
Aldoril Tablets 1910
Atacand HCT 651
Avalide Tablets 888
Avalide Tablets 2874
Benicar HCT Tablets 1044
Diovan HCT Tablets 2196
Dyazide Capsules 1423
Hyzaar 50-12.5 Tablets 1990
Hyzaar 100-12.5 Tablets 1990
Hyzaar 100-25 Tablets 1990
Lopressor HCT 50/25 Tablets 2241
Lopressor HCT 100/25 Tablets 2241
Lopressor HCT 100/50 Tablets 2241
Lotensin HCT Tablets 2246
Micardis HCT Tablets 856
Moduretic Tablets 2028
Prinzide Tablets 2056
Teveten HCT Tablets 1737
Timolide Tablets 2086
Uniretic Tablets 3100

Hydroflumethiazide (NSAIDs can reduce the natriuretic effect of thiazide diuretics in some patients. Patients taking thiazides may have impaired response when taking NSAIDs).
No products indexed under this heading.

Lisinopril (Co-administration of NSAIDs with ACE inhibitors may diminish the antihypertensive effects of ACE inhibitors). Products include:
Prinivil Tablets 2052
Prinzide Tablets 2056

Lithium (NSAIDs can produce an elevation of plasma lithium levels and a reduction in renal lithium clearance; co-administration in healthy subjects has resulted in increased lithium concentration and AUC).
No products indexed under this heading.

Lithium Carbonate (NSAIDs can produce an elevation of plasma lithium levels and a reduction in renal lithium clearance; co-administration in healthy subjects has resulted in increased lithium concentration and AUC). Products include:
Lithobid Tablets 1692

Lithium Citrate (NSAIDs can produce an elevation of plasma lithium levels and a reduction in renal lithium clearance; co-administration in healthy subjects has resulted in increased lithium concentration and AUC).
No products indexed under this heading.

Methotrexate (Caution should be used when NSAIDs are administered concomitantly with methotrexate).
No products indexed under this heading.

Methotrexate Sodium (Caution should be used when NSAIDs are administered concomitantly with methotrexate).
No products indexed under this heading.

Methyclothiazide (NSAIDs can reduce the natriuretic effect of thiazide diuretics in some patients. Patients taking thiazides may have impaired response when taking NSAIDs).
No products indexed under this heading.

Moexipril Hydrochloride (Co-administration of NSAIDs with ACE inhibitors may diminish the antihypertensive effects of ACE inhibitors). Products include:
Uniretic Tablets 3100
Univasc Tablets 3104

Perindopril Erbumine (Co-administration of NSAIDs with ACE inhibitors may diminish the antihypertensive effects of ACE inhibitors). Products include:
Aceon Tablets (2 mg, 4 mg, 8 mg) 3194

Polythiazide (NSAIDs can reduce the natriuretic effect of thiazide diuretics in some patients. Patients taking thiazides may have impaired response when taking NSAIDs).
No products indexed under this heading.

Quinapril Hydrochloride (Co-administration of NSAIDs with ACE inhibitors may diminish the antihypertensive effects of ACE inhibitors).
No products indexed under this heading.

Ramipril (Co-administration of NSAIDs with ACE inhibitors may diminish the antihypertensive effects of ACE inhibitors). Products include:
Altace Capsules 1702

Spirapril Hydrochloride (Co-administration of NSAIDs with ACE inhibitors may diminish the antihypertensive effects of ACE inhibitors).
No products indexed under this heading.

Torsemide (Patients taking loop diuretics may have impaired response when taking NSAIDs). Products include:
Demadex Injection 2759
Demadex Tablets 2759

Trandolapril (Co-administration of NSAIDs with ACE inhibitors may diminish the antihypertensive effects of ACE inhibitors). Products include:
Mavik Tablets 486
Tarka Tablets 524

Warfarin Sodium (Potential for increased risk of bleeding). Products include:
Coumadin for Injection 898
Coumadin Tablets 898

Food Interactions

Food, unspecified (Co-administration with a high-fat breakfast did not affect extent of absorption of meloxicam capsules but led to 22% higher Cmax values; mean Cmax values were achieved between 5 to 6 hours; Mobic tablets can be administered without regard to timing of meals).

MODURETIC TABLETS

(Amiloride Hydrochloride, Hydrochlorothiazide) 2028
May interact with ACE inhibitors, angiotensin-II receptor antagonists, antihypertensives, barbiturates, corticosteroids, cardiac glycosides, oral hypoglycemic agents, insulin, lithium preparations, narcotic analgesics, nondepolarizing neuromuscular blocking agents, non-steroidal anti-inflammatory agents, potassium preparations, potassium sparing diuretics, and certain other agents. Compounds in these categories include:

Acarbose (Hydrochlorothiazide produces hyperglycemia; dosage adjustment of the antidiabetic agent may be required). Products include:
Precose Tablets 751

Acebutolol Hydrochloride (Co-administration with other antihypertensive drugs may result in additive effect or potentiation).
No products indexed under this heading.

ACTH (Intensifies electrolyte depletion particularly hypokalemia).
No products indexed under this heading.

Alfentanil Hydrochloride (Potentiation of orthostatic hypotension).
No products indexed under this heading.

Amlodipine Besylate (Co-administration with other antihypertensive drugs may result in additive effect or potentiation). Products include:
Caduet Tablets 2508
Lotrel Capsules 2249
Norvasc Tablets 2545

Aprobarbital (Potentiation of orthostatic hypotension).
No products indexed under this heading.

Atenolol (Co-administration with other antihypertensive drugs may result in additive effect or potentiation).
No products indexed under this heading.

Atracurium Besylate (Possible increased responsiveness to muscle relaxant).
No products indexed under this heading.

Benazepril Hydrochloride (Co-administration increases the risk of hyperkalemia; potential for additive antihypertensive effect). Products include:
Lotensin Tablets 2243
Lotensin HCT Tablets 2246
Lotrel Capsules 2249

Bendroflumethiazide (Co-administration with other antihypertensive drugs may result in additive effect or potentiation).
No products indexed under this heading.

Betamethasone Acetate (Corticosteroids intensify electrolyte depletion particularly hypokalemia).
No products indexed under this heading.

Betamethasone Sodium Phosphate (Corticosteroids intensify electrolyte depletion particularly hypokalemia).
No products indexed under this heading.

Betaxolol Hydrochloride (Co-administration with other antihypertensive drugs may result in additive effect or potentiation). Products include:
Betoptic S Ophthalmic Suspension 558

Bisoprolol Fumarate (Co-administration with other antihypertensive drugs may result in additive effect or potentiation).
No products indexed under this heading.

Buprenorphine Hydrochloride (Potentiation of orthostatic hypotension). Products include:
Buprenex Injectable 2716
Suboxone Tablets 2717
Subutex Tablets 2717

Butabarbital (Potentiation of orthostatic hypotension).
No products indexed under this heading.

Butalbital (Potentiation of orthostatic hypotension).
No products indexed under this heading.

Candesartan Cilexetil (Co-administration increases the risk of hyperkalemia; potential for additive antihypertensive effect). Products include:

Captopril (Co-administration increases the risk of hyperkalemia; potential for additive antihypertensive effect). Products include:

Carteolol Hydrochloride (Co-administration with other antihypertensive drugs may result in additive effect or potentiation). Products include:

Celecoxib (Co-administration of non-steroidal anti-inflammatory agents can reduce the diuretic, natriuretic, and antihypertensive effects). Products include:

Chlorothiazide (Co-administration with other antihypertensive drugs may result in additive effect or potentiation). Products include:

Chlorothiazide Sodium (Co-administration with other antihypertensive drugs may result in additive effect or potentiation). Products include:

Chlorpropamide (Hydrochlorothiazide produces hyperglycemia; dosage adjustment of the antidiabetic agent may be required).
No products indexed under this heading.

Chlorthalidone (Co-administration with other antihypertensive drugs may result in additive effect or potentiation). Products include:

Cholestyramine (Impairs the absorption of hydrochlorothiazide by binding in the GI tract and reducing the absorption by 85%).
No products indexed under this heading.

Cisatracurium Besylate (Possible increased responsiveness to muscle relaxant). Products include:

Clonidine (Co-administration with other antihypertensive drugs may result in additive effect or potentiation). Products include:

Clonidine Hydrochloride (Co-administration with other antihypertensive drugs may result in additive effect or potentiation). Products include:

Codeine Phosphate (Potentiation of orthostatic hypotension). Products include:

Colestipol Hydrochloride (Impairs the absorption of hydrochlorothiazide by binding in the GI tract and reducing the absorption by 43%).
No products indexed under this heading.

Cortisone Acetate (Corticosteroids intensify electrolyte depletion particularly hypokalemia).
No products indexed under this heading.

Cyclosporine (Co-administration increases the risk of hyperkalemia). Products include:

Deserpidine (Co-administration with other antihypertensive drugs may result in additive effect or potentiation).
No products indexed under this heading.

Deslanoside (Hypokalemia may develop during thiazide therapy and may sensitize or exaggerate the response of the heart to the toxic effects of digitalis, such as increased ventricular irritability).
No products indexed under this heading.

Dexamethasone (Corticosteroids intensify electrolyte depletion particularly hypokalemia). Products include:

Dexamethasone Acetate (Corticosteroids intensify electrolyte depletion particularly hypokalemia).
No products indexed under this heading.

Dexamethasone Sodium Phosphate (Corticosteroids intensify electrolyte depletion particularly hypokalemia).
No products indexed under this heading.

Dezocine (Potentiation of orthostatic hypotension).
No products indexed under this heading.

Diazoxide (Co-administration with other antihypertensive drugs may result in additive effect or potentiation). Products include:

Diclofenac Potassium (Co-administration of non-steroidal anti-inflammatory agents can reduce the diuretic, natriuretic, and antihypertensive effects).
No products indexed under this heading.

Diclofenac Sodium (Co-administration of non-steroidal anti-inflammatory agents can reduce the diuretic, natriuretic, and antihypertensive effects). Products include:

Digitalis Glycoside Preparations (Hypokalemia may develop during thiazide therapy and may sensitize or exaggerate the response of the heart to the toxic effects of digitalis, such as increased ventricular irritability).
No products indexed under this heading.

Digitoxin (Hypokalemia may develop during thiazide therapy and may sensitize or exaggerate the response of the heart to the toxic effects of digitalis, such as increased ventricular irritability).
No products indexed under this heading.

Digoxin (Hypokalemia may develop during thiazide therapy and may sensitize or exaggerate the response of the heart to the toxic effects of digitalis, such as increased ventricular irritability). Products include:

Diltiazem Hydrochloride (Co-administration with other antihypertensive drugs may result in additive effect or potentiation). Products include:

Doxazosin Mesylate (Co-administration with other antihypertensive drugs may result in additive effect or potentiation). Products include:

Enalapril Maleate (Co-administration increases the risk of hyperkalemia; potential for additive antihypertensive effect). Products include:

Enalaprilat (Co-administration increases the risk of hyperkalemia; potential for additive antihypertensive effect).
No products indexed under this heading.

Eprosartan Mesylate (Co-administration increases the risk of hyperkalemia; potential for additive antihypertensive effect). Products include:

Esmolol Hydrochloride (Co-administration with other antihypertensive drugs may result in additive effect or potentiation).
No products indexed under this heading.

Etodolac (Co-administration of non-steroidal anti-inflammatory agents can reduce the diuretic, natriuretic, and antihypertensive effects).
No products indexed under this heading.

Felodipine (Co-administration with other antihypertensive drugs may result in additive effect or potentiation).
No products indexed under this heading.

Fenoprofen Calcium (Co-administration of non-steroidal anti-inflammatory agents can reduce the diuretic, natriuretic, and antihypertensive effects). Products include:

Fentanyl (Potentiation of orthostatic hypotension). Products include:

Fentanyl Citrate (Potentiation of orthostatic hypotension). Products include:

Fludrocortisone Acetate (Corticosteroids intensify electrolyte depletion particularly hypokalemia).
No products indexed under this heading.

Flurbiprofen (Co-administration of non-steroidal anti-inflammatory agents can reduce the diuretic, natriuretic, and antihypertensive effects).
No products indexed under this heading.

Fosinopril Sodium (Co-administration increases the risk of hyperkalemia; potential for additive antihypertensive effect).
No products indexed under this heading.

Furosemide (Co-administration with other antihypertensive drugs may result in additive effect or potentiation). Products include:

Glimepiride (Hydrochlorothiazide produces hyperglycemia; dosage adjustment of the antidiabetic agent may be required). Products include:

Glipizide (Hydrochlorothiazide produces hyperglycemia; dosage adjustment of the antidiabetic agent may be required).
No products indexed under this heading.

Glyburide (Hydrochlorothiazide produces hyperglycemia; dosage adjustment of the antidiabetic agent may be required).
No products indexed under this heading.

Guanabenz Acetate (Co-administration with other antihypertensive drugs may result in additive effect or potentiation).
No products indexed under this heading.

Guanethidine Monosulfate (Co-administration with other antihypertensive drugs may result in additive effect or potentiation).
No products indexed under this heading.

Hydralazine Hydrochloride (Co-administration with other antihypertensive drugs may result in additive effect or potentiation). Products include:

Hydrocodone Bitartrate (Potentiation of orthostatic hypotension). Products include:

Hydrocodone Polistirex (Potentiation of orthostatic hypotension). Products include:

Hydrocortisone (Corticosteroids intensify electrolyte depletion particularly hypokalemia). Products include:

Hydrocortisone Acetate (Corticosteroids intensify electrolyte depletion particularly hypokalemia). Products include:

IMPORTANT NOTE: Always consult each drug listing in the patient's regimen for possible interactions.

Pramosone ... 1161
ProctoFoam-HC ... 3099

Hydrocortisone Sodium Phosphate (Corticosteroids intensify electrolyte depletion particularly hypokalemia).
No products indexed under this heading.

Hydrocortisone Sodium Succinate (Corticosteroids intensify electrolyte depletion particularly hypokalemia).
No products indexed under this heading.

Hydroflumethiazide (Co-administration with other antihypertensive drugs may result in additive effect or potentiation).
No products indexed under this heading.

Hydromorphone Hydrochloride (Potentiation of orthostatic hypotension). Products include:
Dilaudid ... 440
Dilaudid Non-Sterile Powder ... 440
Dilaudid Oral Liquid ... 445
Dilaudid Rectal Suppositories ... 440
Dilaudid Tablets ... 440
Dilaudid Tablets - 8 mg ... 445
Dilaudid-HP ... 442

Ibuprofen (Co-administration of non-steroidal anti-inflammatory agents can reduce the diuretic, natriuretic, and antihypertensive effects). Products include:
Advil Allergy Sinus Caplets ... ▣770
Advil ... ▣674
Children's Advil Oral Suspension ... ▣603
Children's Advil Chewable Tablets ... ▣603
Advil Cold & Sinus ... ▣723
Infants' Advil Concentrated Drops ... ▣604
Infants' Advil Concentrated Drops - White Grape (Dye-Free) ... ▣604
Junior Strength Advil Swallow Tablets ... ▣605
Advil Migraine Liquigels ... ▣608
Advil Multi-Symptom Cold Caplets ... ▣770
Advil PM Caplets ... ▣615
Motrin IB Tablets and Caplets ... 1866
Children's Motrin Oral Suspension ... 1867
Children's Motrin Non-Staining Dye-Free Oral Suspension ... 1867
Children's Motrin Cold Oral Suspension ... 1867
Infants' Motrin Concentrated Drops ... 1867
Infants' Motrin Non-Staining Dye-Free Concentrated Drops ... 1867
Junior Strength Motrin Caplets and Chewable Tablets ... 1867
Vicoprofen Tablets ... 539

Indapamide (Co-administration with other antihypertensive drugs may result in additive effect or potentiation). Products include:
Indapamide Tablets ... 2156

Indomethacin (Co-administration of non-steroidal anti-inflammatory agents can reduce the diuretic, natriuretic, and antihypertensive effects; both indomethacin and amiloride are associated with hyperkalemia, the potential effect on potassium kinetic and renal function should be considered if used concurrently). Products include:
Indocin ... 1995

Indomethacin Sodium Trihydrate (Co-administration of non-steroidal anti-inflammatory agents can reduce the diuretic, natriuretic, and antihypertensive effects; both indomethacin and amiloride are associated with hyperkalemia, the potential effect on potassium kinetic and renal function should be considered if used concurrently). Products include:
Indocin I.V. ... 2465

Insulin, Human, Zinc Suspension (Hydrochlorothiazide produces hyperglycemia; dosage adjustment of the insulin agent may be required). Products include:
Humulin L, 100 Units ... 1794
Humulin U, 100 Units ... 1800

Insulin, Human NPH (Hydrochlorothiazide produces hyperglycemia; dosage adjustment of the insulin agent may be required). Products include:
Humulin N, 100 Units ... 1795
Humulin N Pen ... 1797

Insulin, Human Regular (Hydrochlorothiazide produces hyperglycemia; dosage adjustment of the insulin agent may be required). Products include:
Humulin R, 100 Units ... 1798

Insulin, Human Regular and Human NPH Mixture (Hydrochlorothiazide produces hyperglycemia; dosage adjustment of the insulin agent may be required). Products include:
Humulin 50/50, 100 Units ... 1791
Humulin 70/30 Pen ... 1793

Insulin, NPH (Hydrochlorothiazide produces hyperglycemia; dosage adjustment of the insulin agent may be required).
No products indexed under this heading.

Insulin, Regular (Hydrochlorothiazide produces hyperglycemia; dosage adjustment of the insulin agent may be required).
No products indexed under this heading.

Insulin, Zinc Crystals (Hydrochlorothiazide produces hyperglycemia; dosage adjustment of the insulin agent may be required).
No products indexed under this heading.

Insulin, Zinc Suspension (Hydrochlorothiazide produces hyperglycemia; dosage adjustment of the insulin agent may be required).
No products indexed under this heading.

Insulin Aspart, Human Regular (Hydrochlorothiazide produces hyperglycemia; dosage adjustment of the insulin agent may be required). Products include:
NovoLog Injection ... 2326

Insulin glargine (Hydrochlorothiazide produces hyperglycemia; dosage adjustment of the insulin agent may be required). Products include:
Lantus Injection ... 2909

Insulin Lispro, Human (Hydrochlorothiazide produces hyperglycemia; dosage adjustment of the insulin agent may be required). Products include:
Humalog-Pen ... 1781
Humalog Mix 50/50-Pen ... 1783
Humalog Mix 75/25-Pen ... 1785

Insulin Lispro Protamine, Human (Hydrochlorothiazide produces hyperglycemia; dosage adjustment of the insulin agent may be required). Products include:
Humalog Mix 50/50-Pen ... 1783
Humalog Mix 75/25-Pen ... 1785

Irbesartan (Co-administration increases the risk of hyperkalemia; potential for additive antihypertensive effect). Products include:
Avalide Tablets ... 888
Avalide Tablets ... 2874
Avapro Tablets ... 891
Avapro Tablets ... 2871

Isradipine (Co-administration with other antihypertensive drugs may result in additive effect or potentiation). Products include:
DynaCirc CR Tablets ... 2721

Ketoprofen (Co-administration of non-steroidal anti-inflammatory agents can reduce the diuretic, natriuretic, and antihypertensive effects).
No products indexed under this heading.

Ketorolac Tromethamine (Co-administration of non-steroidal anti-inflammatory agents can reduce the diuretic, natriuretic, and antihypertensive effects). Products include:
Acular Ophthalmic Solution ... ⊙ 565
Acular LS Ophthalmic Solution ... ⊙ 566

Labetalol Hydrochloride (Co-administration with other antihypertensive drugs may result in additive effect or potentiation).
No products indexed under this heading.

Levorphanol Tartrate (Potentiation of orthostatic hypotension).
No products indexed under this heading.

Lisinopril (Co-administration increases the risk of hyperkalemia; potential for additive antihypertensive effect). Products include:
Prinivil Tablets ... 2052
Prinzide Tablets ... 2056

Lithium (Diuretics reduce the renal clearance and add a high risk of lithium toxicity).
No products indexed under this heading.

Lithium Carbonate (Diuretics reduce the renal clearance and add a high risk of lithium toxicity). Products include:
Lithobid Tablets ... 1692

Lithium Citrate (Diuretics reduce the renal clearance and add a high risk of lithium toxicity).
No products indexed under this heading.

Losartan Potassium (Co-administration increases the risk of hyperkalemia; potential for additive antihypertensive effect). Products include:
Cozaar Tablets ... 1935
Hyzaar 50-12.5 Tablets ... 1990
Hyzaar 100-12.5 Tablets ... 1990
Hyzaar 100-25 Tablets ... 1990

Mecamylamine Hydrochloride (Co-administration with other antihypertensive drugs may result in additive effect or potentiation).
No products indexed under this heading.

Meclofenamate Sodium (Co-administration of non-steroidal anti-inflammatory agents can reduce the diuretic, natriuretic, and antihypertensive effects).
No products indexed under this heading.

Mefenamic Acid (Co-administration of non-steroidal anti-inflammatory agents can reduce the diuretic, natriuretic, and antihypertensive effects).
No products indexed under this heading.

Meloxicam (Co-administration of non-steroidal anti-inflammatory agents can reduce the diuretic, natriuretic, and antihypertensive effects). Products include:
Mobic Oral Suspension ... 863
Mobic Tablets ... 863

Meperidine Hydrochloride (Potentiation of orthostatic hypotension).
No products indexed under this heading.

Mephobarbital (Potentiation of orthostatic hypotension).
No products indexed under this heading.

Metformin Hydrochloride (Hydrochlorothiazide produces hyperglycemia; dosage adjustment of the antidiabetic agent may be required). Products include:
ActoPlus Met Tablets ... 3214
Avandamet Tablets ... 1373
Fortamet Extended-Release Tablets ... 3115

Methadone Hydrochloride (Potentiation of orthostatic hypotension).
No products indexed under this heading.

Methyclothiazide (Co-administration with other antihypertensive drugs may result in additive effect or potentiation).
No products indexed under this heading.

Methyldopa (Co-administration with other antihypertensive drugs may result in additive effect or potentiation). Products include:
Aldoril Tablets ... 1910

Methyldopate Hydrochloride (Co-administration with other antihypertensive drugs may result in additive effect or potentiation).
No products indexed under this heading.

Methylprednisolone Acetate (Corticosteroids intensify electrolyte depletion particularly hypokalemia). Products include:
Depo-Medrol Injectable Suspension ... 2617
Depo-Medrol Single-Dose Vial ... 2619

Methylprednisolone Sodium Succinate (Corticosteroids intensify electrolyte depletion particularly hypokalemia).
No products indexed under this heading.

Metocurine Iodide (Possible increased responsiveness to muscle relaxant).
No products indexed under this heading.

Metolazone (Co-administration with other antihypertensive drugs may result in additive effect or potentiation).
No products indexed under this heading.

Metoprolol Succinate (Co-administration with other antihypertensive drugs may result in additive effect or potentiation). Products include:
Toprol-XL Tablets ... 668

Metoprolol Tartrate (Co-administration with other antihypertensive drugs may result in additive effect or potentiation). Products include:
Lopressor Injection ... 2238
Lopressor Tablets ... 2238
Lopressor HCT 50/25 Tablets ... 2241
Lopressor HCT 100/25 Tablets ... 2241
Lopressor HCT 100/50 Tablets ... 2241

Metyrosine (Co-administration with other antihypertensive drugs may result in additive effect or potentiation). Products include:
Demser Capsules ... 1953

Mibefradil Dihydrochloride (Co-administration with other antihypertensive drugs may result in additive effect or potentiation).

No products indexed under this heading.

Miglitol (Hydrochlorothiazide produces hyperglycemia; dosage adjustment of the antidiabetic agent may be required).

No products indexed under this heading.

Minoxidil (Co-administration with other antihypertensive drugs may result in additive effect or potentiation). Products include:

Men's Rogaine Extra Strength
Hair Regrowth Treatment
Topical Solution, Ocean Rush
Scent and Original Unscented ▣◪633
Men's Rogaine Foam Hair
Regrowth Treatment ▣◪633
Women's Rogaine Hair Regrowth
Treatment Topical Solution,
Spring Bloom Scent and
Original Unscented ▣◪634

Mivacurium Chloride (Possible increased responsiveness to muscle relaxant). Products include:

Mivacron Injection 493

Moexipril Hydrochloride (Co-administration increases the risk of hyperkalemia; potential for additive antihypertensive effect). Products include:

Uniretic Tablets 3100
Univasc Tablets 3104

Morphine Sulfate (Potentiation of orthostatic hypotension). Products include:

Avinza Capsules 1741
Kadian Capsules 577
MS Contin Tablets 2701

Nabumetone (Co-administration of non-steroidal anti-inflammatory agents can reduce the diuretic, natriuretic, and antihypertensive effects).

No products indexed under this heading.

Nadolol (Co-administration with other antihypertensive drugs may result in additive effect or potentiation). Products include:

Nadolol Tablets 2159

Naproxen (Co-administration of non-steroidal anti-inflammatory agents can reduce the diuretic, natriuretic, and antihypertensive effects). Products include:

EC-Naprosyn Delayed-Release
Tablets 2761
Naprosyn Suspension 2761
Naprosyn Tablets 2761
Prevacid NapraPAC 3280

Naproxen Sodium (Co-administration of non-steroidal anti-inflammatory agents can reduce the diuretic, natriuretic, and antihypertensive effects). Products include:

Aleve Caplets 742
Aleve Gelcaps 743
Aleve Tablets 743
Aleve Cold & Sinus Caplets 744
Anaprox Tablets 2761
Anaprox DS Tablets 2761

Nicardipine Hydrochloride (Co-administration with other antihypertensive drugs may result in additive effect or potentiation). Products include:

Cardene I.V. 2497

Nifedipine (Co-administration with other antihypertensive drugs may result in additive effect or potentiation). Products include:

Adalat CC Tablets 2964

Nisoldipine (Co-administration with other antihypertensive drugs may result in additive effect or potentiation). Products include:

Sular Tablets 3122

Nitroglycerin (Co-administration with other antihypertensive drugs may result in additive effect or potentiation). Products include:

Nitro-Dur Transdermal Infusion
System 3046
Nitrolingual Pumpspray 3120

Norepinephrine Bitartrate (Possible decreased response to pressor amines).

No products indexed under this heading.

Oxaprozin (Co-administration of non-steroidal anti-inflammatory agents can reduce the diuretic, natriuretic, and antihypertensive effects).

No products indexed under this heading.

Oxycodone Hydrochloride (Potentiation of orthostatic hypotension). Products include:

OxyContin Tablets 2703
OxyFast Oral Concentrate
Solution 2708
OxyIR Capsules 2708
Percocet Tablets 1131
Percodan Tablets 1132

Pancuronium Bromide (Possible increased responsiveness to muscle relaxant).

No products indexed under this heading.

Penbutolol Sulfate (Co-administration with other antihypertensive drugs may result in additive effect or potentiation).

No products indexed under this heading.

Pentobarbital Sodium (Potentiation of orthostatic hypotension). Products include:

Nembutal Sodium Solution, USP 2470

Perindopril Erbumine (Co-administration increases the risk of hyperkalemia; potential for additive antihypertensive effect). Products include:

Aceon Tablets (2 mg, 4 mg,
8 mg) 3194

Phenobarbital (Potentiation of orthostatic hypotension). Products include:

Donnatal Extentabs 2493

Phenoxybenzamine Hydrochloride (Co-administration with other antihypertensive drugs may result in additive effect or potentiation). Products include:

Dibenzyline Capsules 3399

Phentolamine Mesylate (Co-administration with other antihypertensive drugs may result in additive effect or potentiation).

No products indexed under this heading.

Phenylbutazone (Co-administration of non-steroidal anti-inflammatory agents can reduce the diuretic, natriuretic, and antihypertensive effects).

No products indexed under this heading.

Pindolol (Co-administration with other antihypertensive drugs may result in additive effect or potentiation).

No products indexed under this heading.

Pioglitazone Hydrochloride (Hydrochlorothiazide produces hyperglycemia; dosage adjustment of the antidiabetic agent may be required). Products include:

ActoPlus Met Tablets 3214
Actos Tablets 3219
Duetact Tablets 3226

Piroxicam (Co-administration of non-steroidal anti-inflammatory agents can reduce the diuretic, natriuretic, and antihypertensive effects).

No products indexed under this heading.

Polythiazide (Co-administration with other antihypertensive drugs may result in additive effect or potentiation).

No products indexed under this heading.

Potassium Acid Phosphate (Amiloride is associated with hyperkalemia; concurrent use with potassium supplements is contraindicated). Products include:

K-Phos Original (Sodium Free)
Tablets 760

Potassium Bicarbonate (Amiloride is associated with hyperkalemia; concurrent use with potassium supplements is contraindicated).

No products indexed under this heading.

Potassium Chloride (Amiloride is associated with hyperkalemia; concurrent use with potassium supplements is contraindicated). Products include:

Colyte with Flavor Packs for Oral
Solution 3088
HalfLytely and Bisacodyl Tablets
Bowel Prep Kit with Flavors
Packs 881
K-Dur Extended-Release Tablets 3033
K-Lor Oral Solution 474
K-Tab Tablets 475
MoviPrep Oral Solution 2839
TriLyte with Flavor Packs for Oral
Solution 3100

Potassium Citrate (Amiloride is associated with hyperkalemia; concurrent use with potassium supplements is contraindicated). Products include:

Urocit-K Tablets 2144

Potassium Gluconate (Amiloride is associated with hyperkalemia; concurrent use with potassium supplements is contraindicated).

No products indexed under this heading.

Potassium Phosphate (Amiloride is associated with hyperkalemia; concurrent use with potassium supplements is contraindicated). Products include:

K-Phos Neutral Tablets 760

Prazosin Hydrochloride (Co-administration with other antihypertensive drugs may result in additive effect or potentiation).

No products indexed under this heading.

Prednisolone Acetate (Corticosteroids intensify electrolyte depletion particularly hypokalemia). Products include:

Blephamide Ophthalmic Ointment 568
Blephamide Ophthalmic
Suspension 569
Poly-Pred Ophthalmic
Suspension ⊙233
Pred Forte Ophthalmic
Suspension ⊙235
Pred Mild Ophthalmic
Suspension ⊙238
Pred-G Ophthalmic Ointment ⊙237
Pred-G Ophthalmic Suspension ⊙236

Prednisolone Sodium Phosphate (Corticosteroids intensify electrolyte depletion particularly hypokalemia).

No products indexed under this heading.

Prednisolone Tebutate (Corticosteroids intensify electrolyte depletion particularly hypokalemia).

No products indexed under this heading.

Prednisone (Corticosteroids intensify electrolyte depletion particularly hypokalemia).

No products indexed under this heading.

Propoxyphene Hydrochloride (Potentiation of orthostatic hypotension).

No products indexed under this heading.

Propoxyphene Napsylate (Potentiation of orthostatic hypotension).

No products indexed under this heading.

Propranolol Hydrochloride (Co-administration with other antihypertensive drugs may result in additive effect or potentiation). Products include:

Inderal LA Long-Acting Capsules 3429
InnoPran XL Capsules 2723

Quinapril Hydrochloride (Co-administration increases the risk of hyperkalemia; potential for additive antihypertensive effect).

No products indexed under this heading.

Ramipril (Co-administration increases the risk of hyperkalemia; potential for additive antihypertensive effect). Products include:

Altace Capsules 1702

Rapacuronium Bromide (Possible increased responsiveness to muscle relaxant).

No products indexed under this heading.

Rauwolfia Serpentina (Co-administration with other antihypertensive drugs may result in additive effect or potentiation).

No products indexed under this heading.

Remifentanil Hydrochloride (Potentiation of orthostatic hypotension).

No products indexed under this heading.

Repaglinide (Hydrochlorothiazide produces hyperglycemia; dosage adjustment of the antidiabetic agent may be required).

No products indexed under this heading.

Rescinnamine (Co-administration with other antihypertensive drugs may result in additive effect or potentiation).

No products indexed under this heading.

Reserpine (Co-administration with other antihypertensive drugs may result in additive effect or potentiation).

No products indexed under this heading.

Rocuronium Bromide (Possible increased responsiveness to muscle relaxant). Products include:

Zemuron Injection 2346

Rofecoxib (Co-administration of non-steroidal anti-inflammatory agents can reduce the diuretic, natriuretic, and antihypertensive effects).

No products indexed under this heading.

Rosiglitazone Maleate (Hydrochlorothiazide produces hyperglycemia; dosage adjustment of the antidiabetic agent may be required). Products include:

Avandamet Tablets ... 1373
Avandaryl Tablets ... 1379
Avandia Tablets ... 1384

Secobarbital Sodium (Potentiation of orthostatic hypotension).
No products indexed under this heading.

Sodium Nitroprusside (Co-administration with other antihypertensive drugs may result in additive effect or potentiation).
No products indexed under this heading.

Sotalol Hydrochloride (Co-administration with other antihypertensive drugs may result in additive effect or potentiation).
No products indexed under this heading.

Spirapril Hydrochloride (Co-administration increases the risk of hyperkalemia; potential for additive antihypertensive effect).
No products indexed under this heading.

Spironolactone (Amiloride is associated with hyperkalemia; concurrent use with potassium sparing diuretics is contraindicated).
No products indexed under this heading.

Sufentanil Citrate (Potentiation of orthostatic hypotension).
No products indexed under this heading.

Sulindac (Co-administration of non-steroidal anti-inflammatory agents can reduce the diuretic, natriuretic, and antihypertensive effects). Products include:
Clinoril Tablets ... 1924

Tacrolimus (Co-administration increases the risk of hyperkalemia). Products include:
Prograf Capsules and Injection ... 632
Protopic Ointment ... 638

Telmisartan (Co-administration increases the risk of hyperkalemia; potential for additive antihypertensive effect). Products include:
Micardis Tablets ... 854
Micardis HCT Tablets ... 856

Terazosin Hydrochloride (Co-administration with other antihypertensive drugs may result in additive effect or potentiation). Products include:
Hytrin Capsules ... 471

Thiamylal Sodium (Potentiation of orthostatic hypotension).
No products indexed under this heading.

Timolol Maleate (Co-administration with other antihypertensive drugs may result in additive effect or potentiation). Products include:
Blocadren Tablets ... 1916
Cosopt Sterile Ophthalmic Solution ... 1931
Timolide Tablets ... 2086
Timoptic Sterile Ophthalmic Solution ... 2088
Timoptic in Ocudose ... 2091
Timoptic-XE Sterile Ophthalmic Gel Forming Solution ... 2092

Tolazamide (Hydrochlorothiazide produces hyperglycemia; dosage adjustment of the antidiabetic agent may be required).
No products indexed under this heading.

Tolbutamide (Hydrochlorothiazide produces hyperglycemia; dosage adjustment of the antidiabetic agent may be required).
No products indexed under this heading.

Tolmetin Sodium (Co-administration of non-steroidal anti-inflammatory agents can reduce the diuretic, natriuretic, and antihypertensive effects).
No products indexed under this heading.

Torsemide (Co-administration with other antihypertensive drugs may result in additive effect or potentiation). Products include:
Demadex Injection ... 2759
Demadex Tablets ... 2759

Trandolapril (Co-administration increases the risk of hyperkalemia; potential for additive antihypertensive effect). Products include:
Mavik Tablets ... 486
Tarka Tablets ... 524

Triamcinolone (Corticosteroids intensify electrolyte depletion particularly hypokalemia).
No products indexed under this heading.

Triamcinolone Acetonide (Corticosteroids intensify electrolyte depletion particularly hypokalemia). Products include:
Azmacort Inhalation Aerosol ... 1726
Nasacort AQ Nasal Spray ... 2922

Triamcinolone Diacetate (Corticosteroids intensify electrolyte depletion particularly hypokalemia).
No products indexed under this heading.

Triamcinolone Hexacetonide (Corticosteroids intensify electrolyte depletion particularly hypokalemia).
No products indexed under this heading.

Triamterene (Amiloride is associated with hyperkalemia; concurrent use with potassium sparing diuretics is contraindicated). Products include:
Dyazide Capsules ... 1423
Dyrenium Capsules ... 3400

Trimethaphan Camsylate (Co-administration with other antihypertensive drugs may result in additive effect or potentiation).
No products indexed under this heading.

Troglitazone (Hydrochlorothiazide produces hyperglycemia; dosage adjustment of the antidiabetic agent may be required).
No products indexed under this heading.

Tubocurarine Chloride (Possible increased responsiveness to the muscle relaxant).
No products indexed under this heading.

Valdecoxib (Co-administration of non-steroidal anti-inflammatory agents can reduce the diuretic, natriuretic, and antihypertensive effects).
No products indexed under this heading.

Valsartan (Co-administration increases the risk of hyperkalemia; potential for additive antihypertensive effect). Products include:
Diovan Tablets ... 2193
Diovan HCT Tablets ... 2196

Vecuronium Bromide (Possible increased responsiveness to muscle relaxant).
No products indexed under this heading.

Verapamil Hydrochloride (Co-administration with other antihypertensive drugs may result in additive effect or potentiation). Products include:
Covera-HS Tablets ... 3139
Tarka Tablets ... 524
Verelan PM Extended-Release Capsules, Controlled-Onset ... 3106

Food Interactions

Alcohol (Potentiation of orthostatic hypotension).

Diet, potassium-rich (Potential for rapid increases in serum potassium levels).

MOTRIN IB TABLETS AND CAPLETS

(Ibuprofen) ... 1866

May interact with aspirin-acetylsalicylic acid, anticoagulants, corticosteroids, non-steroidal anti-inflammatory agents, and certain other agents. Compounds in these categories include:

Anisindione (Increased risk of stomach bleeding if co-administered with anticoagulants). Products include:
Miradon Tablets ... 3042

Ardeparin Sodium (Increased risk of stomach bleeding if co-administered with anticoagulants).
No products indexed under this heading.

Aspirin (Increased risk of stomach bleeding if co-administered with non-steroidal anti-inflammatory drugs). Products include:
Aggrenox Capsules ... 822
Bayer Aspirin ... 744
BC Allergy Sinus Cold Powder ... ▣ 677
BC Headache Powder ... ▣ 677
Arthritis Strength BC Powder ... ▣ 677
BC Sinus Cold Powder ... ▣ 677
Excedrin Extra Strength Caplets/Tablets/Geltabs ... ▣ 684
Excedrin Migraine Caplets/Tablets/Geltabs ... ▣ 609
Goody's Body Pain Formula Powder ... ▣ 684
Goody's Extra Strength Headache Powders ... ▣ 611
Goody's Extra Strength Pain Relief Tablets ... ▣ 685
Percodan Tablets ... 1132
St. Joseph 81 mg Aspirin Chewable and Enteric Coated Tablets ... 1869

Aspirin, Enteric Coated (Increased risk of stomach bleeding if co-administered with non-steroidal anti-inflammatory drugs).
No products indexed under this heading.

Aspirin Buffered (Increased risk of stomach bleeding if co-administered with non-steroidal anti-inflammatory drugs). Products include:
Bufferin Extra Strength Tablets ... ▣ 678
Bufferin Regular Strength Tablets ... ▣ 678

Betamethasone Acetate (Increased risk of stomach bleeding if co-administered with steroidal drugs).
No products indexed under this heading.

Betamethasone Sodium Phosphate (Increased risk of stomach bleeding if co-administered with steroidal drugs).
No products indexed under this heading.

Celecoxib (Increased risk of stomach bleeding if co-administered with non-steroidal anti-inflammatory drugs). Products include:
Celebrex Capsules ... 3134

Cortisone Acetate (Increased risk of stomach bleeding if co-administered with steroidal drugs).
No products indexed under this heading.

Dalteparin Sodium (Increased risk of stomach bleeding if co-administered with anticoagulants). Products include:
Fragmin Injection ... 1097

Danaparoid Sodium (Increased risk of stomach bleeding if co-administered with anticoagulants).
No products indexed under this heading.

Dexamethasone (Increased risk of stomach bleeding if co-administered with steroidal drugs). Products include:
Ciprodex Otic Suspension ... 559
Decadron Tablets ... 1951
TobraDex Ophthalmic Ointment ... 562
TobraDex Ophthalmic Suspension ... 563

Dexamethasone Acetate (Increased risk of stomach bleeding if co-administered with steroidal drugs).
No products indexed under this heading.

Dexamethasone Sodium Phosphate (Increased risk of stomach bleeding if co-administered with steroidal drugs).
No products indexed under this heading.

Diclofenac Potassium (Increased risk of stomach bleeding if co-administered with non-steroidal anti-inflammatory drugs).
No products indexed under this heading.

Diclofenac Sodium (Increased risk of stomach bleeding if co-administered with non-steroidal anti-inflammatory drugs). Products include:
Arthrotec Tablets ... 3129
Voltaren Ophthalmic Solution ... 2309
Voltaren Tablets ... 2307
Voltaren-XR Tablets ... 2310

Dicumarol (Increased risk of stomach bleeding if co-administered with anticoagulants).
No products indexed under this heading.

Enoxaparin Sodium (Increased risk of stomach bleeding if co-administered with anticoagulants). Products include:
Lovenox Injection ... 2915

Etodolac (Increased risk of stomach bleeding if co-administered with non-steroidal anti-inflammatory drugs).
No products indexed under this heading.

Fenoprofen Calcium (Increased risk of stomach bleeding if co-administered with non-steroidal anti-inflammatory drugs). Products include:
Nalfon Capsules ... 2502

Fludrocortisone Acetate (Increased risk of stomach bleeding if co-administered with steroidal drugs).
No products indexed under this heading.

Flurbiprofen (Increased risk of stomach bleeding if co-administered with non-steroidal anti-inflammatory drugs).
No products indexed under this heading.

Fondaparinux Sodium (Increased risk of stomach bleeding if co-administered with anticoagulants). Products include:
Arixtra Injection ... 1351

Heparin Calcium (Increased risk of stomach bleeding if co-administered with anticoagulants).
No products indexed under this heading.

Heparin Sodium (Increased risk of stomach bleeding if co-administered with anticoagulants).
No products indexed under this heading.

Hydrocortisone (Increased risk of stomach bleeding if co-administered with steroidal drugs). Products include:
Colocort Rectal Suspension, USP (Retention) 100 mg/60 mL 2476
Hydrocortone Tablets 1989
Preparation H Hydrocortisone Cream 646

Hydrocortisone Acetate (Increased risk of stomach bleeding if co-administered with steroidal drugs). Products include:
Analpram-HC 1159
Pramosone 1161
ProctoFoam-HC 3099

Hydrocortisone Sodium Phosphate (Increased risk of stomach bleeding if co-administered with steroidal drugs).
No products indexed under this heading.

Hydrocortisone Sodium Succinate (Increased risk of stomach bleeding if co-administered with steroidal drugs).
No products indexed under this heading.

Indomethacin (Increased risk of stomach bleeding if co-administered with non-steroidal anti-inflammatory drugs). Products include:
Indocin 1995

Indomethacin Sodium Trihydrate (Increased risk of stomach bleeding if co-administered with non-steroidal anti-inflammatory drugs). Products include:
Indocin I.V. 2465

Ketoprofen (Increased risk of stomach bleeding if co-administered with non-steroidal anti-inflammatory drugs).
No products indexed under this heading.

Ketorolac Tromethamine (Increased risk of stomach bleeding if co-administered with non-steroidal anti-inflammatory drugs). Products include:
Acular Ophthalmic Solution 565
Acular LS Ophthalmic Solution 566

Low Molecular Weight Heparins (Increased risk of stomach bleeding if co-administered with anticoagulants).
No products indexed under this heading.

Meclofenamate Sodium (Increased risk of stomach bleeding if co-administered with non-steroidal anti-inflammatory drugs).
No products indexed under this heading.

Mefenamic Acid (Increased risk of stomach bleeding if co-administered with non-steroidal anti-inflammatory drugs).
No products indexed under this heading.

Meloxicam (Increased risk of stomach bleeding if co-administered with non-steroidal anti-inflammatory drugs). Products include:
Mobic Oral Suspension 863
Mobic Tablets 863

Methylprednisolone Acetate (Increased risk of stomach bleeding if co-administered with steroidal drugs). Products include:
Depo-Medrol Injectable Suspension 2617
Depo-Medrol Single-Dose Vial 2619

Methylprednisolone Sodium Succinate (Increased risk of stomach bleeding if co-administered with steroidal drugs).
No products indexed under this heading.

Nabumetone (Increased risk of stomach bleeding if co-administered with non-steroidal anti-inflammatory drugs).
No products indexed under this heading.

Naproxen (Increased risk of stomach bleeding if co-administered with non-steroidal anti-inflammatory drugs). Products include:
EC-Naprosyn Delayed-Release Tablets 2761
Naprosyn Suspension 2761
Naprosyn Tablets 2761
Prevacid NapraPAC 3280

Naproxen Sodium (Increased risk of stomach bleeding if co-administered with non-steroidal anti-inflammatory drugs). Products include:
Aleve Caplets 742
Aleve Gelcaps 743
Aleve Tablets 743
Aleve Cold & Sinus Caplets 744
Anaprox Tablets 2761
Anaprox DS Tablets 2761

Oxaprozin (Increased risk of stomach bleeding if co-administered with non-steroidal anti-inflammatory drugs).
No products indexed under this heading.

Phenylbutazone (Increased risk of stomach bleeding if co-administered with non-steroidal anti-inflammatory drugs).
No products indexed under this heading.

Piroxicam (Increased risk of stomach bleeding if co-administered with non-steroidal anti-inflammatory drugs).
No products indexed under this heading.

Prednisolone Acetate (Increased risk of stomach bleeding if co-administered with steroidal drugs). Products include:
Blephamide Ophthalmic Ointment 568
Blephamide Ophthalmic Suspension.................................. 569
Poly-Pred Ophthalmic Suspension .... ⊙233
Pred Forte Ophthalmic Suspension .... ⊙235
Pred Mild Ophthalmic Suspension .... ⊙238
Pred-G Ophthalmic Ointment .... ⊙237
Pred-G Ophthalmic Suspension ...... ⊙236

Prednisolone Sodium Phosphate (Increased risk of stomach bleeding if co-administered with steroidal drugs).
No products indexed under this heading.

Prednisolone Tebutate (Increased risk of stomach bleeding if co-administered with steroidal drugs).
No products indexed under this heading.

Prednisone (Increased risk of stomach bleeding if co-administered with steroidal drugs).
No products indexed under this heading.

Rofecoxib (Increased risk of stomach bleeding if co-administered with non-steroidal anti-inflammatory drugs).
No products indexed under this heading.

Sulindac (Increased risk of stomach bleeding if co-administered with non-steroidal anti-inflammatory drugs). Products include:
Clinoril Tablets 1924

Tinzaparin Sodium (Increased risk of stomach bleeding if co-administered with anticoagulants).
No products indexed under this heading.

Tolmetin Sodium (Increased risk of stomach bleeding if co-administered with non-steroidal anti-inflammatory drugs).
No products indexed under this heading.

Triamcinolone (Increased risk of stomach bleeding if co-administered with steroidal drugs).
No products indexed under this heading.

Triamcinolone Acetonide (Increased risk of stomach bleeding if co-administered with steroidal drugs). Products include:
Azmacort Inhalation Aerosol 1726
Nasacort AQ Nasal Spray 2922

Triamcinolone Diacetate (Increased risk of stomach bleeding if co-administered with steroidal drugs).
No products indexed under this heading.

Triamcinolone Hexacetonide (Increased risk of stomach bleeding if co-administered with steroidal drugs).
No products indexed under this heading.

Valdecoxib (Increased risk of stomach bleeding if co-administered with non-steroidal anti-inflammatory drugs).
No products indexed under this heading.

Warfarin Sodium (Increased risk of stomach bleeding if co-administered with anticoagulants). Products include:
Coumadin for Injection 898
Coumadin Tablets 898

CHILDREN'S MOTRIN ORAL SUSPENSION

(Ibuprofen) 685

CHILDREN'S MOTRIN NON-STAINING DYE-FREE ORAL SUSPENSION

(Ibuprofen) 685

CHILDREN'S MOTRIN COLD ORAL SUSPENSION

(Ibuprofen, Pseudoephedrine Hydrochloride)................................. 733
May interact with monoamine oxidase inhibitors. Compounds in these categories include:

Isocarboxazid (Concurrent and/or sequential use with MAO inhibitors is not recommended).
No products indexed under this heading.

Moclobemide (Concurrent and/or sequential use with MAO inhibitors is not recommended).
No products indexed under this heading.

Pargyline Hydrochloride (Concurrent and/or sequential use with MAO inhibitors is not recommended).
No products indexed under this heading.

Phenelzine Sulfate (Concurrent and/or sequential use with MAO inhibitors is not recommended).
No products indexed under this heading.

Procarbazine Hydrochloride (Concurrent and/or sequential use with MAO inhibitors is not recommended). Products include:
Matulane Capsules 3191

Selegiline Hydrochloride (Concurrent and/or sequential use with MAO inhibitors is not recommended). Products include:
Eldepryl Capsules 3208
Zelapar Tablets 3372

Tranylcypromine Sulfate (Concurrent and/or sequential use with MAO inhibitors is not recommended). Products include:
Parnate Tablets 1527

CHILDREN'S MOTRIN ORAL SUSPENSION

(Ibuprofen) 1867
None cited in PDR database.

CHILDREN'S MOTRIN NON-STAINING DYE-FREE ORAL SUSPENSION

(Ibuprofen) 1867
See Children's Motrin Oral Suspension

CHILDREN'S MOTRIN COLD ORAL SUSPENSION

(Ibuprofen, Pseudoephedrine Hydrochloride)................................. 1867
May interact with:

See (Motrin Cold & Sinus Caplets).
No products indexed under this heading.

INFANTS' MOTRIN CONCENTRATED DROPS

(Ibuprofen) 1867
None cited in PDR database.

INFANTS' MOTRIN NON-STAINING DYE-FREE CONCENTRATED DROPS

(Ibuprofen) 1867
None cited in PDR database.

JUNIOR STRENGTH MOTRIN CAPLETS AND CHEWABLE TABLETS

(Ibuprofen) 1867
None cited in PDR database.

MOVIPREP ORAL SOLUTION

(Ascorbic Acid, PEG-3350, Potassium Chloride, Sodium Ascorbate, Sodium Chloride, Sodium Sulfate)................................ 2839
May interact with:

Oral Medications, unspecified (Oral medication administered within 1 hour of the start of administration of MoviPrep may be flushed from the gastrointestinal tract and the medication may not be absorbed).
No products indexed under this heading.

MS CONTIN TABLETS

(Morphine Sulfate) 2701
May interact with central nervous system depressants, general anesthetics, hypnotics and sedatives, mixed agonist/antagonist opioid analgesics, neuromuscular blocking agents, phenothiazines, tranquilizers, and certain other agents. Compounds in these categories include:

Alfentanil Hydrochloride (Profound sedation, coma, severe hypotension, respiratory depression).
No products indexed under this heading.

Alprazolam (Profound sedation, coma, severe hypotension, respiratory depression). Products include:
Niravam Orally Disintegrating Tablets 3092

Aprobarbital (Profound sedation, coma, severe hypotension, respiratory depression).
No products indexed under this heading.

Atracurium Besylate (Increased respiratory depression).
No products indexed under this heading.

Buprenorphine Hydrochloride (Mixed agonist/antagonist analgesics may reduce the analgesic effect or may precipitate withdrawal symptoms). Products include:
Buprenex Injectable 2716
Suboxone Tablets 2717
Subutex Tablets 2717

Buspirone Hydrochloride (Profound sedation, coma, severe hypotension, respiratory depression).
No products indexed under this heading.

Butabarbital (Profound sedation, coma, severe hypotension, respiratory depression).
No products indexed under this heading.

Butalbital (Profound sedation, coma, severe hypotension, respiratory depression).
No products indexed under this heading.

Butorphanol Tartrate (Mixed agonist/antagonist analgesics may reduce the analgesic effect or may precipitate withdrawal symptoms).
No products indexed under this heading.

Chlordiazepoxide (Profound sedation, coma, severe hypotension, respiratory depression).
No products indexed under this heading.

Chlordiazepoxide Hydrochloride (Profound sedation, coma, severe hypotension, respiratory depression). Products include:
Librium Capsules 3347

Chlorpromazine (Profound sedation, coma, severe hypotension, respiratory depression).
No products indexed under this heading.

Chlorpromazine Hydrochloride (Profound sedation, coma, severe hypotension, respiratory depression).
No products indexed under this heading.

Chlorprothixene (Profound sedation, coma, severe hypotension, respiratory depression).
No products indexed under this heading.

Chlorprothixene Hydrochloride (Profound sedation, coma, severe hypotension, respiratory depression).
No products indexed under this heading.

Chlorprothixene Lactate (Profound sedation, coma, severe hypotension, respiratory depression).
No products indexed under this heading.

Cisatracurium Besylate (Increased respiratory depression). Products include:
Nimbex Injection 498

Clorazepate Dipotassium (Profound sedation, coma, severe hypotension, respiratory depression). Products include:
Tranxene 2474

Clozapine (Profound sedation, coma, severe hypotension, respiratory depression). Products include:
Clozaril Tablets 2184
FazaClo Orally Disintegrating Tablets 551

Codeine Phosphate (Profound sedation, coma, severe hypotension, respiratory depression). Products include:
Tylenol with Codeine Tablets 2391

Desflurane (Profound sedation, coma, severe hypotension, respiratory depression).
No products indexed under this heading.

Dezocine (Profound sedation, coma, severe hypotension, respiratory depression).
No products indexed under this heading.

Diazepam (Profound sedation, coma, severe hypotension, respiratory depression). Products include:
Diastat Rectal Delivery System 3343
Valium Tablets 2819

Doxacurium Chloride (Increased respiratory depression).
No products indexed under this heading.

Droperidol (Profound sedation, coma, severe hypotension, respiratory depression).
No products indexed under this heading.

Enflurane (Profound sedation, coma, severe hypotension, respiratory depression).
No products indexed under this heading.

Estazolam (Profound sedation, coma, severe hypotension, respiratory depression). Products include:
ProSom Tablets 517

Ethanol (Profound sedation, coma, severe hypotension, respiratory depression).
No products indexed under this heading.

Ethchlorvynol (Profound sedation, coma, severe hypotension, respiratory depression).
No products indexed under this heading.

Ethinamate (Profound sedation, coma, severe hypotension, respiratory depression).
No products indexed under this heading.

Ethyl Alcohol (Profound sedation, coma, severe hypotension, respiratory depression).
No products indexed under this heading.

Fentanyl (Profound sedation, coma, severe hypotension, respiratory depression). Products include:
Duragesic Transdermal System 2373
Ionsys Transdermal System 2379

Fentanyl Citrate (Profound sedation, coma, severe hypotension, respiratory depression). Products include:
Actiq 979

Fluphenazine Decanoate (Profound sedation, coma, severe hypotension, respiratory depression).
No products indexed under this heading.

Fluphenazine Enanthate (Profound sedation, coma, severe hypotension, respiratory depression).
No products indexed under this heading.

Fluphenazine Hydrochloride (Profound sedation, coma, severe hypotension, respiratory depression).
No products indexed under this heading.

Flurazepam Hydrochloride (Profound sedation, coma, severe hypotension, respiratory depression). Products include:
Dalmane Capsules 3342

Glutethimide (Profound sedation, coma, severe hypotension, respiratory depression).
No products indexed under this heading.

Haloperidol (Profound sedation, coma, severe hypotension, respiratory depression).
No products indexed under this heading.

Haloperidol Decanoate (Profound sedation, coma, severe hypotension, respiratory depression).
No products indexed under this heading.

Hydrocodone Bitartrate (Profound sedation, coma, severe hypotension, respiratory depression). Products include:
Hycodan 1116
Hycotuss Expectorant Syrup 1117
Vicodin Tablets 535
Vicodin ES Tablets 536
Vicodin HP Tablets 538
Vicoprofen Tablets 539
Zydone Tablets 1139

Hydrocodone Polistirex (Profound sedation, coma, severe hypotension, respiratory depression). Products include:
Tussionex Pennkinetic Extended-Release Suspension 3327

Hydromorphone Hydrochloride (Profound sedation, coma, severe hypotension, respiratory depression). Products include:
Dilaudid 440
Dilaudid Non-Sterile Powder 440
Dilaudid Oral Liquid 445
Dilaudid Rectal Suppositories 440
Dilaudid Tablets 440
Dilaudid Tablets - 8 mg 445
Dilaudid-HP 442

Hydroxyzine Hydrochloride (Profound sedation, coma, severe hypotension, respiratory depression).
No products indexed under this heading.

Isoflurane (Profound sedation, coma, severe hypotension, respiratory depression).
No products indexed under this heading.

Ketamine Hydrochloride (Profound sedation, coma, severe hypotension, respiratory depression).
No products indexed under this heading.

Levomethadyl Acetate Hydrochloride (Profound sedation, coma, severe hypotension, respiratory depression).
No products indexed under this heading.

Levorphanol Tartrate (Profound sedation, coma, severe hypotension, respiratory depression).
No products indexed under this heading.

Lorazepam (Profound sedation, coma, severe hypotension, respiratory depression).
No products indexed under this heading.

Loxapine Hydrochloride (Profound sedation, coma, severe hypotension, respiratory depression).
No products indexed under this heading.

Loxapine Succinate (Profound sedation, coma, severe hypotension, respiratory depression).
No products indexed under this heading.

Meperidine Hydrochloride (Profound sedation, coma, severe hypotension, respiratory depression).
No products indexed under this heading.

Mephobarbital (Profound sedation, coma, severe hypotension, respiratory depression).
No products indexed under this heading.

Meprobamate (Profound sedation, coma, severe hypotension, respiratory depression).
No products indexed under this heading.

Mesoridazine Besylate (Profound sedation, coma, severe hypotension, respiratory depression).
No products indexed under this heading.

Methadone Hydrochloride (Profound sedation, coma, severe hypotension, respiratory depression).
No products indexed under this heading.

Methohexital Sodium (Profound sedation, coma, severe hypotension, respiratory depression).
No products indexed under this heading.

Methotrimeprazine (Profound sedation, coma, severe hypotension, respiratory depression).
No products indexed under this heading.

Methoxyflurane (Profound sedation, coma, severe hypotension, respiratory depression).
No products indexed under this heading.

Metocurine Iodide (Increased respiratory depression).
No products indexed under this heading.

Midazolam Hydrochloride (Profound sedation, coma, severe hypotension, respiratory depression).
No products indexed under this heading.

Mivacurium Chloride (Increased respiratory depression). Products include:
Mivacron Injection 493

Molindone Hydrochloride (Profound sedation, coma, severe hypotension, respiratory depression). Products include:
Moban Tablets 1119

Nalbuphine Hydrochloride (Mixed agonist/antagonist analgesics may reduce the analgesic effect or may precipitate withdrawal symptoms).
No products indexed under this heading.

Olanzapine (Profound sedation, coma, severe hypotension, respiratory depression). Products include:
Symbyax Capsules 1819
Zyprexa Tablets 1830
Zyprexa IntraMuscular 1830
Zyprexa ZYDIS Orally Disintegrating Tablets 1830

Oxazepam (Profound sedation, coma, severe hypotension, respiratory depression).
No products indexed under this heading.

Oxycodone Hydrochloride (Profound sedation, coma, severe hypotension, respiratory depression). Products include:
OxyContin Tablets 2703
OxyFast Oral Concentrate Solution 2708
OxyIR Capsules 2708
Percocet Tablets 1131
Percodan Tablets 1132

Pancuronium Bromide (Increased respiratory depression).
No products indexed under this heading.

Pentazocine Hydrochloride (Mixed agonist/antagonist analgesics may reduce the analgesic effect or may precipitate withdrawal symptoms).
No products indexed under this heading.

Pentazocine Lactate (Mixed agonist/antagonist analgesics may reduce the analgesic effect or may precipitate withdrawal symptoms).
No products indexed under this heading.

Pentobarbital Sodium (Profound sedation, coma, severe hypotension, respiratory depression). Products include:
Nembutal Sodium Solution, USP 2470

Perphenazine (Profound sedation, coma, severe hypotension, respiratory depression).
No products indexed under this heading.

Phenobarbital (Profound sedation, coma, severe hypotension, respiratory depression). Products include:
Donnatal Extentabs 2493

Prazepam (Profound sedation, coma, severe hypotension, respiratory depression).
No products indexed under this heading.

Prochlorperazine (Profound sedation, coma, severe hypotension, respiratory depression).
No products indexed under this heading.

Promethazine Hydrochloride (Profound sedation, coma, severe hypotension, respiratory depression). Products include:
Phenergan Tablets and Suppositories 3440

Propofol (Profound sedation, coma, severe hypotension, respiratory depression).
No products indexed under this heading.

Propoxyphene Hydrochloride (Profound sedation, coma, severe hypotension, respiratory depression).
No products indexed under this heading.

Propoxyphene Napsylate (Profound sedation, coma, severe hypotension, respiratory depression).
No products indexed under this heading.

Quazepam (Profound sedation, coma, severe hypotension, respiratory depression).
No products indexed under this heading.

Quetiapine Fumarate (Profound sedation, coma, severe hypotension, respiratory depression). Products include:
Seroquel Tablets 690

Ramelteon (Profound sedation, coma, severe hypotension, respiratory depression). Products include:
Rozerem Tablets 3231

Rapacuronium Bromide (Increased respiratory depression).
No products indexed under this heading.

Remifentanil Hydrochloride (Profound sedation, coma, severe hypotension, respiratory depression).
No products indexed under this heading.

Risperidone (Profound sedation, coma, severe hypotension, respiratory depression). Products include:
Risperdal 1676
Risperdal Consta Long-Acting Injection 1682
Risperdal M-Tab Orally Disintegrating Tablets 1676

Rocuronium Bromide (Increased respiratory depression). Products include:
Zemuron Injection 2346

Secobarbital Sodium (Profound sedation, coma, severe hypotension, respiratory depression).
No products indexed under this heading.

Sevoflurane (Profound sedation, coma, severe hypotension, respiratory depression). Products include:
Ultane Liquid for Inhalation 531

Sodium Oxybate (Profound sedation, coma, severe hypotension, respiratory depression). Products include:
Xyrem Oral Solution 1688

Succinylcholine Chloride (Increased respiratory depression).
No products indexed under this heading.

Sufentanil Citrate (Profound sedation, coma, severe hypotension, respiratory depression).
No products indexed under this heading.

Temazepam (Profound sedation, coma, severe hypotension, respiratory depression). Products include:
Restoril Capsules 1860

Thiamylal Sodium (Profound sedation, coma, severe hypotension, respiratory depression).
No products indexed under this heading.

Thioridazine Hydrochloride (Profound sedation, coma, severe hypotension, respiratory depression). Products include:
Thioridazine Hydrochloride Tablets 2163

Thiothixene (Profound sedation, coma, severe hypotension, respiratory depression). Products include:
Thiothixene Capsules 2165

Triazolam (Profound sedation, coma, severe hypotension, respiratory depression).
No products indexed under this heading.

Trifluoperazine Hydrochloride (Profound sedation, coma, severe hypotension, respiratory depression).
No products indexed under this heading.

Vecuronium Bromide (Increased respiratory depression).
No products indexed under this heading.

Zaleplon (Profound sedation, coma, severe hypotension, respiratory depression). Products include:
Sonata Capsules 1717

Ziprasidone Hydrochloride (Profound sedation, coma, severe hypotension, respiratory depression). Products include:
Geodon Capsules 2529

Zolpidem Tartrate (Profound sedation, coma, severe hypotension, respiratory depression). Products include:
Ambien Tablets 2851
Ambien CR Tablets 2855

Food Interactions

Alcohol (Respiratory depression, hypotension and profound sedation or coma may result).

MUCINEX EXTENDED-RELEASE BI-LAYER TABLETS

(Guaifenesin) .... ▣720
None cited in PDR database.

MUCINEX D EXTENDED-RELEASE BI-LAYER TABLETS

(Guaifenesin, Pseudoephedrine Hydrochloride) .... ▣776
May interact with monoamine oxidase inhibitors. Compounds in these categories include:

Isocarboxazid (Concurrent and/or sequential use with MAO inhibitors is not recommended).
No products indexed under this heading.

Moclobemide (Concurrent and/or sequential use with MAO inhibitors is not recommended).
No products indexed under this heading.

Pargyline Hydrochloride (Concurrent and/or sequential use with MAO inhibitors is not recommended).
No products indexed under this heading.

Phenelzine Sulfate (Concurrent and/or sequential use with MAO inhibitors is not recommended).
No products indexed under this heading.

Procarbazine Hydrochloride (Concurrent and/or sequential use with MAO inhibitors is not recommended). Products include:
Matulane Capsules 3191

Selegiline Hydrochloride (Concurrent and/or sequential use with MAO inhibitors is not recommended). Products include:
Eldepryl Capsules 3208
Zelapar Tablets 3372

Tranylcypromine Sulfate (Concurrent and/or sequential use with MAO inhibitors is not recommended). Products include:
Parnate Tablets 1527

MUCINEX DM EXTENDED-RELEASE BI-LAYER TABLETS

(Dextromethorphan Hydrobromide, Guaifenesin) .... ▣720
May interact with monoamine oxidase inhibitors. Compounds in these categories include:

Isocarboxazid (Avoid use with, or for two weeks after stopping, MAOI drugs).
No products indexed under this heading.

Moclobemide (Avoid use with, or for two weeks after stopping, MAOI drugs).
No products indexed under this heading.

Pargyline Hydrochloride (Avoid use with, or for two weeks after stopping, MAOI drugs).
No products indexed under this heading.

Phenelzine Sulfate (Avoid use with, or for two weeks after stopping, MAOI drugs).
No products indexed under this heading.

Procarbazine Hydrochloride (Avoid use with, or for two weeks after stopping, MAOI drugs). Products include:
Matulane Capsules 3191

Selegiline Hydrochloride (Avoid use with, or for two weeks after stopping, MAOI drugs). Products include:
Eldepryl Capsules 3208
Zelapar Tablets 3372

Tranylcypromine Sulfate (Avoid use with, or for two weeks after stopping, MAOI drugs). Products include:
Parnate Tablets 1527

MUMPSVAX

(Mumps Virus Vaccine, Live) 2031
May interact with immunosuppressive agents. Compounds in these categories include:

Azathioprine (Concurrent immunosuppressive therapy is contraindicated).
No products indexed under this heading.

Basiliximab (Concurrent immunosuppressive therapy is contraindicated). Products include:
Simulect for Injection 2284

Cyclosporine (Concurrent immunosuppressive therapy is contraindicated). Products include:
Gengraf Capsules 459
Neoral Oral Solution 2259
Neoral Soft Gelatin Capsules 2259
Restasis Ophthalmic Emulsion 575
Sandimmune 2275

Muromonab-CD3 (Concurrent immunosuppressive therapy is contraindicated). Products include:
Orthoclone OKT3 Sterile Solution 2360

Mycophenolate Mofetil (Concurrent immunosuppressive therapy is contraindicated). Products include:
CellCept Capsules 2747
CellCept Oral Suspension 2747
CellCept Tablets 2747

Sirolimus (Concurrent immunosuppressive therapy is contraindicated). Products include:
Rapamune Oral Solution and Tablets 3475

Tacrolimus (Concurrent immunosuppressive therapy is contraindicated). Products include:
Prograf Capsules and Injection 632
Protopic Ointment 638

MURO 128 OPHTHALMIC OINTMENT
(Sodium Chloride) ⊙253
None cited in PDR database.

MURO 128 OPHTHALMIC SOLUTION 2% AND 5%
(Sodium Chloride) ⊙252
None cited in PDR database.

MUSTARGEN FOR INJECTION
(Mechlorethamine Hydrochloride) 2468
May interact with antineoplastics. Compounds in these categories include:

Altretamine (Hematopoiesis may be further compromised in patients who have been previously treated with chemotherapeutic agents).
No products indexed under this heading.

Anastrozole (Hematopoiesis may be further compromised in patients who have been previously treated with chemotherapeutic agents). Products include:
Arimidex Tablets 673

Asparaginase (Hematopoiesis may be further compromised in patients who have been previously treated with chemotherapeutic agents). Products include:
Elspar for Injection 2463
Elspar for Injection 1960

Bicalutamide (Hematopoiesis may be further compromised in patients who have been previously treated with chemotherapeutic agents).
No products indexed under this heading.

Bleomycin Sulfate (Hematopoiesis may be further compromised in patients who have been previously treated with chemotherapeutic agents).
No products indexed under this heading.

Busulfan (Hematopoiesis may be further compromised in patients who have been previously treated with chemotherapeutic agents). Products include:
I.V. Busulfex 2493
Mleran Tablets 1525

Carboplatin (Hematopoiesis may be further compromised in patients who have been previously treated with chemotherapeutic agents).
No products indexed under this heading.

Carmustine (BCNU) (Hematopoiesis may be further compromised in patients who have been previously treated with chemotherapeutic agents).
No products indexed under this heading.

Chlorambucil (Hematopoiesis may be further compromised in patients who have been previously treated with chemotherapeutic agents). Products include:
Leukeran Tablets 1504

Cisplatin (Hematopoiesis may be further compromised in patients who have been previously treated with chemotherapeutic agents).
No products indexed under this heading.

Cyclophosphamide (Hematopoiesis may be further compromised in patients who have been previously treated with chemotherapeutic agents).
No products indexed under this heading.

Dacarbazine (Hematopoiesis may be further compromised in patients who have been previously treated with chemotherapeutic agents).
No products indexed under this heading.

Daunorubicin Citrate (Hematopoiesis may be further compromised in patients who have been previously treated with chemotherapeutic agents).
No products indexed under this heading.

Daunorubicin Hydrochloride (Hematopoiesis may be further compromised in patients who have been previously treated with chemotherapeutic agents).
No products indexed under this heading.

Denileukin Diftitox (Hematopoiesis may be further compromised in patients who have been previously treated with chemotherapeutic agents). Products include:
Ontak Vials 1745

Docetaxel (Hematopoiesis may be further compromised in patients who have been previously treated with chemotherapeutic agents). Products include:
Taxotere Injection Concentrate 2932

Doxorubicin Hydrochloride (Hematopoiesis may be further compromised in patients who have been previously treated with chemotherapeutic agents).
No products indexed under this heading.

Epirubicin Hydrochloride (Hematopoiesis may be further compromised in patients who have been previously treated with chemotherapeutic agents).
No products indexed under this heading.

Estramustine Phosphate Sodium (Hematopoiesis may be further compromised in patients who have been previously treated with chemotherapeutic agents). Products include:
Emcyt Capsules 2634

Etoposide (Hematopoiesis may be further compromised in patients who have been previously treated with chemotherapeutic agents).
No products indexed under this heading.

Exemestane (Hematopoiesis may be further compromised in patients who have been previously treated with chemotherapeutic agents). Products include:
Aromasin Tablets 2600

Floxuridine (Hematopoiesis may be further compromised in patients who have been previously treated with chemotherapeutic agents).
No products indexed under this heading.

Fluorouracil (Hematopoiesis may be further compromised in patients

who have been previously treated with chemotherapeutic agents). Products include:
Carac Cream, 0.5% 2879
Efudex .. 3363

Flutamide (Hematopoiesis may be further compromised in patients who have been previously treated with chemotherapeutic agents). Products include:
Eulexin Capsules 3009

Gemcitabine Hydrochloride (Hematopoiesis may be further compromised in patients who have been previously treated with chemotherapeutic agents). Products include:
Gemzar for Injection 1771

Hydroxyurea (Hematopoiesis may be further compromised in patients who have been previously treated with chemotherapeutic agents).
No products indexed under this heading.

Idarubicin Hydrochloride (Hematopoiesis may be further compromised in patients who have been previously treated with chemotherapeutic agents).
No products indexed under this heading.

Ifosfamide (Hematopoiesis may be further compromised in patients who have been previously treated with chemotherapeutic agents).
No products indexed under this heading.

Interferon alfa-2a, Recombinant (Hematopoiesis may be further compromised in patients who have been previously treated with chemotherapeutic agents).
No products indexed under this heading.

Interferon alfa-2b, Recombinant (Hematopoiesis may be further compromised in patients who have been previously treated with chemotherapeutic agents). Products include:
Intron A for Injection 3024
Rebetron Combination Therapy 3063

Irinotecan Hydrochloride (Hematopoiesis may be further compromised in patients who have been previously treated with chemotherapeutic agents). Products include:
Camptosar Injection 2604

Levamisole Hydrochloride (Hematopoiesis may be further compromised in patients who have been previously treated with chemotherapeutic agents).
No products indexed under this heading.

Lomustine (CCNU) (Hematopoiesis may be further compromised in patients who have been previously treated with chemotherapeutic agents).
No products indexed under this heading.

Megestrol Acetate (Hematopoiesis may be further compromised in patients who have been previously treated with chemotherapeutic agents). Products include:
Megace ES Oral Suspension 2481

Melphalan (Hematopoiesis may be further compromised in patients who have been previously treated with chemotherapeutic agents). Products include:
Alkeran Tablets 956

Mercaptopurine (Hematopoiesis may be further compromised in patients who have been previously treated with chemotherapeutic agents).
No products indexed under this heading.

Methotrexate Sodium (Hematopoiesis may be further compromised in patients who have been previously treated with chemotherapeutic agents).
No products indexed under this heading.

Mitomycin (Mitomycin-C) (Hematopoiesis may be further compromised in patients who have been previously treated with chemotherapeutic agents).
No products indexed under this heading.

Mitotane (Hematopoiesis may be further compromised in patients who have been previously treated with chemotherapeutic agents).
No products indexed under this heading.

Mitoxantrone Hydrochloride (Hematopoiesis may be further compromised in patients who have been previously treated with chemotherapeutic agents).
No products indexed under this heading.

Paclitaxel (Hematopoiesis may be further compromised in patients who have been previously treated with chemotherapeutic agents).
No products indexed under this heading.

Procarbazine Hydrochloride (Hematopoiesis may be further compromised in patients who have been previously treated with chemotherapeutic agents). Products include:
Matulane Capsules 3191

Streptozocin (Hematopoiesis may be further compromised in patients who have been previously treated with chemotherapeutic agents).
No products indexed under this heading.

Tamoxifen Citrate (Hematopoiesis may be further compromised in patients who have been previously treated with chemotherapeutic agents). Products include:
Soltamox Oral Solution 3527

Teniposide (Hematopoiesis may be further compromised in patients who have been previously treated with chemotherapeutic agents).
No products indexed under this heading.

Thioguanine (Hematopoiesis may be further compromised in patients who have been previously treated with chemotherapeutic agents). Products include:
Tabloid Tablets 1575

Thiotepa (Hematopoiesis may be further compromised in patients who have been previously treated with chemotherapeutic agents).
No products indexed under this heading.

Topotecan Hydrochloride (Hematopoiesis may be further compromised in patients who have been previously treated with chemotherapeutic agents). Products include:
Hycamtin for Injection 1458

Toremifene Citrate (Hematopoiesis may be further compromised in patients who have been previously treated with chemotherapeutic agents).
No products indexed under this heading.

Valrubicin (Hematopoiesis may be further compromised in patients who have been previously treated with chemotherapeutic agents).
No products indexed under this heading.

Vincristine Sulfate (Hematopoiesis may be further compromised in patients who have been previously treated with chemotherapeutic agents).
No products indexed under this heading.

Vinorelbine Tartrate (Hematopoiesis may be further compromised in patients who have been previously treated with chemotherapeutic agents).
No products indexed under this heading.

MY FIRST FLINTSTONES MULTIVITAMIN TABLETS

(Vitamins, Multiple) 814
None cited in PDR database.

MYCAMINE FOR INJECTION

(Micafungin Sodium) 628
May interact with:

Nifedipine (Nifedipine AUC and Cmax were increased by 18% and 42% respectively, in the presence of steady state micafungin sodium compared with nifedipine alone. Patients receiving nifedipine in combination with micafungin sodium should be monitored for nifedipine toxicity and nifedipine dosage should be reduced if necessary). Products include:
Adalat CC Tablets 2964

Sirolimus (Sirolimus AUC and Cmax were increased by 18% and 42% respectively, in the presence of steady state micafungin sodium compared with Sirolimus alone. Patients receiving Sirolimus in combination with micafungin sodium should be monitored for Sirolimus toxicity and Sirolimus dosage should be reduced if necessary). Products include:
Rapamune Oral Solution and Tablets 3475

MYFORTIC TABLETS

(Mycophenolic Acid) 2255
May interact with antacids, bacteriostatic antibiotics, bile acid sequestering agents, oral contraceptives, vaccines, live, and certain other agents. Compounds in these categories include:

Acyclovir (May be taken with mycophenolic acid; however, during the period of treatment, physicians should monitor blood cell counts. Both acyclovir and MPAG concentrations are increased in the presence of renal impairment; their coexistence may compete for tubular secretion and further increase in the concentrations of the two). Products include:
Zovirax 1643
Zovirax Cream 820
Zovirax Ointment 821

Acyclovir Sodium (May be taken with mycophenolic acid; however, during the period of treatment, physicians should monitor blood cell counts. Both acyclovir and MPAG concentrations are increased in the presence of renal impairment; their coexistence may compete for tubular secretion and further increase in the concentrations of the two).
No products indexed under this heading.

Aluminum Carbonate (Absorption of a single dose of mycophenolic acid was decreased when administered to stable renal transplant patients also taking magnesium-aluminum containing antacids. Concurrent use with antacids is not recommended).
No products indexed under this heading.

Aluminum Hydroxide (Absorption of a single dose of mycophenolic acid was decreased when administered to stable renal transplant patients also taking magnesium-aluminum containing antacids. Concurrent use with antacids is not recommended). Products include:
Gaviscon Regular Strength Liquid .. 658
Gaviscon Regular Strength Tablets 658
Gaviscon Extra Strength Liquid 658
Gaviscon Extra Strength Tablets 658
Maalox Regular Strength Antacid/Antigas Liquid 2175
Maalox Max Maximum Strength Antacid/Anti-Gas Liquid 2176

Azathioprine (Given that azathioprine inhibits purine metabolism, it is recommended that mycophenolic acid not be administered concomitantly with azathioprine).
No products indexed under this heading.

Azathioprine Sodium (Given that azathioprine inhibits purine metabolism, it is recommended that mycophenolic acid not be administered concomitantly with azathioprine).
No products indexed under this heading.

BCG Vaccine (During treatment with mycophenolic acid, the use of live attenuated vaccines should be avoided and patients should be advised that vaccinations may be less effective. Influenza vaccination may be of value).
No products indexed under this heading.

Charcoal, Activated (Do not administer mycophenolic acid with agents that may interfere with enterohepatic recirculation, or drugs that may bind bile acids, for example, oral activated charcoal, because of the potential to reduce the efficacy of mycophenolic acid).
No products indexed under this heading.

Chloramphenicol (Drugs that alter the gastrointestinal flora may interact with mycophenolic acid by disrupting enterohepatic recirculation. Interference of MPAG hydrolysis may lead to less mycophenolic acid available for absorption).
No products indexed under this heading.

Chloramphenicol Palmitate (Drugs that alter the gastrointestinal flora may interact with mycophenolic acid by disrupting enterohepatic recirculation. Interference of MPAG hydrolysis may lead to less mycophenolic acid available for absorption).
No products indexed under this heading.

Chloramphenicol Sodium Succinate (Drugs that alter the gastrointestinal flora may interact with mycophenolic acid by disrupting enterohepatic recirculation. Interference of MPAG hydrolysis may lead to less mycophenolic acid available for absorption).
No products indexed under this heading.

Cholestyramine (Do not administer mycophenolic acid with agents that may interfere with enterohepatic recirculation, or drugs that may bind bile acids, for example, bile acid sequestrates, because of the potential to reduce the efficacy of mycophenolic acid).
No products indexed under this heading.

Colesevelam Hydrochloride (Do not administer mycophenolic acid with agents that may interfere with enterohepatic recirculation, or drugs that may bind bile acids, for example, bile acid sequestrates, because of the potential to reduce the efficacy of mycophenolic acid). Products include:
WelChol Tablets 1050

Colestipol Hydrochloride (Do not administer mycophenolic acid with agents that may interfere with enterohepatic recirculation, or drugs that may bind bile acids, for example, bile acid sequestrates, because of the potential to reduce the efficacy of mycophenolic acid).
No products indexed under this heading.

Demeclocycline Hydrochloride (Drugs that alter the gastrointestinal flora may interact with mycophenolic acid by disrupting enterohepatic recirculation. Interference of MPAG hydrolysis may lead to less mycophenolic acid available for absorption).
No products indexed under this heading.

Desogestrel (In a drug-drug interaction study, mean levonorgesterol AUC was decreased by 15% when co-administered with mycophenolate mofetil; therefore, it is recommended that oral contraceptives are co-administered with mycophenolic acid with caution, and additional birth control methods be considered). Products include:
Mircette Tablets 1066

Doxycycline Calcium (Drugs that alter the gastrointestinal flora may interact with mycophenolic acid by disrupting enterohepatic recirculation. Interference of MPAG hydrolysis may lead to less mycophenolic acid available for absorption).
No products indexed under this heading.

Doxycycline Hyclate (Drugs that alter the gastrointestinal flora may interact with mycophenolic acid by disrupting enterohepatic recirculation. Interference of MPAG hydrolysis may lead to less mycophenolic acid available for absorption).
No products indexed under this heading.

Doxycycline Monohydrate (Drugs that alter the gastrointestinal flora may interact with mycophenolic acid by disrupting enterohepatic recirculation. Interference of MPAG hydrolysis may lead to less mycophenolic acid available for absorption). Products include:
Oracea Capsules 1000

Erythromycin (Drugs that alter the gastrointestinal flora may interact with mycophenolic acid by disrupting enterohepatic recirculation. Interference of MPAG hydrolysis may lead to less mycophenolic acid available for absorption). Products include:
Ery-Tab Tablets 449
Erythromycin Base Filmtab Tablets 455
Erythromycin Delayed-Release Capsules, USP 457
PCE Dispertab Tablets 515

Erythromycin Estolate (Drugs that alter the gastrointestinal flora may interact with mycophenolic acid by disrupting enterohepatic recirculation. Interference of MPAG hydrolysis may lead to less mycophenolic acid available for absorption).
No products indexed under this heading.

Erythromycin Ethylsuccinate (Drugs that alter the gastrointestinal flora may interact with mycophenolic acid by disrupting enterohepatic recirculation. Interference of MPAG hydrolysis may lead to less mycophenolic acid available for absorption). Products include:
E.E.S. 451
EryPed 447

Erythromycin Gluceptate (Drugs that alter the gastrointestinal flora may interact with mycophenolic acid by disrupting enterohepatic recirculation. Interference of MPAG hydrolysis may lead to less mycophenolic acid available for absorption).
No products indexed under this heading.

Erythromycin Stearate (Drugs that alter the gastrointestinal flora may interact with mycophenolic acid by disrupting enterohepatic recirculation. Interference of MPAG hydrolysis may lead to less mycophenolic acid available for absorption). Products include:
Erythrocin Stearate Filmtab Tablets 453

Ethinyl Estradiol (In a drug-drug interaction study, mean levonorgesterol AUC was decreased by 15% when co-administered with mycophenolate mofetil; therefore, it is recommended that oral contraceptives are co-administered with mycophenolic acid with caution, and additional birth control methods be considered). Products include:
Mircette Tablets 1066
NuvaRing 2340
Ortho-Cyclen/Ortho Tri-Cyclen 2429
Ortho Evra Transdermal System 2417
Ortho Tri-Cyclen Lo Tablets 2436
Seasonique Tablets 1077
Yasmin 28 Tablets 796
Yaz Tablets 803

Ethynodiol Diacetate (In a drug-drug interaction study, mean levonorgesterol AUC was decreased by 15% when co-administered with mycophenolate mofetil; therefore, it is recommended that oral contraceptives are co-administered with mycophenolic acid with caution, and additional birth control methods be considered).
No products indexed under this heading.

Ganciclovir (May be taken with mycophenolic acid; however, during the period of treatment, physicians should monitor blood cell counts. Both ganciclovir and MPAG concentrations are increased in the presence of renal impairment; their coexistence may compete for tubular secretion and further increase in the concentrations of the two).
No products indexed under this heading.

Ganciclovir Sodium (May be taken with mycophenolic acid; however, during the period of treatment, physicians should monitor blood cell counts. Both ganciclovir and MPAG concentrations are increased in the presence of renal impairment; their coexistence may compete for tubular secretion and further increase in the concentrations of the two).
No products indexed under this heading.

Levonorgestrel (In a drug-drug interaction study, mean levonorgesterol AUC was decreased by 15% when co-administered with mycophenolate mofetil; therefore, it is recommended that oral contraceptives are co-administered with mycophenolic acid with caution, and additional birth control methods be considered). Products include:
Climara Pro Transdermal System 776
Mirena Intrauterine System 787
Plan B Tablets 1076
Seasonique Tablets 1077

Magaldrate (Absorption of a single dose of mycophenolic acid was decreased when administered to stable renal transplant patients also taking magnesium-aluminum containing antacids. Concurrent use with antacids is not recommended).
No products indexed under this heading.

Magnesium Hydroxide (Absorption of a single dose of mycophenolic acid was decreased when administered to stable renal transplant patients also taking magnesium-aluminum containing antacids. Concurrent use with antacids is not recommended). Products include:
Maalox Regular Strength Antacid/Antigas Liquid................. 2175
Maalox Max Maximum Strength Antacid/Anti-Gas Liquid................ 2176
Pepcid Complete Chewable Tablets 1701

Magnesium Oxide (Absorption of a single dose of mycophenolic acid was decreased when administered to stable renal transplant patients also taking magnesium-aluminum containing antacids. Concurrent use with antacids is not recommended). Products include:
Beelith Tablets 759
PremCal Light, Regular, and Extra Strength Tablets................ ▣818

Measles, Mumps, Rubella and Varicella Virus Vaccine Live (During treatment with mycophenolic acid, the use of live attenuated vaccines should be avoided and patients should be advised that vaccinations may be less effective. Influenza vaccination may be of value). Products include:
ProQuad 2064

Measles, Mumps & Rubella Virus Vaccine, Live (During treatment with mycophenolic acid, the use of live attenuated vaccines should be avoided and patients should be advised that vaccinations may be less effective. Influenza vaccination may be of value). Products include:
M-M-R II 2006

Measles & Rubella Virus Vaccine Live (During treatment with mycophenolic acid, the use of live attenuated vaccines should be avoided and patients should be advised that vaccinations may be less effective. Influenza vaccination may be of value).
No products indexed under this heading.

Measles Virus Vaccine Live (During treatment with mycophenolic acid, the use of live attenuated vaccines should be avoided and patients should be advised that vaccinations may be less effective. Influenza vaccination may be of value). Products include:
Attenuvax 1914

Mestranol (In a drug-drug interaction study, mean levonorgesterol AUC was decreased by 15% when co-administered with mycophenolate mofetil; therefore, it is recommended that oral contraceptives are co-administered with mycophenolic acid with caution, and additional birth control methods be considered).
No products indexed under this heading.

Methacycline Hydrochloride (Drugs that alter the gastrointestinal flora may interact with mycophenolic acid by disrupting enterohepatic recirculation. Interference of MPAG hydrolysis may lead to less mycophenolic acid available for absorption).
No products indexed under this heading.

Minocycline Hydrochloride (Drugs that alter the gastrointestinal flora may interact with mycophenolic acid by disrupting enterohepatic recirculation. Interference of MPAG hydrolysis may lead to less mycophenolic acid available for absorption). Products include:
Solodyn Extended Release Tablets 1890

Mumps Virus Vaccine, Live (During treatment with mycophenolic acid, the use of live attenuated vaccines should be avoided and patients should be advised that vaccinations may be less effective. Influenza vaccination may be of value). Products include:
Mumpsvax 2031

Mycophenolate Mofetil (Given that mycophenolate mofetil inhibits purine metabolism, it is recommended that mycophenolic acid not be administered concomitantly with mycophenolate mofetil). Products include:
CellCept Capsules 2747
CellCept Oral Suspension 2747
CellCept Tablets 2747

Mycophenolate Mofetil Hydrochloride (Given that mycophenolate mofetil inhibits purine metabolism, it is recommended that mycophenolic acid not be administered concomitantly with mycophenolate mofetil). Products include:
CellCept Intravenous 2747

Norethindrone (In a drug-drug interaction study, mean levonorgesterol AUC was decreased by 15% when co-administered with mycophenolate mofetil; therefore, it is recommended that oral contraceptives are co-administered with mycophenolic acid with caution, and additional birth control methods be considered). Products include:
Ortho Micronor Tablets 2426

Norethynodrel (In a drug-drug interaction study, mean levonorgesterol AUC was decreased by 15% when co-administered with mycophenolate mofetil; therefore, it is recommended that oral contraceptives are co-administered with mycophenolic acid with caution, and additional birth control methods be considered).
No products indexed under this heading.

Norgestimate (In a drug-drug interaction study, mean levonorgesterol AUC was decreased by 15% when co-administered with mycophenolate mofetil; therefore, it is recommended that oral contraceptives are co-administered with mycophenolic acid with caution, and additional birth control methods be considered). Products include:
Ortho-Cyclen/Ortho Tri-Cyclen 2429
Ortho Tri-Cyclen Lo Tablets 2436

Norgestrel (In a drug-drug interaction study, mean levonorgesterol AUC was decreased by 15% when co-administered with mycophenolate mofetil; therefore, it is recommended that oral contraceptives are co-administered with mycophenolic acid with caution, and additional birth control methods be considered).
No products indexed under this heading.

Oxytetracycline Hydrochloride (Drugs that alter the gastrointestinal flora may interact with mycophenolic acid by disrupting enterohepatic recirculation. Interference of MPAG hydrolysis may lead to less mycophenolic acid available for absorption).
No products indexed under this heading.

Poliovirus Vaccine, Live, Oral, Trivalent, Types 1,2,3 (Sabin) (During treatment with mycophenolic acid, the use of live attenuated vaccines should be avoided and patients should be advised that vaccinations may be less effective. Influenza vaccination may be of value).
No products indexed under this heading.

Rotavirus Vaccine, Live, Oral, Tetravalent (During treatment with mycophenolic acid, the use of live attenuated vaccines should be avoided and patients should be advised that vaccinations may be less effective. Influenza vaccination may be of value).
No products indexed under this heading.

Rubella & Mumps Virus Vaccine Live (During treatment with mycophenolic acid, the use of live attenuated vaccines should be avoided and patients should be advised that vaccinations may be less effective. Influenza vaccination may be of value).
No products indexed under this heading.

Rubella Virus Vaccine Live (During treatment with mycophenolic acid, the use of live attenuated vaccines should be avoided and patients should be advised that vaccinations may be less effective. Influenza vaccination may be of value). Products include:
Meruvax II 2019

Smallpox Vaccine (During treatment with mycophenolic acid, the use of live attenuated vaccines should be avoided and patients should be advised that vaccinations may be less effective. Influenza vaccination may be of value).
No products indexed under this heading.

Sodium Bicarbonate (Absorption of a single dose of mycophenolic acid was decreased when administered to stable renal transplant patients also taking magnesium-aluminum containing antacids. Concurrent use with antacids is not recommended). Products include:
Colyte with Flavor Packs for Oral Solution.. 3088
HalfLytely and Bisacodyl Tablets Bowel Prep Kit with Flavors Packs.. 881
TriLyte with Flavor Packs for Oral Solution.. 3100

Sulfamethizole (Drugs that alter the gastrointestinal flora may interact with mycophenolic acid by disrupting enterohepatic recirculation. Interference of MPAG hydrolysis may lead to less mycophenolic acid available for absorption).
No products indexed under this heading.

Sulfamethoxazole (Drugs that alter the gastrointestinal flora may interact with mycophenolic acid by disrupting enterohepatic recirculation. Interference of MPAG hydrolysis may lead to less mycophenolic acid available for absorption).
No products indexed under this heading.

Sulfisoxazole Acetyl (Drugs that alter the gastrointestinal flora may interact with mycophenolic acid by disrupting enterohepatic recirculation. Interference of MPAG hydrolysis may lead to less mycophenolic acid available for absorption).
No products indexed under this heading.

Tetracycline Hydrochloride (Drugs that alter the gastrointestinal flora may interact with mycophenolic acid by disrupting enterohepatic recirculation. Interference of MPAG hydrolysis may lead to less mycophenolic acid available for absorption).
No products indexed under this heading.

Typhoid Vaccine (During treatment with mycophenolic acid, the use of live attenuated vaccines should be avoided and patients should be advised that vaccinations may be less effective. Influenza vaccination may be of value).
No products indexed under this heading.

Varicella Virus Vaccine Live (During treatment with mycophenolic acid, the use of live attenuated vaccines should be avoided and patients should be advised that vaccinations may be less effective. Influenza vaccination may be of value). Products include:
Varivax 2100

Yellow Fever Vaccine (During treatment with mycophenolic acid, the use of live attenuated vaccines should be avoided and patients should be advised that vaccinations may be less effective. Influenza vaccination may be of value).
No products indexed under this heading.

MYLERAN TABLETS

(Busulfan) 1525
May interact with antineoplastics, cytotoxic drugs, agents associated with myelosuppression, and certain other agents. Compounds in these categories include:

Altretamine (Potential for rare life-threatening hepatic veno-occlusive disease).
No products indexed under this heading.

Anastrozole (Potential for rare life-threatening hepatic veno-occlusive disease). Products include:
Arimidex Tablets 673

Asparaginase (Potential for rare life-threatening hepatic veno-occlusive disease). Products include:
Elspar for Injection 2463
Elspar for Injection 1960

Bicalutamide (Potential for rare life-threatening hepatic veno-occlusive disease).
No products indexed under this heading.

Bleomycin Sulfate (Busulfan-induced pulmonary toxicity may be additive to the effects produced by other cytotoxic agents).
No products indexed under this heading.

Bone Marrow Depressants, unspecified (Additive myelosuppression).
No products indexed under this heading.

Carboplatin (Potential for rare life-threatening hepatic veno-occlusive disease).
No products indexed under this heading.

Carmustine (BCNU) (Potential for rare life-threatening hepatic veno-occlusive disease).
No products indexed under this heading.

Chlorambucil (Potential for rare life-threatening hepatic veno-occlusive disease). Products include:
Leukeran Tablets 1504

Cisplatin (Potential for rare life-threatening hepatic veno-occlusive disease).
No products indexed under this heading.

Cladribine (Busulfan may cause additive myelosuppression when used with other myelosuppressive drugs). Products include:
Leustatin Injection 2357

Cyclophosphamide (Potential for rare life-threatening hepatic veno-occlusive disease; potential for cardiac temponade; co-administration may result in reduced busulfan clearance).
No products indexed under this heading.

Dacarbazine (Potential for rare life-threatening hepatic veno-occlusive disease).
No products indexed under this heading.

Daunorubicin Citrate (Potential for rare life-threatening hepatic veno-occlusive disease).
No products indexed under this heading.

Daunorubicin Citrate Liposome (Busulfan may cause additive myelosuppression when used with other myelosuppressive drugs).
No products indexed under this heading.

Daunorubicin Hydrochloride (Busulfan-induced pulmonary toxicity may be additive to the effects produced by other cytotoxic agents).
No products indexed under this heading.

Denileukin Diftitox (Potential for rare life-threatening hepatic veno-occlusive disease). Products include:
Ontak Vials 1745

Dexrazoxane (Busulfan may cause additive myelosuppression when used with other myelosuppressive drugs). Products include:
Zinecard for Injection 2650

Docetaxel (Potential for rare life-threatening hepatic veno-occlusive disease). Products include:
Taxotere Injection Concentrate 2932

Doxorubicin Hydrochloride (Busulfan-induced pulmonary toxicity may be additive to the effects produced by other cytotoxic agents).
No products indexed under this heading.

Doxorubicin Hydrochloride Liposome (Busulfan may cause additive myelosuppression when used with other myelosuppressive drugs). Products include:
Doxil Injection 2351

Epirubicin Hydrochloride (Busulfan-induced pulmonary toxicity may be additive to the effects produced by other cytotoxic agents).
No products indexed under this heading.

Estramustine Phosphate Sodium (Potential for rare life-threatening hepatic veno-occlusive disease). Products include:
Emcyt Capsules 2634

Etoposide (Potential for rare life-threatening hepatic veno-occlusive disease).
No products indexed under this heading.

Exemestane (Potential for rare life-threatening hepatic veno-occlusive disease). Products include:
Aromasin Tablets 2600

Floxuridine (Potential for rare life-threatening hepatic veno-occlusive disease).
No products indexed under this heading.

Fludarabine Phosphate (Busulfan may cause additive myelosuppression when used with other myelosuppressive drugs).
No products indexed under this heading.

Fluorouracil (Busulfan-induced pulmonary toxicity may be additive to the effects produced by other cytotoxic agents). Products include:
Carac Cream, 0.5% 2879
Efudex 3363

Flutamide (Potential for rare life-threatening hepatic veno-occlusive disease). Products include:
Eulexin Capsules 3009

Gemcitabine Hydrochloride (Potential for rare life-threatening hepatic veno-occlusive disease). Products include:
Gemzar for Injection 1771

Gemtuzumab Ozogamicin (Busulfan may cause additive myelosuppression when used with other myelosuppressive drugs). Products include:
Mylotarg for Injection 3431

Hydroxyurea (Busulfan-induced pulmonary toxicity may be additive to the effects produced by other cytotoxic agents).
No products indexed under this heading.

Idarubicin Hydrochloride (Potential for rare life-threatening hepatic veno-occlusive disease).
No products indexed under this heading.

Ifosfamide (Potential for rare life-threatening hepatic veno-occlusive disease).
No products indexed under this heading.

Interferon alfa-2a, Recombinant (Potential for rare life-threatening hepatic veno-occlusive disease).
No products indexed under this heading.

Interferon alfa-2b, Recombinant (Potential for rare life-threatening hepatic veno-occlusive disease). Products include:
Intron A for Injection 3024
Rebetron Combination Therapy 3063

Irinotecan Hydrochloride (Potential for rare life-threatening hepatic veno-occlusive disease). Products include:
Camptosar Injection 2604

Itraconazole (The concomitant systemic administration of itraconazole to patients receiving high-dose busulfan may result in reduced busulfan clearance. Patients should be monitored for signs of busulfan toxicity when itraconazole is used concomitantly with busulfan).
No products indexed under this heading.

Levamisole Hydrochloride (Potential for rare life-threatening hepatic veno-occlusive disease).
No products indexed under this heading.

Lomustine (CCNU) (Potential for rare life-threatening hepatic veno-occlusive disease).
No products indexed under this heading.

Mechlorethamine Hydrochloride (Potential for rare life-threatening hepatic veno-occlusive disease). Products include:
Mustargen for Injection 2468

Megestrol Acetate (Potential for rare life-threatening hepatic veno-occlusive disease). Products include:
Megace ES Oral Suspension 2481

Melphalan (Potential for rare life-threatening hepatic veno-occlusive disease). Products include:
Alkeran Tablets 956

Melphalan Hydrochloride (Busulfan may cause additive myelosuppression when used with other myelosuppressive drugs). Products include:
Alkeran for Injection 955

Mercaptopurine (Potential for rare life-threatening hepatic veno-occlusive disease).
No products indexed under this heading.

Methotrexate Sodium (Busulfan-induced pulmonary toxicity may be additive to the effects produced by other cytotoxic agents).
No products indexed under this heading.

Metronidazole (The concomitant administration of metronidazole and high-dose busulfan may result in increased trough levels of busulfan and, therefore, it is not recommended). Products include:
Metrogel 1% 1211
MetroGel-Vaginal Gel 1855
Vandazole Vaginal Gel 3338

Metronidazole Benzoate (The concomitant administration of metronidazole and high-dose busulfan may result in increased trough levels of busulfan and, therefore, it is not recommended).
No products indexed under this heading.

Metronidazole Hydrochloride (The concomitant administration of metronidazole and high-dose busulfan may result in increased trough levels of busulfan and, therefore, it is not recommended).
No products indexed under this heading.

Metronidazole Sodium (The concomitant administration of metronidazole and high-dose busulfan may result in increased trough levels of busulfan and, therefore, it is not recommended).
No products indexed under this heading.

Mitomycin (Mitomycin-C) (Potential for rare life-threatening hepatic veno-occlusive disease).
No products indexed under this heading.

Mitotane (Busulfan-induced pulmonary toxicity may be additive to the effects produced by other cytotoxic agents).
No products indexed under this heading.

Mitoxantrone Hydrochloride (Busulfan-induced pulmonary toxicity may be additive to the effects produced by other cytotoxic agents).
No products indexed under this heading.

Oxaliplatin (Potential for rare life-threatening hepatic veno-occlusive disease). Products include:
Eloxatin for Injection 2892

Paclitaxel (Potential for rare life-threatening hepatic veno-occlusive disease).
No products indexed under this heading.

Procarbazine Hydrochloride (Busulfan-induced pulmonary toxicity may be additive to the effects produced by other cytotoxic agents). Products include:
Matulane Capsules 3191

Streptozocin (Potential for rare life-threatening hepatic veno-occlusive disease).
No products indexed under this heading.

Tamoxifen Citrate (Busulfan-induced pulmonary toxicity may be additive to the effects produced by other cytotoxic agents). Products include:

Busulfan (Potential for drug-drug interaction with drugs affected by CYP450 enzymes). Products include:
- I.V. Busulfex 2493
- Myleran Tablets 1525

Caffeine (Potential for drug-drug interaction with drugs affected by CYP450 enzymes). Products include:
- BC Headache Powder 677
- Arthritis Strength BC Powder 677
- Excedrin Extra Strength Caplets/Tablets/Geltabs 684
- Excedrin Migraine Caplets/Tablets/Geltabs 609
- Excedrin Tension Headache Caplets/Tablets/Geltabs 611
- Goody's Extra Strength Headache Powders 611
- Goody's Extra Strength Pain Relief Tablets 685
- Vivarin 602
- Winrgy Dietary Supplement 823

Caffeine Anhydrous (Potential for drug-drug interaction with drugs affected by CYP450 enzymes).
No products indexed under this heading.

Caffeine Citrate (Potential for drug-drug interaction with drugs affected by CYP450 enzymes). Products include:
- Cafcit 1886

Candesartan Cilexetil (Potential for drug-drug interaction with drugs affected by CYP450 enzymes). Products include:
- Atacand Tablets 649
- Atacand HCT 651

Captopril (Potential for drug-drug interaction with drugs affected by CYP450 enzymes). Products include:
- Captopril Tablets 2149

Carbamazepine (Potential for drug-drug interaction with drugs affected by CYP450 enzymes). Products include:
- Carbatrol Capsules 3171
- Equetro Extended-Release Capsules 3180
- Tegretol/Tegretol-XR 2295

Carisoprodol (Potential for drug-drug interaction with drugs affected by CYP450 enzymes).
No products indexed under this heading.

Carvedilol (Potential for drug-drug interaction with drugs affected by CYP450 enzymes). Products include:
- Coreg Tablets 1414

Celecoxib (Potential for drug-drug interaction with drugs affected by CYP450 enzymes). Products include:
- Celebrex Capsules 3134

Cerivastatin Sodium (Potential for drug-drug interaction with drugs affected by CYP450 enzymes).
No products indexed under this heading.

Cevimeline Hydrochloride (Potential for drug-drug interaction with drugs affected by CYP450 enzymes). Products include:
- Evoxac Capsules 1047

Chlordiazepoxide (Potential for drug-drug interaction with drugs affected by CYP450 enzymes).
No products indexed under this heading.

Chlordiazepoxide Hydrochloride (Potential for drug-drug interaction with drugs affected by CYP450 enzymes). Products include:
- Librium Capsules 3347

Chlorpheniramine (Potential for drug-drug interaction with drugs affected by CYP450 enzymes).
No products indexed under this heading.

Chlorpheniramine Maleate (Potential for drug-drug interaction with drugs affected by CYP450 enzymes). Products include:
- Advil Allergy Sinus Caplets 770
- Advil Multi-Symptom Cold Caplets 770
- BC Allergy Sinus Cold Powder 677
- Comtrex Maximum Strength Cold & Cough Day/Night Caplets - Night Formulation 726
- Comtrex Maximum Strength Day/Night Severe Cold & Sinus Caplets - Night Formulation 725
- Contac Cold and Flu Maximum Strength Caplets 728
- Contac Cold and Flu Day and Night Caplets (Night Formulation Only) 727
- Children's Dimetapp Long Acting Cough Plus Cold Syrup 731
- Robitussin Cough & Cold Long-Acting Liquid 735
- Robitussin Cough & Allergy Syrup 736
- Robitussin Cough & Cold Nighttime Liquid 736
- Robitussin Cough, Cold & Flu Nighttime Liquid 738
- Robitussin Pediatric Cough & Cold Long-Acting Liquid 735
- Robitussin Pediatric Cough & Cold Nighttime Liquid 736
- Triaminic Cold & Allergy Liquid 746
- Triaminic Cough & Runny Nose Softchews 748
- Children's Tylenol Plus Flu Oral Suspension 749
- Tylenol Allergy Multi-Symptom Caplets with Cool Burst and Gelcaps 1872
- Children's Tylenol Plus Cold Suspension Liquid 1879
- Children's Tylenol Plus Cough & Runny Nose Suspension Liquid 1879
- Children's Tylenol Plus Flu Suspension Liquid 1881
- Children's Tylenol Plus Multi-Symptom Cold Suspension Liquid 1879
- Tylenol Cold Head Congestion Nighttime Caplets with Cool Burst 1873
- Tylenol Cold Multi-Symptom Nighttime Caplets with Cool Burst 1874
- Tylenol Sinus Congestion & Pain Nighttime Caplets with Cool Burst 1876
- Vicks 44M Cough, Cold & Flu Relief Liquid 2680
- Pediatric Vicks 44m Cough & Cold Relief Liquid 2676
- Children's Vicks NyQuil Cold/Cough Relief 756
- Children's Vicks NyQuil Cold/Cough Relief Liquid 2680
- Zicam Maximum Strength Flu Daytime 768

Chlorpheniramine Polistirex (Potential for drug-drug interaction with drugs affected by CYP450 enzymes). Products include:
- Tussionex Pennkinetic Extended-Release Suspension 3327

Chlorpheniramine Tannate (Potential for drug-drug interaction with drugs affected by CYP450 enzymes).
No products indexed under this heading.

Chlorpromazine (Potential for drug-drug interaction with drugs affected by CYP450 enzymes).
No products indexed under this heading.

Chlorpromazine Hydrochloride (Potential for drug-drug interaction with drugs affected by CYP450 enzymes).
No products indexed under this heading.

Chlorpropamide (Potential for drug-drug interaction with drugs affected by CYP450 enzymes).
No products indexed under this heading.

Cilostazol (Potential for drug-drug interaction with drugs affected by CYP450 enzymes). Products include:
- Pletal Tablets 2455

Cimetidine Hydrochloride (Potential for drug-drug interaction with drugs affected by CYP450 enzymes).
No products indexed under this heading.

Ciprofloxacin (Potential for drug-drug interaction with drugs affected by CYP450 enzymes). Products include:
- Cipro Oral Suspension 2977
- Cipro I.V. 2984
- Cipro XR Tablets 2990
- Ciprodex Otic Suspension 559

Ciprofloxacin Hydrochloride (Potential for drug-drug interaction with drugs affected by CYP450 enzymes). Products include:
- Ciloxan Ophthalmic Ointment 559
- Ciloxan Ophthalmic Solution 206
- Cipro Tablets 2977
- Proquin XR Tablets 1153

Cisapride (Potential for drug-drug interaction with drugs affected by CYP450 enzymes).
No products indexed under this heading.

Citalopram Hydrobromide (Potential for drug-drug interaction with drugs affected by CYP450 enzymes). Products include:
- Celexa 1176

Clarithromycin (Potential for drug-drug interaction with drugs affected by CYP450 enzymes). Products include:
- Biaxin/Biaxin XL 402
- PREVPAC 3284

Clomipramine Hydrochloride (Potential for drug-drug interaction with drugs affected by CYP450 enzymes).
No products indexed under this heading.

Clopidogrel Hydrogen Sulfate (Potential for drug-drug interaction with drugs affected by CYP450 enzymes).
No products indexed under this heading.

Clozapine (Potential for drug-drug interaction with drugs affected by CYP450 enzymes). Products include:
- Clozaril Tablets 2184
- FazaClo Orally Disintegrating Tablets 551

Codeine Phosphate (Potential for drug-drug interaction with drugs affected by CYP450 enzymes). Products include:
- Tylenol with Codeine Tablets 2391

Codeine Sulfate (Potential for drug-drug interaction with drugs affected by CYP450 enzymes).
No products indexed under this heading.

Cyclobenzaprine (Potential for drug-drug interaction with drugs affected by CYP450 enzymes).
No products indexed under this heading.

Cyclobenzaprine Hydrochloride (Potential for drug-drug interaction with drugs affected by CYP450 enzymes).
No products indexed under this heading.

Cyclophosphamide (Potential for drug-drug interaction with drugs affected by CYP450 enzymes).
No products indexed under this heading.

Cyclosporine (Potential for drug-drug interaction with drugs affected by CYP450 enzymes). Products include:
- Gengraf Capsules 459
- Neoral Oral Solution 2259
- Neoral Soft Gelatin Capsules 2259
- Restasis Ophthalmic Emulsion 575
- Sandimmune 2275

Desipramine Hydrochloride (Potential for drug-drug interaction with drugs affected by CYP450 enzymes).
No products indexed under this heading.

Desogestrel (Potential for drug-drug interaction with drugs affected by CYP450 enzymes). Products include:
- Mircette Tablets 1066

Dexamethasone (Potential for drug-drug interaction with drugs affected by CYP450 enzymes). Products include:
- Ciprodex Otic Suspension 559
- Decadron Tablets 1951
- TobraDex Ophthalmic Ointment 562
- TobraDex Ophthalmic Suspension 563

Dexamethasone Acetate (Potential for drug-drug interaction with drugs affected by CYP450 enzymes).
No products indexed under this heading.

Dexamethasone Phosphate (Potential for drug-drug interaction with drugs affected by CYP450 enzymes).
No products indexed under this heading.

Dexamethasone Sodium (Potential for drug-drug interaction with drugs affected by CYP450 enzymes).
No products indexed under this heading.

Dexamethasone Sodium Phosphate (Potential for drug-drug interaction with drugs affected by CYP450 enzymes).
No products indexed under this heading.

Dexfenfluramine Hydrochloride (Potential for drug-drug interaction with drugs affected by CYP450 enzymes).
No products indexed under this heading.

Dextromethorphan (Potential for drug-drug interaction with drugs affected by CYP450 enzymes).
No products indexed under this heading.

Dextromethorphan Hydrobromide (Potential for drug-drug interaction with drugs affected by CYP450 enzymes). Products include:

IMPORTANT NOTE: Always consult each drug listing in the patient's regimen for possible interactions.

Premarin Vaginal Cream 3452
Premphase Tablets 3456
Prempro Tablets 3456

Estrogens, Conjugated, Synthetic A (Potential for drug-drug interaction with drugs affected by CYP450 enzymes).
No products indexed under this heading.

Estrogens, Esterified (Potential for drug-drug interaction with drugs affected by CYP450 enzymes). Products include:
Estratest Tablets 3199
Estratest H.S. Tablets 3199

Ethinyl Estradiol (Potential for drug-drug interaction with drugs affected by CYP450 enzymes). Products include:
Mircette Tablets 1066
NuvaRing 2340
Ortho-Cyclen/Ortho Tri-Cyclen 2429
Ortho Evra Transdermal System 2417
Ortho Tri-Cyclen Lo Tablets 2436
Seasonique Tablets 1077
Yasmin 28 Tablets 796
Yaz Tablets 803

Ethosuximide (Potential for drug-drug interaction with drugs affected by CYP450 enzymes).
No products indexed under this heading.

Ethotoin (Potential for drug-drug interaction with drugs affected by CYP450 enzymes).
No products indexed under this heading.

Ethynodiol Diacetate (Potential for drug-drug interaction with drugs affected by CYP450 enzymes).
No products indexed under this heading.

Etodolac (Potential for drug-drug interaction with drugs affected by CYP450 enzymes).
No products indexed under this heading.

Etoposide (Potential for drug-drug interaction with drugs affected by CYP450 enzymes).
No products indexed under this heading.

Etoposide Phosphate (Potential for drug-drug interaction with drugs affected by CYP450 enzymes).
No products indexed under this heading.

Felbamate (Potential for drug-drug interaction with drugs affected by CYP450 enzymes).
No products indexed under this heading.

Felodipine (Potential for drug-drug interaction with drugs affected by CYP450 enzymes).
No products indexed under this heading.

Fenoprofen Calcium (Potential for drug-drug interaction with drugs affected by CYP450 enzymes). Products include:
Nalfon Capsules 2502

Fentanyl (Potential for drug-drug interaction with drugs affected by CYP450 enzymes). Products include:
Duragesic Transdermal System 2373
Ionsys Transdermal System 2379

Fentanyl Citrate (Potential for drug-drug interaction with drugs affected by CYP450 enzymes). Products include:
Actiq 979

Flecainide Acetate (Potential for drug-drug interaction with drugs affected by CYP450 enzymes). Products include:
Tambocor Tablets 1856

Fluoxetine (Potential for drug-drug interaction with drugs affected by CYP450 enzymes).
No products indexed under this heading.

Fluoxetine Hydrochloride (Potential for drug-drug interaction with drugs affected by CYP450 enzymes). Products include:
Prozac Pulvules and Liquid 1801
Symbyax Capsules 1819

Fluphenazine Decanoate (Potential for drug-drug interaction with drugs affected by CYP450 enzymes).
No products indexed under this heading.

Fluphenazine Enanthate (Potential for drug-drug interaction with drugs affected by CYP450 enzymes).
No products indexed under this heading.

Fluphenazine Hydrochloride (Potential for drug-drug interaction with drugs affected by CYP450 enzymes).
No products indexed under this heading.

Flurbiprofen (Potential for drug-drug interaction with drugs affected by CYP450 enzymes).
No products indexed under this heading.

Flurbiprofen Sodium (Potential for drug-drug interaction with drugs affected by CYP450 enzymes). Products include:
Ocufen Ophthalmic Solution .... ⊙232

Flutamide (Potential for drug-drug interaction with drugs affected by CYP450 enzymes). Products include:
Eulexin Capsules 3009

Fluticasone Propionate (Potential for drug-drug interaction with drugs affected by CYP450 enzymes). Products include:
Advair Diskus 100/50 1308
Advair Diskus 250/50 1308
Advair Diskus 500/50 1308
Advair HFA Inhalation Aerosol 1318
Cutivate Cream 2662
Cutivate Lotion 0.05% 2664
Cutivate Ointment 2665
Flonase Nasal Spray 1440
Flovent Diskus 1443

Fluvastatin Sodium (Potential for drug-drug interaction with drugs affected by CYP450 enzymes). Products include:
Lescol Capsules 2233
Lescol XL Tablets 2233

Fluvoxamine Maleate (Potential for drug-drug interaction with drugs affected by CYP450 enzymes).
No products indexed under this heading.

Formoterol Fumarate (Potential for drug-drug interaction with drugs affected by CYP450 enzymes). Products include:
Foradil Aerolizer 3010

Fosphenytoin (Potential for drug-drug interaction with drugs affected by CYP450 enzymes).
No products indexed under this heading.

Fosphenytoin Sodium (Potential for drug-drug interaction with drugs affected by CYP450 enzymes).
No products indexed under this heading.

Gabapentin (Potential for drug-drug interaction with drugs affected by CYP450 enzymes). Products include:
Neurontin Capsules 2487
Neurontin Oral Solution 2487
Neurontin Tablets 2487

Galantamine Hydrobromide (Potential for drug-drug interaction with drugs affected by CYP450 enzymes). Products include:
Razadyne 2399
Razadyne ER Extended-Release Capsules 2399

Glimepiride (Potential for drug-drug interaction with drugs affected by CYP450 enzymes). Products include:
Avandaryl Tablets 1379
Duetact Tablets 3226

Glipizide (Potential for drug-drug interaction with drugs affected by CYP450 enzymes).
No products indexed under this heading.

Glyburide (Potential for drug-drug interaction with drugs affected by CYP450 enzymes).
No products indexed under this heading.

Grepafloxacin Hydrochloride (Potential for drug-drug interaction with drugs affected by CYP450 enzymes).
No products indexed under this heading.

Haloperidol (Potential for drug-drug interaction with drugs affected by CYP450 enzymes).
No products indexed under this heading.

Haloperidol Decanoate (Potential for drug-drug interaction with drugs affected by CYP450 enzymes).
No products indexed under this heading.

Haloperidol Lactate (Potential for drug-drug interaction with drugs affected by CYP450 enzymes).
No products indexed under this heading.

Hydrocodone Bitartrate (Potential for drug-drug interaction with drugs affected by CYP450 enzymes). Products include:
Hycodan 1116
Hycotuss Expectorant Syrup 1117
Vicodin Tablets 535
Vicodin ES Tablets 536
Vicodin HP Tablets 538
Vicoprofen Tablets 539
Zydone Tablets 1139

Ibuprofen (Potential for drug-drug interaction with drugs affected by CYP450 enzymes). Products include:
Advil Allergy Sinus Caplets 770
Advil 674
Children's Advil Oral Suspension 603
Children's Advil Chewable Tablets 603
Advil Cold & Sinus 723
Infants' Advil Concentrated Drops 604
Infants' Advil Concentrated Drops - White Grape (Dye-Free) 604
Junior Strength Advil Swallow Tablets 605
Advil Migraine Liquigels 608
Advil Multi-Symptom Cold Caplets 770
Advil PM Caplets 615
Motrin IB Tablets and Caplets 1866
Children's Motrin Oral Suspension 1867
Children's Motrin Non-Staining Dye-Free Oral Suspension 1867
Children's Motrin Cold Oral Suspension 1867
Infants' Motrin Concentrated Drops 1867
Infants' Motrin Non-Staining Dye-Free Concentrated Drops 1867
Junior Strength Motrin Caplets and Chewable Tablets 1867
Vicoprofen Tablets 539

Imipramine Hydrochloride (Potential for drug-drug interaction with drugs affected by CYP450 enzymes).
No products indexed under this heading.

Imipramine Pamoate (Potential for drug-drug interaction with drugs affected by CYP450 enzymes).
No products indexed under this heading.

Indinavir Sulfate (Potential for drug-drug interaction with drugs affected by CYP450 enzymes). Products include:
Crixivan Capsules 1940

Indomethacin (Potential for drug-drug interaction with drugs affected by CYP450 enzymes). Products include:
Indocin 1995

Indomethacin Sodium Trihydrate (Potential for drug-drug interaction with drugs affected by CYP450 enzymes). Products include:
Indocin I.V. 2465

Indoramin Hydrochloride (Potential for drug-drug interaction with drugs affected by CYP450 enzymes).
No products indexed under this heading.

Irbesartan (Potential for drug-drug interaction with drugs affected by CYP450 enzymes). Products include:
Avalide Tablets 888
Avalide Tablets 2874
Avapro Tablets 891
Avapro Tablets 2871

Isotretinoin (Potential for drug-drug interaction with drugs affected by CYP450 enzymes). Products include:
Accutane Capsules 2731

Isradipine (Potential for drug-drug interaction with drugs affected by CYP450 enzymes). Products include:
DynaCirc CR Tablets 2721

Itraconazole (Potential for drug-drug interaction with drugs affected by CYP450 enzymes).
No products indexed under this heading.

Ketoconazole (Potential for drug-drug interaction with drugs affected by CYP450 enzymes). Products include:
Nizoral A-D Shampoo, 1% 1868

Ketoprofen (Potential for drug-drug interaction with drugs affected by CYP450 enzymes).
No products indexed under this heading.

Ketorolac Tromethamine (Potential for drug-drug interaction with drugs affected by CYP450 enzymes). Products include:
Acular Ophthalmic Solution 565
Acular LS Ophthalmic Solution 566

Labetalol Hydrochloride (Potential for drug-drug interaction with drugs affected by CYP450 enzymes).
No products indexed under this heading.

Lamotrigine (Potential for drug-drug interaction with drugs affected by CYP450 enzymes). Products include:

Lamictal 1481

Lansoprazole (Potential for drug-drug interaction with drugs affected by CYP450 enzymes). Products include:
Prevacid Delayed-Release Capsules 3271
Prevacid for Delayed-Release Oral Suspension 3271
Prevacid SoluTab Delayed-Release Orally Disintegrating Tablets 3271
Prevacid I.V. for Injection 3277
Prevacid NapraPAC 3280
PREVPAC 3284

Levetiracetam (Potential for drug-drug interaction with drugs affected by CYP450 enzymes). Products include:
Keppra Injection 3320
Keppra Oral Solution 3314
Keppra Tablets 3314

Levobupivacaine Hydrochloride (Potential for drug-drug interaction with drugs affected by CYP450 enzymes).
No products indexed under this heading.

Levonorgestrel (Potential for drug-drug interaction with drugs affected by CYP450 enzymes). Products include:
Climara Pro Transdermal System 776
Mirena Intrauterine System 787
Plan B Tablets 1076
Seasonique Tablets 1077

Lidocaine (Potential for drug-drug interaction with drugs affected by CYP450 enzymes). Products include:
Lidoderm Patch 1118
Synera Topical Patch 1137

Lidocaine Base (Potential for drug-drug interaction with drugs affected by CYP450 enzymes).
No products indexed under this heading.

Lidocaine Hydrochloride (Potential for drug-drug interaction with drugs affected by CYP450 enzymes).
No products indexed under this heading.

Lomefloxacin Hydrochloride (Potential for drug-drug interaction with drugs affected by CYP450 enzymes).
No products indexed under this heading.

Losartan Potassium (Potential for drug-drug interaction with drugs affected by CYP450 enzymes). Products include:
Cozaar Tablets 1935
Hyzaar 50-12.5 Tablets 1990
Hyzaar 100-12.5 Tablets 1990
Hyzaar 100-25 Tablets 1990

Lovastatin (Potential for drug-drug interaction with drugs affected by CYP450 enzymes). Products include:
Advicor Tablets 1722
Altoprev Extended-Release Tablets 3109
Mevacor Tablets 2021

Maprotiline Hydrochloride (Potential for drug-drug interaction with drugs affected by CYP450 enzymes).
No products indexed under this heading.

Meclofenamate Sodium (Potential for drug-drug interaction with drugs affected by CYP450 enzymes).
No products indexed under this heading.

Mefenamic Acid (Potential for drug-drug interaction with drugs affected by CYP450 enzymes).
No products indexed under this heading.

Meloxicam (Potential for drug-drug interaction with drugs affected by CYP450 enzymes). Products include:
Mobic Oral Suspension 863
Mobic Tablets 863

Meperidine Hydrochloride (Potential for drug-drug interaction with drugs affected by CYP450 enzymes).
No products indexed under this heading.

Mephenytoin (Potential for drug-drug interaction with drugs affected by CYP450 enzymes).
No products indexed under this heading.

Mephobarbital (Potential for drug-drug interaction with drugs affected by CYP450 enzymes).
No products indexed under this heading.

Meprobamate (Potential for drug-drug interaction with drugs affected by CYP450 enzymes).
No products indexed under this heading.

Mestranol (Potential for drug-drug interaction with drugs affected by CYP450 enzymes).
No products indexed under this heading.

Metformin Hydrochloride (Potential for drug-drug interaction with drugs affected by CYP450 enzymes). Products include:
ActoPlus Met Tablets 3214
Avandamet Tablets 1373
Fortamet Extended-Release Tablets 3115

Methadone Hydrochloride (Potential for drug-drug interaction with drugs affected by CYP450 enzymes).
No products indexed under this heading.

Methamphetamine Hydrochloride (Potential for drug-drug interaction with drugs affected by CYP450 enzymes). Products include:
Desoxyn Tablets, USP 2462

Methsuximide (Potential for drug-drug interaction with drugs affected by CYP450 enzymes).
No products indexed under this heading.

Metoprolol Succinate (Potential for drug-drug interaction with drugs affected by CYP450 enzymes). Products include:
Toprol-XL Tablets 668

Metoprolol Tartrate (Potential for drug-drug interaction with drugs affected by CYP450 enzymes). Products include:
Lopressor Injection 2238
Lopressor Tablets 2238
Lopressor HCT 50/25 Tablets 2241
Lopressor HCT 100/25 Tablets 2241
Lopressor HCT 100/50 Tablets 2241

Mexiletine Hydrochloride (Potential for drug-drug interaction with drugs affected by CYP450 enzymes).
No products indexed under this heading.

Midazolam Hydrochloride (Potential for drug-drug interaction with drugs affected by CYP450 enzymes).
No products indexed under this heading.

Miglitol (Potential for drug-drug interaction with drugs affected by CYP450 enzymes).
No products indexed under this heading.

Mirtazapine (Potential for drug-drug interaction with drugs affected by CYP450 enzymes).
No products indexed under this heading.

Montelukast Sodium (Potential for drug-drug interaction with drugs affected by CYP450 enzymes). Products include:
Singulair 2077

Morphine Sulfate (Potential for drug-drug interaction with drugs affected by CYP450 enzymes). Products include:
Avinza Capsules 1741
Kadian Capsules 577
MS Contin Tablets 2701

Moxifloxacin Hydrochloride (Potential for drug-drug interaction with drugs affected by CYP450 enzymes). Products include:
Avelox 2970
Vigamox Ophthalmic Solution 564

Nabumetone (Potential for drug-drug interaction with drugs affected by CYP450 enzymes).
No products indexed under this heading.

Nafcillin Sodium (Potential for drug-drug interaction with drugs affected by CYP450 enzymes).
No products indexed under this heading.

Naproxen (Potential for drug-drug interaction with drugs affected by CYP450 enzymes). Products include:
EC-Naprosyn Delayed-Release Tablets 2761
Naprosyn Suspension 2761
Naprosyn Tablets 2761
Prevacid NapraPAC 3280

Naproxen Sodium (Potential for drug-drug interaction with drugs affected by CYP450 enzymes). Products include:
Aleve Caplets 742
Aleve Gelcaps 743
Aleve Tablets 743
Aleve Cold & Sinus Caplets 744
Anaprox Tablets 2761
Anaprox DS Tablets 2761

Nateglinide (Potential for drug-drug interaction with drugs affected by CYP450 enzymes). Products include:
Starlix Tablets 2292

Nefazodone Hydrochloride (Potential for drug-drug interaction with drugs affected by CYP450 enzymes).
No products indexed under this heading.

Nelfinavir Mesylate (Potential for drug-drug interaction with drugs affected by CYP450 enzymes). Products include:
Viracept 2577

Nicardipine (Potential for drug-drug interaction with drugs affected by CYP450 enzymes).
No products indexed under this heading.

Nicardipine Hydrochloride (Potential for drug-drug interaction with drugs affected by CYP450 enzymes). Products include:
Cardene I.V. 2497

Nicotine Polacrilex (Potential for drug-drug interaction with drugs affected by CYP450 enzymes).
No products indexed under this heading.

Nicotine Salicylate (Potential for drug-drug interaction with drugs affected by CYP450 enzymes).
No products indexed under this heading.

Nicotine Sulfate (Potential for drug-drug interaction with drugs affected by CYP450 enzymes).
No products indexed under this heading.

Nifedipine (Potential for drug-drug interaction with drugs affected by CYP450 enzymes). Products include:
Adalat CC Tablets 2964

Nilutamide (Potential for drug-drug interaction with drugs affected by CYP450 enzymes).
No products indexed under this heading.

Nimodipine (Potential for drug-drug interaction with drugs affected by CYP450 enzymes). Products include:
Nimotop Capsules 749

Nisoldipine (Potential for drug-drug interaction with drugs affected by CYP450 enzymes). Products include:
Sular Tablets 3122

Nitrendipine (Potential for drug-drug interaction with drugs affected by CYP450 enzymes).
No products indexed under this heading.

Norethindrone (Potential for drug-drug interaction with drugs affected by CYP450 enzymes). Products include:
Ortho Micronor Tablets 2426

Norethindrone Acetate (Potential for drug-drug interaction with drugs affected by CYP450 enzymes).
No products indexed under this heading.

Norfloxacin (Potential for drug-drug interaction with drugs affected by CYP450 enzymes). Products include:
Noroxin Tablets 2032

Norgestrel (Potential for drug-drug interaction with drugs affected by CYP450 enzymes).
No products indexed under this heading.

Nortriptyline Hydrochloride (Potential for drug-drug interaction with drugs affected by CYP450 enzymes).
No products indexed under this heading.

Ofloxacin (Potential for drug-drug interaction with drugs affected by CYP450 enzymes). Products include:
Floxin Otic Solution 1049

Olanzapine (Potential for drug-drug interaction with drugs affected by CYP450 enzymes). Products include:
Symbyax Capsules 1819
Zyprexa Tablets 1830
Zyprexa IntraMuscular 1830
Zyprexa ZYDIS Orally Disintegrating Tablets 1830

Omeprazole (Potential for drug-drug interaction with drugs affected by CYP450 enzymes). Products include:
- Zegerid Capsules 2958
- Zegerid Powder for Oral Solution 2958

Ondansetron (Potential for drug-drug interaction with drugs affected by CYP450 enzymes). Products include:
- Zofran ODT Orally Disintegrating Tablets 1639

Ondansetron Hydrochloride (Potential for drug-drug interaction with drugs affected by CYP450 enzymes). Products include:
- Zofran Injection 1634
- Zofran 1639

Oxaprozin (Potential for drug-drug interaction with drugs affected by CYP450 enzymes).
No products indexed under this heading.

Oxcarbazepine (Potential for drug-drug interaction with drugs affected by CYP450 enzymes). Products include:
- Trileptal Tablets 2300
- Trileptal Oral Suspension 2300

Oxycodone Hydrochloride (Potential for drug-drug interaction with drugs affected by CYP450 enzymes). Products include:
- OxyContin Tablets 2703
- OxyFast Oral Concentrate Solution 2708
- OxyIR Capsules 2708
- Percocet Tablets 1131
- Percodan Tablets 1132

Paclitaxel (Potential for drug-drug interaction with drugs affected by CYP450 enzymes).
No products indexed under this heading.

Pantoprazole Sodium (Potential for drug-drug interaction with drugs affected by CYP450 enzymes). Products include:
- Protonix I.V. 3472
- Protonix Tablets 3469

Paramethadione (Potential for drug-drug interaction with drugs affected by CYP450 enzymes).
No products indexed under this heading.

Paroxetine Hydrochloride (Potential for drug-drug interaction with drugs affected by CYP450 enzymes). Products include:
- Paxil CR Controlled-Release Tablets 1538
- Paxil 1530

Pentamidine Isethionate (Potential for drug-drug interaction with drugs affected by CYP450 enzymes).
No products indexed under this heading.

Phenacemide (Potential for drug-drug interaction with drugs affected by CYP450 enzymes).
No products indexed under this heading.

Phenobarbital (Potential for drug-drug interaction with drugs affected by CYP450 enzymes). Products include:
- Donnatal Extentabs 2493

Phenobarbital Sodium (Potential for drug-drug interaction with drugs affected by CYP450 enzymes).
No products indexed under this heading.

Phensuximide (Potential for drug-drug interaction with drugs affected by CYP450 enzymes).
No products indexed under this heading.

Phenylbutazone (Potential for drug-drug interaction with drugs affected by CYP450 enzymes).
No products indexed under this heading.

Phenytoin (Potential for drug-drug interaction with drugs affected by CYP450 enzymes).
No products indexed under this heading.

Phenytoin Sodium (Potential for drug-drug interaction with drugs affected by CYP450 enzymes). Products include:
- Phenytek Capsules 2160

Pimozide (Potential for drug-drug interaction with drugs affected by CYP450 enzymes).
No products indexed under this heading.

Pindolol (Potential for drug-drug interaction with drugs affected by CYP450 enzymes).
No products indexed under this heading.

Pioglitazone Hydrochloride (Potential for drug-drug interaction with drugs affected by CYP450 enzymes). Products include:
- ActoPlus Met Tablets 3214
- Actos Tablets 3219
- Duetact Tablets 3226

Piroxicam (Potential for drug-drug interaction with drugs affected by CYP450 enzymes).
No products indexed under this heading.

Polyestradiol Phosphate (Potential for drug-drug interaction with drugs affected by CYP450 enzymes).
No products indexed under this heading.

Primidone (Potential for drug-drug interaction with drugs affected by CYP450 enzymes).
No products indexed under this heading.

Progesterone (Potential for drug-drug interaction with drugs affected by CYP450 enzymes). Products include:
- Prochieve 4% Gel 1003
- Prochieve 8% Gel 1003
- Prometrium Capsules (100 mg, 200 mg) 3203

Proguanil Hydrochloride (Potential for drug-drug interaction with drugs affected by CYP450 enzymes). Products include:
- Malarone Pediatric Tablets 1517
- Malarone Tablets 1517

Propafenone Hydrochloride (Potential for drug-drug interaction with drugs affected by CYP450 enzymes). Products include:
- Rythmol SR Capsules 2727

Propoxyphene Hydrochloride (Potential for drug-drug interaction with drugs affected by CYP450 enzymes).
No products indexed under this heading.

Propoxyphene Napsylate (Potential for drug-drug interaction with drugs affected by CYP450 enzymes).
No products indexed under this heading.

Propranolol Hydrochloride (Potential for drug-drug interaction with drugs affected by CYP450 enzymes). Products include:
- Inderal LA Long-Acting Capsules 3429
- InnoPran XL Capsules 2723

Protriptyline Hydrochloride (Potential for drug-drug interaction with drugs affected by CYP450 enzymes).
No products indexed under this heading.

Quetiapine Fumarate (Potential for drug-drug interaction with drugs affected by CYP450 enzymes). Products include:
- Seroquel Tablets 690

Quinidine Gluconate (Potential for drug-drug interaction with drugs affected by CYP450 enzymes).
No products indexed under this heading.

Quinidine Hydrochloride (Potential for drug-drug interaction with drugs affected by CYP450 enzymes).
No products indexed under this heading.

Quinidine Polygalacturonate (Potential for drug-drug interaction with drugs affected by CYP450 enzymes).
No products indexed under this heading.

Quinidine Sulfate (Potential for drug-drug interaction with drugs affected by CYP450 enzymes).
No products indexed under this heading.

Quinine (Potential for drug-drug interaction with drugs affected by CYP450 enzymes).
No products indexed under this heading.

Quinine Sulfate (Potential for drug-drug interaction with drugs affected by CYP450 enzymes).
No products indexed under this heading.

Rabeprazole Sodium (Potential for drug-drug interaction with drugs affected by CYP450 enzymes). Products include:
- Aciphex Tablets 1090

Repaglinide (Potential for drug-drug interaction with drugs affected by CYP450 enzymes).
No products indexed under this heading.

Rifabutin (Potential for drug-drug interaction with drugs affected by CYP450 enzymes).
No products indexed under this heading.

Riluzole (Potential for drug-drug interaction with drugs affected by CYP450 enzymes). Products include:
- Rilutek Tablets 2930

Risperidone (Potential for drug-drug interaction with drugs affected by CYP450 enzymes). Products include:
- Risperdal 1676
- Risperdal Consta Long-Acting Injection 1682
- Risperdal M-Tab Orally Disintegrating Tablets 1676

Ritonavir (Potential for drug-drug interaction with drugs affected by CYP450 enzymes). Products include:
- Kaletra 476
- Norvir 503

Rofecoxib (Potential for drug-drug interaction with drugs affected by CYP450 enzymes).
No products indexed under this heading.

Ropinirole Hydrochloride (Potential for drug-drug interaction with drugs affected by CYP450 enzymes). Products include:
- Requip Tablets 1555

Ropivacaine Hydrochloride (Potential for drug-drug interaction with drugs affected by CYP450 enzymes).
No products indexed under this heading.

Rosiglitazone Maleate (Potential for drug-drug interaction with drugs affected by CYP450 enzymes). Products include:
- Avandamet Tablets 1373
- Avandaryl Tablets 1379
- Avandia Tablets 1384

Saquinavir (Potential for drug-drug interaction with drugs affected by CYP450 enzymes).
No products indexed under this heading.

Saquinavir Mesylate (Potential for drug-drug interaction with drugs affected by CYP450 enzymes). Products include:
- Invirase 2772

Sertraline Hydrochloride (Potential for drug-drug interaction with drugs affected by CYP450 enzymes). Products include:
- Zoloft 2586

Sildenafil Citrate (Potential for drug-drug interaction with drugs affected by CYP450 enzymes). Products include:
- Revatio Tablets 2557
- Viagra Tablets 2573

Simvastatin (Potential for drug-drug interaction with drugs affected by CYP450 enzymes). Products include:
- Vytorin 10/10 Tablets 2114
- Vytorin 10/10 Tablets 3077
- Vytorin 10/20 Tablets 2114
- Vytorin 10/20 Tablets 3077
- Vytorin 10/40 Tablets 2114
- Vytorin 10/40 Tablets 3077
- Vytorin 10/80 Tablets 2114
- Vytorin 10/80 Tablets 3077
- Zocor Tablets 2105

Sirolimus (Potential for drug-drug interaction with drugs affected by CYP450 enzymes). Products include:
- Rapamune Oral Solution and Tablets 3475

Sulfamethoxazole (Potential for drug-drug interaction with drugs affected by CYP450 enzymes).
No products indexed under this heading.

Sulindac (Potential for drug-drug interaction with drugs affected by CYP450 enzymes). Products include:
- Clinoril Tablets 1924

Suprofen (Potential for drug-drug interaction with drugs affected by CYP450 enzymes).
No products indexed under this heading.

Tacrine Hydrochloride (Potential for drug-drug interaction with drugs affected by CYP450 enzymes).
No products indexed under this heading.

Tacrolimus (Potential for drug-drug interaction with drugs affected by CYP450 enzymes). Products include:

Prograf Capsules and Injection 632
Protopic Ointment 638

Tamoxifen Citrate (Potential for drug-drug interaction with drugs affected by CYP450 enzymes). Products include:
Soltamox Oral Solution 3527

Telmisartan (Potential for drug-drug interaction with drugs affected by CYP450 enzymes). Products include:
Micardis Tablets 854
Micardis HCT Tablets 856

Teniposide (Potential for drug-drug interaction with drugs affected by CYP450 enzymes).
No products indexed under this heading.

Terfenadine (Potential for drug-drug interaction with drugs affected by CYP450 enzymes).
No products indexed under this heading.

Testosterone (Potential for drug-drug interaction with drugs affected by CYP450 enzymes). Products include:
AndroGel 3329
Striant Mucoadhesive 1007
Testim 1% Gel 695

Testosterone Cypionate (Potential for drug-drug interaction with drugs affected by CYP450 enzymes).
No products indexed under this heading.

Testosterone Enanthate (Potential for drug-drug interaction with drugs affected by CYP450 enzymes).
No products indexed under this heading.

Testosterone Propionate (Potential for drug-drug interaction with drugs affected by CYP450 enzymes).
No products indexed under this heading.

Theophylline (Potential for drug-drug interaction with drugs affected by CYP450 enzymes).
No products indexed under this heading.

Theophylline Anhydrous (Potential for drug-drug interaction with drugs affected by CYP450 enzymes). Products include:
Uniphyl Tablets 2710

Theophylline Sodium Glycinate (Potential for drug-drug interaction with drugs affected by CYP450 enzymes).
No products indexed under this heading.

Thioridazine (Potential for drug-drug interaction with drugs affected by CYP450 enzymes).
No products indexed under this heading.

Thioridazine Hydrochloride (Potential for drug-drug interaction with drugs affected by CYP450 enzymes). Products include:
Thioridazine Hydrochloride Tablets 2163

Tiagabine Hydrochloride (Potential for drug-drug interaction with drugs affected by CYP450 enzymes). Products include:
Gabitril Tablets 984

Timolol Maleate (Potential for drug-drug interaction with drugs affected by CYP450 enzymes). Products include:
Blocadren Tablets 1916
Cosopt Sterile Ophthalmic Solution 1931
Timolide Tablets 2086
Timoptic Sterile Ophthalmic Solution 2088
Timoptic in Ocudose 2091
Timoptic-XE Sterile Ophthalmic Gel Forming Solution 2092

Tolazamide (Potential for drug-drug interaction with drugs affected by CYP450 enzymes).
No products indexed under this heading.

Tolbutamide (Potential for drug-drug interaction with drugs affected by CYP450 enzymes).
No products indexed under this heading.

Tolbutamide Sodium (Potential for drug-drug interaction with drugs affected by CYP450 enzymes).
No products indexed under this heading.

Tolmetin Sodium (Potential for drug-drug interaction with drugs affected by CYP450 enzymes).
No products indexed under this heading.

Tolterodine Tartrate (Potential for drug-drug interaction with drugs affected by CYP450 enzymes). Products include:
Detrol Tablets 2628
Detrol LA Capsules 2631

Topiramate (Potential for drug-drug interaction with drugs affected by CYP450 enzymes). Products include:
Topamax Sprinkle Capsules 2404
Topamax Tablets 2404

Torsemide (Potential for drug-drug interaction with drugs affected by CYP450 enzymes). Products include:
Demadex Injection 2759
Demadex Tablets 2759

Tramadol Hydrochloride (Potential for drug-drug interaction with drugs affected by CYP450 enzymes). Products include:
Ultram ER Tablets 2392

Trazodone Hydrochloride (Potential for drug-drug interaction with drugs affected by CYP450 enzymes).
No products indexed under this heading.

Tretinoin (Potential for drug-drug interaction with drugs affected by CYP450 enzymes). Products include:
Tri-Luma Cream 1213
Vesanoid Capsules 2820

Triazolam (Potential for drug-drug interaction with drugs affected by CYP450 enzymes).
No products indexed under this heading.

Trimethadione (Potential for drug-drug interaction with drugs affected by CYP450 enzymes).
No products indexed under this heading.

Trimethaphan Camsylate (Potential for drug-drug interaction with drugs affected by CYP450 enzymes).
No products indexed under this heading.

Trimipramine Maleate (Potential for drug-drug interaction with drugs affected by CYP450 enzymes).
No products indexed under this heading.

Troglitazone (Potential for drug-drug interaction with drugs affected by CYP450 enzymes).
No products indexed under this heading.

Trovafloxacin Mesylate (Potential for drug-drug interaction with drugs affected by CYP450 enzymes).
No products indexed under this heading.

Valdecoxib (Potential for drug-drug interaction with drugs affected by CYP450 enzymes).
No products indexed under this heading.

Valproate Sodium (Potential for drug-drug interaction with drugs affected by CYP450 enzymes). Products include:
Depacon Injection 412

Valproic Acid (Potential for drug-drug interaction with drugs affected by CYP450 enzymes). Products include:
Depakene 417

Valsartan (Potential for drug-drug interaction with drugs affected by CYP450 enzymes). Products include:
Diovan Tablets 2193
Diovan HCT Tablets 2196

Venlafaxine Hydrochloride (Potential for drug-drug interaction with drugs affected by CYP450 enzymes). Products include:
Effexor Tablets 3411
Effexor XR Capsules 3417

Verapamil Hydrochloride (Potential for drug-drug interaction with drugs affected by CYP450 enzymes). Products include:
Covera-HS Tablets 3139
Tarka Tablets 524
Verelan PM Extended-Release Capsules, Controlled-Onset.......... 3106

Vinblastine Sulfate (Potential for drug-drug interaction with drugs affected by CYP450 enzymes).
No products indexed under this heading.

Vincristine Sulfate (Potential for drug-drug interaction with drugs affected by CYP450 enzymes).
No products indexed under this heading.

Vitamin A (Potential for drug-drug interaction with drugs affected by CYP450 enzymes). Products include:
Visutein Capsules 3329

Vitamin A Acetate (Potential for drug-drug interaction with drugs affected by CYP450 enzymes).
No products indexed under this heading.

Voriconazole (Potential for drug-drug interaction with drugs affected by CYP450 enzymes). Products include:
VFEND I.V. 2564
VFEND Oral Suspension 2564
VFEND Tablets 2564

Warfarin Sodium (Potential for drug-drug interaction with drugs affected by CYP450 enzymes). Products include:
Coumadin for Injection 898
Coumadin Tablets 898

Zafirlukast (Potential for drug-drug interaction with drugs affected by CYP450 enzymes). Products include:
Accolate Tablets 671

Zileuton (Potential for drug-drug interaction with drugs affected by CYP450 enzymes). Products include:
Zyflo Tablets 1023

Zolmitriptan (Potential for drug-drug interaction with drugs affected by CYP450 enzymes). Products include:
Zomig Tablets 3519
Zomig Nasal Spray 3523
Zomig-ZMT Tablets 3519

Zonisamide (Potential for drug-drug interaction with drugs affected by CYP450 enzymes). Products include:
Zonegran Capsules 1101

Zopiclone (Potential for drug-drug interaction with drugs affected by CYP450 enzymes).
No products indexed under this heading.

MYOBLOC INJECTION

(Botulinum Toxin Type B) 3192
May interact with aminoglycosides, neuromuscular blocking agents, and certain other agents. Compounds in these categories include:

Amikacin Sulfate (Co-administration with aminoglycosides may potentiate the effect of the toxin).
No products indexed under this heading.

Atracurium Besylate (Co-administration with neuromuscular blocking agents may potentiate the effect of the toxin).
No products indexed under this heading.

Cisatracurium Besylate (Co-administration with neuromuscular blocking agents may potentiate the effect of the toxin). Products include:
Nimbex Injection 498

Doxacurium Chloride (Co-administration with neuromuscular blocking agents may potentiate the effect of the toxin).
No products indexed under this heading.

Gentamicin Sulfate (Co-administration with aminoglycosides may potentiate the effect of the toxin). Products include:
Garamycin Injectable 3014
Pred-G Ophthalmic Ointment .... ⊙237
Pred-G Ophthalmic Suspension ...... ⊙236

Kanamycin Sulfate (Co-administration with aminoglycosides may potentiate the effect of the toxin).
No products indexed under this heading.

Metocurine Iodide (Co-administration with neuromuscular blocking agents may potentiate the effect of the toxin).
No products indexed under this heading.

Mivacurium Chloride (Co-administration with neuromuscular blocking agents may potentiate the effect of the toxin). Products include:
Mivacron Injection 493

Pancuronium Bromide (Co-administration with neuromuscular blocking agents may potentiate the effect of the toxin).
No products indexed under this heading.

Rapacuronium Bromide (Co-administration with neuromuscular blocking agents may potentiate the effect of the toxin).
No products indexed under this heading.

Rocuronium Bromide (Co-administration with neuromuscular blocking agents may potentiate the effect of the toxin). Products include:

Zemuron Injection **2346**

Streptomycin Sulfate (Co-administration with aminoglycosides may potentiate the effect of the toxin).

No products indexed under this heading.

Succinylcholine Chloride (Co-administration with neuromuscular blocking agents may potentiate the effect of the toxin).

No products indexed under this heading.

Tobramycin (Co-administration with aminoglycosides may potentiate the effect of the toxin). Products include:

TOBI Solution for Inhalation **2298**
TobraDex Ophthalmic Ointment **562**
TobraDex Ophthalmic Suspension ... **563**
Zylet Ophthalmic Suspension .... ⊙**259**

Tobramycin Sulfate (Co-administration with aminoglycosides may potentiate the effect of the toxin).

No products indexed under this heading.

Tubocurarine Chloride (Co-administration with curare-like compounds may potentiate the effect of the toxin).

No products indexed under this heading.

Vecuronium Bromide (Co-administration with neuromuscular blocking agents may potentiate the effect of the toxin).

No products indexed under this heading.

MYOZYME FOR INTRAVENOUS INFUSION

(Alglucosidase alfa) **1279**
None cited in PDR database.

NABI-HB

(Hepatitis B Immune Globulin (Human)).. **2169**
May interact with:

Mumps Virus Vaccine, Live (H-BIG may interfere with the immune response to vaccination, therefore, vaccination with live virus vaccine should be deferred until approximately 3 months). Products include:

Mumpsvax **2031**

Rubella & Mumps Virus Vaccine Live (H-BIG may interfere with the immune response to vaccination, therefore, vaccination with live virus vaccine should be deferred until approximately 3 months).

No products indexed under this heading.

Rubella Virus Vaccine Live (H-BIG may interfere with the immune response to vaccination, therefore, vaccination with live virus vaccine should be deferred until approximately 3 months). Products include:

Meruvax II **2019**

NADOLOL TABLETS

(Nadolol) **2159**
May interact with general anesthetics, oral hypoglycemic agents, insulin, and certain other agents. Compounds in these categories include:

Acarbose (Beta-adrenergic blockade may prevent the appearance of premonitory signs and symptoms, such as tachycardia and blood pressure changes, of acute hypoglycemia; beta-blockade also reduces the release of insulin in response to hyperglycemia; adjust dosage of oral antidiabetic drugs). Products include:

Precose Tablets **751**

Chlorpropamide (Beta-adrenergic blockade may prevent the appearance of premonitory signs and symptoms, such as tachycardia and blood pressure changes, of acute hypoglycemia; beta-blockade also reduces the release of insulin in response to hyperglycemia; adjust dosage of oral antidiabetic drugs).

No products indexed under this heading.

Enflurane (Co-administration may result in exaggeration of the hypotension induced by general anesthetics).

No products indexed under this heading.

Epinephrine (Patients with a history of severe anaphylactic reaction to variety of allergens may be more reactive to repeated challenge; potential for unresponsiveness to the usual dose of epinephrine). Products include:

EpiPen **1061**
Primatene Mist **719**
Twinject 0.15 .... **3379**
Twinject 0.3 .... **3378**

Epinephrine Hydrochloride (Patients with a history of severe anaphylactic reaction to variety of allergens may be more reactive to repeated challenge; potential for unresponsiveness to the usual dose of epinephrine).

No products indexed under this heading.

Glimepiride (Beta-adrenergic blockade may prevent the appearance of premonitory signs and symptoms, such as tachycardia and blood pressure changes, of acute hypoglycemia; beta-blockade also reduces the release of insulin in response to hyperglycemia; adjust dosage of oral antidiabetic drugs). Products include:

Avandaryl Tablets **1379**
Duetact Tablets **3226**

Glipizide (Beta-adrenergic blockade may prevent the appearance of premonitory signs and symptoms, such as tachycardia and blood pressure changes, of acute hypoglycemia; beta-blockade also reduces the release of insulin in response to hyperglycemia; adjust dosage of oral antidiabetic drugs).

No products indexed under this heading.

Glyburide (Beta-adrenergic blockade may prevent the appearance of premonitory signs and symptoms, such as tachycardia and blood pressure changes, of acute hypoglycemia; beta-blockade also reduces the release of insulin in response to hyperglycemia; adjust dosage of oral antidiabetic drugs).

No products indexed under this heading.

Insulin, Human, Zinc Suspension (Beta-adrenergic blockade may prevent the appearance of premonitory signs and symptoms, such as tachycardia and blood pressure changes, of acute hypoglycemia; beta-blockade also reduces the release of insulin in response to hyperglycemia; adjust dosage of insulin). Products include:

Humulin L, 100 Units **1794**
Humulin U, 100 Units **1800**

Insulin, Human NPH (Beta-adrenergic blockade may prevent the appearance of premonitory signs and symptoms, such as tachycardia and blood pressure changes, of acute hypoglycemia; beta-blockade also reduces the release of insulin in response to hyperglycemia; adjust dosage of insulin). Products include:

Humulin N, 100 Units **1795**
Humulin N Pen **1797**

Insulin, Human Regular (Beta-adrenergic blockade may prevent the appearance of premonitory signs and symptoms, such as tachycardia and blood pressure changes, of acute hypoglycemia; beta-blockade also reduces the release of insulin in response to hyperglycemia; adjust dosage of insulin). Products include:

Humulin R, 100 Units **1798**

Insulin, Human Regular and Human NPH Mixture (Beta-adrenergic blockade may prevent the appearance of premonitory signs and symptoms, such as tachycardia and blood pressure changes, of acute hypoglycemia; beta-blockade also reduces the release of insulin in response to hyperglycemia; adjust dosage of insulin). Products include:

Humulin 50/50, 100 Units **1791**
Humulin 70/30 Pen **1793**

Insulin, NPH (Beta-adrenergic blockade may prevent the appearance of premonitory signs and symptoms, such as tachycardia and blood pressure changes, of acute hypoglycemia; beta-blockade also reduces the release of insulin in response to hyperglycemia; adjust dosage of insulin).

No products indexed under this heading.

Insulin, Regular (Beta-adrenergic blockade may prevent the appearance of premonitory signs and symptoms, such as tachycardia and blood pressure changes, of acute hypoglycemia; beta-blockade also reduces the release of insulin in response to hyperglycemia; adjust dosage of insulin).

No products indexed under this heading.

Insulin, Zinc Crystals (Beta-adrenergic blockade may prevent the appearance of premonitory signs and symptoms, such as tachycardia and blood pressure changes, of acute hypoglycemia; beta-blockade also reduces the release of insulin in response to hyperglycemia; adjust dosage of insulin).

No products indexed under this heading.

Insulin, Zinc Suspension (Beta-adrenergic blockade may prevent the appearance of premonitory signs and symptoms, such as tachycardia and blood pressure changes, of acute hypoglycemia; beta-blockade also reduces the release of insulin in response to hyperglycemia; adjust dosage of insulin).

No products indexed under this heading.

Insulin Aspart, Human Regular (Beta-adrenergic blockade may prevent the appearance of premonitory signs and symptoms, such as tachycardia and blood pressure changes, of acute hypoglycemia; beta-blockade also reduces the release of insulin in response to hyperglycemia; adjust dosage of insulin). Products include:

NovoLog Injection **2326**

Insulin glargine (Beta-adrenergic blockade may prevent the appearance of premonitory signs and symptoms, such as tachycardia and blood pressure changes, of acute hypoglycemia; beta-blockade also reduces the release of insulin in response to hyperglycemia; adjust dosage of insulin). Products include:

Lantus Injection **2909**

Insulin Lispro, Human (Beta-adrenergic blockade may prevent the appearance of premonitory signs and symptoms, such as tachycardia and blood pressure changes, of acute hypoglycemia; beta-blockade also reduces the release of insulin in response to hyperglycemia; adjust dosage of insulin). Products include:

Humalog-Pen **1781**
Humalog Mix 50/50-Pen **1783**
Humalog Mix 75/25-Pen **1785**

Insulin Lispro Protamine, Human (Beta-adrenergic blockade may prevent the appearance of premonitory signs and symptoms, such as tachycardia and blood pressure changes, of acute hypoglycemia; beta-blockade also reduces the release of insulin in response to hyperglycemia; adjust dosage of insulin). Products include:

Humalog Mix 50/50-Pen **1783**
Humalog Mix 75/25-Pen **1785**

Isoflurane (Co-administration may result in exaggeration of the hypotension induced by general anesthetics).

No products indexed under this heading.

Ketamine Hydrochloride (Co-administration may result in exaggeration of the hypotension induced by general anesthetics).

No products indexed under this heading.

Metformin Hydrochloride (Beta-adrenergic blockade may prevent the appearance of premonitory signs and symptoms, such as tachycardia and blood pressure changes, of acute hypoglycemia; beta-blockade also reduces the release of insulin in response to hyperglycemia; adjust dosage of oral antidiabetic drugs). Products include:

ActoPlus Met Tablets **3214**
Avandamet Tablets **1373**
Fortamet Extended-Release Tablets **3115**

Methohexital Sodium (Co-administration may result in exaggeration of the hypotension induced by general anesthetics).

No products indexed under this heading.

Methoxyflurane (Co-administration may result in exaggeration of the hypotension induced by general anesthetics).

No products indexed under this heading.

Miglitol (Beta-adrenergic blockade may prevent the appearance of premonitory signs and symptoms, such as tachycardia and blood pressure changes, of acute hypoglycemia; beta-blockade also reduces the release of insulin in response to hyperglycemia; adjust dosage of oral antidiabetic drugs).

No products indexed under this heading.

Pioglitazone Hydrochloride (Beta-adrenergic blockade may prevent the appearance of premonitory signs and symptoms, such as tachycardia and blood pressure changes, of acute hypoglycemia; beta-blockade also reduces the release of insulin in response to hyperglycemia; adjust dosage of oral antidiabetic drugs). Products include:

ActoPlus Met Tablets **3214**
Actos Tablets **3219**
Duetact Tablets **3226**

Propofol (Co-administration may result in exaggeration of the hypotension induced by general anesthetics).

No products indexed under this heading.

Repaglinide (Beta-adrenergic blockade may prevent the appearance of premonitory signs and symptoms, such as tachycardia and blood pressure changes, of acute hypoglycemia; beta-blockade also reduces the release of insulin in response to hyperglycemia; adjust dosage of oral antidiabetic drugs).

No products indexed under this heading.

Reserpine (Potential for additive effects resulting in hypotension and/or excessive bradycardia (vertigo, syncope, postural hypotension)).

No products indexed under this heading.

Rosiglitazone Maleate (Beta-adrenergic blockade may prevent the appearance of premonitory signs and symptoms, such as tachycardia and blood pressure changes, of acute hypoglycemia; beta-blockade also reduces the release of insulin in response to hyperglycemia; adjust dosage of oral antidiabetic drugs). Products include:

Avandamet Tablets **1373**
Avandaryl Tablets **1379**
Avandia Tablets **1384**

Sevoflurane (Co-administration may result in exaggeration of the hypotension induced by general anesthetics). Products include:

Ultane Liquid for Inhalation **531**

Tolazamide (Beta-adrenergic blockade may prevent the appearance of premonitory signs and symptoms, such as tachycardia and blood pressure changes, of acute hypoglycemia; beta-blockade also reduces the release of insulin in response to hyperglycemia; adjust dosage of oral antidiabetic drugs).

No products indexed under this heading.

Tolbutamide (Beta-adrenergic blockade may prevent the appearance of premonitory signs and symptoms, such as tachycardia and blood pressure changes, of acute hypoglycemia; beta-blockade also reduces the release of insulin in response to hyperglycemia; adjust dosage of oral antidiabetic drugs).

No products indexed under this heading.

Troglitazone (Beta-adrenergic blockade may prevent the appearance of premonitory signs and symptoms, such as tachycardia and blood pressure changes, of acute hypoglycemia; beta-blockade also reduces the release of insulin in response to hyperglycemia; adjust dosage of oral antidiabetic drugs).

No products indexed under this heading.

NAFTIN CREAM

(Naftifine Hydrochloride) **2126**
None cited in PDR database.

NAFTIN GEL

(Naftifine Hydrochloride) **2126**
None cited in PDR database.

NALFON CAPSULES

(Fenoprofen Calcium) **2502**
May interact with ACE inhibitors, oral anticoagulants, diuretics, hydantoin anticonvulsants, loop diuretics, salicylates, sulfonamides, sulfonylureas, and certain other agents. Compounds in these categories include:

Amiloride Hydrochloride (Fenoprofen calcium may reduce the natriuretic effect of diuretics. This inhibition has been attributed to inhibition of renal prostaglandin synthesis. During concomitant therapy with NSAIDs, the patient should be observed closely for signs of renal failure, as well as to assure diuretic efficacy). Products include:

Midamor Tablets **2026**
Moduretic Tablets **2028**

Anisindione (In patients receiving coumarin-type anticoagulants, the addition of fenoprofen calcium to therapy could prolong the prothrombin time. Patients receiving both drugs should be under careful observation). Products include:

Miradon Tablets **3042**

Aspirin (The co-administration of aspirin decreases the biologic half-life of fenoprofen because of an increase in metabolic clearance that results in a greater amount of hydroxylated fenoprofen in the urine. Although the mechanism of interaction between fenoprofen and aspirin is not totally known, enzyme induction and displacement of fenoprofen from plasma albumin binding sites are possibilities. Because fenoprofen calcium has not been shown to produce any additional effect beyond that obtained with aspirin alone and because aspirin increases the rate of excretion of fenoprofen calcium, concomitant use of fenoprofen calcium and salicylates is not recommended). Products include:

Aggrenox Capsules **822**
Bayer Aspirin **744**
BC Allergy Sinus Cold Powder .... ■**677**
BC Headache Powder .... ■**677**
Arthritis Strength BC Powder .... ■**677**
BC Sinus Cold Powder .... ■**677**
Excedrin Extra Strength Caplets/Tablets/Geltabs .... ■**684**
Excedrin Migraine Caplets/Tablets/Geltabs .... ■**609**
Goody's Body Pain Formula Powder .... ■**684**
Goody's Extra Strength Headache Powders .... ■**611**
Goody's Extra Strength Pain Relief Tablets .... ■**685**
Percodan Tablets **1132**
St. Joseph 81 mg Aspirin Chewable and Enteric Coated Tablets **1869**

Aspirin, Enteric Coated (The co-administration of aspirin decreases the biologic half-life of fenoprofen because of an increase in metabolic clearance that results in a greater amount of hydroxylated fenoprofen in the urine. Although the mechanism of interaction between fenoprofen and aspirin is not totally known, enzyme induction and displacement of fenoprofen from plasma albumin binding sites are possibilities. Because fenoprofen calcium has not been shown to produce any additional effect beyond that obtained with aspirin alone and because aspirin increases the rate of excretion of fenoprofen calcium, concomitant use of fenoprofen calcium and salicylates is not recommended).

No products indexed under this heading.

Aspirin Buffered (The co-administration of aspirin decreases the biologic half-life of fenoprofen because of an increase in metabolic clearance that results in a greater amount of hydroxylated fenoprofen in the urine. Although the mechanism of interaction between fenoprofen and aspirin is not totally known, enzyme induction and displacement of fenoprofen from plasma albumin binding sites are possibilities. Because fenoprofen calcium has not been shown to produce any additional effect beyond that obtained with aspirin alone and because aspirin increases the rate of excretion of fenoprofen calcium, concomitant use of fenoprofen calcium and salicylates is not recommended). Products include:

Bufferin Extra Strength Tablets ...... ■**678**
Bufferin Regular Strength Tablets ... ■**678**

Benazepril Hydrochloride (Reports suggest that NSAIDs may diminish the antihypertensive effect of ACE-inhibitors. This interaction should be given consideration in patients taking NSAIDs concomitantly with ACE-inhibitors). Products include:

Lotensin Tablets **2243**
Lotensin HCT Tablets **2246**
Lotrel Capsules **2249**

Bendroflumethiazide (In vitro studies have shown that fenoprofen, because of its affinity for albumin, may displace from their bindings sites other drugs that are also albumin bound, and this may lead to drug interaction. Theoretically, fenoprofen could likewise be displayed. Patients receiving sulfonylureas should be observed for increased activity of these drugs and, therefore, signs of toxicity from these drugs. Fenoprofen calcium may reduce the natriuretic effect of thiazides. This inhibition has been attributed to inhibition of renal prostaglandin synthesis. During concomitant therapy with NSAIDs, the patient should be observed closely for signs of renal failure, as well as to assure diuretic efficacy).

No products indexed under this heading.

Benzthiazide (Fenoprofen calcium may reduce the natriuretic effect of thiazides. This inhibition has been attributed to inhibition of renal prostaglandin synthesis. During concomitant therapy with NSAIDs, the patient should be observed closely for signs of renal failure, as well as to assure diuretic efficacy).

No products indexed under this heading.

Bumetanide (Fenoprofen calcium may reduce the natriuretic effect of diuretics. This inhibition has been attributed to inhibition of renal prostaglandin synthesis. During concomitant therapy with NSAIDs, the patient should be observed closely for signs of renal failure, as well as to assure diuretic efficacy). Products include:

Bumex Tablets **2746**

Captopril (Reports suggest that NSAIDs may diminish the antihypertensive effect of ACE-inhibitors. This interaction should be given consideration in patients taking NSAIDs concomitantly with ACE-inhibitors). Products include:

Captopril Tablets **2149**

Chlorothiazide (In vitro studies have shown that fenoprofen, because of its affinity for albumin, may displace from their bindings sites other drugs that are also albumin bound, and this may lead to drug interaction. Theoretically, fenoprofen could likewise be displayed. Patients receiving sulfonylureas should be observed for increased activity of these drugs and, therefore, signs of toxicity from these drugs. Fenoprofen calcium may reduce the natriuretic effect of thiazides. This inhibition has been attributed to inhibition of renal prostaglandin synthesis. During concomitant therapy with NSAIDs, the patient should be observed closely for signs of renal failure, as well as to assure diuretic efficacy). Products include:

Diuril Oral Suspension **1954**

Chlorothiazide Sodium (In vitro studies have shown that fenoprofen, because of its affinity for albumin, may displace from their bindings sites other drugs that are also albumin bound, and this may lead to drug interaction. Theoretically, fenoprofen could likewise be displayed. Patients receiving sulfonylureas should be observed for increased activity of these drugs and, therefore, signs of toxicity from these drugs. Fenoprofen calcium may reduce the natriuretic effect of thiazides. This inhibition has been attributed to inhibition of renal prostaglandin synthesis. During concomitant therapy with NSAIDs, the patient should be observed closely for signs of renal failure, as well as to assure diuretic efficacy). Products include:

Diuril Sodium Intravenous **2467**

Chlorpropamide (In vitro studies have shown that fenoprofen, because of its affinity for albumin, may displace from their bindings sites other drugs that are also albumin bound, and this may lead to drug interaction. Theoretically, fenoprofen could likewise be displayed. Patients receiving sulfonamides should be observed for increased activity of these drugs and, therefore, signs of toxicity from these drugs).

No products indexed under this heading.

Chlorthalidone (Fenoprofen calcium may reduce the natriuretic effect of diuretics. This inhibition has been attributed to inhibition of renal prostaglandin synthesis. During concomitant therapy with NSAIDs, the patient should be observed closely for signs of renal failure, as well as to assure diuretic efficacy). Products include:

Clorpres Tablets **2153**

Choline Magnesium Trisalicylate (The co-administration of aspirin decreases the biologic half-life of fenoprofen because of an increase in metabolic clearance that results in a greater amount of hydroxylated fenoprofen in the urine. Although the mechanism of interaction between fenoprofen and aspirin is not totally known, enzyme induction and displacement of fenoprofen from plasma albumin binding sites are possibilities. Because fenoprofen calcium has not been shown to produce any additional effect beyond that obtained with aspirin alone and because aspirin increases the rate of excretion of fenoprofen calcium, concomitant use of fenoprofen calcium and salicylates is not recommended).

No products indexed under this heading.

Dicumarol (In patients receiving coumarin-type anticoagulants, the addition of fenoprofen calcium to therapy could prolong the prothrombin time. Patients receiving both drugs should be under careful observation).

No products indexed under this heading.

Diflunisal (The co-administration of aspirin decreases the biologic half-life of fenoprofen because of an increase in metabolic clearance that results in a greater amount of hydroxylated fenoprofen in the urine. Although the mechanism of interaction between fenoprofen and aspirin is not totally known, enzyme induction and displacement of fenoprofen from plasma albumin binding sites are possibilities. Because fenoprofen calcium has not been shown to produce any additional effect beyond that obtained with aspirin alone and because aspirin increases the rate of excretion of fenoprofen calcium, concomitant use of fenoprofen calcium and salicylates is not recommended). Products include:
Dolobid Tablets 1955

Enalapril Maleate (Reports suggest that NSAIDs may diminish the antihypertensive effect of ACE-inhibitors. This interaction should be given consideration in patients taking NSAIDs concomitantly with ACE-inhibitors). Products include:
Vasotec I.V. Injection 2103

Enalaprilat (Reports suggest that NSAIDs may diminish the antihypertensive effect of ACE-inhibitors. This interaction should be given consideration in patients taking NSAIDs concomitantly with ACE-inhibitors).

No products indexed under this heading.

Ethacrynic Acid (Fenoprofen calcium may reduce the natriuretic effect of diuretics. This inhibition has been attributed to inhibition of renal prostaglandin synthesis. During concomitant therapy with NSAIDs, the patient should be observed closely for signs of renal failure, as well as to assure diuretic efficacy). Products include:
Edecrin Tablets 1959

Ethotoin (In vitro studies have shown that fenoprofen, because of its affinity for albumin, may displace from their binding sites other drugs that are also albumin bound, and this may lead to drug interaction. Theoretically, fenoprofen could likewise be displayed.Patients receiving hydantins should be observed for increased activity drugs and, therefore, signs of toxicity from these drugs).

No products indexed under this heading.

Fosinopril Sodium (Reports suggest that NSAIDs may diminish the antihypertensive effect of ACE-inhibitors. This interaction should be given consideration in patients taking NSAIDs concomitantly with ACE-inhibitors).

No products indexed under this heading.

Fosphenytoin Sodium (In vitro studies have shown that fenoprofen, because of its affinity for albumin,

may displace from their binding sites other drugs that are also albumin bound, and this may lead to drug interaction. Theoretically, fenoprofen could likewise be displayed.Patients receiving hydantins should be observed for increased activity drugs and, therefore, signs of toxicity from these drugs).

No products indexed under this heading.

Furosemide (Fenoprofen calcium may reduce the natriuretic effect of loop diuretics. This inhibition has been attributed to inhibition of renal prostaglandin synthesis. During concomitant therapy with NSAIDs, the patient should be observed closely for signs of renal failure, as well as to assure diuretic efficacy). Products include:
Furosemide Tablets 2154

Glimepiride (In vitro studies have shown that fenoprofen, because of its affinity for albumin, may displace from their bindings sites other drugs that are also albumin bound, and this may lead to drug interaction. Theoretically, fenoprofen could likewise be displayed. Patients receiving sulfonylureas should be observed for increased activity of these drugs and, therefore, signs of toxicity from these drugs). Products include:
Avandaryl Tablets 1379
Duetact Tablets 3226

Glipizide (In vitro studies have shown that fenoprofen, because of its affinity for albumin, may displace from their bindings sites other drugs that are also albumin bound, and this may lead to drug interaction. Theoretically, fenoprofen could likewise be displayed. Patients receiving sulfonamides should be observed for increased activity of these drugs and, therefore, signs of toxicity from these drugs).

No products indexed under this heading.

Glyburide (In vitro studies have shown that fenoprofen, because of its affinity for albumin, may displace from their bindings sites other drugs that are also albumin bound, and this may lead to drug interaction. Theoretically, fenoprofen could likewise be displayed. Patients receiving sulfonamides should be observed for increased activity of these drugs and, therefore, signs of toxicity from these drugs).

No products indexed under this heading.

Hydrochlorothiazide (In vitro studies have shown that fenoprofen, because of its affinity for albumin, may displace from their bindings sites other drugs that are also albumin bound, and this may lead to drug interaction. Theoretically, fenoprofen could likewise be displayed. Patients receiving sulfonylureas should be observed for increased activity of these drugs and, therefore, signs of toxicity from these drugs. Fenoprofen calcium may reduce the natriuretic effect of thiazides. This inhibition has been attributed to inhibition of renal prostaglandin synthesis. During concomitant therapy with NSAIDs, the patient should be observed closely for signs of renal failure, as well as to assure diuretic efficacy). Products include:
Aldoril Tablets 1910
Atacand HCT 651
Avalide Tablets 888

Avalide Tablets 2874
Benicar HCT Tablets 1044
Diovan HCT Tablets 2196
Dyazide Capsules 1423
Hyzaar 50-12.5 Tablets 1990
Hyzaar 100-12.5 Tablets 1990
Hyzaar 100-25 Tablets 1990
Lopressor HCT 50/25 Tablets 2241
Lopressor HCT 100/25 Tablets 2241
Lopressor HCT 100/50 Tablets 2241
Lotensin HCT Tablets 2246
Micardis HCT Tablets 856
Moduretic Tablets 2028
Prinzide Tablets 2056
Teveten HCT Tablets 1737
Timolide Tablets 2086
Uniretic Tablets 3100

Hydroflumethiazide (In vitro studies have shown that fenoprofen, because of its affinity for albumin, may displace from their bindings sites other drugs that are also albumin bound, and this may lead to drug interaction. Theoretically, fenoprofen could likewise be displayed. Patients receiving sulfonylureas should be observed for increased activity of these drugs and, therefore, signs of toxicity from these drugs. Fenoprofen calcium may reduce the natriuretic effect of thiazides. This inhibition has been attributed to inhibition of renal prostaglandin synthesis. During concomitant therapy with NSAIDs, the patient should be observed closely for signs of renal failure, as well as to assure diuretic efficacy).

No products indexed under this heading.

Indapamide (Fenoprofen calcium may reduce the natriuretic effect of diuretics. This inhibition has been attributed to inhibition of renal prostaglandin synthesis. During concomitant therapy with NSAIDs, the patient should be observed closely for signs of renal failure, as well as to assure diuretic efficacy). Products include:
Indapamide Tablets 2156

Lisinopril (Reports suggest that NSAIDs may diminish the antihypertensive effect of ACE-inhibitors. This interaction should be given consideration in patients taking NSAIDs concomitantly with ACE-inhibitors). Products include:
Prinivil Tablets 2052
Prinzide Tablets 2056

Lithium Carbonate (NSAIDs have produced an elevation of plasma lithium levels and a reduction in renal lithium clearance. The mean minimum lithium concentration increased 15% and the renal clearance was decreased by approximately 20%. These effects have been attributed to inhibition of renal prostaglandin synthesis by the NSAID. Thus, when NSAIDs and lithium are administered concurrently, subjects should be observed carefully for signs of lithium toxicity). Products include:
Lithobid Tablets 1692

Lithium Citrate (NSAIDs have produced an elevation of plasma lithium levels and a reduction in renal lithium clearance. The mean minimum lithium concentration increased 15% and the renal clearance was decreased by approximately 20%. These effects have been attributed to inhibition of renal prostaglandin synthesis by the NSAID. Thus, when NSAIDs and lithium are administered concurrently, subjects should be observed carefully for signs of lithi-

um toxicity).

No products indexed under this heading.

Magnesium Salicylate (The co-administration of aspirin decreases the biologic half-life of fenoprofen because of an increase in metabolic clearance that results in a greater amount of hydroxylated fenoprofen in the urine. Although the mechanism of interaction between fenoprofen and aspirin is not totally known, enzyme induction and displacement of fenoprofen from plasma albumin binding sites are possibilities. Because fenoprofen calcium has not been shown to produce any additional effect beyond that obtained with aspirin alone and because aspirin increases the rate of excretion of fenoprofen calcium, concomitant use of fenoprofen calcium and salicylates is not recommended).

No products indexed under this heading.

Mephenytoin (In vitro studies have shown that fenoprofen, because of its affinity for albumin, may displace from their binding sites other drugs that are also albumin bound, and this may lead to drug interaction. Theoretically, fenoprofen could likewise be displayed.Patients receiving hydantins should be observed for increased activity drugs and, therefore, signs of toxicity from these drugs).

No products indexed under this heading.

Methotrexate Sodium (NSAIDs have been reported to competitively inhibit methotrexate accumulation in rabbit kidney slices. This may indicate that they could enhance the toxicity of methotrexate. Caution should be used when NSAIDs are administered concomitantly with methotrexate).

No products indexed under this heading.

Methyclothiazide (In vitro studies have shown that fenoprofen, because of its affinity for albumin, may displace from their bindings sites other drugs that are also albumin bound, and this may lead to drug interaction. Theoretically, fenoprofen could likewise be displayed. Patients receiving sulfonylureas should be observed for increased activity of these drugs and, therefore, signs of toxicity from these drugs. Fenoprofen calcium may reduce the natriuretic effect of thiazides. This inhibition has been attributed to inhibition of renal prostaglandin synthesis. During concomitant therapy with NSAIDs, the patient should be observed closely for signs of renal failure, as well as to assure diuretic efficacy).

No products indexed under this heading.

Metolazone (Fenoprofen calcium may reduce the natriuretic effect of diuretics. This inhibition has been attributed to inhibition of renal prostaglandin synthesis. During concomitant therapy with NSAIDs, the patient should be observed closely for signs of renal failure, as well as to assure diuretic efficacy).

No products indexed under this heading.

Moexipril Hydrochloride (Reports suggest that NSAIDs may diminish the antihypertensive effect of ACE-inhibitors. This interaction should be given consideration in patients taking NSAIDs concomitantly with ACE-inhibitors). Products include:

Perindopril Erbumine (Reports suggest that NSAIDs may diminish the antihypertensive effect of ACE-inhibitors. This interaction should be given consideration in patients taking NSAIDs concomitantly with ACE-inhibitors). Products include:

Phenobarbital (Chronic administration of phenobarbital, a known enzyme inducer, may be associated with a decrease in the plasma half-life of fenoprofen. When phenobarbital is added to or withdrawn from treatment, dosage adjustment of fenoprofen calcium may be required). Products include:

Phenobarbital Sodium (Chronic administration of phenobarbital, a known enzyme inducer, may be associated with a decrease in the plasma half-life of fenoprofen. When phenobarbital is added to or withdrawn from treatment, dosage adjustment of fenoprofen calcium may be required).

No products indexed under this heading.

Phenytoin (In vitro studies have shown that fenoprofen, because of its affinity for albumin, may displace from their binding sites other drugs that are also albumin bound, and this may lead to drug interaction. Theoretically, fenoprofen could likewise be displayed. Patients receiving hydantins should be observed for increased activity drugs and, therefore, signs of toxicity from these drugs).

No products indexed under this heading.

Phenytoin Sodium (In vitro studies have shown that fenoprofen, because of its affinity for albumin, may displace from their binding sites other drugs that are also albumin bound, and this may lead to drug interaction. Theoretically, fenoprofen could likewise be displayed. Patients receiving hydantins should be observed for increased activity drugs and, therefore, signs of toxicity from these drugs). Products include:

Polythiazide (In vitro studies have shown that fenoprofen, because of its affinity for albumin, may displace from their bindings sites other drugs that are also albumin bound, and this may lead to drug interaction. Theoretically, fenoprofen could likewise be displayed. Patients receiving sulfonylureas should be observed for increased activity of these drugs and, therefore, signs of toxicity from these drugs. Fenoprofen calcium may reduce the natriuretic effect of thiazides. This inhibition has been attributed to inhibition of renal prostaglandin synthesis. During concomitant therapy with NSAIDs, the patient should be observed closely for signs of renal failure, as well as to assure diuretic efficacy).

No products indexed under this heading.

Quinapril Hydrochloride (Reports suggest that NSAIDs may diminish the antihypertensive effect of ACE-inhibitors. This interaction should be given consideration in patients taking NSAIDs concomitantly with ACE-inhibitors).

No products indexed under this heading.

Ramipril (Reports suggest that NSAIDs may diminish the antihypertensive effect of ACE-inhibitors. This interaction should be given consideration in patients taking NSAIDs concomitantly with ACE-inhibitors). Products include:

Salsalate (The co-administration of aspirin decreases the biologic half-life of fenoprofen because of an increase in metabolic clearance that results in a greater amount of hydroxylated fenoprofen in the urine. Although the mechanism of interaction between fenoprofen and aspirin is not totally known, enzyme induction and displacement of fenoprofen from plasma albumin binding sites are possibilities. Because fenoprofen calcium has not been shown to produce any additional effect beyond that obtained with aspirin alone and because aspirin increases the rate of excretion of fenoprofen calcium, concomitant use of fenoprofen calcium and salicylates is not recommended).

No products indexed under this heading.

Spirapril Hydrochloride (Reports suggest that NSAIDs may diminish the antihypertensive effect of ACE-inhibitors. This interaction should be given consideration in patients taking NSAIDs concomitantly with ACE-inhibitors).

No products indexed under this heading.

Spironolactone (Fenoprofen calcium may reduce the natriuretic effect of diuretics. This inhibition has been attributed to inhibition of renal prostaglandin synthesis. During concomitant therapy with NSAIDs, the patient should be observed closely for signs of renal failure, as well as to assure diuretic efficacy).

No products indexed under this heading.

Sulfacytine (In vitro studies have shown that fenoprofen, because of its affinity for albumin, may displace from their bindings sites other drugs that are also albumin bound, and this may lead to drug interaction. Theoretically, fenoprofen could likewise be displayed. Patients receiving sulfonamides should be observed for increased activity of these drugs and, therefore, signs of toxicity from these drugs).

No products indexed under this heading.

Sulfamethizole (In vitro studies have shown that fenoprofen, because of its affinity for albumin, may displace from their bindings sites other drugs that are also albumin bound, and this may lead to drug interaction. Theoretically, fenoprofen could likewise be displayed. Patients receiving sulfonamides should be observed for increased activity of these drugs and, therefore, signs of toxicity from these drugs).

No products indexed under this heading.

Sulfamethoxazole (In vitro studies have shown that fenoprofen, because of its affinity for albumin, may displace from their bindings sites other drugs that are also albumin bound, and this may lead to drug interaction. Theoretically, fenoprofen could likewise be displayed. Patients receiving sulfonamides should be observed for increased activity of these drugs and, therefore, signs of toxicity from these drugs).

No products indexed under this heading.

Sulfasalazine (In vitro studies have shown that fenoprofen, because of its affinity for albumin, may displace from their bindings sites other drugs that are also albumin bound, and this may lead to drug interaction. Theoretically, fenoprofen could likewise be displayed. Patients receiving sulfonamides should be observed for increased activity of these drugs and, therefore, signs of toxicity from these drugs).

No products indexed under this heading.

Sulfinpyrazone (In vitro studies have shown that fenoprofen, because of its affinity for albumin, may displace from their bindings sites other drugs that are also albumin bound, and this may lead to drug interaction. Theoretically, fenoprofen could likewise be displayed. Patients receiving sulfonamides should be observed for increased activity of these drugs and, therefore, signs of toxicity from these drugs).

No products indexed under this heading.

Sulfisoxazole Acetyl (In vitro studies have shown that fenoprofen, because of its affinity for albumin, may displace from their bindings sites other drugs that are also albumin bound, and this may lead to drug interaction. Theoretically, fenoprofen could likewise be displayed. Patients receiving sulfonamides should be observed for increased activity of these drugs and, therefore, signs of toxicity from these drugs).

No products indexed under this heading.

Sulfisoxazole Diolamine (In vitro studies have shown that fenoprofen, because of its affinity for albumin, may displace from their bindings sites other drugs that are also albumin bound, and this may lead to drug interaction. Theoretically, fenoprofen could likewise be displayed. Patients receiving sulfonamides should be observed for increased activity of these drugs and, therefore, signs of toxicity from these drugs).

No products indexed under this heading.

Tolazamide (In vitro studies have shown that fenoprofen, because of its affinity for albumin, may displace from their bindings sites other drugs that are also albumin bound, and this may lead to drug interaction. Theoretically, fenoprofen could likewise be displayed. Patients receiving sulfonamides should be observed for increased activity of these drugs and, therefore, signs of toxicity from these drugs).

No products indexed under this heading.

Tolbutamide (In vitro studies have shown that fenoprofen, because of its affinity for albumin, may displace from their bindings sites other drugs that are also albumin bound, and this may lead to drug interaction. Theoretically, fenoprofen could likewise be displayed. Patients receiving sulfonamides should be observed for increased activity of these drugs and, therefore, signs of toxicity from these drugs).

No products indexed under this heading.

Torsemide (Fenoprofen calcium may reduce the natriuretic effect of diuretics. This inhibition has been attributed to inhibition of renal prostaglandin synthesis. During concomitant therapy with NSAIDs, the patient should be observed closely for signs of renal failure, as well as to assure diuretic efficacy). Products include:

Trandolapril (Reports suggest that NSAIDs may diminish the antihypertensive effect of ACE-inhibitors. This interaction should be given consideration in patients taking NSAIDs concomitantly with ACE-inhibitors). Products include:

Triamterene (Fenoprofen calcium may reduce the natriuretic effect of diuretics. This inhibition has been attributed to inhibition of renal prostaglandin synthesis. During concomitant therapy with NSAIDs, the patient should be observed closely for signs of renal failure, as well as to assure diuretic efficacy). Products include:

Trichlormethiazide (In vitro studies have shown that fenoprofen, because of its affinity for albumin, may displace from their bindings sites other drugs that are also albumin bound, and this may lead to drug interaction. Theoretically, fenoprofen could likewise be displayed. Patients receiving sulfonylureas should be observed for increased activity of these drugs and, therefore, signs of toxicity from these drugs. Fenoprofen calcium may reduce the natriuretic effect of thiazides. This inhibition has been attributed to inhibition of renal prostaglandin synthesis. During concomitant therapy with NSAIDs, the patient should be observed closely for signs of renal failure, as well as to assure diuretic efficacy).

No products indexed under this heading.

Warfarin Sodium (In patients receiving coumarin-type anticoagulants, the addition of fenoprofen calcium to therapy could prolong the prothrombin time. Patients receiving both drugs should be under careful observation. The effects of warfarin and NSAIDs on GI bleeding are synergestic, such that users of both drugs together have a risk of serious GI bleeding higher than users of either drug alone). Products include:

NAMENDA ORAL SOLUTION

NAMENDA TABLETS
(Memantine Hydrochloride) 1195
May interact with carbonic anhydrase inhibitors, quinidine, urinary alkalinizing agents, and certain other agents. Compounds in these categories include:

Acetazolamide (Alterations of urine pH towards the alkaline condition by drugs that make the urine alkaline (e.g., carbonic anhydrase inhibitors) may lead to an accumulation of memantine with a possible increase in adverse effects; use with caution).
No products indexed under this heading.

Amantadine Hydrochloride (The combined use of memantine with other NMDA antagonists, like amantadine, has not been systemically evaluated and such use should be approached with caution). Products include:
Symmetrel Tablets 1135

Cimetidine (Co-administration with drugs that use the same renal cationic system, including cimetidine, could potentially result in altered plasma levels of both drugs). Products include:
Tagamet HB 200 Tablets 664

Cimetidine Hydrochloride (Co-administration with drugs that use the same renal cationic system, including cimetidine, could potentially result in altered plasma levels of both drugs).
No products indexed under this heading.

Dextromethorphan (The combined use of memantine with other NMDA antagonists, like dextromethorphan, has not been systemically evaluated and such use should be approached with caution).
No products indexed under this heading.

Dextromethorphan Hydrobromide (The combined use of memantine with other NMDA antagonists, like dextromethorphan, has not been systemically evaluated and such use should be approached with caution). Products include:
Comtrex Maximum Strength Cold & Cough Day/Night Caplets - Day Formulation 726
Comtrex Maximum Strength Cold & Cough Day/Night Caplets - Night Formulation 726
Comtrex Maximum Strength Non-Drowsy Cold & Cough Caplets 725
Children's Dimetapp DM Cold & Cough Elixir 731
Children's Dimetapp Long Acting Cough Plus Cold Syrup 731
Toddler's Dimetapp Cold and Cough Drops 732
Mucinex DM Extended-Release Bi-Layer Tablets 720
Refenesen DM Caplets 721
Robitussin Cough & Cold CF Liquid 735
Robitussin Cough & Cold Long-Acting Liquid 735
Robitussin Cough & Allergy Syrup .. 736
Robitussin Cough & Cold Nighttime Liquid 736
Robitussin Cough & Cold Pediatric Drops 735
Robitussin Cough, Cold & Flu Nighttime Liquid 738
Robitussin Cough & Congestion Liquid 738
Robitussin Cough Gels Long-Acting 737
Robitussin Cough Long Acting Liquid 739
Robitussin Cough DM Syrup 738
Robitussin Cough DM Infant Drops 738
Robitussin Pediatric Cough Long Acting Liquid 739
Robitussin Pediatric Cough & Cold Long-Acting Liquid 735
Robitussin Pediatric Cough & Cold Nighttime Liquid 736
Robitussin Sugar Free Cough 738
TheraFlu Cold & Cough Hot Liquid 740
TheraFlu Warming Relief Daytime Severe Cold 743
TheraFlu Thin Strips Long Acting Cough 744
Triaminic Daytime Cold & Cough Liquid 745
Triaminic Cough & Sore Throat Liquid 747
Triaminic Cough & Runny Nose Softchews 748
Triaminic Thin Strips Cold & Cough 778
Triaminic Infant Thin Strips Decongestant Plus Cough 747
Children's Tylenol Plus Flu Oral Suspension 749
Tylenol Cold Head Congestion Daytime Caplets with Cool Burst and Gelcaps 750
Tylenol Cold Multi-Symptom Daytime Liquid 752
Tylenol Cold Multi-Symptom Severe Daytime Liquid 752
Concentrated Tylenol Infants' Drops Plus Cold & Cough 754
Children's Tylenol Plus Cough & Runny Nose Suspension Liquid 1879
Children's Tylenol Plus Cough & Sore Throat Suspension Liquid 1879
Children's Tylenol Plus Flu Suspension Liquid 1881
Children's Tylenol Plus Multi-Symptom Cold Suspension Liquid 1879
Tylenol Cold Severe Congestion Non-Drowsy Caplets with Cool Burst 1874
Tylenol Cold Head Congestion Daytime Caplets with Cool Burst 1873
Tylenol Cold Head Congestion Nighttime Caplets with Cool Burst 1873
Tylenol Cold Head Congestion Severe Caplets with Cool Burst 1873
Tylenol Cold Multi-Symptom Daytime Caplets with Cool Burst and Gelcaps 1874
Tylenol Cold Multi-Symptom Daytime Liquid with Citrus Burst ... 1874
Tylenol Cold Multi-Symptom Nighttime Caplets with Cool Burst 1874
Tylenol Cold Multi-Symptom Nighttime Liquid with Cool Burst ... 1874
Tylenol Cold Multi-Symptom Severe Caplets with Cool Burst 1874
Tylenol Cold Multi-Symptom Severe Daytime Liquid with Citrus Burst 1874
Tylenol Cough & Sore Throat Daytime Liquid with Cool Burst 1877
Tylenol Cough & Sore Throat Nighttime Liquid with Cool Burst ... 1877
Concentrated Tylenol Infants' Drops Plus Cold and Cough 1879
Vicks 44 Cough Relief Liquid 2679
Vicks 44D Cough & Head Congestion Relief Liquid 2679
Vicks 44E Cough & Chest Congestion Relief Liquid 2679
Pediatric Vicks 44e Cough & Chest Congestion Relief Liquid 2676
Vicks 44M Cough, Cold & Flu Relief Liquid 2680
Pediatric Vicks 44m Cough & Cold Relief Liquid 2676
Vicks DayQuil LiquiCaps/Liquid Multi-Symptom Cold/Flu Relief 761
Vicks DayQuil Multi-Symptom Cold/Flu Relief LiquiCaps 2678
Vicks DayQuil Multi-Symptom Cold/Flu Relief Liquid 2678
Vicks NyQuil Multi-Symptom Cold/Flu Relief Liquid 2681
Children's Vicks NyQuil Cold/Cough Relief 756
Vicks NyQuil Multi-Symptom Cold/Flu Relief LiquiCaps 2681
Vicks NyQuil LiquiCaps/Liquid Multi-Symptom Cold/Flu Relief 763
Vicks NyQuil Cough Liquid 2680
Children's Vicks NyQuil Cold/Cough Relief Liquid 2680
Zicam Cough Max Nighttime Cough Spray 767
Zicam Cough Max Cough Spray 767
Zicam Cough Max Cough Melts 767
Zicam Cough Plus D Cough Spray 767
Zicam Cough Relief Cough Spray ... 767
Zicam Maximum Strength Flu Daytime 768
Zicam Maximum Strength Flu Nighttime 768

Dextromethorphan Polistirex (The combined use of memantine with other NMDA antagonists, like dextromethorphan, has not been systemically evaluated and such use should be approached with caution). Products include:
Delsym Extended-Release Suspension 12 Hour Cough Suppressant 611

Dextromethorphan tannate (The combined use of memantine with other NMDA antagonists, like dextromethorphan, has not been systemically evaluated and such use should be approached with caution).
No products indexed under this heading.

Dichlorphenamide (Alterations of urine pH towards the alkaline condition by drugs that make the urine alkaline (e.g., carbonic anhydrase inhibitors) may lead to an accumulation of memantine with a possible increase in adverse effects; use with caution). Products include:
Daranide Tablets 1950

Dorzolamide Hydrochloride (Alterations of urine pH towards the alkaline condition by drugs that make the urine alkaline (e.g., carbonic anhydrase inhibitors) may lead to an accumulation of memantine with a possible increase in adverse effects; use with caution). Products include:
Cosopt Sterile Ophthalmic Solution 1931
Trusopt Sterile Ophthalmic Solution 2095

Hydrochlorothiazide (Co-administration with drugs that use the same renal cationic system, including hydrochlorothiazide, could potentially result in altered plasma levels of both drugs. The co-administration of memantine and hydrochlorothiazide/triamterene decreased the bioavailability of hydrochlorothiazide by 20%). Products include:
Aldoril Tablets 1910
Atacand HCT 651
Avalide Tablets 888
Avalide Tablets 2874
Benicar HCT Tablets 1044
Diovan HCT Tablets 2196
Dyazide Capsules 1423
Hyzaar 50-12.5 Tablets 1990
Hyzaar 100-12.5 Tablets 1990
Hyzaar 100-25 Tablets 1990
Lopressor HCT 50/25 Tablets 2241
Lopressor HCT 100/25 Tablets 2241
Lopressor HCT 100/50 Tablets 2241
Lotensin HCT Tablets 2246
Micardis HCT Tablets 856
Moduretic Tablets 2028
Prinzide Tablets 2056
Teveten HCT Tablets 1737
Timolide Tablets 2086
Uniretic Tablets 3100

Hydrochlorothiazide Hydrochloride (Co-administration with drugs that use the same renal cationic system, including hydrochlorothiazide, could potentially result in altered plasma levels of both drugs. The co-administration of memantine and hydrochlorothiazide/triamterene decreased the bioavailability of hydrochlorothiazide by 20%).
No products indexed under this heading.

Ketamine (The combined use of memantine with other NMDA antagonists, like ketamine, has not been systemically evaluated and such use should be approached with caution).
No products indexed under this heading.

Ketamine Hydrochloride (The combined use of memantine with other NMDA antagonists, like ketamine, has not been systemically evaluated and such use should be approached with caution).
No products indexed under this heading.

Methazolamide (Alterations of urine pH towards the alkaline condition by drugs that make the urine alkaline (e.g., carbonic anhydrase inhibitors) may lead to an accumulation of memantine with a possible increase in adverse effects; use with caution).
No products indexed under this heading.

Nicotine (Co-administration with drugs that use the same renal cationic system, including nicotine, could potentially result in altered plasma levels of both drugs). Products include:
NicoDerm CQ Clear Patch 622

Nicotine Polacrilex (Co-administration with drugs that use the same renal cationic system, including nicotine, could potentially result in altered plasma levels of both drugs).
No products indexed under this heading.

Nicotine Salicylate (Co-administration with drugs that use the same renal cationic system, including nicotine, could potentially result in altered plasma levels of both drugs).
No products indexed under this heading.

Nicotine Sulfate (Co-administration with drugs that use the same renal cationic system, including nicotine, could potentially result in altered plasma levels of both drugs).
No products indexed under this heading.

Potassium Citrate (Alterations of urine pH towards the alkaline condition by drugs that make the urine alkaline may lead to an accumulation of memantine with a possible increase in adverse effects; use with caution). Products include:
Urocit-K Tablets 2144

Quinidine (Co-administration with drugs that use the same renal cationic system, including quinidine, could potentially result in altered plasma levels of both drugs).
No products indexed under this heading.

Quinidine Gluconate (Co-administration with drugs that use the same renal cationic system, including quinidine, could potentially result in altered plasma levels of both drugs).
No products indexed under this heading.

Quinidine Hydrochloride (Co-administration with drugs that use the same renal cationic system, including quinidine, could potentially result in altered plasma levels of both drugs).
No products indexed under this heading.

Quinidine Polygalacturonate (Co-administration with drugs that use the same renal cationic system, including quinidine, could potentially result in altered plasma levels of both drugs).
No products indexed under this heading.

Quinidine Sulfate (Co-administration with drugs that use the same renal cationic system, including quinidine, could potentially result in altered plasma levels of both drugs).
No products indexed under this heading.

Ranitidine Bismuth Citrate (Co-administration with drugs that use the same renal cationic system, including ranitidine, could potentially result in altered plasma levels of both drugs).
No products indexed under this heading.

Ranitidine Hydrochloride (Co-administration with drugs that use the same renal cationic system, including ranitidine, could potentially result in altered plasma levels of both drugs). Products include:
Zantac 1624
Zantac Injection 1619
Zantac Injection Pharmacy Bulk Package 1622

Sodium Bicarbonate (Alterations of urine pH towards the alkaline condition by drugs that make the urine alkaline (e.g., sodium bicarbonate) may lead to an accumulation of memantine with a possible increase in adverse effects; hence, use with caution). Products include:
Colyte with Flavor Packs for Oral Solution 3088
HalfLytely and Bisacodyl Tablets Bowel Prep Kit with Flavors Packs 881
TriLyte with Flavor Packs for Oral Solution 3100

Sodium Citrate (Alterations of urine pH towards the alkaline condition by drugs that make the urine alkaline may lead to an accumulation of memantine with a possible increase in adverse effects; use with caution).
No products indexed under this heading.

Triamterene (Co-administration with drugs that use the same renal cationic system, including triamterene, could potentially result in altered plasma levels of both drugs. However, co-administration of memantine and hydrochlorothiazide/triamterene did not affect the bioavailability of either memantine or triamterene). Products include:
Dyazide Capsules 1423
Dyrenium Capsules 3400

NAPHCON-A EYE DROPS
(Naphazoline Hydrochloride, Pheniramine Maleate) .... ⊙208
None cited in PDR database.

NAPROSYN SUSPENSION
(Naproxen) 2761
See EC-Naprosyn Delayed-Release Tablets

NAPROSYN TABLETS
(Naproxen) 2761
See EC-Naprosyn Delayed-Release Tablets

NASACORT AQ NASAL SPRAY
(Triamcinolone Acetonide) 2922
None cited in PDR database.

NASAL COMFORT MOISTURE THERAPY SPRAYS - SCENTED AND UNSCENTED
(Sodium Chloride) .... ▣733
None cited in PDR database.

NASONEX NASAL SPRAY
(Mometasone Furoate Monohydrate) 3043
None cited in PDR database.

NATACYN ANTIFUNGAL OPHTHALMIC SUSPENSION
(Natamycin) .... ⊙208
None cited in PDR database.

NATRECOR FOR INJECTION
(Nesiritide) 3127
None cited in PDR database.

NATURAL JOINT CAPSULES
(Dietary Supplement) .... ▣831
None cited in PDR database.

NATURETHROID TABLETS
(Levothyroxine, Liothyronine) 3401
May interact with androgens, corticosteroids, oral anticoagulants, estrogens, oral hypoglycemic agents, insulin, oral contraceptives, salicylates, and certain other agents. Compounds in these categories include:

Acarbose (Initiating thyroid replacement therapy may cause increases in insulin or oral hypoglycemic requirements). Products include:
Precose Tablets 751

Anisindione (Thyroid hormones appear to increase catabolism of vitamin K-dependent clotting factors. If oral anticoagulants are also being given, compensatory increases in clotting factor synthesis are impaired). Products include:
Miradon Tablets 3042

Aspirin (Preparations containing salicylates are known to interfere with laboratory tests performed in patients on thyroid hormone therapy). Products include:
Aggrenox Capsules 822
Bayer Aspirin 744
BC Allergy Sinus Cold Powder .... ▣677
BC Headache Powder .... ▣677
Arthritis Strength BC Powder .... ▣677
BC Sinus Cold Powder .... ▣677
Excedrin Extra Strength Caplets/Tablets/Geltabs .... ▣684
Excedrin Migraine Caplets/Tablets/Geltabs .... ▣609
Goody's Body Pain Formula Powder .... ▣684
Goody's Extra Strength Headache Powders .... ▣611
Goody's Extra Strength Pain Relief Tablets .... ▣685
Percodan Tablets 1132
St. Joseph 81 mg Aspirin Chewable and Enteric Coated Tablets 1869

Aspirin, Enteric Coated (Preparations containing salicylates are known to interfere with laboratory tests performed in patients on thyroid hormone therapy).
No products indexed under this heading.

Aspirin Buffered (Preparations containing salicylates are known to interfere with laboratory tests performed in patients on thyroid hormone therapy). Products include:
Bufferin Extra Strength Tablets .... ▣678
Bufferin Regular Strength Tablets .... ▣678

Betamethasone Acetate (Corticosteroids are known to interfere with laboratory tests performed in patients on thyroid hormone therapy).
No products indexed under this heading.

Betamethasone Sodium Phosphate (Corticosteroids are known to interfere with laboratory tests performed in patients on thyroid hormone therapy).
No products indexed under this heading.

Chlorotrianisene (Patients without a functioning thyroid gland who are on thyroid replacemet therapy may need to increase their thyroid dose if estrogens are given. Estrogens are also known to interfere with laboratory tests performed in patients on thyroid hormone therapy).
No products indexed under this heading.

Chlorpropamide (Initiating thyroid replacement therapy may cause increases in insulin or oral hypoglycemic requirements).
No products indexed under this heading.

Cholestyramine (Cholestyramine binds both levothyroxine and liothyronine in the intestine, thus impairing absorption of these thyroid hormones. Four to five hours should elapse between administration of cholestyramine and thyroid hormones).
No products indexed under this heading.

Choline Magnesium Trisalicylate (Preparations containing salicylates are known to interfere with laboratory tests performed in patients on thyroid hormone therapy).
No products indexed under this heading.

Colestipol (Colestipol binds both levothyroxine and liothyronine in the intestine, thus impairing absorption of these thyroid hormones. Four to five hours should elapse between administration of cholestyramine and thyroid hormones).
No products indexed under this heading.

Colestipol Hydrochloride (Colestipol binds both levothyroxine and liothyronine in the intestine, thus impairing absorption of these thyroid hormones. Four to five hours should elapse between administration of cholestyramine and thyroid hormones).
No products indexed under this heading.

Cortisone Acetate (Corticosteroids are known to interfere with laboratory tests performed in patients on thyroid hormone therapy).
No products indexed under this heading.

Desogestrel (Patients without a functioning thyroid gland who are on thyroid replacemet therapy may need to increase their thyroid dose if estrogens containing oral contraceptives are given. Estrogens containing oral contraceptives are also known to interfere with laboratory tests performed in patients on thyroid hormone therapy). Products include:
Mircette Tablets 1066

Dexamethasone (Corticosteroids are known to interfere with laboratory tests performed in patients on thyroid hormone therapy). Products include:
Ciprodex Otic Suspension 559
Decadron Tablets 1951
TobraDex Ophthalmic Ointment 562
TobraDex Ophthalmic Suspension 563

Dexamethasone Acetate (Corticosteroids are known to interfere with laboratory tests performed in patients on thyroid hormone therapy).
No products indexed under this heading.

Dexamethasone Sodium Phosphate (Corticosteroids are known to interfere with laboratory tests performed in patients on thyroid hormone therapy).
No products indexed under this heading.

Dicumarol (Thyroid hormones appear to increase catabolism of vitamin K-dependent clotting factors. If oral anticoagulants are also being given, compensatory increases in clotting factor synthesis are impaired).
No products indexed under this heading.

Dienestrol (Patients without a functioning thyroid gland who are on thyroid replacemet therapy may need to increase their thyroid dose if estrogens are given. Estrogens are also known to interfere with laboratory tests performed in patients on thyroid hormone therapy).
No products indexed under this heading.

Diethylstilbestrol (Patients without a functioning thyroid gland who are on thyroid replacemet therapy may need to increase their thyroid dose if estrogens are given. Estrogens are also known to interfere with laboratory tests performed in patients on thyroid hormone therapy).
No products indexed under this heading.

Diflunisal (Preparations containing salicylates are known to interfere with laboratory tests performed in patients on thyroid hormone therapy). Products include:
Dolobid Tablets 1955

Estradiol (Patients without a functioning thyroid gland who are on thyroid replacemet therapy may need to increase their thyroid dose if estrogens are given. Estrogens are also known to interfere with laboratory tests performed in patients on thyroid hormone therapy). Products include:
Angeliq Tablets 762
Climara Transdermal System 771
Climara Pro Transdermal System 776

Estrasorb Topical Emulsion 1147
Estring Vaginal Ring 2635
Menostar Transdermal System 782
Vagifem Tablets 2334

Estrogens, Conjugated (Patients without a functioning thyroid gland who are on thyroid replacemet therapy may need to increase their thyroid dose if estrogens are given. Estrogens are also known to interfere with laboratory tests performed in patients on thyroid hormone therapy). Products include:

Premarin Intravenous 3442
Premarin Tablets 3446
Premarin Vaginal Cream 3452
Premphase Tablets 3456
Prempro Tablets 3456

Estrogens, Esterified (Patients without a functioning thyroid gland who are on thyroid replacemet therapy may need to increase their thyroid dose if estrogens are given. Estrogens are also known to interfere with laboratory tests performed in patients on thyroid hormone therapy). Products include:

Estratest Tablets 3199
Estratest H.S. Tablets 3199

Estropipate (Patients without a functioning thyroid gland who are on thyroid replacemet therapy may need to increase their thyroid dose if estrogens are given. Estrogens are also known to interfere with laboratory tests performed in patients on thyroid hormone therapy).

No products indexed under this heading.

Ethinyl Estradiol (Patients without a functioning thyroid gland who are on thyroid replacemet therapy may need to increase their thyroid dose if estrogens are given. Estrogens are also known to interfere with laboratory tests performed in patients on thyroid hormone therapy). Products include:

Mircette Tablets 1066
NuvaRing 2340
Ortho-Cyclen/Ortho Tri-Cyclen 2429
Ortho Evra Transdermal System 2417
Ortho Tri-Cyclen Lo Tablets 2436
Seasonique Tablets 1077
Yasmin 28 Tablets 796
Yaz Tablets 803

Ethynodiol Diacetate (Patients without a functioning thyroid gland who are on thyroid replacemet therapy may need to increase their thyroid dose if estrogens containing oral contraceptives are given. Estrogens containing oral contraceptives are also known to interfere with laboratory tests performed in patients on thyroid hormone therapy).

No products indexed under this heading.

Fludrocortisone Acetate (Corticosteroids are known to interfere with laboratory tests performed in patients on thyroid hormone therapy).

No products indexed under this heading.

Fluoxymesterone (Androgens are known to interfere with laboratory tests performed in patients on thyroid hormone therapy). Products include:

Androxy Tablets 3335

Glimepiride (Initiating thyroid replacement therapy may cause increases in insulin or oral hypoglycemic requirements). Products include:

Avandaryl Tablets 1379
Duetact Tablets 3226

Glipizide (Initiating thyroid replacement therapy may cause increases in insulin or oral hypoglycemic requirements).

No products indexed under this heading.

Glyburide (Initiating thyroid replacement therapy may cause increases in insulin or oral hypoglycemic requirements).

No products indexed under this heading.

Hydrocortisone (Corticosteroids are known to interfere with laboratory tests performed in patients on thryoid hormone therapy). Products include:

Colocort Rectal Suspension, USP (Retention) 100 mg/60 mL.......... 2476
Hydrocortone Tablets 1989
Preparation H Hydrocortisone Cream .... ▣ 646

Hydrocortisone Acetate (Corticosteroids are known to interfere with laboratory tests performed in patients on thryoid hormone therapy). Products include:

Analpram-HC 1159
Pramosone 1161
ProctoFoam-HC 3099

Hydrocortisone Sodium Phosphate (Corticosteroids are known to interfere with laboratory tests performed in patients on thryoid hormone therapy).

No products indexed under this heading.

Hydrocortisone Sodium Succinate (Corticosteroids are known to interfere with laboratory tests performed in patients on thryoid hormone therapy).

No products indexed under this heading.

Insulin, Human, Zinc Suspension (Initiating thyroid replacement therapy may cause increases in insulin or oral hypoglycemic requirements). Products include:

Humulin L, 100 Units 1794
Humulin U, 100 Units 1800

Insulin, Human NPH (Initiating thyroid replacement therapy may cause increases in insulin or oral hypoglycemic requirements). Products include:

Humulin N, 100 Units 1795
Humulin N Pen 1797

Insulin, Human Regular (Initiating thyroid replacement therapy may cause increases in insulin or oral hypoglycemic requirements). Products include:

Humulin R, 100 Units 1798

Insulin, Human Regular and Human NPH Mixture (Initiating thyroid replacement therapy may cause increases in insulin or oral hypoglycemic requirements). Products include:

Humulin 50/50, 100 Units 1791
Humulin 70/30 Pen 1793

Insulin, NPH (Initiating thyroid replacement therapy may cause increases in insulin or oral hypoglycemic requirements).

No products indexed under this heading.

Insulin, Regular (Initiating thyroid replacement therapy may cause increases in insulin or oral hypoglycemic requirements).

No products indexed under this heading.

Insulin, Zinc Crystals (Initiating thyroid replacement therapy may cause increases in insulin or oral hypoglycemic requirements).

No products indexed under this heading.

Insulin, Zinc Suspension (Initiating thyroid replacement therapy may cause increases in insulin or oral hypoglycemic requirements).

No products indexed under this heading.

Insulin Aspart, Human Regular (Initiating thyroid replacement therapy may cause increases in insulin or oral hypoglycemic requirements). Products include:

NovoLog Injection 2326

Insulin glargine (Initiating thyroid replacement therapy may cause increases in insulin or oral hypoglycemic requirements). Products include:

Lantus Injection 2909

Insulin Lispro, Human (Initiating thyroid replacement therapy may cause increases in insulin or oral hypoglycemic requirements). Products include:

Humalog-Pen 1781
Humalog Mix 50/50-Pen 1783
Humalog Mix 75/25-Pen 1785

Insulin Lispro Protamine, Human (Initiating thyroid replacement therapy may cause increases in insulin or oral hypoglycemic requirements). Products include:

Humalog Mix 50/50-Pen 1783
Humalog Mix 75/25-Pen 1785

Iodine Preparations (Iodine-containing preparations are known to interfere with laboratory tests performed in patients on thyroid hormone therapy).

No products indexed under this heading.

Levonorgestrel (Patients without a functioning thyroid gland who are on thyroid replacemet therapy may need to increase their thyroid dose if estrogens containing oral contraceptives are given. Estrogens containing oral contraceptives are also known to interfere with laboratory tests performed in patients on thyroid hormone therapy). Products include:

Climara Pro Transdermal System 776
Mirena Intrauterine System 787
Plan B Tablets 1076
Seasonique Tablets 1077

Magnesium Salicylate (Preparations containing salicylates are known to interfere with laboratory tests performed in patients on thyroid hormone therapy).

No products indexed under this heading.

Mestranol (Patients without a functioning thyroid gland who are on thyroid replacemet therapy may need to increase their thyroid dose if estrogens containing oral contraceptives are given. Estrogens containing oral contraceptives are also known to interfere with laboratory tests performed in patients on thyroid hormone therapy).

No products indexed under this heading.

Metformin Hydrochloride (Initiating thyroid replacement therapy may cause increases in insulin or oral hypoglycemic requirements). Products include:

ActoPlus Met Tablets 3214
Avandamet Tablets 1373

Fortamet Extended-Release Tablets 3115

Methylprednisolone Acetate (Corticosteroids are known to interfere with laboratory tests performed in patients on thryoid hormone therapy). Products include:

Depo-Medrol Injectable Suspension 2617
Depo-Medrol Single-Dose Vial 2619

Methylprednisolone Sodium Succinate (Corticosteroids are known to interfere with laboratory tests performed in patients on thyroid hormone therapy).

No products indexed under this heading.

Methyltestosterone (Androgens are known to interfere with laboratory tests performed in patients on thyroid hormone therapy). Products include:

Estratest Tablets 3199
Estratest H.S. Tablets 3199

Miglitol (Initiating thyroid replacement therapy may cause increases in insulin or oral hypoglycemic requirements).

No products indexed under this heading.

Norethindrone (Patients without a functioning thyroid gland who are on thyroid replacemet therapy may need to increase their thyroid dose if estrogens containing oral contraceptives are given. Estrogens containing oral contraceptives are also known to interfere with laboratory tests performed in patients on thyroid hormone therapy). Products include:

Ortho Micronor Tablets 2426

Norethynodrel (Patients without a functioning thyroid gland who are on thyroid replacemet therapy may need to increase their thyroid dose if estrogens containing oral contraceptives are given. Estrogens containing oral contraceptives are also known to interfere with laboratory tests performed in patients on thyroid hormone therapy).

No products indexed under this heading.

Norgestimate (Patients without a functioning thyroid gland who are on thyroid replacemet therapy may need to increase their thyroid dose if estrogens containing oral contraceptives are given. Estrogens containing oral contraceptives are also known to interfere with laboratory tests performed in patients on thyroid hormone therapy). Products include:

Ortho-Cyclen/Ortho Tri-Cyclen 2429
Ortho Tri-Cyclen Lo Tablets 2436

Norgestrel (Patients without a functioning thyroid gland who are on thyroid replacemet therapy may need to increase their thyroid dose if estrogens containing oral contraceptives are given. Estrogens containing oral contraceptives are also known to interfere with laboratory tests performed in patients on thyroid hormone therapy).

No products indexed under this heading.

Oxandrolone (Androgens are known to interfere with laboratory tests performed in patients on thyroid hormone therapy). Products include:

Oxandrin Tablets 2962

Oxymetholone (Androgens are known to interfere with laboratory tests performed in patients on thyroid hormone therapy).
No products indexed under this heading.

Pioglitazone Hydrochloride (Initiating thyroid replacement therapy may cause increases in insulin or oral hypoglycemic requirements). Products include:
ActoPlus Met Tablets 3214
Actos Tablets 3219
Duetact Tablets 3226

Polyestradiol Phosphate (Patients without a functioning thyroid gland who are on thyroid replacemet therapy may need to increase their thyroid dose if estrogens are given. Estrogens are also known to interfere with laboratory tests performed in patients on thyroid hormone therapy).
No products indexed under this heading.

Prednisolone Acetate (Corticosteroids are known to interfere with laboratory tests performed in patients on thyroid hormone therapy). Products include:
Blephamide Ophthalmic Ointment 568
Blephamide Ophthalmic Suspension 569
Poly-Pred Ophthalmic Suspension .... ⊙233
Pred Forte Ophthalmic Suspension .... ⊙235
Pred Mild Ophthalmic Suspension .... ⊙238
Pred-G Ophthalmic Ointment .... ⊙237
Pred-G Ophthalmic Suspension ...... ⊙236

Prednisolone Sodium Phosphate (Corticosteroids are known to interfere with laboratory tests performed in patients on thyroid hormone therapy).
No products indexed under this heading.

Prednisolone Tebutate (Corticosteroids are known to interfere with laboratory tests performed in patients on thyroid hormone therapy).
No products indexed under this heading.

Prednisone (Corticosteroids are known to interfere with laboratory tests performed in patients on thyroid hormone therapy).
No products indexed under this heading.

Quinestrol (Patients without a functioning thyroid gland who are on thyroid replacemet therapy may need to increase their thyroid dose if estrogens are given. Estrogens are also known to interfere with laboratory tests performed in patients on thyroid hormone therapy).
No products indexed under this heading.

Repaglinide (Initiating thyroid replacement therapy may cause increases in insulin or oral hypoglycemic requirements).
No products indexed under this heading.

Rosiglitazone Maleate (Initiating thyroid replacement therapy may cause increases in insulin or oral hypoglycemic requirements). Products include:
Avandamet Tablets 1373
Avandaryl Tablets 1379
Avandia Tablets 1384

Salsalate (Preparations containing salicylates are known to interfere with laboratory tests performed in patients on thyroid hormone therapy).
No products indexed under this heading.

Stanozolol (Androgens are known to interfere with laboratory tests performed in patients on thyroid hormone therapy).
No products indexed under this heading.

Tolazamide (Initiating thyroid replacement therapy may cause increases in insulin or oral hypoglycemic requirements).
No products indexed under this heading.

Tolbutamide (Initiating thyroid replacement therapy may cause increases in insulin or oral hypoglycemic requirements).
No products indexed under this heading.

Triamcinolone (Corticosteroids are known to interfere with laboratory tests performed in patients on thyroid hormone therapy).
No products indexed under this heading.

Triamcinolone Acetonide (Corticosteroids are known to interfere with laboratory tests performed in patients on thyroid hormone therapy). Products include:
Azmacort Inhalation Aerosol 1726
Nasacort AQ Nasal Spray 2922

Triamcinolone Diacetate (Corticosteroids are known to interfere with laboratory tests performed in patients on thyroid hormone therapy).
No products indexed under this heading.

Triamcinolone Hexacetonide (Corticosteroids are known to interfere with laboratory tests performed in patients on thyroid hormone therapy).
No products indexed under this heading.

Troglitazone (Initiating thyroid replacement therapy may cause increases in insulin or oral hypoglycemic requirements).
No products indexed under this heading.

Warfarin Sodium (Thyroid hormones appear to increase catabolism of vitamin K-dependent clotting factors. If oral anticoagulants are also being given, compensatory increases in clotting factor synthesis are impaired). Products include:
Coumadin for Injection 898
Coumadin Tablets 898

NEMBUTAL SODIUM SOLUTION, USP

(Pentobarbital Sodium) 2470
May interact with central nervous system depressants, corticosteroids, oral anticoagulants, doxycycline, estrogens, monoamine oxidase inhibitors, oral contraceptives, phenytoin, and certain other agents. Compounds in these categories include:

Alfentanil Hydrochloride (Concomitant use of other CNS depressants may produce additive depressant effects).
No products indexed under this heading.

Alprazolam (Concomitant use of other CNS depressants may produce additive depressant effects). Products include:
Niravam Orally Disintegrating Tablets 3092

Anisindione (Barbiturates can induce hepatic microsomal enzymes resulting in increased metabolism and decreased anticoagulant response of oral anticoagulants). Products include:
Miradon Tablets 3042

Aprobarbital (Concomitant use of other CNS depressants may produce additive depressant effects).
No products indexed under this heading.

Betamethasone Acetate (Barbiturates appear to enhance the metabolism of exogenous corticosteroids probably through the induction of hepatic microsomal enzymes).
No products indexed under this heading.

Betamethasone Sodium Phosphate (Barbiturates appear to enhance the metabolism of exogenous corticosteroids probably through the induction of hepatic microsomal enzymes).
No products indexed under this heading.

Buprenorphine Hydrochloride (Concomitant use of other CNS depressants may produce additive depressant effects). Products include:
Buprenex Injectable 2716
Suboxone Tablets 2717
Subutex Tablets 2717

Buspirone Hydrochloride (Concomitant use of other CNS depressants may produce additive depressant effects).
No products indexed under this heading.

Butabarbital (Concomitant use of other CNS depressants may produce additive depressant effects).
No products indexed under this heading.

Butalbital (Concomitant use of other CNS depressants may produce additive depressant effects).
No products indexed under this heading.

Chlordiazepoxide (Concomitant use of other CNS depressants may produce additive depressant effects).
No products indexed under this heading.

Chlordiazepoxide Hydrochloride (Concomitant use of other CNS depressants may produce additive depressant effects). Products include:
Librium Capsules 3347

Chlorotrianisene (Pretreatment with or co-administration of phenobarbital may decrease the effect of estrogen by increasing its metabolism; application of this data to other barbiturates appears valid).
No products indexed under this heading.

Chlorpromazine (Concomitant use of other CNS depressants may produce additive depressant effects).
No products indexed under this heading.

Chlorpromazine Hydrochloride (Concomitant use of other CNS depressants may produce additive depressant effects).
No products indexed under this heading.

Chlorprothixene (Concomitant use of other CNS depressants may produce additive depressant effects).
No products indexed under this heading.

Chlorprothixene Hydrochloride (Concomitant use of other CNS depressants may produce additive depressant effects).
No products indexed under this heading.

Chlorprothixene Lactate (Concomitant use of other CNS depressants may produce additive depressant effects).
No products indexed under this heading.

Clorazepate Dipotassium (Concomitant use of other CNS depressants may produce additive depressant effects). Products include:
Tranxene 2474

Clozapine (Concomitant use of other CNS depressants may produce additive depressant effects). Products include:
Clozaril Tablets 2184
FazaClo Orally Disintegrating Tablets 551

Codeine Phosphate (Concomitant use of other CNS depressants may produce additive depressant effects). Products include:
Tylenol with Codeine Tablets 2391

Cortisone Acetate (Barbiturates appear to enhance the metabolism of exogenous corticosteroids probably through the induction of hepatic microsomal enzymes).
No products indexed under this heading.

Desflurane (Concomitant use of other CNS depressants may produce additive depressant effects).
No products indexed under this heading.

Desogestrel (Pretreatment with or co-administration of phenobarbital may decrease the effect of estrogen by increasing its metabolism; application of this data to other barbiturates appears valid; higher incidence of pregnancy in patients on co-administration). Products include:
Mircette Tablets 1066

Dexamethasone (Barbiturates appear to enhance the metabolism of exogenous corticosteroids probably through the induction of hepatic microsomal enzymes). Products include:
Ciprodex Otic Suspension 559
Decadron Tablets 1951
TobraDex Ophthalmic Ointment 562
TobraDex Ophthalmic Suspension ... 563

Dexamethasone Acetate (Barbiturates appear to enhance the metabolism of exogenous corticosteroids probably through the induction of hepatic microsomal enzymes).
No products indexed under this heading.

Dexamethasone Sodium Phosphate (Barbiturates appear to enhance the metabolism of exogenous corticosteroids probably through the induction of hepatic microsomal enzymes).
No products indexed under this heading.

Dezocine (Concomitant use of other CNS depressants may produce additive depressant effects).
No products indexed under this heading.

Diazepam (Concomitant use of other CNS depressants may produce additive depressant effects). Products include:
Diastat Rectal Delivery System 3343
Valium Tablets 2819

Dicumarol (Barbiturates can induce hepatic microsomal enzymes resulting in increased metabolism and decreased anticoagulant response of oral anticoagulants).
No products indexed under this heading.

Dienestrol (Pretreatment with or co-administration of phenobarbital may decrease the effect of estrogen by increasing its metabolism; application of this data to other barbiturates appears valid).
No products indexed under this heading.

Diethylstilbestrol (Pretreatment with or co-administration of phenobarbital may decrease the effect of estrogen by increasing its metabolism; application of this data to other barbiturates appears valid).
No products indexed under this heading.

Divalproex Sodium (Valproate appears to decrease barbiturate metabolism). Products include:
Depakote Sprinkle Capsules 422
Depakote Tablets 427
Depakote ER Tablets 434

Doxycycline Calcium (Phenobarbital has been shown to shorten the half-life of doxycycline for as long as 2 weeks after barbiturate therapy is discontinued; application of this data to other barbiturates appears valid).
No products indexed under this heading.

Doxycycline Hyclate (Phenobarbital has been shown to shorten the half-life of doxycycline for as long as 2 weeks after barbiturate therapy is discontinued; application of this data to other barbiturates appears valid).
No products indexed under this heading.

Doxycycline Monohydrate (Phenobarbital has been shown to shorten the half-life of doxycycline for as long as 2 weeks after barbiturate therapy is discontinued; application of this data to other barbiturates appears valid). Products include:
Oracea Capsules 1000

Droperidol (Concomitant use of other CNS depressants may produce additive depressant effects).
No products indexed under this heading.

Enflurane (Concomitant use of other CNS depressants may produce additive depressant effects).
No products indexed under this heading.

Estazolam (Concomitant use of other CNS depressants may produce additive depressant effects). Products include:
ProSom Tablets 517

Estradiol (Pretreatment with or co-administration of phenobarbital may decrease the effect of estrogen by increasing its metabolism; application of this data to other barbiturates appears valid). Products include:
Angeliq Tablets 762
Climara Transdermal System 771
Climara Pro Transdermal System 776
Estrasorb Topical Emulsion 1147
Estring Vaginal Ring 2635
Menostar Transdermal System 782
Vagifem Tablets 2334

Estrogens, Conjugated (Pretreatment with or co-administration of phenobarbital may decrease the effect of estrogen by increasing its metabolism; application of this data to other barbiturates appears valid). Products include:
Premarin Intravenous 3442
Premarin Tablets 3446
Premarin Vaginal Cream 3452
Premphase Tablets 3456
Prempro Tablets 3456

Estrogens, Esterified (Pretreatment with or co-administration of phenobarbital may decrease the effect of estrogen by increasing its metabolism; application of this data to other barbiturates appears valid). Products include:
Estratest Tablets 3199
Estratest H.S. Tablets 3199

Estropipate (Pretreatment with or co-administration of phenobarbital may decrease the effect of estrogen by increasing its metabolism; application of this data to other barbiturates appears valid).
No products indexed under this heading.

Ethanol (Concomitant use of other CNS depressants may produce additive depressant effects).
No products indexed under this heading.

Ethchlorvynol (Concomitant use of other CNS depressants may produce additive depressant effects).
No products indexed under this heading.

Ethinamate (Concomitant use of other CNS depressants may produce additive depressant effects).
No products indexed under this heading.

Ethinyl Estradiol (Pretreatment with or co-administration of phenobarbital may decrease the effect of estrogen by increasing its metabolism; application of this data to other barbiturates appears valid; higher incidence of pregnancy in patients on co-administration). Products include:
Mircette Tablets 1066
NuvaRing 2340
Ortho-Cyclen/Ortho Tri-Cyclen 2429
Ortho Evra Transdermal System 2417
Ortho Tri-Cyclen Lo Tablets 2436
Seasonique Tablets 1077
Yasmin 28 Tablets 796
Yaz Tablets 803

Ethyl Alcohol (Concomitant use of other CNS depressants may produce additive depressant effects).
No products indexed under this heading.

Ethynodiol Diacetate (Pretreatment with or co-administration of phenobarbital may decrease the effect of estrogen by increasing its metabolism; application of this data to other barbiturates appears valid; higher incidence of pregnancy in patients on co-administration).
No products indexed under this heading.

Fentanyl (Concomitant use of other CNS depressants may produce additive depressant effects). Products include:
Duragesic Transdermal System 2373
Ionsys Transdermal System 2379

Fentanyl Citrate (Concomitant use of other CNS depressants may produce additive depressant effects). Products include:
Actiq 979

Fludrocortisone Acetate (Barbiturates appear to enhance the metabolism of exogenous corticosteroids probably through the induction of hepatic microsomal enzymes).
No products indexed under this heading.

Fluphenazine Decanoate (Concomitant use of other CNS depressants may produce additive depressant effects).
No products indexed under this heading.

Fluphenazine Enanthate (Concomitant use of other CNS depressants may produce additive depressant effects).
No products indexed under this heading.

Fluphenazine Hydrochloride (Concomitant use of other CNS depressants may produce additive depressant effects).
No products indexed under this heading.

Flurazepam Hydrochloride (Concomitant use of other CNS depressants may produce additive depressant effects). Products include:
Dalmane Capsules 3342

Fosphenytoin Sodium (The effect of barbiturates on the metabolism of phenytoin appears to be variable).
No products indexed under this heading.

Furazolidone (Co-administration with MAO inhibitors prolongs the effects of barbiturates probably because the metabolism of the barbiturate is inhibited).
No products indexed under this heading.

Glutethimide (Concomitant use of other CNS depressants may produce additive depressant effects).
No products indexed under this heading.

Griseofulvin (Phenobarbital appears to interfere with the absorption of orally administered griseofulvin, thus decreasing its blood level; application of this data to other barbiturates appears valid). Products include:
Gris-PEG Tablets 2502

Haloperidol (Concomitant use of other CNS depressants may produce additive depressant effects).
No products indexed under this heading.

Haloperidol Decanoate (Concomitant use of other CNS depressants may produce additive depressant effects).
No products indexed under this heading.

Hydrocodone Bitartrate (Concomitant use of other CNS depressants may produce additive depressant effects). Products include:
Hycodan 1116
Hycotuss Expectorant Syrup 1117
Vicodin Tablets 535
Vicodin ES Tablets 536
Vicodin HP Tablets 538
Vicoprofen Tablets 539
Zydone Tablets 1139

Hydrocodone Polistirex (Concomitant use of other CNS depressants may produce additive depressant effects). Products include:
Tussionex Pennkinetic Extended-Release Suspension 3327

Hydrocortisone (Barbiturates appear to enhance the metabolism of exogenous corticosteroids probably through the induction of hepatic microsomal enzymes). Products include:
Colocort Rectal Suspension, USP (Retention) 100 mg/60 mL 2476
Hydrocortone Tablets 1989
Preparation H Hydrocortisone Cream 646

Hydrocortisone Acetate (Barbiturates appear to enhance the metabolism of exogenous corticosteroids probably through the induction of hepatic microsomal enzymes). Products include:
Analpram-HC 1159
Pramosone 1161
ProctoFoam-HC 3099

Hydrocortisone Sodium Phosphate (Barbiturates appear to enhance the metabolism of exogenous corticosteroids probably through the induction of hepatic microsomal enzymes).
No products indexed under this heading.

Hydrocortisone Sodium Succinate (Barbiturates appear to enhance the metabolism of exogenous corticosteroids probably through the induction of hepatic microsomal enzymes).
No products indexed under this heading.

Hydromorphone Hydrochloride (Concomitant use of other CNS depressants may produce additive depressant effects). Products include:
Dilaudid 440
Dilaudid Non-Sterile Powder 440
Dilaudid Oral Liquid 445
Dilaudid Rectal Suppositories 440
Dilaudid Tablets 440
Dilaudid Tablets - 8 mg 445
Dilaudid-HP 442

Hydroxyzine Hydrochloride (Concomitant use of other CNS depressants may produce additive depressant effects).
No products indexed under this heading.

Isocarboxazid (Co-administration with MAO inhibitors prolongs the effects of barbiturates probably because the metabolism of the barbiturate is inhibited).
No products indexed under this heading.

Isoflurane (Concomitant use of other CNS depressants may produce additive depressant effects).
No products indexed under this heading.

Ketamine Hydrochloride (Concomitant use of other CNS depressants may produce additive depressant effects).
No products indexed under this heading.

Levomethadyl Acetate Hydrochloride (Concomitant use of other CNS depressants may produce additive depressant effects).
No products indexed under this heading.

Levonorgestrel (Pretreatment with or co-administration of phenobarbital may decrease the effect of estrogen by increasing its metabolism; application of this data to other barbiturates appears valid; higher incidence of pregnancy in patients on co-administration). Products include:

IMPORTANT NOTE: Always consult each drug listing in the patient's regimen for possible interactions.

Climara Pro Transdermal System 776
Mirena Intrauterine System 787
Plan B Tablets 1076
Seasonique Tablets 1077

Levorphanol Tartrate (Concomitant use of other CNS depressants may produce additive depressant effects).
No products indexed under this heading.

Lorazepam (Concomitant use of other CNS depressants may produce additive depressant effects).
No products indexed under this heading.

Loxapine Hydrochloride (Concomitant use of other CNS depressants may produce additive depressant effects).
No products indexed under this heading.

Loxapine Succinate (Concomitant use of other CNS depressants may produce additive depressant effects).
No products indexed under this heading.

Meperidine Hydrochloride (Concomitant use of other CNS depressants may produce additive depressant effects).
No products indexed under this heading.

Mephobarbital (Concomitant use of other CNS depressants may produce additive depressant effects).
No products indexed under this heading.

Meprobamate (Concomitant use of other CNS depressants may produce additive depressant effects).
No products indexed under this heading.

Mesoridazine Besylate (Concomitant use of other CNS depressants may produce additive depressant effects).
No products indexed under this heading.

Mestranol (Pretreatment with or co-administration of phenobarbital may decrease the effect of estrogen by increasing its metabolism; application of this data to other barbiturates appears valid; higher incidence of pregnancy in patients on co-administration).
No products indexed under this heading.

Methadone Hydrochloride (Concomitant use of other CNS depressants may produce additive depressant effects).
No products indexed under this heading.

Methohexital Sodium (Concomitant use of other CNS depressants may produce additive depressant effects).
No products indexed under this heading.

Methotrimeprazine (Concomitant use of other CNS depressants may produce additive depressant effects).
No products indexed under this heading.

Methoxyflurane (Concomitant use of other CNS depressants may produce additive depressant effects).
No products indexed under this heading.

Methylprednisolone Acetate (Barbiturates appear to enhance the metabolism of exogenous corticosteroids probably through the induction of hepatic microsomal enzymes). Products include:
Depo-Medrol Injectable Suspension 2617
Depo-Medrol Single-Dose Vial 2619

Methylprednisolone Sodium Succinate (Barbiturates appear to enhance the metabolism of exogenous corticosteroids probably through the induction of hepatic microsomal enzymes).
No products indexed under this heading.

Midazolam Hydrochloride (Concomitant use of other CNS depressants may produce additive depressant effects).
No products indexed under this heading.

Moclobemide (Co-administration with MAO inhibitors prolongs the effects of barbiturates probably because the metabolism of the barbiturate is inhibited).
No products indexed under this heading.

Molindone Hydrochloride (Concomitant use of other CNS depressants may produce additive depressant effects). Products include:
Moban Tablets 1119

Morphine Sulfate (Concomitant use of other CNS depressants may produce additive depressant effects). Products include:
Avinza Capsules 1741
Kadian Capsules 577
MS Contin Tablets 2701

Norethindrone (Pretreatment with or co-administration of phenobarbital may decrease the effect of estrogen by increasing its metabolism; application of this data to other barbiturates appears valid; higher incidence of pregnancy in patients on co-administration). Products include:
Ortho Micronor Tablets 2426

Norethynodrel (Pretreatment with or co-administration of phenobarbital may decrease the effect of estrogen by increasing its metabolism; application of this data to other barbiturates appears valid; higher incidence of pregnancy in patients on co-administration).
No products indexed under this heading.

Norgestimate (Pretreatment with or co-administration of phenobarbital may decrease the effect of estrogen by increasing its metabolism; application of this data to other barbiturates appears valid; higher incidence of pregnancy in patients on co-administration). Products include:
Ortho-Cyclen/Ortho Tri-Cyclen 2429
Ortho Tri-Cyclen Lo Tablets 2436

Norgestrel (Pretreatment with or co-administration of phenobarbital may decrease the effect of estrogen by increasing its metabolism; application of this data to other barbiturates appears valid; higher incidence of pregnancy in patients on co-administration).
No products indexed under this heading.

Olanzapine (Concomitant use of other CNS depressants may produce additive depressant effects). Products include:
Symbyax Capsules 1819
Zyprexa Tablets 1830
Zyprexa IntraMuscular 1830
Zyprexa ZYDIS Orally Disintegrating Tablets 1830

Oxazepam (Concomitant use of other CNS depressants may produce additive depressant effects).
No products indexed under this heading.

Oxycodone Hydrochloride (Concomitant use of other CNS depressants may produce additive depressant effects). Products include:
OxyContin Tablets 2703
OxyFast Oral Concentrate Solution.. 2708
OxyIR Capsules 2708
Percocet Tablets 1131
Percodan Tablets 1132

Pargyline Hydrochloride (Co-administration with MAO inhibitors prolongs the effects of barbiturates probably because the metabolism of the barbiturate is inhibited).
No products indexed under this heading.

Perphenazine (Concomitant use of other CNS depressants may produce additive depressant effects).
No products indexed under this heading.

Phenelzine Sulfate (Co-administration with MAO inhibitors prolongs the effects of barbiturates probably because the metabolism of the barbiturate is inhibited).
No products indexed under this heading.

Phenobarbital (Concomitant use of other CNS depressants may produce additive depressant effects). Products include:
Donnatal Extentabs 2493

Phenytoin (The effect of barbiturates on the metabolism of phenytoin appears to be variable).
No products indexed under this heading.

Phenytoin Sodium (The effect of barbiturates on the metabolism of phenytoin appears to be variable). Products include:
Phenytek Capsules 2160

Polyestradiol Phosphate (Pretreatment with or co-administration of phenobarbital may decrease the effect of estrogen by increasing its metabolism; application of this data to other barbiturates appears valid).
No products indexed under this heading.

Prazepam (Concomitant use of other CNS depressants may produce additive depressant effects).
No products indexed under this heading.

Prednisolone Acetate (Barbiturates appear to enhance the metabolism of exogenous corticosteroids probably through the induction of hepatic microsomal enzymes). Products include:
Blephamide Ophthalmic Ointment 568
Blephamide Ophthalmic Suspension.................................. 569
Poly-Pred Ophthalmic Suspension .... ⊙233
Pred Forte Ophthalmic Suspension .... ⊙235
Pred Mild Ophthalmic Suspension .... ⊙238
Pred-G Ophthalmic Ointment .... ⊙237
Pred-G Ophthalmic Suspension ...... ⊙236

Prednisolone Sodium Phosphate (Barbiturates appear to enhance the metabolism of exogenous corticosteroids probably through the induction of hepatic microsomal enzymes).
No products indexed under this heading.

Prednisolone Tebutate (Barbiturates appear to enhance the metabolism of exogenous corticosteroids probably through the induction of hepatic microsomal enzymes).
No products indexed under this heading.

Prednisone (Barbiturates appear to enhance the metabolism of exogenous corticosteroids probably through the induction of hepatic microsomal enzymes).
No products indexed under this heading.

Procarbazine Hydrochloride (Co-administration with MAO inhibitors prolongs the effects of barbiturates probably because the metabolism of the barbiturate is inhibited). Products include:
Matulane Capsules 3191

Prochlorperazine (Concomitant use of other CNS depressants may produce additive depressant effects).
No products indexed under this heading.

Promethazine Hydrochloride (Concomitant use of other CNS depressants may produce additive depressant effects). Products include:
Phenergan Tablets and Suppositories.............................. 3440

Propofol (Concomitant use of other CNS depressants may produce additive depressant effects).
No products indexed under this heading.

Propoxyphene Hydrochloride (Concomitant use of other CNS depressants may produce additive depressant effects).
No products indexed under this heading.

Propoxyphene Napsylate (Concomitant use of other CNS depressants may produce additive depressant effects).
No products indexed under this heading.

Quazepam (Concomitant use of other CNS depressants may produce additive depressant effects).
No products indexed under this heading.

Quetiapine Fumarate (Concomitant use of other CNS depressants may produce additive depressant effects). Products include:
Seroquel Tablets 690

Quinestrol (Pretreatment with or co-administration of phenobarbital may decrease the effect of estrogen by increasing its metabolism; application of this data to other barbiturates appears valid).
No products indexed under this heading.

Remifentanil Hydrochloride (Concomitant use of other CNS depressants may produce additive depressant effects).
No products indexed under this heading.

Risperidone (Concomitant use of other CNS depressants may produce additive depressant effects). Products include:
Risperdal 1676
Risperdal Consta Long-Acting Injection 1682
Risperdal M-Tab Orally Disintegrating Tablets.................. 1676

Secobarbital Sodium (Concomitant use of other CNS depressants may produce additive depressant effects).
No products indexed under this heading.

Selegiline Hydrochloride (Co-administration with MAO inhibitors prolongs the effects of barbiturates probably because the metabolism of the barbiturate is inhibited). Products include:
Eldepryl Capsules 3208
Zelapar Tablets 3372

Sevoflurane (Concomitant use of other CNS depressants may produce additive depressant effects). Products include:
Ultane Liquid for Inhalation 531

Sufentanil Citrate (Concomitant use of other CNS depressants may produce additive depressant effects).
No products indexed under this heading.

Temazepam (Concomitant use of other CNS depressants may produce additive depressant effects). Products include:
Restoril Capsules 1860

Thiamylal Sodium (Concomitant use of other CNS depressants may produce additive depressant effects).
No products indexed under this heading.

Thioridazine Hydrochloride (Concomitant use of other CNS depressants may produce additive depressant effects). Products include:
Thioridazine Hydrochloride Tablets 2163

Thiothixene (Concomitant use of other CNS depressants may produce additive depressant effects). Products include:
Thiothixene Capsules 2165

Tranylcypromine Sulfate (Co-administration with MAO inhibitors prolongs the effects of barbiturates probably because the metabolism of the barbiturate is inhibited). Products include:
Parnate Tablets 1527

Triamcinolone (Barbiturates appear to enhance the metabolism of exogenous corticosteroids probably through the induction of hepatic microsomal enzymes).
No products indexed under this heading.

Triamcinolone Acetonide (Barbiturates appear to enhance the metabolism of exogenous corticosteroids probably through the induction of hepatic microsomal enzymes). Products include:
Azmacort Inhalation Aerosol 1726
Nasacort AQ Nasal Spray 2922

Triamcinolone Diacetate (Barbiturates appear to enhance the metabolism of exogenous corticosteroids probably through the induction of hepatic microsomal enzymes).
No products indexed under this heading.

Triamcinolone Hexacetonide (Barbiturates appear to enhance the metabolism of exogenous corticosteroids probably through the induction of hepatic microsomal enzymes).
No products indexed under this heading.

Triazolam (Concomitant use of other CNS depressants may produce additive depressant effects).
No products indexed under this heading.

Trifluoperazine Hydrochloride (Concomitant use of other CNS depressants may produce additive depressant effects).
No products indexed under this heading.

Valproate Sodium (Valproate appears to decrease barbiturate metabolism). Products include:
Depacon Injection 412

Valproic Acid (Appears to decrease barbiturate metabolism). Products include:
Depakene 417

Warfarin Sodium (Barbiturates can induce hepatic microsomal enzymes resulting in increased metabolism and decreased anticoagulant response of oral anticoagulants). Products include:
Coumadin for Injection 898
Coumadin Tablets 898

Zaleplon (Concomitant use of other CNS depressants may produce additive depressant effects). Products include:
Sonata Capsules 1717

Ziprasidone Hydrochloride (Concomitant use of other CNS depressants may produce additive depressant effects). Products include:
Geodon Capsules 2529

Zolpidem Tartrate (Concomitant use of other CNS depressants may produce additive depressant effects). Products include:
Ambien Tablets 2851
Ambien CR Tablets 2855

Food Interactions

Alcohol (Concomitant use of other CNS depressants may produce additive depressant effects).

NEOPROFEN INJECTION

(Ibuprofen Lysine) 2472
None cited in PDR database.

NEORAL ORAL SOLUTION

(Cyclosporine) 2259
See Neoral Soft Gelatin Capsules

NEORAL SOFT GELATIN CAPSULES

(Cyclosporine) 2259
May interact with ACE inhibitors, angiotensin-II receptor antagonists, erythromycin, fibrates, HMG-CoA reductase inhibitors, non-steroidal anti-inflammatory agents, oral contraceptives, phenytoin, potassium preparations, protease inhibitors, potassium sparing diuretics, vaccines, live, and certain other agents. Compounds in these categories include:

Allopurinol (Increases cyclosporine concentrations).
No products indexed under this heading.

Amiloride Hydrochloride (Cyclosporine may cause hyperkalemia; concurrent use should be avoided). Products include:
Midamor Tablets 2026
Moduretic Tablets 2028

Amiodarone Hydrochloride (Increases cyclosporine concentrations).
No products indexed under this heading.

Amphotericin B (May potentiate renal dysfunction).
No products indexed under this heading.

Amprenavir (The HIV protease inhibitors are known to inhibit cytochrome P450IIIA and increase the concentration of drugs metabolized by this enzyme system; agents that inhibit this enzyme could decrease metabolism and increase cyclosporine concentrations; this interaction has not been studied; however, care should be exercised). Products include:
Agenerase Capsules 1327
Agenerase Oral Solution 1332

Atorvastatin Calcium (Co-administration may result in myotoxicity; atorvastatin dosage should be reduced according to label recommendations. Atorvastatin needs to be temporarily withheld or discontinued in patients with signs and symptoms of myopathy or those with risk factors predisposing to severe renal injury secondary to rhabdomyolysis). Products include:
Caduet Tablets 2508
Lipitor Tablets 2483

Azapropazon (May potentiate renal dysfunction).
No products indexed under this heading.

Azathioprine (May potentiate renal dysfunction).
No products indexed under this heading.

Azithromycin (Concomitant azithromycin may increase cyclosporine concentrations). Products include:
Zmax for Oral Suspension 2583

BCG Vaccine (The use of live vaccines should be avoided).
No products indexed under this heading.

Benazepril Hydrochloride (Caution is required when cyclosporine is co-administered with potassium-sparing drugs, such as angiotensin-converting enzyme inhibitors). Products include:
Lotensin Tablets 2243
Lotensin HCT Tablets 2246
Lotrel Capsules 2249

Bromocriptine Mesylate (Increases cyclosporine concentrations).
No products indexed under this heading.

Candesartan Cilexetil (Caution is required when cyclosporine is co-administered with potassium-sparing drugs, such as angiotensin II receptor antagonists). Products include:
Atacand Tablets 649
Atacand HCT 651

Captopril (Caution is required when cyclosporine is co-administered with potassium-sparing drugs, such as angiotensin-converting enzyme inhibitors). Products include:
Captopril Tablets 2149

Carbamazepine (Decreases cyclosporine concentrations). Products include:
Carbatrol Capsules 3171
Equetro Extended-Release Capsules 3180
Tegretol/Tegretol-XR 2295

Celecoxib (Co-administration with NSAID's particularly in the setting of dehydration, may potentiate renal dysfunction). Products include:
Celebrex Capsules 3134

Cimetidine (May potentiate renal dysfunction). Products include:
Tagamet HB 200 Tablets .... ▣664

Cimetidine Hydrochloride (May potentiate renal dysfunction).
No products indexed under this heading.

Ciprofloxacin (Concomitant ciprofloxacin may potentiate renal dysfunction). Products include:
Cipro Oral Suspension 2977
Cipro I.V. 2984
Cipro XR Tablets 2990
Ciprodex Otic Suspension 559

Ciprofloxacin Hydrochloride (Concomitant ciprofloxacin may potentiate renal dysfunction). Products include:
Ciloxan Ophthalmic Ointment 559
Ciloxan Ophthalmic Solution .... ⊙206
Cipro Tablets 2977
Proquin XR Tablets 1153

Clarithromycin (Concomitant clarithromycin may increase cyclosporine concentrations). Products include:
Biaxin/Biaxin XL 402
PREVPAC 3284

Clofibrate (Concomitant fibric acid derivatives may potentiate renal dysfunction).
No products indexed under this heading.

Colchicine (Cyclosporine may reduce the clearance of colchicine and enhance the toxic effects of colchicine, such as myopathy and neuropathy, especially in patients with renal dysfunction. Close clinical observation is required during concurrent therapy to enable early detection of colchicine toxicity, followed by reduction of dosage or its withdrawal).
No products indexed under this heading.

Dalfopristin (Co-administration with substrates that inhibit CYP450 3A, such as dalfopristin, could decrease metabolism and increase cyclosporine concentrations).
No products indexed under this heading.

Danazol (Increases cyclosporine concentrations).
No products indexed under this heading.

Desogestrel (Concomitant oral contraceptives may increase cyclosporine concentrations). Products include:
Mircette Tablets 1066

Diclofenac Potassium (Co-administration has been associated with approximate doubling of diclofenac blood levels and occasional reports of reversible decreases in renal function; possible potentiation of renal dysfunction; the dose of diclofenac should be in the lower end of the therapeutic range).
No products indexed under this heading.

Diclofenac Sodium (Co-administration has been associated with approximate doubling of diclofenac blood levels and occasional reports of reversible decreases in renal function; possible potentiation of renal dysfunction; the dose of diclofenac should be in the lower end of the therapeutic range). Products include:
Arthrotec Tablets 3129
Voltaren Ophthalmic Solution 2309
Voltaren Tablets 2307
Voltaren-XR Tablets 2310

Digoxin (Cyclosporine may reduce the clearence of digoxin; severe digitalis toxicity may result. Closed clinical observation is required during concurrent therapy to enable early detection of digitalis toxicity, followed by reduction of dosage or its withdrawal). Products include:

- Lanoxicaps Capsules **1490**
- Lanoxin Injection **1494**
- Lanoxin Injection Pediatric **1497**
- Lanoxin Tablets **1500**

Diltiazem Hydrochloride (Increases cyclosporine concentrations). Products include:

- Cardizem LA Extended Release Tablets **1728**
- Tiazac Capsules **1201**

Enalapril Maleate (Caution is required when cyclosporine is co-administered with potassium-sparing drugs, such as angiotensin-converting enzyme inhibitors). Products include:

- Vasotec I.V. Injection **2103**

Enalaprilat (Caution is required when cyclosporine is co-administered with potassium-sparing drugs, such as angiotensin-converting enzyme inhibitors).

No products indexed under this heading.

Eprosartan Mesylate (Caution is required when cyclosporine is co-administered with potassium-sparing drugs, such as angiotensin II receptor antagonists). Products include:

- Teveten Tablets **1735**
- Teveten HCT Tablets **1737**

Erythromycin (Co-administration with substrates that inhibit CYP450 3A, such as erythromycin, could decrease metabolism and increase cyclosporine concentrations). Products include:

- Ery-Tab Tablets **449**
- Erythromycin Base Filmtab Tablets **455**
- Erythromycin Delayed-Release Capsules, USP **457**
- PCE Dispertab Tablets **515**

Erythromycin Estolate (Co-administration with substrates that inhibit CYP450 3A, such as erythromycin, could decrease metabolism and increase cyclosporine concentrations).

No products indexed under this heading.

Erythromycin Ethylsuccinate (Co-administration with substrates that inhibit CYP450 3A, such as erythromycin, could decrease metabolism and increase cyclosporine concentrations). Products include:

- E.E.S. **451**
- EryPed **447**

Erythromycin Gluceptate (Co-administration with substrates that inhibit CYP450 3A, such as erythromycin, could decrease metabolism and increase cyclosporine concentrations).

No products indexed under this heading.

Erythromycin Lactobionate (Co-administration with substrates that inhibit CYP450 3A, such as erythromycin, could decrease metabolism and increase cyclosporine concentrations).

No products indexed under this heading.

Erythromycin Stearate (Co-administration with substrates that inhibit CYP450 3A, such as erythromycin, could decrease metabolism and increase cyclosporine concentrations). Products include:

- Erythrocin Stearate Filmtab Tablets **453**

Ethinyl Estradiol (Concomitant oral contraceptives may increase cyclosporine concentrations). Products include:

- Mircette Tablets **1066**
- NuvaRing **2340**
- Ortho-Cyclen/Ortho Tri-Cyclen **2429**
- Ortho Evra Transdermal System **2417**
- Ortho Tri-Cyclen Lo Tablets **2436**
- Seasonique Tablets **1077**
- Yasmin 28 Tablets **796**
- Yaz Tablets **803**

Ethynodiol Diacetate (Concomitant oral contraceptives may increase cyclosporine concentrations).

No products indexed under this heading.

Etodolac (Co-administration with NSAID's particularly in the setting of dehydration, may potentiate renal dysfunction).

No products indexed under this heading.

Fenofibrate (Concomitant fibric acid derivatives may potentiate renal dysfunction). Products include:

- Lofibra Tablets **1219**
- Lofibra Capsules **1216**
- Tricor Tablets **527**
- Triglide Tablets **3123**

Fenoprofen Calcium (Co-administration with NSAID's particularly in the setting of dehydration, may potentiate renal dysfunction). Products include:

- Nalfon Capsules **2502**

Fluconazole (Increases cyclosporine concentrations).

No products indexed under this heading.

Flurbiprofen (Co-administration with NSAID's particularly in the setting of dehydration, may potentiate renal dysfunction).

No products indexed under this heading.

Fluvastatin Sodium (Co-administration may rarely result in myotoxicity; fluvastatin dosage should be reduced according to label recommendations. Fluvastatin needs to be temporarily withheld or discontinued in patients with signs and symptoms of myopathy or those with risk factors predisposing to severe renal injury secondary to rhabdomyolysis). Products include:

- Lescol Capsules **2233**
- Lescol XL Tablets **2233**

Fosinopril Sodium (Caution is required when cyclosporine is co-administered with potassium-sparing drugs, such as angiotensin-converting enzyme inhibitors).

No products indexed under this heading.

Fosphenytoin Sodium (Concomitant use may decrease cyclosporine drug levels).

No products indexed under this heading.

Gemfibrozil (Concomitant fibric acid derivatives may potentiate renal dysfunction).

No products indexed under this heading.

Gentamicin Sulfate (May potentiate renal dysfunction). Products include:

- Garamycin Injectable **3014**
- Pred-G Ophthalmic Ointment .... ⊙**237**
- Pred-G Ophthalmic Suspension .... ⊙**236**

Hypericum (Co-administration has been reported to produce a marked reduction in blood cyclosporine concentrations, resulting in subtherapeutic levels, rejection of transplanted organs, and graft loss). Products include:

- Satiete Tablets .... ▣**832**

Ibuprofen (Co-administration with NSAID's particularly in the setting of dehydration, may potentiate renal dysfunction). Products include:

- Advil Allergy Sinus Caplets .... ▣**770**
- Advil .... ▣**674**
- Children's Advil Oral Suspension .... ▣**603**
- Children's Advil Chewable Tablets .. ▣**603**
- Advil Cold & Sinus .... ▣**723**
- Infants' Advil Concentrated Drops .. ▣**604**
- Infants' Advil Concentrated Drops - White Grape (Dye-Free) .... ▣**604**
- Junior Strength Advil Swallow Tablets .... ▣**605**
- Advil Migraine Liquigels .... ▣**608**
- Advil Multi-Symptom Cold Caplets .... ▣**770**
- Advil PM Caplets .... ▣**615**
- Motrin IB Tablets and Caplets **1866**
- Children's Motrin Oral Suspension ... **1867**
- Children's Motrin Non-Staining Dye-Free Oral Suspension **1867**
- Children's Motrin Cold Oral Suspension **1867**
- Infants' Motrin Concentrated Drops **1867**
- Infants' Motrin Non-Staining Dye-Free Concentrated Drops **1867**
- Junior Strength Motrin Caplets and Chewable Tablets **1867**
- Vicoprofen Tablets **539**

Imatinib Mesylate (Concomitant imatinib may increase cyclosporine concentrations). Products include:

- Gleevec Tablets **2227**

Indinavir Sulfate (The HIV protease inhibitors are known to inhibit cytochrome P450IIIA and increase the concentration of drugs metabolized by this enzyme system; agents that inhibit this enzyme could decrease metabolism and increase cyclosporine concentrations; this interaction has not been studied; however, care should be exercised). Products include:

- Crixivan Capsules **1940**

Indomethacin (Co-administration with NSAID's particularly in the setting of dehydration, may potentiate renal dysfunction). Products include:

- Indocin **1995**

Indomethacin Sodium Trihydrate (Co-administration with NSAID's particularly in the setting of dehydration, may potentiate renal dysfunction). Products include:

- Indocin I.V. **2465**

Irbesartan (Caution is required when cyclosporine is co-administered with potassium-sparing drugs, such as angiotensin II receptor antagonists). Products include:

- Avalide Tablets **888**
- Avalide Tablets **2874**
- Avapro Tablets **891**
- Avapro Tablets **2871**

Itraconazole (Increases cyclosporine concentrations).

No products indexed under this heading.

Ketoconazole (May potentiate renal dysfunction; co-administration with substrates that inhibit CYP450 3A, such as ketoconazole, could decrease metabolism and increase cyclosporine concentrations). Products include:

- Nizoral A-D Shampoo, 1% **1868**

Ketoprofen (Co-administration with NSAID's particularly in the setting of dehydration, may potentiate renal dysfunction).

No products indexed under this heading.

Ketorolac Tromethamine (Co-administration with NSAID's particularly in the setting of dehydration, may potentiate renal dysfunction). Products include:

- Acular Ophthalmic Solution **565**
- Acular LS Ophthalmic Solution **566**

Levonorgestrel (Concomitant oral contraceptives may increase cyclosporine concentrations). Products include:

- Climara Pro Transdermal System **776**
- Mirena Intrauterine System **787**
- Plan B Tablets **1076**
- Seasonique Tablets **1077**

Lisinopril (Caution is required when cyclosporine is co-administered with potassium-sparing drugs, such as angiotensin-converting enzyme inhibitors). Products include:

- Prinivil Tablets **2052**
- Prinzide Tablets **2056**

Lopinavir (The HIV protease inhibitors are known to inhibit cytochrome P450IIIA and increase the concentration of drugs metabolized by this enzyme system; agents that inhibit this enzyme could decrease metabolism and increase cyclosporine concentrations; this interaction has not been studied; however, care should be exercised). Products include:

- Kaletra **476**

Losartan Potassium (Caution is required when cyclosporine is co-administered with potassium-sparing drugs, such as angiotensin II receptor antagonists). Products include:

- Cozaar Tablets **1935**
- Hyzaar 50-12.5 Tablets **1990**
- Hyzaar 100-12.5 Tablets **1990**
- Hyzaar 100-25 Tablets **1990**

Lovastatin (Co-administration may results in myotoxicity; lovastatin dosage should be reduced according to label recommendations. Lovastatin needs to be temporarily withheld or discontinued in patients with signs and symptoms of myopathy or those with risk factors predisposing to severe renal injury secondary to rhabdomyolysis). Products include:

- Advicor Tablets **1722**
- Altoprev Extended-Release Tablets **3109**
- Mevacor Tablets **2021**

Measles, Mumps, Rubella and Varicella Virus Vaccine Live (The use of live vaccines should be avoided). Products include:

- ProQuad **2064**

Measles, Mumps & Rubella Virus Vaccine, Live (The use of live vaccines should be avoided). Products include:

- M-M-R II **2006**

Measles & Rubella Virus Vaccine Live (The use of live vaccines should be avoided).

No products indexed under this heading.

Measles Virus Vaccine Live (The use of live vaccines should be avoided). Products include:

- Attenuvax **1914**

Meclofenamate Sodium (Co-administration with NSAID's particularly in the setting of dehydration, may potentiate renal dysfunction).

No products indexed under this heading.

Mefenamic Acid (Co-administration with NSAID's particularly in the setting of dehydration, may potentiate renal dysfunction).
No products indexed under this heading.

Meloxicam (Co-administration with NSAID's particularly in the setting of dehydration, may potentiate renal dysfunction). Products include:
Mobic Oral Suspension 863
Mobic Tablets 863

Melphalan (May potentiate renal dysfunction). Products include:
Alkeran Tablets 956

Mestranol (Concomitant oral contraceptives may increase cyclosporine concentrations).
No products indexed under this heading.

Methotrexate Sodium (Increased risk of developing skin malignancies in psoriasis patients with concurrent use; in rheumatoid arthritis patients, methotrexate concentrations (AUCs) were increased approximately 30% and concentrations (AUCs) of its metabolites were decreased approximately 80%; the clinical significance is unknown).
No products indexed under this heading.

Methylprednisolone (Convulsions have been reported with high doses of methylprednisolone).
No products indexed under this heading.

Methylprednisolone Acetate (Convulsions have been reported with high doses of methylprednisolone). Products include:
Depo-Medrol Injectable Suspension 2617
Depo-Medrol Single-Dose Vial 2619

Methylprednisolone Sodium Succinate (Convulsions have been reported with high doses of methylprednisolone).
No products indexed under this heading.

Metoclopramide Hydrochloride (Increases cyclosporine concentrations).
No products indexed under this heading.

Moexipril Hydrochloride (Caution is required when cyclosporine is co-administered with potassium-sparing drugs, such as angiotensin-converting enzyme inhibitors). Products include:
Uniretic Tablets 3100
Univasc Tablets 3104

Mumps Virus Vaccine, Live (The use of live vaccines should be avoided). Products include:
Mumpsvax 2031

Muromonab-CD3 (Psoriasis patients receiving other immunosuppressive agents, such as muromonab-CD3, should not receive concurrent cyclosporine because of the possibility of excessive immunosuppression). Products include:
Orthoclone OKT3 Sterile Solution 2360

Mycophenolate Mofetil (Psoriasis patients receiving other immunosuppressive agents, such as mycophenolate mofetil, should not receive concurrent cyclosporine because of the possibility of excessive immunosuppression). Products include:
CellCept Capsules 2747
CellCept Oral Suspension 2747
CellCept Tablets 2747

Nabumetone (Co-administration with NSAID's particularly in the setting of dehydration, may potentiate renal dysfunction).
No products indexed under this heading.

Nafcillin Sodium (Decreases cyclosporine concentrations).
No products indexed under this heading.

Naproxen (Concomitant use is associated with additive decreases in renal function with possible potentiation of renal dysfunction). Products include:
EC-Naprosyn Delayed-Release Tablets 2761
Naprosyn Suspension 2761
Naprosyn Tablets 2761
Prevacid NapraPAC 3280

Naproxen Sodium (Concomitant use is associated with additive decreases in renal function with possible potentiation of renal dysfunction). Products include:
Aleve Caplets 742
Aleve Gelcaps 743
Aleve Tablets 743
Aleve Cold & Sinus Caplets 744
Anaprox Tablets 2761
Anaprox DS Tablets 2761

Nelfinavir Mesylate (The HIV protease inhibitors are known to inhibit cytochrome P450IIIA and increase the concentration of drugs metabolized by this enzyme system; agents that inhibit this enzyme could decrease metabolism and increase cyclosporine concentrations; this interaction has not been studied; however, care should be exercised). Products include:
Viracept 2577

Nephrotoxic Drugs (Potential for increased nephrotoxicity; careful monitoring of renal function is required).
No products indexed under this heading.

Nicardipine Hydrochloride (Increases cyclosporine concentrations). Products include:
Cardene I.V. 2497

Nifedipine (Potential for frequent gingival hyperplasia). Products include:
Adalat CC Tablets 2964

Norethindrone (Concomitant oral contraceptives may increase cyclosporine concentrations). Products include:
Ortho Micronor Tablets 2426

Norethynodrel (Concomitant oral contraceptives may increase cyclosporine concentrations).
No products indexed under this heading.

Norgestimate (Concomitant oral contraceptives may increase cyclosporine concentrations). Products include:
Ortho-Cyclen/Ortho Tri-Cyclen 2429
Ortho Tri-Cyclen Lo Tablets 2436

Norgestrel (Concomitant oral contraceptives may increase cyclosporine concentrations).
No products indexed under this heading.

Octreotide Acetate (Decreases cyclosporine concentrations). Products include:
Sandostatin Injection 2278
Sandostatin LAR Depot 2280

Orlistat (Co-administration can result in decreased absorption of cyclosporine; concomitant use should be avoided). Products include:
Xenical Capsules 2831

Oxaprozin (Co-administration with NSAID's particularly in the setting of dehydration, may potentiate renal dysfunction).
No products indexed under this heading.

Perindopril Erbumine (Caution is required when cyclosporine is co-administered with potassium-sparing drugs, such as angiotensin-converting enzyme inhibitors). Products include:
Aceon Tablets (2 mg, 4 mg, 8 mg)... 3194

Phenobarbital (Decreases cyclosporine concentrations). Products include:
Donnatal Extentabs 2493

Phenylbutazone (Co-administration with NSAID's particularly in the setting of dehydration, may potentiate renal dysfunction).
No products indexed under this heading.

Phenytoin (Concomitant use may decrease cyclosporine drug levels).
No products indexed under this heading.

Phenytoin Sodium (Concomitant use may decrease cyclosporine drug levels). Products include:
Phenytek Capsules 2160

Piroxicam (Co-administration with NSAID's particularly in the setting of dehydration, may potentiate renal dysfunction).
No products indexed under this heading.

Poliovirus Vaccine, Live, Oral, Trivalent, Types 1,2,3 (Sabin) (The use of live vaccines should be avoided).
No products indexed under this heading.

Potassium Acid Phosphate (Caution is required when cyclosporine is co-administered with potassium-containing drugs). Products include:
K-Phos Original (Sodium Free) Tablets 760

Potassium Bicarbonate (Caution is required when cyclosporine is co-administered with potassium-containing drugs).
No products indexed under this heading.

Potassium Chloride (Caution is required when cyclosporine is co-administered with potassium-containing drugs). Products include:
Colyte with Flavor Packs for Oral Solution.. 3088
HalfLytely and Bisacodyl Tablets Bowel Prep Kit with Flavors Packs... 881
K-Dur Extended-Relase Tablets 3033
K-Lor Oral Solution 474
K-Tab Tablets 475
MoviPrep Oral Solution 2839
TriLyte with Flavor Packs for Oral Solution.. 3100

Potassium Citrate (Caution is required when cyclosporine is co-administered with potassium-containing drugs). Products include:
Urocit-K Tablets 2144

Potassium Gluconate (Caution is required when cyclosporine is co-administered with potassium-containing drugs).
No products indexed under this heading.

Potassium Phosphate (Caution is required when cyclosporine is co-administered with potassium-containing drugs). Products include:
K-Phos Neutral Tablets 760

Pravastatin Sodium (Co-administration may result in myotoxicity; pravastatin dosage should be reduced according to label recommendations. Pravastatin needs to be temporarily withheld or discontinued in patients with signs and symptoms of myopathy or those with risk factors predisposing to severe renal injury secondary to rhabdomyolysis).
No products indexed under this heading.

Prednisolone (Cyclosporine may reduce the clearance of prednisolone).
No products indexed under this heading.

Prednisolone Acetate (Cyclosporine may reduce the clearance of prednisolone). Products include:
Blephamide Ophthalmic Ointment 568
Blephamide Ophthalmic Suspension.................................. 569
Poly-Pred Ophthalmic Suspension .... ⊙ 233
Pred Forte Ophthalmic Suspension .... ⊙ 235
Pred Mild Ophthalmic Suspension .... ⊙ 238
Pred-G Ophthalmic Ointment .... ⊙ 237
Pred-G Ophthalmic Suspension ...... ⊙ 236

Prednisolone Sodium Phosphate (Cyclosporine may reduce the clearance of prednisolone).
No products indexed under this heading.

Quinapril Hydrochloride (Caution is required when cyclosporine is co-administered with potassium-sparing drugs, such as angiotensin-converting enzyme inhibitors).
No products indexed under this heading.

Quinupristin (Co-administration with substrates that inhibit CYP450 3A, such as quinupristin, could decrease metabolism and increase cyclosporine concentrations).
No products indexed under this heading.

Ramipril (Caution is required when cyclosporine is co-administered with potassium-sparing drugs, such as angiotensin-converting enzyme inhibitors). Products include:
Altace Capsules 1702

Ranitidine Hydrochloride (May potentiate renal dysfunction). Products include:
Zantac 1624
Zantac Injection 1619
Zantac Injection Pharmacy Bulk Package 1622

Rifabutin (Substances that are inducers of cyctochrome P450 activity could increase metabolism and decrease cyclosporine concentrations; rifabutin is known to increase the metabolism of other drugs metabolized by the cytochrome P450; this interaction has not been studied, however, care should be exercised).
No products indexed under this heading.

Rifampin (Decreases cyclosporine concentrations).
No products indexed under this heading.

Ritonavir (The HIV protease inhibitors are known to inhibit cytochrome P450IIIA and increase the concentration of drugs metabolized by this enzyme system; agents that inhibit this enzyme could decrease metabolism and increase cyclosporine concentrations; this interaction has not been studied; however, care should be exercised). Products include:

Kaletra 476
Norvir 503

Rofecoxib (Co-administration with NSAID's particularly in the setting of dehydration, may potentiate renal dysfunction).
No products indexed under this heading.

Rotavirus Vaccine, Live, Oral, Tetravalent (The use of live vaccines should be avoided).
No products indexed under this heading.

Rubella & Mumps Virus Vaccine Live (The use of live vaccines should be avoided).
No products indexed under this heading.

Rubella Virus Vaccine Live (The use of live vaccines should be avoided). Products include:

Meruvax II 2019

Saquinavir (The HIV protease inhibitors are known to inhibit cytochrome P450IIIA and increase the concentration of drugs metabolized by this enzyme system; agents that inhibit this enzyme could decrease metabolism and increase cyclosporine concentrations; this interaction has not been studied; however, care should be exercised).
No products indexed under this heading.

Saquinavir Mesylate (The HIV protease inhibitors are known to inhibit cytochrome P450IIIA and increase the concentration of drugs metabolized by this enzyme system; agents that inhibit this enzyme could decrease metabolism and increase cyclosporine concentrations; this interaction has not been studied; however, care should be exercised). Products include:

Invirase 2772

Simvastatin (Co-administration may result in myotoxicity; simvastation dosage should be reduced according to label recommendations. Simvastatin needs to be temporarily withheld or discontinued in patients with signs and symptoms of myopathy or those with risk factors predisposing to severe renal injury secondary to rhabdomyolysis). Products include:

Vytorin 10/10 Tablets 2114
Vytorin 10/10 Tablets 3077
Vytorin 10/20 Tablets 2114
Vytorin 10/20 Tablets 3077
Vytorin 10/40 Tablets 2114
Vytorin 10/40 Tablets 3077
Vytorin 10/80 Tablets 2114
Vytorin 10/80 Tablets 3077
Zocor Tablets 2105

Sirolimus (Elevations in serum creatinine were observed in studies using sirolimus in combination with full-dose cyclosporine. The effect is often reversible with cyclosporine dose reduction. Simultaneous co-administration of cyclosproine significantly increases blood levels of sirolimus. To minimize increases in sirolimus blood concentrations, it is recommended that sirolimus be given 4 hours after cyclosporine administration). Products include:

Rapamune Oral Solution and Tablets 3475

Smallpox Vaccine (The use of live vaccines should be avoided).
No products indexed under this heading.

Spirapril Hydrochloride (Caution is required when cyclosporine is co-administered with potassium-sparing drugs, such as angiotensin-converting enzyme inhibitors).
No products indexed under this heading.

Spironolactone (Cyclosporine may cause hyperkalemia; concurrent use should be avoided).
No products indexed under this heading.

Sulfamethoxazole (Co-administration with trimethoprim/sulfamethoxazole may potentiate renal dysfunction).
No products indexed under this heading.

Sulfinpyrazone (Concomitant sulfinpyrazone may decrease cyclosporine concentrations).
No products indexed under this heading.

Sulindac (Concomitant use is associated with additive decreases in renal function with possible potentiation of renal dysfunction). Products include:

Clinoril Tablets 1924

Tacrolimus (May potentiate renal dysfunction). Products include:

Prograf Capsules and Injection 632
Protopic Ointment 638

Telmisartan (Caution is required when cyclosporine is co-administered with potassium-sparing drugs, such as angiotensin II receptor antagonists). Products include:

Micardis Tablets 854
Micardis HCT Tablets 856

Terbinafine Hydrochloride (Concomitant terbinafine may decrease cyclosporine concentrations). Products include:

Lamisil Tablets 2232
Lamisil AT Creams (Athlete's Foot & Jock Itch) .... ■643 636

Ticlopidine Hydrochloride (Decreases cyclosporine concentrations). Products include:

Ticlid Tablets 2810

Tobramycin (May potentiate renal dysfunction). Products include:

TOBI Solution for Inhalation 2298
TobraDex Ophthalmic Ointment 562
TobraDex Ophthalmic Suspension ... 563
Zylet Ophthalmic Suspension .... ⊙259

Tobramycin Sulfate (May potentiate renal dysfunction).
No products indexed under this heading.

Tolmetin Sodium (Co-administration with NSAID's particularly in the setting of dehydration, may potentiate renal dysfunction).
No products indexed under this heading.

Trandolapril (Caution is required when cyclosporine is co-administered with potassium-sparing drugs, such as angiotensin-converting enzyme inhibitors). Products include:

Mavik Tablets 486
Tarka Tablets 524

Triamterene (Cyclosporine may cause hyperkalemia; concurrent use should be avoided). Products include:

Dyazide Capsules 1423
Dyrenium Capsules 3400

Trimethoprim (Co-administration with trimethoprim/sulfamethoxazole may potentiate renal dysfunction).
No products indexed under this heading.

Typhoid Vaccine (The use of live vaccines should be avoided).
No products indexed under this heading.

Vaccines (Live) (Vaccination may be less effective).
No products indexed under this heading.

Valdecoxib (Co-administration with NSAID's particularly in the setting of dehydration, may potentiate renal dysfunction).
No products indexed under this heading.

Valsartan (Caution is required when cyclosporine is co-administered with potassium-sparing drugs, such as angiotensin II receptor antagonists). Products include:

Diovan Tablets 2193
Diovan HCT Tablets 2196

Vancomycin Hydrochloride (May potentiate renal dysfunction). Products include:

Vancocin HCl Capsules, USP 3380

Varicella Virus Vaccine Live (The use of live vaccines should be avoided). Products include:

Varivax 2100

Verapamil Hydrochloride (Increases cyclosporine concentrations). Products include:

Covera-HS Tablets 3139
Tarka Tablets 524
Verelan PM Extended-Release Capsules, Controlled-Onset........... 3106

Yellow Fever Vaccine (The use of live vaccines should be avoided).
No products indexed under this heading.

Food Interactions

Diet, high-lipid (A high-fat meal consumed within one-half hour before Neoral administration decreased the AUC by 13% and Cmax by 33%).

Food, unspecified (Administration of food with Neoral decreases the AUC and Cmax).

Grapefruit (Affects the metabolism of cyclosporine and should be avoided).

Grapefruit Juice (Affects the metabolism of cyclosporine and should be avoided).

NEOSPORIN ANTIBIOTIC OINTMENT

(Bacitracin, Neomycin, Polymyxin B Sulfate).. ■643
None cited in PDR database.

NEOSPORIN OPHTHALMIC SOLUTION STERILE

(Gramicidin, Neomycin Sulfate, Polymyxin B Sulfate)......................... ⊙265
May interact with:

Gentamicin (Allergic cross-reactions may occur which could prevent the use of gentamicin for the treatment of future infections).
No products indexed under this heading.

Kanamycin Sulfate (Allergic cross-reactions may occur which could prevent the use of kanamycin for the treatment of future infections).
No products indexed under this heading.

Paromomycin Sulfate (Allergic cross-reactions may occur which could prevent the use of paromomycin for the treatment of future infections).
No products indexed under this heading.

Streptomycin Sulfate (Allergic cross-reactions may occur which could prevent the use of streptomycin for the treatment of future infections).
No products indexed under this heading.

NEOSPORIN + PAIN RELIEF ANTIBIOTIC CREAM AND OINTMENT (MAXIMUM STRENGTH)

(Neomycin, Polymyxin B Sulfate, Pramoxine Hydrochloride)................. ■643
None cited in PDR database.

NEULASTA INJECTION

(Pegfilgrastim) 601
May interact with drugs which potentiate the release of neutrophils. Compounds in these categories include:

Lithium Carbonate (Concurrent use should be undertaken with caution since lithium potentiates the release of neutrophils). Products include:

Lithobid Tablets 1692

Lithium Citrate (Concurrent use should be undertaken with caution since lithium potentiates the release of neutrophils).
No products indexed under this heading.

NEUMEGA FOR INJECTION

(Oprelvekin) 3435
None cited in PDR database.

NEUPOGEN FOR INJECTION

(Filgrastim) 603
May interact with drugs which potentiate the release of neutrophils. Compounds in these categories include:

Lithium Carbonate (Concurrent use should be undertaken with caution since lithium potentiates the release of neutrophils). Products include:

Lithobid Tablets 1692

Lithium Citrate (Concurrent use should be undertaken with caution since lithium potentiates the release of neutrophils).
No products indexed under this heading.

NEURONTIN CAPSULES

(Gabapentin) 2487
May interact with:

Aluminum Hydroxide (Coadministration reduces bioavailability of gabapentin by 20%; gabapentin should be taken at least 2 hours following antacid containing aluminum hydroxide and magnesium hydroxide). Products include:

Gaviscon Regular Strength Liquid .. ■658
Gaviscon Regular Strength Tablets.. ■658
Gaviscon Extra Strength Liquid ...... ■658
Gaviscon Extra Strength Tablets .... ■658
Maalox Regular Strength Antacid/Antigas Liquid................. 2175

Methylprednisolone Sodium Succinate (Topical nonsteroidal anti-inflammatory drugs (NSAIDs), including nepafenac ophthalmic suspension, may slow or delay healing. Topical corticosteroids are known to slow or delay healing. Concomitant use of topical NSAIDs and topical steroids may increase the potential for healing problems).
No products indexed under this heading.

Prednisolone Acetate (Topical nonsteroidal anti-inflammatory drugs (NSAIDs), including nepafenac ophthalmic suspension, may slow or delay healing. Topical corticosteroids are known to slow or delay healing. Concomitant use of topical NSAIDs and topical steroids may increase the potential for healing problems). Products include:
Blephamide Ophthalmic Ointment **568**
Blephamide Ophthalmic Suspension **569**
Poly-Pred Ophthalmic Suspension .... ⊙**233**
Pred Forte Ophthalmic Suspension .... ⊙**235**
Pred Mild Ophthalmic Suspension .... ⊙**238**
Pred-G Ophthalmic Ointment .... ⊙**237**
Pred-G Ophthalmic Suspension .... ⊙**236**

Prednisolone Sodium Phosphate (Topical nonsteroidal anti-inflammatory drugs (NSAIDs), including nepafenac ophthalmic suspension, may slow or delay healing. Topical corticosteroids are known to slow or delay healing. Concomitant use of topical NSAIDs and topical steroids may increase the potential for healing problems).
No products indexed under this heading.

Prednisolone Tebutate (Topical nonsteroidal anti-inflammatory drugs (NSAIDs), including nepafenac ophthalmic suspension, may slow or delay healing. Topical corticosteroids are known to slow or delay healing. Concomitant use of topical NSAIDs and topical steroids may increase the potential for healing problems).
No products indexed under this heading.

Prednisone (Topical nonsteroidal anti-inflammatory drugs (NSAIDs), including nepafenac ophthalmic suspension, may slow or delay healing. Topical corticosteroids are known to slow or delay healing. Concomitant use of topical NSAIDs and topical steroids may increase the potential for healing problems).
No products indexed under this heading.

Tinzaparin Sodium (It is recommended that nepafenac ophthalmic suspension be used with caution in patients who are receiving other medications which may prolong bleeding time).
No products indexed under this heading.

Triamcinolone (Topical nonsteroidal anti-inflammatory drugs (NSAIDs), including nepafenac ophthalmic suspension, may slow or delay healing. Topical corticosteroids are known to slow or delay healing. Concomitant use of topical NSAIDs and topical steroids may increase the potential for healing problems).
No products indexed under this heading.

Triamcinolone Acetonide (Topical nonsteroidal anti-inflammatory drugs (NSAIDs), including nepafenac ophthalmic suspension, may slow or delay healing. Topical corticosteroids are known to slow or delay healing. Concomitant use of topical NSAIDs and topical steroids may increase the potential for healing problems). Products include:
Azmacort Inhalation Aerosol **1726**
Nasacort AQ Nasal Spray **2922**

Triamcinolone Diacetate (Topical nonsteroidal anti-inflammatory drugs (NSAIDs), including nepafenac ophthalmic suspension, may slow or delay healing. Topical corticosteroids are known to slow or delay healing. Concomitant use of topical NSAIDs and topical steroids may increase the potential for healing problems).
No products indexed under this heading.

Triamcinolone Hexacetonide (Topical nonsteroidal anti-inflammatory drugs (NSAIDs), including nepafenac ophthalmic suspension, may slow or delay healing. Topical corticosteroids are known to slow or delay healing. Concomitant use of topical NSAIDs and topical steroids may increase the potential for healing problems).
No products indexed under this heading.

Warfarin Sodium (It is recommended that nepafenac ophthalmic suspension be used with caution in patients who are receiving other medications which may prolong bleeding time). Products include:
Coumadin for Injection **898**
Coumadin Tablets **898**

NEXAVAR TABLETS

(Sorafenib) **746**

May interact with cytochrome p450 2c8 substrates (selected) and certain other agents. Compounds in these categories include:

Amiodarone Hydrochloride (Sorafenib inhibits CYP2B6 and CYP2C8 in vitro. Systemic exposure to substrates of CYP2B6 and CYP2C8 is expected to increase. Caution is recommended when co-administering with these cytochrome P450 substrates).
No products indexed under this heading.

Amitriptyline Hydrochloride (Sorafenib inhibits CYP2B6 and CYP2C8 in vitro. Systemic exposure to substrates of CYP2B6 and CYP2C8 is expected to increase. Caution is recommended when co-administering with these cytochrome P450 substrates).
No products indexed under this heading.

Amoxapine (Sorafenib inhibits CYP2B6 and CYP2C8 in vitro. Systemic exposure to substrates of CYP2B6 and CYP2C8 is expected to increase. Caution is recommended when co-administering with these cytochrome P450 substrates).
No products indexed under this heading.

Benzphetamine Hydrochloride (Sorafenib inhibits CYP2B6 and CYP2C8 in vitro. Systemic exposure to substrates of CYP2B6 and CYP2C8 is expected to increase. Caution is recommended when co-administering with these cytochrome P450 substrates).
No products indexed under this heading.

Carbamazepine (Sorafenib inhibits CYP2B6 and CYP2C8 in vitro. Systemic exposure to substrates of CYP2B6 and CYP2C8 is expected to increase. Caution is recommended when co-administering with these cytochrome P450 substrates). Products include:
Carbatrol Capsules **3171**
Equetro Extended-Release Capsules **3180**
Tegretol/Tegretol-XR **2295**

Clomipramine Hydrochloride (Sorafenib inhibits CYP2B6 and CYP2C8 in vitro. Systemic exposure to substrates of CYP2B6 and CYP2C8 is expected to increase. Caution is recommended when co-administering with these cytochrome P450 substrates).
No products indexed under this heading.

Desipramine Hydrochloride (Sorafenib inhibits CYP2B6 and CYP2C8 in vitro. Systemic exposure to substrates of CYP2B6 and CYP2C8 is expected to increase. Caution is recommended when co-administering with these cytochrome P450 substrates).
No products indexed under this heading.

Diazepam (Sorafenib inhibits CYP2B6 and CYP2C8 in vitro. Systemic exposure to substrates of CYP2B6 and CYP2C8 is expected to increase. Caution is recommended when co-administering with these cytochrome P450 substrates). Products include:
Diastat Rectal Delivery System **3343**
Valium Tablets **2819**

Diclofenac Potassium (Sorafenib inhibits CYP2B6 and CYP2C8 in vitro. Systemic exposure to substrates of CYP2B6 and CYP2C8 is expected to increase. Caution is recommended when co-administering with these cytochrome P450 substrates).
No products indexed under this heading.

Diclofenac Sodium (Sorafenib inhibits CYP2B6 and CYP2C8 in vitro. Systemic exposure to substrates of CYP2B6 and CYP2C8 is expected to increase. Caution is recommended when co-administering with these cytochrome P450 substrates). Products include:
Arthrotec Tablets **3129**
Voltaren Ophthalmic Solution **2309**
Voltaren Tablets **2307**
Voltaren-XR Tablets **2310**

Docetaxel (Sorafenib inhibits CYP2B6 and CYP2C8 in vitro. Systemic exposure to substrates of CYP2B6 and CYP2C8 is expected to increase. Caution is recommended when co-administering with these cytochrome P450 substrates). Products include:
Taxotere Injection Concentrate **2932**

Doxepin Hydrochloride (Sorafenib inhibits CYP2B6 and CYP2C8 in vitro. Systemic exposure to substrates of CYP2B6 and CYP2C8 is expected to increase. Caution is recommended when co-administering with these cytochrome P450 substrates).
No products indexed under this heading.

Doxorubicin Hydrochloride (Concomitant treatment resulted in a 21% increase in the AUC of doxorubicin).
No products indexed under this heading.

Doxorubicin Hydrochloride Liposome (Concomitant treatment resulted in a 21% increase in the AUC of doxorubicin). Products include:
Doxil Injection **2351**

Fluvastatin Sodium (Sorafenib inhibits CYP2B6 and CYP2C8 in vitro. Systemic exposure to substrates of CYP2B6 and CYP2C8 is expected to increase. Caution is recommended when co-administering with these cytochrome P450 substrates). Products include:
Lescol Capsules **2233**
Lescol XL Tablets **2233**

Imipramine Hydrochloride (Sorafenib inhibits CYP2B6 and CYP2C8 in vitro. Systemic exposure to substrates of CYP2B6 and CYP2C8 is expected to increase. Caution is recommended when co-administering with these cytochrome P450 substrates).
No products indexed under this heading.

Imipramine Pamoate (Sorafenib inhibits CYP2B6 and CYP2C8 in vitro. Systemic exposure to substrates of CYP2B6 and CYP2C8 is expected to increase. Caution is recommended when co-administering with these cytochrome P450 substrates).
No products indexed under this heading.

Irinotecan Hydrochloride (When administered with irinotecan, whose active metabolite SN-38 is further metabolized by the UGT1A1 pathway, there was a 67% to 120% increase in the AUC of SN-38 and a 26% to 42% increase in the AUC of irinotecan). Products include:
Camptosar Injection **2604**

Isotretinoin (Sorafenib inhibits CYP2B6 and CYP2C8 in vitro. Systemic exposure to substrates of CYP2B6 and CYP2C8 is expected to increase. Caution is recommended when co-administering with these cytochrome P450 substrates). Products include:
Accutane Capsules **2731**

Maprotiline Hydrochloride (Sorafenib inhibits CYP2B6 and CYP2C8 in vitro. Systemic exposure to substrates of CYP2B6 and CYP2C8 is expected to increase. Caution is recommended when co-administering with these cytochrome P450 substrates).
No products indexed under this heading.

Mephobarbital (Sorafenib inhibits CYP2B6 and CYP2C8 in vitro. Systemic exposure to substrates of CYP2B6 and CYP2C8 is expected to increase. Caution is recommended when co-administering with these cytochrome P450 substrates).
No products indexed under this heading.

Nortriptyline Hydrochloride (Sorafenib inhibits CYP2B6 and CYP2C8 in vitro. Systemic exposure to substrates of CYP2B6 and CYP2C8 is expected to increase. Caution is recommended when co-administering with these cytochrome P450 substrates).
No products indexed under this heading.

Omeprazole (Sorafenib inhibits CYP2B6 and CYP2C8 in vitro. Systemic exposure to substrates of CYP2B6 and CYP2C8 is expected to increase. Caution is recommended when co-administering with these cytochrome P450 substrates). Products include:
Zegerid Capsules **2958**
Zegerid Powder for Oral Solution **2958**

Paclitaxel (Sorafenib inhibits CYP2B6 and CYP2C8 in vitro. Systemic exposure to substrates of CYP2B6 and CYP2C8 is expected to increase. Caution is recommended when co-administering with these cytochrome P450 substrates).
No products indexed under this heading.

Phenytoin (Sorafenib inhibits CYP2B6 and CYP2C8 in vitro. Systemic exposure to substrates of CYP2B6 and CYP2C8 is expected to increase. Caution is recommended when co-administering with these cytochrome P450 substrates).
No products indexed under this heading.

Phenytoin Sodium (Sorafenib inhibits CYP2B6 and CYP2C8 in vitro. Systemic exposure to substrates of CYP2B6 and CYP2C8 is expected to increase. Caution is recommended when co-administering with these cytochrome P450 substrates). Products include:
Phenytek Capsules **2160**

Pioglitazone Hydrochloride (Sorafenib inhibits CYP2B6 and CYP2C8 in vitro. Systemic exposure to substrates of CYP2B6 and CYP2C8 is expected to increase. Caution is recommended when co-administering with these cytochrome P450 substrates). Products include:
ActoPlus Met Tablets **3214**
Actos Tablets **3219**
Duetact Tablets **3226**

Protriptyline Hydrochloride (Sorafenib inhibits CYP2B6 and CYP2C8 in vitro. Systemic exposure to substrates of CYP2B6 and CYP2C8 is expected to increase. Caution is recommended when co-administering with these cytochrome P450 substrates).
No products indexed under this heading.

Repaglinide (Sorafenib inhibits CYP2B6 and CYP2C8 in vitro. Systemic exposure to substrates of CYP2B6 and CYP2C8 is expected to increase. Caution is recommended when co-administering with these cytochrome P450 substrates).
No products indexed under this heading.

Rosiglitazone Maleate (Sorafenib inhibits CYP2B6 and CYP2C8 in vitro. Systemic exposure to substrates of CYP2B6 and CYP2C8 is expected to increase. Caution is recommended when co-administering with these cytochrome P450 substrates). Products include:
Avandamet Tablets **1373**
Avandaryl Tablets **1379**
Avandia Tablets **1384**

Rosiglitazone/Metformin (Sorafenib inhibits CYP2B6 and CYP2C8 in vitro. Systemic exposure to substrates of CYP2B6 and CYP2C8 is expected to increase. Caution is recommended when co-administering with these cytochrome P450 substrates).
No products indexed under this heading.

Tolbutamide (Sorafenib inhibits CYP2B6 and CYP2C8 in vitro. Systemic exposure to substrates of CYP2B6 and CYP2C8 is expected to increase. Caution is recommended when co-administering with these cytochrome P450 substrates).
No products indexed under this heading.

Tolbutamide Sodium (Sorafenib inhibits CYP2B6 and CYP2C8 in vitro. Systemic exposure to substrates of CYP2B6 and CYP2C8 is expected to increase. Caution is recommended when co-administering with these cytochrome P450 substrates).
No products indexed under this heading.

Tretinoin (Sorafenib inhibits CYP2B6 and CYP2C8 in vitro. Systemic exposure to substrates of CYP2B6 and CYP2C8 is expected to increase. Caution is recommended when co-administering with these cytochrome P450 substrates). Products include:
Tri-Luma Cream **1213**
Vesanoid Capsules **2820**

Trimipramine Maleate (Sorafenib inhibits CYP2B6 and CYP2C8 in vitro. Systemic exposure to substrates of CYP2B6 and CYP2C8 is expected to increase. Caution is recommended when co-administering with these cytochrome P450 substrates).
No products indexed under this heading.

Verapamil Hydrochloride (Sorafenib inhibits CYP2B6 and CYP2C8 in vitro. Systemic exposure to substrates of CYP2B6 and CYP2C8 is expected to increase. Caution is recommended when co-administering with these cytochrome P450 substrates). Products include:
Covera-HS Tablets **3139**
Tarka Tablets **524**
Verelan PM Extended-Release Capsules, Controlled-Onset **3106**

Vitamin A (Sorafenib inhibits CYP2B6 and CYP2C8 in vitro. Systemic exposure to substrates of CYP2B6 and CYP2C8 is expected to increase. Caution is recommended when co-administering with these cytochrome P450 substrates). Products include:
Visutein Capsules **3329**

Vitamin A Acetate (Sorafenib inhibits CYP2B6 and CYP2C8 in vitro. Systemic exposure to substrates of CYP2B6 and CYP2C8 is expected to increase. Caution is recommended when co-administering with these cytochrome P450 substrates).
No products indexed under this heading.

Warfarin Sodium (Sorafenib inhibits CYP2B6 and CYP2C8 in vitro. Systemic exposure to substrates of CYP2B6 and CYP2C8 is expected to increase. Caution is recommended when co-administering with these cytochrome P450 substrates). Products include:
Coumadin for Injection **898**
Coumadin Tablets **898**

Zopiclone (Sorafenib inhibits CYP2B6 and CYP2C8 in vitro. Systemic exposure to substrates of CYP2B6 and CYP2C8 is expected to increase. Caution is recommended when co-administering with these cytochrome P450 substrates).
No products indexed under this heading.

NEXIUM DELAYED-RELEASE CAPSULES

(Esomeprazole Magnesium) **655**
May interact with certain other agents. Compounds in these categories include:

Amoxicillin (Co-administration of esomeprazole, clarithromycin, and amoxicillin has resulted in an increase in the plasma levels of esomeprazole and 14-hydroxyclarithromycin; the observed increase in esomeprazole exposure during co-administration with clarithromycin and amoxicillin is not expected to produce safety concerns). Products include:
Amoxil Capsules **1343**
Amoxil Chewable Tablets **1343**
Amoxil Pediatric Drops for Oral Suspension **1343**
Amoxil Powder for Oral Suspension **1343**
Amoxil Tablets **1343**
Augmentin **1360**
Augmentin Tablets **1363**
Augmentin XR Extended-Release Tablets **1369**
Augmentin ES-600 Powder for Oral Suspension **1366**
PREVPAC **3284**

Amoxicillin Trihydrate (Co-administration of esomeprazole, clarithromycin, and amoxicillin has resulted in an increase in the plasma levels of esomeprazole and 14-hydroxyclarithromycin; the observed increase in esomeprazole exposure during co-administration with clarithromycin and amoxicillin is not expected to produce safety concerns).
No products indexed under this heading.

Clarithromycin (Co-administration of esomeprazole, clarithromycin, and amoxicillin has resulted in an increase in the plasma levels of esomeprazole and 14-hydroxyclarithromycin; the observed increase in esomeprazole exposure during co-administration with clarithromycin and amoxicillin is not expected to produce safety concerns). Products include:
Biaxin/Biaxin XL **402**
PREVPAC **3284**

Diazepam (Esomeprazole may interfere with CYP2C19, the major metabolizing enzyme; co-administration of esomeprazole and diazepam, a CYP2C19 substrate, resulted in a 45% decrease in clearance of diazepam; increased plasma levels of diazepam were observed 12 hours after dosing and onwards; however, at that time the plasma levels of diazepam were below the therapeutic interval, and this interaction is unlikely to be of clinical relevance). Products include:
Diastat Rectal Delivery System **3343**
Valium Tablets **2819**

Digoxin (Esomeprazole inhibits gastric acid secretion; therefore, esomeprazole may interfere with the absorption of drugs where gastric pH is an important determinant of bioavailability, such as digoxin). Products include:
Lanoxicaps Capsules **1490**
Lanoxin Injection **1494**
Lanoxin Injection Pediatric **1497**
Lanoxin Tablets **1500**

Ferrous Fumarate (Esomeprazole inhibits gastric acid secretion; therefore, esomeprazole may interfere with the absorption of drugs where gastric pH is an important determinant of bioavailability, such as oral iron salts).
No products indexed under this heading.

Ferrous Gluconate (Esomeprazole inhibits gastric acid secretion; therefore, esomeprazole may interfere with the absorption of drugs where gastric pH is an important determinant of bioavailability, such as oral iron salts).
No products indexed under this heading.

Ferrous Sulfate (Esomeprazole inhibits gastric acid secretion; therefore, esomeprazole may interfere with the absorption of drugs where gastric pH is an important determinant of bioavailability, such as oral iron salts). Products include:
Slow Fe Iron Tablets **818**
Slow Fe with Folic Acid Tablets **819**

Iron (Esomeprazole inhibits gastric acid secretion; therefore, esomeprazole may interfere with the absorption of drugs where gastric pH is an important determinant of bioavailability, such as oral iron salts).
No products indexed under this heading.

Ketoconazole (Esomeprazole inhibits gastric acid secretion; therefore, esomeprazole may interfere with the absorption of drugs where gastric pH is an important determinant of bioavailability, such as ketoconazole). Products include:
Nizoral A-D Shampoo, 1% **1868**

Pimozide (Co-administration of clarithromycin-esomeprazole combination with pimozide is contraindicated; concurrent use of clarithromycin and/or erythromycin with pimozide has resulted in cardiac arrhythmias including QT prolongation, ventricular tachycardia, ventricular fibrillations and torsade de pointes).
No products indexed under this heading.

Polysaccharide Iron Complex (Esomeprazole inhibits gastric acid secretion; therefore, esomeprazole may interfere with the absorption of drugs where gastric pH is an important determinant of bioavailability, such as oral iron salts). Products include:

Nu-Iron 150 Capsules 2127

Warfarin Sodium (Changes in prothrombin measures have been reported among patients on concomitant warfarin and esomeprazole therapy. Increases in INR and prothrombin time may lead to abnormal bleeding and even death. Patients treated with proton pump inhibitors and warfarin concomitantly may need to be monitored for increases in INR and prothrombin time). Products include:

Coumadin for Injection 898
Coumadin Tablets 898

NEXIUM I.V.

(Esomeprazole Sodium) 659

May interact with iron containing oral preparations and certain other agents. Compounds in these categories include:

Atazanavir (Concomitant administration of esomeprazole may reduce the plasma levels of atazanavir).

No products indexed under this heading.

Atazanavir sulfate (Concomitant administration of esomeprazole may reduce the plasma levels of atazanavir). Products include:

Reyataz Capsules 921

Diazepam (Esomeprazole may interfere with CYP2C19, the major metabolizing enzyme; coadministration of esomeprazole and diazepam, a CYP2C19 substrate, resulted in a 45% decrease in clearance of diazepam; increased plasma levels of diazepam were observed 12 hours after dosing and onwards; however, at that time the plasma levels of diazepam were below the therapeutic interval, and this interaction is unlikely to be of clinical relevance). Products include:

Diastat Rectal Delivery System 3343
Valium Tablets 2819

Digoxin (Esomeprazole inhibits gastric acid secretion; therefore, esomeprazole may interfere with the absorption of drugs where gastric pH is an important determinant of bioavailability, such as digoxin). Products include:

Lanoxicaps Capsules 1490
Lanoxin Injection 1494
Lanoxin Injection Pediatric 1497
Lanoxin Tablets 1500

Ferrous Fumarate (Esomeprazole inhibits gastric acid secretion; therefore, esomeprazole may interfere with the absorption of drugs where gastric pH is an important determinant of bioavailability, such as oral iron salts).

No products indexed under this heading.

Ferrous Gluconate (Esomeprazole inhibits gastric acid secretion; therefore, esomeprazole may interfere with the absorption of drugs where gastric pH is an important determinant of bioavailability, such as oral iron salts).

No products indexed under this heading.

Ferrous Sulfate (Esomeprazole inhibits gastric acid secretion; therefore, esomeprazole may interfere with the absorption of drugs where gastric pH is an important determinant of bioavailability, such as oral iron salts). Products include:

Slow Fe Iron Tablets .... ▣818
Slow Fe with Folic Acid Tablets .... ▣819

Iron (Esomeprazole inhibits gastric acid secretion; therefore, esomeprazole may interfere with the absorption of drugs where gastric pH is an important determinant of bioavailability, such as oral iron salts).

No products indexed under this heading.

Ketoconazole (Esomeprazole inhibits gastric acid secretion; therefore, esomeprazole may interfere with the absorption of drugs where gastric pH is an important determinant of bioavailability, such as ketoconazole). Products include:

Nizoral A-D Shampoo, 1% 1868

Pimozide (Co-administration of clarithromycin-esomeprazole combination with pimozide is contraindicated; concurrent use of clarithromycin and/or erythromycin with pimozide has resulted in cardiac arrhythmias including QT prolongation, ventricular tachycardia, ventricular fibrillations and torsade de pointes).

No products indexed under this heading.

Polysaccharide Iron Complex (Esomeprazole inhibits gastric acid secretion; therefore, esomeprazole may interfere with the absorption of drugs where gastric pH is an important determinant of bioavailability, such as oral iron salts). Products include:

Nu-Iron 150 Capsules 2127

Warfarin Sodium (Changes in prothrombin measures have been reported among patients on concomitant warfarin and esomeprazole therapy. Increases in INR and prothrombin time may lead to abnormal bleeding and even death. Patients treated with proton pump inhibitors and warfarin concomitantly may need to be monitored for increases in INR and prothrombin time). Products include:

Coumadin for Injection 898
Coumadin Tablets 898

NIASPAN EXTENDED-RELEASE TABLETS

(Niacin) 1730

May interact with beta blockers, calcium channel blockers, oral anticoagulants, HMG-CoA reductase inhibitors, nitrates and nitrites, and certain other agents. Compounds in these categories include:

Acebutolol Hydrochloride (Co-administration with vasoactive drugs, such as adrenergic blocking agents, may result in postural hypotension, particularly in patients with unstable angina or acute phase of myocardial infarction).

No products indexed under this heading.

Amlodipine Besylate (Co-administration with vasoactive drugs, such as calcium channel blockers, may result in postural hypotension, particularly in patients with unstable angina or acute phase of myocardial infarction). Products include:

Caduet Tablets 2508
Lotrel Capsules 2249
Norvasc Tablets 2545

Amyl Nitrite (Co-administration with vasoactive drugs, such as nitrates, may result in postural hypotension, particularly in patients with unstable angina or acute phase of myocardial infarction).

No products indexed under this heading.

Anisindione (Niacin prolongs prothrombin time; caution should be exercised when used concurrently). Products include:

Miradon Tablets 3042

Aspirin (Concomitant aspirin may decrease the metabolic clearance of nicotinic acid; the clinical relevance of this finding is unclear). Products include:

Aggrenox Capsules 822
Bayer Aspirin 744
BC Allergy Sinus Cold Powder .... ▣677
BC Headache Powder .... ▣677
Arthritis Strength BC Powder .... ▣677
BC Sinus Cold Powder .... ▣677
Excedrin Extra Strength Caplets/Tablets/Geltabs .... ▣684
Excedrin Migraine Caplets/Tablets/Geltabs .... ▣609
Goody's Body Pain Formula Powder .... ▣684
Goody's Extra Strength Headache Powders .... ▣611
Goody's Extra Strength Pain Relief Tablets .... ▣685
Percodan Tablets 1132
St. Joseph 81 mg Aspirin Chewable and Enteric Coated Tablets 1869

Atenolol (Co-administration with vasoactive drugs, such as adrenergic blocking agents, may result in postural hypotension, particularly in patients with unstable angina or acute phase of myocardial infarction).

No products indexed under this heading.

Atorvastatin Calcium (Co-administration of lipid-altering doses (≥ 1 g/day) of niacin and HMG-CoA reductase inhibitors has resulted in rare cases of rhabdomyolysis). Products include:

Caduet Tablets 2508
Lipitor Tablets 2483

Bepridil Hydrochloride (Co-administration with vasoactive drugs, such as calcium channel blockers, may result in postural hypotension, particularly in patients with unstable angina or acute phase of myocardial infarction).

No products indexed under this heading.

Betaxolol Hydrochloride (Co-administration with vasoactive drugs, such as adrenergic blocking agents, may result in postural hypotension, particularly in patients with unstable angina or acute phase of myocardial infarction). Products include:

Betoptic S Ophthalmic Suspension.................................. 558

Bisoprolol Fumarate (Co-administration with vasoactive drugs, such as adrenergic blocking agents, may result in postural hypotension, particularly in patients with unstable angina or acute phase of myocardial infarction).

No products indexed under this heading.

Carteolol Hydrochloride (Co-administration with vasoactive drugs, such as adrenergic blocking agents, may result in postural hypotension, particularly in patients with unstable angina or acute phase of myocardial infarction). Products include:

Carteolol Hydrochloride Ophthalmic Solution USP, 1%....... ⊙249

Cerivastatin Sodium (Co-administration of lipid-altering doses (≥ 1 g/day) of niacin and HMG-CoA reductase inhibitors has resulted in rare cases of rhabdomyolysis).

No products indexed under this heading.

Cholestyramine (*In vitro* study resulted in approximately 10% to 30% of available niacin bound to cholestyramine; 4 to 6 hours or greater should elapse between ingestion of bile acid-binding resins and the administration of Niaspan).

No products indexed under this heading.

Colestipol Hydrochloride (*In vitro* study resulted in approximately 90% of available niacin bound to colestipol; 4 to 6 hours or greater should elapse between ingestion of bile acid-binding resins and the administration of Niaspan).

No products indexed under this heading.

Dicumarol (Niacin prolongs prothrombin time; caution should be exercised when used concurrently).

No products indexed under this heading.

Diltiazem Hydrochloride (Co-administration with vasoactive drugs, such as calcium channel blockers, may result in postural hypotension, particularly in patients with unstable angina or acute phase of myocardial infarction). Products include:

Cardizem LA Extended Release Tablets.. 1728
Tiazac Capsules 1201

Erythrityl Tetranitrate (Co-administration with vasoactive drugs, such as nitrates, may result in postural hypotension, particularly in patients with unstable angina or acute phase of myocardial infarction).

No products indexed under this heading.

Esmolol Hydrochloride (Co-administration with vasoactive drugs, such as adrenergic blocking agents, may result in postural hypotension, particularly in patients with unstable angina or acute phase of myocardial infarction).

No products indexed under this heading.

Felodipine (Co-administration with vasoactive drugs, such as calcium channel blockers, may result in postural hypotension, particularly in patients with unstable angina or acute phase of myocardial infarction).

No products indexed under this heading.

Fluvastatin Sodium (Co-administration of lipid-altering doses (≥ 1 g/day) of niacin and HMG-CoA reductase inhibitors has resulted in rare cases of rhabdomyolysis). Products include:

Lescol Capsules 2233
Lescol XL Tablets 2233

Isosorbide Dinitrate (Co-administration with vasoactive drugs, such as nitrates, may result in postural hypotension, particularly

in patients with unstable angina or acute phase of myocardial infarction). Products include:
BiDil Tablets ... 2171

Isosorbide Mononitrate (Co-administration with vasoactive drugs, such as nitrates, may result in postural hypotension, particularly in patients with unstable angina or acute phase of myocardial infarction). Products include:
Imdur Tablets ... 3018

Isradipine (Co-administration with vasoactive drugs, such as calcium channel blockers, may result in postural hypotension, particularly in patients with unstable angina or acute phase of myocardial infarction). Products include:
DynaCirc CR Tablets ... 2721

Labetalol Hydrochloride (Co-administration with vasoactive drugs, such as adrenergic blocking agents, may result in postural hypotension, particularly in patients with unstable angina or acute phase of myocardial infarction).
No products indexed under this heading.

Levobunolol Hydrochloride (Co-administration with vasoactive drugs, such as adrenergic blocking agents, may result in postural hypotension, particularly in patients with unstable angina or acute phase of myocardial infarction). Products include:
Betagan Ophthalmic Solution, USP ... ⊙220

Lovastatin (Co-administration of lipid-altering doses (≥ 1 g/day) of niacin and HMG-CoA reductase inhibitors has resulted in rare cases of rhabdomyolysis). Products include:
Advicor Tablets ... 1722
Altoprev Extended-Release Tablets ... 3109
Mevacor Tablets ... 2021

Mecamylamine Hydrochloride (Niacin may potentiate the effects of ganglionic blocking agents, such as mecamylamine, resulting in postural hypotension).
No products indexed under this heading.

Metipranolol Hydrochloride (Co-administration with vasoactive drugs, such as adrenergic blocking agents, may result in postural hypotension, particularly in patients with unstable angina or acute phase of myocardial infarction).
No products indexed under this heading.

Metoprolol Succinate (Co-administration with vasoactive drugs, such as adrenergic blocking agents, may result in postural hypotension, particularly in patients with unstable angina or acute phase of myocardial infarction). Products include:
Toprol-XL Tablets ... 668

Metoprolol Tartrate (Co-administration with vasoactive drugs, such as adrenergic blocking agents, may result in postural hypotension, particularly in patients with unstable angina or acute phase of myocardial infarction). Products include:
Lopressor Injection ... 2238
Lopressor Tablets ... 2238
Lopressor HCT 50/25 Tablets ... 2241
Lopressor HCT 100/25 Tablets ... 2241
Lopressor HCT 100/50 Tablets ... 2241

Mibefradil Dihydrochloride (Co-administration with vasoactive drugs, such as calcium channel blockers, may result in postural hypotension, particularly in patients with unstable angina or acute phase of myocardial infarction).
No products indexed under this heading.

Nadolol (Co-administration with vasoactive drugs, such as adrenergic blocking agents, may result in postural hypotension, particularly in patients with unstable angina or acute phase of myocardial infarction). Products include:
Nadolol Tablets ... 2159

Nicardipine Hydrochloride (Co-administration with vasoactive drugs, such as calcium channel blockers, may result in postural hypotension, particularly in patients with unstable angina or acute phase of myocardial infarction). Products include:
Cardene I.V. ... 2497

Nicotinamide (May potentiate the adverse effects of Niaspan). Products include:
Nicomide Tablets ... 1088

Nifedipine (Co-administration with vasoactive drugs, such as calcium channel blockers, may result in postural hypotension, particularly in patients with unstable angina or acute phase of myocardial infarction). Products include:
Adalat CC Tablets ... 2964

Nimodipine (Co-administration with vasoactive drugs, such as calcium channel blockers, may result in postural hypotension, particularly in patients with unstable angina or acute phase of myocardial infarction). Products include:
Nimotop Capsules ... 749

Nisoldipine (Co-administration with vasoactive drugs, such as calcium channel blockers, may result in postural hypotension, particularly in patients with unstable angina or acute phase of myocardial infarction). Products include:
Sular Tablets ... 3122

Nitroglycerin (Co-administration with vasoactive drugs, such as nitrates, may result in postural hypotension, particularly in patients with unstable angina or acute phase of myocardial infarction). Products include:
Nitro-Dur Transdermal Infusion System ... 3046
Nitrolingual Pumpspray ... 3120

Penbutolol Sulfate (Co-administration with vasoactive drugs, such as adrenergic blocking agents, may result in postural hypotension, particularly in patients with unstable angina or acute phase of myocardial infarction).
No products indexed under this heading.

Pentaerythritol Tetranitrate (Co-administration with vasoactive drugs, such as nitrates, may result in postural hypotension, particularly in patients with unstable angina or acute phase of myocardial infarction).
No products indexed under this heading.

Pindolol (Co-administration with vasoactive drugs, such as adrenergic blocking agents, may result in postural hypotension, particularly in patients with unstable angina or acute phase of myocardial infarction).
No products indexed under this heading.

Pravastatin Sodium (Co-administration of lipid-altering doses (≥ 1 g/day) of niacin and HMG-CoA reductase inhibitors has resulted in rare cases of rhabdomyolysis).
No products indexed under this heading.

Propranolol Hydrochloride (Co-administration with vasoactive drugs, such as adrenergic blocking agents, may result in postural hypotension, particularly in patients with unstable angina or acute phase of myocardial infarction). Products include:
Inderal LA Long-Acting Capsules ... 3429
InnoPran XL Capsules ... 2723

Simvastatin (Co-administration of lipid-altering doses (≥ 1 g/day) of niacin and HMG-CoA reductase inhibitors has resulted in rare cases of rhabdomyolysis). Products include:
Vytorin 10/10 Tablets ... 2114
Vytorin 10/10 Tablets ... 3077
Vytorin 10/20 Tablets ... 2114
Vytorin 10/20 Tablets ... 3077
Vytorin 10/40 Tablets ... 2114
Vytorin 10/40 Tablets ... 3077
Vytorin 10/80 Tablets ... 2114
Vytorin 10/80 Tablets ... 3077
Zocor Tablets ... 2105

Sotalol Hydrochloride (Co-administration with vasoactive drugs, such as adrenergic blocking agents, may result in postural hypotension, particularly in patients with unstable angina or acute phase of myocardial infarction).
No products indexed under this heading.

Timolol Hemihydrate (Co-administration with vasoactive drugs, such as adrenergic blocking agents, may result in postural hypotension, particularly in patients with unstable angina or acute phase of myocardial infarction). Products include:
Betimol Ophthalmic Solution ... 3382
Betimol Ophthalmic Solution ... ⊙295

Timolol Maleate (Co-administration with vasoactive drugs, such as adrenergic blocking agents, may result in postural hypotension, particularly in patients with unstable angina or acute phase of myocardial infarction). Products include:
Blocadren Tablets ... 1916
Cosopt Sterile Ophthalmic Solution ... 1931
Timolide Tablets ... 2086
Timoptic Sterile Ophthalmic Solution ... 2088
Timoptic in Ocudose ... 2091
Timoptic-XE Sterile Ophthalmic Gel Forming Solution ... 2092

Verapamil Hydrochloride (Co-administration with vasoactive drugs, such as calcium channel blockers, may result in postural hypotension, particularly in patients with unstable angina or acute phase of myocardial infarction). Products include:
Covera-HS Tablets ... 3139
Tarka Tablets ... 524
Verelan PM Extended-Release Capsules, Controlled-Onset ... 3106

Warfarin Sodium (Niacin prolongs prothrombin time; caution should be exercised when used concurrently). Products include:
Coumadin for Injection ... 898
Coumadin Tablets ... 898

Food Interactions

Alcohol (Concomitant alcohol may increase the side effects of flushing and pruritus and should be avoided around the time of Niaspan ingestion).

Drinks, hot, unspecified (Concomitant hot drinks may increase the side effects of flushing and pruritus and should be avoided around the time of Niaspan ingestion).

NICODERM CQ CLEAR PATCH

(Nicotine) ... 622
See Nicorette Gum

NICOMIDE TABLETS

(Folic Acid, Nicotinamide, Zinc Oxide) ... 1088
May interact with fluoroquinolone antibiotics, tetracyclines, and certain other agents. Compounds in these categories include:

Alatrofloxacin Mesylate (Decreased absorption of oral quinolones).
No products indexed under this heading.

Carbamazepine (Reduced clearance of carbamazepine). Products include:
Carbatrol Capsules ... 3171
Equetro Extended-Release Capsules ... 3180
Tegretol/Tegretol-XR ... 2295

Ciprofloxacin (Decreased absorption of oral quinolones). Products include:
Cipro Oral Suspension ... 2977
Cipro I.V. ... 2984
Cipro XR Tablets ... 2990
Ciprodex Otic Suspension ... 559

Ciprofloxacin Hydrochloride (Decreased absorption of oral quinolones). Products include:
Ciloxan Ophthalmic Ointment ... 559
Ciloxan Ophthalmic Solution ... ⊙206
Cipro Tablets ... 2977
Proquin XR Tablets ... 1153

Demeclocycline Hydrochloride (Decreased absorption of oral tetracyclines).
No products indexed under this heading.

Doxycycline Calcium (Decreased absorption of oral tetracyclines).
No products indexed under this heading.

Doxycycline Hyclate (Decreased absorption of oral tetracyclines).
No products indexed under this heading.

Doxycycline Monohydrate (Decreased absorption of oral tetracyclines). Products include:
Oracea Capsules ... 1000

Enoxacin (Decreased absorption of oral quinolones).
No products indexed under this heading.

Grepafloxacin Hydrochloride (Decreased absorption of oral quinolones).
No products indexed under this heading.

Lomefloxacin Hydrochloride (Decreased absorption of oral quinolones).
No products indexed under this heading.

Methacycline Hydrochloride (Decreased absorption of oral tetracyclines).
No products indexed under this heading.

Minocycline Hydrochloride (Decreased absorption of oral tetracyclines). Products include:
Solodyn Extended Release Tablets 1890

Moxifloxacin Hydrochloride (Decreased absorption of oral quinolones). Products include:
Avelox 2970
Vigamox Ophthalmic Solution 564

Norfloxacin (Decreased absorption of oral quinolones). Products include:
Noroxin Tablets 2032

Ofloxacin (Decreased absorption of oral quinolones). Products include:
Floxin Otic Solution 1049

Oxytetracycline Hydrochloride (Decreased absorption of oral tetracyclines).
No products indexed under this heading.

Primidone (Reduced clearance of primidone).
No products indexed under this heading.

Tetracycline Hydrochloride (Decreased absorption of oral tetracyclines).
No products indexed under this heading.

Trovafloxacin Mesylate (Decreased absorption of oral quinolones).
No products indexed under this heading.

NIMBEX INJECTION

(Cisatracurium Besylate) 498

May interact with aminoglycosides, lithium preparations, local anesthetics, phenytoin, tetracyclines, and certain other agents. Compounds in these categories include:

Amikacin Sulfate (Enhances neuromuscular blocking action).
No products indexed under this heading.

Bacitracin (Enhances neuromuscular blocking action). Products include:
Neosporin Antibiotic Ointment .... ■□643
Polysporin First Aid Antibiotic Ointment .... ■□643

Bupivacaine Hydrochloride (Enhances neuromuscular blocking action).
No products indexed under this heading.

Carbamazepine (Chronic administration of carbamazepine may produce resistance to the neuromuscular blocking action; slightly shorter durations of neuromuscular block may be anticipated). Products include:
Carbatrol Capsules 3171
Equetro Extended-Release Capsules 3180
Tegretol/Tegretol-XR 2295

Chloroprocaine Hydrochloride (Enhances neuromuscular blocking action).
No products indexed under this heading.

Clindamycin Hydrochloride (Enhances neuromuscular blocking action). Products include:
Cleocin Vaginal Ovules 2616

Clindamycin Palmitate Hydrochloride (Enhances neuromuscular blocking action).
No products indexed under this heading.

Clindamycin Phosphate (Enhances neuromuscular blocking action). Products include:
Benzaclin Topical Gel 2877
Clindagel 1203
Evoclin Foam, 1% 1009

Colistimethate Sodium (Enhances neuromuscular blocking action).
No products indexed under this heading.

Colistin Sulfate (Enhances neuromuscular blocking action).
No products indexed under this heading.

Demeclocycline Hydrochloride (Enhances neuromuscular blocking action).
No products indexed under this heading.

Doxycycline Calcium (Enhances neuromuscular blocking action).
No products indexed under this heading.

Doxycycline Hyclate (Enhances neuromuscular blocking action).
No products indexed under this heading.

Doxycycline Monohydrate (Enhances neuromuscular blocking action). Products include:
Oracea Capsules 1000

Enflurane (Enflurane administered with nitrous oxide/oxygen may prolong the clinically effective duration of action of initial and maintenance doses of cisatracurium and decrease the required infusion rate of cisatracurium).
No products indexed under this heading.

Etidocaine Hydrochloride (Enhances neuromuscular blocking action).
No products indexed under this heading.

Fosphenytoin Sodium (Chronic administration of phenytoin may produce resistance to the neuromuscular blocking action; slightly shorter durations of neuromuscular block may be anticipated).
No products indexed under this heading.

Gentamicin Sulfate (Enhances neuromuscular blocking action). Products include:
Garamycin Injectable 3014
Pred-G Ophthalmic Ointment .... ⊙237
Pred-G Ophthalmic Suspension .... ⊙236

Isoflurane (Isoflurane administered with nitrous oxide/oxygen may prolong the clinically effective duration of action of initial and maintenance doses of cisatracurium and decrease the required infusion rate of cisatracurium).
No products indexed under this heading.

Kanamycin Sulfate (Enhances neuromuscular blocking action).
No products indexed under this heading.

Levobupivacaine Hydrochloride (Enhances neuromuscular blocking action).
No products indexed under this heading.

Lidocaine Hydrochloride (Enhances neuromuscular blocking action).
No products indexed under this heading.

Lincomycin Hydrochloride (Enhances neuromuscular blocking action).
No products indexed under this heading.

Lithium (Enhances neuromuscular blocking action).
No products indexed under this heading.

Lithium Carbonate (Enhances neuromuscular blocking action). Products include:
Lithobid Tablets 1692

Lithium Citrate (Enhances neuromuscular blocking action).
No products indexed under this heading.

Magnesium Salts (Enhances neuromuscular blocking action).
No products indexed under this heading.

Mepivacaine Hydrochloride (Enhances neuromuscular blocking action).
No products indexed under this heading.

Methacycline Hydrochloride (Enhances neuromuscular blocking action).
No products indexed under this heading.

Minocycline Hydrochloride (Enhances neuromuscular blocking action). Products include:
Solodyn Extended Release Tablets 1890

Oxytetracycline Hydrochloride (Enhances neuromuscular blocking action).
No products indexed under this heading.

Phenytoin (Chronic administration of phenytoin may produce resistance to the neuromuscular blocking action; slightly shorter durations of neuromuscular block may be anticipated).
No products indexed under this heading.

Phenytoin Sodium (Chronic administration of phenytoin may produce resistance to the neuromuscular blocking action; slightly shorter durations of neuromuscular block may be anticipated). Products include:
Phenytek Capsules 2160

Polymyxin Preparations (Enhances neuromuscular blocking action).
No products indexed under this heading.

Procainamide Hydrochloride (Enhances neuromuscular blocking action).
No products indexed under this heading.

Procaine Hydrochloride (Enhances neuromuscular blocking action).
No products indexed under this heading.

Quinidine Gluconate (Enhances neuromuscular blocking action).
No products indexed under this heading.

Quinidine Polygalacturonate (Enhances neuromuscular blocking action).
No products indexed under this heading.

Quinidine Sulfate (Enhances neuromuscular blocking action).
No products indexed under this heading.

Streptomycin Sulfate (Enhances neuromuscular blocking action).
No products indexed under this heading.

Tetracaine Hydrochloride (Enhances neuromuscular blocking action). Products include:
Cetacaine Topical Anesthetic 999

Tetracycline Hydrochloride (Enhances neuromuscular blocking action).
No products indexed under this heading.

Tobramycin (Enhances neuromuscular blocking action). Products include:
TOBI Solution for Inhalation 2298
TobraDex Ophthalmic Ointment 562
TobraDex Ophthalmic Suspension 563
Zylet Ophthalmic Suspension .... ⊙259

Tobramycin Sulfate (Enhances neuromuscular blocking action).
No products indexed under this heading.

NIMOTOP CAPSULES

(Nimodipine) 749

May interact with antihypertensives, calcium channel blockers, and certain other agents. Compounds in these categories include:

Acebutolol Hydrochloride (Concomitant administration results in intensified effect).
No products indexed under this heading.

Amlodipine Besylate (Possibility of enhanced cardiovascular action). Products include:
Caduet Tablets 2508
Lotrel Capsules 2249
Norvasc Tablets 2545

Atenolol (Concomitant administration results in intensified effect).
No products indexed under this heading.

Benazepril Hydrochloride (Concomitant administration results in intensified effect). Products include:
Lotensin Tablets 2243
Lotensin HCT Tablets 2246
Lotrel Capsules 2249

Bendroflumethiazide (Concomitant administration results in intensified effect).
No products indexed under this heading.

Bepridil Hydrochloride (Possibility of enhanced cardiovascular action).
No products indexed under this heading.

Betaxolol Hydrochloride (Concomitant administration results in intensified effect). Products include:
Betoptic S Ophthalmic Suspension 558

Bisoprolol Fumarate (Concomitant administration results in intensified effect).
No products indexed under this heading.

Candesartan Cilexetil (Concomitant administration results in intensified effect). Products include:
Atacand Tablets 649
Atacand HCT 651

Captopril (Concomitant administration results in intensified effect). Products include:
Captopril Tablets 2149

Carteolol Hydrochloride (Concomitant administration results in intensified effect). Products include:
Carteolol Hydrochloride Ophthalmic Solution USP, 1% .... ⊙249

Chlorothiazide (Concomitant administration results in intensified effect). Products include:
Diuril Oral Suspension 1954

Chlorothiazide Sodium (Concomitant administration results in intensified effect). Products include:
Diuril Sodium Intravenous 2467

Chlorthalidone (Concomitant administration results in intensified effect). Products include:
Clorpres Tablets 2153

Cimetidine (May increase peak nimodipine plasma concentrations and AUC). Products include:
Tagamet HB 200 Tablets .... ▣664

Cimetidine Hydrochloride (May increase peak nimodipine plasma concentrations and AUC).
No products indexed under this heading.

Clonidine (Concomitant administration results in intensified effect). Products include:
Catapres-TTS 844

Clonidine Hydrochloride (Concomitant administration results in intensified effect). Products include:
Catapres Tablets 843
Clorpres Tablets 2153

Deserpidine (Concomitant administration results in intensified effect).
No products indexed under this heading.

Diazoxide (Concomitant administration results in intensified effect). Products include:
Hyperstat I.V. 3017

Diltiazem Hydrochloride (Possibility of enhanced cardiovascular action). Products include:
Cardizem LA Extended Release Tablets 1728
Tiazac Capsules 1201

Doxazosin Mesylate (Concomitant administration results in intensified effect). Products include:
Cardura XL Tablets 2515

Enalapril Maleate (Concomitant administration results in intensified effect). Products include:
Vasotec I.V. Injection 2103

Enalaprilat (Concomitant administration results in intensified effect).
No products indexed under this heading.

Eprosartan Mesylate (Concomitant administration results in intensified effect). Products include:
Teveten Tablets 1735
Teveten HCT Tablets 1737

Esmolol Hydrochloride (Concomitant administration results in intensified effect).
No products indexed under this heading.

Felodipine (Possibility of enhanced cardiovascular action).
No products indexed under this heading.

Fosinopril Sodium (Concomitant administration results in intensified effect).
No products indexed under this heading.

Furosemide (Concomitant administration results in intensified effect). Products include:
Furosemide Tablets 2154

Guanabenz Acetate (Concomitant administration results in intensified effect).
No products indexed under this heading.

Guanethidine Monosulfate (Concomitant administration results in intensified effect).
No products indexed under this heading.

Hydralazine Hydrochloride (Concomitant administration results in intensified effect). Products include:
BiDil Tablets 2171

Hydrochlorothiazide (Concomitant administration results in intensified effect). Products include:
Aldoril Tablets 1910
Atacand HCT 651
Avalide Tablets 888
Avalide Tablets 2874
Benicar HCT Tablets 1044
Diovan HCT Tablets 2196
Dyazide Capsules 1423
Hyzaar 50-12.5 Tablets 1990
Hyzaar 100-12.5 Tablets 1990
Hyzaar 100-25 Tablets 1990
Lopressor HCT 50/25 Tablets 2241
Lopressor HCT 100/25 Tablets 2241
Lopressor HCT 100/50 Tablets 2241
Lotensin HCT Tablets 2246
Micardis HCT Tablets 856
Moduretic Tablets 2028
Prinzide Tablets 2056
Teveten HCT Tablets 1737
Timolide Tablets 2086
Uniretic Tablets 3100

Hydroflumethiazide (Concomitant administration results in intensified effect).
No products indexed under this heading.

Indapamide (Concomitant administration results in intensified effect). Products include:
Indapamide Tablets 2156

Irbesartan (Concomitant administration results in intensified effect). Products include:
Avalide Tablets 888
Avalide Tablets 2874
Avapro Tablets 891
Avapro Tablets 2871

Isradipine (Possibility of enhanced cardiovascular action). Products include:
DynaCirc CR Tablets 2721

Labetalol Hydrochloride (Concomitant administration results in intensified effect).
No products indexed under this heading.

Lisinopril (Concomitant administration results in intensified effect). Products include:
Prinivil Tablets 2052
Prinzide Tablets 2056

Losartan Potassium (Concomitant administration results in intensified effect). Products include:
Cozaar Tablets 1935
Hyzaar 50-12.5 Tablets 1990
Hyzaar 100-12.5 Tablets 1990
Hyzaar 100-25 Tablets 1990

Mecamylamine Hydrochloride (Concomitant administration results in intensified effect).
No products indexed under this heading.

Methyclothiazide (Concomitant administration results in intensified effect).
No products indexed under this heading.

Methyldopa (Concomitant administration results in intensified effect). Products include:
Aldoril Tablets 1910

Methyldopate Hydrochloride (Concomitant administration results in intensified effect).
No products indexed under this heading.

Metolazone (Concomitant administration results in intensified effect).
No products indexed under this heading.

Metoprolol Succinate (Concomitant administration results in intensified effect). Products include:
Toprol-XL Tablets 668

Metoprolol Tartrate (Concomitant administration results in intensified effect). Products include:
Lopressor Injection 2238
Lopressor Tablets 2238
Lopressor HCT 50/25 Tablets 2241
Lopressor HCT 100/25 Tablets 2241
Lopressor HCT 100/50 Tablets 2241

Metyrosine (Concomitant administration results in intensified effect). Products include:
Demser Capsules 1953

Mibefradil Dihydrochloride (Possibility of enhanced cardiovascular action).
No products indexed under this heading.

Minoxidil (Concomitant administration results in intensified effect). Products include:
Men's Rogaine Extra Strength Hair Regrowth Treatment Topical Solution, Ocean Rush Scent and Original Unscented ..... ▣633
Men's Rogaine Foam Hair Regrowth Treatment .... ▣633
Women's Rogaine Hair Regrowth Treatment Topical Solution, Spring Bloom Scent and Original Unscented .... ▣634

Moexipril Hydrochloride (Concomitant administration results in intensified effect). Products include:
Uniretic Tablets 3100
Univasc Tablets 3104

Nadolol (Concomitant administration results in intensified effect). Products include:
Nadolol Tablets 2159

Nicardipine Hydrochloride (Possibility of enhanced cardiovascular action). Products include:
Cardene I.V. 2497

Nifedipine (Possibility of enhanced cardiovascular action). Products include:
Adalat CC Tablets 2964

Nisoldipine (Possibility of enhanced cardiovascular action). Products include:
Sular Tablets 3122

Nitroglycerin (Concomitant administration results in intensified effect). Products include:
Nitro-Dur Transdermal Infusion System 3046
Nitrolingual Pumpspray 3120

Penbutolol Sulfate (Concomitant administration results in intensified effect).
No products indexed under this heading.

Perindopril Erbumine (Concomitant administration results in intensified effect). Products include:
Aceon Tablets (2 mg, 4 mg, 8 mg) 3194

Phenoxybenzamine Hydrochloride (Concomitant administration results in intensified effect). Products include:
Dibenzyline Capsules 3399

Phentolamine Mesylate (Concomitant administration results in intensified effect).
No products indexed under this heading.

Phenytoin (Potential for phenytoin toxicity).
No products indexed under this heading.

Phenytoin Sodium (Potential for phenytoin toxicity). Products include:
Phenytek Capsules 2160

Pindolol (Concomitant administration results in intensified effect).
No products indexed under this heading.

Polythiazide (Concomitant administration results in intensified effect).
No products indexed under this heading.

Prazosin Hydrochloride (Concomitant administration results in intensified effect).
No products indexed under this heading.

Propranolol Hydrochloride (Concomitant administration results in intensified effect). Products include:
Inderal LA Long-Acting Capsules 3429
InnoPran XL Capsules 2723

Quinapril Hydrochloride (Concomitant administration results in intensified effect).
No products indexed under this heading.

Ramipril (Concomitant administration results in intensified effect). Products include:
Altace Capsules 1702

Rauwolfia Serpentina (Concomitant administration results in intensified effect).
No products indexed under this heading.

Rescinnamine (Concomitant administration results in intensified effect).
No products indexed under this heading.

Reserpine (Concomitant administration results in intensified effect).
No products indexed under this heading.

Sodium Nitroprusside (Concomitant administration results in intensified effect).
No products indexed under this heading.

Sotalol Hydrochloride (Concomitant administration results in intensified effect).
No products indexed under this heading.

Spirapril Hydrochloride (Concomitant administration results in intensified effect).
No products indexed under this heading.

Telmisartan (Concomitant administration results in intensified effect). Products include:
Micardis Tablets 854
Micardis HCT Tablets 856

Terazosin Hydrochloride (Concomitant administration results in intensified effect). Products include:
Hytrin Capsules 471

Timolol Maleate (Concomitant administration results in intensified effect). Products include:
Blocadren Tablets 1916
Cosopt Sterile Ophthalmic Solution 1931
Timolide Tablets 2086

Timoptic Sterile Ophthalmic Solution 2088
Timoptic in Ocudose 2091
Timoptic-XE Sterile Ophthalmic Gel Forming Solution 2092

Torsemide (Concomitant administration results in intensified effect). Products include:
Demadex Injection 2759
Demadex Tablets 2759

Trandolapril (Concomitant administration results in intensified effect). Products include:
Mavik Tablets 486
Tarka Tablets 524

Trimethaphan Camsylate (Concomitant administration results in intensified effect).
No products indexed under this heading.

Valsartan (Concomitant administration results in intensified effect). Products include:
Diovan Tablets 2193
Diovan HCT Tablets 2196

Verapamil Hydrochloride (Possibility of enhanced cardiovascular action). Products include:
Covera-HS Tablets 3139
Tarka Tablets 524
Verelan PM Extended-Release Capsules, Controlled-Onset 3106

Food Interactions

Meal, unspecified (Administration of nimodipine capsules following a standard breakfast resulted in 68% lower peak plasma concentration and 38% lower bioavailability).

NIPENT FOR INJECTION

(Pentostatin) 1863
May interact with:

Allopurinol (Both drugs are associated with skin rashes; concomitant therapy in one patient has resulted in a fatal hypersensitivity vasculitis).
No products indexed under this heading.

Carmustine (BCNU) (Co-administration with high dose cyclophosphamide, carmustine, and etoposide has resulted in a report of acute pulmonary edema, hypotension, and death).
No products indexed under this heading.

Cyclophosphamide (Co-administration with high dose cyclophosphamide, carmustine, and etoposide has resulted in a report of acute pulmonary edema, hypotension, and death).
No products indexed under this heading.

Etoposide (Co-administration with high dose cyclophosphamide, carmustine, and etoposide has resulted in a report of acute pulmonary edema, hypotension, and death).
No products indexed under this heading.

Fludarabine Phosphate (Increased risk of fatal pulmonary toxicity; combined use is not recommended).
No products indexed under this heading.

Vidarabine (Enhanced effects of vidarabine and may result in increased adverse reactions associated with each drug).
No products indexed under this heading.

NIRAVAM ORALLY DISINTEGRATING TABLETS

(Alprazolam) 3092
May interact with antacids, antihistamines, central nervous system depressants, cytochrome p450 3a inhibitors (selected), anticonvulsants, histamine H2-receptor antagonists, macrolide antibiotics, oral contraceptives, proton pump inhibitor, psychotropics, and certain other agents. Compounds in these categories include:

Acrivastine (The benzodiazepines, including alprazolam, produce additive CNS depressant effects when co-administered with antihistamines).
No products indexed under this heading.

Alfentanil Hydrochloride (The benzodiazepines, including alprazolam, produce additive CNS depressant effects when co-administered with other drugs which themselves produce CNS depression).
No products indexed under this heading.

Aluminum Carbonate (Because Niravam disintegrates in the presence of saliva and the formulation requires an acidic environment to dissolve, concomitant drugs or diseases that raise stomach pH might slow disintegration or dissolution, resulting in slowed or decreased absorption).
No products indexed under this heading.

Aluminum Hydroxide (Because Niravam disintegrates in the presence of saliva and the formulation requires an acidic environment to dissolve, concomitant drugs or diseases that raise stomach pH might slow disintegration or dissolution, resulting in slowed or decreased absorption). Products include:
Gaviscon Regular Strength Liquid .. ■658
Gaviscon Regular Strength Tablets .... ■658
Gaviscon Extra Strength Liquid .... ■658
Gaviscon Extra Strength Tablets .... ■658
Maalox Regular Strength Antacid/Antigas Liquid 2175
Maalox Max Maximum Strength Antacid/Anti-Gas Liquid 2176

Amiodarone Hydrochloride (Data from in vitro studies of benzodiazepines, other than alprazolam, suggest a possible drug interaction with amiodarone; caution is recommended during co-administration).
No products indexed under this heading.

Amitriptyline Hydrochloride (The benzodiazepines, including alprazolam, produce additive CNS depressant effects when co-administered with other psychotropic medications. If alprazolam is to be combined with other psychotropic agents, careful consideration should be given to the pharmacology of the agents to be employed, particularly with compounds which might potentiate the action of benzodiazepines).
No products indexed under this heading.

Amoxapine (The benzodiazepines, including alprazolam, produce additive CNS depressant effects when co-administered with other psychotropic medications. If alprazolam is to be combined with other psychotropic agents, careful consideration should be given to the pharmacology of the agents to be employed, particularly with compounds which might potentiate the action of benzodiazepines).
No products indexed under this heading.

Amprenavir (The initial step in alprazolam metabolism is hydroxylation catalyzed by cytochrome P450 3A (CYP3A). Drugs which inhibit this metabolic pathway may have a profound effect on the clearance of alprazolam). Products include:
Agenerase Capsules 1327
Agenerase Oral Solution 1332

Aprepitant (The initial step in alprazolam metabolism is hydroxylation catalyzed by cytochrome P450 3A (CYP3A). Drugs which inhibit this metabolic pathway may have a profound effect on the clearance of alprazolam). Products include:
Emend Capsules 1963

Aprobarbital (The benzodiazepines, including alprazolam, produce additive CNS depressant effects when co-administered with other drugs which themselves produce CNS depression).
No products indexed under this heading.

Astemizole (The benzodiazepines, including alprazolam, produce additive CNS depressant effects when co-administered with antihistamines).
No products indexed under this heading.

Azatadine Maleate (The benzodiazepines, including alprazolam, produce additive CNS depressant effects when co-administered with antihistamines).
No products indexed under this heading.

Azithromycin Dihydrate (Available data from clinical studies of benzodiazepines, other than alprazolam, suggest a possible drug interaction with alprazolam and macrolide antibiotics; caution is recommended during co-administration).
No products indexed under this heading.

Belladonna Ergotamine (Data from in vitro studies of benzodiazepines, other than alprazolam, suggest a possible drug interaction with ergotamine; caution is recommended during co-administration).
No products indexed under this heading.

Bromodiphenhydramine Hydrochloride (The benzodiazepines, including alprazolam, produce additive CNS depressant effects when co-administered with antihistamines).
No products indexed under this heading.

Brompheniramine Maleate (The benzodiazepines, including alprazolam, produce additive CNS depressant effects when co-administered with antihistamines). Products include:
Children's Dimetapp Cold & Allergy Elixir .... ■730
Children's Dimetapp Cold & Allergy Chewable Tablets .... ■730
Children's Dimetapp DM Cold & Cough Elixir .... ■731

Buprenorphine Hydrochloride (The benzodiazepines, including alprazolam, produce additive CNS depressant effects when co-administered with other drugs which themselves produce CNS depression). Products include:
Buprenex Injectable 2716
Suboxone Tablets 2717
Subutex Tablets 2717

Buspirone Hydrochloride (The benzodiazepines, including alprazolam, produce additive CNS depressant effects when co-administered with other psychotropic medications. If alprazolam is to be combined with other psychotropic agents, careful consideration should be given to the pharmacology of the agents to be employed, particularly with compounds which might potentiate the action of benzodiazepines).
No products indexed under this heading.

Butabarbital (The benzodiazepines, including alprazolam, produce additive CNS depressant effects when co-administered with other drugs which themselves produce CNS depression).
No products indexed under this heading.

Butalbital (The benzodiazepines, including alprazolam, produce additive CNS depressant effects when co-administered with other drugs which themselves produce CNS depression).
No products indexed under this heading.

Carbamazepine (Carbamazepine can increase alprazolam metabolism and therefore can decrease plasma levels of alprazolam). Products include:
Carbatrol Capsules 3171
Equetro Extended-Release Capsules 3180
Tegretol/Tegretol-XR 2295

Cetirizine Hydrochloride (The benzodiazepines, including alprazolam, produce additive CNS depressant effects when co-administered with antihistamines). Products include:
Zyrtec Chewable Tablets 2594
Zyrtec 2594
Zyrtec-D 12 Hour Extended Release Tablets 2597

Chlordiazepoxide (The benzodiazepines, including alprazolam, produce additive CNS depressant effects when co-administered with other psychotropic medications. If alprazolam is to be combined with other psychotropic agents, careful consideration should be given to the pharmacology of the agents to be employed, particularly with compounds which might potentiate the action of benzodiazepines).
No products indexed under this heading.

Chlordiazepoxide Hydrochloride (The benzodiazepines, including alprazolam, produce additive CNS depressant effects when co-administered with other psychotropic medications. If alprazolam is to be combined with other psychotropic agents, careful consideration should be given to the pharmacology of the agents to be employed, particularly with compounds which might potentiate the action of benzodiazepines). Products include:

Librium Capsules 3347

Chlorpheniramine Maleate (The benzodiazepines, including alprazolam, produce additive CNS depressant effects when co-administered with antihistamines). Products include:

Advil Allergy Sinus Caplets .... ▣770
Advil Multi-Symptom Cold Caplets .... ▣770
BC Allergy Sinus Cold Powder .... ▣677
Comtrex Maximum Strength Cold & Cough Day/Night Caplets - Night Formulation .... ▣726
Comtrex Maximum Strength Day/Night Severe Cold & Sinus Caplets - Night Formulation .... ▣725
Contac Cold and Flu Maximum Strength Caplets .... ▣728
Contac Cold and Flu Day and Night Caplets (Night Formulation Only) .... ▣727
Children's Dimetapp Long Acting Cough Plus Cold Syrup .... ▣731
Robitussin Cough & Cold Long-Acting Liquid .... ▣735
Robitussin Cough & Allergy Syrup .. ▣736
Robitussin Cough & Cold Nighttime Liquid .... ▣736
Robitussin Cough, Cold & Flu Nighttime Liquid .... ▣738
Robitussin Pediatric Cough & Cold Long-Acting Liquid .... ▣735
Robitussin Pediatric Cough & Cold Nighttime Liquid .... ▣736
Triaminic Cold & Allergy Liquid .... ▣746
Triaminic Cough & Runny Nose Softchews .... ▣748
Children's Tylenol Plus Flu Oral Suspension .... ▣749
Tylenol Allergy Multi-Symptom Caplets with Cool Burst and Gelcaps 1872
Children's Tylenol Plus Cold Suspension Liquid 1879
Children's Tylenol Plus Cough & Runny Nose Suspension Liquid 1879
Children's Tylenol Plus Flu Suspension Liquid 1881
Children's Tylenol Plus Multi-Symptom Cold Suspension Liquid 1879
Tylenol Cold Head Congestion Nighttime Caplets with Cool Burst 1873
Tylenol Cold Multi-Symptom Nighttime Caplets with Cool Burst 1874
Tylenol Sinus Congestion & Pain Nighttime Caplets with Cool Burst 1876
Vicks 44M Cough, Cold & Flu Relief Liquid 2680
Pediatric Vicks 44m Cough & Cold Relief Liquid 2676
Children's Vicks NyQuil Cold/Cough Relief .... ▣756
Children's Vicks NyQuil Cold/Cough Relief Liquid 2680
Zicam Maximum Strength Flu Daytime .... ▣768

Chlorpheniramine Polistirex (The benzodiazepines, including alprazolam, produce additive CNS depressant effects when co-administered with antihistamines). Products include:

Tussionex Pennkinetic Extended-Release Suspension 3327

Chlorpheniramine Tannate (The benzodiazepines, including alprazolam, produce additive CNS depressant effects when co-administered with antihistamines).

No products indexed under this heading.

Chlorpromazine (The benzodiazepines, including alprazolam, produce additive CNS depressant effects when co-administered with other psychotropic medications. If alprazolam is to be combined with other psychotropic agents, careful consideration should be given to the pharmacology of the agents to be employed, particularly with compounds which might potentiate the action of benzodiazepines).

No products indexed under this heading.

Chlorpromazine Hydrochloride (The benzodiazepines, including alprazolam, produce additive CNS depressant effects when co-administered with other psychotropic medications. If alprazolam is to be combined with other psychotropic agents, careful consideration should be given to the pharmacology of the agents to be employed, particularly with compounds which might potentiate the action of benzodiazepines).

No products indexed under this heading.

Chlorprothixene (The benzodiazepines, including alprazolam, produce additive CNS depressant effects when co-administered with other psychotropic medications. If alprazolam is to be combined with other psychotropic agents, careful consideration should be given to the pharmacology of the agents to be employed, particularly with compounds which might potentiate the action of benzodiazepines).

No products indexed under this heading.

Chlorprothixene Hydrochloride (The benzodiazepines, including alprazolam, produce additive CNS depressant effects when co-administered with other psychotropic medications. If alprazolam is to be combined with other psychotropic agents, careful consideration should be given to the pharmacology of the agents to be employed, particularly with compounds which might potentiate the action of benzodiazepines).

No products indexed under this heading.

Chlorprothixene Lactate (The benzodiazepines, including alprazolam, produce additive CNS depressant effects when co-administered with other drugs which themselves produce CNS depression).

No products indexed under this heading.

Cimetidine (Because Niravam disintegrates in the presence of saliva and the formulation requires an acidic environment to dissolve, concomitant drugs or diseases that raise stomach pH might slow disintegration or dissolution, resulting in slowed or decreased absorption). Products include:

Tagamet HB 200 Tablets .... ▣664

Cimetidine Hydrochloride (Because Niravam disintegrates in the presence of saliva and the formulation requires an acidic environment to dissolve, concomitant drugs or diseases that raise stomach pH might slow disintegration or dissolution, resulting in slowed or decreased absorption).

No products indexed under this heading.

Ciprofloxacin (The initial step in alprazolam metabolism is hydroxylation catalyzed by cytochrome P450 3A (CYP3A). Drugs which inhibit this metabolic pathway may have a profound effect on the clearance of alprazolam). Products include:

Cipro Oral Suspension 2977
Cipro I.V. 2984
Cipro XR Tablets 2990
Ciprodex Otic Suspension 559

Ciprofloxacin Hydrochloride (The initial step in alprazolam metabolism is hydroxylation catalyzed by cytochrome P450 3A (CYP3A). Drugs which inhibit this metabolic pathway may have a profound effect on the clearance of alprazolam). Products include:

Ciloxan Ophthalmic Ointment 559
Ciloxan Ophthalmic Solution .... ⊙206
Cipro Tablets 2977
Proquin XR Tablets 1153

Clarithromycin (The initial step in alprazolam metabolism is hydroxylation catalyzed by cytochrome P450 3A (CYP3A). Drugs which inhibit this metabolic pathway may have a profound effect on the clearance of alprazolam). Products include:

Biaxin/Biaxin XL 402
PREVPAC 3284

Clemastine Fumarate (The benzodiazepines, including alprazolam, produce additive CNS depressant effects when co-administered with antihistamines).

No products indexed under this heading.

Clorazepate Dipotassium (The benzodiazepines, including alprazolam, produce additive CNS depressant effects when co-administered with other psychotropic medications. If alprazolam is to be combined with other psychotropic agents, careful consideration should be given to the pharmacology of the agents to be employed, particularly with compounds which might potentiate the action of benzodiazepines). Products include:

Tranxene 2474

Clozapine (The benzodiazepines, including alprazolam, produce additive CNS depressant effects when co-administered with other psychotropic medications. If alprazolam is to be combined with other psychotropic agents, careful consideration should be given to the pharmacology of the agents to be employed, particularly with compounds which might potentiate the action of benzodiazepines). Products include:

Clozaril Tablets 2184
FazaClo Orally Disintegrating Tablets 551

Codeine Phosphate (The benzodiazepines, including alprazolam, produce additive CNS depressant effects when co-administered with other drugs which themselves produce CNS depression). Products include:

Tylenol with Codeine Tablets 2391

Cyclosporine (Data from in vitro studies of benzodiazepines, other than alprazolam, suggest a possible drug interaction with cyclosporine; caution is recommended during co-administration). Products include:

Gengraf Capsules 459
Neoral Oral Solution 2259
Neoral Soft Gelatin Capsules 2259
Restasis Ophthalmic Emulsion 575
Sandimmune 2275

Cyproheptadine Hydrochloride (The benzodiazepines, including alprazolam, produce additive CNS depressant effects when co-administered with antihistamines).

No products indexed under this heading.

Delavirdine Mesylate (The initial step in alprazolam metabolism is hydroxylation catalyzed by cytochrome P450 3A (CYP3A). Drugs which inhibit this metabolic pathway may have a profound effect on the clearance of alprazolam). Products include:

Rescriptor Tablets 2551

Desflurane (The benzodiazepines, including alprazolam, produce additive CNS depressant effects when co-administered with other drugs which themselves produce CNS depression).

No products indexed under this heading.

Desipramine Hydrochloride (The steady state plasma concentration of desipramine has been reported to be increased an average of 20% by the concomitant administration of alprazolam in doses up to 4 mg/day. The clinical significance of these changes is unknown).

No products indexed under this heading.

Desogestrel (Co-administration of oral contraceptives increased the maximum plasma concentration of alprazolam by 18%, decreased clearance by 22%, and increased half-life by 29%). Products include:

Mircette Tablets 1066

Dexchlorpheniramine Maleate (The benzodiazepines, including alprazolam, produce additive CNS depressant effects when co-administered with antihistamines).

No products indexed under this heading.

Dezocine (The benzodiazepines, including alprazolam, produce additive CNS depressant effects when co-administered with other drugs which themselves produce CNS depression).

No products indexed under this heading.

Diazepam (The benzodiazepines, including alprazolam, produce additive CNS depressant effects when co-administered with other psychotropic medications. If alprazolam is to be combined with other psychotropic agents, careful consideration should be given to the pharmacology of the agents to be employed, particularly with compounds which might potentiate the action of benzodiazepines). Products include:

Diastat Rectal Delivery System 3343
Valium Tablets 2819

Dihydroergotamine Mesylate (Data from in vitro studies of benzodiazepines other than alprazolam suggest a possible drug interaction with ergotamine; caution is recommended during co-administration). Products include:

Migranal Nasal Spray 3348

Diltiazem Hydrochloride (Available data from clinical studies of benzodiazepines other than alprazolam suggest a possible drug interaction with alprazolam and diltiazem; caution is recommended during co-administration). Products include:

Cardizem LA Extended Release Tablets 1728
Tiazac Capsules 1201

Diltiazem Maleate (Available data from clinical studies of benzodiazepines other than alprazolam suggest a possible drug interaction with alprazolam and diltiazem; caution is recommended during co-administration).

No products indexed under this heading.

Diphenhydramine Citrate (The benzodiazepines, including alprazolam, produce additive CNS depressant effects when co-administered with antihistamines). Products include:

- Advil PM Caplets .... ▣ 615
- Excedrin PM Caplets/Tablets/Geltabs .... ▣ 610
- Goody's PM Powder for Pain with Sleeplessness .... ▣ 612

Diphenhydramine Hydrochloride (The benzodiazepines, including alprazolam, produce additive CNS depressant effects when co-administered with antihistamines). Products include:

- Nytol QuickCaps Caplets .... ▣ 615
- Nytol QuickGels Softgels Maximum Strength .... ▣ 616
- Simply Sleep Caplets 1868
- Sominex Original Formula Tablets .. ▣ 616
- TheraFlu Warming Relief Nighttime Severe Cold .... ▣ 743
- TheraFlu Thin Strips Multi Symptom .... ▣ 744
- Triaminic Nighttime Cold & Cough Liquid .... ▣ 746
- Triaminic Thin Strips Cough & Runny Nose .... ▣ 749
- Extra Strength Tylenol PM Caplets, Vanilla Caplets, Geltabs, Gelcaps and Liquid 1875
- Tylenol Sore Throat Nighttime Liquid with Cool Burst .... ▣ 790
- Tylenol Allergy Multi-Symptom Nighttime Caplets with Cool Burst 1872
- Tylenol Severe Allergy Caplets 1872
- Children's Tylenol Plus Cold & Allergy Suspension Liquid 1878

Diphenylpyraline Hydrochloride (The benzodiazepines, including alprazolam, produce additive CNS depressant effects when co-administered with antihistamines).
No products indexed under this heading.

Dirithromycin (Available data from clinical studies of benzodiazepines, other than alprazolam, suggest a possible drug interaction with alprazolam and macrolide antibiotics; caution is recommended during co-administration).
No products indexed under this heading.

Divalproex Sodium (If alprazolam is to be combined with anticonvulsant drugs, careful consideration should be given to the pharmacology of the agents to be employed, particularly with compounds which might potentiate the action of benzodiazepines. The benzodiazepines, including alprazolam, produce additive CNS depressant effects when co-administered with anticonvulsants). Products include:

- Depakote Sprinkle Capsules 422
- Depakote Tablets 427
- Depakote ER Tablets 434

Doxepin Hydrochloride (The benzodiazepines, including alprazolam, produce additive CNS depressant effects when co-administered with other psychotropic medications. If alprazolam is to be combined with other psychotropic agents, careful consideration should be given to the pharmacology of the agents to be employed, particularly with compounds which might potentiate the action of benzodiazepines).
No products indexed under this heading.

Droperidol (The benzodiazepines, including alprazolam, produce additive CNS depressant effects when co-administered with other psychotropic medications. If alprazolam is to be combined with other psychotropic agents, careful consideration should be given to the pharmacology of the agents to be employed, particularly with compounds which might potentiate the action of benzodiazepines).
No products indexed under this heading.

Efavirenz (The initial step in alprazolam metabolism is hydroxylation catalyzed by cytochrome P450 3A (CYP3A). Drugs which inhibit this metabolic pathway may have a profound effect on the clearance of alprazolam). Products include:

- Atripla Tablets 945
- Sustiva Capsules 930
- Sustiva Tablets 930

Enflurane (The benzodiazepines, including alprazolam, produce additive CNS depressant effects when co-administered with other drugs which themselves produce CNS depression).
No products indexed under this heading.

Ergotamine Tartrate (Data from in vitro studies of benzodiazepines, other than alprazolam, suggest a possible drug interaction with ergotamine; caution is recommended during co-administration).
No products indexed under this heading.

Erythromycin (The initial step in alprazolam metabolism is hydroxylation catalyzed by cytochrome P450 3A (CYP3A). Drugs which inhibit this metabolic pathway may have a profound effect on the clearance of alprazolam). Products include:

- Ery-Tab Tablets 449
- Erythromycin Base Filmtab Tablets 455
- Erythromycin Delayed-Release Capsules, USP 457
- PCE Dispertab Tablets 515

Erythromycin Estolate (Available data from clinical studies of benzodiazepines, other than alprazolam, suggest a possible drug interaction with alprazolam and macrolide antibiotics; caution is recommended during co-administration).
No products indexed under this heading.

Erythromycin Ethylsuccinate (Available data from clinical studies of benzodiazepines, other than alprazolam, suggest a possible drug interaction with alprazolam and macrolide antibiotics; caution is recommended during co-administration). Products include:

- E.E.S. 451
- EryPed 447

Erythromycin Gluceptate (Available data from clinical studies of benzodiazepines, other than alprazolam, suggest a possible drug interaction with alprazolam and macrolide antibiotics; caution is recommended during co-administration).
No products indexed under this heading.

Erythromycin Stearate (Available data from clinical studies of benzodiazepines, other than alprazolam, suggest a possible drug interaction with alprazolam and macrolide antibiotics; caution is recommended during co-administration). Products include:

- Erythrocin Stearate Filmtab Tablets 453

Esomeprazole Magnesium (Because Niravam disintegrates in the presence of saliva and the formulation requires an acidic environment to dissolve, concomitant drugs or diseases that raise stomach pH might slow disintegration or dissolution, resulting in slowed or decreased absorption). Products include:

- Nexium Delayed-Release Capsules 655

Estazolam (The benzodiazepines, including alprazolam, produce additive CNS depressant effects when co-administered with other drugs which themselves produce CNS depression). Products include:

- ProSom Tablets 517

Ethanol (The benzodiazepines, including alprazolam, produce additive CNS depressant effects when co-administered with ethanol).
No products indexed under this heading.

Ethchlorvynol (The benzodiazepines, including alprazolam, produce additive CNS depressant effects when co-administered with other drugs which themselves produce CNS depression).
No products indexed under this heading.

Ethinamate (The benzodiazepines, including alprazolam, produce additive CNS depressant effects when co-administered with other drugs which themselves produce CNS depression).
No products indexed under this heading.

Ethinyl Estradiol (Co-administration of oral contraceptives increased the maximum plasma concentration of alprazolam by 18%, decreased clearance by 22%, and increased half-life by 29%). Products include:

- Mircette Tablets 1066
- NuvaRing 2340
- Ortho-Cyclen/Ortho Tri-Cyclen 2429
- Ortho Evra Transdermal System 2417
- Ortho Tri-Cyclen Lo Tablets 2436
- Seasonique Tablets 1077
- Yasmin 28 Tablets 796
- Yaz Tablets 803

Ethosuximide (If alprazolam is to be combined with anticonvulsant drugs, careful consideration should be given to the pharmacology of the agents to be employed, particularly with compounds which might potentiate the action of benzodiazepines. The benzodiazepines, including alprazolam, produce additive CNS depressant effects when co-administered with anticonvulsants).
No products indexed under this heading.

Ethotoin (If alprazolam is to be combined with anticonvulsant drugs, careful consideration should be given to the pharmacology of the agents to be employed, particularly with compounds which might potentiate the action of benzodiazepines. The benzodiazepines, including alprazolam, produce additive CNS depressant effects when co-administered with anticonvulsants).
No products indexed under this heading.

Ethyl Alcohol (The benzodiazepines, including alprazolam, produce additive CNS depressant effects when co-administered with other drugs which themselves produce CNS depression).
No products indexed under this heading.

Ethynodiol Diacetate (Co-administration of oral contraceptives increased the maximum plasma concentration of alprazolam by 18%, decreased clearance by 22%, and increased half-life by 29%).
No products indexed under this heading.

Famotidine (Because Niravam disintegrates in the presence of saliva and the formulation requires an acidic environment to dissolve, concomitant drugs or diseases that raise stomach pH might slow disintegration or dissolution, resulting in slowed or decreased absorption). Products include:

- Pepcid Injection 2040
- Pepcid 2038
- Pepcid AC Gelcaps 1701
- Pepcid AC Tablets 1701
- Maximum Strength Pepcid AC Tablets 1701
- Pepcid Complete Chewable Tablets 1701

Felbamate (If alprazolam is to be combined with anticonvulsant drugs, careful consideration should be given to the pharmacology of the agents to be employed, particularly with compounds which might potentiate the action of benzodiazepines. The benzodiazepines, including alprazolam, produce additive CNS depressant effects when co-administered with anticonvulsants).
No products indexed under this heading.

Fentanyl (The benzodiazepines, including alprazolam, produce additive CNS depressant effects when co-administered with other drugs which themselves produce CNS depression). Products include:

- Duragesic Transdermal System 2373
- Ionsys Transdermal System 2379

Fentanyl Citrate (The benzodiazepines, including alprazolam, produce additive CNS depressant effects when co-administered with other drugs which themselves produce CNS depression). Products include:

- Actiq 979

Fexofenadine Hydrochloride (The benzodiazepines, including alprazolam, produce additive CNS depressant effects when co-administered with antihistamines). Products include:

- Allegra 2844
- Allegra-D 12 Hour Extended-Release Tablets 2846
- Allegra-D 24 Hour Extended-Release Tablets 2849

Fluconazole (The initial step in alprazolam metabolism is hydroxylation catalyzed by cytochrome P450 3A (CYP3A). Drugs which inhibit this metabolic pathway may have a profound effect on the clearance of alprazolam).
No products indexed under this heading.

Fluoxetine (Co-administration of fluoxetine with alprazolam increased the maximum plasma concentration of alprazolam by 46%, decreased clearance by 21%, increased half-life by 17%, and decreased measured psychomotor performance).
No products indexed under this heading.

Fluoxetine Hydrochloride (Co-administration of fluoxetine with alprazolam increased the maximum plasma concentration of alprazolam by 46%, decreased clearance by 21%, increased half-life by 17%, and decreased measured psychomotor performance). Products include:

Fluphenazine Decanoate (The benzodiazepines, including alprazolam, produce additive CNS depressant effects when co-administered with other psychotropic medications. If alprazolam is to be combined with other psychotropic agents, careful consideration should be given to the pharmacology of the agents to be employed, particularly with compounds which might potentiate the action of benzodiazepines).
No products indexed under this heading.

Fluphenazine Enanthate (The benzodiazepines, including alprazolam, produce additive CNS depressant effects when co-administered with other psychotropic medications. If alprazolam is to be combined with other psychotropic agents, careful consideration should be given to the pharmacology of the agents to be employed, particularly with compounds which might potentiate the action of benzodiazepines).
No products indexed under this heading.

Fluphenazine Hydrochloride (The benzodiazepines, including alprazolam, produce additive CNS depressant effects when co-administered with other psychotropic medications. If alprazolam is to be combined with other psychotropic agents, careful consideration should be given to the pharmacology of the agents to be employed, particularly with compounds which might potentiate the action of benzodiazepines).
No products indexed under this heading.

Flurazepam Hydrochloride (The benzodiazepines, including alprazolam, produce additive CNS depressant effects when co-administered with other drugs which themselves produce CNS depression). Products include:

Fluvoxamine Maleate (The initial step in alprazolam metabolism is hydroxylation catalyzed by cytochrome P450 3A (CYP3A). Drugs which inhibit this metabolic pathway may have a profound effect on the clearance of alprazolam).
No products indexed under this heading.

Fosphenytoin (If alprazolam is to be combined with anticonvulsant drugs, careful consideration should be given to the pharmacology of the agents to be employed, particularly with compounds which might potentiate the action of benzodiazepines. The benzodiazepines, including alprazolam, produce additive CNS depressant effects when co-administered with anticonvulsants).
No products indexed under this heading.

Fosphenytoin Sodium (If alprazolam is to be combined with anticonvulsant drugs, careful consideration should be given to the pharmacology of the agents to be employed, particularly with compounds which might potentiate the action of benzodiazepines. The benzodiazepines, including alprazolam, produce additive CNS depressant effects when co-administered with anticonvulsants).
No products indexed under this heading.

Gabapentin (If alprazolam is to be combined with anticonvulsant drugs, careful consideration should be given to the pharmacology of the agents to be employed, particularly with compounds which might potentiate the action of benzodiazepines. The benzodiazepines, including alprazolam, produce additive CNS depressant effects when co-administered with anticonvulsants). Products include:

Glutethimide (The benzodiazepines, including alprazolam, produce additive CNS depressant effects when co-administered with other drugs which themselves produce CNS depression).
No products indexed under this heading.

Haloperidol (The benzodiazepines, including alprazolam, produce additive CNS depressant effects when co-administered with other psychotropic medications. If alprazolam is to be combined with other psychotropic agents, careful consideration should be given to the pharmacology of the agents to be employed, particularly with compounds which might potentiate the action of benzodiazepines).
No products indexed under this heading.

Haloperidol Decanoate (The benzodiazepines, including alprazolam, produce additive CNS depressant effects when co-administered with other psychotropic medications. If alprazolam is to be combined with other psychotropic agents, careful consideration should be given to the pharmacology of the agents to be employed, particularly with compounds which might potentiate the action of benzodiazepines).
No products indexed under this heading.

Hydrocodone Bitartrate (The benzodiazepines, including alprazolam, produce additive CNS depressant effects when co-administered with other drugs which themselves produce CNS depression). Products include:

Hydrocodone Polistirex (The benzodiazepines, including alprazolam, produce additive CNS depressant effects when co-administered with other drugs which themselves produce CNS depression). Products include:

Hydromorphone Hydrochloride (The benzodiazepines, including alprazolam, produce additive CNS depressant effects when co-administered with other drugs which themselves produce CNS depression). Products include:

Hydroxyzine Hydrochloride (The benzodiazepines, including alprazolam, produce additive CNS depressant effects when co-administered with other psychotropic medications. If alprazolam is to be combined with other psychotropic agents, careful consideration should be given to the pharmacology of the agents to be employed, particularly with compounds which might potentiate the action of benzodiazepines).
No products indexed under this heading.

Imipramine Hydrochloride (The steady state plasma concentration of imipramine has been reported to be increased an average of 31% by the concomitant administration of alprazolam in doses up to 4 mg/day. The clinical significance of these changes is unknown).
No products indexed under this heading.

Imipramine Pamoate (The steady state plasma concentration of imipramine has been reported to be increased an average of 31% by the concomitant administration of alprazolam in doses up to 4 mg/day. The clinical significance of these changes is unknown).
No products indexed under this heading.

Indinavir Sulfate (The initial step in alprazolam metabolism is hydroxylation catalyzed by cytochrome P450 3A (CYP3A). Drugs which inhibit this metabolic pathway may have a profound effect on the clearance of alprazolam). Products include:

Isocarboxazid (The benzodiazepines, including alprazolam, produce additive CNS depressant effects when co-administered with other psychotropic medications. If alprazolam is to be combined with other psychotropic agents, careful consideration should be given to the pharmacology of the agents to be employed, particularly with compounds which might potentiate the action of benzodiazepines).
No products indexed under this heading.

Isoflurane (The benzodiazepines, including alprazolam, produce additive CNS depressant effects when co-administered with other drugs which themselves produce CNS depression).
No products indexed under this heading.

Isoniazid (Available data from clinical studies of benzodiazepines other than alprazolam suggest a possible drug interaction with alprazolam and isoniazid; caution is recommended during co-administration).
No products indexed under this heading.

Itraconazole (Alprazolam is contraindicated with itraconazole since this medication significantly impairs the oxidative metabolism mediated by cytochrome P450 3A (CYP3A)).
No products indexed under this heading.

Ketamine Hydrochloride (The benzodiazepines, including alprazolam, produce additive CNS depressant effects when co-administered with other drugs which themselves produce CNS depression).
No products indexed under this heading.

Ketoconazole (Alprazolam is contraindicated with ketoconazole since this medication significantly impairs the oxidative metabolism mediated by cytochrome P450 3A (CYP3A)). Products include:

Lamotrigine (If alprazolam is to be combined with anticonvulsant drugs, careful consideration should be given to the pharmacology of the agents to be employed, particularly with compounds which might potentiate the action of benzodiazepines. The benzodiazepines, including alprazolam, produce additive CNS depressant effects when co-administered with anticonvulsants). Products include:

Lansoprazole (Because Niravam disintegrates in the presence of saliva and the formulation requires an acidic environment to dissolve, concomitant drugs or diseases that raise stomach pH might slow disintegration or dissolution, resulting in slowed or decreased absorption). Products include:

Levetiracetam (If alprazolam is to be combined with anticonvulsant drugs, careful consideration should be given to the pharmacology of the agents to be employed, particularly with compounds which might potentiate the action of benzodiazepines. The benzodiazepines, including alprazolam, produce additive CNS depressant effects when co-administered with anticonvulsants). Products include:

IMPORTANT NOTE: Always consult each drug listing in the patient's regimen for possible interactions.

Levomethadyl Acetate Hydro-chloride (The benzodiazepines, including alprazolam, produce additive CNS depressant effects when co-administered with other drugs which themselves produce CNS depression).

> No products indexed under this heading.

Levonorgestrel (Co-administration of oral contraceptives increased the maximum plasma concentration of alprazolam by 18%, decreased clearance by 22%, and increased half-life by 29%). Products include:

Levorphanol Tartrate (The benzodiazepines, including alprazolam, produce additive CNS depressant effects when co-administered with other drugs which themselves produce CNS depression).

> No products indexed under this heading.

Lithium Carbonate (The benzodiazepines, including alprazolam, produce additive CNS depressant effects when co-administered with other psychotropic medications. If alprazolam is to be combined with other psychotropic agents, careful consideration should be given to the pharmacology of the agents to be employed, particularly with compounds which might potentiate the action of benzodiazepines). Products include:

Lithium Citrate (The benzodiazepines, including alprazolam, produce additive CNS depressant effects when co-administered with other psychotropic medications. If alprazolam is to be combined with other psychotropic agents, careful consideration should be given to the pharmacology of the agents to be employed, particularly with compounds which might potentiate the action of benzodiazepines).

> No products indexed under this heading.

Lopinavir (The initial step in alprazolam metabolism is hydroxylation catalyzed by cytochrome P450 3A (CYP3A). Drugs which inhibit this metabolic pathway may have a profound effect on the clearance of alprazolam). Products include:

Loratadine (The benzodiazepines, including alprazolam, produce additive CNS depressant effects when co-administered with antihistamines). Products include:

Lorazepam (The benzodiazepines, including alprazolam, produce additive CNS depressant effects when

co-administered with other psychotropic medications. If alprazolam is to be combined with other psychotropic agents, careful consideration should be given to the pharmacology of the agents to be employed, particularly with compounds which might potentiate the action of benzodiazepines).

> No products indexed under this heading.

Loxapine Hydrochloride (The benzodiazepines, including alprazolam, produce additive CNS depressant effects when co-administered with other psychotropic medications. If alprazolam is to be combined with other psychotropic agents, careful consideration should be given to the pharmacology of the agents to be employed, particularly with compounds which might potentiate the action of benzodiazepines).

> No products indexed under this heading.

Loxapine Succinate (The benzodiazepines, including alprazolam, produce additive CNS depressant effects when co-administered with other psychotropic medications. If alprazolam is to be combined with other psychotropic agents, careful consideration should be given to the pharmacology of the agents to be employed, particularly with compounds which might potentiate the action of benzodiazepines).

> No products indexed under this heading.

Magaldrate (Because Niravam disintegrates in the presence of saliva and the formulation requires an acidic environment to dissolve, concomitant drugs or diseases that raise stomach pH might slow disintegration or dissolution, resulting in slowed or decreased absorption).

> No products indexed under this heading.

Magnesium Hydroxide (Because Niravam disintegrates in the presence of saliva and the formulation requires an acidic environment to dissolve, concomitant drugs or diseases that raise stomach pH might slow disintegration or dissolution, resulting in slowed or decreased absorption). Products include:

Magnesium Oxide (Because Niravam disintegrates in the presence of saliva and the formulation requires an acidic environment to dissolve, concomitant drugs or diseases that raise stomach pH might slow disintegration or dissolution, resulting in slowed or decreased absorption). Products include:

Maprotiline Hydrochloride (The benzodiazepines, including alprazolam, produce additive CNS depressant effects when co-administered with other psychotropic medications. If alprazolam is to be combined with other psychotropic agents, careful consideration should

be given to the pharmacology of the agents to be employed, particularly with compounds which might potentiate the action of benzodiazepines).

> No products indexed under this heading.

Meperidine Hydrochloride (The benzodiazepines, including alprazolam, produce additive CNS depressant effects when co-administered with other drugs which themselves produce CNS depression).

> No products indexed under this heading.

Mephenytoin (If alprazolam is to be combined with anticonvulsant drugs, careful consideration should be given to the pharmacology of the agents to be employed, particularly with compounds which might potentiate the action of benzodiazepines. The benzodiazepines, including alprazolam, produce additive CNS depressant effects when co-administered with anticonvulsants).

> No products indexed under this heading.

Mephobarbital (The benzodiazepines, including alprazolam, produce additive CNS depressant effects when co-administered with other drugs which themselves produce CNS depression).

> No products indexed under this heading.

Meprobamate (The benzodiazepines, including alprazolam, produce additive CNS depressant effects when co-administered with other psychotropic medications. If alprazolam is to be combined with other psychotropic agents, careful consideration should be given to the pharmacology of the agents to be employed, particularly with compounds which might potentiate the action of benzodiazepines).

> No products indexed under this heading.

Mesoridazine Besylate (The benzodiazepines, including alprazolam, produce additive CNS depressant effects when co-administered with other psychotropic medications. If alprazolam is to be combined with other psychotropic agents, careful consideration should be given to the pharmacology of the agents to be employed, particularly with compounds which might potentiate the action of benzodiazepines).

> No products indexed under this heading.

Mestranol (Co-administration of oral contraceptives increased the maximum plasma concentration of alprazolam by 18%, decreased clearance by 22%, and increased half-life by 29%).

> No products indexed under this heading.

Methadone Hydrochloride (The benzodiazepines, including alprazolam, produce additive CNS depressant effects when co-administered with other drugs which themselves produce CNS depression).

> No products indexed under this heading.

Methdilazine Hydrochloride (The benzodiazepines, including alprazolam, produce additive CNS depressant effects when co-administered with antihistamines).

> No products indexed under this heading.

Methohexital Sodium (The benzodiazepines, including alprazolam, produce additive CNS depressant effects when co-administered with other drugs which themselves produce CNS depression).

> No products indexed under this heading.

Methotrimeprazine (The benzodiazepines, including alprazolam, produce additive CNS depressant effects when co-administered with other drugs which themselves produce CNS depression).

> No products indexed under this heading.

Methoxyflurane (The benzodiazepines, including alprazolam, produce additive CNS depressant effects when co-administered with other drugs which themselves produce CNS depression).

> No products indexed under this heading.

Methsuximide (If alprazolam is to be combined with anticonvulsant drugs, careful consideration should be given to the pharmacology of the agents to be employed, particularly with compounds which might potentiate the action of benzodiazepines. The benzodiazepines, including alprazolam, produce additive CNS depressant effects when co-administered with anticonvulsants).

> No products indexed under this heading.

Metronidazole (The initial step in alprazolam metabolism is hydroxylation catalyzed by cytochrome P450 3A (CYP3A). Drugs which inhibit this metabolic pathway may have a profound effect on the clearance of alprazolam). Products include:

Metronidazole Benzoate (The initial step in alprazolam metabolism is hydroxylation catalyzed by cytochrome P450 3A (CYP3A). Drugs which inhibit this metabolic pathway may have a profound effect on the clearance of alprazolam).

> No products indexed under this heading.

Metronidazole Hydrochloride (The initial step in alprazolam metabolism is hydroxylation catalyzed by cytochrome P450 3A (CYP3A). Drugs which inhibit this metabolic pathway may have a profound effect on the clearance of alprazolam).

> No products indexed under this heading.

Miconazole (The initial step in alprazolam metabolism is hydroxylation catalyzed by cytochrome P450 3A (CYP3A). Drugs which inhibit this metabolic pathway may have a profound effect on the clearance of alprazolam).

> No products indexed under this heading.

Midazolam Hydrochloride (The benzodiazepines, including alprazolam, produce additive CNS depressant effects when co-administered with other psychotropic medications. If alprazolam is to be combined with other psychotropic agents, careful consideration should be given to the pharmacology of the agents to be employed, particularly with compounds which might potentiate the action of benzodiazepines).

No products indexed under this heading.

Molindone Hydrochloride (The benzodiazepines, including alprazolam, produce additive CNS depressant effects when co-administered with other psychotropic medications. If alprazolam is to be combined with other psychotropic agents, careful consideration should be given to the pharmacology of the agents to be employed, particularly with compounds which might potentiate the action of benzodiazepines). Products include:

Moban Tablets 1119

Morphine Sulfate (The benzodiazepines, including alprazolam, produce additive CNS depressant effects when co-administered with other drugs which themselves produce CNS depression). Products include:

Avinza Capsules 1741
Kadian Capsules 577
MS Contin Tablets 2701

Nefazodone Hydrochloride (The initial step in alprazolam metabolism is hydroxylation catalyzed by cytochrome P450 3A (CYP3A). Drugs which inhibit this metabolic pathway may have a profound effect on the clearance of alprazolam).

No products indexed under this heading.

Nelfinavir Mesylate (The initial step in alprazolam metabolism is hydroxylation catalyzed by cytochrome P450 3A (CYP3A). Drugs which inhibit this metabolic pathway may have a profound effect on the clearance of alprazolam). Products include:

Viracept ... 2577

Nicardipine (Data from in vitro studies of benzodiazepines, other than alprazolam, suggest a possible drug interaction with nicardipine; caution is recommended during co-administration).

No products indexed under this heading.

Nicardipine Hydrochloride (Data from in vitro studies of benzodiazepines, other than alprazolam, suggest a possible drug interaction with nicardipine; caution is recommended during co-administration). Products include:

Cardene I.V. 2497

Nifedipine (Data from in vitro studies of benzodiazepines, other than alprazolam, suggest a possible drug interaction with nifedipine; caution is recommended during co-administration). Products include:

Adalat CC Tablets 2964

Nizatidine (Because Niravam disintegrates in the presence of saliva and the formulation requires an acidic environment to dissolve, concomitant drugs or diseases that raise stomach pH might slow disintegration or dissolution, resulting in slowed or decreased absorption). Products include:

Axid Oral Solution 879

Norethindrone (Co-administration of oral contraceptives increased the maximum plasma concentration of

alprazolam by 18%, decreased clearance by 22%, and increased half-life by 29%). Products include:

Ortho Micronor Tablets 2426

Norethynodrel (Co-administration of oral contraceptives increased the maximum plasma concentration of alprazolam by 18%, decreased clearance by 22%, and increased half-life by 29%).

No products indexed under this heading.

Norfloxacin (The initial step in alprazolam metabolism is hydroxylation catalyzed by cytochrome P450 3A (CYP3A). Drugs which inhibit this metabolic pathway may have a profound effect on the clearance of alprazolam). Products include:

Noroxin Tablets 2032

Norgestimate (Co-administration of oral contraceptives increased the maximum plasma concentration of alprazolam by 18%, decreased clearance by 22%, and increased half-life by 29%). Products include:

Ortho-Cyclen/Ortho Tri-Cyclen 2429
Ortho Tri-Cyclen Lo Tablets 2436

Norgestrel (Co-administration of oral contraceptives increased the maximum plasma concentration of alprazolam by 18%, decreased clearance by 22%, and increased half-life by 29%).

No products indexed under this heading.

Nortriptyline Hydrochloride (The benzodiazepines, including alprazolam, produce additive CNS depressant effects when co-administered with other psychotropic medications. If alprazolam is to be combined with other psychotropic agents, careful consideration should be given to the pharmacology of the agents to be employed, particularly with compounds which might potentiate the action of benzodiazepines).

No products indexed under this heading.

Olanzapine (The benzodiazepines, including alprazolam, produce additive CNS depressant effects when co-administered with other psychotropic medications. If alprazolam is to be combined with other psychotropic agents, careful consideration should be given to the pharmacology of the agents to be employed, particularly with compounds which might potentiate the action of benzodiazepines). Products include:

Symbyax Capsules 1819
Zyprexa Tablets 1830
Zyprexa IntraMuscular 1830
Zyprexa ZYDIS Orally
 Disintegrating Tablets................. 1830

Omeprazole (Because Niravam disintegrates in the presence of saliva and the formulation requires an acidic environment to dissolve, concomitant drugs or diseases that raise stomach pH might slow disintegration or dissolution, resulting in slowed or decreased absorption). Products include:

Zegerid Capsules 2958
Zegerid Powder for Oral Solution 2958

Oxazepam (The benzodiazepines, including alprazolam, produce additive CNS depressant effects when co-administered with other psychotropic medications. If alprazolam is to be combined with other psychotropic agents, careful consideration should be given to the pharmacology of the agents to be employed, particularly with compounds which might potentiate the action of benzodiazepines).

No products indexed under this heading.

Oxcarbazepine (If alprazolam is to be combined with anticonvulsant drugs, careful consideration should be given to the pharmacology of the agents to be employed, particularly with compounds which might potentiate the action of benzodiazepines. The benzodiazepines, including alprazolam, produce additive CNS depressant effects when co-administered with anticonvulsants). Products include:

Trileptal Tablets 2300
Trileptal Oral Suspension 2300

Oxycodone Hydrochloride (The benzodiazepines, including alprazolam, produce additive CNS depressant effects when co-administered with other drugs which themselves produce CNS depression). Products include:

OxyContin Tablets 2703
OxyFast Oral Concentrate
 Solution.................................... 2708
OxyIR Capsules 2708
Percocet Tablets 1131
Percodan Tablets 1132

Pantoprazole Sodium (Because Niravam disintegrates in the presence of saliva and the formulation requires an acidic environment to dissolve, concomitant drugs or diseases that raise stomach pH might slow disintegration or dissolution, resulting in slowed or decreased absorption). Products include:

Protonix I.V. 3472
Protonix Tablets 3469

Paramethadione (If alprazolam is to be combined with anticonvulsant drugs, careful consideration should be given to the pharmacology of the agents to be employed, particularly with compounds which might potentiate the action of benzodiazepines. The benzodiazepines, including alprazolam, produce additive CNS depressant effects when co-administered with anticonvulsants).

No products indexed under this heading.

Paroxetine Hydrochloride (Data from in vitro studies of alprazolam suggest a possible drug interaction with alprazolam and sertraline. However, data from an in vivo drug interaction study involving a single dose of alprazolam 1 mg and steady state doses of sertraline (50 to 150 mg/day) did not reveal any clinically significant changes in the pharmacokinetics of alprazolam; caution is recommended during co-administration). Products include:

Paxil CR Controlled-Release
 Tablets..................................... 1538
Paxil .. 1530

Paroxetine Mesylate (Data from in vitro studies of alprazolam suggest a possible drug interaction with alprazolam and sertraline. However, data from an in vivo drug interaction study involving a single dose of alprazolam 1 mg and steady state

doses of sertraline (50 to 150 mg/day) did not reveal any clinically significant changes in the pharmacokinetics of alprazolam; caution is recommended during co-administration). Products include:

Pexeva Tablets 1694

Pentobarbital Sodium (The benzodiazepines, including alprazolam, produce additive CNS depressant effects when co-administered with other drugs which themselves produce CNS depression). Products include:

Nembutal Sodium Solution, USP 2470

Perphenazine (The benzodiazepines, including alprazolam, produce additive CNS depressant effects when co-administered with other psychotropic medications. If alprazolam is to be combined with other psychotropic agents, careful consideration should be given to the pharmacology of the agents to be employed, particularly with compounds which might potentiate the action of benzodiazepines).

No products indexed under this heading.

Phenacemide (If alprazolam is to be combined with anticonvulsant drugs, careful consideration should be given to the pharmacology of the agents to be employed, particularly with compounds which might potentiate the action of benzodiazepines. The benzodiazepines, including alprazolam, produce additive CNS depressant effects when co-administered with anticonvulsants).

No products indexed under this heading.

Phenelzine Sulfate (The benzodiazepines, including alprazolam, produce additive CNS depressant effects when co-administered with other psychotropic medications. If alprazolam is to be combined with other psychotropic agents, careful consideration should be given to the pharmacology of the agents to be employed, particularly with compounds which might potentiate the action of benzodiazepines).

No products indexed under this heading.

Phenobarbital (If alprazolam is to be combined with anticonvulsant drugs, careful consideration should be given to the pharmacology of the agents to be employed, particularly with compounds which might potentiate the action of benzodiazepines. The benzodiazepines, including alprazolam, produce additive CNS depressant effects when co-administered with anticonvulsants). Products include:

Donnatal Extentabs 2493

Phensuximide (If alprazolam is to be combined with anticonvulsant drugs, careful consideration should be given to the pharmacology of the agents to be employed, particularly with compounds which might potentiate the action of benzodiazepines. The benzodiazepines, including alprazolam, produce additive CNS depressant effects when co-administered with anticonvulsants).

No products indexed under this heading.

Phenytoin (If alprazolam is to be combined with anticonvulsant drugs, careful consideration should be given to the pharmacology of the agents to be employed, particularly with compounds which might potentiate the action of benzodiazepines. The benzodiazepines, including alprazolam, produce additive CNS depressant effects when co-administered with anticonvulsants).

 No products indexed under this heading.

Phenytoin Sodium (If alprazolam is to be combined with anticonvulsant drugs, careful consideration should be given to the pharmacology of the agents to be employed, particularly with compounds which might potentiate the action of benzodiazepines. The benzodiazepines, including alprazolam, produce additive CNS depressant effects when co-administered with anticonvulsants). Products include:

 Phenytek Capsules 2160

Prazepam (The benzodiazepines, including alprazolam, produce additive CNS depressant effects when co-administered with other psychotropic medications. If alprazolam is to be combined with other psychotropic agents, careful consideration should be given to the pharmacology of the agents to be employed, particularly with compounds which might potentiate the action of benzodiazepines).

 No products indexed under this heading.

Primidone (If alprazolam is to be combined with anticonvulsant drugs, careful consideration should be given to the pharmacology of the agents to be employed, particularly with compounds which might potentiate the action of benzodiazepines. The benzodiazepines, including alprazolam, produce additive CNS depressant effects when co-administered with anticonvulsants).

 No products indexed under this heading.

Prochlorperazine (The benzodiazepines, including alprazolam, produce additive CNS depressant effects when co-administered with other psychotropic medications. If alprazolam is to be combined with other psychotropic agents, careful consideration should be given to the pharmacology of the agents to be employed, particularly with compounds which might potentiate the action of benzodiazepines).

 No products indexed under this heading.

Promethazine Hydrochloride (The benzodiazepines, including alprazolam, produce additive CNS depressant effects when co-administered with other psychotropic medications. If alprazolam is to be combined with other psychotropic agents, careful consideration should be given to the pharmacology of the agents to be employed, particularly with compounds which might potentiate the action of benzodiazepines). Products include:

 Phenergan Tablets and Suppositories.............................. 3440

Propofol (The benzodiazepines, including alprazolam, produce additive CNS depressant effects when co-administered with other drugs which themselves produce CNS depression).

 No products indexed under this heading.

Propoxyphene Hydrochloride (Co-administration of propoxyphene decreased the maximum plasma concentration of alprazolam by 6%, decreased clearance by 38%, and increased half-life by 58%).

 No products indexed under this heading.

Propoxyphene Napsylate (Co-administration of propoxyphene decreased the maximum plasma concentration of alprazolam by 6%, decreased clearance by 38%, and increased half-life by 58%).

 No products indexed under this heading.

Protriptyline Hydrochloride (The benzodiazepines, including alprazolam, produce additive CNS depressant effects when co-administered with other psychotropic medications. If alprazolam is to be combined with other psychotropic agents, careful consideration should be given to the pharmacology of the agents to be employed, particularly with compounds which might potentiate the action of benzodiazepines).

 No products indexed under this heading.

Pyrilamine Maleate (The benzodiazepines, including alprazolam, produce additive CNS depressant effects when co-administered with antihistamines).

 No products indexed under this heading.

Pyrilamine Tannate (The benzodiazepines, including alprazolam, produce additive CNS depressant effects when co-administered with antihistamines).

 No products indexed under this heading.

Quazepam (The benzodiazepines, including alprazolam, produce additive CNS depressant effects when co-administered with other drugs which themselves produce CNS depression).

 No products indexed under this heading.

Quetiapine Fumarate (The benzodiazepines, including alprazolam, produce additive CNS depressant effects when co-administered with other psychotropic medications. If alprazolam is to be combined with other psychotropic agents, careful consideration should be given to the pharmacology of the agents to be employed, particularly with compounds which might potentiate the action of benzodiazepines). Products include:

 Seroquel Tablets 690

Quinine (The initial step in alprazolam metabolism is hydroxylation catalyzed by cytochrome P450 3A (CYP3A). Drugs which inhibit this metabolic pathway may have a profound effect on the clearance of alprazolam).

 No products indexed under this heading.

Quinine Sulfate (The initial step in alprazolam metabolism is hydroxylation catalyzed by cytochrome P450 3A (CYP3A). Drugs which inhibit this metabolic pathway may have a profound effect on the clearance of alprazolam).

 No products indexed under this heading.

Rabeprazole Sodium (Because Niravam disintegrates in the presence of saliva and the formulation requires an acidic environment to dissolve, concomitant drugs or diseases that raise stomach pH might slow disintegration or dissolution, resulting in slowed or decreased absorption). Products include:

 Aciphex Tablets 1090

Ranitidine Bismuth Citrate (Because Niravam disintegrates in the presence of saliva and the formulation requires an acidic environment to dissolve, concomitant drugs or diseases that raise stomach pH might slow disintegration or dissolution, resulting in slowed or decreased absorption).

 No products indexed under this heading.

Ranitidine Hydrochloride (Because Niravam disintegrates in the presence of saliva and the formulation requires an acidic environment to dissolve, concomitant drugs or diseases that raise stomach pH might slow disintegration or dissolution, resulting in slowed or decreased absorption). Products include:

 Zantac 1624
 Zantac Injection 1619
 Zantac Injection Pharmacy Bulk Package...................................... 1622

Remifentanil Hydrochloride (The benzodiazepines, including alprazolam, produce additive CNS depressant effects when co-administered with other drugs which themselves produce CNS depression).

 No products indexed under this heading.

Risperidone (The benzodiazepines, including alprazolam, produce additive CNS depressant effects when co-administered with other psychotropic medications. If alprazolam is to be combined with other psychotropic agents, careful consideration should be given to the pharmacology of the agents to be employed, particularly with compounds which might potentiate the action of benzodiazepines). Products include:

 Risperdal 1676
 Risperdal Consta Long-Acting Injection 1682
 Risperdal M-Tab Orally Disintegrating Tablets.................. 1676

Ritonavir (The initial step in alprazolam metabolism is hydroxylation catalyzed by cytochrome P450 3A (CYP3A). Drugs which inhibit this metabolic pathway may have a profound effect on the clearance of alprazolam). Products include:

 Kaletra 476
 Norvir 503

Saquinavir (The initial step in alprazolam metabolism is hydroxylation catalyzed by cytochrome P450 3A (CYP3A). Drugs which inhibit this metabolic pathway may have a profound effect on the clearance of alprazolam).

 No products indexed under this heading.

Saquinavir Mesylate (The initial step in alprazolam metabolism is hydroxylation catalyzed by cytochrome P450 3A (CYP3A). Drugs which inhibit this metabolic pathway may have a profound effect on the clearance of alprazolam). Products include:

 Invirase 2772

Secobarbital Sodium (The benzodiazepines, including alprazolam, produce additive CNS depressant effects when co-administered with other drugs which themselves produce CNS depression).

 No products indexed under this heading.

Sertraline Hydrochloride (Data from in vitro studies of alprazolam suggest a possible drug interaction with alprazolam and sertraline. However, data from an in vivo drug interaction study involving a single dose of alprazolam 1 mg and steady state doses of sertraline (50 to 150 mg/day) did not reveal any clinically significant changes in the pharmacokinetics of alprazolam; caution is recommended during co-administration). Products include:

 Zoloft 2586

Sevoflurane (The benzodiazepines, including alprazolam, produce additive CNS depressant effects when co-administered with other drugs which themselves produce CNS depression). Products include:

 Ultane Liquid for Inhalation 531

Sodium Bicarbonate (Because Niravam disintegrates in the presence of saliva and the formulation requires an acidic environment to dissolve, concomitant drugs or diseases that raise stomach pH might slow disintegration or dissolution, resulting in slowed or decreased absorption). Products include:

 Colyte with Flavor Packs for Oral Solution..................................... 3088
 HalfLytely and Bisacodyl Tablets Bowel Prep Kit with Flavors Packs 881
 TriLyte with Flavor Packs for Oral Solution..................................... 3100

Sodium Oxybate (The benzodiazepines, including alprazolam, produce additive CNS depressant effects when co-administered with other drugs which themselves produce CNS depression). Products include:

 Xyrem Oral Solution 1688

Sufentanil Citrate (The benzodiazepines, including alprazolam, produce additive CNS depressant effects when co-administered with other drugs which themselves produce CNS depression).

 No products indexed under this heading.

Temazepam (The benzodiazepines, including alprazolam, produce additive CNS depressant effects when co-administered with other drugs which themselves produce CNS depression). Products include:

 Restoril Capsules 1860

Terfenadine (The benzodiazepines, including alprazolam, produce additive CNS depressant effects when co-administered with antihistamines).

 No products indexed under this heading.

Thiamylal Sodium (The benzodiazepines, including alprazolam, produce additive CNS depressant effects when co-administered with other drugs which themselves produce CNS depression).
No products indexed under this heading.

Thioridazine Hydrochloride (The benzodiazepines, including alprazolam, produce additive CNS depressant effects when co-administered with other psychotropic medications. If alprazolam is to be combined with other psychotropic agents, careful consideration should be given to the pharmacology of the agents to be employed, particularly with compounds which might potentiate the action of benzodiazepines). Products include:
Thioridazine Hydrochloride Tablets 2163

Thiothixene (The benzodiazepines, including alprazolam, produce additive CNS depressant effects when co-administered with other psychotropic medications. If alprazolam is to be combined with other psychotropic agents, careful consideration should be given to the pharmacology of the agents to be employed, particularly with compounds which might potentiate the action of benzodiazepines). Products include:
Thiothixene Capsules 2165

Tiagabine Hydrochloride (If alprazolam is to be combined with anticonvulsant drugs, careful consideration should be given to the pharmacology of the agents to be employed, particularly with compounds which might potentiate the action of benzodiazepines. The benzodiazepines, including alprazolam, produce additive CNS depressant effects when co-administered with anticonvulsants). Products include:
Gabitril Tablets 984

Topiramate (If alprazolam is to be combined with anticonvulsant drugs, careful consideration should be given to the pharmacology of the agents to be employed, particularly with compounds which might potentiate the action of benzodiazepines. The benzodiazepines, including alprazolam, produce additive CNS depressant effects when co-administered with anticonvulsants). Products include:
Topamax Sprinkle Capsules 2404
Topamax Tablets 2404

Tranylcypromine Sulfate (The benzodiazepines, including alprazolam, produce additive CNS depressant effects when co-administered with other psychotropic medications. If alprazolam is to be combined with other psychotropic agents, careful consideration should be given to the pharmacology of the agents to be employed, particularly with compounds which might potentiate the action of benzodiazepines). Products include:
Parnate Tablets 1527

Triazolam (The benzodiazepines, including alprazolam, produce additive CNS depressant effects when co-administered with other drugs which themselves produce CNS depression).
No products indexed under this heading.

Trifluoperazine Hydrochloride (The benzodiazepines, including alprazolam, produce additive CNS depressant effects when co-administered with other psychotropic medications. If alprazolam is to be combined with other psychotropic agents, careful consideration should be given to the pharmacology of the agents to be employed, particularly with compounds which might potentiate the action of benzodiazepines).
No products indexed under this heading.

Trimeprazine Tartrate (The benzodiazepines, including alprazolam, produce additive CNS depressant effects when co-administered with antihistamines).
No products indexed under this heading.

Trimethadione (If alprazolam is to be combined with anticonvulsant drugs, careful consideration should be given to the pharmacology of the agents to be employed, particularly with compounds which might potentiate the action of benzodiazepines. The benzodiazepines, including alprazolam, produce additive CNS depressant effects when co-administered with anticonvulsants).
No products indexed under this heading.

Trimipramine Maleate (The benzodiazepines, including alprazolam, produce additive CNS depressant effects when co-administered with other psychotropic medications. If alprazolam is to be combined with other psychotropic agents, careful consideration should be given to the pharmacology of the agents to be employed, particularly with compounds which might potentiate the action of benzodiazepines).
No products indexed under this heading.

Tripelennamine Hydrochloride (The benzodiazepines, including alprazolam, produce additive CNS depressant effects when co-administered with antihistamines).
No products indexed under this heading.

Triprolidine Hydrochloride (The benzodiazepines, including alprazolam, produce additive CNS depressant effects when co-administered with antihistamines).
No products indexed under this heading.

Troleandomycin (The initial step in alprazolam metabolism is hydroxylation catalyzed by cytochrome P450 3A (CYP3A). Drugs which inhibit this metabolic pathway may have a profound effect on the clearance of alprazolam).
No products indexed under this heading.

Valproate Sodium (If alprazolam is to be combined with anticonvulsant drugs, careful consideration should be given to the pharmacology of the agents to be employed, particularly with compounds which might potentiate the action of benzodiazepines. The benzodiazepines, including alprazolam, produce additive CNS depressant effects when co-administered with anticonvulsants). Products include:
Depacon Injection 412

Valproic Acid (If alprazolam is to be combined with anticonvulsant drugs, careful consideration should be given to the pharmacology of the agents to be employed, particularly with compounds which might potentiate the action of benzodiazepines. The benzodiazepines, including alprazolam, produce additive CNS depressant effects when co-administered with anticonvulsants). Products include:
Depakene 417

Venlafaxine Hydrochloride (The initial step in alprazolam metabolism is hydroxylation catalyzed by cytochrome P450 3A (CYP3A). Drugs which inhibit this metabolic pathway may have a profound effect on the clearance of alprazolam). Products include:
Effexor Tablets 3411
Effexor XR Capsules 3417

Verapamil Hydrochloride (The initial step in alprazolam metabolism is hydroxylation catalyzed by cytochrome P450 3A (CYP3A). Drugs which inhibit this metabolic pathway may have a profound effect on the clearance of alprazolam). Products include:
Covera-HS Tablets 3139
Tarka Tablets 524
Verelan PM Extended-Release Capsules, Controlled-Onset 3106

Voriconazole (The initial step in alprazolam metabolism is hydroxylation catalyzed by cytochrome P450 3A (CYP3A). Drugs which inhibit this metabolic pathway may have a profound effect on the clearance of alprazolam). Products include:
VFEND I.V. 2564
VFEND Oral Suspension 2564
VFEND Tablets 2564

Zafirlukast (The initial step in alprazolam metabolism is hydroxylation catalyzed by cytochrome P450 3A (CYP3A). Drugs which inhibit this metabolic pathway may have a profound effect on the clearance of alprazolam). Products include:
Accolate Tablets 671

Zaleplon (The benzodiazepines, including alprazolam, produce additive CNS depressant effects when co-administered with other drugs which themselves produce CNS depression). Products include:
Sonata Capsules 1717

Zileuton (The initial step in alprazolam metabolism is hydroxylation catalyzed by cytochrome P450 3A (CYP3A). Drugs which inhibit this metabolic pathway may have a profound effect on the clearance of alprazolam). Products include:
Zyflo Tablets 1023

Ziprasidone Hydrochloride (The benzodiazepines, including alprazolam, produce additive CNS depressant effects when co-administered with other psychotropic medications. If alprazolam is to be combined with other psychotropic agents, careful consideration should be given to the pharmacology of the agents to be employed, particularly with compounds which might potentiate the action of benzodiazepines). Products include:
Geodon Capsules 2529

Zolpidem Tartrate (The benzodiazepines, including alprazolam, produce additive CNS depressant effects when co-administered with other drugs which themselves produce CNS depression). Products include:
Ambien Tablets 2851
Ambien CR Tablets 2855

Zonisamide (If alprazolam is to be combined with anticonvulsant drugs, careful consideration should be given to the pharmacology of the agents to be employed, particularly with compounds which might potentiate the action of benzodiazepines. The benzodiazepines, including alprazolam, produce additive CNS depressant effects when co-administered with anticonvulsants). Products include:
Zonegran Capsules 1101

Food Interactions

Grapefruit (Available data from clinical studies of benzodiazepines, other than alprazolam, suggest a possible drug interaction with alprazolam and grapefruit juice; caution is recommended during co-administration).

Grapefruit Juice (Available data from clinical studies of benzodiazepines, other than alprazolam, suggest a possible drug interaction with alprazolam and grapefruit juice; caution is recommended during co-administration).

NITRO-DUR TRANSDERMAL INFUSION SYSTEM

(Nitroglycerin) 3046
May interact with calcium channel blockers, vasodilators, and certain other agents. Compounds in these categories include:

Amlodipine Besylate (Vasodilating effects of nitroglycerin may be additive with those of other vasodilators). Products include:
Caduet Tablets 2508
Lotrel Capsules 2249
Norvasc Tablets 2545

Amyl Nitrite (Vasodilating effects of nitroglycerin may be additive with those of other vasodilators).
No products indexed under this heading.

Bepridil Hydrochloride (Vasodilating effects of nitroglycerin may be additive with those of other vasodilators).
No products indexed under this heading.

Diazoxide (Vasodilating effects of nitroglycerin may be additive with those of other vasodilators). Products include:
Hyperstat I.V. 3017

Diltiazem Hydrochloride (Vasodilating effects of nitroglycerin may be additive with those of other vasodilators). Products include:
Cardizem LA Extended Release Tablets 1728
Tiazac Capsules 1201

Epoprostenol Sodium (Vasodilating effects of nitroglycerin may be additive with those of other vasodilators).
No products indexed under this heading.

Ethaverine Hydrochloride (Vasodilating effects of nitroglycerin may be additive with those of other vasodilators).
No products indexed under this heading.

Felodipine (Vasodilating effects of nitroglycerin may be additive with those of other vasodilators).
No products indexed under this heading.

Hydralazine Hydrochloride (Vasodilating effects of nitroglycerin may be additive with those of other vasodilators). Products include:
BiDil Tablets 2171

Isosorbide Dinitrate (Vasodilating effects of nitroglycerin may be additive with those of other vasodilators). Products include:
BiDil Tablets 2171

Isosorbide Mononitrate (Vasodilating effects of nitroglycerin may be additive with those of other vasodilators). Products include:
Imdur Tablets 3018

Isoxsuprine Hydrochloride (Vasodilating effects of nitroglycerin may be additive with those of other vasodilators).
No products indexed under this heading.

Isradipine (Vasodilating effects of nitroglycerin may be additive with those of other vasodilators). Products include:
DynaCirc CR Tablets 2721

Mibefradil Dihydrochloride (Vasodilating effects of nitroglycerin may be additive with those of other vasodilators).
No products indexed under this heading.

Minoxidil (Vasodilating effects of nitroglycerin may be additive with those of other vasodilators). Products include:
Men's Rogaine Extra Strength Hair Regrowth Treatment Topical Solution, Ocean Rush Scent and Original Unscented..... ◘ 633
Men's Rogaine Foam Hair Regrowth Treatment..................... ◘ 633
Women's Rogaine Hair Regrowth Treatment Topical Solution, Spring Bloom Scent and Original Unscented...................... ◘ 634

Nicardipine Hydrochloride (Vasodilating effects of nitroglycerin may be additive with those of other vasodilators). Products include:
Cardene I.V. 2497

Nifedipine (Vasodilating effects of nitroglycerin may be additive with those of other vasodilators). Products include:
Adalat CC Tablets 2964

Nimodipine (Vasodilating effects of nitroglycerin may be additive with those of other vasodilators). Products include:
Nimotop Capsules 749

Nisoldipine (Vasodilating effects of nitroglycerin may be additive with those of other vasodilators). Products include:
Sular Tablets 3122

Nitroglycerin, long-acting formulations (Vasodilating effects of nitroglycerin may be additive with those of other vasodilators).
No products indexed under this heading.

Nitroglycerin Intravenous (Vasodilating effects of nitroglycerin may be additive with those of other vasodilators).
No products indexed under this heading.

Papaverine (Vasodilating effects of nitroglycerin may be additive with those of other vasodilators).
No products indexed under this heading.

Papaverine Hydrochloride (Vasodilating effects of nitroglycerin may be additive with those of other vasodilators).
No products indexed under this heading.

Sildenafil Citrate (Amplification of the vasodilatory effects of the nitroglycerin patch by sildenafil can result in severe hypotension). Products include:
Revatio Tablets 2557
Viagra Tablets 2573

Tolazoline Hydrochloride (Vasodilating effects of nitroglycerin may be additive with those of other vasodilators).
No products indexed under this heading.

Verapamil Hydrochloride (Vasodilating effects of nitroglycerin may be additive with those of other vasodilators). Products include:
Covera-HS Tablets 3139
Tarka Tablets 524
Verelan PM Extended-Release Capsules, Controlled-Onset........... 3106

Food Interactions

Alcohol (Enhances sensitivity to the hypotensive effects).

NITROLINGUAL PUMPSPRAY

(Nitroglycerin) 3120
May interact with calcium channel blockers and certain other agents. Compounds in these categories include:

Amlodipine Besylate (Marked symptomatic orthostatic hypotension). Products include:
Caduet Tablets 2508
Lotrel Capsules 2249
Norvasc Tablets 2545

Bepridil Hydrochloride (Marked symptomatic orthostatic hypotension).
No products indexed under this heading.

Diltiazem Hydrochloride (Marked symptomatic orthostatic hypotension). Products include:
Cardizem LA Extended Release Tablets 1728
Tiazac Capsules 1201

Drugs Depending On Vascular Smooth Muscle (Decreased or increased effect).
No products indexed under this heading.

Felodipine (Marked symptomatic orthostatic hypotension).
No products indexed under this heading.

Isradipine (Marked symptomatic orthostatic hypotension). Products include:
DynaCirc CR Tablets 2721

Mibefradil Dihydrochloride (Marked symptomatic orthostatic hypotension).
No products indexed under this heading.

Nicardipine Hydrochloride (Marked symptomatic orthostatic hypotension). Products include:
Cardene I.V. 2497

Nifedipine (Marked symptomatic orthostatic hypotension). Products include:
Adalat CC Tablets 2964

Nimodipine (Marked symptomatic orthostatic hypotension). Products include:
Nimotop Capsules 749

Nisoldipine (Marked symptomatic orthostatic hypotension). Products include:
Sular Tablets 3122

Sildenafil Citrate (Concomitant administration with phosphodiesterase inhibitors can cause severe hypotension. The time, course and dose dependency of this interaction are not known. Concurrent use is contraindicated). Products include:
Revatio Tablets 2557
Viagra Tablets 2573

Tadalafil (Concomitant administration with phosphodiesterase inhibitors can cause severe hypotension. The time, course and dose dependency of this interaction are not known. Concurrent use is contraindicated). Products include:
Cialis Tablets 1838

Vardenafil Hydrochloride (Concomitant administration with phosphodiesterase inhibitors can cause severe hypotension. The time, course and dose dependency of this interaction are not known. Concurrent use is contraindicated). Products include:
Levitra Tablets 3034

Verapamil Hydrochloride (Marked symptomatic orthostatic hypotension). Products include:
Covera-HS Tablets 3139
Tarka Tablets 524
Verelan PM Extended-Release Capsules, Controlled-Onset........... 3106

Food Interactions

Alcohol (Enhanced sensitivity to hypotensive effects).

NIZORAL A-D SHAMPOO, 1%

(Ketoconazole) 1868
None cited in PDR database.

NORDITROPIN CARTRIDGES

(Somatropin) 2323
May interact with corticosteroids, cytochrome p450 3a4 substrates (selected), oral hypoglycemic agents, and insulin. Compounds in these categories include:

Acarbose (In patients with diabetes mellitus requiring drug therapy, the dose of insulin and/or oral agents may require adjustment when somatropin therapy is initiated). Products include:
Precose Tablets 751

Alfentanil Hydrochloride (Data indicates that growth hormone may be an inducer of cytochrome p450 3A4. When growth hormone is administered in combination with drugs known to be metabolized by cytochrome P450 3A4 hepatic enzymes, it is advisable to monitor the clinical effectiveness of such drugs).
No products indexed under this heading.

Alprazolam (Data indicates that growth hormone may be an inducer of cytochrome p450 3A4. When growth hormone is administered in combination with drugs known to be metabolized by cytochrome P450 3A4 hepatic enzymes, it is advisable to monitor the clinical effectiveness of such drugs). Products include:
Niravam Orally Disintegrating Tablets.. 3092

Amitriptyline Hydrochloride (Data indicates that growth hormone may be an inducer of cytochrome p450 3A4. When growth hormone is administered in combination with drugs known to be metabolized by cytochrome P450 3A4 hepatic enzymes, it is advisable to monitor the clinical effectiveness of such drugs).
No products indexed under this heading.

Amlodipine Besylate (Data indicates that growth hormone may be an inducer of cytochrome p450 3A4. When growth hormone is administered in combination with drugs known to be metabolized by cytochrome P450 3A4 hepatic enzymes, it is advisable to monitor the clinical effectiveness of such drugs). Products include:
Caduet Tablets 2508
Lotrel Capsules 2249
Norvasc Tablets 2545

Aprepitant (Data indicates that growth hormone may be an inducer of cytochrome p450 3A4. When growth hormone is administered in combination with drugs known to be metabolized by cytochrome P450 3A4 hepatic enzymes, it is advisable to monitor the clinical effectiveness of such drugs). Products include:
Emend Capsules 1963

Astemizole (Data indicates that growth hormone may be an inducer of cytochrome p450 3A4. When growth hormone is administered in combination with drugs known to be metabolized by cytochrome P450 3A4 hepatic enzymes, it is advisable to monitor the clinical effectiveness of such drugs).
No products indexed under this heading.

Atorvastatin Calcium (Data indicates that growth hormone may be an inducer of cytochrome p450 3A4. When growth hormone is administered in combination with drugs known to be metabolized by cytochrome P450 3A4 hepatic enzymes, it is advisable to monitor the clinical effectiveness of such drugs). Products include:
Caduet Tablets 2508
Lipitor Tablets 2483

Belladonna Ergotamine (Data indicates that growth hormone may be an inducer of cytochrome p450 3A4. When growth hormone is administered in combination with drugs known to be metabolized by cytochrome P450 3A4 hepatic enzymes, it is advisable to monitor the clinical effectiveness of such drugs).
No products indexed under this heading.

Betamethasone Acetate (Concomitant glucocorticoid therapy may inhibit the growth promoting effect of somatropin).
No products indexed under this heading.

Betamethasone Sodium Phosphate (Concomitant glucocorticoid therapy may inhibit the growth promoting effect of somatropin).
No products indexed under this heading.

Buspirone Hydrochloride (Data indicates that growth hormone may be an inducer of cytochrome p450 3A4. When growth hormone is administered in combination with drugs known to be metabolized by cytochrome P450 3A4 hepatic enzymes, it is advisable to monitor the clinical effectiveness of such drugs).
No products indexed under this heading.

Busulfan (Data indicates that growth hormone may be an inducer of cytochrome p450 3A4. When growth hormone is administered in combination with drugs known to be metabolized by cytochrome P450 3A4 hepatic enzymes, it is advisable to monitor the clinical effectiveness of such drugs). Products include:
I.V. Busulfex **2493**
Myleran Tablets **1525**

Carbamazepine (Data indicates that growth hormone may be an inducer of cytochrome p450 3A4. When growth hormone is administered in combination with drugs known to be metabolized by cytochrome P450 3A4 hepatic enzymes, it is advisable to monitor the clinical effectiveness of such drugs). Products include:
Carbatrol Capsules **3171**
Equetro Extended-Release Capsules **3180**
Tegretol/Tegretol-XR **2295**

Cerivastatin Sodium (Data indicates that growth hormone may be an inducer of cytochrome p450 3A4. When growth hormone is administered in combination with drugs known to be metabolized by cytochrome P450 3A4 hepatic enzymes, it is advisable to monitor the clinical effectiveness of such drugs).
No products indexed under this heading.

Chlorpheniramine (Data indicates that growth hormone may be an inducer of cytochrome p450 3A4. When growth hormone is administered in combination with drugs known to be metabolized by cytochrome P450 3A4 hepatic enzymes, it is advisable to monitor the clinical effectiveness of such drugs).
No products indexed under this heading.

Chlorpheniramine Maleate (Data indicates that growth hormone may be an inducer of cytochrome p450 3A4. When growth hormone is administered in combination with drugs known to be metabolized by cytochrome P450 3A4 hepatic enzymes, it is advisable to monitor the clinical effectiveness of such drugs). Products include:
Advil Allergy Sinus Caplets **770**
Advil Multi-Symptom Cold Caplets **770**
BC Allergy Sinus Cold Powder **677**
Comtrex Maximum Strength Cold & Cough Day/Night Caplets - Night Formulation **726**
Comtrex Maximum Strength Day/Night Severe Cold & Sinus Caplets - Night Formulation **725**
Contac Cold and Flu Maximum Strength Caplets **728**
Contac Cold and Flu Day and Night Caplets (Night Formulation Only) **727**
Children's Dimetapp Long Acting Cough Plus Cold Syrup **731**
Robitussin Cough & Cold Long-Acting Liquid **735**
Robitussin Cough & Allergy Syrup .. **736**
Robitussin Cough & Cold Nighttime Liquid **736**
Robitussin Cough, Cold & Flu Nighttime Liquid **738**
Robitussin Pediatric Cough & Cold Long-Acting Liquid **735**
Robitussin Pediatric Cough & Cold Nighttime Liquid **736**
Triaminic Cold & Allergy Liquid **746**
Triaminic Cough & Runny Nose Softchews **748**
Children's Tylenol Plus Flu Oral Suspension **749**
Tylenol Allergy Multi-Symptom Caplets with Cool Burst and Gelcaps **1872**
Children's Tylenol Plus Cold Suspension Liquid **1879**
Children's Tylenol Plus Cough & Runny Nose Suspension Liquid **1879**
Children's Tylenol Plus Flu Suspension Liquid **1881**
Children's Tylenol Plus Multi-Symptom Cold Suspension Liquid **1879**
Tylenol Cold Head Congestion Nighttime Caplets with Cool Burst **1873**
Tylenol Cold Multi-Symptom Nighttime Caplets with Cool Burst **1874**
Tylenol Sinus Congestion & Pain Nighttime Caplets with Cool Burst **1876**
Vicks 44M Cough, Cold & Flu Relief Liquid **2680**
Pediatric Vicks 44m Cough & Cold Relief Liquid **2676**
Children's Vicks NyQuil Cold/Cough Relief **756**
Children's Vicks NyQuil Cold/Cough Relief Liquid **2680**
Zicam Maximum Strength Flu Daytime **768**

Chlorpheniramine Polistirex (Data indicates that growth hormone may be an inducer of cytochrome p450 3A4. When growth hormone is administered in combination with drugs known to be metabolized by cytochrome P450 3A4 hepatic enzymes, it is advisable to monitor the clinical effectiveness of such drugs). Products include:
Tussionex Pennkinetic Extended-Release Suspension **3327**

Chlorpheniramine Tannate (Data indicates that growth hormone may be an inducer of cytochrome p450 3A4. When growth hormone is administered in combination with drugs known to be metabolized by cytochrome P450 3A4 hepatic enzymes, it is advisable to monitor the clinical effectiveness of such drugs).
No products indexed under this heading.

Chlorpropamide (In patients with diabetes mellitus requiring drug therapy, the dose of insulin and/or oral agents may require adjustment when somatropin therapy is initiated).
No products indexed under this heading.

Cisapride (Data indicates that growth hormone may be an inducer of cytochrome p450 3A4. When growth hormone is administered in combination with drugs known to be metabolized by cytochrome P450 3A4 hepatic enzymes, it is advisable to monitor the clinical effectiveness of such drugs).
No products indexed under this heading.

Clarithromycin (Data indicates that growth hormone may be an inducer of cytochrome p450 3A4. When growth hormone is administered in combination with drugs known to be metabolized by cytochrome P450 3A4 hepatic enzymes, it is advisable to monitor the clinical effectiveness of such drugs). Products include:
Biaxin/Biaxin XL **402**
PREVPAC **3284**

Cortisone Acetate (Concomitant glucocorticoid therapy may inhibit the growth promoting effect of somatropin).
No products indexed under this heading.

Cyclosporine (Data indicates that growth hormone may be an inducer of cytochrome p450 3A4. When growth hormone is administered in combination with drugs known to be metabolized by cytochrome P450 3A4 hepatic enzymes, it is advisable to monitor the clinical effectiveness of such drugs). Products include:
Gengraf Capsules **459**
Neoral Oral Solution **2259**
Neoral Soft Gelatin Capsules **2259**
Restasis Ophthalmic Emulsion **575**
Sandimmune **2275**

Desogestrel (Data indicates that growth hormone may be an inducer of cytochrome p450 3A4. When growth hormone is administered in combination with drugs known to be metabolized by cytochrome P450 3A4 hepatic enzymes, it is advisable to monitor the clinical effectiveness of such drugs). Products include:
Mircette Tablets **1066**

Dexamethasone (Concomitant glucocorticoid therapy may inhibit the growth promoting effect of somatropin). Products include:
Ciprodex Otic Suspension **559**
Decadron Tablets **1951**
TobraDex Ophthalmic Ointment **562**
TobraDex Ophthalmic Suspension ... **563**

Dexamethasone Acetate (Concomitant glucocorticoid therapy may inhibit the growth promoting effect of somatropin).
No products indexed under this heading.

Dexamethasone Sodium Phosphate (Concomitant glucocorticoid therapy may inhibit the growth promoting effect of somatropin).
No products indexed under this heading.

Diazepam (Data indicates that growth hormone may be an inducer of cytochrome p450 3A4. When growth hormone is administered in combination with drugs known to be metabolized by cytochrome P450 3A4 hepatic enzymes, it is advisable to monitor the clinical effectiveness of such drugs). Products include:
Diastat Rectal Delivery System **3343**
Valium Tablets **2819**

Dihydroergotamine Mesylate (Data indicates that growth hormone may be an inducer of cytochrome p450 3A4. When growth hormone is administered in combination with drugs known to be metabolized by cytochrome P450 3A4 hepatic enzymes, it is advisable to monitor the clinical effectiveness of such drugs). Products include:
Migranal Nasal Spray **3348**

Diltiazem Hydrochloride (Data indicates that growth hormone may be an inducer of cytochrome p450 3A4. When growth hormone is administered in combination with drugs known to be metabolized by cytochrome P450 3A4 hepatic enzymes, it is advisable to monitor the clinical effectiveness of such drugs). Products include:
Cardizem LA Extended Release Tablets **1728**
Tiazac Capsules **1201**

Diltiazem Maleate (Data indicates that growth hormone may be an inducer of cytochrome p450 3A4. When growth hormone is administered in combination with drugs known to be metabolized by cytochrome P450 3A4 hepatic enzymes, it is advisable to monitor the clinical effectiveness of such drugs).
No products indexed under this heading.

Disopyramide (Data indicates that growth hormone may be an inducer of cytochrome p450 3A4. When growth hormone is administered in combination with drugs known to be metabolized by cytochrome P450 3A4 hepatic enzymes, it is advisable to monitor the clinical effectiveness of such drugs).
No products indexed under this heading.

Disopyramide Phosphate (Data indicates that growth hormone may be an inducer of cytochrome p450 3A4. When growth hormone is administered in combination with drugs known to be metabolized by cytochrome P450 3A4 hepatic enzymes, it is advisable to monitor the clinical effectiveness of such drugs).
No products indexed under this heading.

Disulfiram (Data indicates that growth hormone may be an inducer of cytochrome p450 3A4. When growth hormone is administered in combination with drugs known to be metabolized by cytochrome P450 3A4 hepatic enzymes, it is advisable to monitor the clinical effectiveness of such drugs).
No products indexed under this heading.

Doxorubicin Hydrochloride (Data indicates that growth hormone may be an inducer of cytochrome p450 3A4. When growth hormone is administered in combination with drugs known to be metabolized by cytochrome P450 3A4 hepatic enzymes, it is advisable to monitor the clinical effectiveness of such drugs).
No products indexed under this heading.

Dronabinol (Data indicates that growth hormone may be an inducer of cytochrome p450 3A4. When growth hormone is administered in combination with drugs known to be metabolized by cytochrome P450 3A4 hepatic enzymes, it is advisable to monitor the clinical effectiveness of such drugs). Products include:
Marinol Capsules **3333**

Ergotamine Tartrate (Data indicates that growth hormone may be an inducer of cytochrome p450 3A4. When growth hormone is administered in combination with drugs known to be metabolized by cytochrome P450 3A4 hepatic enzymes, it is advisable to monitor the clinical effectiveness of such drugs).
No products indexed under this heading.

Erythromycin (Data indicates that growth hormone may be an inducer of cytochrome p450 3A4. When growth hormone is administered in combination with drugs known to be metabolized by cytochrome P450

3A4 hepatic enzymes, it is advisable to monitor the clinical effectiveness of such drugs). Products include:

Ery-Tab Tablets 449
Erythromycin Base Filmtab
Tablets 455
Erythromycin Delayed-Release
Capsules, USP 457
PCE Dispertab Tablets 515

Erythromycin Estolate (Data indicates that growth hormone may be an inducer of cytochrome p450 3A4. When growth hormone is administered in combination with drugs known to be metabolized by cytochrome P450 3A4 hepatic enzymes, it is advisable to monitor the clinical effectiveness of such drugs).

No products indexed under this heading.

Erythromycin Ethylsuccinate (Data indicates that growth hormone may be an inducer of cytochrome p450 3A4. When growth hormone is administered in combination with drugs known to be metabolized by cytochrome P450 3A4 hepatic enzymes, it is advisable to monitor the clinical effectiveness of such drugs). Products include:

E.E.S. 451
EryPed 447

Erythromycin Gluceptate (Data indicates that growth hormone may be an inducer of cytochrome p450 3A4. When growth hormone is administered in combination with drugs known to be metabolized by cytochrome P450 3A4 hepatic enzymes, it is advisable to monitor the clinical effectiveness of such drugs).

No products indexed under this heading.

Erythromycin Lactobionate (Data indicates that growth hormone may be an inducer of cytochrome p450 3A4. When growth hormone is administered in combination with drugs known to be metabolized by cytochrome P450 3A4 hepatic enzymes, it is advisable to monitor the clinical effectiveness of such drugs).

No products indexed under this heading.

Erythromycin Stearate (Data indicates that growth hormone may be an inducer of cytochrome p450 3A4. When growth hormone is administered in combination with drugs known to be metabolized by cytochrome P450 3A4 hepatic enzymes, it is advisable to monitor the clinical effectiveness of such drugs). Products include:

Erythrocin Stearate Filmtab
Tablets 453

Estradiol (Data indicates that growth hormone may be an inducer of cytochrome p450 3A4. When growth hormone is administered in combination with drugs known to be metabolized by cytochrome P450 3A4 hepatic enzymes, it is advisable to monitor the clinical effectiveness of such drugs). Products include:

Angeliq Tablets 762
Climara Transdermal System 771
Climara Pro Transdermal System 776
Estrasorb Topical Emulsion 1147
Estring Vaginal Ring 2635
Menostar Transdermal System 782
Vagifem Tablets 2334

Estradiol Benzoate (Data indicates that growth hormone may be an inducer of cytochrome p450 3A4. When growth hormone is administered in combination with drugs known to be metabolized by cytochrome P450 3A4 hepatic enzymes, it is advisable to monitor the clinical effectiveness of such drugs).

No products indexed under this heading.

Estradiol Cypionate (Data indicates that growth hormone may be an inducer of cytochrome p450 3A4. When growth hormone is administered in combination with drugs known to be metabolized by cytochrome P450 3A4 hepatic enzymes, it is advisable to monitor the clinical effectiveness of such drugs).

No products indexed under this heading.

Estradiol Valerate (Data indicates that growth hormone may be an inducer of cytochrome p450 3A4. When growth hormone is administered in combination with drugs known to be metabolized by cytochrome P450 3A4 hepatic enzymes, it is advisable to monitor the clinical effectiveness of such drugs).

No products indexed under this heading.

Ethinyl Estradiol (Data indicates that growth hormone may be an inducer of cytochrome p450 3A4. When growth hormone is administered in combination with drugs known to be metabolized by cytochrome P450 3A4 hepatic enzymes, it is advisable to monitor the clinical effectiveness of such drugs). Products include:

Mircette Tablets 1066
NuvaRing .. 2340
Ortho-Cyclen/Ortho Tri-Cyclen 2429
Ortho Evra Transdermal System 2417
Ortho Tri-Cyclen Lo Tablets 2436
Seasonique Tablets 1077
Yasmin 28 Tablets 796
Yaz Tablets 803

Ethosuximide (Data indicates that growth hormone may be an inducer of cytochrome p450 3A4. When growth hormone is administered in combination with drugs known to be metabolized by cytochrome P450 3A4 hepatic enzymes, it is advisable to monitor the clinical effectiveness of such drugs).

No products indexed under this heading.

Ethynodiol Diacetate (Data indicates that growth hormone may be an inducer of cytochrome p450 3A4. When growth hormone is administered in combination with drugs known to be metabolized by cytochrome P450 3A4 hepatic enzymes, it is advisable to monitor the clinical effectiveness of such drugs).

No products indexed under this heading.

Etoposide (Data indicates that growth hormone may be an inducer of cytochrome p450 3A4. When growth hormone is administered in combination with drugs known to be metabolized by cytochrome P450 3A4 hepatic enzymes, it is advisable to monitor the clinical effectiveness of such drugs).

No products indexed under this heading.

Etoposide Phosphate (Data indicates that growth hormone may be an inducer of cytochrome p450 3A4. When growth hormone is administered in combination with drugs known to be metabolized by cytochrome P450 3A4 hepatic enzymes, it is advisable to monitor the clinical effectiveness of such drugs).

No products indexed under this heading.

Felodipine (Data indicates that growth hormone may be an inducer of cytochrome p450 3A4. When growth hormone is administered in combination with drugs known to be metabolized by cytochrome P450 3A4 hepatic enzymes, it is advisable to monitor the clinical effectiveness of such drugs).

No products indexed under this heading.

Fentanyl (Data indicates that growth hormone may be an inducer of cytochrome p450 3A4. When growth hormone is administered in combination with drugs known to be metabolized by cytochrome P450 3A4 hepatic enzymes, it is advisable to monitor the clinical effectiveness of such drugs). Products include:

Duragesic Transdermal System 2373
Ionsys Transdermal System 2379

Fentanyl Citrate (Data indicates that growth hormone may be an inducer of cytochrome p450 3A4. When growth hormone is administered in combination with drugs known to be metabolized by cytochrome P450 3A4 hepatic enzymes, it is advisable to monitor the clinical effectiveness of such drugs). Products include:

Actiq .. 979

Fludrocortisone Acetate (Concomitant glucocorticoid therapy may inhibit the growth promoting effect of somatropin).

No products indexed under this heading.

Glimepiride (In patients with diabetes mellitus requiring drug therapy, the dose of insulin and/or oral agents may require adjustment when somatropin therapy is initiated). Products include:

Avandaryl Tablets 1379
Duetact Tablets 3226

Glipizide (In patients with diabetes mellitus requiring drug therapy, the dose of insulin and/or oral agents may require adjustment when somatropin therapy is initiated).

No products indexed under this heading.

Glyburide (In patients with diabetes mellitus requiring drug therapy, the dose of insulin and/or oral agents may require adjustment when somatropin therapy is initiated).

No products indexed under this heading.

Haloperidol (Data indicates that growth hormone may be an inducer of cytochrome p450 3A4. When growth hormone is administered in combination with drugs known to be metabolized by cytochrome P450 3A4 hepatic enzymes, it is advisable to monitor the clinical effectiveness of such drugs).

No products indexed under this heading.

Haloperidol Decanoate (Data indicates that growth hormone may be an inducer of cytochrome p450 3A4. When growth hormone is administered in combination with drugs known to be metabolized by cytochrome P450 3A4 hepatic enzymes, it is advisable to monitor the clinical effectiveness of such drugs).

No products indexed under this heading.

Haloperidol Lactate (Data indicates that growth hormone may be an inducer of cytochrome p450 3A4. When growth hormone is administered in combination with drugs known to be metabolized by cytochrome P450 3A4 hepatic enzymes, it is advisable to monitor the clinical effectiveness of such drugs).

No products indexed under this heading.

Hydrocortisone (Concomitant glucocorticoid therapy may inhibit the growth promoting effect of somatropin). Products include:

Colocort Rectal Suspension, USP
(Retention) 100 mg/60 mL........... 2476
Hydrocortone Tablets 1989
Preparation H Hydrocortisone
Cream 🔲646

Hydrocortisone Acetate (Concomitant glucocorticoid therapy may inhibit the growth promoting effect of somatropin). Products include:

Analpram-HC 1159
Pramosone 1161
ProctoFoam-HC 3099

Hydrocortisone Sodium Phosphate (Concomitant glucocorticoid therapy may inhibit the growth promoting effect of somatropin).

No products indexed under this heading.

Hydrocortisone Sodium Succinate (Concomitant glucocorticoid therapy may inhibit the growth promoting effect of somatropin).

No products indexed under this heading.

Indinavir Sulfate (Data indicates that growth hormone may be an inducer of cytochrome p450 3A4. When growth hormone is administered in combination with drugs known to be metabolized by cytochrome P450 3A4 hepatic enzymes, it is advisable to monitor the clinical effectiveness of such drugs). Products include:

Crixivan Capsules 1940

Insulin, Human, Zinc Suspension (In patients with diabetes mellitus requiring drug therapy, the dose of insulin and/or oral agents may require adjustment when somatropin therapy is initiated). Products include:

Humulin L, 100 Units 1794
Humulin U, 100 Units 1800

Insulin, Human NPH (In patients with diabetes mellitus requiring drug therapy, the dose of insulin and/or oral agents may require adjustment when somatropin therapy is initiated). Products include:

Humulin N, 100 Units 1795
Humulin N Pen 1797

Insulin, Human Regular (In patients with diabetes mellitus requiring drug therapy, the dose of insulin and/or oral agents may require adjustment when somatropin therapy is initiated). Products include:

Humulin R, 100 Units 1798

Insulin, Human Regular and Human NPH Mixture (In patients with diabetes mellitus requiring drug therapy, the dose of insulin and/or oral agents may require adjustment when somatropin therapy is initiated). Products include:

Humulin 50/50, 100 Units 1791
Humulin 70/30 Pen 1793

Insulin, NPH (In patients with diabetes mellitus requiring drug therapy, the dose of insulin and/or oral agents may require adjustment when somatropin therapy is initiated).

No products indexed under this heading.

Insulin, Regular (In patients with diabetes mellitus requiring drug therapy, the dose of insulin and/or oral agents may require adjustment when somatropin therapy is initiated).

No products indexed under this heading.

Insulin, Zinc Crystals (In patients with diabetes mellitus requiring drug therapy, the dose of insulin and/or oral agents may require adjustment when somatropin therapy is initiated).

No products indexed under this heading.

Insulin, Zinc Suspension (In patients with diabetes mellitus requiring drug therapy, the dose of insulin and/or oral agents may require adjustment when somatropin therapy is initiated).

No products indexed under this heading.

Insulin Aspart, Human Regular (In patients with diabetes mellitus requiring drug therapy, the dose of insulin and/or oral agents may require adjustment when somatropin therapy is initiated). Products include:

NovoLog Injection 2326

Insulin glargine (In patients with diabetes mellitus requiring drug therapy, the dose of insulin and/or oral agents may require adjustment when somatropin therapy is initiated). Products include:

Lantus Injection 2909

Insulin Lispro, Human (In patients with diabetes mellitus requiring drug therapy, the dose of insulin and/or oral agents may require adjustment when somatropin therapy is initiated). Products include:

Humalog-Pen 1781
Humalog Mix 50/50-Pen 1783
Humalog Mix 75/25-Pen 1785

Insulin Lispro Protamine, Human (In patients with diabetes mellitus requiring drug therapy, the dose of insulin and/or oral agents may require adjustment when somatropin therapy is initiated). Products include:

Humalog Mix 50/50-Pen 1783
Humalog Mix 75/25-Pen 1785

Isradipine (Data indicates that growth hormone may be an inducer of cytochrome p450 3A4. When growth hormone is administered in combination with drugs known to be metabolized by cytochrome P450 3A4 hepatic enzymes, it is advisable to monitor the clinical effectiveness of such drugs). Products include:

DynaCirc CR Tablets 2721

Itraconazole (Data indicates that growth hormone may be an inducer of cytochrome p450 3A4. When growth hormone is administered in combination with drugs known to be metabolized by cytochrome P450 3A4 hepatic enzymes, it is advisable to monitor the clinical effectiveness of such drugs).

No products indexed under this heading.

Ketoconazole (Data indicates that growth hormone may be an inducer of cytochrome p450 3A4. When growth hormone is administered in combination with drugs known to be metabolized by cytochrome P450 3A4 hepatic enzymes, it is advisable to monitor the clinical effectiveness of such drugs). Products include:

Nizoral A-D Shampoo, 1% 1868

Levonorgestrel (Data indicates that growth hormone may be an inducer of cytochrome p450 3A4. When growth hormone is administered in combination with drugs known to be metabolized by cytochrome P450 3A4 hepatic enzymes, it is advisable to monitor the clinical effectiveness of such drugs). Products include:

Climara Pro Transdermal System 776
Mirena Intrauterine System 787
Plan B Tablets 1076
Seasonique Tablets 1077

Lidocaine (Data indicates that growth hormone may be an inducer of cytochrome p450 3A4. When growth hormone is administered in combination with drugs known to be metabolized by cytochrome P450 3A4 hepatic enzymes, it is advisable to monitor the clinical effectiveness of such drugs). Products include:

Lidoderm Patch 1118
Synera Topical Patch 1137

Lidocaine Hydrochloride (Data indicates that growth hormone may be an inducer of cytochrome p450 3A4. When growth hormone is administered in combination with drugs known to be metabolized by cytochrome P450 3A4 hepatic enzymes, it is advisable to monitor the clinical effectiveness of such drugs).

No products indexed under this heading.

Lovastatin (Data indicates that growth hormone may be an inducer of cytochrome p450 3A4. When growth hormone is administered in combination with drugs known to be metabolized by cytochrome P450 3A4 hepatic enzymes, it is advisable to monitor the clinical effectiveness of such drugs). Products include:

Advicor Tablets 1722
Altoprev Extended-Release Tablets 3109
Mevacor Tablets 2021

Mestranol (Data indicates that growth hormone may be an inducer of cytochrome p450 3A4. When growth hormone is administered in combination with drugs known to be metabolized by cytochrome P450 3A4 hepatic enzymes, it is advisable to monitor the clinical effectiveness of such drugs).

No products indexed under this heading.

Metformin Hydrochloride (In patients with diabetes mellitus requiring drug therapy, the dose of insulin and/or oral agents may require adjustment when somatropin therapy is initiated). Products include:

ActoPlus Met Tablets 3214
Avandamet Tablets 1373
Fortamet Extended-Release Tablets 3115

Methadone Hydrochloride (Data indicates that growth hormone may be an inducer of cytochrome p450 3A4. When growth hormone is administered in combination with drugs known to be metabolized by cytochrome P450 3A4 hepatic enzymes, it is advisable to monitor the clinical effectiveness of such drugs).

No products indexed under this heading.

Methylprednisolone Acetate (Concomitant glucocorticoid therapy may inhibit the growth promoting effect of somatropin). Products include:

Depo-Medrol Injectable Suspension 2617
Depo-Medrol Single-Dose Vial 2619

Methylprednisolone Sodium Succinate (Concomitant glucocorticoid therapy may inhibit the growth promoting effect of somatropin).

No products indexed under this heading.

Midazolam Hydrochloride (Data indicates that growth hormone may be an inducer of cytochrome p450 3A4. When growth hormone is administered in combination with drugs known to be metabolized by cytochrome P450 3A4 hepatic enzymes, it is advisable to monitor the clinical effectiveness of such drugs).

No products indexed under this heading.

Miglitol (In patients with diabetes mellitus requiring drug therapy, the dose of insulin and/or oral agents may require adjustment when somatropin therapy is initiated).

No products indexed under this heading.

Nefazodone Hydrochloride (Data indicates that growth hormone may be an inducer of cytochrome p450 3A4. When growth hormone is administered in combination with drugs known to be metabolized by cytochrome P450 3A4 hepatic enzymes, it is advisable to monitor the clinical effectiveness of such drugs).

No products indexed under this heading.

Nelfinavir Mesylate (Data indicates that growth hormone may be an inducer of cytochrome p450 3A4. When growth hormone is administered in combination with drugs known to be metabolized by cytochrome P450 3A4 hepatic enzymes, it is advisable to monitor the clinical effectiveness of such drugs). Products include:

Viracept 2577

Nicardipine Hydrochloride (Data indicates that growth hormone may be an inducer of cytochrome p450 3A4. When growth hormone is administered in combination with drugs known to be metabolized by cytochrome P450 3A4 hepatic enzymes, it is advisable to monitor the clinical effectiveness of such drugs). Products include:

Cardene I.V. 2497

Nifedipine (Data indicates that growth hormone may be an inducer of cytochrome p450 3A4. When growth hormone is administered in combination with drugs known to be metabolized by cytochrome P450 3A4 hepatic enzymes, it is advisable to monitor the clinical effectiveness of such drugs). Products include:

Adalat CC Tablets 2964

Nimodipine (Data indicates that growth hormone may be an inducer of cytochrome p450 3A4. When growth hormone is administered in combination with drugs known to be metabolized by cytochrome P450 3A4 hepatic enzymes, it is advisable to monitor the clinical effectiveness of such drugs). Products include:

Nimotop Capsules 749

Nisoldipine (Data indicates that growth hormone may be an inducer of cytochrome p450 3A4. When growth hormone is administered in combination with drugs known to be metabolized by cytochrome P450 3A4 hepatic enzymes, it is advisable to monitor the clinical effectiveness of such drugs). Products include:

Sular Tablets 3122

Nitrendipine (Data indicates that growth hormone may be an inducer of cytochrome p450 3A4. When growth hormone is administered in combination with drugs known to be metabolized by cytochrome P450 3A4 hepatic enzymes, it is advisable to monitor the clinical effectiveness of such drugs).

No products indexed under this heading.

Norethindrone (Data indicates that growth hormone may be an inducer of cytochrome p450 3A4. When growth hormone is administered in combination with drugs known to be metabolized by cytochrome P450 3A4 hepatic enzymes, it is advisable to monitor the clinical effectiveness of such drugs). Products include:

Ortho Micronor Tablets 2426

Norethindrone Acetate (Data indicates that growth hormone may be an inducer of cytochrome p450 3A4. When growth hormone is administered in combination with drugs known to be metabolized by cytochrome P450 3A4 hepatic enzymes, it is advisable to monitor the clinical effectiveness of such drugs).

No products indexed under this heading.

Norgestrel (Data indicates that growth hormone may be an inducer of cytochrome p450 3A4. When growth hormone is administered in combination with drugs known to be metabolized by cytochrome P450 3A4 hepatic enzymes, it is advisable to monitor the clinical effectiveness of such drugs).

No products indexed under this heading.

Ondansetron (Data indicates that growth hormone may be an inducer of cytochrome p450 3A4. When growth hormone is administered in combination with drugs known to be metabolized by cytochrome P450 3A4 hepatic enzymes, it is advisable to monitor the clinical effectiveness of such drugs). Products include:

Zofran ODT Orally Disintegrating Tablets 1639

Ondansetron Hydrochloride (Data indicates that growth hormone may be an inducer of cytochrome p450 3A4. When growth hormone is administered in combination with drugs known to be metabolized by cytochrome P450 3A4 hepatic

enzymes, it is advisable to monitor the clinical effectiveness of such drugs). Products include:

- Zofran Injection ... **1634**
- Zofran ... **1639**

Paclitaxel (Data indicates that growth hormone may be an inducer of cytochrome p450 3A4. When growth hormone is administered in combination with drugs known to be metabolized by cytochrome P450 3A4 hepatic enzymes, it is advisable to monitor the clinical effectiveness of such drugs).

No products indexed under this heading.

Pimozide (Data indicates that growth hormone may be an inducer of cytochrome p450 3A4. When growth hormone is administered in combination with drugs known to be metabolized by cytochrome P450 3A4 hepatic enzymes, it is advisable to monitor the clinical effectiveness of such drugs).

No products indexed under this heading.

Pioglitazone Hydrochloride (In patients with diabetes mellitus requiring drug therapy, the dose of insulin and/or oral agents may require adjustment when somatropin therapy is initiated). Products include:

- ActoPlus Met Tablets ... **3214**
- Actos Tablets ... **3219**
- Duetact Tablets ... **3226**

Polyestradiol Phosphate (Data indicates that growth hormone may be an inducer of cytochrome p450 3A4. When growth hormone is administered in combination with drugs known to be metabolized by cytochrome P450 3A4 hepatic enzymes, it is advisable to monitor the clinical effectiveness of such drugs).

No products indexed under this heading.

Prednisolone Acetate (Concomitant glucocorticoid therapy may inhibit the growth promoting effect of somatropin). Products include:

- Blephamide Ophthalmic Ointment ... **568**
- Blephamide Ophthalmic Suspension ... **569**
- Poly-Pred Ophthalmic Suspension ... ⊙**233**
- Pred Forte Ophthalmic Suspension ... ⊙**235**
- Pred Mild Ophthalmic Suspension ... ⊙**238**
- Pred-G Ophthalmic Ointment ... ⊙**237**
- Pred-G Ophthalmic Suspension ... ⊙**236**

Prednisolone Sodium Phosphate (Concomitant glucocorticoid therapy may inhibit the growth promoting effect of somatropin).

No products indexed under this heading.

Prednisolone Tebutate (Concomitant glucocorticoid therapy may inhibit the growth promoting effect of somatropin).

No products indexed under this heading.

Prednisone (Concomitant glucocorticoid therapy may inhibit the growth promoting effect of somatropin).

No products indexed under this heading.

Quinidine Gluconate (Data indicates that growth hormone may be an inducer of cytochrome p450 3A4. When growth hormone is administered in combination with drugs known to be metabolized by cytochrome P450 3A4 hepatic enzymes, it is advisable to monitor the clinical effectiveness of such drugs).

No products indexed under this heading.

Quinidine Polygalacturonate (Data indicates that growth hormone may be an inducer of cytochrome p450 3A4. When growth hormone is administered in combination with drugs known to be metabolized by cytochrome P450 3A4 hepatic enzymes, it is advisable to monitor the clinical effectiveness of such drugs).

No products indexed under this heading.

Quinidine Sulfate (Data indicates that growth hormone may be an inducer of cytochrome p450 3A4. When growth hormone is administered in combination with drugs known to be metabolized by cytochrome P450 3A4 hepatic enzymes, it is advisable to monitor the clinical effectiveness of such drugs).

No products indexed under this heading.

Repaglinide (In patients with diabetes mellitus requiring drug therapy, the dose of insulin and/or oral agents may require adjustment when somatropin therapy is initiated).

No products indexed under this heading.

Rifabutin (Data indicates that growth hormone may be an inducer of cytochrome p450 3A4. When growth hormone is administered in combination with drugs known to be metabolized by cytochrome P450 3A4 hepatic enzymes, it is advisable to monitor the clinical effectiveness of such drugs).

No products indexed under this heading.

Ritonavir (Data indicates that growth hormone may be an inducer of cytochrome p450 3A4. When growth hormone is administered in combination with drugs known to be metabolized by cytochrome P450 3A4 hepatic enzymes, it is advisable to monitor the clinical effectiveness of such drugs). Products include:

- Kaletra ... **476**
- Norvir ... **503**

Rosiglitazone Maleate (In patients with diabetes mellitus requiring drug therapy, the dose of insulin and/or oral agents may require adjustment when somatropin therapy is initiated). Products include:

- Avandamet Tablets ... **1373**
- Avandaryl Tablets ... **1379**
- Avandia Tablets ... **1384**

Saquinavir (Data indicates that growth hormone may be an inducer of cytochrome p450 3A4. When growth hormone is administered in combination with drugs known to be metabolized by cytochrome P450 3A4 hepatic enzymes, it is advisable to monitor the clinical effectiveness of such drugs).

No products indexed under this heading.

Saquinavir Mesylate (Data indicates that growth hormone may be an inducer of cytochrome p450 3A4. When growth hormone is administered in combination with drugs known to be metabolized by cytochrome P450 3A4 hepatic enzymes, it is advisable to monitor the clinical effectiveness of such drugs). Products include:

- Invirase ... **2772**

Sertraline Hydrochloride (Data indicates that growth hormone may be an inducer of cytochrome p450 3A4. When growth hormone is administered in combination with drugs known to be metabolized by cytochrome P450 3A4 hepatic enzymes, it is advisable to monitor the clinical effectiveness of such drugs). Products include:

- Zoloft ... **2586**

Sildenafil Citrate (Data indicates that growth hormone may be an inducer of cytochrome p450 3A4. When growth hormone is administered in combination with drugs known to be metabolized by cytochrome P450 3A4 hepatic enzymes, it is advisable to monitor the clinical effectiveness of such drugs). Products include:

- Revatio Tablets ... **2557**
- Viagra Tablets ... **2573**

Simvastatin (Data indicates that growth hormone may be an inducer of cytochrome p450 3A4. When growth hormone is administered in combination with drugs known to be metabolized by cytochrome P450 3A4 hepatic enzymes, it is advisable to monitor the clinical effectiveness of such drugs). Products include:

- Vytorin 10/10 Tablets ... **2114**
- Vytorin 10/10 Tablets ... **3077**
- Vytorin 10/20 Tablets ... **2114**
- Vytorin 10/20 Tablets ... **3077**
- Vytorin 10/40 Tablets ... **2114**
- Vytorin 10/40 Tablets ... **3077**
- Vytorin 10/80 Tablets ... **2114**
- Vytorin 10/80 Tablets ... **3077**
- Zocor Tablets ... **2105**

Sirolimus (Data indicates that growth hormone may be an inducer of cytochrome p450 3A4. When growth hormone is administered in combination with drugs known to be metabolized by cytochrome P450 3A4 hepatic enzymes, it is advisable to monitor the clinical effectiveness of such drugs). Products include:

- Rapamune Oral Solution and Tablets ... **3475**

Tacrolimus (Data indicates that growth hormone may be an inducer of cytochrome p450 3A4. When growth hormone is administered in combination with drugs known to be metabolized by cytochrome P450 3A4 hepatic enzymes, it is advisable to monitor the clinical effectiveness of such drugs). Products include:

- Prograf Capsules and Injection ... **632**
- Protopic Ointment ... **638**

Tamoxifen Citrate (Data indicates that growth hormone may be an inducer of cytochrome p450 3A4. When growth hormone is administered in combination with drugs known to be metabolized by cytochrome P450 3A4 hepatic enzymes, it is advisable to monitor the clinical effectiveness of such drugs). Products include:

- Soltamox Oral Solution ... **3527**

Tiagabine Hydrochloride (Data indicates that growth hormone may be an inducer of cytochrome p450 3A4. When growth hormone is administered in combination with drugs known to be metabolized by cytochrome P450 3A4 hepatic enzymes, it is advisable to monitor the clinical effectiveness of such drugs). Products include:

- Gabitril Tablets ... **984**

Tolazamide (In patients with diabetes mellitus requiring drug therapy, the dose of insulin and/or oral agents may require adjustment when somatropin therapy is initiated).

No products indexed under this heading.

Tolbutamide (In patients with diabetes mellitus requiring drug therapy, the dose of insulin and/or oral agents may require adjustment when somatropin therapy is initiated).

No products indexed under this heading.

Tolterodine Tartrate (Data indicates that growth hormone may be an inducer of cytochrome p450 3A4. When growth hormone is administered in combination with drugs known to be metabolized by cytochrome P450 3A4 hepatic enzymes, it is advisable to monitor the clinical effectiveness of such drugs). Products include:

- Detrol Tablets ... **2628**
- Detrol LA Capsules ... **2631**

Trazodone Hydrochloride (Data indicates that growth hormone may be an inducer of cytochrome p450 3A4. When growth hormone is administered in combination with drugs known to be metabolized by cytochrome P450 3A4 hepatic enzymes, it is advisable to monitor the clinical effectiveness of such drugs).

No products indexed under this heading.

Triamcinolone (Concomitant glucocorticoid therapy may inhibit the growth promoting effect of somatropin).

No products indexed under this heading.

Triamcinolone Acetonide (Concomitant glucocorticoid therapy may inhibit the growth promoting effect of somatropin). Products include:

- Azmacort Inhalation Aerosol ... **1726**
- Nasacort AQ Nasal Spray ... **2922**

Triamcinolone Diacetate (Concomitant glucocorticoid therapy may inhibit the growth promoting effect of somatropin).

No products indexed under this heading.

Triamcinolone Hexacetonide (Concomitant glucocorticoid therapy may inhibit the growth promoting effect of somatropin).

No products indexed under this heading.

Triazolam (Data indicates that growth hormone may be an inducer of cytochrome p450 3A4. When growth hormone is administered in combination with drugs known to be metabolized by cytochrome P450 3A4 hepatic enzymes, it is advisable to monitor the clinical effectiveness of such drugs).

No products indexed under this heading.

Troglitazone (In patients with diabetes mellitus requiring drug therapy, the dose of insulin and/or oral agents may require adjustment when somatropin therapy is initiated).

No products indexed under this heading.

Verapamil Hydrochloride (Data indicates that growth hormone may

be an inducer of cytochrome p450 3A4. When growth hormone is administered in combination with drugs known to be metabolized by cytochrome P450 3A4 hepatic enzymes, it is advisable to monitor the clinical effectiveness of such drugs). Products include:
- Covera-HS Tablets 3139
- Tarka Tablets 524
- Verelan PM Extended-Release Capsules, Controlled-Onset.......... 3106

Vinblastine Sulfate (Data indicates that growth hormone may be an inducer of cytochrome p450 3A4. When growth hormone is administered in combination with drugs known to be metabolized by cytochrome P450 3A4 hepatic enzymes, it is advisable to monitor the clinical effectiveness of such drugs).
No products indexed under this heading.

Vincristine Sulfate (Data indicates that growth hormone may be an inducer of cytochrome p450 3A4. When growth hormone is administered in combination with drugs known to be metabolized by cytochrome P450 3A4 hepatic enzymes, it is advisable to monitor the clinical effectiveness of such drugs).
No products indexed under this heading.

Warfarin Sodium (Data indicates that growth hormone may be an inducer of cytochrome p450 3A4. When growth hormone is administered in combination with drugs known to be metabolized by cytochrome P450 3A4 hepatic enzymes, it is advisable to monitor the clinical effectiveness of such drugs). Products include:
- Coumadin for Injection 898
- Coumadin Tablets 898

NORFLEX INJECTION

(Orphenadrine Citrate) 1856
May interact with:

Propoxyphene Hydrochloride (Concomitant use results in confusion, anxiety and tremors).
No products indexed under this heading.

Propoxyphene Napsylate (Concomitant use results in confusion, anxiety and tremors).
No products indexed under this heading.

NOROXIN TABLETS

(Norfloxacin) 2032
May interact with antacids containing aluminum, calcium and magnesium, class 1A antiarrhythmics, class III antiarrhythmics, corticosteroids, oral anticoagulants, erythromycin, iron containing oral preparations, antipsychotic agents, non-steroidal anti-inflammatory agents, tricyclic antidepressants, xanthines, and certain other agents. Compounds in these categories include:

Aluminum Carbonate (May interfere with absorption resulting in lower serum and urine levels of norfloxacin; antacids should not be administered concomitantly with, or within 2 hours of, the administration of norfloxacin).
No products indexed under this heading.

Aluminum Hydroxide (May interfere with absorption resulting in lower serum and urine levels of norfloxacin; antacids should not be administered concomitantly with, or within 2 hours of, the administration of norfloxacin). Products include:
- Gaviscon Regular Strength Liquid 658
- Gaviscon Regular Strength Tablets 658
- Gaviscon Extra Strength Liquid 658
- Gaviscon Extra Strength Tablets 658
- Maalox Regular Strength Antacid/Antigas Liquid.......... 2175
- Maalox Max Maximum Strength Antacid/Anti-Gas Liquid.......... 2176

Aminophylline (Co-administration of quinolone with theophylline has resulted in elevated plasma levels of theophylline resulting in theophylline-related side effects).
No products indexed under this heading.

Amiodarone Hydrochloride (Risk of developing arrhythmias with norfloxacin may be reduced by avoiding concurrent treatment with class III antiarrhythmic agents).
No products indexed under this heading.

Amitriptyline Hydrochloride (Norfloxacin should be used with caution in subjects receiving drugs that affect the QTc interval, such as tricyclic antidepressants).
No products indexed under this heading.

Amoxapine (Norfloxacin should be used with caution in subjects receiving drugs that affect the QTc interval, such as tricyclic antidepressants).
No products indexed under this heading.

Anisindione (Co-administration may enhance the effects of oral anticoagulants). Products include:
- Miradon Tablets 3042

Aripiprazole (Norfloxacin should be used with caution in subjects receiving drugs that affect the QTc interval, such as antipsychotics). Products include:
- Abilify Oral Solution 882
- Abilify Oral Solution 2450
- Abilify Discmelt Orally Disintegrating Tablets.......... 882
- Abilify Discmelt Orally Disintegrating Tablets.......... 2450
- Abilify Tablets 882
- Abilify Tablets 2450

Betamethasone Acetate (The risk of ruptures of the shoulder, hand or Achilles tendons may be increased in patients receiving concomitant corticosteroids, especially in the elderly).
No products indexed under this heading.

Betamethasone Sodium Phosphate (The risk of ruptures of the shoulder, hand or Achilles tendons may be increased in patients receiving concomitant corticosteroids, especially in the elderly).
No products indexed under this heading.

Bretylium Tosylate (Risk of developing arrhythmias with norfloxacin may be reduced by avoiding concurrent treatment with class III antiarrhythmic agents).
No products indexed under this heading.

Caffeine (Some quinolones have been shown to interfere with the metabolism of caffeine leading to reduced clearance of caffeine and a prolongation of its plasma half-life). Products include:
- BC Headache Powder 677
- Arthritis Strength BC Powder 677
- Excedrin Extra Strength Caplets/Tablets/Geltabs.......... 684
- Excedrin Migraine Caplets/Tablets/Geltabs.......... 609
- Excedrin Tension Headache Caplets/Tablets/Geltabs.......... 611
- Goody's Extra Strength Headache Powders.......... 611
- Goody's Extra Strength Pain Relief Tablets.......... 685
- Vivarin 602
- Winrgy Dietary Supplement.......... 823

Celecoxib (The concomitant administration of a non-steroidal anti-inflammatory drug (NSAID) with a quinolone, including norfloxacin, may increase the risk of CNS stimulation and convulsive seizures. Therefore, norfloxacin should be used with caution in individualsreceiving NSAIDs concomitantly). Products include:
- Celebrex Capsules 3134

Chlorpromazine (Norfloxacin should be used with caution in subjects receiving drugs that affect the QTc interval, such as antipsychotics).
No products indexed under this heading.

Chlorpromazine Hydrochloride (Norfloxacin should be used with caution in subjects receiving drugs that affect the QTc interval, such as antipsychotics).
No products indexed under this heading.

Chlorprothixene (Norfloxacin should be used with caution in subjects receiving drugs that affect the QTc interval, such as antipsychotics).
No products indexed under this heading.

Chlorprothixene Hydrochloride (Norfloxacin should be used with caution in subjects receiving drugs that affect the QTc interval, such as antipsychotics).
No products indexed under this heading.

Cisapride (Norfloxacin should be used with caution in subjects receiving drugs that affect the QTc interval, such as cisapride).
No products indexed under this heading.

Clomipramine Hydrochloride (Norfloxacin should be used with caution in subjects receiving drugs that affect the QTc interval, such as tricyclic antidepressants).
No products indexed under this heading.

Clozapine (Norfloxacin should be used with caution in subjects receiving drugs that affect the QTc interval, such as antipsychotics). Products include:
- Clozaril Tablets 2184
- FazaClo Orally Disintegrating Tablets 551

Cortisone Acetate (The risk of ruptures of the shoulder, hand or Achilles tendons may be increased in patients receiving concomitant corticosteroids, especially in the elderly).
No products indexed under this heading.

Cyclosporine (Co-administration has resulted in elevated serum levels of cyclosporine). Products include:
- Gengraf Capsules 459
- Neoral Oral Solution 2259
- Neoral Soft Gelatin Capsules 2259
- Restasis Ophthalmic Emulsion 575
- Sandimmune 2275

Desipramine Hydrochloride (Norfloxacin should be used with caution in subjects receiving drugs that affect the QTc interval, such as tricyclic antidepressants).
No products indexed under this heading.

Dexamethasone (The risk of ruptures of the shoulder, hand or Achilles tendons may be increased in patients receiving concomitant corticosteroids, especially in the elderly). Products include:
- Ciprodex Otic Suspension 559
- Decadron Tablets 1951
- TobraDex Ophthalmic Ointment 562
- TobraDex Ophthalmic Suspension 563

Dexamethasone Acetate (The risk of ruptures of the shoulder, hand or Achilles tendons may be increased in patients receiving concomitant corticosteroids, especially in the elderly).
No products indexed under this heading.

Dexamethasone Sodium Phosphate (The risk of ruptures of the shoulder, hand or Achilles tendons may be increased in patients receiving concomitant corticosteroids, especially in the elderly).
No products indexed under this heading.

Diclofenac Potassium (The concomitant administration of a non-steroidal anti-inflammatory drug (NSAID) with a quinolone, including norfloxacin, may increase the risk of CNS stimulation and convulsive seizures. Therefore, norfloxacin should be used with caution in individualsreceiving NSAIDs concomitantly).
No products indexed under this heading.

Diclofenac Sodium (The concomitant administration of a non-steroidal anti-inflammatory drug (NSAID) with a quinolone, including norfloxacin, may increase the risk of CNS stimulation and convulsive seizures. Therefore, norfloxacin should be used with caution in individualsreceiving NSAIDs concomitantly). Products include:
- Arthrotec Tablets 3129
- Voltaren Ophthalmic Solution 2309
- Voltaren Tablets 2307
- Voltaren-XR Tablets 2310

Dicumarol (Co-administration may enhance the effects of oral anticoagulants).
No products indexed under this heading.

Didanosine (Co-administration with Videx, didanosine chewable/buffered tablets or the pediatric powder for oral solution may interfere with absorption resulting in lower serum and urine levels of norfloxacin; this combination should not be administered concomitantlyor within 2 hours of administration of norfloxacin).
No products indexed under this heading.

Disopyramide (Risk of developing arrhythmias with norfloxacin may be reduced by avoiding concurrent treatment with class IA antiarrhythmic agents).
No products indexed under this heading.

Doxepin Hydrochloride (Norfloxacin should be used with caution in subjects receiving drugs that affect the QTc interval, such as tricyclic antidepressants).
No products indexed under this heading.

Dyphylline (Co-administration of quinolone with theophylline has resulted in elevated plasma levels of theophylline resulting in theophylline-related side effects).
No products indexed under this heading.

Erythromycin (Norfloxacin should be used with caution in subjects receiving drugs that affect the QTc interval, such as erythromycin). Products include:
Ery-Tab Tablets 449
Erythromycin Base Filmtab Tablets 455
Erythromycin Delayed-Release Capsules, USP 457
PCE Dispertab Tablets 515

Erythromycin Estolate (Norfloxacin should be used with caution in subjects receiving drugs that affect the QTc interval, such as erythromycin).
No products indexed under this heading.

Erythromycin Ethylsuccinate (Norfloxacin should be used with caution in subjects receiving drugs that affect the QTc interval, such as erythromycin). Products include:
E.E.S. 451
EryPed 447

Erythromycin Gluceptate (Norfloxacin should be used with caution in subjects receiving drugs that affect the QTc interval, such as erythromycin).
No products indexed under this heading.

Erythromycin Lactobionate (Norfloxacin should be used with caution in subjects receiving drugs that affect the QTc interval, such as erythromycin).
No products indexed under this heading.

Erythromycin Stearate (Norfloxacin should be used with caution in subjects receiving drugs that affect the QTc interval, such as erythromycin). Products include:
Erythrocin Stearate Filmtab Tablets 453

Etodolac (The concomitant administration of a non-steroidal anti-inflammatory drug (NSAID) with a quinolone, including norfloxacin, may increase the risk of CNS stimulation and convulsive seizures. Therefore, norfloxacin should be used with caution in individualsreceiving NSAIDs concomitantly).
No products indexed under this heading.

Fenoprofen Calcium (The concomitant administration of a non-steroidal anti-inflammatory drug (NSAID) with a quinolone, including norfloxacin, may increase the risk of CNS stimulation and convulsive seizures. Therefore, norfloxacin should be used with caution in individualsreceiving NSAIDs concomitantly). Products include:
Nalfon Capsules 2502

Ferrous Fumarate (May interfere with absorption resulting in lower serum and urine levels of norfloxacin; iron-containing products should not be administered concomitantly with, or within 2 hours of, the administration of norfloxacin).
No products indexed under this heading.

Ferrous Gluconate (May interfere with absorption resulting in lower serum and urine levels of norfloxacin; iron-containing products should not be administered concomitantly with, or within 2 hours of, the administration of norfloxacin).
No products indexed under this heading.

Ferrous Sulfate (May interfere with absorption resulting in lower serum and urine levels of norfloxacin; iron-containing products should not be administered concomitantly with, or within 2 hours of, the administration of norfloxacin). Products include:
Slow Fe Iron Tablets .... ▣ 818
Slow Fe with Folic Acid Tablets .... ▣ 819

Fludrocortisone Acetate (The risk of ruptures of the shoulder, hand or Achilles tendons may be increased in patients receiving concomitant corticosteroids, especially in the elderly).
No products indexed under this heading.

Fluphenazine Decanoate (Norfloxacin should be used with caution in subjects receiving drugs that affect the QTc interval, such as antipsychotics).
No products indexed under this heading.

Fluphenazine Enanthate (Norfloxacin should be used with caution in subjects receiving drugs that affect the QTc interval, such as antipsychotics).
No products indexed under this heading.

Fluphenazine Hydrochloride (Norfloxacin should be used with caution in subjects receiving drugs that affect the QTc interval, such as antipsychotics).
No products indexed under this heading.

Flurbiprofen (The concomitant administration of a non-steroidal anti-inflammatory drug (NSAID) with a quinolone, including norfloxacin, may increase the risk of CNS stimulation and convulsive seizures. Therefore, norfloxacin should be used with caution in individualsreceiving NSAIDs concomitantly).
No products indexed under this heading.

Glyburide (Concomitant administration of norfloxacin with glyburide has rarely resulted in severe hypoglycemia; monitoring of blood glucose is recommended when these agents are co-administered).
No products indexed under this heading.

Haloperidol (Norfloxacin should be used with caution in subjects receiving drugs that affect the QTc interval, such as antipsychotics).
No products indexed under this heading.

Haloperidol Decanoate (Norfloxacin should be used with caution in subjects receiving drugs that affect the QTc interval, such as antipsychotics).
No products indexed under this heading.

Hydrocortisone (The risk of ruptures of the shoulder, hand or Achilles tendons may be increased in patients receiving concomitant corticosteroids, especially in the elderly). Products include:
Colocort Rectal Suspension, USP (Retention) 100 mg/60 mL 2476
Hydrocortone Tablets 1989
Preparation H Hydrocortisone Cream .... ▣ 646

Hydrocortisone Acetate (The risk of ruptures of the shoulder, hand or Achilles tendons may be increased in patients receiving concomitant corticosteroids, especially in the elderly). Products include:
Analpram-HC 1159
Pramosone 1161
ProctoFoam-HC 3099

Hydrocortisone Sodium Phosphate (The risk of ruptures of the shoulder, hand or Achilles tendons may be increased in patients receiving concomitant corticosteroids, especially in the elderly).
No products indexed under this heading.

Hydrocortisone Sodium Succinate (The risk of ruptures of the shoulder, hand or Achilles tendons may be increased in patients receiving concomitant corticosteroids, especially in the elderly).
No products indexed under this heading.

Ibuprofen (The concomitant administration of a non-steroidal anti-inflammatory drug (NSAID) with a quinolone, including norfloxacin, may increase the risk of CNS stimulation and convulsive seizures. Therefore, norfloxacin should be used with caution in individualsreceiving NSAIDs concomitantly). Products include:
Advil Allergy Sinus Caplets .... ▣ 770
Advil .... ▣ 674
Children's Advil Oral Suspension .... ▣ 603
Children's Advil Chewable Tablets .... ▣ 603
Advil Cold & Sinus .... ▣ 723
Infants' Advil Concentrated Drops .... ▣ 604
Infants' Advil Concentrated Drops - White Grape (Dye-Free) .... ▣ 604
Junior Strength Advil Swallow Tablets .... ▣ 605
Advil Migraine Liquigels .... ▣ 608
Advil Multi-Symptom Cold Caplets .... ▣ 770
Advil PM Caplets .... ▣ 615
Motrin IB Tablets and Caplets 1866
Children's Motrin Oral Suspension 1867
Children's Motrin Non-Staining Dye-Free Oral Suspension 1867
Children's Motrin Cold Oral Suspension 1867
Infants' Motrin Concentrated Drops 1867
Infants' Motrin Non-Staining Dye-Free Concentrated Drops 1867
Junior Strength Motrin Caplets and Chewable Tablets 1867
Vicoprofen Tablets 539

Imipramine Hydrochloride (Norfloxacin should be used with caution in subjects receiving drugs that affect the QTc interval, such as tricyclic antidepressants).
No products indexed under this heading.

Imipramine Pamoate (Norfloxacin should be used with caution in subjects receiving drugs that affect the QTc interval, such as tricyclic antidepressants).
No products indexed under this heading.

Indomethacin (The concomitant administration of a non-steroidal anti-inflammatory drug (NSAID) with a quinolone, including norfloxacin, may increase the risk of CNS stimulation and convulsive seizures. Therefore, norfloxacin should be used with caution in individualsreceiving NSAIDs concomitantly). Products include:
Indocin 1995

Indomethacin Sodium Trihydrate (The concomitant administration of a non-steroidal anti-inflammatory drug (NSAID) with a quinolone, including norfloxacin, may increase the risk of CNS stimulation and convulsive seizures. Therefore, norfloxacin should be used with caution in individualsreceiving NSAIDs concomitantly). Products include:
Indocin I.V. 2465

Iron (May interfere with absorption resulting in lower serum and urine levels of norfloxacin; iron-containing products should not be administered concomitantly with, or within 2 hours of, the administration of norfloxacin).
No products indexed under this heading.

Ketoprofen (The concomitant administration of a non-steroidal anti-inflammatory drug (NSAID) with a quinolone, including norfloxacin, may increase the risk of CNS stimulation and convulsive seizures. Therefore, norfloxacin should be used with caution in individualsreceiving NSAIDs concomitantly).
No products indexed under this heading.

Ketorolac Tromethamine (The concomitant administration of a non-steroidal anti-inflammatory drug (NSAID) with a quinolone, including norfloxacin, may increase the risk of CNS stimulation and convulsive seizures. Therefore, norfloxacin should be used with caution in individualsreceiving NSAIDs concomitantly). Products include:
Acular Ophthalmic Solution 565
Acular LS Ophthalmic Solution 566

Lithium Carbonate (Norfloxacin should be used with caution in subjects receiving drugs that affect the QTc interval, such as antipsychotics). Products include:
Lithobid Tablets 1692

Lithium Citrate (Norfloxacin should be used with caution in subjects receiving drugs that affect the QTc interval, such as antipsychotics).
No products indexed under this heading.

Loxapine Hydrochloride (Norfloxacin should be used with caution in subjects receiving drugs that affect the QTc interval, such as antipsychotics).
No products indexed under this heading.

Loxapine Succinate (Norfloxacin should be used with caution in subjects receiving drugs that affect the QTc interval, such as antipsychotics).
No products indexed under this heading.

Magaldrate (May interfere with absorption resulting in lower serum and urine levels of norfloxacin; antacids should not be administered concomitantly with, or within 2 hours of, the administration of norfloxacin).
No products indexed under this heading.

Magnesium Hydroxide (May interfere with absorption resulting in lower serum and urine levels of norfloxacin; antacids should not be administered concomitantly with, or within 2 hours of, the administration of norfloxacin). Products include:
Maalox Regular Strength Antacid/Antigas Liquid 2175
Maalox Max Maximum Strength Antacid/Anti-Gas Liquid 2176
Pepcid Complete Chewable Tablets 1701

Magnesium Oxide (May interfere with absorption resulting in lower serum and urine levels of norfloxacin; antacids should not be administered concomitantly with, or within 2 hours of, the administration of norfloxacin). Products include:
Beelith Tablets 759
PremCal Light, Regular, and Extra Strength Tablets .... ▣818

Maprotiline Hydrochloride (Norfloxacin should be used with caution in subjects receiving drugs that affect the QTc interval, such as tricyclic antidepressants).
No products indexed under this heading.

Meclofenamate Sodium (The concomitant administration of a non-steroidal anti-inflammatory drug (NSAID) with a quinolone, including norfloxacin, may increase the risk of CNS stimulation and convulsive seizures. Therefore, norfloxacin should be used with caution in individualsreceiving NSAIDs concomitantly).
No products indexed under this heading.

Mefenamic Acid (The concomitant administration of a non-steroidal anti-inflammatory drug (NSAID) with a quinolone, including norfloxacin, may increase the risk of CNS stimulation and convulsive seizures. Therefore, norfloxacin should be used with caution in individualsreceiving NSAIDs concomitantly).
No products indexed under this heading.

Meloxicam (The concomitant administration of a non-steroidal anti-inflammatory drug (NSAID) with a quinolone, including norfloxacin, may increase the risk of CNS stimulation and convulsive seizures. Therefore, norfloxacin should be used with caution in individualsreceiving NSAIDs concomitantly). Products include:
Mobic Oral Suspension 863
Mobic Tablets 863

Mesoridazine Besylate (Norfloxacin should be used with caution in subjects receiving drugs that affect the QTc interval, such as antipsychotics).
No products indexed under this heading.

Methotrimeprazine (Norfloxacin should be used with caution in subjects receiving drugs that affect the QTc interval, such as antipsychotics).
No products indexed under this heading.

Methylprednisolone Acetate (The risk of ruptures of the shoulder, hand or Achilles tendons may be increased in patients receiving concomitant corticosteroids, especially in the elderly). Products include:
Depo-Medrol Injectable Suspension 2617
Depo-Medrol Single-Dose Vial 2619

Methylprednisolone Sodium Succinate (The risk of ruptures of the shoulder, hand or Achilles tendons may be increased in patients receiving concomitant corticosteroids, especially in the elderly).
No products indexed under this heading.

Molindone Hydrochloride (Norfloxacin should be used with caution in subjects receiving drugs that affect the QTc interval, such as antipsychotics). Products include:
Moban Tablets 1119

Moricizine Hydrochloride (Risk of developing arrhythmias with norfloxacin may be reduced by avoiding concurrent treatment with class IA antiarrhythmic agents).
No products indexed under this heading.

Nabumetone (The concomitant administration of a non-steroidal anti-inflammatory drug (NSAID) with a quinolone, including norfloxacin, may increase the risk of CNS stimulation and convulsive seizures. Therefore, norfloxacin should be used with caution in individualsreceiving NSAIDs concomitantly).
No products indexed under this heading.

Naproxen (The concomitant administration of a non-steroidal anti-inflammatory drug (NSAID) with a quinolone, including norfloxacin, may increase the risk of CNS stimulation and convulsive seizures. Therefore, norfloxacin should be used with caution in individualsreceiving NSAIDs concomitantly). Products include:
EC-Naprosyn Delayed-Release Tablets 2761
Naprosyn Suspension 2761
Naprosyn Tablets 2761
Prevacid NapraPAC 3280

Naproxen Sodium (The concomitant administration of a non-steroidal anti-inflammatory drug (NSAID) with a quinolone, including norfloxacin, may increase the risk of CNS stimulation and convulsive seizures. Therefore, norfloxacin should be used with caution in individualsreceiving NSAIDs concomitantly). Products include:
Aleve Caplets 742
Aleve Gelcaps 743
Aleve Tablets 743
Aleve Cold & Sinus Caplets 744
Anaprox Tablets 2761
Anaprox DS Tablets 2761

Nitrofurantoin (Nitrofurantoin may antagonize the antibacterial effect of norfloxacin in the urinary tract; concurrent use is not recommended).
No products indexed under this heading.

Nortriptyline Hydrochloride (Norfloxacin should be used with caution in subjects receiving drugs that affect the QTc interval, such as tricyclic antidepressants).
No products indexed under this heading.

Olanzapine (Norfloxacin should be used with caution in subjects receiving drugs that affect the QTc interval, such as antipsychotics).
Products include:
Symbyax Capsules 1819
Zyprexa Tablets 1830
Zyprexa IntraMuscular 1830
Zyprexa ZYDIS Orally Disintegrating Tablets 1830

Oxaprozin (The concomitant administration of a non-steroidal anti-inflammatory drug (NSAID) with a quinolone, including norfloxacin, may increase the risk of CNS stimulation and convulsive seizures. Therefore, norfloxacin should be used with caution in individualsreceiving NSAIDs concomitantly).
No products indexed under this heading.

Perphenazine (Norfloxacin should be used with caution in subjects receiving drugs that affect the QTc interval, such as antipsychotics).
No products indexed under this heading.

Phenylbutazone (The concomitant administration of a non-steroidal anti-inflammatory drug (NSAID) with a quinolone, including norfloxacin, may increase the risk of CNS stimulation and convulsive seizures. Therefore, norfloxacin should be used with caution in individualsreceiving NSAIDs concomitantly).
No products indexed under this heading.

Pimozide (Norfloxacin should be used with caution in subjects receiving drugs that affect the QTc interval, such as antipsychotics).
No products indexed under this heading.

Piroxicam (The concomitant administration of a non-steroidal anti-inflammatory drug (NSAID) with a quinolone, including norfloxacin, may increase the risk of CNS stimulation and convulsive seizures. Therefore, norfloxacin should be used with caution in individualsreceiving NSAIDs concomitantly).
No products indexed under this heading.

Polysaccharide Iron Complex (May interfere with absorption resulting in lower serum and urine levels of norfloxacin; iron-containing products should not be administered concomitantly with, or within 2 hours of, the administration of norfloxacin).
Products include:
Nu-Iron 150 Capsules 2127

Prednisolone Acetate (The risk of ruptures of the shoulder, hand or Achilles tendons may be increased in patients receiving concomitant corticosteroids, especially in the elderly).
Products include:
Blephamide Ophthalmic Ointment 568
Blephamide Ophthalmic Suspension 569
Poly-Pred Ophthalmic Suspension .... ⊙233
Pred Forte Ophthalmic Suspension .... ⊙235
Pred Mild Ophthalmic Suspension .... ⊙238
Pred-G Ophthalmic Ointment .... ⊙237
Pred-G Ophthalmic Suspension .... ⊙236

Prednisolone Sodium Phosphate (The risk of ruptures of the shoulder, hand or Achilles tendons may be increased in patients receiving concomitant corticosteroids, especially in the elderly).
No products indexed under this heading.

Prednisolone Tebutate (The risk of ruptures of the shoulder, hand or Achilles tendons may be increased in patients receiving concomitant corticosteroids, especially in the elderly).
No products indexed under this heading.

Prednisone (The risk of ruptures of the shoulder, hand or Achilles tendons may be increased in patients receiving concomitant corticosteroids, especially in the elderly).
No products indexed under this heading.

Probenecid (Co-administration with probenecid has resulted in diminished urinary excretion).
No products indexed under this heading.

Procainamide (Risk of developing arrhythmias with norfloxacin may be reduced by avoiding concurrent treatment with class IA antiarrhythmic agents).
No products indexed under this heading.

Prochlorperazine (Norfloxacin should be used with caution in subjects receiving drugs that affect the QTc interval, such as antipsychotics).
No products indexed under this heading.

Promethazine Hydrochloride (Norfloxacin should be used with caution in subjects receiving drugs that affect the QTc interval, such as antipsychotics). Products include:
Phenergan Tablets and Suppositories 3440

Protriptyline Hydrochloride (Norfloxacin should be used with caution in subjects receiving drugs that affect the QTc interval, such as tricyclic antidepressants).
No products indexed under this heading.

Quetiapine Fumarate (Norfloxacin should be used with caution in subjects receiving drugs that affect the QTc interval, such as antipsychotics). Products include:
Seroquel Tablets 690

Quinidine (Risk of developing arrhythmias with norfloxacin may be reduced by avoiding concurrent treatment with class IA antiarrhythmic agents).
No products indexed under this heading.

Quinidine Gluconate (Risk of developing arrhythmias with norfloxacin may be reduced by avoiding concurrent treatment with class IA antiarrhythmic agents).
No products indexed under this heading.

Risperidone (Norfloxacin should be used with caution in subjects receiving drugs that affect the QTc interval, such as antipsychotics).
Products include:
Risperdal 1676
Risperdal Consta Long-Acting Injection 1682
Risperdal M-Tab Orally Disintegrating Tablets 1676

Rofecoxib (The concomitant administration of a non-steroidal anti-inflammatory drug (NSAID) with a quinolone, including norfloxacin, may increase the risk of CNS stimulation and convulsive seizures. Therefore, norfloxacin should be used with caution in individualsreceiving NSAIDs concomitantly).
No products indexed under this heading.

Sotalol Hydrochloride (Risk of developing arrhythmias with norfloxacin may be reduced by avoiding concurrent treatment with class III antiarrhythmic agents).
No products indexed under this heading.

Sucralfate (May interfere with absorption resulting in lower serum and urine levels of norfloxacin; sucralfate should not be administered concomitantly with, or within 2 hours of, the administration of norfloxacin). Products include:
Carafate Suspension 701
Carafate Tablets 701

Sulindac (The concomitant administration of a non-steroidal anti-inflammatory drug (NSAID) with a quinolone, including norfloxacin, may increase the risk of CNS stimulation and convulsive seizures. Therefore, norfloxacin should be used with caution in individualsreceiving NSAIDs concomitantly). Products include:

Clinoril Tablets 1924

Theophylline (Co-administration of quinolone with theophylline has resulted in elevated plasma levels of theophylline resulting in theophylline-related side effects).
No products indexed under this heading.

Theophylline Anhydrous (Co-administration of quinolone with theophylline has resulted in elevated plasma levels of theophylline resulting in theophylline-related side effects). Products include:
Uniphyl Tablets 2710

Theophylline Calcium Salicylate (Co-administration of quinolone with theophylline has resulted in elevated plasma levels of theophylline resulting in theophylline-related side effects).
No products indexed under this heading.

Theophylline Dihydroxypropyl (Glyceryl) (Co-administration of quinolone with theophylline has resulted in elevated plasma levels of theophylline resulting in theophylline-related side effects).
No products indexed under this heading.

Theophylline Ethylenediamine (Co-administration of quinolone with theophylline has resulted in elevated plasma levels of theophylline resulting in theophylline-related side effects).
No products indexed under this heading.

Theophylline Sodium Glycinate (Co-administration of quinolone with theophylline has resulted in elevated plasma levels of theophylline resulting in theophylline-related side effects).
No products indexed under this heading.

Thioridazine Hydrochloride (Norfloxacin should be used with caution in subjects receiving drugs that affect the QTc interval, such as antipsychotics). Products include:
Thioridazine Hydrochloride Tablets 2163

Thiothixene (Norfloxacin should be used with caution in subjects receiving drugs that affect the QTc interval, such as antipsychotics). Products include:
Thiothixene Capsules 2165

Tolmetin Sodium (The concomitant administration of a non-steroidal anti-inflammatory drug (NSAID) with a quinolone, including norfloxacin, may increase the risk of CNS stimulation and convulsive seizures. Therefore, norfloxacin should be used with caution in individualsreceiving NSAIDs concomitantly).
No products indexed under this heading.

Triamcinolone (The risk of ruptures of the shoulder, hand or Achilles tendons may be increased in patients receiving concomitant corticosteroids, especially in the elderly).
No products indexed under this heading.

Triamcinolone Acetonide (The risk of ruptures of the shoulder, hand or Achilles tendons may be increased in patients receiving concomitant corticosteroids, especially in the elderly). Products include:
Azmacort Inhalation Aerosol 1726
Nasacort AQ Nasal Spray 2922

Triamcinolone Diacetate (The risk of ruptures of the shoulder, hand or Achilles tendons may be increased in patients receiving concomitant corticosteroids, especially in the elderly).
No products indexed under this heading.

Triamcinolone Hexacetonide (The risk of ruptures of the shoulder, hand or Achilles tendons may be increased in patients receiving concomitant corticosteroids, especially in the elderly).
No products indexed under this heading.

Trifluoperazine Hydrochloride (Norfloxacin should be used with caution in subjects receiving drugs that affect the QTc interval, such as antipsychotics).
No products indexed under this heading.

Trimipramine Maleate (Norfloxacin should be used with caution in subjects receiving drugs that affect the QTc interval, such as tricyclic antidepressants).
No products indexed under this heading.

Valdecoxib (The concomitant administration of a non-steroidal anti-inflammatory drug (NSAID) with a quinolone, including norfloxacin, may increase the risk of CNS stimulation and convulsive seizures. Therefore, norfloxacin should be used with caution in individualsreceiving NSAIDs concomitantly).
No products indexed under this heading.

Warfarin Sodium (Co-administration may enhance the effects of oral anticoagulants). Products include:
Coumadin for Injection 898
Coumadin Tablets 898

Zinc Sulfate (May interfere with absorption resulting in lower serum and urine levels of norfloxacin; zinc-containing oral products should not be administered concomitantly with, or within 2 hours of, the administration of norfloxacin). Products include:
Visine A.C. Seasonal Itching and Redness Relief Drops .... ⊙ 289
Zinc-220 Capsules 580

Ziprasidone Hydrochloride (Norfloxacin should be used with caution in subjects receiving drugs that affect the QTc interval, such as antipsychotics). Products include:
Geodon Capsules 2529

Food Interactions

Dairy products (Avoid simultaneous ingestion; administer norfloxacin at least one hour before or two hours after ingestion of milk and/or other dairy products).

Food, unspecified (Co-administration may decrease the absorption of norfloxacin; administer at least one hour before or two hours after a meal).

NORVASC TABLETS

(Amlodipine Besylate) 2545
None cited in PDR database.

NORVIR SOFT GELATIN CAPSULES

(Ritonavir) 503
May interact with beta blockers, cytochrome p450 3a inducers (selected), dexamethasone, ergot-containing drugs, erythromycin, oral hypoglycemic agents, highly metabolized sedatives and hypnotics, insulin, phenytoin, quinidine, selective serotonin reuptake inhibitors, tricyclic antidepressants, valproate, xanthines, and certain other agents. Compounds in these categories include:

Acarbose (New onset diabetes mellitus, exacerbation of pre-existing diabetes, and hyperglycemia have been reported with protease inhibitors; dosage adjustment of oral hypoglycemic agents may be required). Products include:
Precose Tablets 751

Acebutolol Hydrochloride (Co-administration with beta-blockers has resulted in cardiac and neurologic events).
No products indexed under this heading.

Albendazole (Co-administration results in a possible increase in AUC of albendazole; dosage adjustments may be required). Products include:
Albenza Tablets 1338

Alfentanil Hydrochloride (Co-administration results in a large increase (> 3x) in AUC of alfentanil; dosage adjustments may be required).
No products indexed under this heading.

Alfuzosin Hydrochloride (Co-administration is contraindicated due to the potential for serious reactions such as hypotension). Products include:
Uroxatral Tablets 2943

Allium sativum (Potential for increase in the clearance of ritonavir resulting in decreased ritonavir plasma concentrations).
No products indexed under this heading.

Alprazolam (Co-administration is likely to produce large increases in highly metabolized sedatives and hypnotics resulting in extreme sedation and respiratory depression; concurrent use is contraindicated). Products include:
Niravam Orally Disintegrating Tablets 3092

Aminophylline (Co-administration results in the reduction of the average AUC of theophylline; increased dosage of theophylline may be required and therapeutic monitoring should be considered).
No products indexed under this heading.

Amiodarone Hydrochloride (Co-administration is contraindicated due to potential for serious and/or life-threatening reactions, such as cardiac arrhythmias).
No products indexed under this heading.

Amitriptyline Hydrochloride (Co-administration may result in increased tricyclic antidepressants' plasma concentrations; dose decrease of tricyclics may be needed. Use with caution).
No products indexed under this heading.

Amoxapine (Co-administration may result in increased tricyclic antidepressants' plasma concentrations; dose decrease of tricyclics may be needed. Use with caution).
No products indexed under this heading.

Aprepitant (Potential for increase in the clearance of ritonavir resulting in decreased ritonavir plasma concentrations). Products include:
Emend Capsules 1963

Astemizole (Co-administration is contraindicated due to potential for serious and/or life-threatening reactions, such as cardiac arrhythmias).
No products indexed under this heading.

Atenolol (Co-administration with beta-blockers has resulted in cardiac and neurologic events).
No products indexed under this heading.

Atorvastatin Calcium (Co-administration may result in increased plasma concentrations of atorvastatin calcium; the risk of myopathy, including rhabdomyolysis, may be increased. Dosage adjustment may be needed. Use with caution). Products include:
Caduet Tablets 2508
Lipitor Tablets 2483

Atovaquone (Co-administration may result in decreased atovaquone plasma concentrations; dose increase of atovaquone may be needed. Use with caution). Products include:
Malarone Pediatric Tablets 1517
Malarone Tablets 1517
Mepron Suspension 1521

Bepridil Hydrochloride (Co-administration is contraindicated due to potential for serious and/or life-threatening reactions, such as cardiac arrhythmias).
No products indexed under this heading.

Betaxolol Hydrochloride (Co-administration results in a possible increase in AUC of betaxolol; dosage adjustments may be required). Products include:
Betoptic S Ophthalmic Suspension 558

Bisoprolol Fumarate (Co-administration with beta-blockers has resulted in cardiac and neurologic events).
No products indexed under this heading.

Bromocriptine Mesylate (Co-administration results in a large increase (> 3x) in AUC of bromocriptine; dosage adjustments may be required).
No products indexed under this heading.

Bupropion Hydrochloride (Co-administration may result in increased bupropion plasma concentrations; dose decrease of bupropion may be needed. Use with caution). Products include:
Wellbutrin Tablets 1603
Wellbutrin SR Sustained-Release Tablets 1607
Wellbutrin XL Extended-Release Tablets 1613
Zyban Sustained-Release Tablets 1644

Carbamazepine (Co-administration may result in increased carbamazepine plasma concentrations; dose decrease of carbamazepine may be needed. Use with caution). Products include:
Carbatrol Capsules 3171

Equetro Extended-Release Capsules 3180
Tegretol/Tegretol-XR 2295

Carteolol Hydrochloride (Co-administration with beta-blockers has resulted in cardiac and neurologic events). Products include:
Carteolol Hydrochloride Ophthalmic Solution USP, 1% ..... ⊙ 249

Chloroquine Hydrochloride (Co-administration results in a possible increase in AUC of chloroquine; dosage adjustments may be required).
No products indexed under this heading.

Chloroquine Phosphate (Co-administration results in a possible increase in AUC of chloroquine; dosage adjustments may be required).
No products indexed under this heading.

Chlorpromazine (Co-administration results in a moderate increase (1.5 to 3x) in AUC of chlorpromazine; dosage adjustments may be required).
No products indexed under this heading.

Chlorpromazine Hydrochloride (Co-administration results in a moderate increase (1.5 to 3x) in AUC of chlorpromazine; dosage adjustments may be required).
No products indexed under this heading.

Chlorpropamide (New onset diabetes mellitus, exacerbation of pre-existing diabetes, and hyperglycemia have been reported with protease inhibitors; dosage adjustment of oral hypoglycemic agents may be required).
No products indexed under this heading.

Cisapride (Co-administration is contraindicated due to potential for serious and/or life-threatening reactions, such as cardiac arrhythmias).
No products indexed under this heading.

Citalopram Hydrobromide (Co-administration may result in increased selective serotonin reuptake inhibitors' plasma concentrations; dose decrease of SSRIs may be needed. Use with caution). Products include:
Celexa 1176

Clarithromycin (Co-administration may result in increased clarithromycin concentration; for patients with renal impairment, dosage adjustments should be considered). Products include:
Biaxin/Biaxin XL 402
PREVPAC 3284

Clofibrate (Ritonavir may increase the activity of glucuronosyltransferase; co-administration results in a decrease in AUC of clofibrate; dosage adjustments may be required).
No products indexed under this heading.

Clomipramine Hydrochloride (Co-administration may result in increased tricyclic antidepressants' plasma concentrations; dose decrease of tricyclics may be needed. Use with caution).
No products indexed under this heading.

Clonazepam (Co-administration may result in increased clonazepam plasma concentrations; dose decrease of clonazepam may be needed. Use with caution). Products include:
Klonopin 2778

Clorazepate Dipotassium (Co-administration may result in increased clorazepate plasma concentrations; dose decrease of clorazepate may be needed. Use with caution). Products include:
Tranxene 2474

Clozapine (Ritonavir is expected to produce a large increase in the plasma clozapine concentrations; clozapine has recognized risk to induce hematologic abnormalities; co-administration is contraindicated). Products include:
Clozaril Tablets 2184
FazaClo Orally Disintegrating Tablets 551

Codeine Phosphate (Ritonavir may increase the activity of glucuronosyltransferase; co-administration results in possible decrease in AUC of codeine; possible need for dosage alterations of codeine). Products include:
Tylenol with Codeine Tablets 2391

Cyclophosphamide (An increase in the AUC of cyclophosphamide, activated by CYP, may correspond to a decrease in the AUC of the active metabolite(s) and a possible decrease in efficacy of cyclophosphamide).
No products indexed under this heading.

Cyclosporine (Co-administration may result in increased cyclosporine plasma concentrations; dose decrease of cyclosporine may be needed. Use with caution). Products include:
Gengraf Capsules 459
Neoral Oral Solution 2259
Neoral Soft Gelatin Capsules 2259
Restasis Ophthalmic Emulsion 575
Sandimmune 2275

Daunorubicin Hydrochloride (Co-administration results in a possible increase in AUC of daunorubicin; dosage adjustments may be required).
No products indexed under this heading.

Desipramine Hydrochloride (Co-administration may lead to increased desipramine levels. Dosage reduction and concentration monitoring of desipramine is recommended).
No products indexed under this heading.

Dexamethasone (Co-administration may result in increased dexamethasone plasma concentrations; dose decrease of dexamethasone may be needed. Use with caution). Products include:
Ciprodex Otic Suspension 559
Decadron Tablets 1951
TobraDex Ophthalmic Ointment 562
TobraDex Ophthalmic Suspension 563

Dexamethasone Acetate (Co-administration may result in increased dexamethasone plasma concentrations; dose decrease of dexamethasone may be needed. Use with caution).
No products indexed under this heading.

Dexamethasone Sodium Phosphate (Co-administration may result in increased dexamethasone plasma concentrations; dose decrease of dexamethasone may be needed. Use with caution).
No products indexed under this heading.

Dexfenfluramine Hydrochloride (Co-administration may lead to increased desipramine levels. Dosage reduction and concentration monitoring of desipramine is recommended).
No products indexed under this heading.

Diazepam (Co-administration may result in increased diazepam plasma concentrations; dose decrease of diazepam may be needed. Use with caution). Products include:
Diastat Rectal Delivery System 3343
Valium Tablets 2819

Diclofenac Potassium (Co-administration results in a moderate (1.5 to 3x) increase or decrease in AUC of diclofenac).
No products indexed under this heading.

Diclofenac Sodium (Co-administration results in a moderate (1.5 to 3x) increase or decrease in AUC of diclofenac). Products include:
Arthrotec Tablets 3129
Voltaren Ophthalmic Solution 2309
Voltaren Tablets 2307
Voltaren-XR Tablets 2310

Didanosine (Dosing of these two drugs should be separated by 2.5 hours to avoid formulation incompatability).
No products indexed under this heading.

Dihydroergotamine Mesylate (Co-administration is contraindicated due to potential for serious and/or life-threatening reactions, such as acute ergot toxicity characterized by vasospasm and ischemia of the extremities and other tissues including the CNS). Products include:
Migranal Nasal Spray 3348

Diltiazem Hydrochloride (Co-administration may result in increased diltiazem plasma concentrations; dose decrease of diltiazem may be needed. Use with caution). Products include:
Cardizem LA Extended Release Tablets 1728
Tiazac Capsules 1201

Diphenoxylate Hydrochloride (Ritonavir may increase the activity of glucuronosyltransferase; co-administration results in a decrease in AUC of diphenoxylate; dosage adjustments may be required).
No products indexed under this heading.

Disopyramide Phosphate (Co-administration may result in increased disopyramide plasma concentrations; cardiac and neurologic events have been reported with co-administration. Dosage adjustment may be needed. Use with caution).
No products indexed under this heading.

Disulfiram (Potential for disulfiram-like reactions due to the presence of ethanol in the ritonavir formulations).
No products indexed under this heading.

Divalproex Sodium (Co-administration may result in decreased valproate plasma concentrations; dose increase of valproate may be needed. Use with caution). Products include:
Depakote Sprinkle Capsules 422
Depakote Tablets 427
Depakote ER Tablets 434

Doxazosin Mesylate (Co-administration results in a possible increase in AUC of doxazosin; dosage adjustments may be required). Products include:
Cardura XL Tablets 2515

Doxepin Hydrochloride (Co-administration results in a possible increase in the AUC of doxepin; dosage adjustment of doxepin may be required).
No products indexed under this heading.

Doxorubicin Hydrochloride (Co-administration results in a possible increase in AUC of doxorubicin; dosage adjustments may be required).
No products indexed under this heading.

Dronabinol (Co-administration may result in increased dronabinol plasma concentrations; dose decrease of dronabinol may be needed. Use with caution). Products include:
Marinol Capsules 3333

Dyphylline (Co-administration results in the reduction of the average AUC of theophylline; increased dosage of theophylline may be required and therapeutic monitoring should be considered).
No products indexed under this heading.

Efavirenz (Potential for increase in the clearance of ritonavir resulting in decreased ritonavir plasma concentrations). Products include:
Atripla Tablets 945
Sustiva Capsules 930
Sustiva Tablets 930

Encainide Hydrochloride (Ritonavir is expected to produce a large increase in the plasma concentrations of encainide; concurrent use is contraindicated).
No products indexed under this heading.

Ergonovine Maleate (Co-administration may result in a possible increase in concentrations of ergonovine; in general, concurrent use with ergot alkaloid preparations is contraindicated).
No products indexed under this heading.

Ergotamine Tartrate (Co-administration is contraindicated due to potential for serious and/or life-threatening reactions, such as acute ergot toxicity characterized by vasospasm and ischemia of the extremities and other tissues including the CNS).
No products indexed under this heading.

Erythromycin (Co-administration results in a large increase (> 3x) in AUC of erythromycin; dosage adjustments may be required). Products include:
Ery-Tab Tablets 449
Erythromycin Base Filmtab Tablets 455
Erythromycin Delayed-Release Capsules, USP 457
PCE Dispertab Tablets 515

Erythromycin Estolate (Co-administration results in a large increase (> 3x) in AUC of erythromycin; dosage adjustments may be required).
No products indexed under this heading.

Erythromycin Ethylsuccinate (Co-administration results in a large increase (> 3x) in AUC of erythromycin; dosage adjustments may be required). Products include:
E.E.S. 451

IMPORTANT NOTE: Always consult each drug listing in the patient's regimen for possible interactions.

EryPed 447

Erythromycin Gluceptate (Co-administration results in a large increase (> 3x) in AUC of erythromycin; dosage adjustments may be required).
No products indexed under this heading.

Erythromycin Lactobionate (Co-administration results in a large increase (> 3x) in AUC of erythromycin; dosage adjustments may be required).
No products indexed under this heading.

Erythromycin Stearate (Co-administration results in a large increase (> 3x) in AUC of erythromycin; dosage adjustments may be required). Products include:
Erythrocin Stearate Filmtab Tablets 453

Escitalopram Oxalate (Co-administration may result in increased selective serotonin reuptake inhibitors' plasma concentrations; dose decrease of SSRIs may be needed. Use with caution). Products include:
Lexapro Oral Solution 1190
Lexapro Tablets 1190

Esmolol Hydrochloride (Co-administration with beta-blockers has resulted in cardiac and neurologic events).
No products indexed under this heading.

Estazolam (Co-administration may result in increased estazolam plasma concentrations; dose decrease of estazolam may be needed. Use with caution). Products include:
ProSom Tablets 517

Ethinyl Estradiol (Co-administration may result in the reduction of ethinyl estradiol levels; dosage increase or alternate contraceptive measures should be considered). Products include:
Mircette Tablets 1066
NuvaRing 2340
Ortho-Cyclen/Ortho Tri-Cyclen 2429
Ortho Evra Transdermal System 2417
Ortho Tri-Cyclen Lo Tablets 2436
Seasonique Tablets 1077
Yasmin 28 Tablets 796
Yaz Tablets 803

Ethosuximide (Co-administration may result in increased ethosuximide plasma concentrations; dose decrease of ethosuximide may be needed. Use with caution).
No products indexed under this heading.

Etoposide (Co-administration results in a large increase (> 3x) in AUC of etoposide; dosage adjustments may be required).
No products indexed under this heading.

Fentanyl (Co-administration results in a large increase (> 3x) in AUC of fentanyl; dosage adjustments may be required). Products include:
Duragesic Transdermal System 2373
Ionsys Transdermal System 2379

Fentanyl Citrate (Co-administration results in a large increase (> 3x) in AUC of fentanyl; dosage adjustments may be required). Products include:
Actiq 979

Flecainide Acetate (Co-administration is contraindicated due to potential for serious and/or life-threatening reactions, such as cardiac arrhythmias). Products include:
Tambocor Tablets 1856

Fluconazole (Co-administration has resulted in an increase in AUC and Cmax of ritonavir by 12% and 15%, respectively).
No products indexed under this heading.

Fluoxetine Hydrochloride (Cardiac and neurologic events have been reported when ritonavir has been co-administered with fluoxetine, Co-administration may result in increased selective serotonin reuptake inhibitors' plasma concentrations; dose decrease of SSRIs may be needed. Use with caution). Products include:
Prozac Pulvules and Liquid 1801
Symbyax Capsules 1819

Flurazepam Hydrochloride (Co-administration may result in increased flurazepam plasma concentrations; dose decrease of flurazepam may be needed. Use with caution). Products include:
Dalmane Capsules 3342

Flurbiprofen (Co-administration results in a moderate (1.5 to 3x) increase or decrease in AUC of flurbiprofen).
No products indexed under this heading.

Fluticasone Propionate (Co-administration increases plasma fluticasone proprionate exposures, resulting in significantly decreased serum cortisol concentrations and leading to systemic corticosteroid effects, including Cushing's syndrome and adrenal suppression). Products include:
Advair Diskus 100/50 1308
Advair Diskus 250/50 1308
Advair Diskus 500/50 1308
Advair HFA Inhalation Aerosol 1318
Cutivate Cream 2662
Cutivate Lotion 0.05% 2664
Cutivate Ointment 2665
Flonase Nasal Spray 1440
Flovent Diskus 1443

Fluvastatin Sodium (Co-administration results in a possible increase in AUC of fluvastatin; dosage adjustments may be required). Products include:
Lescol Capsules 2233
Lescol XL Tablets 2233

Fluvoxamine Maleate (Co-administration may result in increased selective serotonin reuptake inhibitors' plasma concentrations; dose decrease of SSRIs may be needed. Use with caution).
No products indexed under this heading.

Fosphenytoin Sodium (Co-administration results in a moderate increase or decrease in AUC of phenytoin; dosage adjustments may be required; potential for increase in the clearance of ritonavir resulting in decreased ritonavir plasma concentrations).
No products indexed under this heading.

Gemfibrozil (Co-administration results in a possible increase in AUC of gemfibrozil; dosage adjustments may be required).
No products indexed under this heading.

Glimepiride (Co-administration results in a moderate increase or decrease in AUC of glimepiride; dosage adjustments may be required). Products include:
Avandaryl Tablets 1379
Duetact Tablets 3226

Glipizide (Co-administration results in a moderate increase or decrease in AUC of glipizide; dosage adjustments may be required).
No products indexed under this heading.

Glyburide (Co-administration results in a moderate increase or decrease in AUC of glyburide; dosage adjustments may be required).
No products indexed under this heading.

Haloperidol (Co-administration results in a moderate increase (1.5 to 3x) in AUC of haloperidol; dosage adjustments may be required).
No products indexed under this heading.

Haloperidol Decanoate (Co-administration results in a moderate increase (1.5 to 3x) in AUC of haloperidol; dosage adjustments may be required).
No products indexed under this heading.

Hydrocodone Bitartrate (Co-administration results in a moderate increase (1.5 to 3x) in AUC of hydrocodone; dosage adjustments may be required). Products include:
Hycodan 1116
Hycotuss Expectorant Syrup 1117
Vicodin Tablets 535
Vicodin ES Tablets 536
Vicodin HP Tablets 538
Vicoprofen Tablets 539
Zydone Tablets 1139

Hydromorphone Hydrochloride (Ritonavir may increase the activity of glucuronosyltransferase; co-administration results in possible decrease in AUC of hydromorphone; possible need for dosage alterations of hydromorphone). Products include:
Dilaudid 440
Dilaudid Non-Sterile Powder 440
Dilaudid Oral Liquid 445
Dilaudid Rectal Suppositories 440
Dilaudid Tablets 440
Dilaudid Tablets - 8 mg 445
Dilaudid-HP 442

Hypericum (May lead to loss of virologic response and possible resistance to ritonavir or to the class of protease inhibitors). Products include:
Satiete Tablets .... ■832

Ibuprofen (Co-administration results in a moderate (1.5 to 3x) increase or decrease in AUC of ibuprofen). Products include:
Advil Allergy Sinus Caplets .... ■770
Advil .... ■674
Children's Advil Oral Suspension .... ■603
Children's Advil Chewable Tablets .... ■603
Advil Cold & Sinus .... ■723
Infants' Advil Concentrated Drops .... ■604
Infants' Advil Concentrated Drops - White Grape (Dye-Free) .... ■604
Junior Strength Advil Swallow Tablets .... ■605
Advil Migraine Liquigels .... ■608
Advil Multi-Symptom Cold Caplets .... ■770
Advil PM Caplets .... ■615
Motrin IB Tablets and Caplets 1866
Children's Motrin Oral Suspension 1867
Children's Motrin Non-Staining Dye-Free Oral Suspension 1867
Children's Motrin Cold Oral Suspension 1867
Infants' Motrin Concentrated Drops 1867
Infants' Motrin Non-Staining Dye-Free Concentrated Drops 1867
Junior Strength Motrin Caplets and Chewable Tablets 1867
Vicoprofen Tablets 539

Ifosfamide (An increase in the AUC of ifosfamide, activated by CYP, may correspond to a decrease in the AUC of the active metabolite(s) and a possible decrease in efficacy of ifosfamide).
No products indexed under this heading.

Imipramine Hydrochloride (Co-administration may result in increased tricyclic antidepressants' plasma concentrations; dose decrease of tricyclics may be needed. Use with caution).
No products indexed under this heading.

Imipramine Pamoate (Co-administration may result in increased tricyclic antidepressants' plasma concentrations; dose decrease of tricyclics may be needed. Use with caution).
No products indexed under this heading.

Indinavir Sulfate (When co-administered with reduced doses of indinavir, ritonavir increased indinavir concentration, decreased Cmax, and increased Cmin; appropriate doses for this combination with respect to efficacy and safety have not been established). Products include:
Crixivan Capsules 1940

Indomethacin (Co-administration results in a moderate (1.5 to 3x) increase or decrease in AUC of indomethacin). Products include:
Indocin 1995

Insulin, Human, Zinc Suspension (New onset diabetes mellitus, exacerbation of pre-existing diabetes, and hyperglycemia have been reported with protease inhibitors; dosage adjustment of insulin may be required). Products include:
Humulin L, 100 Units 1794
Humulin U, 100 Units 1800

Insulin, Human NPH (New onset diabetes mellitus, exacerbation of pre-existing diabetes, and hyperglycemia have been reported with protease inhibitors; dosage adjustment of insulin may be required). Products include:
Humulin N, 100 Units 1795
Humulin N Pen 1797

Insulin, Human Regular (New onset diabetes mellitus, exacerbation of pre-existing diabetes, and hyperglycemia have been reported with protease inhibitors; dosage adjustment of insulin may be required). Products include:
Humulin R, 100 Units 1798

Insulin, Human Regular and Human NPH Mixture (New onset diabetes mellitus, exacerbation of pre-existing diabetes, and hyperglycemia have been reported with protease inhibitors; dosage adjustment of insulin may be required). Products include:
Humulin 50/50, 100 Units 1791
Humulin 70/30 Pen 1793

Insulin, NPH (New onset diabetes mellitus, exacerbation of pre-existing diabetes, and hyperglycemia have been reported with protease inhibitors; dosage adjustment of insulin may be required).
No products indexed under this heading.

Insulin, Regular (New onset diabetes mellitus, exacerbation of pre-existing diabetes, and hyperglycemia have been reported with protease inhibitors; dosage adjustment of insulin may be required).
No products indexed under this heading.

Insulin, Zinc Crystals (New onset diabetes mellitus, exacerbation of pre-existing diabetes, and hyperglycemia have been reported with protease inhibitors; dosage adjustment of insulin may be required).
No products indexed under this heading.

Insulin, Zinc Suspension (New onset diabetes mellitus, exacerbation of pre-existing diabetes, and hyperglycemia have been reported with protease inhibitors; dosage adjustment of insulin may be required).
No products indexed under this heading.

Insulin Aspart, Human Regular (New onset diabetes mellitus, exacerbation of pre-existing diabetes, and hyperglycemia have been reported with protease inhibitors; dosage adjustment of insulin may be required). Products include:
NovoLog Injection 2326

Insulin glargine (New onset diabetes mellitus, exacerbation of pre-existing diabetes, and hyperglycemia have been reported with protease inhibitors; dosage adjustment of insulin may be required). Products include:
Lantus Injection 2909

Insulin Lispro, Human (New onset diabetes mellitus, exacerbation of pre-existing diabetes, and hyperglycemia have been reported with protease inhibitors; dosage adjustment of insulin may be required). Products include:
Humalog-Pen 1781
Humalog Mix 50/50-Pen 1783
Humalog Mix 75/25-Pen 1785

Insulin Lispro Protamine, Human (New onset diabetes mellitus, exacerbation of pre-existing diabetes, and hyperglycemia have been reported with protease inhibitors; dosage adjustment of insulin may be required). Products include:
Humalog Mix 50/50-Pen 1783
Humalog Mix 75/25-Pen 1785

Itraconazole (Co-administration may result in a possible increase in plasma concentrations of itraconazole; dosage adjustment may be required. Use with caution).
No products indexed under this heading.

Ketoconazole (Co-administration may result in increased ketoconazole concentration; high doses of ketoconazole (>200 mg/day) are not recommended). Products include:
Nizoral A-D Shampoo, 1% 1868

Ketoprofen (Ritonavir may increase the activity of glucuronosyltransferase; co-administration results in possible decrease in AUC of ketoprofen; possible need for dosage alterations of ketoprofen).
No products indexed under this heading.

Ketorolac Tromethamine (Ritonavir may increase the activity of glucuronosyltransferase; co-administration results in possible decrease in AUC of ketorolac; possible need for dosage alterations of ketorolac). Products include:
Acular Ophthalmic Solution 565
Acular LS Ophthalmic Solution 566

Labetalol Hydrochloride (Co-administration with beta-blockers has resulted in cardiac and neurologic events).
No products indexed under this heading.

Lamotrigine (Co-administration may result in decreased lamotrigine plasma concentrations; dose increase of lamotrigine may be needed. Use with caution). Products include:
Lamictal 1481

Lansoprazole (Co-administration results in a moderate increase or decrease in AUC of lansoprazole; dosage adjustments may be required). Products include:
Prevacid Delayed-Release Capsules 3271
Prevacid for Delayed-Release Oral Suspension 3271
Prevacid SoluTab Delayed-Release Orally Disintegrating Tablets 3271
Prevacid I.V. for Injection 3277
Prevacid NapraPAC 3280
PREVPAC 3284

Levobunolol Hydrochloride (Co-administration with beta-blockers has resulted in cardiac and neurologic events). Products include:
Betagan Ophthalmic Solution, USP .... ⊙220

Lidocaine Hydrochloride (Co-administration may result in an increase in plasma concentrations of lidocaine; dosage adjustments may be required. Use with caution).
No products indexed under this heading.

Loperamide Hydrochloride (Co-administration results in a decrease in AUC of loperamide). Products include:
Imodium A-D Liquid and Caplets 1865
Imodium Advanced Caplets and Chewable Tablets 1866

Loratadine (Ritonavir is expected to produce a large increase (> 3x) in the plasma concentrations of loratadine; dosage adjustments may be required). Products include:
Alavert Allergy & Sinus D-12 Hour Tablets .... ▣771
Alavert .... ▣771
Children's Claritin Allergy Oral Solution .... ▣771
Claritin Non-Drowsy 24 Hour Tablets .... ▣772
Claritin Reditabs 24 Hour Non-Drowsy Tablets .... ▣772
Claritin-D Non-Drowsy 12 Hour Tablets .... ▣772
Claritin-D Non-Drowsy 24 Hour Tablets .... ▣772

Lorazepam (Ritonavir may increase the activity of glucuronosyltransferase; co-administration results in a decrease in AUC of lorazepam; dosage adjustments may be required).
No products indexed under this heading.

Losartan Potassium (Co-administration results in a moderate increase or decrease in AUC of losartan; dosage adjustments may be required). Products include:
Cozaar Tablets 1935
Hyzaar 50-12.5 Tablets 1990
Hyzaar 100-12.5 Tablets 1990
Hyzaar 100-25 Tablets 1990

Lovastatin (Co-administration results in increased plasma concentrations of lovastatin; the risk of myopathy, including rhabdomyolysis, may be increased). Products include:
Advicor Tablets 1722
Altoprev Extended-Release Tablets 3109
Mevacor Tablets 2021

Maprotiline Hydrochloride (Co-administration may result in increased tricyclic antidepressants' plasma concentrations; dose decrease of tricyclics may be needed. Use with caution).
No products indexed under this heading.

Meperidine Hydrochloride (Co-administration results in decreased meperidine concentration and increased normeperidine concentration; dosage increase and long-term use of meperidine with ritonavir are not recommended due to the increased concentrations of the metabolite normeperidine which has both analgesic activity and CNS stimulant activity, such as seizures).
No products indexed under this heading.

Metformin Hydrochloride (New onset diabetes mellitus, exacerbation of pre-existing diabetes, and hyperglycemia have been reported with protease inhibitors; dosage adjustment of oral hypoglycemic agents may be required). Products include:
ActoPlus Met Tablets 3214
Avandamet Tablets 1373
Fortamet Extended-Release Tablets 3115

Methadone Hydrochloride (Co-administration may result may result in decreased methadone concentration; dosage increase of methadone may be considered).
No products indexed under this heading.

Methamphetamine Hydrochloride (Co-administration may result in increased methamphetamine plasma concentrations; dose decrease of methamphetamine may be needed. Use with caution). Products include:
Desoxyn Tablets, USP 2462

Methylergonovine Maleate (Co-administration is contraindicated due to potential for serious and/or life-threatening reactions, such as acute ergot toxicity characterized by vasospasm and ischemia of the extremities and other tissues including the CNS).
No products indexed under this heading.

Methylphenidate Hydrochloride (Co-administration results in a possible increase in AUC of methylphenidate; dosage adjustments may be required). Products include:
Concerta Extended-Release Tablets 1881
Metadate CD Capsules 3323
Ritalin Hydrochloride Tablets 2269
Ritalin LA Capsules 2271
Ritalin-SR Tablets 2269

Methysergide Maleate (Co-administration is contraindicated due to potential for serious and/or life-threatening reactions, such as acute ergot toxicity characterized by vasospasm and ischemia of the extremities and other tissues including the CNS).
No products indexed under this heading.

Metipranolol Hydrochloride (Co-administration with beta-blockers has resulted in cardiac and neurologic events).
No products indexed under this heading.

Metoclopramide Hydrochloride (Ritonavir may increase the activity of glucuronosyltransferase; co-administration results in a decrease in AUC of metoclopramide; dosage adjustments may be required).
No products indexed under this heading.

Metoprolol Succinate (Co-administration may result in increased metoprolol plasma concentrations; cardiac and neurologic events have been reported with co-administration. Dosage adjustment may be needed. Use with caution). Products include:
Toprol-XL Tablets 668

Metoprolol Tartrate (Co-administration may result in increased metoprolol plasma concentrations; cardiac and neurologic events have been reported with co-administration. Dosage adjustment may be needed. Use with caution). Products include:
Lopressor Injection 2238
Lopressor Tablets 2238
Lopressor HCT 50/25 Tablets 2241
Lopressor HCT 100/25 Tablets 2241
Lopressor HCT 100/50 Tablets 2241

Metronidazole (Potential for disulfiram-like reactions due to the presence of ethanol in the ritonavir formulations). Products include:
Metrogel 1% 1211
MetroGel-Vaginal Gel 1855
Vandazole Vaginal Gel 3338

Metronidazole Hydrochloride (Potential for disulfiram-like reactions due to the presence of ethanol in the ritonavir formulations).
No products indexed under this heading.

Mexiletine Hydrochloride (Co-administration may result in increased mexiletine plasma concentrations; cardiac and neurologic events have been reported with co-administration. Dosage adjustment may be needed. Use with caution).
No products indexed under this heading.

Miconazole (Co-administration results in a possible increase in AUC of miconazole; dosage adjustments may be required).
No products indexed under this heading.

Miconazole Nitrate (Co-administration results in a possible increase in AUC of miconazole; dosage adjustments may be required). Products include:
Desenex .... ▣635
Desenex Jock Itch Spray Powder .... ▣635

Midazolam Hydrochloride (Co-administration is contraindicated due to potential for prolonged or increased sedation and/or respiratory depression).
No products indexed under this heading.

Miglitol (New onset diabetes mellitus, exacerbation of pre-existing diabetes, and hyperglycemia have been reported with protease inhibitors; dosage adjustment of oral hypoglycemic agents may be required).
No products indexed under this heading.

Modafinil (Potential for increase in the clearance of ritonavir resulting in decreased ritonavir plasma concentrations). Products include:
Provigil Tablets 988

Morphine Sulfate (Ritonavir may increase the activity of glucuronosyltransferase; co-administration results in possible decrease in AUC of morphine; possible need for dosage alterations of morphine). Products include:
Avinza Capsules 1741
Kadian Capsules 577
MS Contin Tablets 2701

Nadolol (Co-administration with beta-blockers has resulted in cardiac and neurologic events). Products include:
Nadolol Tablets 2159

Naproxen (Ritonavir may increase the activity of glucuronosyltransferase; co-administration results in possible decrease in AUC of naproxen; possible need for dosage alterations of naproxen). Products include:
EC-Naprosyn Delayed-Release
Tablets ... 2761
Naprosyn Suspension 2761
Naprosyn Tablets 2761
Prevacid NapraPAC 3280

Naproxen Sodium (Ritonavir may increase the activity of glucuronosyltransferase; co-administration results in possible decrease in AUC of naproxen; possible need for dosage alterations of naproxen). Products include:
Aleve Caplets 742
Aleve Gelcaps 743
Aleve Tablets 743
Aleve Cold & Sinus Caplets 744
Anaprox Tablets 2761
Anaprox DS Tablets 2761

Nefazodone Hydrochloride (Co-administration may result in increased nefazodone plasma concentrations; cardiac and neurologic events have been reported with co-administration. Dosage adjustment may be needed. Use with caution).
No products indexed under this heading.

Nevirapine (Co-administration may result in a possible increase in concentrations of nevirapine). Products include:
Viramune Oral Suspension 873
Viramune Tablets 873

Nifedipine (Co-administration may result in increased nifedipine plasma concentrations; dose decrease of nifedipine may be needed. Use with caution). Products include:
Adalat CC Tablets 2964

Nitrendipine (Co-administration results in a large increase (> 3x) in AUC of nitrendipine; dosage adjustments may be required).
No products indexed under this heading.

Nortriptyline Hydrochloride (Co-administration may result in increased tricyclic antidepressants' plasma concentrations; dose decrease of tricyclics may be needed. Use with caution).
No products indexed under this heading.

Omeprazole (Co-administration results in a moderate increase or decrease in AUC of omeprazole; dosage adjustments may be required). Products include:
Zegerid Capsules 2958
Zegerid Powder for Oral Solution 2958

Ondansetron Hydrochloride (Co-administration results in a large increase (> 3x) in AUC of ondansetron; dosage adjustments may be required). Products include:
Zofran Injection 1634
Zofran .. 1639

Oxazepam (Ritonavir may increase the activity of glucuronosyltransferase; co-administration results in a decrease in AUC of oxazepam; dosage adjustments may be required).
No products indexed under this heading.

Oxycodone Hydrochloride (Co-administration results in a moderate increase (1.5 to 3x) in AUC of oxycodone; dosage adjustments may be required). Products include:
OxyContin Tablets 2703
OxyFast Oral Concentrate
Solution .. 2708
OxyIR Capsules 2708
Percocet Tablets 1131
Percodan Tablets 1132

Paclitaxel (Co-administration results in a large increase (> 3x) in AUC of paclitaxel; dosage adjustments may be required).
No products indexed under this heading.

Paroxetine Hydrochloride (Co-administration results in a moderate increase (1.5 to 3x) in AUC of paroxetine; dosage adjustments may be required). Products include:
Paxil CR Controlled-Release
Tablets ... 1538
Paxil .. 1530

Penbutolol Sulfate (Co-administration results in a possible increase in AUC of penbutolol; dosage adjustments may be required).
No products indexed under this heading.

Pentoxifylline (Co-administration results in a possible increase in AUC of pentoxifylline; dosage adjustments may be required).
No products indexed under this heading.

Perphenazine (Co-administration may result in increased perphenazine plasma concentrations; dose decrease of perphenazine may be needed).
No products indexed under this heading.

Phenobarbital (Co-administration results in a possible increase in AUC of phenobarbital; dosage adjustments may be required; potential for increase in the clearance of ritonavir resulting in decreased ritonavir plasma concentrations). Products include:
Donnatal Extentabs 2493

Phenytoin (Co-administration may result in decreased phenytoin plasma concentrations; dose increase of phenytoin may be needed. Use with caution).
No products indexed under this heading.

Phenytoin Sodium (Co-administration may result in decreased phenytoin plasma concentrations; dose increase of phenytoin may be needed. Use with caution). Products include:
Phenytek Capsules 2160

Pimozide (Co-administration is contraindicated due to potential for serious and/or life-threatening reactions, such as cardiac arrhythmias).
No products indexed under this heading.

Pindolol (Co-administration results in a possible increase in AUC of pindolol; dosage adjustments may be required).
No products indexed under this heading.

Pioglitazone Hydrochloride (New onset diabetes mellitus, exacerbation of pre-existing diabetes, and hyperglycemia have been reported with protease inhibitors; dosage adjustment of oral hypoglycemic agents may be required). Products include:
ActoPlus Met Tablets 3214
Actos Tablets 3219
Duetact Tablets 3226

Piroxicam (Ritonavir is expected to produce a large increase in the plasma concentrations of piroxicam; concurrent use is contraindicated).
No products indexed under this heading.

Pravastatin Sodium (Co-administration results in a large increase (> 3x) in AUC of pravastatin; dosage adjustments may be required).
No products indexed under this heading.

Prazosin Hydrochloride (Co-administration results in a possible increase in AUC of prazosin; dosage adjustments may be required).
No products indexed under this heading.

Prednisone (Co-administration may result in increased prednisone plasma concentrations; dose decrease of prednisone may be needed. Use with caution).
No products indexed under this heading.

Primaquine Phosphate (Co-administration results in a possible increase in AUC of primaquine; dosage adjustments may be required).
No products indexed under this heading.

Prochlorperazine (Co-administration results in a possible increase in AUC of prochlorperazine; dosage adjustments may be required).
No products indexed under this heading.

Proguanil (Co-administration results in a moderate increase or decrease in AUC of proguanil; dosage adjustments may be required).
No products indexed under this heading.

Promethazine Hydrochloride (Co-administration results in a possible increase in AUC of promethazine; dosage adjustments may be required). Products include:
Phenergan Tablets and
Suppositories 3440

Propafenone Hydrochloride (Co-administration is contraindicated due to potential for serious and/or life-threatening reactions, such as cardiac arrhythmias). Products include:
Rythmol SR Capsules 2727

Propofol (Ritonavir may increase the activity of glucuronosyltransferase; co-administration results in a decrease in AUC of propofol; dosage adjustments may be required).
No products indexed under this heading.

Propoxyphene Hydrochloride (Ritonavir may produce an increase in the plasma concentrations of propoxyphene. Dosage adjustment may be needed. Use with caution).
No products indexed under this heading.

Propoxyphene Napsylate (Ritonavir may produce an increase in the plasma concentrations of propoxyphene. Dosage adjustment may be needed. Use with caution).
No products indexed under this heading.

Propranolol Hydrochloride (Co-administration results in a moderate increase (1.5 to 3x) in AUC of propranolol; dosage adjustments may be required). Products include:
Inderal LA Long-Acting Capsules 3429
InnoPran XL Capsules 2723

Protriptyline Hydrochloride (Co-administration may result in increased tricyclic antidepressants' plasma concentrations; dose decrease of tricyclics may be needed. Use with caution).
No products indexed under this heading.

Pyrimethamine (Co-administration results in a possible increase in AUC of pyrimethamine; dosage adjustments may be required). Products include:
Daraprim Tablets 1419
Fansidar Tablets 2765

Quinidine (Co-administration is contraindicated due to potential for serious and/or life-threatening reactions, such as cardiac arrhythmias).
No products indexed under this heading.

Quinidine Gluconate (Co-administration is contraindicated due to potential for serious and/or life-threatening reactions, such as cardiac arrhythmias).
No products indexed under this heading.

Quinidine Hydrochloride (Co-administration is contraindicated due to potential for serious and/or life-threatening reactions, such as cardiac arrhythmias).
No products indexed under this heading.

Quinidine Polygalacturonate (Co-administration is contraindicated due to potential for serious and/or life-threatening reactions, such as cardiac arrhythmias).
No products indexed under this heading.

Quinidine Sulfate (Co-administration is contraindicated due to potential for serious and/or life-threatening reactions, such as cardiac arrhythmias).
No products indexed under this heading.

Quinine Sulfate (Co-administration may result in increased quinine plasma concentrations; dose decrease of quinine may be needed. Use with caution).
No products indexed under this heading.

Repaglinide (New onset diabetes mellitus, exacerbation of pre-existing diabetes, and hyperglycemia have been reported with protease inhibitors; dosage adjustment of oral hypoglycemic agents may be required).
No products indexed under this heading.

Rifabutin (Co-administration results in increased rifabutin and rifabutin metabolite concentration; dosage reduction of rifabutin by at least three-quarters of the usual dose of 300 mg/day is recommended).
No products indexed under this heading.

Rifampicin (Potential for increase in the clearance of ritonavir resulting in decreased ritonavir plasma concentrations).
No products indexed under this heading.

Rifampin (Co-administration has resulted in decreased ritonavir concentration leading to loss of virologic response. Consider alternate anti-myobacterial agents).
No products indexed under this heading.

Rifapentine (Potential for increase in the clearance of ritonavir resulting in decreased ritonavir plasma concentrations).
No products indexed under this heading.

Risperidone (Co-administration may result in increased risperidone plasma concentrations; dose decrease of risperidone may be needed. Use with caution). Products include:
Risperdal 1676
Risperdal Consta Long-Acting Injection 1682
Risperdal M-Tab Orally Disintegrating Tablets 1676

Rosiglitazone Maleate (New onset diabetes mellitus, exacerbation of pre-existing diabetes, and hyperglycemia have been reported with protease inhibitors; dosage adjustment of oral hypoglycemic agents may be required). Products include:
Avandamet Tablets 1373
Avandaryl Tablets 1379
Avandia Tablets 1384

Saquinavir (When co-administered with reduced doses of saquinavir and ritonavir increased saquinavir concentration, increased AUC, Cmax, and Cmin have resulted).
No products indexed under this heading.

Saquinavir Mesylate (When co-administered with reduced doses of saquinavir and ritonavir, increased saquinavir concentration, increased AUC, Cmax, and Cmin have resulted). Products include:
Invirase 2772

Sertraline Hydrochloride (Co-administration results in a large increase (> 3x) in AUC of sertraline; dosage adjustments may be required). Products include:
Zoloft 2586

Sildenafil Citrate (Co-administration is expected to substantially increase PDE 5 inhibitor concentrations and may result in an increase in adverse events, including hypotension, syncope, visual changes, and prolonged erection). Products include:
Revatio Tablets 2557
Viagra Tablets 2573

Simvastatin (Co-administration results in increased plasma concentrations of simvastatin; the risk of myopathy, including rhabdomyolysis, may be increased). Products include:
Vytorin 10/10 Tablets 2114
Vytorin 10/10 Tablets 3077
Vytorin 10/20 Tablets 2114
Vytorin 10/20 Tablets 3077
Vytorin 10/40 Tablets 2114
Vytorin 10/40 Tablets 3077
Vytorin 10/80 Tablets 2114
Vytorin 10/80 Tablets 3077
Zocor Tablets 2105

Sirolimus (Co-administration may result in increased sirolimus plasma concentrations; dose decrease of sirolimus may be needed. Use with caution). Products include:
Rapamune Oral Solution and Tablets 3475

Sotalol Hydrochloride (Co-administration with beta-blockers has resulted in cardiac and neurologic events).
No products indexed under this heading.

Sulfamethoxazole (Co-administration with a combination tablet containing sulfamethoxazole and trimethoprim has resulted in decreased AUC of sulfamethoxazole by 20% and no change in AUC).
No products indexed under this heading.

Tacrolimus (Co-administration may result in increased tacrolimus plasma concentrations; dose decrease of tacrolimus may be needed. Use with caution). Products include:
Prograf Capsules and Injection 632
Protopic Ointment 638

Tadalafil (Co-administration is expected to substantially increase PDE 5 inhibitor concentrations and may result in an increase in adverse events, including hypotension, syncope, visual changes, and prolonged erection). Products include:
Cialis Tablets 1838

Tamoxifen Citrate (Co-administration results in a large increase (> 3x) in AUC of tamoxifen; dosage adjustments may be required). Products include:
Soltamox Oral Solution 3527

Temazepam (Ritonavir may increase the activity of glucuronosyltransferase; co-administration results in a decrease in AUC of temazepam; dosage adjustments may be required). Products include:
Restoril Capsules 1860

Terazosin Hydrochloride (Co-administration results in a possible increase in AUC of terazosin; dosage adjustments may be required). Products include:
Hytrin Capsules 471

Terfenadine (Co-administration is contraindicated due to potential for serious and/or life-threatening reactions, such as cardiac arrhythmias).
No products indexed under this heading.

Theophylline (Co-administration results in the reduction of the average AUC of theophylline; increased dosage of theophylline may be required and therapeutic monitoring should be considered).
No products indexed under this heading.

Theophylline Anhydrous (Co-administration results in the reduction of the average AUC of theophylline; increased dosage of theophylline may be required and therapeutic monitoring should be considered). Products include:
Uniphyl Tablets 2710

Theophylline Calcium Salicylate (Co-administration results in the reduction of the average AUC of theophylline; increased dosage of theophylline may be required and therapeutic monitoring should be considered).
No products indexed under this heading.

Theophylline Dihydroxypropyl (Glyceryl) (Co-administration results in the reduction of the average AUC of theophylline; increased dosage of theophylline may be required and therapeutic monitoring should be considered).
No products indexed under this heading.

Theophylline Ethylenediamine (Co-administration results in the reduction of the average AUC of theophylline; increased dosage of theophylline may be required and therapeutic monitoring should be considered).
No products indexed under this heading.

Theophylline Sodium Glycinate (Co-administration results in the reduction of the average AUC of theophylline; increased dosage of theophylline may be required and therapeutic monitoring should be considered).
No products indexed under this heading.

Thioridazine Hydrochloride (Co-administration may result in increased thioridazine plasma concentrations; dose decrease of thioridazine may be needed. Use with caution). Products include:
Thioridazine Hydrochloride Tablets 2163

Timolol Hemihydrate (Co-administration may result in increased timolol plasma concentrations; cardiac and neurologic events have been reported with co-administration. Dosage adjustment may be needed. Use with caution). Products include:
Betimol Ophthalmic Solution 3382
Betimol Ophthalmic Solution .... ⊙ 295

Timolol Maleate (Co-administration may result in increased timolol plasma concentrations; dosage adjustment may be needed). Products include:
Blocadren Tablets 1916
Cosopt Sterile Ophthalmic Solution 1931
Timolide Tablets 2086
Timoptic Sterile Ophthalmic Solution 2088
Timoptic in Ocudose 2091
Timoptic-XE Sterile Ophthalmic Gel Forming Solution 2092

Tocainide Hydrochloride (Co-administration results in a possible increase in AUC of tocainide; dosage adjustments may be required).
No products indexed under this heading.

Tolazamide (New onset diabetes mellitus, exacerbation of pre-existing diabetes, and hyperglycemia have been reported with protease inhibitors; dosage adjustment of oral hypoglycemic agents may be required).
No products indexed under this heading.

Tolbutamide (Co-administration results in a moderate increase or decrease in AUC of tolbutamide; dosage adjustments may be required).
No products indexed under this heading.

Tramadol Hydrochloride (Co-administration may result in an increase in AUC of tramadol; dosage adjustments may be required. Use with caution). Products include:
Ultram ER Tablets 2392

Trazodone Hydrochloride (Co-administration results in a large increase (> 3x) in AUC of trazodone; dosage adjustments may be required).
No products indexed under this heading.

Triazolam (Co-administration is contraindicated due to potential for prolonged or increased sedation and/or respiratory depression).
No products indexed under this heading.

Trimethoprim (Co-administration with a combination tablet containing sulfamethoxazole and trimethoprim has resulted in increased AUC of trimethoprim by 20% and no change in AUC of ritonavir).
No products indexed under this heading.

Trimipramine Maleate (Co-administration may result in increased tricyclic antidepressants' plasma concentrations; dose decrease of tricyclics may be needed. Use with caution).
No products indexed under this heading.

Troglitazone (New onset diabetes mellitus, exacerbation of pre-existing diabetes, and hyperglycemia have been reported with protease inhibitors; dosage adjustment of oral hypoglycemic agents may be required).
No products indexed under this heading.

Valproate Sodium (Co-administration may result in decreased valproate plasma concentrations; dose increase of valproate may be needed. Use with caution). Products include:
Depacon Injection 412

Valproic Acid (Co-administration may result in decreased valproate plasma concentrations; dose increase of valproate may be needed. Use with caution). Products include:
Depakene 417

Vardenafil Hydrochloride (Co-administration is expected to substantially increase PDE 5 inhibitor concentrations and may result in an increase in adverse events, including hypotension, syncope, visual changes, and prolonged erection). Products include:
Levitra Tablets 3034

Venlafaxine Hydrochloride (Co-administration results in a moderate increase (1.5 to 3x) in AUC of venlafaxine; dosage adjustments may be required). Products include:
Effexor Tablets 3411
Effexor XR Capsules 3417

Verapamil Hydrochloride (Co-administration may result in increased verapamil plasma concentrations; dose decrease of verapamil may be needed. Use with caution). Products include:

Covera-HS Tablets 3139
Tarka Tablets 524
Verelan PM Extended-Release Capsules, Controlled-Onset 3106

Vinblastine Sulfate (Co-administration results in a large increase (> 3x) in AUC of vinblastine; dosage adjustments may be required).
No products indexed under this heading.

Vincristine Sulfate (Co-administration results in a large increase (> 3x) in AUC of vincristine; dosage adjustments may be required).
No products indexed under this heading.

Voriconazole (Co-administration is contraindicated due to significant decreases in voriconazole plasma concentrations and may lead to loss of antifungal response). Products include:

VFEND I.V. 2564
VFEND Oral Suspension 2564
VFEND Tablets 2564

Warfarin Sodium (Co-administration may result in decreased warfarin plasma concentrations; initial frequent monitoring of the INR during ritonavir and nartarin co-administration is indicated). Products include:

Coumadin for Injection 898
Coumadin Tablets 898

Zidovudine (Co-administration has resulted in decreased AUC and Cmax of zidovudine by 25% and 27%, respectively, and no change in ritonavir AUC and/or Cmax). Products include:

Combivir Tablets 1411
Retrovir 1560
Retrovir IV Infusion 1564
Trizivir Tablets 1589

Zolpidem Tartrate (Co-administration may result in increased zolpidem plasma concentrations; dose decrease of zolpidem may be needed. Use with caution). Products include:

Ambien Tablets 2851
Ambien CR Tablets 2855

Food Interactions

Meal, unspecified (Relative to fasting conditions, the extent of absorption of ritonavir from capsule formulation was 15% higher when administered with a meal; decreased peak ritonavir concentrations when oral solution was given under non-fasting condition).

NORVIR ORAL SOLUTION

(Ritonavir) 503
See Norvir Soft Gelatin Capsules

NOVOLOG INJECTION

(Insulin Aspart, Human Regular) 2326
May interact with ACE inhibitors, beta blockers, corticosteroids, diuretics, fibrates, oral hypoglycemic agents, lithium preparations, monoamine oxidase inhibitors, oral contraceptives, phenothiazines, salicylates, sympathomimetics, thyroid preparations, and certain other agents. Compounds in these categories include:

Acarbose (May increase the blood-glucose-lowering effect and susceptibility to hypoglycemia). Products include:

Precose Tablets 751

Acebutolol Hydrochloride (Beta-blockers may either potentiate or weaken the blood-glucose-lowering effect of insulin; signs of hypoglycemia may be reduced or absent with co-administration).
No products indexed under this heading.

Albuterol (Sympathomimetic agents may reduce the blood-glucose-lowering effect of insulin). Products include:

Proventil Inhalation Aerosol 3053

Albuterol Sulfate (Sympathomimetic agents may reduce the blood-glucose-lowering effect of insulin). Products include:

AccuNeb Inhalation Solution 1055
Combivent Inhalation Aerosol 847
DuoNeb Inhalation Solution 1058
ProAir HFA Inhalation Aerosol 3300
Proventil Inhalation Solution 0.083% 3055
Proventil HFA Inhalation Aerosol 3056
Ventolin HFA Inhalation Aerosol 1600
VoSpire ER Tablets 1052

Amiloride Hydrochloride (Diuretics may reduce the blood-glucose-lowering effect of insulin). Products include:

Midamor Tablets 2026
Moduretic Tablets 2028

Aspirin (May increase the blood-glucose-lowering effect and susceptibility to hypoglycemia). Products include:

Aggrenox Capsules 822
Bayer Aspirin 744
BC Allergy Sinus Cold Powder .... ■677
BC Headache Powder .... ■677
Arthritis Strength BC Powder .... ■677
BC Sinus Cold Powder .... ■677
Excedrin Extra Strength Caplets/Tablets/Geltabs .... ■684
Excedrin Migraine Caplets/Tablets/Geltabs .... ■609
Goody's Body Pain Formula Powder .... ■684
Goody's Extra Strength Headache Powders .... ■611
Goody's Extra Strength Pain Relief Tablets .... ■685
Percodan Tablets 1132
St. Joseph 81 mg Aspirin Chewable and Enteric Coated Tablets 1869

Aspirin, Enteric Coated (May increase the blood-glucose-lowering effect and susceptibility to hypoglycemia).
No products indexed under this heading.

Aspirin Buffered (May increase the blood-glucose-lowering effect and susceptibility to hypoglycemia). Products include:

Bufferin Extra Strength Tablets .... ■678
Bufferin Regular Strength Tablets .... ■678

Atenolol (Beta-blockers may either potentiate or weaken the blood-glucose-lowering effect of insulin; signs of hypoglycemia may be reduced or absent with co-administration).
No products indexed under this heading.

Benazepril Hydrochloride (May increase the blood-glucose-lowering effect and susceptibility to hypoglycemia). Products include:

Lotensin Tablets 2243
Lotensin HCT Tablets 2246
Lotrel Capsules 2249

Bendroflumethiazide (Diuretics may reduce the blood-glucose-lowering effect of insulin).
No products indexed under this heading.

Betamethasone Acetate (Co-administration with corticosteroids may reduce the blood-glucose-lowering effect of insulin).
No products indexed under this heading.

Betamethasone Sodium Phosphate (Co-administration with corticosteroids may reduce the blood-glucose-lowering effect of insulin).
No products indexed under this heading.

Betaxolol Hydrochloride (Beta-blockers may either potentiate or weaken the blood-glucose-lowering effect of insulin; signs of hypoglycemia may be reduced or absent with co-administration). Products include:

Betoptic S Ophthalmic Suspension 558

Bisoprolol Fumarate (Beta-blockers may either potentiate or weaken the blood-glucose-lowering effect of insulin; signs of hypoglycemia may be reduced or absent with co-administration).
No products indexed under this heading.

Bumetanide (Diuretics may reduce the blood-glucose-lowering effect of insulin). Products include:

Bumex Tablets 2746

Captopril (May increase the blood-glucose-lowering effect and susceptibility to hypoglycemia). Products include:

Captopril Tablets 2149

Carteolol Hydrochloride (Beta-blockers may either potentiate or weaken the blood-glucose-lowering effect of insulin; signs of hypoglycemia may be reduced or absent with co-administration). Products include:

Carteolol Hydrochloride Ophthalmic Solution USP, 1% .... ⊙249

Chlorothiazide (Diuretics may reduce the blood-glucose-lowering effect of insulin). Products include:

Diuril Oral Suspension 1954

Chlorothiazide Sodium (Diuretics may reduce the blood-glucose-lowering effect of insulin). Products include:

Diuril Sodium Intravenous 2467

Chlorpromazine (Phenothiazine derivatives may reduce the blood-glucose-lowering effect of insulin).
No products indexed under this heading.

Chlorpromazine Hydrochloride (Phenothiazine derivatives may reduce the blood-glucose-lowering effect of insulin).
No products indexed under this heading.

Chlorpropamide (May increase the blood-glucose-lowering effect and susceptibility to hypoglycemia).
No products indexed under this heading.

Chlorthalidone (Diuretics may reduce the blood-glucose-lowering effect of insulin). Products include:

Clorpres Tablets 2153

Choline Magnesium Trisalicylate (May increase the blood-glucose-lowering effect and susceptibility to hypoglycemia).
No products indexed under this heading.

Clofibrate (May increase the blood-glucose-lowering effect and susceptibility to hypoglycemia).
No products indexed under this heading.

Clonidine (Signs of hypoglycemia may be reduced or absent with co-administration). Products include:

Catapres-TTS 844

Clonidine Hydrochloride (Signs of hypoglycemia may be reduced or absent with co-administration). Products include:

Catapres Tablets 843
Clorpres Tablets 2153

Cortisone Acetate (Co-administration with corticosteroids may reduce the blood-glucose-lowering effect of insulin).
No products indexed under this heading.

Danazol (May reduce the blood-glucose-lowering effect of insulin).
No products indexed under this heading.

Desogestrel (Oral contraceptives may reduce the blood-glucose-lowering effect of insulin). Products include:

Mircette Tablets 1066

Dexamethasone (Co-administration with corticosteroids may reduce the blood-glucose-lowering effect of insulin). Products include:

Ciprodex Otic Suspension 559
Decadron Tablets 1951
TobraDex Ophthalmic Ointment 562
TobraDex Ophthalmic Suspension 563

Dexamethasone Acetate (Co-administration with corticosteroids may reduce the blood-glucose-lowering effect of insulin).
No products indexed under this heading.

Dexamethasone Sodium Phosphate (Co-administration with corticosteroids may reduce the blood-glucose-lowering effect of insulin).
No products indexed under this heading.

Diflunisal (May increase the blood-glucose-lowering effect and susceptibility to hypoglycemia). Products include:

Dolobid Tablets 1955

Disopyramide Phosphate (May increase the blood-glucose-lowering effect and susceptibility to hypoglycemia).
No products indexed under this heading.

Dobutamine Hydrochloride (Sympathomimetic agents may reduce the blood-glucose-lowering effect of insulin).
No products indexed under this heading.

Dopamine Hydrochloride (Sympathomimetic agents may reduce the blood-glucose-lowering effect of insulin).
No products indexed under this heading.

Enalapril Maleate (May increase the blood-glucose-lowering effect and susceptibility to hypoglycemia). Products include:

Vasotec I.V. Injection 2103

Enalaprilat (May increase the blood-glucose-lowering effect and susceptibility to hypoglycemia).
No products indexed under this heading.

Ephedrine Hydrochloride (Sympathomimetic agents may reduce the blood-glucose-lowering effect of insulin).
No products indexed under this heading.

Ephedrine Sulfate (Sympathomimetic agents may reduce the blood-glucose-lowering effect of insulin).
No products indexed under this heading.

Ephedrine Tannate (Sympathomimetic agents may reduce the blood-glucose-lowering effect of insulin).
No products indexed under this heading.

Epinephrine (Sympathomimetic agents may reduce the blood-glucose-lowering effect of insulin). Products include:
EpiPen 1061
Primatene Mist 719
Twinject 0.15 3379
Twinject 0.3 3378

Epinephrine Bitartrate (Sympathomimetic agents may reduce the blood-glucose-lowering effect of insulin).
No products indexed under this heading.

Epinephrine Hydrochloride (Sympathomimetic agents may reduce the blood-glucose-lowering effect of insulin).
No products indexed under this heading.

Esmolol Hydrochloride (Beta-blockers may either potentiate or weaken the blood-glucose-lowering effect of insulin; signs of hypoglycemia may be reduced or absent with co-administration).
No products indexed under this heading.

Ethacrynic Acid (Diuretics may reduce the blood-glucose-lowering effect of insulin). Products include:
Edecrin Tablets 1959

Ethinyl Estradiol (Oral contraceptives may reduce the blood-glucose-lowering effect of insulin). Products include:
Mircette Tablets 1066
NuvaRing 2340
Ortho-Cyclen/Ortho Tri-Cyclen 2429
Ortho Evra Transdermal System 2417
Ortho Tri-Cyclen Lo Tablets 2436
Seasonique Tablets 1077
Yasmin 28 Tablets 796
Yaz Tablets 803

Ethynodiol Diacetate (Oral contraceptives may reduce the blood-glucose-lowering effect of insulin).
No products indexed under this heading.

Fenofibrate (May increase the blood-glucose-lowering effect and susceptibility to hypoglycemia). Products include:
Lofibra Tablets 1219
Lofibra Capsules 1216
Tricor Tablets 527
Triglide Tablets 3123

Fludrocortisone Acetate (Co-administration with corticosteroids may reduce the blood-glucose-lowering effect of insulin).
No products indexed under this heading.

Fluoxetine Hydrochloride (May increase the blood-glucose-lowering effect and susceptibility to hypoglycemia). Products include:
Prozac Pulvules and Liquid 1801
Symbyax Capsules 1819

Fluphenazine Decanoate (Phenothiazine derivatives may reduce the blood-glucose-lowering effect of insulin).
No products indexed under this heading.

Fluphenazine Enanthate (Phenothiazine derivatives may reduce the blood-glucose-lowering effect of insulin).
No products indexed under this heading.

Fluphenazine Hydrochloride (Phenothiazine derivatives may reduce the blood-glucose-lowering effect of insulin).
No products indexed under this heading.

Fosinopril Sodium (May increase the blood-glucose-lowering effect and susceptibility to hypoglycemia).
No products indexed under this heading.

Furosemide (Diuretics may reduce the blood-glucose-lowering effect of insulin). Products include:
Furosemide Tablets 2154

Gemfibrozil (May increase the blood-glucose-lowering effect and susceptibility to hypoglycemia).
No products indexed under this heading.

Glimepiride (May increase the blood-glucose-lowering effect and susceptibility to hypoglycemia). Products include:
Avandaryl Tablets 1379
Duetact Tablets 3226

Glipizide (May increase the blood-glucose-lowering effect and susceptibility to hypoglycemia).
No products indexed under this heading.

Glyburide (May increase the blood-glucose-lowering effect and susceptibility to hypoglycemia).
No products indexed under this heading.

Guanethidine Monosulfate (Signs of hypoglycemia may be reduced or absent with co-administration).
No products indexed under this heading.

Hydrochlorothiazide (Diuretics may reduce the blood-glucose-lowering effect of insulin). Products include:
Aldoril Tablets 1910
Atacand HCT 651
Avalide Tablets 888
Avalide Tablets 2874
Benicar HCT Tablets 1044
Diovan HCT Tablets 2196
Dyazide Capsules 1423
Hyzaar 50-12.5 Tablets 1990
Hyzaar 100-12.5 Tablets 1990
Hyzaar 100-25 Tablets 1990
Lopressor HCT 50/25 Tablets 2241
Lopressor HCT 100/25 Tablets 2241
Lopressor HCT 100/50 Tablets 2241
Lotensin HCT Tablets 2246
Micardis HCT Tablets 856
Moduretic Tablets 2028
Prinzide Tablets 2056
Teveten HCT Tablets 1737
Timolide Tablets 2086
Uniretic Tablets 3100

Hydrocortisone (Co-administration with corticosteroids may reduce the blood-glucose-lowering effect of insulin). Products include:
Colocort Rectal Suspension, USP (Retention) 100 mg/60 mL 2476
Hydrocortone Tablets 1989
Preparation H Hydrocortisone Cream 646

Hydrocortisone Acetate (Co-administration with corticosteroids may reduce the blood-glucose-lowering effect of insulin). Products include:
Analpram-HC 1159
Pramosone 1161
ProctoFoam-HC 3099

Hydrocortisone Sodium Phosphate (Co-administration with corticosteroids may reduce the blood-glucose-lowering effect of insulin).
No products indexed under this heading.

Hydrocortisone Sodium Succinate (Co-administration with corticosteroids may reduce the blood-glucose-lowering effect of insulin).
No products indexed under this heading.

Hydroflumethiazide (Diuretics may reduce the blood-glucose-lowering effect of insulin).
No products indexed under this heading.

Indapamide (Diuretics may reduce the blood-glucose-lowering effect of insulin). Products include:
Indapamide Tablets 2156

Isocarboxazid (May increase the blood-glucose-lowering effect and susceptibility to hypoglycemia).
No products indexed under this heading.

Isoniazid (May reduce the blood-glucose-lowering effect of insulin).
No products indexed under this heading.

Isoproterenol Hydrochloride (Sympathomimetic agents may reduce the blood-glucose-lowering effect of insulin).
No products indexed under this heading.

Isoproterenol Sulfate (Sympathomimetic agents may reduce the blood-glucose-lowering effect of insulin).
No products indexed under this heading.

Labetalol Hydrochloride (Beta-blockers may either potentiate or weaken the blood-glucose-lowering effect of insulin; signs of hypoglycemia may be reduced or absent with co-administration).
No products indexed under this heading.

Levalbuterol Hydrochloride (Sympathomimetic agents may reduce the blood-glucose-lowering effect of insulin). Products include:
Xopenex Inhalation Solution 3146
Xopenex Inhalation Solution Concentrate 3150

Levobunolol Hydrochloride (Beta-blockers may either potentiate or weaken the blood-glucose-lowering effect of insulin; signs of hypoglycemia may be reduced or absent with co-administration). Products include:
Betagan Ophthalmic Solution, USP .... ⊙220

Levonorgestrel (Oral contraceptives may reduce the blood-glucose-lowering effect of insulin). Products include:
Climara Pro Transdermal System 776
Mirena Intrauterine System 787
Plan B Tablets 1076
Seasonique Tablets 1077

Levothyroxine Sodium (May reduce the blood-glucose-lowering effect of insulin). Products include:
Levothroid Tablets 1186
Levoxyl Tablets 1712
Synthroid Tablets 520
Westhroid Tablets 3403

Liothyronine Sodium (May reduce the blood-glucose-lowering effect of insulin). Products include:
Cytomel Tablets 1710
Westhroid Tablets 3403

Liotrix (May reduce the blood-glucose-lowering effect of insulin). Products include:
Thyrolar Tablets 1199

Lisinopril (May increase the blood-glucose-lowering effect and susceptibility to hypoglycemia). Products include:
Prinivil Tablets 2052
Prinzide Tablets 2056

Lithium (May either potentiate or weaken the blood-glucose-lowering effect of insulin).
No products indexed under this heading.

Lithium Carbonate (May either potentiate or weaken the blood-glucose-lowering effect of insulin). Products include:
Lithobid Tablets 1692

Lithium Citrate (May either potentiate or weaken the blood-glucose-lowering effect of insulin).
No products indexed under this heading.

Magnesium Salicylate (May increase the blood-glucose-lowering effect and susceptibility to hypoglycemia).
No products indexed under this heading.

Mesoridazine Besylate (Phenothiazine derivatives may reduce the blood-glucose-lowering effect of insulin).
No products indexed under this heading.

Mestranol (Oral contraceptives may reduce the blood-glucose-lowering effect of insulin).
No products indexed under this heading.

Metaproterenol Sulfate (Sympathomimetic agents may reduce the blood-glucose-lowering effect of insulin). Products include:
Alupent Inhalation Aerosol 826

Metaraminol Bitartrate (Sympathomimetic agents may reduce the blood-glucose-lowering effect of insulin).
No products indexed under this heading.

Metformin Hydrochloride (May increase the blood-glucose-lowering effect and susceptibility to hypoglycemia). Products include:
ActoPlus Met Tablets 3214
Avandamet Tablets 1373
Fortamet Extended-Release Tablets 3115

Methotrimeprazine (Phenothiazine derivatives may reduce the blood-glucose-lowering effect of insulin).
No products indexed under this heading.

Methoxamine Hydrochloride (Sympathomimetic agents may reduce the blood-glucose-lowering effect of insulin).
No products indexed under this heading.

Methyclothiazide (Diuretics may reduce the blood-glucose-lowering effect of insulin).
No products indexed under this heading.

Methylprednisolone Acetate (Co-administration with corticosteroids may reduce the blood-glucose-lowering effect of insulin). Products include:
Depo-Medrol Injectable Suspension 2617
Depo-Medrol Single-Dose Vial 2619

IMPORTANT NOTE: Always consult each drug listing in the patient's regimen for possible interactions.

Prochlorperazine (Phenothiazine derivatives may reduce the blood-glucose-lowering effect of insulin).
No products indexed under this heading.

Promethazine Hydrochloride (Phenothiazine derivatives may reduce the blood-glucose-lowering effect of insulin). Products include:
Phenergan Tablets and Suppositories 3440

Propoxyphene Hydrochloride (May increase the blood-glucose-lowering effect and susceptibility to hypoglycemia).
No products indexed under this heading.

Propoxyphene Napsylate (May increase the blood-glucose-lowering effect and susceptibility to hypoglycemia).
No products indexed under this heading.

Propranolol Hydrochloride (Beta-blockers may either potentiate or weaken the blood-glucose-lowering effect of insulin; signs of hypoglycemia may be reduced or absent with co-administration). Products include:
Inderal LA Long-Acting Capsules 3429
InnoPran XL Capsules 2723

Pseudoephedrine Hydrochloride (Sympathomimetic agents may reduce the blood-glucose-lowering effect of insulin). Products include:
Advil Allergy Sinus Caplets .... ▣770
Advil Cold & Sinus .... ▣723
Advil Multi-Symptom Cold Caplets .... ▣770
Aleve Cold & Sinus Caplets 744
Allegra-D 12 Hour Extended-Release Tablets 2846
Allegra-D 24 Hour Extended-Release Tablets 2849
BC Cold Powder .... ▣677
Comtrex Maximum Strength Cold & Cough Day/Night Caplets - Day Formulation .... ▣726
Comtrex Maximum Strength Cold & Cough Day/Night Caplets - Night Formulation .... ▣726
Children's Motrin Cold Oral Suspension 1867
Mucinex D Extended-Release Bi-Layer Tablets .... ▣776
Robitussin Cough & Cold CF Liquid .... ▣735
Robitussin Cough & Cold Pediatric Drops .... ▣735
Tylenol Sinus Congestion & Pain Nighttime Caplets with Cool Burst .... ▣778
Tylenol Cold Severe Congestion Non-Drowsy Caplets with Cool Burst 1874
Tylenol Sinus Severe Congestion Caplets with Cool Burst 1876
Vicks 44D Cough & Head Congestion Relief Liquid 2679
Vicks 44M Cough, Cold & Flu Relief Liquid 2680
Vicks DayQuil Multi-Symptom Cold/Flu Relief LiquiCaps 2678
Vicks DayQuil Multi-Symptom Cold/Flu Relief Liquid 2678
Vicks NyQuil Multi-Symptom Cold/Flu Relief Liquid 2681
Vicks NyQuil Multi-Symptom Cold/Flu Relief LiquiCaps 2681
Children's Vicks NyQuil Cold/Cough Relief Liquid 2680
Zyrtec-D 12 Hour Extended Release Tablets 2597

Pseudoephedrine Sulfate (Sympathomimetic agents may reduce the blood-glucose-lowering effect of insulin). Products include:
Alavert Allergy & Sinus D-12 Hour Tablets .... ▣771
Clarinex-D 24-Hour Extended-Release Tablets 2998
Claritin-D Non-Drowsy 12 Hour Tablets .... ▣772
Claritin-D Non-Drowsy 24 Hour Tablets .... ▣772

Quinapril Hydrochloride (May increase the blood-glucose-lowering effect and susceptibility to hypoglycemia).
No products indexed under this heading.

Ramipril (May increase the blood-glucose-lowering effect and susceptibility to hypoglycemia). Products include:
Altace Capsules 1702

Repaglinide (May increase the blood-glucose-lowering effect and susceptibility to hypoglycemia).
No products indexed under this heading.

Reserpine (Signs of hypoglycemia may be reduced or absent with co-administration).
No products indexed under this heading.

Rosiglitazone Maleate (May increase the blood-glucose-lowering effect and susceptibility to hypoglycemia). Products include:
Avandamet Tablets 1373
Avandaryl Tablets 1379
Avandia Tablets 1384

Salmeterol Xinafoate (Sympathomimetic agents may reduce the blood-glucose-lowering effect of insulin). Products include:
Advair Diskus 100/50 1308
Advair Diskus 250/50 1308
Advair Diskus 500/50 1308
Advair HFA Inhalation Aerosol 1318
Serevent Diskus 1568

Salsalate (May increase the blood-glucose-lowering effect and susceptibility to hypoglycemia).
No products indexed under this heading.

Selegiline Hydrochloride (May increase the blood-glucose-lowering effect and susceptibility to hypoglycemia). Products include:
Eldepryl Capsules 3208
Zelapar Tablets 3372

Somatropin (May reduce the blood-glucose-lowering effect of insulin). Products include:
Genotropin Lyophilized Powder 2638
Humatrope Vials and Cartridges 1787
Norditropin Cartridges 2323
Nutropin for Injection 1239
Nutropin AQ Injection 1243
Nutropin AQ Pen 1243
Nutropin AQ Pen Cartridge 1243

Sotalol Hydrochloride (Beta-blockers may either potentiate or weaken the blood-glucose-lowering effect of insulin; signs of hypoglycemia may be reduced or absent with co-administration).
No products indexed under this heading.

Spirapril Hydrochloride (May increase the blood-glucose-lowering effect and susceptibility to hypoglycemia).
No products indexed under this heading.

Spironolactone (Diuretics may reduce the blood-glucose-lowering effect of insulin).
No products indexed under this heading.

Sulfamethoxazole (Co-administration with sulfonamide antibiotics may increase the blood-glucose-lowering effect and susceptibility to hypoglycemia).
No products indexed under this heading.

Sulfisoxazole Acetyl (Co-administration with sulfonamide antibiotics may increase the blood-glucose-lowering effect and susceptibility to hypoglycemia).
No products indexed under this heading.

Terbutaline Sulfate (Sympathomimetic agents may reduce the blood-glucose-lowering effect of insulin).
No products indexed under this heading.

Thioridazine Hydrochloride (Phenothiazine derivatives may reduce the blood-glucose-lowering effect of insulin). Products include:
Thioridazine Hydrochloride Tablets 2163

Thyroglobulin (May reduce the blood-glucose-lowering effect of insulin).
No products indexed under this heading.

Thyroid (May reduce the blood-glucose-lowering effect of insulin).
No products indexed under this heading.

Thyroxine (May reduce the blood-glucose-lowering effect of insulin).
No products indexed under this heading.

Thyroxine Sodium (May reduce the blood-glucose-lowering effect of insulin).
No products indexed under this heading.

Timolol Hemihydrate (Beta-blockers may either potentiate or weaken the blood-glucose-lowering effect of insulin; signs of hypoglycemia may be reduced or absent with co-administration). Products include:
Betimol Ophthalmic Solution 3382
Betimol Ophthalmic Solution .... ⊙295

Timolol Maleate (Beta-blockers may either potentiate or weaken the blood-glucose-lowering effect of insulin; signs of hypoglycemia may be reduced or absent with co-administration). Products include:
Blocadren Tablets 1916
Cosopt Sterile Ophthalmic Solution 1931
Timolide Tablets 2086
Timoptic Sterile Ophthalmic Solution 2088
Timoptic in Ocudose 2091
Timoptic-XE Sterile Ophthalmic Gel Forming Solution 2092

Tolazamide (May increase the blood-glucose-lowering effect and susceptibility to hypoglycemia).
No products indexed under this heading.

Tolbutamide (May increase the blood-glucose-lowering effect and susceptibility to hypoglycemia).
No products indexed under this heading.

Torsemide (Diuretics may reduce the blood-glucose-lowering effect of insulin). Products include:
Demadex Injection 2759
Demadex Tablets 2759

Trandolapril (May increase the blood-glucose-lowering effect and susceptibility to hypoglycemia). Products include:
Mavik Tablets 486
Tarka Tablets 524

Tranylcypromine Sulfate (May increase the blood-glucose-lowering effect and susceptibility to hypoglycemia). Products include:
Parnate Tablets 1527

Triamcinolone (Co-administration with corticosteroids may reduce the blood-glucose-lowering effect of insulin).
No products indexed under this heading.

Triamcinolone Acetonide (Co-administration with corticosteroids may reduce the blood-glucose-lowering effect of insulin). Products include:
Azmacort Inhalation Aerosol 1726
Nasacort AQ Nasal Spray 2922

Triamcinolone Diacetate (Co-administration with corticosteroids may reduce the blood-glucose-lowering effect of insulin).
No products indexed under this heading.

Triamcinolone Hexacetonide (Co-administration with corticosteroids may reduce the blood-glucose-lowering effect of insulin).
No products indexed under this heading.

Triamterene (Diuretics may reduce the blood-glucose-lowering effect of insulin). Products include:
Dyazide Capsules 1423
Dyrenium Capsules 3400

Trifluoperazine Hydrochloride (Phenothiazine derivatives may reduce the blood-glucose-lowering effect of insulin).
No products indexed under this heading.

Troglitazone (May increase the blood-glucose-lowering effect and susceptibility to hypoglycemia).
No products indexed under this heading.

Food Interactions

Alcohol (May either potentiate or weaken the blood-glucose-lowering effect of insulin).

NOVOLOG MIX 70/30

(Insulin Aspart, Human, Insulin Aspart Protamine, Human) 2328
May interact with ACE inhibitors, beta blockers, corticosteroids, diuretics, estrogens, fibrates, monoamine oxidase inhibitors, oral contraceptives, phenothiazines, progestins, sulfonamides, sympathomimetics, thyroid preparations, and certain other agents. Compounds in these categories include:

Acebutolol Hydrochloride (May potentiate or weaken the blood-glucose-lowering effect of insulin. The signs of hypoglycemia may be reduced or absent.).
No products indexed under this heading.

Albuterol (Substances that may reduce the blood-glucose-lowering effect). Products include:
Proventil Inhalation Aerosol 3053

Albuterol Sulfate (Substances that may reduce the blood-glucose-lowering effect). Products include:
AccuNeb Inhalation Solution 1055
Combivent Inhalation Aerosol 847
DuoNeb Inhalation Solution 1058
ProAir HFA Inhalation Aerosol 3300
Proventil Inhalation Solution 0.083% 3055
Proventil HFA Inhalation Aerosol 3056
Ventolin HFA Inhalation Aerosol 1600
VoSpire ER Tablets 1052

Amiloride Hydrochloride (Substances that may reduce the blood-glucose-lowering effect). Products include:
Midamor Tablets 2026

Moduretic Tablets 2028

Atenolol (May potentiate or weaken the blood-glucose-lowering effect of insulin. The signs of hypoglycemia may be reduced or absent.).
No products indexed under this heading.

Benazepril Hydrochloride (Substances that may increase the blood-glucose-lowering effect and susceptibility to hypoglycemia). Products include:
Lotensin Tablets 2243
Lotensin HCT Tablets 2246
Lotrel Capsules 2249

Bendroflumethiazide (Substances that may increase the blood-glucose-lowering effect and susceptibility to hypoglycemia).
No products indexed under this heading.

Betamethasone Acetate (Substances that may reduce the blood-glucose-lowering effect).
No products indexed under this heading.

Betamethasone Sodium Phosphate (Substances that may reduce the blood-glucose-lowering effect).
No products indexed under this heading.

Betaxolol Hydrochloride (May potentiate or weaken the blood-glucose-lowering effect of insulin. The signs of hypoglycemia may be reduced or absent). Products include:
Betoptic S Ophthalmic Suspension 558

Bisoprolol Fumarate (May potentiate or weaken the blood-glucose-lowering effect of insulin. The signs of hypoglycemia may be reduced or absent.).
No products indexed under this heading.

Bumetanide (Substances that may reduce the blood-glucose-lowering effect). Products include:
Bumex Tablets 2746

Captopril (Substances that may increase the blood-glucose-lowering effect and susceptibility to hypoglycemia). Products include:
Captopril Tablets 2149

Carteolol Hydrochloride (May potentiate or weaken the blood-glucose-lowering effect of insulin. The signs of hypoglycemia may be reduced or absent). Products include:
Carteolol Hydrochloride Ophthalmic Solution USP, 1%...... ⊙249

Chlorothiazide (Substances that may increase the blood-glucose-lowering effect and susceptibility to hypoglycemia). Products include:
Diuril Oral Suspension 1954

Chlorothiazide Sodium (Substances that may increase the blood-glucose-lowering effect and susceptibility to hypoglycemia). Products include:
Diuril Sodium Intravenous 2467

Chlorotrianisene (Substances that may reduce the blood-glucose-lowering effect).
No products indexed under this heading.

Chlorpromazine (Substances that may reduce the blood-glucose-lowering effect).
No products indexed under this heading.

Chlorpromazine Hydrochloride (Substances that may reduce the blood-glucose-lowering effect).
No products indexed under this heading.

Chlorpropamide (Substances that may increase the blood-glucose-lowering effect and susceptibility to hypoglycemia).
No products indexed under this heading.

Chlorthalidone (Substances that may reduce the blood-glucose-lowering effect). Products include:
Clorpres Tablets 2153

Clofibrate (Substances that may increase the blood-glucose-lowering effect and susceptibility to hypoglycemia).
No products indexed under this heading.

Clonidine Hydrochloride (May potentiate or weaken the blood-glucose-lowering effect of insulin. The signs of hypoglycemia may be reduced or absent). Products include:
Catapres Tablets 843
Clorpres Tablets 2153

Cortisone Acetate (Substances that may reduce the blood-glucose-lowering effect).
No products indexed under this heading.

Danazol (Substances that may reduce the blood-glucose-lowering effect).
No products indexed under this heading.

Desogestrel (Substances that may reduce the blood-glucose-lowering effect). Products include:
Mircette Tablets 1066

Dexamethasone (Substances that may reduce the blood-glucose-lowering effect). Products include:
Ciprodex Otic Suspension 559
Decadron Tablets 1951
TobraDex Ophthalmic Ointment 562
TobraDex Ophthalmic Suspension ... 563

Dexamethasone Acetate (Substances that may reduce the blood-glucose-lowering effect).
No products indexed under this heading.

Dexamethasone Sodium Phosphate (Substances that may reduce the blood-glucose-lowering effect).
No products indexed under this heading.

Dienestrol (Substances that may reduce the blood-glucose-lowering effect).
No products indexed under this heading.

Diethylstilbestrol (Substances that may reduce the blood-glucose-lowering effect).
No products indexed under this heading.

Disopyramide Phosphate (Substances that may increase the blood-glucose-lowering effect and susceptibility to hypoglycemia).
No products indexed under this heading.

Dobutamine Hydrochloride (Substances that may reduce the blood-glucose-lowering effect).
No products indexed under this heading.

Dopamine Hydrochloride (Substances that may reduce the blood-glucose-lowering effect).
No products indexed under this heading.

Enalapril Maleate (Substances that may increase the blood-glucose-lowering effect and susceptibility to hypoglycemia). Products include:
Vasotec I.V. Injection 2103

Enalaprilat (Substances that may increase the blood-glucose-lowering effect and susceptibility to hypoglycemia).
No products indexed under this heading.

Ephedrine Hydrochloride (Substances that may reduce the blood-glucose-lowering effect).
No products indexed under this heading.

Ephedrine Sulfate (Substances that may reduce the blood-glucose-lowering effect).
No products indexed under this heading.

Ephedrine Tannate (Substances that may reduce the blood-glucose-lowering effect).
No products indexed under this heading.

Epinephrine (Substances that may reduce the blood-glucose-lowering effect). Products include:
EpiPen 1061
Primatene Mist .... ▣719
Twinject 0.15 3379
Twinject 0.3 3378

Epinephrine Bitartrate (Substances that may reduce the blood-glucose-lowering effect).
No products indexed under this heading.

Epinephrine Hydrochloride (Substances that may reduce the blood-glucose-lowering effect).
No products indexed under this heading.

Esmolol Hydrochloride (May potentiate or weaken the blood-glucose-lowering effect of insulin. The signs of hypoglycemia may be reduced or absent.).
No products indexed under this heading.

Estradiol (Substances that may reduce the blood-glucose-lowering effect). Products include:
Angeliq Tablets 762
Climara Transdermal System 771
Climara Pro Transdermal System 776
Estrasorb Topical Emulsion 1147
Estring Vaginal Ring 2635
Menostar Transdermal System 782
Vagifem Tablets 2334

Estrogens, Conjugated (Substances that may reduce the blood-glucose-lowering effect). Products include:
Premarin Intravenous 3442
Premarin Tablets 3446
Premarin Vaginal Cream 3452
Premphase Tablets 3456
Prempro Tablets 3456

Estrogens, Esterified (Substances that may reduce the blood-glucose-lowering effect). Products include:
Estratest Tablets 3199
Estratest H.S. Tablets 3199

Estropipate (Substances that may reduce the blood-glucose-lowering effect).
No products indexed under this heading.

Ethacrynic Acid (Substances that may reduce the blood-glucose-lowering effect). Products include:
Edecrin Tablets 1959

Ethinyl Estradiol (Substances that may reduce the blood-glucose-lowering effect). Products include:
Mircette Tablets 1066
NuvaRing 2340
Ortho-Cyclen/Ortho Tri-Cyclen 2429
Ortho Evra Transdermal System 2417
Ortho Tri-Cyclen Lo Tablets 2436
Seasonique Tablets 1077
Yasmin 28 Tablets 796
Yaz Tablets 803

Ethynodiol Diacetate (Substances that may reduce the blood-glucose-lowering effect).
No products indexed under this heading.

Fenofibrate (Substances that may increase the blood-glucose-lowering effect and susceptibility to hypoglycemia). Products include:
Lofibra Tablets 1219
Lofibra Capsules 1216
Tricor Tablets 527
Triglide Tablets 3123

Fludrocortisone Acetate (Substances that may reduce the blood-glucose-lowering effect).
No products indexed under this heading.

Fluoxetine Hydrochloride (Substances that may increase the blood-glucose-lowering effect and susceptibility to hypoglycemia). Products include:
Prozac Pulvules and Liquid 1801
Symbyax Capsules 1819

Fluphenazine Decanoate (Substances that may reduce the blood-glucose-lowering effect).
No products indexed under this heading.

Fluphenazine Enanthate (Substances that may reduce the blood-glucose-lowering effect).
No products indexed under this heading.

Fluphenazine Hydrochloride (Substances that may reduce the blood-glucose-lowering effect).
No products indexed under this heading.

Fosinopril Sodium (Substances that may increase the blood-glucose-lowering effect and susceptibility to hypoglycemia).
No products indexed under this heading.

Furosemide (Substances that may reduce the blood-glucose-lowering effect). Products include:
Furosemide Tablets 2154

Gemfibrozil (Substances that may increase the blood-glucose-lowering effect and susceptibility to hypoglycemia).
No products indexed under this heading.

Glipizide (Substances that may increase the blood-glucose-lowering effect and susceptibility to hypoglycemia).
No products indexed under this heading.

Glyburide (Substances that may increase the blood-glucose-lowering effect and susceptibility to hypoglycemia).
No products indexed under this heading.

Guanethidine Monosulfate (The signs of hypoglycemia may be reduced or absent when under the influence of guanethidine).
No products indexed under this heading.

Hydrochlorothiazide (Substances that may increase the blood-glucose-lowering effect and susceptibility to hypoglycemia). Products include:

Hydrocortisone (Substances that may reduce the blood-glucose-lowering effect). Products include:

Hydrocortisone Acetate (Substances that may reduce the blood-glucose-lowering effect). Products include:

Hydrocortisone Sodium Phosphate (Substances that may reduce the blood-glucose-lowering effect).
No products indexed under this heading.

Hydrocortisone Sodium Succinate (Substances that may reduce the blood-glucose-lowering effect).
No products indexed under this heading.

Hydroflumethiazide (Substances that may increase the blood-glucose-lowering effect and susceptibility to hypoglycemia).
No products indexed under this heading.

Indapamide (Substances that may reduce the blood-glucose-lowering effect). Products include:

Isocarboxazid (Substances that may increase the blood-glucose-lowering effect and susceptibility to hypoglycemia).
No products indexed under this heading.

Isoniazid (Substances that may reduce the blood-glucose-lowering effect).
No products indexed under this heading.

Isoproterenol Hydrochloride (Substances that may reduce the blood-glucose-lowering effect).
No products indexed under this heading.

Isoproterenol Sulfate (Substances that may reduce the blood-glucose-lowering effect).
No products indexed under this heading.

Labetalol Hydrochloride (May potentiate or weaken the blood-glucose-lowering effect of insulin. The signs of hypoglycemia may be reduced or absent.).
No products indexed under this heading.

Levalbuterol Hydrochloride (Substances that may reduce the blood-glucose-lowering effect). Products include:

Levobunolol Hydrochloride (May potentiate or weaken the blood-glucose-lowering effect of insulin. The signs of hypoglycemia may be reduced or absent). Products include:

Levonorgestrel (Substances that may reduce the blood-glucose-lowering effect). Products include:

Levothyroxine Sodium (Substances that may reduce the blood-glucose-lowering effect). Products include:

Liothyronine Sodium (Substances that may reduce the blood-glucose-lowering effect). Products include:

Liotrix (Substances that may reduce the blood-glucose-lowering effect). Products include:

Lisinopril (Substances that may increase the blood-glucose-lowering effect and susceptibility to hypoglycemia). Products include:

Lithium Carbonate (May potentiate or weaken the blood-glucose-lowering effect of insulin). Products include:

Lithium Citrate (May potentiate or weaken the blood-glucose-lowering effect of insulin).
No products indexed under this heading.

Medroxyprogesterone Acetate (Substances that may reduce the blood-glucose-lowering effect). Products include:

Megestrol Acetate (Substances that may reduce the blood-glucose-lowering effect). Products include:

Mesoridazine Besylate (Substances that may reduce the blood-glucose-lowering effect).
No products indexed under this heading.

Mestranol (Substances that may reduce the blood-glucose-lowering effect).
No products indexed under this heading.

Metaproterenol Sulfate (Substances that may reduce the blood-glucose-lowering effect). Products include:

Metaraminol Bitartrate (Substances that may reduce the blood-glucose-lowering effect).
No products indexed under this heading.

Methotrimeprazine (Substances that may reduce the blood-glucose-lowering effect).
No products indexed under this heading.

Methoxamine Hydrochloride (Substances that may reduce the blood-glucose-lowering effect).
No products indexed under this heading.

Methyclothiazide (Substances that may increase the blood-glucose-lowering effect and susceptibility to hypoglycemia).
No products indexed under this heading.

Methylprednisolone Acetate (Substances that may reduce the blood-glucose-lowering effect). Products include:

Methylprednisolone Sodium Succinate (Substances that may reduce the blood-glucose-lowering effect).
No products indexed under this heading.

Metipranolol Hydrochloride (May potentiate or weaken the blood-glucose-lowering effect of insulin. The signs of hypoglycemia may be reduced or absent.).
No products indexed under this heading.

Metolazone (Substances that may reduce the blood-glucose-lowering effect).
No products indexed under this heading.

Metoprolol Succinate (May potentiate or weaken the blood-glucose-lowering effect of insulin. The signs of hypoglycemia may be reduced or absent). Products include:

Metoprolol Tartrate (May potentiate or weaken the blood-glucose-lowering effect of insulin. The signs of hypoglycemia may be reduced or absent). Products include:

Moclobemide (Substances that may increase the blood-glucose-lowering effect and susceptibility to hypoglycemia).
No products indexed under this heading.

Moexipril Hydrochloride (Substances that may increase the blood-glucose-lowering effect and susceptibility to hypoglycemia). Products include:

Nadolol (May potentiate or weaken the blood-glucose-lowering effect of insulin. The signs of hypoglycemia may be reduced or absent). Products include:

Niacin (Substances that may reduce the blood-glucose-lowering effect). Products include:

Norepinephrine Bitartrate (Substances that may reduce the blood-glucose-lowering effect).
No products indexed under this heading.

Norethindrone (Substances that may reduce the blood-glucose-lowering effect). Products include:

Norethynodrel (Substances that may reduce the blood-glucose-lowering effect).
No products indexed under this heading.

Norgestimate (Substances that may reduce the blood-glucose-lowering effect). Products include:

Norgestrel (Substances that may reduce the blood-glucose-lowering effect).
No products indexed under this heading.

Octreotide Acetate (Substances that may increase the blood-glucose-lowering effect and susceptibility to hypoglycemia). Products include:

Pargyline Hydrochloride (Substances that may increase the blood-glucose-lowering effect and susceptibility to hypoglycemia).
No products indexed under this heading.

Penbutolol Sulfate (May potentiate or weaken the blood-glucose-lowering effect of insulin. The signs of hypoglycemia may be reduced or absent.).
No products indexed under this heading.

Pentamidine Isethionate (May cause hypoglycemia, which may sometimes be followed by hyperglycemia).
No products indexed under this heading.

Perindopril Erbumine (Substances that may increase the blood-glucose-lowering effect and susceptibility to hypoglycemia). Products include:

Perphenazine (Substances that may reduce the blood-glucose-lowering effect).
No products indexed under this heading.

Phenelzine Sulfate (Substances that may increase the blood-glucose-lowering effect and susceptibility to hypoglycemia).
No products indexed under this heading.

Phenylephrine Bitartrate (Substances that may reduce the blood-glucose-lowering effect).
No products indexed under this heading.

Phenylephrine Hydrochloride (Substances that may reduce the blood-glucose-lowering effect). Products include:

IMPORTANT NOTE: Always consult each drug listing in the patient's regimen for possible interactions.

Phenylephrine Tannate (Substances that may reduce the blood-glucose-lowering effect).
 No products indexed under this heading.

Phenylpropanolamine Hydrochloride (Substances that may reduce the blood-glucose-lowering effect).
 No products indexed under this heading.

Pindolol (May potentiate or weaken the blood-glucose-lowering effect of insulin. The signs of hypoglycemia may be reduced or absent.).
 No products indexed under this heading.

Pirbuterol Acetate (Substances that may reduce the blood-glucose-lowering effect). Products include:
 Maxair Autohaler 1852

Polyestradiol Phosphate (Substances that may reduce the blood-glucose-lowering effect).
 No products indexed under this heading.

Polythiazide (Substances that may increase the blood-glucose-lowering effect and susceptibility to hypoglycemia).
 No products indexed under this heading.

Prednisolone Acetate (Substances that may reduce the blood-glucose-lowering effect). Products include:
 Blephamide Ophthalmic Ointment 568
 Blephamide Ophthalmic Suspension.................................. 569
 Poly-Pred Ophthalmic Suspension ⊙233
 Pred Forte Ophthalmic Suspension ⊙235
 Pred Mild Ophthalmic Suspension ⊙238
 Pred-G Ophthalmic Ointment ⊙237
 Pred-G Ophthalmic Suspension ⊙236

Prednisolone Sodium Phosphate (Substances that may reduce the blood-glucose-lowering effect).
 No products indexed under this heading.

Prednisolone Tebutate (Substances that may reduce the blood-glucose-lowering effect).
 No products indexed under this heading.

Prednisone (Substances that may reduce the blood-glucose-lowering effect).
 No products indexed under this heading.

Procarbazine Hydrochloride (Substances that may increase the

blood-glucose-lowering effect and susceptibility to hypoglycemia).
Products include:
 Matulane Capsules 3191

Prochlorperazine (Substances that may reduce the blood-glucose-lowering effect).
 No products indexed under this heading.

Promethazine Hydrochloride (Substances that may reduce the blood-glucose-lowering effect). Products include:
 Phenergan Tablets and Suppositories................................ 3440

Propoxyphene Hydrochloride (Substances that may increase the blood-glucose-lowering effect and susceptibility to hypoglycemia).
 No products indexed under this heading.

Propoxyphene Napsylate (Substances that may increase the blood-glucose-lowering effect and susceptibility to hypoglycemia).
 No products indexed under this heading.

Propranolol Hydrochloride (May potentiate or weaken the blood-glucose-lowering effect of insulin. The signs of hypoglycemia may be reduced or absent). Products include:
 Inderal LA Long-Acting Capsules 3429
 InnoPran XL Capsules 2723

Pseudoephedrine Hydrochloride (Substances that may reduce the blood-glucose-lowering effect). Products include:
 Advil Allergy Sinus Caplets ▣□770
 Advil Cold & Sinus ▣□723
 Advil Multi-Symptom Cold Caplets................................ ▣□770
 Aleve Cold & Sinus Caplets 744
 Allegra-D 12 Hour Extended-Release Tablets............. 2846
 Allegra-D 24 Hour Extended-Release Tablets............. 2849
 BC Cold Powder ▣□677
 Comtrex Maximum Strength Cold & Cough Day/Night Caplets - Day Formulation....................... ▣□726
 Comtrex Maximum Strength Cold & Cough Day/Night Caplets - Night Formulation..................... ▣□726
 Children's Motrin Cold Oral Suspension............................. 1867
 Mucinex D Extended-Release Bi-Layer Tablets........................ ▣□776
 Robitussin Cough & Cold CF Liquid................................ ▣□735
 Robitussin Cough & Cold Pediatric Drops......................... ▣□735
 Tylenol Sinus Congestion & Pain Nighttime Caplets with Cool Burst................................ ▣□778
 Tylenol Cold Severe Congestion Non-Drowsy Caplets with Cool Burst................................ 1874
 Tylenol Sinus Severe Congestion Caplets with Cool Burst 1876
 Vicks 44D Cough & Head Congestion Relief Liquid............. 2679
 Vicks 44M Cough, Cold & Flu Relief Liquid........................... 2680
 Vicks DayQuil Multi-Symptom Cold/Flu Relief LiquiCaps............. 2678
 Vicks DayQuil Multi-Symptom Cold/Flu Relief Liquid.................. 2678
 Vicks NyQuil Multi-Symptom Cold/Flu Relief Liquid.................. 2681
 Vicks NyQuil Multi-Symptom Cold/Flu Relief LiquiCaps............. 2681
 Children's Vicks NyQuil Cold/Cough Relief Liquid.............. 2680
 Zyrtec-D 12 Hour Extended Release Tablets....................... 2597

Pseudoephedrine Sulfate (Substances that may reduce the blood-glucose-lowering effect). Products include:

Alavert Allergy & Sinus D-12 Hour Tablets................................ ▣□771
Clarinex-D 24-Hour Extended-Release Tablets............. 2998
Claritin-D Non-Drowsy 12 Hour Tablets................................ ▣□772
Claritin-D Non-Drowsy 24 Hour Tablets................................ ▣□772

Quinapril Hydrochloride (Substances that may increase the blood-glucose-lowering effect and susceptibility to hypoglycemia).
 No products indexed under this heading.

Quinestrol (Substances that may reduce the blood-glucose-lowering effect).
 No products indexed under this heading.

Ramipril (Substances that may increase the blood-glucose-lowering effect and susceptibility to hypoglycemia). Products include:
 Altace Capsules 1702

Reserpine (The signs of hypoglycemia may be reduced or absent when under the influence of reserpine).
 No products indexed under this heading.

Salmeterol Xinafoate (Substances that may reduce the blood-glucose-lowering effect). Products include:
 Advair Diskus 100/50 1308
 Advair Diskus 250/50 1308
 Advair Diskus 500/50 1308
 Advair HFA Inhalation Aerosol 1318
 Serevent Diskus 1568

Selegiline Hydrochloride (Substances that may increase the blood-glucose-lowering effect and susceptibility to hypoglycemia). Products include:
 Eldepryl Capsules 3208
 Zelapar Tablets 3372

Somatropin (Substances that may reduce the blood-glucose-lowering effect). Products include:
 Genotropin Lyophilized Powder 2638
 Humatrope Vials and Cartridges 1787
 Norditropin Cartridges 2323
 Nutropin for Injection 1239
 Nutropin AQ Injection 1243
 Nutropin AQ Pen 1243
 Nutropin AQ Pen Cartridge 1243

Sotalol Hydrochloride (May potentiate or weaken the blood-glucose-lowering effect of insulin. The signs of hypoglycemia may be reduced or absent).
 No products indexed under this heading.

Spirapril Hydrochloride (Substances that may increase the blood-glucose-lowering effect and susceptibility to hypoglycemia).
 No products indexed under this heading.

Spironolactone (Substances that may reduce the blood-glucose-lowering effect).
 No products indexed under this heading.

Sulfacytine (Substances that may increase the blood-glucose-lowering effect and susceptibility to hypoglycemia).
 No products indexed under this heading.

Sulfamethizole (Substances that may increase the blood-glucose-lowering effect and susceptibility to hypoglycemia).
 No products indexed under this heading.

Sulfamethoxazole (Substances that may increase the blood-glucose-lowering effect and susceptibility to hypoglycemia).
No products indexed under this heading.

Sulfasalazine (Substances that may increase the blood-glucose-lowering effect and susceptibility to hypoglycemia).
No products indexed under this heading.

Sulfinpyrazone (Substances that may increase the blood-glucose-lowering effect and susceptibility to hypoglycemia).
No products indexed under this heading.

Sulfisoxazole Acetyl (Substances that may increase the blood-glucose-lowering effect and susceptibility to hypoglycemia).
No products indexed under this heading.

Sulfisoxazole Diolamine (Substances that may increase the blood-glucose-lowering effect and susceptibility to hypoglycemia).
No products indexed under this heading.

Terbutaline Sulfate (Substances that may reduce the blood-glucose-lowering effect).
No products indexed under this heading.

Thioridazine Hydrochloride (Substances that may reduce the blood-glucose-lowering effect). Products include:
Thioridazine Hydrochloride Tablets **2163**

Thyroglobulin (Substances that may reduce the blood-glucose-lowering effect).
No products indexed under this heading.

Thyroid (Substances that may reduce the blood-glucose-lowering effect).
No products indexed under this heading.

Thyroxine (Substances that may reduce the blood-glucose-lowering effect).
No products indexed under this heading.

Thyroxine Sodium (Substances that may reduce the blood-glucose-lowering effect).
No products indexed under this heading.

Timolol Hemihydrate (May potentiate or weaken the blood-glucose-lowering effect of insulin. The signs of hypoglycemia may be reduced or absent). Products include:
Betimol Ophthalmic Solution **3382**
Betimol Ophthalmic Solution .... ⊙**295**

Timolol Maleate (May potentiate or weaken the blood-glucose-lowering effect of insulin. The signs of hypoglycemia may be reduced or absent). Products include:
Blocadren Tablets **1916**
Cosopt Sterile Ophthalmic Solution **1931**
Timolide Tablets **2086**
Timoptic Sterile Ophthalmic Solution **2088**
Timoptic in Ocudose **2091**
Timoptic-XE Sterile Ophthalmic Gel Forming Solution **2092**

Tolazamide (Substances that may increase the blood-glucose-lowering effect and susceptibility to hypoglycemia).
No products indexed under this heading.

Tolbutamide (Substances that may increase the blood-glucose-lowering effect and susceptibility to hypoglycemia).
No products indexed under this heading.

Torsemide (Substances that may reduce the blood-glucose-lowering effect). Products include:
Demadex Injection **2759**
Demadex Tablets **2759**

Trandolapril (Substances that may increase the blood-glucose-lowering effect and susceptibility to hypoglycemia). Products include:
Mavik Tablets **486**
Tarka Tablets **524**

Tranylcypromine Sulfate (Substances that may increase the blood-glucose-lowering effect and susceptibility to hypoglycemia). Products include:
Parnate Tablets **1527**

Triamcinolone (Substances that may reduce the blood-glucose-lowering effect).
No products indexed under this heading.

Triamcinolone Acetonide (Substances that may reduce the blood-glucose-lowering effect). Products include:
Azmacort Inhalation Aerosol **1726**
Nasacort AQ Nasal Spray **2922**

Triamcinolone Diacetate (Substances that may reduce the blood-glucose-lowering effect).
No products indexed under this heading.

Triamcinolone Hexacetonide (Substances that may reduce the blood-glucose-lowering effect).
No products indexed under this heading.

Triamterene (Substances that may reduce the blood-glucose-lowering effect). Products include:
Dyazide Capsules **1423**
Dyrenium Capsules **3400**

Trifluoperazine Hydrochloride (Substances that may reduce the blood-glucose-lowering effect).
No products indexed under this heading.

NOVOSEVEN
(Antihemophilic Factor (Recombinant)) **2331**
None cited in PDR database.

NU-IRON 150 CAPSULES
(Polysaccharide Iron Complex) **2127**
None cited in PDR database.

NUMORPHAN INJECTION
(Oxymorphone Hydrochloride) **1120**
May interact with anticholinergics, central nervous system depressants, general anesthetics, hypnotics and sedatives, monoamine oxidase inhibitors, narcotic analgesics, phenothiazines, tranquilizers, tricyclic antidepressants, and certain other agents. Compounds in these categories include:

Alfentanil Hydrochloride (Concomitant use may produce additive CNS depressant effects).
No products indexed under this heading.

Alprazolam (Concomitant use may produce additive CNS depressant effects). Products include:
Niravam Orally Disintegrating Tablets **3092**

Amitriptyline Hydrochloride (Concomitant use may produce additive CNS depressant effects).
No products indexed under this heading.

Amoxapine (Concomitant use may produce additive CNS depressant effects).
No products indexed under this heading.

Aprobarbital (Concomitant use may produce additive CNS depressant effects).
No products indexed under this heading.

Atropine Sulfate (Co-administration of anticholinergics and opiod analgesics may result in increased risk of urinary retention and/or severe constipation and paralytic ileus). Products include:
Donnatal Extentabs **2493**

Belladonna Alkaloids (Co-administration of anticholinergics and opiod analgesics may result in increased risk of urinary retention and/or severe constipation and paralytic ileus). Products include:
Hyland's Teething Tablets .... ⊡**830**

Benztropine Mesylate (Co-administration of anticholinergics and opiod analgesics may result in increased risk of urinary retention and/or severe constipation and paralytic ileus).
No products indexed under this heading.

Biperiden Hydrochloride (Co-administration of anticholinergics and opiod analgesics may result in increased risk of urinary retention and/or severe constipation and paralytic ileus).
No products indexed under this heading.

Buprenorphine Hydrochloride (Concomitant use may produce additive CNS depressant effects). Products include:
Buprenex Injectable **2716**
Suboxone Tablets **2717**
Subutex Tablets **2717**

Buspirone Hydrochloride (Concomitant use may produce additive CNS depressant effects).
No products indexed under this heading.

Butabarbital (Concomitant use may produce additive CNS depressant effects).
No products indexed under this heading.

Butalbital (Concomitant use may produce additive CNS depressant effects).
No products indexed under this heading.

Chlordiazepoxide (Concomitant use may produce additive CNS depressant effects).
No products indexed under this heading.

Chlordiazepoxide Hydrochloride (Concomitant use may produce additive CNS depressant effects). Products include:
Librium Capsules **3347**

Chlorpromazine (Concomitant use may produce additive CNS depressant effects).
No products indexed under this heading.

Chlorpromazine Hydrochloride (Concomitant use may produce additive CNS depressant effects).
No products indexed under this heading.

Chlorprothixene (Concomitant use may produce additive CNS depressant effects).
No products indexed under this heading.

Chlorprothixene Hydrochloride (Concomitant use may produce additive CNS depressant effects).
No products indexed under this heading.

Chlorprothixene Lactate (Concomitant use may produce additive CNS depressant effects).
No products indexed under this heading.

Cimetidine (Co-administration of cimetidine and opioid analgesics has resulted in confusion, disorientation, respiratory depression, apnea, and seizures; no clear-cut cause and effect relationship was established). Products include:
Tagamet HB 200 Tablets .... ⊡**664**

Cimetidine Hydrochloride (Co-administration of cimetidine and opioid analgesics has resulted in confusion, disorientation, respiratory depression, apnea, and seizures; no clear-cut cause and effect relationship was established).
No products indexed under this heading.

Clidinium Bromide (Co-administration of anticholinergics and opiod analgesics may result in increased risk of urinary retention and/or severe constipation and paralytic ileus).
No products indexed under this heading.

Clomipramine Hydrochloride (Concomitant use may produce additive CNS depressant effects).
No products indexed under this heading.

Clorazepate Dipotassium (Concomitant use may produce additive CNS depressant effects). Products include:
Tranxene **2474**

Clozapine (Concomitant use may produce additive CNS depressant effects). Products include:
Clozaril Tablets **2184**
FazaClo Orally Disintegrating Tablets **551**

Codeine Phosphate (Concomitant use may produce additive CNS depressant effects). Products include:
Tylenol with Codeine Tablets **2391**

Desflurane (Concomitant use may produce additive CNS depressant effects).
No products indexed under this heading.

Desipramine Hydrochloride (Concomitant use may produce additive CNS depressant effects).
No products indexed under this heading.

Dezocine (Concomitant use may produce additive CNS depressant effects).
No products indexed under this heading.

Diazepam (Concomitant use may produce additive CNS depressant effects). Products include:
Diastat Rectal Delivery System **3343**
Valium Tablets **2819**

Dicyclomine Hydrochloride (Co-administration of anticholinergics and opioid analgesics may result in increased risk of urinary retention and/or severe constipation and paralytic ileus). Products include:
Bentyl Capsules ... 697
Bentyl Injection ... 697
Bentyl Syrup ... 697
Bentyl Tablets ... 697

Doxepin Hydrochloride (Concomitant use may produce additive CNS depressant effects).
No products indexed under this heading.

Droperidol (Concomitant use may produce additive CNS depressant effects).
No products indexed under this heading.

Enflurane (Concomitant use may produce additive CNS depressant effects).
No products indexed under this heading.

Estazolam (Concomitant use may produce additive CNS depressant effects). Products include:
ProSom Tablets ... 517

Ethanol (Concomitant use may produce additive CNS depressant effects).
No products indexed under this heading.

Ethchlorvynol (Concomitant use may produce additive CNS depressant effects).
No products indexed under this heading.

Ethinamate (Concomitant use may produce additive CNS depressant effects).
No products indexed under this heading.

Ethyl Alcohol (Concomitant use may produce additive CNS depressant effects).
No products indexed under this heading.

Fentanyl (Concomitant use may produce additive CNS depressant effects). Products include:
Duragesic Transdermal System ... 2373
Ionsys Transdermal System ... 2379

Fentanyl Citrate (Concomitant use may produce additive CNS depressant effects). Products include:
Actiq ... 979

Fluphenazine Decanoate (Concomitant use may produce additive CNS depressant effects).
No products indexed under this heading.

Fluphenazine Enanthate (Concomitant use may produce additive CNS depressant effects).
No products indexed under this heading.

Fluphenazine Hydrochloride (Concomitant use may produce additive CNS depressant effects).
No products indexed under this heading.

Flurazepam Hydrochloride (Concomitant use may produce additive CNS depressant effects). Products include:
Dalmane Capsules ... 3342

Glutethimide (Concomitant use may produce additive CNS depressant effects).
No products indexed under this heading.

Glycopyrrolate (Co-administration of anticholinergics and opioid analgesics may result in increased risk of urinary retention and/or severe constipation and paralytic ileus).
No products indexed under this heading.

Haloperidol (Concomitant use may produce additive CNS depressant effects).
No products indexed under this heading.

Haloperidol Decanoate (Concomitant use may produce additive CNS depressant effects).
No products indexed under this heading.

Hydrocodone Bitartrate (Concomitant use may produce additive CNS depressant effects). Products include:
Hycodan ... 1116
Hycotuss Expectorant Syrup ... 1117
Vicodin Tablets ... 535
Vicodin ES Tablets ... 536
Vicodin HP Tablets ... 538
Vicoprofen Tablets ... 539
Zydone Tablets ... 1139

Hydrocodone Polistirex (Concomitant use may produce additive CNS depressant effects). Products include:
Tussionex Pennkinetic Extended-Release Suspension ... 3327

Hydromorphone Hydrochloride (Concomitant use may produce additive CNS depressant effects). Products include:
Dilaudid ... 440
Dilaudid Non-Sterile Powder ... 440
Dilaudid Oral Liquid ... 445
Dilaudid Rectal Suppositories ... 440
Dilaudid Tablets ... 440
Dilaudid Tablets - 8 mg ... 445
Dilaudid-HP ... 442

Hydroxyzine Hydrochloride (Concomitant use may produce additive CNS depressant effects).
No products indexed under this heading.

Hyoscyamine (Co-administration of anticholinergics and opioid analgesics may result in increased risk of urinary retention and/or severe constipation and paralytic ileus).
No products indexed under this heading.

Hyoscyamine Sulfate (Co-administration of anticholinergics and opioid analgesics may result in increased risk of urinary retention and/or severe constipation and paralytic ileus). Products include:
Donnatal Extentabs ... 2493
Prosed/DS Tablets ... 1157

Imipramine Hydrochloride (Concomitant use may produce additive CNS depressant effects).
No products indexed under this heading.

Imipramine Pamoate (Concomitant use may produce additive CNS depressant effects).
No products indexed under this heading.

Ipratropium Bromide (Co-administration of anticholinergics and opioid analgesics may result in increased risk of urinary retention and/or severe constipation and paralytic ileus). Products include:
Atrovent Inhalation Solution ... 835
Atrovent HFA Inhalation Aerosol ... 841
Atrovent Nasal Spray 0.03% ... 837
Atrovent Nasal Spray 0.06% ... 839
Combivent Inhalation Aerosol ... 847
DuoNeb Inhalation Solution ... 1058

Isocarboxazid (Concomitant use may produce additive CNS depressant effects).
No products indexed under this heading.

Isoflurane (Concomitant use may produce additive CNS depressant effects).
No products indexed under this heading.

Ketamine Hydrochloride (Concomitant use may produce additive CNS depressant effects).
No products indexed under this heading.

Levomethadyl Acetate Hydrochloride (Concomitant use may produce additive CNS depressant effects).
No products indexed under this heading.

Levorphanol Tartrate (Concomitant use may produce additive CNS depressant effects).
No products indexed under this heading.

Lorazepam (Concomitant use may produce additive CNS depressant effects).
No products indexed under this heading.

Loxapine Hydrochloride (Concomitant use may produce additive CNS depressant effects).
No products indexed under this heading.

Loxapine Succinate (Concomitant use may produce additive CNS depressant effects).
No products indexed under this heading.

Maprotiline Hydrochloride (Concomitant use may produce additive CNS depressant effects).
No products indexed under this heading.

Mepenzolate Bromide (Co-administration of anticholinergics and opioid analgesics may result in increased risk of urinary retention and/or severe constipation and paralytic ileus).
No products indexed under this heading.

Meperidine Hydrochloride (Concomitant use may produce additive CNS depressant effects).
No products indexed under this heading.

Mephobarbital (Concomitant use may produce additive CNS depressant effects).
No products indexed under this heading.

Meprobamate (Concomitant use may produce additive CNS depressant effects).
No products indexed under this heading.

Mesoridazine Besylate (Concomitant use may produce additive CNS depressant effects).
No products indexed under this heading.

Methadone Hydrochloride (Concomitant use may produce additive CNS depressant effects).
No products indexed under this heading.

Methohexital Sodium (Concomitant use may produce additive CNS depressant effects).
No products indexed under this heading.

Methotrimeprazine (Concomitant use may produce additive CNS depressant effects).
No products indexed under this heading.

Methoxyflurane (Concomitant use may produce additive CNS depressant effects).
No products indexed under this heading.

Midazolam Hydrochloride (Concomitant use may produce additive CNS depressant effects).
No products indexed under this heading.

Moclobemide (Concomitant use may produce additive CNS depressant effects).
No products indexed under this heading.

Molindone Hydrochloride (Concomitant use may produce additive CNS depressant effects). Products include:
Moban Tablets ... 1119

Morphine Sulfate (Concomitant use may produce additive CNS depressant effects). Products include:
Avinza Capsules ... 1741
Kadian Capsules ... 577
MS Contin Tablets ... 2701

Nortriptyline Hydrochloride (Concomitant use may produce additive CNS depressant effects).
No products indexed under this heading.

Olanzapine (Concomitant use may produce additive CNS depressant effects). Products include:
Symbyax Capsules ... 1819
Zyprexa Tablets ... 1830
Zyprexa IntraMuscular ... 1830
Zyprexa ZYDIS Orally Disintegrating Tablets ... 1830

Oxazepam (Concomitant use may produce additive CNS depressant effects).
No products indexed under this heading.

Oxybutynin Chloride (Co-administration of anticholinergics and opioid analgesics may result in increased risk of urinary retention and/or severe constipation and paralytic ileus). Products include:
Ditropan XL Extended-Release Tablets ... 2413

Oxycodone Hydrochloride (Concomitant use may produce additive CNS depressant effects). Products include:
OxyContin Tablets ... 2703
OxyFast Oral Concentrate Solution ... 2708
OxyIR Capsules ... 2708
Percocet Tablets ... 1131
Percodan Tablets ... 1132

Pargyline Hydrochloride (Concomitant use may produce additive CNS depressant effects).
No products indexed under this heading.

Pentobarbital Sodium (Concomitant use may produce additive CNS depressant effects). Products include:
Nembutal Sodium Solution, USP ... 2470

Perphenazine (Concomitant use may produce additive CNS depressant effects).
No products indexed under this heading.

Phenelzine Sulfate (Concomitant use may produce additive CNS depressant effects).
No products indexed under this heading.

Phenobarbital (Concomitant use may produce additive CNS depressant effects). Products include:
Donnatal Extentabs 2493

Prazepam (Concomitant use may produce additive CNS depressant effects).
No products indexed under this heading.

Procarbazine Hydrochloride (Concomitant use may produce additive CNS depressant effects). Products include:
Matulane Capsules 3191

Prochlorperazine (Concomitant use may produce additive CNS depressant effects).
No products indexed under this heading.

Procyclidine Hydrochloride (Co-administration of anticholinergics and opiod analgesics may result in increased risk of urinary retention and/or severe constipation and paralytic ileus).
No products indexed under this heading.

Promethazine Hydrochloride (Concomitant use may produce additive CNS depressant effects). Products include:
Phenergan Tablets and Suppositories 3440

Propantheline Bromide (Co-administration of anticholinergics and opiod analgesics may result in increased risk of urinary retention and/or severe constipation and paralytic ileus).
No products indexed under this heading.

Propofol (Co-administration has resulted in increased incidence of bradycardia; concomitant use may produce additive CNS depressant effects).
No products indexed under this heading.

Propoxyphene Hydrochloride (Concomitant use may produce additive CNS depressant effects).
No products indexed under this heading.

Propoxyphene Napsylate (Concomitant use may produce additive CNS depressant effects).
No products indexed under this heading.

Protriptyline Hydrochloride (Concomitant use may produce additive CNS depressant effects).
No products indexed under this heading.

Quazepam (Concomitant use may produce additive CNS depressant effects).
No products indexed under this heading.

Quetiapine Fumarate (Concomitant use may produce additive CNS depressant effects). Products include:
Seroquel Tablets 690

Ramelteon (Concomitant use may produce additive CNS depressant effects). Products include:
Rozerem Tablets 3231

Remifentanil Hydrochloride (Concomitant use may produce additive CNS depressant effects).
No products indexed under this heading.

Risperidone (Concomitant use may produce additive CNS depressant effects). Products include:
Risperdal 1676
Risperdal Consta Long-Acting Injection 1682
Risperdal M-Tab Orally Disintegrating Tablets 1676

Scopolamine (Co-administration of anticholinergics and opiod analgesics may result in increased risk of urinary retention and/or severe constipation and paralytic ileus). Products include:
Transderm Scōp Transdermal Therapeutic System 2177

Scopolamine Hydrobromide (Co-administration of anticholinergics and opiod analgesics may result in increased risk of urinary retention and/or severe constipation and paralytic ileus). Products include:
Donnatal Extentabs 2493

Secobarbital Sodium (Concomitant use may produce additive CNS depressant effects).
No products indexed under this heading.

Selegiline Hydrochloride (Concomitant use may produce additive CNS depressant effects). Products include:
Eldepryl Capsules 3208
Zelapar Tablets 3372

Sevoflurane (Concomitant use may produce additive CNS depressant effects). Products include:
Ultane Liquid for Inhalation 531

Sodium Oxybate (Concomitant use may produce additive CNS depressant effects). Products include:
Xyrem Oral Solution 1688

Sufentanil Citrate (Concomitant use may produce additive CNS depressant effects).
No products indexed under this heading.

Temazepam (Concomitant use may produce additive CNS depressant effects). Products include:
Restoril Capsules 1860

Thiamylal Sodium (Concomitant use may produce additive CNS depressant effects).
No products indexed under this heading.

Thioridazine Hydrochloride (Concomitant use may produce additive CNS depressant effects). Products include:
Thioridazine Hydrochloride Tablets 2163

Thiothixene (Concomitant use may produce additive CNS depressant effects). Products include:
Thiothixene Capsules 2165

Tolterodine Tartrate (Co-administration of anticholinergics and opiod analgesics may result in increased risk of urinary retention and/or severe constipation and paralytic ileus). Products include:
Detrol Tablets 2628
Detrol LA Capsules 2631

Tranylcypromine Sulfate (Concomitant use may produce additive CNS depressant effects). Products include:
Parnate Tablets 1527

Triazolam (Concomitant use may produce additive CNS depressant effects).
No products indexed under this heading.

Tridihexethyl Chloride (Co-administration of anticholinergics and opiod analgesics may result in increased risk of urinary retention and/or severe constipation and paralytic ileus).
No products indexed under this heading.

Trifluoperazine Hydrochloride (Concomitant use may produce additive CNS depressant effects).
No products indexed under this heading.

Trihexyphenidyl Hydrochloride (Co-administration of anticholinergics and opiod analgesics may result in increased risk of urinary retention and/or severe constipation and paralytic ileus).
No products indexed under this heading.

Trimipramine Maleate (Concomitant use may produce additive CNS depressant effects).
No products indexed under this heading.

Zaleplon (Concomitant use may produce additive CNS depressant effects). Products include:
Sonata Capsules 1717

Ziprasidone Hydrochloride (Concomitant use may produce additive CNS depressant effects). Products include:
Geodon Capsules 2529

Zolpidem Tartrate (Concomitant use may produce additive CNS depressant effects). Products include:
Ambien Tablets 2851
Ambien CR Tablets 2855

Food Interactions

Alcohol (Concomitant use may produce additive CNS depressant effects).

NUTROPIN FOR INJECTION
(Somatropin) 1239
May interact with corticosteroids, phenytoin, and certain other agents. Compounds in these categories include:

Betamethasone Acetate (Excessive glucocorticoid therapy will inhibit the growth-promoting effect of human growth hormone).
No products indexed under this heading.

Betamethasone Sodium Phosphate (Excessive glucocorticoid therapy will inhibit the growth-promoting effect of human growth hormone).
No products indexed under this heading.

Carbamazepine (Limited published data suggests that growth hormone treatment increased CYP450 mediated antipyrine clearance in man; therefore, growth hormone administration may alter the clearance of compounds known to be metabolized by CYP450 liver enzymes, such as anticonvulsanta including carbamazepine). Products include:
Carbatrol Capsules 3171
Equetro Extended-Release Capsules 3180
Tegretol/Tegretol-XR 2295

Cortisone Acetate (Excessive glucocorticoid therapy will inhibit the growth-promoting effect of human growth hormone).
No products indexed under this heading.

Cyclosporine (Limited published data suggests that growth hormone treatment increases CYP450 mediated antipyrine clearance in man, therefore, growth hormone administration may alter the clearance of compounds known to be metabolized by CYP450 liver enzymes, such as cyclosporine). Products include:
Gengraf Capsules 459
Neoral Oral Solution 2259
Neoral Soft Gelatin Capsules 2259
Restasis Ophthalmic Emulsion 575
Sandimmune 2275

Dexamethasone (Excessive glucocorticoid therapy will inhibit the growth-promoting effect of human growth hormone). Products include:
Ciprodex Otic Suspension 559
Decadron Tablets 1951
TobraDex Ophthalmic Ointment 562
TobraDex Ophthalmic Suspension 563

Dexamethasone Acetate (Excessive glucocorticoid therapy will inhibit the growth-promoting effect of human growth hormone).
No products indexed under this heading.

Dexamethasone Sodium Phosphate (Excessive glucocorticoid therapy will inhibit the growth-promoting effect of human growth hormone).
No products indexed under this heading.

Fludrocortisone Acetate (Excessive glucocorticoid therapy will inhibit the growth-promoting effect of human growth hormone).
No products indexed under this heading.

Fosphenytoin Sodium (Limited published data suggests that growth hormone treatment increases CYP450 mediated antipyrine clearance in man; therefore, growth hormone administration may alter the clearance of compounds known to be metabolized by CYP450 liver enzymes, such as anticonvulsants, including phenytoin).
No products indexed under this heading.

Hydrocortisone (Excessive glucocorticoid therapy will inhibit the growth-promoting effect of human growth hormone). Products include:
Colocort Rectal Suspension, USP (Retention) 100 mg/60 mL 2476
Hydrocortone Tablets 1989
Preparation H Hydrocortisone Cream 646

Hydrocortisone Acetate (Excessive glucocorticoid therapy will inhibit the growth-promoting effect of human growth hormone). Products include:
Analpram-HC 1159
Pramosone 1161
ProctoFoam-HC 3099

Hydrocortisone Sodium Phosphate (Excessive glucocorticoid therapy will inhibit the growth-promoting effect of human growth hormone).
No products indexed under this heading.

Hydrocortisone Sodium Succinate (Excessive glucocorticoid therapy will inhibit the growth-promoting effect of human growth hormone).
No products indexed under this heading.

Methylprednisolone Acetate (Excessive glucocorticoid therapy will inhibit the growth-promoting effect of human growth hormone). Products include:
Depo-Medrol Injectable Suspension 2617
Depo-Medrol Single-Dose Vial 2619

Methylprednisolone Sodium Succinate (Excessive glucocorticoid therapy will inhibit the growth-promoting effect of human growth hormone).
No products indexed under this heading.

Phenytoin (Limited published data suggests that growth hormone treatment increases CYP450 mediated antipyrine clearance in man; therefore, growth hormone administration may alter the clearance of compounds known to be metabolized by CYP450 liver enzymes, such as anticonvulsants, including phenytoin).
No products indexed under this heading.

Phenytoin Sodium (Limited published data suggests that growth hormone treatment increases CYP450 mediated antipyrine clearance in man; therefore, growth hormone administration may alter the clearance of compounds known to be metabolized by CYP450 liver enzymes, such as anticonvulsants, including phenytoin). Products include:
Phenytek Capsules 2160

Prednisolone Acetate (Excessive glucocorticoid therapy will inhibit the growth-promoting effect of human growth hormone). Products include:
Blephamide Ophthalmic Ointment 568
Blephamide Ophthalmic Suspension 569
Poly-Pred Ophthalmic Suspension .... ⊙233
Pred Forte Ophthalmic Suspension .... ⊙235
Pred Mild Ophthalmic Suspension .... ⊙238
Pred-G Ophthalmic Ointment .... ⊙237
Pred-G Ophthalmic Suspension .... ⊙236

Prednisolone Sodium Phosphate (Excessive glucocorticoid therapy will inhibit the growth-promoting effect of human growth hormone).
No products indexed under this heading.

Prednisolone Tebutate (Excessive glucocorticoid therapy will inhibit the growth-promoting effect of human growth hormone).
No products indexed under this heading.

Prednisone (Excessive glucocorticoid therapy will inhibit the growth-promoting effect of human growth hormone).
No products indexed under this heading.

Triamcinolone (Excessive glucocorticoid therapy will inhibit the growth-promoting effect of human growth hormone).
No products indexed under this heading.

Triamcinolone Acetonide (Excessive glucocorticoid therapy will inhibit the growth-promoting effect of human growth hormone). Products include:
Azmacort Inhalation Aerosol 1726
Nasacort AQ Nasal Spray 2922

Triamcinolone Diacetate (Excessive glucocorticoid therapy will inhibit the growth-promoting effect of human growth hormone).
No products indexed under this heading.

Triamcinolone Hexacetonide (Excessive glucocorticoid therapy will inhibit the growth-promoting effect of human growth hormone).
No products indexed under this heading.

NUTROPIN AQ INJECTION

(Somatropin) 1243
See Nutropin for Injection

NUTROPIN AQ PEN

(Somatropin) 1243
See Nutropin for Injection

NUTROPIN AQ PEN CARTRIDGE

(Somatropin) 1243
See Nutropin for Injection

NUVARING

(Ethinyl Estradiol, Etonogestrel) 2340
May interact with azole antifungals, barbiturates, cytochrome p450 3a4 inhibitors (selected), anticonvulsants, protease inhibitors, theophyllines, and certain other agents. Compounds in these categories include:

Acetaminophen (Acetaminophen may increase plasma ethinyl estradiol levels. Decreased plasma concentrations of acetaminophen have been noted when administered with oral contraceptives). Products include:
Comtrex Maximum Strength Cold & Cough Day/Night Caplets - Day Formulation .... ▣726
Comtrex Maximum Strength Cold & Cough Day/Night Caplets - Night Formulation .... ▣726
Comtrex Maximum Strength Non-Drowsy Cold & Cough Caplets .... ▣725
Comtrex Maximum Strength Day/Night Severe Cold & Sinus Caplets - Day Formulation .... ▣725
Comtrex Maximum Strength Day/Night Severe Cold & Sinus Caplets - Night Formulation .... ▣725
Contac Cold and Flu Maximum Strength Caplets .... ▣728
Contac Cold and Flu Day and Night Caplets (Day Formulation Only) .... ▣727
Contac Cold and Flu Day and Night Caplets (Night Formulation Only) .... ▣727
Contac Cold and Flu Non-Drowsy Caplets .... ▣728
Excedrin Extra Strength Caplets/Tablets/Geltabs .... ▣684
Excedrin Migraine Caplets/Tablets/Geltabs .... ▣609
Excedrin PM Caplets/Tablets/Geltabs .... ▣610
Excedrin Sinus Headache Caplets/Tablets .... ▣610
Excedrin Tension Headache Caplets/Tablets/Geltabs .... ▣611
Goody's Body Pain Formula Powder .... ▣684
Goody's Extra Strength Headache Powders .... ▣611
Goody's Extra Strength Pain Relief Tablets .... ▣685
Goody's PM Powder for Pain with Sleeplessness .... ▣612
Percocet Tablets 1131
Robitussin Cough, Cold & Flu Nighttime Liquid .... ▣738
TheraFlu Cold & Sore Throat Hot Liquid .... ▣741
TheraFlu Flu & Chest Congestion Hot Liquid .... ▣741
TheraFlu Flu & Sore Throat Hot Liquid .... ▣742
TheraFlu Daytime Severe Cold Hot Liquid .... ▣742
TheraFlu Nighttime Severe Cold Hot Liquid .... ▣740
TheraFlu Warming Relief Daytime Severe Cold .... ▣743
TheraFlu Warming Relief Nighttime Severe Cold .... ▣743
Triaminic Cough & Sore Throat Liquid .... ▣747
Regular Strength Tylenol Tablets 1870
Children's Tylenol with Flavor Creator .... ▣679
Children's Tylenol Plus Flu Oral Suspension .... ▣749
Tylenol Cold Head Congestion Daytime Caplets with Cool Burst and Gelcaps .... ▣750
Tylenol Cold Multi-Symptom Daytime Liquid .... ▣752
Tylenol Cold Multi-Symptom Severe Daytime Liquid .... ▣752
Tylenol 8 Hour Extended Release Caplets 1870
Tylenol 1870
Extra Strength Tylenol PM Caplets, Vanilla Caplets, Geltabs, Gelcaps and Liquid 1875
Extra Strength Tylenol Rapid Release Gels 1870
Concentrated Tylenol Infants' Drops Plus Cold & Cough .... ▣754
Tylenol with Codeine Tablets 2391
Tylenol Allergy Multi-Symptom Caplets with Cool Burst and Gelcaps 1872
Tylenol Allergy Multi-Symptom Nighttime Caplets with Cool Burst 1872
Tylenol Severe Allergy Caplets 1872
Tylenol Arthritis Pain Extended Release Caplets and Geltabs 1870
Tylenol Chest Congestion Caplets with Cool Burst 1872
Tylenol Chest Congestion Liquid with Cool Burst 1872
Children's Tylenol Suspension Liquid and Meltaways 1878
Children's Tylenol Plus Cold Suspension Liquid 1879
Children's Tylenol Plus Cold & Allergy Suspension Liquid 1878
Children's Tylenol Plus Cough & Runny Nose Suspension Liquid 1879
Children's Tylenol Plus Cough & Sore Throat Suspension Liquid 1879
Children's Tylenol Suspension with Flavor Creator 1878
Children's Tylenol Plus Flu Suspension Liquid 1881
Children's Tylenol Plus Multi-Symptom Cold Suspension Liquid 1879
Tylenol Cold Severe Congestion Non-Drowsy Caplets with Cool Burst 1874
Tylenol Cold Head Congestion Daytime Caplets with Cool Burst 1873
Tylenol Cold Head Congestion Nighttime Caplets with Cool Burst 1873
Tylenol Cold Head Congestion Severe Caplets with Cool Burst 1873
Tylenol Cold Multi-Symptom Daytime Caplets with Cool Burst and Gelcaps 1874
Tylenol Cold Multi-Symptom Daytime Liquid with Citrus Burst 1874
Tylenol Cold Multi-Symptom Nighttime Caplets with Cool Burst 1874
Tylenol Cold Multi-Symptom Nighttime Liquid with Cool Burst 1874
Tylenol Cold Multi-Symptom Severe Caplets with Cool Burst 1874
Tylenol Cold Multi-Symptom Severe Daytime Liquid with Citrus Burst 1874
Tylenol Cough & Sore Throat Daytime Liquid with Cool Burst 1877
Tylenol Cough & Sore Throat Nighttime Liquid with Cool Burst 1877
Concentrated Tylenol Infants' Drops 1878
Concentrated Tylenol Infants' Drops Plus Cold 1879
Concentrated Tylenol Infants' Drops Plus Cold and Cough 1879
Jr. Tylenol Meltaways 1878
Tylenol Sinus Severe Congestion Caplets with Cool Burst 1876
Tylenol Sinus Congestion & Pain Daytime Caplets with Cool Burst and Gelcaps 1876
Tylenol Sinus Congestion & Pain Nighttime Caplets with Cool Burst 1876
Tylenol Sinus Congestion & Pain Severe Caplets with Cool Burst 1876
Tylenol Sore Throat Daytime Liquid with Cool Burst 1877
Tylenol Sore Throat Nighttime Liquid with Cool Burst 1877
Women's Tylenol Menstrual Relief Caplets 1877
Vicks 44M Cough, Cold & Flu Relief Liquid 2680
Vicks DayQuil LiquiCaps/Liquid Multi-Symptom Cold/Flu Relief .... ▣761
Vicks DayQuil Multi-Symptom Cold/Flu Relief LiquiCaps 2678
Vicks DayQuil Multi-Symptom Cold/Flu Relief Liquid 2678
Vicks NyQuil Multi-Symptom Cold/Flu Relief Liquid 2681
Vicks NyQuil Multi-Symptom Cold/Flu Relief LiquiCaps 2681
Vicks NyQuil LiquiCaps/Liquid Multi-Symptom Cold/Flu Relief .... ▣763
Vicodin Tablets 535
Vicodin ES Tablets 536
Vicodin HP Tablets 538
Zicam Maximum Strength Flu Daytime .... ▣768
Zicam Maximum Strength Flu Nighttime .... ▣768
Zydone Tablets 1139

Acetazolamide (CYP3A4 inhibitors may increase plasma hormone levels).
No products indexed under this heading.

Amiodarone Hydrochloride (CYP3A4 inhibitors may increase plasma hormone levels).
No products indexed under this heading.

Amprenavir (Several of the anti-HIV protease inhibitors have been studied with co-administration of oral combination hormonal contraceptives; significant changes (increases and decreases) in the mean AUC of the estrogen and progestin have been noted in some cases. The efficacy and safety of oral contraceptive products may be affected; it is not known whether this applies to NuvaRing). Products include:
Agenerase Capsules 1327
Agenerase Oral Solution 1332

Anastrozole (CYP3A4 inhibitors may increase plasma hormone levels). Products include:
Arimidex Tablets 673

Aprepitant (CYP3A4 inhibitors may increase plasma hormone levels). Products include:
Emend Capsules 1963

Aprobarbital (Contraceptive effectiveness may be reduced when hormonal contraceptives are co-administered with drugs that increase the metabolism of contraceptive steroids. This could result in unintended pregnancy or breakthrough bleeding. Women may need to use anadditional contraceptive method).
No products indexed under this heading.

Ascorbic Acid (Ascorbic acid may increase plasma ethinyl estradiol levels). Products include:

MoviPrep Oral Solution 2839

Atorvastatin Calcium (Co-administration of atorvastatin and certain oral contraceptives containing ethinyl estradiol increase AUC values for ethinyl estradiol by approximately 20%). Products include:

Caduet Tablets 2508
Lipitor Tablets 2483

Butabarbital (Contraceptive effectiveness may be reduced when hormonal contraceptives are co-administered with drugs that increase the metabolism of contraceptive steroids. This could result in unintended pregnancy or breakthrough bleeding. Women may need to use anadditional contraceptive method).

No products indexed under this heading.

Butalbital (Contraceptive effectiveness may be reduced when hormonal contraceptives are co-administered with drugs that increase the metabolism of contraceptive steroids. This could result in unintended pregnancy or breakthrough bleeding. Women may need to use anadditional contraceptive method).

No products indexed under this heading.

Carbamazepine (Contraceptive effectiveness may be reduced when hormonal contraceptives are co-administered with some anticonvulsants and other drugs that increase the metabolism of contraceptive steroids. This could result in unintended pregnancy or breakthrough bleeding. Women may need to use an additional contraceptive method). Products include:

Carbatrol Capsules 3171
Equetro Extended-Release Capsules 3180
Tegretol/Tegretol-XR 2295

Cimetidine (CYP3A4 inhibitors may increase plasma hormone levels). Products include:

Tagamet HB 200 Tablets 664

Cimetidine Hydrochloride (CYP3A4 inhibitors may increase plasma hormone levels).

No products indexed under this heading.

Ciprofloxacin (CYP3A4 inhibitors may increase plasma hormone levels). Products include:

Cipro Oral Suspension 2977
Cipro I.V. 2984
Cipro XR Tablets 2990
Ciprodex Otic Suspension 559

Clarithromycin (CYP3A4 inhibitors may increase plasma hormone levels). Products include:

Biaxin/Biaxin XL 402
PREVPAC 3284

Clofibric Acid (Increased clearance of clofibric acid have been noted when administered with oral contraceptives).

No products indexed under this heading.

Clotrimazole (Contraceptive effectiveness may be reduced when hormonal contraceptives are co-administered with some antifungals and other drugs that increase the metabolism of contraceptive steroids. This could result in unintended pregnancy or breakthrough bleeding. Women may need to use an additional contraceptive method). Products include:

Desenex Athlete's Foot Cream 635
Lotrimin 3039
Lotrisone 3040

Cyclosporine (Combination hormonal contraceptives containing some synthetic estrogens may inhibit the metabolism of other compounds. Increased plasma concentrations of cyclosporine have been reported with concomitant administration of oral contraceptives). Products include:

Gengraf Capsules 459
Neoral Oral Solution 2259
Neoral Soft Gelatin Capsules 2259
Restasis Ophthalmic Emulsion 575
Sandimmune 2275

Dalfopristin (CYP3A4 inhibitors may increase plasma hormone levels).

No products indexed under this heading.

Danazol (CYP3A4 inhibitors may increase plasma hormone levels).

No products indexed under this heading.

Delavirdine Mesylate (CYP3A4 inhibitors may increase plasma hormone levels). Products include:

Rescriptor Tablets 2551

Diltiazem Hydrochloride (CYP3A4 inhibitors may increase plasma hormone levels). Products include:

Cardizem LA Extended Release Tablets 1728
Tiazac Capsules 1201

Diltiazem Maleate (CYP3A4 inhibitors may increase plasma hormone levels).

No products indexed under this heading.

Divalproex Sodium (Contraceptive effectiveness may be reduced when hormonal contraceptives are co-administered with some anticonvulsants and other drugs that increase the metabolism of contraceptive steroids. This could result in unintended pregnancy or breakthrough bleeding. Women may need to use an additional contraceptive method). Products include:

Depakote Sprinkle Capsules 422
Depakote Tablets 427
Depakote ER Tablets 434

Efavirenz (CYP3A4 inhibitors may increase plasma hormone levels). Products include:

Atripla Tablets 945
Sustiva Capsules 930
Sustiva Tablets 930

Erythromycin (CYP3A4 inhibitors may increase plasma hormone levels). Products include:

Ery-Tab Tablets 449
Erythromycin Base Filmtab Tablets 455
Erythromycin Delayed-Release Capsules, USP 457
PCE Dispertab Tablets 515

Erythromycin Estolate (CYP3A4 inhibitors may increase plasma hormone levels).

No products indexed under this heading.

Erythromycin Ethylsuccinate (CYP3A4 inhibitors may increase plasma hormone levels). Products include:

E.E.S. 451
EryPed 447

Erythromycin Gluceptate (CYP3A4 inhibitors may increase plasma hormone levels).

No products indexed under this heading.

Erythromycin Lactobionate (CYP3A4 inhibitors may increase plasma hormone levels).

No products indexed under this heading.

Erythromycin Stearate (CYP3A4 inhibitors may increase plasma hormone levels). Products include:

Erythrocin Stearate Filmtab Tablets 453

Esomeprazole Magnesium (CYP3A4 inhibitors may increase plasma hormone levels). Products include:

Nexium Delayed-Release Capsules 655

Ethosuximide (Contraceptive effectiveness may be reduced when hormonal contraceptives are co-administered with some anticonvulsants and other drugs that increase the metabolism of contraceptive steroids. This could result in unintended pregnancy or breakthrough bleeding. Women may need to use an additional contraceptive method).

No products indexed under this heading.

Ethotoin (Contraceptive effectiveness may be reduced when hormonal contraceptives are co-administered with some anticonvulsants and other drugs that increase the metabolism of contraceptive steroids. This could result in unintended pregnancy or breakthrough bleeding. Women may need to use an additional contraceptive method).

No products indexed under this heading.

Felbamate (Contraceptive effectiveness may be reduced when hormonal contraceptives are co-administered with some anticonvulsants and other drugs that increase the metabolism of contraceptive steroids. This could result in unintended pregnancy or breakthrough bleeding. Women may need to use an additional contraceptive method).

No products indexed under this heading.

Fluconazole (Contraceptive effectiveness may be reduced when hormonal contraceptives are co-administered with some antifungals and other drugs that increase the metabolism of contraceptive steroids. This could result in unintended pregnancy or breakthrough bleeding. Women may need to use an additional contraceptive method).

No products indexed under this heading.

Fluoxetine Hydrochloride (CYP3A4 inhibitors may increase plasma hormone levels). Products include:

Prozac Pulvules and Liquid 1801
Symbyax Capsules 1819

Fluvoxamine Maleate (CYP3A4 inhibitors may increase plasma hormone levels).

No products indexed under this heading.

Fosamprenavir Calcium (CYP3A4 inhibitors may increase plasma hormone levels). Products include:

Lexiva Tablets 1505

Fosphenytoin (Contraceptive effectiveness may be reduced when hormonal contraceptives are co-administered with some anticonvulsants and other drugs that increase the metabolism of contraceptive steroids. This could result in unintended pregnancy or breakthrough bleeding. Women may need to use an additional contraceptive method).

No products indexed under this heading.

Fosphenytoin Sodium (Contraceptive effectiveness may be reduced when hormonal contraceptives are co-administered with some anticonvulsants and other drugs that increase the metabolism of contraceptive steroids. This could result in unintended pregnancy or breakthrough bleeding. Women may need to use an additional contraceptive method).

No products indexed under this heading.

Gabapentin (Contraceptive effectiveness may be reduced when hormonal contraceptives are co-administered with some anticonvulsants and other drugs that increase the metabolism of contraceptive steroids. This could result in unintended pregnancy or breakthrough bleeding. Women may need to use an additional contraceptive method). Products include:

Neurontin Capsules 2487
Neurontin Oral Solution 2487
Neurontin Tablets 2487

Griseofulvin (Contraceptive effectiveness may be reduced when hormonal contraceptives are co-administered with drugs that increase the metabolism of contraceptive steroids. This could result in unintended pregnancy or breakthrough bleeding. Women may need to use an additional contraceptive method). Products include:

Gris-PEG Tablets 2502

Hypericum (Herbal products containing St. John's Wort may induce hepatic enzymes (cytochrome P450) and p-glycoprotein transporter and may reduce the effectiveness of contraceptive steroids. This may also result in breakthrough bleeding). Products include:

Satiete Tablets 832

Indinavir Sulfate (Several of the anti-HIV protease inhibitors have been studied with co-administration of oral combination hormonal contraceptives; significant changes (increases and decreases) in the mean AUC of the estrogen and progestin have been noted in some cases. The efficacy and safety of oral contraceptive products may be affected; it is not known whether this applies to NuvaRing). Products include:

Crixivan Capsules 1940

Isoniazid (CYP3A4 inhibitors may increase plasma hormone levels).

No products indexed under this heading.

Itraconazole (Contraceptive effectiveness may be reduced when hormonal contraceptives are co-administered with some antifungals and other drugs that increase the metabolism of contraceptive steroids. This could result in unintended pregnancy or breakthrough bleeding. Women may need to use an additional contraceptive method).

No products indexed under this heading.

Ketoconazole (Contraceptive effectiveness may be reduced when hormonal contraceptives are co-administered with some antifungals and other drugs that increase the metabolism of contraceptive steroids. This could result in unintended pregnancy or breakthrough bleeding. Women may need to use an additional contraceptive method). Products include:

Nizoral A-D Shampoo, 1% **1868**

Lamotrigine (Contraceptive effectiveness may be reduced when hormonal contraceptives are co-administered with some anticonvulsants and other drugs that increase the metabolism of contraceptive steroids. This could result in unintended pregnancy or breakthrough bleeding. Women may need to use an additional contraceptive method). Products include:

Lamictal **1481**

Levetiracetam (Contraceptive effectiveness may be reduced when hormonal contraceptives are co-administered with some anticonvulsants and other drugs that increase the metabolism of contraceptive steroids. This could result in unintended pregnancy or breakthrough bleeding. Women may need to use an additional contraceptive method). Products include:

Keppra Injection **3320**
Keppra Oral Solution **3314**
Keppra Tablets **3314**

Lopinavir (Several of the anti-HIV protease inhibitors have been studied with co-administration of oral combination hormonal contraceptives; significant changes (increases and decreases) in the mean AUC of the estrogen and progestin have been noted in some cases. The efficacy and safety of oral contraceptive products may be affected; it is not known whether this applies to NuvaRing). Products include:

Kaletra **476**

Loratadine (CYP3A4 inhibitors may increase plasma hormone levels). Products include:

Alavert Allergy & Sinus D-12 Hour Tablets .... ▣**771**
Alavert .... ▣**771**
Children's Claritin Allergy Oral Solution .... ▣**771**
Claritin Non-Drowsy 24 Hour Tablets .... ▣**772**
Claritin Reditabs 24 Hour Non-Drowsy Tablets .... ▣**772**
Claritin-D Non-Drowsy 12 Hour Tablets .... ▣**772**
Claritin-D Non-Drowsy 24 Hour Tablets .... ▣**772**

Mephenytoin (Contraceptive effectiveness may be reduced when hormonal contraceptives are co-administered with some anticonvulsants and other drugs that increase the metabolism of contraceptive steroids. This could result in unintended pregnancy or breakthrough bleeding. Women may need to use an additional contraceptive method).

No products indexed under this heading.

Mephobarbital (Contraceptive effectiveness may be reduced when hormonal contraceptives are co-administered with drugs that increase the metabolism of contraceptive steroids. This could result in unintended pregnancy or breakthrough bleeding. Women may need to use anadditional contraceptive method).

No products indexed under this heading.

Methsuximide (Contraceptive effectiveness may be reduced when hormonal contraceptives are co-administered with some anticonvulsants and other drugs that increase the metabolism of contraceptive steroids. This could result in unintended pregnancy or breakthrough bleeding. Women may need to use an additional contraceptive method).

No products indexed under this heading.

Metronidazole (CYP3A4 inhibitors may increase plasma hormone levels). Products include:

Metrogel 1% **1211**
MetroGel-Vaginal Gel **1855**
Vandazole Vaginal Gel **3338**

Metronidazole Benzoate (CYP3A4 inhibitors may increase plasma hormone levels).

No products indexed under this heading.

Metronidazole Hydrochloride (CYP3A4 inhibitors may increase plasma hormone levels).

No products indexed under this heading.

Miconazole (Contraceptive effectiveness may be reduced when hormonal contraceptives are co-administered with some antifungals and other drugs that increase the metabolism of contraceptive steroids. This could result in unintended pregnancy or breakthrough bleeding. Women may need to use an additional contraceptive method).

No products indexed under this heading.

Miconazole Nitrate (Co-administration of vaginal miconazole nitrate increases the serum concentrations of etonogestrel and ethinyl estradiol by up to 40%). Products include:

Desenex .... ▣**635**
Desenex Jock Itch Spray Powder ... ▣**635**

Modafinil (Contraceptive effectiveness may be reduced when hormonal contraceptives are co-administered with drugs that increase the metabolism of contraceptive steroids. This could result in unintended pregnancy or breakthrough bleeding. Women may need to use an additional contraceptive method). Products include:

Provigil Tablets **988**

Morphine Sulfate (Increased clearance of morphine has been noted when administered with oral contraceptives). Products include:

Avinza Capsules **1741**
Kadian Capsules **577**
MS Contin Tablets **2701**

Nefazodone Hydrochloride (CYP3A4 inhibitors may increase plasma hormone levels).

No products indexed under this heading.

Nelfinavir Mesylate (Several of the anti-HIV protease inhibitors have been studied with co-administration of oral combination hormonal contraceptives; significant changes (increases and decreases) in the mean AUC of the estrogen and progestin have been noted in some cases. The efficacy and safety of oral contraceptive products may be affected; it is not known whether this applies to NuvaRing). Products include:

Viracept **2577**

Nevirapine (CYP3A4 inhibitors may increase plasma hormone levels). Products include:

Viramune Oral Suspension **873**
Viramune Tablets **873**

Niacinamide (CYP3A4 inhibitors may increase plasma hormone levels).

No products indexed under this heading.

Nicotinamide (CYP3A4 inhibitors may increase plasma hormone levels). Products include:

Nicomide Tablets **1088**

Nifedipine (CYP3A4 inhibitors may increase plasma hormone levels). Products include:

Adalat CC Tablets **2964**

Norfloxacin (CYP3A4 inhibitors may increase plasma hormone levels). Products include:

Noroxin Tablets **2032**

Omeprazole (CYP3A4 inhibitors may increase plasma hormone levels). Products include:

Zegerid Capsules **2958**
Zegerid Powder for Oral Solution **2958**

Oxcarbazepine (Contraceptive effectiveness may be reduced when hormonal contraceptives are co-administered with some anticonvulsants and other drugs that increase the metabolism of contraceptive steroids. This could result in unintended pregnancy or breakthrough bleeding. Women may need to use an additional contraceptive method). Products include:

Trileptal Tablets **2300**
Trileptal Oral Suspension **2300**

Oxiconazole Nitrate (Contraceptive effectiveness may be reduced when hormonal contraceptives are co-administered with some antifungals and other drugs that increase the metabolism of contraceptive steroids. This could result in unintended pregnancy or breakthrough bleeding. Women may need to use an additional contraceptive method). Products include:

Oxistat **2667**

Paramethadione (Contraceptive effectiveness may be reduced when hormonal contraceptives are co-administered with some anticonvulsants and other drugs that increase the metabolism of contraceptive steroids. This could result in unintended pregnancy or breakthrough bleeding. Women may need to use an additional contraceptive method).

No products indexed under this heading.

Paroxetine Hydrochloride (CYP3A4 inhibitors may increase plasma hormone levels). Products include:

Paxil CR Controlled-Release Tablets **1538**
Paxil **1530**

Pentobarbital Sodium (Contraceptive effectiveness may be reduced when hormonal contraceptives are co-administered with drugs that increase the metabolism of contraceptive steroids. This could result in unintended pregnancy or breakthrough bleeding. Women may need to use anadditional contraceptive method). Products include:

Nembutal Sodium Solution, USP **2470**

Phenacemide (Contraceptive effectiveness may be reduced when hormonal contraceptives are co-administered with some anticonvulsants and other drugs that increase the metabolism of contraceptive steroids. This could result in unintended pregnancy or breakthrough bleeding. Women may need to use an additional contraceptive method).

No products indexed under this heading.

Phenobarbital (Contraceptive effectiveness may be reduced when hormonal contraceptives are co-administered with some anticonvulsants and other drugs that increase the metabolism of contraceptive steroids. This could result in unintended pregnancy or breakthrough bleeding. Women may need to use an additional contraceptive method). Products include:

Donnatal Extentabs **2493**

Phensuximide (Contraceptive effectiveness may be reduced when hormonal contraceptives are co-administered with some anticonvulsants and other drugs that increase the metabolism of contraceptive steroids. This could result in unintended pregnancy or breakthrough bleeding. Women may need to use an additional contraceptive method).

No products indexed under this heading.

Phenylbutazone (Contraceptive effectiveness may be reduced when hormonal contraceptives are co-administered with drugs that increase the metabolism of contraceptive steroids. This could result in unintended pregnancy or breakthrough bleeding. Women may need to use an additional contraceptive method).

No products indexed under this heading.

Phenytoin (Contraceptive effectiveness may be reduced when hormonal contraceptives are co-administered with some anticonvulsants and other drugs that increase the metabolism of contraceptive steroids. This could result in unintended pregnancy or breakthrough bleeding. Women may need to use an additional contraceptive method).
No products indexed under this heading.

Phenytoin Sodium (Contraceptive effectiveness may be reduced when hormonal contraceptives are co-administered with some anticonvulsants and other drugs that increase the metabolism of contraceptive steroids. This could result in unintended pregnancy or breakthrough bleeding. Women may need to use an additional contraceptive method). Products include:
Phenytek Capsules 2160

Prednisolone (Combination hormonal contraceptives containing some synthetic estrogens may inhibit the metabolism of other compounds. Increased plasma concentrations of prednisolone have been reported with concomitant administration of oral contraceptives).
No products indexed under this heading.

Prednisolone Acetate (Combination hormonal contraceptives containing some synthetic estrogens may inhibit the metabolism of other compounds. Increased plasma concentrations of prednisolone have been reported with concomitant administration of oral contraceptives). Products include:
Blephamide Ophthalmic Ointment 568
Blephamide Ophthalmic Suspension 569
Poly-Pred Ophthalmic Suspension .... ⊙233
Pred Forte Ophthalmic Suspension .... ⊙235
Pred Mild Ophthalmic Suspension .... ⊙238
Pred-G Ophthalmic Ointment .... ⊙237
Pred-G Ophthalmic Suspension ...... ⊙236

Prednisolone Sodium Phosphate (Combination hormonal contraceptives containing some synthetic estrogens may inhibit the metabolism of other compounds. Increased plasma concentrations of prednisolone have been reported with concomitant administration of oral contraceptives).
No products indexed under this heading.

Prednisolone Tebutate (Combination hormonal contraceptives containing some synthetic estrogens may inhibit the metabolism of other compounds. Increased plasma concentrations of prednisolone have been reported with concomitant administration of oral contraceptives).
No products indexed under this heading.

Primidone (Contraceptive effectiveness may be reduced when hormonal contraceptives are co-administered with some anticonvulsants and other drugs that increase the metabolism of contraceptive steroids. This could result in unintended pregnancy or breakthrough bleeding. Women may need to use an additional contraceptive method).
No products indexed under this heading.

Propoxyphene Hydrochloride (CYP3A4 inhibitors may increase plasma hormone levels).
No products indexed under this heading.

Propoxyphene Napsylate (CYP3A4 inhibitors may increase plasma hormone levels).
No products indexed under this heading.

Quinidine (CYP3A4 inhibitors may increase plasma hormone levels).
No products indexed under this heading.

Quinidine Hydrochloride (CYP3A4 inhibitors may increase plasma hormone levels).
No products indexed under this heading.

Quinidine Polygalacturonate (CYP3A4 inhibitors may increase plasma hormone levels).
No products indexed under this heading.

Quinidine Sulfate (CYP3A4 inhibitors may increase plasma hormone levels).
No products indexed under this heading.

Quinine (CYP3A4 inhibitors may increase plasma hormone levels).
No products indexed under this heading.

Quinine Sulfate (CYP3A4 inhibitors may increase plasma hormone levels).
No products indexed under this heading.

Quinupristin (CYP3A4 inhibitors may increase plasma hormone levels).
No products indexed under this heading.

Ranitidine Bismuth Citrate (CYP3A4 inhibitors may increase plasma hormone levels).
No products indexed under this heading.

Ranitidine Hydrochloride (CYP3A4 inhibitors may increase plasma hormone levels). Products include:
Zantac 1624
Zantac Injection 1619
Zantac Injection Pharmacy Bulk Package 1622

Rifampin (Contraceptive effectiveness may be reduced when hormonal contraceptives are co-administered with drugs that increase the metabolism of contraceptive steroids. This could result in unintended pregnancy or breakthrough bleeding. Women may need to use an additional contraceptive method).
No products indexed under this heading.

Ritonavir (Several of the anti-HIV protease inhibitors have been studied with co-administration of oral combination hormonal contraceptives; significant changes (increases and decreases) in the mean AUC of the estrogen and progestin have been noted in some cases. The efficacy and safety of oral contraceptive products may be affected; it is not known whether this applies to NuvaRing). Products include:
Kaletra 476
Norvir 503

Salicylic Acid (Increased clearance of salicylic acid has been noted when administered with oral contraceptives).
No products indexed under this heading.

Saquinavir (Several of the anti-HIV protease inhibitors have been studied with co-administration of oral combination hormonal contraceptives; significant changes (increases and decreases) in the mean AUC of the estrogen and progestin have been noted in some cases. The efficacy and safety of oral contraceptive products may be affected; it is not known whether this applies to NuvaRing).
No products indexed under this heading.

Saquinavir Mesylate (Several of the anti-HIV protease inhibitors have been studied with co-administration of oral combination hormonal contraceptives; significant changes (increases and decreases) in the mean AUC of the estrogen and progestin have been noted in some cases. The efficacy and safety of oral contraceptive products may be affected; it is not known whether this applies to NuvaRing). Products include:
Invirase 2772

Secobarbital Sodium (Contraceptive effectiveness may be reduced when hormonal contraceptives are co-administered with drugs that increase the metabolism of contraceptive steroids. This could result in unintended pregnancy or breakthrough bleeding. Women may need to use anadditional contraceptive method).
No products indexed under this heading.

Sertraline Hydrochloride (CYP3A4 inhibitors may increase plasma hormone levels). Products include:
Zoloft 2586

Telithromycin (CYP3A4 inhibitors may increase plasma hormone levels). Products include:
Ketek Tablets 2903

Temazepam (Increased clearance of temazepam has been noted when administered with oral contraceptives). Products include:
Restoril Capsules 1860

Terconazole (Contraceptive effectiveness may be reduced when hormonal contraceptives are co-administered with some antifungals and other drugs that increase the metabolism of contraceptive steroids. This could result in unintended pregnancy or breakthrough bleeding. Women may need to use an additional contraceptive method).
No products indexed under this heading.

Theophylline (Combination hormonal contraceptives containing some synthetic estrogens may inhibit the metabolism of other compounds. Increased plasma concentrations of theophylline have been reported with concomitant administration of oral contraceptives).
No products indexed under this heading.

Theophylline Anhydrous (Combination hormonal contraceptives containing some synthetic estrogens may inhibit the metabolism of other compounds. Increased plasma concentrations of theophylline have been reported with concomitant administration of oral contraceptives). Products include:
Uniphyl Tablets 2710

Theophylline Calcium Salicylate (Combination hormonal contraceptives containing some synthetic estrogens may inhibit the metabolism of other compounds. Increased plasma concentrations of theophylline have been reported with concomitant administration of oral contraceptives).
No products indexed under this heading.

Theophylline Dihydroxypropyl (Glyceryl) (Combination hormonal contraceptives containing some synthetic estrogens may inhibit the metabolism of other compounds. Increased plasma concentrations of theophylline have been reported with concomitant administration of oral contraceptives).
No products indexed under this heading.

Theophylline Ethylenediamine (Combination hormonal contraceptives containing some synthetic estrogens may inhibit the metabolism of other compounds. Increased plasma concentrations of theophylline have been reported with concomitant administration of oral contraceptives).
No products indexed under this heading.

Theophylline Sodium Glycinate (Combination hormonal contraceptives containing some synthetic estrogens may inhibit the metabolism of other compounds. Increased plasma concentrations of theophylline have been reported with concomitant administration of oral contraceptives).
No products indexed under this heading.

Thiamylal Sodium (Contraceptive effectiveness may be reduced when hormonal contraceptives are co-administered with drugs that increase the metabolism of contraceptive steroids. This could result in unintended pregnancy or breakthrough bleeding. Women may need to use anadditional contraceptive method).
No products indexed under this heading.

Tiagabine Hydrochloride (Contraceptive effectiveness may be reduced when hormonal contraceptives are co-administered with some anticonvulsants and other drugs that increase the metabolism of contraceptive steroids. This could result in unintended pregnancy or breakthrough bleeding. Women may need to use an additional contraceptive method). Products include:
Gabitril Tablets 984

Topiramate (Contraceptive effectiveness may be reduced when hormonal contraceptives are co-administered with some anticonvulsants and other drugs that increase the metabolism of contraceptive steroids. This could result in unintended pregnancy or breakthrough bleeding. Women may need to use an additional contraceptive method). Products include:
Topamax Sprinkle Capsules 2404
Topamax Tablets 2404

Trimethadione (Contraceptive effectiveness may be reduced when hormonal contraceptives are co-administered with some anticonvulsants and other drugs that increase the metabolism of contraceptive steroids. This could result in unintended pregnancy or breakthrough bleeding. Women may need to use an additional contraceptive method).
No products indexed under this heading.

Troglitazone (CYP3A4 inhibitors may increase plasma hormone levels).
No products indexed under this heading.

Troleandomycin (CYP3A4 inhibitors may increase plasma hormone levels).
No products indexed under this heading.

Valproate Sodium (Contraceptive effectiveness may be reduced when hormonal contraceptives are co-administered with some anticonvulsants and other drugs that increase the metabolism of contraceptive steroids. This could result in unintended pregnancy or breakthrough bleeding. Women may need to use an additional contraceptive method). Products include:
Depacon Injection 412

Valproic Acid (Contraceptive effectiveness may be reduced when hormonal contraceptives are co-administered with some anticonvulsants and other drugs that increase the metabolism of contraceptive steroids. This could result in unintended pregnancy or breakthrough bleeding. Women may need to use an additional contraceptive method). Products include:
Depakene 417

Verapamil Hydrochloride (CYP3A4 inhibitors may increase plasma hormone levels). Products include:
Covera-HS Tablets 3139
Tarka Tablets 524
Verelan PM Extended-Release Capsules, Controlled-Onset.......... 3106

Vitamin C (Ascorbic acid may increase plasma ethinyl estradiol levels). Products include:
Bausch & Lomb Ocuvite Adult Eye Vitamin and Mineral Supplement Soft Gels .... ▣706
Bausch & Lomb Ocuvite Adult 50+ Eye Vitamin and Mineral Supplement Soft Gels .... ▣706
Ocuvite Adult Vitamin and Mineral Supplement................................ ⊙253
Ocuvite Adult 50+ Vitamin and Mineral Supplement..................... ⊙253
Peridin-C Vitamin C Supplement ..... ▣818

Voriconazole (CYP3A4 inhibitors may increase plasma hormone levels). Products include:
VFEND I.V. 2564
VFEND Oral Suspension 2564
VFEND Tablets 2564

Zafirlukast (CYP3A4 inhibitors may increase plasma hormone levels). Products include:
Accolate Tablets 671

Zileuton (CYP3A4 inhibitors may increase plasma hormone levels). Products include:
Zyflo Tablets 1023

Zonisamide (Contraceptive effectiveness may be reduced when hormonal contraceptives are co-administered with some anticonvulsants and other drugs that increase the metabolism of contraceptive steroids. This could result in unintended pregnancy or breakthrough bleeding. Women may need to use an additional contraceptive method). Products include:
Zonegran Capsules 1101

Food Interactions

Grapefruit (CYP3A4 inhibitors may increase plasma hormone levels).

Grapefruit Juice (CYP3A4 inhibitors may increase plasma hormone levels).

NYSTOP TOPICAL POWDER USP

(Nystatin) 2478
None cited in PDR database.

NYTOL QUICKCAPS CAPLETS

(Diphenhydramine Hydrochloride) ..... ▣615
See Nytol QuickGels Softgels Maximum Strength

NYTOL QUICKGELS SOFTGELS MAXIMUM STRENGTH

(Diphenhydramine Hydrochloride) ..... ▣616
May interact with central nervous system depressants, monoamine oxidase inhibitors, and certain other agents. Compounds in these categories include:

Alfentanil Hydrochloride (Concurrent use with CNS depressant will heighten the depressant effect of Nytol).
No products indexed under this heading.

Alprazolam (Concurrent use with CNS depressant will heighten the depressant effect of Nytol). Products include:
Niravam Orally Disintegrating Tablets 3092

Aprobarbital (Concurrent use with CNS depressant will heighten the depressant effect of Nytol).
No products indexed under this heading.

Buprenorphine Hydrochloride (Concurrent use with CNS depressant will heighten the depressant effect of Nytol). Products include:
Buprenex Injectable 2716
Suboxone Tablets 2717
Subutex Tablets 2717

Buspirone Hydrochloride (Concurrent use with CNS depressant will heighten the depressant effect of Nytol).
No products indexed under this heading.

Butabarbital (Concurrent use with CNS depressant will heighten the depressant effect of Nytol).
No products indexed under this heading.

Butalbital (Concurrent use with CNS depressant will heighten the depressant effect of Nytol).
No products indexed under this heading.

Chlordiazepoxide (Concurrent use with CNS depressant will heighten the depressant effect of Nytol).
No products indexed under this heading.

Chlordiazepoxide Hydrochloride (Concurrent use with CNS depressant will heighten the depressant effect of Nytol). Products include:
Librium Capsules 3347

Chlorpromazine (Concurrent use with CNS depressant will heighten the depressant effect of Nytol).
No products indexed under this heading.

Chlorpromazine Hydrochloride (Concurrent use with CNS depressant will heighten the depressant effect of Nytol).
No products indexed under this heading.

Chlorprothixene (Concurrent use with CNS depressant will heighten the depressant effect of Nytol).
No products indexed under this heading.

Chlorprothixene Hydrochloride (Concurrent use with CNS depressant will heighten the depressant effect of Nytol).
No products indexed under this heading.

Chlorprothixene Lactate (Concurrent use with CNS depressant will heighten the depressant effect of Nytol).
No products indexed under this heading.

Clorazepate Dipotassium (Concurrent use with CNS depressant will heighten the depressant effect of Nytol). Products include:
Tranxene 2474

Clozapine (Concurrent use with CNS depressant will heighten the depressant effect of Nytol). Products include:
Clozaril Tablets 2184
FazaClo Orally Disintegrating Tablets 551

Codeine Phosphate (Concurrent use with CNS depressant will heighten the depressant effect of Nytol). Products include:
Tylenol with Codeine Tablets 2391

Desflurane (Concurrent use with CNS depressant will heighten the depressant effect of Nytol).
No products indexed under this heading.

Dezocine (Concurrent use with CNS depressant will heighten the depressant effect of Nytol).
No products indexed under this heading.

Diazepam (Concurrent use with CNS depressant will heighten the depressant effect of Nytol). Products include:
Diastat Rectal Delivery System 3343
Valium Tablets 2819

Droperidol (Concurrent use with CNS depressant will heighten the depressant effect of Nytol).
No products indexed under this heading.

Enflurane (Concurrent use with CNS depressant will heighten the depressant effect of Nytol).
No products indexed under this heading.

Estazolam (Concurrent use with CNS depressant will heighten the depressant effect of Nytol). Products include:
ProSom Tablets 517

Ethanol (Concurrent use with CNS depressant will heighten the depressant effect of Nytol).
No products indexed under this heading.

Ethchlorvynol (Concurrent use with CNS depressant will heighten the depressant effect of Nytol).
No products indexed under this heading.

Ethinamate (Concurrent use with CNS depressant will heighten the depressant effect of Nytol).
No products indexed under this heading.

Ethyl Alcohol (Concurrent use with CNS depressant will heighten the depressant effect of Nytol).
No products indexed under this heading.

Fentanyl (Concurrent use with CNS depressant will heighten the depressant effect of Nytol). Products include:
Duragesic Transdermal System 2373
Ionsys Transdermal System 2379

Fentanyl Citrate (Concurrent use with CNS depressant will heighten the depressant effect of Nytol). Products include:
Actiq 979

Fluphenazine Decanoate (Concurrent use with CNS depressant will heighten the depressant effect of Nytol).
No products indexed under this heading.

Fluphenazine Enanthate (Concurrent use with CNS depressant will heighten the depressant effect of Nytol).
No products indexed under this heading.

Fluphenazine Hydrochloride (Concurrent use with CNS depressant will heighten the depressant effect of Nytol).
No products indexed under this heading.

Flurazepam Hydrochloride (Concurrent use with CNS depressant will heighten the depressant effect of Nytol). Products include:
Dalmane Capsules 3342

Glutethimide (Concurrent use with CNS depressant will heighten the depressant effect of Nytol).
No products indexed under this heading.

Haloperidol (Concurrent use with CNS depressant will heighten the depressant effect of Nytol).
No products indexed under this heading.

Haloperidol Decanoate (Concurrent use with CNS depressant will heighten the depressant effect of Nytol).
No products indexed under this heading.

Hydrocodone Bitartrate (Concurrent use with CNS depressant will heighten the depressant effect of Nytol). Products include:
Hycodan 1116
Hycotuss Expectorant Syrup 1117
Vicodin Tablets 535
Vicodin ES Tablets 536
Vicodin HP Tablets 538
Vicoprofen Tablets 539
Zydone Tablets 1139

Hydrocodone Polistirex (Concurrent use with CNS depressant will heighten the depressant effect of Nytol). Products include:
Tussionex Pennkinetic Extended-Release Suspension...... 3327

Hydromorphone Hydrochloride (Concurrent use with CNS depressant will heighten the depressant effect of Nytol). Products include:
Dilaudid 440
Dilaudid Non-Sterile Powder 440
Dilaudid Oral Liquid 445
Dilaudid Rectal Suppositories 440
Dilaudid Tablets 440
Dilaudid Tablets - 8 mg 445

Food Interactions

Alcohol (Concurrent use will heighten the depressant effect of Nytol; avoid alcoholic beverages while taking this product).

OCUFEN OPHTHALMIC SOLUTION

(Flurbiprofen Sodium) ☉232
May interact with:

Acetylcholine Chloride (There have been reports that acetylcholine chloride is ineffective when used in patients treated with ophthalmic flurbiprofen).

No products indexed under this heading.

Carbachol (There have been reports that carbachol is ineffective when used in patients treated with ophthalmic flurbiprofen).

No products indexed under this heading.

OCUVITE ADULT VITAMIN AND MINERAL SUPPLEMENT

(Copper, Lutein, Omega-3 Acids, Vitamin C, Vitamin E, Vitamins with Minerals, Zinc Oxide)................. ☉253
None cited in PDR database.

IMPORTANT NOTE: Always consult each drug listing in the patient's regimen for possible interactions.

OCUVITE ADULT 50+ VITAMIN AND MINERAL SUPPLEMENT
(Copper, Lutein, Omega-3 Acids, Vitamin C, Vitamin E, Vitamins with Minerals, Zinc Oxide) .... ⊙253
None cited in PDR database.

OCUVITE LUTEIN VITAMIN AND MINERAL SUPPLEMENT
(Lutein, Vitamins with Minerals) .... ⊙254
None cited in PDR database.

OLUX FOAM
(Clobetasol Propionate) 1012
None cited in PDR database.

OMACOR CAPSULES
(Omega-3-acid ethyl esters) 2725
May interact with anticoagulants and oral anticoagulants. Compounds in these categories include:

Anisindione (Some studies with omega-3-acids demonstrated prolongation of bleeding time. Patients receiving treatment with omega-3-acid ethyl esters and anticoagulants should be monitored periodically). Products include:
Miradon Tablets 3042

Ardeparin Sodium (Some studies with omega-3-acids demonstrated prolongation of bleeding time. Patients receiving treatment with omega-3-acid ethyl esters and anticoagulants should be monitored periodically).
No products indexed under this heading.

Dalteparin Sodium (Some studies with omega-3-acids demonstrated prolongation of bleeding time. Patients receiving treatment with omega-3-acid ethyl esters and anticoagulants should be monitored periodically). Products include:
Fragmin Injection 1097

Danaparoid Sodium (Some studies with omega-3-acids demonstrated prolongation of bleeding time. Patients receiving treatment with omega-3-acid ethyl esters and anticoagulants should be monitored periodically).
No products indexed under this heading.

Dicumarol (Some studies with omega-3-acids demonstrated prolongation of bleeding time. Patients receiving treatment with omega-3-acid ethyl esters and anticoagulants should be monitored periodically).
No products indexed under this heading.

Enoxaparin Sodium (Some studies with omega-3-acids demonstrated prolongation of bleeding time. Patients receiving treatment with omega-3-acid ethyl esters and anticoagulants should be monitored periodically). Products include:
Lovenox Injection 2915

Fondaparinux Sodium (Some studies with omega-3-acids demonstrated prolongation of bleeding time. Patients receiving treatment with omega-3-acid ethyl esters and anticoagulants should be monitored periodically). Products include:
Arixtra Injection 1351

Heparin Calcium (Some studies with omega-3-acids demonstrated prolongation of bleeding time. Patients receiving treatment with omega-3-acid ethyl esters and anticoagulants should be monitored periodically).
No products indexed under this heading.

Heparin Sodium (Some studies with omega-3-acids demonstrated prolongation of bleeding time. Patients receiving treatment with omega-3-acid ethyl esters and anticoagulants should be monitored periodically).
No products indexed under this heading.

Low Molecular Weight Heparins (Some studies with omega-3-acids demonstrated prolongation of bleeding time. Patients receiving treatment with omega-3-acid ethyl esters and anticoagulants should be monitored periodically).
No products indexed under this heading.

Tinzaparin Sodium (Some studies with omega-3-acids demonstrated prolongation of bleeding time. Patients receiving treatment with omega-3-acid ethyl esters and anticoagulants should be monitored periodically).
No products indexed under this heading.

Warfarin Sodium (Some studies with omega-3-acids demonstrated prolongation of bleeding time. Patients receiving treatment with omega-3-acid ethyl esters and anticoagulants should be monitored periodically). Products include:
Coumadin for Injection 898
Coumadin Tablets 898

OMNICEF CAPSULES
(Cefdinir) 511
May interact with antacids containing aluminum, calcium and magnesium, iron containing oral preparations, and certain other agents. Compounds in these categories include:

Aluminum Carbonate (Antacids (aluminum- or magnesium-containing) interfere with the absorption of cefdinir; Omnicef should be taken at least 2 hours before or after the antacids).
No products indexed under this heading.

Aluminum Hydroxide (Antacids (aluminum- or magnesium-containing) interfere with the absorption of cefdinir; Omnicef should be taken at least 2 hours before or after the antacids). Products include:
Gaviscon Regular Strength Liquid .. ■658
Gaviscon Regular Strength Tablets....................................... ■658
Gaviscon Extra Strength Liquid ...... ■658
Gaviscon Extra Strength Tablets .... ■658
Maalox Regular Strength Antacid/Antigas Liquid................. 2175
Maalox Max Maximum Strength Antacid/Anti-Gas Liquid................ 2176

Ferrous Fumarate (Iron supplements, including multivitamins that contain iron, interfere with the absorption of cefdinir; Omnicef should be taken at least 2 hours before or after the administration of iron-containing products).
No products indexed under this heading.

Ferrous Gluconate (Iron supplements, including multivitamins that contain iron, interfere with the absorption of cefdinir; Omnicef should be taken at least 2 hours before or after the administration of iron-containing products).
No products indexed under this heading.

Ferrous Sulfate (Iron supplements, including multivitamins that contain iron, interfere with the absorption of cefdinir; Omnicef should be taken at least 2 hours before or after the administration of iron-containing products). Products include:
Slow Fe Iron Tablets .... ■818
Slow Fe with Folic Acid Tablets .... ■819

Iron (Iron supplements, including multivitamins that contain iron, interfere with the absorption of cefdinir; Omnicef should be taken at least 2 hours before or after the administration of iron-containing products).
No products indexed under this heading.

Magaldrate (Antacids (aluminum- or magnesium-containing) interfere with the absorption of cefdinir; Omnicef should be taken at least 2 hours before or after the antacids).
No products indexed under this heading.

Magnesium Hydroxide (Antacids (aluminum- or magnesium-containing) interfere with the absorption of cefdinir; Omnicef should be taken at least 2 hours before or after the antacids). Products include:
Maalox Regular Strength Antacid/Antigas Liquid................. 2175
Maalox Max Maximum Strength Antacid/Anti-Gas Liquid................ 2176
Pepcid Complete Chewable Tablets 1701

Magnesium Oxide (Antacids (aluminum- or magnesium-containing) interfere with the absorption of cefdinir; Omnicef should be taken at least 2 hours before or after the antacids). Products include:
Beelith Tablets 759
PremCal Light, Regular, and Extra Strength Tablets................ ■818

Polysaccharide Iron Complex (Iron supplements, including multivitamins that contain iron, interfere with the absorption of cefdinir; Omnicef should be taken at least 2 hours before or after the administration of iron-containing products). Products include:
Nu-Iron 150 Capsules 2127

Probenecid (Inhibits renal excretion of cefdinir, resulting in an approximate doubling in AUC, a 54% increase in peak cefdinir plasma levels, and a 50% prolongation in the apparent elimination).
No products indexed under this heading.

Food Interactions

Food, unspecified (Although Cmax and AUC of cefdinir absorption from capsules are reduced by 44% and 33%, respectively, when given with a high-fat meal, the magnitude of these reductions is not likely to be clinically significant; therefore, cefdinir may be taken without regard to food).

OMNICEF FOR ORAL SUSPENSION
(Cefdinir) 511
See Omnicef Capsules

ONCASPAR
(Pegaspargase) 1145
May interact with antineoplastics, anticoagulants, non-steroidal anti-inflammatory agents, highly protein bound drugs (selected), and certain other agents. Compounds in these categories include:

Altretamine (Potential for unspecified unfavorable interactions).
No products indexed under this heading.

Amiodarone Hydrochloride (Depletion of serum proteins by pegaspargase may increase the toxicity of other drugs which are protein bound).
No products indexed under this heading.

Amitriptyline Hydrochloride (Depletion of serum proteins by pegaspargase may increase the toxicity of other drugs which are protein bound).
No products indexed under this heading.

Anastrozole (Potential for unspecified unfavorable interactions). Products include:
Arimidex Tablets 673

Anisindione (Increased risk of bleeding and/or thrombosis). Products include:
Miradon Tablets 3042

Ardeparin Sodium (Increased risk of bleeding and/or thrombosis).
No products indexed under this heading.

Asparaginase (Potential for unspecified unfavorable interactions). Products include:
Elspar for Injection 2463
Elspar for Injection 1960

Aspirin (Increased risk of bleeding and/or thrombosis). Products include:
Aggrenox Capsules 822
Bayer Aspirin 744
BC Allergy Sinus Cold Powder .... ■677
BC Headache Powder .... ■677
Arthritis Strength BC Powder .... ■677
BC Sinus Cold Powder .... ■677
Excedrin Extra Strength Caplets/Tablets/Geltabs............ ■684
Excedrin Migraine Caplets/Tablets/Geltabs............ ■609
Goody's Body Pain Formula Powder....................................... ■684
Goody's Extra Strength Headache Powders.................. ■611
Goody's Extra Strength Pain Relief Tablets........................... ■685
Percodan Tablets 1132
St. Joseph 81 mg Aspirin Chewable and Enteric Coated Tablets.. 1869

Atovaquone (Depletion of serum proteins by pegaspargase may increase the toxicity of other drugs which are protein bound). Products include:
Malarone Pediatric Tablets 1517
Malarone Tablets 1517
Mepron Suspension 1521

Bicalutamide (Potential for unspecified unfavorable interactions).
No products indexed under this heading.

Bleomycin Sulfate (Potential for unspecified unfavorable interactions).
No products indexed under this heading.

Busulfan (Potential for unspecified unfavorable interactions). Products include:
I.V. Busulfex 2493

Myleran Tablets ... 1525

Carboplatin (Potential for unspecified unfavorable interactions).
No products indexed under this heading.

Carmustine (BCNU) (Potential for unspecified unfavorable interactions).
No products indexed under this heading.

Cefonicid Sodium (Depletion of serum proteins by pegaspargase may increase the toxicity of other drugs which are protein bound).
No products indexed under this heading.

Celecoxib (Increased risk of bleeding and/or thrombosis). Products include:
Celebrex Capsules ... 3134

Chlorambucil (Potential for unspecified unfavorable interactions). Products include:
Leukeran Tablets ... 1504

Chlordiazepoxide (Depletion of serum proteins by pegaspargase may increase the toxicity of other drugs which are protein bound).
No products indexed under this heading.

Chlordiazepoxide Hydrochloride (Depletion of serum proteins by pegaspargase may increase the toxicity of other drugs which are protein bound). Products include:
Librium Capsules ... 3347

Chlorpromazine (Depletion of serum proteins by pegaspargase may increase the toxicity of other drugs which are protein bound).
No products indexed under this heading.

Chlorpromazine Hydrochloride (Depletion of serum proteins by pegaspargase may increase the toxicity of other drugs which are protein bound).
No products indexed under this heading.

Cisplatin (Potential for unspecified unfavorable interactions).
No products indexed under this heading.

Clomipramine Hydrochloride (Depletion of serum proteins by pegaspargase may increase the toxicity of other drugs which are protein bound).
No products indexed under this heading.

Clozapine (Depletion of serum proteins by pegaspargase may increase the toxicity of other drugs which are protein bound). Products include:
Clozaril Tablets ... 2184
FazaClo Orally Disintegrating Tablets ... 551

Cyclophosphamide (Potential for unspecified unfavorable interactions).
No products indexed under this heading.

Cyclosporine (Depletion of serum proteins by pegaspargase may increase the toxicity of other drugs which are protein bound). Products include:
Gengraf Capsules ... 459
Neoral Oral Solution ... 2259
Neoral Soft Gelatin Capsules ... 2259
Restasis Ophthalmic Emulsion ... 575
Sandimmune ... 2275

Dacarbazine (Potential for unspecified unfavorable interactions).
No products indexed under this heading.

Dalteparin Sodium (Increased risk of bleeding and/or thrombosis). Products include:
Fragmin Injection ... 1097

Danaparoid Sodium (Increased risk of bleeding and/or thrombosis).
No products indexed under this heading.

Daunorubicin Citrate (Potential for unspecified unfavorable interactions).
No products indexed under this heading.

Daunorubicin Hydrochloride (Potential for unspecified unfavorable interactions).
No products indexed under this heading.

Denileukin Diftitox (Potential for unspecified unfavorable interactions). Products include:
Ontak Vials ... 1745

Diazepam (Depletion of serum proteins by pegaspargase may increase the toxicity of other drugs which are protein bound). Products include:
Diastat Rectal Delivery System ... 3343
Valium Tablets ... 2819

Diclofenac Potassium (Depletion of serum proteins by pegaspargase may increase the toxicity of other drugs which are protein bound; increased risk of bleeding and/or thrombosis).
No products indexed under this heading.

Diclofenac Sodium (Depletion of serum proteins by pegaspargase may increase the toxicity of other drugs which are protein bound; increased risk of bleeding and/or thrombosis). Products include:
Arthrotec Tablets ... 3129
Voltaren Ophthalmic Solution ... 2309
Voltaren Tablets ... 2307
Voltaren-XR Tablets ... 2310

Dicumarol (Increased risk of bleeding and/or thrombosis).
No products indexed under this heading.

Dipyridamole (Depletion of serum proteins by pegaspargase may increase the toxicity of other drugs which are protein bound). Products include:
Aggrenox Capsules ... 822
Persantine Tablets ... 868

Docetaxel (Potential for unspecified unfavorable interactions). Products include:
Taxotere Injection Concentrate ... 2932

Doxorubicin Hydrochloride (Potential for unspecified unfavorable interactions).
No products indexed under this heading.

Enoxaparin Sodium (Increased risk of bleeding and/or thrombosis). Products include:
Lovenox Injection ... 2915

Epirubicin Hydrochloride (Potential for unspecified unfavorable interactions).
No products indexed under this heading.

Estramustine Phosphate Sodium (Potential for unspecified unfavorable interactions). Products include:
Emcyt Capsules ... 2634

Etodolac (Increased risk of bleeding and/or thrombosis).
No products indexed under this heading.

Etoposide (Potential for unspecified unfavorable interactions).
No products indexed under this heading.

Exemestane (Potential for unspecified unfavorable interactions). Products include:
Aromasin Tablets ... 2600

Fenoprofen Calcium (Depletion of serum proteins by pegaspargase may increase the toxicity of other drugs which are protein bound; increased risk of bleeding and/or thrombosis). Products include:
Nalfon Capsules ... 2502

Floxuridine (Potential for unspecified unfavorable interactions).
No products indexed under this heading.

Fluorouracil (Potential for unspecified unfavorable interactions). Products include:
Carac Cream, 0.5% ... 2879
Efudex ... 3363

Flurazepam Hydrochloride (Depletion of serum proteins by pegaspargase may increase the toxicity of other drugs which are protein bound). Products include:
Dalmane Capsules ... 3342

Flurbiprofen (Depletion of serum proteins by pegaspargase may increase the toxicity of other drugs which are protein bound; increased risk of bleeding and/or thrombosis).
No products indexed under this heading.

Flutamide (Potential for unspecified unfavorable interactions). Products include:
Eulexin Capsules ... 3009

Fondaparinux Sodium (Increased risk of bleeding and/or thrombosis). Products include:
Arixtra Injection ... 1351

Gemcitabine Hydrochloride (Potential for unspecified unfavorable interactions). Products include:
Gemzar for Injection ... 1771

Glipizide (Depletion of serum proteins by pegaspargase may increase the toxicity of other drugs which are protein bound).
No products indexed under this heading.

Heparin Calcium (Increased risk of bleeding and/or thrombosis).
No products indexed under this heading.

Heparin Sodium (Increased risk of bleeding and/or thrombosis).
No products indexed under this heading.

Hydroxyurea (Potential for unspecified unfavorable interactions).
No products indexed under this heading.

Ibuprofen (Depletion of serum proteins by pegaspargase may increase the toxicity of other drugs which are protein bound; increased risk of bleeding and/or thrombosis). Products include:
Advil Allergy Sinus Caplets ... 770
Advil ... 674
Children's Advil Oral Suspension ... 603
Children's Advil Chewable Tablets ... 603
Advil Cold & Sinus ... 723
Infants' Advil Concentrated Drops ... 604
Infants' Advil Concentrated Drops - White Grape (Dye-Free) ... 604
Junior Strength Advil Swallow Tablets ... 605
Advil Migraine Liquigels ... 608
Advil Multi-Symptom Cold Caplets ... 770
Advil PM Caplets ... 615
Motrin IB Tablets and Caplets ... 1866
Children's Motrin Oral Suspension ... 1867
Children's Motrin Non-Staining Dye-Free Oral Suspension ... 1867
Children's Motrin Cold Oral Suspension ... 1867
Infants' Motrin Concentrated Drops ... 1867
Infants' Motrin Non-Staining Dye-Free Concentrated Drops ... 1867
Junior Strength Motrin Caplets and Chewable Tablets ... 1867
Vicoprofen Tablets ... 539

Idarubicin Hydrochloride (Potential for unspecified unfavorable interactions).
No products indexed under this heading.

Ifosfamide (Potential for unspecified unfavorable interactions).
No products indexed under this heading.

Imipramine Hydrochloride (Depletion of serum proteins by pegaspargase may increase the toxicity of other drugs which are protein bound).
No products indexed under this heading.

Imipramine Pamoate (Depletion of serum proteins by pegaspargase may increase the toxicity of other drugs which are protein bound).
No products indexed under this heading.

Indomethacin (Depletion of serum proteins by pegaspargase may increase the toxicity of other drugs which are protein bound; increased risk of bleeding and/or thrombosis). Products include:
Indocin ... 1995

Indomethacin Sodium Trihydrate (Depletion of serum proteins by pegaspargase may increase the toxicity of other drugs which are protein bound; increased risk of bleeding and/or thrombosis). Products include:
Indocin I.V. ... 2465

Interferon alfa-2a, Recombinant (Potential for unspecified unfavorable interactions).
No products indexed under this heading.

Interferon alfa-2b, Recombinant (Potential for unspecified unfavorable interactions). Products include:
Intron A for Injection ... 3024
Rebetron Combination Therapy ... 3063

Irinotecan Hydrochloride (Potential for unspecified unfavorable interactions). Products include:
Camptosar Injection ... 2604

Ketoprofen (Depletion of serum proteins by pegaspargase may increase the toxicity of other drugs which are protein bound; increased risk of bleeding and/or thrombosis).
No products indexed under this heading.

Ketorolac Tromethamine (Depletion of serum proteins by pegaspargase may increase the toxicity of other drugs which are protein bound; increased risk of bleeding and/or thrombosis). Products include:
Acular Ophthalmic Solution ... 565
Acular LS Ophthalmic Solution ... 566

Levamisole Hydrochloride (Potential for unspecified unfavorable interactions).
No products indexed under this heading.

IMPORTANT NOTE: Always consult each drug listing in the patient's regimen for possible interactions.

Lomustine (CCNU) (Potential for unspecified unfavorable interactions).
No products indexed under this heading.

Low Molecular Weight Heparins (Increased risk of bleeding and/or thrombosis).
No products indexed under this heading.

Mechlorethamine Hydrochloride (Potential for unspecified unfavorable interactions). Products include:
Mustargen for Injection 2468

Meclofenamate Sodium (Depletion of serum proteins by pegaspargase may increase the toxicity of other drugs which are protein bound; increased risk of bleeding and/or thrombosis).
No products indexed under this heading.

Mefenamic Acid (Depletion of serum proteins by pegaspargase may increase the toxicity of other drugs which are protein bound; increased risk of bleeding and/or thrombosis).
No products indexed under this heading.

Megestrol Acetate (Potential for unspecified unfavorable interactions). Products include:
Megace ES Oral Suspension 2481

Meloxicam (Increased risk of bleeding and/or thrombosis). Products include:
Mobic Oral Suspension 863
Mobic Tablets 863

Melphalan (Potential for unspecified unfavorable interactions). Products include:
Alkeran Tablets 956

Mercaptopurine (Potential for unspecified unfavorable interactions).
No products indexed under this heading.

Methotrexate Sodium (Pegaspargase inhibits protein synthesis and cell replication and thus interferes with the action of methotrexate which requires cell replication for its lethal effect; potential for unspecified unfavorable interactions).
No products indexed under this heading.

Midazolam Hydrochloride (Depletion of serum proteins by pegaspargase may increase the toxicity of other drugs which are protein bound).
No products indexed under this heading.

Mitomycin (Mitomycin-C) (Potential for unspecified unfavorable interactions).
No products indexed under this heading.

Mitotane (Potential for unspecified unfavorable interactions).
No products indexed under this heading.

Mitoxantrone Hydrochloride (Potential for unspecified unfavorable interactions).
No products indexed under this heading.

Nabumetone (Increased risk of bleeding and/or thrombosis).
No products indexed under this heading.

Naproxen (Depletion of serum proteins by pegaspargase may increase the toxicity of other drugs which are protein bound; increased risk of bleeding and/or thrombosis). Products include:
EC-Naprosyn Delayed-Release Tablets 2761
Naprosyn Suspension 2761
Naprosyn Tablets 2761
Prevacid NapraPAC 3280

Naproxen Sodium (Depletion of serum proteins by pegaspargase may increase the toxicity of other drugs which are protein bound; increased risk of bleeding and/or thrombosis). Products include:
Aleve Caplets 742
Aleve Gelcaps 743
Aleve Tablets 743
Aleve Cold & Sinus Caplets 744
Anaprox Tablets 2761
Anaprox DS Tablets 2761

Nortriptyline Hydrochloride (Depletion of serum proteins by pegaspargase may increase the toxicity of other drugs which are protein bound).
No products indexed under this heading.

Oxaliplatin (Potential for unspecified unfavorable interactions). Products include:
Eloxatin for Injection 2892

Oxaprozin (Depletion of serum proteins by pegaspargase may increase the toxicity of other drugs which are protein bound; increased risk of bleeding and/or thrombosis).
No products indexed under this heading.

Oxazepam (Depletion of serum proteins by pegaspargase may increase the toxicity of other drugs which are protein bound).
No products indexed under this heading.

Paclitaxel (Potential for unspecified unfavorable interactions).
No products indexed under this heading.

Phenylbutazone (Depletion of serum proteins by pegaspargase may increase the toxicity of other drugs which are protein bound; increased risk of bleeding and/or thrombosis).
No products indexed under this heading.

Piroxicam (Depletion of serum proteins by pegaspargase may increase the toxicity of other drugs which are protein bound; increased risk of bleeding and/or thrombosis).
No products indexed under this heading.

Procarbazine Hydrochloride (Potential for unspecified unfavorable interactions). Products include:
Matulane Capsules 3191

Propranolol Hydrochloride (Depletion of serum proteins by pegaspargase may increase the toxicity of other drugs which are protein bound). Products include:
Inderal LA Long-Acting Capsules 3429
InnoPran XL Capsules 2723

Rofecoxib (Increased risk of bleeding and/or thrombosis).
No products indexed under this heading.

Streptozocin (Potential for unspecified unfavorable interactions).
No products indexed under this heading.

Sulindac (Depletion of serum proteins by pegaspargase may increase the toxicity of other drugs which are protein bound; increased risk of bleeding and/or thrombosis). Products include:
Clinoril Tablets 1924

Tamoxifen Citrate (Potential for unspecified unfavorable interactions). Products include:
Soltamox Oral Solution 3527

Temazepam (Depletion of serum proteins by pegaspargase may increase the toxicity of other drugs which are protein bound). Products include:
Restoril Capsules 1860

Teniposide (Potential for unspecified unfavorable interactions).
No products indexed under this heading.

Thioguanine (Potential for unspecified unfavorable interactions). Products include:
Tabloid Tablets 1575

Thiotepa (Potential for unspecified unfavorable interactions).
No products indexed under this heading.

Tinzaparin Sodium (Increased risk of bleeding and/or thrombosis).
No products indexed under this heading.

Tolbutamide (Depletion of serum proteins by pegaspargase may increase the toxicity of other drugs which are protein bound).
No products indexed under this heading.

Tolmetin Sodium (Depletion of serum proteins by pegaspargase may increase the toxicity of other drugs which are protein bound; increased risk of bleeding and/or thrombosis).
No products indexed under this heading.

Topotecan Hydrochloride (Potential for unspecified unfavorable interactions). Products include:
Hycamtin for Injection 1458

Toremifene Citrate (Potential for unspecified unfavorable interactions).
No products indexed under this heading.

Trimipramine Maleate (Depletion of serum proteins by pegaspargase may increase the toxicity of other drugs which are protein bound).
No products indexed under this heading.

Valdecoxib (Increased risk of bleeding and/or thrombosis).
No products indexed under this heading.

Valrubicin (Potential for unspecified unfavorable interactions).
No products indexed under this heading.

Vincristine Sulfate (Potential for unspecified unfavorable interactions).
No products indexed under this heading.

Vinorelbine Tartrate (Potential for unspecified unfavorable interactions).
No products indexed under this heading.

Warfarin Sodium (Depletion of serum proteins by pegaspargase may increase the toxicity of other drugs which are protein bound; increased risk of bleeding and/or thrombosis). Products include:
Coumadin for Injection 898
Coumadin Tablets 898

ONE-A-DAY CHOLESTEROL PLUS TABLETS

(Multivitamins with Minerals) .... ▣815
None cited in PDR database.

ONE-A-DAY MEN'S HEALTH FORMULA TABLETS

(Fish Oils, Multivitamins with Minerals, Soy-containing dietary supplements).................................. ▣815
None cited in PDR database.

ONE-A-DAY WEIGHT SMART TABLETS

(Green Tea Extract, Herbals with Vitamins & Minerals, Vitamins with Minerals)... ▣816
None cited in PDR database.

ONE-A-DAY WOMEN'S TABLETS

(Vitamins with Minerals) .... ▣816
None cited in PDR database.

ONTAK VIALS

(Denileukin Diftitox) 1745
None cited in PDR database.

OPANA TABLETS

(Oxymorphone Hydrochloride) 1122
May interact with anesthetics, anticholinergics, hypnotics and sedatives, monoamine oxidase inhibitors, mixed agonist/antagonist opioid analgesics, narcotic analgesics, phenothiazines, tranquilizers, and certain other agents. Compounds in these categories include:

Alfentanil Hydrochloride (The concomitant use of other CNS depressants including sedatives, hypnotics, tranquilizers, general anesthetics, phenothiazines, other opioids, and alcohol may produce additive CNS depressant effects. Additive effects resulting in respiratory depression, hypotension, profound sedation or coma may result if these drugs are taken in combination with the usual doses of oxymorphone hydrochloride).
No products indexed under this heading.

Alprazolam (The concomitant use of other CNS depressants including sedatives, hypnotics, tranquilizers, general anesthetics, phenothiazines, other opioids, and alcohol may produce additive CNS depressant effects. Additive effects resulting in respiratory depression, hypotension, profound sedation or coma may result if these drugs are taken in combination with the usual doses of oxymorphone hydrochloride). Products include:
Niravam Orally Disintegrating Tablets 3092

Atropine Sulfate (Anticholinergics or other medications with anticholinergic activity when used concurrently with opioid analgesics may result in increased risk of urinary retention and/or severe constipation, which may lead to paralytic ileus). Products include:
Donnatal Extentabs 2493

Belladonna Alkaloids (Anticholinergics or other medications with anticholinergic activity when used concurrently with opioid analgesics may result in increased risk of urinary retention and/or severe constipation, which may lead to paralytic ileus). Products include:
Hyland's Teething Tablets .... ▣830

Benztropine Mesylate (Anticholinergics or other medications with anticholinergic activity when used concurrently with opioid analgesics may result in increased risk of urinary retention and/or severe constipation, which may lead to paralytic ileus).

No products indexed under this heading.

Biperiden Hydrochloride (Anticholinergics or other medications with anticholinergic activity when used concurrently with opioid analgesics may result in increased risk of urinary retention and/or severe constipation, which may lead to paralytic ileus).

No products indexed under this heading.

Buprenorphine Hydrochloride (The concomitant use of other CNS depressants including sedatives, hypnotics, tranquilizers, general anesthetics, phenothiazines, other opioids, and alcohol may produce additive CNS depressant effects. Additive effects resulting in respiratory depression, hypotension, profound sedation or coma may result if these drugs are taken in combination with the usual doses of oxymorphone hydrochloride). Products include:

Buspirone Hydrochloride (The concomitant use of other CNS depressants including sedatives, hypnotics, tranquilizers, general anesthetics, phenothiazines, other opioids, and alcohol may produce additive CNS depressant effects. Additive effects resulting in respiratory depression, hypotension, profound sedation or coma may result if these drugs are taken in combination with the usual doses of oxymorphone hydrochloride).

No products indexed under this heading.

Butorphanol Tartrate (Agonist/antagonist analgesics should not be administered to patients who have received or are receiving a course of therapy with pure opioid agonist analgesic, such as oxymorphone hydrochloride. In this situation, mixed agonist/antagonist analgesics may reduce the analgesic effect of oxymorphone hydrochloride and/or may precipitate withdrawal symptoms).

No products indexed under this heading.

Chlordiazepoxide (The concomitant use of other CNS depressants including sedatives, hypnotics, tranquilizers, general anesthetics, phenothiazines, other opioids, and alcohol may produce additive CNS depressant effects. Additive effects resulting in respiratory depression, hypotension, profound sedation or coma may result if these drugs are taken in combination with the usual doses of oxymorphone hydrochloride).

No products indexed under this heading.

Chlordiazepoxide Hydrochloride (The concomitant use of other CNS depressants including sedatives, hypnotics, tranquilizers, general anesthetics, phenothiazines, other opioids, and alcohol may produce additive CNS depressant effects.

Additive effects resulting in respiratory depression, hypotension, profound sedation or coma may result if these drugs are taken in combination with the usual doses of oxymorphone hydrochloride). Products include:

Chlorpromazine (The concomitant use of other CNS depressants including sedatives, hypnotics, tranquilizers, general anesthetics, phenothiazines, other opioids, and alcohol may produce additive CNS depressant effects. Additive effects resulting in respiratory depression, hypotension, profound sedation or coma may result if these drugs are taken in combination with the usual doses of oxymorphone hydrochloride).

No products indexed under this heading.

Chlorpromazine Hydrochloride (The concomitant use of other CNS depressants including sedatives, hypnotics, tranquilizers, general anesthetics, phenothiazines, other opioids, and alcohol may produce additive CNS depressant effects. Additive effects resulting in respiratory depression, hypotension, profound sedation or coma may result if these drugs are taken in combination with the usual doses of oxymorphone hydrochloride).

No products indexed under this heading.

Chlorprothixene (The concomitant use of other CNS depressants including sedatives, hypnotics, tranquilizers, general anesthetics, phenothiazines, other opioids, and alcohol may produce additive CNS depressant effects. Additive effects resulting in respiratory depression, hypotension, profound sedation or coma may result if these drugs are taken in combination with the usual doses of oxymorphone hydrochloride).

No products indexed under this heading.

Chlorprothixene Hydrochloride (The concomitant use of other CNS depressants including sedatives, hypnotics, tranquilizers, general anesthetics, phenothiazines, other opioids, and alcohol may produce additive CNS depressant effects. Additive effects resulting in respiratory depression, hypotension, profound sedation or coma may result if these drugs are taken in combination with the usual doses of oxymorphone hydrochloride).

No products indexed under this heading.

Clidinium Bromide (Anticholinergics or other medications with anticholinergic activity when used concurrently with opioid analgesics may result in increased risk of urinary retention and/or severe constipation, which may lead to paralytic ileus).

No products indexed under this heading.

Clorazepate Dipotassium (The concomitant use of other CNS depressants including sedatives, hypnotics, tranquilizers, general anesthetics, phenothiazines, other opioids, and alcohol may produce additive CNS depressant effects. Additive effects resulting in respiratory depression, hypotension, profound sedation or coma may result if

these drugs are taken in combination with the usual doses of oxymorphone hydrochloride). Products include:

Codeine Phosphate (The concomitant use of other CNS depressants including sedatives, hypnotics, tranquilizers, general anesthetics, phenothiazines, other opioids, and alcohol may produce additive CNS depressant effects. Additive effects resulting in respiratory depression, hypotension, profound sedation or coma may result if these drugs are taken in combination with the usual doses of oxymorphone hydrochloride). Products include:

Dezocine (The concomitant use of other CNS depressants including sedatives, hypnotics, tranquilizers, general anesthetics, phenothiazines, other opioids, and alcohol may produce additive CNS depressant effects. Additive effects resulting in respiratory depression, hypotension, profound sedation or coma may result if these drugs are taken in combination with the usual doses of oxymorphone hydrochloride).

No products indexed under this heading.

Diazepam (The concomitant use of other CNS depressants including sedatives, hypnotics, tranquilizers, general anesthetics, phenothiazines, other opioids, and alcohol may produce additive CNS depressant effects. Additive effects resulting in respiratory depression, hypotension, profound sedation or coma may result if these drugs are taken in combination with the usual doses of oxymorphone hydrochloride). Products include:

Dicyclomine Hydrochloride (Anticholinergics or other medications with anticholinergic activity when used concurrently with opioid analgesics may result in increased risk of urinary retention and/or severe constipation, which may lead to paralytic ileus). Products include:

Droperidol (The concomitant use of other CNS depressants including sedatives, hypnotics, tranquilizers, general anesthetics, phenothiazines, other opioids, and alcohol may produce additive CNS depressant effects. Additive effects resulting in respiratory depression, hypotension, profound sedation or coma may result if these drugs are taken in combination with the usual doses of oxymorphone hydrochloride).

No products indexed under this heading.

Enflurane (The concomitant use of other CNS depressants including sedatives, hypnotics, tranquilizers, general anesthetics, phenothiazines, other opioids, and alcohol may produce additive CNS depressant effects. Additive effects resulting in respiratory depression, hypotension, profound sedation or coma may result if these drugs are taken in combination with the usual doses of oxymorphone hydrochloride).

No products indexed under this heading.

Estazolam (The concomitant use of other CNS depressants including sedatives, hypnotics, tranquilizers, general anesthetics, phenothiazines, other opioids, and alcohol may produce additive CNS depressant effects. Additive effects resulting in respiratory depression, hypotension, profound sedation or coma may result if these drugs are taken in combination with the usual doses of oxymorphone hydrochloride). Products include:

Ethchlorvynol (The concomitant use of other CNS depressants including sedatives, hypnotics, tranquilizers, general anesthetics, phenothiazines, other opioids, and alcohol may produce additive CNS depressant effects. Additive effects resulting in respiratory depression, hypotension, profound sedation or coma may result if these drugs are taken in combination with the usual doses of oxymorphone hydrochloride).

No products indexed under this heading.

Ethinamate (The concomitant use of other CNS depressants including sedatives, hypnotics, tranquilizers, general anesthetics, phenothiazines, other opioids, and alcohol may produce additive CNS depressant effects. Additive effects resulting in respiratory depression, hypotension, profound sedation or coma may result if these drugs are taken in combination with the usual doses of oxymorphone hydrochloride).

No products indexed under this heading.

Fentanyl (The concomitant use of other CNS depressants including sedatives, hypnotics, tranquilizers, general anesthetics, phenothiazines, other opioids, and alcohol may produce additive CNS depressant effects. Additive effects resulting in respiratory depression, hypotension, profound sedation or coma may result if these drugs are taken in combination with the usual doses of oxymorphone hydrochloride). Products include:

Fentanyl Citrate (The concomitant use of other CNS depressants including sedatives, hypnotics, tranquilizers, general anesthetics, phenothiazines, other opioids, and alcohol may produce additive CNS depressant effects. Additive effects resulting in respiratory depression, hypotension, profound sedation or coma may result if these drugs are taken in combination with the usual doses of oxymorphone hydrochloride). Products include:

Fluphenazine Decanoate (The concomitant use of other CNS depressants including sedatives, hypnotics, tranquilizers, general anesthetics, phenothiazines, other opioids, and alcohol may produce additive CNS depressant effects. Additive effects resulting in respiratory depression, hypotension, profound sedation or coma may result if these drugs are taken in combination with the usual doses of oxymorphone hydrochloride).

No products indexed under this heading.

IMPORTANT NOTE: Always consult each drug listing in the patient's regimen for possible interactions.

Fluphenazine Enanthate (The concomitant use of other CNS depressants including sedatives, hypnotics, tranquilizers, general anesthetics, phenothiazines, other opioids, and alcohol may produce additive CNS depressant effects. Additive effects resulting in respiratory depression, hypotension, profound sedation or coma may result if these drugs are taken in combination with the usual doses of oxymorphone hydrochloride).

No products indexed under this heading.

Fluphenazine Hydrochloride (The concomitant use of other CNS depressants including sedatives, hypnotics, tranquilizers, general anesthetics, phenothiazines, other opioids, and alcohol may produce additive CNS depressant effects. Additive effects resulting in respiratory depression, hypotension, profound sedation or coma may result if these drugs are taken in combination with the usual doses of oxymorphone hydrochloride).

No products indexed under this heading.

Flurazepam Hydrochloride (The concomitant use of other CNS depressants including sedatives, hypnotics, tranquilizers, general anesthetics, phenothiazines, other opioids, and alcohol may produce additive CNS depressant effects. Additive effects resulting in respiratory depression, hypotension, profound sedation or coma may result if these drugs are taken in combination with the usual doses of oxymorphone hydrochloride). Products include:

' Dalmane Capsules 3342

Glutethimide (The concomitant use of other CNS depressants including sedatives, hypnotics, tranquilizers, general anesthetics, phenothiazines, other opioids, and alcohol may produce additive CNS depressant effects. Additive effects resulting in respiratory depression, hypotension, profound sedation or coma may result if these drugs are taken in combination with the usual doses of oxymorphone hydrochloride).

No products indexed under this heading.

Glycopyrrolate (Anticholinergics or other medications with anticholinergic activity when used concurrently with opioid analgesics may result in increased risk of urinary retention and/or severe constipation, which may lead to paralytic ileus).

No products indexed under this heading.

Haloperidol (The concomitant use of other CNS depressants including sedatives, hypnotics, tranquilizers, general anesthetics, phenothiazines, other opioids, and alcohol may produce additive CNS depressant effects. Additive effects resulting in respiratory depression, hypotension, profound sedation or coma may result if these drugs are taken in combination with the usual doses of oxymorphone hydrochloride).

No products indexed under this heading.

Haloperidol Decanoate (The concomitant use of other CNS depressants including sedatives, hypnotics, tranquilizers, general anesthetics, phenothiazines, other opioids, and alcohol may produce additive CNS

depressant effects. Additive effects resulting in respiratory depression, hypotension, profound sedation or coma may result if these drugs are taken in combination with the usual doses of oxymorphone hydrochloride).

No products indexed under this heading.

Halothane (The concomitant use of other CNS depressants including sedatives, hypnotics, tranquilizers, general anesthetics, phenothiazines, other opioids, and alcohol may produce additive CNS depressant effects. Additive effects resulting in respiratory depression, hypotension, profound sedation or coma may result if these drugs are taken in combination with the usual doses of oxymorphone hydrochloride).

No products indexed under this heading.

Hydrocodone Bitartrate (The concomitant use of other CNS depressants including sedatives, hypnotics, tranquilizers, general anesthetics, phenothiazines, other opioids, and alcohol may produce additive CNS depressant effects. Additive effects resulting in respiratory depression, hypotension, profound sedation or coma may result if these drugs are taken in combination with the usual doses of oxymorphone hydrochloride). Products include:

Hycodan ... 1116
Hycotuss Expectorant Syrup 1117
Vicodin Tablets 535
Vicodin ES Tablets 536
Vicodin HP Tablets 538
Vicoprofen Tablets 539
Zydone Tablets 1139

Hydrocodone Polistirex (The concomitant use of other CNS depressants including sedatives, hypnotics, tranquilizers, general anesthetics, phenothiazines, other opioids, and alcohol may produce additive CNS depressant effects. Additive effects resulting in respiratory depression, hypotension, profound sedation or coma may result if these drugs are taken in combination with the usual doses of oxymorphone hydrochloride). Products include:

Tussionex Pennkinetic
 Extended-Release Suspension 3327

Hydromorphone Hydrochloride (The concomitant use of other CNS depressants including sedatives, hypnotics, tranquilizers, general anesthetics, phenothiazines, other opioids, and alcohol may produce additive CNS depressant effects. Additive effects resulting in respiratory depression, hypotension, profound sedation or coma may result if these drugs are taken in combination with the usual doses of oxymorphone hydrochloride). Products include:

Dilaudid ... 440
Dilaudid Non-Sterile Powder 440
Dilaudid Oral Liquid 445
Dilaudid Rectal Suppositories 440
Dilaudid Tablets 440
Dilaudid Tablets - 8 mg 445
Dilaudid-HP 442

Hydroxyzine Hydrochloride (The concomitant use of other CNS depressants including sedatives, hypnotics, tranquilizers, general anesthetics, phenothiazines, other opioids, and alcohol may produce additive CNS depressant effects. Additive effects resulting in respiratory depression, hypotension, pro-

found sedation or coma may result if these drugs are taken in combination with the usual doses of oxymorphone hydrochloride).

No products indexed under this heading.

Hyoscyamine (Anticholinergics or other medications with anticholinergic activity when used concurrently with opioid analgesics may result in increased risk of urinary retention and/or severe constipation, which may lead to paralytic ileus).

No products indexed under this heading.

Hyoscyamine Sulfate (Anticholinergics or other medications with anticholinergic activity when used concurrently with opioid analgesics may result in increased risk of urinary retention and/or severe constipation, which may lead to paralytic ileus). Products include:

Donnatal Extentabs 2493
Prosed/DS Tablets 1157

Ipratropium Bromide (Anticholinergics or other medications with anticholinergic activity when used concurrently with opioid analgesics may result in increased risk of urinary retention and/or severe constipation, which may lead to paralytic ileus). Products include:

Atrovent Inhalation Solution 835
Atrovent HFA Inhalation Aerosol 841
Atrovent Nasal Spray 0.03% 837
Atrovent Nasal Spray 0.06% 839
Combivent Inhalation Aerosol 847
DuoNeb Inhalation Solution 1058

Isocarboxazid (No specific interaction between oxymorphone and monoamine oxidase inhibitors has been observed, but caution in the use of any opioid in patients taking this class of drugs is appropriate).

No products indexed under this heading.

Isoflurane (The concomitant use of other CNS depressants including sedatives, hypnotics, tranquilizers, general anesthetics, phenothiazines, other opioids, and alcohol may produce additive CNS depressant effects. Additive effects resulting in respiratory depression, hypotension, profound sedation or coma may result if these drugs are taken in combination with the usual doses of oxymorphone hydrochloride).

No products indexed under this heading.

Ketamine Hydrochloride (The concomitant use of other CNS depressants including sedatives, hypnotics, tranquilizers, general anesthetics, phenothiazines, other opioids, and alcohol may produce additive CNS depressant effects. Additive effects resulting in respiratory depression, hypotension, profound sedation or coma may result if these drugs are taken in combination with the usual doses of oxymorphone hydrochloride).

No products indexed under this heading.

Levorphanol Tartrate (The concomitant use of other CNS depressants including sedatives, hypnotics, tranquilizers, general anesthetics, phenothiazines, other opioids, and alcohol may produce additive CNS depressant effects. Additive effects resulting in respiratory depression, hypotension, profound sedation or coma may result if these drugs are taken in combination with the usual doses of oxymorphone

hydrochloride).

No products indexed under this heading.

Lorazepam (The concomitant use of other CNS depressants including sedatives, hypnotics, tranquilizers, general anesthetics, phenothiazines, other opioids, and alcohol may produce additive CNS depressant effects. Additive effects resulting in respiratory depression, hypotension, profound sedation or coma may result if these drugs are taken in combination with the usual doses of oxymorphone hydrochloride).

No products indexed under this heading.

Loxapine Hydrochloride (The concomitant use of other CNS depressants including sedatives, hypnotics, tranquilizers, general anesthetics, phenothiazines, other opioids, and alcohol may produce additive CNS depressant effects. Additive effects resulting in respiratory depression, hypotension, profound sedation or coma may result if these drugs are taken in combination with the usual doses of oxymorphone hydrochloride).

No products indexed under this heading.

Loxapine Succinate (The concomitant use of other CNS depressants including sedatives, hypnotics, tranquilizers, general anesthetics, phenothiazines, other opioids, and alcohol may produce additive CNS depressant effects. Additive effects resulting in respiratory depression, hypotension, profound sedation or coma may result if these drugs are taken in combination with the usual doses of oxymorphone hydrochloride).

No products indexed under this heading.

Mepenzolate Bromide (Anticholinergics or other medications with anticholinergic activity when used concurrently with opioid analgesics may result in increased risk of urinary retention and/or severe constipation, which may lead to paralytic ileus).

No products indexed under this heading.

Meperidine Hydrochloride (The concomitant use of other CNS depressants including sedatives, hypnotics, tranquilizers, general anesthetics, phenothiazines, other opioids, and alcohol may produce additive CNS depressant effects. Additive effects resulting in respiratory depression, hypotension, profound sedation or coma may result if these drugs are taken in combination with the usual doses of oxymorphone hydrochloride).

No products indexed under this heading.

Meprobamate (The concomitant use of other CNS depressants including sedatives, hypnotics, tranquilizers, general anesthetics, phenothiazines, other opioids, and alcohol may produce additive CNS depressant effects. Additive effects resulting in respiratory depression, hypotension, profound sedation or coma may result if these drugs are taken in combination with the usual doses of oxymorphone hydrochloride).

No products indexed under this heading.

Mesoridazine Besylate (The concomitant use of other CNS depressants including sedatives, hypnotics, tranquilizers, general anesthetics, phenothiazines, other opioids, and alcohol may produce additive CNS depressant effects. Additive effects resulting in respiratory depression, hypotension, profound sedation or coma may result if these drugs are taken in combination with the usual doses of oxymorphone hydrochloride).

No products indexed under this heading.

Methadone Hydrochloride (The concomitant use of other CNS depressants including sedatives, hypnotics, tranquilizers, general anesthetics, phenothiazines, other opioids, and alcohol may produce additive CNS depressant effects. Additive effects resulting in respiratory depression, hypotension, profound sedation or coma may result if these drugs are taken in combination with the usual doses of oxymorphone hydrochloride).

No products indexed under this heading.

Methohexital Sodium (The concomitant use of other CNS depressants including sedatives, hypnotics, tranquilizers, general anesthetics, phenothiazines, other opioids, and alcohol may produce additive CNS depressant effects. Additive effects resulting in respiratory depression, hypotension, profound sedation or coma may result if these drugs are taken in combination with the usual doses of oxymorphone hydrochloride).

No products indexed under this heading.

Methotrimeprazine (The concomitant use of other CNS depressants including sedatives, hypnotics, tranquilizers, general anesthetics, phenothiazines, other opioids, and alcohol may produce additive CNS depressant effects. Additive effects resulting in respiratory depression, hypotension, profound sedation or coma may result if these drugs are taken in combination with the usual doses of oxymorphone hydrochloride).

No products indexed under this heading.

Midazolam Hydrochloride (The concomitant use of other CNS depressants including sedatives, hypnotics, tranquilizers, general anesthetics, phenothiazines, other opioids, and alcohol may produce additive CNS depressant effects. Additive effects resulting in respiratory depression, hypotension, profound sedation or coma may result if these drugs are taken in combination with the usual doses of oxymorphone hydrochloride).

No products indexed under this heading.

Moclobemide (No specific interaction between oxymorphone and monoamine oxidase inhibitors has been observed, but caution in the use of any opioid in patients taking this class of drugs is appropriate).

No products indexed under this heading.

Molindone Hydrochloride (The concomitant use of other CNS depressants including sedatives, hypnotics, tranquilizers, general anesthetics, phenothiazines, other

opioids, and alcohol may produce additive CNS depressant effects. Additive effects resulting in respiratory depression, hypotension, profound sedation or coma may result if these drugs are taken in combination with the usual doses of oxymorphone hydrochloride). Products include:

Moban Tablets 1119

Morphine Sulfate (The concomitant use of other CNS depressants including sedatives, hypnotics, tranquilizers, general anesthetics, phenothiazines, other opioids, and alcohol may produce additive CNS depressant effects. Additive effects resulting in respiratory depression, hypotension, profound sedation or coma may result if these drugs are taken in combination with the usual doses of oxymorphone hydrochloride). Products include:

Avinza Capsules 1741
Kadian Capsules 577
MS Contin Tablets 2701

Nalbuphine Hydrochloride (Agonist/antagonist analgesics should not be administered to patients who have received or are receiving a course of therapy with pure opioid agonist analgesic, such as oxymorphone hydrochloride. In this situation, mixed agonist/antagonist analgesics may reduce the analgesic effect of oxymorphone hydrochloride and/or may precipitate withdrawal symptoms).

No products indexed under this heading.

Oxazepam (The concomitant use of other CNS depressants including sedatives, hypnotics, tranquilizers, general anesthetics, phenothiazines, other opioids, and alcohol may produce additive CNS depressant effects. Additive effects resulting in respiratory depression, hypotension, profound sedation or coma may result if these drugs are taken in combination with the usual doses of oxymorphone hydrochloride).

No products indexed under this heading.

Oxybutynin Chloride (Anticholinergics or other medications with anticholinergic activity when used concurrently with opioid analgesics may result in increased risk of urinary retention and/or severe constipation, which may lead to paralytic ileus). Products include:

Ditropan XL Extended-Release
Tablets ... 2413

Oxycodone Hydrochloride (The concomitant use of other CNS depressants including sedatives, hypnotics, tranquilizers, general anesthetics, phenothiazines, other opioids, and alcohol may produce additive CNS depressant effects. Additive effects resulting in respiratory depression, hypotension, profound sedation or coma may result if these drugs are taken in combination with the usual doses of oxymorphone hydrochloride). Products include:

OxyContin Tablets 2703
OxyFast Oral Concentrate
Solution 2708
OxyIR Capsules 2708
Percocet Tablets 1131
Percodan Tablets 1132

Pargyline Hydrochloride (No specific interaction between oxymorphone and monoamine oxidase inhibitors has been observed, but caution in the use of any opioid in patients taking this class of drugs is appropriate).

No products indexed under this heading.

Pentazocine Hydrochloride (Agonist/antagonist analgesics should not be administered to patients who have received or are receiving a course of therapy with pure opioid agonist analgesic, such as oxymorphone hydrochloride. In this situation, mixed agonist/antagonist analgesics may reduce the analgesic effect of oxymorphone hydrochloride and/or may precipitate withdrawal symptoms).

No products indexed under this heading.

Pentazocine Lactate (Agonist/antagonist analgesics should not be administered to patients who have received or are receiving a course of therapy with pure opioid agonist analgesic, such as oxymorphone hydrochloride. In this situation, mixed agonist/antagonist analgesics may reduce the analgesic effect of oxymorphone hydrochloride and/or may precipitate withdrawal symptoms).

No products indexed under this heading.

Perphenazine (The concomitant use of other CNS depressants including sedatives, hypnotics, tranquilizers, general anesthetics, phenothiazines, other opioids, and alcohol may produce additive CNS depressant effects. Additive effects resulting in respiratory depression, hypotension, profound sedation or coma may result if these drugs are taken in combination with the usual doses of oxymorphone hydrochloride).

No products indexed under this heading.

Phenelzine Sulfate (No specific interaction between oxymorphone and monoamine oxidase inhibitors has been observed, but caution in the use of any opioid in patients taking this class of drugs is appropriate).

No products indexed under this heading.

Prazepam (The concomitant use of other CNS depressants including sedatives, hypnotics, tranquilizers, general anesthetics, phenothiazines, other opioids, and alcohol may produce additive CNS depressant effects. Additive effects resulting in respiratory depression, hypotension, profound sedation or coma may result if these drugs are taken in combination with the usual doses of oxymorphone hydrochloride).

No products indexed under this heading.

Procarbazine Hydrochloride (No specific interaction between oxymorphone and monoamine oxidase inhibitors has been observed, but caution in the use of any opioid in patients taking this class of drugs is appropriate). Products include:

Matulane Capsules 3191

Prochlorperazine (The concomitant use of other CNS depressants including sedatives, hypnotics, tranquilizers, general anesthetics, phe-

nothiazines, other opioids, and alcohol may produce additive CNS depressant effects. Additive effects resulting in respiratory depression, hypotension, profound sedation or coma may result if these drugs are taken in combination with the usual doses of oxymorphone hydrochloride).

No products indexed under this heading.

Procyclidine Hydrochloride (Anticholinergics or other medications with anticholinergic activity when used concurrently with opioid analgesics may result in increased risk of urinary retention and/or severe constipation, which may lead to paralytic ileus).

No products indexed under this heading.

Promethazine Hydrochloride (The concomitant use of other CNS depressants including sedatives, hypnotics, tranquilizers, general anesthetics, phenothiazines, other opioids, and alcohol may produce additive CNS depressant effects. Additive effects resulting in respiratory depression, hypotension, profound sedation or coma may result if these drugs are taken in combination with the usual doses of oxymorphone hydrochloride). Products include:

Phenergan Tablets and
Suppositories 3440

Propantheline Bromide (Anticholinergics or other medications with anticholinergic activity when used concurrently with opioid analgesics may result in increased risk of urinary retention and/or severe constipation, which may lead to paralytic ileus).

No products indexed under this heading.

Propofol (The concomitant use of other CNS depressants including sedatives, hypnotics, tranquilizers, general anesthetics, phenothiazines, other opioids, and alcohol may produce additive CNS depressant effects. Additive effects resulting in respiratory depression, hypotension, profound sedation or coma may result if these drugs are taken in combination with the usual doses of oxymorphone hydrochloride).

No products indexed under this heading.

Propoxyphene Hydrochloride (The concomitant use of other CNS depressants including sedatives, hypnotics, tranquilizers, general anesthetics, phenothiazines, other opioids, and alcohol may produce additive CNS depressant effects. Additive effects resulting in respiratory depression, hypotension, profound sedation or coma may result if these drugs are taken in combination with the usual doses of oxymorphone hydrochloride).

No products indexed under this heading.

Propoxyphene Napsylate (The concomitant use of other CNS depressants including sedatives, hypnotics, tranquilizers, general anesthetics, phenothiazines, other opioids, and alcohol may produce additive CNS depressant effects. Additive effects resulting in respiratory depression, hypotension, profound sedation or coma may result if these drugs are taken in combination with the usual doses of oxymor-

IMPORTANT NOTE: Always consult each drug listing in the patient's regimen for possible interactions.

phone hydrochloride).
No products indexed under this heading.

Quazepam (The concomitant use of other CNS depressants including sedatives, hypnotics, tranquilizers, general anesthetics, phenothiazines, other opioids, and alcohol may produce additive CNS depressant effects. Additive effects resulting in respiratory depression, hypotension, profound sedation or coma may result if these drugs are taken in combination with the usual doses of oxymorphone hydrochloride).
No products indexed under this heading.

Ramelteon (The concomitant use of other CNS depressants including sedatives, hypnotics, tranquilizers, general anesthetics, phenothiazines, other opioids, and alcohol may produce additive CNS depressant effects. Additive effects resulting in respiratory depression, hypotension, profound sedation or coma may result if these drugs are taken in combination with the usual doses of oxymorphone hydrochloride). Products include:
Rozerem Tablets 3231

Remifentanil Hydrochloride (The concomitant use of other CNS depressants including sedatives, hypnotics, tranquilizers, general anesthetics, phenothiazines, other opioids, and alcohol may produce additive CNS depressant effects. Additive effects resulting in respiratory depression, hypotension, profound sedation or coma may result if these drugs are taken in combination with the usual doses of oxymorphone hydrochloride).
No products indexed under this heading.

Scopolamine (Anticholinergics or other medications with anticholinergic activity when used concurrently with opioid analgesics may result in increased risk of urinary retention and/or severe constipation, which may lead to paralytic ileus). Products include:
Transderm Scōp Transdermal Therapeutic System 2177

Scopolamine Hydrobromide (Anticholinergics or other medications with anticholinergic activity when used concurrently with opioid analgesics may result in increased risk of urinary retention and/or severe constipation, which may lead to paralytic ileus). Products include:
Donnatal Extentabs 2493

Secobarbital Sodium (The concomitant use of other CNS depressants including sedatives, hypnotics, tranquilizers, general anesthetics, phenothiazines, other opioids, and alcohol may produce additive CNS depressant effects. Additive effects resulting in respiratory depression, hypotension, profound sedation or coma may result if these drugs are taken in combination with the usual doses of oxymorphone hydrochloride).
No products indexed under this heading.

Selegiline Hydrochloride (No specific interaction between oxymorphone and monoamine oxidase inhibitors has been observed, but caution in the use of any opioid in patients taking this class of drugs is appropriate). Products include:
Eldepryl Capsules 3208
Zelapar Tablets 3372

Sufentanil Citrate (The concomitant use of other CNS depressants including sedatives, hypnotics, tranquilizers, general anesthetics, phenothiazines, other opioids, and alcohol may produce additive CNS depressant effects. Additive effects resulting in respiratory depression, hypotension, profound sedation or coma may result if these drugs are taken in combination with the usual doses of oxymorphone hydrochloride).
No products indexed under this heading.

Temazepam (The concomitant use of other CNS depressants including sedatives, hypnotics, tranquilizers, general anesthetics, phenothiazines, other opioids, and alcohol may produce additive CNS depressant effects. Additive effects resulting in respiratory depression, hypotension, profound sedation or coma may result if these drugs are taken in combination with the usual doses of oxymorphone hydrochloride). Products include:
Restoril Capsules 1860

Thiamylal Sodium (The concomitant use of other CNS depressants including sedatives, hypnotics, tranquilizers, general anesthetics, phenothiazines, other opioids, and alcohol may produce additive CNS depressant effects. Additive effects resulting in respiratory depression, hypotension, profound sedation or coma may result if these drugs are taken in combination with the usual doses of oxymorphone hydrochloride).
No products indexed under this heading.

Thioridazine Hydrochloride (The concomitant use of other CNS depressants including sedatives, hypnotics, tranquilizers, general anesthetics, phenothiazines, other opioids, and alcohol may produce additive CNS depressant effects. Additive effects resulting in respiratory depression, hypotension, profound sedation or coma may result if these drugs are taken in combination with the usual doses of oxymorphone hydrochloride). Products include:
Thioridazine Hydrochloride Tablets 2163

Thiothixene (The concomitant use of other CNS depressants including sedatives, hypnotics, tranquilizers, general anesthetics, phenothiazines, other opioids, and alcohol may produce additive CNS depressant effects. Additive effects resulting in respiratory depression, hypotension, profound sedation or coma may result if these drugs are taken in combination with the usual doses of oxymorphone hydrochloride). Products include:
Thiothixene Capsules 2165

Tolterodine Tartrate (Anticholinergics or other medications with anticholinergic activity when used concurrently with opioid analgesics may result in increased risk of urinary retention and/or severe constipation, which may lead to paralytic ileus). Products include:
Detrol Tablets 2628
Detrol LA Capsules 2631

Tranylcypromine Sulfate (No specific interaction between oxymorphone and monoamine oxidase inhibitors has been observed, but caution in the use of any opioid in patients taking this class of drugs is appropriate). Products include:
Parnate Tablets 1527

Triazolam (The concomitant use of other CNS depressants including sedatives, hypnotics, tranquilizers, general anesthetics, phenothiazines, other opioids, and alcohol may produce additive CNS depressant effects. Additive effects resulting in respiratory depression, hypotension, profound sedation or coma may result if these drugs are taken in combination with the usual doses of oxymorphone hydrochloride).
No products indexed under this heading.

Tridihexethyl Chloride (Anticholinergics or other medications with anticholinergic activity when used concurrently with opioid analgesics may result in increased risk of urinary retention and/or severe constipation, which may lead to paralytic ileus).
No products indexed under this heading.

Trifluoperazine Hydrochloride (The concomitant use of other CNS depressants including sedatives, hypnotics, tranquilizers, general anesthetics, phenothiazines, other opioids, and alcohol may produce additive CNS depressant effects. Additive effects resulting in respiratory depression, hypotension, profound sedation or coma may result if these drugs are taken in combination with the usual doses of oxymorphone hydrochloride).
No products indexed under this heading.

Trihexyphenidyl Hydrochloride (Anticholinergics or other medications with anticholinergic activity when used concurrently with opioid analgesics may result in increased risk of urinary retention and/or severe constipation, which may lead to paralytic ileus).
No products indexed under this heading.

Zaleplon (The concomitant use of other CNS depressants including sedatives, hypnotics, tranquilizers, general anesthetics, phenothiazines, other opioids, and alcohol may produce additive CNS depressant effects. Additive effects resulting in respiratory depression, hypotension, profound sedation or coma may result if these drugs are taken in combination with the usual doses of oxymorphone hydrochloride). Products include:
Sonata Capsules 1717

Zolpidem Tartrate (The concomitant use of other CNS depressants including sedatives, hypnotics, tranquilizers, general anesthetics, phenothiazines, other opioids, and alcohol may produce additive CNS depressant effects. Additive effects resulting in respiratory depression, hypotension, profound sedation or coma may result if these drugs are taken in combination with the usual doses of oxymorphone hydrochloride). Products include:
Ambien Tablets 2851
Ambien CR Tablets 2855

Food Interactions

Alcohol (The concomitant use of other CNS depressants including sedatives, hypnotics, tranquilizers, general anesthetics, phenothiazines, other opioids, and alcohol may produce additive CNS depressant effects. Additive effects resulting in respiratory depression, hypotension, profound sedation or coma may result if these drugs are taken in combination with the usual doses of oxymorphone hydrochloride).

OPANA ER TABLETS
(Oxymorphone Hydrochloride) 1126
See Opana Tablets

OPHTHETIC OPHTHALMIC SOLUTION
(Proparacaine Hydrochloride) .... ⊙232
None cited in PDR database.

OPTIPRANOLOL METIPRANOLOL OPHTHALMIC SOLUTION 0.3%
(Metipranolol) .... ⊙256
May interact with adrenergic augmenting psychotropics, beta blockers, calcium channel blockers, cardiac glycosides, and certain other agents. Compounds in these categories include:

Acebutolol Hydrochloride (Co-administration with oral beta blockers may result in additive effects or systemic beta blockade).
No products indexed under this heading.

Amlodipine Besylate (Co-administration with oral or intravenous calcium channel antagonists may result in possible precipitation of left ventricular failure and hypotension). Products include:
Caduet Tablets 2508
Lotrel Capsules 2249
Norvasc Tablets 2545

Atenolol (Co-administration with oral beta blockers may result in additive effects or systemic beta blockade).
No products indexed under this heading.

Bepridil Hydrochloride (Co-administration with oral or intravenous calcium channel antagonists may result in possible precipitation of left ventricular failure and hypotension).
No products indexed under this heading.

Betaxolol Hydrochloride (Co-administration with oral beta blockers may result in additive effects or systemic beta blockade). Products include:
Betoptic S Ophthalmic Suspension................................ 558

Bisoprolol Fumarate (Co-administration with oral beta blockers may result in additive effects or systemic beta blockade).
No products indexed under this heading.

Carteolol Hydrochloride (Co-administration with oral beta blockers may result in additive effects or systemic beta blockade). Products include:
Carteolol Hydrochloride Ophthalmic Solution USP, 1%....... ⊙249

Deserpidine (Possible additive effects and production of hypotension and/or bradycardia when beta blocker is concurrently used with catecholamine-depleting drugs).
No products indexed under this heading.

Deslanoside (Concomitant use of beta blockers with digitalis and calcium channel blockers may result in additive effects in prolonging atrioventricular conduction time).
No products indexed under this heading.

Digitalis Glycoside Preparations (Concomitant use of beta blockers with digitalis and calcium channel blockers may result in additive effects in prolonging atrioventricular conduction time).
No products indexed under this heading.

Digitoxin (Concomitant use of beta blockers with digitalis and calcium channel blockers may result in additive effects in prolonging atrioventricular conduction time).
No products indexed under this heading.

Digoxin (Concomitant use of beta blockers with digitalis and calcium channel blockers may result in additive effects in prolonging atrioventricular conduction time). Products include:
Lanoxicaps Capsules 1490
Lanoxin Injection 1494
Lanoxin Injection Pediatric 1497
Lanoxin Tablets 1500

Diltiazem Hydrochloride (Co-administration with oral or intravenous calcium channel antagonists may result in possible precipitation of left ventricular failure and hypotension). Products include:
Cardizem LA Extended Release Tablets 1728
Tiazac Capsules 1201

Epinephrine (Concurrent use in patients with history of atopy or severe anaphylactic reaction to allergens may be unresponsive to the usual doses of epinephrine used to treat anaphylactic reaction). Products include:
EpiPen 1061
Primatene Mist .... ▣ 719
Twinject 0.15 3379
Twinject 0.3 3378

Epinephrine Hydrochloride (Concurrent use in patients with history of atopy or severe anaphylactic reaction to allergens may be unresponsive to the usual doses of epinephrine used to treat anaphylactic reaction).
No products indexed under this heading.

Esmolol Hydrochloride (Co-administration with oral beta blockers may result in additive effects or systemic beta blockade).
No products indexed under this heading.

Felodipine (Co-administration with oral or intravenous calcium channel antagonists may result in possible precipitation of left ventricular failure and hypotension).
No products indexed under this heading.

Isocarboxazid (Exercise caution when used concurrently with adrenergic psychotropic drugs).
No products indexed under this heading.

Isradipine (Co-administration with oral or intravenous calcium channel antagonists may result in possible precipitation of left ventricular failure and hypotension). Products include:
DynaCirc CR Tablets 2721

Labetalol Hydrochloride (Co-administration with oral beta blockers may result in additive effects or systemic beta blockade).
No products indexed under this heading.

Levobunolol Hydrochloride (Co-administration with oral beta blockers may result in additive effects or systemic beta blockade). Products include:
Betagan Ophthalmic Solution, USP .... ⊙ 220

Metoprolol Succinate (Co-administration with oral beta blockers may result in additive effects or systemic beta blockade). Products include:
Toprol-XL Tablets 668

Metoprolol Tartrate (Co-administration with oral beta blockers may result in additive effects or systemic beta blockade). Products include:
Lopressor Injection 2238
Lopressor Tablets 2238
Lopressor HCT 50/25 Tablets 2241
Lopressor HCT 100/25 Tablets 2241
Lopressor HCT 100/50 Tablets 2241

Mibefradil Dihydrochloride (Co-administration with oral or intravenous calcium channel antagonists may result in possible precipitation of left ventricular failure and hypotension).
No products indexed under this heading.

Nadolol (Co-administration with oral beta blockers may result in additive effects or systemic beta blockade). Products include:
Nadolol Tablets 2159

Nicardipine Hydrochloride (Co-administration with oral or intravenous calcium channel antagonists may result in possible precipitation of left ventricular failure and hypotension). Products include:
Cardene I.V. 2497

Nifedipine (Co-administration with oral or intravenous calcium channel antagonists may result in possible precipitation of left ventricular failure and hypotension). Products include:
Adalat CC Tablets 2964

Nimodipine (Co-administration with oral or intravenous calcium channel antagonists may result in possible precipitation of left ventricular failure and hypotension). Products include:
Nimotop Capsules 749

Nisoldipine (Co-administration with oral or intravenous calcium channel antagonists may result in possible precipitation of left ventricular failure and hypotension). Products include:
Sular Tablets 3122

Pargyline Hydrochloride (Exercise caution when used concurrently with adrenergic psychotropic drugs).
No products indexed under this heading.

Penbutolol Sulfate (Co-administration with oral beta blockers may result in additive effects or systemic beta blockade).
No products indexed under this heading.

Phenelzine Sulfate (Exercise caution when used concurrently with adrenergic psychotropic drugs).
No products indexed under this heading.

Pindolol (Co-administration with oral beta blockers may result in additive effects or systemic beta blockade).
No products indexed under this heading.

Propranolol Hydrochloride (Co-administration with oral beta blockers may result in additive effects or systemic beta blockade). Products include:
Inderal LA Long-Acting Capsules 3429
InnoPran XL Capsules 2723

Rauwolfia Serpentina (Possible additive effects and production of hypotension and/or bradycardia when beta blocker is concurrently used with catecholamine-depleting drugs).
No products indexed under this heading.

Rescinnamine (Possible additive effects and production of hypotension and/or bradycardia when beta blocker is concurrently used with catecholamine-depleting drugs).
No products indexed under this heading.

Reserpine (Possible additive effects and production of hypotension and/or bradycardia when beta blocker is concurrently used with catecholamine-depleting drugs).
No products indexed under this heading.

Sotalol Hydrochloride (Co-administration with oral beta blockers may result in additive effects or systemic beta blockade).
No products indexed under this heading.

Timolol Hemihydrate (Co-administration with oral beta blockers may result in additive effects or systemic beta blockade). Products include:
Betimol Ophthalmic Solution 3382
Betimol Ophthalmic Solution .... ⊙ 295

Timolol Maleate (Co-administration with oral beta blockers may result in additive effects or systemic beta blockade). Products include:
Blocadren Tablets 1916
Cosopt Sterile Ophthalmic Solution 1931
Timolide Tablets 2086
Timoptic Sterile Ophthalmic Solution 2088
Timoptic in Ocudose 2091
Timoptic-XE Sterile Ophthalmic Gel Forming Solution 2092

Tranylcypromine Sulfate (Exercise caution when used concurrently with adrenergic psychotropic drugs). Products include:
Parnate Tablets 1527

Verapamil Hydrochloride (Co-administration with oral or intravenous calcium channel antagonists may result in possible precipitation of left ventricular failure and hypotension). Products include:
Covera-HS Tablets 3139
Tarka Tablets 524
Verelan PM Extended-Release Capsules, Controlled-Onset 3106

OPTIVAR OPHTHALMIC SOLUTION

(Azelastine Hydrochloride) .... ⊙ 267

ORACEA CAPSULES

(Doxycycline Monohydrate) 1000

May interact with antacids, antacids containing aluminum, calcium and magnesium, anticoagulants, oral anticoagulants, iron containing oral preparations, magnesium-containing antacids, oral contraceptives, proton pump inhibitor, retinoids, and certain other agents. Compounds in these categories include:

Adapalene (There have been reports of pseudotumor cerebri (benign intracranial hypertension) associated with the concomitant use of isotretinoin and tetracyclines. Since both oral retinoids, including isotretinoin and acitretin, and the tetracyclines, primarily minocycline, can cause increased intracranial pressure, the concurrent use of an oral retinoid and a tetracycline should be avoided). Products include:
Differin Cream 1210
Differin Gel 1211

Aluminum Carbonate (Absorption of tetracyclines is impaired by bismuth subsalicylate, proton pump inhibitors, antacids containing aluminum, calcium, or magnesium and iron-containing preparations).
No products indexed under this heading.

Aluminum Hydroxide (Absorption of tetracyclines is impaired by bismuth subsalicylate, proton pump inhibitors, antacids containing aluminum, calcium, or magnesium and iron-containing preparations). Products include:
Gaviscon Regular Strength Liquid .... ▣ 658
Gaviscon Regular Strength Tablets .... ▣ 658
Gaviscon Extra Strength Liquid .... ▣ 658
Gaviscon Extra Strength Tablets .... ▣ 658
Maalox Regular Strength Antacid/Antigas Liquid 2175
Maalox Max Maximum Strength Antacid/Anti-Gas Liquid 2176

Anisindione (Because tetracyclines have been shown to depress plasma prothrombin activity, patients who are on anticoagulant therapy may require downward adjustment of their anticoagulant dosage). Products include:
Miradon Tablets 3042

Ardeparin Sodium (Because tetracyclines have been shown to depress plasma prothrombin activity, patients who are on anticoagulant therapy may require downward adjustment of their anticoagulant dosage).
No products indexed under this heading.

Bismuth Subsalicylate (Absorption of tetracyclines is impaired by bismuth subsalicylate, proton pump inhibitors, antacids containing aluminum, calcium or magnesium and iron-containing preparations). Products include:
Maalox Maximum Strength Total Stomach Relief Peppermint Liquid .... ▣ 660
Maalox Maximum Strength Total Stomach Relief Strawberry Liquid .... ▣ 672
Pepto-Bismol Original Liquid, Maximum Strength Liquid, Original and Cherry Tablets, Chewable Tablets and Easy-To-Swallow Caplets 2676
Pepto-Bismol Maximum Strength Liquid .... ▣ 672

Dalteparin Sodium (Because tetracyclines have been shown to depress plasma prothrombin activity, patients who are on anticoagulant therapy may require downward adjustment of their anticoagulant dosage). Products include:

Fragmin Injection 1097

Danaparoid Sodium (Because tetracyclines have been shown to depress plasma prothrombin activity, patients who are on anticoagulant therapy may require downward adjustment of their anticoagulant dosage).

No products indexed under this heading.

Desogestrel (Doxycycline may interfere with the effectiveness of low dose oral contraceptives. To avoid contraceptive failure, females are advised to use a second form of contraceptive during treatment with doxycycline). Products include:

Mircette Tablets 1066

Dicumarol (Because tetracyclines have been shown to depress plasma prothrombin activity, patients who are on anticoagulant therapy may require downward adjustment of their anticoagulant dosage).

No products indexed under this heading.

Enoxaparin Sodium (Because tetracyclines have been shown to depress plasma prothrombin activity, patients who are on anticoagulant therapy may require downward adjustment of their anticoagulant dosage). Products include:

Lovenox Injection 2915

Esomeprazole Magnesium (Absorption of tetracyclines is impaired by bismuth subsalicylate, proton pump inhibitors, antacids containing aluminum, calcium, or magnesium and iron-containing preparations). Products include:

Nexium Delayed-Release Capsules 655

Ethinyl Estradiol (Doxycycline may interfere with the effectiveness of low dose oral contraceptives. To avoid contraceptive failure, females are advised to use a second form of contraceptive during treatment with doxycycline). Products include:

Mircette Tablets 1066
NuvaRing 2340
Ortho-Cyclen/Ortho Tri-Cyclen 2429
Ortho Evra Transdermal System 2417
Ortho Tri-Cyclen Lo Tablets 2436
Seasonique Tablets 1077
Yasmin 28 Tablets 796
Yaz Tablets 803

Ethynodiol Diacetate (Doxycycline may interfere with the effectiveness of low dose oral contraceptives. To avoid contraceptive failure, females are advised to use a second form of contraceptive during treatment with doxycycline).

No products indexed under this heading.

Etretinate (There have been reports of pseudotumor cerebri (benign intracranial hypertension) associated with the concomitant use of isotretinoin and tetracyclines. Since both oral retinoids, including isotretinoin and acitretin, and the tetracyclines, primarily minocycline, can cause increased intracranial pressure, the concurrent use of an oral retinoid and a tetracycline should be avoided).

No products indexed under this heading.

Ferrous Fumarate (Absorption of tetracyclines is impaired by bismuth subsalicylate, proton pump inhibitors, antacids containing aluminum, calcium, or magnesium and iron-containing preparations).

No products indexed under this heading.

Ferrous Gluconate (Absorption of tetracyclines is impaired by bismuth subsalicylate, proton pump inhibitors, antacids containing aluminum, calcium, or magnesium and iron-containing preparations).

No products indexed under this heading.

Ferrous Sulfate (Absorption of tetracyclines is impaired by bismuth subsalicylate, proton pump inhibitors, antacids containing aluminum, calcium, or magnesium and iron-containing preparations). Products include:

Slow Fe Iron Tablets .... ▣818
Slow Fe with Folic Acid Tablets .... ▣819

Fondaparinux Sodium (Because tetracyclines have been shown to depress plasma prothrombin activity, patients who are on anticoagulant therapy may require downward adjustment of their anticoagulant dosage). Products include:

Arixtra Injection 1351

Heparin Calcium (Because tetracyclines have been shown to depress plasma prothrombin activity, patients who are on anticoagulant therapy may require downward adjustment of their anticoagulant dosage).

No products indexed under this heading.

Heparin Sodium (Because tetracyclines have been shown to depress plasma prothrombin activity, patients who are on anticoagulant therapy may require downward adjustment of their anticoagulant dosage).

No products indexed under this heading.

Iron (Absorption of tetracyclines is impaired by bismuth subsalicylate, proton pump inhibitors, antacids containing aluminum, calcium, or magnesium and iron-containing preparations).

No products indexed under this heading.

Isotretinoin (There have been reports of pseudotumor cerebri (benign intracranial hypertension) associated with the concomitant use of isotretinoin and tetracyclines. Since both oral retinoids, including isotretinoin and acitretin, and the tetracyclines, primarily minocycline, can cause increased intracranial pressure, the concurrent use of an oral retinoid and a tetracycline should be avoided). Products include:

Accutane Capsules 2731

Lansoprazole (Absorption of tetracyclines is impaired by bismuth subsalicylate, proton pump inhibitors, antacids containing aluminum, calcium, or magnesium and iron-containing preparations). Products include:

Prevacid Delayed-Release Capsules 3271
Prevacid for Delayed-Release Oral Suspension 3271
Prevacid SoluTab Delayed-Release Orally Disintegrating Tablets 3271
Prevacid I.V. for Injection 3277
Prevacid NapraPAC 3280
PREVPAC 3284

Levonorgestrel (Doxycycline may interfere with the effectiveness of low dose oral contraceptives. To avoid contraceptive failure, females are advised to use a second form of contraceptive during treatment with doxycycline). Products include:

Climara Pro Transdermal System 776
Mirena Intrauterine System 787
Plan B Tablets 1076
Seasonique Tablets 1077

Low Molecular Weight Heparins (Because tetracyclines have been shown to depress plasma prothrombin activity, patients who are on anticoagulant therapy may require downward adjustment of their anticoagulant dosage).

No products indexed under this heading.

Magaldrate (Absorption of tetracyclines is impaired by bismuth subsalicylate, proton pump inhibitors, antacids containing aluminum, calcium, or magnesium and iron-containing preparations).

No products indexed under this heading.

Magnesium Carbonate (Absorption of tetracyclines is impaired by bismuth subsalicylate, proton pump inhibitors, antacids containing aluminum, calcium, or magnesium and iron-containing preparations). Products include:

Gaviscon Regular Strength Liquid .... ▣658
Gaviscon Extra Strength Liquid .... ▣658
Gaviscon Extra Strength Tablets .... ▣658

Magnesium Hydroxide (Absorption of tetracyclines is impaired by bismuth subsalicylate, proton pump inhibitors, antacids containing aluminum, calcium, or magnesium and iron-containing preparations). Products include:

Maalox Regular Strength Antacid/Antigas Liquid 2175
Maalox Max Maximum Strength Antacid/Anti-Gas Liquid 2176
Pepcid Complete Chewable Tablets 1701

Magnesium Oxide (Absorption of tetracyclines is impaired by bismuth subsalicylate, proton pump inhibitors, antacids containing aluminum, calcium, or magnesium and iron-containing preparations). Products include:

Beelith Tablets 759
PremCal Light, Regular, and Extra Strength Tablets .... ▣818

Magnesium Trisilicate (Absorption of tetracyclines is impaired by bismuth subsalicylate, proton pump inhibitors, antacids containing aluminum, calcium, or magnesium and iron-containing preparations). Products include:

Gaviscon Regular Strength Tablets .... ▣658

Mestranol (Doxycycline may interfere with the effectiveness of low dose oral contraceptives. To avoid contraceptive failure, females are advised to use a second form of contraceptive during treatment with doxycycline).

No products indexed under this heading.

Methoxyflurane (The concurrent use of tetracycline and methoxyflurane has been reported to result in fatal renal toxicity).

No products indexed under this heading.

Norethindrone (Doxycycline may interfere with the effectiveness of low dose oral contraceptives. To avoid contraceptive failure, females are advised to use a second form of contraceptive during treatment with doxycycline). Products include:

Ortho Micronor Tablets 2426

Norethynodrel (Doxycycline may interfere with the effectiveness of low dose oral contraceptives. To avoid contraceptive failure, females are advised to use a second form of contraceptive during treatment with doxycycline).

No products indexed under this heading.

Norgestimate (Doxycycline may interfere with the effectiveness of low dose oral contraceptives. To avoid contraceptive failure, females are advised to use a second form of contraceptive during treatment with doxycycline). Products include:

Ortho-Cyclen/Ortho Tri-Cyclen 2429
Ortho Tri-Cyclen Lo Tablets 2436

Norgestrel (Doxycycline may interfere with the effectiveness of low dose oral contraceptives. To avoid contraceptive failure, females are advised to use a second form of contraceptive during treatment with doxycycline).

No products indexed under this heading.

Omeprazole (Absorption of tetracyclines is impaired by bismuth subsalicylate, proton pump inhibitors, antacids containing aluminum, calcium, or magnesium and iron-containing preparations). Products include:

Zegerid Capsules 2958
Zegerid Powder for Oral Solution 2958

Pantoprazole Sodium (Absorption of tetracyclines is impaired by bismuth subsalicylate, proton pump inhibitors, antacids containing aluminum, calcium, or magnesium and iron-containing preparations). Products include:

Protonix I.V. 3472
Protonix Tablets 3469

Penicillin, Potassium Phenoxymethyl (Since bacteriostatic drugs may interfere with the bactericidal action of penicillin, it is advisable to avoid giving tetracycline-class drugs in conjunction with penicillin).

No products indexed under this heading.

Penicillin G Benzathine (Since bacteriostatic drugs may interfere with the bactericidal action of penicillin, it is advisable to avoid giving tetracycline-class drugs in conjunction with penicillin). Products include:

Bicillin C-R Injectable Suspension 1706

Penicillin G Dibenzylethyenediamine (Since bacteriostatic drugs may interfere with the bactericidal action of penicillin, it is advisable to avoid giving tetracycline-class drugs in conjunction with penicillin).

No products indexed under this heading.

Penicillin G Potassium (Since bacteriostatic drugs may interfere with the bactericidal action of penicillin, it is advisable to avoid giving tetracycline-class drugs in conjunction with penicillin).

No products indexed under this heading.

Penicillin G Procaine (Since bacteriostatic drugs may interfere with the bactericidal action of penicillin, it is advisable to avoid giving tetracycline-class drugs in conjunction with penicillin). Products include:

Bicillin C-R Injectable Suspension 1706

Penicillin G Sodium (Since bacteriostatic drugs may interfere with the bactericidal action of penicillin, it is advisable to avoid giving tetracycline-class drugs in conjunction with penicillin).

No products indexed under this heading.

Penicillin V (Since bacteriostatic drugs may interfere with the bactericidal action of penicillin, it is advisable to avoid giving tetracycline-class drugs in conjunction with penicillin).

No products indexed under this heading.

Penicillin V Potassium (Since bacteriostatic drugs may interfere with the bactericidal action of penicillin, it is advisable to avoid giving tetracycline-class drugs in conjunction with penicillin).

No products indexed under this heading.

Polysaccharide Iron Complex (Absorption of tetracyclines is impaired by bismuth subsalicylate, proton pump inhibitors, antacids containing aluminum, calcium, or magnesium and iron-containing preparations). Products include:

Nu-Iron 150 Capsules 2127

Rabeprazole Sodium (Absorption of tetracyclines is impaired by bismuth subsalicylate, proton pump inhibitors, antacids containing aluminum, calcium, or magnesium and iron-containing preparations). Products include:

Aciphex Tablets 1090

Sodium Bicarbonate (Absorption of tetracyclines is impaired by bismuth subsalicylate, proton pump inhibitors, antacids containing aluminum, calcium, or magnesium and iron-containing preparations). Products include:

Colyte with Flavor Packs for Oral Solution....................................... 3088

HalfLytely and Bisacodyl Tablets Bowel Prep Kit with Flavors Packs... 881

TriLyte with Flavor Packs for Oral Solution....................................... 3100

Tazarotene (There have been reports of pseudotumor cerebri (benign intracranial hypertension) associated with the concomitant use of isotretinoin and tetracyclines. Since both oral retinoids, including isotretinoin and acitretin, and the tetracyclines, primarily minocycline, can cause increased intracranial pressure, the concurrent use of an oral retinoid and a tetracycline should be avoided).

No products indexed under this heading.

Tinzaparin Sodium (Because tetracyclines have been shown to depress plasma prothrombin activity, patients who are on anticoagulant therapy may require downward adjustment of their anticoagulant dosage).

No products indexed under this heading.

Tretinoin (There have been reports of pseudotumor cerebri (benign intracranial hypertension) associated with the concomitant use of isotretinoin and tetracyclines. Since both oral retinoids, including isotretinoin and acitretin, and the tetracyclines, primarily minocycline, can cause increased intracranial pressure, the concurrent use of an oral retinoid and a tetracycline should be avoided). Products include:

Tri-Luma Cream 1213

Vesanoid Capsules 2820

Warfarin Sodium (Because tetracyclines have been shown to depress plasma prothrombin activity, patients who are on anticoagulant therapy may require downward adjustment of their anticoagulant dosage). Products include:

Coumadin for Injection 898

Coumadin Tablets 898

ORENCIA POWDER FOR INTRAVENOUS INFUSION

(Abatacept) 914

May interact with TNF antagonists, vaccines, live, and certain other agents. Compounds in these categories include:

Adalimumab (Concurrent administration of TNF antagonists with abatacept has been associated with an increased risk of serious infections and no significant additional efficacy over use of the TNF antagonists alone. Concurrent therapy with abatacept and TNF antagonists is not recommended). Products include:

Humira Injection 466

Anakinra (There is insufficient experience to assess the safety and efficacy of abatacept concurrently administered with anakinra. Concurrent use is not recommended). Products include:

Kineret Injection 599

BCG Vaccine (Avoid administration of live vaccines).

No products indexed under this heading.

Etanercept (Concurrent administration of TNF antagonists with abatacept has been associated with an increased risk of serious infections and no significant additional efficacy over use of the TNF antagonists alone. Concurrent therapy with abatacept and TNF antagonists is not recommended). Products include:

Enbrel for Injection 584

Infliximab (Concurrent administration of TNF antagonists with abatacept has been associated with an increased risk of serious infections and no significant additional efficacy over use of the TNF antagonists alone. Concurrent therapy with abatacept and TNF antagonists is not recommended). Products include:

Remicade for IV Injection 971

Measles, Mumps, Rubella and Varicella Virus Vaccine Live (Avoid administration of live vaccines). Products include:

ProQuad 2064

Measles, Mumps & Rubella Virus Vaccine, Live (Avoid administration of live vaccines). Products include:

M-M-R II 2006

Measles & Rubella Virus Vaccine Live (Avoid administration of live vaccines).

No products indexed under this heading.

Measles Virus Vaccine Live (Avoid administration of live vaccines). Products include:

Attenuvax 1914

Mumps Virus Vaccine, Live (Avoid administration of live vaccines). Products include:

Mumpsvax 2031

Poliovirus Vaccine, Live, Oral, Trivalent, Types 1,2,3 (Sabin) (Avoid administration of live vaccines).

No products indexed under this heading.

Rotavirus Vaccine, Live, Oral, Tetravalent (Avoid administration of live vaccines).

No products indexed under this heading.

Rubella & Mumps Virus Vaccine Live (Avoid administration of live vaccines).

No products indexed under this heading.

Rubella Virus Vaccine Live (Avoid administration of live vaccines). Products include:

Meruvax II 2019

Smallpox Vaccine (Avoid administration of live vaccines).

No products indexed under this heading.

Typhoid Vaccine (Avoid administration of live vaccines).

No products indexed under this heading.

Varicella Virus Vaccine Live (Avoid administration of live vaccines). Products include:

Varivax 2100

Yellow Fever Vaccine (Avoid administration of live vaccines).

No products indexed under this heading.

ORTHO-CYCLEN TABLETS

(Ethinyl Estradiol, Norgestimate) 2429

May interact with barbiturates, phenytoin, tetracyclines, and certain other agents. Compounds in these categories include:

Ampicillin (Potential for reduced efficacy and increased incidence of breakthrough bleeding and menstrual irregularities with concomitant use).

No products indexed under this heading.

Ampicillin Sodium (Potential for reduced efficacy and increased incidence of breakthrough bleeding and menstrual irregularities with concomitant use).

No products indexed under this heading.

Aprobarbital (Potential for reduced efficacy and increased incidence of breakthrough bleeding and menstrual irregularities with concomitant use).

No products indexed under this heading.

Butabarbital (Potential for reduced efficacy and increased incidence of breakthrough bleeding and menstrual irregularities with concomitant use).

No products indexed under this heading.

Butalbital (Potential for reduced efficacy and increased incidence of breakthrough bleeding and menstrual irregularities with concomitant use).

No products indexed under this heading.

Carbamazepine (Potential for reduced efficacy and increased incidence of breakthrough bleeding and menstrual irregularities with concomitant use). Products include:

Carbatrol Capsules 3171

Equetro Extended-Release Capsules 3180

Tegretol/Tegretol-XR 2295

Demeclocycline Hydrochloride (Potential for reduced efficacy and increased incidence of breakthrough bleeding and menstrual irregularities with concomitant use).

No products indexed under this heading.

Doxycycline Calcium (Potential for reduced efficacy and increased incidence of breakthrough bleeding and menstrual irregularities with concomitant use).

No products indexed under this heading.

Doxycycline Hyclate (Potential for reduced efficacy and increased incidence of breakthrough bleeding and menstrual irregularities with concomitant use).

No products indexed under this heading.

Doxycycline Monohydrate (Potential for reduced efficacy and increased incidence of breakthrough bleeding and menstrual irregularities with concomitant use). Products include:

Oracea Capsules 1000

Fosphenytoin Sodium (Potential for reduced efficacy and increased incidence of breakthrough bleeding and menstrual irregularities with concomitant use).

No products indexed under this heading.

Griseofulvin (Potential for reduced efficacy and increased incidence of breakthrough bleeding and menstrual irregularities with concomitant use). Products include:

Gris-PEG Tablets 2502

Hypericum (Co-administration of hormonal contraceptives and St. John's Wort containing herbal supplements has resulted in breakthrough bleeding shortly after starting St. John's Wort and pregnancies have been reported with concomitant therapy in some patients). Products include:

Satiete Tablets 832

Mephobarbital (Potential for reduced efficacy and increased incidence of breakthrough bleeding and menstrual irregularities with concomitant use).

No products indexed under this heading.

Methacycline Hydrochloride (Potential for reduced efficacy and increased incidence of breakthrough bleeding and menstrual irregularities with concomitant use).

No products indexed under this heading.

Minocycline Hydrochloride (Potential for reduced efficacy and increased incidence of breakthrough bleeding and menstrual irregularities with concomitant use). Products include:

Solodyn Extended Release Tablets 1890

Oxytetracycline Hydrochloride (Potential for reduced efficacy and increased incidence of breakthrough bleeding and menstrual irregularities with concomitant use).

No products indexed under this heading.

Pentobarbital Sodium (Potential for reduced efficacy and increased

incidence of breakthrough bleeding and menstrual irregularities with concomitant use). Products include:
Nembutal Sodium Solution, USP 2470

Phenobarbital (Potential for reduced efficacy and increased incidence of breakthrough bleeding and menstrual irregularities with concomitant use). Products include:
Donnatal Extentabs 2493

Phenylbutazone (Potential for reduced efficacy and increased incidence of breakthrough bleeding and menstrual irregularities with concomitant use).
No products indexed under this heading.

Phenytoin (Potential for reduced efficacy and increased incidence of breakthrough bleeding and menstrual irregularities with concomitant use).
No products indexed under this heading.

Phenytoin Sodium (Potential for reduced efficacy and increased incidence of breakthrough bleeding and menstrual irregularities with concomitant use). Products include:
Phenytek Capsules 2160

Rifampin (Co-administration has been associated with reduced efficacy and increased incidence of breakthrough bleeding and menstrual irregularities).
No products indexed under this heading.

Secobarbital Sodium (Potential for reduced efficacy and increased incidence of breakthrough bleeding and menstrual irregularities with concomitant use).
No products indexed under this heading.

Tetracycline Hydrochloride (Potential for reduced efficacy and increased incidence of breakthrough bleeding and menstrual irregularities with concomitant use).
No products indexed under this heading.

Thiamylal Sodium (Potential for reduced efficacy and increased incidence of breakthrough bleeding and menstrual irregularities with concomitant use).
No products indexed under this heading.

Topiramate (Co-administration may result in reduced efficacy and increased incidence of breakthrough bleeding and menstrual irregularities). Products include:
Topamax Sprinkle Capsules 2404
Topamax Tablets 2404

ORTHO EVRA TRANSDERMAL SYSTEM

(Ethinyl Estradiol, Norelgestromin) 2417
May interact with barbiturates, phenytoin, prednisolone, protease inhibitors, xanthines, and certain other agents. Compounds in these categories include:

Acetaminophen (Co-administration with certain oral contraceptives containing ethinyl estradiol increases plasma ethinyl estradiol levels possibly by inhibition of conjugation; decreased plasma levels of acetaminophen). Products include:
Comtrex Maximum Strength Cold & Cough Day/Night Caplets - Day Formulation .... ▣726
Comtrex Maximum Strength Cold & Cough Day/Night Caplets - Night Formulation .... ▣726
Comtrex Maximum Strength Non-Drowsy Cold & Cough Caplets .... ▣725
Comtrex Maximum Strength Day/Night Severe Cold & Sinus Caplets - Day Formulation .... ▣725
Comtrex Maximum Strength Day/Night Severe Cold & Sinus Caplets - Night Formulation .... ▣725
Contac Cold and Flu Maximum Strength Caplets .... ▣728
Contac Cold and Flu Day and Night Caplets (Day Formulation Only) .... ▣727
Contac Cold and Flu Day and Night Caplets (Night Formulation Only) .... ▣727
Contac Cold and Flu Non-Drowsy Caplets .... ▣728
Excedrin Extra Strength Caplets/Tablets/Geltabs .... ▣684
Excedrin Migraine Caplets/Tablets/Geltabs .... ▣609
Excedrin PM Caplets/Tablets/Geltabs .... ▣610
Excedrin Sinus Headache Caplets/Tablets .... ▣610
Excedrin Tension Headache Caplets/Tablets/Geltabs .... ▣611
Goody's Body Pain Formula Powder .... ▣684
Goody's Extra Strength Headache Powders .... ▣611
Goody's Extra Strength Pain Relief Tablets .... ▣685
Goody's PM Powder for Pain with Sleeplessness .... ▣612
Percocet Tablets 1131
Robitussin Cough, Cold & Flu Nighttime Liquid .... ▣738
TheraFlu Cold & Sore Throat Hot Liquid .... ▣741
TheraFlu Flu & Chest Congestion Hot Liquid .... ▣741
TheraFlu Flu & Sore Throat Hot Liquid .... ▣742
TheraFlu Daytime Severe Cold Hot Liquid .... ▣742
TheraFlu Nighttime Severe Cold Hot Liquid .... ▣740
TheraFlu Warming Relief Daytime Severe Cold .... ▣743
TheraFlu Warming Relief Nighttime Severe Cold .... ▣743
Triaminic Cough & Sore Throat Liquid .... ▣747
Regular Strength Tylenol Tablets 1870
Children's Tylenol with Flavor Creator .... ▣679
Children's Tylenol Plus Flu Oral Suspension .... ▣749
Tylenol Cold Head Congestion Daytime Caplets with Cool Burst and Gelcaps .... ▣750
Tylenol Cold Multi-Symptom Daytime Liquid .... ▣752
Tylenol Cold Multi-Symptom Severe Daytime Liquid .... ▣752
Tylenol 8 Hour Extended Release Caplets 1870
Tylenol 1870
Extra Strength Tylenol PM Caplets, Vanilla Caplets, Geltabs, Gelcaps and Liquid.......... 1875
Extra Strength Tylenol Rapid Release Gels 1870
Concentrated Tylenol Infants' Drops Plus Cold & Cough........... ▣754
Tylenol with Codeine Tablets 2391
Tylenol Allergy Multi-Symptom Caplets with Cool Burst and Gelcaps 1872
Tylenol Allergy Multi-Symptom Nighttime Caplets with Cool Burst 1872
Tylenol Severe Allergy Caplets 1872
Tylenol Arthritis Pain Extended Release Caplets and Geltabs 1870
Tylenol Chest Congestion Caplets with Cool Burst 1872
Tylenol Chest Congestion Liquid with Cool Burst 1872
Children's Tylenol Suspension Liquid and Meltaways 1878
Children's Tylenol Plus Cold Suspension Liquid 1879
Children's Tylenol Plus Cold & Allergy Suspension Liquid 1878
Children's Tylenol Plus Cough & Runny Nose Suspension Liquid 1879
Children's Tylenol Plus Cough & Sore Throat Suspension Liquid 1879
Children's Tylenol Suspension with Flavor Creator 1878
Children's Tylenol Plus Flu Suspension Liquid 1881
Children's Tylenol Plus Multi-Symptom Cold Suspension Liquid 1879
Tylenol Cold Severe Congestion Non-Drowsy Caplets with Cool Burst 1874
Tylenol Cold Head Congestion Daytime Caplets with Cool Burst 1873
Tylenol Cold Head Congestion Nighttime Caplets with Cool Burst 1873
Tylenol Cold Head Congestion Severe Caplets with Cool Burst..... 1873
Tylenol Cold Multi-Symptom Daytime Caplets with Cool Burst and Gelcaps 1874
Tylenol Cold Multi-Symptom Daytime Liquid with Citrus Burst ... 1874
Tylenol Cold Multi-Symptom Nighttime Caplets with Cool Burst 1874
Tylenol Cold Multi-Symptom Nighttime Liquid with Cool Burst ... 1874
Tylenol Cold Multi-Symptom Severe Caplets with Cool Burst..... 1874
Tylenol Cold Multi-Symptom Severe Daytime Liquid with Citrus Burst 1874
Tylenol Cough & Sore Throat Daytime Liquid with Cool Burst...... 1877
Tylenol Cough & Sore Throat Nighttime Liquid with Cool Burst ... 1877
Concentrated Tylenol Infants' Drops 1878
Concentrated Tylenol Infants' Drops Plus Cold 1879
Concentrated Tylenol Infants' Drops Plus Cold and Cough 1879
Jr. Tylenol Meltaways 1878
Tylenol Sinus Severe Congestion Caplets with Cool Burst 1876
Tylenol Sinus Congestion & Pain Daytime Caplets with Cool Burst and Gelcaps 1876
Tylenol Sinus Congestion & Pain Nighttime Caplets with Cool Burst 1876
Tylenol Sinus Congestion & Pain Severe Caplets with Cool Burst..... 1876
Tylenol Sore Throat Daytime Liquid with Cool Burst.................. 1877
Tylenol Sore Throat Nighttime Liquid with Cool Burst.................. 1877
Women's Tylenol Menstrual Relief Caplets.. 1877
Vicks 44M Cough, Cold & Flu Relief Liquid.................................. 2680
Vicks DayQuil LiquiCaps/Liquid Multi-Symptom Cold/Flu Relief..... ▣761
Vicks DayQuil Multi-Symptom Cold/Flu Relief LiquiCaps............. 2678
Vicks DayQuil Multi-Symptom Cold/Flu Relief Liquid.................. 2678
Vicks NyQuil Multi-Symptom Cold/Flu Relief Liquid.................. 2681
Vicks NyQuil Multi-Symptom Cold/Flu Relief LiquiCaps............. 2681
Vicks NyQuil LiquiCaps/Liquid Multi-Symptom Cold/Flu Relief..... ▣763
Vicodin Tablets 535
Vicodin ES Tablets 536
Vicodin HP Tablets 538
Zicam Maximum Strength Flu Daytime.. ▣768
Zicam Maximum Strength Flu Nighttime.................................... ▣768
Zydone Tablets 1139

Aminophylline (Co-administration increases the plasma concentrations of theophylline).
No products indexed under this heading.

Ampicillin (Increases the metabolism of contraceptive steroids resulting in reduced contraceptive effectiveness which could precipitate unintended pregnancy).
No products indexed under this heading.

Ampicillin Sodium (Increases the metabolism of contraceptive steroids resulting in reduced contraceptive effectiveness which could precipitate unintended pregnancy).
No products indexed under this heading.

Amprenavir (Several of the protease inhibitors have induced significant changes in the AUC of the estrogen and progestins in some cases; it is not known if this applies to Ortho Evra). Products include:
Agenerase Capsules 1327
Agenerase Oral Solution 1332

Aprobarbital (Barbiturates increase the metabolism of contraceptive steroids resulting in reduced contraceptive effectiveness which could precipitate unintended pregnancy).
No products indexed under this heading.

Atorvastatin Calcium (Co-administration with certain oral contraceptives containing ethinyl estradiol increases AUC values for ethinyl estradiol by approximately 20%). Products include:
Caduet Tablets 2508
Lipitor Tablets 2483

Butabarbital (Barbiturates increase the metabolism of contraceptive steroids resulting in reduced contraceptive effectiveness which could precipitate unintended pregnancy).
No products indexed under this heading.

Butalbital (Barbiturates increase the metabolism of contraceptive steroids resulting in reduced contraceptive effectiveness which could precipitate unintended pregnancy).
No products indexed under this heading.

Carbamazepine (Increases the metabolism of contraceptive steroids resulting in reduced contraceptive effectiveness which could precipitate unintended pregnancy). Products include:
Carbatrol Capsules 3171
Equetro Extended-Release Capsules 3180
Tegretol/Tegretol-XR 2295

Clofibrate (Increased clearance of clofibric acid).
No products indexed under this heading.

Cyclosporine (Co-administration increases the plasma concentrations of cyclosporine). Products include:
Gengraf Capsules 459
Neoral Oral Solution 2259
Neoral Soft Gelatin Capsules 2259
Restasis Ophthalmic Emulsion 575
Sandimmune 2275

Dyphylline (Co-administration increases the plasma concentrations of theophylline).
No products indexed under this heading.

Fosphenytoin Sodium (Increases the metabolism of contraceptive steroids resulting in reduced contraceptive effectiveness which could precipitate unintended pregnancy).
No products indexed under this heading.

Griseofulvin (Increases the metabolism of contraceptive steroids result-

ing in reduced contraceptive effectiveness which could precipitate unintended pregnancy). Products include:
Gris-PEG Tablets 2502

Hypericum (May induce hepatic enzymes and p-glycoprotein transporter and may reduce the effectiveness of contraceptive steroids which may result in breakthrough bleeding). Products include:
Satiete Tablets .... ▣832

Indinavir Sulfate (Several of the protease inhibitors have induced significant changes in the AUC of the estrogen and progestins in some cases; it is not known if this applies to Ortho Evra). Products include:
Crixivan Capsules 1940

Itraconazole (Co-administration with CYP 3A4 inhibitors may increase plasma hormone levels).
No products indexed under this heading.

Ketoconazole (Co-administration with CYP 3A4 inhibitors may increase plasma hormone levels). Products include:
Nizoral A-D Shampoo, 1% 1868

Lopinavir (Several of the protease inhibitors have induced significant changes in the AUC of the estrogen and progestins in some cases; it is not known if this applies to Ortho Evra). Products include:
Kaletra 476

Mephobarbital (Barbiturates increase the metabolism of contraceptive steroids resulting in reduced contraceptive effectiveness which could precipitate unintended pregnancy).
No products indexed under this heading.

Morphine Sulfate (Increased clearance of morphine). Products include:
Avinza Capsules 1741
Kadian Capsules 577
MS Contin Tablets 2701

Nelfinavir Mesylate (Several of the protease inhibitors have induced significant changes in the AUC of the estrogen and progestins in some cases; it is not known if this applies to Ortho Evra). Products include:
Viracept 2577

Pentobarbital Sodium (Barbiturates increase the metabolism of contraceptive steroids resulting in reduced contraceptive effectiveness which could precipitate unintended pregnancy). Products include:
Nembutal Sodium Solution, USP 2470

Phenobarbital (Barbiturates increase the metabolism of contraceptive steroids resulting in reduced contraceptive effectiveness which could precipitate unintended pregnancy). Products include:
Donnatal Extentabs 2493

Phenylbutazone (Increases the metabolism of contraceptive steroids resulting in reduced contraceptive effectiveness which could precipitate unintended pregnancy).
No products indexed under this heading.

Phenytoin (Increases the metabolism of contraceptive steroids resulting in reduced contraceptive effectiveness which could precipitate unintended pregnancy).
No products indexed under this heading.

Phenytoin Sodium (Increases the metabolism of contraceptive steroids resulting in reduced contraceptive effectiveness which could precipitate unintended pregnancy). Products include:
Phenytek Capsules 2160

Prednisolone (Co-administration increases the plasma concentrations of prednisolone).
No products indexed under this heading.

Prednisolone Acetate (Co-administration increases the plasma concentrations of prednisolone). Products include:
Blephamide Ophthalmic Ointment 568
Blephamide Ophthalmic Suspension 569
Poly-Pred Ophthalmic Suspension .... ⊙233
Pred Forte Ophthalmic Suspension .... ⊙235
Pred Mild Ophthalmic Suspension .... ⊙238
Pred-G Ophthalmic Ointment .... ⊙237
Pred-G Ophthalmic Suspension ...... ⊙236

Prednisolone Sodium Phosphate (Co-administration increases the plasma concentrations of prednisolone).
No products indexed under this heading.

Prednisolone Tebutate (Co-administration increases the plasma concentrations of prednisolone).
No products indexed under this heading.

Rifampin (Increases the metabolism of contraceptive steroids resulting in reduced contraceptive effectiveness which could precipitate unintended pregnancy).
No products indexed under this heading.

Ritonavir (Several of the protease inhibitors have induced significant changes in the AUC of the estrogen and progestins in some cases; it is not known if this applies to Ortho Evra). Products include:
Kaletra 476
Norvir 503

Salicylic Acid (Increased clearance of salicylic acid).
No products indexed under this heading.

Saquinavir (Several of the protease inhibitors have induced significant changes in the AUC of the estrogen and progestins in some cases; it is not known if this applies to Ortho Evra).
No products indexed under this heading.

Saquinavir Mesylate (Several of the protease inhibitors have induced significant changes in the AUC of the estrogen and progestins in some cases; it is not known if this applies to Ortho Evra). Products include:
Invirase 2772

Secobarbital Sodium (Barbiturates increase the metabolism of contraceptive steroids resulting in reduced contraceptive effectiveness which could precipitate unintended pregnancy).
No products indexed under this heading.

Temazepam (Increased clearance of temazepam). Products include:
Restoril Capsules 1860

Theophylline (Co-administration increases the plasma concentrations of theophylline).
No products indexed under this heading.

Theophylline Anhydrous (Co-administration increases the plasma concentrations of theophylline). Products include:
Uniphyl Tablets 2710

Theophylline Calcium Salicylate (Co-administration increases the plasma concentrations of theophylline).
No products indexed under this heading.

Theophylline Dihydroxypropyl (Glyceryl) (Co-administration increases the plasma concentrations of theophylline).
No products indexed under this heading.

Theophylline Ethylenediamine (Co-administration increases the plasma concentrations of theophylline).
No products indexed under this heading.

Theophylline Sodium Glycinate (Co-administration increases the plasma concentrations of theophylline).
No products indexed under this heading.

Thiamylal Sodium (Barbiturates increase the metabolism of contraceptive steroids resulting in reduced contraceptive effectiveness which could precipitate unintended pregnancy).
No products indexed under this heading.

Topiramate (Increases the metabolism of contraceptive steroids resulting in reduced contraceptive effectiveness which could precipitate unintended pregnancy). Products include:
Topamax Sprinkle Capsules 2404
Topamax Tablets 2404

Vitamin C (Co-administration with certain oral contraceptives containing ethinyl estradiol increases plasma ethinyl estradiol levels possibly by inhibition of conjugation). Products include:
Bausch & Lomb Ocuvite Adult Eye Vitamin and Mineral Supplement Soft Gels .... ▣706
Bausch & Lomb Ocuvite Adult 50+ Eye Vitamin and Mineral Supplement Soft Gels .... ▣706
Ocuvite Adult Vitamin and Mineral Supplement .... ⊙253
Ocuvite Adult 50+ Vitamin and Mineral Supplement .... ⊙253
Peridin-C Vitamin C Supplement ..... ▣818

ORTHO MICRONOR TABLETS

(Norethindrone) 2426
May interact with barbiturates, phenytoin, and certain other agents. Compounds in these categories include:

Aprobarbital (The effectiveness of progestin-only oral contraceptives is reduced by hepatic enzyme-inducing agents such as barbiturates).
No products indexed under this heading.

Butabarbital (The effectiveness of progestin-only oral contraceptives is reduced by hepatic enzyme-inducing agents such as barbiturates).
No products indexed under this heading.

Butalbital (The effectiveness of progestin-only oral contraceptives is reduced by hepatic enzyme-inducing agents such as barbiturates).
No products indexed under this heading.

Carbamazepine (The effectiveness of progestin-only oral contraceptives is reduced by hepatic enzyme-inducing agents such as carbamazepine). Products include:
Carbatrol Capsules 3171
Equetro Extended-Release Capsules 3180
Tegretol/Tegretol-XR 2295

Fosphenytoin Sodium (The effectiveness of progestin-only oral contraceptives is reduced by hepatic enzyme-inducing agents such as phenytoin).
No products indexed under this heading.

Mephobarbital (The effectiveness of progestin-only oral contraceptives is reduced by hepatic enzyme-inducing agents such as barbiturates).
No products indexed under this heading.

Pentobarbital Sodium (The effectiveness of progestin-only oral contraceptives is reduced by hepatic enzyme-inducing agents such as barbiturates). Products include:
Nembutal Sodium Solution, USP 2470

Phenobarbital (The effectiveness of progestin-only oral contraceptives is reduced by hepatic enzyme-inducing agents such as barbiturates). Products include:
Donnatal Extentabs 2493

Phenytoin (The effectiveness of progestin-only oral contraceptives is reduced by hepatic enzyme-inducing agents such as phenytoin).
No products indexed under this heading.

Phenytoin Sodium (The effectiveness of progestin-only oral contraceptives is reduced by hepatic enzyme-inducing agents such as phenytoin). Products include:
Phenytek Capsules 2160

Rifampin (The effectiveness of progestin-only oral contraceptives is reduced by hepatic enzyme-inducing agents such as rifampin).
No products indexed under this heading.

Secobarbital Sodium (The effectiveness of progestin-only oral contraceptives is reduced by hepatic enzyme-inducing agents such as barbiturates).
No products indexed under this heading.

Thiamylal Sodium (The effectiveness of progestin-only oral contraceptives is reduced by hepatic enzyme-inducing agents such as barbiturates).
No products indexed under this heading.

ORTHO TRI-CYCLEN TABLETS

(Ethinyl Estradiol, Norgestimate) 2429
See Ortho Tri-Cyclen Lo Tablets

ORTHO TRI-CYCLEN LO TABLETS

(Ethinyl Estradiol, Norgestimate) 2436
May interact with barbiturates, phenytoin, prednisolone, protease inhibitors, tetracyclines, xanthines, and certain other agents. Compounds in these categories include:

Acetaminophen (Co-administration with certain oral contraceptives containing ethinyl estradiol increases plasma ethinyl estradiol levels possibly by inhibition of conjugation; decreased plasma levels of acetaminophen). Products include:

Comtrex Maximum Strength Cold & Cough Day/Night Caplets - Day Formulation .... ▣ 726
Comtrex Maximum Strength Cold & Cough Day/Night Caplets - Night Formulation .... ▣ 726
Comtrex Maximum Strength Non-Drowsy Cold & Cough Caplets .... ▣ 725
Comtrex Maximum Strength Day/Night Severe Cold & Sinus Caplets - Day Formulation .... ▣ 725
Comtrex Maximum Strength Day/Night Severe Cold & Sinus Caplets - Night Formulation .... ▣ 725
Contac Cold and Flu Maximum Strength Caplets .... ▣ 728
Contac Cold and Flu Day and Night Caplets (Day Formulation Only) .... ▣ 727
Contac Cold and Flu Day and Night Caplets (Night Formulation Only) .... ▣ 727
Contac Cold and Flu Non-Drowsy Caplets .... ▣ 728
Excedrin Extra Strength Caplets/Tablets/Geltabs .... ▣ 684
Excedrin Migraine Caplets/Tablets/Geltabs .... ▣ 609
Excedrin PM Caplets/Tablets/Geltabs .... ▣ 610
Excedrin Sinus Headache Caplets/Tablets .... ▣ 610
Excedrin Tension Headache Caplets/Tablets/Geltabs .... ▣ 611
Goody's Body Pain Formula Powder .... ▣ 684
Goody's Extra Strength Headache Powders .... ▣ 611
Goody's Extra Strength Pain Relief Tablets .... ▣ 685
Goody's PM Powder for Pain with Sleeplessness .... ▣ 612
Percocet Tablets 1131
Robitussin Cough, Cold & Flu Nighttime Liquid .... ▣ 738
TheraFlu Cold & Sore Throat Hot Liquid .... ▣ 741
TheraFlu Flu & Chest Congestion Hot Liquid .... ▣ 741
TheraFlu Flu & Sore Throat Hot Liquid .... ▣ 742
TheraFlu Daytime Severe Cold Hot Liquid .... ▣ 742
TheraFlu Nighttime Severe Cold Hot Liquid .... ▣ 740
TheraFlu Warming Relief Daytime Severe Cold .... ▣ 743
TheraFlu Warming Relief Nighttime Severe Cold .... ▣ 743
Triaminic Cough & Sore Throat Liquid .... ▣ 747
Regular Strength Tylenol Tablets 1870
Children's Tylenol with Flavor Creator .... ▣ 679
Children's Tylenol Plus Flu Oral Suspension .... ▣ 749
Tylenol Cold Head Congestion Daytime Caplets with Cool Burst and Gelcaps .... ▣ 750
Tylenol Cold Multi-Symptom Daytime Liquid .... ▣ 752
Tylenol Cold Multi-Symptom Severe Daytime Liquid .... ▣ 752
Tylenol 8 Hour Extended Release Caplets 1870
Tylenol 1870
Extra Strength Tylenol PM Caplets, Vanilla Caplets, Geltabs, Gelcaps and Liquid 1875
Extra Strength Tylenol Rapid Release Gels 1870
Concentrated Tylenol Infants' Drops Plus Cold & Cough .... ▣ 754
Tylenol with Codeine Tablets 2391
Tylenol Allergy Multi-Symptom Caplets with Cool Burst and Gelcaps 1872
Tylenol Allergy Multi-Symptom Nighttime Caplets with Cool Burst 1872
Tylenol Severe Allergy Caplets 1872
Tylenol Arthritis Pain Extended Release Caplets and Geltabs 1870
Tylenol Chest Congestion Caplets with Cool Burst 1872
Tylenol Chest Congestion Liquid with Cool Burst 1872
Children's Tylenol Suspension Liquid and Meltaways 1878
Children's Tylenol Plus Cold Suspension Liquid 1879
Children's Tylenol Plus Cold & Allergy Suspension Liquid 1878
Children's Tylenol Plus Cough & Runny Nose Suspension Liquid 1879
Children's Tylenol Plus Cough & Sore Throat Suspension Liquid 1879
Children's Tylenol Suspension with Flavor Creator 1878
Children's Tylenol Plus Flu Suspension Liquid 1881
Children's Tylenol Plus Multi-Symptom Cold Suspension Liquid 1879
Tylenol Cold Severe Congestion Non-Drowsy Caplets with Cool Burst 1874
Tylenol Cold Head Congestion Daytime Caplets with Cool Burst 1873
Tylenol Cold Head Congestion Nighttime Caplets with Cool Burst 1873
Tylenol Cold Head Congestion Severe Caplets with Cool Burst 1873
Tylenol Cold Multi-Symptom Daytime Caplets with Cool Burst and Gelcaps 1874
Tylenol Cold Multi-Symptom Daytime Liquid with Citrus Burst 1874
Tylenol Cold Multi-Symptom Nighttime Caplets with Cool Burst 1874
Tylenol Cold Multi-Symptom Nighttime Liquid with Cool Burst 1874
Tylenol Cold Multi-Symptom Severe Caplets with Cool Burst 1874
Tylenol Cold Multi-Symptom Severe Daytime Liquid with Citrus Burst 1874
Tylenol Cough & Sore Throat Daytime Liquid with Cool Burst 1877
Tylenol Cough & Sore Throat Nighttime Liquid with Cool Burst 1877
Concentrated Tylenol Infants' Drops 1878
Concentrated Tylenol Infants' Drops Plus Cold 1879
Concentrated Tylenol Infants' Drops Plus Cold and Cough 1879
Jr. Tylenol Meltaways 1878
Tylenol Sinus Severe Congestion Caplets with Cool Burst 1876
Tylenol Sinus Congestion & Pain Daytime Caplets with Cool Burst and Gelcaps 1876
Tylenol Sinus Congestion & Pain Nighttime Caplets with Cool Burst 1876
Tylenol Sinus Congestion & Pain Severe Caplets with Cool Burst 1876
Tylenol Sore Throat Daytime Liquid with Cool Burst 1877
Tylenol Sore Throat Nighttime Liquid with Cool Burst 1877
Women's Tylenol Menstrual Relief Caplets 1877
Vicks 44M Cough, Cold & Flu Relief Liquid 2680
Vicks DayQuil LiquiCaps/Liquid Multi-Symptom Cold/Flu Relief .... ▣ 761
Vicks DayQuil Multi-Symptom Cold/Flu Relief LiquiCaps 2678
Vicks DayQuil Multi-Symptom Cold/Flu Relief Liquid 2678
Vicks NyQuil Multi-Symptom Cold/Flu Relief Liquid 2681
Vicks NyQuil Multi-Symptom Cold/Flu Relief LiquiCaps 2681
Vicks NyQuil LiquiCaps/Liquid Multi-Symptom Cold/Flu Relief .... ▣ 763
Vicodin Tablets 535
Vicodin ES Tablets 536
Vicodin HP Tablets 538
Zicam Maximum Strength Flu Daytime .... ▣ 768
Zicam Maximum Strength Flu Nighttime .... ▣ 768
Zydone Tablets 1139

Aminophylline (Co-administration increases the plasma concentrations of theophylline).
No products indexed under this heading.

Ampicillin (Several cases of contraceptive failure and breakthrough bleeding have been reported in the literature with concomitant administration of antibiotics, such as tetracyclines. However, clinical pharmacology studies investigating drug interaction between combined oral contraceptives and tetracyclines have reported inconsistent results).
No products indexed under this heading.

Ampicillin Sodium (Several cases of contraceptive failure and breakthrough bleeding have been reported in the literature with concomitant administration of antibiotics, such as tetracyclines. However, clinical pharmacology studies investigating drug interaction between combined oral contraceptives and tetracyclines have reported inconsistent results).
No products indexed under this heading.

Amprenavir (Several of the protease inhibitors have induced significant changes in the AUC of the estrogen and progestins in some cases; co-administration may affect safety and efficacy of oral contraceptives). Products include:
Agenerase Capsules 1327
Agenerase Oral Solution 1332

Aprobarbital (Barbiturates increase the metabolism of contraceptive steroids resulting in reduced contraceptive effectiveness and this could precipitate unintended pregnancy or breakthrough bleeding).
No products indexed under this heading.

Atorvastatin Calcium (Co-administration with certain oral contraceptives containing ethinyl estradiol increases AUC values for ethinyl estradiol by approximately 20%). Products include:
Caduet Tablets 2508
Lipitor Tablets 2483

Butabarbital (Barbiturates increase the metabolism of contraceptive steroids resulting in reduced contraceptive effectiveness and this could precipitate unintended pregnancy or breakthrough bleeding).
No products indexed under this heading.

Butalbital (Barbiturates increase the metabolism of contraceptive steroids resulting in reduced contraceptive effectiveness and this could precipitate unintended pregnancy or breakthrough bleeding).
No products indexed under this heading.

Carbamazepine (Increases the metabolism of contraceptive steroids resulting in reduced contraceptive effectiveness and this could precipitate unintended pregnancy or breakthrough bleeding). Products include:
Carbatrol Capsules 3171
Equetro Extended-Release Capsules 3180
Tegretol/Tegretol-XR 2295

Clofibrate (Increased clearance of clofibric acid).
No products indexed under this heading.

Cyclosporine (Co-administration increases the plasma concentrations of cyclosporine). Products include:
Gengraf Capsules 459
Neoral Oral Solution 2259
Neoral Soft Gelatin Capsules 2259
Restasis Ophthalmic Emulsion 575
Sandimmune 2275

Demeclocycline Hydrochloride (Several cases of contraceptive failure and breakthrough bleeding have been reported in the literature with concomitant administration of antibiotics, such as tetracyclines. However, clinical pharmacology studies investigating drug interaction between combined oral contraceptives and tetracyclines have reported inconsistent results).
No products indexed under this heading.

Doxycycline Calcium (Several cases of contraceptive failure and breakthrough bleeding have been reported in the literature with concomitant administration of antibiotics, such as tetracyclines. However, clinical pharmacology studies investigating drug interaction between combined oral contraceptives and tetracyclines have reported inconsistent results).
No products indexed under this heading.

Doxycycline Hyclate (Several cases of contraceptive failure and breakthrough bleeding have been reported in the literature with concomitant administration of antibiotics, such as tetracyclines. However, clinical pharmacology studies investigating drug interaction between combined oral contraceptives and tetracyclines have reported inconsistent results).
No products indexed under this heading.

Doxycycline Monohydrate (Several cases of contraceptive failure and breakthrough bleeding have been reported in the literature with concomitant administration of antibiotics, such as tetracyclines. However, clinical pharmacology studies investigating drug interaction between combined oral contraceptives and tetracyclines have reported inconsistent results). Products include:
Oracea Capsules 1000

Dyphylline (Co-administration increases the plasma concentrations of theophylline).
No products indexed under this heading.

Felbamate (Increases the metabolism of contraceptive steroids resulting in reduced contraceptive effectiveness and this could precipitate unintended pregnancy or breakthrough bleeding).
No products indexed under this heading.

Fosphenytoin Sodium (Increases the metabolism of contraceptive steroids resulting in reduced contraceptive effectiveness and this could precipitate unintended pregnancy or breakthrough bleeding).
No products indexed under this heading.

Griseofulvin (Increases the metabolism of contraceptive steroids resulting in reduced contraceptive effectiveness and this could precipitate unintended pregnancy or breakthrough bleeding). Products include:
Gris-PEG Tablets 2502

Hypericum (May induce hepatic enzymes and p-glycoprotein transporter and may reduce the effectiveness of contraceptive steroids and this may result in breakthrough bleeding). Products include:

Satiete Tablets 832

Indinavir Sulfate (Several of the protease inhibitors have induced significant changes in the AUC of the estrogen and progestins in some cases; co-administration may affect safety and efficacy of oral contraceptives). Products include:
Crixivan Capsules 1940

Itraconazole (Co-administration with CYP 3A4 inhibitors may increase plasma hormone levels).
No products indexed under this heading.

Ketoconazole (Co-administration with CYP 3A4 inhibitors may increase plasma hormone levels). Products include:
Nizoral A-D Shampoo, 1% 1868

Lopinavir (Several of the protease inhibitors have induced significant changes in the AUC of the estrogen and progestins in some cases; co-administration may affect safety and efficacy of oral contraceptives). Products include:
Kaletra 476

Mephobarbital (Barbiturates increase the metabolism of contraceptive steroids resulting in reduced contraceptive effectiveness and this could precipitate unintended pregnancy or breakthrough bleeding).
No products indexed under this heading.

Methacycline Hydrochloride (Several cases of contraceptive failure and breakthrough bleeding have been reported in the literature with concomitant administration of antibiotics, such as tetracyclines. However, clinical pharmacology studies investigating drug interaction between combined oral contraceptives and tetracyclines have reported inconsistent results).
No products indexed under this heading.

Minocycline Hydrochloride (Several cases of contraceptive failure and breakthrough bleeding have been reported in the literature with concomitant administration of antibiotics, such as tetracyclines. However, clinical pharmacology studies investigating drug interaction between combined oral contraceptives and tetracyclines have reported inconsistent results). Products include:
Solodyn Extended Release Tablets 1890

Morphine Sulfate (Increased clearance of morphine). Products include:
Avinza Capsules 1741
Kadian Capsules 577
MS Contin Tablets 2701

Nelfinavir Mesylate (Several of the protease inhibitors have induced significant changes in the AUC of the estrogen and progestins in some cases; co-administration may affect safety and efficacy of oral contraceptives). Products include:
Viracept 2577

Oxcarbazepine (Increases the metabolism of contraceptive steroids resulting in reduced contraceptive effectiveness and this could precipitate unintended pregnancy or breakthrough bleeding). Products include:
Trileptal Tablets 2300
Trileptal Oral Suspension 2300

Oxytetracycline Hydrochloride (Several cases of contraceptive failure and breakthrough bleeding have been reported in the literature with concomitant administration of antibiotics, such as tetracyclines. However, clinical pharmacology studies investigating drug interaction between combined oral contraceptives and tetracyclines have reported inconsistent results).
No products indexed under this heading.

Pentobarbital Sodium (Barbiturates increase the metabolism of contraceptive steroids resulting in reduced contraceptive effectiveness and this could precipitate unintended pregnancy or breakthrough bleeding). Products include:
Nembutal Sodium Solution, USP 2470

Phenobarbital (Barbiturates increase the metabolism of contraceptive steroids resulting in reduced contraceptive effectiveness and this could precipitate unintended pregnancy or breakthrough bleeding). Products include:
Donnatal Extentabs 2493

Phenylbutazone (Increases the metabolism of contraceptive steroids resulting in reduced contraceptive effectiveness and this could precipitate unintended pregnancy or breakthrough bleeding).
No products indexed under this heading.

Phenytoin (Increases the metabolism of contraceptive steroids resulting in reduced contraceptive effectiveness and this could precipitate unintended pregnancy or breakthrough bleeding).
No products indexed under this heading.

Phenytoin Sodium (Increases the metabolism of contraceptive steroids resulting in reduced contraceptive effectiveness and this could precipitate unintended pregnancy or breakthrough bleeding). Products include:
Phenytek Capsules 2160

Prednisolone (Co-administration increases the plasma concentrations of prednisolone).
No products indexed under this heading.

Prednisolone Acetate (Co-administration increases the plasma concentrations of prednisolone). Products include:
Blephamide Ophthalmic Ointment 568
Blephamide Ophthalmic Suspension................................. 569
Poly-Pred Ophthalmic Suspension .... ⊙233
Pred Forte Ophthalmic Suspension .... ⊙235
Pred Mild Ophthalmic Suspension .... ⊙238
Pred-G Ophthalmic Ointment .... ⊙237
Pred-G Ophthalmic Suspension ...... ⊙236

Prednisolone Sodium Phosphate (Co-administration increases the plasma concentrations of prednisolone).
No products indexed under this heading.

Prednisolone Tebutate (Co-administration increases the plasma concentrations of prednisolone).
No products indexed under this heading.

Rifampin (Increases the metabolism of contraceptive steroids resulting in reduced contraceptive effectiveness and this could precipitate unintended pregnancy or breakthrough bleeding).
No products indexed under this heading.

Ritonavir (Several of the protease inhibitors have induced significant changes in the AUC of the estrogen and progestins in some cases; co-administration may affect safety and efficacy of oral contraceptives). Products include:
Kaletra 476
Norvir 503

Salicylic Acid (Increased clearance of salicylic acid).
No products indexed under this heading.

Saquinavir (Several of the protease inhibitors have induced significant changes in the AUC of the estrogen and progestins in some cases; co-administration may affect safety and efficacy of oral contraceptives).
No products indexed under this heading.

Saquinavir Mesylate (Several of the protease inhibitors have induced significant changes in the AUC of the estrogen and progestins in some cases; co-administration may affect safety and efficacy of oral contraceptives). Products include:
Invirase 2772

Secobarbital Sodium (Barbiturates increase the metabolism of contraceptive steroids resulting in reduced contraceptive effectiveness and this could precipitate unintended pregnancy or breakthrough bleeding).
No products indexed under this heading.

Temazepam (Increased clearance of temazepam). Products include:
Restoril Capsules 1860

Tetracycline Hydrochloride (Several cases of contraceptive failure and breakthrough bleeding have been reported in the literature with concomitant administration of antibiotics, such as tetracyclines. However, clinical pharmacology studies investigating drug interaction between combined oral contraceptives and tetracyclines have reported inconsistent results).
No products indexed under this heading.

Theophylline (Co-administration increases the plasma concentrations of theophylline).
No products indexed under this heading.

Theophylline Anhydrous (Co-administration increases the plasma concentrations of theophylline). Products include:
Uniphyl Tablets 2710

Theophylline Calcium Salicylate (Co-administration increases the plasma concentrations of theophylline).
No products indexed under this heading.

Theophylline Dihydroxypropyl (Glyceryl) (Co-administration increases the plasma concentrations of theophylline).
No products indexed under this heading.

Theophylline Ethylenediamine (Co-administration increases the plasma concentrations of theophylline).
No products indexed under this heading.

Theophylline Sodium Glycinate (Co-administration increases the plasma concentrations of theophylline).
No products indexed under this heading.

Thiamylal Sodium (Barbiturates increase the metabolism of contraceptive steroids resulting in reduced contraceptive effectiveness and this could precipitate unintended pregnancy or breakthrough bleeding).
No products indexed under this heading.

Topiramate (Increases the metabolism of contraceptive steroids resulting in reduced contraceptive effectiveness and this could precipitate unintended pregnancy or breakthrough bleeding). Products include:
Topamax Sprinkle Capsules 2404
Topamax Tablets 2404

Vitamin C (Co-administration with certain oral contraceptives containing ethinyl estradiol increases plasma ethinyl estradiol levels possibly by inhibition of conjugation). Products include:
Bausch & Lomb Ocuvite Adult Eye Vitamin and Mineral Supplement Soft Gels 706
Bausch & Lomb Ocuvite Adult 50+ Eye Vitamin and Mineral Supplement Soft Gels 706
Ocuvite Adult Vitamin and Mineral Supplement................................ ⊙253
Ocuvite Adult 50+ Vitamin and Mineral Supplement.................... ⊙253
Peridin-C Vitamin C Supplement 818

ORTHOCLONE OKT3 STERILE SOLUTION

(Muromonab-CD3) 2360
May interact with corticosteroids and certain other agents. Compounds in these categories include:

Azathioprine (Infection or malignancies have been reported with azathioprine alone and in conjunction with muromonab-CD3).
No products indexed under this heading.

Betamethasone Acetate (Psychosis and infection have been reported in patients treated with corticosteroids alone and in conjunction with muromonab-CD3).
No products indexed under this heading.

Betamethasone Sodium Phosphate (Psychosis and infection have been reported in patients treated with corticosteroids alone and in conjunction with muromonab-CD3).
No products indexed under this heading.

Cortisone Acetate (Psychosis and infection have been reported in patients treated with corticosteroids alone and in conjunction with muromonab-CD3).
No products indexed under this heading.

Cyclosporine (Seizures, encephalopathy, infections, malignancies, and thrombotic events have been reported in patients receiving cyclosporine alone and in conjunction with muromonab-CD3). Products include:
Gengraf Capsules 459

Neoral Oral Solution 2259
Neoral Soft Gelatin Capsules 2259
Restasis Ophthalmic Emulsion 575
Sandimmune 2275

Dexamethasone (Psychosis and infection have been reported in patients treated with corticosteroids alone and in conjunction with muromonab-CD3). Products include:
Ciprodex Otic Suspension 559
Decadron Tablets 1951
TobraDex Ophthalmic Ointment 562
TobraDex Ophthalmic Suspension ... 563

Dexamethasone Acetate (Psychosis and infection have been reported in patients treated with corticosteroids alone and in conjunction with muromonab-CD3).
No products indexed under this heading.

Dexamethasone Sodium Phosphate (Psychosis and infection have been reported in patients treated with corticosteroids alone and in conjunction with muromonab-CD3).
No products indexed under this heading.

Fludrocortisone Acetate (Psychosis and infection have been reported in patients treated with corticosteroids alone and in conjunction with muromonab-CD3).
No products indexed under this heading.

Hydrocortisone (Psychosis and infection have been reported in patients treated with corticosteroids alone and in conjunction with muromonab-CD3). Products include:
Colocort Rectal Suspension, USP (Retention) 100 mg/60 mL........... 2476
Hydrocortone Tablets 1989
Preparation H Hydrocortisone Cream .... ▣646

Hydrocortisone Acetate (Psychosis and infection have been reported in patients treated with corticosteroids alone and in conjunction with muromonab-CD3). Products include:
Analpram-HC 1159
Pramosone 1161
ProctoFoam-HC 3099

Hydrocortisone Sodium Phosphate (Psychosis and infection have been reported in patients treated with corticosteroids alone and in conjunction with muromonab-CD3).
No products indexed under this heading.

Hydrocortisone Sodium Succinate (Psychosis and infection have been reported in patients treated with corticosteroids alone and in conjunction with muromonab-CD3).
No products indexed under this heading.

Indomethacin (Encephalopathy and other CNS effects have been reported in patients treated with indomethacin alone and in conjunction with muromonab-CD3). Products include:
Indocin 1995

Indomethacin Sodium Trihydrate (Encephalopathy and other CNS effects have been reported in patients treated with indomethacin alone and in conjunction with muromonab-CD3). Products include:
Indocin I.V. 2465

Methylprednisolone Acetate (Psychosis and infection have been reported in patients treated with corticosteroids alone and in conjunction with muromonab-CD3). Products include:
Depo-Medrol Injectable Suspension 2617
Depo-Medrol Single-Dose Vial 2619

Methylprednisolone Sodium Succinate (Psychosis and infection have been reported in patients treated with corticosteroids alone and in conjunction with muromonab-CD3).
No products indexed under this heading.

Prednisolone Acetate (Psychosis and infection have been reported in patients treated with corticosteroids alone and in conjunction with muromonab-CD3). Products include:
Blephamide Ophthalmic Ointment 568
Blephamide Ophthalmic Suspension................................. 569
Poly-Pred Ophthalmic Suspension .... ⊙233
Pred Forte Ophthalmic Suspension .... ⊙235
Pred Mild Ophthalmic Suspension .... ⊙238
Pred-G Ophthalmic Ointment .... ⊙237
Pred-G Ophthalmic Suspension ...... ⊙236

Prednisolone Sodium Phosphate (Psychosis and infection have been reported in patients treated with corticosteroids alone and in conjunction with muromonab-CD3).
No products indexed under this heading.

Prednisolone Tebutate (Psychosis and infection have been reported in patients treated with corticosteroids alone and in conjunction with muromonab-CD3).
No products indexed under this heading.

Prednisone (Psychosis and infection have been reported in patients treated with corticosteroids alone and in conjunction with muromonab-CD3).
No products indexed under this heading.

Triamcinolone (Psychosis and infection have been reported in patients treated with corticosteroids alone and in conjunction with muromonab-CD3).
No products indexed under this heading.

Triamcinolone Acetonide (Psychosis and infection have been reported in patients treated with corticosteroids alone and in conjunction with muromonab-CD3). Products include:
Azmacort Inhalation Aerosol 1726
Nasacort AQ Nasal Spray 2922

Triamcinolone Diacetate (Psychosis and infection have been reported in patients treated with corticosteroids alone and in conjunction with muromonab-CD3).
No products indexed under this heading.

Triamcinolone Hexacetonide (Psychosis and infection have been reported in patients treated with corticosteroids alone and in conjunction with muromonab-CD3).
No products indexed under this heading.

OS-CAL CHEWABLE TABLETS

(Calcium Carbonate) .... ▣818
None cited in PDR database.

OS-CAL 250 + D TABLETS

(Calcium, Vitamin D) .... ▣817
None cited in PDR database.

OS-CAL 500 TABLETS

(Calcium) .... ▣817
None cited in PDR database.

OS-CAL 500 + D TABLETS

(Calcium, Vitamin D) .... ▣817
None cited in PDR database.

OSMOPREP TABLETS

(Sodium Phosphate) 2840
May interact with:

Oral Medications, unspecified (Medications administered in close proximity to OsmoPrep tablets may not be absorbed from the gastrointestinal tract due to the rapid intestinal peristalsis and watery diarrhea induced by the purgative agent).
No products indexed under this heading.

OVIDE .5% LOTION

(Malathion) 3290
None cited in PDR database.

OXANDRIN TABLETS

(Oxandrolone) 2962
May interact with corticosteroids, oral anticoagulants, oral hypoglycemic agents, and certain other agents. Compounds in these categories include:

Acarbose (Oxandrolone may inhibit the metabolism of oral hypoglycemic agents). Products include:
Precose Tablets 751

ACTH (In patients with edema, co-administration with ACTH may increase the edema).
No products indexed under this heading.

Anisindione (Concurrent dosing of oxandrolone and warfarin may result in unexpectedly large increases in the INR or prothrombin time (PT). When oxandrolone is prescribed to patients being treated with warfarin, doses of warfarin may need to be decreased significantlyto maintain the desirable INR level and diminish the risk of potentially serious bleeding. Furthermore, in patients receiving both drugs, careful monitoring of the PT or INR and adjustment of the warfarin dosage if indicated are recommended when the oxandrolone dose is changed or discontinued. Patients should be closely monitored for signs and symptoms of occult bleeding). Products include:
Miradon Tablets 3042

Betamethasone Acetate (In patients with edema, co-administration with adrenal cortical steroids may increase the edema).
No products indexed under this heading.

Betamethasone Sodium Phosphate (In patients with edema, co-administration with adrenal cortical steroids may increase the edema).
No products indexed under this heading.

Chlorpropamide (Oxandrolone may inhibit the metabolism of oral hypoglycemic agents).
No products indexed under this heading.

Cortisone Acetate (In patients with edema, co-administration with adrenal cortical steroids may increase the edema).
No products indexed under this heading.

Dexamethasone (In patients with edema, co-administration with adrenal cortical steroids may increase the edema). Products include:
Ciprodex Otic Suspension 559
Decadron Tablets 1951
TobraDex Ophthalmic Ointment 562
TobraDex Ophthalmic Suspension ... 563

Dexamethasone Acetate (In patients with edema, co-administration with adrenal cortical steroids may increase the edema).
No products indexed under this heading.

Dexamethasone Sodium Phosphate (In patients with edema, co-administration with adrenal cortical steroids may increase the edema).
No products indexed under this heading.

Dicumarol (Concurrent dosing of oxandrolone and warfarin may result in unexpectedly large increases in the INR or prothrombin time (PT). When oxandrolone is prescribed to patients being treated with warfarin, doses of warfarin may need to be decreased significantlyto maintain the desirable INR level and diminish the risk of potentially serious bleeding. Furthermore, in patients receiving both drugs, careful monitoring of the PT or INR and adjustment of the warfarin dosage if indicated are recommended when the oxandrolone dose is changed or discontinued. Patients should be closely monitored for signs and symptoms of occult bleeding).
No products indexed under this heading.

Fludrocortisone Acetate (In patients with edema, co-administration with adrenal cortical steroids may increase the edema).
No products indexed under this heading.

Glimepiride (Oxandrolone may inhibit the metabolism of oral hypoglycemic agents). Products include:
Avandaryl Tablets 1379
Duetact Tablets 3226

Glipizide (Oxandrolone may inhibit the metabolism of oral hypoglycemic agents).
No products indexed under this heading.

Glyburide (Oxandrolone may inhibit the metabolism of oral hypoglycemic agents).
No products indexed under this heading.

Hydrocortisone (In patients with edema, co-administration with adrenal cortical steroids may increase the edema). Products include:
Colocort Rectal Suspension, USP (Retention) 100 mg/60 mL........... 2476
Hydrocortone Tablets 1989
Preparation H Hydrocortisone Cream .... ▣646

Hydrocortisone Acetate (In patients with edema, co-administration with adrenal cortical steroids may increase the edema). Products include:
Analpram-HC 1159
Pramosone 1161
ProctoFoam-HC 3099

Hydrocortisone Sodium Phosphate (In patients with edema, co-administration with adrenal cortical steroids may increase the edema).
No products indexed under this heading.

Hydrocortisone Sodium Succinate (In patients with edema, co-administration with adrenal cortical steroids may increase the edema).
No products indexed under this heading.

Metformin Hydrochloride (Oxandrolone may inhibit the metabolism of oral hypoglycemic agents). Products include:
- ActoPlus Met Tablets 3214
- Avandamet Tablets 1373
- Fortamet Extended-Release Tablets 3115

Methylprednisolone Acetate (In patients with edema, co-administration with adrenal cortical steroids may increase the edema). Products include:
- Depo-Medrol Injectable Suspension 2617
- Depo-Medrol Single-Dose Vial 2619

Methylprednisolone Sodium Succinate (In patients with edema, co-administration with adrenal cortical steroids may increase the edema).
No products indexed under this heading.

Miglitol (Oxandrolone may inhibit the metabolism of oral hypoglycemic agents).
No products indexed under this heading.

Pioglitazone Hydrochloride (Oxandrolone may inhibit the metabolism of oral hypoglycemic agents). Products include:
- ActoPlus Met Tablets 3214
- Actos Tablets 3219
- Duetact Tablets 3226

Prednisolone Acetate (In patients with edema, co-administration with adrenal cortical steroids may increase the edema). Products include:
- Blephamide Ophthalmic Ointment 568
- Blephamide Ophthalmic Suspension 569
- Poly-Pred Ophthalmic Suspension .... ⊙233
- Pred Forte Ophthalmic Suspension .... ⊙235
- Pred Mild Ophthalmic Suspension .... ⊙238
- Pred-G Ophthalmic Ointment .... ⊙237
- Pred-G Ophthalmic Suspension ...... ⊙236

Prednisolone Sodium Phosphate (In patients with edema, co-administration with adrenal cortical steroids may increase the edema).
No products indexed under this heading.

Prednisolone Tebutate (In patients with edema, co-administration with adrenal cortical steroids may increase the edema).
No products indexed under this heading.

Prednisone (In patients with edema, co-administration with adrenal cortical steroids may increase the edema).
No products indexed under this heading.

Repaglinide (Oxandrolone may inhibit the metabolism of oral hypoglycemic agents).
No products indexed under this heading.

Rosiglitazone Maleate (Oxandrolone may inhibit the metabolism of oral hypoglycemic agents). Products include:
- Avandamet Tablets 1373
- Avandaryl Tablets 1379
- Avandia Tablets 1384

Tolazamide (Oxandrolone may inhibit the metabolism of oral hypoglycemic agents).
No products indexed under this heading.

Tolbutamide (Oxandrolone may inhibit the metabolism of oral hypoglycemic agents).
No products indexed under this heading.

Triamcinolone (In patients with edema, co-administration with adrenal cortical steroids may increase the edema).
No products indexed under this heading.

Triamcinolone Acetonide (In patients with edema, co-administration with adrenal cortical steroids may increase the edema). Products include:
- Azmacort Inhalation Aerosol 1726
- Nasacort AQ Nasal Spray 2922

Triamcinolone Diacetate (In patients with edema, co-administration with adrenal cortical steroids may increase the edema).
No products indexed under this heading.

Triamcinolone Hexacetonide (In patients with edema, co-administration with adrenal cortical steroids may increase the edema).
No products indexed under this heading.

Troglitazone (Oxandrolone may inhibit the metabolism of oral hypoglycemic agents).
No products indexed under this heading.

Warfarin Sodium (Concurrent dosing of oxandrolone and warfarin may result in unexpectedly large increases in the INR or prothrombin time (PT). When oxandrolone is prescribed to patients being treated with warfarin, doses of warfarin may need to be decreased significantlyto maintain the desirable INR level and diminish the risk of potentially serious bleeding. Furthermore, in patients receiving both drugs, careful monitoring of the PT or INR and adjustment of the warfarin dosage if indicated are recommended when the oxandrolone dose is changed or discontinued. Patients should be closely monitored for signs and symptoms of occult bleeding). Products include:
- Coumadin for Injection 898
- Coumadin Tablets 898

OXISTAT CREAM
(Oxiconazole Nitrate) 2667
None cited in PDR database.

OXISTAT LOTION
(Oxiconazole Nitrate) 2667
None cited in PDR database.

OXSORALEN LOTION 1%
(Methoxsalen) 3352
May interact with phenothiazines, sulfonamides, tetracyclines, thiazides, and certain other agents. Compounds in these categories include:

Anthralin (Possible photosensitivity effects). Products include:
- Psoriatec Cream 1089

Bendroflumethiazide (Possible photosensitivity effects).
No products indexed under this heading.

Chlorothiazide (Possible photosensitivity effects). Products include:
- Diuril Oral Suspension 1954

Chlorothiazide Sodium (Possible photosensitivity effects). Products include:
- Diuril Sodium Intravenous 2467

Chlorpromazine (Possible photosensitivity effects).
No products indexed under this heading.

Chlorpromazine Hydrochloride (Possible photosensitivity effects).
No products indexed under this heading.

Chlorpropamide (Possible photosensitivity effects).
No products indexed under this heading.

Coal Tar (Possible photosensitivity effects).
No products indexed under this heading.

Demeclocycline Hydrochloride (Possible photosensitivity effects).
No products indexed under this heading.

Doxycycline Calcium (Possible photosensitivity effects).
No products indexed under this heading.

Doxycycline Hyclate (Possible photosensitivity effects).
No products indexed under this heading.

Doxycycline Monohydrate (Possible photosensitivity effects). Products include:
- Oracea Capsules 1000

Fluphenazine Decanoate (Possible photosensitivity effects).
No products indexed under this heading.

Fluphenazine Enanthate (Possible photosensitivity effects).
No products indexed under this heading.

Fluphenazine Hydrochloride (Possible photosensitivity effects).
No products indexed under this heading.

Glipizide (Possible photosensitivity effects).
No products indexed under this heading.

Glyburide (Possible photosensitivity effects).
No products indexed under this heading.

Griseofulvin (Possible photosensitivity effects). Products include:
- Gris-PEG Tablets 2502

Hydrochlorothiazide (Possible photosensitivity effects). Products include:
- Aldoril Tablets 1910
- Atacand HCT 651
- Avalide Tablets 888
- Avalide Tablets 2874
- Benicar HCT Tablets 1044
- Diovan HCT Tablets 2196
- Dyazide Capsules 1423
- Hyzaar 50-12.5 Tablets 1990
- Hyzaar 100-12.5 Tablets 1990
- Hyzaar 100-25 Tablets 1990
- Lopressor HCT 50/25 Tablets 2241
- Lopressor HCT 100/25 Tablets 2241
- Lopressor HCT 100/50 Tablets 2241
- Lotensin HCT Tablets 2246
- Micardis HCT Tablets 856
- Moduretic Tablets 2028
- Prinzide Tablets 2056
- Teveten HCT Tablets 1737
- Timolide Tablets 2086
- Uniretic Tablets 3100

Hydroflumethiazide (Possible photosensitivity effects).
No products indexed under this heading.

Mesoridazine Besylate (Possible photosensitivity effects).
No products indexed under this heading.

Methacycline Hydrochloride (Possible photosensitivity effects).
No products indexed under this heading.

Methotrimeprazine (Possible photosensitivity effects).
No products indexed under this heading.

Methyclothiazide (Possible photosensitivity effects).
No products indexed under this heading.

Methylene Blue (Possible photosensitivity effects). Products include:
- Prosed/DS Tablets 1157

Minocycline Hydrochloride (Possible photosensitivity effects). Products include:
- Solodyn Extended Release Tablets 1890

Nalidixic Acid (Possible photosensitivity effects).
No products indexed under this heading.

Oxytetracycline (Possible photosensitivity effects).
No products indexed under this heading.

Oxytetracycline Hydrochloride (Possible photosensitivity effects).
No products indexed under this heading.

Perphenazine (Possible photosensitivity effects).
No products indexed under this heading.

Polythiazide (Possible photosensitivity effects).
No products indexed under this heading.

Prochlorperazine (Possible photosensitivity effects).
No products indexed under this heading.

Promethazine Hydrochloride (Possible photosensitivity effects). Products include:
- Phenergan Tablets and Suppositories 3440

Sulfacytine (Possible photosensitivity effects).
No products indexed under this heading.

Sulfamethizole (Possible photosensitivity effects).
No products indexed under this heading.

Sulfamethoxazole (Possible photosensitivity effects).
No products indexed under this heading.

Sulfasalazine (Possible photosensitivity effects).
No products indexed under this heading.

Sulfinpyrazone (Possible photosensitivity effects).
No products indexed under this heading.

Sulfisoxazole Acetyl (Possible photosensitivity effects).
No products indexed under this heading.

Sulfisoxazole Diolamine (Possible photosensitivity effects).
No products indexed under this heading.

Tetracycline Hydrochloride (Possible photosensitivity effects).
No products indexed under this heading.

Thioridazine Hydrochloride (Possible photosensitivity effects). Products include:

Thioridazine Hydrochloride Tablets 2163

Tolazamide (Possible photosensitivity effects).
No products indexed under this heading.

Tolbutamide (Possible photosensitivity effects).
No products indexed under this heading.

Trifluoperazine Hydrochloride (Possible photosensitivity effects).
No products indexed under this heading.

OXSORALEN-ULTRA CAPSULES

(Methoxsalen) 3353

May interact with phenothiazines, sulfonamides, tetracyclines, thiazides, and certain other agents. Compounds in these categories include:

Anthralin (Possible photosensitivity effects). Products include:
Psoriatec Cream 1089

Bendroflumethiazide (Possible photosensitivity effects).
No products indexed under this heading.

Chlorothiazide (Possible photosensitivity effects). Products include:
Diuril Oral Suspension 1954

Chlorothiazide Sodium (Possible photosensitivity effects). Products include:
Diuril Sodium Intravenous 2467

Chlorpromazine (Possible photosensitivity effects).
No products indexed under this heading.

Chlorpromazine Hydrochloride (Possible photosensitivity effects).
No products indexed under this heading.

Chlorpropamide (Possible photosensitivity effects).
No products indexed under this heading.

Coal Tar (Possible photosensitivity effects).
No products indexed under this heading.

Demeclocycline Hydrochloride (Possible photosensitivity effects).
No products indexed under this heading.

Doxycycline Calcium (Possible photosensitivity effects).
No products indexed under this heading.

Doxycycline Hyclate (Possible photosensitivity effects).
No products indexed under this heading.

Doxycycline Monohydrate (Possible photosensitivity effects). Products include:
Oracea Capsules 1000

Fluphenazine Decanoate (Possible photosensitivity effects).
No products indexed under this heading.

Fluphenazine Enanthate (Possible photosensitivity effects).
No products indexed under this heading.

Fluphenazine Hydrochloride (Possible photosensitivity effects).
No products indexed under this heading.

Glipizide (Possible photosensitivity effects).
No products indexed under this heading.

Glyburide (Possible photosensitivity effects).
No products indexed under this heading.

Griseofulvin (Possible photosensitivity effects). Products include:
Gris-PEG Tablets 2502

Hydrochlorothiazide (Possible photosensitivity effects). Products include:
Aldoril Tablets 1910
Atacand HCT 651
Avalide Tablets 888
Avalide Tablets 2874
Benicar HCT Tablets 1044
Diovan HCT Tablets 2196
Dyazide Capsules 1423
Hyzaar 50-12.5 Tablets 1990
Hyzaar 100-12.5 Tablets 1990
Hyzaar 100-25 Tablets 1990
Lopressor HCT 50/25 Tablets 2241
Lopressor HCT 100/25 Tablets 2241
Lopressor HCT 100/50 Tablets 2241
Lotensin HCT Tablets 2246
Micardis HCT Tablets 856
Moduretic Tablets 2028
Prinzide Tablets 2056
Teveten HCT Tablets 1737
Timolide Tablets 2086
Uniretic Tablets 3100

Hydroflumethiazide (Possible photosensitivity effects).
No products indexed under this heading.

Mesoridazine Besylate (Possible photosensitivity effects).
No products indexed under this heading.

Methacycline Hydrochloride (Possible photosensitivity effects).
No products indexed under this heading.

Methotrimeprazine (Possible photosensitivity effects).
No products indexed under this heading.

Methyclothiazide (Possible photosensitivity effects).
No products indexed under this heading.

Methylene Blue (Possible photosensitivity effects). Products include:
Prosed/DS Tablets 1157

Minocycline Hydrochloride (Possible photosensitivity effects). Products include:
Solodyn Extended Release Tablets 1890

Nalidixic Acid (Possible photosensitivity effects).
No products indexed under this heading.

Oxytetracycline (Possible photosensitivity effects).
No products indexed under this heading.

Oxytetracycline Hydrochloride (Possible photosensitivity effects).
No products indexed under this heading.

Perphenazine (Possible photosensitivity effects).
No products indexed under this heading.

Polythiazide (Possible photosensitivity effects).
No products indexed under this heading.

Prochlorperazine (Possible photosensitivity effects).
No products indexed under this heading.

Promethazine Hydrochloride (Possible photosensitivity effects). Products include:
Phenergan Tablets and Suppositories 3440

Sulfacytine (Possible photosensitivity effects).
No products indexed under this heading.

Sulfamethizole (Possible photosensitivity effects).
No products indexed under this heading.

Sulfamethoxazole (Possible photosensitivity effects).
No products indexed under this heading.

Sulfasalazine (Possible photosensitivity effects).
No products indexed under this heading.

Sulfinpyrazone (Possible photosensitivity effects).
No products indexed under this heading.

Sulfisoxazole Acetyl (Possible photosensitivity effects).
No products indexed under this heading.

Sulfisoxazole Diolamine (Possible photosensitivity effects).
No products indexed under this heading.

Tetracycline Hydrochloride (Possible photosensitivity effects).
No products indexed under this heading.

Thioridazine Hydrochloride (Possible photosensitivity effects). Products include:
Thioridazine Hydrochloride Tablets 2163

Tolazamide (Possible photosensitivity effects).
No products indexed under this heading.

Tolbutamide (Possible photosensitivity effects).
No products indexed under this heading.

Trifluoperazine Hydrochloride (Possible photosensitivity effects).
No products indexed under this heading.

OXYCONTIN TABLETS

(Oxycodone Hydrochloride) 2703

May interact with central nervous system depressants, general anesthetics, hypnotics and sedatives, mixed agonist/antagonist opioid analgesics, phenothiazines, tranquilizers, and certain other agents. Compounds in these categories include:

Alfentanil Hydrochloride (Concurrent use with the usual dose of OxyContin may result in respiratory depression, profound sedation or coma; reduced dosage (1/3 to 1/2 of the usual dosage) may be necessary).
No products indexed under this heading.

Alprazolam (Concurrent use with the usual dose of OxyContin may result in respiratory depression, profound sedation or coma; reduced dosage (1/3 to 1/2 of the usual dosage) may be necessary). Products include:
Niravam Orally Disintegrating Tablets 3092

Aprobarbital (Concurrent use with the usual dose of OxyContin may result in respiratory depression, profound sedation or coma; reduced dosage (1/3 to 1/2 of the usual dosage) may be necessary).
No products indexed under this heading.

Buprenorphine Hydrochloride (Mixed agonist/antagonist analgesics may reduce the analgesic effect of oxycodone and/or may precipitate withdrawal symptoms). Products include:
Buprenex Injectable 2716
Suboxone Tablets 2717
Subutex Tablets 2717

Buspirone Hydrochloride (Concurrent use with the usual dose of OxyContin may result in respiratory depression, profound sedation or coma; reduced dosage (1/3 to 1/2 of the usual dosage) may be necessary).
No products indexed under this heading.

Butabarbital (Concurrent use with the usual dose of OxyContin may result in respiratory depression, profound sedation or coma; reduced dosage (1/3 to 1/2 of the usual dosage) may be necessary).
No products indexed under this heading.

Butalbital (Concurrent use with the usual dose of OxyContin may result in respiratory depression, profound sedation or coma; reduced dosage (1/3 to 1/2 of the usual dosage) may be necessary).
No products indexed under this heading.

Butorphanol Tartrate (Mixed agonist/antagonist analgesics may reduce the analgesic effect of oxycodone and/or may precipitate withdrawal symptoms).
No products indexed under this heading.

Chlordiazepoxide (Concurrent use with the usual dose of OxyContin may result in respiratory depression, profound sedation or coma; reduced dosage (1/3 to 1/2 of the usual dosage) may be necessary).
No products indexed under this heading.

Chlordiazepoxide Hydrochloride (Concurrent use with the usual dose of OxyContin may result in respiratory depression, profound sedation or coma; reduced dosage (1/3 to 1/2 of the usual dosage) may be necessary). Products include:
Librium Capsules 3347

Chlorpromazine (Concurrent use with the usual dose of OxyContin may result in respiratory depression, profound sedation or coma; reduced dosage (1/3 to 1/2 of the usual dosage) may be necessary).
No products indexed under this heading.

Chlorpromazine Hydrochloride (Concurrent use with the usual dose of OxyContin may result in respiratory depression, profound sedation or coma; reduced dosage (1/3 to 1/2 of the usual dosage) may be necessary).
No products indexed under this heading.

Chlorprothixene (Concurrent use with the usual dose of OxyContin may result in respiratory depression, profound sedation or coma; reduced dosage (1/3 to 1/2 of the usual dosage) may be necessary).
No products indexed under this heading.

Chlorprothixene Hydrochloride (Concurrent use with the usual dose of OxyContin may result in respiratory depression, profound sedation or coma; reduced dosage (1/3 to 1/2 of the usual dosage) may be necessary).
No products indexed under this heading.

Chlorprothixene Lactate (Concurrent use with the usual dose of OxyContin may result in respiratory depression, profound sedation or coma; reduced dosage (1/3 to 1/2 of the usual dosage) may be necessary).
No products indexed under this heading.

Clorazepate Dipotassium (Concurrent use with the usual dose of OxyContin may result in respiratory depression, profound sedation or coma; reduced dosage (1/3 to 1/2 of the usual dosage) may be necessary). Products include:
Tranxene 2474

Clozapine (Concurrent use with the usual dose of OxyContin may result in respiratory depression, profound sedation or coma; reduced dosage (1/3 to 1/2 of the usual dosage) may be necessary). Products include:
Clozaril Tablets 2184
FazaClo Orally Disintegrating Tablets 551

Codeine Phosphate (Concurrent use with the usual dose of OxyContin may result in respiratory depression, profound sedation or coma; reduced dosage (1/3 to 1/2 of the usual dosage) may be necessary). Products include:
Tylenol with Codeine Tablets 2391

Desflurane (Concurrent use with the usual dose of OxyContin may result in respiratory depression, profound sedation or coma; reduced dosage (1/3 to 1/2 of the usual dosage) may be necessary).
No products indexed under this heading.

Dezocine (Concurrent use with the usual dose of OxyContin may result in respiratory depression, profound sedation or coma; reduced dosage (1/3 to 1/2 of the usual dosage) may be necessary).
No products indexed under this heading.

Diazepam (Concurrent use with the usual dose of OxyContin may result in respiratory depression, profound sedation or coma; reduced dosage (1/3 to 1/2 of the usual dosage) may be necessary). Products include:
Diastat Rectal Delivery System 3343
Valium Tablets 2819

Droperidol (Concurrent use with the usual dose of OxyContin may result in respiratory depression, profound sedation or coma; reduced dosage (1/3 to 1/2 of the usual dosage) may be necessary).
No products indexed under this heading.

Enflurane (Concurrent use with the usual dose of OxyContin may result in respiratory depression, profound sedation or coma; reduced dosage (1/3 to 1/2 of the usual dosage) may be necessary).
No products indexed under this heading.

Estazolam (Concurrent use with the usual dose of OxyContin may result in respiratory depression, profound sedation or coma; reduced dosage (1/3 to 1/2 of the usual dosage) may be necessary). Products include:
ProSom Tablets 517

Ethanol (Concurrent use with the usual dose of OxyContin may result in respiratory depression, profound sedation or coma; reduced dosage (1/3 to 1/2 of the usual dosage) may be necessary).
No products indexed under this heading.

Ethchlorvynol (Concurrent use with the usual dose of OxyContin may result in respiratory depression, profound sedation or coma; reduced dosage (1/3 to 1/2 of the usual dosage) may be necessary).
No products indexed under this heading.

Ethinamate (Concurrent use with the usual dose of OxyContin may result in respiratory depression, profound sedation or coma; reduced dosage (1/3 to 1/2 of the usual dosage) may be necessary).
No products indexed under this heading.

Ethyl Alcohol (Concurrent use with the usual dose of OxyContin may result in respiratory depression, profound sedation or coma; reduced dosage (1/3 to 1/2 of the usual dosage) may be necessary).
No products indexed under this heading.

Fentanyl (Concurrent use with the usual dose of OxyContin may result in respiratory depression, profound sedation or coma; reduced dosage (1/3 to 1/2 of the usual dosage) may be necessary). Products include:
Duragesic Transdermal System 2373
Ionsys Transdermal System 2379

Fentanyl Citrate (Concurrent use with the usual dose of OxyContin may result in respiratory depression, profound sedation or coma; reduced dosage (1/3 to 1/2 of the usual dosage) may be necessary). Products include:
Actiq 979

Fluphenazine Decanoate (Concurrent use with the usual dose of OxyContin may result in respiratory depression, profound sedation or coma; reduced dosage (1/3 to 1/2 of the usual dosage) may be necessary).
No products indexed under this heading.

Fluphenazine Enanthate (Concurrent use with the usual dose of OxyContin may result in respiratory depression, profound sedation or coma; reduced dosage (1/3 to 1/2 of the usual dosage) may be necessary).
No products indexed under this heading.

Fluphenazine Hydrochloride (Concurrent use with the usual dose of OxyContin may result in respiratory depression, profound sedation or coma; reduced dosage (1/3 to 1/2 of the usual dosage) may be necessary).
No products indexed under this heading.

Flurazepam Hydrochloride (Concurrent use with the usual dose of OxyContin may result in respiratory depression, profound sedation or coma; reduced dosage (1/3 to 1/2 of the usual dosage) may be necessary). Products include:
Dalmane Capsules 3342

Glutethimide (Concurrent use with the usual dose of OxyContin may result in respiratory depression, profound sedation or coma; reduced dosage (1/3 to 1/2 of the usual dosage) may be necessary).
No products indexed under this heading.

Haloperidol (Concurrent use with the usual dose of OxyContin may result in respiratory depression, profound sedation or coma; reduced dosage (1/3 to 1/2 of the usual dosage) may be necessary).
No products indexed under this heading.

Haloperidol Decanoate (Concurrent use with the usual dose of OxyContin may result in respiratory depression, profound sedation or coma; reduced dosage (1/3 to 1/2 of the usual dosage) may be necessary).
No products indexed under this heading.

Hydrocodone Bitartrate (Concurrent use with the usual dose of OxyContin may result in respiratory depression, profound sedation or coma; reduced dosage (1/3 to 1/2 of the usual dosage) may be necessary). Products include:
Hycodan 1116
Hycotuss Expectorant Syrup 1117
Vicodin Tablets 535
Vicodin ES Tablets 536
Vicodin HP Tablets 538
Vicoprofen Tablets 539
Zydone Tablets 1139

Hydrocodone Polistirex (Concurrent use with the usual dose of OxyContin may result in respiratory depression, profound sedation or coma; reduced dosage (1/3 to 1/2 of the usual dosage) may be necessary). Products include:
Tussionex Pennkinetic Extended-Release Suspension 3327

Hydromorphone Hydrochloride (Concurrent use with the usual dose of OxyContin may result in respiratory depression, profound sedation or coma; reduced dosage (1/3 to 1/2 of the usual dosage) may be necessary). Products include:
Dilaudid 440
Dilaudid Non-Sterile Powder 440
Dilaudid Oral Liquid 445
Dilaudid Rectal Suppositories 440
Dilaudid Tablets 440
Dilaudid Tablets - 8 mg 445
Dilaudid-HP 442

Hydroxyzine Hydrochloride (Concurrent use with the usual dose of OxyContin may result in respiratory depression, profound sedation or coma; reduced dosage (1/3 to 1/2 of the usual dosage) may be necessary).
No products indexed under this heading.

Isoflurane (Concurrent use with the usual dose of OxyContin may result in respiratory depression, profound sedation or coma; reduced dosage (1/3 to 1/2 of the usual dosage) may be necessary).
No products indexed under this heading.

Ketamine Hydrochloride (Concurrent use with the usual dose of OxyContin may result in respiratory depression, profound sedation or coma; reduced dosage (1/3 to 1/2 of the usual dosage) may be necessary).
No products indexed under this heading.

Levomethadyl Acetate Hydrochloride (Concurrent use with the usual dose of OxyContin may result in respiratory depression, profound sedation or coma; reduced dosage (1/3 to 1/2 of the usual dosage) may be necessary).
No products indexed under this heading.

Levorphanol Tartrate (Concurrent use with the usual dose of OxyContin may result in respiratory depression, profound sedation or coma; reduced dosage (1/3 to 1/2 of the usual dosage) may be necessary).
No products indexed under this heading.

Lorazepam (Concurrent use with the usual dose of OxyContin may result in respiratory depression, profound sedation or coma; reduced dosage (1/3 to 1/2 of the usual dosage) may be necessary).
No products indexed under this heading.

Loxapine Hydrochloride (Concurrent use with the usual dose of OxyContin may result in respiratory depression, profound sedation or coma; reduced dosage (1/3 to 1/2 of the usual dosage) may be necessary).
No products indexed under this heading.

Loxapine Succinate (Concurrent use with the usual dose of OxyContin may result in respiratory depression, profound sedation or coma; reduced dosage (1/3 to 1/2 of the usual dosage) may be necessary).
No products indexed under this heading.

Meperidine Hydrochloride (Concurrent use with the usual dose of OxyContin may result in respiratory depression, profound sedation or coma; reduced dosage (1/3 to 1/2 of the usual dosage) may be necessary).
No products indexed under this heading.

Mephobarbital (Concurrent use with the usual dose of OxyContin may result in respiratory depression, profound sedation or coma; reduced dosage (1/3 to 1/2 of the usual dosage) may be necessary).
No products indexed under this heading.

Meprobamate (Concurrent use with the usual dose of OxyContin may result in respiratory depression, profound sedation or coma; reduced dosage (1/3 to 1/2 of the usual dosage) may be necessary).
No products indexed under this heading.

Mesoridazine Besylate (Concurrent use with the usual dose of OxyContin may result in respiratory depression, profound sedation or coma; reduced dosage (1/3 to 1/2 of the usual dosage) may be necessary).
No products indexed under this heading.

Methadone Hydrochloride (Concurrent use with the usual dose of OxyContin may result in respiratory depression, profound sedation or coma; reduced dosage (1/3 to 1/2 of the usual dosage) may be necessary).
　No products indexed under this heading.

Methohexital Sodium (Concurrent use with the usual dose of OxyContin may result in respiratory depression, profound sedation or coma; reduced dosage (1/3 to 1/2 of the usual dosage) may be necessary).
　No products indexed under this heading.

Methotrimeprazine (Concurrent use with the usual dose of OxyContin may result in respiratory depression, profound sedation or coma; reduced dosage (1/3 to 1/2 of the usual dosage) may be necessary).
　No products indexed under this heading.

Methoxyflurane (Concurrent use with the usual dose of OxyContin may result in respiratory depression, profound sedation or coma; reduced dosage (1/3 to 1/2 of the usual dosage) may be necessary).
　No products indexed under this heading.

Midazolam Hydrochloride (Concurrent use with the usual dose of OxyContin may result in respiratory depression, profound sedation or coma; reduced dosage (1/3 to 1/2 of the usual dosage) may be necessary).
　No products indexed under this heading.

Molindone Hydrochloride (Concurrent use with the usual dose of OxyContin may result in respiratory depression, profound sedation or coma; reduced dosage (1/3 to 1/2 of the usual dosage) may be necessary). Products include:

Morphine Sulfate (Concurrent use with the usual dose of OxyContin may result in respiratory depression, profound sedation or coma; reduced dosage (1/3 to 1/2 of the usual dosage) may be necessary). Products include:

Nalbuphine Hydrochloride (Mixed agonist/antagonist analgesics may reduce the analgesic effect of oxycodone and/or may precipitate withdrawal symptoms).
　No products indexed under this heading.

Olanzapine (Concurrent use with the usual dose of OxyContin may result in respiratory depression, profound sedation or coma; reduced dosage (1/3 to 1/2 of the usual dosage) may be necessary). Products include:

Oxazepam (Concurrent use with the usual dose of OxyContin may result in respiratory depression, profound sedation or coma; reduced dosage (1/3 to 1/2 of the usual dosage) may be necessary).
　No products indexed under this heading.

Pentazocine Hydrochloride (Mixed agonist/antagonist analgesics may reduce the analgesic effect of oxycodone and/or may precipitate withdrawal symptoms).
　No products indexed under this heading.

Pentazocine Lactate (Mixed agonist/antagonist analgesics may reduce the analgesic effect of oxycodone and/or may precipitate withdrawal symptoms).
　No products indexed under this heading.

Pentobarbital Sodium (Concurrent use with the usual dose of OxyContin may result in respiratory depression, profound sedation or coma; reduced dosage (1/3 to 1/2 of the usual dosage) may be necessary). Products include:

Perphenazine (Concurrent use with the usual dose of OxyContin may result in respiratory depression, profound sedation or coma; reduced dosage (1/3 to 1/2 of the usual dosage) may be necessary).
　No products indexed under this heading.

Phenobarbital (Concurrent use with the usual dose of OxyContin may result in respiratory depression, profound sedation or coma; reduced dosage (1/3 to 1/2 of the usual dosage) may be necessary). Products include:

Prazepam (Concurrent use with the usual dose of OxyContin may result in respiratory depression, profound sedation or coma; reduced dosage (1/3 to 1/2 of the usual dosage) may be necessary).
　No products indexed under this heading.

Prochlorperazine (Concurrent use with the usual dose of OxyContin may result in respiratory depression, profound sedation or coma; reduced dosage (1/3 to 1/2 of the usual dosage) may be necessary).
　No products indexed under this heading.

Promethazine Hydrochloride (Concurrent use with the usual dose of OxyContin may result in respiratory depression, profound sedation or coma; reduced dosage (1/3 to 1/2 of the usual dosage) may be necessary). Products include:

Propofol (Concurrent use with the usual dose of OxyContin may result in respiratory depression, profound sedation or coma; reduced dosage (1/3 to 1/2 of the usual dosage) may be necessary).
　No products indexed under this heading.

Propoxyphene Hydrochloride (Concurrent use with the usual dose of OxyContin may result in respiratory depression, profound sedation or coma; reduced dosage (1/3 to 1/2 of the usual dosage) may be necessary).
　No products indexed under this heading.

Propoxyphene Napsylate (Concurrent use with the usual dose of OxyContin may result in respiratory depression, profound sedation or coma; reduced dosage (1/3 to 1/2 of the usual dosage) may be necessary).
　No products indexed under this heading.

Quazepam (Concurrent use with the usual dose of OxyContin may result in respiratory depression, profound sedation or coma; reduced dosage (1/3 to 1/2 of the usual dosage) may be necessary).
　No products indexed under this heading.

Quetiapine Fumarate (Concurrent use with the usual dose of OxyContin may result in respiratory depression, profound sedation or coma; reduced dosage (1/3 to 1/2 of the usual dosage) may be necessary). Products include:

Ramelteon (Concurrent use with the usual dose of OxyContin may result in respiratory depression, profound sedation or coma; reduced dosage (1/3 to 1/2 of the usual dosage) may be necessary). Products include:

Remifentanil Hydrochloride (Concurrent use with the usual dose of OxyContin may result in respiratory depression, profound sedation or coma; reduced dosage (1/3 to 1/2 of the usual dosage) may be necessary).
　No products indexed under this heading.

Risperidone (Concurrent use with the usual dose of OxyContin may result in respiratory depression, profound sedation or coma; reduced dosage (1/3 to 1/2 of the usual dosage) may be necessary). Products include:

Secobarbital Sodium (Concurrent use with the usual dose of OxyContin may result in respiratory depression, profound sedation or coma; reduced dosage (1/3 to 1/2 of the usual dosage) may be necessary).
　No products indexed under this heading.

Sevoflurane (Concurrent use with the usual dose of OxyContin may result in respiratory depression, profound sedation or coma; reduced dosage (1/3 to 1/2 of the usual dosage) may be necessary). Products include:

Sufentanil Citrate (Concurrent use with the usual dose of OxyContin may result in respiratory depression, profound sedation or coma; reduced dosage (1/3 to 1/2 of the usual dosage) may be necessary).
　No products indexed under this heading.

Temazepam (Concurrent use with the usual dose of OxyContin may result in respiratory depression, profound sedation or coma; reduced dosage (1/3 to 1/2 of the usual dosage) may be necessary). Products include:

Thiamylal Sodium (Concurrent use with the usual dose of OxyContin may result in respiratory depression, profound sedation or coma; reduced dosage (1/3 to 1/2 of the usual dosage) may be necessary).
　No products indexed under this heading.

Thioridazine Hydrochloride (Concurrent use with the usual dose of OxyContin may result in respiratory depression, profound sedation or coma; reduced dosage (1/3 to 1/2 of the usual dosage) may be necessary). Products include:

Thiothixene (Concurrent use with the usual dose of OxyContin may result in respiratory depression, profound sedation or coma; reduced dosage (1/3 to 1/2 of the usual dosage) may be necessary). Products include:

Triazolam (Concurrent use with the usual dose of OxyContin may result in respiratory depression, profound sedation or coma; reduced dosage (1/3 to 1/2 of the usual dosage) may be necessary).
　No products indexed under this heading.

Trifluoperazine Hydrochloride (Concurrent use with the usual dose of OxyContin may result in respiratory depression, profound sedation or coma; reduced dosage (1/3 to 1/2 of the usual dosage) may be necessary).
　No products indexed under this heading.

Zaleplon (Concurrent use with the usual dose of OxyContin may result in respiratory depression, profound sedation or coma; reduced dosage (1/3 to 1/2 of the usual dosage) may be necessary). Products include:

Ziprasidone Hydrochloride (Concurrent use with the usual dose of OxyContin may result in respiratory depression, profound sedation or coma; reduced dosage (1/3 to 1/2 of the usual dosage) may be necessary). Products include:

Zolpidem Tartrate (Concurrent use with the usual dose of OxyContin may result in respiratory depression, profound sedation or coma; reduced dosage (1/3 to 1/2 of the usual dosage) may be necessary). Products include:

Food Interactions

Alcohol (Concurrent use with the usual dose of OxyContin may result in respiratory depression, profound sedation or coma).

OXYFAST ORAL CONCENTRATE SOLUTION

See OxyIR Capsules

OXYIR CAPSULES

(Oxycodone Hydrochloride) 2708

May interact with central nervous system depressants, general anesthetics, hypnotics and sedatives, mixed agonist/antagonist opioid analgesics, narcotic analgesics, phenothiazines, tranquilizers, and certain other agents. Compounds in these categories include:

Alfentanil Hydrochloride (Concomitant use may exhibit an additive CNS depression).
No products indexed under this heading.

Alprazolam (Concomitant use may exhibit an additive CNS depression). Products include:
Niravam Orally Disintegrating Tablets 3092

Aprobarbital (Concomitant use may exhibit an additive CNS depression).
No products indexed under this heading.

Buprenorphine Hydrochloride (Co-administration with mixed agonist/antagonist analgesics may reduce the analgesic effect of oxycodone and/or may precipitate withdrawal symptoms). Products include:
Buprenex Injectable 2716
Suboxone Tablets 2717
Subutex Tablets 2717

Buspirone Hydrochloride (Concomitant use may exhibit an additive CNS depression).
No products indexed under this heading.

Butabarbital (Concomitant use may exhibit an additive CNS depression).
No products indexed under this heading.

Butalbital (Concomitant use may exhibit an additive CNS depression).
No products indexed under this heading.

Butorphanol Tartrate (Co-administration with mixed agonist/antagonist analgesics may reduce the analgesic effect of oxycodone and/or may precipitate withdrawal symptoms).
No products indexed under this heading.

Chlordiazepoxide (Concomitant use may exhibit an additive CNS depression).
No products indexed under this heading.

Chlordiazepoxide Hydrochloride (Concomitant use may exhibit an additive CNS depression). Products include:
Librium Capsules 3347

Chlorpromazine (Concomitant use may exhibit an additive CNS depression).
No products indexed under this heading.

Chlorpromazine Hydrochloride (Concomitant use may exhibit an additive CNS depression).
No products indexed under this heading.

Chlorprothixene (Concomitant use may exhibit an additive CNS depression).
No products indexed under this heading.

Chlorprothixene Hydrochloride (Concomitant use may exhibit an additive CNS depression).
No products indexed under this heading.

Chlorprothixene Lactate (Concomitant use may exhibit an additive CNS depression).
No products indexed under this heading.

Clorazepate Dipotassium (Concomitant use may exhibit an additive CNS depression). Products include:
Tranxene 2474

Clozapine (Concomitant use may exhibit an additive CNS depression). Products include:
Clozaril Tablets 2184
FazaClo Orally Disintegrating Tablets 551

Codeine Phosphate (Concomitant use may exhibit an additive CNS depression). Products include:
Tylenol with Codeine Tablets 2391

Desflurane (Concomitant use may exhibit an additive CNS depression).
No products indexed under this heading.

Dezocine (Concomitant use may exhibit an additive CNS depression).
No products indexed under this heading.

Diazepam (Concomitant use may exhibit an additive CNS depression). Products include:
Diastat Rectal Delivery System 3343
Valium Tablets 2819

Droperidol (Concomitant use may exhibit an additive CNS depression).
No products indexed under this heading.

Enflurane (Concomitant use may exhibit an additive CNS depression).
No products indexed under this heading.

Estazolam (Concomitant use may exhibit an additive CNS depression). Products include:
ProSom Tablets 517

Ethanol (Concomitant use may exhibit an additive CNS depression).
No products indexed under this heading.

Ethchlorvynol (Concomitant use may exhibit an additive CNS depression).
No products indexed under this heading.

Ethinamate (Concomitant use may exhibit an additive CNS depression).
No products indexed under this heading.

Ethyl Alcohol (Concomitant use may exhibit an additive CNS depression).
No products indexed under this heading.

Fentanyl (Concomitant use may exhibit an additive CNS depression). Products include:
Duragesic Transdermal System 2373
Ionsys Transdermal System 2379

Fentanyl Citrate (Concomitant use may exhibit an additive CNS depression). Products include:
Actiq 979

Fluphenazine Decanoate (Concomitant use may exhibit an additive CNS depression).
No products indexed under this heading.

Fluphenazine Enanthate (Concomitant use may exhibit an additive CNS depression).
No products indexed under this heading.

Fluphenazine Hydrochloride (Concomitant use may exhibit an additive CNS depression).
No products indexed under this heading.

Flurazepam Hydrochloride (Concomitant use may exhibit an additive CNS depression). Products include:
Dalmane Capsules 3342

Glutethimide (Concomitant use may exhibit an additive CNS depression).
No products indexed under this heading.

Haloperidol (Concomitant use may exhibit an additive CNS depression).
No products indexed under this heading.

Haloperidol Decanoate (Concomitant use may exhibit an additive CNS depression).
No products indexed under this heading.

Hydrocodone Bitartrate (Concomitant use may exhibit an additive CNS depression). Products include:
Hycodan 1116
Hycotuss Expectorant Syrup 1117
Vicodin Tablets 535
Vicodin ES Tablets 536
Vicodin HP Tablets 538
Vicoprofen Tablets 539
Zydone Tablets 1139

Hydrocodone Polistirex (Concomitant use may exhibit an additive CNS depression). Products include:
Tussionex Pennkinetic Extended-Release Suspension 3327

Hydromorphone Hydrochloride (Concomitant use may exhibit an additive CNS depression). Products include:
Dilaudid 440
Dilaudid Non-Sterile Powder 440
Dilaudid Oral Liquid 445
Dilaudid Rectal Suppositories 440
Dilaudid Tablets 440
Dilaudid Tablets - 8 mg 445
Dilaudid-HP 442

Hydroxyzine Hydrochloride (Concomitant use may exhibit an additive CNS depression).
No products indexed under this heading.

Isoflurane (Concomitant use may exhibit an additive CNS depression).
No products indexed under this heading.

Ketamine Hydrochloride (Concomitant use may exhibit an additive CNS depression).
No products indexed under this heading.

Levomethadyl Acetate Hydrochloride (Concomitant use may exhibit an additive CNS depression).
No products indexed under this heading.

Levorphanol Tartrate (Concomitant use may exhibit an additive CNS depression).
No products indexed under this heading.

Lorazepam (Concomitant use may exhibit an additive CNS depression).
No products indexed under this heading.

Loxapine Hydrochloride (Concomitant use may exhibit an additive CNS depression).
No products indexed under this heading.

Loxapine Succinate (Concomitant use may exhibit an additive CNS depression).
No products indexed under this heading.

Meperidine Hydrochloride (Concomitant use may exhibit an additive CNS depression).
No products indexed under this heading.

Mephobarbital (Concomitant use may exhibit an additive CNS depression).
No products indexed under this heading.

Meprobamate (Concomitant use may exhibit an additive CNS depression).
No products indexed under this heading.

Mesoridazine Besylate (Concomitant use may exhibit an additive CNS depression).
No products indexed under this heading.

Methadone Hydrochloride (Concomitant use may exhibit an additive CNS depression).
No products indexed under this heading.

Methohexital Sodium (Concomitant use may exhibit an additive CNS depression).
No products indexed under this heading.

Methotrimeprazine (Concomitant use may exhibit an additive CNS depression).
No products indexed under this heading.

Methoxyflurane (Concomitant use may exhibit an additive CNS depression).
No products indexed under this heading.

Midazolam Hydrochloride (Concomitant use may exhibit an additive CNS depression).
No products indexed under this heading.

Molindone Hydrochloride (Concomitant use may exhibit an additive CNS depression). Products include:
Moban Tablets 1119

Morphine Sulfate (Concomitant use may exhibit an additive CNS depression). Products include:
Avinza Capsules 1741
Kadian Capsules 577
MS Contin Tablets 2701

Nalbuphine Hydrochloride (Co-administration with mixed agonist/antagonist analgesics may reduce the analgesic effect of oxycodone and/or may precipitate withdrawal symptoms).
No products indexed under this heading.

Olanzapine (Concomitant use may exhibit an additive CNS depression). Products include:
Symbyax Capsules 1819
Zyprexa Tablets 1830
Zyprexa IntraMuscular 1830
Zyprexa ZYDIS Orally Disintegrating Tablets 1830

Oxazepam (Concomitant use may exhibit an additive CNS depression).
No products indexed under this heading.

Pentazocine Hydrochloride (Co-administration with mixed agonist/antagonist analgesics may reduce the analgesic effect of oxycodone and/or may precipitate withdrawal symptoms).
No products indexed under this heading.

Pentazocine Lactate (Co-administration with mixed agonist/antagonist analgesics may reduce the analgesic effect of oxycodone and/or may precipitate withdrawal symptoms).
No products indexed under this heading.

Pentobarbital Sodium (Concomitant use may exhibit an additive CNS depression). Products include:
Nembutal Sodium Solution, USP 2470

Perphenazine (Concomitant use may exhibit an additive CNS depression).
No products indexed under this heading.

Phenobarbital (Concomitant use may exhibit an additive CNS depression). Products include:
Donnatal Extentabs 2493

Prazepam (Concomitant use may exhibit an additive CNS depression).
No products indexed under this heading.

Prochlorperazine (Concomitant use may exhibit an additive CNS depression).
No products indexed under this heading.

Promethazine Hydrochloride (Concomitant use may exhibit an additive CNS depression). Products include:
Phenergan Tablets and Suppositories......................... 3440

Propofol (Concomitant use may exhibit an additive CNS depression).
No products indexed under this heading.

Propoxyphene Hydrochloride (Concomitant use may exhibit an additive CNS depression).
No products indexed under this heading.

Propoxyphene Napsylate (Concomitant use may exhibit an additive CNS depression).
No products indexed under this heading.

Quazepam (Concomitant use may exhibit an additive CNS depression).
No products indexed under this heading.

Quetiapine Fumarate (Concomitant use may exhibit an additive CNS depression). Products include:
Seroquel Tablets 690

Ramelteon (Concomitant use may exhibit an additive CNS depression). Products include:
Rozerem Tablets 3231

Remifentanil Hydrochloride (Concomitant use may exhibit an additive CNS depression).
No products indexed under this heading.

Risperidone (Concomitant use may exhibit an additive CNS depression). Products include:
Risperdal 1676
Risperdal Consta Long-Acting Injection 1682
Risperdal M-Tab Orally Disintegrating Tablets.................. 1676

Secobarbital Sodium (Concomitant use may exhibit an additive CNS depression).
No products indexed under this heading.

Sevoflurane (Concomitant use may exhibit an additive CNS depression). Products include:
Ultane Liquid for Inhalation 531

Sufentanil Citrate (Concomitant use may exhibit an additive CNS depression).
No products indexed under this heading.

Temazepam (Concomitant use may exhibit an additive CNS depression). Products include:
Restoril Capsules 1860

Thiamylal Sodium (Concomitant use may exhibit an additive CNS depression).
No products indexed under this heading.

Thioridazine Hydrochloride (Concomitant use may exhibit an additive CNS depression). Products include:
Thioridazine Hydrochloride Tablets 2163

Thiothixene (Concomitant use may exhibit an additive CNS depression). Products include:
Thiothixene Capsules 2165

Triazolam (Concomitant use may exhibit an additive CNS depression).
No products indexed under this heading.

Trifluoperazine Hydrochloride (Concomitant use may exhibit an additive CNS depression).
No products indexed under this heading.

Zaleplon (Concomitant use may exhibit an additive CNS depression). Products include:
Sonata Capsules 1717

Ziprasidone Hydrochloride (Concomitant use may exhibit an additive CNS depression). Products include:
Geodon Capsules 2529

Zolpidem Tartrate (Concomitant use may exhibit an additive CNS depression). Products include:
Ambien Tablets 2851
Ambien CR Tablets 2855

Food Interactions

Alcohol (Concomitant use may exhibit an additive CNS depression).

OXYTROL TRANSDERMAL SYSTEM

(Oxybutynin) 3392
May interact with anticholinergics, bisphosphonates, and certain other agents. Compounds in these categories include:

Alendronate Sodium (Concurrent use with drugs that can cause or exacerbate esophagitis, such as biphosphonates, should be undertaken with caution). Products include:
Fosamax ... 1969
Fosamax Plus D Tablets 1977

Atropine Sulfate (Co-administration of oxybutynin with other anticholinergic drugs may increase the frequency and/or severity of anticholinergic side effects such as dry mouth, constipation, drowsiness and others). Products include:
Donnatal Extentabs 2493

Belladonna Alkaloids (Co-administration of oxybutynin with other anticholinergic drugs may increase the frequency and/or severity of anticholinergic side effects such as dry mouth, constipation, drowsiness and others). Products include:
Hyland's Teething Tablets ▣830

Benztropine Mesylate (Co-administration of oxybutynin with other anticholinergic drugs may increase the frequency and/or severity of anticholinergic side effects such as dry mouth, constipation, drowsiness and others).
No products indexed under this heading.

Biperiden Hydrochloride (Co-administration of oxybutynin with other anticholinergic drugs may increase the frequency and/or severity of anticholinergic side effects such as dry mouth, constipation, drowsiness and others).
No products indexed under this heading.

Clidinium Bromide (Co-administration of oxybutynin with other anticholinergic drugs may increase the frequency and/or severity of anticholinergic side effects such as dry mouth, constipation, drowsiness and others).
No products indexed under this heading.

Dicyclomine Hydrochloride (Co-administration of oxybutynin with other anticholinergic drugs may increase the frequency and/or severity of anticholinergic side effects such as dry mouth, constipation, drowsiness and others). Products include:
Bentyl Capsules 697
Bentyl Injection 697
Bentyl Syrup 697
Bentyl Tablets 697

Etidronate Disodium (Concurrent use with drugs that can cause or exacerbate esophagitis, such as biphosphonates, should be undertaken with caution). Products include:
Didronel Tablets 2697

Glycopyrrolate (Co-administration of oxybutynin with other anticholinergic drugs may increase the frequency and/or severity of anticholinergic side effects such as dry mouth, constipation, drowsiness and others).
No products indexed under this heading.

Hyoscyamine (Co-administration of oxybutynin with other anticholinergic drugs may increase the frequency and/or severity of anticholinergic side effects such as dry mouth, constipation, drowsiness and others).
No products indexed under this heading.

Hyoscyamine Sulfate (Co-administration of oxybutynin with other anticholinergic drugs may increase the frequency and/or severity of anticholinergic side effects such as dry mouth, constipation, drowsiness and others). Products include:
Donnatal Extentabs 2493
Prosed/DS Tablets 1157

Ipratropium Bromide (Co-administration of oxybutynin with other anticholinergic drugs may increase the frequency and/or severity of anticholinergic side effects such as dry mouth, constipation, drowsiness and others). Products include:
Atrovent Inhalation Solution 835
Atrovent HFA Inhalation Aerosol 841
Atrovent Nasal Spray 0.03% 837
Atrovent Nasal Spray 0.06% 839
Combivent Inhalation Aerosol 847
DuoNeb Inhalation Solution 1058

Mepenzolate Bromide (Co-administration of oxybutynin with other anticholinergic drugs may increase the frequency and/or severity of anticholinergic side effects such as dry mouth, constipation, drowsiness and others).
No products indexed under this heading.

Procyclidine Hydrochloride (Co-administration of oxybutynin with other anticholinergic drugs may increase the frequency and/or severity of anticholinergic side effects such as dry mouth, constipation, drowsiness and others).
No products indexed under this heading.

Propantheline Bromide (Co-administration of oxybutynin with other anticholinergic drugs may increase the frequency and/or severity of anticholinergic side effects such as dry mouth, constipation, drowsiness and others).
No products indexed under this heading.

Risedronate Sodium (Concurrent use with drugs that can cause or exacerbate esophagitis, such as biphosphonates, should be undertaken with caution). Products include:
Actonel Tablets 2683
Actonel with Calcium Tablets 2688

Scopolamine (Co-administration of oxybutynin with other anticholinergic drugs may increase the frequency and/or severity of anticholinergic side effects such as dry mouth, constipation, drowsiness and others). Products include:
Transderm Scōp Transdermal Therapeutic System 2177

Scopolamine Hydrobromide (Co-administration of oxybutynin with other anticholinergic drugs may increase the frequency and/or severity of anticholinergic side effects such as dry mouth, constipation, drowsiness and others). Products include:
Donnatal Extentabs 2493

Tiludronate Disodium (Concurrent use with drugs that can cause or exacerbate esophagitis, such as biphosphonates, should be undertaken with caution).
No products indexed under this heading.

Tolterodine Tartrate (Co-administration of oxybutynin with other anticholinergic drugs may increase the frequency and/or severity of anticholinergic side effects such as dry mouth, constipation, drowsiness and others). Products include:
Detrol Tablets 2628
Detrol LA Capsules 2631

Tridihexethyl Chloride (Co-administration of oxybutynin with other anticholinergic drugs may increase the frequency and/or severity of anticholinergic side effects such as dry mouth, constipation, drowsiness and others).
No products indexed under this heading.

Trihexyphenidyl Hydrochloride (Co-administration of oxybutynin with other anticholinergic drugs may increase the frequency and/or severity of anticholinergic side effects such as dry mouth, constipation, drowsiness and others).
No products indexed under this heading.

Food Interactions

Alcohol (May enhance drowsiness caused by anticholinergic agents such as oxybutynin).

(▣ Described in PDR For Nonprescription Drugs)

(☉ Described in PDR For Ophthalmic Medicines™)

PADDOCK NYSTATIN USP FOR ORAL SUSPENSION
(Nystatin) 2478
None cited in PDR database.

PANAFIL OINTMENT
(Chlorophyllin Copper Complex Sodium, Papain, Urea) 1663
May interact with:

Heavy metal salts, unspecified (Papain may be inactivated by the salts of heavy metals).
No products indexed under this heading.

Hydrogen Peroxide (May inactivate papain).
No products indexed under this heading.

PANAFIL SE SPRAY EMULSION
(Chlorophyllin Copper Complex Sodium, Papain, Urea) 1663
See Panafil Ointment

PANCREASE MT CAPSULES
(Pancrelipase) 1885
None cited in PDR database.

PANHEMATIN FOR INJECTION
(Hemin) 2473
May interact with barbiturates, oral anticoagulants, and estrogens. Compounds in these categories include:

Anisindione (Hemin exhibits transient, mild anticoagulant effects, therefore, concurrent anticoagulant therapy should be avoided). Products include:
Miradon Tablets 3042

Aprobarbital (Hemin inhibits the enzyme delta-aminolevulinic acid synthetase; concurrent use with drugs that increase the activity of delta-aminolevulinic acid synthetase, such as barbiturates, should be avoided).
No products indexed under this heading.

Butabarbital (Hemin inhibits the enzyme delta-aminolevulinic acid synthetase; concurrent use with drugs that increase the activity of delta-aminolevulinic acid synthetase, such as barbiturates, should be avoided).
No products indexed under this heading.

Butalbital (Hemin inhibits the enzyme delta-aminolevulinic acid synthetase; concurrent use with drugs that increase the activity of delta-aminolevulinic acid synthetase, such as barbiturates, should be avoided).
No products indexed under this heading.

Chlorotrianisene (Hemin inhibits the enzyme delta-aminolevulinic acid synthetase; concurrent use with drugs that increase the activity of delta-aminolevulinic acid synthetase, such as estrogens, should be avoided).
No products indexed under this heading.

Dicumarol (Hemin exhibits transient, mild anticoagulant effects, therefore, concurrent anticoagulant therapy should be avoided).
No products indexed under this heading.

Dienestrol (Hemin inhibits the enzyme delta-aminolevulinic acid synthetase; concurrent use with drugs that increase the activity of delta-aminolevulinic acid synthetase, such as estrogens, should be avoided).
No products indexed under this heading.

Diethylstilbestrol (Hemin inhibits the enzyme delta-aminolevulinic acid synthetase; concurrent use with drugs that increase the activity of delta-aminolevulinic acid synthetase, such as estrogens, should be avoided).
No products indexed under this heading.

Estradiol (Hemin inhibits the enzyme delta-aminolevulinic acid synthetase; concurrent use with drugs that increase the activity of delta-aminolevulinic acid synthetase, such as estrogens, should be avoided). Products include:
Angeliq Tablets 762
Climara Transdermal System 771
Climara Pro Transdermal System 776
Estrasorb Topical Emulsion 1147
Estring Vaginal Ring 2635
Menostar Transdermal System 782
Vagifem Tablets 2334

Estrogens, Conjugated (Hemin inhibits the enzyme delta-aminolevulinic acid synthetase; concurrent use with drugs that increase the activity of delta-aminolevulinic acid synthetase, such as estrogens, should be avoided). Products include:
Premarin Intravenous 3442
Premarin Tablets 3446
Premarin Vaginal Cream 3452
Premphase Tablets 3456
Prempro Tablets 3456

Estrogens, Esterified (Hemin inhibits the enzyme delta-aminolevulinic acid synthetase; concurrent use with drugs that increase the activity of delta-aminolevulinic acid synthetase, such as estrogens, should be avoided). Products include:
Estratest Tablets 3199
Estratest H.S. Tablets 3199

Estropipate (Hemin inhibits the enzyme delta-aminolevulinic acid synthetase; concurrent use with drugs that increase the activity of delta-aminolevulinic acid synthetase, such as estrogens, should be avoided).
No products indexed under this heading.

Ethinyl Estradiol (Hemin inhibits the enzyme delta-aminolevulinic acid synthetase; concurrent use with drugs that increase the activity of delta-aminolevulinic acid synthetase, such as estrogens, should be avoided). Products include:
Mircette Tablets 1066
NuvaRing 2340
Ortho-Cyclen/Ortho Tri-Cyclen 2429
Ortho Evra Transdermal System 2417
Ortho Tri-Cyclen Lo Tablets 2436
Seasonique Tablets 1077
Yasmin 28 Tablets 796
Yaz Tablets 803

Mephobarbital (Hemin inhibits the enzyme delta-aminolevulinic acid synthetase; concurrent use with drugs that increase the activity of delta-aminolevulinic acid synthetase, such as barbiturates, should be avoided).
No products indexed under this heading.

Pentobarbital Sodium (Hemin inhibits the enzyme delta-aminolevulinic acid synthetase; concurrent use with drugs that increase the activity of delta-aminolevulinic acid synthetase, such as barbiturates, should be avoided). Products include:
Nembutal Sodium Solution, USP 2470

Phenobarbital (Hemin inhibits the enzyme delta-aminolevulinic acid synthetase; concurrent use with drugs that increase the activity of delta-aminolevulinic acid synthetase, such as barbiturates, should be avoided). Products include:
Donnatal Extentabs 2493

Polyestradiol Phosphate (Hemin inhibits the enzyme delta-aminolevulinic acid synthetase; concurrent use with drugs that increase the activity of delta-aminolevulinic acid synthetase, such as estrogens, should be avoided).
No products indexed under this heading.

Quinestrol (Hemin inhibits the enzyme delta-aminolevulinic acid synthetase; concurrent use with drugs that increase the activity of delta-aminolevulinic acid synthetase, such as estrogens, should be avoided).
No products indexed under this heading.

Secobarbital Sodium (Hemin inhibits the enzyme delta-aminolevulinic acid synthetase; concurrent use with drugs that increase the activity of delta-aminolevulinic acid synthetase, such as barbiturates, should be avoided).
No products indexed under this heading.

Thiamylal Sodium (Hemin inhibits the enzyme delta-aminolevulinic acid synthetase; concurrent use with drugs that increase the activity of delta-aminolevulinic acid synthetase, such as barbiturates, should be avoided).
No products indexed under this heading.

Warfarin Sodium (Hemin exhibits transient, mild anticoagulant effects, therefore, concurrent anticoagulant therapy should be avoided). Products include:
Coumadin for Injection 898
Coumadin Tablets 898

PANRETIN GEL
(Alitretinoin) 1747
May interact with:

DEET (N,N-diethyl-m-toluamide) (Avoid DEET (N,N-diethyl-m-toluamide) containing products (e.g., insect repellent). Alitretinoin may increase DEET toxicity).
No products indexed under this heading.

PARAGARD T 380A INTRAUTERINE COPPER CONTRACEPTIVE
(Copper, Intrauterine) 1073
None cited in PDR database.

PARCOPA ORALLY DISINTEGRATING TABLETS
(Carbidopa, Levodopa) 3097
May interact with antihypertensives, dopamine D2 antagonists, iron salts, nonselective MAO inhibitors, phenytoin, tricyclic antidepressants, and certain other agents. Compounds in these categories include:

Acebutolol Hydrochloride (Symptomatic postural hypotension has occurred with concomitant use; therefore, when therapy with carbidopa/levodopa is started, dosage adjustment of the antihypertensive drug may be required).
No products indexed under this heading.

Amitriptyline Hydrochloride (There have been rare reports of adverse reactions, including hypertension and dyskinesia, resulting from the concomitant use of tricyclic antidepressants and carbidopa/levodopa).
No products indexed under this heading.

Amlodipine Besylate (Symptomatic postural hypotension has occurred with concomitant use; therefore, when therapy with carbidopa/levodopa is started, dosage adjustment of the antihypertensive drug may be required). Products include:
Caduet Tablets 2508
Lotrel Capsules 2249
Norvasc Tablets 2545

Amoxapine (There have been rare reports of adverse reactions, including hypertension and dyskinesia, resulting from the concomitant use of tricyclic antidepressants and carbidopa/levodopa).
No products indexed under this heading.

Atenolol (Symptomatic postural hypotension has occurred with concomitant use; therefore, when therapy with carbidopa/levodopa is started, dosage adjustment of the antihypertensive drug may be required).
No products indexed under this heading.

Benazepril Hydrochloride (Symptomatic postural hypotension has occurred with concomitant use; therefore, when therapy with carbidopa/levodopa is started, dosage adjustment of the antihypertensive drug may be required). Products include:
Lotensin Tablets 2243
Lotensin HCT Tablets 2246
Lotrel Capsules 2249

Bendroflumethiazide (Symptomatic postural hypotension has occurred with concomitant use; therefore, when therapy with carbidopa/levodopa is started, dosage adjustment of the antihypertensive drug may be required).
No products indexed under this heading.

Betaxolol Hydrochloride (Symptomatic postural hypotension has occurred with concomitant use; therefore, when therapy with carbidopa/levodopa is started, dosage adjustment of the antihypertensive drug may be required). Products include:
Betoptic S Ophthalmic Suspension 558

Bisoprolol Fumarate (Symptomatic postural hypotension has occurred with concomitant use; therefore, when therapy with carbidopa/levodopa is started, dosage adjustment of the antihypertensive drug may be required).
No products indexed under this heading.

Candesartan Cilexetil (Symptomatic postural hypotension has occurred with concomitant use; therefore, when therapy with carbidopa/levodopa is started, dosage adjustment of the antihypertensive drug may be required). Products include:
Atacand Tablets 649
Atacand HCT 651

Captopril (Symptomatic postural hypotension has occurred with concomitant use; therefore, when therapy with carbidopa/levodopa is started, dosage adjustment of the antihypertensive drug may be required). Products include:
Captopril Tablets 2149

Carteolol Hydrochloride (Symptomatic postural hypotension has occurred with concomitant use; therefore, when therapy with carbidopa/levodopa is started, dosage adjustment of the antihypertensive drug may be required). Products include:
Carteolol Hydrochloride Ophthalmic Solution USP, 1%.......⊙249

Chlorothiazide (Symptomatic postural hypotension has occurred with concomitant use; therefore, when therapy with carbidopa/levodopa is started, dosage adjustment of the antihypertensive drug may be required). Products include:
Diuril Oral Suspension 1954

Chlorothiazide Sodium (Symptomatic postural hypotension has occurred with concomitant use; therefore, when therapy with carbidopa/levodopa is started, dosage adjustment of the antihypertensive drug may be required). Products include:
Diuril Sodium Intravenous 2467

Chlorpromazine (Dopamine D2 receptor antagonists may reduce the therapeutic effects of levodopa).
No products indexed under this heading.

Chlorpromazine Hydrochloride (Dopamine D2 receptor antagonists may reduce the therapeutic effects of levodopa).
No products indexed under this heading.

Chlorprothixene (Dopamine D2 receptor antagonists may reduce the therapeutic effects of levodopa).
No products indexed under this heading.

Chlorprothixene Hydrochloride (Dopamine D2 receptor antagonists may reduce the therapeutic effects of levodopa).
No products indexed under this heading.

Chlorthalidone (Symptomatic postural hypotension has occurred with concomitant use; therefore, when therapy with carbidopa/levodopa is started, dosage adjustment of the antihypertensive drug may be required). Products include:
Clorpres Tablets 2153

Clomipramine Hydrochloride (There have been rare reports of adverse reactions, including hypertension and dyskinesia, resulting from the concomitant use of tricyclic antidepressants and carbidopa/levodopa).
No products indexed under this heading.

Clonidine (Symptomatic postural hypotension has occurred with concomitant use; therefore, when therapy with carbidopa/levodopa is started, dosage adjustment of the antihypertensive drug may be required). Products include:
Catapres-TTS 844

Clonidine Hydrochloride (Symptomatic postural hypotension has occurred with concomitant use; therefore, when therapy with carbidopa/levodopa is started, dosage adjustment of the antihypertensive drug may be required). Products include:
Catapres Tablets 843
Clorpres Tablets 2153

Deserpidine (Symptomatic postural hypotension has occurred with concomitant use; therefore, when therapy with carbidopa/levodopa is started, dosage adjustment of the antihypertensive drug may be required).
No products indexed under this heading.

Desipramine Hydrochloride (There have been rare reports of adverse reactions, including hypertension and dyskinesia, resulting from the concomitant use of tricyclic antidepressants and carbidopa/levodopa).
No products indexed under this heading.

Diazoxide (Symptomatic postural hypotension has occurred with concomitant use; therefore, when therapy with carbidopa/levodopa is started, dosage adjustment of the antihypertensive drug may be required). Products include:
Hyperstat I.V. 3017

Diltiazem Hydrochloride (Symptomatic postural hypotension has occurred with concomitant use; therefore, when therapy with carbidopa/levodopa is started, dosage adjustment of the antihypertensive drug may be required). Products include:
Cardizem LA Extended Release Tablets 1728
Tiazac Capsules 1201

Doxazosin Mesylate (Symptomatic postural hypotension has occurred with concomitant use; therefore, when therapy with carbidopa/levodopa is started, dosage adjustment of the antihypertensive drug may be required). Products include:
Cardura XL Tablets 2515

Doxepin Hydrochloride (There have been rare reports of adverse reactions, including hypertension and dyskinesia, resulting from the concomitant use of tricyclic antidepressants and carbidopa/levodopa).
No products indexed under this heading.

Enalapril Maleate (Symptomatic postural hypotension has occurred with concomitant use; therefore, when therapy with carbidopa/levodopa is started, dosage adjustment of the antihypertensive drug may be required). Products include:
Vasotec I.V. Injection 2103

Enalaprilat (Symptomatic postural hypotension has occurred with concomitant use; therefore, when therapy with carbidopa/levodopa is started, dosage adjustment of the antihypertensive drug may be required).
No products indexed under this heading.

Eprosartan Mesylate (Symptomatic postural hypotension has occurred with concomitant use; therefore, when therapy with carbidopa/levodopa is started, dosage adjustment of the antihypertensive drug may be required). Products include:
Teveten Tablets 1735
Teveten HCT Tablets 1737

Esmolol Hydrochloride (Symptomatic postural hypotension has occurred with concomitant use; therefore, when therapy with carbidopa/levodopa is started, dosage adjustment of the antihypertensive drug may be required).
No products indexed under this heading.

Felodipine (Symptomatic postural hypotension has occurred with concomitant use; therefore, when therapy with carbidopa/levodopa is started, dosage adjustment of the antihypertensive drug may be required).
No products indexed under this heading.

Ferrous Fumarate (Iron salts may reduce the bioavailability of levodopa and carbidopa. The clinical relevance is unclear).
No products indexed under this heading.

Ferrous Gluconate (Iron salts may reduce the bioavailability of levodopa and carbidopa. The clinical relevance is unclear).
No products indexed under this heading.

Ferrous Sulfate (Iron salts may reduce the bioavailability of levodopa and carbidopa. The clinical relevance is unclear). Products include:
Slow Fe Iron Tablets .... ■818
Slow Fe with Folic Acid Tablets .... ■819

Fluphenazine Decanoate (Dopamine D2 receptor antagonists may reduce the therapeutic effects of levodopa).
No products indexed under this heading.

Fluphenazine Enanthate (Dopamine D2 receptor antagonists may reduce the therapeutic effects of levodopa).
No products indexed under this heading.

Fluphenazine Hydrochloride (Dopamine D2 receptor antagonists may reduce the therapeutic effects of levodopa).
No products indexed under this heading.

Fosinopril Sodium (Symptomatic postural hypotension has occurred with concomitant use; therefore, when therapy with carbidopa/levodopa is started, dosage adjustment of the antihypertensive drug may be required).
No products indexed under this heading.

Fosphenytoin Sodium (The beneficial effects of levodopa in Parkinson's disease have been reported to be reversed by phenytoin).
No products indexed under this heading.

Furosemide (Symptomatic postural hypotension has occurred with concomitant use; therefore, when therapy with carbidopa/levodopa is started, dosage adjustment of the antihypertensive drug may be required). Products include:
Furosemide Tablets 2154

Guanabenz Acetate (Symptomatic postural hypotension has occurred with concomitant use; therefore, when therapy with carbidopa/levodopa is started, dosage adjustment of the antihypertensive drug may be required).
No products indexed under this heading.

Guanethidine Monosulfate (Symptomatic postural hypotension has occurred with concomitant use; therefore, when therapy with carbidopa/levodopa is started, dosage adjustment of the antihypertensive drug may be required).
No products indexed under this heading.

Haloperidol (Dopamine D2 receptor antagonists may reduce the therapeutic effects of levodopa).
No products indexed under this heading.

Haloperidol Decanoate (Dopamine D2 receptor antagonists may reduce the therapeutic effects of levodopa).
No products indexed under this heading.

Hydralazine Hydrochloride (Symptomatic postural hypotension has occurred with concomitant use; therefore, when therapy with carbidopa/levodopa is started, dosage adjustment of the antihypertensive drug may be required). Products include:
BiDil Tablets 2171

Hydrochlorothiazide (Symptomatic postural hypotension has occurred with concomitant use; therefore, when therapy with carbidopa/levodopa is started, dosage adjustment of the antihypertensive drug may be required). Products include:
Aldoril Tablets 1910
Atacand HCT 651
Avalide Tablets 888
Avalide Tablets 2874
Benicar HCT Tablets 1044
Diovan HCT Tablets 2196
Dyazide Capsules 1423
Hyzaar 50-12.5 Tablets 1990
Hyzaar 100-12.5 Tablets 1990
Hyzaar 100-25 Tablets 1990
Lopressor HCT 50/25 Tablets 2241
Lopressor HCT 100/25 Tablets 2241
Lopressor HCT 100/50 Tablets 2241
Lotensin HCT Tablets 2246
Micardis HCT Tablets 856
Moduretic Tablets 2028
Prinzide Tablets 2056
Teveten HCT Tablets 1737
Timolide Tablets 2086
Uniretic Tablets 3100

Hydroflumethiazide (Symptomatic postural hypotension has occurred with concomitant use; therefore, when therapy with carbidopa/levodopa is started, dosage adjustment of the antihypertensive drug may be required).
No products indexed under this heading.

Imipramine Hydrochloride (There have been rare reports of adverse reactions, including hypertension and dyskinesia, resulting from the concomitant use of tricyclic antidepressants and carbidopa/levodopa).

No products indexed under this heading.

Imipramine Pamoate (There have been rare reports of adverse reactions, including hypertension and dyskinesia, resulting from the concomitant use of tricyclic antidepressants and carbidopa/levodopa).

No products indexed under this heading.

Indapamide (Symptomatic postural hypotension has occurred with concomitant use; therefore, when therapy with carbidopa/levodopa is started, dosage adjustment of the antihypertensive drug may be required). Products include:

Irbesartan (Symptomatic postural hypotension has occurred with concomitant use; therefore, when therapy with carbidopa/levodopa is started, dosage adjustment of the antihypertensive drug may be required). Products include:

Iron (Iron salts may reduce the bioavailability of levodopa and carbidopa. The clinical relevance is unclear).

No products indexed under this heading.

Iron, Peptonized (Iron salts may reduce the bioavailability of levodopa and carbidopa. The clinical relevance is unclear).

No products indexed under this heading.

Iron Cacodylate (Iron salts may reduce the bioavailability of levodopa and carbidopa. The clinical relevance is unclear).

No products indexed under this heading.

Iron Carbonyl (Iron salts may reduce the bioavailability of levodopa and carbidopa. The clinical relevance is unclear).

No products indexed under this heading.

Iron Dextran (Iron salts may reduce the bioavailability of levodopa and carbidopa. The clinical relevance is unclear). Products include:

Iron Polysaccharide Complex (Iron salts may reduce the bioavailability of levodopa and carbidopa. The clinical relevance is unclear).

No products indexed under this heading.

Iron Sucrose (Iron salts may reduce the bioavailability of levodopa and carbidopa. The clinical relevance is unclear).

No products indexed under this heading.

Iron Supplements (Iron salts may reduce the bioavailability of levodopa and carbidopa. The clinical relevance is unclear).

No products indexed under this heading.

Isocarboxazid (Nonselective MAO inhibitors must be discontinued at least two weeks prior to initiating therapy with carbidopa/levodopa; concurrent use is contraindicated).

No products indexed under this heading.

Isoniazid (Isoniazid may reduce the therapeutic effects of levodopa).

No products indexed under this heading.

Isradipine (Symptomatic postural hypotension has occurred with concomitant use; therefore, when therapy with carbidopa/levodopa is started, dosage adjustment of the antihypertensive drug may be required). Products include:

Labetalol Hydrochloride (Symptomatic postural hypotension has occurred with concomitant use; therefore, when therapy with carbidopa/levodopa is started, dosage adjustment of the antihypertensive drug may be required).

No products indexed under this heading.

Lisinopril (Symptomatic postural hypotension has occurred with concomitant use; therefore, when therapy with carbidopa/levodopa is started, dosage adjustment of the antihypertensive drug may be required). Products include:

Losartan Potassium (Symptomatic postural hypotension has occurred with concomitant use; therefore, when therapy with carbidopa/levodopa is started, dosage adjustment of the antihypertensive drug may be required). Products include:

Loxapine Hydrochloride (Dopamine D2 receptor antagonists may reduce the therapeutic effects of levodopa).

No products indexed under this heading.

Loxapine Succinate (Dopamine D2 receptor antagonists may reduce the therapeutic effects of levodopa).

No products indexed under this heading.

Maprotiline Hydrochloride (There have been rare reports of adverse reactions, including hypertension and dyskinesia, resulting from the concomitant use of tricyclic antidepressants and carbidopa/levodopa).

No products indexed under this heading.

Mecamylamine Hydrochloride (Symptomatic postural hypotension has occurred with concomitant use; therefore, when therapy with carbidopa/levodopa is started, dosage adjustment of the antihypertensive drug may be required).

No products indexed under this heading.

Mesoridazine Besylate (Dopamine D2 receptor antagonists may reduce the therapeutic effects of levodopa).

No products indexed under this heading.

Methotrimeprazine (Dopamine D2 receptor antagonists may reduce the therapeutic effects of levodopa).

No products indexed under this heading.

Methyclothiazide (Symptomatic postural hypotension has occurred with concomitant use; therefore, when therapy with carbidopa/levodopa is started, dosage adjustment of the antihypertensive drug may be required).

No products indexed under this heading.

Methyldopa (Symptomatic postural hypotension has occurred with concomitant use; therefore, when therapy with carbidopa/levodopa is started, dosage adjustment of the antihypertensive drug may be required). Products include:

Methyldopate Hydrochloride (Symptomatic postural hypotension has occurred with concomitant use; therefore, when therapy with carbidopa/levodopa is started, dosage adjustment of the antihypertensive drug may be required).

No products indexed under this heading.

Metoclopramide Hydrochloride (Metoclopramine may increase the bioavailability of levodopa by increasing gastric emptying and may also adversely affect disease control by its dopamine receptor antagonistic properties).

No products indexed under this heading.

Metolazone (Symptomatic postural hypotension has occurred with concomitant use; therefore, when therapy with carbidopa/levodopa is started, dosage adjustment of the antihypertensive drug may be required).

No products indexed under this heading.

Metoprolol Succinate (Symptomatic postural hypotension has occurred with concomitant use; therefore, when therapy with carbidopa/levodopa is started, dosage adjustment of the antihypertensive drug may be required). Products include:

Metoprolol Tartrate (Symptomatic postural hypotension has occurred with concomitant use; therefore, when therapy with carbidopa/levodopa is started, dosage adjustment of the antihypertensive drug may be required). Products include:

Metyrosine (Symptomatic postural hypotension has occurred with concomitant use; therefore, when therapy with carbidopa/levodopa is started, dosage adjustment of the antihypertensive drug may be required). Products include:

Mibefradil Dihydrochloride (Symptomatic postural hypotension has occurred with concomitant use; therefore, when therapy with carbidopa/levodopa is started, dosage adjustment of the antihypertensive drug may be required).

No products indexed under this heading.

Minoxidil (Symptomatic postural hypotension has occurred with concomitant use; therefore, when therapy with carbidopa/levodopa is start-

ed, dosage adjustment of the antihypertensive drug may be required). Products include:

Moexipril Hydrochloride (Symptomatic postural hypotension has occurred with concomitant use; therefore, when therapy with carbidopa/levodopa is started, dosage adjustment of the antihypertensive drug may be required). Products include:

Molindone Hydrochloride (Dopamine D2 receptor antagonists may reduce the therapeutic effects of levodopa). Products include:

Nadolol (Symptomatic postural hypotension has occurred with concomitant use; therefore, when therapy with carbidopa/levodopa is started, dosage adjustment of the antihypertensive drug may be required). Products include:

Nicardipine Hydrochloride (Symptomatic postural hypotension has occurred with concomitant use; therefore, when therapy with carbidopa/levodopa is started, dosage adjustment of the antihypertensive drug may be required). Products include:

Nifedipine (Symptomatic postural hypotension has occurred with concomitant use; therefore, when therapy with carbidopa/levodopa is started, dosage adjustment of the antihypertensive drug may be required). Products include:

Nisoldipine (Symptomatic postural hypotension has occurred with concomitant use; therefore, when therapy with carbidopa/levodopa is started, dosage adjustment of the antihypertensive drug may be required). Products include:

Nitroglycerin (Symptomatic postural hypotension has occurred with concomitant use; therefore, when therapy with carbidopa/levodopa is started, dosage adjustment of the antihypertensive drug may be required). Products include:

Nortriptyline Hydrochloride (There have been rare reports of adverse reactions, including hypertension and dyskinesia, resulting from the concomitant use of tricyclic antidepressants and carbidopa/levodopa).

No products indexed under this heading.

Papaverine (The beneficial effects of levodopa in Parkinson's disease have been reported to be reversed by papaverine).

No products indexed under this heading.

Papaverine Hydrochloride (The beneficial effects of levodopa in Parkinson's disease have been reported to be reversed by papaverine).
No products indexed under this heading.

Pargyline Hydrochloride (Nonselective MAO inhibitors must be discontinued at least two weeks prior to initiating therapy with carbidopa/levodopa; concurrent use is contraindicated).
No products indexed under this heading.

Penbutolol Sulfate (Symptomatic postural hypotension has occurred with concomitant use; therefore, when therapy with carbidopa/levodopa is started, dosage adjustment of the antihypertensive drug may be required).
No products indexed under this heading.

Perindopril Erbumine (Symptomatic postural hypotension has occurred with concomitant use; therefore, when therapy with carbidopa/levodopa is started, dosage adjustment of the antihypertensive drug may be required). Products include:
Aceon Tablets (2 mg, 4 mg, 8 mg) 3194

Perphenazine (Dopamine D2 receptor antagonists may reduce the therapeutic effects of levodopa).
No products indexed under this heading.

Phenelzine Sulfate (Nonselective MAO inhibitors must be discontinued at least two weeks prior to initiating therapy with carbidopa/levodopa; concurrent use is contraindicated).
No products indexed under this heading.

Phenoxybenzamine Hydrochloride (Symptomatic postural hypotension has occurred with concomitant use; therefore, when therapy with carbidopa/levodopa is started, dosage adjustment of the antihypertensive drug may be required). Products include:
Dibenzyline Capsules 3399

Phentolamine Mesylate (Symptomatic postural hypotension has occurred with concomitant use; therefore, when therapy with carbidopa/levodopa is started, dosage adjustment of the antihypertensive drug may be required).
No products indexed under this heading.

Phenytoin (The beneficial effects of levodopa in Parkinson's disease have been reported to be reversed by phenytoin).
No products indexed under this heading.

Phenytoin Sodium (The beneficial effects of levodopa in Parkinson's disease have been reported to be reversed by phenytoin). Products include:
Phenytek Capsules 2160

Pindolol (Symptomatic postural hypotension has occurred with concomitant use; therefore, when therapy with carbidopa/levodopa is started, dosage adjustment of the antihypertensive drug may be required).
No products indexed under this heading.

Polysaccharide Iron Complex (Iron salts may reduce the bioavailability of levodopa and carbidopa. The clinical relevance is unclear). Products include:
Nu-Iron 150 Capsules 2127

Polythiazide (Symptomatic postural hypotension has occurred with concomitant use; therefore, when therapy with carbidopa/levodopa is started, dosage adjustment of the antihypertensive drug may be required).
No products indexed under this heading.

Prazosin Hydrochloride (Symptomatic postural hypotension has occurred with concomitant use; therefore, when therapy with carbidopa/levodopa is started, dosage adjustment of the antihypertensive drug may be required).
No products indexed under this heading.

Procarbazine Hydrochloride (Nonselective MAO inhibitors must be discontinued at least two weeks prior to initiating therapy with carbidopa/levodopa; concurrent use is contraindicated). Products include:
Matulane Capsules 3191

Prochlorperazine (Dopamine D2 receptor antagonists may reduce the therapeutic effects of levodopa).
No products indexed under this heading.

Promethazine Hydrochloride (Dopamine D2 receptor antagonists may reduce the therapeutic effects of levodopa). Products include:
Phenergan Tablets and Suppositories 3440

Propranolol Hydrochloride (Symptomatic postural hypotension has occurred with concomitant use; therefore, when therapy with carbidopa/levodopa is started, dosage adjustment of the antihypertensive drug may be required). Products include:
Inderal LA Long-Acting Capsules 3429
InnoPran XL Capsules 2723

Protriptyline Hydrochloride (There have been rare reports of adverse reactions, including hypertension and dyskinesia, resulting from the concomitant use of tricyclic antidepressants and carbidopa/levodopa).
No products indexed under this heading.

Quetiapine Fumarate (Dopamine D2 receptor antagonists may reduce the therapeutic effects of levodopa). Products include:
Seroquel Tablets 690

Quinapril Hydrochloride (Symptomatic postural hypotension has occurred with concomitant use; therefore, when therapy with carbidopa/levodopa is started, dosage adjustment of the antihypertensive drug may be required).
No products indexed under this heading.

Ramipril (Symptomatic postural hypotension has occurred with concomitant use; therefore, when therapy with carbidopa/levodopa is started, dosage adjustment of the antihypertensive drug may be required). Products include:
Altace Capsules 1702

Rauwolfia Serpentina (Symptomatic postural hypotension has occurred with concomitant use; therefore, when therapy with carbidopa/levodopa is started, dosage adjustment of the antihypertensive drug may be required).
No products indexed under this heading.

Rescinnamine (Symptomatic postural hypotension has occurred with concomitant use; therefore, when therapy with carbidopa/levodopa is started, dosage adjustment of the antihypertensive drug may be required).
No products indexed under this heading.

Reserpine (Symptomatic postural hypotension has occurred with concomitant use; therefore, when therapy with carbidopa/levodopa is started, dosage adjustment of the antihypertensive drug may be required).
No products indexed under this heading.

Risperidone (Dopamine D2 receptor antagonists may reduce the therapeutic effects of levodopa). Products include:
Risperdal 1676
Risperdal Consta Long-Acting Injection 1682
Risperdal M-Tab Orally Disintegrating Tablets 1676

Selegiline Hydrochloride (Concomitant therapy with selegiline may be associated with severe orthostatic hypotension not attributable to carbidopa/levodopa alone). Products include:
Eldepryl Capsules 3208
Zelapar Tablets 3372

Sodium Nitroprusside (Symptomatic postural hypotension has occurred with concomitant use; therefore, when therapy with carbidopa/levodopa is started, dosage adjustment of the antihypertensive drug may be required).
No products indexed under this heading.

Sotalol Hydrochloride (Symptomatic postural hypotension has occurred with concomitant use; therefore, when therapy with carbidopa/levodopa is started, dosage adjustment of the antihypertensive drug may be required).
No products indexed under this heading.

Spirapril Hydrochloride (Symptomatic postural hypotension has occurred with concomitant use; therefore, when therapy with carbidopa/levodopa is started, dosage adjustment of the antihypertensive drug may be required).
No products indexed under this heading.

Telmisartan (Symptomatic postural hypotension has occurred with concomitant use; therefore, when therapy with carbidopa/levodopa is started, dosage adjustment of the antihypertensive drug may be required). Products include:
Micardis Tablets 854
Micardis HCT Tablets 856

Terazosin Hydrochloride (Symptomatic postural hypotension has occurred with concomitant use; therefore, when therapy with carbidopa/levodopa is started, dosage adjustment of the antihypertensive drug may be required). Products include:
Hytrin Capsules 471

Thioridazine Hydrochloride (Dopamine D2 receptor antagonists may reduce the therapeutic effects of levodopa). Products include:
Thioridazine Hydrochloride Tablets 2163

Thiothixene (Dopamine D2 receptor antagonists may reduce the therapeutic effects of levodopa). Products include:
Thiothixene Capsules 2165

Timolol Maleate (Symptomatic postural hypotension has occurred with concomitant use; therefore, when therapy with carbidopa/levodopa is started, dosage adjustment of the antihypertensive drug may be required). Products include:
Blocadren Tablets 1916
Cosopt Sterile Ophthalmic Solution 1931
Timolide Tablets 2086
Timoptic Sterile Ophthalmic Solution 2088
Timoptic in Ocudose 2091
Timoptic-XE Sterile Ophthalmic Gel Forming Solution 2092

Torsemide (Symptomatic postural hypotension has occurred with concomitant use; therefore, when therapy with carbidopa/levodopa is started, dosage adjustment of the antihypertensive drug may be required). Products include:
Demadex Injection 2759
Demadex Tablets 2759

Trandolapril (Symptomatic postural hypotension has occurred with concomitant use; therefore, when therapy with carbidopa/levodopa is started, dosage adjustment of the antihypertensive drug may be required). Products include:
Mavik Tablets 486
Tarka Tablets 524

Tranylcypromine Sulfate (Nonselective MAO inhibitors must be discontinued at least two weeks prior to initiating therapy with carbidopa/levodopa; concurrent use is contraindicated). Products include:
Parnate Tablets 1527

Trifluoperazine Hydrochloride (Dopamine D2 receptor antagonists may reduce the therapeutic effects of levodopa).
No products indexed under this heading.

Trimethaphan Camsylate (Symptomatic postural hypotension has occurred with concomitant use; therefore, when therapy with carbidopa/levodopa is started, dosage adjustment of the antihypertensive drug may be required).
No products indexed under this heading.

Trimipramine Maleate (There have been rare reports of adverse reactions, including hypertension and dyskinesia, resulting from the concomitant use of tricyclic antidepressants and carbidopa/levodopa).
No products indexed under this heading.

Valsartan (Symptomatic postural hypotension has occurred with concomitant use; therefore, when therapy with carbidopa/levodopa is started, dosage adjustment of the antihypertensive drug may be required). Products include:
Diovan Tablets 2193
Diovan HCT Tablets 2196

Verapamil Hydrochloride (Symptomatic postural hypotension has occurred with concomitant use; therefore, when therapy with carbidopa/levodopa is started, dosage adjustment of the antihypertensive drug may be required). Products include:
- Covera-HS Tablets 3139
- Tarka Tablets 524
- Verelan PM Extended-Release Capsules, Controlled-Onset 3106

PARNATE TABLETS

(Tranylcypromine Sulfate) 1527

May interact with alpha adrenergic stimulants, amphetamines, anesthetics, anorexiants, antihistamines, antihypertensives, anticholinergic-type antiparkinsonism drugs, dibenzazepines, diuretics, oral hypoglycemic agents, hypnotics and sedatives, insulin, monoamine oxidase inhibitors, narcotic analgesics, phenothiazines, selective serotonin reuptake inhibitors, sympathomimetics, tricyclic antidepressants, and certain other agents. Compounds in these categories include:

Acarbose (Some MAO inhibitors have contributed to hypoglycemic episodes in diabetic patients receiving oral hypoglycemic agents). Products include:
- Precose Tablets 751

Acebutolol Hydrochloride (Concurrent use with hypotensive agents is contraindicated; a marked potentiating effect on these classes of drugs has been reported).
No products indexed under this heading.

Acrivastine (Concurrent use is contraindicated).
No products indexed under this heading.

Albuterol (Concurrent and/or sequential use is contraindicated; combination therapy may precipitate hypertension, headache and related symptoms). Products include:
- Proventil Inhalation Aerosol 3053

Albuterol Sulfate (Concurrent and/or sequential use is contraindicated; combination therapy may precipitate hypertension, headache and related symptoms). Products include:
- AccuNeb Inhalation Solution 1055
- Combivent Inhalation Aerosol 847
- DuoNeb Inhalation Solution 1058
- ProAir HFA Inhalation Aerosol 3300
- Proventil Inhalation Solution 0.083% 3055
- Proventil HFA Inhalation Aerosol 3056
- Ventolin HFA Inhalation Aerosol 1600
- VoSpire ER Tablets 1052

Alfentanil Hydrochloride (Concurrent use is contraindicated; a marked potentiating effect on these classes of drugs has been reported).
No products indexed under this heading.

Amiloride Hydrochloride (Concurrent use with hypotensive agents is contraindicated; a marked potentiating effect on these classes of drugs has been reported). Products include:
- Midamor Tablets 2026
- Moduretic Tablets 2028

Amitriptyline Hydrochloride (Concurrent use with dibenzazepine-related entities may result in hypertensive crises or severe convulsive seizures; concurrent and/or sequential use is contraindicated).
No products indexed under this heading.

Amlodipine Besylate (Concurrent use with hypotensive agents is contraindicated; a marked potentiating effect on these classes of drugs has been reported). Products include:
- Caduet Tablets 2508
- Lotrel Capsules 2249
- Norvasc Tablets 2545

Amoxapine (Concurrent use with dibenzazepine-related entities may result in hypertensive crises or severe convulsive seizures; concurrent and/or sequential use is contraindicated).
No products indexed under this heading.

Amphetamine Resins (Concurrent and/or sequential use is contraindicated).
No products indexed under this heading.

Amphetamine Sulfate (Concurrent and/or sequential use is contraindicated). Products include:
- Adderall Tablets 3164
- Adderall XR Capsules 3166

Astemizole (Concurrent use is contraindicated).
No products indexed under this heading.

Atenolol (Concurrent use with hypotensive agents is contraindicated; a marked potentiating effect on these classes of drugs has been reported).
No products indexed under this heading.

Azatadine Maleate (Concurrent use is contraindicated).
No products indexed under this heading.

Benazepril Hydrochloride (Concurrent use with hypotensive agents is contraindicated; a marked potentiating effect on these classes of drugs has been reported). Products include:
- Lotensin Tablets 2243
- Lotensin HCT Tablets 2246
- Lotrel Capsules 2249

Bendroflumethiazide (Concurrent use with hypotensive agents is contraindicated; a marked potentiating effect on these classes of drugs has been reported).
No products indexed under this heading.

Benzphetamine Hydrochloride (Concurrent and/or sequential use is contraindicated).
No products indexed under this heading.

Benztropine Mesylate (Anti-Parkinsonism drugs should be used with caution in patients receiving Parnate since severe reactions have been reported).
No products indexed under this heading.

Betaxolol Hydrochloride (Concurrent use with hypotensive agents is contraindicated; a marked potentiating effect on these classes of drugs has been reported). Products include:
- Betoptic S Ophthalmic Suspension 558

Biperiden Hydrochloride (Anti-Parkinsonism drugs should be used with caution in patients receiving Parnate since severe reactions have been reported).
No products indexed under this heading.

Bisoprolol Fumarate (Concurrent use with hypotensive agents is contraindicated; a marked potentiating effect on these classes of drugs has been reported).
No products indexed under this heading.

Bromodiphenhydramine Hydrochloride (Concurrent use is contraindicated).
No products indexed under this heading.

Brompheniramine Maleate (Concurrent use is contraindicated). Products include:
- Children's Dimetapp Cold & Allergy Elixir .... ■730
- Children's Dimetapp Cold & Allergy Chewable Tablets .... ■730
- Children's Dimetapp DM Cold & Cough Elixir .... ■731

Bumetanide (Concurrent use with hypotensive agents is contraindicated; a marked potentiating effect on these classes of drugs has been reported). Products include:
- Bumex Tablets 2746

Buprenorphine Hydrochloride (Concurrent use is contraindicated; a marked potentiating effect on these classes of drugs has been reported). Products include:
- Buprenex Injectable 2716
- Suboxone Tablets 2717
- Subutex Tablets 2717

Bupropion Hydrochloride (Concurrent use is contraindicated; at least 14 days should elapse between discontinuation of an MAO inhibitor and initiation of treatment with bupropion). Products include:
- Wellbutrin Tablets 1603
- Wellbutrin SR Sustained-Release Tablets 1607
- Wellbutrin XL Extended-Release Tablets 1613
- Zyban Sustained-Release Tablets 1644

Buspirone Hydrochloride (Concurrent use of buspirone and an MAO inhibitor has resulted in several cases of hypertension; concurrent use is contraindicated; at least 10 days should elapse between the discontinuation of Parnate and the initiation of buspirone).
No products indexed under this heading.

Caffeine (Excessive use of caffeine in any form is contraindicated). Products include:
- BC Headache Powder .... ■677
- Arthritis Strength BC Powder .... ■677
- Excedrin Extra Strength Caplets/Tablets/Geltabs .... ■684
- Excedrin Migraine Caplets/Tablets/Geltabs .... ■609
- Excedrin Tension Headache Caplets/Tablets/Geltabs .... ■611
- Goody's Extra Strength Headache Powders .... ■611
- Goody's Extra Strength Pain Relief Tablets .... ■685
- Vivarin .... ■602
- Winrgy Dietary Supplement .... ■823

Candesartan Cilexetil (Concurrent use with hypotensive agents is contraindicated; a marked potentiating effect on these classes of drugs has been reported). Products include:
- Atacand Tablets 649
- Atacand HCT 651

Captopril (Concurrent use with hypotensive agents is contraindicated; a marked potentiating effect on these classes of drugs has been reported). Products include:
- Captopril Tablets 2149

Carbamazepine (Concurrent use with dibenzazepine-related entities may result in hypertensive crises or severe convulsive seizures; concurrent and/or sequential use is contraindicated). Products include:
- Carbatrol Capsules 3171
- Equetro Extended-Release Capsules 3180
- Tegretol/Tegretol-XR 2295

Carteolol Hydrochloride (Concurrent use with hypotensive agents is contraindicated; a marked potentiating effect on these classes of drugs has been reported). Products include:
- Carteolol Hydrochloride Ophthalmic Solution USP, 1% .... ⊙249

Cetirizine Hydrochloride (Concurrent use is contraindicated). Products include:
- Zyrtec Chewable Tablets 2594
- Zyrtec 2594
- Zyrtec-D 12 Hour Extended Release Tablets 2597

Chlorothiazide (Concurrent use with hypotensive agents is contraindicated; a marked potentiating effect on these classes of drugs has been reported). Products include:
- Diuril Oral Suspension 1954

Chlorothiazide Sodium (Concurrent use with hypotensive agents is contraindicated; a marked potentiating effect on these classes of drugs has been reported). Products include:
- Diuril Sodium Intravenous 2467

Chlorpheniramine Maleate (Concurrent use is contraindicated). Products include:
- Advil Allergy Sinus Caplets .... ■770
- Advil Multi-Symptom Cold Caplets .... ■770
- BC Allergy Sinus Cold Powder .... ■677
- Comtrex Maximum Strength Cold & Cough Day/Night Caplets - Night Formulation .... ■726
- Comtrex Maximum Strength Day/Night Severe Cold & Sinus Caplets - Night Formulation .... ■725
- Contac Cold and Flu Maximum Strength Caplets .... ■728
- Contac Cold and Flu Day and Night Caplets (Night Formulation Only) .... ■727
- Children's Dimetapp Long Acting Cough Plus Cold Syrup .... ■731
- Robitussin Cough & Cold Long-Acting Liquid .... ■735
- Robitussin Cough & Allergy Syrup .. ■736
- Robitussin Cough & Cold Nighttime Liquid .... ■736
- Robitussin Cough, Cold & Flu Nighttime Liquid .... ■738
- Robitussin Pediatric Cough & Cold Long-Acting Liquid .... ■735
- Robitussin Pediatric Cough & Cold Nighttime Liquid .... ■736
- Triaminic Cold & Allergy Liquid .... ■746
- Triaminic Cough & Runny Nose Softchews .... ■748
- Children's Tylenol Plus Flu Oral Suspension .... ■749
- Tylenol Allergy Multi-Symptom Caplets with Cool Burst and Gelcaps 1872
- Children's Tylenol Plus Cold Suspension Liquid 1879
- Children's Tylenol Plus Cough & Runny Nose Suspension Liquid 1879
- Children's Tylenol Plus Flu Suspension Liquid 1881
- Children's Tylenol Plus Multi-Symptom Cold Suspension Liquid 1879
- Tylenol Cold Head Congestion Nighttime Caplets with Cool Burst 1873
- Tylenol Cold Multi-Symptom Nighttime Caplets with Cool Burst 1874
- Tylenol Sinus Congestion & Pain Nighttime Caplets with Cool Burst 1876

Vicks 44M Cough, Cold & Flu Relief Liquid 2680
Pediatric Vicks 44m Cough & Cold Relief Liquid 2676
Children's Vicks NyQuil Cold/Cough Relief .... ▣756
Children's Vicks NyQuil Cold/Cough Relief Liquid 2680
Zicam Maximum Strength Flu Daytime .... ▣768

Chlorpheniramine Polistirex (Concurrent use is contraindicated). Products include:
Tussionex Pennkinetic Extended-Release Suspension 3327

Chlorpheniramine Tannate (Concurrent use is contraindicated).
No products indexed under this heading.

Chlorpromazine (Possibility of additive hypotensive effects).
No products indexed under this heading.

Chlorpromazine Hydrochloride (Possibility of additive hypotensive effects).
No products indexed under this heading.

Chlorpropamide (Some MAO inhibitors have contributed to hypoglycemic episodes in diabetic patients receiving oral hypoglycemic agents).
No products indexed under this heading.

Chlorthalidone (Concurrent use with hypotensive agents is contraindicated; a marked potentiating effect on these classes of drugs has been reported). Products include:
Clorpres Tablets 2153

Citalopram Hydrobromide (Concurrent and/or sequential use is contraindicated; potential for serious, sometimes fatal, reactions including hyperthermia, rigidity, myoclonus, and other toxicities). Products include:
Celexa 1176

Clemastine Fumarate (Concurrent use is contraindicated).
No products indexed under this heading.

Clomipramine Hydrochloride (Concurrent use with dibenzazepine-related entities may result in hypertensive crises or severe convulsive seizures; concurrent and/or sequential use is contraindicated).
No products indexed under this heading.

Clonidine (Concurrent use with hypotensive agents is contraindicated; a marked potentiating effect on these classes of drugs has been reported). Products include:
Catapres-TTS 844

Clonidine Hydrochloride (Concurrent use with hypotensive agents is contraindicated; a marked potentiating effect on these classes of drugs has been reported). Products include:
Catapres Tablets 843
Clorpres Tablets 2153

Clozapine (Concurrent use with dibenzazepine-related entities may result in hypertensive crises or severe convulsive seizures; concurrent and/or sequential use is contraindicated). Products include:
Clozaril Tablets 2184
FazaClo Orally Disintegrating Tablets 551

Cocaine Hydrochloride (Concurrent use is contraindicated).
No products indexed under this heading.

Codeine Phosphate (Concurrent use is contraindicated; a marked potentiating effect on these classes of drugs has been reported). Products include:
Tylenol with Codeine Tablets 2391

Cyclobenzaprine Hydrochloride (Concurrent use with dibenzazepine-related entities may result in hypertensive crises or severe convulsive seizures; concurrent and/or sequential use is contraindicated).
No products indexed under this heading.

Cyproheptadine Hydrochloride (Concurrent use is contraindicated).
No products indexed under this heading.

Deserpidine (Concurrent use with hypotensive agents is contraindicated; a marked potentiating effect on these classes of drugs has been reported).
No products indexed under this heading.

Desipramine Hydrochloride (Concurrent use with dibenzazepine-related entities may result in hypertensive crises or severe convulsive seizures; concurrent and/or sequential use is contraindicated).
No products indexed under this heading.

Dexchlorpheniramine Maleate (Concurrent use is contraindicated).
No products indexed under this heading.

Dexfenfluramine Hydrochloride (Co-administration with dexfenfluramine, a serotonin releaser and reuptake inhibitor, is contraindicated).
No products indexed under this heading.

Dextroamphetamine Sulfate (Concurrent and/or sequential use is contraindicated). Products include:
Adderall Tablets 3164
Adderall XR Capsules 3166
Dexedrine 1420
DextroStat Tablets 3179

Dextromethorphan Hydrobromide (The combination of dextromethorphan and MAO inhibitors has been reported to cause brief episodes of psychosis or bizzare behavior; concurrent use is contraindicated). Products include:
Comtrex Maximum Strength Cold & Cough Day/Night Caplets - Day Formulation .... ▣726
Comtrex Maximum Strength Cold & Cough Day/Night Caplets - Night Formulation .... ▣726
Comtrex Maximum Strength Non-Drowsy Cold & Cough Caplets .... ▣725
Children's Dimetapp DM Cold & Cough Elixir .... ▣731
Children's Dimetapp Long Acting Cough Plus Cold Syrup .... ▣731
Toddler's Dimetapp Cold and Cough Drops .... ▣732
Mucinex DM Extended-Release Bi-Layer Tablets .... ▣720
Refenesen DM Caplets .... ▣721
Robitussin Cough & Cold CF Liquid .... ▣735
Robitussin Cough & Cold Long-Acting Liquid .... ▣735
Robitussin Cough & Allergy Syrup .... ▣736
Robitussin Cough & Cold Nighttime Liquid .... ▣736
Robitussin Cough & Cold Pediatric Drops .... ▣735
Robitussin Cough, Cold & Flu Nighttime Liquid .... ▣738
Robitussin Cough & Congestion Liquid .... ▣738
Robitussin Cough Gels Long-Acting .... ▣737
Robitussin Cough Long Acting Liquid .... ▣739
Robitussin Cough DM Syrup .... ▣738
Robitussin Cough DM Infant Drops .... ▣738
Robitussin Pediatric Cough Long Acting Liquid .... ▣739
Robitussin Pediatric Cough & Cold Long-Acting Liquid .... ▣735
Robitussin Pediatric Cough & Cold Nighttime Liquid .... ▣736
Robitussin Sugar Free Cough .... ▣738
TheraFlu Cold & Cough Hot Liquid .... ▣740
TheraFlu Warming Relief Daytime Severe Cold .... ▣743
TheraFlu Thin Strips Long Acting Cough .... ▣744
Triaminic Daytime Cold & Cough Liquid .... ▣745
Triaminic Cough & Sore Throat Liquid .... ▣747
Triaminic Cough & Runny Nose Softchews .... ▣748
Triaminic Thin Strips Cold & Cough .... ▣778
Triaminic Infant Thin Strips Decongestant Plus Cough .... ▣747
Children's Tylenol Plus Flu Oral Suspension .... ▣749
Tylenol Cold Head Congestion Daytime Caplets with Cool Burst and Gelcaps .... ▣750
Tylenol Cold Multi-Symptom Daytime Liquid .... ▣752
Tylenol Cold Multi-Symptom Severe Daytime Liquid .... ▣752
Concentrated Tylenol Infants' Drops Plus Cold & Cough .... ▣754
Children's Tylenol Plus Cough & Runny Nose Suspension Liquid 1879
Children's Tylenol Plus Cough & Sore Throat Suspension Liquid 1879
Children's Tylenol Plus Flu Suspension Liquid 1881
Children's Tylenol Plus Multi-Symptom Cold Suspension Liquid 1879
Tylenol Cold Severe Congestion Non-Drowsy Caplets with Cool Burst 1874
Tylenol Cold Head Congestion Daytime Caplets with Cool Burst 1873
Tylenol Cold Head Congestion Nighttime Caplets with Cool Burst 1873
Tylenol Cold Head Congestion Severe Caplets with Cool Burst 1873
Tylenol Cold Multi-Symptom Daytime Caplets with Cool Burst and Gelcaps 1874
Tylenol Cold Multi-Symptom Daytime Liquid with Citrus Burst 1874
Tylenol Cold Multi-Symptom Nighttime Caplets with Cool Burst 1874
Tylenol Cold Multi-Symptom Nighttime Liquid with Cool Burst 1874
Tylenol Cold Multi-Symptom Severe Caplets with Cool Burst 1874
Tylenol Cold Multi-Symptom Severe Daytime Liquid with Citrus Burst 1874
Tylenol Cough & Sore Throat Daytime Liquid with Cool Burst 1877
Tylenol Cough & Sore Throat Nighttime Liquid with Cool Burst 1877
Concentrated Tylenol Infants' Drops Plus Cold and Cough 1879
Vicks 44 Cough Relief Liquid 2679
Vicks 44D Cough & Head Congestion Relief Liquid 2679
Vicks 44E Cough & Chest Congestion Relief Liquid 2679
Pediatric Vicks 44e Cough & Chest Congestion Relief Liquid 2676
Vicks 44M Cough, Cold & Flu Relief Liquid 2680
Pediatric Vicks 44m Cough & Cold Relief Liquid 2676
Vicks DayQuil LiquiCaps/Liquid Multi-Symptom Cold/Flu Relief .... ▣761
Vicks DayQuil Multi-Symptom Cold/Flu Relief LiquiCaps 2678
Vicks DayQuil Multi-Symptom Cold/Flu Relief Liquid 2678
Vicks NyQuil Multi-Symptom Cold/Flu Relief Liquid 2681
Children's Vicks NyQuil Cold/Cough Relief .... ▣756
Vicks NyQuil Multi-Symptom Cold/Flu Relief LiquiCaps 2681
Vicks NyQuil LiquiCaps/Liquid Multi-Symptom Cold/Flu Relief .... ▣763
Vicks NyQuil Cough Liquid 2680
Children's Vicks NyQuil Cold/Cough Relief Liquid 2680
Zicam Cough Max Nighttime Cough Spray .... ▣767
Zicam Cough Max Cough Spray .... ▣767
Zicam Cough Max Cough Melts .... ▣767
Zicam Cough Plus D Cough Spray .... ▣767
Zicam Cough Relief Cough Spray .... ▣767
Zicam Maximum Strength Flu Daytime .... ▣768
Zicam Maximum Strength Flu Nighttime .... ▣768

Dextromethorphan Polistirex (The combination of dextromethorphan and MAO inhibitors has been reported to cause brief episodes of psychosis or bizzare behavior; concurrent use is contraindicated). Products include:
Delsym Extended-Release Suspension 12 Hour Cough Suppressant .... ▣611

Dezocine (Concurrent use is contraindicated; a marked potentiating effect on these classes of drugs has been reported).
No products indexed under this heading.

Diazoxide (Concurrent use with hypotensive agents is contraindicated; a marked potentiating effect on these classes of drugs has been reported). Products include:
Hyperstat I.V. 3017

Diethylpropion Hydrochloride (Concurrent and/or sequential use is contraindicated).
No products indexed under this heading.

Diltiazem Hydrochloride (Concurrent use with hypotensive agents is contraindicated; a marked potentiating effect on these classes of drugs has been reported). Products include:
Cardizem LA Extended Release Tablets 1728
Tiazac Capsules 1201

Diphenhydramine Citrate (Concurrent use is contraindicated). Products include:
Advil PM Caplets .... ▣615
Excedrin PM Caplets/Tablets/Geltabs .... ▣610
Goody's PM Powder for Pain with Sleeplessness .... ▣612

Diphenhydramine Hydrochloride (Anti-Parkinsonism drugs should be used with caution in patients receiving Parnate since severe reactions have been reported). Products include:
Nytol QuickCaps Caplets .... ▣615
Nytol QuickGels Softgels Maximum Strength .... ▣616
Simply Sleep Caplets 1868
Sominex Original Formula Tablets .... ▣616
TheraFlu Warming Relief Nighttime Severe Cold .... ▣743
TheraFlu Thin Strips Multi Symptom .... ▣744
Triaminic Nighttime Cold & Cough Liquid .... ▣746
Triaminic Thin Strips Cough & Runny Nose .... ▣749

Diphenylpyraline Hydrochloride
(Concurrent use is contraindicated).
No products indexed under this
heading.

Disulfiram (Concurrent use requires
caution; co-administration in animal
models has resulted in severe toxicity, including convulsions and death).
No products indexed under this
heading.

Dobutamine Hydrochloride (Concurrent and/or sequential use is contraindicated; combination therapy
may precipitate hypertension, headache and related symptoms).
No products indexed under this
heading.

Dopamine Hydrochloride (Concurrent and/or sequential use is contraindicated; combination therapy
may precipitate hypertension, headache and related symptoms).
No products indexed under this
heading.

Doxazosin Mesylate (Concurrent
use with hypotensive agents is contraindicated; a marked potentiating
effect on these classes of drugs has
been reported). Products include:
Cardura XL Tablets 2515

Doxepin Hydrochloride (Concurrent use with dibenzazepine-related
entities may result in hypertensive
crises or severe convulsive seizures;
concurrent and/or sequential use is
contraindicated).
No products indexed under this
heading.

Enalapril Maleate (Concurrent use
with hypotensive agents is contraindicated; a marked potentiating
effect on these classes of drugs has
been reported). Products include:
Vasotec I.V. Injection 2103

Enalaprilat (Concurrent use with
hypotensive agents is contraindicated; a marked potentiating effect
on these classes of drugs has been
reported).
No products indexed under this
heading.

Enflurane (Patients taking tranylcypromine should not undergo elective
surgery requiring general anesthesia; the possible combined hypotensive effects of tranylcypromine
should be kept in mind; Parnate
should be discontinued at least 10
days prior to elective surgery).
No products indexed under this
heading.

Ephedrine Hydrochloride (Concurrent and/or sequential use is contraindicated; combination therapy
may precipitate hypertension, headache and related symptoms).
No products indexed under this
heading.

Ephedrine Sulfate (Concurrent
and/or sequential use is contraindicated; combination therapy may precipitate hypertension, headache and
related symptoms).
No products indexed under this
heading.

Ephedrine Tannate (Concurrent
and/or sequential use is contraindicated; combination therapy may precipitate hypertension, headache and
related symptoms).
No products indexed under this
heading.

Epinephrine (Concurrent and/or
sequential use is contraindicated;
combination therapy may precipitate
hypertension, headache and related
symptoms). Products include:
EpiPen ... 1061
Primatene Mist ▣□719
Twinject 0.15 3379
Twinject 0.3 3378

Epinephrine Bitartrate (Concurrent and/or sequential use is contraindicated; combination therapy may
precipitate hypertension, headache
and related symptoms).
No products indexed under this
heading.

Epinephrine Hydrochloride (Concurrent and/or sequential use is contraindicated; combination therapy
may precipitate hypertension, headache and related symptoms).
No products indexed under this
heading.

Eprosartan Mesylate (Concurrent
use with hypotensive agents is contraindicated; a marked potentiating
effect on these classes of drugs has
been reported). Products include:
Teveten Tablets 1735
Teveten HCT Tablets 1737

Escitalopram Oxalate (Concurrent
and/or sequential use is contraindicated; potential for serious, sometimes fatal, reactions including
hyperthermia, rigidity, myoclonus,
and other toxicities). Products
include:
Lexapro Oral Solution 1190
Lexapro Tablets 1190

Esmolol Hydrochloride (Concurrent use with hypotensive agents is
contraindicated; a marked potentiating effect on these classes of drugs
has been reported).
No products indexed under this
heading.

Estazolam (Concurrent use is contraindicated). Products include:
ProSom Tablets 517

Ethacrynic Acid (Concurrent use
with hypotensive agents is contraindicated; a marked potentiating
effect on these classes of drugs has
been reported). Products include:
Edecrin Tablets 1959

Ethchlorvynol (Concurrent use is
contraindicated).
No products indexed under this
heading.

Ethinamate (Concurrent use is
contraindicated).
No products indexed under this
heading.

Felodipine (Concurrent use with
hypotensive agents is contraindicated; a marked potentiating effect
on these classes of drugs has been
reported).
No products indexed under this
heading.

Fenfluramine Hydrochloride
(Concurrent and/or sequential use is
contraindicated).
No products indexed under this
heading.

Fentanyl (Concurrent use is contraindicated; a marked potentiating
effect on these classes of drugs has
been reported). Products include:

Duragesic Transdermal System 2373
Ionsys Transdermal System 2379

Fentanyl Citrate (Concurrent use
is contraindicated; a marked potentiating effect on these classes of
drugs has been reported). Products
include:
Actiq ... 979

Fexofenadine Hydrochloride
(Concurrent use is contraindicated).
Products include:
Allegra .. 2844
Allegra-D 12 Hour
Extended-Release Tablets............. 2846
Allegra-D 24 Hour
Extended-Release Tablets............. 2849

Fluoxetine Hydrochloride (Concurrent use has resulted in serious,
sometimes fatal, reactions, including
hyperthermia, rigidity, myoclonus,
autonomic instability with possible
rapid fluctuations of vital signs and
mental status; concurrent use is contraindicated; at least 5 weeks should
be allowed after stopping fluoxetine
before starting an MAO inhibitor).
Products include:
Prozac Pulvules and Liquid 1801
Symbyax Capsules 1819

Fluphenazine Decanoate (Possibility of additive hypotensive effects).
No products indexed under this
heading.

Fluphenazine Enanthate (Possibility of additive hypotensive effects).
No products indexed under this
heading.

Fluphenazine Hydrochloride
(Possibility of additive hypotensive
effects).
No products indexed under this
heading.

Flurazepam Hydrochloride (Con-
current use is contraindicated).
Products include:
Dalmane Capsules 3342

Fluvoxamine Maleate (Concurrent
and/or sequential use is contraindicated; potential for serious, sometimes fatal, reactions including
hyperthermia, rigidity, myoclonus,
and other toxicities).
No products indexed under this
heading.

Fosinopril Sodium (Concurrent use
with hypotensive agents is contraindicated; a marked potentiating
effect on these classes of drugs has
been reported).
No products indexed under this
heading.

Furazolidone (Concurrent use with
another MAO inhibitor may result in
hypertensive crises or severe convulsive seizures; concurrent and/or
sequential use is contraindicated).
No products indexed under this
heading.

Furosemide (Concurrent use with
hypotensive agents is contraindicated; a marked potentiating effect
on these classes of drugs has been
reported). Products include:
Furosemide Tablets 2154

Glimepiride (Some MAO inhibitors
have contributed to hypoglycemic
episodes in diabetic patients receiving oral hypoglycemic agents).
Products include:
Avandaryl Tablets 1379
Duetact Tablets 3226

Glipizide (Some MAO inhibitors
have contributed to hypoglycemic
episodes in diabetic patients receiving oral hypoglycemic agents).
No products indexed under this
heading.

Glutethimide (Concurrent use is
contraindicated).
No products indexed under this
heading.

Glyburide (Some MAO inhibitors
have contributed to hypoglycemic
episodes in diabetic patients receiving oral hypoglycemic agents).
No products indexed under this
heading.

Guanabenz Acetate (Concurrent
use with hypotensive agents is contraindicated; a marked potentiating
effect on these classes of drugs has
been reported).
No products indexed under this
heading.

Guanethidine Monosulfate (Concurrent and/or sequential use is contraindicated; combination therapy
may precipitate hypertension, headache and related symptoms).
No products indexed under this
heading.

Halothane (Patients taking tranylcypromine should not undergo elective
surgery requiring general anesthesia; the possible combined hypotensive effects of tranylcypromine
should be kept in mind; Parnate
should be discontinued at least 10
days prior to elective surgery).
No products indexed under this
heading.

Hydralazine Hydrochloride (Concurrent use with hypotensive agents
is contraindicated; a marked potentiating effect on these classes of
drugs has been reported). Products
include:
BiDil Tablets 2171

Hydrochlorothiazide (Concurrent
use with hypotensive agents is con-
traindicated; a marked potentiating
effect on these classes of drugs has
been reported). Products include:
Aldoril Tablets 1910
Atacand HCT 651
Avalide Tablets 888
Avalide Tablets 2874
Benicar HCT Tablets 1044
Diovan HCT Tablets 2196
Dyazide Capsules 1423
Hyzaar 50-12.5 Tablets 1990
Hyzaar 100-12.5 Tablets 1990
Hyzaar 100-25 Tablets 1990
Lopressor HCT 50/25 Tablets 2241
Lopressor HCT 100/25 Tablets 2241
Lopressor HCT 100/50 Tablets 2241
Lotensin HCT Tablets 2246
Micardis HCT Tablets 856
Moduretic Tablets 2028
Prinzide Tablets 2056
Teveten HCT Tablets 1737
Timolide Tablets 2086
Uniretic Tablets 3100

Hydrocodone Bitartrate (Concur-
rent use is contraindicated; a
marked potentiating effect on these
classes of drugs has been reported).
Products include:
Hycodan ... 1116
Hycotuss Expectorant Syrup 1117
Vicodin Tablets 535
Vicodin ES Tablets 536
Vicodin HP Tablets 538
Vicoprofen Tablets 539
Zydone Tablets 1139

Hydrocodone Polistirex (Concurrent use is contraindicated; a
marked potentiating effect on these
classes of drugs has been reported).
Products include:
Tussionex Pennkinetic
Extended-Release Suspension 3327

IMPORTANT NOTE: Always consult each drug listing in the patient's regimen for possible interactions.

Hydroflumethiazide (Concurrent use with hypotensive agents is contraindicated; a marked potentiating effect on these classes of drugs has been reported).
No products indexed under this heading.

Hydromorphone Hydrochloride (Concurrent use is contraindicated; a marked potentiating effect on these classes of drugs has been reported).
Products include:
- Dilaudid 440
- Dilaudid Non-Sterile Powder 440
- Dilaudid Oral Liquid 445
- Dilaudid Rectal Suppositories 440
- Dilaudid Tablets 440
- Dilaudid Tablets - 8 mg 445
- Dilaudid-HP 442

Imipramine Hydrochloride (Concurrent use with dibenzazepine-related entities may result in hypertensive crises or severe convulsive seizures; concurrent and/or sequential use is contraindicated).
No products indexed under this heading.

Imipramine Pamoate (Concurrent use with dibenzazepine-related entities may result in hypertensive crises or severe convulsive seizures; concurrent and/or sequential use is contraindicated).
No products indexed under this heading.

Indapamide (Concurrent use with hypotensive agents is contraindicated; a marked potentiating effect on these classes of drugs has been reported). Products include:
- Indapamide Tablets 2156

Insulin, Human, Zinc Suspension (Some MAO inhibitors have contributed to hypoglycemic episodes in diabetic patients receiving insulin).
Products include:
- Humulin L, 100 Units 1794
- Humulin U, 100 Units 1800

Insulin, Human NPH (Some MAO inhibitors have contributed to hypoglycemic episodes in diabetic patients receiving insulin). Products include:
- Humulin N, 100 Units 1795
- Humulin N Pen 1797

Insulin, Human Regular (Some MAO inhibitors have contributed to hypoglycemic episodes in diabetic patients receiving insulin). Products include:
- Humulin R, 100 Units 1798

Insulin, Human Regular and Human NPH Mixture (Some MAO inhibitors have contributed to hypoglycemic episodes in diabetic patients receiving insulin). Products include:
- Humulin 50/50, 100 Units 1791
- Humulin 70/30 Pen 1793

Insulin, NPH (Some MAO inhibitors have contributed to hypoglycemic episodes in diabetic patients receiving insulin).
No products indexed under this heading.

Insulin, Regular (Some MAO inhibitors have contributed to hypoglycemic episodes in diabetic patients receiving insulin).
No products indexed under this heading.

Insulin, Zinc Crystals (Some MAO inhibitors have contributed to hypoglycemic episodes in diabetic patients receiving insulin).
No products indexed under this heading.

Insulin, Zinc Suspension (Some MAO inhibitors have contributed to hypoglycemic episodes in diabetic patients receiving insulin).
No products indexed under this heading.

Insulin Aspart, Human Regular (Some MAO inhibitors have contributed to hypoglycemic episodes in diabetic patients receiving insulin).
Products include:
- NovoLog Injection 2326

Insulin glargine (Some MAO inhibitors have contributed to hypoglycemic episodes in diabetic patients receiving insulin). Products include:
- Lantus Injection 2909

Insulin Lispro, Human (Some MAO inhibitors have contributed to hypoglycemic episodes in diabetic patients receiving insulin). Products include:
- Humalog-Pen 1781
- Humalog Mix 50/50-Pen 1783
- Humalog Mix 75/25-Pen 1785

Insulin Lispro Protamine, Human (Some MAO inhibitors have contributed to hypoglycemic episodes in diabetic patients receiving insulin).
Products include:
- Humalog Mix 50/50-Pen 1783
- Humalog Mix 75/25-Pen 1785

Irbesartan (Concurrent use with hypotensive agents is contraindicated; a marked potentiating effect on these classes of drugs has been reported). Products include:
- Avalide Tablets 888
- Avalide Tablets 2874
- Avapro Tablets 891
- Avapro Tablets 2871

Isocarboxazid (Concurrent use with another MAO inhibitor may result in hypertensive crises or severe convulsive seizures; concurrent and/or sequential use is contraindicated).
No products indexed under this heading.

Isoflurane (Patients taking tranylcypromine should not undergo elective surgery requiring general anesthesia; the possible combined hypotensive effects of tranylcypromine should be kept in mind; Parnate should be discontinued at least 10 days prior to elective surgery).
No products indexed under this heading.

Isoproterenol Hydrochloride (Concurrent and/or sequential use is contraindicated; combination therapy may precipitate hypertension, headache and related symptoms).
No products indexed under this heading.

Isoproterenol Sulfate (Concurrent and/or sequential use is contraindicated; combination therapy may precipitate hypertension, headache and related symptoms).
No products indexed under this heading.

Isradipine (Concurrent use with hypotensive agents is contraindicated; a marked potentiating effect on these classes of drugs has been reported). Products include:
- DynaCirc CR Tablets 2721

Ketamine Hydrochloride (Patients taking tranylcypromine should not undergo elective surgery requiring general anesthesia; the possible combined hypotensive effects of tranylcypromine should be kept in mind; Parnate should be discontinued at least 10 days prior to elective surgery).
No products indexed under this heading.

Labetalol Hydrochloride (Concurrent use with hypotensive agents is contraindicated; a marked potentiating effect on these classes of drugs has been reported).
No products indexed under this heading.

Levalbuterol Hydrochloride (Concurrent and/or sequential use is contraindicated; combination therapy may precipitate hypertension, headache and related symptoms).
Products include:
- Xopenex Inhalation Solution 3146
- Xopenex Inhalation Solution Concentrate 3150

Levodopa (Concurrent and/or sequential use is contraindicated; combination therapy may precipitate hypertension, headache and related symptoms). Products include:
- Parcopa Orally Disintegrating Tablets 3097
- Stalevo Tablets 2287

Levorphanol Tartrate (Concurrent use is contraindicated; a marked potentiating effect on these classes of drugs has been reported).
No products indexed under this heading.

Lisinopril (Concurrent use with hypotensive agents is contraindicated; a marked potentiating effect on these classes of drugs has been reported). Products include:
- Prinivil Tablets 2052
- Prinzide Tablets 2056

Loratadine (Concurrent use is contraindicated). Products include:
- Alavert Allergy & Sinus D-12 Hour Tablets .... ▣ 771
- Alavert .... ▣ 771
- Children's Claritin Allergy Oral Solution .... ▣ 771
- Claritin Non-Drowsy 24 Hour Tablets .... ▣ 772
- Claritin Reditabs 24 Hour Non-Drowsy Tablets .... ▣ 772
- Claritin-D Non-Drowsy 12 Hour Tablets .... ▣ 772
- Claritin-D Non-Drowsy 24 Hour Tablets .... ▣ 772

Lorazepam (Concurrent use is contraindicated).
No products indexed under this heading.

Losartan Potassium (Concurrent use with hypotensive agents is contraindicated; a marked potentiating effect on these classes of drugs has been reported). Products include:
- Cozaar Tablets 1935
- Hyzaar 50-12.5 Tablets 1990
- Hyzaar 100-12.5 Tablets 1990
- Hyzaar 100-25 Tablets 1990

Maprotiline Hydrochloride (Concurrent use with dibenzazepine-related entities may result in hypertensive crises or severe convulsive seizures; concurrent and/or sequential use is contraindicated).
No products indexed under this heading.

Mazindol (Concurrent and/or sequential use is contraindicated).
No products indexed under this heading.

Mecamylamine Hydrochloride (Concurrent use with hypotensive agents is contraindicated; a marked potentiating effect on these classes of drugs has been reported).
No products indexed under this heading.

Meperidine Hydrochloride (Concomitant use or within 2 or 3 weeks following MAOI therapy is contraindicated; serious reactions including coma, severe hypertension or hypotension, convulsion, severe respiratory depression, malignant hyperplexia, excitation, peripheral vascular collapse, and death have been reported with combined use).
No products indexed under this heading.

Mesoridazine Besylate (Possibility of additive hypotensive effects).
No products indexed under this heading.

Metaproterenol Sulfate (Concurrent and/or sequential use is contraindicated; combination therapy may precipitate hypertension, headache and related symptoms). Products include:
- Alupent Inhalation Aerosol 826

Metaraminol Bitartrate (Concurrent and/or sequential use is contraindicated; combination therapy may precipitate hypertension, headache and related symptoms).
No products indexed under this heading.

Metformin Hydrochloride (Some MAO inhibitors have contributed to hypoglycemic episodes in diabetic patients receiving oral hypoglycemic agents). Products include:
- ActoPlus Met Tablets 3214
- Avandamet Tablets 1373
- Fortamet Extended-Release Tablets 3115

Methadone Hydrochloride (Concurrent use is contraindicated; a marked potentiating effect on these classes of drugs has been reported).
No products indexed under this heading.

Methamphetamine Hydrochloride (Concurrent and/or sequential use is contraindicated). Products include:
- Desoxyn Tablets, USP 2462

Methdilazine Hydrochloride (Concurrent use is contraindicated).
No products indexed under this heading.

Methohexital Sodium (Patients taking tranylcypromine should not undergo elective surgery requiring general anesthesia; the possible combined hypotensive effects of tranylcypromine should be kept in mind; Parnate should be discontinued at least 10 days prior to elective surgery).
No products indexed under this heading.

Methotrimeprazine (Possibility of additive hypotensive effects).
No products indexed under this heading.

Methoxamine Hydrochloride (Concurrent and/or sequential use is contraindicated; combination therapy may precipitate hypertension, headache and related symptoms).
No products indexed under this heading.

Methyclothiazide (Concurrent use with hypotensive agents is contraindicated; a marked potentiating effect on these classes of drugs has been reported).
No products indexed under this heading.

Methyldopa (Concurrent and/or sequential use is contraindicated; combination therapy may precipitate hypertension, headache and related symptoms). Products include:
Aldoril Tablets 1910

Methyldopate Hydrochloride (Concurrent and/or sequential use is contraindicated; combination therapy may precipitate hypertension, headache and related symptoms).
No products indexed under this heading.

Metolazone (Concurrent use with hypotensive agents is contraindicated; a marked potentiating effect on these classes of drugs has been reported).
No products indexed under this heading.

Metoprolol Succinate (Concurrent use with hypotensive agents is contraindicated; a marked potentiating effect on these classes of drugs has been reported). Products include:
Toprol-XL Tablets 668

Metoprolol Tartrate (Concurrent use with hypotensive agents is contraindicated; a marked potentiating effect on these classes of drugs has been reported). Products include:
Lopressor Injection 2238
Lopressor Tablets 2238
Lopressor HCT 50/25 Tablets 2241
Lopressor HCT 100/25 Tablets 2241
Lopressor HCT 100/50 Tablets 2241

Metrizamide (Concurrent use with drugs which lower seizure threshold, including MAO inhibitors, should not be used with metrizamide).
No products indexed under this heading.

Metyrosine (Concurrent use with hypotensive agents is contraindicated; a marked potentiating effect on these classes of drugs has been reported). Products include:
Demser Capsules 1953

Mibefradil Dihydrochloride (Concurrent use with hypotensive agents is contraindicated; a marked potentiating effect on these classes of drugs has been reported).
No products indexed under this heading.

Midazolam Hydrochloride (Patients taking tranylcypromine should not undergo elective surgery requiring general anesthesia; the possible combined hypotensive effects of tranylcypromine should be kept in mind; Parnate should be discontinued at least 10 days prior to elective surgery).
No products indexed under this heading.

Miglitol (Some MAO inhibitors have contributed to hypoglycemic episodes in diabetic patients receiving oral hypoglycemic agents).
No products indexed under this heading.

Minoxidil (Concurrent use with hypotensive agents is contraindicated; a marked potentiating effect on these classes of drugs has been reported). Products include:
Men's Rogaine Extra Strength Hair Regrowth Treatment Topical Solution, Ocean Rush Scent and Original Unscented 633
Men's Rogaine Foam Hair Regrowth Treatment 633
Women's Rogaine Hair Regrowth Treatment Topical Solution, Spring Bloom Scent and Original Unscented 634

Moclobemide (Concurrent use with another MAO inhibitor may result in hypertensive crises or severe convulsive seizures; concurrent and/or sequential use is contraindicated).
No products indexed under this heading.

Moexipril Hydrochloride (Concurrent use with hypotensive agents is contraindicated; a marked potentiating effect on these classes of drugs has been reported). Products include:
Uniretic Tablets 3100
Univasc Tablets 3104

Morphine Sulfate (Concurrent use is contraindicated; a marked potentiating effect on these classes of drugs has been reported). Products include:
Avinza Capsules 1741
Kadian Capsules 577
MS Contin Tablets 2701

Nadolol (Concurrent use with hypotensive agents is contraindicated; a marked potentiating effect on these classes of drugs has been reported). Products include:
Nadolol Tablets 2159

Naphazoline Hydrochloride (Concurrent and/or sequential use is contraindicated; combination therapy may precipitate hypertension, headache and related symptoms). Products include:
Albalon Ophthalmic Solution .... ⊙218
Naphcon-A Eye Drops .... ⊙208
Visine-A Eye Allergy Relief Eye Drops .... ⊙289

Nicardipine Hydrochloride (Concurrent use with hypotensive agents is contraindicated; a marked potentiating effect on these classes of drugs has been reported). Products include:
Cardene I.V. 2497

Nifedipine (Concurrent use with hypotensive agents is contraindicated; a marked potentiating effect on these classes of drugs has been reported). Products include:
Adalat CC Tablets 2964

Nisoldipine (Concurrent use with hypotensive agents is contraindicated; a marked potentiating effect on these classes of drugs has been reported). Products include:
Sular Tablets 3122

Nitroglycerin (Concurrent use with hypotensive agents is contraindicated; a marked potentiating effect on these classes of drugs has been reported). Products include:
Nitro-Dur Transdermal Infusion System 3046
Nitrolingual Pumpspray 3120

Norepinephrine Bitartrate (Concurrent and/or sequential use is contraindicated; combination therapy may precipitate hypertension, headache and related symptoms).
No products indexed under this heading.

Nortriptyline Hydrochloride (Concurrent use with dibenzazepine-related entities may result in hypertensive crises or severe convulsive seizures; concurrent and/or sequential use is contraindicated).
No products indexed under this heading.

Oxycodone Hydrochloride (Concurrent use is contraindicated; a marked potentiating effect on these classes of drugs has been reported). Products include:
OxyContin Tablets 2703
OxyFast Oral Concentrate Solution 2708
OxyIR Capsules 2708
Percocet Tablets 1131
Percodan Tablets 1132

Oxymetazoline Hydrochloride (Concurrent and/or sequential use is contraindicated; combination therapy may precipitate hypertension, headache and related symptoms). Products include:
Vicks Sinex Nasal Spray and Ultra Fine Mist for Sinus Relief 2681
Vicks Sinex 12-Hour Nasal Spray and Ultra Fine Mist for Sinus Relief 2681
Visine L.R. Long Lasting Eye Drops .... ⊙290
Zicam Extreme Congestion Relief 767
Zicam Intense Sinus Relief 767

Pargyline Hydrochloride (Concurrent use with another MAO inhibitor may result in hypertensive crises or severe convulsive seizures; concurrent and/or sequential use is contraindicated).
No products indexed under this heading.

Paroxetine Hydrochloride (Concurrent and/or sequential use is contraindicated; potential for serious, sometimes fatal, reactions including hyperthermia, rigidity, myoclonus, and other toxicities; at least 2 weeks should be allowed after stopping paroxetine before starting an MAO inhibitor). Products include:
Paxil CR Controlled-Release Tablets 1538
Paxil 1530

Penbutolol Sulfate (Concurrent use with hypotensive agents is contraindicated; a marked potentiating effect on these classes of drugs has been reported).
No products indexed under this heading.

Perindopril Erbumine (Concurrent use with hypotensive agents is contraindicated; a marked potentiating effect on these classes of drugs has been reported). Products include:
Aceon Tablets (2 mg, 4 mg, 8 mg) 3194

Perphenazine (Possibility of additive hypotensive effects).
No products indexed under this heading.

Phendimetrazine Tartrate (Concurrent and/or sequential use is contraindicated).
No products indexed under this heading.

Phenelzine Sulfate (Concurrent use with another MAO inhibitor may result in hypertensive crises or severe convulsive seizures; concurrent and/or sequential use is contraindicated).
No products indexed under this heading.

Phenmetrazine Hydrochloride (Concurrent and/or sequential use is contraindicated).
No products indexed under this heading.

Phenoxybenzamine Hydrochloride (Concurrent use with hypotensive agents is contraindicated; a marked potentiating effect on these classes of drugs has been reported). Products include:
Dibenzyline Capsules 3399

Phentolamine Mesylate (Concurrent use with hypotensive agents is contraindicated; a marked potentiating effect on these classes of drugs has been reported).
No products indexed under this heading.

Phenylephrine Bitartrate (Concurrent and/or sequential use is contraindicated; combination therapy may precipitate hypertension, headache and related symptoms).
No products indexed under this heading.

Phenylephrine Hydrochloride (Concurrent and/or sequential use is contraindicated; combination therapy may precipitate hypertension, headache and related symptoms). Products include:
Comtrex Maximum Strength Non-Drowsy Cold & Cough Caplets 725
Comtrex Maximum Strength Day/Night Severe Cold & Sinus Caplets - Day Formulation 725
Comtrex Maximum Strength Day/Night Severe Cold & Sinus Caplets - Night Formulation 725
Contac Cold and Flu Maximum Strength Caplets 728
Contac Cold and Flu Day and Night Caplets (Day Formulation Only) 727
Contac Cold and Flu Day and Night Caplets (Night Formulation Only) 727
Contac Cold and Flu Non-Drowsy Caplets 728
Contac-D Cold Non-Drowsy Tablets 729
Children's Dimetapp Cold & Allergy Elixir 730
Children's Dimetapp Cold & Allergy Chewable Tablets 730
Children's Dimetapp DM Cold & Cough Elixir 731
Toddler's Dimetapp Cold and Cough Drops 732
Excedrin Sinus Headache Caplets/Tablets 610
4-Way Fast Acting Nasal Spray 775
4-Way Menthol Nasal Spray 775
Preparation H Maximum Strength Cream 666
Preparation H Cooling Gel 666
Preparation H 666
Refenesen PE Caplets 721
Robitussin Cough & Allergy Syrup 736
Robitussin Cough & Cold Nighttime Liquid 736
Robitussin Cough, Cold & Flu Nighttime Liquid 738
Robitussin Head & Chest Congestion PE Syrup 739
Robitussin Pediatric Cough & Cold Nighttime Liquid 736
TheraFlu Cold & Cough Hot Liquid 740
TheraFlu Cold & Sore Throat Hot Liquid 741
TheraFlu Flu & Sore Throat Hot Liquid 742
TheraFlu Daytime Severe Cold Hot Liquid 742
TheraFlu Nighttime Severe Cold Hot Liquid 740
TheraFlu Warming Relief Daytime Severe Cold 743
TheraFlu Warming Relief Nighttime Severe Cold 743

Triaminic Chest & Nasal Congestion Liquid ▣ 746
Triaminic Cold & Allergy Liquid ▣ 746
Triaminic Daytime Cold & Cough Liquid ▣ 745
Triaminic Nighttime Cold & Cough Liquid ▣ 746
Triaminic Thin Strips Cold ▣ 748
Triaminic Thin Strips Cold & Cough ▣ 778
Triaminic Infant Thin Strips Decongestant ▣ 747
Triaminic Infant Thin Strips Decongestant Plus Cough ▣ 747
Children's Tylenol Plus Flu Oral Suspension ▣ 749
Tylenol Cold Head Congestion Daytime Caplets with Cool Burst and Gelcaps ▣ 750
Tylenol Cold Multi-Symptom Daytime Liquid ▣ 752
Tylenol Cold Multi-Symptom Severe Daytime Liquid ▣ 752
Concentrated Tylenol Infants' Drops Plus Cold & Cough ▣ 754
Tylenol Allergy Multi-Symptom Caplets with Cool Burst and Gelcaps 1872
Tylenol Allergy Multi-Symptom Nighttime Caplets with Cool Burst 1872
Children's Tylenol Plus Cold Suspension Liquid 1879
Children's Tylenol Plus Cold & Allergy Suspension Liquid 1878
Children's Tylenol Plus Flu Suspension Liquid 1881
Children's Tylenol Plus Multi-Symptom Cold Suspension Liquid 1879
Tylenol Cold Head Congestion Daytime Caplets with Cool Burst 1873
Tylenol Cold Head Congestion Nighttime Caplets with Cool Burst 1873
Tylenol Cold Head Congestion Severe Caplets with Cool Burst 1873
Tylenol Cold Multi-Symptom Daytime Caplets with Cool Burst and Gelcaps 1874
Tylenol Cold Multi-Symptom Daytime Liquid with Citrus Burst 1874
Tylenol Cold Multi-Symptom Nighttime Caplets with Cool Burst 1874
Tylenol Cold Multi-Symptom Nighttime Liquid with Cool Burst 1874
Tylenol Cold Multi-Symptom Severe Caplets with Cool Burst 1874
Tylenol Cold Multi-Symptom Severe Daytime Liquid with Citrus Burst 1874
Tylenol Sinus Congestion & Pain Daytime Caplets with Cool Burst and Gelcaps 1876
Tylenol Sinus Congestion & Pain Nighttime Caplets with Cool Burst 1876
Tylenol Sinus Congestion & Pain Severe Caplets with Cool Burst 1876
Vicks 44D Cough & Head Congestion Relief Liquid ▣ 760
Vicks DayQuil LiquiCaps/Liquid Multi-Symptom Cold/Flu Relief ▣ 761
Zicam Cough Plus D Cough Spray ▣ 767

Phenylephrine Tannate (Concurrent and/or sequential use is contraindicated; combination therapy may precipitate hypertension, headache and related symptoms).
No products indexed under this heading.

Phenylpropanolamine Hydrochloride (Concurrent and/or sequential use is contraindicated; combination therapy may precipitate hypertension, headache and related symptoms).
No products indexed under this heading.

Pindolol (Concurrent use with hypotensive agents is contraindicated; a marked potentiating effect on these classes of drugs has been reported).
No products indexed under this heading.

Pioglitazone Hydrochloride (Some MAO inhibitors have contributed to hypoglycemic episodes in diabetic patients receiving oral hypoglycemic agents). Products include:
ActoPlus Met Tablets 3214
Actos Tablets 3219
Duetact Tablets 3226

Pirbuterol Acetate (Concurrent and/or sequential use is contraindicated; combination therapy may precipitate hypertension, headache and related symptoms). Products include:
Maxair Autohaler 1852

Polythiazide (Concurrent use with hypotensive agents is contraindicated; a marked potentiating effect on these classes of drugs has been reported).
No products indexed under this heading.

Prazosin Hydrochloride (Concurrent use with hypotensive agents is contraindicated; a marked potentiating effect on these classes of drugs has been reported).
No products indexed under this heading.

Procarbazine Hydrochloride (Concurrent use with another MAO inhibitor may result in hypertensive crises or severe convulsive seizures; concurrent and/or sequential use is contraindicated). Products include:
Matulane Capsules 3191

Prochlorperazine (Possibility of additive hypotensive effects).
No products indexed under this heading.

Procyclidine Hydrochloride (Anti-Parkinsonism drugs should be used with caution in patients receiving Parnate since severe reactions have been reported).
No products indexed under this heading.

Promethazine Hydrochloride (Concurrent use is contraindicated). Products include:
Phenergan Tablets and Suppositories 3440

Propofol (Patients taking tranylcypromine should not undergo elective surgery requiring general anesthesia; the possible combined hypotensive effects of tranylcypromine should be kept in mind; Parnate should be discontinued at least 10 days prior to elective surgery).
No products indexed under this heading.

Propoxyphene Hydrochloride (Concurrent use is contraindicated; a marked potentiating effect on these classes of drugs has been reported).
No products indexed under this heading.

Propoxyphene Napsylate (Concurrent use is contraindicated; a marked potentiating effect on these classes of drugs has been reported).
No products indexed under this heading.

Propranolol Hydrochloride (Concurrent use with hypotensive agents is contraindicated; a marked potentiating effect on these classes of drugs has been reported). Products include:
Inderal LA Long-Acting Capsules 3429
InnoPran XL Capsules 2723

Protriptyline Hydrochloride (Concurrent use with dibenzazepine-related entities may result in hypertensive crises or severe convulsive seizures; concurrent and/or sequential use is contraindicated).
No products indexed under this heading.

Pseudoephedrine Hydrochloride (Concurrent and/or sequential use is contraindicated; combination therapy may precipitate hypertension, headache and related symptoms). Products include:
Advil Allergy Sinus Caplets ▣ 770
Advil Cold & Sinus ▣ 723
Advil Multi-Symptom Cold Caplets ▣ 770
Aleve Cold & Sinus Caplets 744
Allegra-D 12 Hour Extended-Release Tablets 2846
Allegra-D 24 Hour Extended-Release Tablets 2849
BC Cold Powder ▣ 677
Comtrex Maximum Strength Cold & Cough Day/Night Caplets - Day Formulation ▣ 726
Comtrex Maximum Strength Cold & Cough Day/Night Caplets - Night Formulation ▣ 726
Children's Motrin Cold Oral Suspension 1867
Mucinex D Extended-Release Bi-Layer Tablets ▣ 776
Robitussin Cough & Cold CF Liquid ▣ 735
Robitussin Cough & Cold Pediatric Drops ▣ 735
Tylenol Sinus Congestion & Pain Nighttime Caplets with Cool Burst ▣ 778
Tylenol Cold Severe Congestion Non-Drowsy Caplets with Cool Burst 1874
Tylenol Sinus Severe Congestion Caplets with Cool Burst 1876
Vicks 44D Cough & Head Congestion Relief Liquid 2679
Vicks 44M Cough, Cold & Flu Relief Liquid 2680
Vicks DayQuil Multi-Symptom Cold/Flu Relief LiquiCaps 2678
Vicks DayQuil Multi-Symptom Cold/Flu Relief Liquid 2678
Vicks NyQuil Multi-Symptom Cold/Flu Relief Liquid 2681
Vicks NyQuil Multi-Symptom Cold/Flu Relief LiquiCaps 2681
Children's Vicks NyQuil Cold/Cough Relief Liquid 2680
Zyrtec-D 12 Hour Extended Release Tablets 2597

Pseudoephedrine Sulfate (Concurrent and/or sequential use is contraindicated; combination therapy may precipitate hypertension, headache and related symptoms). Products include:
Alavert Allergy & Sinus D-12 Hour Tablets ▣ 771
Clarinex-D 24-Hour Extended-Release Tablets 2998
Claritin-D Non-Drowsy 12 Hour Tablets ▣ 772
Claritin-D Non-Drowsy 24 Hour Tablets ▣ 772

Pyrilamine Maleate (Concurrent use is contraindicated).
No products indexed under this heading.

Pyrilamine Tannate (Concurrent use is contraindicated).
No products indexed under this heading.

Quazepam (Concurrent use is contraindicated).
No products indexed under this heading.

Quinapril Hydrochloride (Concurrent use with hypotensive agents is contraindicated; a marked potentiating effect on these classes of drugs has been reported).
No products indexed under this heading.

Ramelteon (Concurrent use is contraindicated). Products include:
Rozerem Tablets 3231

Ramipril (Concurrent use with hypotensive agents is contraindicated; a marked potentiating effect on these classes of drugs has been reported). Products include:
Altace Capsules 1702

Rauwolfia Serpentina (Concurrent use with hypotensive agents is contraindicated; a marked potentiating effect on these classes of drugs has been reported).
No products indexed under this heading.

Remifentanil Hydrochloride (Concurrent use is contraindicated; a marked potentiating effect on these classes of drugs has been reported).
No products indexed under this heading.

Repaglinide (Some MAO inhibitors have contributed to hypoglycemic episodes in diabetic patients receiving oral hypoglycemic agents).
No products indexed under this heading.

Rescinnamine (Concurrent use with hypotensive agents is contraindicated; a marked potentiating effect on these classes of drugs has been reported).
No products indexed under this heading.

Reserpine (Concurrent and/or sequential use is contraindicated; combination therapy may precipitate hypertension, headache and related symptoms).
No products indexed under this heading.

Rosiglitazone Maleate (Some MAO inhibitors have contributed to hypoglycemic episodes in diabetic patients receiving oral hypoglycemic agents). Products include:
Avandamet Tablets 1373
Avandaryl Tablets 1379
Avandia Tablets 1384

Salmeterol Xinafoate (Concurrent and/or sequential use is contraindicated; combination therapy may precipitate hypertension, headache and related symptoms). Products include:
Advair Diskus 100/50 1308
Advair Diskus 250/50 1308
Advair Diskus 500/50 1308
Advair HFA Inhalation Aerosol 1318
Serevent Diskus 1568

Secobarbital Sodium (Concurrent use is contraindicated).
No products indexed under this heading.

Selegiline Hydrochloride (Concurrent use with another MAO inhibitor may result in hypertensive crises or severe convulsive seizures; concurrent and/or sequential use is contraindicated). Products include:
Eldepryl Capsules 3208
Zelapar Tablets 3372

Sertraline Hydrochloride (Concurrent and/or sequential use is contraindicated; potential for serious, sometimes fatal, reactions, including hyperthermia, rigidity, myoclonus, and other toxicities; at least 2 weeks

should be allowed after stopping sertraline before starting an MAOinhibitor). Products include:
Zoloft 2586

Sibutramine Hydrochloride Monohydrate (Concurrent and/or sequential use is contraindicated). Products include:
Meridia Capsules 489

Sodium Nitroprusside (Concurrent use with hypotensive agents is contraindicated; a marked potentiating effect on these classes of drugs has been reported).
No products indexed under this heading.

Sotalol Hydrochloride (Concurrent use with hypotensive agents is contraindicated; a marked potentiating effect on these classes of drugs has been reported).
No products indexed under this heading.

Spirapril Hydrochloride (Concurrent use with hypotensive agents is contraindicated; a marked potentiating effect on these classes of drugs has been reported).
No products indexed under this heading.

Spironolactone (Concurrent use with hypotensive agents is contraindicated; a marked potentiating effect on these classes of drugs has been reported).
No products indexed under this heading.

Sufentanil Citrate (Concurrent use is contraindicated; a marked potentiating effect on these classes of drugs has been reported).
No products indexed under this heading.

Telmisartan (Concurrent use with hypotensive agents is contraindicated; a marked potentiating effect on these classes of drugs has been reported). Products include:
Micardis Tablets 854
Micardis HCT Tablets 856

Temazepam (Concurrent use is contraindicated). Products include:
Restoril Capsules 1860

Terazosin Hydrochloride (Concurrent use with hypotensive agents is contraindicated; a marked potentiating effect on these classes of drugs has been reported). Products include:
Hytrin Capsules 471

Terbutaline Sulfate (Concurrent and/or sequential use is contraindicated; combination therapy may precipitate hypertension, headache and related symptoms).
No products indexed under this heading.

Terfenadine (Concurrent use is contraindicated).
No products indexed under this heading.

Tetrahydrozoline Hydrochloride (Concurrent and/or sequential use is contraindicated; combination therapy may precipitate hypertension, headache and related symptoms). Products include:
Visine Original Eye Drops .... ⊙290
Visine A.C. Seasonal Itching and Redness Relief Drops .... ⊙289
Advanced Relief Visine Eye Drops ... ⊙288

Thiamylal Sodium (Patients taking tranylcypromine should not undergo elective surgery requiring general anesthesia; the possible combined hypotensive effects of tranylcypromine should be kept in mind; Parnate should be discontinued at least 10 days prior to elective surgery).
No products indexed under this heading.

Thioridazine Hydrochloride (Possibility of additive hypotensive effects). Products include:
Thioridazine Hydrochloride Tablets 2163

Timolol Maleate (Concurrent use with hypotensive agents is contraindicated; a marked potentiating effect on these classes of drugs has been reported). Products include:
Blocadren Tablets 1916
Cosopt Sterile Ophthalmic Solution 1931
Timolide Tablets 2086
Timoptic Sterile Ophthalmic Solution 2088
Timoptic in Ocudose 2091
Timoptic-XE Sterile Ophthalmic Gel Forming Solution 2092

Tolazamide (Some MAO inhibitors have contributed to hypoglycemic episodes in diabetic patients receiving oral hypoglycemic agents).
No products indexed under this heading.

Tolbutamide (Some MAO inhibitors have contributed to hypoglycemic episodes in diabetic patients receiving oral hypoglycemic agents).
No products indexed under this heading.

Torsemide (Concurrent use with hypotensive agents is contraindicated; a marked potentiating effect on these classes of drugs has been reported). Products include:
Demadex Injection 2759
Demadex Tablets 2759

Trandolapril (Concurrent use with hypotensive agents is contraindicated; a marked potentiating effect on these classes of drugs has been reported). Products include:
Mavik Tablets 486
Tarka Tablets 524

Triamterene (Concurrent use with hypotensive agents is contraindicated; a marked potentiating effect on these classes of drugs has been reported). Products include:
Dyazide Capsules 1423
Dyrenium Capsules 3400

Triazolam (Concurrent use is contraindicated).
No products indexed under this heading.

Tridihexethyl Chloride (Anti-Parkinsonism drugs should be used with caution in patients receiving Parnate since severe reactions have been reported).
No products indexed under this heading.

Trifluoperazine Hydrochloride (Possibility of additive hypotensive effects).
No products indexed under this heading.

Trihexyphenidyl Hydrochloride (Anti-Parkinsonism drugs should be used with caution in patients receiving Parnate since severe reactions have been reported).
No products indexed under this heading.

Trimeprazine Tartrate (Concurrent use is contraindicated).
No products indexed under this heading.

Trimethaphan Camsylate (Concurrent use with hypotensive agents is contraindicated; a marked potentiating effect on these classes of drugs has been reported).
No products indexed under this heading.

Trimipramine Maleate (Concurrent use with dibenzazepine-related entities may result in hypertensive crises or severe convulsive seizures; concurrent and/or sequential use is contraindicated).
No products indexed under this heading.

Tripelennamine Hydrochloride (Concurrent use is contraindicated).
No products indexed under this heading.

Triprolidine Hydrochloride (Concurrent use is contraindicated).
No products indexed under this heading.

Troglitazone (Some MAO inhibitors have contributed to hypoglycemic episodes in diabetic patients receiving oral hypoglycemic agents).
No products indexed under this heading.

L-Tryptophan (Concurrent and/or sequential use is contraindicated; combination therapy may precipitate hypertension, disorientation, memory impairment, other neurologic and behavioral changes, headache and related symptoms). Products include:
L-Tryptophan Capsules 2145

Tyramine (Concurrent use is contraindicated).
No products indexed under this heading.

Valsartan (Concurrent use with hypotensive agents is contraindicated; a marked potentiating effect on these classes of drugs has been reported). Products include:
Diovan Tablets 2193
Diovan HCT Tablets 2196

Verapamil Hydrochloride (Concurrent use with hypotensive agents is contraindicated; a marked potentiating effect on these classes of drugs has been reported). Products include:
Covera-HS Tablets 3139
Tarka Tablets 524
Verelan PM Extended-Release Capsules, Controlled-Onset 3106

Zaleplon (Concurrent use is contraindicated). Products include:
Sonata Capsules 1717

Zolpidem Tartrate (Concurrent use is contraindicated). Products include:
Ambien Tablets 2851
Ambien CR Tablets 2855

Food Interactions

Alcohol (Concurrent use is contraindicated; a marked potentiating effect on alcohol has been reported).

Anchovies (Potential for hypertensive crisis; concurrent use is contraindicated).

Avocados (Potential for hypertensive crisis; concurrent use is contraindicated).

Bananas (Potential for hypertensive crisis; concurrent use is contraindicated).

Beans, broad (Potential for hypertensive crisis; concurrent use is contraindicated).

Beans, Fava (Potential for hypertensive crisis; concurrent use is contraindicated).

Beer, alcohol-free (Potential for hypertensive crisis; concurrent use is contraindicated).

Beer, unspecified (Potential for hypertensive crisis; concurrent use is contraindicated).

Beverages, caffeine-containing (Potential for hypertensive crisis; concurrent use is contraindicated).

Caviar (Potential for hypertensive crisis; concurrent use is contraindicated).

Cheese, aged (Potential for hypertensive crisis; concurrent use is contraindicated).

Cheese, strong, unpasteurized (Potential for hypertensive crisis; concurrent use is contraindicated).

Cheese, unspecified (Potential for hypertensive crisis; concurrent use is contraindicated).

Chocolate (Potential for hypertensive crisis; concurrent use is contraindicated).

Cream, sour (Potential for hypertensive crisis; concurrent use is contraindicated).

Figs, canned (Potential for hypertensive crisis; concurrent use is contraindicated).

Food with high concentration of tyramine (Potential for hypertensive crisis; concurrent use is contraindicated).

Fruits, dried (Potential for hypertensive crisis; concurrent use is contraindicated).

Fruits, overripe (Potential for hypertensive crisis; concurrent use is contraindicated).

Herring, pickled (Potential for hypertensive crisis; concurrent use is contraindicated).

Liqueurs (Potential for hypertensive crisis; concurrent use is contraindicated).

Liver (Potential for hypertensive crisis; concurrent use is contraindicated).

Meat extracts (Potential for hypertensive crisis; concurrent use is contraindicated).

Meat prepared with tenderizers (Potential for hypertensive crisis; concurrent use is contraindicated).

Prunes (Potential for hypertensive crisis; concurrent use is contraindicated).

Raisins (Potential for hypertensive crisis; concurrent use is contraindicated).

Raspberries (Potential for hypertensive crisis; concurrent use is contraindicated).

Sauerkraut (Potential for hypertensive crisis; concurrent use is contraindicated).

Sherry (Potential for hypertensive crisis; concurrent use is contraindicated).

Soy Sauce (Potential for hypertensive crisis; concurrent use is contraindicated).

Wine, Chianti (Potential for hypertensive crisis; concurrent use is contraindicated).

Yeast Extract (Potential for hypertensive crisis; concurrent use is contraindicated).

Yogurt (Potential for hypertensive crisis; concurrent use is contraindicated).

PASER GRANULES
(Aminosalicylic Acid) 1674
May interact with:

Digoxin (Potential for reduced digoxin levels). Products include:
Lanoxicaps Capsules 1490
Lanoxin Injection 1494
Lanoxin Injection Pediatric 1497
Lanoxin Tablets 1500

Isoniazid (Concurrent use with a rapidly available form of aminosalicylic acid has been reported to produce a 20% reduction in the acetylation of INH; the lower serum levels produced by delayed release preparation will result in a reduced effect on the acetylation of INH).
No products indexed under this heading.

Rifampin (May block the absorption of rifampin; PASER granules do not contain excipient that blocks the absorption).
No products indexed under this heading.

Vitamin B_{12} (Reduced absorption of vitamin B_{12} with clinically significant erythrocyte abnormalities developing after depletion). Products include:
Animi-3 Capsules 2492
Authia Cream 3404
Bevitamel Tablets 3404
Folgard RX Tablets 3337

PATANOL OPHTHALMIC SOLUTION
(Olopatadine Hydrochloride) 561
None cited in PDR database.

PAXIL CR CONTROLLED-RELEASE TABLETS
(Paroxetine Hydrochloride) 1538
See Paxil Tablets

PAXIL ORAL SUSPENSION
(Paroxetine Hydrochloride) 1530
See Paxil Tablets

PAXIL TABLETS
(Paroxetine Hydrochloride) 1530
May interact with anticoagulants, cytochrome p450 2d6 inhibitors (selected), cytochrome p450 2d6 substrates (selected), lithium preparations, monoamine oxidase inhibitors, non-steroidal anti-inflammatory agents, phenothiazines, phenytoin, highly protein bound drugs (selected), serotoninergic agents, selective serotonin reuptake inhibitors, tricyclic antidepressants, triptans, xanthines, and certain other agents. Compounds in these categories include:

Almotriptan Malate (There have been rare postmarketing reports of serotonin syndrome with the use of an SSRI and a triptan. If concomitant use of paroxetine hydrochloride with a triptan is clinically warranted, careful observation of the patient is advised, particularly during treatment initiation and dose increases). Products include:
Axert Tablets 2396

Aminophylline (There have been reports of elevated theophylline levels associated with co-administration; monitor theophylline levels when these drugs are concurrently administered).
No products indexed under this heading.

Amiodarone Hydrochloride (Paroxetine is metabolized by the cytochrome P450 isoenzyme CYP2D6. Therefore, co-administration of paroxetine with other drugs that inhibit this enzyme should be approached with caution).
No products indexed under this heading.

Amitriptyline Hydrochloride (Caution is indicated in the co-administration of tricyclic antidepressants with paroxetine because paroxetine may inhibit TCA metabolism. Plasma TCA concentrations may need to be monitored and the dose of TCA may need to be reduced if a TCA is co-administered with paroxetine).
No products indexed under this heading.

Amoxapine (Caution is indicated in the co-administration of tricyclic antidepressants with paroxetine because paroxetine may inhibit TCA metabolism. Plasma TCA concentrations may need to be monitored and the dose of TCA may need to be reduced if a TCA is co-administered with paroxetine).
No products indexed under this heading.

Amphetamine Aspartate (Paroxetine may significantly inhibit the activity of the cytochrome P450 2D6 isoenzyme. Concomitant use of paroxetine with other drugs metabolized by cytochrome CYP2D6 has not been formally studied but may require lower doses than usually prescribed for either paroxetine or the other drug. Therefore, co-administration of paroxetine with other drugs that are metabolized by this isozyme should be approached with caution). Products include:
Adderall Tablets 3164
Adderall XR Capsules 3166

Amphetamine Aspartate Monohydrate (Paroxetine may significantly inhibit the activity of the cytochrome P450 2D6 isoenzyme. Concomitant use of paroxetine with other drugs metabolized by cytochrome CYP2D6 has not been formally studied but may require lower doses than usually prescribed for either paroxetine or the other drug. Therefore, co-administration of paroxetine with other drugs that are metabolized by this isozyme should be approached with caution).
No products indexed under this heading.

Amphetamine Sulfate (Paroxetine may significantly inhibit the activity of the cytochrome P450 2D6 isoenzyme. Concomitant use of paroxetine with other drugs metabolized by cytochrome CYP2D6 has not been formally studied but may require lower doses than usually prescribed for either paroxetine or the other drug. Therefore, co-administration of paroxetine with other drugs that are metabolized by this isozyme should be approached with caution). Products include:
Adderall Tablets 3164
Adderall XR Capsules 3166

Anisindione (The combined use of psychotropic drugs that interfere with serotonin reuptake and drugs that affect coagulation has been associated with an increased risk of bleeding; concomitant administration should be undertaken with caution). Products include:
Miradon Tablets 3042

Ardeparin Sodium (The combined use of psychotropic drugs that interfere with serotonin reuptake and drugs that affect coagulation has been associated with an increased risk of bleeding; concomitant administration should be undertaken with caution).
No products indexed under this heading.

Aspirin (The combined use of psychotropic drugs that interfere with serotonin reuptake and drugs that affect coagulation has been associated with an increased risk of bleeding). Products include:
Aggrenox Capsules 822
Bayer Aspirin 744
BC Allergy Sinus Cold Powder .... ▣ 677
BC Headache Powder .... ▣ 677
Arthritis Strength BC Powder .... ▣ 677
BC Sinus Cold Powder .... ▣ 677
Excedrin Extra Strength Caplets/Tablets/Geltabs .... ▣ 684
Excedrin Migraine Caplets/Tablets/Geltabs .... ▣ 609
Goody's Body Pain Formula Powder .... ▣ 684
Goody's Extra Strength Headache Powders .... ▣ 611
Goody's Extra Strength Pain Relief Tablets .... ▣ 685
Percodan Tablets 1132
St. Joseph 81 mg Aspirin Chewable and Enteric Coated Tablets 1869

Aspirin, Enteric Coated (The combined use of psychotropic drugs that interfere with serotonin reuptake and drugs that affect coagulation has been associated with an increased risk of bleeding).
No products indexed under this heading.

Aspirin Buffered (The combined use of psychotropic drugs that interfere with serotonin reuptake and drugs that affect coagulation has been associated with an increased risk of bleeding). Products include:
Bufferin Extra Strength Tablets ...... ▣ 678
Bufferin Regular Strength Tablets ... ▣ 678

Atomoxetine Hydrochloride (Paroxetine may significantly inhibit the activity of the cytochrome P450 2D6 isoenzyme. Concomitant use of paroxetine with other drugs metabolized by cytochrome CYP2D6 has not been formally studied but may require lower doses than usually prescribed for either paroxetine or the other drug. Therefore, co-administration of paroxetine with other drugs that are metabolized by this isozyme should be approached with caution). Products include:
Strattera Capsules 1814

Atovaquone (Co-administration with another drug that is highly protein bound may increase free concentrations of the other drug or paroxetine potentially resulting in adverse events). Products include:
Malarone Pediatric Tablets 1517
Malarone Tablets 1517
Mepron Suspension 1521

Bisoprolol Fumarate (Paroxetine may significantly inhibit the activity of the cytochrome P450 2D6 isoenzyme. Concomitant use of paroxetine with other drugs metabolized by cytochrome CYP2D6 has not been formally studied but may require lower doses than usually prescribed for either paroxetine or the other drug. Therefore, co-administration of paroxetine with other drugs that are metabolized by this isozyme should be approached with caution).
No products indexed under this heading.

Bupropion Hydrochloride (Paroxetine is metabolized by the cytochrome P450 isoenzyme CYP2D6. Therefore, co-administration of paroxetine with other drugs that inhibit this enzyme should be approached with caution). Products include:
Wellbutrin Tablets 1603
Wellbutrin SR Sustained-Release Tablets 1607
Wellbutrin XL Extended-Release Tablets 1613
Zyban Sustained-Release Tablets 1644

Captopril (Paroxetine may significantly inhibit the activity of the cytochrome P450 2D6 isoenzyme. Concomitant use of paroxetine with other drugs metabolized by cytochrome CYP2D6 has not been formally studied but may require lower doses than usually prescribed for either paroxetine or the other drug. Therefore, co-administration of paroxetine with other drugs that are metabolized by this isozyme should be approached with caution). Products include:
Captopril Tablets 2149

Carvedilol (Paroxetine may significantly inhibit the activity of the cytochrome P450 2D6 isoenzyme. Concomitant use of paroxetine with other drugs metabolized by cytochrome CYP2D6 has not been formally studied but may require lower doses than usually prescribed for either paroxetine or the other drug. Therefore, co-administration of paroxetine with other drugs that are metabolized by this isozyme should be approached with caution). Products include:
Coreg Tablets 1414

Cefonicid Sodium (Co-administration with another drug that is highly protein bound may increase free concentrations of the other drug or paroxetine potentially resulting in adverse events).
No products indexed under this heading.

Celecoxib (Paroxetine is metabolized by the cytochrome P450 isoenzyme CYP2D6. Therefore, co-administration of paroxetine with other drugs that inhibit this enzyme should be approached with caution). Products include:
Celebrex Capsules 3134

Cevimeline Hydrochloride (Paroxetine may significantly inhibit the activity of the cytochrome P450 2D6 isoenzyme. Concomitant use of paroxetine with other drugs metabolized by cytochrome CYP2D6 has not been formally studied but may require lower doses than usually prescribed for either paroxetine or the other drug. Therefore, co-administration of paroxetine with other drugs that are metabolized by this isozyme should be approached with caution). Products include:
Evoxac Capsules 1047

Chlordiazepoxide (Co-administration with another drug that is highly protein bound may increase free concentrations of the other drug or paroxetine potentially resulting in adverse events).
No products indexed under this heading.

Chlordiazepoxide Hydrochloride (Co-administration with another drug that is highly protein bound may increase free concentrations of the other drug or paroxetine potentially resulting in adverse events). Products include:

- Librium Capsules 3347

Chloroquine Hydrochloride (Paroxetine is metabolized by the cytochrome P450 isoenzyme CYP2D6. Therefore, co-administration of paroxetine with other drugs that inhibit this enzyme should be approached with caution).

No products indexed under this heading.

Chloroquine Phosphate (Paroxetine is metabolized by the cytochrome P450 isoenzyme CYP2D6. Therefore, co-administration of paroxetine with other drugs that inhibit this enzyme should be approached with caution).

No products indexed under this heading.

Chlorpheniramine (Paroxetine is metabolized by the cytochrome P450 isoenzyme CYP2D6. Therefore, co-administration of paroxetine with other drugs that inhibit this enzyme should be approached with caution).

No products indexed under this heading.

Chlorpheniramine Maleate (Paroxetine is metabolized by the cytochrome P450 isoenzyme CYP2D6. Therefore, co-administration of paroxetine with other drugs that inhibit this enzyme should be approached with caution). Products include:

- Advil Allergy Sinus Caplets 770
- Advil Multi-Symptom Cold Caplets 770
- BC Allergy Sinus Cold Powder 677
- Comtrex Maximum Strength Cold & Cough Day/Night Caplets - Night Formulation 726
- Comtrex Maximum Strength Day/Night Severe Cold & Sinus Caplets - Night Formulation 725
- Contac Cold and Flu Maximum Strength Caplets 728
- Contac Cold and Flu Day and Night Caplets (Night Formulation Only) 727
- Children's Dimetapp Long Acting Cough Plus Cold Syrup 731
- Robitussin Cough & Cold Long-Acting Liquid 735
- Robitussin Cough & Allergy Syrup .. 736
- Robitussin Cough & Cold Nighttime Liquid 736
- Robitussin Cough, Cold & Flu Nighttime Liquid 738
- Robitussin Pediatric Cough & Cold Long-Acting Liquid 735
- Robitussin Pediatric Cough & Cold Nighttime Liquid 736
- Triaminic Cold & Allergy Liquid 746
- Triaminic Cough & Runny Nose Softchews 748
- Children's Tylenol Plus Flu Oral Suspension 749
- Tylenol Allergy Multi-Symptom Caplets with Cool Burst and Gelcaps 1872
- Children's Tylenol Plus Cold Suspension Liquid 1879
- Children's Tylenol Plus Cough & Runny Nose Suspension Liquid 1879
- Children's Tylenol Plus Flu Suspension Liquid 1881
- Children's Tylenol Plus Multi-Symptom Cold Suspension Liquid 1879
- Tylenol Cold Head Congestion Nighttime Caplets with Cool Burst 1873
- Tylenol Cold Multi-Symptom Nighttime Caplets with Cool Burst 1874
- Tylenol Sinus Congestion & Pain Nighttime Caplets with Cool Burst 1876
- Vicks 44M Cough, Cold & Flu Relief Liquid 2680
- Pediatric Vicks 44m Cough & Cold Relief Liquid 2676
- Children's Vicks NyQuil Cold/Cough Relief 756
- Children's Vicks NyQuil Cold/Cough Relief Liquid 2680
- Zicam Maximum Strength Flu Daytime 768

Chlorpheniramine Polistirex (Paroxetine is metabolized by the cytochrome P450 isoenzyme CYP2D6. Therefore, co-administration of paroxetine with other drugs that inhibit this enzyme should be approached with caution). Products include:

- Tussionex Pennkinetic Extended-Release Suspension 3327

Chlorpheniramine Tannate (Paroxetine is metabolized by the cytochrome P450 isoenzyme CYP2D6. Therefore, co-administration of paroxetine with other drugs that inhibit this enzyme should be approached with caution).

No products indexed under this heading.

Chlorpromazine (Paroxetine may significantly inhibit the activity of cytochrome P450 2D6 isoenzyme. Concomitant use of paroxetine with other drugs metabolized by cytochrome CYP2D6 has not been formally studied but may require lower doses than usually prescribed for either paroxetine or the other drug. Therefore, co-administration of paroxetine with other drugs that are metabolized by this isozyme should be approached with caution).

No products indexed under this heading.

Chlorpromazine Hydrochloride (Paroxetine may significantly inhibit the activity of cytochrome P450 2D6 isoenzyme. Concomitant use of paroxetine with other drugs metabolized by cytochrome CYP2D6 has not been formally studied but may require lower doses than usually prescribed for either paroxetine or the other drug. Therefore, co-administration of paroxetine with other drugs that are metabolized by this isozyme should be approached with caution).

No products indexed under this heading.

Chlorpropamide (Paroxetine may significantly inhibit the activity of the cytochrome P450 2D6 isoenzyme. Concomitant use of paroxetine with other drugs metabolized by cytochrome CYP2D6 has not been formally studied but may require lower doses than usually prescribed for either paroxetine or the other drug. Therefore, co-administration of paroxetine with other drugs that are metabolized by this isozyme should be approached with caution).

No products indexed under this heading.

Cimetidine (Co-administration with oral cimetidine has resulted in an increase in steady-state plasma concentrations of paroxetine). Products include:

- Tagamet HB 200 Tablets 664

Cimetidine Hydrochloride (Co-administration with oral cimetidine has resulted in an increase in steady-state plasma concentrations of paroxetine).

No products indexed under this heading.

Citalopram Hydrobromide (Paroxetine is metabolized by the cytochrome P450 isoenzyme CYP2D6. Therefore, co-administration of paroxetine with other drugs that inhibit this enzyme should be approached with caution). Products include:

- Celexa 1176

Clomipramine Hydrochloride (Caution is indicated in the co-administration of tricyclic antidepressants with paroxetine because paroxetine may inhibit TCA metabolism. Plasma TCA concentrations may need to be monitored and the dose of TCA may need to be reduced if a TCA is co-administered with paroxetine).

No products indexed under this heading.

Clozapine (Paroxetine may significantly inhibit the activity of the cytochrome P450 2D6 isoenzyme. Concomitant use of paroxetine with other drugs metabolized by cytochrome CYP2D6 has not been formally studied but may require lower doses than usually prescribed for either paroxetine or the other drug. Therefore, co-administration of paroxetine with other drugs that are metabolized by this isozyme should be approached with caution). Products include:

- Clozaril Tablets 2184
- FazaClo Orally Disintegrating Tablets 551

Cocaine Hydrochloride (Paroxetine is metabolized by the cytochrome P450 isoenzyme CYP2D6. Therefore, co-administration of paroxetine with other drugs that inhibit this enzyme should be approached with caution).

No products indexed under this heading.

Codeine Phosphate (Paroxetine may significantly inhibit the activity of the cytochrome P450 2D6 isoenzyme. Concomitant use of paroxetine with other drugs metabolized by cytochrome CYP2D6 has not been formally studied but may require lower doses than usually prescribed for either paroxetine or the other drug. Therefore, co-administration of paroxetine with other drugs that are metabolized by this isozyme should be approached with caution). Products include:

- Tylenol with Codeine Tablets 2391

Codeine Sulfate (Paroxetine may significantly inhibit the activity of the cytochrome P450 2D6 isoenzyme. Concomitant use of paroxetine with other drugs metabolized by cytochrome CYP2D6 has not been formally studied but may require lower doses than usually prescribed for either paroxetine or the other drug. Therefore, co-administration of paroxetine with other drugs that are metabolized by this isozyme should be approached with caution).

No products indexed under this heading.

Cyclobenzaprine Hydrochloride (Paroxetine may significantly inhibit the activity of the cytochrome P450 2D6 isoenzyme. Concomitant use of paroxetine with other drugs metabolized by cytochrome CYP2D6 has not been formally studied but may require lower doses than usually prescribed for either paroxetine or the other drug. Therefore, co-administration of paroxetine with other drugs that are metabolized by this isozyme should be approached with caution).

No products indexed under this heading.

Cyclosporine (Co-administration with another drug that is highly protein bound may increase free concentrations of the other drug or paroxetine potentially resulting in adverse events). Products include:

- Gengraf Capsules 459
- Neoral Oral Solution 2259
- Neoral Soft Gelatin Capsules 2259
- Restasis Ophthalmic Emulsion 575
- Sandimmune 2275

Dalteparin Sodium (The combined use of psychotropic drugs that interfere with serotonin reuptake and drugs that affect coagulation has been associated with an increased risk of bleeding; concomitant administration should be undertaken with caution). Products include:

- Fragmin Injection 1097

Danaparoid Sodium (The combined use of psychotropic drugs that interfere with serotonin reuptake and drugs that affect coagulation has been associated with an increased risk of bleeding; concomitant administration should be undertaken with caution).

No products indexed under this heading.

Desipramine Hydrochloride (Co-administration with desipramine has resulted in an increase in Cmax, AUC and T1/2 by an average of approximately two-, five- and three-fold, respectively).

No products indexed under this heading.

Dexfenfluramine Hydrochloride (Paroxetine may significantly inhibit the activity of the cytochrome P450 2D6 isoenzyme. Concomitant use of paroxetine with other drugs metabolized by cytochrome CYP2D6 has not been formally studied but may require lower doses than usually prescribed for either paroxetine or the other drug. Therefore, co-administration of paroxetine with other drugs that are metabolized by this isozyme should be approached with caution).

No products indexed under this heading.

Dextromethorphan Hydrobromide (Paroxetine may significantly inhibit the activity of the cytochrome P450 2D6 isoenzyme. Concomitant use of paroxetine with other drugs metabolized by cytochrome CYP2D6 has not been formally studied but may require lower doses than usually prescribed for either paroxetine or the other drug. Therefore, co-administration of paroxetine with other drugs that are metabolized by this isozyme should be approached with caution). Products include:

- Comtrex Maximum Strength Cold & Cough Day/Night Caplets - Day Formulation 726
- Comtrex Maximum Strength Cold & Cough Day/Night Caplets - Night Formulation 726
- Comtrex Maximum Strength Non-Drowsy Cold & Cough Caplets 725
- Children's Dimetapp DM Cold & Cough Elixir 731
- Children's Dimetapp Long Acting Cough Plus Cold Syrup 731
- Toddler's Dimetapp Cold and Cough Drops 732
- Mucinex DM Extended-Release Bi-Layer Tablets 720

Refenesen DM Caplets .... ▣ 721
Robitussin Cough & Cold CF Liquid .... ▣ 735
Robitussin Cough & Cold Long-Acting Liquid .... ▣ 735
Robitussin Cough & Allergy Syrup .. ▣ 736
Robitussin Cough & Cold Nighttime Liquid .... ▣ 736
Robitussin Cough & Cold Pediatric Drops .... ▣ 735
Robitussin Cough, Cold & Flu Nighttime Liquid .... ▣ 738
Robitussin Cough & Congestion Liquid .... ▣ 738
Robitussin Cough Gels Long-Acting .... ▣ 737
Robitussin Cough Long Acting Liquid .... ▣ 739
Robitussin Cough DM Syrup .... ▣ 738
Robitussin Cough DM Infant Drops .... ▣ 738
Robitussin Pediatric Cough Long Acting Liquid .... ▣ 739
Robitussin Pediatric Cough & Cold Long-Acting Liquid .... ▣ 735
Robitussin Pediatric Cough & Cold Nighttime Liquid .... ▣ 736
Robitussin Sugar Free Cough .... ▣ 738
TheraFlu Cold & Cough Hot Liquid .... ▣ 740
TheraFlu Warming Relief Daytime Severe Cold .... ▣ 743
TheraFlu Thin Strips Long Acting Cough .... ▣ 744
Triaminic Daytime Cold & Cough Liquid .... ▣ 745
Triaminic Cough & Sore Throat Liquid .... ▣ 747
Triaminic Cough & Runny Nose Softchews .... ▣ 748
Triaminic Thin Strips Cold & Cough .... ▣ 778
Triaminic Infant Thin Strips Decongestant Plus Cough .... ▣ 747
Children's Tylenol Plus Flu Oral Suspension .... ▣ 749
Tylenol Cold Head Congestion Daytime Caplets with Cool Burst and Gelcaps .... ▣ 750
Tylenol Cold Multi-Symptom Daytime Liquid .... ▣ 752
Tylenol Cold Multi-Symptom Severe Daytime Liquid .... ▣ 752
Concentrated Tylenol Infants' Drops Plus Cold & Cough .... ▣ 754
Children's Tylenol Plus Cough & Runny Nose Suspension Liquid 1879
Children's Tylenol Plus Cough & Sore Throat Suspension Liquid 1879
Children's Tylenol Plus Flu Suspension Liquid 1881
Children's Tylenol Plus Multi-Symptom Cold Suspension Liquid 1879
Tylenol Cold Severe Congestion Non-Drowsy Caplets with Cool Burst 1874
Tylenol Cold Head Congestion Daytime Caplets with Cool Burst 1873
Tylenol Cold Head Congestion Nighttime Caplets with Cool Burst 1873
Tylenol Cold Head Congestion Severe Caplets with Cool Burst 1873
Tylenol Cold Multi-Symptom Daytime Caplets with Cool Burst and Gelcaps 1874
Tylenol Cold Multi-Symptom Daytime Liquid with Citrus Burst ... 1874
Tylenol Cold Multi-Symptom Nighttime Caplets with Cool Burst 1874
Tylenol Cold Multi-Symptom Nighttime Liquid with Cool Burst ... 1874
Tylenol Cold Multi-Symptom Severe Caplets with Cool Burst 1874
Tylenol Cold Multi-Symptom Severe Daytime Liquid with Citrus Burst 1874
Tylenol Cough & Sore Throat Daytime Liquid with Cool Burst 1877
Tylenol Cough & Sore Throat Nighttime Liquid with Cool Burst ... 1877
Concentrated Tylenol Infants' Drops Plus Cold and Cough 1879
Vicks 44 Cough Relief Liquid 2679
Vicks 44D Cough & Head Congestion Relief Liquid 2679
Vicks 44E Cough & Chest Congestion Relief Liquid 2679
Pediatric Vicks 44e Cough & Chest Congestion Relief Liquid 2676
Vicks 44M Cough, Cold & Flu Relief Liquid 2680
Pediatric Vicks 44m Cough & Cold Relief Liquid 2676
Vicks DayQuil LiquiCaps/Liquid Multi-Symptom Cold/Flu Relief ..... ▣ 761
Vicks DayQuil Multi-Symptom Cold/Flu Relief LiquiCaps 2678
Vicks DayQuil Multi-Symptom Cold/Flu Relief Liquid 2678
Vicks NyQuil Multi-Symptom Cold/Flu Relief Liquid 2681
Children's Vicks NyQuil Cold/Cough Relief .... ▣ 756
Vicks NyQuil Multi-Symptom Cold/Flu Relief LiquiCaps 2681
Vicks NyQuil LiquiCaps/Liquid Multi-Symptom Cold/Flu Relief ..... ▣ 763
Vicks NyQuil Cough Liquid 2680
Children's Vicks NyQuil Cold/Cough Relief Liquid 2680
Zicam Cough Max Nighttime Cough Spray .... ▣ 767
Zicam Cough Max Cough Spray ..... ▣ 767
Zicam Cough Max Cough Melts ...... ▣ 767
Zicam Cough Plus D Cough Spray .... ▣ 767
Zicam Cough Relief Cough Spray ... ▣ 767
Zicam Maximum Strength Flu Daytime .... ▣ 768
Zicam Maximum Strength Flu Nighttime .... ▣ 768

Dextromethorphan Polistirex (Paroxetine may significantly inhibit the activity of the cytochrome P450 2D6 isoenzyme. Concomitant use of paroxetine with other drugs metabolized by cytochrome CYP2D6 has not been formally studied but may require lower doses than usually prescribed for either paroxetine or the other drug. Therefore, co-administration of paroxetine with other drugs that are metabolized by this isozyme should be approached with caution). Products include:
Delsym Extended-Release Suspension 12 Hour Cough Suppressant .... ▣ 611

Diazepam (Co-administration with another drug that is highly protein bound may increase free concentrations of the other drug or paroxetine potentially resulting in adverse events). Products include:
Diastat Rectal Delivery System 3343
Valium Tablets 2819

Diclofenac Potassium (The combined use of psychotropic drugs that interfere with serotonin reuptake and drugs that affect coagulation has been associated with an increased risk of bleeding).
No products indexed under this heading.

Diclofenac Sodium (The combined use of psychotropic drugs that interfere with serotonin reuptake and drugs that affect coagulation has been associated with an increased risk of bleeding). Products include:
Arthrotec Tablets 3129
Voltaren Ophthalmic Solution 2309
Voltaren Tablets 2307
Voltaren-XR Tablets 2310

Dicumarol (The combined use of psychotropic drugs that interfere with serotonin reuptake and drugs that affect coagulation has been associated with an increased risk of bleeding; concomitant administration should be undertaken with caution).
No products indexed under this heading.

Digoxin (The steady-state pharmacokinetics of paroxetine was not altered when administered with digoxin at steady state. Mean digoxin AUC at steady state decreased by 15% in the presence of paroxetine. Since there is little clinical experience, the concurrent administration of paroxetine and digoxin should be undertaken with caution). Products include:
Lanoxicaps Capsules 1490
Lanoxin Injection 1494
Lanoxin Injection Pediatric 1497
Lanoxin Tablets 1500

Diphenhydramine (Paroxetine is metabolized by the cytochrome P450 isoenzyme CYP2D6. Therefore, co-administration of paroxetine with other drugs that inhibit this enzyme should be approached with caution). Products include:
Tylenol Sore Throat Nighttime Liquid with Cool Burst 1877

Diphenhydramine Hydrochloride (Paroxetine is metabolized by the cytochrome P450 isoenzyme CYP2D6. Therefore, co-administration of paroxetine with other drugs that inhibit this enzyme should be approached with caution). Products include:
Nytol QuickCaps Caplets .... ▣ 615
Nytol QuickGels Softgels Maximum Strength .... ▣ 616
Simply Sleep Caplets 1868
Sominex Original Formula Tablets .. ▣ 616
TheraFlu Warming Relief Nighttime Severe Cold .... ▣ 743
TheraFlu Thin Strips Multi Symptom .... ▣ 744
Triaminic Nighttime Cold & Cough Liquid .... ▣ 746
Triaminic Thin Strips Cough & Runny Nose .... ▣ 749
Extra Strength Tylenol PM Caplets, Vanilla Caplets, Geltabs, Gelcaps and Liquid 1875
Tylenol Sore Throat Nighttime Liquid with Cool Burst .... ▣ 790
Tylenol Allergy Multi-Symptom Nighttime Caplets with Cool Burst 1872
Tylenol Severe Allergy Caplets 1872
Children's Tylenol Plus Cold & Allergy Suspension Liquid 1878

Dipyridamole (Co-administration with another drug that is highly protein bound may increase free concentrations of the other drug or paroxetine potentially resulting in adverse events). Products include:
Aggrenox Capsules 822
Persantine Tablets 868

Dolasetron Mesylate (Paroxetine may significantly inhibit the activity of the cytochrome P450 2D6 isoenzyme. Concomitant use of paroxetine with other drugs metabolized by cytochrome CYP2D6 has not been formally studied but may require lower doses than usually prescribed for either paroxetine or the other drug. Therefore, co-administration of paroxetine with other drugs that are metabolized by this isozyme should be approached with caution). Products include:
Anzemet Injection 2859
Anzemet Tablets 2862

Donepezil Hydrochloride (Paroxetine may significantly inhibit the activity of the cytochrome P450 2D6 isoenzyme. Concomitant use of paroxetine with other drugs metabolized by cytochrome CYP2D6 has not been formally studied but may require lower doses than usually prescribed for either paroxetine or the other drug. Therefore, co-administration of paroxetine with other drugs that are metabolized by this isozyme should be approached with caution). Products include:
Aricept Tablets 1094
Aricept ODT Tablets 1094

Doxepin Hydrochloride (Caution is indicated in the co-administration of tricyclic antidepressants with paroxetine because paroxetine may inhibit TCA metabolism. Plasma TCA concentrations may need to be monitored and the dose of TCA may need to be reduced if a TCA is co-administered with paroxetine).
No products indexed under this heading.

Dyphylline (There have been reports of elevated theophylline levels associated with co-administration; monitor theophylline levels when these drugs are concurrently administered).
No products indexed under this heading.

Eletriptan Hydrobromide (There have been rare postmarketing reports of serotonin syndrome with the use of an SSRI and a triptan. If concomitant use of paroxetine hydrochloride with a triptan is clinically warranted, careful observation of the patient is advised, particularly during treatment initiation and dose increases). Products include:
Relpax Tablets 2548

Encainide Hydrochloride (Paroxetine may significantly inhibit the activity of the cytochrome P450 2D6 isoenzyme. Concomitant use of paroxetine with other drugs metabolized by cytochrome CYP2D6 has not been formally studied but may require lower doses than usually prescribed for either paroxetine or the other drug. Therefore, co-administration of paroxetine with other drugs that are metabolized by this isozyme should be approached with caution).
No products indexed under this heading.

Enoxaparin Sodium (The combined use of psychotropic drugs that interfere with serotonin reuptake and drugs that affect coagulation has been associated with an increased risk of bleeding; concomitant administration should be undertaken with caution). Products include:
Lovenox Injection 2915

Escitalopram Oxalate (Paroxetine is metabolized by the cytochrome P450 isoenzyme CYP2D6. Therefore, co-administration of paroxetine with other drugs that inhibit this enzyme should be approached with caution). Products include:
Lexapro Oral Solution 1190
Lexapro Tablets 1190

Etodolac (The combined use of psychotropic drugs that interfere with serotonin reuptake and drugs that affect coagulation has been associated with an increased risk of bleeding).
No products indexed under this heading.

Fenoprofen Calcium (The combined use of psychotropic drugs that interfere with serotonin reuptake and drugs that affect coagulation has been associated with an increased risk of bleeding). Products include:
Nalfon Capsules 2502

Fentanyl (Paroxetine may significantly inhibit the activity of the cytochrome P450 2D6 isoenzyme. Concomitant use of paroxetine with other drugs metabolized by cytochrome CYP2D6 has not been formally studied but may require lower doses than usually prescribed for either paroxetine or the other drug. Therefore, co-administration of paroxetine with other drugs that are metabolized by this isozyme should be approached with caution). Products include:

- Duragesic Transdermal System **2373**
- Ionsys Transdermal System **2379**

Fentanyl Citrate (Paroxetine may significantly inhibit the activity of the cytochrome P450 2D6 isoenzyme. Concomitant use of paroxetine with other drugs metabolized by cytochrome CYP2D6 has not been formally studied but may require lower doses than usually prescribed for either paroxetine or the other drug. Therefore, co-administration of paroxetine with other drugs that are metabolized by this isozyme should be approached with caution). Products include:

- Actiq **979**

Flecainide Acetate (Paroxetine may significantly inhibit the activity of the cytochrome P450 2D6 isoenzyme. Concomitant use of paroxetine with other drugs metabolized by cytochrome CYP2D6 has not been formally studied but may require lower doses than usually prescribed for either paroxetine or the other drug. Therefore, co-administration of paroxetine with other drugs that are metabolized by this isozyme should be approached with caution). Products include:

- Tambocor Tablets **1856**

Fluoxetine (Paroxetine is metabolized by the cytochrome P450 isoenzyme CYP2D6. Therefore, co-administration of paroxetine with other drugs that inhibit this enzyme should be approached with caution).

No products indexed under this heading.

Fluoxetine Hydrochloride (Paroxetine is metabolized by the cytochrome P450 isoenzyme CYP2D6. Therefore, co-administration of paroxetine with other drugs that inhibit this enzyme should be approached with caution). Products include:

- Prozac Pulvules and Liquid **1801**
- Symbyax Capsules **1819**

Fluphenazine Decanoate (Paroxetine is metabolized by the cytochrome P450 isoenzyme CYP2D6. Therefore, co-administration of paroxetine with other drugs that inhibit this enzyme should be approached with caution).

No products indexed under this heading.

Fluphenazine Enanthate (Paroxetine is metabolized by the cytochrome P450 isoenzyme CYP2D6. Therefore, co-administration of paroxetine with other drugs that inhibit this enzyme should be approached with caution).

No products indexed under this heading.

Fluphenazine Hydrochloride (Paroxetine is metabolized by the cytochrome P450 isoenzyme CYP2D6. Therefore, co-administration of paroxetine with other drugs that inhibit this enzyme should be approached with caution).

No products indexed under this heading.

Flurazepam Hydrochloride (Co-administration with another drug that is highly protein bound may increase free concentrations of the other drug or paroxetine potentially resulting in adverse events). Products include:

- Dalmane Capsules **3342**

Flurbiprofen (The combined use of psychotropic drugs that interfere with serotonin reuptake and drugs that affect coagulation has been associated with an increased risk of bleeding).

No products indexed under this heading.

Fluvoxamine Maleate (Paroxetine is metabolized by the cytochrome P450 isoenzyme CYP2D6. Therefore, co-administration of paroxetine with other drugs that inhibit this enzyme should be approached with caution).

No products indexed under this heading.

Fondaparinux Sodium (The combined use of psychotropic drugs that interfere with serotonin reuptake and drugs that affect coagulation has been associated with an increased risk of bleeding; concomitant administration should be undertaken with caution). Products include:

- Arixtra Injection **1351**

Formoterol Fumarate (Paroxetine may significantly inhibit the activity of the cytochrome P450 2D6 isoenzyme. Concomitant use of paroxetine with other drugs metabolized by cytochrome CYP2D6 has not been formally studied but may require lower doses than usually prescribed for either paroxetine or the other drug. Therefore, co-administration of paroxetine with other drugs that are metabolized by this isozyme should be approached with caution). Products include:

- Foradil Aerolizer **3010**

Fosamprenavir Calcium (Co-administration of fosamprenavir with paroxetine significantly decreased plasma levels of paroxetine. Any dose adjustment should be guided by clinical effect (tolerability and efficacy)). Products include:

- Lexiva Tablets **1505**

Fosphenytoin Sodium (Co-administration has resulted in reduction of paroxetine AUC and T1/2; potential for elevated phenytoin levels or slight reduction in phenytoin AUC).

No products indexed under this heading.

Frovatriptan Succinate (There have been rare postmarketing reports of serotonin syndrome with the use of an SSRI and a triptan. If concomitant use of paroxetine hydrochloride with a triptan is clinically warranted, careful observation of the patient is advised, particularly during treatment initiation and dose increases). Products include:

- Frova Tablets **1113**

Galantamine Hydrobromide (Paroxetine may significantly inhibit the activity of the cytochrome P450 2D6 isoenzyme. Concomitant use of paroxetine with other drugs metabolized by cytochrome CYP2D6 has not been formally studied but may require lower doses than usually prescribed for either paroxetine or the other drug. Therefore, co-administration of paroxetine with other drugs that are metabolized by this isozyme should be approached with caution). Products include:

- Razadyne **2399**
- Razadyne ER Extended-Release Capsules **2399**

Glipizide (Co-administration with another drug that is highly protein bound may increase free concentrations of the other drug or paroxetine potentially resulting in adverse events).

No products indexed under this heading.

Halofantrine Hydrochloride (Paroxetine is metabolized by the cytochrome P450 isoenzyme CYP2D6. Therefore, co-administration of paroxetine with other drugs that inhibit this enzyme should be approached with caution).

No products indexed under this heading.

Haloperidol (Paroxetine is metabolized by the cytochrome P450 isoenzyme CYP2D6. Therefore, co-administration of paroxetine with other drugs that inhibit this enzyme should be approached with caution).

No products indexed under this heading.

Haloperidol Decanoate (Paroxetine is metabolized by the cytochrome P450 isoenzyme CYP2D6. Therefore, co-administration of paroxetine with other drugs that inhibit this enzyme should be approached with caution).

No products indexed under this heading.

Heparin Calcium (The combined use of psychotropic drugs that interfere with serotonin reuptake and drugs that affect coagulation has been associated with an increased risk of bleeding; concomitant administration should be undertaken with caution).

No products indexed under this heading.

Heparin Sodium (The combined use of psychotropic drugs that interfere with serotonin reuptake and drugs that affect coagulation has been associated with an increased risk of bleeding; concomitant administration should be undertaken with caution).

No products indexed under this heading.

Hydrocodone Bitartrate (Paroxetine may significantly inhibit the activity of the cytochrome P450 2D6 isoenzyme. Concomitant use of paroxetine with other drugs metabolized by cytochrome CYP2D6 has not been formally studied but may require lower doses than usually prescribed for either paroxetine or the other drug. Therefore, co-administration of paroxetine with other drugs that are metabolized by this isozyme should be approached with caution). Products include:

- Hycodan **1116**
- Hycotuss Expectorant Syrup **1117**
- Vicodin Tablets **535**
- Vicodin ES Tablets **536**
- Vicodin HP Tablets **538**
- Vicoprofen Tablets **539**
- Zydone Tablets **1139**

Hydroxychloroquine Sulfate (Paroxetine is metabolized by the cytochrome P450 isoenzyme CYP2D6. Therefore, co-administration of paroxetine with other drugs that inhibit this enzyme should be approached with caution).

No products indexed under this heading.

Hypericum (Based on the mechanism of action of paroxetine and the potential for serotonin syndrome, caution is advised when paroxetine hydrochloride is co-administered with other drugs or agents that may affect the serotonergic neurotransmitter systems, such as St. John's Wort). Products include:

- Satiete Tablets **832**

Ibuprofen (The combined use of psychotropic drugs that interfere with serotonin reuptake and drugs that affect coagulation has been associated with an increased risk of bleeding). Products include:

- Advil Allergy Sinus Caplets **770**
- Advil **674**
- Children's Advil Oral Suspension **603**
- Children's Advil Chewable Tablets .. **603**
- Advil Cold & Sinus **723**
- Infants' Advil Concentrated Drops .. **604**
- Infants' Advil Concentrated Drops - White Grape (Dye-Free)............. **604**
- Junior Strength Advil Swallow Tablets.. **605**
- Advil Migraine Liquigels **608**
- Advil Multi-Symptom Cold Caplets... **770**
- Advil PM Caplets **615**
- Motrin IB Tablets and Caplets **1866**
- Children's Motrin Oral Suspension ... **1867**
- Children's Motrin Non-Staining Dye-Free Oral Suspension............ **1867**
- Children's Motrin Cold Oral Suspension **1867**
- Infants' Motrin Concentrated Drops.. **1867**
- Infants' Motrin Non-Staining Dye-Free Concentrated Drops....... **1867**
- Junior Strength Motrin Caplets and Chewable Tablets.................. **1867**
- Vicoprofen Tablets **539**

Imatinib Mesylate (Paroxetine is metabolized by the cytochrome P450 isoenzyme CYP2D6. Therefore, co-administration of paroxetine with other drugs that inhibit this enzyme should be approached with caution). Products include:

- Gleevec Tablets **2227**

Imipramine Hydrochloride (Caution is indicated in the co-administration of tricyclic antidepressants with paroxetine because paroxetine may inhibit TCA metabolism. Plasma TCA concentrations may need to be monitored and the dose of TCA may need to be reduced if a TCA is co-administered with paroxetine).

No products indexed under this heading.

Imipramine Pamoate (Caution is indicated in the co-administration of tricyclic antidepressants with paroxetine because paroxetine may inhibit TCA metabolism. Plasma TCA concentrations may need to be monitored and the dose of TCA may need to be reduced if a TCA is co-administered with paroxetine).

No products indexed under this heading.

Indomethacin (The combined use of psychotropic drugs that interfere with serotonin reuptake and drugs that affect coagulation has been associated with an increased risk of bleeding). Products include:

Indomethacin Sodium Trihydrate (The combined use of psychotropic drugs that interfere with serotonin reuptake and drugs that affect coagulation has been associated with an increased risk of bleeding). Products include:

Indoramin Hydrochloride (Paroxetine may significantly inhibit the activity of the cytochrome P450 2D6 isoenzyme. Concomitant use of paroxetine with other drugs metabolized by cytochrome CYP2D6 has not been formally studied but may require lower doses than usually prescribed for either paroxetine or the other drug. Therefore, co-administration of paroxetine with other drugs that are metabolized by this isozyme should be approached with caution).

 No products indexed under this heading.

Isocarboxazid (Concomitant use of paroxetine hydrochloride and MAOIs intended to treat depression is contraindicated. Potential for serious and/or fatal reactions, including hyperthermia, rigidity, myoclonus, and other serious reactions; therefore, it is recommended that paroxetine hydrochloride not be used in combination with an MAOI, or within 14 days of discontinuing treatment with an MAOI. At least 2 weeks should be allowed after stopping paroxetine hydrochloride before starting an MAOI).

 No products indexed under this heading.

Ketoprofen (The combined use of psychotropic drugs that interfere with serotonin reuptake and drugs that affect coagulation has been associated with an increased risk of bleeding).

 No products indexed under this heading.

Ketorolac Tromethamine (The combined use of psychotropic drugs that interfere with serotonin reuptake and drugs that affect coagulation has been associated with an increased risk of bleeding). Products include:

Labetalol Hydrochloride (Paroxetine may significantly inhibit the activity of the cytochrome P450 2D6 isoenzyme. Concomitant use of paroxetine with other drugs metabolized by cytochrome CYP2D6 has not been formally studied but may require lower doses than usually prescribed for either paroxetine or the other drug. Therefore, co-administration of paroxetine with other drugs that are metabolized by this isozyme should be approached with caution).

 No products indexed under this heading.

Lidocaine (Paroxetine may significantly inhibit the activity of the cytochrome P450 2D6 isoenzyme. Concomitant use of paroxetine with other drugs metabolized by cytochrome CYP2D6 has not been formally studied but may require lower doses than usually prescribed for either paroxetine or the other drug. Therefore, co-administration of paroxetine with other drugs that are

metabolized by this isozyme should be approached with caution). Products include:

Lidocaine Hydrochloride (Paroxetine may significantly inhibit the activity of the cytochrome P450 2D6 isoenzyme. Concomitant use of paroxetine with other drugs metabolized by cytochrome CYP2D6 has not been formally studied but may require lower doses than usually prescribed for either paroxetine or the other drug. Therefore, co-administration of paroxetine with other drugs that are metabolized by this isozyme should be approached with caution).

 No products indexed under this heading.

Linezolid (Based on the mechanism of action of paroxetine and the potential for serotonin syndrome, caution is advised when paroxetine hydrochloride is co-administered with other drugs or agents that may affect the serotonergic neurotransmitter systems, such as linezolid). Products include:

Lithium (A multiple-dose study has shown that there is no pharmacokinetic interaction between paroxetine and lithium carbonate. However, due to the potential for serotonin syndrome, caution is advised when paroxetine is co-administered with lithium).

 No products indexed under this heading.

Lithium Carbonate (A multiple-dose study has shown that there is no pharmacokinetic interaction between paroxetine and lithium carbonate. However, due to the potential for serotonin syndrome, caution is advised when paroxetine is co-administered with lithium). Products include:

Lithium Citrate (A multiple-dose study has shown that there is no pharmacokinetic interaction between paroxetine and lithium carbonate. However, due to the potential for serotonin syndrome, caution is advised when paroxetine is co-administered with lithium).

 No products indexed under this heading.

Low Molecular Weight Heparins (The combined use of psychotropic drugs that interfere with serotonin reuptake and drugs that affect coagulation has been associated with an increased risk of bleeding; concomitant administration should be undertaken with caution).

 No products indexed under this heading.

Maprotiline Hydrochloride (Caution is indicated in the co-administration of tricyclic antidepressants with paroxetine because paroxetine may inhibit TCA metabolism. Plasma TCA concentrations may need to be monitored and the dose of TCA may need to be reduced if a TCA is co-administered with paroxetine).

 No products indexed under this heading.

Meclofenamate Sodium (The combined use of psychotropic drugs that interfere with serotonin reuptake and drugs that affect coagulation has been associated with an increased risk of bleeding).

 No products indexed under this heading.

Mefenamic Acid (The combined use of psychotropic drugs that interfere with serotonin reuptake and drugs that affect coagulation has been associated with an increased risk of bleeding).

 No products indexed under this heading.

Meloxicam (The combined use of psychotropic drugs that interfere with serotonin reuptake and drugs that affect coagulation has been associated with an increased risk of bleeding). Products include:

Meperidine Hydrochloride (Paroxetine may significantly inhibit the activity of the cytochrome P450 2D6 isoenzyme. Concomitant use of paroxetine with other drugs metabolized by cytochrome CYP2D6 has not been formally studied but may require lower doses than usually prescribed for either paroxetine or the other drug. Therefore, co-administration of paroxetine with other drugs that are metabolized by this isozyme should be approached with caution).

 No products indexed under this heading.

Mesoridazine Besylate (Paroxetine may significantly inhibit the activity of cytochrome P450 2D6 isoenzyme. Concomitant use of paroxetine with other drugs metabolized by cytochrome CYP2D6 has not been formally studied but may require lower doses than usually prescribed for either paroxetine or the other drug. Therefore, co-administration of paroxetine with other drugs that are metabolized by this isozyme should be approached with caution).

 No products indexed under this heading.

Methadone Hydrochloride (Paroxetine is metabolized by the cytochrome P450 isoenzyme CYP2D6. Therefore, co-administration of paroxetine with other drugs that inhibit this enzyme should be approached with caution).

 No products indexed under this heading.

Methamphetamine Hydrochloride (Paroxetine may significantly inhibit the activity of the cytochrome P450 2D6 isoenzyme. Concomitant use of paroxetine with other drugs metabolized by cytochrome CYP2D6 has not been formally studied but may require lower doses than usually prescribed for either paroxetine or the other drug. Therefore, co-administration of paroxetine with other drugs that are metabolized by this isozyme should be approached with caution). Products include:

Methotrimeprazine (Paroxetine may significantly inhibit the activity of cytochrome P450 2D6 isoenzyme. Concomitant use of paroxetine with other drugs metabolized by cytochrome CYP2D6 has not been formally studied but may require lower

doses than usually prescribed for either paroxetine or the other drug. Therefore, co-administration of paroxetine with other drugs that are metabolized by this isozyme should be approached with caution).

 No products indexed under this heading.

Metoprolol Succinate (There has been a case report of severe hypotension when immediate-release paroxetine was added to chronic metoprolol treatment). Products include:

Metoprolol Tartrate (There has been a case report of severe hypotension when immediate-release paroxetine was added to chronic metoprolol treatment). Products include:

Mexiletine Hydrochloride (Paroxetine may significantly inhibit the activity of the cytochrome P450 2D6 isoenzyme. Concomitant use of paroxetine with other drugs metabolized by cytochrome CYP2D6 has not been formally studied but may require lower doses than usually prescribed for either paroxetine or the other drug. Therefore, co-administration of paroxetine with other drugs that are metabolized by this isozyme should be approached with caution).

 No products indexed under this heading.

Mibefradil Dihydrochloride (Paroxetine is metabolized by the cytochrome P450 isoenzyme CYP2D6. Therefore, co-administration of paroxetine with other drugs that inhibit this enzyme should be approached with caution).

 No products indexed under this heading.

Midazolam Hydrochloride (Co-administration with another drug that is highly protein bound may increase free concentrations of the other drug or paroxetine potentially resulting in adverse events).

 No products indexed under this heading.

Mirtazapine (Paroxetine may significantly inhibit the activity of the cytochrome P450 2D6 isoenzyme. Concomitant use of paroxetine with other drugs metabolized by cytochrome CYP2D6 has not been formally studied but may require lower doses than usually prescribed for either paroxetine or the other drug. Therefore, co-administration of paroxetine with other drugs that are metabolized by this isozyme should be approached with caution).

 No products indexed under this heading.

Moclobemide (Concomitant use of paroxetine hydrochloride and MAOIs intended to treat depression is contraindicated. Potential for serious and/or fatal reactions, including hyperthermia, rigidity, myoclonus, and other serious reactions; therefore, it is recommended that paroxetine hydrochloride not be used in combination with an MAOI, or within 14 days of discontinuing treatment with an MAOI. At least 2 weeks should be allowed after stopping paroxetine hydrochloride before starting an MAOI).

No products indexed under this heading.

Morphine Sulfate (Paroxetine may significantly inhibit the activity of the cytochrome P450 2D6 isoenzyme. Concomitant use of paroxetine with other drugs metabolized by cytochrome CYP2D6 has not been formally studied but may require lower doses than usually prescribed for either paroxetine or the other drug. Therefore, co-administration of paroxetine with other drugs that are metabolized by this isozyme should be approached with caution). Products include:

Avinza Capsules	1741
Kadian Capsules	577
MS Contin Tablets	2701

Nabumetone (The combined use of psychotropic drugs that interfere with serotonin reuptake and drugs that affect coagulation has been associated with an increased risk of bleeding).

No products indexed under this heading.

Naproxen (The combined use of psychotropic drugs that interfere with serotonin reuptake and drugs that affect coagulation has been associated with an increased risk of bleeding). Products include:

EC-Naprosyn Delayed-Release Tablets	2761
Naprosyn Suspension	2761
Naprosyn Tablets	2761
Prevacid NapraPAC	3280

Naproxen Sodium (The combined use of psychotropic drugs that interfere with serotonin reuptake and drugs that affect coagulation has been associated with an increased risk of bleeding). Products include:

Aleve Caplets	742
Aleve Gelcaps	743
Aleve Tablets	743
Aleve Cold & Sinus Caplets	744
Anaprox Tablets	2761
Anaprox DS Tablets	2761

Naratriptan Hydrochloride (There have been rare postmarketing reports of serotonin syndrome with the use of an SSRI and a triptan. If concomitant use of paroxetine hydrochloride with a triptan is clinically warranted, careful observation of the patient is advised, particularly during treatment initiation and dose increases). Products include:

Amerge Tablets	1339

Nelfinavir Mesylate (Paroxetine may significantly inhibit the activity of the cytochrome P450 2D6 isoenzyme. Concomitant use of paroxetine with other drugs metabolized by cytochrome CYP2D6 has not been formally studied but may require lower doses than usually prescribed for either paroxetine or the other drug. Therefore, co-administration of paroxetine with other drugs that are metabolized by this isozyme should be approached with caution). Products include:

Viracept	2577

Nortriptyline Hydrochloride (Caution is indicated in the co-administration of tricyclic antidepressants with paroxetine because paroxetine may inhibit TCA metabolism. Plasma TCA concentrations may need to be monitored and the dose of TCA may need to be reduced if a TCA is co-administered with paroxetine).

No products indexed under this heading.

Olanzapine (Paroxetine may significantly inhibit the activity of the cytochrome P450 2D6 isoenzyme. Concomitant use of paroxetine with other drugs metabolized by cytochrome CYP2D6 has not been formally studied but may require lower doses than usually prescribed for either paroxetine or the other drug. Therefore, co-administration of paroxetine with other drugs that are metabolized by this isozyme should be approached with caution). Products include:

Symbyax Capsules	1819
Zyprexa Tablets	1830
Zyprexa IntraMuscular	1830
Zyprexa ZYDIS Orally Disintegrating Tablets	1830

Omeprazole (Paroxetine may significantly inhibit the activity of the cytochrome P450 2D6 isoenzyme. Concomitant use of paroxetine with other drugs metabolized by cytochrome CYP2D6 has not been formally studied but may require lower doses than usually prescribed for either paroxetine or the other drug. Therefore, co-administration of paroxetine with other drugs that are metabolized by this isozyme should be approached with caution). Products include:

Zegerid Capsules	2958
Zegerid Powder for Oral Solution	2958

Ondansetron (Paroxetine may significantly inhibit the activity of the cytochrome P450 2D6 isoenzyme. Concomitant use of paroxetine with other drugs metabolized by cytochrome CYP2D6 has not been formally studied but may require lower doses than usually prescribed for either paroxetine or the other drug. Therefore, co-administration of paroxetine with other drugs that are metabolized by this isozyme should be approached with caution). Products include:

Zofran ODT Orally Disintegrating Tablets	1639

Ondansetron Hydrochloride (Paroxetine may significantly inhibit the activity of the cytochrome P450 2D6 isoenzyme. Concomitant use of paroxetine with other drugs metabolized by cytochrome CYP2D6 has not been formally studied but may require lower doses than usually prescribed for either paroxetine or the other drug. Therefore, co-administration of paroxetine with other drugs that are metabolized by this isozyme should be approached with caution). Products include:

Zofran Injection	1634
Zofran	1639

Oxaprozin (The combined use of psychotropic drugs that interfere with serotonin reuptake and drugs that affect coagulation has been associated with an increased risk of bleeding).

No products indexed under this heading.

Oxazepam (Co-administration with another drug that is highly protein bound may increase free concentrations of the other drug or paroxetine potentially resulting in adverse events).

No products indexed under this heading.

Oxycodone Hydrochloride (Paroxetine may significantly inhibit the activity of the cytochrome P450 2D6 isoenzyme. Concomitant use of paroxetine with other drugs metabolized

by cytochrome CYP2D6 has not been formally studied but may require lower doses than usually prescribed for either paroxetine or the other drug. Therefore, co-administration of paroxetine with other drugs that are metabolized by this isozyme should be approached with caution). Products include:

OxyContin Tablets	2703
OxyFast Oral Concentrate Solution	2708
OxyIR Capsules	2708
Percocet Tablets	1131
Percodan Tablets	1132

Paclitaxel (Paroxetine may significantly inhibit the activity of the cytochrome P450 2D6 isoenzyme. Concomitant use of paroxetine with other drugs metabolized by cytochrome CYP2D6 has not been formally studied but may require lower doses than usually prescribed for either paroxetine or the other drug. Therefore, co-administration of paroxetine with other drugs that are metabolized by this isozyme should be approached with caution).

No products indexed under this heading.

Pargyline Hydrochloride (Concomitant use of paroxetine hydrochloride and MAOIs intended to treat depression is contraindicated. Potential for serious and/or fatal reactions, including hyperthermia, rigidity, myoclonus, and other serious reactions; therefore, it is recommended that paroxetine hydrochloride not be used in combination with an MAOI, or within 14 days of discontinuing treatment with an MAOI. At least 2 weeks should be allowed after stopping paroxetine hydrochloride before starting an MAOI).

No products indexed under this heading.

Perphenazine (Paroxetine is metabolized by the cytochrome P450 isoenzyme CYP2D6. Therefore, co-administration of paroxetine with other drugs that inhibit this enzyme should be approached with caution).

No products indexed under this heading.

Phenelzine Sulfate (Concomitant use of paroxetine hydrochloride and MAOIs intended to treat depression is contraindicated. Potential for serious and/or fatal reactions, including hyperthermia, rigidity, myoclonus, and other serious reactions; therefore, it is recommended that paroxetine hydrochloride not be used in combination with an MAOI, or within 14 days of discontinuing treatment with an MAOI. At least 2 weeks should be allowed after stopping paroxetine hydrochloride before starting an MAOI).

No products indexed under this heading.

Phenobarbital (Co-administration has resulted in reduction of paroxetine AUC and T1/2). Products include:

Donnatal Extentabs	2493

Phenylbutazone (The combined use of psychotropic drugs that interfere with serotonin reuptake and drugs that affect coagulation has been associated with an increased risk of bleeding).

No products indexed under this heading.

Phenytoin (Co-administration has resulted in reduction of paroxetine AUC and T1/2; potential for elevated phenytoin levels or slight reduction in phenytoin AUC).

No products indexed under this heading.

Phenytoin Sodium (Co-administration has resulted in reduction of paroxetine AUC and T1/2; potential for elevated phenytoin levels or slight reduction in phenytoin AUC). Products include:

Phenytek Capsules	2160

Pimozide (Due to the narrow therapeutic index of pimozide and its known ability to prolong the QT interval, concomitant use of pimozide and paroxetine hydrocholoride is contraindicated).

No products indexed under this heading.

Pindolol (Paroxetine may significantly inhibit the activity of the cytochrome P450 2D6 isoenzyme. Concomitant use of paroxetine with other drugs metabolized by cytochrome CYP2D6 has not been formally studied but may require lower doses than usually prescribed for either paroxetine or the other drug. Therefore, co-administration of paroxetine with other drugs that are metabolized by this isozyme should be approached with caution).

No products indexed under this heading.

Piroxicam (The combined use of psychotropic drugs that interfere with serotonin reuptake and drugs that affect coagulation has been associated with an increased risk of bleeding).

No products indexed under this heading.

Procarbazine Hydrochloride (Concomitant use of paroxetine hydrochloride and MAOIs intended to treat depression is contraindicated. Potential for serious and/or fatal reactions, including hyperthermia, rigidity, myoclonus, and other serious reactions; therefore, it is recommended that paroxetine hydrochloride not be used in combination with an MAOI, or within 14 days of discontinuing treatment with an MAOI. At least 2 weeks should be allowed after stopping paroxetine hydrochloride before starting an MAOI). Products include:

Matulane Capsules	3191

Prochlorperazine (Paroxetine may significantly inhibit the activity of cytochrome P450 2D6 isoenzyme. Concomitant use of paroxetine with other drugs metabolized by cytochrome CYP2D6 has not been formally studied but may require lower doses than usually prescribed for either paroxetine or the other drug. Therefore, co-administration of paroxetine with other drugs that are metabolized by this isozyme should be approached with caution).

No products indexed under this heading.

Procyclidine Hydrochloride (Increased steady-state AUC, Cmax and Cmin values of procyclidine with concurrent use).

No products indexed under this heading.

Promethazine Hydrochloride (Paroxetine may significantly inhibit the activity of cytochrome P450 2D6 isoenzyme. Concomitant use of par-

IMPORTANT NOTE: Always consult each drug listing in the patient's regimen for possible interactions.

oxetine with other drugs metabolized by cytochrome CYP2D6 has not been formally studied but may require lower doses than usually prescribed for either paroxetine or the other drug. Therefore, co-administration of paroxetine with other drugs that are metabolized by this isozyme should be approached with caution). Products include:

Phenergan Tablets and Suppositories 3440

Propafenone Hydrochloride (Paroxetine is metabolized by the cytochrome P450 isoenzyme CYP2D6. Therefore, co-administration of paroxetine with other drugs that inhibit this enzyme should be approached with caution). Products include:

Rythmol SR Capsules 2727

Propoxyphene Hydrochloride (Paroxetine is metabolized by the cytochrome P450 isoenzyme CYP2D6. Therefore, co-administration of paroxetine with other drugs that inhibit this enzyme should be approached with caution).

No products indexed under this heading.

Propoxyphene Napsylate (Paroxetine is metabolized by the cytochrome P450 isoenzyme CYP2D6. Therefore, co-administration of paroxetine with other drugs that inhibit this enzyme should be approached with caution).

No products indexed under this heading.

Propranolol Hydrochloride (Paroxetine may significantly inhibit the activity of the cytochrome P450 2D6 isoenzyme. Concomitant use of paroxetine with other drugs metabolized by cytochrome CYP2D6 has not been formally studied but may require lower doses than usually prescribed for either paroxetine or the other drug. Therefore, co-administration of paroxetine with other drugs that are metabolized by this isozyme should be approached with caution). Products include:

Inderal LA Long-Acting Capsules 3429
InnoPran XL Capsules 2723

Protriptyline Hydrochloride (Caution is indicated in the co-administration of tricyclic antidepressants with paroxetine because paroxetine may inhibit TCA metabolism. Plasma TCA concentrations may need to be monitored and the dose of TCA may need to be reduced if a TCA is co-administered with paroxetine).

No products indexed under this heading.

Quetiapine Fumarate (Paroxetine may significantly inhibit the activity of the cytochrome P450 2D6 isoenzyme. Concomitant use of paroxetine with other drugs metabolized by cytochrome CYP2D6 has not been formally studied but may require lower doses than usually prescribed for either paroxetine or the other drug. Therefore, co-administration of paroxetine with other drugs that are metabolized by this isozyme should be approached with caution). Products include:

Seroquel Tablets 690

Quinacrine Hydrochloride (Paroxetine is metabolized by the cytochrome P450 isoenzyme CYP2D6. Therefore, co-administration of paroxetine with other drugs that inhibit this enzyme should be approached with caution).

No products indexed under this heading.

Quinidine Gluconate (Paroxetine is metabolized by the cytochrome P450 isoenzyme CYP2D6. Therefore, co-administration of paroxetine with other drugs that inhibit this enzyme should be approached with caution).

No products indexed under this heading.

Quinidine Hydrochloride (Paroxetine is metabolized by the cytochrome P450 isoenzyme CYP2D6. Therefore, co-administration of paroxetine with other drugs that inhibit this enzyme should be approached with caution).

No products indexed under this heading.

Quinidine Polygalacturonate (Paroxetine is metabolized by the cytochrome P450 isoenzyme CYP2D6. Therefore, co-administration of paroxetine with other drugs that inhibit this enzyme should be approached with caution).

No products indexed under this heading.

Quinidine Sulfate (Paroxetine is metabolized by the cytochrome P450 isoenzyme CYP2D6. Therefore, co-administration of paroxetine with other drugs that inhibit this enzyme should be approached with caution).

No products indexed under this heading.

Ranitidine Bismuth Citrate (Paroxetine is metabolized by the cytochrome P450 isoenzyme CYP2D6. Therefore, co-administration of paroxetine with other drugs that inhibit this enzyme should be approached with caution).

No products indexed under this heading.

Ranitidine Hydrochloride (Paroxetine is metabolized by the cytochrome P450 isoenzyme CYP2D6. Therefore, co-administration of paroxetine with other drugs that inhibit this enzyme should be approached with caution). Products include:

Zantac 1624
Zantac Injection 1619
Zantac Injection Pharmacy Bulk Package 1622

Risperidone (Paroxetine may significantly inhibit the activity of the cytochrome P450 2D6 isoenzyme. Concomitant use of paroxetine with other drugs metabolized by cytochrome CYP2D6 has not been formally studied but may require lower doses than usually prescribed for either paroxetine or the other drug. Therefore, co-administration of paroxetine with other drugs that are metabolized by this isozyme should be approached with caution). Products include:

Risperdal 1676
Risperdal Consta Long-Acting Injection 1682
Risperdal M-Tab Orally Disintegrating Tablets 1676

Ritonavir (Co-administration of ritonavir with paroxetine significantly decreased plasma levels of paroxetine. Any dose adjustment should be guided by clinical effect (tolerability and efficacy)). Products include:

Kaletra 476
Norvir 503

Rizatriptan Benzoate (There have been rare postmarketing reports of serotonin syndrome with the use of an SSRI and a triptan. If concomitant use of paroxetine hydrochloride with a triptan is clinically warranted, careful observation of the patient is advised, particularly during treatment initiation and dose increases). Products include:

Maxalt Tablets 2008
Maxalt-MLT Orally Disintegrating Tablets 2008

Rofecoxib (The combined use of psychotropic drugs that interfere with serotonin reuptake and drugs that affect coagulation has been associated with an increased risk of bleeding).

No products indexed under this heading.

Selegiline Hydrochloride (Concomitant use of paroxetine hydrochloride and MAOIs intended to treat depression is contraindicated. Potential for serious and/or fatal reactions, including hyperthermia, rigidity, myoclonus, and other serious reactions; therefore, it is recommended that paroxetine hydrochloride not be used in combination with an MAOI, or within 14 days of discontinuing treatment with an MAOI. At least 2 weeks should be allowed after stopping paroxetine hydrochloride before starting an MAOI). Products include:

Eldepryl Capsules 3208
Zelapar Tablets 3372

Sertraline Hydrochloride (Paroxetine is metabolized by the cytochrome P450 isoenzyme CYP2D6. Therefore, co-administration of paroxetine with other drugs that inhibit this enzyme should be approached with caution). Products include:

Zoloft 2586

Sulindac (The combined use of psychotropic drugs that interfere with serotonin reuptake and drugs that affect coagulation has been associated with an increased risk of bleeding). Products include:

Clinoril Tablets 1924

Sumatriptan (Co-administration of a selective serotonin reuptake inhibitor (SSRI) and sumatriptan has resulted in weakness, hyperreflexia, and incoordination). Products include:

Imitrex Nasal Spray 1467

Sumatriptan Succinate (Co-administration of a selective serotonin reuptake inhibitor (SSRI) and sumatriptan has resulted in weakness, hyperreflexia, and incoordination). Products include:

Imitrex Injection 1463
Imitrex Tablets 1471

Tamoxifen Citrate (Paroxetine may significantly inhibit the activity of the cytochrome P450 2D6 isoenzyme. Concomitant use of paroxetine with other drugs metabolized by cytochrome CYP2D6 has not been formally studied but may require lower doses than usually prescribed for either paroxetine or the other drug. Therefore, co-administration of paroxetine with other drugs that are metabolized by this isozyme should be approached with caution). Products include:

Soltamox Oral Solution 3527

Temazepam (Co-administration with another drug that is highly protein bound may increase free concentrations of the other drug or paroxetine potentially resulting in adverse events). Products include:

Restoril Capsules 1860

Teniposide (Paroxetine may significantly inhibit the activity of the cytochrome P450 2D6 isoenzyme. Concomitant use of paroxetine with other drugs metabolized by cytochrome CYP2D6 has not been formally studied but may require lower doses than usually prescribed for either paroxetine or the other drug. Therefore, co-administration of paroxetine with other drugs that are metabolized by this isozyme should be approached with caution).

No products indexed under this heading.

Terbinafine Hydrochloride (Paroxetine is metabolized by the cytochrome P450 isoenzyme CYP2D6. Therefore, co-administration of paroxetine with other drugs that inhibit this enzyme should be approached with caution). Products include:

Lamisil Tablets 2232
Lamisil AT Creams (Athlete's Foot & Jock Itch) .... ▣ 636

Testosterone (Paroxetine may significantly inhibit the activity of the cytochrome P450 2D6 isoenzyme. Concomitant use of paroxetine with other drugs metabolized by cytochrome CYP2D6 has not been formally studied but may require lower doses than usually prescribed for either paroxetine or the other drug. Therefore, co-administration of paroxetine with other drugs that are metabolized by this isozyme should be approached with caution). Products include:

AndroGel 3329
Striant Mucoadhesive 1007
Testim 1% Gel 695

Testosterone Cypionate (Paroxetine may significantly inhibit the activity of the cytochrome P450 2D6 isoenzyme. Concomitant use of paroxetine with other drugs metabolized by cytochrome CYP2D6 has not been formally studied but may require lower doses than usually prescribed for either paroxetine or the other drug. Therefore, co-administration of paroxetine with other drugs that are metabolized by this isozyme should be approached with caution).

No products indexed under this heading.

Testosterone Enanthate (Paroxetine may significantly inhibit the activity of the cytochrome P450 2D6 isoenzyme. Concomitant use of paroxetine with other drugs metabolized by cytochrome CYP2D6 has not been formally studied but may require lower doses than usually prescribed for either paroxetine or the other drug. Therefore, co-administration of paroxetine with other drugs that are metabolized by this isozyme should be approached with caution).

No products indexed under this heading.

Testosterone Propionate (Paroxetine may significantly inhibit the activity of the cytochrome P450 2D6 isoenzyme. Concomitant use of paroxetine with other drugs metabolized by cytochrome CYP2D6 has not

been formally studied but may require lower doses than usually prescribed for either paroxetine or the other drug. Therefore, co-administration of paroxetine with other drugs that are metabolized by this isozyme should be approached with caution).
No products indexed under this heading.

Theophylline (There have been reports of elevated theophylline levels associated with co-administration; monitor theophylline levels when these drugs are concurrently administered).
No products indexed under this heading.

Theophylline Anhydrous (There have been reports of elevated theophylline levels associated with co-administration; monitor theophylline levels when these drugs are concurrently administered). Products include:
Uniphyl Tablets 2710

Theophylline Calcium Salicylate (There have been reports of elevated theophylline levels associated with co-administration; monitor theophylline levels when these drugs are concurrently administered).
No products indexed under this heading.

Theophylline Dihydroxypropyl (Glyceryl) (There have been reports of elevated theophylline levels associated with co-administration; monitor theophylline levels when these drugs are concurrently administered).
No products indexed under this heading.

Theophylline Ethylenediamine (There have been reports of elevated theophylline levels associated with co-administration; monitor theophylline levels when these drugs are concurrently administered).
No products indexed under this heading.

Theophylline Sodium Glycinate (There have been reports of elevated theophylline levels associated with co-administration; monitor theophylline levels when these drugs are concurrently administered).
No products indexed under this heading.

Thioridazine (Co-administration of drugs which inhibit CYP450IID6, such as paroxetine, will elevate plasma levels of thioridazine because thioridazine administration produces a dose-related prolongation of the QTc interval which is associated with serious ventricular arrhythmias, such as torsade de pointes-type arrhythmias, and sudden death; concurrent use is contraindicated).
No products indexed under this heading.

Thioridazine Hydrochloride (Co-administration of drugs which inhibit CYP450IID6, such as paroxetine, will elevate plasma levels of thioridazine because thioridazine administration produces a dose-related prolongation of the QTc interval which is associated with serious ventricular arrhythmias, such as torsade de pointes-type arrhythmias, and sudden death; concurrent use is contraindicated). Products include:
Thioridazine Hydrochloride Tablets 2163

Timolol Maleate (Paroxetine may significantly inhibit the activity of the cytochrome P450 2D6 isoenzyme. Concomitant use of paroxetine with other drugs metabolized by cytochrome CYP2D6 has not been formally studied but may require lower doses than usually prescribed for either paroxetine or the other drug. Therefore, co-administration of paroxetine with other drugs that are metabolized by this isozyme should be approached with caution). Products include:
Blocadren Tablets 1916
Cosopt Sterile Ophthalmic Solution 1931
Timolide Tablets 2086
Timoptic Sterile Ophthalmic Solution 2088
Timoptic in Ocudose 2091
Timoptic-XE Sterile Ophthalmic Gel Forming Solution 2092

Tinzaparin Sodium (The combined use of psychotropic drugs that interfere with serotonin reuptake and drugs that affect coagulation has been associated with an increased risk of bleeding; concomitant administration should be undertaken with caution).
No products indexed under this heading.

Tolbutamide (Co-administration with another drug that is highly protein bound may increase free concentrations of the other drug or paroxetine potentially resulting in adverse events).
No products indexed under this heading.

Tolmetin Sodium (The combined use of psychotropic drugs that interfere with serotonin reuptake and drugs that affect coagulation has been associated with an increased risk of bleeding).
No products indexed under this heading.

Tolterodine Tartrate (Paroxetine may significantly inhibit the activity of the cytochrome P450 2D6 isoenzyme. Concomitant use of paroxetine with other drugs metabolized by cytochrome CYP2D6 has not been formally studied but may require lower doses than usually prescribed for either paroxetine or the other drug. Therefore, co-administration of paroxetine with other drugs that are metabolized by this isozyme should be approached with caution). Products include:
Detrol Tablets 2628
Detrol LA Capsules 2631

Tramadol Hydrochloride (Based on the mechanism of action of paroxetine and the potential for serotonin syndrome, caution is advised when paroxetine hydrochloride is co-administered with other drugs or agents that may affect the serotonergic neurotransmitter systems, such as tramadol). Products include:
Ultram ER Tablets 2392

Tranylcypromine Sulfate (Concomitant use of paroxetine hydrochloride and MAOIs intended to treat depression is contraindicated. Potential for serious and/or fatal reactions, including hyperthermia, rigidity, myoclonus, and other serious reactions; therefore, it is recommended that paroxetine hydrochloride not be used in combination with an MAOI, or within 14 days of discontinuing treatment with an MAOI. At least 2 weeks should be allowed after stopping paroxetine hydrochloride before starting an MAOI). Products include:
Parnate Tablets 1527

Trazodone Hydrochloride (Paroxetine may significantly inhibit the activity of the cytochrome P450 2D6 isoenzyme. Concomitant use of paroxetine with other drugs metabolized by cytochrome CYP2D6 has not been formally studied but may require lower doses than usually prescribed for either paroxetine or the other drug. Therefore, co-administration of paroxetine with other drugs that are metabolized by this isozyme should be approached with caution).
No products indexed under this heading.

Triazolam (Paroxetine may significantly inhibit the activity of the cytochrome P450 2D6 isoenzyme. Concomitant use of paroxetine with other drugs metabolized by cytochrome CYP2D6 has not been formally studied but may require lower doses than usually prescribed for either paroxetine or the other drug. Therefore, co-administration of paroxetine with other drugs that are metabolized by this isozyme should be approached with caution).
No products indexed under this heading.

Trifluoperazine Hydrochloride (Paroxetine may significantly inhibit the activity of cytochrome P450 2D6 isoenzyme. Concomitant use of paroxetine with other drugs metabolized by cytochrome CYP2D6 has not been formally studied but may require lower doses than usually prescribed for either paroxetine or the other drug. Therefore, co-administration of paroxetine with other drugs that are metabolized by this isozyme should be approached with caution).
No products indexed under this heading.

Trimipramine Maleate (Caution is indicated in the co-administration of tricyclic antidepressants with paroxetine because paroxetine may inhibit TCA metabolism. Plasma TCA concentrations may need to be monitored and the dose of TCA may need to be reduced if a TCA is co-administered with paroxetine).
No products indexed under this heading.

L-Tryptophan (Potential for headache, nausea, sweating and dizziness; concomitant use is not recommended). Products include:
L-Tryptophan Capsules 2145

Valdecoxib (The combined use of psychotropic drugs that interfere with serotonin reuptake and drugs that affect coagulation has been associated with an increased risk of bleeding).
No products indexed under this heading.

Venlafaxine Hydrochloride (Paroxetine may significantly inhibit the activity of the cytochrome P450 2D6 isoenzyme. Concomitant use of paroxetine with other drugs metabolized by cytochrome CYP2D6 has not been formally studied but may require lower doses than usually prescribed for either paroxetine or the other drug. Therefore, co-administration of paroxetine with other drugs that are metabolized by this isozyme should be approached with caution). Products include:
Effexor Tablets 3411
Effexor XR Capsules 3417

Vinblastine Sulfate (Paroxetine may significantly inhibit the activity of the cytochrome P450 2D6 isoenzyme. Concomitant use of paroxetine with other drugs metabolized by cytochrome CYP2D6 has not been formally studied but may require lower doses than usually prescribed for either paroxetine or the other drug. Therefore, co-administration of paroxetine with other drugs that are metabolized by this isozyme should be approached with caution).
No products indexed under this heading.

Warfarin Sodium (Preliminary data suggest that there may be a pharmacodynamic interaction (that causes an increased bleeding diathesis in the face of unaltered prothrombin time) between paroxetine and warfarin. Since there is little clinical experience, the concomitant administration of paroxetine and warfarin should be undertaken with caution). Products include:
Coumadin for Injection 898
Coumadin Tablets 898

Zolmitriptan (There have been rare postmarketing reports of serotonin syndrome with the use of an SSRI and a triptan. If concomitant use of paroxetine hydrochloride with a triptan is clinically warranted, careful observation of the patient is advised, particularly during treatment initiation and dose increases). Products include:
Zomig Tablets 3519
Zomig Nasal Spray 3523
Zomig-ZMT Tablets 3519

Zonisamide (Paroxetine may significantly inhibit the activity of the cytochrome P450 2D6 isoenzyme. Concomitant use of paroxetine with other drugs metabolized by cytochrome CYP2D6 has not been formally studied but may require lower doses than usually prescribed for either paroxetine or the other drug. Therefore, co-administration of paroxetine with other drugs that are metabolized by this isozyme should be approached with caution). Products include:
Zonegran Capsules 1101

Food Interactions

Alcohol (Concurrent use should be avoided).

Food, unspecified (Co-administration with food resulted in a slight increase (6%) in AUC, but Cmax was 29% greater; time to reach peak plasma concentration decreased from 6.4 hours post-dosing to 4.9 hours).

PCE DISPERTAB TABLETS

(Erythromycin) 515
May interact with oral anticoagulants, HMG-CoA reductase inhibitors, phenytoin, triazolobenzodiazepines, valproate, xanthines, and certain other agents. Compounds in these categories include:

Alfentanil Hydrochloride (Concurrent use of erythromycin in patients receiving drugs metabolized by the cytochrome P450 system may be associated with elevation in serum levels of alfentanil).
No products indexed under this heading.

Alprazolam (Erythromycin has been reported to decrease the clearance of triazolam and midazolam; may increase the pharmacologic effect of these benzodiazepines). Products include:
Niravam Orally Disintegrating Tablets 3092

Aminophylline (Co-administration in patients who are receiving high doses of theophylline may be associated with an increase in serum theophylline levels and potential theophylline toxicity).
No products indexed under this heading.

Anisindione (Co-administration has resulted in increased anticoagulant effects). Products include:
Miradon Tablets 3042

Astemizole (Concurrent use of erythromycin in patients receiving astemizole has been reported to significantly alter the metabolism of astemizole; rare cases of cardiovascular adverse events, including prolonged QT interval, cardiac arrest, torsade de pointes, and other ventricular arrhythmias have been reported; co-administration is contraindicated).
No products indexed under this heading.

Atorvastatin Calcium (Erythromycin has been reported to increase concentrations of HMG-CoA reductase inhibitors (e.g. lovastatin and simvastatin); rare reports of rhabdomyolysis have been reported in patients taking these drugs concomitantly). Products include:
Caduet Tablets 2508
Lipitor Tablets 2483

Bromocriptine Mesylate (Concurrent use of erythromycin in patients receiving drugs metabolized by the cytochrome P450 system may be associated with elevation in serum levels of bromocriptine).
No products indexed under this heading.

Carbamazepine (Concurrent use of erythromycin in patients receiving drugs metabolized by the cytochrome P450 system may be associated with elevation in serum levels of carbamazepine). Products include:
Carbatrol Capsules 3171
Equetro Extended-Release Capsules 3180
Tegretol/Tegretol-XR 2295

Cerivastatin Sodium (Erythromycin has been reported to increase concentrations of HMG-CoA reductase inhibitors (e.g. lovastatin and simvastatin); rare reports of rhabdomyolysis have been reported in patients taking these drugs concomitantly).
No products indexed under this heading.

Cisapride (Concurrent use of erythromycin in patients receiving cisapride has been reported to inhibit the metabolism of cisapride; cases of cardiovascular adverse events, including prolonged QT interval, torsade de pointes, ventricular tachycardia, and ventricular fibrillation have been reported; co-administration is contraindicated).
No products indexed under this heading.

Cyclosporine (Concurrent use of erythromycin in patients receiving drugs metabolized by the cytochrome P450 system may be associated with elevation in serum levels of cyclosporine). Products include:
Gengraf Capsules 459
Neoral Oral Solution 2259
Neoral Soft Gelatin Capsules 2259
Restasis Ophthalmic Emulsion 575
Sandimmune 2275

Dicumarol (Co-administration has resulted in increased anticoagulant effects).
No products indexed under this heading.

Digoxin (Co-administration has been reported to result in elevated digoxin serum levels). Products include:
Lanoxicaps Capsules 1490
Lanoxin Injection 1494
Lanoxin Injection Pediatric 1497
Lanoxin Tablets 1500

Dihydroergotamine Mesylate (Co-administration has been associated in some patients with acute ergot toxicity characterized by severe peripheral vasospasm and dysesthesia). Products include:
Migranal Nasal Spray 3348

Disopyramide Phosphate (Concurrent use of erythromycin in patients receiving drugs metabolized by the cytochrome P450 system may be associated with elevation in serum levels of disopyramide).
No products indexed under this heading.

Divalproex Sodium (There have been reports of interactions of erythromycin with drugs not thought to be metabolized by CYP3A, including valproate). Products include:
Depakote Sprinkle Capsules 422
Depakote Tablets 427
Depakote ER Tablets 434

Dyphylline (Co-administration in patients who are receiving high doses of theophylline may be associated with an increase in serum theophylline levels and potential theophylline toxicity).
No products indexed under this heading.

Ergotamine Tartrate (Co-administration has been associated in some patients with acute ergot toxicity characterized by severe peripheral vasospasm and dysethesia).
No products indexed under this heading.

Fluvastatin Sodium (Erythromycin has been reported to increase concentrations of HMG-CoA reductase inhibitors (e.g. lovastatin and simvastatin); rare reports of rhabdomyolysis have been reported in patients taking these drugs concomitantly). Products include:
Lescol Capsules 2233
Lescol XL Tablets 2233

Fosphenytoin Sodium (There have been reports of interactions of erythromycin with drugs not thought to be metabolized by CYP3A, including phenytoin).
No products indexed under this heading.

Hexobarbital (There have been reports of interactions of erythromycin with drugs not thought to be metabolized by CYP3A, including hexobarbital).
No products indexed under this heading.

Lovastatin (Erythromycin has been reported to increase concentrations of HMG-CoA reductase inhibitors (e.g. lovastatin and simvastatin); rare reports of rhabdomyolysis have been reported in patients taking these drugs concomitantly). Products include:
Advicor Tablets 1722
Altoprev Extended-Release Tablets 3109
Mevacor Tablets 2021

Midazolam Hydrochloride (Erythromycin has been reported to decrease the clearance of triazolam and midazolam; may increase the pharmacologic effect of these benzodiazepines).
No products indexed under this heading.

Phenytoin (There have been reports of interactions of erythromycin with drugs not thought to be metabolized by CYP3A, including phenytoin).
No products indexed under this heading.

Phenytoin Sodium (There have been reports of interactions of erythromycin with drugs not thought to be metabolized by CYP3A, including phenytoin). Products include:
Phenytek Capsules 2160

Pimozide (Concurrent use of erythromycin in patients receiving drugs metabolized by the cytochrome P450 system may be associated with elevation in serum levels of pimozide; co-administration is contraindicated).
No products indexed under this heading.

Pravastatin Sodium (Erythromycin has been reported to increase concentrations of HMG-CoA reductase inhibitors (e.g. lovastatin and simvastatin); rare reports of rhabdomyolysis have been reported in patients taking these drugs concomitantly).
No products indexed under this heading.

Sildenafil Citrate (Erythromycin has been reported to increase the systemic exposure (AUC) of sildenafil). Products include:
Revatio Tablets 2557
Viagra Tablets 2573

Simvastatin (Erythromycin has been reported to increase concentrations of HMG-CoA reductase inhibitors (e.g. lovastatin and simvastatin); rare reports of rhabdomyolysis have been reported in patients taking these drugs concomitantly). Products include:
Vytorin 10/10 Tablets 2114
Vytorin 10/10 Tablets 3077
Vytorin 10/20 Tablets 2114
Vytorin 10/20 Tablets 3077
Vytorin 10/40 Tablets 2114
Vytorin 10/40 Tablets 3077
Vytorin 10/80 Tablets 2114
Vytorin 10/80 Tablets 3077
Zocor Tablets 2105

Tacrolimus (Concurrent use of erythromycin in patients receiving drugs metabolized by the cytochrome P450 system may be associated with elevation in serum levels of tacrolimus). Products include:
Prograf Capsules and Injection 632
Protopic Ointment 638

Terfenadine (Concurrent use of erythromycin in patients receiving terfenadine has been reported to significantly alter the metabolism of terfenadine; rare cases of cardiovascular adverse events, including prolonged QT interval, cardiac arrest, torsade de pointes, other ventricular arrhythmias, and death have been reported; co-administration is contraindicated).
No products indexed under this heading.

Theophylline (Co-administration in patients who are receiving high doses of theophylline may be associated with an increase in serum theophylline levels and potential theophylline toxicity).
No products indexed under this heading.

Theophylline Anhydrous (Co-administration in patients who are receiving high doses of theophylline may be associated with an increase in serum theophylline levels and potential theophylline toxicity). Products include:
Uniphyl Tablets 2710

Theophylline Calcium Salicylate (Co-administration in patients who are receiving high doses of theophylline may be associated with an increase in serum theophylline levels and potential theophylline toxicity).
No products indexed under this heading.

Theophylline Dihydroxypropyl (Glyceryl) (Co-administration in patients who are receiving high doses of theophylline may be associated with an increase in serum theophylline levels and potential theophylline toxicity).
No products indexed under this heading.

Theophylline Ethylenediamine (Co-administration in patients who are receiving high doses of theophylline may be associated with an increase in serum theophylline levels and potential theophylline toxicity).
No products indexed under this heading.

Theophylline Sodium Glycinate (Co-administration in patients who are receiving high doses of theophylline may be associated with an increase in serum theophylline levels and potential theophylline toxicity).
No products indexed under this heading.

Triazolam (Erythromycin has been reported to decrease the clearance of triazolam and midazolam; may increase the pharmacologic effect of these benzodiazepines).
No products indexed under this heading.

Valproate Sodium (There have been reports of interactions of erythromycin with drugs not thought to be metabolized by CYP3A, including valproate). Products include:
Depacon Injection 412

Valproic Acid (There have been reports of interactions of erythromycin with drugs not thought to be metabolized by CYP3A, including valproate). Products include:
Depakene 417

Warfarin Sodium (Co-administration has resulted in increased anticoagulant effects). Products include:
Coumadin for Injection 898

Coumadin Tablets 898

Food Interactions

Meal, unspecified (Presence of food results in lower blood levels; optimal blood levels are obtained when PCE is given in the fasting state (at least ½ hour and preferably 2 hours before meals)).

PEDIARIX VACCINE

(Diphtheria & Tetanus Toxoids and Pertussis Vaccine Adsorbed, Hepatitis B Vaccine, Recombinant, Poliovirus Vaccine Inactivated, Trivalent Types 1,2,3)........................... **1548**
May interact with alkylating agents, antimetabolites, corticosteroids, cytotoxic drugs, immunosuppressive agents, and certain other agents. Compounds in these categories include:

Azathioprine (May reduce immune response to vaccines. When administered to patients who are receiving immunosuppressive therapy, who have an immunodeficiency disorder, or who have received a recent injection of immune globulin, an adequate immunologic response may not be obtained.).
 No products indexed under this heading.

Basiliximab (May reduce immune response to vaccines. When administered to patients who are receiving immunosuppressive therapy, who have an immunodeficiency disorder, or who have received a recent injection of immune globulin, an adequate immunologic response may not be obtained). Products include:
 Simulect for Injection **2284**

Betamethasone Acetate (May reduce immune response to vaccines. When administered to patients who are receiving immunosuppressive therapy, who have an immunodeficiency disorder, or who have received a recent injection of immune globulin, an adequate immunologic response may not be obtained.).
 No products indexed under this heading.

Betamethasone Sodium Phosphate (May reduce immune response to vaccines. When administered to patients who are receiving immunosuppressive therapy, who have an immunodeficiency disorder, or who have received a recent injection of immune globulin, an adequate immunologic response may not be obtained.).
 No products indexed under this heading.

Bleomycin Sulfate (May reduce immune response to vaccines. When administered to patients who are receiving immunosuppressive therapy, who have an immunodeficiency disorder, or who have received a recent injection of immune globulin, an adequate immunologic response may not be obtained.).
 No products indexed under this heading.

Busulfan (May reduce immune response to vaccines. When administered to patients who are receiving immunosuppressive therapy, who have an immunodeficiency disorder, or who have received a recent injection of immune globulin, an adequate immunologic response may not be obtained). Products include:

I.V. Busulfex 2493
Myleran Tablets 1525

Capecitabine (May reduce immune response to vaccines. When administered to patients who are receiving immunosuppressive therapy, who have an immunodeficiency disorder, or who have received a recent injection of immune globulin, an adequate immunologic response may not be obtained). Products include:
 Xeloda Tablets 2822

Carmustine (BCNU) (May reduce immune response to vaccines. When administered to patients who are receiving immunosuppressive therapy, who have an immunodeficiency disorder, or who have received a recent injection of immune globulin, an adequate immunologic response may not be obtained.).
 No products indexed under this heading.

Chlorambucil (May reduce immune response to vaccines. When administered to patients who are receiving immunosuppressive therapy, who have an immunodeficiency disorder, or who have received a recent injection of immune globulin, an adequate immunologic response may not be obtained). Products include:
 Leukeran Tablets 1504

Cladribine (May reduce immune response to vaccines. When administered to patients who are receiving immunosuppressive therapy, who have an immunodeficiency disorder, or who have received a recent injection of immune globulin, an adequate immunologic response may not be obtained). Products include:
 Leustatin Injection 2357

Cortisone Acetate (May reduce immune response to vaccines. When administered to patients who are receiving immunosuppressive therapy, who have an immunodeficiency disorder, or who have received a recent injection of immune globulin, an adequate immunologic response may not be obtained.).
 No products indexed under this heading.

Cyclophosphamide (May reduce immune response to vaccines. When administered to patients who are receiving immunosuppressive therapy, who have an immunodeficiency disorder, or who have received a recent injection of immune globulin, an adequate immunologic response may not be obtained.).
 No products indexed under this heading.

Cyclosporine (May reduce immune response to vaccines. When administered to patients who are receiving immunosuppressive therapy, who have an immunodeficiency disorder, or who have received a recent injection of immune globulin, an adequate immunologic response may not be obtained). Products include:
Gengraf Capsules 459
Neoral Oral Solution 2259
Neoral Soft Gelatin Capsules 2259
Restasis Ophthalmic Emulsion 575
Sandimmune 2275

Cytarabine (May reduce immune response to vaccines. When administered to patients who are receiving immunosuppressive therapy, who have an immunodeficiency disorder, or who have received a recent injection of immune globulin, an adequate immunologic response may not be obtained.).
 No products indexed under this heading.

Dacarbazine (May reduce immune response to vaccines. When administered to patients who are receiving immunosuppressive therapy, who have an immunodeficiency disorder, or who have received a recent injection of immune globulin, an adequate immunologic response may not be obtained.).
 No products indexed under this heading.

Daunorubicin Hydrochloride (May reduce immune response to vaccines. When administered to patients who are receiving immunosuppressive therapy, who have an immunodeficiency disorder, or who have received a recent injection of immune globulin, an adequate immunologic response may not be obtained.).
 No products indexed under this heading.

Dexamethasone (May reduce immune response to vaccines. When administered to patients who are receiving immunosuppressive therapy, who have an immunodeficiency disorder, or who have received a recent injection of immune globulin, an adequate immunologic response may not be obtained.). Products include:
Ciprodex Otic Suspension 559
Decadron Tablets 1951
TobraDex Ophthalmic Ointment 562
TobraDex Ophthalmic Suspension ... 563

Dexamethasone Acetate (May reduce immune response to vaccines. When administered to patients who are receiving immunosuppressive therapy, who have an immunodeficiency disorder, or who have received a recent injection of immune globulin, an adequate immunologic response may not be obtained.).
 No products indexed under this heading.

Dexamethasone Sodium Phosphate (May reduce immune response to vaccines. When administered to patients who are receiving immunosuppressive therapy, who have an immunodeficiency disorder, or who have received a recent injection of immune globulin, an adequate immunologic response may not be obtained.).
 No products indexed under this heading.

Doxorubicin Hydrochloride (May reduce immune response to vaccines. When administered to patients who are receiving immunosuppressive therapy, who have an immunodeficiency disorder, or who have received a recent injection of immune globulin, an adequate immunologic response may not be obtained.).
 No products indexed under this heading.

Epirubicin Hydrochloride (May reduce immune response to vaccines. When administered to patients who are receiving immunosuppressive therapy, who have an immunodeficiency disorder, or who have received a recent injection of immune globulin, an adequate immunologic response may not be obtained.).
 No products indexed under this heading.

Floxuridine (May reduce immune response to vaccines. When administered to patients who are receiving immunosuppressive therapy, who have an immunodeficiency disorder, or who have received a recent injection of immune globulin, an adequate immunologic response may not be obtained.).
 No products indexed under this heading.

Fludarabine Phosphate (May reduce immune response to vaccines. When administered to patients who are receiving immunosuppressive therapy, who have an immunodeficiency disorder, or who have received a recent injection of immune globulin, an adequate immunologic response may not be obtained.).
 No products indexed under this heading.

Fludrocortisone Acetate (May reduce immune response to vaccines. When administered to patients who are receiving immunosuppressive therapy, who have an immunodeficiency disorder, or who have received a recent injection of immune globulin, an adequate immunologic response may not be obtained.).
 No products indexed under this heading.

Fluorouracil (May reduce immune response to vaccines. When administered to patients who are receiving immunosuppressive therapy, who have an immunodeficiency disorder, or who have received a recent injection of immune globulin, an adequate immunologic response may not be obtained.). Products include:
Carac Cream, 0.5% 2879
Efudex ... 3363

Gemcitabine Hydrochloride (May reduce immune response to vaccines. When administered to patients who are receiving immunosuppressive therapy, who have an immunodeficiency disorder, or who have received a recent injection of immune globulin, an adequate immunologic response may not be obtained.). Products include:
 Gemzar for Injection 1771

Hydrocortisone (May reduce immune response to vaccines. When administered to patients who are receiving immunosuppressive therapy, who have an immunodeficiency disorder, or who have received a recent injection of immune globulin, an adequate immunologic response may not be obtained.). Products include:
Colocort Rectal Suspension, USP (Retention) 100 mg/60 mL........... 2476
Hydrocortone Tablets 1989
Preparation H Hydrocortisone Cream .. 646

Hydrocortisone Acetate (May reduce immune response to vaccines. When administered to patients

IMPORTANT NOTE: Always consult each drug listing in the patient's regimen for possible interactions.

who are receiving immunosuppressive therapy, who have an immunodeficiency disorder, or who have received a recent injection of immune globulin, an adequate immunologic response may not be obtained). Products include:

Analpram-HC 1159
Pramosone 1161
ProctoFoam-HC 3099

Hydrocortisone Sodium Phosphate (May reduce immune response to vaccines. When administered to patients who are receiving immunosuppressive therapy, who have an immunodeficiency disorder, or who have received a recent injection of immune globulin, an adequate immunologic response may not be obtained.).

No products indexed under this heading.

Hydrocortisone Sodium Succinate (May reduce immune response to vaccines. When administered to patients who are receiving immunosuppressive therapy, who have an immunodeficiency disorder, or who have received a recent injection of immune globulin, an adequate immunologic response may not be obtained.).

No products indexed under this heading.

Hydroxyurea (May reduce immune response to vaccines. When administered to patients who are receiving immunosuppressive therapy, who have an immunodeficiency disorder, or who have received a recent injection of immune globulin, an adequate immunologic response may not be obtained.).

No products indexed under this heading.

Immune Globulin Intravenous (Human) (May reduce immune response to vaccines. When administered to patients who are receiving immunosuppressive therapy, who have an immunodeficiency disorder, or who have received a recent injection of immune globulin, an adequate immunologic response may not be obtained). Products include:

Carimune NF 3499
Gammagard Liquid 721
Gammagard S/D 724
Gamunex Immune Globulin I.V., 10% 3235

Lomustine (CCNU) (May reduce immune response to vaccines. When administered to patients who are receiving immunosuppressive therapy, who have an immunodeficiency disorder, or who have received a recent injection of immune globulin, an adequate immunologic response may not be obtained.).

No products indexed under this heading.

Mechlorethamine Hydrochloride (May reduce immune response to vaccines. When administered to patients who are receiving immunosuppressive therapy, who have an immunodeficiency disorder, or who have received a recent injection of immune globulin, an adequate immunologic response may not be obtained). Products include:

Mustargen for Injection 2468

Melphalan (May reduce immune response to vaccines. When administered to patients who are receiving immunosuppressive therapy, who have an immunodeficiency disorder, or who have received a recent injection of immune globulin, an adequate immunologic response may not be obtained). Products include:

Alkeran Tablets 956

Mercaptopurine (May reduce immune response to vaccines. When administered to patients who are receiving immunosuppressive therapy, who have an immunodeficiency disorder, or who have received a recent injection of immune globulin, an adequate immunologic response may not be obtained.).

No products indexed under this heading.

Methotrexate (May reduce immune response to vaccines. When administered to patients who are receiving immunosuppressive therapy, who have an immunodeficiency disorder, or who have received a recent injection of immune globulin, an adequate immunologic response may not be obtained.).

No products indexed under this heading.

Methotrexate Sodium (May reduce immune response to vaccines. When administered to patients who are receiving immunosuppressive therapy, who have an immunodeficiency disorder, or who have received a recent injection of immune globulin, an adequate immunologic response may not be obtained.).

No products indexed under this heading.

Methylprednisolone Acetate (May reduce immune response to vaccines. When administered to patients who are receiving immunosuppressive therapy, who have an immunodeficiency disorder, or who have received a recent injection of immune globulin, an adequate immunologic response may not be obtained). Products include:

Depo-Medrol Injectable Suspension 2617
Depo-Medrol Single-Dose Vial 2619

Methylprednisolone Sodium Succinate (May reduce immune response to vaccines. When administered to patients who are receiving immunosuppressive therapy, who have an immunodeficiency disorder, or who have received a recent injection of immune globulin, an adequate immunologic response may not be obtained.).

No products indexed under this heading.

Mitotane (May reduce immune response to vaccines. When administered to patients who are receiving immunosuppressive therapy, who have an immunodeficiency disorder, or who have received a recent injection of immune globulin, an adequate immunologic response may not be obtained.).

No products indexed under this heading.

Mitoxantrone Hydrochloride (May reduce immune response to vaccines. When administered to patients who are receiving immunosuppressive therapy, who have an immunodeficiency disorder, or who have received a recent injection of immune globulin, an adequate immunologic response may not be obtained.).

No products indexed under this heading.

Muromonab-CD3 (May reduce immune response to vaccines. When administered to patients who are receiving immunosuppressive therapy, who have an immunodeficiency disorder, or who have received a recent injection of immune globulin, an adequate immunologic response may not be obtained). Products include:

Orthoclone OKT3 Sterile Solution 2360

Mycophenolate Mofetil (May reduce immune response to vaccines. When administered to patients who are receiving immunosuppressive therapy, who have an immunodeficiency disorder, or who have received a recent injection of immune globulin, an adequate immunologic response may not be obtained). Products include:

CellCept Capsules 2747
CellCept Oral Suspension 2747
CellCept Tablets 2747

Pentostatin (May reduce immune response to vaccines. When administered to patients who are receiving immunosuppressive therapy, who have an immunodeficiency disorder, or who have received a recent injection of immune globulin, an adequate immunologic response may not be obtained). Products include:

Nipent for Injection 1863

Prednisolone Acetate (May reduce immune response to vaccines. When administered to patients who are receiving immunosuppressive therapy, who have an immunodeficiency disorder, or who have received a recent injection of immune globulin, an adequate immunologic response may not be obtained). Products include:

Blephamide Ophthalmic Ointment 568
Blephamide Ophthalmic Suspension 569
Poly-Pred Ophthalmic Suspension .... ⊙233
Pred Forte Ophthalmic Suspension .... ⊙235
Pred Mild Ophthalmic Suspension .... ⊙238
Pred-G Ophthalmic Ointment .... ⊙237
Pred-G Ophthalmic Suspension ...... ⊙236

Prednisolone Sodium Phosphate (May reduce immune response to vaccines. When administered to patients who are receiving immunosuppressive therapy, who have an immunodeficiency disorder, or who have received a recent injection of immune globulin, an adequate immunologic response may not be obtained.).

No products indexed under this heading.

Prednisolone Tebutate (May reduce immune response to vaccines. When administered to patients who are receiving immunosuppressive therapy, who have an immunodeficiency disorder, or who have received a recent injection of immune globulin, an adequate immunologic response may not be obtained.).

No products indexed under this heading.

Prednisone (May reduce immune response to vaccines. When administered to patients who are receiving immunosuppressive therapy, who have an immunodeficiency disorder, or who have received a recent injection of immune globulin, an adequate immunologic response may not be obtained.).

No products indexed under this heading.

Procarbazine Hydrochloride (May reduce immune response to vaccines. When administered to patients who are receiving immunosuppressive therapy, who have an immunodeficiency disorder, or who have received a recent injection of immune globulin, an adequate immunologic response may not be obtained). Products include:

Matulane Capsules 3191

Sirolimus (May reduce immune response to vaccines. When administered to patients who are receiving immunosuppressive therapy, who have an immunodeficiency disorder, or who have received a recent injection of immune globulin, an adequate immunologic response may not be obtained). Products include:

Rapamune Oral Solution and Tablets 3475

Tacrolimus (May reduce immune response to vaccines. When administered to patients who are receiving immunosuppressive therapy, who have an immunodeficiency disorder, or who have received a recent injection of immune globulin, an adequate immunologic response may not be obtained). Products include:

Prograf Capsules and Injection 632
Protopic Ointment 638

Tamoxifen Citrate (May reduce immune response to vaccines. When administered to patients who are receiving immunosuppressive therapy, who have an immunodeficiency disorder, or who have received a recent injection of immune globulin, an adequate immunologic response may not be obtained). Products include:

Soltamox Oral Solution 3527

Thioguanine (May reduce immune response to vaccines. When administered to patients who are receiving immunosuppressive therapy, who have an immunodeficiency disorder, or who have received a recent injection of immune globulin, an adequate immunologic response may not be obtained). Products include:

Tabloid Tablets 1575

Thiotepa (May reduce immune response to vaccines. When administered to patients who are receiving immunosuppressive therapy, who have an immunodeficiency disorder, or who have received a recent injection of immune globulin, an adequate immunologic response may not be obtained.).

No products indexed under this heading.

Triamcinolone (May reduce immune response to vaccines. When administered to patients who are receiving immunosuppressive therapy, who have an immunodeficiency disorder, or who have received a recent injection of immune globulin, an adequate immunologic response may not be obtained.).

No products indexed under this heading.

Triamcinolone Acetonide (May reduce immune response to vaccines. When administered to patients who are receiving immunosuppressive therapy, who have an immunodeficiency disorder, or who have received a recent injection of immune globulin, an adequate immunologic response may not be obtained). Products include:

Azmacort Inhalation Aerosol 1726

Nasacort AQ Nasal Spray 2922

Triamcinolone Diacetate (May reduce immune response to vaccines. When administered to patients who are receiving immunosuppressive therapy, who have an immunodeficiency disorder, or who have received a recent injection of immune globulin, an adequate immunologic response may not be obtained.).

No products indexed under this heading.

Triamcinolone Hexacetonide (May reduce immune response to vaccines. When administered to patients who are receiving immunosuppressive therapy, who have an immunodeficiency disorder, or who have received a recent injection of immune globulin, an adequate immunologic response may not be obtained.).

No products indexed under this heading.

Vincristine Sulfate (May reduce immune response to vaccines. When administered to patients who are receiving immunosuppressive therapy, who have an immunodeficiency disorder, or who have received a recent injection of immune globulin, an adequate immunologic response may not be obtained.).

No products indexed under this heading.

LIQUID PEDVAXHIB

(Haemophilus B Conjugate Vaccine).. 2035

None cited in PDR database.

PEGASYS

(Peginterferon alfa-2a) 2789

May interact with theophyllines and certain other agents. Compounds in these categories include:

Methadone Hydrochloride (In a study of HCV patients concomitantly receiving methadone, treatment with peginterferon alfa-2a once weekly for four weeks was associated with methadone levels that were 10%-15% higher than at baseline. Therefore, patients should be monitored for signs and symptoms of methadone toxicity during co-administration).

No products indexed under this heading.

Theophylline (Inhibition of CYP450 1A2 and a 25% increase in theophylline AUC; monitor theophylline levels and consider appropriate dose adjustments).

No products indexed under this heading.

Theophylline Anhydrous (Inhibition of CYP450 1A2 and a 25% increase in theophylline AUC; monitor theophylline levels and consider appropriate dose adjustments). Products include:

Uniphyl Tablets 2710

Theophylline Calcium Salicylate (Inhibition of CYP450 1A2 and a 25% increase in theophylline AUC; monitor theophylline levels and consider appropriate dose adjustments).

No products indexed under this heading.

Theophylline Dihydroxypropyl (Glyceryl) (Inhibition of CYP450 1A2 and a 25% increase in theophylline AUC; monitor theophylline levels and consider appropriate dose adjustments).

No products indexed under this heading.

Theophylline Ethylenediamine (Inhibition of CYP450 1A2 and a 25% increase in theophylline AUC; monitor theophylline levels and consider appropriate dose adjustments).

No products indexed under this heading.

Theophylline Sodium Glycinate (Inhibition of CYP450 1A2 and a 25% increase in theophylline AUC; monitor theophylline levels and consider appropriate dose adjustments).

No products indexed under this heading.

Zidovudine (Co-administration of zidovudine and Pegasys/Copegus develops sever neutropenia and severe anemia more frequently than similar patients not receiving zidovudine (neutropenia 15% vs. 9%) (anemia 5% vs. 1%)). Products include:

Combivir Tablets 1411
Retrovir 1560
Retrovir IV Infusion 1564
Trizivir Tablets 1589

PEG-INTRON POWDER FOR INJECTION

(Peginterferon Alfa-2b) 3048

May interact with:

Methadone Hydrochloride (In a pharmacokinetic study of 18 chronic hepatitis C patients concomitantly receiving methadone, treatment with PEG-Intron once weekly for four weeks was associated with a mean increase of 16% in methadone AUC. In two out of 18 patients, methadone AUC doubled. The clinical significance of this finding is unknown, however, patients should be monitored for the signs and symptoms of increased narcotic effect).

No products indexed under this heading.

PENLAC NAIL LACQUER, TOPICAL SOLUTION, 8%

(Ciclopirox) 2924

None cited in PDR database.

PENTASA CAPSULES

(Mesalamine) 3185

None cited in PDR database.

PEPCID AC TABLETS AND GELCAPS

(Famotidine) 661

May interact with antacids, antacids containing aluminum, calcium and magnesium, nonabsorbable antacids, and magnesium-containing antacids. Compounds in these categories include:

Aluminum Carbonate (Do not use with other acid reducers).

No products indexed under this heading.

Aluminum Hydroxide (Do not use with other acid reducers). Products include:

Gaviscon Regular Strength Liquid .. 658
Gaviscon Regular Strength Tablets.................................... 658
Gaviscon Extra Strength Liquid 658
Gaviscon Extra Strength Tablets 658
Maalox Regular Strength Antacid/Antigas Liquid................. 2175
Maalox Max Maximum Strength Antacid/Anti-Gas Liquid................ 2176

Calcium Carbonate (Do not use with other acid reducers). Products include:

Actonel with Calcium Tablets 2688
Calcet Tablets 2138
Caltrate 600 PLUS 809
Caltrate 600 + D Tablets 809
D-Cal Chewable Caplets 812
Gas-X with Maalox 656
Maalox Regular Strength Antacid Chewable Tablets 2177
Maalox Max Maximum Strength Antacid/Antigas Chewable Tablets 2176
Maalox Max Maximum Strength Chewable Tablets........................ 660
Os-Cal Chewable Tablets 818
Pepcid Complete Chewable Tablets 1701
Children's Pepto 2674
PremCal Light, Regular, and Extra Strength Tablets................ 818
Tums 664

Magaldrate (Do not use with other acid reducers).

No products indexed under this heading.

Magnesium Carbonate (Do not use with other acid reducers). Products include:

Gaviscon Regular Strength Liquid .. 658
Gaviscon Extra Strength Liquid 658
Gaviscon Extra Strength Tablets 658

Magnesium Hydroxide (Do not use with other acid reducers). Products include:

Maalox Regular Strength Antacid/Antigas Liquid................. 2175
Maalox Max Maximum Strength Antacid/Anti-Gas Liquid................ 2176
Pepcid Complete Chewable Tablets 1701

Magnesium Oxide (Do not use with other acid reducers). Products include:

Beelith Tablets 759
PremCal Light, Regular, and Extra Strength Tablets................ 818

Magnesium Trisilicate (Do not use with other acid reducers). Products include:

Gaviscon Regular Strength Tablets.. 658

Sodium Bicarbonate (Do not use with other acid reducers). Products include:

Colyte with Flavor Packs for Oral Solution... 3088
HalfLytely and Bisacodyl Tablets Bowel Prep Kit with Flavors Packs.. 881
TriLyte with Flavor Packs for Oral Solution... 3100

MAXIMUM STRENGTH PEPCID AC TABLETS

(Famotidine) 661

See Pepcid AC Tablets and Gelcaps

PEPCID COMPLETE CHEWABLE TABLETS

(Calcium Carbonate, Famotidine, Magnesium Hydroxide)..................... 662

May interact with:

Prescription Drugs, unspecified (Antacids contained in Pepcid Complete may interact with certain prescription drugs).

No products indexed under this heading.

PEPCID INJECTION

(Famotidine) 2040

None cited in PDR database.

PEPCID INJECTION PREMIXED

(Famotidine) 2040

None cited in PDR database.

PEPCID FOR ORAL SUSPENSION

(Famotidine) 2038

May interact with antacids and certain other agents. Compounds in these categories include:

Aluminum Carbonate (Bioavailability may be slightly decreased by antacids).

No products indexed under this heading.

Aluminum Hydroxide (Bioavailability may be slightly decreased by antacids). Products include:

Gaviscon Regular Strength Liquid .. 658
Gaviscon Regular Strength Tablets.. 658
Gaviscon Extra Strength Liquid 658
Gaviscon Extra Strength Tablets 658
Maalox Regular Strength Antacid/Antigas Liquid................. 2175
Maalox Max Maximum Strength Antacid/Anti-Gas Liquid................ 2176

Magaldrate (Bioavailability may be slightly decreased by antacids).

No products indexed under this heading.

Magnesium Hydroxide (Bioavailability may be slightly decreased by antacids). Products include:

Maalox Regular Strength Antacid/Antigas Liquid................. 2175
Maalox Max Maximum Strength Antacid/Anti-Gas Liquid................ 2176
Pepcid Complete Chewable Tablets 1701

Magnesium Oxide (Bioavailability may be slightly decreased by antacids). Products include:

Beelith Tablets 759
PremCal Light, Regular, and Extra Strength Tablets................ 818

Sodium Bicarbonate (Bioavailability may be slightly decreased by antacids). Products include:

Colyte with Flavor Packs for Oral Solution... 3088
HalfLytely and Bisacodyl Tablets Bowel Prep Kit with Flavors Packs.. 881
TriLyte with Flavor Packs for Oral Solution... 3100

Food Interactions

Food, unspecified (Bioavailability may be slightly increased by antacids).

PEPCID TABLETS

(Famotidine) 2038

See Pepcid for Oral Suspension

PEPCID AC GELCAPS

(Famotidine) 1701

None cited in PDR database.

PEPCID AC TABLETS

(Famotidine) 1701

None cited in PDR database.

MAXIMUM STRENGTH PEPCID AC TABLETS

(Famotidine) 1701

None cited in PDR database.

PEPCID COMPLETE CHEWABLE TABLETS

(Calcium Carbonate, Famotidine, Magnesium Hydroxide)...................... 1701

May interact with:

Prescription Drugs, unspecified (Antacids contained in Pepcid Complete may interact with certain prescription drugs).

No products indexed under this heading.

CHILDREN'S PEPTO

(Calcium Carbonate) 662

None cited in PDR database.

PEPTO-BISMOL ORIGINAL LIQUID, MAXIMUM STRENGTH LIQUID, ORIGINAL AND CHERRY TABLETS, CHEWABLE TABLETS AND EASY-TO-SWALLOW CAPLETS

(Bismuth Subsalicylate) 2676

May interact with oral anticoagulants, antigout agents, and oral hypoglycemic agents. Compounds in these categories include:

Acarbose (Concurrent use should be undertaken with physician's supervision). Products include:
Precose Tablets 751

Allopurinol (Concurrent use should be undertaken with physician's supervision).
No products indexed under this heading.

Anisindione (Concurrent use should be undertaken with physician's supervision). Products include:
Miradon Tablets 3042

Chlorpropamide (Concurrent use should be undertaken with physician's supervision).
No products indexed under this heading.

Dicumarol (Concurrent use should be undertaken with physician's supervision).
No products indexed under this heading.

Glimepiride (Concurrent use should be undertaken with physician's supervision). Products include:
Avandaryl Tablets 1379
Duetact Tablets 3226

Glipizide (Concurrent use should be undertaken with physician's supervision).
No products indexed under this heading.

Glyburide (Concurrent use should be undertaken with physician's supervision).
No products indexed under this heading.

Metformin Hydrochloride (Concurrent use should be undertaken with physician's supervision). Products include:
ActoPlus Met Tablets 3214
Avandamet Tablets 1373
Fortamet Extended-Release Tablets 3115

Miglitol (Concurrent use should be undertaken with physician's supervision).
No products indexed under this heading.

Pioglitazone Hydrochloride (Concurrent use should be undertaken with physician's supervision). Products include:
ActoPlus Met Tablets 3214
Actos Tablets 3219
Duetact Tablets 3226

Probenecid (Concurrent use should be undertaken with physician's supervision).
No products indexed under this heading.

Repaglinide (Concurrent use should be undertaken with physician's supervision).
No products indexed under this heading.

Rosiglitazone Maleate (Concurrent use should be undertaken with physician's supervision). Products include:
Avandamet Tablets 1373
Avandaryl Tablets 1379
Avandia Tablets 1384

Sulfinpyrazone (Concurrent use should be undertaken with physician's supervision).
No products indexed under this heading.

Tolazamide (Concurrent use should be undertaken with physician's supervision).
No products indexed under this heading.

Tolbutamide (Concurrent use should be undertaken with physician's supervision).
No products indexed under this heading.

Troglitazone (Concurrent use should be undertaken with physician's supervision).
No products indexed under this heading.

Warfarin Sodium (Concurrent use should be undertaken with physician's supervision). Products include:
Coumadin for Injection 898
Coumadin Tablets 898

PEPTO-BISMOL MAXIMUM STRENGTH LIQUID

(Bismuth Subsalicylate) .... ▣672

May interact with oral anticoagulants, antigout agents, and oral hypoglycemic agents. Compounds in these categories include:

Acarbose (Use cautiously). Products include:
Precose Tablets 751

Allopurinol (Use cautiously).
No products indexed under this heading.

Anisindione (Use cautiously). Products include:
Miradon Tablets 3042

Chlorpropamide (Use cautiously).
No products indexed under this heading.

Dicumarol (Use cautiously).
No products indexed under this heading.

Glimepiride (Use cautiously). Products include:
Avandaryl Tablets 1379
Duetact Tablets 3226

Glipizide (Use cautiously).
No products indexed under this heading.

Glyburide (Use cautiously).
No products indexed under this heading.

Metformin Hydrochloride (Use cautiously). Products include:
ActoPlus Met Tablets 3214
Avandamet Tablets 1373
Fortamet Extended-Release Tablets 3115

Miglitol (Use cautiously).
No products indexed under this heading.

Pioglitazone Hydrochloride (Use cautiously). Products include:
ActoPlus Met Tablets 3214
Actos Tablets 3219
Duetact Tablets 3226

Probenecid (Use cautiously).
No products indexed under this heading.

Repaglinide (Use cautiously).
No products indexed under this heading.

Rosiglitazone Maleate (Use cautiously). Products include:
Avandamet Tablets 1373
Avandaryl Tablets 1379
Avandia Tablets 1384

Sulfinpyrazone (Use cautiously).
No products indexed under this heading.

Tolazamide (Use cautiously).
No products indexed under this heading.

Tolbutamide (Use cautiously).
No products indexed under this heading.

Troglitazone (Use cautiously).
No products indexed under this heading.

Warfarin Sodium (Use cautiously). Products include:
Coumadin for Injection 898
Coumadin Tablets 898

CHILDREN'S PEPTO

(Calcium Carbonate) 2674

None cited in PDR database.

PERCOCET TABLETS

(Acetaminophen, Oxycodone Hydrochloride) 1131

May interact with anticholinergics, central nervous system depressants, general anesthetics, hypnotics and sedatives, monoamine oxidase inhibitors, narcotic analgesics, phenothiazines, tranquilizers, tricyclic antidepressants, and certain other agents. Compounds in these categories include:

Alfentanil Hydrochloride (Additive CNS depression; dose of one or both agents should be reduced).
No products indexed under this heading.

Alprazolam (Additive CNS depression; dose of one or both agents should be reduced). Products include:
Niravam Orally Disintegrating Tablets 3092

Amitriptyline Hydrochloride (Increased effect of antidepressant or oxycodone).
No products indexed under this heading.

Amoxapine (Increased effect of antidepressant or oxycodone).
No products indexed under this heading.

Aprobarbital (Additive CNS depression; dose of one or both agents should be reduced).
No products indexed under this heading.

Atropine Sulfate (May produce paralytic ileus). Products include:
Donnatal Extentabs 2493

Belladonna Alkaloids (May produce paralytic ileus). Products include:
Hyland's Teething Tablets .... ▣830

Benztropine Mesylate (May produce paralytic ileus).
No products indexed under this heading.

Biperiden Hydrochloride (May produce paralytic ileus).
No products indexed under this heading.

Buprenorphine Hydrochloride (Additive CNS depression; dose of one or both agents should be reduced). Products include:
Buprenex Injectable 2716
Suboxone Tablets 2717
Subutex Tablets 2717

Buspirone Hydrochloride (Additive CNS depression; dose of one or both agents should be reduced).
No products indexed under this heading.

Butabarbital (Additive CNS depression; dose of one or both agents should be reduced).
No products indexed under this heading.

Butalbital (Additive CNS depression; dose of one or both agents should be reduced).
No products indexed under this heading.

Chlordiazepoxide (Additive CNS depression; dose of one or both agents should be reduced).
No products indexed under this heading.

Chlordiazepoxide Hydrochloride (Additive CNS depression; dose of one or both agents should be reduced). Products include:
Librium Capsules 3347

Chlorpromazine (Additive CNS depression; dose of one or both agents should be reduced).
No products indexed under this heading.

Chlorpromazine Hydrochloride (Additive CNS depression; dose of one or both agents should be reduced).
No products indexed under this heading.

Chlorprothixene (Additive CNS depression; dose of one or both agents should be reduced).
No products indexed under this heading.

Chlorprothixene Hydrochloride (Additive CNS depression; dose of one or both agents should be reduced).
No products indexed under this heading.

Chlorprothixene Lactate (Additive CNS depression; dose of one or both agents should be reduced).
No products indexed under this heading.

Clidinium Bromide (May produce paralytic ileus).
No products indexed under this heading.

Clomipramine Hydrochloride (Increased effect of antidepressant or oxycodone).
No products indexed under this heading.

Clorazepate Dipotassium (Additive CNS depression; dose of one or both agents should be reduced). Products include:
Tranxene 2474

Clozapine (Additive CNS depression; dose of one or both agents should be reduced). Products include:
Clozaril Tablets 2184
FazaClo Orally Disintegrating Tablets 551

Codeine Phosphate (Additive CNS depression; dose of one or both agents should be reduced). Products include:
Tylenol with Codeine Tablets 2391

Desflurane (Additive CNS depression; dose of one or both agents should be reduced).
No products indexed under this heading.

Desipramine Hydrochloride (Increased effect of antidepressant or oxycodone).

No products indexed under this heading.

Dezocine (Additive CNS depression; dose of one or both agents should be reduced).

No products indexed under this heading.

Diazepam (Additive CNS depression; dose of one or both agents should be reduced). Products include:

Diastat Rectal Delivery System 3343
Valium Tablets 2819

Dicyclomine Hydrochloride (May produce paralytic ileus). Products include:

Bentyl Capsules 697
Bentyl Injection 697
Bentyl Syrup 697
Bentyl Tablets 697

Doxepin Hydrochloride (Increased effect of antidepressant or oxycodone).

No products indexed under this heading.

Droperidol (Additive CNS depression; dose of one or both agents should be reduced).

No products indexed under this heading.

Enflurane (Additive CNS depression; dose of one or both agents should be reduced).

No products indexed under this heading.

Estazolam (Additive CNS depression; dose of one or both agents should be reduced). Products include:

ProSom Tablets 517

Ethanol (Additive CNS depression; dose of one or both agents should be reduced).

No products indexed under this heading.

Ethchlorvynol (Additive CNS depression; dose of one or both agents should be reduced).

No products indexed under this heading.

Ethinamate (Additive CNS depression; dose of one or both agents should be reduced).

No products indexed under this heading.

Ethopropazine Hydrochloride (May produce paralytic ileus).

No products indexed under this heading.

Ethyl Alcohol (Additive CNS depression; dose of one or both agents should be reduced).

No products indexed under this heading.

Fentanyl (Additive CNS depression; dose of one or both agents should be reduced). Products include:

Duragesic Transdermal System 2373
Ionsys Transdermal System 2379

Fentanyl Citrate (Additive CNS depression; dose of one or both agents should be reduced). Products include:

Actiq ... 979

Fluphenazine Decanoate (Additive CNS depression; dose of one or both agents should be reduced).

No products indexed under this heading.

Fluphenazine Enanthate (Additive CNS depression; dose of one or both agents should be reduced).

No products indexed under this heading.

Fluphenazine Hydrochloride (Additive CNS depression; dose of one or both agents should be reduced).

No products indexed under this heading.

Flurazepam Hydrochloride (Additive CNS depression; dose of one or both agents should be reduced). Products include:

Dalmane Capsules 3342

Glutethimide (Additive CNS depression; dose of one or both agents should be reduced).

No products indexed under this heading.

Glycopyrrolate (May produce paralytic ileus).

No products indexed under this heading.

Haloperidol (Additive CNS depression; dose of one or both agents should be reduced).

No products indexed under this heading.

Haloperidol Decanoate (Additive CNS depression; dose of one or both agents should be reduced).

No products indexed under this heading.

Hydrocodone Bitartrate (Additive CNS depression; dose of one or both agents should be reduced). Products include:

Hycodan .. 1116
Hycotuss Expectorant Syrup 1117
Vicodin Tablets 535
Vicodin ES Tablets 536
Vicodin HP Tablets 538
Vicoprofen Tablets 539
Zydone Tablets 1139

Hydrocodone Polistirex (Additive CNS depression; dose of one or both agents should be reduced). Products include:

Tussionex Pennkinetic
 Extended-Release Suspension 3327

Hydromorphone Hydrochloride (Additive CNS depression; dose of one or both agents should be reduced). Products include:

Dilaudid ... 440
Dilaudid Non-Sterile Powder 440
Dilaudid Oral Liquid 445
Dilaudid Rectal Suppositories 440
Dilaudid Tablets 440
Dilaudid Tablets - 8 mg 445
Dilaudid-HP 442

Hydroxyzine Hydrochloride (Additive CNS depression; dose of one or both agents should be reduced).

No products indexed under this heading.

Hyoscyamine (May produce paralytic ileus).

No products indexed under this heading.

Hyoscyamine Sulfate (May produce paralytic ileus). Products include:

Donnatal Extentabs 2493
Prosed/DS Tablets 1157

Imipramine Hydrochloride (Increased effect of antidepressant or oxycodone).

No products indexed under this heading.

Imipramine Pamoate (Increased effect of antidepressant or oxycodone).

No products indexed under this heading.

Ipratropium Bromide (May produce paralytic ileus). Products include:

Atrovent Inhalation Solution 835
Atrovent HFA Inhalation Aerosol 841
Atrovent Nasal Spray 0.03% 837
Atrovent Nasal Spray 0.06% 839
Combivent Inhalation Aerosol 847
DuoNeb Inhalation Solution 1058

Isocarboxazid (Increased effect of either oxycodone or MAO inhibitor).

No products indexed under this heading.

Isoflurane (Additive CNS depression; dose of one or both agents should be reduced).

No products indexed under this heading.

Ketamine Hydrochloride (Additive CNS depression; dose of one or both agents should be reduced).

No products indexed under this heading.

Levomethadyl Acetate Hydrochloride (Additive CNS depression; dose of one or both agents should be reduced).

No products indexed under this heading.

Levorphanol Tartrate (Additive CNS depression; dose of one or both agents should be reduced).

No products indexed under this heading.

Lorazepam (Additive CNS depression; dose of one or both agents should be reduced).

No products indexed under this heading.

Loxapine Hydrochloride (Additive CNS depression; dose of one or both agents should be reduced).

No products indexed under this heading.

Loxapine Succinate (Additive CNS depression; dose of one or both agents should be reduced).

No products indexed under this heading.

Maprotiline Hydrochloride (Increased effect of antidepressant or oxycodone).

No products indexed under this heading.

Mepenzolate Bromide (May produce paralytic ileus).

No products indexed under this heading.

Meperidine Hydrochloride (Additive CNS depression; dose of one or both agents should be reduced).

No products indexed under this heading.

Mephobarbital (Additive CNS depression; dose of one or both agents should be reduced).

No products indexed under this heading.

Meprobamate (Additive CNS depression; dose of one or both agents should be reduced).

No products indexed under this heading.

Mesoridazine Besylate (Additive CNS depression; dose of one or both agents should be reduced).

No products indexed under this heading.

Methadone Hydrochloride (Additive CNS depression; dose of one or both agents should be reduced).

No products indexed under this heading.

Methohexital Sodium (Additive CNS depression; dose of one or both agents should be reduced).

No products indexed under this heading.

Methotrimeprazine (Additive CNS depression; dose of one or both agents should be reduced).

No products indexed under this heading.

Methoxyflurane (Additive CNS depression; dose of one or both agents should be reduced).

No products indexed under this heading.

Midazolam Hydrochloride (Additive CNS depression; dose of one or both agents should be reduced).

No products indexed under this heading.

Moclobemide (Increased effect of either oxycodone or MAO inhibitor).

No products indexed under this heading.

Molindone Hydrochloride (Additive CNS depression; dose of one or both agents should be reduced). Products include:

Moban Tablets 1119

Morphine Sulfate (Additive CNS depression; dose of one or both agents should be reduced). Products include:

Avinza Capsules 1741
Kadian Capsules 577
MS Contin Tablets 2701

Nortriptyline Hydrochloride (Increased effect of antidepressant or oxycodone).

No products indexed under this heading.

Olanzapine (Additive CNS depression; dose of one or both agents should be reduced). Products include:

Symbyax Capsules 1819
Zyprexa Tablets 1830
Zyprexa IntraMuscular 1830
Zyprexa ZYDIS Orally
 Disintegrating Tablets 1830

Oxazepam (Additive CNS depression; dose of one or both agents should be reduced; increased effect of antidepressant).

No products indexed under this heading.

Oxybutynin Chloride (May produce paralytic ileus). Products include:

Ditropan XL Extended-Release
 Tablets 2413

Oxyphenonium Bromide (May produce paralytic ileus).

No products indexed under this heading.

Pargyline Hydrochloride (Increased effect of either oxycodone or MAO inhibitor).

No products indexed under this heading.

Pentobarbital Sodium (Additive CNS depression; dose of one or both agents should be reduced). Products include:

Nembutal Sodium Solution, USP 2470

Perphenazine (Additive CNS depression; dose of one or both agents should be reduced).

No products indexed under this heading.

IMPORTANT NOTE: Always consult each drug listing in the patient's regimen for possible interactions.

Phenelzine Sulfate (Increased effect of either oxycodone or MAO inhibitor).
No products indexed under this heading.

Phenobarbital (Additive CNS depression; dose of one or both agents should be reduced). Products include:
Donnatal Extentabs 2493

Prazepam (Additive CNS depression; dose of one or both agents should be reduced).
No products indexed under this heading.

Procarbazine Hydrochloride (Increased effect of either oxycodone or MAO inhibitor). Products include:
Matulane Capsules 3191

Prochlorperazine (Additive CNS depression; dose of one or both agents should be reduced).
No products indexed under this heading.

Procyclidine Hydrochloride (May produce paralytic ileus).
No products indexed under this heading.

Promethazine Hydrochloride (Additive CNS depression; dose of one or both agents should be reduced). Products include:
Phenergan Tablets and Suppositories 3440

Propantheline Bromide (May produce paralytic ileus).
No products indexed under this heading.

Propofol (Additive CNS depression; dose of one or both agents should be reduced).
No products indexed under this heading.

Propoxyphene Hydrochloride (Additive CNS depression; dose of one or both agents should be reduced).
No products indexed under this heading.

Propoxyphene Napsylate (Additive CNS depression; dose of one or both agents should be reduced).
No products indexed under this heading.

Protriptyline Hydrochloride (Increased effect of antidepressant or oxycodone).
No products indexed under this heading.

Quazepam (Additive CNS depression; dose of one or both agents should be reduced).
No products indexed under this heading.

Quetiapine Fumarate (Additive CNS depression; dose of one or both agents should be reduced). Products include:
Seroquel Tablets 690

Ramelteon (Additive CNS depression; dose of one or both agents should be reduced). Products include:
Rozerem Tablets 3231

Remifentanil Hydrochloride (Additive CNS depression; dose of one or both agents should be reduced).
No products indexed under this heading.

Risperidone (Additive CNS depression; dose of one or both agents should be reduced). Products include:
Risperdal 1676
Risperdal Consta Long-Acting Injection 1682
Risperdal M-Tab Orally Disintegrating Tablets 1676

Scopolamine (May produce paralytic ileus). Products include:
Transderm Scōp Transdermal Therapeutic System 2177

Scopolamine Hydrobromide (May produce paralytic ileus). Products include:
Donnatal Extentabs 2493

Secobarbital Sodium (Additive CNS depression; dose of one or both agents should be reduced).
No products indexed under this heading.

Selegiline Hydrochloride (Increased effect of either oxycodone or MAO inhibitor). Products include:
Eldepryl Capsules 3208
Zelapar Tablets 3372

Sevoflurane (Additive CNS depression; dose of one or both agents should be reduced). Products include:
Ultane Liquid for Inhalation 531

Sodium Oxybate (Additive CNS depression; dose of one or both agents should be reduced). Products include:
Xyrem Oral Solution 1688

Sufentanil Citrate (Additive CNS depression; dose of one or both agents should be reduced).
No products indexed under this heading.

Temazepam (Additive CNS depression; dose of one or both agents should be reduced). Products include:
Restoril Capsules 1860

Thiamylal Sodium (Additive CNS depression; dose of one or both agents should be reduced).
No products indexed under this heading.

Thioridazine Hydrochloride (Additive CNS depression; dose of one or both agents should be reduced). Products include:
Thioridazine Hydrochloride Tablets 2163

Thiothixene (Additive CNS depression; dose of one or both agents should be reduced). Products include:
Thiothixene Capsules 2165

Tolterodine Tartrate (May produce paralytic ileus). Products include:
Detrol Tablets 2628
Detrol LA Capsules 2631

Tranylcypromine Sulfate (Increased effect of either oxycodone or MAO inhibitor). Products include:
Parnate Tablets 1527

Triazolam (Additive CNS depression; dose of one or both agents should be reduced).
No products indexed under this heading.

Tridihexethyl Chloride (May produce paralytic ileus).
No products indexed under this heading.

Trifluoperazine Hydrochloride (Additive CNS depression; dose of one or both agents should be reduced).
No products indexed under this heading.

Trihexyphenidyl Hydrochloride (May produce paralytic ileus).
No products indexed under this heading.

Trimipramine Maleate (Increased effect of antidepressant or oxycodone).
No products indexed under this heading.

Zaleplon (Additive CNS depression; dose of one or both agents should be reduced). Products include:
Sonata Capsules 1717

Ziprasidone Hydrochloride (Additive CNS depression; dose of one or both agents should be reduced). Products include:
Geodon Capsules 2529

Zolpidem Tartrate (Additive CNS depression; dose of one or both agents should be reduced). Products include:
Ambien Tablets 2851
Ambien CR Tablets 2855

Food Interactions

Alcohol (Additive CNS depression).

PERCODAN TABLETS

(Aspirin, Oxycodone Hydrochloride) ... 1132
May interact with ACE inhibitors, beta blockers, central nervous system depressants, anticoagulants, diuretics, anticonvulsants, general anesthetics, antigout agents, oral hypoglycemic agents, hypnotics and sedatives, mixed agonist/antagonist opioid analgesics, narcotic analgesics, non-steroidal anti-inflammatory agents, phenothiazines, tranquilizers, and certain other agents. Compounds in these categories include:

Acarbose (Aspirin may increase the serum glucose-lowering action of insulin and sulfonylureas leading to hypoglycemia). Products include:
Precose Tablets 751

Acebutolol Hydrochloride (The hypotensive effects of beta blockers may be diminished by concomitant administration of aspirin).
No products indexed under this heading.

Acetazolamide (Concurrent use of acetazolamide can lead to high serum levels of acetazolamide and toxicity).
No products indexed under this heading.

Acetazolamide Sodium (Concurrent use of acetazolamide can lead to high serum levels of acetazolamide and toxicity).
No products indexed under this heading.

Alfentanil Hydrochloride (Additive CNS depression).
No products indexed under this heading.

Allopurinol (Salicylates antagonize the uricosuric action of uricosuric agents).
No products indexed under this heading.

Alprazolam (Additive CNS depression). Products include:
Niravam Orally Disintegrating Tablets 3092

Amiloride Hydrochloride (The effectiveness of diuretics in patients with underlying renal or cardiovascular disease may by diminished by the concomitant administration of aspirin). Products include:
Midamor Tablets 2026
Moduretic Tablets 2028

Anisindione (Enhanced effect of anticoagulant). Products include:
Miradon Tablets 3042

Aprobarbital (Additive CNS depression).
No products indexed under this heading.

Ardeparin Sodium (Enhanced effect of anticoagulant).
No products indexed under this heading.

Atenolol (The hypotensive effects of beta blockers may be diminished by concomitant administration of aspirin).
No products indexed under this heading.

Benazepril Hydrochloride (Reports suggested that NSAIDs may diminish the hyponatremic and hypotensive effect of ACE inhibitors). Products include:
Lotensin Tablets 2243
Lotensin HCT Tablets 2246
Lotrel Capsules 2249

Bendroflumethiazide (The effectiveness of diuretics in patients with underlying renal or cardiovascular disease may by diminished by the concomitant administration of aspirin).
No products indexed under this heading.

Betaxolol Hydrochloride (The hypotensive effects of beta blockers may be diminished by concomitant administration of aspirin). Products include:
Betoptic S Ophthalmic Suspension........................ 558

Bisoprolol Fumarate (The hypotensive effects of beta blockers may be diminished by concomitant administration of aspirin).
No products indexed under this heading.

Bumetanide (The effectiveness of diuretics in patients with underlying renal or cardiovascular disease may by diminished by the concomitant administration of aspirin). Products include:
Bumex Tablets 2746

Buprenorphine Hydrochloride (Additive CNS depression). Products include:
Buprenex Injectable 2716
Suboxone Tablets 2717
Subutex Tablets 2717

Buspirone Hydrochloride (Additive CNS depression).
No products indexed under this heading.

Butabarbital (Additive CNS depression).
No products indexed under this heading.

Butalbital (Additive CNS depression).
No products indexed under this heading.

Butorphanol Tartrate (Agonist/antagonist analgesics may reduce the analgesic effect of oxycodone or may precipitate withdrawal symptoms).
No products indexed under this heading.

Captopril (Reports suggested that NSAIDs may diminish the hyponatremic and hypotensive effect of ACE inhibitors). Products include:
Captopril Tablets 2149

Carbamazepine (Salicylate can displace protein-bound phenytoin and valproic acid, leading to a decrease in the total concentration of phenytoin and an increase in serum valproic acid levels). Products include:

Carteolol Hydrochloride (The hypotensive effects of beta blockers may be diminished by concomitant administration of aspirin). Products include:

Celecoxib (The concurrent use of aspirin with other NSAIDs should be avoided because this may increase bleeding or lead to decreased renal function). Products include:

Chlordiazepoxide (Additive CNS depression).

No products indexed under this heading.

Chlordiazepoxide Hydrochloride (Additive CNS depression). Products include:

Chlorothiazide (The effectiveness of diuretics in patients with underlying renal or cardiovascular disease may by diminished by the concomitant administration of aspirin). Products include:

Chlorothiazide Sodium (The effectiveness of diuretics in patients with underlying renal or cardiovascular disease may by diminished by the concomitant administration of aspirin). Products include:

Chlorpromazine (Additive CNS depression).

No products indexed under this heading.

Chlorpromazine Hydrochloride (Additive CNS depression).

No products indexed under this heading.

Chlorpropamide (Aspirin may increase the serum glucose-lowering action of insulin and sulfonylureas leading to hypoglycemia).

No products indexed under this heading.

Chlorprothixene (Additive CNS depression).

No products indexed under this heading.

Chlorprothixene Hydrochloride (Additive CNS depression).

No products indexed under this heading.

Chlorprothixene Lactate (Additive CNS depression).

No products indexed under this heading.

Chlorthalidone (The effectiveness of diuretics in patients with underlying renal or cardiovascular disease may by diminished by the concomitant administration of aspirin). Products include:

Clorazepate Dipotassium (Additive CNS depression). Products include:

Clozapine (Additive CNS depression). Products include:

Codeine Phosphate (Additive CNS depression). Products include:

Dalteparin Sodium (Enhanced effect of anticoagulant). Products include:

Danaparoid Sodium (Enhanced effect of anticoagulant).

No products indexed under this heading.

Desflurane (Additive CNS depression).

No products indexed under this heading.

Dezocine (Additive CNS depression).

No products indexed under this heading.

Diazepam (Additive CNS depression). Products include:

Diclofenac Potassium (The concurrent use of aspirin with other NSAIDs should be avoided because this may increase bleeding or lead to decreased renal function).

No products indexed under this heading.

Diclofenac Sodium (The concurrent use of aspirin with other NSAIDs should be avoided because this may increase bleeding or lead to decreased renal function). Products include:

Dicumarol (Enhanced effect of anticoagulant).

No products indexed under this heading.

Divalproex Sodium (Salicylate can displace protein-bound phenytoin and valproic acid, leading to a decrease in the total concentration of phenytoin and an increase in serum valproic acid levels). Products include:

Droperidol (Additive CNS depression).

No products indexed under this heading.

Enalapril Maleate (Reports suggested that NSAIDs may diminish the hyponatremic and hypotensive effect of ACE inhibitors). Products include:

Enalaprilat (Reports suggested that NSAIDs may diminish the hyponatremic and hypotensive effect of ACE inhibitors).

No products indexed under this heading.

Enflurane (Additive CNS depression).

No products indexed under this heading.

Enoxaparin Sodium (Enhanced effect of anticoagulant). Products include:

Esmolol Hydrochloride (The hypotensive effects of beta blockers may be diminished by concomitant administration of aspirin).

No products indexed under this heading.

Estazolam (Additive CNS depression). Products include:

Ethacrynic Acid (The effectiveness of diuretics in patients with underly-

ing renal or cardiovascular disease may by diminished by the concomitant administration of aspirin). Products include:

Ethanol (Additive CNS depression).

No products indexed under this heading.

Ethchlorvynol (Additive CNS depression).

No products indexed under this heading.

Ethinamate (Additive CNS depression).

No products indexed under this heading.

Ethosuximide (Salicylate can displace protein-bound phenytoin and valproic acid, leading to a decrease in the total concentration of phenytoin and an increase in serum valproic acid levels).

No products indexed under this heading.

Ethotoin (Salicylate can displace protein-bound phenytoin and valproic acid, leading to a decrease in the total concentration of phenytoin and an increase in serum valproic acid levels).

No products indexed under this heading.

Ethyl Alcohol (Additive CNS depression).

No products indexed under this heading.

Etodolac (The concurrent use of aspirin with other NSAIDs should be avoided because this may increase bleeding or lead to decreased renal function).

No products indexed under this heading.

Felbamate (Salicylate can displace protein-bound phenytoin and valproic acid, leading to a decrease in the total concentration of phenytoin and an increase in serum valproic acid levels).

No products indexed under this heading.

Fenoprofen Calcium (The concurrent use of aspirin with other NSAIDs should be avoided because this may increase bleeding or lead to decreased renal function). Products include:

Fentanyl (Additive CNS depression). Products include:

Fentanyl Citrate (Additive CNS depression). Products include:

Fluphenazine Decanoate (Additive CNS depression).

No products indexed under this heading.

Fluphenazine Enanthate (Additive CNS depression).

No products indexed under this heading.

Fluphenazine Hydrochloride (Additive CNS depression).

No products indexed under this heading.

Flurazepam Hydrochloride (Additive CNS depression). Products include:

Flurbiprofen (The concurrent use of aspirin with other NSAIDs should be avoided because this may increase bleeding or lead to decreased renal function).

No products indexed under this heading.

Fondaparinux Sodium (Enhanced effect of anticoagulant). Products include:

Fosinopril Sodium (Reports suggested that NSAIDs may diminish the hyponatremic and hypotensive effect of ACE inhibitors).

No products indexed under this heading.

Fosphenytoin (Salicylate can displace protein-bound phenytoin and valproic acid, leading to a decrease in the total concentration of phenytoin and an increase in serum valproic acid levels).

No products indexed under this heading.

Fosphenytoin Sodium (Salicylate can displace protein-bound phenytoin and valproic acid, leading to a decrease in the total concentration of phenytoin and an increase in serum valproic acid levels).

No products indexed under this heading.

Furosemide (The effectiveness of diuretics in patients with underlying renal or cardiovascular disease may by diminished by the concomitant administration of aspirin). Products include:

Gabapentin (Salicylate can displace protein-bound phenytoin and valproic acid, leading to a decrease in the total concentration of phenytoin and an increase in serum valproic acid levels). Products include:

Glimepiride (Aspirin may increase the serum glucose-lowering action of insulin and sulfonylureas leading to hypoglycemia). Products include:

Glipizide (Aspirin may increase the serum glucose-lowering action of insulin and sulfonylureas leading to hypoglycemia).

No products indexed under this heading.

Glutethimide (Additive CNS depression).

No products indexed under this heading.

Glyburide (Aspirin may increase the serum glucose-lowering action of insulin and sulfonylureas leading to hypoglycemia).

No products indexed under this heading.

Haloperidol (Additive CNS depression).

No products indexed under this heading.

Haloperidol Decanoate (Additive CNS depression).

No products indexed under this heading.

Heparin Calcium (Enhanced effect of anticoagulant).

No products indexed under this heading.

Heparin Sodium (Enhanced effect of anticoagulant).

No products indexed under this heading.

IMPORTANT NOTE: Always consult each drug listing in the patient's regimen for possible interactions.

Hydrochlorothiazide (The effectiveness of diuretics in patients with underlying renal or cardiovascular disease may by diminished by the concomitant administration of aspirin). Products include:
- Aldoril Tablets 1910
- Atacand HCT 651
- Avalide Tablets 888
- Avalide Tablets 2874
- Benicar HCT Tablets 1044
- Diovan HCT Tablets 2196
- Dyazide Capsules 1423
- Hyzaar 50-12.5 Tablets 1990
- Hyzaar 100-12.5 Tablets 1990
- Hyzaar 100-25 Tablets 1990
- Lopressor HCT 50/25 Tablets 2241
- Lopressor HCT 100/25 Tablets 2241
- Lopressor HCT 100/50 Tablets 2241
- Lotensin HCT Tablets 2246
- Micardis HCT Tablets 856
- Moduretic Tablets 2028
- Prinzide Tablets 2056
- Teveten HCT Tablets 1737
- Timolide Tablets 2086
- Uniretic Tablets 3100

Hydrocodone Bitartrate (Additive CNS depression). Products include:
- Hycodan 1116
- Hycotuss Expectorant Syrup 1117
- Vicodin Tablets 535
- Vicodin ES Tablets 536
- Vicodin HP Tablets 538
- Vicoprofen Tablets 539
- Zydone Tablets 1139

Hydrocodone Polistirex (Additive CNS depression). Products include:
- Tussionex Pennkinetic Extended-Release Suspension 3327

Hydroflumethiazide (The effectiveness of diuretics in patients with underlying renal or cardiovascular disease may by diminished by the concomitant administration of aspirin).
No products indexed under this heading.

Hydromorphone Hydrochloride (Additive CNS depression). Products include:
- Dilaudid 440
- Dilaudid Non-Sterile Powder 440
- Dilaudid Oral Liquid 445
- Dilaudid Rectal Suppositories 440
- Dilaudid Tablets 440
- Dilaudid Tablets - 8 mg 445
- Dilaudid-HP 442

Hydroxyzine Hydrochloride (Additive CNS depression).
No products indexed under this heading.

Ibuprofen (The concurrent use of aspirin with other NSAIDs should be avoided because this may increase bleeding or lead to decreased renal function). Products include:
- Advil Allergy Sinus Caplets .... ▣770
- Advil .... ▣674
- Children's Advil Oral Suspension .... ▣603
- Children's Advil Chewable Tablets .... ▣603
- Advil Cold & Sinus .... ▣723
- Infants' Advil Concentrated Drops .... ▣604
- Infants' Advil Concentrated Drops - White Grape (Dye-Free) .... ▣604
- Junior Strength Advil Swallow Tablets .... ▣605
- Advil Migraine Liquigels .... ▣608
- Advil Multi-Symptom Cold Caplets .... ▣770
- Advil PM Caplets .... ▣615
- Motrin IB Tablets and Caplets 1866
- Children's Motrin Oral Suspension 1867
- Children's Motrin Non-Staining Dye-Free Oral Suspension 1867
- Children's Motrin Cold Oral Suspension 1867
- Infants' Motrin Concentrated Drops 1867
- Infants' Motrin Non-Staining Dye-Free Concentrated Drops 1867
- Junior Strength Motrin Caplets and Chewable Tablets 1867
- Vicoprofen Tablets 539

Indapamide (The effectiveness of diuretics in patients with underlying renal or cardiovascular disease may by diminished by the concomitant administration of aspirin). Products include:
- Indapamide Tablets 2156

Indomethacin (The concurrent use of aspirin with other NSAIDs should be avoided because this may increase bleeding or lead to decreased renal function). Products include:
- Indocin 1995

Indomethacin Sodium Trihydrate (The concurrent use of aspirin with other NSAIDs should be avoided because this may increase bleeding or lead to decreased renal function). Products include:
- Indocin I.V. 2465

Isoflurane (Additive CNS depression).
No products indexed under this heading.

Ketamine Hydrochloride (Additive CNS depression).
No products indexed under this heading.

Ketoprofen (The concurrent use of aspirin with other NSAIDs should be avoided because this may increase bleeding or lead to decreased renal function).
No products indexed under this heading.

Ketorolac Tromethamine (The concurrent use of aspirin with other NSAIDs should be avoided because this may increase bleeding or lead to decreased renal function). Products include:
- Acular Ophthalmic Solution 565
- Acular LS Ophthalmic Solution 566

Labetalol Hydrochloride (The hypotensive effects of beta blockers may be diminished by concomitant administration of aspirin).
No products indexed under this heading.

Lamotrigine (Salicylate can displace protein-bound phenytoin and valproic acid, leading to a decrease in the total concentration of phenytoin and an increase in serum valproic acid levels). Products include:
- Lamictal 1481

Levetiracetam (Salicylate can displace protein-bound phenytoin and valproic acid, leading to a decrease in the total concentration of phenytoin and an increase in serum valproic acid levels). Products include:
- Keppra Injection 3320
- Keppra Oral Solution 3314
- Keppra Tablets 3314

Levobunolol Hydrochloride (The hypotensive effects of beta blockers may be diminished by concomitant administration of aspirin). Products include:
- Betagan Ophthalmic Solution, USP .... ⊙220

Levomethadyl Acetate Hydrochloride (Additive CNS depression).
No products indexed under this heading.

Levorphanol Tartrate (Additive CNS depression).
No products indexed under this heading.

Lisinopril (Reports suggested that NSAIDs may diminish the hyponatremic and hypotensive effect of ACE inhibitors). Products include:
- Prinivil Tablets 2052
- Prinzide Tablets 2056

Lorazepam (Additive CNS depression).
No products indexed under this heading.

Low Molecular Weight Heparins (Enhanced effect of anticoagulant).
No products indexed under this heading.

Loxapine Hydrochloride (Additive CNS depression).
No products indexed under this heading.

Loxapine Succinate (Additive CNS depression).
No products indexed under this heading.

Meclofenamate Sodium (The concurrent use of aspirin with other NSAIDs should be avoided because this may increase bleeding or lead to decreased renal function).
No products indexed under this heading.

Mefenamic Acid (The concurrent use of aspirin with other NSAIDs should be avoided because this may increase bleeding or lead to decreased renal function).
No products indexed under this heading.

Meloxicam (The concurrent use of aspirin with other NSAIDs should be avoided because this may increase bleeding or lead to decreased renal function). Products include:
- Mobic Oral Suspension 863
- Mobic Tablets 863

Meperidine Hydrochloride (Additive CNS depression).
No products indexed under this heading.

Mephenytoin (Salicylate can displace protein-bound phenytoin and valproic acid, leading to a decrease in the total concentration of phenytoin and an increase in serum valproic acid levels).
No products indexed under this heading.

Mephobarbital (Additive CNS depression).
No products indexed under this heading.

Meprobamate (Additive CNS depression).
No products indexed under this heading.

Mesoridazine Besylate (Additive CNS depression).
No products indexed under this heading.

Metformin Hydrochloride (Aspirin may increase the serum glucose-lowering action of insulin and sulfonylureas leading to hypoglycemia). Products include:
- ActoPlus Met Tablets 3214
- Avandamet Tablets 1373
- Fortamet Extended-Release Tablets 3115

Methadone Hydrochloride (Additive CNS depression).
No products indexed under this heading.

Methohexital Sodium (Additive CNS depression).
No products indexed under this heading.

Methotrexate (Salicylate can inhibit renal clearance of methotrexate, leading to bone marrow toxicity, especially in the elderly or renal impaired).
No products indexed under this heading.

Methotrexate Sodium (Salicylate can inhibit renal clearance of methotrexate, leading to bone marrow toxicity, especially in the elderly or renal impaired).
No products indexed under this heading.

Methotrimeprazine (Additive CNS depression).
No products indexed under this heading.

Methoxyflurane (Additive CNS depression).
No products indexed under this heading.

Methsuximide (Salicylate can displace protein-bound phenytoin and valproic acid, leading to a decrease in the total concentration of phenytoin and an increase in serum valproic acid levels).
No products indexed under this heading.

Methyclothiazide (The effectiveness of diuretics in patients with underlying renal or cardiovascular disease may by diminished by the concomitant administration of aspirin).
No products indexed under this heading.

Metipranolol Hydrochloride (The hypotensive effects of beta blockers may be diminished by concomitant administration of aspirin).
No products indexed under this heading.

Metolazone (The effectiveness of diuretics in patients with underlying renal or cardiovascular disease may by diminished by the concomitant administration of aspirin).
No products indexed under this heading.

Metoprolol Succinate (The hypotensive effects of beta blockers may be diminished by concomitant administration of aspirin). Products include:
- Toprol-XL Tablets 668

Metoprolol Tartrate (The hypotensive effects of beta blockers may be diminished by concomitant administration of aspirin). Products include:
- Lopressor Injection 2238
- Lopressor Tablets 2238
- Lopressor HCT 50/25 Tablets 2241
- Lopressor HCT 100/25 Tablets 2241
- Lopressor HCT 100/50 Tablets 2241

Midazolam Hydrochloride (Additive CNS depression).
No products indexed under this heading.

Miglitol (Aspirin may increase the serum glucose-lowering action of insulin and sulfonylureas leading to hypoglycemia).
No products indexed under this heading.

Moexipril Hydrochloride (Reports suggested that NSAIDs may diminish the hyponatremic and hypotensive effect of ACE inhibitors). Products include:
- Uniretic Tablets 3100
- Univasc Tablets 3104

Molindone Hydrochloride (Additive CNS depression). Products include:

Moban Tablets 1119

Morphine Sulfate (Additive CNS depression). Products include:
Avinza Capsules 1741
Kadian Capsules 577
MS Contin Tablets 2701

Nabumetone (The concurrent use of aspirin with other NSAIDs should be avoided because this may increase bleeding or lead to decreased renal function).
No products indexed under this heading.

Nadolol (The hypotensive effects of beta blockers may be diminished by concomitant administration of aspirin). Products include:
Nadolol Tablets 2159

Nalbuphine Hydrochloride (Agonist/antagonist analgesics may reduce the analgesic effect of oxycodone or may precipitate withdrawal symptoms).
No products indexed under this heading.

Naproxen (The concurrent use of aspirin with other NSAIDs should be avoided because this may increase bleeding or lead to decreased renal function). Products include:
EC-Naprosyn Delayed-Release Tablets 2761
Naprosyn Suspension 2761
Naprosyn Tablets 2761
Prevacid NapraPAC 3280

Naproxen Sodium (The concurrent use of aspirin with other NSAIDs should be avoided because this may increase bleeding or lead to decreased renal function). Products include:
Aleve Caplets 742
Aleve Gelcaps 743
Aleve Tablets 743
Aleve Cold & Sinus Caplets 744
Anaprox Tablets 2761
Anaprox DS Tablets 2761

Olanzapine (Additive CNS depression). Products include:
Symbyax Capsules 1819
Zyprexa Tablets 1830
Zyprexa IntraMuscular 1830
Zyprexa ZYDIS Orally Disintegrating Tablets 1830

Oxaprozin (The concurrent use of aspirin with other NSAIDs should be avoided because this may increase bleeding or lead to decreased renal function).
No products indexed under this heading.

Oxazepam (Additive CNS depression).
No products indexed under this heading.

Oxcarbazepine (Salicylate can displace protein-bound phenytoin and valproic acid, leading to a decrease in the total concentration of phenytoin and an increase in serum valproic acid levels). Products include:
Trileptal Tablets 2300
Trileptal Oral Suspension 2300

Paramethadione (Salicylate can displace protein-bound phenytoin and valproic acid, leading to a decrease in the total concentration of phenytoin and an increase in serum valproic acid levels).
No products indexed under this heading.

Penbutolol Sulfate (The hypotensive effects of beta blockers may be diminished by concomitant administration of aspirin).
No products indexed under this heading.

Pentazocine Hydrochloride (Agonist/antagonist analgesics may reduce the analgesic effect of oxycodone or may precipitate withdrawal symptoms).
No products indexed under this heading.

Pentazocine Lactate (Agonist/antagonist analgesics may reduce the analgesic effect of oxycodone or may precipitate withdrawal symptoms).
No products indexed under this heading.

Pentobarbital Sodium (Additive CNS depression). Products include:
Nembutal Sodium Solution, USP 2470

Perindopril Erbumine (Reports suggested that NSAIDs may diminish the hyponatremic and hypotensive effect of ACE inhibitors). Products include:
Aceon Tablets (2 mg, 4 mg, 8 mg) 3194

Perphenazine (Additive CNS depression).
No products indexed under this heading.

Phenacemide (Salicylate can displace protein-bound phenytoin and valproic acid, leading to a decrease in the total concentration of phenytoin and an increase in serum valproic acid levels).
No products indexed under this heading.

Phenobarbital (Additive CNS depression). Products include:
Donnatal Extentabs 2493

Phensuximide (Salicylate can displace protein-bound phenytoin and valproic acid, leading to a decrease in the total concentration of phenytoin and an increase in serum valproic acid levels).
No products indexed under this heading.

Phenylbutazone (The concurrent use of aspirin with other NSAIDs should be avoided because this may increase bleeding or lead to decreased renal function).
No products indexed under this heading.

Phenytoin (Salicylate can displace protein-bound phenytoin and valproic acid, leading to a decrease in the total concentration of phenytoin and an increase in serum valproic acid levels).
No products indexed under this heading.

Phenytoin Sodium (Salicylate can displace protein-bound phenytoin and valproic acid, leading to a decrease in the total concentration of phenytoin and an increase in serum valproic acid levels). Products include:
Phenytek Capsules 2160

Pindolol (The hypotensive effects of beta blockers may be diminished by concomitant administration of aspirin).
No products indexed under this heading.

Pioglitazone Hydrochloride (Aspirin may increase the serum glucose-lowering action of insulin and sulfonylureas leading to hypoglycemia). Products include:
ActoPlus Met Tablets 3214
Actos Tablets 3219
Duetact Tablets 3226

Piroxicam (The concurrent use of aspirin with other NSAIDs should be avoided because this may increase bleeding or lead to decreased renal function).
No products indexed under this heading.

Polythiazide (The effectiveness of diuretics in patients with underlying renal or cardiovascular disease may by diminished by the concomitant administration of aspirin).
No products indexed under this heading.

Prazepam (Additive CNS depression).
No products indexed under this heading.

Primidone (Salicylate can displace protein-bound phenytoin and valproic acid, leading to a decrease in the total concentration of phenytoin and an increase in serum valproic acid levels).
No products indexed under this heading.

Probenecid (Aspirin may inhibit the uricosuric effects).
No products indexed under this heading.

Prochlorperazine (Additive CNS depression).
No products indexed under this heading.

Promethazine Hydrochloride (Additive CNS depression). Products include:
Phenergan Tablets and Suppositories 3440

Propofol (Additive CNS depression).
No products indexed under this heading.

Propoxyphene Hydrochloride (Additive CNS depression).
No products indexed under this heading.

Propoxyphene Napsylate (Additive CNS depression).
No products indexed under this heading.

Propranolol Hydrochloride (The hypotensive effects of beta blockers may be diminished by concomitant administration of aspirin). Products include:
Inderal LA Long-Acting Capsules 3429
InnoPran XL Capsules 2723

Quazepam (Additive CNS depression).
No products indexed under this heading.

Quetiapine Fumarate (Additive CNS depression). Products include:
Seroquel Tablets 690

Quinapril Hydrochloride (Reports suggested that NSAIDs may diminish the hyponatremic and hypotensive effect of ACE inhibitors).
No products indexed under this heading.

Ramelteon (Additive CNS depression). Products include:
Rozerem Tablets 3231

Ramipril (Reports suggested that NSAIDs may diminish the hyponatremic and hypotensive effect of ACE inhibitors). Products include:
Altace Capsules 1702

Remifentanil Hydrochloride (Additive CNS depression).
No products indexed under this heading.

Repaglinide (Aspirin may increase the serum glucose-lowering action of insulin and sulfonylureas leading to hypoglycemia).
No products indexed under this heading.

Risperidone (Additive CNS depression). Products include:
Risperdal 1676
Risperdal Consta Long-Acting Injection 1682
Risperdal M-Tab Orally Disintegrating Tablets 1676

Rofecoxib (The concurrent use of aspirin with other NSAIDs should be avoided because this may increase bleeding or lead to decreased renal function).
No products indexed under this heading.

Rosiglitazone Maleate (Aspirin may increase the serum glucose-lowering action of insulin and sulfonylureas leading to hypoglycemia). Products include:
Avandamet Tablets 1373
Avandaryl Tablets 1379
Avandia Tablets 1384

Secobarbital Sodium (Additive CNS depression).
No products indexed under this heading.

Sevoflurane (Additive CNS depression). Products include:
Ultane Liquid for Inhalation 531

Sodium Oxybate (Additive CNS depression). Products include:
Xyrem Oral Solution 1688

Sotalol Hydrochloride (The hypotensive effects of beta blockers may be diminished by concomitant administration of aspirin).
No products indexed under this heading.

Spirapril Hydrochloride (Reports suggested that NSAIDs may diminish the hyponatremic and hypotensive effect of ACE inhibitors).
No products indexed under this heading.

Spironolactone (The effectiveness of diuretics in patients with underlying renal or cardiovascular disease may by diminished by the concomitant administration of aspirin).
No products indexed under this heading.

Sufentanil Citrate (Additive CNS depression).
No products indexed under this heading.

Sulfinpyrazone (Aspirin may inhibit the uricosuric effects).
No products indexed under this heading.

Sulindac (The concurrent use of aspirin with other NSAIDs should be avoided because this may increase bleeding or lead to decreased renal function). Products include:
Clinoril Tablets 1924

Temazepam (Additive CNS depression). Products include:
Restoril Capsules 1860

Thiamylal Sodium (Additive CNS depression).
No products indexed under this heading.

Thioridazine Hydrochloride (Additive CNS depression). Products include:
Thioridazine Hydrochloride Tablets 2163

Thiothixene (Additive CNS depression). Products include:
Thiothixene Capsules 2165

Tiagabine Hydrochloride (Salicylate can displace protein-bound phenytoin and valproic acid, leading to a decrease in the total concentration of phenytoin and an increase in serum valproic acid levels). Products include:
Gabitril Tablets 984

Timolol Hemihydrate (The hypotensive effects of beta blockers may be diminished by concomitant administration of aspirin). Products include:
Betimol Ophthalmic Solution 3382
Betimol Ophthalmic Solution .... ⊙295

Timolol Maleate (The hypotensive effects of beta blockers may be diminished by concomitant administration of aspirin). Products include:
Blocadren Tablets 1916
Cosopt Sterile Ophthalmic Solution...................................... 1931
Timolide Tablets 2086
Timoptic Sterile Ophthalmic Solution...................................... 2088
Timoptic in Ocudose 2091
Timoptic-XE Sterile Ophthalmic Gel Forming Solution.................. 2092

Tinzaparin Sodium (Enhanced effect of anticoagulant).
No products indexed under this heading.

Tolazamide (Aspirin may increase the serum glucose-lowering action of insulin and sulfonylureas leading to hypoglycemia).
No products indexed under this heading.

Tolbutamide (Aspirin may increase the serum glucose-lowering action of insulin and sulfonylureas leading to hypoglycemia).
No products indexed under this heading.

Tolmetin Sodium (The concurrent use of aspirin with other NSAIDs should be avoided because this may increase bleeding or lead to decreased renal function).
No products indexed under this heading.

Topiramate (Salicylate can displace protein-bound phenytoin and valproic acid, leading to a decrease in the total concentration of phenytoin and an increase in serum valproic acid levels). Products include:
Topamax Sprinkle Capsules 2404
Topamax Tablets 2404

Torsemide (The effectiveness of diuretics in patients with underlying renal or cardiovascular disease may by diminished by the concomitant administration of aspirin). Products include:
Demadex Injection 2759
Demadex Tablets 2759

Trandolapril (Reports suggested that NSAIDs may diminish the hyponatremic and hypotensive effect of ACE inhibitors). Products include:
Mavik Tablets 486
Tarka Tablets 524

Triamterene (The effectiveness of diuretics in patients with underlying renal or cardiovascular disease may by diminished by the concomitant administration of aspirin). Products include:
Dyazide Capsules 1423
Dyrenium Capsules 3400

Triazolam (Additive CNS depression).
No products indexed under this heading.

Trifluoperazine Hydrochloride (Additive CNS depression).
No products indexed under this heading.

Trimethadione (Salicylate can displace protein-bound phenytoin and valproic acid, leading to a decrease in the total concentration of phenytoin and an increase in serum valproic acid levels).
No products indexed under this heading.

Troglitazone (Aspirin may increase the serum glucose-lowering action of insulin and sulfonylureas leading to hypoglycemia).
No products indexed under this heading.

Valdecoxib (The concurrent use of aspirin with other NSAIDs should be avoided because this may increase bleeding or lead to decreased renal function).
No products indexed under this heading.

Valproate Sodium (Salicylate can displace protein-bound phenytoin and valproic acid, leading to a decrease in the total concentration of phenytoin and an increase in serum valproic acid levels). Products include:
Depacon Injection 412

Valproic Acid (Salicylate can displace protein-bound phenytoin and valproic acid, leading to a decrease in the total concentration of phenytoin and an increase in serum valproic acid levels). Products include:
Depakene 417

Warfarin Sodium (Enhanced effect of anticoagulant). Products include:
Coumadin for Injection 898
Coumadin Tablets 898

Zaleplon (Additive CNS depression). Products include:
Sonata Capsules 1717

Ziprasidone Hydrochloride (Additive CNS depression). Products include:
Geodon Capsules 2529

Zolpidem Tartrate (Additive CNS depression). Products include:
Ambien Tablets 2851
Ambien CR Tablets 2855

Zonisamide (Salicylate can displace protein-bound phenytoin and valproic acid, leading to a decrease in the total concentration of phenytoin and an increase in serum valproic acid levels). Products include:
Zonegran Capsules 1101

Food Interactions

Alcohol (Additive CNS depression).

PERIDIN-C VITAMIN C SUPPLEMENT

(Bioflavonoids, Hesperidin Complex, Hesperidin Methyl Chalcone, Vitamin C)........................ ▣818
None cited in PDR database.

PERMAX TABLETS

(Pergolide Mesylate) 3356
May interact with dopamine antagonists, central nervous system depressants, and certain other agents. Compounds in these categories include:

Alfentanil Hydrochloride (Pergolide may cause somnolence; concurrent use with CNS depressants may result in additive sedative effects).
No products indexed under this heading.

Alprazolam (Pergolide may cause somnolence; concurrent use with CNS depressants may result in additive sedative effects). Products include:
Niravam Orally Disintegrating Tablets 3092

Aprobarbital (Pergolide may cause somnolence; concurrent use with CNS depressants may result in additive sedative effects).
No products indexed under this heading.

Buprenorphine Hydrochloride (Pergolide may cause somnolence; concurrent use with CNS depressants may result in additive sedative effects). Products include:
Buprenex Injectable 2716
Suboxone Tablets 2717
Subutex Tablets 2717

Buspirone Hydrochloride (Pergolide may cause somnolence; concurrent use with CNS depressants may result in additive sedative effects).
No products indexed under this heading.

Butabarbital (Pergolide may cause somnolence; concurrent use with CNS depressants may result in additive sedative effects).
No products indexed under this heading.

Butalbital (Pergolide may cause somnolence; concurrent use with CNS depressants may result in additive sedative effects).
No products indexed under this heading.

Chlordiazepoxide (Pergolide may cause somnolence; concurrent use with CNS depressants may result in additive sedative effects).
No products indexed under this heading.

Chlordiazepoxide Hydrochloride (Pergolide may cause somnolence; concurrent use with CNS depressants may result in additive sedative effects). Products include:
Librium Capsules 3347

Chlorpromazine (May diminish the effectiveness of Permax; caution should be exercised if co-administered).
No products indexed under this heading.

Chlorpromazine Hydrochloride (Concurrent use with dopamine antagonists may diminish the effectiveness of pergolide).
No products indexed under this heading.

Chlorprothixene (Pergolide may cause somnolence; concurrent use with CNS depressants may result in additive sedative effects).
No products indexed under this heading.

Chlorprothixene Hydrochloride (Pergolide may cause somnolence; concurrent use with CNS depressants may result in additive sedative effects).
No products indexed under this heading.

Chlorprothixene Lactate (Pergolide may cause somnolence; concurrent use with CNS depressants may result in additive sedative effects).
No products indexed under this heading.

Clorazepate Dipotassium (Pergolide may cause somnolence; concurrent use with CNS depressants may result in additive sedative effects). Products include:
Tranxene 2474

Clozapine (Concurrent use with dopamine antagonists may diminish the effectiveness of pergolide). Products include:
Clozaril Tablets 2184
FazaClo Orally Disintegrating Tablets 551

Codeine Phosphate (Pergolide may cause somnolence; concurrent use with CNS depressants may result in additive sedative effects). Products include:
Tylenol with Codeine Tablets 2391

Desflurane (Pergolide may cause somnolence; concurrent use with CNS depressants may result in additive sedative effects).
No products indexed under this heading.

Dezocine (Pergolide may cause somnolence; concurrent use with CNS depressants may result in additive sedative effects).
No products indexed under this heading.

Diazepam (Pergolide may cause somnolence; concurrent use with CNS depressants may result in additive sedative effects). Products include:
Diastat Rectal Delivery System 3343
Valium Tablets 2819

Droperidol (Pergolide may cause somnolence; concurrent use with CNS depressants may result in additive sedative effects).
No products indexed under this heading.

Enflurane (Pergolide may cause somnolence; concurrent use with CNS depressants may result in additive sedative effects).
No products indexed under this heading.

Estazolam (Pergolide may cause somnolence; concurrent use with CNS depressants may result in additive sedative effects). Products include:
ProSom Tablets 517

Ethanol (Pergolide may cause somnolence; concurrent use with CNS depressants may result in additive sedative effects).
No products indexed under this heading.

Ethchlorvynol (Pergolide may cause somnolence; concurrent use with CNS depressants may result in additive sedative effects).
No products indexed under this heading.

Ethinamate (Pergolide may cause somnolence; concurrent use with CNS depressants may result in additive sedative effects).
No products indexed under this heading.

Ethyl Alcohol (Pergolide may cause somnolence; concurrent use with CNS depressants may result in additive sedative effects).
No products indexed under this heading.

Fentanyl (Pergolide may cause somnolence; concurrent use with CNS depressants may result in additive sedative effects). Products include:
Duragesic Transdermal System 2373
Ionsys Transdermal System 2379

Fentanyl Citrate (Pergolide may cause somnolence; concurrent use with CNS depressants may result in additive sedative effects). Products include:

Fluphenazine Decanoate (Concurrent use with dopamine antagonists may diminish the effectiveness of pergolide).
No products indexed under this heading.

Fluphenazine Enanthate (Concurrent use with dopamine antagonists may diminish the effectiveness of pergolide).
No products indexed under this heading.

Fluphenazine Hydrochloride (Concurrent use with dopamine antagonists may diminish the effectiveness of pergolide).
No products indexed under this heading.

Flurazepam Hydrochloride (Pergolide may cause somnolence; concurrent use with CNS depressants may result in additive sedative effects). Products include:

Glutethimide (Pergolide may cause somnolence; concurrent use with CNS depressants may result in additive sedative effects).
No products indexed under this heading.

Haloperidol (Concurrent use with dopamine antagonists may diminish the effectiveness of pergolide).
No products indexed under this heading.

Haloperidol Decanoate (Concurrent use with dopamine antagonists may diminish the effectiveness of pergolide).
No products indexed under this heading.

Hydrocodone Bitartrate (Pergolide may cause somnolence; concurrent use with CNS depressants may result in additive sedative effects). Products include:

Hydrocodone Polistirex (Pergolide may cause somnolence; concurrent use with CNS depressants may result in additive sedative effects). Products include:

Hydromorphone Hydrochloride (Pergolide may cause somnolence; concurrent use with CNS depressants may result in additive sedative effects). Products include:

Hydroxyzine Hydrochloride (Pergolide may cause somnolence; concurrent use with CNS depressants may result in additive sedative effects).
No products indexed under this heading.

Isoflurane (Pergolide may cause somnolence; concurrent use with CNS depressants may result in additive sedative effects).
No products indexed under this heading.

Ketamine Hydrochloride (Pergolide may cause somnolence; concurrent use with CNS depressants may result in additive sedative effects).
No products indexed under this heading.

Levodopa (Concomitant use may cause and/or exacerbate pre-existing states of confusion and hallucination). Products include:

Levomethadyl Acetate Hydrochloride (Pergolide may cause somnolence; concurrent use with CNS depressants may result in additive sedative effects).
No products indexed under this heading.

Levorphanol Tartrate (Pergolide may cause somnolence; concurrent use with CNS depressants may result in additive sedative effects).
No products indexed under this heading.

Lorazepam (Pergolide may cause somnolence; concurrent use with CNS depressants may result in additive sedative effects).
No products indexed under this heading.

Loxapine Hydrochloride (Pergolide may cause somnolence; concurrent use with CNS depressants may result in additive sedative effects).
No products indexed under this heading.

Loxapine Succinate (Pergolide may cause somnolence; concurrent use with CNS depressants may result in additive sedative effects).
No products indexed under this heading.

Meperidine Hydrochloride (Pergolide may cause somnolence; concurrent use with CNS depressants may result in additive sedative effects).
No products indexed under this heading.

Mephobarbital (Pergolide may cause somnolence; concurrent use with CNS depressants may result in additive sedative effects).
No products indexed under this heading.

Meprobamate (Pergolide may cause somnolence; concurrent use with CNS depressants may result in additive sedative effects).
No products indexed under this heading.

Mesoridazine Besylate (Concurrent use with dopamine antagonists may diminish the effectiveness of pergolide).
No products indexed under this heading.

Methadone Hydrochloride (Pergolide may cause somnolence; concurrent use with CNS depressants may result in additive sedative effects).
No products indexed under this heading.

Methohexital Sodium (Pergolide may cause somnolence; concurrent use with CNS depressants may result in additive sedative effects).
No products indexed under this heading.

Methotrimeprazine (Concurrent use with dopamine antagonists may diminish the effectiveness of pergolide).
No products indexed under this heading.

Methoxyflurane (Pergolide may cause somnolence; concurrent use with CNS depressants may result in additive sedative effects).
No products indexed under this heading.

Metoclopramide Hydrochloride (Concurrent use with dopamine antagonists may diminish the effectiveness of pergolide).
No products indexed under this heading.

Midazolam Hydrochloride (Pergolide may cause somnolence; concurrent use with CNS depressants may result in additive sedative effects).
No products indexed under this heading.

Molindone Hydrochloride (Pergolide may cause somnolence; concurrent use with CNS depressants may result in additive sedative effects). Products include:

Morphine Sulfate (Pergolide may cause somnolence; concurrent use with CNS depressants may result in additive sedative effects). Products include:

Olanzapine (Concurrent use with dopamine antagonists may diminish the effectiveness of pergolide). Products include:

Oxazepam (Pergolide may cause somnolence; concurrent use with CNS depressants may result in additive sedative effects).
No products indexed under this heading.

Oxycodone Hydrochloride (Pergolide may cause somnolence; concurrent use with CNS depressants may result in additive sedative effects). Products include:

Pentobarbital Sodium (Pergolide may cause somnolence; concurrent use with CNS depressants may result in additive sedative effects). Products include:

Perphenazine (Concurrent use with dopamine antagonists may diminish the effectiveness of pergolide).
No products indexed under this heading.

Phenobarbital (Pergolide may cause somnolence; concurrent use with CNS depressants may result in additive sedative effects). Products

Pimozide (Concurrent use with dopamine antagonists may diminish the effectiveness of pergolide).
No products indexed under this heading.

Prazepam (Pergolide may cause somnolence; concurrent use with CNS depressants may result in additive sedative effects).
No products indexed under this heading.

Prochlorperazine (Concurrent use with dopamine antagonists may diminish the effectiveness of pergolide).
No products indexed under this heading.

Promethazine Hydrochloride (Concurrent use with dopamine antagonists may diminish the effectiveness of pergolide). Products include:

Propofol (Pergolide may cause somnolence; concurrent use with CNS depressants may result in additive sedative effects).
No products indexed under this heading.

Propoxyphene Hydrochloride (Pergolide may cause somnolence; concurrent use with CNS depressants may result in additive sedative effects).
No products indexed under this heading.

Propoxyphene Napsylate (Pergolide may cause somnolence; concurrent use with CNS depressants may result in additive sedative effects).
No products indexed under this heading.

Quazepam (Pergolide may cause somnolence; concurrent use with CNS depressants may result in additive sedative effects).
No products indexed under this heading.

Quetiapine Fumarate (Concurrent use with dopamine antagonists may diminish the effectiveness of pergolide). Products include:

Remifentanil Hydrochloride (Pergolide may cause somnolence; concurrent use with CNS depressants may result in additive sedative effects).
No products indexed under this heading.

Risperidone (Pergolide may cause somnolence; concurrent use with CNS depressants may result in additive sedative effects). Products include:

Secobarbital Sodium (Pergolide may cause somnolence; concurrent use with CNS depressants may result in additive sedative effects).
No products indexed under this heading.

Sevoflurane (Pergolide may cause somnolence; concurrent use with CNS depressants may result in additive sedative effects). Products include:

Sodium Oxybate (Pergolide may cause somnolence; concurrent use with CNS depressants may result in additive sedative effects). Products include:

Xyrem Oral Solution 1688

Sufentanil Citrate (Pergolide may cause somnolence; concurrent use with CNS depressants may result in additive sedative effects).

No products indexed under this heading.

Temazepam (Pergolide may cause somnolence; concurrent use with CNS depressants may result in additive sedative effects). Products include:

Restoril Capsules 1860

Thiamylal Sodium (Pergolide may cause somnolence; concurrent use with CNS depressants may result in additive sedative effects).

No products indexed under this heading.

Thioridazine Hydrochloride (Concurrent use with dopamine antagonists may diminish the effectiveness of pergolide). Products include:

Thioridazine Hydrochloride Tablets 2163

Thiothixene (May diminish the effectiveness of Permax). Products include:

Thiothixene Capsules 2165

Triazolam (Pergolide may cause somnolence; concurrent use with CNS depressants may result in additive sedative effects).

No products indexed under this heading.

Trifluoperazine Hydrochloride (Concurrent use with dopamine antagonists may diminish the effectiveness of pergolide).

No products indexed under this heading.

Zaleplon (Pergolide may cause somnolence; concurrent use with CNS depressants may result in additive sedative effects). Products include:

Sonata Capsules 1717

Ziprasidone Hydrochloride (Pergolide may cause somnolence; concurrent use with CNS depressants may result in additive sedative effects). Products include:

Geodon Capsules 2529

Zolpidem Tartrate (Pergolide may cause somnolence; concurrent use with CNS depressants may result in additive sedative effects). Products include:

Ambien Tablets 2851
Ambien CR Tablets 2855

Food Interactions

Alcohol (Pergolide may cause somnolence; concurrent use with alcohol may result in additive sedative effects).

PERMETHRIN LOTION

(Permethrin) .... ■641
None cited in PDR database.

PERSANTINE TABLETS

(Dipyridamole) 868
May interact with anticholinesterase drugs and certain other agents. Compounds in these categories include:

Adenosine (Dipyridamole has been reported to increase the plasma levels and cardiovascular effects of adenosine. Adjustment of adenosine dosage may be necessary). Products include:

Adenocard Injection 617
Adenoscan 619

Donepezil Hydrochloride (Dipyridamole may counteract the anticholinesterase effect of cholinesterase inhibitors, thereby potentially aggravating myasthenia gravis). Products include:

Aricept Tablets 1094
Aricept ODT Tablets 1094

Galantamine Hydrobromide (Dipyridamole may counteract the anticholinesterase effect of cholinesterase inhibitors, thereby potentially aggravating myasthenia gravis). Products include:

Razadyne 2399
Razadyne ER Extended-Release Capsules 2399

Neostigmine Bromide (Dipyridamole may counteract the anticholinesterase effect of cholinesterase inhibitors, thereby potentially aggravating myasthenia gravis).

No products indexed under this heading.

Neostigmine Methylsulfate (Dipyridamole may counteract the anticholinesterase effect of cholinesterase inhibitors, thereby potentially aggravating myasthenia gravis).

No products indexed under this heading.

Pyridostigmine Bromide (Dipyridamole may counteract the anticholinesterase effect of cholinesterase inhibitors, thereby potentially aggravating myasthenia gravis).

No products indexed under this heading.

Rivastigmine Tartrate (Dipyridamole may counteract the anticholinesterase effect of cholinesterase inhibitors, thereby potentially aggravating myasthenia gravis). Products include:

Exelon Capsules 2206
Exelon Oral Solution 2206

Tacrine Hydrochloride (Dipyridamole may counteract the anticholinesterase effect of cholinesterase inhibitors, thereby potentially aggravating myasthenia gravis).

No products indexed under this heading.

PEXEVA TABLETS

(Paroxetine Mesylate) 1694
May interact with 5HT1-receptor agonists, anticoagulants, cytochrome p450 2d6 substrates (selected), lithium preparations, monoamine oxidase inhibitors, non-steroidal anti-inflammatory agents, highly protein bound drugs (selected), serotoninergic agents, selective serotonin reuptake inhibitors, tricyclic antidepressants, and certain other agents. Compounds in these categories include:

Amiodarone Hydrochloride (Because paroxetine is highly bound to plasma proteins, co-administration of Pexeva with another highly protein bound drug may cause increased free concentrations of Pexeva or the other drug, potentially resulting in adverse events).

No products indexed under this heading.

Amitriptyline Hydrochloride (Co-administration of Pexeva with other drugs metabolized by CYP 2D6 isoenzyme and inhibitors should be approached with caution. Paroxetine and thioriadazine should not be co-administered due to risk of serious ventricular arrhythmias and sudden death).

No products indexed under this heading.

Amoxapine (Paroxetine may inhibit the metabolism of tricyclic antidepressants (TCA), reduce TCA dose if administered together).

No products indexed under this heading.

Amphetamine Aspartate (Co-administration of Pexeva with other drugs metabolized by CYP 2D6 isoenzyme and inhibitors should be approached with caution. Paroxetine and thioriadazine should not be co-administered due to risk of serious ventricular arrhythmias and sudden death). Products include:

Adderall Tablets 3164
Adderall XR Capsules 3166

Amphetamine Aspartate Monohydrate (Co-administration of Pexeva with other drugs metabolized by CYP 2D6 isoenzyme and inhibitors should be approached with caution. Paroxetine and thioriadazine should not be co-administered due to risk of serious ventricular arrhythmias and sudden death).

No products indexed under this heading.

Amphetamine Sulfate (Co-administration of Pexeva with other drugs metabolized by CYP 2D6 isoenzyme and inhibitors should be approached with caution. Paroxetine and thioriadazine should not be co-administered due to risk of serious ventricular arrhythmias and sudden death). Products include:

Adderall Tablets 3164
Adderall XR Capsules 3166

Anisindione (Concurrent use of psychotropic drugs that interfere with serotonin reuptake and the occurence of upper gastrointestinal bleeding with drugs that interfere with hemostasis potentiate the risk of bleeding). Products include:

Miradon Tablets 3042

Ardeparin Sodium (Concurrent use of psychotropic drugs that interfere with serotonin reuptake and the occurence of upper gastrointestinal bleeding with drugs that interfere with hemostasis potentiate the risk of bleeding).

No products indexed under this heading.

Aspirin (Concurrent use of psychotropic drugs that interfere with serotonin reuptake and the occurence of upper gastrointestinal bleeding with aspirin potentiate the risk of bleeding). Products include:

Aggrenox Capsules 822
Bayer Aspirin 744
BC Allergy Sinus Cold Powder .... ■677
BC Headache Powder .... ■677
Arthritis Strength BC Powder .... ■677
BC Sinus Cold Powder .... ■677
Excedrin Extra Strength Caplets/Tablets/Geltabs .... ■684
Excedrin Migraine Caplets/Tablets/Geltabs .... ■609
Goody's Body Pain Formula Powder .... ■684
Goody's Extra Strength Headache Powders .... ■611
Goody's Extra Strength Pain Relief Tablets .... ■685
Percodan Tablets 1132
St. Joseph 81 mg Aspirin Chewable and Enteric Coated Tablets 1869

Aspirin, Enteric Coated (Concurrent use of psychotropic drugs that interfere with serotonin reuptake and the occurence of upper gastrointestinal bleeding with aspirin potentiate the risk of bleeding).

No products indexed under this heading.

Aspirin Buffered (Concurrent use of psychotropic drugs that interfere with serotonin reuptake and the occurence of upper gastrointestinal bleeding with aspirin potentiate the risk of bleeding). Products include:

Bufferin Extra Strength Tablets ...... ■678
Bufferin Regular Strength Tablets ... ■678

Atomoxetine Hydrochloride (Co-administration of Pexeva with other drugs metabolized by CYP 2D6 isoenzyme and inhibitors should be approached with caution. Paroxetine and thioriadazine should not be co-administered due to risk of serious ventricular arrhythmias and sudden death). Products include:

Strattera Capsules 1814

Atovaquone (Because paroxetine is highly bound to plasma proteins, co-administration of Pexeva with another highly protein bound drug may cause increased free concentrations of Pexeva or the other drug, potentially resulting in adverse events). Products include:

Malarone Pediatric Tablets 1517
Malarone Tablets 1517
Mepron Suspension 1521

Bisoprolol Fumarate (Co-administration of Pexeva with other drugs metabolized by CYP 2D6 isoenzyme and inhibitors should be approached with caution. Paroxetine and thioriadazine should not be co-administered due to risk of serious ventricular arrhythmias and sudden death).

No products indexed under this heading.

Captopril (Co-administration of Pexeva with other drugs metabolized by CYP 2D6 isoenzyme and inhibitors should be approached with caution. Paroxetine and thioriadazine should not be co-administered due to risk of serious ventricular arrhythmias and sudden death). Products include:

Captopril Tablets 2149

Carvedilol (Co-administration of Pexeva with other drugs metabolized by CYP 2D6 isoenzyme and inhibitors should be approached with caution. Paroxetine and thioriadazine should not be co-administered due to risk of serious ventricular arrhythmias and sudden death). Products include:

Coreg Tablets 1414

Cefonicid Sodium (Because paroxetine is highly bound to plasma proteins, co-administration of Pexeva with another highly protein bound drug may cause increased free concentrations of Pexeva or the other drug, potentially resulting in adverse events).

No products indexed under this heading.

Celecoxib (Because paroxetine is highly bound to plasma proteins, co-administration of Pexeva with another highly protein bound drug may cause increased free concentra-

tions of Pexeva or the other drug, potentially resulting in adverse events). Products include:
Celebrex Capsules 3134

Cevimeline Hydrochloride (Co-administration of Pexeva with other drugs metabolized by CYP 2D6 isoenzyme and inhibitors should be approached with caution. Paroxetine and thioriadazine should not be co-administered due to risk of serious ventricular arrhythmias and sudden death). Products include:
Evoxac Capsules 1047

Chlordiazepoxide (Because paroxetine is highly bound to plasma proteins, co-administration of Pexeva with another highly protein bound drug may cause increased free concentrations of Pexeva or the other drug, potentially resulting in adverse events).
No products indexed under this heading.

Chlordiazepoxide Hydrochloride (Because paroxetine is highly bound to plasma proteins, co-administration of Pexeva with another highly protein bound drug may cause increased free concentrations of Pexeva or the other drug, potentially resulting in adverse events). Products include:
Librium Capsules 3347

Chlorpromazine (Co-administration of Pexeva with other drugs metabolized by CYP 2D6 isoenzyme and inhibitors should be approached with caution. Paroxetine and thioriadazine should not be co-administered due to risk of serious ventricular arrhythmias and sudden death).
No products indexed under this heading.

Chlorpromazine Hydrochloride (Co-administration of Pexeva with other drugs metabolized by CYP 2D6 isoenzyme and inhibitors should be approached with caution. Paroxetine and thioriadazine should not be co-administered due to risk of serious ventricular arrhythmias and sudden death).
No products indexed under this heading.

Chlorpropamide (Co-administration of Pexeva with other drugs metabolized by CYP 2D6 isoenzyme and inhibitors should be approached with caution. Paroxetine and thioriadazine should not be co-administered due to risk of serious ventricular arrhythmias and sudden death).
No products indexed under this heading.

Cimetidine (Steady-state plasma concentrations of paroxetine were increased by approximately 50% during co-administration with oral cimetidine). Products include:
Tagamet HB 200 Tablets 664

Citalopram Hydrobromide (Based on the mechanism of action of paroxetine and the potential for serotonin syndrome, caution is advised when paroxetine is co-administered with other drugs or agents that may affect the serotonergic neurotransmitter system, such as serotonin reuptake inhibitors). Products include:
Celexa 1176

Clomipramine Hydrochloride (Co-administration of Pexeva with other drugs metabolized by CYP 2D6 isoenzyme and inhibitors should be approached with caution. Paroxetine and thioriadazine should not be co-administered due to risk of serious ventricular arrhythmias and sudden death).
No products indexed under this heading.

Clozapine (Co-administration of Pexeva with other drugs metabolized by CYP 2D6 isoenzyme and inhibitors should be approached with caution. Paroxetine and thioriadazine should not be co-administered due to risk of serious ventricular arrhythmias and sudden death). Products include:
Clozaril Tablets 2184
FazaClo Orally Disintegrating Tablets 551

Codeine Phosphate (Co-administration of Pexeva with other drugs metabolized by CYP 2D6 isoenzyme and inhibitors should be approached with caution. Paroxetine and thioriadazine should not be co-administered due to risk of serious ventricular arrhythmias and sudden death). Products include:
Tylenol with Codeine Tablets 2391

Codeine Sulfate (Co-administration of Pexeva with other drugs metabolized by CYP 2D6 isoenzyme and inhibitors should be approached with caution. Paroxetine and thioriadazine should not be co-administered due to risk of serious ventricular arrhythmias and sudden death).
No products indexed under this heading.

Cyclobenzaprine Hydrochloride (Co-administration of Pexeva with other drugs metabolized by CYP 2D6 isoenzyme and inhibitors should be approached with caution. Paroxetine and thioriadazine should not be co-administered due to risk of serious ventricular arrhythmias and sudden death).
No products indexed under this heading.

Cyclosporine (Because paroxetine is highly bound to plasma proteins, co-administration of Pexeva with another highly protein bound drug may cause increased free concentrations of Pexeva or the other drug, potentially resulting in adverse events). Products include:
Gengraf Capsules 459
Neoral Oral Solution 2259
Neoral Soft Gelatin Capsules 2259
Restasis Ophthalmic Emulsion 575
Sandimmune 2275

Dalteparin Sodium (Concurrent use of psychotropic drugs that interfere with serotonin reuptake and the occurence of upper gastrointestinal bleeding with drugs that interfere with hemostasis potentiate the risk of bleeding). Products include:
Fragmin Injection 1097

Danaparoid Sodium (Concurrent use of psychotropic drugs that interfere with serotonin reuptake and the occurence of upper gastrointestinal bleeding with drugs that interfere with hemostasis potentiate the risk of bleeding).
No products indexed under this heading.

Desipramine Hydrochloride (Co-administration of Pexeva with other drugs metabolized by CYP 2D6 isoenzyme and inhibitors should be approached with caution. Paroxetine and thioriadazine should not be co-administered due to risk of serious ventricular arrhythmias and sudden death).
No products indexed under this heading.

Dexfenfluramine Hydrochloride (Co-administration of Pexeva with other drugs metabolized by CYP 2D6 isoenzyme and inhibitors should be approached with caution. Paroxetine and thioriadazine should not be co-administered due to risk of serious ventricular arrhythmias and sudden death).
No products indexed under this heading.

Dextromethorphan Hydrobromide (Co-administration of Pexeva with other drugs metabolized by CYP 2D6 isoenzyme and inhibitors should be approached with caution. Paroxetine and thioriadazine should not be co-administered due to risk of serious ventricular arrhythmias and sudden death). Products include:
Comtrex Maximum Strength Cold & Cough Day/Night Caplets - Day Formulation 726
Comtrex Maximum Strength Cold & Cough Day/Night Caplets - Night Formulation 726
Comtrex Maximum Strength Non-Drowsy Cold & Cough Caplets 725
Children's Dimetapp DM Cold & Cough Elixir 731
Children's Dimetapp Long Acting Cough Plus Cold Syrup 731
Toddler's Dimetapp Cold and Cough Drops 732
Mucinex DM Extended-Release Bi-Layer Tablets 720
Refenesen DM Caplets 721
Robitussin Cough & Cold CF Liquid 735
Robitussin Cough & Cold Long-Acting Liquid 735
Robitussin Cough & Allergy Syrup .. 736
Robitussin Cough & Cold Nighttime Liquid 736
Robitussin Cough & Cold Pediatric Drops 735
Robitussin Cough, Cold & Flu Nighttime Liquid 738
Robitussin Cough & Congestion Liquid 738
Robitussin Cough Gels Long-Acting 737
Robitussin Cough Long Acting Liquid 739
Robitussin Cough DM Syrup 738
Robitussin Cough DM Infant Drops 738
Robitussin Pediatric Cough Long Acting Liquid 739
Robitussin Pediatric Cough & Cold Long-Acting Liquid 735
Robitussin Pediatric Cough & Cold Nighttime Liquid 736
Robitussin Sugar Free Cough 738
TheraFlu Cold & Cough Hot Liquid 740
TheraFlu Warming Relief Daytime Severe Cold 743
TheraFlu Thin Strips Long Acting Cough 744
Triaminic Daytime Cold & Cough Liquid 745
Triaminic Cough & Sore Throat Liquid 747
Triaminic Cough & Runny Nose Softchews 748
Triaminic Thin Strips Cold & Cough 778
Triaminic Infant Thin Strips Decongestant Plus Cough 747
Children's Tylenol Plus Flu Oral Suspension 749
Tylenol Cold Head Congestion Daytime Caplets with Cool Burst and Gelcaps 750
Tylenol Cold Multi-Symptom Daytime Liquid 752
Tylenol Cold Multi-Symptom Severe Daytime Liquid 752
Concentrated Tylenol Infants' Drops Plus Cold & Cough 754
Children's Tylenol Plus Cough & Runny Nose Suspension Liquid 1879
Children's Tylenol Plus Cough & Sore Throat Suspension Liquid 1879
Children's Tylenol Plus Flu Suspension Liquid 1881
Children's Tylenol Plus Multi-Symptom Cold Suspension Liquid 1879
Tylenol Cold Severe Congestion Non-Drowsy Caplets with Cool Burst 1874
Tylenol Cold Head Congestion Daytime Caplets with Cool Burst 1873
Tylenol Cold Head Congestion Nighttime Caplets with Cool Burst 1873
Tylenol Cold Head Congestion Severe Caplets with Cool Burst..... 1873
Tylenol Cold Multi-Symptom Daytime Caplets with Cool Burst and Gelcaps 1874
Tylenol Cold Multi-Symptom Daytime Liquid with Citrus Burst ... 1874
Tylenol Cold Multi-Symptom Nighttime Caplets with Cool Burst 1874
Tylenol Cold Multi-Symptom Nighttime Liquid with Cool Burst ... 1874
Tylenol Cold Multi-Symptom Severe Caplets with Cool Burst..... 1874
Tylenol Cold Multi-Symptom Severe Daytime Liquid with Citrus Burst 1874
Tylenol Cough & Sore Throat Daytime Liquid with Cool Burst...... 1877
Tylenol Cough & Sore Throat Nighttime Liquid with Cool Burst ... 1877
Concentrated Tylenol Infants' Drops Plus Cold and Cough 1879
Vicks 44 Cough Relief Liquid 2679
Vicks 44D Cough & Head Congestion Relief Liquid 2679
Vicks 44E Cough & Chest Congestion Relief Liquid 2679
Pediatric Vicks 44e Cough & Chest Congestion Relief Liquid...... 2676
Vicks 44M Cough, Cold & Flu Relief Liquid 2680
Pediatric Vicks 44m Cough & Cold Relief Liquid 2676
Vicks DayQuil LiquiCaps/Liquid Multi-Symptom Cold/Flu Relief..... 761
Vicks DayQuil Multi-Symptom Cold/Flu Relief LiquiCaps 2678
Vicks DayQuil Multi-Symptom Cold/Flu Relief Liquid 2678
Vicks NyQuil Multi-Symptom Cold/Flu Relief Liquid 2681
Children's Vicks NyQuil Cold/Cough Relief 756
Vicks NyQuil Multi-Symptom Cold/Flu Relief LiquiCaps 2681
Vicks NyQuil LiquiCaps/Liquid Multi-Symptom Cold/Flu Relief..... 763
Vicks NyQuil Cough Liquid 2680
Children's Vicks NyQuil Cold/Cough Relief Liquid 2680
Zicam Cough Max Nighttime Cough Spray 767
Zicam Cough Max Cough Spray 767
Zicam Cough Max Cough Melts 767
Zicam Cough Plus D Cough Spray 767
Zicam Cough Relief Cough Spray ... 767
Zicam Maximum Strength Flu Daytime 768
Zicam Maximum Strength Flu Nighttime 768

Dextromethorphan Polistirex (Co-administration of Pexeva with other drugs metabolized by CYP 2D6 isoenzyme and inhibitors should be approached with caution. Paroxetine and thioriadazine should not be

IMPORTANT NOTE: Always consult each drug listing in the patient's regimen for possible interactions.

co-administered due to risk of serious ventricular arrhythmias and sudden death). Products include:
- Delsym Extended-Release Suspension 12 Hour Cough Suppressant .... ■611

Diazepam (Because paroxetine is highly bound to plasma proteins, co-administration of Pexeva with another highly protein bound drug may cause increased free concentrations of Pexeva or the other drug, potentially resulting in adverse events). Products include:
- Diastat Rectal Delivery System 3343
- Valium Tablets 2819

Diclofenac Potassium (Because paroxetine is highly bound to plasma proteins, co-administration of Pexeva with another highly protein bound drug may cause increased free concentrations of Pexeva or the other drug, potentially resulting in adverse events).
No products indexed under this heading.

Diclofenac Sodium (Because paroxetine is highly bound to plasma proteins, co-administration of Pexeva with another highly protein bound drug may cause increased free concentrations of Pexeva or the other drug, potentially resulting in adverse events). Products include:
- Arthrotec Tablets 3129
- Voltaren Ophthalmic Solution 2309
- Voltaren Tablets 2307
- Voltaren-XR Tablets 2310

Dicumarol (Concurrent use of psychotropic drugs that interfere with serotonin reuptake and the occurence of upper gastrointestinal bleeding with drugs that interfere with hemostasis potentiate the risk of bleeding).
No products indexed under this heading.

Digoxin (Mean digoxin AUC at steady state decreased in the presence of paroxetine). Products include:
- Lanoxicaps Capsules 1490
- Lanoxin Injection 1494
- Lanoxin Injection Pediatric 1497
- Lanoxin Tablets 1500

3-Diphenylacrylate (Based on the mechanism of action of paroxetine and the potential for serotonin syndrome, caution is advised when paroxetine is co-administered with other drugs or agents that may affect the serotonergic neurotransmitter system, such as triptans).
No products indexed under this heading.

Dipyridamole (Because paroxetine is highly bound to plasma proteins, co-administration of Pexeva with another highly protein bound drug may cause increased free concentrations of Pexeva or the other drug, potentially resulting in adverse events). Products include:
- Aggrenox Capsules 822
- Persantine Tablets 868

Dolasetron Mesylate (Co-administration of Pexeva with other drugs metabolized by CYP 2D6 isoenzyme and inhibitors should be approached with caution. Paroxetine and thioriadazine should not be co-administered due to risk of serious ventricular arrhythmias and sudden death). Products include:
- Anzemet Injection 2859
- Anzemet Tablets 2862

Donepezil Hydrochloride (Co-administration of Pexeva with other drugs metabolized by CYP 2D6 isoenzyme and inhibitors should be approached with caution. Paroxetine and thioriadazine should not be co-administered due to risk of serious ventricular arrhythmias and sudden death). Products include:
- Aricept Tablets 1094
- Aricept ODT Tablets 1094

Doxepin Hydrochloride (Co-administration of Pexeva with other drugs metabolized by CYP 2D6 isoenzyme and inhibitors should be approached with caution. Paroxetine and thioriadazine should not be co-administered due to risk of serious ventricular arrhythmias and sudden death).
No products indexed under this heading.

Encainide Hydrochloride (Co-administration of Pexeva with other drugs metabolized by CYP 2D6 isoenzyme and inhibitors should be approached with caution. Paroxetine and thioriadazine should not be co-administered due to risk of serious ventricular arrhythmias and sudden death).
No products indexed under this heading.

Enoxaparin Sodium (Concurrent use of psychotropic drugs that interfere with serotonin reuptake and the occurence of upper gastrointestinal bleeding with drugs that interfere with hemostasis potentiate the risk of bleeding). Products include:
- Lovenox Injection 2915

Escitalopram Oxalate (Based on the mechanism of action of paroxetine and the potential for serotonin syndrome, caution is advised when paroxetine is co-administered with other drugs or agents that may affect the serotonergic neurotransmitter system, such as serotonin reuptake inhibitors). Products include:
- Lexapro Oral Solution 1190
- Lexapro Tablets 1190

Etodolac (Concurrent use of psychotropic drugs that interfere with serotonin reuptake and the occurence of upper gastrointestinal bleeding with an NSAID potentiate the risk of bleeding).
No products indexed under this heading.

Fenoprofen Calcium (Because paroxetine is highly bound to plasma proteins, co-administration of Pexeva with another highly protein bound drug may cause increased free concentrations of Pexeva or the other drug, potentially resulting in adverse events). Products include:
- Nalfon Capsules 2502

Fentanyl (Co-administration of Pexeva with other drugs metabolized by CYP 2D6 isoenzyme and inhibitors should be approached with caution. Paroxetine and thioriadazine should not be co-administered due to risk of serious ventricular arrhythmias and sudden death). Products include:
- Duragesic Transdermal System 2373
- Ionsys Transdermal System 2379

Fentanyl Citrate (Co-administration of Pexeva with other drugs metabolized by CYP 2D6 isoenzyme and inhibitors should be approached with caution. Paroxetine and thioriadazine should not be co-administered due to risk of serious ventricular arrhythmias and sudden death). Products include:
- Actiq 979

Flecainide Acetate (Co-administration of Pexeva with other drugs metabolized by CYP 2D6 isoenzyme and inhibitors should be approached with caution. Paroxetine and thioriadazine should not be co-administered due to risk of serious ventricular arrhythmias and sudden death). Products include:
- Tambocor Tablets 1856

Fluoxetine (Co-administration of Pexeva with other drugs metabolized by CYP 2D6 isoenzyme and inhibitors should be approached with caution. Paroxetine and thioriadazine should not be co-administered due to risk of serious ventricular arrhythmias and sudden death).
No products indexed under this heading.

Fluoxetine Hydrochloride (Co-administration of Pexeva with other drugs metabolized by CYP 2D6 isoenzyme and inhibitors should be approached with caution. Paroxetine and thioriadazine should not be co-administered due to risk of serious ventricular arrhythmias and sudden death). Products include:
- Prozac Pulvules and Liquid 1801
- Symbyax Capsules 1819

Fluphenazine Decanoate (Co-administration of Pexeva with other drugs metabolized by CYP 2D6 isoenzyme and inhibitors should be approached with caution. Paroxetine and thioriadazine should not be co-administered due to risk of serious ventricular arrhythmias and sudden death).
No products indexed under this heading.

Fluphenazine Enanthate (Co-administration of Pexeva with other drugs metabolized by CYP 2D6 isoenzyme and inhibitors should be approached with caution. Paroxetine and thioriadazine should not be co-administered due to risk of serious ventricular arrhythmias and sudden death).
No products indexed under this heading.

Fluphenazine Hydrochloride (Co-administration of Pexeva with other drugs metabolized by CYP 2D6 isoenzyme and inhibitors should be approached with caution. Paroxetine and thioriadazine should not be co-administered due to risk of serious ventricular arrhythmias and sudden death).
No products indexed under this heading.

Flurazepam Hydrochloride (Because paroxetine is highly bound to plasma proteins, co-administration of Pexeva with another highly protein bound drug may cause increased free concentrations of Pexeva or the other drug, potentially resulting in adverse events). Products include:
- Dalmane Capsules 3342

Flurbiprofen (Because paroxetine is highly bound to plasma proteins, co-administration of Pexeva with another highly protein bound drug may cause increased free concentrations of Pexeva or the other drug, potentially resulting in adverse events).
No products indexed under this heading.

Fluvoxamine Maleate (Co-administration of Pexeva with other drugs metabolized by CYP 2D6 isoenzyme and inhibitors should be approached with caution. Paroxetine and thioriadazine should not be co-administered due to risk of serious ventricular arrhythmias and sudden death).
No products indexed under this heading.

Fondaparinux Sodium (Concurrent use of psychotropic drugs that interfere with serotonin reuptake and the occurence of upper gastrointestinal bleeding with drugs that interfere with hemostasis potentiate the risk of bleeding). Products include:
- Arixtra Injection 1351

Formoterol Fumarate (Co-administration of Pexeva with other drugs metabolized by CYP 2D6 isoenzyme and inhibitors should be approached with caution. Paroxetine and thioriadazine should not be co-administered due to risk of serious ventricular arrhythmias and sudden death). Products include:
- Foradil Aerolizer 3010

Fosamprenavir Calcium (Co-administration of fosamprenavir/ritonavir with paroxetine significantly decreased plasma levels of paroxetine. Any dose adjustment should be guided by clinical effect (tolerability and efficacy)). Products include:
- Lexiva Tablets 1505

Galantamine Hydrobromide (Co-administration of Pexeva with other drugs metabolized by CYP 2D6 isoenzyme and inhibitors should be approached with caution. Paroxetine and thioriadazine should not be co-administered due to risk of serious ventricular arrhythmias and sudden death). Products include:
- Razadyne 2399
- Razadyne ER Extended-Release Capsules 2399

Glipizide (Because paroxetine is highly bound to plasma proteins, co-administration of Pexeva with another highly protein bound drug may cause increased free concentrations of Pexeva or the other drug, potentially resulting in adverse events).
No products indexed under this heading.

Haloperidol (Co-administration of Pexeva with other drugs metabolized by CYP 2D6 isoenzyme and inhibitors should be approached with caution. Paroxetine and thioriadazine should not be co-administered due to risk of serious ventricular arrhythmias and sudden death).
No products indexed under this heading.

Haloperidol Decanoate (Co-administration of Pexeva with other drugs metabolized by CYP 2D6 isoenzyme and inhibitors should be approached with caution. Paroxetine and thioriadazine should not be co-administered due to risk of serious ventricular arrhythmias and sudden death).
No products indexed under this heading.

Heparin Calcium (Concurrent use of psychotropic drugs that interfere with serotonin reuptake and the occurence of upper gastrointestinal bleeding with drugs that interfere with hemostasis potentiate the risk of bleeding).
No products indexed under this heading.

Heparin Sodium (Concurrent use of psychotropic drugs that interfere with serotonin reuptake and the occurence of upper gastrointestinal bleeding with drugs that interfere with hemostasis potentiate the risk of bleeding).
No products indexed under this heading.

Hydrocodone Bitartrate (Co-administration of Pexeva with other drugs metabolized by CYP 2D6 isoenzyme and inhibitors should be approached with caution. Paroxetine and thioriadazine should not be co-administered due to risk of serious ventricular arrhythmias and sudden death). Products include:
Hycodan **1116**
Hycotuss Expectorant Syrup **1117**
Vicodin Tablets **535**
Vicodin ES Tablets **536**
Vicodin HP Tablets **538**
Vicoprofen Tablets **539**
Zydone Tablets **1139**

Hypericum (Based on the mechanism of action of paroxetine and the potential for serotonin syndrome, caution is advised when paroxetine is co-administered with other drugs or agents that may affect the serotonergic neurotransmitter system, such as St. John's Wort). Products include:
Satiete Tablets **832**

Hypericum Perforatum (Based on the mechanism of action of paroxetine and the potential for serotonin syndrome, caution is advised when paroxetine is co-administered with other drugs or agents that may affect the serotonergic neurotransmitter system, such as St. John's Wort).
No products indexed under this heading.

Ibuprofen (Because paroxetine is highly bound to plasma proteins, co-administration of Pexeva with another highly protein bound drug may cause increased free concentrations of Pexeva or the other drug, potentially resulting in adverse events). Products include:
Advil Allergy Sinus Caplets **770**
Advil **674**
Children's Advil Oral Suspension **603**
Children's Advil Chewable Tablets **603**
Advil Cold & Sinus **723**
Infants' Advil Concentrated Drops **604**
Infants' Advil Concentrated Drops - White Grape (Dye-Free) **604**
Junior Strength Advil Swallow Tablets **605**
Advil Migraine Liquigels **608**
Advil Multi-Symptom Cold Caplets **770**
Advil PM Caplets **615**
Motrin IB Tablets and Caplets **1866**
Children's Motrin Oral Suspension **1867**
Children's Motrin Non-Staining Dye-Free Oral Suspension **1867**
Children's Motrin Cold Oral Suspension **1867**
Infants' Motrin Concentrated Drops **1867**
Infants' Motrin Non-Staining Dye-Free Concentrated Drops **1867**
Junior Strength Motrin Caplets and Chewable Tablets **1867**
Vicoprofen Tablets **539**

Imipramine Hydrochloride (Co-administration of Pexeva with other drugs metabolized by CYP 2D6 isoenzyme and inhibitors should be approached with caution. Paroxetine and thioriadazine should not be co-administered due to risk of serious ventricular arrhythmias and sudden death).
No products indexed under this heading.

Imipramine Pamoate (Co-administration of Pexeva with other drugs metabolized by CYP 2D6 isoenzyme and inhibitors should be approached with caution. Paroxetine and thioriadazine should not be co-administered due to risk of serious ventricular arrhythmias and sudden death).
No products indexed under this heading.

Indomethacin (Because paroxetine is highly bound to plasma proteins, co-administration of Pexeva with another highly protein bound drug may cause increased free concentrations of Pexeva or the other drug, potentially resulting in adverse events). Products include:
Indocin **1995**

Indomethacin Sodium Trihydrate (Because paroxetine is highly bound to plasma proteins, co-administration of Pexeva with another highly protein bound drug may cause increased free concentrations of Pexeva or the other drug, potentially resulting in adverse events). Products include:
Indocin I.V. **2465**

Indoramin Hydrochloride (Co-administration of Pexeva with other drugs metabolized by CYP 2D6 isoenzyme and inhibitors should be approached with caution. Paroxetine and thioriadazine should not be co-administered due to risk of serious ventricular arrhythmias and sudden death).
No products indexed under this heading.

Isocarboxazid (In patients receiving another serotonin reuptake inhibitor drug in combination with a monoamine oxidase inhibitor (MAOI), there have been reports of serious, sometimes fatal, reactions including hyperthermia, rigidity, myoclonus, autonomic instability with possible rapid fluctuations of vital signs, and mental status changes that include extreme agitation progressing to delirium and coma. Paroxetine should not be used in combination with a MAOI, or within 14 days of discontinuing treatment with a MAOI).
No products indexed under this heading.

Ketoprofen (Because paroxetine is highly bound to plasma proteins, co-administration of Pexeva with another highly protein bound drug may cause increased free concentrations of Pexeva or the other drug, potentially resulting in adverse events).
No products indexed under this heading.

Ketorolac Tromethamine (Because paroxetine is highly bound to plasma proteins, co-administration of Pexeva with another highly protein bound drug may cause increased free concentrations of Pexeva or the other drug, potentially resulting in adverse events). Products include:
Acular Ophthalmic Solution **565**
Acular LS Ophthalmic Solution **566**

Labetalol Hydrochloride (Co-administration of Pexeva with other drugs metabolized by CYP 2D6 isoenzyme and inhibitors should be approached with caution. Paroxetine and thioriadazine should not be co-administered due to risk of serious ventricular arrhythmias and sudden death).
No products indexed under this heading.

Lidocaine (Co-administration of Pexeva with other drugs metabolized by CYP 2D6 isoenzyme and inhibitors should be approached with caution. Paroxetine and thioriadazine should not be co-administered due to risk of serious ventricular arrhythmias and sudden death). Products include:
Lidoderm Patch **1118**
Synera Topical Patch **1137**

Lidocaine Hydrochloride (Co-administration of Pexeva with other drugs metabolized by CYP 2D6 isoenzyme and inhibitors should be approached with caution. Paroxetine and thioriadazine should not be co-administered due to risk of serious ventricular arrhythmias and sudden death).
No products indexed under this heading.

Linezolid (Based on the mechanism of action of paroxetine and the potential for serotonin syndrome, caution is advised when paroxetine is co-administered with other drugs or agents that may affect the serotonergic neurotransmitter system, such as linezolid (an antibiotic which is a reversible non-selective MAOI)). Products include:
Zyvox **2652**

Lithium (The concurrent administration of paroxetine and lithium should be taken with caution).
No products indexed under this heading.

Lithium Carbonate (Based on the mechanism of action of paroxetine and the potential for serotonin syndrome, caution is advised when paroxetine is co-administered with other drugs or agents that may affect the serotonergic neurotransmitter system, such as lithium). Products include:
Lithobid Tablets **1692**

Lithium Citrate (Based on the mechanism of action of paroxetine and the potential for serotonin syndrome, caution is advised when paroxetine is co-administered with other drugs or agents that may affect the serotonergic neurotransmitter system, such as lithium).
No products indexed under this heading.

Low Molecular Weight Heparins (Concurrent use of psychotropic drugs that interfere with serotonin reuptake and the occurence of upper gastrointestinal bleeding with drugs that interfere with hemostasis potentiate the risk of bleeding).
No products indexed under this heading.

Maprotiline Hydrochloride (Co-administration of Pexeva with other drugs metabolized by CYP 2D6 isoenzyme and inhibitors should be approached with caution. Paroxetine and thioriadazine should not be co-administered due to risk of serious ventricular arrhythmias and sudden death).
No products indexed under this heading.

Meclofenamate Sodium (Because paroxetine is highly bound to plasma proteins, co-administration of Pexeva with another highly protein bound drug may cause increased free concentrations of Pexeva or the other drug, potentially resulting in adverse events).
No products indexed under this heading.

Mefenamic Acid (Because paroxetine is highly bound to plasma proteins, co-administration of Pexeva with another highly protein bound drug may cause increased free concentrations of Pexeva or the other drug, potentially resulting in adverse events).
No products indexed under this heading.

Meloxicam (Concurrent use of psychotropic drugs that interfere with serotonin reuptake and the occurence of upper gastrointestinal bleeding with an NSAID potentiate the risk of bleeding). Products include:
Mobic Oral Suspension **863**
Mobic Tablets **863**

Meperidine Hydrochloride (Co-administration of Pexeva with other drugs metabolized by CYP 2D6 isoenzyme and inhibitors should be approached with caution. Paroxetine and thioriadazine should not be co-administered due to risk of serious ventricular arrhythmias and sudden death).
No products indexed under this heading.

Methadone Hydrochloride (Co-administration of Pexeva with other drugs metabolized by CYP 2D6 isoenzyme and inhibitors should be approached with caution. Paroxetine and thioriadazine should not be co-administered due to risk of serious ventricular arrhythmias and sudden death).
No products indexed under this heading.

Methamphetamine Hydrochloride (Co-administration of Pexeva with other drugs metabolized by CYP 2D6 isoenzyme and inhibitors should be approached with caution. Paroxetine and thioriadazine should not be co-administered due to risk of serious ventricular arrhythmias and sudden death). Products include:
Desoxyn Tablets, USP **2462**

Metoprolol Succinate (Co-administration of Pexeva with other drugs metabolized by CYP 2D6 isoenzyme and inhibitors should be approached with caution. Paroxetine and thioriadazine should not be co-administered due to risk of serious ventricular arrhythmias and sudden death). Products include:
Toprol-XL Tablets **668**

Metoprolol Tartrate (Co-administration of Pexeva with other drugs metabolized by CYP 2D6 isoenzyme and inhibitors should be approached with caution. Paroxetine and thioriadazine should not be co-administered due to risk of serious ventricular arrhythmias and sudden death). Products include:
Lopressor Injection **2238**
Lopressor Tablets **2238**
Lopressor HCT 50/25 Tablets **2241**
Lopressor HCT 100/25 Tablets **2241**
Lopressor HCT 100/50 Tablets **2241**

Mexiletine Hydrochloride (Co-administration of Pexeva with other drugs metabolized by CYP 2D6 isoenzyme and inhibitors should be approached with caution. Paroxetine and thioriadazine should not be co-administered due to risk of serious ventricular arrhythmias and sudden death).

No products indexed under this heading.

Midazolam Hydrochloride (Because paroxetine is highly bound to plasma proteins, co-administration of Pexeva with another highly protein bound drug may cause increased free concentrations of Pexeva or the other drug, potentially resulting in adverse events).

No products indexed under this heading.

Mirtazapine (Co-administration of Pexeva with other drugs metabolized by CYP 2D6 isoenzyme and inhibitors should be approached with caution. Paroxetine and thioriadazine should not be co-administered due to risk of serious ventricular arrhythmias and sudden death).

No products indexed under this heading.

Moclobemide (In patients receiving another serotonin reuptake inhibitor drug in combination with a monoamine oxidase inhibitor (MAOI), there have been reports of serious, sometimes fatal, reactions including hyperthermia, rigidity, myoclonus, autonomic instability with possible rapid fluctuations of vital signs, and mental status changes that include extreme agitation progressing to delirium and coma. Paroxetine should not be used in combination with a MAOI, or within 14 days of discontinuing treatment with a MAOI).

No products indexed under this heading.

Morphine Sulfate (Co-administration of Pexeva with other drugs metabolized by CYP 2D6 isoenzyme and inhibitors should be approached with caution. Paroxetine and thioriadazine should not be co-administered due to risk of serious ventricular arrhythmias and sudden death). Products include:

Avinza Capsules 1741
Kadian Capsules 577
MS Contin Tablets 2701

Nabumetone (Concurrent use of psychotropic drugs that interfere with serotonin reuptake and the occurence of upper gastrointestinal bleeding with an NSAID potentiate the risk of bleeding).

No products indexed under this heading.

Naproxen (Because paroxetine is highly bound to plasma proteins, co-administration of Pexeva with another highly protein bound drug may cause increased free concentrations of Pexeva or the other drug, potentially resulting in adverse events). Products include:

EC-Naprosyn Delayed-Release
Tablets ... 2761
Naprosyn Suspension 2761
Naprosyn Tablets 2761
Prevacid NapraPAC 3280

Naproxen Sodium (Because paroxetine is highly bound to plasma proteins, co-administration of Pexeva with another highly protein bound drug may cause increased free con-

centrations of Pexeva or the other drug, potentially resulting in adverse events). Products include:

Aleve Caplets 742
Aleve Gelcaps 743
Aleve Tablets 743
Aleve Cold & Sinus Caplets 744
Anaprox Tablets 2761
Anaprox DS Tablets 2761

Naratriptan Hydrochloride
(Based on the mechanism of action of paroxetine and the potential for serotonin syndrome, caution is advised when paroxetine is co-administered with other drugs or agents that may affect the serotonergic neurotransmitter system, such as triptans). Products include:

Amerge Tablets 1339

Nelfinavir Mesylate (Co-administration of Pexeva with other drugs metabolized by CYP 2D6 isoenzyme and inhibitors should be approached with caution. Paroxetine and thioriadazine should not be co-administered due to risk of serious ventricular arrhythmias and sudden death). Products include:

Viracept ... 2577

Nortriptyline Hydrochloride (Co-administration of Pexeva with other drugs metabolized by CYP 2D6 isoenzyme and inhibitors should be approached with caution. Paroxetine and thioriadazine should not be co-administered due to risk of serious ventricular arrhythmias and sudden death).

No products indexed under this heading.

Olanzapine (Co-administration of Pexeva with other drugs metabolized by CYP 2D6 isoenzyme and inhibitors should be approached with caution. Paroxetine and thioriadazine should not be co-administered due to risk of serious ventricular arrhythmias and sudden death). Products include:

Symbyax Capsules 1819
Zyprexa Tablets 1830
Zyprexa IntraMuscular 1830
Zyprexa ZYDIS Orally
Disintegrating Tablets.................. 1830

Omeprazole (Co-administration of Pexeva with other drugs metabolized by CYP 2D6 isoenzyme and inhibitors should be approached with caution. Paroxetine and thioriadazine should not be co-administered due to risk of serious ventricular arrhythmias and sudden death). Products include:

Zegerid Capsules 2958
Zegerid Powder for Oral Solution 2958

Ondansetron (Co-administration of Pexeva with other drugs metabolized by CYP 2D6 isoenzyme and inhibitors should be approached with caution. Paroxetine and thioriadazine should not be co-administered due to risk of serious ventricular arrhythmias and sudden death). Products include:

Zofran ODT Orally Disintegrating
Tablets ... 1639

Ondansetron Hydrochloride (Co-administration of Pexeva with other drugs metabolized by CYP 2D6 isoenzyme and inhibitors should be approached with caution. Paroxetine and thioriadazine should not be co-administered due to risk of serious ventricular arrhythmias and sudden death). Products include:

Zofran Injection 1634
Zofran .. 1639

Oxaprozin (Because paroxetine is highly bound to plasma proteins, co-administration of Pexeva with another highly protein bound drug may cause increased free concentrations of Pexeva or the other drug, potentially resulting in adverse events).

No products indexed under this heading.

Oxazepam (Because paroxetine is highly bound to plasma proteins, co-administration of Pexeva with another highly protein bound drug may cause increased free concentrations of Pexeva or the other drug, potentially resulting in adverse events).

No products indexed under this heading.

Oxycodone Hydrochloride (Co-administration of Pexeva with other drugs metabolized by CYP 2D6 isoenzyme and inhibitors should be approached with caution. Paroxetine and thioriadazine should not be co-administered due to risk of serious ventricular arrhythmias and sudden death). Products include:

OxyContin Tablets 2703
OxyFast Oral Concentrate
Solution 2708
OxyIR Capsules 2708
Percocet Tablets 1131
Percodan Tablets 1132

Paclitaxel (Co-administration of Pexeva with other drugs metabolized by CYP 2D6 isoenzyme and inhibitors should be approached with caution. Paroxetine and thioriadazine should not be co-administered due to risk of serious ventricular arrhythmias and sudden death).

No products indexed under this heading.

Pargyline Hydrochloride (In patients receiving another serotonin reuptake inhibitor drug in combination with a monoamine oxidase inhibitor (MAOI), there have been reports of serious, sometimes fatal, reactions including hyperthermia, rigidity, myoclonus, autonomic instability with possible rapid fluctuations of vital signs, and mental status changes that include extreme agitation progressing to delirium and coma. Paroxetine should not be used in combination with a MAOI, or within 14 days of discontinuing treatment with a MAOI).

No products indexed under this heading.

Paroxetine Hydrochloride (Paroxetine mesylate and paroxetine hydrochloride should not be co-administered because they contain the same active ingredient).
Products include:

Paxil CR Controlled-Release
Tablets .. 1538
Paxil .. 1530

Phenelzine Sulfate (In patients receiving another serotonin reuptake inhibitor drug in combination with a monoamine oxidase inhibitor (MAOI), there have been reports of serious, sometimes fatal, reactions including hyperthermia, rigidity, myoclonus, autonomic instability with possible rapid fluctuations of vital signs, and mental status changes that include extreme agitation progressing to delirium and coma. Paroxetine should not be used in combination with a MAOI, or within 14 days of discontinuing treatment with a

MAOI).

No products indexed under this heading.

Phenobarbital (Paroxetine AUC and T1/2 were reduced when co-administered with phenobarbital). Products include:

Donnatal Extentabs 2493

Phenylbutazone (Because paroxetine is highly bound to plasma proteins, co-administration of Pexeva with another highly protein bound drug may cause increased free concentrations of Pexeva or the other drug, potentially resulting in adverse events).

No products indexed under this heading.

Phenytoin (At phenytoin steady state concentrations, paroxetine AUC and T1/2 were reduced compared to paroxetime administered alone. When phenytoin was administered at paroxetine steady state, the AUC of phenytoin was also slightly reduced. No initial dose adjustments are necessary when administered together).

No products indexed under this heading.

Pimozide (Due to the narrow therapeutic index of pimozide and its known ability to prolong the QT interval, concomitant use of pimozide and paroxetine mesylate is contraindicated).

No products indexed under this heading.

Pindolol (Co-administration of Pexeva with other drugs metabolized by CYP 2D6 isoenzyme and inhibitors should be approached with caution. Paroxetine and thioriadazine should not be co-administered due to risk of serious ventricular arrhythmias and sudden death).

No products indexed under this heading.

Piroxicam (Because paroxetine is highly bound to plasma proteins, co-administration of Pexeva with another highly protein bound drug may cause increased free concentrations of Pexeva or the other drug, potentially resulting in adverse events).

No products indexed under this heading.

Procarbazine Hydrochloride (In patients receiving another serotonin reuptake inhibitor drug in combination with a monoamine oxidase inhibitor (MAOI), there have been reports of serious, sometimes fatal, reactions including hyperthermia, rigidity, myoclonus, autonomic instability with possible rapid fluctuations of vital signs, and mental status changes that include extreme agitation progressing to delirium and coma. Paroxetine should not be used in combination with a MAOI, or within 14 days of discontinuing treatment with a MAOI). Products include:

Matulane Capsules 3191

Procyclidine Hydrochloride (Daily dosing of paroxetine increased steady-state AUC0-24, Cmax and Cmin values of procyclidine. If anticholinergic effects are seen, the dose of procyclidine should be reduced).

No products indexed under this heading.

Propafenone Hydrochloride (Co-administration of Pexeva with other drugs metabolized by CYP 2D6 isoenzyme and inhibitors should be approached with caution. Paroxetine and thioriadazine should not be co-administered due to risk of serious ventricular arrhythmias and sudden death). Products include:

Propoxyphene Hydrochloride (Co-administration of Pexeva with other drugs metabolized by CYP 2D6 isoenzyme and inhibitors should be approached with caution. Paroxetine and thioriadazine should not be co-administered due to risk of serious ventricular arrhythmias and sudden death).
No products indexed under this heading.

Propoxyphene Napsylate (Co-administration of Pexeva with other drugs metabolized by CYP 2D6 isoenzyme and inhibitors should be approached with caution. Paroxetine and thioriadazine should not be co-administered due to risk of serious ventricular arrhythmias and sudden death).
No products indexed under this heading.

Propranolol Hydrochloride (Co-administration of Pexeva with other drugs metabolized by CYP 2D6 isoenzyme and inhibitors should be approached with caution. Paroxetine and thioriadazine should not be co-administered due to risk of serious ventricular arrhythmias and sudden death). Products include:

Protriptyline Hydrochloride (Paroxetine may inhibit the metabolism of tricyclic antidepressants (TCA), reduce TCA dose if administered together).
No products indexed under this heading.

Quetiapine Fumarate (Co-administration of Pexeva with other drugs metabolized by CYP 2D6 isoenzyme and inhibitors should be approached with caution. Paroxetine and thioriadazine should not be co-administered due to risk of serious ventricular arrhythmias and sudden death). Products include:

Quinidine Gluconate (Co-administration of Pexeva with other drugs metabolized by CYP 2D6 isoenzyme and inhibitors should be approached with caution. Paroxetine and thioriadazine should not be co-administered due to risk of serious ventricular arrhythmias and sudden death).
No products indexed under this heading.

Quinidine Hydrochloride (Co-administration of Pexeva with other drugs metabolized by CYP 2D6 isoenzyme and inhibitors should be approached with caution. Paroxetine and thioriadazine should not be co-administered due to risk of serious ventricular arrhythmias and sudden death).
No products indexed under this heading.

Quinidine Polygalacturonate (Co-administration of Pexeva with other drugs metabolized by CYP 2D6 isoenzyme and inhibitors should be approached with caution. Paroxetine and thioriadazine should not be co-administered due to risk of serious ventricular arrhythmias and sudden death).
No products indexed under this heading.

Quinidine Sulfate (Co-administration of Pexeva with other drugs metabolized by CYP 2D6 isoenzyme and inhibitors should be approached with caution. Paroxetine and thioriadazine should not be co-administered due to risk of serious ventricular arrhythmias and sudden death).
No products indexed under this heading.

Risperidone (Co-administration of Pexeva with other drugs metabolized by CYP 2D6 isoenzyme and inhibitors should be approached with caution. Paroxetine and thioriadazine should not be co-administered due to risk of serious ventricular arrhythmias and sudden death). Products include:

Ritonavir (Co-administration of fosamprenavir/ritonavir with paroxetine significantly decreased plasma levels of paroxetine. Any dose adjustment should be guided by clinical effect (tolerability and efficacy)). Products include:

Rizatriptan Benzoate (Based on the mechanism of action of paroxetine and the potential for serotonin syndrome, caution is advised when paroxetine is co-administered with other drugs or agents that may affect the serotonergic neurotransmitter system, such as triptans). Products include:

Rofecoxib (Concurrent use of psychotropic drugs that interfere with serotonin reuptake and the occurence of upper gastrointestinal bleeding with an NSAID potentiate the risk of bleeding).
No products indexed under this heading.

Selegiline Hydrochloride (In patients receiving another serotonin reuptake inhibitor drug in combination with a monoamine oxidase inhibitor (MAOI), there have been reports of serious, sometimes fatal, reactions including hyperthermia, rigidity, myoclonus, autonomic instability with possible rapid fluctuations of vital signs, and mental status changes that include extreme agitation progressing to delirium and coma. Paroxetine should not be used in combination with a MAOI, or within 14 days of discontinuing treatment with a MAOI). Products include:

Sertraline Hydrochloride (Based on the mechanism of action of paroxetine and the potential for serotonin syndrome, caution is advised when paroxetine is co-administered

with other drugs or agents that may affect the serotonergic neurotransmitter system, such as serotonin reuptake inhibitors). Products include:

Sulindac (Because paroxetine is highly bound to plasma proteins, co-administration of Pexeva with another highly protein bound drug may cause increased free concentrations of Pexeva or the other drug, potentially resulting in adverse events). Products include:

Sumatriptan (Reports of patients with weakness, hyperreflexia, and incoordination following the use of a selective serotonin reuptake inhibitor and sumatriptan). Products include:

Sumatriptan Succinate (Based on the mechanism of action of paroxetine and the potential for serotonin syndrome, caution is advised when paroxetine is co-administered with other drugs or agents that may affect the serotonergic neurotransmitter system, such as triptans). Products include:

Tamoxifen Citrate (Co-administration of Pexeva with other drugs metabolized by CYP 2D6 isoenzyme and inhibitors should be approached with caution. Paroxetine and thioriadazine should not be co-administered due to risk of serious ventricular arrhythmias and sudden death). Products include:

Temazepam (Because paroxetine is highly bound to plasma proteins, co-administration of Pexeva with another highly protein bound drug may cause increased free concentrations of Pexeva or the other drug, potentially resulting in adverse events). Products include:

Teniposide (Co-administration of Pexeva with other drugs metabolized by CYP 2D6 isoenzyme and inhibitors should be approached with caution. Paroxetine and thioriadazine should not be co-administered due to risk of serious ventricular arrhythmias and sudden death).
No products indexed under this heading.

Testosterone (Co-administration of Pexeva with other drugs metabolized by CYP 2D6 isoenzyme and inhibitors should be approached with caution. Paroxetine and thioriadazine should not be co-administered due to risk of serious ventricular arrhythmias and sudden death). Products include:

Testosterone Cypionate (Co-administration of Pexeva with other drugs metabolized by CYP 2D6 isoenzyme and inhibitors should be approached with caution. Paroxetine and thioriadazine should not be co-administered due to risk of serious ventricular arrhythmias and sudden death).
No products indexed under this heading.

Testosterone Enanthate (Co-administration of Pexeva with other drugs metabolized by CYP 2D6 isoenzyme and inhibitors should be approached with caution. Paroxetine and thioriadazine should not be co-administered due to risk of serious ventricular arrhythmias and sudden death).
No products indexed under this heading.

Testosterone Propionate (Co-administration of Pexeva with other drugs metabolized by CYP 2D6 isoenzyme and inhibitors should be approached with caution. Paroxetine and thioriadazine should not be co-administered due to risk of serious ventricular arrhythmias and sudden death).
No products indexed under this heading.

Theophylline (Reports of elevated theophylline levels associated with paroxetine treatment. Monitor theophylline levels when these drugs are concurrently administered).
No products indexed under this heading.

Thioridazine (Thioridazine produces prolongation of the QTc interval, which is associated with serious ventricular arrhythmias, such as torsade de pointes-type arrhythmias, and sudden death. Drugs which inhibit P4502D6, such as paroxetine, will elevate plasma levels of thioridazine).
No products indexed under this heading.

Thioridazine Hydrochloride (Thioridazine produces prolongation of the QTc interval, which is associated with serious ventricular arrhythmias, such as torsade de pointes-type arrhythmias, and sudden death. Drugs which inhibit P4502D6, such as paroxetine, will elevate plasma levels of thioridazine). Products include:

Timolol Maleate (Co-administration of Pexeva with other drugs metabolized by CYP 2D6 isoenzyme and inhibitors should be approached with caution. Paroxetine and thioriadazine should not be co-administered due to risk of serious ventricular arrhythmias and sudden death). Products include:

Tinzaparin Sodium (Concurrent use of psychotropic drugs that interfere with serotonin reuptake and the occurence of upper gastrointestinal bleeding with drugs that interfere with hemostasis potentiate the risk of bleeding).
No products indexed under this heading.

Tolbutamide (Because paroxetine is highly bound to plasma proteins, co-administration of Pexeva with another highly protein bound drug may cause increased free concentrations of Pexeva or the other drug, potentially resulting in adverse events).
No products indexed under this heading.

IMPORTANT NOTE: Always consult each drug listing in the patient's regimen for possible interactions.

Tolmetin Sodium (Because paroxetine is highly bound to plasma proteins, co-administration of Pexeva with another highly protein bound drug may cause increased free concentrations of Pexeva or the other drug, potentially resulting in adverse events).
No products indexed under this heading.

Tolterodine Tartrate (Co-administration of Pexeva with other drugs metabolized by CYP 2D6 isoenzyme and inhibitors should be approached with caution. Paroxetine and thioriadazine should not be co-administered due to risk of serious ventricular arrhythmias and sudden death). Products include:
Detrol Tablets 2628
Detrol LA Capsules 2631

Tramadol Hydrochloride (Co-administration of Pexeva with other drugs metabolized by CYP 2D6 isoenzyme and inhibitors should be approached with caution. Paroxetine and thioriadazine should not be co-administered due to risk of serious ventricular arrhythmias and sudden death). Products include:
Ultram ER Tablets 2392

Tranylcypromine Sulfate (In patients receiving another serotonin reuptake inhibitor drug in combination with a monoamine oxidase inhibitor (MAOI), there have been reports of serious, sometimes fatal, reactions including hyperthermia, rigidity, myoclonus, autonomic instability with possible rapid fluctuations of vital signs, and mental status changes that include extreme agitation progressing to delirium and coma. Paroxetine should not be used in combination with a MAOI, or within 14 days of discontinuing treatment with a MAOI). Products include:
Parnate Tablets 1527

Trazodone Hydrochloride (Co-administration of Pexeva with other drugs metabolized by CYP 2D6 isoenzyme and inhibitors should be approached with caution. Paroxetine and thioriadazine should not be co-administered due to risk of serious ventricular arrhythmias and sudden death).
No products indexed under this heading.

Triazolam (Co-administration of Pexeva with other drugs metabolized by CYP 2D6 isoenzyme and inhibitors should be approached with caution. Paroxetine and thioriadazine should not be co-administered due to risk of serious ventricular arrhythmias and sudden death).
No products indexed under this heading.

Trimipramine Maleate (Co-administration of Pexeva with other drugs metabolized by CYP 2D6 isoenzyme and inhibitors should be approached with caution. Paroxetine and thioriadazine should not be co-administered due to risk of serious ventricular arrhythmias and sudden death).
No products indexed under this heading.

Tryptophan (As with other serotonin reuptake inhibitors, an interaction between paroxetine and tryptophan may occur when they are co-administered. Adverse experiences, consisting of headache, nausea, sweating, and dizziness have been reported).
No products indexed under this heading.

Valdecoxib (Concurrent use of psychotropic drugs that interfere with serotonin reuptake and the occurence of upper gastrointestinal bleeding with an NSAID potentiate the risk of bleeding).
No products indexed under this heading.

Venlafaxine Hydrochloride (Co-administration of Pexeva with other drugs metabolized by CYP 2D6 isoenzyme and inhibitors should be approached with caution. Paroxetine and thioriadazine should not be co-administered due to risk of serious ventricular arrhythmias and sudden death). Products include:
Effexor Tablets 3411
Effexor XR Capsules 3417

Vinblastine Sulfate (Co-administration of Pexeva with other drugs metabolized by CYP 2D6 isoenzyme and inhibitors should be approached with caution. Paroxetine and thioriadazine should not be co-administered due to risk of serious ventricular arrhythmias and sudden death).
No products indexed under this heading.

Warfarin Sodium (Potential for pharmacodynamic interaction that causes an increased bleeding diathesis in the face of unaltered prothrombin time). Products include:
Coumadin for Injection 898
Coumadin Tablets 898

Zolmitriptan (Based on the mechanism of action of paroxetine and the potential for serotonin syndrome, caution is advised when paroxetine is co-administered with other drugs or agents that may affect the serotonergic neurotransmitter system, such as triptans). Products include:
Zomig Tablets 3519
Zomig Nasal Spray 3523
Zomig-ZMT Tablets 3519

Zonisamide (Co-administration of Pexeva with other drugs metabolized by CYP 2D6 isoenzyme and inhibitors should be approached with caution. Paroxetine and thioriadazine should not be co-administered due to risk of serious ventricular arrhythmias and sudden death). Products include:
Zonegran Capsules 1101

Food Interactions

Alcohol (Avoid the use of alcohol while taking Pexeva).

PHAZYME-125 MG QUICK DISSOLVE CHEWABLE TABLETS

(Simethicone) .... ▣657
None cited in PDR database.

PHAZYME-180 MG ULTRA STRENGTH SOFTGELS

(Simethicone) .... ▣657
None cited in PDR database.

PHENERGAN TABLETS AND SUPPOSITORIES

(Promethazine Hydrochloride) 3440
May interact with anticholinergics, barbiturates, central nervous system depressants, monoamine oxidase inhibitors, narcotic analgesics, tricyclic antidepressants, and certain other agents. Compounds in these categories include:

Alfentanil Hydrochloride (Promethazine may increase, prolong, or intensify the sedative action of other CNS depressants; when co-administered with narcotics, the dose of narcotics should be reduced by at least one-quarter to one-half; excessive amount of promethazine relative to narcotic may lead to restlessness and motor hyperactivity in the patient with pain).
No products indexed under this heading.

Alprazolam (Promethazine may increase, prolong, or intensify the sedative action of other CNS depressants; concurrent use should be avoided with other CNS depressants or administered in reduced dosage to patient receiving promethazine). Products include:
Niravam Orally Disintegrating Tablets 3092

Amitriptyline Hydrochloride (Promethazine may increase, prolong, or intensify the sedative action of other CNS depressants; concurrent use should be avoided with tricyclic antidepressants or administered in reduced dosage to patient receiving promethazine).
No products indexed under this heading.

Amoxapine (Promethazine may increase, prolong, or intensify the sedative action of other CNS depressants; concurrent use should be avoided with tricyclic antidepressants or administered in reduced dosage to patient receiving promethazine).
No products indexed under this heading.

Aprobarbital (Promethazine may increase, prolong, or intensify the sedative action of other CNS depressants; when co-administered with barbiturates, the dose of barbiturates should be reduced by one-quarter to one-half).
No products indexed under this heading.

Atropine Sulfate (Co-administration with agents with anticholinergic properties should be undertaken with caution). Products include:
Donnatal Extentabs 2493

Belladonna Alkaloids (Co-administration with agents with anticholinergic properties should be undertaken with caution). Products include:
Hyland's Teething Tablets .... ▣830

Benztropine Mesylate (Co-administration with agents with anticholinergic properties should be undertaken with caution).
No products indexed under this heading.

Biperiden Hydrochloride (Co-administration with agents with anticholinergic properties should be undertaken with caution).
No products indexed under this heading.

Buprenorphine Hydrochloride (Promethazine may increase, prolong, or intensify the sedative action of other CNS depressants; when co-administered with narcotics, the dose of narcotics should be reduced by at least one-quarter to one-half; excessive amount of promethazine relative to narcotic may lead to restlessness and motor hyperactivity in the patient with pain). Products include:
Buprenex Injectable 2716
Suboxone Tablets 2717
Subutex Tablets 2717

Buspirone Hydrochloride (Promethazine may increase, prolong, or intensify the sedative action of other CNS depressants; concurrent use should be avoided with other CNS depressants or administered in reduced dosage to patient receiving promethazine).
No products indexed under this heading.

Butabarbital (Promethazine may increase, prolong, or intensify the sedative action of other CNS depressants; when co-administered with barbiturates, the dose of barbiturates should be reduced by one-quarter to one-half).
No products indexed under this heading.

Butalbital (Promethazine may increase, prolong, or intensify the sedative action of other CNS depressants; when co-administered with barbiturates, the dose of barbiturates should be reduced by one-quarter to one-half).
No products indexed under this heading.

Chlordiazepoxide (Promethazine may increase, prolong, or intensify the sedative action of other CNS depressants; concurrent use should be avoided with other CNS depressants or administered in reduced dosage to patient receiving promethazine).
No products indexed under this heading.

Chlordiazepoxide Hydrochloride (Promethazine may increase, prolong, or intensify the sedative action of other CNS depressants; concurrent use should be avoided with other CNS depressants or administered in reduced dosage to patient receiving promethazine). Products include:
Librium Capsules 3347

Chlorpromazine (Promethazine may increase, prolong, or intensify the sedative action of other CNS depressants; concurrent use should be avoided with other CNS depressants or administered in reduced dosage to patient receiving promethazine).
No products indexed under this heading.

Chlorpromazine Hydrochloride (Promethazine may increase, prolong, or intensify the sedative action of other CNS depressants; concurrent use should be avoided with other CNS depressants or administered in reduced dosage to patient receiving promethazine).
No products indexed under this heading.

Chlorprothixene (Promethazine may increase, prolong, or intensify the sedative action of other CNS depressants; concurrent use should be avoided with other CNS depressants or administered in reduced dosage to patient receiving promethazine).

No products indexed under this heading.

Chlorprothixene Hydrochloride (Promethazine may increase, prolong, or intensify the sedative action of other CNS depressants; concurrent use should be avoided with other CNS depressants or administered in reduced dosage to patient receiving promethazine).

No products indexed under this heading.

Chlorprothixene Lactate (Promethazine may increase, prolong, or intensify the sedative action of other CNS depressants; concurrent use should be avoided with other CNS depressants or administered in reduced dosage to patient receiving promethazine).

No products indexed under this heading.

Clidinium Bromide (Co-administration with agents with anticholinergic properties should be undertaken with caution).

No products indexed under this heading.

Clomipramine Hydrochloride (Promethazine may increase, prolong, or intensify the sedative action of other CNS depressants; concurrent use should be avoided with tricyclic antidepressants or administered in reduced dosage to patient receiving promethazine).

No products indexed under this heading.

Clorazepate Dipotassium (Promethazine may increase, prolong, or intensify the sedative action of other CNS depressants; concurrent use should be avoided with other CNS depressants or administered in reduced dosage to patient receiving promethazine). Products include:

Clozapine (Promethazine may increase, prolong, or intensify the sedative action of other CNS depressants; concurrent use should be avoided with other CNS depressants or administered in reduced dosage to patient receiving promethazine). Products include:

Codeine Phosphate (Promethazine may increase, prolong, or intensify the sedative action of other CNS depressants; when co-administered with narcotics, the dose of narcotics should be reduced by at least one-quarter to one-half; excessive amount of promethazine relative to narcotic may lead to restlessness and motor hyperactivity in the patient with pain). Products include:

Desflurane (Promethazine may increase, prolong, or intensify the sedative action of other CNS depressants; concurrent use should be avoided with other CNS depressants or administered in reduced dosage to patient receiving promethazine).

No products indexed under this heading.

Desipramine Hydrochloride (Promethazine may increase, prolong, or intensify the sedative action of other CNS depressants; concurrent use should be avoided with tricyclic antidepressants or administered in reduced dosage to patient receiving promethazine).

No products indexed under this heading.

Dezocine (Promethazine may increase, prolong, or intensify the sedative action of other CNS depressants; when co-administered with narcotics, the dose of narcotics should be reduced by at least one-quarter to one-half; excessive amount of promethazine relative to narcotic may lead to restlessness and motor hyperactivity in the patient with pain).

No products indexed under this heading.

Diazepam (Promethazine may increase, prolong, or intensify the sedative action of other CNS depressants; concurrent use should be avoided with other CNS depressants or administered in reduced dosage to patient receiving promethazine). Products include:

Dicyclomine Hydrochloride (Co-administration with agents with anticholinergic properties should be undertaken with caution). Products include:

Doxepin Hydrochloride (Promethazine may increase, prolong, or intensify the sedative action of other CNS depressants; concurrent use should be avoided with tricyclic antidepressants or administered in reduced dosage to patient receiving promethazine).

No products indexed under this heading.

Droperidol (Promethazine may increase, prolong, or intensify the sedative action of other CNS depressants; concurrent use should be avoided with other CNS depressants or administered in reduced dosage to patient receiving promethazine).

No products indexed under this heading.

Enflurane (Promethazine may increase, prolong, or intensify the sedative action of other CNS depressants; concurrent use should be avoided with other CNS depressants or administered in reduced dosage to patient receiving promethazine).

No products indexed under this heading.

Estazolam (Promethazine may increase, prolong, or intensify the sedative action of other CNS depressants; concurrent use should be avoided with other CNS depressants or administered in reduced dosage to patient receiving promethazine). Products include:

Ethanol (Promethazine may increase, prolong, or intensify the sedative action of other CNS depressants; concurrent use should be avoided with other CNS depressants or administered in reduced dosage to patient receiving promethazine).

No products indexed under this heading.

Ethchlorvynol (Promethazine may increase, prolong, or intensify the sedative action of other CNS depressants; concurrent use should be avoided with other CNS depressants or administered in reduced dosage to patient receiving promethazine).

No products indexed under this heading.

Ethinamate (Promethazine may increase, prolong, or intensify the sedative action of other CNS depressants; concurrent use should be avoided with other CNS depressants or administered in reduced dosage to patient receiving promethazine).

No products indexed under this heading.

Ethyl Alcohol (Promethazine may increase, prolong, or intensify the sedative action of other CNS depressants; concurrent use should be avoided with other CNS depressants or administered in reduced dosage to patient receiving promethazine).

No products indexed under this heading.

Fentanyl (Promethazine may increase, prolong, or intensify the sedative action of other CNS depressants; when co-administered with narcotics, the dose of narcotics should be reduced by at least one-quarter to one-half; excessive amount of promethazine relative to narcotic may lead to restlessness and motor hyperactivity in the patient with pain). Products include:

Fentanyl Citrate (Promethazine may increase, prolong, or intensify the sedative action of other CNS depressants; when co-administered with narcotics, the dose of narcotics should be reduced by at least one-quarter to one-half; excessive amount of promethazine relative to narcotic may lead to restlessness and motor hyperactivity in the patient with pain). Products include:

Fluphenazine Decanoate (Promethazine may increase, prolong, or intensify the sedative action of other CNS depressants; concurrent use should be avoided with other CNS depressants or administered in reduced dosage to patient receiving promethazine).

No products indexed under this heading.

Fluphenazine Enanthate (Promethazine may increase, prolong, or intensify the sedative action of other CNS depressants; concurrent use should be avoided with other CNS depressants or administered in reduced dosage to patient receiving promethazine).

No products indexed under this heading.

Fluphenazine Hydrochloride (Promethazine may increase, prolong, or intensify the sedative action of other CNS depressants; concurrent use should be avoided with other CNS depressants or administered in reduced dosage to patient receiving promethazine).

No products indexed under this heading.

Flurazepam Hydrochloride (Promethazine may increase, prolong, or intensify the sedative action of other CNS depressants; concurrent use should be avoided with other CNS

depressants or administered in reduced dosage to patient receiving promethazine). Products include:

Glutethimide (Promethazine may increase, prolong, or intensify the sedative action of other CNS depressants; concurrent use should be avoided with other CNS depressants or administered in reduced dosage to patient receiving promethazine).

No products indexed under this heading.

Glycopyrrolate (Co-administration with agents with anticholinergic properties should be undertaken with caution).

No products indexed under this heading.

Haloperidol (Promethazine may increase, prolong, or intensify the sedative action of other CNS depressants; concurrent use should be avoided with other CNS depressants or administered in reduced dosage to patient receiving promethazine).

No products indexed under this heading.

Haloperidol Decanoate (Promethazine may increase, prolong, or intensify the sedative action of other CNS depressants; concurrent use should be avoided with other CNS depressants or administered in reduced dosage to patient receiving promethazine).

No products indexed under this heading.

Hydrocodone Bitartrate (Promethazine may increase, prolong, or intensify the sedative action of other CNS depressants; when co-administered with narcotics, the dose of narcotics should be reduced by at least one-quarter to one-half; excessive amount of promethazine relative to narcotic may lead to restlessness and motor hyperactivity in the patient with pain). Products include:

Hydrocodone Polistirex (Promethazine may increase, prolong, or intensify the sedative action of other CNS depressants; when co-administered with narcotics, the dose of narcotics should be reduced by at least one-quarter to one-half; excessive amount of promethazine relative to narcotic may lead to restlessness and motor hyperactivity in the patient with pain). Products include:

Hydromorphone Hydrochloride (Promethazine may increase, prolong, or intensify the sedative action of other CNS depressants; when co-administered with narcotics, the dose of narcotics should be reduced by at least one-quarter to one-half; excessive amount of promethazine relative to narcotic may lead to restlessness and motor hyperactivity in the patient with pain). Products include:

IMPORTANT NOTE: Always consult each drug listing in the patient's regimen for possible interactions.

Hydroxyzine Hydrochloride (Promethazine may increase, prolong, or intensify the sedative action of other CNS depressants; concurrent use should be avoided with other CNS depressants or administered in reduced dosage to patient receiving promethazine).
No products indexed under this heading.

Hyoscyamine (Co-administration with agents with anticholinergic properties should be undertaken with caution).
No products indexed under this heading.

Hyoscyamine Sulfate (Co-administration with agents with anticholinergic properties should be undertaken with caution). Products include:

Imipramine Hydrochloride (Promethazine may increase, prolong, or intensify the sedative action of other CNS depressants; concurrent use should be avoided with tricyclic antidepressants or administered in reduced dosage to patient receiving promethazine).
No products indexed under this heading.

Imipramine Pamoate (Promethazine may increase, prolong, or intensify the sedative action of other CNS depressants; concurrent use should be avoided with tricyclic antidepressants or administered in reduced dosage to patient receiving promethazine).
No products indexed under this heading.

Ipratropium Bromide (Co-administration with agents with anticholinergic properties should be undertaken with caution). Products include:

Isocarboxazid (Co-administration of phenothiazines with MAO inhibitors may increase the incidence of extrapyramidal effects).
No products indexed under this heading.

Isoflurane (Promethazine may increase, prolong, or intensify the sedative action of other CNS depressants; concurrent use should be avoided with other CNS depressants or administered in reduced dosage to patient receiving promethazine).
No products indexed under this heading.

Ketamine Hydrochloride (Promethazine may increase, prolong, or intensify the sedative action of other CNS depressants; concurrent use should be avoided with other CNS depressants or administered in reduced dosage to patient receiving promethazine).
No products indexed under this heading.

Levomethadyl Acetate Hydrochloride (Promethazine may increase, prolong, or intensify the sedative action of other CNS depressants; concurrent use should be avoided with other CNS depressants or administered in reduced dosage to patient receiving promethazine).
No products indexed under this heading.

Levorphanol Tartrate (Promethazine may increase, prolong, or intensify the sedative action of other CNS depressants; when co-administered with narcotics, the dose of narcotics should be reduced by at least one-quarter to one-half; excessive amount of promethazine relative to narcotic may lead to restlessness and motor hyperactivity in the patient with pain).
No products indexed under this heading.

Lorazepam (Promethazine may increase, prolong, or intensify the sedative action of other CNS depressants; concurrent use should be avoided with other CNS depressants or administered in reduced dosage to patient receiving promethazine).
No products indexed under this heading.

Loxapine Hydrochloride (Promethazine may increase, prolong, or intensify the sedative action of other CNS depressants; concurrent use should be avoided with other CNS depressants or administered in reduced dosage to patient receiving promethazine).
No products indexed under this heading.

Loxapine Succinate (Promethazine may increase, prolong, or intensify the sedative action of other CNS depressants; concurrent use should be avoided with other CNS depressants or administered in reduced dosage to patient receiving promethazine).
No products indexed under this heading.

Maprotiline Hydrochloride (Promethazine may increase, prolong, or intensify the sedative action of other CNS depressants; concurrent use should be avoided with tricyclic antidepressants or administered in reduced dosage to patient receiving promethazine).
No products indexed under this heading.

Mepenzolate Bromide (Co-administration with agents with anticholinergic properties should be undertaken with caution).
No products indexed under this heading.

Meperidine Hydrochloride (Promethazine may increase, prolong, or intensify the sedative action of other CNS depressants; when co-administered with narcotics, the dose of narcotics should be reduced by at least one-quarter to one-half; excessive amount of promethazine relative to narcotic may lead to restlessness and motor hyperactivity in the patient with pain).
No products indexed under this heading.

Mephobarbital (Promethazine may increase, prolong, or intensify the sedative action of other CNS depressants; when co-administered with barbiturates, the dose of barbiturates should be reduced by one-quarter to one-half).
No products indexed under this heading.

Meprobamate (Promethazine may increase, prolong, or intensify the sedative action of other CNS depressants; concurrent use should be avoided with other CNS depressants or administered in reduced dosage to patient receiving promethazine).
No products indexed under this heading.

Mesoridazine Besylate (Promethazine may increase, prolong, or intensify the sedative action of other CNS depressants; concurrent use should be avoided with other CNS depressants or administered in reduced dosage to patient receiving promethazine).
No products indexed under this heading.

Methadone Hydrochloride (Promethazine may increase, prolong, or intensify the sedative action of other CNS depressants; when co-administered with narcotics, the dose of narcotics should be reduced by at least one-quarter to one-half; excessive amount of promethazine relative to narcotic may lead to restlessness and motor hyperactivity in the patient with pain).
No products indexed under this heading.

Methohexital Sodium (Promethazine may increase, prolong, or intensify the sedative action of other CNS depressants; concurrent use should be avoided with other CNS depressants or administered in reduced dosage to patient receiving promethazine).
No products indexed under this heading.

Methotrimeprazine (Promethazine may increase, prolong, or intensify the sedative action of other CNS depressants; concurrent use should be avoided with other CNS depressants or administered in reduced dosage to patient receiving promethazine).
No products indexed under this heading.

Methoxyflurane (Promethazine may increase, prolong, or intensify the sedative action of other CNS depressants; concurrent use should be avoided with other CNS depressants or administered in reduced dosage to patient receiving promethazine).
No products indexed under this heading.

Midazolam Hydrochloride (Promethazine may increase, prolong, or intensify the sedative action of other CNS depressants; concurrent use should be avoided with other CNS depressants or administered in reduced dosage to patient receiving promethazine).
No products indexed under this heading.

Moclobemide (Co-administration of phenothiazines with MAO inhibitors may increase the incidence of extrapyramidal effects).
No products indexed under this heading.

Molindone Hydrochloride (Promethazine may increase, prolong, or intensify the sedative action of other CNS depressants; concurrent use should be avoided with other CNS depressants or administered in reduced dosage to patient receiving promethazine). Products include:

Morphine Sulfate (Promethazine may increase, prolong, or intensify the sedative action of other CNS depressants; when co-administered with narcotics, the dose of narcotics should be reduced by at least one-quarter to one-half; excessive amount of promethazine relative to narcotic may lead to restlessness and motor hyperactivity in the patient with pain). Products include:

Nortriptyline Hydrochloride (Promethazine may increase, prolong, or intensify the sedative action of other CNS depressants; concurrent use should be avoided with tricyclic antidepressants or administered in reduced dosage to patient receiving promethazine).
No products indexed under this heading.

Olanzapine (Promethazine may increase, prolong, or intensify the sedative action of other CNS depressants; concurrent use should be avoided with other CNS depressants or administered in reduced dosage to patient receiving promethazine). Products include:

Oxazepam (Promethazine may increase, prolong, or intensify the sedative action of other CNS depressants; concurrent use should be avoided with other CNS depressants or administered in reduced dosage to patient receiving promethazine).
No products indexed under this heading.

Oxybutynin Chloride (Co-administration with agents with anticholinergic properties should be undertaken with caution). Products include:

Oxycodone Hydrochloride (Promethazine may increase, prolong, or intensify the sedative action of other CNS depressants; when co-administered with narcotics, the dose of narcotics should be reduced by at least one-quarter to one-half; excessive amount of promethazine relative to narcotic may lead to restlessness and motor hyperactivity in the patient with pain). Products include:

Pargyline Hydrochloride (Co-administration of phenothiazines with MAO inhibitors may increase the incidence of extrapyramidal effects).
No products indexed under this heading.

Pentobarbital Sodium (Promethazine may increase, prolong, or intensify the sedative action of other CNS depressants; when co-administered with barbiturates, the dose of barbiturates should be reduced by one-quarter to one-half). Products include:

Nembutal Sodium Solution, USP **2470**

Perphenazine (Promethazine may increase, prolong, or intensify the sedative action of other CNS depressants; concurrent use should be avoided with other CNS depressants or administered in reduced dosage to patient receiving promethazine).

No products indexed under this heading.

Phenelzine Sulfate (Co-administration of phenothiazines with MAO inhibitors may increase the incidence of extrapyramidal effects).

No products indexed under this heading.

Phenobarbital (Promethazine may increase, prolong, or intensify the sedative action of other CNS depressants; when co-administered with barbiturates, the dose of barbiturates should be reduced by one-quarter to one-half). Products include:

Donnatal Extentabs **2493**

Prazepam (Promethazine may increase, prolong, or intensify the sedative action of other CNS depressants; concurrent use should be avoided with other CNS depressants or administered in reduced dosage to patient receiving promethazine).

No products indexed under this heading.

Procarbazine Hydrochloride (Co-administration of phenothiazines with MAO inhibitors may increase the incidence of extrapyramidal effects). Products include:

Matulane Capsules **3191**

Prochlorperazine (Promethazine may increase, prolong, or intensify the sedative action of other CNS depressants; concurrent use should be avoided with other CNS depressants or administered in reduced dosage to patient receiving promethazine).

No products indexed under this heading.

Procyclidine Hydrochloride (Co-administration with agents with anticholinergic properties should be undertaken with caution).

No products indexed under this heading.

Propantheline Bromide (Co-administration with agents with anticholinergic properties should be undertaken with caution).

No products indexed under this heading.

Propofol (Promethazine may increase, prolong, or intensify the sedative action of other CNS depressants; concurrent use should be avoided with other CNS depressants or administered in reduced dosage to patient receiving promethazine).

No products indexed under this heading.

Propoxyphene Hydrochloride (Promethazine may increase, prolong, or intensify the sedative action of other CNS depressants; when co-administered with narcotics, the dose of narcotics should be reduced by at least one-quarter to one-half; excessive amount of promethazine relative to narcotic may lead to restlessness and motor hyperactivity in the patient with pain).

No products indexed under this heading.

Propoxyphene Napsylate (Promethazine may increase, prolong, or intensify the sedative action of other CNS depressants; when co-administered with narcotics, the dose of narcotics should be reduced by at least one-quarter to one-half; excessive amount of promethazine relative to narcotic may lead to restlessness and motor hyperactivity in the patient with pain).

No products indexed under this heading.

Protriptyline Hydrochloride (Promethazine may increase, prolong, or intensify the sedative action of other CNS depressants; concurrent use should be avoided with tricyclic antidepressants or administered in reduced dosage to patient receiving promethazine).

No products indexed under this heading.

Quazepam (Promethazine may increase, prolong, or intensify the sedative action of other CNS depressants; concurrent use should be avoided with other CNS depressants or administered in reduced dosage to patient receiving promethazine).

No products indexed under this heading.

Quetiapine Fumarate (Promethazine may increase, prolong, or intensify the sedative action of other CNS depressants; concurrent use should be avoided with other CNS depressants or administered in reduced dosage to patient receiving promethazine). Products include:

Seroquel Tablets **690**

Remifentanil Hydrochloride (Promethazine may increase, prolong, or intensify the sedative action of other CNS depressants; when co-administered with narcotics, the dose of narcotics should be reduced by at least one-quarter to one-half; excessive amount of promethazine relative to narcotic may lead to restlessness and motor hyperactivity in the patient with pain).

No products indexed under this heading.

Risperidone (Promethazine may increase, prolong, or intensify the sedative action of other CNS depressants; concurrent use should be avoided with other CNS depressants or administered in reduced dosage to patient receiving promethazine). Products include:

Risperdal **1676**
Risperdal Consta Long-Acting Injection **1682**
Risperdal M-Tab Orally Disintegrating Tablets.................. **1676**

Scopolamine (Co-administration with agents with anticholinergic properties should be undertaken with caution). Products include:

Transderm Scōp Transdermal Therapeutic System **2177**

Scopolamine Hydrobromide (Co-administration with agents with anticholinergic properties should be undertaken with caution). Products include:

Donnatal Extentabs **2493**

Secobarbital Sodium (Promethazine may increase, prolong, or intensify the sedative action of other CNS depressants; when co-administered with barbiturates, the dose of barbiturates should be reduced by one-quarter to one-half).

No products indexed under this heading.

Selegiline Hydrochloride (Co-administration of phenothiazines with MAO inhibitors may increase the incidence of extrapyramidal effects). Products include:

Eldepryl Capsules **3208**
Zelapar Tablets **3372**

Sevoflurane (Promethazine may increase, prolong, or intensify the sedative action of other CNS depressants; concurrent use should be avoided with other CNS depressants or administered in reduced dosage to patient receiving promethazine). Products include:

Ultane Liquid for Inhalation **531**

Sufentanil Citrate (Promethazine may increase, prolong, or intensify the sedative action of other CNS depressants; when co-administered with narcotics, the dose of narcotics should be reduced by at least one-quarter to one-half; excessive amount of promethazine relative to narcotic may lead to restlessness and motor hyperactivity in the patient with pain).

No products indexed under this heading.

Temazepam (Promethazine may increase, prolong, or intensify the sedative action of other CNS depressants; concurrent use should be avoided with other CNS depressants or administered in reduced dosage to patient receiving promethazine). Products include:

Restoril Capsules **1860**

Thiamylal Sodium (Promethazine may increase, prolong, or intensify the sedative action of other CNS depressants; when co-administered with barbiturates, the dose of barbiturates should be reduced by one-quarter to one-half).

No products indexed under this heading.

Thioridazine Hydrochloride (Promethazine may increase, prolong, or intensify the sedative action of other CNS depressants; concurrent use should be avoided with other CNS depressants or administered in reduced dosage to patient receiving promethazine). Products include:

Thioridazine Hydrochloride Tablets.. **2163**

Thiothixene (Promethazine may increase, prolong, or intensify the sedative action of other CNS depressants; concurrent use should be avoided with other CNS depressants or administered in reduced dosage to patient receiving promethazine). Products include:

Thiothixene Capsules **2165**

Tolterodine Tartrate (Co-administration with agents with anticholinergic properties should be undertaken with caution). Products include:

Detrol Tablets **2628**
Detrol LA Capsules **2631**

Tranylcypromine Sulfate (Co-administration of phenothiazines with MAO inhibitors may increase the incidence of extrapyramidal effects). Products include:

Parnate Tablets **1527**

Triazolam (Promethazine may increase, prolong, or intensify the sedative action of other CNS depressants; concurrent use should be avoided with other CNS depressants or administered in reduced dosage to patient receiving promethazine).

No products indexed under this heading.

Tridihexethyl Chloride (Co-administration with agents with anticholinergic properties should be undertaken with caution).

No products indexed under this heading.

Trifluoperazine Hydrochloride (Promethazine may increase, prolong, or intensify the sedative action of other CNS depressants; concurrent use should be avoided with other CNS depressants or administered in reduced dosage to patient receiving promethazine).

No products indexed under this heading.

Trihexyphenidyl Hydrochloride (Co-administration with agents with anticholinergic properties should be undertaken with caution).

No products indexed under this heading.

Trimipramine Maleate (Promethazine may increase, prolong, or intensify the sedative action of other CNS depressants; concurrent use should be avoided with tricyclic antidepressants or administered in reduced dosage to patient receiving promethazine).

No products indexed under this heading.

Zaleplon (Promethazine may increase, prolong, or intensify the sedative action of other CNS depressants; concurrent use should be avoided with other CNS depressants or administered in reduced dosage to patient receiving promethazine). Products include:

Sonata Capsules **1717**

Ziprasidone Hydrochloride (Promethazine may increase, prolong, or intensify the sedative action of other CNS depressants; concurrent use should be avoided with other CNS depressants or administered in reduced dosage to patient receiving promethazine). Products include:

Geodon Capsules **2529**

Zolpidem Tartrate (Promethazine may increase, prolong, or intensify the sedative action of other CNS depressants; concurrent use should be avoided with other CNS depressants or administered in reduced dosage to patient receiving promethazine). Products include:

Ambien Tablets **2851**
Ambien CR Tablets **2855**

Food Interactions

Alcohol (Promethazine may increase, prolong, or intensify the sedative action of other CNS depressants, such as alcohol).

PHENYTEK CAPSULES
(Phenytoin Sodium) **2160**
May interact with chloramphenicol, corticosteroids, oral anticoagulants, doxycycline, estrogens, histamine H2-receptor antagonists, oral contraceptives, phenothiazines, quinidine, salicylates, succinimides, tricyclic antidepressants, valproate, xanthines, and certain other agents. Compounds in these categories include:

Aminophylline (Phenytoin impairs efficacy of theophylline).
No products indexed under this heading.

Amiodarone Hydrochloride (May increase phenytoin serum levels).
No products indexed under this heading.

Amitriptyline Hydrochloride (Tricyclic antidepressants may precipitate seizures in susceptible patients and phenytoin dosage may need to be adjusted).
No products indexed under this heading.

Amoxapine (Tricyclic antidepressants may precipitate seizures in susceptible patients and phenytoin dosage may need to be adjusted).
No products indexed under this heading.

Anisindione (Phenytoin impairs efficacy of oral anticoagulants). Products include:
Miradon Tablets **3042**

Aspirin (May increase phenytoin serum levels). Products include:
Aggrenox Capsules **822**
Bayer Aspirin **744**
BC Allergy Sinus Cold Powder .... ▣**677**
BC Headache Powder .... ▣**677**
Arthritis Strength BC Powder .... ▣**677**
BC Sinus Cold Powder .... ▣**677**
Excedrin Extra Strength Caplets/Tablets/Geltabs .... ▣**684**
Excedrin Migraine Caplets/Tablets/Geltabs .... ▣**609**
Goody's Body Pain Formula Powder .... ▣**684**
Goody's Extra Strength Headache Powders .... ▣**611**
Goody's Extra Strength Pain Relief Tablets .... ▣**685**
Percodan Tablets **1132**
St. Joseph 81 mg Aspirin Chewable and Enteric Coated Tablets **1869**

Aspirin, Enteric Coated (May increase phenytoin serum levels).
No products indexed under this heading.

Aspirin Buffered (May increase phenytoin serum levels). Products include:
Bufferin Extra Strength Tablets .... ▣**678**
Bufferin Regular Strength Tablets .... ▣**678**

Betamethasone Acetate (Phenytoin impairs efficacy of corticosteroids).
No products indexed under this heading.

Betamethasone Sodium Phosphate (Phenytoin impairs efficacy of corticosteroids).
No products indexed under this heading.

Calcium Carbonate (Ingestion times of phenytoin and antacid preparations containing calcium should be staggered in patients with low phenytoin levels to prevent absorption problems). Products include:
Actonel with Calcium Tablets **2688**
Calcet Tablets **2138**
Caltrate 600 PLUS .... ▣**809**
Caltrate 600 + D Tablets .... ▣**809**
D-Cal Chewable Caplets .... ▣**812**
Gas-X with Maalox .... ▣**656**
Maalox Regular Strength Antacid Chewable Tablets **2177**
Maalox Max Maximum Strength Antacid/Antigas Chewable Tablets **2176**
Maalox Max Maximum Strength Chewable Tablets .... ▣**660**
Os-Cal Chewable Tablets .... ▣**818**
Pepcid Complete Chewable Tablets **1701**
Children's Pepto **2674**
PremCal Light, Regular, and Extra Strength Tablets .... ▣**818**
Tums .... ▣**664**

Carbamazepine (May increase phenytoin serum levels). Products include:
Carbatrol Capsules **3171**
Equetro Extended-Release Capsules **3180**
Tegretol/Tegretol-XR **2295**

Chloramphenicol (May increase phenytoin serum levels).
No products indexed under this heading.

Chloramphenicol Palmitate (May increase phenytoin serum levels).
No products indexed under this heading.

Chloramphenicol Sodium Succinate (May increase phenytoin serum levels).
No products indexed under this heading.

Chlordiazepoxide (May increase phenytoin serum levels).
No products indexed under this heading.

Chlordiazepoxide Hydrochloride (May increase phenytoin serum levels). Products include:
Librium Capsules **3347**

Chlorotrianisene (May increase phenytoin serum levels; phenytoin impairs efficacy of estrogens).
No products indexed under this heading.

Chlorpromazine (Phenothiazines may increase phenytoin serum levels).
No products indexed under this heading.

Chlorpromazine Hydrochloride (Phenothiazines may increase phenytoin serum levels).
No products indexed under this heading.

Choline Magnesium Trisalicylate (May increase phenytoin serum levels).
No products indexed under this heading.

Cimetidine (May increase phenytoin serum levels). Products include:
Tagamet HB 200 Tablets .... ▣**664**

Cimetidine Hydrochloride (May increase phenytoin serum levels).
No products indexed under this heading.

Clomipramine Hydrochloride (Tricyclic antidepressants may precipitate seizures in susceptible patients and phenytoin dosage may need to be adjusted).
No products indexed under this heading.

Cortisone Acetate (Phenytoin impairs efficacy of corticosteroids).
No products indexed under this heading.

Desipramine Hydrochloride (Tricyclic antidepressants may precipitate seizures in susceptible patients and phenytoin dosage may need to be adjusted).
No products indexed under this heading.

Desogestrel (Phenytoin impairs efficacy of oral contraceptives). Products include:
Mircette Tablets **1066**

Dexamethasone (Phenytoin impairs efficacy of corticosteroids). Products include:
Ciprodex Otic Suspension **559**
Decadron Tablets **1951**
TobraDex Ophthalmic Ointment **562**
TobraDex Ophthalmic Suspension **563**

Dexamethasone Acetate (Phenytoin impairs efficacy of corticosteroids).
No products indexed under this heading.

Dexamethasone Sodium Phosphate (Phenytoin impairs efficacy of corticosteroids).
No products indexed under this heading.

Diazepam (May increase phenytoin serum levels). Products include:
Diastat Rectal Delivery System **3343**
Valium Tablets **2819**

Dicumarol (May increase phenytoin serum levels; phenytoin impairs efficacy of oral anticoagulants).
No products indexed under this heading.

Dienestrol (May increase phenytoin serum levels; phenytoin impairs efficacy of estrogens).
No products indexed under this heading.

Diethylstilbestrol (May increase phenytoin serum levels; phenytoin impairs efficacy of estrogens).
No products indexed under this heading.

Diflunisal (May increase phenytoin serum levels). Products include:
Dolobid Tablets **1955**

Digitoxin (Phenytoin impairs efficacy of digitoxin).
No products indexed under this heading.

Disulfiram (May increase phenytoin serum levels).
No products indexed under this heading.

Divalproex Sodium (May decrease or increase phenytoin serum levels; the effect of phenytoin on valproate serum levels is unpredictable). Products include:
Depakote Sprinkle Capsules **422**
Depakote Tablets **427**
Depakote ER Tablets **434**

Doxepin Hydrochloride (Tricyclic antidepressants may precipitate seizures in susceptible patients and phenytoin dosage may need to be adjusted).
No products indexed under this heading.

Doxycycline Calcium (Phenytoin impairs efficacy of doxycycline).
No products indexed under this heading.

Doxycycline Hyclate (Phenytoin impairs efficacy of doxycycline).
No products indexed under this heading.

Doxycycline Monohydrate (Phenytoin impairs efficacy of doxycycline). Products include:
Oracea Capsules **1000**

Dyphylline (Phenytoin impairs efficacy of theophylline).
No products indexed under this heading.

Estradiol (May increase phenytoin serum levels; phenytoin impairs efficacy of estrogens). Products include:
Angeliq Tablets **762**
Climara Transdermal System **771**
Climara Pro Transdermal System **776**
Estrasorb Topical Emulsion **1147**
Estring Vaginal Ring **2635**
Menostar Transdermal System **782**
Vagifem Tablets **2334**

Estrogens, Conjugated (May increase phenytoin serum levels; phenytoin impairs efficacy of estrogens). Products include:
Premarin Intravenous **3442**
Premarin Tablets **3446**
Premarin Vaginal Cream **3452**
Premphase Tablets **3456**
Prempro Tablets **3456**

Estrogens, Esterified (May increase phenytoin serum levels; phenytoin impairs efficacy of estrogens). Products include:
Estratest Tablets **3199**
Estratest H.S. Tablets **3199**

Estropipate (May increase phenytoin serum levels; phenytoin impairs efficacy of estrogens).
No products indexed under this heading.

Ethinyl Estradiol (May increase phenytoin serum levels; phenytoin impairs efficacy of estrogens). Products include:
Mircette Tablets **1066**
NuvaRing **2340**
Ortho-Cyclen/Ortho Tri-Cyclen **2429**
Ortho Evra Transdermal System **2417**
Ortho Tri-Cyclen Lo Tablets **2436**
Seasonique Tablets **1077**
Yasmin 28 Tablets **796**
Yaz Tablets **803**

Ethosuximide (May increase phenytoin serum levels).
No products indexed under this heading.

Ethynodiol Diacetate (Phenytoin impairs efficacy of oral contraceptives).
No products indexed under this heading.

Famotidine (May increase phenytoin serum levels). Products include:
Pepcid Injection **2040**
Pepcid **2038**
Pepcid AC Gelcaps **1701**
Pepcid AC Tablets **1701**
Maximum Strength Pepcid AC Tablets **1701**
Pepcid Complete Chewable Tablets **1701**

Fludrocortisone Acetate (Phenytoin impairs efficacy of corticosteroids).
No products indexed under this heading.

Fluphenazine Decanoate (Phenothiazines may increase phenytoin serum levels).
No products indexed under this heading.

Fluphenazine Enanthate (Phenothiazines may increase phenytoin serum levels).
No products indexed under this heading.

Fluphenazine Hydrochloride (Phenothiazines may increase phenytoin serum levels).
No products indexed under this heading.

Furosemide (Phenytoin impairs efficacy of furosemide). Products include:
Furosemide Tablets 2154

Halothane (May increase phenytoin serum levels).
No products indexed under this heading.

Hydrocortisone (Phenytoin impairs efficacy of corticosteroids). Products include:
Colocort Rectal Suspension, USP (Retention) 100 mg/60 mL.......... 2476
Hydrocortone Tablets 1989
Preparation H Hydrocortisone Cream .... ■ 646

Hydrocortisone Acetate (Phenytoin impairs efficacy of corticosteroids). Products include:
Analpram-HC 1159
Pramosone 1161
ProctoFoam-HC 3099

Hydrocortisone Sodium Phosphate (Phenytoin impairs efficacy of corticosteroids).
No products indexed under this heading.

Hydrocortisone Sodium Succinate (Phenytoin impairs efficacy of corticosteroids).
No products indexed under this heading.

Imipramine Hydrochloride (Tricyclic antidepressants may precipitate seizures in susceptible patients and phenytoin dosage may need to be adjusted).
No products indexed under this heading.

Imipramine Pamoate (Tricyclic antidepressants may precipitate seizures in susceptible patients and phenytoin dosage may need to be adjusted).
No products indexed under this heading.

Isoniazid (May increase phenytoin serum levels).
No products indexed under this heading.

Levonorgestrel (Phenytoin impairs efficacy of oral contraceptives). Products include:
Climara Pro Transdermal System 776
Mirena Intrauterine System 787
Plan B Tablets 1076
Seasonique Tablets 1077

Magnesium Salicylate (May increase phenytoin serum levels).
No products indexed under this heading.

Maprotiline Hydrochloride (Tricyclic antidepressants may precipitate seizures in susceptible patients and phenytoin dosage may need to be adjusted).
No products indexed under this heading.

Mesoridazine Besylate (Phenothiazines may increase phenytoin serum levels).
No products indexed under this heading.

Mestranol (Phenytoin impairs efficacy of oral contraceptives).
No products indexed under this heading.

Methotrimeprazine (Phenothiazines may increase phenytoin serum levels).
No products indexed under this heading.

Methsuximide (May increase phenytoin serum levels).
No products indexed under this heading.

Methylphenidate Hydrochloride (May increase phenytoin serum levels). Products include:
Concerta Extended-Release Tablets 1881
Metadate CD Capsules 3323
Ritalin Hydrochloride Tablets 2269
Ritalin LA Capsules 2271
Ritalin-SR Tablets 2269

Methylprednisolone Acetate (Phenytoin impairs efficacy of corticosteroids). Products include:
Depo-Medrol Injectable Suspension 2617
Depo-Medrol Single-Dose Vial 2619

Methylprednisolone Sodium Succinate (Phenytoin impairs efficacy of corticosteroids).
No products indexed under this heading.

Molindone Hydrochloride (Contains calcium ions which may decrease phenytoin serum levels). Products include:
Moban Tablets 1119

Nizatidine (May increase phenytoin serum levels). Products include:
Axid Oral Solution 879

Norethindrone (Phenytoin impairs efficacy of oral contraceptives). Products include:
Ortho Micronor Tablets 2426

Norethynodrel (Phenytoin impairs efficacy of oral contraceptives).
No products indexed under this heading.

Norgestimate (Phenytoin impairs efficacy of oral contraceptives). Products include:
Ortho-Cyclen/Ortho Tri-Cyclen 2429
Ortho Tri-Cyclen Lo Tablets 2436

Norgestrel (Phenytoin impairs efficacy of oral contraceptives).
No products indexed under this heading.

Nortriptyline Hydrochloride (Tricyclic antidepressants may precipitate seizures in susceptible patients and phenytoin dosage may need to be adjusted).
No products indexed under this heading.

Perphenazine (Phenothiazines may increase phenytoin serum levels).
No products indexed under this heading.

Phenobarbital (May decrease or increase phenytoin serum levels; the effect of phenytoin on phenobarbital serum levels is unpredictable). Products include:
Donnatal Extentabs 2493

Phensuximide (May increase phenytoin serum levels).
No products indexed under this heading.

Phenylbutazone (May increase phenytoin serum levels).
No products indexed under this heading.

Polyestradiol Phosphate (May increase phenytoin serum levels; phenytoin impairs efficacy of estrogens).
No products indexed under this heading.

Prednisolone Acetate (Phenytoin impairs efficacy of corticosteroids). Products include:
Blephamide Ophthalmic Ointment 568
Blephamide Ophthalmic Suspension.................................. 569
Poly-Pred Ophthalmic Suspension .... ⊙ 233
Pred Forte Ophthalmic Suspension .... ⊙ 235
Pred Mild Ophthalmic Suspension .... ⊙ 238
Pred-G Ophthalmic Ointment .... ⊙ 237
Pred-G Ophthalmic Suspension ...... ⊙ 236

Prednisolone Sodium Phosphate (Phenytoin impairs efficacy of corticosteroids).
No products indexed under this heading.

Prednisolone Tebutate (Phenytoin impairs efficacy of corticosteroids).
No products indexed under this heading.

Prednisone (Phenytoin impairs efficacy of corticosteroids).
No products indexed under this heading.

Prochlorperazine (Phenothiazines may increase phenytoin serum levels).
No products indexed under this heading.

Promethazine Hydrochloride (Phenothiazines may increase phenytoin serum levels). Products include:
Phenergan Tablets and Suppositories............................. 3440

Protriptyline Hydrochloride (Tricyclic antidepressants may precipitate seizures in susceptible patients and phenytoin dosage may need to be adjusted).
No products indexed under this heading.

Quinestrol (May increase phenytoin serum levels; phenytoin impairs efficacy of estrogens).
No products indexed under this heading.

Quinidine (Phenytoin impairs efficacy of quinidine).
No products indexed under this heading.

Quinidine Gluconate (Phenytoin impairs efficacy of quinidine).
No products indexed under this heading.

Quinidine Hydrochloride (Phenytoin impairs efficacy of quinidine).
No products indexed under this heading.

Quinidine Polygalacturonate (Phenytoin impairs efficacy of quinidine).
No products indexed under this heading.

Quinidine Sulfate (Phenytoin impairs efficacy of quinidine).
No products indexed under this heading.

Ranitidine Bismuth Citrate (May increase phenytoin serum levels).
No products indexed under this heading.

Ranitidine Hydrochloride (May increase phenytoin serum levels). Products include:
Zantac 1624
Zantac Injection 1619
Zantac Injection Pharmacy Bulk Package.................................... 1622

Reserpine (May increase phenytoin serum levels).
No products indexed under this heading.

Rifampin (Phenytoin impairs efficacy of rifampin).
No products indexed under this heading.

Salsalate (May increase phenytoin serum levels).
No products indexed under this heading.

Sucralfate (May increase phenytoin serum levels). Products include:
Carafate Suspension 701
Carafate Tablets 701

Sulfamethizole (May increase phenytoin serum levels).
No products indexed under this heading.

Sulfamethoxazole (May increase phenytoin serum levels).
No products indexed under this heading.

Sulfisoxazole Acetyl (May increase phenytoin serum levels).
No products indexed under this heading.

Theophylline (Phenytoin impairs efficacy of theophylline).
No products indexed under this heading.

Theophylline Anhydrous (Phenytoin impairs efficacy of theophylline). Products include:
Uniphyl Tablets 2710

Theophylline Calcium Salicylate (Phenytoin impairs efficacy of theophylline).
No products indexed under this heading.

Theophylline Dihydroxypropyl (Glyceryl) (Phenytoin impairs efficacy of theophylline).
No products indexed under this heading.

Theophylline Ethylenediamine (Phenytoin impairs efficacy of theophylline).
No products indexed under this heading.

Theophylline Sodium Glycinate (Phenytoin impairs efficacy of theophylline).
No products indexed under this heading.

Thioridazine Hydrochloride (Phenothiazines may increase phenytoin serum levels). Products include:
Thioridazine Hydrochloride Tablets 2163

Tolbutamide (May increase phenytoin serum levels).
No products indexed under this heading.

Trazodone Hydrochloride (May increase phenytoin serum levels).
No products indexed under this heading.

Triamcinolone (Phenytoin impairs efficacy of corticosteroids).
No products indexed under this heading.

Triamcinolone Acetonide (Phenytoin impairs efficacy of corticosteroids). Products include:
Azmacort Inhalation Aerosol 1726
Nasacort AQ Nasal Spray 2922

Triamcinolone Diacetate (Phenytoin impairs efficacy of corticosteroids).
No products indexed under this heading.

Triamcinolone Hexacetonide (Phenytoin impairs efficacy of corticosteroids).
No products indexed under this heading.

Trifluoperazine Hydrochloride (Phenothiazines may increase phenytoin serum levels).
No products indexed under this heading.

Trimipramine Maleate (Tricyclic antidepressants may precipitate seizures in susceptible patients and phenytoin dosage may need to be adjusted).
No products indexed under this heading.

Valproate Sodium (May decrease or increase phenytoin serum levels; the effect of phenytoin on valproate serum levels is unpredictable). Products include:
Depacon Injection 412

Valproic Acid (May decrease or increase phenytoin serum levels; the effect of phenytoin on valproate serum levels is unpredictable). Products include:
Depakene 417

Vitamin D (Phenytoin impairs efficacy of vitamin D). Products include:
Active Calcium Tablets 3339
Caltrate 600 PLUS .... ■809
Caltrate 600 + D Tablets .... ■809
D-Cal Chewable Caplets .... ■812
Os-Cal 250 + D Tablets .... ■817
Os-Cal 500 + D Tablets .... ■817

Warfarin Sodium (Phenytoin impairs efficacy of oral anticoagulants). Products include:
Coumadin for Injection 898
Coumadin Tablets 898

Food Interactions

Alcohol (Acute alcohol intake may increase phenytoin serum levels; chronic alcohol abuse may decrease phenytoin serum levels).

PHOSLO GELCAPS

(Calcium Acetate) 2169

May interact with calcium preparations, cardiac glycosides, tetracyclines, and certain other agents. Compounds in these categories include:

Antacids, unspecified (Concurrent use should be avoided).
No products indexed under this heading.

Calcium Carbonate (Potential for increased risk of hypercalcemia; concurrent use with other calcium supplements is not recommended). Products include:
Actonel with Calcium Tablets 2688
Calcet Tablets 2138
Caltrate 600 PLUS .... ■809
Caltrate 600 + D Tablets .... ■809
D-Cal Chewable Caplets .... ■812
Gas-X with Maalox .... ■656
Maalox Regular Strength Antacid Chewable Tablets 2177
Maalox Max Maximum Strength Antacid/Antigas Chewable Tablets 2176
Maalox Max Maximum Strength Chewable Tablets .... ■660
Os-Cal Chewable Tablets .... ■818
Pepcid Complete Chewable Tablets 1701
Children's Pepto 2674
PremCal Light, Regular, and Extra Strength Tablets .... ■818
Tums .... ■664

Calcium Chloride (Potential for increased risk of hypercalcemia; concurrent use with other calcium supplements is not recommended).
No products indexed under this heading.

Calcium Citrate (Potential for increased risk of hypercalcemia; concurrent use with other calcium supplements is not recommended). Products include:
Active Calcium Tablets 3339
Citracal Caplets .... ■703
Citracal Lemon Cream Creamy Bites 2139
Citracal Prenatal + DHA Tablets and Capsules 2139

Calcium Glubionate (Potential for increased risk of hypercalcemia; concurrent use with other calcium supplements is not recommended).
No products indexed under this heading.

Demeclocycline Hydrochloride (Bioavailability of oral tetracyclines may be decreased).
No products indexed under this heading.

Deslanoside (Hypercalcemia may precipitate cardiac arrhythmia).
No products indexed under this heading.

Digitalis Glycoside Preparations (Hypercalcemia may precipitate cardiac arrhythmia).
No products indexed under this heading.

Digitoxin (Hypercalcemia may precipitate cardiac arrhythmia).
No products indexed under this heading.

Digoxin (Hypercalcemia may precipitate cardiac arrhythmia). Products include:
Lanoxicaps Capsules 1490
Lanoxin Injection 1494
Lanoxin Injection Pediatric 1497
Lanoxin Tablets 1500

Doxycycline Calcium (Bioavailability of oral tetracyclines may be decreased).
No products indexed under this heading.

Doxycycline Hyclate (Bioavailability of oral tetracyclines may be decreased).
No products indexed under this heading.

Doxycycline Monohydrate (Bioavailability of oral tetracyclines may be decreased). Products include:
Oracea Capsules 1000

Methacycline Hydrochloride (Bioavailability of oral tetracyclines may be decreased).
No products indexed under this heading.

Minocycline Hydrochloride (Bioavailability of oral tetracyclines may be decreased). Products include:
Solodyn Extended Release Tablets 1890

Oxytetracycline Hydrochloride (Bioavailability of oral tetracyclines may be decreased).
No products indexed under this heading.

Tetracycline Hydrochloride (Bioavailability of oral tetracyclines may be decreased).
No products indexed under this heading.

PHOTOFRIN FOR INJECTION

(Porfimer Sodium) 702

May interact with calcium channel blockers, glucocorticoids, drugs known to be photosensitizers, inhibitors of endogenous prostaglandin synthesis, and certain other agents. Compounds in these categories include:

Acetazolamide (Co-administration with other photosensitizing agents could increase the photosensitivity reactions).
No products indexed under this heading.

Acitretin (Co-administration with other photosensitizing agents could increase the photosensitivity reactions). Products include:
Soriatane Capsules 1013

Alatrofloxacin Mesylate (Co-administration with other photosensitizing agents could increase the photosensitivity reactions).
No products indexed under this heading.

Allopurinol (Could interfere with porfimer photodynamic therapy).
No products indexed under this heading.

Amlodipine Besylate (Could interfere with porfimer photodynamic therapy). Products include:
Caduet Tablets 2508
Lotrel Capsules 2249
Norvasc Tablets 2545

Anthralin (Co-administration with other photosensitizing agents could increase the photosensitivity reactions). Products include:
Psoriatec Cream 1089

Aspirin (Some prostaglandin synthesis inhibitors could interfere with porfimer photodynamic therapy). Products include:
Aggrenox Capsules 822
Bayer Aspirin 744
BC Allergy Sinus Cold Powder .... ■677
BC Headache Powder .... ■677
Arthritis Strength BC Powder .... ■677
BC Sinus Cold Powder .... ■677
Excedrin Extra Strength Caplets/Tablets/Geltabs .... ■684
Excedrin Migraine Caplets/Tablets/Geltabs .... ■609
Goody's Body Pain Formula Powder .... ■684
Goody's Extra Strength Headache Powders .... ■611
Goody's Extra Strength Pain Relief Tablets .... ■685
Percodan Tablets 1132
St. Joseph 81 mg Aspirin Chewable and Enteric Coated Tablets 1869

Bendroflumethiazide (Co-administration with other photosensitizing agents could increase the photosensitivity reactions).
No products indexed under this heading.

Bepridil Hydrochloride (Could interfere with porfimer photodynamic therapy).
No products indexed under this heading.

Beta-Carotene (Compounds that quench active oxygen species or scavenge radicals, such as b-carotene, would be expected to decrease photodynamic therapy; no human data available to support or rebut this possibility).
No products indexed under this heading.

Betamethasone Acetate (Glucocorticoid hormone given before or concomitantly with photodynamic therapy may decrease the efficacy of the treatment).
No products indexed under this heading.

Betamethasone Sodium Phosphate (Glucocorticoid hormone given before or concomitantly with photodynamic therapy may decrease the efficacy of the treatment).
No products indexed under this heading.

Celecoxib (Some prostaglandin synthesis inhibitors could interfere with porfimer photodynamic therapy). Products include:
Celebrex Capsules 3134

Chlorothiazide (Co-administration with other photosensitizing agents could increase the photosensitivity reactions). Products include:
Diuril Oral Suspension 1954

Chlorothiazide Sodium (Co-administration with other photosensitizing agents could increase the photosensitivity reactions). Products include:
Diuril Sodium Intravenous 2467

Chlorpromazine (Co-administration with other photosensitizing agents could increase the photosensitivity reactions).
No products indexed under this heading.

Chlorpromazine Hydrochloride (Co-administration with other photosensitizing agents could increase the photosensitivity reactions).
No products indexed under this heading.

Chlorpropamide (Co-administration with other photosensitizing agents could increase the photosensitivity reactions).
No products indexed under this heading.

Ciprofloxacin (Co-administration with other photosensitizing agents could increase the photosensitivity reactions). Products include:
Cipro Oral Suspension 2977
Cipro I.V. 2984
Cipro XR Tablets 2990
Ciprodex Otic Suspension 559

Ciprofloxacin Hydrochloride (Co-administration with other photosensitizing agents could increase the photosensitivity reactions). Products include:
Ciloxan Ophthalmic Ointment 559
Ciloxan Ophthalmic Solution .... ⊙206
Cipro Tablets 2977
Proquin XR Tablets 1153

Coal Tar (Co-administration with other photosensitizing agents could increase the photosensitivity reactions).
No products indexed under this heading.

Cortisone Acetate (Glucocorticoid hormone given before or concomitantly with photodynamic therapy may decrease the efficacy of the treatment).
No products indexed under this heading.

Demeclocycline Hydrochloride (Co-administration with other photosensitizing agents could increase the photosensitivity reactions).
No products indexed under this heading.

Dexamethasone (Glucocorticoid hormone given before or concomitantly with photodynamic therapy may decrease the efficacy of the treatment). Products include:
Ciprodex Otic Suspension 559
Decadron Tablets 1951
TobraDex Ophthalmic Ointment 562
TobraDex Ophthalmic Suspension 563

Dexamethasone Acetate (Glucocorticoid hormone given before or concomitantly with photodynamic therapy may decrease the efficacy of the treatment).
No products indexed under this heading.

Dexamethasone Sodium Phosphate (Glucocorticoid hormone given before or concomitantly with photodynamic therapy may decrease the efficacy of the treatment).
No products indexed under this heading.

Diclofenac Potassium (Some prostaglandin synthesis inhibitors could interfere with porfimer photodynamic therapy).
No products indexed under this heading.

Diclofenac Sodium (Some prostaglandin synthesis inhibitors could interfere with porfimer photodynamic therapy). Products include:
Arthrotec Tablets **3129**
Voltaren Ophthalmic Solution **2309**
Voltaren Tablets **2307**
Voltaren-XR Tablets **2310**

Diltiazem Hydrochloride (Could interfere with porfimer photodynamic therapy). Products include:
Cardizem LA Extended Release Tablets **1728**
Tiazac Capsules **1201**

Dimethyl Sulfoxide (Compounds that quench active oxygen species or scavenge radicals, such as DMSO, would be expected to decrease photodynamic therapy; no human data available to support or rebut this possibility).
No products indexed under this heading.

Doxycycline Calcium (Co-administration with other photosensitizing agents could increase the photosensitivity reactions).
No products indexed under this heading.

Doxycycline Hyclate (Co-administration with other photosensitizing agents could increase the photosensitivity reactions).
No products indexed under this heading.

Doxycycline Monohydrate (Co-administration with other photosensitizing agents could increase the photosensitivity reactions). Products include:
Oracea Capsules **1000**

Enoxacin (Co-administration with other photosensitizing agents could increase the photosensitivity reactions).
No products indexed under this heading.

Felodipine (Could interfere with porfimer photodynamic therapy).
No products indexed under this heading.

Fenoprofen Calcium (Some prostaglandin synthesis inhibitors could interfere with porfimer photodynamic therapy). Products include:
Nalfon Capsules **2502**

Fludrocortisone Acetate (Glucocorticoid hormone given before or concomitantly with photodynamic therapy may decrease the efficacy of the treatment).
No products indexed under this heading.

Fluphenazine Decanoate (Co-administration with other photosensitizing agents could increase the photosensitivity reactions).
No products indexed under this heading.

Fluphenazine Enanthate (Co-administration with other photosensitizing agents could increase the photosensitivity reactions).
No products indexed under this heading.

Fluphenazine Hydrochloride (Co-administration with other photosensitizing agents could increase the photosensitivity reactions).
No products indexed under this heading.

Flurbiprofen (Some prostaglandin synthesis inhibitors could interfere with porfimer photodynamic therapy).
No products indexed under this heading.

Furosemide (Co-administration with other photosensitizing agents could increase the photosensitivity reactions). Products include:
Furosemide Tablets **2154**

Glipizide (Co-administration with other photosensitizing agents could increase the photosensitivity reactions).
No products indexed under this heading.

Glyburide (Co-administration with other photosensitizing agents could increase the photosensitivity reactions).
No products indexed under this heading.

Grepafloxacin Hydrochloride (Co-administration with other photosensitizing agents could increase the photosensitivity reactions).
No products indexed under this heading.

Griseofulvin (Co-administration with other photosensitizing agents could increase the photosensitivity reactions). Products include:
Gris-PEG Tablets **2502**

Hydrochlorothiazide (Co-administration with other photosensitizing agents could increase the photosensitivity reactions). Products include:
Aldoril Tablets **1910**
Atacand HCT **651**
Avalide Tablets **888**
Avalide Tablets **2874**
Benicar HCT Tablets **1044**
Diovan HCT Tablets **2196**
Dyazide Capsules **1423**
Hyzaar 50-12.5 Tablets **1990**
Hyzaar 100-12.5 Tablets **1990**
Hyzaar 100-25 Tablets **1990**
Lopressor HCT 50/25 Tablets **2241**
Lopressor HCT 100/25 Tablets **2241**
Lopressor HCT 100/50 Tablets **2241**
Lotensin HCT Tablets **2246**
Micardis HCT Tablets **856**
Moduretic Tablets **2028**
Prinzide Tablets **2056**
Teveten HCT Tablets **1737**
Timolide Tablets **2086**
Uniretic Tablets **3100**

Hydrocortisone (Glucocorticoid hormone given before or concomitantly with photodynamic therapy may decrease the efficacy of the treatment). Products include:
Colocort Rectal Suspension, USP (Retention) 100 mg/60 mL **2476**
Hydrocortone Tablets **1989**
Preparation H Hydrocortisone Cream **646**

Hydrocortisone Acetate (Glucocorticoid hormone given before or concomitantly with photodynamic therapy may decrease the efficacy of the treatment). Products include:
Analpram-HC **1159**
Pramosone **1161**
ProctoFoam-HC **3099**

Hydrocortisone Sodium Phosphate (Glucocorticoid hormone given before or concomitantly with photodynamic therapy may decrease the efficacy of the treatment).
No products indexed under this heading.

Hydrocortisone Sodium Succinate (Glucocorticoid hormone given before or concomitantly with photodynamic therapy may decrease the efficacy of the treatment).
No products indexed under this heading.

Hydroflumethiazide (Co-administration with other photosensitizing agents could increase the photosensitivity reactions).
No products indexed under this heading.

Ibuprofen (Some prostaglandin synthesis inhibitors could interfere with porfimer photodynamic therapy). Products include:
Advil Allergy Sinus Caplets **770**
Advil **674**
Children's Advil Oral Suspension **603**
Children's Advil Chewable Tablets **603**
Advil Cold & Sinus **723**
Infants' Advil Concentrated Drops **604**
Infants' Advil Concentrated Drops - White Grape (Dye-Free) **604**
Junior Strength Advil Swallow Tablets **605**
Advil Migraine Liquigels **608**
Advil Multi-Symptom Cold Caplets **770**
Advil PM Caplets **615**
Motrin IB Tablets and Caplets **1866**
Children's Motrin Oral Suspension **1867**
Children's Motrin Non-Staining Dye-Free Oral Suspension **1867**
Children's Motrin Cold Oral Suspension **1867**
Infants' Motrin Concentrated Drops **1867**
Infants' Motrin Non-Staining Dye-Free Concentrated Drops **1867**
Junior Strength Motrin Caplets and Chewable Tablets **1867**
Vicoprofen Tablets **539**

Indomethacin (Some prostaglandin synthesis inhibitors could interfere with porfimer photodynamic therapy). Products include:
Indocin **1995**

Indomethacin Sodium Trihydrate (Some prostaglandin synthesis inhibitors could interfere with porfimer photodynamic therapy). Products include:
Indocin I.V. **2465**

Isradipine (Could interfere with porfimer photodynamic therapy). Products include:
DynaCirc CR Tablets **2721**

Ketoprofen (Some prostaglandin synthesis inhibitors could interfere with porfimer photodynamic therapy).
No products indexed under this heading.

Lomefloxacin Hydrochloride (Co-administration with other photosensitizing agents could increase the photosensitivity reactions).
No products indexed under this heading.

Mannitol (Compounds that quench active oxygen species or scavenge radicals, such as mannitol, would be expected to decrease photodynamic therapy; no human data available to support or rebut this possibility).
No products indexed under this heading.

Meclofenamate Sodium (Some prostaglandin synthesis inhibitors could interfere with porfimer photodynamic therapy).
No products indexed under this heading.

Mefenamic Acid (Some prostaglandin synthesis inhibitors could interfere with porfimer photodynamic therapy).
No products indexed under this heading.

Mesoridazine Besylate (Co-administration with other photosensitizing agents could increase the photosensitivity reactions).
No products indexed under this heading.

Metabromsalan (Co-administration with other photosensitizing agents could increase the photosensitivity reactions).
No products indexed under this heading.

Methacycline Hydrochloride (Co-administration with other photosensitizing agents could increase the photosensitivity reactions).
No products indexed under this heading.

Methotrimeprazine (Co-administration with other photosensitizing agents could increase the photosensitivity reactions).
No products indexed under this heading.

Methyclothiazide (Co-administration with other photosensitizing agents could increase the photosensitivity reactions).
No products indexed under this heading.

Methylprednisolone Acetate (Glucocorticoid hormone given before or concomitantly with photodynamic therapy may decrease the efficacy of the treatment). Products include:
Depo-Medrol Injectable Suspension **2617**
Depo-Medrol Single-Dose Vial **2619**

Methylprednisolone Sodium Succinate (Glucocorticoid hormone given before or concomitantly with photodynamic therapy may decrease the efficacy of the treatment).
No products indexed under this heading.

Mibefradil Dihydrochloride (Could interfere with porfimer photodynamic therapy).
No products indexed under this heading.

Minocycline Hydrochloride (Co-administration with other photosensitizing agents could increase the photosensitivity reactions). Products include:
Solodyn Extended Release Tablets **1890**

Nalidixic Acid (Co-administration with other photosensitizing agents could increase the photosensitivity reactions).
No products indexed under this heading.

Naproxen (Some prostaglandin synthesis inhibitors could interfere with porfimer photodynamic therapy). Products include:
EC-Naprosyn Delayed-Release Tablets **2761**
Naprosyn Suspension **2761**
Naprosyn Tablets **2761**
Prevacid NapraPAC **3280**

Naproxen Sodium (Some prostaglandin synthesis inhibitors could interfere with porfimer photodynamic therapy). Products include:
- Aleve Caplets 742
- Aleve Gelcaps 743
- Aleve Tablets 743
- Aleve Cold & Sinus Caplets 744
- Anaprox Tablets 2761
- Anaprox DS Tablets 2761

Nicardipine Hydrochloride (Could interfere with porfimer photodynamic therapy). Products include:
- Cardene I.V. 2497

Nifedipine (Could interfere with porfimer photodynamic therapy). Products include:
- Adalat CC Tablets 2964

Nimodipine (Could interfere with porfimer photodynamic therapy). Products include:
- Nimotop Capsules 749

Nisoldipine (Could interfere with porfimer photodynamic therapy). Products include:
- Sular Tablets 3122

Norfloxacin (Co-administration with other photosensitizing agents could increase the photosensitivity reactions). Products include:
- Noroxin Tablets 2032

Ofloxacin (Co-administration with other photosensitizing agents could increase the photosensitivity reactions). Products include:
- Floxin Otic Solution 1049

Oxytetracycline Hydrochloride (Co-administration with other photosensitizing agents could increase the photosensitivity reactions).
No products indexed under this heading.

Perphenazine (Co-administration with other photosensitizing agents could increase the photosensitivity reactions).
No products indexed under this heading.

Phenylbutazone (Some prostaglandin synthesis inhibitors could interfere with porfimer photodynamic therapy).
No products indexed under this heading.

Piroxicam (Some prostaglandin synthesis inhibitors could interfere with porfimer photodynamic therapy).
No products indexed under this heading.

Polythiazide (Co-administration with other photosensitizing agents could increase the photosensitivity reactions).
No products indexed under this heading.

Prednisolone Acetate (Glucocorticoid hormone given before or concomitantly with photodynamic therapy may decrease the efficacy of the treatment). Products include:
- Blephamide Ophthalmic Ointment 568
- Blephamide Ophthalmic Suspension 569
- Poly-Pred Ophthalmic Suspension ..... ⊙233
- Pred Forte Ophthalmic Suspension ..... ⊙235
- Pred Mild Ophthalmic Suspension ..... ⊙238
- Pred-G Ophthalmic Ointment ..... ⊙237
- Pred-G Ophthalmic Suspension ..... ⊙236

Prednisolone Sodium Phosphate (Glucocorticoid hormone given before or concomitantly with photodynamic therapy may decrease the efficacy of the treatment).
No products indexed under this heading.

Prednisolone Tebutate (Glucocorticoid hormone given before or concomitantly with photodynamic therapy may decrease the efficacy of the treatment).
No products indexed under this heading.

Prednisone (Glucocorticoid hormone given before or concomitantly with photodynamic therapy may decrease the efficacy of the treatment).
No products indexed under this heading.

Prochlorperazine (Co-administration with other photosensitizing agents could increase the photosensitivity reactions).
No products indexed under this heading.

Promethazine Hydrochloride (Co-administration with other photosensitizing agents could increase the photosensitivity reactions). Products include:
- Phenergan Tablets and Suppositories 3440

Sulfamethizole (Co-administration with other photosensitizing agents could increase the photosensitivity reactions).
No products indexed under this heading.

Sulfamethoxazole (Co-administration with other photosensitizing agents could increase the photosensitivity reactions).
No products indexed under this heading.

Sulfasalazine (Co-administration with other photosensitizing agents could increase the photosensitivity reactions).
No products indexed under this heading.

Sulfinpyrazone (Co-administration with other photosensitizing agents could increase the photosensitivity reactions).
No products indexed under this heading.

Sulfisoxazole Acetyl (Co-administration with other photosensitizing agents could increase the photosensitivity reactions).
No products indexed under this heading.

Sulfisoxazole Diolamine (Co-administration with other photosensitizing agents could increase the photosensitivity reactions).
No products indexed under this heading.

Sulindac (Some prostaglandin synthesis inhibitors could interfere with porfimer photodynamic therapy). Products include:
- Clinoril Tablets 1924

Tetrachlorosalicylanilide (Co-administration with other photosensitizing agents could increase the photosensitivity reactions).
No products indexed under this heading.

Tetracycline Hydrochloride (Co-administration with other photosensitizing agents could increase the photosensitivity reactions).
No products indexed under this heading.

Thioridazine Hydrochloride (Co-administration with other photosensitizing agents could increase the photosensitivity reactions). Products include:
- Thioridazine Hydrochloride Tablets 2163

Tolazamide (Co-administration with other photosensitizing agents could increase the photosensitivity reactions).
No products indexed under this heading.

Tolbutamide (Co-administration with other photosensitizing agents could increase the photosensitivity reactions).
No products indexed under this heading.

Tolmetin Sodium (Some prostaglandin synthesis inhibitors could interfere with porfimer photodynamic therapy).
No products indexed under this heading.

Triamcinolone (Glucocorticoid hormone given before or concomitantly with photodynamic therapy may decrease the efficacy of the treatment).
No products indexed under this heading.

Triamcinolone Acetonide (Glucocorticoid hormone given before or concomitantly with photodynamic therapy may decrease the efficacy of the treatment). Products include:
- Azmacort Inhalation Aerosol 1726
- Nasacort AQ Nasal Spray 2922

Triamcinolone Diacetate (Glucocorticoid hormone given before or concomitantly with photodynamic therapy may decrease the efficacy of the treatment).
No products indexed under this heading.

Triamcinolone Hexacetonide (Glucocorticoid hormone given before or concomitantly with photodynamic therapy may decrease the efficacy of the treatment).
No products indexed under this heading.

Trifluoperazine Hydrochloride (Co-administration with other photosensitizing agents could increase the photosensitivity reactions).
No products indexed under this heading.

Trovafloxacin Mesylate (Co-administration with other photosensitizing agents could increase the photosensitivity reactions).
No products indexed under this heading.

Verapamil Hydrochloride (Could interfere with porfimer photodynamic therapy). Products include:
- Covera-HS Tablets 3139
- Tarka Tablets 524
- Verelan PM Extended-Release Capsules, Controlled-Onset 3106

Food Interactions

Alcohol (Compounds that quench active oxygen species or scavenge radicals, such as ethanol, would be expected to decrease photodynamic therapy; no human data available to support or rebut this possibility).

PHYTO-VITE TABLETS

(Antioxidants, Bioflavonoids, Ginkgo biloba, Herbals with Vitamins & Minerals) ..... ⊡831
None cited in PDR database.

PLAN B TABLETS

(Levonorgestrel) 1076
May interact with barbiturates and hepatic microsomal enzyme inducers. Compounds in these categories include:

Aprobarbital (Hepatic enzyme-inducing drugs (e.g., barbiturates) may reduce the effectiveness of low-dose progestin-only pills).
No products indexed under this heading.

Butabarbital (Hepatic enzyme-inducing drugs (e.g., barbiturates) may reduce the effectiveness of low-dose progestin-only pills).
No products indexed under this heading.

Butalbital (Hepatic enzyme-inducing drugs (e.g., barbiturates) may reduce the effectiveness of low-dose progestin-only pills).
No products indexed under this heading.

Carbamazepine (Hepatic enzyme-inducing drugs may reduce the effectiveness of low-dose progestin-only pills). Products include:
- Carbatrol Capsules 3171
- Equetro Extended-Release Capsules 3180
- Tegretol/Tegretol-XR 2295

Chlorpropamide (Hepatic enzyme-inducing drugs may reduce the effectiveness of low-dose progestin-only pills).
No products indexed under this heading.

Ethanol (Hepatic enzyme-inducing drugs may reduce the effectiveness of low-dose progestin-only pills).
No products indexed under this heading.

Fosphenytoin Sodium (Hepatic enzyme-inducing drugs may reduce the effectiveness of low-dose progestin-only pills).
No products indexed under this heading.

Glipizide (Hepatic enzyme-inducing drugs may reduce the effectiveness of low-dose progestin-only pills).
No products indexed under this heading.

Glyburide (Hepatic enzyme-inducing drugs may reduce the effectiveness of low-dose progestin-only pills).
No products indexed under this heading.

Mephobarbital (Hepatic enzyme-inducing drugs (e.g., barbiturates) may reduce the effectiveness of low-dose progestin-only pills).
No products indexed under this heading.

Pentobarbital Sodium (Hepatic enzyme-inducing drugs (e.g., barbiturates) may reduce the effectiveness of low-dose progestin-only pills). Products include:
- Nembutal Sodium Solution, USP 2470

Phenobarbital (Hepatic enzyme-inducing drugs may reduce the effectiveness of low-dose progestin-only pills). Products include:
- Donnatal Extentabs 2493

Phenylbutazone (Hepatic enzyme-inducing drugs may reduce the effectiveness of low-dose progestin-only pills).
No products indexed under this heading.

Phenytoin (Hepatic enzyme-inducing drugs may reduce the effectiveness of low-dose progestin-only pills).
No products indexed under this heading.

Phenytoin Sodium (Hepatic enzyme-inducing drugs may reduce the effectiveness of low-dose progestin-only pills). Products include:
Phenytek Capsules 2160

Rifampin (Hepatic enzyme-inducing drugs may reduce the effectiveness of low-dose progestin-only pills).
No products indexed under this heading.

Rifapentine (Hepatic enzyme-inducing drugs may reduce the effectiveness of low-dose progestin-only pills).
No products indexed under this heading.

Secobarbital Sodium (Hepatic enzyme-inducing drugs (e.g., barbiturates) may reduce the effectiveness of low-dose progestin-only pills).
No products indexed under this heading.

Thiamylal Sodium (Hepatic enzyme-inducing drugs (e.g., barbiturates) may reduce the effectiveness of low-dose progestin-only pills).
No products indexed under this heading.

Tolazamide (Hepatic enzyme-inducing drugs may reduce the effectiveness of low-dose progestin-only pills).
No products indexed under this heading.

Tolbutamide (Hepatic enzyme-inducing drugs may reduce the effectiveness of low-dose progestin-only pills).
No products indexed under this heading.

PLASBUMIN-5

(Albumin (human)) 3251
None cited in PDR database.

PLASBUMIN-20

(Albumin (human)) 3252
None cited in PDR database.

PLASBUMIN-25

(Albumin (human)) 3253
None cited in PDR database.

PLASMANATE

(Plasma Protein Fraction (Human)) 3255
None cited in PDR database.

PLAVIX TABLETS

(Clopidogrel Bisulfate) 917
May interact with aspirin-acetylsalicylic acid, non-steroidal anti-inflammatory agents, phenytoin, and certain other agents. Compounds in these categories include:

Aspirin (Clopidogrel potentiates the effect of aspirin on collagen-induced platelet aggregation; co-administration did not significantly increase the prolongation of bleeding time induced by clopidogrel but has increased major bleeding). Products include:
Aggrenox Capsules 822
Bayer Aspirin 744
BC Allergy Sinus Cold Powder 677
BC Headache Powder 677
Arthritis Strength BC Powder 677
BC Sinus Cold Powder 677
Excedrin Extra Strength Caplets/Tablets/Geltabs 684
Excedrin Migraine Caplets/Tablets/Geltabs 609
Goody's Body Pain Formula Powder 684
Goody's Extra Strength Headache Powders.................... 611
Goody's Extra Strength Pain Relief Tablets 685
Percodan Tablets 1132
St. Joseph 81 mg Aspirin Chewable and Enteric Coated Tablets 1869

Aspirin, Enteric Coated (Clopidogrel potentiates the effect of aspirin on collagen-induced platelet aggregation; co-administration did not significantly increase the prolongation of bleeding time induced by clopidogrel but has increased major bleeding).
No products indexed under this heading.

Aspirin Buffered (Clopidogrel potentiates the effect of aspirin on collagen-induced platelet aggregation; co-administration did not significantly increase the prolongation of bleeding time induced by clopidogrel but has increased major bleeding). Products include:
Bufferin Extra Strength Tablets 678
Bufferin Regular Strength Tablets ... 678

Celecoxib (Co-administration can be associated with increased occult gastrointestinal blood loss; at high concentrations in vitro, clopidogrel inhibits P450IIC9; accordingly, it may interfere with the metabolism of many non-steroidal anti-inflammatory agents). Products include:
Celebrex Capsules 3134

Diclofenac Potassium (Co-administration can be associated with increased occult gastrointestinal blood loss; at high concentrations in vitro, clopidogrel inhibits P450IIC9; accordingly, it may interfere with the metabolism of many non-steroidal anti-inflammatory agents).
No products indexed under this heading.

Diclofenac Sodium (Co-administration can be associated with increased occult gastrointestinal blood loss; at high concentrations in vitro, clopidogrel inhibits P450IIC9; accordingly, it may interfere with the metabolism of many non-steroidal anti-inflammatory agents). Products include:
Arthrotec Tablets 3129
Voltaren Ophthalmic Solution 2309
Voltaren Tablets 2307
Voltaren-XR Tablets 2310

Etodolac (Co-administration can be associated with increased occult gastrointestinal blood loss; at high concentrations in vitro, clopidogrel inhibits P450IIC9; accordingly, it may interfere with the metabolism of many non-steroidal anti-inflammatory agents).
No products indexed under this heading.

Fenoprofen Calcium (Co-administration can be associated with increased occult gastrointestinal blood loss; at high concentrations in vitro, clopidogrel inhibits P450IIC9; accordingly, it may interfere with the metabolism of many non-steroidal anti-inflammatory agents). Products include:
Nalfon Capsules 2502

Flurbiprofen (Co-administration can be associated with increased occult gastrointestinal blood loss; at high concentrations in vitro, clopidogrel inhibits P450IIC9; accordingly, it may interfere with the metabolism of many non-steroidal anti-inflammatory agents).
No products indexed under this heading.

Fluvastatin Sodium (At high concentrations in vitro, clopidogrel inhibits P450IIC9; accordingly, it may interfere with the metabolism of fluvastatin). Products include:
Lescol Capsules 2233
Lescol XL Tablets 2233

Fosphenytoin Sodium (At high concentrations in vitro, clopidogrel inhibits P450IIC9; accordingly, it may interfere with the metabolism of phenytoin).
No products indexed under this heading.

Heparin Sodium (Co-administration should be undertaken with caution; concomitant heparin has no effect on inhibition of platelet aggregation induced by clopidogrel).
No products indexed under this heading.

Ibuprofen (Co-administration can be associated with increased occult gastrointestinal blood loss; at high concentrations in vitro, clopidogrel inhibits P450IIC9; accordingly, it may interfere with the metabolism of many non-steroidal anti-inflammatory agents). Products include:
Advil Allergy Sinus Caplets 770
Advil 674
Children's Advil Oral Suspension 603
Children's Advil Chewable Tablets .. 603
Advil Cold & Sinus 723
Infants' Advil Concentrated Drops .. 604
Infants' Advil Concentrated Drops - White Grape (Dye-Free)............. 604
Junior Strength Advil Swallow Tablets.. 605
Advil Migraine Liquigels 608
Advil Multi-Symptom Cold Caplets....................................... 770
Advil PM Caplets 615
Motrin IB Tablets and Caplets 1866
Children's Motrin Oral Suspension ... 1867
Children's Motrin Non-Staining Dye-Free Oral Suspension............ 1867
Children's Motrin Cold Oral Suspension 1867
Infants' Motrin Concentrated Drops 1867
Infants' Motrin Non-Staining Dye-Free Concentrated Drops....... 1867
Junior Strength Motrin Caplets and Chewable Tablets.................. 1867
Vicoprofen Tablets 539

Indomethacin (Co-administration can be associated with increased occult gastrointestinal blood loss; at high concentrations in vitro, clopidogrel inhibits P450IIC9; accordingly, it may interfere with the metabolism of many non-steroidal anti-inflammatory agents). Products include:
Indocin 1995

Indomethacin Sodium Trihydrate (Co-administration can be associated with increased occult gastrointestinal blood loss; at high concentrations in vitro, clopidogrel inhibits P450IIC9; accordingly, it may interfere with the metabolism of many non-steroidal anti-inflammatory agents). Products include:
Indocin I.V. 2465

Ketoprofen (Co-administration can be associated with increased occult gastrointestinal blood loss; at high concentrations in vitro, clopidogrel inhibits P450IIC9; accordingly, it may interfere with the metabolism of many non-steroidal anti-inflammatory agents).
No products indexed under this heading.

Ketorolac Tromethamine (Co-administration can be associated with increased occult gastrointestinal blood loss; at high concentrations in vitro, clopidogrel inhibits P450IIC9; accordingly, it may interfere with the metabolism of many non-steroidal anti-inflammatory agents). Products include:
Acular Ophthalmic Solution 565
Acular LS Ophthalmic Solution 566

Meclofenamate Sodium (Co-administration can be associated with increased occult gastrointestinal blood loss; at high concentrations in vitro, clopidogrel inhibits P450IIC9; accordingly, it may interfere with the metabolism of many non-steroidal anti-inflammatory agents).
No products indexed under this heading.

Mefenamic Acid (Co-administration can be associated with increased occult gastrointestinal blood loss; at high concentrations in vitro, clopidogrel inhibits P450IIC9; accordingly, it may interfere with the metabolism of many non-steroidal anti-inflammatory agents).
No products indexed under this heading.

Meloxicam (Co-administration can be associated with increased occult gastrointestinal blood loss; at high concentrations in vitro, clopidogrel inhibits P450IIC9; accordingly, it may interfere with the metabolism of many non-steroidal anti-inflammatory agents). Products include:
Mobic Oral Suspension 863
Mobic Tablets 863

Nabumetone (Co-administration can be associated with increased occult gastrointestinal blood loss; at high concentrations in vitro, clopidogrel inhibits P450IIC9; accordingly, it may interfere with the metabolism of many non-steroidal anti-inflammatory agents).
No products indexed under this heading.

Naproxen (Co-administration can be associated with increased occult gastrointestinal blood loss; at high concentrations in vitro, clopidogrel inhibits P450IIC9; accordingly, it may interfere with the metabolism of many non-steroidal anti-inflammatory agents). Products include:
EC-Naprosyn Delayed-Release Tablets.. 2761
Naprosyn Suspension 2761
Naprosyn Tablets 2761
Prevacid NapraPAC 3280

Naproxen Sodium (Co-administration can be associated with increased occult gastrointestinal blood loss; at high concentrations in vitro, clopidogrel inhibits P450IIC9; accordingly, it may interfere with the metabolism of many non-steroidal anti-inflammatory agents). Products include:
Aleve Caplets 742

Aleve Gelcaps 743
Aleve Tablets 743
Aleve Cold & Sinus Caplets 744
Anaprox Tablets 2761
Anaprox DS Tablets 2761

Oxaprozin (Co-administration can be associated with increased occult gastrointestinal blood loss; at high concentrations in vitro, clopidogrel inhibits P450IIC9; accordingly, it may interfere with the metabolism of many non-steroidal anti-inflammatory agents).
No products indexed under this heading.

Phenylbutazone (Co-administration can be associated with increased occult gastrointestinal blood loss; at high concentrations in vitro, clopidogrel inhibits P450IIC9; accordingly, it may interfere with the metabolism of many non-steroidal anti-inflammatory agents).
No products indexed under this heading.

Phenytoin (At high concentrations in vitro, clopidogrel inhibits P450IIC9; accordingly, it may interfere with the metabolism of phenytoin).
No products indexed under this heading.

Phenytoin Sodium (At high concentrations in vitro, clopidogrel inhibits P450IIC9; accordingly, it may interfere with the metabolism of phenytoin). Products include:
Phenytek Capsules 2160

Piroxicam (Co-administration can be associated with increased occult gastrointestinal blood loss; at high concentrations in vitro, clopidogrel inhibits P450IIC9; accordingly, it may interfere with the metabolism of many non-steroidal anti-inflammatory agents).
No products indexed under this heading.

Rofecoxib (Co-administration can be associated with increased occult gastrointestinal blood loss; at high concentrations in vitro, clopidogrel inhibits P450IIC9; accordingly, it may interfere with the metabolism of many non-steroidal anti-inflammatory agents).
No products indexed under this heading.

Sulindac (Co-administration can be associated with increased occult gastrointestinal blood loss; at high concentrations in vitro, clopidogrel inhibits P450IIC9; accordingly, it may interfere with the metabolism of many non-steroidal anti-inflammatory agents). Products include:
Clinoril Tablets 1924

Tamoxifen Citrate (At high concentrations in vitro, clopidogrel inhibits P450IIC9; accordingly, it may interfere with the metabolism of tamoxifen). Products include:
Soltamox Oral Solution 3527

Tolbutamide (At high concentrations in vitro, clopidogrel inhibits P450IIC9; accordingly, it may interfere with the metabolism of tolbutamide).
No products indexed under this heading.

Tolmetin Sodium (Co-administration can be associated with increased occult gastrointestinal blood loss; at high concentrations in vitro, clopidogrel inhibits P450IIC9; accordingly, it may interfere with the metabolism of many non-steroidal anti-inflammatory agents).
No products indexed under this heading.

Torsemide (At high concentrations in vitro, clopidogrel inhibits P450IIC9; accordingly, it may interfere with the metabolism of torsemide). Products include:
Demadex Injection 2759
Demadex Tablets 2759

Valdecoxib (Co-administration can be associated with increased occult gastrointestinal blood loss; at high concentrations in vitro, clopidogrel inhibits P450IIC9; accordingly, it may interfere with the metabolism of many non-steroidal anti-inflammatory agents).
No products indexed under this heading.

Warfarin Sodium (Co-administration should be undertaken with caution due to the increased risk of bleeding; at high concentrations in vitro, clopidogrel inhibits P450IIC9; accordingly, it may interfere with the metabolism of warfarin). Products include:
Coumadin for Injection 898
Coumadin Tablets 898

PLAVIX TABLETS

(Clopidogrel Bisulfate) 2926
May interact with non-steroidal anti-inflammatory agents, phenytoin, and certain other agents. Compounds in these categories include:

Aspirin (Clopidogrel potentiates the effect of aspirin on collagen-induced platelet aggregation). Products include:
Aggrenox Capsules 822
Bayer Aspirin 744
BC Allergy Sinus Cold Powder .... ■677
BC Headache Powder .... ■677
Arthritis Strength BC Powder .... ■677
BC Sinus Cold Powder .... ■677
Excedrin Extra Strength Caplets/Tablets/Geltabs .... ■684
Excedrin Migraine Caplets/Tablets/Geltabs .... ■609
Goody's Body Pain Formula Powder .... ■684
Goody's Extra Strength Headache Powders .... ■611
Goody's Extra Strength Pain Relief Tablets .... ■685
Percodan Tablets 1132
St. Joseph 81 mg Aspirin Chewable and Enteric Coated Tablets 1869

Celecoxib (Co-administration can be associated with increased occult gastrointestinal blood loss; at high concentrations in vitro, clopidogrel inhibits P450IIC9; accordingly, it may interfere with the metabolism of many non-steroidal anti-inflammatory agents. Use caution when co-adminstering with clopidogrel). Products include:
Celebrex Capsules 3134

Diclofenac Potassium (Co-administration can be associated with increased occult gastrointestinal blood loss; at high concentrations in vitro, clopidogrel inhibits P450IIC9; accordingly, it may interfere with the metabolism of many non-steroidal anti-inflammatory agents. Use caution when co-adminstering with clopidrogel).
No products indexed under this heading.

Diclofenac Sodium (Co-administration can be associated with increased occult gastrointestinal blood loss; at high concentrations in vitro, clopidogrel inhibits P450IIC9; accordingly, it may interfere with the metabolism of many non-steroidal anti-inflammatory agents. Use caution when co-adminstering with clopidrogel). Products include:
Arthrotec Tablets 3129
Voltaren Ophthalmic Solution 2309
Voltaren Tablets 2307
Voltaren-XR Tablets 2310

Etodolac (Co-administration can be associated with increased occult gastrointestinal blood loss; at high concentrations in vitro, clopidogrel inhibits P450IIC9; accordingly, it may interfere with the metabolism of many non-steroidal anti-inflammatory agents. Use caution when co-adminstering with clopidrogel).
No products indexed under this heading.

Fenoprofen Calcium (Co-administration can be associated with increased occult gastrointestinal blood loss; at high concentrations in vitro, clopidogrel inhibits P450IIC9; accordingly, it may interfere with the metabolism of many non-steroidal anti-inflammatory agents. Use caution when co-adminstering with clopidrogel). Products include:
Nalfon Capsules 2502

Flurbiprofen (Co-administration can be associated with increased occult gastrointestinal blood loss; at high concentrations in vitro, clopidogrel inhibits P450IIC9; accordingly, it may interfere with the metabolism of many non-steroidal anti-inflammatory agents. Use caution when co-adminstering with clopidrogel).
No products indexed under this heading.

Fluvastatin Sodium (At high concentrations in vitro, clopidogrel inhibits P450IIC9; accordingly, it may interfere with the metabolism of fluvastatin. Use caution when co-administering with clopidrogel). Products include:
Lescol Capsules 2233
Lescol XL Tablets 2233

Fosphenytoin Sodium (At high concentrations in vitro, clopidogrel inhibits P450IIC9; accordingly, it may interfere with the metabolism of phenytoin. Use caution when co-administering with clopidrogel).
No products indexed under this heading.

Ibuprofen (Co-administration can be associated with increased occult gastrointestinal blood loss; at high concentrations in vitro, clopidogrel inhibits P450IIC9; accordingly, it may interfere with the metabolism of many non-steroidal anti-inflammatory agents. Use caution when co-adminstering with clopidrogel). Products include:
Advil Allergy Sinus Caplets .... ■770
Advil .... ■674
Children's Advil Oral Suspension .... ■603
Children's Advil Chewable Tablets .. ■603
Advil Cold & Sinus .... ■723
Infants' Advil Concentrated Drops .. ■604
Infants' Advil Concentrated Drops - White Grape (Dye-Free)............ ■604
Junior Strength Advil Swallow Tablets.. ■605
Advil Migraine Liquigels .... ■608
Advil Multi-Symptom Cold Caplets.. ■770
Advil PM Caplets .... ■615
Motrin IB Tablets and Caplets 1866
Children's Motrin Oral Suspension ... 1867
Children's Motrin Non-Staining Dye-Free Oral Suspension............... 1867
Children's Motrin Cold Oral Suspension 1867
Infants' Motrin Concentrated Drops 1867
Infants' Motrin Non-Staining Dye-Free Concentrated Drops....... 1867
Junior Strength Motrin Caplets and Chewable Tablets................. 1867
Vicoprofen Tablets 539

Indomethacin (Co-administration can be associated with increased occult gastrointestinal blood loss; at high concentrations in vitro, clopidogrel inhibits P450IIC9; accordingly, it may interfere with the metabolism of many non-steroidal anti-inflammatory agents. Use caution when co-adminstering with clopidrogel). Products include:
Indocin 1995

Indomethacin Sodium Trihydrate (Co-administration can be associated with increased occult gastrointestinal blood loss; at high concentrations in vitro, clopidogrel inhibits P450IIC9; accordingly, it may interfere with the metabolism of many non-steroidal anti-inflammatory agents. Use caution when co-adminstering with clopidrogel). Products include:
Indocin I.V. 2465

Ketoprofen (Co-administration can be associated with increased occult gastrointestinal blood loss; at high concentrations in vitro, clopidogrel inhibits P450IIC9; accordingly, it may interfere with the metabolism of many non-steroidal anti-inflammatory agents. Use caution when co-adminstering with clopidrogel).
No products indexed under this heading.

Ketorolac Tromethamine (Co-administration can be associated with increased occult gastrointestinal blood loss; at high concentrations in vitro, clopidogrel inhibits P450IIC9; accordingly, it may interfere with the metabolism of many non-steroidal anti-inflammatory agents. Use caution when co-adminstering with clopidrogel). Products include:
Acular Ophthalmic Solution 565
Acular LS Ophthalmic Solution 566

Meclofenamate Sodium (Co-administration can be associated with increased occult gastrointestinal blood loss; at high concentrations in vitro, clopidogrel inhibits P450IIC9; accordingly, it may interfere with the metabolism of many non-steroidal anti-inflammatory agents. Use caution when co-adminstering with clopidrogel).
No products indexed under this heading.

Mefenamic Acid (Co-administration can be associated with increased occult gastrointestinal blood loss; at high concentrations in vitro, clopidogrel inhibits P450IIC9; accordingly, it may interfere with the metabolism of many non-steroidal anti-inflammatory agents. Use caution when co-adminstering with clopidrogel).
No products indexed under this heading.

Meloxicam (Co-administration can be associated with increased occult gastrointestinal blood loss; at high concentrations in vitro, clopidogrel inhibits P450IIC9; accordingly, it may interfere with the metabolism of many non-steroidal anti-inflammatory agents. Use caution when co-adminstering with clopidrogel).
Products include:
Mobic Oral Suspension 863
Mobic Tablets 863

Nabumetone (Co-administration can be associated with increased occult gastrointestinal blood loss; at high concentrations in vitro, clopidogrel inhibits P450IIC9; accordingly, it may interfere with the metabolism of many non-steroidal anti-inflammatory agents. Use caution when co-adminstering with clopidrogel).
No products indexed under this heading.

Naproxen (Co-administration can be associated with increased occult gastrointestinal blood loss; at high concentrations in vitro, clopidogrel inhibits P450IIC9; accordingly, it may interfere with the metabolism of many non-steroidal anti-inflammatory agents. Use caution when co-adminstering with clopidrogel).
Products include:
EC-Naprosyn Delayed-Release Tablets 2761
Naprosyn Suspension 2761
Naprosyn Tablets 2761
Prevacid NapraPAC 3280

Naproxen Sodium (Co-administration can be associated with increased occult gastrointestinal blood loss; at high concentrations in vitro, clopidogrel inhibits P450IIC9; accordingly, it may interfere with the metabolism of many non-steroidal anti-inflammatory agents. Use caution when co-adminstering with clopidrogel).
Products include:
Aleve Caplets 742
Aleve Gelcaps 743
Aleve Tablets 743
Aleve Cold & Sinus Caplets 744
Anaprox Tablets 2761
Anaprox DS Tablets 2761

Oxaprozin (Co-administration can be associated with increased occult gastrointestinal blood loss; at high concentrations in vitro, clopidogrel inhibits P450IIC9; accordingly, it may interfere with the metabolism of many non-steroidal anti-inflammatory agents. Use caution when co-adminstering with clopidrogel).
No products indexed under this heading.

Phenylbutazone (Co-administration can be associated with increased occult gastrointestinal blood loss; at high concentrations in vitro, clopidogrel inhibits P450IIC9; accordingly, it may interfere with the metabolism of many non-steroidal anti-inflammatory agents. Use caution when co-adminstering with clopidrogel).
No products indexed under this heading.

Phenytoin (At high concentrations in vitro, clopidogrel inhibits P450IIC9; accordingly, it may interfere with the metabolism of phenytoin. Use caution when co-administering with clopidrogel).
No products indexed under this heading.

Phenytoin Sodium (At high concentrations in vitro, clopidogrel inhibits P450IIC9; accordingly, it may interfere with the metabolism of phenytoin. Use caution when co-administering with clopidrogel).
Products include:
Phenytek Capsules 2160

Piroxicam (Co-administration can be associated with increased occult gastrointestinal blood loss; at high concentrations in vitro, clopidogrel inhibits P450IIC9; accordingly, it may interfere with the metabolism of many non-steroidal anti-inflammatory agents. Use caution when co-adminstering with clopidrogel).
No products indexed under this heading.

Rofecoxib (Co-administration can be associated with increased occult gastrointestinal blood loss; at high concentrations in vitro, clopidogrel inhibits P450IIC9; accordingly, it may interfere with the metabolism of many non-steroidal anti-inflammatory agents. Use caution when co-adminstering with clopidrogel).
No products indexed under this heading.

Sulindac (Co-administration can be associated with increased occult gastrointestinal blood loss; at high concentrations in vitro, clopidogrel inhibits P450IIC9; accordingly, it may interfere with the metabolism of many non-steroidal anti-inflammatory agents. Use caution when co-adminstering with clopidrogel).
Products include:
Clinoril Tablets 1924

Tamoxifen Citrate (At high concentrations in vitro, clopidogrel inhibits P450IIC9; accordingly, it may interfere with the metabolism of tamoxifen. Use caution when co-administering with clopidrogel).
Products include:
Soltamox Oral Solution 3527

Tolbutamide (At high concentrations in vitro, clopidogrel inhibits P450IIC9; accordingly, it may interfere with the metabolism of tolbutamide. Use caution when co-administering with clopidrogel).
No products indexed under this heading.

Tolmetin Sodium (Co-administration can be associated with increased occult gastrointestinal blood loss; at high concentrations in vitro, clopidogrel inhibits P450IIC9; accordingly, it may interfere with the metabolism of many non-steroidal anti-inflammatory agents. Use caution when co-adminstering with clopidrogel).
No products indexed under this heading.

Torsemide (At high concentrations in vitro, clopidogrel inhibits P450IIC9; accordingly, it may interfere with the metabolism of torsemide. Use caution when co-administering with clopidrogel).
Products include:
Demadex Injection 2759
Demadex Tablets 2759

Valdecoxib (Co-administration can be associated with increased occult gastrointestinal blood loss; at high concentrations in vitro, clopidogrel inhibits P450IIC9; accordingly, it may interfere with the metabolism of many non-steroidal anti-inflammatory agents. Use caution when co-adminstering with clopidrogel).
No products indexed under this heading.

Warfarin Sodium (Because of the increased risk of bleeding, the concomitant administration of warfarin with clopidrogel should be undertaken with caution). Products include:
Coumadin for Injection 898
Coumadin Tablets 898

PLETAL TABLETS

(Cilostazol) 2455
May interact with cytochrome p450 2c9 inhibitors (selected), cytochrome p450 3a4 inhibitors (selected), erythromycin, platelet inhibitors, and certain other agents. Compounds in these categories include:

Acetazolamide (A reduced dose of cilostazol should be considered when taken concomitantly with CYP3A4 inhibitors).
No products indexed under this heading.

Amiodarone Hydrochloride (A reduced dose of cilostazol should be considered when taken concomitantly with CYP3A4 inhibitors).
No products indexed under this heading.

Amprenavir (A reduced dose of cilostazol should be considered when taken concomitantly with CYP3A4 inhibitors). Products include:
Agenerase Capsules 1327
Agenerase Oral Solution 1332

Anastrozole (A reduced dose of cilostazol should be considered when taken concomitantly with CYP3A4 inhibitors). Products include:
Arimidex Tablets 673

Aprepitant (A reduced dose of cilostazol should be considered when taken concomitantly with CYP3A4 inhibitors). Products include:
Emend Capsules 1963

Aspirin (Short-term (less than or equal to 4 days) co-administration has shown a 22% to 37% increase in inhibition of ADP-induced ex vivo platelet aggregation compared to aspirin alone; no clinically significant impact on bleeding time, PT, or aPTT was noted; there was no apparent greater incidence of hemorrhagic adverse effects in patients on cilostazol and aspirin compared to patients taking placebo and aspirin).
Products include:
Aggrenox Capsules 822
Bayer Aspirin 744
BC Allergy Sinus Cold Powder 677
BC Headache Powder 677
Arthritis Strength BC Powder 677
BC Sinus Cold Powder 677
Excedrin Extra Strength Caplets/Tablets/Geltabs 684
Excedrin Migraine Caplets/Tablets/Geltabs 609
Goody's Body Pain Formula Powder 684
Goody's Extra Strength Headache Powders 611
Goody's Extra Strength Pain Relief Tablets 685
Percodan Tablets 1132
St. Joseph 81 mg Aspirin Chewable and Enteric Coated Tablets 1869

Aspirin, Enteric Coated (Caution is advised in patients receiving both cilostazol and any other antiplatelet agent).
No products indexed under this heading.

Aspirin Buffered (Caution is advised in patients receiving both cilostazol and any other antiplatelet agent). Products include:
Bufferin Extra Strength Tablets 678
Bufferin Regular Strength Tablets ... 678

Azlocillin Sodium (Caution is advised in patients receiving both cilostazol and any other antiplatelet agent).
No products indexed under this heading.

Bendroflumethiazide (A reduced dose of cilostazol should be considered when taken concomitantly with CYP2C19 inhibitors).
No products indexed under this heading.

Carbenicillin Indanyl Sodium (Caution is advised in patients receiving both cilostazol and any other antiplatelet agent).
No products indexed under this heading.

Chloramphenicol (A reduced dose of cilostazol should be considered when taken concomitantly with CYP2C19 inhibitors).
No products indexed under this heading.

Chlorothiazide (A reduced dose of cilostazol should be considered when taken concomitantly with CYP2C19 inhibitors). Products include:
Diuril Oral Suspension 1954

Chlorothiazide Sodium (A reduced dose of cilostazol should be considered when taken concomitantly with CYP2C19 inhibitors).
Products include:
Diuril Sodium Intravenous 2467

Chlorpropamide (A reduced dose of cilostazol should be considered when taken concomitantly with CYP2C19 inhibitors).
No products indexed under this heading.

Choline Magnesium Trisalicylate (Caution is advised in patients receiving both cilostazol and any other antiplatelet agent).
No products indexed under this heading.

Cimetidine (A reduced dose of cilostazol should be considered when taken concomitantly with CYP3A4 inhibitors). Products include:
Tagamet HB 200 Tablets 664

Cimetidine Hydrochloride (A reduced dose of cilostazol should be considered when taken concomitantly with CYP3A4 inhibitors).
No products indexed under this heading.

Ciprofloxacin (A reduced dose of cilostazol should be considered when taken concomitantly with CYP3A4 inhibitors). Products include:

Cipro Oral Suspension 2977
Cipro I.V. 2984
Cipro XR Tablets 2990
Ciprodex Otic Suspension 559

Clarithromycin (Co-administration of cilostazol with moderate inhibitors of CYP3A4, such as clarithromycin, a macrolide antibiotic, may result in significant increases in the systemic exposure of cilostazol and/or its major metabolites; caution should be exercised if concurrently used). Products include:
Biaxin/Biaxin XL 402
PREVPAC 3284

Clopidogrel Bisulfate (Althought it cannot be determined whether there was an additive effect on bleeding times during concomitant administration, caution should be advised for checking bleeding times). Products include:
Plavix Tablets 917
Plavix Tablets 2926

Clopidogrel Hydrogen Sulfate (Althought it cannot be determined whether there was an additive effect on bleeding times during concomitant administration, caution should be advised for checking bleeding times).
No products indexed under this heading.

Clotrimazole (A reduced dose of cilostazol should be considered when taken concomitantly with CYP3A4 inhibitors). Products include:
Desenex Athlete's Foot Cream .... ▣635
Lotrimin 3039
Lotrisone 3040

Cyclosporine (A reduced dose of cilostazol should be considered when taken concomitantly with CYP3A4 inhibitors). Products include:
Gengraf Capsules 459
Neoral Oral Solution 2259
Neoral Soft Gelatin Capsules 2259
Restasis Ophthalmic Emulsion 575
Sandimmune 2275

Dalfopristin (A reduced dose of cilostazol should be considered when taken concomitantly with CYP3A4 inhibitors).
No products indexed under this heading.

Danazol (A reduced dose of cilostazol should be considered when taken concomitantly with CYP3A4 inhibitors).
No products indexed under this heading.

Delavirdine Mesylate (A reduced dose of cilostazol should be considered when taken concomitantly with CYP3A4 inhibitors). Products include:
Rescriptor Tablets 2551

Diclofenac Potassium (A reduced dose of cilostazol should be considered when taken concomitantly with CYP2C19 inhibitors).
No products indexed under this heading.

Diclofenac Sodium (A reduced dose of cilostazol should be considered when taken concomitantly with CYP2C19 inhibitors). Products include:
Arthrotec Tablets 3129
Voltaren Ophthalmic Solution 2309
Voltaren Tablets 2307
Voltaren-XR Tablets 2310

Diflunisal (Caution is advised in patients receiving both cilostazol and any other antiplatelet agent). Products include:
Dolobid Tablets 1955

Diltiazem Hydrochloride (Co-administration of cilostazol with moderate inhibitors of CYP3A4, such as diltiazem, has been shown to increase cilostazol plasma concentrations by approximately 30%). Products include:
Cardizem LA Extended Release Tablets 1728
Tiazac Capsules 1201

Diltiazem Maleate (Co-administration of cilostazol with moderate inhibitors of CYP3A4, such as diltiazem, has been shown to increase cilostazol plasma concentrations by approximately 30%).
No products indexed under this heading.

Dipyridamole (Caution is advised in patients receiving both cilostazol and any other antiplatelet agent). Products include:
Aggrenox Capsules 822
Persantine Tablets 868

Disulfiram (A reduced dose of cilostazol should be considered when taken concomitantly with CYP2C19 inhibitors).
No products indexed under this heading.

Efavirenz (A reduced dose of cilostazol should be considered when taken concomitantly with CYP2C19 inhibitors). Products include:
Atripla Tablets 945
Sustiva Capsules 930
Sustiva Tablets 930

Erythromycin (Co-administration of cilostazol with moderately strong inhibitors of CYP3A4, such as erythromycin, significantly increases the systemic exposure of cilostazol and/or its major metabolites; caution should be exercised if concurrently used). Products include:
Ery-Tab Tablets 449
Erythromycin Base Filmtab Tablets 455
Erythromycin Delayed-Release Capsules, USP 457
PCE Dispertab Tablets 515

Erythromycin Estolate (Co-administration of cilostazol with moderately strong inhibitors of CYP3A4, such as erythromycin, significantly increases the systemic exposure of cilostazol and/or its major metabolites; caution should be exercised if concurrently used).
No products indexed under this heading.

Erythromycin Ethylsuccinate (Co-administration of cilostazol with moderately strong inhibitors of CYP3A4, such as erythromycin, significantly increases the systemic exposure of cilostazol and/or its major metabolites; caution should be exercised if concurrently used). Products include:
E.E.S. 451
EryPed 447

Erythromycin Gluceptate (Co-administration of cilostazol with moderately strong inhibitors of CYP3A4, such as erythromycin, significantly increases the systemic exposure of cilostazol and/or its major metabolites; caution should be exercised if concurrently used).
No products indexed under this heading.

Erythromycin Lactobionate (Co-administration of cilostazol with moderately strong inhibitors of CYP3A4, such as erythromycin, significantly increases the systemic exposure of cilostazol and/or its major metabolites; caution should be exercised if concurrently used).
No products indexed under this heading.

Erythromycin Stearate (Co-administration of cilostazol with moderately strong inhibitors of CYP3A4, such as erythromycin, significantly increases the systemic exposure of cilostazol and/or its major metabolites; caution should be exercised if concurrently used). Products include:
Erythrocin Stearate Filmtab Tablets 453

Esomeprazole Magnesium (A reduced dose of cilostazol should be considered when taken concomitantly with CYP3A4 inhibitors). Products include:
Nexium Delayed-Release Capsules 655

Fenofibrate (A reduced dose of cilostazol should be considered when taken concomitantly with CYP2C19 inhibitors). Products include:
Lofibra Tablets 1219
Lofibra Capsules 1216
Tricor Tablets 527
Triglide Tablets 3123

Fenoprofen Calcium (Caution is advised in patients receiving both cilostazol and any other antiplatelet agent). Products include:
Nalfon Capsules 2502

Fluconazole (Co-administration of cilostazol with strong inhibitors of CYP3A4, such as fluconazole, would be expected to cause an increase in cilostazol Cmax and AUC).
No products indexed under this heading.

Fluorouracil (A reduced dose of cilostazol should be considered when taken concomitantly with CYP2C19 inhibitors). Products include:
Carac Cream, 0.5% 2879
Efudex 3363

Fluoxetine Hydrochloride (Co-administration of cilostazol with strong inhibitors of CYP3A4, such as fluoxetine, would be expected to cause an increase in cilostazol Cmax and AUC). Products include:
Prozac Pulvules and Liquid 1801
Symbyax Capsules 1819

Flurbiprofen (A reduced dose of cilostazol should be considered when taken concomitantly with CYP2C19 inhibitors).
No products indexed under this heading.

Flurbiprofen Sodium (A reduced dose of cilostazol should be considered when taken concomitantly with CYP2C19 inhibitors). Products include:
Ocufen Ophthalmic Solution .... ⊙232

Fluvastatin Sodium (A reduced dose of cilostazol should be considered when taken concomitantly with CYP2C19 inhibitors). Products include:
Lescol Capsules 2233
Lescol XL Tablets 2233

Fluvoxamine Maleate (Co-administration of cilostazol with strong inhibitors of CYP3A4, such as fluvoxamine, would be expected to cause an increase in cilostazol Cmax and AUC).
No products indexed under this heading.

Fosamprenavir Calcium (A reduced dose of cilostazol should be considered when taken concomitantly with CYP3A4 inhibitors). Products include:
Lexiva Tablets 1505

Gemfibrozil (A reduced dose of cilostazol should be considered when taken concomitantly with CYP2C19 inhibitors).
No products indexed under this heading.

Glipizide (A reduced dose of cilostazol should be considered when taken concomitantly with CYP2C19 inhibitors).
No products indexed under this heading.

Glyburide (A reduced dose of cilostazol should be considered when taken concomitantly with CYP2C19 inhibitors).
No products indexed under this heading.

Hydrochlorothiazide (A reduced dose of cilostazol should be considered when taken concomitantly with CYP2C19 inhibitors). Products include:
Aldoril Tablets 1910
Atacand HCT 651
Avalide Tablets 888
Avalide Tablets 2874
Benicar HCT Tablets 1044
Diovan HCT Tablets 2196
Dyazide Capsules 1423
Hyzaar 50-12.5 Tablets 1990
Hyzaar 100-12.5 Tablets 1990
Hyzaar 100-25 Tablets 1990
Lopressor HCT 50/25 Tablets 2241
Lopressor HCT 100/25 Tablets 2241
Lopressor HCT 100/50 Tablets 2241
Lotensin HCT Tablets 2246
Micardis HCT Tablets 856
Moduretic Tablets 2028
Prinzide Tablets 2056
Teveten HCT Tablets 1737
Timolide Tablets 2086
Uniretic Tablets 3100

Hydroflumethiazide (A reduced dose of cilostazol should be considered when taken concomitantly with CYP2C19 inhibitors).
No products indexed under this heading.

Ibuprofen (Caution is advised in patients receiving both cilostazol and any other antiplatelet agent). Products include:
Advil Allergy Sinus Caplets .... ▣770
Advil .... ▣674
Children's Advil Oral Suspension .... ▣603
Children's Advil Chewable Tablets .... ▣603
Advil Cold & Sinus .... ▣723
Infants' Advil Concentrated Drops .... ▣604
Infants' Advil Concentrated Drops - White Grape (Dye-Free) .... ▣604
Junior Strength Advil Swallow Tablets .... ▣605
Advil Migraine Liquigels .... ▣608
Advil Multi-Symptom Cold Caplets .... ▣770
Advil PM Caplets .... ▣615
Motrin IB Tablets and Caplets 1866
Children's Motrin Oral Suspension 1867
Children's Motrin Non-Staining Dye-Free Oral Suspension 1867
Children's Motrin Cold Oral Suspension 1867
Infants' Motrin Concentrated Drops 1867

Infants' Motrin Non-Staining Dye-Free Concentrated Drops....... 1867
Junior Strength Motrin Caplets and Chewable Tablets.................. 1867
Vicoprofen Tablets 539

Imatinib Mesylate (A reduced dose of cilostazol should be considered when taken concomitantly with CYP2C19 inhibitors). Products include:
Gleevec Tablets 2227

Indinavir Sulfate (A reduced dose of cilostazol should be considered when taken concomitantly with CYP3A4 inhibitors). Products include:
Crixivan Capsules 1940

Indomethacin (Caution is advised in patients receiving both cilostazol and any other antiplatelet agent). Products include:
Indocin 1995

Indomethacin Sodium Trihydrate (Caution is advised in patients receiving both cilostazol and any other antiplatelet agent). Products include:
Indocin I.V. 2465

Isoniazid (A reduced dose of cilostazol should be considered when taken concomitantly with CYP2C19 inhibitors).
No products indexed under this heading.

Itraconazole (Co-administration of cilostazol with strong inhibitors of CYP3A4, such as itraconazole, would be expected to cause an increase in cilostazol Cmax and AUC).
No products indexed under this heading.

Ketoconazole (Co-administration of cilostazol with strong inhibitors of CYP3A4, such as ketoconazole increased cilostazol Cmax and AUC). Products include:
Nizoral A-D Shampoo, 1%................ 1868

Ketoprofen (A reduced dose of cilostazol should be considered when taken concomitantly with CYP2C19 inhibitors).
No products indexed under this heading.

Leflunomide (A reduced dose of cilostazol should be considered when taken concomitantly with CYP2C19 inhibitors).
No products indexed under this heading.

Lopinavir (A reduced dose of cilostazol should be considered when taken concomitantly with CYP3A4 inhibitors). Products include:
Kaletra 476

Loratadine (A reduced dose of cilostazol should be considered when taken concomitantly with CYP3A4 inhibitors). Products include:
Alavert Allergy & Sinus D-12 Hour Tablets.. 771
Alavert 771
Children's Claritin Allergy Oral Solution 771
Claritin Non-Drowsy 24 Hour Tablets.. 772
Claritin Reditabs 24 Hour Non-Drowsy Tablets.................... 772
Claritin-D Non-Drowsy 12 Hour Tablets.. 772
Claritin-D Non-Drowsy 24 Hour Tablets.. 772

Lovastatin (A reduced dose of cilostazol should be considered when taken concomitantly with CYP2C19 inhibitors). Products include:
Advicor Tablets 1722
Altoprev Extended-Release Tablets 3109
Mevacor Tablets 2021

Magnesium Salicylate (Caution is advised in patients receiving both cilostazol and any other antiplatelet agent).
No products indexed under this heading.

Meclofenamate Sodium (Caution is advised in patients receiving both cilostazol and any other antiplatelet agent).
No products indexed under this heading.

Mefenamic Acid (Caution is advised in patients receiving both cilostazol and any other antiplatelet agent).
No products indexed under this heading.

Methyclothiazide (A reduced dose of cilostazol should be considered when taken concomitantly with CYP2C19 inhibitors).
No products indexed under this heading.

Metronidazole (A reduced dose of cilostazol should be considered when taken concomitantly with CYP2C19 inhibitors). Products include:
Metrogel 1% 1211
MetroGel-Vaginal Gel 1855
Vandazole Vaginal Gel 3338

Metronidazole Benzoate (A reduced dose of cilostazol should be considered when taken concomitantly with CYP3A4 inhibitors).
No products indexed under this heading.

Metronidazole Hydrochloride (A reduced dose of cilostazol should be considered when taken concomitantly with CYP2C19 inhibitors).
No products indexed under this heading.

Mezlocillin Sodium (Caution is advised in patients receiving both cilostazol and any other antiplatelet agent).
No products indexed under this heading.

Miconazole (Co-administration of cilostazol with strong inhibitors of CYP3A4, such as miconazole, would be expected to cause an increase in Cmax and AUC).
No products indexed under this heading.

Miconazole Nitrate (A reduced dose of cilostazol should be considered when taken concomitantly with CYP3A4 inhibitors). Products include:
Desenex 635
Desenex Jock Itch Spray Powder ... 635

Modafinil (A reduced dose of cilostazol should be considered when taken concomitantly with CYP2C19 inhibitors). Products include:
Provigil Tablets 988

Nafcillin Sodium (Caution is advised in patients receiving both cilostazol and any other antiplatelet agent).
No products indexed under this heading.

Naproxen (Caution is advised in patients receiving both cilostazol and any other antiplatelet agent). Products include:
EC-Naprosyn Delayed-Release Tablets 2761
Naprosyn Suspension 2761
Naprosyn Tablets 2761
Prevacid NapraPAC 3280

Naproxen Sodium (Caution is advised in patients receiving both cilostazol and any other antiplatelet agent). Products include:
Aleve Caplets 742
Aleve Gelcaps 743
Aleve Tablets 743
Aleve Cold & Sinus Caplets 744
Anaprox Tablets 2761
Anaprox DS Tablets 2761

Nefazodone Hydrochloride (Co-administration of cilostazol with strong inhibitors of CYP3A4, such as nefazodone, would be expected to cause an increase cilostazol Cmax and AUC).
No products indexed under this heading.

Nelfinavir Mesylate (A reduced dose of cilostazol should be considered when taken concomitantly with CYP3A4 inhibitors). Products include:
Viracept 2577

Nevirapine (A reduced dose of cilostazol should be considered when taken concomitantly with CYP3A4 inhibitors). Products include:
Viramune Oral Suspension 873
Viramune Tablets 873

Niacinamide (A reduced dose of cilostazol should be considered when taken concomitantly with CYP3A4 inhibitors).
No products indexed under this heading.

Nicotinamide (A reduced dose of cilostazol should be considered when taken concomitantly with CYP3A4 inhibitors). Products include:
Nicomide Tablets 1088

Nifedipine (A reduced dose of cilostazol should be considered when taken concomitantly with CYP3A4 inhibitors). Products include:
Adalat CC Tablets 2964

Norfloxacin (A reduced dose of cilostazol should be considered when taken concomitantly with CYP3A4 inhibitors). Products include:
Noroxin Tablets 2032

Omeprazole (Co-administration with potent inhibitors of CYP2C19, such as omeprazole, has increased the systemic exposure to 3,4 dehydro-cilostazol by 69%). Products include:
Zegerid Capsules 2958
Zegerid Powder for Oral Solution 2958

Oxiconazole Nitrate (A reduced dose of cilostazol should be considered when taken concomitantly with CYP2C19 inhibitors). Products include:
Oxistat 2667

Paroxetine Hydrochloride (A reduced dose of cilostazol should be considered when taken concomitantly with CYP2C19 inhibitors). Products include:
Paxil CR Controlled-Release Tablets 1538
Paxil 1530

Penicillin G Benzathine (Caution is advised in patients receiving both cilostazol and any other antiplatelet agent). Products include:
Bicillin C-R Injectable Suspension 1706

Penicillin G Procaine (Caution is advised in patients receiving both cilostazol and any other antiplatelet agent). Products include:
Bicillin C-R Injectable Suspension 1706

Phenylbutazone (A reduced dose of cilostazol should be considered when taken concomitantly with CYP2C19 inhibitors).
No products indexed under this heading.

Piroxicam (Caution is advised in patients receiving both cilostazol and any other antiplatelet agent).
No products indexed under this heading.

Polythiazide (A reduced dose of cilostazol should be considered when taken concomitantly with CYP2C19 inhibitors).
No products indexed under this heading.

Propoxyphene Hydrochloride (A reduced dose of cilostazol should be considered when taken concomitantly with CYP3A4 inhibitors).
No products indexed under this heading.

Propoxyphene Napsylate (A reduced dose of cilostazol should be considered when taken concomitantly with CYP3A4 inhibitors).
No products indexed under this heading.

Quinidine (A reduced dose of cilostazol should be considered when taken concomitantly with CYP3A4 inhibitors).
No products indexed under this heading.

Quinidine Hydrochloride (A reduced dose of cilostazol should be considered when taken concomitantly with CYP3A4 inhibitors).
No products indexed under this heading.

Quinidine Polygalacturonate (A reduced dose of cilostazol should be considered when taken concomitantly with CYP3A4 inhibitors).
No products indexed under this heading.

Quinidine Sulfate (A reduced dose of cilostazol should be considered when taken concomitantly with CYP3A4 inhibitors).
No products indexed under this heading.

Quinine (A reduced dose of cilostazol should be considered when taken concomitantly with CYP3A4 inhibitors).
No products indexed under this heading.

Quinine Sulfate (A reduced dose of cilostazol should be considered when taken concomitantly with CYP3A4 inhibitors).
No products indexed under this heading.

Quinupristin (A reduced dose of cilostazol should be considered when taken concomitantly with CYP3A4 inhibitors).
No products indexed under this heading.

Ranitidine Bismuth Citrate (A reduced dose of cilostazol should be considered when taken concomitantly with CYP3A4 inhibitors).
No products indexed under this heading.

Ranitidine Hydrochloride (A reduced dose of cilostazol should be considered when taken concomitantly with CYP3A4 inhibitors). Products include:
Zantac 1624
Zantac Injection 1619
Zantac Injection Pharmacy Bulk Package....................................... 1622

IMPORTANT NOTE: Always consult each drug listing in the patient's regimen for possible interactions.

Ritonavir (A reduced dose of cilostazol should be considered when taken concomitantly with CYP2C19 inhibitors). Products include:
- Kaletra ... 476
- Norvir ... 503

Salsalate (Caution is advised in patients receiving both cilostazol and any other antiplatelet agent).
No products indexed under this heading.

Saquinavir (A reduced dose of cilostazol should be considered when taken concomitantly with CYP3A4 inhibitors).
No products indexed under this heading.

Saquinavir Mesylate (A reduced dose of cilostazol should be considered when taken concomitantly with CYP3A4 inhibitors). Products include:
- Invirase ... 2772

Sertraline Hydrochloride (Co-administration of cilostazol with strong inhibitors of CYP3A4, such as sertraline, would be expected to cause an increase in cilostazol Cmax and AUC). Products include:
- Zoloft ... 2586

Sulfacytine (A reduced dose of cilostazol should be considered when taken concomitantly with CYP2C19 inhibitors).
No products indexed under this heading.

Sulfamethizole (A reduced dose of cilostazol should be considered when taken concomitantly with CYP2C19 inhibitors).
No products indexed under this heading.

Sulfamethoxazole (A reduced dose of cilostazol should be considered when taken concomitantly with CYP2C19 inhibitors).
No products indexed under this heading.

Sulfasalazine (A reduced dose of cilostazol should be considered when taken concomitantly with CYP2C19 inhibitors).
No products indexed under this heading.

Sulfinpyrazone (A reduced dose of cilostazol should be considered when taken concomitantly with CYP2C19 inhibitors).
No products indexed under this heading.

Sulfisoxazole Acetyl (A reduced dose of cilostazol should be considered when taken concomitantly with CYP2C19 inhibitors).
No products indexed under this heading.

Sulfisoxazole Diolamine (A reduced dose of cilostazol should be considered when taken concomitantly with CYP2C19 inhibitors).
No products indexed under this heading.

Sulindac (Caution is advised in patients receiving both cilostazol and any other antiplatelet agent). Products include:
- Clinoril Tablets ... 1924

Telithromycin (A reduced dose of cilostazol should be considered when taken concomitantly with CYP3A4 inhibitors). Products include:
- Ketek Tablets ... 2903

Terconazole (A reduced dose of cilostazol should be considered when taken concomitantly with CYP2C19 inhibitors).
No products indexed under this heading.

Ticarcillin Disodium (Caution is advised in patients receiving both cilostazol and any other antiplatelet agent). Products include:
- Timentin ADD-Vantage ... 1580
- Timentin Injection Galaxy Container ... 1583
- Timentin IV Infusion ... 1577
- Timentin Pharmacy Bulk Package ... 1586

Ticlopidine Hydrochloride (A reduced dose of cilostazol should be considered when taken concomitantly with CYP2C19 inhibitors). Products include:
- Ticlid Tablets ... 2810

Tolazamide (A reduced dose of cilostazol should be considered when taken concomitantly with CYP2C19 inhibitors).
No products indexed under this heading.

Tolbutamide (A reduced dose of cilostazol should be considered when taken concomitantly with CYP2C19 inhibitors).
No products indexed under this heading.

Tolbutamide Sodium (A reduced dose of cilostazol should be considered when taken concomitantly with CYP2C19 inhibitors).
No products indexed under this heading.

Tolmetin Sodium (Caution is advised in patients receiving both cilostazol and any other antiplatelet agent).
No products indexed under this heading.

Troglitazone (A reduced dose of cilostazol should be considered when taken concomitantly with CYP2C19 inhibitors).
No products indexed under this heading.

Troleandomycin (A reduced dose of cilostazol should be considered when taken concomitantly with CYP3A4 inhibitors).
No products indexed under this heading.

Valproate Sodium (A reduced dose of cilostazol should be considered when taken concomitantly with CYP3A4 inhibitors). Products include:
- Depacon Injection ... 412

Verapamil Hydrochloride (A reduced dose of cilostazol should be considered when taken concomitantly with CYP3A4 inhibitors). Products include:
- Covera-HS Tablets ... 3139
- Tarka Tablets ... 524
- Verelan PM Extended-Release Capsules, Controlled-Onset ... 3106

Voriconazole (A reduced dose of cilostazol should be considered when taken concomitantly with CYP3A4 inhibitors). Products include:
- VFEND I.V. ... 2564
- VFEND Oral Suspension ... 2564
- VFEND Tablets ... 2564

Zafirlukast (A reduced dose of cilostazol should be considered when taken concomitantly with CYP2C19 inhibitors). Products include:
- Accolate Tablets ... 671

Zileuton (A reduced dose of cilostazol should be considered when taken concomitantly with CYP3A4 inhibitors). Products include:
- Zyflo Tablets ... 1023

Food Interactions

Food, unspecified (Co-administration with a high-fat meal increases absorption, with an approximately 90% increase in Cmax and a 25% increase in AUC; patients should be advised to take Pletal at least one hour before or two hours after breakfast and dinner).

Grapefruit (A reduced dose of cilostazol should be considered when taken concomitantly with CYP3A4 inhibitors).

Grapefruit Juice (Co-administration of cilostazol with inhibitors of CYP3A4, such as grapefruit juice, increase cilostazol plasma concentration by 50%; concurrent consumption of grapefruit juice should be avoided).

PLEXION CLEANSER
(Sodium Sulfacetamide, Sulfur) ... 1889
None cited in PDR database.

PLEXION CLEANSING CLOTHS
(Sodium Sulfacetamide, Sulfur) ... 1889
None cited in PDR database.

PLEXION SCT
(Sodium Sulfacetamide, Sulfur) ... 1889
None cited in PDR database.

PLEXION TOPICAL SUSPENSION
(Sodium Sulfacetamide, Sulfur) ... 1889
None cited in PDR database.

PLUS WITH AMBROTOSE COMPLEX CAPLETS
(Amino Acid Preparations) ... ▣831
None cited in PDR database.

PNEUMOVAX 23
(Pneumococcal Vaccine, Polyvalent) ... 2043
May interact with:

Azathioprine (Co-administration of vaccine in patients receiving immunosuppressive therapy may not result in expected serum antibody response; potential impairment of future immune responses to pneumococcal antigens may occur).
No products indexed under this heading.

Cyclosporine (Co-administration of vaccine in patients receiving immunosuppressive therapy may not result in expected serum antibody response; potential impairment of future immune responses to pneumococcal antigens may occur). Products include:
- Gengraf Capsules ... 459
- Neoral Oral Solution ... 2259
- Neoral Soft Gelatin Capsules ... 2259
- Restasis Ophthalmic Emulsion ... 575
- Sandimmune ... 2275

Muromonab-CD3 (Co-administration of vaccine in patients receiving immunosuppressive therapy may not result in expected serum antibody response; potential impairment of future immune responses to pneumococcal antigens may occur). Products include:
- Orthoclone OKT3 Sterile Solution ... 2360

Mycophenolate Mofetil (Co-administration of vaccine in patients receiving immunosuppressive therapy may not result in expected serum antibody response; potential impairment of future immune responses to pneumococcal antigens may occur). Products include:
- CellCept Capsules ... 2747
- CellCept Oral Suspension ... 2747
- CellCept Tablets ... 2747

Tacrolimus (Co-administration of vaccine in patients receiving immunosuppressive therapy may not result in expected serum antibody response; potential impairment of future immune responses to pneumococcal antigens may occur). Products include:
- Prograf Capsules and Injection ... 632
- Protopic Ointment ... 638

PODOCON-25 LIQUID
(Podophyllin, Tincture of Benzoin) ... 2478
None cited in PDR database.

POLY-PRED OPHTHALMIC SUSPENSION
(Neomycin Sulfate, Polymyxin B Sulfate, Prednisolone Acetate) ... ⊙233
None cited in PDR database.

POLYSPORIN FIRST AID ANTIBIOTIC OINTMENT
(Bacitracin, Polymyxin B Sulfate) ... ▣643
None cited in PDR database.

POLYTRIM OPHTHALMIC SOLUTION
(Polymyxin B Sulfate, Trimethoprim Sulfate) ... 574
None cited in PDR database.

POTABA CAPSULES
(Aminobenzoate Potassium) ... 1650
May interact with sulfonamides. Compounds in these categories include:

Bendroflumethiazide (Co-administration with sulfonamides is contraindicated).
No products indexed under this heading.

Chlorothiazide (Co-administration with sulfonamides is contraindicated). Products include:
- Diuril Oral Suspension ... 1954

Chlorothiazide Sodium (Co-administration with sulfonamides is contraindicated). Products include:
- Diuril Sodium Intravenous ... 2467

Chlorpropamide (Co-administration with sulfonamides is contraindicated).
No products indexed under this heading.

Glipizide (Co-administration with sulfonamides is contraindicated).
No products indexed under this heading.

Glyburide (Co-administration with sulfonamides is contraindicated).
No products indexed under this heading.

Hydrochlorothiazide (Co-administration with sulfonamides is contraindicated). Products include:
- Aldoril Tablets ... 1910
- Atacand HCT ... 651
- Avalide Tablets ... 888
- Avalide Tablets ... 2874
- Benicar HCT Tablets ... 1044
- Diovan HCT Tablets ... 2196
- Dyazide Capsules ... 1423
- Hyzaar 50-12.5 Tablets ... 1990
- Hyzaar 100-12.5 Tablets ... 1990
- Hyzaar 100-25 Tablets ... 1990
- Lopressor HCT 50/25 Tablets ... 2241
- Lopressor HCT 100/25 Tablets ... 2241
- Lopressor HCT 100/50 Tablets ... 2241
- Lotensin HCT Tablets ... 2246
- Micardis HCT Tablets ... 856
- Moduretic Tablets ... 2028
- Prinzide Tablets ... 2056

Teveten HCT Tablets 1737
Timolide Tablets 2086
Uniretic Tablets 3100

Hydroflumethiazide (Co-administration with sulfonamides is contraindicated).
No products indexed under this heading.

Methyclothiazide (Co-administration with sulfonamides is contraindicated).
No products indexed under this heading.

Polythiazide (Co-administration with sulfonamides is contraindicated).
No products indexed under this heading.

Sulfacytine (Co-administration with sulfonamides is contraindicated).
No products indexed under this heading.

Sulfamethizole (Co-administration with sulfonamides is contraindicated).
No products indexed under this heading.

Sulfamethoxazole (Co-administration with sulfonamides is contraindicated).
No products indexed under this heading.

Sulfasalazine (Co-administration with sulfonamides is contraindicated).
No products indexed under this heading.

Sulfinpyrazone (Co-administration with sulfonamides is contraindicated).
No products indexed under this heading.

Sulfisoxazole Acetyl (Co-administration with sulfonamides is contraindicated).
No products indexed under this heading.

Sulfisoxazole Diolamine (Co-administration with sulfonamides is contraindicated).
No products indexed under this heading.

Tolazamide (Co-administration with sulfonamides is contraindicated).
No products indexed under this heading.

Tolbutamide (Co-administration with sulfonamides is contraindicated).
No products indexed under this heading.

POTABA ENVULES

(Aminobenzoate Potassium) 1650
See Potaba Capsules

POTABA TABLETS

(Aminobenzoate Potassium) 1650
See Potaba Capsules

PRAMOSONE CREAM 1% AND 2.5%

(Hydrocortisone Acetate, Pramoxine Hydrochloride).................. 1161
None cited in PDR database.

PRAMOSONE LOTION 1% AND 2.5%

(Hydrocortisone Acetate, Pramoxine Hydrochloride).................. 1161
See Pramosone Cream 1% and 2.5%

PRAMOSONE OINTMENT 1% AND 2.5%

(Hydrocortisone Acetate, Pramoxine Hydrochloride).................. 1161
See Pramosone Cream 1% and 2.5%

PRECOSE TABLETS

(Acarbose) 751
May interact with calcium channel blockers, corticosteroids, estrogens, oral contraceptives, phenothiazines, phenytoin, sympathomimetics, thiazides, thyroid preparations, and certain other agents. Compounds in these categories include:

Albuterol (Sympathomimetics tend to produce hyperglycemia leading to loss of control; patients on concurrent therapy should be closely observed for loss of control). Products include:
Proventil Inhalation Aerosol 3053

Albuterol Sulfate (Sympathomimetics tend to produce hyperglycemia leading to loss of control; patients on concurrent therapy should be closely observed for loss of control). Products include:
AccuNeb Inhalation Solution 1055
Combivent Inhalation Aerosol 847
DuoNeb Inhalation Solution 1058
ProAir HFA Inhalation Aerosol 3300
Proventil Inhalation Solution 0.083%.. 3055
Proventil HFA Inhalation Aerosol 3056
Ventolin HFA Inhalation Aerosol 1600
VoSpire ER Tablets 1052

Amlodipine Besylate (Calcium channel blockers tend to produce hyperglycemia leading to loss of control; patients on concurrent therapy should be closely observed for loss of control). Products include:
Caduet Tablets 2508
Lotrel Capsules 2249
Norvasc Tablets 2545

Amylase (Amylase, a carbohydrate splitting enzyme, may reduce the effect of acarbose and should not be taken concurrently).
No products indexed under this heading.

Bendroflumethiazide (Thiazide diuretics tend to produce hyperglycemia leading to loss of control; patients on concurrent therapy should be closely observed for loss of control).
No products indexed under this heading.

Bepridil Hydrochloride (Calcium channel blockers tend to produce hyperglycemia leading to loss of control; patients on concurrent therapy should be closely observed for loss of control).
No products indexed under this heading.

Betamethasone Acetate (Corticosteroids tend to produce hyperglycemia leading to loss of control; patients on concurrent therapy should be closely observed for loss of control).
No products indexed under this heading.

Betamethasone Sodium Phosphate (Corticosteroids tend to produce hyperglycemia leading to loss of control; patients on concurrent therapy should be closely observed for loss of control).
No products indexed under this heading.

Charcoal, Activated (Charcoal, an intestinal adsorbent, may reduce the effect of acarbose and should not be taken concurrently).
No products indexed under this heading.

Chlorothiazide (Thiazide diuretics tend to produce hyperglycemia leading to loss of control; patients on concurrent therapy should be closely observed for loss of control). Products include:
Diuril Oral Suspension 1954

Chlorothiazide Sodium (Thiazide diuretics tend to produce hyperglycemia leading to loss of control; patients on concurrent therapy should be closely observed for loss of control). Products include:
Diuril Sodium Intravenous 2467

Chlorotrianisene (Estrogens tend to produce hyperglycemia leading to loss of control; patients on concurrent therapy should be closely observed for loss of control).
No products indexed under this heading.

Chlorpromazine (Phenothiazines tend to produce hyperglycemia leading to loss of control; patients on concurrent therapy should be closely observed for loss of control).
No products indexed under this heading.

Chlorpromazine Hydrochloride (Phenothiazines tend to produce hyperglycemia leading to loss of control; patients on concurrent therapy should be closely observed for loss of control).
No products indexed under this heading.

Cortisone Acetate (Corticosteroids tend to produce hyperglycemia leading to loss of control; patients on concurrent therapy should be closely observed for loss of control).
No products indexed under this heading.

Desogestrel (Oral contraceptives tend to produce hyperglycemia leading to loss of control; patients on concurrent therapy should be closely observed for loss of control). Products include:
Mircette Tablets 1066

Dexamethasone (Corticosteroids tend to produce hyperglycemia leading to loss of control; patients on concurrent therapy should be closely observed for loss of control). Products include:
Ciprodex Otic Suspension 559
Decadron Tablets 1951
TobraDex Ophthalmic Ointment 562
TobraDex Ophthalmic Suspension 563

Dexamethasone Acetate (Corticosteroids tend to produce hyperglycemia leading to loss of control; patients on concurrent therapy should be closely observed for loss of control).
No products indexed under this heading.

Dexamethasone Sodium Phosphate (Corticosteroids tend to produce hyperglycemia leading to loss of control; patients on concurrent therapy should be closely observed for loss of control).
No products indexed under this heading.

Dienestrol (Estrogens tend to produce hyperglycemia leading to loss of control; patients on concurrent therapy should be closely observed for loss of control).
No products indexed under this heading.

Diethylstilbestrol (Estrogens tend to produce hyperglycemia leading to loss of control; patients on concurrent therapy should be closely observed for loss of control).
No products indexed under this heading.

Digoxin (Precose has been shown to change the bioavailability of digoxin when they are co-administered, which may require digoxin dose adjustment). Products include:
Lanoxicaps Capsules 1490
Lanoxin Injection 1494
Lanoxin Injection Pediatric 1497
Lanoxin Tablets 1500

Diltiazem Hydrochloride (Calcium channel blockers tend to produce hyperglycemia leading to loss of control; patients on concurrent therapy should be closely observed for loss of control). Products include:
Cardizem LA Extended Release Tablets 1728
Tiazac Capsules 1201

Dobutamine Hydrochloride (Sympathomimetics tend to produce hyperglycemia leading to loss of control; patients on concurrent therapy should be closely observed for loss of control).
No products indexed under this heading.

Dopamine Hydrochloride (Sympathomimetics tend to produce hyperglycemia leading to loss of control; patients on concurrent therapy should be closely observed for loss of control).
No products indexed under this heading.

Ephedrine Hydrochloride (Sympathomimetics tend to produce hyperglycemia leading to loss of control; patients on concurrent therapy should be closely observed for loss of control).
No products indexed under this heading.

Ephedrine Sulfate (Sympathomimetics tend to produce hyperglycemia leading to loss of control; patients on concurrent therapy should be closely observed for loss of control).
No products indexed under this heading.

Ephedrine Tannate (Sympathomimetics tend to produce hyperglycemia leading to loss of control; patients on concurrent therapy should be closely observed for loss of control).
No products indexed under this heading.

Epinephrine (Sympathomimetics tend to produce hyperglycemia leading to loss of control; patients on concurrent therapy should be closely observed for loss of control). Products include:
EpiPen 1061
Primatene Mist 719
Twinject 0.15 3379
Twinject 0.3 3378

Epinephrine Bitartrate (Sympathomimetics tend to produce hyperglycemia leading to loss of control; patients on concurrent therapy should be closely observed for loss of control).
No products indexed under this heading.

Epinephrine Hydrochloride (Sympathomimetics tend to produce hyperglycemia leading to loss of control; patients on concurrent therapy should be closely observed for loss of control).
No products indexed under this heading.

Estradiol (Estrogens tend to produce hyperglycemia leading to loss of control; patients on concurrent therapy should be closely observed for loss of control). Products include:
Angeliq Tablets ... 762
Climara Transdermal System ... 771
Climara Pro Transdermal System ... 776
Estrasorb Topical Emulsion ... 1147
Estring Vaginal Ring ... 2635
Menostar Transdermal System ... 782
Vagifem Tablets ... 2334

Estrogens, Conjugated (Estrogens tend to produce hyperglycemia leading to loss of control; patients on concurrent therapy should be closely observed for loss of control). Products include:
Premarin Intravenous ... 3442
Premarin Tablets ... 3446
Premarin Vaginal Cream ... 3452
Premphase Tablets ... 3456
Prempro Tablets ... 3456

Estrogens, Esterified (Estrogens tend to produce hyperglycemia leading to loss of control; patients on concurrent therapy should be closely observed for loss of control). Products include:
Estratest Tablets ... 3199
Estratest H.S. Tablets ... 3199

Estropipate (Estrogens tend to produce hyperglycemia leading to loss of control; patients on concurrent therapy should be closely observed for loss of control).
No products indexed under this heading.

Ethinyl Estradiol (Estrogens tend to produce hyperglycemia leading to loss of control; patients on concurrent therapy should be closely observed for loss of control). Products include:
Mircette Tablets ... 1066
NuvaRing ... 2340
Ortho-Cyclen/Ortho Tri-Cyclen ... 2429
Ortho Evra Transdermal System ... 2417
Ortho Tri-Cyclen Lo Tablets ... 2436
Seasonique Tablets ... 1077
Yasmin 28 Tablets ... 796
Yaz Tablets ... 803

Ethynodiol Diacetate (Oral contraceptives tend to produce hyperglycemia leading to loss of control; patients on concurrent therapy should be closely observed for loss of control).
No products indexed under this heading.

Felodipine (Calcium channel blockers tend to produce hyperglycemia leading to loss of control; patients on concurrent therapy should be closely observed for loss of control).
No products indexed under this heading.

Fludrocortisone Acetate (Corticosteroids tend to produce hyperglycemia leading to loss of control; patients on concurrent therapy should be closely observed for loss of control).
No products indexed under this heading.

Fluphenazine Decanoate (Phenothiazines tend to produce hyperglycemia leading to loss of control; patients on concurrent therapy should be closely observed for loss of control).
No products indexed under this heading.

Fluphenazine Enanthate (Phenothiazines tend to produce hyperglycemia leading to loss of control; patients on concurrent therapy should be closely observed for loss of control).
No products indexed under this heading.

Fluphenazine Hydrochloride (Phenothiazines tend to produce hyperglycemia leading to loss of control; patients on concurrent therapy should be closely observed for loss of control).
No products indexed under this heading.

Fosphenytoin Sodium (Phenytoin tends to produce hyperglycemia leading to loss of control; patients on concurrent therapy should be closely observed for loss of control).
No products indexed under this heading.

Hydrochlorothiazide (Thiazide diuretics tend to produce hyperglycemia leading to loss of control; patients on concurrent therapy should be closely observed for loss of control). Products include:
Aldoril Tablets ... 1910
Atacand HCT ... 651
Avalide Tablets ... 888
Avalide Tablets ... 2874
Benicar HCT Tablets ... 1044
Diovan HCT Tablets ... 2196
Dyazide Capsules ... 1423
Hyzaar 50-12.5 Tablets ... 1990
Hyzaar 100-12.5 Tablets ... 1990
Hyzaar 100-25 Tablets ... 1990
Lopressor HCT 50/25 Tablets ... 2241
Lopressor HCT 100/25 Tablets ... 2241
Lopressor HCT 100/50 Tablets ... 2241
Lotensin HCT Tablets ... 2246
Micardis HCT Tablets ... 856
Moduretic Tablets ... 2028
Prinzide Tablets ... 2056
Teveten HCT Tablets ... 1737
Timolide Tablets ... 2086
Uniretic Tablets ... 3100

Hydrocortisone (Corticosteroids tend to produce hyperglycemia leading to loss of control; patients on concurrent therapy should be closely observed for loss of control). Products include:
Colocort Rectal Suspension, USP (Retention) 100 mg/60 mL ... 2476
Hydrocortone Tablets ... 1989
Preparation H Hydrocortisone Cream ... ▣ 646

Hydrocortisone Acetate (Corticosteroids tend to produce hyperglycemia leading to loss of control; patients on concurrent therapy should be closely observed for loss of control). Products include:
Analpram-HC ... 1159
Pramosone ... 1161
ProctoFoam-HC ... 3099

Hydrocortisone Sodium Phosphate (Corticosteroids tend to produce hyperglycemia leading to loss of control; patients on concurrent therapy should be closely observed for loss of control).
No products indexed under this heading.

Hydrocortisone Sodium Succinate (Corticosteroids tend to produce hyperglycemia leading to loss of control; patients on concurrent therapy should be closely observed for loss of control).
No products indexed under this heading.

Hydroflumethiazide (Thiazide diuretics tend to produce hyperglycemia leading to loss of control; patients on concurrent therapy should be closely observed for loss of control).
No products indexed under this heading.

Isoniazid (Isoniazid tends to produce hyperglycemia leading to loss of control; patients on concurrent therapy should be closely observed for loss of control).
No products indexed under this heading.

Isoproterenol Hydrochloride (Sympathomimetics tend to produce hyperglycemia leading to loss of control; patients on concurrent therapy should be closely observed for loss of control).
No products indexed under this heading.

Isoproterenol Sulfate (Sympathomimetics tend to produce hyperglycemia leading to loss of control; patients on concurrent therapy should be closely observed for loss of control).
No products indexed under this heading.

Isradipine (Calcium channel blockers tend to produce hyperglycemia leading to loss of control; patients on concurrent therapy should be closely observed for loss of control). Products include:
DynaCirc CR Tablets ... 2721

Levalbuterol Hydrochloride (Sympathomimetics tend to produce hyperglycemia leading to loss of control; patients on concurrent therapy should be closely observed for loss of control). Products include:
Xopenex Inhalation Solution ... 3146
Xopenex Inhalation Solution Concentrate ... 3150

Levonorgestrel (Oral contraceptives tend to produce hyperglycemia leading to loss of control; patients on concurrent therapy should be closely observed for loss of control). Products include:
Climara Pro Transdermal System ... 776
Mirena Intrauterine System ... 787
Plan B Tablets ... 1076
Seasonique Tablets ... 1077

Levothyroxine Sodium (Thyroid products tend to produce hyperglycemia leading to loss of control; patients on concurrent therapy should be closely observed for loss of control). Products include:
Levothroid Tablets ... 1186
Levoxyl Tablets ... 1712
Synthroid Tablets ... 520
Westhroid Tablets ... 3403

Liothyronine Sodium (Thyroid products tend to produce hyperglycemia leading to loss of control; patients on concurrent therapy should be closely observed for loss of control). Products include:
Cytomel Tablets ... 1710
Westhroid Tablets ... 3403

Liotrix (Thyroid products tend to produce hyperglycemia leading to loss of control; patients on concurrent therapy should be closely observed for loss of control). Products include:
Thyrolar Tablets ... 1199

Mesoridazine Besylate (Phenothiazines tend to produce hyperglycemia leading to loss of control; patients on concurrent therapy should be closely observed for loss of control).
No products indexed under this heading.

Mestranol (Oral contraceptives tend to produce hyperglycemia leading to loss of control; patients on concurrent therapy should be closely observed for loss of control).
No products indexed under this heading.

Metaproterenol Sulfate (Sympathomimetics tend to produce hyperglycemia leading to loss of control; patients on concurrent therapy should be closely observed for loss of control). Products include:
Alupent Inhalation Aerosol ... 826

Metaraminol Bitartrate (Sympathomimetics tend to produce hyperglycemia leading to loss of control; patients on concurrent therapy should be closely observed for loss of control).
No products indexed under this heading.

Methotrimeprazine (Phenothiazines tend to produce hyperglycemia leading to loss of control; patients on concurrent therapy should be closely observed for loss of control).
No products indexed under this heading.

Methoxamine Hydrochloride (Sympathomimetics tend to produce hyperglycemia leading to loss of control; patients on concurrent therapy should be closely observed for loss of control).
No products indexed under this heading.

Methyclothiazide (Thiazide diuretics tend to produce hyperglycemia leading to loss of control; patients on concurrent therapy should be closely observed for loss of control).
No products indexed under this heading.

Methylprednisolone Acetate (Corticosteroids tend to produce hyperglycemia leading to loss of control; patients on concurrent therapy should be closely observed for loss of control). Products include:
Depo-Medrol Injectable Suspension ... 2617
Depo-Medrol Single-Dose Vial ... 2619

Methylprednisolone Sodium Succinate (Corticosteroids tend to produce hyperglycemia leading to loss of control; patients on concurrent therapy should be closely observed for loss of control).
No products indexed under this heading.

Mibefradil Dihydrochloride (Calcium channel blockers tend to produce hyperglycemia leading to loss of control; patients on concurrent therapy should be closely observed for loss of control).
No products indexed under this heading.

Nicardipine Hydrochloride (Calcium channel blockers tend to produce hyperglycemia leading to loss of control; patients on concurrent therapy should be closely observed for loss of control). Products include:
Cardene I.V. ... 2497

Nicotinic Acid (Nicotinic acid tends to produce hyperglycemia leading to loss of control; patients on concurrent therapy should be closely observed for loss of control).
No products indexed under this heading.

Nifedipine (Calcium channel blockers tend to produce hyperglycemia leading to loss of control; patients on concurrent therapy should be closely observed for loss of control). Products include:
Adalat CC Tablets ... 2964

Nimodipine (Calcium channel blockers tend to produce hyperglycemia leading to loss of control; patients on concurrent therapy should be closely observed for loss of control). Products include:
Nimotop Capsules ... 749

Nisoldipine (Calcium channel blockers tend to produce hyperglycemia leading to loss of control; patients on concurrent therapy should be closely observed for loss of control). Products include:
Sular Tablets ... 3122

Norepinephrine Bitartrate (Sympathomimetics tend to produce hyperglycemia leading to loss of control; patients on concurrent therapy should be closely observed for loss of control).
No products indexed under this heading.

Norethindrone (Oral contraceptives tend to produce hyperglycemia leading to loss of control; patients on concurrent therapy should be closely observed for loss of control). Products include:
Ortho Micronor Tablets ... 2426

Norethynodrel (Oral contraceptives tend to produce hyperglycemia leading to loss of control; patients on concurrent therapy should be closely observed for loss of control).
No products indexed under this heading.

Norgestimate (Oral contraceptives tend to produce hyperglycemia leading to loss of control; patients on concurrent therapy should be closely observed for loss of control). Products include:
Ortho-Cyclen/Ortho Tri-Cyclen ... 2429
Ortho Tri-Cyclen Lo Tablets ... 2436

Norgestrel (Oral contraceptives tend to produce hyperglycemia leading to loss of control; patients on concurrent therapy should be closely observed for loss of control).
No products indexed under this heading.

Pancreatin (Pancreatin, a carbohydrate splitting enzyme, may reduce the effect of acarbose and should not be taken concurrently).
No products indexed under this heading.

Perphenazine (Phenothiazines tend to produce hyperglycemia leading to loss of control; patients on concurrent therapy should be closely observed for loss of control).
No products indexed under this heading.

Phenylephrine Bitartrate (Sympathomimetics tend to produce hyperglycemia leading to loss of control; patients on concurrent therapy should be closely observed for loss of control).
No products indexed under this heading.

Phenylephrine Hydrochloride (Sympathomimetics tend to produce hyperglycemia leading to loss of control; patients on concurrent therapy should be closely observed for loss of control). Products include:
Comtrex Maximum Strength Non-Drowsy Cold & Cough Caplets ... 725
Comtrex Maximum Strength Day/Night Severe Cold & Sinus Caplets - Day Formulation ... 725
Comtrex Maximum Strength Day/Night Severe Cold & Sinus Caplets - Night Formulation ... 725
Contac Cold and Flu Maximum Strength Caplets ... 728
Contac Cold and Flu Day and Night Caplets (Day Formulation Only) ... 727
Contac Cold and Flu Day and Night Caplets (Night Formulation Only) ... 727
Contac Cold and Flu Non-Drowsy Caplets ... 728
Contac-D Cold Non-Drowsy Tablets ... 729
Children's Dimetapp Cold & Allergy Elixir ... 730
Children's Dimetapp Cold & Allergy Chewable Tablets ... 730
Children's Dimetapp DM Cold & Cough Elixir ... 731
Toddler's Dimetapp Cold and Cough Drops ... 732
Excedrin Sinus Headache Caplets/Tablets ... 610
4-Way Fast Acting Nasal Spray ... 775
4-Way Menthol Nasal Spray ... 775
Preparation H Maximum Strength Cream ... 666
Preparation H Cooling Gel ... 666
Preparation H ... 666
Refenesen PE Caplets ... 721
Robitussin Cough & Allergy Syrup .. 736
Robitussin Cough & Cold Nighttime Liquid ... 736
Robitussin Cough, Cold & Flu Nighttime Liquid ... 738
Robitussin Head & Chest Congestion PE Syrup ... 739
Robitussin Pediatric Cough & Cold Nighttime Liquid ... 736
TheraFlu Cold & Cough Hot Liquid ... 740
TheraFlu Cold & Sore Throat Hot Liquid ... 741
TheraFlu Flu & Sore Throat Hot Liquid ... 742
TheraFlu Daytime Severe Cold Hot Liquid ... 742
TheraFlu Nighttime Severe Cold Hot Liquid ... 740
TheraFlu Warming Relief Daytime Severe Cold ... 743
TheraFlu Warming Relief Nighttime Severe Cold ... 743
Triaminic Chest & Nasal Congestion Liquid ... 746
Triaminic Cold & Allergy Liquid ... 746
Triaminic Daytime Cold & Cough Liquid ... 745
Triaminic Nighttime Cold & Cough Liquid ... 746
Triaminic Thin Strips Cold ... 748
Triaminic Thin Strips Cold & Cough ... 778
Triaminic Infant Thin Strips Decongestant ... 747
Triaminic Infant Thin Strips Decongestant Plus Cough ... 747
Children's Tylenol Plus Flu Oral Suspension ... 749
Tylenol Cold Head Congestion Daytime Caplets with Cool Burst and Gelcaps ... 750
Tylenol Cold Multi-Symptom Daytime Liquid ... 752
Tylenol Cold Multi-Symptom Severe Daytime Liquid ... 752
Concentrated Tylenol Infants' Drops Plus Cold & Cough ... 754
Tylenol Allergy Multi-Symptom Caplets with Cool Burst and Gelcaps ... 1872
Tylenol Allergy Multi-Symptom Nighttime Caplets with Cool Burst ... 1872
Children's Tylenol Plus Cold Suspension Liquid ... 1879
Children's Tylenol Plus Cold & Allergy Suspension Liquid ... 1878
Children's Tylenol Plus Flu Suspension Liquid ... 1881
Children's Tylenol Plus Multi-Symptom Cold Suspension Liquid ... 1879
Tylenol Cold Head Congestion Daytime Caplets with Cool Burst ... 1873
Tylenol Cold Head Congestion Nighttime Caplets with Cool Burst ... 1873
Tylenol Cold Head Congestion Severe Caplets with Cool Burst ... 1873
Tylenol Cold Multi-Symptom Daytime Caplets with Cool Burst and Gelcaps ... 1874
Tylenol Cold Multi-Symptom Daytime Liquid with Citrus Burst ... 1874
Tylenol Cold Multi-Symptom Nighttime Caplets with Cool Burst ... 1874
Tylenol Cold Multi-Symptom Nighttime Liquid with Cool Burst ... 1874
Tylenol Cold Multi-Symptom Severe Caplets with Cool Burst ... 1874
Tylenol Cold Multi-Symptom Severe Daytime Liquid with Citrus Burst ... 1874
Tylenol Sinus Congestion & Pain Daytime Caplets with Cool Burst and Gelcaps ... 1876
Tylenol Sinus Congestion & Pain Nighttime Caplets with Cool Burst ... 1876
Tylenol Sinus Congestion & Pain Severe Caplets with Cool Burst ... 1876
Vicks 44D Cough & Head Congestion Relief Liquid ... 760
Vicks DayQuil LiquiCaps/Liquid Multi-Symptom Cold/Flu Relief ... 761
Zicam Cough Plus D Cough Spray ... 767

Phenylephrine Tannate (Sympathomimetics tend to produce hyperglycemia leading to loss of control; patients on concurrent therapy should be closely observed for loss of control).
No products indexed under this heading.

Phenylpropanolamine Hydrochloride (Sympathomimetics tend to produce hyperglycemia leading to loss of control; patients on concurrent therapy should be closely observed for loss of control).
No products indexed under this heading.

Phenytoin (Phenytoin tends to produce hyperglycemia leading to loss of control; patients on concurrent therapy should be closely observed for loss of control).
No products indexed under this heading.

Phenytoin Sodium (Phenytoin tends to produce hyperglycemia leading to loss of control; patients on concurrent therapy should be closely observed for loss of control). Products include:
Phenytek Capsules ... 2160

Pirbuterol Acetate (Sympathomimetics tend to produce hyperglycemia leading to loss of control; patients on concurrent therapy should be closely observed for loss of control). Products include:
Maxair Autohaler ... 1852

Polyestradiol Phosphate (Estrogens tend to produce hyperglycemia leading to loss of control; patients on concurrent therapy should be closely observed for loss of control).
No products indexed under this heading.

Polythiazide (Thiazide diuretics tend to produce hyperglycemia leading to loss of control; patients on concurrent therapy should be closely observed for loss of control).
No products indexed under this heading.

Prednisolone Acetate (Corticosteroids tend to produce hyperglycemia leading to loss of control; patients on concurrent therapy should be closely observed for loss of control). Products include:
Blephamide Ophthalmic Ointment 568
Blephamide Ophthalmic Suspension ... 569
Poly-Pred Ophthalmic Suspension ... ⊙233
Pred Forte Ophthalmic Suspension ... ⊙235
Pred Mild Ophthalmic Suspension ... ⊙238
Pred-G Ophthalmic Ointment ... ⊙237
Pred-G Ophthalmic Suspension ... ⊙236

Prednisolone Sodium Phosphate (Corticosteroids tend to produce hyperglycemia leading to loss of control; patients on concurrent therapy should be closely observed for loss of control).
No products indexed under this heading.

Prednisolone Tebutate (Corticosteroids tend to produce hyperglycemia leading to loss of control; patients on concurrent therapy should be closely observed for loss of control).
No products indexed under this heading.

Prednisone (Corticosteroids tend to produce hyperglycemia leading to loss of control; patients on concurrent therapy should be closely observed for loss of control).
No products indexed under this heading.

Prochlorperazine (Phenothiazines tend to produce hyperglycemia leading to loss of control; patients on concurrent therapy should be closely observed for loss of control).
No products indexed under this heading.

Promethazine Hydrochloride (Phenothiazines tend to produce hyperglycemia leading to loss of control; patients on concurrent therapy should be closely observed for loss of control). Products include:
Phenergan Tablets and Suppositories ... 3440

Pseudoephedrine Hydrochloride (Sympathomimetics tend to produce hyperglycemia leading to loss of control; patients on concurrent therapy should be closely observed for loss of control). Products include:
Advil Allergy Sinus Caplets ... 770
Advil Cold & Sinus ... 723
Advil Multi-Symptom Cold Caplets ... 770
Aleve Cold & Sinus Caplets ... 744

Allegra-D 12 Hour Extended-Release Tablets 2846
Allegra-D 24 Hour Extended-Release Tablets 2849
BC Cold Powder .... ▣677
Comtrex Maximum Strength Cold & Cough Day/Night Caplets - Day Formulation .... ▣726
Comtrex Maximum Strength Cold & Cough Day/Night Caplets - Night Formulation .... ▣726
Children's Motrin Cold Oral Suspension 1867
Mucinex D Extended-Release Bi-Layer Tablets .... ▣776
Robitussin Cough & Cold CF Liquid .... ▣735
Robitussin Cough & Cold Pediatric Drops .... ▣735
Tylenol Sinus Congestion & Pain Nighttime Caplets with Cool Burst .... ▣778
Tylenol Cold Severe Congestion Non-Drowsy Caplets with Cool Burst 1874
Tylenol Sinus Severe Congestion Caplets with Cool Burst 1876
Vicks 44D Cough & Head Congestion Relief Liquid 2679
Vicks 44M Cough, Cold & Flu Relief Liquid 2680
Vicks DayQuil Multi-Symptom Cold/Flu Relief LiquiCaps 2678
Vicks DayQuil Multi-Symptom Cold/Flu Relief Liquid 2678
Vicks NyQuil Multi-Symptom Cold/Flu Relief Liquid 2681
Vicks NyQuil Multi-Symptom Cold/Flu Relief LiquiCaps 2681
Children's Vicks NyQuil Cold/Cough Relief Liquid 2680
Zyrtec-D 12 Hour Extended Release Tablets 2597

Pseudoephedrine Sulfate (Sympathomimetics tend to produce hyperglycemia leading to loss of control; patients on concurrent therapy should be closely observed for loss of control). Products include:
Alavert Allergy & Sinus D-12 Hour Tablets .... ▣771
Clarinex-D 24-Hour Extended-Release Tablets 2998
Claritin-D Non-Drowsy 12 Hour Tablets .... ▣772
Claritin-D Non-Drowsy 24 Hour Tablets .... ▣772

Quinestrol (Estrogens tend to produce hyperglycemia leading to loss of control; patients on concurrent therapy should be closely observed for loss of control).
No products indexed under this heading.

Salmeterol Xinafoate (Sympathomimetics tend to produce hyperglycemia leading to loss of control; patients on concurrent therapy should be closely observed for loss of control). Products include:
Advair Diskus 100/50 1308
Advair Diskus 250/50 1308
Advair Diskus 500/50 1308
Advair HFA Inhalation Aerosol 1318
Serevent Diskus 1568

Terbutaline Sulfate (Sympathomimetics tend to produce hyperglycemia leading to loss of control; patients on concurrent therapy should be closely observed for loss of control).
No products indexed under this heading.

Thioridazine Hydrochloride (Phenothiazines tend to produce hyperglycemia leading to loss of control; patients on concurrent therapy should be closely observed for loss of control). Products include:
Thioridazine Hydrochloride Tablets 2163

Thyroglobulin (Thyroid products tend to produce hyperglycemia leading to loss of control; patients on concurrent therapy should be closely observed for loss of control).
No products indexed under this heading.

Thyroid (Thyroid products tend to produce hyperglycemia leading to loss of control; patients on concurrent therapy should be closely observed for loss of control).
No products indexed under this heading.

Thyroxine (Thyroid products tend to produce hyperglycemia leading to loss of control; patients on concurrent therapy should be closely observed for loss of control).
No products indexed under this heading.

Thyroxine Sodium (Thyroid products tend to produce hyperglycemia leading to loss of control; patients on concurrent therapy should be closely observed for loss of control).
No products indexed under this heading.

Triamcinolone (Corticosteroids tend to produce hyperglycemia leading to loss of control; patients on concurrent therapy should be closely observed for loss of control).
No products indexed under this heading.

Triamcinolone Acetonide (Corticosteroids tend to produce hyperglycemia leading to loss of control; patients on concurrent therapy should be closely observed for loss of control). Products include:
Azmacort Inhalation Aerosol 1726
Nasacort AQ Nasal Spray 2922

Triamcinolone Diacetate (Corticosteroids tend to produce hyperglycemia leading to loss of control; patients on concurrent therapy should be closely observed for loss of control).
No products indexed under this heading.

Triamcinolone Hexacetonide (Corticosteroids tend to produce hyperglycemia leading to loss of control; patients on concurrent therapy should be closely observed for loss of control).
No products indexed under this heading.

Trifluoperazine Hydrochloride (Phenothiazines tend to produce hyperglycemia leading to loss of control; patients on concurrent therapy should be closely observed for loss of control).
No products indexed under this heading.

Verapamil Hydrochloride (Calcium channel blockers tend to produce hyperglycemia leading to loss of control; patients on concurrent therapy should be closely observed for loss of control). Products include:
Covera-HS Tablets 3139
Tarka Tablets 524
Verelan PM Extended-Release Capsules, Controlled-Onset 3106

PRED FORTE OPHTHALMIC SUSPENSION

(Prednisolone Acetate) .... ⊙235
None cited in PDR database.

PRED MILD OPHTHALMIC SUSPENSION

(Prednisolone Acetate) .... ⊙238
None cited in PDR database.

PRED-G OPHTHALMIC OINTMENT

(Gentamicin Sulfate, Prednisolone Acetate) .... ⊙237
None cited in PDR database.

PRED-G OPHTHALMIC SUSPENSION

(Gentamicin Sulfate, Prednisolone Acetate) .... ⊙236
None cited in PDR database.

PREMARIN INTRAVENOUS

(Estrogens, Conjugated) 3442
See Premarin Tablets

PREMARIN TABLETS

(Estrogens, Conjugated) 3446
May interact with cytochrome p450 3a4 inducers (selected), cytochrome p450 3a4 inhibitors (selected), and certain other agents. Compounds in these categories include:

Acetazolamide (Co-administration of inhibitors of CYP3A4 with estrogens may affect estrogen drug metabolism. Inhibitors of CYP3A4 may increase plasma concentrations of estrogens and may result in side effects).
No products indexed under this heading.

Allium sativum (Co-administration of inducers of CYP3A4 with estrogens may affect estrogen drug metabolism. Inducers of CYP3A4 may reduce plasma concentrations of estrogens, possibly resulting in a decrease in therapeutic effects and/or changes in the uterine bleeding profile).
No products indexed under this heading.

Amiodarone Hydrochloride (Co-administration of inhibitors of CYP3A4 with estrogens may affect estrogen drug metabolism. Inhibitors of CYP3A4 may increase plasma concentrations of estrogens and may result in side effects).
No products indexed under this heading.

Amprenavir (Co-administration of inhibitors of CYP3A4 with estrogens may affect estrogen drug metabolism. Inhibitors of CYP3A4 may increase plasma concentrations of estrogens and may result in side effects). Products include:
Agenerase Capsules 1327
Agenerase Oral Solution 1332

Anastrozole (Co-administration of inhibitors of CYP3A4 with estrogens may affect estrogen drug metabolism. Inhibitors of CYP3A4 may increase plasma concentrations of estrogens and may result in side effects). Products include:
Arimidex Tablets 673

Aprepitant (Co-administration of inducers of CYP3A4 with estrogens may affect estrogen drug metabolism. Inducers of CYP3A4 may reduce plasma concentrations of estrogens, possibly resulting in a decrease in therapeutic effects and/or changes in the uterine bleeding profile). Products include:
Emend Capsules 1963

Betamethasone Acetate (Co-administration of inducers of CYP3A4 with estrogens may affect estrogen drug metabolism. Inducers of CYP3A4 may reduce plasma concentrations of estrogens, possibly resulting in a decrease in therapeutic effects and/or changes in the uterine bleeding profile).
No products indexed under this heading.

Betamethasone Sodium Phosphate (Co-administration of inducers of CYP3A4 with estrogens may affect estrogen drug metabolism. Inducers of CYP3A4 may reduce plasma concentrations of estrogens, possibly resulting in a decrease in therapeutic effects and/or changes in the uterine bleeding profile).
No products indexed under this heading.

Carbamazepine (Co-administration of inducers of CYP3A4 with estrogens may affect estrogen drug metabolism. Inducers of CYP3A4 may reduce plasma concentrations of estrogens, possibly resulting in a decrease in therapeutic effects and/or changes in the uterine bleeding profile). Products include:
Carbatrol Capsules 3171
Equetro Extended-Release Capsules 3180
Tegretol/Tegretol-XR 2295

Cimetidine (Co-administration of inhibitors of CYP3A4 with estrogens may affect estrogen drug metabolism. Inhibitors of CYP3A4 may increase plasma concentrations of estrogens and may result in side effects). Products include:
Tagamet HB 200 Tablets .... ▣664

Cimetidine Hydrochloride (Co-administration of inhibitors of CYP3A4 with estrogens may affect estrogen drug metabolism. Inhibitors of CYP3A4 may increase plasma concentrations of estrogens and may result in side effects).
No products indexed under this heading.

Ciprofloxacin (Co-administration of inhibitors of CYP3A4 with estrogens may affect estrogen drug metabolism. Inhibitors of CYP3A4 may increase plasma concentrations of estrogens and may result in side effects). Products include:
Cipro Oral Suspension 2977
Cipro I.V. 2984
Cipro XR Tablets 2990
Ciprodex Otic Suspension 559

Ciprofloxacin Hydrochloride (Co-administration of inducers of CYP3A4 with estrogens may affect estrogen drug metabolism. Inducers of CYP3A4 may reduce plasma concentrations of estrogens, possibly resulting in a decrease in therapeutic effects and/or changes in the uterine bleeding profile). Products include:
Ciloxan Ophthalmic Ointment 559
Ciloxan Ophthalmic Solution .... ⊙206
Cipro Tablets 2977
Proquin XR Tablets 1153

Cisplatin (Co-administration of inducers of CYP3A4 with estrogens may affect estrogen drug metabolism. Inducers of CYP3A4 may reduce plasma concentrations of estrogens, possibly resulting in a decrease in therapeutic effects and/or changes in the uterine bleeding profile).
No products indexed under this heading.

Clarithromycin (Co-administration of inhibitors of CYP3A4 with estrogens may affect estrogen drug metabolism. Inhibitors of CYP3A4 may increase plasma concentrations of estrogens and may result in side effects). Products include:

Biaxin/Biaxin XL 402
PREVPAC 3284

Clotrimazole (Co-administration of inhibitors of CYP3A4 with estrogens may affect estrogen drug metabolism. Inhibitors of CYP3A4 may increase plasma concentrations of estrogens and may result in side effects). Products include:

Desenex Athlete's Foot Cream 635
Lotrimin 3039
Lotrisone 3040

Cortisone Acetate (Co-administration of inducers of CYP3A4 with estrogens may affect estrogen drug metabolism. Inducers of CYP3A4 may reduce plasma concentrations of estrogens, possibly resulting in a decrease in therapeutic effects and/or changes in the uterine bleeding profile).

No products indexed under this heading.

Cyclosporine (Co-administration of inhibitors of CYP3A4 with estrogens may affect estrogen drug metabolism. Inhibitors of CYP3A4 may increase plasma concentrations of estrogens and may result in side effects). Products include:

Gengraf Capsules 459
Neoral Oral Solution 2259
Neoral Soft Gelatin Capsules 2259
Restasis Ophthalmic Emulsion 575
Sandimmune 2275

Dalfopristin (Co-administration of inhibitors of CYP3A4 with estrogens may affect estrogen drug metabolism. Inhibitors of CYP3A4 may increase plasma concentrations of estrogens and may result in side effects).

No products indexed under this heading.

Danazol (Co-administration of inhibitors of CYP3A4 with estrogens may affect estrogen drug metabolism. Inhibitors of CYP3A4 may increase plasma concentrations of estrogens and may result in side effects).

No products indexed under this heading.

Delavirdine Mesylate (Co-administration of inhibitors of CYP3A4 with estrogens may affect estrogen drug metabolism. Inhibitors of CYP3A4 may increase plasma concentrations of estrogens and may result in side effects). Products include:

Rescriptor Tablets 2551

Dexamethasone (Co-administration of inducers of CYP3A4 with estrogens may affect estrogen drug metabolism. Inducers of CYP3A4 may reduce plasma concentrations of estrogens, possibly resulting in a decrease in therapeutic effects and/or changes in the uterine bleeding profile). Products include:

Ciprodex Otic Suspension 559
Decadron Tablets 1951
TobraDex Ophthalmic Ointment 562
TobraDex Ophthalmic Suspension ... 563

Dexamethasone Acetate (Co-administration of inducers of CYP3A4 with estrogens may affect estrogen drug metabolism. Inducers of CYP3A4 may reduce plasma concentrations of estrogens, possibly resulting in a decrease in therapeutic effects and/or changes in the uterine bleeding profile).

No products indexed under this heading.

Dexamethasone Sodium Phosphate (Co-administration of inducers of CYP3A4 with estrogens may affect estrogen drug metabolism. Inducers of CYP3A4 may reduce plasma concentrations of estrogens, possibly resulting in a decrease in therapeutic effects and/or changes in the uterine bleeding profile).

No products indexed under this heading.

Diltiazem Hydrochloride (Co-administration of inhibitors of CYP3A4 with estrogens may affect estrogen drug metabolism. Inhibitors of CYP3A4 may increase plasma concentrations of estrogens and may result in side effects). Products include:

Cardizem LA Extended Release Tablets 1728
Tiazac Capsules 1201

Diltiazem Maleate (Co-administration of inhibitors of CYP3A4 with estrogens may affect estrogen drug metabolism. Inhibitors of CYP3A4 may increase plasma concentrations of estrogens and may result in side effects).

No products indexed under this heading.

Doxorubicin Hydrochloride (Co-administration of inducers of CYP3A4 with estrogens may affect estrogen drug metabolism. Inducers of CYP3A4 may reduce plasma concentrations of estrogens, possibly resulting in a decrease in therapeutic effects and/or changes in the uterine bleeding profile).

No products indexed under this heading.

Efavirenz (Co-administration of inducers of CYP3A4 with estrogens may affect estrogen drug metabolism. Inducers of CYP3A4 may reduce plasma concentrations of estrogens, possibly resulting in a decrease in therapeutic effects and/or changes in the uterine bleeding profile). Products include:

Atripla Tablets 945
Sustiva Capsules 930
Sustiva Tablets 930

Erythromycin (Co-administration of inhibitors of CYP3A4 with estrogens may affect estrogen drug metabolism. Inhibitors of CYP3A4 may increase plasma concentrations of estrogens and may result in side effects). Products include:

Ery-Tab Tablets 449
Erythromycin Base Filmtab Tablets 455
Erythromycin Delayed-Release Capsules, USP............................. 457
PCE Dispertab Tablets 515

Erythromycin Estolate (Co-administration of inhibitors of CYP3A4 with estrogens may affect estrogen drug metabolism. Inhibitors of CYP3A4 may increase plasma concentrations of estrogens and may result in side effects).

No products indexed under this heading.

Erythromycin Ethylsuccinate (Co-administration of inhibitors of CYP3A4 with estrogens may affect estrogen drug metabolism. Inhibitors of CYP3A4 may increase plasma concentrations of estrogens and may result in side effects). Products include:

E.E.S. 451
EryPed 447

Erythromycin Gluceptate (Co-administration of inhibitors of CYP3A4 with estrogens may affect estrogen drug metabolism. Inhibitors of CYP3A4 may increase plasma concentrations of estrogens and may result in side effects).

No products indexed under this heading.

Erythromycin Lactobionate (Co-administration of inhibitors of CYP3A4 with estrogens may affect estrogen drug metabolism. Inhibitors of CYP3A4 may increase plasma concentrations of estrogens and may result in side effects).

No products indexed under this heading.

Erythromycin Stearate (Co-administration of inhibitors of CYP3A4 with estrogens may affect estrogen drug metabolism. Inhibitors of CYP3A4 may increase plasma concentrations of estrogens and may result in side effects). Products include:

Erythrocin Stearate Filmtab Tablets 453

Esomeprazole Magnesium (Co-administration of inhibitors of CYP3A4 with estrogens may affect estrogen drug metabolism. Inhibitors of CYP3A4 may increase plasma concentrations of estrogens and may result in side effects). Products include:

Nexium Delayed-Release Capsules 655

Ethosuximide (Co-administration of inducers of CYP3A4 with estrogens may affect estrogen drug metabolism. Inducers of CYP3A4 may reduce plasma concentrations of estrogens, possibly resulting in a decrease in therapeutic effects and/or changes in the uterine bleeding profile).

No products indexed under this heading.

Felbamate (Co-administration of inducers of CYP3A4 with estrogens may affect estrogen drug metabolism. Inducers of CYP3A4 may reduce plasma concentrations of estrogens, possibly resulting in a decrease in therapeutic effects and/or changes in the uterine bleeding profile).

No products indexed under this heading.

Fluconazole (Co-administration of inhibitors of CYP3A4 with estrogens may affect estrogen drug metabolism. Inhibitors of CYP3A4 may increase plasma concentrations of estrogens and may result in side effects).

No products indexed under this heading.

Fludrocortisone Acetate (Co-administration of inducers of CYP3A4 with estrogens may affect estrogen drug metabolism. Inducers of CYP3A4 may reduce plasma concentrations of estrogens, possibly resulting in a decrease in therapeutic effects and/or changes in the uterine bleeding profile).

No products indexed under this heading.

Fluoxetine Hydrochloride (Co-administration of inhibitors of CYP3A4 with estrogens may affect estrogen drug metabolism. Inhibitors of CYP3A4 may increase plasma concentrations of estrogens and may result in side effects). Products include:

Prozac Pulvules and Liquid 1801
Symbyax Capsules 1819

Fluvoxamine Maleate (Co-administration of inhibitors of CYP3A4 with estrogens may affect estrogen drug metabolism. Inhibitors of CYP3A4 may increase plasma concentrations of estrogens and may result in side effects).

No products indexed under this heading.

Fosamprenavir Calcium (Co-administration of inhibitors of CYP3A4 with estrogens may affect estrogen drug metabolism. Inhibitors of CYP3A4 may increase plasma concentrations of estrogens and may result in side effects). Products include:

Lexiva Tablets 1505

Fosphenytoin Sodium (Co-administration of inducers of CYP3A4 with estrogens may affect estrogen drug metabolism. Inducers of CYP3A4 may reduce plasma concentrations of estrogens, possibly resulting in a decrease in therapeutic effects and/or changes in the uterine bleeding profile).

No products indexed under this heading.

Garlic Extract (Co-administration of inducers of CYP3A4 with estrogens may affect estrogen drug metabolism. Inducers of CYP3A4 may reduce plasma concentrations of estrogens, possibly resulting in a decrease in therapeutic effects and/or changes in the uterine bleeding profile).

No products indexed under this heading.

Garlic Oil (Co-administration of inducers of CYP3A4 with estrogens may affect estrogen drug metabolism. Inducers of CYP3A4 may reduce plasma concentrations of estrogens, possibly resulting in a decrease in therapeutic effects and/or changes in the uterine bleeding profile).

No products indexed under this heading.

Hydrocortisone (Co-administration of inducers of CYP3A4 with estrogens may affect estrogen drug metabolism. Inducers of CYP3A4 may reduce plasma concentrations of estrogens, possibly resulting in a decrease in therapeutic effects and/or changes in the uterine bleeding profile). Products include:

Colocort Rectal Suspension, USP (Retention) 100 mg/60 mL........... 2476
Hydrocortone Tablets 1989
Preparation H Hydrocortisone Cream 646

Hydrocortisone Acetate (Co-administration of inducers of CYP3A4 with estrogens may affect estrogen drug metabolism. Inducers of CYP3A4 may reduce plasma concentrations of estrogens, possibly resulting in a decrease in therapeutic effects and/or changes in the uterine bleeding profile). Products include:

Analpram-HC 1159
Pramosone 1161
ProctoFoam-HC 3099

Hydrocortisone Butyrate (Co-administration of inducers of CYP3A4 with estrogens may affect estrogen drug metabolism. Inducers of CYP3A4 may reduce plasma concentrations of estrogens, possibly resulting in a decrease in therapeutic effects and/or changes in the uterine bleeding profile). Products include:

Locoid Lipocream Cream 1160

Hydrocortisone Cypionate (Co-administration of inducers of CYP3A4 with estrogens may affect estrogen drug metabolism. Inducers of CYP3A4 may reduce plasma concentrations of estrogens, possibly resulting in a decrease in therapeutic effects and/or changes in the uterine bleeding profile).

No products indexed under this heading.

Hydrocortisone Hemisuccinate (Co-administration of inducers of CYP3A4 with estrogens may affect estrogen drug metabolism. Inducers of CYP3A4 may reduce plasma concentrations of estrogens, possibly resulting in a decrease in therapeutic effects and/or changes in the uterine bleeding profile).

No products indexed under this heading.

Hydrocortisone Probutate (Co-administration of inducers of CYP3A4 with estrogens may affect estrogen drug metabolism. Inducers of CYP3A4 may reduce plasma concentrations of estrogens, possibly resulting in a decrease in therapeutic effects and/or changes in the uterine bleeding profile).

No products indexed under this heading.

Hydrocortisone Sodium Phosphate (Co-administration of inducers of CYP3A4 with estrogens may affect estrogen drug metabolism. Inducers of CYP3A4 may reduce plasma concentrations of estrogens, possibly resulting in a decrease in therapeutic effects and/or changes in the uterine bleeding profile).

No products indexed under this heading.

Hydrocortisone Sodium Succinate (Co-administration of inducers of CYP3A4 with estrogens may affect estrogen drug metabolism. Inducers of CYP3A4 may reduce plasma concentrations of estrogens, possibly resulting in a decrease in therapeutic effects and/or changes in the uterine bleeding profile).

No products indexed under this heading.

Hydrocortisone Valerate (Co-administration of inducers of CYP3A4 with estrogens may affect estrogen drug metabolism. Inducers of CYP3A4 may reduce plasma concentrations of estrogens, possibly resulting in a decrease in therapeutic effects and/or changes in the uterine bleeding profile).

No products indexed under this heading.

Hypericum (Co-administration of inducers of CYP3A4 with estrogens may affect estrogen drug metabolism. Inducers of CYP3A4 may reduce plasma concentrations of estrogens, possibly resulting in a decrease in therapeutic effects and/or changes in the uterine bleeding profile). Products include:

Satiete Tablets .... ▣832

Hypericum Perforatum (Co-administration of inducers of CYP3A4 with estrogens may affect estrogen drug metabolism. Inducers of CYP3A4 may reduce plasma concentrations of estrogens, possibly resulting in a decrease in therapeutic effects and/or changes in the uterine bleeding profile).

No products indexed under this heading.

Indinavir Sulfate (Co-administration of inhibitors of CYP3A4 with estrogens may affect estrogen drug metabolism. Inhibitors of CYP3A4 may increase plasma concentrations of estrogens and may result in side effects). Products include:

Crixivan Capsules 1940

Isoniazid (Co-administration of inhibitors of CYP3A4 with estrogens may affect estrogen drug metabolism. Inhibitors of CYP3A4 may increase plasma concentrations of estrogens and may result in side effects).

No products indexed under this heading.

Itraconazole (Co-administration of inhibitors of CYP3A4 with estrogens may affect estrogen drug metabolism. Inhibitors of CYP3A4 may increase plasma concentrations of estrogens and may result in side effects).

No products indexed under this heading.

Ketoconazole (Co-administration of inhibitors of CYP3A4 with estrogens may affect estrogen drug metabolism. Inhibitors of CYP3A4 may increase plasma concentrations of estrogens and may result in side effects). Products include:

Nizoral A-D Shampoo, 1% 1868

Lopinavir (Co-administration of inhibitors of CYP3A4 with estrogens may affect estrogen drug metabolism. Inhibitors of CYP3A4 may increase plasma concentrations of estrogens and may result in side effects). Products include:

Kaletra 476

Loratadine (Co-administration of inhibitors of CYP3A4 with estrogens may affect estrogen drug metabolism. Inhibitors of CYP3A4 may increase plasma concentrations of estrogens and may result in side effects). Products include:

Alavert Allergy & Sinus D-12 Hour Tablets .... ▣771
Alavert .... ▣771
Children's Claritin Allergy Oral Solution .... ▣771
Claritin Non-Drowsy 24 Hour Tablets .... ▣772
Claritin Reditabs 24 Hour Non-Drowsy Tablets .... ▣772
Claritin-D Non-Drowsy 12 Hour Tablets .... ▣772
Claritin-D Non-Drowsy 24 Hour Tablets .... ▣772

Mephenytoin (Co-administration of inducers of CYP3A4 with estrogens may affect estrogen drug metabolism. Inducers of CYP3A4 may reduce plasma concentrations of estrogens, possibly resulting in a decrease in therapeutic effects and/or changes in the uterine bleeding profile).

No products indexed under this heading.

Methsuximide (Co-administration of inducers of CYP3A4 with estrogens may affect estrogen drug metabolism. Inducers of CYP3A4 may reduce plasma concentrations of estrogens, possibly resulting in a decrease in therapeutic effects and/or changes in the uterine bleeding profile).

No products indexed under this heading.

Methylprednisolone (Co-administration of inducers of CYP3A4 with estrogens may affect estrogen drug metabolism. Inducers of CYP3A4 may reduce plasma concentrations of estrogens, possibly resulting in a decrease in therapeutic effects and/or changes in the uterine bleeding profile).

No products indexed under this heading.

Methylprednisolone Acetate (Co-administration of inducers of CYP3A4 with estrogens may affect estrogen drug metabolism. Inducers of CYP3A4 may reduce plasma concentrations of estrogens, possibly resulting in a decrease in therapeutic effects and/or changes in the uterine bleeding profile). Products include:

Depo-Medrol Injectable Suspension 2617
Depo-Medrol Single-Dose Vial 2619

Methylprednisolone Sodium Succinate (Co-administration of inducers of CYP3A4 with estrogens may affect estrogen drug metabolism. Inducers of CYP3A4 may reduce plasma concentrations of estrogens, possibly resulting in a decrease in therapeutic effects and/or changes in the uterine bleeding profile).

No products indexed under this heading.

Metronidazole (Co-administration of inhibitors of CYP3A4 with estrogens may affect estrogen drug metabolism. Inhibitors of CYP3A4 may increase plasma concentrations of estrogens and may result in side effects). Products include:

Metrogel 1% 1211
MetroGel-Vaginal Gel 1855
Vandazole Vaginal Gel 3338

Metronidazole Benzoate (Co-administration of inhibitors of CYP3A4 with estrogens may affect estrogen drug metabolism. Inhibitors of CYP3A4 may increase plasma concentrations of estrogens and may result in side effects).

No products indexed under this heading.

Metronidazole Hydrochloride (Co-administration of inhibitors of CYP3A4 with estrogens may affect estrogen drug metabolism. Inhibitors of CYP3A4 may increase plasma concentrations of estrogens and may result in side effects).

No products indexed under this heading.

Miconazole (Co-administration of inhibitors of CYP3A4 with estrogens may affect estrogen drug metabolism. Inhibitors of CYP3A4 may increase plasma concentrations of estrogens and may result in side effects).

No products indexed under this heading.

Miconazole Nitrate (Co-administration of inhibitors of CYP3A4 with estrogens may affect estrogen drug metabolism. Inhibitors of CYP3A4 may increase plasma concentrations of estrogens and may result in side effects). Products include:

Desenex .... ▣635
Desenex Jock Itch Spray Powder ... ▣635

Modafinil (Co-administration of inducers of CYP3A4 with estrogens may affect estrogen drug metabolism. Inducers of CYP3A4 may reduce plasma concentrations of estrogens, possibly resulting in a decrease in therapeutic effects and/or changes in the uterine bleeding profile). Products include:

Provigil Tablets 988

Nefazodone Hydrochloride (Co-administration of inhibitors of CYP3A4 with estrogens may affect estrogen drug metabolism. Inhibitors of CYP3A4 may increase plasma concentrations of estrogens and may result in side effects).

No products indexed under this heading.

Nelfinavir Mesylate (Co-administration of inhibitors of CYP3A4 with estrogens may affect estrogen drug metabolism. Inhibitors of CYP3A4 may increase plasma concentrations of estrogens and may result in side effects). Products include:

Viracept 2577

Nevirapine (Co-administration of inducers of CYP3A4 with estrogens may affect estrogen drug metabolism. Inducers of CYP3A4 may reduce plasma concentrations of estrogens, possibly resulting in a decrease in therapeutic effects and/or changes in the uterine bleeding profile). Products include:

Viramune Oral Suspension 873
Viramune Tablets 873

Niacinamide (Co-administration of inhibitors of CYP3A4 with estrogens may affect estrogen drug metabolism. Inhibitors of CYP3A4 may increase plasma concentrations of estrogens and may result in side effects).

No products indexed under this heading.

Nicotinamide (Co-administration of inhibitors of CYP3A4 with estrogens may affect estrogen drug metabolism. Inhibitors of CYP3A4 may increase plasma concentrations of estrogens and may result in side effects). Products include:

Nicomide Tablets 1088

Nifedipine (Co-administration of inhibitors of CYP3A4 with estrogens may affect estrogen drug metabolismlism. Inhibitors of CYP3A4 may increase plasma concentrations of estrogens and may result in side effects). Products include:

Adalat CC Tablets 2964

Norfloxacin (Co-administration of inhibitors of CYP3A4 with estrogens may affect estrogen drug metabolism. Inhibitors of CYP3A4 may increase plasma concentrations of estrogens and may result in side effects). Products include:

Noroxin Tablets 2032

Omeprazole (Co-administration of inhibitors of CYP3A4 with estrogens may affect estrogen drug metabolism. Inhibitors of CYP3A4 may increase plasma concentrations of estrogens and may result in side effects). Products include:

Zegerid Capsules 2958
Zegerid Powder for Oral Solution 2958

Oxcarbazepine (Co-administration of inducers of CYP3A4 with estrogens may affect estrogen drug metabolism. Inducers of CYP3A4 may reduce plasma concentrations of estrogens, possibly resulting in a decrease in therapeutic effects and/or changes in the uterine bleeding profile). Products include:

Trileptal Tablets 2300
Trileptal Oral Suspension 2300

Paroxetine Hydrochloride (Co-administration of inhibitors of CYP3A4 with estrogens may affect estrogen drug metabolism. Inhibitors of CYP3A4 may increase plasma concentrations of estrogens and may result in side effects). Products include:

Paxil CR Controlled-Release Tablets 1538
Paxil 1530

Phenobarbital (Co-administration of inducers of CYP3A4 with estrogens may affect estrogen drug metabolism. Inducers of CYP3A4 may reduce plasma concentrations of estrogens, possibly resulting in a decrease in therapeutic effects and/or changes in the uterine bleeding profile). Products include:

Donnatal Extentabs 2493

Phenobarbital Sodium (Co-administration of inducers of CYP3A4 with estrogens may affect estrogen drug metabolism. Inducers of CYP3A4 may reduce plasma concentrations of estrogens, possibly resulting in a decrease in therapeutic effects and/or changes in the uterine bleeding profile).

No products indexed under this heading.

Phenytoin (Co-administration of inducers of CYP3A4 with estrogens may affect estrogen drug metabolism. Inducers of CYP3A4 may reduce plasma concentrations of estrogens, possibly resulting in a decrease in therapeutic effects and/or changes in the uterine bleeding profile).

No products indexed under this heading.

Phenytoin Sodium (Co-administration of inducers of CYP3A4 with estrogens may affect estrogen drug metabolism. Inducers of CYP3A4 may reduce plasma concentrations of estrogens, possibly resulting in a decrease in therapeutic effects and/or changes in the uterine bleeding profile). Products include:

Phenytek Capsules 2160

Prednisolone Acetate (Co-administration of inducers of CYP3A4 with estrogens may affect estrogen drug metabolism. Inducers of CYP3A4 may reduce plasma concentrations of estrogens, possibly resulting in a decrease in therapeutic effects and/or changes in the uterine bleeding profile). Products include:

Blephamide Ophthalmic Ointment 568
Blephamide Ophthalmic Suspension 569
Poly-Pred Ophthalmic Suspension .... ⊙ 233
Pred Forte Ophthalmic Suspension .... ⊙ 235
Pred Mild Ophthalmic Suspension .... ⊙ 238
Pred-G Ophthalmic Ointment .... ⊙ 237
Pred-G Ophthalmic Suspension ...... ⊙ 236

Prednisolone Sodium Phosphate (Co-administration of inducers of CYP3A4 with estrogens may affect estrogen drug metabolism. Inducers of CYP3A4 may reduce plasma concentrations of estrogens, possibly resulting in a decrease in therapeutic effects and/or changes in the uterine bleeding profile).

No products indexed under this heading.

Prednisolone Tebutate (Co-administration of inducers of CYP3A4 with estrogens may affect estrogen drug metabolism. Inducers of CYP3A4 may reduce plasma concentrations of estrogens, possibly resulting in a decrease in therapeutic effects and/or changes in the uterine bleeding profile).

No products indexed under this heading.

Prednisone (Co-administration of inducers of CYP3A4 with estrogens may affect estrogen drug metabolism. Inducers of CYP3A4 may reduce plasma concentrations of estrogens, possibly resulting in a decrease in therapeutic effects and/or changes in the uterine bleeding profile).

No products indexed under this heading.

Primidone (Co-administration of inducers of CYP3A4 with estrogens may affect estrogen drug metabolism. Inducers of CYP3A4 may reduce plasma concentrations of estrogens, possibly resulting in a decrease in therapeutic effects and/or changes in the uterine bleeding profile).

No products indexed under this heading.

Propoxyphene Hydrochloride (Co-administration of inhibitors of CYP3A4 with estrogens may affect estrogen drug metabolism. Inhibitors of CYP3A4 may increase plasma concentrations of estrogens and may result in side effects).

No products indexed under this heading.

Propoxyphene Napsylate (Co-administration of inhibitors of CYP3A4 with estrogens may affect estrogen drug metabolism. Inhibitors of CYP3A4 may increase plasma concentrations of estrogens and may result in side effects).

No products indexed under this heading.

Quinidine (Co-administration of inhibitors of CYP3A4 with estrogens may affect estrogen drug metabolism. Inhibitors of CYP3A4 may increase plasma concentrations of estrogens and may result in side effects).

No products indexed under this heading.

Quinidine Hydrochloride (Co-administration of inhibitors of CYP3A4 with estrogens may affect estrogen drug metabolism. Inhibitors of CYP3A4 may increase plasma concentrations of estrogens and may result in side effects).

No products indexed under this heading.

Quinidine Polygalacturonate (Co-administration of inhibitors of CYP3A4 with estrogens may affect estrogen drug metabolism. Inhibitors of CYP3A4 may increase plasma concentrations of estrogens and may result in side effects).

No products indexed under this heading.

Quinidine Sulfate (Co-administration of inhibitors of CYP3A4 with estrogens may affect estrogen drug metabolism. Inhibitors of CYP3A4 may increase plasma concentrations of estrogens and may result in side effects).

No products indexed under this heading.

Quinine (Co-administration of inhibitors of CYP3A4 with estrogens may affect estrogen drug metabolism. Inhibitors of CYP3A4 may increase plasma concentrations of estrogens and may result in side effects).

No products indexed under this heading.

Quinine Sulfate (Co-administration of inhibitors of CYP3A4 with estrogens may affect estrogen drug metabolism. Inhibitors of CYP3A4 may increase plasma concentrations of estrogens and may result in side effects).

No products indexed under this heading.

Quinupristin (Co-administration of inhibitors of CYP3A4 with estrogens may affect estrogen drug metabolism. Inhibitors of CYP3A4 may increase plasma concentrations of estrogens and may result in side effects).

No products indexed under this heading.

Ranitidine Bismuth Citrate (Co-administration of inhibitors of CYP3A4 with estrogens may affect estrogen drug metabolism. Inhibitors of CYP3A4 may increase plasma concentrations of estrogens and may result in side effects).

No products indexed under this heading.

Ranitidine Hydrochloride (Co-administration of inhibitors of CYP3A4 with estrogens may affect estrogen drug metabolism. Inhibitors of CYP3A4 may increase plasma concentrations of estrogens and may result in side effects). Products include:

Zantac 1624
Zantac Injection 1619
Zantac Injection Pharmacy Bulk Package 1622

Rifabutin (Co-administration of inducers of CYP3A4 with estrogens may affect estrogen drug metabolism. Inducers of CYP3A4 may reduce plasma concentrations of estrogens, possibly resulting in a decrease in therapeutic effects and/or changes in the uterine bleeding profile).

No products indexed under this heading.

Rifampicin (Co-administration of inducers of CYP3A4 with estrogens may affect estrogen drug metabolism. Inducers of CYP3A4 may reduce plasma concentrations of estrogens, possibly resulting in a decrease in therapeutic effects and/or changes in the uterine bleeding profile).

No products indexed under this heading.

Rifampin (Co-administration of inducers of CYP3A4 with estrogens may affect estrogen drug metabolism. Inducers of CYP3A4 may reduce plasma concentrations of estrogens, possibly resulting in a decrease in therapeutic effects and/or changes in the uterine bleeding profile).

No products indexed under this heading.

Rifapentine (Co-administration of inducers of CYP3A4 with estrogens may affect estrogen drug metabolism. Inducers of CYP3A4 may reduce plasma concentrations of estrogens, possibly resulting in a decrease in therapeutic effects and/or changes in the uterine bleeding profile).

No products indexed under this heading.

Ritonavir (Co-administration of inhibitors of CYP3A4 with estrogens may affect estrogen drug metabolism. Inhibitors of CYP3A4 may increase plasma concentrations of estrogens and may result in side effects). Products include:

Kaletra 476
Norvir 503

Saquinavir (Co-administration of inhibitors of CYP3A4 with estrogens may affect estrogen drug metabolism. Inhibitors of CYP3A4 may increase plasma concentrations of estrogens and may result in side effects).

No products indexed under this heading.

Saquinavir Mesylate (Co-administration of inhibitors of CYP3A4 with estrogens may affect estrogen drug metabolism. Inhibitors of CYP3A4 may increase plasma concentrations of estrogens and may result in side effects). Products include:

Invirase 2772

Sertraline Hydrochloride (Co-administration of inhibitors of CYP3A4 with estrogens may affect estrogen drug metabolism. Inhibitors of CYP3A4 may increase plasma concentrations of estrogens and may result in side effects). Products include:

Zoloft 2586

Sulfinpyrazone (Co-administration of inducers of CYP3A4 with estrogens may affect estrogen drug metabolism. Inducers of CYP3A4 may reduce plasma concentrations of estrogens, possibly resulting in a decrease in therapeutic effects and/or changes in the uterine bleeding profile).
No products indexed under this heading.

Telithromycin (Co-administration of inhibitors of CYP3A4 with estrogens may affect estrogen drug metabolism. Inhibitors of CYP3A4 may increase plasma concentrations of estrogens and may result in side effects). Products include:
Ketek Tablets **2903**

Theophylline (Co-administration of inducers of CYP3A4 with estrogens may affect estrogen drug metabolism. Inducers of CYP3A4 may reduce plasma concentrations of estrogens, possibly resulting in a decrease in therapeutic effects and/or changes in the uterine bleeding profile).
No products indexed under this heading.

Triamcinolone (Co-administration of inducers of CYP3A4 with estrogens may affect estrogen drug metabolism. Inducers of CYP3A4 may reduce plasma concentrations of estrogens, possibly resulting in a decrease in therapeutic effects and/or changes in the uterine bleeding profile).
No products indexed under this heading.

Triamcinolone Acetonide (Co-administration of inducers of CYP3A4 with estrogens may affect estrogen drug metabolism. Inducers of CYP3A4 may reduce plasma concentrations of estrogens, possibly resulting in a decrease in therapeutic effects and/or changes in the uterine bleeding profile). Products include:
Azmacort Inhalation Aerosol **1726**
Nasacort AQ Nasal Spray **2922**

Triamcinolone Diacetate (Co-administration of inducers of CYP3A4 with estrogens may affect estrogen drug metabolism. Inducers of CYP3A4 may reduce plasma concentrations of estrogens, possibly resulting in a decrease in therapeutic effects and/or changes in the uterine bleeding profile).
No products indexed under this heading.

Triamcinolone Hexacetonide (Co-administration of inducers of CYP3A4 with estrogens may affect estrogen drug metabolism. Inducers of CYP3A4 may reduce plasma concentrations of estrogens, possibly resulting in a decrease in therapeutic effects and/or changes in the uterine bleeding profile).
No products indexed under this heading.

Troglitazone (Co-administration of inducers of CYP3A4 with estrogens may affect estrogen drug metabolism. Inducers of CYP3A4 may reduce plasma concentrations of estrogens, possibly resulting in a decrease in therapeutic effects and/or changes in the uterine bleeding profile).
No products indexed under this heading.

Troleandomycin (Co-administration of inhibitors of CYP3A4 with estrogens may affect estrogen drug metabolism. Inhibitors of CYP3A4 may increase plasma concentrations of estrogens and may result in side effects).
No products indexed under this heading.

Valproate Sodium (Co-administration of inhibitors of CYP3A4 with estrogens may affect estrogen drug metabolism. Inhibitors of CYP3A4 may increase plasma concentrations of estrogens and may result in side effects). Products include:
Depacon Injection **412**

Verapamil Hydrochloride (Co-administration of inhibitors of CYP3A4 with estrogens may affect estrogen drug metabolism. Inhibitors of CYP3A4 may increase plasma concentrations of estrogens and may result in side effects). Products include:
Covera-HS Tablets **3139**
Tarka Tablets **524**
Verelan PM Extended-Release Capsules, Controlled-Onset.......... **3106**

Voriconazole (Co-administration of inhibitors of CYP3A4 with estrogens may affect estrogen drug metabolism. Inhibitors of CYP3A4 may increase plasma concentrations of estrogens and may result in side effects). Products include:
VFEND I.V. **2564**
VFEND Oral Suspension **2564**
VFEND Tablets **2564**

Zafirlukast (Co-administration of inhibitors of CYP3A4 with estrogens may affect estrogen drug metabolism. Inhibitors of CYP3A4 may increase plasma concentrations of estrogens and may result in side effects). Products include:
Accolate Tablets **671**

Zileuton (Co-administration of inhibitors of CYP3A4 with estrogens may affect estrogen drug metabolism. Inhibitors of CYP3A4 may increase plasma concentrations of estrogens and may result in side effects). Products include:
Zyflo Tablets **1023**

Food Interactions

Grapefruit (Co-administration of inhibitors of CYP3A4 with estrogens may affect estrogen drug metabolism. Inhibitors of CYP3A4 may increase plasma concentrations of estrogens and may result in side effects).

Grapefruit Juice (Co-administration of grapefruit juice with estrogens may increase plasma concentrations of estrogens and may result in side effects).

PREMARIN VAGINAL CREAM

(Estrogens, Conjugated) **3452**
See Premarin Tablets

PREMCAL LIGHT, REGULAR, AND EXTRA STRENGTH TABLETS

(Calcium Carbonate, Magnesium Oxide, Vitamin D_3)............................ ▣**818**
None cited in PDR database.

PREMPHASE TABLETS

(Estrogens, Conjugated, Medroxyprogesterone Acetate)........... **3456**
May interact with cytochrome p450 3a4 inducers (selected), cytochrome p450 3a4 inhibitors (selected), and certain other agents. Compounds in these categories include:

Acetazolamide (Co-administration of estrogens with inhibitors of CYP3A4 may increase plasma concentrations of estrogens and may result in side effects).
No products indexed under this heading.

Allium sativum (Co-administration of estrogens with inducers of CYP3A4 may reduce plasma concentrations of estrogens, possibly resulting in a decrease in therapeutic effects and/or changes in the uterine bleeding profile).
No products indexed under this heading.

Aminoglutethimide (Aminoglutethimide administered concomitantly with medroxyprogesterone acetate (MPA) may significantly depress the bioavailability of MPA).
No products indexed under this heading.

Amiodarone Hydrochloride (Co-administration of estrogens with inhibitors of CYP3A4 may increase plasma concentrations of estrogens and may result in side effects).
No products indexed under this heading.

Amprenavir (Co-administration of estrogens with inhibitors of CYP3A4 may increase plasma concentrations of estrogens and may result in side effects). Products include:
Agenerase Capsules **1327**
Agenerase Oral Solution **1332**

Anastrozole (Co-administration of estrogens with inhibitors of CYP3A4 may increase plasma concentrations of estrogens and may result in side effects). Products include:
Arimidex Tablets **673**

Aprepitant (Co-administration of estrogens with inducers of CYP3A4 may reduce plasma concentrations of estrogens, possibly resulting in a decrease in therapeutic effects and/or changes in the uterine bleeding profile). Products include:
Emend Capsules **1963**

Betamethasone Acetate (Co-administration of estrogens with inducers of CYP3A4 may reduce plasma concentrations of estrogens, possibly resulting in a decrease in therapeutic effects and/or changes in the uterine bleeding profile).
No products indexed under this heading.

Betamethasone Sodium Phosphate (Co-administration of estrogens with inducers of CYP3A4 may reduce plasma concentrations of estrogens, possibly resulting in a decrease in therapeutic effects and/or changes in the uterine bleeding profile).
No products indexed under this heading.

Carbamazepine (Co-administration of estrogens with inducers of CYP3A4 may reduce plasma concentrations of estrogens, possibly resulting in a decrease in therapeutic effects and/or changes in the uterine bleeding profile). Products include:
Carbatrol Capsules **3171**
Equetro Extended-Release Capsules **3180**
Tegretol/Tegretol-XR **2295**

Cimetidine (Co-administration of estrogens with inhibitors of CYP3A4 may increase plasma concentrations of estrogens and may result in side effects). Products include:
Tagamet HB 200 Tablets .... ▣**664**

Cimetidine Hydrochloride (Co-administration of estrogens with inhibitors of CYP3A4 may increase plasma concentrations of estrogens and may result in side effects).
No products indexed under this heading.

Ciprofloxacin (Co-administration of estrogens with inhibitors of CYP3A4 may increase plasma concentrations of estrogens and may result in side effects). Products include:
Cipro Oral Suspension **2977**
Cipro I.V. **2984**
Cipro XR Tablets **2990**
Ciprodex Otic Suspension **559**

Ciprofloxacin Hydrochloride (Co-administration of estrogens with inducers of CYP3A4 may reduce plasma concentrations of estrogens, possibly resulting in a decrease in therapeutic effects and/or changes in the uterine bleeding profile). Products include:
Ciloxan Ophthalmic Ointment **559**
Ciloxan Ophthalmic Solution .... ⊙**206**
Cipro Tablets **2977**
Proquin XR Tablets **1153**

Cisplatin (Co-administration of estrogens with inducers of CYP3A4 may reduce plasma concentrations of estrogens, possibly resulting in a decrease in therapeutic effects and/or changes in the uterine bleeding profile).
No products indexed under this heading.

Clarithromycin (Co-administration of estrogens with inhibitors of CYP3A4 may increase plasma concentrations of estrogens and may result in side effects). Products include:
Biaxin/Biaxin XL **402**
PREVPAC **3284**

Clotrimazole (Co-administration of estrogens with inhibitors of CYP3A4 may increase plasma concentrations of estrogens and may result in side effects). Products include:
Desenex Athlete's Foot Cream .... ▣**635**
Lotrimin **3039**
Lotrisone **3040**

Cortisone Acetate (Co-administration of estrogens with inducers of CYP3A4 may reduce plasma concentrations of estrogens, possibly resulting in a decrease in therapeutic effects and/or changes in the uterine bleeding profile).
No products indexed under this heading.

Cyclosporine (Co-administration of estrogens with inhibitors of CYP3A4 may increase plasma concentrations of estrogens and may result in side effects). Products include:
Gengraf Capsules **459**
Neoral Oral Solution **2259**
Neoral Soft Gelatin Capsules **2259**
Restasis Ophthalmic Emulsion **575**
Sandimmune **2275**

Dalfopristin (Co-administration of estrogens with inhibitors of CYP3A4 may increase plasma concentrations of estrogens and may result in side effects).
No products indexed under this heading.

Danazol (Co-administration of estrogens with inhibitors of CYP3A4 may increase plasma concentrations of estrogens and may result in side effects).
No products indexed under this heading.

Delavirdine Mesylate (Co-administration of estrogens with inhibitors of CYP3A4 may increase plasma concentrations of estrogens and may result in side effects). Products include:

Dexamethasone (Co-administration of estrogens with inducers of CYP3A4 may reduce plasma concentrations of estrogens, possibly resulting in a decrease in therapeutic effects and/or changes in the uterine bleeding profile). Products include:

Dexamethasone Acetate (Co-administration of estrogens with inducers of CYP3A4 may reduce plasma concentrations of estrogens, possibly resulting in a decrease in therapeutic effects and/or changes in the uterine bleeding profile).
No products indexed under this heading.

Dexamethasone Sodium Phosphate (Co-administration of estrogens with inducers of CYP3A4 may reduce plasma concentrations of estrogens, possibly resulting in a decrease in therapeutic effects and/or changes in the uterine bleeding profile).
No products indexed under this heading.

Diltiazem Hydrochloride (Co-administration of estrogens with inhibitors of CYP3A4 may increase plasma concentrations of estrogens and may result in side effects). Products include:

Diltiazem Maleate (Co-administration of estrogens with inhibitors of CYP3A4 may increase plasma concentrations of estrogens and may result in side effects).
No products indexed under this heading.

Doxorubicin Hydrochloride (Co-administration of estrogens with inducers of CYP3A4 may reduce plasma concentrations of estrogens, possibly resulting in a decrease in therapeutic effects and/or changes in the uterine bleeding profile).
No products indexed under this heading.

Efavirenz (Co-administration of estrogens with inducers of CYP3A4 may reduce plasma concentrations of estrogens, possibly resulting in a decrease in therapeutic effects and/or changes in the uterine bleeding profile). Products include:

Erythromycin (Co-administration of estrogens with inhibitors of CYP3A4 may increase plasma concentrations of estrogens and may result in side effects). Products include:

Erythromycin Estolate (Co-administration of estrogens with inhibitors of CYP3A4 may increase plasma concentrations of estrogens and may result in side effects).
No products indexed under this heading.

Erythromycin Ethylsuccinate (Co-administration of estrogens with inhibitors of CYP3A4 may increase plasma concentrations of estrogens and may result in side effects). Products include:

Erythromycin Gluceptate (Co-administration of estrogens with inhibitors of CYP3A4 may increase plasma concentrations of estrogens and may result in side effects).
No products indexed under this heading.

Erythromycin Lactobionate (Co-administration of estrogens with inhibitors of CYP3A4 may increase plasma concentrations of estrogens and may result in side effects).
No products indexed under this heading.

Erythromycin Stearate (Co-administration of estrogens with inhibitors of CYP3A4 may increase plasma concentrations of estrogens and may result in side effects). Products include:

Esomeprazole Magnesium (Co-administration of estrogens with inhibitors of CYP3A4 may increase plasma concentrations of estrogens and may result in side effects). Products include:

Ethosuximide (Co-administration of estrogens with inducers of CYP3A4 may reduce plasma concentrations of estrogens, possibly resulting in a decrease in therapeutic effects and/or changes in the uterine bleeding profile).
No products indexed under this heading.

Felbamate (Co-administration of estrogens with inducers of CYP3A4 may reduce plasma concentrations of estrogens, possibly resulting in a decrease in therapeutic effects and/or changes in the uterine bleeding profile).
No products indexed under this heading.

Fluconazole (Co-administration of estrogens with inhibitors of CYP3A4 may increase plasma concentrations of estrogens and may result in side effects).
No products indexed under this heading.

Fludrocortisone Acetate (Co-administration of estrogens with inducers of CYP3A4 may reduce plasma concentrations of estrogens, possibly resulting in a decrease in therapeutic effects and/or changes in the uterine bleeding profile).
No products indexed under this heading.

Fluoxetine Hydrochloride (Co-administration of estrogens with inhibitors of CYP3A4 may increase plasma concentrations of estrogens and may result in side effects). Products include:

Fluvoxamine Maleate (Co-administration of estrogens with inhibitors of CYP3A4 may increase plasma concentrations of estrogens and may result in side effects).
No products indexed under this heading.

Fosamprenavir Calcium (Co-administration of estrogens with inhibitors of CYP3A4 may increase plasma concentrations of estrogens and may result in side effects). Products include:

Fosphenytoin Sodium (Co-administration of estrogens with inducers of CYP3A4 may reduce plasma concentrations of estrogens, possibly resulting in a decrease in therapeutic effects and/or changes in the uterine bleeding profile).
No products indexed under this heading.

Garlic Extract (Co-administration of estrogens with inducers of CYP3A4 may reduce plasma concentrations of estrogens, possibly resulting in a decrease in therapeutic effects and/or changes in the uterine bleeding profile).
No products indexed under this heading.

Garlic Oil (Co-administration of estrogens with inducers of CYP3A4 may reduce plasma concentrations of estrogens, possibly resulting in a decrease in therapeutic effects and/or changes in the uterine bleeding profile).
No products indexed under this heading.

Hydrocortisone (Co-administration of estrogens with inducers of CYP3A4 may reduce plasma concentrations of estrogens, possibly resulting in a decrease in therapeutic effects and/or changes in the uterine bleeding profile). Products include:

Hydrocortisone Acetate (Co-administration of estrogens with inducers of CYP3A4 may reduce plasma concentrations of estrogens, possibly resulting in a decrease in therapeutic effects and/or changes in the uterine bleeding profile). Products include:

Hydrocortisone Butyrate (Co-administration of estrogens with inducers of CYP3A4 may reduce plasma concentrations of estrogens, possibly resulting in a decrease in

therapeutic effects and/or changes in the uterine bleeding profile). Products include:

Hydrocortisone Cypionate (Co-administration of estrogens with inducers of CYP3A4 may reduce plasma concentrations of estrogens, possibly resulting in a decrease in therapeutic effects and/or changes in the uterine bleeding profile).
No products indexed under this heading.

Hydrocortisone Hemisuccinate (Co-administration of estrogens with inducers of CYP3A4 may reduce plasma concentrations of estrogens, possibly resulting in a decrease in therapeutic effects and/or changes in the uterine bleeding profile).
No products indexed under this heading.

Hydrocortisone Probutate (Co-administration of estrogens with inducers of CYP3A4 may reduce plasma concentrations of estrogens, possibly resulting in a decrease in therapeutic effects and/or changes in the uterine bleeding profile).
No products indexed under this heading.

Hydrocortisone Sodium Phosphate (Co-administration of estrogens with inducers of CYP3A4 may reduce plasma concentrations of estrogens, possibly resulting in a decrease in therapeutic effects and/or changes in the uterine bleeding profile).
No products indexed under this heading.

Hydrocortisone Sodium Succinate (Co-administration of estrogens with inducers of CYP3A4 may reduce plasma concentrations of estrogens, possibly resulting in a decrease in therapeutic effects and/or changes in the uterine bleeding profile).
No products indexed under this heading.

Hydrocortisone Valerate (Co-administration of estrogens with inducers of CYP3A4 may reduce plasma concentrations of estrogens, possibly resulting in a decrease in therapeutic effects and/or changes in the uterine bleeding profile).
No products indexed under this heading.

Hypericum (Co-administration of estrogens with inducers of CYP3A4 may reduce plasma concentrations of estrogens, possibly resulting in a decrease in therapeutic effects and/or changes in the uterine bleeding profile). Products include:

Hypericum Perforatum (Co-administration of estrogens with inducers of CYP3A4 may reduce plasma concentrations of estrogens, possibly resulting in a decrease in therapeutic effects and/or changes in the uterine bleeding profile).
No products indexed under this heading.

Indinavir Sulfate (Co-administration of estrogens with inhibitors of CYP3A4 may increase plasma concentrations of estrogens and may result in side effects). Products include:

IMPORTANT NOTE: Always consult each drug listing in the patient's regimen for possible interactions.

Isoniazid (Co-administration of estrogens with inhibitors of CYP3A4 may increase plasma concentrations of estrogens and may result in side effects).
No products indexed under this heading.

Itraconazole (Co-administration of estrogens with inhibitors of CYP3A4 may increase plasma concentrations of estrogens and may result in side effects).
No products indexed under this heading.

Ketoconazole (Co-administration of estrogens with inhibitors of CYP3A4 may increase plasma concentrations of estrogens and may result in side effects). Products include:
Nizoral A-D Shampoo, 1% 1868

Lopinavir (Co-administration of estrogens with inhibitors of CYP3A4 may increase plasma concentrations of estrogens and may result in side effects). Products include:
Kaletra 476

Loratadine (Co-administration of estrogens with inhibitors of CYP3A4 may increase plasma concentrations of estrogens and may result in side effects). Products include:
Alavert Allergy & Sinus D-12 Hour Tablets .... ■771
Alavert .... ■771
Children's Claritin Allergy Oral Solution .... ■771
Claritin Non-Drowsy 24 Hour Tablets .... ■772
Claritin Reditabs 24 Hour Non-Drowsy Tablets .... ■772
Claritin-D Non-Drowsy 12 Hour Tablets .... ■772
Claritin-D Non-Drowsy 24 Hour Tablets .... ■772

Mephenytoin (Co-administration of estrogens with inducers of CYP3A4 may reduce plasma concentrations of estrogens, possibly resulting in a decrease in therapeutic effects and/or changes in the uterine bleeding profile).
No products indexed under this heading.

Methsuximide (Co-administration of estrogens with inducers of CYP3A4 may reduce plasma concentrations of estrogens, possibly resulting in a decrease in therapeutic effects and/or changes in the uterine bleeding profile).
No products indexed under this heading.

Methylprednisolone (Co-administration of estrogens with inducers of CYP3A4 may reduce plasma concentrations of estrogens, possibly resulting in a decrease in therapeutic effects and/or changes in the uterine bleeding profile).
No products indexed under this heading.

Methylprednisolone Acetate (Co-administration of estrogens with inducers of CYP3A4 may reduce plasma concentrations of estrogens, possibly resulting in a decrease in therapeutic effects and/or changes in the uterine bleeding profile). Products include:
Depo-Medrol Injectable Suspension 2617
Depo-Medrol Single-Dose Vial 2619

Methylprednisolone Sodium Succinate (Co-administration of estrogens with inducers of CYP3A4 may reduce plasma concentrations of estrogens, possibly resulting in a decrease in therapeutic effects and/or changes in the uterine bleeding profile).
No products indexed under this heading.

Metronidazole (Co-administration of estrogens with inhibitors of CYP3A4 may increase plasma concentrations of estrogens and may result in side effects). Products include:
Metrogel 1% 1211
MetroGel-Vaginal Gel 1855
Vandazole Vaginal Gel 3338

Metronidazole Benzoate (Co-administration of estrogens with inhibitors of CYP3A4 may increase plasma concentrations of estrogens and may result in side effects).
No products indexed under this heading.

Metronidazole Hydrochloride (Co-administration of estrogens with inhibitors of CYP3A4 may increase plasma concentrations of estrogens and may result in side effects).
No products indexed under this heading.

Miconazole (Co-administration of estrogens with inhibitors of CYP3A4 may increase plasma concentrations of estrogens and may result in side effects).
No products indexed under this heading.

Miconazole Nitrate (Co-administration of estrogens with inhibitors of CYP3A4 may increase plasma concentrations of estrogens and may result in side effects). Products include:
Desenex .... ■635
Desenex Jock Itch Spray Powder ... ■635

Modafinil (Co-administration of estrogens with inducers of CYP3A4 may reduce plasma concentrations of estrogens, possibly resulting in a decrease in therapeutic effects and/or changes in the uterine bleeding profile). Products include:
Provigil Tablets 988

Nefazodone Hydrochloride (Co-administration of estrogens with inhibitors of CYP3A4 may increase plasma concentrations of estrogens and may result in side effects).
No products indexed under this heading.

Nelfinavir Mesylate (Co-administration of estrogens with inhibitors of CYP3A4 may increase plasma concentrations of estrogens and may result in side effects). Products include:
Viracept 2577

Nevirapine (Co-administration of estrogens with inducers of CYP3A4 may reduce plasma concentrations of estrogens, possibly resulting in a decrease in therapeutic effects and/or changes in the uterine bleeding profile). Products include:
Viramune Oral Suspension 873
Viramune Tablets 873

Niacinamide (Co-administration of estrogens with inhibitors of CYP3A4 may increase plasma concentrations of estrogens and may result in side effects).
No products indexed under this heading.

Nicotinamide (Co-administration of estrogens with inhibitors of CYP3A4 may increase plasma concentrations of estrogens and may result in side effects). Products include:
Nicomide Tablets 1088

Nifedipine (Co-administration of estrogens with inhibitors of CYP3A4 may increase plasma concentrations of estrogens and may result in side effects). Products include:
Adalat CC Tablets 2964

Norfloxacin (Co-administration of estrogens with inhibitors of CYP3A4 may increase plasma concentrations of estrogens and may result in side effects). Products include:
Noroxin Tablets 2032

Omeprazole (Co-administration of estrogens with inhibitors of CYP3A4 may increase plasma concentrations of estrogens and may result in side effects). Products include:
Zegerid Capsules 2958
Zegerid Powder for Oral Solution 2958

Oxcarbazepine (Co-administration of estrogens with inducers of CYP3A4 may reduce plasma concentrations of estrogens, possibly resulting in a decrease in therapeutic effects and/or changes in the uterine bleeding profile). Products include:
Trileptal Tablets 2300
Trileptal Oral Suspension 2300

Paroxetine Hydrochloride (Co-administration of estrogens with inhibitors of CYP3A4 may increase plasma concentrations of estrogens and may result in side effects). Products include:
Paxil CR Controlled-Release Tablets 1538
Paxil 1530

Phenobarbital (Co-administration of estrogens with inducers of CYP3A4 may reduce plasma concentrations of estrogens, possibly resulting in a decrease in therapeutic effects and/or changes in the uterine bleeding profile). Products include:
Donnatal Extentabs 2493

Phenobarbital Sodium (Co-administration of estrogens with inducers of CYP3A4 may reduce plasma concentrations of estrogens, possibly resulting in a decrease in therapeutic effects and/or changes in the uterine bleeding profile).
No products indexed under this heading.

Phenytoin (Co-administration of estrogens with inducers of CYP3A4 may reduce plasma concentrations of estrogens, possibly resulting in a decrease in therapeutic effects and/or changes in the uterine bleeding profile).
No products indexed under this heading.

Phenytoin Sodium (Co-administration of estrogens with inducers of CYP3A4 may reduce plasma concentrations of estrogens, possibly resulting in a decrease in therapeutic effects and/or changes in the uterine bleeding profile). Products include:
Phenytek Capsules 2160

Prednisolone Acetate (Co-administration of estrogens with inducers of CYP3A4 may reduce plasma concentrations of estrogens, possibly resulting in a decrease in therapeutic effects and/or changes in the uterine bleeding profile). Products include:
Blephamide Ophthalmic Ointment 568
Blephamide Ophthalmic Suspension 569
Poly-Pred Ophthalmic Suspension .... ⊙233
Pred Forte Ophthalmic Suspension .... ⊙235
Pred Mild Ophthalmic Suspension .... ⊙238
Pred-G Ophthalmic Ointment .... ⊙237
Pred-G Ophthalmic Suspension ...... ⊙236

Prednisolone Sodium Phosphate (Co-administration of estrogens with inducers of CYP3A4 may reduce plasma concentrations of estrogens, possibly resulting in a decrease in therapeutic effects and/or changes in the uterine bleeding profile).
No products indexed under this heading.

Prednisolone Tebutate (Co-administration of estrogens with inducers of CYP3A4 may reduce plasma concentrations of estrogens, possibly resulting in a decrease in therapeutic effects and/or changes in the uterine bleeding profile).
No products indexed under this heading.

Prednisone (Co-administration of estrogens with inducers of CYP3A4 may reduce plasma concentrations of estrogens, possibly resulting in a decrease in therapeutic effects and/or changes in the uterine bleeding profile).
No products indexed under this heading.

Primidone (Co-administration of estrogens with inducers of CYP3A4 may reduce plasma concentrations of estrogens, possibly resulting in a decrease in therapeutic effects and/or changes in the uterine bleeding profile).
No products indexed under this heading.

Propoxyphene Hydrochloride (Co-administration of estrogens with inhibitors of CYP3A4 may increase plasma concentrations of estrogens and may result in side effects).
No products indexed under this heading.

Propoxyphene Napsylate (Co-administration of estrogens with inhibitors of CYP3A4 may increase plasma concentrations of estrogens and may result in side effects).
No products indexed under this heading.

Quinidine (Co-administration of estrogens with inhibitors of CYP3A4 may increase plasma concentrations of estrogens and may result in side effects).
No products indexed under this heading.

Quinidine Hydrochloride (Co-administration of estrogens with inhibitors of CYP3A4 may increase plasma concentrations of estrogens and may result in side effects).
No products indexed under this heading.

Quinidine Polygalacturonate (Co-administration of estrogens with inhibitors of CYP3A4 may increase plasma concentrations of estrogens and may result in side effects).
No products indexed under this heading.

Quinidine Sulfate (Co-administration of estrogens with inhibitors of CYP3A4 may increase plasma concentrations of estrogens and may result in side effects).

No products indexed under this heading.

Quinine (Co-administration of estrogens with inhibitors of CYP3A4 may increase plasma concentrations of estrogens and may result in side effects).

No products indexed under this heading.

Quinine Sulfate (Co-administration of estrogens with inhibitors of CYP3A4 may increase plasma concentrations of estrogens and may result in side effects).

No products indexed under this heading.

Quinupristin (Co-administration of estrogens with inhibitors of CYP3A4 may increase plasma concentrations of estrogens and may result in side effects).

No products indexed under this heading.

Ranitidine Bismuth Citrate (Co-administration of estrogens with inhibitors of CYP3A4 may increase plasma concentrations of estrogens and may result in side effects).

No products indexed under this heading.

Ranitidine Hydrochloride (Co-administration of estrogens with inhibitors of CYP3A4 may increase plasma concentrations of estrogens and may result in side effects). Products include:

Rifabutin (Co-administration of estrogens with inducers of CYP3A4 may reduce plasma concentrations of estrogens, possibly resulting in a decrease in therapeutic effects and/or changes in the uterine bleeding profile).

No products indexed under this heading.

Rifampicin (Co-administration of estrogens with inducers of CYP3A4 may reduce plasma concentrations of estrogens, possibly resulting in a decrease in therapeutic effects and/or changes in the uterine bleeding profile).

No products indexed under this heading.

Rifampin (Co-administration of estrogens with inducers of CYP3A4 may reduce plasma concentrations of estrogens, possibly resulting in a decrease in therapeutic effects and/or changes in the uterine bleeding profile).

No products indexed under this heading.

Rifapentine (Co-administration of estrogens with inducers of CYP3A4 may reduce plasma concentrations of estrogens, possibly resulting in a decrease in therapeutic effects and/or changes in the uterine bleeding profile).

No products indexed under this heading.

Ritonavir (Co-administration of estrogens with inhibitors of CYP3A4 may increase plasma concentrations of estrogens and may result in side effects). Products include:

Saquinavir (Co-administration of estrogens with inhibitors of CYP3A4 may increase plasma concentrations of estrogens and may result in side effects).

No products indexed under this heading.

Saquinavir Mesylate (Co-administration of estrogens with inhibitors of CYP3A4 may increase plasma concentrations of estrogens and may result in side effects). Products include:

Sertraline Hydrochloride (Co-administration of estrogens with inhibitors of CYP3A4 may increase plasma concentrations of estrogens and may result in side effects). Products include:

Sulfinpyrazone (Co-administration of estrogens with inducers of CYP3A4 may reduce plasma concentrations of estrogens, possibly resulting in a decrease in therapeutic effects and/or changes in the uterine bleeding profile).

No products indexed under this heading.

Telithromycin (Co-administration of estrogens with inhibitors of CYP3A4 may increase plasma concentrations of estrogens and may result in side effects). Products include:

Theophylline (Co-administration of estrogens with inducers of CYP3A4 may reduce plasma concentrations of estrogens, possibly resulting in a decrease in therapeutic effects and/or changes in the uterine bleeding profile).

No products indexed under this heading.

Triamcinolone (Co-administration of estrogens with inducers of CYP3A4 may reduce plasma concentrations of estrogens, possibly resulting in a decrease in therapeutic effects and/or changes in the uterine bleeding profile).

No products indexed under this heading.

Triamcinolone Acetonide (Co-administration of estrogens with inducers of CYP3A4 may reduce plasma concentrations of estrogens, possibly resulting in a decrease in therapeutic effects and/or changes in the uterine bleeding profile). Products include:

Triamcinolone Diacetate (Co-administration of estrogens with inducers of CYP3A4 may reduce plasma concentrations of estrogens, possibly resulting in a decrease in therapeutic effects and/or changes in the uterine bleeding profile).

No products indexed under this heading.

Triamcinolone Hexacetonide (Co-administration of estrogens with inducers of CYP3A4 may reduce plasma concentrations of estrogens, possibly resulting in a decrease in therapeutic effects and/or changes in the uterine bleeding profile).

No products indexed under this heading.

Troglitazone (Co-administration of estrogens with inducers of CYP3A4 may reduce plasma concentrations of estrogens, possibly resulting in a decrease in therapeutic effects and/or changes in the uterine bleeding profile).

No products indexed under this heading.

Troleandomycin (Co-administration of estrogens with inhibitors of CYP3A4 may increase plasma concentrations of estrogens and may result in side effects).

No products indexed under this heading.

Valproate Sodium (Co-administration of estrogens with inhibitors of CYP3A4 may increase plasma concentrations of estrogens and may result in side effects). Products include:

Verapamil Hydrochloride (Co-administration of estrogens with inhibitors of CYP3A4 may increase plasma concentrations of estrogens and may result in side effects). Products include:

Voriconazole (Co-administration of estrogens with inhibitors of CYP3A4 may increase plasma concentrations of estrogens and may result in side effects). Products include:

Zafirlukast (Co-administration of estrogens with inhibitors of CYP3A4 may increase plasma concentrations of estrogens and may result in side effects). Products include:

Zileuton (Co-administration of estrogens with inhibitors of CYP3A4 may increase plasma concentrations of estrogens and may result in side effects). Products include:

Food Interactions

Food, unspecified (Administration with a high fat breakfast decreased total estrone Cmax and increased total equilin Cmax compared to fasting state, no other effect on rate or extent of absorption; administration with food doubles MPA Cmax and increases MPA AUC).

Grapefruit (Co-administration of estrogens with inhibitors of CYP3A4 may increase plasma concentrations of estrogens and may result in side effects).

Grapefruit Juice (Co-administration of estrogens with inhibitors of CYP3A4, such as grapefruit juice, may increase plasma concentrations of estrogens and may result in side effects).

PREMPRO TABLETS

(Estrogens, Conjugated, Medroxyprogesterone Acetate).......... 3456
May interact with cytochrome p450 3a4 inducers (selected), cytochrome p450 3a4 inhibitors (selected), and certain other agents. Compounds in these categories include:

Acetazolamide (Co-administration of estrogens with inhibitors of CYP3A4 may increase plasma concentrations of estrogens and may result in side effects).

No products indexed under this heading.

Allium sativum (Co-administration of estrogens with inducers of CYP3A4 may reduce plasma concentrations of estrogens, possibly resulting in a decrease in therapeutic effects and/or changes in the uterine bleeding profile).

No products indexed under this heading.

Aminoglutethimide (Aminoglutethimide administered concomitantly with medroxyprogesterone acetate (MPA) may significantly depress the bioavailability of MPA).

No products indexed under this heading.

Amiodarone Hydrochloride (Co-administration of estrogens with inhibitors of CYP3A4 may increase plasma concentrations of estrogens and may result in side effects).

No products indexed under this heading.

Amprenavir (Co-administration of estrogens with inhibitors of CYP3A4 may increase plasma concentrations of estrogens and may result in side effects). Products include:

Anastrozole (Co-administration of estrogens with inhibitors of CYP3A4 may increase plasma concentrations of estrogens and may result in side effects). Products include:

Aprepitant (Co-administration of estrogens with inducers of CYP3A4 may reduce plasma concentrations of estrogens, possibly resulting in a decrease in therapeutic effects and/or changes in the uterine bleeding profile). Products include:

Betamethasone Acetate (Co-administration of estrogens with inducers of CYP3A4 may reduce plasma concentrations of estrogens, possibly resulting in a decrease in therapeutic effects and/or changes in the uterine bleeding profile).

No products indexed under this heading.

Betamethasone Sodium Phosphate (Co-administration of estrogens with inducers of CYP3A4 may reduce plasma concentrations of estrogens, possibly resulting in a decrease in therapeutic effects and/or changes in the uterine bleeding profile).

No products indexed under this heading.

Carbamazepine (Co-administration of estrogens with inducers of CYP3A4 may reduce plasma concentrations of estrogens, possibly resulting in a decrease in therapeutic effects and/or changes in the uterine bleeding profile). Products include:

Cimetidine (Co-administration of estrogens with inhibitors of CYP3A4 may increase plasma concentrations of estrogens and may result in side effects). Products include:

IMPORTANT NOTE: Always consult each drug listing in the patient's regimen for possible interactions.

Cimetidine Hydrochloride (Co-administration of estrogens with inhibitors of CYP3A4 may increase plasma concentrations of estrogens and may result in side effects).
No products indexed under this heading.

Ciprofloxacin (Co-administration of estrogens with inhibitors of CYP3A4 may increase plasma concentrations of estrogens and may result in side effects). Products include:
Cipro Oral Suspension 2977
Cipro I.V. 2984
Cipro XR Tablets 2990
Ciprodex Otic Suspension 559

Ciprofloxacin Hydrochloride (Co-administration of estrogens with inducers of CYP3A4 may reduce plasma concentrations of estrogens, possibly resulting in a decrease in therapeutic effects and/or changes in the uterine bleeding profile).
Products include:
Ciloxan Ophthalmic Ointment 559
Ciloxan Ophthalmic Solution .... ⊙206
Cipro Tablets 2977
Proquin XR Tablets 1153

Cisplatin (Co-administration of estrogens with inducers of CYP3A4 may reduce plasma concentrations of estrogens, possibly resulting in a decrease in therapeutic effects and/or changes in the uterine bleeding profile).
No products indexed under this heading.

Clarithromycin (Co-administration of estrogens with inhibitors of CYP3A4 may increase plasma concentrations of estrogens and may result in side effects). Products include:
Biaxin/Biaxin XL 402
PREVPAC 3284

Clotrimazole (Co-administration of estrogens with inhibitors of CYP3A4 may increase plasma concentrations of estrogens and may result in side effects). Products include:
Desenex Athlete's Foot Cream .... ▣635
Lotrimin 3039
Lotrisone 3040

Cortisone Acetate (Co-administration of estrogens with inducers of CYP3A4 may reduce plasma concentrations of estrogens, possibly resulting in a decrease in therapeutic effects and/or changes in the uterine bleeding profile).
No products indexed under this heading.

Cyclosporine (Co-administration of estrogens with inhibitors of CYP3A4 may increase plasma concentrations of estrogens and may result in side effects). Products include:
Gengraf Capsules 459
Neoral Oral Solution 2259
Neoral Soft Gelatin Capsules 2259
Restasis Ophthalmic Emulsion 575
Sandimmune 2275

Dalfopristin (Co-administration of estrogens with inhibitors of CYP3A4 may increase plasma concentrations of estrogens and may result in side effects).
No products indexed under this heading.

Danazol (Co-administration of estrogens with inhibitors of CYP3A4 may increase plasma concentrations of estrogens and may result in side effects).
No products indexed under this heading.

Delavirdine Mesylate (Co-administration of estrogens with inhibitors of CYP3A4 may increase plasma concentrations of estrogens and may result in side effects).
Products include:
Rescriptor Tablets 2551

Dexamethasone (Co-administration of estrogens with inducers of CYP3A4 may reduce plasma concentrations of estrogens, possibly resulting in a decrease in therapeutic effects and/or changes in the uterine bleeding profile).
Products include:
Ciprodex Otic Suspension 559
Decadron Tablets 1951
TobraDex Ophthalmic Ointment 562
TobraDex Ophthalmic Suspension 563

Dexamethasone Acetate (Co-administration of estrogens with inducers of CYP3A4 may reduce plasma concentrations of estrogens, possibly resulting in a decrease in therapeutic effects and/or changes in the uterine bleeding profile).
No products indexed under this heading.

Dexamethasone Sodium Phosphate (Co-administration of estrogens with inducers of CYP3A4 may reduce plasma concentrations of estrogens, possibly resulting in a decrease in therapeutic effects and/or changes in the uterine bleeding profile).
No products indexed under this heading.

Diltiazem Hydrochloride (Co-administration of estrogens with inhibitors of CYP3A4 may increase plasma concentrations of estrogens and may result in side effects).
Products include:
Cardizem LA Extended Release Tablets 1728
Tiazac Capsules 1201

Diltiazem Maleate (Co-administration of estrogens with inhibitors of CYP3A4 may increase plasma concentrations of estrogens and may result in side effects).
No products indexed under this heading.

Doxorubicin Hydrochloride (Co-administration of estrogens with inducers of CYP3A4 may reduce plasma concentrations of estrogens, possibly resulting in a decrease in therapeutic effects and/or changes in the uterine bleeding profile).
No products indexed under this heading.

Efavirenz (Co-administration of estrogens with inducers of CYP3A4 may reduce plasma concentrations of estrogens, possibly resulting in a decrease in therapeutic effects and/or changes in the uterine bleeding profile). Products include:
Atripla Tablets 945
Sustiva Capsules 930
Sustiva Tablets 930

Erythromycin (Co-administration of estrogens with inhibitors of CYP3A4 may increase plasma concentrations of estrogens and may result in side effects). Products include:
Ery-Tab Tablets 449
Erythromycin Base Filmtab Tablets 455
Erythromycin Delayed-Release Capsules, USP 457
PCE Dispertab Tablets 515

Erythromycin Estolate (Co-administration of estrogens with inhibitors of CYP3A4 may increase plasma concentrations of estrogens and may result in side effects).
No products indexed under this heading.

Erythromycin Ethylsuccinate (Co-administration of estrogens with inhibitors of CYP3A4 may increase plasma concentrations of estrogens and may result in side effects).
Products include:
E.E.S. 451
EryPed 447

Erythromycin Gluceptate (Co-administration of estrogens with inhibitors of CYP3A4 may increase plasma concentrations of estrogens and may result in side effects).
No products indexed under this heading.

Erythromycin Lactobionate (Co-administration of estrogens with inhibitors of CYP3A4 may increase plasma concentrations of estrogens and may result in side effects).
No products indexed under this heading.

Erythromycin Stearate (Co-administration of estrogens with inhibitors of CYP3A4 may increase plasma concentrations of estrogens and may result in side effects).
Products include:
Erythrocin Stearate Filmtab Tablets 453

Esomeprazole Magnesium (Co-administration of estrogens with inhibitors of CYP3A4 may increase plasma concentrations of estrogens and may result in side effects).
Products include:
Nexium Delayed-Release Capsules 655

Ethosuximide (Co-administration of estrogens with inducers of CYP3A4 may reduce plasma concentrations of estrogens, possibly resulting in a decrease in therapeutic effects and/or changes in the uterine bleeding profile).
No products indexed under this heading.

Felbamate (Co-administration of estrogens with inducers of CYP3A4 may reduce plasma concentrations of estrogens, possibly resulting in a decrease in therapeutic effects and/or changes in the uterine bleeding profile).
No products indexed under this heading.

Fluconazole (Co-administration of estrogens with inhibitors of CYP3A4 may increase plasma concentrations of estrogens and may result in side effects).
No products indexed under this heading.

Fludrocortisone Acetate (Co-administration of estrogens with inducers of CYP3A4 may reduce plasma concentrations of estrogens, possibly resulting in a decrease in therapeutic effects and/or changes in the uterine bleeding profile).
No products indexed under this heading.

Fluoxetine Hydrochloride (Co-administration of estrogens with inhibitors of CYP3A4 may increase plasma concentrations of estrogens and may result in side effects).
Products include:
Prozac Pulvules and Liquid 1801
Symbyax Capsules 1819

Fluvoxamine Maleate (Co-administration of estrogens with inhibitors of CYP3A4 may increase plasma concentrations of estrogens and may result in side effects).
No products indexed under this heading.

Fosamprenavir Calcium (Co-administration of estrogens with inhibitors of CYP3A4 may increase plasma concentrations of estrogens and may result in side effects).
Products include:
Lexiva Tablets 1505

Fosphenytoin Sodium (Co-administration of estrogens with inducers of CYP3A4 may reduce plasma concentrations of estrogens, possibly resulting in a decrease in therapeutic effects and/or changes in the uterine bleeding profile).
No products indexed under this heading.

Garlic Extract (Co-administration of estrogens with inducers of CYP3A4 may reduce plasma concentrations of estrogens, possibly resulting in a decrease in therapeutic effects and/or changes in the uterine bleeding profile).
No products indexed under this heading.

Garlic Oil (Co-administration of estrogens with inducers of CYP3A4 may reduce plasma concentrations of estrogens, possibly resulting in a decrease in therapeutic effects and/or changes in the uterine bleeding profile).
No products indexed under this heading.

Hydrocortisone (Co-administration of estrogens with inducers of CYP3A4 may reduce plasma concentrations of estrogens, possibly resulting in a decrease in therapeutic effects and/or changes in the uterine bleeding profile). Products include:
Colocort Rectal Suspension, USP (Retention) 100 mg/60 mL 2476
Hydrocortone Tablets 1989
Preparation H Hydrocortisone Cream .... ▣646

Hydrocortisone Acetate (Co-administration of estrogens with inducers of CYP3A4 may reduce plasma concentrations of estrogens, possibly resulting in a decrease in therapeutic effects and/or changes in the uterine bleeding profile).
Products include:
Analpram-HC 1159
Pramosone 1161
ProctoFoam-HC 3099

Hydrocortisone Butyrate (Co-administration of estrogens with inducers of CYP3A4 may reduce plasma concentrations of estrogens, possibly resulting in a decrease in therapeutic effects and/or changes in the uterine bleeding profile).
Products include:
Locoid Lipocream Cream 1160

Hydrocortisone Cypionate (Co-administration of estrogens with inducers of CYP3A4 may reduce plasma concentrations of estrogens, possibly resulting in a decrease in therapeutic effects and/or changes in the uterine bleeding profile).
No products indexed under this heading.

Hydrocortisone Hemisuccinate (Co-administration of estrogens with inducers of CYP3A4 may reduce plasma concentrations of estrogens, possibly resulting in a decrease in therapeutic effects and/or changes in the uterine bleeding profile).
No products indexed under this heading.

Hydrocortisone Probutate (Co-administration of estrogens with inducers of CYP3A4 may reduce plasma concentrations of estrogens, possibly resulting in a decrease in therapeutic effects and/or changes in the uterine bleeding profile).
No products indexed under this heading.

Hydrocortisone Sodium Phosphate (Co-administration of estrogens with inducers of CYP3A4 may reduce plasma concentrations of estrogens, possibly resulting in a decrease in therapeutic effects and/or changes in the uterine bleeding profile).
No products indexed under this heading.

Hydrocortisone Sodium Succinate (Co-administration of estrogens with inducers of CYP3A4 may reduce plasma concentrations of estrogens, possibly resulting in a decrease in therapeutic effects and/or changes in the uterine bleeding profile).
No products indexed under this heading.

Hydrocortisone Valerate (Co-administration of estrogens with inducers of CYP3A4 may reduce plasma concentrations of estrogens, possibly resulting in a decrease in therapeutic effects and/or changes in the uterine bleeding profile).
No products indexed under this heading.

Hypericum (Co-administration of estrogens with inducers of CYP3A4 may reduce plasma concentrations of estrogens, possibly resulting in a decrease in therapeutic effects and/or changes in the uterine bleeding profile). Products include:
Satiete Tablets .... ▣832

Hypericum Perforatum (Co-administration of estrogens with inducers of CYP3A4 may reduce plasma concentrations of estrogens, possibly resulting in a decrease in therapeutic effects and/or changes in the uterine bleeding profile).
No products indexed under this heading.

Indinavir Sulfate (Co-administration of estrogens with inhibitors of CYP3A4 may increase plasma concentrations of estrogens and may result in side effects). Products include:
Crixivan Capsules 1940

Isoniazid (Co-administration of estrogens with inhibitors of CYP3A4 may increase plasma concentrations of estrogens and may result in side effects).
No products indexed under this heading.

Itraconazole (Co-administration of estrogens with inhibitors of CYP3A4 may increase plasma concentrations of estrogens and may result in side effects).
No products indexed under this heading.

Ketoconazole (Co-administration of estrogens with inhibitors of CYP3A4 may increase plasma concentrations of estrogens and may result in side effects). Products include:
Nizoral A-D Shampoo, 1% 1868

Lopinavir (Co-administration of estrogens with inhibitors of CYP3A4 may increase plasma concentrations of estrogens and may result in side effects). Products include:
Kaletra 476

Loratadine (Co-administration of estrogens with inhibitors of CYP3A4 may increase plasma concentrations of estrogens and may result in side effects). Products include:
Alavert Allergy & Sinus D-12 Hour Tablets .... ▣771
Alavert .... ▣771
Children's Claritin Allergy Oral Solution .... ▣771
Claritin Non-Drowsy 24 Hour Tablets .... ▣772
Claritin Reditabs 24 Hour Non-Drowsy Tablets .... ▣772
Claritin-D Non-Drowsy 12 Hour Tablets .... ▣772
Claritin-D Non-Drowsy 24 Hour Tablets .... ▣772

Mephenytoin (Co-administration of estrogens with inducers of CYP3A4 may reduce plasma concentrations of estrogens, possibly resulting in a decrease in therapeutic effects and/or changes in the uterine bleeding profile).
No products indexed under this heading.

Methsuximide (Co-administration of estrogens with inducers of CYP3A4 may reduce plasma concentrations of estrogens, possibly resulting in a decrease in therapeutic effects and/or changes in the uterine bleeding profile).
No products indexed under this heading.

Methylprednisolone (Co-administration of estrogens with inducers of CYP3A4 may reduce plasma concentrations of estrogens, possibly resulting in a decrease in therapeutic effects and/or changes in the uterine bleeding profile).
No products indexed under this heading.

Methylprednisolone Acetate (Co-administration of estrogens with inducers of CYP3A4 may reduce plasma concentrations of estrogens, possibly resulting in a decrease in therapeutic effects and/or changes in the uterine bleeding profile). Products include:
Depo-Medrol Injectable Suspension 2617
Depo-Medrol Single-Dose Vial 2619

Methylprednisolone Sodium Succinate (Co-administration of estrogens with inducers of CYP3A4 may reduce plasma concentrations of estrogens, possibly resulting in a decrease in therapeutic effects and/or changes in the uterine bleeding profile).
No products indexed under this heading.

Metronidazole (Co-administration of estrogens with inhibitors of CYP3A4 may increase plasma concentrations of estrogens and may result in side effects). Products include:
Metrogel 1% 1211
MetroGel-Vaginal Gel 1855
Vandazole Vaginal Gel 3338

Metronidazole Benzoate (Co-administration of estrogens with inhibitors of CYP3A4 may increase plasma concentrations of estrogens and may result in side effects).
No products indexed under this heading.

Metronidazole Hydrochloride (Co-administration of estrogens with inhibitors of CYP3A4 may increase plasma concentrations of estrogens and may result in side effects).
No products indexed under this heading.

Miconazole (Co-administration of estrogens with inhibitors of CYP3A4 may increase plasma concentrations of estrogens and may result in side effects).
No products indexed under this heading.

Miconazole Nitrate (Co-administration of estrogens with inhibitors of CYP3A4 may increase plasma concentrations of estrogens and may result in side effects). Products include:
Desenex .... ▣635
Desenex Jock Itch Spray Powder ... ▣635

Modafinil (Co-administration of estrogens with inducers of CYP3A4 may reduce plasma concentrations of estrogens, possibly resulting in a decrease in therapeutic effects and/or changes in the uterine bleeding profile). Products include:
Provigil Tablets 988

Nefazodone Hydrochloride (Co-administration of estrogens with inhibitors of CYP3A4 may increase plasma concentrations of estrogens and may result in side effects).
No products indexed under this heading.

Nelfinavir Mesylate (Co-administration of estrogens with inhibitors of CYP3A4 may increase plasma concentrations of estrogens and may result in side effects). Products include:
Viracept 2577

Nevirapine (Co-administration of estrogens with inducers of CYP3A4 may reduce plasma concentrations of estrogens, possibly resulting in a decrease in therapeutic effects and/or changes in the uterine bleeding profile). Products include:
Viramune Oral Suspension 873
Viramune Tablets 873

Niacinamide (Co-administration of estrogens with inhibitors of CYP3A4 may increase plasma concentrations of estrogens and may result in side effects).
No products indexed under this heading.

Nicotinamide (Co-administration of estrogens with inhibitors of CYP3A4 may increase plasma concentrations of estrogens and may result in side effects). Products include:
Nicomide Tablets 1088

Nifedipine (Co-administration of estrogens with inhibitors of CYP3A4 may increase plasma concentrations of estrogens and may result in side effects). Products include:
Adalat CC Tablets 2964

Norfloxacin (Co-administration of estrogens with inhibitors of CYP3A4 may increase plasma concentrations of estrogens and may result in side effects). Products include:
Noroxin Tablets 2032

Omeprazole (Co-administration of estrogens with inhibitors of CYP3A4 may increase plasma concentrations of estrogens and may result in side effects). Products include:
Zegerid Capsules 2958
Zegerid Powder for Oral Solution 2958

Oxcarbazepine (Co-administration of estrogens with inducers of CYP3A4 may reduce plasma concentrations of estrogens, possibly resulting in a decrease in therapeutic effects and/or changes in the uterine bleeding profile). Products include:
Trileptal Tablets 2300
Trileptal Oral Suspension 2300

Paroxetine Hydrochloride (Co-administration of estrogens with inhibitors of CYP3A4 may increase plasma concentrations of estrogens and may result in side effects). Products include:
Paxil CR Controlled-Release Tablets 1538
Paxil 1530

Phenobarbital (Co-administration of estrogens with inducers of CYP3A4 may reduce plasma concentrations of estrogens, possibly resulting in a decrease in therapeutic effects and/or changes in the uterine bleeding profile). Products include:
Donnatal Extentabs 2493

Phenobarbital Sodium (Co-administration of estrogens with inducers of CYP3A4 may reduce plasma concentrations of estrogens, possibly resulting in a decrease in therapeutic effects and/or changes in the uterine bleeding profile).
No products indexed under this heading.

Phenytoin (Co-administration of estrogens with inducers of CYP3A4 may reduce plasma concentrations of estrogens, possibly resulting in a decrease in therapeutic effects and/or changes in the uterine bleeding profile).
No products indexed under this heading.

Phenytoin Sodium (Co-administration of estrogens with inducers of CYP3A4 may reduce plasma concentrations of estrogens, possibly resulting in a decrease in therapeutic effects and/or changes in the uterine bleeding profile). Products include:
Phenytek Capsules 2160

Prednisolone Acetate (Co-administration of estrogens with inducers of CYP3A4 may reduce plasma concentrations of estrogens, possibly resulting in a decrease in therapeutic effects and/or changes in the uterine bleeding profile). Products include:
Blephamide Ophthalmic Ointment 568
Blephamide Ophthalmic Suspension 569
Poly-Pred Ophthalmic Suspension .... ⊙233
Pred Forte Ophthalmic Suspension .... ⊙235
Pred Mild Ophthalmic Suspension .... ⊙238
Pred-G Ophthalmic Ointment .... ⊙237
Pred-G Ophthalmic Suspension ...... ⊙236

Prednisolone Sodium Phosphate (Co-administration of estrogens with inducers of CYP3A4 may reduce plasma concentrations of estrogens, possibly resulting in a decrease in therapeutic effects and/or changes in the uterine bleeding profile).
No products indexed under this heading.

Prednisolone Tebutate (Co-administration of estrogens with inducers of CYP3A4 may reduce plasma concentrations of estrogens, possibly resulting in a decrease in therapeutic effects and/or changes in the uterine bleeding profile).
No products indexed under this heading.

Prednisone (Co-administration of estrogens with inducers of CYP3A4 may reduce plasma concentrations of estrogens, possibly resulting in a decrease in therapeutic effects and/or changes in the uterine bleeding profile).
No products indexed under this heading.

Primidone (Co-administration of estrogens with inducers of CYP3A4 may reduce plasma concentrations of estrogens, possibly resulting in a decrease in therapeutic effects and/or changes in the uterine bleeding profile).
No products indexed under this heading.

Propoxyphene Hydrochloride (Co-administration of estrogens with inhibitors of CYP3A4 may increase plasma concentrations of estrogens and may result in side effects).
No products indexed under this heading.

Propoxyphene Napsylate (Co-administration of estrogens with inhibitors of CYP3A4 may increase plasma concentrations of estrogens and may result in side effects).
No products indexed under this heading.

Quinidine (Co-administration of estrogens with inhibitors of CYP3A4 may increase plasma concentrations of estrogens and may result in side effects).
No products indexed under this heading.

Quinidine Hydrochloride (Co-administration of estrogens with inhibitors of CYP3A4 may increase plasma concentrations of estrogens and may result in side effects).
No products indexed under this heading.

Quinidine Polygalacturonate (Co-administration of estrogens with inhibitors of CYP3A4 may increase plasma concentrations of estrogens and may result in side effects).
No products indexed under this heading.

Quinidine Sulfate (Co-administration of estrogens with inhibitors of CYP3A4 may increase plasma concentrations of estrogens and may result in side effects).
No products indexed under this heading.

Quinine (Co-administration of estrogens with inhibitors of CYP3A4 may increase plasma concentrations of estrogens and may result in side effects).
No products indexed under this heading.

Quinine Sulfate (Co-administration of estrogens with inhibitors of CYP3A4 may increase plasma concentrations of estrogens and may result in side effects).
No products indexed under this heading.

Quinupristin (Co-administration of estrogens with inhibitors of CYP3A4 may increase plasma concentrations of estrogens and may result in side effects).
No products indexed under this heading.

Ranitidine Bismuth Citrate (Co-administration of estrogens with inhibitors of CYP3A4 may increase plasma concentrations of estrogens and may result in side effects).
No products indexed under this heading.

Ranitidine Hydrochloride (Co-administration of estrogens with inhibitors of CYP3A4 may increase plasma concentrations of estrogens and may result in side effects).
Products include:
Zantac 1624
Zantac Injection 1619
Zantac Injection Pharmacy Bulk Package 1622

Rifabutin (Co-administration of estrogens with inducers of CYP3A4 may reduce plasma concentrations of estrogens, possibly resulting in a decrease in therapeutic effects and/or changes in the uterine bleeding profile).
No products indexed under this heading.

Rifampicin (Co-administration of estrogens with inducers of CYP3A4 may reduce plasma concentrations of estrogens, possibly resulting in a decrease in therapeutic effects and/or changes in the uterine bleeding profile).
No products indexed under this heading.

Rifampin (Co-administration of estrogens with inducers of CYP3A4 may reduce plasma concentrations of estrogens, possibly resulting in a decrease in therapeutic effects and/or changes in the uterine bleeding profile).
No products indexed under this heading.

Rifapentine (Co-administration of estrogens with inducers of CYP3A4 may reduce plasma concentrations of estrogens, possibly resulting in a decrease in therapeutic effects and/or changes in the uterine bleeding profile).
No products indexed under this heading.

Ritonavir (Co-administration of estrogens with inhibitors of CYP3A4 may increase plasma concentrations of estrogens and may result in side effects). Products include:
Kaletra 476
Norvir 503

Saquinavir (Co-administration of estrogens with inhibitors of CYP3A4 may increase plasma concentrations of estrogens and may result in side effects).
No products indexed under this heading.

Saquinavir Mesylate (Co-administration of estrogens with inhibitors of CYP3A4 may increase plasma concentrations of estrogens and may result in side effects).
Products include:
Invirase 2772

Sertraline Hydrochloride (Co-administration of estrogens with inhibitors of CYP3A4 may increase plasma concentrations of estrogens and may result in side effects).
Products include:
Zoloft 2586

Sulfinpyrazone (Co-administration of estrogens with inducers of CYP3A4 may reduce plasma concentrations of estrogens, possibly resulting in a decrease in therapeutic effects and/or changes in the uterine bleeding profile).
No products indexed under this heading.

Telithromycin (Co-administration of estrogens with inhibitors of CYP3A4 may increase plasma concentrations of estrogens and may result in side effects). Products include:
Ketek Tablets 2903

Theophylline (Co-administration of estrogens with inducers of CYP3A4 may reduce plasma concentrations of estrogens, possibly resulting in a decrease in therapeutic effects and/or changes in the uterine bleeding profile).
No products indexed under this heading.

Triamcinolone (Co-administration of estrogens with inducers of CYP3A4 may reduce plasma concentrations of estrogens, possibly resulting in a decrease in therapeutic effects and/or changes in the uterine bleeding profile).
No products indexed under this heading.

Triamcinolone Acetonide (Co-administration of estrogens with inducers of CYP3A4 may reduce plasma concentrations of estrogens, possibly resulting in a decrease in therapeutic effects and/or changes in the uterine bleeding profile).
Products include:
Azmacort Inhalation Aerosol 1726
Nasacort AQ Nasal Spray 2922

Triamcinolone Diacetate (Co-administration of estrogens with inducers of CYP3A4 may reduce plasma concentrations of estrogens, possibly resulting in a decrease in therapeutic effects and/or changes in the uterine bleeding profile).
No products indexed under this heading.

Triamcinolone Hexacetonide (Co-administration of estrogens with inducers of CYP3A4 may reduce plasma concentrations of estrogens, possibly resulting in a decrease in therapeutic effects and/or changes in the uterine bleeding profile).
No products indexed under this heading.

Troglitazone (Co-administration of estrogens with inducers of CYP3A4 may reduce plasma concentrations of estrogens, possibly resulting in a decrease in therapeutic effects and/or changes in the uterine bleeding profile).
No products indexed under this heading.

Troleandomycin (Co-administration of estrogens with inhibitors of CYP3A4 may increase plasma concentrations of estrogens and may result in side effects).
No products indexed under this heading.

Valproate Sodium (Co-administration of estrogens with inhibitors of CYP3A4 may increase plasma concentrations of estrogens and may result in side effects).
Products include:
Depacon Injection 412

Verapamil Hydrochloride (Co-administration of estrogens with inhibitors of CYP3A4 may increase plasma concentrations of estrogens and may result in side effects).
Products include:
Covera-HS Tablets 3139
Tarka Tablets 524
Verelan PM Extended-Release Capsules, Controlled-Onset 3106

Voriconazole (Co-administration of estrogens with inhibitors of CYP3A4 may increase plasma concentrations of estrogens and may result in side effects). Products include:
VFEND I.V. 2564
VFEND Oral Suspension 2564
VFEND Tablets 2564

Zafirlukast (Co-administration of estrogens with inhibitors of CYP3A4 may increase plasma concentrations of estrogens and may result in side effects). Products include:
Accolate Tablets 671

Zileuton (Co-administration of estrogens with inhibitors of CYP3A4 may increase plasma concentrations of estrogens and may result in side effects). Products include:
Zyflo Tablets 1023

Food Interactions

Food, unspecified (Administration with food decreased Cmax of total estrone compared to fasting state, no other effect on rate or extent of absorption; administration with food doubles MPA Cmax and increases MPA AUC).

Grapefruit (Co-administration of estrogens with inhibitors of CYP3A4 may increase plasma concentrations of estrogens and may result in side effects).

Grapefruit Juice (Co-administration of estrogens with inhibitors of CYP3A4, such as grapefruit juice, may increase plasma concentrations of estrogens and may result in side effects).

PRENATE ELITE TABLETS
(Vitamins, Prenatal) 3121
None cited in PDR database.

PREPARATION H MAXIMUM STRENGTH CREAM
(Glycerin, Petrolatum, Phenylephrine Hydrochloride, Pramoxine Hydrochloride) .... ■ 666
None cited in PDR database.

PREPARATION H COOLING GEL
(Phenylephrine Hydrochloride) .... ■ 666
None cited in PDR database.

PREPARATION H HYDROCORTISONE CREAM
(Hydrocortisone) .... ■ 646
None cited in PDR database.

PREPARATION H OINTMENT
(Mineral Oil, Petrolatum, Phenylephrine Hydrochloride, Shark Liver Oil) .... ■ 666
None cited in PDR database.

PREPARATION H SUPPOSITORIES
(Cocoa Butter, Phenylephrine Hydrochloride, Shark Liver Oil)........... 666
None cited in PDR database.

PREPARATION H MEDICATED WIPES
(Witch Hazel) 667
None cited in PDR database.

PREVACID DELAYED-RELEASE CAPSULES
(Lansoprazole) 3271
May interact with iron containing oral preparations, absorption of drugs where gastric ph is an important determinant in their bioavailability, xanthines, and certain other agents. Compounds in these categories include:

Aminophylline (Co-administration has resulted in a minor increase (10%) in the clearance of theophylline; this interaction is unlikely to be of clinical concern, nonetheless, monitor blood levels).
No products indexed under this heading.

Astemizole (There have been post-marketing reports of drug interactions when clarithromycin and/or erythromycin are co-administered with cisapride, pimozide, astemizole or terfenadine resulting in cardiac arrhythmias most likely due to inhibition of metabolism of these drugs by erythromycin and clarithromycin. Fatalities have been reported).
No products indexed under this heading.

Bacampicillin Hydrochloride (Lansoprazole causes a profound and long-lasting inhibition of gastric acid secretion; therefore, it is theoretically possible that it may interfere with the oral absorption of drugs where gastric pH is an important determinant of bioavailability).
No products indexed under this heading.

Cisapride (There have been post-marketing reports of drug interactions when clarithromycin and/or erythromycin are co-administered with cisapride, pimozide, astemizole or terfenadine resulting in cardiac arrhythmias most likely due to inhibition of metabolism of these drugs by erythromycin and clarithromycin. Fatalities have been reported).
No products indexed under this heading.

Digoxin (Lansoprazole causes a profound and long-lasting inhibition of gastric acid secretion; therefore, it is theoretically possible that it may interfere with the oral absorption of drugs where gastric pH is an important determinant of bioavailability, such as digoxin). Products include:
Lanoxicaps Capsules 1490
Lanoxin Injection 1494
Lanoxin Injection Pediatric 1497
Lanoxin Tablets 1500

Dyphylline (Co-administration has resulted in a minor increase (10%) in the clearance of theophylline; this interaction is unlikely to be of clinical concern, nonetheless, monitor blood levels).
No products indexed under this heading.

Ferrous Fumarate (Lansoprazole causes a profound and long-lasting inhibition of gastric acid secretion; therefore, it is theoretically possible that it may interfere with the absorption of drugs, such as iron salts, where gastric pH is an important determinant of bioavailability).
No products indexed under this heading.

Ferrous Gluconate (Lansoprazole causes a profound and long-lasting inhibition of gastric acid secretion; therefore, it is theoretically possible that it may interfere with the absorption of drugs, such as iron salts, where gastric pH is an important determinant of bioavailability).
No products indexed under this heading.

Ferrous Sulfate (Lansoprazole causes a profound and long-lasting inhibition of gastric acid secretion; therefore, it is theoretically possible that it may interfere with the absorption of drugs, such as iron salts, where gastric pH is an important determinant of bioavailability). Products include:
Slow Fe Iron Tablets 818
Slow Fe with Folic Acid Tablets 819

Iron (Lansoprazole causes a profound and long-lasting inhibition of gastric acid secretion; therefore, it is theoretically possible that it may interfere with the absorption of drugs, such as iron salts, where gastric pH is an important determinant of bioavailability).
No products indexed under this heading.

Ketoconazole (Lansoprazole causes a profound and long-lasting inhibition of gastric acid secretion; therefore, it is theoretically possible that it may interfere with the oral absorption of drugs where gastric pH is an important determinant of bioavailability). Products include:
Nizoral A-D Shampoo, 1% 1868

Pimozide (There have been post-marketing reports of drug interactions when clarithromycin and/or erythromycin are co-administered with cisapride, pimozide, astemizole or terfenadine resulting in cardiac arrhythmias most likely due to inhibition of metabolism of these drugs by erythromycin and clarithromycin. Fatalities have been reported).
No products indexed under this heading.

Polysaccharide Iron Complex (Lansoprazole causes a profound and long-lasting inhibition of gastric acid secretion; therefore, it is theoretically possible that it may interfere with the absorption of drugs, such as iron salts, where gastric pH is an important determinant of bioavailability). Products include:
Nu-Iron 150 Capsules 2127

Sucralfate (Co-administration delays absorption and reduces bioavailability of lansoprazole by about 30%; therefore, lansoprazole should be taken at least 30 minutes prior to sucralfate). Products include:
Carafate Suspension 701
Carafate Tablets 701

Terfenadine (There have been post-marketing reports of drug interactions when clarithromycin and/or erythromycin are co-administered with cisapride, pimozide, astemizole or terfenadine resulting in cardiac arrhythmias most likely due to inhibition of metabolism of these drugs by erythromycin and clarithromycin. Fatalities have been reported).
No products indexed under this heading.

Theophylline (Co-administration has resulted in a minor increase (10%) in the clearance of theophylline; this interaction is unlikely to be of clinical concern, nonetheless, monitor blood levels).
No products indexed under this heading.

Theophylline Anhydrous (Co-administration has resulted in a minor increase (10%) in the clearance of theophylline; this interaction is unlikely to be of clinical concern, nonetheless, monitor blood levels). Products include:
Uniphyl Tablets 2710

Theophylline Calcium Salicylate (Co-administration has resulted in a minor increase (10%) in the clearance of theophylline; this interaction is unlikely to be of clinical concern, nonetheless, monitor blood levels).
No products indexed under this heading.

Theophylline Dihydroxypropyl (Glyceryl) (Co-administration has resulted in a minor increase (10%) in the clearance of theophylline; this interaction is unlikely to be of clinical concern, nonetheless, monitor blood levels).
No products indexed under this heading.

Theophylline Ethylenediamine (Co-administration has resulted in a minor increase (10%) in the clearance of theophylline; this interaction is unlikely to be of clinical concern, nonetheless, monitor blood levels).
No products indexed under this heading.

Theophylline Sodium Glycinate (Co-administration has resulted in a minor increase (10%) in the clearance of theophylline; this interaction is unlikely to be of clinical concern, nonetheless, monitor blood levels).
No products indexed under this heading.

Food Interactions

Food, unspecified (Cmax and AUC are diminished by about 50% if the drug is given 30 minutes after food as opposed to the fasting condition; Prevacid should be taken before eating).

PREVACID FOR DELAYED-RELEASE ORAL SUSPENSION
(Lansoprazole) 3271
See Prevacid Delayed-Release Capsules

PREVACID SOLUTAB DELAYED-RELEASE ORALLY DISINTEGRATING TABLETS
(Lansoprazole) 3271
See Prevacid Delayed-Release Capsules

PREVACID I.V. FOR INJECTION
(Lansoprazole) 3277
May interact with iron salts, absorption of drugs where gastric ph is an important determinant in their bioavailability, xanthines, and certain other agents. Compounds in these categories include:

Aminophylline (Co-administration has resulted in a minor increase (10%) in the clearance of theophylline; this interaction is unlikely to be of clinical concern; nonetheless, monitor blood levels).
No products indexed under this heading.

Bacampicillin Hydrochloride (Lansoprazole causes a profound and long-lasting inhibition of gastric acid secretion; therefore, it is theoretically possible that it may interfere with the absorption of drugs where gastric pH is an important determinant of bioavailability).
No products indexed under this heading.

Digoxin (Lansoprazole causes a profound and long-lasting inhibition of gastric acid secretion; therefore, it is theoretically possible that it may interfere with the absorption of drugs where gastric pH is an important determinant of bioavailability, such as digoxin). Products include:
Lanoxicaps Capsules 1490
Lanoxin Injection 1494
Lanoxin Injection Pediatric 1497
Lanoxin Tablets 1500

Dyphylline (Co-administration has resulted in a minor increase (10%) in the clearance of theophylline; this interaction is unlikely to be of clinical concern; nonetheless, monitor blood levels).
No products indexed under this heading.

Ferrous Fumarate (Lansoprazole causes a profound and long-lasting inhibition of gastric acid secretion; therefore, it is theoretically possible that it may interfere with the absorption of drugs, such as iron salts, where gastric pH is an important determinant of bioavailability).
No products indexed under this heading.

Ferrous Gluconate (Lansoprazole causes a profound and long-lasting inhibition of gastric acid secretion; therefore, it is theoretically possible that it may interfere with the absorption of drugs, such as iron salts, where gastric pH is an important determinant of bioavailability).
No products indexed under this heading.

Ferrous Sulfate (Lansoprazole causes a profound and long-lasting inhibition of gastric acid secretion; therefore, it is theoretically possible that it may interfere with the absorption of drugs, such as iron salts, where gastric pH is an important determinant of bioavailability). Products include:
Slow Fe Iron Tablets 818
Slow Fe with Folic Acid Tablets 819

Iron (Lansoprazole causes a profound and long-lasting inhibition of gastric acid secretion; therefore, it is theoretically possible that it may interfere with the absorption of drugs, such as iron salts, where gastric pH is an important determinant of bioavailability).
No products indexed under this heading.

Iron, Peptonized (Lansoprazole causes a profound and long-lasting inhibition of gastric acid secretion; therefore, it is theoretically possible that it may interfere with the absorption of drugs, such as iron salts, where gastric pH is an important determinant of bioavailability).
No products indexed under this heading.

Iron Cacodylate (Lansoprazole causes a profound and long-lasting inhibition of gastric acid secretion; therefore, it is theoretically possible that it may interfere with the absorption of drugs, such as iron salts, where gastric pH is an important determinant of bioavailability).
No products indexed under this heading.

Iron Carbonyl (Lansoprazole causes a profound and long-lasting inhibition of gastric acid secretion; therefore, it is theoretically possible that it may interfere with the absorption of drugs, such as iron salts, where gastric pH is an important determinant of bioavailability).
No products indexed under this heading.

Iron Dextran (Lansoprazole causes a profound and long-lasting inhibition of gastric acid secretion; therefore, it is theoretically possible that it may interfere with the absorption of drugs, such as iron salts, where gastric pH is an important determinant of bioavailability). Products include:
Infed Injection 3390

Iron Polysaccharide Complex (Lansoprazole causes a profound and long-lasting inhibition of gastric acid secretion; therefore, it is theoretically possible that it may interfere with the absorption of drugs, such as iron salts, where gastric pH is an important determinant of bioavailability).
No products indexed under this heading.

Iron Sucrose (Lansoprazole causes a profound and long-lasting inhibition of gastric acid secretion; therefore, it is theoretically possible that it may interfere with the absorption of drugs, such as iron salts, where gastric pH is an important determinant of bioavailability).
No products indexed under this heading.

Iron Supplements (Lansoprazole causes a profound and long-lasting inhibition of gastric acid secretion; therefore, it is theoretically possible that it may interfere with the absorption of drugs, such as iron salts, where gastric pH is an important determinant of bioavailability).
No products indexed under this heading.

Ketoconazole (Lansoprazole causes a profound and long-lasting inhibition of gastric acid secretion; therefore, it is theoretically possible that it may interfere with the absorption of drugs where gastric pH is an important determinant of bioavailability). Products include:
Nizoral A-D Shampoo, 1% 1868

Polysaccharide Iron Complex (Lansoprazole causes a profound and long-lasting inhibition of gastric acid secretion; therefore, it is theoretically possible that it may interfere with the absorption of drugs, such as iron salts, where gastric pH is an important determinant of bioavailability). Products include:
Nu-Iron 150 Capsules 2127

Theophylline (Co-administration has resulted in a minor increase (10%) in the clearance of theophylline; this interaction is unlikely to be of clinical concern; nonetheless, monitor blood levels).
No products indexed under this heading.

Theophylline Anhydrous (Co-administration has resulted in a minor increase (10%) in the clearance of theophylline; this interaction is unlikely to be of clinical concern; nonetheless, monitor blood levels). Products include:
Uniphyl Tablets 2710

Theophylline Calcium Salicylate (Co-administration has resulted in a minor increase (10%) in the clearance of theophylline; this interaction is unlikely to be of clinical concern; nonetheless, monitor blood levels).
No products indexed under this heading.

Theophylline Dihydroxypropyl (Glyceryl) (Co-administration has resulted in a minor increase (10%) in the clearance of theophylline; this interaction is unlikely to be of clinical concern; nonetheless, monitor blood levels).
No products indexed under this heading.

Theophylline Ethylenediamine (Co-administration has resulted in a minor increase (10%) in the clearance of theophylline; this interaction is unlikely to be of clinical concern; nonetheless, monitor blood levels).
No products indexed under this heading.

Theophylline Sodium Glycinate (Co-administration has resulted in a minor increase (10%) in the clearance of theophylline; this interaction is unlikely to be of clinical concern; nonetheless, monitor blood levels).
No products indexed under this heading.

Warfarin Sodium (There have been reports of increased International Normalized Ratio (INR) and prothrombin time in patients receiving proton pump inhibitors, including lansoprazole, and warfarin concomitantly). Products include:
Coumadin for Injection 898
Coumadin Tablets 898

PREVACID NAPRAPAC 375

(Lansoprazole, Naproxen) 3280
May interact with ACE inhibitors, beta blockers, oral anticoagulants, hydantoin anticonvulsants, lithium preparations, absorption of drugs where gastric ph is an important determinant in their bioavailability, highly protein bound drugs (selected), sulfonamides, sulfonylureas, and certain other agents. Compounds in these categories include:

Acebutolol Hydrochloride (Naproxen can reduce the antihypertensive effect of beta-blockers).
No products indexed under this heading.

Amiodarone Hydrochloride (In vitro studies have shown that naproxen anion, because of its affinity for protein, may displace from their binding sites other drugs that are also albumin-bound).
No products indexed under this heading.

Amitriptyline Hydrochloride (In vitro studies have shown that naproxen anion, because of its affinity for protein, may displace from their binding sites other drugs that are also albumin-bound).
No products indexed under this heading.

Anisindione (Short-term studies have failed to show any significant effects of concurrent use on prothrombin time; caution is advised since interactions have been seen with other NSAIDs). Products include:
Miradon Tablets 3042

Aspirin (Concomitant administration of naproxen and aspirin is not recommended because naproxen is displaced from its binding sites resulting in lower plasma concentrations and peak plasma levels). Products include:
Aggrenox Capsules 822
Bayer Aspirin 744
BC Allergy Sinus Cold Powder .... ▣677
BC Headache Powder .... ▣677
Arthritis Strength BC Powder .... ▣677
BC Sinus Cold Powder .... ▣677
Excedrin Extra Strength Caplets/Tablets/Geltabs .... ▣684
Excedrin Migraine Caplets/Tablets/Geltabs .... ▣609
Goody's Body Pain Formula Powder .... ▣684
Goody's Extra Strength Headache Powders.................... ▣611
Goody's Extra Strength Pain Relief Tablets .... ▣685
Percodan Tablets 1132
St. Joseph 81 mg Aspirin Chewable and Enteric Coated Tablets 1869

Atenolol (Naproxen can reduce the antihypertensive effect of beta-blockers).
No products indexed under this heading.

Atovaquone (In vitro studies have shown that naproxen anion, because of its affinity for protein, may displace from their binding sites other drugs that are also albumin-bound). Products include:
Malarone Pediatric Tablets 1517
Malarone Tablets 1517
Mepron Suspension 1521

Bacampicillin Hydrochloride (Lansoprazole causes a profound and long-lasting inhibition of gastric acid secretion; therefore, it is theoretically possible that lansoprazole may interfere with the absorption of drugs where gastric pH is an important determinant of bioavailability).
No products indexed under this heading.

Benazepril Hydrochloride (Co-administration of NSAIDs and ACE inhibitors may potentiate renal disease states). Products include:
Lotensin Tablets 2243
Lotensin HCT Tablets 2246
Lotrel Capsules 2249

Bendroflumethiazide (Observe signs for sulfonamide toxicity).
No products indexed under this heading.

Betaxolol Hydrochloride (Naproxen can reduce the antihypertensive effect of beta-blockers). Products include:
Betoptic S Ophthalmic Suspension................................. 558

Bisoprolol Fumarate (Naproxen can reduce the antihypertensive effect of beta-blockers).
No products indexed under this heading.

Captopril (Co-administration of NSAIDs and ACE inhibitors may potentiate renal disease states). Products include:
Captopril Tablets 2149

Carteolol Hydrochloride (Naproxen can reduce the antihypertensive effect of beta-blockers). Products include:
Carteolol Hydrochloride Ophthalmic Solution USP, 1%....... ⊙249

Cefonicid Sodium (In vitro studies have shown that naproxen anion, because of its affinity for protein, may displace from their binding sites other drugs that are also albumin-bound).
No products indexed under this heading.

Celecoxib (In vitro studies have shown that naproxen anion, because of its affinity for protein, may displace from their binding sites other drugs that are also albumin-bound). Products include:
Celebrex Capsules 3134

Chlordiazepoxide (In vitro studies have shown that naproxen anion, because of its affinity for protein, may displace from their binding sites other drugs that are also albumin-bound).
No products indexed under this heading.

Chlordiazepoxide Hydrochloride (In vitro studies have shown that naproxen anion, because of its affinity for protein, may displace from their binding sites other drugs that are also albumin-bound). Products include:
Librium Capsules 3347

Chlorothiazide (Observe signs for sulfonamide toxicity). Products include:
Diuril Oral Suspension 1954

Chlorothiazide Sodium (Observe signs for sulfonamide toxicity). Products include:
Diuril Sodium Intravenous 2467

Chlorpromazine (In vitro studies have shown that naproxen anion, because of its affinity for protein, may displace from their binding sites other drugs that are also albumin-bound).
No products indexed under this heading.

Chlorpromazine Hydrochloride (In vitro studies have shown that naproxen anion, because of its affinity for protein, may displace from their binding sites other drugs that are also albumin-bound).
No products indexed under this heading.

Chlorpropamide (Observe signs for sulfonamide toxicity).
No products indexed under this heading.

Clomipramine Hydrochloride (In vitro studies have shown that naproxen anion, because of its affinity for protein, may displace from their binding sites other drugs that are also albumin-bound).
No products indexed under this heading.

Clozapine (In vitro studies have shown that naproxen anion, because of its affinity for protein, may displace from their binding sites other drugs that are also albumin-bound). Products include:
Clozaril Tablets 2184

FazaClo Orally Disintegrating Tablets ... 551

Cyclosporine (In vitro studies have shown that naproxen anion, because of its affinity for protein, may displace from their binding sites other drugs that are also albumin-bound). Products include:
- Gengraf Capsules ... 459
- Neoral Oral Solution ... 2259
- Neoral Soft Gelatin Capsules ... 2259
- Restasis Ophthalmic Emulsion ... 575
- Sandimmune ... 2275

Diazepam (In vitro studies have shown that naproxen anion, because of its affinity for protein, may displace from their binding sites other drugs that are also albumin-bound). Products include:
- Diastat Rectal Delivery System ... 3343
- Valium Tablets ... 2819

Diclofenac Potassium (In vitro studies have shown that naproxen anion, because of its affinity for protein, may displace from their binding sites other drugs that are also albumin-bound).
No products indexed under this heading.

Diclofenac Sodium (In vitro studies have shown that naproxen anion, because of its affinity for protein, may displace from their binding sites other drugs that are also albumin-bound). Products include:
- Arthrotec Tablets ... 3129
- Voltaren Ophthalmic Solution ... 2309
- Voltaren Tablets ... 2307
- Voltaren-XR Tablets ... 2310

Dicumarol (Short-term studies have failed to show any significant effects of concurrent use on prothrombin time; caution is advised since interactions have been seen with other NSAIDs).
No products indexed under this heading.

Dipyridamole (In vitro studies have shown that naproxen anion, because of its affinity for protein, may displace from their binding sites other drugs that are also albumin-bound). Products include:
- Aggrenox Capsules ... 822
- Persantine Tablets ... 868

Enalapril Maleate (Co-administration of NSAIDs and ACE inhibitors may potentiate renal disease states). Products include:
- Vasotec I.V. Injection ... 2103

Enalaprilat (Co-administration of NSAIDs and ACE inhibitors may potentiate renal disease states).
No products indexed under this heading.

Esmolol Hydrochloride (Naproxen can reduce the antihypertensive effect of beta-blockers).
No products indexed under this heading.

Ethotoin (Observe signs for hydantoin toxicity).
No products indexed under this heading.

Fenoprofen Calcium (In vitro studies have shown that naproxen anion, because of its affinity for protein, may displace from their binding sites other drugs that are also albumin-bound). Products include:
- Nalfon Capsules ... 2502

Ferrous Fumarate (Lansoprazole causes a profound and long-lasting inhibition of gastric acid secretion; therefore, it is theoretically possible that lansoprazole may interfere with the absorption of drugs where gastric pH is an important determinant of bioavailability).
No products indexed under this heading.

Ferrous Gluconate (Lansoprazole causes a profound and long-lasting inhibition of gastric acid secretion; therefore, it is theoretically possible that lansoprazole may interfere with the absorption of drugs where gastric pH is an important determinant of bioavailability).
No products indexed under this heading.

Ferrous Sulfate (Lansoprazole causes a profound and long-lasting inhibition of gastric acid secretion; therefore, it is theoretically possible that lansoprazole may interfere with the absorption of drugs where gastric pH is an important determinant of bioavailability). Products include:
- Slow Fe Iron Tablets ... ▣818
- Slow Fe with Folic Acid Tablets ... ▣819

Flurazepam Hydrochloride (In vitro studies have shown that naproxen anion, because of its affinity for protein, may displace from their binding sites other drugs that are also albumin-bound). Products include:
- Dalmane Capsules ... 3342

Flurbiprofen (In vitro studies have shown that naproxen anion, because of its affinity for protein, may displace from their binding sites other drugs that are also albumin-bound).
No products indexed under this heading.

Fosinopril Sodium (Co-administration of NSAIDs and ACE inhibitors may potentiate renal disease states).
No products indexed under this heading.

Fosphenytoin Sodium (Observe signs for hydantoin toxicity).
No products indexed under this heading.

Furosemide (The natriuretic effect of furosemide has been reported to be inhibited by some NSAIDs). Products include:
- Furosemide Tablets ... 2154

Glimepiride (Observe signs for sulfonylurea toxicity). Products include:
- Avandaryl Tablets ... 1379
- Duetact Tablets ... 3226

Glipizide (Observe signs for sulfonamide toxicity).
No products indexed under this heading.

Glyburide (Observe signs for sulfonamide toxicity).
No products indexed under this heading.

Hydrochlorothiazide (Observe signs for sulfonamide toxicity). Products include:
- Aldoril Tablets ... 1910
- Atacand HCT ... 651
- Avalide Tablets ... 888
- Avalide Tablets ... 2874
- Benicar HCT Tablets ... 1044
- Diovan HCT Tablets ... 2196
- Dyazide Capsules ... 1423
- Hyzaar 50-12.5 Tablets ... 1990
- Hyzaar 100-12.5 Tablets ... 1990
- Hyzaar 100-25 Tablets ... 1990
- Lopressor HCT 50/25 Tablets ... 2241
- Lopressor HCT 100/25 Tablets ... 2241
- Lopressor HCT 100/50 Tablets ... 2241
- Lotensin HCT Tablets ... 2246
- Micardis HCT Tablets ... 856
- Moduretic Tablets ... 2028
- Prinzide Tablets ... 2056
- Teveten HCT Tablets ... 1737
- Timolide Tablets ... 2086
- Uniretic Tablets ... 3100

Hydroflumethiazide (Observe signs for sulfonamide toxicity).
No products indexed under this heading.

Ibuprofen (In vitro studies have shown that naproxen anion, because of its affinity for protein, may displace from their binding sites other drugs that are also albumin-bound). Products include:
- Advil Allergy Sinus Caplets ... ▣770
- Advil ... ▣674
- Children's Advil Oral Suspension ... ▣603
- Children's Advil Chewable Tablets ... ▣603
- Advil Cold & Sinus ... ▣723
- Infants' Advil Concentrated Drops ... ▣604
- Infants' Advil Concentrated Drops - White Grape (Dye-Free) ... ▣604
- Junior Strength Advil Swallow Tablets ... ▣605
- Advil Migraine Liquigels ... ▣608
- Advil Multi-Symptom Cold Caplets ... ▣770
- Advil PM Caplets ... ▣615
- Motrin IB Tablets and Caplets ... 1866
- Children's Motrin Oral Suspension ... 1867
- Children's Motrin Non-Staining Dye-Free Oral Suspension ... 1867
- Children's Motrin Cold Oral Suspension ... 1867
- Infants' Motrin Concentrated Drops ... 1867
- Infants' Motrin Non-Staining Dye-Free Concentrated Drops ... 1867
- Junior Strength Motrin Caplets and Chewable Tablets ... 1867
- Vicoprofen Tablets ... 539

Imipramine Hydrochloride (In vitro studies have shown that naproxen anion, because of its affinity for protein, may displace from their binding sites other drugs that are also albumin-bound).
No products indexed under this heading.

Imipramine Pamoate (In vitro studies have shown that naproxen anion, because of its affinity for protein, may displace from their binding sites other drugs that are also albumin-bound).
No products indexed under this heading.

Indomethacin (In vitro studies have shown that naproxen anion, because of its affinity for protein, may displace from their binding sites other drugs that are also albumin-bound). Products include:
- Indocin ... 1995

Indomethacin Sodium Trihydrate (In vitro studies have shown that naproxen anion, because of its affinity for protein, may displace from their binding sites other drugs that are also albumin-bound). Products include:
- Indocin I.V. ... 2465

Ketoconazole (Lansoprazole causes a profound and long-lasting inhibition of gastric acid secretion; therefore, it is theoretically possible that lansoprazole may interfere with the absorption of drugs where gastric pH is an important determinant of bioavailability). Products include:
- Nizoral A-D Shampoo, 1% ... 1868

Ketoprofen (In vitro studies have shown that naproxen anion, because of its affinity for protein, may displace from their binding sites other drugs that are also albumin-bound).
No products indexed under this heading.

Ketorolac Tromethamine (In vitro studies have shown that naproxen anion, because of its affinity for protein, may displace from their binding sites other drugs that are also albumin-bound). Products include:
- Acular Ophthalmic Solution ... 565
- Acular LS Ophthalmic Solution ... 566

Labetalol Hydrochloride (Naproxen can reduce the antihypertensive effect of beta-blockers).
No products indexed under this heading.

Levobunolol Hydrochloride (Naproxen can reduce the antihypertensive effect of beta-blockers). Products include:
- Betagan Ophthalmic Solution, USP ... ⊙220

Lisinopril (Co-administration of NSAIDs and ACE inhibitors may potentiate renal disease states). Products include:
- Prinivil Tablets ... 2052
- Prinzide Tablets ... 2056

Lithium (Inhibition of renal lithium clearance leading to increases in plasma lithium concentrations has been reported with naproxen).
No products indexed under this heading.

Lithium Carbonate (Inhibition of renal lithium clearance leading to increases in plasma lithium concentrations has been reported with naproxen). Products include:
- Lithobid Tablets ... 1692

Lithium Citrate (Inhibition of renal lithium clearance leading to increases in plasma lithium concentrations has been reported with naproxen).
No products indexed under this heading.

Meclofenamate Sodium (In vitro studies have shown that naproxen anion, because of its affinity for protein, may displace from their binding sites other drugs that are also albumin-bound).
No products indexed under this heading.

Mefenamic Acid (In vitro studies have shown that naproxen anion, because of its affinity for protein, may displace from their binding sites other drugs that are also albumin-bound).
No products indexed under this heading.

Mephenytoin (Observe signs for hydantoin toxicity).
No products indexed under this heading.

Methotrexate Sodium (Naproxen has been reported to reduce the tubular secretion of methotrexate in an animal model, possibly increasing the toxicity of methotrexate; caution is recommended).
No products indexed under this heading.

Methyclothiazide (Observe signs for sulfonamide toxicity).
No products indexed under this heading.

Metipranolol Hydrochloride
(Naproxen can reduce the antihypertensive effect of beta-blockers).
No products indexed under this heading.

Metoprolol Succinate (Naproxen can reduce the antihypertensive effect of beta-blockers). Products include:
Toprol-XL Tablets 668

Metoprolol Tartrate (Naproxen can reduce the antihypertensive effect of beta-blockers). Products include:
Lopressor Injection 2238
Lopressor Tablets 2238
Lopressor HCT 50/25 Tablets 2241
Lopressor HCT 100/25 Tablets 2241
Lopressor HCT 100/50 Tablets 2241

Midazolam Hydrochloride (In vitro studies have shown that naproxen anion, because of its affinity for protein, may displace from their binding sites other drugs that are also albumin-bound).
No products indexed under this heading.

Moexipril Hydrochloride (Co-administration of NSAIDs and ACE inhibitors may potentiate renal disease states). Products include:
Uniretic Tablets 3100
Univasc Tablets 3104

Nadolol (Naproxen can reduce the antihypertensive effect of beta-blockers). Products include:
Nadolol Tablets 2159

Naproxen Sodium (In vitro studies have shown that naproxen anion, because of its affinity for protein, may displace from their binding sites other drugs that are also albumin-bound). Products include:
Aleve Caplets 742
Aleve Gelcaps 743
Aleve Tablets 743
Aleve Cold & Sinus Caplets 744
Anaprox Tablets 2761
Anaprox DS Tablets 2761

Nortriptyline Hydrochloride (In vitro studies have shown that naproxen anion, because of its affinity for protein, may displace from their binding sites other drugs that are also albumin-bound).
No products indexed under this heading.

Oxaprozin (In vitro studies have shown that naproxen anion, because of its affinity for protein, may displace from their binding sites other drugs that are also albumin-bound).
No products indexed under this heading.

Oxazepam (In vitro studies have shown that naproxen anion, because of its affinity for protein, may displace from their binding sites other drugs that are also albumin-bound).
No products indexed under this heading.

Penbutolol Sulfate (Naproxen can reduce the antihypertensive effect of beta-blockers).
No products indexed under this heading.

Perindopril Erbumine (Co-administration of NSAIDs and ACE inhibitors may potentiate renal disease states). Products include:
Aceon Tablets (2 mg, 4 mg, 8 mg) 3194

Phenylbutazone (In vitro studies have shown that naproxen anion, because of its affinity for protein, may displace from their binding sites other drugs that are also albumin-bound).
No products indexed under this heading.

Phenytoin (Observe signs for hydantoin toxicity).
No products indexed under this heading.

Phenytoin Sodium (Observe signs for hydantoin toxicity). Products include:
Phenytek Capsules 2160

Pindolol (Naproxen can reduce the antihypertensive effect of beta-blockers).
No products indexed under this heading.

Piroxicam (In vitro studies have shown that naproxen anion, because of its affinity for protein, may displace from their binding sites other drugs that are also albumin-bound).
No products indexed under this heading.

Polythiazide (Observe signs for sulfonamide toxicity).
No products indexed under this heading.

Probenecid (Probenecid given concurrently increases naproxen anion plasma levels and extends its plasma half-life significantly).
No products indexed under this heading.

Propranolol Hydrochloride
(Naproxen can reduce the antihypertensive effect of beta-blockers). Products include:
Inderal LA Long-Acting Capsules 3429
InnoPran XL Capsules 2723

Quinapril Hydrochloride (Co-administration of NSAIDs and ACE inhibitors may potentiate renal disease states).
No products indexed under this heading.

Ramipril (Co-administration of NSAIDs and ACE inhibitors may potentiate renal disease states). Products include:
Altace Capsules 1702

Sotalol Hydrochloride (Naproxen can reduce the antihypertensive effect of beta-blockers).
No products indexed under this heading.

Spirapril Hydrochloride (Co-administration of NSAIDs and ACE inhibitors may potentiate renal disease states).
No products indexed under this heading.

Sucralfate (In a single-crossover study examining lansoprazole 30 mg given concomitantly with sucralfate 1 gram, absorption was delayed and bioavailability was reduced by 17%; therefore, lansoprazole should be taken at least 30 minutes prior to sucralfate). Products include:
Carafate Suspension 701
Carafate Tablets 701

Sulfacytine (Observe signs for sulfonamide toxicity).
No products indexed under this heading.

Sulfamethizole (Observe signs for sulfonamide toxicity).
No products indexed under this heading.

Sulfamethoxazole (Observe signs for sulfonamide toxicity).
No products indexed under this heading.

Sulfasalazine (Observe signs for sulfonamide toxicity).
No products indexed under this heading.

Sulfinpyrazone (Observe signs for sulfonamide toxicity).
No products indexed under this heading.

Sulfisoxazole Acetyl (Observe signs for sulfonamide toxicity).
No products indexed under this heading.

Sulfisoxazole Diolamine (Observe signs for sulfonamide toxicity).
No products indexed under this heading.

Sulindac (In vitro studies have shown that naproxen anion, because of its affinity for protein, may displace from their binding sites other drugs that are also albumin-bound). Products include:
Clinoril Tablets 1924

Temazepam (In vitro studies have shown that naproxen anion, because of its affinity for protein, may displace from their binding sites other drugs that are also albumin-bound). Products include:
Restoril Capsules 1860

Theophylline (Co-administration resulted in a minor increase (10%) in the clearance of theophylline; this interaction is unlikely to be of clinical concern; nonetheless, patients may require additional titration of their theophylline dosage when lansoprazole is started or stopped).
No products indexed under this heading.

Theophylline Anhydrous (Co-administration resulted in a minor increase (10%) in the clearance of theophylline; this interaction is unlikely to be of clinical concern; nonetheless, patients may require additional titration of their theophylline dosage when lansoprazole is started or stopped). Products include:
Uniphyl Tablets 2710

Theophylline Calcium Salicylate
(Co-administration resulted in a minor increase (10%) in the clearance of theophylline; this interaction is unlikely to be of clinical concern; nonetheless, patients may require additional titration of their theophylline dosage when lansoprazole is started or stopped).
No products indexed under this heading.

Theophylline Dihydroxypropyl (Glyceryl) (Co-administration resulted in a minor increase (10%) in the clearance of theophylline; this interaction is unlikely to be of clinical concern; nonetheless, patients may require additional titration of their theophylline dosage when lansoprazole is started or stopped).
No products indexed under this heading.

Theophylline Ethylenediamine
(Co-administration resulted in a minor increase (10%) in the clearance of theophylline; this interaction is unlikely to be of clinical concern, nonetheless patients may require additional titration of their theophylline dosage when lansoprazole is started or stopped).
No products indexed under this heading.

Theophylline Sodium Glycinate
(Co-administration resulted in a minor increase (10%) in the clearance of theophylline; this interaction is unlikely to be of clinical concern; nonetheless, patients may require additional titration of their theophylline dosage when lansoprazole is started or stopped).
No products indexed under this heading.

Timolol Hemihydrate (Naproxen can reduce the antihypertensive effect of beta-blockers). Products include:
Betimol Ophthalmic Solution 3382
Betimol Ophthalmic Solution ⊙295

Timolol Maleate (Naproxen can reduce the antihypertensive effect of beta-blockers). Products include:
Blocadren Tablets 1916
Cosopt Sterile Ophthalmic Solution 1931
Timolide Tablets 2086
Timoptic Sterile Ophthalmic Solution 2088
Timoptic in Ocudose 2091
Timoptic-XE Sterile Ophthalmic Gel Forming Solution 2092

Tolazamide (Observe signs for sulfonamide toxicity).
No products indexed under this heading.

Tolbutamide (Observe signs for sulfonamide toxicity).
No products indexed under this heading.

Tolmetin Sodium (In vitro studies have shown that naproxen anion, because of its affinity for protein, may displace from their binding sites other drugs that are also albumin-bound).
No products indexed under this heading.

Trandolapril (Co-administration of NSAIDs and ACE inhibitors may potentiate renal disease states). Products include:
Mavik Tablets 486
Tarka Tablets 524

Trimipramine Maleate (In vitro studies have shown that naproxen anion, because of its affinity for protein, may displace from their binding sites other drugs that are also albumin-bound).
No products indexed under this heading.

Warfarin Sodium (There have been reports of increased INR and prothrombin time in patients receiving proton pump inhibitors, including lansoprazole, and warfarin concomitantly; monitor for these increases). Products include:
Coumadin for Injection 898
Coumadin Tablets 898

PREVACID NAPRAPAC 500
(Lansoprazole, Naproxen) 3280
See Prevacid NapraPAC 375

PREVNAR FOR INJECTION
(Pneumococcal vaccine, diphtheria conjugate).. 3463
May interact with alkylating agents, antimetabolites, anticoagulants, corticosteroids, cytotoxic drugs, and immunosuppressive agents. Compounds in these categories include:

Anisindione (Prevnar should be given with caution to children on anticoagulant therapy). Products include:
Miradon Tablets 3042

Ardeparin Sodium (Prevnar should be given with caution to children on anticoagulant therapy).
No products indexed under this heading.

Azathioprine (Children receiving immunosuppressive therapy may not respond optimally to active immunization).
No products indexed under this heading.

Basiliximab (Children receiving immunosuppressive therapy may not respond optimally to active immunization). Products include:
Simulect for Injection 2284

Betamethasone Acetate (Children receiving large doses of corticosteroids for immunosuppressive therapy may not respond optimally to active immunization).
No products indexed under this heading.

Betamethasone Sodium Phosphate (Children receiving large doses of corticosteroids for immunosuppressive therapy may not respond optimally to active immunization).
No products indexed under this heading.

Bleomycin Sulfate (Children receiving cytotoxic agents may not respond optimally to active immunization).
No products indexed under this heading.

Busulfan (Children receiving alkylating agents may not respond optimally to active immunization). Products include:
I.V. Busulfex 2493
Myleran Tablets 1525

Capecitabine (Children receiving antimetabolite agents may not respond optimally to active immunization). Products include:
Xeloda Tablets 2822

Carmustine (BCNU) (Children receiving alkylating agents may not respond optimally to active immunization).
No products indexed under this heading.

Chlorambucil (Children receiving alkylating agents may not respond optimally to active immunization). Products include:
Leukeran Tablets 1504

Cladribine (Children receiving antimetabolite agents may not respond optimally to active immunization). Products include:
Leustatin Injection 2357

Cortisone Acetate (Children receiving large doses of corticosteroids for immunosuppressive therapy may not respond optimally to active immunization).
No products indexed under this heading.

Cyclophosphamide (Children receiving cytotoxic agents may not respond optimally to active immunization).
No products indexed under this heading.

Cyclosporine (Children receiving immunosuppressive therapy may not respond optimally to active immunization). Products include:
Gengraf Capsules 459
Neoral Oral Solution 2259
Neoral Soft Gelatin Capsules 2259
Restasis Ophthalmic Emulsion 575
Sandimmune 2275

Cytarabine (Children receiving antimetabolite agents may not respond optimally to active immunization).
No products indexed under this heading.

Dacarbazine (Children receiving alkylating agents may not respond optimally to active immunization).
No products indexed under this heading.

Dalteparin Sodium (Prevnar should be given with caution to children on anticoagulant therapy). Products include:
Fragmin Injection 1097

Danaparoid Sodium (Prevnar should be given with caution to children on anticoagulant therapy).
No products indexed under this heading.

Daunorubicin Hydrochloride (Children receiving cytotoxic agents may not respond optimally to active immunization).
No products indexed under this heading.

Dexamethasone (Children receiving large doses of corticosteroids for immunosuppressive therapy may not respond optimally to active immunization). Products include:
Ciprodex Otic Suspension 559
Decadron Tablets 1951
TobraDex Ophthalmic Ointment 562
TobraDex Ophthalmic Suspension ... 563

Dexamethasone Acetate (Children receiving large doses of corticosteroids for immunosuppressive therapy may not respond optimally to active immunization).
No products indexed under this heading.

Dexamethasone Sodium Phosphate (Children receiving large doses of corticosteroids for immunosuppressive therapy may not respond optimally to active immunization).
No products indexed under this heading.

Dicumarol (Prevnar should be given with caution to children on anticoagulant therapy).
No products indexed under this heading.

Doxorubicin Hydrochloride (Children receiving cytotoxic agents may not respond optimally to active immunization).
No products indexed under this heading.

Enoxaparin Sodium (Prevnar should be given with caution to children on anticoagulant therapy). Products include:
Lovenox Injection 2915

Epirubicin Hydrochloride (Children receiving cytotoxic agents may not respond optimally to active immunization).
No products indexed under this heading.

Floxuridine (Children receiving antimetabolite agents may not respond optimally to active immunization).
No products indexed under this heading.

Fludarabine Phosphate (Children receiving antimetabolite agents may not respond optimally to active immunization).
No products indexed under this heading.

Fludrocortisone Acetate (Children receiving large doses of corticosteroids for immunosuppressive therapy may not respond optimally to active immunization).
No products indexed under this heading.

Fluorouracil (Children receiving cytotoxic agents may not respond optimally to active immunization). Products include:
Carac Cream, 0.5% 2879
Efudex 3363

Fondaparinux Sodium (Prevnar should be given with caution to children on anticoagulant therapy). Products include:
Arixtra Injection 1351

Gemcitabine Hydrochloride (Children receiving antimetabolite agents may not respond optimally to active immunization). Products include:
Gemzar for Injection 1771

Heparin Calcium (Prevnar should be given with caution to children on anticoagulant therapy).
No products indexed under this heading.

Heparin Sodium (Prevnar should be given with caution to children on anticoagulant therapy).
No products indexed under this heading.

Hydrocortisone (Children receiving large doses of corticosteroids for immunosuppressive therapy may not respond optimally to active immunization). Products include:
Colocort Rectal Suspension, USP
(Retention) 100 mg/60 mL 2476
Hydrocortone Tablets 1989
Preparation H Hydrocortisone
Cream ▣646

Hydrocortisone Acetate (Children receiving large doses of corticosteroids for immunosuppressive therapy may not respond optimally to active immunization). Products include:
Analpram-HC 1159
Pramosone 1161
ProctoFoam-HC 3099

Hydrocortisone Sodium Phosphate (Children receiving large doses of corticosteroids for immunosuppressive therapy may not respond optimally to active immunization).
No products indexed under this heading.

Hydrocortisone Sodium Succinate (Children receiving large doses of corticosteroids for immunosuppressive therapy may not respond optimally to active immunization).
No products indexed under this heading.

Hydroxyurea (Children receiving cytotoxic agents may not respond optimally to active immunization).
No products indexed under this heading.

Lomustine (CCNU) (Children receiving alkylating agents may not respond optimally to active immunization).
No products indexed under this heading.

Low Molecular Weight Heparins (Prevnar should be given with caution to children on anticoagulant therapy).
No products indexed under this heading.

Mechlorethamine Hydrochloride (Children receiving alkylating agents may not respond optimally to active immunization). Products include:

Mustargen for Injection 2468

Melphalan (Children receiving alkylating agents may not respond optimally to active immunization). Products include:
Alkeran Tablets 956

Mercaptopurine (Children receiving antimetabolite agents may not respond optimally to active immunization).
No products indexed under this heading.

Methotrexate (Children receiving antimetabolite agents may not respond optimally to active immunization).
No products indexed under this heading.

Methotrexate Sodium (Children receiving cytotoxic agents may not respond optimally to active immunization).
No products indexed under this heading.

Methylprednisolone Acetate (Children receiving large doses of corticosteroids for immunosuppressive therapy may not respond optimally to active immunization). Products include:
Depo-Medrol Injectable
Suspension 2617
Depo-Medrol Single-Dose Vial 2619

Methylprednisolone Sodium Succinate (Children receiving large doses of corticosteroids for immunosuppressive therapy may not respond optimally to active immunization).
No products indexed under this heading.

Mitotane (Children receiving cytotoxic agents may not respond optimally to active immunization).
No products indexed under this heading.

Mitoxantrone Hydrochloride (Children receiving cytotoxic agents may not respond optimally to active immunization).
No products indexed under this heading.

Muromonab-CD3 (Children receiving immunosuppressive therapy may not respond optimally to active immunization). Products include:
Orthoclone OKT3 Sterile Solution 2360

Mycophenolate Mofetil (Children receiving immunosuppressive therapy may not respond optimally to active immunization). Products include:
CellCept Capsules 2747
CellCept Oral Suspension 2747
CellCept Tablets 2747

Pentostatin (Children receiving antimetabolite agents may not respond optimally to active immunization). Products include:
Nipent for Injection 1863

Prednisolone Acetate (Children receiving large doses of corticosteroids for immunosuppressive therapy may not respond optimally to active immunization). Products include:
Blephamide Ophthalmic Ointment 568
Blephamide Ophthalmic
Suspension 569
Poly-Pred Ophthalmic
Suspension ⊙233
Pred Forte Ophthalmic
Suspension ⊙235
Pred Mild Ophthalmic
Suspension ⊙238
Pred-G Ophthalmic Ointment ⊙237
Pred-G Ophthalmic Suspension ⊙236

IMPORTANT NOTE: Always consult each drug listing in the patient's regimen for possible interactions.

Prednisolone Sodium Phosphate (Children receiving large doses of corticosteroids for immunosuppressive therapy may not respond optimally to active immunization).
No products indexed under this heading.

Prednisolone Tebutate (Children receiving large doses of corticosteroids for immunosuppressive therapy may not respond optimally to active immunization).
No products indexed under this heading.

Prednisone (Children receiving large doses of corticosteroids for immunosuppressive therapy may not respond optimally to active immunization).
No products indexed under this heading.

Procarbazine Hydrochloride (Children receiving cytotoxic agents may not respond optimally to active immunization). Products include:
Matulane Capsules 3191

Sirolimus (Children receiving immunosuppressive therapy may not respond optimally to active immunization). Products include:
Rapamune Oral Solution and Tablets 3475

Tacrolimus (Children receiving immunosuppressive therapy may not respond optimally to active immunization). Products include:
Prograf Capsules and Injection 632
Protopic Ointment 638

Tamoxifen Citrate (Children receiving cytotoxic agents may not respond optimally to active immunization). Products include:
Soltamox Oral Solution 3527

Thioguanine (Children receiving antimetabolite agents may not respond optimally to active immunization). Products include:
Tabloid Tablets 1575

Thiotepa (Children receiving alkylating agents may not respond optimally to active immunization).
No products indexed under this heading.

Tinzaparin Sodium (Prevnar should be given with caution to children on anticoagulant therapy).
No products indexed under this heading.

Triamcinolone (Children receiving large doses of corticosteroids for immunosuppressive therapy may not respond optimally to active immunization).
No products indexed under this heading.

Triamcinolone Acetonide (Children receiving large doses of corticosteroids for immunosuppressive therapy may not respond optimally to active immunization). Products include:
Azmacort Inhalation Aerosol 1726
Nasacort AQ Nasal Spray 2922

Triamcinolone Diacetate (Children receiving large doses of corticosteroids for immunosuppressive therapy may not respond optimally to active immunization).
No products indexed under this heading.

Triamcinolone Hexacetonide (Children receiving large doses of corticosteroids for immunosuppressive therapy may not respond optimally to active immunization).
No products indexed under this heading.

Vincristine Sulfate (Children receiving cytotoxic agents may not respond optimally to active immunization).
No products indexed under this heading.

Warfarin Sodium (Prevnar should be given with caution to children on anticoagulant therapy). Products include:
Coumadin for Injection 898
Coumadin Tablets 898

PREVPAC

(Amoxicillin, Clarithromycin, Lansoprazole).................................. 3284

May interact with antiarrhythmics, oral anticoagulants, HMG-CoA reductase inhibitors, oral hypoglycemic agents, insulin, iron containing oral preparations, absorption of drugs where gastric ph is an important determinant in their bioavailability, phenytoin, triazolobenzodiazepines, valproate, xanthines, and certain other agents. Compounds in these categories include:

Acarbose (Co-administration has resulted in rare reports of hypoglycemia, some of which occurred in patients taking oral hypoglycemia agents). Products include:
Precose Tablets 751

Acebutolol Hydrochloride (There have been post-marketing reports of torsade de pointes occurring with concurrent use of clarithromycin and quinidine or dispyramide. Electrocardiograms should be monitored for QTc prolongation during co-administration of clarithromycin with these drugs).
No products indexed under this heading.

Adenosine (There have been post-marketing reports of torsade de pointes occurring with concurrent use of clarithromycin and quinidine or dispyramide. Electrocardiograms should be monitored for QTc prolongation during co-administration of clarithromycin with these drugs). Products include:
Adenocard Injection 617
Adenoscan 619

Alfentanil Hydrochloride (There have been reports of CYP3A-based interactions of clarithromycin with alfentanil).
No products indexed under this heading.

Alprazolam (Erythromycin, another macrolide antibiotic, has been reported to decrease the clearance of triazolam and midazolam, and thus, may increase the pharmacologic effect of these benzodiazepines). Products include:
Niravam Orally Disintegrating Tablets 3092

Aminophylline (Co-administration of theophylline with clarithromycin in patients who are receiving high doses of theophylline may be associated with an increase in serum theophylline levels and potential theophylline toxicity).
No products indexed under this heading.

Amiodarone Hydrochloride (There have been post-marketing reports of torsade de pointes occurring with concurrent use of clarithromycin and quinidine or dispyramide. Electrocardiograms should be monitored for QTc prolongation during co-administration of clarithromycin with these drugs).
No products indexed under this heading.

Anisindione (Co-administration of clarithromycin with oral anticoagulants may result in the potentiation of oral coagulant effects). Products include:
Miradon Tablets 3042

Astemizole (Concomitant administration of Prevpac with astemizole is contraindicated. There have been post-marketing reports of drug interactions when clarithromycin is co-administered with astemizole resulting in cardiac arrhythmias (QT prolongation, ventricular tachycardia, ventricular fibrillation, and torsade de pointes) most likely due to inhibition of metabolism of these drugs by clarithromycin. Fatalities have been reported).
No products indexed under this heading.

Atorvastatin Calcium (Clarithromycin has been reported to increase concentrations of HMG-CoA reductase inhibitors. Rare reports of rhabdomyolysis have been reported in patients taking these drugs concomitantly). Products include:
Caduet Tablets 2508
Lipitor Tablets 2483

Bacampicillin Hydrochloride (Lansoprazole causes a profound and long lasting inhibition of gastric secretion; therefore, it is theoretically possible that it may interfere with oral absorption of drugs where gastric pH is an important determinant of bioavailability).
No products indexed under this heading.

Bretylium Tosylate (There have been post-marketing reports of torsade de pointes occurring with concurrent use of clarithromycin and quinidine or dispyramide. Electrocardiograms should be monitored for QTc prolongation during co-administration of clarithromycin with these drugs).
No products indexed under this heading.

Bromocriptine Mesylate (There have been reports of CYP3A-based interactions of clarithromycin with bromocriptine).
No products indexed under this heading.

Carbamazepine (There have been reports of CYP3A-based interactions of clarithromycin with carbamazepine). Products include:
Carbatrol Capsules 3171
Equetro Extended-Release Capsules 3180
Tegretol/Tegretol-XR 2295

Cerivastatin Sodium (Clarithromycin has been reported to increase concentrations of HMG-CoA reductase inhibitors. Rare reports of rhabdomyolysis have been reported in patients taking these drugs concomitantly).
No products indexed under this heading.

Chlorpropamide (Co-administration has resulted in rare reports of hypoglycemia, some of which occurred in patients taking oral hypoglycemia agents).
No products indexed under this heading.

Cilostazol (There have been reports of CYP3A-based interactions of clarithromycin with cilostazol). Products include:
Pletal Tablets 2455

Cisapride (Concomitant administration of Prevpac with cisapride is contraindicated. There have been post-marketing reports of drug interactions when clarithromycin is co-administered with cisapride resulting in cardiac arrhythmias (QT prolongation, ventricular tachycardia, ventricular fibrillation, and torsade de pointes) most likely due to inhibition of metabolism of these drugs by clarithromycin. Fatalities have been reported).
No products indexed under this heading.

Cyclosporine (There have been reports of CYP3A-based interactions of clarithromycin with cyclosporine). Products include:
Gengraf Capsules 459
Neoral Oral Solution 2259
Neoral Soft Gelatin Capsules 2259
Restasis Ophthalmic Emulsion 575
Sandimmune 2275

Dicumarol (Co-administration of clarithromycin with oral anticoagulants may result in the potentiation of oral coagulant effects).
No products indexed under this heading.

Digoxin (Co-administration of clarithromycin and digoxin has resulted in elevated digoxin serum concentrations resulting in clinical signs of digoxin toxicity including potentially fatal arrhythmias; lansoprazole causes profound and long-lasting inhibition of gastric acid secretion; therefore, it is theoretically possible that it may interfere with the absorption of drugs, such as digoxin, where gastric pH is an important determinant of bioavailability). Products include:
Lanoxicaps Capsules 1490
Lanoxin Injection 1494
Lanoxin Injection Pediatric 1497
Lanoxin Tablets 1500

Dihydroergotamine Mesylate (Co-administration of clarithromycin or erythromycin with dihydroergotamine has been associated in some patients with acute ergot toxicity characterized by severe peripheral vasospasm and dysesthesia). Products include:
Migranal Nasal Spray 3348

Disopyramide Phosphate (There have been reports of CYP3A-based interactions of clarithromycin with disopyramide).
No products indexed under this heading.

Divalproex Sodium (Concurrent use of erythromycin or clarithromycin in patients receiving drugs metabolized by the cytochrome P450 system may be associated with elevation in serum levels of valproate). Products include:
Depakote Sprinkle Capsules 422
Depakote Tablets 427
Depakote ER Tablets 434

Dofetilide (There have been post-marketing reports of torsade de pointes occurring with concurrent use of clarithromycin and quinidine or dispyramide. Electrocardiograms should be monitored for QTc prolongation during co-administration of clarithromycin with these drugs).
No products indexed under this heading.

Dyphylline (Co-administration of theophylline with clarithromycin in patients who are receiving high doses of theophylline may be associated with an increase in serum theophylline levels and potential theophylline toxicity).
No products indexed under this heading.

Ergotamine Tartrate (Co-administration of clarithromycin or erythromycin with ergotamine has been associated in some patients with acute ergot toxicity characterized by severe peripheral vasospasm and dysesthesia).
No products indexed under this heading.

Ferrous Fumarate (Lansoprazole causes a profound and long-lasting inhibition of gastric acid secretion; therefore, it is theoretically possible that it may interfere with the absorption of drugs, such as iron salts, where gastric pH is an important determinant of bioavailability).
No products indexed under this heading.

Ferrous Gluconate (Lansoprazole causes a profound and long-lasting inhibition of gastric acid secretion; therefore, it is theoretically possible that it may interfere with the absorption of drugs, such as iron salts, where gastric pH is an important determinant of bioavailability).
No products indexed under this heading.

Ferrous Sulfate (Lansoprazole causes a profound and long-lasting inhibition of gastric acid secretion; therefore, it is theoretically possible that it may interfere with the absorption of drugs, such as iron salts, where gastric pH is an important determinant of bioavailability). Products include:
Slow Fe Iron Tablets **818**
Slow Fe with Folic Acid Tablets **819**

Flecainide Acetate (There have been post-marketing reports of torsade de pointes occurring with concurrent use of clarithromycin and quinidine or dispyramide. Electrocardiograms should be monitored for QTc prolongation during co-administration of clarithromycin with these drugs). Products include:
Tambocor Tablets **1856**

Fluvastatin Sodium (Clarithromycin has been reported to increase concentrations of HMG-CoA reductase inhibitors. Rare reports of rhabdomyolysis have been reported in patients taking these drugs concomitantly). Products include:
Lescol Capsules **2233**
Lescol XL Tablets **2233**

Fosphenytoin Sodium (Concurrent use of erythromycin or clarithromycin in patients receiving drugs metabolized by the cytochrome P450 system may be associated with elevation in serum levels of phenytoin).
No products indexed under this heading.

Glimepiride (Co-administration has resulted in rare reports of hypoglycemia, some of which occurred in patients taking oral hypoglycemia agents). Products include:
Avandaryl Tablets **1379**
Duetact Tablets **3226**

Glipizide (Co-administration has resulted in rare reports of hypoglycemia, some of which occurred in patients taking oral hypoglycemia agents).
No products indexed under this heading.

Glyburide (Co-administration has resulted in rare reports of hypoglycemia, some of which occurred in patients taking oral hypoglycemia agents).
No products indexed under this heading.

Hexobarbital (Concurrent use of clarithromycin and hexobarbital may be associated with an elevation in the serum levels of hexobarbital).
No products indexed under this heading.

Insulin, Human, Zinc Suspension (Co-administration has resulted in rare reports of hypoglycemia, some of which occurred in patients taking insulin). Products include:
Humulin L, 100 Units **1794**
Humulin U, 100 Units **1800**

Insulin, Human NPH (Co-administration has resulted in rare reports of hypoglycemia, some of which occurred in patients taking insulin). Products include:
Humulin N, 100 Units **1795**
Humulin N Pen **1797**

Insulin, Human Regular (Co-administration has resulted in rare reports of hypoglycemia, some of which occurred in patients taking insulin). Products include:
Humulin R, 100 Units **1798**

Insulin, Human Regular and Human NPH Mixture (Co-administration has resulted in rare reports of hypoglycemia, some of which occurred in patients taking insulin). Products include:
Humulin 50/50, 100 Units **1791**
Humulin 70/30 Pen **1793**

Insulin, NPH (Co-administration has resulted in rare reports of hypoglycemia, some of which occurred in patients taking insulin).
No products indexed under this heading.

Insulin, Regular (Co-administration has resulted in rare reports of hypoglycemia, some of which occurred in patients taking insulin).
No products indexed under this heading.

Insulin, Zinc Crystals (Co-administration has resulted in rare reports of hypoglycemia, some of which occurred in patients taking insulin).
No products indexed under this heading.

Insulin, Zinc Suspension (Co-administration has resulted in rare reports of hypoglycemia, some of which occurred in patients taking insulin).
No products indexed under this heading.

Insulin Aspart, Human Regular (Co-administration has resulted in rare reports of hypoglycemia, some of which occurred in patients taking insulin). Products include:
NovoLog Injection **2326**

Insulin glargine (Co-administration has resulted in rare reports of hypoglycemia, some of which occurred in patients taking insulin). Products include:
Lantus Injection **2909**

Insulin Lispro, Human (Co-administration has resulted in rare reports of hypoglycemia, some of which occurred in patients taking insulin). Products include:
Humalog-Pen **1781**
Humalog Mix 50/50-Pen **1783**
Humalog Mix 75/25-Pen **1785**

Insulin Lispro Protamine, Human (Co-administration has resulted in rare reports of hypoglycemia, some of which occurred in patients taking insulin). Products include:
Humalog Mix 50/50-Pen **1783**
Humalog Mix 75/25-Pen **1785**

Iron (Lansoprazole causes a profound and long-lasting inhibition of gastric acid secretion; therefore, it is theoretically possible that it may interfere with the absorption of drugs, such as iron salts, where gastric pH is an important determinant of bioavailability).
No products indexed under this heading.

Ketoconazole (Lansoprazole causes a profound and long lasting inhibition of gastric secretion; therefore, it is theoretically possible that it may interfere with oral absorption of drugs where gastric pH is an important determinant of bioavailability). Products include:
Nizoral A-D Shampoo, 1% **1868**

Lidocaine Hydrochloride (There have been post-marketing reports of torsade de pointes occurring with concurrent use of clarithromycin and quinidine or dispyramide. Electrocardiograms should be monitored for QTc prolongation during co-administration of clarithromycin with these drugs).
No products indexed under this heading.

Lovastatin (Clarithromycin has been reported to increase concentrations of HMG-CoA reductase inhibitors. Rare reports of rhabdomyolysis have been reported in patients taking these drugs concomitantly). Products include:
Advicor Tablets **1722**
Altoprev Extended-Release Tablets **3109**
Mevacor Tablets **2021**

Metformin Hydrochloride (Co-administration has resulted in rare reports of hypoglycemia, some of which occurred in patients taking oral hypoglycemia agents). Products include:
ActoPlus Met Tablets **3214**
Avandamet Tablets **1373**
Fortamet Extended-Release Tablets **3115**

Methylprednisolone (There have been reports of CYP3A-based interactions of clarithromycin with methyprednisolone).
No products indexed under this heading.

Mexiletine Hydrochloride (There have been post-marketing reports of torsade de pointes occurring with concurrent use of clarithromycin and quinidine or dispyramide. Electrocardiograms should be monitored for QTc prolongation during co-administration of clarithromycin with these drugs).
No products indexed under this heading.

Midazolam Hydrochloride (Erythromycin, another macrolide antibiotic, has been reported to decrease the clearance of triazolam and midazolam, and thus, may increase the pharmacologic effect of these benzodiazepines).
No products indexed under this heading.

Miglitol (Co-administration has resulted in rare reports of hypoglycemia, some of which occurred in patients taking oral hypoglycemia agents).
No products indexed under this heading.

Moricizine Hydrochloride (There have been post-marketing reports of torsade de pointes occurring with concurrent use of clarithromycin and quinidine or dispyramide. Electrocardiograms should be monitored for QTc prolongation during co-administration of clarithromycin with these drugs).
No products indexed under this heading.

Phenytoin (Concurrent use of erythromycin or clarithromycin in patients receiving drugs metabolized by the cytochrome P450 system may be associated with elevation in serum levels of phenytoin).
No products indexed under this heading.

Phenytoin Sodium (Concurrent use of erythromycin or clarithromycin in patients receiving drugs metabolized by the cytochrome P450 system may be associated with elevation in serum levels of phenytoin). Products include:
Phenytek Capsules **2160**

Pimozide (Concomitant administration of Prevpac with pimozide is contraindicated. There have been post-marketing reports of drug interactions when clarithromycin is co-administered with pimozide resulting in cardiac arrhythmias (QT prolongation, ventricular tachycardia, ventricular fibrillation, and torsade de pointes) most likely due to inhibition of metabolism of these drugs by clarithromycin. Fatalities have been reported).
No products indexed under this heading.

Pioglitazone Hydrochloride (Co-administration has resulted in rare reports of hypoglycemia, some of which occurred in patients taking oral hypoglycemia agents). Products include:
ActoPlus Met Tablets **3214**
Actos Tablets **3219**
Duetact Tablets **3226**

Polysaccharide Iron Complex (Lansoprazole causes a profound and long-lasting inhibition of gastric acid secretion; therefore, it is theoretically possible that it may interfere with the absorption of drugs, such as iron salts, where gastric pH is an important determinant of bioavailability). Products include:

Nu-Iron 150 Capsules 2127

Pravastatin Sodium (Clarithromycin has been reported to increase concentrations of HMG-CoA reductase inhibitors. Rare reports of rhabdomyolysis have been reported in patients taking these drugs concomitantly).
No products indexed under this heading.

Probenecid (Probenecid decreases the renal tubular secretion of amoxicillin. Concurrent use may result in increased and prolonged blood levels of amoxicillin).
No products indexed under this heading.

Procainamide Hydrochloride (There have been post-marketing reports of torsade de pointes occurring with concurrent use of clarithromycin and quinidine or dispyramide. Electrocardiograms should be monitored for QTc prolongation during co-administration of clarithromycin with these drugs).
No products indexed under this heading.

Propafenone Hydrochloride (There have been post-marketing reports of torsade de pointes occurring with concurrent use of clarithromycin and quinidine or dispyramide. Electrocardiograms should be monitored for QTc prolongation during co-administration of clarithromycin with these drugs). Products include:
Rythmol SR Capsules 2727

Propranolol Hydrochloride (There have been post-marketing reports of torsade de pointes occurring with concurrent use of clarithromycin and quinidine or dispyramide. Electrocardiograms should be monitored for QTc prolongation during co-administration of clarithromycin with these drugs). Products include:
Inderal LA Long-Acting Capsules 3429
InnoPran XL Capsules 2723

Quinidine (There have been reports of CYP3A-based interactions of clarithromycin with quinidine).
No products indexed under this heading.

Quinidine Gluconate (There have been post-marketing reports of torsade de pointes occurring with concurrent use of clarithromycin and quinidine or dispyramide. Electrocardiograms should be monitored for QTc prolongation during co-administration of clarithromycin with these drugs).
No products indexed under this heading.

Quinidine Polygalacturonate (There have been post-marketing reports of torsade de pointes occurring with concurrent use of clarithromycin and quinidine or dispyramide. Electrocardiograms should be monitored for QTc prolongation during co-administration of clarithromycin with these drugs).
No products indexed under this heading.

Quinidine Sulfate (There have been post-marketing reports of torsade de pointes occurring with concurrent use of clarithromycin and quinidine or dispyramide. Electrocardiograms should be monitored for QTc prolongation during co-administration of clarithromycin with these drugs).
No products indexed under this heading.

Repaglinide (Co-administration has resulted in rare reports of hypoglycemia, some of which occurred in patients taking oral hypoglycemia agents).
No products indexed under this heading.

Rifabutin (There have been reports of CYP3A-based interactions of clarithromycin with rifabutin).
No products indexed under this heading.

Rosiglitazone Maleate (Co-administration has resulted in rare reports of hypoglycemia, some of which occurred in patients taking oral hypoglycemia agents). Products include:
Avandamet Tablets 1373
Avandaryl Tablets 1379
Avandia Tablets 1384

Sildenafil Citrate (Erythromycin, another macrolide antibiotic, has been reported to increase the systemic exposure (AUC) of sildenafil. A similar interaction may occur with clarithromycin; reduction of sildenafil dosage should be considered). Products include:
Revatio Tablets 2557
Viagra Tablets 2573

Simvastatin (Clarithromycin has been reported to increase concentrations of HMG-CoA reductase inhibitors. Rare reports of rhabdomyolysis have been reported in patients taking these drugs concomitantly). Products include:
Vytorin 10/10 Tablets 2114
Vytorin 10/10 Tablets 3077
Vytorin 10/20 Tablets 2114
Vytorin 10/20 Tablets 3077
Vytorin 10/40 Tablets 2114
Vytorin 10/40 Tablets 3077
Vytorin 10/80 Tablets 2114
Vytorin 10/80 Tablets 3077
Zocor Tablets 2105

Sotalol Hydrochloride (There have been post-marketing reports of torsade de pointes occurring with concurrent use of clarithromycin and quinidine or dispyramide. Electrocardiograms should be monitored for QTc prolongation during co-administration of clarithromycin with these drugs).
No products indexed under this heading.

Sucralfate (Co-administration delays absorption and reduces bioavailability by about 30%; therefore, lansoprazole should be taken at least 30 minutes prior to sucralfate). Products include:
Carafate Suspension 701
Carafate Tablets 701

Tacrolimus (There have been reports of CYP3A-based interactions of clarithromycin with tacrolimus). Products include:
Prograf Capsules and Injection 632
Protopic Ointment 638

Terfenadine (Concomitant administration of Prevpac with terfenadine is contraindicated. There have been post-marketing reports of drug interactions when clarithromycin is co-administered with terfenadine resulting in cardiac arrhythmias (QT prolongation, ventricular tachycardia, ventricular fibrillation, and torsade de pointes) most likely due to inhibition of metabolism of these drugs by clarithromycin. Fatalities have been reported).
No products indexed under this heading.

Theophylline (Co-administration of theophylline with clarithromycin in patients who are receiving high doses of theophylline may be associated with an increase in serum theophylline levels and potential theophylline toxicity).
No products indexed under this heading.

Theophylline Anhydrous (Co-administration of theophylline with clarithromycin in patients who are receiving high doses of theophylline may be associated with an increase in serum theophylline levels and potential theophylline toxicity). Products include:
Uniphyl Tablets 2710

Theophylline Calcium Salicylate (Co-administration of theophylline with clarithromycin in patients who are receiving high doses of theophylline may be associated with an increase in serum theophylline levels and potential theophylline toxicity).
No products indexed under this heading.

Theophylline Dihydroxypropyl (Glyceryl) (Co-administration of theophylline with clarithromycin in patients who are receiving high doses of theophylline may be associated with an increase in serum theophylline levels and potential theophylline toxicity).
No products indexed under this heading.

Theophylline Ethylenediamine (Co-administration of theophylline with clarithromycin in patients who are receiving high doses of theophylline may be associated with an increase in serum theophylline levels and potential theophylline toxicity).
No products indexed under this heading.

Theophylline Sodium Glycinate (Co-administration of theophylline with clarithromycin in patients who are receiving high doses of theophylline may be associated with an increase in serum theophylline levels and potential theophylline toxicity).
No products indexed under this heading.

Tocainide Hydrochloride (There have been post-marketing reports of torsade de pointes occurring with concurrent use of clarithromycin and quinidine or dispyramide. Electrocardiograms should be monitored for QTc prolongation during co-administration of clarithromycin with these drugs).
No products indexed under this heading.

Tolazamide (Co-administration has resulted in rare reports of hypoglycemia, some of which occurred in patients taking oral hypoglycemia agents).
No products indexed under this heading.

Tolbutamide (Co-administration has resulted in rare reports of hypoglycemia, some of which occurred in patients taking oral hypoglycemia agents).
No products indexed under this heading.

Triazolam (Concomitant use of clarithromycin and triazolam has resulted in CNS effects (somnolence and confusion) and drug interactions).
No products indexed under this heading.

Troglitazone (Co-administration has resulted in rare reports of hypoglycemia, some of which occurred in patients taking oral hypoglycemia agents).
No products indexed under this heading.

Valproate Sodium (Concurrent use of erythromycin or clarithromycin in patients receiving drugs metabolized by the cytochrome P450 system may be associated with elevation in serum levels of valproate). Products include:
Depacon Injection 412

Valproic Acid (Concurrent use of erythromycin or clarithromycin in patients receiving drugs metabolized by the cytochrome P450 system may be associated with elevation in serum levels of valproate). Products include:
Depakene 417

Verapamil Hydrochloride (There have been post-marketing reports of torsade de pointes occurring with concurrent use of clarithromycin and quinidine or dispyramide. Electrocardiograms should be monitored for QTc prolongation during co-administration of clarithromycin with these drugs). Products include:
Covera-HS Tablets 3139
Tarka Tablets 524
Verelan PM Extended-Release Capsules, Controlled-Onset........... 3106

Warfarin Sodium (Co-administration of clarithromycin with oral anticoagulants may result in the potentiation of oral coagulant effects. Co-administration of warfarin and proton pump inhibitors, including Prevacid, has resulted in increased International Normalized Ratio (INR) and prothrombin time). Products include:
Coumadin for Injection 898
Coumadin Tablets 898

Food Interactions

Food, unspecified (Both Cmax and AUC are diminished by about 50% if the lansoprazole is given 30 minutes after food as opposed to the fasting condition).

PREZISTA TABLETS

(Darunavir) 3306

May interact with calcium channel blockers, cytochrome p450 3a inducers (selected), cytochrome p450 3a substrates (selected), protease inhibitors, and certain other agents. Compounds in these categories include:

Alfentanil Hydrochloride (Darunavir and ritonavir are both inhibitors of CYP3A. Co-administration of darunavir and ritonavir with drugs primarily metabolized by CYP3A may result in increased plasma concentrations of such drugs, which could increase or prolong their therapeutic effect and adverse events).
No products indexed under this heading.

Allium sativum (Darunavir and ritonavir are metabolized by CYP3A. Drugs that induce CYP3A activity would be expected to increase the clearance of darunavir and ritonavir, resulting in lowered plasma concentrations of darunavir and ritonavir. Co-administration of darunavir and ritonavir and other drugs that inhibit CYP3A may decrease the clearance of darunavir and ritonavir and may

result in increased plasma concentrations of darunavir and ritonavir).
No products indexed under this heading.

Alprazolam (Darunavir and ritonavir are both inhibitors of CYP3A. Co-administration of darunavir and ritonavir with drugs primarily metabolized by CYP3A may result in increased plasma concentrations of such drugs, which could increase or prolong their therapeutic effect and adverse events). Products include:
Niravam Orally Disintegrating Tablets **3092**

Aminophylline (Darunavir and ritonavir are both inhibitors of CYP3A. Co-administration of darunavir and ritonavir with drugs primarily metabolized by CYP3A may result in increased plasma concentrations of such drugs, which could increase or prolong their therapeutic effect and adverse events).
No products indexed under this heading.

Amiodarone Hydrochloride (Concentrations of bepridil, lidocaine, quinidine and amiodarone may be increased when co-administered with darunavir/rtv. Caution is warranted and therapeutic concentration monitoring, if available, is recommended for antiarrhythmics when co-administered with darunavir/rtv).
No products indexed under this heading.

Amitriptyline Hydrochloride (Darunavir and ritonavir are both inhibitors of CYP3A. Co-administration of darunavir and ritonavir with drugs primarily metabolized by CYP3A may result in increased plasma concentrations of such drugs, which could increase or prolong their therapeutic effect and adverse events).
No products indexed under this heading.

Amlodipine Besylate (Darunavir and ritonavir are both inhibitors of CYP3A. Co-administration of darunavir and ritonavir with drugs primarily metabolized by CYP3A may result in increased plasma concentrations of such drugs, which could increase or prolong their therapeutic effect and adverse events). Products include:
Caduet Tablets **2508**
Lotrel Capsules **2249**
Norvasc Tablets **2545**

Amprenavir (The co-administration of darunavir/rtv and PIs other than lopinavir/ritonavir, saquinavir, atazanavir, and indinavir has not been studied. Therefore, such co-administration is not recommended). Products include:
Agenerase Capsules **1327**
Agenerase Oral Solution **1332**

Aprepitant (Darunavir and ritonavir are both inhibitors of CYP3A. Co-administration of darunavir and ritonavir with drugs primarily metabolized by CYP3A may result in increased plasma concentrations of such drugs, which could increase or prolong their therapeutic effect and adverse events). Products include:
Emend Capsules **1963**

Astemizole (Astemizole is contraindicated due to a potential for serious and/or life-threatening reactions such as cardiac arrhythmias).
No products indexed under this heading.

Atorvastatin Calcium (When atorvastatin and darunavir/rtv is co-administered, it is recommended to start with the lowest possible dose of atorvastatin with careful monitoring. A gradual dose increase of atorvastatin may be considered based on the clinical response). Products include:
Caduet Tablets **2508**
Lipitor Tablets **2483**

Bepridil Hydrochloride (Concentrations of bepridil, lidocaine, quinidine and amiodarone may be increased when co-administered with darunavir/rtv. Caution is warranted and therapeutic concentration monitoring, if available, is recommended for antiarrhythmics when co-administered with darunavir/rtv).
No products indexed under this heading.

Buspirone Hydrochloride (Darunavir and ritonavir are both inhibitors of CYP3A. Co-administration of darunavir and ritonavir with drugs primarily metabolized by CYP3A may result in increased plasma concentrations of such drugs, which could increase or prolong their therapeutic effect and adverse events).
No products indexed under this heading.

Busulfan (Darunavir and ritonavir are both inhibitors of CYP3A. Co-administration of darunavir and ritonavir with drugs primarily metabolized by CYP3A may result in increased plasma concentrations of such drugs, which could increase or prolong their therapeutic effect and adverse events). Products include:
I.V. Busulfex **2493**
Myleran Tablets **1525**

Carbamazepine (Darunavir and ritonavir are both inhibitors of CYP3A. Co-administration of darunavir and ritonavir with drugs primarily metabolized by CYP3A may result in increased plasma concentrations of such drugs, which could increase or prolong their therapeutic effect and adverse events). Products include:
Carbatrol Capsules **3171**
Equetro Extended-Release Capsules **3180**
Tegretol/Tegretol-XR **2295**

Cerivastatin Sodium (Darunavir and ritonavir are both inhibitors of CYP3A. Co-administration of darunavir and ritonavir with drugs primarily metabolized by CYP3A may result in increased plasma concentrations of such drugs, which could increase or prolong their therapeutic effect and adverse events).
No products indexed under this heading.

Chlorpheniramine (Darunavir and ritonavir are both inhibitors of CYP3A. Co-administration of darunavir and ritonavir with drugs primarily metabolized by CYP3A may result in increased plasma concentrations of such drugs, which could increase or prolong their therapeutic effect and adverse events).
No products indexed under this heading.

Chlorpheniramine Maleate (Darunavir and ritonavir are both inhibitors of CYP3A. Co-administration of darunavir and ritonavir with drugs primarily metabolized by CYP3A may result in increased plasma concentrations of such drugs, which could increase or prolong their therapeutic effect and adverse events). Products include:
Advil Allergy Sinus Caplets **770**
Advil Multi-Symptom Cold Caplets **770**
BC Allergy Sinus Cold Powder **677**
Comtrex Maximum Strength Cold & Cough Day/Night Caplets - Night Formulation **726**
Comtrex Maximum Strength Day/Night Severe Cold & Sinus Caplets - Night Formulation **725**
Contac Cold and Flu Maximum Strength Caplets **728**
Contac Cold and Flu Day and Night Caplets (Night Formulation Only) **727**
Children's Dimetapp Long Acting Cough Plus Cold Syrup **731**
Robitussin Cough & Cold Long-Acting Liquid **735**
Robitussin Cough & Allergy Syrup **736**
Robitussin Cough & Cold Nighttime Liquid **736**
Robitussin Cough, Cold & Flu Nighttime Liquid **738**
Robitussin Pediatric Cough & Cold Long-Acting Liquid **735**
Robitussin Pediatric Cough & Cold Nighttime Liquid **736**
Triaminic Cold & Allergy Liquid **746**
Triaminic Cough & Runny Nose Softchews **748**
Children's Tylenol Plus Flu Oral Suspension **749**
Tylenol Allergy Multi-Symptom Caplets with Cool Burst and Gelcaps **1872**
Children's Tylenol Plus Cold Suspension Liquid **1879**
Children's Tylenol Plus Cough & Runny Nose Suspension Liquid **1879**
Children's Tylenol Plus Flu Suspension Liquid **1881**
Children's Tylenol Plus Multi-Symptom Cold Suspension Liquid **1879**
Tylenol Cold Head Congestion Nighttime Caplets with Cool Burst **1873**
Tylenol Cold Multi-Symptom Nighttime Caplets with Cool Burst **1874**
Tylenol Sinus Congestion & Pain Nighttime Caplets with Cool Burst **1876**
Vicks 44M Cough, Cold & Flu Relief Liquid **2680**
Pediatric Vicks 44m Cough & Cold Relief Liquid **2676**
Children's Vicks NyQuil Cold/Cough Relief **756**
Children's Vicks NyQuil Cold/Cough Relief Liquid **2680**
Zicam Maximum Strength Flu Daytime **768**

Chlorpheniramine Polistirex (Darunavir and ritonavir are both inhibitors of CYP3A. Co-administration of darunavir and ritonavir with drugs primarily metabolized by CYP3A may result in increased plasma concentrations of such drugs, which could increase or prolong their therapeutic effect and adverse events). Products include:
Tussionex Pennkinetic Extended-Release Suspension **3327**

Chlorpheniramine Tannate (Darunavir and ritonavir are both inhibitors of CYP3A. Co-administration of darunavir and ritonavir with drugs primarily metabolized by CYP3A may result in increased plasma concentrations of such drugs, which could increase or prolong their therapeutic effect and adverse events).
No products indexed under this heading.

Cisapride (Cisapride is contraindicated due to a potential for serious and/or life-threatening reactions such as cardiac arrhythmias).
No products indexed under this heading.

Clarithromycin (Darunavir and ritonavir are both inhibitors of CYP3A. Co-administration of darunavir and ritonavir with drugs primarily metabolized by CYP3A may result in increased plasma concentrations of such drugs, which could increase or prolong their therapeutic effect and adverse events). Products include:
Biaxin/Biaxin XL **402**
PREVPAC **3284**

Cyclosporine (Plasma concentrations of cyclosporine, tacrolimus or sirolimus may be increased when co-administered with darunavir/rtv. Therapeutic concentration monitoring of the immunosuppressive agent is recommended for immunosuppressant agents when co-administeredwith darunavir/rtv). Products include:
Gengraf Capsules **459**
Neoral Oral Solution **2259**
Neoral Soft Gelatin Capsules **2259**
Restasis Ophthalmic Emulsion **575**
Sandimmune **2275**

Desogestrel (Darunavir and ritonavir are both inhibitors of CYP3A. Co-administration of darunavir and ritonavir with drugs primarily metabolized by CYP3A may result in increased plasma concentrations of such drugs, which could increase or prolong their therapeutic effect and adverse events). Products include:
Mircette Tablets **1066**

Dexamethasone (Darunavir and ritonavir are both inhibitors of CYP3A. Co-administration of darunavir and ritonavir with drugs primarily metabolized by CYP3A may result in increased plasma concentrations of such drugs, which could increase or prolong their therapeutic effect and adverse events). Products include:
Ciprodex Otic Suspension **559**
Decadron Tablets **1951**
TobraDex Ophthalmic Ointment **562**
TobraDex Ophthalmic Suspension **563**

Dexamethasone Acetate (Darunavir and ritonavir are both inhibitors of CYP3A. Co-administration of darunavir and ritonavir with drugs primarily metabolized by CYP3A may result in increased plasma concentrations of such drugs, which could increase or prolong their therapeutic effect and adverse events).
No products indexed under this heading.

Dexamethasone Phosphate (Darunavir and ritonavir are both inhibitors of CYP3A. Co-administration of darunavir and ritonavir with drugs primarily metabolized by CYP3A may result in increased plasma concentrations of such drugs, which could increase or prolong their therapeutic effect and adverse events).
No products indexed under this heading.

Dexamethasone Sodium
(Darunavir and ritonavir are both inhibitors of CYP3A. Co-administration of darunavir and ritonavir with drugs primarily metabolized by CYP3A may result in increased plasma concentrations of such drugs, which could increase or prolong their therapeutic effect and adverse events).
No products indexed under this heading.

Dexamethasone Sodium Phosphate (Darunavir and ritonavir are both inhibitors of CYP3A. Co-administration of darunavir and ritonavir with drugs primarily metabolized by CYP3A may result in increased plasma concentrations of such drugs, which could increase or prolong their therapeutic effect and adverse events).
No products indexed under this heading.

Diazepam (Darunavir and ritonavir are both inhibitors of CYP3A. Co-administration of darunavir and ritonavir with drugs primarily metabolized by CYP3A may result in increased plasma concentrations of such drugs, which could increase or prolong their therapeutic effect and adverse events). Products include:
Diastat Rectal Delivery System **3343**
Valium Tablets **2819**

Didanosine (It is recommended that didanosine be administered on an empty stomach. Therefore, didanosine should be administered one hour before or two hours after darunavir/rtv (which are administered with food)).
No products indexed under this heading.

Dihydroergotamine Mesylate
(Dihydroergotamine mesylate is contraindicated due to a potential for serious and/or life-threatening reactions such as acute ergot toxicity characterized by peripheral vasospasm and ischemia of the extremities and other tissues). Products include:
Migranal Nasal Spray **3348**

Diltiazem Hydrochloride
(Darunavir and ritonavir are both inhibitors of CYP3A. Co-administration of darunavir and ritonavir with drugs primarily metabolized by CYP3A may result in increased plasma concentrations of such drugs, which could increase or prolong their therapeutic effect and adverse events). Products include:
Cardizem LA Extended Release Tablets **1728**
Tiazac Capsules **1201**

Diltiazem Maleate (Darunavir and ritonavir are both inhibitors of CYP3A. Co-administration of darunavir and ritonavir with drugs primarily metabolized by CYP3A may result in increased plasma concentrations of such drugs, which could increase or prolong their therapeutic effect and adverse events).
No products indexed under this heading.

Disopyramide Phosphate
(Darunavir and ritonavir are both inhibitors of CYP3A. Co-administration of darunavir and ritonavir with drugs primarily metabolized by CYP3A may result in increased plasma concentrations of such drugs, which could increase or prolong their therapeutic effect and adverse events).
No products indexed under this heading.

Doxorubicin Hydrochloride
(Darunavir and ritonavir are both inhibitors of CYP3A. Co-administration of darunavir and ritonavir with drugs primarily metabolized by CYP3A may result in increased plasma concentrations of such drugs, which could increase or prolong their therapeutic effect and adverse events).
No products indexed under this heading.

Dronabinol (Darunavir and ritonavir are both inhibitors of CYP3A. Co-administration of darunavir and ritonavir with drugs primarily metabolized by CYP3A may result in increased plasma concentrations of such drugs, which could increase or prolong their therapeutic effect and adverse events). Products include:
Marinol Capsules **3333**

Dyphylline (Darunavir and ritonavir are both inhibitors of CYP3A. Co-administration of darunavir and ritonavir with drugs primarily metabolized by CYP3A may result in increased plasma concentrations of such drugs, which could increase or prolong their therapeutic effect and adverse events).
No products indexed under this heading.

Efavirenz (Co-administration of darunavir/rtv and efavirenz decreased darunavir AUC by 13% and Cmin by 31%. The AUC of efavirenz increased by 21% and Cmin increased by 17%. The clinical significance has not been established. The combination of darunavir/rtv and efavirenz should be used with caution). Products include:
Atripla Tablets **945**
Sustiva Capsules **930**
Sustiva Tablets **930**

Ergonovine Maleate (Ergonovine maleate is contraindicated due to a potential for serious and/or life-threatening reactions such as acute ergot toxicity characterized by peripheral vasospasm and ischemia of the extremities and other tissues).
No products indexed under this heading.

Ergotamine Tartrate (Ergotamine tartrate is contraindicated due to a potential for serious and/or life-threatening reactions such as acute ergot toxicity characterized by peripheral vasospasm and ischemia of the extremities and other tissues).
No products indexed under this heading.

Erythromycin (Darunavir and ritonavir are both inhibitors of CYP3A. Co-administration of darunavir and ritonavir with drugs primarily metabolized by CYP3A may result in increased plasma concentrations of such drugs, which could increase or prolong their therapeutic effect and adverse events). Products include:
Ery-Tab Tablets **449**
Erythromycin Base Filmtab Tablets **455**
Erythromycin Delayed-Release Capsules, USP **457**
PCE Dispertab Tablets **515**

Erythromycin Estolate (Darunavir and ritonavir are both inhibitors of CYP3A. Co-administration of darunavir and ritonavir with drugs primarily metabolized by CYP3A may result in increased plasma concentrations of such drugs, which could increase or prolong their therapeutic effect and adverse events).
No products indexed under this heading.

Erythromycin Ethylsuccinate
(Darunavir and ritonavir are both inhibitors of CYP3A. Co-administration of darunavir and ritonavir with drugs primarily metabolized by CYP3A may result in increased plasma concentrations of such drugs, which could increase or prolong their therapeutic effect and adverse events). Products include:
E.E.S. **451**
EryPed **447**

Erythromycin Gluceptate
(Darunavir and ritonavir are both inhibitors of CYP3A. Co-administration of darunavir and ritonavir with drugs primarily metabolized by CYP3A may result in increased plasma concentrations of such drugs, which could increase or prolong their therapeutic effect and adverse events).
No products indexed under this heading.

Erythromycin Lactobionate
(Darunavir and ritonavir are both inhibitors of CYP3A. Co-administration of darunavir and ritonavir with drugs primarily metabolized by CYP3A may result in increased plasma concentrations of such drugs, which could increase or prolong their therapeutic effect and adverse events).
No products indexed under this heading.

Erythromycin Stearate (Darunavir and ritonavir are both inhibitors of CYP3A. Co-administration of darunavir and ritonavir with drugs primarily metabolized by CYP3A may result in increased plasma concentrations of such drugs, which could increase or prolong their therapeutic effect and adverse events). Products include:
Erythrocin Stearate Filmtab Tablets ... **453**

Estrogen (Darunavir and ritonavir are both inhibitors of CYP3A. Co-administration of darunavir and ritonavir with drugs primarily metabolized by CYP3A may result in increased plasma concentrations of such drugs, which could increase or prolong their therapeutic effect and adverse events).
No products indexed under this heading.

Estrogens, Conjugated (Darunavir and ritonavir are both inhibitors of CYP3A. Co-administration of darunavir and ritonavir with drugs primarily metabolized by CYP3A may result in increased plasma concentrations of such drugs, which could increase or prolong their therapeutic effect and adverse events). Products include:
Premarin Intravenous **3442**
Premarin Tablets **3446**
Premarin Vaginal Cream **3452**
Premphase Tablets **3456**
Prempro Tablets **3456**

Estrogens, Conjugated, Synthetic A (Darunavir and ritonavir are both inhibitors of CYP3A. Co-administration of darunavir and ritonavir with drugs primarily metabolized by CYP3A may result in increased plasma concentrations of such drugs, which could increase or prolong their therapeutic effect and adverse events).
No products indexed under this heading.

Estrogens, Esterified (Darunavir and ritonavir are both inhibitors of CYP3A. Co-administration of darunavir and ritonavir with drugs primarily metabolized by CYP3A may result in increased plasma concentrations of such drugs, which could increase or prolong their therapeutic effect and adverse events). Products include:
Estratest Tablets **3199**
Estratest H.S. Tablets **3199**

Ethinyl Estradiol (Plasma concentrations of ethinyl estradiol may be decreased due to induction of its metabolism by ritonavir. Alternative or additional contraceptive measures should be used when estrogen-based contraceptives are co-administered with darunavir/rtv). Products include:
Mircette Tablets **1066**
NuvaRing **2340**
Ortho-Cyclen/Ortho Tri-Cyclen **2429**
Ortho Evra Transdermal System **2417**
Ortho Tri-Cyclen Lo Tablets **2436**
Seasonique Tablets **1077**
Yasmin 28 Tablets **796**
Yaz Tablets **803**

Ethosuximide (Darunavir and ritonavir are both inhibitors of CYP3A. Co-administration of darunavir and ritonavir with drugs primarily metabolized by CYP3A may result in increased plasma concentrations of such drugs, which could increase or prolong their therapeutic effect and adverse events).
No products indexed under this heading.

Ethynodiol Diacetate (Darunavir and ritonavir are both inhibitors of CYP3A. Co-administration of darunavir and ritonavir with drugs primarily metabolized by CYP3A may result in increased plasma concentrations of such drugs, which could increase or prolong their therapeutic effect and adverse events).
No products indexed under this heading.

Etoposide (Darunavir and ritonavir are both inhibitors of CYP3A. Co-administration of darunavir and ritonavir with drugs primarily metabolized by CYP3A may result in increased plasma concentrations of such drugs, which could increase or prolong their therapeutic effect and adverse events).
No products indexed under this heading.

Etoposide Phosphate (Darunavir and ritonavir are both inhibitors of CYP3A. Co-administration of darunavir and ritonavir with drugs primarily metabolized by CYP3A may result in increased plasma concentrations of such drugs, which could increase or prolong their therapeutic effect and adverse events).
No products indexed under this heading.

Felodipine (Darunavir and ritonavir are both inhibitors of CYP3A. Co-administration of darunavir and ritonavir with drugs primarily metabolized by CYP3A may result in increased plasma concentrations of such drugs, which could increase or prolong their therapeutic effect and adverse events).

No products indexed under this heading.

Fentanyl (Darunavir and ritonavir are both inhibitors of CYP3A. Co-administration of darunavir and ritonavir with drugs primarily metabolized by CYP3A may result in increased plasma concentrations of such drugs, which could increase or prolong their therapeutic effect and adverse events). Products include:

Duragesic Transdermal System 2373
Ionsys Transdermal System 2379

Fentanyl Citrate (Darunavir and ritonavir are both inhibitors of CYP3A. Co-administration of darunavir and ritonavir with drugs primarily metabolized by CYP3A may result in increased plasma concentrations of such drugs, which could increase or prolong their therapeutic effect and adverse events). Products include:

Actiq 979

Fluticasone Propionate (Concomitant use of inhaled fluticasone propionate and darunavir/rtv may increase plasma concentrations of fluticasone propionate. Alternatives should be considered, particularly for long term use). Products include:

Advair Diskus 100/50 1308
Advair Diskus 250/50 1308
Advair Diskus 500/50 1308
Advair HFA Inhalation Aerosol 1318
Cutivate Cream 2662
Cutivate Lotion 0.05% 2664
Cutivate Ointment 2665
Flonase Nasal Spray 1440
Flovent Diskus 1443

Glyburide (Darunavir and ritonavir are both inhibitors of CYP3A. Co-administration of darunavir and ritonavir with drugs primarily metabolized by CYP3A may result in increased plasma concentrations of such drugs, which could increase or prolong their therapeutic effect and adverse events).

No products indexed under this heading.

Haloperidol (Darunavir and ritonavir are both inhibitors of CYP3A. Co-administration of darunavir and ritonavir with drugs primarily metabolized by CYP3A may result in increased plasma concentrations of such drugs, which could increase or prolong their therapeutic effect and adverse events).

No products indexed under this heading.

Haloperidol Decanoate (Darunavir and ritonavir are both inhibitors of CYP3A. Co-administration of darunavir and ritonavir with drugs primarily metabolized by CYP3A may result in increased plasma concentrations of such drugs, which could increase or prolong their therapeutic effect and adverse events).

No products indexed under this heading.

Hypericum Perforatum (Darunavir should not be used concomitantly with products containing hypericum perforatum because co-administration may cause significant decreases in darunavir plasma concentrations. This may result in loss of therapeutic effect to darunavir).

No products indexed under this heading.

Imipramine Hydrochloride (Darunavir and ritonavir are both inhibitors of CYP3A. Co-administration of darunavir and ritonavir with drugs primarily metabolized by CYP3A may result in increased plasma concentrations of such drugs, which could increase or prolong their therapeutic effect and adverse events).

No products indexed under this heading.

Imipramine Pamoate (Darunavir and ritonavir are both inhibitors of CYP3A. Co-administration of darunavir and ritonavir with drugs primarily metabolized by CYP3A may result in increased plasma concentrations of such drugs, which could increase or prolong their therapeutic effect and adverse events).

No products indexed under this heading.

Indinavir Sulfate (Darunavir and ritonavir are both inhibitors of CYP3A. Co-administration of darunavir and ritonavir with drugs primarily metabolized by CYP3A may result in increased plasma concentrations of such drugs, which could increase or prolong their therapeutic effect and adverse events). Products include:

Crixivan Capsules 1940

Isradipine (Darunavir and ritonavir are both inhibitors of CYP3A. Co-administration of darunavir and ritonavir with drugs primarily metabolized by CYP3A may result in increased plasma concentrations of such drugs, which could increase or prolong their therapeutic effect and adverse events). Products include:

DynaCirc CR Tablets 2721

Itraconazole (Darunavir and ritonavir are both inhibitors of CYP3A. Co-administration of darunavir and ritonavir with drugs primarily metabolized by CYP3A may result in increased plasma concentrations of such drugs, which could increase or prolong their therapeutic effect and adverse events).

No products indexed under this heading.

Ketoconazole (Darunavir and ritonavir are both inhibitors of CYP3A. Co-administration of darunavir and ritonavir with drugs primarily metabolized by CYP3A may result in increased plasma concentrations of such drugs, which could increase or prolong their therapeutic effect and adverse events). Products include:

Nizoral A-D Shampoo, 1% 1868

Levonorgestrel (Darunavir and ritonavir are both inhibitors of CYP3A. Co-administration of darunavir and ritonavir with drugs primarily metabolized by CYP3A may result in increased plasma concentrations of such drugs, which could increase or prolong their therapeutic effect and adverse events). Products include:

Climara Pro Transdermal System 776

Mirena Intrauterine System 787
Plan B Tablets 1076
Seasonique Tablets 1077

Lidocaine (Concentrations of bepridil, lidocaine, quinidine and amiodarone may be increased when co-administered with darunavir/rtv. Caution is warranted and therapeutic concentration monitoring, if available, is recommended for antiarrhythmics when co-administered with darunavir/rtv). Products include:

Lidoderm Patch 1118
Synera Topical Patch 1137

Lidocaine Base (Concentrations of bepridil, lidocaine, quinidine and amiodarone may be increased when co-administered with darunavir/rtv. Caution is warranted and therapeutic concentration monitoring, if available, is recommended for antiarrhythmics when co-administered with darunavir/rtv).

No products indexed under this heading.

Lidocaine Hydrochloride (Concentrations of bepridil, lidocaine, quinidine and amiodarone may be increased when co-administered with darunavir/rtv. Caution is warranted and therapeutic concentration monitoring, if available, is recommended for antiarrhythmics when co-administered with darunavir/rtv).

No products indexed under this heading.

Lopinavir (Due to a decrease in the exposure (AUC) of darunavir by 53%, appropriate doses of the combination have not been established. Hence, it is not recommended to co-administer lopinavir/ritonavir and darunavir, with or without an additional low dose of ritonavir). Products include:

Kaletra 476

Lovastatin (Concomitant use may raise the potential for serious reactions such as risk of myopathy including rhabdomyolysis). Products include:

Advicor Tablets 1722
Altoprev Extended-Release Tablets 3109
Mevacor Tablets 2021

Mestranol (Darunavir and ritonavir are both inhibitors of CYP3A. Co-administration of darunavir and ritonavir with drugs primarily metabolized by CYP3A may result in increased plasma concentrations of such drugs, which could increase or prolong their therapeutic effect and adverse events).

No products indexed under this heading.

Methadone Hydrochloride (When methadone is co-administered with darunavir/rtv, patients should be monitored for opiate abstinence syndrome, as ritonavir is known to induce the metabolism of methadone, leading to a decrease in its plasma concentrations. An increase in methadone dosage may be considered based on the clinical response).

No products indexed under this heading.

Methylergonovine Maleate (Methylergonovine maleate is contraindicated due to a potential for serious and/or life-threatening reactions such as acute ergot toxicity characterized by peripheral vasospasm and ischemia of the extremities and other tissues).

No products indexed under this heading.

Mibefradil Dihydrochloride (Plasma concentrations of calcium channel blockers (e.g. felodipine, nifedipine, nicardipine) may increase when darunavir/rtv are co-administered. Caution is warranted and clinical monitoring of patients is recommended).

No products indexed under this heading.

Midazolam Hydrochloride (Midazolam hydrochloride is contraindicated due to a potential for serious and/or life-threatening reactions such as prolonged or increased sedation or respiratory depression).

No products indexed under this heading.

Modafinil (Darunavir and ritonavir are metabolized by CYP3A. Drugs that induce CYP3A activity would be expected to increase the clearance of darunavir and ritonavir, resulting in lowered plasma concentrations of darunavir and ritonavir. Co-administration of darunavir and ritonavir and other drugs that inhibit CYP3A may decrease the clearance of darunavir and ritonavir and may result in increased plasma concentrations of darunavir and ritonavir). Products include:

Provigil Tablets 988

Nefazodone Hydrochloride (Darunavir and ritonavir are both inhibitors of CYP3A. Co-administration of darunavir and ritonavir with drugs primarily metabolized by CYP3A may result in increased plasma concentrations of such drugs, which could increase or prolong their therapeutic effect and adverse events).

No products indexed under this heading.

Nelfinavir Mesylate (Darunavir and ritonavir are both inhibitors of CYP3A. Co-administration of darunavir and ritonavir with drugs primarily metabolized by CYP3A may result in increased plasma concentrations of such drugs, which could increase or prolong their therapeutic effect and adverse events). Products include:

Viracept 2577

Nevirapine (Darunavir and ritonavir are metabolized by CYP3A. Drugs that induce CYP3A activity would be expected to increase the clearance of darunavir and ritonavir, resulting in lowered plasma concentrations of darunavir and ritonavir. Co-administration of darunavir and ritonavir and other drugs that inhibit CYP3A may decrease the clearance of darunavir and ritonavir and may result in increased plasma concentrations of darunavir and ritonavir). Products include:

Viramune Oral Suspension 873
Viramune Tablets 873

Nicardipine (Darunavir and ritonavir are both inhibitors of CYP3A. Co-administration of darunavir and ritonavir with drugs primarily metabolized by CYP3A may result in increased plasma concentrations of such drugs, which could increase or prolong their therapeutic effect and adverse events).

No products indexed under this heading.

Nicardipine Hydrochloride (Darunavir and ritonavir are both inhibitors of CYP3A. Co-administration of darunavir and ritonavir with drugs primarily metab-

IMPORTANT NOTE: Always consult each drug listing in the patient's regimen for possible interactions.

olized by CYP3A may result in increased plasma concentrations of such drugs, which could increase or prolong their therapeutic effect and adverse events). Products include:

Cardene I.V. 2497

Nifedipine (Darunavir and ritonavir are both inhibitors of CYP3A. Co-administration of darunavir and ritonavir with drugs primarily metabolized by CYP3A may result in increased plasma concentrations of such drugs, which could increase or prolong their therapeutic effect and adverse events). Products include:

Adalat CC Tablets 2964

Nimodipine (Darunavir and ritonavir are both inhibitors of CYP3A. Co-administration of darunavir and ritonavir with drugs primarily metabolized by CYP3A may result in increased plasma concentrations of such drugs, which could increase or prolong their therapeutic effect and adverse events). Products include:

Nimotop Capsules 749

Nisoldipine (Darunavir and ritonavir are both inhibitors of CYP3A. Co-administration of darunavir and ritonavir with drugs primarily metabolized by CYP3A may result in increased plasma concentrations of such drugs, which could increase or prolong their therapeutic effect and adverse events). Products include:

Sular Tablets 3122

Norethindrone (Plasma concentrations of ethinyl estradiol may be decreased due to induction of its metabolism by ritonavir. Alternative or additional contraceptive measures should be used when estrogen-based contraceptives are co-administered with darunavir/rtv). Products include:

Ortho Micronor Tablets 2426

Norethindrone Acetate (Plasma concentrations of ethinyl estradiol may be decreased due to induction of its metabolism by ritonavir. Alternative or additional contraceptive measures should be used when estrogen-based contraceptives are co-administered with darunavir/rtv).

No products indexed under this heading.

Norgestrel (Darunavir and ritonavir are both inhibitors of CYP3A. Co-administration of darunavir and ritonavir with drugs primarily metabolized by CYP3A may result in increased plasma concentrations of such drugs, which could increase or prolong their therapeutic effect and adverse events).

No products indexed under this heading.

Ondansetron Hydrochloride (Darunavir and ritonavir are both inhibitors of CYP3A. Co-administration of darunavir and ritonavir with drugs primarily metabolized by CYP3A may result in increased plasma concentrations of such drugs, which could increase or prolong their therapeutic effect and adverse events). Products include:

Zofran Injection 1634
Zofran 1639

Paclitaxel (Darunavir and ritonavir are both inhibitors of CYP3A. Co-administration of darunavir and ritonavir with drugs primarily metabolized by CYP3A may result in increased plasma concentrations of such drugs, which could increase or prolong their therapeutic effect and adverse events).

No products indexed under this heading.

Paroxetine Hydrochloride (If sertraline or paroxetine is co-administered with darunavir/rtv, the recommended approach is a carfeul dose titration of the SSRI based on a clinical assessment of antidepressant response. In addition, patients on a stable dose of sertraline or paroxetine who start treatment with darunavir/rtv should be monitored for antidepressant response). Products include:

Paxil CR Controlled-Release Tablets 1538
Paxil 1530

Paroxetine Mesylate (If sertraline or paroxetine is co-administered with darunavir/rtv, the recommended approach is a carfeul dose titration of the SSRI based on a clinical assessment of antidepressant response. In addition, patients on a stable dose of sertraline or paroxetine who start treatment with darunavir/rtv should be monitored for antidepressant response). Products include:

Pexeva Tablets 1694

Phenobarbital (Darunavir and ritonavir are metabolized by CYP3A. Drugs that induce CYP3A activity would be expected to increase the clearance of darunavir and ritonavir, resulting in lowered plasma concentrations of darunavir and ritonavir. Co-administration of darunavir and ritonavir and other drugs that inhibit CYP3A may decrease the clearance of darunavir and ritonavir and may result in increased plasma concentrations of darunavir and ritonavir). Products include:

Donnatal Extentabs 2493

Phenytoin (Darunavir and ritonavir are metabolized by CYP3A. Drugs that induce CYP3A activity would be expected to increase the clearance of darunavir and ritonavir, resulting in lowered plasma concentrations of darunavir and ritonavir. Co-administration of darunavir and ritonavir and other drugs that inhibit CYP3A may decrease the clearance of darunavir and ritonavir and may result in increased plasma concentrations of darunavir and ritonavir).

No products indexed under this heading.

Phenytoin Sodium (Darunavir and ritonavir are metabolized by CYP3A. Drugs that induce CYP3A activity would be expected to increase the clearance of darunavir and ritonavir, resulting in lowered plasma concentrations of darunavir and ritonavir. Co-administration of darunavir and ritonavir and other drugs that inhibit CYP3A may decrease the clearance of darunavir and ritonavir and may result in increased plasma concentrations of darunavir and ritonavir). Products include:

Phenytek Capsules 2160

Pimozide (Pimozide is contraindicated due to the potential for serious and/or life-threatening reactions such as cardiac arrhythmias).

No products indexed under this heading.

Pravastatin Sodium (When darunavir/rtv was administered with pravastatin, the mean increase in pravastatin AUC was 81%. However, pravastatin AUC increased by up to 5-fold in some subjects. The mechanism of the interaction is not known).

No products indexed under this heading.

Quinidine (Concentrations of bepridil, lidocaine, quinidine and amiodarone may be increased when co-administered with darunavir/rtv. Caution is warranted and therapeutic concentration monitoring, if available, is recommended for antiarrhythmics when co-administered with darunavir/rtv).

No products indexed under this heading.

Quinidine Gluconate (Concentrations of bepridil, lidocaine, quinidine and amiodarone may be increased when co-administered with darunavir/rtv. Caution is warranted and therapeutic concentration monitoring, if available, is recommended for antiarrhythmics when co-administered with darunavir/rtv).

No products indexed under this heading.

Quinidine Hydrochloride (Concentrations of bepridil, lidocaine, quinidine and amiodarone may be increased when co-administered with darunavir/rtv. Caution is warranted and therapeutic concentration monitoring, if available, is recommended for antiarrhythmics when co-administered with darunavir/rtv).

No products indexed under this heading.

Quinidine Polygalacturonate (Concentrations of bepridil, lidocaine, quinidine and amiodarone may be increased when co-administered with darunavir/rtv. Caution is warranted and therapeutic concentration monitoring, if available, is recommended for antiarrhythmics when co-administered with darunavir/rtv).

No products indexed under this heading.

Quinidine Sulfate (Concentrations of bepridil, lidocaine, quinidine and amiodarone may be increased when co-administered with darunavir/rtv. Caution is warranted and therapeutic concentration monitoring, if available, is recommended for antiarrhythmics when co-administered with darunavir/rtv).

No products indexed under this heading.

Quinine (Darunavir and ritonavir are both inhibitors of CYP3A. Co-administration of darunavir and ritonavir with drugs primarily metabolized by CYP3A may result in increased plasma concentrations of such drugs, which could increase or prolong their therapeutic effect and adverse events).

No products indexed under this heading.

Quinine Sulfate (Darunavir and ritonavir are both inhibitors of CYP3A. Co-administration of darunavir and ritonavir with drugs primarily metabolized by CYP3A may result in increased plasma concentrations of such drugs, which could increase or prolong their therapeutic effect and adverse events).

No products indexed under this heading.

Rifabutin (Darunavir and ritonavir are both inhibitors of CYP3A. Co-administration of darunavir and ritonavir with drugs primarily metabolized by CYP3A may result in increased plasma concentrations of such drugs, which could increase or prolong their therapeutic effect and adverse events).

No products indexed under this heading.

Rifampicin (Darunavir and ritonavir are metabolized by CYP3A. Drugs that induce CYP3A activity would be expected to increase the clearance of darunavir and ritonavir, resulting in lowered plasma concentrations of darunavir and ritonavir. Co-administration of darunavir and ritonavir and other drugs that inhibit CYP3A may decrease the clearance of darunavir and ritonavir and may result in increased plasma concentrations of darunavir and ritonavir).

No products indexed under this heading.

Rifampin (Darunavir and ritonavir are metabolized by CYP3A. Drugs that induce CYP3A activity would be expected to increase the clearance of darunavir and ritonavir, resulting in lowered plasma concentrations of darunavir and ritonavir. Co-administration of darunavir and ritonavir and other drugs that inhibit CYP3A may decrease the clearance of darunavir and ritonavir and may result in increased plasma concentrations of darunavir and ritonavir).

No products indexed under this heading.

Rifapentine (Darunavir and ritonavir are metabolized by CYP3A. Drugs that induce CYP3A activity would be expected to increase the clearance of darunavir and ritonavir, resulting in lowered plasma concentrations of darunavir and ritonavir. Co-administration of darunavir and ritonavir and other drugs that inhibit CYP3A may decrease the clearance of darunavir and ritonavir and may result in increased plasma concentrations of darunavir and ritonavir).

No products indexed under this heading.

Ritonavir (Darunavir and ritonavir are both inhibitors of CYP3A. Co-administration of darunavir and ritonavir with drugs primarily metabolized by CYP3A may result in increased plasma concentrations of such drugs, which could increase or prolong their therapeutic effect and adverse events). Products include:

Kaletra 476
Norvir 503

Saquinavir (Due to a decrease in the exposure (AUC) of darunavir by 26%, appropriate doses of the combination have not been established. Hence, it is not recommended to co-administer saquinavir and darunavir, with or without an additional low dose of ritonavir).

No products indexed under this heading.

Saquinavir Mesylate (Due to a decrease in the exposure (AUC) of darunavir by 26%, appropriate doses of the combination have not been established. Hence, it is not recommended to co-administer lopinavir/ritonavir and darunavir, with or without an additional low dose of ritonavir). Products include:

Sertraline Hydrochloride (If sertraline or paroxetine is co-administered with darunavir/rtv, the recommended approach is a carfeul dose titration of the SSRI based on a clinical assessment of antidepressant response. In addition, patients on a stable dose of sertraline or paroxetine who start treatment with darunavir/rtv should be monitored for antidepressant response). Products include:

Sildenafil Citrate (Darunavir and ritonavir are both inhibitors of CYP3A. Co-administration of darunavir and ritonavir with drugs primarily metabolized by CYP3A may result in increased plasma concentrations of such drugs, which could increase or prolong their therapeutic effect and adverse events). Products include:

Simvastatin (Concomitant use may raise the potential for serious reactions such as risk of myopathy including rhabdomyolysis). Products include:

Sirolimus (Plasma concentrations of cyclosporine, tacrolimus or sirolimus may be increased when co-administered with darunavir/rtv. Therapeutic concentration monitoring of the immunosuppressive agent is recommended for immunosuppressant agents when co-administeredwith darunavir/rtv). Products include:

Tacrolimus (Plasma concentrations of cyclosporine, tacrolimus or sirolimus may be increased when co-administered with darunavir/rtv. Therapeutic concentration monitoring of the immunosuppressive agent is recommended for immunosuppressant agents when co-administeredwith darunavir/rtv). Products include:

Tadalafil (Concomitant use of PDE-5 inhibitors with darunavir/rtv should be done with caution. If concomitant use of darunavir/rtv with vardenafil or tadalafil is required, vardenafil at a single dose not exceeding 2.5 mg dose in 72 hours, or tadaladil at a singledose not exceeding 10 mg in 72 hours, is recommended). Products include:

Tamoxifen Citrate (Darunavir and ritonavir are both inhibitors of CYP3A. Co-administration of darunavir and ritonavir with drugs

primarily metabolized by CYP3A may result in increased plasma concentrations of such drugs, which could increase or prolong their therapeutic effect and adverse events). Products include:

Terfenadine (Terfenadine is contraindicated due to a potential for serious and/or life-threatening reactions such as cardiac arrhythmias). No products indexed under this heading.

Testosterone (Darunavir and ritonavir are both inhibitors of CYP3A. Co-administration of darunavir and ritonavir with drugs primarily metabolized by CYP3A may result in increased plasma concentrations of such drugs, which could increase or prolong their therapeutic effect and adverse events). Products include:

Testosterone Cypionate (Darunavir and ritonavir are both inhibitors of CYP3A. Co-administration of darunavir and ritonavir with drugs primarily metabolized by CYP3A may result in increased plasma concentrations of such drugs, which could increase or prolong their therapeutic effect and adverse events). No products indexed under this heading.

Testosterone Enanthate (Darunavir and ritonavir are both inhibitors of CYP3A. Co-administration of darunavir and ritonavir with drugs primarily metabolized by CYP3A may result in increased plasma concentrations of such drugs, which could increase or prolong their therapeutic effect and adverse events). No products indexed under this heading.

Testosterone Propionate (Darunavir and ritonavir are both inhibitors of CYP3A. Co-administration of darunavir and ritonavir with drugs primarily metabolized by CYP3A may result in increased plasma concentrations of such drugs, which could increase or prolong their therapeutic effect and adverse events). No products indexed under this heading.

Theophylline (Darunavir and ritonavir are both inhibitors of CYP3A. Co-administration of darunavir and ritonavir with drugs primarily metabolized by CYP3A may result in increased plasma concentrations of such drugs, which could increase or prolong their therapeutic effect and adverse events). No products indexed under this heading.

Theophylline Anhydrous (Darunavir and ritonavir are both inhibitors of CYP3A. Co-administration of darunavir and ritonavir with drugs primarily metabolized by CYP3A may result in increased plasma concentrations of such drugs, which could increase or prolong their therapeutic effect and adverse events). Products include:

Theophylline Calcium Salicylate (Darunavir and ritonavir are both inhibitors of CYP3A. Co-administration of darunavir and ritonavir with drugs primarily metabolized by CYP3A may result in increased plasma concentrations of such drugs, which could increase or prolong their therapeutic effect and adverse events). No products indexed under this heading.

Theophylline Sodium Glycinate (Darunavir and ritonavir are both inhibitors of CYP3A. Co-administration of darunavir and ritonavir with drugs primarily metabolized by CYP3A may result in increased plasma concentrations of such drugs, which could increase or prolong their therapeutic effect and adverse events). No products indexed under this heading.

Tiagabine Hydrochloride (Darunavir and ritonavir are both inhibitors of CYP3A. Co-administration of darunavir and ritonavir with drugs primarily metabolized by CYP3A may result in increased plasma concentrations of such drugs, which could increase or prolong their therapeutic effect and adverse events). Products include:

Tolterodine Tartrate (Darunavir and ritonavir are both inhibitors of CYP3A. Co-administration of darunavir and ritonavir with drugs primarily metabolized by CYP3A may result in increased plasma concentrations of such drugs, which could increase or prolong their therapeutic effect and adverse events). Products include:

Trazodone Hydrochloride (Darunavir and ritonavir are both inhibitors of CYP3A. Co-administration of darunavir and ritonavir with drugs primarily metabolized by CYP3A may result in increased plasma concentrations of such drugs, which could increase or prolong their therapeutic effect and adverse events). No products indexed under this heading.

Triazolam (Triazolam is contraindicated due to a potential for serious and/or life-threatening reactions such as prolonged or increased sedation or respiratory depression). No products indexed under this heading.

Vardenafil Hydrochloride (Concomitant use of PDE-5 inhibitors with darunavir/rtv should be done with caution. If concomitant use of darunavir/rtv with vardenafil or tadalafil is required, vardenafil at a single dose not exceeding 2.5 mg dose in 72 hours, or tadaladil at a singledose not exceeding 10 mg in 72 hours, is recommended). Products include:

Venlafaxine Hydrochloride (Darunavir and ritonavir are both inhibitors of CYP3A. Co-administration of darunavir and ritonavir with drugs primarily metabolized by CYP3A may result in increased plasma concentrations of such drugs, which could increase or prolong their therapeutic effect and adverse events). Products include:

Verapamil Hydrochloride (Darunavir and ritonavir are both inhibitors of CYP3A. Co-administration of darunavir and ritonavir with drugs primarily metabolized by CYP3A may result in increased plasma concentrations of such drugs, which could increase or prolong their therapeutic effect and adverse events). Products include:

Vinblastine Sulfate (Darunavir and ritonavir are both inhibitors of CYP3A. Co-administration of darunavir and ritonavir with drugs primarily metabolized by CYP3A may result in increased plasma concentrations of such drugs, which could increase or prolong their therapeutic effect and adverse events). No products indexed under this heading.

Vincristine Sulfate (Darunavir and ritonavir are both inhibitors of CYP3A. Co-administration of darunavir and ritonavir with drugs primarily metabolized by CYP3A may result in increased plasma concentrations of such drugs, which could increase or prolong their therapeutic effect and adverse events). No products indexed under this heading.

Warfarin Sodium (Warfarin concentrations may be affected when co-administered with darunavir/rtv. It is recommended that the international normalized ratio (INR) be monitored when warfarin is combined with darunavir/rtv). Products include:

PRILOSEC OTC DELAYED-RELEASE TABLETS

(Omeprazole magnesium) 2677
May interact with benzodiazepines, iron containing oral preparations, phenytoin, and certain other agents. Compounds in these categories include:

Alprazolam (Potential for metabolism interaction via cytochrome P450 system). Products include:

Astemizole (Co-administration of omeprazole-clarithromycin combination with astemizole is not recommended because clarithromycin, like erythromycin, is also metabolized by cytochrome P450 and there have been reports of QT prolongation and torsade de pointes with concurrent use of erythromycin and astemizole). No products indexed under this heading.

Bacampicillin Hydrochloride (Omeprazole may interfere with gastric absorption of drugs, such as ampicillin esters, where gastric pH is an important determinant of their bioavailability). No products indexed under this heading.

Chlordiazepoxide (Potential for metabolism interaction via cytochrome P450 system). No products indexed under this heading.

Chlordiazepoxide Hydrochloride (Potential for metabolism interaction via cytochrome P450 system). Products include:
Librium Capsules 3347

Cisapride (Co-administration of omeprazole-clarithromycin combination with cisapride has resulted in cardiac arrhythmias, including QT prolongation, ventricular tachycardia and fibrillation and torsade de points, and fatalities; concomitant use of clarithromycin and cisapride is contraindicated).
No products indexed under this heading.

Clarithromycin (Co-administration may result in increases in plasma levels of omeprazole, clarithromycin, and 14-hydroxy-clarithromycin). Products include:
Biaxin/Biaxin XL 402
PREVPAC 3284

Clonazepam (Potential for metabolism interaction via cytochrome P450 system). Products include:
Klonopin 2778

Clorazepate Dipotassium (Potential for metabolism interaction via cytochrome P450 system). Products include:
Tranxene 2474

Cyclosporine (Potential for metabolism interaction via cytochrome P450 system). Products include:
Gengraf Capsules 459
Neoral Oral Solution 2259
Neoral Soft Gelatin Capsules 2259
Restasis Ophthalmic Emulsion 575
Sandimmune 2275

Diazepam (Potential for metabolism interaction via cytochrome P450 system; prolonged elimination of diazepam). Products include:
Diastat Rectal Delivery System 3343
Valium Tablets 2819

Disulfiram (Potential for metabolism interaction via cytochrome P450 system).
No products indexed under this heading.

Estazolam (Potential for metabolism interaction via cytochrome P450 system). Products include:
ProSom Tablets 517

Ferrous Fumarate (Omeprazole may interfere with gastric absorption of drugs, such as iron salts, where gastric pH is an important determinant of their bioavailability).
No products indexed under this heading.

Ferrous Gluconate (Omeprazole may interfere with gastric absorption of drugs, such as iron salts, where gastric pH is an important determinant of their bioavailability).
No products indexed under this heading.

Ferrous Sulfate (Omeprazole may interfere with gastric absorption of drugs, such as iron salts, where gastric pH is an important determinant of their bioavailability). Products include:
Slow Fe Iron Tablets .... ▣818
Slow Fe with Folic Acid Tablets .... ▣819

Flurazepam Hydrochloride (Potential for metabolism interaction via cytochrome P450 system). Products include:
Dalmane Capsules 3342

Fosphenytoin Sodium (Prolonged elimination of phenytoin).
No products indexed under this heading.

Halazepam (Potential for metabolism interaction via cytochrome P450 system).
No products indexed under this heading.

Iron (Omeprazole may interfere with gastric absorption of drugs, such as iron salts, where gastric pH is an important determinant of their bioavailability).
No products indexed under this heading.

Ketoconazole (Omeprazole may interfere with gastric absorption of drugs, such as ketoconazole, where gastric pH is an important determinant of their bioavailability). Products include:
Nizoral A-D Shampoo, 1% 1868

Lorazepam (Potential for metabolism interaction via cytochrome P450 system).
No products indexed under this heading.

Midazolam Hydrochloride (Potential for metabolism interaction via cytochrome P450 system).
No products indexed under this heading.

Oxazepam (Potential for metabolism interaction via cytochrome P450 system).
No products indexed under this heading.

Phenytoin (Prolonged elimination of phenytoin).
No products indexed under this heading.

Phenytoin Sodium (Prolonged elimination of phenytoin). Products include:
Phenytek Capsules 2160

Pimozide (Co-administration of omeprazole-clarithromycin combination with pimozide has resulted in cardiac arrhythmias, including QT prolongation, ventricular tachycardia and fibrillation and torsade de points, and fatalities; concomitant use of clarithromycin and pimozide is contraindicated).
No products indexed under this heading.

Polysaccharide Iron Complex (Omeprazole may interfere with gastric absorption of drugs, such as iron salts, where gastric pH is an important determinant of their bioavailability). Products include:
Nu-Iron 150 Capsules 2127

Prazepam (Potential for metabolism interaction via cytochrome P450 system).
No products indexed under this heading.

Quazepam (Potential for metabolism interaction via cytochrome P450 system).
No products indexed under this heading.

Temazepam (Potential for metabolism interaction via cytochrome P450 system). Products include:
Restoril Capsules 1860

Terfenadine (Co-administration of omeprazole-clarithromycin combination with terfenadine has resulted in cardiac arrhythmias, including QT prolongation, ventricular tachycardia and fibrillation and torsade de points, and fatalities; concomitant use of clarithromycin and terfenadine is contraindicated).
No products indexed under this heading.

Triazolam (Potential for metabolism interaction via cytochrome P450 system).
No products indexed under this heading.

Warfarin Sodium (Prolonged elimination of warfarin). Products include:
Coumadin for Injection 898
Coumadin Tablets 898

Food Interactions

Food, unspecified (Absorption begins only after the granules leave the stomach; Prilosec should be taken before eating).

PRIMATENE MIST

(Epinephrine) .... ▣719
May interact with:

Caffeine (Avoid caffeine-containing foods or beverages). Products include:
BC Headache Powder .... ▣677
Arthritis Strength BC Powder .... ▣677
Excedrin Extra Strength Caplets/Tablets/Geltabs .... ▣684
Excedrin Migraine Caplets/Tablets/Geltabs .... ▣609
Excedrin Tension Headache Caplets/Tablets/Geltabs .... ▣611
Goody's Extra Strength Headache Powders .... ▣611
Goody's Extra Strength Pain Relief Tablets .... ▣685
Vivarin .... ▣602
Winrgy Dietary Supplement .... ▣823

Dietary Supplement (Avoid dietary supplements containing ingredients reported or claimed to have a stimulant effect). Products include:
COLD-fX Capsules 1000
4-Way Saline Nasal Spray .... ▣775
Hyland's Complete Flu Care 4 Kids Tablets .... ▣732
Hyland's Restful Legs Tablets .... ▣829
Hyland's Sniffles 'N Sneezes 4 Kids Tablets .... ▣732
Natural Joint Capsules .... ▣831
Proflavanol 90 Tablets 3339
Sen-Sei-Ro Liquid Gold 1740
Sen-Sei-Ro Powder Gold 1741
Tahitian Noni Liquid .... ▣834
Wobenzym Tablets 1862

PRIMAXIN I.M.

(Cilastatin Sodium, Imipenem) 2045
See Primaxin I.V.

PRIMAXIN I.V.

(Cilastatin Sodium, Imipenem) 2048
May interact with:

Ganciclovir Sodium (Concomitant administration may result in generalized seizures).
No products indexed under this heading.

Probenecid (Concomitant administration results in only minimal increase in plasma levels of imipenem; concomitant administration not recommended).
No products indexed under this heading.

PRINIVIL TABLETS

(Lisinopril) 2052
May interact with diuretics, oral hypoglycemic agents, insulin, lithium preparations, non-steroidal anti-inflammatory agents, potassium preparations, potassium sparing diuretics, thiazides, and certain other agents. Compounds in these categories include:

Acarbose (Epidemiological studies have suggested that concomitant administration of ACE inhibitors and antidiabetic medicines (insulins, oral hypoglycemic agents) may cause an increased blood-glucose-lowering effect with risk of hypoglycemia. This phenomenon appeared to be more likely to occur during the first weeks of combined treatment and in patients with renal impairment. In diabetic patients treated with oral antidiabetic agents or insulin, glycemic control should be closely monitored for hypoglycemia, especially during the first month of treatment with an ACE inhibitor). Products include:
Precose Tablets 751

Amiloride Hydrochloride (Use of lisinopril with potassium-sparing diuretics (such as spironolactone, triamterene or amiloride), potassium supplements or potassium-containing salt substitutes may lead to significant increases in serum potassium. Therefore, if concomitant use of these agents is indicated because of demonstrated hypokalemia, they should be used with caution and with frequent monitoring of serum potassium. Potassium-sparing agents should generally not be used in patients with heart failure who are receiving lisinopril). Products include:
Midamor Tablets 2026
Moduretic Tablets 2028

Bendroflumethiazide (Thiazide-induced potassium loss attenuated; possibility of excessive reduction in blood pressure).
No products indexed under this heading.

Bumetanide (Possibility of excessive reduction in blood pressure). Products include:
Bumex Tablets 2746

Celecoxib (Co-administration in some patients with compromised renal function who are being treated with NSAIDs may result in a further deterioration of renal function). Products include:
Celebrex Capsules 3134

Chlorothiazide (Thiazide-induced potassium loss attenuated; possibility of excessive reduction in blood pressure). Products include:
Diuril Oral Suspension 1954

Chlorothiazide Sodium (Thiazide-induced potassium loss attenuated; possibility of excessive reduction in blood pressure). Products include:
Diuril Sodium Intravenous 2467

Chlorpropamide (Epidemiological studies have suggested that concomitant administration of ACE inhibitors and antidiabetic medicines (insulins, oral hypoglycemic agents) may cause an increased blood-glucose-lowering effect with risk of hypoglycemia. This phenomenon appeared to be more likely to occur during the first weeks of combined treatment and in patients with renal impairment. In diabetic patients treated with oral antidiabetic agents or insulin, glycemic control should be closely monitored for hypoglycemia, especially during the first month of treatment with an ACE inhibitor).
No products indexed under this heading.

Chlorthalidone (Possibility of excessive reduction in blood pressure). Products include:
Clorpres Tablets 2153

Diclofenac Potassium (Co-administration in some patients with compromised renal function who are being treated with NSAIDs may result in a further deterioration of renal function).

No products indexed under this heading.

Diclofenac Sodium (Co-administration in some patients with compromised renal function who are being treated with NSAIDs may result in a further deterioration of renal function). Products include:

Arthrotec Tablets ... **3129**
Voltaren Ophthalmic Solution ... **2309**
Voltaren Tablets ... **2307**
Voltaren-XR Tablets ... **2310**

Eplerenone (Use of lisinopril with potassium-sparing diuretics (such as spironolactone, triamterene or amiloride), potassium supplements or potassium-containing salt substitutes may lead to significant increases in serum potassium. Therefore, if concomitant use of these agents is indicated because of demonstrated hypokalemia, they should be used with caution and with frequent monitoring of serum potassium. Potassium-sparing agents should generally not be used in patients with heart failure who are receiving lisinopril). Products include:

Inspra Tablets ... **2536**

Ethacrynic Acid (Possibility of excessive reduction in blood pressure). Products include:

Edecrin Tablets ... **1959**

Etodolac (Co-administration in some patients with compromised renal function who are being treated with NSAIDs may result in a further deterioration of renal function).

No products indexed under this heading.

Fenoprofen Calcium (Co-administration in some patients with compromised renal function who are being treated with NSAIDs may result in a further deterioration of renal function). Products include:

Nalfon Capsules ... **2502**

Flurbiprofen (Co-administration in some patients with compromised renal function who are being treated with NSAIDs may result in a further deterioration of renal function).

No products indexed under this heading.

Furosemide (Possibility of excessive reduction in blood pressure). Products include:

Furosemide Tablets ... **2154**

Glimepiride (Epidemiological studies have suggested that concomitant administration of ACE inhibitors and antidiabetic medicines (insulins, oral hypoglycemic agents) may cause an increased blood-glucose-lowering effect with risk of hypoglycemia. This phenomenon appeared to be more likely to occur during the first weeks of combined treatment and in patients with renal impairment. In diabetic patients treated with oral antidiabetic agents or insulin, glycemic control should be closely monitored for hypoglycemia, especially during the first month of treatment with an ACE inhibitor). Products include:

Avandaryl Tablets ... **1379**
Duetact Tablets ... **3226**

Glipizide (Epidemiological studies have suggested that concomitant administration of ACE inhibitors and antidiabetic medicines (insulins, oral hypoglycemic agents) may cause an increased blood-glucose-lowering effect with risk of hypoglycemia. This phenomenon appeared to be more likely to occur during the first weeks of combined treatment and in patients with renal impairment. In diabetic patients treated with oral antidiabetic agents or insulin, glycemic control should be closely monitored for hypoglycemia, especially during the first month of treatment with an ACE inhibitor).

No products indexed under this heading.

Glyburide (Epidemiological studies have suggested that concomitant administration of ACE inhibitors and antidiabetic medicines (insulins, oral hypoglycemic agents) may cause an increased blood-glucose-lowering effect with risk of hypoglycemia. This phenomenon appeared to be more likely to occur during the first weeks of combined treatment and in patients with renal impairment. In diabetic patients treated with oral antidiabetic agents or insulin, glycemic control should be closely monitored for hypoglycemia, especially during the first month of treatment with an ACE inhibitor).

No products indexed under this heading.

Gold Sodium Thiomalate (Nitroid reactions (symptoms include facial flushing, nausea, vomiting and hypotension) have been reported rarely in patients on therapy with injectable gold and concomitant ACE inhibitor therapy including lisinopril).

No products indexed under this heading.

Gold Therapy (Nitroid reactions (symptoms include facial flushing, nausea, vomiting and hypotension) have been reported rarely in patients on therapy with injectable gold and concomitant ACE inhibitor therapy including lisinopril).

No products indexed under this heading.

Hydrochlorothiazide (Thiazide-induced potassium loss attenuated; possibility of excessive reduction in blood pressure). Products include:

Aldoril Tablets ... **1910**
Atacand HCT ... **651**
Avalide Tablets ... **888**
Avalide Tablets ... **2874**
Benicar HCT Tablets ... **1044**
Diovan HCT Tablets ... **2196**
Dyazide Capsules ... **1423**
Hyzaar 50-12.5 Tablets ... **1990**
Hyzaar 100-12.5 Tablets ... **1990**
Hyzaar 100-25 Tablets ... **1990**
Lopressor HCT 50/25 Tablets ... **2241**
Lopressor HCT 100/25 Tablets ... **2241**
Lopressor HCT 100/50 Tablets ... **2241**
Lotensin HCT Tablets ... **2246**
Micardis HCT Tablets ... **856**
Moduretic Tablets ... **2028**
Prinzide Tablets ... **2056**
Teveten HCT Tablets ... **1737**
Timolide Tablets ... **2086**
Uniretic Tablets ... **3100**

Hydroflumethiazide (Thiazide-induced potassium loss attenuated; possibility of excessive reduction in blood pressure).

No products indexed under this heading.

Ibuprofen (Co-administration in some patients with compromised renal function who are being treated with NSAIDs may result in a further deterioration of renal function). Products include:

Advil Allergy Sinus Caplets ... **770**
Advil ... **674**
Children's Advil Oral Suspension ... **603**
Children's Advil Chewable Tablets ... **603**
Advil Cold & Sinus ... **723**
Infants' Advil Concentrated Drops ... **604**
Infants' Advil Concentrated Drops - White Grape (Dye-Free) ... **604**
Junior Strength Advil Swallow Tablets ... **605**
Advil Migraine Liquigels ... **608**
Advil Multi-Symptom Cold Caplets ... **770**
Advil PM Caplets ... **615**
Motrin IB Tablets and Caplets ... **1866**
Children's Motrin Oral Suspension ... **1867**
Children's Motrin Non-Staining Dye-Free Oral Suspension ... **1867**
Children's Motrin Cold Oral Suspension ... **1867**
Infants' Motrin Concentrated Drops ... **1867**
Infants' Motrin Non-Staining Dye-Free Concentrated Drops ... **1867**
Junior Strength Motrin Caplets and Chewable Tablets ... **1867**
Vicoprofen Tablets ... **539**

Indapamide (Possibility of excessive reduction in blood pressure). Products include:

Indapamide Tablets ... **2156**

Indomethacin (Co-administration in some patients with compromised renal function who are being treated with NSAIDs may result in a further deterioration of renal function. In a study, the use of indomethacin was associated with a reduced antihypertensive effect, although the difference between lisinopril alone to lisinopril given concomitantly with indomethacin was not significant). Products include:

Indocin ... **1995**

Indomethacin Sodium Trihydrate (Co-administration in some patients with compromised renal function who are being treated with NSAIDs may result in a further deterioration of renal function). Products include:

Indocin I.V. ... **2465**

Insulin, Human, Zinc Suspension (Epidemiological studies have suggested that concomitant administration of ACE inhibitors and antidiabetic medicines (insulins, oral hypoglycemic agents) may cause an increased blood-glucose-lowering effect with risk of hypoglycemia. This phenomenon appeared to be more likely to occur during the first weeks of combined treatment and in patients with renal impairment. In diabetic patients treated with oral antidiabetic agents or insulin, glycemic control should be closely monitored for hypoglycemia, especially during the first month of treatment with an ACE inhibitor). Products include:

Humulin L, 100 Units ... **1794**
Humulin U, 100 Units ... **1800**

Insulin, Human NPH (Epidemiological studies have suggested that concomitant administration of ACE inhibitors and antidiabetic medicines (insulins, oral hypoglycemic agents) may cause an increased blood-glucose-lowering effect with risk of hypoglycemia. This phenomenon appeared to be more likely to occur during the first weeks of combined treatment and in patients with renal impairment. In diabetic patients treated with oral antidiabetic agents or insulin, glycemic control should be closely monitored for hypoglycemia, especially during the first month of treatment with an ACE inhibitor). Products include:

Humulin N, 100 Units ... **1795**
Humulin N Pen ... **1797**

Insulin, Human Regular (Epidemiological studies have suggested that concomitant administration of ACE inhibitors and antidiabetic medicines (insulins, oral hypoglycemic agents) may cause an increased blood-glucose-lowering effect with risk of hypoglycemia. This phenomenon appeared to be more likely to occur during the first weeks of combined treatment and in patients with renal impairment. In diabetic patients treated with oral antidiabetic agents or insulin, glycemic control should be closely monitored for hypoglycemia, especially during the first month of treatment with an ACE inhibitor). Products include:

Humulin R, 100 Units ... **1798**

Insulin, Human Regular and Human NPH Mixture (Epidemiological studies have suggested that concomitant administration of ACE inhibitors and antidiabetic medicines (insulins, oral hypoglycemic agents) may cause an increased blood-glucose-lowering effect with risk of hypoglycemia. This phenomenon appeared to be more likely to occur during the first weeks of combined treatment and in patients with renal impairment. In diabetic patients treated with oral antidiabetic agents or insulin, glycemic control should be closely monitored for hypoglycemia, especially during the first month of treatment with an ACE inhibitor). Products include:

Humulin 50/50, 100 Units ... **1791**
Humulin 70/30 Pen ... **1793**

Insulin, NPH (Epidemiological studies have suggested that concomitant administration of ACE inhibitors and antidiabetic medicines (insulins, oral hypoglycemic agents) may cause an increased blood-glucose-lowering effect with risk of hypoglycemia. This phenomenon appeared to be more likely to occur during the first weeks of combined treatment and in patients with renal impairment. In diabetic patients treated with oral antidiabetic agents or insulin, glycemic control should be closely monitored for hypoglycemia, especially during the first month of treatment with an ACE inhibitor).

No products indexed under this heading.

Insulin, Regular (Epidemiological studies have suggested that concomitant administration of ACE inhibitors and antidiabetic medicines (insulins, oral hypoglycemic agents) may cause an increased blood-glucose-lowering effect with risk of hypoglycemia. This phenomenon appeared to be more likely to occur during the first weeks of combined treatment and in patients with renal impairment. In diabetic patients treated with oral antidiabetic agents or insulin, glycemic control should be closely monitored for hypoglycemia, especially during the first month of treatment with an ACE inhibitor).

No products indexed under this heading.

Insulin, Zinc Crystals (Epidemiological studies have suggested that concomitant administration of ACE inhibitors and antidiabetic medicines (insulins, oral hypoglycemic agents) may cause an increased blood-glucose-lowering effect with risk of hypoglycemia. This phenomenon appeared to be more likely to occur during the first weeks of combined treatment and in patients with renal impairment. In diabetic patients treated with oral antidiabetic agents or insulin, glycemic control should be closely monitored for hypoglycemia, especially during the first month of treatment with an ACE inhibitor).

No products indexed under this heading.

Insulin, Zinc Suspension (Epidemiological studies have suggested that concomitant administration of ACE inhibitors and antidiabetic medicines (insulins, oral hypoglycemic agents) may cause an increased blood-glucose-lowering effect with risk of hypoglycemia. This phenomenon appeared to be more likely to occur during the first weeks of combined treatment and in patients with renal impairment. In diabetic patients treated with oral antidiabetic agents or insulin, glycemic control should be closely monitored during the first month of treatment with an ACE inhibitor).

No products indexed under this heading.

Insulin Aspart, Human Regular (Epidemiological studies have suggested that concomitant administration of ACE inhibitors and antidiabetic medicines (insulins, oral hypoglycemic agents) may cause an increased blood-glucose-lowering effect with risk of hypoglycemia. This phenomenon appeared to be more likely to occur during the first weeks of combined treatment and in patients with renal impairment. In diabetic patients treated with oral antidiabetic agents or insulin, glycemic control should be closely monitored for hypoglycemia, especially during the first month of treatment with an ACE inhibitor). Products include:

Insulin glargine (Epidemiological studies have suggested that concomitant administration of ACE inhibitors and antidiabetic medicines (insulins, oral hypoglycemic agents) may cause an increased blood-glucose-lowering effect with risk of hypoglycemia. This phenomenon appeared to be more likely to occur during the first weeks of combined treatment and in patients with renal impairment. In diabetic patients treated with oral antidiabetic agents or insulin, glycemic control should be closely monitored for hypoglycemia, especially during the first month of treatment with an ACE inhibitor). Products include:

Insulin Lispro, Human (Epidemiological studies have suggested that concomitant administration of ACE inhibitors and antidiabetic medicines (insulins, oral hypoglycemic agents) may cause an increased blood-glucose-lowering effect with risk of hypoglycemia. This phenomenon appeared to be more likely to occur during the first weeks of combined treatment and in patients with renal impairment. In diabetic patients treated with oral antidiabetic agents or insulin, glycemic control should be closely monitored for hypoglyce-

mia, especially during the first month of treatment with an ACE inhibitor). Products include:

Insulin Lispro Protamine, Human (Epidemiological studies have suggested that concomitant administration of ACE inhibitors and antidiabetic medicines (insulins, oral hypoglycemic agents) may cause an increased blood-glucose-lowering effect with risk of hypoglycemia. This phenomenon appeared to be more likely to occur during the first weeks of combined treatment and in patients with renal impairment. In diabetic patients treated with oral antidiabetic agents or insulin, glycemic control should be closely monitored for hypoglycemia, especially during the first month of treatment with an ACE inhibitor). Products include:

Ketoprofen (Co-administration in some patients with compromised renal function who are being treated with NSAIDs may result in a further deterioration of renal function).

No products indexed under this heading.

Ketorolac Tromethamine (Co-administration in some patients with compromised renal function who are being treated with NSAIDs may result in a further deterioration of renal function). Products include:

Lithium (Potential for reversible lithium toxicity; frequent monitoring of lithium levels is recommended).

No products indexed under this heading.

Lithium Carbonate (Potential for reversible lithium toxicity; frequent monitoring of lithium levels is recommended). Products include:

Lithium Citrate (Potential for reversible lithium toxicity; frequent monitoring of lithium levels is recommended).

No products indexed under this heading.

Meclofenamate Sodium (Co-administration in some patients with compromised renal function who are being treated with NSAIDs may result in a further deterioration of renal function).

No products indexed under this heading.

Mefenamic Acid (Co-administration in some patients with compromised renal function who are being treated with NSAIDs may result in a further deterioration of renal function).

No products indexed under this heading.

Meloxicam (Co-administration in some patients with compromised renal function who are being treated with NSAIDs may result in a further deterioration of renal function). Products include:

Metformin Hydrochloride (Epidemiological studies have suggested that concomitant administration of ACE inhibitors and antidiabetic medicines (insulins, oral hypoglycemic

agents) may cause an increased blood-glucose-lowering effect with risk of hypoglycemia. This phenomenon appeared to be more likely to occur during the first weeks of combined treatment and in patients with renal impairment. In diabetic patients treated with oral antidiabetic agents or insulin, glycemic control should be closely monitored for hypoglycemia, especially during the first month of treatment with an ACE inhibitor). Products include:

Methyclothiazide (Thiazide-induced potassium loss attenuated; possibility of excessive reduction in blood pressure).

No products indexed under this heading.

Metolazone (Possibility of excessive reduction in blood pressure).

No products indexed under this heading.

Miglitol (Epidemiological studies have suggested that concomitant administration of ACE inhibitors and antidiabetic medicines (insulins, oral hypoglycemic agents) may cause an increased blood-glucose-lowering effect with risk of hypoglycemia. This phenomenon appeared to be more likely to occur during the first weeks of combined treatment and in patients with renal impairment. In diabetic patients treated with oral antidiabetic agents or insulin, glycemic control should be closely monitored for hypoglycemia, especially during the first month of treatment with an ACE inhibitor).

No products indexed under this heading.

Nabumetone (Co-administration in some patients with compromised renal function who are being treated with NSAIDs may result in a further deterioration of renal function).

No products indexed under this heading.

Naproxen (Co-administration in some patients with compromised renal function who are being treated with NSAIDs may result in a further deterioration of renal function). Products include:

Naproxen Sodium (Co-administration in some patients with compromised renal function who are being treated with NSAIDs may result in a further deterioration of renal function). Products include:

Oxaprozin (Co-administration in some patients with compromised renal function who are being treated with NSAIDs may result in a further deterioration of renal function).

No products indexed under this heading.

Phenylbutazone (Co-administration in some patients with compromised renal function who are being treated with NSAIDs may result in a further deterioration of renal function).

No products indexed under this heading.

Pioglitazone Hydrochloride (Epidemiological studies have suggested that concomitant administration of ACE inhibitors and antidiabetic medicines (insulins, oral hypoglycemic agents) may cause an increased blood-glucose-lowering effect with risk of hypoglycemia. This phenomenon appeared to be more likely to occur during the first weeks of combined treatment and in patients with renal impairment. In diabetic patients treated with oral antidiabetic agents or insulin, glycemic control should be closely monitored for hypoglycemia, especially during the first month of treatment with an ACE inhibitor). Products include:

Piroxicam (Co-administration in some patients with compromised renal function who are being treated with NSAIDs may result in a further deterioration of renal function).

No products indexed under this heading.

Polythiazide (Thiazide-induced potassium loss attenuated; possibility of excessive reduction in blood pressure).

No products indexed under this heading.

Potassium Acid Phosphate (Use of lisinopril with potassium-sparing diuretics (such as spironolactone, triamterene or amiloride), potassium supplements or potassium-containing salt substitutes may lead to significant increases in serum potassium. Therefore, if concomitant use of these agents is indicated because of demonstrated hypokalemia, they should be used with caution and with frequent monitoring of serum potassium. Potassium-sparing agents should generally not be used in patients with heart failure who are receiving lisinopril). Products include:

Potassium Bicarbonate (Use of lisinopril with potassium-sparing diuretics (such as spironolactone, triamterene or amiloride), potassium supplements or potassium-containing salt substitutes may lead to significant increases in serum potassium. Therefore, if concomitant use of these agents is indicated because of demonstrated hypokalemia, they should be used with caution and with frequent monitoring of serum potassium. Potassium-sparing agents should generally not be used in patients with heart failure who are receiving lisinopril).

No products indexed under this heading.

Potassium Chloride (Use of lisinopril with potassium-sparing diuretics (such as spironolactone, triamterene or amiloride), potassium supplements or potassium-containing salt substitutes may lead to significant increases in serum potassium. Therefore, if concomitant use of these agents is indicated because of demonstrated hypokalemia, they should be used with caution and with frequent monitoring of serum potassium. Potassium-sparing agents should generally not be used in patients with heart failure who are receiving lisinopril). Products include:

Potassium Citrate (Use of lisinopril with potassium-sparing diuretics (such as spironolactone, triamterene or amiloride), potassium supplements or potassium-containing salt substitutes may lead to significant increases in serum potassium. Therefore, if concomitant use of these agents is indicated because of demonstrated hypokalemia, they should be used with caution and with frequent monitoring of serum potassium. Potassium-sparing agents should generally not be used in patients with heart failure who are receiving lisinopril). Products include:

Potassium Gluconate (Use of lisinopril with potassium-sparing diuretics (such as spironolactone, triamterene or amiloride), potassium supplements or potassium-containing salt substitutes may lead to significant increases in serum potassium. Therefore, if concomitant use of these agents is indicated because of demonstrated hypokalemia, they should be used with caution and with frequent monitoring of serum potassium. Potassium-sparing agents should generally not be used in patients with heart failure who are receiving lisinopril).

No products indexed under this heading.

Potassium Phosphate (Use of lisinopril with potassium-sparing diuretics (such as spironolactone, triamterene or amiloride), potassium supplements or potassium-containing salt substitutes may lead to significant increases in serum potassium. Therefore, if concomitant use of these agents is indicated because of demonstrated hypokalemia, they should be used with caution and with frequent monitoring of serum potassium. Potassium-sparing agents should generally not be used in patients with heart failure who are receiving lisinopril). Products include:

Repaglinide (Epidemiological studies have suggested that concomitant administration of ACE inhibitors and antidiabetic medicines (insulins, oral hypoglycemic agents) may cause an increased blood-glucose-lowering effect with risk of hypoglycemia. This phenomenon appeared to be more likely to occur during the first weeks of combined treatment and in patients with renal impairment. In diabetic patients treated with oral antidiabetic agents or insulin, glycemic control should be closely monitored for hypoglycemia, especially during the first month of treatment

with an ACE inhibitor).

No products indexed under this heading.

Rofecoxib (Co-administration in some patients with compromised renal function who are being treated with NSAIDs may result in a further deterioration of renal function).

No products indexed under this heading.

Rosiglitazone Maleate (Epidemiological studies have suggested that concomitant administration of ACE inhibitors and antidiabetic medicines (insulins, oral hypoglycemic agents) may cause an increased blood-glucose-lowering effect with risk of hypoglycemia. This phenomenon appeared to be more likely to occur during the first weeks of combined treatment and in patients with renal impairment. In diabetic patients treated with oral antidiabetic agents or insulin, glycemic control should be closely monitored for hypoglycemia, especially during the first month of treatment with an ACE inhibitor). Products include:

Spironolactone (Use of lisinopril with potassium-sparing diuretics (such as spironolactone, triamterene or amiloride), potassium supplements or potassium-containing salt substitutes may lead to significant increases in serum potassium. Therefore, if concomitant use of these agents is indicated because of demonstrated hypokalemia, they should be used with caution and with frequent monitoring of serum potassium. Potassium-sparing agents should generally not be used in patients with heart failure who are receiving lisinopril).

No products indexed under this heading.

Sulindac (Co-administration in some patients with compromised renal function who are being treated with NSAIDs may result in a further deterioration of renal function). Products include:

Tolazamide (Epidemiological studies have suggested that concomitant administration of ACE inhibitors and antidiabetic medicines (insulins, oral hypoglycemic agents) may cause an increased blood-glucose-lowering effect with risk of hypoglycemia. This phenomenon appeared to be more likely to occur during the first weeks of combined treatment and in patients with renal impairment. In diabetic patients treated with oral antidiabetic agents or insulin, glycemic control should be closely monitored for hypoglycemia, especially during the first month of treatment with an ACE inhibitor).

No products indexed under this heading.

Tolbutamide (Epidemiological studies have suggested that concomitant administration of ACE inhibitors and antidiabetic medicines (insulins, oral hypoglycemic agents) may cause an increased blood-glucose-lowering effect with risk of hypoglycemia. This phenomenon appeared to be more likely to occur during the first weeks of combined treatment and in patients with renal impairment. In diabetic patients treated with oral antidiabetic agents or insulin, glyce-

mic control should be closely monitored for hypoglycemia, especially during the first month of treatment with an ACE inhibitor).

No products indexed under this heading.

Tolmetin Sodium (Co-administration in some patients with compromised renal function who are being treated with NSAIDs may result in a further deterioration of renal function).

No products indexed under this heading.

Torsemide (Possibility of excessive reduction in blood pressure). Products include:

Triamterene (Use of lisinopril with potassium-sparing diuretics (such as spironolactone, triamterene or amiloride), potassium supplements or potassium-containing salt substitutes may lead to significant increases in serum potassium. Therefore, if concomitant use of these agents is indicated because of demonstrated hypokalemia, they should be used with caution and with frequent monitoring of serum potassium. Potassium-sparing agents should generally not be used in patients with heart failure who are receiving lisinopril). Products include:

Troglitazone (Epidemiological studies have suggested that concomitant administration of ACE inhibitors and antidiabetic medicines (insulins, oral hypoglycemic agents) may cause an increased blood-glucose-lowering effect with risk of hypoglycemia. This phenomenon appeared to be more likely to occur during the first weeks of combined treatment and in patients with renal impairment. In diabetic patients treated with oral antidiabetic agents or insulin, glycemic control should be closely monitored for hypoglycemia, especially during the first month of treatment with an ACE inhibitor).

No products indexed under this heading.

Valdecoxib (Co-administration in some patients with compromised renal function who are being treated with NSAIDs may result in a further deterioration of renal function).

No products indexed under this heading.

Food Interactions

Salt Substitutes, Potassium-Containing (Use of lisinopril with potassium-sparing diuretics (such as spironolactone, triamterene or amiloride), potassium supplements or potassium-containing salt substitutes may lead to significant increases in serum potassium. Therefore, if concomitant use of these agents is indicated because of demonstrated hypokalemia, they should be used with caution and with frequent monitoring of serum potassium. Potassium-sparing agents should generally not be used in patients with heart failure who are receiving lisinopril).

PRINZIDE TABLETS

May interact with antihypertensives, barbiturates, corticosteroids, diuretics, cardiac glycosides, oral hypoglycemic agents, insulin, lithium preparations, narcotic analgesics, nondepolarizing neuromuscular blocking agents, non-steroidal anti-inflammatory agents, potassium preparations, potassium sparing diuretics, and certain other agents. Compounds in these categories include:

Acarbose (Hyperglycemia may occur with thiazide diuretics; dosage adjustment of oral hypoglycemic agents may be required). Products include:

Acebutolol Hydrochloride (Co-administration of thiazide and other antihypertensive agents can lead to additive effect or potentiation).

No products indexed under this heading.

ACTH (Co-administration of thiazide diuretics with ACTH intensifies electrolyte depletion, particularly potassium).

No products indexed under this heading.

Alfentanil Hydrochloride (Co-administration of thiazide and narcotics may potentiate orthostatic hypotension).

No products indexed under this heading.

Amiloride Hydrochloride (Risk factors for the development of hyperkalemia include the concomitant use of potassium-sparing diuretics, potassium supplements and/or potassium-containing salt substitutes. Hyperkalemia can cause serious, sometimes, fatal, arrhythmias. Prinzide should be used cautiously, if at all, with these agents and with frequent monitoring of serum potassium). Products include:

Amlodipine Besylate (Co-administration of thiazide and other antihypertensive agents can lead to additive effect or potentiation). Products include:

Aprobarbital (Co-administration of thiazide and barbiturates may potentiate orthostatic hypotension).

No products indexed under this heading.

Atenolol (Co-administration of thiazide and other antihypertensive agents can lead to additive effect or potentiation).

No products indexed under this heading.

Atracurium Besylate (Co-administration with nondepolarizing skeletal muscle relaxants may result in possible increased responsiveness to the muscle relaxant).

No products indexed under this heading.

Benazepril Hydrochloride (Co-administration of thiazide and other antihypertensive agents can lead to additive effect or potentiation). Products include:

IMPORTANT NOTE: Always consult each drug listing in the patient's regimen for possible interactions.

Bendroflumethiazide (Co-administration of lisinopril in patients on diuretics, especially those in whom diuretic therapy was recently instituted, may occasionally experience excessive hypotension; antihypertensive effects of lisinopril are augmented by antihypertensive agents that cause renin release).
No products indexed under this heading.

Betamethasone Acetate (Co-administration of thiazide diuretics with corticosteroids intensifies electrolyte depletion, particularly potassium).
No products indexed under this heading.

Betamethasone Sodium Phosphate (Co-administration of thiazide diuretics with corticosteroids intensifies electrolyte depletion, particularly potassium).
No products indexed under this heading.

Betaxolol Hydrochloride (Co-administration of thiazide and other antihypertensive agents can lead to additive effect or potentiation). Products include:
Betoptic S Ophthalmic Suspension 558

Bisoprolol Fumarate (Co-administration of thiazide and other antihypertensive agents can lead to additive effect or potentiation).
No products indexed under this heading.

Bumetanide (Co-administration of lisinopril in patients on diuretics, especially those in whom diuretic therapy was recently instituted, may occasionally experience excessive hypotension; antihypertensive effects of lisinopril are augmented by antihypertensive agents that cause renin release). Products include:
Bumex Tablets 2746

Buprenorphine Hydrochloride (Co-administration of thiazide and narcotics may potentiate orthostatic hypotension). Products include:
Buprenex Injectable 2716
Suboxone Tablets 2717
Subutex Tablets 2717

Butabarbital (Co-administration of thiazide and barbiturates may potentiate orthostatic hypotension).
No products indexed under this heading.

Butalbital (Co-administration of thiazide and barbiturates may potentiate orthostatic hypotension).
No products indexed under this heading.

Candesartan Cilexetil (Co-administration of thiazide and other antihypertensive agents can lead to additive effect or potentiation). Products include:
Atacand Tablets 649
Atacand HCT 651

Captopril (Co-administration of thiazide and other antihypertensive agents can lead to additive effect or potentiation). Products include:
Captopril Tablets 2149

Carteolol Hydrochloride (Co-administration of thiazide and other antihypertensive agents can lead to additive effect or potentiation). Products include:
Carteolol Hydrochloride Ophthalmic Solution USP, 1%........ ⊙249

Celecoxib (Co-administration in some patients with compromised renal function who are being treated with NSAIDs may result in a further deterioration of renal function: NSAID may reduce the diuretic, natriuretic and antihypertensive effects of thiazide). Products include:
Celebrex Capsules 3134

Chlorothiazide (Co-administration of lisinopril in patients on diuretics, especially those in whom diuretic therapy was recently instituted, may occasionally experience excessive hypotension; antihypertensive effects of lisinopril are augmented by antihypertensive agents that cause renin release). Products include:
Diuril Oral Suspension 1954

Chlorothiazide Sodium (Co-administration of lisinopril in patients on diuretics, especially those in whom diuretic therapy was recently instituted, may occasionally experience excessive hypotension; antihypertensive effects of lisinopril are augmented by antihypertensive agents that cause renin release). Products include:
Diuril Sodium Intravenous 2467

Chlorpropamide (Hyperglycemia may occur with thiazide diuretics; dosage adjustment of oral hypoglycemic agents may be required).
No products indexed under this heading.

Chlorthalidone (Co-administration of lisinopril in patients on diuretics, especially those in whom diuretic therapy was recently instituted, may occasionally experience excessive hypotension; antihypertensive effects of lisinopril are augmented by antihypertensive agents that cause renin release). Products include:
Clorpres Tablets 2153

Cholestyramine (Absorption of hydrochlorothiazide is impaired in the presence of anionic exchange resins; these resins bind the hydrochlorothiazide and reduce its absorption from GI tract).
No products indexed under this heading.

Cisatracurium Besylate (Co-administration with nondepolarizing skeletal muscle relaxants may result in possible increased responsiveness to the muscle relaxant). Products include:
Nimbex Injection 498

Clonidine (Co-administration of thiazide and other antihypertensive agents can lead to additive effect or potentiation). Products include:
Catapres-TTS 844

Clonidine Hydrochloride (Co-administration of thiazide and other antihypertensive agents can lead to additive effect or potentiation). Products include:
Catapres Tablets 843
Clorpres Tablets 2153

Codeine Phosphate (Co-administration of thiazide and narcotics may potentiate orthostatic hypotension). Products include:
Tylenol with Codeine Tablets 2391

Colestipol Hydrochloride (Absorption of hydrochlorothiazide is impaired in the presence of anionic exchange resins; these resins bind the hydrochlorothiazide and reduce its absorption from GI tract).
No products indexed under this heading.

Cortisone Acetate (Co-administration of thiazide diuretics with corticosteroids intensifies electrolyte depletion, particularly potassium).
No products indexed under this heading.

Deserpidine (Co-administration of thiazide and other antihypertensive agents can lead to additive effect or potentiation).
No products indexed under this heading.

Deslanoside (Hypokalemia induced by thiazide diuretics may cause cardiac arrhythmia and may also sensitize or exaggerate the response to the heart to the toxic effects of digitalis, such as ventricular irritability).
No products indexed under this heading.

Dexamethasone (Co-administration of thiazide diuretics with corticosteroids intensifies electrolyte depletion, particularly potassium). Products include:
Ciprodex Otic Suspension 559
Decadron Tablets 1951
TobraDex Ophthalmic Ointment 562
TobraDex Ophthalmic Suspension ... 563

Dexamethasone Acetate (Co-administration of thiazide diuretics with corticosteroids intensifies electrolyte depletion, particularly potassium).
No products indexed under this heading.

Dexamethasone Sodium Phosphate (Co-administration of thiazide diuretics with corticosteroids intensifies electrolyte depletion, particularly potassium).
No products indexed under this heading.

Dezocine (Co-administration of thiazide and narcotics may potentiate orthostatic hypotension).
No products indexed under this heading.

Diazoxide (Co-administration of thiazide and other antihypertensive agents can lead to additive effect or potentiation). Products include:
Hyperstat I.V. 3017

Diclofenac Potassium (Co-administration in some patients with compromised renal function who are being treated with NSAIDs may result in a further deterioration of renal function: NSAID may reduce the diuretic, natriuretic and antihypertensive effects of thiazide).
No products indexed under this heading.

Diclofenac Sodium (Co-administration in some patients with compromised renal function who are being treated with NSAIDs may result in a further deterioration of renal function: NSAID may reduce the diuretic, natriuretic and antihypertensive effects of thiazide). Products include:
Arthrotec Tablets 3129
Voltaren Ophthalmic Solution 2309
Voltaren Tablets 2307
Voltaren-XR Tablets 2310

Digitalis Glycoside Preparations (Hypokalemia induced by thiazide diuretics may cause cardiac arrhythmia and may also sensitize or exaggerate the response to the heart to the toxic effects of digitalis, such as ventricular irritability).
No products indexed under this heading.

Digitoxin (Hypokalemia induced by thiazide diuretics may cause cardiac arrhythmia and may also sensitize or exaggerate the response to the heart to the toxic effects of digitalis, such as ventricular irritability).
No products indexed under this heading.

Digoxin (Hypokalemia induced by thiazide diuretics may cause cardiac arrhythmia and may also sensitize or exaggerate the response to the heart to the toxic effects of digitalis, such as ventricular irritability). Products include:
Lanoxicaps Capsules 1490
Lanoxin Injection 1494
Lanoxin Injection Pediatric 1497
Lanoxin Tablets 1500

Diltiazem Hydrochloride (Co-administration of thiazide and other antihypertensive agents can lead to additive effect or potentiation). Products include:
Cardizem LA Extended Release Tablets 1728
Tiazac Capsules 1201

Doxazosin Mesylate (Co-administration of thiazide and other antihypertensive agents can lead to additive effect or potentiation). Products include:
Cardura XL Tablets 2515

Enalapril Maleate (Co-administration of thiazide and other antihypertensive agents can lead to additive effect or potentiation). Products include:
Vasotec I.V. Injection 2103

Enalaprilat (Co-administration of thiazide and other antihypertensive agents can lead to additive effect or potentiation).
No products indexed under this heading.

Eplerenone (Use of lisinopril with potassium-sparing diuretics (such as spironolactone, triamterene or amiloride), potassium supplements or potassium-containing salt substitutes may lead to significant increases in serum potassium. Therefore, if concomitant use of these agents is indicated because of demonstrated hypokalemia, they should be used with caution and with frequent monitoring of serum potassium. Potassium-sparing agents should generally not be used in patients with heart failure who are receiving lisinopril). Products include:
Inspra Tablets 2536

Eprosartan Mesylate (Co-administration of thiazide and other antihypertensive agents can lead to additive effect or potentiation). Products include:
Teveten Tablets 1735
Teveten HCT Tablets 1737

Esmolol Hydrochloride (Co-administration of thiazide and other antihypertensive agents can lead to additive effect or potentiation).
No products indexed under this heading.

Ethacrynic Acid (Co-administration of lisinopril in patients on diuretics, especially those in whom diuretic therapy was recently instituted, may occasionally experience excessive hypotension; antihypertensive effects of lisinopril are augmented by antihypertensive agents that cause renin release). Products include:
Edecrin Tablets 1959

Etodolac (Co-administration in some patients with compromised renal function who are being treated with NSAIDs may result in a further deterioration of renal function: NSAID may reduce the diuretic, natriuretic and antihypertensive effects of thiazide).
No products indexed under this heading.

Felodipine (Co-administration of thiazide and other antihypertensive agents can lead to additive effect or potentiation).
No products indexed under this heading.

Fenoprofen Calcium (Co-administration in some patients with compromised renal function who are being treated with NSAIDs may result in a further deterioration of renal function: NSAID may reduce the diuretic, natriuretic and antihypertensive effects of thiazide). Products include:
Nalfon Capsules ... 2502

Fentanyl (Co-administration of thiazide and narcotics may potentiate orthostatic hypotension). Products include:
Duragesic Transdermal System ... 2373
Ionsys Transdermal System ... 2379

Fentanyl Citrate (Co-administration of thiazide and narcotics may potentiate orthostatic hypotension). Products include:
Actiq ... 979

Fludrocortisone Acetate (Co-administration of thiazide diuretics with corticosteroids intensifies electrolyte depletion, particularly potassium).
No products indexed under this heading.

Flurbiprofen (Co-administration in some patients with compromised renal function who are being treated with NSAIDs may result in a further deterioration of renal function: NSAID may reduce the diuretic, natriuretic and antihypertensive effects of thiazide).
No products indexed under this heading.

Fosinopril Sodium (Co-administration of thiazide and other antihypertensive agents can lead to additive effect or potentiation).
No products indexed under this heading.

Furosemide (Co-administration of lisinopril in patients on diuretics, especially those in whom diuretic therapy was recently instituted, may occasionally experience excessive hypotension; antihypertensive effects of lisinopril are augmented by antihypertensive agents that cause renin release). Products include:
Furosemide Tablets ... 2154

Glimepiride (Hyperglycemia may occur with thiazide diuretics; dosage adjustment of oral hypoglycemic agents may be required). Products include:
Avandaryl Tablets ... 1379
Duetact Tablets ... 3226

Glipizide (Hyperglycemia may occur with thiazide diuretics; dosage adjustment of oral hypoglycemic agents may be required).
No products indexed under this heading.

Glyburide (Hyperglycemia may occur with thiazide diuretics; dosage adjustment of oral hypoglycemic agents may be required).
No products indexed under this heading.

Guanabenz Acetate (Co-administration of thiazide and other antihypertensive agents can lead to additive effect or potentiation).
No products indexed under this heading.

Guanethidine Monosulfate (Co-administration of thiazide and other antihypertensive agents can lead to additive effect or potentiation).
No products indexed under this heading.

Hydralazine Hydrochloride (Co-administration of thiazide and other antihypertensive agents can lead to additive effect or potentiation). Products include:
BiDil Tablets ... 2171

Hydrocodone Bitartrate (Co-administration of thiazide and narcotics may potentiate orthostatic hypotension). Products include:
Hycodan ... 1116
Hycotuss Expectorant Syrup ... 1117
Vicodin Tablets ... 535
Vicodin ES Tablets ... 536
Vicodin HP Tablets ... 538
Vicoprofen Tablets ... 539
Zydone Tablets ... 1139

Hydrocodone Polistirex (Co-administration of thiazide and narcotics may potentiate orthostatic hypotension). Products include:
Tussionex Pennkinetic Extended-Release Suspension ... 3327

Hydrocortisone (Co-administration of thiazide diuretics with corticosteroids intensifies electrolyte depletion, particularly potassium). Products include:
Colocort Rectal Suspension, USP (Retention) 100 mg/60 mL ... 2476
Hydrocortone Tablets ... 1989
Preparation H Hydrocortisone Cream ... 646

Hydrocortisone Acetate (Co-administration of thiazide diuretics with corticosteroids intensifies electrolyte depletion, particularly potassium). Products include:
Analpram-HC ... 1159
Pramosone ... 1161
ProctoFoam-HC ... 3099

Hydrocortisone Sodium Phosphate (Co-administration of thiazide diuretics with corticosteroids intensifies electrolyte depletion, particularly potassium).
No products indexed under this heading.

Hydrocortisone Sodium Succinate (Co-administration of thiazide diuretics with corticosteroids intensifies electrolyte depletion, particularly potassium).
No products indexed under this heading.

Hydroflumethiazide (Co-administration of lisinopril in patients on diuretics, especially those in whom diuretic therapy was recently instituted, may occasionally experience excessive hypotension; antihypertensive effects of lisinopril are augmented by antihypertensive agents that cause renin release).
No products indexed under this heading.

Hydromorphone Hydrochloride (Co-administration of thiazide and narcotics may potentiate orthostatic hypotension). Products include:
Dilaudid ... 440
Dilaudid Non-Sterile Powder ... 440
Dilaudid Oral Liquid ... 445
Dilaudid Rectal Suppositories ... 440
Dilaudid Tablets ... 440
Dilaudid Tablets - 8 mg ... 445
Dilaudid-HP ... 442

Ibuprofen (Co-administration in some patients with compromised renal function who are being treated with NSAIDs may result in a further deterioration of renal function: NSAID may reduce the diuretic, natriuretic and antihypertensive effects of thiazide). Products include:
Advil Allergy Sinus Caplets ... 770
Advil ... 674
Children's Advil Oral Suspension ... 603
Children's Advil Chewable Tablets ... 603
Advil Cold & Sinus ... 723
Infants' Advil Concentrated Drops ... 604
Infants' Advil Concentrated Drops - White Grape (Dye-Free) ... 604
Junior Strength Advil Swallow Tablets ... 605
Advil Migraine Liquigels ... 608
Advil Multi-Symptom Cold Caplets ... 770
Advil PM Caplets ... 615
Motrin IB Tablets and Caplets ... 1866
Children's Motrin Oral Suspension ... 1867
Children's Motrin Non-Staining Dye-Free Oral Suspension ... 1867
Children's Motrin Cold Oral Suspension ... 1867
Infants' Motrin Concentrated Drops ... 1867
Infants' Motrin Non-Staining Dye-Free Concentrated Drops ... 1867
Junior Strength Motrin Caplets and Chewable Tablets ... 1867
Vicoprofen Tablets ... 539

Indapamide (Co-administration of lisinopril in patients on diuretics, especially those in whom diuretic therapy was recently instituted, may occasionally experience excessive hypotension; antihypertensive effects of lisinopril are augmented by antihypertensive agents that cause renin release). Products include:
Indapamide Tablets ... 2156

Indomethacin (Co-administration in some patients with compromised renal function who are being treated with NSAIDs may result in a further deterioration of renal function: NSAID may reduce the diuretic, natriuretic and antihypertensive effects of thiazide). Products include:
Indocin ... 1995

Indomethacin Sodium Trihydrate (Co-administration in some patients with compromised renal function who are being treated with NSAIDs may result in a further deterioration of renal function: NSAID may reduce the diuretic, natriuretic and antihypertensive effects of thiazide). Products include:
Indocin I.V. ... 2465

Insulin, Human, Zinc Suspension (Hyperglycemia may occur with thiazide diuretics; dosage adjustment of insulin may be required). Products include:
Humulin L, 100 Units ... 1794
Humulin U, 100 Units ... 1800

Insulin, Human NPH (Hyperglycemia may occur with thiazide diuretics; dosage adjustment of insulin may be required). Products include:
Humulin N, 100 Units ... 1795
Humulin N Pen ... 1797

Insulin, Human Regular (Hyperglycemia may occur with thiazide diuretics; dosage adjustment of insulin may be required). Products include:
Humulin R, 100 Units ... 1798

Insulin, Human Regular and Human NPH Mixture (Hyperglycemia may occur with thiazide diuretics; dosage adjustment of insulin may be required). Products include:
Humulin 50/50, 100 Units ... 1791
Humulin 70/30 Pen ... 1793

Insulin, NPH (Hyperglycemia may occur with thiazide diuretics; dosage adjustment of insulin may be required).
No products indexed under this heading.

Insulin, Regular (Hyperglycemia may occur with thiazide diuretics; dosage adjustment of insulin may be required).
No products indexed under this heading.

Insulin, Zinc Crystals (Hyperglycemia may occur with thiazide diuretics; dosage adjustment of insulin may be required).
No products indexed under this heading.

Insulin, Zinc Suspension (Hyperglycemia may occur with thiazide diuretics; dosage adjustment of insulin may be required).
No products indexed under this heading.

Insulin Aspart, Human Regular (Hyperglycemia may occur with thiazide diuretics; dosage adjustment of insulin may be required). Products include:
NovoLog Injection ... 2326

Insulin glargine (Hyperglycemia may occur with thiazide diuretics; dosage adjustment of insulin may be required). Products include:
Lantus Injection ... 2909

Insulin Lispro, Human (Hyperglycemia may occur with thiazide diuretics; dosage adjustment of insulin may be required). Products include:
Humalog-Pen ... 1781
Humalog Mix 50/50-Pen ... 1783
Humalog Mix 75/25-Pen ... 1785

Insulin Lispro Protamine, Human (Hyperglycemia may occur with thiazide diuretics; dosage adjustment of insulin may be required). Products include:
Humalog Mix 50/50-Pen ... 1783
Humalog Mix 75/25-Pen ... 1785

Irbesartan (Co-administration of thiazide and other antihypertensive agents can lead to additive effect or potentiation). Products include:
Avalide Tablets ... 888
Avalide Tablets ... 2874
Avapro Tablets ... 891
Avapro Tablets ... 2871

Isradipine (Co-administration of thiazide and other antihypertensive agents can lead to additive effect or potentiation). Products include:
DynaCirc CR Tablets ... 2721

Ketoprofen (Co-administration in some patients with compromised renal function who are being treated with NSAIDs may result in a further deterioration of renal function: NSAID may reduce the diuretic, natriuretic and antihypertensive effects of thiazide).
No products indexed under this heading.

Ketorolac Tromethamine (Co-administration in some patients with compromised renal function who are being treated with NSAIDs may result in a further deterioration of renal function: NSAID may reduce the diuretic, natriuretic and antihypertensive effects of thiazide). Products include:

Acular Ophthalmic Solution 565
Acular LS Ophthalmic Solution 566

Labetalol Hydrochloride (Co-administration of thiazide and other antihypertensive agents can lead to additive effect or potentiation).

No products indexed under this heading.

Levorphanol Tartrate (Co-administration of thiazide and narcotics may potentiate orthostatic hypotension).

No products indexed under this heading.

Lithium (Co-administration of lithium with drugs that cause elimination of sodium, including ACE inhibitors, can lead to lithium toxicity; diuretics can reduce renal clearance of lithium and add a high risk of lithium toxicity).

No products indexed under this heading.

Lithium Carbonate (Co-administration of lithium with drugs that cause elimination of sodium, including ACE inhibitors, can lead to lithium toxicity; diuretics can reduce renal clearance of lithium and add a high risk of lithium toxicity). Products include:

Lithobid Tablets 1692

Lithium Citrate (Co-administration of lithium with drugs that cause elimination of sodium, including ACE inhibitors, can lead to lithium toxicity; diuretics can reduce renal clearance of lithium and add a high risk of lithium toxicity).

No products indexed under this heading.

Losartan Potassium (Co-administration of thiazide and other antihypertensive agents can lead to additive effect or potentiation). Products include:

Cozaar Tablets 1935
Hyzaar 50-12.5 Tablets 1990
Hyzaar 100-12.5 Tablets 1990
Hyzaar 100-25 Tablets 1990

Mecamylamine Hydrochloride (Co-administration of thiazide and other antihypertensive agents can lead to additive effect or potentiation).

No products indexed under this heading.

Meclofenamate Sodium (Co-administration in some patients with compromised renal function who are being treated with NSAIDs may result in a further deterioration of renal function: NSAID may reduce the diuretic, natriuretic and antihypertensive effects of thiazide).

No products indexed under this heading.

Mefenamic Acid (Co-administration in some patients with compromised renal function who are being treated with NSAIDs may result in a further deterioration of renal function: NSAID may reduce the diuretic, natriuretic and antihypertensive effects of thiazide).

No products indexed under this heading.

Meloxicam (Co-administration in some patients with compromised renal function who are being treated with NSAIDs may result in a further deterioration of renal function: NSAID may reduce the diuretic, natriuretic and antihypertensive effects of thiazide). Products include:

Mobic Oral Suspension 863
Mobic Tablets 863

Meperidine Hydrochloride (Co-administration of thiazide and narcotics may potentiate orthostatic hypotension).

No products indexed under this heading.

Mephobarbital (Co-administration of thiazide and barbiturates may potentiate orthostatic hypotension).

No products indexed under this heading.

Metformin Hydrochloride (Hyperglycemia may occur with thiazide diuretics; dosage adjustment of oral hypoglycemic agents may be required). Products include:

ActoPlus Met Tablets 3214
Avandamet Tablets 1373
Fortamet Extended-Release Tablets 3115

Methadone Hydrochloride (Co-administration of thiazide and narcotics may potentiate orthostatic hypotension).

No products indexed under this heading.

Methyclothiazide (Co-administration of lisinopril in patients on diuretics, especially those in whom diuretic therapy was recently instituted, may occasionally experience excessive hypotension; antihypertensive effects of lisinopril are augmented by antihypertensive agents that cause renin release).

No products indexed under this heading.

Methyldopa (Co-administration of thiazide and other antihypertensive agents can lead to additive effect or potentiation). Products include:

Aldoril Tablets 1910

Methyldopate Hydrochloride (Co-administration of thiazide and other antihypertensive agents can lead to additive effect or potentiation).

No products indexed under this heading.

Methylprednisolone Acetate (Co-administration of thiazide diuretics with corticosteroids intensifies electrolyte depletion, particularly potassium). Products include:

Depo-Medrol Injectable Suspension 2617
Depo-Medrol Single-Dose Vial 2619

Methylprednisolone Sodium Succinate (Co-administration of thiazide diuretics with corticosteroids intensifies electrolyte depletion, particularly potassium).

No products indexed under this heading.

Metocurine Iodide (Co-administration with nondepolarizing skeletal muscle relaxants may result in possible increased responsiveness to the muscle relaxant).

No products indexed under this heading.

Metolazone (Co-administration of lisinopril in patients on diuretics, especially those in whom diuretic therapy was recently instituted, may occasionally experience excessive hypotension; antihypertensive effects of lisinopril are augmented by antihypertensive agents that cause renin release).

No products indexed under this heading.

Metoprolol Succinate (Co-administration of thiazide and other antihypertensive agents can lead to additive effect or potentiation). Products include:

Toprol-XL Tablets 668

Metoprolol Tartrate (Co-administration of thiazide and other antihypertensive agents can lead to additive effect or potentiation). Products include:

Lopressor Injection 2238
Lopressor Tablets 2238
Lopressor HCT 50/25 Tablets 2241
Lopressor HCT 100/25 Tablets 2241
Lopressor HCT 100/50 Tablets 2241

Metyrosine (Co-administration of thiazide and other antihypertensive agents can lead to additive effect or potentiation). Products include:

Demser Capsules 1953

Mibefradil Dihydrochloride (Co-administration of thiazide and other antihypertensive agents can lead to additive effect or potentiation).

No products indexed under this heading.

Miglitol (Hyperglycemia may occur with thiazide diuretics; dosage adjustment of oral hypoglycemic agents may be required).

No products indexed under this heading.

Minoxidil (Co-administration of thiazide and other antihypertensive agents can lead to additive effect or potentiation). Products include:

Men's Rogaine Extra Strength Hair Regrowth Treatment Topical Solution, Ocean Rush Scent and Original Unscented ..... ◘ 633
Men's Rogaine Foam Hair Regrowth Treatment.................. ◘ 633
Women's Rogaine Hair Regrowth Treatment Topical Solution, Spring Bloom Scent and Original Unscented..................... ◘ 634

Mivacurium Chloride (Co-administration with nondepolarizing skeletal muscle relaxants may result in possible increased responsiveness to the muscle relaxant). Products include:

Mivacron Injection 493

Moexipril Hydrochloride (Co-administration of thiazide and other antihypertensive agents can lead to additive effect or potentiation). Products include:

Uniretic Tablets 3100
Univasc Tablets 3104

Morphine Sulfate (Co-administration of thiazide and narcotics may potentiate orthostatic hypotension). Products include:

Avinza Capsules 1741
Kadian Capsules 577
MS Contin Tablets 2701

Nabumetone (Co-administration in some patients with compromised renal function who are being treated with NSAIDs may result in a further deterioration of renal function: NSAID may reduce the diuretic, natriuretic and antihypertensive effects of thiazide).

No products indexed under this heading.

Nadolol (Co-administration of thiazide and other antihypertensive agents can lead to additive effect or potentiation). Products include:

Nadolol Tablets 2159

Naproxen (Co-administration in some patients with compromised renal function who are being treated with NSAIDs may result in a further deterioration of renal function: NSAID may reduce the diuretic, natriuretic and antihypertensive effects of thiazide). Products include:

EC-Naprosyn Delayed-Release Tablets 2761
Naprosyn Suspension 2761
Naprosyn Tablets 2761
Prevacid NapraPAC 3280

Naproxen Sodium (Co-administration in some patients with compromised renal function who are being treated with NSAIDs may result in a further deterioration of renal function: NSAID may reduce the diuretic, natriuretic and antihypertensive effects of thiazide). Products include:

Aleve Caplets 742
Aleve Gelcaps 743
Aleve Tablets 743
Aleve Cold & Sinus Caplets 744
Anaprox Tablets 2761
Anaprox DS Tablets 2761

Nicardipine Hydrochloride (Co-administration of thiazide and other antihypertensive agents can lead to additive effect or potentiation). Products include:

Cardene I.V. 2497

Nifedipine (Co-administration of thiazide and other antihypertensive agents can lead to additive effect or potentiation). Products include:

Adalat CC Tablets 2964

Nisoldipine (Co-administration of thiazide and other antihypertensive agents can lead to additive effect or potentiation). Products include:

Sular Tablets 3122

Nitroglycerin (Co-administration of thiazide and other antihypertensive agents can lead to additive effect or potentiation). Products include:

Nitro-Dur Transdermal Infusion System... 3046
Nitrolingual Pumpspray 3120

Norepinephrine Bitartrate (Possible decreased response to pressor amines but not sufficient to preclude pressor amine use).

No products indexed under this heading.

Oxaprozin (Co-administration in some patients with compromised renal function who are being treated with NSAIDs may result in a further deterioration of renal function: NSAID may reduce the diuretic, natriuretic and antihypertensive effects of thiazide).

No products indexed under this heading.

Oxycodone Hydrochloride (Co-administration of thiazide and narcotics may potentiate orthostatic hypotension). Products include:

OxyContin Tablets 2703
OxyFast Oral Concentrate Solution....................................... 2708
OxyIR Capsules 2708
Percocet Tablets 1131
Percodan Tablets 1132

Pancuronium Bromide (Co-administration with nondepolarizing skeletal muscle relaxants may result in possible increased responsiveness to the muscle relaxant).

No products indexed under this heading.

Penbutolol Sulfate (Co-administration of thiazide and other antihypertensive agents can lead to additive effect or potentiation).

No products indexed under this heading.

Pentobarbital Sodium (Co-administration of thiazide and barbiturates may potentiate orthostatic hypotension). Products include:
Nembutal Sodium Solution, USP 2470

Perindopril Erbumine (Co-administration of thiazide and other antihypertensive agents can lead to additive effect or potentiation). Products include:
Aceon Tablets (2 mg, 4 mg, 8 mg) 3194

Phenobarbital (Co-administration of thiazide and barbiturates may potentiate orthostatic hypotension). Products include:
Donnatal Extentabs 2493

Phenoxybenzamine Hydrochloride (Co-administration of thiazide and other antihypertensive agents can lead to additive effect or potentiation). Products include:
Dibenzyline Capsules 3399

Phentolamine Mesylate (Co-administration of thiazide and other antihypertensive agents can lead to additive effect or potentiation).
No products indexed under this heading.

Phenylbutazone (Co-administration in some patients with compromised renal function who are being treated with NSAIDs may result in a further deterioration of renal function: NSAID may reduce the diuretic, natriuretic and antihypertensive effects of thiazide).
No products indexed under this heading.

Pindolol (Co-administration of thiazide and other antihypertensive agents can lead to additive effect or potentiation).
No products indexed under this heading.

Pioglitazone Hydrochloride (Hyperglycemia may occur with thiazide diuretics; dosage adjustment of oral hypoglycemic agents may be required). Products include:
ActoPlus Met Tablets 3214
Actos Tablets 3219
Duetact Tablets 3226

Piroxicam (Co-administration in some patients with compromised renal function who are being treated with NSAIDs may result in a further deterioration of renal function: NSAID may reduce the diuretic, natriuretic and antihypertensive effects of thiazide).
No products indexed under this heading.

Polythiazide (Co-administration of lisinopril in patients on diuretics, especially those in whom diuretic therapy was recently instituted, may occasionally experience excessive hypotension; antihypertensive effects of lisinopril are augmented by antihypertensive agents that cause renin release).
No products indexed under this heading.

Potassium Acid Phosphate (Risk factors for the development of hyperkalemia include the concomitant use of potassium-sparing diuretics, potassium supplements and/or potassium-containing salt substitutes. Hyperkalemia can cause serious, sometimes, fatal, arrhythmias. Prinzide should be used cautiously, if at all, with these agents and with frequent monitoring of serum potassium). Products include:
K-Phos Original (Sodium Free) Tablets 760

Potassium Bicarbonate (Risk factors for the development of hyperkalemia include the concomitant use of potassium-sparing diuretics, potassium supplements and/or potassium-containing salt substitutes. Hyperkalemia can cause serious, sometimes, fatal, arrhythmias. Prinzide should be used cautiously, if at all, with these agents and with frequent monitoring of serum potassium).
No products indexed under this heading.

Potassium Chloride (Risk factors for the development of hyperkalemia include the concomitant use of potassium-sparing diuretics, potassium supplements and/or potassium-containing salt substitutes. Hyperkalemia can cause serious, sometimes, fatal, arrhythmias. Prinzide should be used cautiously, if at all, with these agents and with frequent monitoring of serum potassium). Products include:
Colyte with Flavor Packs for Oral Solution 3088
HalfLytely and Bisacodyl Tablets Bowel Prep Kit with Flavors Packs 881
K-Dur Extended-Relase Tablets 3033
K-Lor Oral Solution 474
K-Tab Tablets 475
MoviPrep Oral Solution 2839
TriLyte with Flavor Packs for Oral Solution 3100

Potassium Citrate (Risk factors for the development of hyperkalemia include the concomitant use of potassium-sparing diuretics, potassium supplements and/or potassium-containing salt substitutes. Hyperkalemia can cause serious, sometimes, fatal, arrhythmias. Prinzide should be used cautiously, if at all, with these agents and with frequent monitoring of serum potassium). Products include:
Urocit-K Tablets 2144

Potassium Gluconate (Risk factors for the development of hyperkalemia include the concomitant use of potassium-sparing diuretics, potassium supplements and/or potassium-containing salt substitutes. Hyperkalemia can cause serious, sometimes, fatal, arrhythmias. Prinzide should be used cautiously, if at all, with these agents and with frequent monitoring of serum potassium).
No products indexed under this heading.

Potassium Phosphate (Risk factors for the development of hyperkalemia include the concomitant use of potassium-sparing diuretics, potassium supplements and/or potassium-containing salt substitutes. Hyperkalemia can cause serious, sometimes, fatal, arrhythmias. Prinzide should be used cautiously, if at all, with these agents and with frequent monitoring of serum potassium). Products include:
K-Phos Neutral Tablets 760

Prazosin Hydrochloride (Co-administration of thiazide and other antihypertensive agents can lead to additive effect or potentiation).
No products indexed under this heading.

Prednisolone Acetate (Co-administration of thiazide diuretics with corticosteroids intensifies electrolyte depletion, particularly potassium). Products include:
Blephamide Ophthalmic Ointment 568
Blephamide Ophthalmic Suspension 569
Poly-Pred Ophthalmic Suspension .... ⊙233
Pred Forte Ophthalmic Suspension .... ⊙235
Pred Mild Ophthalmic Suspension .... ⊙238
Pred-G Ophthalmic Ointment .... ⊙237
Pred-G Ophthalmic Suspension .... ⊙236

Prednisolone Sodium Phosphate (Co-administration of thiazide diuretics with corticosteroids intensifies electrolyte depletion, particularly potassium).
No products indexed under this heading.

Prednisolone Tebutate (Co-administration of thiazide diuretics with corticosteroids intensifies electrolyte depletion, particularly potassium).
No products indexed under this heading.

Prednisone (Co-administration of thiazide diuretics with corticosteroids intensifies electrolyte depletion, particularly potassium).
No products indexed under this heading.

Propoxyphene Hydrochloride (Co-administration of thiazide and narcotics may potentiate orthostatic hypotension).
No products indexed under this heading.

Propoxyphene Napsylate (Co-administration of thiazide and narcotics may potentiate orthostatic hypotension).
No products indexed under this heading.

Propranolol Hydrochloride (Co-administration of thiazide and other antihypertensive agents can lead to additive effect or potentiation). Products include:
Inderal LA Long-Acting Capsules 3429
InnoPran XL Capsules 2723

Quinapril Hydrochloride (Co-administration of thiazide and other antihypertensive agents can lead to additive effect or potentiation).
No products indexed under this heading.

Ramipril (Co-administration of thiazide and other antihypertensive agents can lead to additive effect or potentiation). Products include:
Altace Capsules 1702

Rapacuronium Bromide (Co-administration with nondepolarizing skeletal muscle relaxants may result in possible increased responsiveness to the muscle relaxant).
No products indexed under this heading.

Rauwolfia Serpentina (Co-administration of thiazide and other antihypertensive agents can lead to additive effect or potentiation).
No products indexed under this heading.

Remifentanil Hydrochloride (Co-administration of thiazide and narcotics may potentiate orthostatic hypotension).
No products indexed under this heading.

Repaglinide (Hyperglycemia may occur with thiazide diuretics; dosage adjustment of oral hypoglycemic agents may be required).
No products indexed under this heading.

Rescinnamine (Co-administration of thiazide and other antihypertensive agents can lead to additive effect or potentiation).
No products indexed under this heading.

Reserpine (Co-administration of thiazide and other antihypertensive agents can lead to additive effect or potentiation).
No products indexed under this heading.

Rocuronium Bromide (Co-administration with nondepolarizing skeletal muscle relaxants may result in possible increased responsiveness to the muscle relaxant). Products include:
Zemuron Injection 2346

Rofecoxib (Co-administration in some patients with compromised renal function who are being treated with NSAIDs may result in a further deterioration of renal function: NSAID may reduce the diuretic, natriuretic and antihypertensive effects of thiazide).
No products indexed under this heading.

Rosiglitazone Maleate (Hyperglycemia may occur with thiazide diuretics; dosage adjustment of oral hypoglycemic agents may be required). Products include:
Avandamet Tablets 1373
Avandaryl Tablets 1379
Avandia Tablets 1384

Secobarbital Sodium (Co-administration of thiazide and barbiturates may potentiate orthostatic hypotension).
No products indexed under this heading.

Sodium Nitroprusside (Co-administration of thiazide and other antihypertensive agents can lead to additive effect or potentiation).
No products indexed under this heading.

Sotalol Hydrochloride (Co-administration of thiazide and other antihypertensive agents can lead to additive effect or potentiation).
No products indexed under this heading.

Spirapril Hydrochloride (Co-administration of thiazide and other antihypertensive agents can lead to additive effect or potentiation).
No products indexed under this heading.

Spironolactone (Risk factors for the development of hyperkalemia include the concomitant use of potassium-sparing diuretics, potassium supplements and/or potassium-containing salt substitutes. Hyperkalemia can cause serious, sometimes, fatal, arrhythmias. Prinzide should be used cautiously, if at all, with these agents and with frequent monitoring of serum potassium).
No products indexed under this heading.

Sufentanil Citrate (Co-administration of thiazide and narcotics may potentiate orthostatic hypotension).
No products indexed under this heading.

Sulindac (Co-administration in some patients with compromised renal function who are being treated with NSAIDs may result in a further deterioration of renal function: NSAID may reduce the diuretic, natriuretic and antihypertensive effects of thiazide). Products include:
Clinoril Tablets 1924

Telmisartan (Co-administration of thiazide and other antihypertensive agents can lead to additive effect or potentiation). Products include:
Micardis Tablets 854
Micardis HCT Tablets 856

Terazosin Hydrochloride (Co-administration of thiazide and other antihypertensive agents can lead to additive effect or potentiation). Products include:
Hytrin Capsules 471

Thiamylal Sodium (Co-administration of thiazide and barbiturates may potentiate orthostatic hypotension).
No products indexed under this heading.

Timolol Maleate (Co-administration of thiazide and other antihypertensive agents can lead to additive effect or potentiation). Products include:
Blocadren Tablets 1916
Cosopt Sterile Ophthalmic Solution........ 1931
Timolide Tablets 2086
Timoptic Sterile Ophthalmic Solution........ 2088
Timoptic in Ocudose 2091
Timoptic-XE Sterile Ophthalmic Gel Forming Solution........ 2092

Tolazamide (Hyperglycemia may occur with thiazide diuretics; dosage adjustment of oral hypoglycemic agents may be required).
No products indexed under this heading.

Tolbutamide (Hyperglycemia may occur with thiazide diuretics; dosage adjustment of oral hypoglycemic agents may be required).
No products indexed under this heading.

Tolmetin Sodium (Co-administration in some patients with compromised renal function who are being treated with NSAIDs may result in a further deterioration of renal function: NSAID may reduce the diuretic, natriuretic and antihypertensive effects of thiazide).
No products indexed under this heading.

Torsemide (Co-administration of lisinopril in patients on diuretics, especially those in whom diuretic therapy was recently instituted, may occasionally experience excessive hypotension; antihypertensive effects of lisinopril are augmented by antihypertensive agents that cause renin release). Products include:
Demadex Injection 2759
Demadex Tablets 2759

Trandolapril (Co-administration of thiazide and other antihypertensive agents can lead to additive effect or potentiation). Products include:
Mavik Tablets 486
Tarka Tablets 524

Triamcinolone (Co-administration of thiazide diuretics with corticosteroids intensifies electrolyte depletion, particularly potassium).
No products indexed under this heading.

Triamcinolone Acetonide (Co-administration of thiazide diuretics with corticosteroids intensifies electrolyte depletion, particularly potassium). Products include:
Azmacort Inhalation Aerosol 1726
Nasacort AQ Nasal Spray 2922

Triamcinolone Diacetate (Co-administration of thiazide diuretics with corticosteroids intensifies electrolyte depletion, particularly potassium).
No products indexed under this heading.

Triamcinolone Hexacetonide (Co-administration of thiazide diuretics with corticosteroids intensifies electrolyte depletion, particularly potassium).
No products indexed under this heading.

Triamterene (Risk factors for the development of hyperkalemia include the concomitant use of potassium-sparing diuretics, potassium supplements and/or potassium-containing salt substitutes. Hyperkalemia can cause serious, sometimes, fatal, arrhythmias. Prinzide should be used cautiously, if at all, with these agents and with frequent monitoring of serum potassium). Products include:
Dyazide Capsules 1423
Dyrenium Capsules 3400

Trimethaphan Camsylate (Co-administration of thiazide and other antihypertensive agents can lead to additive effect or potentiation).
No products indexed under this heading.

Troglitazone (Hyperglycemia may occur with thiazide diuretics; dosage adjustment of oral hypoglycemic agents may be required).
No products indexed under this heading.

Valdecoxib (Co-administration in some patients with compromised renal function who are being treated with NSAIDs may result in a further deterioration of renal function: NSAID may reduce the diuretic, natriuretic and antihypertensive effects of thiazide).
No products indexed under this heading.

Valsartan (Co-administration of thiazide and other antihypertensive agents can lead to additive effect or potentiation). Products include:
Diovan Tablets 2193
Diovan HCT Tablets 2196

Vecuronium Bromide (Co-administration with nondepolarizing skeletal muscle relaxants may result in possible increased responsiveness to the muscle relaxant).
No products indexed under this heading.

Verapamil Hydrochloride (Co-administration of thiazide and other antihypertensive agents can lead to additive effect or potentiation). Products include:
Covera-HS Tablets 3139
Tarka Tablets 524
Verelan PM Extended-Release Capsules, Controlled-Onset........ 3106

Food Interactions

Alcohol (Co-administration of thiazide and alcohol may potentiate orthostatic hypotension).

Salt Substitutes, Potassium-Containing (Risk factors for the development of hyperkalemia include the concomitant use of potassium-sparing diuretics, potassium supplements and/or potassium-containing salt substitutes. Hyperkalemia can cause serious, sometimes, fatal, arrhythmias. Prinzide should be used cautiously, if at all, with these agents and with frequent monitoring of serum potassium).

PROAIR HFA INHALATION AEROSOL

(Albuterol Sulfate) 3300

May interact with beta blockers, monoamine oxidase inhibitors, non-potassium-sparing diuretics, sympathomimetic aerosol bronchodilators, tricyclic antidepressants, and certain other agents. Compounds in these categories include:

Acebutolol Hydrochloride (Beta-adrenergic-receptor blocking agents not only block the pulmonary effect of beta-agonists, such as albuterol sulfate, but may produce severe bronchospasm in asthmatic patients. Therefore, patients with asthma should not normally be treated with beta-blockers. However, under certain circumstances, e.g., as prophylaxis after myocardial infarction, there may be no acceptable alternatives to the use of beta-adrenergic-blocking agents in patients with asthma. In this setting, cardioselective beta-blockers should be considered, although they should be administered with caution).
No products indexed under this heading.

Albuterol (Other short-acting sympathomimetic aerosol bronchodilators should not be used concomitantly with albuterol sulfate. If additional adrenergic drugs are to be administered by any route, they should be used with caution to avoid deleterious cardiovascular effects). Products include:
Proventil Inhalation Aerosol 3053

Amitriptyline Hydrochloride (Albuterol sulfate should be administered with extreme caution to patients being treated with monoamine oxidase inhibitors or tricyclic antidepressants, or within 2 weeks of discontinuation of such agents, because the action of albuterol on the cardiovascular system may be potentiated).
No products indexed under this heading.

Amoxapine (Albuterol sulfate should be administered with extreme caution to patients being treated with monoamine oxidase inhibitors or tricyclic antidepressants, or within 2 weeks of discontinuation of such agents, because the action of albuterol on the cardiovascular system may be potentiated).
No products indexed under this heading.

Atenolol (Beta-adrenergic-receptor blocking agents not only block the pulmonary effect of beta-agonists, such as albuterol sulfate, but may produce severe bronchospasm in asthmatic patients. Therefore, patients with asthma should not normally be treated with beta-blockers. However, under certain circumstances, e.g., as prophylaxis after myocardial infarction, there may be no acceptable alternatives to the use of beta-adrenergic-blocking agents in patients with asthma. In this setting, cardioselective beta-blockers should be considered, although they should be administered with caution).
No products indexed under this heading.

Bendroflumethiazide (The ECG changes and/or hypokalemia which may result from the administration of non-potassium sparing diuretics (such as loop or thiazide diuretics) can be acutely worsened by beta-agonists, especially when the recommended dose of beta-agonist is exceeded. Although the clinical significance of these effects is not known, caution is advised in the co-administration of beta-agonists with non-potassium sparing diuretics).
No products indexed under this heading.

Betaxolol Hydrochloride (Beta-adrenergic-receptor blocking agents not only block the pulmonary effect of beta-agonists, such as albuterol sulfate, but may produce severe bronchospasm in asthmatic patients. Therefore, patients with asthma should not normally be treated with beta-blockers. However, under certain circumstances, e.g., as prophylaxis after myocardial infarction, there may be no acceptable alternatives to the use of beta-adrenergic-blocking agents in patients with asthma. In this setting, cardioselective beta-blockers should be considered, although they should be administered with caution). Products include:
Betoptic S Ophthalmic Suspension........ 558

Bisoprolol Fumarate (Beta-adrenergic-receptor blocking agents not only block the pulmonary effect of beta-agonists, such as albuterol sulfate, but may produce severe bronchospasm in asthmatic patients. Therefore, patients with asthma should not normally be treated with beta-blockers. However, under certain circumstances, e.g., as prophylaxis after myocardial infarction, there may be no acceptable alternatives to the use of beta-adrenergic-blocking agents in patients with asthma. In this setting, cardioselective beta-blockers should be considered, although they should be administered with caution).
No products indexed under this heading.

Bitolterol Mesylate (Other short-acting sympathomimetic aerosol bronchodilators should not be used concomitantly with albuterol sulfate. If additional adrenergic drugs are to be administered by any route, they should be used with caution to avoid deleterious cardiovascular effects).
No products indexed under this heading.

Bumetanide (The ECG changes and/or hypokalemia which may result from the administration of non-potassium sparing diuretics (such as loop or thiazide diuretics) can be acutely worsened by beta-agonists, especially when the recommended dose of beta-agonist is exceeded. Although the clinical significance of these effects is not known, caution is advised in the co-administration of beta-agonists with non-potassium sparing diuretics). Products include:
Bumex Tablets 2746

Carteolol Hydrochloride (Beta-adrenergic-receptor blocking agents not only block the pulmonary effect of beta-agonists, such as albuterol sulfate, but may produce severe bronchospasm in asthmatic patients. Therefore, patients with asthma should not normally be treated with beta-blockers. However, under certain circumstances, e.g., as prophylaxis after myocardial infarction, there may be no acceptable alternatives to the use of beta-adrenergic-blocking agents in patients with asthma. In this setting, cardioselective beta-blockers should be considered, although they should be administered with caution). Products include:

Carteolol Hydrochloride Ophthalmic Solution USP, 1%...... ⊙249

Chlorothiazide (The ECG changes and/or hypokalemia which may result from the administration of non-potassium sparing diuretics (such as loop or thiazide diuretics) can be acutely worsened by beta-agonists, especially when the recommended dose of beta-agonist is exceeded. Although the clinical significance of these effects is not known, caution is advised in the co-administration of beta-agonists with non-potassium sparing diuretics). Products include:

Diuril Oral Suspension 1954

Chlorothiazide Sodium (The ECG changes and/or hypokalemia which may result from the administration of non-potassium sparing diuretics (such as loop or thiazide diuretics) can be acutely worsened by beta-agonists, especially when the recommended dose of beta-agonist is exceeded. Although the clinical significance of these effects is not known, caution is advised in the co-administration of beta-agonists with non-potassium sparing diuretics). Products include:

Diuril Sodium Intravenous 2467

Clomipramine Hydrochloride (Albuterol sulfate should be administered with extreme caution to patients being treated with monoamine oxidase inhibitors or tricyclic antidepressants, or within 2 weeks of discontinuation of such agents, because the action of albuterol on the cardiovascular system may be potentiated).

No products indexed under this heading.

Desipramine Hydrochloride (Albuterol sulfate should be administered with extreme caution to patients being treated with monoamine oxidase inhibitors or tricyclic antidepressants, or within 2 weeks of discontinuation of such agents, because the action of albuterol on the cardiovascular system may be potentiated).

No products indexed under this heading.

Digoxin (Mean decreases of 16% and 22% in serum digoxin levels were demonstrated after single dose intravenous and oral administration of albuterol, respectively, to normal volunteers who had received digoxin for 10 days. The clinical significance of these findings for patients with obstructive airway disease who are receiving albuterol and digoxin on a chronic basis is unclear. Nevertheless, it would be prudent to carefully evaluate the serum digoxin levels in patients who are currently receiving digoxin and albuterol sulfate). Products include:

Lanoxicaps Capsules 1490
Lanoxin Injection 1494
Lanoxin Injection Pediatric 1497
Lanoxin Tablets 1500

Doxepin Hydrochloride (Albuterol sulfate should be administered with extreme caution to patients being treated with monoamine oxidase inhibitors or tricyclic antidepressants, or within 2 weeks of discontinuation of such agents, because the action of albuterol on the cardiovascular system may be potentiated).

No products indexed under this heading.

Esmolol Hydrochloride (Beta-adrenergic-receptor blocking agents not only block the pulmonary effect of beta-agonists, such as albuterol sulfate, but may produce severe bronchospasm in asthmatic patients. Therefore, patients with asthma should not normally be treated with beta-blockers. However, under certain circumstances, e.g., as prophylaxis after myocardial infarction, there may be no acceptable alternatives to the use of beta-adrenergic-blocking agents in patients with asthma. In this setting, cardioselective beta-blockers should be considered, although they should be administered with caution).

No products indexed under this heading.

Ethacrynic Acid (The ECG changes and/or hypokalemia which may result from the administration of non-potassium sparing diuretics (such as loop or thiazide diuretics) can be acutely worsened by beta-agonists, especially when the recommended dose of beta-agonist is exceeded. Although the clinical significance of these effects is not known, caution is advised in the co-administration of beta-agonists with non-potassium sparing diuretics). Products include:

Edecrin Tablets 1959

Furosemide (The ECG changes and/or hypokalemia which may result from the administration of non-potassium sparing diuretics (such as loop or thiazide diuretics) can be acutely worsened by beta-agonists, especially when the recommended dose of beta-agonist is exceeded. Although the clinical significance of these effects is not known, caution is advised in the co-administration of beta-agonists with non-potassium sparing diuretics). Products include:

Furosemide Tablets 2154

Hydrochlorothiazide (The ECG changes and/or hypokalemia which may result from the administration of non-potassium sparing diuretics (such as loop or thiazide diuretics) can be acutely worsened by beta-agonists, especially when the recommended dose of beta-agonist is exceeded. Although the clinical significance of these effects is not known, caution is advised in the co-administration of beta-agonists with non-potassium sparing diuretics). Products include:

Aldoril Tablets 1910
Atacand HCT 651
Avalide Tablets 888
Avalide Tablets 2874
Benicar HCT Tablets 1044
Diovan HCT Tablets 2196
Dyazide Capsules 1423
Hyzaar 50-12.5 Tablets 1990
Hyzaar 100-12.5 Tablets 1990
Hyzaar 100-25 Tablets 1990
Lopressor HCT 50/25 Tablets 2241
Lopressor HCT 100/25 Tablets 2241
Lopressor HCT 100/50 Tablets 2241
Lotensin HCT Tablets 2246
Micardis HCT Tablets 856
Moduretic Tablets 2028
Prinzide Tablets 2056
Teveten HCT Tablets 1737
Timolide Tablets 2086
Uniretic Tablets 3100

Hydroflumethiazide (The ECG changes and/or hypokalemia which may result from the administration of non-potassium sparing diuretics (such as loop or thiazide diuretics) can be acutely worsened by beta-agonists, especially when the recommended dose of beta-agonist is exceeded. Although the clinical significance of these effects is not known, caution is advised in the co-administration of beta-agonists with non-potassium sparing diuretics).

No products indexed under this heading.

Imipramine Hydrochloride (Albuterol sulfate should be administered with extreme caution to patients being treated with monoamine oxidase inhibitors or tricyclic antidepressants, or within 2 weeks of discontinuation of such agents, because the action of albuterol on the cardiovascular system may be potentiated).

No products indexed under this heading.

Imipramine Pamoate (Albuterol sulfate should be administered with extreme caution to patients being treated with monoamine oxidase inhibitors or tricyclic antidepressants, or within 2 weeks of discontinuation of such agents, because the action of albuterol on the cardiovascular system may be potentiated).

No products indexed under this heading.

Isocarboxazid (Albuterol sulfate should be administered with extreme caution to patients being treated with monoamine oxidase inhibitors or tricyclic antidepressants, or within 2 weeks of discontinuation of such agents, because the action of albuterol on the cardiovascular system may be potentiated).

No products indexed under this heading.

Isoetharine (Other short-acting sympathomimetic aerosol bronchodilators should not be used concomitantly with albuterol sulfate. If additional adrenergic drugs are to be administered by any route, they should be used with caution to avoid deleterious cardiovascular effects).

No products indexed under this heading.

Isoproterenol Hydrochloride (Other short-acting sympathomimetic aerosol bronchodilators should not be used concomitantly with albuterol sulfate. If additional adrenergic drugs are to be administered by any route, they should be used with caution to avoid deleterious cardiovascular effects).

No products indexed under this heading.

Labetalol Hydrochloride (Beta-adrenergic-receptor blocking agents not only block the pulmonary effect of beta-agonists, such as albuterol sulfate, but may produce severe bronchospasm in asthmatic patients. Therefore, patients with asthma should not normally be treated with beta-blockers. However, under certain circumstances, e.g., as prophylaxis after myocardial infarction, there may be no acceptable alternatives to the use of beta-adrenergic-blocking agents in patients with asthma. In this setting, cardioselective beta-blockers should be considered, although they should be administered with caution).

No products indexed under this heading.

Levalbuterol Hydrochloride (Other short-acting sympathomimetic aerosol bronchodilators should not be used concomitantly with albuterol sulfate. If additional adrenergic drugs are to be administered by any route, they should be used with caution to avoid deleterious cardiovascular effects). Products include:

Xopenex Inhalation Solution 3146
Xopenex Inhalation Solution Concentrate 3150

Levobunolol Hydrochloride (Beta-adrenergic-receptor blocking agents not only block the pulmonary effect of beta-agonists, such as albuterol sulfate, but may produce severe bronchospasm in asthmatic patients. Therefore, patients with asthma should not normally be treated with beta-blockers. However, under certain circumstances, e.g., as prophylaxis after myocardial infarction, there may be no acceptable alternatives to the use of beta-adrenergic-blocking agents in patients with asthma. In this setting, cardioselective beta-blockers should be considered, although they should be administered with caution). Products include:

Betagan Ophthalmic Solution, USP.. ⊙220

Maprotiline Hydrochloride (Albuterol sulfate should be administered with extreme caution to patients being treated with monoamine oxidase inhibitors or tricyclic antidepressants, or within 2 weeks of discontinuation of such agents, because the action of albuterol on the cardiovascular system may be potentiated).

No products indexed under this heading.

Metaproterenol Sulfate (Other short-acting sympathomimetic aerosol bronchodilators should not be used concomitantly with albuterol sulfate. If additional adrenergic drugs are to be administered by any route, they should be used with caution to avoid deleterious cardiovascular effects). Products include:

Alupent Inhalation Aerosol 826

Methyclothiazide (The ECG changes and/or hypokalemia which may result from the administration of non-potassium sparing diuretics (such as loop or thiazide diuretics) can be acutely worsened by beta-agonists, especially when the recommended dose of beta-agonist is exceeded. Although the clinical significance of these effects is not known, caution is advised in the co-administration of beta-agonists with non-potassium sparing diuretics).

No products indexed under this heading.

Metipranolol Hydrochloride (Beta-adrenergic-receptor blocking agents not only block the pulmonary effect of beta-agonists, such as albuterol sulfate, but may produce severe bronchospasm in asthmatic patients. Therefore, patients with asthma should not normally be treated with beta-blockers. However, under certain circumstances, e.g., as prophylaxis after myocardial infarction, there may be no acceptable alternatives to the use of beta-adrenergic-blocking agents in patients with asthma. In this setting, cardioselective beta-blockers should be considered, although they should be administered with caution).

No products indexed under this heading.

Metoprolol Succinate (Beta-adrenergic-receptor blocking agents not only block the pulmonary effect of beta-agonists, such as albuterol sulfate, but may produce severe bronchospasm in asthmatic patients. Therefore, patients with asthma should not normally be treated with beta-blockers. However, under certain circumstances, e.g., as prophylaxis after myocardial infarction, there may be no acceptable alternatives to the use of beta-adrenergic-blocking agents in patients with asthma. In this setting, cardioselective beta-blockers should be considered, although they should be administered with caution). Products include:

Toprol-XL Tablets 668

Metoprolol Tartrate (Beta-adrenergic-receptor blocking agents not only block the pulmonary effect of beta-agonists, such as albuterol sulfate, but may produce severe bronchospasm in asthmatic patients. Therefore, patients with asthma should not normally be treated with beta-blockers. However, under certain circumstances, e.g., as prophylaxis after myocardial infarction, there may be no acceptable alternatives to the use of beta-adrenergic-blocking agents in patients with asthma. In this setting, cardioselective beta-blockers should be considered, although they should be administered with caution). Products include:

Lopressor Injection 2238
Lopressor Tablets 2238
Lopressor HCT 50/25 Tablets 2241
Lopressor HCT 100/25 Tablets 2241
Lopressor HCT 100/50 Tablets 2241

Moclobemide (Albuterol sulfate should be administered with extreme caution to patients being treated with monoamine oxidase inhibitors or tricyclic antidepressants, or within 2 weeks of discontinuation of such agents, because the action of albuterol on the cardiovascular system may be potentiated).

No products indexed under this heading.

Nadolol (Beta-adrenergic-receptor blocking agents not only block the pulmonary effect of beta-agonists, such as albuterol sulfate, but may produce severe bronchospasm in asthmatic patients. Therefore, patients with asthma should not normally be treated with beta-blockers. However, under certain circumstances, e.g., as prophylaxis after myocardial infarction, there may be no acceptable alternatives to the use of beta-adrenergic-blocking agents in patients with asthma. In this setting, cardioselective beta-blockers should be considered, although they should be administered with caution). Products include:

Nadolol Tablets 2159

Nortriptyline Hydrochloride (Albuterol sulfate should be administered with extreme caution to patients being treated with monoamine oxidase inhibitors or tricyclic antidepressants, or within 2 weeks of discontinuation of such agents, because the action of albuterol on the cardiovascular system may be potentiated).

No products indexed under this heading.

Pargyline Hydrochloride (Albuterol sulfate should be administered with extreme caution to patients being treated with monoamine oxidase inhibitors or tricyclic antidepressants, or within 2 weeks of discontinuation of such agents, because the action of albuterol on the cardiovascular system may be potentiated).

No products indexed under this heading.

Penbutolol Sulfate (Beta-adrenergic-receptor blocking agents not only block the pulmonary effect of beta-agonists, such as albuterol sulfate, but may produce severe bronchospasm in asthmatic patients. Therefore, patients with asthma should not normally be treated with beta-blockers. However, under certain circumstances, e.g., as prophylaxis after myocardial infarction, there may be no acceptable alternatives to the use of beta-adrenergic-blocking agents in patients with asthma. In this setting, cardioselective beta-blockers should be considered, although they should be administered with caution).

No products indexed under this heading.

Phenelzine Sulfate (Albuterol sulfate should be administered with extreme caution to patients being treated with monoamine oxidase inhibitors or tricyclic antidepressants, or within 2 weeks of discontinuation of such agents, because the action of albuterol on the cardiovascular system may be potentiated).

No products indexed under this heading.

Pindolol (Beta-adrenergic-receptor blocking agents not only block the pulmonary effect of beta-agonists, such as albuterol sulfate, but may produce severe bronchospasm in asthmatic patients. Therefore, patients with asthma should not normally be treated with beta-blockers. However, under certain circumstances, e.g., as prophylaxis after myocardial infarction, there may be no acceptable alternatives to the use of beta-adrenergic-blocking agents in patients with asthma. In this setting, cardioselective beta-blockers should be considered, although they should be administered with caution).

No products indexed under this heading.

Pirbuterol Acetate (Other short-acting sympathomimetic aerosol bronchodilators should not be used concomitantly with albuterol sulfate. If additional adrenergic drugs are to be administered by any route, they should be used with caution to avoid deleterious cardiovascular effects). Products include:

Maxair Autohaler 1852

Polythiazide (The ECG changes and/or hypokalemia which may result from the administration of non-potassium sparing diuretics (such as loop or thiazide diuretics) can be acutely worsened by beta-agonists, especially when the recommended dose of beta-agonist is exceeded. Although the clinical significance of these effects is not known, caution is advised in the co-administration of beta-agonists with non-potassium sparing diuretics).

No products indexed under this heading.

Procarbazine Hydrochloride (Albuterol sulfate should be administered with extreme caution to patients being treated with monoamine oxidase inhibitors or tricyclic antidepressants, or within 2 weeks of discontinuation of such agents, because the action of albuterol on the cardiovascular system may be potentiated). Products include:

Matulane Capsules 3191

Propranolol Hydrochloride (Beta-adrenergic-receptor blocking agents not only block the pulmonary effect of beta-agonists, such as albuterol sulfate, but may produce severe bronchospasm in asthmatic patients. Therefore, patients with asthma should not normally be treated with beta-blockers. However, under certain circumstances, e.g., as prophylaxis after myocardial infarction, there may be no acceptable alternatives to the use of beta-adrenergic-blocking agents in patients with asthma. In this setting, cardioselective beta-blockers should be considered, although they should be administered with caution). Products include:

Inderal LA Long-Acting Capsules 3429
InnoPran XL Capsules 2723

Protriptyline Hydrochloride (Albuterol sulfate should be administered with extreme caution to patients being treated with monoamine oxidase inhibitors or tricyclic antidepressants, or within 2 weeks of discontinuation of such agents, because the action of albuterol on the cardiovascular system may be potentiated).

No products indexed under this heading.

Salmeterol Xinafoate (Other short-acting sympathomimetic aerosol bronchodilators should not be used concomitantly with albuterol sulfate. If additional adrenergic drugs are to be administered by any route, they should be used with caution to avoid deleterious cardiovascular effects). Products include:

Advair Diskus 100/50 1308
Advair Diskus 250/50 1308
Advair Diskus 500/50 1308
Advair HFA Inhalation Aerosol 1318
Serevent Diskus 1568

Selegiline Hydrochloride (Albuterol sulfate should be administered with extreme caution to patients being treated with monoamine oxidase inhibitors or tricyclic antidepressants, or within 2 weeks of discontinuation of such agents, because the action of albuterol on the cardiovascular system may be potentiated). Products include:

Eldepryl Capsules 3208
Zelapar Tablets 3372

Sotalol Hydrochloride (Beta-adrenergic-receptor blocking agents not only block the pulmonary effect of beta-agonists, such as albuterol sulfate, but may produce severe bronchospasm in asthmatic patients. Therefore, patients with asthma should not normally be treated with beta-blockers. However, under certain circumstances, e.g., as prophylaxis after myocardial infarction, there may be no acceptable alternatives to the use of beta-adrenergic-blocking agents in patients with asthma. In this setting, cardioselective beta-blockers should be considered, although they should be administered with caution).

No products indexed under this heading.

Terbutaline Sulfate (Other short-acting sympathomimetic aerosol bronchodilators should not be used concomitantly with albuterol sulfate. If additional adrenergic drugs are to be administered by any route, they should be used with caution to avoid deleterious cardiovascular effects).

No products indexed under this heading.

Timolol Hemihydrate (Beta-adrenergic-receptor blocking agents not only block the pulmonary effect of beta-agonists, such as albuterol sulfate, but may produce severe bronchospasm in asthmatic patients. Therefore, patients with asthma should not normally be treated with beta-blockers. However, under certain circumstances, e.g., as prophylaxis after myocardial infarction, there may be no acceptable alternatives to the use of beta-adrenergic-blocking agents in patients with asthma. In this setting, cardioselective beta-blockers should be considered, although they should be administered with caution). Products include:

Betimol Ophthalmic Solution 3382
Betimol Ophthalmic Solution .... ⊙295

Timolol Maleate (Beta-adrenergic-receptor blocking agents not only block the pulmonary effect of beta-agonists, such as albuterol sulfate, but may produce severe bronchospasm in asthmatic patients. Therefore, patients with asthma should not normally be treated with beta-blockers. However, under certain circumstances, e.g., as prophylaxis after myocardial infarction, there may be no acceptable alternatives to the use of beta-adrenergic-blocking agents in patients with asthma. In this setting, cardioselective beta-blockers should be considered, although they should be administered with caution). Products include:

Blocadren Tablets 1916
Cosopt Sterile Ophthalmic Solution 1931
Timolide Tablets 2086
Timoptic Sterile Ophthalmic Solution 2088
Timoptic in Ocudose 2091
Timoptic-XE Sterile Ophthalmic Gel Forming Solution 2092

Torsemide (The ECG changes and/or hypokalemia which may result from the administration of non-potassium sparing diuretics (such as loop or thiazide diuretics) can be acutely worsened by beta-agonists, especially when the recommended dose of beta-agonist is exceeded. Although the clinical significance of these effects is not known, caution is advised in the co-administration of beta-agonists with non-potassium sparing diuretics). Products include:

Demadex Injection 2759
Demadex Tablets 2759

Tranylcypromine Sulfate (Albuterol sulfate should be administered with extreme caution to patients being treated with monoamine oxidase inhibitors or tricyclic antidepressants, or within 2 weeks of discontinuation of such agents, because the action of albuterol on the cardiovascular system may be potentiated). Products include:
- Parnate Tablets 1527

Trimipramine Maleate (Albuterol sulfate should be administered with extreme caution to patients being treated with monoamine oxidase inhibitors or tricyclic antidepressants, or within 2 weeks of discontinuation of such agents, because the action of albuterol on the cardiovascular system may be potentiated).
- No products indexed under this heading.

PROAMATINE TABLETS

(Midodrine Hydrochloride) 3186

May interact with alpha adrenergic blockers, cardiac glycosides, quinidine, and certain other agents. Compounds in these categories include:

Cimetidine (The high renal clearance of desglymidodrine is due to active tubular secretion by the base-secreting system also responsible for the secretion of cimetidine; possibility of drug interaction exists with co-administration). Products include:
- Tagamet HB 200 Tablets ..... ■664

Deslanoside (Co-administration with cardiac glycosides may enhance or precipitate bradycardia, AV block or arrhythmia).
- No products indexed under this heading.

Digitalis Glycoside Preparations (Co-administration with cardiac glycosides may enhance or precipitate bradycardia, AV block, or arrhythmia).
- No products indexed under this heading.

Digitoxin (Co-administration with cardiac glycosides may enhance or precipitate bradycardia, AV block or arrhythmia).
- No products indexed under this heading.

Digoxin (Co-administration with cardiac glycosides may enhance or precipitate bradycardia, AV block or arrhythmia). Products include:
- Lanoxicaps Capsules 1490
- Lanoxin Injection 1494
- Lanoxin Injection Pediatric 1497
- Lanoxin Tablets 1500

Dihydroergotamine Mesylate (Co-administration with alpha-adrenergic receptor stimulants may enhance or potentiate pressor effects of midodrine). Products include:
- Migranal Nasal Spray 3348

Doxazosin Mesylate (Alpha adrenergic blocking agents can antagonize the effects of midodrine). Products include:
- Cardura XL Tablets 2515

Ephedrine Hydrochloride (Co-administration with alpha-adrenergic receptor stimulants may enhance or potentiate pressor effects of midodrine).
- No products indexed under this heading.

Ephedrine Sulfate (Co-administration with alpha-adrenergic receptor stimulants may enhance or potentiate pressor effects of midodrine).
- No products indexed under this heading.

Ephedrine Tannate (Co-administration with alpha-adrenergic receptor stimulants may enhance or potentiate pressor effects of midodrine).
- No products indexed under this heading.

Flecainide Acetate (The high renal clearance of desglymidodrine is due to active tubular secretion by the base-secreting system also responsible for the secretion of flecainide; possibility of drug interaction exists with co-administration). Products include:
- Tambocor Tablets 1856

Fludrocortisone Acetate (Co-administration with salt-retaining steroid therapy increases the potential for supine hypertension; this can be minimized by reducing the dose of fludrocortisone or decreasing salt intake).
- No products indexed under this heading.

Metformin (The high renal clearance of desglymidodrine is due to active tubular secretion by the base-secreting system also responsible for the secretion of metformin; possibility of drug interaction exists with co-administration).
- No products indexed under this heading.

Phenylephrine Hydrochloride (Co-administration with alpha-adrenergic receptor stimulants may enhance or potentiate pressor effects of midodrine). Products include:
- Comtrex Maximum Strength Non-Drowsy Cold & Cough Caplets ..... ■725
- Comtrex Maximum Strength Day/Night Severe Cold & Sinus Caplets - Day Formulation ..... ■725
- Comtrex Maximum Strength Day/Night Severe Cold & Sinus Caplets - Night Formulation ..... ■725
- Contac Cold and Flu Maximum Strength Caplets ..... ■728
- Contac Cold and Flu Day and Night Caplets (Day Formulation Only) ..... ■727
- Contac Cold and Flu Day and Night Caplets (Night Formulation Only) ..... ■727
- Contac Cold and Flu Non-Drowsy Caplets ..... ■728
- Contac-D Cold Non-Drowsy Tablets ..... ■729
- Children's Dimetapp Cold & Allergy Elixir ..... ■730
- Children's Dimetapp Cold & Allergy Chewable Tablets ..... ■730
- Children's Dimetapp DM Cold & Cough Elixir ..... ■731
- Toddler's Dimetapp Cold and Cough Drops ..... ■732
- Excedrin Sinus Headache Caplets/Tablets ..... ■610
- 4-Way Fast Acting Nasal Spray ..... ■775
- 4-Way Menthol Nasal Spray ..... ■775
- Preparation H Maximum Strength Cream ..... ■666
- Preparation H Cooling Gel ..... ■666
- Preparation H ..... ■666
- Refenesen PE Caplets ..... ■721
- Robitussin Cough & Allergy Syrup ..... ■736
- Robitussin Cough & Cold Nighttime Liquid ..... ■736
- Robitussin Cough, Cold & Flu Nighttime Liquid ..... ■738
- Robitussin Head & Chest Congestion PE Syrup ..... ■739
- Robitussin Pediatric Cough & Cold Nighttime Liquid ..... ■736
- TheraFlu Cold & Cough Hot Liquid ..... ■740
- TheraFlu Cold & Sore Throat Hot Liquid ..... ■741
- TheraFlu Flu & Sore Throat Hot Liquid ..... ■742
- TheraFlu Daytime Severe Cold Hot Liquid ..... ■742
- TheraFlu Nighttime Severe Cold Hot Liquid ..... ■740
- TheraFlu Warming Relief Daytime Severe Cold ..... ■743
- TheraFlu Warming Relief Nighttime Severe Cold ..... ■743
- Triaminic Chest & Nasal Congestion Liquid ..... ■746
- Triaminic Cold & Allergy Liquid ..... ■746
- Triaminic Daytime Cold & Cough Liquid ..... ■745
- Triaminic Nighttime Cold & Cough Liquid ..... ■746
- Triaminic Thin Strips Cold ..... ■748
- Triaminic Thin Strips Cold & Cough ..... ■778
- Triaminic Infant Thin Strips Decongestant ..... ■747
- Triaminic Infant Thin Strips Decongestant Plus Cough ..... ■747
- Children's Tylenol Plus Flu Oral Suspension ..... ■749
- Tylenol Cold Head Congestion Daytime Caplets with Cool Burst and Gelcaps ..... ■750
- Tylenol Cold Multi-Symptom Daytime Liquid ..... ■752
- Tylenol Cold Multi-Symptom Severe Daytime Liquid ..... ■752
- Concentrated Tylenol Infants' Drops Plus Cold & Cough ..... ■754
- Tylenol Allergy Multi-Symptom Caplets with Cool Burst and Gelcaps 1872
- Tylenol Allergy Multi-Symptom Nighttime Caplets with Cool Burst 1872
- Children's Tylenol Plus Cold Suspension Liquid 1879
- Children's Tylenol Plus Cold & Allergy Suspension Liquid 1878
- Children's Tylenol Plus Flu Suspension Liquid 1881
- Children's Tylenol Plus Multi-Symptom Cold Suspension Liquid 1879
- Tylenol Cold Head Congestion Daytime Caplets with Cool Burst 1873
- Tylenol Cold Head Congestion Nighttime Caplets with Cool Burst 1873
- Tylenol Cold Head Congestion Severe Caplets with Cool Burst 1873
- Tylenol Cold Multi-Symptom Daytime Caplets with Cool Burst and Gelcaps 1874
- Tylenol Cold Multi-Symptom Daytime Liquid with Citrus Burst 1874
- Tylenol Cold Multi-Symptom Nighttime Caplets with Cool Burst 1874
- Tylenol Cold Multi-Symptom Nighttime Liquid with Cool Burst 1874
- Tylenol Cold Multi-Symptom Severe Caplets with Cool Burst 1874
- Tylenol Cold Multi-Symptom Severe Daytime Liquid with Citrus Burst 1874
- Tylenol Sinus Congestion & Pain Daytime Caplets with Cool Burst and Gelcaps 1876
- Tylenol Sinus Congestion & Pain Nighttime Caplets with Cool Burst 1876
- Tylenol Sinus Congestion & Pain Severe Caplets with Cool Burst 1876
- Vicks 44D Cough & Head Congestion Relief Liquid ..... ■760
- Vicks DayQuil LiquiCaps/Liquid Multi-Symptom Cold/Flu Relief ..... ■761
- Zicam Cough Plus D Cough Spray ..... ■767

Phenylephrine Tannate (Co-administration with alpha-adrenergic receptor stimulants may enhance or potentiate pressor effects of midodrine).
- No products indexed under this heading.

Prazosin Hydrochloride (Alpha adrenergic blocking agents can antagonize the effects of midodrine).
- No products indexed under this heading.

Procainamide Hydrochloride (The high renal clearance of desglymidodrine is due to active tubular secretion by the base-secreting system also responsible for the secretion of procainamide; possibility of drug interaction exists with co-administration).
- No products indexed under this heading.

Pseudoephedrine Hydrochloride (Co-administration with alpha-adrenergic receptor stimulants may enhance or potentiate pressor effects of midodrine). Products include:
- Advil Allergy Sinus Caplets ..... ■770
- Advil Cold & Sinus ..... ■723
- Advil Multi-Symptom Cold Caplets ..... ■770
- Aleve Cold & Sinus Caplets 744
- Allegra-D 12 Hour Extended-Release Tablets 2846
- Allegra-D 24 Hour Extended-Release Tablets 2849
- BC Cold Powder ..... ■677
- Comtrex Maximum Strength Cold & Cough Day/Night Caplets - Day Formulation ..... ■726
- Comtrex Maximum Strength Cold & Cough Day/Night Caplets - Night Formulation ..... ■726
- Children's Motrin Cold Oral Suspension 1867
- Mucinex D Extended-Release Bi-Layer Tablets ..... ■776
- Robitussin Cough & Cold CF Liquid ..... ■735
- Robitussin Cough & Cold Pediatric Drops ..... ■735
- Tylenol Sinus Congestion & Pain Nighttime Caplets with Cool Burst ..... ■778
- Tylenol Cold Severe Congestion Non-Drowsy Caplets with Cool Burst 1874
- Tylenol Sinus Severe Congestion Caplets with Cool Burst 1876
- Vicks 44D Cough & Head Congestion Relief Liquid 2679
- Vicks 44M Cough, Cold & Flu Relief Liquid 2680
- Vicks DayQuil Multi-Symptom Cold/Flu Relief LiquiCaps 2678
- Vicks DayQuil Multi-Symptom Cold/Flu Relief Liquid 2678
- Vicks NyQuil Multi-Symptom Cold/Flu Relief Liquid 2681
- Vicks NyQuil Multi-Symptom Cold/Flu Relief LiquiCaps 2681
- Children's Vicks NyQuil Cold/Cough Relief Liquid 2680
- Zyrtec-D 12 Hour Extended Release Tablets 2597

Pseudoephedrine Sulfate (Co-administration with alpha-adrenergic receptor stimulants may enhance or potentiate pressor effects of midodrine). Products include:
- Alavert Allergy & Sinus D-12 Hour Tablets ..... ■771
- Clarinex-D 24-Hour Extended-Release Tablets 2998
- Claritin-D Non-Drowsy 12 Hour Tablets ..... ■772
- Claritin-D Non-Drowsy 24 Hour Tablets ..... ■772

Quinidine (The high renal clearance of desglymidodrine is due to active tubular secretion by the base-secreting system also responsible for the secretion of quinidine; possibility of drug interaction exists with co-administration).
No products indexed under this heading.

Quinidine Gluconate (The high renal clearance of desglymidodrine is due to active tubular secretion by the base-secreting system also responsible for the secretion of quinidine; possibility of drug interaction exists with co-administration).
No products indexed under this heading.

Quinidine Hydrochloride (The high renal clearance of desglymidodrine is due to active tubular secretion by the base-secreting system also responsible for the secretion of quinidine; possibility of drug interaction exists with co-administration).
No products indexed under this heading.

Quinidine Polygalacturonate (The high renal clearance of desglymidodrine is due to active tubular secretion by the base-secreting system also responsible for the secretion of quinidine; possibility of drug interaction exists with co-administration).
No products indexed under this heading.

Quinidine Sulfate (The high renal clearance of desglymidodrine is due to active tubular secretion by the base-secreting system also responsible for the secretion of quinidine; possibility of drug interaction exists with co-administration).
No products indexed under this heading.

Ranitidine Hydrochloride (The high renal clearance of desglymidodrine is due to active tubular secretion by the base-secreting system also responsible for the secretion of ranitidine; possibility of drug interaction exists with co-administration). Products include:
Zantac **1624**
Zantac Injection **1619**
Zantac Injection Pharmacy Bulk Package **1622**

Tamsulosin Hydrochloride (Alpha adrenergic blocking agents can antagonize the effects of midodrine). Products include:
Flomax Capsules **850**

Terazosin Hydrochloride (Alpha adrenergic blocking agents can antagonize the effects of midodrine). Products include:
Hytrin Capsules **471**

Triamterene (The high renal clearance of desglymidodrine is due to active tubular secretion by the base-secreting system also responsible for the secretion of triamterene; possibility of drug interaction exists with co-administration). Products include:
Dyazide Capsules **1423**
Dyrenium Capsules **3400**

PROCHIEVE 4% GEL
(Progesterone) **1003**
None cited in PDR database.

PROCHIEVE 8% GEL
(Progesterone) **1003**
None cited in PDR database.

PROCOSA II TABLETS
(Glucosamine Sulfate) **3339**
None cited in PDR database.

PROCRIT FOR INJECTION
(Epoetin Alfa) **2364**
None cited in PDR database.

PROCTOFOAM-HC
(Hydrocortisone Acetate, Pramoxine Hydrochloride) **3099**
None cited in PDR database.

PROFILNINE SD, FACTOR IX COMPLEX (HUMAN)
(Factor IX Complex) **1660**
None cited in PDR database.

PROFLAVANOL 90 TABLETS
(Dietary Supplement) **3339**
None cited in PDR database.

PROGRAF CAPSULES AND INJECTION
(Tacrolimus) **632**
May interact with aminoglycosides, calcium channel blockers, cytochrome p450 3a inducers (selected), cytochrome p450 3a inhibitors (selected), erythromycin, methylprednisolone, phenytoin, protease inhibitors, potassium sparing diuretics, vaccines, live, and certain other agents. Compounds in these categories include:

Allium sativum (Since tacrolimus is metabolized mainly by the CYP3A enzyme systems, drugs known to induce these enzymes may result in an increased metabolism of tacrolimus or decreased bioavailability as indicated by decreased whole blood or plasma concentrations. Monitoring of blood concentrations and appropriate dosage adjustments are essential when such drugs are used concomitantly).
No products indexed under this heading.

Aluminum Hydroxide (Co-administration has resulted in a 21% increase in the mean tacrolimus AUC and a 10% decrease in the Cmax). Products include:
Gaviscon Regular Strength Liquid .... ■658
Gaviscon Regular Strength Tablets .... ■658
Gaviscon Extra Strength Liquid .... ■658
Gaviscon Extra Strength Tablets .... ■658
Maalox Regular Strength Antacid/Antigas Liquid **2175**
Maalox Max Maximum Strength Antacid/Anti-Gas Liquid **2176**

Amikacin Sulfate (Potential for additive or synergistic impairment of renal function).
No products indexed under this heading.

Amiloride Hydrochloride (Mild to severe hyperkalemia has been reported with tacrolimus; concurrent use with potassium-sparing diuretics should be avoided). Products include:
Midamor Tablets **2026**
Moduretic Tablets **2028**

Amiodarone Hydrochloride (Since tacrolimus is metabolized mainly by the CYP3A enzyme systems, substances known to inhibit these enzymes may decrease the metabolism or increase bioavailability of tacrolimus as indicated by increased whole blood or plasma concentrations. Monitoringof blood concentrations and appropriate dosage adjustments are essential when such drugs are used concomitantly).
No products indexed under this heading.

Amlodipine Besylate (While calcium-channel blocking agents can be effective in treating tacrolimus-associated hypertension, care should be taken since interference with tacrolimus metabolism may require dosage reduction). Products include:
Caduet Tablets **2508**
Lotrel Capsules **2249**
Norvasc Tablets **2545**

Amphotericin B (Potential for additive or synergistic impairment of renal function).
No products indexed under this heading.

Amprenavir (Co-administration with drugs known to inhibit CYP3A enzyme systems, such as protease inhibitors, may increase tacrolimus blood concentrations). Products include:
Agenerase Capsules **1327**
Agenerase Oral Solution **1332**

Aprepitant (Since tacrolimus is metabolized mainly by the CYP3A enzyme systems, substances known to inhibit these enzymes may decrease the metabolism or increase bioavailability of tacrolimus as indicated by increased whole blood or plasma concentrations. Monitoringof blood concentrations and appropriate dosage adjustments are essential when such drugs are used concomitantly). Products include:
Emend Capsules **1963**

BCG Vaccine (Immunosupressants may affect vaccination. Therefore, during treatment with tacrolimus, vaccination may be less effective. The use of live vaccines should be avoided).
No products indexed under this heading.

Bepridil Hydrochloride (While calcium-channel blocking agents can be effective in treating tacrolimus-associated hypertension, care should be taken since interference with tacrolimus metabolism may require dosage reduction).
No products indexed under this heading.

Bromocriptine Mesylate (Co-administration with drugs known to inhibit CYP3A enzyme systems, such as bromocriptine, may increase tacrolimus blood concentrations).
No products indexed under this heading.

Carbamazepine (Co-administration with drugs known to induce CYP3A enzyme systems, such as carbamazepine, may result in increased metabolism of tacrolimus and decreased blood or plasma concentrations). Products include:
Carbatrol Capsules **3171**
Equetro Extended-Release Capsules **3180**
Tegretol/Tegretol-XR **2295**

Caspofungin acetate (Co-administration has resulted in a significant decrease in oral tacrolimus blood concentrations). Products include:
Cancidas for Injection **1918**

Chloramphenicol (Co-administration with drugs known to inhibit CYP3A enzyme systems, such as chloramphenicol, may increase tacrolimus blood concentrations).
No products indexed under this heading.

Chloramphenicol Palmitate (Co-administration with drugs known to inhibit CYP3A enzyme systems, such as chloramphenicol, may increase tacrolimus blood concentrations).
No products indexed under this heading.

Chloramphenicol Sodium Succinate (Co-administration with drugs known to inhibit CYP3A enzyme systems, such as chloramphenicol, may increase tacrolimus blood concentrations).
No products indexed under this heading.

Cimetidine (Co-administration with drugs known to inhibit CYP3A enzyme systems, such as cimetidine, may increase tacrolimus blood concentrations). Products include:
Tagamet HB 200 Tablets .... ■**664**

Cimetidine Hydrochloride (Co-administration with drugs known to inhibit CYP3A enzyme systems, such as cimetidine, may increase tacrolimus blood concentrations).
No products indexed under this heading.

Ciprofloxacin (Since tacrolimus is metabolized mainly by the CYP3A enzyme systems, substances known to inhibit these enzymes may decrease the metabolism or increase bioavailability of tacrolimus as indicated by increased whole blood or plasma concentrations. Monitoringof blood concentrations and appropriate dosage adjustments are essential when such drugs are used concomitantly). Products include:
Cipro Oral Suspension **2977**
Cipro I.V. **2984**
Cipro XR Tablets **2990**
Ciprodex Otic Suspension **559**

Ciprofloxacin Hydrochloride (Since tacrolimus is metabolized mainly by the CYP3A enzyme systems, substances known to inhibit these enzymes may decrease the metabolism or increase bioavailability of tacrolimus as indicated by increased whole blood or plasma concentrations. Monitoringof blood concentrations and appropriate dosage adjustments are essential when such drugs are used concomitantly). Products include:
Ciloxan Ophthalmic Ointment **559**
Ciloxan Ophthalmic Solution .... ⊙**206**
Cipro Tablets **2977**
Proquin XR Tablets **1153**

Cisapride (Co-administration with drugs known to inhibit CYP3A enzyme systems, such as cisapride, may increase tacrolimus blood concentrations).
No products indexed under this heading.

Cisplatin (Potential for additive or synergistic impairment of renal function).
No products indexed under this heading.

Clarithromycin (Co-administration with drugs known to inhibit CYP3A enzyme systems, such as clarithromycin, may increase tacrolimus blood concentrations). Products include:
Biaxin/Biaxin XL **402**
PREVPAC **3284**

Clotrimazole (Co-administration with drugs known to inhibit CYP3A enzyme systems, such as clotrimazole, may increase tacrolimus blood concentrations). Products include:

Desenex Athlete's Foot Cream 635
Lotrimin 3039
Lotrisone 3040

Cyclosporine (Increases tacrolimus blood levels resulting in additive/synergistic nephrotoxicity; Prograf should not be used simultaneously with cyclosporine; Prograf or cyclosporine should be discontinued at least 24 hours or more prior to initiating the other). Products include:

Gengraf Capsules 459
Neoral Oral Solution 2259
Neoral Soft Gelatin Capsules 2259
Restasis Ophthalmic Emulsion 575
Sandimmune 2275

Danazol (Co-administration with drugs known to inhibit CYP3A enzyme systems, such as danazol, may increase tacrolimus blood concentrations).

No products indexed under this heading.

Delavirdine Mesylate (Since tacrolimus is metabolized mainly by the CYP3A enzyme systems, substances known to inhibit these enzymes may decrease the metabolism or increase bioavailability of tacrolimus as indicated by increased whole blood or plasma concentrations. Monitoringof blood concentrations and appropriate dosage adjustments are essential when such drugs are used concomitantly). Products include:

Rescriptor Tablets 2551

Dexamethasone (Since tacrolimus is metabolized mainly by the CYP3A enzyme systems, drugs known to induce these enzymes may result in an increased metabolism of tacrolimus or decreased bioavailability as indicated by decreased whole blood or plasma concentrations. Monitoring of blood concentrations and appropriate dosage adjustments are essential when such drugs are used concomitantly). Products include:

Ciprodex Otic Suspension 559
Decadron Tablets 1951
TobraDex Ophthalmic Ointment 562
TobraDex Ophthalmic Suspension ... 563

Diltiazem Hydrochloride (Co-administration with drugs known to inhibit CYP3A enzyme systems, such as diltiazem, may increase tacrolimus blood concentrations). Products include:

Cardizem LA Extended Release Tablets 1728
Tiazac Capsules 1201

Diltiazem Maleate (Since tacrolimus is metabolized mainly by the CYP3A enzyme systems, substances known to inhibit these enzymes may decrease the metabolism or increase bioavailability of tacrolimus as indicated by increased whole blood or plasma concentrations. Monitoringof blood concentrations and appropriate dosage adjustments are essential when such drugs are used concomitantly).

No products indexed under this heading.

Efavirenz (Since tacrolimus is metabolized mainly by the CYP3A enzyme systems, substances known to inhibit these enzymes may decrease the metabolism or increase bioavailability of tacrolimus as indicated by increased whole blood or plasma concentrations. Monitoringof blood concentrations and appropriate dosage adjustments are essential when such drugs are used concomitantly). Products include:

Atripla Tablets 945
Sustiva Capsules 930
Sustiva Tablets 930

Erythromycin (Co-administration with drugs known to inhibit CYP3A enzyme systems, such as erythromycin, may increase tacrolimus blood concentrations). Products include:

Ery-Tab Tablets 449
Erythromycin Base Filmtab Tablets 455
Erythromycin Delayed-Release Capsules, USP 457
PCE Dispertab Tablets 515

Erythromycin Estolate (Co-administration with drugs known to inhibit CYP3A enzyme systems, such as erythromycin, may increase tacrolimus blood concentrations).

No products indexed under this heading.

Erythromycin Ethylsuccinate (Co-administration with drugs known to inhibit CYP3A enzyme systems, such as erythromycin, may increase tacrolimus blood concentrations). Products include:

E.E.S. 451
EryPed 447

Erythromycin Gluceptate (Co-administration with drugs known to inhibit CYP3A enzyme systems, such as erythromycin, may increase tacrolimus blood concentrations).

No products indexed under this heading.

Erythromycin Lactobionate (Co-administration with drugs known to inhibit CYP3A enzyme systems, such as erythromycin, may increase tacrolimus blood concentrations).

No products indexed under this heading.

Erythromycin Stearate (Co-administration with drugs known to inhibit CYP3A enzyme systems, such as erythromycin, may increase tacrolimus blood concentrations). Products include:

Erythrocin Stearate Filmtab Tablets 453

Ethinyl Estradiol (May increase tacrolimus blood concentrations). Products include:

Mircette Tablets 1066
NuvaRing 2340
Ortho-Cyclen/Ortho Tri-Cyclen 2429
Ortho Evra Transdermal System 2417
Ortho Tri-Cyclen Lo Tablets 2436
Seasonique Tablets 1077
Yasmin 28 Tablets 796
Yaz Tablets 803

Ethosuximide (Since tacrolimus is metabolized mainly by the CYP3A enzyme systems, drugs known to induce these enzymes may result in an increased metabolism of tacrolimus or decreased bioavailability as indicated by decreased whole blood or plasma concentrations. Monitoring of blood concentrations and appropriate dosage adjustments are essential when such drugs are used concomitantly).

No products indexed under this heading.

Felodipine (While calcium-channel blocking agents can be effective in treating tacrolimus-associated hypertension, care should be taken since interference with tacrolimus metabolism may require dosage reduction).

No products indexed under this heading.

Fluconazole (Co-administration with drugs known to inhibit CYP3A enzyme systems, such as fluconazole, may increase tacrolimus blood concentrations).

No products indexed under this heading.

Fluoxetine (Since tacrolimus is metabolized mainly by the CYP3A enzyme systems, substances known to inhibit these enzymes may decrease the metabolism or increase bioavailability of tacrolimus as indicated by increased whole blood or plasma concentrations. Monitoringof blood concentrations and appropriate dosage adjustments are essential when such drugs are used concomitantly).

No products indexed under this heading.

Fluoxetine Hydrochloride (Since tacrolimus is metabolized mainly by the CYP3A enzyme systems, substances known to inhibit these enzymes may decrease the metabolism or increase bioavailability of tacrolimus as indicated by increased whole blood or plasma concentrations. Monitoringof blood concentrations and appropriate dosage adjustments are essential when such drugs are used concomitantly). Products include:

Prozac Pulvules and Liquid 1801
Symbyax Capsules 1819

Fluvoxamine Maleate (Since tacrolimus is metabolized mainly by the CYP3A enzyme systems, substances known to inhibit these enzymes may decrease the metabolism or increase bioavailability of tacrolimus as indicated by increased whole blood or plasma concentrations. Monitoringof blood concentrations and appropriate dosage adjustments are essential when such drugs are used concomitantly).

No products indexed under this heading.

Fosphenytoin Sodium (Co-administration may result in increased metabolism of tacrolimus and decreased plasma levels; tacrolimus may increase the plasma phenytoin levels).

No products indexed under this heading.

Ganciclovir (May increase nephrotoxicity).

No products indexed under this heading.

Ganciclovir Sodium (May increase nephrotoxicity).

No products indexed under this heading.

Gentamicin Sulfate (Potential for additive or synergistic impairment of renal function). Products include:

Garamycin Injectable 3014
Pred-G Ophthalmic Ointment .... ⊙237
Pred-G Ophthalmic Suspension .... ⊙236

Hypericum (Co-administration with St. John's Wort may result in decreased tacrolimus blood concentrations). Products include:

Satiete Tablets 832

Indinavir Sulfate (Co-administration with drugs known to inhibit CYP3A enzyme systems, such as protease inhibitors, may increase tacrolimus blood concentrations). Products include:

Crixivan Capsules 1940

Isoniazid (Since tacrolimus is metabolized mainly by the CYP3A enzyme systems, substances known to inhibit these enzymes may decrease the metabolism or increase bioavailability of tacrolimus as indicated by increased whole blood or plasma concentrations. Monitoringof blood concentrations and appropriate dosage adjustments are essential when such drugs are used concomitantly).

No products indexed under this heading.

Isradipine (While calcium-channel blocking agents can be effective in treating tacrolimus-associated hypertension, care should be taken since interference with tacrolimus metabolism may require dosage reduction). Products include:

DynaCirc CR Tablets 2721

Itraconazole (Co-administration with drugs known to inhibit CYP3A enzyme systems, such as itraconazole, may increase tacrolimus blood concentrations).

No products indexed under this heading.

Kanamycin Sulfate (Potential for additive or synergistic impairment of renal function).

No products indexed under this heading.

Ketoconazole (Co-administration has resulted in a significant increase in tacrolimus bioavailability and significant decrease in clearance; overall IV clearance of tacrolimus was not significantly changed by ketoconazole, although it was highly variable between patients). Products include:

Nizoral A-D Shampoo, 1% 1868

Lopinavir (Co-administration with drugs known to inhibit CYP3A enzyme systems, such as protease inhibitors, may increase tacrolimus blood concentrations). Products include:

Kaletra 476

Magnesium Hydroxide (Co-administration has resulted in a 21% increase in the mean tacrolimus AUC and a 10% decrease in the Cmax). Products include:

Maalox Regular Strength Antacid/Antigas Liquid 2175
Maalox Max Maximum Strength Antacid/Anti-Gas Liquid 2176
Pepcid Complete Chewable Tablets 1701

Measles, Mumps, Rubella and Varicella Virus Vaccine Live (Immunosupressants may affect vaccination. Therefore, during treatment with tacrolimus, vaccination may be less effective. The use of live vaccines should be avoided). Products include:

ProQuad 2064

Measles, Mumps & Rubella Virus Vaccine, Live (During treatment with tacrolimus, vaccination may be less effective). Products include:

M-M-R II 2006

Measles & Rubella Virus Vaccine Live (During treatment with tacrolimus, vaccination may be less effective).

No products indexed under this heading.

Measles Virus Vaccine Live (During treatment with tacrolimus, vaccination may be less effective). Products include:

Attenuvax **1914**

Methylprednisolone (May increase tacrolimus blood concentrations).
No products indexed under this heading.

Methylprednisolone Acetate (May increase tacrolimus blood concentrations). Products include:
Depo-Medrol Injectable Suspension **2617**
Depo-Medrol Single-Dose Vial **2619**

Methylprednisolone Sodium Succinate (May increase tacrolimus blood concentrations).
No products indexed under this heading.

Metoclopramide Hydrochloride (Co-administration with drugs known to inhibit CYP3A enzyme systems, such as metoclopramide, may increase tacrolimus blood concentrations).
No products indexed under this heading.

Metronidazole (Since tacrolimus is metabolized mainly by the CYP3A enzyme systems, substances known to inhibit these enzymes may decrease the metabolism or increase bioavailability of tacrolimus as indicated by increased whole blood or plasma concentrations. Monitoringof blood concentrations and appropriate dosage adjustments are essential when such drugs are used concomitantly). Products include:
Metrogel 1% **1211**
MetroGel-Vaginal Gel **1855**
Vandazole Vaginal Gel **3338**

Metronidazole Benzoate (Since tacrolimus is metabolized mainly by the CYP3A enzyme systems, substances known to inhibit these enzymes may decrease the metabolism or increase bioavailability of tacrolimus as indicated by increased whole blood or plasma concentrations. Monitoringof blood concentrations and appropriate dosage adjustments are essential when such drugs are used concomitantly).
No products indexed under this heading.

Metronidazole Hydrochloride (Since tacrolimus is metabolized mainly by the CYP3A enzyme systems, substances known to inhibit these enzymes may decrease the metabolism or increase bioavailability of tacrolimus as indicated by increased whole blood or plasma concentrations. Monitoringof blood concentrations and appropriate dosage adjustments are essential when such drugs are used concomitantly).
No products indexed under this heading.

Mibefradil Dihydrochloride (While calcium-channel blocking agents can be effective in treating tacrolimus-associated hypertension, care should be taken since interference with tacrolimus metabolism may require dosage reduction).
No products indexed under this heading.

Miconazole (Since tacrolimus is metabolized mainly by the CYP3A enzyme systems, substances known to inhibit these enzymes may decrease the metabolism or increase bioavailability of tacrolimus as indicated by increased whole blood or plasma concentrations. Monitoringof blood concentrations and appropriate dosage adjustments are essential when such drugs are used concomitantly).
No products indexed under this heading.

Modafinil (Since tacrolimus is metabolized mainly by the CYP3A enzyme systems, drugs known to induce these enzymes may result in an increased metabolism of tacrolimus or decreased bioavailability as indicated by decreased whole blood or plasma concentrations. Monitoring of blood concentrations and appropriate dosage adjustments are essential when such drugs are used concomitantly). Products include:
Provigil Tablets **988**

Mumps Virus Vaccine, Live (Immunosupressants may affect vaccination. Therefore, during treatment with tacrolimus, vaccination may be less effective. The use of live vaccines should be avoided). Products include:
Mumpsvax **2031**

Nefazodone Hydrochloride (May increase tacrolimus blood concentrations).
No products indexed under this heading.

Nelfinavir Mesylate (Co-administration has resulted in a significant increase in oral tacrolimus blood concentrations). Products include:
Viracept **2577**

Nevirapine (Since tacrolimus is metabolized mainly by the CYP3A enzyme systems, drugs known to induce these enzymes may result in an increased metabolism of tacrolimus or decreased bioavailability as indicated by decreased whole blood or plasma concentrations. Monitoring of blood concentrations and appropriate dosage adjustments are essential when such drugs are used concomitantly). Products include:
Viramune Oral Suspension **873**
Viramune Tablets **873**

Nicardipine Hydrochloride (Co-administration with drugs known to inhibit CYP3A enzyme systems, such as nicardipine, may increase tacrolimus blood concentrations). Products include:
Cardene I.V. **2497**

Nifedipine (Co-administration with drugs known to inhibit CYP3A enzyme systems, such as nifedipine, may increase tacrolimus blood concentrations). Products include:
Adalat CC Tablets **2964**

Nimodipine (While calcium-channel blocking agents can be effective in treating tacrolimus-associated hypertension, care should be taken since interference with tacrolimus metabolism may require dosage reduction). Products include:
Nimotop Capsules **749**

Nisoldipine (While calcium-channel blocking agents can be effective in treating tacrolimus-associated hypertension, care should be taken since interference with tacrolimus metabolism may require dosage reduction). Products include:
Sular Tablets **3122**

Norfloxacin (Since tacrolimus is metabolized mainly by the CYP3A enzyme systems, substances known to inhibit these enzymes may decrease the metabolism or increase bioavailability of tacrolimus as indicated by increased whole blood or plasma concentrations. Monitoringof blood concentrations and appropriate dosage adjustments are essential when such drugs are used concomitantly). Products include:
Noroxin Tablets **2032**

Omeprazole (May increase tacrolimus blood concentrations). Products include:
Zegerid Capsules **2958**
Zegerid Powder for Oral Solution **2958**

Paroxetine Hydrochloride (Since tacrolimus is metabolized mainly by the CYP3A enzyme systems, substances known to inhibit these enzymes may decrease the metabolism or increase bioavailability of tacrolimus as indicated by increased whole blood or plasma concentrations. Monitoringof blood concentrations and appropriate dosage adjustments are essential when such drugs are used concomitantly). Products include:
Paxil CR Controlled-Release Tablets **1538**
Paxil **1530**

Phenobarbital (Co-administration with drugs known to induce CYP3A enzyme systems, such as phenobarbital, may result in increased metabolism of tacrolimus and decreased blood or plasma concentrations). Products include:
Donnatal Extentabs **2493**

Phenytoin (Co-administration may result in increased metabolism of tacrolimus and decreased plasma levels; tacrolimus may increase the plasma phenytoin levels).
No products indexed under this heading.

Phenytoin Sodium (Co-administration may result in increased metabolism of tacrolimus and decreased plasma levels; tacrolimus may increase the plasma phenytoin levels). Products include:
Phenytek Capsules **2160**

Poliovirus Vaccine, Live, Oral, Trivalent, Types 1,2,3 (Sabin) (During treatment with tacrolimus, vaccination may be less effective).
No products indexed under this heading.

Poliovirus Vaccine Inactivated, Trivalent Types 1,2,3 (During treatment with tacrolimus, vaccination may be less effective). Products include:
Pediarix Vaccine **1548**

Quinine (Since tacrolimus is metabolized mainly by the CYP3A enzyme systems, substances known to inhibit these enzymes may decrease the metabolism or increase bioavailability of tacrolimus as indicated by increased whole blood or plasma concentrations. Monitoringof blood concentrations and appropriate dosage adjustments are essential when such drugs are used concomitantly).
No products indexed under this heading.

Quinine Sulfate (Since tacrolimus is metabolized mainly by the CYP3A enzyme systems, substances known to inhibit these enzymes may decrease the metabolism or increase bioavailability of tacrolimus as indicated by increased whole blood or plasma concentrations. Monitoringof blood concentrations and appropriate dosage adjustments are essential when such drugs are used concomitantly).
No products indexed under this heading.

Rifabutin (Co-administration with drugs known to induce CYP3A enzyme systems, such as rifabutin, may result in increased metabolism of tacrolimus and decreased blood or plasma concentrations).
No products indexed under this heading.

Rifampicin (Since tacrolimus is metabolized mainly by the CYP3A enzyme systems, drugs known to induce these enzymes may result in an increased metabolism of tacrolimus or decreased bioavailability as indicated by decreased whole blood or plasma concentrations. Monitoring of blood concentrations and appropriate dosage adjustments are essential when such drugs are used concomitantly).
No products indexed under this heading.

Rifampin (Co-administration has resulted in a significant decrease in oral tacrolimus bioavailability and significant increase in clearance).
No products indexed under this heading.

Rifapentine (Since tacrolimus is metabolized mainly by the CYP3A enzyme systems, drugs known to induce these enzymes may result in an increased metabolism of tacrolimus or decreased bioavailability as indicated by decreased whole blood or plasma concentrations. Monitoring of blood concentrations and appropriate dosage adjustments are essential when such drugs are used concomitantly).
No products indexed under this heading.

Ritonavir (Co-administration with drugs known to inhibit CYP3A enzyme systems, such as protease inhibitors, may increase tacrolimus blood concentrations). Products include:
Kaletra **476**
Norvir **503**

Rotavirus Vaccine, Live, Oral, Tetravalent (Immunosupressants may affect vaccination. Therefore, during treatment with tacrolimus, vaccination may be less effective. The use of live vaccines should be avoided).
No products indexed under this heading.

Rubella & Mumps Virus Vaccine Live (Immunosupressants may affect vaccination. Therefore, during treatment with tacrolimus, vaccination may be less effective. The use of live vaccines should be avoided).
No products indexed under this heading.

Rubella Virus Vaccine Live (Immunosupressants may affect vaccination. Therefore, during treatment with tacrolimus, vaccination may be less effective. The use of live vaccines should be avoided). Products include:

Meruvax II 2019

Saquinavir (Co-administration with drugs known to inhibit CYP3A enzyme systems, such as protease inhibitors, may increase tacrolimus blood concentrations).

No products indexed under this heading.

Saquinavir Mesylate (Co-administration with drugs known to inhibit CYP3A enzyme systems, such as protease inhibitors, may increase tacrolimus blood concentrations). Products include:

Invirase 2772

Sertraline Hydrochloride (Since tacrolimus is metabolized mainly by the CYP3A enzyme systems, substances known to inhibit these enzymes may decrease the metabolism or increase bioavailability of tacrolimus as indicated by increased whole blood or plasma concentrations. Monitoringof blood concentrations and appropriate dosage adjustments are essential when such drugs are used concomitantly). Products include:

Zoloft 2586

Sirolimus (Co-administration has resulted in a 30% decrease in oral tacrolimus AUC(0-12) and Cmin). Products include:

Rapamune Oral Solution and Tablets 3475

Smallpox Vaccine (Immunosupressants may affect vaccination. Therefore, during treatment with tacrolimus, vaccination may be less effective. The use of live vaccines should be avoided).

No products indexed under this heading.

Spironolactone (Mild to severe hyperkalemia has been reported with tacrolimus; concurrent use with potassium-sparing diuretics should be avoided).

No products indexed under this heading.

Streptomycin Sulfate (Potential for additive or synergistic impairment of renal function).

No products indexed under this heading.

Tobramycin (Potential for additive or synergistic impairment of renal function). Products include:

TOBI Solution for Inhalation 2298
TobraDex Ophthalmic Ointment 562
TobraDex Ophthalmic Suspension ... 563
Zylet Ophthalmic Suspension .... ⊙ 259

Tobramycin Sulfate (Potential for additive or synergistic impairment of renal function).

No products indexed under this heading.

Triamterene (Mild to severe hyperkalemia has been reported with tacrolimus; concurrent use with potassium-sparing diuretics should be avoided). Products include:

Dyazide Capsules 1423
Dyrenium Capsules 3400

Troleandomycin (Co-administration with drugs known to inhibit CYP3A enzyme systems, such as troleandomycin, may increase tacrolimus blood concentrations).

No products indexed under this heading.

Typhoid Vaccine (Immunosupressants may affect vaccination. Therefore, during treatment with tacrolimus, vaccination may be less effective. The use of live vaccines should be avoided).

No products indexed under this heading.

Typhoid Vaccine Live Oral TY21a (During treatment with tacrolimus, vaccination may be less effective). Products include:

Vivotif 819

Vaccines (Live) (During treatment with tacrolimus, vaccination may be less effective).

No products indexed under this heading.

Varicella Virus Vaccine Live (Immunosupressants may affect vaccination. Therefore, during treatment with tacrolimus, vaccination may be less effective. The use of live vaccines should be avoided). Products include:

Varivax 2100

Venlafaxine Hydrochloride (Since tacrolimus is metabolized mainly by the CYP3A enzyme systems, substances known to inhibit these enzymes may decrease the metabolism or increase bioavailability of tacrolimus as indicated by increased whole blood or plasma concentrations. Monitoringof blood concentrations and appropriate dosage adjustments are essential when such drugs are used concomitantly). Products include:

Effexor Tablets 3411
Effexor XR Capsules 3417

Verapamil Hydrochloride (Co-administration with drugs known to inhibit CYP3A enzyme systems, such as verapamil, may increase tacrolimus blood concentrations). Products include:

Covera-HS Tablets 3139
Tarka Tablets 524
Verelan PM Extended-Release Capsules, Controlled-Onset........ 3106

Voriconazole (Co-administration with drugs known to inhibit CYP3A enzyme systems, such as voriconazole, may increase tacrolimus blood concentrations). Products include:

VFEND I.V. 2564
VFEND Oral Suspension 2564
VFEND Tablets 2564

Yellow Fever Vaccine (During treatment with tacrolimus, vaccination may be less effective).

No products indexed under this heading.

Zafirlukast (Since tacrolimus is metabolized mainly by the CYP3A enzyme systems, substances known to inhibit these enzymes may decrease the metabolism or increase bioavailability of tacrolimus as indicated by increased whole blood or plasma concentrations. Monitoringof blood concentrations and appropriate dosage adjustments are essential when such drugs are used concomitantly). Products include:

Accolate Tablets 671

Zileuton (Since tacrolimus is metabolized mainly by the CYP3A enzyme systems, substances known to inhibit these enzymes may decrease the metabolism or increase bioavailability of tacrolimus as indicated by increased whole blood or plasma concentrations. Monitoringof blood concentrations and appropriate dosage adjustments are essential when such drugs are used concomitantly). Products include:

Zyflo Tablets 1023

Food Interactions

Food, unspecified (The presence and composition of food has decreased both the rate and extent of tacrolimus absorption; this effect was most pronounced with a high-fat meal; the rate and extent of tacrolimus absorption were greatest under fasted conditions).

Grapefruit (Since tacrolimus is metabolized mainly by the CYP3A enzyme systems, substances known to inhibit these enzymes may decrease the metabolism or increase bioavailability of tacrolimus as indicated by increased whole blood or plasma concentrations. Monitoringof blood concentrations and appropriate dosage adjustments are essential when such drugs are used concomitantly).

Grapefruit Juice (Co-administered grapefruit juice has been reported to increase tacrolimus blood trough concentrations in liver transplant patients; grapefruit juice should be avoided).

PROLASTIN

(Alpha$_1$-Proteinase Inhibitor (Human))........ 3255

None cited in PDR database.

PROLEUKIN FOR INJECTION

(Aldesleukin) 2266

May interact with aminoglycosides, antihypertensives, beta blockers, cytotoxic drugs, glucocorticoids, hypnotics and sedatives, narcotic analgesics, radiographic iodinated contrast media, tranquilizers, and certain other agents. Compounds in these categories include:

Acebutolol Hydrochloride (May potentiate the hypotension seen with aldesleukin).

No products indexed under this heading.

Alfentanil Hydrochloride (Potential for unspecified effect on central nervous function).

No products indexed under this heading.

Alprazolam (Potential for unspecified effect on central nervous function). Products include:

Niravam Orally Disintegrating Tablets 3092

Amikacin Sulfate (Potential for increased nephrotoxicity).

No products indexed under this heading.

Amlodipine Besylate (May potentiate the hypotension seen with aldesleukin). Products include:

Caduet Tablets 2508
Lotrel Capsules 2249
Norvasc Tablets 2545

Asparaginase (Potential for increased hepatic toxicity). Products include:

Elspar for Injection 2463
Elspar for Injection 1960

Atenolol (May potentiate the hypotension seen with aldesleukin).

No products indexed under this heading.

Benazepril Hydrochloride (May potentiate the hypotension seen with aldesleukin). Products include:

Lotensin Tablets 2243
Lotensin HCT Tablets 2246
Lotrel Capsules 2249

Bendroflumethiazide (May potentiate the hypotension seen with aldesleukin).

No products indexed under this heading.

Betamethasone Acetate (May reduce the antitumor effectiveness of aldesleukin).

No products indexed under this heading.

Betamethasone Sodium Phosphate (May reduce the antitumor effectiveness of aldesleukin).

No products indexed under this heading.

Betaxolol Hydrochloride (May potentiate the hypotension seen with aldesleukin). Products include:

Betoptic S Ophthalmic Suspension........ 558

Bisoprolol Fumarate (May potentiate the hypotension seen with aldesleukin).

No products indexed under this heading.

Bleomycin Sulfate (Potential for increased myelotoxicity).

No products indexed under this heading.

Buprenorphine Hydrochloride (Potential for unspecified effect on central nervous function). Products include:

Buprenex Injectable 2716
Suboxone Tablets 2717
Subutex Tablets 2717

Buspirone Hydrochloride (Potential for unspecified effect on central nervous function).

No products indexed under this heading.

Candesartan Cilexetil (May potentiate the hypotension seen with aldesleukin). Products include:

Atacand Tablets 649
Atacand HCT 651

Captopril (May potentiate the hypotension seen with aldesleukin). Products include:

Captopril Tablets 2149

Carteolol Hydrochloride (May potentiate the hypotension seen with aldesleukin). Products include:

Carteolol Hydrochloride Ophthalmic Solution USP, 1%....... ⊙ 249

Chlordiazepoxide (Potential for unspecified effect on central nervous function).

No products indexed under this heading.

Chlordiazepoxide Hydrochloride (Potential for unspecified effect on central nervous function). Products include:

Librium Capsules 3347

Chlorothiazide (May potentiate the hypotension seen with aldesleukin). Products include:

Diuril Oral Suspension 1954

Chlorothiazide Sodium (May potentiate the hypotension seen with aldesleukin). Products include:

Diuril Sodium Intravenous 2467

Chlorpromazine (Potential for unspecified effect on central nervous function).

No products indexed under this heading.

Chlorpromazine Hydrochloride (Potential for unspecified effect on central nervous function).

No products indexed under this heading.

Chlorprothixene (Potential for unspecified effect on central nervous function).

No products indexed under this heading.

Chlorprothixene Hydrochloride (Potential for unspecified effect on central nervous function).

No products indexed under this heading.

Chlorthalidone (May potentiate the hypotension seen with aldesleukin). Products include:
Clorpres Tablets 2153

Clonidine (May potentiate the hypotension seen with aldesleukin). Products include:
Catapres-TTS 844

Clonidine Hydrochloride (May potentiate the hypotension seen with aldesleukin). Products include:
Catapres Tablets 843
Clorpres Tablets 2153

Clorazepate Dipotassium (Potential for unspecified effect on central nervous function). Products include:
Tranxene 2474

Codeine Phosphate (Potential for unspecified effect on central nervous function). Products include:
Tylenol with Codeine Tablets 2391

Cortisone Acetate (May reduce the antitumor effectiveness of aldesleukin).

No products indexed under this heading.

Cyclophosphamide (Potential for increased myelotoxicity).

No products indexed under this heading.

Daunorubicin Hydrochloride (Potential for increased myelotoxicity).

No products indexed under this heading.

Deserpidine (May potentiate the hypotension seen with aldesleukin).

No products indexed under this heading.

Dexamethasone (May reduce the antitumor effectiveness of aldesleukin). Products include:
Ciprodex Otic Suspension 559
Decadron Tablets 1951
TobraDex Ophthalmic Ointment 562
TobraDex Ophthalmic Suspension ... 563

Dexamethasone Acetate (May reduce the antitumor effectiveness of aldesleukin).

No products indexed under this heading.

Dexamethasone Sodium Phosphate (May reduce the antitumor effectiveness of aldesleukin).

No products indexed under this heading.

Dezocine (Potential for unspecified effect on central nervous function).

No products indexed under this heading.

Diatrizoate Meglumine (Potential for delayed adverse reactions to iodinated contrast media including fever, chills, nausea, vomiting, pruritus, rash, diarrhea, hypotension, edema, and oliguria).

No products indexed under this heading.

Diatrizoate Sodium (Potential for delayed adverse reactions to iodinated contrast media including fever, chills, nausea, vomiting, pruritus, rash, diarrhea, hypotension, edema, and oliguria).

No products indexed under this heading.

Diazepam (Potential for unspecified effect on central nervous function). Products include:
Diastat Rectal Delivery System 3343
Valium Tablets 2819

Diazoxide (May potentiate the hypotension seen with aldesleukin). Products include:
Hyperstat I.V. 3017

Diltiazem Hydrochloride (May potentiate the hypotension seen with aldesleukin). Products include:
Cardizem LA Extended Release
 Tablets 1728
Tiazac Capsules 1201

Doxazosin Mesylate (May potentiate the hypotension seen with aldesleukin). Products include:
Cardura XL Tablets 2515

Doxorubicin Hydrochloride (Potential for increased cardiotoxicity and myelotoxicity).

No products indexed under this heading.

Droperidol (Potential for unspecified effect on central nervous function).

No products indexed under this heading.

Enalapril Maleate (May potentiate the hypotension seen with aldesleukin). Products include:
Vasotec I.V. Injection 2103

Enalaprilat (May potentiate the hypotension seen with aldesleukin).

No products indexed under this heading.

Epirubicin Hydrochloride (Potential for increased myelotoxicity).

No products indexed under this heading.

Eprosartan Mesylate (May potentiate the hypotension seen with aldesleukin). Products include:
Teveten Tablets 1735
Teveten HCT Tablets 1737

Esmolol Hydrochloride (May potentiate the hypotension seen with aldesleukin).

No products indexed under this heading.

Estazolam (Potential for unspecified effect on central nervous function). Products include:
ProSom Tablets 517

Ethchlorvynol (Potential for unspecified effect on central nervous function).

No products indexed under this heading.

Ethinamate (Potential for unspecified effect on central nervous function).

No products indexed under this heading.

Ethiodized Oil (Potential for delayed adverse reactions to iodinated contrast media including fever, chills, nausea, vomiting, pruritus, rash, diarrhea, hypotension, edema, and oliguria).

No products indexed under this heading.

Felodipine (May potentiate the hypotension seen with aldesleukin).

No products indexed under this heading.

Fentanyl (Potential for unspecified effect on central nervous function). Products include:
Duragesic Transdermal System 2373
Ionsys Transdermal System 2379

Fentanyl Citrate (Potential for unspecified effect on central nervous function). Products include:

Actiq 979

Fludrocortisone Acetate (May reduce the antitumor effectiveness of aldesleukin).

No products indexed under this heading.

Fluorouracil (Potential for increased myelotoxicity). Products include:
Carac Cream, 0.5% 2879
Efudex 3363

Fluphenazine Decanoate (Potential for unspecified effect on central nervous function).

No products indexed under this heading.

Fluphenazine Enanthate (Potential for unspecified effect on central nervous function).

No products indexed under this heading.

Fluphenazine Hydrochloride (Potential for unspecified effect on central nervous function).

No products indexed under this heading.

Flurazepam Hydrochloride (Potential for unspecified effect on central nervous function). Products include:
Dalmane Capsules 3342

Fosinopril Sodium (May potentiate the hypotension seen with aldesleukin).

No products indexed under this heading.

Furosemide (May potentiate the hypotension seen with aldesleukin). Products include:
Furosemide Tablets 2154

Gadopentetate Dimeglumine (Potential for delayed adverse reactions to iodinated contrast media including fever, chills, nausea, vomiting, pruritus, rash, diarrhea, hypotension, edema, and oliguria).

No products indexed under this heading.

Gentamicin Sulfate (Potential for increased nephrotoxicity). Products include:
Garamycin Injectable 3014
Pred-G Ophthalmic Ointment ⊙ 237
Pred-G Ophthalmic Suspension ⊙ 236

Glutethimide (Potential for unspecified effect on central nervous function).

No products indexed under this heading.

Guanabenz Acetate (May potentiate the hypotension seen with aldesleukin).

No products indexed under this heading.

Guanethidine Monosulfate (May potentiate the hypotension seen with aldesleukin).

No products indexed under this heading.

Haloperidol (Potential for unspecified effect on central nervous function).

No products indexed under this heading.

Haloperidol Decanoate (Potential for unspecified effect on central nervous function).

No products indexed under this heading.

Hepatotoxic Drugs, unspecified (Potential for increased hepatic toxicity).

No products indexed under this heading.

Hydralazine Hydrochloride (May potentiate the hypotension seen with aldesleukin). Products include:
BiDil Tablets 2171

Hydrochlorothiazide (May potentiate the hypotension seen with aldesleukin). Products include:
Aldoril Tablets 1910
Atacand HCT 651
Avalide Tablets 888
Avalide Tablets 2874
Benicar HCT Tablets 1044
Diovan HCT Tablets 2196
Dyazide Capsules 1423
Hyzaar 50-12.5 Tablets 1990
Hyzaar 100-12.5 Tablets 1990
Hyzaar 100-25 Tablets 1990
Lopressor HCT 50/25 Tablets 2241
Lopressor HCT 100/25 Tablets 2241
Lopressor HCT 100/50 Tablets 2241
Lotensin HCT Tablets 2246
Micardis HCT Tablets 856
Moduretic Tablets 2028
Prinzide Tablets 2056
Teveten HCT Tablets 1737
Timolide Tablets 2086
Uniretic Tablets 3100

Hydrocodone Bitartrate (Potential for unspecified effect on central nervous function). Products include:
Hycodan 1116
Hycotuss Expectorant Syrup 1117
Vicodin Tablets 535
Vicodin ES Tablets 536
Vicodin HP Tablets 538
Vicoprofen Tablets 539
Zydone Tablets 1139

Hydrocodone Polistirex (Potential for unspecified effect on central nervous function). Products include:
Tussionex Pennkinetic
 Extended-Release Suspension 3327

Hydrocortisone (May reduce the antitumor effectiveness of aldesleukin). Products include:
Colocort Rectal Suspension, USP
 (Retention) 100 mg/60 mL........... 2476
Hydrocortone Tablets 1989
Preparation H Hydrocortisone
 Cream ▣646

Hydrocortisone Acetate (May reduce the antitumor effectiveness of aldesleukin). Products include:
Analpram-HC 1159
Pramosone 1161
ProctoFoam-HC 3099

Hydrocortisone Sodium Phosphate (May reduce the antitumor effectiveness of aldesleukin).

No products indexed under this heading.

Hydrocortisone Sodium Succinate (May reduce the antitumor effectiveness of aldesleukin).

No products indexed under this heading.

Hydroflumethiazide (May potentiate the hypotension seen with aldesleukin).

No products indexed under this heading.

Hydromorphone Hydrochloride (Potential for unspecified effect on central nervous function). Products include:
Dilaudid 440
Dilaudid Non-Sterile Powder 440
Dilaudid Oral Liquid 445
Dilaudid Rectal Suppositories 440
Dilaudid Tablets 440
Dilaudid Tablets - 8 mg 445
Dilaudid-HP 442

Hydroxyurea (Potential for increased myelotoxicity).

No products indexed under this heading.

Hydroxyzine Hydrochloride (Potential for unspecified effect on central nervous function).
No products indexed under this heading.

Indapamide (May potentiate the hypotension seen with aldesleukin). Products include:
Indapamide Tablets 2156

Indomethacin (Potential for increased nephrotoxicity). Products include:
Indocin 1995

Interferon alfa-2a, Recombinant (Co-administration of Proleukin and interferon-alfa has resulted in increased incidence of myocardial injury, including myocardial infarction, myocarditis, ventricular hypokinesia, and severe rhabdomyolysis; exacerbation or the initial presentation of a number of autoimmune and inflammatory disorders has been observed with concurrent use).
No products indexed under this heading.

Interferon alfa-2b, Recombinant (Co-administration of Proleukin and interferon-alfa has resulted in increased incidence of myocardial injury, including myocardial infarction, myocarditis, ventricular hypokinesia, and severe rhabdomyolysis; exacerbation or the initial presentation of a number of autoimmune and inflammatory disorders has been observed with concurrent use). Products include:
Intron A for Injection 3024
Rebetron Combination Therapy 3063

Iodamide Meglumine (Potential for delayed adverse reactions to iodinated contrast media including fever, chills, nausea, vomiting, pruritus, rash, diarrhea, hypotension, edema, and oliguria).
No products indexed under this heading.

Iohexol (Potential for delayed adverse reactions to iodinated contrast media including fever, chills, nausea, vomiting, pruritus, rash, diarrhea, hypotension, edema, and oliguria).
No products indexed under this heading.

Iopamidol (Potential for delayed adverse reactions to iodinated contrast media including fever, chills, nausea, vomiting, pruritus, rash, diarrhea, hypotension, edema, and oliguria).
No products indexed under this heading.

Iopanoic Acid (Potential for delayed adverse reactions to iodinated contrast media including fever, chills, nausea, vomiting, pruritus, rash, diarrhea, hypotension, edema, and oliguria).
No products indexed under this heading.

Iothalamate Meglumine (Potential for delayed adverse reactions to iodinated contrast media including fever, chills, nausea, vomiting, pruritus, rash, diarrhea, hypotension, edema, and oliguria).
No products indexed under this heading.

Ioxaglate Meglumine (Potential for delayed adverse reactions to iodinated contrast media including fever, chills, nausea, vomiting, pruritus, rash, diarrhea, hypotension, edema, and oliguria).
No products indexed under this heading.

Ioxaglate Sodium (Potential for delayed adverse reactions to iodinated contrast media including fever, chills, nausea, vomiting, pruritus, rash, diarrhea, hypotension, edema, and oliguria).
No products indexed under this heading.

Irbesartan (May potentiate the hypotension seen with aldesleukin). Products include:
Avalide Tablets 888
Avalide Tablets 2874
Avapro Tablets 891
Avapro Tablets 2871

Isradipine (May potentiate the hypotension seen with aldesleukin). Products include:
DynaCirc CR Tablets 2721

Kanamycin Sulfate (Potential for increased nephrotoxicity).
No products indexed under this heading.

Labetalol Hydrochloride (May potentiate the hypotension seen with aldesleukin).
No products indexed under this heading.

Levobunolol Hydrochloride (May potentiate the hypotension seen with aldesleukin). Products include:
Betagan Ophthalmic Solution, USP.. ⊙ 220

Levorphanol Tartrate (Potential for unspecified effect on central nervous function).
No products indexed under this heading.

Lisinopril (May potentiate the hypotension seen with aldesleukin). Products include:
Prinivil Tablets 2052
Prinzide Tablets 2056

Lorazepam (Potential for unspecified effect on central nervous function).
No products indexed under this heading.

Losartan Potassium (May potentiate the hypotension seen with aldesleukin). Products include:
Cozaar Tablets 1935
Hyzaar 50-12.5 Tablets 1990
Hyzaar 100-12.5 Tablets 1990
Hyzaar 100-25 Tablets 1990

Loxapine Hydrochloride (Potential for unspecified effect on central nervous function).
No products indexed under this heading.

Loxapine Succinate (Potential for unspecified effect on central nervous function).
No products indexed under this heading.

Mecamylamine Hydrochloride (May potentiate the hypotension seen with aldesleukin).
No products indexed under this heading.

Meperidine Hydrochloride (Potential for unspecified effect on central nervous function).
No products indexed under this heading.

Meprobamate (Potential for unspecified effect on central nervous function).
No products indexed under this heading.

Mesoridazine Besylate (Potential for unspecified effect on central nervous function).
No products indexed under this heading.

Methadone Hydrochloride (Potential for unspecified effect on central nervous function).
No products indexed under this heading.

Methotrexate Sodium (Potential for increased hepatic toxicity and myelotoxicity).
No products indexed under this heading.

Methyclothiazide (May potentiate the hypotension seen with aldesleukin).
No products indexed under this heading.

Methyldopa (May potentiate the hypotension seen with aldesleukin). Products include:
Aldoril Tablets 1910

Methyldopate Hydrochloride (May potentiate the hypotension seen with aldesleukin).
No products indexed under this heading.

Methylprednisolone Acetate (May reduce the antitumor effectiveness of aldesleukin). Products include:
Depo-Medrol Injectable Suspension 2617
Depo-Medrol Single-Dose Vial 2619

Methylprednisolone Sodium Succinate (May reduce the antitumor effectiveness of aldesleukin).
No products indexed under this heading.

Metipranolol Hydrochloride (May potentiate the hypotension seen with aldesleukin).
No products indexed under this heading.

Metolazone (May potentiate the hypotension seen with aldesleukin).
No products indexed under this heading.

Metoprolol Succinate (May potentiate the hypotension seen with aldesleukin). Products include:
Toprol-XL Tablets 668

Metoprolol Tartrate (May potentiate the hypotension seen with aldesleukin). Products include:
Lopressor Injection 2238
Lopressor Tablets 2238
Lopressor HCT 50/25 Tablets 2241
Lopressor HCT 100/25 Tablets 2241
Lopressor HCT 100/50 Tablets 2241

Metyrosine (May potentiate the hypotension seen with aldesleukin). Products include:
Demser Capsules 1953

Mibefradil Dihydrochloride (May potentiate the hypotension seen with aldesleukin).
No products indexed under this heading.

Midazolam Hydrochloride (Potential for unspecified effect on central nervous function).
No products indexed under this heading.

Minoxidil (May potentiate the hypotension seen with aldesleukin). Products include:
Men's Rogaine Extra Strength Hair Regrowth Treatment Topical Solution, Ocean Rush Scent and Original Unscented ..... ▣ 633
Men's Rogaine Foam Hair Regrowth Treatment..................... ▣ 633
Women's Rogaine Hair Regrowth Treatment Topical Solution, Spring Bloom Scent and Original Unscented.............................. ▣ 634

Mitotane (Potential for increased myelotoxicity).
No products indexed under this heading.

Mitoxantrone Hydrochloride (Potential for increased myelotoxicity).
No products indexed under this heading.

Moexipril Hydrochloride (May potentiate the hypotension seen with aldesleukin). Products include:
Uniretic Tablets 3100
Univasc Tablets 3104

Molindone Hydrochloride (Potential for unspecified effect on central nervous function). Products include:
Moban Tablets 1119

Morphine Sulfate (Potential for unspecified effect on central nervous function). Products include:
Avinza Capsules 1741
Kadian Capsules 577
MS Contin Tablets 2701

Nadolol (May potentiate the hypotension seen with aldesleukin). Products include:
Nadolol Tablets 2159

Nephrotoxic Drugs (Potential for increased nephrotoxicity).
No products indexed under this heading.

Nicardipine Hydrochloride (May potentiate the hypotension seen with aldesleukin). Products include:
Cardene I.V. 2497

Nifedipine (May potentiate the hypotension seen with aldesleukin). Products include:
Adalat CC Tablets 2964

Nisoldipine (May potentiate the hypotension seen with aldesleukin). Products include:
Sular Tablets 3122

Nitroglycerin (May potentiate the hypotension seen with aldesleukin). Products include:
Nitro-Dur Transdermal Infusion System.. 3046
Nitrolingual Pumpspray 3120

Oxazepam (Potential for unspecified effect on central nervous function).
No products indexed under this heading.

Oxycodone Hydrochloride (Potential for unspecified effect on central nervous function). Products include:
OxyContin Tablets 2703
OxyFast Oral Concentrate Solution.. 2708
OxyIR Capsules 2708
Percocet Tablets 1131
Percodan Tablets 1132

Penbutolol Sulfate (May potentiate the hypotension seen with aldesleukin).
No products indexed under this heading.

Perindopril Erbumine (May potentiate the hypotension seen with aldesleukin). Products include:
Aceon Tablets (2 mg, 4 mg, 8 mg)... 3194

IMPORTANT NOTE: Always consult each drug listing in the patient's regimen for possible interactions.

Perphenazine (Potential for unspecified effect on central nervous function).
No products indexed under this heading.

Phenoxybenzamine Hydrochloride (May potentiate the hypotension seen with aldesleukin). Products include:
Dibenzyline Capsules **3399**

Phentolamine Mesylate (May potentiate the hypotension seen with aldesleukin).
No products indexed under this heading.

Pindolol (May potentiate the hypotension seen with aldesleukin).
No products indexed under this heading.

Polythiazide (May potentiate the hypotension seen with aldesleukin).
No products indexed under this heading.

Prazepam (Potential for unspecified effect on central nervous function).
No products indexed under this heading.

Prazosin Hydrochloride (May potentiate the hypotension seen with aldesleukin).
No products indexed under this heading.

Prednisolone Acetate (May reduce the antitumor effectiveness of aldesleukin). Products include:
Blephamide Ophthalmic Ointment **568**
Blephamide Ophthalmic Suspension **569**
Poly-Pred Ophthalmic Suspension .... ⊙**233**
Pred Forte Ophthalmic Suspension .... ⊙**235**
Pred Mild Ophthalmic Suspension .... ⊙**238**
Pred-G Ophthalmic Ointment .... ⊙**237**
Pred-G Ophthalmic Suspension ...... ⊙**236**

Prednisolone Sodium Phosphate (May reduce the antitumor effectiveness of aldesleukin).
No products indexed under this heading.

Prednisolone Tebutate (May reduce the antitumor effectiveness of aldesleukin).
No products indexed under this heading.

Prednisone (May reduce the antitumor effectiveness of aldesleukin).
No products indexed under this heading.

Procarbazine Hydrochloride (Potential for increased myelotoxicity). Products include:
Matulane Capsules **3191**

Prochlorperazine (Potential for unspecified effect on central nervous function).
No products indexed under this heading.

Promethazine Hydrochloride (Potential for unspecified effect on central nervous function). Products include:
Phenergan Tablets and Suppositories **3440**

Propofol (Potential for unspecified effect on central nervous function).
No products indexed under this heading.

Propoxyphene Hydrochloride (Potential for unspecified effect on central nervous function).
No products indexed under this heading.

Propoxyphene Napsylate (Potential for unspecified effect on central nervous function).
No products indexed under this heading.

Propranolol Hydrochloride (May potentiate the hypotension seen with aldesleukin). Products include:
Inderal LA Long-Acting Capsules **3429**
InnoPran XL Capsules **2723**

Quazepam (Potential for unspecified effect on central nervous function).
No products indexed under this heading.

Quinapril Hydrochloride (May potentiate the hypotension seen with aldesleukin).
No products indexed under this heading.

Ramelteon (Potential for unspecified effect on central nervous function). Products include:
Rozerem Tablets **3231**

Ramipril (May potentiate the hypotension seen with aldesleukin). Products include:
Altace Capsules **1702**

Rauwolfia Serpentina (May potentiate the hypotension seen with aldesleukin).
No products indexed under this heading.

Remifentanil Hydrochloride (Potential for unspecified effect on central nervous function).
No products indexed under this heading.

Rescinnamine (May potentiate the hypotension seen with aldesleukin).
No products indexed under this heading.

Reserpine (May potentiate the hypotension seen with aldesleukin).
No products indexed under this heading.

Secobarbital Sodium (Potential for unspecified effect on central nervous function).
No products indexed under this heading.

Sodium Nitroprusside (May potentiate the hypotension seen with aldesleukin).
No products indexed under this heading.

Sotalol Hydrochloride (May potentiate the hypotension seen with aldesleukin).
No products indexed under this heading.

Spirapril Hydrochloride (May potentiate the hypotension seen with aldesleukin).
No products indexed under this heading.

Streptomycin Sulfate (Potential for increased nephrotoxicity).
No products indexed under this heading.

Sufentanil Citrate (Potential for unspecified effect on central nervous function).
No products indexed under this heading.

Tamoxifen Citrate (Potential for increased myelotoxicity). Products include:
Soltamox Oral Solution **3527**

Telmisartan (May potentiate the hypotension seen with aldesleukin). Products include:
Micardis Tablets **854**
Micardis HCT Tablets **856**

Temazepam (Potential for unspecified effect on central nervous function). Products include:
Restoril Capsules **1860**

Terazosin Hydrochloride (May potentiate the hypotension seen with aldesleukin). Products include:
Hytrin Capsules **471**

Thioridazine Hydrochloride (Potential for unspecified effect on central nervous function). Products include:
Thioridazine Hydrochloride Tablets **2163**

Thiothixene (Potential for unspecified effect on central nervous function). Products include:
Thiothixene Capsules **2165**

Timolol Hemihydrate (May potentiate the hypotension seen with aldesleukin). Products include:
Betimol Ophthalmic Solution **3382**
Betimol Ophthalmic Solution .... ⊙**295**

Timolol Maleate (May potentiate the hypotension seen with aldesleukin). Products include:
Blocadren Tablets **1916**
Cosopt Sterile Ophthalmic Solution **1931**
Timolide Tablets **2086**
Timoptic Sterile Ophthalmic Solution **2088**
Timoptic in Ocudose **2091**
Timoptic-XE Sterile Ophthalmic Gel Forming Solution **2092**

Tobramycin (Potential for increased nephrotoxicity). Products include:
TOBI Solution for Inhalation **2298**
TobraDex Ophthalmic Ointment **562**
TobraDex Ophthalmic Suspension ... **563**
Zylet Ophthalmic Suspension .... ⊙**259**

Tobramycin Sulfate (Potential for increased nephrotoxicity).
No products indexed under this heading.

Torsemide (May potentiate the hypotension seen with aldesleukin). Products include:
Demadex Injection **2759**
Demadex Tablets **2759**

Trandolapril (May potentiate the hypotension seen with aldesleukin). Products include:
Mavik Tablets **486**
Tarka Tablets **524**

Triamcinolone (May reduce the antitumor effectiveness of aldesleukin).
No products indexed under this heading.

Triamcinolone Acetonide (May reduce the antitumor effectiveness of aldesleukin). Products include:
Azmacort Inhalation Aerosol **1726**
Nasacort AQ Nasal Spray **2922**

Triamcinolone Diacetate (May reduce the antitumor effectiveness of aldesleukin).
No products indexed under this heading.

Triamcinolone Hexacetonide (May reduce the antitumor effectiveness of aldesleukin).
No products indexed under this heading.

Triazolam (Potential for unspecified effect on central nervous function).
No products indexed under this heading.

Trifluoperazine Hydrochloride (Potential for unspecified effect on central nervous function).
No products indexed under this heading.

Trimethaphan Camsylate (May potentiate the hypotension seen with aldesleukin).
No products indexed under this heading.

Tyropanoate Sodium (Potential for delayed adverse reactions to iodinated contrast media including fever, chills, nausea, vomiting, pruritus, rash, diarrhea, hypotension, edema, and oliguria).
No products indexed under this heading.

Valsartan (May potentiate the hypotension seen with aldesleukin). Products include:
Diovan Tablets **2193**
Diovan HCT Tablets **2196**

Verapamil Hydrochloride (May potentiate the hypotension seen with aldesleukin). Products include:
Covera-HS Tablets **3139**
Tarka Tablets **524**
Verelan PM Extended-Release Capsules, Controlled-Onset........... **3106**

Vincristine Sulfate (Potential for increased myelotoxicity).
No products indexed under this heading.

Zaleplon (Potential for unspecified effect on central nervous function). Products include:
Sonata Capsules **1717**

Zolpidem Tartrate (Potential for unspecified effect on central nervous function). Products include:
Ambien Tablets **2851**
Ambien CR Tablets **2855**

PROMETRIUM CAPSULES (100 MG, 200 MG)

(Progesterone) **3203**
May interact with:

Estrogens, Conjugated (Co-administration has resulted in an increase in total estrone and equilin concentrations and decrease in circulating 17β estradiol concentrations). Products include:
Premarin Intravenous **3442**
Premarin Tablets **3446**
Premarin Vaginal Cream **3452**
Premphase Tablets **3456**
Prempro Tablets **3456**

Ketoconazole (The metabolism of progesterone by human liver microsomes is inhibited by ketoconazole, a known inhibitor of CYP4503A4; the clinical relevance of the in vitro findings is unknown). Products include:
Nizoral A-D Shampoo, 1% **1868**

Food Interactions

Food, unspecified (Concomitant food ingestion increases the bioavailability of Prometrium Capsules relative to the fasting state).

PRONUTRA PROTEIN SUPPLEMENT

(Vitamins with Minerals, Whey Protein Isolate) **1668**
None cited in PDR database.

PROPECIA TABLETS

(Finasteride) **2060**
None cited in PDR database.

PROPINE OPHTHALMIC SOLUTION

(Dipivefrin Hydrochloride) .... ⊙**239**
None cited in PDR database.

PROQUAD
(Measles, Mumps, Rubella and Varicella Virus Vaccine Live) ... 2064
May interact with corticosteroids, immunosuppressive agents, salicylates, and certain other agents. Compounds in these categories include:

Aspirin (Reye's syndrome has been reported following the use of salicylates during wild-type varicella infection. Vaccine recipients should avoid use of salicylates for 6 weeks after vaccination with Measles, Mumps, Rubella, and Varicella Virus Vaccine, Live). Products include:
- Aggrenox Capsules ... 822
- Bayer Aspirin ... 744
- BC Allergy Sinus Cold Powder ... 677
- BC Headache Powder ... 677
- Arthritis Strength BC Powder ... 677
- BC Sinus Cold Powder ... 677
- Excedrin Extra Strength Caplets/Tablets/Geltabs ... 684
- Excedrin Migraine Caplets/Tablets/Geltabs ... 609
- Goody's Body Pain Formula Powder ... 684
- Goody's Extra Strength Headache Powders ... 611
- Goody's Extra Strength Pain Relief Tablets ... 685
- Percodan Tablets ... 1132
- St. Joseph 81 mg Aspirin Chewable and Enteric Coated Tablets ... 1869

Aspirin, Enteric Coated (Reye's syndrome has been reported following the use of salicylates during wild-type varicella infection. Vaccine recipients should avoid use of salicylates for 6 weeks after vaccination with Measles, Mumps, Rubella, and Varicella Virus Vaccine, Live).
No products indexed under this heading.

Aspirin Buffered (Reye's syndrome has been reported following the use of salicylates during wild-type varicella infection. Vaccine recipients should avoid use of salicylates for 6 weeks after vaccination with Measles, Mumps, Rubella, and Varicella Virus Vaccine, Live). Products include:
- Bufferin Extra Strength Tablets ... 678
- Bufferin Regular Strength Tablets ... 678

Azathioprine (Measles, Mumps, Rubella, and Varicella Virus Vaccine, Live may be used in individuals who are receiving topical corticosteroids or low-dose corticosteroids for asthma prophylaxis or replacement therapy, (e.g., for Addison's disease). Measles, Mumps, Rubella, and Varicella Virus Vaccine, Live should not be given to individuals receiving immunosuppressive doses of corticosteroids or other immunosuppressive drugs).
No products indexed under this heading.

Basiliximab (Measles, Mumps, Rubella, and Varicella Virus Vaccine, Live may be used in individuals who are receiving topical corticosteroids or low-dose corticosteroids for asthma prophylaxis or replacement therapy, (e.g., for Addison's disease). Measles, Mumps, Rubella, and Varicella Virus Vaccine, Live should not be given to individuals receiving immunosuppressive doses of corticosteroids or other immunosuppressive drugs). Products include:
- Simulect for Injection ... 2284

Betamethasone Acetate (Measles, Mumps, Rubella, and Varicella Virus Vaccine, Live may be used in individuals who are receiving topical corticosteroids or low-dose corticosteroids for asthma prophylaxis or replacement therapy, (e.g., for Addison's disease). Measles, Mumps, Rubella, and Varicella Virus Vaccine, Live should not be given to individuals receiving immunosuppressive doses of corticosteroids or other immunosuppressive drugs).
No products indexed under this heading.

Betamethasone Sodium Phosphate (Measles, Mumps, Rubella, and Varicella Virus Vaccine, Live may be used in individuals who are receiving topical corticosteroids or low-dose corticosteroids for asthma prophylaxis or replacement therapy, (e.g., for Addison's disease). Measles, Mumps, Rubella, and Varicella Virus Vaccine, Live should not be given to individuals receiving immunosuppressive doses of corticosteroids or other immunosuppressive drugs).
No products indexed under this heading.

Choline Magnesium Trisalicylate (Reye's syndrome has been reported following the use of salicylates during wild-type varicella infection. Vaccine recipients should avoid use of salicylates for 6 weeks after vaccination with Measles, Mumps, Rubella, and Varicella Virus Vaccine, Live).
No products indexed under this heading.

Cortisone Acetate (Measles, Mumps, Rubella, and Varicella Virus Vaccine, Live may be used in individuals who are receiving topical corticosteroids or low-dose corticosteroids for asthma prophylaxis or replacement therapy, (e.g., for Addison's disease). Measles, Mumps, Rubella, and Varicella Virus Vaccine, Live should not be given to individuals receiving immunosuppressive doses of corticosteroids or other immunosuppressive drugs).
No products indexed under this heading.

Cyclosporine (Measles, Mumps, Rubella, and Varicella Virus Vaccine, Live may be used in individuals who are receiving topical corticosteroids or low-dose corticosteroids for asthma prophylaxis or replacement therapy, (e.g., for Addison's disease). Measles, Mumps, Rubella, and Varicella Virus Vaccine, Live should not be given to individuals receiving immunosuppressive doses of corticosteroids or other immunosuppressive drugs). Products include:
- Gengraf Capsules ... 459
- Neoral Oral Solution ... 2259
- Neoral Soft Gelatin Capsules ... 2259
- Restasis Ophthalmic Emulsion ... 575
- Sandimmune ... 2275

Dexamethasone (Measles, Mumps, Rubella, and Varicella Virus Vaccine, Live may be used in individuals who are receiving topical corticosteroids or low-dose corticosteroids for asthma prophylaxis or replacement therapy, (e.g., for Addison's disease). Measles, Mumps, Rubella, and Varicella Virus Vaccine, Live should not be given to individuals receiving immunosuppressive doses of corticosteroids or other immunosuppressive drugs). Products include:
- Ciprodex Otic Suspension ... 559
- Decadron Tablets ... 1951
- TobraDex Ophthalmic Ointment ... 562
- TobraDex Ophthalmic Suspension ... 563

Dexamethasone Acetate (Measles, Mumps, Rubella, and Varicella Virus Vaccine, Live may be used in individuals who are receiving topical corticosteroids or low-dose corticosteroids for asthma prophylaxis or replacement therapy, (e.g., for Addison's disease). Measles, Mumps, Rubella, and Varicella Virus Vaccine, Live should not be given to individuals receiving immunosuppressive doses of corticosteroids or other immunosuppressive drugs).
No products indexed under this heading.

Dexamethasone Sodium Phosphate (Measles, Mumps, Rubella, and Varicella Virus Vaccine, Live may be used in individuals who are receiving topical corticosteroids or low-dose corticosteroids for asthma prophylaxis or replacement therapy, (e.g., for Addison's disease). Measles, Mumps, Rubella, and Varicella Virus Vaccine, Live should not be given to individuals receiving immunosuppressive doses of corticosteroids or other immunosuppressive drugs).
No products indexed under this heading.

Diflunisal (Reye's syndrome has been reported following the use of salicylates during wild-type varicella infection. Vaccine recipients should avoid use of salicylates for 6 weeks after vaccination with Measles, Mumps, Rubella, and Varicella Virus Vaccine, Live). Products include:
- Dolobid Tablets ... 1955

Fludrocortisone Acetate (Measles, Mumps, Rubella, and Varicella Virus Vaccine, Live may be used in individuals who are receiving topical corticosteroids or low-dose corticosteroids for asthma prophylaxis or replacement therapy, (e.g., for Addison's disease). Measles, Mumps, Rubella, and Varicella Virus Vaccine, Live should not be given to individuals receiving immunosuppressive doses of corticosteroids or other immunosuppressive drugs).
No products indexed under this heading.

Globulin, Immune (Human) (Immune globulins administered concomitantly with Measles, Mumps, Rubella, and Varicella Virus Vaccine, Live may interfere with the expected immune response. Vaccination should be deferred for at least 3 months following blood plasma transfusions, or administration of immune globulins (IG)). Products include:
- Flebogamma 5%, Immune Globulin Intravenous (Human) ... 1658
- GamaSTAN ... 3234

Hydrocortisone (Measles, Mumps, Rubella, and Varicella Virus Vaccine, Live may be used in individuals who are receiving topical corticosteroids or low-dose corticosteroids for asthma prophylaxis or replacement therapy, (e.g., for Addison's disease). Measles, Mumps, Rubella, and Varicella Virus Vaccine, Live should not be given to individuals receiving immunosuppressive doses of corticosteroids or other immunosuppressive drugs). Products include:
- Colocort Rectal Suspension, USP (Retention) 100 mg/60 mL ... 2476
- Hydrocortone Tablets ... 1989
- Preparation H Hydrocortisone Cream ... 646

Hydrocortisone Acetate (Measles, Mumps, Rubella, and Varicella Virus Vaccine, Live may be used in individuals who are receiving topical corticosteroids or low-dose corticosteroids for asthma prophylaxis or replacement therapy, (e.g., for Addison's disease). Measles, Mumps, Rubella, and Varicella Virus Vaccine, Live should not be given to individuals receiving immunosuppressive doses of corticosteroids or other immunosuppressive drugs).
Products include:
- Analpram-HC ... 1159
- Pramosone ... 1161
- ProctoFoam-HC ... 3099

Hydrocortisone Sodium Phosphate (Measles, Mumps, Rubella, and Varicella Virus Vaccine, Live may be used in individuals who are receiving topical corticosteroids or low-dose corticosteroids for asthma prophylaxis or replacement therapy, (e.g., for Addison's disease). Measles, Mumps, Rubella, and Varicella Virus Vaccine, Live should not be given to individuals receiving immunosuppressive doses of corticosteroids or other immunosuppressive drugs).
No products indexed under this heading.

Hydrocortisone Sodium Succinate (Measles, Mumps, Rubella, and Varicella Virus Vaccine, Live may be used in individuals who are receiving topical corticosteroids or low-dose corticosteroids for asthma prophylaxis or replacement therapy, (e.g., for Addison's disease). Measles, Mumps, Rubella, and Varicella Virus Vaccine, Live should not be given to individuals receiving immunosuppressive doses of corticosteroids or other immunosuppressive drugs).
No products indexed under this heading.

Magnesium Salicylate (Reye's syndrome has been reported following the use of salicylates during wild-type varicella infection. Vaccine recipients should avoid use of salicylates for 6 weeks after vaccination with Measles, Mumps, Rubella, and Varicella Virus Vaccine, Live).
No products indexed under this heading.

Methylprednisolone Acetate (Measles, Mumps, Rubella, and Varicella Virus Vaccine, Live may be used in individuals who are receiving topical corticosteroids or low-dose corticosteroids for asthma prophylaxis or replacement therapy, (e.g., for Addison's disease). Measles, Mumps, Rubella, and Varicella Virus Vaccine, Live should not be given to individuals receiving immunosuppressive doses of corticosteroids or other immunosuppressive drugs).
Products include:
- Depo-Medrol Injectable Suspension ... 2617
- Depo-Medrol Single-Dose Vial ... 2619

Methylprednisolone Sodium Succinate (Measles, Mumps, Rubella, and Varicella Virus Vaccine, Live may be used in individuals who are receiving topical corticosteroids or low-dose corticosteroids for asthma prophylaxis or replacement therapy, (e.g., for Addison's disease). Measles, Mumps, Rubella, and Varicella Virus Vaccine, Live should not be given to individuals receiving immunosuppressive doses of corticosteroids or other immunosuppressive

drugs).
No products indexed under this heading.

Muromonab-CD3 (Measles, Mumps, Rubella, and Varicella Virus Vaccine, Live may be used in individuals who are receiving topical corticosteroids or low-dose corticosteroids for asthma prophylaxis or replacement therapy, (e.g., for Addison's disease). Measles, Mumps, Rubella, and Varicella Virus Vaccine, Live should not be given to individuals receiving immunosuppressive doses of corticosteroids or other immunosuppressive drugs).
Products include:
Orthoclone OKT3 Sterile Solution 2360

Mycophenolate Mofetil (Measles, Mumps, Rubella, and Varicella Virus Vaccine, Live may be used in individuals who are receiving topical corticosteroids or low-dose corticosteroids for asthma prophylaxis or replacement therapy, (e.g., for Addison's disease). Measles, Mumps, Rubella, and Varicella Virus Vaccine, Live should not be given to individuals receiving immunosuppressive doses of corticosteroids or other immunosuppressive drugs).
Products include:
CellCept Capsules 2747
CellCept Oral Suspension 2747
CellCept Tablets 2747

Prednisolone Acetate (Measles, Mumps, Rubella, and Varicella Virus Vaccine, Live may be used in individuals who are receiving topical corticosteroids or low-dose corticosteroids for asthma prophylaxis or replacement therapy, (e.g., for Addison's disease). Measles, Mumps, Rubella, and Varicella Virus Vaccine, Live should not be given to individuals receiving immunosuppressive doses of corticosteroids or other immunosuppressive drugs).
Products include:
Blephamide Ophthalmic Ointment 568
Blephamide Ophthalmic Suspension.................................. 569
Poly-Pred Ophthalmic Suspension .... ⊙ 233
Pred Forte Ophthalmic Suspension .... ⊙ 235
Pred Mild Ophthalmic Suspension .... ⊙ 238
Pred-G Ophthalmic Ointment .... ⊙ 237
Pred-G Ophthalmic Suspension ...... ⊙ 236

Prednisolone Sodium Phosphate (Measles, Mumps, Rubella, and Varicella Virus Vaccine, Live may be used in individuals who are receiving topical corticosteroids or low-dose corticosteroids for asthma prophylaxis or replacement therapy, (e.g., for Addison's disease). Measles, Mumps, Rubella, and Varicella Virus Vaccine, Live should not be given to individuals receiving immunosuppressive doses of corticosteroids or other immunosuppressive drugs).
No products indexed under this heading.

Prednisolone Tebutate (Measles, Mumps, Rubella, and Varicella Virus Vaccine, Live may be used in individuals who are receiving topical corticosteroids or low-dose corticosteroids for asthma prophylaxis or replacement therapy, (e.g., for Addison's disease). Measles, Mumps, Rubella, and Varicella Virus Vaccine, Live should not be given to individuals receiving immunosuppressive doses of corticosteroids or other immunosuppressive drugs).
No products indexed under this heading.

Prednisone (Measles, Mumps, Rubella, and Varicella Virus Vaccine, Live may be used in individuals who are receiving topical corticosteroids or low-dose corticosteroids for asthma prophylaxis or replacement therapy, (e.g., for Addison's disease). Measles, Mumps, Rubella, and Varicella Virus Vaccine, Live should not be given to individuals receiving immunosuppressive doses of corticosteroids or other immunosuppressive drugs).
No products indexed under this heading.

Salsalate (Reye's syndrome has been reported following the use of salicylates during wild-type varicella infection. Vaccine recipients should avoid use of salicylates for 6 weeks after vaccination with Measles, Mumps, Rubella, and Varicella Virus Vaccine, Live).
No products indexed under this heading.

Sirolimus (Measles, Mumps, Rubella, and Varicella Virus Vaccine, Live may be used in individuals who are receiving topical corticosteroids or low-dose corticosteroids for asthma prophylaxis or replacement therapy, (e.g., for Addison's disease). Measles, Mumps, Rubella, and Varicella Virus Vaccine, Live should not be given to individuals receiving immunosuppressive doses of corticosteroids or other immunosuppressive drugs). Products include:
Rapamune Oral Solution and Tablets 3475

Tacrolimus (Measles, Mumps, Rubella, and Varicella Virus Vaccine, Live may be used in individuals who are receiving topical corticosteroids or low-dose corticosteroids for asthma prophylaxis or replacement therapy, (e.g., for Addison's disease). Measles, Mumps, Rubella, and Varicella Virus Vaccine, Live should not be given to individuals receiving immunosuppressive doses of corticosteroids or other immunosuppressive drugs). Products include:
Prograf Capsules and Injection 632
Protopic Ointment 638

Triamcinolone (Measles, Mumps, Rubella, and Varicella Virus Vaccine, Live may be used in individuals who are receiving topical corticosteroids or low-dose corticosteroids for asthma prophylaxis or replacement therapy, (e.g., for Addison's disease). Measles, Mumps, Rubella, and Varicella Virus Vaccine, Live should not be given to individuals receiving immunosuppressive doses of corticosteroids or other immunosuppressive drugs).
No products indexed under this heading.

Triamcinolone Acetonide (Measles, Mumps, Rubella, and Varicella Virus Vaccine, Live may be used in individuals who are receiving topical corticosteroids or low-dose corticosteroids for asthma prophylaxis or replacement therapy, (e.g., for Addison's disease). Measles, Mumps, Rubella, and Varicella Virus Vaccine, Live should not be given to individuals receiving immunosuppressive doses of corticosteroids or other immunosuppressive drugs).
Products include:
Azmacort Inhalation Aerosol 1726
Nasacort AQ Nasal Spray 2922

Triamcinolone Diacetate (Measles, Mumps, Rubella, and Varicella Virus Vaccine, Live may be used in individuals who are receiving topical corticosteroids or low-dose corticosteroids for asthma prophylaxis or replacement therapy, (e.g., for Addison's disease). Measles, Mumps, Rubella, and Varicella Virus Vaccine, Live should not be given to individuals receiving immunosuppressive doses of corticosteroids or other immunosuppressive drugs).
No products indexed under this heading.

Triamcinolone Hexacetonide (Measles, Mumps, Rubella, and Varicella Virus Vaccine, Live may be used in individuals who are receiving topical corticosteroids or low-dose corticosteroids for asthma prophylaxis or replacement therapy, (e.g., for Addison's disease). Measles, Mumps, Rubella, and Varicella Virus Vaccine, Live should not be given to individuals receiving immunosuppressive doses of corticosteroids or other immunosuppressive drugs).
No products indexed under this heading.

PROQUIN XR TABLETS

(Ciprofloxacin Hydrochloride) 1153
May interact with cations, oral anticoagulants, non-steroidal anti-inflammatory agents, phenytoin, theophyllines, and certain other agents. Compounds in these categories include:

Aluminum-containing Compounds, unspecified (Concurrent administration of a quinolone, including ciprofloxacin, with multivalent cation-containing products such as magnesium or aluminum antacids, sucralfate, VIDEX (didanosine) chewable/buffered tablets or pediatric powder, or products containing calcium, iron, or zinc may substantially decrease the absorption of ciprofloxacin, resulting in serum and urine levels considerably lower than desired. Ciprofloxacin extended-release tablets should be administered at least 4 hours before or 2 hours after these products. This time window is different than for other oral formulations of ciprofloxacin, which are usually administered 2 hours before or 6 hours after antacids).
No products indexed under this heading.

Anisindione (Quinolones have been reported to enhance the effects of the oral anticoagulant warfarin or its derivatives. When these products are administered concomitantly, prothrombin time or other suitable coagulation tests should be monitored).
Products include:
Miradon Tablets 3042

Caffeine (Some quinolones, including ciprofloxacin, have also been shown to interfere with the metabolism of caffeine. This may lead to reduced clearance of caffeine and a prolongation of its serum half-life).
Products include:
BC Headache Powder .... ▣ 677
Arthritis Strength BC Powder .... ▣ 677
Excedrin Extra Strength Caplets/Tablets/Geltabs............ ▣ 684
Excedrin Migraine Caplets/Tablets/Geltabs............ ▣ 609
Excedrin Tension Headache Caplets/Tablets/Geltabs............ ▣ 611
Goody's Extra Strength Headache Powders.................... ▣ 611
Goody's Extra Strength Pain Relief Tablets............................ ▣ 685
Vivarin .... ▣ 602
Winrgy Dietary Supplement........... ▣ 823

Calcium (Concurrent administration of a quinolone, including ciprofloxacin, with multivalent cation-containing products such as magnesium or aluminum antacids, sucralfate, VIDEX (didanosine) chewable/buffered tablets or pediatric powder, or products containing calcium, iron, or zinc may substantially decrease the absorption of ciprofloxacin, resulting in serum and urine levels considerably lower than desired. Ciprofloxacin extended-release tablets should be administered at least 4 hours before or 2 hours after these products. This time window is different than for other oral formulations of ciprofloxacin, which are usually administered 2 hours before or 6 hours after antacids). Products include:
Os-Cal 250 + D Tablets .... ▣ 817
Os-Cal 500 Tablets .... ▣ 817
Os-Cal 500 + D Tablets .... ▣ 817

Celecoxib (These drugs in combination with very high doses of quinolones have been shown to provoke convulsions in preclinical studies).
Products include:
Celebrex Capsules 3134

Cyclosporine (Some quinolones, including ciprofloxacin, have been associated with transient elevations in serum creatinine in patients receiving cyclosporine concomitantly).
Products include:
Gengraf Capsules 459
Neoral Oral Solution 2259
Neoral Soft Gelatin Capsules 2259
Restasis Ophthalmic Emulsion 575
Sandimmune 2275

Diclofenac Potassium (These drugs in combination with very high doses of quinolones have been shown to provoke convulsions in preclinical studies).
No products indexed under this heading.

Diclofenac Sodium (These drugs in combination with very high doses of quinolones have been shown to provoke convulsions in preclinical studies). Products include:
Arthrotec Tablets 3129
Voltaren Ophthalmic Solution 2309
Voltaren Tablets 2307
Voltaren-XR Tablets 2310

Dicumarol (Quinolones have been reported to enhance the effects of the oral anticoagulant warfarin or its derivatives. When these products are administered concomitantly, prothrombin time or other suitable coagulation tests should be monitored).
No products indexed under this heading.

Etodolac (These drugs in combination with very high doses of quinolones have been shown to provoke convulsions in preclinical studies).
No products indexed under this heading.

Fenoprofen Calcium (These drugs in combination with very high doses of quinolones have been shown to provoke convulsions in preclinical studies). Products include:
Nalfon Capsules 2502

Flurbiprofen (These drugs in combination with very high doses of quinolones have been shown to provoke convulsions in preclinical studies).
No products indexed under this heading.

Fosphenytoin Sodium (Altered serum levels of phenytoin (increased and decreased) have been reported in patients receiving concomitant ciprofloxacin).
No products indexed under this heading.

Glyburide (The concomitant administration of ciprofloxacin with the sulfonylurea glyburide has, on rare occasions, resulted in severe hypoglycemia).
No products indexed under this heading.

Ibuprofen (These drugs in combination with very high doses of quinolones have been shown to provoke convulsions in preclinical studies). Products include:
Advil Allergy Sinus Caplets 770
Advil 674
Children's Advil Oral Suspension 603
Children's Advil Chewable Tablets .. 603
Advil Cold & Sinus 723
Infants' Advil Concentrated Drops .. 604
Infants' Advil Concentrated Drops - White Grape (Dye-Free) 604
Junior Strength Advil Swallow Tablets 605
Advil Migraine Liquigels 608
Advil Multi-Symptom Cold Caplets 770
Advil PM Caplets 615
Motrin IB Tablets and Caplets 1866
Children's Motrin Oral Suspension ... 1867
Children's Motrin Non-Staining Dye-Free Oral Suspension 1867
Children's Motrin Cold Oral Suspension 1867
Infants' Motrin Concentrated Drops 1867
Infants' Motrin Non-Staining Dye-Free Concentrated Drops 1867
Junior Strength Motrin Caplets and Chewable Tablets 1867
Vicoprofen Tablets 539

Indomethacin (These drugs in combination with very high doses of quinolones have been shown to provoke convulsions in preclinical studies). Products include:
Indocin 1995

Indomethacin Sodium Trihydrate (These drugs in combination with very high doses of quinolones have been shown to provoke convulsions in preclinical studies). Products include:
Indocin I.V. 2465

Iron (Concurrent administration of a quinolone, including ciprofloxacin, with multivalent cation-containing products such as magnesium or aluminum antacids, sucralfate, VIDEX (didanosine) chewable/buffered tablets or pediatric powder, or products containing calcium, iron, or zinc may substantially decrease the absorption of ciprofloxacin, resulting in serum and urine levels considerably lower than desired. Ciprofloxacin extended-release tablets should be administered at least 4 hours before or 2 hours after these products. This time window is different than for other oral formulations of ciprofloxacin, which are usually administered 2 hours before or 6 hours after antacids).
No products indexed under this heading.

Ketoprofen (These drugs in combination with very high doses of quinolones have been shown to provoke convulsions in preclinical studies).
No products indexed under this heading.

Ketorolac Tromethamine (These drugs in combination with very high doses of quinolones have been shown to provoke convulsions in preclinical studies). Products include:
Acular Ophthalmic Solution 565
Acular LS Ophthalmic Solution 566

Magnesium (Concurrent administration of a quinolone, including ciprofloxacin, with multivalent cation-containing products such as magnesium or aluminum antacids, sucralfate, VIDEX (didanosine) chewable/buffered tablets or pediatric powder, or products containing calcium, iron, or zinc may substantially decrease the absorption of ciprofloxacin, resulting in serum and urine levels considerably lower than desired. Ciprofloxacin extended-release tablets should be administered at least 4 hours before or 2 hours after these products. This time window is different than for other oral formulations of ciprofloxacin, which are usually administered 2 hours before or 6 hours after antacids).
No products indexed under this heading.

Meclofenamate Sodium (These drugs in combination with very high doses of quinolones have been shown to provoke convulsions in preclinical studies).
No products indexed under this heading.

Mefenamic Acid (These drugs in combination with very high doses of quinolones have been shown to provoke convulsions in preclinical studies).
No products indexed under this heading.

Meloxicam (These drugs in combination with very high doses of quinolones have been shown to provoke convulsions in preclinical studies). Products include:
Mobic Oral Suspension 863
Mobic Tablets 863

Methotrexate (Renal tubular transport of methotrexate may be inhibited by concomitant administration of ciprofloxacin, potentially leading to increased plasma levels of methotrexate. This might increase the risk of methotrexate toxic reactions. Therefore, patients under methotrexate therapy should be carefully monitored when concomitant ciprofloxacin therapy is indicated).
No products indexed under this heading.

Nabumetone (These drugs in combination with very high doses of quinolones have been shown to provoke convulsions in preclinical studies).
No products indexed under this heading.

Naproxen (These drugs in combination with very high doses of quinolones have been shown to provoke convulsions in preclinical studies). Products include:
EC-Naprosyn Delayed-Release Tablets 2761
Naprosyn Suspension 2761
Naprosyn Tablets 2761
Prevacid NapraPAC 3280

Naproxen Sodium (These drugs in combination with very high doses of quinolones have been shown to provoke convulsions in preclinical studies). Products include:
Aleve Caplets 742
Aleve Gelcaps 743
Aleve Tablets 743
Aleve Cold & Sinus Caplets 744
Anaprox Tablets 2761
Anaprox DS Tablets 2761

Oxaprozin (These drugs in combination with very high doses of quinolones have been shown to provoke convulsions in preclinical studies).
No products indexed under this heading.

Phenylbutazone (These drugs in combination with very high doses of quinolones have been shown to provoke convulsions in preclinical studies).
No products indexed under this heading.

Phenytoin (Altered serum levels of phenytoin (increased and decreased) have been reported in patients receiving concomitant ciprofloxacin).
No products indexed under this heading.

Phenytoin Sodium (Altered serum levels of phenytoin (increased and decreased) have been reported in patients receiving concomitant ciprofloxacin). Products include:
Phenytek Capsules 2160

Piroxicam (These drugs in combination with very high doses of quinolones have been shown to provoke convulsions in preclinical studies).
No products indexed under this heading.

Probenecid (Probenecid interferes with renal tubular secretion of ciprofloxacin and produces an increase in the level of ciprofloxacin in serum).
No products indexed under this heading.

Rofecoxib (These drugs in combination with very high doses of quinolones have been shown to provoke convulsions in preclinical studies).
No products indexed under this heading.

Sulindac (These drugs in combination with very high doses of quinolones have been shown to provoke convulsions in preclinical studies). Products include:
Clinoril Tablets 1924

Theophylline (As with some other quinolones, concurrent administration of ciprofloxacin with theophylline may lead to elevated serum concentrations of theophylline and prolongation of its elimination half-life. This may result in increased risk of theophylline-related adverse reactions. If concomitant use cannot be avoided, serum levels of theophylline should be monitored and dosage adjustments made as appropriate).
No products indexed under this heading.

Theophylline Anhydrous (As with some other quinolones, concurrent administration of ciprofloxacin with theophylline may lead to elevated serum concentrations of theophylline and prolongation of its elimination half-life. This may result in increased risk of theophylline-related adverse reactions. If concomitant use cannot be avoided, serum levels of theophylline should be monitored and dosage adjustments made as appropriate). Products include:
Uniphyl Tablets 2710

Theophylline Calcium Salicylate (As with some other quinolones, concurrent administration of ciprofloxacin with theophylline may lead to elevated serum concentrations of theophylline and prolongation of its elimination half-life. This may result in increased risk of theophylline-related adverse reactions. If concomitant use cannot be avoided, serum levels of theophylline should be monitored and dosage adjustments made as appropriate).
No products indexed under this heading.

Theophylline Dihydroxypropyl (Glyceryl) (As with some other quinolones, concurrent administration of ciprofloxacin with theophylline may lead to elevated serum concentrations of theophylline and prolongation of its elimination half-life. This may result in increased risk of theophylline-related adverse reactions. If concomitant use cannot be avoided, serum levels of theophylline should be monitored and dosage adjustments made as appropriate).
No products indexed under this heading.

Theophylline Ethylenediamine (As with some other quinolones, concurrent administration of ciprofloxacin with theophylline may lead to elevated serum concentrations of theophylline and prolongation of its elimination half-life. This may result in increased risk of theophylline-related adverse reactions. If concomitant use cannot be avoided, serum levels of theophylline should be monitored and dosage adjustments made as appropriate).
No products indexed under this heading.

Theophylline Sodium Glycinate (As with some other quinolones, concurrent administration of ciprofloxacin with theophylline may lead to elevated serum concentrations of theophylline and prolongation of its elimination half-life. This may result in increased risk of theophylline-related adverse reactions. If concomitant use cannot be avoided, serum levels of theophylline should be monitored and dosage adjustments made as appropriate).
No products indexed under this heading.

Tolmetin Sodium (These drugs in combination with very high doses of quinolones have been shown to provoke convulsions in preclinical studies).
No products indexed under this heading.

Valdecoxib (These drugs in combination with very high doses of quinolones have been shown to provoke convulsions in preclinical studies).
No products indexed under this heading.

Warfarin Sodium (Quinolones have been reported to enhance the effects of the oral anticoagulant warfarin or its derivatives. When these products are administered concomitantly, prothrombin time or other suitable coagulation tests should be monitored). Products include:
Coumadin for Injection 898
Coumadin Tablets 898

Zinc (Concurrent administration of a quinolone, including ciprofloxacin, with multivalent cation-containing products such as magnesium or aluminum antacids, sucralfate, VIDEX (didanosine) chewable/buffered tablets or pediatric powder, or products containing calcium, iron, or zinc may substantially decrease the absorption of ciprofloxacin, resulting in serum and urine levels considerably lower than desired. Ciprofloxacin extended-release tablets should be administered at least 4 hours before or 2 hours after these products. This time window is different than for other oral formulations of ciprofloxacin, which are usually administered 2 hours before or 6 hours after antacids). Products include:

Visutein Capsules 3329

PROSCAR TABLETS

(Finasteride) 2067

None cited in PDR database.

PROSED/DS TABLETS

(Benzoic Acid, Hyoscyamine Sulfate, Methenamine, Methylene Blue, Phenyl Salicylate)....................... 1157

May interact with antacids, antimuscarinic drugs, monoamine oxidase inhibitors, narcotic analgesics, sulfonamides, thiazides, urinary alkalinizing agents, and certain other agents. Compounds in these categories include:

Alfentanil Hydrochloride (Concurrent use may result in increased risk of severe constipation).

No products indexed under this heading.

Aluminum Carbonate (Concurrent use may reduce absorption of hyocyamine resulting in decreased therapeutic effectiveness. Concurrent use with antacids may cause urine to become alkaline reducing the effectiveness of methenamine by inhibiting its conversion to formaldehyde.Doses of these medications should be spaced 1 hour apart from doses of hyocyamine).

No products indexed under this heading.

Aluminum Hydroxide (Concurrent use may reduce absorption of hyocyamine resulting in decreased therapeutic effectiveness. Concurrent use with antacids may cause urine to become alkaline reducing the effectiveness of methenamine by inhibiting its conversion to formaldehyde.Doses of these medications should be spaced 1 hour apart from doses of hyocyamine). Products include:

Gaviscon Regular Strength Liquid .. ■ 658
Gaviscon Regular Strength Tablets .... ■ 658
Gaviscon Extra Strength Liquid ...... ■ 658
Gaviscon Extra Strength Tablets ..... ■ 658
Maalox Regular Strength Antacid/Antigas Liquid.................. 2175
Maalox Max Maximum Strength Antacid/Anti-Gas Liquid................. 2176

Atropine Sulfate (Concurrent use may reduce absorption of hyoscyamine resulting in decreased therapeutic effectiveness. Concurrent use with antacids may cause urine to become alkaline reducing the effectiveness of methenamine by inhibiting its conversion to formaldehyde.Doses of these medications should be spaced 1 hour apart from doses of hyoscyamine). Products include:

Donnatal Extentabs 2493

Belladonna Alkaloids (Concurrent use may reduce absorption of hyoscyamine resulting in decreased therapeutic effectiveness. Concurrent use with antacids may cause urine to become alkaline reducing the effectiveness of methenamine by inhibiting its conversion to formaldehyde.Doses of these medications should be spaced 1 hour apart from doses of hyoscyamine). Products include:

Hyland's Teething Tablets .... ■ 830

Bendroflumethiazide (May cause the urine to become alkaline reducing the effectiveness of methenamine by inhibiting its conversion to formaldehyde).

No products indexed under this heading.

Buprenorphine Hydrochloride (Concurrent use may result in increased risk of severe constipation). Products include:

Buprenex Injectable 2716
Suboxone Tablets 2717
Subutex Tablets 2717

Chlorothiazide (May cause the urine to become alkaline reducing the effectiveness of methenamine by inhibiting its conversion to formaldehyde). Products include:

Diuril Oral Suspension 1954

Chlorothiazide Sodium (May cause the urine to become alkaline reducing the effectiveness of methenamine by inhibiting its conversion to formaldehyde). Products include:

Diuril Sodium Intravenous 2467

Chlorpropamide (These drugs may precipitate with formaldehyde in the urine increasing the danger of crystalluria).

No products indexed under this heading.

Clidinium Bromide (Concurrent use may reduce absorption of hyoscyamine resulting in decreased therapeutic effectiveness. Concurrent use with antacids may cause urine to become alkaline reducing the effectiveness of methenamine by inhibiting its conversion to formaldehyde.Doses of these medications should be spaced 1 hour apart from doses of hyoscyamine).

No products indexed under this heading.

Codeine Phosphate (Concurrent use may result in increased risk of severe constipation). Products include:

Tylenol with Codeine Tablets 2391

Dezocine (Concurrent use may result in increased risk of severe constipation).

No products indexed under this heading.

Dicyclomine Hydrochloride (Concurrent use may reduce absorption of hyoscyamine resulting in decreased therapeutic effectiveness. Concurrent use with antacids may cause urine to become alkaline reducing the effectiveness of methenamine by inhibiting its conversion to formaldehyde.Doses of these medications should be spaced 1 hour apart from doses of hyoscyamine). Products include:

Bentyl Capsules 697
Bentyl Injection 697
Bentyl Syrup 697
Bentyl Tablets 697

Diphenoxylate Hydrochloride (Concurrent use may reduce absorption of hyoscyamine resulting in decreased therapeutic effectiveness. Doses of these medications should be spaced 1 hour apart from doses of hyoscyamine).

No products indexed under this heading.

Fentanyl (Concurrent use may result in increased risk of severe constipation). Products include:

Duragesic Transdermal System 2373
Ionsys Transdermal System 2379

Fentanyl Citrate (Concurrent use may result in increased risk of severe constipation). Products include:

Actiq 979

Glipizide (These drugs may precipitate with formaldehyde in the urine increasing the danger of crystalluria).

No products indexed under this heading.

Glyburide (These drugs may precipitate with formaldehyde in the urine increasing the danger of crystalluria).

No products indexed under this heading.

Glycopyrrolate (Concurrent use may reduce absorption of hyoscyamine resulting in decreased therapeutic effectiveness. Concurrent use with antacids may cause urine to become alkaline reducing the effectiveness of methenamine by inhibiting its conversion to formaldehyde.Doses of these medications should be spaced 1 hour apart from doses of hyoscyamine).

No products indexed under this heading.

Hydrochlorothiazide (May cause the urine to become alkaline reducing the effectiveness of methenamine by inhibiting its conversion to formaldehyde). Products include:

Aldoril Tablets 1910
Atacand HCT 651
Avalide Tablets 888
Avalide Tablets 2874
Benicar HCT Tablets 1044
Diovan HCT Tablets 2196
Dyazide Capsules 1423
Hyzaar 50-12.5 Tablets 1990
Hyzaar 100-12.5 Tablets 1990
Hyzaar 100-25 Tablets 1990
Lopressor HCT 50/25 Tablets 2241
Lopressor HCT 100/25 Tablets 2241
Lopressor HCT 100/50 Tablets 2241
Lotensin HCT Tablets 2246
Micardis HCT Tablets 856
Moduretic Tablets 2028
Prinzide Tablets 2056
Teveten HCT Tablets 1737
Timolide Tablets 2086
Uniretic Tablets 3100

Hydrocodone Bitartrate (Concurrent use may result in increased risk of severe constipation). Products include:

Hycodan 1116
Hycotuss Expectorant Syrup 1117
Vicodin Tablets 535
Vicodin ES Tablets 536
Vicodin HP Tablets 538
Vicoprofen Tablets 539
Zydone Tablets 1139

Hydrocodone Polistirex (Concurrent use may result in increased risk of severe constipation). Products include:

Tussionex Pennkinetic Extended-Release Suspension 3327

Hydroflumethiazide (May cause the urine to become alkaline reducing the effectiveness of methenamine by inhibiting its conversion to formaldehyde).

No products indexed under this heading.

Hydromorphone Hydrochloride (Concurrent use may result in increased risk of severe constipation). Products include:

Dilaudid 440
Dilaudid Non Sterile Powder 440
Dilaudid Oral Liquid 445
Dilaudid Rectal Suppositories 440
Dilaudid Tablets 440
Dilaudid Tablets - 8 mg 445
Dilaudid-HP 442

Hyoscyamine (Concurrent use may reduce absorption of hyoscyamine resulting in decreased therapeutic effectiveness. Concurrent use with antacids may cause urine to become alkaline reducing the effectiveness of methenamine by inhibiting its conversion to formaldehyde.Doses of these medications should be spaced 1 hour apart from doses of hyoscyamine).

No products indexed under this heading.

Ipratropium Bromide (Concurrent use may reduce absorption of hyoscyamine resulting in decreased therapeutic effectiveness. Concurrent use with antacids may cause urine to become alkaline reducing the effectiveness of methenamine by inhibiting its conversion to formaldehyde.Doses of these medications should be spaced 1 hour apart from doses of hyoscyamine). Products include:

Atrovent Inhalation Solution 835
Atrovent HFA Inhalation Aerosol 841
Atrovent Nasal Spray 0.03% 837
Atrovent Nasal Spray 0.06% 839
Combivent Inhalation Aerosol 847
DuoNeb Inhalation Solution 1058

Isocarboxazid (Concurrent use with hyoscyamine may intensify antimuscarinic side effects).

No products indexed under this heading.

Ketoconazole (Hyoscyamine may cause increased gastrointestinal pH. Concurrent administration with hyoscyamine may result in marked reduction in the aborption of ketoconazole. Patients should be advised to take this combination at least 2 hours after ketoconazole). Products include:

Nizoral A-D Shampoo, 1% 1868

Levorphanol Tartrate (Concurrent use may result in increased risk of severe constipation).

No products indexed under this heading.

Loperamide Hydrochloride (Concurrent use may reduce absorption of hyoscyamine resulting in decreased therapeutic effectiveness. Doses of these medications should be spaced 1 hour apart from doses of hyoscyamine). Products include:

Imodium A-D Liquid and Caplets 1865
Imodium Advanced Caplets and Chewable Tablets 1866

Magaldrate (Concurrent use may reduce absorption of hyocyamine resulting in decreased therapeutic effectiveness. Concurrent use with antacids may cause urine to become alkaline reducing the effectiveness of methenamine by inhibiting its conversion to formaldehyde.Doses of these medications should be spaced 1 hour apart from doses of hyocyamine).
No products indexed under this heading.

Magnesium Hydroxide (Concurrent use may reduce absorption of hyocyamine resulting in decreased therapeutic effectiveness. Concurrent use with antacids may cause urine to become alkaline reducing the effectiveness of methenamine by inhibiting its conversion to formaldehyde.Doses of these medications should be spaced 1 hour apart from doses of hyocyamine). Products include:
Maalox Regular Strength Antacid/Antigas Liquid 2175
Maalox Max Maximum Strength Antacid/Anti-Gas Liquid 2176
Pepcid Complete Chewable Tablets 1701

Magnesium Oxide (Concurrent use may reduce absorption of hyocyamine resulting in decreased therapeutic effectiveness. Concurrent use with antacids may cause urine to become alkaline reducing the effectiveness of methenamine by inhibiting its conversion to formaldehyde.Doses of these medications should be spaced 1 hour apart from doses of hyocyamine). Products include:
Beelith Tablets 759
PremCal Light, Regular, and Extra Strength Tablets 818

Mepenzolate Bromide (Concurrent use may reduce absorption of hyoscyamine resulting in decreased therapeutic effectiveness. Concurrent use with antacids may cause urine to become alkaline reducing the effectiveness of methenamine by inhibiting its conversion to formaldehyde.Doses of these medications should be spaced 1 hour apart from doses of hyoscyamine).
No products indexed under this heading.

Meperidine Hydrochloride (Concurrent use may result in increased risk of severe constipation).
No products indexed under this heading.

Methadone Hydrochloride (Concurrent use may result in increased risk of severe constipation).
No products indexed under this heading.

Methyclothiazide (May cause the urine to become alkaline reducing the effectiveness of methenamine by inhibiting its conversion to formaldehyde).
No products indexed under this heading.

Moclobemide (Concurrent use with hyoscyamine may intensify antimuscarinic side effects).
No products indexed under this heading.

Morphine Sulfate (Concurrent use may result in increased risk of severe constipation). Products include:
Avinza Capsules 1741
Kadian Capsules 577
MS Contin Tablets 2701

Neostigmine Bromide (Concurrent use with hyoscyamine may further reduce intestinal motility, therefore, caution is recommended).
No products indexed under this heading.

Neostigmine Methylsulfate (Concurrent use with hyoscyamine may further reduce intestinal motility, therefore, caution is recommended).
No products indexed under this heading.

Oxycodone Hydrochloride (Concurrent use may result in increased risk of severe constipation). Products include:
OxyContin Tablets 2703
OxyFast Oral Concentrate Solution 2708
OxyIR Capsules 2708
Percocet Tablets 1131
Percodan Tablets 1132

Oxyphenonium Bromide (Concurrent use may reduce absorption of hyoscyamine resulting in decreased therapeutic effectiveness. Concurrent use with antacids may cause urine to become alkaline reducing the effectiveness of methenamine by inhibiting its conversion to formaldehyde.Doses of these medications should be spaced 1 hour apart from doses of hyoscyamine).
No products indexed under this heading.

Pargyline Hydrochloride (Concurrent use with hyoscyamine may intensify antimuscarinic side effects).
No products indexed under this heading.

Phenelzine Sulfate (Concurrent use with hyoscyamine may intensify antimuscarinic side effects).
No products indexed under this heading.

Polythiazide (May cause the urine to become alkaline reducing the effectiveness of methenamine by inhibiting its conversion to formaldehyde).
No products indexed under this heading.

Potassium Citrate (May cause the urine to become alkaline reducing the effectiveness of methenamine by inhibiting its conversion to formaldehyde). Products include:
Urocit-K Tablets 2144

Procarbazine Hydrochloride (Concurrent use with hyoscyamine may intensify antimuscarinic side effects). Products include:
Matulane Capsules 3191

Propantheline Bromide (Concurrent use may reduce absorption of hyoscyamine resulting in decreased therapeutic effectiveness. Concurrent use with antacids may cause urine to become alkaline reducing the effectiveness of methenamine by inhibiting its conversion to formaldehyde.Doses of these medications should be spaced 1 hour apart from doses of hyoscyamine).
No products indexed under this heading.

Propoxyphene Hydrochloride (Concurrent use may result in increased risk of severe constipation).
No products indexed under this heading.

Propoxyphene Napsylate (Concurrent use may result in increased risk of severe constipation).
No products indexed under this heading.

Pyridostigmine Bromide (Concurrent use with hyoscyamine may further reduce intestinal motility, therefore, caution is recommended).
No products indexed under this heading.

Remifentanil Hydrochloride (Concurrent use may result in increased risk of severe constipation).
No products indexed under this heading.

Scopolamine (Concurrent use may reduce absorption of hyoscyamine resulting in decreased therapeutic effectiveness. Concurrent use with antacids may cause urine to become alkaline reducing the effectiveness of methenamine by inhibiting its conversion to formaldehyde.Doses of these medications should be spaced 1 hour apart from doses of hyoscyamine). Products include:
Transderm Scōp Transdermal Therapeutic System 2177

Scopolamine Hydrobromide (Concurrent use may reduce absorption of hyoscyamine resulting in decreased therapeutic effectiveness. Concurrent use with antacids may cause urine to become alkaline reducing the effectiveness of methenamine by inhibiting its conversion to formaldehyde.Doses of these medications should be spaced 1 hour apart from doses of hyoscyamine). Products include:
Donnatal Extentabs 2493

Selegiline Hydrochloride (Concurrent use with hyoscyamine may intensify antimuscarinic side effects). Products include:
Eldepryl Capsules 3208
Zelapar Tablets 3372

Sodium Bicarbonate (May cause the urine to become alkaline reducing the effectiveness of methenamine by inhibiting its conversion to formaldehyde). Products include:
Colyte with Flavor Packs for Oral Solution 3088
HalfLytely and Bisacodyl Tablets Bowel Prep Kit with Flavors Packs 881
TriLyte with Flavor Packs for Oral Solution 3100

Sodium Citrate (May cause the urine to become alkaline reducing the effectiveness of methenamine by inhibiting its conversion to formaldehyde).
No products indexed under this heading.

Sufentanil Citrate (Concurrent use may result in increased risk of severe constipation).
No products indexed under this heading.

Sulfacytine (These drugs may precipitate with formaldehyde in the urine increasing the danger of crystalluria).
No products indexed under this heading.

Sulfamethizole (These drugs may precipitate with formaldehyde in the urine increasing the danger of crystalluria).
No products indexed under this heading.

Sulfamethoxazole (These drugs may precipitate with formaldehyde in the urine increasing the danger of crystalluria).
No products indexed under this heading.

Sulfasalazine (These drugs may precipitate with formaldehyde in the urine increasing the danger of crystalluria).
No products indexed under this heading.

Sulfinpyrazone (These drugs may precipitate with formaldehyde in the urine increasing the danger of crystalluria).
No products indexed under this heading.

Sulfisoxazole Acetyl (These drugs may precipitate with formaldehyde in the urine increasing the danger of crystalluria).
No products indexed under this heading.

Sulfisoxazole Diolamine (These drugs may precipitate with formaldehyde in the urine increasing the danger of crystalluria).
No products indexed under this heading.

Tolazamide (These drugs may precipitate with formaldehyde in the urine increasing the danger of crystalluria).
No products indexed under this heading.

Tolbutamide (These drugs may precipitate with formaldehyde in the urine increasing the danger of crystalluria).
No products indexed under this heading.

Tolterodine Tartrate (Concurrent use may reduce absorption of hyoscyamine resulting in decreased therapeutic effectiveness. Concurrent use with antacids may cause urine to become alkaline reducing the effectiveness of methenamine by inhibiting its conversion to formaldehyde.Doses of these medications should be spaced 1 hour apart from doses of hyoscyamine). Products include:
Detrol Tablets 2628
Detrol LA Capsules 2631

Tranylcypromine Sulfate (Concurrent use with hyoscyamine may intensify antimuscarinic side effects). Products include:
Parnate Tablets 1527

Tridihexethyl Chloride (Concurrent use may reduce absorption of hyoscyamine resulting in decreased therapeutic effectiveness. Concurrent use with antacids may cause urine to become alkaline reducing the effectiveness of methenamine by inhibiting its conversion to formaldehyde.Doses of these medications should be spaced 1 hour apart from doses of hyoscyamine).
No products indexed under this heading.

PROSOM TABLETS

(Estazolam) 517

May interact with antihistamines, barbiturates, central nervous system depressants, anticonvulsants, erythromycin, monoamine oxidase inhibitors, narcotic analgesics, phenothiazines, phenytoin, psychotropics, and certain other agents. Compounds in these categories include:

Acrivastine (Co-administration may result in increased CNS depression).
No products indexed under this heading.

Alfentanil Hydrochloride (Co-administration may result in increased CNS depression).
No products indexed under this heading.

Alprazolam (Co-administration may result in increased CNS depression). Products include:
- Niravam Orally Disintegrating Tablets ... 3092

Amitriptyline Hydrochloride (Co-administration may result in increased CNS depression).
No products indexed under this heading.

Amoxapine (Co-administration may result in increased CNS depression).
No products indexed under this heading.

Aprobarbital (Potent CYP3A inducers, such as barbiturates, would be expected to decrease plasma estazolam concentrations and may potentiate the action of estazolam).
No products indexed under this heading.

Astemizole (Co-administration may result in increased CNS depression).
No products indexed under this heading.

Azatadine Maleate (Co-administration may result in increased CNS depression).
No products indexed under this heading.

Bromodiphenhydramine Hydrochloride (Co-administration may result in increased CNS depression).
No products indexed under this heading.

Brompheniramine Maleate (Co-administration may result in increased CNS depression). Products include:
- Children's Dimetapp Cold & Allergy Elixir ... ▣730
- Children's Dimetapp Cold & Allergy Chewable Tablets ... ▣730
- Children's Dimetapp DM Cold & Cough Elixir ... ▣731

Buprenorphine Hydrochloride (Co-administration may result in increased CNS depression). Products include:
- Buprenex Injectable ... 2716
- Suboxone Tablets ... 2717
- Subutex Tablets ... 2717

Buspirone Hydrochloride (Co-administration may result in increased CNS depression).
No products indexed under this heading.

Butabarbital (Potent CYP3A inducers, such as barbiturates, would be expected to decrease plasma estazolam concentrations and may potentiate the action of estazolam).
No products indexed under this heading.

Butalbital (Potent CYP3A inducers, such as barbiturates, would be expected to decrease plasma estazolam concentrations and may potentiate the action of estazolam).
No products indexed under this heading.

Carbamazepine (Potent CYP3A inducers, such as carbamazepine, would be expected to decrease plasma estazolam concentrations and may potentiate the action of estazolam). Products include:
- Carbatrol Capsules ... 3171
- Equetro Extended-Release Capsules ... 3180
- Tegretol/Tegretol-XR ... 2295

Cetirizine Hydrochloride (Co-administration may result in increased CNS depression). Products include:
- Zyrtec Chewable Tablets ... 2594
- Zyrtec ... 2594
- Zyrtec-D 12 Hour Extended Release Tablets ... 2597

Chlordiazepoxide (Co-administration may result in increased CNS depression).
No products indexed under this heading.

Chlordiazepoxide Hydrochloride (Co-administration may result in increased CNS depression). Products include:
- Librium Capsules ... 3347

Chlorpheniramine Maleate (Co-administration may result in increased CNS depression). Products include:
- Advil Allergy Sinus Caplets ... ▣770
- Advil Multi-Symptom Cold Caplets ... ▣770
- BC Allergy Sinus Cold Powder ... ▣677
- Comtrex Maximum Strength Cold & Cough Day/Night Caplets - Night Formulation ... ▣726
- Comtrex Maximum Strength Day/Night Severe Cold & Sinus Caplets - Night Formulation ... ▣725
- Contac Cold and Flu Maximum Strength Caplets ... ▣728
- Contac Cold and Flu Day and Night Caplets (Night Formulation Only) ... ▣727
- Children's Dimetapp Long Acting Cough Plus Cold Syrup ... ▣731
- Robitussin Cough & Cold Long-Acting Liquid ... ▣735
- Robitussin Cough & Allergy Syrup .. ▣736
- Robitussin Cough & Cold Nighttime Liquid ... ▣736
- Robitussin Cough, Cold & Flu Nighttime Liquid ... ▣738
- Robitussin Pediatric Cough & Cold Long-Acting Liquid ... ▣735
- Robitussin Pediatric Cough & Cold Nighttime Liquid ... ▣736
- Triaminic Cold & Allergy Liquid ... ▣746
- Triaminic Cough & Runny Nose Softchews ... ▣748
- Children's Tylenol Plus Flu Oral Suspension ... ▣749
- Tylenol Allergy Multi-Symptom Caplets with Cool Burst and Gelcaps ... 1872
- Children's Tylenol Plus Cold Suspension Liquid ... 1879
- Children's Tylenol Plus Cough & Runny Nose Suspension Liquid ... 1879
- Children's Tylenol Plus Flu Suspension Liquid ... 1881
- Children's Tylenol Plus Multi-Symptom Cold Suspension Liquid ... 1879
- Tylenol Cold Head Congestion Nighttime Caplets with Cool Burst ... 1873
- Tylenol Cold Multi-Symptom Nighttime Caplets with Cool Burst ... 1874
- Tylenol Sinus Congestion & Pain Nighttime Caplets with Cool Burst ... 1876
- Vicks 44M Cough, Cold & Flu Relief Liquid ... 2680
- Pediatric Vicks 44m Cough & Cold Relief Liquid ... 2676
- Children's Vicks NyQuil Cold/Cough Relief ... ▣756
- Children's Vicks NyQuil Cold/Cough Relief Liquid ... 2680
- Zicam Maximum Strength Flu Daytime ... ▣768

Chlorpheniramine Polistirex (Co-administration may result in increased CNS depression). Products include:
- Tussionex Pennkinetic Extended-Release Suspension ... 3327

Chlorpheniramine Tannate (Co-administration may result in increased CNS depression).
No products indexed under this heading.

Chlorpromazine (Co-administration may result in increased CNS depression).
No products indexed under this heading.

Chlorpromazine Hydrochloride (Co-administration may result in increased CNS depression).
No products indexed under this heading.

Chlorprothixene (Co-administration may result in increased CNS depression).
No products indexed under this heading.

Chlorprothixene Hydrochloride (Co-administration may result in increased CNS depression).
No products indexed under this heading.

Chlorprothixene Lactate (Co-administration may result in increased CNS depression).
No products indexed under this heading.

Cimetidine (CYP3A inhibitors, such as cimetidine, would be expected to increase plasma estazolam concentrations). Products include:
- Tagamet HB 200 Tablets ... ▣664

Cimetidine Hydrochloride (CYP3A inhibitors, such as cimetidine, would be expected to increase plasma estazolam concentrations).
No products indexed under this heading.

Clemastine Fumarate (Co-administration may result in increased CNS depression).
No products indexed under this heading.

Clonazepam (Co-administration may result in increased CNS depression). Products include:
- Klonopin ... 2778

Clorazepate Dipotassium (Co-administration may result in increased CNS depression). Products include:
- Tranxene ... 2474

Clozapine (Co-administration may result in increased CNS depression). Products include:
- Clozaril Tablets ... 2184
- FazaClo Orally Disintegrating Tablets ... 551

Codeine Phosphate (Co-administration may result in increased CNS depression). Products include:
- Tylenol with Codeine Tablets ... 2391

Cyproheptadine Hydrochloride (Co-administration may result in increased CNS depression).
No products indexed under this heading.

Desflurane (Co-administration may result in increased CNS depression).
No products indexed under this heading.

Desipramine Hydrochloride (Co-administration may result in increased CNS depression).
No products indexed under this heading.

Dexchlorpheniramine Maleate (Co-administration may result in increased CNS depression).
No products indexed under this heading.

Dezocine (Co-administration may result in increased CNS depression).
No products indexed under this heading.

Diazepam (Co-administration may result in increased CNS depression). Products include:
- Diastat Rectal Delivery System ... 3343
- Valium Tablets ... 2819

Diltiazem Hydrochloride (CYP3A inhibitors, such as diltiazem, would be expected to increase plasma estazolam concentrations). Products include:
- Cardizem LA Extended Release Tablets ... 1728
- Tiazac Capsules ... 1201

Diltiazem Maleate (CYP3A inhibitors, such as diltiazem, would be expected to increase plasma estazolam concentrations).
No products indexed under this heading.

Diphenhydramine Citrate (Co-administration may result in increased CNS depression). Products include:
- Advil PM Caplets ... ▣615
- Excedrin PM Caplets/Tablets/Geltabs ... ▣610
- Goody's PM Powder for Pain with Sleeplessness ... ▣612

Diphenhydramine Hydrochloride (Co-administration may result in increased CNS depression). Products include:
- Nytol QuickCaps Caplets ... ▣615
- Nytol QuickGels Softgels Maximum Strength ... ▣616
- Simply Sleep Caplets ... 1868
- Sominex Original Formula Tablets .. ▣616
- TheraFlu Warming Relief Nighttime Severe Cold ... ▣743
- TheraFlu Thin Strips Multi Symptom ... ▣744
- Triaminic Nighttime Cold & Cough Liquid ... ▣746
- Triaminic Thin Strips Cough & Runny Nose ... ▣749
- Extra Strength Tylenol PM Caplets, Vanilla Caplets, Geltabs, Gelcaps and Liquid ... 1875
- Tylenol Sore Throat Nighttime Liquid with Cool Burst ... ▣790
- Tylenol Allergy Multi-Symptom Nighttime Caplets with Cool Burst ... 1872
- Tylenol Severe Allergy Caplets ... 1872
- Children's Tylenol Plus Cold & Allergy Suspension Liquid ... 1878

Diphenylpyraline Hydrochloride (Co-administration may result in increased CNS depression).
No products indexed under this heading.

Divalproex Sodium (Co-administration may result in increased CNS depression). Products include:
- Depakote Sprinkle Capsules ... 422
- Depakote Tablets ... 427
- Depakote ER Tablets ... 434

Doxepin Hydrochloride (Co-administration may result in increased CNS depression).
No products indexed under this heading.

Droperidol (Co-administration may result in increased CNS depression).
No products indexed under this heading.

Enflurane (Co-administration may result in increased CNS depression).
No products indexed under this heading.

Erythromycin Estolate (Potent CYP3A inhibitors, such as erythromycin, would be expected to increase plasma estazolam concentrations).
No products indexed under this heading.

Erythromycin Ethylsuccinate (Potent CYP3A inhibitors, such as

erythromycin, would be expected to increase plasma estazolam concentrations). Products include:
- E.E.S. 451
- EryPed 447

Erythromycin Gluceptate (Potent CYP3A inhibitors, such as erythromycin, would be expected to increase plasma estazolam concentrations).
No products indexed under this heading.

Erythromycin Lactobionate (Potent CYP3A inhibitors, such as erythromycin, would be expected to increase plasma estazolam concentrations).
No products indexed under this heading.

Erythromycin Stearate (Potent CYP3A inhibitors, such as erythromycin, would be expected to increase plasma estazolam concentrations). Products include:
- Erythrocin Stearate Filmtab Tablets 453

Ethanol (Co-administration may result in increased CNS depression).
No products indexed under this heading.

Ethchlorvynol (Co-administration may result in increased CNS depression).
No products indexed under this heading.

Ethinamate (Co-administration may result in increased CNS depression).
No products indexed under this heading.

Ethosuximide (Co-administration may result in increased CNS depression).
No products indexed under this heading.

Ethotoin (Co-administration may result in increased CNS depression).
No products indexed under this heading.

Ethyl Alcohol (Co-administration may result in increased CNS depression).
No products indexed under this heading.

Felbamate (Co-administration may result in increased CNS depression).
No products indexed under this heading.

Fentanyl (Co-administration may result in increased CNS depression). Products include:
- Duragesic Transdermal System 2373
- Ionsys Transdermal System 2379

Fentanyl Citrate (Co-administration may result in increased CNS depression). Products include:
- Actiq 979

Fexofenadine Hydrochloride (Co-administration may result in increased CNS depression). Products include:
- Allegra 2844
- Allegra-D 12 Hour Extended-Release Tablets 2846
- Allegra-D 24 Hour Extended-Release Tablets 2849

Fluphenazine Decanoate (Co-administration may result in increased CNS depression).
No products indexed under this heading.

Fluphenazine Enanthate (Co-administration may result in increased CNS depression).
No products indexed under this heading.

Fluphenazine Hydrochloride (Co-administration may result in increased CNS depression).
No products indexed under this heading.

Flurazepam Hydrochloride (Co-administration may result in increased CNS depression). Products include:
- Dalmane Capsules 3342

Fluvoxamine (Potent CYP3A inhibitors, such as fluvoxamine, would be expected to increase plasma estazolam concentrations).
No products indexed under this heading.

Fluvoxamine Maleate (Potent CYP3A inhibitors, such as fluvoxamine, would be expected to increase plasma estazolam concentrations).
No products indexed under this heading.

Fosphenytoin (Co-administration may result in increased CNS depression).
No products indexed under this heading.

Fosphenytoin Sodium (Potent CYP3A inducers, such as phenytoin, would be expected to decrease plasma estazolam concentrations and may potentiate the action of estazolam).
No products indexed under this heading.

Gabapentin (Co-administration may result in increased CNS depression). Products include:
- Neurontin Capsules 2487
- Neurontin Oral Solution 2487
- Neurontin Tablets 2487

Glutethimide (Co-administration may result in increased CNS depression).
No products indexed under this heading.

Haloperidol (Co-administration may result in increased CNS depression).
No products indexed under this heading.

Haloperidol Decanoate (Co-administration may result in increased CNS depression).
No products indexed under this heading.

Hydrocodone Bitartrate (Co-administration may result in increased CNS depression). Products include:
- Hycodan 1116
- Hycotuss Expectorant Syrup 1117
- Vicodin Tablets 535
- Vicodin ES Tablets 536
- Vicodin HP Tablets 538
- Vicoprofen Tablets 539
- Zydone Tablets 1139

Hydrocodone Polistirex (Co-administration may result in increased CNS depression). Products include:
- Tussionex Pennkinetic Extended-Release Suspension 3327

Hydromorphone Hydrochloride (Co-administration may result in increased CNS depression). Products include:
- Dilaudid 440
- Dilaudid Non-Sterile Powder 440
- Dilaudid Oral Liquid 445
- Dilaudid Rectal Suppositories 440
- Dilaudid Tablets 440
- Dilaudid Tablets - 8 mg 445
- Dilaudid-HP 442

Hydroxyzine Hydrochloride (Co-administration may result in increased CNS depression).
No products indexed under this heading.

Imipramine Hydrochloride (Co-administration may result in increased CNS depression).
No products indexed under this heading.

Imipramine Pamoate (Co-administration may result in increased CNS depression).
No products indexed under this heading.

Isocarboxazid (Co-administration may result in increased CNS depression).
No products indexed under this heading.

Isoflurane (Co-administration may result in increased CNS depression).
No products indexed under this heading.

Isoniazid (CYP3A inhibitors, such as diltiazem isoniazid, would be expected to increase plasma estazolam concentrations).
No products indexed under this heading.

Itraconazole (Potent CYP3A inhibitors, such as itraconazole, would be expected to increase plasma estazolam concentrations; estazolam should be avoided in patients receiving itraconazole).
No products indexed under this heading.

Ketamine Hydrochloride (Co-administration may result in increased CNS depression).
No products indexed under this heading.

Ketoconazole (Potent CYP3A inhibitors, such as ketoconazole, would be expected to increase plasma estazolam concentrations; estazolam should be avoided in patients receiving ketoconazole). Products include:
- Nizoral A-D Shampoo, 1% 1868

Lamotrigine (Co-administration may result in increased CNS depression). Products include:
- Lamictal 1481

Levetiracetam (Co-administration may result in increased CNS depression). Products include:
- Keppra Injection 3320
- Keppra Oral Solution 3314
- Keppra Tablets 3314

Levomethadyl Acetate Hydrochloride (Co-administration may result in increased CNS depression).
No products indexed under this heading.

Levorphanol Tartrate (Co-administration may result in increased CNS depression).
No products indexed under this heading.

Lithium Carbonate (Co-administration may result in increased CNS depression). Products include:
- Lithobid Tablets 1692

Lithium Citrate (Co-administration may result in increased CNS depression).
No products indexed under this heading.

Loratadine (Co-administration may result in increased CNS depression). Products include:
- Alavert Allergy & Sinus D-12 Hour Tablets 771
- Alavert 771
- Children's Claritin Allergy Oral Solution 771
- Claritin Non-Drowsy 24 Hour Tablets 772
- Claritin Reditabs 24 Hour Non-Drowsy Tablets 772
- Claritin-D Non-Drowsy 12 Hour Tablets 772
- Claritin-D Non-Drowsy 24 Hour Tablets 772

Lorazepam (Co-administration may result in increased CNS depression).
No products indexed under this heading.

Loxapine Hydrochloride (Co-administration may result in increased CNS depression).
No products indexed under this heading.

Loxapine Succinate (Co-administration may result in increased CNS depression).
No products indexed under this heading.

Maprotiline Hydrochloride (Co-administration may result in increased CNS depression).
No products indexed under this heading.

Meperidine Hydrochloride (Co-administration may result in increased CNS depression).
No products indexed under this heading.

Mephenytoin (Co-administration may result in increased CNS depression).
No products indexed under this heading.

Mephobarbital (Potent CYP3A inducers, such as barbiturates, would be expected to decrease plasma estazolam concentrations and may potentiate the action of estazolam).
No products indexed under this heading.

Meprobamate (Co-administration may result in increased CNS depression).
No products indexed under this heading.

Mesoridazine Besylate (Co-administration may result in increased CNS depression).
No products indexed under this heading.

Methadone Hydrochloride (Co-administration may result in increased CNS depression).
No products indexed under this heading.

Methdilazine Hydrochloride (Co-administration may result in increased CNS depression).
No products indexed under this heading.

Methohexital Sodium (Co-administration may result in increased CNS depression).
No products indexed under this heading.

Methotrimeprazine (Co-administration may result in increased CNS depression).
No products indexed under this heading.

Methoxyflurane (Co-administration may result in increased CNS depression).
No products indexed under this heading.

IMPORTANT NOTE: Always consult each drug listing in the patient's regimen for possible interactions.

Methsuximide (Co-administration may result in increased CNS depression).

No products indexed under this heading.

Midazolam Hydrochloride (Co-administration may result in increased CNS depression).

No products indexed under this heading.

Moclobemide (Co-administration with MAO inhibitors may result in increased CNS depression).

No products indexed under this heading.

Molindone Hydrochloride (Co-administration may result in increased CNS depression). Products include:

Moban Tablets 1119

Morphine Sulfate (Co-administration may result in increased CNS depression). Products include:

Avinza Capsules 1741
Kadian Capsules 577
MS Contin Tablets 2701

Nefazodone Hydrochloride (Potent CYP3A inhibitors, such as nefazodone, would be expected to increase plasma estazolam concentrations).

No products indexed under this heading.

Nortriptyline Hydrochloride (Co-administration may result in increased CNS depression).

No products indexed under this heading.

Olanzapine (Co-administration may result in increased CNS depression). Products include:

Symbyax Capsules 1819
Zyprexa Tablets 1830
Zyprexa IntraMuscular 1830
Zyprexa ZYDIS Orally
Disintegrating Tablets 1830

Oxazepam (Co-administration may result in increased CNS depression).

No products indexed under this heading.

Oxcarbazepine (Co-administration may result in increased CNS depression). Products include:

Trileptal Tablets 2300
Trileptal Oral Suspension 2300

Oxycodone Hydrochloride (Co-administration may result in increased CNS depression). Products include:

OxyContin Tablets 2703
OxyFast Oral Concentrate
Solution 2708
OxyIR Capsules 2708
Percocet Tablets 1131
Percodan Tablets 1132

Paramethadione (Co-administration may result in increased CNS depression).

No products indexed under this heading.

Pargyline Hydrochloride (Co-administration with MAO inhibitors may result in increased CNS depression).

No products indexed under this heading.

Pentobarbital Sodium (Potent CYP3A inducers, such as barbiturates, would be expected to decrease plasma estazolam concentrations and may potentiate the action of estazolam). Products include:

Nembutal Sodium Solution, USP 2470

Perphenazine (Co-administration may result in increased CNS depression).

No products indexed under this heading.

Phenacemide (Co-administration may result in increased CNS depression).

No products indexed under this heading.

Phenelzine Sulfate (Co-administration may result in increased CNS depression).

No products indexed under this heading.

Phenobarbital (Potent CYP3A inducers, such as barbiturates, would be expected to decrease plasma estazolam concentrations and may potentiate the action of estazolam). Products include:

Donnatal Extentabs 2493

Phensuximide (Co-administration may result in increased CNS depression).

No products indexed under this heading.

Phenytoin (Potent CYP3A inducers, such as phenytoin, would be expected to decrease plasma estazolam concentrations and may potentiate the action of estazolam).

No products indexed under this heading.

Phenytoin Sodium (Potent CYP3A inducers, such as phenytoin, would be expected to decrease plasma estazolam concentrations and may potentiate the action of estazolam). Products include:

Phenytek Capsules 2160

Prazepam (Co-administration may result in increased CNS depression).

No products indexed under this heading.

Primidone (Co-administration may result in increased CNS depression).

No products indexed under this heading.

Procarbazine Hydrochloride (Co-administration with MAO inhibitors may result in increased CNS depression). Products include:

Matulane Capsules 3191

Prochlorperazine (Co-administration may result in increased CNS depression).

No products indexed under this heading.

Promethazine Hydrochloride (Co-administration may result in increased CNS depression). Products include:

Phenergan Tablets and
Suppositories............................... 3440

Propofol (Co-administration may result in increased CNS depression).

No products indexed under this heading.

Propoxyphene Hydrochloride (Co-administration may result in increased CNS depression).

No products indexed under this heading.

Propoxyphene Napsylate (Co-administration may result in increased CNS depression).

No products indexed under this heading.

Protriptyline Hydrochloride (Co-administration may result in increased CNS depression).

No products indexed under this heading.

Pyrilamine Maleate (Co-administration may result in increased CNS depression).

No products indexed under this heading.

Pyrilamine Tannate (Co-administration may result in increased CNS depression).

No products indexed under this heading.

Quazepam (Co-administration may result in increased CNS depression).

No products indexed under this heading.

Quetiapine Fumarate (Co-administration may result in increased CNS depression). Products include:

Seroquel Tablets 690

Remifentanil Hydrochloride (Co-administration may result in increased CNS depression).

No products indexed under this heading.

Rifampin (Potent CYP3A inducers, such as rifampin, would be expected to decrease plasma estazolam concentrations).

No products indexed under this heading.

Risperidone (Co-administration may result in increased CNS depression). Products include:

Risperdal .. 1676
Risperdal Consta Long-Acting
Injection 1682
Risperdal M-Tab Orally
Disintegrating Tablets 1676

Secobarbital Sodium (Potent CYP3A inducers, such as barbiturates, would be expected to decrease plasma estazolam concentrations and may potentiate the action of estazolam).

No products indexed under this heading.

Selegiline Hydrochloride (Co-administration with MAO inhibitors may result in increased CNS depression). Products include:

Eldepryl Capsules 3208
Zelapar Tablets 3372

Sevoflurane (Co-administration may result in increased CNS depression). Products include:

Ultane Liquid for Inhalation 531

Sodium Oxybate (Co-administration may result in increased CNS depression). Products include:

Xyrem Oral Solution 1688

Sufentanil Citrate (Co-administration may result in increased CNS depression).

No products indexed under this heading.

Temazepam (Co-administration may result in increased CNS depression). Products include:

Restoril Capsules 1860

Terfenadine (Co-administration may result in increased CNS depression).

No products indexed under this heading.

Thiamylal Sodium (Potent CYP3A inducers, such as barbiturates, would be expected to decrease plasma estazolam concentrations and may potentiate the action of estazolam).

No products indexed under this heading.

Thioridazine Hydrochloride (Co-administration may result in increased CNS depression). Products include:

Thioridazine Hydrochloride
Tablets .. 2163

Thiothixene (Co-administration may result in increased CNS depression). Products include:

Thiothixene Capsules 2165

Tiagabine Hydrochloride (Co-administration may result in increased CNS depression). Products include:

Gabitril Tablets 984

Topiramate (Co-administration may result in increased CNS depression). Products include:

Topamax Sprinkle Capsules 2404
Topamax Tablets 2404

Tranylcypromine Sulfate (Co-administration may result in increased CNS depression). Products include:

Parnate Tablets 1527

Triazolam (Co-administration may result in increased CNS depression).

No products indexed under this heading.

Trifluoperazine Hydrochloride (Co-administration may result in increased CNS depression).

No products indexed under this heading.

Trimeprazine Tartrate (Co-administration may result in increased CNS depression).

No products indexed under this heading.

Trimethadione (Co-administration may result in increased CNS depression).

No products indexed under this heading.

Trimipramine Maleate (Co-administration may result in increased CNS depression).

No products indexed under this heading.

Tripelennamine Hydrochloride (Co-administration may result in increased CNS depression).

No products indexed under this heading.

Triprolidine Hydrochloride (Co-administration may result in increased CNS depression).

No products indexed under this heading.

Valproate Sodium (Co-administration may result in increased CNS depression). Products include:

Depacon Injection 412

Valproic Acid (Co-administration may result in increased CNS depression). Products include:

Depakene .. 417

Zaleplon (Co-administration may result in increased CNS depression). Products include:

Sonata Capsules 1717

Ziprasidone Hydrochloride (Co-administration may result in increased CNS depression). Products include:

Geodon Capsules 2529

Zolpidem Tartrate (Co-administration may result in increased CNS depression). Products include:

Ambien Tablets 2851
Ambien CR Tablets 2855

Zonisamide (Co-administration may result in increased CNS depression). Products include:

Zonegran Capsules 1101

Food Interactions

Alcohol (Co-administration may result in increased CNS depression).

PROSTASCINT KIT
(Capromab Pendetide) **1037**

May interact with antiandrogens. Compounds in these categories include:

Bicalutamide (The effect of surgical and/or medical androgen ablation on the imaging performance of Indium In 111 capromab pendetide has not been studied. Preliminary data suggest hormone ablation may increase PSMA expression, with concurrent decrease in tumor expression of PSA. The use of capromab pendetide in this patient population cannot be recommended at this time).

No products indexed under this heading.

Flutamide (The effect of surgical and/or medical androgen ablation on the imaging performance of Indium In 111 capromab pendetide has not been studied. Preliminary data suggest hormone ablation may increase PSMA expression, with concurrent decrease in tumor expression of PSA. The use of capromab pendetide in this patient population cannot be recommended at this time). Products include:

Eulexin Capsules **3009**

Nilutamide (The effect of surgical and/or medical androgen ablation on the imaging performance of Indium In 111 capromab pendetide has not been studied. Preliminary data suggest hormone ablation may increase PSMA expression, with concurrent decrease in tumor expression of PSA. The use of capromab pendetide in this patient population cannot be recommended at this time).

No products indexed under this heading.

PROTONIX I.V.
(Pantoprazole Sodium) **3472**

See Protonix Tablets

PROTONIX TABLETS
(Pantoprazole Sodium) **3469**

May interact with iron containing oral preparations and certain other agents. Compounds in these categories include:

Bacampicillin Hydrochloride (Pantoprazole produces sustained inhibition of gastric acid secretion; pantoprazole may interfere with the absorption of certain drugs, such as ampicillin esters, where gastric pH is an important determinant of the bioavailability).

No products indexed under this heading.

Ferrous Fumarate (Pantoprazole produces sustained inhibition of gastric acid secretion; pantoprazole may interfere with the absorption of certain drugs, such as iron salts, where gastric pH is an important determinant of the bioavailability).

No products indexed under this heading.

Ferrous Gluconate (Pantoprazole produces sustained inhibition of gastric acid secretion; pantoprazole may interfere with the absorption of certain drugs, such as iron salts, where gastric pH is an important determinant of the bioavailability).

No products indexed under this heading.

Ferrous Sulfate (Pantoprazole produces sustained inhibition of gastric acid secretion; pantoprazole may interfere with the absorption of certain drugs, such as iron salts, where gastric pH is an important determinant of the bioavailability). Products include:

Slow Fe Iron Tablets **818**

Slow Fe with Folic Acid Tablets **819**

Iron (Pantoprazole produces sustained inhibition of gastric acid secretion; pantoprazole may interfere with the absorption of certain drugs, such as iron salts, where gastric pH is an important determinant of the bioavailability).

No products indexed under this heading.

Ketoconazole (Pantoprazole produces sustained inhibition of gastric acid secretion; pantoprazole may interfere with the absorption of certain drugs, such as ketoconazole, where gastric pH is an important determinant of the bioavailability). Products include:

Nizoral A-D Shampoo, 1% **1868**

Polysaccharide Iron Complex (Pantoprazole produces sustained inhibition of gastric acid secretion; pantoprazole may interfere with the absorption of certain drugs, such as iron salts, where gastric pH is an important determinant of the bioavailability). Products include:

Nu-Iron 150 Capsules **2127**

Warfarin Sodium (There have been reports of increased INR and prothrombin time in patients receiving proton pump inhibitors, including pantoprazole and warfarin concomitantly. Patients treated with proton pump inhibitors and warfarin concomitantly should be monitored for increases in INR and prothrombin time). Products include:

Coumadin for Injection **898**

Coumadin Tablets **898**

PROTOPIC OINTMENT
(Tacrolimus) **638**

May interact with calcium channel blockers, erythromycin, and certain other agents. Compounds in these categories include:

Amlodipine Besylate (Co-administration of known CYP3A4 inhibitors, such as calcium channel blockers, in patients with widespread and/or erythrodermic disease should be done with caution; based on its minimal extent of absorption, interactions of Protopic Ointment with systemically administered drugs are unlikely to occur but cannot be ruled out). Products include:

Caduet Tablets **2508**

Lotrel Capsules **2249**

Norvasc Tablets **2545**

Bepridil Hydrochloride (Co-administration of known CYP3A4 inhibitors, such as calcium channel blockers, in patients with widespread and/or erythrodermic disease should be done with caution; based on its minimal extent of absorption, interactions of Protopic Ointment with systemically administered drugs are unlikely to occur but cannot be ruled out).

No products indexed under this heading.

Cimetidine (Co-administration of known CYP3A4 inhibitors, such as cimetidine, in patients with widespread and/or erythrodermic disease should be done with caution; based on its minimal extent of absorption, interactions of Protopic Ointment with systemically administered drugs are unlikely to occur but cannot be ruled out). Products include:

Tagamet HB 200 Tablets **664**

Cimetidine Hydrochloride (Co-administration of known CYP3A4 inhibitors, such as cimetidine, in patients with widespread and/or erythrodermic disease should be done with caution; based on its minimal extent of absorption, interactions of Protopic Ointment with systemically administered drugs are unlikely to occur but cannot be ruled out).

No products indexed under this heading.

Diltiazem Hydrochloride (Co-administration of known CYP3A4 inhibitors, such as calcium channel blockers, in patients with widespread and/or erythrodermic disease should be done with caution; based on its minimal extent of absorption, interactions of Protopic Ointment with systemically administered drugs are unlikely to occur but cannot be ruled out). Products include:

Cardizem LA Extended Release Tablets **1728**

Tiazac Capsules **1201**

Erythromycin (Co-administration of known CYP3A4 inhibitors, such as erythromycin, in patients with widespread and/or erythrodermic disease should be done with caution; based on its minimal extent of absorption, interactions of Protopic Ointment with systemically administered drugs are unlikely to occur but cannot be ruled out). Products include:

Ery-Tab Tablets **449**

Erythromycin Base Filmtab Tablets **455**

Erythromycin Delayed-Release Capsules, USP **457**

PCE Dispertab Tablets **515**

Erythromycin Estolate (Co-administration of known CYP3A4 inhibitors, such as erythromycin, in patients with widespread and/or erythrodermic disease should be done with caution; based on its minimal extent of absorption, interactions of Protopic Ointment with systemically administered drugs are unlikely to occur but cannot be ruled out).

No products indexed under this heading.

Erythromycin Ethylsuccinate (Co-administration of known CYP3A4 inhibitors, such as erythromycin, in patients with widespread and/or erythrodermic disease should be done with caution; based on its minimal extent of absorption, interactions of Protopic Ointment with systemically administered drugs are unlikely to occur but cannot be ruled out). Products include:

E.E.S. **451**

EryPed **447**

Erythromycin Gluceptate (Co-administration of known CYP3A4 inhibitors, such as erythromycin, in patients with widespread and/or erythrodermic disease should be done with caution; based on its minimal extent of absorption, interactions of Protopic Ointment with systemically administered drugs are unlikely to occur but cannot be ruled out).

No products indexed under this heading.

Erythromycin Lactobionate (Co-administration of known CYP3A4 inhibitors, such as erythromycin, in patients with widespread and/or erythrodermic disease should be done with caution; based on its minimal extent of absorption, interactions of Protopic Ointment with systemically administered drugs are unlikely to occur but cannot be ruled out).

No products indexed under this heading.

Erythromycin Stearate (Co-administration of known CYP3A4 inhibitors, such as erythromycin, in patients with widespread and/or erythrodermic disease should be done with caution; based on its minimal extent of absorption, interactions of Protopic Ointment with systemically administered drugs are unlikely to occur but cannot be ruled out). Products include:

Erythrocin Stearate Filmtab Tablets **453**

Felodipine (Co-administration of known CYP3A4 inhibitors, such as calcium channel blockers, in patients with widespread and/or erythrodermic disease should be done with caution; based on its minimal extent of absorption, interactions of Protopic Ointment with systemically administered drugs are unlikely to occur but cannot be ruled out).

No products indexed under this heading.

Fluconazole (Co-administration of known CYP3A4 inhibitors, such as fluconazole, in patients with widespread and/or erythrodermic disease should be done with caution; based on its minimal extent of absorption, interactions of Protopic Ointment with systemically administered drugs are unlikely to occur but cannot be ruled out).

No products indexed under this heading.

Isradipine (Co-administration of known CYP3A4 inhibitors, such as calcium channel blockers, in patients with widespread and/or erythrodermic disease should be done with caution; based on its minimal extent of absorption, interactions of Protopic Ointment with systemically administered drugs are unlikely to occur but cannot be ruled out). Products include:

DynaCirc CR Tablets **2721**

Itraconazole (Co-administration of known CYP3A4 inhibitors, such as itraconazole, in patients with widespread and/or erythrodermic disease should be done with caution; based on its minimal extent of absorption, interactions of Protopic Ointment with systemically administered drugs are unlikely to occur but cannot be ruled out).

No products indexed under this heading.

Ketoconazole (Co-administration of known CYP3A4 inhibitors, such as ketoconazole, in patients with widespread and/or erythrodermic disease should be done with caution; based on its minimal extent of absorption, interactions of Protopic Ointment with systemically administered drugs are unlikely to occur but cannot be ruled out). Products include:

Nizoral A-D Shampoo, 1% **1868**

Mibefradil Dihydrochloride (Co-administration of known CYP3A4 inhibitors, such as calcium channel blockers, in patients with widespread and/or erythrodermic disease should be done with caution; based on its minimal extent of absorption, interactions of Protopic Ointment with systemically administered drugs are unlikely to occur but cannot be ruled out).
No products indexed under this heading.

Nicardipine Hydrochloride (Co-administration of known CYP3A4 inhibitors, such as calcium channel blockers, in patients with widespread and/or erythrodermic disease should be done with caution; based on its minimal extent of absorption, interactions of Protopic Ointment with systemically administered drugs are unlikely to occur but cannot be ruled out). Products include:
Cardene I.V. 2497

Nifedipine (Co-administration of known CYP3A4 inhibitors, such as calcium channel blockers, in patients with widespread and/or erythrodermic disease should be done with caution; based on its minimal extent of absorption, interactions of Protopic Ointment with systemically administered drugs are unlikely to occur but cannot be ruled out). Products include:
Adalat CC Tablets 2964

Nimodipine (Co-administration of known CYP3A4 inhibitors, such as calcium channel blockers, in patients with widespread and/or erythrodermic disease should be done with caution; based on its minimal extent of absorption, interactions of Protopic Ointment with systemically administered drugs are unlikely to occur but cannot be ruled out). Products include:
Nimotop Capsules 749

Nisoldipine (Co-administration of known CYP3A4 inhibitors, such as calcium channel blockers, in patients with widespread and/or erythrodermic disease should be done with caution; based on its minimal extent of absorption, interactions of Protopic Ointment with systemically administered drugs are unlikely to occur but cannot be ruled out). Products include:
Sular Tablets 3122

Verapamil Hydrochloride (Co-administration of known CYP3A4 inhibitors, such as calcium channel blockers, in patients with widespread and/or erythrodermic disease should be done with caution; based on its minimal extent of absorption, interactions of Protopic Ointment with systemically administered drugs are unlikely to occur but cannot be ruled out). Products include:
Covera-HS Tablets 3139
Tarka Tablets 524
Verelan PM Extended-Release Capsules, Controlled-Onset 3106

PROVENTIL INHALATION AEROSOL

(Albuterol) 3053

May interact with beta blockers, drugs that lower serum potassium (selected), loop diuretics, monoamine oxidase inhibitors, nonpotassium-sparing diuretics, thiazides, tricyclic antidepressants, and certain other agents. Compounds in these categories include:

Acebutolol Hydrochloride (Beta-adrenergic receptor blocking agents not only block the pulmonary effect of beta-agonists, such as albuterol, but may produce severe bronchospasm in asthmatic patients. Therefore, patients with asthma should not normally be treated with beta-blockers. However, under certain circumstances, (e.g., as prophylaxis after myocardial infarction) there may be no acceptable alternatives to the use of beta-adrenergic-blocking agents in patients with asthma. In this setting, cardioselective beta-blockers should be considered, although they should be administered with caution).
No products indexed under this heading.

Amitriptyline Hydrochloride (Albuterol should be administered with extreme caution to patients being treated with tricyclic antidepressants, or within 2 weeks of discontinuation of such agents, because of action of albuterol on the cardiovascular system may be potentiated).
No products indexed under this heading.

Amoxapine (Albuterol should be administered with extreme caution to patients being treated with tricyclic antidepressants, or within 2 weeks of discontinuation of such agents, because of action of albuterol on the cardiovascular system may be potentiated).
No products indexed under this heading.

Atenolol (Beta-adrenergic receptor blocking agents not only block the pulmonary effect of beta-agonists, such as albuterol, but may produce severe bronchospasm in asthmatic patients. Therefore, patients with asthma should not normally be treated with beta-blockers. However, under certain circumstances, (e.g., as prophylaxis after myocardial infarction) there may be no acceptable alternatives to the use of beta-adrenergic-blocking agents in patients with asthma. In this setting, cardioselective beta-blockers should be considered, although they should be administered with caution).
No products indexed under this heading.

Bendroflumethiazide (Potential for additive hypokalemic effect with concurrent use).
No products indexed under this heading.

Betamethasone Acetate (Potential for additive hypokalemic effect with concurrent use).
No products indexed under this heading.

Betamethasone Sodium Phosphate (Potential for additive hypokalemic effect with concurrent use).
No products indexed under this heading.

Betaxolol Hydrochloride (Beta-adrenergic receptor blocking agents not only block the pulmonary effect of beta-agonists, such as albuterol, but may produce severe bronchospasm in asthmatic patients. Therefore, patients with asthma should not normally be treated with beta-blockers. However, under certain circumstances, (e.g., as prophylaxis after myocardial infarction) there may be no acceptable alternatives to the use of beta-adrenergic-blocking agents in patients with asthma. In this setting, cardioselective beta-blockers should be considered, although they should be administered with caution). Products include:
Betoptic S Ophthalmic Suspension 558

Bisoprolol Fumarate (Beta-adrenergic receptor blocking agents not only block the pulmonary effect of beta-agonists, such as albuterol, but may produce severe bronchospasm in asthmatic patients. Therefore, patients with asthma should not normally be treated with beta-blockers. However, under certain circumstances, (e.g., as prophylaxis after myocardial infarction) there may be no acceptable alternatives to the use of beta-adrenergic-blocking agents in patients with asthma. In this setting, cardioselective beta-blockers should be considered, although they should be administered with caution).
No products indexed under this heading.

Bumetanide (The ECG changes and/or hypokalemia which may result from the administration of non-potassium sparing diuretics (such as loop or thiazide diuretics) can be acutely worsened by beta agonists, especially when the recommended dose of the beta agonist is exceeded. Although the clinical significance of these effects is not known, caution is advised in the co-administration of beta agonists with non-potassium sparing diuretics). Products include:
Bumex Tablets 2746

Carteolol Hydrochloride (Beta-adrenergic receptor blocking agents not only block the pulmonary effect of beta-agonists, such as albuterol, but may produce severe bronchospasm in asthmatic patients. Therefore, patients with asthma should not normally be treated with beta-blockers. However, under certain circumstances, (e.g., as prophylaxis after myocardial infarction) there may be no acceptable alternatives to the use of beta-adrenergic-blocking agents in patients with asthma. In this setting, cardioselective beta-blockers should be considered, although they should be administered with caution). Products include:
Carteolol Hydrochloride Ophthalmic Solution USP, 1% .... ⊙249

Chlorothiazide (Potential for additive hypokalemic effect with concurrent use). Products include:
Diuril Oral Suspension 1954

Chlorothiazide Sodium (Potential for additive hypokalemic effect with concurrent use). Products include:
Diuril Sodium Intravenous 2467

Clomipramine Hydrochloride (Albuterol should be administered with extreme caution to patients being treated with tricyclic antidepressants, or within 2 weeks of discontinuation of such agents, because of action of albuterol on the cardiovascular system may be potentiated).
No products indexed under this heading.

Cortisone Acetate (Potential for additive hypokalemic effect with concurrent use).
No products indexed under this heading.

Desipramine Hydrochloride (Albuterol should be administered with extreme caution to patients being treated with tricyclic antidepressants, or within 2 weeks of discontinuation of such agents, because of action of albuterol on the cardiovascular system may be potentiated).
No products indexed under this heading.

Dexamethasone (Potential for additive hypokalemic effect with concurrent use). Products include:
Ciprodex Otic Suspension 559
Decadron Tablets 1951
TobraDex Ophthalmic Ointment 562
TobraDex Ophthalmic Suspension 563

Dexamethasone Acetate (Potential for additive hypokalemic effect with concurrent use).
No products indexed under this heading.

Dexamethasone Sodium Phosphate (Potential for additive hypokalemic effect with concurrent use).
No products indexed under this heading.

Digoxin (Mean decreases of 16% and 22% in serum digoxin levels were demonstrated after single-dose intravenous and oral administration of albuterol, respectively, to normal volunteers who had received digoxin for 10 days. The clinical significance of these findings for patients with obstructive airway disease who are receiving albuterol and digoxin on a chronic basis is unclear; nevertheless, it would be prudent to carefully evaluate the serum digoxin levels in patients who are currently receiving digoxin and albuterol). Products include:
Lanoxicaps Capsules 1490
Lanoxin Injection 1494
Lanoxin Injection Pediatric 1497
Lanoxin Tablets 1500

Doxepin Hydrochloride (Albuterol should be administered with extreme caution to patients being treated with tricyclic antidepressants, or within 2 weeks of discontinuation of such agents, because of action of albuterol on the cardiovascular system may be potentiated).
No products indexed under this heading.

Esmolol Hydrochloride (Beta-adrenergic receptor blocking agents not only block the pulmonary effect of beta-agonists, such as albuterol, but may produce severe bronchospasm in asthmatic patients. Therefore, patients with asthma should not normally be treated with beta-blockers. However, under certain circumstances, (e.g., as prophylaxis after myocardial infarction) there may be no acceptable alternatives to the use of beta-adrenergic-blocking agents in patients with asthma. In this setting, cardioselective beta-blockers should be considered, although they should be administered with caution).
No products indexed under this heading.

Ethacrynic Acid (The ECG changes and/or hypokalemia which may result from the administration of non-potassium sparing diuretics (such as loop or thiazide diuretics) can be acutely worsened by beta agonists, especially when the recommended dose of the beta agonist is exceeded. Although the clinical significance of these effects is not known, caution is advised in the co-administration of beta agonists with non-potassium sparing diuretics). Products include:

Edecrin Tablets 1959

Furosemide (The ECG changes and/or hypokalemia which may result from the administration of non-potassium sparing diuretics (such as loop or thiazide diuretics) can be acutely worsened by beta agonists, especially when the recommended dose of the beta agonist is exceeded. Although the clinical significance of these effects is not known, caution is advised in the co-administration of beta agonists with non-potassium sparing diuretics). Products include:

Furosemide Tablets 2154

Hydrochlorothiazide (Potential for additive hypokalemic effect with concurrent use). Products include:

Aldoril Tablets 1910
Atacand HCT 651
Avalide Tablets 888
Avalide Tablets 2874
Benicar HCT Tablets 1044
Diovan HCT Tablets 2196
Dyazide Capsules 1423
Hyzaar 50-12.5 Tablets 1990
Hyzaar 100-12.5 Tablets 1990
Hyzaar 100-25 Tablets 1990
Lopressor HCT 50/25 Tablets 2241
Lopressor HCT 100/25 Tablets 2241
Lopressor HCT 100/50 Tablets 2241
Lotensin HCT Tablets 2246
Micardis HCT Tablets 856
Moduretic Tablets 2028
Prinzide Tablets 2056
Teveten HCT Tablets 1737
Timolide Tablets 2086
Uniretic Tablets 3100

Hydrocortisone (Potential for additive hypokalemic effect with concurrent use). Products include:

Colocort Rectal Suspension, USP (Retention) 100 mg/60 mL........... 2476
Hydrocortone Tablets 1989
Preparation H Hydrocortisone Cream 646

Hydrocortisone Acetate (Potential for additive hypokalemic effect with concurrent use). Products include:

Analpram-HC 1159
Pramosone 1161
ProctoFoam-HC 3099

Hydrocortisone Sodium Phosphate (Potential for additive hypokalemic effect with concurrent use).

No products indexed under this heading.

Hydrocortisone Sodium Succinate (Potential for additive hypokalemic effect with concurrent use).

No products indexed under this heading.

Hydroflumethiazide (Potential for additive hypokalemic effect with concurrent use).

No products indexed under this heading.

Imipramine Hydrochloride (Albuterol should be administered with extreme caution to patients being treated with tricyclic antidepressants, or within 2 weeks of discontinuation of such agents, because of action of albuterol on the cardiovascular system may be potentiated).

No products indexed under this heading.

Imipramine Pamoate (Albuterol should be administered with extreme caution to patients being treated with tricyclic antidepressants, or within 2 weeks of discontinuation of such agents, because of action of albuterol on the cardiovascular system may be potentiated).

No products indexed under this heading.

Isocarboxazid (Albuterol should be administered with extreme caution to patients being treated with monoamine oxidase inhibitors, or within 2 weeks of discontinuation of such agents, because of action of albuterol on the cardiovascular system may be potentiated).

No products indexed under this heading.

Labetalol Hydrochloride (Beta-adrenergic receptor blocking agents not only block the pulmonary effect of beta-agonists, such as albuterol, but may produce severe bronchospasm in asthmatic patients. Therefore, patients with asthma should not normally be treated with beta-blockers. However, under certain circumstances, (e.g., as prophylaxis after myocardial infarction) there may be no acceptable alternatives to the use of beta-adrenergic-blocking agents in patients with asthma. In this setting, cardioselective beta-blockers should be considered, although they should be administered with caution).

No products indexed under this heading.

Levobunolol Hydrochloride (Beta-adrenergic receptor blocking agents not only block the pulmonary effect of beta-agonists, such as albuterol, but may produce severe bronchospasm in asthmatic patients. Therefore, patients with asthma should not normally be treated with beta-blockers. However, under certain circumstances, (e.g., as prophylaxis after myocardial infarction) there may be no acceptable alternatives to the use of beta-adrenergic-blocking agents in patients with asthma. In this setting, cardioselective beta-blockers should be considered, although they should be administered with caution). Products include:

Betagan Ophthalmic Solution, USP.. ⊙220

Maprotiline Hydrochloride (Albuterol should be administered with extreme caution to patients being treated with tricyclic antidepressants, or within 2 weeks of discontinuation of such agents, because of action of albuterol on the cardiovascular system may be potentiated).

No products indexed under this heading.

Methyclothiazide (Potential for additive hypokalemic effect with concurrent use).

No products indexed under this heading.

Methylprednisolone Acetate (Potential for additive hypokalemic effect with concurrent use). Products include:

Depo-Medrol Injectable Suspension 2617
Depo-Medrol Single-Dose Vial 2619

Methylprednisolone Sodium Succinate (Potential for additive hypokalemic effect with concurrent use).

No products indexed under this heading.

Metipranolol Hydrochloride (Beta-adrenergic receptor blocking agents not only block the pulmonary effect of beta-agonists, such as albuterol, but may produce severe bronchospasm in asthmatic patients. Therefore, patients with asthma should not normally be treated with beta-blockers. However, under certain circumstances, (e.g., as prophylaxis after myocardial infarction) there may be no acceptable alternatives to the use of beta-adrenergic-blocking agents in patients with asthma. In this setting, cardioselective beta-blockers should be considered, although they should be administered with caution).

No products indexed under this heading.

Metoprolol Succinate (Beta-adrenergic receptor blocking agents not only block the pulmonary effect of beta-agonists, such as albuterol, but may produce severe bronchospasm in asthmatic patients. Therefore, patients with asthma should not normally be treated with beta-blockers. However, under certain circumstances, (e.g., as prophylaxis after myocardial infarction) there may be no acceptable alternatives to the use of beta-adrenergic-blocking agents in patients with asthma. In this setting, cardioselective beta-blockers should be considered, although they should be administered with caution). Products include:

Toprol-XL Tablets 668

Metoprolol Tartrate (Beta-adrenergic receptor blocking agents not only block the pulmonary effect of beta-agonists, such as albuterol, but may produce severe bronchospasm in asthmatic patients. Therefore, patients with asthma should not normally be treated with beta-blockers. However, under certain circumstances, (e.g., as prophylaxis after myocardial infarction) there may be no acceptable alternatives to the use of beta-adrenergic-blocking agents in patients with asthma. In this setting, cardioselective beta-blockers should be considered, although they should be administered with caution). Products include:

Lopressor Injection 2238
Lopressor Tablets 2238
Lopressor HCT 50/25 Tablets 2241
Lopressor HCT 100/25 Tablets 2241
Lopressor HCT 100/50 Tablets 2241

Moclobemide (Albuterol should be administered with extreme caution to patients being treated with monoamine oxidase inhibitors, or within 2 weeks of discontinuation of such agents, because of action of albuterol on the cardiovascular system may be potentiated).

No products indexed under this heading.

Nadolol (Beta-adrenergic receptor blocking agents not only block the pulmonary effect of beta-agonists, such as albuterol, but may produce severe bronchospasm in asthmatic patients. Therefore, patients with asthma should not normally be treated with beta-blockers. However, under certain circumstances, (e.g., as prophylaxis after myocardial infarction) there may be no acceptable alternatives to the use of beta-adrenergic-blocking agents in patients with asthma. In this setting, cardioselective beta-blockers should be considered, although they should be administered with caution). Products include:

Nadolol Tablets 2159

Nortriptyline Hydrochloride (Albuterol should be administered with extreme caution to patients being treated with tricyclic antidepressants, or within 2 weeks of discontinuation of such agents, because of action of albuterol on the cardiovascular system may be potentiated).

No products indexed under this heading.

Pargyline Hydrochloride (Albuterol should be administered with extreme caution to patients being treated with monoamine oxidase inhibitors, or within 2 weeks of discontinuation of such agents, because of action of albuterol on the cardiovascular system may be potentiated).

No products indexed under this heading.

Penbutolol Sulfate (Beta-adrenergic receptor blocking agents not only block the pulmonary effect of beta-agonists, such as albuterol, but may produce severe bronchospasm in asthmatic patients. Therefore, patients with asthma should not normally be treated with beta-blockers. However, under certain circumstances, (e.g., as prophylaxis after myocardial infarction) there may be no acceptable alternatives to the use of beta-adrenergic-blocking agents in patients with asthma. In this setting, cardioselective beta-blockers should be considered, although they should be administered with caution).

No products indexed under this heading.

Phenelzine Sulfate (Albuterol should be administered with extreme caution to patients being treated with monoamine oxidase inhibitors, or within 2 weeks of discontinuation of such agents, because of action of albuterol on the cardiovascular system may be potentiated).

No products indexed under this heading.

Pindolol (Beta-adrenergic receptor blocking agents not only block the pulmonary effect of beta-agonists, such as albuterol, but may produce severe bronchospasm in asthmatic patients. Therefore, patients with asthma should not normally be treated with beta-blockers. However, under certain circumstances, (e.g., as prophylaxis after myocardial infarction) there may be no acceptable alternatives to the use of beta-adrenergic-blocking agents in patients with asthma. In this setting, cardioselective beta-blockers should be considered, although they should be administered with caution).

No products indexed under this heading.

Polythiazide (Potential for additive hypokalemic effect with concurrent use).

No products indexed under this heading.

Prednisolone Acetate (Potential for additive hypokalemic effect with concurrent use). Products include:

Blephamide Ophthalmic Ointment 568
Blephamide Ophthalmic Suspension 569
Poly-Pred Ophthalmic Suspension .... ⊙233
Pred Forte Ophthalmic Suspension .... ⊙235
Pred Mild Ophthalmic Suspension .... ⊙238
Pred-G Ophthalmic Ointment .... ⊙237
Pred-G Ophthalmic Suspension .... ⊙236

Prednisolone Sodium Phosphate (Potential for additive hypokalemic effect with concurrent use).
No products indexed under this heading.

Prednisolone Tebutate (Potential for additive hypokalemic effect with concurrent use).
No products indexed under this heading.

Prednisone (Potential for additive hypokalemic effect with concurrent use).
No products indexed under this heading.

Procarbazine Hydrochloride (Albuterol should be administered with extreme caution to patients being treated with monoamine oxidase inhibitors, or within 2 weeks of discontinuation of such agents, because of action of albuterol on the cardiovascular system may be potentiated). Products include:
Matulane Capsules 3191

Propranolol Hydrochloride (Beta-adrenergic receptor blocking agents not only block the pulmonary effect of beta-agonists, such as albuterol, but may produce severe bronchospasm in asthmatic patients. Therefore, patients with asthma should not normally be treated with beta-blockers. However, under certain circumstances, (e.g., as prophylaxis after myocardial infarction) there may be no acceptable alternatives to the use of beta-adrenergic-blocking agents in patients with asthma. In this setting, cardioselective beta-blockers should be considered, although they should be administered with caution). Products include:
Inderal LA Long-Acting Capsules 3429
InnoPran XL Capsules 2723

Protriptyline Hydrochloride (Albuterol should be administered with extreme caution to patients being treated with tricyclic antidepressants, or within 2 weeks of discontinuation of such agents, because of action of albuterol on the cardiovascular system may be potentiated).
No products indexed under this heading.

Selegiline Hydrochloride (Albuterol should be administered with extreme caution to patients being treated with monoamine oxidase inhibitors, or within 2 weeks of discontinuation of such agents, because of action of albuterol on the cardiovascular system may be potentiated). Products include:
Eldepryl Capsules 3208
Zelapar Tablets 3372

Sotalol Hydrochloride (Beta-adrenergic receptor blocking agents not only block the pulmonary effect of beta-agonists, such as albuterol, but may produce severe bronchospasm in asthmatic patients. Therefore, patients with asthma should not normally be treated with beta-blockers. However, under certain circumstances, (e.g., as prophylaxis after myocardial infarction) there may be no acceptable alternatives to the use of beta-adrenergic-blocking agents in patients with asthma. In this setting, cardioselective beta-blockers should be considered, although they should be administered with caution).
No products indexed under this heading.

Timolol Hemihydrate (Beta-adrenergic receptor blocking agents not only block the pulmonary effect of beta-agonists, such as albuterol, but may produce severe bronchospasm in asthmatic patients. Therefore, patients with asthma should not normally be treated with beta-blockers. However, under certain circumstances, (e.g., as prophylaxis after myocardial infarction) there may be no acceptable alternatives to the use of beta-adrenergic-blocking agents in patients with asthma. In this setting, cardioselective beta-blockers should be considered, although they should be administered with caution). Products include:
Betimol Ophthalmic Solution 3382
Betimol Ophthalmic Solution .... ⊙295

Timolol Maleate (Beta-adrenergic receptor blocking agents not only block the pulmonary effect of beta-agonists, such as albuterol, but may produce severe bronchospasm in asthmatic patients. Therefore, patients with asthma should not normally be treated with beta-blockers. However, under certain circumstances, (e.g., as prophylaxis after myocardial infarction) there may be no acceptable alternatives to the use of beta-adrenergic-blocking agents in patients with asthma. In this setting, cardioselective beta-blockers should be considered, although they should be administered with caution). Products include:
Blocadren Tablets 1916
Cosopt Sterile Ophthalmic Solution 1931
Timolide Tablets 2086
Timoptic Sterile Ophthalmic Solution 2088
Timoptic in Ocudose 2091
Timoptic-XE Sterile Ophthalmic Gel Forming Solution 2092

Torsemide (The ECG changes and/or hypokalemia which may result from the administration of non-potassium sparing diuretics (such as loop or thiazide diuretics) can be acutely worsened by beta agonists, especially when the recommended dose of the beta agonist is exceeded. Although the clinical significance of these effects is not known, caution is advised in the co-administration of beta agonists with non-potassium sparing diuretics). Products include:
Demadex Injection 2759
Demadex Tablets 2759

Tranylcypromine Sulfate (Albuterol should be administered with extreme caution to patients being treated with monoamine oxidase inhibitors, or within 2 weeks of discontinuation of such agents, because of action of albuterol on the cardiovascular system may be potentiated). Products include:
Parnate Tablets 1527

Triamcinolone (Potential for additive hypokalemic effect with concurrent use).
No products indexed under this heading.

Triamcinolone Acetonide (Potential for additive hypokalemic effect with concurrent use). Products include:
Azmacort Inhalation Aerosol 1726
Nasacort AQ Nasal Spray 2922

Triamcinolone Diacetate (Potential for additive hypokalemic effect with concurrent use).
No products indexed under this heading.

Triamcinolone Hexacetonide (Potential for additive hypokalemic effect with concurrent use).
No products indexed under this heading.

Trimipramine Maleate (Albuterol should be administered with extreme caution to patients being treated with tricyclic antidepressants, or within 2 weeks of discontinuation of such agents, because of action of albuterol on the cardiovascular system may be potentiated).
No products indexed under this heading.

PROVENTIL INHALATION SOLUTION 0.083%

(Albuterol Sulfate) 3055
May interact with:

See (Proventil Inhalation Aerosol).
No products indexed under this heading.

PROVENTIL HFA INHALATION AEROSOL

(Albuterol Sulfate) 3056
May interact with beta blockers, loop diuretics, monoamine oxidase inhibitors, nonpotassium-sparing diuretics, thiazides, tricyclic antidepressants, and certain other agents. Compounds in these categories include:

Acebutolol Hydrochloride (Co-administration with beta adrenergic blocking agent blocks the pulmonary effect of beta agonists and may produce severe bronchospasm in asthmatic patients; co-administer with caution).
No products indexed under this heading.

Amitriptyline Hydrochloride (Action of albuterol on the cardiovascular system may be potentiated by tricyclic antidepressants; co-administer with caution).
No products indexed under this heading.

Amoxapine (Action of albuterol on the cardiovascular system may be potentiated by tricyclic antidepressants; co-administer with caution).
No products indexed under this heading.

Atenolol (Co-administration with beta adrenergic blocking agent blocks the pulmonary effect of beta agonists and may produce severe bronchospasm in asthmatic patients; co-administer with caution).
No products indexed under this heading.

Bendroflumethiazide (The ECG changes and hypokalemia which may result from administration of nonpotassium-sparing diuretics can be acutely worsened by beta agonists. Caution is advised in the co-administration of beta agonists with nonpotassium-sparing diuretics).
No products indexed under this heading.

Betaxolol Hydrochloride (Co-administration with beta adrenergic blocking agent blocks the pulmonary effect of beta agonists and may produce severe bronchospasm in asthmatic patients; co-administer with caution). Products include:
Betoptic S Ophthalmic Suspension 558

Bisoprolol Fumarate (Co-administration with beta adrenergic blocking agent blocks the pulmonary effect of beta agonists and may produce severe bronchospasm in asthmatic patients; co-administer with caution).
No products indexed under this heading.

Bumetanide (The ECG changes and hypokalemia which may result from administration of nonpotassium-sparing diuretics can be acutely worsened by beta agonists. Caution is advised in the co-administration of beta agonists with nonpotassium-sparing diuretics). Products include:
Bumex Tablets 2746

Carteolol Hydrochloride (Co-administration with beta adrenergic blocking agent blocks the pulmonary effect of beta agonists and may produce severe bronchospasm in asthmatic patients; co-administer with caution). Products include:
Carteolol Hydrochloride Ophthalmic Solution USP, 1% .... ⊙249

Chlorothiazide (The ECG changes and hypokalemia which may result from administration of nonpotassium-sparing diuretics can be acutely worsened by beta agonists. Caution is advised in the co-administration of beta agonists with nonpotassium-sparing diuretics). Products include:
Diuril Oral Suspension 1954

Chlorothiazide Sodium (The ECG changes and hypokalemia which may result from administration of nonpotassium-sparing diuretics can be acutely worsened by beta agonists. Caution is advised in the co-administration of beta agonists with nonpotassium-sparing diuretics). Products include:
Diuril Sodium Intravenous 2467

Clomipramine Hydrochloride (Action of albuterol on the cardiovascular system may be potentiated by tricyclic antidepressants; co-administer with caution).
No products indexed under this heading.

Desipramine Hydrochloride (Action of albuterol on the cardiovascular system may be potentiated by tricyclic antidepressants; co-administer with caution).
No products indexed under this heading.

Digoxin (Mean decreases in serum digoxin levels have been demonstrated with intravenous and oral albuterol). Products include:
Lanoxicaps Capsules 1490
Lanoxin Injection 1494
Lanoxin Injection Pediatric 1497
Lanoxin Tablets 1500

Doxepin Hydrochloride (Action of albuterol on the cardiovascular system may be potentiated by tricyclic antidepressants; co-administer with caution).
No products indexed under this heading.

Esmolol Hydrochloride (Co-administration with beta adrenergic blocking agent blocks the pulmonary effect of beta agonists and may produce severe bronchospasm in asthmatic patients; co-administer with caution).
No products indexed under this heading.

Ethacrynic Acid (The ECG changes and hypokalemia which may result from administration of nonpotassium-sparing diuretics can be acutely worsened by beta agonists. Caution is advised in the co-administration of beta agonists with nonpotassium-sparing diuretics). Products include:
Edecrin Tablets **1959**

Furosemide (The ECG changes and hypokalemia which may result from administration of nonpotassium-sparing diuretics can be acutely worsened by beta agonists. Caution is advised in the co-administration of beta agonists with nonpotassium-sparing diuretics). Products include:
Furosemide Tablets **2154**

Hydrochlorothiazide (The ECG changes and hypokalemia which may result from administration of nonpotassium-sparing diuretics can be acutely worsened by beta agonists. Caution is advised in the co-administration of beta agonists with nonpotassium-sparing diuretics). Products include:
Aldoril Tablets **1910**
Atacand HCT **651**
Avalide Tablets **888**
Avalide Tablets **2874**
Benicar HCT Tablets **1044**
Diovan HCT Tablets **2196**
Dyazide Capsules **1423**
Hyzaar 50-12.5 Tablets **1990**
Hyzaar 100-12.5 Tablets **1990**
Hyzaar 100-25 Tablets **1990**
Lopressor HCT 50/25 Tablets **2241**
Lopressor HCT 100/25 Tablets **2241**
Lopressor HCT 100/50 Tablets **2241**
Lotensin HCT Tablets **2246**
Micardis HCT Tablets **856**
Moduretic Tablets **2028**
Prinzide Tablets **2056**
Teveten HCT Tablets **1737**
Timolide Tablets **2086**
Uniretic Tablets **3100**

Hydroflumethiazide (The ECG changes and hypokalemia which may result from administration of nonpotassium-sparing diuretics can be acutely worsened by beta agonists. Caution is advised in the co-administration of beta agonists with nonpotassium-sparing diuretics).
No products indexed under this heading.

Imipramine Hydrochloride (Action of albuterol on the cardiovascular system may be potentiated by tricyclic antidepressants; co-administer with caution).
No products indexed under this heading.

Imipramine Pamoate (Action of albuterol on the cardiovascular system may be potentiated by tricyclic antidepressants; co-administer with caution).
No products indexed under this heading.

Isocarboxazid (Action of albuterol on the cardiovascular system may be potentiated by MAO inhibitors; co-administer with caution).
No products indexed under this heading.

Labetalol Hydrochloride (Co-administration with beta adrenergic blocking agent blocks the pulmonary effect of beta agonists and may produce severe bronchospasm in asthmatic patients; co-administer with caution).
No products indexed under this heading.

Levobunolol Hydrochloride (Co-administration with beta adrenergic blocking agent blocks the pulmonary effect of beta agonists and may produce severe bronchospasm in asthmatic patients; co-administer with caution). Products include:
Betagan Ophthalmic Solution, USP .... ⊙ **220**

Maprotiline Hydrochloride (Action of albuterol on the cardiovascular system may be potentiated by tricyclic antidepressants; co-administer with caution).
No products indexed under this heading.

Methyclothiazide (The ECG changes and hypokalemia which may result from administration of nonpotassium-sparing diuretics can be acutely worsened by beta agonists. Caution is advised in the co-administration of beta agonists with nonpotassium-sparing diuretics).
No products indexed under this heading.

Metipranolol Hydrochloride (Co-administration with beta adrenergic blocking agent blocks the pulmonary effect of beta agonists and may produce severe bronchospasm in asthmatic patients; co-administer with caution).
No products indexed under this heading.

Metoprolol Succinate (Co-administration with beta adrenergic blocking agent blocks the pulmonary effect of beta agonists and may produce severe bronchospasm in asthmatic patients; co-administer with caution). Products include:
Toprol-XL Tablets **668**

Metoprolol Tartrate (Co-administration with beta adrenergic blocking agent blocks the pulmonary effect of beta agonists and may produce severe bronchospasm in asthmatic patients; co-administer with caution). Products include:
Lopressor Injection **2238**
Lopressor Tablets **2238**
Lopressor HCT 50/25 Tablets **2241**
Lopressor HCT 100/25 Tablets **2241**
Lopressor HCT 100/50 Tablets **2241**

Moclobemide (Action of albuterol on the cardiovascular system may be potentiated by MAO inhibitors; co-administer with caution).
No products indexed under this heading.

Nadolol (Co-administration with beta adrenergic blocking agent blocks the pulmonary effect of beta agonists and may produce severe bronchospasm in asthmatic patients; co-administer with caution). Products include:
Nadolol Tablets **2159**

Nortriptyline Hydrochloride (Action of albuterol on the cardiovascular system may be potentiated by tricyclic antidepressants; co-administer with caution).
No products indexed under this heading.

Pargyline Hydrochloride (Action of albuterol on the cardiovascular system may be potentiated by MAO inhibitors; co-administer with caution).
No products indexed under this heading.

Penbutolol Sulfate (Co-administration with beta adrenergic blocking agent blocks the pulmonary effect of beta agonists and may produce severe bronchospasm in asthmatic patients; co-administer with caution).
No products indexed under this heading.

Phenelzine Sulfate (Action of albuterol on the cardiovascular system may be potentiated by MAO inhibitors; co-administer with caution).
No products indexed under this heading.

Pindolol (Co-administration with beta adrenergic blocking agent blocks the pulmonary effect of beta agonists and may produce severe bronchospasm in asthmatic patients; co-administer with caution).
No products indexed under this heading.

Polythiazide (The ECG changes and hypokalemia which may result from administration of nonpotassium-sparing diuretics can be acutely worsened by beta agonists. Caution is advised in the co-administration of beta agonists with nonpotassium-sparing diuretics).
No products indexed under this heading.

Procarbazine Hydrochloride (Action of albuterol on the cardiovascular system may be potentiated by MAO inhibitors; co-administer with caution). Products include:
Matulane Capsules **3191**

Propranolol Hydrochloride (Co-administration with beta adrenergic blocking agent blocks the pulmonary effect of beta agonists and may produce severe bronchospasm in asthmatic patients; co-administer with caution). Products include:
Inderal LA Long-Acting Capsules **3429**
InnoPran XL Capsules **2723**

Protriptyline Hydrochloride (Action of albuterol on the cardiovascular system may be potentiated by tricyclic antidepressants; co-administer with caution).
No products indexed under this heading.

Selegiline Hydrochloride (Action of albuterol on the cardiovascular system may be potentiated by MAO inhibitors; co-administer with caution). Products include:
Eldepryl Capsules **3208**
Zelapar Tablets **3372**

Sotalol Hydrochloride (Co-administration with beta adrenergic blocking agent blocks the pulmonary effect of beta agonists and may produce severe bronchospasm in asthmatic patients; co-administer with caution).
No products indexed under this heading.

Timolol Hemihydrate (Co-administration with beta adrenergic blocking agent blocks the pulmonary effect of beta agonists and may produce severe bronchospasm in asthmatic patients; co-administer with caution). Products include:
Betimol Ophthalmic Solution **3382**
Betimol Ophthalmic Solution .... ⊙ **295**

Timolol Maleate (Co-administration with beta adrenergic blocking agent blocks the pulmonary effect of beta agonists and may produce severe bronchospasm in asthmatic patients; co-administer with caution). Products include:
Blocadren Tablets **1916**
Cosopt Sterile Ophthalmic Solution **1931**
Timolide Tablets **2086**
Timoptic Sterile Ophthalmic Solution **2088**
Timoptic in Ocudose **2091**
Timoptic-XE Sterile Ophthalmic Gel Forming Solution **2092**

Torsemide (The ECG changes and hypokalemia which may result from administration of nonpotassium-sparing diuretics can be acutely worsened by beta agonists. Caution is advised in the co-administration of beta agonists with nonpotassium-sparing diuretics). Products include:
Demadex Injection **2759**
Demadex Tablets **2759**

Tranylcypromine Sulfate (Action of albuterol on the cardiovascular system may be potentiated by MAO inhibitors; co-administer with caution). Products include:
Parnate Tablets **1527**

Trimipramine Maleate (Action of albuterol on the cardiovascular system may be potentiated by tricyclic antidepressants; co-administer with caution).
No products indexed under this heading.

PROVIGIL TABLETS

(Modafinil) **988**

May interact with cytochrome p450 2c9 substrates (selected), cytochrome p450 3a4 inducers (selected), cytochrome p450 3a4 inhibitors (selected), cytochrome p450 3a4 substrates (selected), monoamine oxidase inhibitors, oral contraceptives, phenytoin, selective serotonin reuptake inhibitors, tricyclic antidepressants, xanthines, and certain other agents. Compounds in these categories include:

Acarbose (An apparent concentration-related suppression of CYP2C9 activity was observed in human hepatocytes after exposure to modafinil in vitro suggesting that there is a potential for a metabolic interaction between modafinil and substrates of CYP2C9). Products include:
Precose Tablets **751**

Acetazolamide (Co-administration of potent inhibitors of CYP3A4 could alter the plasma levels of modafinil).
No products indexed under this heading.

Alfentanil Hydrochloride (Chronic administration of modafinil can increase the elimination of substrates of CYP3A4. Dose adjustments may be necessary for patients being treated with these and similar medications).
No products indexed under this heading.

Allium sativum (Co-administration of potent inducers of CYP3A4 could alter the plasma levels of modafinil).
No products indexed under this heading.

Alprazolam (Chronic administration of modafinil can increase the elimination of substrates of CYP3A4. Dose adjustments may be necessary for

patients being treated with these and similar medications). Products include:
Niravam Orally Disintegrating Tablets 3092

Aminophylline (Chronic administration of modafinil may cause modest induction of CYP3A4, thus reducing the levels, to a lesser degree, of co-administered substrate for that enzyme system, such as theophylline).
No products indexed under this heading.

Amiodarone Hydrochloride (Co-administration of potent inhibitors of CYP3A4 could alter the plasma levels of modafinil).
No products indexed under this heading.

Amitriptyline Hydrochloride (CYP2C19 provides an ancillary pathway for the metabolism of certain tricyclic antidepressants that are primarily metabolized by CYP2D6. In tricyclic-treated patients deficient in CYP2D6, the amount of metabolism by CYP2C19 may be substantially increased. Modafinil may cause elevation of the levels of these tricyclics in this subset of patients. A reduction in the dose of tricyclic agents might be needed in these patients).
No products indexed under this heading.

Amlodipine Besylate (Chronic administration of modafinil can increase the elimination of substrates of CYP3A4. Dose adjustments may be necessary for patients being treated with these and similar medications). Products include:
Caduet Tablets 2508
Lotrel Capsules 2249
Norvasc Tablets 2545

Amoxapine (CYP2C19 provides an ancillary pathway for the metabolism of certain tricyclic antidepressants that are primarily metabolized by CYP2D6. In tricyclic-treated patients deficient in CYP2D6, the amount of metabolism by CYP2C19 may be substantially increased. Modafinil may cause elevation of the levels of these tricyclics in this subset of patients. A reduction in the dose of tricyclic agents might be needed in these patients).
No products indexed under this heading.

Amprenavir (Co-administration of potent inhibitors of CYP3A4 could alter the plasma levels of modafinil). Products include:
Agenerase Capsules 1327
Agenerase Oral Solution 1332

Anastrozole (Co-administration of potent inhibitors of CYP3A4 could alter the plasma levels of modafinil). Products include:
Arimidex Tablets 673

Aprepitant (Chronic administration of modafinil can increase the elimination of substrates of CYP3A4. Dose adjustments may be necessary for patients being treated with these and similar medications). Products include:
Emend Capsules 1963

Astemizole (Chronic administration of modafinil can increase the elimination of substrates of CYP3A4. Dose adjustments may be necessary for patients being treated with these and similar medications).
No products indexed under this heading.

Atorvastatin Calcium (Chronic administration of modafinil can increase the elimination of substrates of CYP3A4. Dose adjustments may be necessary for patients being treated with these and similar medications). Products include:
Caduet Tablets 2508
Lipitor Tablets 2483

Belladonna Ergotamine (Chronic administration of modafinil can increase the elimination of substrates of CYP3A4. Dose adjustments may be necessary for patients being treated with these and similar medications).
No products indexed under this heading.

Betamethasone Acetate (Co-administration of potent inducers of CYP3A4 could alter the plasma levels of modafinil).
No products indexed under this heading.

Betamethasone Sodium Phosphate (Co-administration of potent inducers of CYP3A4 could alter the plasma levels of modafinil).
No products indexed under this heading.

Buspirone Hydrochloride (Chronic administration of modafinil can increase the elimination of substrates of CYP3A4. Dose adjustments may be necessary for patients being treated with these and similar medications).
No products indexed under this heading.

Busulfan (Chronic administration of modafinil can increase the elimination of substrates of CYP3A4. Dose adjustments may be necessary for patients being treated with these and similar medications). Products include:
I.V. Busulfex 2493
Myleran Tablets 1525

Candesartan Cilexetil (An apparent concentration-related suppression of CYP2C9 activity was observed in human hepatocytes after exposure to modafinil in vitro suggesting that there is a potential for a metabolic interaction between modafinil and substrates of CYP2C9). Products include:
Atacand Tablets 649
Atacand HCT 651

Carbamazepine (Chronic administration of modafinil may cause induction of its metabolism; co-administration of potent inducers of CYP3A4, such as carbamazepine, could alter the levels of modafinil due to the partial involvement of that enzyme in the metabolic elimination of the compound). Products include:
Carbatrol Capsules 3171
Equetro Extended-Release Capsules 3180
Tegretol/Tegretol-XR 2295

Carvedilol (An apparent concentration-related suppression of CYP2C9 activity was observed in human hepatocytes after exposure to modafinil in vitro suggesting that there is a potential for a metabolic interaction between modafinil and substrates of CYP2C9). Products include:
Coreg Tablets 1414

Celecoxib (An apparent concentration-related suppression of CYP2C9 activity was observed in human hepatocytes after exposure to modafinil in vitro suggesting that there is a potential for a metabolic interaction between modafinil and substrates of CYP2C9). Products include:
Celebrex Capsules 3134

Cerivastatin Sodium (Chronic administration of modafinil can increase the elimination of substrates of CYP3A4. Dose adjustments may be necessary for patients being treated with these and similar medications).
No products indexed under this heading.

Chlorpheniramine (Chronic administration of modafinil can increase the elimination of substrates of CYP3A4. Dose adjustments may be necessary for patients being treated with these and similar medications).
No products indexed under this heading.

Chlorpheniramine Maleate (Chronic administration of modafinil can increase the elimination of substrates of CYP3A4. Dose adjustments may be necessary for patients being treated with these and similar medications). Products include:
Advil Allergy Sinus Caplets .... ▣770
Advil Multi-Symptom Cold Caplets .... ▣770
BC Allergy Sinus Cold Powder .... ▣677
Comtrex Maximum Strength Cold & Cough Day/Night Caplets - Night Formulation .... ▣726
Comtrex Maximum Strength Day/Night Severe Cold & Sinus Caplets - Night Formulation .... ▣725
Contac Cold and Flu Maximum Strength Caplets .... ▣728
Contac Cold and Flu Day and Night Caplets (Night Formulation Only) .... ▣727
Children's Dimetapp Long Acting Cough Plus Cold Syrup .... ▣731
Robitussin Cough & Cold Long-Acting Liquid .... ▣735
Robitussin Cough & Allergy Syrup .. ▣736
Robitussin Cough & Cold Nighttime Liquid .... ▣736
Robitussin Cough, Cold & Flu Nighttime Liquid .... ▣738
Robitussin Pediatric Cough & Cold Long-Acting Liquid .... ▣735
Robitussin Pediatric Cough & Cold Nighttime Liquid .... ▣736
Triaminic Cold & Allergy Liquid .... ▣746
Triaminic Cough & Runny Nose Softchews .... ▣748
Children's Tylenol Plus Flu Oral Suspension .... ▣749
Tylenol Allergy Multi-Symptom Caplets with Cool Burst and Gelcaps 1872
Children's Tylenol Plus Cold Suspension Liquid 1879
Children's Tylenol Plus Cough & Runny Nose Suspension Liquid 1879
Children's Tylenol Plus Flu Suspension Liquid 1881
Children's Tylenol Plus Multi-Symptom Cold Suspension Liquid 1879
Tylenol Cold Head Congestion Nighttime Caplets with Cool Burst 1873
Tylenol Cold Multi-Symptom Nighttime Caplets with Cool Burst 1874
Tylenol Sinus Congestion & Pain Nighttime Caplets with Cool Burst 1876
Vicks 44M Cough, Cold & Flu Relief Liquid 2680
Pediatric Vicks 44m Cough & Cold Relief Liquid 2676
Children's Vicks NyQuil Cold/Cough Relief .... ▣756
Children's Vicks NyQuil Cold/Cough Relief Liquid 2680
Zicam Maximum Strength Flu Daytime .... ▣768

Chlorpheniramine Polistirex (Chronic administration of modafinil can increase the elimination of substrates of CYP3A4. Dose adjustments may be necessary for patients being treated with these and similar medications). Products include:
Tussionex Pennkinetic Extended-Release Suspension 3327

Chlorpheniramine Tannate (Chronic administration of modafinil can increase the elimination of substrates of CYP3A4. Dose adjustments may be necessary for patients being treated with these and similar medications).
No products indexed under this heading.

Chlorpropamide (An apparent concentration-related suppression of CYP2C9 activity was observed in human hepatocytes after exposure to modafinil in vitro suggesting that there is a potential for a metabolic interaction between modafinil and substrates of CYP2C9).
No products indexed under this heading.

Cimetidine (Co-administration of potent inhibitors of CYP3A4 could alter the plasma levels of modafinil). Products include:
Tagamet HB 200 Tablets .... ▣664

Cimetidine Hydrochloride (Co-administration of potent inhibitors of CYP3A4 could alter the plasma levels of modafinil).
No products indexed under this heading.

Ciprofloxacin (Co-administration of potent inhibitors of CYP3A4 could alter the plasma levels of modafinil). Products include:
Cipro Oral Suspension 2977
Cipro I.V. 2984
Cipro XR Tablets 2990
Ciprodex Otic Suspension 559

Ciprofloxacin Hydrochloride (Co-administration of potent inducers of CYP3A4 could alter the plasma levels of modafinil). Products include:
Ciloxan Ophthalmic Ointment 559
Ciloxan Ophthalmic Solution .... ⊙206
Cipro Tablets 2977
Proquin XR Tablets 1153

Cisapride (Chronic administration of modafinil can increase the elimination of substrates of CYP3A4. Dose adjustments may be necessary for patients being treated with these and similar medications).
No products indexed under this heading.

Cisplatin (Co-administration of potent inducers of CYP3A4 could alter the plasma levels of modafinil).
No products indexed under this heading.

Citalopram Hydrobromide (Modafinil is a reversible inhibitor of the CYP2C19; the levels of CYP2D6 substrates, such as selective serotonin reuptake inhibitors, which have ancillary routes of elimination through CYP2D6, may be increased by co-administration of modafinil). Products include:

Celexa 1176

Clarithromycin (Chronic administration of modafinil can increase the
elimination of substrates of CYP3A4.
Dose adjustments may be necessary
for patients being treated with these
and similar medications. Products
include:
 Biaxin/Biaxin XL 402
 PREVPAC 3284

Clomipramine Hydrochloride
(Co-administration has resulted in
one incident of increased levels of
clomipramine and its active metabolite desmethylclomipramine).
 No products indexed under this
 heading.

Clotrimazole (Co-administration of
potent inhibitors of CYP3A4 could
alter the plasma levels of modafinil).
Products include:
 Desenex Athlete's Foot Cream ▧635
 Lotrimin 3039
 Lotrisone 3040

Cortisone Acetate (Co-
administration of potent inducers of
CYP3A4 could alter the plasma levels of modafinil).
 No products indexed under this
 heading.

Cyclosporine (One case of an inter-
action between modafinil and
cyclosporine has been reported.
After one month of administration of
200mg/day of modafinil, cyclospo-
rine blood levels were decreased by
50%). Products include:
 Gengraf Capsules 459
 Neoral Oral Solution 2259
 Neoral Soft Gelatin Capsules 2259
 Restasis Ophthalmic Emulsion 575
 Sandimmune 2275

Dalfopristin (Co-administration of
potent inhibitors of CYP3A4 could
alter the plasma levels of modafinil).
 No products indexed under this
 heading.

Danazol (Co-administration of
potent inhibitors of CYP3A4 could
alter the plasma levels of modafinil).
 No products indexed under this
 heading.

Delavirdine Mesylate (Co-
administration of potent inhibitors of
CYP3A4 could alter the plasma levels of modafinil). Products include:
 Rescriptor Tablets 2551

Desipramine Hydrochloride
(CYP2C19 provides an ancillary pathway for the metabolism of certain
tricyclic antidepressants that are
primarily metabolized by CYP2D6. In
tricyclic-treated patients deficient in
CYP2D6, the amount of metabolism
by CYP2C19 may be substantially
increased. Modafinil may cause elevation of the levels of these tricyclics
in this subset of patients. A reduction in the dose of tricyclic agents
might be needed in these patients).
 No products indexed under this
 heading.

Desogestrel (The effectiveness of
steroidal contraceptives may be
reduced when used with modafinil
tablets and for one month after discontinuation of therapy. Alternative
or concomitant methods of contraception are recommended for
patients treated with modafinil tablets and for one month after discontinuation of modafinil). Products
include:
 Mircette Tablets 1066

Dexamethasone (Co-
administration of potent inducers of
CYP3A4 could alter the plasma lev-
els of modafinil). Products include:
 Ciprodex Otic Suspension 559
 Decadron Tablets 1951
 TobraDex Ophthalmic Ointment 562
 TobraDex Ophthalmic Suspension ... 563

Dexamethasone Acetate (Co-
administration of potent inducers of
CYP3A4 could alter the plasma levels of modafinil).
 No products indexed under this
 heading.

**Dexamethasone Sodium Phos-
phate** (Co-administration of potent
inducers of CYP3A4 could alter the
plasma levels of modafinil).
 No products indexed under this
 heading.

Dextroamphetamine (Absorption
of modafinil may be delayed by
approximately one hour when co-
administered with
dextroamphetamine).
 No products indexed under this
 heading.

**Dextroamphetamine Saccha-
rate** (Absorption of modafinil may be
delayed by approximately one hour
when co-administered with dextroamphetamine). Products include:
 Adderall Tablets 3164
 Adderall XR Capsules 3166

Dextroamphetamine Sulfate
(Absorption of modafinil may be
delayed by approximately one hour
when co-administered with dextroam-
phetamine). Products include:
 Adderall Tablets 3164
 Adderall XR Capsules 3166
 Dexedrine 1420
 DextroStat Tablets 3179

Dextromethorphan (An apparent
concentration-related suppression of
CYP2C9 activity was observed in
human hepatocytes after exposure
to modafinil in vitro suggesting that
there is a potential for a metabolic
interaction between modafinil and
substrates of CYP2C9).
 No products indexed under this
 heading.

Diazepam (Modafinil is a reversible
inhibitor of the CYP2C19; co-
administration with drugs that are
largely eliminated via this pathway,
such as diazepam, may increase the
circulating levels of diazepam).
Products include:
 Diastat Rectal Delivery System 3343
 Valium Tablets 2819

Diclofenac Potassium (An apparent concentration-related suppression of CYP2C9 activity was
observed in human hepatocytes
after exposure to modafinil in vitro
suggesting that there is a potential
for a metabolic interaction between
modafinil and substrates of
CYP2C9).
 No products indexed under this
 heading.

Diclofenac Sodium (An apparent
concentration-related suppression of
CYP2C9 activity was observed in
human hepatocytes after exposure
to modafinil in vitro suggesting that
there is a potential for a metabolic
interaction between modafinil and
substrates of CYP2C9). Products
include:
 Arthrotec Tablets 3129
 Voltaren Ophthalmic Solution 2309
 Voltaren Tablets 2307
 Voltaren-XR Tablets 2310

Dihydroergotamine Mesylate
(Chronic administration of modafinil
can increase the elimination of substrates of CYP3A4. Dose adjustments may be necessary for
patients being treated with these and
similar medications). Products
include:
 Migranal Nasal Spray 3348

Diltiazem Hydrochloride (Chronic
administration of modafinil can
increase the elimination of substrates of CYP3A4. Dose adjustments may be necessary for
patients being treated with these and
similar medications). Products
include:
 Cardizem LA Extended Release
 Tablets 1728
 Tiazac Capsules 1201

Diltiazem Maleate (Chronic administration of modafinil can increase
the elimination of substrates of
CYP3A4. Dose adjustments may be
necessary for patients being treated
with these and similar medications).
 No products indexed under this
 heading.

Disopyramide (Chronic administration of modafinil can increase the
elimination of substrates of CYP3A4.
Dose adjustments may be necessary
for patients being treated with these
and similar medications).
 No products indexed under this
 heading.

Disopyramide Phosphate (Chronic administration of modafinil can
increase the elimination of substrates of CYP3A4. Dose adjustments may be necessary for
patients being treated with these and
similar medications).
 No products indexed under this
 heading.

Disulfiram (Chronic administration
of modafinil can increase the elimination of substrates of CYP3A4. Dose
adjustments may be necessary for
patients being treated with these and
similar medications).
 No products indexed under this
 heading.

Doxepin Hydrochloride
(CYP2C19 provides an ancillary pathway for the metabolism of certain
tricyclic antidepressants that are
primarily metabolized by CYP2D6. In
tricyclic-treated patients deficient in
CYP2D6, the amount of metabolism
by CYP2C19 may be substantially
increased. Modafinil may cause elevation of the levels of these tricyclics
in this subset of patients. A reduction in the dose of tricyclic agents
might be needed in these patients).
 No products indexed under this
 heading.

Doxorubicin Hydrochloride
(Chronic administration of modafinil
can increase the elimination of substrates of CYP3A4. Dose adjustments may be necessary for
patients being treated with these and
similar medications).
 No products indexed under this
 heading.

Dronabinol (Chronic administration
of modafinil can increase the elimination of substrates of CYP3A4. Dose
adjustments may be necessary for
patients being treated with these and
similar medications). Products
include:
 Marinol Capsules 3333

Dyphylline (Chronic administration
of modafinil may cause modest
induction of CYP3A4, thus reducing
the levels, to a lesser degree, of
co-administered substrate for that
enzyme system, such as
theophylline).
 No products indexed under this
 heading.

Efavirenz (Co-administration of
potent inducers of CYP3A4 could
alter the plasma levels of modafinil).
Products include:
 Atripla Tablets 945
 Sustiva Capsules 930
 Sustiva Tablets 930

Eprosartan Mesylate (An apparent
concentration-related suppression of
CYP2C9 activity was observed in
human hepatocytes after exposure
to modafinil in vitro suggesting that
there is a potential for a metabolic
interaction between modafinil and
substrates of CYP2C9). Products
include:
 Teveten Tablets 1735
 Teveten HCT Tablets 1737

Ergotamine Tartrate (Chronic
administration of modafinil can
increase the elimination of substrates of CYP3A4. Dose adjustments may be necessary for
patients being treated with these and
similar medications).
 No products indexed under this
 heading.

Erythromycin (Chronic administra-
tion of modafinil can increase the
elimination of substrates of CYP3A4.
Dose adjustments may be necessary
for patients being treated with these
and similar medications). Products
include:
 Ery-Tab Tablets 449
 Erythromycin Base Filmtab
 Tablets 455
 Erythromycin Delayed-Release
 Capsules, USP 457
 PCE Dispertab Tablets 515

Erythromycin Estolate (Chronic
administration of modafinil can
increase the elimination of substrates of CYP3A4. Dose adjustments may be necessary for
patients being treated with these and
similar medications).
 No products indexed under this
 heading.

Erythromycin Ethylsuccinate
(Chronic administration of modafinil
can increase the elimination of substrates of CYP3A4. Dose adjustments may be necessary for
patients being treated with these and
similar medications). Products
include:
 E.E.S. 451
 EryPed 447

Erythromycin Gluceptate (Chronic administration of modafinil can
increase the elimination of substrates of CYP3A4. Dose adjustments may be necessary for
patients being treated with these and
similar medications).
 No products indexed under this
 heading.

Erythromycin Lactobionate
(Chronic administration of modafinil
can increase the elimination of substrates of CYP3A4. Dose adjustments may be necessary for
patients being treated with these and
similar medications).
 No products indexed under this
 heading.

Erythromycin Stearate (Chronic
administration of modafinil can

increase the elimination of substrates of CYP3A4. Dose adjustments may be necessary for patients being treated with these and similar medications). Products include:

Erythrocin Stearate Filmtab Tablets 453

Escitalopram Oxalate (Modafinil is a reversible inhibitor of the CYP2C19; the levels of CYP2D6 substrates, such as selective serotonin reuptake inhibitors, which have ancillary routes of elimination through CYP2D6, may be increased by co-administration of modafinil). Products include:

Lexapro Oral Solution 1190
Lexapro Tablets 1190

Esomeprazole Magnesium (Co-administration of potent inhibitors of CYP3A4 could alter the plasma levels of modafinil). Products include:

Nexium Delayed-Release Capsules 655

Estradiol (Chronic administration of modafinil can increase the elimination of substrates of CYP3A4. Dose adjustments may be necessary for patients being treated with these and similar medications). Products include:

Angeliq Tablets 762
Climara Transdermal System 771
Climara Pro Transdermal System 776
Estrasorb Topical Emulsion 1147
Estring Vaginal Ring 2635
Menostar Transdermal System 782
Vagifem Tablets 2334

Estradiol Benzoate (Chronic administration of modafinil can increase the elimination of substrates of CYP3A4. Dose adjustments may be necessary for patients being treated with these and similar medications).

No products indexed under this heading.

Estradiol Cypionate (Chronic administration of modafinil can increase the elimination of substrates of CYP3A4. Dose adjustments may be necessary for patients being treated with these and similar medications).

No products indexed under this heading.

Estradiol Valerate (Chronic administration of modafinil can increase the elimination of substrates of CYP3A4. Dose adjustments may be necessary for patients being treated with these and similar medications).

No products indexed under this heading.

Ethinyl Estradiol (Administration of modafinil to female volunteers resulted in a mean 11% decrease in Cmax and an 18% decrease in AUC of ethinyl estradiol. There was no apparent change in the elimination rate of ethinyl estradiol). Products include:

Mircette Tablets 1066
NuvaRing 2340
Ortho-Cyclen/Ortho Tri-Cyclen 2429
Ortho Evra Transdermal System 2417
Ortho Tri-Cyclen Lo Tablets 2436
Seasonique Tablets 1077
Yasmin 28 Tablets 796
Yaz Tablets 803

Ethosuximide (Chronic administration of modafinil can increase the elimination of substrates of CYP3A4. Dose adjustments may be necessary for patients being treated with these and similar medications).

No products indexed under this heading.

Ethynodiol Diacetate (The effectiveness of steroidal contraceptives may be reduced when used with modafinil tablets and for one month after discontinuation of therapy. Alternative or concomitant methods of contraception are recommended for patients treated with modafinil tablets and for one month after discontinuation of modafinil).

No products indexed under this heading.

Etodolac (An apparent concentration-related suppression of CYP2C9 activity was observed in human hepatocytes after exposure to modafinil in vitro suggesting that there is a potential for a metabolic interaction between modafinil and substrates of CYP2C9).

No products indexed under this heading.

Etoposide (Chronic administration of modafinil can increase the elimination of substrates of CYP3A4. Dose adjustments may be necessary for patients being treated with these and similar medications).

No products indexed under this heading.

Etoposide Phosphate (Chronic administration of modafinil can increase the elimination of substrates of CYP3A4. Dose adjustments may be necessary for patients being treated with these and similar medications).

No products indexed under this heading.

Felbamate (Co-administration of potent inducers of CYP3A4 could alter the plasma levels of modafinil).

No products indexed under this heading.

Felodipine (Chronic administration of modafinil can increase the elimination of substrates of CYP3A4. Dose adjustments may be necessary for patients being treated with these and similar medications).

No products indexed under this heading.

Fenoprofen Calcium (An apparent concentration-related suppression of CYP2C9 activity was observed in human hepatocytes after exposure to modafinil in vitro suggesting that there is a potential for a metabolic interaction between modafinil and substrates of CYP2C9). Products include:

Nalfon Capsules 2502

Fentanyl (Chronic administration of modafinil can increase the elimination of substrates of CYP3A4. Dose adjustments may be necessary for patients being treated with these and similar medications). Products include:

Duragesic Transdermal System 2373
Ionsys Transdermal System 2379

Fentanyl Citrate (Chronic administration of modafinil can increase the elimination of substrates of CYP3A4. Dose adjustments may be necessary for patients being treated with these and similar medications). Products include:

Actiq 979

Fluconazole (Co-administration of potent inhibitors of CYP3A4 could alter the plasma levels of modafinil).

No products indexed under this heading.

Fludrocortisone Acetate (Co-administration of potent inducers of CYP3A4 could alter the plasma levels of modafinil).

No products indexed under this heading.

Fluoxetine Hydrochloride (Modafinil is a reversible inhibitor of the CYP2C19; the levels of CYP2D6 substrates, such as selective serotonin reuptake inhibitors, which have ancillary routes of elimination through CYP2D6, may be increased by co-administration of modafinil). Products include:

Prozac Pulvules and Liquid 1801
Symbyax Capsules 1819

Flurbiprofen (An apparent concentration-related suppression of CYP2C9 activity was observed in human hepatocytes after exposure to modafinil in vitro suggesting that there is a potential for a metabolic interaction between modafinil and substrates of CYP2C9).

No products indexed under this heading.

Flurbiprofen Sodium (An apparent concentration-related suppression of CYP2C9 activity was observed in human hepatocytes after exposure to modafinil in vitro suggesting that there is a potential for a metabolic interaction between modafinil and substrates of CYP2C9). Products include:

Ocufen Ophthalmic Solution .... ⊙232

Fluvastatin Sodium (An apparent concentration-related suppression of CYP2C9 activity was observed in human hepatocytes after exposure to modafinil in vitro suggesting that there is a potential for a metabolic interaction between modafinil and substrates of CYP2C9). Products include:

Lescol Capsules 2233
Lescol XL Tablets 2233

Fluvoxamine Maleate (Modafinil is a reversible inhibitor of the CYP2C19; the levels of CYP2D6 substrates, such as selective serotonin reuptake inhibitors, which have ancillary routes of elimination through CYP2D6, may be increased by co-administration of modafinil).

No products indexed under this heading.

Fosamprenavir Calcium (Co-administration of potent inhibitors of CYP3A4 could alter the plasma levels of modafinil). Products include:

Lexiva Tablets 1505

Fosphenytoin Sodium (Modafinil is a reversible inhibitor of the CYP2C19; co-administration with drugs that are largely eliminated via this pathway, such as phenytoin, may increase the circulating levels of phenytoin).

No products indexed under this heading.

Garlic Extract (Co-administration of potent inducers of CYP3A4 could alter the plasma levels of modafinil).

No products indexed under this heading.

Garlic Oil (Co-administration of potent inducers of CYP3A4 could alter the plasma levels of modafinil).

No products indexed under this heading.

Glimepiride (An apparent concentration-related suppression of CYP2C9 activity was observed in human hepatocytes after exposure to modafinil in vitro suggesting that there is a potential for a metabolic interaction between modafinil and substrates of CYP2C9). Products include:

Avandaryl Tablets 1379
Duetact Tablets 3226

Glipizide (An apparent concentration-related suppression of CYP2C9 activity was observed in human hepatocytes after exposure to modafinil in vitro suggesting that there is a potential for a metabolic interaction between modafinil and substrates of CYP2C9).

No products indexed under this heading.

Haloperidol (Chronic administration of modafinil can increase the elimination of substrates of CYP3A4. Dose adjustments may be necessary for patients being treated with these and similar medications).

No products indexed under this heading.

Haloperidol Decanoate (Chronic administration of modafinil can increase the elimination of substrates of CYP3A4. Dose adjustments may be necessary for patients being treated with these and similar medications).

No products indexed under this heading.

Haloperidol Lactate (Chronic administration of modafinil can increase the elimination of substrates of CYP3A4. Dose adjustments may be necessary for patients being treated with these and similar medications).

No products indexed under this heading.

Hydrocortisone (Co-administration of potent inducers of CYP3A4 could alter the plasma levels of modafinil). Products include:

Colocort Rectal Suspension, USP (Retention) 100 mg/60 mL 2476
Hydrocortone Tablets 1989
Preparation H Hydrocortisone Cream .... ▣646

Hydrocortisone Acetate (Co-administration of potent inducers of CYP3A4 could alter the plasma levels of modafinil). Products include:

Analpram-HC 1159
Pramosone 1161
ProctoFoam-HC 3099

Hydrocortisone Butyrate (Co-administration of potent inducers of CYP3A4 could alter the plasma levels of modafinil). Products include:

Locoid Lipocream Cream 1160

Hydrocortisone Cypionate (Co-administration of potent inducers of CYP3A4 could alter the plasma levels of modafinil).

No products indexed under this heading.

Hydrocortisone Hemisuccinate (Co-administration of potent inducers of CYP3A4 could alter the plasma levels of modafinil).

No products indexed under this heading.

Hydrocortisone Probutate (Co-administration of potent inducers of CYP3A4 could alter the plasma levels of modafinil).

No products indexed under this heading.

Hydrocortisone Sodium Phosphate (Co-administration of potent inducers of CYP3A4 could alter the plasma levels of modafinil).

No products indexed under this heading.

Hydrocortisone Sodium Succinate (Co-administration of potent inducers of CYP3A4 could alter the plasma levels of modafinil).
No products indexed under this heading.

Hydrocortisone Valerate (Co-administration of potent inducers of CYP3A4 could alter the plasma levels of modafinil).
No products indexed under this heading.

Hypericum (Co-administration of potent inducers of CYP3A4 could alter the plasma levels of modafinil). Products include:
Satiete Tablets 832

Hypericum Perforatum (Co-administration of potent inducers of CYP3A4 could alter the plasma levels of modafinil).
No products indexed under this heading.

Ibuprofen (An apparent concentration-related suppression of CYP2C9 activity was observed in human hepatocytes after exposure to modafinil in vitro suggesting that there is a potential for a metabolic interaction between modafinil and substrates of CYP2C9). Products include:
Advil Allergy Sinus Caplets 770
Advil 674
Children's Advil Oral Suspension 603
Children's Advil Chewable Tablets 603
Advil Cold & Sinus 723
Infants' Advil Concentrated Drops 604
Infants' Advil Concentrated Drops - White Grape (Dye-Free) 604
Junior Strength Advil Swallow Tablets 605
Advil Migraine Liquigels 608
Advil Multi-Symptom Cold Caplets 770
Advil PM Caplets 615
Motrin IB Tablets and Caplets 1866
Children's Motrin Oral Suspension 1867
Children's Motrin Non-Staining Dye-Free Oral Suspension 1867
Children's Motrin Cold Oral Suspension 1867
Infants' Motrin Concentrated Drops 1867
Infants' Motrin Non-Staining Dye-Free Concentrated Drops 1867
Junior Strength Motrin Caplets and Chewable Tablets 1867
Vicoprofen Tablets 539

Imipramine Hydrochloride (CYP2C19 provides an ancillary pathway for the metabolism of certain tricyclic antidepressants that are primarily metabolized by CYP2D6. In tricyclic-treated patients deficient in CYP2D6, the amount of metabolism by CYP2C19 may be substantially increased. Modafinil may cause elevation of the levels of these tricyclics in this subset of patients. A reduction in the dose of tricyclic agents might be needed in these patients).
No products indexed under this heading.

Imipramine Pamoate (CYP2C19 provides an ancillary pathway for the metabolism of certain tricyclic antidepressants that are primarily metabolized by CYP2D6. In tricyclic-treated patients deficient in CYP2D6, the amount of metabolism by CYP2C19 may be substantially increased. Modafinil may cause elevation of the levels of these tricyclics in this subset of patients. A reduction in the dose of tricyclic agents might be needed in these patients).
No products indexed under this heading.

Indinavir Sulfate (Chronic administration of modafinil can increase the elimination of substrates of CYP3A4. Dose adjustments may be necessary for patients being treated with these and similar medications). Products include:
Crixivan Capsules 1940

Indomethacin (An apparent concentration-related suppression of CYP2C9 activity was observed in human hepatocytes after exposure to modafinil in vitro suggesting that there is a potential for a metabolic interaction between modafinil and substrates of CYP2C9). Products include:
Indocin 1995

Indomethacin Sodium Trihydrate (An apparent concentration-related suppression of CYP2C9 activity was observed in human hepatocytes after exposure to modafinil in vitro suggesting that there is a potential for a metabolic interaction between modafinil and substrates of CYP2C9). Products include:
Indocin I.V. 2465

Irbesartan (An apparent concentration-related suppression of CYP2C9 activity was observed in human hepatocytes after exposure to modafinil in vitro suggesting that there is a potential for a metabolic interaction between modafinil and substrates of CYP2C9). Products include:
Avalide Tablets 888
Avalide Tablets 2874
Avapro Tablets 891
Avapro Tablets 2871

Isocarboxazid (Co-administration requires caution; no interaction studies have been performed).
No products indexed under this heading.

Isoniazid (Co-administration of potent inhibitors of CYP3A4 could alter the plasma levels of modafinil).
No products indexed under this heading.

Isradipine (Chronic administration of modafinil can increase the elimination of substrates of CYP3A4. Dose adjustments may be necessary for patients being treated with these and similar medications). Products include:
DynaCirc CR Tablets 2721

Itraconazole (Chronic administration of modafinil may cause induction of its metabolism; co-administration of potent inhibitors of CYP3A4, such as itraconazole, could alter the levels of modafinil due to the partial involvement of that enzyme in the metabolic elimination of the compound).
No products indexed under this heading.

Ketoconazole (Chronic administration of modafinil may cause induction of its metabolism; co-administration of potent inhibitors of CYP3A4, such as ketoconazole, could alter the levels of modafinil due to the partial involvement of that enzyme in the metabolic elimination of the compound). Products include:
Nizoral A-D Shampoo, 1% 1868

Ketoprofen (An apparent concentration-related suppression of CYP2C9 activity was observed in human hepatocytes after exposure to modafinil in vitro suggesting that there is a potential for a metabolic interaction between modafinil and substrates of CYP2C9).
No products indexed under this heading.

Ketorolac Tromethamine (An apparent concentration-related suppression of CYP2C9 activity was observed in human hepatocytes after exposure to modafinil in vitro suggesting that there is a potential for a metabolic interaction between modafinil and substrates of CYP2C9). Products include:
Acular Ophthalmic Solution 565
Acular LS Ophthalmic Solution 566

Lansoprazole (An apparent concentration-related suppression of CYP2C9 activity was observed in human hepatocytes after exposure to modafinil in vitro suggesting that there is a potential for a metabolic interaction between modafinil and substrates of CYP2C9). Products include:
Prevacid Delayed-Release Capsules 3271
Prevacid for Delayed-Release Oral Suspension 3271
Prevacid SoluTab Delayed-Release Orally Disintegrating Tablets 3271
Prevacid I.V. for Injection 3277
Prevacid NapraPAC 3280
PREVPAC 3284

Levonorgestrel (The effectiveness of steroidal contraceptives may be reduced when used with modafinil tablets and for one month after discontinuation of therapy. Alternative or concomitant methods of contraception are recommended for patients treated with modafinil tablets and for one month after discontinuation of modafinil). Products include:
Climara Pro Transdermal System 776
Mirena Intrauterine System 787
Plan B Tablets 1076
Seasonique Tablets 1077

Lidocaine (Chronic administration of modafinil can increase the elimination of substrates of CYP3A4. Dose adjustments may be necessary for patients being treated with these and similar medications). Products include:
Lidoderm Patch 1118
Synera Topical Patch 1137

Lidocaine Hydrochloride (Chronic administration of modafinil can increase the elimination of substrates of CYP3A4. Dose adjustments may be necessary for patients being treated with these and similar medications).
No products indexed under this heading.

Lopinavir (Co-administration of potent inhibitors of CYP3A4 could alter the plasma levels of modafinil). Products include:
Kaletra 476

Loratadine (Co-administration of potent inhibitors of CYP3A4 could alter the plasma levels of modafinil). Products include:
Alavert Allergy & Sinus D-12 Hour Tablets 771
Alavert 771
Children's Claritin Allergy Oral Solution 771
Claritin Non-Drowsy 24 Hour Tablets 772
Claritin Reditabs 24 Hour Non-Drowsy Tablets 772
Claritin-D Non-Drowsy 12 Hour Tablets 772
Claritin-D Non-Drowsy 24 Hour Tablets 772

Losartan Potassium (An apparent concentration-related suppression of CYP2C9 activity was observed in human hepatocytes after exposure to modafinil in vitro suggesting that there is a potential for a metabolic interaction between modafinil and substrates of CYP2C9). Products include:
Cozaar Tablets 1935
Hyzaar 50-12.5 Tablets 1990
Hyzaar 100-12.5 Tablets 1990
Hyzaar 100-25 Tablets 1990

Lovastatin (Chronic administration of modafinil can increase the elimination of substrates of CYP3A4. Dose adjustments may be necessary for patients being treated with these and similar medications). Products include:
Advicor Tablets 1722
Altoprev Extended-Release Tablets 3109
Mevacor Tablets 2021

Maprotiline Hydrochloride (CYP2C19 provides an ancillary pathway for the metabolism of certain tricyclic antidepressants that are primarily metabolized by CYP2D6. In tricyclic-treated patients deficient in CYP2D6, the amount of metabolism by CYP2C19 may be substantially increased. Modafinil may cause elevation of the levels of these tricyclics in this subset of patients. A reduction in the dose of tricyclic agents might be needed in these patients).
No products indexed under this heading.

Meclofenamate Sodium (An apparent concentration-related suppression of CYP2C9 activity was observed in human hepatocytes after exposure to modafinil in vitro suggesting that there is a potential for a metabolic interaction between modafinil and substrates of CYP2C9).
No products indexed under this heading.

Mefenamic Acid (An apparent concentration-related suppression of CYP2C9 activity was observed in human hepatocytes after exposure to modafinil in vitro suggesting that there is a potential for a metabolic interaction between modafinil and substrates of CYP2C9).
No products indexed under this heading.

Meloxicam (An apparent concentration-related suppression of CYP2C9 activity was observed in human hepatocytes after exposure to modafinil in vitro suggesting that there is a potential for a metabolic interaction between modafinil and substrates of CYP2C9). Products include:
Mobic Oral Suspension 863
Mobic Tablets 863

Mephenytoin (Co-administration of potent inducers of CYP3A4 could alter the plasma levels of modafinil).
No products indexed under this heading.

Mestranol (The effectiveness of steroidal contraceptives may be reduced when used with modafinil tablets and for one month after discontinuation of therapy. Alternative or concomitant methods of contraception are recommended for patients treated with modafinil tablets and for one month after discontinuation of modafinil).
No products indexed under this heading.

Metformin Hydrochloride (An apparent concentration-related suppression of CYP2C9 activity was observed in human hepatocytes after exposure to modafinil in vitro suggesting that there is a potential for a metabolic interaction between modafinil and substrates of CYP2C9). Products include:
ActoPlus Met Tablets ... 3214
Avandamet Tablets ... 1373
Fortamet Extended-Release Tablets ... 3115

Methadone Hydrochloride (Chronic administration of modafinil can increase the elimination of substrates of CYP3A4. Dose adjustments may be necessary for patients being treated with these and similar medications).
No products indexed under this heading.

Methsuximide (Co-administration of potent inducers of CYP3A4 could alter the plasma levels of modafinil).
No products indexed under this heading.

Methylphenidate Hydrochloride (May delay absorption of modafinil by approximately one hour; no significant alterations in pharmacokinetics of either drug). Products include:
Concerta Extended-Release Tablets ... 1881
Metadate CD Capsules ... 3323
Ritalin Hydrochloride Tablets ... 2269
Ritalin LA Capsules ... 2271
Ritalin-SR Tablets ... 2269

Methylprednisolone (Co-administration of potent inducers of CYP3A4 could alter the plasma levels of modafinil).
No products indexed under this heading.

Methylprednisolone Acetate (Co-administration of potent inducers of CYP3A4 could alter the plasma levels of modafinil). Products include:
Depo-Medrol Injectable Suspension ... 2617
Depo-Medrol Single-Dose Vial ... 2619

Methylprednisolone Sodium Succinate (Co-administration of potent inducers of CYP3A4 could alter the plasma levels of modafinil).
No products indexed under this heading.

Metronidazole (Co-administration of potent inhibitors of CYP3A4 could alter the plasma levels of modafinil). Products include:
Metrogel 1% ... 1211
MetroGel-Vaginal Gel ... 1855
Vandazole Vaginal Gel ... 3338

Metronidazole Benzoate (Co-administration of potent inhibitors of CYP3A4 could alter the plasma levels of modafinil).
No products indexed under this heading.

Metronidazole Hydrochloride (Co-administration of potent inhibitors of CYP3A4 could alter the plasma levels of modafinil).
No products indexed under this heading.

Miconazole (Co-administration of potent inhibitors of CYP3A4 could alter the plasma levels of modafinil).
No products indexed under this heading.

Miconazole Nitrate (Co-administration of potent inhibitors of CYP3A4 could alter the plasma levels of modafinil). Products include:
Desenex ... ▣635
Desenex Jock Itch Spray Powder ... ▣635

Midazolam Hydrochloride (Chronic administration of modafinil can increase the elimination of substrates of CYP3A4. Dose adjustments may be necessary for patients being treated with these and similar medications).
No products indexed under this heading.

Miglitol (An apparent concentration-related suppression of CYP2C9 activity was observed in human hepatocytes after exposure to modafinil in vitro suggesting that there is a potential for a metabolic interaction between modafinil and substrates of CYP2C9).
No products indexed under this heading.

Mirtazapine (An apparent concentration-related suppression of CYP2C9 activity was observed in human hepatocytes after exposure to modafinil in vitro suggesting that there is a potential for a metabolic interaction between modafinil and substrates of CYP2C9).
No products indexed under this heading.

Moclobemide (Co-administration requires caution; no interaction studies have been performed).
No products indexed under this heading.

Montelukast Sodium (An apparent concentration-related suppression of CYP2C9 activity was observed in human hepatocytes after exposure to modafinil in vitro suggesting that there is a potential for a metabolic interaction between modafinil and substrates of CYP2C9). Products include:
Singulair ... 2077

Nabumetone (An apparent concentration-related suppression of CYP2C9 activity was observed in human hepatocytes after exposure to modafinil in vitro suggesting that there is a potential for a metabolic interaction between modafinil and substrates of CYP2C9).
No products indexed under this heading.

Naproxen (An apparent concentration-related suppression of CYP2C9 activity was observed in human hepatocytes after exposure to modafinil in vitro suggesting that there is a potential for a metabolic interaction between modafinil and substrates of CYP2C9). Products include:
EC-Naprosyn Delayed-Release Tablets ... 2761
Naprosyn Suspension ... 2761
Naprosyn Tablets ... 2761
Prevacid NapraPAC ... 3280

Naproxen Sodium (An apparent concentration-related suppression of CYP2C9 activity was observed in human hepatocytes after exposure to modafinil in vitro suggesting that there is a potential for a metabolic interaction between modafinil and substrates of CYP2C9). Products include:
Aleve Caplets ... 742
Aleve Gelcaps ... 743
Aleve Tablets ... 743
Aleve Cold & Sinus Caplets ... 744
Anaprox Tablets ... 2761
Anaprox DS Tablets ... 2761

Nateglinide (An apparent concentration-related suppression of CYP2C9 activity was observed in human hepatocytes after exposure to modafinil in vitro suggesting that there is a potential for a metabolic interaction between modafinil and substrates of CYP2C9). Products include:
Starlix Tablets ... 2292

Nefazodone Hydrochloride (Chronic administration of modafinil can increase the elimination of substrates of CYP3A4. Dose adjustments may be necessary for patients being treated with these and similar medications).
No products indexed under this heading.

Nelfinavir Mesylate (Chronic administration of modafinil can increase the elimination of substrates of CYP3A4. Dose adjustments may be necessary for patients being treated with these and similar medications). Products include:
Viracept ... 2577

Nevirapine (Co-administration of potent inducers of CYP3A4 could alter the plasma levels of modafinil). Products include:
Viramune Oral Suspension ... 873
Viramune Tablets ... 873

Niacinamide (Co-administration of potent inhibitors of CYP3A4 could alter the plasma levels of modafinil).
No products indexed under this heading.

Nicardipine Hydrochloride (Chronic administration of modafinil can increase the elimination of substrates of CYP3A4. Dose adjustments may be necessary for patients being treated with these and similar medications). Products include:
Cardene I.V. ... 2497

Nicotinamide (Co-administration of potent inhibitors of CYP3A4 could alter the plasma levels of modafinil). Products include:
Nicomide Tablets ... 1088

Nifedipine (Chronic administration of modafinil can increase the elimination of substrates of CYP3A4. Dose adjustments may be necessary for patients being treated with these and similar medications). Products include:
Adalat CC Tablets ... 2964

Nimodipine (Chronic administration of modafinil can increase the elimination of substrates of CYP3A4. Dose adjustments may be necessary for patients being treated with these and similar medications). Products include:
Nimotop Capsules ... 749

Nisoldipine (Chronic administration of modafinil can increase the elimination of substrates of CYP3A4. Dose adjustments may be necessary for patients being treated with these and similar medications). Products include:
Sular Tablets ... 3122

Nitrendipine (Chronic administration of modafinil can increase the elimination of substrates of CYP3A4. Dose adjustments may be necessary for patients being treated with these and similar medications).
No products indexed under this heading.

Norethindrone (The effectiveness of steroidal contraceptives may be reduced when used with modafinil tablets and for one month after discontinuation of therapy. Alternative or concomitant methods of contraception are recommended for patients treated with modafinil tablets and for one month after discontinuation of modafinil). Products include:
Ortho Micronor Tablets ... 2426

Norethindrone Acetate (Chronic administration of modafinil can increase the elimination of substrates of CYP3A4. Dose adjustments may be necessary for patients being treated with these and similar medications).
No products indexed under this heading.

Norethynodrel (The effectiveness of steroidal contraceptives may be reduced when used with modafinil tablets and for one month after discontinuation of therapy. Alternative or concomitant methods of contraception are recommended for patients treated with modafinil tablets and for one month after discontinuation of modafinil).
No products indexed under this heading.

Norfloxacin (Co-administration of potent inhibitors of CYP3A4 could alter the plasma levels of modafinil). Products include:
Noroxin Tablets ... 2032

Norgestimate (The effectiveness of steroidal contraceptives may be reduced when used with modafinil tablets and for one month after discontinuation of therapy. Alternative or concomitant methods of contraception are recommended for patients treated with modafinil tablets and for one month after discontinuation of modafinil). Products include:
Ortho-Cyclen/Ortho Tri-Cyclen ... 2429
Ortho Tri-Cyclen Lo Tablets ... 2436

Norgestrel (The effectiveness of steroidal contraceptives may be reduced when used with modafinil tablets and for one month after discontinuation of therapy. Alternative or concomitant methods of contraception are recommended for patients treated with modafinil tablets and for one month after discontinuation of modafinil).
No products indexed under this heading.

Nortriptyline Hydrochloride (CYP2C19 provides an ancillary pathway for the metabolism of certain tricyclic antidepressants that are primarily metabolized by CYP2D6. In tricyclic-treated patients deficient in CYP2D6, the amount of metabolism by CYP2C19 may be substantially increased. Modafinil may cause elevation of the levels of these tricyclics in this subset of patients. A reduction in the dose of tricyclic agents might be needed in these patients).
No products indexed under this heading.

Omeprazole (An apparent concentration-related suppression of CYP2C9 activity was observed in human hepatocytes after exposure to modafinil in vitro suggesting that there is a potential for a metabolic interaction between modafinil and substrates of CYP2C9). Products include:
- Zegerid Capsules ... 2958
- Zegerid Powder for Oral Solution ... 2958

Ondansetron (Chronic administration of modafinil can increase the elimination of substrates of CYP3A4. Dose adjustments may be necessary for patients being treated with these and similar medications). Products include:
- Zofran ODT Orally Disintegrating Tablets ... 1639

Ondansetron Hydrochloride (Chronic administration of modafinil can increase the elimination of substrates of CYP3A4. Dose adjustments may be necessary for patients being treated with these and similar medications). Products include:
- Zofran Injection ... 1634
- Zofran ... 1639

Oxaprozin (An apparent concentration-related suppression of CYP2C9 activity was observed in human hepatocytes after exposure to modafinil in vitro suggesting that there is a potential for a metabolic interaction between modafinil and substrates of CYP2C9).
No products indexed under this heading.

Oxcarbazepine (Co-administration of potent inducers of CYP3A4 could alter the plasma levels of modafinil). Products include:
- Trileptal Tablets ... 2300
- Trileptal Oral Suspension ... 2300

Paclitaxel (Chronic administration of modafinil can increase the elimination of substrates of CYP3A4. Dose adjustments may be necessary for patients being treated with these and similar medications).
No products indexed under this heading.

Pargyline Hydrochloride (Co-administration requires caution; no interaction studies have been performed).
No products indexed under this heading.

Paroxetine Hydrochloride (Modafinil is a reversible inhibitor of the CYP2C19; the levels of CYP2D6 substrates, such as selective serotonin reuptake inhibitors, which have ancillary routes of elimination through CYP2D6, may be increased by co-administration of modafinil). Products include:
- Paxil CR Controlled-Release Tablets ... 1538
- Paxil ... 1530

Phenelzine Sulfate (Co-administration requires caution; no interaction studies have been performed).
No products indexed under this heading.

Phenobarbital (Chronic administration of modafinil may cause induction of its metabolism; co-administration of potent inducers of CYP3A4, such as phenobarbital, could alter the levels of modafinil due to the partial involvement of that enzyme in the metabolic elimination of the compound). Products include:
- Donnatal Extentabs ... 2493

Phenobarbital Sodium (Co-administration of potent inducers of CYP3A4 could alter the plasma levels of modafinil).
No products indexed under this heading.

Phenylbutazone (An apparent concentration-related suppression of CYP2C9 activity was observed in human hepatocytes after exposure to modafinil in vitro suggesting that there is a potential for a metabolic interaction between modafinil and substrates of CYP2C9).
No products indexed under this heading.

Phenytoin (Modafinil is a reversible inhibitor of the CYP2C19; co-administration with drugs that are largely eliminated via this pathway, such as phenytoin, may increase the circulating levels of phenytoin).
No products indexed under this heading.

Phenytoin Sodium (Modafinil is a reversible inhibitor of the CYP2C19; co-administration with drugs that are largely eliminated via this pathway, such as phenytoin, may increase the circulating levels of phenytoin). Products include:
- Phenytek Capsules ... 2160

Pimozide (Chronic administration of modafinil can increase the elimination of substrates of CYP3A4. Dose adjustments may be necessary for patients being treated with these and similar medications).
No products indexed under this heading.

Pioglitazone Hydrochloride (An apparent concentration-related suppression of CYP2C9 activity was observed in human hepatocytes after exposure to modafinil in vitro suggesting that there is a potential for a metabolic interaction between modafinil and substrates of CYP2C9). Products include:
- ActoPlus Met Tablets ... 3214
- Actos Tablets ... 3219
- Duetact Tablets ... 3226

Piroxicam (An apparent concentration-related suppression of CYP2C9 activity was observed in human hepatocytes after exposure to modafinil in vitro suggesting that there is a potential for a metabolic interaction between modafinil and substrates of CYP2C9).
No products indexed under this heading.

Polyestradiol Phosphate (Chronic administration of modafinil can increase the elimination of substrates of CYP3A4. Dose adjustments may be necessary for patients being treated with these and similar medications).
No products indexed under this heading.

Prednisolone Acetate (Co-administration of potent inducers of CYP3A4 could alter the plasma levels of modafinil). Products include:
- Blephamide Ophthalmic Ointment ... 568
- Blephamide Ophthalmic Suspension ... 569
- Poly-Pred Ophthalmic Suspension ... ⊙ 233
- Pred Forte Ophthalmic Suspension ... ⊙ 235
- Pred Mild Ophthalmic Suspension ... ⊙ 238
- Pred-G Ophthalmic Ointment ... ⊙ 237
- Pred-G Ophthalmic Suspension ... ⊙ 236

Prednisolone Sodium Phosphate (Co-administration of potent inducers of CYP3A4 could alter the plasma levels of modafinil).
No products indexed under this heading.

Prednisolone Tebutate (Co-administration of potent inducers of CYP3A4 could alter the plasma levels of modafinil).
No products indexed under this heading.

Prednisone (Co-administration of potent inducers of CYP3A4 could alter the plasma levels of modafinil).
No products indexed under this heading.

Primidone (Co-administration of potent inducers of CYP3A4 could alter the plasma levels of modafinil).
No products indexed under this heading.

Procarbazine Hydrochloride (Co-administration requires caution; no interaction studies have been performed). Products include:
- Matulane Capsules ... 3191

Propoxyphene Hydrochloride (Co-administration of potent inhibitors of CYP3A4 could alter the plasma levels of modafinil).
No products indexed under this heading.

Propoxyphene Napsylate (Co-administration of potent inhibitors of CYP3A4 could alter the plasma levels of modafinil).
No products indexed under this heading.

Propranolol Hydrochloride (Modafinil is a reversible inhibitor of the CYP2C19; co-administration with drugs that are largely eliminated via this pathway, such as propranolol, may increase the circulating levels of propranolol). Products include:
- Inderal LA Long-Acting Capsules ... 3429
- InnoPran XL Capsules ... 2723

Protriptyline Hydrochloride (CYP2C19 provides an ancillary pathway for the metabolism of certain tricyclic antidepressants that are primarily metabolized by CYP2D6. In tricyclic-treated patients deficient in CYP2D6, the amount of metabolism by CYP2C19 may be substantially increased. Modafinil may cause elevation of the levels of these tricyclics in this subset of patients. A reduction in the dose of tricyclic agents might be needed in these patients).
No products indexed under this heading.

Quinidine (Co-administration of potent inhibitors of CYP3A4 could alter the plasma levels of modafinil).
No products indexed under this heading.

Quinidine Gluconate (Chronic administration of modafinil can increase the elimination of substrates of CYP3A4. Dose adjustments may be necessary for patients being treated with these and similar medications).
No products indexed under this heading.

Quinidine Hydrochloride (Co-administration of potent inhibitors of CYP3A4 could alter the plasma levels of modafinil).
No products indexed under this heading.

Quinidine Polygalacturonate (Chronic administration of modafinil can increase the elimination of substrates of CYP3A4. Dose adjustments may be necessary for patients being treated with these and similar medications).
No products indexed under this heading.

Quinidine Sulfate (Chronic administration of modafinil can increase the elimination of substrates of CYP3A4. Dose adjustments may be necessary for patients being treated with these and similar medications).
No products indexed under this heading.

Quinine (Co-administration of potent inhibitors of CYP3A4 could alter the plasma levels of modafinil).
No products indexed under this heading.

Quinine Sulfate (Co-administration of potent inhibitors of CYP3A4 could alter the plasma levels of modafinil).
No products indexed under this heading.

Quinupristin (Co-administration of potent inhibitors of CYP3A4 could alter the plasma levels of modafinil).
No products indexed under this heading.

Ranitidine Bismuth Citrate (Co-administration of potent inhibitors of CYP3A4 could alter the plasma levels of modafinil).
No products indexed under this heading.

Ranitidine Hydrochloride (Co-administration of potent inhibitors of CYP3A4 could alter the plasma levels of modafinil). Products include:
- Zantac ... 1624
- Zantac Injection ... 1619
- Zantac Injection Pharmacy Bulk Package ... 1622

Repaglinide (An apparent concentration-related suppression of CYP2C9 activity was observed in human hepatocytes after exposure to modafinil in vitro suggesting that there is a potential for a metabolic interaction between modafinil and substrates of CYP2C9).
No products indexed under this heading.

Rifabutin (Chronic administration of modafinil can increase the elimination of substrates of CYP3A4. Dose adjustments may be necessary for patients being treated with these and similar medications).
No products indexed under this heading.

Rifampicin (Co-administration of potent inducers of CYP3A4 could alter the plasma levels of modafinil).
No products indexed under this heading.

Rifampin (Chronic administration of modafinil may cause induction of its metabolism; co-administration of potent inducers of CYP3A4, such as rifampin, could alter the levels of modafinil due to the partial involvement of that enzyme in the metabolic elimination of the compound).
No products indexed under this heading.

Rifapentine (Co-administration of potent inducers of CYP3A4 could alter the plasma levels of modafinil).
No products indexed under this heading.

Ritonavir (Chronic administration of modafinil can increase the elimination of substrates of CYP3A4. Dose adjustments may be necessary for patients being treated with these and similar medications). Products include:

Kaletra 476
Norvir 503

Rofecoxib (An apparent concentration-related suppression of CYP2C9 activity was observed in human hepatocytes after exposure to modafinil in vitro suggesting that there is a potential for a metabolic interaction between modafinil and substrates of CYP2C9).

No products indexed under this heading.

Rosiglitazone Maleate (An apparent concentration-related suppression of CYP2C9 activity was observed in human hepatocytes after exposure to modafinil in vitro suggesting that there is a potential for a metabolic interaction between modafinil and substrates of CYP2C9). Products include:

Avandamet Tablets 1373
Avandaryl Tablets 1379
Avandia Tablets 1384

Saquinavir (Chronic administration of modafinil can increase the elimination of substrates of CYP3A4. Dose adjustments may be necessary for patients being treated with these and similar medications).

No products indexed under this heading.

Saquinavir Mesylate (Chronic administration of modafinil can increase the elimination of substrates of CYP3A4. Dose adjustments may be necessary for patients being treated with these and similar medications). Products include:

Invirase 2772

Selegiline Hydrochloride (Co-administration requires caution; no interaction studies have been performed). Products include:

Eldepryl Capsules 3208
Zelapar Tablets 3372

Sertraline Hydrochloride (Modafinil is a reversible inhibitor of the CYP2C19; the levels of CYP2D6 substrates, such as selective serotonin reuptake inhibitors, which have ancillary routes of elimination through CYP2D6, may be increased by co-administration of modafinil). Products include:

Zoloft 2586

Sildenafil Citrate (Chronic administration of modafinil can increase the elimination of substrates of CYP3A4. Dose adjustments may be necessary for patients being treated with these and similar medications). Products include:

Revatio Tablets 2557
Viagra Tablets 2573

Simvastatin (Chronic administration of modafinil can increase the elimination of substrates of CYP3A4. Dose adjustments may be necessary for patients being treated with these and similar medications). Products include:

Vytorin 10/10 Tablets 2114
Vytorin 10/10 Tablets 3077
Vytorin 10/20 Tablets 2114
Vytorin 10/20 Tablets 3077
Vytorin 10/40 Tablets 2114
Vytorin 10/40 Tablets 3077
Vytorin 10/80 Tablets 2114
Vytorin 10/80 Tablets 3077
Zocor Tablets 2105

Sirolimus (Chronic administration of modafinil can increase the elimination of substrates of CYP3A4. Dose adjustments may be necessary for patients being treated with these and similar medications). Products include:

Rapamune Oral Solution and Tablets 3475

Sulfamethoxazole (An apparent concentration-related suppression of CYP2C9 activity was observed in human hepatocytes after exposure to modafinil in vitro suggesting that there is a potential for a metabolic interaction between modafinil and substrates of CYP2C9).

No products indexed under this heading.

Sulfinpyrazone (Co-administration of potent inducers of CYP3A4 could alter the plasma levels of modafinil).

No products indexed under this heading.

Sulindac (An apparent concentration-related suppression of CYP2C9 activity was observed in human hepatocytes after exposure to modafinil in vitro suggesting that there is a potential for a metabolic interaction between modafinil and substrates of CYP2C9). Products include:

Clinoril Tablets 1924

Suprofen (An apparent concentration-related suppression of CYP2C9 activity was observed in human hepatocytes after exposure to modafinil in vitro suggesting that there is a potential for a metabolic interaction between modafinil and substrates of CYP2C9).

No products indexed under this heading.

Tacrolimus (Chronic administration of modafinil can increase the elimination of substrates of CYP3A4. Dose adjustments may be necessary for patients being treated with these and similar medications). Products include:

Prograf Capsules and Injection 632
Protopic Ointment 638

Tamoxifen Citrate (Chronic administration of modafinil can increase the elimination of substrates of CYP3A4. Dose adjustments may be necessary for patients being treated with these and similar medications). Products include:

Soltamox Oral Solution 3527

Telithromycin (Co-administration of potent inhibitors of CYP3A4 could alter the plasma levels of modafinil). Products include:

Ketek Tablets 2903

Telmisartan (An apparent concentration-related suppression of CYP2C9 activity was observed in human hepatocytes after exposure to modafinil in vitro suggesting that there is a potential for a metabolic interaction between modafinil and substrates of CYP2C9). Products include:

Micardis Tablets 854
Micardis HCT Tablets 856

Theophylline (Chronic administration of modafinil may cause modest induction of CYP3A4, thus reducing the levels, to a lesser degree, of co-administered substrate for that enzyme system, such as theophylline).

No products indexed under this heading.

Theophylline Anhydrous (Chronic administration of modafinil may cause modest induction of CYP3A4, thus reducing the levels, to a lesser degree, of co-administered substrate for that enzyme system, such as theophylline). Products include:

Uniphyl Tablets 2710

Theophylline Calcium Salicylate (Chronic administration of modafinil may cause modest induction of CYP3A4, thus reducing the levels, to a lesser degree, of co-administered substrate for that enzyme system, such as theophylline).

No products indexed under this heading.

Theophylline Dihydroxypropyl (Glyceryl) (Chronic administration of modafinil may cause modest induction of CYP3A4, thus reducing the levels, to a lesser degree, of co-administered substrate for that enzyme system, such as theophylline).

No products indexed under this heading.

Theophylline Ethylenediamine (Chronic administration of modafinil may cause modest induction of CYP3A4, thus reducing the levels, to a lesser degree, of co-administered substrate for that enzyme system, such as theophylline).

No products indexed under this heading.

Theophylline Sodium Glycinate (Chronic administration of modafinil may cause modest induction of CYP3A4, thus reducing the levels, to a lesser degree, of co-administered substrate for that enzyme system, such as theophylline).

No products indexed under this heading.

Tiagabine Hydrochloride (Chronic administration of modafinil can increase the elimination of substrates of CYP3A4. Dose adjustments may be necessary for patients being treated with these and similar medications). Products include:

Gabitril Tablets 984

Tolazamide (An apparent concentration-related suppression of CYP2C9 activity was observed in human hepatocytes after exposure to modafinil in vitro suggesting that there is a potential for a metabolic interaction between modafinil and substrates of CYP2C9).

No products indexed under this heading.

Tolbutamide (An apparent concentration-related suppression of CYP2C9 activity was observed in human hepatocytes after exposure to modafinil in vitro suggesting that there is a potential for a metabolic interaction between modafinil and substrates of CYP2C9).

No products indexed under this heading.

Tolbutamide Sodium (An apparent concentration-related suppression of CYP2C9 activity was observed in human hepatocytes after exposure to modafinil in vitro suggesting that there is a potential for a metabolic interaction between modafinil and substrates of CYP2C9).

No products indexed under this heading.

Tolmetin Sodium (An apparent concentration-related suppression of CYP2C9 activity was observed in human hepatocytes after exposure to modafinil in vitro suggesting that there is a potential for a metabolic interaction between modafinil and substrates of CYP2C9).

No products indexed under this heading.

Tolterodine Tartrate (Chronic administration of modafinil can increase the elimination of substrates of CYP3A4. Dose adjustments may be necessary for patients being treated with these and similar medications). Products include:

Detrol Tablets 2628
Detrol LA Capsules 2631

Torsemide (An apparent concentration-related suppression of CYP2C9 activity was observed in human hepatocytes after exposure to modafinil in vitro suggesting that there is a potential for a metabolic interaction between modafinil and substrates of CYP2C9). Products include:

Demadex Injection 2759
Demadex Tablets 2759

Tranylcypromine Sulfate (Co-administration requires caution; no interaction studies have been performed). Products include:

Parnate Tablets 1527

Trazodone Hydrochloride (Chronic administration of modafinil can increase the elimination of substrates of CYP3A4. Dose adjustments may be necessary for patients being treated with these and similar medications).

No products indexed under this heading.

Triamcinolone (Co-administration of potent inducers of CYP3A4 could alter the plasma levels of modafinil).

No products indexed under this heading.

Triamcinolone Acetonide (Co-administration of potent inducers of CYP3A4 could alter the plasma levels of modafinil). Products include:

Azmacort Inhalation Aerosol 1726
Nasacort AQ Nasal Spray 2922

Triamcinolone Diacetate (Co-administration of potent inducers of CYP3A4 could alter the plasma levels of modafinil).

No products indexed under this heading.

Triamcinolone Hexacetonide (Co-administration of potent inducers of CYP3A4 could alter the plasma levels of modafinil).

No products indexed under this heading.

Triazolam (When modafinil was administered concurrently with triazolam, mean Cmax and AUC of triazolam were decreased by 42% and 59%, respectively, and its elimination half-life was decreased by approximately an hour after the modafinil treatment).

No products indexed under this heading.

Trimipramine Maleate (CYP2C19 provides an ancillary pathway for the metabolism of certain tricyclic antidepressants that are primarily metabolized by CYP2D6. In tricyclic-treated patients deficient in CYP2D6, the amount of metabolism by CYP2C19 may be substantially increased. Modafinil may cause ele-

vation of the levels of these tricyclics in this subset of patients. A reduction in the dose of tricyclic agents might be needed in these patients).
No products indexed under this heading.

Troglitazone (An apparent concentration-related suppression of CYP2C9 activity was observed in human hepatocytes after exposure to modafinil in vitro suggesting that there is a potential for a metabolic interaction between modafinil and substrates of CYP2C9).
No products indexed under this heading.

Troleandomycin (Co-administration of potent inhibitors of CYP3A4 could alter the plasma levels of modafinil).
No products indexed under this heading.

Valdecoxib (An apparent concentration-related suppression of CYP2C9 activity was observed in human hepatocytes after exposure to modafinil in vitro suggesting that there is a potential for a metabolic interaction between modafinil and substrates of CYP2C9).
No products indexed under this heading.

Valproate Sodium (Co-administration of potent inhibitors of CYP3A4 could alter the plasma levels of modafinil). Products include:
Depacon Injection 412

Valsartan (An apparent concentration-related suppression of CYP2C9 activity was observed in human hepatocytes after exposure to modafinil in vitro suggesting that there is a potential for a metabolic interaction between modafinil and substrates of CYP2C9). Products include:
Diovan Tablets 2193
Diovan HCT Tablets 2196

Verapamil Hydrochloride (Chronic administration of modafinil can increase the elimination of substrates of CYP3A4. Dose adjustments may be necessary for patients being treated with these and similar medications). Products include:
Covera-HS Tablets 3139
Tarka Tablets 524
Verelan PM Extended-Release Capsules, Controlled-Onset........... 3106

Vinblastine Sulfate (Chronic administration of modafinil can increase the elimination of substrates of CYP3A4. Dose adjustments may be necessary for patients being treated with these and similar medications).
No products indexed under this heading.

Vincristine Sulfate (Chronic administration of modafinil can increase the elimination of substrates of CYP3A4. Dose adjustments may be necessary for patients being treated with these and similar medications).
No products indexed under this heading.

Voriconazole (An apparent concentration-related suppression of CYP2C9 activity was observed in human hepatocytes after exposure to modafinil in vitro suggesting that there is a potential for a metabolic interaction between modafinil and substrates of CYP2C9). Products include:
VFEND I.V. 2564
VFEND Oral Suspension 2564
VFEND Tablets 2564

Warfarin Sodium (There were no significant changes in the pharmacokinetic profile of warfarin in healthy subjects given a single dose of warfarin following chronic administration of modafinil relative to the profiles in subjects given placebo. However, more frequent monitoring of prothrombin times/INR is advisable whenever modafinil is co-administered with warfarin). Products include:
Coumadin for Injection 898
Coumadin Tablets 898

Zafirlukast (An apparent concentration-related suppression of CYP2C9 activity was observed in human hepatocytes after exposure to modafinil in vitro suggesting that there is a potential for a metabolic interaction between modafinil and substrates of CYP2C9). Products include:
Accolate Tablets 671

Zileuton (An apparent concentration-related suppression of CYP2C9 activity was observed in human hepatocytes after exposure to modafinil in vitro suggesting that there is a potential for a metabolic interaction between modafinil and substrates of CYP2C9). Products include:
Zyflo Tablets 1023

Food Interactions

Alcohol (The use of modafinil in combination with alcohol has not been studied. It is advisable to avoid alcohol while taking modafinil).

Food, unspecified (Delays the absorption (tmax) by approximately one hour; no effect on overall bioavailability).

Grapefruit (Co-administration of potent inhibitors of CYP3A4 could alter the plasma levels of modafinil).

Grapefruit Juice (Co-administration of potent inhibitors of CYP3A4 could alter the plasma levels of modafinil).

PROVOCHOLINE POWDER FOR INHALATION

(Methacholine Chloride) 2127
None cited in PDR database.

PROZAC PULVULES AND LIQUID

(Fluoxetine Hydrochloride) 1801
May interact with anticoagulants, cytochrome p450 2d6 substrates (selected), oral hypoglycemic agents, insulin, lithium preparations, monoamine oxidase inhibitors, non-steroidal anti-inflammatory agents, phenytoin, tricyclic antidepressants, and certain other agents. Compounds in these categories include:

Acarbose (Fluoxetine may alter glycemic control in diabetics; hypoglycemia has occurred during therapy with fluoxetine and hyperglycemia has developed following discontinuation of the drug; hypoglycemia dosage may need to be adjusted). Products include:
Precose Tablets 751

Alprazolam (Co-administration has resulted in increased alprazolam plasma concentrations and further psychomotor performance decrement due to increased alprazolam levels). Products include:
Niravam Orally Disintegrating Tablets 3092

Amitriptyline Hydrochloride (Fluoxetine inhibits the activity of P450 IID6 isoenzyme making normal metabolizers resemble poor metabolizers; therapy with drugs that are predominantly metabolized by the P450 IID6 isoenzyme, such as tricyclic antidepressants, and have a relatively narrow therapeutic index should be initiated at low end of the dose range if a patient is receiving fluoxetine concurrently or has taken it in the previous 5 weeks).
No products indexed under this heading.

Amoxapine (Fluoxetine inhibits the activity of P450 IID6 isoenzyme making normal metabolizers resemble poor metabolizers; therapy with drugs that are predominantly metabolized by the P450 IID6 isoenzyme, such as tricyclic antidepressants, and have a relatively narrow therapeutic index should be initiated at low end of the dose range if a patient is receiving fluoxetine concurrently or has taken it in the previous 5 weeks).
No products indexed under this heading.

Amphetamine Aspartate (If fluoxetine is added to the treatment regimen of a patient already receiving a drug metabolized by CYP2D6, the need for decreased dose of the original medication should be considered. Fluoxetine is metabolized by this isoenzyme; thus, both the pharmacokinetic properties and relative proportion of metabolites are altered in poor metabolizers of CYP2D6). Products include:
Adderall Tablets 3164
Adderall XR Capsules 3166

Amphetamine Aspartate Monohydrate (If fluoxetine is added to the treatment regimen of a patient already receiving a drug metabolized by CYP2D6, the need for decreased dose of the original medication should be considered. Fluoxetine is metabolized by this isoenzyme; thus, both the pharmacokinetic properties and relative proportion of metabolites are altered in poor metabolizers of CYP2D6).
No products indexed under this heading.

Amphetamine Sulfate (If fluoxetine is added to the treatment regimen of a patient already receiving a drug metabolized by CYP2D6, the need for decreased dose of the original medication should be considered. Fluoxetine is metabolized by this isoenzyme; thus, both the pharmacokinetic properties and relative proportion of metabolites are altered in poor metabolizers of CYP2D6). Products include:
Adderall Tablets 3164
Adderall XR Capsules 3166

Anisindione (Concurrent use of fluoxetine with drugs that affect coagulation may potentiate the risk of bleeding). Products include:
Miradon Tablets 3042

Ardeparin Sodium (Concurrent use of fluoxetine with drugs that affect coagulation may potentiate the risk of bleeding).
No products indexed under this heading.

Aspirin (Concurrent use of fluoxetine with aspirin potentiated the risk of upper gastrointestinal bleeding and there is a reason to believe that bleeding at other sites may be similarly potentiated. Combined use of psychotropic drugs that interfere with serotonin reuptake and aspirin has been associated with an increased risk of bleeding). Products include:
Aggrenox Capsules 822
Bayer Aspirin 744
BC Allergy Sinus Cold Powder 677
BC Headache Powder 677
Arthritis Strength BC Powder 677
BC Sinus Cold Powder 677
Excedrin Extra Strength Caplets/Tablets/Geltabs 684
Excedrin Migraine Caplets/Tablets/Geltabs 609
Goody's Body Pain Formula Powder 684
Goody's Extra Strength Headache Powders..................... 611
Goody's Extra Strength Pain Relief Tablets 685
Percodan Tablets 1132
St. Joseph 81 mg Aspirin Chewable and Enteric Coated Tablets 1869

Aspirin, Enteric Coated (Concurrent use of fluoxetine with aspirin potentiated the risk of upper gastrointestinal bleeding and there is a reason to believe that bleeding at other sites may be similarly potentiated. Combined use of psychotropic drugs that interfere with serotonin reuptake and aspirin has been associated with an increased risk of bleeding).
No products indexed under this heading.

Aspirin Buffered (Concurrent use of fluoxetine with aspirin potentiated the risk of upper gastrointestinal bleeding and there is a reason to believe that bleeding at other sites may be similarly potentiated. Combined use of psychotropic drugs that interfere with serotonin reuptake and aspirin has been associated with an increased risk of bleeding). Products include:
Bufferin Extra Strength Tablets 678
Bufferin Regular Strength Tablets ... 678

Atomoxetine Hydrochloride (If fluoxetine is added to the treatment regimen of a patient already receiving a drug metabolized by CYP2D6, the need for decreased dose of the original medication should be considered. Fluoxetine is metabolized by this isoenzyme; thus, both the pharmacokinetic properties and relative proportion of metabolites are altered in poor metabolizers of CYP2D6). Products include:
Strattera Capsules 1814

Bisoprolol Fumarate (If fluoxetine is added to the treatment regimen of a patient already receiving a drug metabolized by CYP2D6, the need for decreased dose of the original medication should be considered. Fluoxetine is metabolized by this isoenzyme; thus, both the pharmacokinetic properties and relative proportion of metabolites are altered in poor metabolizers of CYP2D6).
No products indexed under this heading.

Captopril (If fluoxetine is added to the treatment regimen of a patient already receiving a drug metabolized by CYP2D6, the need for decreased dose of the original medication should be considered. Fluoxetine is metabolized by this isoenzyme; thus, both the pharmacokinetic properties and relative proportion of metabolites are altered in poor metabolizers of CYP2D6). Products include:
Captopril Tablets 2149

Carbamazepine (Patients stable on doses of carbamazepine have developed elevated plasma carbamazepine concentrations and clinical anticonvulsant toxicity following initiation of concomitant fluoxetine therapy). Products include:

Carbatrol Capsules 3171
Equetro Extended-Release Capsules 3180
Tegretol/Tegretol-XR 2295

Carvedilol (If fluoxetine is added to the treatment regimen of a patient already receiving a drug metabolized by CYP2D6, the need for decreased dose of the original medication should be considered. Fluoxetine is metabolized by this isoenzyme; thus, both the pharmacokinetic properties and relative proportion of metabolites are altered in poor metabolizers of CYP2D6). Products include:

Coreg Tablets 1414

Celecoxib (Concurrent use of fluoxetine with an NSAID potentiated the risk of upper gastrointestinal bleeding and there is a reason to believe that bleeding at other sites may be similarly potentiated. Combined use of psychotropic drugs that interfere with serotonin reuptake and NSAIDs have been associated with an increased risk of bleeding). Products include:

Celebrex Capsules 3134

Cevimeline Hydrochloride (If fluoxetine is added to the treatment regimen of a patient already receiving a drug metabolized by CYP2D6, the need for decreased dose of the original medication should be considered. Fluoxetine is metabolized by this isoenzyme; thus, both the pharmacokinetic properties and relative proportion of metabolites are altered in poor metabolizers of CYP2D6). Products include:

Evoxac Capsules 1047

Chlorpromazine (If fluoxetine is added to the treatment regimen of a patient already receiving a drug metabolized by CYP2D6, the need for decreased dose of the original medication should be considered. Fluoxetine is metabolized by this isoenzyme; thus, both the pharmacokinetic properties and relative proportion of metabolites are altered in poor metabolizers of CYP2D6).

No products indexed under this heading.

Chlorpromazine Hydrochloride (If fluoxetine is added to the treatment regimen of a patient already receiving a drug metabolized by CYP2D6, the need for decreased dose of the original medication should be considered. Fluoxetine is metabolized by this isoenzyme; thus, both the pharmacokinetic properties and relative proportion of metabolites are altered in poor metabolizers of CYP2D6).

No products indexed under this heading.

Chlorpropamide (Fluoxetine may alter glycemic control in diabetics; hypoglycemia has occurred during therapy with fluoxetine and hyperglycemia has developed following discontinuation of the drug; hypoglycemia dosage may need to be adjusted).

No products indexed under this heading.

Clomipramine Hydrochloride (Fluoxetine inhibits the activity of P450 IID6 isoenzyme making normal metabolizers resemble poor metabolizers; therapy with drugs that are predominantly metabolized by the P450 IID6 isoenzyme, such as tricyclic antidepressants, and have a relatively narrow therapeutic index should be initiated at low end of the dose range if a patient is receiving fluoxetine concurrently or has taken it in the previous 5 weeks).

No products indexed under this heading.

Clozapine (Co-administration of SSRIs, fluoxetine, and antipsychotics, such as clozapine, has resulted in elevation of blood levels of clozapine). Products include:

Clozaril Tablets 2184
FazaClo Orally Disintegrating Tablets 551

Codeine Phosphate (If fluoxetine is added to the treatment regimen of a patient already receiving a drug metabolized by CYP2D6, the need for decreased dose of the original medication should be considered. Fluoxetine is metabolized by this isoenzyme; thus, both the pharmacokinetic properties and relative proportion of metabolites are altered in poor metabolizers of CYP2D6). Products include:

Tylenol with Codeine Tablets 2391

Codeine Sulfate (If fluoxetine is added to the treatment regimen of a patient already receiving a drug metabolized by CYP2D6, the need for decreased dose of the original medication should be considered. Fluoxetine is metabolized by this isoenzyme; thus, both the pharmacokinetic properties and relative proportion of metabolites are altered in poor metabolizers of CYP2D6).

No products indexed under this heading.

Cyclobenzaprine Hydrochloride (If fluoxetine is added to the treatment regimen of a patient already receiving a drug metabolized by CYP2D6, the need for decreased dose of the original medication should be considered. Fluoxetine is metabolized by this isoenzyme; thus, both the pharmacokinetic properties and relative proportion of metabolites are altered in poor metabolizers of CYP2D6).

No products indexed under this heading.

Dalteparin Sodium (Concurrent use of fluoxetine with drugs that affect coagulation may potentiate the risk of bleeding). Products include:

Fragmin Injection 1097

Danaparoid Sodium (Concurrent use of fluoxetine with drugs that affect coagulation may potentiate the risk of bleeding).

No products indexed under this heading.

Desipramine Hydrochloride (Fluoxetine inhibits the activity of P450 IID6 isoenzyme making normal metabolizers resemble poor metabolizers; therapy with drugs that are predominantly metabolized by the P450 IID6 isoenzyme, such as tricyclic antidepressants, and have a relatively narrow therapeutic index should be initiated at low end of the dose range if a patient is receiving fluoxetine concurrently or has taken it in the previous 5 weeks).

No products indexed under this heading.

Dexfenfluramine Hydrochloride (If fluoxetine is added to the treatment regimen of a patient already receiving a drug metabolized by CYP2D6, the need for decreased dose of the original medication should be considered. Fluoxetine is metabolized by this isoenzyme; thus, both the pharmacokinetic properties and relative proportion of metabolites are altered in poor metabolizers of CYP2D6).

No products indexed under this heading.

Dextromethorphan Hydrobromide (If fluoxetine is added to the treatment regimen of a patient already receiving a drug metabolized by CYP2D6, the need for decreased dose of the original medication should be considered. Fluoxetine is metabolized by this isoenzyme; thus, both the pharmacokinetic properties and relative proportion of metabolites are altered in poor metabolizers of CYP2D6). Products include:

Comtrex Maximum Strength Cold & Cough Day/Night Caplets - Day Formulation .... ▣ 726
Comtrex Maximum Strength Cold & Cough Day/Night Caplets - Night Formulation .... ▣ 726
Comtrex Maximum Strength Non-Drowsy Cold & Cough Caplets .... ▣ 725
Children's Dimetapp DM Cold & Cough Elixir .... ▣ 731
Children's Dimetapp Long Acting Cough Plus Cold Syrup .... ▣ 731
Toddler's Dimetapp Cold and Cough Drops .... ▣ 732
Mucinex DM Extended-Release Bi-Layer Tablets .... ▣ 720
Refenesen DM Caplets .... ▣ 721
Robitussin Cough & Cold CF Liquid .... ▣ 735
Robitussin Cough & Cold Long-Acting Liquid .... ▣ 735
Robitussin Cough & Allergy Syrup .. ▣ 736
Robitussin Cough & Cold Nighttime Liquid .... ▣ 736
Robitussin Cough & Cold Pediatric Drops .... ▣ 735
Robitussin Cough, Cold & Flu Nighttime Liquid .... ▣ 738
Robitussin Cough & Congestion Liquid .... ▣ 738
Robitussin Cough Gels Long-Acting .... ▣ 737
Robitussin Cough Long Acting Liquid .... ▣ 739
Robitussin Cough DM Syrup .... ▣ 738
Robitussin Cough DM Infant Drops .... ▣ 738
Robitussin Pediatric Cough Long Acting Liquid .... ▣ 739
Robitussin Pediatric Cough & Cold Long-Acting Liquid .... ▣ 735
Robitussin Pediatric Cough & Cold Nighttime Liquid .... ▣ 736
Robitussin Sugar Free Cough .... ▣ 738
TheraFlu Cold & Cough Hot Liquid .... ▣ 740
TheraFlu Warming Relief Daytime Severe Cold .... ▣ 743
TheraFlu Thin Strips Long Acting Cough .... ▣ 744
Triaminic Daytime Cold & Cough Liquid .... ▣ 745
Triaminic Cough & Sore Throat Liquid .... ▣ 747
Triaminic Cough & Runny Nose Softchews .... ▣ 748
Triaminic Thin Strips Cold & Cough .... ▣ 778
Triaminic Infant Thin Strips Decongestant Plus Cough .... ▣ 747
Children's Tylenol Plus Flu Oral Suspension .... ▣ 749
Tylenol Cold Head Congestion Daytime Caplets with Cool Burst and Gelcaps .... ▣ 750
Tylenol Cold Multi-Symptom Daytime Liquid .... ▣ 752
Tylenol Cold Multi-Symptom Severe Daytime Liquid .... ▣ 752
Concentrated Tylenol Infants' Drops Plus Cold & Cough .... ▣ 754
Children's Tylenol Plus Cough & Runny Nose Suspension Liquid 1879
Children's Tylenol Plus Cough & Sore Throat Suspension Liquid 1879
Children's Tylenol Plus Flu Suspension Liquid 1881
Children's Tylenol Plus Multi-Symptom Cold Suspension Liquid 1879
Tylenol Cold Severe Congestion Non-Drowsy Caplets with Cool Burst 1874
Tylenol Cold Head Congestion Daytime Caplets with Cool Burst 1873
Tylenol Cold Head Congestion Nighttime Caplets with Cool Burst 1873
Tylenol Cold Head Congestion Severe Caplets with Cool Burst 1873
Tylenol Cold Multi-Symptom Daytime Caplets with Cool Burst and Gelcaps 1874
Tylenol Cold Multi-Symptom Daytime Liquid with Citrus Burst ... 1874
Tylenol Cold Multi-Symptom Nighttime Caplets with Cool Burst 1874
Tylenol Cold Multi-Symptom Nighttime Liquid with Cool Burst ... 1874
Tylenol Cold Multi-Symptom Severe Caplets with Cool Burst 1874
Tylenol Cold Multi-Symptom Severe Daytime Liquid with Citrus Burst 1874
Tylenol Cough & Sore Throat Daytime Liquid with Cool Burst 1877
Tylenol Cough & Sore Throat Nighttime Liquid with Cool Burst ... 1877
Concentrated Tylenol Infants' Drops Plus Cold and Cough 1879
Vicks 44 Cough Relief Liquid 2679
Vicks 44D Cough & Head Congestion Relief Liquid 2679
Vicks 44E Cough & Chest Congestion Relief Liquid 2679
Pediatric Vicks 44e Cough & Chest Congestion Relief Liquid 2676
Vicks 44M Cough, Cold & Flu Relief Liquid 2680
Pediatric Vicks 44m Cough & Cold Relief Liquid 2676
Vicks DayQuil LiquiCaps/Liquid Multi-Symptom Cold/Flu Relief ..... ▣ 761
Vicks DayQuil Multi-Symptom Cold/Flu Relief LiquiCaps 2678
Vicks DayQuil Multi-Symptom Cold/Flu Relief Liquid 2678
Vicks NyQuil Multi-Symptom Cold/Flu Relief Liquid 2681
Children's Vicks NyQuil Cold/Cough Relief .... ▣ 756
Vicks NyQuil Multi-Symptom Cold/Flu Relief LiquiCaps 2681
Vicks NyQuil LiquiCaps/Liquid Multi-Symptom Cold/Flu Relief ..... ▣ 763
Vicks NyQuil Cough Liquid 2680
Children's Vicks NyQuil Cold/Cough Relief Liquid 2680
Zicam Cough Max Nighttime Cough Spray .... ▣ 767
Zicam Cough Max Cough Spray ..... ▣ 767
Zicam Cough Max Cough Melts ...... ▣ 767
Zicam Cough Plus D Cough Spray .... ▣ 767
Zicam Cough Relief Cough Spray ... ▣ 767
Zicam Maximum Strength Flu Daytime .... ▣ 768
Zicam Maximum Strength Flu Nighttime .... ▣ 768

Dextromethorphan Polistirex (If fluoxetine is added to the treatment regimen of a patient already receiving a drug metabolized by CYP2D6, the need for decreased dose of the original medication should be considered. Fluoxetine is metabolized by this isoenzyme; thus, both the pharmacokinetic properties and relative proportion of metabolites are altered in poor metabolizers of CYP2D6). Products include:

Delsym Extended-Release Suspension 12 Hour Cough Suppressant 611

Diazepam (Co-administration results in prolonged half-life of diazepam). Products include:

Diastat Rectal Delivery System 3343
Valium Tablets 2819

Diclofenac Potassium (Concurrent use of fluoxetine with an NSAID potentiated the risk of upper gastrointestinal bleeding and there is a reason to believe that bleeding at other sites may be similarly potentiated. Combined use of psychotropic drugs that interfere with serotonin reuptake and NSAIDs have been associated with an increased risk of bleeding).

No products indexed under this heading.

Diclofenac Sodium (Concurrent use of fluoxetine with an NSAID potentiated the risk of upper gastrointestinal bleeding and there is a reason to believe that bleeding at other sites may be similarly potentiated. Combined use of psychotropic drugs that interfere with serotonin reuptake and NSAIDs have been associated with an increased risk of bleeding). Products include:

Arthrotec Tablets 3129
Voltaren Ophthalmic Solution 2309
Voltaren Tablets 2307
Voltaren-XR Tablets 2310

Dicumarol (Concurrent use of fluoxetine with drugs that affect coagulation may potentiate the risk of bleeding).

No products indexed under this heading.

Digitoxin (Fluoxetine is tightly bound to protein; co-administration may cause shift in plasma concentrations resulting in potential adverse effects).

No products indexed under this heading.

Dolasetron Mesylate (If fluoxetine is added to the treatment regimen of a patient already receiving a drug metabolized by CYP2D6, the need for decreased dose of the original medication should be considered. Fluoxetine is metabolized by this isoenzyme; thus, both the pharmacokinetic properties and relative proportion of metabolites are altered in poor metabolizers of CYP2D6). Products include:

Anzemet Injection 2859
Anzemet Tablets 2862

Donepezil Hydrochloride (If fluoxetine is added to the treatment regimen of a patient already receiving a drug metabolized by CYP2D6, the need for decreased dose of the original medication should be considered. Fluoxetine is metabolized by this isoenzyme; thus, both the pharmacokinetic properties and relative proportion of metabolites are altered in poor metabolizers of CYP2D6). Products include:

Aricept Tablets 1094
Aricept ODT Tablets 1094

Doxepin Hydrochloride (Fluoxetine inhibits the activity of P450 IID6 isoenzyme making normal metabolizers resemble poor metabolizers; therapy with drugs that are predominantly metabolized by the P450 IID6 isoenzyme, such as tricyclic antidepressants, and have a relatively narrow therapeutic index should be initiated at low end of the dose range if a patient is receiving fluoxetine concurrently or has taken it in the previous 5 weeks).

No products indexed under this heading.

Encainide Hydrochloride (If fluoxetine is added to the treatment regimen of a patient already receiving a drug metabolized by CYP2D6, the need for decreased dose of the original medication should be considered. Fluoxetine is metabolized by this isoenzyme; thus, both the pharmacokinetic properties and relative proportion of metabolites are altered in poor metabolizers of CYP2D6).

No products indexed under this heading.

Enoxaparin Sodium (Concurrent use of fluoxetine with drugs that affect coagulation may potentiate the risk of bleeding). Products include:

Lovenox Injection 2915

Etodolac (Concurrent use of fluoxetine with an NSAID potentiated the risk of upper gastrointestinal bleeding and there is a reason to believe that bleeding at other sites may be similarly potentiated. Combined use of psychotropic drugs that interfere with serotonin reuptake and NSAIDs have been associated with an increased risk of bleeding).

No products indexed under this heading.

Fenoprofen Calcium (Concurrent use of fluoxetine with an NSAID potentiated the risk of upper gastrointestinal bleeding and there is a reason to believe that bleeding at other sites may be similarly potentiated. Combined use of psychotropic drugs that interfere with serotonin reuptake and NSAIDs have been associated with an increased risk of bleeding). Products include:

Nalfon Capsules 2502

Fentanyl (If fluoxetine is added to the treatment regimen of a patient already receiving a drug metabolized by CYP2D6, the need for decreased dose of the original medication should be considered. Fluoxetine is metabolized by this isoenzyme; thus, both the pharmacokinetic properties and relative proportion of metabolites are altered in poor metabolizers of CYP2D6). Products include:

Duragesic Transdermal System 2373
Ionsys Transdermal System 2379

Fentanyl Citrate (If fluoxetine is added to the treatment regimen of a patient already receiving a drug metabolized by CYP2D6, the need for decreased dose of the original medication should be considered. Fluoxetine is metabolized by this isoenzyme; thus, both the pharmacokinetic properties and relative proportion of metabolites are altered in poor metabolizers of CYP2D6). Products include:

Actiq 979

Flecainide Acetate (Fluoxetine inhibits the activity of P450 IID6 isoenzyme making normal metabolizers resemble poor metabolizers; therapy with drugs that are predominantly metabolized by the P450 IID6 isoenzyme, such as flecainide, and have a relatively narrow therapeutic index should be initiated at low end of the dose range if a patient is receiving fluoxetine concurrently or has taken it in the previous 5 weeks). Products include:

Tambocor Tablets 1856

Fluoxetine (If fluoxetine is added to the treatment regimen of a patient already receiving a drug metabolized by CYP2D6, the need for decreased dose of the original medication should be considered. Fluoxetine is metabolized by this isoenzyme; thus, both the pharmacokinetic properties and relative proportion of metabolites are altered in poor metabolizers of CYP2D6).

No products indexed under this heading.

Fluphenazine Decanoate (If fluoxetine is added to the treatment regimen of a patient already receiving a drug metabolized by CYP2D6, the need for decreased dose of the original medication should be considered. Fluoxetine is metabolized by this isoenzyme; thus, both the pharmacokinetic properties and relative proportion of metabolites are altered in poor metabolizers of CYP2D6).

No products indexed under this heading.

Fluphenazine Enanthate (If fluoxetine is added to the treatment regimen of a patient already receiving a drug metabolized by CYP2D6, the need for decreased dose of the original medication should be considered. Fluoxetine is metabolized by this isoenzyme; thus, both the pharmacokinetic properties and relative proportion of metabolites are altered in poor metabolizers of CYP2D6).

No products indexed under this heading.

Fluphenazine Hydrochloride (If fluoxetine is added to the treatment regimen of a patient already receiving a drug metabolized by CYP2D6, the need for decreased dose of the original medication should be considered. Fluoxetine is metabolized by this isoenzyme; thus, both the pharmacokinetic properties and relative proportion of metabolites are altered in poor metabolizers of CYP2D6).

No products indexed under this heading.

Flurbiprofen (Concurrent use of fluoxetine with an NSAID potentiated the risk of upper gastrointestinal bleeding and there is a reason to believe that bleeding at other sites may be similarly potentiated. Combined use of psychotropic drugs that interfere with serotonin reuptake and NSAIDs have been associated with an increased risk of bleeding).

No products indexed under this heading.

Fluvoxamine Maleate (If fluoxetine is added to the treatment regimen of a patient already receiving a drug metabolized by CYP2D6, the need for decreased dose of the original medication should be considered. Fluoxetine is metabolized by this isoenzyme; thus, both the pharmacokinetic properties and relative proportion of metabolites are altered in poor metabolizers of CYP2D6).

No products indexed under this heading.

Fondaparinux Sodium (Concurrent use of fluoxetine with drugs that affect coagulation may potentiate the risk of bleeding). Products include:

Arixtra Injection 1351

Formoterol Fumarate (If fluoxetine is added to the treatment regimen of a patient already receiving a drug metabolized by CYP2D6, the need for decreased dose of the original medication should be considered. Fluoxetine is metabolized by this isoenzyme; thus, both the pharmacokinetic properties and relative proportion of metabolites are altered in poor metabolizers of CYP2D6). Products include:

Foradil Aerolizer 3010

Fosphenytoin Sodium (Patients stable on doses of phenytoin have developed elevated plasma phenytoin concentrations and clinical anticonvulsant toxicity following initiation of concomitant fluoxetine therapy).

No products indexed under this heading.

Galantamine Hydrobromide (If fluoxetine is added to the treatment regimen of a patient already receiving a drug metabolized by CYP2D6, the need for decreased dose of the original medication should be considered. Fluoxetine is metabolized by this isoenzyme; thus, both the pharmacokinetic properties and relative proportion of metabolites are altered in poor metabolizers of CYP2D6). Products include:

Razadyne 2399
Razadyne ER Extended-Release Capsules 2399

Glimepiride (Fluoxetine may alter glycemic control in diabetics; hypoglycemia has occurred during therapy with fluoxetine and hyperglycemia has developed following discontinuation of the drug; hypoglycemia dosage may need to be adjusted). Products include:

Avandaryl Tablets 1379
Duetact Tablets 3226

Glipizide (Fluoxetine may alter glycemic control in diabetics; hypoglycemia has occurred during therapy with fluoxetine and hyperglycemia has developed following discontinuation of the drug; hypoglycemia dosage may need to be adjusted).

No products indexed under this heading.

Glyburide (Fluoxetine may alter glycemic control in diabetics; hypoglycemia has occurred during therapy with fluoxetine and hyperglycemia has developed following discontinuation of the drug; hypoglycemia dosage may need to be adjusted).

No products indexed under this heading.

Haloperidol (Co-administration of SSRIs, fluoxetine, and antipsychotics, such as haloperidol, has resulted in elevation of blood levels of haloperidol).

No products indexed under this heading.

Haloperidol Decanoate (Co-administration of SSRIs, fluoxetine, and antipsychotics, such as haloperidol, has resulted in elevation of blood levels of haloperidol).

No products indexed under this heading.

Heparin Calcium (Concurrent use of fluoxetine with drugs that affect coagulation may potentiate the risk of bleeding).

No products indexed under this heading.

Heparin Sodium (Concurrent use of fluoxetine with drugs that affect coagulation may potentiate the risk of bleeding).

No products indexed under this heading.

Hydrocodone Bitartrate (If fluoxetine is added to the treatment regimen of a patient already receiving a drug metabolized by CYP2D6, the need for decreased dose of the original medication should be considered. Fluoxetine is metabolized by this isoenzyme; thus, both the pharmacokinetic properties and relative proportion of metabolites are altered in poor metabolizers of CYP2D6). Products include:

- Hycodan 1116
- Hycotuss Expectorant Syrup 1117
- Vicodin Tablets 535
- Vicodin ES Tablets 536
- Vicodin HP Tablets 538
- Vicoprofen Tablets 539
- Zydone Tablets 1139

Ibuprofen (Concurrent use of fluoxetine with an NSAID potentiated the risk of upper gastrointestinal bleeding and there is a reason to believe that bleeding at other sites may be similarly potentiated. Combined use of psychotropic drugs that interfere with serotonin reuptake and NSAIDs have been associated with an increased risk of bleeding). Products include:

- Advil Allergy Sinus Caplets .... ■ 770
- Advil .... ■ 674
- Children's Advil Oral Suspension .... ■ 603
- Children's Advil Chewable Tablets .. ■ 603
- Advil Cold & Sinus .... ■ 723
- Infants' Advil Concentrated Drops .. ■ 604
- Infants' Advil Concentrated Drops - White Grape (Dye-Free)............. ■ 604
- Junior Strength Advil Swallow Tablets... ■ 605
- Advil Migraine Liquigels .... ■ 608
- Advil Multi-Symptom Cold Caplets.. ■ 770
- Advil PM Caplets .... ■ 615
- Motrin IB Tablets and Caplets 1866
- Children's Motrin Oral Suspension ... 1867
- Children's Motrin Non-Staining Dye-Free Oral Suspension............. 1867
- Children's Motrin Cold Oral Suspension 1867
- Infants' Motrin Concentrated Drops... 1867
- Infants' Motrin Non-Staining Dye-Free Concentrated Drops....... 1867
- Junior Strength Motrin Caplets and Chewable Tablets................... 1867
- Vicoprofen Tablets 539

Imipramine Hydrochloride (Fluoxetine inhibits the activity of P450 IID6 isoenzyme making normal metabolizers resemble poor metabolizers; therapy with drugs that are predominantly metabolized by the P450 IID6 isoenzyme, such as tricyclic antidepressants, and have a relatively narrow therapeutic index should be initiated at low end of the dose range if a patient is receiving fluoxetine concurrently or has taken it in the previous 5 weeks).
No products indexed under this heading.

Imipramine Pamoate (Fluoxetine inhibits the activity of P450 IID6 isoenzyme making normal metabolizers resemble poor metabolizers; therapy with drugs that are predominantly metabolized by the P450 IID6 isoenzyme, such as tricyclic antidepressants, and have a relatively narrow therapeutic index should be initiated at low end of the dose range if a patient is receiving fluoxetine concurrently or has taken it in the previous 5 weeks).
No products indexed under this heading.

Indomethacin (Concurrent use of fluoxetine with an NSAID potentiated the risk of upper gastrointestinal bleeding and there is a reason to believe that bleeding at other sites may be similarly potentiated. Combined use of psychotropic drugs that interfere with serotonin reuptake and NSAIDs have been associated with an increased risk of bleeding). Products include:

- Indocin 1995

Indomethacin Sodium Trihydrate (Concurrent use of fluoxetine with an NSAID potentiated the risk of upper gastrointestinal bleeding and there is a reason to believe that bleeding at other sites may be similarly potentiated. Combined use of psychotropic drugs that interfere with serotonin reuptake and NSAIDs have been associated with an increased risk of bleeding). Products include:

- Indocin I.V. 2465

Indoramin Hydrochloride (If fluoxetine is added to the treatment regimen of a patient already receiving a drug metabolized by CYP2D6, the need for decreased dose of the original medication should be considered. Fluoxetine is metabolized by this isoenzyme; thus, both the pharmacokinetic properties and relative proportion of metabolites are altered in poor metabolizers of CYP2D6).
No products indexed under this heading.

Insulin, Human, Zinc Suspension (Fluoxetine may alter glycemic control in diabetics; hypoglycemia has occurred during therapy with fluoxetine and hyperglycemia has developed following discontinuation of the drug; insulin dosage may need to be adjusted). Products include:

- Humulin L, 100 Units 1794
- Humulin U, 100 Units 1800

Insulin, Human NPH (Fluoxetine may alter glycemic control in diabetics; hypoglycemia has occurred during therapy with fluoxetine and hyperglycemia has developed following discontinuation of the drug; insulin dosage may need to be adjusted). Products include:

- Humulin N, 100 Units 1795
- Humulin N Pen 1797

Insulin, Human Regular (Fluoxetine may alter glycemic control in diabetics; hypoglycemia has occurred during therapy with fluoxetine and hyperglycemia has developed following discontinuation of the drug; insulin dosage may need to be adjusted). Products include:

- Humulin R, 100 Units 1798

Insulin, Human Regular and Human NPH Mixture (Fluoxetine may alter glycemic control in diabetics; hypoglycemia has occurred during therapy with fluoxetine and hyperglycemia has developed following discontinuation of the drug; insulin dosage may need to be adjusted). Products include:

- Humulin 50/50, 100 Units 1791
- Humulin 70/30 Pen 1793

Insulin, NPH (Fluoxetine may alter glycemic control in diabetics; hypoglycemia has occurred during therapy with fluoxetine and hyperglycemia has developed following discontinuation of the drug; insulin dosage may need to be adjusted).
No products indexed under this heading.

Insulin, Regular (Fluoxetine may alter glycemic control in diabetics; hypoglycemia has occurred during therapy with fluoxetine and hyperglycemia has developed following discontinuation of the drug; insulin dosage may need to be adjusted).
No products indexed under this heading.

Insulin, Zinc Crystals (Fluoxetine may alter glycemic control in diabetics; hypoglycemia has occurred during therapy with fluoxetine and hyperglycemia has developed following discontinuation of the drug; insulin dosage may need to be adjusted).
No products indexed under this heading.

Insulin, Zinc Suspension (Fluoxetine may alter glycemic control in diabetics; hypoglycemia has occurred during therapy with fluoxetine and hyperglycemia has developed following discontinuation of the drug; insulin dosage may need to be adjusted).
No products indexed under this heading.

Insulin Aspart, Human Regular (Fluoxetine may alter glycemic control in diabetics; hypoglycemia has occurred during therapy with fluoxetine and hyperglycemia has developed following discontinuation of the drug; insulin dosage may need to be adjusted). Products include:

- NovoLog Injection 2326

Insulin glargine (Fluoxetine may alter glycemic control in diabetics; hypoglycemia has occurred during therapy with fluoxetine and hyperglycemia has developed following discontinuation of the drug; insulin dosage may need to be adjusted). Products include:

- Lantus Injection 2909

Insulin Lispro, Human (Fluoxetine may alter glycemic control in diabetics; hypoglycemia has occurred during therapy with fluoxetine and hyperglycemia has developed following discontinuation of the drug; insulin dosage may need to be adjusted). Products include:

- Humalog-Pen 1781
- Humalog Mix 50/50-Pen 1783
- Humalog Mix 75/25-Pen 1785

Insulin Lispro Protamine, Human (Fluoxetine may alter glycemic control in diabetics; hypoglycemia has occurred during therapy with fluoxetine and hyperglycemia has developed following discontinuation of the drug; insulin dosage may need to be adjusted). Products include:

- Humalog Mix 50/50-Pen 1783
- Humalog Mix 75/25-Pen 1785

Isocarboxazid (Co-administration with MAO inhibitors has resulted in serious, sometimes fatal, reactions, including hyperthermia, rigidity, extreme agitation, delirium, coma, and features resembling neuroleptic malignant syndrome; concurrent and/or sequential use is contraindicated).
No products indexed under this heading.

Ketoprofen (Concurrent use of fluoxetine with an NSAID potentiated the risk of upper gastrointestinal bleeding and there is a reason to believe that bleeding at other sites may be similarly potentiated. Combined use of psychotropic drugs that interfere with serotonin reuptake and NSAIDs have been associated with an increased risk of bleeding).
No products indexed under this heading.

Ketorolac Tromethamine (Concurrent use of fluoxetine with an NSAID potentiated the risk of upper gastrointestinal bleeding and there is a reason to believe that bleeding at other sites may be similarly potentiated. Combined use of psychotropic drugs that interfere with serotonin reuptake and NSAIDs have been associated with an increased risk of bleeding). Products include:

- Acular Ophthalmic Solution 565
- Acular LS Ophthalmic Solution 566

Labetalol Hydrochloride (If fluoxetine is added to the treatment regimen of a patient already receiving a drug metabolized by CYP2D6, the need for decreased dose of the original medication should be considered. Fluoxetine is metabolized by this isoenzyme; thus, both the pharmacokinetic properties and relative proportion of metabolites are altered in poor metabolizers of CYP2D6).
No products indexed under this heading.

Lidocaine (If fluoxetine is added to the treatment regimen of a patient already receiving a drug metabolized by CYP2D6, the need for decreased dose of the original medication should be considered. Fluoxetine is metabolized by this isoenzyme; thus, both the pharmacokinetic properties and relative proportion of metabolites are altered in poor metabolizers of CYP2D6). Products include:

- Lidoderm Patch 1118
- Synera Topical Patch 1137

Lidocaine Hydrochloride (If fluoxetine is added to the treatment regimen of a patient already receiving a drug metabolized by CYP2D6, the need for decreased dose of the original medication should be considered. Fluoxetine is metabolized by this isoenzyme; thus, both the pharmacokinetic properties and relative proportion of metabolites are altered in poor metabolizers of CYP2D6).
No products indexed under this heading.

Lithium (Co-administration has resulted in reports of both increased and decreased lithium levels; cases of lithium toxicity have been reported).
No products indexed under this heading.

Lithium Carbonate (Co-administration has resulted in reports of both increased and decreased lithium levels; cases of lithium toxicity have been reported). Products include:

- Lithobid Tablets 1692

Lithium Citrate (Co-administration has resulted in reports of both increased and decreased lithium levels; cases of lithium toxicity have been reported).
No products indexed under this heading.

Low Molecular Weight Heparins (Concurrent use of fluoxetine with drugs that affect coagulation may potentiate the risk of bleeding).

No products indexed under this heading.

Maprotiline Hydrochloride (Fluoxetine inhibits the activity of P450 IID6 isoenzyme making normal metabolizers resemble poor metabolizers; therapy with drugs that are predominantly metabolized by the P450 IID6 isoenzyme, such as tricyclic antidepressants, and have a relatively narrow therapeutic index should be initiated at low end of the dose range if a patient is receiving fluoxetine concurrently or has taken it in the previous 5 weeks).

No products indexed under this heading.

Meclofenamate Sodium (Concurrent use of fluoxetine with an NSAID potentiated the risk of upper gastrointestinal bleeding and there is a reason to believe that bleeding at other sites may be similarly potentiated. Combined use of psychotropic drugs that interfere with serotonin reuptake and NSAIDs have been associated with an increased risk of bleeding).

No products indexed under this heading.

Mefenamic Acid (Concurrent use of fluoxetine with an NSAID potentiated the risk of upper gastrointestinal bleeding and there is a reason to believe that bleeding at other sites may be similarly potentiated. Combined use of psychotropic drugs that interfere with serotonin reuptake and NSAIDs have been associated with an increased risk of bleeding).

No products indexed under this heading.

Meloxicam (Concurrent use of fluoxetine with an NSAID potentiated the risk of upper gastrointestinal bleeding and there is a reason to believe that bleeding at other sites may be similarly potentiated. Combined use of psychotropic drugs that interfere with serotonin reuptake and NSAIDs have been associated with an increased risk of bleeding). Products include:

Mobic Oral Suspension **863**
Mobic Tablets **863**

Meperidine Hydrochloride (If fluoxetine is added to the treatment regimen of a patient already receiving a drug metabolized by CYP2D6, the need for decreased dose of the original medication should be considered. Fluoxetine is metabolized by this isoenzyme; thus, both the pharmacokinetic properties and relative proportion of metabolites are altered in poor metabolizers of CYP2D6).

No products indexed under this heading.

Metformin Hydrochloride (Fluoxetine may alter glycemic control in diabetics; hypoglycemia has occurred during therapy with fluoxetine and hyperglycemia has developed following discontinuation of the drug; hypoglycemia dosage may need to be adjusted). Products include:

ActoPlus Met Tablets **3214**
Avandamet Tablets **1373**
Fortamet Extended-Release Tablets.. **3115**

Methadone Hydrochloride (If fluoxetine is added to the treatment regimen of a patient already receiving a drug metabolized by CYP2D6, the need for decreased dose of the original medication should be considered. Fluoxetine is metabolized by this isoenzyme; thus, both the pharmacokinetic properties and relative proportion of metabolites are altered in poor metabolizers of CYP2D6).

No products indexed under this heading.

Methamphetamine Hydrochloride (If fluoxetine is added to the treatment regimen of a patient already receiving a drug metabolized by CYP2D6, the need for decreased dose of the original medication should be considered. Fluoxetine is metabolized by this isoenzyme; thus, both the pharmacokinetic properties and relative proportion of metabolites are altered in poor metabolizers of CYP2D6). Products include:

Desoxyn Tablets, USP **2462**

Metoprolol Succinate (If fluoxetine is added to the treatment regimen of a patient already receiving a drug metabolized by CYP2D6, the need for decreased dose of the original medication should be considered. Fluoxetine is metabolized by this isoenzyme; thus, both the pharmacokinetic properties and relative proportion of metabolites are altered in poor metabolizers of CYP2D6). Products include:

Toprol-XL Tablets **668**

Metoprolol Tartrate (If fluoxetine is added to the treatment regimen of a patient already receiving a drug metabolized by CYP2D6, the need for decreased dose of the original medication should be considered. Fluoxetine is metabolized by this isoenzyme; thus, both the pharmacokinetic properties and relative proportion of metabolites are altered in poor metabolizers of CYP2D6). Products include:

Lopressor Injection **2238**
Lopressor Tablets **2238**
Lopressor HCT 50/25 Tablets **2241**
Lopressor HCT 100/25 Tablets **2241**
Lopressor HCT 100/50 Tablets **2241**

Mexiletine Hydrochloride (If fluoxetine is added to the treatment regimen of a patient already receiving a drug metabolized by CYP2D6, the need for decreased dose of the original medication should be considered. Fluoxetine is metabolized by this isoenzyme; thus, both the pharmacokinetic properties and relative proportion of metabolites are altered in poor metabolizers of CYP2D6).

No products indexed under this heading.

Miglitol (Fluoxetine may alter glycemic control in diabetics; hypoglycemia has occurred during therapy with fluoxetine and hyperglycemia has developed following discontinuation of the drug; hypoglycemia dosage may need to be adjusted).

No products indexed under this heading.

Mirtazapine (If fluoxetine is added to the treatment regimen of a patient already receiving a drug metabolized by CYP2D6, the need for decreased dose of the original medication should be considered. Fluoxetine is metabolized by this isoenzyme; thus, both the pharmacokinetic properties and relative proportion of metabolites are altered in poor metabolizers of CYP2D6).

No products indexed under this heading.

Moclobemide (Co-administration with MAO inhibitors has resulted in serious, sometimes fatal, reactions, including hyperthermia, rigidity, extreme agitation, delirium, coma, and features resembling neuroleptic malignant syndrome; concurrent and/or sequential use is contraindicated).

No products indexed under this heading.

Morphine Sulfate (If fluoxetine is added to the treatment regimen of a patient already receiving a drug metabolized by CYP2D6, the need for decreased dose of the original medication should be considered. Fluoxetine is metabolized by this isoenzyme; thus, both the pharmacokinetic properties and relative proportion of metabolites are altered in poor metabolizers of CYP2D6). Products include:

Avinza Capsules **1741**
Kadian Capsules **577**
MS Contin Tablets **2701**

Nabumetone (Concurrent use of fluoxetine with an NSAID potentiated the risk of upper gastrointestinal bleeding and there is a reason to believe that bleeding at other sites may be similarly potentiated. Combined use of psychotropic drugs that interfere with serotonin reuptake and NSAIDs have been associated with an increased risk of bleeding).

No products indexed under this heading.

Naproxen (Concurrent use of fluoxetine with an NSAID potentiated the risk of upper gastrointestinal bleeding and there is a reason to believe that bleeding at other sites may be similarly potentiated. Combined use of psychotropic drugs that interfere with serotonin reuptake and NSAIDs have been associated with an increased risk of bleeding). Products include:

EC-Naprosyn Delayed-Release Tablets.. **2761**
Naprosyn Suspension **2761**
Naprosyn Tablets **2761**
Prevacid NapraPAC **3280**

Naproxen Sodium (Concurrent use of fluoxetine with an NSAID potentiated the risk of upper gastrointestinal bleeding and there is a reason to believe that bleeding at other sites may be similarly potentiated. Combined use of psychotropic drugs that interfere with serotonin reuptake and NSAIDs have been associated with an increased risk of bleeding). Products include:

Aleve Caplets **742**
Aleve Gelcaps **743**
Aleve Tablets **743**
Aleve Cold & Sinus Caplets **744**
Anaprox Tablets **2761**
Anaprox DS Tablets **2761**

Nelfinavir Mesylate (If fluoxetine is added to the treatment regimen of a patient already receiving a drug metabolized by CYP2D6, the need

for decreased dose of the original medication should be considered. Fluoxetine is metabolized by this isoenzyme; thus, both the pharmacokinetic properties and relative proportion of metabolites are altered in poor metabolizers of CYP2D6). Products include:

Viracept .. **2577**

Nortriptyline Hydrochloride (Fluoxetine inhibits the activity of P450 IID6 isoenzyme making normal metabolizers resemble poor metabolizers; therapy with drugs that are predominantly metabolized by the P450 IID6 isoenzyme, such as tricyclic antidepressants, and have a relatively narrow therapeutic index should be initiated at low end of the dose range if a patient is receiving fluoxetine concurrently or has taken it in the previous 5 weeks).

No products indexed under this heading.

Olanzapine (If fluoxetine is added to the treatment regimen of a patient already receiving a drug metabolized by CYP2D6, the need for decreased dose of the original medication should be considered. Fluoxetine is metabolized by this isoenzyme; thus, both the pharmacokinetic properties and relative proportion of metabolites are altered in poor metabolizers of CYP2D6). Products include:

Symbyax Capsules **1819**
Zyprexa Tablets **1830**
Zyprexa IntraMuscular **1830**
Zyprexa ZYDIS Orally Disintegrating Tablets.................. **1830**

Omeprazole (If fluoxetine is added to the treatment regimen of a patient already receiving a drug metabolized by CYP2D6, the need for decreased dose of the original medication should be considered. Fluoxetine is metabolized by this isoenzyme; thus, both the pharmacokinetic properties and relative proportion of metabolites are altered in poor metabolizers of CYP2D6). Products include:

Zegerid Capsules **2958**
Zegerid Powder for Oral Solution **2958**

Ondansetron (If fluoxetine is added to the treatment regimen of a patient already receiving a drug metabolized by CYP2D6, the need for decreased dose of the original medication should be considered. Fluoxetine is metabolized by this isoenzyme; thus, both the pharmacokinetic properties and relative proportion of metabolites are altered in poor metabolizers of CYP2D6). Products include:

Zofran ODT Orally Disintegrating Tablets.. **1639**

Ondansetron Hydrochloride (If fluoxetine is added to the treatment regimen of a patient already receiving a drug metabolized by CYP2D6, the need for decreased dose of the original medication should be considered. Fluoxetine is metabolized by this isoenzyme; thus, both the pharmacokinetic properties and relative proportion of metabolites are altered in poor metabolizers of CYP2D6). Products include:

Zofran Injection **1634**
Zofran ... **1639**

IMPORTANT NOTE: Always consult each drug listing in the patient's regimen for possible interactions.

Oxaprozin (Concurrent use of fluoxetine with an NSAID potentiated the risk of upper gastrointestinal bleeding and there is a reason to believe that bleeding at other sites may be similarly potentiated. Combined use of psychotropic drugs that interfere with serotonin reuptake and NSAIDs have been associated with an increased risk of bleeding).

No products indexed under this heading.

Oxycodone Hydrochloride (If fluoxetine is added to the treatment regimen of a patient already receiving a drug metabolized by CYP2D6, the need for decreased dose of the original medication should be considered. Fluoxetine is metabolized by this isoenzyme; thus, both the pharmacokinetic properties and relative proportion of metabolites are altered in poor metabolizers of CYP2D6). Products include:

Paclitaxel (If fluoxetine is added to the treatment regimen of a patient already receiving a drug metabolized by CYP2D6, the need for decreased dose of the original medication should be considered. Fluoxetine is metabolized by this isoenzyme; thus, both the pharmacokinetic properties and relative proportion of metabolites are altered in poor metabolizers of CYP2D6).

No products indexed under this heading.

Pargyline Hydrochloride (Co-administration with MAO inhibitors has resulted in serious, sometimes fatal, reactions, including hyperthermia, rigidity, extreme agitation, delirium, coma, and features resembling neuroleptic malignant syndrome; concurrent and/or sequential use is contraindicated).

No products indexed under this heading.

Paroxetine Hydrochloride (If fluoxetine is added to the treatment regimen of a patient already receiving a drug metabolized by CYP2D6, the need for decreased dose of the original medication should be considered. Fluoxetine is metabolized by this isoenzyme; thus, both the pharmacokinetic properties and relative proportion of metabolites are altered in poor metabolizers of CYP2D6). Products include:

Phenelzine Sulfate (Co-administration with MAO inhibitors has resulted in serious, sometimes fatal, reactions, including hyperthermia, rigidity, extreme agitation, delirium, coma, and features resembling neuroleptic malignant syndrome; concurrent and/or sequential use is contraindicated).

No products indexed under this heading.

Phenylbutazone (Concurrent use of fluoxetine with an NSAID potentiated the risk of upper gastrointestinal bleeding and there is a reason to believe that bleeding at other sites may be similarly potentiated. Combined use of psychotropic drugs that interfere with serotonin reuptake and NSAIDs have been associated with an increased risk of bleeding).

No products indexed under this heading.

Phenytoin (Patients stable on doses of phenytoin have developed elevated plasma phenytoin concentrations and clinical anticonvulsant toxicity following initiation of concomitant fluoxetine therapy).

No products indexed under this heading.

Phenytoin Sodium (Patients stable on doses of phenytoin have developed elevated plasma phenytoin concentrations and clinical anticonvulsant toxicity following initiation of concomitant fluoxetine therapy). Products include:

Pimozide (Co-administration has resulted in a single case report of possible additive effects of pimozide leading to bradycardia).

No products indexed under this heading.

Pindolol (If fluoxetine is added to the treatment regimen of a patient already receiving a drug metabolized by CYP2D6, the need for decreased dose of the original medication should be considered. Fluoxetine is metabolized by this isoenzyme; thus, both the pharmacokinetic properties and relative proportion of metabolites are altered in poor metabolizers of CYP2D6).

No products indexed under this heading.

Pioglitazone Hydrochloride (Fluoxetine may alter glycemic control in diabetics; hypoglycemia has occurred during therapy with fluoxetine and hyperglycemia has developed following discontinuation of the drug; hypoglycemia dosage may need to be adjusted). Products include:

Piroxicam (Concurrent use of fluoxetine with an NSAID potentiated the risk of upper gastrointestinal bleeding and there is a reason to believe that bleeding at other sites may be similarly potentiated. Combined use of psychotropic drugs that interfere with serotonin reuptake and NSAIDs have been associated with an increased risk of bleeding).

No products indexed under this heading.

Procarbazine Hydrochloride (Co-administration with MAO inhibitors has resulted in serious, sometimes fatal, reactions, including hyperthermia, rigidity, extreme agitation, delirium, coma, and features resembling neuroleptic malignant syndrome; concurrent and/or sequential use is contraindicated). Products include:

Propafenone Hydrochloride (If fluoxetine is added to the treatment regimen of a patient already receiving a drug metabolized by CYP2D6, the need for decreased dose of the original medication should be considered. Fluoxetine is metabolized by this isoenzyme; thus, both the pharmacokinetic properties and relative proportion of metabolites are altered in poor metabolizers of CYP2D6). Products include:

Propoxyphene Hydrochloride (If fluoxetine is added to the treatment regimen of a patient already receiving a drug metabolized by CYP2D6, the need for decreased dose of the original medication should be considered. Fluoxetine is metabolized by this isoenzyme; thus, both the pharmacokinetic properties and relative proportion of metabolites are altered in poor metabolizers of CYP2D6).

No products indexed under this heading.

Propoxyphene Napsylate (If fluoxetine is added to the treatment regimen of a patient already receiving a drug metabolized by CYP2D6, the need for decreased dose of the original medication should be considered. Fluoxetine is metabolized by this isoenzyme; thus, both the pharmacokinetic properties and relative proportion of metabolites are altered in poor metabolizers of CYP2D6).

No products indexed under this heading.

Propranolol Hydrochloride (If fluoxetine is added to the treatment regimen of a patient already receiving a drug metabolized by CYP2D6, the need for decreased dose of the original medication should be considered. Fluoxetine is metabolized by this isoenzyme; thus, both the pharmacokinetic properties and relative proportion of metabolites are altered in poor metabolizers of CYP2D6). Products include:

Protriptyline Hydrochloride (Fluoxetine inhibits the activity of P450 IID6 isoenzyme making normal metabolizers resemble poor metabolizers; therapy with drugs that are predominantly metabolized by the P450 IID6 isoenzyme, such as tricyclic antidepressants, and have a relatively narrow therapeutic index should be initiated at low end of the dose range if a patient is receiving fluoxetine concurrently or has taken it in the previous 5 weeks).

No products indexed under this heading.

Quetiapine Fumarate (If fluoxetine is added to the treatment regimen of a patient already receiving a drug metabolized by CYP2D6, the need for decreased dose of the original medication should be considered. Fluoxetine is metabolized by this isoenzyme; thus, both the pharmacokinetic properties and relative proportion of metabolites are altered in poor metabolizers of CYP2D6). Products include:

Quinidine Gluconate (If fluoxetine is added to the treatment regimen of a patient already receiving a drug metabolized by CYP2D6, the need for decreased dose of the original medication should be considered. Fluoxetine is metabolized by this isoenzyme; thus, both the pharmacokinetic properties and relative proportion of metabolites are altered in poor metabolizers of CYP2D6).

No products indexed under this heading.

Quinidine Hydrochloride (If fluoxetine is added to the treatment regimen of a patient already receiving a drug metabolized by CYP2D6, the need for decreased dose of the original medication should be considered. Fluoxetine is metabolized by this isoenzyme; thus, both the pharmacokinetic properties and relative proportion of metabolites are altered in poor metabolizers of CYP2D6).

No products indexed under this heading.

Quinidine Polygalacturonate (If fluoxetine is added to the treatment regimen of a patient already receiving a drug metabolized by CYP2D6, the need for decreased dose of the original medication should be considered. Fluoxetine is metabolized by this isoenzyme; thus, both the pharmacokinetic properties and relative proportion of metabolites are altered in poor metabolizers of CYP2D6).

No products indexed under this heading.

Quinidine Sulfate (If fluoxetine is added to the treatment regimen of a patient already receiving a drug metabolized by CYP2D6, the need for decreased dose of the original medication should be considered. Fluoxetine is metabolized by this isoenzyme; thus, both the pharmacokinetic properties and relative proportion of metabolites are altered in poor metabolizers of CYP2D6).

No products indexed under this heading.

Repaglinide (Fluoxetine may alter glycemic control in diabetics; hypoglycemia has occurred during therapy with fluoxetine and hyperglycemia has developed following discontinuation of the drug; hypoglycemia dosage may need to be adjusted).

No products indexed under this heading.

Risperidone (If fluoxetine is added to the treatment regimen of a patient already receiving a drug metabolized by CYP2D6, the need for decreased dose of the original medication should be considered. Fluoxetine is metabolized by this isoenzyme; thus, both the pharmacokinetic properties and relative proportion of metabolites are altered in poor metabolizers of CYP2D6). Products include:

Ritonavir (If fluoxetine is added to the treatment regimen of a patient already receiving a drug metabolized by CYP2D6, the need for decreased dose of the original medication should be considered. Fluoxetine is metabolized by this isoenzyme; thus, both the pharmacokinetic properties and relative proportion of metabolites are altered in poor metabolizers of CYP2D6). Products include:

Rofecoxib (Concurrent use of fluoxetine with an NSAID potentiated the risk of upper gastrointestinal bleeding and there is a reason to believe that bleeding at other sites may be similarly potentiated. Combined use of psychotropic drugs that interfere with serotonin reuptake and NSAIDs have been associated with an increased risk of bleeding).

No products indexed under this heading.

Rosiglitazone Maleate (Fluoxetine may alter glycemic control in diabetics; hypoglycemia has occurred during therapy with fluoxetine and hyperglycemia has developed following discontinuation of the drug; hypoglycemia dosage may need to be adjusted). Products include:

Avandamet Tablets 1373
Avandaryl Tablets 1379
Avandia Tablets 1384

Selegiline Hydrochloride (Co-administration with MAO inhibitors has resulted in serious, sometimes fatal, reactions, including hyperthermia, rigidity, extreme agitation, delirium, coma, and features resembling neuroleptic malignant syndrome; concurrent and/or sequential use is contraindicated). Products include:

Eldepryl Capsules 3208
Zelapar Tablets 3372

Sulindac (Concurrent use of fluoxetine with an NSAID potentiated the risk of upper gastrointestinal bleeding and there is a reason to believe that bleeding at other sites may be similarly potentiated. Combined use of psychotropic drugs that interfere with serotonin reuptake and NSAIDs have been associated with an increased risk of bleeding). Products include:

Clinoril Tablets 1924

Sumatriptan (Co-administration of SSRIs and sumatriptan has resulted in weakness, hyperreflexia, and incoordination). Products include:

Imitrex Nasal Spray 1467

Sumatriptan Succinate (Co-administration of SSRIs and sumatriptan has resulted in weakness, hyperreflexia, and incoordination). Products include:

Imitrex Injection 1463
Imitrex Tablets 1471

Tamoxifen Citrate (If fluoxetine is added to the treatment regimen of a patient already receiving a drug metabolized by CYP2D6, the need for decreased dose of the original medication should be considered. Fluoxetine is metabolized by this isoenzyme; thus, both the pharmacokinetic properties and relative proportion of metabolites are altered in poor metabolizers of CYP2D6). Products include:

Soltamox Oral Solution 3527

Teniposide (If fluoxetine is added to the treatment regimen of a patient already receiving a drug metabolized by CYP2D6, the need for decreased dose of the original medication should be considered. Fluoxetine is metabolized by this isoenzyme; thus, both the pharmacokinetic properties and relative proportion of metabolites are altered in poor metabolizers of CYP2D6).

No products indexed under this heading.

Testosterone (If fluoxetine is added to the treatment regimen of a patient already receiving a drug metabolized by CYP2D6, the need for decreased dose of the original medication should be considered. Fluoxetine is metabolized by this isoenzyme; thus, both the pharmacokinetic properties and relative proportion of metabolites are altered in poor metabolizers of CYP2D6). Products include:

AndroGel 3329
Striant Mucoadhesive 1007
Testim 1% Gel 695

Testosterone Cypionate (If fluoxetine is added to the treatment regimen of a patient already receiving a drug metabolized by CYP2D6, the need for decreased dose of the original medication should be considered. Fluoxetine is metabolized by this isoenzyme; thus, both the pharmacokinetic properties and relative proportion of metabolites are altered in poor metabolizers of CYP2D6).

No products indexed under this heading.

Testosterone Enanthate (If fluoxetine is added to the treatment regimen of a patient already receiving a drug metabolized by CYP2D6, the need for decreased dose of the original medication should be considered. Fluoxetine is metabolized by this isoenzyme; thus, both the pharmacokinetic properties and relative proportion of metabolites are altered in poor metabolizers of CYP2D6).

No products indexed under this heading.

Testosterone Propionate (If fluoxetine is added to the treatment regimen of a patient already receiving a drug metabolized by CYP2D6, the need for decreased dose of the original medication should be considered. Fluoxetine is metabolized by this isoenzyme; thus, both the pharmacokinetic properties and relative proportion of metabolites are altered in poor metabolizers of CYP2D6).

No products indexed under this heading.

Thioridazine (If fluoxetine is added to the treatment regimen of a patient already receiving a drug metabolized by CYP2D6, the need for decreased dose of the original medication should be considered. Fluoxetine is metabolized by this isoenzyme; thus, both the pharmacokinetic properties and relative proportion of metabolites are altered in poor metabolizers of CYP2D6).

No products indexed under this heading.

Thioridazine Hydrochloride (Co-administration of fluoxetine with thioridazine has produced a 2.4-fold higher Cmax and a 4.5-fold higher AUC for thioridazine; because thioridazine administration produces a dose-related prolongation of the QTc interval, which is associated with serious ventricular arrhythmias such as torsade de pointes-type arrhythmias and sudden death; concurrent and/or sequential use within a minimum of 5 weeks of Prozac is contraindicated). Products include:

Thioridazine Hydrochloride Tablets 2163

Timolol Maleate (If fluoxetine is added to the treatment regimen of a patient already receiving a drug metabolized by CYP2D6, the need for decreased dose of the original medication should be considered. Fluoxetine is metabolized by this isoenzyme; thus, both the pharmacokinetic properties and relative proportion of metabolites are altered in poor metabolizers of CYP2D6). Products include:

Blocadren Tablets 1916
Cosopt Sterile Ophthalmic Solution 1931
Timolide Tablets 2086
Timoptic Sterile Ophthalmic Solution 2088
Timoptic in Ocudose 2091
Timoptic-XE Sterile Ophthalmic Gel Forming Solution 2092

Tinzaparin Sodium (Concurrent use of fluoxetine with drugs that affect coagulation may potentiate the risk of bleeding).

No products indexed under this heading.

Tolazamide (Fluoxetine may alter glycemic control in diabetics; hypoglycemia has occurred during therapy with fluoxetine and hyperglycemia has developed following discontinuation of the drug; hypoglycemia dosage may need to be adjusted).

No products indexed under this heading.

Tolbutamide (Fluoxetine may alter glycemic control in diabetics; hypoglycemia has occurred during therapy with fluoxetine and hyperglycemia has developed following discontinuation of the drug; hypoglycemia dosage may need to be adjusted).

No products indexed under this heading.

Tolmetin Sodium (Concurrent use of fluoxetine with an NSAID potentiated the risk of upper gastrointestinal bleeding and there is a reason to believe that bleeding at other sites may be similarly potentiated. Combined use of psychotropic drugs that interfere with serotonin reuptake and NSAIDs have been associated with an increased risk of bleeding).

No products indexed under this heading.

Tolterodine Tartrate (If fluoxetine is added to the treatment regimen of a patient already receiving a drug metabolized by CYP2D6, the need for decreased dose of the original medication should be considered. Fluoxetine is metabolized by this isoenzyme; thus, both the pharmacokinetic properties and relative proportion of metabolites are altered in poor metabolizers of CYP2D6). Products include:

Detrol Tablets 2628
Detrol LA Capsules 2631

Tramadol Hydrochloride (If fluoxetine is added to the treatment regimen of a patient already receiving a drug metabolized by CYP2D6, the need for decreased dose of the original medication should be considered. Fluoxetine is metabolized by this isoenzyme; thus, both the pharmacokinetic properties and relative proportion of metabolites are altered in poor metabolizers of CYP2D6). Products include:

Ultram ER Tablets 2392

Tranylcypromine Sulfate (Co-administration with MAO inhibitors has resulted in serious, sometimes fatal, reactions, including hyperthermia, rigidity, extreme agitation, delirium, coma, and features resembling neuroleptic malignant syndrome; concurrent and/or sequential use is contraindicated). Products include:

Parnate Tablets 1527

Trazodone Hydrochloride (If fluoxetine is added to the treatment regimen of a patient already receiving a drug metabolized by CYP2D6, the need for decreased dose of the original medication should be considered. Fluoxetine is metabolized by this isoenzyme; thus, both the pharmacokinetic properties and relative proportion of metabolites are altered in poor metabolizers of CYP2D6).

No products indexed under this heading.

Triazolam (If fluoxetine is added to the treatment regimen of a patient already receiving a drug metabolized by CYP2D6, the need for decreased dose of the original medication should be considered. Fluoxetine is metabolized by this isoenzyme; thus, both the pharmacokinetic properties and relative proportion of metabolites are altered in poor metabolizers of CYP2D6).

No products indexed under this heading.

Trimipramine Maleate (Fluoxetine inhibits the activity of P450 IID6 isoenzyme making normal metabolizers resemble poor metabolizers; therapy with drugs that are predominantly metabolized by the P450 IID6 isoenzyme, such as tricyclic antidepressants, and have a relatively narrow therapeutic index should be initiated at low end of the dose range if a patient is receiving fluoxetine concurrently or has taken it in the previous 5 weeks).

No products indexed under this heading.

Troglitazone (Fluoxetine may alter glycemic control in diabetics; hypoglycemia has occurred during therapy with fluoxetine and hyperglycemia has developed following discontinuation of the drug; hypoglycemia dosage may need to be adjusted).

No products indexed under this heading.

L-Tryptophan (Co-administration has resulted in adverse reactions, including agitation, restlessness, and gastrointestinal distress). Products include:

L-Tryptophan Capsules 2145

Valdecoxib (Concurrent use of fluoxetine with an NSAID potentiated the risk of upper gastrointestinal bleeding and there is a reason to believe that bleeding at other sites may be similarly potentiated. Combined use of psychotropic drugs that interfere with serotonin reuptake and NSAIDs have been associated with an increased risk of bleeding).

No products indexed under this heading.

Venlafaxine Hydrochloride (If fluoxetine is added to the treatment regimen of a patient already receiving a drug metabolized by CYP2D6, the need for decreased dose of the original medication should be considered. Fluoxetine is metabolized by this isoenzyme; thus, both the pharmacokinetic properties and relative proportion of metabolites are altered in poor metabolizers of CYP2D6). Products include:

Effexor Tablets 3411
Effexor XR Capsules 3417

Vinblastine Sulfate (Fluoxetine inhibits the activity of P450 IID6 isoenzyme making normal metabolizers resemble poor metabolizers; therapy with drugs that are predominantly metabolized by the P450 IID6 isoenzyme such as vinblastine, and have a relatively narrow therapeutic index, should be initiated at low end of the dose range if a patient is receiving fluoxetine concurrently or has taken it in the previous 5 weeks).

No products indexed under this heading.

Warfarin Sodium (Altered anticoagulant effects, including increased bleeding, have been reported with concomitant use. Patients on warfarin therapy should receive coagula-

tion monitoring when fluoxetine is initiated or stopped). Products include:
Coumadin for Injection 898
Coumadin Tablets 898

Zonisamide (If fluoxetine is added to the treatment regimen of a patient already receiving a drug metabolized by CYP2D6, the need for decreased dose of the original medication should be considered. Fluoxetine is metabolized by this isoenzyme; thus, both the pharmacokinetic properties and relative proportion of metabolites are altered in poor metabolizers of CYP2D6). Products include:
Zonegran Capsules 1101

Food Interactions

Alcohol (Concurrent use with CNS active agents, such as alcohol, requires caution).

Food, unspecified (May delay absorption of fluoxetine inconsequentially; Prozac may be administered with or without food).

PSORIATEC CREAM

(Anthralin) 1089
None cited in PDR database.

PULMICORT RESPULES

(Budesonide) 661
May interact with cytochrome p450 3a4 inhibitors (selected) and certain other agents. Compounds in these categories include:

Acetazolamide (Concomitant administration of budesonide with known inhibitors of CYP3A4 may inhibit the metabolism of, and increase the systemic exposure to, budesonide; care should be exercised).
No products indexed under this heading.

Amiodarone Hydrochloride (Concomitant administration of budesonide with known inhibitors of CYP3A4 may inhibit the metabolism of, and increase the systemic exposure to, budesonide; care should be exercised).
No products indexed under this heading.

Amprenavir (Concomitant administration of budesonide with known inhibitors of CYP3A4 may inhibit the metabolism of, and increase the systemic exposure to, budesonide; care should be exercised). Products include:
Agenerase Capsules 1327
Agenerase Oral Solution 1332

Anastrozole (Concomitant administration of budesonide with known inhibitors of CYP3A4 may inhibit the metabolism of, and increase the systemic exposure to, budesonide; care should be exercised). Products include:
Arimidex Tablets 673

Aprepitant (Concomitant administration of budesonide with known inhibitors of CYP3A4 may inhibit the metabolism of, and increase the systemic exposure to, budesonide; care should be exercised). Products include:
Emend Capsules 1963

Cimetidine (Co-administration of budesonide with cimetidine caused a slight decrease in budesonide clearance and a corresponding increase in its oral bioavailability). Products include:
Tagamet HB 200 Tablets .... ▣664

Cimetidine Hydrochloride (Concomitant administration of budesonide with known inhibitors of CYP3A4 may inhibit the metabolism of, and increase the systemic exposure to, budesonide; care should be exercised).
No products indexed under this heading.

Ciprofloxacin (Concomitant administration of budesonide with known inhibitors of CYP3A4 may inhibit the metabolism of, and increase the systemic exposure to, budesonide; care should be exercised). Products include:
Cipro Oral Suspension 2977
Cipro I.V. 2984
Cipro XR Tablets 2990
Ciprodex Otic Suspension 559

Clarithromycin (Concomitant administration of budesonide with known inhibitors of CYP3A4 may inhibit the metabolism of, and increase the systemic exposure to, budesonide; care should be exercised). Products include:
Biaxin/Biaxin XL 402
PREVPAC 3284

Clotrimazole (Concomitant administration of budesonide with known inhibitors of CYP3A4 may inhibit the metabolism of, and increase the systemic exposure to, budesonide; care should be exercised). Products include:
Desenex Athlete's Foot Cream .... ▣635
Lotrimin 3039
Lotrisone 3040

Cyclosporine (Concomitant administration of budesonide with known inhibitors of CYP3A4 may inhibit the metabolism of, and increase the systemic exposure to, budesonide; care should be exercised). Products include:
Gengraf Capsules 459
Neoral Oral Solution 2259
Neoral Soft Gelatin Capsules 2259
Restasis Ophthalmic Emulsion 575
Sandimmune 2275

Dalfopristin (Concomitant administration of budesonide with known inhibitors of CYP3A4 may inhibit the metabolism of, and increase the systemic exposure to, budesonide; care should be exercised).
No products indexed under this heading.

Danazol (Concomitant administration of budesonide with known inhibitors of CYP3A4 may inhibit the metabolism of, and increase the systemic exposure to, budesonide; care should be exercised).
No products indexed under this heading.

Delavirdine Mesylate (Concomitant administration of budesonide with known inhibitors of CYP3A4 may inhibit the metabolism of, and increase the systemic exposure to, budesonide; care should be exercised). Products include:
Rescriptor Tablets 2551

Diltiazem Hydrochloride (Concomitant administration of budesonide with known inhibitors of CYP3A4 may inhibit the metabolism of, and increase the systemic exposure to, budesonide; care should be exercised). Products include:
Cardizem LA Extended Release Tablets 1728
Tiazac Capsules 1201

Diltiazem Maleate (Concomitant administration of budesonide with known inhibitors of CYP3A4 may inhibit the metabolism of, and increase the systemic exposure to, budesonide; care should be exercised).
No products indexed under this heading.

Efavirenz (Concomitant administration of budesonide with known inhibitors of CYP3A4 may inhibit the metabolism of, and increase the systemic exposure to, budesonide; care should be exercised). Products include:
Atripla Tablets 945
Sustiva Capsules 930
Sustiva Tablets 930

Erythromycin (Concomitant administration of budesonide with known inhibitors of CYP3A4 may inhibit the metabolism of, and increase the systemic exposure to, budesonide; care should be exercised). Products include:
Ery-Tab Tablets 449
Erythromycin Base Filmtab Tablets 455
Erythromycin Delayed-Release Capsules, USP 457
PCE Dispertab Tablets 515

Erythromycin Estolate (Concomitant administration of budesonide with known inhibitors of CYP3A4 may inhibit the metabolism of, and increase the systemic exposure to, budesonide; care should be exercised).
No products indexed under this heading.

Erythromycin Ethylsuccinate (Concomitant administration of budesonide with known inhibitors of CYP3A4 may inhibit the metabolism of, and increase the systemic exposure to, budesonide; care should be exercised). Products include:
E.E.S. 451
EryPed 447

Erythromycin Gluceptate (Concomitant administration of budesonide with known inhibitors of CYP3A4 may inhibit the metabolism of, and increase the systemic exposure to, budesonide; care should be exercised).
No products indexed under this heading.

Erythromycin Lactobionate (Concomitant administration of budesonide with known inhibitors of CYP3A4 may inhibit the metabolism of, and increase the systemic exposure to, budesonide; care should be exercised).
No products indexed under this heading.

Erythromycin Stearate (Concomitant administration of budesonide with known inhibitors of CYP3A4 may inhibit the metabolism of, and increase the systemic exposure to, budesonide; care should be exercised). Products include:
Erythrocin Stearate Filmtab Tablets 453

Esomeprazole Magnesium (Concomitant administration of budesonide with known inhibitors of CYP3A4 may inhibit the metabolism of, and increase the systemic exposure to, budesonide; care should be exercised). Products include:
Nexium Delayed-Release Capsules 655

Fluconazole (Concomitant administration of budesonide with known inhibitors of CYP3A4 may inhibit the metabolism of, and increase the systemic exposure to, budesonide; care should be exercised).
No products indexed under this heading.

Fluoxetine Hydrochloride (Concomitant administration of budesonide with known inhibitors of CYP3A4 may inhibit the metabolism of, and increase the systemic exposure to, budesonide; care should be exercised). Products include:
Prozac Pulvules and Liquid 1801
Symbyax Capsules 1819

Fluvoxamine Maleate (Concomitant administration of budesonide with known inhibitors of CYP3A4 may inhibit the metabolism of, and increase the systemic exposure to, budesonide; care should be exercised).
No products indexed under this heading.

Fosamprenavir Calcium (Concomitant administration of budesonide with known inhibitors of CYP3A4 may inhibit the metabolism of, and increase the systemic exposure to, budesonide; care should be exercised). Products include:
Lexiva Tablets 1505

Indinavir Sulfate (Concomitant administration of budesonide with known inhibitors of CYP3A4 may inhibit the metabolism of, and increase the systemic exposure to, budesonide; care should be exercised). Products include:
Crixivan Capsules 1940

Isoniazid (Concomitant administration of budesonide with known inhibitors of CYP3A4 may inhibit the metabolism of, and increase the systemic exposure to, budesonide; care should be exercised).
No products indexed under this heading.

Itraconazole (Concomitant administration of budesonide with known inhibitors of CYP3A4 may inhibit the metabolism of, and increase the systemic exposure to, budesonide; care should be exercised).
No products indexed under this heading.

Ketoconazole (Concomitant administration of budesonide with known inhibitors of CYP3A4 may inhibit the metabolism of, and increase the systemic exposure to, budesonide; care should be exercised). Products include:
Nizoral A-D Shampoo, 1% 1868

Lopinavir (Concomitant administration of budesonide with known inhibitors of CYP3A4 may inhibit the metabolism of, and increase the systemic exposure to, budesonide; care should be exercised). Products include:
Kaletra 476

Loratadine (Concomitant administration of budesonide with known inhibitors of CYP3A4 may inhibit the metabolism of, and increase the systemic exposure to, budesonide; care should be exercised). Products include:
Alavert Allergy & Sinus D-12 Hour Tablets .... ▣771
Alavert .... ▣771
Children's Claritin Allergy Oral Solution .... ▣771

Claritin Non-Drowsy 24 Hour Tablets 772
Claritin Reditabs 24 Hour Non-Drowsy Tablets 772
Claritin-D Non-Drowsy 12 Hour Tablets 772
Claritin-D Non-Drowsy 24 Hour Tablets 772

Metronidazole (Concomitant administration of budesonide with known inhibitors of CYP3A4 may inhibit the metabolism of, and increase the systemic exposure to, budesonide; care should be exercised). Products include:
Metrogel 1% 1211
MetroGel-Vaginal Gel 1855
Vandazole Vaginal Gel 3338

Metronidazole Benzoate (Concomitant administration of budesonide with known inhibitors of CYP3A4 may inhibit the metabolism of, and increase the systemic exposure to, budesonide; care should be exercised).
No products indexed under this heading.

Metronidazole Hydrochloride (Concomitant administration of budesonide with known inhibitors of CYP3A4 may inhibit the metabolism of, and increase the systemic exposure to, budesonide; care should be exercised).
No products indexed under this heading.

Miconazole (Concomitant administration of budesonide with known inhibitors of CYP3A4 may inhibit the metabolism of, and increase the systemic exposure to, budesonide; care should be exercised).
No products indexed under this heading.

Miconazole Nitrate (Concomitant administration of budesonide with known inhibitors of CYP3A4 may inhibit the metabolism of, and increase the systemic exposure to, budesonide; care should be exercised). Products include:
Desenex 635
Desenex Jock Itch Spray Powder 635

Nefazodone Hydrochloride (Concomitant administration of budesonide with known inhibitors of CYP3A4 may inhibit the metabolism of, and increase the systemic exposure to, budesonide; care should be exercised).
No products indexed under this heading.

Nelfinavir Mesylate (Concomitant administration of budesonide with known inhibitors of CYP3A4 may inhibit the metabolism of, and increase the systemic exposure to, budesonide; care should be exercised). Products include:
Viracept 2577

Nevirapine (Concomitant administration of budesonide with known inhibitors of CYP3A4 may inhibit the metabolism of, and increase the systemic exposure to, budesonide; care should be exercised). Products include:
Viramune Oral Suspension 873
Viramune Tablets 873

Niacinamide (Concomitant administration of budesonide with known inhibitors of CYP3A4 may inhibit the metabolism of, and increase the systemic exposure to, budesonide; care should be exercised).
No products indexed under this heading.

Nicotinamide (Concomitant administration of budesonide with known inhibitors of CYP3A4 may inhibit the metabolism of, and increase the systemic exposure to, budesonide; care should be exercised). Products include:
Nicomide Tablets 1088

Nifedipine (Concomitant administration of budesonide with known inhibitors of CYP3A4 may inhibit the metabolism of, and increase the systemic exposure to, budesonide; care should be exercised). Products include:
Adalat CC Tablets 2964

Norfloxacin (Concomitant administration of budesonide with known inhibitors of CYP3A4 may inhibit the metabolism of, and increase the systemic exposure to, budesonide; care should be exercised). Products include:
Noroxin Tablets 2032

Omeprazole (Concomitant administration of budesonide with known inhibitors of CYP3A4 may inhibit the metabolism of, and increase the systemic exposure to, budesonide; care should be exercised). Products include:
Zegerid Capsules 2958
Zegerid Powder for Oral Solution 2958

Paroxetine Hydrochloride (Concomitant administration of budesonide with known inhibitors of CYP3A4 may inhibit the metabolism of, and increase the systemic exposure to, budesonide; care should be exercised). Products include:
Paxil CR Controlled-Release Tablets 1538
Paxil 1530

Propoxyphene Hydrochloride (Concomitant administration of budesonide with known inhibitors of CYP3A4 may inhibit the metabolism of, and increase the systemic exposure to, budesonide; care should be exercised).
No products indexed under this heading.

Propoxyphene Napsylate (Concomitant administration of budesonide with known inhibitors of CYP3A4 may inhibit the metabolism of, and increase the systemic exposure to, budesonide; care should be exercised).
No products indexed under this heading.

Quinidine (Concomitant administration of budesonide with known inhibitors of CYP3A4 may inhibit the metabolism of, and increase the systemic exposure to, budesonide; care should be exercised).
No products indexed under this heading.

Quinidine Hydrochloride (Concomitant administration of budesonide with known inhibitors of CYP3A4 may inhibit the metabolism of, and increase the systemic exposure to, budesonide; care should be exercised).
No products indexed under this heading.

Quinidine Polygalacturonate (Concomitant administration of budesonide with known inhibitors of CYP3A4 may inhibit the metabolism of, and increase the systemic exposure to, budesonide; care should be exercised).
No products indexed under this heading.

Quinidine Sulfate (Concomitant administration of budesonide with known inhibitors of CYP3A4 may inhibit the metabolism of, and increase the systemic exposure to, budesonide; care should be exercised).
No products indexed under this heading.

Quinine (Concomitant administration of budesonide with known inhibitors of CYP3A4 may inhibit the metabolism of, and increase the systemic exposure to, budesonide; care should be exercised).
No products indexed under this heading.

Quinine Sulfate (Concomitant administration of budesonide with known inhibitors of CYP3A4 may inhibit the metabolism of, and increase the systemic exposure to, budesonide; care should be exercised).
No products indexed under this heading.

Quinupristin (Concomitant administration of budesonide with known inhibitors of CYP3A4 may inhibit the metabolism of, and increase the systemic exposure to, budesonide; care should be exercised).
No products indexed under this heading.

Ranitidine Bismuth Citrate (Concomitant administration of budesonide with known inhibitors of CYP3A4 may inhibit the metabolism of, and increase the systemic exposure to, budesonide; care should be exercised).
No products indexed under this heading.

Ranitidine Hydrochloride (Concomitant administration of budesonide with known inhibitors of CYP3A4 may inhibit the metabolism of, and increase the systemic exposure to, budesonide; care should be exercised). Products include:
Zantac 1624
Zantac Injection 1619
Zantac Injection Pharmacy Bulk Package 1622

Ritonavir (Concomitant administration of budesonide with known inhibitors of CYP3A4 may inhibit the metabolism of, and increase the systemic exposure to, budesonide; care should be exercised). Products include:
Kaletra 476
Norvir 503

Saquinavir (Concomitant administration of budesonide with known inhibitors of CYP3A4 may inhibit the metabolism of, and increase the systemic exposure to, budesonide; care should be exercised).
No products indexed under this heading.

Saquinavir Mesylate (Concomitant administration of budesonide with known inhibitors of CYP3A4 may inhibit the metabolism of, and increase the systemic exposure to, budesonide; care should be exercised). Products include:
Invirase 2772

Sertraline Hydrochloride (Concomitant administration of budesonide with known inhibitors of CYP3A4 may inhibit the metabolism of, and increase the systemic exposure to, budesonide; care should be exercised). Products include:
Zoloft 2586

Telithromycin (Concomitant administration of budesonide with known inhibitors of CYP3A4 may inhibit the metabolism of, and increase the systemic exposure to, budesonide; care should be exercised). Products include:
Ketek Tablets 2903

Troglitazone (Concomitant administration of budesonide with known inhibitors of CYP3A4 may inhibit the metabolism of, and increase the systemic exposure to, budesonide; care should be exercised).
No products indexed under this heading.

Troleandomycin (Concomitant administration of budesonide with known inhibitors of CYP3A4 may inhibit the metabolism of, and increase the systemic exposure to, budesonide; care should be exercised).
No products indexed under this heading.

Valproate Sodium (Concomitant administration of budesonide with known inhibitors of CYP3A4 may inhibit the metabolism of, and increase the systemic exposure to, budesonide; care should be exercised). Products include:
Depacon Injection 412

Verapamil Hydrochloride (Concomitant administration of budesonide with known inhibitors of CYP3A4 may inhibit the metabolism of, and increase the systemic exposure to, budesonide; care should be exercised). Products include:
Covera-HS Tablets 3139
Tarka Tablets 524
Verelan PM Extended-Release Capsules, Controlled-Onset 3106

Voriconazole (Concomitant administration of budesonide with known inhibitors of CYP3A4 may inhibit the metabolism of, and increase the systemic exposure to, budesonide; care should be exercised). Products include:
VFEND I.V. 2564
VFEND Oral Suspension 2564
VFEND Tablets 2564

Zafirlukast (Concomitant administration of budesonide with known inhibitors of CYP3A4 may inhibit the metabolism of, and increase the systemic exposure to, budesonide; care should be exercised). Products include:
Accolate Tablets 671

Zileuton (Concomitant administration of budesonide with known inhibitors of CYP3A4 may inhibit the metabolism of, and increase the systemic exposure to, budesonide; care should be exercised). Products include:
Zyflo Tablets 1023

Food Interactions

Grapefruit (Concomitant administration of budesonide with known inhibitors of CYP3A4 may inhibit the metabolism of, and increase the systemic exposure to, budesonide; care should be exercised).

Grapefruit Juice (Concomitant administration of budesonide with known inhibitors of CYP3A4 may inhibit the metabolism of, and increase the systemic exposure to, budesonide; care should be exercised).

PULMOZYME INHALATION SOLUTION

(Dornase Alfa) 1248
None cited in PDR database.

PURE GARDENS CREAM
(Herbals with Vitamins) .... ▣832
None cited in PDR database.

PURETRIM MEDITERRANEAN WELLNESS SHAKE
(Antioxidants, Fatty Acids, Rice Protein) .... ▣818
None cited in PDR database.

QUADRAMET INJECTION
(Samarium Lexidronam Pentasodium) 1040
May interact with antineoplastics and certain other agents. Compounds in these categories include:

Altretamine (The potential for additive bone marrow toxicity of Samarium lexidronam pentasodium with chemotherapy or external beam radiation has not been studied. Samarium lexidronam pentasodium should not be given concurrently with chemotherapy or external beam radiation therapy unless the benefit outweighs the risks. Samarium lexidronam pentasodium should not be given after either of these treatments until there has been time for adequate marrow recovery).
No products indexed under this heading.

Anastrozole (The potential for additive bone marrow toxicity of Samarium lexidronam pentasodium with chemotherapy or external beam radiation has not been studied. Samarium lexidronam pentasodium should not be given concurrently with chemotherapy or external beam radiation therapy unless the benefit outweighs the risks. Samarium lexidronam pentasodium should not be given after either of these treatments until there has been time for adequate marrow recovery).
Products include:
Arimidex Tablets 673

Asparaginase (The potential for additive bone marrow toxicity of Samarium lexidronam pentasodium with chemotherapy or external beam radiation has not been studied. Samarium lexidronam pentasodium should not be given concurrently with chemotherapy or external beam radiation therapy unless the benefit outweighs the risks. Samarium lexidronam pentasodium should not be given after either of these treatments until there has been time for adequate marrow recovery).
Products include:
Elspar for Injection 2463
Elspar for Injection 1960

Bicalutamide (The potential for additive bone marrow toxicity of Samarium lexidronam pentasodium with chemotherapy or external beam radiation has not been studied. Samarium lexidronam pentasodium should not be given concurrently with chemotherapy or external beam radiation therapy unless the benefit outweighs the risks. Samarium lexidronam pentasodium should not be given after either of these treatments until there has been time for adequate marrow recovery).
No products indexed under this heading.

Bleomycin Sulfate (The potential for additive bone marrow toxicity of Samarium lexidronam pentasodium with chemotherapy or external beam radiation has not been studied. Samarium lexidronam pentasodium should not be given concurrently with chemotherapy or external beam radiation therapy unless the benefit outweighs the risks. Samarium lexidronam pentasodium should not be given after either of these treatments until there has been time for adequate marrow recovery).
No products indexed under this heading.

Busulfan (The potential for additive bone marrow toxicity of Samarium lexidronam pentasodium with chemotherapy or external beam radiation has not been studied. Samarium lexidronam pentasodium should not be given concurrently with chemotherapy or external beam radiation therapy unless the benefit outweighs the risks. Samarium lexidronam pentasodium should not be given after either of these treatments until there has been time for adequate marrow recovery). Products include:
I.V. Busulfex 2493
Myleran Tablets 1525

Carboplatin (The potential for additive bone marrow toxicity of Samarium lexidronam pentasodium with chemotherapy or external beam radiation has not been studied. Samarium lexidronam pentasodium should not be given concurrently with chemotherapy or external beam radiation therapy unless the benefit outweighs the risks. Samarium lexidronam pentasodium should not be given after either of these treatments until there has been time for adequate marrow recovery).
No products indexed under this heading.

Carmustine (BCNU) (The potential for additive bone marrow toxicity of Samarium lexidronam pentasodium with chemotherapy or external beam radiation has not been studied. Samarium lexidronam pentasodium should not be given concurrently with chemotherapy or external beam radiation therapy unless the benefit outweighs the risks. Samarium lexidronam pentasodium should not be given after either of these treatments until there has been time for adequate marrow recovery).
No products indexed under this heading.

Chlorambucil (The potential for additive bone marrow toxicity of Samarium lexidronam pentasodium with chemotherapy or external beam radiation has not been studied. Samarium lexidronam pentasodium should not be given concurrently with chemotherapy or external beam radiation therapy unless the benefit outweighs the risks. Samarium lexidronam pentasodium should not be given after either of these treatments until there has been time for adequate marrow recovery).
Products include:
Leukeran Tablets 1504

Cisplatin (The potential for additive bone marrow toxicity of Samarium lexidronam pentasodium with chemotherapy or external beam radiation has not been studied. Samarium lexidronam pentasodium should not be given concurrently with chemotherapy or external beam radiation therapy unless the benefit outweighs the risks. Samarium lexidronam pentasodium should not be given after either of these treatments until there has been time for adequate marrow recovery).
No products indexed under this heading.

Cyclophosphamide (The potential for additive bone marrow toxicity of Samarium lexidronam pentasodium with chemotherapy or external beam radiation has not been studied. Samarium lexidronam pentasodium should not be given concurrently with chemotherapy or external beam radiation therapy unless the benefit outweighs the risks. Samarium lexidronam pentasodium should not be given after either of these treatments until there has been time for adequate marrow recovery).
No products indexed under this heading.

Dacarbazine (The potential for additive bone marrow toxicity of Samarium lexidronam pentasodium with chemotherapy or external beam radiation has not been studied. Samarium lexidronam pentasodium should not be given concurrently with chemotherapy or external beam radiation therapy unless the benefit outweighs the risks. Samarium lexidronam pentasodium should not be given after either of these treatments until there has been time for adequate marrow recovery).
No products indexed under this heading.

Daunorubicin Citrate (The potential for additive bone marrow toxicity of Samarium lexidronam pentasodium with chemotherapy or external beam radiation has not been studied. Samarium lexidronam pentasodium should not be given concurrently with chemotherapy or external beam radiation therapy unless the benefit outweighs the risks. Samarium lexidronam pentasodium should not be given after either of these treatments until there has been time for adequate marrow recovery).
No products indexed under this heading.

Daunorubicin Hydrochloride (The potential for additive bone marrow toxicity of Samarium lexidronam pentasodium with chemotherapy or external beam radiation has not been studied. Samarium lexidronam pentasodium should not be given concurrently with chemotherapy or external beam radiation therapy unless the benefit outweighs the risks. Samarium lexidronam pentasodium should not be given after either of these treatments until there has been time for adequate marrow recovery).
No products indexed under this heading.

Denileukin Diftitox (The potential for additive bone marrow toxicity of Samarium lexidronam pentasodium with chemotherapy or external beam radiation has not been studied. Samarium lexidronam pentasodium should not be given concurrently with chemotherapy or external beam radiation therapy unless the benefit outweighs the risks. Samarium lexidronam pentasodium should not be given after either of these treatments until there has been time for adequate marrow recovery).
Products include:
Ontak Vials 1745

Docetaxel (The potential for additive bone marrow toxicity of Samarium lexidronam pentasodium with chemotherapy or external beam radiation has not been studied. Samarium lexidronam pentasodium should not be given concurrently with chemotherapy or external beam radiation therapy unless the benefit outweighs the risks. Samarium lexidronam pentasodium should not be given after either of these treatments until there has been time for adequate marrow recovery).
Products include:
Taxotere Injection Concentrate 2932

Doxorubicin Hydrochloride (The potential for additive bone marrow toxicity of Samarium lexidronam pentasodium with chemotherapy or external beam radiation has not been studied. Samarium lexidronam pentasodium should not be given concurrently with chemotherapy or external beam radiation therapy unless the benefit outweighs the risks. Samarium lexidronam pentasodium should not be given after either of these treatments until there has been time for adequate marrow recovery).
No products indexed under this heading.

Epirubicin Hydrochloride (The potential for additive bone marrow toxicity of Samarium lexidronam pentasodium with chemotherapy or external beam radiation has not been studied. Samarium lexidronam pentasodium should not be given concurrently with chemotherapy or external beam radiation therapy unless the benefit outweighs the risks. Samarium lexidronam pentasodium should not be given after either of these treatments until there has been time for adequate marrow recovery).
No products indexed under this heading.

Estramustine Phosphate Sodium (The potential for additive bone marrow toxicity of Samarium lexidronam pentasodium with chemotherapy or external beam radiation has not been studied. Samarium lexidronam pentasodium should not be given concurrently with chemotherapy or external beam radiation therapy unless the benefit outweighs the risks. Samarium lexidronam pentasodium should not be given after either of these treatments until there has been time for adequate marrow recovery). Products include:
Emcyt Capsules 2634

Etoposide (The potential for additive bone marrow toxicity of Samarium lexidronam pentasodium with chemotherapy or external beam radiation has not been studied. Samarium lexidronam pentasodium should not be given concurrently with chemotherapy or external beam radiation therapy unless the benefit outweighs the risks. Samarium lexidronam pentasodium should not be given after either of these treatments until there has been time for adequate marrow recovery).
No products indexed under this heading.

Exemestane (The potential for additive bone marrow toxicity of Samarium lexidronam pentasodium with chemotherapy or external beam radiation has not been studied. Samarium lexidronam pentasodium should not be given concurrently with chemotherapy or external beam radiation therapy unless the benefit outweighs the risks. Samarium lexidronam pentasodium should not be given after either of these treatments until there has been time for adequate marrow recovery). Products include:

Aromasin Tablets 2600

Floxuridine (The potential for additive bone marrow toxicity of Samarium lexidronam pentasodium with chemotherapy or external beam radiation has not been studied. Samarium lexidronam pentasodium should not be given concurrently with chemotherapy or external beam radiation therapy unless the benefit outweighs the risks. Samarium lexidronam pentasodium should not be given after either of these treatments until there has been time for adequate marrow recovery).

No products indexed under this heading.

Fluorouracil (The potential for additive bone marrow toxicity of Samarium lexidronam pentasodium with chemotherapy or external beam radiation has not been studied. Samarium lexidronam pentasodium should not be given concurrently with chemotherapy or external beam radiation therapy unless the benefit outweighs the risks. Samarium lexidronam pentasodium should not be given after either of these treatments until there has been time for adequate marrow recovery). Products include:

Carac Cream, 0.5% 2879
Efudex 3363

Flutamide (The potential for additive bone marrow toxicity of Samarium lexidronam pentasodium with chemotherapy or external beam radiation has not been studied. Samarium lexidronam pentasodium should not be given concurrently with chemotherapy or external beam radiation therapy unless the benefit outweighs the risks. Samarium lexidronam pentasodium should not be given after either of these treatments until there has been time for adequate marrow recovery). Products include:

Eulexin Capsules 3009

Gemcitabine Hydrochloride (The potential for additive bone marrow toxicity of Samarium lexidronam pentasodium with chemotherapy or external beam radiation has not been studied. Samarium lexidronam pentasodium should not be given concurrently with chemotherapy or external beam radiation therapy unless the benefit outweighs the risks. Samarium lexidronam pentasodium should not be given after either of these treatments until there has been time for adequate marrow recovery). Products include:

Gemzar for Injection 1771

Hydroxyurea (The potential for additive bone marrow toxicity of Samarium lexidronam pentasodium with chemotherapy or external beam radiation has not been studied. Samarium lexidronam pentasodium should not be given concurrently with chemotherapy or external beam radiation therapy unless the benefit outweighs the risks. Samarium lexidronam pentasodium should not be given after either of these treatments until there has been time for adequate marrow recovery).

No products indexed under this heading.

Idarubicin Hydrochloride (The potential for additive bone marrow toxicity of Samarium lexidronam pentasodium with chemotherapy or external beam radiation has not been studied. Samarium lexidronam pentasodium should not be given concurrently with chemotherapy or external beam radiation therapy unless the benefit outweighs the risks. Samarium lexidronam pentasodium should not be given after either of these treatments until there has been time for adequate marrow recovery).

No products indexed under this heading.

Ifosfamide (The potential for additive bone marrow toxicity of Samarium lexidronam pentasodium with chemotherapy or external beam radiation has not been studied. Samarium lexidronam pentasodium should not be given concurrently with chemotherapy or external beam radiation therapy unless the benefit outweighs the risks. Samarium lexidronam pentasodium should not be given after either of these treatments until there has been time for adequate marrow recovery).

No products indexed under this heading.

Interferon alfa-2a, Recombinant (The potential for additive bone marrow toxicity of Samarium lexidronam pentasodium with chemotherapy or external beam radiation has not been studied. Samarium lexidronam pentasodium should not be given concurrently with chemotherapy or external beam radiation therapy unless the benefit outweighs the risks. Samarium lexidronam pentasodium should not be given after either of these treatments until there has been time for adequate marrow recovery).

No products indexed under this heading.

Interferon alfa-2b, Recombinant (The potential for additive bone marrow toxicity of Samarium lexidronam pentasodium with chemotherapy or external beam radiation has not been studied. Samarium lexidronam pentasodium should not be given concurrently with chemotherapy or external beam radiation therapy unless the benefit outweighs the risks. Samarium lexidronam pentasodium should not be given after either of these treatments until there has been time for adequate marrow recovery). Products include:

Intron A for Injection 3024
Rebetron Combination Therapy 3063

Irinotecan Hydrochloride (The potential for additive bone marrow toxicity of Samarium lexidronam pentasodium with chemotherapy or external beam radiation has not been studied. Samarium lexidronam pentasodium should not be given concurrently with chemotherapy or external beam radiation therapy unless the benefit outweighs the risks. Samarium lexidronam pentasodium should not be given after either of these treatments until there has been time for adequate marrow recovery). Products include:

Camptosar Injection 2604

Levamisole Hydrochloride (The potential for additive bone marrow toxicity of Samarium lexidronam pentasodium with chemotherapy or external beam radiation has not been studied. Samarium lexidronam pentasodium should not be given concurrently with chemotherapy or external beam radiation therapy unless the benefit outweighs the risks. Samarium lexidronam pentasodium should not be given after either of these treatments until there has been time for adequate marrow recovery).

No products indexed under this heading.

Lomustine (CCNU) (The potential for additive bone marrow toxicity of Samarium lexidronam pentasodium with chemotherapy or external beam radiation has not been studied. Samarium lexidronam pentasodium should not be given concurrently with chemotherapy or external beam radiation therapy unless the benefit outweighs the risks. Samarium lexidronam pentasodium should not be given after either of these treatments until there has been time for adequate marrow recovery).

No products indexed under this heading.

Mechlorethamine Hydrochloride (The potential for additive bone marrow toxicity of Samarium lexidronam pentasodium with chemotherapy or external beam radiation has not been studied. Samarium lexidronam pentasodium should not be given concurrently with chemotherapy or external beam radiation therapy unless the benefit outweighs the risks. Samarium lexidronam pentasodium should not be given after either of these treatments until there has been time for adequate marrow recovery). Products include:

Mustargen for Injection 2468

Megestrol Acetate (The potential for additive bone marrow toxicity of Samarium lexidronam pentasodium with chemotherapy or external beam radiation has not been studied. Samarium lexidronam pentasodium should not be given concurrently with chemotherapy or external beam radiation therapy unless the benefit outweighs the risks. Samarium lexidronam pentasodium should not be given after either of these treatments until there has been time for adequate marrow recovery). Products include:

Megace ES Oral Suspension 2481

Melphalan (The potential for additive bone marrow toxicity of Samarium lexidronam pentasodium with chemotherapy or external beam radiation has not been studied. Samarium lexidronam pentasodium should not be given concurrently with chemotherapy or external beam radiation therapy unless the benefit outweighs the risks. Samarium lexidronam pentasodium should not be given after either of these treatments until there has been time for adequate marrow recovery). Products include:

Alkeran Tablets 956

Mercaptopurine (The potential for additive bone marrow toxicity of Samarium lexidronam pentasodium with chemotherapy or external beam radiation has not been studied. Samarium lexidronam pentasodium should not be given concurrently with chemotherapy or external beam radiation therapy unless the benefit outweighs the risks. Samarium lexidronam pentasodium should not be given after either of these treatments until there has been time for adequate marrow recovery).

No products indexed under this heading.

Methotrexate Sodium (The potential for additive bone marrow toxicity of Samarium lexidronam pentasodium with chemotherapy or external beam radiation has not been studied. Samarium lexidronam pentasodium should not be given concurrently with chemotherapy or external beam radiation therapy unless the benefit outweighs the risks. Samarium lexidronam pentasodium should not be given after either of these treatments until there has been time for adequate marrow recovery).

No products indexed under this heading.

Mitomycin (Mitomycin-C) (The potential for additive bone marrow toxicity of Samarium lexidronam pentasodium with chemotherapy or external beam radiation has not been studied. Samarium lexidronam pentasodium should not be given concurrently with chemotherapy or external beam radiation therapy unless the benefit outweighs the risks. Samarium lexidronam pentasodium should not be given after either of these treatments until there has been time for adequate marrow recovery).

No products indexed under this heading.

Mitotane (The potential for additive bone marrow toxicity of Samarium lexidronam pentasodium with chemotherapy or external beam radiation has not been studied. Samarium lexidronam pentasodium should not be given concurrently with chemotherapy or external beam radiation therapy unless the benefit outweighs the risks. Samarium lexidronam pentasodium should not be given after either of these treatments until there has been time for adequate marrow recovery).

No products indexed under this heading.

Mitoxantrone Hydrochloride (The potential for additive bone marrow toxicity of Samarium lexidronam pentasodium with chemotherapy or external beam radiation has not been studied. Samarium lexidronam pentasodium should not be given concurrently with chemotherapy or external beam radiation therapy unless the benefit outweighs the risks. Samarium lexidronam pentasodium should not be given after either of these treatments until there has been time for adequate marrow recovery).

No products indexed under this heading.

Oxaliplatin (The potential for additive bone marrow toxicity of Samarium lexidronam pentasodium with chemotherapy or external beam radiation has not been studied. Samarium lexidronam pentasodium should not be given concurrently with chemotherapy or external beam radiation therapy unless the benefit outweighs the risks. Samarium lexidronam pentasodium should not be given after either of these treatments until there has been time for adequate marrow recovery). Products include:

Eloxatin for Injection 2892

Paclitaxel (The potential for additive bone marrow toxicity of Samari-

um lexidronam pentasodium with chemotherapy or external beam radiation has not been studied. Samarium lexidronam pentasodium should not be given concurrently with chemotherapy or external beam radiation therapy unless the benefit outweighs the risks. Samarium lexidronam pentasodium should not be given after either of these treatments until there has been time for adequate marrow recovery).
No products indexed under this heading.

Procarbazine Hydrochloride (The potential for additive bone marrow toxicity of Samarium lexidronam pentasodium with chemotherapy or external beam radiation has not been studied. Samarium lexidronam pentasodium should not be given concurrently with chemotherapy or external beam radiation therapy unless the benefit outweighs the risks. Samarium lexidronam pentasodium should not be given after either of these treatments until there has been time for adequate marrow recovery). Products include:
Matulane Capsules 3191

Radiation (The potential for additive bone marrow toxicity of Samarium lexidronam pentasodium with chemotherapy or external beam radiation has not been studied. Samarium lexidronam pentasodium should not be given concurrently with chemotherapy or external beam radiation therapy unless the benefit outweighs the risks. Samarium lexidronam pentasodium should not be given after either of these treatments until there has been time for adequate marrow recovery).
No products indexed under this heading.

Streptozocin (The potential for additive bone marrow toxicity of Samarium lexidronam pentasodium with chemotherapy or external beam radiation has not been studied. Samarium lexidronam pentasodium should not be given concurrently with chemotherapy or external beam radiation therapy unless the benefit outweighs the risks. Samarium lexidronam pentasodium should not be given after either of these treatments until there has been time for adequate marrow recovery).
No products indexed under this heading.

Tamoxifen Citrate (The potential for additive bone marrow toxicity of Samarium lexidronam pentasodium with chemotherapy or external beam radiation has not been studied. Samarium lexidronam pentasodium should not be given concurrently with chemotherapy or external beam radiation therapy unless the benefit outweighs the risks. Samarium lexidronam pentasodium should not be given after either of these treatments until there has been time for adequate marrow recovery). Products include:
Soltamox Oral Solution 3527

Teniposide (The potential for additive bone marrow toxicity of Samarium lexidronam pentasodium with chemotherapy or external beam radiation has not been studied. Samarium lexidronam pentasodium should not be given concurrently with chemotherapy or external beam radiation therapy unless the benefit outweighs the risks. Samarium lexidronam pentasodium should not be given after either of these treatments until there has been time for adequate marrow recovery).
No products indexed under this heading.

Thioguanine (The potential for additive bone marrow toxicity of Samarium lexidronam pentasodium with chemotherapy or external beam radiation has not been studied. Samarium lexidronam pentasodium should not be given concurrently with chemotherapy or external beam radiation therapy unless the benefit outweighs the risks. Samarium lexidronam pentasodium should not be given after either of these treatments until there has been time for adequate marrow recovery). Products include:
Tabloid Tablets 1575

Thiotepa (The potential for additive bone marrow toxicity of Samarium lexidronam pentasodium with chemotherapy or external beam radiation has not been studied. Samarium lexidronam pentasodium should not be given concurrently with chemotherapy or external beam radiation therapy unless the benefit outweighs the risks. Samarium lexidronam pentasodium should not be given after either of these treatments until there has been time for adequate marrow recovery).
No products indexed under this heading.

Topotecan Hydrochloride (The potential for additive bone marrow toxicity of Samarium lexidronam pentasodium with chemotherapy or external beam radiation has not been studied. Samarium lexidronam pentasodium should not be given concurrently with chemotherapy or external beam radiation therapy unless the benefit outweighs the risks. Samarium lexidronam pentasodium should not be given after either of these treatments until there has been time for adequate marrow recovery). Products include:
Hycamtin for Injection 1458

Toremifene Citrate (The potential for additive bone marrow toxicity of Samarium lexidronam pentasodium with chemotherapy or external beam radiation has not been studied. Samarium lexidronam pentasodium should not be given concurrently with chemotherapy or external beam radiation therapy unless the benefit outweighs the risks. Samarium lexidronam pentasodium should not be given after either of these treatments until there has been time for adequate marrow recovery).
No products indexed under this heading.

Valrubicin (The potential for additive bone marrow toxicity of Samarium lexidronam pentasodium with chemotherapy or external beam radiation has not been studied. Samarium lexidronam pentasodium should not be given concurrently with chemotherapy or external beam radiation therapy unless the benefit outweighs the risks. Samarium lexidronam pentasodium should not be given after either of these treatments until there has been time for adequate marrow recovery).
No products indexed under this heading.

Vincristine Sulfate (The potential for additive bone marrow toxicity of Samarium lexidronam pentasodium with chemotherapy or external beam radiation has not been studied. Samarium lexidronam pentasodium should not be given concurrently with chemotherapy or external beam radiation therapy unless the benefit outweighs the risks. Samarium lexidronam pentasodium should not be given after either of these treatments until there has been time for adequate marrow recovery).
No products indexed under this heading.

Vinorelbine Tartrate (The potential for additive bone marrow toxicity of Samarium lexidronam pentasodium with chemotherapy or external beam radiation has not been studied. Samarium lexidronam pentasodium should not be given concurrently with chemotherapy or external beam radiation therapy unless the benefit outweighs the risks. Samarium lexidronam pentasodium should not be given after either of these treatments until there has been time for adequate marrow recovery).
No products indexed under this heading.

QUIXIN OPHTHALMIC SOLUTION

(Levofloxacin) 3383
May interact with xanthines and certain other agents. Compounds in these categories include:

Aminophylline (Systemic administration of some quinolones has been shown to elevate plasma concentrations of theophylline).
No products indexed under this heading.

Caffeine (Systemic administration of some quinolones has been shown to interfere with the metabolism of caffeine). Products include:
BC Headache Powder .... ▣677
Arthritis Strength BC Powder .... ▣677
Excedrin Extra Strength Caplets/Tablets/Geltabs .... ▣684
Excedrin Migraine Caplets/Tablets/Geltabs .... ▣609
Excedrin Tension Headache Caplets/Tablets/Geltabs .... ▣611
Goody's Extra Strength Headache Powders .... ▣611
Goody's Extra Strength Pain Relief Tablets .... ▣685
Vivarin .... ▣602
Winrgy Dietary Supplement .... ▣823

Caffeine Citrate (Systemic administration of some quinolones has been shown to interfere with the metabolism of caffeine). Products include:
Cafcit 1886

Cyclosporine (Systemic administration of some quinolones has been associated with transient elevations of serum creatinine in patients receiving systemic cyclosporine concomitantly). Products include:
Gengraf Capsules 459
Neoral Oral Solution 2259
Neoral Soft Gelatin Capsules 2259
Restasis Ophthalmic Emulsion 575
Sandimmune 2275

Dyphylline (Systemic administration of some quinolones has been shown to elevate plasma concentrations of theophylline).
No products indexed under this heading.

Theophylline (Systemic administration of some quinolones has been shown to elevate plasma concentrations of theophylline).
No products indexed under this heading.

Theophylline Anhydrous (Systemic administration of some quinolones has been shown to elevate plasma concentrations of theophylline). Products include:
Uniphyl Tablets 2710

Theophylline Calcium Salicylate (Systemic administration of some quinolones has been shown to elevate plasma concentrations of theophylline).
No products indexed under this heading.

Theophylline Dihydroxypropyl (Glyceryl) (Systemic administration of some quinolones has been shown to elevate plasma concentrations of theophylline).
No products indexed under this heading.

Theophylline Ethylenediamine (Systemic administration of some quinolones has been shown to elevate plasma concentrations of theophylline).
No products indexed under this heading.

Theophylline Sodium Glycinate (Systemic administration of some quinolones has been shown to elevate plasma concentrations of theophylline).
No products indexed under this heading.

Warfarin Sodium (Systemic administration of some quinolones has been shown to enhance the effects of the oral anticoagulant warfarin). Products include:
Coumadin for Injection 898
Coumadin Tablets 898

QVAR INHALATION AEROSOL

(Beclomethasone Dipropionate) 3303
None cited in PDR database.

RANEXA TABLETS

(Ranolazine) 1035
May interact with class 1A antiarrhythmics, class III antiarrhythmics, azole antifungals, cytochrome p450 2d6 substrates (selected), cytochrome p450 3a inhibitors (selected), macrolide antibiotics, antipsychotic agents, protease inhibitors, drugs that prolong the QT interval, tricyclic antidepressants, and certain other agents. Compounds in these categories include:

Amiodarone Hydrochloride (Ranolazine has been shown to prolong the QTc interval in a dose-related manner. Because of possible additive effects on the QT interval, ranolazine is contraindicated with drugs that prolong the QTc interval).
No products indexed under this heading.

Amitriptyline Hydrochloride (Ranolazine has been shown to prolong the QTc interval in a dose-related manner. Because of possible additive effects on the QT interval, ranolazine is contraindicated with drugs that prolong the QTc interval).
No products indexed under this heading.

Amoxapine (Ranolazine has been shown to prolong the QTc interval in a dose-related manner. Because of possible additive effects on the QT interval, ranolazine is contraindicated with drugs that prolong the QTc interval).
No products indexed under this heading.

Amphetamine Aspartate (Ranolazine can inhibit the activity of CYP2D6 and, thus, the metabolism of drugs that are mainly metabolized by this enzyme may be impaired and exposure to these drugs increased. The dose of such drugs may have to be reduced when ranolazine is co-administered). Products include:
Adderall Tablets 3164
Adderall XR Capsules 3166

Amphetamine Aspartate Monohydrate (Ranolazine can inhibit the activity of CYP2D6 and, thus, the metabolism of drugs that are mainly metabolized by this enzyme may be impaired and exposure to these drugs increased. The dose of such drugs may have to be reduced when ranolazine is co-administered).
No products indexed under this heading.

Amphetamine Sulfate (Ranolazine can inhibit the activity of CYP2D6 and, thus, the metabolism of drugs that are mainly metabolized by this enzyme may be impaired and exposure to these drugs increased. The dose of such drugs may have to be reduced when ranolazine is co-administered). Products include:
Adderall Tablets 3164
Adderall XR Capsules 3166

Amprenavir (Ranolazine is primarily metabolized by CYP3A. Use of ranolazine with potent or moderately potent inhibitors of CYP3A, such as HIV protease inhibitors, is contraindicated because concomitant administration will increase ranolazine plasma levels and QTc prolongation). Products include:
Agenerase Capsules 1327
Agenerase Oral Solution 1332

Aprepitant (Ranolazine is primarily metabolized by CYP3A. Use of ranolazine with potent or moderately potent inhibitors of CYP3A is contraindicated because concomitant administration will increase ranolazine plasma levels and QTc prolongation). Products include:
Emend Capsules 1963

Aripiprazole (Ranolazine has been shown to prolong the QTc interval in a dose-related manner. Because of possible additive effects on the QT interval, ranolazine is contraindicated with drugs that prolong the QTc interval, such as antipsychotics. Ranolazine can inhibit the activity of CYP2D6 and, thus, the metabolism of drugs that are mainly metabolized by this enzyme, such as some antipsychotics, may be impaired and exposure to these drugs increased). Products include:
Abilify Oral Solution 882
Abilify Oral Solution 2450
Abilify Discmelt Orally Disintegrating Tablets 882
Abilify Discmelt Orally Disintegrating Tablets 2450
Abilify Tablets 882
Abilify Tablets 2450

Astemizole (Ranolazine has been shown to prolong the QTc interval in a dose-related manner. Because of possible additive effects on the QT interval, ranolazine is contraindicated with drugs that prolong the QTc interval).
No products indexed under this heading.

Atomoxetine Hydrochloride (Ranolazine can inhibit the activity of CYP2D6 and, thus, the metabolism of drugs that are mainly metabolized by this enzyme may be impaired and exposure to these drugs increased. The dose of such drugs may have to be reduced when ranolazine is co-administered). Products include:
Strattera Capsules 1814

Azithromycin Dihydrate (Ranolazine is primarily metabolized by CYP3A. Use of ranolazine with potent or moderately potent inhibitors of CYP3A, such as macrolide antibiotics, is contraindicated because concomitant administration will increase ranolazine plasma levels and QTc prolongation).
No products indexed under this heading.

Bisoprolol Fumarate (Ranolazine can inhibit the activity of CYP2D6 and, thus, the metabolism of drugs that are mainly metabolized by this enzyme may be impaired and exposure to these drugs increased. The dose of such drugs may have to be reduced when ranolazine is co-administered).
No products indexed under this heading.

Bretylium Tosylate (Ranolazine has been shown to prolong the QTc interval in a dose-related manner. Because of possible additive effects on the QT interval, ranolazine is contraindicated with drugs that prolong the QTc interval).
No products indexed under this heading.

Captopril (Ranolazine can inhibit the activity of CYP2D6 and, thus, the metabolism of drugs that are mainly metabolized by this enzyme may be impaired and exposure to these drugs increased. The dose of such drugs may have to be reduced when ranolazine is co-administered). Products include:
Captopril Tablets 2149

Carvedilol (Ranolazine can inhibit the activity of CYP2D6 and, thus, the metabolism of drugs that are mainly metabolized by this enzyme may be impaired and exposure to these drugs increased. The dose of such drugs may have to be reduced when ranolazine is co-administered). Products include:
Coreg Tablets 1414

Cevimeline Hydrochloride (Ranolazine can inhibit the activity of CYP2D6 and, thus, the metabolism of drugs that are mainly metabolized by this enzyme may be impaired and exposure to these drugs increased. The dose of such drugs may have to be reduced when ranolazine is co-administered). Products include:
Evoxac Capsules 1047

Chlorpromazine (Ranolazine has been shown to prolong the QTc interval in a dose-related manner. Because of possible additive effects on the QT interval, ranolazine is contraindicated with drugs that prolong the QTc interval).
No products indexed under this heading.

Chlorpromazine Hydrochloride (Ranolazine has been shown to prolong the QTc interval in a dose-related manner. Because of possible additive effects on the QT interval, ranolazine is contraindicated with drugs that prolong the QTc interval).
No products indexed under this heading.

Chlorpropamide (Ranolazine can inhibit the activity of CYP2D6 and, thus, the metabolism of drugs that are mainly metabolized by this enzyme may be impaired and exposure to these drugs increased. The dose of such drugs may have to be reduced when ranolazine is co-administered).
No products indexed under this heading.

Chlorprothixene (Ranolazine has been shown to prolong the QTc interval in a dose-related manner. Because of possible additive effects on the QT interval, ranolazine is contraindicated with drugs that prolong the QTc interval, such as antipsychotics. Ranolazine can inhibit the activity of CYP2D6 and, thus, the metabolism of drugs that are mainly metabolized by this enzyme, such as some antipsychotics, may be impaired and exposure to these drugs increased).
No products indexed under this heading.

Chlorprothixene Hydrochloride (Ranolazine has been shown to prolong the QTc interval in a dose-related manner. Because of possible additive effects on the QT interval, ranolazine is contraindicated with drugs that prolong the QTc interval, such as antipsychotics. Ranolazine can inhibit the activity of CYP2D6 and, thus, the metabolism of drugs that are mainly metabolized by this enzyme, such as some antipsychotics, may be impaired and exposure to these drugs increased).
No products indexed under this heading.

Cimetidine (Ranolazine is primarily metabolized by CYP3A. Use of ranolazine with potent or moderately potent inhibitors of CYP3A is contraindicated because concomitant administration will increase ranolazine plasma levels and QTc prolongation). Products include:
Tagamet HB 200 Tablets 664

Cimetidine Hydrochloride (Ranolazine is primarily metabolized by CYP3A. Use of ranolazine with potent or moderately potent inhibitors of CYP3A is contraindicated because concomitant administration will increase ranolazine plasma levels and QTc prolongation).
No products indexed under this heading.

Ciprofloxacin (Ranolazine is primarily metabolized by CYP3A. Use of ranolazine with potent or moderately potent inhibitors of CYP3A is contraindicated because concomitant administration will increase ranolazine plasma levels and QTc prolongation). Products include:
Cipro Oral Suspension 2977
Cipro I.V. 2984
Cipro XR Tablets 2990
Ciprodex Otic Suspension 559

Ciprofloxacin Hydrochloride (Ranolazine is primarily metabolized by CYP3A. Use of ranolazine with potent or moderately potent inhibitors of CYP3A is contraindicated because concomitant administration will increase ranolazine plasma levels and QTc prolongation). Products include:
Ciloxan Ophthalmic Ointment 559
Ciloxan Ophthalmic Solution .... ⊙ 206
Cipro Tablets 2977
Proquin XR Tablets 1153

Clarithromycin (Ranolazine is primarily metabolized by CYP3A. Use of ranolazine with potent or moderately potent inhibitors of CYP3A, such as macrolide antibiotics, is contraindicated because concomitant administration will increase ranolazine plasma levels and QTc prolongation). Products include:
Biaxin/Biaxin XL 402
PREVPAC 3284

Clomipramine Hydrochloride (Ranolazine has been shown to prolong the QTc interval in a dose-related manner. Because of possible additive effects on the QT interval, ranolazine is contraindicated with drugs that prolong the QTc interval).
No products indexed under this heading.

Clotrimazole (Ranolazine is primarily metabolized by CYP3A. Use of ranolazine with potent or moderately potent inhibitors of CYP3A, such as ketoconazole and other azole antifungals, is contraindicated because concomitant administration will increase ranolazine plasma levels and QTc prolongation). Products include:
Desenex Athlete's Foot Cream 635
Lotrimin 3039
Lotrisone 3040

Clozapine (Ranolazine has been shown to prolong the QTc interval in a dose-related manner. Because of possible additive effects on the QT interval, ranolazine is contraindicated with drugs that prolong the QTc interval, such as antipsychotics. Ranolazine can inhibit the activity of CYP2D6 and, thus, the metabolism of drugs that are mainly metabolized by this enzyme, such as some antipsychotics, may be impaired and exposure to these drugs increased). Products include:
Clozaril Tablets 2184
FazaClo Orally Disintegrating Tablets 551

Codeine Phosphate (Ranolazine can inhibit the activity of CYP2D6 and, thus, the metabolism of drugs that are mainly metabolized by this enzyme may be impaired and exposure to these drugs increased. The dose of such drugs may have to be reduced when ranolazine is co-administered). Products include:
Tylenol with Codeine Tablets 2391

Codeine Sulfate (Ranolazine can inhibit the activity of CYP2D6 and, thus, the metabolism of drugs that are mainly metabolized by this enzyme may be impaired and exposure to these drugs increased. The dose of such drugs may have to be reduced when ranolazine is co-administered).
No products indexed under this heading.

Cyclobenzaprine Hydrochloride (Ranolazine can inhibit the activity of CYP2D6 and, thus, the metabolism of drugs that are mainly metabolized by this enzyme may be impaired and exposure to these drugs increased. The dose of such drugs may have to be reduced when ranolazine is co-administered).
No products indexed under this heading.

Cyclosporine (Ranolazine is primarily metabolized by CYP3A. Use of ranolazine with potent or moderately potent inhibitors of CYP3A is contraindicated because concomitant administration will increase ranolazine plasma levels and QTc prolongation). Products include:
Gengraf Capsules ... 459
Neoral Oral Solution ... 2259
Neoral Soft Gelatin Capsules ... 2259
Restasis Ophthalmic Emulsion ... 575
Sandimmune ... 2275

Delavirdine Mesylate (Ranolazine is primarily metabolized by CYP3A. Use of ranolazine with potent or moderately potent inhibitors of CYP3A is contraindicated because concomitant administration will increase ranolazine plasma levels and QTc prolongation). Products include:
Rescriptor Tablets ... 2551

Desipramine Hydrochloride (Ranolazine has been shown to prolong the QTc interval in a dose-related manner. Because of possible additive effects on the QT interval, ranolazine is contraindicated with drugs that prolong the QTc interval).
No products indexed under this heading.

Dexfenfluramine Hydrochloride (Ranolazine can inhibit the activity of CYP2D6 and, thus, the metabolism of drugs that are mainly metabolized by this enzyme may be impaired and exposure to these drugs increased. The dose of such drugs may have to be reduced when ranolazine is co-administered).
No products indexed under this heading.

Dextromethorphan Hydrobromide (Ranolazine can inhibit the activity of CYP2D6 and, thus, the metabolism of drugs that are mainly metabolized by this enzyme may be impaired and exposure to these drugs increased. The dose of such drugs may have to be reduced when ranolazine is co-administered). Products include:
Comtrex Maximum Strength Cold & Cough Day/Night Caplets - Day Formulation ... ▣726
Comtrex Maximum Strength Cold & Cough Day/Night Caplets - Night Formulation ... ▣726
Comtrex Maximum Strength Non-Drowsy Cold & Cough Caplets ... ▣725
Children's Dimetapp DM Cold & Cough Elixir ... ▣731
Children's Dimetapp Long Acting Cough Plus Cold Syrup ... ▣731
Toddler's Dimetapp Cold and Cough Drops ... ▣732
Mucinex DM Extended-Release Bi-Layer Tablets ... ▣720
Refenesen DM Caplets ... ▣721
Robitussin Cough & Cold CF Liquid ... ▣735
Robitussin Cough & Cold Long-Acting Liquid ... ▣735
Robitussin Cough & Allergy Syrup ... ▣736
Robitussin Cough & Cold Nighttime Liquid ... ▣736
Robitussin Cough & Cold Pediatric Drops ... ▣735
Robitussin Cough, Cold & Flu Nighttime Liquid ... ▣738
Robitussin Cough & Congestion Liquid ... ▣738
Robitussin Cough Gels Long-Acting ... ▣737
Robitussin Cough Long Acting Liquid ... ▣739
Robitussin Cough DM Syrup ... ▣738
Robitussin Cough DM Infant Drops ... ▣738
Robitussin Pediatric Cough Long Acting Liquid ... ▣739
Robitussin Pediatric Cough & Cold Long-Acting Liquid ... ▣735
Robitussin Pediatric Cough & Cold Nighttime Liquid ... ▣736
Robitussin Sugar Free Cough ... ▣738
TheraFlu Cold & Cough Hot Liquid ... ▣740
TheraFlu Warming Relief Daytime Severe Cold ... ▣743
TheraFlu Thin Strips Long Acting Cough ... ▣744
Triaminic Daytime Cold & Cough Liquid ... ▣745
Triaminic Cough & Sore Throat Liquid ... ▣747
Triaminic Cough & Runny Nose Softchews ... ▣748
Triaminic Thin Strips Cold & Cough ... ▣778
Triaminic Infant Thin Strips Decongestant Plus Cough ... ▣747
Children's Tylenol Plus Flu Oral Suspension ... ▣749
Tylenol Cold Head Congestion Daytime Caplets with Cool Burst and Gelcaps ... ▣750
Tylenol Cold Multi-Symptom Daytime Liquid ... ▣752
Tylenol Cold Multi-Symptom Severe Daytime Liquid ... ▣752
Concentrated Tylenol Infants' Drops Plus Cold & Cough ... ▣754
Children's Tylenol Plus Cough & Runny Nose Suspension Liquid ... 1879
Children's Tylenol Plus Cough & Sore Throat Suspension Liquid ... 1879
Children's Tylenol Plus Flu Suspension Liquid ... 1881
Children's Tylenol Plus Multi-Symptom Cold Suspension Liquid ... 1879
Tylenol Cold Severe Congestion Non-Drowsy Caplets with Cool Burst ... 1874
Tylenol Cold Head Congestion Daytime Caplets with Cool Burst ... 1873
Tylenol Cold Head Congestion Nighttime Caplets with Cool Burst ... 1873
Tylenol Cold Head Congestion Severe Caplets with Cool Burst ... 1873
Tylenol Cold Multi-Symptom Daytime Caplets with Cool Burst and Gelcaps ... 1874
Tylenol Cold Multi-Symptom Daytime Liquid with Citrus Burst ... 1874
Tylenol Cold Multi-Symptom Nighttime Caplets with Cool Burst ... 1874
Tylenol Cold Multi-Symptom Nighttime Liquid with Cool Burst ... 1874
Tylenol Cold Multi-Symptom Severe Caplets with Cool Burst ... 1874
Tylenol Cold Multi-Symptom Severe Daytime Liquid with Citrus Burst ... 1874
Tylenol Cough & Sore Throat Daytime Liquid with Cool Burst ... 1877
Tylenol Cough & Sore Throat Nighttime Liquid with Cool Burst ... 1877
Concentrated Tylenol Infants' Drops Plus Cold and Cough ... 1879
Vicks 44 Cough Relief Liquid ... 2679
Vicks 44D Cough & Head Congestion Relief Liquid ... 2679
Vicks 44E Cough & Chest Congestion Relief Liquid ... 2679
Pediatric Vicks 44e Cough & Chest Congestion Relief Liquid ... 2676
Vicks 44M Cough, Cold & Flu Relief Liquid ... 2680
Pediatric Vicks 44m Cough & Cold Relief Liquid ... 2676
Vicks DayQuil LiquiCaps/Liquid Multi-Symptom Cold/Flu Relief ... ▣761
Vicks DayQuil Multi-Symptom Cold/Flu Relief LiquiCaps ... 2678
Vicks DayQuil Multi-Symptom Cold/Flu Relief Liquid ... 2678
Vicks NyQuil Multi-Symptom Cold/Flu Relief Liquid ... 2681
Children's Vicks NyQuil Cold/Cough Relief ... ▣756
Vicks NyQuil Multi-Symptom Cold/Flu Relief LiquiCaps ... 2681
Vicks NyQuil LiquiCaps/Liquid Multi-Symptom Cold/Flu Relief ... ▣763
Vicks NyQuil Cough Liquid ... 2680
Children's Vicks NyQuil Cold/Cough Relief Liquid ... 2680
Zicam Cough Max Nighttime Cough Spray ... ▣767
Zicam Cough Max Cough Spray ... ▣767
Zicam Cough Max Cough Melts ... ▣767
Zicam Cough Plus D Cough Spray ... ▣767
Zicam Cough Relief Cough Spray ... ▣767
Zicam Maximum Strength Flu Daytime ... ▣768
Zicam Maximum Strength Flu Nighttime ... ▣768

Dextromethorphan Polistirex (Ranolazine can inhibit the activity of CYP2D6 and, thus, the metabolism of drugs that are mainly metabolized by this enzyme may be impaired and exposure to these drugs increased. The dose of such drugs may have to be reduced when ranolazine is co-administered). Products include:
Delsym Extended-Release Suspension 12 Hour Cough Suppressant ... ▣611

Digoxin (As a result of an interaction at the P-gp level, co-administration of ranolazine and digoxin results in a 1.5-fold elevation of digoxin plasma concentrations. The dose of digoxin and other P-gp substrates may have to be reduced when ranolazine is co-administered with digoxin). Products include:
Lanoxicaps Capsules ... 1490
Lanoxin Injection ... 1494
Lanoxin Injection Pediatric ... 1497
Lanoxin Tablets ... 1500

Diltiazem Hydrochloride (Ranolazine is primarily metabolized by CYP3A. Use of ranolazine with potent or moderately potent inhibitors of CYP3A is contraindicated because concomitant administration will increase ranolazine plasma levels and QTc prolongation). Products include:
Cardizem LA Extended Release Tablets ... 1728
Tiazac Capsules ... 1201

Diltiazem Maleate (Ranolazine is primarily metabolized by CYP3A. Use of ranolazine with potent or moderately potent inhibitors of CYP3A is contraindicated because concomitant administration will increase ranolazine plasma levels and QTc prolongation).
No products indexed under this heading.

Dirithromycin (Ranolazine is primarily metabolized by CYP3A. Use of ranolazine with potent or moderately potent inhibitors of CYP3A, such as macrolide antibiotics, is contraindicated because concomitant administration will increase ranolazine plasma levels and QTc prolongation).
No products indexed under this heading.

Disopyramide (Ranolazine has been shown to prolong the QTc interval in a dose-related manner. Because of possible additive effects on the QT interval, ranolazine is contraindicated with drugs that prolong the QTc interval, such as Class 1A antiarrhythmics).
No products indexed under this heading.

Disopyramide Phosphate (Ranolazine has been shown to prolong the QTc interval in a dose-related manner. Because of possible additive effects on the QT interval, ranolazine is contraindicated with drugs that prolong the QTc interval).
No products indexed under this heading.

Dofetilide (Ranolazine has been shown to prolong the QTc interval in a dose-related manner. Because of possible additive effects on the QT interval, ranolazine is contraindicated with drugs that prolong the QTc interval).
No products indexed under this heading.

Dolasetron Mesylate (Ranolazine can inhibit the activity of CYP2D6 and, thus, the metabolism of drugs that are mainly metabolized by this enzyme may be impaired and exposure to these drugs increased. The dose of such drugs may have to be reduced when ranolazine is co-administered). Products include:
Anzemet Injection ... 2859
Anzemet Tablets ... 2862

Donepezil Hydrochloride (Ranolazine can inhibit the activity of CYP2D6 and, thus, the metabolism of drugs that are mainly metabolized by this enzyme may be impaired and exposure to these drugs increased. The dose of such drugs may have to be reduced when ranolazine is co-administered). Products include:
Aricept Tablets ... 1094
Aricept ODT Tablets ... 1094

Doxepin Hydrochloride (Ranolazine has been shown to prolong the QTc interval in a dose-related manner. Because of possible additive effects on the QT interval, ranolazine is contraindicated with drugs that prolong the QTc interval).
No products indexed under this heading.

Efavirenz (Ranolazine is primarily metabolized by CYP3A. Use of ranolazine with potent or moderately potent inhibitors of CYP3A is contraindicated because concomitant administration will increase ranolazine plasma levels and QTc prolongation). Products include:
Atripla Tablets ... 945
Sustiva Capsules ... 930
Sustiva Tablets ... 930

Encainide Hydrochloride (Ranolazine can inhibit the activity of CYP2D6 and, thus, the metabolism of drugs that are mainly metabolized by this enzyme may be impaired and exposure to these drugs increased. The dose of such drugs may have to be reduced when ranolazine is co-administered).
No products indexed under this heading.

Erythromycin (Ranolazine is primarily metabolized by CYP3A. Use of ranolazine with potent or moderately potent inhibitors of CYP3A, such as macrolide antibiotics, is contraindicated because concomitant administration will increase ranolazine plasma levels and QTc prolongation). Products include:
Ery-Tab Tablets 449
Erythromycin Base Filmtab Tablets 455
Erythromycin Delayed-Release Capsules, USP 457
PCE Dispertab Tablets 515

Erythromycin Estolate (Ranolazine is primarily metabolized by CYP3A. Use of ranolazine with potent or moderately potent inhibitors of CYP3A, such as macrolide antibiotics, is contraindicated because concomitant administration will increase ranolazine plasma levels and QTc prolongation).
No products indexed under this heading.

Erythromycin Ethylsuccinate (Ranolazine is primarily metabolized by CYP3A. Use of ranolazine with potent or moderately potent inhibitors of CYP3A, such as macrolide antibiotics, is contraindicated because concomitant administration will increase ranolazine plasma levels and QTc prolongation). Products include:
E.E.S. 451
EryPed 447

Erythromycin Gluceptate (Ranolazine is primarily metabolized by CYP3A. Use of ranolazine with potent or moderately potent inhibitors of CYP3A, such as macrolide antibiotics, is contraindicated because concomitant administration will increase ranolazine plasma levels and QTc prolongation).
No products indexed under this heading.

Erythromycin Stearate (Ranolazine is primarily metabolized by CYP3A. Use of ranolazine with potent or moderately potent inhibitors of CYP3A, such as macrolide antibiotics, is contraindicated because concomitant administration will increase ranolazine plasma levels and QTc prolongation). Products include:
Erythrocin Stearate Filmtab Tablets 453

Fentanyl (Ranolazine can inhibit the activity of CYP2D6 and, thus, the metabolism of drugs that are mainly metabolized by this enzyme may be impaired and exposure to these drugs increased. The dose of such drugs may have to be reduced when ranolazine is co-administered). Products include:
Duragesic Transdermal System 2373
Ionsys Transdermal System 2379

Fentanyl Citrate (Ranolazine can inhibit the activity of CYP2D6 and, thus, the metabolism of drugs that are mainly metabolized by this enzyme may be impaired and exposure to these drugs increased. The dose of such drugs may have to be reduced when ranolazine is co-administered). Products include:
Actiq 979

Flecainide Acetate (Ranolazine has been shown to prolong the QTc interval in a dose-related manner. Because of possible additive effects on the QT interval, ranolazine is contraindicated with drugs that prolong the QTc interval). Products include:
Tambocor Tablets 1856

Fluconazole (Ranolazine is primarily metabolized by CYP3A. Use of ranolazine with potent or moderately potent inhibitors of CYP3A, such as ketoconazole and other azole antifungals, is contraindicated because concomitant administration will increase ranolazine plasma levels and QTc prolongation).
No products indexed under this heading.

Fluoxetine (Ranolazine is primarily metabolized by CYP3A. Use of ranolazine with potent or moderately potent inhibitors of CYP3A is contraindicated because concomitant administration will increase ranolazine plasma levels and QTc prolongation).
No products indexed under this heading.

Fluoxetine Hydrochloride (Ranolazine is primarily metabolized by CYP3A. Use of ranolazine with potent or moderately potent inhibitors of CYP3A is contraindicated because concomitant administration will increase ranolazine plasma levels and QTc prolongation). Products include:
Prozac Pulvules and Liquid 1801
Symbyax Capsules 1819

Fluphenazine Decanoate (Ranolazine has been shown to prolong the QTc interval in a dose-related manner. Because of possible additive effects on the QT interval, ranolazine is contraindicated with drugs that prolong the QTc interval).
No products indexed under this heading.

Fluphenazine Enanthate (Ranolazine has been shown to prolong the QTc interval in a dose-related manner. Because of possible additive effects on the QT interval, ranolazine is contraindicated with drugs that prolong the QTc interval).
No products indexed under this heading.

Fluphenazine Hydrochloride (Ranolazine has been shown to prolong the QTc interval in a dose-related manner. Because of possible additive effects on the QT interval, ranolazine is contraindicated with drugs that prolong the QTc interval).
No products indexed under this heading.

Fluvoxamine Maleate (Ranolazine is primarily metabolized by CYP3A. Use of ranolazine with potent or moderately potent inhibitors of CYP3A is contraindicated because concomitant administration will increase ranolazine plasma levels and QTc prolongation).
No products indexed under this heading.

Formoterol Fumarate (Ranolazine can inhibit the activity of CYP2D6 and, thus, the metabolism of drugs that are mainly metabolized by this enzyme may be impaired and exposure to these drugs increased. The dose of such drugs may have to be reduced when ranolazine is co-administered). Products include:
Foradil Aerolizer 3010

Galantamine Hydrobromide (Ranolazine can inhibit the activity of CYP2D6 and, thus, the metabolism of drugs that are mainly metabolized by this enzyme may be impaired and exposure to these drugs increased. The dose of such drugs may have to be reduced when ranolazine is co-administered). Products include:
Razadyne 2399
Razadyne ER Extended-Release Capsules 2399

Haloperidol (Ranolazine has been shown to prolong the QTc interval in a dose-related manner. Because of possible additive effects on the QT interval, ranolazine is contraindicated with drugs that prolong the QTc interval, such as antipsychotics. Ranolazine can inhibit the activity of CYP2D6 and, thus, the metabolism of drugs that are mainly metabolized by this enzyme, such as some antipsychotics, may be impaired and exposure to these drugs increased).
No products indexed under this heading.

Haloperidol Decanoate (Ranolazine has been shown to prolong the QTc interval in a dose-related manner. Because of possible additive effects on the QT interval, ranolazine is contraindicated with drugs that prolong the QTc interval, such as antipsychotics. Ranolazine can inhibit the activity of CYP2D6 and, thus, the metabolism of drugs that are mainly metabolized by this enzyme, such as some antipsychotics, may be impaired and exposure to these drugs increased).
No products indexed under this heading.

Hydrocodone Bitartrate (Ranolazine can inhibit the activity of CYP2D6 and, thus, the metabolism of drugs that are mainly metabolized by this enzyme may be impaired and exposure to these drugs increased. The dose of such drugs may have to be reduced when ranolazine is co-administered). Products include:
Hycodan 1116
Hycotuss Expectorant Syrup 1117
Vicodin Tablets 535
Vicodin ES Tablets 536
Vicodin HP Tablets 538
Vicoprofen Tablets 539
Zydone Tablets 1139

Imipramine Hydrochloride (Ranolazine has been shown to prolong the QTc interval in a dose-related manner. Because of possible additive effects on the QT interval, ranolazine is contraindicated with drugs that prolong the QTc interval).
No products indexed under this heading.

Imipramine Pamoate (Ranolazine has been shown to prolong the QTc interval in a dose-related manner. Because of possible additive effects on the QT interval, ranolazine is contraindicated with drugs that prolong the QTc interval).
No products indexed under this heading.

Indinavir Sulfate (Ranolazine is primarily metabolized by CYP3A. Use of ranolazine with potent or moderately potent inhibitors of CYP3A, such as HIV protease inhibitors, is contraindicated because concomitant administration will increase ranolazine plasma levels and QTc prolongation). Products include:
Crixivan Capsules 1940

Indoramin Hydrochloride (Ranolazine can inhibit the activity of CYP2D6 and, thus, the metabolism of drugs that are mainly metabolized by this enzyme may be impaired and exposure to these drugs increased. The dose of such drugs may have to be reduced when ranolazine is co-administered).
No products indexed under this heading.

Isoniazid (Ranolazine is primarily metabolized by CYP3A. Use of ranolazine with potent or moderately potent inhibitors of CYP3A is contraindicated because concomitant administration will increase ranolazine plasma levels and QTc prolongation).
No products indexed under this heading.

Itraconazole (Ranolazine is primarily metabolized by CYP3A. Use of ranolazine with potent or moderately potent inhibitors of CYP3A, such as ketoconazole and other azole antifungals, is contraindicated because concomitant administration will increase ranolazine plasma levels and QTc prolongation).
No products indexed under this heading.

Ketoconazole (Ranolazine is primarily metabolized by CYP3A. Use of ranolazine with potent or moderately potent inhibitors of CYP3A, such as ketoconazole and other azole antifungals, is contraindicated because concomitant administration will increase ranolazine plasma levels and QTc prolongation). Products include:
Nizoral A-D Shampoo, 1% 1868

Labetalol Hydrochloride (Ranolazine can inhibit the activity of CYP2D6 and, thus, the metabolism of drugs that are mainly metabolized by this enzyme may be impaired and exposure to these drugs increased. The dose of such drugs may have to be reduced when ranolazine is co-administered).
No products indexed under this heading.

Lidocaine (Ranolazine can inhibit the activity of CYP2D6 and, thus, the metabolism of drugs that are mainly metabolized by this enzyme may be impaired and exposure to these drugs increased. The dose of such drugs may have to be reduced when ranolazine is co-administered). Products include:
Lidoderm Patch 1118
Synera Topical Patch 1137

Lidocaine Hydrochloride (Ranolazine has been shown to prolong the QTc interval in a dose-related manner. Because of possible additive effects on the QT interval, ranolazine is contraindicated with drugs that prolong the QTc interval).
No products indexed under this heading.

Lithium Carbonate (Ranolazine has been shown to prolong the QTc interval in a dose-related manner. Because of possible additive effects on the QT interval, ranolazine is contraindicated with drugs that prolong the QTc interval, such as antipsychotics. Ranolazine can inhibit the activity of CYP2D6 and, thus, the metabolism of drugs that are mainly metabolized by this enzyme, such as some antipsychotics, may be impaired and exposure to these drugs increased). Products include:

Lithium Citrate (Ranolazine has been shown to prolong the QTc interval in a dose-related manner. Because of possible additive effects on the QT interval, ranolazine is contraindicated with drugs that prolong the QT interval, such as antipsychotics. Ranolazine can inhibit the activity of CYP2D6 and, thus, the metabolism of drugs that are mainly metabolized by this enzyme, such as some antipsychotics, may be impaired and exposure to these drugs increased).

No products indexed under this heading.

Lopinavir (Ranolazine is primarily metabolized by CYP3A. Use of ranolazine with potent or moderately potent inhibitors of CYP3A, such as HIV protease inhibitors, is contraindicated because concomitant administration will increase ranolazine plasma levels and QTc prolongation). Products include:

Loxapine Hydrochloride (Ranolazine has been shown to prolong the QTc interval in a dose-related manner. Because of possible additive effects on the QT interval, ranolazine is contraindicated with drugs that prolong the QTc interval, such as antipsychotics. Ranolazine can inhibit the activity of CYP2D6 and, thus, the metabolism of drugs that are mainly metabolized by this enzyme, such as some antipsychotics, may be impaired and exposure to these drugs increased).

No products indexed under this heading.

Loxapine Succinate (Ranolazine has been shown to prolong the QTc interval in a dose-related manner. Because of possible additive effects on the QT interval, ranolazine is contraindicated with drugs that prolong the QTc interval, such as antipsychotics. Ranolazine can inhibit the activity of CYP2D6 and, thus, the metabolism of drugs that are mainly metabolized by this enzyme, such as some antipsychotics, may be impaired and exposure to these drugs increased).

No products indexed under this heading.

Maprotiline Hydrochloride (Ranolazine has been shown to prolong the QTc interval in a dose-related manner. Because of possible additive effects on the QT interval, ranolazine is contraindicated with drugs that prolong the QTc interval).

No products indexed under this heading.

Meperidine Hydrochloride (Ranolazine can inhibit the activity of CYP2D6 and, thus, the metabolism of drugs that are mainly metabolized by this enzyme may be impaired and exposure to these drugs increased. The dose of such drugs may have to be reduced when ranolazine is co-administered).

No products indexed under this heading.

Mesoridazine Besylate (Ranolazine has been shown to prolong the QTc interval in a dose-related manner. Because of possible additive effects on the QT interval, ranolazine is contraindicated with drugs that prolong the QTc interval).

No products indexed under this heading.

Methadone Hydrochloride (Ranolazine can inhibit the activity of CYP2D6 and, thus, the metabolism of drugs that are mainly metabolized by this enzyme may be impaired and exposure to these drugs increased. The dose of such drugs may have to be reduced when ranolazine is co-administered).

No products indexed under this heading.

Methamphetamine Hydrochloride (Ranolazine can inhibit the activity of CYP2D6 and, thus, the metabolism of drugs that are mainly metabolized by this enzyme may be impaired and exposure to these drugs increased. The dose of such drugs may have to be reduced when ranolazine is co-administered). Products include:

Methotrimeprazine (Ranolazine has been shown to prolong the QTc interval in a dose-related manner. Because of possible additive effects on the QT interval, ranolazine is contraindicated with drugs that prolong the QTc interval, such as antipsychotics. Ranolazine can inhibit the activity of CYP2D6 and, thus, the metabolism of drugs that are mainly metabolized by this enzyme, such as some antipsychotics, may be impaired and exposure to these drugs increased).

No products indexed under this heading.

Metoprolol Succinate (Ranolazine can inhibit the activity of CYP2D6 and, thus, the metabolism of drugs that are mainly metabolized by this enzyme may be impaired and exposure to these drugs increased. The dose of such drugs may have to be reduced when ranolazine is co-administered). Products include:

Metoprolol Tartrate (Ranolazine can inhibit the activity of CYP2D6 and, thus, the metabolism of drugs that are mainly metabolized by this enzyme may be impaired and exposure to these drugs increased. The dose of such drugs may have to be reduced when ranolazine is co-administered). Products include:

Metronidazole (Ranolazine is primarily metabolized by CYP3A. Use of ranolazine with potent or moderately potent inhibitors of CYP3A is contraindicated because concomitant administration will increase ranolazine plasma levels and QTc prolongation). Products include:

Metronidazole Benzoate (Ranolazine is primarily metabolized by CYP3A. Use of ranolazine with potent or moderately potent inhibitors of CYP3A is contraindicated because concomitant administration will increase ranolazine plasma levels and QTc prolongation).

No products indexed under this heading.

Metronidazole Hydrochloride (Ranolazine is primarily metabolized by CYP3A. Use of ranolazine with potent or moderately potent inhibitors of CYP3A is contraindicated because concomitant administration will increase ranolazine plasma levels and QTc prolongation).

No products indexed under this heading.

Mexiletine Hydrochloride (Ranolazine has been shown to prolong the QTc interval in a dose-related manner. Because of possible additive effects on the QT interval, ranolazine is contraindicated with drugs that prolong the QTc interval).

No products indexed under this heading.

Miconazole (Ranolazine is primarily metabolized by CYP3A. Use of ranolazine with potent or moderately potent inhibitors of CYP3A, such as ketoconazole and other azole antifungals, is contraindicated because concomitant administration will increase ranolazine plasma levels and QTc prolongation).

No products indexed under this heading.

Mirtazapine (Ranolazine can inhibit the activity of CYP2D6 and, thus, the metabolism of drugs that are mainly metabolized by this enzyme may be impaired and exposure to these drugs increased. The dose of such drugs may have to be reduced when ranolazine is co-administered).

No products indexed under this heading.

Molindone Hydrochloride (Ranolazine has been shown to prolong the QTc interval in a dose-related manner. Because of possible additive effects on the QT interval, ranolazine is contraindicated with drugs that prolong the QTc interval, such as antipsychotics. Ranolazine can inhibit the activity of CYP2D6 and, thus, the metabolism of drugs that are mainly metabolized by this enzyme, such as some antipsychotics, may be impaired and exposure to these drugs increased). Products include:

Moricizine Hydrochloride (Ranolazine has been shown to prolong the QTc interval in a dose-related manner. Because of possible additive effects on the QT interval, ranolazine is contraindicated with drugs that prolong the QTc interval, such as Class 1A antiarrhythmics).

No products indexed under this heading.

Morphine Sulfate (Ranolazine can inhibit the activity of CYP2D6 and, thus, the metabolism of drugs that are mainly metabolized by this enzyme may be impaired and exposure to these drugs increased. The dose of such drugs may have to be reduced when ranolazine is co-administered). Products include:

Nefazodone Hydrochloride (Ranolazine is primarily metabolized by CYP3A. Use of ranolazine with potent or moderately potent inhibitors of CYP3A is contraindicated because concomitant administration will increase ranolazine plasma levels and QTc prolongation).

No products indexed under this heading.

Nelfinavir Mesylate (Ranolazine is primarily metabolized by CYP3A. Use of ranolazine with potent or moderately potent inhibitors of CYP3A, such as HIV protease inhibitors, is contraindicated because concomitant administration will increase ranolazine plasma levels and QTc prolongation). Products include:

Nifedipine (Ranolazine is primarily metabolized by CYP3A. Use of ranolazine with potent or moderately potent inhibitors of CYP3A is contraindicated because concomitant administration will increase ranolazine plasma levels and QTc prolongation). Products include:

Norfloxacin (Ranolazine is primarily metabolized by CYP3A. Use of ranolazine with potent or moderately potent inhibitors of CYP3A is contraindicated because concomitant administration will increase ranolazine plasma levels and QTc prolongation). Products include:

Nortriptyline Hydrochloride (Ranolazine has been shown to prolong the QTc interval in a dose-related manner. Because of possible additive effects on the QT interval, ranolazine is contraindicated with drugs that prolong the QTc interval).

No products indexed under this heading.

Olanzapine (Ranolazine has been shown to prolong the QTc interval in a dose-related manner. Because of possible additive effects on the QT interval, ranolazine is contraindicated with drugs that prolong the QTc interval, such as antipsychotics. Ranolazine can inhibit the activity of CYP2D6 and, thus, the metabolism of drugs that are mainly metabolized by this enzyme, such as some antipsychotics, may be impaired and exposure to these drugs increased). Products include:

Omeprazole (Ranolazine can inhibit the activity of CYP2D6 and, thus, the metabolism of drugs that are mainly metabolized by this enzyme may be impaired and exposure to these drugs increased. The dose of such drugs may have to be reduced when ranolazine is co-administered). Products include:

Ondansetron (Ranolazine can inhibit the activity of CYP2D6 and, thus, the metabolism of drugs that are mainly metabolized by this enzyme may be impaired and exposure to these drugs increased. The dose of such drugs may have to be reduced when ranolazine is co-administered). Products include:

Zofran ODT Orally Disintegrating Tablets .. **1639**

Ondansetron Hydrochloride (Ranolazine can inhibit the activity of CYP2D6 and, thus, the metabolism of drugs that are mainly metabolized by this enzyme may be impaired and exposure to these drugs increased. The dose of such drugs may have to be reduced when ranolazine is co-administered). Products include:

Zofran Injection **1634**
Zofran .. **1639**

Oxiconazole Nitrate (Ranolazine is primarily metabolized by CYP3A. Use of ranolazine with potent or moderately potent inhibitors of CYP3A, such as ketoconazole and other azole antifungals, is contraindicated because concomitant administration will increase ranolazine plasma levels and QTc prolongation). Products include:

Oxistat ... **2667**

Oxycodone Hydrochloride (Ranolazine can inhibit the activity of CYP2D6 and, thus, the metabolism of drugs that are mainly metabolized by this enzyme may be impaired and exposure to these drugs increased. The dose of such drugs may have to be reduced when ranolazine is co-administered). Products include:

OxyContin Tablets **2703**
OxyFast Oral Concentrate Solution... **2708**
OxyIR Capsules **2708**
Percocet Tablets **1131**
Percodan Tablets **1132**

Paclitaxel (Ranolazine can inhibit the activity of CYP2D6 and, thus, the metabolism of drugs that are mainly metabolized by this enzyme may be impaired and exposure to these drugs increased. The dose of such drugs may have to be reduced when ranolazine is co-administered).

No products indexed under this heading.

Paroxetine Hydrochloride (Paroxetine, a potent inhibitor of CYP2D6, increased average steady-state plasma concentrations of ranolazine 1.2-fold. No dose adjustment of ranolazine is required in patients treated with paroxetine or other CYP2D6 inhibitors). Products include:

Paxil CR Controlled-Release Tablets .. **1538**
Paxil ... **1530**

Paroxetine Mesylate (Paroxetine, a potent inhibitor of CYP2D6, increased average steady-state plasma concentrations of ranolazine 1.2-fold. No dose adjustment of ranolazine is required in patients treated with paroxetine or other CYP2D6 inhibitors). Products include:

Pexeva Tablets **1694**

Perphenazine (Ranolazine has been shown to prolong the QTc interval in a dose-related manner. Because of possible additive effects on the QT interval, ranolazine is contraindicated with drugs that prolong the QTc interval).

No products indexed under this heading.

Pimozide (Ranolazine has been shown to prolong the QTc interval in a dose-related manner. Because of possible additive effects on the QT interval, ranolazine is contraindicated with drugs that prolong the QTc interval, such as antipsychotics. Ranolazine can inhibit the activity of

CYP2D6 and, thus, the metabolism of drugs that are mainly metabolized by this enzyme, such as some antipsychotics, may be impaired and exposure to these drugs increased).

No products indexed under this heading.

Pindolol (Ranolazine can inhibit the activity of CYP2D6 and, thus, the metabolism of drugs that are mainly metabolized by this enzyme may be impaired and exposure to these drugs increased. The dose of such drugs may have to be reduced when ranolazine is co-administered).

No products indexed under this heading.

Procainamide (Ranolazine has been shown to prolong the QTc interval in a dose-related manner. Because of possible additive effects on the QT interval, ranolazine is contraindicated with drugs that prolong the QTc interval, such as Class 1A antiarrhythmics).

No products indexed under this heading.

Procainamide Hydrochloride (Ranolazine has been shown to prolong the QTc interval in a dose-related manner. Because of possible additive effects on the QT interval, ranolazine is contraindicated with drugs that prolong the QTc interval).

No products indexed under this heading.

Prochlorperazine (Ranolazine has been shown to prolong the QTc interval in a dose-related manner. Because of possible additive effects on the QT interval, ranolazine is contraindicated with drugs that prolong the QTc interval).

No products indexed under this heading.

Promethazine Hydrochloride (Ranolazine has been shown to prolong the QTc interval in a dose-related manner. Because of possible additive effects on the QT interval, ranolazine is contraindicated with drugs that prolong the QTc interval). Products include:

Phenergan Tablets and Suppositories............................... **3440**

Propafenone Hydrochloride (Ranolazine has been shown to prolong the QTc interval in a dose-related manner. Because of possible additive effects on the QT interval, ranolazine is contraindicated with drugs that prolong the QTc interval). Products include:

Rythmol SR Capsules **2727**

Propoxyphene Hydrochloride (Ranolazine can inhibit the activity of CYP2D6 and, thus, the metabolism of drugs that are mainly metabolized by this enzyme may be impaired and exposure to these drugs increased. The dose of such drugs may have to be reduced when ranolazine is co-administered).

No products indexed under this heading.

Propoxyphene Napsylate (Ranolazine can inhibit the activity of CYP2D6 and, thus, the metabolism of drugs that are mainly metabolized by this enzyme may be impaired and exposure to these drugs increased. The dose of such drugs may have to be reduced when ranolazine is co-administered).

No products indexed under this heading.

Propranolol Hydrochloride (Ranolazine can inhibit the activity of CYP2D6 and, thus, the metabolism of drugs that are mainly metabolized by this enzyme may be impaired and exposure to these drugs increased. The dose of such drugs may have to be reduced when ranolazine is co-administered). Products include:

Inderal LA Long-Acting Capsules **3429**
InnoPran XL Capsules **2723**

Protriptyline Hydrochloride (Ranolazine has been shown to prolong the QTc interval in a dose-related manner. Because of possible additive effects on the QT interval, ranolazine is contraindicated with drugs that prolong the QTc interval).

No products indexed under this heading.

Quetiapine Fumarate (Ranolazine has been shown to prolong the QTc interval in a dose-related manner. Because of possible additive effects on the QT interval, ranolazine is contraindicated with drugs that prolong the QTc interval, such as antipsychotics. Ranolazine can inhibit the activity of CYP2D6 and, thus, the metabolism of drugs that are mainly metabolized by this enzyme, such as some antipsychotics, may be impaired and exposure to these drugs increased). Products include:

Seroquel Tablets **690**

Quinidine (Ranolazine has been shown to prolong the QTc interval in a dose-related manner. Because of possible additive effects on the QT interval, ranolazine is contraindicated with drugs that prolong the QTc interval, such as Class 1A antiarrhythmics).

No products indexed under this heading.

Quinidine Gluconate (Ranolazine has been shown to prolong the QTc interval in a dose-related manner. Because of possible additive effects on the QT interval, ranolazine is contraindicated with drugs that prolong the QTc interval).

No products indexed under this heading.

Quinidine Hydrochloride (Ranolazine can inhibit the activity of CYP2D6 and, thus, the metabolism of drugs that are mainly metabolized by this enzyme may be impaired and exposure to these drugs increased. The dose of such drugs may have to be reduced when ranolazine is co-administered).

No products indexed under this heading.

Quinidine Polygalacturonate (Ranolazine has been shown to prolong the QTc interval in a dose-related manner. Because of possible additive effects on the QT interval, ranolazine is contraindicated with drugs that prolong the QTc interval).

No products indexed under this heading.

Quinidine Sulfate (Ranolazine has been shown to prolong the QTc interval in a dose-related manner. Because of possible additive effects on the QT interval, ranolazine is contraindicated with drugs that prolong the QTc interval).

No products indexed under this heading.

Quinine (Ranolazine is primarily metabolized by CYP3A. Use of ranolazine with potent or moderately potent inhibitors of CYP3A is contraindicated because concomitant administration will increase ranolazine plasma levels and QTc prolongation).

No products indexed under this heading.

Quinine Sulfate (Ranolazine is primarily metabolized by CYP3A. Use of ranolazine with potent or moderately potent inhibitors of CYP3A is contraindicated because concomitant administration will increase ranolazine plasma levels and QTc prolongation).

No products indexed under this heading.

Risperidone (Ranolazine has been shown to prolong the QTc interval in a dose-related manner. Because of possible additive effects on the QT interval, ranolazine is contraindicated with drugs that prolong the QTc interval, such as antipsychotics. Ranolazine can inhibit the activity of CYP2D6 and, thus, the metabolism of drugs that are mainly metabolized by this enzyme, such as some antipsychotics, may be impaired and exposure to these drugs increased). Products include:

Risperdal ... **1676**
Risperdal Consta Long-Acting Injection **1682**
Risperdal M-Tab Orally Disintegrating Tablets.................. **1676**

Ritonavir (Ranolazine is primarily metabolized by CYP3A. Use of ranolazine with potent or moderately potent inhibitors of CYP3A, such as HIV protease inhibitors, is contraindicated because concomitant administration will increase ranolazine plasma levels and QTc prolongation). Products include:

Kaletra ... **476**
Norvir ... **503**

Saquinavir (Ranolazine is primarily metabolized by CYP3A. Use of ranolazine with potent or moderately potent inhibitors of CYP3A, such as HIV protease inhibitors, is contraindicated because concomitant administration will increase ranolazine plasma levels and QTc prolongation).

No products indexed under this heading.

Saquinavir Mesylate (Ranolazine is primarily metabolized by CYP3A. Use of ranolazine with potent or moderately potent inhibitors of CYP3A, such as HIV protease inhibitors, is contraindicated because concomitant administration will increase ranolazine plasma levels and QTc prolongation). Products include:

Invirase .. **2772**

Sertraline Hydrochloride (Ranolazine is primarily metabolized by CYP3A. Use of ranolazine with potent or moderately potent inhibitors of CYP3A is contraindicated because concomitant administration will increase ranolazine plasma levels and QTc prolongation). Products include:

Zoloft ... **2586**

Simvastatin (Co-administration of ranolazine and simvastatin results in about a 2-fold increase in plasma concentrations of simvastatin and its active metabolite. The dose of simvastatin and other P-gp substrates

IMPORTANT NOTE: Always consult each drug listing in the patient's regimen for possible interactions.

may have to be reduced when ranolazine is co-administered with simvastatin). Products include:

Sotalol Hydrochloride (Ranolazine
has been shown to prolong the QTc
interval in a dose-related manner.
Because of possible additive effects
on the QT interval, ranolazine is contraindicated with drugs that prolong
the QTc interval, such as Class III
antiarrhythmics).

No products indexed under this
heading.

Tamoxifen Citrate (Ranolazine can
inhibit the activity of CYP2D6 and,
thus, the metabolism of drugs that
are mainly metabolized by this
enzyme may be impaired and exposure to these drugs increased. The
dose of such drugs may have to be
reduced when ranolazine is co-
administered). Products include:

Teniposide (Ranolazine can inhibit
the activity of CYP2D6 and, thus, the
metabolism of drugs that are mainly
metabolized by this enzyme may be
impaired and exposure to these
drugs increased. The dose of such
drugs may have to be reduced when
ranolazine is co-administered).

No products indexed under this
heading.

Terconazole (Ranolazine is primarily metabolized by CYP3A. Use of
ranolazine with potent or moderately
potent inhibitors of CYP3A, such as
ketoconazole and other azole antifungals, is contraindicated because
concomitant administration will
increase ranolazine plasma levels
and QTc prolongation).

No products indexed under this
heading.

Testosterone (Ranolazine can inhibit the activity of CYP2D6 and, thus,
the metabolism of drugs that are
mainly metabolized by this enzyme
may be impaired and exposure to
these drugs increased. The dose of
such drugs may have to be reduced
when ranolazine is co-administered).
Products include:

Testosterone Cypionate (Ranolazine can inhibit the activity of
CYP2D6 and, thus, the metabolism
of drugs that are mainly metabolized
by this enzyme may be impaired and
exposure to these drugs increased.
The dose of such drugs may have to
be reduced when ranolazine is
co-administered).

No products indexed under this
heading.

Testosterone Enanthate (Ranolazine can inhibit the activity of
CYP2D6 and, thus, the metabolism
of drugs that are mainly metabolized
by this enzyme may be impaired and
exposure to these drugs increased.
The dose of such drugs may have to
be reduced when ranolazine is
co-administered).

No products indexed under this
heading.

Testosterone Propionate (Ranolazine can inhibit the activity of
CYP2D6 and, thus, the metabolism
of drugs that are mainly metabolized
by this enzyme may be impaired and
exposure to these drugs increased.
The dose of such drugs may have to
be reduced when ranolazine is
co-administered).

No products indexed under this
heading.

Thioridazine (Ranolazine can inhibit
the activity of CYP2D6 and, thus, the
metabolism of drugs that are mainly
metabolized by this enzyme may be
impaired and exposure to these
drugs increased. The dose of such
drugs may have to be reduced when
ranolazine is co-administered).

No products indexed under this
heading.

Thioridazine Hydrochloride
(Ranolazine has been shown to prolong the QTc interval in a dose-
related manner. Because of possible
additive effects on the QT interval,
ranolazine is contraindicated with
drugs that prolong the QTc interval).
Products include:

Thiothixene (Ranolazine has been
shown to prolong the QTc interval in
a dose-related manner. Because of
possible additive effects on the QT
interval, ranolazine is contraindicated with drugs that prolong the
QTc interval, such as antipsychotics.
Ranolazine can inhibit the activity of
CYP2D6 and, thus, the metabolism
of drugs that are mainly metabolized
by this enzyme, such as some antipsychotics, may be impaired and
exposure to these drugs increased).
Products include:

Timolol Maleate (Ranolazine can
inhibit the activity of CYP2D6 and,
thus, the metabolism of drugs that
are mainly metabolized by this
enzyme may be impaired and exposure to these drugs increased. The
dose of such drugs may have to be
reduced when ranolazine is co-
administered). Products include:

Tocainide Hydrochloride (Ranolazine has been shown to prolong the
QTc interval in a dose-related manner. Because of possible additive
effects on the QT interval, ranolazine
is contraindicated with drugs that
prolong the QTc interval).

No products indexed under this
heading.

Tolterodine Tartrate (Ranolazine
can inhibit the activity of CYP2D6
and, thus, the metabolism of drugs
that are mainly metabolized by this
enzyme may be impaired and exposure to these drugs increased. The
dose of such drugs may have to be
reduced when ranolazine is co-
administered). Products include:

Tramadol Hydrochloride (Ranolazine can inhibit the activity of
CYP2D6 and, thus, the metabolism
of drugs that are mainly metabolized

by this enzyme may be impaired and
exposure to these drugs increased.
The dose of such drugs may have to
be reduced when ranolazine is co-
administered). Products include:

Trazodone Hydrochloride (Ranolazine can inhibit the activity of
CYP2D6 and, thus, the metabolism
of drugs that are mainly metabolized
by this enzyme may be impaired and
exposure to these drugs increased.
The dose of such drugs may have to
be reduced when ranolazine is
co-administered).

No products indexed under this
heading.

Triazolam (Ranolazine can inhibit
the activity of CYP2D6 and, thus, the
metabolism of drugs that are mainly
metabolized by this enzyme may be
impaired and exposure to these
drugs increased. The dose of such
drugs may have to be reduced when
ranolazine is co-administered).

No products indexed under this
heading.

Trifluoperazine Hydrochloride
(Ranolazine has been shown to prolong the QTc interval in a dose-
related manner. Because of possible
additive effects on the QT interval,
ranolazine is contraindicated with
drugs that prolong the QTc interval).

No products indexed under this
heading.

Trimipramine Maleate (Ranolazine has been shown to prolong the
QTc interval in a dose-related manner. Because of possible additive
effects on the QT interval, ranolazine
is contraindicated with drugs that
prolong the QTc interval).

No products indexed under this
heading.

Troleandomycin (Ranolazine is
primarily metabolized by CYP3A.
Use of ranolazine with potent or
moderately potent inhibitors of
CYP3A, such as macrolide antibiotics, is contraindicated because concomitant administration will increase
ranolazine plasma levels and QTc
prolongation).

No products indexed under this
heading.

Venlafaxine Hydrochloride (Ranolazine is primarily metabolized by
CYP3A. Use of ranolazine with
potent or moderately potent inhibitors of CYP3A is contraindicated
because concomitant administration
will increase ranolazine plasma levels and QTc prolongation). Products
include:

Verapamil Hydrochloride (Ranolazine is primarily metabolized by
CYP3A. Use of ranolazine with
potent or moderately potent inhibitors of CYP3A is contraindicated
because concomitant administration
will increase ranolazine plasma levels and QTc prolongation). Products
include:

Vinblastine Sulfate (Ranolazine
can inhibit the activity of CYP2D6
and, thus, the metabolism of drugs
that are mainly metabolized by this
enzyme may be impaired and exposure to these drugs increased. The
dose of such drugs may have to be
reduced when ranolazine is
co-administered).

No products indexed under this
heading.

Voriconazole (Ranolazine is primarily metabolized by CYP3A. Use of
ranolazine with potent or moderately
potent inhibitors of CYP3A is contraindicated because concomitant
administration will increase ranolazine plasma levels and QTc prolongation). Products include:

Zafirlukast (Ranolazine is primarily
metabolized by CYP3A. Use of ranolazine with potent or moderately
potent inhibitors of CYP3A is contraindicated because concomitant
administration will increase ranolazine plasma levels and QTc prolongation). Products include:

Zileuton (Ranolazine is primarily
metabolized by CYP3A. Use of ranolazine with potent or moderately
potent inhibitors of CYP3A is contraindicated because concomitant
administration will increase ranolazine plasma levels and QTc prolongation). Products include:

Ziprasidone Hydrochloride (Ranolazine has been shown to prolong the
QTc interval in a dose-related
manner. Because of possible additive effects on the QT interval, ranolazine is contraindicated with drugs
that prolong the QTc interval).
Products include:

Zonisamide (Ranolazine can inhibit
the activity of CYP2D6 and, thus, the
metabolism of drugs that are mainly
metabolized by this enzyme may be
impaired and exposure to these
drugs increased. The dose of such
drugs may have to be reduced when
ranolazine is co-administered).
Products include:

Food Interactions

Grapefruit (Ranolazine is primarily
metabolized by CYP3A. Use of ranolazine with potent or moderately potent
inhibitors of CYP3A, such as grapefruit
juice or grapefruit containing products,
is contraindicated because concomitant
administration will increase ranolazine
plasma levels and QTc prolongation).

Grapefruit Juice (Ranolazine is primarily metabolized by CYP3A. Use of ranolazine with potent or moderately potent
inhibitors of CYP3A, such as grapefruit
juice or grapefruit containing products,
is contraindicated because concomitant
administration will increase ranolazine
plasma levels and QTc prolongation).

RANICLOR TABLETS, CHEWABLE

(Cefaclor Monohydrate) 2505
May interact with oral anticoagulants. Compounds in these categories include:

Anisindione (There have been
reports of increased anticoagulant
effect when cefaclor and oral anticoagulants were administered concomitantly). Products include:

Miradon Tablets 3042

Dicumarol (There have been reports of increased anticoagulant effect when cefaclor and oral anticoagulants were administered concomitantly).

No products indexed under this heading.

Warfarin Sodium (There have been reports of increased anticoagulant effect when cefaclor and oral anticoagulants were administered concomitantly). Products include:

Coumadin for Injection 898
Coumadin Tablets 898

RAPAMUNE ORAL SOLUTION AND TABLETS

(Sirolimus) 3475

May interact with ACE inhibitors, cytochrome p450 3a4 inducers (selected), cytochrome p450 3a4 inhibitors (selected), cytochrome p450 3a4 substrates (selected), erythromycin, fibrates, glycoprotein (GP) IIb/IIIa inhibitors, HMG-CoA reductase inhibitors, phenytoin, protease inhibitors, vaccines, live, and certain other agents. Compounds in these categories include:

Abciximab (Strong inhibitors of P-gp significantly decrease the metabolism of sirolimus and increase sirolimus concentrations). Products include:

ReoPro Vials 1809

Acetazolamide (Sirolimus is extensively metabolized by the CYP3A4 isoenzyme in the gut wall and liver. Co-administration with inhibitors of CYP3A4 may decrease the metabolism of sirolimus and increase sirolimus levels. Co-administration with strong inducers of CYP3A4 is not recommended).

No products indexed under this heading.

Alfentanil Hydrochloride (Care should be exercised when drugs or other substances metabolized by CYP3A4 are administered concomitantly with sirolimus).

No products indexed under this heading.

Allium sativum (Sirolimus is extensively metabolized by the CYP3A4 isoenzyme in the gut wall and liver. Co-administration with inducers of CYP3A4 may increase the metabolism of sirolimus and decrease sirolimus levels. Co-administration with strong inducers of CYP3A4 is not recommended).

No products indexed under this heading.

Alprazolam (Care should be exercised when drugs or other substances metabolized by CYP3A4 are administered concomitantly with sirolimus). Products include:

Niravam Orally Disintegrating Tablets 3092

Amiodarone Hydrochloride (Sirolimus is extensively metabolized by the CYP3A4 isoenzyme in the gut wall and liver. Co-administration with inhibitors of CYP3A4 may decrease the metabolism of sirolimus and increase sirolimus levels. Co-administration with strong inducers of CYP3A4 is not recommended).

No products indexed under this heading.

Amitriptyline Hydrochloride (Care should be exercised when drugs or other substances metabolized by CYP3A4 are administered concomitantly with sirolimus).

No products indexed under this heading.

Amlodipine Besylate (Care should be exercised when drugs or other substances metabolized by CYP3A4 are administered concomitantly with sirolimus). Products include:

Caduet Tablets 2508
Lotrel Capsules 2249
Norvasc Tablets 2545

Amprenavir (Sirolimus is extensively metabolized by the CYP3A4 isoenzyme in the gut wall and liver. Co-administration with inhibitors of CYP3A4 may decrease the metabolism of sirolimus and increase sirolimus levels. Co-administration with strong inducers of CYP3A4 is not recommended). Products include:

Agenerase Capsules 1327
Agenerase Oral Solution 1332

Anastrozole (Sirolimus is extensively metabolized by the CYP3A4 isoenzyme in the gut wall and liver. Co-administration with inhibitors of CYP3A4 may decrease the metabolism of sirolimus and increase sirolimus levels. Co-administration with strong inducers of CYP3A4 is not recommended). Products include:

Arimidex Tablets 673

Aprepitant (Sirolimus is extensively metabolized by the CYP3A4 isoenzyme in the gut wall and liver. Co-administration with inhibitors of CYP3A4 may decrease the metabolism of sirolimus and increase sirolimus levels. Co-administration with strong inducers of CYP3A4 is not recommended). Products include:

Emend Capsules 1963

Astemizole (Care should be exercised when drugs or other substances metabolized by CYP3A4 are administered concomitantly with sirolimus).

No products indexed under this heading.

Atorvastatin Calcium (Co-administration of sirolimus with cyclosporine in conjunction with HMG-CoA reductase inhibitors should be monitored for the possible development of rhabdomyolysis; in clinical trials, the concurrent use of sirolimus and HMG-CoA reductase inhibitors was well tolerated). Products include:

Caduet Tablets 2508
Lipitor Tablets 2483

BCG Vaccine (During treatment with sirolimus, vaccination may be less effective. The use of live vaccinations should be avoided).

No products indexed under this heading.

Belladonna Ergotamine (Care should be exercised when drugs or other substances metabolized by CYP3A4 are administered concomitantly with sirolimus).

No products indexed under this heading.

Benazepril Hydrochloride (In rare cases, the concomitant administration of sirolimus and ACE inhibitors has resulted in angioneurotic edema-type reactions). Products include:

Lotensin Tablets 2243
Lotensin HCT Tablets 2246
Lotrel Capsules 2249

Betamethasone Acetate (Sirolimus is extensively metabolized by the CYP3A4 isoenzyme in the gut wall and liver. Co-administration with inducers of CYP3A4 may increase the metabolism of sirolimus and decrease sirolimus levels. Co-administration with strong inducers of CYP3A4 is not recommended).

No products indexed under this heading.

Betamethasone Sodium Phosphate (Sirolimus is extensively metabolized by the CYP3A4 isoenzyme in the gut wall and liver. Co-administration with inducers of CYP3A4 may increase the metabolism of sirolimus and decrease sirolimus levels. Co-administration with strong inducers of CYP3A4 is not recommended).

No products indexed under this heading.

Bromocriptine Mesylate (Sirolimus is extensively metabolized by the CYP3A4 isoenzyme; co-administration with inhibitors of CYP3A4, such as bromocriptine, may decrease the metabolism of sirolimus and increase the plasma levels of sirolimus).

No products indexed under this heading.

Buspirone Hydrochloride (Care should be exercised when drugs or other substances metabolized by CYP3A4 are administered concomitantly with sirolimus).

No products indexed under this heading.

Busulfan (Care should be exercised when drugs or other substances metabolized by CYP3A4 are administered concomitantly with sirolimus). Products include:

I.V. Busulfex 2493
Myleran Tablets 1525

Captopril (In rare cases, the concomitant administration of sirolimus and ACE inhibitors has resulted in angioneurotic edema-type reactions). Products include:

Captopril Tablets 2149

Carbamazepine (Sirolimus is extensively metabolized by the CYP3A4 isoenzyme; co-administration with inducers of CYP3A4, such as carbamazepine, may increase the metabolism of sirolimus and decrease the plasma levels of sirolimus). Products include:

Carbatrol Capsules 3171
Equetro Extended-Release Capsules 3180
Tegretol/Tegretol-XR 2295

Cerivastatin Sodium (Co-administration of sirolimus with cyclosporine in conjunction with HMG-CoA reductase inhibitors should be monitored for the possible development of rhabdomyolysis; in clinical trials, the concurrent use of sirolimus and HMG-CoA reductase inhibitors was well tolerated).

No products indexed under this heading.

Chlorpheniramine (Care should be exercised when drugs or other substances metabolized by CYP3A4 are administered concomitantly with sirolimus).

No products indexed under this heading.

Chlorpheniramine Maleate (Care should be exercised when drugs or other substances metabolized by CYP3A4 are administered concomitantly with sirolimus). Products include:

Advil Allergy Sinus Caplets 770
Advil Multi-Symptom Cold Caplets 770
BC Allergy Sinus Cold Powder 677
Comtrex Maximum Strength Cold & Cough Day/Night Caplets - Night Formulation 726
Comtrex Maximum Strength Day/Night Severe Cold & Sinus Caplets - Night Formulation 725
Contac Cold and Flu Maximum Strength Caplets 728
Contac Cold and Flu Day and Night Caplets (Night Formulation Only) 727
Children's Dimetapp Long Acting Cough Plus Cold Syrup 731
Robitussin Cough & Cold Long-Acting Liquid 735
Robitussin Cough & Allergy Syrup .. 736
Robitussin Cough & Cold Nighttime Liquid 736
Robitussin Cough, Cold & Flu Nighttime Liquid 738
Robitussin Pediatric Cough & Cold Long-Acting Liquid 735
Robitussin Pediatric Cough & Cold Nighttime Liquid 736
Triaminic Cold & Allergy Liquid 746
Triaminic Cough & Runny Nose Softchews 748
Children's Tylenol Plus Flu Oral Suspension 749
Tylenol Allergy Multi-Symptom Caplets with Cool Burst and Gelcaps 1872
Children's Tylenol Plus Cold Suspension Liquid 1879
Children's Tylenol Plus Cough & Runny Nose Suspension Liquid 1879
Children's Tylenol Plus Flu Suspension Liquid 1881
Children's Tylenol Plus Multi-Symptom Cold Suspension Liquid 1879
Tylenol Cold Head Congestion Nighttime Caplets with Cool Burst 1873
Tylenol Cold Multi-Symptom Nighttime Caplets with Cool Burst 1874
Tylenol Sinus Congestion & Pain Nighttime Caplets with Cool Burst 1876
Vicks 44M Cough, Cold & Flu Relief Liquid 2680
Pediatric Vicks 44m Cough & Cold Relief Liquid 2676
Children's Vicks NyQuil Cold/Cough Relief 756
Children's Vicks NyQuil Cold/Cough Relief Liquid 2680
Zicam Maximum Strength Flu Daytime 768

Chlorpheniramine Polistirex (Care should be exercised when drugs or other substances metabolized by CYP3A4 are administered concomitantly with sirolimus). Products include:

Tussionex Pennkinetic Extended-Release Suspension 3327

Chlorpheniramine Tannate (Care should be exercised when drugs or other substances metabolized by CYP3A4 are administered concomitantly with sirolimus).

No products indexed under this heading.

Cimetidine (Sirolimus is extensively metabolized by the CYP3A4 isoenzyme; co-administration with inhibitors of CYP3A4, such as cimetidine, may decrease the metabolism of sirolimus and increase the plasma levels of sirolimus). Products include:

Tagamet HB 200 Tablets 664

Cimetidine Hydrochloride (Sirolimus is extensively metabolized by the CYP3A4 isoenzyme; co-administration with inhibitors of CYP3A4, such as cimetidine, may decrease the metabolism of sirolimus and increase the plasma levels of sirolimus).
No products indexed under this heading.

Ciprofloxacin (Sirolimus is extensively metabolized by the CYP3A4 isoenzyme in the gut wall and liver. Co-administration with inhibitors of CYP3A4 may decrease the metabolism of sirolimus and increase sirolimus levels. Co-administration with strong inducers of CYP3A4 is not recommended). Products include:
Cipro Oral Suspension 2977
Cipro I.V. 2984
Cipro XR Tablets 2990
Ciprodex Otic Suspension 559

Ciprofloxacin Hydrochloride (Sirolimus is extensively metabolized by the CYP3A4 isoenzyme in the gut wall and liver. Co-administration with inducers of CYP3A4 may increase the metabolism of sirolimus and decrease sirolimus levels. Co-administration with strong inducers of CYP3A4 is not recommended). Products include:
Ciloxan Ophthalmic Ointment 559
Ciloxan Ophthalmic Solution .... ⊙206
Cipro Tablets 2977
Proquin XR Tablets 1153

Cisapride (Sirolimus is extensively metabolized by the CYP3A4 isoenzyme; co-administration with inhibitors of CYP3A4, such as cisapride, may decrease the metabolism of sirolimus and increase the plasma levels of sirolimus).
No products indexed under this heading.

Cisplatin (Sirolimus is extensively metabolized by the CYP3A4 isoenzyme in the gut wall and liver. Co-administration with inducers of CYP3A4 may increase the metabolism of sirolimus and decrease sirolimus levels. Co-administration with strong inducers of CYP3A4 is not recommended).
No products indexed under this heading.

Clarithromycin (Sirolimus is extensively metabolized by the CYP3A4 isoenzyme; co-administration with inhibitors of CYP3A4, such as clarithromycin, may decrease the metabolism of sirolimus and increase the plasma levels of sirolimus). Products include:
Biaxin/Biaxin XL 402
PREVPAC 3284

Clofibrate (Co-administration of sirolimus with cyclosporine in conjunction with fibrates should be monitored for the possible development of rhabdomyolysis; in clinical trials, the concurrent use of sirolimus and fibrates was well tolerated).
No products indexed under this heading.

Clotrimazole (Co-administration of sirolimus and clotrimazole may increase sirolimus blood concentrations). Products include:
Desenex Athlete's Foot Cream .... ■635
Lotrimin 3039
Lotrisone 3040

Cortisone Acetate (Sirolimus is extensively metabolized by the CYP3A4 isoenzyme in the gut wall and liver. Co-administration with inducers of CYP3A4 may increase the metabolism of sirolimus and decrease sirolimus levels. Co-administration with strong inducers of CYP3A4 is not recommended).
No products indexed under this heading.

Cyclosporine (Co-administration of sirolimus simultaneously with cyclosporine capsules modified results in increased AUC and Cmax relative to sirolimus alone; because of the effect of cyclosporine capsules, modified, it is recommended that sirolimus should be taken 4 hours after cyclosporine oral solution modified and/or cyclosporine modified capsules; combination use is associated with hepatic artery thrombosis (HAT); the safety and efficacy of sirolimus has not been established in liver transplant patients and, therefore, such use is not recommended). Products include:
Gengraf Capsules 459
Neoral Oral Solution 2259
Neoral Soft Gelatin Capsules 2259
Restasis Ophthalmic Emulsion 575
Sandimmune 2275

Dalfopristin (Sirolimus is extensively metabolized by the CYP3A4 isoenzyme in the gut wall and liver. Co-administration with inhibitors of CYP3A4 may decrease the metabolism of sirolimus and increase sirolimus levels. Co-administration with strong inducers of CYP3A4 is not recommended).
No products indexed under this heading.

Danazol (Sirolimus is extensively metabolized by the CYP3A4 isoenzyme; co-administration with inhibitors of CYP3A4, such as danazol, may decrease the metabolism of sirolimus and increase the plasma levels of sirolimus).
No products indexed under this heading.

Delavirdine Mesylate (Sirolimus is extensively metabolized by the CYP3A4 isoenzyme in the gut wall and liver. Co-administration with inhibitors of CYP3A4 may decrease the metabolism of sirolimus and increase sirolimus levels. Co-administration with strong inducers of CYP3A4 is not recommended). Products include:
Rescriptor Tablets 2551

Desogestrel (Care should be exercised when drugs or other substances metabolized by CYP3A4 are administered concomitantly with sirolimus). Products include:
Mircette Tablets 1066

Dexamethasone (Sirolimus is extensively metabolized by the CYP3A4 isoenzyme in the gut wall and liver. Co-administration with inducers of CYP3A4 may increase the metabolism of sirolimus and decrease sirolimus levels. Co-administration with strong inducers of CYP3A4 is not recommended). Products include:
Ciprodex Otic Suspension 559
Decadron Tablets 1951
TobraDex Ophthalmic Ointment 562
TobraDex Ophthalmic Suspension 563

Dexamethasone Acetate (Sirolimus is extensively metabolized by the CYP3A4 isoenzyme in the gut wall and liver. Co-administration with inducers of CYP3A4 may increase the metabolism of sirolimus and decrease sirolimus levels. Co-administration with strong inducers of CYP3A4 is not recommended).
No products indexed under this heading.

Dexamethasone Sodium Phosphate (Sirolimus is extensively metabolized by the CYP3A4 isoenzyme in the gut wall and liver. Co-administration with inducers of CYP3A4 may increase the metabolism of sirolimus and decrease sirolimus levels. Co-administration with strong inducers of CYP3A4 is not recommended).
No products indexed under this heading.

Diazepam (Care should be exercised when drugs or other substances metabolized by CYP3A4 are administered concomitantly with sirolimus). Products include:
Diastat Rectal Delivery System 3343
Valium Tablets 2819

Dihydroergotamine Mesylate (Care should be exercised when drugs or other substances metabolized by CYP3A4 are administered concomitantly with sirolimus). Products include:
Migranal Nasal Spray 3348

Diltiazem Hydrochloride (Co-administration in healthy individuals significantly affects the bioavailability of sirolimus; monitor sirolimus levels; a dose adjustment may be necessary). Products include:
Cardizem LA Extended Release Tablets 1728
Tiazac Capsules 1201

Diltiazem Maleate (Sirolimus is extensively metabolized by the CYP3A4 isoenzyme in the gut wall and liver. Co-administration with inhibitors of CYP3A4 may decrease the metabolism of sirolimus and increase sirolimus levels. Co-administration with strong inducers of CYP3A4 is not recommended).
No products indexed under this heading.

Disopyramide (Care should be exercised when drugs or other substances metabolized by CYP3A4 are administered concomitantly with sirolimus).
No products indexed under this heading.

Disopyramide Phosphate (Care should be exercised when drugs or other substances metabolized by CYP3A4 are administered concomitantly with sirolimus).
No products indexed under this heading.

Disulfiram (Care should be exercised when drugs or other substances metabolized by CYP3A4 are administered concomitantly with sirolimus).
No products indexed under this heading.

Doxorubicin Hydrochloride (Sirolimus is extensively metabolized by the CYP3A4 isoenzyme in the gut wall and liver. Co-administration with inducers of CYP3A4 may increase the metabolism of sirolimus and decrease sirolimus levels. Co-administration with strong inducers of CYP3A4 is not recommended).
No products indexed under this heading.

Dronabinol (Care should be exercised when drugs or other substances metabolized by CYP3A4 are administered concomitantly with sirolimus). Products include:
Marinol Capsules 3333

Efavirenz (Sirolimus is extensively metabolized by the CYP3A4 isoenzyme in the gut wall and liver. Co-administration with inhibitors of CYP3A4 may decrease the metabolism of sirolimus and increase sirolimus levels. Co-administration with strong inducers of CYP3A4 is not recommended). Products include:
Atripla Tablets 945
Sustiva Capsules 930
Sustiva Tablets 930

Enalapril Maleate (In rare cases, the concomitant administration of sirolimus and ACE inhibitors has resulted in angioneurotic edema-type reactions). Products include:
Vasotec I.V. Injection 2103

Enalaprilat (In rare cases, the concomitant administration of sirolimus and ACE inhibitors has resulted in angioneurotic edema-type reactions).
No products indexed under this heading.

Eptifibatide (Strong inhibitors of P-gp significantly decrease the metabolism of sirolimus and increase sirolimus concentrations). Products include:
Integrilin Injection 3020

Ergotamine Tartrate (Care should be exercised when drugs or other substances metabolized by CYP3A4 are administered concomitantly with sirolimus).
No products indexed under this heading.

Erythromycin (Sirolimus is extensively metabolized by the CYP3A4 isoenzyme; co-administration with inhibitors of CYP3A4, such as erythromycin, may decrease the metabolism of sirolimus and increase the plasma levels of sirolimus. Co-administration of sirolimus oral solution or tablets and erythromycin is not recommended). Products include:
Ery-Tab Tablets 449
Erythromycin Base Filmtab Tablets 455
Erythromycin Delayed-Release Capsules, USP 457
PCE Dispertab Tablets 515

Erythromycin Estolate (Sirolimus is extensively metabolized by the CYP3A4 isoenzyme; co-administration with inhibitors of CYP3A4, such as erythromycin, may decrease the metabolism of sirolimus and increase the plasma levels of sirolimus. Co-administration of sirolimus oral solution or tablets and erythromycin is not recommended).
No products indexed under this heading.

Erythromycin Ethylsuccinate (Sirolimus is extensively metabolized by the CYP3A4 isoenzyme; co-administration with inhibitors of CYP3A4, such as erythromycin, may decrease the metabolism of sirolimus and increase the plasma levels of sirolimus. Co-administration of sirolimus oral solution or tablets and erythromycin is not recommended). Products include:
E.E.S. 451
EryPed 447

Erythromycin Gluceptate (Sirolimus is extensively metabolized by the CYP3A4 isoenzyme; co-administration with inhibitors of CYP3A4, such as erythromycin, may decrease the metabolism of sirolimus and increase the plasma levels of sirolimus. Co-administration of sirolimus oral solution or tablets and erythromycin is not recommended).
No products indexed under this heading.

Erythromycin Lactobionate (Sirolimus is extensively metabolized by the CYP3A4 isoenzyme; co-administration with inhibitors of CYP3A4, such as erythromycin, may decrease the metabolism of sirolimus and increase the plasma levels of sirolimus. Co-administration of sirolimus oral solution or tablets and erythromycin is not recommended).
No products indexed under this heading.

Erythromycin Stearate (Sirolimus is extensively metabolized by the CYP3A4 isoenzyme; co-administration with inhibitors of CYP3A4, such as erythromycin, may decrease the metabolism of sirolimus and increase the plasma levels of sirolimus. Co-administration of sirolimus oral solution or tablets and erythromycin is not recommended). Products include:
Erythrocin Stearate Filmtab Tablets **453**

Esomeprazole Magnesium (Sirolimus is extensively metabolized by the CYP3A4 isoenzyme in the gut wall and liver. Co-administration with inhibitors of CYP3A4 may decrease the metabolism of sirolimus and increase sirolimus levels. Co-administration with strong inducers of CYP3A4 is not recommended). Products include:
Nexium Delayed-Release Capsules **655**

Estradiol (Care should be exercised when drugs or other substances metabolized by CYP3A4 are administered concomitantly with sirolimus). Products include:
Angeliq Tablets **762**
Climara Transdermal System **771**
Climara Pro Transdermal System **776**
Estrasorb Topical Emulsion **1147**
Estring Vaginal Ring **2635**
Menostar Transdermal System **782**
Vagifem Tablets **2334**

Estradiol Benzoate (Care should be exercised when drugs or other substances metabolized by CYP3A4 are administered concomitantly with sirolimus).
No products indexed under this heading.

Estradiol Cypionate (Care should be exercised when drugs or other substances metabolized by CYP3A4 are administered concomitantly with sirolimus).
No products indexed under this heading.

Estradiol Valerate (Care should be exercised when drugs or other substances metabolized by CYP3A4 are administered concomitantly with sirolimus).
No products indexed under this heading.

Ethinyl Estradiol (Care should be exercised when drugs or other substances metabolized by CYP3A4 are administered concomitantly with sirolimus). Products include:
Mircette Tablets **1066**
NuvaRing **2340**
Ortho-Cyclen/Ortho Tri-Cyclen **2429**
Ortho Evra Transdermal System **2417**
Ortho Tri-Cyclen Lo Tablets **2436**
Seasonique Tablets **1077**
Yasmin 28 Tablets **796**
Yaz Tablets **803**

Ethosuximide (Sirolimus is extensively metabolized by the CYP3A4 isoenzyme in the gut wall and liver. Co-administration with inducers of CYP3A4 may increase the metabolism of sirolimus and decrease sirolimus levels. Co-administration with strong inducers of CYP3A4 is not recommended).
No products indexed under this heading.

Ethynodiol Diacetate (Care should be exercised when drugs or other substances metabolized by CYP3A4 are administered concomitantly with sirolimus).
No products indexed under this heading.

Etoposide (Care should be exercised when drugs or other substances metabolized by CYP3A4 are administered concomitantly with sirolimus).
No products indexed under this heading.

Etoposide Phosphate (Care should be exercised when drugs or other substances metabolized by CYP3A4 are administered concomitantly with sirolimus).
No products indexed under this heading.

Felbamate (Sirolimus is extensively metabolized by the CYP3A4 isoenzyme in the gut wall and liver. Co-administration with inducers of CYP3A4 may increase the metabolism of sirolimus and decrease sirolimus levels. Co-administration with strong inducers of CYP3A4 is not recommended).
No products indexed under this heading.

Felodipine (Care should be exercised when drugs or other substances metabolized by CYP3A4 are administered concomitantly with sirolimus).
No products indexed under this heading.

Fenofibrate (Co-administration of sirolimus with cyclosporine in conjunction with fibrates should be monitored for the possible development of rhabdomyolysis; in clinical trials, the concurrent use of sirolimus and fibrates was well tolerated). Products include:
Lofibra Tablets **1219**
Lofibra Capsules **1216**
Tricor Tablets **527**
Triglide Tablets **3123**

Fentanyl (Care should be exercised when drugs or other substances metabolized by CYP3A4 are administered concomitantly with sirolimus). Products include:
Duragesic Transdermal System **2373**
Ionsys Transdermal System **2379**

Fentanyl Citrate (Care should be exercised when drugs or other substances metabolized by CYP3A4 are administered concomitantly with sirolimus). Products include:
Actiq **979**

Fluconazole (Sirolimus is extensively metabolized by the CYP3A4 isoenzyme; co-administration with inhibitors of CYP3A4, such as fluconazole, may decrease the metabolism of sirolimus and increase the plasma levels of sirolimus).
No products indexed under this heading.

Fludrocortisone Acetate (Sirolimus is extensively metabolized by the CYP3A4 isoenzyme in the gut wall and liver. Co-administration with inducers of CYP3A4 may increase the metabolism of sirolimus and decrease sirolimus levels. Co-administration with strong inducers of CYP3A4 is not recommended).
No products indexed under this heading.

Fluoxetine Hydrochloride (Sirolimus is extensively metabolized by the CYP3A4 isoenzyme in the gut wall and liver. Co-administration with inhibitors of CYP3A4 may decrease the metabolism of sirolimus and increase sirolimus levels. Co-administration with strong inducers of CYP3A4 is not recommended). Products include:
Prozac Pulvules and Liquid **1801**
Symbyax Capsules **1819**

Fluvastatin Sodium (Co-administration of sirolimus with cyclosporine in conjunction with HMG-CoA reductase inhibitors should be monitored for the possible development of rhabdomyolysis; in clinical trials, the concurrent use of sirolimus and HMG-CoA reductase inhibitors was well tolerated). Products include:
Lescol Capsules **2233**
Lescol XL Tablets **2233**

Fluvoxamine Maleate (Sirolimus is extensively metabolized by the CYP3A4 isoenzyme in the gut wall and liver. Co-administration with inhibitors of CYP3A4 may decrease the metabolism of sirolimus and increase sirolimus levels. Co-administration with strong inducers of CYP3A4 is not recommended).
No products indexed under this heading.

Fosamprenavir Calcium (Sirolimus is extensively metabolized by the CYP3A4 isoenzyme in the gut wall and liver. Co-administration with inhibitors of CYP3A4 may decrease the metabolism of sirolimus and increase sirolimus levels. Co-administration with strong inducers of CYP3A4 is not recommended). Products include:
Lexiva Tablets **1505**

Fosinopril Sodium (In rare cases, the concomitant administration of sirolimus and ACE inhibitors has resulted in angioneurotic edema-type reactions).
No products indexed under this heading.

Fosphenytoin Sodium (Sirolimus is extensively metabolized by the CYP3A4 isoenzyme; co-administration with inducers of CYP3A4, such as phenytoin, may increase the metabolism of sirolimus and decrease the plasma levels of sirolimus).
No products indexed under this heading.

Garlic Extract (Sirolimus is extensively metabolized by the CYP3A4 isoenzyme in the gut wall and liver. Co-administration with inducers of CYP3A4 may increase the metabolism of sirolimus and decrease sirolimus levels. Co-administration with strong inducers of CYP3A4 is not recommended).
No products indexed under this heading.

Garlic Oil (Sirolimus is extensively metabolized by the CYP3A4 isoenzyme in the gut wall and liver. Co-administration with inducers of CYP3A4 may increase the metabolism of sirolimus and decrease sirolimus levels. Co-administration with strong inducers of CYP3A4 is not recommended).
No products indexed under this heading.

Gemfibrozil (Co-administration of sirolimus with cyclosporine in conjunction with fibrates should be monitored for the possible development of rhabdomyolysis; in clinical trials, the concurrent use of sirolimus and fibrates was well tolerated).
No products indexed under this heading.

Haloperidol (Care should be exercised when drugs or other substances metabolized by CYP3A4 are administered concomitantly with sirolimus).
No products indexed under this heading.

Haloperidol Decanoate (Care should be exercised when drugs or other substances metabolized by CYP3A4 are administered concomitantly with sirolimus).
No products indexed under this heading.

Haloperidol Lactate (Care should be exercised when drugs or other substances metabolized by CYP3A4 are administered concomitantly with sirolimus).
No products indexed under this heading.

Hydrocortisone (Sirolimus is extensively metabolized by the CYP3A4 isoenzyme in the gut wall and liver. Co-administration with inducers of CYP3A4 may increase the metabolism of sirolimus and decrease sirolimus levels. Co-administration with strong inducers of CYP3A4 is not recommended). Products include:
Colocort Rectal Suspension, USP (Retention) 100 mg/60 mL **2476**
Hydrocortone Tablets **1989**
Preparation H Hydrocortisone Cream **646**

Hydrocortisone Acetate (Sirolimus is extensively metabolized by the CYP3A4 isoenzyme in the gut wall and liver. Co-administration with inducers of CYP3A4 may increase the metabolism of sirolimus and decrease sirolimus levels. Co-administration with strong inducers of CYP3A4 is not recommended). Products include:
Analpram-HC **1159**
Pramosone **1161**
ProctoFoam-HC **3099**

Hydrocortisone Butyrate (Sirolimus is extensively metabolized by the CYP3A4 isoenzyme in the gut wall and liver. Co-administration with inducers of CYP3A4 may increase the metabolism of sirolimus and decrease sirolimus levels. Co-administration with strong inducers of CYP3A4 is not recommended). Products include:

Locoid Lipocream Cream 1160

Hydrocortisone Cypionate (Sirolimus is extensively metabolized by the CYP3A4 isoenzyme in the gut wall and liver. Co-administration with inducers of CYP3A4 may increase the metabolism of sirolimus and decrease sirolimus levels. Co-administration with strong inducers of CYP3A4 is not recommended).

No products indexed under this heading.

Hydrocortisone Hemisuccinate (Sirolimus is extensively metabolized by the CYP3A4 isoenzyme in the gut wall and liver. Co-administration with inducers of CYP3A4 may increase the metabolism of sirolimus and decrease sirolimus levels. Co-administration with strong inducers of CYP3A4 is not recommended).

No products indexed under this heading.

Hydrocortisone Probutate (Sirolimus is extensively metabolized by the CYP3A4 isoenzyme in the gut wall and liver. Co-administration with inducers of CYP3A4 may increase the metabolism of sirolimus and decrease sirolimus levels. Co-administration with strong inducers of CYP3A4 is not recommended).

No products indexed under this heading.

Hydrocortisone Sodium Phosphate (Sirolimus is extensively metabolized by the CYP3A4 isoenzyme in the gut wall and liver. Co-administration with inducers of CYP3A4 may increase the metabolism of sirolimus and decrease sirolimus levels. Co-administration with strong inducers of CYP3A4 is not recommended).

No products indexed under this heading.

Hydrocortisone Sodium Succinate (Sirolimus is extensively metabolized by the CYP3A4 isoenzyme in the gut wall and liver. Co-administration with inducers of CYP3A4 may increase the metabolism of sirolimus and decrease sirolimus levels. Co-administration with strong inducers of CYP3A4 is not recommended).

No products indexed under this heading.

Hydrocortisone Valerate (Sirolimus is extensively metabolized by the CYP3A4 isoenzyme in the gut wall and liver. Co-administration with inducers of CYP3A4 may increase the metabolism of sirolimus and decrease sirolimus levels. Co-administration with strong inducers of CYP3A4 is not recommended).

No products indexed under this heading.

Hypericum (Potential for reduced sirolimus levels). Products include:

Satiete Tablets ⊞⊙832

Hypericum Perforatum (Sirolimus is extensively metabolized by the CYP3A4 isoenzyme in the gut wall and liver. Co-administration with inducers of CYP3A4 may increase the metabolism of sirolimus and decrease sirolimus levels. Co-administration with strong inducers of CYP3A4 is not recommended).

No products indexed under this heading.

Indinavir Sulfate (Sirolimus is extensively metabolized by the CYP3A4 isoenzyme in the gut wall and liver. Co-administration with inhibitors of CYP3A4 may decrease the metabolism of sirolimus and increase sirolimus levels. Co-administration with strong inducers of CYP3A4 is not recommended). Products include:

Crixivan Capsules 1940

Isoniazid (Sirolimus is extensively metabolized by the CYP3A4 isoenzyme in the gut wall and liver. Co-administration with inhibitors of CYP3A4 may decrease the metabolism of sirolimus and increase sirolimus levels. Co-administration with strong inducers of CYP3A4 is not recommended).

No products indexed under this heading.

Isradipine (Care should be exercised when drugs or other substances metabolized by CYP3A4 are administered concomitantly with sirolimus). Products include:

DynaCirc CR Tablets 2721

Itraconazole (Sirolimus is extensively metabolized by the CYP3A4 isoenzyme; co-administration with inhibitors of CYP3A4, such as itraconazole, may decrease the metabolism of sirolimus and increase the plasma levels of sirolimus).

No products indexed under this heading.

Ketoconazole (Multiple-dose ketoconazole administration significantly affected the rate and extent of absorption and sirolimus exposure; sirolimus should not be co-administered with ketoconazole). Products include:

Nizoral A-D Shampoo, 1% 1868

Levonorgestrel (Care should be exercised when drugs or other substances metabolized by CYP3A4 are administered concomitantly with sirolimus). Products include:

Climara Pro Transdermal System 776
Mirena Intrauterine System 787
Plan B Tablets 1076
Seasonique Tablets 1077

Lidocaine (Care should be exercised when drugs or other substances metabolized by CYP3A4 are administered concomitantly with sirolimus). Products include:

Lidoderm Patch 1118
Synera Topical Patch 1137

Lidocaine Hydrochloride (Care should be exercised when drugs or other substances metabolized by CYP3A4 are administered concomitantly with sirolimus).

No products indexed under this heading.

Lisinopril (In rare cases, the concomitant administration of sirolimus and ACE inhibitors has resulted in angioneurotic edema-type reactions). Products include:

Prinivil Tablets 2052
Prinzide Tablets 2056

Lopinavir (Sirolimus is extensively metabolized by the CYP3A4 isoenzyme in the gut wall and liver. Co-administration with inhibitors of CYP3A4 may decrease the metabolism of sirolimus and increase sirolimus levels. Co-administration with strong inducers of CYP3A4 is not recommended). Products include:

Kaletra ... 476

Loratadine (Sirolimus is extensively metabolized by the CYP3A4 isoen-

zyme in the gut wall and liver. Co-administration with inhibitors of CYP3A4 may decrease the metabolism of sirolimus and increase sirolimus levels. Co-administration with strong inducers of CYP3A4 is not recommended). Products include:

Alavert Allergy & Sinus D-12 Hour Tablets.. ⊞⊙771
Alavert .. ⊞⊙771
Children's Claritin Allergy Oral Solution ⊞⊙771
Claritin Non-Drowsy 24 Hour Tablets.. ⊞⊙772
Claritin Reditabs 24 Hour Non-Drowsy Tablets ⊞⊙772
Claritin-D Non-Drowsy 12 Hour Tablets.. ⊞⊙772
Claritin-D Non-Drowsy 24 Hour Tablets.. ⊞⊙772

Lovastatin (Co-administration of sirolimus with cyclosporine in conjunction with HMG-CoA reductase inhibitors should be monitored for the possible development of rhabdomyolysis; in clinical trials, the concurrent use of sirolimus and HMG-CoA reductase inhibitors was well tolerated). Products include:

Advicor Tablets 1722
Altoprev Extended-Release Tablets...................................... 3109
Mevacor Tablets 2021

Measles, Mumps, Rubella and Varicella Virus Vaccine Live (During treatment with sirolimus, vaccination may be less effective. The use of live vaccinations should be avoided). Products include:

ProQuad 2064

Measles, Mumps & Rubella Virus Vaccine, Live (During treatment with sirolimus, vaccination may be less effective. The use of live vaccinations should be avoided). Products include:

M-M-R II 2006

Measles & Rubella Virus Vaccine Live (During treatment with sirolimus, vaccination may be less effective. The use of live vaccinations should be avoided).

No products indexed under this heading.

Measles Virus Vaccine Live (During treatment with sirolimus, vaccination may be less effective. The use of live vaccinations should be avoided). Products include:

Attenuvax 1914

Mephenytoin (Sirolimus is extensively metabolized by the CYP3A4 isoenzyme in the gut wall and liver. Co-administration with inducers of CYP3A4 may increase the metabolism of sirolimus and decrease sirolimus levels. Co-administration with strong inducers of CYP3A4 is not recommended).

No products indexed under this heading.

Mestranol (Care should be exercised when drugs or other substances metabolized by CYP3A4 are administered concomitantly with sirolimus).

No products indexed under this heading.

Methadone Hydrochloride (Care should be exercised when drugs or other substances metabolized by CYP3A4 are administered concomitantly with sirolimus).

No products indexed under this heading.

Methsuximide (Sirolimus is extensively metabolized by the CYP3A4 isoenzyme in the gut wall and liver. Co-administration with inducers of CYP3A4 may increase the metabolism of sirolimus and decrease sirolimus levels. Co-administration with strong inducers of CYP3A4 is not recommended).

No products indexed under this heading.

Methylprednisolone (Sirolimus is extensively metabolized by the CYP3A4 isoenzyme in the gut wall and liver. Co-administration with inducers of CYP3A4 may increase the metabolism of sirolimus and decrease sirolimus levels. Co-administration with strong inducers of CYP3A4 is not recommended).

No products indexed under this heading.

Methylprednisolone Acetate (Sirolimus is extensively metabolized by the CYP3A4 isoenzyme in the gut wall and liver. Co-administration with inducers of CYP3A4 may increase the metabolism of sirolimus and decrease sirolimus levels. Co-administration with strong inducers of CYP3A4 is not recommended). Products include:

Depo-Medrol Injectable Suspension 2617
Depo-Medrol Single-Dose Vial 2619

Methylprednisolone Sodium Succinate (Sirolimus is extensively metabolized by the CYP3A4 isoenzyme in the gut wall and liver. Co-administration with inducers of CYP3A4 may increase the metabolism of sirolimus and decrease sirolimus levels. Co-administration with strong inducers of CYP3A4 is not recommended).

No products indexed under this heading.

Metoclopramide Hydrochloride (Sirolimus is extensively metabolized by the CYP3A4 isoenzyme; co-administration with inhibitors of CYP3A4, such as metoclopramide, may decrease the metabolism of sirolimus and increase the plasma levels of sirolimus).

No products indexed under this heading.

Metronidazole (Sirolimus is extensively metabolized by the CYP3A4 isoenzyme in the gut wall and liver. Co-administration with inhibitors of CYP3A4 may decrease the metabolism of sirolimus and increase sirolimus levels. Co-administration with strong inducers of CYP3A4 is not recommended). Products include:

Metrogel 1% 1211
MetroGel-Vaginal Gel 1855
Vandazole Vaginal Gel 3338

Metronidazole Benzoate (Sirolimus is extensively metabolized by the CYP3A4 isoenzyme in the gut wall and liver. Co-administration with inhibitors of CYP3A4 may decrease the metabolism of sirolimus and increase sirolimus levels. Co-administration with strong inducers of CYP3A4 is not recommended).

No products indexed under this heading.

Metronidazole Hydrochloride (Sirolimus is extensively metabolized by the CYP3A4 isoenzyme in the gut wall and liver. Co-administration with inhibitors of CYP3A4 may decrease the metabolism of sirolimus and increase sirolimus levels. Co-administration with strong inducers of CYP3A4 is not recommended).
No products indexed under this heading.

Miconazole (Sirolimus is extensively metabolized by the CYP3A4 isoenzyme in the gut wall and liver. Co-administration with inhibitors of CYP3A4 may decrease the metabolism of sirolimus and increase sirolimus levels. Co-administration with strong inducers of CYP3A4 is not recommended).
No products indexed under this heading.

Miconazole Nitrate (Sirolimus is extensively metabolized by the CYP3A4 isoenzyme in the gut wall and liver. Co-administration with inhibitors of CYP3A4 may decrease the metabolism of sirolimus and increase sirolimus levels. Co-administration with strong inducers of CYP3A4 is not recommended). Products include:
Desenex ▣◻635
Desenex Jock Itch Spray Powder ... ▣◻635

Midazolam Hydrochloride (Care should be exercised when drugs or other substances metabolized by CYP3A4 are administered concomitantly with sirolimus).
No products indexed under this heading.

Modafinil (Sirolimus is extensively metabolized by the CYP3A4 isoenzyme in the gut wall and liver. Co-administration with inducers of CYP3A4 may increase the metabolism of sirolimus and decrease sirolimus levels. Co-administration with strong inducers of CYP3A4 is not recommended). Products include:
Provigil Tablets 988

Moexipril Hydrochloride (In rare cases, the concomitant administration of sirolimus and ACE inhibitors has resulted in angioneurotic edema-type reactions). Products include:
Uniretic Tablets 3100
Univasc Tablets 3104

Mumps Virus Vaccine, Live (During treatment with sirolimus, vaccination may be less effective. The use of live vaccinations should be avoided). Products include:
Mumpsvax 2031

Nefazodone Hydrochloride (Sirolimus is extensively metabolized by the CYP3A4 isoenzyme in the gut wall and liver. Co-administration with inhibitors of CYP3A4 may decrease the metabolism of sirolimus and increase sirolimus levels. Co-administration with strong inducers of CYP3A4 is not recommended).
No products indexed under this heading.

Nelfinavir Mesylate (Sirolimus is extensively metabolized by the CYP3A4 isoenzyme in the gut wall and liver. Co-administration with inhibitors of CYP3A4 may decrease the metabolism of sirolimus and increase sirolimus levels. Co-administration with strong inducers of CYP3A4 is not recommended). Products include:
Viracept 2577

Nevirapine (Sirolimus is extensively metabolized by the CYP3A4 isoenzyme in the gut wall and liver. Co-administration with inhibitors of CYP3A4 may decrease the metabolism of sirolimus and increase sirolimus levels. Co-administration with strong inducers of CYP3A4 is not recommended). Products include:
Viramune Oral Suspension 873
Viramune Tablets 873

Niacinamide (Sirolimus is extensively metabolized by the CYP3A4 isoenzyme in the gut wall and liver. Co-administration with inhibitors of CYP3A4 may decrease the metabolism of sirolimus and increase sirolimus levels. Co-administration with strong inducers of CYP3A4 is not recommended).
No products indexed under this heading.

Nicardipine Hydrochloride (Sirolimus is extensively metabolized by the CYP3A4 isoenzyme; co-administration with inhibitors of CYP3A4, such as nicardipine, may decrease the metabolism of sirolimus and increase the plasma levels of sirolimus). Products include:
Cardene I.V. 2497

Nicotinamide (Sirolimus is extensively metabolized by the CYP3A4 isoenzyme in the gut wall and liver. Co-administration with inhibitors of CYP3A4 may decrease the metabolism of sirolimus and increase sirolimus levels. Co-administration with strong inducers of CYP3A4 is not recommended). Products include:
Nicomide Tablets 1088

Nifedipine (Sirolimus is extensively metabolized by the CYP3A4 isoenzyme in the gut wall and liver. Co-administration with inhibitors of CYP3A4 may decrease the metabolism of sirolimus and increase sirolimus levels. Co-administration with strong inducers of CYP3A4 is not recommended). Products include:
Adalat CC Tablets 2964

Nimodipine (Care should be exercised when drugs or other substances metabolized by CYP3A4 are administered concomitantly with sirolimus). Products include:
Nimotop Capsules 749

Nisoldipine (Care should be exercised when drugs or other substances metabolized by CYP3A4 are administered concomitantly with sirolimus). Products include:
Sular Tablets 3122

Nitrendipine (Care should be exercised when drugs or other substances metabolized by CYP3A4 are administered concomitantly with sirolimus).
No products indexed under this heading.

Norethindrone (Care should be exercised when drugs or other substances metabolized by CYP3A4 are administered concomitantly with sirolimus). Products include:
Ortho Micronor Tablets 2426

Norethindrone Acetate (Care should be exercised when drugs or other substances metabolized by CYP3A4 are administered concomitantly with sirolimus).
No products indexed under this heading.

Norfloxacin (Sirolimus is extensively metabolized by the CYP3A4 isoenzyme in the gut wall and liver. Co-administration with inhibitors of

CYP3A4 may decrease the metabolism of sirolimus and increase sirolimus levels. Co-administration with strong inducers of CYP3A4 is not recommended). Products include:
Noroxin Tablets 2032

Norgestrel (Care should be exercised when drugs or other substances metabolized by CYP3A4 are administered concomitantly with sirolimus).
No products indexed under this heading.

Omeprazole (Sirolimus is extensively metabolized by the CYP3A4 isoenzyme in the gut wall and liver. Co-administration with inhibitors of CYP3A4 may decrease the metabolism of sirolimus and increase sirolimus levels. Co-administration with strong inducers of CYP3A4 is not recommended). Products include:
Zegerid Capsules 2958
Zegerid Powder for Oral Solution 2958

Ondansetron (Care should be exercised when drugs or other substances metabolized by CYP3A4 are administered concomitantly with sirolimus). Products include:
Zofran ODT Orally Disintegrating Tablets .. 1639

Ondansetron Hydrochloride (Care should be exercised when drugs or other substances metabolized by CYP3A4 are administered concomitantly with sirolimus). Products include:
Zofran Injection 1634
Zofran 1639

Oxcarbazepine (Sirolimus is extensively metabolized by the CYP3A4 isoenzyme in the gut wall and liver. Co-administration with inducers of CYP3A4 may increase the metabolism of sirolimus and decrease sirolimus levels. Co-administration with strong inducers of CYP3A4 is not recommended). Products include:
Trileptal Tablets 2300
Trileptal Oral Suspension 2300

Paclitaxel (Care should be exercised when drugs or other substances metabolized by CYP3A4 are administered concomitantly with sirolimus).
No products indexed under this heading.

Paroxetine Hydrochloride (Sirolimus is extensively metabolized by the CYP3A4 isoenzyme in the gut wall and liver. Co-administration with inhibitors of CYP3A4 may decrease the metabolism of sirolimus and increase sirolimus levels. Co-administration with strong inducers of CYP3A4 is not recommended). Products include:
Paxil CR Controlled-Release Tablets ... 1538
Paxil ... 1530

Perindopril Erbumine (In rare cases, the concomitant administration of sirolimus and ACE inhibitors has resulted in angioneurotic edema-type reactions). Products include:
Aceon Tablets (2 mg, 4 mg, 8 mg) 3194

Phenobarbital (Sirolimus is extensively metabolized by the CYP3A4 isoenzyme; co-administration with inducers of CYP3A4, such as phenobarbital, may increase the metabolism of sirolimus and decrease the plasma levels of sirolimus). Products include:
Donnatal Extentabs 2493

Phenobarbital Sodium (Sirolimus is extensively metabolized by the CYP3A4 isoenzyme in the gut wall and liver. Co-administration with inducers of CYP3A4 may increase the metabolism of sirolimus and decrease sirolimus levels. Co-administration with strong inducers of CYP3A4 is not recommended).
No products indexed under this heading.

Phenytoin (Sirolimus is extensively metabolized by the CYP3A4 isoenzyme; co-administration with inducers of CYP3A4, such as phenytoin, may increase the metabolism of sirolimus and decrease the plasma levels of sirolimus).
No products indexed under this heading.

Phenytoin Sodium (Sirolimus is extensively metabolized by the CYP3A4 isoenzyme; co-administration with inducers of CYP3A4, such as phenytoin, may increase the metabolism of sirolimus and decrease the plasma levels of sirolimus). Products include:
Phenytek Capsules 2160

Pimozide (Care should be exercised when drugs or other substances metabolized by CYP3A4 are administered concomitantly with sirolimus).
No products indexed under this heading.

Poliovirus Vaccine, Live, Oral, Trivalent, Types 1,2,3 (Sabin) (During treatment with sirolimus, vaccination may be less effective. The use of live vaccinations should be avoided).
No products indexed under this heading.

Polyestradiol Phosphate (Care should be exercised when drugs or other substances metabolized by CYP3A4 are administered concomitantly with sirolimus).
No products indexed under this heading.

Pravastatin Sodium (Co-administration of sirolimus with cyclosporine in conjunction with HMG-CoA reductase inhibitors should be monitored for the possible development of rhabdomyolysis; in clinical trials, the concurrent use of sirolimus and HMG-CoA reductase inhibitors was well tolerated).
No products indexed under this heading.

Prednisolone Acetate (Sirolimus is extensively metabolized by the CYP3A4 isoenzyme in the gut wall and liver. Co-administration with inducers of CYP3A4 may increase the metabolism of sirolimus and decrease sirolimus levels. Co-administration with strong inducers of CYP3A4 is not recommended). Products include:
Blephamide Ophthalmic Ointment 568
Blephamide Ophthalmic Suspension................................. 569
Poly-Pred Ophthalmic Suspension............................... ⊙233
Pred Forte Ophthalmic Suspension ⊙235
Pred Mild Ophthalmic Suspension ⊙238
Pred-G Ophthalmic Ointment ⊙237
Pred-G Ophthalmic Suspension ⊙236

IMPORTANT NOTE: Always consult each drug listing in the patient's regimen for possible interactions.

Prednisolone Sodium Phosphate (Sirolimus is extensively metabolized by the CYP3A4 isoenzyme in the gut wall and liver. Co-administration with inducers of CYP3A4 may increase the metabolism of sirolimus and decrease sirolimus levels. Co-administration with strong inducers of CYP3A4 is not recommended).
 No products indexed under this heading.

Prednisolone Tebutate (Sirolimus is extensively metabolized by the CYP3A4 isoenzyme in the gut wall and liver. Co-administration with inducers of CYP3A4 may increase the metabolism of sirolimus and decrease sirolimus levels. Co-administration with strong inducers of CYP3A4 is not recommended).
 No products indexed under this heading.

Prednisone (Sirolimus is extensively metabolized by the CYP3A4 isoenzyme in the gut wall and liver. Co-administration with inducers of CYP3A4 may increase the metabolism of sirolimus and decrease sirolimus levels. Co-administration with strong inducers of CYP3A4 is not recommended).
 No products indexed under this heading.

Primidone (Sirolimus is extensively metabolized by the CYP3A4 isoenzyme in the gut wall and liver. Co-administration with inducers of CYP3A4 may increase the metabolism of sirolimus and decrease sirolimus levels. Co-administration with strong inducers of CYP3A4 is not recommended).
 No products indexed under this heading.

Propoxyphene Hydrochloride (Sirolimus is extensively metabolized by the CYP3A4 isoenzyme in the gut wall and liver. Co-administration with inhibitors of CYP3A4 may decrease the metabolism of sirolimus and increase sirolimus levels. Co-administration with strong inducers of CYP3A4 is not recommended).
 No products indexed under this heading.

Propoxyphene Napsylate (Sirolimus is extensively metabolized by the CYP3A4 isoenzyme in the gut wall and liver. Co-administration with inhibitors of CYP3A4 may decrease the metabolism of sirolimus and increase sirolimus levels. Co-administration with strong inducers of CYP3A4 is not recommended).
 No products indexed under this heading.

Quinapril Hydrochloride (In rare cases, the concomitant administration of sirolimus and ACE inhibitors has resulted in angioneurotic edema-type reactions).
 No products indexed under this heading.

Quinidine (Sirolimus is extensively metabolized by the CYP3A4 isoenzyme in the gut wall and liver. Co-administration with inhibitors of CYP3A4 may decrease the metabolism of sirolimus and increase sirolimus levels. Co-administration with strong inducers of CYP3A4 is not recommended).
 No products indexed under this heading.

Quinidine Gluconate (Care should be exercised when drugs or other substances metabolized by CYP3A4 are administered concomitantly with sirolimus).
 No products indexed under this heading.

Quinidine Hydrochloride (Sirolimus is extensively metabolized by the CYP3A4 isoenzyme in the gut wall and liver. Co-administration with inhibitors of CYP3A4 may decrease the metabolism of sirolimus and increase sirolimus levels. Co-administration with strong inducers of CYP3A4 is not recommended).
 No products indexed under this heading.

Quinidine Polygalacturonate (Sirolimus is extensively metabolized by the CYP3A4 isoenzyme in the gut wall and liver. Co-administration with inhibitors of CYP3A4 may decrease the metabolism of sirolimus and increase sirolimus levels. Co-administration with strong inducers of CYP3A4 is not recommended).
 No products indexed under this heading.

Quinidine Sulfate (Sirolimus is extensively metabolized by the CYP3A4 isoenzyme in the gut wall and liver. Co-administration with inhibitors of CYP3A4 may decrease the metabolism of sirolimus and increase sirolimus levels. Co-administration with strong inducers of CYP3A4 is not recommended).
 No products indexed under this heading.

Quinine (Sirolimus is extensively metabolized by the CYP3A4 isoenzyme in the gut wall and liver. Co-administration with inhibitors of CYP3A4 may decrease the metabolism of sirolimus and increase sirolimus levels. Co-administration with strong inducers of CYP3A4 is not recommended).
 No products indexed under this heading.

Quinine Sulfate (Sirolimus is extensively metabolized by the CYP3A4 isoenzyme in the gut wall and liver. Co-administration with inhibitors of CYP3A4 may decrease the metabolism of sirolimus and increase sirolimus levels. Co-administration with strong inducers of CYP3A4 is not recommended).
 No products indexed under this heading.

Quinupristin (Sirolimus is extensively metabolized by the CYP3A4 isoenzyme in the gut wall and liver. Co-administration with inhibitors of CYP3A4 may decrease the metabolism of sirolimus and increase sirolimus levels. Co-administration with strong inducers of CYP3A4 is not recommended).
 No products indexed under this heading.

Ramipril (In rare cases, the concomitant administration of sirolimus and ACE inhibitors has resulted in angioneurotic edema-type reactions). Products include:
 Altace Capsules 1702

Ranitidine Bismuth Citrate (Sirolimus is extensively metabolized by the CYP3A4 isoenzyme in the gut wall and liver. Co-administration with inhibitors of CYP3A4 may decrease the metabolism of sirolimus and increase sirolimus levels. Co-administration with strong inducers of CYP3A4 is not recommended).
 No products indexed under this heading.

Ranitidine Hydrochloride (Sirolimus is extensively metabolized by the CYP3A4 isoenzyme in the gut wall and liver. Co-administration with inhibitors of CYP3A4 may decrease the metabolism of sirolimus and increase sirolimus levels. Co-administration with strong inducers of CYP3A4 is not recommended). Products include:
 Zantac .. 1624
 Zantac Injection 1619
 Zantac Injection Pharmacy Bulk
 Package.................................... 1622

Rifabutin (Sirolimus is extensively metabolized by the CYP3A4 isoenzyme; co-administration with inducers of CYP3A4, such as rifabutin, may increase the metabolism of sirolimus and decrease the plasma levels of sirolimus).
 No products indexed under this heading.

Rifampicin (Sirolimus is extensively metabolized by the CYP3A4 isoenzyme in the gut wall and liver. Co-administration with inducers of CYP3A4 may increase the metabolism of sirolimus and decrease sirolimus levels. Co-administration with strong inducers of CYP3A4 is not recommended).
 No products indexed under this heading.

Rifampin (Pretreatment with multiple doses of rifampin greatly increased sirolimus oral dose clearance resulting in mean decrease in AUC and Cmax. Co-administration of sirolimus oral solution or tablets and rifampin is not recommended and alternative therapeutic agents with less enzyme induction potential than rifampin should be considered).
 No products indexed under this heading.

Rifapentine (Sirolimus is extensively metabolized by the CYP3A4 isoenzyme; co-administration with inducers of CYP3A4, such as rifapentine, may increase the metabolism of sirolimus and decrease the plasma levels of sirolimus).
 No products indexed under this heading.

Ritonavir (Sirolimus is extensively metabolized by the CYP3A4 isoenzyme in the gut wall and liver. Co-administration with inhibitors of CYP3A4 may decrease the metabolism of sirolimus and increase sirolimus levels. Co-administration with strong inducers of CYP3A4 is not recommended). Products include:
 Kaletra .. 476
 Norvir .. 503

Rotavirus Vaccine, Live, Oral, Tetravalent (During treatment with sirolimus, vaccination may be less effective. The use of live vaccinations should be avoided).
 No products indexed under this heading.

Rubella & Mumps Virus Vaccine Live (During treatment with sirolimus, vaccination may be less effective. The use of live vaccinations should be avoided).
 No products indexed under this heading.

Rubella Virus Vaccine Live (During treatment with sirolimus, vaccination may be less effective. The use of live vaccinations should be avoided). Products include:
 Meruvax II 2019

Saquinavir (Sirolimus is extensively metabolized by the CYP3A4 isoenzyme in the gut wall and liver. Co-administration with inhibitors of CYP3A4 may decrease the metabolism of sirolimus and increase sirolimus levels. Co-administration with strong inducers of CYP3A4 is not recommended).
 No products indexed under this heading.

Saquinavir Mesylate (Sirolimus is extensively metabolized by the CYP3A4 isoenzyme in the gut wall and liver. Co-administration with inhibitors of CYP3A4 may decrease the metabolism of sirolimus and increase sirolimus levels. Co-administration with strong inducers of CYP3A4 is not recommended). Products include:
 Invirase .. 2772

Sertraline Hydrochloride (Sirolimus is extensively metabolized by the CYP3A4 isoenzyme in the gut wall and liver. Co-administration with inhibitors of CYP3A4 may decrease the metabolism of sirolimus and increase sirolimus levels. Co-administration with strong inducers of CYP3A4 is not recommended). Products include:
 Zoloft ... 2586

Sildenafil Citrate (Care should be exercised when drugs or other substances metabolized by CYP3A4 are administered concomitantly with sirolimus). Products include:
 Revatio Tablets 2557
 Viagra Tablets 2573

Simvastatin (Co-administration of sirolimus with cyclosporine in conjunction with HMG-CoA reductase inhibitors should be monitored for the possible development of rhabdomyolysis; in clinical trials, the concurrent use of sirolimus and HMG-CoA reductase inhibitors was well tolerated). Products include:
 Vytorin 10/10 Tablets 2114
 Vytorin 10/10 Tablets 3077
 Vytorin 10/20 Tablets 2114
 Vytorin 10/20 Tablets 3077
 Vytorin 10/40 Tablets 2114
 Vytorin 10/40 Tablets 3077
 Vytorin 10/80 Tablets 2114
 Vytorin 10/80 Tablets 3077
 Zocor Tablets 2105

Smallpox Vaccine (During treatment with sirolimus, vaccination may be less effective. The use of live vaccinations should be avoided).
 No products indexed under this heading.

Spirapril Hydrochloride (In rare cases, the concomitant administration of sirolimus and ACE inhibitors has resulted in angioneurotic edema-type reactions).
 No products indexed under this heading.

Sulfinpyrazone (Sirolimus is extensively metabolized by the CYP3A4 isoenzyme in the gut wall and liver. Co-administration with inducers of CYP3A4 may increase the metabolism of sirolimus and decrease sirolimus levels. Co-administration with strong inducers of CYP3A4 is not recommended).
No products indexed under this heading.

Tacrolimus (Co-administration was associated with excess mortality and graft loss in de novo liver transplant recipients; combination use is associated with hepatic artery thrombosis (HAT); the safety and efficacy of Rapamune has not been established in liver transplant patients; therefore, such use is not recommended). Products include:
Prograf Capsules and Injection 632
Protopic Ointment 638

Tamoxifen Citrate (Care should be exercised when drugs or other substances metabolized by CYP3A4 are administered concomitantly with sirolimus). Products include:
Soltamox Oral Solution 3527

Telithromycin (Sirolimus is extensively metabolized by the CYP3A4 isoenzyme in the gut wall and liver. Co-administration with inhibitors of CYP3A4 may decrease the metabolism of sirolimus and increase sirolimus levels. Co-administration with strong inducers of CYP3A4 is not recommended). Products include:
Ketek Tablets 2903

Theophylline (Sirolimus is extensively metabolized by the CYP3A4 isoenzyme in the gut wall and liver. Co-administration with inducers of CYP3A4 may increase the metabolism of sirolimus and decrease sirolimus levels. Co-administration with strong inducers of CYP3A4 is not recommended).
No products indexed under this heading.

Tiagabine Hydrochloride (Care should be exercised when drugs or other substances metabolized by CYP3A4 are administered concomitantly with sirolimus). Products include:
Gabitril Tablets 984

Tirofiban Hydrochloride (Strong inhibitors of P-gp significantly decrease the metabolism of sirolimus and increase sirolimus concentrations). Products include:
Aggrastat 1907

Tolterodine Tartrate (Care should be exercised when drugs or other substances metabolized by CYP3A4 are administered concomitantly with sirolimus). Products include:
Detrol Tablets 2628
Detrol LA Capsules 2631

Trandolapril (In rare cases, the concomitant administration of sirolimus and ACE inhibitors has resulted in angioneurotic edema-type reactions). Products include:
Mavik Tablets 486
Tarka Tablets 524

Trazodone Hydrochloride (Care should be exercised when drugs or other substances metabolized by CYP3A4 are administered concomitantly with sirolimus).
No products indexed under this heading.

Triamcinolone (Sirolimus is extensively metabolized by the CYP3A4 isoenzyme in the gut wall and liver. Co-administration with inducers of CYP3A4 may increase the metabolism of sirolimus and decrease sirolimus levels. Co-administration with strong inducers of CYP3A4 is not recommended).
No products indexed under this heading.

Triamcinolone Acetonide (Sirolimus is extensively metabolized by the CYP3A4 isoenzyme in the gut wall and liver. Co-administration with inducers of CYP3A4 may increase the metabolism of sirolimus and decrease sirolimus levels. Co-administration with strong inducers of CYP3A4 is not recommended). Products include:
Azmacort Inhalation Aerosol 1726
Nasacort AQ Nasal Spray 2922

Triamcinolone Diacetate (Sirolimus is extensively metabolized by the CYP3A4 isoenzyme in the gut wall and liver. Co-administration with inducers of CYP3A4 may increase the metabolism of sirolimus and decrease sirolimus levels. Co-administration with strong inducers of CYP3A4 is not recommended).
No products indexed under this heading.

Triamcinolone Hexacetonide (Sirolimus is extensively metabolized by the CYP3A4 isoenzyme in the gut wall and liver. Co-administration with inducers of CYP3A4 may increase the metabolism of sirolimus and decrease sirolimus levels. Co-administration with strong inducers of CYP3A4 is not recommended).
No products indexed under this heading.

Triazolam (Care should be exercised when drugs or other substances metabolized by CYP3A4 are administered concomitantly with sirolimus).
No products indexed under this heading.

Troglitazone (Sirolimus is extensively metabolized by the CYP3A4 isoenzyme in the gut wall and liver. Co-administration with inhibitors of CYP3A4 may decrease the metabolism of sirolimus and increase sirolimus levels. Co-administration with strong inducers of CYP3A4 is not recommended).
No products indexed under this heading.

Troleandomycin (Sirolimus is extensively metabolized by the CYP3A4 isoenzyme; co-administration with inhibitors of CYP3A4, such as troleandomycin, may decrease the metabolism of sirolimus and increase the plasma levels of sirolimus).
No products indexed under this heading.

Typhoid Vaccine (During treatment with sirolimus, vaccination may be less effective. The use of live vaccinations should be avoided).
No products indexed under this heading.

Valproate Sodium (Sirolimus is extensively metabolized by the CYP3A4 isoenzyme in the gut wall and liver. Co-administration with inhibitors of CYP3A4 may decrease the metabolism of sirolimus and increase sirolimus levels. Co-administration with strong inducers of CYP3A4 is not recommended). Products include:
Depacon Injection 412

Varicella Virus Vaccine Live (During treatment with sirolimus, vaccination may be less effective. The use of live vaccinations should be avoided). Products include:
Varivax 2100

Verapamil Hydrochloride (Sirolimus is extensively metabolized by the CYP3A4 isoenzyme; co-administration with inhibitors of CYP3A4, such as verapamil, may decrease the metabolism of sirolimus and increase the plasma levels of sirolimus. Concentrations of sirolimus should be monitored and a dose adjustment may be necessary when co-administered with verapamil). Products include:
Covera-HS Tablets 3139
Tarka Tablets 524
Verelan PM Extended-Release Capsules, Controlled-Onset 3106

Vinblastine Sulfate (Care should be exercised when drugs or other substances metabolized by CYP3A4 are administered concomitantly with sirolimus).
No products indexed under this heading.

Vincristine Sulfate (Care should be exercised when drugs or other substances metabolized by CYP3A4 are administered concomitantly with sirolimus).
No products indexed under this heading.

Voriconazole (Sirolimus is extensively metabolized by the CYP3A4 isoenzyme in the gut wall and liver. Co-administration with inhibitors of CYP3A4 may decrease the metabolism of sirolimus and increase sirolimus levels. Co-administration with strong inducers of CYP3A4 is not recommended). Products include:
VFEND I.V. 2564
VFEND Oral Suspension 2564
VFEND Tablets 2564

Warfarin Sodium (Care should be exercised when drugs or other substances metabolized by CYP3A4 are administered concomitantly with sirolimus). Products include:
Coumadin for Injection 898
Coumadin Tablets 898

Yellow Fever Vaccine (During treatment with sirolimus, vaccination may be less effective. The use of live vaccinations should be avoided).
No products indexed under this heading.

Zafirlukast (Sirolimus is extensively metabolized by the CYP3A4 isoenzyme in the gut wall and liver. Co-administration with inhibitors of CYP3A4 may decrease the metabolism of sirolimus and increase sirolimus levels. Co-administration with strong inducers of CYP3A4 is not recommended). Products include:
Accolate Tablets 671

Zileuton (Sirolimus is extensively metabolized by the CYP3A4 isoenzyme in the gut wall and liver. Co-administration with inhibitors of CYP3A4 may decrease the metabolism of sirolimus and increase sirolimus levels. Co-administration with strong inducers of CYP3A4 is not recommended). Products include:
Zyflo Tablets 1023

Food Interactions

Food, unspecified (A high-fat meal altered the bioavailability characteristics of sirolimus compared to fasting; 34% decrease in the peak blood sirolimus concentration, a 3.5-fold increase in the time-to-peak concentration and 35% increase in total exposure; to minimize variability, Rapamune should be taken consistently with or without food).

Grapefruit (Sirolimus is extensively metabolized by the CYP3A4 isoenzyme in the gut wall and liver. Co-administration with inhibitors of CYP3A4 may decrease the metabolism of sirolimus and increase sirolimus levels. Co-administration with strong inducers of CYP3A4 is not recommended).

Grapefruit Juice (Induces CYP3A4-mediated metabolism of sirolimus; Rapamune must not be administered or diluted with grapefruit juice).

RAPTIVA FOR INJECTION

(Efalizumab) 1250
May interact with immunosuppressive agents and vaccines, live. Compounds in these categories include:

Azathioprine (Patients receiving other immunosuppressive agents should not receive concurrent therapy with efalizumab because of the possibility of increased risk of infections and malignancies).
No products indexed under this heading.

Basiliximab (Patients receiving other immunosuppressive agents should not receive concurrent therapy with efalizumab because of the possibility of increased risk of infections and malignancies). Products include:
Simulect for Injection 2284

BCG Vaccine (Acellular, live and live-attenuated vaccines should not be administered during efalizumab treatment).
No products indexed under this heading.

Cyclosporine (Patients receiving other immunosuppressive agents should not receive concurrent therapy with efalizumab because of the possibility of increased risk of infections and malignancies). Products include:
Gengraf Capsules 459
Neoral Oral Solution 2259
Neoral Soft Gelatin Capsules 2259
Restasis Ophthalmic Emulsion 575
Sandimmune 2275

Measles, Mumps, Rubella and Varicella Virus Vaccine Live (Acellular, live and live-attenuated vaccines should not be administered during efalizumab treatment). Products include:
ProQuad 2064

Measles, Mumps & Rubella Virus Vaccine, Live (Acellular, live and live-attenuated vaccines should not be administered during efalizumab treatment). Products include:
M-M-R II 2006

Measles & Rubella Virus Vaccine Live (Acellular, live and live-attenuated vaccines should not be administered during efalizumab treatment).
No products indexed under this heading.

Measles Virus Vaccine Live (Acellular, live and live-attenuated vaccines should not be administered during efalizumab treatment). Products include:

Attenuvax ... **1914**

Mumps Virus Vaccine, Live (Acellular, live and live-attenuated vaccines should not be administered during efalizumab treatment). Products include:

Mumpsvax ... **2031**

Muromonab-CD3 (Patients receiving other immunosuppressive agents should not receive concurrent therapy with efalizumab because of the possibility of increased risk of infections and malignancies). Products include:

Orthoclone OKT3 Sterile Solution ... **2360**

Mycophenolate Mofetil (Patients receiving other immunosuppressive agents should not receive concurrent therapy with efalizumab because of the possibility of increased risk of infections and malignancies). Products include:

CellCept Capsules ... **2747**
CellCept Oral Suspension ... **2747**
CellCept Tablets ... **2747**

Poliovirus Vaccine, Live, Oral, Trivalent, Types 1,2,3 (Sabin) (Acellular, live and live-attenuated vaccines should not be administered during efalizumab treatment).

No products indexed under this heading.

Rotavirus Vaccine, Live, Oral, Tetravalent (Acellular, live and live-attenuated vaccines should not be administered during efalizumab treatment).

No products indexed under this heading.

Rubella & Mumps Virus Vaccine Live (Acellular, live and live-attenuated vaccines should not be administered during efalizumab treatment).

No products indexed under this heading.

Rubella Virus Vaccine Live (Acellular, live and live-attenuated vaccines should not be administered during efalizumab treatment). Products include:

Meruvax II ... **2019**

Sirolimus (Patients receiving other immunosuppressive agents should not receive concurrent therapy with efalizumab because of the possibility of increased risk of infections and malignancies). Products include:

Rapamune Oral Solution and Tablets ... **3475**

Smallpox Vaccine (Acellular, live and live-attenuated vaccines should not be administered during efalizumab treatment).

No products indexed under this heading.

Tacrolimus (Patients receiving other immunosuppressive agents should not receive concurrent therapy with efalizumab because of the possibility of increased risk of infections and malignancies). Products include:

Prograf Capsules and Injection ... **632**
Protopic Ointment ... **638**

Typhoid Vaccine (Acellular, live and live-attenuated vaccines should not be administered during efalizumab treatment).

No products indexed under this heading.

Varicella Virus Vaccine Live (Acellular, live and live-attenuated vaccines should not be administered during efalizumab treatment). Products include:

Varivax ... **2100**

Yellow Fever Vaccine (Acellular, live and live-attenuated vaccines should not be administered during efalizumab treatment).

No products indexed under this heading.

RAZADYNE ORAL SOLUTION

(Galantamine Hydrobromide) ... **2399**
See Razadyne Tablets

RAZADYNE TABLETS

(Galantamine Hydrobromide) ... **2399**
May interact with anticholinergics, cholinergic agents, erythromycin, neuromuscular blocking agents, nonsteroidal anti-inflammatory agents, and certain other agents. Compounds in these categories include:

Atracurium Besylate (Galantamine is a cholinesterase inhibitor; co-administration with neuromuscular blocking agents may exaggerate neuromuscular blockade).

No products indexed under this heading.

Atropine Sulfate (Galantamine has the potential to interfere with the activity of anticholinergic agents). Products include:

Donnatal Extentabs ... **2493**

Belladonna Alkaloids (Galantamine has the potential to interfere with the activity of anticholinergic agents). Products include:

Hyland's Teething Tablets ... ▣**830**

Benztropine Mesylate (Galantamine has the potential to interfere with the activity of anticholinergic agents).

No products indexed under this heading.

Bethanechol Chloride (Co-administration with other cholinesterase inhibitors or cholinergic agonists may result in a synergistic effect).

No products indexed under this heading.

Biperiden Hydrochloride (Galantamine has the potential to interfere with the activity of anticholinergic agents).

No products indexed under this heading.

Celecoxib (Cholinomimetics, such as galantamine, may be expected to increase gastric acid secretion; therefore, co-administration in patients with increased risk of developing gastric ulcers or bleeding, such as patients on NSAIDs, should be closely monitored). Products include:

Celebrex Capsules ... **3134**

Cevimeline Hydrochloride (Co-administration with other cholinesterase inhibitors or cholinergic agonists may result in a synergistic effect). Products include:

Evoxac Capsules ... **1047**

Cimetidine (Co-administration with cimetidine has resulted in increased bioavailability galantamine by approximately 16%). Products include:

Tagamet HB 200 Tablets ... ▣**664**

Cimetidine Hydrochloride (Co-administration with cimetidine has resulted in increased bioavailability galantamine by approximately 16%).

No products indexed under this heading.

Cisatracurium Besylate (Galantamine is a cholinesterase inhibitor; co-administration with neuromuscular blocking agents may exaggerate neuromuscular blockade). Products include:

Nimbex Injection ... **498**

Clidinium Bromide (Galantamine has the potential to interfere with the activity of anticholinergic agents).

No products indexed under this heading.

Diclofenac Potassium (Cholinomimetics, such as galantamine, may be expected to increase gastric acid secretion; therefore, co-administration in patients with increased risk of developing gastric ulcers or bleeding, such as patients on NSAIDs, should be closely monitored).

No products indexed under this heading.

Diclofenac Sodium (Cholinomimetics, such as galantamine, may be expected to increase gastric acid secretion; therefore, co-administration in patients with increased risk of developing gastric ulcers or bleeding, such as patients on NSAIDs, should be closely monitored). Products include:

Arthrotec Tablets ... **3129**
Voltaren Ophthalmic Solution ... **2309**
Voltaren Tablets ... **2307**
Voltaren-XR Tablets ... **2310**

Dicyclomine Hydrochloride (Galantamine has the potential to interfere with the activity of anticholinergic agents). Products include:

Bentyl Capsules ... **697**
Bentyl Injection ... **697**
Bentyl Syrup ... **697**
Bentyl Tablets ... **697**

Digoxin (Co-administration in a healthy subject has resulted in 2nd and 3rd degree heart block and bradycardia). Products include:

Lanoxicaps Capsules ... **1490**
Lanoxin Injection ... **1494**
Lanoxin Injection Pediatric ... **1497**
Lanoxin Tablets ... **1500**

Donepezil Hydrochloride (Co-administration with other cholinesterase inhibitors or cholinergic agonists may result in a synergistic effect). Products include:

Aricept Tablets ... **1094**
Aricept ODT Tablets ... **1094**

Doxacurium Chloride (Galantamine is a cholinesterase inhibitor; co-administration with neuromuscular blocking agents may exaggerate neuromuscular blockade).

No products indexed under this heading.

Edrophonium Chloride (Co-administration with other cholinesterase inhibitors or cholinergic agonists may result in a synergistic effect).

No products indexed under this heading.

Erythromycin (Co-administration with a moderate inhibitor of CYP3A4, such as erythromycin, increases the AUC of galantamine by 10%). Products include:

Ery-Tab Tablets ... **449**
Erythromycin Base Filmtab Tablets ... **455**
Erythromycin Delayed-Release Capsules, USP ... **457**
PCE Dispertab Tablets ... **515**

Erythromycin Estolate (Co-administration with a moderate inhibitor of CYP3A4, such as erythromycin, increases the AUC of galantamine by 10%).

No products indexed under this heading.

Erythromycin Ethylsuccinate (Co-administration with a moderate inhibitor of CYP3A4, such as erythromycin, increases the AUC of galantamine by 10%). Products include:

E.E.S. ... **451**
EryPed ... **447**

Erythromycin Gluceptate (Co-administration with a moderate inhibitor of CYP3A4, such as erythromycin, increases the AUC of galantamine by 10%).

No products indexed under this heading.

Erythromycin Lactobionate (Co-administration with a moderate inhibitor of CYP3A4, such as erythromycin, increases the AUC of galantamine by 10%).

No products indexed under this heading.

Erythromycin Stearate (Co-administration with a moderate inhibitor of CYP3A4, such as erythromycin, increases the AUC of galantamine by 10%). Products include:

Erythrocin Stearate Filmtab Tablets ... **453**

Etodolac (Cholinomimetics, such as galantamine, may be expected to increase gastric acid secretion; therefore, co-administration in patients with increased risk of developing gastric ulcers or bleeding, such as patients on NSAIDs, should be closely monitored).

No products indexed under this heading.

Fenoprofen Calcium (Cholinomimetics, such as galantamine, may be expected to increase gastric acid secretion; therefore, co-administration in patients with increased risk of developing gastric ulcers or bleeding, such as patients on NSAIDs, should be closely monitored). Products include:

Nalfon Capsules ... **2502**

Flurbiprofen (Cholinomimetics, such as galantamine, may be expected to increase gastric acid secretion; therefore, co-administration in patients with increased risk of developing gastric ulcers or bleeding, such as patients on NSAIDs, should be closely monitored).

No products indexed under this heading.

Glycopyrrolate (Galantamine has the potential to interfere with the activity of anticholinergic agents).

No products indexed under this heading.

Hyoscyamine (Galantamine has the potential to interfere with the activity of anticholinergic agents).

No products indexed under this heading.

Hyoscyamine Sulfate (Galantamine has the potential to interfere with the activity of anticholinergic agents). Products include:

Donnatal Extentabs ... **2493**
Prosed/DS Tablets ... **1157**

Ibuprofen (Cholinomimetics, such as galantamine, may be expected to increase gastric acid secretion; therefore, co-administration in patients with increased risk of developing gastric ulcers or bleeding, such as patients on NSAIDs, should be closely monitored). Products include:

Advil Allergy Sinus Caplets ... ▣**770**
Advil ... ▣**674**

Children's Advil Oral Suspension 603
Children's Advil Chewable Tablets .. 603
Advil Cold & Sinus 723
Infants' Advil Concentrated Drops .. 604
Infants' Advil Concentrated Drops - White Grape (Dye-Free)............. 604
Junior Strength Advil Swallow Tablets.. 605
Advil Migraine Liquigels 608
Advil Multi-Symptom Cold Caplets.. 770
Advil PM Caplets 615
Motrin IB Tablets and Caplets 1866
Children's Motrin Oral Suspension ... 1867
Children's Motrin Non-Staining Dye-Free Oral Suspension............ 1867
Children's Motrin Cold Oral Suspension 1867
Infants' Motrin Concentrated Drops... 1867
Infants' Motrin Non-Staining Dye-Free Concentrated Drops....... 1867
Junior Strength Motrin Caplets and Chewable Tablets................... 1867
Vicoprofen Tablets 539

Indomethacin (Cholinomimetics, such as galantamine, may be expected to increase gastric acid secretion; therefore, co-administration in patients with increased risk of developing gastric ulcers or bleeding, such as patients on NSAIDs, should be closely monitored). Products include:
Indocin 1995

Indomethacin Sodium Trihydrate (Cholinomimetics, such as galantamine, may be expected to increase gastric acid secretion; therefore, co-administration in patients with increased risk of developing gastric ulcers or bleeding, such as patients on NSAIDs, should be closely monitored). Products include:
Indocin I.V. 2465

Ipratropium Bromide (Galantamine has the potential to interfere with the activity of anticholinergic agents). Products include:
Atrovent Inhalation Solution 835
Atrovent HFA Inhalation Aerosol 841
Atrovent Nasal Spray 0.03%............ 837
Atrovent Nasal Spray 0.06%............ 839
Combivent Inhalation Aerosol 847
DuoNeb Inhalation Solution 1058

Ketoconazole (Co-administration with a potent inhibitor of CYP3A4, such as ketoconazole, increases the AUC of galantamine by 30%). Products include:
Nizoral A-D Shampoo, 1%............... 1868

Ketoprofen (Cholinomimetics, such as galantamine, may be expected to increase gastric acid secretion; therefore, co-administration in patients with increased risk of developing gastric ulcers or bleeding, such as patients on NSAIDs, should be closely monitored).
No products indexed under this heading.

Ketorolac Tromethamine (Cholinomimetics, such as galantamine, may be expected to increase gastric acid secretion; therefore, co-administration in patients with increased risk of developing gastric ulcers or bleeding, such as patients on NSAIDs, should be closely monitored). Products include:
Acular Ophthalmic Solution 565
Acular LS Ophthalmic Solution 566

Meclofenamate Sodium (Cholinomimetics, such as galantamine, may be expected to increase gastric acid secretion; therefore, co-administration in patients with increased risk of developing gastric ulcers or bleeding, such as patients on NSAIDs, should be closely monitored).
No products indexed under this heading.

Mefenamic Acid (Cholinomimetics, such as galantamine, may be expected to increase gastric acid secretion; therefore, co-administration in patients with increased risk of developing gastric ulcers or bleeding, such as patients on NSAIDs, should be closely monitored).
No products indexed under this heading.

Meloxicam (Cholinomimetics, such as galantamine, may be expected to increase gastric acid secretion; therefore, co-administration in patients with increased risk of developing gastric ulcers or bleeding, such as patients on NSAIDs, should be closely monitored). Products include:
Mobic Oral Suspension 863
Mobic Tablets 863

Mepenzolate Bromide (Galantamine has the potential to interfere with the activity of anticholinergic agents).
No products indexed under this heading.

Metocurine Iodide (Galantamine is a cholinesterase inhibitor; co-administration with neuromuscular blocking agents may exaggerate neuromuscular blockade).
No products indexed under this heading.

Mivacurium Chloride (Galantamine is a cholinesterase inhibitor; co-administration with neuromuscular blocking agents may exaggerate neuromuscular blockade). Products include:
Mivacron Injection 493

Nabumetone (Cholinomimetics, such as galantamine, may be expected to increase gastric acid secretion; therefore, co-administration in patients with increased risk of developing gastric ulcers or bleeding, such as patients on NSAIDs, should be closely monitored).
No products indexed under this heading.

Naproxen (Cholinomimetics, such as galantamine, may be expected to increase gastric acid secretion; therefore, co-administration in patients with increased risk of developing gastric ulcers or bleeding, such as patients on NSAIDs, should be closely monitored). Products include:
EC-Naprosyn Delayed-Release Tablets...................................... 2761
Naprosyn Suspension 2761
Naprosyn Tablets 2761
Prevacid NapraPAC 3280

Naproxen Sodium (Cholinomimetics, such as galantamine, may be expected to increase gastric acid secretion; therefore, co-administration in patients with increased risk of developing gastric ulcers or bleeding, such as patients on NSAIDs, should be closely monitored). Products include:
Aleve Caplets 742
Aleve Gelcaps 743
Aleve Tablets 743
Aleve Cold & Sinus Caplets 744
Anaprox Tablets 2761
Anaprox DS Tablets 2761

Neostigmine Bromide (Co-administration with other cholinesterase inhibitors or cholinergic agonists may result in a synergistic effect).
No products indexed under this heading.

Neostigmine Methylsulfate (Co-administration with other cholinesterase inhibitors or cholinergic agonists may result in a synergistic effect).
No products indexed under this heading.

Oxaprozin (Cholinomimetics, such as galantamine, may be expected to increase gastric acid secretion; therefore, co-administration in patients with increased risk of developing gastric ulcers or bleeding, such as patients on NSAIDs, should be closely monitored).
No products indexed under this heading.

Oxybutynin Chloride (Galantamine has the potential to interfere with the activity of anticholinergic agents). Products include:
Ditropan XL Extended-Release Tablets.. 2413

Pancuronium Bromide (Galantamine is a cholinesterase inhibitor; co-administration with neuromuscular blocking agents may exaggerate neuromuscular blockade).
No products indexed under this heading.

Paroxetine Hydrochloride (Co-administration with a strong inhibitor of CYP2D6, such as paroxetine results in increased AUC of galantamine by 40%). Products include:
Paxil CR Controlled-Release Tablets.. 1538
Paxil 1530

Phenylbutazone (Cholinomimetics, such as galantamine, may be expected to increase gastric acid secretion; therefore, co-administration in patients with increased risk of developing gastric ulcers or bleeding, such as patients on NSAIDs, should be closely monitored).
No products indexed under this heading.

Piroxicam (Cholinomimetics, such as galantamine, may be expected to increase gastric acid secretion; therefore, co-administration in patients with increased risk of developing gastric ulcers or bleeding, such as patients on NSAIDs, should be closely monitored).
No products indexed under this heading.

Procyclidine Hydrochloride (Galantamine has the potential to interfere with the activity of anticholinergic agents).
No products indexed under this heading.

Propantheline Bromide (Galantamine has the potential to interfere with the activity of anticholinergic agents).
No products indexed under this heading.

Pyridostigmine Bromide (Co-administration with other cholinesterase inhibitors or cholinergic agonists may result in a synergistic effect).
No products indexed under this heading.

Rapacuronium Bromide (Galantamine is a cholinesterase inhibitor; co-administration with neuromuscular blocking agents may exaggerate neuromuscular blockade).
No products indexed under this heading.

Rivastigmine Tartrate (Co-administration with other cholinesterase inhibitors or cholinergic agonists may result in a synergistic effect). Products include:
Exelon Capsules 2206
Exelon Oral Solution 2206

Rocuronium Bromide (Galantamine is a cholinesterase inhibitor; co-administration with neuromuscular blocking agents may exaggerate neuromuscular blockade). Products include:
Zemuron Injection 2346

Rofecoxib (Cholinomimetics, such as galantamine, may be expected to increase gastric acid secretion; therefore, co-administration in patients with increased risk of developing gastric ulcers or bleeding, such as patients on NSAIDs, should be closely monitored).
No products indexed under this heading.

Scopolamine (Galantamine has the potential to interfere with the activity of anticholinergic agents). Products include:
Transderm Scōp Transdermal Therapeutic System 2177

Scopolamine Hydrobromide (Galantamine has the potential to interfere with the activity of anticholinergic agents). Products include:
Donnatal Extentabs 2493

Succinylcholine Chloride (Galantamine is a cholinesterase inhibitor; co-administration with neuromuscular blocking agents may exaggerate neuromuscular blockade).
No products indexed under this heading.

Sulindac (Cholinomimetics, such as galantamine, may be expected to increase gastric acid secretion; therefore, co-administration in patients with increased risk of developing gastric ulcers or bleeding, such as patients on NSAIDs, should be closely monitored). Products include:
Clinoril Tablets 1924

Tacrine Hydrochloride (Co-administration with other cholinesterase inhibitors or cholinergic agonists may result in a synergistic effect).
No products indexed under this heading.

Tolmetin Sodium (Cholinomimetics, such as galantamine, may be expected to increase gastric acid secretion; therefore, co-administration in patients with increased risk of developing gastric ulcers or bleeding, such as patients on NSAIDs, should be closely monitored).
No products indexed under this heading.

Tolterodine Tartrate (Galantamine has the potential to interfere with the activity of anticholinergic agents). Products include:
Detrol Tablets 2628
Detrol LA Capsules 2631

Tridihexethyl Chloride (Galantamine has the potential to interfere with the activity of anticholinergic agents).
No products indexed under this heading.

Trihexyphenidyl Hydrochloride (Galantamine has the potential to interfere with the activity of anticholinergic agents).
No products indexed under this heading.

Valdecoxib (Cholinomimetics, such as galantamine, may be expected to increase gastric acid secretion; therefore, co-administration in patients with increased risk of developing gastric ulcers or bleeding, such as patients on NSAIDs, should be closely monitored).
No products indexed under this heading.

Vecuronium Bromide (Galantamine is a cholinesterase inhibitor; co-administration with neuromuscular blocking agents may exaggerate neuromuscular blockade).
No products indexed under this heading.

RAZADYNE ER EXTENDED-RELEASE CAPSULES

(Galantamine Hydrobromide) 2399
See Razadyne Tablets

REBETOL CAPSULES

(Ribavirin) 3058
May interact with antacids. Compounds in these categories include:

Aluminum Carbonate (Co-administration of ribavirin capsules with an antacid containing magnesium, aluminum and simethicone resulted in a 14% decrease in mean ribavirin AUC. The clinical relevance of results from this study is unknown).
No products indexed under this heading.

Aluminum Hydroxide (Co-administration of ribavirin capsules with an antacid containing magnesium, aluminum and simethicone resulted in a 14% decrease in mean ribavirin AUC. The clinical relevance of results from this study is unknown). Products include:
Gaviscon Regular Strength Liquid .. (■) 658
Gaviscon Regular Strength Tablets.. (■) 658
Gaviscon Extra Strength Liquid ...... (■) 658
Gaviscon Extra Strength Tablets .... (■) 658
Maalox Regular Strength Antacid/Antigas Liquid................. 2175
Maalox Max Maximum Strength Antacid/Anti-Gas Liquid................ 2176

Magaldrate (Co-administration of ribavirin capsules with an antacid containing magnesium, aluminum and simethicone resulted in a 14% decrease in mean ribavirin AUC. The clinical relevance of results from this study is unknown).
No products indexed under this heading.

Magnesium Hydroxide (Co-administration of ribavirin capsules with an antacid containing magnesium, aluminum and simethicone resulted in a 14% decrease in mean ribavirin AUC. The clinical relevance of results from this study is unknown). Products include:
Maalox Regular Strength Antacid/Antigas Liquid................. 2175
Maalox Max Maximum Strength Antacid/Anti-Gas Liquid................ 2176
Pepcid Complete Chewable Tablets.. 1701

Magnesium Oxide (Co-administration of ribavirin capsules with an antacid containing magnesium, aluminum and simethicone resulted in a 14% decrease in mean ribavirin AUC. The clinical relevance of results from this study is unknown). Products include:
Beelith Tablets 759
PremCal Light, Regular, and Extra Strength Tablets................ (■) 818

Sodium Bicarbonate (Co-administration of ribavirin capsules with an antacid containing magnesium, aluminum and simethicone resulted in a 14% decrease in mean ribavirin AUC. The clinical relevance of results from this study is unknown). Products include:
Colyte with Flavor Packs for Oral Solution.. 3088
HalfLytely and Bisacodyl Tablets Bowel Prep Kit with Flavors Packs.. 881
TriLyte with Flavor Packs for Oral Solution.. 3100

REBETOL ORAL SOLUTION

(Ribavirin) 3058
May interact with:

See (Rebetol Capsules).
No products indexed under this heading.

REBETRON COMBINATION THERAPY

(Interferon alfa-2b, Recombinant, Ribavirin).. 3063
May interact with:

Abacavir Sulfate (Administration of nucleoside analogues has resulted in fatal and nonfatal lactic acidosis; co-administration of ribavirin and nucleoside analogues should be undertaken with caution and only if the potential benefit outweighs the potential risks). Products include:
Epzicom Tablets 1436
Trizivir Tablets 1589
Ziagen 1626

Didanosine (Administration of nucleoside analogues has resulted in fatal and nonfatal lactic acidosis; co-administration of ribavirin and nucleoside analogues should be undertaken with caution and only if the potential benefit outweighs the potential risks. Exposure to didanosine or its active metabolite is increased when didanosine is co-administered with ribavirin, which could cause or worsen clinical toxicities).
No products indexed under this heading.

Lamivudine (Administration of nucleoside analogues has resulted in fatal and nonfatal lactic acidosis; co-administration of ribavirin and nucleoside analogues should be undertaken with caution and only if the potential benefit outweighs the potential risks). Products include:
Combivir Tablets 1411
Epivir 1427
Epivir-HBV 1432
Epzicom Tablets 1436
Trizivir Tablets 1589

Magnesium Hydroxide (Co-administration with an antacid containing magnesium, aluminum, and simethicone resulted in a 14% decrease in ribavirin AUC; the clinical relevance of results from this single-dose study is unknown). Products include:
Maalox Regular Strength Antacid/Antigas Liquid................. 2175
Maalox Max Maximum Strength Antacid/Anti-Gas Liquid................ 2176
Pepcid Complete Chewable Tablets.. 1701

Stavudine (Administration of nucleoside analogues has resulted in fatal and nonfatal lactic acidosis; co-administration of ribavirin and nucleoside analogues should be undertaken with caution and only if the potential benefit outweighs the potential risks. Ribavirin may antagonize the in-vitro antiviral activity of stavudine against HIV; co-administer with caution).
No products indexed under this heading.

Zalacitabine (Administration of nucleoside analogues has resulted in fatal and nonfatal lactic acidosis; co-administration of ribavirin and nucleoside analogues should be undertaken with caution and only if the potential benefit outweighs the potential risks).
No products indexed under this heading.

Zidovudine (Administration of nucleoside analogues has resulted in fatal and nonfatal lactic acidosis; co-administration of ribavirin and nucleoside analogues should be undertaken with caution and only if the potential benefit outweighs the potential risks. Ribavirin may antagonize the in-vitro antiviral activity of zidovudine against HIV; co-administer with caution). Products include:
Combivir Tablets 1411
Retrovir 1560
Retrovir IV Infusion 1564
Trizivir Tablets 1589

Food Interactions

Food, unspecified (Both AUC and Cmax increased by 70% when Rebetron was administered with a high-fat meal in a single-dose pharmacokinetic study; there are insufficient data to address the clinical relevance of these results).

REBIF PREFILLED SYRINGE FOR INJECTION

(Interferon Beta-1a) 3159
May interact with agents associated with myelosuppression. Compounds in these categories include:

Altretamine (Due to its potential to cause neutropenia and lymphopenia, proper monitoring of patients is required if interferon beta-1 is given in combination with myelosuppressive agents).
No products indexed under this heading.

Busulfan (Due to its potential to cause neutropenia and lymphopenia, proper monitoring of patients is required if interferon beta-1 is given in combination with myelosuppressive agents). Products include:
I.V. Busulfex 2493
Myleran Tablets 1525

Chlorambucil (Due to its potential to cause neutropenia and lymphopenia, proper monitoring of patients is required if interferon beta-1 is given in combination with myelosuppressive agents). Products include:
Leukeran Tablets 1504

Cladribine (Due to its potential to cause neutropenia and lymphopenia, proper monitoring of patients is required if interferon beta-1 is given in combination with myelosuppressive agents). Products include:
Leustatin Injection 2357

Daunorubicin Citrate Liposome (Due to its potential to cause neutropenia and lymphopenia, proper monitoring of patients is required if interferon beta-1 is given in combination with myelosuppressive agents).
No products indexed under this heading.

Daunorubicin Hydrochloride (Due to its potential to cause neutropenia and lymphopenia, proper monitoring of patients is required if interferon beta-1 is given in combination with myelosuppressive agents).
No products indexed under this heading.

Dexrazoxane (Due to its potential to cause neutropenia and lymphopenia, proper monitoring of patients is required if interferon beta-1 is given in combination with myelosuppressive agents). Products include:
Zinecard for Injection 2650

Doxorubicin Hydrochloride (Due to its potential to cause neutropenia and lymphopenia, proper monitoring of patients is required if interferon beta-1 is given in combination with myelosuppressive agents).
No products indexed under this heading.

Doxorubicin Hydrochloride Liposome (Due to its potential to cause neutropenia and lymphopenia, proper monitoring of patients is required if interferon beta-1 is given in combination with myelosuppressive agents). Products include:
Doxil Injection 2351

Fludarabine Phosphate (Due to its potential to cause neutropenia and lymphopenia, proper monitoring of patients is required if interferon beta-1 is given in combination with myelosuppressive agents).
No products indexed under this heading.

Gemcitabine Hydrochloride (Due to its potential to cause neutropenia and lymphopenia, proper monitoring of patients is required if interferon beta-1 is given in combination with myelosuppressive agents). Products include:
Gemzar for Injection 1771

Gemtuzumab Ozogamicin (Due to its potential to cause neutropenia and lymphopenia, proper monitoring of patients is required if interferon beta-1 is given in combination with myelosuppressive agents). Products include:
Mylotarg for Injection 3431

Idarubicin Hydrochloride (Due to its potential to cause neutropenia and lymphopenia, proper monitoring of patients is required if interferon beta-1 is given in combination with myelosuppressive agents).
No products indexed under this heading.

Interferon alfa-2a, Recombinant (Due to its potential to cause neutropenia and lymphopenia, proper monitoring of patients is required if interferon beta-1 is given in combination with myelosuppressive agents).
No products indexed under this heading.

Irinotecan Hydrochloride (Due to its potential to cause neutropenia and lymphopenia, proper monitoring of patients is required if interferon beta-1 is given in combination with myelosuppressive agents). Products include:
- Camptosar Injection 2604

Melphalan Hydrochloride (Due to its potential to cause neutropenia and lymphopenia, proper monitoring of patients is required if interferon beta-1 is given in combination with myelosuppressive agents). Products include:
- Alkeran for Injection 955

Mercaptopurine (Due to its potential to cause neutropenia and lymphopenia, proper monitoring of patients is required if interferon beta-1 is given in combination with myelosuppressive agents).
- No products indexed under this heading.

Mitoxantrone Hydrochloride (Due to its potential to cause neutropenia and lymphopenia, proper monitoring of patients is required if interferon beta-1 is given in combination with myelosuppressive agents).
- No products indexed under this heading.

Temozolomide (Due to its potential to cause neutropenia and lymphopenia, proper monitoring of patients is required if interferon beta-1 is given in combination with myelosuppressive agents). Products include:
- Temodar Capsules 3073

Thioguanine (Due to its potential to cause neutropenia and lymphopenia, proper monitoring of patients is required if interferon beta-1 is given in combination with myelosuppressive agents). Products include:
- Tabloid Tablets 1575

Vinorelbine Tartrate (Due to its potential to cause neutropenia and lymphopenia, proper monitoring of patients is required if interferon beta-1 is given in combination with myelosuppressive agents).
- No products indexed under this heading.

RECOMBINATE

(Antihemophilic Factor (Recombinant)) 729
None cited in PDR database.

RECOMBIVAX HB

(Hepatitis B Vaccine, Recombinant) ... 2071
None cited in PDR database.

REESE'S PINWORM TREATMENTS

(Pyrantel Pamoate) 670
None cited in PDR database.

REFACTO VIALS

(Antihemophilic Factor (Recombinant)) 3484
None cited in PDR database.

REFENESEN 400 CAPLETS

(Guaifenesin) 721
None cited in PDR database.

REFENESEN DM CAPLETS

(Dextromethorphan Hydrobromide, Guaifenesin) 721
None cited in PDR database.

REFENESEN PE CAPLETS

(Guaifenesin, Phenylephrine Hydrochloride) 721
None cited in PDR database.

REFLUDAN FOR INJECTION

(Lepirudin) 792

May interact with oral anticoagulants, non-steroidal anti-inflammatory agents, thrombolytics, and certain other agents. Compounds in these categories include:

Alteplase (Concomitant therapy with thrombolytics may increase the risk of bleeding complications and considerably enhance the effect of Refludan on aPTT prolongation). Products include:
- Activase I.V. 1223
- Cathflo Activase 1231

Anisindione (Concomitant therapy with oral anticoagulants may increase the risk of bleeding). Products include:
- Miradon Tablets 3042

Anistreplase (Concomitant therapy with thrombolytics may increase the risk of bleeding complications and considerably enhance the effect of Refludan on aPTT prolongation).
- No products indexed under this heading.

Aspirin (Concomitant therapy with drugs that affect platelet function, such as aspirin, may increase the risk of bleeding). Products include:
- Aggrenox Capsules 822
- Bayer Aspirin 744
- BC Allergy Sinus Cold Powder 677
- BC Headache Powder 677
- Arthritis Strength BC Powder 677
- BC Sinus Cold Powder 677
- Excedrin Extra Strength Caplets/Tablets/Geltabs 684
- Excedrin Migraine Caplets/Tablets/Geltabs 609
- Goody's Body Pain Formula Powder 684
- Goody's Extra Strength Headache Powders 611
- Goody's Extra Strength Pain Relief Tablets 685
- Percodan Tablets 1132
- St. Joseph 81 mg Aspirin Chewable and Enteric Coated Tablets 1869

Celecoxib (Concomitant therapy with drugs that affect platelet function, such as non-steroid anti-inflammatory agents, may increase the risk of bleeding). Products include:
- Celebrex Capsules 3134

Clopidogrel Bisulfate (Concomitant therapy with drugs that affect platelet function, such as clopidogrel, may increase the risk of bleeding). Products include:
- Plavix Tablets 917
- Plavix Tablets 2926

Diclofenac Potassium (Concomitant therapy with drugs that affect platelet function, such as non-steroid anti-inflammatory agents, may increase the risk of bleeding).
- No products indexed under this heading.

Diclofenac Sodium (Concomitant therapy with drugs that affect platelet function, such as non-steroid anti-inflammatory agents, may increase the risk of bleeding). Products include:
- Arthrotec Tablets 3129
- Voltaren Ophthalmic Solution 2309
- Voltaren Tablets 2307
- Voltaren-XR Tablets 2310

Dicumarol (Concomitant therapy with oral anticoagulants may increase the risk of bleeding).
- No products indexed under this heading.

Dipyridamole (Concomitant therapy with drugs that affect platelet function, such as dipyridamole, may increase the risk of bleeding). Products include:
- Aggrenox Capsules 822
- Persantine Tablets 868

Etodolac (Concomitant therapy with drugs that affect platelet function, such as non-steroid anti-inflammatory agents, may increase the risk of bleeding).
- No products indexed under this heading.

Fenoprofen Calcium (Concomitant therapy with drugs that affect platelet function, such as non-steroid anti-inflammatory agents, may increase the risk of bleeding). Products include:
- Nalfon Capsules 2502

Flurbiprofen (Concomitant therapy with drugs that affect platelet function, such as non-steroid anti-inflammatory agents, may increase the risk of bleeding).
- No products indexed under this heading.

Ibuprofen (Concomitant therapy with drugs that affect platelet function, such as non-steroid anti-inflammatory agents, may increase the risk of bleeding). Products include:
- Advil Allergy Sinus Caplets 770
- Advil 674
- Children's Advil Oral Suspension 603
- Children's Advil Chewable Tablets 603
- Advil Cold & Sinus 723
- Infants' Advil Concentrated Drops 604
- Infants' Advil Concentrated Drops - White Grape (Dye-Free) 604
- Junior Strength Advil Swallow Tablets 605
- Advil Migraine Liquigels 608
- Advil Multi-Symptom Cold Caplets 770
- Advil PM Caplets 615
- Motrin IB Tablets and Caplets 1866
- Children's Motrin Oral Suspension ... 1867
- Children's Motrin Non-Staining Dye-Free Oral Suspension 1867
- Children's Motrin Cold Oral Suspension 1867
- Infants' Motrin Concentrated Drops 1867
- Infants' Motrin Non-Staining Dye-Free Concentrated Drops 1867
- Junior Strength Motrin Caplets and Chewable Tablets 1867
- Vicoprofen Tablets 539

Indomethacin (Concomitant therapy with drugs that affect platelet function, such as non-steroid anti-inflammatory agents, may increase the risk of bleeding). Products include:
- Indocin 1995

Indomethacin Sodium Trihydrate (Concomitant therapy with drugs that affect platelet function, such as non-steroid anti-inflammatory agents, may increase the risk of bleeding). Products include:
- Indocin I.V. 2465

Ketoprofen (Concomitant therapy with drugs that affect platelet function, such as non-steroid anti-inflammatory agents, may increase the risk of bleeding).
- No products indexed under this heading.

Ketorolac Tromethamine (Concomitant therapy with drugs that affect platelet function, such as non-steroid anti-inflammatory agents, may increase the risk of bleeding). Products include:
- Acular Ophthalmic Solution 565
- Acular LS Ophthalmic Solution 566

Meclofenamate Sodium (Concomitant therapy with drugs that affect platelet function, such as non-steroid anti-inflammatory agents, may increase the risk of bleeding).
- No products indexed under this heading.

Mefenamic Acid (Concomitant therapy with drugs that affect platelet function, such as non-steroid anti-inflammatory agents, may increase the risk of bleeding).
- No products indexed under this heading.

Meloxicam (Concomitant therapy with drugs that affect platelet function, such as non-steroid anti-inflammatory agents, may increase the risk of bleeding). Products include:
- Mobic Oral Suspension 863
- Mobic Tablets 863

Nabumetone (Concomitant therapy with drugs that affect platelet function, such as non-steroid anti-inflammatory agents, may increase the risk of bleeding).
- No products indexed under this heading.

Naproxen (Concomitant therapy with drugs that affect platelet function, such as non-steroid anti-inflammatory agents, may increase the risk of bleeding). Products include:
- EC-Naprosyn Delayed-Release Tablets 2761
- Naprosyn Suspension 2761
- Naprosyn Tablets 2761
- Prevacid NapraPAC 3280

Naproxen Sodium (Concomitant therapy with drugs that affect platelet function, such as non-steroid anti-inflammatory agents, may increase the risk of bleeding). Products include:
- Aleve Caplets 742
- Aleve Gelcaps 743
- Aleve Tablets 743
- Aleve Cold & Sinus Caplets 744
- Anaprox Tablets 2761
- Anaprox DS Tablets 2761

Oxaprozin (Concomitant therapy with drugs that affect platelet function, such as non-steroid anti-inflammatory agents, may increase the risk of bleeding).
- No products indexed under this heading.

Phenylbutazone (Concomitant therapy with drugs that affect platelet function, such as non-steroid anti-inflammatory agents, may increase the risk of bleeding).
- No products indexed under this heading.

Piroxicam (Concomitant therapy with drugs that affect platelet function, such as non-steroid anti-inflammatory agents, may increase the risk of bleeding).
- No products indexed under this heading.

Reteplase (Concomitant therapy with thrombolytics may increase the risk of bleeding complications and considerably enhance the effect of Refludan on aPTT prolongation). Products include:
- Retavase 2499

Rofecoxib (Concomitant therapy with drugs that affect platelet function, such as non-steroid anti-inflammatory agents, may increase the risk of bleeding).
- No products indexed under this heading.

IMPORTANT NOTE: Always consult each drug listing in the patient's regimen for possible interactions.

Streptokinase (Concomitant therapy with thrombolytics may increase the risk of bleeding complications and considerably enhance the effect of Refludan on aPTT prolongation).
No products indexed under this heading.

Sulindac (Concomitant therapy with drugs that affect platelet function, such as non-steroid anti-inflammatory agents, may increase the risk of bleeding). Products include:
Clinoril Tablets 1924

Tolmetin Sodium (Concomitant therapy with drugs that affect platelet function, such as non-steroid anti-inflammatory agents, may increase the risk of bleeding).
No products indexed under this heading.

Urokinase (Concomitant therapy with thrombolytics may increase the risk of bleeding complications and considerably enhance the effect of Refludan on aPTT prolongation).
No products indexed under this heading.

Valdecoxib (Concomitant therapy with drugs that affect platelet function, such as non-steroid anti-inflammatory agents, may increase the risk of bleeding).
No products indexed under this heading.

Warfarin Sodium (Concomitant therapy with oral anticoagulants may increase the risk of bleeding). Products include:
Coumadin for Injection 898
Coumadin Tablets 898

REFRESH CELLUVISC LUBRICANT EYE DROPS
(Carboxymethylcellulose Sodium) ..... ⊙240
None cited in PDR database.

REFRESH ENDURA LUBRICANT EYE DROPS
(Glycerin, Polysorbate 80) .... ⊙240
None cited in PDR database.

REFRESH LIQUIGEL LUBRICANT EYE DROPS
(Carboxymethylcellulose Sodium) ..... ⊙241
None cited in PDR database.

REFRESH PLUS LUBRICANT EYE DROPS
(Carboxymethylcellulose Sodium) ..... ⊙241
None cited in PDR database.

REFRESH P.M. LUBRICANT EYE OINTMENT
(Mineral Oil, Petrolatum, White) .... ⊙241
None cited in PDR database.

REFRESH TEARS LUBRICANT EYE DROPS
(Carboxymethylcellulose Sodium) ..... ⊙241
None cited in PDR database.

REISHIMAX CAPSULES
(Ganoderma lucinum mushroom extract).. 2672
May interact with immunosuppressive agents. Compounds in these categories include:

Azathioprine (Concurrent use with immunosuppressive agents requires consultation with a physician).
No products indexed under this heading.

Basiliximab (Concurrent use with immunosuppressive agents requires consultation with a physician). Products include:
Simulect for Injection 2284

Cyclosporine (Concurrent use with immunosuppressive agents requires consultation with a physician). Products include:
Gengraf Capsules 459
Neoral Oral Solution 2259
Neoral Soft Gelatin Capsules 2259
Restasis Ophthalmic Emulsion 575
Sandimmune 2275

Muromonab-CD3 (Concurrent use with immunosuppressive agents requires consultation with a physician). Products include:
Orthoclone OKT3 Sterile Solution 2360

Mycophenolate Mofetil (Concurrent use with immunosuppressive agents requires consultation with a physician). Products include:
CellCept Capsules 2747
CellCept Oral Suspension 2747
CellCept Tablets 2747

Sirolimus (Concurrent use with immunosuppressive agents requires consultation with a physician). Products include:
Rapamune Oral Solution and Tablets 3475

Tacrolimus (Concurrent use with immunosuppressive agents requires consultation with a physician). Products include:
Prograf Capsules and Injection 632
Protopic Ointment 638

RELENZA ROTADISK
(Zanamivir) 1552
May interact with:

Influenza Virus Vaccine Live, Intranasal (Because of potential interference between zanamivir and the influenza virus vaccine live, it is advisable that the influenza virus vaccine live not be administered until 24 hours after cessation of zanamivir and that zanamivir not be administered until 2weeks after the administration of influenza virus vaccine live unless medically indicated).
No products indexed under this heading.

RELPAX TABLETS
(Eletriptan Hydrobromide) 2548
May interact with 5HT1-receptor agonists, cytochrome p450 3a4 inhibitors (selected), ergot-containing drugs, and selective serotonin reuptake inhibitors. Compounds in these categories include:

Acetazolamide (Eletriptan should not be used within 72 hours of drugs that have demonstrated potent CYP3A4 inhibition).
No products indexed under this heading.

Amiodarone Hydrochloride (Eletriptan should not be used within 72 hours of drugs that have demonstrated potent CYP3A4 inhibition).
No products indexed under this heading.

Amprenavir (Eletriptan should not be used within 72 hours of drugs that have demonstrated potent CYP3A4 inhibition). Products include:
Agenerase Capsules 1327
Agenerase Oral Solution 1332

Anastrozole (Eletriptan should not be used within 72 hours of drugs that have demonstrated potent CYP3A4 inhibition). Products include:
Arimidex Tablets 673

Aprepitant (Eletriptan should not be used within 72 hours of drugs that have demonstrated potent CYP3A4 inhibition). Products include:
Emend Capsules 1963

Cimetidine (Eletriptan should not be used within 72 hours of drugs that have demonstrated potent CYP3A4 inhibition). Products include:
Tagamet HB 200 Tablets .... ▣664

Cimetidine Hydrochloride (Eletriptan should not be used within 72 hours of drugs that have demonstrated potent CYP3A4 inhibition).
No products indexed under this heading.

Ciprofloxacin (Eletriptan should not be used within 72 hours of drugs that have demonstrated potent CYP3A4 inhibition). Products include:
Cipro Oral Suspension 2977
Cipro I.V. 2984
Cipro XR Tablets 2990
Ciprodex Otic Suspension 559

Citalopram Hydrobromide (Selective serotonin reuptake inhibitors (SSRI) have been reported, rarely, to cause weakness, hyperreflexia, and incoordination when co-administered with 5-HT agonists. If concomitant treatment with eletriptan and an SSRI is clinically warranted, appropriate observation of the patient is advised). Products include:
Celexa 1176

Clarithromycin (Eletriptan should not be used within 72 hours of drugs that have demonstrated potent CYP3A4 inhibition). Products include:
Biaxin/Biaxin XL 402
PREVPAC 3284

Clotrimazole (Eletriptan should not be used within 72 hours of drugs that have demonstrated potent CYP3A4 inhibition). Products include:
Desenex Athlete's Foot Cream .... ▣635
Lotrimin 3039
Lotrisone 3040

Cyclosporine (Eletriptan should not be used within 72 hours of drugs that have demonstrated potent CYP3A4 inhibition). Products include:
Gengraf Capsules 459
Neoral Oral Solution 2259
Neoral Soft Gelatin Capsules 2259
Restasis Ophthalmic Emulsion 575
Sandimmune 2275

Dalfopristin (Eletriptan should not be used within 72 hours of drugs that have demonstrated potent CYP3A4 inhibition).
No products indexed under this heading.

Danazol (Eletriptan should not be used within 72 hours of drugs that have demonstrated potent CYP3A4 inhibition).
No products indexed under this heading.

Delavirdine Mesylate (Eletriptan should not be used within 72 hours of drugs that have demonstrated potent CYP3A4 inhibition). Products include:
Rescriptor Tablets 2551

Dihydroergotamine Mesylate (Ergot-containing drugs have been reported to cause prolonged vasospastic reactions. Because these effects may be additive, use of ergotamine-containing or ergot-type medications and eletriptan within 24 hours of each other is not recommended). Products include:
Migranal Nasal Spray 3348

Diltiazem Hydrochloride (Eletriptan should not be used within 72 hours of drugs that have demonstrated potent CYP3A4 inhibition). Products include:
Cardizem LA Extended Release Tablets 1728
Tiazac Capsules 1201

Diltiazem Maleate (Eletriptan should not be used within 72 hours of drugs that have demonstrated potent CYP3A4 inhibition).
No products indexed under this heading.

Efavirenz (Eletriptan should not be used within 72 hours of drugs that have demonstrated potent CYP3A4 inhibition). Products include:
Atripla Tablets 945
Sustiva Capsules 930
Sustiva Tablets 930

Ergonovine Maleate (Ergot-containing drugs have been reported to cause prolonged vasospastic reactions. Because these effects may be additive, use of ergotamine-containing or ergot-type medications and eletriptan within 24 hours of each other is not recommended.).
No products indexed under this heading.

Ergotamine Tartrate (Ergot-containing drugs have been reported to cause prolonged vasospastic reactions. Because these effects may be additive, use of ergotamine-containing or ergot-type medications and eletriptan within 24 hours of each other is not recommended.).
No products indexed under this heading.

Erythromycin (Eletriptan should not be used within 72 hours of drugs that have demonstrated potent CYP3A4 inhibition). Products include:
Ery-Tab Tablets 449
Erythromycin Base Filmtab Tablets 455
Erythromycin Delayed-Release Capsules, USP............................. 457
PCE Dispertab Tablets 515

Erythromycin Estolate (Eletriptan should not be used within 72 hours of drugs that have demonstrated potent CYP3A4 inhibition).
No products indexed under this heading.

Erythromycin Ethylsuccinate (Eletriptan should not be used within 72 hours of drugs that have demonstrated potent CYP3A4 inhibition). Products include:
E.E.S. 451
EryPed 447

Erythromycin Gluceptate (Eletriptan should not be used within 72 hours of drugs that have demonstrated potent CYP3A4 inhibition).
No products indexed under this heading.

Erythromycin Lactobionate (Eletriptan should not be used within 72 hours of drugs that have demonstrated potent CYP3A4 inhibition).
No products indexed under this heading.

Erythromycin Stearate (Eletriptan should not be used within 72 hours of drugs that have demonstrated potent CYP3A4 inhibition). Products include:
Erythrocin Stearate Filmtab Tablets 453

Escitalopram Oxalate (Selective serotonin reuptake inhibitors (SSRI) have been reported, rarely, to cause weakness, hyperreflexia, and incoordination when co-administered with 5-HT agonists. If concomitant treatment with eletriptan and an SSRI is clinically warranted, appropriate observation of the patient is advised). Products include:

Lexapro Oral Solution 1190
Lexapro Tablets 1190

Esomeprazole Magnesium (Eletriptan should not be used within 72 hours of drugs that have demonstrated potent CYP3A4 inhibition). Products include:
Nexium Delayed-Release Capsules 655

Fluconazole (Eletriptan should not be used within 72 hours of drugs that have demonstrated potent CYP3A4 inhibition).
No products indexed under this heading.

Fluoxetine Hydrochloride (Eletriptan should not be used within 72 hours of drugs that have demonstrated potent CYP3A4 inhibition). Products include:
Prozac Pulvules and Liquid 1801
Symbyax Capsules 1819

Fluvoxamine Maleate (Eletriptan should not be used within 72 hours of drugs that have demonstrated potent CYP3A4 inhibition).
No products indexed under this heading.

Fosamprenavir Calcium (Eletriptan should not be used within 72 hours of drugs that have demonstrated potent CYP3A4 inhibition). Products include:
Lexiva Tablets 1505

Indinavir Sulfate (Eletriptan should not be used within 72 hours of drugs that have demonstrated potent CYP3A4 inhibition). Products include:
Crixivan Capsules 1940

Isoniazid (Eletriptan should not be used within 72 hours of drugs that have demonstrated potent CYP3A4 inhibition).
No products indexed under this heading.

Itraconazole (Eletriptan should not be used within 72 hours of drugs that have demonstrated potent CYP3A4 inhibition).
No products indexed under this heading.

Ketoconazole (Eletriptan should not be used within 72 hours of drugs that have demonstrated potent CYP3A4 inhibition). Products include:
Nizoral A-D Shampoo, 1% 1868

Lopinavir (Eletriptan should not be used within 72 hours of drugs that have demonstrated potent CYP3A4 inhibition). Products include:
Kaletra 476

Loratadine (Eletriptan should not be used within 72 hours of drugs that have demonstrated potent CYP3A4 inhibition). Products include:
Alavert Allergy & Sinus D-12 Hour Tablets.. 771
Alavert 771
Children's Claritin Allergy Oral Solution 771
Claritin Non-Drowsy 24 Hour Tablets.. 772
Claritin Reditabs 24 Hour Non-Drowsy Tablets 772
Claritin-D Non-Drowsy 12 Hour Tablets.. 772
Claritin-D Non-Drowsy 24 Hour Tablets.. 772

Methylergonovine Maleate (Ergot-containing drugs have been reported to cause prolonged vasospastic reactions. Because these effects may be additive, use of ergotamine-containing or ergot-type medications and eletriptan within 24 hours of each other is not recommended.).
No products indexed under this heading.

Methysergide Maleate (Ergot-containing drugs have been reported to cause prolonged vasospastic reactions. Because these effects may be additive, use of ergotamine-containing or ergot-type medications and eletriptan within 24 hours of each other is not recommended.).
No products indexed under this heading.

Metronidazole (Eletriptan should not be used within 72 hours of drugs that have demonstrated potent CYP3A4 inhibition). Products include:
Metrogel 1% 1211
MetroGel-Vaginal Gel 1855
Vandazole Vaginal Gel 3338

Metronidazole Benzoate (Eletriptan should not be used within 72 hours of drugs that have demonstrated potent CYP3A4 inhibition).
No products indexed under this heading.

Metronidazole Hydrochloride (Eletriptan should not be used within 72 hours of drugs that have demonstrated potent CYP3A4 inhibition).
No products indexed under this heading.

Miconazole (Eletriptan should not be used within 72 hours of drugs that have demonstrated potent CYP3A4 inhibition).
No products indexed under this heading.

Miconazole Nitrate (Eletriptan should not be used within 72 hours of drugs that have demonstrated potent CYP3A4 inhibition). Products include:
Desenex 635
Desenex Jock Itch Spray Powder ... 635

Naratriptan Hydrochloride (Concomitant use of other 5-HT1 agonists within 24 hours of eletriptan treatment is not recommended). Products include:
Amerge Tablets 1339

Nefazodone Hydrochloride (Eletriptan should not be used within 72 hours of drugs that have demonstrated potent CYP3A4 inhibition).
No products indexed under this heading.

Nelfinavir Mesylate (Eletriptan should not be used within 72 hours of drugs that have demonstrated potent CYP3A4 inhibition). Products include:
Viracept 2577

Nevirapine (Eletriptan should not be used within 72 hours of drugs that have demonstrated potent CYP3A4 inhibition). Products include:
Viramune Oral Suspension 873
Viramune Tablets 873

Niacinamide (Eletriptan should not be used within 72 hours of drugs that have demonstrated potent CYP3A4 inhibition).
No products indexed under this heading.

Nicotinamide (Eletriptan should not be used within 72 hours of drugs that have demonstrated potent CYP3A4 inhibition). Products include:
Nicomide Tablets 1088

Nifedipine (Eletriptan should not be used within 72 hours of drugs that have demonstrated potent CYP3A4 inhibition). Products include:
Adalat CC Tablets 2964

Norfloxacin (Eletriptan should not be used within 72 hours of drugs that have demonstrated potent CYP3A4 inhibition). Products include:
Noroxin Tablets 2032

Omeprazole (Eletriptan should not be used within 72 hours of drugs that have demonstrated potent CYP3A4 inhibition). Products include:
Zegerid Capsules 2958
Zegerid Powder for Oral Solution 2958

Paroxetine Hydrochloride (Eletriptan should not be used within 72 hours of drugs that have demonstrated potent CYP3A4 inhibition). Products include:
Paxil CR Controlled-Release Tablets 1538
Paxil 1530

Propoxyphene Hydrochloride (Eletriptan should not be used within 72 hours of drugs that have demonstrated potent CYP3A4 inhibition).
No products indexed under this heading.

Propoxyphene Napsylate (Eletriptan should not be used within 72 hours of drugs that have demonstrated potent CYP3A4 inhibition).
No products indexed under this heading.

Propranolol Hydrochloride (The Cmax and AUC of eletriptan were increased by 10 and 33% respectively in the presence of propranolol. No interactive increases in blood pressure were observed. No dosage adjustment appears to be needed for patients taking propranolol). Products include:
Inderal LA Long-Acting Capsules 3429
InnoPran XL Capsules 2723

Quinidine (Eletriptan should not be used within 72 hours of drugs that have demonstrated potent CYP3A4 inhibition).
No products indexed under this heading.

Quinidine Hydrochloride (Eletriptan should not be used within 72 hours of drugs that have demonstrated potent CYP3A4 inhibition).
No products indexed under this heading.

Quinidine Polygalacturonate (Eletriptan should not be used within 72 hours of drugs that have demonstrated potent CYP3A4 inhibition).
No products indexed under this heading.

Quinidine Sulfate (Eletriptan should not be used within 72 hours of drugs that have demonstrated potent CYP3A4 inhibition).
No products indexed under this heading.

Quinine (Eletriptan should not be used within 72 hours of drugs that have demonstrated potent CYP3A4 inhibition).
No products indexed under this heading.

Quinine Sulfate (Eletriptan should not be used within 72 hours of drugs that have demonstrated potent CYP3A4 inhibition).
No products indexed under this heading.

Quinupristin (Eletriptan should not be used within 72 hours of drugs that have demonstrated potent CYP3A4 inhibition).
No products indexed under this heading.

Ranitidine Bismuth Citrate (Eletriptan should not be used within 72 hours of drugs that have demonstrated potent CYP3A4 inhibition).
No products indexed under this heading.

Ranitidine Hydrochloride (Eletriptan should not be used within 72 hours of drugs that have demonstrated potent CYP3A4 inhibition). Products include:
Zantac 1624
Zantac Injection 1619
Zantac Injection Pharmacy Bulk Package 1622

Ritonavir (Eletriptan should not be used within 72 hours of drugs that have demonstrated potent CYP3A4 inhibition). Products include:
Kaletra 476
Norvir 503

Rizatriptan Benzoate (Concomitant use of other 5-HT1 agonists within 24 hours of eletriptan treatment is not recommended). Products include:
Maxalt Tablets 2008
Maxalt-MLT Orally Disintegrating Tablets 2008

Saquinavir (Eletriptan should not be used within 72 hours of drugs that have demonstrated potent CYP3A4 inhibition).
No products indexed under this heading.

Saquinavir Mesylate (Eletriptan should not be used within 72 hours of drugs that have demonstrated potent CYP3A4 inhibition). Products include:
Invirase 2772

Sertraline Hydrochloride (Eletriptan should not be used within 72 hours of drugs that have demonstrated potent CYP3A4 inhibition). Products include:
Zoloft 2586

Sumatriptan (Concomitant use of other 5-HT1 agonists within 24 hours of eletriptan treatment is not recommended). Products include:
Imitrex Nasal Spray 1467

Sumatriptan Succinate (Concomitant use of other 5-HT1 agonists within 24 hours of eletriptan treatment is not recommended). Products include:
Imitrex Injection 1463
Imitrex Tablets 1471

Telithromycin (Eletriptan should not be used within 72 hours of drugs that have demonstrated potent CYP3A4 inhibition). Products include:
Ketek Tablets 2903

Troglitazone (Eletriptan should not be used within 72 hours of drugs that have demonstrated potent CYP3A4 inhibition).
No products indexed under this heading.

Troleandomycin (Eletriptan should not be used within 72 hours of drugs that have demonstrated potent CYP3A4 inhibition).
No products indexed under this heading.

Valproate Sodium (Eletriptan should not be used within 72 hours of drugs that have demonstrated potent CYP3A4 inhibition). Products include:

Depacon Injection 412

Verapamil Hydrochloride (Eletriptan should not be used within 72 hours of drugs that have demonstrated potent CYP3A4 inhibition). Products include:
- Covera-HS Tablets 3139
- Tarka Tablets 524
- Verelan PM Extended-Release Capsules, Controlled-Onset 3106

Voriconazole (Eletriptan should not be used within 72 hours of drugs that have demonstrated potent CYP3A4 inhibition). Products include:
- VFEND I.V. 2564
- VFEND Oral Suspension 2564
- VFEND Tablets 2564

Zafirlukast (Eletriptan should not be used within 72 hours of drugs that have demonstrated potent CYP3A4 inhibition). Products include:
- Accolate Tablets 671

Zileuton (Eletriptan should not be used within 72 hours of drugs that have demonstrated potent CYP3A4 inhibition). Products include:
- Zyflo Tablets 1023

Zolmitriptan (Concomitant use of other 5-HT1 agonists within 24 hours of eletriptan treatment is not recommended). Products include:
- Zomig Tablets 3519
- Zomig Nasal Spray 3523
- Zomig-ZMT Tablets 3519

Food Interactions

Grapefruit (Eletriptan should not be used within 72 hours of drugs that have demonstrated potent CYP3A4 inhibition).

Grapefruit Juice (Eletriptan should not be used within 72 hours of drugs that have demonstrated potent CYP3A4 inhibition).

REMICADE FOR IV INJECTION

(Infliximab) 971

May interact with:

2-Amino-6-Mercaptopurine (Rare postmarketing cases of hepatosplenic T-cell lymphoma have been reported in adolescent and young adult patients with Crohns's disease treated with remicade; all of these hepatosplenic T-cell lymphomas with remicade have occurred in patients on concomitant treatment with azathioprine or 6-mercaptopurine).
- No products indexed under this heading.

Anakinra (Serious infections were seen with concurrent use of anakinra and another TNF2-blocking agent, etanercept. Similar toxicities may also result from the combination of anakinra and other TNF2-blocking agents; therefore, concurrent use of anakinra and infliximab is not recommended). Products include:
- Kineret Injection 599

Azathioprine (Rare postmarketing cases of hepatosplenic T-cell lymphoma have been reported in adolescent and young adult patients with Crohns's disease treated with remicade; all of these hepatosplenic T-cell lymphomas with remicade have occurred in patients on concomitant treatment with azathioprine or 6-mercaptopurine).
- No products indexed under this heading.

Azathioprine Sodium (Rare postmarketing cases of hepatosplenic T-cell lymphoma have been reported in adolescent and young adult patients with Crohns's disease treated with remicade; all of these hepatosplenic T-cell lymphomas with remicade have occurred in patients on concomitant treatment with azathioprine or 6-mercaptopurine).
- No products indexed under this heading.

Mercaptopurine (Rare postmarketing cases of hepatosplenic T-cell lymphoma have been reported in adolescent and young adult patients with Crohns's disease treated with remicade; all of these hepatosplenic T-cell lymphomas with remicade have occurred in patients on concomitant treatment with azathioprine or 6-mercaptopurine).
- No products indexed under this heading.

RENAGEL TABLETS

(Sevelamer Hydrochloride) 1282

May interact with:

Ciprofloxacin (Co-administration may decrease the bioavailability of ciprofloxacin by approximately 50%). Products include:
- Cipro Oral Suspension 2977
- Cipro I.V. 2984
- Cipro XR Tablets 2990
- Ciprodex Otic Suspension 559

REOPRO VIALS

(Abciximab) 1809

May interact with anticoagulants, oral anticoagulants, non-steroidal anti-inflammatory agents, thrombolytics, and certain other agents. Compounds in these categories include:

Alteplase (Co-administration with thrombolytics may be associated with an increase in bleeding). Products include:
- Activase I.V. 1223
- Cathflo Activase 1231

Anisindione (Co-administration of oral anticoagulants within seven days is contraindicated unless prothrombin time is less than or equal to 1.2 times control; concurrent use with other anticoagulant agents may be associated with an increase in bleeding). Products include:
- Miradon Tablets 3042

Anistreplase (Co-administration with thrombolytics may be associated with an increase in bleeding).
- No products indexed under this heading.

Ardeparin Sodium (Co-administration with other anticoagulant agents may be associated with an increase in bleeding).
- No products indexed under this heading.

Aspirin (Co-administration with antiplatelet agents, such as aspirin, may be associated with an increase in bleeding). Products include:
- Aggrenox Capsules 822
- Bayer Aspirin 744
- BC Allergy Sinus Cold Powder .... ▣677
- BC Headache Powder .... ▣677
- Arthritis Strength BC Powder .... ▣677
- BC Sinus Cold Powder .... ▣677
- Excedrin Extra Strength Caplets/Tablets/Geltabs .... ▣684
- Excedrin Migraine Caplets/Tablets/Geltabs .... ▣609
- Goody's Body Pain Formula Powder .... ▣684
- Goody's Extra Strength Headache Powders .... ▣611
- Goody's Extra Strength Pain Relief Tablets .... ▣685
- Percodan Tablets 1132
- St. Joseph 81 mg Aspirin Chewable and Enteric Coated Tablets 1869

Celecoxib (Co-administration with antiplatelet agents, such as non-steroidal anti-inflammatory agents, may be associated with an increase in bleeding). Products include:
- Celebrex Capsules 3134

Clopidogrel Bisulfate (Co-administration with antiplatelet agents, such as clopidogrel, may be associated with an increase in bleeding). Products include:
- Plavix Tablets 917
- Plavix Tablets 2926

Dalteparin Sodium (Co-administration with other anticoagulant agents may be associated with an increase in bleeding). Products include:
- Fragmin Injection 1097

Danaparoid Sodium (Co-administration with other anticoagulant agents may be associated with an increase in bleeding).
- No products indexed under this heading.

Dextran (Co-administration with intravenous dextran before percutaneous coronary intervention, or intent to use it during an intervention is contraindicated).
- No products indexed under this heading.

Diclofenac Potassium (Co-administration with antiplatelet agents, such as non-steroidal anti-inflammatory agents, may be associated with an increase in bleeding).
- No products indexed under this heading.

Diclofenac Sodium (Co-administration with antiplatelet agents, such as non-steroidal anti-inflammatory agents, may be associated with an increase in bleeding). Products include:
- Arthrotec Tablets 3129
- Voltaren Ophthalmic Solution 2309
- Voltaren Tablets 2307
- Voltaren-XR Tablets 2310

Dicumarol (Co-administration of oral anticoagulants within seven days is contraindicated unless prothrombin time is less than or equal to 1.2 times control; concurrent use with other anticoagulant agents may be associated with an increase in bleeding).
- No products indexed under this heading.

Dipyridamole (Co-administration with antiplatelet agents, such as dipyridamole, may be associated with an increase in bleeding). Products include:
- Aggrenox Capsules 822
- Persantine Tablets 868

Enoxaparin Sodium (Co-administration with other anticoagulant agents may be associated with an increase in bleeding). Products include:
- Lovenox Injection 2915

Etodolac (Co-administration with antiplatelet agents, such as non-steroidal anti-inflammatory agents, may be associated with an increase in bleeding).
- No products indexed under this heading.

Fenoprofen Calcium (Co-administration with antiplatelet agents, such as non-steroidal anti-inflammatory agents, may be associated with an increase in bleeding). Products include:
- Nalfon Capsules 2502

Flurbiprofen (Co-administration with antiplatelet agents, such as non-steroidal anti-inflammatory agents, may be associated with an increase in bleeding).
- No products indexed under this heading.

Fondaparinux Sodium (Co-administration with other anticoagulant agents may be associated with an increase in bleeding). Products include:
- Arixtra Injection 1351

Heparin Calcium (Co-administration with other anticoagulant agents may be associated with an increase in bleeding).
- No products indexed under this heading.

Heparin Sodium (Co-administration with other anticoagulant agents may be associated with an increase in bleeding).
- No products indexed under this heading.

Ibuprofen (Co-administration with antiplatelet agents, such as non-steroidal anti-inflammatory agents, may be associated with an increase in bleeding). Products include:
- Advil Allergy Sinus Caplets .... ▣770
- Advil .... ▣674
- Children's Advil Oral Suspension .... ▣603
- Children's Advil Chewable Tablets .... ▣603
- Advil Cold & Sinus .... ▣723
- Infants' Advil Concentrated Drops .... ▣604
- Infants' Advil Concentrated Drops - White Grape (Dye-Free) .... ▣604
- Junior Strength Advil Swallow Tablets .... ▣605
- Advil Migraine Liquigels .... ▣608
- Advil Multi-Symptom Cold Caplets .... ▣770
- Advil PM Caplets .... ▣615
- Motrin IB Tablets and Caplets 1866
- Children's Motrin Oral Suspension 1867
- Children's Motrin Non-Staining Dye-Free Oral Suspension 1867
- Children's Motrin Cold Oral Suspension 1867
- Infants' Motrin Concentrated Drops 1867
- Infants' Motrin Non-Staining Dye-Free Concentrated Drops 1867
- Junior Strength Motrin Caplets and Chewable Tablets 1867
- Vicoprofen Tablets 539

Indomethacin (Co-administration with antiplatelet agents, such as non-steroidal anti-inflammatory agents, may be associated with an increase in bleeding). Products include:
- Indocin 1995

Indomethacin Sodium Trihydrate (Co-administration with antiplatelet agents, such as non-steroidal anti-inflammatory agents, may be associated with an increase in bleeding). Products include:
- Indocin I.V. 2465

Ketoprofen (Co-administration with antiplatelet agents, such as non-steroidal anti-inflammatory agents, may be associated with an increase in bleeding).
- No products indexed under this heading.

Ketorolac Tromethamine (Co-administration with antiplatelet agents, such as non-steroidal anti-in-

flammatory agents, may be associated with an increase in bleeding). Products include:
- Acular Ophthalmic Solution 565
- Acular LS Ophthalmic Solution 566

Low Molecular Weight Heparins (Co-administration with other anticoagulant agents may be associated with an increase in bleeding).
No products indexed under this heading.

Meclofenamate Sodium (Co-administration with antiplatelet agents, such as non-steroidal anti-inflammatory agents, may be associated with an increase in bleeding).
No products indexed under this heading.

Mefenamic Acid (Co-administration with antiplatelet agents, such as non-steroidal anti-inflammatory agents, may be associated with an increase in bleeding).
No products indexed under this heading.

Meloxicam (Co-administration with antiplatelet agents, such as non-steroidal anti-inflammatory agents, may be associated with an increase in bleeding). Products include:
- Mobic Oral Suspension 863
- Mobic Tablets 863

Nabumetone (Co-administration with antiplatelet agents, such as non-steroidal anti-inflammatory agents, may be associated with an increase in bleeding).
No products indexed under this heading.

Naproxen (Co-administration with antiplatelet agents, such as non-steroidal anti-inflammatory agents, may be associated with an increase in bleeding). Products include:
- EC-Naprosyn Delayed-Release Tablets 2761
- Naprosyn Suspension 2761
- Naprosyn Tablets 2761
- Prevacid NapraPAC 3280

Naproxen Sodium (Co-administration with antiplatelet agents, such as non-steroidal anti-inflammatory agents, may be associated with an increase in bleeding). Products include:
- Aleve Caplets 742
- Aleve Gelcaps 743
- Aleve Tablets 743
- Aleve Cold & Sinus Caplets 744
- Anaprox Tablets 2761
- Anaprox DS Tablets 2761

Oxaprozin (Co-administration with antiplatelet agents, such as non-steroidal anti-inflammatory agents, may be associated with an increase in bleeding).
No products indexed under this heading.

Phenylbutazone (Co-administration with antiplatelet agents, such as non-steroidal anti-inflammatory agents, may be associated with an increase in bleeding).
No products indexed under this heading.

Piroxicam (Co-administration with antiplatelet agents, such as non-steroidal anti-inflammatory agents, may be associated with an increase in bleeding).
No products indexed under this heading.

Reteplase (Co-administration with thrombolytics may be associated with an increase in bleeding). Products include:
- Retavase 2499

Rofecoxib (Co-administration with antiplatelet agents, such as non-steroidal anti-inflammatory agents, may be associated with an increase in bleeding).
No products indexed under this heading.

Streptokinase (Co-administration with thrombolytics may be associated with an increase in bleeding).
No products indexed under this heading.

Sulindac (Co-administration with antiplatelet agents, such as non-steroidal anti-inflammatory agents, may be associated with an increase in bleeding). Products include:
- Clinoril Tablets 1924

Ticlopidine Hydrochloride (Co-administration with antiplatelet agents, such as ticlopidine, may be associated with an increase in bleeding). Products include:
- Ticlid Tablets 2810

Tinzaparin Sodium (Co-administration with other anticoagulant agents may be associated with an increase in bleeding).
No products indexed under this heading.

Tolmetin Sodium (Co-administration with antiplatelet agents, such as non-steroidal anti-inflammatory agents, may be associated with an increase in bleeding).
No products indexed under this heading.

Urokinase (Co-administration with thrombolytics may be associated with an increase in bleeding).
No products indexed under this heading.

Valdecoxib (Co-administration with antiplatelet agents, such as non-steroidal anti-inflammatory agents, may be associated with an increase in bleeding).
No products indexed under this heading.

Warfarin Sodium (Co-administration of oral anticoagulants within seven days is contraindicated unless prothrombin time is less than or equal to 1.2 times control; concurrent use with other anticoagulant agents may be associated with an increase in bleeding). Products include:
- Coumadin for Injection 898
- Coumadin Tablets 898

REQUIP TABLETS

(Ropinirole Hydrochloride) 1555

May interact with central nervous system depressants, cytochrome p450 1a2 inhibitors (selected), cytochrome p450 1a2 substrates (selected), antidepressant drugs, dopamine D2 antagonists, estrogens, hypnotics and sedatives, sedating antihistamines, and certain other agents. Compounds in these categories include:

Acetaminophen (CYP1A2 was the major enzyme responsible for the metabolism of ropinirole There is thus the potential for substrates or inhibitors of this enzyme when co-administered with ropinirole to alter its clearance). Products include:
- Comtrex Maximum Strength Cold & Cough Day/Night Caplets - Day Formulation 726
- Comtrex Maximum Strength Cold & Cough Day/Night Caplets - Night Formulation 726
- Comtrex Maximum Strength Non-Drowsy Cold & Cough Caplets 725
- Comtrex Maximum Strength Day/Night Severe Cold & Sinus Caplets - Day Formulation 725
- Comtrex Maximum Strength Day/Night Severe Cold & Sinus Caplets - Night Formulation 725
- Contac Cold and Flu Maximum Strength Caplets 728
- Contac Cold and Flu Day and Night Caplets (Day Formulation Only) 727
- Contac Cold and Flu Day and Night Caplets (Night Formulation Only) 727
- Contac Cold and Flu Non-Drowsy Caplets 728
- Excedrin Extra Strength Caplets/Tablets/Geltabs 684
- Excedrin Migraine Caplets/Tablets/Geltabs 609
- Excedrin PM Caplets/Tablets/Geltabs 610
- Excedrin Sinus Headache Caplets/Tablets 610
- Excedrin Tension Headache Caplets/Tablets/Geltabs 611
- Goody's Body Pain Formula Powder 684
- Goody's Extra Strength Headache Powders 611
- Goody's Extra Strength Pain Relief Tablets 685
- Goody's PM Powder for Pain with Sleeplessness 612
- Percocet Tablets 1131
- Robitussin Cough, Cold & Flu Nighttime Liquid 738
- TheraFlu Cold & Sore Throat Hot Liquid 741
- TheraFlu Flu & Chest Congestion Hot Liquid 741
- TheraFlu Flu & Sore Throat Hot Liquid 742
- TheraFlu Daytime Severe Cold Hot Liquid 742
- TheraFlu Nighttime Severe Cold Hot Liquid 740
- TheraFlu Warming Relief Daytime Severe Cold 743
- TheraFlu Warming Relief Nighttime Severe Cold 743
- Triaminic Cough & Sore Throat Liquid 747
- Regular Strength Tylenol Tablets 1870
- Children's Tylenol with Flavor Creator 679
- Children's Tylenol Plus Flu Oral Suspension 749
- Tylenol Cold Head Congestion Daytime Caplets with Cool Burst and Gelcaps 750
- Tylenol Cold Multi-Symptom Daytime Liquid 752
- Tylenol Cold Multi-Symptom Severe Daytime Liquid 752
- Tylenol 8 Hour Extended Release Caplets 1870
- Tylenol 1870
- Extra Strength Tylenol PM Caplets, Vanilla Caplets, Geltabs, Gelcaps and Liquid.......... 1875
- Extra Strength Tylenol Rapid Release Gels 1870
- Concentrated Tylenol Infants' Drops Plus Cold & Cough.............. 754
- Tylenol with Codeine Tablets 2391
- Tylenol Allergy Multi-Symptom Caplets with Cool Burst and Gelcaps 1872
- Tylenol Allergy Multi-Symptom Nighttime Caplets with Cool Burst 1872
- Tylenol Severe Allergy Caplets 1872
- Tylenol Arthritis Pain Extended Release Caplets and Geltabs 1870
- Tylenol Chest Congestion Caplets with Cool Burst 1872
- Tylenol Chest Congestion Liquid with Cool Burst 1872
- Children's Tylenol Suspension Liquid and Meltaways................... 1878
- Children's Tylenol Plus Cold Suspension Liquid 1879
- Children's Tylenol Plus Cold & Allergy Suspension Liquid 1878
- Children's Tylenol Plus Cough & Runny Nose Suspension Liquid 1879
- Children's Tylenol Plus Cough & Sore Throat Suspension Liquid 1879
- Children's Tylenol Suspension with Flavor Creator 1878
- Children's Tylenol Plus Flu Suspension Liquid 1881
- Children's Tylenol Plus Multi-Symptom Cold Suspension Liquid 1879
- Tylenol Cold Severe Congestion Non-Drowsy Caplets with Cool Burst 1874
- Tylenol Cold Head Congestion Daytime Caplets with Cool Burst 1873
- Tylenol Cold Head Congestion Nighttime Caplets with Cool Burst 1873
- Tylenol Cold Head Congestion Severe Caplets with Cool Burst..... 1873
- Tylenol Cold Multi-Symptom Daytime Caplets with Cool Burst and Gelcaps........................ 1874
- Tylenol Cold Multi-Symptom Daytime Liquid with Citrus Burst... 1874
- Tylenol Cold Multi-Symptom Nighttime Caplets with Cool Burst 1874
- Tylenol Cold Multi-Symptom Nighttime Liquid with Cool Burst... 1874
- Tylenol Cold Multi-Symptom Severe Caplets with Cool Burst..... 1874
- Tylenol Cold Multi-Symptom Severe Daytime Liquid with Citrus Burst 1874
- Tylenol Cough & Sore Throat Daytime Liquid with Cool Burst...... 1877
- Tylenol Cough & Sore Throat Nighttime Liquid with Cool Burst... 1877
- Concentrated Tylenol Infants' Drops 1878
- Concentrated Tylenol Infants' Drops Plus Cold.......................... 1879
- Concentrated Tylenol Infants' Drops Plus Cold and Cough 1879
- Jr. Tylenol Meltaways 1878
- Tylenol Sinus Severe Congestion Caplets with Cool Burst 1876
- Tylenol Sinus Congestion & Pain Daytime Caplets with Cool Burst and Gelcaps........................ 1876
- Tylenol Sinus Congestion & Pain Nighttime Caplets with Cool Burst 1876
- Tylenol Sinus Congestion & Pain Severe Caplets with Cool Burst..... 1876
- Tylenol Sore Throat Daytime Liquid with Cool Burst.................. 1877
- Tylenol Sore Throat Nighttime Liquid with Cool Burst.................. 1877
- Women's Tylenol Menstrual Relief Caplets.. 1877
- Vicks 44M Cough, Cold & Flu Relief Liquid................................. 2680
- Vicks DayQuil LiquiCaps/Liquid Multi-Symptom Cold/Flu Relief..... 761
- Vicks DayQuil Multi-Symptom Cold/Flu Relief LiquiCaps 2678
- Vicks DayQuil Multi-Symptom Cold/Flu Relief Liquid.................. 2678
- Vicks NyQuil Multi-Symptom Cold/Flu Relief Liquid.................... 2681
- Vicks NyQuil Multi-Symptom Cold/Flu Relief LiquiCaps............. 2681
- Vicks NyQuil LiquiCaps/Liquid Multi-Symptom Cold/Flu Relief..... 763
- Vicodin Tablets 535
- Vicodin ES Tablets 536
- Vicodin HP Tablets 538
- Zicam Maximum Strength Flu Daytime... 768
- Zicam Maximum Strength Flu Nighttime.. 768
- Zydone Tablets 1139

Acrivastine (Possible additive sedative effects).
No products indexed under this heading.

Alatrofloxacin Mesylate (If therapy with a drug known to be a potent inhibitor of CYP1A2 is stopped or started during treatment with ropinirole hydrochloride, adjustment of the dose of ropinirole hydrocholoride may be required).
No products indexed under this heading.

Alfentanil Hydrochloride (Possible additive sedative effects).
No products indexed under this heading.

Alprazolam (Possible additive sedative effects). Products include:
Niravam Orally Disintegrating Tablets ... 3092

Amiodarone Hydrochloride (If therapy with a drug known to be a potent inhibitor of CYP1A2 is stopped or started during treatment with ropinirole hydrochloride, adjustment of the dose of ropinirole hydrocholoride may be required).
No products indexed under this heading.

Amitriptyline Hydrochloride (Possible additive sedative effects).
No products indexed under this heading.

Amoxapine (Possible additive sedative effects).
No products indexed under this heading.

Anagrelide Hydrochloride (CYP1A2 was the major enzyme responsible for the metabolism of ropinirole There is thus the potential for substrates or inhibitors of this enzyme when co-administered with ropinirole to alter its clearance). Products include:
Agrylin Capsules ... 3169

Anastrozole (If therapy with a drug known to be a potent inhibitor of CYP1A2 is stopped or started during treatment with ropinirole hydrochloride, adjustment of the dose of ropinirole hydrocholoride may be required). Products include:
Arimidex Tablets ... 673

Aprobarbital (Possible additive sedative effects).
No products indexed under this heading.

Azatadine Maleate (Possible additive sedative effects).
No products indexed under this heading.

Bromodiphenhydramine Hydrochloride (Possible additive sedative effects).
No products indexed under this heading.

Brompheniramine Maleate (Possible additive sedative effects). Products include:
Children's Dimetapp Cold & Allergy Elixir ... ▣730
Children's Dimetapp Cold & Allergy Chewable Tablets ... ▣730
Children's Dimetapp DM Cold & Cough Elixir ... ▣731

Buprenorphine Hydrochloride (Possible additive sedative effects). Products include:
Buprenex Injectable ... 2716
Suboxone Tablets ... 2717
Subutex Tablets ... 2717

Bupropion Hydrochloride (Possible additive sedative effects). Products include:
Wellbutrin Tablets ... 1603
Wellbutrin SR Sustained-Release Tablets ... 1607
Wellbutrin XL Extended-Release Tablets ... 1613
Zyban Sustained-Release Tablets ... 1644

Buspirone Hydrochloride (Possible additive sedative effects).
No products indexed under this heading.

Butabarbital (Possible additive sedative effects).
No products indexed under this heading.

Butalbital (Possible additive sedative effects).
No products indexed under this heading.

Caffeine (CYP1A2 was the major enzyme responsible for the metabolism of ropinirole There is thus the potential for substrates or inhibitors of this enzyme when co-administered with ropinirole to alter its clearance). Products include:
BC Headache Powder ... ▣677
Arthritis Strength BC Powder ... ▣677
Excedrin Extra Strength Caplets/Tablets/Geltabs ... ▣684
Excedrin Migraine Caplets/Tablets/Geltabs ... ▣609
Excedrin Tension Headache Caplets/Tablets/Geltabs ... ▣611
Goody's Extra Strength Headache Powders ... ▣611
Goody's Extra Strength Pain Relief Tablets ... ▣685
Vivarin ... ▣602
Winrgy Dietary Supplement ... ▣823

Caffeine Anhydrous (CYP1A2 was the major enzyme responsible for the metabolism of ropinirole There is thus the potential for substrates or inhibitors of this enzyme when co-administered with ropinirole to alter its clearance).
No products indexed under this heading.

Chlordiazepoxide (Possible additive sedative effects).
No products indexed under this heading.

Chlordiazepoxide Hydrochloride (Possible additive sedative effects). Products include:
Librium Capsules ... 3347

Chlorotrianisene (Population pharmacokinetic analysis revealed that estrogens (mainly ethinyl estradiol) reduced the oral clearance of ropinirole by 36%. Dosage adjustment may not be needed for ropinirole patients on estrogen therapy unless estrogen therapy is stopped or started during treatment with ropinirole).
No products indexed under this heading.

Chlorpheniramine Maleate (Possible additive sedative effects). Products include:
Advil Allergy Sinus Caplets ... ▣770
Advil Multi-Symptom Cold Caplets ... ▣770
BC Allergy Sinus Cold Powder ... ▣677
Comtrex Maximum Strength Cold & Cough Day/Night Caplets - Night Formulation ... ▣726
Comtrex Maximum Strength Day/Night Severe Cold & Sinus Caplets - Night Formulation ... ▣725
Contac Cold and Flu Maximum Strength Caplets ... ▣728
Contac Cold and Flu Day and Night Caplets (Night Formulation Only) ... ▣727
Children's Dimetapp Long Acting Cough Plus Cold Syrup ... ▣731
Robitussin Cough & Cold Long-Acting Liquid ... ▣735
Robitussin Cough & Allergy Syrup .. ▣736
Robitussin Cough & Cold Nighttime Liquid ... ▣736
Robitussin Cough, Cold & Flu Nighttime Liquid ... ▣738
Robitussin Pediatric Cough & Cold Long-Acting Liquid ... ▣735
Robitussin Pediatric Cough & Cold Nighttime Liquid ... ▣736
Triaminic Cold & Allergy Liquid ... ▣746
Triaminic Cough & Runny Nose Softchews ... ▣748
Children's Tylenol Plus Flu Oral Suspension ... ▣749
Tylenol Allergy Multi-Symptom Caplets with Cool Burst and Gelcaps ... 1872
Children's Tylenol Plus Cold Suspension Liquid ... 1879
Children's Tylenol Plus Cough & Runny Nose Suspension Liquid ... 1879
Children's Tylenol Plus Flu Suspension Liquid ... 1881
Children's Tylenol Plus Multi-Symptom Cold Suspension Liquid ... 1879
Tylenol Cold Head Congestion Nighttime Caplets with Cool Burst ... 1873
Tylenol Cold Multi-Symptom Nighttime Caplets with Cool Burst ... 1874
Tylenol Sinus Congestion & Pain Nighttime Caplets with Cool Burst ... 1876
Vicks 44M Cough, Cold & Flu Relief Liquid ... 2680
Pediatric Vicks 44m Cough & Cold Relief Liquid ... 2676
Children's Vicks NyQuil Cold/Cough Relief ... ▣756
Children's Vicks NyQuil Cold/Cough Relief Liquid ... 2680
Zicam Maximum Strength Flu Daytime ... ▣768

Chlorpheniramine Polistirex (Possible additive sedative effects). Products include:
Tussionex Pennkinetic Extended-Release Suspension ... 3327

Chlorpheniramine Tannate (Possible additive sedative effects).
No products indexed under this heading.

Chlorpromazine (Co-administration with dopamine antagonists may diminish the effectiveness of ropinirole).
No products indexed under this heading.

Chlorpromazine Hydrochloride (Co-administration with dopamine antagonists may diminish the effectiveness of ropinirole).
No products indexed under this heading.

Chlorprothixene (Co-administration with dopamine antagonists may diminish the effectiveness of ropinirole).
No products indexed under this heading.

Chlorprothixene Hydrochloride (Co-administration with dopamine antagonists may diminish the effectiveness of ropinirole).
No products indexed under this heading.

Chlorprothixene Lactate (Possible additive sedative effects).
No products indexed under this heading.

Cimetidine (If therapy with a drug known to be a potent inhibitor of CYP1A2 is stopped or started during treatment with ropinirole hydrochloride, adjustment of the dose of ropinirole hydrocholoride may be required). Products include:
Tagamet HB 200 Tablets ... ▣664

Cimetidine Hydrochloride (If therapy with a drug known to be a potent inhibitor of CYP1A2 is stopped or started during treatment with ropinirole hydrochloride, adjustment of the dose of ropinirole hydrocholoride may be required).
No products indexed under this heading.

Ciprofloxacin (Co-administration increases ropinirole AUC by 84% on average and Cmax by 60%). Products include:
Cipro Oral Suspension ... 2977
Cipro I.V. ... 2984
Cipro XR Tablets ... 2990
Ciprodex Otic Suspension ... 559

Ciprofloxacin Hydrochloride (Co-administration increases ropinirole AUC by 84% on average and Cmax by 60%). Products include:
Ciloxan Ophthalmic Ointment ... 559
Ciloxan Ophthalmic Solution ... ⊙206
Cipro Tablets ... 2977
Proquin XR Tablets ... 1153

Citalopram Hydrobromide (Possible additive sedative effects). Products include:
Celexa ... 1176

Clarithromycin (If therapy with a drug known to be a potent inhibitor of CYP1A2 is stopped or started during treatment with ropinirole hydrochloride, adjustment of the dose of ropinirole hydrocholoride may be required). Products include:
Biaxin/Biaxin XL ... 402
PREVPAC ... 3284

Clemastine Fumarate (Possible additive sedative effects).
No products indexed under this heading.

Clomipramine Hydrochloride (CYP1A2 was the major enzyme responsible for the metabolism of ropinirole There is thus the potential for substrates or inhibitors of this enzyme when co-administered with ropinirole to alter its clearance).
No products indexed under this heading.

Clopidogrel Bisulfate (CYP1A2 was the major enzyme responsible for the metabolism of ropinirole There is thus the potential for substrates or inhibitors of this enzyme when co-administered with ropinirole to alter its clearance). Products include:
Plavix Tablets ... 917
Plavix Tablets ... 2926

Clorazepate Dipotassium (Possible additive sedative effects). Products include:
Tranxene ... 2474

Clozapine (Possible additive sedative effects). Products include:
Clozaril Tablets ... 2184
FazaClo Orally Disintegrating Tablets ... 551

Codeine Phosphate (Possible additive sedative effects). Products include:
Tylenol with Codeine Tablets ... 2391

Cyclobenzaprine (CYP1A2 was the major enzyme responsible for the metabolism of ropinirole There is thus the potential for substrates or inhibitors of this enzyme when co-administered with ropinirole to alter its clearance).
No products indexed under this heading.

Cyclobenzaprine Hydrochloride (CYP1A2 was the major enzyme responsible for the metabolism of ropinirole There is thus the potential for substrates or inhibitors of this enzyme when co-administered with ropinirole to alter its clearance).
No products indexed under this heading.

Cyproheptadine Hydrochloride (Possible additive sedative effects).
No products indexed under this heading.

Desflurane (Possible additive sedative effects).
No products indexed under this heading.

Desipramine Hydrochloride (Possible additive sedative effects).
No products indexed under this heading.

Desogestrel (If therapy with a drug known to be a potent inhibitor of CYP1A2 is stopped or started during treatment with ropinirole hydrochloride, adjustment of the dose of ropinirole hydrocholoride may be required). Products include:
Mircette Tablets ... **1066**

Dexchlorpheniramine Maleate (Possible additive sedative effects).
No products indexed under this heading.

Dezocine (Possible additive sedative effects).
No products indexed under this heading.

Diazepam (Possible additive sedative effects). Products include:
Diastat Rectal Delivery System ... **3343**
Valium Tablets ... **2819**

Dienestrol (Population pharmacokinetic analysis revealed that estrogens (mainly ethinyl estradiol) reduced the oral clearance of ropinirole by 36%. Dosage adjustment may not be needed for ropinirole patients on estrogen therapy unless estrogen therapy is stopped or started during treatment with ropinirole).
No products indexed under this heading.

Diethylstilbestrol (Population pharmacokinetic analysis revealed that estrogens (mainly ethinyl estradiol) reduced the oral clearance of ropinirole by 36%. Dosage adjustment may not be needed for ropinirole patients on estrogen therapy unless estrogen therapy is stopped or started during treatment with ropinirole).
No products indexed under this heading.

Diltiazem Hydrochloride (CYP1A2 was the major enzyme responsible for the metabolism of ropinirole There is thus the potential for substrates or inhibitors of this enzyme when co-administered with ropinirole to alter its clearance). Products include:
Cardizem LA Extended Release Tablets ... **1728**
Tiazac Capsules ... **1201**

Diltiazem Maleate (CYP1A2 was the major enzyme responsible for the metabolism of ropinirole There is thus the potential for substrates or inhibitors of this enzyme when co-administered with ropinirole to alter its clearance).
No products indexed under this heading.

Diphenhydramine Citrate (Possible additive sedative effects). Products include:
Advil PM Caplets ... **615**
Excedrin PM Caplets/Tablets/Geltabs ... **610**
Goody's PM Powder for Pain with Sleeplessness ... **612**

Diphenhydramine Hydrochloride (Possible additive sedative effects). Products include:
Nytol QuickCaps Caplets ... **615**
Nytol QuickGels Softgels Maximum Strength ... **616**
Simply Sleep Caplets ... **1868**
Sominex Original Formula Tablets .. **616**
TheraFlu Warming Relief Nighttime Severe Cold ... **743**
TheraFlu Thin Strips Multi Symptom ... **744**
Triaminic Nighttime Cold & Cough Liquid ... **746**
Triaminic Thin Strips Cough & Runny Nose ... **749**
Extra Strength Tylenol PM Caplets, Vanilla Caplets, Geltabs, Gelcaps and Liquid ... **1875**
Tylenol Sore Throat Nighttime Liquid with Cool Burst ... **790**
Tylenol Allergy Multi-Symptom Nighttime Caplets with Cool Burst ... **1872**
Tylenol Severe Allergy Caplets ... **1872**
Children's Tylenol Plus Cold & Allergy Suspension Liquid ... **1878**

Diphenylpyraline Hydrochloride (Possible additive sedative effects).
No products indexed under this heading.

Doxepin Hydrochloride (Possible additive sedative effects).
No products indexed under this heading.

Droperidol (Possible additive sedative effects).
No products indexed under this heading.

Enflurane (Possible additive sedative effects).
No products indexed under this heading.

Enoxacin (If therapy with a drug known to be a potent inhibitor of CYP1A2 is stopped or started during treatment with ropinirole hydrochloride, adjustment of the dose of ropinirole hydrocholoride may be required).
No products indexed under this heading.

Erythromycin (CYP1A2 was the major enzyme responsible for the metabolism of ropinirole There is thus the potential for substrates or inhibitors of this enzyme when co-administered with ropinirole to alter its clearance). Products include:
Ery-Tab Tablets ... **449**
Erythromycin Base Filmtab Tablets ... **455**
Erythromycin Delayed-Release Capsules, USP ... **457**
PCE Dispertab Tablets ... **515**

Erythromycin Estolate (CYP1A2 was the major enzyme responsible for the metabolism of ropinirole There is thus the potential for substrates or inhibitors of this enzyme when co-administered with ropinirole to alter its clearance).
No products indexed under this heading.

Erythromycin Ethylsuccinate (CYP1A2 was the major enzyme responsible for the metabolism of ropinirole There is thus the potential for substrates or inhibitors of this enzyme when co-administered with ropinirole to alter its clearance). Products include:
E.E.S. ... **451**
EryPed ... **447**

Erythromycin Gluceptate (CYP1A2 was the major enzyme responsible for the metabolism of ropinirole There is thus the potential for substrates or inhibitors of this enzyme when co-administered with ropinirole to alter its clearance).
No products indexed under this heading.

Erythromycin Lactobionate (CYP1A2 was the major enzyme responsible for the metabolism of ropinirole There is thus the potential for substrates or inhibitors of this enzyme when co-administered with ropinirole to alter its clearance).
No products indexed under this heading.

Erythromycin Stearate (CYP1A2 was the major enzyme responsible for the metabolism of ropinirole There is thus the potential for substrates or inhibitors of this enzyme when co-administered with ropinirole to alter its clearance). Products include:
Erythrocin Stearate Filmtab Tablets ... **453**

Escitalopram Oxalate (Possible additive sedative effects). Products include:
Lexapro Oral Solution ... **1190**
Lexapro Tablets ... **1190**

Estazolam (Possible additive sedative effects). Products include:
ProSom Tablets ... **517**

Estradiol (Population pharmacokinetic analysis revealed that estrogens (mainly ethinyl estradiol) reduced the oral clearance of ropinirole by 36%. Dosage adjustment may not be needed for ropinirole patients on estrogen therapy unless estrogen therapy is stopped or started during treatment with ropinirole). Products include:
Angeliq Tablets ... **762**
Climara Transdermal System ... **771**
Climara Pro Transdermal System **776**
Estrasorb Topical Emulsion ... **1147**
Estring Vaginal Ring ... **2635**
Menostar Transdermal System ... **782**
Vagifem Tablets ... **2334**

Estradiol Benzoate (CYP1A2 was the major enzyme responsible for the metabolism of ropinirole There is thus the potential for substrates or inhibitors of this enzyme when co-administered with ropinirole to alter its clearance).
No products indexed under this heading.

Estradiol Cypionate (CYP1A2 was the major enzyme responsible for the metabolism of ropinirole There is thus the potential for substrates or inhibitors of this enzyme when co-administered with ropinirole to alter its clearance).
No products indexed under this heading.

Estrogens, Conjugated (Population pharmacokinetic analysis revealed that estrogens (mainly ethinyl estradiol) reduced the oral clearance of ropinirole by 36%. Dosage adjustment may not be needed for ropinirole patients on estrogen therapy unless estrogen therapy is stopped or started during treatment with ropinirole). Products include:
Premarin Intravenous ... **3442**
Premarin Tablets ... **3446**
Premarin Vaginal Cream ... **3452**
Premphase Tablets ... **3456**
Prempro Tablets ... **3456**

Estrogens, Esterified (Population pharmacokinetic analysis revealed that estrogens (mainly ethinyl estradiol) reduced the oral clearance of ropinirole by 36%. Dosage adjustment may not be needed for ropinirole patients on estrogen therapy unless estrogen therapy is stopped or started during treatment with ropinirole). Products include:
Estratest Tablets ... **3199**
Estratest H.S. Tablets ... **3199**

Estropipate (Population pharmacokinetic analysis revealed that estrogens (mainly ethinyl estradiol) reduced the oral clearance of ropinirole by 36%. Dosage adjustment may not be needed for ropinirole patients on estrogen therapy unless estrogen therapy is stopped or started during treatment with ropinirole).
No products indexed under this heading.

Ethanol (Possible additive sedative effects).
No products indexed under this heading.

Ethchlorvynol (Possible additive sedative effects).
No products indexed under this heading.

Ethinamate (Possible additive sedative effects).
No products indexed under this heading.

Ethinyl Estradiol (Reduces the oral clearance of ropinirole by 36%). Products include:
Mircette Tablets ... **1066**
NuvaRing ... **2340**
Ortho-Cyclen/Ortho Tri-Cyclen ... **2429**
Ortho Evra Transdermal System ... **2417**
Ortho Tri-Cyclen Lo Tablets ... **2436**
Seasonique Tablets ... **1077**
Yasmin 28 Tablets ... **796**
Yaz Tablets ... **803**

Ethyl Alcohol (Possible additive sedative effects).
No products indexed under this heading.

Fentanyl (Possible additive sedative effects). Products include:
Duragesic Transdermal System ... **2373**
Ionsys Transdermal System ... **2379**

Fentanyl Citrate (Possible additive sedative effects). Products include:
Actiq ... **979**

Fluoxetine Hydrochloride (Possible additive sedative effects). Products include:
Prozac Pulvules and Liquid ... **1801**
Symbyax Capsules ... **1819**

Fluphenazine Decanoate (Co-administration with dopamine antagonists may diminish the effectiveness of ropinirole).
No products indexed under this heading.

Fluphenazine Enanthate (Co-administration with dopamine antagonists may diminish the effectiveness of ropinirole).
No products indexed under this heading.

Fluphenazine Hydrochloride (Co-administration with dopamine antagonists may diminish the effectiveness of ropinirole).
No products indexed under this heading.

Flurazepam Hydrochloride (Possible additive sedative effects). Products include:
Dalmane Capsules ... **3342**

Flutamide (CYP1A2 was the major enzyme responsible for the metabolism of ropinirole There is thus the potential for substrates or inhibitors

of this enzyme when co-administered with ropinirole to alter its clearance). Products include:

Fluticasone Propionate (CYP1A2 was the major enzyme responsible for the metabolism of ropinirole There is thus the potential for substrates or inhibitors of this enzyme when co-administered with ropinirole to alter its clearance). Products include:

Fluvoxamine (If therapy with a drug known to be a potent inhibitor of CYP1A2 is stopped or started during treatment with ropinirole hydrochloride, adjustment of the dose of ropinirole hydrocholoride may be required).

No products indexed under this heading.

Fluvoxamine Maleate (If therapy with a drug known to be a potent inhibitor of CYP1A2 is stopped or started during treatment with ropinirole hydrochloride, adjustment of the dose of ropinirole hydrocholoride may be required).

No products indexed under this heading.

Gatifloxacin (If therapy with a drug known to be a potent inhibitor of CYP1A2 is stopped or started during treatment with ropinirole hydrochloride, adjustment of the dose of ropinirole hydrocholoride may be required). Products include:

Gemifloxacin Mesylate (If therapy with a drug known to be a potent inhibitor of CYP1A2 is stopped or started during treatment with ropinirole hydrochloride, adjustment of the dose of ropinirole hydrocholoride may be required).

No products indexed under this heading.

Glutethimide (Possible additive sedative effects).

No products indexed under this heading.

Grepafloxacin Hydrochloride (If therapy with a drug known to be a potent inhibitor of CYP1A2 is stopped or started during treatment with ropinirole hydrochloride, adjustment of the dose of ropinirole hydrocholoride may be required).

No products indexed under this heading.

Haloperidol (Co-administration with dopamine antagonists may diminish the effectiveness of ropinirole).

No products indexed under this heading.

Haloperidol Decanoate (Co-administration with dopamine antagonists may diminish the effectiveness of ropinirole).

No products indexed under this heading.

Haloperidol Lactate (CYP1A2 was the major enzyme responsible for the metabolism of ropinirole There is thus the potential for substrates or inhibitors of this enzyme when co-administered with ropinirole to alter its clearance).

No products indexed under this heading.

Hydrocodone Bitartrate (Possible additive sedative effects). Products include:

Hydrocodone Polistirex (Possible additive sedative effects). Products include:

Hydromorphone Hydrochloride (Possible additive sedative effects). Products include:

Hydroxyzine Hydrochloride (Possible additive sedative effects).

No products indexed under this heading.

Imipramine Hydrochloride (Possible additive sedative effects).

No products indexed under this heading.

Imipramine Pamoate (Possible additive sedative effects).

No products indexed under this heading.

Isocarboxazid (Possible additive sedative effects).

No products indexed under this heading.

Isoflurane (Possible additive sedative effects).

No products indexed under this heading.

Isoniazid (If therapy with a drug known to be a potent inhibitor of CYP1A2 is stopped or started during treatment with ropinirole hydrochloride, adjustment of the dose of ropinirole hydrocholoride may be required).

No products indexed under this heading.

Ketamine Hydrochloride (Possible additive sedative effects).

No products indexed under this heading.

Ketoconazole (If therapy with a drug known to be a potent inhibitor of CYP1A2 is stopped or started during treatment with ropinirole hydrochloride, adjustment of the dose of ropinirole hydrocholoride may be required). Products include:

Levobupivacaine Hydrochloride (CYP1A2 was the major enzyme responsible for the metabolism of ropinirole There is thus the potential for substrates or inhibitors of this enzyme when co-administered with ropinirole to alter its clearance).

No products indexed under this heading.

Levodopa (Ropinirole may potentiate the dopaminergic effects of L-dopa and may cause and/or exacer-

bate pre-existing dyskinesia; increased mean steady state of L-dopa by 20%). Products include:

Levofloxacin (If therapy with a drug known to be a potent inhibitor of CYP1A2 is stopped or started during treatment with ropinirole hydrochloride, adjustment of the dose of ropinirole hydrocholoride may be required). Products include:

Levomethadyl Acetate Hydrochloride (Possible additive sedative effects).

No products indexed under this heading.

Levonorgestrel (If therapy with a drug known to be a potent inhibitor of CYP1A2 is stopped or started during treatment with ropinirole hydrochloride, adjustment of the dose of ropinirole hydrocholoride may be required). Products include:

Levorphanol Tartrate (Possible additive sedative effects).

No products indexed under this heading.

Lomefloxacin Hydrochloride (If therapy with a drug known to be a potent inhibitor of CYP1A2 is stopped or started during treatment with ropinirole hydrochloride, adjustment of the dose of ropinirole hydrocholoride may be required).

No products indexed under this heading.

Lorazepam (Possible additive sedative effects).

No products indexed under this heading.

Loxapine Hydrochloride (Co-administration with dopamine antagonists may diminish the effectiveness of ropinirole).

No products indexed under this heading.

Loxapine Succinate (Co-administration with dopamine antagonists may diminish the effectiveness of ropinirole).

No products indexed under this heading.

Maprotiline Hydrochloride (Possible additive sedative effects).

No products indexed under this heading.

Meperidine Hydrochloride (Possible additive sedative effects).

No products indexed under this heading.

Mephobarbital (Possible additive sedative effects).

No products indexed under this heading.

Meprobamate (Possible additive sedative effects).

No products indexed under this heading.

Mesoridazine Besylate (Co-administration with dopamine antagonists may diminish the effectiveness of ropinirole).

No products indexed under this heading.

Mestranol (If therapy with a drug known to be a potent inhibitor of CYP1A2 is stopped or started during treatment with ropinirole hydrochloride, adjustment of the dose of ropinirole hydrocholoride may be required).

No products indexed under this heading.

Methadone Hydrochloride (Possible additive sedative effects).

No products indexed under this heading.

Methdilazine Hydrochloride (Possible additive sedative effects).

No products indexed under this heading.

Methohexital Sodium (Possible additive sedative effects).

No products indexed under this heading.

Methotrimeprazine (Co-administration with dopamine antagonists may diminish the effectiveness of ropinirole).

No products indexed under this heading.

Methoxsalen (If therapy with a drug known to be a potent inhibitor of CYP1A2 is stopped or started during treatment with ropinirole hydrochloride, adjustment of the dose of ropinirole hydrocholoride may be required). Products include:

Methoxyflurane (Possible additive sedative effects).

No products indexed under this heading.

Metoclopramide Hydrochloride (Co-administration with dopamine antagonists may diminish the effectiveness of ropinirole).

No products indexed under this heading.

Mexiletine Hydrochloride (If therapy with a drug known to be a potent inhibitor of CYP1A2 is stopped or started during treatment with ropinirole hydrochloride, adjustment of the dose of ropinirole hydrochloride may be required).

No products indexed under this heading.

Mibefradil Dihydrochloride (If therapy with a drug known to be a potent inhibitor of CYP1A2 is stopped or started during treatment with ropinirole hydrochloride, adjustment of the dose of ropinirole hydrocholoride may be required).

No products indexed under this heading.

Midazolam Hydrochloride (Possible additive sedative effects).

No products indexed under this heading.

Mirtazapine (Possible additive sedative effects).

No products indexed under this heading.

Molindone Hydrochloride (Co-administration with dopamine antagonists may diminish the effectiveness of ropinirole). Products include:

Morphine Sulfate (Possible additive sedative effects). Products include:

Moxifloxacin Hydrochloride (If therapy with a drug known to be a potent inhibitor of CYP1A2 is stopped or started during treatment with ropinirole hydrochloride, adjustment of the dose of ropinirole hydrocholoride may be required). Products include:

Nafcillin Sodium (CYP1A2 was the major enzyme responsible for the metabolism of ropinirole There is thus the potential for substrates or inhibitors of this enzyme when co-administered with ropinirole to alter its clearance).

No products indexed under this heading.

Nalidixic Acid (If therapy with a drug known to be a potent inhibitor of CYP1A2 is stopped or started during treatment with ropinirole hydrochloride, adjustment of the dose of ropinirole hydrocholoride may be required).

No products indexed under this heading.

Naproxen (CYP1A2 was the major enzyme responsible for the metabolism of ropinirole There is thus the potential for substrates or inhibitors of this enzyme when co-administered with ropinirole to alter its clearance). Products include:

Naproxen Sodium (CYP1A2 was the major enzyme responsible for the metabolism of ropinirole There is thus the potential for substrates or inhibitors of this enzyme when co-administered with ropinirole to alter its clearance). Products include:

Nefazodone Hydrochloride (Possible additive sedative effects).

No products indexed under this heading.

Nicotine Polacrilex (CYP1A2 was the major enzyme responsible for the metabolism of ropinirole There is thus the potential for substrates or inhibitors of this enzyme when co-administered with ropinirole to alter its clearance).

No products indexed under this heading.

Nicotine Salicylate (CYP1A2 was the major enzyme responsible for the metabolism of ropinirole There is thus the potential for substrates or inhibitors of this enzyme when co-administered with ropinirole to alter its clearance).

No products indexed under this heading.

Nicotine Sulfate (CYP1A2 was the major enzyme responsible for the metabolism of ropinirole There is thus the potential for substrates or inhibitors of this enzyme when co-administered with ropinirole to alter its clearance).

No products indexed under this heading.

Norethindrone (If therapy with a drug known to be a potent inhibitor of CYP1A2 is stopped or started during treatment with ropinirole hydrochloride, adjustment of the

dose of ropinirole hydrocholoride may be required). Products include:

Norethindrone Acetate (CYP1A2 was the major enzyme responsible for the metabolism of ropinirole There is thus the potential for substrates or inhibitors of this enzyme when co-administered with ropinirole to alter its clearance).

No products indexed under this heading.

Norfloxacin (If therapy with a drug known to be a potent inhibitor of CYP1A2 is stopped or started during treatment with ropinirole hydrochloride, adjustment of the dose of ropinirole hydrochloride may be required). Products include:

Norgestrel (If therapy with a drug known to be a potent inhibitor of CYP1A2 is stopped or started during treatment with ropinirole hydrochloride, adjustment of the dose of ropinirole hydrocholoride may be required).

No products indexed under this heading.

Nortriptyline Hydrochloride (Possible additive sedative effects).

No products indexed under this heading.

Ofloxacin (If therapy with a drug known to be a potent inhibitor of CYP1A2 is stopped or started during treatment with ropinirole hydrochloride, adjustment of the dose of ropinirole hydrocholoride may be required). Products include:

Olanzapine (Possible additive sedative effects). Products include:

Omeprazole (If therapy with a drug known to be a potent inhibitor of CYP1A2 is stopped or started during treatment with ropinirole hydrochloride, adjustment of the dose of ropinirole hydrocholoride may be required). Products include:

Ondansetron (CYP1A2 was the major enzyme responsible for the metabolism of ropinirole There is thus the potential for substrates or inhibitors of this enzyme when co-administered with ropinirole to alter its clearance). Products include:

Ondansetron Hydrochloride (CYP1A2 was the major enzyme responsible for the metabolism of ropinirole There is thus the potential for substrates or inhibitors of this enzyme when co-administered with ropinirole to alter its clearance). Products include:

Oxazepam (Possible additive sedative effects).

No products indexed under this heading.

Oxycodone Hydrochloride (Possible additive sedative effects). Products include:

Paroxetine Hydrochloride (Possible additive sedative effects). Products include:

Pentobarbital Sodium (Possible additive sedative effects). Products include:

Perphenazine (Co-administration with dopamine antagonists may diminish the effectiveness of ropinirole).

No products indexed under this heading.

Phenelzine Sulfate (Possible additive sedative effects).

No products indexed under this heading.

Phenobarbital (Possible additive sedative effects). Products include:

Phenobarbital Sodium (CYP1A2 was the major enzyme responsible for the metabolism of ropinirole There is thus the potential for substrates or inhibitors of this enzyme when co-administered with ropinirole to alter its clearance).

No products indexed under this heading.

Phenytoin Sodium (CYP1A2 was the major enzyme responsible for the metabolism of ropinirole There is thus the potential for substrates or inhibitors of this enzyme when co-administered with ropinirole to alter its clearance). Products include:

Polyestradiol Phosphate (Population pharmacokinetic analysis revealed that estrogens (mainly ethinyl estradiol) reduced the oral clearance of ropinirole by 36%. Dosage adjustment may not be needed for ropinirole patients on estrogen therapy unless estrogen therapy is stopped or started during treatment with ropinirole).

No products indexed under this heading.

Prazepam (Possible additive sedative effects).

No products indexed under this heading.

Prochlorperazine (Co-administration with dopamine antagonists may diminish the effectiveness of ropinirole).

No products indexed under this heading.

Promethazine Hydrochloride (Co-administration with dopamine antagonists may diminish the effectiveness of ropinirole). Products include:

Propafenone Hydrochloride (CYP1A2 was the major enzyme responsible for the metabolism of ropinirole There is thus the potential for substrates or inhibitors of this enzyme when co-administered with ropinirole to alter its clearance). Products include:

Propofol (Possible additive sedative effects).

No products indexed under this heading.

Propoxyphene Hydrochloride (Possible additive sedative effects).

No products indexed under this heading.

Propoxyphene Napsylate (Possible additive sedative effects).

No products indexed under this heading.

Propranolol Hydrochloride (CYP1A2 was the major enzyme responsible for the metabolism of ropinirole There is thus the potential for substrates or inhibitors of this enzyme when co-administered with ropinirole to alter its clearance). Products include:

Protriptyline Hydrochloride (Possible additive sedative effects).

No products indexed under this heading.

Pyrilamine Maleate (Possible additive sedative effects).

No products indexed under this heading.

Pyrilamine Tannate (Possible additive sedative effects).

No products indexed under this heading.

Quazepam (Possible additive sedative effects).

No products indexed under this heading.

Quetiapine Fumarate (Co-administration with dopamine antagonists may diminish the effectiveness of ropinirole). Products include:

Quinestrol (Population pharmacokinetic analysis revealed that estrogens (mainly ethinyl estradiol) reduced the oral clearance of ropinirole by 36%. Dosage adjustment may not be needed for ropinirole patients on estrogen therapy unless estrogen therapy is stopped or started during treatment with ropinirole).

No products indexed under this heading.

Ramelteon (Possible additive sedative effects). Products include:

Ranitidine Hydrochloride (If therapy with a drug known to be a potent inhibitor of CYP1A2 is stopped or started during treatment with ropinirole hydrochloride, adjustment of the dose of ropinirole hydrocholoride may be required). Products include:

Remifentanil Hydrochloride (Possible additive sedative effects).

No products indexed under this heading.

Riluzole (CYP1A2 was the major enzyme responsible for the metabolism of ropinirole There is thus the potential for substrates or inhibitors of this enzyme when co-administered with ropinirole to alter its clearance). Products include:

Risperidone (Co-administration with dopamine antagonists may diminish the effectiveness of ropinirole). Products include:

Ritonavir (If therapy with a drug known to be a potent inhibitor of CYP1A2 is stopped or started during treatment with ropinirole hydrochloride, adjustment of the dose of ropinirole hydrocholoride may be required). Products include:
Kaletra 476
Norvir 503

Ropivacaine Hydrochloride (CYP1A2 was the major enzyme responsible for the metabolism of ropinirole There is thus the potential for substrates or inhibitors of this enzyme when co-administered with ropinirole to alter its clearance).
No products indexed under this heading.

Secobarbital Sodium (Possible additive sedative effects).
No products indexed under this heading.

Sertraline Hydrochloride (Possible additive sedative effects). Products include:
Zoloft 2586

Sevoflurane (Possible additive sedative effects). Products include:
Ultane Liquid for Inhalation 531

Sodium Oxybate (Possible additive sedative effects). Products include:
Xyrem Oral Solution 1688

Sparfloxacin (If therapy with a drug known to be a potent inhibitor of CYP1A2 is stopped or started during treatment with ropinirole hydrochloride, adjustment of the dose of ropinirole hydrocholoride may be required).
No products indexed under this heading.

Sufentanil Citrate (Possible additive sedative effects).
No products indexed under this heading.

Tacrine Hydrochloride (If therapy with a drug known to be a potent inhibitor of CYP1A2 is stopped or started during treatment with ropinirole hydrochloride, adjustment of the dose of ropinirole hydrocholoride may be required).
No products indexed under this heading.

Tamoxifen Citrate (CYP1A2 was the major enzyme responsible for the metabolism of ropinirole There is thus the potential for substrates or inhibitors of this enzyme when co-administered with ropinirole to alter its clearance). Products include:
Soltamox Oral Solution 3527

Temazepam (Possible additive sedative effects). Products include:
Restoril Capsules 1860

Theophylline (CYP1A2 was the major enzyme responsible for the metabolism of ropinirole There is thus the potential for substrates or inhibitors of this enzyme when co-administered with ropinirole to alter its clearance).
No products indexed under this heading.

Theophylline Anhydrous (CYP1A2 was the major enzyme responsible for the metabolism of ropinirole There is thus the potential for substrates or inhibitors of this enzyme when co-administered with ropinirole to alter its clearance). Products include:
Uniphyl Tablets 2710

Thiamylal Sodium (Possible additive sedative effects).
No products indexed under this heading.

Thioridazine Hydrochloride (Co-administration with dopamine antagonists may diminish the effectiveness of ropinirole). Products include:
Thioridazine Hydrochloride Tablets 2163

Thiothixene (Co-administration with dopamine antagonists may diminish the effectiveness of ropinirole). Products include:
Thiothixene Capsules 2165

Ticlopidine Hydrochloride (If therapy with a drug known to be a potent inhibitor of CYP1A2 is stopped or started during treatment with ropinirole hydrochloride, adjustment of the dose of ropinirole hydrocholoride may be required). Products include:
Ticlid Tablets 2810

Tobacco (Decreases ropinirole Cmax by 30% and decreases AUC by 38%).
No products indexed under this heading.

Tranylcypromine Sulfate (Possible additive sedative effects). Products include:
Parnate Tablets 1527

Trazodone Hydrochloride (Possible additive sedative effects).
No products indexed under this heading.

Triazolam (Possible additive sedative effects).
No products indexed under this heading.

Trifluoperazine Hydrochloride (Co-administration with dopamine antagonists may diminish the effectiveness of ropinirole).
No products indexed under this heading.

Trimeprazine Tartrate (Possible additive sedative effects).
No products indexed under this heading.

Trimethaphan Camsylate (CYP1A2 was the major enzyme responsible for the metabolism of ropinirole There is thus the potential for substrates or inhibitors of this enzyme when co-administered with ropinirole to alter its clearance).
No products indexed under this heading.

Trimipramine Maleate (Possible additive sedative effects).
No products indexed under this heading.

Tripelennamine Hydrochloride (Possible additive sedative effects).
No products indexed under this heading.

Triprolidine Hydrochloride (Possible additive sedative effects).
No products indexed under this heading.

Troleandomycin (If therapy with a drug known to be a potent inhibitor of CYP1A2 is stopped or started during treatment with ropinirole hydrochloride, adjustment of the dose of ropinirole hydrocholoride may be required).
No products indexed under this heading.

Trovafloxacin Mesylate (If therapy with a drug known to be a potent inhibitor of CYP1A2 is stopped or started during treatment with ropinirole hydrochloride, adjustment of the dose of ropinirole hydrocholoride may be required).
No products indexed under this heading.

Venlafaxine Hydrochloride (Possible additive sedative effects). Products include:
Effexor Tablets 3411
Effexor XR Capsules 3417

Verapamil Hydrochloride (CYP1A2 was the major enzyme responsible for the metabolism of ropinirole There is thus the potential for substrates or inhibitors of this enzyme when co-administered with ropinirole to alter its clearance). Products include:
Covera-HS Tablets 3139
Tarka Tablets 524
Verelan PM Extended-Release Capsules, Controlled-Onset 3106

Warfarin Sodium (CYP1A2 was the major enzyme responsible for the metabolism of ropinirole There is thus the potential for substrates or inhibitors of this enzyme when co-administered with ropinirole to alter its clearance). Products include:
Coumadin for Injection 898
Coumadin Tablets 898

Zaleplon (Possible additive sedative effects). Products include:
Sonata Capsules 1717

Zileuton (If therapy with a drug known to be a potent inhibitor of CYP1A2 is stopped or started during treatment with ropinirole hydrochloride, adjustment of the dose of ropinirole hydrocholoride may be required). Products include:
Zyflo Tablets 1023

Ziprasidone Hydrochloride (Possible additive sedative effects). Products include:
Geodon Capsules 2529

Zolmitriptan (CYP1A2 was the major enzyme responsible for the metabolism of ropinirole There is thus the potential for substrates or inhibitors of this enzyme when co-administered with ropinirole to alter its clearance). Products include:
Zomig Tablets 3519
Zomig Nasal Spray 3523
Zomig-ZMT Tablets 3519

Zolpidem Tartrate (Possible additive sedative effects). Products include:
Ambien Tablets 2851
Ambien CR Tablets 2855

Food Interactions

Alcohol (Possible additive sedative effects).

Food, unspecified (Food does not affect the extent of absorption of ropinirole, although Tmax is increased by 2.5 hours and Cmax is decreased by 25% when taken with a high fat meal).

Grapefruit Juice (If therapy with a drug known to be a potent inhibitor of CYP1A2 is stopped or started during treatment with ropinirole hydrochloride, adjustment of the dose of ropinirole hydrocholoride may be required).

RESCRIPTOR TABLETS

(Delavirdine Mesylate) 2551
May interact with amphetamines, antacids, cytochrome p450 3a inducers (selected), cytochrome p450 3a inhibitors (selected), cytochrome p450 3a substrates (selected), dexamethasone, dihydropyridine calcium channel blockers, ergot-containing drugs, histamine H2-receptor antagonists, phenytoin, proton pump inhibitor, quinidine, and certain other agents. Compounds in these categories include:

Alfentanil Hydrochloride (Co-administration with drugs primarily metabolized by CYP3A may result in increased plasma concentrations of the coadministered drug that could increase or prolong both its therapeutic or adverse effects).
No products indexed under this heading.

Allium sativum (Co-administration with drugs that induce CYP3A may decrease delavirdine plasma concentrations and reduce its therapeutic effect).
No products indexed under this heading.

Alprazolam (Co-administration with drugs that are highly dependent on CYP3A for clearance and for which elevated plasma levels are associated with serious and/or life threatening events, such as prolonged or increased sedation or respiratory depression, is contraindicated). Products include:
Niravam Orally Disintegrating Tablets 3092

Aluminum Carbonate (Co-administration with antacids results in decreased delavirdine concentrations because of reduced absorption; patients taking antacids should be advised to take them at least one hour apart).
No products indexed under this heading.

Aluminum Hydroxide (Co-administration with antacids results in decreased delavirdine concentrations because of reduced absorption; patients taking antacids should be advised to take them at least one hour apart). Products include:
Gaviscon Regular Strength Liquid .. ▣ 658
Gaviscon Regular Strength Tablets .... ▣ 658
Gaviscon Extra Strength Liquid ...... ▣ 658
Gaviscon Extra Strength Tablets .... ▣ 658
Maalox Regular Strength Antacid/Antigas Liquid 2175
Maalox Max Maximum Strength Antacid/Anti-Gas Liquid................ 2176

Aminophylline (Co-administration with drugs primarily metabolized by CYP3A may result in increased plasma concentrations of the coadministered drug that could increase or prolong both its therapeutic or adverse effects).
No products indexed under this heading.

Amiodarone Hydrochloride (Co-administration with drugs that inhibit CYP3A may increase delavirdine plasma concentrations).
No products indexed under this heading.

Amitriptyline Hydrochloride (Co-administration with drugs primarily metabolized by CYP3A may result in increased plasma concentrations of the coadministered drug that could increase or prolong both its therapeutic or adverse effects).
No products indexed under this heading.

Amlodipine Besylate (Co-administration results in increased dihydropyridine calcium channel blocker concentrations). Products include:
- Caduet Tablets ... 2508
- Lotrel Capsules ... 2249
- Norvasc Tablets ... 2545

Amphetamine Resins (Co-administration results in increased amphetamine concentrations).
No products indexed under this heading.

Amphetamine Sulfate (Co-administration results in increased amphetamine concentrations). Products include:
- Adderall Tablets ... 3164
- Adderall XR Capsules ... 3166

Amprenavir (Co-administration results in increased amprenavir concentrations). Products include:
- Agenerase Capsules ... 1327
- Agenerase Oral Solution ... 1332

Aprepitant (Co-administration with drugs that induce CYP3A may decrease delavirdine plasma concentrations and reduce its therapeutic effect). Products include:
- Emend Capsules ... 1963

Astemizole (Co-administration with drugs that are highly dependent on CYP3A for clearance and for which elevated plasma levels are associated with serious and/or life-threatening events, such as cardiac arrhythmias; concurrent use is contraindicated).
No products indexed under this heading.

Atorvastatin Calcium (The risk of myopathy, including rhabdomolysis, may be increased with concurrent use). Products include:
- Caduet Tablets ... 2508
- Lipitor Tablets ... 2483

Bepridil Hydrochloride (Co-administration results in increased bepridil concentrations; increased bepridil exposure may be associated with life-threatening reactions such as cardiac arrhythmias).
No products indexed under this heading.

Buspirone Hydrochloride (Co-administration with drugs primarily metabolized by CYP3A may result in increased plasma concentrations of the coadministered drug that could increase or prolong both its therapeutic or adverse effects).
No products indexed under this heading.

Busulfan (Co-administration with drugs primarily metabolized by CYP3A may result in increased plasma concentrations of the coadministered drug that could increase or prolong both its therapeutic or adverse effects). Products include:
- I.V. Busulfex ... 2493
- Myleran Tablets ... 1525

Carbamazepine (May lead to loss of virologic response and possible resistance to delavirdine or the class of non-nucleoside reverse transcriptase inhibitors). Products include:
- Carbatrol Capsules ... 3171
- Equetro Extended-Release Capsules ... 3180
- Tegretol/Tegretol-XR ... 2295

Cerivastatin Sodium (The risk of myopathy, including rhabdomyolysis, may be increased with concurrent use).
No products indexed under this heading.

Chlorpheniramine (Co-administration with drugs primarily metabolized by CYP3A may result in increased plasma concentrations of the coadministered drug that could increase or prolong both its therapeutic or adverse effects).
No products indexed under this heading.

Chlorpheniramine Maleate (Co-administration with drugs primarily metabolized by CYP3A may result in increased plasma concentrations of the coadministered drug that could increase or prolong both its therapeutic or adverse effects). Products include:
- Advil Allergy Sinus Caplets ... 770
- Advil Multi-Symptom Cold Caplets ... 770
- BC Allergy Sinus Cold Powder ... 677
- Comtrex Maximum Strength Cold & Cough Day/Night Caplets - Night Formulation ... 726
- Comtrex Maximum Strength Day/Night Severe Cold & Sinus Caplets - Night Formulation ... 725
- Contac Cold and Flu Maximum Strength Caplets ... 728
- Contac Cold and Flu Day and Night Caplets (Night Formulation Only) ... 727
- Children's Dimetapp Long Acting Cough Plus Cold Syrup ... 731
- Robitussin Cough & Cold Long-Acting Liquid ... 735
- Robitussin Cough & Allergy Syrup .. 736
- Robitussin Cough & Cold Nighttime Liquid ... 736
- Robitussin Cough, Cold & Flu Nighttime Liquid ... 738
- Robitussin Pediatric Cough & Cold Long-Acting Liquid ... 735
- Robitussin Pediatric Cough & Cold Nighttime Liquid ... 736
- Triaminic Cold & Allergy Liquid ... 746
- Triaminic Cough & Runny Nose Softchews ... 748
- Children's Tylenol Plus Flu Oral Suspension ... 749
- Tylenol Allergy Multi-Symptom Caplets with Cool Burst and Gelcaps ... 1872
- Children's Tylenol Plus Cold Suspension Liquid ... 1879
- Children's Tylenol Plus Cough & Runny Nose Suspension Liquid ... 1879
- Children's Tylenol Plus Flu Suspension Liquid ... 1881
- Children's Tylenol Plus Multi-Symptom Cold Suspension Liquid ... 1879
- Tylenol Cold Head Congestion Nighttime Caplets with Cool Burst ... 1873
- Tylenol Cold Multi-Symptom Nighttime Caplets with Cool Burst ... 1874
- Tylenol Sinus Congestion & Pain Nighttime Caplets with Cool Burst ... 1876
- Vicks 44M Cough, Cold & Flu Relief Liquid ... 2680
- Pediatric Vicks 44m Cough & Cold Relief Liquid ... 2676
- Children's Vicks NyQuil Cold/Cough Relief ... 756
- Children's Vicks NyQuil Cold/Cough Relief Liquid ... 2680
- Zicam Maximum Strength Flu Daytime ... 768

Chlorpheniramine Polistirex (Co-administration with drugs primarily metabolized by CYP3A may result in increased plasma concentrations of the coadministered drug that could increase or prolong both its therapeutic or adverse effects). Products include:
- Tussionex Pennkinetic Extended-Release Suspension ... 3327

Chlorpheniramine Tannate (Co-administration with drugs primarily metabolized by CYP3A may result in increased plasma concentrations of the coadministered drug that could increase or prolong both its therapeutic or adverse effects).
No products indexed under this heading.

Cimetidine (H2 antagonists increase gastric pH and may reduce the absorption of delavirdine; chronic use of these drugs with delavirdine is not recommended). Products include:
- Tagamet HB 200 Tablets ... 664

Cimetidine Hydrochloride (H2 antagonists increase gastric pH and may reduce the absorption of delavirdine; chronic use of these drugs with delavirdine is not recommended).
No products indexed under this heading.

Ciprofloxacin (Co-administration with drugs that inhibit CYP3A may increase delavirdine plasma concentrations). Products include:
- Cipro Oral Suspension ... 2977
- Cipro I.V. ... 2984
- Cipro XR Tablets ... 2990
- Ciprodex Otic Suspension ... 559

Ciprofloxacin Hydrochloride (Co-administration with drugs that inhibit CYP3A may increase delavirdine plasma concentrations). Products include:
- Ciloxan Ophthalmic Ointment ... 559
- Ciloxan Ophthalmic Solution ... ⊙ 206
- Cipro Tablets ... 2977
- Proquin XR Tablets ... 1153

Cisapride (Co-administration with drugs that are highly dependent on CYP3A for clearance and for which elevated plasma levels are associated with serious and/or life-threatening events, such as cardiac arrthythmias, is contraindicated).
No products indexed under this heading.

Clarithromycin (Co-administrations results in increased clarithromycin concentrations). Products include:
- Biaxin/Biaxin XL ... 402
- PREVPAC ... 3284

Cyclosporine (Co-administration results in increased cyclosporine concentrations). Products include:
- Gengraf Capsules ... 459
- Neoral Oral Solution ... 2259
- Neoral Soft Gelatin Capsules ... 2259
- Restasis Ophthalmic Emulsion ... 575
- Sandimmune ... 2275

Desogestrel (Co-administration with drugs primarily metabolized by CYP3A may result in increased plasma concentrations of the coadministered drug that could increase or prolong both its therapeutic or adverse effects). Products include:
- Mircette Tablets ... 1066

Dexamethasone (Co-administration results in decreased delavirdine concentrations). Products include:
- Ciprodex Otic Suspension ... 559
- Decadron Tablets ... 1951
- TobraDex Ophthalmic Ointment ... 562
- TobraDex Ophthalmic Suspension ... 563

Dexamethasone Acetate (Co-administration results in decreased delavirdine concentrations).
No products indexed under this heading.

Dexamethasone Phosphate (Co-administration with drugs primarily metabolized by CYP3A may result in increased plasma concentrations of the coadministered drug that could increase or prolong both its therapeutic or adverse effects).
No products indexed under this heading.

Dexamethasone Sodium (Co-administration with drugs primarily metabolized by CYP3A may result in increased plasma concentrations of the coadministered drug that could increase or prolong both its therapeutic or adverse effects).
No products indexed under this heading.

Dexamethasone Sodium Phosphate (Co-administration results in decreased delavirdine concentrations).
No products indexed under this heading.

Dextroamphetamine Sulfate (Co-administration results in increased amphetamine concentrations). Products include:
- Adderall Tablets ... 3164
- Adderall XR Capsules ... 3166
- Dexedrine ... 1420
- DextroStat Tablets ... 3179

Diazepam (Co-administration with drugs primarily metabolized by CYP3A may result in increased plasma concentrations of the coadministered drug that could increase or prolong both its therapeutic or adverse effects). Products include:
- Diastat Rectal Delivery System ... 3343
- Valium Tablets ... 2819

Didanosine (Co-administration results in decreased didanosine and delavirdine plasma concentrations; administration of didanosine (buffered tablets) and delavirdine should be separated by at least one hour).
No products indexed under this heading.

Dihydroergotamine Mesylate (Co-administration with drugs that are highly dependent on CYP3A for clearance and for which elevated plasma levels are associated with serious and/or life-threatening events, such as acute ergot toxicity characterized by peripheral vasospasm and ischemiaof the extremities, is contraindicated). Products include:
- Migranal Nasal Spray ... 3348

Diltiazem Hydrochloride (Co-administration results in increased calcium channel blocker concentrations). Products include:
- Cardizem LA Extended Release Tablets ... 1728
- Tiazac Capsules ... 1201

Diltiazem Maleate (Co-administration with drugs that inhibit CYP3A may increase delavirdine plasma concentrations).
No products indexed under this heading.

IMPORTANT NOTE: Always consult each drug listing in the patient's regimen for possible interactions.

Disopyramide Phosphate (Co-administration with drugs primarily metabolized by CYP3A may result in increased plasma concentrations of the coadministered drug that could increase or prolong both its therapeutic or adverse effects).
No products indexed under this heading.

Doxorubicin Hydrochloride (Co-administration with drugs primarily metabolized by CYP3A may result in increased plasma concentrations of the coadministered drug that could increase or prolong both its therapeutic or adverse effects).
No products indexed under this heading.

Dronabinol (Co-administration with drugs primarily metabolized by CYP3A may result in increased plasma concentrations of the coadministered drug that could increase or prolong both its therapeutic or adverse effects). Products include:
Marinol Capsules ... 3333

Dyphylline (Co-administration with drugs primarily metabolized by CYP3A may result in increased plasma concentrations of the coadministered drug that could increase or prolong both its therapeutic or adverse effects).
No products indexed under this heading.

Efavirenz (Co-administration with drugs that induce CYP3A may decrease delavirdine plasma concentrations and reduce its therapeutic effect). Products include:
Atripla Tablets ... 945
Sustiva Capsules ... 930
Sustiva Tablets ... 930

Ergonovine Maleate (Co-administration with drugs that are highly dependent on CYP3A for clearance and for which elevated plasma levels are associated with serious and/or life-threatening events, such as acute ergot toxicity characterized by peripheral vasospasm and ischemiaof the extremities, is contraindicated).
No products indexed under this heading.

Ergotamine Tartrate (Co-administration with drugs that are highly dependent on CYP3A for clearance and for which elevated plasma levels are associated with serious and/or life-threatening events, such as acute ergot toxicity characterized by peripheral vasospasm and ischemiaof the extremities, is contraindicated).
No products indexed under this heading.

Erythromycin (Co-administration with drugs that inhibit CYP3A may increase delavirdine plasma concentrations). Products include:
Ery-Tab Tablets ... 449
Erythromycin Base Filmtab Tablets ... 455
Erythromycin Delayed-Release Capsules, USP ... 457
PCE Dispertab Tablets ... 515

Erythromycin Estolate (Co-administration with drugs primarily metabolized by CYP3A may result in increased plasma concentrations of the coadministered drug that could increase or prolong both its therapeutic or adverse effects).
No products indexed under this heading.

Erythromycin Ethylsuccinate (Co-administration with drugs primarily metabolized by CYP3A may result in increased plasma concentrations of the coadministered drug that could increase or prolong both its therapeutic or adverse effects). Products include:
E.E.S. ... 451
EryPed ... 447

Erythromycin Gluceptate (Co-administration with drugs primarily metabolized by CYP3A may result in increased plasma concentrations of the coadministered drug that could increase or prolong both its therapeutic or adverse effects).
No products indexed under this heading.

Erythromycin Lactobionate (Co-administration with drugs primarily metabolized by CYP3A may result in increased plasma concentrations of the coadministered drug that could increase or prolong both its therapeutic or adverse effects).
No products indexed under this heading.

Erythromycin Stearate (Co-administration with drugs primarily metabolized by CYP3A may result in increased plasma concentrations of the coadministered drug that could increase or prolong both its therapeutic or adverse effects). Products include:
Erythrocin Stearate Filmtab Tablets ... 453

Esomeprazole Magnesium (Proton pump inhibitors increase gastric pH and may reduce the absorption of delavirdine; chronic use of these drugs with delavirdine is not recommended). Products include:
Nexium Delayed-Release Capsules ... 655

Estrogen (Co-administration with drugs primarily metabolized by CYP3A may result in increased plasma concentrations of the coadministered drug that could increase or prolong both its therapeutic or adverse effects).
No products indexed under this heading.

Estrogens, Conjugated (Co-administration with drugs primarily metabolized by CYP3A may result in increased plasma concentrations of the coadministered drug that could increase or prolong both its therapeutic or adverse effects). Products include:
Premarin Intravenous ... 3442
Premarin Tablets ... 3446
Premarin Vaginal Cream ... 3452
Premphase Tablets ... 3456
Prempro Tablets ... 3456

Estrogens, Conjugated, Synthetic A (Co-administration with drugs primarily metabolized by CYP3A may result in increased plasma concentrations of the coadministered drug that could increase or prolong both its therapeutic or adverse effects).
No products indexed under this heading.

Estrogens, Esterified (Co-administration with drugs primarily metabolized by CYP3A may result in increased plasma concentrations of the coadministered drug that could increase or prolong both its therapeutic or adverse effects). Products include:
Estratest Tablets ... 3199
Estratest H.S. Tablets ... 3199

Ethinyl Estradiol (Co-administration results in increased ethinyl estradiol concentrations). Products include:
Mircette Tablets ... 1066
NuvaRing ... 2340
Ortho-Cyclen/Ortho Tri-Cyclen ... 2429
Ortho Evra Transdermal System ... 2417
Ortho Tri-Cyclen Lo Tablets ... 2436
Seasonique Tablets ... 1077
Yasmin 28 Tablets ... 796
Yaz Tablets ... 803

Ethosuximide (Co-administration with drugs that induce CYP3A may decrease delavirdine plasma concentrations and reduce its therapeutic effect).
No products indexed under this heading.

Ethynodiol Diacetate (Co-administration with drugs primarily metabolized by CYP3A may result in increased plasma concentrations of the coadministered drug that could increase or prolong both its therapeutic or adverse effects).
No products indexed under this heading.

Etoposide (Co-administration with drugs primarily metabolized by CYP3A may result in increased plasma concentrations of the coadministered drug that could increase or prolong both its therapeutic or adverse effects).
No products indexed under this heading.

Etoposide Phosphate (Co-administration with drugs primarily metabolized by CYP3A may result in increased plasma concentrations of the coadministered drug that could increase or prolong both its therapeutic or adverse effects).
No products indexed under this heading.

Famotidine (H2 antagonists increase gastric pH and may reduce the absorption of delavirdine; chronic use of these drugs with delavirdine is not recommended). Products include:
Pepcid Injection ... 2040
Pepcid ... 2038
Pepcid AC Gelcaps ... 1701
Pepcid AC Tablets ... 1701
Maximum Strength Pepcid AC Tablets ... 1701
Pepcid Complete Chewable Tablets ... 1701

Felodipine (Co-administration results in increased dihydropyridine calcium channel blocker concentrations).
No products indexed under this heading.

Fentanyl (Co-administration with drugs primarily metabolized by CYP3A may result in increased plasma concentrations of the coadministered drug that could increase or prolong both its therapeutic or adverse effects). Products include:
Duragesic Transdermal System ... 2373
Ionsys Transdermal System ... 2379

Fentanyl Citrate (Co-administration with drugs primarily metabolized by CYP3A may result in increased plasma concentrations of the coadministered drug that could increase or prolong both its therapeutic or adverse effects). Products include:
Actiq ... 979

Flecainide Acetate (Co-administration results in increased flecainide concentrations). Products include:
Tambocor Tablets ... 1856

Fluconazole (Co-administration with drugs that inhibit CYP3A may increase delavirdine plasma concentrations).
No products indexed under this heading.

Fluoxetine (Co-administration with drugs that inhibit CYP3A may increase delavirdine plasma concentrations).
No products indexed under this heading.

Fluoxetine Hydrochloride (Co-administration with drugs that inhibit CYP3A may increase delavirdine plasma concentrations). Products include:
Prozac Pulvules and Liquid ... 1801
Symbyax Capsules ... 1819

Fluticasone Propionate (Co-administration results in increased fluticasone propionate concentrations; consider alternatives to fluticasone propionate, particularly for long-term use). Products include:
Advair Diskus 100/50 ... 1308
Advair Diskus 250/50 ... 1308
Advair Diskus 500/50 ... 1308
Advair HFA Inhalation Aerosol ... 1318
Cutivate Cream ... 2662
Cutivate Lotion 0.05% ... 2664
Cutivate Ointment ... 2665
Flonase Nasal Spray ... 1440
Flovent Diskus ... 1443

Fluticasone Propionate HFA (Co-administration results in increased fluticasone propionate concentrations; consider alternatives to fluticasone propionate, particularly for long-term use). Products include:
Flovent HFA ... 1447

Fluvastatin Sodium (Co-administration results in increased fluvastatin concentrations). Products include:
Lescol Capsules ... 2233
Lescol XL Tablets ... 2233

Fluvoxamine Maleate (Co-administration with drugs that inhibit CYP3A may increase delavirdine plasma concentrations).
No products indexed under this heading.

Fosphenytoin Sodium (May lead to loss of virologic response and possible resistance to delavirdine or the class of non-nucleoside reverse transcriptase inhibitors).
No products indexed under this heading.

Glyburide (Co-administration with drugs primarily metabolized by CYP3A may result in increased plasma concentrations of the coadministered drug that could increase or prolong both its therapeutic or adverse effects).
No products indexed under this heading.

Haloperidol (Co-administration with drugs primarily metabolized by CYP3A may result in increased plasma concentrations of the coadministered drug that could increase or prolong both its therapeutic or adverse effects).
No products indexed under this heading.

Haloperidol Decanoate (Co-administration with drugs primarily metabolized by CYP3A may result in increased plasma concentrations of the coadministered drug that could increase or prolong both its therapeutic or adverse effects).
No products indexed under this heading.

Hypericum (Co-administration with St. John's Wort or St. John's Wort-containing products and delavirdine is expected to substantially decrease delavirdine's concentrations and may result in suboptimal levels of delavirdine and lead to loss of virologic response). Products include:
- Satiete Tablets 832

Imipramine Hydrochloride (Co-administration with drugs primarily metabolized by CYP3A may result in increased plasma concentrations of the coadministered drug that could increase or prolong both its therapeutic or adverse effects).
No products indexed under this heading.

Imipramine Pamoate (Co-administration with drugs primarily metabolized by CYP3A may result in increased plasma concentrations of the coadministered drug that could increase or prolong both its therapeutic or adverse effects).
No products indexed under this heading.

Indinavir Sulfate (Co-administration results in increased indinavir concentrations; a dose reduction of indinavir to 600 mg t.i.d. should be considered when used concurrently). Products include:
- Crixivan Capsules 1940

Isoniazid (Co-administration with drugs that inhibit CYP3A may increase delavirdine plasma concentrations).
No products indexed under this heading.

Isradipine (Co-administration results in increased dihydropyridine calcium channel blocker concentrations). Products include:
- DynaCirc CR Tablets 2721

Itraconazole (Co-administration with drugs that inhibit CYP3A may increase delavirdine plasma concentrations).
No products indexed under this heading.

Ketoconazole (Co-administration with drugs that inhibit CYP3A may increase delavirdine plasma concentrations). Products include:
- Nizoral A-D Shampoo, 1% 1868

Lansoprazole (Proton pump inhibitors increase gastric pH and may reduce the absorption of delavirdine; chronic use of these drugs with delavirdine is not recommended). Products include:
- Prevacid Delayed-Release Capsules 3271
- Prevacid for Delayed-Release Oral Suspension 3271
- Prevacid SoluTab Delayed-Release Orally Disintegrating Tablets 3271
- Prevacid I.V. for Injection 3277
- Prevacid NapraPAC 3280
- PREVPAC 3284

Levonorgestrel (Co-administration with drugs primarily metabolized by CYP3A may result in increased plasma concentrations of the coadministered drug that could increase or prolong both its therapeutic or adverse effects). Products include:
- Climara Pro Transdermal System 776
- Mirena Intrauterine System 787
- Plan B Tablets 1076
- Seasonique Tablets 1077

Lidocaine (Co-administration with drugs primarily metabolized by CYP3A may result in increased plasma concentrations of the coadministered drug that could increase or prolong both its therapeutic or adverse effects). Products include:
- Lidoderm Patch 1118
- Synera Topical Patch 1137

Lidocaine Hydrochloride (Co-administration results in increased systemic lidocaine concentrations).
No products indexed under this heading.

Lopinavir (Co-administration results in increased lopinavir concentrations). Products include:
- Kaletra 476

Lovastatin (Potential for serious reactions such as myopathy including rhabdomyolysis; concurrent use is not recommended). Products include:
- Advicor Tablets 1722
- Altoprev Extended-Release Tablets 3109
- Mevacor Tablets 2021

Magaldrate (Co-administration with antacids results in decreased delavirdine concentrations because of reduced absorption; patients taking antacids should be advised to take them at least one hour apart).
No products indexed under this heading.

Magnesium Hydroxide (Co-administration with antacids results in decreased delavirdine concentrations because of reduced absorption; patients taking antacids should be advised to take them at least one hour apart). Products include:
- Maalox Regular Strength Antacid/Antigas Liquid 2175
- Maalox Max Maximum Strength Antacid/Anti-Gas Liquid 2176
- Pepcid Complete Chewable Tablets 1701

Magnesium Oxide (Co-administration with antacids results in decreased delavirdine concentrations because of reduced absorption; patients taking antacids should be advised to take them at least one hour apart). Products include:
- Beelith Tablets 759
- PremCal Light, Regular, and Extra Strength Tablets 818

Mestranol (Co-administration with drugs primarily metabolized by CYP3A may result in increased plasma concentrations of the coadministered drug that could increase or prolong both its therapeutic or adverse effects).
No products indexed under this heading.

Methadone Hydrochloride (Co-administration results in increased methadone concentrations).
No products indexed under this heading.

Methamphetamine Hydrochloride (Co-administration results in increased amphetamine concentrations). Products include:
- Desoxyn Tablets, USP 2462

Methylergonovine Maleate (Co-administration with drugs that are highly dependent on CYP3A for clearance and for which elevated plasma levels are associated with serious and/or life-threatening events, such as acute ergot toxicity characterized by peripheral vasospasm and ischemiaof the extremities, is contraindicated).
No products indexed under this heading.

Methysergide Maleate (Co-administration with drugs that are highly dependent on CYP3A for clearance and for which elevated plasma levels are associated with serious and/or life-threatening events, such as acute ergot toxicity characterized by peripheral vasospasm and ischemiaof the extremities, is contraindicated).
No products indexed under this heading.

Metronidazole (Co-administration with drugs that inhibit CYP3A may increase delavirdine plasma concentrations). Products include:
- Metrogel 1% 1211
- MetroGel-Vaginal Gel 1855
- Vandazole Vaginal Gel 3338

Metronidazole Benzoate (Co-administration with drugs that inhibit CYP3A may increase delavirdine plasma concentrations).
No products indexed under this heading.

Metronidazole Hydrochloride (Co-administration with drugs that inhibit CYP3A may increase delavirdine plasma concentrations).
No products indexed under this heading.

Miconazole (Co-administration with drugs that inhibit CYP3A may increase delavirdine plasma concentrations).
No products indexed under this heading.

Midazolam Hydrochloride (Co-administration with drugs that are highly dependent on CYP3A for clearance and for which elevated plasma levels are associated with serious and/or life-threatening events, such as cardiac arrhythmias, is contraindicated).
No products indexed under this heading.

Modafinil (Co-administration with drugs that induce CYP3A may decrease delavirdine plasma concentrations and reduce its therapeutic effect). Products include:
- Provigil Tablets 988

Nefazodone Hydrochloride (Co-administration with drugs that inhibit CYP3A may increase delavirdine plasma concentrations).
No products indexed under this heading.

Nelfinavir Mesylate (Co-administration results in increased nelfinavir concentrations and decreased delavirdine concentrations). Products include:
- Viracept 2577

Nevirapine (Co-administration with drugs that induce CYP3A may decrease delavirdine plasma concentrations and reduce its therapeutic effect). Products include:
- Viramune Oral Suspension 873
- Viramune Tablets 873

Nicardipine (Co-administration with drugs primarily metabolized by CYP3A may result in increased plasma concentrations of the coadministered drug that could increase or prolong both its therapeutic or adverse effects).
No products indexed under this heading.

Nicardipine Hydrochloride (Co-administration results in increased dihydropyridine calcium channel blocker concentrations). Products include:
- Cardene I.V. 2497

Nifedipine (Co-administration results in increased dihydropyridine calcium channel blocker concentrations). Products include:
- Adalat CC Tablets 2964

Nimodipine (Co-administration results in increased dihydropyridine calcium channel blocker concentrations). Products include:
- Nimotop Capsules 749

Nisoldipine (Co-adminstration results in increased calcium channel blocker concentrations). Products include:
- Sular Tablets 3122

Nizatidine (H2 antagonists increase gastric pH and may reduce the absorption of delavirdine; chronic use of these drugs with delavirdine is not recommended). Products include:
- Axid Oral Solution 879

Norethindrone (Co-administration with drugs primarily metabolized by CYP3A may result in increased plasma concentrations of the coadministered drug that could increase or prolong both its therapeutic or adverse effects). Products include:
- Ortho Micronor Tablets 2426

Norfloxacin (Co-administration with drugs that inhibit CYP3A may increase delavirdine plasma concentrations). Products include:
- Noroxin Tablets 2032

Norgestrel (Co-administration with drugs primarily metabolized by CYP3A may result in increased plasma concentrations of the coadministered drug that could increase or prolong both its therapeutic or adverse effects).
No products indexed under this heading.

Omeprazole (Proton pump inhibitors increase gastric pH and may reduce the absorption of delavirdine; chronic use of these drugs with delavirdine is not recommended). Products include:
- Zegerid Capsules 2958
- Zegerid Powder for Oral Solution 2958

Ondansetron Hydrochloride (Co-administration with drugs primarily metabolized by CYP3A may result in increased plasma concentrations of the coadministered drug that could increase or prolong both its therapeutic or adverse effects). Products include:
- Zofran Injection 1634
- Zofran 1639

Paclitaxel (Co-administration with drugs primarily metabolized by CYP3A may result in increased plasma concentrations of the coadministered drug that could increase or prolong both its therapeutic or adverse effects).
No products indexed under this heading.

Pantoprazole Sodium (Proton pump inhibitors increase gastric pH and may reduce the absorption of delavirdine; chronic use of these drugs with delavirdine is not recommended). Products include:
- Protonix I.V. 3472
- Protonix Tablets 3469

Paroxetine Hydrochloride (Co-administration with drugs that inhibit CYP3A may increase delavirdine plasma concentrations). Products include:
- Paxil CR Controlled-Release Tablets 1538

Paxil 1530

Phenobarbital (May lead to loss of virologic response and possible resistance to delavirdine or the class of non-nucleoside reverse transcriptase inhibitors). Products include:

Donnatal Extentabs 2493

Phenytoin (May lead to loss of virologic response and possible resistance to delavirdine or the class of non-nucleoside reverse transcriptase inhibitors).

No products indexed under this heading.

Phenytoin Sodium (May lead to loss of virologic response and possible resistance to delavirdine or the class of non-nucleoside reverse transcriptase inhibitors). Products include:

Phenytek Capsules 2160

Pimozide (Co-administration with drugs that are highly dependent on CYP3A for clearance and for which elevated plasma levels are associated with serious and/or life-threatening events, such as cardiac arrhythmias, is contraindicated).

No products indexed under this heading.

Propafenone Hydrochloride (Co-administration results in increased propafenone concentrations). Products include:

Rythmol SR Capsules 2727

Quinidine (Co-administration results in increased quinidine concentrations).

No products indexed under this heading.

Quinidine Gluconate (Co-administration results in increased quinidine concentrations).

No products indexed under this heading.

Quinidine Hydrochloride (Co-administration results in increased quinidine concentrations).

No products indexed under this heading.

Quinidine Polygalacturonate (Co-administration results in increased quinidine concentrations).

No products indexed under this heading.

Quinidine Sulfate (Co-administration results in increased quinidine concentrations).

No products indexed under this heading.

Quinine (Co-administration with drugs that inhibit CYP3A may increase delavirdine plasma concentrations).

No products indexed under this heading.

Quinine Sulfate (Co-administration with drugs that inhibit CYP3A may increase delavirdine plasma concentrations).

No products indexed under this heading.

Rabeprazole Sodium (Proton pump inhibitors increase gastric pH and may reduce the absorption of delavirdine; chronic use of these drugs with delavirdine is not recommended). Products include:

Aciphex Tablets 1090

Ranitidine Bismuth Citrate (H2 antagonists increase gastric pH and may reduce the absorption of delavirdine; chronic use of these drugs with delavirdine is not recommended).

No products indexed under this heading.

Ranitidine Hydrochloride (H2 antagonists increase gastric pH and may reduce the absorption of delavirdine; chronic use of these drugs with delavirdine is not recommended). Products include:

Zantac 1624
Zantac Injection 1619
Zantac Injection Pharmacy Bulk Package 1622

Rapamycin (Co-administration results in increased rapamycin concentrations).

No products indexed under this heading.

Rifabutin (May lead to loss of virologic response and possible resistance to delavirdine or the class of non-nucleoside reverse transcriptase inhibitors or other co-administered antiviral drugs).

No products indexed under this heading.

Rifampicin (Co-administration with drugs that induce CYP3A may decrease delavirdine plasma concentrations and reduce its therapeutic effect).

No products indexed under this heading.

Rifampin (May lead to loss or virologic response and possible resistance to delavirdine or the class of non-nucleoside reverse transcriptase inhibitors or other co-administered antiviral drugs).

No products indexed under this heading.

Rifapentine (Co-administration with drugs that induce CYP3A may decrease delavirdine plasma concentrations and reduce its therapeutic effect).

No products indexed under this heading.

Ritonavir (Co-administration results in increased ritonavir concentrations). Products include:

Kaletra 476
Norvir 503

Saquinavir (Co-administration results in increased saquinavir concentrations).

No products indexed under this heading.

Saquinavir Mesylate (Co-administration results in increased saquinavir concentrations). Products include:

Invirase 2772

Sertraline Hydrochloride (Co-administration with drugs that inhibit CYP3A may increase delavirdine plasma concentrations). Products include:

Zoloft 2586

Sildenafil Citrate (Co-administration is expected to substantially increase sildenafil concentrations and may result in an increase in sildenafil-associated adverse events, including hypotension, visual changes, and priapism). Products include:

Revatio Tablets 2557
Viagra Tablets 2573

Simvastatin (Potential for serious reactions such as myopathy including rhabdomyolysis; concurrent use is not recommended). Products include:

Vytorin 10/10 Tablets 2114
Vytorin 10/10 Tablets 3077
Vytorin 10/20 Tablets 2114
Vytorin 10/20 Tablets 3077
Vytorin 10/40 Tablets 2114
Vytorin 10/40 Tablets 3077
Vytorin 10/80 Tablets 2114
Vytorin 10/80 Tablets 3077
Zocor Tablets 2105

Sirolimus (Co-administration with drugs primarily metabolized by CYP3A may result in increased plasma concentrations of the coadministered drug that could increase or prolong both its therapeutic or adverse effects). Products include:

Rapamune Oral Solution and Tablets 3475

Sodium Bicarbonate (Co-administration with antacids results in decreased delavirdine concentrations because of reduced absorption; patients taking antacids should be advised to take them at least one hour apart). Products include:

Colyte with Flavor Packs for Oral Solution 3088
HalfLytely and Bisacodyl Tablets Bowel Prep Kit with Flavors Packs 881
TriLyte with Flavor Packs for Oral Solution 3100

Tacrolimus (Co-administration results in increased tacrolimus concentrations). Products include:

Prograf Capsules and Injection 632
Protopic Ointment 638

Tamoxifen Citrate (Co-administration with drugs primarily metabolized by CYP3A may result in increased plasma concentrations of the coadministered drug that could increase or prolong both its therapeutic or adverse effects). Products include:

Soltamox Oral Solution 3527

Terfenadine (Co-administration with drugs that are highly dependent on CYP3A for clearance and for which elevated plasma levels are associated with serious and/or life-threatening events, such as cardiac arrhythmias, is contraindicated).

No products indexed under this heading.

Testosterone (Co-administration with drugs primarily metabolized by CYP3A may result in increased plasma concentrations of the coadministered drug that could increase or prolong both its therapeutic or adverse effects). Products include:

AndroGel 3329
Striant Mucoadhesive 1007
Testim 1% Gel 695

Testosterone Cypionate (Co-administration with drugs primarily metabolized by CYP3A may result in increased plasma concentrations of the coadministered drug that could increase or prolong both its therapeutic or adverse effects).

No products indexed under this heading.

Testosterone Enanthate (Co-administration with drugs primarily metabolized by CYP3A may result in increased plasma concentrations of the coadministered drug that could increase or prolong both its therapeutic or adverse effects).

No products indexed under this heading.

Testosterone Propionate (Co-administration with drugs primarily metabolized by CYP3A may result in increased plasma concentrations of the coadministered drug that could increase or prolong both its therapeutic or adverse effects).

No products indexed under this heading.

Theophylline (Co-administration with drugs primarily metabolized by CYP3A may result in increased plasma concentrations of the coadministered drug that could increase or prolong both its therapeutic or adverse effects).

No products indexed under this heading.

Theophylline Anhydrous (Co-administration with drugs primarily metabolized by CYP3A may result in increased plasma concentrations of the coadministered drug that could increase or prolong both its therapeutic or adverse effects). Products include:

Uniphyl Tablets 2710

Theophylline Calcium Salicylate (Co-administration with drugs primarily metabolized by CYP3A may result in increased plasma concentrations of the coadministered drug that could increase or prolong both its therapeutic or adverse effects).

No products indexed under this heading.

Theophylline Sodium Glycinate (Co-administration with drugs primarily metabolized by CYP3A may result in increased plasma concentrations of the coadministered drug that could increase or prolong both its therapeutic or adverse effects).

No products indexed under this heading.

Tiagabine Hydrochloride (Co-administration with drugs primarily metabolized by CYP3A may result in increased plasma concentrations of the coadministered drug that could increase or prolong both its therapeutic or adverse effects). Products include:

Gabitril Tablets 984

Tolterodine Tartrate (Co-administration with drugs primarily metabolized by CYP3A may result in increased plasma concentrations of the coadministered drug that could increase or prolong both its therapeutic or adverse effects). Products include:

Detrol Tablets 2628
Detrol LA Capsules 2631

Trazodone Hydrochloride (Co-administration results in increased trazodone concentrations; a lower dose of trazadone should be considered).

No products indexed under this heading.

Triazolam (Co-administration with drugs that are highly dependent on CYP3A for clearance and for which elevated plasma levels are associated with serious and/or life-threatening events, such as prolonged or increased sedation or respiratory depression, is contraindicated).

No products indexed under this heading.

Troleandomycin (Co-administration with drugs that inhibit CYP3A may increase delavirdine plasma concentrations).
No products indexed under this heading.

Venlafaxine Hydrochloride (Co-administration with drugs that inhibit CYP3A may increase delavirdine plasma concentrations). Products include:
Effexor Tablets 3411
Effexor XR Capsules 3417

Verapamil Hydrochloride (Co-administration results in increased calcium channel blocker concentrations). Products include:
Covera-HS Tablets 3139
Tarka Tablets 524
Verelan PM Extended-Release Capsules, Controlled-Onset 3106

Vinblastine Sulfate (Co-administration with drugs primarily metabolized by CYP3A may result in increased plasma concentrations of the coadministered drug that could increase or prolong both its therapeutic or adverse effects).
No products indexed under this heading.

Vincristine Sulfate (Co-administration with drugs primarily metabolized by CYP3A may result in increased plasma concentrations of the coadministered drug that could increase or prolong both its therapeutic or adverse effects).
No products indexed under this heading.

Voriconazole (Co-administration with drugs that inhibit CYP3A may increase delavirdine plasma concentrations). Products include:
VFEND I.V. 2564
VFEND Oral Suspension 2564
VFEND Tablets 2564

Warfarin Sodium (Co-administration results in increased warfarin concentrations). Products include:
Coumadin for Injection 898
Coumadin Tablets 898

Zafirlukast (Co-administration with drugs that inhibit CYP3A may increase delavirdine plasma concentrations). Products include:
Accolate Tablets 671

Zileuton (Co-administration with drugs that inhibit CYP3A may increase delavirdine plasma concentrations). Products include:
Zyflo Tablets 1023

Food Interactions

Grapefruit (Co-administration with drugs that inhibit CYP3A may increase delavirdine plasma concentrations).

RESTASIS OPHTHALMIC EMULSION

(Cyclosporine) 575
None cited in PDR database.

RESTORIL CAPSULES

(Temazepam) 1860
None cited in PDR database.

RETAVASE

(Reteplase) 2499
May interact with vitamin K antagonists and certain other agents. Compounds in these categories include:

Abciximab (Drugs that alter platelet function, such as abciximab, may increase the risk of bleeding if administered prior to or after reteplase therapy). Products include:
ReoPro Vials 1809

Aspirin (Drugs that alter platelet function, such as aspirin, may increase the risk of bleeding if administered prior to or after reteplase therapy). Products include:
Aggrenox Capsules 822
Bayer Aspirin 744
BC Allergy Sinus Cold Powder 677
BC Headache Powder 677
Arthritis Strength BC Powder 677
BC Sinus Cold Powder 677
Excedrin Extra Strength Caplets/Tablets/Geltabs 684
Excedrin Migraine Caplets/Tablets/Geltabs 609
Goody's Body Pain Formula Powder 684
Goody's Extra Strength Headache Powders 611
Goody's Extra Strength Pain Relief Tablets 685
Percodan Tablets 1132
St. Joseph 81 mg Aspirin Chewable and Enteric Coated Tablets 1869

Clopidogrel Bisulfate (Drugs that alter platelet function, such as clopidogrel, may increase the risk of bleeding if administered prior to or after reteplase therapy). Products include:
Plavix Tablets 917
Plavix Tablets 2926

Dicumarol (Co-administration increases the risk of bleeding).
No products indexed under this heading.

Dipyridamole (Drugs that alter platelet function, such as dipyridamole, may increase the risk of bleeding if administered prior to or after reteplase therapy). Products include:
Aggrenox Capsules 822
Persantine Tablets 868

Eptifibatide (Drugs that alter platelet function, such as eptifibatide, may increase the risk of bleeding if administered prior to or after reteplase therapy). Products include:
Integrilin Injection 3020

Ticlopidine Hydrochloride (Drugs that alter platelet function, such as ticlopidine, may increase the risk of bleeding if administered prior to or after reteplase therapy). Products include:
Ticlid Tablets 2810

Tirofiban Hydrochloride (Drugs that alter platelet function, such as tirofiban, may increase the risk of bleeding if administered prior to or after reteplase therapy). Products include:
Aggrastat 1907

Warfarin Sodium (Co-administration increases the risk of bleeding). Products include:
Coumadin for Injection 898
Coumadin Tablets 898

RETISERT IMPLANT

(Fluocinolone Acetonide) .... ⊙258
None cited in PDR database.

RETROVIR CAPSULES

(Zidovudine) 1560
May interact with cytotoxic drugs, Interferon alpha, phenytoin, valproate, and certain other agents. Compounds in these categories include:

Atovaquone (Co-administration results in increased AUC of zidovudine; routine dose modification of zidovudine is not warranted). Products include:
Malarone Pediatric Tablets 1517
Malarone Tablets 1517
Mepron Suspension 1521

Bleomycin Sulfate (Co-administration with cytotoxic agents may increase the hematologic toxicity of zidovudine).
No products indexed under this heading.

Bone Marrow Suppressants, unspecified (May increase the hematologic toxicity of zidovudine).
No products indexed under this heading.

Cyclophosphamide (Co-administration with cytotoxic agents may increase the hematologic toxicity of zidovudine).
No products indexed under this heading.

Daunorubicin Hydrochloride (Co-administration with cytotoxic agents may increase the hematologic toxicity of zidovudine).
No products indexed under this heading.

Divalproex Sodium (Co-administration results in increased AUC of zidovudine by 80%; routine dose modification of zidovudine is not warranted unless patient is experiencing pronounced anemia or other severe zidovudine-associated events). Products include:
Depakote Sprinkle Capsules 422
Depakote Tablets 427
Depakote ER Tablets 434

Doxorubicin Hydrochloride (Concomitant use should be avoided since an antagonistic relationship has been demonstrated).
No products indexed under this heading.

Epirubicin Hydrochloride (Co-administration with cytotoxic agents may increase the hematologic toxicity of zidovudine).
No products indexed under this heading.

Fluconazole (Co-administration results in increased AUC of zidovudine by 74%; routine dose modification of zidovudine is not warranted unless patient is experiencing pronounced anemia or other severe zidovudine-associated events).
No products indexed under this heading.

Fluorouracil (Co-administration with cytotoxic agents may increase the hematologic toxicity of zidovudine). Products include:
Carac Cream, 0.5% 2879
Efudex 3363

Fosphenytoin Sodium (Co-administration has resulted in low phenytoin levels in some patients and a high level in one case; a 30% decrease in oral zidovudine clearance was observed with phenytoin).
No products indexed under this heading.

Ganciclovir Sodium (May increase the hematologic toxicity of zidovudine).
No products indexed under this heading.

Hydroxyurea (Co-administration with cytotoxic agents may increase the hematologic toxicity of zidovudine).
No products indexed under this heading.

Interferon alfa-2a, Recombinant (Hepatic decompensation (some fatal) has occurred in HIV/HCV co-infected patients receiving combination antiretroviral therapy for HIV and interferon alfa and ribavirin. Patients receiving interferon alfa with or without ribavirin and zidovudine shouldbe closely monitored for treatment-associated toxicities, especially neutropenia, anemia and hepatic decompensation. Discontinuation of zidovudine should be considered as medically appropriate. Dose reduction or discontinuation of interferon alfa, ribavirin or both should also be considered if worsening of clinical toxicities are observed, including hepatic decompensation (e.g., Childs Pugh greater than 6)).
No products indexed under this heading.

Interferon alfa-2b, Recombinant (Hepatic decompensation (some fatal) has occurred in HIV/HCV co-infected patients receiving combination antiretroviral therapy for HIV and interferon alfa and ribavirin. Patients receiving interferon alfa with or without ribavirin and zidovudine shouldbe closely monitored for treatment-associated toxicities, especially neutropenia, anemia and hepatic decompensation. Discontinuation of zidovudine should be considered as medically appropriate. Dose reduction or discontinuation of interferon alfa, ribavirin or both should also be considered if worsening of clinical toxicities are observed, including hepatic decompensation (e.g., Childs Pugh greater than 6)). Products include:
Intron A for Injection 3024
Rebetron Combination Therapy 3063

Interferon alfa-N3 (Human Leukocyte Derived) (Hepatic decompensation (some fatal) has occurred in HIV/HCV co-infected patients receiving combination antiretroviral therapy for HIV and interferon alfa and ribavirin. Patients receiving interferon alfa with or without ribavirin and zidovudine shouldbe closely monitored for treatment-associated toxicities, especially neutropenia, anemia and hepatic decompensation. Discontinuation of zidovudine should be considered as medically appropriate. Dose reduction or discontinuation of interferon alfa, ribavirin or both should also be considered if worsening of clinical toxicities are observed, including hepatic decompensation (e.g., Childs Pugh greater than 6)). Products include:
Alferon N Injection 1665

Methadone Hydrochloride (Co-administration results in increased AUC of zidovudine; routine dose modification of zidovudine is not warranted).
No products indexed under this heading.

Methotrexate Sodium (Co-administration with cytotoxic agents may increase the hematologic toxicity of zidovudine).
No products indexed under this heading.

Mitotane (Co-administration with cytotoxic agents may increase the hematologic toxicity of zidovudine).
No products indexed under this heading.

Mitoxantrone Hydrochloride (Co-administration with cytotoxic agents may increase the hematologic toxicity of zidovudine).
No products indexed under this heading.

Nelfinavir Mesylate (Co-administration results in decreased

AUC of zidovudine; routine dose modification of zidovudine is not warranted). Products include:
- Viracept 2577

Peginterferon Alfa-2b (May increase the hematologic toxicity of zidovudine). Products include:
- PEG-Intron Powder for Injection 3048

Phenytoin (Co-administration has resulted in low phenytoin levels in some patients and a high level in one case; a 30% decrease in oral zidovudine clearance was observed with phenytoin).
- No products indexed under this heading.

Phenytoin Sodium (Co-administration has resulted in low phenytoin levels in some patients and a high level in one case; a 30% decrease in oral zidovudine clearance was observed with phenytoin). Products include:
- Phenytek Capsules 2160

Probenecid (Co-administration results in increased AUC of zidovudine by 106%; routine dose modification of zidovudine is not warranted unless patient is experiencing pronounced anemia or other severe zidovudine-associated events).
- No products indexed under this heading.

Procarbazine Hydrochloride (Co-administration with cytotoxic agents may increase the hematologic toxicity of zidovudine). Products include:
- Matulane Capsules 3191

Ribavirin (Antagonizes the in vitro antiviral activity of zidovudine against HIV; concomitant use should be avoided). Products include:
- Copegus Tablets 2754
- Rebetol 3058
- Rebetron Combination Therapy 3063
- Ribavirin, USP Capsules 3068
- Virazole for Inhalation Solution 3370

Rifampin (Co-administration results in decreased AUC of zidovudine; routine dose modification of zidovudine is not warranted).
- No products indexed under this heading.

Ritonavir (Co-administration results in decreased AUC of zidovudine; routine dose modification of zidovudine is not warranted). Products include:
- Kaletra 476
- Norvir 503

Stavudine (Concomitant use should be avoided since an antagonistic relationship has been demonstrated in vitro).
- No products indexed under this heading.

Tamoxifen Citrate (Co-administration with cytotoxic agents may increase the hematologic toxicity of zidovudine). Products include:
- Soltamox Oral Solution 3527

Valproate Sodium (Co-administration results in increased AUC of zidovudine by 80%; routine dose modification of zidovudine is not warranted unless patient is experiencing pronounced anemia or other severe zidovudine-associated events). Products include:
- Depacon Injection 412

Valproic Acid (Co-administration results in increased AUC of zidovudine by 80%; routine dose modification of zidovudine is not warranted unless patient is experiencing pronounced anemia or other severe zidovudine-associated events). Products include:
- Depakene 417

Vincristine Sulfate (Co-administration with cytotoxic agents may increase the hematologic toxicity of zidovudine).
- No products indexed under this heading.

RETROVIR IV INFUSION

(Zidovudine) 1564

See Retrovir Capsules

RETROVIR SYRUP

(Zidovudine) 1560

See Retrovir Capsules

RETROVIR TABLETS

(Zidovudine) 1560

See Retrovir Capsules

REVATIO TABLETS

(Sildenafil Citrate) 2557

May interact with cytochrome p450 2c9 inducers (selected), cytochrome p450 2c9 inhibitors (selected), cytochrome p450 3a4 inducers (selected), cytochrome p450 3a4 inhibitors (selected), nitrates and nitrites, vitamin K antagonists, and certain other agents. Compounds in these categories include:

Acetazolamide (Sildenafil metabolism is principally mediated by the CYP3A4 (major route) and CYP2C9 (minor route) cytochrome P450 isoforms. Therefore, inhibitors of these isoenzymes may reduce sildenafil clearance).
- No products indexed under this heading.

Allium sativum (Sildenafil metabolism is principally mediated by the CYP3A4 (major route) and CYP2C9 (minor route) cytochrome P450 isoforms. Therefore, inducers of these isoenzymes may increase sildenafil clearance).
- No products indexed under this heading.

Amiodarone Hydrochloride (Sildenafil metabolism is principally mediated by the CYP3A4 (major route) and CYP2C9 (minor route) cytochrome P450 isoforms. Therefore, inhibitors of these isoenzymes may reduce sildenafil clearance).
- No products indexed under this heading.

Amlodipine Besylate (When sildenafil 100 mg oral was co-administered with amlodipine, 5 mg or 10 mg oral, to hypertensive patients, the mean additional reduction on supine blood pressure was 8mmHg systolic and 7mmHg diastolic). Products include:
- Caduet Tablets 2508
- Lotrel Capsules 2249
- Norvasc Tablets 2545

Amprenavir (Sildenafil metabolism is principally mediated by the CYP3A4 (major route) and CYP2C9 (minor route) cytochrome P450 isoforms. Therefore, inhibitors of these isoenzymes may reduce sildenafil clearance). Products include:
- Agenerase Capsules 1327
- Agenerase Oral Solution 1332

Amyl Nitrite (Consistent with its known effect on the nitric oxide/cGMP pathway, sildenafil was shown to potentiate the hypotensive effects of nitrates, and its administration to patients who are using organic nitrates, either regularly and/or intermittently, in any form is therefore contraindicated).
- No products indexed under this heading.

Anastrozole (Sildenafil metabolism is principally mediated by the CYP3A4 (major route) and CYP2C9 (minor route) cytochrome P450 isoforms. Therefore, inhibitors of these isoenzymes may reduce sildenafil clearance). Products include:
- Arimidex Tablets 673

Aprepitant (Sildenafil metabolism is principally mediated by the CYP3A4 (major route) and CYP2C9 (minor route) cytochrome P450 isoforms. Therefore, inducers of these isoenzymes may increase sildenafil clearance). Products include:
- Emend Capsules 1963

Bendroflumethiazide (Sildenafil metabolism is principally mediated by the CYP3A4 (major route) and CYP2C9 (minor route) cytochrome P450 isoforms. Therefore, inhibitors of these isoenzymes may reduce sildenafil clearance).
- No products indexed under this heading.

Betamethasone Acetate (Sildenafil metabolism is principally mediated by the CYP3A4 (major route) and CYP2C9 (minor route) cytochrome P450 isoforms. Therefore, inducers of these isoenzymes may increase sildenafil clearance).
- No products indexed under this heading.

Betamethasone Sodium Phosphate (Sildenafil metabolism is principally mediated by the CYP3A4 (major route) and CYP2C9 (minor route) cytochrome P450 isoforms. Therefore, inducers of these isoenzymes may increase sildenafil clearance).
- No products indexed under this heading.

Bosentan (Co-administration of sildenafil at steady state (80 mg t.i.d.) with the endothelin receptor antagonist bosentan (a moderate inducer of CYP3A4, CYP2C9 and possibly of cytochrome p450 2C19) at steady state (125 mg b.i.d.) resulted in a 63% decrease of sildenafil AUC and a 55% decrease in sildenafil Cmax). Products include:
- Tracleer Tablets 545

Carbamazepine (Sildenafil metabolism is principally mediated by the CYP3A4 (major route) and CYP2C9 (minor route) cytochrome P450 isoforms. Therefore, inducers of these isoenzymes may increase sildenafil clearance). Products include:
- Carbatrol Capsules 3171
- Equetro Extended-Release Capsules 3180
- Tegretol/Tegretol-XR 2295

Chloramphenicol (Sildenafil metabolism is principally mediated by the CYP3A4 (major route) and CYP2C9 (minor route) cytochrome P450 isoforms. Therefore, inhibitors of these isoenzymes may reduce sildenafil clearance).
- No products indexed under this heading.

Chlorothiazide (Sildenafil metabolism is principally mediated by the CYP3A4 (major route) and CYP2C9 (minor route) cytochrome P450 isoforms. Therefore, inhibitors of these isoenzymes may reduce sildenafil clearance). Products include:
- Diuril Oral Suspension 1954

Chlorothiazide Sodium (Sildenafil metabolism is principally mediated by the CYP3A4 (major route) and CYP2C9 (minor route) cytochrome P450 isoforms. Therefore, inhibitors of these isoenzymes may reduce sildenafil clearance). Products include:
- Diuril Sodium Intravenous 2467

Chlorpropamide (Sildenafil metabolism is principally mediated by the CYP3A4 (major route) and CYP2C9 (minor route) cytochrome P450 isoforms. Therefore, inhibitors of these isoenzymes may reduce sildenafil clearance).
- No products indexed under this heading.

Cimetidine (Cimetidine (800mg), a non-specific CYP inhibitor, caused a 56% increase in plasma sildenafil concentrations when co-administered with sildenafil (50 mg) to healthy volunteers). Products include:
- Tagamet HB 200 Tablets .... ▣664

Cimetidine Hydrochloride (Sildenafil metabolism is principally mediated by the CYP3A4 (major route) and CYP2C9 (minor route) cytochrome P450 isoforms. Therefore, inhibitors of these isoenzymes may reduce sildenafil clearance).
- No products indexed under this heading.

Ciprofloxacin (Sildenafil metabolism is principally mediated by the CYP3A4 (major route) and CYP2C9 (minor route) cytochrome P450 isoforms. Therefore, inhibitors of these isoenzymes may reduce sildenafil clearance). Products include:
- Cipro Oral Suspension 2977
- Cipro I.V. 2984
- Cipro XR Tablets 2990
- Ciprodex Otic Suspension 559

Ciprofloxacin Hydrochloride (Sildenafil metabolism is principally mediated by the CYP3A4 (major route) and CYP2C9 (minor route) cytochrome P450 isoforms. Therefore, inducers of these isoenzymes may increase sildenafil clearance). Products include:
- Ciloxan Ophthalmic Ointment 559
- Ciloxan Ophthalmic Solution .... ⊙206
- Cipro Tablets 2977
- Proquin XR Tablets 1153

Cisplatin (Sildenafil metabolism is principally mediated by the CYP3A4 (major route) and CYP2C9 (minor route) cytochrome P450 isoforms. Therefore, inducers of these isoenzymes may increase sildenafil clearance).
- No products indexed under this heading.

Clarithromycin (Sildenafil metabolism is principally mediated by the CYP3A4 (major route) and CYP2C9 (minor route) cytochrome P450 isoforms. Therefore, inhibitors of these isoenzymes may reduce sildenafil clearance). Products include:
- Biaxin/Biaxin XL 402
- PREVPAC 3284

Clopidogrel Hydrogen Sulfate (Sildenafil metabolism is principally mediated by the CYP3A4 (major route) and CYP2C9 (minor route) cytochrome P450 isoforms. Therefore, inhibitors of these isoenzymes may reduce sildenafil clearance).
No products indexed under this heading.

Clotrimazole (Sildenafil metabolism is principally mediated by the CYP3A4 (major route) and CYP2C9 (minor route) cytochrome P450 isoforms. Therefore, inhibitors of these isoenzymes may reduce sildenafil clearance). Products include:
Desenex Athlete's Foot Cream 635
Lotrimin 3039
Lotrisone 3040

Cortisone Acetate (Sildenafil metabolism is principally mediated by the CYP3A4 (major route) and CYP2C9 (minor route) cytochrome P450 isoforms. Therefore, inducers of these isoenzymes may increase sildenafil clearance).
No products indexed under this heading.

Cyclosporine (Sildenafil metabolism is principally mediated by the CYP3A4 (major route) and CYP2C9 (minor route) cytochrome P450 isoforms. Therefore, inhibitors of these isoenzymes may reduce sildenafil clearance). Products include:
Gengraf Capsules 459
Neoral Oral Solution 2259
Neoral Soft Gelatin Capsules 2259
Restasis Ophthalmic Emulsion 575
Sandimmune 2275

Dalfopristin (Sildenafil metabolism is principally mediated by the CYP3A4 (major route) and CYP2C9 (minor route) cytochrome P450 isoforms. Therefore, inhibitors of these isoenzymes may reduce sildenafil clearance).
No products indexed under this heading.

Danazol (Sildenafil metabolism is principally mediated by the CYP3A4 (major route) and CYP2C9 (minor route) cytochrome P450 isoforms. Therefore, inhibitors of these isoenzymes may reduce sildenafil clearance).
No products indexed under this heading.

Delavirdine Mesylate (Sildenafil metabolism is principally mediated by the CYP3A4 (major route) and CYP2C9 (minor route) cytochrome P450 isoforms. Therefore, inhibitors of these isoenzymes may reduce sildenafil clearance). Products include:
Rescriptor Tablets 2551

Dexamethasone (Sildenafil metabolism is principally mediated by the CYP3A4 (major route) and CYP2C9 (minor route) cytochrome P450 isoforms. Therefore, inducers of these isoenzymes may increase sildenafil clearance). Products include:
Ciprodex Otic Suspension 559
Decadron Tablets 1951
TobraDex Ophthalmic Ointment 562
TobraDex Ophthalmic Suspension 563

Dexamethasone Acetate (Sildenafil metabolism is principally mediated by the CYP3A4 (major route) and CYP2C9 (minor route) cytochrome P450 isoforms. Therefore, inducers of these isoenzymes may increase sildenafil clearance).
No products indexed under this heading.

Dexamethasone Sodium Phosphate (Sildenafil metabolism is principally mediated by the CYP3A4 (major route) and CYP2C9 (minor route) cytochrome P450 isoforms. Therefore, inducers of these isoenzymes may increase sildenafil clearance).
No products indexed under this heading.

Diclofenac Potassium (Sildenafil metabolism is principally mediated by the CYP3A4 (major route) and CYP2C9 (minor route) cytochrome P450 isoforms. Therefore, inhibitors of these isoenzymes may reduce sildenafil clearance).
No products indexed under this heading.

Diclofenac Sodium (Sildenafil metabolism is principally mediated by the CYP3A4 (major route) and CYP2C9 (minor route) cytochrome P450 isoforms. Therefore, inhibitors of these isoenzymes may reduce sildenafil clearance). Products include:
Arthrotec Tablets 3129
Voltaren Ophthalmic Solution 2309
Voltaren Tablets 2307
Voltaren-XR Tablets 2310

Dicumarol (In pulmonary arterial hypertension (PAH) patients, the concomitant use of vitamin K antagonists and sildenafil resulted in a greater incidence of reports of bleeding (primarily epistaxis) versus placebo).
No products indexed under this heading.

Diltiazem Hydrochloride (Sildenafil metabolism is principally mediated by the CYP3A4 (major route) and CYP2C9 (minor route) cytochrome P450 isoforms. Therefore, inhibitors of these isoenzymes may reduce sildenafil clearance). Products include:
Cardizem LA Extended Release Tablets 1728
Tiazac Capsules 1201

Diltiazem Maleate (Sildenafil metabolism is principally mediated by the CYP3A4 (major route) and CYP2C9 (minor route) cytochrome P450 isoforms. Therefore, inhibitors of these isoenzymes may reduce sildenafil clearance).
No products indexed under this heading.

Disulfiram (Sildenafil metabolism is principally mediated by the CYP3A4 (major route) and CYP2C9 (minor route) cytochrome P450 isoforms. Therefore, inhibitors of these isoenzymes may reduce sildenafil clearance).
No products indexed under this heading.

Doxazosin Mesylate (In drug-drug interaction studies, co-administration of sildenafil (25 mg, 50mg, or 100mg) and the alpha-blocker doxazosin (4 mg or 8mg) in patients with benign prostatic hyperplasia (BPH) stabilized on doxazosin therapy resulted in mean additional reduction of supine systolic and diastolic blood pressure of 7/7 mmHg, 9/5 mmHg and 8/4 mmHg, respectively, were observed. Mean additional reductions of standing blood pressure of 6/6 mmHg, 11/4 mmHg and 4/5 mmHg, respectively, were also observed. There were infrequent reports of patients who experienced symptomatic postural hypotension. These reports included dizziness and light-headedness, but not syncope). Products include:
Cardura XL Tablets 2515

Doxorubicin Hydrochloride (Sildenafil metabolism is principally mediated by the CYP3A4 (major route) and CYP2C9 (minor route) cytochrome P450 isoforms. Therefore, inducers of these isoenzymes may increase sildenafil clearance).
No products indexed under this heading.

Efavirenz (Sildenafil metabolism is principally mediated by the CYP3A4 (major route) and CYP2C9 (minor route) cytochrome P450 isoforms. Therefore, inhibitors of these isoenzymes may reduce sildenafil clearance). Products include:
Atripla Tablets 945
Sustiva Capsules 930
Sustiva Tablets 930

Erythrityl Tetranitrate (Consistent with its known effect on the nitric oxide/cGMP pathway, sildenafil was shown to potentiate the hypotensive effects of nitrates, and its administration to patients who are using organic nitrates, either regularly and/or intermittently, in any form is therefore contraindicated).
No products indexed under this heading.

Erythromycin (When a single 100 mg dose of sildenafil was co-administered with erythromycin, a CYP3A4 inhibitor, at steady state (500 mg twice daily (b.i.d.) for 5 days), there was a 182% increase in sildenafil systemic exposure (AUC)). Products include:
Ery-Tab Tablets 449
Erythromycin Base Filmtab Tablets 455
Erythromycin Delayed-Release Capsules, USP 457
PCE Dispertab Tablets 515

Erythromycin Estolate (Sildenafil metabolism is principally mediated by the CYP3A4 (major route) and CYP2C9 (minor route) cytochrome P450 isoforms. Therefore, inhibitors of these isoenzymes may reduce sildenafil clearance).
No products indexed under this heading.

Erythromycin Ethylsuccinate (Sildenafil metabolism is principally mediated by the CYP3A4 (major route) and CYP2C9 (minor route) cytochrome P450 isoforms. Therefore, inhibitors of these isoenzymes may reduce sildenafil clearance). Products include:
E.E.S. 451
EryPed 447

Erythromycin Gluceptate (Sildenafil metabolism is principally mediated by the CYP3A4 (major route) and CYP2C9 (minor route) cytochrome P450 isoforms. Therefore, inhibitors of these isoenzymes may reduce sildenafil clearance).
No products indexed under this heading.

Erythromycin Lactobionate (Sildenafil metabolism is principally mediated by the CYP3A4 (major route) and CYP2C9 (minor route) cytochrome P450 isoforms. Therefore, inhibitors of these isoenzymes may reduce sildenafil clearance).
No products indexed under this heading.

Erythromycin Stearate (Sildenafil metabolism is principally mediated by the CYP3A4 (major route) and CYP2C9 (minor route) cytochrome P450 isoforms. Therefore, inhibitors of these isoenzymes may reduce sildenafil clearance). Products include:
Erythrocin Stearate Filmtab Tablets 453

Esomeprazole Magnesium (Sildenafil metabolism is principally mediated by the CYP3A4 (major route) and CYP2C9 (minor route) cytochrome P450 isoforms. Therefore, inhibitors of these isoenzymes may reduce sildenafil clearance). Products include:
Nexium Delayed-Release Capsules 655

Ethosuximide (Sildenafil metabolism is principally mediated by the CYP3A4 (major route) and CYP2C9 (minor route) cytochrome P450 isoforms. Therefore, inducers of these isoenzymes may increase sildenafil clearance).
No products indexed under this heading.

Felbamate (Sildenafil metabolism is principally mediated by the CYP3A4 (major route) and CYP2C9 (minor route) cytochrome P450 isoforms. Therefore, inducers of these isoenzymes may increase sildenafil clearance).
No products indexed under this heading.

Fenofibrate (Sildenafil metabolism is principally mediated by the CYP3A4 (major route) and CYP2C9 (minor route) cytochrome P450 isoforms. Therefore, inhibitors of these isoenzymes may reduce sildenafil clearance). Products include:
Lofibra Tablets 1219
Lofibra Capsules 1216
Tricor Tablets 527
Triglide Tablets 3123

Fluconazole (Sildenafil metabolism is principally mediated by the CYP3A4 (major route) and CYP2C9 (minor route) cytochrome P450 isoforms. Therefore, inhibitors of these isoenzymes may reduce sildenafil clearance).
No products indexed under this heading.

Fludrocortisone Acetate (Sildenafil metabolism is principally mediated by the CYP3A4 (major route) and CYP2C9 (minor route) cytochrome P450 isoforms. Therefore, inducers of these isoenzymes may increase sildenafil clearance).
No products indexed under this heading.

Fluorouracil (Sildenafil metabolism is principally mediated by the CYP3A4 (major route) and CYP2C9 (minor route) cytochrome P450 isoforms. Therefore, inhibitors of these isoenzymes may reduce sildenafil clearance). Products include:
Carac Cream, 0.5% 2879
Efudex 3363

Fluoxetine Hydrochloride (Sildenafil metabolism is principally mediated by the CYP3A4 (major route) and CYP2C9 (minor route) cytochrome P450 isoforms. Therefore, inhibitors of these isoenzymes may reduce sildenafil clearance). Products include:
Prozac Pulvules and Liquid 1801
Symbyax Capsules 1819

Flurbiprofen (Sildenafil metabolism is principally mediated by the CYP3A4 (major route) and CYP2C9 (minor route) cytochrome P450 isoforms. Therefore, inhibitors of these isoenzymes may reduce sildenafil clearance).

No products indexed under this heading.

Flurbiprofen Sodium (Sildenafil metabolism is principally mediated by the CYP3A4 (major route) and CYP2C9 (minor route) cytochrome P450 isoforms. Therefore, inhibitors of these isoenzymes may reduce sildenafil clearance). Products include:

Fluvastatin Sodium (Sildenafil metabolism is principally mediated by the CYP3A4 (major route) and CYP2C9 (minor route) cytochrome P450 isoforms. Therefore, inhibitors of these isoenzymes may reduce sildenafil clearance). Products include:

Fluvoxamine Maleate (Sildenafil metabolism is principally mediated by the CYP3A4 (major route) and CYP2C9 (minor route) cytochrome P450 isoforms. Therefore, inhibitors of these isoenzymes may reduce sildenafil clearance).

No products indexed under this heading.

Fosamprenavir Calcium (Sildenafil metabolism is principally mediated by the CYP3A4 (major route) and CYP2C9 (minor route) cytochrome P450 isoforms. Therefore, inhibitors of these isoenzymes may reduce sildenafil clearance). Products include:

Fosphenytoin Sodium (Sildenafil metabolism is principally mediated by the CYP3A4 (major route) and CYP2C9 (minor route) cytochrome P450 isoforms. Therefore, inducers of these isoenzymes may increase sildenafil clearance).

No products indexed under this heading.

Garlic Extract (Sildenafil metabolism is principally mediated by the CYP3A4 (major route) and CYP2C9 (minor route) cytochrome P450 isoforms. Therefore, inducers of these isoenzymes may increase sildenafil clearance).

No products indexed under this heading.

Garlic Oil (Sildenafil metabolism is principally mediated by the CYP3A4 (major route) and CYP2C9 (minor route) cytochrome P450 isoforms. Therefore, inducers of these isoenzymes may increase sildenafil clearance).

No products indexed under this heading.

Gemfibrozil (Sildenafil metabolism is principally mediated by the CYP3A4 (major route) and CYP2C9 (minor route) cytochrome P450 isoforms. Therefore, inhibitors of these isoenzymes may reduce sildenafil clearance).

No products indexed under this heading.

Glipizide (Sildenafil metabolism is principally mediated by the CYP3A4 (major route) and CYP2C9 (minor route) cytochrome P450 isoforms. Therefore, inhibitors of these isoenzymes may reduce sildenafil clearance).

No products indexed under this heading.

Glyburide (Sildenafil metabolism is principally mediated by the CYP3A4 (major route) and CYP2C9 (minor route) cytochrome P450 isoforms. Therefore, inhibitors of these isoenzymes may reduce sildenafil clearance).

No products indexed under this heading.

Hydrochlorothiazide (Sildenafil metabolism is principally mediated by the CYP3A4 (major route) and CYP2C9 (minor route) cytochrome P450 isoforms. Therefore, inhibitors of these isoenzymes may reduce sildenafil clearance). Products include:

Hydrocortisone (Sildenafil metabolism is principally mediated by the CYP3A4 (major route) and CYP2C9 (minor route) cytochrome P450 isoforms. Therefore, inducers of these isoenzymes may increase sildenafil clearance). Products include:

Hydrocortisone Acetate (Sildenafil metabolism is principally mediated by the CYP3A4 (major route) and CYP2C9 (minor route) cytochrome P450 isoforms. Therefore, inducers of these isoenzymes may increase sildenafil clearance). Products include:

Hydrocortisone Butyrate (Sildenafil metabolism is principally mediated by the CYP3A4 (major route) and CYP2C9 (minor route) cytochrome P450 isoforms. Therefore, inducers of these isoenzymes may increase sildenafil clearance). Products include:

Hydrocortisone Cypionate (Sildenafil metabolism is principally mediated by the CYP3A4 (major route) and CYP2C9 (minor route) cytochrome P450 isoforms. Therefore, inducers of these isoenzymes may increase sildenafil clearance).

No products indexed under this heading.

Hydrocortisone Hemisuccinate (Sildenafil metabolism is principally mediated by the CYP3A4 (major route) and CYP2C9 (minor route) cytochrome P450 isoforms. Therefore, inducers of these isoenzymes may increase sildenafil clearance).

No products indexed under this heading.

Hydrocortisone Probutate (Sildenafil metabolism is principally mediated by the CYP3A4 (major route) and CYP2C9 (minor route) cytochrome P450 isoforms. Therefore, inducers of these isoenzymes may increase sildenafil clearance).

No products indexed under this heading.

Hydrocortisone Sodium Phosphate (Sildenafil metabolism is principally mediated by the CYP3A4 (major route) and CYP2C9 (minor route) cytochrome P450 isoforms. Therefore, inducers of these isoenzymes may increase sildenafil clearance).

No products indexed under this heading.

Hydrocortisone Sodium Succinate (Sildenafil metabolism is principally mediated by the CYP3A4 (major route) and CYP2C9 (minor route) cytochrome P450 isoforms. Therefore, inducers of these isoenzymes may increase sildenafil clearance).

No products indexed under this heading.

Hydrocortisone Valerate (Sildenafil metabolism is principally mediated by the CYP3A4 (major route) and CYP2C9 (minor route) cytochrome P450 isoforms. Therefore, inducers of these isoenzymes may increase sildenafil clearance).

No products indexed under this heading.

Hydroflumethiazide (Sildenafil metabolism is principally mediated by the CYP3A4 (major route) and CYP2C9 (minor route) cytochrome P450 isoforms. Therefore, inhibitors of these isoenzymes may reduce sildenafil clearance).

No products indexed under this heading.

Hypericum (Sildenafil metabolism is principally mediated by the CYP3A4 (major route) and CYP2C9 (minor route) cytochrome P450 isoforms. Therefore, inducers of these isoenzymes may increase sildenafil clearance). Products include:

Hypericum Perforatum (Sildenafil metabolism is principally mediated by the CYP3A4 (major route) and CYP2C9 (minor route) cytochrome P450 isoforms. Therefore, inducers of these isoenzymes may increase sildenafil clearance).

No products indexed under this heading.

Imatinib Mesylate (Sildenafil metabolism is principally mediated by the CYP3A4 (major route) and CYP2C9 (minor route) cytochrome P450 isoforms. Therefore, inhibitors of these isoenzymes may reduce sildenafil clearance). Products include:

Indinavir Sulfate (Sildenafil metabolism is principally mediated by the CYP3A4 (major route) and CYP2C9 (minor route) cytochrome P450 iso-

forms. Therefore, inhibitors of these isoenzymes may reduce sildenafil clearance). Products include:

Isoniazid (Sildenafil metabolism is principally mediated by the CYP3A4 (major route) and CYP2C9 (minor route) cytochrome P450 isoforms. Therefore, inhibitors of these isoenzymes may reduce sildenafil clearance).

No products indexed under this heading.

Isosorbide Dinitrate (Consistent with its known effect on the nitric oxide/cGMP pathway, sildenafil was shown to potentiate the hypotensive effects of nitrates, and its administration to patients who are using organic nitrates, either regularly and/or intermittently, in any form is therefore contraindicated). Products include:

Isosorbide Mononitrate (Consistent with its known effect on the nitric oxide/cGMP pathway, sildenafil was shown to potentiate the hypotensive effects of nitrates, and its administration to patients who are using organic nitrates, either regularly and/or intermittently, in any form is therefore contraindicated). Products include:

Itraconazole (Sildenafil metabolism is principally mediated by the CYP3A4 (major route) and CYP2C9 (minor route) cytochrome P450 isoforms. Therefore, inhibitors of these isoenzymes may reduce sildenafil clearance).

No products indexed under this heading.

Ketoconazole (Sildenafil metabolism is principally mediated by the CYP3A4 (major route) and CYP2C9 (minor route) cytochrome P450 isoforms. Therefore, inhibitors of these isoenzymes may reduce sildenafil clearance). Products include:

Ketoprofen (Sildenafil metabolism is principally mediated by the CYP3A4 (major route) and CYP2C9 (minor route) cytochrome P450 isoforms. Therefore, inhibitors of these isoenzymes may reduce sildenafil clearance).

No products indexed under this heading.

Leflunomide (Sildenafil metabolism is principally mediated by the CYP3A4 (major route) and CYP2C9 (minor route) cytochrome P450 isoforms. Therefore, inhibitors of these isoenzymes may reduce sildenafil clearance).

No products indexed under this heading.

Lopinavir (Sildenafil metabolism is principally mediated by the CYP3A4 (major route) and CYP2C9 (minor route) cytochrome P450 isoforms. Therefore, inhibitors of these isoenzymes may reduce sildenafil clearance). Products include:

Loratadine (Sildenafil metabolism is principally mediated by the CYP3A4 (major route) and CYP2C9 (minor route) cytochrome P450 isoforms. Therefore, inhibitors of these isoenzymes may reduce sildenafil clearance). Products include:

Alavert ... 771
Children's Claritin Allergy Oral Solution ... 771
Claritin Non-Drowsy 24 Hour Tablets ... 772
Claritin Reditabs 24 Hour Non-Drowsy Tablets ... 772
Claritin-D Non-Drowsy 12 Hour Tablets ... 772
Claritin-D Non-Drowsy 24 Hour Tablets ... 772

Lovastatin (Sildenafil metabolism is principally mediated by the CYP3A4 (major route) and CYP2C9 (minor route) cytochrome P450 isoforms. Therefore, inhibitors of these isoenzymes may reduce sildenafil clearance). Products include:
Advicor Tablets ... **1722**
Altoprev Extended-Release Tablets ... **3109**
Mevacor Tablets ... **2021**

Mephenytoin (Sildenafil metabolism is principally mediated by the CYP3A4 (major route) and CYP2C9 (minor route) cytochrome P450 isoforms. Therefore, inducers of these isoenzymes may increase sildenafil clearance).
No products indexed under this heading.

Methsuximide (Sildenafil metabolism is principally mediated by the CYP3A4 (major route) and CYP2C9 (minor route) cytochrome P450 isoforms. Therefore, inducers of these isoenzymes may increase sildenafil clearance).
No products indexed under this heading.

Methyclothiazide (Sildenafil metabolism is principally mediated by the CYP3A4 (major route) and CYP2C9 (minor route) cytochrome P450 isoforms. Therefore, inhibitors of these isoenzymes may reduce sildenafil clearance).
No products indexed under this heading.

Methylprednisolone (Sildenafil metabolism is principally mediated by the CYP3A4 (major route) and CYP2C9 (minor route) cytochrome P450 isoforms. Therefore, inducers of these isoenzymes may increase sildenafil clearance).
No products indexed under this heading.

Methylprednisolone Acetate (Sildenafil metabolism is principally mediated by the CYP3A4 (major route) and CYP2C9 (minor route) cytochrome P450 isoforms. Therefore, inducers of these isoenzymes may increase sildenafil clearance). Products include:
Depo-Medrol Injectable Suspension ... **2617**
Depo-Medrol Single-Dose Vial ... **2619**

Methylprednisolone Sodium Succinate (Sildenafil metabolism is principally mediated by the CYP3A4 (major route) and CYP2C9 (minor route) cytochrome P450 isoforms. Therefore, inducers of these isoenzymes may increase sildenafil clearance).
No products indexed under this heading.

Metronidazole (Sildenafil metabolism is principally mediated by the CYP3A4 (major route) and CYP2C9 (minor route) cytochrome P450 isoforms. Therefore, inhibitors of these isoenzymes may reduce sildenafil clearance). Products include:
Metrogel 1% ... **1211**
MetroGel-Vaginal Gel ... **1855**
Vandazole Vaginal Gel ... **3338**

Metronidazole Benzoate (Sildenafil metabolism is principally mediated by the CYP3A4 (major route) and CYP2C9 (minor route) cytochrome P450 isoforms. Therefore, inhibitors of these isoenzymes may reduce sildenafil clearance).
No products indexed under this heading.

Metronidazole Hydrochloride (Sildenafil metabolism is principally mediated by the CYP3A4 (major route) and CYP2C9 (minor route) cytochrome P450 isoforms. Therefore, inhibitors of these isoenzymes may reduce sildenafil clearance).
No products indexed under this heading.

Miconazole (Sildenafil metabolism is principally mediated by the CYP3A4 (major route) and CYP2C9 (minor route) cytochrome P450 isoforms. Therefore, inhibitors of these isoenzymes may reduce sildenafil clearance).
No products indexed under this heading.

Miconazole Nitrate (Sildenafil metabolism is principally mediated by the CYP3A4 (major route) and CYP2C9 (minor route) cytochrome P450 isoforms. Therefore, inhibitors of these isoenzymes may reduce sildenafil clearance). Products include:
Desenex ... 635
Desenex Jock Itch Spray Powder ... 635

Modafinil (Sildenafil metabolism is principally mediated by the CYP3A4 (major route) and CYP2C9 (minor route) cytochrome P450 isoforms. Therefore, inhibitors of these isoenzymes may reduce sildenafil clearance). Products include:
Provigil Tablets ... **988**

Nefazodone Hydrochloride (Sildenafil metabolism is principally mediated by the CYP3A4 (major route) and CYP2C9 (minor route) cytochrome P450 isoforms. Therefore, inhibitors of these isoenzymes may reduce sildenafil clearance).
No products indexed under this heading.

Nelfinavir Mesylate (Sildenafil metabolism is principally mediated by the CYP3A4 (major route) and CYP2C9 (minor route) cytochrome P450 isoforms. Therefore, inhibitors of these isoenzymes may reduce sildenafil clearance). Products include:
Viracept ... **2577**

Nevirapine (Sildenafil metabolism is principally mediated by the CYP3A4 (major route) and CYP2C9 (minor route) cytochrome P450 isoforms. Therefore, inducers of these isoenzymes may increase sildenafil clearance). Products include:
Viramune Oral Suspension ... **873**
Viramune Tablets ... **873**

Niacinamide (Sildenafil metabolism is principally mediated by the CYP3A4 (major route) and CYP2C9 (minor route) cytochrome P450 isoforms. Therefore, inhibitors of these isoenzymes may reduce sildenafil clearance).
No products indexed under this heading.

Nicotinamide (Sildenafil metabolism is principally mediated by the CYP3A4 (major route) and CYP2C9 (minor route) cytochrome P450 isoforms. Therefore, inhibitors of these isoenzymes may reduce sildenafil clearance). Products include:
Nicomide Tablets ... **1088**

Nifedipine (Sildenafil metabolism is principally mediated by the CYP3A4 (major route) and CYP2C9 (minor route) cytochrome P450 isoforms. Therefore, inhibitors of these isoenzymes may reduce sildenafil clearance). Products include:
Adalat CC Tablets ... **2964**

Nitroglycerin (Consistent with its known effect on the nitric oxide/cGMP pathway, sildenafil was shown to potentiate the hypotensive effects of nitrates, and its administration to patients who are using organic nitrates, either regularly and/or intermittently, in any form is therefore contraindicated). Products include:
Nitro-Dur Transdermal Infusion System ... **3046**
Nitrolingual Pumpspray ... **3120**

Norfloxacin (Sildenafil metabolism is principally mediated by the CYP3A4 (major route) and CYP2C9 (minor route) cytochrome P450 isoforms. Therefore, inhibitors of these isoenzymes may reduce sildenafil clearance). Products include:
Noroxin Tablets ... **2032**

Omeprazole (Sildenafil metabolism is principally mediated by the CYP3A4 (major route) and CYP2C9 (minor route) cytochrome P450 isoforms. Therefore, inhibitors of these isoenzymes may reduce sildenafil clearance). Products include:
Zegerid Capsules ... **2958**
Zegerid Powder for Oral Solution ... **2958**

Oxcarbazepine (Sildenafil metabolism is principally mediated by the CYP3A4 (major route) and CYP2C9 (minor route) cytochrome P450 isoforms. Therefore, inducers of these isoenzymes may increase sildenafil clearance). Products include:
Trileptal Tablets ... **2300**
Trileptal Oral Suspension ... **2300**

Oxiconazole Nitrate (Sildenafil metabolism is principally mediated by the CYP3A4 (major route) and CYP2C9 (minor route) cytochrome P450 isoforms. Therefore, inhibitors of these isoenzymes may reduce sildenafil clearance). Products include:
Oxistat ... **2667**

Paroxetine Hydrochloride (Sildenafil metabolism is principally mediated by the CYP3A4 (major route) and CYP2C9 (minor route) cytochrome P450 isoforms. Therefore, inhibitors of these isoenzymes may reduce sildenafil clearance). Products include:
Paxil CR Controlled-Release Tablets ... **1538**
Paxil ... **1530**

Pentaerythritol Tetranitrate (Consistent with its known effect on the nitric oxide/cGMP pathway, sildenafil was shown to potentiate the hypotensive effects of nitrates, and its administration to patients who are using organic nitrates, either regularly and/or intermittently, in any form is therefore contraindicated).
No products indexed under this heading.

Phenobarbital (Sildenafil metabolism is principally mediated by the CYP3A4 (major route) and CYP2C9 (minor route) cytochrome P450 isoforms. Therefore, inducers of these isoenzymes may increase sildenafil clearance). Products include:
Donnatal Extentabs ... **2493**

Phenobarbital Sodium (Sildenafil metabolism is principally mediated by the CYP3A4 (major route) and CYP2C9 (minor route) cytochrome P450 isoforms. Therefore, inducers of these isoenzymes may increase sildenafil clearance).
No products indexed under this heading.

Phenylbutazone (Sildenafil metabolism is principally mediated by the CYP3A4 (major route) and CYP2C9 (minor route) cytochrome P450 isoforms. Therefore, inhibitors of these isoenzymes may reduce sildenafil clearance).
No products indexed under this heading.

Phenytoin (Sildenafil metabolism is principally mediated by the CYP3A4 (major route) and CYP2C9 (minor route) cytochrome P450 isoforms. Therefore, inducers of these isoenzymes may increase sildenafil clearance).
No products indexed under this heading.

Phenytoin Sodium (Sildenafil metabolism is principally mediated by the CYP3A4 (major route) and CYP2C9 (minor route) cytochrome P450 isoforms. Therefore, inducers of these isoenzymes may increase sildenafil clearance). Products include:
Phenytek Capsules ... **2160**

Polythiazide (Sildenafil metabolism is principally mediated by the CYP3A4 (major route) and CYP2C9 (minor route) cytochrome P450 isoforms. Therefore, inhibitors of these isoenzymes may reduce sildenafil clearance).
No products indexed under this heading.

Prednisolone Acetate (Sildenafil metabolism is principally mediated by the CYP3A4 (major route) and CYP2C9 (minor route) cytochrome P450 isoforms. Therefore, inducers of these isoenzymes may increase sildenafil clearance). Products include:
Blephamide Ophthalmic Ointment ... **568**
Blephamide Ophthalmic Suspension ... **569**
Poly-Pred Ophthalmic Suspension ... ⊙ **233**
Pred Forte Ophthalmic Suspension ... ⊙ **235**
Pred Mild Ophthalmic Suspension ... ⊙ **238**
Pred-G Ophthalmic Ointment ... ⊙ **237**
Pred-G Ophthalmic Suspension ... ⊙ **236**

Prednisolone Sodium Phosphate (Sildenafil metabolism is principally mediated by the CYP3A4 (major route) and CYP2C9 (minor route) cytochrome P450 isoforms. Therefore, inducers of these isoenzymes may increase sildenafil clearance).
No products indexed under this heading.

Prednisolone Tebutate (Sildenafil metabolism is principally mediated by the CYP3A4 (major route) and CYP2C9 (minor route) cytochrome P450 isoforms. Therefore, inducers of these isoenzymes may increase sildenafil clearance).
No products indexed under this heading.

Prednisone (Sildenafil metabolism is principally mediated by the CYP3A4 (major route) and CYP2C9 (minor route) cytochrome P450 isoforms. Therefore, inducers of these isoenzymes may increase sildenafil clearance).
 No products indexed under this heading.

Primidone (Sildenafil metabolism is principally mediated by the CYP3A4 (major route) and CYP2C9 (minor route) cytochrome P450 isoforms. Therefore, inducers of these isoenzymes may increase sildenafil clearance).
 No products indexed under this heading.

Propoxyphene Hydrochloride (Sildenafil metabolism is principally mediated by the CYP3A4 (major route) and CYP2C9 (minor route) cytochrome P450 isoforms. Therefore, inhibitors of these isoenzymes may reduce sildenafil clearance).
 No products indexed under this heading.

Propoxyphene Napsylate (Sildenafil metabolism is principally mediated by the CYP3A4 (major route) and CYP2C9 (minor route) cytochrome P450 isoforms. Therefore, inhibitors of these isoenzymes may reduce sildenafil clearance).
 No products indexed under this heading.

Quinidine (Sildenafil metabolism is principally mediated by the CYP3A4 (major route) and CYP2C9 (minor route) cytochrome P450 isoforms. Therefore, inhibitors of these isoenzymes may reduce sildenafil clearance).
 No products indexed under this heading.

Quinidine Hydrochloride (Sildenafil metabolism is principally mediated by the CYP3A4 (major route) and CYP2C9 (minor route) cytochrome P450 isoforms. Therefore, inhibitors of these isoenzymes may reduce sildenafil clearance).
 No products indexed under this heading.

Quinidine Polygalacturonate (Sildenafil metabolism is principally mediated by the CYP3A4 (major route) and CYP2C9 (minor route) cytochrome P450 isoforms. Therefore, inhibitors of these isoenzymes may reduce sildenafil clearance).
 No products indexed under this heading.

Quinidine Sulfate (Sildenafil metabolism is principally mediated by the CYP3A4 (major route) and CYP2C9 (minor route) cytochrome P450 isoforms. Therefore, inhibitors of these isoenzymes may reduce sildenafil clearance).
 No products indexed under this heading.

Quinine (Sildenafil metabolism is principally mediated by the CYP3A4 (major route) and CYP2C9 (minor route) cytochrome P450 isoforms. Therefore, inhibitors of these isoenzymes may reduce sildenafil clearance).
 No products indexed under this heading.

Quinine Sulfate (Sildenafil metabolism is principally mediated by the CYP3A4 (major route) and CYP2C9 (minor route) cytochrome P450 isoforms. Therefore, inhibitors of these isoenzymes may reduce sildenafil clearance).
 No products indexed under this heading.

Quinupristin (Sildenafil metabolism is principally mediated by the CYP3A4 (major route) and CYP2C9 (minor route) cytochrome P450 isoforms. Therefore, inhibitors of these isoenzymes may reduce sildenafil clearance).
 No products indexed under this heading.

Ranitidine Bismuth Citrate (Sildenafil metabolism is principally mediated by the CYP3A4 (major route) and CYP2C9 (minor route) cytochrome P450 isoforms. Therefore, inhibitors of these isoenzymes may reduce sildenafil clearance).
 No products indexed under this heading.

Ranitidine Hydrochloride (Sildenafil metabolism is principally mediated by the CYP3A4 (major route) and CYP2C9 (minor route) cytochrome P450 isoforms. Therefore, inhibitors of these isoenzymes may reduce sildenafil clearance).
Products include:

Zantac ... 1624
Zantac Injection 1619
Zantac Injection Pharmacy Bulk
 Package 1622

Rifabutin (Sildenafil metabolism is principally mediated by the CYP3A4 (major route) and CYP2C9 (minor route) cytochrome P450 isoforms. Therefore, inducers of these isoenzymes may increase sildenafil clearance).
 No products indexed under this heading.

Rifampicin (Sildenafil metabolism is principally mediated by the CYP3A4 (major route) and CYP2C9 (minor route) cytochrome P450 isoforms. Therefore, inducers of these isoenzymes may increase sildenafil clearance).
 No products indexed under this heading.

Rifampin (Sildenafil metabolism is principally mediated by the CYP3A4 (major route) and CYP2C9 (minor route) cytochrome P450 isoforms. Therefore, inducers of these isoenzymes may increase sildenafil clearance).
 No products indexed under this heading.

Rifapentine (Sildenafil metabolism is principally mediated by the CYP3A4 (major route) and CYP2C9 (minor route) cytochrome P450 isoforms. Therefore, inducers of these isoenzymes may increase sildenafil clearance).
 No products indexed under this heading.

Ritonavir (In a study in healthy volunteers, co-administration of the HIV protease inhibitor ritonavir, a potent CYP3A4 inhibitor, at steady state (500 mg b.i.d.) with sildenafil (100 mg single dose) resulted in a 300% (4-fold) increase in sildenafil Cmax and a 1000% (11-fold) increase in sildenafil plasma AUC. At 24 hours, the plasma levels of sildenafil were still approximately 200 ng/mL, compared to approxi-

mately 5 ng/mL when sildenafil was dosed alone. This is consistent with ritonavir's marked effects on a broad range of P450 substrates). Products include:

Kaletra ... 476
Norvir ... 503

Saquinavir (In a study performed in healthy volunteers, co-administration of the HIV protease inhibitor saquinavier, a CYP3A4 inhibitor, at steady state (1200 mg t.i.d.) with sildenafil (100 mg single dose) resulted in a 140% increase in sildenafil Cmax and a 210% increase in sildenafil AUC).
 No products indexed under this heading.

Saquinavir Mesylate (Sildenafil metabolism is principally mediated by the CYP3A4 (major route) and CYP2C9 (minor route) cytochrome P450 isoforms. Therefore, inhibitors of these isoenzymes may reduce sildenafil clearance). Products include:

Invirase ... 2772

Secobarbital Sodium (Sildenafil metabolism is principally mediated by the CYP3A4 (major route) and CYP2C9 (minor route) cytochrome P450 isoforms. Therefore, inducers of these isoenzymes may increase sildenafil clearance).
 No products indexed under this heading.

Sertraline Hydrochloride (Sildenafil metabolism is principally mediated by the CYP3A4 (major route) and CYP2C9 (minor route) cytochrome P450 isoforms. Therefore, inhibitors of these isoenzymes may reduce sildenafil clearance). Products include:

Zoloft .. 2586

Sulfacytine (Sildenafil metabolism is principally mediated by the CYP3A4 (major route) and CYP2C9 (minor route) cytochrome P450 isoforms. Therefore, inhibitors of these isoenzymes may reduce sildenafil clearance).
 No products indexed under this heading.

Sulfamethizole (Sildenafil metabolism is principally mediated by the CYP3A4 (major route) and CYP2C9 (minor route) cytochrome P450 isoforms. Therefore, inhibitors of these isoenzymes may reduce sildenafil clearance).
 No products indexed under this heading.

Sulfamethoxazole (Sildenafil metabolism is principally mediated by the CYP3A4 (major route) and CYP2C9 (minor route) cytochrome P450 isoforms. Therefore, inhibitors of these isoenzymes may reduce sildenafil clearance).
 No products indexed under this heading.

Sulfasalazine (Sildenafil metabolism is principally mediated by the CYP3A4 (major route) and CYP2C9 (minor route) cytochrome P450 isoforms. Therefore, inhibitors of these isoenzymes may reduce sildenafil clearance).
 No products indexed under this heading.

Sulfinpyrazone (Sildenafil metabolism is principally mediated by the CYP3A4 (major route) and CYP2C9 (minor route) cytochrome P450 isoforms. Therefore, inhibitors of these isoenzymes may reduce sildenafil clearance).
 No products indexed under this heading.

Sulfisoxazole Acetyl (Sildenafil metabolism is principally mediated by the CYP3A4 (major route) and CYP2C9 (minor route) cytochrome P450 isoforms. Therefore, inhibitors of these isoenzymes may reduce sildenafil clearance).
 No products indexed under this heading.

Sulfisoxazole Diolamine (Sildenafil metabolism is principally mediated by the CYP3A4 (major route) and CYP2C9 (minor route) cytochrome P450 isoforms. Therefore, inhibitors of these isoenzymes may reduce sildenafil clearance).
 No products indexed under this heading.

Telithromycin (Sildenafil metabolism is principally mediated by the CYP3A4 (major route) and CYP2C9 (minor route) cytochrome P450 isoforms. Therefore, inhibitors of these isoenzymes may reduce sildenafil clearance). Products include:

Ketek Tablets 2903

Terconazole (Sildenafil metabolism is principally mediated by the CYP3A4 (major route) and CYP2C9 (minor route) cytochrome P450 isoforms. Therefore, inhibitors of these isoenzymes may reduce sildenafil clearance).
 No products indexed under this heading.

Theophylline (Sildenafil metabolism is principally mediated by the CYP3A4 (major route) and CYP2C9 (minor route) cytochrome P450 isoforms. Therefore, inducers of these isoenzymes may increase sildenafil clearance).
 No products indexed under this heading.

Ticlopidine Hydrochloride (Sildenafil metabolism is principally mediated by the CYP3A4 (major route) and CYP2C9 (minor route) cytochrome P450 isoforms. Therefore, inhibitors of these isoenzymes may reduce sildenafil clearance). Products include:

Ticlid Tablets 2810

Tolazamide (Sildenafil metabolism is principally mediated by the CYP3A4 (major route) and CYP2C9 (minor route) cytochrome P450 isoforms. Therefore, inhibitors of these isoenzymes may reduce sildenafil clearance).
 No products indexed under this heading.

Tolbutamide (Sildenafil metabolism is principally mediated by the CYP3A4 (major route) and CYP2C9 (minor route) cytochrome P450 isoforms. Therefore, inhibitors of these isoenzymes may reduce sildenafil clearance).
 No products indexed under this heading.

Tolbutamide Sodium (Sildenafil metabolism is principally mediated by the CYP3A4 (major route) and CYP2C9 (minor route) cytochrome P450 isoforms. Therefore, inhibitors of these isoenzymes may reduce sildenafil clearance).

No products indexed under this heading.

Triamcinolone (Sildenafil metabolism is principally mediated by the CYP3A4 (major route) and CYP2C9 (minor route) cytochrome P450 isoforms. Therefore, inducers of these isoenzymes may increase sildenafil clearance).

No products indexed under this heading.

Triamcinolone Acetonide (Sildenafil metabolism is principally mediated by the CYP3A4 (major route) and CYP2C9 (minor route) cytochrome P450 isoforms. Therefore, inducers of these isoenzymes may increase sildenafil clearance). Products include:

Triamcinolone Diacetate (Sildenafil metabolism is principally mediated by the CYP3A4 (major route) and CYP2C9 (minor route) cytochrome P450 isoforms. Therefore, inducers of these isoenzymes may increase sildenafil clearance).

No products indexed under this heading.

Triamcinolone Hexacetonide (Sildenafil metabolism is principally mediated by the CYP3A4 (major route) and CYP2C9 (minor route) cytochrome P450 isoforms. Therefore, inducers of these isoenzymes may increase sildenafil clearance).

No products indexed under this heading.

Troglitazone (Sildenafil metabolism is principally mediated by the CYP3A4 (major route) and CYP2C9 (minor route) cytochrome P450 isoforms. Therefore, inhibitors of these isoenzymes may reduce sildenafil clearance).

No products indexed under this heading.

Troleandomycin (Sildenafil metabolism is principally mediated by the CYP3A4 (major route) and CYP2C9 (minor route) cytochrome P450 isoforms. Therefore, inhibitors of these isoenzymes may reduce sildenafil clearance).

No products indexed under this heading.

Valproate Sodium (Sildenafil metabolism is principally mediated by the CYP3A4 (major route) and CYP2C9 (minor route) cytochrome P450 isoforms. Therefore, inhibitors of these isoenzymes may reduce sildenafil clearance). Products include:

Verapamil Hydrochloride (Sildenafil metabolism is principally mediated by the CYP3A4 (major route) and CYP2C9 (minor route) cytochrome P450 isoforms. Therefore, inhibitors of these isoenzymes may reduce sildenafil clearance). Products include:

Voriconazole (Sildenafil metabolism is principally mediated by the CYP3A4 (major route) and CYP2C9 (minor route) cytochrome P450 isoforms. Therefore, inhibitors of these isoenzymes may reduce sildenafil clearance). Products include:

Warfarin Sodium (In pulmonary arterial hypertension (PAH) patients, the concomitant use of vitamin K antagonists and sildenafil resulted in a greater incidence of reports of bleeding (primarily epistaxis) versus placebo). Products include:

Zafirlukast (Sildenafil metabolism is principally mediated by the CYP3A4 (major route) and CYP2C9 (minor route) cytochrome P450 isoforms. Therefore, inhibitors of these isoenzymes may reduce sildenafil clearance). Products include:

Zileuton (Sildenafil metabolism is principally mediated by the CYP3A4 (major route) and CYP2C9 (minor route) cytochrome P450 isoforms. Therefore, inhibitors of these isoenzymes may reduce sildenafil clearance). Products include:

Food Interactions

Grapefruit (Sildenafil metabolism is principally mediated by the CYP3A4 (major route) and CYP2C9 (minor route) cytochrome P450 isoforms. Therefore, inhibitors of these isoenzymes may reduce sildenafil clearance).

Grapefruit Juice (Sildenafil metabolism is principally mediated by the CYP3A4 (major route) and CYP2C9 (minor route) cytochrome P450 isoforms. Therefore, inhibitors of these isoenzymes may reduce sildenafil clearance).

REVLIMID CAPSULES

None cited in PDR database.

REYATAZ CAPSULES

May interact with antacids, cytochrome p450 1a2 substrates (selected), cytochrome p450 2c9 substrates (selected), cytochrome p450 3a inducers (selected), cytochrome p450 3a inhibitors (selected), ergot-containing drugs, histamine H2-receptor antagonists, immunosuppressive agents, oral contraceptives, protease inhibitors, proton pump inhibitor, and certain other agents. Compounds in these categories include:

Acarbose (Atazanavir sulfate competitively inhibits CYP1A2 and CYP2C9. There is a potential drug-drug interaction between atazanavir sulfate and CYP1A2 or CYP2C9 substrates). Products include:

Acetaminophen (Atazanavir sulfate competitively inhibits CYP1A2 and CYP2C9. There is a potential drug-drug interaction between atazanavir sulfate and CYP1A2 or CYP2C9 substrates). Products include:

Alatrofloxacin Mesylate (Atazanavir sulfate competitively inhibits CYP1A2 and CYP2C9. There is a potential drug-drug interaction between atazanavir sulfate and CYP1A2 or CYP2C9 substrates).

No products indexed under this heading.

Allium sativum (Drugs that induce CYP3A activity may increase the clearance of atazanavir sulfate, resulting in lowered plasma concentrations).
No products indexed under this heading.

Aluminum Carbonate (Reduced plasma concentrations of atazanavir are expected if antacids, including buffered medications, are administered with atazanavir sulfate. Atazanavir sulfate should be administered 2 hours before or 1 hour after these medications).
No products indexed under this heading.

Aluminum Hydroxide (Reduced plasma concentrations of atazanavir are expected if antacids, including buffered medications, are administered with atazanavir sulfate. Atazanavir sulfate should be administered 2 hours before or 1 hour after these medications). Products include:
- Gaviscon Regular Strength Liquid .. ▣658
- Gaviscon Regular Strength Tablets .... ▣658
- Gaviscon Extra Strength Liquid ...... ▣658
- Gaviscon Extra Strength Tablets .... ▣658
- Maalox Regular Strength Antacid/Antigas Liquid 2175
- Maalox Max Maximum Strength Antacid/Anti-Gas Liquid 2176

Amiodarone Hydrochloride (Co-administration with atazanavir sulfate has the potential to produce serious and/or life-threatening adverse events and has not been studied. Caution is warranted and therapeutic concentration monitoring of these drugs is recommended if they are used concomitantly with atazanavir sulfate.).
No products indexed under this heading.

Amitriptyline Hydrochloride (Atazanavir sulfate competitively inhibits CYP1A2 and CYP2C9. There is a potential drug-drug interaction between atazanavir sulfate and CYP1A2 or CYP2C9 substrates).
No products indexed under this heading.

Amoxapine (Atazanavir sulfate competitively inhibits CYP1A2 and CYP2C9. There is a potential drug-drug interaction between atazanavir sulfate and CYP1A2 or CYP2C9 substrates).
No products indexed under this heading.

Amprenavir (Co- administration of atazanavir sulfate/ritonavir and other protease inhibitors would be expected to increase exposure to the other protease inhibitors; co-administration is not recommended). Products include:
- Agenerase Capsules 1327
- Agenerase Oral Solution 1332

Anagrelide Hydrochloride (Atazanavir sulfate competitively inhibits CYP1A2 and CYP2C9. There is a potential drug-drug interaction between atazanavir sulfate and CYP1A2 or CYP2C9 substrates). Products include:
- Agrylin Capsules 3169

Aprepitant (Drugs that induce CYP3A activity may increase the clearance of atazanavir sulfate, resulting in lowered plasma concentrations). Products include:
- Emend Capsules 1963

Atorvastatin Calcium (The risk of myopathy, including rhabdomyolysis, may be increased when protease inhibitors, including atazanavir sulfate, are used in combination with atorvastatin. Caution should be exercised). Products include:
- Caduet Tablets 2508
- Lipitor Tablets 2483

Azathioprine (Therapeutic concentration monitoring is recommended for immunosuppressant agents when co-administered with atazanavir sulfate).
No products indexed under this heading.

Basiliximab (Therapeutic concentration monitoring is recommended for immunosuppressant agents when co-administered with atazanavir sulfate). Products include:
- Simulect for Injection 2284

Bepridil Hydrochloride (Co-administration with atazanavir sulfate has the potential to produce serious and/or life-threatening adverse events and has not been studied. Caution is warranted and therapeutic concentration monitoring of these drugs is recommended if they are used concomitantly with atazanavir sulfate).
No products indexed under this heading.

Caffeine (Atazanavir sulfate competitively inhibits CYP1A2 and CYP2C9. There is a potential drug-drug interaction between atazanavir sulfate and CYP1A2 or CYP2C9 substrates). Products include:
- BC Headache Powder .... ▣677
- Arthritis Strength BC Powder .... ▣677
- Excedrin Extra Strength Caplets/Tablets/Geltabs .... ▣684
- Excedrin Migraine Caplets/Tablets/Geltabs .... ▣609
- Excedrin Tension Headache Caplets/Tablets/Geltabs .... ▣611
- Goody's Extra Strength Headache Powders .... ▣611
- Goody's Extra Strength Pain Relief Tablets .... ▣685
- Vivarin .... ▣602
- Winrgy Dietary Supplement .... ▣823

Caffeine Anhydrous (Atazanavir sulfate competitively inhibits CYP1A2 and CYP2C9. There is a potential drug-drug interaction between atazanavir sulfate and CYP1A2 or CYP2C9 substrates).
No products indexed under this heading.

Candesartan Cilexetil (Atazanavir sulfate competitively inhibits CYP1A2 and CYP2C9. There is a potential drug-drug interaction between atazanavir sulfate and CYP1A2 or CYP2C9 substrates). Products include:
- Atacand Tablets 649
- Atacand HCT 651

Carbamazepine (Drugs that induce CYP3A activity may increase the clearance of atazanavir sulfate, resulting in lowered plasma concentrations). Products include:
- Carbatrol Capsules 3171
- Equetro Extended-Release Capsules 3180
- Tegretol/Tegretol-XR 2295

Carvedilol (Atazanavir sulfate competitively inhibits CYP1A2 and CYP2C9. There is a potential drug-drug interaction between atazanavir sulfate and CYP1A2 or CYP2C9 substrates). Products include:
- Coreg Tablets 1414

Celecoxib (Atazanavir sulfate competitively inhibits CYP1A2 and CYP2C9. There is a potential drug-drug interaction between atazanavir sulfate and CYP1A2 or CYP2C9 substrates). Products include:
- Celebrex Capsules 3134

Chlordiazepoxide (Atazanavir sulfate competitively inhibits CYP1A2 and CYP2C9. There is a potential drug-drug interaction between atazanavir sulfate and CYP1A2 or CYP2C9 substrates).
No products indexed under this heading.

Chlordiazepoxide Hydrochloride (Atazanavir sulfate competitively inhibits CYP1A2 and CYP2C9. There is a potential drug-drug interaction between atazanavir sulfate and CYP1A2 or CYP2C9 substrates). Products include:
- Librium Capsules 3347

Chlorpropamide (Atazanavir sulfate competitively inhibits CYP1A2 and CYP2C9. There is a potential drug-drug interaction between atazanavir sulfate and CYP1A2 or CYP2C9 substrates).
No products indexed under this heading.

Cimetidine (Reduced plasma concentrations of atazanavir are expected if H2-receptor antagonists are administered with atazanavir sulfate. This may result in loss of therapeutic effect and development of resistance. To lessen the effect of H2-receptor antagonists on atazanavir exposure, it is recommended that an H2-receptor antagonist and atazanavir sulfate be administered as far apart as possible, preferably 12 hours apart). Products include:
- Tagamet HB 200 Tablets .... ▣664

Cimetidine Hydrochloride (Reduced plasma concentrations of atazanavir are expected if H2-receptor antagonists are administered with atazanavir sulfate. This may result in loss of therapeutic effect and development of resistance. To lessen the effect of H2-receptor antagonists on atazanavir exposure, it is recommended that an H2-receptor antagonist and atazanavir sulfate be administered as far apart as possible, preferably 12 hours apart).
No products indexed under this heading.

Ciprofloxacin (Atazanavir sulfate competitively inhibits CYP1A2 and CYP2C9. There is a potential drug-drug interaction between atazanavir sulfate and CYP1A2 or CYP2C9 substrates). Products include:
- Cipro Oral Suspension 2977
- Cipro I.V. 2984
- Cipro XR Tablets 2990
- Ciprodex Otic Suspension 559

Ciprofloxacin Hydrochloride (Atazanavir sulfate competitively inhibits CYP1A2 and CYP2C9. There is a potential drug-drug interaction between atazanavir sulfate and CYP1A2 or CYP2C9 substrates). Products include:
- Ciloxan Ophthalmic Ointment 559
- Ciloxan Ophthalmic Solution .... ⊙206
- Cipro Tablets 2977
- Proquin XR Tablets 1153

Cisapride (Contraindicated due to potential for serious and/or life-threatening reactions such as cardiac arrhythmias).
No products indexed under this heading.

Clarithromycin (Increased concentrations of clarithromycin may cause QTc prolongations; therefore, a dose reduction of clarithromycin by 50% should be considered when it is co-administered with atazanavir sulfate. In addition, concentrations of the active metabolite 14-OH clarithromycin are significantly reduced; consider alternative therapy for indications other than infections due to Mycobacterium Avium Complex). Products include:
- Biaxin/Biaxin XL 402
- PREVPAC 3284

Clomipramine Hydrochloride (Atazanavir sulfate competitively inhibits CYP1A2 and CYP2C9. There is a potential drug-drug interaction between atazanavir sulfate and CYP1A2 or CYP2C9 substrates).
No products indexed under this heading.

Clopidogrel Bisulfate (Atazanavir sulfate competitively inhibits CYP1A2 and CYP2C9. There is a potential drug-drug interaction between atazanavir sulfate and CYP1A2 or CYP2C9 substrates). Products include:
- Plavix Tablets 917
- Plavix Tablets 2926

Clozapine (Atazanavir sulfate competitively inhibits CYP1A2 and CYP2C9. There is a potential drug-drug interaction between atazanavir sulfate and CYP1A2 or CYP2C9 substrates). Products include:
- Clozaril Tablets 2184
- FazaClo Orally Disintegrating Tablets 551

Cyclobenzaprine (Atazanavir sulfate competitively inhibits CYP1A2 and CYP2C9. There is a potential drug-drug interaction between atazanavir sulfate and CYP1A2 or CYP2C9 substrates).
No products indexed under this heading.

Cyclobenzaprine Hydrochloride (Atazanavir sulfate competitively inhibits CYP1A2 and CYP2C9. There is a potential drug-drug interaction between atazanavir sulfate and CYP1A2 or CYP2C9 substrates).
No products indexed under this heading.

Cyclosporine (Therapeutic concentration monitoring is recommended for immunosuppressant agents when co-administered with atazanavir sulfate). Products include:
- Gengraf Capsules 459
- Neoral Oral Solution 2259
- Neoral Soft Gelatin Capsules 2259
- Restasis Ophthalmic Emulsion 575
- Sandimmune 2275

Delavirdine Mesylate (Co-administration of atazanavir sulfate and other drugs that inhibit CYP3A may increase atazanavir sulfate plasma concentrations). Products include:
- Rescriptor Tablets 2551

Desipramine Hydrochloride (Atazanavir sulfate competitively inhibits CYP1A2 and CYP2C9. There is a potential drug-drug interaction between atazanavir sulfate and CYP1A2 or CYP2C9 substrates).
No products indexed under this heading.

Desogestrel (Because contraceptive steriod concentrations may be altered when atazanavir sulfate or atazanavir sulfate/ritonavir is co-administered with oral contraceptives or with the contraceptive

patch, alternate methods of non-hormonal contraception are recommended). Products include:
Mircette Tablets 1066

Dexamethasone (Drugs that induce CYP3A activity may increase the clearance of atazanavir sulfate, resulting in lowered plasma concentrations). Products include:
Ciprodex Otic Suspension 559
Decadron Tablets 1951
TobraDex Ophthalmic Ointment 562
TobraDex Ophthalmic Suspension ... 563

Dextromethorphan (Atazanavir sulfate competitively inhibits CYP1A2 and CYP2C9. There is a potential drug-drug interaction between atazanavir sulfate and CYP1A2 or CYP2C9 substrates).
No products indexed under this heading.

Diazepam (Atazanavir sulfate competitively inhibits CYP1A2 and CYP2C9. There is a potential drug-drug interaction between atazanavir sulfate and CYP1A2 or CYP2C9 substrates). Products include:
Diastat Rectal Delivery System 3343
Valium Tablets 2819

Diclofenac Potassium (Atazanavir sulfate competitively inhibits CYP1A2 and CYP2C9. There is a potential drug-drug interaction between atazanavir sulfate and CYP1A2 or CYP2C9 substrates).
No products indexed under this heading.

Diclofenac Sodium (Atazanavir sulfate competitively inhibits CYP1A2 and CYP2C9. There is a potential drug-drug interaction between atazanavir sulfate and CYP1A2 or CYP2C9 substrates). Products include:
Arthrotec Tablets 3129
Voltaren Ophthalmic Solution 2309
Voltaren Tablets 2307
Voltaren-XR Tablets 2310

Didanosine (Presumably due to the increase in gastric pH caused by buffers in the didanosine buffered tablets, exposure to atazanavir sulfate was markedly decreased. Atazanavir sulfate should be given 2 hours before or 1 hour after didanosine buffered formulations. Didanosine EC capsules and atazanavir should also be given at different times).
No products indexed under this heading.

Dihydroergotamine Mesylate (Contraindicated due to potential for serious and/or life-threatening events such as acute ergot toxicity characterized by peripheral vasospasm and ischemia of the extremities and other tissues). Products include:
Migranal Nasal Spray 3348

Diltiazem Hydrochloride (Concomitant administration may lead to increased levels of diltiazem and desacetyl-diltiazem; therefore, caution is warranted and dose reduction of diltiazem by 50% should be considered. ECG monitoring is also recommended). Products include:
Cardizem LA Extended Release Tablets 1728
Tiazac Capsules 1201

Diltiazem Maleate (Atazanavir sulfate competitively inhibits CYP1A2 and CYP2C9. There is a potential drug-drug interaction between atazanavir sulfate and CYP1A2 or CYP2C9 substrates).
No products indexed under this heading.

Doxepin Hydrochloride (Atazanavir sulfate competitively inhibits CYP1A2 and CYP2C9. There is a potential drug-drug interaction between atazanavir sulfate and CYP1A2 or CYP2C9 substrates).
No products indexed under this heading.

Dronabinol (Atazanavir sulfate competitively inhibits CYP1A2 and CYP2C9. There is a potential drug-drug interaction between atazanavir sulfate and CYP1A2 or CYP2C9 substrates). Products include:
Marinol Capsules 3333

Efavirenz (If atazanavir sulfate is to be co-administered with efavirenz, which decreases atazanavir exposure, it is recommended that atazanavir sulfate 300mg with ritonavir 100mg be co-administered with efavirenz 600mg, as this combination results in atazanavir exposure that approximates the mean exposure to atazanavir produced by 400mg of atazanavir sulfate alone. Atazanavir sulfate without ritonavir should not be co-administered with efavirenz). Products include:
Atripla Tablets 945
Sustiva Capsules 930
Sustiva Tablets 930

Enoxacin (Atazanavir sulfate competitively inhibits CYP1A2 and CYP2C9. There is a potential drug-drug interaction between atazanavir sulfate and CYP1A2 or CYP2C9 substrates).
No products indexed under this heading.

Eprosartan Mesylate (Atazanavir sulfate competitively inhibits CYP1A2 and CYP2C9. There is a potential drug-drug interaction between atazanavir sulfate and CYP1A2 or CYP2C9 substrates). Products include:
Teveten Tablets 1735
Teveten HCT Tablets 1737

Ergonovine Maleate (Contraindicated due to potential for serious and/or life-threatening events such as acute ergot toxicity characterized by peripheral vasospasm and ischemia of the extremities and other tissues).
No products indexed under this heading.

Ergotamine Tartrate (Contraindicated due to potential for serious and/or life-threatening events such as acute ergot toxicity characterized by peripheral vasospasm and ischemia of the extremities and other tissues).
No products indexed under this heading.

Erythromycin (Atazanavir sulfate competitively inhibits CYP1A2 and CYP2C9. There is a potential drug-drug interaction between atazanavir sulfate and CYP1A2 or CYP2C9 substrates). Products include:
Ery-Tab Tablets 449
Erythromycin Base Filmtab Tablets 455
Erythromycin Delayed-Release Capsules, USP 457
PCE Dispertab Tablets 515

Erythromycin Estolate (Atazanavir sulfate competitively inhibits CYP1A2 and CYP2C9. There is a potential drug-drug interaction between atazanavir sulfate and CYP1A2 or CYP2C9 substrates).
No products indexed under this heading.

Erythromycin Ethylsuccinate (Atazanavir sulfate competitively inhibits CYP1A2 and CYP2C9. There is a potential drug-drug interaction between atazanavir sulfate and CYP1A2 or CYP2C9 substrates). Products include:
E.E.S. 451
EryPed 447

Erythromycin Gluceptate (Atazanavir sulfate competitively inhibits CYP1A2 and CYP2C9. There is a potential drug-drug interaction between atazanavir sulfate and CYP1A2 or CYP2C9 substrates).
No products indexed under this heading.

Erythromycin Lactobionate (Atazanavir sulfate competitively inhibits CYP1A2 and CYP2C9. There is a potential drug-drug interaction between atazanavir sulfate and CYP1A2 or CYP2C9 substrates).
No products indexed under this heading.

Erythromycin Stearate (Atazanavir sulfate competitively inhibits CYP1A2 and CYP2C9. There is a potential drug-drug interaction between atazanavir sulfate and CYP1A2 or CYP2C9 substrates). Products include:
Erythrocin Stearate Filmtab Tablets 453

Esomeprazole Magnesium (Concomitant use of atazanavir sulfate and proton-pump inhibitors is not recommended. Co-administration of atazanavir sulfate with proton-pump inhibitors is expected to substantially decrease atazanavir sulfate plasma concentrations and reduce its therapeutic effect). Products include:
Nexium Delayed-Release Capsules 655

Estradiol (Atazanavir sulfate competitively inhibits CYP1A2 and CYP2C9. There is a potential drug-drug interaction between atazanavir sulfate and CYP1A2 or CYP2C9 substrates). Products include:
Angeliq Tablets 762
Climara Transdermal System 771
Climara Pro Transdermal System 776
Estrasorb Topical Emulsion 1147
Estring Vaginal Ring 2635
Menostar Transdermal System 782
Vagifem Tablets 2334

Estradiol Benzoate (Atazanavir sulfate competitively inhibits CYP1A2 and CYP2C9. There is a potential drug-drug interaction between atazanavir sulfate and CYP1A2 or CYP2C9 substrates).
No products indexed under this heading.

Estradiol Cypionate (Atazanavir sulfate competitively inhibits CYP1A2 and CYP2C9. There is a potential drug-drug interaction between atazanavir sulfate and CYP1A2 or CYP2C9 substrates).
No products indexed under this heading.

Ethinyl Estradiol (Because contraceptive steriod concentrations may be altered when atazanavir sulfate or atazanavir sulfate/ritonavir is co-administered with oral contraceptives or with the contraceptive patch, alternate methods of non-hormonal contraception are recommended). Products include:
Mircette Tablets 1066
NuvaRing 2340
Ortho-Cyclen/Ortho Tri-Cyclen 2429
Ortho Evra Transdermal System 2417
Ortho Tri-Cyclen Lo Tablets 2436
Seasonique Tablets 1077
Yasmin 28 Tablets 796
Yaz Tablets 803

Ethosuximide (Drugs that induce CYP3A activity may increase the clearance of atazanavir sulfate, resulting in lowered plasma concentrations).
No products indexed under this heading.

Ethynodiol Diacetate (Because contraceptive steriod concentrations may be altered when atazanavir sulfate or atazanavir sulfate/ritonavir is co-administered with oral contraceptives or with the contraceptive patch, alternate methods of non-hormonal contraception are recommended).
No products indexed under this heading.

Etodolac (Atazanavir sulfate competitively inhibits CYP1A2 and CYP2C9. There is a potential drug-drug interaction between atazanavir sulfate and CYP1A2 or CYP2C9 substrates).
No products indexed under this heading.

Famotidine (Reduced plasma concentrations of atazanavir are expected if H2-receptor antagonists are administered with atazanavir sulfate. This may result in loss of therapeutic effect and development of resistance. To lessen the effect of H2-receptor antagonists on atazanavir exposure, it is recommended that an H2-receptor antagonist and atazanavir sulfate be administered as far apart as possible, preferably 12 hours apart). Products include:
Pepcid Injection 2040
Pepcid 2038
Pepcid AC Gelcaps 1701
Pepcid AC Tablets 1701
Maximum Strength Pepcid AC Tablets 1701
Pepcid Complete Chewable Tablets 1701

Fenoprofen Calcium (Atazanavir sulfate competitively inhibits CYP1A2 and CYP2C9. There is a potential drug-drug interaction between atazanavir sulfate and CYP1A2 or CYP2C9 substrates). Products include:
Nalfon Capsules 2502

Fluconazole (Co-administration of atazanavir sulfate and other drugs that inhibit CYP3A may increase atazanavir sulfate plasma concentrations).
No products indexed under this heading.

Fluoxetine (Co-administration of atazanavir sulfate and other drugs that inhibit CYP3A may increase atazanavir sulfate plasma concentrations).
No products indexed under this heading.

Fluoxetine Hydrochloride (Atazanavir sulfate competitively inhibits CYP1A2 and CYP2C9. There is a potential drug-drug interaction between atazanavir sulfate and CYP1A2 or CYP2C9 substrates). Products include:
Prozac Pulvules and Liquid 1801
Symbyax Capsules 1819

Flurbiprofen (Atazanavir sulfate competitively inhibits CYP1A2 and CYP2C9. There is a potential drug-drug interaction between atazanavir sulfate and CYP1A2 or CYP2C9 substrates).
No products indexed under this heading.

Flurbiprofen Sodium (Atazanavir sulfate competitively inhibits CYP1A2 and CYP2C9. There is a potential drug-drug interaction between atazanavir sulfate and CYP1A2 or CYP2C9 substrates). Products include:
Ocufen Ophthalmic Solution .... ⊙232

Flutamide (Atazanavir sulfate competitively inhibits CYP1A2 and CYP2C9. There is a potential drug-drug interaction between atazanavir sulfate and CYP1A2 or CYP2C9 substrates). Products include:
Eulexin Capsules 3009

Fluticasone Propionate (A study has shown that ritonavir significantly increases plasma fluticasone propionate exposures, resulting in significantly decreased serum cortisol concentrations. Concomitant use of atazanavir with ritonavir and fluticasone propionate is expected to produce the same effects. Systemic corticosteroid effects, including Cushing's syndrome and adrenal suppression have been reported during postmarketing use in patients receiving ritonavir and inhaled or intranasally administered fluticasone propionate. Therefore, co-administration of fluticasone propionate and atazanavir/ritonavir is not recommended unless the potential benefit to the patient outweighs the risk of systemic corticosteroid side effects). Products include:
Advair Diskus 100/50 1308
Advair Diskus 250/50 1308
Advair Diskus 500/50 1308
Advair HFA Inhalation Aerosol 1318
Cutivate Cream 2662
Cutivate Lotion 0.05% 2664
Cutivate Ointment 2665
Flonase Nasal Spray 1440
Flovent Diskus 1443

Fluticasone Propionate HFA (A study has shown that ritonavir significantly increases plasma fluticasone propionate exposures, resulting in significantly decreased serum cortisol concentrations. Concomitant use of atazanavir with ritonavir and fluticasone propionate is expected to produce the same effects. Systemic corticosteroid effects, including Cushing's syndrome and adrenal suppression have been reported during postmarketing use in patients receiving ritonavir and inhaled or intranasally administered fluticasone propionate. Therefore, co-administration of fluticasone propionate and atazanavir/ritonavir is not recommended unless the potential benefit to the patient outweighs the risk of systemic corticosteroid side effects). Products include:
Flovent HFA 1447

Fluvastatin Sodium (Atazanavir sulfate competitively inhibits CYP1A2 and CYP2C9. There is a potential drug-drug interaction between atazanavir sulfate and CYP1A2 or CYP2C9 substrates). Products include:
Lescol Capsules 2233
Lescol XL Tablets 2233

Fluvoxamine Maleate (Atazanavir sulfate competitively inhibits CYP1A2 and CYP2C9. There is a potential drug-drug interaction between atazanavir sulfate and CYP1A2 or CYP2C9 substrates).
No products indexed under this heading.

Glimepiride (Atazanavir sulfate competitively inhibits CYP1A2 and CYP2C9. There is a potential drug-drug interaction between atazanavir sulfate and CYP1A2 or CYP2C9 substrates). Products include:
Avandaryl Tablets 1379
Duetact Tablets 3226

Glipizide (Atazanavir sulfate competitively inhibits CYP1A2 and CYP2C9. There is a potential drug-drug interaction between atazanavir sulfate and CYP1A2 or CYP2C9 substrates).
No products indexed under this heading.

Grepafloxacin Hydrochloride (Atazanavir sulfate competitively inhibits CYP1A2 and CYP2C9. There is a potential drug-drug interaction between atazanavir sulfate and CYP1A2 or CYP2C9 substrates).
No products indexed under this heading.

Haloperidol (Atazanavir sulfate competitively inhibits CYP1A2 and CYP2C9. There is a potential drug-drug interaction between atazanavir sulfate and CYP1A2 or CYP2C9 substrates).
No products indexed under this heading.

Haloperidol Decanoate (Atazanavir sulfate competitively inhibits CYP1A2 and CYP2C9. There is a potential drug-drug interaction between atazanavir sulfate and CYP1A2 or CYP2C9 substrates).
No products indexed under this heading.

Haloperidol Lactate (Atazanavir sulfate competitively inhibits CYP1A2 and CYP2C9. There is a potential drug-drug interaction between atazanavir sulfate and CYP1A2 or CYP2C9 substrates).
No products indexed under this heading.

Hypericum Perforatum (Concomitant use of atazanavir sulfate and St. John's Wort, or products containing St. John's Wort, is not recommended. Co-administration of protease inhibitors with St. John's Wort is expected to substantially decrease concentrations of the protease inhibitor and may result in suboptimal levels of atazanavir sulfate and lead to loss of virologic response and possible resistance to atazanavir sulfate or to the class of protease inhibitors).
No products indexed under this heading.

Ibuprofen (Atazanavir sulfate competitively inhibits CYP1A2 and CYP2C9. There is a potential drug-drug interaction between atazanavir sulfate and CYP1A2 or CYP2C9 substrates). Products include:
Advil Allergy Sinus Caplets .... ■770
Advil .... ■674
Children's Advil Oral Suspension .... ■603
Children's Advil Chewable Tablets .. ■603
Advil Cold & Sinus .... ■723
Infants' Advil Concentrated Drops .. ■604
Infants' Advil Concentrated Drops - White Grape (Dye-Free) .... ■604
Junior Strength Advil Swallow Tablets .... ■605
Advil Migraine Liquigels .... ■608
Advil Multi-Symptom Cold Caplets .... ■770
Advil PM Caplets .... ■615
Motrin IB Tablets and Caplets 1866
Children's Motrin Oral Suspension ... 1867
Children's Motrin Non-Staining Dye-Free Oral Suspension 1867
Children's Motrin Cold Oral Suspension 1867
Infants' Motrin Concentrated Drops 1867
Infants' Motrin Non-Staining Dye-Free Concentrated Drops 1867
Junior Strength Motrin Caplets and Chewable Tablets 1867
Vicoprofen Tablets 539

Imipramine Hydrochloride (Atazanavir sulfate competitively inhibits CYP1A2 and CYP2C9. There is a potential drug-drug interaction between atazanavir sulfate and CYP1A2 or CYP2C9 substrates).
No products indexed under this heading.

Imipramine Pamoate (Atazanavir sulfate competitively inhibits CYP1A2 and CYP2C9. There is a potential drug-drug interaction between atazanavir sulfate and CYP1A2 or CYP2C9 substrates).
No products indexed under this heading.

Indinavir Sulfate (Both atazanavir sulfate and indinavir are associated with indirect hyperbilirubinemia. Combinations of these drugs have not been studied and co-administration is not recommended). Products include:
Crixivan Capsules 1940

Indomethacin (Atazanavir sulfate competitively inhibits CYP1A2 and CYP2C9. There is a potential drug-drug interaction between atazanavir sulfate and CYP1A2 or CYP2C9 substrates). Products include:
Indocin 1995

Indomethacin Sodium Trihydrate (Atazanavir sulfate competitively inhibits CYP1A2 and CYP2C9. There is a potential drug-drug interaction between atazanavir sulfate and CYP1A2 or CYP2C9 substrates). Products include:
Indocin I.V. 2465

Irbesartan (Atazanavir sulfate competitively inhibits CYP1A2 and CYP2C9. There is a potential drug-drug interaction between atazanavir sulfate and CYP1A2 or CYP2C9 substrates). Products include:
Avalide Tablets 888
Avalide Tablets 2874
Avapro Tablets 891
Avapro Tablets 2871

Irinotecan Hydrochloride (Atazanavir inhibits UGT and may interfere with the metabolism of irinotecan, resulting in increased irinotecan toxicity). Products include:
Camptosar Injection 2604

Isoniazid (Co-administration of atazanavir sulfate and other drugs that inhibit CYP3A may increase atazanavir sulfate plasma concentrations).
No products indexed under this heading.

Itraconazole (Due to the effect of ritonavir on ketoconazole, high doses of ketoconazole and itraconazole (greater than 200 mg/day) should be used cautiously with atazanavir sulfate/ritonavir).
No products indexed under this heading.

Ketoconazole (Due to the effect of ritonavir on ketoconazole, high doses of ketoconazole and itraconazole (greater than 200 mg/day) should be used cautiously with atazanavir sulfate/ritonavir). Products include:
Nizoral A-D Shampoo, 1% 1868

Ketoprofen (Atazanavir sulfate competitively inhibits CYP1A2 and CYP2C9. There is a potential drug-drug interaction between atazanavir sulfate and CYP1A2 or CYP2C9 substrates).
No products indexed under this heading.

Ketorolac Tromethamine (Atazanavir sulfate competitively inhibits CYP1A2 and CYP2C9. There is a potential drug-drug interaction between atazanavir sulfate and CYP1A2 or CYP2C9 substrates). Products include:
Acular Ophthalmic Solution 565
Acular LS Ophthalmic Solution 566

Lansoprazole (Concomitant use of atazanavir sulfate and proton-pump inhibitors is not recommended. Co-administration of atazanavir sulfate with proton-pump inhibitors is expected to substantially decrease atazanavir sulfate plasma concentrations and reduce its therapeutic effect). Products include:
Prevacid Delayed-Release Capsules 3271
Prevacid for Delayed-Release Oral Suspension 3271
Prevacid SoluTab Delayed-Release Orally Disintegrating Tablets 3271
Prevacid I.V. for Injection 3277
Prevacid NapraPAC 3280
PREVPAC 3284

Levobupivacaine Hydrochloride (Atazanavir sulfate competitively inhibits CYP1A2 and CYP2C9. There is a potential drug-drug interaction between atazanavir sulfate and CYP1A2 or CYP2C9 substrates).
No products indexed under this heading.

Levonorgestrel (Because contraceptive steriod concentrations may be altered when atazanavir sulfate or atazanavir sulfate/ritonavir is co-administered with oral contraceptives or with the contraceptive patch, alternate methods of non-hormonal contraception are recommended). Products include:
Climara Pro Transdermal System 776
Mirena Intrauterine System 787
Plan B Tablets 1076
Seasonique Tablets 1077

Lidocaine (Co-administration with atazanavir sulfate has the potential to produce serious and/or life-threatening adverse events and has not been studied. Caution is warranted and therapeutic concentration monitoring of these drugs is recommended if they are used concomitantly with atazanavir sulfate). Products include:
Lidoderm Patch 1118
Synera Topical Patch 1137

Lidocaine Hydrochloride (Co-administration with atazanavir sulfate has the potential to produce serious and/or life-threatening adverse events and has not been studied. Caution is warranted and therapeutic concentration monitoring of these drugs is recommended if they are used concomitantly with atazanavir sulfate).
No products indexed under this heading.

Lomefloxacin Hydrochloride (Atazanavir sulfate competitively inhibits CYP1A2 and CYP2C9. There is a potential drug-drug interaction between atazanavir sulfate and CYP1A2 or CYP2C9 substrates).
No products indexed under this heading.

Lopinavir (Co- administration of atazanavir sulfate/ritonavir and other protease inhibitors would be expected to increase exposure to the other protease inhibitors; co-administration is not recommended). Products include:
Kaletra **476**

Losartan Potassium (Atazanavir sulfate competitively inhibits CYP1A2 and CYP2C9. There is a potential drug-drug interaction between atazanavir sulfate and CYP1A2 or CYP2C9 substrates). Products include:
Cozaar Tablets **1935**
Hyzaar 50-12.5 Tablets **1990**
Hyzaar 100-12.5 Tablets **1990**
Hyzaar 100-25 Tablets **1990**

Lovastatin (Concomitant use of atazanavir sulfate with lovastatin is not recommended. Caution should be exercised if HIV protease inhibitors, including atazanavir sulfate, are used concurrently with other HMG-CoA reductase inhibitors that are also metabolized by theCYP3A4 pathway. The risk of myopathy, including rhabdomyolysis, may be increased when HIV protease inhibitors, including atazanavir sulfate, are used in combination with these drugs). Products include:
Advicor Tablets **1722**
Altoprev Extended-Release Tablets **3109**
Mevacor Tablets **2021**

Magaldrate (Reduced plasma concentrations of atazanavir are expected if antacids, including buffered medications, are administered with atazanavir sulfate. Atazanavir sulfate should be administered 2 hours before or 1 hour after these medications).
No products indexed under this heading.

Magnesium Hydroxide (Reduced plasma concentrations of atazanavir are expected if antacids, including buffered medications, are administered with atazanavir sulfate. Atazanavir sulfate should be administered 2 hours before or 1 hour after these medications). Products include:
Maalox Regular Strength Antacid/Antigas Liquid **2175**
Maalox Max Maximum Strength Antacid/Anti-Gas Liquid **2176**
Pepcid Complete Chewable Tablets **1701**

Magnesium Oxide (Reduced plasma concentrations of atazanavir are expected if antacids, including buffered medications, are administered with atazanavir sulfate. Atazanavir sulfate should be administered 2 hours before or 1 hour after these medications). Products include:
Beelith Tablets **759**
PremCal Light, Regular, and Extra Strength Tablets **818**

Maprotiline Hydrochloride (Atazanavir sulfate competitively inhibits CYP1A2 and CYP2C9. There is a potential drug-drug interaction between atazanavir sulfate and CYP1A2 or CYP2C9 substrates).
No products indexed under this heading.

Meclofenamate Sodium (Atazanavir sulfate competitively inhibits CYP1A2 and CYP2C9. There is a potential drug-drug interaction between atazanavir sulfate and CYP1A2 or CYP2C9 substrates).
No products indexed under this heading.

Mefenamic Acid (Atazanavir sulfate competitively inhibits CYP1A2 and CYP2C9. There is a potential drug-drug interaction between atazanavir sulfate and CYP1A2 or CYP2C9 substrates).
No products indexed under this heading.

Meloxicam (Atazanavir sulfate competitively inhibits CYP1A2 and CYP2C9. There is a potential drug-drug interaction between atazanavir sulfate and CYP1A2 or CYP2C9 substrates). Products include:
Mobic Oral Suspension **863**
Mobic Tablets **863**

Mestranol (Because contraceptive steriod concentrations may be altered when atazanavir sulfate or atazanavir sulfate/ritonavir is co-administered with oral contraceptives or with the contraceptive patch, alternate methods of non-hormonal contraception are recommended).
No products indexed under this heading.

Metformin Hydrochloride (Atazanavir sulfate competitively inhibits CYP1A2 and CYP2C9. There is a potential drug-drug interaction between atazanavir sulfate and CYP1A2 or CYP2C9 substrates). Products include:
ActoPlus Met Tablets **3214**
Avandamet Tablets **1373**
Fortamet Extended-Release Tablets **3115**

Methadone Hydrochloride (Atazanavir sulfate competitively inhibits CYP1A2 and CYP2C9. There is a potential drug-drug interaction between atazanavir sulfate and CYP1A2 or CYP2C9 substrates).
No products indexed under this heading.

Methylergonovine Maleate (Contraindicated due to potential for serious and/or life-threatening events such as acute ergot toxicity characterized by peripheral vasospasm and ischemia of the extremities and other tissues).
No products indexed under this heading.

Methysergide Maleate (Contraindicated due to potential for serious and/or life-threatening events such as acute ergot toxicity characterized by peripheral vasospasm and ischemia of the extremities and other tissues).
No products indexed under this heading.

Metronidazole (Co-administration of atazanavir sulfate and other drugs that inhibit CYP3A may increase atazanavir sulfate plasma concentrations). Products include:
Metrogel 1% **1211**
MetroGel-Vaginal Gel **1855**
Vandazole Vaginal Gel **3338**

Metronidazole Benzoate (Co-administration of atazanavir sulfate and other drugs that inhibit CYP3A may increase atazanavir sulfate plasma concentrations).
No products indexed under this heading.

Metronidazole Hydrochloride (Co-administration of atazanavir sulfate and other drugs that inhibit CYP3A may increase atazanavir sulfate plasma concentrations).
No products indexed under this heading.

Mexiletine Hydrochloride (Atazanavir sulfate competitively inhibits CYP1A2 and CYP2C9. There is a potential drug-drug interaction between atazanavir sulfate and CYP1A2 or CYP2C9 substrates).
No products indexed under this heading.

Miconazole (Co-administration of atazanavir sulfate and other drugs that inhibit CYP3A may increase atazanavir sulfate plasma concentrations).
No products indexed under this heading.

Midazolam Hydrochloride (Contraindicated due to potential for serious and/or life-threatening events, such as prolonged or increased sedation or respiratory depression).
No products indexed under this heading.

Miglitol (Atazanavir sulfate competitively inhibits CYP1A2 and CYP2C9. There is a potential drug-drug interaction between atazanavir sulfate and CYP1A2 or CYP2C9 substrates).
No products indexed under this heading.

Mirtazapine (Atazanavir sulfate competitively inhibits CYP1A2 and CYP2C9. There is a potential drug-drug interaction between atazanavir sulfate and CYP1A2 or CYP2C9 substrates).
No products indexed under this heading.

Modafinil (Drugs that induce CYP3A activity may increase the clearance of atazanavir sulfate, resulting in lowered plasma concentrations). Products include:
Provigil Tablets **988**

Montelukast Sodium (Atazanavir sulfate competitively inhibits CYP1A2 and CYP2C9. There is a potential drug-drug interaction between atazanavir sulfate and CYP1A2 or CYP2C9 substrates). Products include:
Singulair **2077**

Moxifloxacin Hydrochloride (Atazanavir sulfate competitively inhibits CYP1A2 and CYP2C9. There is a potential drug-drug interaction between atazanavir sulfate and CYP1A2 or CYP2C9 substrates). Products include:
Avelox **2970**
Vigamox Ophthalmic Solution **564**

Muromonab-CD3 (Therapeutic concentration monitoring is recommended for immunosuppressant agents when co-administered with atazanavir sulfate). Products include:
Orthoclone OKT3 Sterile Solution **2360**

Mycophenolate Mofetil (Therapeutic concentration monitoring is recommended for immunosuppressant agents when co-administered with atazanavir sulfate). Products include:
CellCept Capsules **2747**
CellCept Oral Suspension **2747**
CellCept Tablets **2747**

Nabumetone (Atazanavir sulfate competitively inhibits CYP1A2 and CYP2C9. There is a potential drug-drug interaction between atazanavir sulfate and CYP1A2 or CYP2C9 substrates).
No products indexed under this heading.

Nafcillin Sodium (Atazanavir sulfate competitively inhibits CYP1A2 and CYP2C9. There is a potential drug-drug interaction between atazanavir sulfate and CYP1A2 or CYP2C9 substrates).
No products indexed under this heading.

Naproxen (Atazanavir sulfate competitively inhibits CYP1A2 and CYP2C9. There is a potential drug-drug interaction between atazanavir sulfate and CYP1A2 or CYP2C9 substrates). Products include:
EC-Naprosyn Delayed-Release Tablets **2761**
Naprosyn Suspension **2761**
Naprosyn Tablets **2761**
Prevacid NapraPAC **3280**

Naproxen Sodium (Atazanavir sulfate competitively inhibits CYP1A2 and CYP2C9. There is a potential drug-drug interaction between atazanavir sulfate and CYP1A2 or CYP2C9 substrates). Products include:
Aleve Caplets **742**
Aleve Gelcaps **743**
Aleve Tablets **743**
Aleve Cold & Sinus Caplets **744**
Anaprox Tablets **2761**
Anaprox DS Tablets **2761**

Nateglinide (Atazanavir sulfate competitively inhibits CYP1A2 and CYP2C9. There is a potential drug-drug interaction between atazanavir sulfate and CYP1A2 or CYP2C9 substrates). Products include:
Starlix Tablets **2292**

Nefazodone Hydrochloride (Co-administration of atazanavir sulfate and other drugs that inhibit CYP3A may increase atazanavir sulfate plasma concentrations).
No products indexed under this heading.

Nelfinavir Mesylate (Co- administration of atazanavir sulfate/ritonavir and other protease inhibitors would be expected to increase exposure to the other protease inhibitors; co-administration is not recommended). Products include:
Viracept **2577**

Nevirapine (Nevirapine, an inducer of CYP3A, is expected to decrease atazanavir sulfate exposure. In the absence of data, co-administration is not recommended). Products include:
Viramune Oral Suspension **873**
Viramune Tablets **873**

Nicotine Polacrilex (Atazanavir sulfate competitively inhibits CYP1A2 and CYP2C9. There is a potential drug-drug interaction between atazanavir sulfate and CYP1A2 or CYP2C9 substrates).
No products indexed under this heading.

Nicotine Salicylate (Atazanavir sulfate competitively inhibits CYP1A2 and CYP2C9. There is a potential drug-drug interaction between atazanavir sulfate and CYP1A2 or CYP2C9 substrates).
No products indexed under this heading.

Nicotine Sulfate (Atazanavir sulfate competitively inhibits CYP1A2 and CYP2C9. There is a potential drug-drug interaction between atazanavir sulfate and CYP1A2 or CYP2C9 substrates).
No products indexed under this heading.

Nifedipine (Co-administration of atazanavir sulfate and other drugs that inhibit CYP3A may increase atazanavir sulfate plasma concentrations). Products include:
Adalat CC Tablets **2964**

Nizatidine (Reduced plasma concentrations of atazanavir are expected if H2-receptor antagonists are administered with atazanavir sulfate. This may result in loss of therapeutic effect and development of resistance. To lessen the effect of H2-receptor antagonists on atazanavir exposure, it is recommended that an H2-receptor antagonist and atazanavir sulfate be administered as far apart as possible, preferably 12 hours apart). Products include:
Axid Oral Solution **879**

Norethindrone (Because contraceptive steriod concentrations may be altered when atazanavir sulfate or atazanavir sulfate/ritonavir is co-administered with oral contraceptives or with the contraceptive patch, alternate methods of non-hormonal contraception are recommended). Products include:
Ortho Micronor Tablets **2426**

Norethindrone Acetate (Atazanavir sulfate competitively inhibits CYP1A2 and CYP2C9. There is a potential drug-drug interaction between atazanavir sulfate and CYP1A2 or CYP2C9 substrates).
No products indexed under this heading.

Norethynodrel (Because contraceptive steriod concentrations may be altered when atazanavir sulfate or atazanavir sulfate/ritonavir is co-administered with oral contraceptives or with the contraceptive patch, alternate methods of non-hormonal contraception are recommended).
No products indexed under this heading.

Norfloxacin (Atazanavir sulfate competitively inhibits CYP1A2 and CYP2C9. There is a potential drug-drug interaction between atazanavir sulfate and CYP1A2 or CYP2C9 substrates). Products include:
Noroxin Tablets **2032**

Norgestimate (Because contraceptive steriod concentrations may be altered when atazanavir sulfate or atazanavir sulfate/ritonavir is co-administered with oral contraceptives or with the contraceptive patch, alternate methods of non-hormonal contraception are recommended). Products include:
Ortho-Cyclen/Ortho Tri-Cyclen **2429**
Ortho Tri-Cyclen Lo Tablets **2436**

Norgestrel (Because contraceptive steriod concentrations may be altered when atazanavir sulfate or atazanavir sulfate/ritonavir is co-administered with oral contraceptives or with the contraceptive patch, alternate methods of non-hormonal contraception are recommended).
No products indexed under this heading.

Nortriptyline Hydrochloride (Atazanavir sulfate competitively inhibits CYP1A2 and CYP2C9. There is a potential drug-drug interaction between atazanavir sulfate and CYP1A2 or CYP2C9 substrates).
No products indexed under this heading.

Ofloxacin (Atazanavir sulfate competitively inhibits CYP1A2 and CYP2C9. There is a potential drug-drug interaction between atazanavir sulfate and CYP1A2 or CYP2C9 substrates). Products include:
Floxin Otic Solution **1049**

Olanzapine (Atazanavir sulfate competitively inhibits CYP1A2 and CYP2C9. There is a potential drug-drug interaction between atazanavir sulfate and CYP1A2 or CYP2C9 substrates). Products include:
Symbyax Capsules **1819**
Zyprexa Tablets **1830**
Zyprexa IntraMuscular **1830**
Zyprexa ZYDIS Orally Disintegrating Tablets **1830**

Omeprazole (Concomitant use of atazanavir sulfate and proton-pump inhibitors is not recommended. Co-administration of atazanavir sulfate with proton-pump inhibitors is expected to substantially decrease atazanavir sulfate plasma concentrations and reduce its therapeutic effect). Products include:
Zegerid Capsules **2958**
Zegerid Powder for Oral Solution **2958**

Ondansetron (Atazanavir sulfate competitively inhibits CYP1A2 and CYP2C9. There is a potential drug-drug interaction between atazanavir sulfate and CYP1A2 or CYP2C9 substrates). Products include:
Zofran ODT Orally Disintegrating Tablets **1639**

Ondansetron Hydrochloride (Atazanavir sulfate competitively inhibits CYP1A2 and CYP2C9. There is a potential drug-drug interaction between atazanavir sulfate and CYP1A2 or CYP2C9 substrates). Products include:
Zofran Injection **1634**
Zofran **1639**

Oxaprozin (Atazanavir sulfate competitively inhibits CYP1A2 and CYP2C9. There is a potential drug-drug interaction between atazanavir sulfate and CYP1A2 or CYP2C9 substrates).
No products indexed under this heading.

Pantoprazole Sodium (Concomitant use of atazanavir sulfate and proton-pump inhibitors is not recommended. Co-administration of atazanavir sulfate with proton-pump inhibitors is expected to substantially decrease atazanavir sulfate plasma concentrations and reduce its therapeutic effect). Products include:
Protonix I.V. **3472**
Protonix Tablets **3469**

Paroxetine Hydrochloride (Co-administration of atazanavir sulfate and other drugs that inhibit CYP3A may increase atazanavir sulfate plasma concentrations). Products include:
Paxil CR Controlled-Release Tablets **1538**
Paxil **1530**

Phenobarbital (Drugs that induce CYP3A activity may increase the clearance of atazanavir sulfate, resulting in lowered plasma concentrations). Products include:
Donnatal Extentabs **2493**

Phenobarbital Sodium (Atazanavir sulfate competitively inhibits CYP1A2 and CYP2C9. There is a potential drug-drug interaction between atazanavir sulfate and CYP1A2 or CYP2C9 substrates).
No products indexed under this heading.

Phenylbutazone (Atazanavir sulfate competitively inhibits CYP1A2 and CYP2C9. There is a potential drug-drug interaction between atazanavir sulfate and CYP1A2 or CYP2C9 substrates).
No products indexed under this heading.

Phenytoin (Drugs that induce CYP3A activity may increase the clearance of atazanavir sulfate, resulting in lowered plasma concentrations).
No products indexed under this heading.

Phenytoin Sodium (Atazanavir sulfate competitively inhibits CYP1A2 and CYP2C9. There is a potential drug-drug interaction between atazanavir sulfate and CYP1A2 or CYP2C9 substrates). Products include:
Phenytek Capsules **2160**

Pimozide (Contraindicated due to potential for serious and/or life-threatening reactions, such as cardiac arrhythmias).
No products indexed under this heading.

Pioglitazone Hydrochloride (Atazanavir sulfate competitively inhibits CYP1A2 and CYP2C9. There is a potential drug-drug interaction between atazanavir sulfate and CYP1A2 or CYP2C9 substrates). Products include:
ActoPlus Met Tablets **3214**
Actos Tablets **3219**
Duetact Tablets **3226**

Piroxicam (Atazanavir sulfate competitively inhibits CYP1A2 and CYP2C9. There is a potential drug-drug interaction between atazanavir sulfate and CYP1A2 or CYP2C9 substrates).
No products indexed under this heading.

Propafenone Hydrochloride (Atazanavir sulfate competitively inhibits CYP1A2 and CYP2C9. There is a potential drug-drug interaction between atazanavir sulfate and CYP1A2 or CYP2C9 substrates). Products include:
Rythmol SR Capsules **2727**

Propranolol Hydrochloride (Atazanavir sulfate competitively inhibits CYP1A2 and CYP2C9. There is a potential drug-drug interaction between atazanavir sulfate and CYP1A2 or CYP2C9 substrates). Products include:
Inderal LA Long-Acting Capsules **3429**
InnoPran XL Capsules **2723**

Protriptyline Hydrochloride (Atazanavir sulfate competitively inhibits CYP1A2 and CYP2C9. There is a potential drug-drug interaction between atazanavir sulfate and CYP1A2 or CYP2C9 substrates).
No products indexed under this heading.

Quinidine (Co-administration with atazanavir sulfate has the potential to produce serious and/or life-threatening adverse events and has not been studied. Caution is warranted and therapeutic concentration monitoring of these drugs is recommended if they are used concomitantly with atazanavir sulfate).
No products indexed under this heading.

Quinidine Gluconate (Co-administration with atazanavir sulfate has the potential to produce serious and/or life-threatening adverse events and has not been studied. Caution is warranted and therapeutic concentration monitoring of these drugs is recommended if they are used concomitantly with atazanavir sulfate).
No products indexed under this heading.

Quinidine Hydrochloride (Co-administration with atazanavir sulfate has the potential to produce serious and/or life-threatening adverse events and has not been studied. Concentration monitoring of these drugs is recommended if they are used concomitantly with atazanavir sulfate).
No products indexed under this heading.

Quinidine Polygalacturonate (Co-administration with atazanavir sulfate has the potential to produce serious and/or life-threatening adverse events and has not been studied. Caution is warranted and therapeutic concentration monitoring of these drugs is recommended if they are used concomitantly with atazanavir sulfate).
No products indexed under this heading.

Quinidine Sulfate (Co-administration with atazanavir sulfate has the potential to produce serious and/or life-threatening adverse events and has not been studied. Caution is warranted and therapeutic concentration monitoring of these drugs is recommended if they are used concomitantly with atazanavir sulfate).
No products indexed under this heading.

Quinine (Co-administration of atazanavir sulfate and other drugs that inhibit CYP3A may increase atazanavir sulfate plasma concentrations).
No products indexed under this heading.

Quinine Sulfate (Co-administration of atazanavir sulfate and other drugs that inhibit CYP3A may increase atazanavir sulfate plasma concentrations).
No products indexed under this heading.

Rabeprazole Sodium (Concomitant use of atazanavir sulfate and proton-pump inhibitors is not recommended. Co-administration of atazanavir sulfate with proton-pump inhibitors is expected to substantially decrease atazanavir sulfate plasma concentrations and reduce its therapeutic effect). Products include:
Aciphex Tablets **1090**

Ranitidine Bismuth Citrate (Reduced plasma concentrations of atazanavir are expected if H2-receptor antagonists are administered with atazanavir sulfate. This may result in loss of therapeutic effect and development of resistance. To lessen the effect of H2-receptor antagonists on atazanavir exposure, it is recommended that an H2-receptor antagonist and atazanavir sulfate be administered as far apart as possible, preferably 12 hours apart).

No products indexed under this heading.

Ranitidine Hydrochloride (Reduced plasma concentrations of atazanavir are expected if H2-receptor antagonists are administered with atazanavir sulfate. This may result in loss of therapeutic effect and development of resistance. To lessen the effect of H2-receptor antagonists on atazanavir exposure, it is recommended that an H2-receptor antagonist and atazanavir sulfate be administered as far apart as possible, preferably 12 hours apart). Products include:

Zantac 1624
Zantac Injection 1619
Zantac Injection Pharmacy Bulk Package 1622

Repaglinide (Atazanavir sulfate competitively inhibits CYP1A2 and CYP2C9. There is a potential drug-drug interaction between atazanavir sulfate and CYP1A2 or CYP2C9 substrates).

No products indexed under this heading.

Rifabutin (A rifabutin dose reduction of up to 75% (e.g., 150mg every other day or three times a week) is recommended).

No products indexed under this heading.

Rifampicin (Drugs that induce CYP3A activity may increase the clearance of atazanavir sulfate, resulting in lowered plasma concentrations).

No products indexed under this heading.

Rifampin (Co-administration of atazanavir sulfate and drugs that induce CYP3A, such as rifampin, may decrease atazanavir plasma concentrations and reduce its therapeutic effect. Rifampin decreases plasma concentrations and AUC of most protease inhibitors by about 90%. This may result in loss of theraputic effect and development of resistance).

No products indexed under this heading.

Rifapentine (Drugs that induce CYP3A activity may increase the clearance of atazanavir sulfate, resulting in lowered plasma concentrations).

No products indexed under this heading.

Riluzole (Atazanavir sulfate competitively inhibits CYP1A2 and CYP2C9. There is a potential drug-drug interaction between atazanavir sulfate and CYP1A2 or CYP2C9 substrates). Products include:

Rilutek Tablets 2930

Ritonavir (If atazanavir sulfate is co-administered with ritonavir, it is recommended that atazanavir sulfate 300 mg once daily be given with ritonavir 100 mg once daily with food). Products include:

Kaletra 476
Norvir 503

Rofecoxib (Atazanavir sulfate competitively inhibits CYP1A2 and CYP2C9. There is a potential drug-drug interaction between atazanavir sulfate and CYP1A2 or CYP2C9 substrates).

No products indexed under this heading.

Ropinirole Hydrochloride (Atazanavir sulfate competitively inhibits CYP1A2 and CYP2C9. There is a potential drug-drug interaction between atazanavir sulfate and CYP1A2 or CYP2C9 substrates). Products include:

Requip Tablets 1555

Ropivacaine Hydrochloride (Atazanavir sulfate competitively inhibits CYP1A2 and CYP2C9. There is a potential drug-drug interaction between atazanavir sulfate and CYP1A2 or CYP2C9 substrates).

No products indexed under this heading.

Rosiglitazone Maleate (Atazanavir sulfate competitively inhibits CYP1A2 and CYP2C9. There is a potential drug-drug interaction between atazanavir sulfate and CYP1A2 or CYP2C9 substrates). Products include:

Avandamet Tablets 1373
Avandaryl Tablets 1379
Avandia Tablets 1384

Saquinavir (Saquinavir 1200 mg co-administered with atazanavir sulfate 400 mg and tenofovir 300 mg (all given once daily) plus nucleoside analogue reverse transcriptase inhibitors did not provide adequate efficacy).

No products indexed under this heading.

Saquinavir Mesylate (Saquinavir 1200 mg co-administered with atazanavir sulfate 400 mg and tenofovir 300 mg (all given once daily) plus nucleoside analogue reverse transcriptase inhibitors did not provide adequate efficacy). Products include:

Invirase 2772

Sertraline Hydrochloride (Co-administration of atazanavir sulfate and other drugs that inhibit CYP3A may increase atazanavir sulfate plasma concentrations). Products include:

Zoloft 2586

Sildenafil Citrate (Co-administration may result in an increase in PDE5 inhibitor-associated adverse events, including hypertension, visual changes, and priapism. Use sildenafil with caution at reduced doses of 25 mg every 48 hours with increased monitoring for adverse events). Products include:

Revatio Tablets 2557
Viagra Tablets 2573

Simvastatin (Concomitant use of atazanavir sulfate with simvastatin is not recommended. Caution should be exercised if HIV protease inhibitors, including atazanavir sulfate, are used concurrently with other HMG-CoA reductase inhibitors that are also metabolized by the CYP3A4 pathway. The risk of myopathy, including rhabdomyolysis, may be increased when HIV protease inhibitors, including atazanavir sulfate, are used in combination with these drugs). Products include:

Vytorin 10/10 Tablets 2114
Vytorin 10/10 Tablets 3077
Vytorin 10/20 Tablets 2114
Vytorin 10/20 Tablets 3077
Vytorin 10/40 Tablets 2114
Vytorin 10/40 Tablets 3077
Vytorin 10/80 Tablets 2114
Vytorin 10/80 Tablets 3077
Zocor Tablets 2105

Sirolimus (Therapeutic concentration monitoring is recommended for immunosuppressant agents when co-administered with atazanavir sulfate). Products include:

Rapamune Oral Solution and Tablets 3475

Sodium Bicarbonate (Reduced plasma concentrations of atazanavir are expected if antacids, including buffered medications, are administered with atazanavir sulfate. Atazanavir sulfate should be administered 2 hours before or 1 hour after these medications). Products include:

Colyte with Flavor Packs for Oral Solution 3088
HalfLytely and Bisacodyl Tablets Bowel Prep Kit with Flavors Packs 881
TriLyte with Flavor Packs for Oral Solution 3100

Sulfamethoxazole (Atazanavir sulfate competitively inhibits CYP1A2 and CYP2C9. There is a potential drug-drug interaction between atazanavir sulfate and CYP1A2 or CYP2C9 substrates).

No products indexed under this heading.

Sulindac (Atazanavir sulfate competitively inhibits CYP1A2 and CYP2C9. There is a potential drug-drug interaction between atazanavir sulfate and CYP1A2 or CYP2C9 substrates). Products include:

Clinoril Tablets 1924

Suprofen (Atazanavir sulfate competitively inhibits CYP1A2 and CYP2C9. There is a potential drug-drug interaction between atazanavir sulfate and CYP1A2 or CYP2C9 substrates).

No products indexed under this heading.

Tacrine Hydrochloride (Atazanavir sulfate competitively inhibits CYP1A2 and CYP2C9. There is a potential drug-drug interaction between atazanavir sulfate and CYP1A2 or CYP2C9 substrates).

No products indexed under this heading.

Tacrolimus (Therapeutic concentration monitoring is recommended for immunosuppressant agents when co-administered with atazanavir sulfate). Products include:

Prograf Capsules and Injection 632
Protopic Ointment 638

Tadalafil (Co-administration may result in an increase in PDE5 inhibitor-associated adverse events, including hypertension, visual changes, and priapism. Use tadalafil with caution at reduced doses of 10 mg every 72 hours with increased monitoring of adverse events). Products include:

Cialis Tablets 1838

Tamoxifen Citrate (Atazanavir sulfate competitively inhibits CYP1A2 and CYP2C9. There is a potential drug-drug interaction between atazanavir sulfate and CYP1A2 or CYP2C9 substrates). Products include:

Soltamox Oral Solution 3527

Telmisartan (Atazanavir sulfate competitively inhibits CYP1A2 and CYP2C9. There is a potential drug-drug interaction between atazanavir sulfate and CYP1A2 or CYP2C9 substrates). Products include:

Micardis Tablets 854
Micardis HCT Tablets 856

Tenofovir Disoproxil Fumarate (Tenofovir may decrease the AUC and Cmin of atazanavir sulfate, while atazanavir sulfate increases tenofovir concentrations. It is recommended to administer tenofovir 300 mg with atazanavir sulfate 300 mg and ritonavir 100 mg as a single dose). Products include:

Atripla Tablets 945
Truvada Tablets 1296
Viread Tablets 1301

Theophylline (Atazanavir sulfate competitively inhibits CYP1A2 and CYP2C9. There is a potential drug-drug interaction between atazanavir sulfate and CYP1A2 or CYP2C9 substrates).

No products indexed under this heading.

Theophylline Anhydrous (Atazanavir sulfate competitively inhibits CYP1A2 and CYP2C9. There is a potential drug-drug interaction between atazanavir sulfate and CYP1A2 or CYP2C9 substrates). Products include:

Uniphyl Tablets 2710

Tolazamide (Atazanavir sulfate competitively inhibits CYP1A2 and CYP2C9. There is a potential drug-drug interaction between atazanavir sulfate and CYP1A2 or CYP2C9 substrates).

No products indexed under this heading.

Tolbutamide (Atazanavir sulfate competitively inhibits CYP1A2 and CYP2C9. There is a potential drug-drug interaction between atazanavir sulfate and CYP1A2 or CYP2C9 substrates).

No products indexed under this heading.

Tolbutamide Sodium (Atazanavir sulfate competitively inhibits CYP1A2 and CYP2C9. There is a potential drug-drug interaction between atazanavir sulfate and CYP1A2 or CYP2C9 substrates).

No products indexed under this heading.

Tolmetin Sodium (Atazanavir sulfate competitively inhibits CYP1A2 and CYP2C9. There is a potential drug-drug interaction between atazanavir sulfate and CYP1A2 or CYP2C9 substrates).

No products indexed under this heading.

Torsemide (Atazanavir sulfate competitively inhibits CYP1A2 and CYP2C9. There is a potential drug-drug interaction between atazanavir sulfate and CYP1A2 or CYP2C9 substrates). Products include:

Demadex Injection 2759
Demadex Tablets 2759

Trazodone Hydrochloride (Concomitant use will increase plasma concentration of trazodone).

No products indexed under this heading.

Triazolam (Contraindicated due to potential for serious and/or life-threatening events, such as prolonged or increased sedation or respiratory depression).

No products indexed under this heading.

IMPORTANT NOTE: Always consult each drug listing in the patient's regimen for possible interactions.

Trimethaphan Camsylate (Atazanavir sulfate competitively inhibits CYP1A2 and CYP2C9. There is a potential drug-drug interaction between atazanavir sulfate and CYP1A2 or CYP2C9 substrates).
No products indexed under this heading.

Trimipramine Maleate (Atazanavir sulfate competitively inhibits CYP1A2 and CYP2C9. There is a potential drug-drug interaction between atazanavir sulfate and CYP1A2 or CYP2C9 substrates).
No products indexed under this heading.

Troglitazone (Atazanavir sulfate competitively inhibits CYP1A2 and CYP2C9. There is a potential drug-drug interaction between atazanavir sulfate and CYP1A2 or CYP2C9 substrates).
No products indexed under this heading.

Troleandomycin (Co-administration of atazanavir sulfate and other drugs that inhibit CYP3A may increase atazanavir sulfate plasma concentrations).
No products indexed under this heading.

Trovafloxacin Mesylate (Atazanavir sulfate competitively inhibits CYP1A2 and CYP2C9. There is a potential drug-drug interaction between atazanavir sulfate and CYP1A2 or CYP2C9 substrates).
No products indexed under this heading.

Valdecoxib (Atazanavir sulfate competitively inhibits CYP1A2 and CYP2C9. There is a potential drug-drug interaction between atazanavir sulfate and CYP1A2 or CYP2C9 substrates).
No products indexed under this heading.

Valsartan (Atazanavir sulfate competitively inhibits CYP1A2 and CYP2C9. There is a potential drug-drug interaction between atazanavir sulfate and CYP1A2 or CYP2C9 substrates). Products include:
Diovan Tablets 2193
Diovan HCT Tablets 2196

Vardenafil Hydrochloride (Co-administration may result in an increase in PDE5 inhibitor-associated adverse events, including hypertension, visual changes, and priapism. Use vardenafil with caution at reduced doses of no more than 2.5 mg every 72 hours with increased monitoring of adverse events). Products include:
Levitra Tablets 3034

Venlafaxine Hydrochloride (Co-administration of atazanavir sulfate and other drugs that inhibit CYP3A may increase atazanavir sulfate plasma concentrations). Products include:
Effexor Tablets 3411
Effexor XR Capsules 3417

Verapamil Hydrochloride (Atazanavir sulfate competitively inhibits CYP1A2 and CYP2C9. There is a potential drug-drug interaction between atazanavir sulfate and CYP1A2 or CYP2C9 substrates). Products include:
Covera-HS Tablets 3139
Tarka Tablets 524
Verelan PM Extended-Release Capsules, Controlled-Onset 3106

Voriconazole (Voriconazole with ritonavir 400 mg every 12 hours decreased voriconazole steady state AUC by 82%; therefore, voriconazole should not be co-administered with atazanavir sulfate/ritonavir. Co-administration of voriconazole with atazanavir sulfate (without ritonavir) may increase atazanavir sulfate concentrations; however, no data are available). Products include:
VFEND I.V. 2564
VFEND Oral Suspension 2564
VFEND Tablets 2564

Warfarin Sodium (Atazanavir sulfate competitively inhibits CYP1A2 and CYP2C9. There is a potential drug-drug interaction between atazanavir sulfate and CYP1A2 or CYP2C9 substrates). Products include:
Coumadin for Injection 898
Coumadin Tablets 898

Zafirlukast (Atazanavir sulfate competitively inhibits CYP1A2 and CYP2C9. There is a potential drug-drug interaction between atazanavir sulfate and CYP1A2 or CYP2C9 substrates). Products include:
Accolate Tablets 671

Zileuton (Atazanavir sulfate competitively inhibits CYP1A2 and CYP2C9. There is a potential drug-drug interaction between atazanavir sulfate and CYP1A2 or CYP2C9 substrates). Products include:
Zyflo Tablets 1023

Zolmitriptan (Atazanavir sulfate competitively inhibits CYP1A2 and CYP2C9. There is a potential drug-drug interaction between atazanavir sulfate and CYP1A2 or CYP2C9 substrates). Products include:
Zomig Tablets 3519
Zomig Nasal Spray 3523
Zomig-ZMT Tablets 3519

Food Interactions

Grapefruit (Co-administration of atazanavir sulfate and other drugs that inhibit CYP3A may increase atazanavir sulfate plasma concentrations).

R-GENE 10 FOR INTRAVENOUS USE

(Arginine Hydrochloride) 2641
None cited in PDR database.

RHINOCORT AQUA NASAL SPRAY

(Budesonide) 665
May interact with cytochrome p450 3a4 inhibitors (selected) and certain other agents. Compounds in these categories include:

Acetazolamide (Co-administration with inhibitors of CYP4503A4 may inhibit the metabolism of, and increase the systemic exposure to budesonide).
No products indexed under this heading.

Amiodarone Hydrochloride (Co-administration with inhibitors of CYP4503A4 may inhibit the metabolism of, and increase the systemic exposure to budesonide).
No products indexed under this heading.

Amprenavir (Co-administration with inhibitors of CYP4503A4 may inhibit the metabolism of, and increase the systemic exposure to budesonide). Products include:
Agenerase Capsules 1327
Agenerase Oral Solution 1332

Anastrozole (Co-administration with inhibitors of CYP4503A4 may inhibit the metabolism of, and increase the systemic exposure to budesonide). Products include:
Arimidex Tablets 673

Aprepitant (Co-administration with inhibitors of CYP4503A4 may inhibit the metabolism of, and increase the systemic exposure to budesonide). Products include:
Emend Capsules 1963

Cimetidine (Co-administration with inhibitors of CYP4501A2, such as cimetidine, caused a slight decrease in budesonide clearance and corresponding increase in its oral bioavailability). Products include:
Tagamet HB 200 Tablets .... ▣ 664

Cimetidine Hydrochloride (Co-administration with inhibitors of CYP4501A2, such as cimetidine, caused a slight decrease in budesonide clearance and corresponding increase in its oral bioavailability).
No products indexed under this heading.

Ciprofloxacin (Co-administration with inhibitors of CYP4503A4 may inhibit the metabolism of, and increase the systemic exposure to budesonide). Products include:
Cipro Oral Suspension 2977
Cipro I.V. 2984
Cipro XR Tablets 2990
Ciprodex Otic Suspension 559

Clarithromycin (Co-administration with inhibitors of CYP4503A4 may inhibit the metabolism of, and increase the systemic exposure to budesonide). Products include:
Biaxin/Biaxin XL 402
PREVPAC 3284

Clotrimazole (Co-administration with inhibitors of CYP4503A4 may inhibit the metabolism of, and increase the systemic exposure to budesonide). Products include:
Desenex Athlete's Foot Cream .... ▣ 635
Lotrimin 3039
Lotrisone 3040

Cyclosporine (Co-administration with inhibitors of CYP4503A4 may inhibit the metabolism of, and increase the systemic exposure to budesonide). Products include:
Gengraf Capsules 459
Neoral Oral Solution 2259
Neoral Soft Gelatin Capsules 2259
Restasis Ophthalmic Emulsion 575
Sandimmune 2275

Dalfopristin (Co-administration with inhibitors of CYP4503A4 may inhibit the metabolism of, and increase the systemic exposure to budesonide).
No products indexed under this heading.

Danazol (Co-administration with inhibitors of CYP4503A4 may inhibit the metabolism of, and increase the systemic exposure to budesonide).
No products indexed under this heading.

Delavirdine Mesylate (Co-administration with inhibitors of CYP4503A4 may inhibit the metabolism of, and increase the systemic exposure to budesonide). Products include:
Rescriptor Tablets 2551

Diltiazem Hydrochloride (Co-administration with inhibitors of CYP4503A4 may inhibit the metabolism of, and increase the systemic exposure to budesonide). Products include:
Cardizem LA Extended Release Tablets 1728
Tiazac Capsules 1201

Diltiazem Maleate (Co-administration with inhibitors of CYP4503A4 may inhibit the metabolism of, and increase the systemic exposure to budesonide).
No products indexed under this heading.

Efavirenz (Co-administration with inhibitors of CYP4503A4 may inhibit the metabolism of, and increase the systemic exposure to budesonide). Products include:
Atripla Tablets 945
Sustiva Capsules 930
Sustiva Tablets 930

Erythromycin (Co-administration with inhibitors of CYP4503A4 may inhibit the metabolism of, and increase the systemic exposure to budesonide). Products include:
Ery-Tab Tablets 449
Erythromycin Base Filmtab Tablets 455
Erythromycin Delayed-Release Capsules, USP 457
PCE Dispertab Tablets 515

Erythromycin Estolate (Co-administration with inhibitors of CYP4503A4 may inhibit the metabolism of, and increase the systemic exposure to budesonide).
No products indexed under this heading.

Erythromycin Ethylsuccinate (Co-administration with inhibitors of CYP4503A4 may inhibit the metabolism of, and increase the systemic exposure to budesonide). Products include:
E.E.S. 451
EryPed 447

Erythromycin Gluceptate (Co-administration with inhibitors of CYP4503A4 may inhibit the metabolism of, and increase the systemic exposure to budesonide).
No products indexed under this heading.

Erythromycin Lactobionate (Co-administration with inhibitors of CYP4503A4 may inhibit the metabolism of, and increase the systemic exposure to budesonide).
No products indexed under this heading.

Erythromycin Stearate (Co-administration with inhibitors of CYP4503A4 may inhibit the metabolism of, and increase the systemic exposure to budesonide). Products include:
Erythrocin Stearate Filmtab Tablets 453

Esomeprazole Magnesium (Co-administration with inhibitors of CYP4503A4 may inhibit the metabolism of, and increase the systemic exposure to budesonide). Products include:
Nexium Delayed-Release Capsules 655

Fluconazole (Co-administration with inhibitors of CYP4503A4 may inhibit the metabolism of, and increase the systemic exposure to budesonide).
No products indexed under this heading.

Fluoxetine Hydrochloride (Co-administration with inhibitors of CYP4503A4 may inhibit the metabolism of, and increase the systemic exposure to budesonide). Products include:
Prozac Pulvules and Liquid 1801
Symbyax Capsules 1819

Fluvoxamine Maleate (Co-administration with inhibitors of CYP4503A4 may inhibit the metabolism of, and increase the systemic exposure to budesonide).
 No products indexed under this heading.

Fosamprenavir Calcium (Co-administration with inhibitors of CYP4503A4 may inhibit the metabolism of, and increase the systemic exposure to budesonide). Products include:

Indinavir Sulfate (Co-administration with inhibitors of CYP4503A4 may inhibit the metabolism of, and increase the systemic exposure to budesonide). Products include:

Isoniazid (Co-administration with inhibitors of CYP4503A4 may inhibit the metabolism of, and increase the systemic exposure to budesonide).
 No products indexed under this heading.

Itraconazole (Co-administration with inhibitors of CYP4503A4 may inhibit the metabolism of, and increase the systemic exposure to budesonide).
 No products indexed under this heading.

Ketoconazole (The main route of metabolism of budesonide is via CYP4503A4; co-administration with a potent inhibitor of CYP4503A4, such as ketoconazole, has resulted in increased plasma concentration of orally administered budesonide). Products include:

Lopinavir (Co-administration with inhibitors of CYP4503A4 may inhibit the metabolism of, and increase the systemic exposure to budesonide). Products include:

Loratadine (Co-administration with inhibitors of CYP4503A4 may inhibit the metabolism of, and increase the systemic exposure to budesonide). Products include:

Metronidazole (Co-administration with inhibitors of CYP4503A4 may inhibit the metabolism of, and increase the systemic exposure to budesonide). Products include:

Metronidazole Benzoate (Co-administration with inhibitors of CYP4503A4 may inhibit the metabolism of, and increase the systemic exposure to budesonide).
 No products indexed under this heading.

Metronidazole Hydrochloride (Co-administration with inhibitors of CYP4503A4 may inhibit the metabolism of, and increase the systemic exposure to budesonide).
 No products indexed under this heading.

Miconazole (Co-administration with inhibitors of CYP4503A4 may inhibit the metabolism of, and increase the systemic exposure to budesonide).
 No products indexed under this heading.

Miconazole Nitrate (Co-administration with inhibitors of CYP4503A4 may inhibit the metabolism of, and increase the systemic exposure to budesonide). Products include:

Nefazodone Hydrochloride (Co-administration with inhibitors of CYP4503A4 may inhibit the metabolism of, and increase the systemic exposure to budesonide).
 No products indexed under this heading.

Nelfinavir Mesylate (Co-administration with inhibitors of CYP4503A4 may inhibit the metabolism of, and increase the systemic exposure to budesonide). Products include:

Nevirapine (Co-administration with inhibitors of CYP4503A4 may inhibit the metabolism of, and increase the systemic exposure to budesonide). Products include:

Niacinamide (Co-administration with inhibitors of CYP4503A4 may inhibit the metabolism of, and increase the systemic exposure to budesonide).
 No products indexed under this heading.

Nicotinamide (Co-administration with inhibitors of CYP4503A4 may inhibit the metabolism of, and increase the systemic exposure to budesonide). Products include:

Nifedipine (Co-administration with inhibitors of CYP4503A4 may inhibit the metabolism of, and increase the systemic exposure to budesonide). Products include:

Norfloxacin (Co-administration with inhibitors of CYP4503A4 may inhibit the metabolism of, and increase the systemic exposure to budesonide). Products include:

Omeprazole (Co-administration with inhibitors of CYP4503A4 may inhibit the metabolism of, and increase the systemic exposure to budesonide). Products include:

Paroxetine Hydrochloride (Co-administration with inhibitors of CYP4503A4 may inhibit the metabolism of, and increase the systemic exposure to budesonide). Products include:

Propoxyphene Hydrochloride (Co-administration with inhibitors of CYP4503A4 may inhibit the metabolism of, and increase the systemic exposure to budesonide).
 No products indexed under this heading.

Propoxyphene Napsylate (Co-administration with inhibitors of CYP4503A4 may inhibit the metabolism of, and increase the systemic exposure to budesonide).
 No products indexed under this heading.

Quinidine (Co-administration with inhibitors of CYP4503A4 may inhibit the metabolism of, and increase the systemic exposure to budesonide).
 No products indexed under this heading.

Quinidine Hydrochloride (Co-administration with inhibitors of CYP4503A4 may inhibit the metabolism of, and increase the systemic exposure to budesonide).
 No products indexed under this heading.

Quinidine Polygalacturonate (Co-administration with inhibitors of CYP4503A4 may inhibit the metabolism of, and increase the systemic exposure to budesonide).
 No products indexed under this heading.

Quinidine Sulfate (Co-administration with inhibitors of CYP4503A4 may inhibit the metabolism of, and increase the systemic exposure to budesonide).
 No products indexed under this heading.

Quinine (Co-administration with inhibitors of CYP4503A4 may inhibit the metabolism of, and increase the systemic exposure to budesonide).
 No products indexed under this heading.

Quinine Sulfate (Co-administration with inhibitors of CYP4503A4 may inhibit the metabolism of, and increase the systemic exposure to budesonide).
 No products indexed under this heading.

Quinupristin (Co-administration with inhibitors of CYP4503A4 may inhibit the metabolism of, and increase the systemic exposure to budesonide).
 No products indexed under this heading.

Ranitidine Bismuth Citrate (Co-administration with inhibitors of CYP4503A4 may inhibit the metabolism of, and increase the systemic exposure to budesonide).
 No products indexed under this heading.

Ranitidine Hydrochloride (Co-administration with inhibitors of CYP4503A4 may inhibit the metabolism of, and increase the systemic exposure to budesonide). Products include:

Ritonavir (Co-administration with inhibitors of CYP4503A4 may inhibit the metabolism of, and increase the systemic exposure to budesonide). Products include:

Saquinavir (Co-administration with inhibitors of CYP4503A4 may inhibit the metabolism of, and increase the systemic exposure to budesonide).
 No products indexed under this heading.

Saquinavir Mesylate (Co-administration with inhibitors of CYP4503A4 may inhibit the metabolism of, and increase the systemic exposure to budesonide). Products include:

Sertraline Hydrochloride (Co-administration with inhibitors of CYP4503A4 may inhibit the metabolism of, and increase the systemic exposure to budesonide). Products include:

Telithromycin (Co-administration with inhibitors of CYP4503A4 may inhibit the metabolism of, and increase the systemic exposure to budesonide). Products include:

Troglitazone (Co-administration with inhibitors of CYP4503A4 may inhibit the metabolism of, and increase the systemic exposure to budesonide).
 No products indexed under this heading.

Troleandomycin (Co-administration with inhibitors of CYP4503A4 may inhibit the metabolism of, and increase the systemic exposure to budesonide).
 No products indexed under this heading.

Valproate Sodium (Co-administration with inhibitors of CYP4503A4 may inhibit the metabolism of, and increase the systemic exposure to budesonide). Products include:

Verapamil Hydrochloride (Co-administration with inhibitors of CYP4503A4 may inhibit the metabolism of, and increase the systemic exposure to budesonide). Products include:

Voriconazole (Co-administration with inhibitors of CYP4503A4 may inhibit the metabolism of, and increase the systemic exposure to budesonide). Products include:

Zafirlukast (Co-administration with inhibitors of CYP4503A4 may inhibit the metabolism of, and increase the systemic exposure to budesonide). Products include:

Zileuton (Co-administration with inhibitors of CYP4503A4 may inhibit the metabolism of, and increase the systemic exposure to budesonide). Products include:

Food Interactions

Grapefruit (Co-administration with inhibitors of CYP4503A4 may inhibit the metabolism of, and increase the systemic exposure to budesonide).

Grapefruit Juice (Co-administration with inhibitors of CYP4503A4 may inhibit the metabolism of, and increase the systemic exposure to budesonide).

IMPORTANT NOTE: Always consult each drug listing in the patient's regimen for possible interactions.

RHOGAM ULTRA-FILTERED
(Rh_o (D) Immune Globulin (Human)) 2371
None cited in PDR database.

RHOPHYLAC
(Rh_o (D) Immune Globulin (Human)) 3505
May interact with:

Measles, Mumps & Rubella Virus Vaccine, Live (Active immunization with live virus vaccines should be postponed until 3 months after the last administration of immunoglobin, as the efficacy of the vaccine may be impaired). Products include:
M-M-R II 2006

Measles & Rubella Virus Vaccine Live (Active immunization with live virus vaccines should be postponed until 3 months after the last administration of immunoglobin, as the efficacy of the vaccine may be impaired).
No products indexed under this heading.

Measles Virus Vaccine Live (Active immunization with live virus vaccines should be postponed until 3 months after the last administration of immunoglobin, as the efficacy of the vaccine may be impaired). Products include:
Attenuvax 1914

Mumps Virus Vaccine, Live (Active immunization with live virus vaccines should be postponed until 3 months after the last administration of immunoglobin, as the efficacy of the vaccine may be impaired). Products include:
Mumpsvax 2031

Rubella & Mumps Virus Vaccine Live (Active immunization with live virus vaccines should be postponed until 3 months after the last administration of immunoglobin, as the efficacy of the vaccine may be impaired).
No products indexed under this heading.

Rubella Virus Vaccine Live (Active immunization with live virus vaccines should be postponed until 3 months after the last administration of immunoglobin, as the efficacy of the vaccine may be impaired). Products include:
Meruvax II 2019

Varicella Virus Vaccine Live (Active immunization with live virus vaccines should be postponed until 3 months after the last administration of immunoglobin, as the efficacy of the vaccine may be impaired). Products include:
Varivax 2100

RIBAVIRIN, USP CAPSULES
(Ribavirin) 3068
May interact with:

Didanosine (Exposure to didanosine or its active metabolite (dideoxyadenosine 5' - triphosphate) is increased when didanosine is co-administered with ribavirin, which could cause or worsen clinical toxicities. Co-administration of ribavirin and didanosine is not recommended).
No products indexed under this heading.

Stavudine (Ribavirin has been shown in vitro to inhibit phosphorylation of zidovudine and stavudine which could lead to decreased antiretroviral activity. Therefore, concomitant use of ribavirin with either of these drugs should be used with caution).
No products indexed under this heading.

Zidovudine (Ribavirin has been shown in vitro to inhibit phosphorylation of zidovudine and stavudine which could lead to decreased antiretroviral activity. Therefore, concomitant use of ribavirin with either of these drugs should be used with caution). Products include:
Combivir Tablets 1411
Retrovir 1560
Retrovir IV Infusion 1564
Trizivir Tablets 1589

RILUTEK TABLETS
(Riluzole) 2930
May interact with quinolones, xanthines, and certain other agents. Compounds in these categories include:

Alatrofloxacin Mesylate (Potential inhibitors of CYP1A2, such as quinolones, could decrease the rate of riluzole elimination).
No products indexed under this heading.

Allopurinol (Riluzole induces hepatic injury; ALS patients on concomitant hepatotoxic drugs, such as allopurinol, were excluded in the clinical trials; if such combination is used, practitioner should exercise caution).
No products indexed under this heading.

Aminophylline (Potential inhibitors of CYP1A2, such as theophylline, could decrease the rate of riluzole elimination).
No products indexed under this heading.

Amitriptyline Hydrochloride (Potential inhibitors of CYP1A2, such as amitriptyline, could decrease the rate of riluzole elimination).
No products indexed under this heading.

Caffeine (Potential inhibitors of CYP1A2, such as caffeine, could decrease the rate of riluzole elimination). Products include:
BC Headache Powder .... ▣677
Arthritis Strength BC Powder .... ▣677
Excedrin Extra Strength Caplets/Tablets/Geltabs .... ▣684
Excedrin Migraine Caplets/Tablets/Geltabs .... ▣609
Excedrin Tension Headache Caplets/Tablets/Geltabs .... ▣611
Goody's Extra Strength Headache Powders .... ▣611
Goody's Extra Strength Pain Relief Tablets .... ▣685
Vivarin .... ▣602
Winrgy Dietary Supplement .... ▣823

Ciprofloxacin (Potential inhibitors of CYP1A2, such as quinolones, could decrease the rate of riluzole elimination). Products include:
Cipro Oral Suspension 2977
Cipro I.V. 2984
Cipro XR Tablets 2990
Ciprodex Otic Suspension 559

Ciprofloxacin Hydrochloride (Potential inhibitors of CYP1A2, such as quinolones, could decrease the rate of riluzole elimination). Products include:
Ciloxan Ophthalmic Ointment 559
Ciloxan Ophthalmic Solution .... ⊙206
Cipro Tablets 2977
Proquin XR Tablets 1153

Dyphylline (Potential inhibitors of CYP1A2, such as theophylline, could decrease the rate of riluzole elimination).
No products indexed under this heading.

Enoxacin (Potential inhibitors of CYP1A2, such as quinolones, could decrease the rate of riluzole elimination).
No products indexed under this heading.

Grepafloxacin Hydrochloride (Potential inhibitors of CYP1A2, such as quinolones, could decrease the rate of riluzole elimination).
No products indexed under this heading.

Lomefloxacin Hydrochloride (Potential inhibitors of CYP1A2, such as quinolones, could decrease the rate of riluzole elimination).
No products indexed under this heading.

Methyldopa (Riluzole induces hepatic injury; ALS patients on concomitant hepatotoxic drugs, such as methyldopa, were excluded in the clinical trials; if such combination is used, practitioner should exercise caution). Products include:
Aldoril Tablets 1910

Moxifloxacin Hydrochloride (Potential inhibitors of CYP1A2, such as quinolones, could decrease the rate of riluzole elimination). Products include:
Avelox 2970
Vigamox Ophthalmic Solution 564

Norfloxacin (Potential inhibitors of CYP1A2, such as quinolones, could decrease the rate of riluzole elimination). Products include:
Noroxin Tablets 2032

Ofloxacin (Potential inhibitors of CYP1A2, such as quinolones, could decrease the rate of riluzole elimination). Products include:
Floxin Otic Solution 1049

Omeprazole (Potential inducers of CYP1A2, such as theophylline, could increase the rate of riluzole elimination). Products include:
Zegerid Capsules 2958
Zegerid Powder for Oral Solution 2958

Phenacetin (Potential inhibitors of CYP1A2, such as phenacetin, could decrease the rate of riluzole elimination).
No products indexed under this heading.

Rifampin (Potential inducers of CYP1A2, such as theophylline, could increase the rate of riluzole elimination).
No products indexed under this heading.

Sulfasalazine (Riluzole induces hepatic injury; ALS patients on concomitant hepatotoxic drugs, such as sulfasalazine, were excluded in the clinical trials; if such combination is used, practitioner should exercise caution).
No products indexed under this heading.

Tacrine Hydrochloride (CYP1A2 is the principal isoenzyme involved in the initial oxidative metabolism of riluzole; potential interaction may occur when co-administered with other agents, such as tacrine, which are also metabolized primarily by CYP1A2).
No products indexed under this heading.

Theophylline (Potential inhibitors of CYP1A2, such as theophylline, could decrease the rate of riluzole elimination).
No products indexed under this heading.

Theophylline Anhydrous (Potential inhibitors of CYP1A2, such as theophylline, could decrease the rate of riluzole elimination). Products include:
Uniphyl Tablets 2710

Theophylline Calcium Salicylate (Potential inhibitors of CYP1A2, such as theophylline, could decrease the rate of riluzole elimination).
No products indexed under this heading.

Theophylline Dihydroxypropyl (Glyceryl) (Potential inhibitors of CYP1A2, such as theophylline, could decrease the rate of riluzole elimination).
No products indexed under this heading.

Theophylline Ethylenediamine (Potential inhibitors of CYP1A2, such as theophylline, could decrease the rate of riluzole elimination).
No products indexed under this heading.

Theophylline Sodium Glycinate (Potential inhibitors of CYP1A2, such as theophylline, could decrease the rate of riluzole elimination).
No products indexed under this heading.

Trovafloxacin Mesylate (Potential inhibitors of CYP1A2, such as quinolones, could decrease the rate of riluzole elimination).
No products indexed under this heading.

Food Interactions

Alcohol (Alcohol may increase the risk of hepatotoxicity; patients on riluzole should be discouraged from drinking excessive amounts of alcohol).

Diet, high-lipid (Co-administration with high-fat meal decreases absorption, reduces AUC by about 20% and peak blood levels by about 45%).

Food, charcoal-broiled (Potential inducers of CYP1A2, such as charcoal-broiled food, could increase the rate of riluzole elimination).

RISPERDAL ORAL SOLUTION
(Risperidone) 1676
See Risperdal Tablets

RISPERDAL TABLETS

(Risperidone) 1676
May interact with antihypertensives, central nervous system depressants, central nervous system stimulants, cytochrome p450 2d6 inhibitors (selected), dopamine agonists, hepatic microsomal enzyme inducers, and certain other agents. Compounds in these categories include:

Acebutolol Hydrochloride (Because of its potential for inducing hypotension, risperidone may enhance the hypotensive effects of other therapeutic agents with this potential).
 No products indexed under this heading.

Alfentanil Hydrochloride (Given the primary CNS effects of risperidone, caution should be used if taken in combination with other centrally-acting drugs).
 No products indexed under this heading.

Alprazolam (Given the primary CNS effects of risperidone, caution should be used if taken in combination with other centrally-acting drugs). Products include:
 Niravam Orally Disintegrating Tablets 3092

Amiodarone Hydrochloride (Risperidone is metabolized to 9-hydroxyrisperidone by CYP2D6. Drug interactions that reduce the metabolism of risperidone to 9-hydroxyrisperidone would increase the plasma concentrations of risperidone and lower the concentrations of 9-hydroxyrisperidone).
 No products indexed under this heading.

Amitriptyline Hydrochloride (Risperidone is metabolized to 9-hydroxyrisperidone by CYP2D6. Drug interactions that reduce the metabolism of risperidone to 9-hydroxyrisperidone would increase the plasma concentrations of risperidone and lower the concentrations of 9-hydroxyrisperidone).
 No products indexed under this heading.

Amlodipine Besylate (Because of its potential for inducing hypotension, risperidone may enhance the hypotensive effects of other therapeutic agents with this potential). Products include:
 Caduet Tablets 2508
 Lotrel Capsules 2249
 Norvasc Tablets 2545

Amoxapine (Risperidone is metabolized to 9-hydroxyrisperidone by CYP2D6. Drug interactions that reduce the metabolism of risperidone to 9-hydroxyrisperidone would increase the plasma concentrations of risperidone and lower the concentrations of 9-hydroxyrisperidone).
 No products indexed under this heading.

Amphetamine Resins (Given the primary CNS effects of risperdone, caution should be taken with other centrally-acting drugs).
 No products indexed under this heading.

Aprobarbital (Given the primary CNS effects of risperidone, caution should be used if taken in combination with other centrally-acting drugs).
 No products indexed under this heading.

Atenolol (Because of its potential for inducing hypotension, risperidone may enhance the hypotensive effects of other therapeutic agents with this potential).
 No products indexed under this heading.

Benazepril Hydrochloride (Because of its potential for inducing hypotension, risperidone may enhance the hypotensive effects of other therapeutic agents with this potential). Products include:
 Lotensin Tablets 2243
 Lotensin HCT Tablets 2246
 Lotrel Capsules 2249

Bendroflumethiazide (Because of its potential for inducing hypotension, risperidone may enhance the hypotensive effects of other therapeutic agents with this potential).
 No products indexed under this heading.

Betaxolol Hydrochloride (Because of its potential for inducing hypotension, risperidone may enhance the hypotensive effects of other therapeutic agents with this potential). Products include:
 Betoptic S Ophthalmic Suspension................................. 558

Bisoprolol Fumarate (Because of its potential for inducing hypotension, risperidone may enhance the hypotensive effects of other therapeutic agents with this potential).
 No products indexed under this heading.

Bromocriptine Mesylate (Risperidone may antagonize the effect of dopamine agonists).
 No products indexed under this heading.

Buprenorphine Hydrochloride (Given the primary CNS effects of risperidone, caution should be used if taken in combination with other centrally-acting drugs). Products include:
 Buprenex Injectable 2716
 Suboxone Tablets 2717
 Subutex Tablets 2717

Bupropion Hydrochloride (Risperidone is metabolized to 9-hydroxyrisperidone by CYP2D6. Drug interactions that reduce the metabolism of risperidone to 9-hydroxyrisperidone would increase the plasma concentrations of risperidone and lower the concentrations of 9-hydroxyrisperidone). Products include:
 Wellbutrin Tablets 1603
 Wellbutrin SR Sustained-Release Tablets... 1607
 Wellbutrin XL Extended-Release Tablets... 1613
 Zyban Sustained-Release Tablets 1644

Buspirone Hydrochloride (Given the primary CNS effects of risperidone, caution should be used if taken in combination with other centrally-acting drugs).
 No products indexed under this heading.

Butabarbital (Given the primary CNS effects of risperidone, caution should be used if taken in combination with other centrally-acting drugs).
 No products indexed under this heading.

Butalbital (Given the primary CNS effects of risperidone, caution should be used if taken in combination with other centrally-acting drugs).
 No products indexed under this heading.

Candesartan Cilexetil (Because of its potential for inducing hypotension, risperidone may enhance the hypotensive effects of other therapeutic agents with this potential). Products include:
 Atacand Tablets 649
 Atacand HCT 651

Captopril (Because of its potential for inducing hypotension, risperidone may enhance the hypotensive effects of other therapeutic agents with this potential). Products include:
 Captopril Tablets 2149

Carbamazepine (During co-administration, the plasma concentrations of risperidone and its pharmacologically active metabolite, 9-hydroxyrisperidone, were decreased by about 50%. Plasma concentrations of carbamazepine did not appear to be affected. The dose of risperidone may need to be titrated accordingly for patients receiving carbamazepine, particularly during initiation or discontinuation of carbamazepine therapy). Products include:
 Carbatrol Capsules 3171
 Equetro Extended-Release Capsules...................................... 3180
 Tegretol/Tegretol-XR 2295

Carteolol Hydrochloride (Because of its potential for inducing hypotension, risperidone may enhance the hypotensive effects of other therapeutic agents with this potential). Products include:
 Carteolol Hydrochloride Ophthalmic Solution USP, 1%....... ⊙249

Celecoxib (Risperidone is metabolized to 9-hydroxyrisperidone by CYP2D6. Drug interactions that reduce the metabolism of risperidone to 9-hydroxyrisperidone would increase the plasma concentrations of risperidone and lower the concentrations of 9-hydroxyrisperidone). Products include:
 Celebrex Capsules 3134

Chlordiazepoxide (Given the primary CNS effects of risperidone, caution should be used if taken in combination with other centrally-acting drugs).
 No products indexed under this heading.

Chlordiazepoxide Hydrochloride (Given the primary CNS effects of risperidone, caution should be used if taken in combination with other centrally-acting drugs). Products include:
 Librium Capsules 3347

Chloroquine Hydrochloride (Risperidone is metabolized to 9-hydroxyrisperidone by CYP2D6. Drug interactions that reduce the metabolism of risperidone to 9-hydroxyrisperidone would increase the plasma concentrations of risperidone and lower the concentrations of 9-hydroxyrisperidone).
 No products indexed under this heading.

Chloroquine Phosphate (Risperidone is metabolized to 9-hydroxyrisperidone by CYP2D6. Drug interactions that reduce the metabolism of risperidone to 9-hydroxyrisperidone would increase the plasma concentrations of risperidone and lower the concentrations of 9-hydroxyrisperidone).
 No products indexed under this heading.

Chlorothiazide (Because of its potential for inducing hypotension, risperidone may enhance the hypotensive effects of other therapeutic agents with this potential). Products include:
 Diuril Oral Suspension 1954

Chlorothiazide Sodium (Because of its potential for inducing hypotension, risperidone may enhance the hypotensive effects of other therapeutic agents with this potential). Products include:
 Diuril Sodium Intravenous 2467

Chlorpheniramine (Risperidone is metabolized to 9-hydroxyrisperidone by CYP2D6. Drug interactions that reduce the metabolism of risperidone to 9-hydroxyrisperidone would increase the plasma concentrations of risperidone and lower the concentrations of 9-hydroxyrisperidone).
 No products indexed under this heading.

Chlorpheniramine Maleate (Risperidone is metabolized to 9-hydroxyrisperidone by CYP2D6. Drug interactions that reduce the metabolism of risperidone to 9-hydroxyrisperidone would increase the plasma concentrations of risperidone and lower the concentrations of 9-hydroxyrisperidone). Products include:
 Advil Allergy Sinus Caplets ▣□770
 Advil Multi-Symptom Cold Caplets...................................... ▣□770
 BC Allergy Sinus Cold Powder ▣□677
 Comtrex Maximum Strength Cold & Cough Day/Night Caplets - Night Formulation ▣□726
 Comtrex Maximum Strength Day/Night Severe Cold & Sinus Caplets - Night Formulation......... ▣□725
 Contac Cold and Flu Maximum Strength Caplets ▣□728
 Contac Cold and Flu Day and Night Caplets (Night Formulation Only)...................... ▣□727
 Children's Dimetapp Long Acting Cough Plus Cold Syrup................ ▣□731
 Robitussin Cough & Cold Long-Acting Liquid................... ▣□735
 Robitussin Cough & Allergy Syrup .. ▣□736
 Robitussin Cough & Cold Nighttime Liquid...................... ▣□736
 Robitussin Cough, Cold & Flu Nighttime Liquid...................... ▣□738
 Robitussin Pediatric Cough & Cold Long-Acting Liquid............ ▣□735
 Robitussin Pediatric Cough & Cold Nighttime Liquid................ ▣□736
 Triaminic Cold & Allergy Liquid ▣□746
 Triaminic Cough & Runny Nose Softchews ▣□748
 Children's Tylenol Plus Flu Oral Suspension.............................. ▣□749
 Tylenol Allergy Multi-Symptom Caplets with Cool Burst and Gelcaps................................... 1872
 Children's Tylenol Plus Cold Suspension Liquid 1879
 Children's Tylenol Plus Cough & Runny Nose Suspension Liquid..... 1879
 Children's Tylenol Plus Flu Suspension Liquid 1881
 Children's Tylenol Plus Multi-Symptom Cold Suspension Liquid 1879

IMPORTANT NOTE: Always consult each drug listing in the patient's regimen for possible interactions.

Tylenol Cold Head Congestion Nighttime Caplets with Cool Burst 1873
Tylenol Cold Multi-Symptom Nighttime Caplets with Cool Burst 1874
Tylenol Sinus Congestion & Pain Nighttime Caplets with Cool Burst 1876
Vicks 44M Cough, Cold & Flu Relief Liquid 2680
Pediatric Vicks 44m Cough & Cold Relief Liquid 2676
Children's Vicks NyQuil Cold/Cough Relief .... ■756
Children's Vicks NyQuil Cold/Cough Relief Liquid 2680
Zicam Maximum Strength Flu Daytime .... ■768

Chlorpheniramine Polistirex (Risperidone is metabolized to 9-hydroxyrisperidone by CYP2D6. Drug interactions that reduce the metabolism of risperidone to 9-hydroxyrisperidone would increase the plasma concentrations of risperidone and lower the concentrations of 9-hydroxyrisperidone). Products include:
Tussionex Pennkinetic Extended-Release Suspension 3327

Chlorpheniramine Tannate (Risperidone is metabolized to 9-hydroxyrisperidone by CYP2D6. Drug interactions that reduce the metabolism of risperidone to 9-hydroxyrisperidone would increase the plasma concentrations of risperidone and lower the concentrations of 9-hydroxyrisperidone).
No products indexed under this heading.

Chlorpromazine (Given the primary CNS effects of risperidone, caution should be used if taken in combination with other centrally-acting drugs).
No products indexed under this heading.

Chlorpromazine Hydrochloride (Given the primary CNS effects of risperidone, caution should be used if taken in combination with other centrally-acting drugs).
No products indexed under this heading.

Chlorpropamide (Co-administration of known enzyme inducers (e.g., phenytoin, rifampin and phenobarbital) with risperidone may cause decreases in the combined plasma concentrations of risperidone and 9-hydroxyrisperidone, which could lead to decreased efficacy. The dose of risperidone may need to be adjusted accordingly, particularly during the initiation or discontinuation of therapy with enzyme inducers).
No products indexed under this heading.

Chlorprothixene (Given the primary CNS effects of risperidone, caution should be used if taken in combination with other centrally-acting drugs).
No products indexed under this heading.

Chlorprothixene Hydrochloride (Given the primary CNS effects of risperidone, caution should be used if taken in combination with other centrally-acting drugs).
No products indexed under this heading.

Chlorprothixene Lactate (Given the primary CNS effects of risperidone, caution should be used if taken in combination with other centrally-acting drugs).
No products indexed under this heading.

Chlorthalidone (Because of its potential for inducing hypotension, risperidone may enhance the hypotensive effects of other therapeutic agents with this potential). Products include:
Clorpres Tablets 2153

Cimetidine (Cimetidine increased the bioavailability of risperidone, but only marginally increased the plasma concentration of the active antipsychotic fraction). Products include:
Tagamet HB 200 Tablets .... ■664

Cimetidine Hydrochloride (Cimetidine increased the bioavailability of risperidone, but only marginally increased the plasma concentration of the active anti-psychotic fraction).
No products indexed under this heading.

Citalopram Hydrobromide (Risperidone is metabolized to 9-hydroxyrisperidone by CYP2D6. Drug interactions that reduce the metabolism of risperidone to 9-hydroxyrisperidone would increase the plasma concentrations of risperidone and lower the concentrations of 9-hydroxyrisperidone). Products include:
Celexa 1176

Clomipramine Hydrochloride (Risperidone is metabolized to 9-hydroxyrisperidone by CYP2D6. Drug interactions that reduce the metabolism of risperidone to 9-hydroxyrisperidone would increase the plasma concentrations of risperidone and lower the concentrations of 9-hydroxyrisperidone).
No products indexed under this heading.

Clonidine (Because of its potential for inducing hypotension, risperidone may enhance the hypotensive effects of other therapeutic agents with this potential). Products include:
Catapres-TTS 844

Clonidine Hydrochloride (Because of its potential for inducing hypotension, risperidone may enhance the hypotensive effects of other therapeutic agents with this potential). Products include:
Catapres Tablets 843
Clorpres Tablets 2153

Clorazepate Dipotassium (Given the primary CNS effects of risperidone, caution should be used if taken in combination with other centrally-acting drugs). Products include:
Tranxene 2474

Clozapine (Chronic administration of clozapine with risperidone may decrease the clearance of risperidone). Products include:
Clozaril Tablets 2184
FazaClo Orally Disintegrating Tablets 551

CNS-Active Drugs, unspecified (Given the primary CNS effects of risperidone, caution should be taken if used with centrally-acting drugs).
No products indexed under this heading.

Cocaine Hydrochloride (Risperidone is metabolized to 9-hydroxyrisperidone by CYP2D6. Drug interactions that reduce the metabolism of risperidone to 9-hydroxyrisperidone would increase the plasma concentrations of risperidone and lower the concentrations of 9-hydroxyrisperidone).
No products indexed under this heading.

Codeine Phosphate (Given the primary CNS effects of risperidone, caution should be used if taken in combination with other centrally-acting drugs). Products include:
Tylenol with Codeine Tablets 2391

Deserpidine (Because of its potential for inducing hypotension, risperidone may enhance the hypotensive effects of other therapeutic agents with this potential).
No products indexed under this heading.

Desflurane (Given the primary CNS effects of risperidone, caution should be used if taken in combination with other centrally-acting drugs).
No products indexed under this heading.

Desipramine Hydrochloride (Risperidone is metabolized to 9-hydroxyrisperidone by CYP2D6. Drug interactions that reduce the metabolism of risperidone to 9-hydroxyrisperidone would increase the plasma concentrations of risperidone and lower the concentrations of 9-hydroxyrisperidone).
No products indexed under this heading.

Dextroamphetamine Sulfate (Given the primary CNS effects of risperdone, caution should be taken with other centrally-acting drugs). Products include:
Adderall Tablets 3164
Adderall XR Capsules 3166
Dexedrine 1420
DextroStat Tablets 3179

Dezocine (Given the primary CNS effects of risperidone, caution should be used if taken in combination with other centrally-acting drugs).
No products indexed under this heading.

Diazepam (Given the primary CNS effects of risperidone, caution should be used if taken in combination with other centrally-acting drugs). Products include:
Diastat Rectal Delivery System 3343
Valium Tablets 2819

Diazoxide (Because of its potential for inducing hypotension, risperidone may enhance the hypotensive effects of other therapeutic agents with this potential). Products include:
Hyperstat I.V. 3017

Diltiazem Hydrochloride (Because of its potential for inducing hypotension, risperidone may enhance the hypotensive effects of other therapeutic agents with this potential). Products include:
Cardizem LA Extended Release Tablets 1728
Tiazac Capsules 1201

Diphenhydramine (Risperidone is metabolized to 9-hydroxyrisperidone by CYP2D6. Drug interactions that reduce the metabolism of risperidone to 9-hydroxyrisperidone would increase the plasma concentrations of risperidone and lower the concentrations of 9-hydroxyrisperidone). Products include:
Tylenol Sore Throat Nighttime Liquid with Cool Burst 1877

Diphenhydramine Hydrochloride (Risperidone is metabolized to 9-hydroxyrisperidone by CYP2D6. Drug interactions that reduce the metabolism of risperidone to 9-hydroxyrisperidone would increase the plasma concentrations of risperidone and lower the concentrations of 9-hydroxyrisperidone). Products include:
Nytol QuickCaps Caplets .... ■615
Nytol QuickGels Softgels Maximum Strength .... ■616
Simply Sleep Caplets 1868
Sominex Original Formula Tablets .. ■616
TheraFlu Warming Relief Nighttime Severe Cold .... ■743
TheraFlu Thin Strips Multi Symptom .... ■744
Triaminic Nighttime Cold & Cough Liquid .... ■746
Triaminic Thin Strips Cough & Runny Nose .... ■749
Extra Strength Tylenol PM Caplets, Vanilla Caplets, Geltabs, Gelcaps and Liquid 1875
Tylenol Sore Throat Nighttime Liquid with Cool Burst .... ■790
Tylenol Allergy Multi-Symptom Nighttime Caplets with Cool Burst 1872
Tylenol Severe Allergy Caplets 1872
Children's Tylenol Plus Cold & Allergy Suspension Liquid 1878

Dopamine Hydrochloride (Risperidone may antagonize the effect of dopamine agonists).
No products indexed under this heading.

Doxazosin Mesylate (Because of its potential for inducing hypotension, risperidone may enhance the hypotensive effects of other therapeutic agents with this potential). Products include:
Cardura XL Tablets 2515

Doxepin Hydrochloride (Risperidone is metabolized to 9-hydroxyrisperidone by CYP2D6. Drug interactions that reduce the metabolism of risperidone to 9-hydroxyrisperidone would increase the plasma concentrations of risperidone and lower the concentrations of 9-hydroxyrisperidone).
No products indexed under this heading.

Droperidol (Given the primary CNS effects of risperidone, caution should be used if taken in combination with other centrally-acting drugs).
No products indexed under this heading.

Enalapril Maleate (Because of its potential for inducing hypotension, risperidone may enhance the hypotensive effects of other therapeutic agents with this potential). Products include:
Vasotec I.V. Injection 2103

Enalaprilat (Because of its potential for inducing hypotension, risperidone may enhance the hypotensive effects of other therapeutic agents with this potential).
No products indexed under this heading.

Enflurane (Given the primary CNS effects of risperidone, caution should be used if taken in combination with other centrally-acting drugs).
No products indexed under this heading.

Eprosartan Mesylate (Because of its potential for inducing hypotension, risperidone may enhance the hypotensive effects of other therapeutic agents with this potential). Products include:

Escitalopram Oxalate (Risperidone is metabolized to 9-hydroxyrisperidone by CYP2D6. Drug interactions that reduce the metabolism of risperidone to 9-hydroxyrisperidone would increase the plasma concentrations of risperidone and lower the concentrations of 9-hydroxyrisperidone). Products include:

Esmolol Hydrochloride (Because of its potential for inducing hypotension, risperidone may enhance the hypotensive effects of other therapeutic agents with this potential).

No products indexed under this heading.

Estazolam (Given the primary CNS effects of risperidone, caution should be used if taken in combination with other centrally-acting drugs). Products include:

Ethanol (Co-administration of known enzyme inducers (e.g., phenytoin, rifampin and phenobarbital) with risperidone may cause decreases in the combined plasma concentrations of risperidone and 9-hydroxyrisperidone, which could lead to decreased efficacy. The dose of risperidone may need to be adjusted accordingly, particularly during the initiation or discontinuation of therapy with enzyme inducers).

No products indexed under this heading.

Ethchlorvynol (Given the primary CNS effects of risperidone, caution should be used if taken in combination with other centrally-acting drugs).

No products indexed under this heading.

Ethinamate (Given the primary CNS effects of risperidone, caution should be used if taken in combination with other centrally-acting drugs).

No products indexed under this heading.

Ethyl Alcohol (Given the primary CNS effects of risperidone, caution should be used if taken in combination with other centrally-acting drugs).

No products indexed under this heading.

Felodipine (Because of its potential for inducing hypotension, risperidone may enhance the hypotensive effects of other therapeutic agents with this potential).

No products indexed under this heading.

Fentanyl (Given the primary CNS effects of risperidone, caution should be used if taken in combination with other centrally-acting drugs). Products include:

Fentanyl Citrate (Given the primary CNS effects of risperidone, cau-

tion should be used if taken in combination with other centrally-acting drugs). Products include:

Fluoxetine (Risperidone is metabolized to 9-hydroxyrisperidone by CYP2D6. Drug interactions that reduce the metabolism of risperidone to 9-hydroxyrisperidone would increase the plasma concentrations of risperidone and lower the concentrations of 9-hydroxyrisperidone).

No products indexed under this heading.

Fluoxetine Hydrochloride (Fluoxetine (20mg QD) has been shown to increase the plasma concentration of risperidone 2.5- to 2.8- fold, while the plasma concentration of 9-hydroxyrisperidone was not affected. When concomitant fluoxetine is initiated or discontinued, the dosage of risperidone should be re-evaluated). Products include:

Fluphenazine Decanoate (Given the primary CNS effects of risperidone, caution should be used if taken in combination with other centrally-acting drugs).

No products indexed under this heading.

Fluphenazine Enanthate (Given the primary CNS effects of risperidone, caution should be used if taken in combination with other centrally-acting drugs).

No products indexed under this heading.

Fluphenazine Hydrochloride (Given the primary CNS effects of risperidone, caution should be used if taken in combination with other centrally-acting drugs).

No products indexed under this heading.

Flurazepam Hydrochloride (Given the primary CNS effects of risperidone, caution should be used if taken in combination with other centrally-acting drugs). Products include:

Fluvoxamine Maleate (Risperidone is metabolized to 9-hydroxyrisperidone by CYP2D6. Drug interactions that reduce the metabolism of risperidone to 9-hydroxyrisperidone would increase the plasma concentrations of risperidone and lower the concentrations of 9-hydroxyrisperidone).

No products indexed under this heading.

Fosinopril Sodium (Because of its potential for inducing hypotension, risperidone may enhance the hypotensive effects of other therapeutic agents with this potential).

No products indexed under this heading.

Fosphenytoin Sodium (Co-administration of known enzyme inducers (e.g., phenytoin, rifampin and phenobarbital) with risperidone may cause decreases in the combined plasma concentrations of risperidone and 9-hydroxyrisperidone, which could lead to decreased efficacy. The dose of risperidone may need to be adjusted accordingly, particularly during the initiation or discontinuation of therapy with enzyme inducers).

No products indexed under this heading.

Furosemide (In placebo-controlled trials in elderly patients with dementia-related psychosis, a higher incidence of mortality was observed in patients treated with furosemide plus risperdone (7.3%; mean age 89 years, range 75-97) when compared to patients treated with risperdone alone (3.1%; mean age 84 years, range 70-96) or furosemide alone (4.1%; mean age 80 years, range 67-90). The increase in mortality in patients treated with furosemide plus risperidone was observed in 2 of the 4 clinical trials). Products include:

Glipizide (Co-administration of known enzyme inducers (e.g., phenytoin, rifampin and phenobarbital) with risperidone may cause decreases in the combined plasma concentrations of risperidone and 9-hydroxyrisperidone, which could lead to decreased efficacy. The dose of risperidone may need to be adjusted accordingly, particularly during the initiation or discontinuation of therapy with enzyme inducers).

No products indexed under this heading.

Glutethimide (Given the primary CNS effects of risperidone, caution should be used if taken in combination with other centrally-acting drugs).

No products indexed under this heading.

Glyburide (Co-administration of known enzyme inducers (e.g., phenytoin, rifampin and phenobarbital) with risperidone may cause decreases in the combined plasma concentrations of risperidone and 9-hydroxyrisperidone, which could lead to decreased efficacy. The dose of risperidone may need to be adjusted accordingly, particularly during the initiation or discontinuation of therapy with enzyme inducers).

No products indexed under this heading.

Guanabenz Acetate (Because of its potential for inducing hypotension, risperidone may enhance the hypotensive effects of other therapeutic agents with this potential).

No products indexed under this heading.

Guanethidine Monosulfate (Because of its potential for inducing hypotension, risperidone may enhance the hypotensive effects of other therapeutic agents with this potential).

No products indexed under this heading.

Halofantrine Hydrochloride (Risperidone is metabolized to 9-hydroxyrisperidone by CYP2D6. Drug interactions that reduce the metabolism of risperidone to 9-hydroxyrisperidone would increase the plasma concentrations of risperidone and lower the concentrations of 9-hydroxyrisperidone).

No products indexed under this heading.

Haloperidol (Given the primary CNS effects of risperidone, caution should be used if taken in combination with other centrally-acting drugs).

No products indexed under this heading.

Haloperidol Decanoate (Given the primary CNS effects of risperidone, caution should be used if taken in combination with other centrally-acting drugs).

No products indexed under this heading.

Hydralazine Hydrochloride (Because of its potential for inducing hypotension, risperidone may enhance the hypotensive effects of other therapeutic agents with this potential). Products include:

Hydrochlorothiazide (Because of its potential for inducing hypotension, risperidone may enhance the hypotensive effects of other therapeutic agents with this potential). Products include:

Hydrocodone Bitartrate (Given the primary CNS effects of risperidone, caution should be used if taken in combination with other centrally-acting drugs). Products include:

Hydrocodone Polistirex (Given the primary CNS effects of risperidone, caution should be used if taken in combination with other centrally-acting drugs). Products include:

Hydroflumethiazide (Because of its potential for inducing hypotension, risperidone may enhance the hypotensive effects of other therapeutic agents with this potential).

No products indexed under this heading.

Hydromorphone Hydrochloride (Given the primary CNS effects of risperidone, caution should be used if taken in combination with other centrally-acting drugs). Products include:

Hydroxychloroquine Sulfate (Risperidone is metabolized to 9-hydroxyrisperidone by CYP2D6. Drug interactions that reduce the metabolism of risperidone to 9-hydroxyrisperidone would increase the plasma concentrations of risperidone and lower the concentrations of 9-hydroxyrisperidone).
No products indexed under this heading.

Hydroxyzine Hydrochloride (Given the primary CNS effects of risperidone, caution should be used if taken in combination with other centrally-acting drugs).
No products indexed under this heading.

Imatinib Mesylate (Risperidone is metabolized to 9-hydroxyrisperidone by CYP2D6. Drug interactions that reduce the metabolism of risperidone to 9-hydroxyrisperidone would increase the plasma concentrations of risperidone and lower the concentrations of 9-hydroxyrisperidone). Products include:
Gleevec Tablets **2227**

Imipramine Hydrochloride (Risperidone is metabolized to 9-hydroxyrisperidone by CYP2D6. Drug interactions that reduce the metabolism of risperidone to 9-hydroxyrisperidone would increase the plasma concentrations of risperidone and lower the concentrations of 9-hydroxyrisperidone).
No products indexed under this heading.

Imipramine Pamoate (Risperidone is metabolized to 9-hydroxyrisperidone by CYP2D6. Drug interactions that reduce the metabolism of risperidone to 9-hydroxyrisperidone would increase the plasma concentrations of risperidone and lower the concentrations of 9-hydroxyrisperidone).
No products indexed under this heading.

Indapamide (Because of its potential for inducing hypotension, risperidone may enhance the hypotensive effects of other therapeutic agents with this potential). Products include:
Indapamide Tablets **2156**

Irbesartan (Because of its potential for inducing hypotension, risperidone may enhance the hypotensive effects of other therapeutic agents with this potential). Products include:
Avalide Tablets **888**
Avalide Tablets **2874**
Avapro Tablets **891**
Avapro Tablets **2871**

Isoflurane (Given the primary CNS effects of risperidone, caution should be used if taken in combination with other centrally-acting drugs).
No products indexed under this heading.

Isradipine (Because of its potential for inducing hypotension, risperidone may enhance the hypotensive effects of other therapeutic agents with this potential). Products include:
DynaCirc CR Tablets **2721**

Ketamine Hydrochloride (Given the primary CNS effects of risperidone, caution should be used if taken in combination with other centrally-acting drugs).
No products indexed under this heading.

Labetalol Hydrochloride (Because of its potential for inducing hypotension, risperidone may enhance the hypotensive effects of other therapeutic agents with this potential).
No products indexed under this heading.

Levodopa (Risperidone may antagonize the effect of levodopa). Products include:
Parcopa Orally Disintegrating Tablets **3097**
Stalevo Tablets **2287**

Levomethadyl Acetate Hydrochloride (Given the primary CNS effects of risperidone, caution should be used if taken in combination with other centrally-acting drugs).
No products indexed under this heading.

Levorphanol Tartrate (Given the primary CNS effects of risperidone, caution should be used if taken in combination with other centrally-acting drugs).
No products indexed under this heading.

Lisinopril (Because of its potential for inducing hypotension, risperidone may enhance the hypotensive effects of other therapeutic agents with this potential). Products include:
Prinivil Tablets **2052**
Prinzide Tablets **2056**

Lorazepam (Given the primary CNS effects of risperidone, caution should be used if taken in combination with other centrally-acting drugs).
No products indexed under this heading.

Losartan Potassium (Because of its potential for inducing hypotension, risperidone may enhance the hypotensive effects of other therapeutic agents with this potential). Products include:
Cozaar Tablets **1935**
Hyzaar 50-12.5 Tablets **1990**
Hyzaar 100-12.5 Tablets **1990**
Hyzaar 100-25 Tablets **1990**

Loxapine Hydrochloride (Given the primary CNS effects of risperidone, caution should be used if taken in combination with other centrally-acting drugs).
No products indexed under this heading.

Loxapine Succinate (Given the primary CNS effects of risperidone, caution should be used if taken in combination with other centrally-acting drugs).
No products indexed under this heading.

Maprotiline Hydrochloride (Risperidone is metabolized to 9-hydroxyrisperidone by CYP2D6. Drug interactions that reduce the metabolism of risperidone to 9-hydroxyrisperidone would increase the plasma concentrations of risperidone and lower the concentrations of 9-hydroxyrisperidone).
No products indexed under this heading.

Mecamylamine Hydrochloride (Because of its potential for inducing hypotension, risperidone may enhance the hypotensive effects of other therapeutic agents with this potential).
No products indexed under this heading.

Meperidine Hydrochloride (Given the primary CNS effects of risperidone, caution should be used if taken in combination with other centrally-acting drugs).
No products indexed under this heading.

Mephobarbital (Given the primary CNS effects of risperidone, caution should be used if taken in combination with other centrally-acting drugs).
No products indexed under this heading.

Meprobamate (Given the primary CNS effects of risperidone, caution should be used if taken in combination with other centrally-acting drugs).
No products indexed under this heading.

Mesoridazine Besylate (Given the primary CNS effects of risperidone, caution should be used if taken in combination with other centrally-acting drugs).
No products indexed under this heading.

Methadone Hydrochloride (Given the primary CNS effects of risperidone, caution should be used if taken in combination with other centrally-acting drugs).
No products indexed under this heading.

Methamphetamine Hydrochloride (Given the primary CNS effects of risperdone, caution should be taken with other centrally-acting drugs). Products include:
Desoxyn Tablets, USP **2462**

Methohexital Sodium (Given the primary CNS effects of risperidone, caution should be used if taken in combination with other centrally-acting drugs).
No products indexed under this heading.

Methotrimeprazine (Given the primary CNS effects of risperidone, caution should be used if taken in combination with other centrally-acting drugs).
No products indexed under this heading.

Methoxyflurane (Given the primary CNS effects of risperidone, caution should be used if taken in combination with other centrally-acting drugs).
No products indexed under this heading.

Methyclothiazide (Because of its potential for inducing hypotension, risperidone may enhance the hypotensive effects of other therapeutic agents with this potential).
No products indexed under this heading.

Methyldopa (Because of its potential for inducing hypotension, risperidone may enhance the hypotensive effects of other therapeutic agents with this potential). Products include:
Aldoril Tablets **1910**

Methyldopate Hydrochloride (Because of its potential for inducing hypotension, risperidone may enhance the hypotensive effects of other therapeutic agents with this potential).
No products indexed under this heading.

Methylphenidate (Given the primary CNS effects of risperdone, caution should be taken with other centrally-acting drugs). Products include:
Daytrana Transdermal Patch **3174**

Methylphenidate Hydrochloride (Given the primary CNS effects of risperdone, caution should be taken with other centrally-acting drugs). Products include:
Concerta Extended-Release Tablets **1881**
Metadate CD Capsules **3323**
Ritalin Hydrochloride Tablets **2269**
Ritalin LA Capsules **2271**
Ritalin-SR Tablets **2269**

Metolazone (Because of its potential for inducing hypotension, risperidone may enhance the hypotensive effects of other therapeutic agents with this potential).
No products indexed under this heading.

Metoprolol Succinate (Because of its potential for inducing hypotension, risperidone may enhance the hypotensive effects of other therapeutic agents with this potential). Products include:
Toprol-XL Tablets **668**

Metoprolol Tartrate (Because of its potential for inducing hypotension, risperidone may enhance the hypotensive effects of other therapeutic agents with this potential). Products include:
Lopressor Injection **2238**
Lopressor Tablets **2238**
Lopressor HCT 50/25 Tablets **2241**
Lopressor HCT 100/25 Tablets **2241**
Lopressor HCT 100/50 Tablets **2241**

Metyrosine (Because of its potential for inducing hypotension, risperidone may enhance the hypotensive effects of other therapeutic agents with this potential). Products include:
Demser Capsules **1953**

Mibefradil Dihydrochloride (Because of its potential for inducing hypotension, risperidone may enhance the hypotensive effects of other therapeutic agents with this potential).
No products indexed under this heading.

Midazolam Hydrochloride (Given the primary CNS effects of risperidone, caution should be used if taken in combination with other centrally-acting drugs).
No products indexed under this heading.

Minoxidil (Because of its potential for inducing hypotension, risperidone may enhance the hypotensive effects of other therapeutic agents with this potential). Products include:
Men's Rogaine Extra Strength Hair Regrowth Treatment Topical Solution, Ocean Rush Scent and Original Unscented ..... ▣ **633**
Men's Rogaine Foam Hair Regrowth Treatment.................... ▣ **633**
Women's Rogaine Hair Regrowth Treatment Topical Solution, Spring Bloom Scent and Original Unscented...................... ▣ **634**

Moclobemide (Risperidone is metabolized to 9-hydroxyrisperidone by CYP2D6. Drug interactions that reduce the metabolism of risperidone to 9-hydroxyrisperidone would increase the plasma concentrations of risperidone and lower the concentrations of 9-hydroxyrisperidone).
No products indexed under this heading.

Moexipril Hydrochloride (Because of its potential for inducing hypotension, risperidone may enhance the hypotensive effects of other therapeutic agents with this potential). Products include:

Molindone Hydrochloride (Given the primary CNS effects of risperidone, caution should be used if taken in combination with other centrally-acting drugs). Products include:

Morphine Sulfate (Given the primary CNS effects of risperidone, caution should be used if taken in combination with other centrally-acting drugs). Products include:

Nadolol (Because of its potential for inducing hypotension, risperidone may enhance the hypotensive effects of other therapeutic agents with this potential). Products include:

Nicardipine Hydrochloride (Because of its potential for inducing hypotension, risperidone may enhance the hypotensive effects of other therapeutic agents with this potential). Products include:

Nifedipine (Because of its potential for inducing hypotension, risperidone may enhance the hypotensive effects of other therapeutic agents with this potential). Products include:

Nisoldipine (Because of its potential for inducing hypotension, risperidone may enhance the hypotensive effects of other therapeutic agents with this potential). Products include:

Nitroglycerin (Because of its potential for inducing hypotension, risperidone may enhance the hypotensive effects of other therapeutic agents with this potential). Products include:

Nortriptyline Hydrochloride (Risperidone is metabolized to 9-hydroxyrisperidone by CYP2D6. Drug interactions that reduce the metabolism of risperidone to 9-hydroxyrisperidone would increase the plasma concentrations of risperidone and lower the concentrations of 9-hydroxyrisperidone).

No products indexed under this heading.

Olanzapine (Given the primary CNS effects of risperidone, caution should be used if taken in combination with other centrally-acting drugs). Products include:

Oxazepam (Given the primary CNS effects of risperidone, caution should be used if taken in combination with other centrally-acting drugs).

No products indexed under this heading.

Oxycodone Hydrochloride (Given the primary CNS effects of risperidone, caution should be used if taken in combination with other centrally-acting drugs). Products include:

Paroxetine Hydrochloride (Paroxetine (20mg QD) has been shown to increase the plasma concentration of risperidone 3- to 9-fold and lower the concentration of 9-hydroxyrisperidone an average of 13%. When concomitant paroxetine is initiated or discontinued, the dosage of risperidone should be re-evaluated). Products include:

Pemoline (Given the primary CNS effects of risperdone, caution should be taken with other centrally-acting drugs).

No products indexed under this heading.

Penbutolol Sulfate (Because of its potential for inducing hypotension, risperidone may enhance the hypotensive effects of other therapeutic agents with this potential).

No products indexed under this heading.

Pentobarbital Sodium (Given the primary CNS effects of risperidone, caution should be used if taken in combination with other centrally-acting drugs). Products include:

Pergolide Mesylate (Risperidone may antagonize the effect of dopamine agonists). Products include:

Perindopril Erbumine (Because of its potential for inducing hypotension, risperidone may enhance the hypotensive effects of other therapeutic agents with this potential). Products include:

Perphenazine (Given the primary CNS effects of risperidone, caution should be used if taken in combination with other centrally-acting drugs).

No products indexed under this heading.

Phenobarbital (Co-administration of known enzyme inducers (e.g., phenytoin, rifampin and phenobarbital) with risperidone may cause decreases in the combined plasma concentrations of risperidone and 9-hydroxyrisperidone, which could lead to decreased efficacy. The dose of risperidone may need to be adjusted accordingly, particularly during the initiation or discontinuation of therapy with enzyme inducers). Products include:

Phenoxybenzamine Hydrochloride (Because of its potential for inducing hypotension, risperidone may enhance the hypotensive effects of other therapeutic agents with this potential). Products include:

Phentolamine Mesylate (Because of its potential for inducing hypotension, risperidone may enhance the hypotensive effects of other therapeutic agents with this potential).

No products indexed under this heading.

Phenylbutazone (Co-administration of known enzyme inducers (e.g., phenytoin, rifampin and phenobarbi-

tal) with risperidone may cause decreases in the combined plasma concentrations of risperidone and 9-hydroxyrisperidone, which could lead to decreased efficacy. The dose of risperidone may need to be adjusted accordingly, particularly during the initiation or discontinuation of therapy with enzyme inducers).

No products indexed under this heading.

Phenytoin (Co-administration of known enzyme inducers (e.g., phenytoin, rifampin and phenobarbital) with risperidone may cause decreases in the combined plasma concentrations of risperidone and 9-hydroxyrisperidone, which could lead to decreased efficacy. The dose of risperidone may need to be adjusted accordingly, particularly during the initiation or discontinuation of therapy with enzyme inducers).

No products indexed under this heading.

Phenytoin Sodium (Co-administration of known enzyme inducers (e.g., phenytoin, rifampin and phenobarbital) with risperidone may cause decreases in the combined plasma concentrations of risperidone and 9-hydroxyrisperidone, which could lead to decreased efficacy. The dose of risperidone may need to be adjusted accordingly, particularly during the initiation or discontinuation of therapy with enzyme inducers). Products include:

Pindolol (Because of its potential for inducing hypotension, risperidone may enhance the hypotensive effects of other therapeutic agents with this potential).

No products indexed under this heading.

Polythiazide (Because of its potential for inducing hypotension, risperidone may enhance the hypotensive effects of other therapeutic agents with this potential).

No products indexed under this heading.

Pramipexole Dihydrochloride (Risperidone may antagonize the effect of dopamine agonists). Products include:

Prazepam (Given the primary CNS effects of risperidone, caution should be used if taken in combination with other centrally-acting drugs).

No products indexed under this heading.

Prazosin Hydrochloride (Because of its potential for inducing hypotension, risperidone may enhance the hypotensive effects of other therapeutic agents with this potential).

No products indexed under this heading.

Prochlorperazine (Given the primary CNS effects of risperidone, caution should be used if taken in combination with other centrally-acting drugs).

No products indexed under this heading.

Promethazine Hydrochloride (Given the primary CNS effects of risperidone, caution should be used if taken in combination with other centrally-acting drugs). Products include:

Propafenone Hydrochloride (Risperidone is metabolized to 9-hydroxyrisperidone by CYP2D6. Drug interactions that reduce the metabolism of risperidone to 9-hydroxyrisperidone would increase the plasma concentrations of risperidone and lower the concentrations of 9-hydroxyrisperidone). Products include:

Propofol (Given the primary CNS effects of risperidone, caution should be used if taken in combination with other centrally-acting drugs).

No products indexed under this heading.

Propoxyphene Hydrochloride (Given the primary CNS effects of risperidone, caution should be used if taken in combination with other centrally-acting drugs).

No products indexed under this heading.

Propoxyphene Napsylate (Given the primary CNS effects of risperidone, caution should be used if taken in combination with other centrally-acting drugs).

No products indexed under this heading.

Propranolol Hydrochloride (Because of its potential for inducing hypotension, risperidone may enhance the hypotensive effects of other therapeutic agents with this potential). Products include:

Protriptyline Hydrochloride (Risperidone is metabolized to 9-hydroxyrisperidone by CYP2D6. Drug interactions that reduce the metabolism of risperidone to 9-hydroxyrisperidone would increase the plasma concentrations of risperidone and lower the concentrations of 9-hydroxyrisperidone).

No products indexed under this heading.

Quazepam (Given the primary CNS effects of risperidone, caution should be used if taken in combination with other centrally-acting drugs).

No products indexed under this heading.

Quetiapine Fumarate (Given the primary CNS effects of risperidone, caution should be used if taken in combination with other centrally-acting drugs). Products include:

Quinacrine Hydrochloride (Risperidone is metabolized to 9-hydroxyrisperidone by CYP2D6. Drug interactions that reduce the metabolism of risperidone to 9-hydroxyrisperidone would increase the plasma concentrations of risperidone and lower the concentrations of 9-hydroxyrisperidone).

No products indexed under this heading.

Quinapril Hydrochloride (Because of its potential for inducing hypotension, risperidone may enhance the hypotensive effects of other therapeutic agents with this potential).

No products indexed under this heading.

IMPORTANT NOTE: Always consult each drug listing in the patient's regimen for possible interactions.

Quinidine Gluconate (Risperidone is metabolized to 9-hydroxyrisperidone by CYP2D6. Drug interactions that reduce the metabolism of risperidone to 9-hydroxyrisperidone would increase the plasma concentrations of risperidone and lower the concentrations of 9-hydroxyrisperidone).
No products indexed under this heading.

Quinidine Hydrochloride (Risperidone is metabolized to 9-hydroxyrisperidone by CYP2D6. Drug interactions that reduce the metabolism of risperidone to 9-hydroxyrisperidone would increase the plasma concentrations of risperidone and lower the concentrations of 9-hydroxyrisperidone).
No products indexed under this heading.

Quinidine Polygalacturonate (Risperidone is metabolized to 9-hydroxyrisperidone by CYP2D6. Drug interactions that reduce the metabolism of risperidone to 9-hydroxyrisperidone would increase the plasma concentrations of risperidone and lower the concentrations of 9-hydroxyrisperidone).
No products indexed under this heading.

Quinidine Sulfate (Risperidone is metabolized to 9-hydroxyrisperidone by CYP2D6. Drug interactions that reduce the metabolism of risperidone to 9-hydroxyrisperidone would increase the plasma concentrations of risperidone and lower the concentrations of 9-hydroxyrisperidone).
No products indexed under this heading.

Ramipril (Because of its potential for inducing hypotension, risperidone may enhance the hypotensive effects of other therapeutic agents with this potential). Products include:
Altace Capsules ... 1702

Ranitidine Bismuth Citrate (Cimetidine increased the bioavailability of risperidone, but only marginally increased the plasma concentration of the active anti-psychotic fraction).
No products indexed under this heading.

Ranitidine Hydrochloride (Cimetidine increased the bioavailability of risperidone, but only marginally increased the plasma concentration of the active anti-psychotic fraction). Products include:
Zantac ... 1624
Zantac Injection ... 1619
Zantac Injection Pharmacy Bulk Package ... 1622

Rauwolfia Serpentina (Because of its potential for inducing hypotension, risperidone may enhance the hypotensive effects of other therapeutic agents with this potential).
No products indexed under this heading.

Remifentanil Hydrochloride (Given the primary CNS effects of risperidone, caution should be used if taken in combination with other centrally-acting drugs).
No products indexed under this heading.

Rescinnamine (Because of its potential for inducing hypotension, risperidone may enhance the hypotensive effects of other therapeutic agents with this potential).
No products indexed under this heading.

Reserpine (Because of its potential for inducing hypotension, risperidone may enhance the hypotensive effects of other therapeutic agents with this potential).
No products indexed under this heading.

Rifampin (Co-administration of known enzyme inducers (e.g., phenytoin, rifampin and phenobarbital) with risperidone may cause decreases in the combined plasma concentrations of risperidone and 9-hydroxyrisperidone, which could lead to decreased efficacy. The dose of risperidone may need to be adjusted accordingly, particularly during the initiation or discontinuation of therapy with enzyme inducers).
No products indexed under this heading.

Rifapentine (Co-administration of known enzyme inducers (e.g., phenytoin, rifampin and phenobarbital) with risperidone may cause decreases in the combined plasma concentrations of risperidone and 9-hydroxyrisperidone, which could lead to decreased efficacy. The dose of risperidone may need to be adjusted accordingly, particularly during the initiation or discontinuation of therapy with enzyme inducers).
No products indexed under this heading.

Ritonavir (Risperidone is metabolized to 9-hydroxyrisperidone by CYP2D6. Drug interactions that reduce the metabolism of risperidone to 9-hydroxyrisperidone would increase the plasma concentrations of risperidone and lower the concentrations of 9-hydroxyrisperidone). Products include:
Kaletra ... 476
Norvir ... 503

Ropinirole Hydrochloride (Risperidone may antagonize the effect of dopamine agonists). Products include:
Requip Tablets ... 1555

Secobarbital Sodium (Given the primary CNS effects of risperidone, caution should be used if taken in combination with other centrally-acting drugs).
No products indexed under this heading.

Sertraline Hydrochloride (Risperidone is metabolized to 9-hydroxyrisperidone by CYP2D6. Drug interactions that reduce the metabolism of risperidone to 9-hydroxyrisperidone would increase the plasma concentrations of risperidone and lower the concentrations of 9-hydroxyrisperidone). Products include:
Zoloft ... 2586

Sevoflurane (Given the primary CNS effects of risperidone, caution should be used if taken in combination with other centrally-acting drugs). Products include:
Ultane Liquid for Inhalation ... 531

Sodium Nitroprusside (Because of its potential for inducing hypotension, risperidone may enhance the hypotensive effects of other therapeutic agents with this potential).
No products indexed under this heading.

Sodium Oxybate (Given the primary CNS effects of risperidone, caution should be used if taken in combination with other centrally-acting drugs). Products include:
Xyrem Oral Solution ... 1688

Sotalol Hydrochloride (Because of its potential for inducing hypotension, risperidone may enhance the hypotensive effects of other therapeutic agents with this potential).
No products indexed under this heading.

Spirapril Hydrochloride (Because of its potential for inducing hypotension, risperidone may enhance the hypotensive effects of other therapeutic agents with this potential).
No products indexed under this heading.

Sufentanil Citrate (Given the primary CNS effects of risperidone, caution should be used if taken in combination with other centrally-acting drugs).
No products indexed under this heading.

Telmisartan (Because of its potential for inducing hypotension, risperidone may enhance the hypotensive effects of other therapeutic agents with this potential). Products include:
Micardis Tablets ... 854
Micardis HCT Tablets ... 856

Temazepam (Given the primary CNS effects of risperidone, caution should be used if taken in combination with other centrally-acting drugs). Products include:
Restoril Capsules ... 1860

Terazosin Hydrochloride (Because of its potential for inducing hypotension, risperidone may enhance the hypotensive effects of other therapeutic agents with this potential). Products include:
Hytrin Capsules ... 471

Terbinafine Hydrochloride (Risperidone is metabolized to 9-hydroxyrisperidone by CYP2D6. Drug interactions that reduce the metabolism of risperidone to 9-hydroxyrisperidone would increase the plasma concentrations of risperidone and lower the concentrations of 9-hydroxyrisperidone). Products include:
Lamisil Tablets ... 2232
Lamisil AT Creams (Athlete's Foot & Jock Itch) ... ▣636

Thiamylal Sodium (Given the primary CNS effects of risperidone, caution should be used if taken in combination with other centrally-acting drugs).
No products indexed under this heading.

Thioridazine Hydrochloride (Given the primary CNS effects of risperidone, caution should be used if taken in combination with other centrally-acting drugs). Products include:
Thioridazine Hydrochloride Tablets ... 2163

Thiothixene (Given the primary CNS effects of risperidone, caution should be used if taken in combination with other centrally-acting drugs). Products include:
Thiothixene Capsules ... 2165

Timolol Maleate (Because of its potential for inducing hypotension, risperidone may enhance the hypotensive effects of other therapeutic agents with this potential). Products include:
Blocadren Tablets ... 1916
Cosopt Sterile Ophthalmic Solution ... 1931
Timolide Tablets ... 2086
Timoptic Sterile Ophthalmic Solution ... 2088
Timoptic in Ocudose ... 2091
Timoptic-XE Sterile Ophthalmic Gel Forming Solution ... 2092

Tolazamide (Co-administration of known enzyme inducers (e.g., phenytoin, rifampin and phenobarbital) with risperidone may cause decreases in the combined plasma concentrations of risperidone and 9-hydroxyrisperidone, which could lead to decreased efficacy. The dose of risperidone may need to be adjusted accordingly, particularly during the initiation or discontinuation of therapy with enzyme inducers).
No products indexed under this heading.

Tolbutamide (Co-administration of known enzyme inducers (e.g., phenytoin, rifampin and phenobarbital) with risperidone may cause decreases in the combined plasma concentrations of risperidone and 9-hydroxyrisperidone, which could lead to decreased efficacy. The dose of risperidone may need to be adjusted accordingly, particularly during the initiation or discontinuation of therapy with enzyme inducers).
No products indexed under this heading.

Torsemide (Because of its potential for inducing hypotension, risperidone may enhance the hypotensive effects of other therapeutic agents with this potential). Products include:
Demadex Injection ... 2759
Demadex Tablets ... 2759

Trandolapril (Because of its potential for inducing hypotension, risperidone may enhance the hypotensive effects of other therapeutic agents with this potential). Products include:
Mavik Tablets ... 486
Tarka Tablets ... 524

Triazolam (Given the primary CNS effects of risperidone, caution should be used if taken in combination with other centrally-acting drugs).
No products indexed under this heading.

Trifluoperazine Hydrochloride (Given the primary CNS effects of risperidone, caution should be used if taken in combination with other centrally-acting drugs).
No products indexed under this heading.

Trimethaphan Camsylate (Because of its potential for inducing hypotension, risperidone may enhance the hypotensive effects of other therapeutic agents with this potential).
No products indexed under this heading.

Trimipramine Maleate (Risperidone is metabolized to 9-hydroxyrisperidone by CYP2D6. Drug interactions that reduce the metabolism of risperidone to 9-hydroxyrisperidone would increase the plasma concentrations of risperidone and lower the concentrations of 9-hydroxyrisperidone).
No products indexed under this heading.

Valproate Sodium (Repeated oral doses of risperidone (4mg QD) did not affect the pre-dose or average plasma concentrations exposure (AUC) of valproate (1000 mg/day in three divided doses) compared to placebo (n=21). However, there was a 20% increase of valproate peak plasma concentration (Cmax) after concomitant administration of risperidone). Products include:

Depacon Injection 412

Valsartan (Because of its potential for inducing hypotension, risperidone may enhance the hypotensive effects of other therapeutic agents with this potential). Products include:

Diovan Tablets 2193
Diovan HCT Tablets 2196

Verapamil Hydrochloride (Because of its potential for inducing hypotension, risperidone may enhance the hypotensive effects of other therapeutic agents with this potential). Products include:

Covera-HS Tablets 3139
Tarka Tablets 524
Verelan PM Extended-Release Capsules, Controlled-Onset 3106

Zaleplon (Given the primary CNS effects of risperidone, caution should be used if taken in combination with other centrally-acting drugs). Products include:

Sonata Capsules 1717

Ziprasidone Hydrochloride (Given the primary CNS effects of risperidone, caution should be used if taken in combination with other centrally-acting drugs). Products include:

Geodon Capsules 2529

Zolpidem Tartrate (Given the primary CNS effects of risperidone, caution should be used if taken in combination with other centrally-acting drugs). Products include:

Ambien Tablets 2851
Ambien CR Tablets 2855

Food Interactions

Alcohol (Caution should be used when risperidone is taken in combination with alcohol).

RISPERDAL CONSTA LONG-ACTING INJECTION

(Risperidone) 1682
See Risperdal Tablets

RISPERDAL M-TAB ORALLY DISINTEGRATING TABLETS

(Risperidone) 1676
See Risperdal Tablets

RITALIN HYDROCHLORIDE TABLETS

(Methylphenidate Hydrochloride) 2269
May interact with oral anticoagulants, anticonvulsants, monoamine oxidase inhibitors, tricyclic antidepressants, vasopressors, and certain other agents. Compounds in these categories include:

Amitriptyline Hydrochloride (Human pharmacologic studies have shown that racemic methylphenidate may inhibit the metabolism of coumarin anticoagulants, anticonvulsants (e.g., phenobarbital, phenytoin, primidone), and tricyclic drugs (e.g., imipramine, clomipramine, desipramine). It may be necessary to adjust the dosage and monitor plasma drug concentration (or, in case of coumarin, coagulation times), when initiating or discontinuing

methylphenidate).
No products indexed under this heading.

Amoxapine (Human pharmacologic studies have shown that racemic methylphenidate may inhibit the metabolism of coumarin anticoagulants, anticonvulsants (e.g., phenobarbital, phenytoin, primidone), and tricyclic drugs (e.g., imipramine, clomipramine, desipramine). It may be necessary to adjust the dosage and monitor plasma drug concentration (or, in case of coumarin, coagulation times), when initiating or discontinuing methylphenidate).
No products indexed under this heading.

Anisindione (Human pharmacologic studies have shown that racemic methylphenidate may inhibit the metabolism of coumarin anticoagulants, anticonvulsants (e.g., phenobarbital, phenytoin, primidone), and tricyclic drugs (e.g., imipramine, clomipramine, desipramine). It may be necessary to adjust the dosage and monitor plasma drug concentration (or, in case of coumarin, coagulation times), when initiating or discontinuing methylphenidate). Products include:

Miradon Tablets 3042

Carbamazepine (Human pharmacologic studies have shown that racemic methylphenidate may inhibit the metabolism of coumarin anticoagulants, anticonvulsants (e.g., phenobarbital, phenytoin, primidone), and tricyclic drugs (e.g., imipramine, clomipramine, desipramine). It may be necessary to adjust the dosage and monitor plasma drug concentration (or, in case of coumarin, coagulation times), when initiating or discontinuing methylphenidate). Products include:

Carbatrol Capsules 3171
Equetro Extended-Release Capsules 3180
Tegretol/Tegretol-XR 2295

Clomipramine Hydrochloride (Human pharmacologic studies have shown that racemic methylphenidate may inhibit the metabolism of coumarin anticoagulants, anticonvulsants (e.g., phenobarbital, phenytoin, primidone), and tricyclic drugs (e.g., imipramine, clomipramine, desipramine). It may be necessary to adjust the dosage and monitor plasma drug concentration (or, in case of coumarin, coagulation times), when initiating or discontinuing methylphenidate).
No products indexed under this heading.

Clonidine (Serious adverse events have been reported in concomitant use with clonidine). Products include:

Catapres-TTS 844

Desipramine Hydrochloride (Human pharmacologic studies have shown that racemic methylphenidate may inhibit the metabolism of coumarin anticoagulants, anticonvulsants (e.g., phenobarbital, phenytoin, primidone), and tricyclic drugs (e.g., imipramine, clomipramine, desipramine). It may be necessary to adjust the dosage and monitor plasma drug concentration (or, in case of coumarin, coagulation times), when initiating or discontinuing methylphenidate).
No products indexed under this heading.

Dicumarol (Human pharmacologic studies have shown that racemic methylphenidate may inhibit the metabolism of coumarin anticoagulants, anticonvulsants (e.g., phenobarbital, phenytoin, primidone), and tricyclic drugs (e.g., imipramine, clomipramine, desipramine). It may be necessary to adjust the dosage and monitor plasma drug concentration (or, in case of coumarin, coagulation times), when initiating or discontinuing methylphenidate).
No products indexed under this heading.

Divalproex Sodium (Human pharmacologic studies have shown that racemic methylphenidate may inhibit the metabolism of coumarin anticoagulants, anticonvulsants (e.g., phenobarbital, phenytoin, primidone), and tricyclic drugs (e.g., imipramine, clomipramine, desipramine). It may be necessary to adjust the dosage and monitor plasma drug concentration (or, in case of coumarin, coagulation times), when initiating or discontinuing methylphenidate). Products include:

Depakote Sprinkle Capsules 422
Depakote Tablets 427
Depakote ER Tablets 434

Dobutamine (Because of possible effects on blood pressure, Methylphenidate should be used cautiously with pressor agents).
No products indexed under this heading.

Dobutamine Hydrochloride (Because of possible effects on blood pressure, Methylphenidate should be used cautiously with pressor agents).
No products indexed under this heading.

Dopamine Hydrochloride (Because of possible effects on blood pressure, Methylphenidate should be used cautiously with pressor agents).
No products indexed under this heading.

Doxepin Hydrochloride (Human pharmacologic studies have shown that racemic methylphenidate may inhibit the metabolism of coumarin anticoagulants, anticonvulsants (e.g., phenobarbital, phenytoin, primidone), and tricyclic drugs (e.g., imipramine, clomipramine, desipramine). It may be necessary to adjust the dosage and monitor plasma drug concentration (or, in case of coumarin, coagulation times), when initiating or discontinuing methylphenidate).
No products indexed under this heading.

Ephedrine Sulfate (Because of possible effects on blood pressure, Methylphenidate should be used cautiously with pressor agents).
No products indexed under this heading.

Epinephrine Bitartrate (Because of possible effects on blood pressure, Methylphenidate should be used cautiously with pressor agents).
No products indexed under this heading.

Epinephrine Hydrochloride (Because of possible effects on blood pressure, Methylphenidate should be used cautiously with pressor agents).
No products indexed under this heading.

Ethosuximide (Human pharmacologic studies have shown that racemic methylphenidate may inhibit the metabolism of coumarin anticoagulants, anticonvulsants (e.g., phenobarbital, phenytoin, primidone), and tricyclic drugs (e.g., imipramine, clomipramine, desipramine). It may be necessary to adjust the dosage and monitor plasma drug concentration (or, in case of coumarin, coagulation times), when initiating or discontinuing methylphenidate).
No products indexed under this heading.

Ethotoin (Human pharmacologic studies have shown that racemic methylphenidate may inhibit the metabolism of coumarin anticoagulants, anticonvulsants (e.g., phenobarbital, phenytoin, primidone), and tricyclic drugs (e.g., imipramine, clomipramine, desipramine). It may be necessary to adjust the dosage and monitor plasma drug concentration (or, in case of coumarin, coagulation times), when initiating or discontinuing methylphenidate).
No products indexed under this heading.

Felbamate (Human pharmacologic studies have shown that racemic methylphenidate may inhibit the metabolism of coumarin anticoagulants, anticonvulsants (e.g., phenobarbital, phenytoin, primidone), and tricyclic drugs (e.g., imipramine, clomipramine, desipramine). It may be necessary to adjust the dosage and monitor plasma drug concentration (or, in case of coumarin, coagulation times), when initiating or discontinuing methylphenidate).
No products indexed under this heading.

Fosphenytoin (Human pharmacologic studies have shown that racemic methylphenidate may inhibit the metabolism of coumarin anticoagulants, anticonvulsants (e.g., phenobarbital, phenytoin, primidone), and tricyclic drugs (e.g., imipramine, clomipramine, desipramine). It may be necessary to adjust the dosage and monitor plasma drug concentration (or, in case of coumarin, coagulation times), when initiating or discontinuing methylphenidate).
No products indexed under this heading.

Fosphenytoin Sodium (Human pharmacologic studies have shown that racemic methylphenidate may inhibit the metabolism of coumarin anticoagulants, anticonvulsants (e.g., phenobarbital, phenytoin, primidone), and tricyclic drugs (e.g., imipramine, clomipramine, desipramine). It may be necessary to adjust the dosage and monitor plasma drug concentration (or, in case of coumarin, coagulation times), when initiating or discontinuing methylphenidate).
No products indexed under this heading.

Gabapentin (Human pharmacologic studies have shown that racemic methylphenidate may inhibit the metabolism of coumarin anticoagulants, anticonvulsants (e.g., phenobarbital, phenytoin, primidone), and tricyclic drugs (e.g., imipramine, clomipramine, desipramine). It may be necessary to adjust the dosage and monitor plasma drug concentration (or, in case of coumarin, coagulation times), when initiating or discontinuing methylphenidate).

Products include:

Imipramine Hydrochloride
(Human pharmacologic studies have shown that racemic methylphenidate may inhibit the metabolism of coumarin anticoagulants, anticonvulsants (e.g., phenobarbital, phenytoin, primidone), and tricyclic drugs (e.g., imipramine, clomipramine, desipramine). It may be necessary to adjust the dosage and monitor plasma drug concentration (or, in case of coumarin, coagulation times), when initiating or discontinuing methylphenidate).

No products indexed under this heading.

Imipramine Pamoate (Human pharmacologic studies have shown that racemic methylphenidate may inhibit the metabolism of coumarin anticoagulants, anticonvulsants (e.g., phenobarbital, phenytoin, primidone), and tricyclic drugs (e.g., imipramine, clomipramine, desipramine). It may be necessary to adjust the dosage and monitor plasma drug concentration (or, in case of coumarin, coagulation times), when initiating or discontinuing methylphenidate).

No products indexed under this heading.

Isocarboxazid (Methylphenidate should not be used in patients being treated with MAO Inhibitors).

No products indexed under this heading.

Isoproterenol Hydrochloride
(Because of possible effects on blood pressure, Methylphenidate should be used cautiously with pressor agents).

No products indexed under this heading.

Isoproterenol Sulfate (Because of possible effects on blood pressure, Methylphenidate should be used cautiously with pressor agents).

No products indexed under this heading.

Lamotrigine (Human pharmacologic studies have shown that racemic methylphenidate may inhibit the metabolism of coumarin anticoagulants, anticonvulsants (e.g., phenobarbital, phenytoin, primidone), and tricyclic drugs (e.g., imipramine, clomipramine, desipramine). It may be necessary to adjust the dosage and monitor plasma drug concentration (or, in case of coumarin, coagulation times), when initiating or discontinuing methylphenidate).

Products include:

Levetiracetam (Human pharmacologic studies have shown that racemic methylphenidate may inhibit the metabolism of coumarin anticoagulants, anticonvulsants (e.g., phenobarbital, phenytoin, primidone), and tricyclic drugs (e.g., imipramine, clomipramine, desipramine). It may be necessary to adjust the dosage and monitor plasma drug concentration (or, in case of coumarin, coagulation times), when initiating or discontinuing methylphenidate).

Products include:

Maprotiline Hydrochloride
(Human pharmacologic studies have shown that racemic methylphenidate may inhibit the metabolism of coumarin anticoagulants, anticonvulsants (e.g., phenobarbital, phenytoin, primidone), and tricyclic drugs (e.g., imipramine, clomipramine, desipramine). It may be necessary to adjust the dosage and monitor plasma drug concentration (or, in case of coumarin, coagulation times), when initiating or discontinuing methylphenidate).

No products indexed under this heading.

Mephentermine Sulfate (Because of possible effects on blood pressure, Methylphenidate should be used cautiously with pressor agents).

No products indexed under this heading.

Mephenytoin (Human pharmacologic studies have shown that racemic methylphenidate may inhibit the metabolism of coumarin anticoagulants, anticonvulsants (e.g., phenobarbital, phenytoin, primidone), and tricyclic drugs (e.g., imipramine, clomipramine, desipramine). It may be necessary to adjust the dosage and monitor plasma drug concentration (or, in case of coumarin, coagulation times), when initiating or discontinuing methylphenidate).

No products indexed under this heading.

Metaraminol Bitartrate (Because of possible effects on blood pressure, Methylphenidate should be used cautiously with pressor agents).

No products indexed under this heading.

Methoxamine Hydrochloride
(Because of possible effects on blood pressure, Methylphenidate should be used cautiously with pressor agents).

No products indexed under this heading.

Methsuximide (Human pharmacologic studies have shown that racemic methylphenidate may inhibit the metabolism of coumarin anticoagulants, anticonvulsants (e.g., phenobarbital, phenytoin, primidone), and tricyclic drugs (e.g., imipramine, clomipramine, desipramine). It may be necessary to adjust the dosage and monitor plasma drug concentration (or, in case of coumarin, coagulation times), when initiating or discontinuing methylphenidate).

No products indexed under this heading.

Moclobemide (Methylphenidate should not be used in patients treated with MAO Inhibitors).

No products indexed under this heading.

Norepinephrine Bitartrate
(Because of possible effects on blood pressure, Methylphenidate should be used cautiously with pressor agents).

No products indexed under this heading.

Nortriptyline Hydrochloride
(Human pharmacologic studies have shown that racemic methylphenidate may inhibit the metabolism of coumarin anticoagulants, anticonvulsants (e.g., phenobarbital, phenytoin, primidone), and tricyclic drugs

(e.g., imipramine, clomipramine, desipramine). It may be necessary to adjust the dosage and monitor plasma drug concentration (or, in case of coumarin, coagulation times), when initiating or discontinuing methylphenidate).

No products indexed under this heading.

Oxcarbazepine (Human pharmacologic studies have shown that racemic methylphenidate may inhibit the metabolism of coumarin anticoagulants, anticonvulsants (e.g., phenobarbital, phenytoin, primidone), and tricyclic drugs (e.g., imipramine, clomipramine, desipramine). It may be necessary to adjust the dosage and monitor plasma drug concentration (or, in case of coumarin, coagulation times), when initiating or discontinuing methylphenidate).

Products include:

Paramethadione (Human pharmacologic studies have shown that racemic methylphenidate may inhibit the metabolism of coumarin anticoagulants, anticonvulsants (e.g., phenobarbital, phenytoin, primidone), and tricyclic drugs (e.g., imipramine, clomipramine, desipramine). It may be necessary to adjust the dosage and monitor plasma drug concentration (or, in case of coumarin, coagulation times), when initiating or discontinuing methylphenidate).

No products indexed under this heading.

Pargyline Hydrochloride (Methylphenidate should not be used in patients being treated with MAO Inhibitors).

No products indexed under this heading.

Phenacemide (Human pharmacologic studies have shown that racemic methylphenidate may inhibit the metabolism of coumarin anticoagulants, anticonvulsants (e.g., phenobarbital, phenytoin, primidone), and tricyclic drugs (e.g., imipramine, clomipramine, desipramine). It may be necessary to adjust the dosage and monitor plasma drug concentration (or, in case of coumarin, coagulation times), when initiating or discontinuing methylphenidate).

No products indexed under this heading.

Phenelzine Sulfate (Methylphenidate should not be used in patients being treated with MAO Inhibitors).

No products indexed under this heading.

Phenobarbital (Human pharmacologic studies have shown that racemic methylphenidate may inhibit the metabolism of coumarin anticoagulants, anticonvulsants (e.g., phenobarbital, phenytoin, primidone), and tricyclic drugs (e.g., imipramine, clomipramine, desipramine). It may be necessary to adjust the dosage and monitor plasma drug concentration (or, in case of coumarin, coagulation times), when initiating or discontinuing methylphenidate).

Products include:

Phensuximide (Human pharmacologic studies have shown that racemic methylphenidate may inhibit the metabolism of coumarin anticoagulants, anticonvulsants (e.g., phenobarbital, phenytoin, primidone), and

tricyclic drugs (e.g., imipramine, clomipramine, desipramine). It may be necessary to adjust the dosage and monitor plasma drug concentration (or, in case of coumarin, coagulation times), when initiating or discontinuing methylphenidate).

No products indexed under this heading.

Phenylephrine Hydrochloride
(Because of possible effects on blood pressure, Methylphenidate should be used cautiously with pressor agents). Products include:

Tylenol Cold Multi-Symptom Severe Daytime Liquid 752
Concentrated Tylenol Infants' Drops Plus Cold & Cough 754
Tylenol Allergy Multi-Symptom Caplets with Cool Burst and Gelcaps 1872
Tylenol Allergy Multi-Symptom Nighttime Caplets with Cool Burst 1872
Children's Tylenol Plus Cold Suspension Liquid 1879
Children's Tylenol Plus Cold & Allergy Suspension Liquid 1878
Children's Tylenol Plus Flu Suspension Liquid 1881
Children's Tylenol Plus Multi-Symptom Cold Suspension Liquid 1879
Tylenol Cold Head Congestion Daytime Caplets with Cool Burst 1873
Tylenol Cold Head Congestion Nighttime Caplets with Cool Burst 1873
Tylenol Cold Head Congestion Severe Caplets with Cool Burst..... 1873
Tylenol Cold Multi-Symptom Daytime Caplets with Cool Burst and Gelcaps 1874
Tylenol Cold Multi-Symptom Daytime Liquid with Citrus Burst ... 1874
Tylenol Cold Multi-Symptom Nighttime Caplets with Cool Burst 1874
Tylenol Cold Multi-Symptom Nighttime Liquid with Cool Burst ... 1874
Tylenol Cold Multi-Symptom Severe Caplets with Cool Burst..... 1874
Tylenol Cold Multi-Symptom Severe Daytime Liquid with Citrus Burst 1874
Tylenol Sinus Congestion & Pain Daytime Caplets with Cool Burst and Gelcaps 1876
Tylenol Sinus Congestion & Pain Nighttime Caplets with Cool Burst 1876
Tylenol Sinus Congestion & Pain Severe Caplets with Cool Burst..... 1876
Vicks 44D Cough & Head Congestion Relief Liquid 760
Vicks DayQuil LiquiCaps/Liquid Multi-Symptom Cold/Flu Relief..... 761
Zicam Cough Plus D Cough Spray 767

Phenytoin (Human pharmacologic studies have shown that racemic methylphenidate may inhibit the metabolism of coumarin anticoagulants, anticonvulsants (e.g., phenobarbital, phenytoin, primidone), and tricyclic drugs (e.g., imipramine, clomipramine, desipramine). It may be necessary to adjust the dosage and monitor plasma drug concentration (or, in case of coumarin, coagulation times), when initiating or discontinuing methylphenidate).
No products indexed under this heading.

Phenytoin Sodium (Human pharmacologic studies have shown that racemic methylphenidate may inhibit the metabolism of coumarin anticoagulants, anticonvulsants (e.g., phenobarbital, phenytoin, primidone), and tricyclic drugs (e.g., imipramine, clomipramine, desipramine). It may be necessary to adjust the dosage and monitor plasma drug concentration (or, in case of coumarin, coagulation times), when initiating or discontinuing methylphenidate). Products include:
Phenytek Capsules 2160

Primidone (Human pharmacologic studies have shown that racemic methylphenidate may inhibit the metabolism of coumarin anticoagulants, anticonvulsants (e.g., phenobarbital, phenytoin, primidone), and tricyclic drugs (e.g., imipramine, clomipramine, desipramine). It may be necessary to adjust the dosage and monitor plasma drug concentration (or, in case of coumarin, coagulation times), when initiating or discontinuing methylphenidate).
No products indexed under this heading.

Procarbazine Hydrochloride (Methylphenidate should not be used in patients being treated with MAO Inhibitors). Products include:
Matulane Capsules 3191

Protriptyline Hydrochloride (Human pharmacologic studies have shown that racemic methylphenidate may inhibit the metabolism of coumarin anticoagulants, anticonvulsants (e.g., phenobarbital, phenytoin, primidone), and tricyclic drugs (e.g., imipramine, clomipramine, desipramine). It may be necessary to adjust the dosage and monitor plasma drug concentration (or, in case of coumarin, coagulation times), when initiating or discontinuing methylphenidate).
No products indexed under this heading.

Selegiline Hydrochloride (Methylphenidate should not be used in patients being treated with MAO Inhibitors). Products include:
Eldepryl Capsules 3208
Zelapar Tablets 3372

Tiagabine Hydrochloride (Human pharmacologic studies have shown that racemic methylphenidate may inhibit the metabolism of coumarin anticoagulants, anticonvulsants (e.g., phenobarbital, phenytoin, primidone), and tricyclic drugs (e.g., imipramine, clomipramine, desipramine). It may be necessary to adjust the dosage and monitor plasma drug concentration (or, in case of coumarin, coagulation times), when initiating or discontinuing methylphenidate). Products include:
Gabitril Tablets 984

Topiramate (Human pharmacologic studies have shown that racemic methylphenidate may inhibit the metabolism of coumarin anticoagulants, anticonvulsants (e.g., phenobarbital, phenytoin, primidone), and tricyclic drugs (e.g., imipramine, clomipramine, desipramine). It may be necessary to adjust the dosage and monitor plasma drug concentration (or, in case of coumarin, coagulation times), when initiating or discontinuing methylphenidate). Products include:
Topamax Sprinkle Capsules 2404
Topamax Tablets 2404

Tranylcypromine Sulfate (Methylphenidate should not be used in patients being treated with MAO Inhibitors). Products include:
Parnate Tablets 1527

Trimethadione (Human pharmacologic studies have shown that racemic methylphenidate may inhibit the metabolism of coumarin anticoagulants, anticonvulsants (e.g., phenobarbital, phenytoin, primidone), and tricyclic drugs (e.g., imipramine, clomipramine, desipramine). It may be necessary to adjust the dosage and monitor plasma drug concentration (or, in case of coumarin, coagulation times), when initiating or discontinuing methylphenidate).
No products indexed under this heading.

Trimipramine Maleate (Human pharmacologic studies have shown that racemic methylphenidate may inhibit the metabolism of coumarin anticoagulants, anticonvulsants (e.g., phenobarbital, phenytoin, primidone), and tricyclic drugs (e.g., imipramine, clomipramine, desipramine). It may be necessary to adjust the dosage and monitor plasma drug concentration (or, in case of coumarin, coagulation times), when initiating or discontinuing methylphenidate).
No products indexed under this heading.

Valproate Sodium (Human pharmacologic studies have shown that racemic methylphenidate may inhibit the metabolism of coumarin anticoagulants, anticonvulsants (e.g., phenobarbital, phenytoin, primidone), and tricyclic drugs (e.g., imipramine, clomipramine, desipramine). It may be necessary to adjust the dosage and monitor plasma drug concentration (or, in case of coumarin, coagulation times), when initiating or discontinuing methylphenidate). Products include:
Depacon Injection 412

Valproic Acid (Human pharmacologic studies have shown that racemic methylphenidate may inhibit the metabolism of coumarin anticoagulants, anticonvulsants (e.g., phenobarbital, phenytoin, primidone), and tricyclic drugs (e.g., imipramine, clomipramine, desipramine). It may be necessary to adjust the dosage and monitor plasma drug concentration (or, in case of coumarin, coagulation times), when initiating or discontinuing methylphenidate). Products include:
Depakene 417

Warfarin Sodium (Human pharmacologic studies have shown that racemic methylphenidate may inhibit the metabolism of coumarin anticoagulants, anticonvulsants (e.g., phenobarbital, phenytoin, primidone), and tricyclic drugs (e.g., imipramine, clomipramine, desipramine). It may be necessary to adjust the dosage and monitor plasma drug concentration (or, in case of coumarin, coagulation times), when initiating or discontinuing methylphenidate). Products include:
Coumadin for Injection 898
Coumadin Tablets 898

Zonisamide (Human pharmacologic studies have shown that racemic methylphenidate may inhibit the metabolism of coumarin anticoagulants, anticonvulsants (e.g., phenobarbital, phenytoin, primidone), and tricyclic drugs (e.g., imipramine, clomipramine, desipramine). It may be necessary to adjust the dosage and monitor plasma drug concentration (or, in case of coumarin, coagulation times), when initiating or discontinuing methylphenidate). Products include:
Zonegran Capsules 1101

RITALIN LA CAPSULES

(Methylphenidate Hydrochloride) 2271
May interact with antacids, oral anticoagulants, histamine H2-receptor antagonists, monoamine oxidase inhibitors, phenytoin, proton pump inhibitor, tricyclic antidepressants, vasopressors, and certain other agents. Compounds in these categories include:

Aluminum Carbonate (Since the modified release characteristics of Ritalin LA are pH dependent, the co-administration of antacids could alter the release of methylphenidate).
No products indexed under this heading.

Aluminum Hydroxide (Since the modified release characteristics of Ritalin LA are pH dependent, the co-administration of antacids could alter the release of methylphenidate). Products include:
Gaviscon Regular Strength Liquid .. 658
Gaviscon Regular Strength Tablets 658
Gaviscon Extra Strength Liquid 658
Gaviscon Extra Strength Tablets 658
Maalox Regular Strength Antacid/Antigas Liquid 2175
Maalox Max Maximum Strength Antacid/Anti-Gas Liquid 2176

Amitriptyline Hydrochloride (Methylphenidate inhibits the metabolism of tricyclic antidepressants).
No products indexed under this heading.

Amoxapine (Methylphenidate inhibits the metabolism of tricyclic antidepressants).
No products indexed under this heading.

Anisindione (Methylphenidate inhibits the metabolism of coumarin anticoagulants). Products include:
Miradon Tablets 3042

Cimetidine (Since the modified release characteristics of Ritalin LA are pH dependent, the co-administration of acid suppressants could alter the release of methylphenidate). Products include:
Tagamet HB 200 Tablets 664

Cimetidine Hydrochloride (Since the modified release characteristics of Ritalin LA are pH dependent, the co-administration of acid suppressants could alter the release of methylphenidate).
No products indexed under this heading.

Clomipramine Hydrochloride (Methylphenidate inhibits the metabolism of tricyclic antidepressants).
No products indexed under this heading.

Clonidine (Co-administration has resulted in serious adverse events). Products include:
Catapres-TTS 844

Clonidine Hydrochloride (Co-administration has resulted in serious adverse events). Products include:
Catapres Tablets 843
Clorpres Tablets 2153

Desipramine Hydrochloride (Methylphenidate inhibits the metabolism of tricyclic antidepressants).
No products indexed under this heading.

Dicumarol (Methylphenidate inhibits the metabolism of coumarin anticoagulants).
No products indexed under this heading.

Dobutamine (Possible additive effects on blood pressure with pressor agents if used concurrently).
No products indexed under this heading.

Dobutamine Hydrochloride (Possible additive effects on blood pressure with pressor agents if used concurrently).
No products indexed under this heading.

Dopamine Hydrochloride (Possible additive effects on blood pressure with pressor agents if used concurrently).
No products indexed under this heading.

Doxepin Hydrochloride (Methylphenidate inhibits the metabolism of tricyclic antidepressants).
No products indexed under this heading.

Ephedrine Sulfate (Possible additive effects on blood pressure with pressor agents if used concurrently).
No products indexed under this heading.

Epinephrine Bitartrate (Possible additive effects on blood pressure with pressor agents if used concurrently).
No products indexed under this heading.

Epinephrine Hydrochloride (Possible additive effects on blood pressure with pressor agents if used concurrently).
No products indexed under this heading.

Esomeprazole Magnesium (Since the modified release characteristics of Ritalin LA are pH dependent, the co-administration of acid suppressants could alter the release of methylphenidate). Products include:
- Nexium Delayed-Release Capsules 655

Famotidine (Since the modified release characteristics of Ritalin LA are pH dependent, the co-administration of acid suppressants could alter the release of methylphenidate). Products include:
- Pepcid Injection 2040
- Pepcid 2038
- Pepcid AC Gelcaps 1701
- Pepcid AC Tablets 1701
- Maximum Strength Pepcid AC Tablets 1701
- Pepcid Complete Chewable Tablets 1701

Fosphenytoin Sodium (Methylphenidate inhibits the metabolism of phenytoin).
No products indexed under this heading.

Guanethidine Monosulfate (Decreased hypotensive effect of guanethidine).
No products indexed under this heading.

Imipramine Hydrochloride (Methylphenidate inhibits the metabolism of tricyclic antidepressants).
No products indexed under this heading.

Imipramine Pamoate (Methylphenidate inhibits the metabolism of tricyclic antidepressants).
No products indexed under this heading.

Isocarboxazid (Concurrent and/or sequential use with MAO inhibitors may result in hypertensive crises; concurrent use or use within 14 days following discontinuation of an MAO inhibitor is contraindicated).
No products indexed under this heading.

Isoproterenol Hydrochloride (Possible additive effects on blood pressure with pressor agents if used concurrently).
No products indexed under this heading.

Isoproterenol Sulfate (Possible additive effects on blood pressure with pressor agents if used concurrently).
No products indexed under this heading.

Lansoprazole (Since the modified release characteristics of Ritalin LA are pH dependent, the co-administration of acid suppressants could alter the release of methylphenidate). Products include:
- Prevacid Delayed-Release Capsules 3271
- Prevacid for Delayed-Release Oral Suspension 3271
- Prevacid SoluTab Delayed-Release Orally Disintegrating Tablets 3271
- Prevacid I.V. for Injection 3277
- Prevacid NapraPAC 3280
- PREVPAC 3284

Magaldrate (Since the modified release characteristics of Ritalin LA are pH dependent, the co-administration of antacids could alter the release of methylphenidate).
No products indexed under this heading.

Magnesium Hydroxide (Since the modified release characteristics of Ritalin LA are pH dependent, the co-administration of antacids could alter the release of methylphenidate). Products include:
- Maalox Regular Strength Antacid/Antigas Liquid 2175
- Maalox Max Maximum Strength Antacid/Anti-Gas Liquid 2176
- Pepcid Complete Chewable Tablets 1701

Magnesium Oxide (Since the modified release characteristics of Ritalin LA are pH dependent, the co-administration of antacids could alter the release of methylphenidate). Products include:
- Beelith Tablets 759
- PremCal Light, Regular, and Extra Strength Tablets .... ■ 818

Maprotiline Hydrochloride (Methylphenidate inhibits the metabolism of tricyclic antidepressants).
No products indexed under this heading.

Mephentermine Sulfate (Possible additive effects on blood pressure with pressor agents if used concurrently).
No products indexed under this heading.

Metaraminol Bitartrate (Possible additive effects on blood pressure with pressor agents if used concurrently).
No products indexed under this heading.

Methoxamine Hydrochloride (Possible additive effects on blood pressure with pressor agents if used concurrently).
No products indexed under this heading.

Moclobemide (Concurrent and/or sequential use with MAO inhibitors may result in hypertensive crises; concurrent use or use within 14 days following discontinuation of an MAO inhibitor is contraindicated).
No products indexed under this heading.

Nizatidine (Since the modified release characteristics of Ritalin LA are pH dependent, the co-administration of acid suppressants could alter the release of methylphenidate). Products include:
- Axid Oral Solution 879

Norepinephrine Bitartrate (Possible additive effects on blood pressure with pressor agents if used concurrently).
No products indexed under this heading.

Nortriptyline Hydrochloride (Methylphenidate inhibits the metabolism of tricyclic antidepressants).
No products indexed under this heading.

Omeprazole (Since the modified release characteristics of Ritalin LA are pH dependent, the co-administration of acid suppressants could alter the release of methylphenidate). Products include:
- Zegerid Capsules 2958
- Zegerid Powder for Oral Solution 2958

Pantoprazole Sodium (Since the modified release characteristics of Ritalin LA are pH dependent, the co-administration of acid suppressants could alter the release of methylphenidate). Products include:
- Protonix I.V. 3472
- Protonix Tablets 3469

Pargyline Hydrochloride (Concurrent and/or sequential use with MAO inhibitors may result in hypertensive crises; concurrent use or use within 14 days following discontinuation of an MAO inhibitor is contraindicated).
No products indexed under this heading.

Phenelzine Sulfate (Concurrent and/or sequential use with MAO inhibitors may result in hypertensive crises; concurrent use or use within 14 days following discontinuation of an MAO inhibitor is contraindicated).
No products indexed under this heading.

Phenobarbital (Methylphenidate inhibits the metabolism of phenobarbital). Products include:
- Donnatal Extentabs 2493

Phenylephrine Hydrochloride (Possible additive effects on blood pressure with pressor agents if used concurrently). Products include:
- Comtrex Maximum Strength Non-Drowsy Cold & Cough Caplets .... ■ 725
- Comtrex Maximum Strength Day/Night Severe Cold & Sinus Caplets - Day Formulation .... ■ 725
- Comtrex Maximum Strength Day/Night Severe Cold & Sinus Caplets - Night Formulation .... ■ 725
- Contac Cold and Flu Maximum Strength Caplets .... ■ 728
- Contac Cold and Flu Day and Night Caplets (Day Formulation Only) .... ■ 727
- Contac Cold and Flu Day and Night Caplets (Night Formulation Only) .... ■ 727
- Contac Cold and Flu Non-Drowsy Caplets .... ■ 728
- Contac-D Cold Non-Drowsy Tablets .... ■ 729
- Children's Dimetapp Cold & Allergy Elixir .... ■ 730
- Children's Dimetapp Cold & Allergy Chewable Tablets .... ■ 730
- Children's Dimetapp DM Cold & Cough Elixir .... ■ 731
- Toddler's Dimetapp Cold and Cough Drops .... ■ 732
- Excedrin Sinus Headache Caplets/Tablets .... ■ 610
- 4-Way Fast Acting Nasal Spray .... ■ 775
- 4-Way Menthol Nasal Spray .... ■ 775
- Preparation H Maximum Strength Cream .... ■ 666
- Preparation H Cooling Gel .... ■ 666
- Preparation H .... ■ 666
- Refenesen PE Caplets .... ■ 721
- Robitussin Cough & Allergy Syrup .... ■ 736
- Robitussin Cough & Cold Nighttime Liquid .... ■ 736
- Robitussin Cough, Cold & Flu Nighttime Liquid .... ■ 738
- Robitussin Head & Chest Congestion PE Syrup .... ■ 739
- Robitussin Pediatric Cough & Cold Nighttime Liquid .... ■ 736
- TheraFlu Cold & Cough Hot Liquid .... ■ 740
- TheraFlu Cold & Sore Throat Hot Liquid .... ■ 741
- TheraFlu Flu & Sore Throat Hot Liquid .... ■ 742
- TheraFlu Daytime Severe Cold Hot Liquid .... ■ 742
- TheraFlu Nighttime Severe Cold Hot Liquid .... ■ 740
- TheraFlu Warming Relief Daytime Severe Cold .... ■ 743
- TheraFlu Warming Relief Nighttime Severe Cold .... ■ 743
- Triaminic Chest & Nasal Congestion Liquid .... ■ 746
- Triaminic Cold & Allergy Liquid .... ■ 746
- Triaminic Daytime Cold & Cough Liquid .... ■ 745
- Triaminic Nighttime Cold & Cough Liquid .... ■ 746
- Triaminic Thin Strips Cold .... ■ 748
- Triaminic Thin Strips Cold & Cough .... ■ 778
- Triaminic Infant Thin Strips Decongestant .... ■ 747
- Triaminic Infant Thin Strips Decongestant Plus Cough .... ■ 747
- Children's Tylenol Plus Flu Oral Suspension .... ■ 749
- Tylenol Cold Head Congestion Daytime Caplets with Cool Burst and Gelcaps .... ■ 750
- Tylenol Cold Multi-Symptom Daytime Liquid .... ■ 752
- Tylenol Cold Multi-Symptom Severe Daytime Liquid .... ■ 752
- Concentrated Tylenol Infants' Drops Plus Cold & Cough .... ■ 754
- Tylenol Allergy Multi-Symptom Caplets with Cool Burst and Gelcaps 1872
- Tylenol Allergy Multi-Symptom Nighttime Caplets with Cool Burst 1872
- Children's Tylenol Plus Cold Suspension Liquid 1879
- Children's Tylenol Plus Cold & Allergy Suspension Liquid 1878
- Children's Tylenol Plus Flu Suspension Liquid 1881
- Children's Tylenol Plus Multi-Symptom Cold Suspension Liquid 1879
- Tylenol Cold Head Congestion Daytime Caplets with Cool Burst 1873
- Tylenol Cold Head Congestion Nighttime Caplets with Cool Burst 1873
- Tylenol Cold Head Congestion Severe Caplets with Cool Burst 1873
- Tylenol Cold Multi-Symptom Daytime Caplets with Cool Burst and Gelcaps 1874
- Tylenol Cold Multi-Symptom Daytime Liquid with Citrus Burst 1874
- Tylenol Cold Multi-Symptom Nighttime Caplets with Cool Burst 1874
- Tylenol Cold Multi-Symptom Nighttime Liquid with Cool Burst 1874
- Tylenol Cold Multi-Symptom Severe Caplets with Cool Burst 1874

Tylenol Cold Multi-Symptom Severe Daytime Liquid with Citrus Burst 1874
Tylenol Sinus Congestion & Pain Daytime Caplets with Cool Burst and Gelcaps 1876
Tylenol Sinus Congestion & Pain Nighttime Caplets with Cool Burst 1876
Tylenol Sinus Congestion & Pain Severe Caplets with Cool Burst 1876
Vicks 44D Cough & Head Congestion Relief Liquid 760
Vicks DayQuil LiquiCaps/Liquid Multi-Symptom Cold/Flu Relief 761
Zicam Cough Plus D Cough Spray 767

Phenytoin (Methylphenidate inhibits the metabolism of phenytoin).
No products indexed under this heading.

Phenytoin Sodium (Methylphenidate inhibits the metabolism of phenytoin). Products include:
Phenytek Capsules 2160

Primidone (Methylphenidate inhibits the metabolism of primidone).
No products indexed under this heading.

Procarbazine Hydrochloride (Concurrent and/or sequential use with MAO inhibitors may result in hypertensive crises; concurrent use or use within 14 days following discontinuation of an MAO inhibitor is contraindicated). Products include:
Matulane Capsules 3191

Protriptyline Hydrochloride (Methylphenidate inhibits the metabolism of tricyclic antidepressants).
No products indexed under this heading.

Rabeprazole Sodium (Since the modified release characteristics of Ritalin LA are pH dependent, the co-administration of acid suppressants could alter the release of methylphenidate). Products include:
Aciphex Tablets 1090

Ranitidine Bismuth Citrate (Since the modified release characteristics of Ritalin LA are pH dependent, the co-administration of acid suppressants could alter the release of methylphenidate).
No products indexed under this heading.

Ranitidine Hydrochloride (Since the modified release characteristics of Ritalin LA are pH dependent, the co-administration of acid suppressants could alter the release of methylphenidate). Products include:
Zantac 1624
Zantac Injection 1619
Zantac Injection Pharmacy Bulk Package 1622

Selegiline Hydrochloride (Concurrent and/or sequential use with MAO inhibitors may result in hypertensive crises; concurrent use or use within 14 days following discontinuation of an MAO inhibitor is contraindicated). Products include:
Eldepryl Capsules 3208
Zelapar Tablets 3372

Sodium Bicarbonate (Since the modified release characteristics of Ritalin LA are pH dependent, the co-administration of antacids could alter the release of methylphenidate). Products include:
Colyte with Flavor Packs for Oral Solution 3088
HalfLytely and Bisacodyl Tablets Bowel Prep Kit with Flavors Packs 881
TriLyte with Flavor Packs for Oral Solution 3100

Tranylcypromine Sulfate (Concurrent and/or sequential use with MAO inhibitors may result in hypertensive crises; concurrent use or use within 14 days following discontinuation of an MAO inhibitor is contraindicated). Products include:
Parnate Tablets 1527

Trimipramine Maleate (Methylphenidate inhibits the metabolism of tricyclic antidepressants).
No products indexed under this heading.

Venlafaxine Hydrochloride (Co-administration of venlafaxine in a patient stabilized on methylphenidate has resulted in an NMS-like event within 45 minutes of ingestion of venlafaxine; it is uncertain whether this case represented a drug-drug interaction, a response to either drug alone, or some other cause). Products include:
Effexor Tablets 3411
Effexor XR Capsules 3417

Warfarin Sodium (Methylphenidate inhibits the metabolism of coumarin anticoagulants). Products include:
Coumadin for Injection 898
Coumadin Tablets 898

Food Interactions

Food, unspecified (When Ritalin LA was administered with a high fat breakfast to adults, Ritalin LA had a longer lag time until absorption began and variable delays in the time until the peak concentration, the time until the interpeak minimum, and the time until the second peak; administration times relative to meals and meal composition may need to be individually titrated).

RITALIN-SR TABLETS

(Methylphenidate Hydrochloride) 2269
See Ritalin Hydrochloride Tablets

RITUXAN I.V.

(Rituximab) 1254
May interact with vaccines, live. Compounds in these categories include:

BCG Vaccine (Vaccination with live virus vaccines is not recommended).
No products indexed under this heading.

Measles, Mumps, Rubella and Varicella Virus Vaccine Live (Vaccination with live virus vaccines is not recommended). Products include:
ProQuad 2064

Measles, Mumps & Rubella Virus Vaccine, Live (Vaccination with live virus vaccines is not recommended). Products include:
M-M-R II 2006

Measles & Rubella Virus Vaccine Live (Vaccination with live virus vaccines is not recommended).
No products indexed under this heading.

Measles Virus Vaccine Live (Vaccination with live virus vaccines is not recommended). Products include:
Attenuvax 1914

Mumps Virus Vaccine, Live (Vaccination with live virus vaccines is not recommended). Products include:
Mumpsvax 2031

Poliovirus Vaccine, Live, Oral, Trivalent, Types 1,2,3 (Sabin) (Vaccination with live virus vaccines is not recommended).
No products indexed under this heading.

Rotavirus Vaccine, Live, Oral, Tetravalent (Vaccination with live virus vaccines is not recommended).
No products indexed under this heading.

Rubella & Mumps Virus Vaccine Live (Vaccination with live virus vaccines is not recommended).
No products indexed under this heading.

Rubella Virus Vaccine Live (Vaccination with live virus vaccines is not recommended). Products include:
Meruvax II 2019

Smallpox Vaccine (Vaccination with live virus vaccines is not recommended).
No products indexed under this heading.

Typhoid Vaccine (Vaccination with live virus vaccines is not recommended).
No products indexed under this heading.

Varicella Virus Vaccine Live (Vaccination with live virus vaccines is not recommended). Products include:
Varivax 2100

Yellow Fever Vaccine (Vaccination with live virus vaccines is not recommended).
No products indexed under this heading.

ROBITUSSIN CHEST CONGESTION LIQUID

(Guaifenesin) 721
None cited in PDR database.

ROBITUSSIN COUGH & COLD CF LIQUID

(Dextromethorphan Hydrobromide, Guaifenesin, Pseudoephedrine Hydrochloride) 735
May interact with monoamine oxidase inhibitors. Compounds in these categories include:

Isocarboxazid (Concurrent and/or sequential use with MAO inhibitors is not recommended).
No products indexed under this heading.

Moclobemide (Concurrent and/or sequential use with MAO inhibitors is not recommended).
No products indexed under this heading.

Pargyline Hydrochloride (Concurrent and/or sequential use with MAO inhibitors is not recommended).
No products indexed under this heading.

Phenelzine Sulfate (Concurrent and/or sequential use with MAO inhibitors is not recommended).
No products indexed under this heading.

Procarbazine Hydrochloride (Concurrent and/or sequential use with MAO inhibitors is not recommended). Products include:
Matulane Capsules 3191

Selegiline Hydrochloride (Concurrent and/or sequential use with MAO inhibitors is not recommended). Products include:
Eldepryl Capsules 3208
Zelapar Tablets 3372

Tranylcypromine Sulfate (Concurrent and/or sequential use with MAO inhibitors is not recommended). Products include:
Parnate Tablets 1527

ROBITUSSIN COUGH & COLD LONG-ACTING LIQUID

(Chlorpheniramine Maleate, Dextromethorphan Hydrobromide) 735
May interact with hypnotics and sedatives, monoamine oxidase inhibitors, tranquilizers, and certain other agents. Compounds in these categories include:

Alprazolam (Concurrent use of tranquilizers may increase the drowsiness effect). Products include:
Niravam Orally Disintegrating Tablets 3092

Buspirone Hydrochloride (Concurrent use of tranquilizers may increase the drowsiness effect).
No products indexed under this heading.

Chlordiazepoxide (Concurrent use of tranquilizers may increase the drowsiness effect).
No products indexed under this heading.

Chlordiazepoxide Hydrochloride (Concurrent use of tranquilizers may increase the drowsiness effect). Products include:
Librium Capsules 3347

Chlorpromazine (Concurrent use of tranquilizers may increase the drowsiness effect).
No products indexed under this heading.

Chlorpromazine Hydrochloride (Concurrent use of tranquilizers may increase the drowsiness effect).
No products indexed under this heading.

Chlorprothixene (Concurrent use of tranquilizers may increase the drowsiness effect).
No products indexed under this heading.

Chlorprothixene Hydrochloride (Concurrent use of tranquilizers may increase the drowsiness effect).
No products indexed under this heading.

Clorazepate Dipotassium (Concurrent use of tranquilizers may increase the drowsiness effect). Products include:
Tranxene 2474

Diazepam (Concurrent use of tranquilizers may increase the drowsiness effect). Products include:
Diastat Rectal Delivery System 3343
Valium Tablets 2819

Droperidol (Concurrent use of tranquilizers may increase the drowsiness effect).
No products indexed under this heading.

Estazolam (Concurrent use of sedatives may increase the drowsiness effect). Products include:
ProSom Tablets 517

Ethchlorvynol (Concurrent use of sedatives may increase the drowsiness effect).
No products indexed under this heading.

Ethinamate (Concurrent use of sedatives may increase the drowsiness effect).
No products indexed under this heading.

Fluphenazine Decanoate (Concurrent use of tranquilizers may increase the drowsiness effect).
No products indexed under this heading.

Fluphenazine Enanthate (Concurrent use of tranquilizers may increase the drowsiness effect).
No products indexed under this heading.

Fluphenazine Hydrochloride (Concurrent use of tranquilizers may increase the drowsiness effect).
No products indexed under this heading.

Flurazepam Hydrochloride (Concurrent use of sedatives may increase the drowsiness effect). Products include:
Dalmane Capsules 3342

Glutethimide (Concurrent use of sedatives may increase the drowsiness effect).
No products indexed under this heading.

Haloperidol (Concurrent use of tranquilizers may increase the drowsiness effect).
No products indexed under this heading.

Haloperidol Decanoate (Concurrent use of tranquilizers may increase the drowsiness effect).
No products indexed under this heading.

Hydroxyzine Hydrochloride (Concurrent use of tranquilizers may increase the drowsiness effect).
No products indexed under this heading.

Isocarboxazid (Concurrent and/or sequential use with MAO inhibitors is not recommended).
No products indexed under this heading.

Lorazepam (Concurrent use of sedatives may increase the drowsiness effect).
No products indexed under this heading.

Loxapine Hydrochloride (Concurrent use of tranquilizers may increase the drowsiness effect).
No products indexed under this heading.

Loxapine Succinate (Concurrent use of tranquilizers may increase the drowsiness effect).
No products indexed under this heading.

Meprobamate (Concurrent use of tranquilizers may increase the drowsiness effect).
No products indexed under this heading.

Mesoridazine Besylate (Concurrent use of tranquilizers may increase the drowsiness effect).
No products indexed under this heading.

Midazolam Hydrochloride (Concurrent use of sedatives may increase the drowsiness effect).
No products indexed under this heading.

Moclobemide (Concurrent and/or sequential use with MAO inhibitors is not recommended).
No products indexed under this heading.

Molindone Hydrochloride (Concurrent use of tranquilizers may increase the drowsiness effect). Products include:
Moban Tablets 1119

Oxazepam (Concurrent use of tranquilizers may increase the drowsiness effect).
No products indexed under this heading.

Pargyline Hydrochloride (Concurrent and/or sequential use with MAO inhibitors is not recommended).
No products indexed under this heading.

Perphenazine (Concurrent use of tranquilizers may increase the drowsiness effect).
No products indexed under this heading.

Phenelzine Sulfate (Concurrent and/or sequential use with MAO inhibitors is not recommended).
No products indexed under this heading.

Prazepam (Concurrent use of tranquilizers may increase the drowsiness effect).
No products indexed under this heading.

Procarbazine Hydrochloride (Concurrent and/or sequential use with MAO inhibitors is not recommended). Products include:
Matulane Capsules 3191

Prochlorperazine (Concurrent use of tranquilizers may increase the drowsiness effect).
No products indexed under this heading.

Promethazine Hydrochloride (Concurrent use of tranquilizers may increase the drowsiness effect). Products include:
Phenergan Tablets and Suppositories............................... 3440

Propofol (Concurrent use of sedatives may increase the drowsiness effect).
No products indexed under this heading.

Quazepam (Concurrent use of sedatives may increase the drowsiness effect).
No products indexed under this heading.

Ramelteon (Concurrent use of sedatives may increase the drowsiness effect). Products include:
Rozerem Tablets 3231

Secobarbital Sodium (Concurrent use of sedatives may increase the drowsiness effect).
No products indexed under this heading.

Selegiline Hydrochloride (Concurrent and/or sequential use with MAO inhibitors is not recommended). Products include:
Eldepryl Capsules 3208
Zelapar Tablets 3372

Temazepam (Concurrent use of sedatives may increase the drowsiness effect). Products include:
Restoril Capsules 1860

Thioridazine Hydrochloride (Concurrent use of tranquilizers may increase the drowsiness effect). Products include:
Thioridazine Hydrochloride Tablets ... 2163

Thiothixene (Concurrent use of tranquilizers may increase the drowsiness effect). Products include:
Thiothixene Capsules 2165

Tranylcypromine Sulfate (Concurrent and/or sequential use with MAO inhibitors is not recommended). Products include:
Parnate Tablets 1527

Triazolam (Concurrent use of sedatives may increase the drowsiness effect).
No products indexed under this heading.

Trifluoperazine Hydrochloride (Concurrent use of tranquilizers may increase the drowsiness effect).
No products indexed under this heading.

Zaleplon (Concurrent use of sedatives may increase the drowsiness effect). Products include:
Sonata Capsules 1717

Zolpidem Tartrate (Concurrent use of sedatives may increase the drowsiness effect). Products include:
Ambien Tablets 2851
Ambien CR Tablets 2855

Food Interactions

Alcohol (Avoid alcoholic beverages. Consumption of alcohol may increase the drowsiness effect).

ROBITUSSIN COUGH & ALLERGY SYRUP

(Chlorpheniramine Maleate, Dextromethorphan Hydrobromide, Phenylephrine Hydrochloride)............ ▣ 736
May interact with hypnotics and sedatives, monoamine oxidase inhibitors, tranquilizers, and certain other agents. Compounds in these categories include:

Alprazolam (May increase drowsiness effect). Products include:
Niravam Orally Disintegrating Tablets .. 3092

Buspirone Hydrochloride (May increase drowsiness effect).
No products indexed under this heading.

Chlordiazepoxide (May increase drowsiness effect).
No products indexed under this heading.

Chlordiazepoxide Hydrochloride (May increase drowsiness effect). Products include:
Librium Capsules 3347

Chlorpromazine (May increase drowsiness effect).
No products indexed under this heading.

Chlorpromazine Hydrochloride (May increase drowsiness effect).
No products indexed under this heading.

Chlorprothixene (May increase drowsiness effect).
No products indexed under this heading.

Chlorprothixene Hydrochloride (May increase drowsiness effect).
No products indexed under this heading.

Clorazepate Dipotassium (May increase drowsiness effect). Products include:
Tranxene 2474

Diazepam (May increase drowsiness effect). Products include:
Diastat Rectal Delivery System 3343
Valium Tablets 2819

Droperidol (May increase drowsiness effect).
No products indexed under this heading.

Estazolam (May increase drowsiness effect). Products include:
ProSom Tablets 517

Ethchlorvynol (May increase drowsiness effect).
No products indexed under this heading.

Ethinamate (May increase drowsiness effect).
No products indexed under this heading.

Fluphenazine Decanoate (May increase drowsiness effect).
No products indexed under this heading.

Fluphenazine Enanthate (May increase drowsiness effect).
No products indexed under this heading.

Fluphenazine Hydrochloride (May increase drowsiness effect).
No products indexed under this heading.

Flurazepam Hydrochloride (May increase drowsiness effect). Products include:
Dalmane Capsules 3342

Glutethimide (May increase drowsiness effect).
No products indexed under this heading.

Haloperidol (May increase drowsiness effect).
No products indexed under this heading.

Haloperidol Decanoate (May increase drowsiness effect).
No products indexed under this heading.

Hydroxyzine Hydrochloride (May increase drowsiness effect).
No products indexed under this heading.

Isocarboxazid (Concurrent or sequential use with MAO inhibitors is not recommended).
No products indexed under this heading.

Lorazepam (May increase drowsiness effect).
No products indexed under this heading.

Loxapine Hydrochloride (May increase drowsiness effect).
No products indexed under this heading.

Loxapine Succinate (May increase drowsiness effect).
No products indexed under this heading.

Meprobamate (May increase drowsiness effect).
No products indexed under this heading.

Mesoridazine Besylate (May increase drowsiness effect).
No products indexed under this heading.

Midazolam Hydrochloride (May increase drowsiness effect).
No products indexed under this heading.

Moclobemide (Concurrent or sequential use with MAO inhibitors is not recommended).
No products indexed under this heading.

Molindone Hydrochloride (May increase drowsiness effect). Products include:
Moban Tablets 1119

Oxazepam (May increase drowsiness effect).
No products indexed under this heading.

Pargyline Hydrochloride (Concurrent or sequential use with MAO inhibitors is not recommended).
No products indexed under this heading.

Perphenazine (May increase drowsiness effect).
No products indexed under this heading.

Phenelzine Sulfate (Concurrent or sequential use with MAO inhibitors is not recommended).
No products indexed under this heading.

Prazepam (May increase drowsiness effect).
No products indexed under this heading.

Procarbazine Hydrochloride (Concurrent or sequential use with MAO inhibitors is not recommended). Products include:
Matulane Capsules 3191

Prochlorperazine (May increase drowsiness effect).
No products indexed under this heading.

Promethazine Hydrochloride (May increase drowsiness effect). Products include:
Phenergan Tablets and Suppositories 3440

Propofol (May increase drowsiness effect).
No products indexed under this heading.

Quazepam (May increase drowsiness effect).
No products indexed under this heading.

Ramelteon (May increase drowsiness effect). Products include:
Rozerem Tablets 3231

Secobarbital Sodium (May increase drowsiness effect).
No products indexed under this heading.

Selegiline Hydrochloride (Concurrent or sequential use with MAO inhibitors is not recommended). Products include:
Eldepryl Capsules 3208
Zelapar Tablets 3372

Temazepam (May increase drowsiness effect). Products include:
Restoril Capsules 1860

Thioridazine Hydrochloride (May increase drowsiness effect). Products include:
Thioridazine Hydrochloride Tablets 2163

Thiothixene (May increase drowsiness effect). Products include:
Thiothixene Capsules 2165

Tranylcypromine Sulfate (Concurrent or sequential use with MAO inhibitors is not recommended). Products include:
Parnate Tablets 1527

Triazolam (May increase drowsiness effect).
No products indexed under this heading.

Trifluoperazine Hydrochloride (May increase drowsiness effect).
No products indexed under this heading.

Zaleplon (May increase drowsiness effect). Products include:
Sonata Capsules 1717

Zolpidem Tartrate (May increase drowsiness effect). Products include:
Ambien Tablets 2851
Ambien CR Tablets 2855

Food Interactions

Alcohol (Avoid alcoholic beverages when using this product).

ROBITUSSIN COUGH & COLD NIGHTTIME LIQUID

(Chlorpheniramine Maleate, Dextromethorphan Hydrobromide, Phenylephrine Hydrochloride)........... 736
May interact with hypnotics and sedatives, monoamine oxidase inhibitors, tranquilizers, and certain other agents. Compounds in these categories include:

Alprazolam (May increase drowsiness effect). Products include:
Niravam Orally Disintegrating Tablets 3092

Buspirone Hydrochloride (May increase drowsiness effect).
No products indexed under this heading.

Chlordiazepoxide (May increase drowsiness effect).
No products indexed under this heading.

Chlordiazepoxide Hydrochloride (May increase drowsiness effect). Products include:
Librium Capsules 3347

Chlorpromazine (May increase drowsiness effect).
No products indexed under this heading.

Chlorpromazine Hydrochloride (May increase drowsiness effect).
No products indexed under this heading.

Chlorprothixene (May increase drowsiness effect).
No products indexed under this heading.

Chlorprothixene Hydrochloride (May increase drowsiness effect).
No products indexed under this heading.

Clorazepate Dipotassium (May increase drowsiness effect). Products include:
Tranxene 2474

Diazepam (May increase drowsiness effect). Products include:
Diastat Rectal Delivery System 3343
Valium Tablets 2819

Droperidol (May increase drowsiness effect).
No products indexed under this heading.

Estazolam (May increase drowsiness effect). Products include:
ProSom Tablets 517

Ethchlorvynol (May increase drowsiness effect).
No products indexed under this heading.

Ethinamate (May increase drowsiness effect).
No products indexed under this heading.

Fluphenazine Decanoate (May increase drowsiness effect).
No products indexed under this heading.

Fluphenazine Enanthate (May increase drowsiness effect).
No products indexed under this heading.

Fluphenazine Hydrochloride (May increase drowsiness effect).
No products indexed under this heading.

Flurazepam Hydrochloride (May increase drowsiness effect). Products include:
Dalmane Capsules 3342

Glutethimide (May increase drowsiness effect).
No products indexed under this heading.

Haloperidol (May increase drowsiness effect).
No products indexed under this heading.

Haloperidol Decanoate (May increase drowsiness effect).
No products indexed under this heading.

Hydroxyzine Hydrochloride (May increase drowsiness effect).
No products indexed under this heading.

Isocarboxazid (Concurrent or sequential use with MAO inhibitors is not recommended).
No products indexed under this heading.

Lorazepam (May increase drowsiness effect).
No products indexed under this heading.

Loxapine Hydrochloride (May increase drowsiness effect).
No products indexed under this heading.

Loxapine Succinate (May increase drowsiness effect).
No products indexed under this heading.

Meprobamate (May increase drowsiness effect).
No products indexed under this heading.

Mesoridazine Besylate (May increase drowsiness effect).
No products indexed under this heading.

Midazolam Hydrochloride (May increase drowsiness effect).
No products indexed under this heading.

Moclobemide (Concurrent or sequential use with MAO inhibitors is not recommended).
No products indexed under this heading.

Molindone Hydrochloride (May increase drowsiness effect). Products include:
Moban Tablets 1119

Oxazepam (May increase drowsiness effect).
No products indexed under this heading.

Pargyline Hydrochloride (Concurrent or sequential use with MAO inhibitors is not recommended).
No products indexed under this heading.

Perphenazine (May increase drowsiness effect).
No products indexed under this heading.

Phenelzine Sulfate (Concurrent or sequential use with MAO inhibitors is not recommended).
No products indexed under this heading.

Prazepam (May increase drowsiness effect).
No products indexed under this heading.

Procarbazine Hydrochloride (Concurrent or sequential use with MAO inhibitors is not recommended). Products include:
Matulane Capsules 3191

Prochlorperazine (May increase drowsiness effect).
No products indexed under this heading.

Promethazine Hydrochloride (May increase drowsiness effect). Products include:
Phenergan Tablets and Suppositories 3440

Propofol (May increase drowsiness effect).
No products indexed under this heading.

Quazepam (May increase drowsiness effect).
No products indexed under this heading.

Ramelteon (May increase drowsiness effect). Products include:
Rozerem Tablets 3231

Secobarbital Sodium (May increase drowsiness effect).
No products indexed under this heading.

Selegiline Hydrochloride (Concurrent or sequential use with MAO inhibitors is not recommended). Products include:
Eldepryl Capsules 3208
Zelapar Tablets 3372

Temazepam (May increase drowsiness effect). Products include:
Restoril Capsules 1860

Thioridazine Hydrochloride (May increase drowsiness effect). Products include:
Thioridazine Hydrochloride Tablets 2163

Thiothixene (May increase drowsiness effect). Products include:
Thiothixene Capsules 2165

Tranylcypromine Sulfate (Concurrent or sequential use with MAO inhibitors is not recommended). Products include:
Parnate Tablets 1527

Triazolam (May increase drowsiness effect).
No products indexed under this heading.

Trifluoperazine Hydrochloride (May increase drowsiness effect).
No products indexed under this heading.

Zaleplon (May increase drowsiness effect). Products include:
Sonata Capsules 1717

Zolpidem Tartrate (May increase drowsiness effect). Products include:
Ambien Tablets 2851
Ambien CR Tablets 2855

Food Interactions

Alcohol (Avoid alcoholic beverages when using this product).

ROBITUSSIN COUGH & COLD PEDIATRIC DROPS

(Dextromethorphan Hydrobromide, Guaifenesin, Pseudoephedrine Hydrochloride)...... 735
See Robitussin Head & Chest Congestion PE Syrup

ROBITUSSIN COUGH, COLD & FLU NIGHTTIME LIQUID

(Acetaminophen, Chlorpheniramine Maleate, Dextromethorphan Hydrobromide, Phenylephrine Hydrochloride)........... 738
May interact with hypnotics and sedatives, monoamine oxidase inhibitors, tranquilizers, and certain other agents. Compounds in these categories include:

Alprazolam (May increase drowsiness). Products include:
Niravam Orally Disintegrating Tablets 3092

Buspirone Hydrochloride (May increase drowsiness).
No products indexed under this heading.

Chlordiazepoxide (May increase drowsiness).
No products indexed under this heading.

Chlordiazepoxide Hydrochloride (May increase drowsiness). Products include:
Librium Capsules 3347

Chlorpromazine (May increase drowsiness).
No products indexed under this heading.

Chlorpromazine Hydrochloride (May increase drowsiness).
No products indexed under this heading.

Chlorprothixene (May increase drowsiness).
No products indexed under this heading.

Chlorprothixene Hydrochloride (May increase drowsiness).
No products indexed under this heading.

Clorazepate Dipotassium (May increase drowsiness). Products include:
Tranxene ... 2474

Diazepam (May increase drowsiness). Products include:
Diastat Rectal Delivery System 3343
Valium Tablets 2819

Droperidol (May increase drowsiness).
No products indexed under this heading.

Estazolam (May increase drowsiness). Products include:
ProSom Tablets 517

Ethchlorvynol (May increase drowsiness).
No products indexed under this heading.

Ethinamate (May increase drowsiness).
No products indexed under this heading.

Fluphenazine Decanoate (May increase drowsiness).
No products indexed under this heading.

Fluphenazine Enanthate (May increase drowsiness).
No products indexed under this heading.

Fluphenazine Hydrochloride (May increase drowsiness).
No products indexed under this heading.

Flurazepam Hydrochloride (May increase drowsiness). Products include:
Dalmane Capsules 3342

Glutethimide (May increase drowsiness).
No products indexed under this heading.

Haloperidol (May increase drowsiness).
No products indexed under this heading.

Haloperidol Decanoate (May increase drowsiness).
No products indexed under this heading.

Hydroxyzine Hydrochloride (May increase drowsiness).
No products indexed under this heading.

Isocarboxazid (Concurrent and/or sequential use with MAO inhibitors is not recommended).
No products indexed under this heading.

Lorazepam (May increase drowsiness).
No products indexed under this heading.

Loxapine Hydrochloride (May increase drowsiness).
No products indexed under this heading.

Loxapine Succinate (May increase drowsiness).
No products indexed under this heading.

Meprobamate (May increase drowsiness).
No products indexed under this heading.

Mesoridazine Besylate (May increase drowsiness).
No products indexed under this heading.

Midazolam Hydrochloride (May increase drowsiness).
No products indexed under this heading.

Moclobemide (Concurrent and/or sequential use with MAO inhibitors is not recommended).
No products indexed under this heading.

Molindone Hydrochloride (May increase drowsiness). Products include:
Moban Tablets 1119

Oxazepam (May increase drowsiness).
No products indexed under this heading.

Pargyline Hydrochloride (Concurrent and/or sequential use with MAO inhibitors is not recommended).
No products indexed under this heading.

Perphenazine (May increase drowsiness).
No products indexed under this heading.

Phenelzine Sulfate (Concurrent and/or sequential use with MAO inhibitors is not recommended).
No products indexed under this heading.

Prazepam (May increase drowsiness).
No products indexed under this heading.

Procarbazine Hydrochloride (Concurrent and/or sequential use with MAO inhibitors is not recommended). Products include:
Matulane Capsules 3191

Prochlorperazine (May increase drowsiness).
No products indexed under this heading.

Promethazine Hydrochloride (May increase drowsiness). Products include:
Phenergan Tablets and Suppositories 3440

Propofol (May increase drowsiness).
No products indexed under this heading.

Quazepam (May increase drowsiness).
No products indexed under this heading.

Ramelteon (May increase drowsiness). Products include:
Rozerem Tablets 3231

Secobarbital Sodium (May increase drowsiness).
No products indexed under this heading.

Selegiline Hydrochloride (Concurrent and/or sequential use with MAO inhibitors is not recommended). Products include:
Eldepryl Capsules 3208
Zelapar Tablets 3372

Temazepam (May increase drowsiness). Products include:
Restoril Capsules 1860

Thioridazine Hydrochloride (May increase drowsiness). Products include:
Thioridazine Hydrochloride Tablets .. 2163

Thiothixene (May increase drowsiness). Products include:
Thiothixene Capsules 2165

Tranylcypromine Sulfate (Concurrent and/or sequential use with MAO inhibitors is not recommended). Products include:
Parnate Tablets 1527

Triazolam (May increase drowsiness).
No products indexed under this heading.

Trifluoperazine Hydrochloride (May increase drowsiness).
No products indexed under this heading.

Zaleplon (May increase drowsiness). Products include:
Sonata Capsules 1717

Zolpidem Tartrate (May increase drowsiness). Products include:
Ambien Tablets 2851
Ambien CR Tablets 2855

Food Interactions

Alcohol (Chronic heavy alcohol users, 3 or more drinks per day, should consult their physicians for advice on when and how they should take pain relievers/ fever reducers including acetaminophen; increases drowsiness effect).

ROBITUSSIN COUGH & CONGESTION LIQUID

(Dextromethorphan Hydrobromide, Guaifenesin).............. ■◻738
May interact with monoamine oxidase inhibitors. Compounds in these categories include:

Isocarboxazid (Concurrent and/or sequential use with MAO inhibitors is not recommended).
No products indexed under this heading.

Moclobemide (Concurrent and/or sequential use with MAO inhibitors is not recommended).
No products indexed under this heading.

Pargyline Hydrochloride (Concurrent and/or sequential use with MAO inhibitors is not recommended).
No products indexed under this heading.

Phenelzine Sulfate (Concurrent and/or sequential use with MAO inhibitors is not recommended).
No products indexed under this heading.

Procarbazine Hydrochloride (Concurrent and/or sequential use with MAO inhibitors is not recommended). Products include:
Matulane Capsules 3191

Selegiline Hydrochloride (Concurrent and/or sequential use with MAO inhibitors is not recommended). Products include:
Eldepryl Capsules 3208
Zelapar Tablets 3372

Tranylcypromine Sulfate (Concurrent and/or sequential use with MAO inhibitors is not recommended). Products include:
Parnate Tablets 1527

ROBITUSSIN COUGH GELS LONG-ACTING

(Dextromethorphan Hydrobromide)................................... ■◻737
May interact with monoamine oxidase inhibitors. Compounds in these categories include:

Isocarboxazid (Concurrent or sequential use with MAO inhibitors is not recommended).
No products indexed under this heading.

Moclobemide (Concurrent or sequential use with MAO inhibitors is not recommended).
No products indexed under this heading.

Pargyline Hydrochloride (Concurrent or sequential use with MAO inhibitors is not recommended).
No products indexed under this heading.

Phenelzine Sulfate (Concurrent or sequential use with MAO inhibitors is not recommended).
No products indexed under this heading.

Procarbazine Hydrochloride (Concurrent or sequential use with MAO inhibitors is not recommended). Products include:
Matulane Capsules 3191

Selegiline Hydrochloride (Concurrent or sequential use with MAO inhibitors is not recommended). Products include:
Eldepryl Capsules 3208
Zelapar Tablets 3372

Tranylcypromine Sulfate (Concurrent or sequential use with MAO inhibitors is not recommended). Products include:
Parnate Tablets 1527

ROBITUSSIN COUGH LONG ACTING LIQUID

(Dextromethorphan Hydrobromide)................................... ■◻739
See Robitussin Pediatric Cough Long Acting Liquid

ROBITUSSIN COUGH DM SYRUP

(Dextromethorphan Hydrobromide, Guaifenesin).............. ■◻738
May interact with monoamine oxidase inhibitors. Compounds in these categories include:

Isocarboxazid (Concurrent and/or sequential use with MAO inhibitors is not recommended).
No products indexed under this heading.

Moclobemide (Concurrent and/or sequential use with MAO inhibitors is not recommended).
No products indexed under this heading.

Pargyline Hydrochloride (Concurrent and/or sequential use with MAO inhibitors is not recommended).
No products indexed under this heading.

Phenelzine Sulfate (Concurrent and/or sequential use with MAO inhibitors is not recommended).
No products indexed under this heading.

Procarbazine Hydrochloride
(Concurrent and/or sequential use with MAO inhibitors is not recommended). Products include:
Matulane Capsules 3191

Selegiline Hydrochloride (Concurrent and/or sequential use with MAO inhibitors is not recommended). Products include:
Eldepryl Capsules 3208
Zelapar Tablets 3372

Tranylcypromine Sulfate (Concurrent and/or sequential use with MAO inhibitors is not recommended). Products include:
Parnate Tablets 1527

ROBITUSSIN COUGH DM INFANT DROPS

(Dextromethorphan Hydrobromide, Guaifenesin)............. ▣▫738
See Robitussin Cough DM Syrup

ROBITUSSIN COUGH DROPS MENTHOL, CHERRY, AND HONEY-LEMON

(Menthol) ▣▫737
None cited in PDR database.

ROBITUSSIN HONEY COUGH DROPS

(Menthol) ▣▫737
None cited in PDR database.

ROBITUSSIN SUGAR FREE THROAT DROPS

(Menthol) ▣▫737
None cited in PDR database.

ROBITUSSIN HEAD & CHEST CONGESTION PE SYRUP

(Guaifenesin, Phenylephrine Hydrochloride)................................. ▣▫739
May interact with monoamine oxidase inhibitors. Compounds in these categories include:

Isocarboxazid (Concurrent and/or sequential use with MAO inhibitors is not recommended).
No products indexed under this heading.

Moclobemide (Concurrent and/or sequential use with MAO inhibitors is not recommended).
No products indexed under this heading.

Pargyline Hydrochloride (Concurrent and/or sequential use with MAO inhibitors is not recommended).
No products indexed under this heading.

Phenelzine Sulfate (Concurrent and/or sequential use with MAO inhibitors is not recommended).
No products indexed under this heading.

Procarbazine Hydrochloride
(Concurrent and/or sequential use with MAO inhibitors is not recommended). Products include:
Matulane Capsules 3191

Selegiline Hydrochloride (Concurrent and/or sequential use with MAO inhibitors is not recommended). Products include:
Eldepryl Capsules 3208
Zelapar Tablets 3372

Tranylcypromine Sulfate (Concurrent and/or sequential use with MAO inhibitors is not recommended). Products include:
Parnate Tablets 1527

ROBITUSSIN PEDIATRIC COUGH LONG ACTING LIQUID

(Dextromethorphan Hydrobromide)................................. ▣▫739
May interact with monoamine oxidase inhibitors. Compounds in these categories include:

Isocarboxazid (Concurrent and/or sequential use with MAO inhibitors should be avoided).
No products indexed under this heading.

Moclobemide (Concurrent and/or sequential use with MAO inhibitors should be avoided).
No products indexed under this heading.

Pargyline Hydrochloride (Concurrent and/or sequential use with MAO inhibitors should be avoided).
No products indexed under this heading.

Phenelzine Sulfate (Concurrent and/or sequential use with MAO inhibitors should be avoided).
No products indexed under this heading.

Procarbazine Hydrochloride
(Concurrent and/or sequential use with MAO inhibitors should be avoided). Products include:
Matulane Capsules 3191

Selegiline Hydrochloride (Concurrent and/or sequential use with MAO inhibitors should be avoided). Products include:
Eldepryl Capsules 3208
Zelapar Tablets 3372

Tranylcypromine Sulfate (Concurrent and/or sequential use with MAO inhibitors should be avoided). Products include:
Parnate Tablets 1527

ROBITUSSIN PEDIATRIC COUGH & COLD LONG-ACTING LIQUID

(Chlorpheniramine Maleate, Dextromethorphan Hydrobromide).... ▣▫735
See Robitussin Cough & Cold Long-Acting Liquid

ROBITUSSIN PEDIATRIC COUGH & COLD NIGHTTIME LIQUID

(Chlorpheniramine Maleate, Dextromethorphan Hydrobromide, Phenylephrine Hydrochloride)........... ▣▫736
May interact with hypnotics and sedatives, monoamine oxidase inhibitors, tranquilizers, and certain other agents. Compounds in these categories include:

Alprazolam (May increase drowsiness effect). Products include:
Niravam Orally Disintegrating Tablets....................................... 3092

Buspirone Hydrochloride (May increase drowsiness effect).
No products indexed under this heading.

Chlordiazepoxide (May increase drowsiness effect).
No products indexed under this heading.

Chlordiazepoxide Hydrochloride (May increase drowsiness effect). Products include:
Librium Capsules 3347

Chlorpromazine (May increase drowsiness effect).
No products indexed under this heading.

Chlorpromazine Hydrochloride (May increase drowsiness effect).
No products indexed under this heading.

Chlorprothixene (May increase drowsiness effect).
No products indexed under this heading.

Chlorprothixene Hydrochloride (May increase drowsiness effect).
No products indexed under this heading.

Clorazepate Dipotassium (May increase drowsiness effect). Products include:
Tranxene 2474

Diazepam (May increase drowsiness effect). Products include:
Diastat Rectal Delivery System 3343
Valium Tablets 2819

Droperidol (May increase drowsiness effect).
No products indexed under this heading.

Estazolam (May increase drowsiness effect). Products include:
ProSom Tablets 517

Ethchlorvynol (May increase drowsiness effect).
No products indexed under this heading.

Ethinamate (May increase drowsiness effect).
No products indexed under this heading.

Fluphenazine Decanoate (May increase drowsiness effect).
No products indexed under this heading.

Fluphenazine Enanthate (May increase drowsiness effect).
No products indexed under this heading.

Fluphenazine Hydrochloride (May increase drowsiness effect).
No products indexed under this heading.

Flurazepam Hydrochloride (May increase drowsiness effect). Products include:
Dalmane Capsules 3342

Glutethimide (May increase drowsiness effect).
No products indexed under this heading.

Haloperidol (May increase drowsiness effect).
No products indexed under this heading.

Haloperidol Decanoate (May increase drowsiness effect).
No products indexed under this heading.

Hydroxyzine Hydrochloride (May increase drowsiness effect).
No products indexed under this heading.

Isocarboxazid (Concurrent or sequential use with MAO inhibitors is not recommended).
No products indexed under this heading.

Lorazepam (May increase drowsiness effect).
No products indexed under this heading.

Loxapine Hydrochloride (May increase drowsiness effect).
No products indexed under this heading.

Loxapine Succinate (May increase drowsiness effect).
No products indexed under this heading.

Meprobamate (May increase drowsiness effect).
No products indexed under this heading.

Mesoridazine Besylate (May increase drowsiness effect).
No products indexed under this heading.

Midazolam Hydrochloride (May increase drowsiness effect).
No products indexed under this heading.

Moclobemide (Concurrent or sequential use with MAO inhibitors is not recommended).
No products indexed under this heading.

Molindone Hydrochloride (May increase drowsiness effect). Products include:
Moban Tablets 1119

Oxazepam (May increase drowsiness effect).
No products indexed under this heading.

Pargyline Hydrochloride (Concurrent or sequential use with MAO inhibitors is not recommended).
No products indexed under this heading.

Perphenazine (May increase drowsiness effect).
No products indexed under this heading.

Phenelzine Sulfate (Concurrent or sequential use with MAO inhibitors is not recommended).
No products indexed under this heading.

Prazepam (May increase drowsiness effect).
No products indexed under this heading.

Procarbazine Hydrochloride
(Concurrent or sequential use with MAO inhibitors is not recommended). Products include:
Matulane Capsules 3191

Prochlorperazine (May increase drowsiness effect).
No products indexed under this heading.

Promethazine Hydrochloride (May increase drowsiness effect). Products include:
Phenergan Tablets and Suppositories............................... 3440

Propofol (May increase drowsiness effect).
No products indexed under this heading.

Quazepam (May increase drowsiness effect).
No products indexed under this heading.

Ramelteon (May increase drowsiness effect). Products include:
Rozerem Tablets 3231

Secobarbital Sodium (May increase drowsiness effect).
No products indexed under this heading.

Selegiline Hydrochloride (Concurrent or sequential use with MAO inhibitors is not recommended). Products include:
Eldepryl Capsules 3208
Zelapar Tablets 3372

Temazepam (May increase drowsiness effect). Products include:
Restoril Capsules 1860

Thioridazine Hydrochloride (May increase drowsiness effect). Products include:

IMPORTANT NOTE: Always consult each drug listing in the patient's regimen for possible interactions.

Thioridazine Hydrochloride Tablets 2163

Thiothixene (May increase drowsiness effect). Products include:

Thiothixene Capsules 2165

Tranylcypromine Sulfate (Concurrent or sequential use with MAO inhibitors is not recommended). Products include:

Parnate Tablets 1527

Triazolam (May increase drowsiness effect).

No products indexed under this heading.

Trifluoperazine Hydrochloride (May increase drowsiness effect).

No products indexed under this heading.

Zaleplon (May increase drowsiness effect). Products include:

Sonata Capsules 1717

Zolpidem Tartrate (May increase drowsiness effect). Products include:

Ambien Tablets 2851
Ambien CR Tablets 2855

Food Interactions

Alcohol (Avoid alcoholic beverages when using this product).

ROBITUSSIN SUGAR FREE COUGH

(Dextromethorphan Hydrobromide, Guaifenesin) .... ■738

May interact with monoamine oxidase inhibitors. Compounds in these categories include:

Isocarboxazid (Concurrent and/or sequential use with MAO inhibitors is not recommended).

No products indexed under this heading.

Moclobemide (Concurrent and/or sequential use with MAO inhibitors is not recommended).

No products indexed under this heading.

Pargyline Hydrochloride (Concurrent and/or sequential use with MAO inhibitors is not recommended).

No products indexed under this heading.

Phenelzine Sulfate (Concurrent and/or sequential use with MAO inhibitors is not recommended).

No products indexed under this heading.

Procarbazine Hydrochloride (Concurrent and/or sequential use with MAO inhibitors is not recommended). Products include:

Matulane Capsules 3191

Selegiline Hydrochloride (Concurrent and/or sequential use with MAO inhibitors is not recommended). Products include:

Eldepryl Capsules 3208
Zelapar Tablets 3372

Tranylcypromine Sulfate (Concurrent and/or sequential use with MAO inhibitors is not recommended). Products include:

Parnate Tablets 1527

ROCALTROL CAPSULES

(Calcitriol) 2798

May interact with calcium preparations, corticosteroids, cardiac glycosides, magnesium-containing antacids, phenytoin, phosphate-binding agents, and thiazides. Compounds in these categories include:

Antacids, magnesium-containing (Magnesium-containing preparations (e.g., antacids) may cause hypermagnesemia and should therefore not be taken during therapy with calcitriol by patients on chronic renal dialysis).

No products indexed under this heading.

Bendroflumethiazide (Thiazides are known to induce hypercalcemia by the reduction of calcium excretion in urine. Some reports have shown that the concomitant administration of thiazides with calcitriol causes hypercalcemia. Therefore, precaution should be taken when co-administration is necessary).

No products indexed under this heading.

Betamethasone Acetate (A relationship of functional antagonism exists between vitamin D analogues, which promote calcium absorption, and corticosteroids, which inhibit calcium absorption).

No products indexed under this heading.

Betamethasone Sodium Phosphate (A relationship of functional antagonism exists between vitamin D analogues, which promote calcium absorption, and corticosteroids, which inhibit calcium absorption).

No products indexed under this heading.

Calcium (Uncontrolled intake of additional calcium-containing preparations should be avoided). Products include:

Os-Cal 250 + D Tablets .... ■817
Os-Cal 500 Tablets .... ■817
Os-Cal 500 + D Tablets .... ■817

Calcium, intravenous (Uncontrolled intake of additional calcium-containing preparations should be avoided).

No products indexed under this heading.

Calcium (Oyster Shell) (Uncontrolled intake of additional calcium-containing preparations should be avoided).

No products indexed under this heading.

Calcium Acetate (Uncontrolled intake of additional calcium-containing preparations should be avoided). Products include:

PhosLo GelCaps 2169

Calcium Ascorbate (Uncontrolled intake of additional calcium-containing preparations should be avoided).

No products indexed under this heading.

Calcium Carbaspirin (Uncontrolled intake of additional calcium-containing preparations should be avoided).

No products indexed under this heading.

Calcium Carbonate (Uncontrolled intake of additional calcium-containing preparations should be avoided). Products include:

Actonel with Calcium Tablets 2688
Calcet Tablets 2138
Caltrate 600 PLUS .... ■809
Caltrate 600 + D Tablets .... ■809
D-Cal Chewable Caplets .... ■812
Gas-X with Maalox .... ■656
Maalox Regular Strength Antacid Chewable Tablets 2177
Maalox Max Maximum Strength Antacid/Antigas Chewable Tablets 2176
Maalox Max Maximum Strength Chewable Tablets .... ■660
Os-Cal Chewable Tablets .... ■818
Pepcid Complete Chewable Tablets 1701
Children's Pepto 2674
PremCal Light, Regular, and Extra Strength Tablets .... ■818
Tums .... ■664

Calcium Carbonate, Precipitated (Uncontrolled intake of additional calcium-containing preparations should be avoided).

No products indexed under this heading.

Calcium Caseinate (Uncontrolled intake of additional calcium-containing preparations should be avoided).

No products indexed under this heading.

Calcium Chloride (Uncontrolled intake of additional calcium-containing preparations should be avoided).

No products indexed under this heading.

Calcium Citrate (Uncontrolled intake of additional calcium-containing preparations should be avoided). Products include:

Active Calcium Tablets 3339
Citracal Caplets .... ■703
Citracal Lemon Cream Creamy Bites 2139
Citracal Prenatal + DHA Tablets and Capsules 2139

Calcium Glubionate (Uncontrolled intake of additional calcium-containing preparations should be avoided).

No products indexed under this heading.

Calcium Gluconate (Uncontrolled intake of additional calcium-containing preparations should be avoided). Products include:

Calcet Tablets 2138

Calcium Lactate (Uncontrolled intake of additional calcium-containing preparations should be avoided). Products include:

Calcet Tablets 2138

Calcium Phosphate (Uncontrolled intake of additional calcium-containing preparations should be avoided).

No products indexed under this heading.

Calcium Phosphate, Dibasic (Uncontrolled intake of additional calcium-containing preparations should be avoided).

No products indexed under this heading.

Calcium Phosphate, Tribasic (Uncontrolled intake of additional calcium-containing preparations should be avoided).

No products indexed under this heading.

Calcium Phosphorus Preparations (Uncontrolled intake of additional calcium-containing preparations should be avoided).

No products indexed under this heading.

Calcium Polycarbophil (Uncontrolled intake of additional calcium-containing preparations should be avoided). Products include:

FiberCon Caplets .... ■650

Calcium Salts (Uncontrolled intake of additional calcium-containing preparations should be avoided).

No products indexed under this heading.

Chlorothiazide (Thiazides are known to induce hypercalcemia by the reduction of calcium excretion in urine. Some reports have shown that the concomitant administration of thiazides with calcitriol causes hypercalcemia. Therefore, precaution should be taken when co-administration is necessary). Products include:

Diuril Oral Suspension 1954

Chlorothiazide Sodium (Thiazides are known to induce hypercalcemia by the reduction of calcium excretion in urine. Some reports have shown that the concomitant administration of thiazides with calcitriol causes hypercalcemia. Therefore, precaution should be taken when co-administration is necessary). Products include:

Diuril Sodium Intravenous 2467

Cholestyramine (Cholestryramine has been reported to reduce intestinal absorption of fat-soluble vitamins; as such it may impair intestinal absorption of calcitriol).

No products indexed under this heading.

Cortisone Acetate (A relationship of functional antagonism exists between vitamin D analogues, which promote calcium absorption, and corticosteroids, which inhibit calcium absorption).

No products indexed under this heading.

Deslanoside (Calcitriol dosage must be determined with care in patients undergoing treamtent with digitalis, as hypercalcemia in such patients may precipitate cardiac arrhythmias).

No products indexed under this heading.

Dexamethasone (A relationship of functional antagonism exists between vitamin D analogues, which promote calcium absorption, and corticosteroids, which inhibit calcium absorption). Products include:

Ciprodex Otic Suspension 559
Decadron Tablets 1951
TobraDex Ophthalmic Ointment 562
TobraDex Ophthalmic Suspension ... 563

Dexamethasone Acetate (A relationship of functional antagonism exists between vitamin D analogues, which promote calcium absorption, and corticosteroids, which inhibit calcium absorption).

No products indexed under this heading.

Dexamethasone Sodium Phosphate (A relationship of functional antagonism exists between vitamin D analogues, which promote calcium absorption, and corticosteroids, which inhibit calcium absorption).

No products indexed under this heading.

Digitalis Glycoside Preparations (Calcitriol dosage must be determined with care in patients undergoing treamtent with digitalis, as hypercalcemia in such patients may precipitate cardiac arrhythmias).

No products indexed under this heading.

Digitoxin (Calcitriol dosage must be determined with care in patients undergoing treamtent with digitalis, as hypercalcemia in such patients may precipitate cardiac arrhythmias).

No products indexed under this heading.

Digoxin (Calcitriol dosage must be determined with care in patients undergoing treamtent with digitalis, as hypercalcemia in such patients may precipitate cardiac arrhythmias). Products include:

Lanoxicaps Capsules 1490
Lanoxin Injection 1494
Lanoxin Injection Pediatric 1497
Lanoxin Tablets 1500

Fludrocortisone Acetate (A relationship of functional antagonism exists between vitamin D analogues, which promote calcium absorption, and corticosteroids, which inhibit calcium absorption).

No products indexed under this heading.

Fosphenytoin Sodium (The co-administration of phenytoin will not affect plasma concentrations of calcitriol, but may reduce endogenous plasma levels of 25(OH)D3 by accelerating metabolism. Since blood level of calcitriol will be reduced, higher doses of calcitriol may be necessary if these drugs are administered simultaneously).

No products indexed under this heading.

Hydrochlorothiazide (Thiazides are known to induce hypercalcemia by the reduction of calcium excretion in urine. Some reports have shown that the concomitant administration of thiazides with calcitriol causes hypercalcemia. Therefore, precaution should be taken when co-administration is necessary). Products include:

Aldoril Tablets 1910
Atacand HCT 651
Avalide Tablets 888
Avalide Tablets 2874
Benicar HCT Tablets 1044
Diovan HCT Tablets 2196
Dyazide Capsules 1423
Hyzaar 50-12.5 Tablets 1990
Hyzaar 100-12.5 Tablets 1990
Hyzaar 100-25 Tablets 1990
Lopressor HCT 50/25 Tablets 2241
Lopressor HCT 100/25 Tablets 2241
Lopressor HCT 100/50 Tablets 2241
Lotensin HCT Tablets 2246
Micardis HCT Tablets 856
Moduretic Tablets 2028
Prinzide Tablets 2056
Teveten HCT Tablets 1737
Timolide Tablets 2086
Uniretic Tablets 3100

Hydrocortisone (A relationship of functional antagonism exists between vitamin D analogues, which promote calcium absorption, and corticosteroids, which inhibit calcium absorption). Products include:

Colocort Rectal Suspension, USP (Retention) 100 mg/60 mL 2476
Hydrocortone Tablets 1989
Preparation H Hydrocortisone Cream 646

Hydrocortisone Acetate (A relationship of functional antagonism exists between vitamin D analogues, which promote calcium absorption, and corticosteroids, which inhibit calcium absorption). Products include:

Analpram-HC 1159
Pramosone 1161
ProctoFoam-HC 3099

Hydrocortisone Sodium Phosphate (A relationship of functional antagonism exists between vitamin D analogues, which promote calcium absorption, and corticosteroids, which inhibit calcium absorption).

No products indexed under this heading.

Hydrocortisone Sodium Succinate (A relationship of functional antagonism exists between vitamin D analogues, which promote calcium absorption, and corticosteroids, which inhibit calcium absorption).

No products indexed under this heading.

Hydroflumethiazide (Thiazides are known to induce hypercalcemia by the reduction of calcium excretion in urine. Some reports have shown that the concomitant administration of thiazides with calcitriol causes hypercalcemia. Therefore, precaution should be taken when co-administration is necessary).

No products indexed under this heading.

Ketoconazole (Ketoconazole may inhibit both synthetic and catabolic enzymes of calcitriol. Reductions in serum endogenous calcitriol concentrations have been observed following the administration of 300 mg/day to 1200 mg/day ketoconazole for a week to healthy men. However, in vivo dug interaction studies of ketoconazole with calcitriol have not been investigated). Products include:

Nizoral A-D Shampoo, 1% 1868

Lanthanum Carbonate (Since calcitriol has an effect on phosphate transport in the intestine, kidneys and bones, the dosage of phosphate-binding agents must be adjusted in accordance with the serum phosphate concentration). Products include:

Fosrenol Chewable Tablets 3183

Laxatives, magnesium-containing (Magnesium-containing preparations may cause hypermagnesemia and should therefore not be taken during therapy with calcitriol by patients on chronic renal dialysis).

No products indexed under this heading.

Magaldrate (Magnesium-containing preparations (e.g., antacids) may cause hypermagnesemia and should therefore not be taken during therapy with calcitriol by patients on chronic renal dialysis).

No products indexed under this heading.

Magnesium (Magnesium-containing preparations may cause hypermagnesemia and should therefore not be taken during therapy with calcitriol by patients on chronic renal dialysis).

No products indexed under this heading.

Magnesium Carbonate (Magnesium-containing preparations may cause hypermagnesemia and should therefore not be taken during therapy with calcitriol by patients on chronic renal dialysis). Products include:

Gaviscon Regular Strength Liquid 658
Gaviscon Extra Strength Liquid 658
Gaviscon Extra Strength Tablets 658

Magnesium Chloride (Magnesium-containing preparations may cause hypermagnesemia and should therefore not be taken during therapy with calcitriol by patients on chronic renal dialysis).

No products indexed under this heading.

Magnesium Citrate (Magnesium-containing preparations may cause hypermagnesemia and should therefore not be taken during therapy with calcitriol by patients on chronic renal dialysis).

No products indexed under this heading.

Magnesium Gluconate (Magnesium-containing preparations may cause hypermagnesemia and should therefore not be taken during therapy with calcitriol by patients on chronic renal dialysis).

No products indexed under this heading.

Magnesium Hydroxide (Magnesium-containing preparations may cause hypermagnesemia and should therefore not be taken during therapy with calcitriol by patients on chronic renal dialysis). Products include:

Maalox Regular Strength Antacid/Antigas Liquid 2175
Maalox Max Maximum Strength Antacid/Anti-Gas Liquid 2176
Pepcid Complete Chewable Tablets 1701

Magnesium Lactate (Magnesium-containing preparations may cause hypermagnesemia and should therefore not be taken during therapy with calcitriol by patients on chronic renal dialysis).

No products indexed under this heading.

Magnesium Oxide (Magnesium-containing preparations may cause hypermagnesemia and should therefore not be taken during therapy with calcitriol by patients on chronic renal dialysis). Products include:

Beelith Tablets 759
PremCal Light, Regular, and Extra Strength Tablets 818

Magnesium Salicylate (Magnesium-containing preparations may cause hypermagnesemia and should therefore not be taken during therapy with calcitriol by patients on chronic renal dialysis).

No products indexed under this heading.

Magnesium Salicylate Tetrahydrate (Magnesium-containing preparations may cause hypermagnesemia and should therefore not be taken during therapy with calcitriol by patients on chronic renal dialysis).

No products indexed under this heading.

Magnesium Salts (Magnesium-containing preparations may cause hypermagnesemia and should therefore not be taken during therapy with calcitriol by patients on chronic renal dialysis).

No products indexed under this heading.

Magnesium Sulfate (Magnesium-containing preparations may cause hypermagnesemia and should therefore not be taken during therapy with calcitriol by patients on chronic renal dialysis).

No products indexed under this heading.

Magnesium Trisilicate (Magnesium-containing preparations may cause hypermagnesemia and should therefore not be taken during therapy with calcitriol by patients on chronic renal dialysis). Products include:

Gaviscon Regular Strength Tablets 658

Methyclothiazide (Thiazides are known to induce hypercalcemia by the reduction of calcium excretion in urine. Some reports have shown that the concomitant administration of thiazides with calcitriol causes hypercalcemia. Therefore, precaution should be taken when co-administration is necessary).

No products indexed under this heading.

Methylprednisolone Acetate (A relationship of functional antagonism exists between vitamin D analogues, which promote calcium absorption, and corticosteroids, which inhibit calcium absorption). Products include:

Depo-Medrol Injectable Suspension 2617
Depo-Medrol Single-Dose Vial 2619

Methylprednisolone Sodium Succinate (A relationship of functional antagonism exists between vitamin D analogues, which promote calcium absorption, and corticosteroids, which inhibit calcium absorption).

No products indexed under this heading.

Phenobarbital (The co-administration of phenobarbital will not affect plasma concentrations of calcitriol, but may reduce endogenous plasma levels of 25(OH)D3 by accelerating metabolism. Since blood level of calcitriol will be reduced, higher doses of calcitriol may be necessary if these drugs are administered simultaneously). Products include:

Donnatal Extentabs 2493

Phenobarbital Sodium (The co-administration of phenobarbital will not affect plasma concentrations of calcitrol, but may reduce endogenous plasma levels of 25(OH)D3 by accelerating metabolism. Since blood level of calcitriol will be reduced, higher doses of calcitriol may benecessary if these drugs are administered simultaneously).

No products indexed under this heading.

Phenytoin (The co-administration of phenytoin will not affect plasma concentrations of calcitriol, but may reduce endogenous plasma levels of 25(OH)D3 by accelerating metabolism. Since blood level of calcitriol will be reduced, higher doses of calcitriol may be necessary if these drugs are administered simultaneously).

No products indexed under this heading.

Phenytoin Sodium (The co-administration of phenytoin will not affect plasma concentrations of calcitriol, but may reduce endogenous plasma levels of 25(OH)D3 by accelerating metabolism. Since blood level of calcitriol will be reduced, higher doses of calcitriol may be necessary if these drugs are administered simultaneously). Products include:

Phenytek Capsules 2160

Polythiazide (Thiazides are known to induce hypercalcemia by the reduction of calcium excretion in urine. Some reports have shown that the concomitant administration of thiazides with calcitriol causes hypercalcemia. Therefore, precaution should be taken when co-administration is necessary).
No products indexed under this heading.

Prednisolone Acetate (A relationship of functional antagonism exists between vitamin D analogues, which promote calcium absorption, and corticosteroids, which inhibit calcium absorption). Products include:
Blephamide Ophthalmic Ointment 568
Blephamide Ophthalmic Suspension 569
Poly-Pred Ophthalmic Suspension .... ⊙233
Pred Forte Ophthalmic Suspension .... ⊙235
Pred Mild Ophthalmic Suspension .... ⊙238
Pred-G Ophthalmic Ointment .... ⊙237
Pred-G Ophthalmic Suspension ...... ⊙236

Prednisolone Sodium Phosphate (A relationship of functional antagonism exists between vitamin D analogues, which promote calcium absorption, and corticosteroids, which inhibit calcium absorption).
No products indexed under this heading.

Prednisolone Tebutate (A relationship of functional antagonism exists between vitamin D analogues, which promote calcium absorption, and corticosteroids, which inhibit calcium absorption).
No products indexed under this heading.

Prednisone (A relationship of functional antagonism exists between vitamin D analogues, which promote calcium absorption, and corticosteroids, which inhibit calcium absorption).
No products indexed under this heading.

Sevelamer Hydrochloride (Since calcitriol has an effect on phosphate transport in the intestine, kidneys and bones, the dosage of phosphate-binding agents must be adjusted in accordance with the serum phosphate concentration). Products include:
Renagel Tablets 1282

Triamcinolone (A relationship of functional antagonism exists between vitamin D analogues, which promote calcium absorption, and corticosteroids, which inhibit calcium absorption).
No products indexed under this heading.

Triamcinolone Acetonide (A relationship of functional antagonism exists between vitamin D analogues, which promote calcium absorption, and corticosteroids, which inhibit calcium absorption). Products include:
Azmacort Inhalation Aerosol 1726
Nasacort AQ Nasal Spray 2922

Triamcinolone Diacetate (A relationship of functional antagonism exists between vitamin D analogues, which promote calcium absorption, and corticosteroids, which inhibit calcium absorption).
No products indexed under this heading.

Triamcinolone Hexacetonide (A relationship of functional antagonism exists between vitamin D analogues, which promote calcium absorption, and corticosteroids, which inhibit calcium absorption).
No products indexed under this heading.

Vitamin D (Since calcitriol is the most potent active metabolite of vitamin D3, pharmacological doses of vitamin D and its derivatives should be withheld during treatment with calcitriol to avoid possible additive effects of hypercalcemia). Products include:
Active Calcium Tablets 3339
Caltrate 600 PLUS .... ■□809
Caltrate 600 + D Tablets .... ■□809
D-Cal Chewable Caplets .... ■□812
Os-Cal 250 + D Tablets .... ■□817
Os-Cal 500 + D Tablets .... ■□817

ROCALTROL ORAL SOLUTION

(Calcitriol) 2798
See Rocaltrol Capsules

ROCEPHIN INJECTABLE VIALS, ADD-VANTAGE, GALAXY, BULK

(Ceftriaxone Sodium) 2800
None cited in PDR database.

MEN'S ROGAINE EXTRA STRENGTH HAIR REGROWTH TREATMENT TOPICAL SOLUTION, OCEAN RUSH SCENT AND ORIGINAL UNSCENTED

(Minoxidil) .... ■□633
None cited in PDR database.

MEN'S ROGAINE FOAM HAIR REGROWTH TREATMENT

(Minoxidil) .... ■□633
None cited in PDR database.

WOMEN'S ROGAINE HAIR REGROWTH TREATMENT TOPICAL SOLUTION, SPRING BLOOM SCENT AND ORIGINAL UNSCENTED

(Minoxidil) .... ■□634
None cited in PDR database.

ROMAZICON INJECTION

(Flumazenil) 2804
May interact with antidepressant drugs, neuromuscular blocking agents, and certain other agents. Compounds in these categories include:

Amitriptyline Hydrochloride (Toxic effects of cyclic antidepressant may emerge with the reversal of the benzodiazepine effect).
No products indexed under this heading.

Amoxapine (Toxic effects of cyclic antidepressants may emerge with the reversal of the benzodiazepine effect).
No products indexed under this heading.

Atracurium Besylate (Romazicon should not be used until the effects of neuromuscular blockade have been fully reversed).
No products indexed under this heading.

Bupropion Hydrochloride (Toxic effects of cyclic antidepressants may emerge with the reversal of the benzodiazepine effect). Products include:
Wellbutrin Tablets 1603
Wellbutrin SR Sustained-Release Tablets 1607
Wellbutrin XL Extended-Release Tablets 1613
Zyban Sustained-Release Tablets 1644

Cisatracurium Besylate (Romazicon should not be used until the effects of neuromuscular blockade have been fully reversed). Products include:
Nimbex Injection 498

Citalopram Hydrobromide (Toxic effects of cyclic antidepressants may emerge with the reversal of the benzodiazepine effect). Products include:
Celexa 1176

Desipramine Hydrochloride (Toxic effects of cyclic antidepressants may emerge with the reversal of the benzodiazepine effect).
No products indexed under this heading.

Doxacurium Chloride (Romazicon should not be used until the effects of neuromuscular blockade have been fully reversed).
No products indexed under this heading.

Doxepin Hydrochloride (Toxic effects of cyclic antidepressants may emerge with the reversal of the benzodiazepine effect).
No products indexed under this heading.

Escitalopram Oxalate (Toxic effects of cyclic antidepressants may emerge with the reversal of the benzodiazepine effect). Products include:
Lexapro Oral Solution 1190
Lexapro Tablets 1190

Fluoxetine Hydrochloride (Toxic effects of cyclic antidepressants may emerge with the reversal of the benzodiazepine effect). Products include:
Prozac Pulvules and Liquid 1801
Symbyax Capsules 1819

Imipramine Hydrochloride (Toxic effects of cyclic antidepressants may emerge with the reversal of the benzodiazepine effect).
No products indexed under this heading.

Imipramine Pamoate (Toxic effects of cyclic antidepressants may emerge with the reversal of the benzodiazepine effect).
No products indexed under this heading.

Isocarboxazid (Toxic effects of cyclic antidepressants may emerge with the reversal of the benzodiazepine effect).
No products indexed under this heading.

Maprotiline Hydrochloride (Toxic effects of cyclic antidepressants may emerge with the reversal of the benzodiazepine effect).
No products indexed under this heading.

Metocurine Iodide (Romazicon should not be used until the effects of neuromuscular blockade have been fully reversed).
No products indexed under this heading.

Mirtazapine (Toxic effects of cyclic antidepressants may emerge with the reversal of the benzodiazepine effect).
No products indexed under this heading.

Mivacurium Chloride (Romazicon should not be used until the effects of neuromuscular blockade have been fully reversed). Products include:
Mivacron Injection 493

Nefazodone Hydrochloride (Toxic effects of cyclic antidepressants may emerge with the reversal of the benzodiazepine effect).
No products indexed under this heading.

Nortriptyline Hydrochloride (Toxic effects of cyclic antidepressants may emerge with the reversal of the benzodiazepine effect).
No products indexed under this heading.

Pancuronium Bromide (Romazicon should not be used until the effects of neuromuscular blockade have been fully reversed).
No products indexed under this heading.

Paroxetine Hydrochloride (Toxic effects of cyclic antidepressants may emerge with the reversal of the benzodiazepine effect). Products include:
Paxil CR Controlled-Release Tablets 1538
Paxil 1530

Phenelzine Sulfate (Toxic effects of cyclic antidepressants may emerge with the reversal of the benzodiazepine effect).
No products indexed under this heading.

Protriptyline Hydrochloride (Toxic effects of cyclic antidepressants may emerge with the reversal of the benzodiazepine effect).
No products indexed under this heading.

Rapacuronium Bromide (Romazicon should not be used until the effects of neuromuscular blockade have been fully reversed).
No products indexed under this heading.

Rocuronium Bromide (Romazicon should not be used until the effects of neuromuscular blockade have been fully reversed). Products include:
Zemuron Injection 2346

Sertraline Hydrochloride (Toxic effects of cyclic antidepressants may emerge with the reversal of the benzodiazepine effect). Products include:
Zoloft 2586

Succinylcholine Chloride (Romazicon should not be used until the effects of neuromuscular blockade have been fully reversed).
No products indexed under this heading.

Tranylcypromine Sulfate (Toxic effects of cyclic antidepressants may emerge with the reversal of the benzodiazepine effect). Products include:
Parnate Tablets 1527

Trazodone Hydrochloride (Toxic effects of cyclic antidepressants may emerge with the reversal of the benzodiazepine effect).
No products indexed under this heading.

Trimipramine Maleate (Toxic effects of cyclic antidepressants may emerge with the reversal of the benzodiazepine effect).
No products indexed under this heading.

Vecuronium Bromide (Romazicon should not be used until the effects of neuromuscular blockade have been fully reversed).
No products indexed under this heading.

Venlafaxine Hydrochloride (Toxic effects of cyclic antidepressants may emerge with the reversal of the benzodiazepine effect). Products include:
Effexor Tablets 3411
Effexor XR Capsules 3417

Food Interactions

Food, unspecified (Ingestion of food during an IV infusion results in a 50% increase in clearance).

ROSAC CREAM WITH SUNSCREENS

(Sodium Sulfacetamide, Sulfur) 3213
None cited in PDR database.

ROTATEQ

(Rotavirus vaccine, live, oral, pentavalent) 2074
May interact with alkylating agents, antimetabolites, corticosteroids, and cytotoxic drugs. Compounds in these categories include:

Betamethasone Acetate (Immunosuppressive therapies including corticosteroids (used in greater than physiologic doses) may reduce the immune response to vaccines).
No products indexed under this heading.

Betamethasone Sodium Phosphate (Immunosuppressive therapies including corticosteroids (used in greater than physiologic doses) may reduce the immune response to vaccines).
No products indexed under this heading.

Bleomycin Sulfate (Immunosuppressive therapies including cytotoxic drugs may reduce the immune response to vaccines).
No products indexed under this heading.

Busulfan (Immunosuppressive therapies including alkylating agents may reduce the immune response to vaccines). Products include:
I.V. Busulfex 2493
Myleran Tablets 1525

Capecitabine (Immunosuppresive therapies including antimetabolites may reduce the immune response to vaccines). Products include:
Xeloda Tablets 2822

Carmustine (BCNU) (Immunosuppressive therapies including alkylating agents may reduce the immune response to vaccines).
No products indexed under this heading.

Chlorambucil (Immunosuppressive therapies including alkylating agents may reduce the immune response to vaccines). Products include:
Leukeran Tablets 1504

Cladribine (Immunosuppresive therapies including antimetabolites may reduce the immune response to vaccines). Products include:
Leustatin Injection 2357

Cortisone Acetate (Immunosuppressive therapies including corticosteroids (used in greater than physiologic doses) may reduce the immune response to vaccines).
No products indexed under this heading.

Cyclophosphamide (Immunosuppressive therapies including alkylating agents may reduce the immune response to vaccines).
No products indexed under this heading.

Cytarabine (Immunosuppresive therapies including antimetabolites may reduce the immune response to vaccines).
No products indexed under this heading.

Dacarbazine (Immunosuppressive therapies including alkylating agents may reduce the immune response to vaccines).
No products indexed under this heading.

Daunorubicin Hydrochloride (Immunosuppressive therapies including cytotoxic drugs may reduce the immune response to vaccines).
No products indexed under this heading.

Dexamethasone (Immunosuppressive therapies including corticosteroids (used in greater than physiologic doses) may reduce the immune response to vaccines). Products include:
Ciprodex Otic Suspension 559
Decadron Tablets 1951
TobraDex Ophthalmic Ointment 562
TobraDex Ophthalmic Suspension ... 563

Dexamethasone Acetate (Immunosuppressive therapies including corticosteroids (used in greater than physiologic doses) may reduce the immune response to vaccines).
No products indexed under this heading.

Dexamethasone Sodium Phosphate (Immunosuppressive therapies including corticosteroids (used in greater than physiologic doses) may reduce the immune response to vaccines).
No products indexed under this heading.

Doxorubicin Hydrochloride (Immunosuppressive therapies including cytotoxic drugs may reduce the immune response to vaccines).
No products indexed under this heading.

Epirubicin Hydrochloride (Immunosuppressive therapies including cytotoxic drugs may reduce the immune response to vaccines).
No products indexed under this heading.

Floxuridine (Immunosuppresive therapies including antimetabolites may reduce the immune response to vaccines).
No products indexed under this heading.

Fludarabine Phosphate (Immunosuppresive therapies including antimetabolites may reduce the immune response to vaccines).
No products indexed under this heading.

Fludrocortisone Acetate (Immunosuppressive therapies including corticosteroids (used in greater than physiologic doses) may reduce the immune response to vaccines).
No products indexed under this heading.

Fluorouracil (Immunosuppresive therapies including antimetabolites may reduce the immune response to vaccines). Products include:
Carac Cream, 0.5% 2879
Efudex 3363

Gemcitabine Hydrochloride (Immunosuppresive therapies including antimetabolites may reduce the immune response to vaccines). Products include:
Gemzar for Injection 1771

Hydrocortisone (Immunosuppressive therapies including corticosteroids (used in greater than physiologic doses) may reduce the immune response to vaccines). Products include:
Colocort Rectal Suspension, USP (Retention) 100 mg/60 mL 2476
Hydrocortone Tablets 1989
Preparation H Hydrocortisone Cream .... ⊡646

Hydrocortisone Acetate (Immunosuppressive therapies including corticosteroids (used in greater than physiologic doses) may reduce the immune response to vaccines). Products include:
Analpram-HC 1159
Pramosone 1161
ProctoFoam-HC 3099

Hydrocortisone Sodium Phosphate (Immunosuppressive therapies including corticosteroids (used in greater than physiologic doses) may reduce the immune response to vaccines).
No products indexed under this heading.

Hydrocortisone Sodium Succinate (Immunosuppressive therapies including corticosteroids (used in greater than physiologic doses) may reduce the immune response to vaccines).
No products indexed under this heading.

Hydroxyurea (Immunosuppressive therapies including cytotoxic drugs may reduce the immune response to vaccines).
No products indexed under this heading.

Lomustine (CCNU) (Immunosuppressive therapies including alkylating agents may reduce the immune response to vaccines).
No products indexed under this heading.

Mechlorethamine Hydrochloride (Immunosuppressive therapies including alkylating agents may reduce the immune response to vaccines). Products include:
Mustargen for Injection 2468

Melphalan (Immunosuppressive therapies including alkylating agents may reduce the immune response to vaccines). Products include:
Alkeran Tablets 956

Mercaptopurine (Immunosuppresive therapies including antimetabolites may reduce the immune response to vaccines).
No products indexed under this heading.

Methotrexate (Immunosuppresive therapies including antimetabolites may reduce the immune response to vaccines).
No products indexed under this heading.

Methotrexate Sodium (Immunosuppressive therapies including cytotoxic drugs may reduce the immune response to vaccines).
No products indexed under this heading.

Methylprednisolone Acetate (Immunosuppressive therapies including corticosteroids (used in greater than physiologic doses) may reduce the immune response to vaccines). Products include:
Depo-Medrol Injectable Suspension 2617
Depo-Medrol Single-Dose Vial 2619

Methylprednisolone Sodium Succinate (Immunosuppressive therapies including corticosteroids (used in greater than physiologic doses) may reduce the immune response to vaccines).
No products indexed under this heading.

Mitotane (Immunosuppressive therapies including cytotoxic drugs may reduce the immune response to vaccines).
No products indexed under this heading.

Mitoxantrone Hydrochloride (Immunosuppressive therapies including cytotoxic drugs may reduce the immune response to vaccines).
No products indexed under this heading.

Pentostatin (Immunosuppresive therapies including antimetabolites may reduce the immune response to vaccines). Products include:
Nipent for Injection 1863

Prednisolone Acetate (Immunosuppressive therapies including corticosteroids (used in greater than physiologic doses) may reduce the immune response to vaccines). Products include:
Blephamide Ophthalmic Ointment 568
Blephamide Ophthalmic Suspension 569
Poly-Pred Ophthalmic Suspension .... ⊙233
Pred Forte Ophthalmic Suspension .... ⊙235
Pred Mild Ophthalmic Suspension .... ⊙238
Pred-G Ophthalmic Ointment .... ⊙237
Pred-G Ophthalmic Suspension ...... ⊙236

Prednisolone Sodium Phosphate (Immunosuppressive therapies including corticosteroids (used in greater than physiologic doses) may reduce the immune response to vaccines).
No products indexed under this heading.

Prednisolone Tebutate (Immunosuppressive therapies including corticosteroids (used in greater than physiologic doses) may reduce the immune response to vaccines).
No products indexed under this heading.

Prednisone (Immunosuppressive therapies including corticosteroids (used in greater than physiologic doses) may reduce the immune response to vaccines).
No products indexed under this heading.

Procarbazine Hydrochloride (Immunosuppressive therapies

including cytotoxic drugs may reduce the immune response to vaccines). Products include:

Matulane Capsules 3191

Tamoxifen Citrate (Immunosuppressive therapies including cytotoxic drugs may reduce the immune response to vaccines). Products include:

Soltamox Oral Solution 3527

Thioguanine (Immunosuppresive therapies including antimetabolites may reduce the immune response to vaccines). Products include:

Tabloid Tablets 1575

Thiotepa (Immunosuppressive therapies including alkylating agents may reduce the immune response to vaccines).

No products indexed under this heading.

Triamcinolone (Immunosuppressive therapies including corticosteroids (used in greater than physiologic doses) may reduce the immune response to vaccines).

No products indexed under this heading.

Triamcinolone Acetonide (Immunosuppressive therapies including corticosteroids (used in greater than physiologic doses) may reduce the immune response to vaccines). Products include:

Azmacort Inhalation Aerosol 1726
Nasacort AQ Nasal Spray 2922

Triamcinolone Diacetate (Immunosuppressive therapies including corticosteroids (used in greater than physiologic doses) may reduce the immune response to vaccines).

No products indexed under this heading.

Triamcinolone Hexacetonide (Immunosuppressive therapies including corticosteroids (used in greater than physiologic doses) may reduce the immune response to vaccines).

No products indexed under this heading.

Vincristine Sulfate (Immunosuppressive therapies including cytotoxic drugs may reduce the immune response to vaccines).

No products indexed under this heading.

ROZEREM TABLETS

(Ramelteon) 3231
May interact with cytochrome p450 1a2 inducers (selected), cytochrome p450 1a2 inhibitors (selected), cytochrome p450 2c8 inducers (selected), cytochrome p450 2c9 inducers (selected), cytochrome p450 2c9 inhibitors (selected), cytochrome p450 2d6 inducers (selected), cytochrome p450 3a4 inducers (selected), cytochrome p450 3a4 inhibitors (selected), cytochrome p450 3a inducers (selected), and certain other agents. Compounds in these categories include:

Acetazolamide (Ramelteon should be administered with caution in subjects taking strong CYP2C9 inhibitors such as fluconazole).

No products indexed under this heading.

Alatrofloxacin Mesylate (Ramelteon should be administered with caution in subjects taking strong CYP2C9 inhibitors such as fluconazole).

No products indexed under this heading.

Allium sativum (Efficacy may be reduced when ramelteon is used in combination with strong CYP enzyme inducers such as rifampin).

No products indexed under this heading.

Amiodarone Hydrochloride (Ramelteon should be administered with caution in subjects taking strong CYP2C9 inhibitors such as fluconazole).

No products indexed under this heading.

Amprenavir (Ramelteon should be administered with caution in subjects taking strong CYP2C9 inhibitors such as fluconazole). Products include:

Agenerase Capsules 1327
Agenerase Oral Solution 1332

Anastrozole (Ramelteon should be administered with caution in subjects taking strong CYP2C9 inhibitors such as fluconazole). Products include:

Arimidex Tablets 673

Aprepitant (Ramelteon should be administered with caution in subjects taking strong CYP2C9 inhibitors such as fluconazole). Products include:

Emend Capsules 1963

Bendroflumethiazide (Ramelteon should be administered with caution in subjects taking strong CYP2C9 inhibitors such as fluconazole).

No products indexed under this heading.

Betamethasone Acetate (Efficacy may be reduced when ramelteon is used in combination with strong CYP enzyme inducers such as rifampin).

No products indexed under this heading.

Betamethasone Sodium Phosphate (Efficacy may be reduced when ramelteon is used in combination with strong CYP enzyme inducers such as rifampin).

No products indexed under this heading.

Carbamazepine (Efficacy may be reduced when ramelteon is used in combination with strong CYP enzyme inducers such as rifampin). Products include:

Carbatrol Capsules 3171
Equetro Extended-Release
Capsules 3180
Tegretol/Tegretol-XR 2295

Chloramphenicol (Ramelteon should be administered with caution in subjects taking strong CYP2C9 inhibitors such as fluconazole).

No products indexed under this heading.

Chlorothiazide (Ramelteon should be administered with caution in subjects taking strong CYP2C9 inhibitors such as fluconazole). Products include:

Diuril Oral Suspension 1954

Chlorothiazide Sodium (Ramelteon should be administered with caution in subjects taking strong CYP2C9 inhibitors such as fluconazole). Products include:

Diuril Sodium Intravenous 2467

Chlorpropamide (Ramelteon should be administered with caution in subjects taking strong CYP2C9 inhibitors such as fluconazole).

No products indexed under this heading.

Cimetidine (Ramelteon should be administered with caution in subjects

taking strong CYP2C9 inhibitors such as fluconazole). Products include:

Tagamet HB 200 Tablets ▣664

Cimetidine Hydrochloride (Ramelteon should be administered with caution in subjects taking strong CYP2C9 inhibitors such as fluconazole).

No products indexed under this heading.

Ciprofloxacin (Ramelteon should be administered with caution in subjects taking strong CYP2C9 inhibitors such as fluconazole). Products include:

Cipro Oral Suspension 2977
Cipro I.V. 2984
Cipro XR Tablets 2990
Ciprodex Otic Suspension 559

Ciprofloxacin Hydrochloride (Ramelteon should be administered with caution in subjects taking strong CYP2C9 inhibitors such as fluconazole). Products include:

Ciloxan Ophthalmic Ointment 559
Ciloxan Ophthalmic Solution ⊙206
Cipro Tablets 2977
Proquin XR Tablets 1153

Cisplatin (Efficacy may be reduced when ramelteon is used in combination with strong CYP enzyme inducers such as rifampin).

No products indexed under this heading.

Citalopram Hydrobromide (Efficacy may be reduced when ramelteon is used in combination with strong CYP enzyme inducers such as rifampin). Products include:

Celexa .. 1176

Clarithromycin (Ramelteon should be administered with caution in subjects taking strong CYP2C9 inhibitors such as fluconazole). Products include:

Biaxin/Biaxin XL 402
PREVPAC 3284

Clopidogrel Hydrogen Sulfate (Ramelteon should be administered with caution in subjects taking strong CYP2C9 inhibitors such as fluconazole).

No products indexed under this heading.

Clotrimazole (Ramelteon should be administered with caution in subjects taking strong CYP2C9 inhibitors such as fluconazole). Products include:

Desenex Athlete's Foot Cream ▣635
Lotrimin 3039
Lotrisone 3040

Cortisone Acetate (Efficacy may be reduced when ramelteon is used in combination with strong CYP enzyme inducers such as rifampin).

No products indexed under this heading.

Cyclosporine (Ramelteon should be administered with caution in subjects taking strong CYP2C9 inhibitors such as fluconazole). Products include:

Gengraf Capsules 459
Neoral Oral Solution 2259
Neoral Soft Gelatin Capsules 2259
Restasis Ophthalmic Emulsion 575
Sandimmune 2275

Dalfopristin (Ramelteon should be administered with caution in subjects taking strong CYP2C9 inhibitors such as fluconazole).

No products indexed under this heading.

Danazol (Ramelteon should be administered with caution in subjects taking strong CYP2C9 inhibitors such as fluconazole).

No products indexed under this heading.

Delavirdine Mesylate (Ramelteon should be administered with caution in subjects taking strong CYP2C9 inhibitors such as fluconazole). Products include:

Rescriptor Tablets 2551

Desogestrel (Ramelteon should be administered with caution in subjects taking strong CYP2C9 inhibitors such as fluconazole). Products include:

Mircette Tablets 1066

Dexamethasone (Efficacy may be reduced when ramelteon is used in combination with strong CYP enzyme inducers such as rifampin). Products include:

Ciprodex Otic Suspension 559
Decadron Tablets 1951
TobraDex Ophthalmic Ointment 562
TobraDex Ophthalmic Suspension ... 563

Dexamethasone Acetate (Efficacy may be reduced when ramelteon is used in combination with strong CYP enzyme inducers such as rifampin).

No products indexed under this heading.

Dexamethasone Sodium Phosphate (Efficacy may be reduced when ramelteon is used in combination with strong CYP enzyme inducers such as rifampin).

No products indexed under this heading.

Diclofenac Potassium (Ramelteon should be administered with caution in subjects taking strong CYP2C9 inhibitors such as fluconazole).

No products indexed under this heading.

Diclofenac Sodium (Ramelteon should be administered with caution in subjects taking strong CYP2C9 inhibitors such as fluconazole). Products include:

Arthrotec Tablets 3129
Voltaren Ophthalmic Solution 2309
Voltaren Tablets 2307
Voltaren-XR Tablets 2310

Diltiazem Hydrochloride (Ramelteon should be administered with caution in subjects taking strong CYP2C9 inhibitors such as fluconazole). Products include:

Cardizem LA Extended Release
Tablets 1728
Tiazac Capsules 1201

Diltiazem Maleate (Ramelteon should be administered with caution in subjects taking strong CYP2C9 inhibitors such as fluconazole).

No products indexed under this heading.

Disulfiram (Ramelteon should be administered with caution in subjects taking strong CYP2C9 inhibitors such as fluconazole).

No products indexed under this heading.

Doxorubicin Hydrochloride (Efficacy may be reduced when ramelteon is used in combination with strong CYP enzyme inducers such as rifampin).

No products indexed under this heading.

Efavirenz (Ramelteon should be administered with caution in subjects

taking strong CYP2C9 inhibitors such as fluconazole). Products include:
- Atripla Tablets 945
- Sustiva Capsules 930
- Sustiva Tablets 930

Enoxacin (Ramelteon should be administered with caution in subjects taking strong CYP2C9 inhibitors such as fluconazole).
No products indexed under this heading.

Erythromycin (Ramelteon should be administered with caution in subjects taking strong CYP2C9 inhibitors such as fluconazole). Products include:
- Ery-Tab Tablets 449
- Erythromycin Base Filmtab Tablets 455
- Erythromycin Delayed-Release Capsules, USP 457
- PCE Dispertab Tablets 515

Erythromycin Estolate (Ramelteon should be administered with caution in subjects taking strong CYP2C9 inhibitors such as fluconazole).
No products indexed under this heading.

Erythromycin Ethylsuccinate (Ramelteon should be administered with caution in subjects taking strong CYP2C9 inhibitors such as fluconazole). Products include:
- E.E.S. 451
- EryPed 447

Erythromycin Gluceptate (Ramelteon should be administered with caution in subjects taking strong CYP2C9 inhibitors such as fluconazole).
No products indexed under this heading.

Erythromycin Lactobionate (Ramelteon should be administered with caution in subjects taking strong CYP2C9 inhibitors such as fluconazole).
No products indexed under this heading.

Erythromycin Stearate (Ramelteon should be administered with caution in subjects taking strong CYP2C9 inhibitors such as fluconazole). Products include:
- Erythrocin Stearate Filmtab Tablets 453

Esomeprazole Magnesium (Ramelteon should be administered with caution in subjects taking strong CYP2C9 inhibitors such as fluconazole). Products include:
- Nexium Delayed-Release Capsules 655

Ethanol (Efficacy may be reduced when ramelteon is used in combination with strong CYP enzyme inducers such as rifampin).
No products indexed under this heading.

Ethinyl Estradiol (Ramelteon should be administered with caution in subjects taking strong CYP2C9 inhibitors such as fluconazole). Products include:
- Mircette Tablets 1066
- NuvaRing 2340
- Ortho-Cyclen/Ortho Tri-Cyclen 2429
- Ortho Evra Transdermal System 2417
- Ortho Tri-Cyclen Lo Tablets 2436
- Seasonique Tablets 1077
- Yasmin 28 Tablets 796
- Yaz Tablets 803

Ethosuximide (Efficacy may be reduced when ramelteon is used in combination with strong CYP enzyme inducers such as rifampin).
No products indexed under this heading.

Felbamate (Efficacy may be reduced when ramelteon is used in combination with strong CYP enzyme inducers such as rifampin).
No products indexed under this heading.

Fenofibrate (Ramelteon should be administered with caution in subjects taking strong CYP2C9 inhibitors such as fluconazole). Products include:
- Lofibra Tablets 1219
- Lofibra Capsules 1216
- Tricor Tablets 527
- Triglide Tablets 3123

Fluconazole (The total and peak systemic exposure (AUC 0-inf and Cmax) of ramelteon after a single 16 mg dose of ramelteon was increased by approximately 150% when administered with fluconazole. Similar increases were also seen in M-II exposure. Ramelteon should be administered with caution in subjects taking strong CYP2C9 inhibitors such as fluconazole).
No products indexed under this heading.

Fludrocortisone Acetate (Efficacy may be reduced when ramelteon is used in combination with strong CYP enzyme inducers such as rifampin).
No products indexed under this heading.

Fluorouracil (Ramelteon should be administered with caution in subjects taking strong CYP2C9 inhibitors such as fluconazole). Products include:
- Carac Cream, 0.5% 2879
- Efudex 3363

Fluoxetine Hydrochloride (Ramelteon should be administered with caution in subjects taking strong CYP2C9 inhibitors such as fluconazole). Products include:
- Prozac Pulvules and Liquid 1801
- Symbyax Capsules 1819

Flurbiprofen (Ramelteon should be administered with caution in subjects taking strong CYP2C9 inhibitors such as fluconazole).
No products indexed under this heading.

Flurbiprofen Sodium (Ramelteon should be administered with caution in subjects taking strong CYP2C9 inhibitors such as fluconazole). Products include:
- Ocufen Ophthalmic Solution .... ⊙232

Fluvastatin Sodium (Ramelteon should be administered with caution in subjects taking strong CYP2C9 inhibitors such as fluconazole). Products include:
- Lescol Capsules 2233
- Lescol XL Tablets 2233

Fluvoxamine (When fluvoxamine 100 mg twice daily was administered for 3 days prior to single-dose co-administration of ramelteon 16 mg and fluvoxamine, the AUC 0-inf for ramelteon increased approximately 190-fold, and the Cmax increased approximately 70-fold, compared to ramelteon administered alone. Ramelteon should not be used in combination with fluvoxamine. Other less potent CYP1A2 inhibitors have not been adequately studied. Ramelteon should be administered with caution to patients taking less strong CYP1A2 inhibitors).
No products indexed under this heading.

Fluvoxamine Maleate (Ramelteon should be administered with caution in subjects taking strong CYP2C9 inhibitors such as fluconazole).
No products indexed under this heading.

Fosamprenavir Calcium (Ramelteon should be administered with caution in subjects taking strong CYP2C9 inhibitors such as fluconazole). Products include:
- Lexiva Tablets 1505

Fosphenytoin Sodium (Efficacy may be reduced when ramelteon is used in combination with strong CYP enzyme inducers such as rifampin).
No products indexed under this heading.

Garlic Extract (Efficacy may be reduced when ramelteon is used in combination with strong CYP enzyme inducers such as rifampin).
No products indexed under this heading.

Garlic Oil (Efficacy may be reduced when ramelteon is used in combination with strong CYP enzyme inducers such as rifampin).
No products indexed under this heading.

Gatifloxacin (Ramelteon should be administered with caution in subjects taking strong CYP2C9 inhibitors such as fluconazole). Products include:
- Tequin Injection 938
- Tequin Injection in 5% Dextrose 938
- Tequin Tablets 938
- Zymar Ophthalmic Solution 575

Gemfibrozil (Ramelteon should be administered with caution in subjects taking strong CYP2C9 inhibitors such as fluconazole).
No products indexed under this heading.

Gemifloxacin Mesylate (Ramelteon should be administered with caution in subjects taking strong CYP2C9 inhibitors such as fluconazole).
No products indexed under this heading.

Glipizide (Ramelteon should be administered with caution in subjects taking strong CYP2C9 inhibitors such as fluconazole).
No products indexed under this heading.

Glyburide (Ramelteon should be administered with caution in subjects taking strong CYP2C9 inhibitors such as fluconazole).
No products indexed under this heading.

Grepafloxacin Hydrochloride (Ramelteon should be administered with caution in subjects taking strong CYP2C9 inhibitors such as fluconazole).
No products indexed under this heading.

Hydrochlorothiazide (Ramelteon should be administered with caution in subjects taking strong CYP2C9 inhibitors such as fluconazole). Products include:
- Aldoril Tablets 1910
- Atacand HCT 651
- Avalide Tablets 888
- Avalide Tablets 2874
- Benicar HCT Tablets 1044
- Diovan HCT Tablets 2196
- Dyazide Capsules 1423
- Hyzaar 50-12.5 Tablets 1990
- Hyzaar 100-12.5 Tablets 1990
- Hyzaar 100-25 Tablets 1990
- Lopressor HCT 50/25 Tablets 2241
- Lopressor HCT 100/25 Tablets 2241
- Lopressor HCT 100/50 Tablets 2241
- Lotensin HCT Tablets 2246
- Micardis HCT Tablets 856
- Moduretic Tablets 2028
- Prinzide Tablets 2056
- Teveten HCT Tablets 1737
- Timolide Tablets 2086
- Uniretic Tablets 3100

Hydrocortisone (Efficacy may be reduced when ramelteon is used in combination with strong CYP enzyme inducers such as rifampin). Products include:
- Colocort Rectal Suspension, USP (Retention) 100 mg/60 mL 2476
- Hydrocortone Tablets 1989
- Preparation H Hydrocortisone Cream .... ■646

Hydrocortisone Acetate (Efficacy may be reduced when ramelteon is used in combination with strong CYP enzyme inducers such as rifampin). Products include:
- Analpram-HC 1159
- Pramosone 1161
- ProctoFoam-HC 3099

Hydrocortisone Butyrate (Efficacy may be reduced when ramelteon is used in combination with strong CYP enzyme inducers such as rifampin). Products include:
- Locoid Lipocream Cream 1160

Hydrocortisone Cypionate (Efficacy may be reduced when ramelteon is used in combination with strong CYP enzyme inducers such as rifampin).
No products indexed under this heading.

Hydrocortisone Hemisuccinate (Efficacy may be reduced when ramelteon is used in combination with strong CYP enzyme inducers such as rifampin).
No products indexed under this heading.

Hydrocortisone Probutate (Efficacy may be reduced when ramelteon is used in combination with strong CYP enzyme inducers such as rifampin).
No products indexed under this heading.

Hydrocortisone Sodium Phosphate (Efficacy may be reduced when ramelteon is used in combination with strong CYP enzyme inducers such as rifampin).
No products indexed under this heading.

Hydrocortisone Sodium Succinate (Efficacy may be reduced when ramelteon is used in combination with strong CYP enzyme inducers such as rifampin).
No products indexed under this heading.

Hydrocortisone Valerate (Efficacy may be reduced when ramelteon is used in combination with strong CYP enzyme inducers such as rifampin).
No products indexed under this heading.

Hydroflumethiazide (Ramelteon should be administered with caution in subjects taking strong CYP2C9 inhibitors such as fluconazole).
No products indexed under this heading.

Hypericum (Efficacy may be reduced when ramelteon is used in combination with strong CYP enzyme inducers such as rifampin). Products include:

Satiete Tablets .... ▣832

Hypericum Perforatum (Efficacy may be reduced when ramelteon is used in combination with strong CYP enzyme inducers such as rifampin).

No products indexed under this heading.

Imatinib Mesylate (Ramelteon should be administered with caution in subjects taking strong CYP2C9 inhibitors such as fluconazole). Products include:

Gleevec Tablets 2227

Indinavir Sulfate (Ramelteon should be administered with caution in subjects taking strong CYP2C9 inhibitors such as fluconazole). Products include:

Crixivan Capsules 1940

Insulin (Efficacy may be reduced when ramelteon is used in combination with strong CYP enzyme inducers such as rifampin).

No products indexed under this heading.

Isoniazid (Ramelteon should be administered with caution in subjects taking strong CYP2C9 inhibitors such as fluconazole).

No products indexed under this heading.

Itraconazole (Ramelteon should be administered with caution in subjects taking strong CYP2C9 inhibitors such as fluconazole).

No products indexed under this heading.

Ketoconazole (The AUC 0-inf and Cmax of ramelteon increased by approximately 84% and 36%, respectively, when a single 16 mg dose of ramelteon was administered on the fourth day of ketoconazole 200 mg twice daily administration, compared to administration of rameltenonalone. Similar increases were seen in M-II pharmacokinetic variables. Ramelteon should be administered with caution in subjects taking strong CYP3A4 inhibitors such as ketoconazole). Products include:

Nizoral A-D Shampoo, 1% 1868

Ketoprofen (Ramelteon should be administered with caution in subjects taking strong CYP2C9 inhibitors such as fluconazole).

No products indexed under this heading.

Lansoprazole (Efficacy may be reduced when ramelteon is used in combination with strong CYP enzyme inducers such as rifampin). Products include:

Prevacid Delayed-Release Capsules 3271
Prevacid for Delayed-Release Oral Suspension 3271
Prevacid SoluTab Delayed-Release Orally Disintegrating Tablets 3271
Prevacid I.V. for Injection 3277
Prevacid NapraPAC 3280
PREVPAC 3284

Leflunomide (Ramelteon should be administered with caution in subjects taking strong CYP2C9 inhibitors such as fluconazole).

No products indexed under this heading.

Levofloxacin (Ramelteon should be administered with caution in subjects taking strong CYP2C9 inhibitors such as fluconazole). Products include:

Levaquin 2384
Levaquin in 5% Dextrose Injection 2384
Quixin Ophthalmic Solution 3383

Levonorgestrel (Ramelteon should be administered with caution in subjects taking strong CYP2C9 inhibitors such as fluconazole). Products include:

Climara Pro Transdermal System 776
Mirena Intrauterine System 787
Plan B Tablets 1076
Seasonique Tablets 1077

Lomefloxacin Hydrochloride (Ramelteon should be administered with caution in subjects taking strong CYP2C9 inhibitors such as fluconazole).

No products indexed under this heading.

Lopinavir (Ramelteon should be administered with caution in subjects taking strong CYP2C9 inhibitors such as fluconazole). Products include:

Kaletra 476

Loratadine (Ramelteon should be administered with caution in subjects taking strong CYP2C9 inhibitors such as fluconazole). Products include:

Alavert Allergy & Sinus D-12 Hour Tablets .... ▣771
Alavert .... ▣771
Children's Claritin Allergy Oral Solution .... ▣771
Claritin Non-Drowsy 24 Hour Tablets .... ▣772
Claritin Reditabs 24 Hour Non-Drowsy Tablets .... ▣772
Claritin-D Non-Drowsy 12 Hour Tablets .... ▣772
Claritin-D Non-Drowsy 24 Hour Tablets .... ▣772

Lovastatin (Ramelteon should be administered with caution in subjects taking strong CYP2C9 inhibitors such as fluconazole). Products include:

Advicor Tablets 1722
Altoprev Extended-Release Tablets 3109
Mevacor Tablets 2021

Mephenytoin (Efficacy may be reduced when ramelteon is used in combination with strong CYP enzyme inducers such as rifampin).

No products indexed under this heading.

Mestranol (Ramelteon should be administered with caution in subjects taking strong CYP2C9 inhibitors such as fluconazole).

No products indexed under this heading.

Methoxsalen (Ramelteon should be administered with caution in subjects taking strong CYP2C9 inhibitors such as fluconazole). Products include:

Oxsoralen Lotion 1% 3352
Oxsoralen-Ultra Capsules 3353

Methsuximide (Efficacy may be reduced when ramelteon is used in combination with strong CYP enzyme inducers such as rifampin).

No products indexed under this heading.

Methyclothiazide (Ramelteon should be administered with caution in subjects taking strong CYP2C9 inhibitors such as fluconazole).

No products indexed under this heading.

Methylprednisolone (Efficacy may be reduced when ramelteon is used in combination with strong CYP enzyme inducers such as rifampin).

No products indexed under this heading.

Methylprednisolone Acetate (Efficacy may be reduced when ramelteon is used in combination with strong CYP enzyme inducers such as rifampin). Products include:

Depo-Medrol Injectable Suspension 2617
Depo-Medrol Single-Dose Vial 2619

Methylprednisolone Sodium Succinate (Efficacy may be reduced when ramelteon is used in combination with strong CYP enzyme inducers such as rifampin).

No products indexed under this heading.

Metronidazole (Ramelteon should be administered with caution in subjects taking strong CYP2C9 inhibitors such as fluconazole). Products include:

Metrogel 1% 1211
MetroGel-Vaginal Gel 1855
Vandazole Vaginal Gel 3338

Metronidazole Benzoate (Ramelteon should be administered with caution in subjects taking strong CYP2C9 inhibitors such as fluconazole).

No products indexed under this heading.

Metronidazole Hydrochloride (Ramelteon should be administered with caution in subjects taking strong CYP2C9 inhibitors such as fluconazole).

No products indexed under this heading.

Mexiletine Hydrochloride (Ramelteon should be administered with caution in subjects taking strong CYP2C9 inhibitors such as fluconazole).

No products indexed under this heading.

Mibefradil Dihydrochloride (Ramelteon should be administered with caution in subjects taking strong CYP2C9 inhibitors such as fluconazole).

No products indexed under this heading.

Miconazole (Ramelteon should be administered with caution in subjects taking strong CYP2C9 inhibitors such as fluconazole).

No products indexed under this heading.

Miconazole Nitrate (Ramelteon should be administered with caution in subjects taking strong CYP2C9 inhibitors such as fluconazole). Products include:

Desenex .... ▣635
Desenex Jock Itch Spray Powder .... ▣635

Modafinil (Ramelteon should be administered with caution in subjects taking strong CYP2C9 inhibitors such as fluconazole). Products include:

Provigil Tablets 988

Moxifloxacin Hydrochloride (Ramelteon should be administered with caution in subjects taking strong CYP2C9 inhibitors such as fluconazole). Products include:

Avelox 2970
Vigamox Ophthalmic Solution 564

Nafcillin Sodium (Efficacy may be reduced when ramelteon is used in combination with strong CYP enzyme inducers such as rifampin).

No products indexed under this heading.

Nalidixic Acid (Ramelteon should be administered with caution in subjects taking strong CYP2C9 inhibitors such as fluconazole).

No products indexed under this heading.

Nefazodone Hydrochloride (Ramelteon should be administered with caution in subjects taking strong CYP2C9 inhibitors such as fluconazole).

No products indexed under this heading.

Nelfinavir Mesylate (Ramelteon should be administered with caution in subjects taking strong CYP2C9 inhibitors such as fluconazole). Products include:

Viracept 2577

Nevirapine (Ramelteon should be administered with caution in subjects taking strong CYP2C9 inhibitors such as fluconazole). Products include:

Viramune Oral Suspension 873
Viramune Tablets 873

Niacinamide (Ramelteon should be administered with caution in subjects taking strong CYP2C9 inhibitors such as fluconazole).

No products indexed under this heading.

Nicotinamide (Ramelteon should be administered with caution in subjects taking strong CYP2C9 inhibitors such as fluconazole). Products include:

Nicomide Tablets 1088

Nicotine (Efficacy may be reduced when ramelteon is used in combination with strong CYP enzyme inducers such as rifampin). Products include:

NicoDerm CQ Clear Patch .... ▣622

Nicotine Polacrilex (Efficacy may be reduced when ramelteon is used in combination with strong CYP enzyme inducers such as rifampin).

No products indexed under this heading.

Nicotine Salicylate (Efficacy may be reduced when ramelteon is used in combination with strong CYP enzyme inducers such as rifampin).

No products indexed under this heading.

Nicotine Sulfate (Efficacy may be reduced when ramelteon is used in combination with strong CYP enzyme inducers such as rifampin).

No products indexed under this heading.

Nifedipine (Ramelteon should be administered with caution in subjects taking strong CYP2C9 inhibitors such as fluconazole). Products include:

Adalat CC Tablets 2964

Norethindrone (Ramelteon should be administered with caution in subjects taking strong CYP2C9 inhibitors such as fluconazole). Products include:

Ortho Micronor Tablets 2426

Norfloxacin (Ramelteon should be administered with caution in subjects taking strong CYP2C9 inhibitors such as fluconazole). Products include:

Noroxin Tablets 2032

Norgestrel (Ramelteon should be administered with caution in subjects taking strong CYP2C9 inhibitors such as fluconazole).

No products indexed under this heading.

Ofloxacin (Ramelteon should be administered with caution in subjects taking strong CYP2C9 inhibitors such as fluconazole). Products include:

Omeprazole (Ramelteon should be administered with caution in subjects taking strong CYP2C9 inhibitors such as fluconazole). Products include:

Oxcarbazepine (Efficacy may be reduced when ramelteon is used in combination with strong CYP enzyme inducers such as rifampin). Products include:

Oxiconazole Nitrate (Ramelteon should be administered with caution in subjects taking strong CYP2C9 inhibitors such as fluconazole). Products include:

Paroxetine Hydrochloride (Ramelteon should be administered with caution in subjects taking strong CYP2C9 inhibitors such as fluconazole). Products include:

Phenobarbital (Efficacy may be reduced when ramelteon is used in combination with strong CYP enzyme inducers such as rifampin). Products include:

Phenobarbital Sodium (Efficacy may be reduced when ramelteon is used in combination with strong CYP enzyme inducers such as rifampin).
No products indexed under this heading.

Phenylbutazone (Ramelteon should be administered with caution in subjects taking strong CYP2C9 inhibitors such as fluconazole).
No products indexed under this heading.

Phenytoin (Efficacy may be reduced when ramelteon is used in combination with strong CYP enzyme inducers such as rifampin).
No products indexed under this heading.

Phenytoin Sodium (Efficacy may be reduced when ramelteon is used in combination with strong CYP enzyme inducers such as rifampin). Products include:

Polythiazide (Ramelteon should be administered with caution in subjects taking strong CYP2C9 inhibitors such as fluconazole).
No products indexed under this heading.

Prednisolone Acetate (Efficacy may be reduced when ramelteon is used in combination with strong CYP enzyme inducers such as rifampin). Products include:

Prednisolone Sodium Phosphate (Efficacy may be reduced when ramelteon is used in combination with strong CYP enzyme inducers such as rifampin).
No products indexed under this heading.

Prednisolone Tebutate (Efficacy may be reduced when ramelteon is used in combination with strong CYP enzyme inducers such as rifampin).
No products indexed under this heading.

Prednisone (Efficacy may be reduced when ramelteon is used in combination with strong CYP enzyme inducers such as rifampin).
No products indexed under this heading.

Primidone (Efficacy may be reduced when ramelteon is used in combination with strong CYP enzyme inducers such as rifampin).
No products indexed under this heading.

Propoxyphene Hydrochloride (Ramelteon should be administered with caution in subjects taking strong CYP2C9 inhibitors such as fluconazole).
No products indexed under this heading.

Propoxyphene Napsylate (Ramelteon should be administered with caution in subjects taking strong CYP2C9 inhibitors such as fluconazole).
No products indexed under this heading.

Quinidine (Ramelteon should be administered with caution in subjects taking strong CYP2C9 inhibitors such as fluconazole).
No products indexed under this heading.

Quinidine Hydrochloride (Ramelteon should be administered with caution in subjects taking strong CYP2C9 inhibitors such as fluconazole).
No products indexed under this heading.

Quinidine Polygalacturonate (Ramelteon should be administered with caution in subjects taking strong CYP2C9 inhibitors such as fluconazole).
No products indexed under this heading.

Quinidine Sulfate (Ramelteon should be administered with caution in subjects taking strong CYP2C9 inhibitors such as fluconazole).
No products indexed under this heading.

Quinine (Ramelteon should be administered with caution in subjects taking strong CYP2C9 inhibitors such as fluconazole).
No products indexed under this heading.

Quinine Sulfate (Ramelteon should be administered with caution in subjects taking strong CYP2C9 inhibitors such as fluconazole).
No products indexed under this heading.

Quinupristin (Ramelteon should be administered with caution in subjects taking strong CYP2C9 inhibitors such as fluconazole).
No products indexed under this heading.

Ranitidine Bismuth Citrate (Ramelteon should be administered with caution in subjects taking strong CYP2C9 inhibitors such as fluconazole).
No products indexed under this heading.

Ranitidine Hydrochloride (Ramelteon should be administered with caution in subjects taking strong CYP2C9 inhibitors such as fluconazole). Products include:

Rifabutin (Efficacy may be reduced when ramelteon is used in combination with strong CYP enzyme inducers such as rifampin).
No products indexed under this heading.

Rifampicin (Efficacy may be reduced when ramelteon is used in combination with strong CYP enzyme inducers such as rifampin).
No products indexed under this heading.

Rifampin (Administration of rifampin 600 mg once daily for 11 days resulted in a mean decrease of approximately 80% (40% to 90%) in total exposure to ramelteon and metabolite M-II, (both AUC 0-inf and Cmax) after a single 32 mg dose of ramelteon. Efficacy may be reduced when ramelteon is used in combination with strong CYP enzyme inducers such as rifampin).
No products indexed under this heading.

Rifapentine (Efficacy may be reduced when ramelteon is used in combination with strong CYP enzyme inducers such as rifampin).
No products indexed under this heading.

Ritonavir (Ramelteon should be administered with caution in subjects taking strong CYP2C9 inhibitors such as fluconazole). Products include:

Saquinavir (Ramelteon should be administered with caution in subjects taking strong CYP2C9 inhibitors such as fluconazole).
No products indexed under this heading.

Saquinavir Mesylate (Ramelteon should be administered with caution in subjects taking strong CYP2C9 inhibitors such as fluconazole). Products include:

Secobarbital Sodium (Efficacy may be reduced when ramelteon is used in combination with strong CYP enzyme inducers such as rifampin).
No products indexed under this heading.

Sertraline Hydrochloride (Ramelteon should be administered with caution in subjects taking strong CYP2C9 inhibitors such as fluconazole). Products include:

Sparfloxacin (Ramelteon should be administered with caution in subjects taking strong CYP2C9 inhibitors such as fluconazole).
No products indexed under this heading.

Sulfacytine (Ramelteon should be administered with caution in subjects taking strong CYP2C9 inhibitors such as fluconazole).
No products indexed under this heading.

Sulfamethizole (Ramelteon should be administered with caution in subjects taking strong CYP2C9 inhibitors such as fluconazole).
No products indexed under this heading.

Sulfamethoxazole (Ramelteon should be administered with caution in subjects taking strong CYP2C9 inhibitors such as fluconazole).
No products indexed under this heading.

Sulfasalazine (Ramelteon should be administered with caution in subjects taking strong CYP2C9 inhibitors such as fluconazole).
No products indexed under this heading.

Sulfinpyrazone (Ramelteon should be administered with caution in subjects taking strong CYP2C9 inhibitors such as fluconazole).
No products indexed under this heading.

Sulfisoxazole Acetyl (Ramelteon should be administered with caution in subjects taking strong CYP2C9 inhibitors such as fluconazole).
No products indexed under this heading.

Sulfisoxazole Diolamine (Ramelteon should be administered with caution in subjects taking strong CYP2C9 inhibitors such as fluconazole).
No products indexed under this heading.

Tacrine Hydrochloride (Ramelteon should be administered with caution in subjects taking strong CYP2C9 inhibitors such as fluconazole).
No products indexed under this heading.

Telithromycin (Ramelteon should be administered with caution in subjects taking strong CYP2C9 inhibitors such as fluconazole). Products include:

Terconazole (Ramelteon should be administered with caution in subjects taking strong CYP2C9 inhibitors such as fluconazole).
No products indexed under this heading.

Theophylline (Efficacy may be reduced when ramelteon is used in combination with strong CYP enzyme inducers such as rifampin).
No products indexed under this heading.

Ticlopidine Hydrochloride (Ramelteon should be administered with caution in subjects taking strong CYP2C9 inhibitors such as fluconazole). Products include:

Tobacco (Efficacy may be reduced when ramelteon is used in combination with strong CYP enzyme inducers such as rifampin).
No products indexed under this heading.

Tolazamide (Ramelteon should be administered with caution in subjects taking strong CYP2C9 inhibitors such as fluconazole).
No products indexed under this heading.

IMPORTANT NOTE: Always consult each drug listing in the patient's regimen for possible interactions.

Tolbutamide (Ramelteon should be administered with caution in subjects taking strong CYP2C9 inhibitors such as fluconazole).
No products indexed under this heading.

Tolbutamide Sodium (Ramelteon should be administered with caution in subjects taking strong CYP2C9 inhibitors such as fluconazole).
No products indexed under this heading.

Triamcinolone (Efficacy may be reduced when ramelteon is used in combination with strong CYP enzyme inducers such as rifampin).
No products indexed under this heading.

Triamcinolone Acetonide (Efficacy may be reduced when ramelteon is used in combination with strong CYP enzyme inducers such as rifampin). Products include:
Azmacort Inhalation Aerosol 1726
Nasacort AQ Nasal Spray 2922

Triamcinolone Diacetate (Efficacy may be reduced when ramelteon is used in combination with strong CYP enzyme inducers such as rifampin).
No products indexed under this heading.

Triamcinolone Hexacetonide (Efficacy may be reduced when ramelteon is used in combination with strong CYP enzyme inducers such as rifampin).
No products indexed under this heading.

Troglitazone (Ramelteon should be administered with caution in subjects taking strong CYP2C9 inhibitors such as fluconazole).
No products indexed under this heading.

Troleandomycin (Ramelteon should be administered with caution in subjects taking strong CYP2C9 inhibitors such as fluconazole).
No products indexed under this heading.

Trovafloxacin Mesylate (Ramelteon should be administered with caution in subjects taking strong CYP2C9 inhibitors such as fluconazole).
No products indexed under this heading.

Valproate Sodium (Ramelteon should be administered with caution in subjects taking strong CYP2C9 inhibitors such as fluconazole). Products include:
Depacon Injection 412

Verapamil Hydrochloride (Ramelteon should be administered with caution in subjects taking strong CYP2C9 inhibitors such as fluconazole). Products include:
Covera-HS Tablets 3139
Tarka Tablets 524
Verelan PM Extended-Release Capsules, Controlled-Onset.......... 3106

Voriconazole (Ramelteon should be administered with caution in subjects taking strong CYP2C9 inhibitors such as fluconazole). Products include:
VFEND I.V. 2564
VFEND Oral Suspension 2564
VFEND Tablets 2564

Zafirlukast (Ramelteon should be administered with caution in subjects taking strong CYP2C9 inhibitors such as fluconazole). Products include:
Accolate Tablets 671

Zileuton (Ramelteon should be administered with caution in subjects taking strong CYP2C9 inhibitors such as fluconazole). Products include:
Zyflo Tablets 1023

Food Interactions

Alcohol (With single-dose, daytime co-administration of ramelteon 32 mg and alcohol (0.6 g/kg), there were no clinically meaningful or statistically significant effects on peak or total exposure to ramelteon. However, an additive effect was seen on some measures of psychomotor performance (ie. the Digit Symbol Substitution Test, the Psychomotor Vigilance Task Test, and a Visual Analog Scale of sedation) at some post-dose time points. No additive effect was seen on the Delayed Word Recognition Test. Because alcohol by itself impairs performance, and the intended effect of ramelteon is to promote sleep, patients should be cautioned not to consume alcohol when using ramelteon).

Broccoli (Efficacy may be reduced when ramelteon is used in combination with strong CYP enzyme inducers such as rifampin).

Brussel Sprouts (Efficacy may be reduced when ramelteon is used in combination with strong CYP enzyme inducers such as rifampin).

Charbroiled Food (Efficacy may be reduced when ramelteon is used in combination with strong CYP enzyme inducers such as rifampin).

Grapefruit (Ramelteon should be administered with caution in subjects taking strong CYP2C9 inhibitors such as fluconazole).

Grapefruit Juice (Ramelteon should be administered with caution in subjects taking strong CYP2C9 inhibitors such as fluconazole).

RYTHMOL SR CAPSULES

(Propafenone Hydrochloride) 2727
May interact with class 1A antiarrhythmics, class III antiarrhythmics, cytochrome p450 1a2 inhibitors (selected), cytochrome p450 2d6 inhibitors (selected), cytochrome p450 3a4 inhibitors (selected), cardiac glycosides, local anesthetics, macrolide antibiotics, drugs that prolong the QT interval, quinidine, xanthines, and certain other agents. Compounds in these categories include:

Acetazolamide (Drugs that inhibit CYP3A4 might lead to increased plasma levels of propafenone; patients should be closely monitored and the propafenone dose adjusted accordingly).
No products indexed under this heading.

Alatrofloxacin Mesylate (Drugs that inhibit CYP1A2 might lead to increased plasma levels of propafenone; patients should be closely monitored and the propafenone dose adjusted accordingly).
No products indexed under this heading.

Aminophylline (Combined therapy may result in an increase in theophylline concentration with the development of theophylline toxicity).
No products indexed under this heading.

Amiodarone Hydrochloride (The use of propafenone in conjunction with other drugs that prolong the QT interval has not been extensively studied and is not recommended).
No products indexed under this heading.

Amitriptyline Hydrochloride (The use of propafenone in conjunction with other drugs that prolong the QT interval has not been extensively studied and is not recommended).
No products indexed under this heading.

Amoxapine (The use of propafenone in conjunction with other drugs that prolong the QT interval has not been extensively studied and is not recommended).
No products indexed under this heading.

Amprenavir (Drugs that inhibit CYP3A4 might lead to increased plasma levels of propafenone; patients should be closely monitored and the propafenone dose adjusted accordingly). Products include:
Agenerase Capsules 1327
Agenerase Oral Solution 1332

Anastrozole (Drugs that inhibit CYP1A2 might lead to increased plasma levels of propafenone; patients should be closely monitored and the propafenone dose adjusted accordingly). Products include:
Arimidex Tablets 673

Aprepitant (Drugs that inhibit CYP3A4 might lead to increased plasma levels of propafenone; patients should be closely monitored and the propafenone dose adjusted accordingly). Products include:
Emend Capsules 1963

Astemizole (The use of propafenone in conjunction with other drugs that prolong the QT interval has not been extensively studied and is not recommended).
No products indexed under this heading.

Azithromycin Dihydrate (The use of propafenone in conjunction with other drugs that prolong the QT interval has not been extensively studied and is not recommended).
No products indexed under this heading.

Bepridil Hydrochloride (The use of propafenone in conjunction with other drugs that prolong the QT interval has not been extensively studied and is not recommended).
No products indexed under this heading.

Bretylium Tosylate (The use of propafenone in conjunction with other drugs that prolong the QT interval has not been extensively studied and is not recommended).
No products indexed under this heading.

Bupivacaine Hydrochloride (Concomitant use of local anesthetics may increase the risk of CNS side effects).
No products indexed under this heading.

Bupropion Hydrochloride (Drugs that inhibit CYP2D6 might lead to increased plasma levels of propafenone; patients should be closely monitored and the propafenone dose adjusted accordingly). Products include:
Wellbutrin Tablets 1603
Wellbutrin SR Sustained-Release Tablets 1607
Wellbutrin XL Extended-Release Tablets 1613
Zyban Sustained-Release Tablets 1644

Celecoxib (Drugs that inhibit CYP2D6 might lead to increased plasma levels of propafenone; patients should be closely monitored and the propafenone dose adjusted accordingly). Products include:
Celebrex Capsules 3134

Chloroprocaine Hydrochloride (Concomitant use of local anesthetics may increase the risk of CNS side effects).
No products indexed under this heading.

Chloroquine Hydrochloride (Drugs that inhibit CYP2D6 might lead to increased plasma levels of propafenone; patients should be closely monitored and the propafenone dose adjusted accordingly).
No products indexed under this heading.

Chloroquine Phosphate (Drugs that inhibit CYP2D6 might lead to increased plasma levels of propafenone; patients should be closely monitored and the propafenone dose adjusted accordingly).
No products indexed under this heading.

Chlorpheniramine (Drugs that inhibit CYP2D6 might lead to increased plasma levels of propafenone; patients should be closely monitored and the propafenone dose adjusted accordingly).
No products indexed under this heading.

Chlorpheniramine Maleate (Drugs that inhibit CYP2D6 might lead to increased plasma levels of propafenone; patients should be closely monitored and the propafenone dose adjusted accordingly). Products include:
Advil Allergy Sinus Caplets .... ■ 770
Advil Multi-Symptom Cold Caplets .... ■ 770
BC Allergy Sinus Cold Powder .... ■ 677
Comtrex Maximum Strength Cold & Cough Day/Night Caplets - Night Formulation .... ■ 726
Comtrex Maximum Strength Day/Night Severe Cold & Sinus Caplets - Night Formulation .... ■ 725
Contac Cold and Flu Maximum Strength Caplets......................... ■ 728
Contac Cold and Flu Day and Night Caplets (Night Formulation Only)........................ ■ 727
Children's Dimetapp Long Acting Cough Plus Cold Syrup................ ■ 731
Robitussin Cough & Cold Long-Acting Liquid .... ■ 735
Robitussin Cough & Allergy Syrup .. ■ 736
Robitussin Cough & Cold Nighttime Liquid............................ ■ 736
Robitussin Cough, Cold & Flu Nighttime Liquid............................ ■ 738
Robitussin Pediatric Cough & Cold Long-Acting Liquid............... ■ 735
Robitussin Pediatric Cough & Cold Nighttime Liquid................... ■ 736
Triaminic Cold & Allergy Liquid .... ■ 746
Triaminic Cough & Runny Nose Softchews .... ■ 748
Children's Tylenol Plus Flu Oral Suspension................................... ■ 749
Tylenol Allergy Multi-Symptom Caplets with Cool Burst and Gelcaps.. 1872
Children's Tylenol Plus Cold Suspension Liquid 1879
Children's Tylenol Plus Cough & Runny Nose Suspension Liquid..... 1879
Children's Tylenol Plus Flu Suspension Liquid 1881

Chlorpheniramine Polistirex
(Drugs that inhibit CYP2D6 might
lead to increased plasma levels of
propafenone; patients should be
closely monitored and the propafenone dose adjusted accordingly). Products include:

Chlorpheniramine Tannate
(Drugs that inhibit CYP2D6 might
lead to increased plasma levels of
propafenone; patients should be
closely monitored and the propafenone dose adjusted
accordingly).
 No products indexed under this
 heading.

Chlorpromazine (The use of propafenone in conjunction with other
drugs that prolong the QT interval
has not been extensively studied and
is not recommended).
 No products indexed under this
 heading.

Chlorpromazine Hydrochloride
(The use of propafenone in conjunction with other drugs that prolong
the QT interval has not been extensively studied and is not
recommended).
 No products indexed under this
 heading.

Cimetidine (Increases steady-state
plasma concentrations with no
detectable changes in electrocardiographic parameters). Products
include:

Cimetidine Hydrochloride
(Increases steady-state plasma concentrations with no detectable
changes in electrocardiographic
parameters).
 No products indexed under this
 heading.

Ciprofloxacin (Drugs that inhibit
CYP1A2 might lead to increased
plasma levels of propafenone;
patients should be closely monitored
and the propafenone dose adjusted
accordingly). Products include:

Ciprofloxacin Hydrochloride
(Drugs that inhibit CYP1A2 might
lead to increased plasma levels of
propafenone; patients should be
closely monitored and the propafenone dose adjusted accordingly). Products include:

Cisapride (The use of propafenone
in conjunction with other drugs that
prolong the QT interval has not been
extensively studied and is not
recommended).
 No products indexed under this
 heading.

Citalopram Hydrobromide (Drugs
that inhibit CYP2D6 might lead to
increased plasma levels of propafenone; patients should be closely
monitored and the propafenone dose
adjusted accordingly). Products
include:

Clarithromycin (The use of propafenone in conjunction with other
drugs that prolong the QT interval
has not been extensively studied and
is not recommended). Products
include:

Clomipramine Hydrochloride
(The use of propafenone in conjunction with other drugs that prolong
the QT interval has not been extensively studied and is not
recommended).
 No products indexed under this
 heading.

Clotrimazole (Drugs that inhibit
CYP3A4 might lead to increased
plasma levels of propafenone;
patients should be closely monitored
and the propafenone dose adjusted
accordingly). Products include:

Cocaine Hydrochloride (Drugs
that inhibit CYP2D6 might lead to
increased plasma levels of propafenone; patients should be closely
monitored and the propafenone dose
adjusted accordingly).
 No products indexed under this
 heading.

Cyclosporine (Propafenone therapy may increase levels of cyclosporine). Products include:

Dalfopristin (Drugs that inhibit
CYP3A4 might lead to increased
plasma levels of propafenone;
patients should be closely monitored
and the propafenone dose adjusted
accordingly).
 No products indexed under this
 heading.

Danazol (Drugs that inhibit CYP3A4
might lead to increased plasma levels of propafenone; patients should
be closely monitored and the propafenone dose adjusted
accordingly).
 No products indexed under this
 heading.

Delavirdine Mesylate (Drugs that
inhibit CYP3A4 might lead to
increased plasma levels of propafenone; patients should be closely
monitored and the propafenone dose
adjusted accordingly). Products
include:

Desipramine Hydrochloride (Co-
administration may result in elevated
serum desipramine levels).
 No products indexed under this
 heading.

Deslanoside (Potential for elevated
digoxin levels; dosage reduction of
digitalis may be necessary).
 No products indexed under this
 heading.

Desogestrel (Drugs that inhibit
CYP1A2 might lead to increased
plasma levels of propafenone;
patients should be closely monitored
and the propafenone dose adjusted
accordingly). Products include:

Digitalis Glycoside Preparations
(Potential for elevated digoxin levels;
dosage reduction of digitalis may be
necessary).
 No products indexed under this
 heading.

Digitoxin (Potential for elevated
digoxin levels; dosage reduction of
digitalis may be necessary).•
 No products indexed under this
 heading.

Digoxin (Potential for elevated
digoxin levels; dosage reduction of
digitalis may be necessary).
Products include:

Diltiazem Hydrochloride (Drugs
that inhibit CYP3A4 might lead to
increased plasma levels of propafenone; patients should be closely
monitored and the propafenone dose
adjusted accordingly). Products
include:

Diltiazem Maleate (Drugs that
inhibit CYP3A4 might lead to
increased plasma levels of propafenone; patients should be
monitored and the propafenone dose
adjusted accordingly).
 No products indexed under this
 heading.

Diphenhydramine (Drugs that
inhibit CYP2D6 might lead to
increased plasma levels of propafenone; patients should be closely
monitored and the propafenone dose
adjusted accordingly). Products
include:

Diphenhydramine Hydrochloride
(Drugs that inhibit CYP2D6 might
lead to increased plasma levels of
propafenone; patients should be
closely monitored and the propafenone dose adjusted accordingly). Products include:

Dirithromycin (The use of propafenone in conjunction with other
drugs that prolong the QT interval
has not been extensively studied and
is not recommended).
 No products indexed under this
 heading.

Disopyramide (Class Ia antiarrythmic agents should be withheld for at
least five half-lives prior to dosing
with extended release propafenone.
The use of propafenone with Class Ia
antiarrhythmic agents is not
recommended).
 No products indexed under this
 heading.

Disopyramide Phosphate (The
use of propafenone in conjunction
with other drugs that prolong the QT
interval has not been extensively
studied and is not recommended).
 No products indexed under this
 heading.

Dofetilide (The use of propafenone
in conjunction with other drugs that
prolong the QT interval has not been
extensively studied and is not
recommended).
 No products indexed under this
 heading.

Doxepin Hydrochloride (The use
of propafenone in conjunction with
other drugs that prolong the QT
interval has not been extensively
studied and is not recommended).
 No products indexed under this
 heading.

Dyphilline (Combined therapy may
result in an increase in theophylline
concentration with the development
of theophylline toxicity).
 No products indexed under this
 heading.

Efavirenz (Drugs that inhibit
CYP3A4 might lead to increased
plasma levels of propafenone;
patients should be closely monitored
and the propafenone dose adjusted
accordingly). Products include:

Enoxacin (Drugs that inhibit
CYP1A2 might lead to increased
plasma levels of propafenone;
patients should be closely monitored
and the propafenone dose adjusted
accordingly).
 No products indexed under this
 heading.

Erythromycin (The use of propafenone in conjunction with other
drugs that prolong the QT interval
has not been extensively studied and
is not recommended). Products
include:

Erythromycin Estolate (The use of
propafenone in conjunction with other drugs that prolong the QT interval
has not been extensively studied and
is not recommended).
 No products indexed under this
 heading.

Erythromycin Ethylsuccinate
(The use of propafenone in conjunction with other drugs that prolong
the QT interval has not been extensively studied and is not recommended). Products include:

IMPORTANT NOTE: Always consult each drug listing in the patient's regimen for possible interactions.

Erythromycin Gluceptate (The use of propafenone in conjunction with other drugs that prolong the QT interval has not been extensively studied and is not recommended).

No products indexed under this heading.

Erythromycin Lactobionate (Drugs that inhibit CYP3A4 might lead to increased plasma levels of propafenone; patients should be closely monitored and the propafenone dose adjusted accordingly).

No products indexed under this heading.

Erythromycin Stearate (The use of propafenone in conjunction with other drugs that prolong the QT interval has not been extensively studied and is not recommended). Products include:

Escitalopram Oxalate (Drugs that inhibit CYP2D6 might lead to increased plasma levels of propafenone; patients should be closely monitored and the propafenone dose adjusted accordingly). Products include:

Esomeprazole Magnesium (Drugs that inhibit CYP3A4 might lead to increased plasma levels of propafenone; patients should be closely monitored and the propafenone dose adjusted accordingly). Products include:

Ethinyl Estradiol (Drugs that inhibit CYP1A2 might lead to increased plasma levels of propafenone; patients should be closely monitored and the propafenone dose adjusted accordingly). Products include:

Etidocaine Hydrochloride (Concomitant use of local anesthetics may increase the risk of CNS side effects).

No products indexed under this heading.

Flecainide Acetate (The use of propafenone in conjunction with other drugs that prolong the QT interval has not been extensively studied and is not recommended). Products include:

Fluconazole (Drugs that inhibit CYP3A4 might lead to increased plasma levels of propafenone; patients should be closely monitored and the propafenone dose adjusted accordingly).

No products indexed under this heading.

Fluoxetine (Drugs that inhibit CYP2D6 might lead to increased plasma levels of propafenone; patients should be closely monitored and the propafenone dose adjusted accordingly).

No products indexed under this heading.

Fluoxetine Hydrochloride (Drugs that inhibit CYP2D6 might lead to increased plasma levels of pro-

pafenone; patients should be closely monitored and the propafenone dose adjusted accordingly). Products include:

Fluphenazine Decanoate (The use of propafenone in conjunction with other drugs that prolong the QT interval has not been extensively studied and is not recommended).

No products indexed under this heading.

Fluphenazine Enanthate (The use of propafenone in conjunction with other drugs that prolong the QT interval has not been extensively studied and is not recommended).

No products indexed under this heading.

Fluphenazine Hydrochloride (The use of propafenone in conjunction with other drugs that prolong the QT interval has not been extensively studied and is not recommended).

No products indexed under this heading.

Fluvoxamine (Drugs that inhibit CYP1A2 might lead to increased plasma levels of propafenone; patients should be closely monitored and the propafenone dose adjusted accordingly).

No products indexed under this heading.

Fluvoxamine Maleate (Drugs that inhibit CYP2D6 might lead to increased plasma levels of propafenone; patients should be closely monitored and the propafenone dose adjusted accordingly).

No products indexed under this heading.

Fosamprenavir Calcium (Drugs that inhibit CYP3A4 might lead to increased plasma levels of propafenone; patients should be closely monitored and the propafenone dose adjusted accordingly). Products include:

Gatifloxacin (Drugs that inhibit CYP1A2 might lead to increased plasma levels of propafenone; patients should be closely monitored and the propafenone dose adjusted accordingly). Products include:

Gemifloxacin Mesylate (Drugs that inhibit CYP1A2 might lead to increased plasma levels of propafenone; patients should be closely monitored and the propafenone dose adjusted accordingly).

No products indexed under this heading.

Grepafloxacin Hydrochloride (Drugs that inhibit CYP1A2 might lead to increased plasma levels of propafenone; patients should be closely monitored and the propafenone dose adjusted accordingly).

No products indexed under this heading.

Halofantrine Hydrochloride (Drugs that inhibit CYP2D6 might lead to increased plasma levels of propafenone; patients should be closely monitored and the propafenone dose adjusted accordingly).

No products indexed under this heading.

Haloperidol (Drugs that inhibit CYP2D6 might lead to increased plasma levels of propafenone; patients should be closely monitored and the propafenone dose adjusted accordingly).

No products indexed under this heading.

Haloperidol Decanoate (Drugs that inhibit CYP2D6 might lead to increased plasma levels of propafenone; patients should be closely monitored and the propafenone dose adjusted accordingly).

No products indexed under this heading.

Hydroxychloroquine Sulfate (Drugs that inhibit CYP2D6 might lead to increased plasma levels of propafenone; patients should be closely monitored and the propafenone dose adjusted accordingly).

No products indexed under this heading.

Imatinib Mesylate (Drugs that inhibit CYP2D6 might lead to increased plasma levels of propafenone; patients should be closely monitored and the propafenone dose adjusted accordingly). Products include:

Imipramine Hydrochloride (The use of propafenone in conjunction with other drugs that prolong the QT interval has not been extensively studied and is not recommended).

No products indexed under this heading.

Imipramine Pamoate (The use of propafenone in conjunction with other drugs that prolong the QT interval has not been extensively studied and is not recommended).

No products indexed under this heading.

Indinavir Sulfate (Drugs that inhibit CYP3A4 might lead to increased plasma levels of propafenone; patients should be closely monitored and the propafenone dose adjusted accordingly). Products include:

Isoniazid (Drugs that inhibit CYP1A2 might lead to increased plasma levels of propafenone; patients should be closely monitored and the propafenone dose adjusted accordingly).

No products indexed under this heading.

Itraconazole (Drugs that inhibit CYP3A4 might lead to increased plasma levels of propafenone; patients should be closely monitored and the propafenone dose adjusted accordingly).

No products indexed under this heading.

Ketoconazole (Drugs that inhibit CYP1A2 might lead to increased plasma levels of propafenone; patients should be closely monitored and the propafenone dose adjusted accordingly). Products include:

Levobupivacaine Hydrochloride (Concomitant use of local anesthetics may increase the risk of CNS side effects).

No products indexed under this heading.

Levofloxacin (Drugs that inhibit CYP1A2 might lead to increased plasma levels of propafenone;

patients should be closely monitored and the propafenone dose adjusted accordingly). Products include:

Levonorgestrel (Drugs that inhibit CYP1A2 might lead to increased plasma levels of propafenone; patients should be closely monitored and the propafenone dose adjusted accordingly). Products include:

Lidocaine Hydrochloride (The use of propafenone in conjunction with other drugs that prolong the QT interval has not been extensively studied and is not recommended).

No products indexed under this heading.

Lomefloxacin Hydrochloride (Drugs that inhibit CYP1A2 might lead to increased plasma levels of propafenone; patients should be closely monitored and the propafenone dose adjusted accordingly).

No products indexed under this heading.

Lopinavir (Drugs that inhibit CYP3A4 might lead to increased plasma levels of propafenone; patients should be closely monitored and the propafenone dose adjusted accordingly). Products include:

Loratadine (Drugs that inhibit CYP3A4 might lead to increased plasma levels of propafenone; patients should be closely monitored and the propafenone dose adjusted accordingly). Products include:

Maprotiline Hydrochloride (The use of propafenone in conjunction with other drugs that prolong the QT interval has not been extensively studied and is not recommended).

No products indexed under this heading.

Mepivacaine Hydrochloride (Concomitant use of local anesthetics may increase the risk of CNS side effects).

No products indexed under this heading.

Mesoridazine Besylate (The use of propafenone in conjunction with other drugs that prolong the QT interval has not been extensively studied and is not recommended).

No products indexed under this heading.

Mestranol (Drugs that inhibit CYP1A2 might lead to increased plasma levels of propafenone; patients should be closely monitored and the propafenone dose adjusted accordingly).

No products indexed under this heading.

Methadone Hydrochloride (Drugs that inhibit CYP2D6 might lead to increased plasma levels of propafenone; patients should be closely monitored and the propafenone dose adjusted accordingly).
No products indexed under this heading.

Methoxsalen (Drugs that inhibit CYP1A2 might lead to increased plasma levels of propafenone; patients should be closely monitored and the propafenone dose adjusted accordingly). Products include:
Oxsoralen Lotion 1% 3352
Oxsoralen-Ultra Capsules 3353

Metoprolol Succinate (Co-administration can result in substantial increases in metoprolol concentration and elimination half-life; increased plasma levels of metoprolol could overcome its cardioselectivity). Products include:
Toprol-XL Tablets 668

Metoprolol Tartrate (Co-administration can result in substantial increases in metoprolol concentration and elimination half-life; increased plasma levels of metoprolol could overcome its cardioselectivity). Products include:
Lopressor Injection 2238
Lopressor Tablets 2238
Lopressor HCT 50/25 Tablets 2241
Lopressor HCT 100/25 Tablets 2241
Lopressor HCT 100/50 Tablets 2241

Metronidazole (Drugs that inhibit CYP3A4 might lead to increased plasma levels of propafenone; patients should be closely monitored and the propafenone dose adjusted accordingly). Products include:
Metrogel 1% 1211
MetroGel-Vaginal Gel 1855
Vandazole Vaginal Gel 3338

Metronidazole Benzoate (Drugs that inhibit CYP3A4 might lead to increased plasma levels of propafenone; patients should be closely monitored and the propafenone dose adjusted accordingly).
No products indexed under this heading.

Metronidazole Hydrochloride (Drugs that inhibit CYP3A4 might lead to increased plasma levels of propafenone; patients should be closely monitored and the propafenone dose adjusted accordingly).
No products indexed under this heading.

Mexiletine Hydrochloride (The use of propafenone in conjunction with other drugs that prolong the QT interval has not been extensively studied and is not recommended).
No products indexed under this heading.

Mibefradil Dihydrochloride (Drugs that inhibit CYP2D6 might lead to increased plasma levels of propafenone; patients should be closely monitored and the propafenone dose adjusted accordingly).
No products indexed under this heading.

Miconazole (Drugs that inhibit CYP3A4 might lead to increased plasma levels of propafenone; patients should be closely monitored and the propafenone dose adjusted accordingly).
No products indexed under this heading.

Miconazole Nitrate (Drugs that inhibit CYP3A4 might lead to increased plasma levels of propafenone; patients should be closely monitored and the propafenone dose adjusted accordingly). Products include:
Desenex 635
Desenex Jock Itch Spray Powder 635

Moclobemide (Drugs that inhibit CYP2D6 might lead to increased plasma levels of propafenone; patients should be closely monitored and the propafenone dose adjusted accordingly).
No products indexed under this heading.

Moricizine Hydrochloride (Class Ia antiarrythmic agents should be withheld for at least five half-lives prior to dosing with extended release propafenone. The use of propafenone with Class Ia antiarrythmic agents is not recommended).
No products indexed under this heading.

Moxifloxacin Hydrochloride (Drugs that inhibit CYP1A2 might lead to increased plasma levels of propafenone; patients should be closely monitored and the propafenone dose adjusted accordingly). Products include:
Avelox 2970
Vigamox Ophthalmic Solution 564

Nalidixic Acid (Drugs that inhibit CYP1A2 might lead to increased plasma levels of propafenone; patients should be closely monitored and the propafenone dose adjusted accordingly).
No products indexed under this heading.

Nefazodone Hydrochloride (Drugs that inhibit CYP3A4 might lead to increased plasma levels of propafenone; patients should be closely monitored and the propafenone dose adjusted accordingly).
No products indexed under this heading.

Nelfinavir Mesylate (Drugs that inhibit CYP3A4 might lead to increased plasma levels of propafenone; patients should be closely monitored and the propafenone dose adjusted accordingly). Products include:
Viracept 2577

Nevirapine (Drugs that inhibit CYP3A4 might lead to increased plasma levels of propafenone; patients should be closely monitored and the propafenone dose adjusted accordingly). Products include:
Viramune Oral Suspension 873
Viramune Tablets 873

Niacinamide (Drugs that inhibit CYP3A4 might lead to increased plasma levels of propafenone; patients should be closely monitored and the propafenone dose adjusted accordingly).
No products indexed under this heading.

Nicotinamide (Drugs that inhibit CYP3A4 might lead to increased plasma levels of propafenone; patients should be closely monitored and the propafenone dose adjusted accordingly). Products include:
Nicomide Tablets 1088

Nifedipine (Drugs that inhibit CYP3A4 might lead to increased plasma levels of propafenone; patients should be closely monitored and the propafenone dose adjusted accordingly). Products include:
Adalat CC Tablets 2964

Norethindrone (Drugs that inhibit CYP1A2 might lead to increased plasma levels of propafenone; patients should be closely monitored and the propafenone dose adjusted accordingly). Products include:
Ortho Micronor Tablets 2426

Norfloxacin (Drugs that inhibit CYP1A2 might lead to increased plasma levels of propafenone; patients should be closely monitored and the propafenone dose adjusted accordingly). Products include:
Noroxin Tablets 2032

Norgestrel (Drugs that inhibit CYP1A2 might lead to increased plasma levels of propafenone; patients should be closely monitored and the propafenone dose adjusted accordingly).
No products indexed under this heading.

Nortriptyline Hydrochloride (The use of propafenone in conjunction with other drugs that prolong the QT interval has not been extensively studied and is not recommended).
No products indexed under this heading.

Ofloxacin (Drugs that inhibit CYP1A2 might lead to increased plasma levels of propafenone; patients should be closely monitored and the propafenone dose adjusted accordingly). Products include:
Floxin Otic Solution 1049

Omeprazole (Drugs that inhibit CYP1A2 might lead to increased plasma levels of propafenone; patients should be closely monitored and the propafenone dose adjusted accordingly). Products include:
Zegerid Capsules 2958
Zegerid Powder for Oral Solution 2958

Paroxetine Hydrochloride (Drugs that inhibit CYP2D6 might lead to increased plasma levels of propafenone; patients should be closely monitored and the propafenone dose adjusted accordingly). Products include:
Paxil CR Controlled-Release Tablets 1538
Paxil 1530

Perphenazine (The use of propafenone in conjunction with other drugs that prolong the QT interval has not been extensively studied and is not recommended).
No products indexed under this heading.

Procainamide (Class Ia antiarrythmic agents should be withheld for at least five half-lives prior to dosing with extended release propafenone. The use of propafenone with Class Ia antiarrythmic agents is not recommended).
No products indexed under this heading.

Procainamide Hydrochloride (The use of propafenone in conjunction with other drugs that prolong the QT interval has not been extensively studied and is not recommended).
No products indexed under this heading.

Procaine Hydrochloride (Concomitant use of local anesthetics may increase the risk of CNS side effects).
No products indexed under this heading.

Prochlorperazine (The use of propafenone in conjunction with other drugs that prolong the QT interval has not been extensively studied and is not recommended).
No products indexed under this heading.

Promethazine Hydrochloride (The use of propafenone in conjunction with other drugs that prolong the QT interval has not been extensively studied and is not recommended). Products include:
Phenergan Tablets and Suppositories 3440

Propoxyphene Hydrochloride (Drugs that inhibit CYP2D6 might lead to increased plasma levels of propafenone; patients should be closely monitored and the propafenone dose adjusted accordingly).
No products indexed under this heading.

Propoxyphene Napsylate (Drugs that inhibit CYP2D6 might lead to increased plasma levels of propafenone; patients should be closely monitored and the propafenone dose adjusted accordingly).
No products indexed under this heading.

Propranolol Hydrochloride (Co-administration has resulted in substantial increases in propranolol concentration and elimination half-life). Products include:
Inderal LA Long-Acting Capsules 3429
InnoPran XL Capsules 2723

Protriptyline Hydrochloride (The use of propafenone in conjunction with other drugs that prolong the QT interval has not been extensively studied and is not recommended).
No products indexed under this heading.

Quinacrine Hydrochloride (Drugs that inhibit CYP2D6 might lead to increased plasma levels of propafenone; patients should be closely monitored and the propafenone dose adjusted accordingly).
No products indexed under this heading.

Quinidine (Class Ia antiarrythmic agents should be withheld for at least five half-lives prior to dosing with extended release propafenone. The use of propafenone with Class Ia antiarrythmic agents is not recommended).
No products indexed under this heading.

Quinidine Gluconate (The use of propafenone in conjunction with other drugs that prolong the QT interval has not been extensively studied and is not recommended).
No products indexed under this heading.

Quinidine Hydrochloride (Small doses of quinidine completely inhibit the hydroxylation metabolic pathway, making all patients, in effect, slow metabolizers; there is too little information to recommend concomitant use).
No products indexed under this heading.

Quinidine Polygalacturonate (The use of propafenone in conjunction with other drugs that prolong the QT interval has not been extensively studied and is not recommended).
No products indexed under this heading.

Quinidine Sulfate (The use of propafenone in conjunction with other drugs that prolong the QT interval has not been extensively studied and is not recommended).

 No products indexed under this heading.

Quinine (Drugs that inhibit CYP3A4 might lead to increased plasma levels of propafenone; patients should be closely monitored and the propafenone dose adjusted accordingly).

 No products indexed under this heading.

Quinine Sulfate (Drugs that inhibit CYP3A4 might lead to increased plasma levels of propafenone; patients should be closely monitored and the propafenone dose adjusted accordingly).

 No products indexed under this heading.

Quinupristin (Drugs that inhibit CYP3A4 might lead to increased plasma levels of propafenone; patients should be closely monitored and the propafenone dose adjusted accordingly).

 No products indexed under this heading.

Ranitidine Bismuth Citrate (Drugs that inhibit CYP2D6 might lead to increased plasma levels of propafenone; patients should be closely monitored and the propafenone dose adjusted accordingly).

 No products indexed under this heading.

Ranitidine Hydrochloride (Drugs that inhibit CYP2D6 might lead to increased plasma levels of propafenone; patients should be closely monitored and the propafenone dose adjusted accordingly). Products include:

Rifampin (May accelerate the metabolism and decrease the plasma levels and antiarythmic efficacy of propafenone).

 No products indexed under this heading.

Ritonavir (Drugs that inhibit CYP2D6 might lead to increased plasma levels of propafenone; patients should be closely monitored and the propafenone dose adjusted accordingly). Products include:

Saquinavir (Drugs that inhibit CYP3A4 might lead to increased plasma levels of propafenone; patients should be closely monitored and the propafenone dose adjusted accordingly).

 No products indexed under this heading.

Saquinavir Mesylate (Drugs that inhibit CYP3A4 might lead to increased plasma levels of propafenone; patients should be closely monitored and the propafenone dose adjusted accordingly). Products include:

Sertraline Hydrochloride (Drugs that inhibit CYP2D6 might lead to increased plasma levels of propafenone; patients should be closely

monitored and the propafenone dose adjusted accordingly). Products include:

Sotalol Hydrochloride (Class III antiarrythmic agents should be withheld for at least five half-lives prior to dosing with extended release propafenone. The use of propafenone with Class III antiarrythmic agents is not recommended).

 No products indexed under this heading.

Sparfloxacin (Drugs that inhibit CYP1A2 might lead to increased plasma levels of propafenone; patients should be closely monitored and the propafenone dose adjusted accordingly).

 No products indexed under this heading.

Tacrine Hydrochloride (Drugs that inhibit CYP1A2 might lead to increased plasma levels of propafenone; patients should be closely monitored and the propafenone dose adjusted accordingly).

 No products indexed under this heading.

Telithromycin (Drugs that inhibit CYP3A4 might lead to increased plasma levels of propafenone; patients should be closely monitored and the propafenone dose adjusted accordingly). Products include:

Terbinafine Hydrochloride (Drugs that inhibit CYP2D6 might lead to increased plasma levels of propafenone; patients should be closely monitored and the propafenone dose adjusted accordingly). Products include:

Tetracaine Hydrochloride (Concomitant use of local anesthetics may increase the risk of CNS side effects). Products include:

Theophylline (Combined therapy may result in an increase in theophylline concentration with the development of theophylline toxicity).

 No products indexed under this heading.

Theophylline Anhydrous (Combined therapy may result in an increase in theophylline concentration with the development of theophylline toxicity). Products include:

Theophylline Calcium Salicylate (Combined therapy may result in an increase in theophylline concentration with the development of theophylline toxicity).

 No products indexed under this heading.

Theophylline Dihydroxypropyl (Glyceryl) (Combined therapy may result in an increase in theophylline concentration with the development of theophylline toxicity).

 No products indexed under this heading.

Theophylline Ethylenediamine (Combined therapy may result in an increase in theophylline concentration with the development of theophylline toxicity).

 No products indexed under this heading.

Theophylline Sodium Glycinate (Combined therapy may result in an increase in theophylline concentration with the development of theophylline toxicity).

 No products indexed under this heading.

Thioridazine Hydrochloride (The use of propafenone in conjunction with other drugs that prolong the QT interval has not been extensively studied and is not recommended). Products include:

Ticlopidine Hydrochloride (Drugs that inhibit CYP1A2 might lead to increased plasma levels of propafenone; patients should be closely monitored and the propafenone dose adjusted accordingly). Products include:

Tocainide Hydrochloride (The use of propafenone in conjunction with other drugs that prolong the QT interval has not been extensively studied and is not recommended).

 No products indexed under this heading.

Trifluoperazine Hydrochloride (The use of propafenone in conjunction with other drugs that prolong the QT interval has not been extensively studied and is not recommended).

 No products indexed under this heading.

Trimipramine Maleate (The use of propafenone in conjunction with other drugs that prolong the QT interval has not been extensively studied and is not recommended).

 No products indexed under this heading.

Troglitazone (Drugs that inhibit CYP3A4 might lead to increased plasma levels of propafenone; patients should be closely monitored and the propafenone dose adjusted accordingly).

 No products indexed under this heading.

Troleandomycin (The use of propafenone in conjunction with other drugs that prolong the QT interval has not been extensively studied and is not recommended).

 No products indexed under this heading.

Trovafloxacin Mesylate (Drugs that inhibit CYP1A2 might lead to increased plasma levels of propafenone; patients should be closely monitored and the propafenone dose adjusted accordingly).

 No products indexed under this heading.

Valproate Sodium (Drugs that inhibit CYP3A4 might lead to increased plasma levels of propafenone; patients should be closely monitored and the propafenone dose adjusted accordingly). Products include:

Verapamil Hydrochloride (Drugs that inhibit CYP3A4 might lead to increased plasma levels of propafenone; patients should be closely monitored and the propafenone dose adjusted accordingly). Products include:

Voriconazole (Drugs that inhibit CYP3A4 might lead to increased plasma levels of propafenone; patients should be closely monitored and the propafenone dose adjusted accordingly). Products include:

Warfarin Sodium (Increase in mean steady-state plasma levels of warfarin resulting in increased prothrombin time). Products include:

Zafirlukast (Drugs that inhibit CYP3A4 might lead to increased plasma levels of propafenone; patients should be closely monitored and the propafenone dose adjusted accordingly). Products include:

Zileuton (Drugs that inhibit CYP1A2 might lead to increased plasma levels of propafenone; patients should be closely monitored and the propafenone dose adjusted accordingly). Products include:

Ziprasidone Hydrochloride (The use of propafenone in conjunction with other drugs that prolong the QT interval has not been extensively studied and is not recommended). Products include:

Food Interactions

Food, unspecified (Increased peak blood level and bioavailability in a single dose study).

Grapefruit (Drugs that inhibit CYP3A4 might lead to increased plasma levels of propafenone; patients should be closely monitored and the propafenone dose adjusted accordingly).

Grapefruit Juice (Drugs that inhibit CYP1A2 might lead to increased plasma levels of propafenone; patients should be closely monitored and the propafenone dose adjusted accordingly).

SANCTURA TABLETS

May interact with anticholinergics and certain other agents. Compounds in these categories include:

Atropine Sulfate (The concomitant use of trospium with other anticholinergic agents that produce dry mouth, constipation, and other anticholinergic pharmacological effects, may increase the frequency and/or severity of such effects). Products include:

Belladonna Alkaloids (The concomitant use of trospium with other anticholinergic agents that produce dry mouth, constipation, and other anticholinergic pharmacological effects, may increase the frequency and/or severity of such effects). Products include:

Benztropine Mesylate (The concomitant use of trospium with other anticholinergic agents that produce dry mouth, constipation, and other anticholinergic pharmacological effects, may increase the frequency and/or severity of such effects).

 No products indexed under this heading.

Biperiden Hydrochloride (The concomitant use of trospium with other anticholinergic agents that produce dry mouth, constipation, and other anticholinergic pharmacological effects, may increase the frequency and/or severity of such effects).
No products indexed under this heading.

Clidinium Bromide (The concomitant use of trospium with other anticholinergic agents that produce dry mouth, constipation, and other anticholinergic pharmacological effects, may increase the frequency and/or severity of such effects).
No products indexed under this heading.

Dicyclomine Hydrochloride (The concomitant use of trospium with other anticholinergic agents that produce dry mouth, constipation, and other anticholinergic pharmacological effects, may increase the frequency and/or severity of such effects). Products include:
Bentyl Capsules 697
Bentyl Injection 697
Bentyl Syrup 697
Bentyl Tablets 697

Digoxin (Co-administration with drugs that are eliminated by active renal tubular secretion, like digoxin, may increase the serum concentration of trospium and/or the co-administered drug, due to competition for this elimination pathway). Products include:
Lanoxicaps Capsules 1490
Lanoxin Injection 1494
Lanoxin Injection Pediatric 1497
Lanoxin Tablets 1500

Glycopyrrolate (The concomitant use of trospium with other anticholinergic agents that produce dry mouth, constipation, and other anticholinergic pharmacological effects, may increase the frequency and/or severity of such effects).
No products indexed under this heading.

Hyoscyamine (The concomitant use of trospium with other anticholinergic agents that produce dry mouth, constipation, and other anticholinergic pharmacological effects, may increase the frequency and/or severity of such effects).
No products indexed under this heading.

Hyoscyamine Sulfate (The concomitant use of trospium with other anticholinergic agents that produce dry mouth, constipation, and other anticholinergic pharmacological effects, may increase the frequency and/or severity of such effects). Products include:
Donnatal Extentabs 2493
Prosed/DS Tablets 1157

Ipratropium Bromide (The concomitant use of trospium with other anticholinergic agents that produce dry mouth, constipation, and other anticholinergic pharmacological effects, may increase the frequency and/or severity of such effects). Products include:
Atrovent Inhalation Solution 835
Atrovent HFA Inhalation Aerosol 841
Atrovent Nasal Spray 0.03% 837
Atrovent Nasal Spray 0.06% 839
Combivent Inhalation Aerosol 847
DuoNeb Inhalation Solution 1058

Mepenzolate Bromide (The concomitant use of trospium with other anticholinergic agents that produce dry mouth, constipation, and other anticholinergic pharmacological effects, may increase the frequency and/or severity of such effects).
No products indexed under this heading.

Metformin (Co-administration with drugs that are eliminated by active renal tubular secretion, like metformin, may increase the serum concentration of trospium and/or the co-administered drug, due to competition for this elimination pathway).
No products indexed under this heading.

Metformin Hydrochloride (Co-administration with drugs that are eliminated by active renal tubular secretion, like metformin, may increase the serum concentration of trospium and/or the co-administered drug, due to competition for this elimination pathway). Products include:
ActoPlus Met Tablets 3214
Avandamet Tablets 1373
Fortamet Extended-Release Tablets 3115

Morphine Sulfate (Co-administration with drugs that are eliminated by active renal tubular secretion, like morphine, may increase the serum concentration of trospium and/or the co-administered drug, due to competition for this elimination pathway). Products include:
Avinza Capsules 1741
Kadian Capsules 577
MS Contin Tablets 2701

Oxybutynin Chloride (The concomitant use of trospium with other anticholinergic agents that produce dry mouth, constipation, and other anticholinergic pharmacological effects, may increase the frequency and/or severity of such effects). Products include:
Ditropan XL Extended-Release Tablets 2413

Pancuronium Bromide (Co-administration with drugs that are eliminated by active renal tubular secretion, like pancuronium, may increase the serum concentration of trospium and/or the co-administered drug, due to competition for this elimination pathway).
No products indexed under this heading.

Procainamide (Co-administration with drugs that are eliminated by active renal tubular secretion, like procainamide, may increase the serum concentration of trospium and/or the co-administered drug, due to competition for this elimination pathway).
No products indexed under this heading.

Procainamide Hydrochloride (Co-administration with drugs that are eliminated by active renal tubular secretion, like procainamide, may increase the serum concentration of trospium and/or the co-administered drug, due to competition for this elimination pathway).
No products indexed under this heading.

Procyclidine Hydrochloride (The concomitant use of trospium with other anticholinergic agents that produce dry mouth, constipation, and other anticholinergic pharmacological effects, may increase the frequency and/or severity of such effects).
No products indexed under this heading.

Propantheline Bromide (The concomitant use of trospium with other anticholinergic agents that produce dry mouth, constipation, and other anticholinergic pharmacological effects, may increase the frequency and/or severity of such effects).
No products indexed under this heading.

Scopolamine (The concomitant use of trospium with other anticholinergic agents that produce dry mouth, constipation, and other anticholinergic pharmacological effects, may increase the frequency and/or severity of such effects). Products include:
Transderm Scōp Transdermal Therapeutic System 2177

Scopolamine Hydrobromide (The concomitant use of trospium with other anticholinergic agents that produce dry mouth, constipation, and other anticholinergic pharmacological effects, may increase the frequency and/or severity of such effects). Products include:
Donnatal Extentabs 2493

Tenofovir Disoproxil Fumarate (Co-administration with drugs that are eliminated by active renal tubular secretion, like tenofovir, may increase the serum concentration of trospium and/or the co-administered drug, due to competition for this elimination pathway). Products include:
Atripla Tablets 945
Truvada Tablets 1296
Viread Tablets 1301

Tolterodine Tartrate (The concomitant use of trospium with other anticholinergic agents that produce dry mouth, constipation, and other anticholinergic pharmacological effects, may increase the frequency and/or severity of such effects). Products include:
Detrol Tablets 2628
Detrol LA Capsules 2631

Tridihexethyl Chloride (The concomitant use of trospium with other anticholinergic agents that produce dry mouth, constipation, and other anticholinergic pharmacological effects, may increase the frequency and/or severity of such effects).
No products indexed under this heading.

Trihexyphenidyl Hydrochloride (The concomitant use of trospium with other anticholinergic agents that produce dry mouth, constipation, and other anticholinergic pharmacological effects, may increase the frequency and/or severity of such effects).
No products indexed under this heading.

Vancomycin Hydrochloride (Co-administration with drugs that are eliminated by active renal tubular secretion, like vancomycin, may increase the serum concentration of trospium and/or the co-administered drug, due to competition for this elimination pathway). Products include:
Vancocin HCl Capsules, USP 3380

SANDIMMUNE ORAL SOLUTION

(Cyclosporine) 2275
See Sandimmune I.V. Ampuls for Infusion

SANDIMMUNE I.V. AMPULS FOR INFUSION

(Cyclosporine) 2275
May interact with ACE inhibitors, angiotensin-II receptor antagonists, erythromycin, fibrates, HMG-CoA reductase inhibitors, methylprednisolone, non-steroidal anti-inflammatory agents, oral contraceptives, phenytoin, potassium preparations, prednisolone, protease inhibitors, potassium sparing diuretics, vaccines, live, and certain other agents. Compounds in these categories include:

Allopurinol (Increases cyclosporine concentrations).
No products indexed under this heading.

Amiloride Hydrochloride (Cyclosporine may cause hyperkalemia; concurrent use should be avoided). Products include:
Midamor Tablets 2026
Moduretic Tablets 2028

Amiodarone Hydrochloride (Increases cyclosporine concentrations).
No products indexed under this heading.

Amphotericin B (May potentiate renal dysfunction).
No products indexed under this heading.

Amprenavir (The HIV protease inhibitors are known to inhibit CYP450 3A and, thus, could potentially increase the concentrations of cyclosporine). Products include:
Agenerase Capsules 1327
Agenerase Oral Solution 1332

Antibiotics, unspecified (Potential synergies of nephrotoxicity may occur).
No products indexed under this heading.

Atorvastatin Calcium (Cyclosporine may reduce the clearance of HMG-CoA reductase inhibitors (statins). Literature and postmarketing cases of myotoxicity, including muscle pain and weakness, myositis, and rhabdomyolysis have been reported with concomitant administration of cyclosporine and atorvastatin. When concurrently administered with cyclosporine, the dosage of atorvastatin should be reduced. Statin therapy needs to be temporarily withheld or discontinued in patients with signs/symptoms of myopathy or those with risk factors predisposing to severe renal injury). Products include:
Caduet Tablets 2508
Lipitor Tablets 2483

Azapropazon (May potentiate renal dysfunction).
No products indexed under this heading.

Azithromycin (Concomitant azithromycin may increase cyclosporine concentrations). Products include:
Zmax for Oral Suspension 2583

BCG Vaccine (During treatment with cyclosporine, vaccination may be less effective; the use of live vaccines should be avoided).
No products indexed under this heading.

Benazepril Hydrochloride (Caution is required when cyclosporine is co-administered with potassium-sparing drugs, such as angiotensin-converting enzyme inhibitors). Products include:

Bromocriptine Mesylate
(Increases cyclosporine levels; dosage adjustments are essential).

No products indexed under this heading.

Candesartan Cilexetil (Caution is required when cyclosporine is co-administered with potassium-sparing drugs, such as angiotensin II receptor antagonists). Products include:

Captopril (Caution is required when cyclosporine is co-administered with potassium-sparing drugs, such as angiotensin-converting enzyme inhibitors). Products include:

Carbamazepine (Decreases cyclosporine plasma concentrations; dosage adjustments are essential). Products include:

Celecoxib (Co-administration with NSAID's, particularly in the setting of dehydration, may potentiate renal dysfunction). Products include:

Cerivastatin Sodium (Literature and post-marketing cases of myotoxicity, including muscle pain and weakness, myositis, and rhabdomyolysis, have been reported with concomitant administration of cyclosporine with lovastatin, simvastatin, atorvastatin, pravastatin, and rarely, fluvastatin. When concurrently administered with cyclosporine, the dosage of these statins should be reduced according to label recommendations. Statin therapy needs to be temporarily withheld or discontinued in patients with signs and symptoms of myopathy or those with risk factors predisposing to severe renal injury, including renal failure, secondary to rhabomyolysis).

No products indexed under this heading.

Cimetidine (May potentiate renal dysfunction). Products include:

Cimetidine Hydrochloride (May potentiate renal dysfunction).

No products indexed under this heading.

Ciprofloxacin (Concomitant ciprofloxacin may potentiate renal dysfunction). Products include:

Ciprofloxacin Hydrochloride (Concomitant ciprofloxacin may potentiate renal dysfunction). Products include:

Clarithromycin (Concomitant clarithromycin may increase cyclosporine concentrations). Products include:

Clofibrate (Concomitant fibric acid derivatives may potentiate renal dysfunction).

No products indexed under this heading.

Colchicine (Co-administration results in increased cyclosporine concentrations and potentiation of renal dysfunction. Cyclosporine may reduce the clearance of colchicine. There are reports on the potential of cyclosporine to enhance the toxic effects of colchicine, such as myopathy and neuropathy, especially in patients with renal dysfunction. If colchicine is used concurrently with cyclosporine, close clinical observation is required).

No products indexed under this heading.

Dalfopristin (Co-administration with substrates that inhibit CYP450 3A, such as dalfopristin, could decrease metabolism and increase cyclosporine concentrations).

No products indexed under this heading.

Danazol (Increases cyclosporine plasma concentrations; dosage adjustments are essential).

No products indexed under this heading.

Desogestrel (Concomitant oral contraceptives may increase cyclosporine concentrations). Products include:

Diclofenac Potassium (Co-administration with NSAID's, particularly in the setting of dehydration, may potentiate renal dysfunction).

No products indexed under this heading.

Diclofenac Sodium (Co-administration with NSAID's, particularly in the setting of dehydration, may potentiate renal dysfunction). Products include:

Digoxin (Reduced clearance of digoxin and potential for severe digitalis toxicity. If digoxin is used concurrently with cyclosporine, close clinical observation is required). Products include:

Diltiazem Hydrochloride (Increases cyclosporine plasma concentrations; dosage adjustments are essential). Products include:

Enalapril Maleate (Caution is required when cyclosporine is co-administered with potassium-sparing drugs, such as angiotensin-converting enzyme inhibitors). Products include:

Enalaprilat (Caution is required when cyclosporine is co-administered with potassium-sparing drugs, such as angiotensin-converting enzyme inhibitors).

No products indexed under this heading.

Eprosartan Mesylate (Caution is required when cyclosporine is co-

administered with potassium-sparing drugs, such as angiotensin II receptor antagonists). Products include:

Erythromycin (Co-administration with substrates that inhibit CYP450 3A, such as erythromycin, could decrease metabolism and increase cyclosporine concentrations). Products include:

Erythromycin Estolate (Co-administration with substrates that inhibit CYP450 3A, such as erythromycin, could decrease metabolism and increase cyclosporine concentrations).

No products indexed under this heading.

Erythromycin Ethylsuccinate (Co-administration with substrates that inhibit CYP450 3A, such as erythromycin, could decrease metabolism and increase cyclosporine concentrations). Products include:

Erythromycin Gluceptate (Co-administration with substrates that inhibit CYP450 3A, such as erythromycin, could decrease metabolism and increase cyclosporine concentrations).

No products indexed under this heading.

Erythromycin Lactobionate (Co-administration with substrates that inhibit CYP450 3A, such as erythromycin, could decrease metabolism and increase cyclosporine concentrations).

No products indexed under this heading.

Erythromycin Stearate (Co-administration with substrates that inhibit CYP450 3A, such as erythromycin, could decrease metabolism and increase cyclosporine concentrations). Products include:

Ethinyl Estradiol (Concomitant oral contraceptives may increase cyclosporine concentrations). Products include:

Ethynodiol Diacetate (Concomitant oral contraceptives may increase cyclosporine concentrations).

No products indexed under this heading.

Etodolac (Co-administration with NSAID's, particularly in the setting of dehydration, may potentiate renal dysfunction).

No products indexed under this heading.

Fenofibrate (Concomitant fibric acid derivatives may potentiate renal dysfunction). Products include:

Fenoprofen Calcium (Co-administration with NSAID's, particularly in the setting of dehydration, may potentiate renal dysfunction). Products include:

Fluconazole (Increases cyclosporine levels; dosage adjustments are essential).

No products indexed under this heading.

Flurbiprofen (Co-administration with NSAID's, particularly in the setting of dehydration, may potentiate renal dysfunction).

No products indexed under this heading.

Fluvastatin Sodium (Cyclosporine may reduce the clearance of HMG-CoA reductase inhibitors (statins). Literature and postmarketing cases of myotoxicity, including muscle pain and weakness, myositis, and rhabdomyolysis have been reported with concomitant administration of cyclosporine and fluvastatin. When concurrently administered with cyclosporine, the dosage of fluvastatin should be reduced. Statin therapy needs to be temporarily withheld or discontinued in patients with signs/symptoms of myopathy or those with risk factors predisposing to severe renal injury). Products include:

Fosinopril Sodium (Caution is required when cyclosporine is co-administered with potassium-sparing drugs, such as angiotensin-converting enzyme inhibitors).

No products indexed under this heading.

Fosphenytoin Sodium (Co-administration with agents that are known to induce CYP450 system, such as phenytoin, will increase hepatic metabolism and decrease cyclosporine levels).

No products indexed under this heading.

Gemfibrozil (Concomitant fibric acid derivatives may potentiate renal dysfunction).

No products indexed under this heading.

Gentamicin Sulfate (May potentiate renal dysfunction). Products include:

Hypericum (Co-administration has been reported to produce a marked reduction in blood cyclosporine concentrations, resulting in subtherapeutic levels, rejection of transplanted organs, and graft loss). Products include:

Ibuprofen (Co-administration with NSAID's, particularly in the setting of dehydration, may potentiate renal dysfunction). Products include:

Advil Multi-Symptom Cold Caplets 770
Advil PM Caplets 615
Motrin IB Tablets and Caplets 1866
Children's Motrin Oral Suspension ... 1867
Children's Motrin Non-Staining Dye-Free Oral Suspension 1867
Children's Motrin Cold Oral Suspension 1867
Infants' Motrin Concentrated Drops 1867
Infants' Motrin Non-Staining Dye-Free Concentrated Drops 1867
Junior Strength Motrin Caplets and Chewable Tablets 1867
Vicoprofen Tablets 539

Imatinib Mesylate (Concomitant imatinib may increase cyclosporine concentrations). Products include:
Gleevec Tablets 2227

Immune Globulin Intravenous (Human) (Increases susceptibility to infection). Products include:
Carimune NF 3499
Gammagard Liquid 721
Gammagard S/D 724
Gamunex Immune Globulin I.V., 10% 3235

Indinavir Sulfate (The HIV protease inhibitors are known to inhibit CYP450 3A and, thus, could potentially increase the concentrations of cyclosporine). Products include:
Crixivan Capsules 1940

Indomethacin (Co-administration with NSAID's, particularly in the setting of dehydration, may potentiate renal dysfunction). Products include:
Indocin 1995

Indomethacin Sodium Trihydrate (Co-administration with NSAID's, particularly in the setting of dehydration, may potentiate renal dysfunction). Products include:
Indocin I.V. 2465

Irbesartan (Caution is required when cyclosporine is co-administered with potassium-sparing drugs, such as angiotensin II receptor antagonists). Products include:
Avalide Tablets 888
Avalide Tablets 2874
Avapro Tablets 891
Avapro Tablets 2871

Itraconazole (Increases cyclosporine levels; dosage adjustments are essential).
No products indexed under this heading.

Ketoconazole (May potentiate renal dysfunction; co-administration with substrates that inhibit CYP450 3A, such as ketoconazole, could decrease metabolism and increase cyclosporine concentrations). Products include:
Nizoral A-D Shampoo, 1% 1868

Ketoprofen (Co-administration with NSAID's, particularly in the setting of dehydration, may potentiate renal dysfunction).
No products indexed under this heading.

Ketorolac Tromethamine (Co-administration with NSAID's, particularly in the setting of dehydration, may potentiate renal dysfunction). Products include:
Acular Ophthalmic Solution 565
Acular LS Ophthalmic Solution 566

Levonorgestrel (Concomitant oral contraceptives may increase cyclosporine concentrations). Products include:
Climara Pro Transdermal System 776
Mirena Intrauterine System 787
Plan B Tablets 1076
Seasonique Tablets 1077

Lisinopril (Caution is required when cyclosporine is co-administered with potassium-sparing drugs, such as angiotensin-converting enzyme inhibitors). Products include:
Prinivil Tablets 2052
Prinzide Tablets 2056

Lopinavir (The HIV protease inhibitors are known to inhibit CYP450 3A and, thus, could potentially increase the concentrations of cyclosporine). Products include:
Kaletra 476

Losartan Potassium (Caution is required when cyclosporine is co-administered with potassium-sparing drugs, such as angiotensin II receptor antagonists). Products include:
Cozaar Tablets 1935
Hyzaar 50-12.5 Tablets 1990
Hyzaar 100-12.5 Tablets 1990
Hyzaar 100-25 Tablets 1990

Lovastatin (Cyclosporine may reduce the clearance of HMG-CoA reductase inhibitors (statins). Literature and postmarketing cases of myotoxicity, including muscle pain and weakness, myositis, and rhabdomyolysis have been reported with concomitant administration of cyclosporine and lovastatin. When concurrently administered with cyclosporine, the dosage of lovastatin should be reduced. Statin therapy needs to be temporarily withheld or discontinued in patients with signs/symptoms of myopathy or those with risk factors predisposing to severe renal injury). Products include:
Advicor Tablets 1722
Altoprev Extended-Release Tablets 3109
Mevacor Tablets 2021

Measles, Mumps, Rubella and Varicella Virus Vaccine Live (During treatment with cyclosporine, vaccination may be less effective; the use of live vaccines should be avoided). Products include:
ProQuad 2064

Measles, Mumps & Rubella Virus Vaccine, Live (During treatment with cyclosporine, vaccination may be less effective; the use of live vaccines should be avoided). Products include:
M-M-R II 2006

Measles & Rubella Virus Vaccine Live (During treatment with cyclosporine, vaccination may be less effective; the use of live vaccines should be avoided).
No products indexed under this heading.

Measles Virus Vaccine Live (During treatment with cyclosporine, vaccination may be less effective; the use of live vaccines should be avoided). Products include:
Attenuvax 1914

Meclofenamate Sodium (Co-administration with NSAID's, particularly in the setting of dehydration, may potentiate renal dysfunction).
No products indexed under this heading.

Mefenamic Acid (Co-administration with NSAID's, particularly in the setting of dehydration, may potentiate renal dysfunction).
No products indexed under this heading.

Meloxicam (Co-administration with NSAID's, particularly in the setting of dehydration, may potentiate renal dysfunction). Products include:
Mobic Oral Suspension 863
Mobic Tablets 863

Melphalan (May potentiate renal dysfunction). Products include:
Alkeran Tablets 956

Mestranol (Concomitant oral contraceptives may increase cyclosporine concentrations).
No products indexed under this heading.

Methotrexate Sodium (Co-administration in rheumatoid arthritis patients has resulted in increased AUC of methotrexate by approximately 30% and concentration of its metabolite decreased by approximately 80%; the clinical significance is not known).
No products indexed under this heading.

Methylprednisolone (Co-administration with agents that are known to inhibit CYP450 system, such as methylprednisolone, will decrease hepatic metabolism and increase cyclosporine levels; convulsions have been reported with concomitant high doses of methylprednisolone).
No products indexed under this heading.

Methylprednisolone Acetate (Co-administration with agents that are known to inhibit CYP450 system, such as methylprednisolone, will decrease hepatic metabolism and increase cyclosporine levels; convulsions have been reported with concomitant high doses of methylprednisolone). Products include:
Depo-Medrol Injectable Suspension 2617
Depo-Medrol Single-Dose Vial 2619

Methylprednisolone Sodium Succinate (Co-administration with agents that are known to inhibit CYP450 system, such as methylprednisolone, will decrease hepatic metabolism and increase cyclosporine levels; convulsions have been reported with concomitant high doses of methylprednisolone).
No products indexed under this heading.

Metoclopramide Hydrochloride (Increases cyclosporine levels; dosage adjustments are essential).
No products indexed under this heading.

Moexipril Hydrochloride (Caution is required when cyclosporine is co-administered with potassium-sparing drugs, such as angiotensin-converting enzyme inhibitors). Products include:
Uniretic Tablets 3100
Univasc Tablets 3104

Mumps Virus Vaccine, Live (During treatment with cyclosporine, vaccination may be less effective; the use of live vaccines should be avoided). Products include:
Mumpsvax 2031

Muromonab-CD3 (Increased susceptibility to infection and increased risk for development of lymphomas and malignancies). Products include:
Orthoclone OKT3 Sterile Solution 2360

Nabumetone (Co-administration with NSAID's, particularly in the setting of dehydration, may potentiate renal dysfunction).
No products indexed under this heading.

Nafcillin Sodium (Decreases cyclosporine concentrations).
No products indexed under this heading.

Naproxen (Co-administration with NSAID's, particularly in the setting of dehydration, may potentiate renal dysfunction). Products include:
EC-Naprosyn Delayed-Release Tablets 2761
Naprosyn Suspension 2761
Naprosyn Tablets 2761
Prevacid NapraPAC 3280

Naproxen Sodium (Co-administration with NSAID's, particularly in the setting of dehydration, may potentiate renal dysfunction). Products include:
Aleve Caplets 742
Aleve Gelcaps 743
Aleve Tablets 743
Aleve Cold & Sinus Caplets 744
Anaprox Tablets 2761
Anaprox DS Tablets 2761

Nelfinavir Mesylate (The HIV protease inhibitors are known to inhibit CYP450 3A and, thus, could potentially increase the concentrations of cyclosporine). Products include:
Viracept 2577

Nephrotoxic Drugs (Potential synergics of nephrotoxicity).
No products indexed under this heading.

Nicardipine Hydrochloride (Increases cyclosporine plasma concentrations; dosage adjustments are essential). Products include:
Cardene I.V. 2497

Nifedipine (Potential for frequent gingival hyperplasia). Products include:
Adalat CC Tablets 2964

Norethindrone (Concomitant oral contraceptives may increase cyclosporine concentrations). Products include:
Ortho Micronor Tablets 2426

Norethynodrel (Concomitant oral contraceptives may increase cyclosporine concentrations).
No products indexed under this heading.

Norgestimate (Concomitant oral contraceptives may increase cyclosporine concentrations). Products include:
Ortho-Cyclen/Ortho Tri-Cyclen 2429
Ortho Tri-Cyclen Lo Tablets 2436

Norgestrel (Concomitant oral contraceptives may increase cyclosporine concentrations).
No products indexed under this heading.

Octreotide Acetate (Decreases cyclosporine concentrations). Products include:
Sandostatin Injection 2278
Sandostatin LAR Depot 2280

Orlistat (Co-administration can result in decreased absorption of cyclosporine; concomitant use should be avoided). Products include:
Xenical Capsules 2831

Oxaprozin (Co-administration with NSAID's, particularly in the setting of dehydration, may potentiate renal dysfunction).
No products indexed under this heading.

Perindopril Erbumine (Caution is required when cyclosporine is co-administered with potassium-sparing drugs, such as angiotensin-converting enzyme inhibitors). Products include:

Aceon Tablets (2 mg, 4 mg, 8 mg) 3194

Phenobarbital (Decreases cyclosporine plasma levels; dosage adjustments are essential). Products include:
Donnatal Extentabs 2493

Phenylbutazone (Co-administration with NSAID's, particularly in the setting of dehydration, may potentiate renal dysfunction).
No products indexed under this heading.

Phenytoin (Co-administration with agents that are known to induce CYP450 system, such as phenytoin, will increase hepatic metabolism and decrease cyclosporine levels).
No products indexed under this heading.

Phenytoin Sodium (Co-administration with agents that are known to induce CYP450 system, such as phenytoin, will increase hepatic metabolism and decrease cyclosporine levels). Products include:
Phenytek Capsules 2160

Piroxicam (Co-administration with NSAID's, particularly in the setting of dehydration, may potentiate renal dysfunction).
No products indexed under this heading.

Poliovirus Vaccine, Live, Oral, Trivalent, Types 1,2,3 (Sabin) (During treatment with cyclosporine, vaccination may be less effective; the use of live vaccines should be avoided).
No products indexed under this heading.

Potassium Acid Phosphate (Caution is required when cyclosporine in co-administered with potassium-containing drugs). Products include:
K-Phos Original (Sodium Free) Tablets 760

Potassium Bicarbonate (Caution is required when cyclosporine in co-administered with potassium-containing drugs).
No products indexed under this heading.

Potassium Chloride (Caution is required when cyclosporine in co-administered with potassium-containing drugs). Products include:
Colyte with Flavor Packs for Oral Solution 3088
HalfLytely and Bisacodyl Tablets Bowel Prep Kit with Flavors Packs 881
K-Dur Extended-Relase Tablets 3033
K-Lor Oral Solution 474
K-Tab Tablets 475
MoviPrep Oral Solution 2839
TriLyte with Flavor Packs for Oral Solution 3100

Potassium Citrate (Caution is required when cyclosporine in co-administered with potassium-containing drugs). Products include:
Urocit-K Tablets 2144

Potassium Gluconate (Caution is required when cyclosporine in co-administered with potassium-containing drugs).
No products indexed under this heading.

Potassium Phosphate (Caution is required when cyclosporine in co-administered with potassium-containing drugs). Products include:
K-Phos Neutral Tablets 760

Pravastatin Sodium (Cyclosporine may reduce the clearance of HMG-CoA reductase inhibitors (statins). Literature and postmarketing cases of myotoxicity, including muscle pain and weakness, myositis, and rhabdomyolysis have been reported with concomitant administration of cyclosporine and pravastatin. When concurrently administered with cyclosporine, the dosage of pravastatin should be reduced. Statin therapy needs to be temporarily withheld or discontinued in patients with signs/symptoms of myopathy or those with risk factors predisposing to severe renal injury).
No products indexed under this heading.

Prednisolone (Co-administration results in reduced clearance of prednisolone).
No products indexed under this heading.

Prednisolone Acetate (Co-administration results in reduced clearance of prednisolone). Products include:
Blephamide Ophthalmic Ointment 568
Blephamide Ophthalmic Suspension 569
Poly-Pred Ophthalmic Suspension .... ⊙233
Pred Forte Ophthalmic Suspension .... ⊙235
Pred Mild Ophthalmic Suspension .... ⊙238
Pred-G Ophthalmic Ointment .... ⊙237
Pred-G Ophthalmic Suspension .... ⊙236

Prednisolone Sodium Phosphate (Co-administration results in reduced clearance of prednisolone).
No products indexed under this heading.

Prednisolone Tebutate (Co-administration results in reduced clearance of prednisolone).
No products indexed under this heading.

Quinapril Hydrochloride (Caution is required when cyclosporine is co-administered with potassium-sparing drugs, such as angiotensin-converting enzyme inhibitors).
No products indexed under this heading.

Quinupristin (Co-administration with substrates that inhibit CYP450 3A, such as quinupristine, could decrease metabolism and increase cyclosporine concentrations).
No products indexed under this heading.

Ramipril (Caution is required when cyclosporine is co-administered with potassium-sparing drugs, such as angiotensin-converting enzyme inhibitors). Products include:
Altace Capsules 1702

Ranitidine Hydrochloride (May potentiate renal dysfunction). Products include:
Zantac 1624
Zantac Injection 1619
Zantac Injection Pharmacy Bulk Package 1622

Rifabutin (Rifabutin is known to increase the metabolism of other drugs metabolized by CYP450 system; the interaction between cyclosporine and rifabutin has not been studied; care should be exercised).
No products indexed under this heading.

Rifampin (Decreases cyclosporine plasma levels; dosage adjustments are essential).
No products indexed under this heading.

Ritonavir (The HIV protease inhibitors are known to inhibit CYP450 3A and, thus, could potentially increase the concentrations of cyclosporine). Products include:
Kaletra 476
Norvir 503

Rofecoxib (Co-administration with NSAID's, particularly in the setting of dehydration, may potentiate renal dysfunction).
No products indexed under this heading.

Rotavirus Vaccine, Live, Oral, Tetravalent (During treatment with cyclosporine, vaccination may be less effective; the use of live vaccines should be avoided).
No products indexed under this heading.

Rubella & Mumps Virus Vaccine Live (During treatment with cyclosporine, vaccination may be less effective; the use of live vaccines should be avoided).
No products indexed under this heading.

Rubella Virus Vaccine Live (During treatment with cyclosporine, vaccination may be less effective; the use of live vaccines should be avoided). Products include:
Meruvax II 2019

Saquinavir (The HIV protease inhibitors are known to inhibit CYP450 3A and, thus, could potentially increase the concentrations of cyclosporine).
No products indexed under this heading.

Saquinavir Mesylate (The HIV protease inhibitors are known to inhibit CYP450 3A and, thus, could potentially increase the concentrations of cyclosporine). Products include:
Invirase 2772

Simvastatin (Cyclosporine may reduce the clearance of HMG-CoA reductase inhibitors (statins). Literature and postmarketing cases of myotoxicity, including muscle pain and weakness, myositis, and rhabdomyolysis have been reported with concomitant administration of cyclosporine and simvastatin. When concurrently administered with cyclosporine, the dosage of simvastatin should be reduced. Statin therapy needs to be temporarily withheld or discontinued in patients with signs/symptoms of myopathy or those with risk factors predisposing to severe renal injury). Products include:
Vytorin 10/10 Tablets 2114
Vytorin 10/10 Tablets 3077
Vytorin 10/20 Tablets 2114
Vytorin 10/20 Tablets 3077
Vytorin 10/40 Tablets 2114
Vytorin 10/40 Tablets 3077
Vytorin 10/80 Tablets 2114
Vytorin 10/80 Tablets 3077
Zocor Tablets 2105

Sirolimus (Elevations in serum creatinine were observed in studies using sirolimus in combination with full-dose cyclosporine. The effect is often reversible with cyclosporine dose reduction. Simultaneous co-administration of cyclosproine significantly increases blood levels of sirolimus. To minimize increases in sirolimus blood concentrations, it is recommended that sirolimus be given 4 hours after cyclosporine administration). Products include:
Rapamune Oral Solution and Tablets 3475

Smallpox Vaccine (During treatment with cyclosporine, vaccination may be less effective; the use of live vaccines should be avoided).
No products indexed under this heading.

Spirapril Hydrochloride (Caution is required when cyclosporine is co-administered with potassium-sparing drugs, such as angiotensin-converting enzyme inhibitors).
No products indexed under this heading.

Spironolactone (Cyclosporine may cause hyperkalemia; concurrent use should be avoided).
No products indexed under this heading.

Sulfamethoxazole (May potentiate renal dysfunction).
No products indexed under this heading.

Sulfinpyrazone (Concomitant sulfinpyrazone may decrease cyclosporine concentrations).
No products indexed under this heading.

Sulindac (Co-administration with NSAID's, particularly in the setting of dehydration, may potentiate renal dysfunction). Products include:
Clinoril Tablets 1924

Tacrolimus (May potentiate renal dysfunction). Products include:
Prograf Capsules and Injection 632
Protopic Ointment 638

Telmisartan (Caution is required when cyclosporine is co-administered with potassium-sparing drugs, such as angiotensin II receptor antagonists). Products include:
Micardis Tablets 854
Micardis HCT Tablets 856

Terbinafine Hydrochloride (Concomitant terbinafine may decrease cyclosporine concentrations). Products include:
Lamisil Tablets 2232
Lamisil AT Creams (Athlete's Foot & Jock Itch) .... ▣636

Ticlopidine Hydrochloride (Decreases cyclosporine concentrations). Products include:
Ticlid Tablets 2810

Tobramycin (May potentiate renal dysfunction). Products include:
TOBI Solution for Inhalation 2298
TobraDex Ophthalmic Ointment 562
TobraDex Ophthalmic Suspension 563
Zylet Ophthalmic Suspension .... ⊙259

Tobramycin Sulfate (May potentiate renal dysfunction).
No products indexed under this heading.

Tolmetin Sodium (Co-administration with NSAID's, particularly in the setting of dehydration, may potentiate renal dysfunction).
No products indexed under this heading.

Trandolapril (Caution is required when cyclosporine is co-administered with potassium-sparing drugs, such as angiotensin-converting enzyme inhibitors). Products include:
Mavik Tablets 486
Tarka Tablets 524

Triamterene (Cyclosporine may cause hyperkalemia; concurrent use should be avoided). Products include:
Dyazide Capsules 1423
Dyrenium Capsules 3400

Trimethoprim (May potentiate renal dysfunction).
No products indexed under this heading.

Typhoid Vaccine (During treatment with cyclosporine, vaccination may be less effective; the use of live vaccines should be avoided).
No products indexed under this heading.

Valdecoxib (Co-administration with NSAID's, particularly in the setting of dehydration, may potentiate renal dysfunction).
No products indexed under this heading.

Valsartan (Caution is required when cyclosporine is co-administered with potassium-sparing drugs, such as angiotensin II receptor antagonists). Products include:
Diovan Tablets 2193
Diovan HCT Tablets 2196

Vancomycin Hydrochloride (May potentiate renal dysfunction). Products include:
Vancocin HCl Capsules, USP 3380

Varicella Virus Vaccine Live (During treatment with cyclosporine, vaccination may be less effective; the use of live vaccines should be avoided). Products include:
Varivax 2100

Verapamil Hydrochloride (Increases cyclosporine levels; dosage adjustments are essential). Products include:
Covera-HS Tablets 3139
Tarka Tablets 524
Verelan PM Extended-Release Capsules, Controlled-Onset 3106

Yellow Fever Vaccine (During treatment with cyclosporine, vaccination may be less effective; the use of live vaccines should be avoided).
No products indexed under this heading.

Food Interactions

Grapefruit (Co-administration results in increased blood concentrations of cyclosporine; concurrent use should be avoided).

Grapefruit Juice (Co-administration results in increased blood concentrations of cyclosporine; concurrent use should be avoided).

SANDIMMUNE SOFT GELATIN CAPSULES

(Cyclosporine) 2275
See Sandimmune I.V. Ampuls for Infusion

SANDOSTATIN INJECTION

(Octreotide Acetate) 2278
See Sandostatin LAR Depot

SANDOSTATIN LAR DEPOT

(Octreotide Acetate) 2280
May interact with beta blockers, calcium channel blockers, cytochrome p450 3a4 substrates (selected), oral hypoglycemic agents, insulin, and certain other agents. Compounds in these categories include:

Acarbose (Octreotide causes hypo- and hyperglycemia in some patients; dosage adjustments of oral hypoglycemic agents may be required). Products include:
Precose Tablets 751

Acebutolol Hydrochloride (Adjustment of the dosage of beta blockers may be required).
No products indexed under this heading.

Alfentanil Hydrochloride (Data indicates that somatostatin analogs might decrease the metabolic clearance of compounds known to be metabolized by cytochrome P450 enzymes, which may be due to the suppression of growth hormones. Since it cannot be excluded that octreotide may have this effect, other drugs mainly metabolized by CYP3A4, and which have a low therapeutic index should therefore be used with caution).
No products indexed under this heading.

Alprazolam (Data indicates that somatostatin analogs might decrease the metabolic clearance of compounds known to be metabolized by cytochrome P450 enzymes, which may be due to the suppression of growth hormones. Since it cannot be excluded that octreotide may have this effect, other drugs mainly metabolized by CYP3A4, and which have a low therapeutic index should therefore be used with caution). Products include:
Niravam Orally Disintegrating Tablets 3092

Amitriptyline Hydrochloride (Data indicates that somatostatin analogs might decrease the metabolic clearance of compounds known to be metabolized by cytochrome P450 enzymes, which may be due to the suppression of growth hormones. Since it cannot be excluded that octreotide may have this effect, other drugs mainly metabolized by CYP3A4, and which have a low therapeutic index should therefore be used with caution).
No products indexed under this heading.

Amlodipine Besylate (Adjustment of the dosage of calcium channel blocker may be required). Products include:
Caduet Tablets 2508
Lotrel Capsules 2249
Norvasc Tablets 2545

Aprepitant (Data indicates that somatostatin analogs might decrease the metabolic clearance of compounds known to be metabolized by cytochrome P450 enzymes, which may be due to the suppression of growth hormones. Since it cannot be excluded that octreotide may have this effect, other drugs mainly metabolized by CYP3A4, and which have a low therapeutic index should therefore be used with caution). Products include:
Emend Capsules 1963

Astemizole (Data indicates that somatostatin analogs might decrease the metabolic clearance of compounds known to be metabolized by cytochrome P450 enzymes, which may be due to the suppression of growth hormones. Since it cannot be excluded that octreotide may have this effect, other drugs mainly metabolized by CYP3A4, and which have a low therapeutic index should therefore be used with caution).
No products indexed under this heading.

Atenolol (Adjustment of the dosage of beta blockers may be required).
No products indexed under this heading.

Atorvastatin Calcium (Data indicates that somatostatin analogs might decrease the metabolic clearance of compounds known to be metabolized by cytochrome P450 enzymes, which may be due to the suppression of growth hormones. Since it cannot be excluded that octreotide may have this effect, other drugs mainly metabolized by CYP3A4, and which have a low therapeutic index should therefore be used with caution). Products include:
Caduet Tablets 2508
Lipitor Tablets 2483

Belladonna Ergotamine (Data indicates that somatostatin analogs might decrease the metabolic clearance of compounds known to be metabolized by cytochrome P450 enzymes, which may be due to the suppression of growth hormones. Since it cannot be excluded that octreotide may have this effect, other drugs mainly metabolized by CYP3A4, and which have a low therapeutic index should therefore be used with caution).
No products indexed under this heading.

Bepridil Hydrochloride (Adjustment of the dosage of calcium channel blocker may be required).
No products indexed under this heading.

Betaxolol Hydrochloride (Adjustment of the dosage of beta blockers may be required). Products include:
Betoptic S Ophthalmic Suspension 558

Bisoprolol Fumarate (Adjustment of the dosage of beta blockers may be required).
No products indexed under this heading.

Bromocriptine Mesylate (Co-administration increases the availability of bromocriptine).
No products indexed under this heading.

Buspirone Hydrochloride (Data indicates that somatostatin analogs might decrease the metabolic clearance of compounds known to be metabolized by cytochrome P450 enzymes, which may be due to the suppression of growth hormones. Since it cannot be excluded that octreotide may have this effect, other drugs mainly metabolized by CYP3A4, and which have a low therapeutic index should therefore be used with caution).
No products indexed under this heading.

Busulfan (Data indicates that somatostatin analogs might decrease the metabolic clearance of compounds known to be metabolized by cytochrome P450 enzymes, which may be due to the suppression of growth hormones. Since it cannot be excluded that octreotide may have this effect, other drugs mainly metabolized by CYP3A4, and which have a low therapeutic index should therefore be used with caution). Products include:
I.V. Busulfex 2493
Myleran Tablets 1525

Carbamazepine (Data indicates that somatostatin analogs might decrease the metabolic clearance of compounds known to be metabolized by cytochrome P450 enzymes, which may be due to the suppression of growth hormones. Since it cannot be excluded that octreotide may have this effect, other drugs mainly metabolized by CYP3A4, and which have a low therapeutic index should therefore be used with caution). Products include:
Carbatrol Capsules 3171
Equetro Extended-Release Capsules 3180
Tegretol/Tegretol-XR 2295

Carteolol Hydrochloride (Adjustment of the dosage of beta blockers may be required). Products include:
Carteolol Hydrochloride Ophthalmic Solution USP, 1% .... ⊙ 249

Cerivastatin Sodium (Data indicates that somatostatin analogs might decrease the metabolic clearance of compounds known to be metabolized by cytochrome P450 enzymes, which may be due to the suppression of growth hormones. Since it cannot be excluded that octreotide may have this effect, other drugs mainly metabolized by CYP3A4, and which have a low therapeutic index should therefore be used with caution).
No products indexed under this heading.

Chlorpheniramine (Data indicates that somatostatin analogs might decrease the metabolic clearance of compounds known to be metabolized by cytochrome P450 enzymes, which may be due to the suppression of growth hormones. Since it cannot be excluded that octreotide may have this effect, other drugs mainly metabolized by CYP3A4, and which have a low therapeutic index should therefore be used with caution).
No products indexed under this heading.

Chlorpheniramine Maleate (Data indicates that somatostatin analogs might decrease the metabolic clearance of compounds known to be metabolized by cytochrome P450 enzymes, which may be due to the suppression of growth hormones. Since it cannot be excluded that octreotide may have this effect, other drugs mainly metabolized by CYP3A4, and which have a low therapeutic index should therefore be used with caution). Products include:
Advil Allergy Sinus Caplets 770
Advil Multi-Symptom Cold Caplets 770
BC Allergy Sinus Cold Powder 677
Comtrex Maximum Strength Cold & Cough Day/Night Caplets - Night Formulation 726
Comtrex Maximum Strength Day/Night Severe Cold & Sinus Caplets - Night Formulation 725
Contac Cold and Flu Maximum Strength Caplets 728
Contac Cold and Flu Day and Night Caplets (Night Formulation Only) 727
Children's Dimetapp Long Acting Cough Plus Cold Syrup 731
Robitussin Cough & Cold Long-Acting Liquid 735
Robitussin Cough & Allergy Syrup 736
Robitussin Cough & Cold Nighttime Liquid 736
Robitussin Cough, Cold & Flu Nighttime Liquid 738
Robitussin Pediatric Cough & Cold Long-Acting Liquid 735
Robitussin Pediatric Cough & Cold Nighttime Liquid 736
Triaminic Cold & Allergy Liquid 746
Triaminic Cough & Runny Nose Softchews 748
Children's Tylenol Plus Flu Oral Suspension 749
Tylenol Allergy Multi-Symptom Caplets with Cool Burst and Gelcaps 1872

Children's Tylenol Plus Cold Suspension Liquid 1879
Children's Tylenol Plus Cough & Runny Nose Suspension Liquid 1879
Children's Tylenol Plus Flu Suspension Liquid 1881
Children's Tylenol Plus Multi-Symptom Cold Suspension Liquid 1879
Tylenol Cold Head Congestion Nighttime Caplets with Cool Burst 1873
Tylenol Cold Multi-Symptom Nighttime Caplets with Cool Burst 1874
Tylenol Sinus Congestion & Pain Nighttime Caplets with Cool Burst 1876
Vicks 44M Cough, Cold & Flu Relief Liquid 2680
Pediatric Vicks 44m Cough & Cold Relief Liquid 2676
Children's Vicks NyQuil Cold/Cough Relief .... ▣ 756
Children's Vicks NyQuil Cold/Cough Relief Liquid 2680
Zicam Maximum Strength Flu Daytime .... ▣ 768

Chlorpheniramine Polistirex (Data indicates that somatostatin analogs might decrease the metabolic clearance of compounds known to be metabolized by cytochrome P450 enzymes, which may be due to the suppression of growth hormones. Since it cannot be excluded that octreotide may have this effect, other drugs mainly metabolized by CYP3A4, and which have a low therapeutic index should therefore be used with caution). Products include:
Tussionex Pennkinetic Extended-Release Suspension 3327

Chlorpheniramine Tannate (Data indicates that somatostatin analogs might decrease the metabolic clearance of compounds known to be metabolized by cytochrome P450 enzymes, which may be due to the suppression of growth hormones. Since it cannot be excluded that octreotide may have this effect, other drugs mainly metabolized by CYP3A4, and which have a low therapeutic index should therefore be used with caution).
No products indexed under this heading.

Chlorpropamide (Octreotide causes hypo- and hyperglycemia in some patients; dosage adjustments of oral hypoglycemic agents may be required).
No products indexed under this heading.

Cisapride (Data indicates that somatostatin analogs might decrease the metabolic clearance of compounds known to be metabolized by cytochrome P450 enzymes, which may be due to the suppression of growth hormones. Since it cannot be excluded that octreotide may have this effect, other drugs mainly metabolized by CYP3A4, and which have a low therapeutic index should therefore be used with caution).
No products indexed under this heading.

Clarithromycin (Data indicates that somatostatin analogs might decrease the metabolic clearance of compounds known to be metabolized by cytochrome P450 enzymes, which may be due to the suppression of growth hormones. Since it cannot be excluded that octreotide may have this effect, other drugs mainly metabolized by CYP3A4, and which have a low therapeutic index should therefore be used with caution). Products include:
Biaxin/Biaxin XL 402
PREVPAC 3284

Cyclosporine (Co-administration may decrease blood levels of cyclosporine and may result in transplant rejection). Products include:
Gengraf Capsules 459
Neoral Oral Solution 2259
Neoral Soft Gelatin Capsules 2259
Restasis Ophthalmic Emulsion 575
Sandimmune 2275

Desogestrel (Data indicates that somatostatin analogs might decrease the metabolic clearance of compounds known to be metabolized by cytochrome P450 enzymes, which may be due to the suppression of growth hormones. Since it cannot be excluded that octreotide may have this effect, other drugs mainly metabolized by CYP3A4, and which have a low therapeutic index should therefore be used with caution). Products include:
Mircette Tablets 1066

Diazepam (Data indicates that somatostatin analogs might decrease the metabolic clearance of compounds known to be metabolized by cytochrome P450 enzymes, which may be due to the suppression of growth hormones. Since it cannot be excluded that octreotide may have this effect, other drugs mainly metabolized by CYP3A4, and which have a low therapeutic index should therefore be used with caution). Products include:
Diastat Rectal Delivery System 3343
Valium Tablets 2819

Diazoxide (Adjustment of the dosage of diazoxide may be required). Products include:
Hyperstat I.V. 3017

Dihydroergotamine Mesylate (Data indicates that somatostatin analogs might decrease the metabolic clearance of compounds known to be metabolized by cytochrome P450 enzymes, which may be due to the suppression of growth hormones. Since it cannot be excluded that octreotide may have this effect, other drugs mainly metabolized by CYP3A4, and which have a low therapeutic index should therefore be used with caution). Products include:
Migranal Nasal Spray 3348

Diltiazem Hydrochloride (Adjustment of the dosage of calcium channel blocker may be required). Products include:
Cardizem LA Extended Release Tablets 1728
Tiazac Capsules 1201

Diltiazem Maleate (Data indicates that somatostatin analogs might decrease the metabolic clearance of compounds known to be metabolized by cytochrome P450 enzymes, which may be due to the suppression of growth hormones. Since it cannot be excluded that octreotide may have this effect, other drugs mainly metabolized by CYP3A4, and which have a low therapeutic index should therefore be used with caution).
No products indexed under this heading.

Disopyramide (Data indicates that somatostatin analogs might decrease the metabolic clearance of compounds known to be metabolized by cytochrome P450 enzymes, which may be due to the suppression of growth hormones. Since it cannot be excluded that octreotide may have this effect, other drugs mainly metabolized by CYP3A4, and which have a low therapeutic index should therefore be used with caution).
No products indexed under this heading.

Disopyramide Phosphate (Data indicates that somatostatin analogs might decrease the metabolic clearance of compounds known to be metabolized by cytochrome P450 enzymes, which may be due to the suppression of growth hormones. Since it cannot be excluded that octreotide may have this effect, other drugs mainly metabolized by CYP3A4, and which have a low therapeutic index should therefore be used with caution).
No products indexed under this heading.

Disulfiram (Data indicates that somatostatin analogs might decrease the metabolic clearance of compounds known to be metabolized by cytochrome P450 enzymes, which may be due to the suppression of growth hormones. Since it cannot be excluded that octreotide may have this effect, other drugs mainly metabolized by CYP3A4, and which have a low therapeutic index should therefore be used with caution).
No products indexed under this heading.

Doxorubicin Hydrochloride (Data indicates that somatostatin analogs might decrease the metabolic clearance of compounds known to be metabolized by cytochrome P450 enzymes, which may be due to the suppression of growth hormones. Since it cannot be excluded that octreotide may have this effect, other drugs mainly metabolized by CYP3A4, and which have a low therapeutic index should therefore be used with caution).
No products indexed under this heading.

Dronabinol (Data indicates that somatostatin analogs might decrease the metabolic clearance of compounds known to be metabolized by cytochrome P450 enzymes, which may be due to the suppression of growth hormones. Since it cannot be excluded that octreotide may have this effect, other drugs mainly metabolized by CYP3A4, and which have a low therapeutic index should therefore be used with caution). Products include:
Marinol Capsules 3333

Ergotamine Tartrate (Data indicates that somatostatin analogs might decrease the metabolic clearance of compounds known to be metabolized by cytochrome P450 enzymes, which may be due to the suppression of growth hormones. Since it cannot be excluded that octreotide may have this effect, other drugs mainly metabolized by CYP3A4, and which have a low therapeutic index should therefore be used with caution).
No products indexed under this heading.

Erythromycin (Data indicates that somatostatin analogs might decrease the metabolic clearance of compounds known to be metabolized by cytochrome P450 enzymes, which may be due to the suppression of growth hormones. Since it cannot be excluded that octreotide may have this effect, other drugs mainly metabolized by CYP3A4, and which have a low therapeutic index should therefore be used with caution). Products include:
Ery-Tab Tablets 449
Erythromycin Base Filmtab Tablets 455
Erythromycin Delayed-Release Capsules, USP 457
PCE Dispertab Tablets 515

Erythromycin Estolate (Data indicates that somatostatin analogs might decrease the metabolic clearance of compounds known to be metabolized by cytochrome P450 enzymes, which may be due to the suppression of growth hormones. Since it cannot be excluded that octreotide may have this effect, other drugs mainly metabolized by CYP3A4, and which have a low therapeutic index should therefore be used with caution).
No products indexed under this heading.

Erythromycin Ethylsuccinate (Data indicates that somatostatin analogs might decrease the metabolic clearance of compounds known to be metabolized by cytochrome P450 enzymes, which may be due to the suppression of growth hormones. Since it cannot be excluded that octreotide may have this effect, other drugs mainly metabolized by CYP3A4, and which have a low therapeutic index should therefore be used with caution). Products include:
E.E.S. 451
EryPed 447

Erythromycin Gluceptate (Data indicates that somatostatin analogs might decrease the metabolic clearance of compounds known to be metabolized by cytochrome P450 enzymes, which may be due to the suppression of growth hormones. Since it cannot be excluded that octreotide may have this effect, other drugs mainly metabolized by CYP3A4, and which have a low therapeutic index should therefore be used with caution).
No products indexed under this heading.

Erythromycin Lactobionate (Data indicates that somatostatin analogs might decrease the metabolic clearance of compounds known to be metabolized by cytochrome P450 enzymes, which may be due to the suppression of growth hormones. Since it cannot be excluded that octreotide may have this effect, other drugs mainly metabolized by CYP3A4, and which have a low therapeutic index should therefore be used with caution).
No products indexed under this heading.

Erythromycin Stearate (Data indicates that somatostatin analogs might decrease the metabolic clearance of compounds known to be metabolized by cytochrome P450 enzymes, which may be due to the suppression of growth hormones. Since it cannot be excluded that octreotide may have this effect, other drugs mainly metabolized by CYP3A4, and which have a low therapeutic index should therefore be used with caution). Products include:

Esmolol Hydrochloride (Adjustment of the dosage of beta blockers may be required).

No products indexed under this heading.

Estradiol (Data indicates that somatostatin analogs might decrease the metabolic clearance of compounds known to be metabolized by cytochrome P450 enzymes, which may be due to the suppression of growth hormones. Since it cannot be excluded that octreotide may have this effect, other drugs mainly metabolized by CYP3A4, and which have a low therapeutic index should therefore be used with caution). Products include:

Estradiol Benzoate (Data indicates that somatostatin analogs might decrease the metabolic clearance of compounds known to be metabolized by cytochrome P450 enzymes, which may be due to the suppression of growth hormones. Since it cannot be excluded that octreotide may have this effect, other drugs mainly metabolized by CYP3A4, and which have a low therapeutic index should therefore be used with caution).

No products indexed under this heading.

Estradiol Cypionate (Data indicates that somatostatin analogs might decrease the metabolic clearance of compounds known to be metabolized by cytochrome P450 enzymes, which may be due to the suppression of growth hormones. Since it cannot be excluded that octreotide may have this effect, other drugs mainly metabolized by CYP3A4, and which have a low therapeutic index should therefore be used with caution).

No products indexed under this heading.

Estradiol Valerate (Data indicates that somatostatin analogs might decrease the metabolic clearance of compounds known to be metabolized by cytochrome P450 enzymes, which may be due to the suppression of growth hormones. Since it cannot be excluded that octreotide may have this effect, other drugs mainly metabolized by CYP3A4, and which have a low therapeutic index should therefore be used with caution).

No products indexed under this heading.

Ethinyl Estradiol (Data indicates that somatostatin analogs might decrease the metabolic clearance of compounds known to be metabolized by cytochrome P450 enzymes, which may be due to the suppression of growth hormones. Since it cannot be excluded that octreotide may have this effect, other drugs mainly metabolized by CYP3A4, and which have a low therapeutic index should therefore be used with caution). Products include:

Ethosuximide (Data indicates that somatostatin analogs might decrease the metabolic clearance of compounds known to be metabolized by cytochrome P450 enzymes, which may be due to the suppression of growth hormones. Since it cannot be excluded that octreotide may have this effect, other drugs mainly metabolized by CYP3A4, and which have a low therapeutic index should therefore be used with caution).

No products indexed under this heading.

Ethynodiol Diacetate (Data indicates that somatostatin analogs might decrease the metabolic clearance of compounds known to be metabolized by cytochrome P450 enzymes, which may be due to the suppression of growth hormones. Since it cannot be excluded that octreotide may have this effect, other drugs mainly metabolized by CYP3A4, and which have a low therapeutic index should therefore be used with caution).

No products indexed under this heading.

Etoposide (Data indicates that somatostatin analogs might decrease the metabolic clearance of compounds known to be metabolized by cytochrome P450 enzymes, which may be due to the suppression of growth hormones. Since it cannot be excluded that octreotide may have this effect, other drugs mainly metabolized by CYP3A4, and which have a low therapeutic index should therefore be used with caution).

No products indexed under this heading.

Etoposide Phosphate (Data indicates that somatostatin analogs might decrease the metabolic clearance of compounds known to be metabolized by cytochrome P450 enzymes, which may be due to the suppression of growth hormones. Since it cannot be excluded that octreotide may have this effect, other drugs mainly metabolized by CYP3A4, and which have a low therapeutic index should therefore be used with caution).

No products indexed under this heading.

Felodipine (Adjustment of the dosage of calcium channel blocker may be required).

No products indexed under this heading.

Fentanyl (Data indicates that somatostatin analogs might decrease the metabolic clearance of compounds known to be metabolized by cytochrome P450 enzymes, which may be due to the suppression of growth hormones. Since it cannot be excluded that octreotide may have this effect, other drugs mainly metabolized by CYP3A4, and which have a low therapeutic index should therefore be used with caution). Products include:

Fentanyl Citrate (Data indicates that somatostatin analogs might decrease the metabolic clearance of compounds known to be metabolized by cytochrome P450 enzymes, which may be due to the suppression of growth hormones. Since it cannot be excluded that octreotide may have this effect, other drugs mainly metabolized by CYP3A4, and which have a low therapeutic index should therefore be used with caution). Products include:

Glimepiride (Octreotide causes hypo- and hyperglycemia in some patients; dosage adjustments of oral hypoglycemic agents may be required). Products include:

Glipizide (Octreotide causes hypo- and hyperglycemia in some patients; dosage adjustments of oral hypoglycemic agents may be required).

No products indexed under this heading.

Glyburide (Octreotide causes hypo- and hyperglycemia in some patients; dosage adjustments of oral hypoglycemic agents may be required).

No products indexed under this heading.

Haloperidol (Data indicates that somatostatin analogs might decrease the metabolic clearance of compounds known to be metabolized by cytochrome P450 enzymes, which may be due to the suppression of growth hormones. Since it cannot be excluded that octreotide may have this effect, other drugs mainly metabolized by CYP3A4, and which have a low therapeutic index should therefore be used with caution).

No products indexed under this heading.

Haloperidol Decanoate (Data indicates that somatostatin analogs might decrease the metabolic clearance of compounds known to be metabolized by cytochrome P450 enzymes, which may be due to the suppression of growth hormones. Since it cannot be excluded that octreotide may have this effect, other drugs mainly metabolized by CYP3A4, and which have a low therapeutic index should therefore be used with caution).

No products indexed under this heading.

Haloperidol Lactate (Data indicates that somatostatin analogs might decrease the metabolic clearance of compounds known to be metabolized by cytochrome P450 enzymes, which may be due to the suppression of growth hormones. Since it cannot be excluded that octreotide may have this effect, other drugs mainly metabolized by CYP3A4, and which have a low therapeutic index should therefore be used with caution).

No products indexed under this heading.

Indinavir Sulfate (Data indicates that somatostatin analogs might decrease the metabolic clearance of compounds known to be metabolized by cytochrome P450 enzymes, which may be due to the suppression of growth hormones. Since it cannot be excluded that octreotide may have this effect, other drugs mainly metabolized by CYP3A4, and

which have a low therapeutic index should therefore be used with caution). Products include:

Insulin, Human, Zinc Suspension (Octreotide causes hypo- and hyperglycemia in some patients; insulin dosage adjustments may be required). Products include:

Insulin, Human NPH (Octreotide causes hypo- and hyperglycemia in some patients; insulin dosage adjustments may be required). Products include:

Insulin, Human Regular (Octreotide causes hypo- and hyperglycemia in some patients; insulin dosage adjustments may be required). Products include:

Insulin, Human Regular and Human NPH Mixture (Octreotide causes hypo- and hyperglycemia in some patients; insulin dosage adjustments may be required). Products include:

Insulin, NPH (Octreotide causes hypo- and hyperglycemia in some patients; insulin dosage adjustments may be required).

No products indexed under this heading.

Insulin, Regular (Octreotide causes hypo- and hyperglycemia in some patients; insulin dosage adjustments may be required).

No products indexed under this heading.

Insulin, Zinc Crystals (Octreotide causes hypo- and hyperglycemia in some patients; insulin dosage adjustments may be required).

No products indexed under this heading.

Insulin, Zinc Suspension (Octreotide causes hypo- and hyperglycemia in some patients; insulin dosage adjustments may be required).

No products indexed under this heading.

Insulin Aspart, Human Regular (Octreotide causes hypo- and hyperglycemia in some patients; insulin dosage adjustments may be required). Products include:

Insulin glargine (Octreotide causes hypo- and hyperglycemia in some patients; insulin dosage adjustments may be required). Products include:

Insulin Lispro, Human (Octreotide causes hypo- and hyperglycemia in some patients; insulin dosage adjustments may be required). Products include:

Insulin Lispro Protamine, Human (Octreotide causes hypo- and hyperglycemia in some patients; insulin dosage adjustments may be required). Products include:

Isradipine (Adjustment of the dosage of calcium channel blocker may be required). Products include:

IMPORTANT NOTE: Always consult each drug listing in the patient's regimen for possible interactions.

Itraconazole (Data indicates that somatostatin analogs might decrease the metabolic clearance of compounds known to be metabolized by cytochrome P450 enzymes, which may be due to the suppression of growth hormones. Since it cannot be excluded that octreotide may have this effect, other drugs mainly metabolized by CYP3A4, and which have a low therapeutic index should therefore be used with caution).
No products indexed under this heading.

Ketoconazole (Data indicates that somatostatin analogs might decrease the metabolic clearance of compounds known to be metabolized by cytochrome P450 enzymes, which may be due to the suppression of growth hormones. Since it cannot be excluded that octreotide may have this effect, other drugs mainly metabolized by CYP3A4, and which have a low therapeutic index should therefore be used with caution). Products include:
Nizoral A-D Shampoo, 1% 1868

Labetalol Hydrochloride (Adjustment of the dosage of beta blockers may be required).
No products indexed under this heading.

Levobunolol Hydrochloride (Adjustment of the dosage of beta blockers may be required). Products include:
Betagan Ophthalmic Solution, USP .... ⊙220

Levonorgestrel (Data indicates that somatostatin analogs might decrease the metabolic clearance of compounds known to be metabolized by cytochrome P450 enzymes, which may be due to the suppression of growth hormones. Since it cannot be excluded that octreotide may have this effect, other drugs mainly metabolized by CYP3A4, and which have a low therapeutic index should therefore be used with caution). Products include:
Climara Pro Transdermal System 776
Mirena Intrauterine System 787
Plan B Tablets 1076
Seasonique Tablets 1077

Lidocaine (Data indicates that somatostatin analogs might decrease the metabolic clearance of compounds known to be metabolized by cytochrome P450 enzymes, which may be due to the suppression of growth hormones. Since it cannot be excluded that octreotide may have this effect, other drugs mainly metabolized by CYP3A4, and which have a low therapeutic index should therefore be used with caution). Products include:
Lidoderm Patch 1118
Synera Topical Patch 1137

Lidocaine Hydrochloride (Data indicates that somatostatin analogs might decrease the metabolic clearance of compounds known to be metabolized by cytochrome P450 enzymes, which may be due to the suppression of growth hormones. Since it cannot be excluded that octreotide may have this effect, other drugs mainly metabolized by CYP3A4, and which have a low therapeutic index should therefore be used with caution).
No products indexed under this heading.

Lovastatin (Data indicates that somatostatin analogs might decrease the metabolic clearance of compounds known to be metabolized by cytochrome P450 enzymes, which may be due to the suppression of growth hormones. Since it cannot be excluded that octreotide may have this effect, other drugs mainly metabolized by CYP3A4, and which have a low therapeutic index should therefore be used with caution). Products include:
Advicor Tablets 1722
Altoprev Extended-Release Tablets 3109
Mevacor Tablets 2021

Mestranol (Data indicates that somatostatin analogs might decrease the metabolic clearance of compounds known to be metabolized by cytochrome P450 enzymes, which may be due to the suppression of growth hormones. Since it cannot be excluded that octreotide may have this effect, other drugs mainly metabolized by CYP3A4, and which have a low therapeutic index should therefore be used with caution).
No products indexed under this heading.

Metformin Hydrochloride (Octreotide causes hypo- and hyperglycemia in some patients; dosage adjustments of oral hypoglycemic agents may be required). Products include:
ActoPlus Met Tablets 3214
Avandamet Tablets 1373
Fortamet Extended-Release Tablets 3115

Methadone Hydrochloride (Data indicates that somatostatin analogs might decrease the metabolic clearance of compounds known to be metabolized by cytochrome P450 enzymes, which may be due to the suppression of growth hormones. Since it cannot be excluded that octreotide may have this effect, other drugs mainly metabolized by CYP3A4, and which have a low therapeutic index should therefore be used with caution).
No products indexed under this heading.

Metipranolol Hydrochloride (Adjustment of the dosage of beta blockers may be required).
No products indexed under this heading.

Metoprolol Succinate (Adjustment of the dosage of beta blockers may be required). Products include:
Toprol-XL Tablets 668

Metoprolol Tartrate (Adjustment of the dosage of beta blockers may be required). Products include:
Lopressor Injection 2238
Lopressor Tablets 2238
Lopressor HCT 50/25 Tablets 2241
Lopressor HCT 100/25 Tablets 2241
Lopressor HCT 100/50 Tablets 2241

Mibefradil Dihydrochloride (Adjustment of the dosage of calcium channel blocker may be required).
No products indexed under this heading.

Midazolam Hydrochloride (Data indicates that somatostatin analogs might decrease the metabolic clearance of compounds known to be metabolized by cytochrome P450 enzymes, which may be due to the suppression of growth hormones. Since it cannot be excluded that octreotide may have this effect, other drugs mainly metabolized by CYP3A4, and which have a low therapeutic index should therefore be used with caution).
No products indexed under this heading.

Miglitol (Octreotide causes hypo- and hyperglycemia in some patients; dosage adjustments of oral hypoglycemic agents may be required).
No products indexed under this heading.

Nadolol (Adjustment of the dosage of beta blockers may be required). Products include:
Nadolol Tablets 2159

Nefazodone Hydrochloride (Data indicates that somatostatin analogs might decrease the metabolic clearance of compounds known to be metabolized by cytochrome P450 enzymes, which may be due to the suppression of growth hormones. Since it cannot be excluded that octreotide may have this effect, other drugs mainly metabolized by CYP3A4, and which have a low therapeutic index should therefore be used with caution).
No products indexed under this heading.

Nelfinavir Mesylate (Data indicates that somatostatin analogs might decrease the metabolic clearance of compounds known to be metabolized by cytochrome P450 enzymes, which may be due to the suppression of growth hormones. Since it cannot be excluded that octreotide may have this effect, other drugs mainly metabolized by CYP3A4, and which have a low therapeutic index should therefore be used with caution). Products include:
Viracept 2577

Nicardipine Hydrochloride (Adjustment of the dosage of calcium channel blocker may be required). Products include:
Cardene I.V. 2497

Nifedipine (Adjustment of the dosage of calcium channel blocker may be required). Products include:
Adalat CC Tablets 2964

Nimodipine (Adjustment of the dosage of calcium channel blocker may be required). Products include:
Nimotop Capsules 749

Nisoldipine (Adjustment of the dosage of calcium channel blocker may be required). Products include:
Sular Tablets 3122

Nitrendipine (Data indicates that somatostatin analogs might decrease the metabolic clearance of compounds known to be metabolized by cytochrome P450 enzymes, which may be due to the suppression of growth hormones. Since it cannot be excluded that octreotide may have this effect, other drugs mainly metabolized by CYP3A4, and which have a low therapeutic index should therefore be used with caution).
No products indexed under this heading.

Norethindrone (Data indicates that somatostatin analogs might decrease the metabolic clearance of compounds known to be metabolized by cytochrome P450 enzymes, which may be due to the suppression of growth hormones. Since it cannot be excluded that octreotide may have this effect, other drugs mainly metabolized by CYP3A4, and which have a low therapeutic index should therefore be used with caution). Products include:
Ortho Micronor Tablets 2426

Norethindrone Acetate (Data indicates that somatostatin analogs might decrease the metabolic clearance of compounds known to be metabolized by cytochrome P450 enzymes, which may be due to the suppression of growth hormones. Since it cannot be excluded that octreotide may have this effect, other drugs mainly metabolized by CYP3A4, and which have a low therapeutic index should therefore be used with caution).
No products indexed under this heading.

Norgestrel (Data indicates that somatostatin analogs might decrease the metabolic clearance of compounds known to be metabolized by cytochrome P450 enzymes, which may be due to the suppression of growth hormones. Since it cannot be excluded that octreotide may have this effect, other drugs mainly metabolized by CYP3A4, and which have a low therapeutic index should therefore be used with caution).
No products indexed under this heading.

Ondansetron (Data indicates that somatostatin analogs might decrease the metabolic clearance of compounds known to be metabolized by cytochrome P450 enzymes, which may be due to the suppression of growth hormones. Since it cannot be excluded that octreotide may have this effect, other drugs mainly metabolized by CYP3A4, and which have a low therapeutic index should therefore be used with caution). Products include:
Zofran ODT Orally Disintegrating Tablets 1639

Ondansetron Hydrochloride (Data indicates that somatostatin analogs might decrease the metabolic clearance of compounds known to be metabolized by cytochrome P450 enzymes, which may be due to the suppression of growth hormones. Since it cannot be excluded that octreotide may have this effect, other drugs mainly metabolized by CYP3A4, and which have a low therapeutic index should therefore be used with caution). Products include:
Zofran Injection 1634
Zofran 1639

Paclitaxel (Data indicates that somatostatin analogs might decrease the metabolic clearance of compounds known to be metabolized by cytochrome P450 enzymes, which may be due to the suppression of growth hormones. Since it cannot be excluded that octreotide may have this effect, other drugs mainly metabolized by CYP3A4, and which have a low therapeutic index should therefore be used with caution).
No products indexed under this heading.

Penbutolol Sulfate (Adjustment of the dosage of beta blockers may be required).
No products indexed under this heading.

Pimozide (Data indicates that somatostatin analogs might decrease the metabolic clearance of compounds known to be metabolized by cytochrome P450 enzymes, which may be due to the suppression of growth hormones. Since it cannot be excluded that octreotide may have this effect, other drugs mainly metabolized by CYP3A4, and which have a low therapeutic index should therefore be used with caution).

 No products indexed under this heading.

Pindolol (Adjustment of the dosage of beta blockers may be required).

 No products indexed under this heading.

Pioglitazone Hydrochloride (Octreotide causes hypo- and hyperglycemia in some patients; dosage adjustments of oral hypoglycemic agents may be required). Products include:

ActoPlus Met Tablets	3214
Actos Tablets	3219
Duetact Tablets	3226

Polyestradiol Phosphate (Data indicates that somatostatin analogs might decrease the metabolic clearance of compounds known to be metabolized by cytochrome P450 enzymes, which may be due to the suppression of growth hormones. Since it cannot be excluded that octreotide may have this effect, other drugs mainly metabolized by CYP3A4, and which have a low therapeutic index should therefore be used with caution).

 No products indexed under this heading.

Propranolol Hydrochloride (Adjustment of the dosage of beta blockers may be required). Products include:

Inderal LA Long-Acting Capsules	3429
InnoPran XL Capsules	2723

Quinidine (Use caution with drugs mainly metabolized by CYP3A4 and which have a low therapeutic index. Data indicate that somatostatin analogs might decrease the metabolic clearance of compounds metabolized by CYP450 enzymes).

 No products indexed under this heading.

Quinidine Gluconate (Use caution with drugs mainly metabolized by CYP3A4 and which have a low therapeutic index. Data indicate that somatostatin analogs might decrease the metabolic clearance of compounds metabolized by CYP450 enzymes).

 No products indexed under this heading.

Quinidine Hydrochloride (Use caution with drugs mainly metabolized by CYP3A4 and which have a low therapeutic index. Data indicate that somatostatin analogs might decrease the metabolic clearance of compounds metabolized by CYP450 enzymes).

 No products indexed under this heading.

Quinidine Polygalacturonate (Use caution with drugs mainly metabolized by CYP3A4 and which have a low therapeutic index. Data indicate that somatostatin analogs might decrease the metabolic clearance of compounds metabolized by CYP450 enzymes).

 No products indexed under this heading.

Quinidine Sulfate (Use caution with drugs mainly metabolized by CYP3A4 and which have a low therapeutic index. Data indicate that somatostatin analogs might decrease the metabolic clearance of compounds metabolized by CYP450 enzymes).

 No products indexed under this heading.

Repaglinide (Octreotide causes hypo- and hyperglycemia in some patients; dosage adjustments of oral hypoglycemic agents may be required).

 No products indexed under this heading.

Rifabutin (Data indicates that somatostatin analogs might decrease the metabolic clearance of compounds known to be metabolized by cytochrome P450 enzymes, which may be due to the suppression of growth hormones. Since it cannot be excluded that octreotide may have this effect, other drugs mainly metabolized by CYP3A4, and which have a low therapeutic index should therefore be used with caution).

 No products indexed under this heading.

Ritonavir (Data indicates that somatostatin analogs might decrease the metabolic clearance of compounds known to be metabolized by cytochrome P450 enzymes, which may be due to the suppression of growth hormones. Since it cannot be excluded that octreotide may have this effect, other drugs mainly metabolized by CYP3A4, and which have a low therapeutic index should therefore be used with caution). Products include:

Kaletra	476
Norvir	503

Rosiglitazone Maleate (Octreotide causes hypo- and hyperglycemia in some patients; dosage adjustments of oral hypoglycemic agents may be required). Products include:

Avandamet Tablets	1373
Avandaryl Tablets	1379
Avandia Tablets	1384

Saquinavir (Data indicates that somatostatin analogs might decrease the metabolic clearance of compounds known to be metabolized by cytochrome P450 enzymes, which may be due to the suppression of growth hormones. Since it cannot be excluded that octreotide may have this effect, other drugs mainly metabolized by CYP3A4, and which have a low therapeutic index should therefore be used with caution).

 No products indexed under this heading.

Saquinavir Mesylate (Data indicates that somatostatin analogs might decrease the metabolic clearance of compounds known to be metabolized by cytochrome P450 enzymes, which may be due to the suppression of growth hormones. Since it cannot be excluded that octreotide may have this effect, other drugs mainly metabolized by CYP3A4, and which have a low therapeutic index should therefore be used with caution). Products include:

Invirase	2772

Sertraline Hydrochloride (Data indicates that somatostatin analogs might decrease the metabolic clearance of compounds known to be metabolized by cytochrome P450 enzymes, which may be due to the suppression of growth hormones. Since it cannot be excluded that octreotide may have this effect, other drugs mainly metabolized by CYP3A4, and which have a low therapeutic index should therefore be used with caution). Products include:

Zoloft	2586

Sildenafil Citrate (Data indicates that somatostatin analogs might decrease the metabolic clearance of compounds known to be metabolized by cytochrome P450 enzymes, which may be due to the suppression of growth hormones. Since it cannot be excluded that octreotide may have this effect, other drugs mainly metabolized by CYP3A4, and which have a low therapeutic index should therefore be used with caution). Products include:

Revatio Tablets	2557
Viagra Tablets	2573

Simvastatin (Data indicates that somatostatin analogs might decrease the metabolic clearance of compounds known to be metabolized by cytochrome P450 enzymes, which may be due to the suppression of growth hormones. Since it cannot be excluded that octreotide may have this effect, other drugs mainly metabolized by CYP3A4, and which have a low therapeutic index should therefore be used with caution). Products include:

Vytorin 10/10 Tablets	2114
Vytorin 10/10 Tablets	3077
Vytorin 10/20 Tablets	2114
Vytorin 10/20 Tablets	3077
Vytorin 10/40 Tablets	2114
Vytorin 10/40 Tablets	3077
Vytorin 10/80 Tablets	2114
Vytorin 10/80 Tablets	3077
Zocor Tablets	2105

Sirolimus (Data indicates that somatostatin analogs might decrease the metabolic clearance of compounds known to be metabolized by cytochrome P450 enzymes, which may be due to the suppression of growth hormones. Since it cannot be excluded that octreotide may have this effect, other drugs mainly metabolized by CYP3A4, and which have a low therapeutic index should therefore be used with caution). Products include:

Rapamune Oral Solution and Tablets	3475

Sotalol Hydrochloride (Adjustment of the dosage of beta blockers may be required).

 No products indexed under this heading.

Tacrolimus (Data indicates that somatostatin analogs might decrease the metabolic clearance of compounds known to be metabolized by cytochrome P450 enzymes, which may be due to the suppression of growth hormones. Since it cannot be excluded that octreotide may have this effect, other drugs mainly metabolized by CYP3A4, and which have a low therapeutic index should therefore be used with caution). Products include:

Prograf Capsules and Injection	632
Protopic Ointment	638

Tamoxifen Citrate (Data indicates that somatostatin analogs might decrease the metabolic clearance of compounds known to be metabolized by cytochrome P450 enzymes, which may be due to the suppres-

sion of growth hormones. Since it cannot be excluded that octreotide may have this effect, other drugs mainly metabolized by CYP3A4, and which have a low therapeutic index should therefore be used with caution). Products include:

Soltamox Oral Solution	3527

Terfenadine (Use caution with drugs mainly metabolized by CYP3A4 and which have a low therapeutic index. Data indicate that somatostatin analogs might decrease the metabolic clearance of compounds metabolized by CYP450 enzymes).

 No products indexed under this heading.

Tiagabine Hydrochloride (Data indicates that somatostatin analogs might decrease the metabolic clearance of compounds known to be metabolized by cytochrome P450 enzymes, which may be due to the suppression of growth hormones. Since it cannot be excluded that octreotide may have this effect, other drugs mainly metabolized by CYP3A4, and which have a low therapeutic index should therefore be used with caution). Products include:

Gabitril Tablets	984

Timolol Hemihydrate (Adjustment of the dosage of beta blockers may be required). Products include:

Betimol Ophthalmic Solution	3382
Betimol Ophthalmic Solution	⊙ 295

Timolol Maleate (Adjustment of the dosage of beta blockers may be required). Products include:

Blocadren Tablets	1916
Cosopt Sterile Ophthalmic Solution	1931
Timolide Tablets	2086
Timoptic Sterile Ophthalmic Solution	2088
Timoptic in Ocudose	2091
Timoptic-XE Sterile Ophthalmic Gel Forming Solution	2092

Tolazamide (Octreotide causes hypo- and hyperglycemia in some patients; dosage adjustments of oral hypoglycemic agents may be required).

 No products indexed under this heading.

Tolbutamide (Octreotide causes hypo- and hyperglycemia in some patients; dosage adjustments of oral hypoglycemic agents may be required).

 No products indexed under this heading.

Tolterodine Tartrate (Data indicates that somatostatin analogs might decrease the metabolic clearance of compounds known to be metabolized by cytochrome P450 enzymes, which may be due to the suppression of growth hormones. Since it cannot be excluded that octreotide may have this effect, other drugs mainly metabolized by CYP3A4, and which have a low therapeutic index should therefore be used with caution). Products include:

Detrol Tablets	2628
Detrol LA Capsules	2631

Trazodone Hydrochloride (Data indicates that somatostatin analogs might decrease the metabolic clearance of compounds known to be metabolized by cytochrome P450 enzymes, which may be due to the suppression of growth hormones. Since it cannot be excluded that octreotide may have this effect, other drugs mainly metabolized by

CYP3A4, and which have a low therapeutic index should therefore be used with caution).
No products indexed under this heading.

Triazolam (Data indicates that somatostatin analogs might decrease the metabolic clearance of compounds known to be metabolized by cytochrome P450 enzymes, which may be due to the suppression of growth hormones. Since it cannot be excluded that octreotide may have this effect, other drugs mainly metabolized by CYP3A4, and which have a low therapeutic index should therefore be used with caution).
No products indexed under this heading.

Troglitazone (Octreotide causes hypo- and hyperglycemia in some patients; dosage adjustments of oral hypoglycemic agents may be required).
No products indexed under this heading.

Verapamil Hydrochloride (Adjustment of the dosage of calcium channel blocker may be required).
Products include:
- Covera-HS Tablets 3139
- Tarka Tablets 524
- Verelan PM Extended-Release Capsules, Controlled-Onset 3106

Vinblastine Sulfate (Data indicates that somatostatin analogs might decrease the metabolic clearance of compounds known to be metabolized by cytochrome P450 enzymes, which may be due to the suppression of growth hormones. Since it cannot be excluded that octreotide may have this effect, other drugs mainly metabolized by CYP3A4, and which have a low therapeutic index should therefore be used with caution).
No products indexed under this heading.

Vincristine Sulfate (Data indicates that somatostatin analogs might decrease the metabolic clearance of compounds known to be metabolized by cytochrome P450 enzymes, which may be due to the suppression of growth hormones. Since it cannot be excluded that octreotide may have this effect, other drugs mainly metabolized by CYP3A4, and which have a low therapeutic index should therefore be used with caution).
No products indexed under this heading.

Warfarin Sodium (Data indicates that somatostatin analogs might decrease the metabolic clearance of compounds known to be metabolized by cytochrome P450 enzymes, which may be due to the suppression of growth hormones. Since it cannot be excluded that octreotide may have this effect, other drugs mainly metabolized by CYP3A4, and which have a low therapeutic index should therefore be used with caution). Products include:
- Coumadin for Injection 898
- Coumadin Tablets 898

SATIETE TABLETS

(Amino Acid Preparations, Ginkgo biloba, Herbals with Vitamins & Minerals, Hypericum) .... ▣832
May interact with anorexiants, monoamine oxidase inhibitors, selective serotonin reuptake inhibitors, and tricyclic antidepressants. Compounds in these categories include:

Amitriptyline Hydrochloride (Concurrent use with tricyclic antidepressants is not recommended).
No products indexed under this heading.

Amoxapine (Concurrent use with tricyclic antidepressants is not recommended).
No products indexed under this heading.

Amphetamine Resins (Concurrent use with prescription diet drugs is not recommended).
No products indexed under this heading.

Benzphetamine Hydrochloride (Concurrent use with prescription diet drugs is not recommended).
No products indexed under this heading.

Citalopram Hydrobromide (Concurrent use with SSRI antidepressants is not recommended).
Products include:
- Celexa 1176

Clomipramine Hydrochloride (Concurrent use with tricyclic antidepressants is not recommended).
No products indexed under this heading.

Desipramine Hydrochloride (Concurrent use with tricyclic antidepressants is not recommended).
No products indexed under this heading.

Dextroamphetamine Sulfate (Concurrent use with prescription diet drugs is not recommended).
Products include:
- Adderall Tablets 3164
- Adderall XR Capsules 3166
- Dexedrine 1420
- DextroStat Tablets 3179

Diethylpropion Hydrochloride (Concurrent use with prescription diet drugs is not recommended).
No products indexed under this heading.

Doxepin Hydrochloride (Concurrent use with tricyclic antidepressants is not recommended).
No products indexed under this heading.

Escitalopram Oxalate (Concurrent use with SSRI antidepressants is not recommended). Products include:
- Lexapro Oral Solution 1190
- Lexapro Tablets 1190

Fenfluramine Hydrochloride (Concurrent use with prescription diet drugs is not recommended).
No products indexed under this heading.

Fluoxetine Hydrochloride (Concurrent use with SSRI antidepressants is not recommended).
Products include:
- Prozac Pulvules and Liquid 1801
- Symbyax Capsules 1819

Fluvoxamine Maleate (Concurrent use with SSRI antidepressants is not recommended).
No products indexed under this heading.

Imipramine Hydrochloride (Concurrent use with tricyclic antidepressants is not recommended).
No products indexed under this heading.

Imipramine Pamoate (Concurrent use with tricyclic antidepressants is not recommended).
No products indexed under this heading.

Isocarboxazid (Concurrent use with MAO inhibitors is not recommended).
No products indexed under this heading.

Maprotiline Hydrochloride (Concurrent use with tricyclic antidepressants is not recommended).
No products indexed under this heading.

Mazindol (Concurrent use with prescription diet drugs is not recommended).
No products indexed under this heading.

Methamphetamine Hydrochloride (Concurrent use with prescription diet drugs is not recommended).
Products include:
- Desoxyn Tablets, USP 2462

Moclobemide (Concurrent use with MAO inhibitors is not recommended).
No products indexed under this heading.

Nortriptyline Hydrochloride (Concurrent use with tricyclic antidepressants is not recommended).
No products indexed under this heading.

Pargyline Hydrochloride (Concurrent use with MAO inhibitors is not recommended).
No products indexed under this heading.

Paroxetine Hydrochloride (Concurrent use with SSRI antidepressants is not recommended).
Products include:
- Paxil CR Controlled-Release Tablets 1538
- Paxil 1530

Phendimetrazine Tartrate (Concurrent use with prescription diet drugs is not recommended).
No products indexed under this heading.

Phenelzine Sulfate (Concurrent use with MAO inhibitors is not recommended).
No products indexed under this heading.

Phenmetrazine Hydrochloride (Concurrent use with prescription diet drugs is not recommended).
No products indexed under this heading.

Procarbazine Hydrochloride (Concurrent use with MAO inhibitors is not recommended). Products include:
- Matulane Capsules 3191

Protriptyline Hydrochloride (Concurrent use with tricyclic antidepressants is not recommended).
No products indexed under this heading.

Selegiline Hydrochloride (Concurrent use with MAO inhibitors is not recommended). Products include:
- Eldepryl Capsules 3208
- Zelapar Tablets 3372

Sertraline Hydrochloride (Concurrent use with SSRI antidepressants is not recommended).
Products include:
- Zoloft 2586

Sibutramine Hydrochloride Monohydrate (Concurrent use with prescription diet drugs is not recommended). Products include:
- Meridia Capsules 489

Tranylcypromine Sulfate (Concurrent use with MAO inhibitors is not recommended). Products include:
- Parnate Tablets 1527

Trimipramine Maleate (Concurrent use with tricyclic antidepressants is not recommended).
No products indexed under this heading.

SEASONIQUE TABLETS

(Ethinyl Estradiol, Levonorgestrel) 1077
May interact with barbiturates, cytochrome p450 3a4 inhibitors (selected), phenytoin, prednisolone, protease inhibitors, salicylates, tetracyclines, theophyllines, and certain other agents. Compounds in these categories include:

Acetaminophen (Acetaminophen may increase plasma ethinyl estradiol levels, possibly by inhibition of conjugation. Decreased plasma concentrations of acetaminophen have been noted when co-administered with combination oral contraceptives). Products include:
- Comtrex Maximum Strength Cold & Cough Day/Night Caplets - Day Formulation .... ▣726
- Comtrex Maximum Strength Cold & Cough Day/Night Caplets - Night Formulation .... ▣726
- Comtrex Maximum Strength Non-Drowsy Cold & Cough Caplets .... ▣725
- Comtrex Maximum Strength Day/Night Severe Cold & Sinus Caplets - Day Formulation .... ▣725
- Comtrex Maximum Strength Day/Night Severe Cold & Sinus Caplets - Night Formulation .... ▣725
- Contac Cold and Flu Maximum Strength Caplets .... ▣728
- Contac Cold and Flu Day and Night Caplets (Day Formulation Only) .... ▣727
- Contac Cold and Flu Day and Night Caplets (Night Formulation Only) .... ▣727
- Contac Cold and Flu Non-Drowsy Caplets .... ▣728
- Excedrin Extra Strength Caplets/Tablets/Geltabs .... ▣684
- Excedrin Migraine Caplets/Tablets/Geltabs .... ▣609
- Excedrin PM Caplets/Tablets/Geltabs .... ▣610
- Excedrin Sinus Headache Caplets/Tablets .... ▣610
- Excedrin Tension Headache Caplets/Tablets/Geltabs .... ▣611
- Goody's Body Pain Formula Powder .... ▣684
- Goody's Extra Strength Headache Powders .... ▣611
- Goody's Extra Strength Pain Relief Tablets .... ▣685
- Goody's PM Powder for Pain with Sleeplessness .... ▣612
- Percocet Tablets 1131
- Robitussin Cough, Cold & Flu Nighttime Liquid .... ▣738
- TheraFlu Cold & Sore Throat Hot Liquid .... ▣741
- TheraFlu Flu & Chest Congestion Hot Liquid .... ▣741
- TheraFlu Flu & Sore Throat Hot Liquid .... ▣742
- TheraFlu Daytime Severe Cold Hot Liquid .... ▣742
- TheraFlu Nighttime Severe Cold Hot Liquid .... ▣740
- TheraFlu Warming Relief Daytime Severe Cold .... ▣743
- TheraFlu Warming Relief Nighttime Severe Cold .... ▣743

Acetazolamide (CYP3A4 inhibitors may increase plasma ethinyl estradiol levels).

No products indexed under this heading.

Amiodarone Hydrochloride (CYP3A4 inhibitors may increase plasma ethinyl estradiol levels).

No products indexed under this heading.

Ampicillin (Several cases of contraceptive failure and breakthrough bleeding have been reported in the literature with concomitant administration of antibiotics, such as ampicillin; however, clinical pharmacology studies investigating drug interactions between combined oral contraceptives and these antibiotics have reported inconsistent results).

No products indexed under this heading.

Ampicillin Sodium (Several cases of contraceptive failure and breakthrough bleeding have been reported in the literature with concomitant administration of antibiotics, such as ampicillin; however, clinical pharmacology studies investigating drug interactions between combined oral contraceptives and these antibiotics have reported inconsistent results).

No products indexed under this heading.

Ampicillin Trihydrate (Several cases of contraceptive failure and breakthrough bleeding have been reported in the literature with concomitant administration of antibiotics, such as ampicillin; however, clinical pharmacology studies investigating drug interactions between combined oral contraceptives and these antibiotics have reported inconsistent results).

No products indexed under this heading.

Amprenavir (Several protease inhibitors have been studied with co-administration of oral combination hormonal contraceptives with significant changes (increase and decrease) in the plasma levels of the estrogen and progestin being noted in some cases). Products include:

Anastrozole (CYP3A4 inhibitors may increase plasma ethinyl estradiol levels). Products include:

Aprepitant (CYP3A4 inhibitors may increase plasma ethinyl estradiol levels). Products include:

Aprobarbitai (Contraceptive effectivness may be reduced when hormonal contraceptives are co-administered with drugs that increase the metabolism of contraceptive steroids, such as barbiturates).

No products indexed under this heading.

Ascorbic Acid (Ascorbic acid may increase plasma ethinyl estradiol levels, possibly by inhibition of conjugation). Products include:

Aspirin (Increased clearance of salicylic acid due to induction of conjugation has been noted when co-administered with combination oral contraceptives). Products include:

Aspirin, Enteric Coated (Increased clearance of salicylic acid due to induction of conjugation has been noted when co-administered with combination oral contraceptives).

No products indexed under this heading.

Aspirin Buffered (Increased clearance of salicylic acid due to induction of conjugation has been noted when co-administered with combination oral contraceptives). Products include:

Atorvastatin Calcium (Co-administration of atorvastatin and certain combination oral contraceptives containing ethinyl estradiol increase AUC values for ethinyl estradiol by approximately 20%). Products include:

Butabarbital (Contraceptive effectivness may be reduced when hormonal contraceptives are co-administered with drugs that increase the metabolism of contraceptive steroids, such as barbiturates).

No products indexed under this heading.

Butalbital (Contraceptive effectivness may be reduced when hormonal contraceptives are co-administered with drugs that increase the metabolism of contraceptive steroids, such as barbiturates).

No products indexed under this heading.

Carbamazepine (Contraceptive effectiveness may be reduced when hormonal contraceptives are co-administered with drugs that increase the metabolism of contraceptive steroids, such as carbamazepine). Products include:

Choline Magnesium Trisalicylate (Increased clearance of salicylic acid due to induction of conjugation has been noted when co-administered with combination oral contraceptives).

No products indexed under this heading.

Cimetidine (CYP3A4 inhibitors may increase plasma ethinyl estradiol levels). Products include:

Cimetidine Hydrochloride (CYP3A4 inhibitors may increase plasma ethinyl estradiol levels).

No products indexed under this heading.

Ciprofloxacin (CYP3A4 inhibitors may increase plasma ethinyl estradiol levels). Products include:

Clarithromycin (CYP3A4 inhibitors may increase plasma ethinyl estradiol levels). Products include:

Clotrimazole (CYP3A4 inhibitors may increase plasma ethinyl estradiol levels). Products include:

Cyclosporine (Combination hormonal contraceptives containing some synthetic estrogens (e.g. ethinyl estradiol) may inhibit the metabolism of other compounds. Increased plasma concentrations of cyclosporine have been reported with concomitant administration of combination oral contraceptives). Products include:

Dalfopristin (CYP3A4 inhibitors may increase plasma ethinyl estradiol levels).

No products indexed under this heading.

Danazol (CYP3A4 inhibitors may increase plasma ethinyl estradiol levels).

No products indexed under this heading.

Delavirdine Mesylate (CYP3A4 inhibitors may increase plasma ethinyl estradiol levels). Products include:

IMPORTANT NOTE: Always consult each drug listing in the patient's regimen for possible interactions.

Demeclocycline Hydrochloride
(Several cases of contraceptive failure and breakthrough bleeding have been reported in the literature concomitant administration of antibiotics, such as tetracyclines; however, clinical pharmacology studies investigating drug interactions between combined oral contraceptives and these antibiotics have reported inconsistent results).
No products indexed under this heading.

Diflunisal (Increased clearance of salicylic acid due to induction of conjugation has been noted when co-administered with combination oral contraceptives). Products include:
Dolobid Tablets 1955

Diltiazem Hydrochloride (CYP3A4 inhibitors may increase plasma ethinyl estradiol levels). Products include:
Cardizem LA Extended Release Tablets .. 1728
Tiazac Capsules 1201

Diltiazem Maleate (CYP3A4 inhibitors may increase plasma ethinyl estradiol levels).
No products indexed under this heading.

Doxycycline Calcium (Several cases of contraceptive failure and breakthrough bleeding have been reported in the literature concomitant administration of antibiotics, such as tetracyclines; however, clinical pharmacology studies investigating drug interactions between combined oral contraceptives and these antibiotics have reported inconsistent results).
No products indexed under this heading.

Doxycycline Hyclate (Several cases of contraceptive failure and breakthrough bleeding have been reported in the literature concomitant administration of antibiotics, such as tetracyclines; however, clinical pharmacology studies investigating drug interactions between combined oral contraceptives and these antibiotics have reported inconsistent results).
No products indexed under this heading.

Doxycycline Monohydrate (Several cases of contraceptive failure and breakthrough bleeding have been reported in the literature concomitant administration of antibiotics, such as tetracyclines; however, clinical pharmacology studies investigating drug interactions between combined oral contraceptives and these antibiotics have reported inconsistent results). Products include:
Oracea Capsules 1000

Efavirenz (CYP3A4 inhibitors may increase plasma ethinyl estradiol levels). Products include:
Atripla Tablets 945
Sustiva Capsules 930
Sustiva Tablets 930

Erythromycin (CYP3A4 inhibitors may increase plasma ethinyl estradiol levels). Products include:
Ery-Tab Tablets 449
Erythromycin Base Filmtab Tablets .. 455
Erythromycin Delayed-Release Capsules, USP 457
PCE Dispertab Tablets 515

Erythromycin Estolate (CYP3A4 inhibitors may increase plasma ethinyl estradiol levels).
No products indexed under this heading.

Erythromycin Ethylsuccinate (CYP3A4 inhibitors may increase plasma ethinyl estradiol levels). Products include:
E.E.S. ... 451
EryPed ... 447

Erythromycin Gluceptate (CYP3A4 inhibitors may increase plasma ethinyl estradiol levels).
No products indexed under this heading.

Erythromycin Lactobionate (CYP3A4 inhibitors may increase plasma ethinyl estradiol levels).
No products indexed under this heading.

Erythromycin Stearate (CYP3A4 inhibitors may increase plasma ethinyl estradiol levels). Products include:
Erythrocin Stearate Filmtab Tablets .. 453

Esomeprazole Magnesium (CYP3A4 inhibitors may increase plasma ethinyl estradiol levels). Products include:
Nexium Delayed-Release Capsules 655

Felbamate (Contraceptive effectiveness may be reduced when hormonal contraceptives are co-administered with drugs that increase the metabolism of contraceptive steroids, such as felbamate).
No products indexed under this heading.

Fluconazole (CYP3A4 inhibitors may increase plasma ethinyl estradiol levels).
No products indexed under this heading.

Fluoxetine Hydrochloride (CYP3A4 inhibitors may increase plasma ethinyl estradiol levels). Products include:
Prozac Pulvules and Liquid 1801
Symbyax Capsules 1819

Fluvoxamine Maleate (CYP3A4 inhibitors may increase plasma ethinyl estradiol levels).
No products indexed under this heading.

Fosamprenavir Calcium (CYP3A4 inhibitors may increase plasma ethinyl estradiol levels). Products include:
Lexiva Tablets 1505

Fosphenytoin Sodium (Contraceptive effectiveness may be reduced when hormonal contraceptives are co-administered with drugs that increase the metabolism of contraceptive steroids, such as phenytoin).
No products indexed under this heading.

Griseofulvin (Contraceptive effectiveness may be reduced when hormonal contraceptives are co-administered with drugs that increase the metabolism of contraceptive steroids, such as griseofulvin). Products include:
Gris-PEG Tablets 2502

Hypericum (Herbal products containing St. John's Wort (hypericum perforatum) may induce hepatic enzymes (cytochrome p450) and p-glycoprotein transporter and may reduce the effectiveness of contraceptive steroids. This may also result in breakthrough bleeding). Products include:

Satiete Tablets ■□832

Hypericum Perforatum (Herbal products containing St. John's Wort (hypericum perforatum) may induce hepatic enzymes (cytochrome p450) and p-glycoprotein transporter and may reduce the effectiveness of contraceptive steroids. This may also result in breakthrough bleeding).
No products indexed under this heading.

Indinavir Sulfate (Several protease inhibitors have been studied with co-administration of oral combination hormonal contraceptives with significant changes (increase and decrease) in the plasma levels of the estrogen and progestin being noted in some cases). Products include:
Crixivan Capsules 1940

Isoniazid (CYP3A4 inhibitors may increase plasma ethinyl estradiol levels).
No products indexed under this heading.

Itraconazole (CYP3A4 inhibitors may increase plasma ethinyl estradiol levels).
No products indexed under this heading.

Ketoconazole (CYP3A4 inhibitors may increase plasma ethinyl estradiol levels). Products include:
Nizoral A-D Shampoo, 1% 1868

Lopinavir (Several protease inhibitors have been studied with co-administration of oral combination hormonal contraceptives with significant changes (increase and decrease) in the plasma levels of the estrogen and progestin being noted in some cases). Products include:
Kaletra ... 476

Loratadine (CYP3A4 inhibitors may increase plasma ethinyl estradiol levels). Products include:
Alavert Allergy & Sinus D-12 Hour Tablets ■□771
Alavert .. ■□771
Children's Claritin Allergy Oral Solution ■□771
Claritin Non-Drowsy 24 Hour Tablets ■□772
Claritin Reditabs 24 Hour Non-Drowsy Tablets ■□772
Claritin-D Non-Drowsy 12 Hour Tablets ■□772
Claritin-D Non-Drowsy 24 Hour Tablets ■□772

Magnesium Salicylate (Increased clearance of salicylic acid due to induction of conjugation has been noted when co-administered with combination oral contraceptives).
No products indexed under this heading.

Mephobarbital (Contraceptive effectiveness may be reduced when hormonal contraceptives are co-administered with drugs that increase the metabolism of contraceptive steroids, such as barbiturates).
No products indexed under this heading.

Methacycline Hydrochloride (Several cases of contraceptive failure and breakthrough bleeding have been reported in the literature concomitant administration of antibiotics, such as tetracyclines; however, clinical pharmacology studies investigating drug interactions between combined oral contraceptives and these antibiotics have reported inconsistent results).
No products indexed under this heading.

Metronidazole (CYP3A4 inhibitors may increase plasma ethinyl estradiol levels). Products include:
Metrogel 1% 1211
MetroGel-Vaginal Gel 1855
Vandazole Vaginal Gel 3338

Metronidazole Benzoate (CYP3A4 inhibitors may increase plasma ethinyl estradiol levels).
No products indexed under this heading.

Metronidazole Hydrochloride (CYP3A4 inhibitors may increase plasma ethinyl estradiol levels).
No products indexed under this heading.

Miconazole (CYP3A4 inhibitors may increase plasma ethinyl estradiol levels).
No products indexed under this heading.

Miconazole Nitrate (CYP3A4 inhibitors may increase plasma ethinyl estradiol levels). Products include:
Desenex ■□635
Desenex Jock Itch Spray Powder ... ■□635

Minocycline Hydrochloride (Several cases of contraceptive failure and breakthrough bleeding have been reported in the literature concomitant administration of antibiotics, such as tetracyclines; however, clinical pharmacology studies investigating drug interactions between combined oral contraceptives and these antibiotics have reported inconsistent results). Products include:
Solodyn Extended Release Tablets .. 1890

Nefazodone Hydrochloride (CYP3A4 inhibitors may increase plasma ethinyl estradiol levels).
No products indexed under this heading.

Nelfinavir Mesylate (Several protease inhibitors have been studied with co-administration of oral combination hormonal contraceptives with significant changes (increase and decrease) in the plasma levels of the estrogen and progestin being noted in some cases). Products include:
Viracept 2577

Nevirapine (CYP3A4 inhibitors may increase plasma ethinyl estradiol levels). Products include:
Viramune Oral Suspension 873
Viramune Tablets 873

Niacinamide (CYP3A4 inhibitors may increase plasma ethinyl estradiol levels).
No products indexed under this heading.

Nicotinamide (CYP3A4 inhibitors may increase plasma ethinyl estradiol levels). Products include:
Nicomide Tablets 1088

Nifedipine (CYP3A4 inhibitors may increase plasma ethinyl estradiol levels). Products include:
Adalat CC Tablets 2964

Norfloxacin (CYP3A4 inhibitors may increase plasma ethinyl estradiol levels). Products include:
Noroxin Tablets 2032

Omeprazole (CYP3A4 inhibitors may increase plasma ethinyl estradiol levels). Products include:
Zegerid Capsules 2958
Zegerid Powder for Oral Solution 2958

Oxcarbazepine (Contraceptive effectiveness may be reduced when hormonal contraceptives are co-administered with drugs that increase the metabolism of contraceptive steroids, such as oxcarbazepine). Products include:

- Trileptal Tablets 2300
- Trileptal Oral Suspension 2300

Oxytetracycline Hydrochloride (Several cases of contraceptive failure and breakthrough bleeding have been reported in the literature concomitant administration of antibiotics, such as tetracyclines; however, clinical pharmacology studies investigating drug interactions between combined oral contraceptives and these antibiotics have reported inconsistent results).

No products indexed under this heading.

Paroxetine Hydrochloride (CYP3A4 inhibitors may increase plasma ethinyl estradiol levels). Products include:

- Paxil CR Controlled-Release Tablets 1538
- Paxil 1530

Pentobarbital Sodium (Contraceptive effectivness may be reduced when hormonal contraceptives are co-administered with drugs that increase the metabolism of contraceptive steroids, such as barbiturates). Products include:

- Nembutal Sodium Solution, USP 2470

Phenobarbital (Contraceptive effectivness may be reduced when hormonal contraceptives are co-administered with drugs that increase the metabolism of contraceptive steroids, such as barbiturates). Products include:

- Donnatal Extentabs 2493

Phenytoin (Contraceptive effectivness may be reduced when hormonal contraceptives are co-administered with drugs that increase the metabolism of contraceptive steroids, such as phenytoin).

No products indexed under this heading.

Phenytoin Sodium (Contraceptive effectivness may be reduced when hormonal contraceptives are co-administered with drugs that increase the metabolism of contraceptive steroids, such as phenytoin). Products include:

- Phenytek Capsules 2160

Prednisolone (Combination hormonal contraceptives containing some synthetic estrogens (e.g. ethinyl estradiol) may inhibit the metabolism of other compounds. Increased plasma concentrations of prednisolone have been reported with concomitant adminstration of combination oral contraceptives).

No products indexed under this heading.

Prednisolone Acetate (Combination hormonal contraceptives containing some synthetic estrogens (e.g. ethinyl estradiol) may inhibit the metabolism of other compounds. Increased plasma concentrations of prednisolone have been reported with concomitant adminstration of combination oral contraceptives). Products include:

- Blephamide Ophthalmic Ointment 568
- Blephamide Ophthalmic Suspension 569
- Poly-Pred Ophthalmic Suspension .... ⊙233
- Pred Forte Ophthalmic Suspension .... ⊙235
- Pred Mild Ophthalmic Suspension .... ⊙238
- Pred-G Ophthalmic Ointment .... ⊙237
- Pred-G Ophthalmic Suspension ...... ⊙236

Prednisolone Sodium Phosphate (Combination hormonal contraceptives containing some synthetic estrogens (e.g. ethinyl estradiol) may inhibit the metabolism of other compounds. Increased plasma concentrations of prednisolone have been reported with concomitant adminstration of combination oral contraceptives).

No products indexed under this heading.

Prednisolone Tebutate (Combination hormonal contraceptives containing some synthetic estrogens (e.g. ethinyl estradiol) may inhibit the metabolism of other compounds. Increased plasma concentrations of prednisolone have been reported with concomitant adminstration of combination oral contraceptives).

No products indexed under this heading.

Propoxyphene Hydrochloride (CYP3A4 inhibitors may increase plasma ethinyl estradiol levels).

No products indexed under this heading.

Propoxyphene Napsylate (CYP3A4 inhibitors may increase plasma ethinyl estradiol levels).

No products indexed under this heading.

Quinidine (CYP3A4 inhibitors may increase plasma ethinyl estradiol levels).

No products indexed under this heading.

Quinidine Hydrochloride (CYP3A4 inhibitors may increase plasma ethinyl estradiol levels).

No products indexed under this heading.

Quinidine Polygalacturonate (CYP3A4 inhibitors may increase plasma ethinyl estradiol levels).

No products indexed under this heading.

Quinidine Sulfate (CYP3A4 inhibitors may increase plasma ethinyl estradiol levels).

No products indexed under this heading.

Quinine (CYP3A4 inhibitors may increase plasma ethinyl estradiol levels).

No products indexed under this heading.

Quinine Sulfate (CYP3A4 inhibitors may increase plasma ethinyl estradiol levels).

No products indexed under this heading.

Quinupristin (CYP3A4 inhibitors may increase plasma ethinyl estradiol levels).

No products indexed under this heading.

Ranitidine Bismuth Citrate (CYP3A4 inhibitors may increase plasma ethinyl estradiol levels).

No products indexed under this heading.

Ranitidine Hydrochloride (CYP3A4 inhibitors may increase plasma ethinyl estradiol levels). Products include:

- Zantac 1624
- Zantac Injection 1619
- Zantac Injection Pharmacy Bulk Package 1622

Rifampin (Contraceptive effectiveness may be reduced when hormonal contraceptives are co-administered with drugs that increase the metabolism of contraceptive steroids, such as rifampin).

No products indexed under this heading.

Ritonavir (Several protease inhibitors have been studied with co-administration of oral combination hormonal contraceptives with significant changes (increase and decrease) in the plasma levels of the estrogen and progestin being noted in some cases). Products include:

- Kaletra 476
- Norvir 503

Salsalate (Increased clearance of salicylic acid due to induction of conjugation has been noted when co-administered with combination oral contraceptives).

No products indexed under this heading.

Saquinavir (Several protease inhibitors have been studied with co-administration of oral combination hormonal contraceptives with significant changes (increase and decrease) in the plasma levels of the estrogen and progestin being noted in some cases).

No products indexed under this heading.

Saquinavir Mesylate (Several protease inhibitors have been studied with co-administration of oral combination hormonal contraceptives with significant changes (increase and decrease) in the plasma levels of the estrogen and progestin being noted in some cases). Products include:

- Invirase 2772

Secobarbital Sodium (Contraceptive effectivness may be reduced when hormonal contraceptives are co-administered with drugs that increase the metabolism of contraceptive steroids, such as barbiturates).

No products indexed under this heading.

Sertraline Hydrochloride (CYP3A4 inhibitors may increase plasma ethinyl estradiol levels). Products include:

- Zoloft 2586

Telithromycin (CYP3A4 inhibitors may increase plasma ethinyl estradiol levels). Products include:

- Ketek Tablets 2903

Temazepam (Increased clearance of temazepam due to induction of conjugation has been noted when co-administered with combination oral contraceptives). Products include:

- Restoril Capsules 1860

Tetracycline Hydrochloride (Several cases of contraceptive failure and breakthrough bleeding have been reported in the literature concomitant administration of antibiotics, such as tetracyclines; however, clinical pharmacology studies investigating drug interactions between combined oral contraceptives and these antibiotics have reported inconsistent results).

No products indexed under this heading.

Theophylline (Combination hormonal contraceptives containing some synthetic estrogens (e.g. ethinyl estradiol) may inhibit the metabolism of other compounds. Increased plasma concentrations of theophylline have been reported with concomitant administration of combination oral contraceptives).

No products indexed under this heading.

Theophylline Anhydrous (Combination hormonal contraceptives containing some synthetic estrogens (e.g. ethinyl estradiol) may inhibit the metabolism of other compounds. Increased plasma concentrations of theophylline have been reported with concomitant administration of combination oral contraceptives). Products include:

- Uniphyl Tablets 2710

Theophylline Calcium Salicylate (Combination hormonal contraceptives containing some synthetic estrogens (e.g. ethinyl estradiol) may inhibit the metabolism of other compounds. Increased plasma concentrations of theophylline have been reported with concomitant administration of combination oral contraceptives).

No products indexed under this heading.

Theophylline Dihydroxypropyl (Glyceryl) (Combination hormonal contraceptives containing some synthetic estrogens (e.g. ethinyl estradiol) may inhibit the metabolism of other compounds. Increased plasma concentrations of theophylline have been reported with concomitant administration of combination oral contraceptives).

No products indexed under this heading.

Theophylline Ethylenediamine (Combination hormonal contraceptives containing some synthetic estrogens (e.g. ethinyl estradiol) may inhibit the metabolism of other compounds. Increased plasma concentrations of theophylline have been reported with concomitant administration of combination oral contraceptives).

No products indexed under this heading.

Theophylline Sodium Glycinate (Combination hormonal contraceptives containing some synthetic estrogens (e.g. ethinyl estradiol) may inhibit the metabolism of other compounds. Increased plasma concentrations of theophylline have been reported with concomitant administration of combination oral contraceptives).

No products indexed under this heading.

Thiamylal Sodium (Contraceptive effectivness may be reduced when hormonal contraceptives are co-administered with drugs that increase the metabolism of contraceptive steroids, such as barbiturates).

No products indexed under this heading.

Topiramate (Contraceptive effectiveness may be reduced when hormonal contraceptives are co-administered with drugs that increase the metabolism of contraceptive steroids, such as topiramate). Products include:

- Topamax Sprinkle Capsules 2404

Topamax Tablets 2404

Troglitazone (CYP3A4 inhibitors may increase plasma ethinyl estradiol levels).
No products indexed under this heading.

Troleandomycin (CYP3A4 inhibitors may increase plasma ethinyl estradiol levels).
No products indexed under this heading.

Valproate Sodium (CYP3A4 inhibitors may increase plasma ethinyl estradiol levels). Products include:
Depacon Injection 412

Verapamil Hydrochloride (CYP3A4 inhibitors may increase plasma ethinyl estradiol levels). Products include:
Covera-HS Tablets 3139
Tarka Tablets 524
Verelan PM Extended-Release Capsules, Controlled-Onset 3106

Vitamin C (Ascorbic acid may increase plasma ethinyl estradiol levels, possibly by inhibition of conjugation). Products include:
Bausch & Lomb Ocuvite Adult Eye Vitamin and Mineral Supplement Soft Gels .... ▣706
Bausch & Lomb Ocuvite Adult 50+ Eye Vitamin and Mineral Supplement Soft Gels .... ▣706
Ocuvite Adult Vitamin and Mineral Supplement .... ⊙253
Ocuvite Adult 50+ Vitamin and Mineral Supplement .... ⊙253
Peridin-C Vitamin C Supplement .... ▣818

Voriconazole (CYP3A4 inhibitors may increase plasma ethinyl estradiol levels). Products include:
VFEND I.V. 2564
VFEND Oral Suspension 2564
VFEND Tablets 2564

Zafirlukast (CYP3A4 inhibitors may increase plasma ethinyl estradiol levels). Products include:
Accolate Tablets 671

Zileuton (CYP3A4 inhibitors may increase plasma ethinyl estradiol levels). Products include:
Zyflo Tablets 1023

Food Interactions

Grapefruit (CYP3A4 inhibitors may increase plasma ethinyl estradiol levels).

Grapefruit Juice (CYP3A4 inhibitors may increase plasma ethinyl estradiol levels).

SEN-SEI-RO LIQUID GOLD

(Dietary Supplement) 1740
None cited in PDR database.

SEN-SEI-RO POWDER GOLD

(Dietary Supplement) 1741
None cited in PDR database.

SENSIPAR TABLETS

(Cinacalcet Hydrochloride) 608
May interact with cytochrome p450 2d6 substrates (selected), cytochrome p450 3a inhibitors (selected), and certain other agents. Compounds in these categories include:

Amiodarone Hydrochloride (Since cinacalcet hydrochloride is metabolized in part by CYP3A4, dose adjustment of cinacalcet hydrochloride may be required and PTH and serum calcium concentrations closely monitored if a patient initiates or discontinues therapy with a strong CYP3A4 inhibitor).
No products indexed under this heading.

Amitriptyline Hydrochloride (Administration of 25mg or 100mg cinacalcet with 50mg amitriptyline increased amitriptyline exposure and nortriptyline (active metabolite) exposure by approximately 20% in CYP2D6 extensive metabolizers. Cinacalcet hydrochloride is a strong in vitro inhibitor of CYP2D6. Therefore, dose adjustments of concomitant medications that are predominantly metabolized by CYP2D6 and have a narrow therapeutic index may be required).
No products indexed under this heading.

Amphetamine Aspartate (Cinacalcet hydrochloride is a strong in vitro inhibitor of CYP2D6. Therefore, dose adjustments of concomitant medications that are predominantly metabolized by CYP2D6 and have a narrow therapeutic index may be required). Products include:
Adderall Tablets 3164
Adderall XR Capsules 3166

Amphetamine Aspartate Monohydrate (Cinacalcet hydrochloride is a strong in vitro inhibitor of CYP2D6. Therefore, dose adjustments of concomitant medications that are predominantly metabolized by CYP2D6 and have a narrow therapeutic index may be required).
No products indexed under this heading.

Amphetamine Sulfate (Cinacalcet hydrochloride is a strong in vitro inhibitor of CYP2D6. Therefore, dose adjustments of concomitant medications that are predominantly metabolized by CYP2D6 and have a narrow therapeutic index may be required). Products include:
Adderall Tablets 3164
Adderall XR Capsules 3166

Amprenavir (Since cinacalcet hydrochloride is metabolized in part by CYP3A4, dose adjustment of cinacalcet hydrochloride may be required and PTH and serum calcium concentrations closely monitored if a patient initiates or discontinues therapy with a strong CYP3A4 inhibitor). Products include:
Agenerase Capsules 1327
Agenerase Oral Solution 1332

Aprepitant (Since cinacalcet hydrochloride is metabolized in part by CYP3A4, dose adjustment of cinacalcet hydrochloride may be required and PTH and serum calcium concentrations closely monitored if a patient initiates or discontinues therapy with a strong CYP3A4 inhibitor). Products include:
Emend Capsules 1963

Atomoxetine Hydrochloride (Cinacalcet hydrochloride is a strong in vitro inhibitor of CYP2D6. Therefore, dose adjustments of concomitant medications that are predominantly metabolized by CYP2D6 and have a narrow therapeutic index may be required). Products include:
Strattera Capsules 1814

Bisoprolol Fumarate (Cinacalcet hydrochloride is a strong in vitro inhibitor of CYP2D6. Therefore, dose adjustments of concomitant medications that are predominantly metabolized by CYP2D6 and have a narrow therapeutic index may be required).
No products indexed under this heading.

Captopril (Cinacalcet hydrochloride is a strong in vitro inhibitor of CYP2D6. Therefore, dose adjustments of concomitant medications that are predominantly metabolized by CYP2D6 and have a narrow therapeutic index may be required). Products include:
Captopril Tablets 2149

Carvedilol (Cinacalcet hydrochloride is a strong in vitro inhibitor of CYP2D6. Therefore, dose adjustments of concomitant medications that are predominantly metabolized by CYP2D6 and have a narrow therapeutic index may be required). Products include:
Coreg Tablets 1414

Cevimeline Hydrochloride (Cinacalcet hydrochloride is a strong in vitro inhibitor of CYP2D6. Therefore, dose adjustments of concomitant medications that are predominantly metabolized by CYP2D6 and have a narrow therapeutic index may be required). Products include:
Evoxac Capsules 1047

Chlorpromazine (Cinacalcet hydrochloride is a strong in vitro inhibitor of CYP2D6. Therefore, dose adjustments of concomitant medications that are predominantly metabolized by CYP2D6 and have a narrow therapeutic index may be required).
No products indexed under this heading.

Chlorpromazine Hydrochloride (Cinacalcet hydrochloride is a strong in vitro inhibitor of CYP2D6. Therefore, dose adjustments of concomitant medications that are predominantly metabolized by CYP2D6 and have a narrow therapeutic index may be required).
No products indexed under this heading.

Chlorpropamide (Cinacalcet hydrochloride is a strong in vitro inhibitor of CYP2D6. Therefore, dose adjustments of concomitant medications that are predominantly metabolized by CYP2D6 and have a narrow therapeutic index may be required).
No products indexed under this heading.

Cimetidine (Since cinacalcet hydrochloride is metabolized in part by CYP3A4, dose adjustment of cinacalcet hydrochloride may be required and PTH and serum calcium concentrations closely monitored if a patient initiates or discontinues therapy with a strong CYP3A4 inhibitor). Products include:
Tagamet HB 200 Tablets .... ▣664

Cimetidine Hydrochloride (Since cinacalcet hydrochloride is metabolized in part by CYP3A4, dose adjustment of cinacalcet hydrochloride may be required and PTH and serum calcium concentrations closely monitored if a patient initiates or discontinues therapy with a strong CYP3A4 inhibitor).
No products indexed under this heading.

Ciprofloxacin (Since cinacalcet hydrochloride is metabolized in part by CYP3A4, dose adjustment of cinacalcet hydrochloride may be required and PTH and serum calcium concentrations closely monitored if a patient initiates or discontinues therapy with a strong CYP3A4 inhibitor). Products include:
Cipro Oral Suspension 2977
Cipro I.V. 2984
Cipro XR Tablets 2990
Ciprodex Otic Suspension 559

Ciprofloxacin Hydrochloride (Since cinacalcet hydrochloride is metabolized in part by CYP3A4, dose adjustment of cinacalcet hydrochloride may be required and PTH and serum calcium concentrations closely monitored if a patient initiates or discontinues therapy with a strong CYP3A4 inhibitor). Products include:
Ciloxan Ophthalmic Ointment 559
Ciloxan Ophthalmic Solution .... ⊙206
Cipro Tablets 2977
Proquin XR Tablets 1153

Clarithromycin (Since cinacalcet hydrochloride is metabolized in part by CYP3A4, dose adjustment of cinacalcet hydrochloride may be required and PTH and serum calcium concentrations closely monitored if a patient initiates or discontinues therapy with a strong CYP3A4 inhibitor). Products include:
Biaxin/Biaxin XL 402
PREVPAC 3284

Clomipramine Hydrochloride (Cinacalcet hydrochloride is a strong in vitro inhibitor of CYP2D6. Therefore, dose adjustments of concomitant medications that are predominantly metabolized by CYP2D6 and have a narrow therapeutic index may be required).
No products indexed under this heading.

Clozapine (Cinacalcet hydrochloride is a strong in vitro inhibitor of CYP2D6. Therefore, dose adjustments of concomitant medications that are predominantly metabolized by CYP2D6 and have a narrow therapeutic index may be required). Products include:
Clozaril Tablets 2184
FazaClo Orally Disintegrating Tablets 551

Codeine Phosphate (Cinacalcet hydrochloride is a strong in vitro inhibitor of CYP2D6. Therefore, dose adjustments of concomitant medications that are predominantly metabolized by CYP2D6 and have a narrow therapeutic index may be required). Products include:
Tylenol with Codeine Tablets 2391

Codeine Sulfate (Cinacalcet hydrochloride is a strong in vitro inhibitor of CYP2D6. Therefore, dose adjustments of concomitant medications that are predominantly metabolized by CYP2D6 and have a narrow therapeutic index may be required).
No products indexed under this heading.

Cyclobenzaprine Hydrochloride (Cinacalcet hydrochloride is a strong in vitro inhibitor of CYP2D6. Therefore, dose adjustments of concomitant medications that are predominantly metabolized by CYP2D6 and have a narrow therapeutic index may be required).
No products indexed under this heading.

Cyclosporine (Since cinacalcet hydrochloride is metabolized in part by CYP3A4, dose adjustment of cinacalcet hydrochloride may be required and PTH and serum calcium concentrations closely monitored if a patient initiates or discontinues therapy with a strong CYP3A4 inhibitor). Products include:
Gengraf Capsules 459
Neoral Oral Solution 2259
Neoral Soft Gelatin Capsules 2259
Restasis Ophthalmic Emulsion 575
Sandimmune 2275

Delavirdine Mesylate (Since cinacalcet hydrochloride is metabolized in part by CYP3A4, dose adjustment of cinacalcet hydrochloride may be required and PTH and serum calcium concentrations closely monitored if a patient initiates or discontinues therapy with a strong CYP3A4 inhibitor). Products include:
- Rescriptor Tablets ... 2551

Desipramine Hydrochloride (Cinacalcet hydrochloride is a strong in vitro inhibitor of CYP2D6. Therefore, dose adjustments of concomitant medications that are predominantly metabolized by CYP2D6 and have a narrow therapeutic index may be required).
- No products indexed under this heading.

Dexfenfluramine Hydrochloride (Cinacalcet hydrochloride is a strong in vitro inhibitor of CYP2D6. Therefore, dose adjustments of concomitant medications that are predominantly metabolized by CYP2D6 and have a narrow therapeutic index may be required).
- No products indexed under this heading.

Dextromethorphan Hydrobromide (Cinacalcet hydrochloride is a strong in vitro inhibitor of CYP2D6. Therefore, dose adjustments of concomitant medications that are predominantly metabolized by CYP2D6 and have a narrow therapeutic index may be required). Products include:
- Comtrex Maximum Strength Cold & Cough Day/Night Caplets - Day Formulation ... ■726
- Comtrex Maximum Strength Cold & Cough Day/Night Caplets - Night Formulation ... ■726
- Comtrex Maximum Strength Non-Drowsy Cold & Cough Caplets ... ■725
- Children's Dimetapp DM Cold & Cough Elixir ... ■731
- Children's Dimetapp Long Acting Cough Plus Cold Syrup ... ■731
- Toddler's Dimetapp Cold and Cough Drops ... ■732
- Mucinex DM Extended-Release Bi-Layer Tablets ... ■720
- Refenesen DM Caplets ... ■721
- Robitussin Cough & Cold CF Liquid ... ■735
- Robitussin Cough & Cold Long-Acting Liquid ... ■735
- Robitussin Cough & Allergy Syrup .. ■736
- Robitussin Cough & Cold Nighttime Liquid ... ■736
- Robitussin Cough & Cold Pediatric Drops ... ■735
- Robitussin Cough, Cold & Flu Nighttime Liquid ... ■738
- Robitussin Cough & Congestion Liquid ... ■738
- Robitussin Cough Gels Long-Acting ... ■737
- Robitussin Cough Long Acting Liquid ... ■739
- Robitussin Cough DM Syrup ... ■738
- Robitussin Cough DM Infant Drops ... ■738
- Robitussin Pediatric Cough Long Acting Liquid ... ■739
- Robitussin Pediatric Cough & Cold Long-Acting Liquid ... ■735
- Robitussin Pediatric Cough & Cold Nighttime Liquid ... ■736
- Robitussin Sugar Free Cough ... ■738
- TheraFlu Cold & Cough Hot Liquid ... ■740
- TheraFlu Warming Relief Daytime Severe Cold ... ■743
- TheraFlu Thin Strips Long Acting Cough ... ■744
- Triaminic Daytime Cold & Cough Liquid ... ■745
- Triaminic Cough & Sore Throat Liquid ... ■747
- Triaminic Cough & Runny Nose Softchews ... ■748
- Triaminic Thin Strips Cold & Cough ... ■778
- Triaminic Infant Thin Strips Decongestant Plus Cough ... ■747
- Children's Tylenol Plus Flu Oral Suspension ... ■749
- Tylenol Cold Head Congestion Daytime Caplets with Cool Burst and Gelcaps ... ■750
- Tylenol Cold Multi-Symptom Daytime Liquid ... ■752
- Tylenol Cold Multi-Symptom Severe Daytime Liquid ... ■752
- Concentrated Tylenol Infants' Drops Plus Cold & Cough ... ■754
- Children's Tylenol Plus Cough & Runny Nose Suspension Liquid ... 1879
- Children's Tylenol Plus Cough & Sore Throat Suspension Liquid ... 1879
- Children's Tylenol Plus Flu Suspension Liquid ... 1881
- Children's Tylenol Plus Multi-Symptom Cold Suspension Liquid ... 1879
- Tylenol Cold Severe Congestion Non-Drowsy Caplets with Cool Burst ... 1874
- Tylenol Cold Head Congestion Daytime Caplets with Cool Burst ... 1873
- Tylenol Cold Head Congestion Nighttime Caplets with Cool Burst ... 1873
- Tylenol Cold Head Congestion Severe Caplets with Cool Burst ... 1873
- Tylenol Cold Multi-Symptom Daytime Caplets with Cool Burst and Gelcaps ... 1874
- Tylenol Cold Multi-Symptom Daytime Liquid with Citrus Burst ... 1874
- Tylenol Cold Multi-Symptom Nighttime Caplets with Cool Burst ... 1874
- Tylenol Cold Multi-Symptom Nighttime Liquid with Cool Burst ... 1874
- Tylenol Cold Multi-Symptom Severe Caplets with Cool Burst ... 1874
- Tylenol Cold Multi-Symptom Severe Daytime Liquid with Citrus Burst ... 1874
- Tylenol Cough & Sore Throat Daytime Liquid with Cool Burst ... 1877
- Tylenol Cough & Sore Throat Nighttime Liquid with Cool Burst ... 1877
- Concentrated Tylenol Infants' Drops Plus Cold and Cough ... 1879
- Vicks 44 Cough Relief Liquid ... 2679
- Vicks 44D Cough & Head Congestion Relief Liquid ... 2679
- Vicks 44E Cough & Chest Congestion Relief Liquid ... 2679
- Pediatric Vicks 44e Cough & Chest Congestion Relief Liquid ... 2676
- Vicks 44M Cough, Cold & Flu Relief Liquid ... 2680
- Pediatric Vicks 44m Cough & Cold Relief Liquid ... 2676
- Vicks DayQuil LiquiCaps/Liquid Multi-Symptom Cold/Flu Relief ... ■761
- Vicks DayQuil Multi-Symptom Cold/Flu Relief LiquiCaps ... 2678
- Vicks DayQuil Multi-Symptom Cold/Flu Relief Liquid ... 2678
- Vicks NyQuil Multi-Symptom Cold/Flu Relief Liquid ... 2681
- Children's Vicks NyQuil Cold/Cough Relief ... ■756
- Vicks NyQuil Multi-Symptom Cold/Flu Relief LiquiCaps ... 2681
- Vicks NyQuil LiquiCaps/Liquid Multi-Symptom Cold/Flu Relief ... ■763
- Vicks NyQuil Cough Liquid ... 2680
- Children's Vicks NyQuil Cold/Cough Relief Liquid ... 2680
- Zicam Cough Max Nighttime Cough Spray ... ■767
- Zicam Cough Max Cough Spray ... ■767
- Zicam Cough Max Cough Melts ... ■767
- Zicam Cough Plus D Cough Spray ... ■767
- Zicam Cough Relief Cough Spray ... ■767
- Zicam Maximum Strength Flu Daytime ... ■768
- Zicam Maximum Strength Flu Nighttime ... ■768

Dextromethorphan Polistirex (Cinacalcet hydrochloride is a strong in vitro inhibitor of CYP2D6. Therefore, dose adjustments of concomitant medications that are predominantly metabolized by CYP2D6 and have a narrow therapeutic index may be required). Products include:
- Delsym Extended-Release Suspension 12 Hour Cough Suppressant ... ■611

Diltiazem Hydrochloride (Since cinacalcet hydrochloride is metabolized in part by CYP3A4, dose adjustment of cinacalcet hydrochloride may be required and PTH and serum calcium concentrations closely monitored if a patient initiates or discontinues therapy with a strong CYP3A4 inhibitor). Products include:
- Cardizem LA Extended Release Tablets ... 1728
- Tiazac Capsules ... 1201

Diltiazem Maleate (Since cinacalcet hydrochloride is metabolized in part by CYP3A4, dose adjustment of cinacalcet hydrochloride may be required and PTH and serum calcium concentrations closely monitored if a patient initiates or discontinues therapy with a strong CYP3A4 inhibitor).
- No products indexed under this heading.

Dolasetron Mesylate (Cinacalcet hydrochloride is a strong in vitro inhibitor of CYP2D6. Therefore, dose adjustments of concomitant medications that are predominantly metabolized by CYP2D6 and have a narrow therapeutic index may be required). Products include:
- Anzemet Injection ... 2859
- Anzemet Tablets ... 2862

Donepezil Hydrochloride (Cinacalcet hydrochloride is a strong in vitro inhibitor of CYP2D6. Therefore, dose adjustments of concomitant medications that are predominantly metabolized by CYP2D6 and have a narrow therapeutic index may be required). Products include:
- Aricept Tablets ... 1094
- Aricept ODT Tablets ... 1094

Doxepin Hydrochloride (Cinacalcet hydrochloride is a strong in vitro inhibitor of CYP2D6. Therefore, dose adjustments of concomitant medications that are predominantly metabolized by CYP2D6 and have a narrow therapeutic index may be required).
- No products indexed under this heading.

Efavirenz (Since cinacalcet hydrochloride is metabolized in part by CYP3A4, dose adjustment of cinacalcet hydrochloride may be required and PTH and serum calcium concentrations closely monitored if a patient initiates or discontinues therapy with a strong CYP3A4 inhibitor). Products include:
- Atripla Tablets ... 945
- Sustiva Capsules ... 930
- Sustiva Tablets ... 930

Encainide Hydrochloride (Cinacalcet hydrochloride is a strong in vitro inhibitor of CYP2D6. Therefore, dose adjustments of concomitant medications that are predominantly metabolized by CYP2D6 and have a narrow therapeutic index may be required).
- No products indexed under this heading.

Erythromycin (Since cinacalcet hydrochloride is metabolized in part by CYP3A4, dose adjustment of cinacalcet hydrochloride may be required and PTH and serum calcium concentrations closely monitored if a patient initiates or discontinues therapy with a strong CYP3A4 inhibitor). Products include:
- Ery-Tab Tablets ... 449
- Erythromycin Base Filmtab Tablets ... 455
- Erythromycin Delayed-Release Capsules, USP ... 457
- PCE Dispertab Tablets ... 515

Fentanyl (Cinacalcet hydrochloride is a strong in vitro inhibitor of CYP2D6. Therefore, dose adjustments of concomitant medications that are predominantly metabolized by CYP2D6 and have a narrow therapeutic index may be required). Products include:
- Duragesic Transdermal System ... 2373
- Ionsys Transdermal System ... 2379

Fentanyl Citrate (Cinacalcet hydrochloride is a strong in vitro inhibitor of CYP2D6. Therefore, dose adjustments of concomitant medications that are predominantly metabolized by CYP2D6 and have a narrow therapeutic index may be required). Products include:
- Actiq ... 979

Flecainide Acetate (Cinacalcet hydrochloride is a strong in vitro inhibitor of CYP2D6. Therefore, dose adjustments of concomitant medications that are predominantly metabolized by CYP2D6 and have a narrow therapeutic index may be required). Products include:
- Tambocor Tablets ... 1856

Fluconazole (Since cinacalcet hydrochloride is metabolized in part by CYP3A4, dose adjustment of cinacalcet hydrochloride may be required and PTH and serum calcium concentrations closely monitored if a patient initiates or discontinues therapy with a strong CYP3A4 inhibitor).
- No products indexed under this heading.

Fluoxetine (Cinacalcet hydrochloride is a strong in vitro inhibitor of CYP2D6. Therefore, dose adjustments of concomitant medications that are predominantly metabolized by CYP2D6 and have a narrow therapeutic index may be required).
- No products indexed under this heading.

Fluoxetine Hydrochloride (Cinacalcet hydrochloride is a strong in vitro inhibitor of CYP2D6. Therefore, dose adjustments of concomitant medications that are predominantly metabolized by CYP2D6 and have a narrow therapeutic index may be required). Products include:
- Prozac Pulvules and Liquid ... 1801
- Symbyax Capsules ... 1819

Fluphenazine Decanoate (Cinacalcet hydrochloride is a strong in vitro inhibitor of CYP2D6. Therefore, dose adjustments of concomitant medications that are predominantly metabolized by CYP2D6 and have a narrow therapeutic index may be required).
- No products indexed under this heading.

Fluphenazine Enanthate (Cinacalcet hydrochloride is a strong in vitro inhibitor of CYP2D6. Therefore, dose adjustments of concomitant medications that are predominantly metabolized by CYP2D6 and have a narrow therapeutic index may be required).
- No products indexed under this heading.

Fluphenazine Hydrochloride
(Cinacalcet hydrochloride is a strong
in vitro inhibitor of CYP2D6. Therefore, dose adjustments of concomitant medications that are predominantly metabolized by CYP2D6 and
have a narrow therapeutic index may
be required).
 No products indexed under this
 heading.

Fluvoxamine Maleate (Cinacalcet
hydrochloride is a strong in vitro
inhibitor of CYP2D6. Therefore, dose
adjustments of concomitant medications that are predominantly metabolized by CYP2D6 and have a narrow
therapeutic index may be required).
 No products indexed under this
 heading.

Formoterol Fumarate (Cinacalcet
hydrochloride is a strong in vitro
inhibitor of CYP2D6. Therefore, dose
adjustments of concomitant medications that are predominantly metabolized by CYP2D6 and have a narrow
therapeutic index may be required).
Products include:
 Foradil Aerolizer 3010

Galantamine Hydrobromide
(Cinacalcet hydrochloride is a strong
in vitro inhibitor of CYP2D6. Therefore, dose adjustments of concomitant medications that are predominantly metabolized by CYP2D6 and
have a narrow therapeutic index may
be required). Products include:
 Razadyne .. 2399
 Razadyne ER Extended-Release
 Capsules ... 2399

Haloperidol (Cinacalcet hydrochloride is a strong in vitro inhibitor of
CYP2D6. Therefore, dose adjustments of concomitant medications
that are predominantly metabolized
by CYP2D6 and have a narrow therapeutic index may be required).
 No products indexed under this
 heading.

Haloperidol Decanoate (Cinacalcet hydrochloride is a strong in vitro
inhibitor of CYP2D6. Therefore, dose
adjustments of concomitant medications that are predominantly metabolized by CYP2D6 and have a narrow
therapeutic index may be required).
 No products indexed under this
 heading.

Hydrocodone Bitartrate (Cinacal-
cet hydrochloride is a strong in vitro
inhibitor of CYP2D6. Therefore, dose
adjustments of concomitant medica-
tions that are predominantly metabo-
lized by CYP2D6 and have a narrow
therapeutic index may be required).
Products include:
 Hycodan .. 1116
 Hycotuss Expectorant Syrup 1117
 Vicodin Tablets 535
 Vicodin ES Tablets 536
 Vicodin HP Tablets 538
 Vicoprofen Tablets 539
 Zydone Tablets 1139

Imipramine Hydrochloride (Cinacalcet hydrochloride is a strong in
vitro inhibitor of CYP2D6. Therefore,
dose adjustments of concomitant
medications that are predominantly
metabolized by CYP2D6 and have a
narrow therapeutic index may be
required).
 No products indexed under this
 heading.

Imipramine Pamoate (Cinacalcet
hydrochloride is a strong in vitro
inhibitor of CYP2D6. Therefore, dose
adjustments of concomitant medications that are predominantly metabolized by CYP2D6 and have a narrow
therapeutic index may be required).
 No products indexed under this
 heading.

Indinavir Sulfate (Since cinacalcet
hydrochloride is metabolized in part
by CYP3A4, dose adjustment of
cinacalcet hydrochloride may be
required and PTH and serum calcium
concentrations closely monitored if a
patient initiates or discontinues therapy with a strong CYP3A4 inhibitor).
Products include:
 Crixivan Capsules 1940

Indoramin Hydrochloride (Cinacalcet hydrochloride is a strong in
vitro inhibitor of CYP2D6. Therefore,
dose adjustments of concomitant
medications that are predominantly
metabolized by CYP2D6 and have a
narrow therapeutic index may be
required).
 No products indexed under this
 heading.

Isoniazid (Since cinacalcet hydrochloride is metabolized in part by
CYP3A4, dose adjustment of cinacalcet hydrochloride may be required
and PTH and serum calcium concentrations closely monitored if a
patient initiates or discontinues therapy with a strong CYP3A4 inhibitor).
 No products indexed under this
 heading.

Itraconazole (Since cinacalcet
hydrochloride is metabolized in part
by CYP3A4, dose adjustment of
cinacalcet hydrochloride may be
required and PTH and serum calcium
concentrations closely monitored if a
patient initiates or discontinues therapy with a strong CYP3A4 inhibitor).
 No products indexed under this
 heading.

Ketoconazole (Co-administration of
ketoconazole, a strong inhibitor of
CYP3A4, increased cinacalcet exposure following a single 90 mg dose
of cinacalcet hydrochloride by 2.3
fold. Since cinacalcet hydrochloride
is metabolized in part by CYP3A4,
dose adjustment of cinacalcet hydrochloride may be required and PTH
and serum calcium concentrations
closely monitored if a patient initiates or discontinues therapy with a
strong CYP3A4 inhibitor). Products
include:
 Nizoral A-D Shampoo, 1% 1868

Labetalol Hydrochloride (Cinacalcet hydrochloride is a strong in vitro
inhibitor of CYP2D6. Therefore, dose
adjustments of concomitant medications that are predominantly metabolized by CYP2D6 and have a narrow
therapeutic index may be required).
 No products indexed under this
 heading.

Lidocaine (Cinacalcet hydrochloride
is a strong in vitro inhibitor of
CYP2D6. Therefore, dose adjustments of concomitant medications
that are predominantly metabolized
by CYP2D6 and have a narrow therapeutic index may be required).
Products include:
 Lidoderm Patch 1118
 Synera Topical Patch 1137

Lidocaine Hydrochloride (Cinacalcet hydrochloride is a strong in vitro
inhibitor of CYP2D6. Therefore, dose
adjustments of concomitant medications that are predominantly metabolized by CYP2D6 and have a narrow
therapeutic index may be required).
 No products indexed under this
 heading.

Lopinavir (Since cinacalcet hydrochloride is metabolized in part by
CYP3A4, dose adjustment of cinacalcet hydrochloride may be required
and PTH and serum calcium concentrations closely monitored if a
patient initiates or discontinues therapy with a strong CYP3A4 inhibitor).
Products include:
 Kaletra ... 476

Maprotiline Hydrochloride (Cinacalcet hydrochloride is a strong in
vitro inhibitor of CYP2D6. Therefore,
dose adjustments of concomitant
medications that are predominantly
metabolized by CYP2D6 and have a
narrow therapeutic index may be
required).
 No products indexed under this
 heading.

Meperidine Hydrochloride (Cinacalcet hydrochloride is a strong in
vitro inhibitor of CYP2D6. Therefore,
dose adjustments of concomitant
medications that are predominantly
metabolized by CYP2D6 and have a
narrow therapeutic index may be
required).
 No products indexed under this
 heading.

Methadone Hydrochloride (Cinacalcet hydrochloride is a strong in
vitro inhibitor of CYP2D6. Therefore,
dose adjustments of concomitant
medications that are predominantly
metabolized by CYP2D6 and have a
narrow therapeutic index may be
required).
 No products indexed under this
 heading.

**Methamphetamine Hydrochlo-
ride** (Cinacalcet hydrochloride is a
strong in vitro inhibitor of CYP2D6.
Therefore, dose adjustments of concomitant medications that are predominantly metabolized by CYP2D6
and have a narrow therapeutic index
may be required). Products include:
 Desoxyn Tablets, USP 2462

Metoprolol Succinate (Cinacalcet
hydrochloride is a strong in vitro
inhibitor of CYP2D6. Therefore, dose
adjustments of concomitant medications that are predominantly metabolized by CYP2D6 and have a narrow
therapeutic index may be required).
Products include:
 Toprol-XL Tablets 668

Metoprolol Tartrate (Cinacalcet
hydrochloride is a strong in vitro
inhibitor of CYP2D6. Therefore, dose
adjustments of concomitant medications that are predominantly metabolized by CYP2D6 and have a narrow
therapeutic index may be required).
Products include:
 Lopressor Injection 2238
 Lopressor Tablets 2238
 Lopressor HCT 50/25 Tablets 2241
 Lopressor HCT 100/25 Tablets 2241
 Lopressor HCT 100/50 Tablets 2241

Metronidazole (Since cinacalcet
hydrochloride is metabolized in part
by CYP3A4, dose adjustment of
cinacalcet hydrochloride may be
required and PTH and serum calcium
concentrations closely monitored if a

patient initiates or discontinues ther-
apy with a strong CYP3A4 inhibitor).
Products include:
 Metrogel 1% 1211
 MetroGel-Vaginal Gel 1855
 Vandazole Vaginal Gel 3338

Metronidazole Benzoate (Since
cinacalcet hydrochloride is metabolized in part by CYP3A4, dose adjustment of cinacalcet hydrochloride
may be required and PTH and serum
calcium concentrations closely monitored if a patient initiates or discontinues therapy with a strong CYP3A4
inhibitor).
 No products indexed under this
 heading.

Metronidazole Hydrochloride
(Since cinacalcet hydrochloride is
metabolized in part by CYP3A4,
dose adjustment of cinacalcet hydrochloride may be required and PTH
and serum calcium concentrations
closely monitored if a patient initiates or discontinues therapy with a
strong CYP3A4 inhibitor).
 No products indexed under this
 heading.

Mexiletine Hydrochloride (Cinacalcet hydrochloride is a strong in
vitro inhibitor of CYP2D6. Therefore,
dose adjustments of concomitant
medications that are predominantly
metabolized by CYP2D6 and have a
narrow therapeutic index may be
required).
 No products indexed under this
 heading.

Miconazole (Since cinacalcet
hydrochloride is metabolized in part
by CYP3A4, dose adjustment of
cinacalcet hydrochloride may be
required and PTH and serum calcium
concentrations closely monitored if a
patient initiates or discontinues therapy with a strong CYP3A4 inhibitor).
 No products indexed under this
 heading.

Mirtazapine (Cinacalcet hydrochloride is a strong in vitro inhibitor of
CYP2D6. Therefore, dose adjustments of concomitant medications
that are predominantly metabolized
by CYP2D6 and have a narrow therapeutic index may be required).
 No products indexed under this
 heading.

Morphine Sulfate (Cinacalcet
hydrochloride is a strong in vitro
inhibitor of CYP2D6. Therefore, dose
adjustments of concomitant medications that are predominantly metabolized by CYP2D6 and have a narrow
therapeutic index may be required).
Products include:
 Avinza Capsules 1741
 Kadian Capsules 577
 MS Contin Tablets 2701

Nefazodone Hydrochloride
(Since cinacalcet hydrochloride is
metabolized in part by CYP3A4,
dose adjustment of cinacalcet hydrochloride may be required and PTH
and serum calcium concentrations
closely monitored if a patient initiates or discontinues therapy with a
strong CYP3A4 inhibitor).
 No products indexed under this
 heading.

Nelfinavir Mesylate (Cinacalcet
hydrochloride is a strong in vitro
inhibitor of CYP2D6. Therefore, dose
adjustments of concomitant medications that are predominantly metabolized by CYP2D6 and have a narrow
therapeutic index may be required).
Products include:

Viracept 2577

Nifedipine (Since cinacalcet hydrochloride is metabolized in part by CYP3A4, dose adjustment of cinacalcet hydrochloride may be required and PTH and serum calcium concentrations closely monitored if a patient initiates or discontinues therapy with a strong CYP3A4 inhibitor). Products include:

Adalat CC Tablets 2964

Norfloxacin (Since cinacalcet hydrochloride is metabolized in part by CYP3A4, dose adjustment of cinacalcet hydrochloride may be required and PTH and serum calcium concentrations closely monitored if a patient initiates or discontinues therapy with a strong CYP3A4 inhibitor). Products include:

Noroxin Tablets 2032

Nortriptyline Hydrochloride (Cinacalcet hydrochloride is a strong in vitro inhibitor of CYP2D6. Therefore, dose adjustments of concomitant medications that are predominantly metabolized by CYP2D6 and have a narrow therapeutic index may be required).

No products indexed under this heading.

Olanzapine (Cinacalcet hydrochloride is a strong in vitro inhibitor of CYP2D6. Therefore, dose adjustments of concomitant medications that are predominantly metabolized by CYP2D6 and have a narrow therapeutic index may be required). Products include:

Symbyax Capsules 1819
Zyprexa Tablets 1830
Zyprexa IntraMuscular 1830
Zyprexa ZYDIS Orally Disintegrating Tablets 1830

Omeprazole (Cinacalcet hydrochloride is a strong in vitro inhibitor of CYP2D6. Therefore, dose adjustments of concomitant medications that are predominantly metabolized by CYP2D6 and have a narrow therapeutic index may be required). Products include:

Zegerid Capsules 2958
Zegerid Powder for Oral Solution 2958

Ondansetron (Cinacalcet hydrochloride is a strong in vitro inhibitor of CYP2D6. Therefore, dose adjustments of concomitant medications that are predominantly metabolized by CYP2D6 and have a narrow therapeutic index may be required). Products include:

Zofran ODT Orally Disintegrating Tablets 1639

Ondansetron Hydrochloride (Cinacalcet hydrochloride is a strong in vitro inhibitor of CYP2D6. Therefore, dose adjustments of concomitant medications that are predominantly metabolized by CYP2D6 and have a narrow therapeutic index may be required). Products include:

Zofran Injection 1634
Zofran 1639

Oxycodone Hydrochloride (Cinacalcet hydrochloride is a strong in vitro inhibitor of CYP2D6. Therefore, dose adjustments of concomitant medications that are predominantly metabolized by CYP2D6 and have a narrow therapeutic index may be required). Products include:

OxyContin Tablets 2703
OxyFast Oral Concentrate Solution 2708
OxyIR Capsules 2708
Percocet Tablets 1131
Percodan Tablets 1132

Paclitaxel (Cinacalcet hydrochloride is a strong in vitro inhibitor of CYP2D6. Therefore, dose adjustments of concomitant medications that are predominantly metabolized by CYP2D6 and have a narrow therapeutic index may be required).

No products indexed under this heading.

Paroxetine Hydrochloride (Cinacalcet hydrochloride is a strong in vitro inhibitor of CYP2D6. Therefore, dose adjustments of concomitant medications that are predominantly metabolized by CYP2D6 and have a narrow therapeutic index may be required). Products include:

Paxil CR Controlled-Release Tablets 1538
Paxil 1530

Pindolol (Cinacalcet hydrochloride is a strong in vitro inhibitor of CYP2D6. Therefore, dose adjustments of concomitant medications that are predominantly metabolized by CYP2D6 and have a narrow therapeutic index may be required).

No products indexed under this heading.

Propafenone Hydrochloride (Cinacalcet hydrochloride is a strong in vitro inhibitor of CYP2D6. Therefore, dose adjustments of concomitant medications that are predominantly metabolized by CYP2D6 and have a narrow therapeutic index may be required). Products include:

Rythmol SR Capsules 2727

Propoxyphene Hydrochloride (Cinacalcet hydrochloride is a strong in vitro inhibitor of CYP2D6. Therefore, dose adjustments of concomitant medications that are predominantly metabolized by CYP2D6 and have a narrow therapeutic index may be required).

No products indexed under this heading.

Propoxyphene Napsylate (Cinacalcet hydrochloride is a strong in vitro inhibitor of CYP2D6. Therefore, dose adjustments of concomitant medications that are predominantly metabolized by CYP2D6 and have a narrow therapeutic index may be required).

No products indexed under this heading.

Propranolol Hydrochloride (Cinacalcet hydrochloride is a strong in vitro inhibitor of CYP2D6. Therefore, dose adjustments of concomitant medications that are predominantly metabolized by CYP2D6 and have a narrow therapeutic index may be required). Products include:

Inderal LA Long-Acting Capsules 3429
InnoPran XL Capsules 2723

Quetiapine Fumarate (Cinacalcet hydrochloride is a strong in vitro inhibitor of CYP2D6. Therefore, dose adjustments of concomitant medications that are predominantly metabolized by CYP2D6 and have a narrow therapeutic index may be required). Products include:

Seroquel Tablets 690

Quinidine Gluconate (Cinacalcet hydrochloride is a strong in vitro inhibitor of CYP2D6. Therefore, dose adjustments of concomitant medications that are predominantly metabolized by CYP2D6 and have a narrow therapeutic index may be required).

No products indexed under this heading.

Quinidine Hydrochloride (Cinacalcet hydrochloride is a strong in vitro inhibitor of CYP2D6. Therefore, dose adjustments of concomitant medications that are predominantly metabolized by CYP2D6 and have a narrow therapeutic index may be required).

No products indexed under this heading.

Quinidine Polygalacturonate (Cinacalcet hydrochloride is a strong in vitro inhibitor of CYP2D6. Therefore, dose adjustments of concomitant medications that are predominantly metabolized by CYP2D6 and have a narrow therapeutic index may be required).

No products indexed under this heading.

Quinidine Sulfate (Cinacalcet hydrochloride is a strong in vitro inhibitor of CYP2D6. Therefore, dose adjustments of concomitant medications that are predominantly metabolized by CYP2D6 and have a narrow therapeutic index may be required).

No products indexed under this heading.

Quinine (Since cinacalcet hydrochloride is metabolized in part by CYP3A4, dose adjustment of cinacalcet hydrochloride may be required and PTH and serum calcium concentrations closely monitored if a patient initiates or discontinues therapy with a strong CYP3A4 inhibitor).

No products indexed under this heading.

Quinine Sulfate (Since cinacalcet hydrochloride is metabolized in part by CYP3A4, dose adjustment of cinacalcet hydrochloride may be required and PTH and serum calcium concentrations closely monitored if a patient initiates or discontinues therapy with a strong CYP3A4 inhibitor).

No products indexed under this heading.

Risperidone (Cinacalcet hydrochloride is a strong in vitro inhibitor of CYP2D6. Therefore, dose adjustments of concomitant medications that are predominantly metabolized by CYP2D6 and have a narrow therapeutic index may be required). Products include:

Risperdal 1676
Risperdal Consta Long-Acting Injection 1682
Risperdal M-Tab Orally Disintegrating Tablets 1676

Ritonavir (Cinacalcet hydrochloride is a strong in vitro inhibitor of CYP2D6. Therefore, dose adjustments of concomitant medications that are predominantly metabolized by CYP2D6 and have a narrow therapeutic index may be required). Products include:

Kaletra 476
Norvir 503

Saquinavir (Since cinacalcet hydrochloride is metabolized in part by CYP3A4, dose adjustment of cinacalcet hydrochloride may be required and PTH and serum calcium concentrations closely monitored if a patient initiates or discontinues therapy with a strong CYP3A4 inhibitor).

No products indexed under this heading.

Saquinavir Mesylate (Since cinacalcet hydrochloride is metabolized in part by CYP3A4, dose adjustment of cinacalcet hydrochloride may be required and PTH and serum calcium concentrations closely monitored if a patient initiates or discontinues therapy with a strong CYP3A4 inhibitor). Products include:

Invirase 2772

Sertraline Hydrochloride (Since cinacalcet hydrochloride is metabolized in part by CYP3A4, dose adjustment of cinacalcet hydrochloride may be required and PTH and serum calcium concentrations closely monitored if a patient initiates or discontinues therapy with a strong CYP3A4 inhibitor). Products include:

Zoloft 2586

Tamoxifen Citrate (Cinacalcet hydrochloride is a strong in vitro inhibitor of CYP2D6. Therefore, dose adjustments of concomitant medications that are predominantly metabolized by CYP2D6 and have a narrow therapeutic index may be required). Products include:

Soltamox Oral Solution 3527

Teniposide (Cinacalcet hydrochloride is a strong in vitro inhibitor of CYP2D6. Therefore, dose adjustments of concomitant medications that are predominantly metabolized by CYP2D6 and have a narrow therapeutic index may be required).

No products indexed under this heading.

Testosterone (Cinacalcet hydrochloride is a strong in vitro inhibitor of CYP2D6. Therefore, dose adjustments of concomitant medications that are predominantly metabolized by CYP2D6 and have a narrow therapeutic index may be required). Products include:

AndroGel 3329
Striant Mucoadhesive 1007
Testim 1% Gel 695

Testosterone Cypionate (Cinacalcet hydrochloride is a strong in vitro inhibitor of CYP2D6. Therefore, dose adjustments of concomitant medications that are predominantly metabolized by CYP2D6 and have a narrow therapeutic index may be required).

No products indexed under this heading.

Testosterone Enanthate (Cinacalcet hydrochloride is a strong in vitro inhibitor of CYP2D6. Therefore, dose adjustments of concomitant medications that are predominantly metabolized by CYP2D6 and have a narrow therapeutic index may be required).

No products indexed under this heading.

Testosterone Propionate (Cinacalcet hydrochloride is a strong in vitro inhibitor of CYP2D6. Therefore, dose adjustments of concomitant medications that are predominantly metabolized by CYP2D6 and have a narrow therapeutic index may be required).

No products indexed under this heading.

Thioridazine (Cinacalcet hydrochloride is a strong in vitro inhibitor of CYP2D6. Therefore, dose adjustments of concomitant medications that are predominantly metabolized by CYP2D6 and have a narrow therapeutic index may be required).

No products indexed under this heading.

Thioridazine Hydrochloride (Cinacalcet hydrochloride is a strong in vitro inhibitor of CYP2D6. Therefore, dose adjustments of concomitant medications that are predominantly metabolized by CYP2D6 and have a narrow therapeutic index may be required). Products include:

Thioridazine Hydrochloride Tablets 2163

Timolol Maleate (Cinacalcet hydrochloride is a strong in vitro inhibitor of CYP2D6. Therefore, dose adjustments of concomitant medications that are predominantly metabolized by CYP2D6 and have a narrow therapeutic index may be required). Products include:
- Blocadren Tablets 1916
- Cosopt Sterile Ophthalmic Solution 1931
- Timolide Tablets 2086
- Timoptic Sterile Ophthalmic Solution 2088
- Timoptic in Ocudose 2091
- Timoptic-XE Sterile Ophthalmic Gel Forming Solution 2092

Tolterodine Tartrate (Cinacalcet hydrochloride is a strong in vitro inhibitor of CYP2D6. Therefore, dose adjustments of concomitant medications that are predominantly metabolized by CYP2D6 and have a narrow therapeutic index may be required). Products include:
- Detrol Tablets 2628
- Detrol LA Capsules 2631

Tramadol Hydrochloride (Cinacalcet hydrochloride is a strong in vitro inhibitor of CYP2D6. Therefore, dose adjustments of concomitant medications that are predominantly metabolized by CYP2D6 and have a narrow therapeutic index may be required). Products include:
- Ultram ER Tablets 2392

Trazodone Hydrochloride (Cinacalcet hydrochloride is a strong in vitro inhibitor of CYP2D6. Therefore, dose adjustments of concomitant medications that are predominantly metabolized by CYP2D6 and have a narrow therapeutic index may be required).
No products indexed under this heading.

Triazolam (Cinacalcet hydrochloride is a strong in vitro inhibitor of CYP2D6. Therefore, dose adjustments of concomitant medications that are predominantly metabolized by CYP2D6 and have a narrow therapeutic index may be required).
No products indexed under this heading.

Trimipramine Maleate (Cinacalcet hydrochloride is a strong in vitro inhibitor of CYP2D6. Therefore, dose adjustments of concomitant medications that are predominantly metabolized by CYP2D6 and have a narrow therapeutic index may be required).
No products indexed under this heading.

Troleandomycin (Since cinacalcet hydrochloride is metabolized in part by CYP3A4, dose adjustment of cinacalcet hydrochloride may be required and PTH and serum calcium concentrations closely monitored if a patient initiates or discontinues therapy with a strong CYP3A4 inhibitor).
No products indexed under this heading.

Venlafaxine Hydrochloride (Cinacalcet hydrochloride is a strong in vitro inhibitor of CYP2D6. Therefore, dose adjustments of concomitant medications that are predominantly metabolized by CYP2D6 and have a narrow therapeutic index may be required). Products include:
- Effexor Tablets 3411
- Effexor XR Capsules 3417

Verapamil Hydrochloride (Since cinacalcet hydrochloride is metabolized in part by CYP3A4, dose adjustment of cinacalcet hydrochloride may be required and PTH and serum calcium concentrations closely monitored if a patient initiates or discontinues therapy with a strong CYP3A4 inhibitor). Products include:
- Covera-HS Tablets 3139
- Tarka Tablets 524
- Verelan PM Extended-Release Capsules, Controlled-Onset 3106

Vinblastine Sulfate (Cinacalcet hydrochloride is a strong in vitro inhibitor of CYP2D6. Therefore, dose adjustments of concomitant medications that are predominantly metabolized by CYP2D6 and have a narrow therapeutic index may be required).
No products indexed under this heading.

Voriconazole (Since cinacalcet hydrochloride is metabolized in part by CYP3A4, dose adjustment of cinacalcet hydrochloride may be required and PTH and serum calcium concentrations closely monitored if a patient initiates or discontinues therapy with a strong CYP3A4 inhibitor). Products include:
- VFEND I.V. 2564
- VFEND Oral Suspension 2564
- VFEND Tablets 2564

Zafirlukast (Since cinacalcet hydrochloride is metabolized in part by CYP3A4, dose adjustment of cinacalcet hydrochloride may be required and PTH and serum calcium concentrations closely monitored if a patient initiates or discontinues therapy with a strong CYP3A4 inhibitor). Products include:
- Accolate Tablets 671

Zileuton (Since cinacalcet hydrochloride is metabolized in part by CYP3A4, dose adjustment of cinacalcet hydrochloride may be required and PTH and serum calcium concentrations closely monitored if a patient initiates or discontinues therapy with a strong CYP3A4 inhibitor). Products include:
- Zyflo Tablets 1023

Zonisamide (Cinacalcet hydrochloride is a strong in vitro inhibitor of CYP2D6. Therefore, dose adjustments of concomitant medications that are predominantly metabolized by CYP2D6 and have a narrow therapeutic index may be required). Products include:
- Zonegran Capsules 1101

Food Interactions

Grapefruit (Since cinacalcet hydrochloride is metabolized in part by CYP3A4, dose adjustment of cinacalcet hydrochloride may be required and PTH and serum calcium concentrations closely monitored if a patient initiates or discontinues therapy with a strong CYP3A4 inhibitor).

SENSODYNE ORIGINAL FLAVOR

(Potassium Nitrate, Sodium Fluoride) .... ■□711
None cited in PDR database.

SENSODYNE COOL GEL

(Potassium Nitrate, Sodium Fluoride) .... ■□711
None cited in PDR database.

SENSODYNE EXTRA WHITENING

(Potassium Nitrate, Sodium Monofluorophosphate) .... ■□711
None cited in PDR database.

SENSODYNE FRESH IMPACT

(Potassium Nitrate, Sodium Fluoride) .... ■□711
None cited in PDR database.

SENSODYNE FRESH MINT

(Potassium Nitrate, Sodium Fluoride) .... ■□711
None cited in PDR database.

SENSODYNE TARTAR CONTROL

(Potassium Nitrate, Sodium Fluoride) .... ■□711
None cited in PDR database.

SENSODYNE TARTAR CONTROL PLUS WHITENING

(Potassium Nitrate, Sodium Fluoride) .... ■□711
None cited in PDR database.

SENSODYNE WITH BAKING SODA

(Potassium Nitrate, Sodium Fluoride) .... ■□711
None cited in PDR database.

SEREVENT DISKUS

(Salmeterol Xinafoate) 1568
May interact with beta blockers, monoamine oxidase inhibitors, nonpotassium-sparing diuretics, and tricyclic antidepressants. Compounds in these categories include:

Acebutolol Hydrochloride (Beta-adrenergic blockers may produce severe bronchospasm in asthmatic patients, however, beta blockers do not block the pulmonary effect of beta-agonists).
No products indexed under this heading.

Amitriptyline Hydrochloride (The action of salmeterol on the vascular system may be potentiated by tricyclic antidepressant).
No products indexed under this heading.

Amoxapine (The action of salmeterol on the vascular system may be potentiated by tricyclic antidepressant).
No products indexed under this heading.

Atenolol (Beta-adrenergic blockers may produce severe bronchospasm in asthmatic patients, however, beta blockers do not block the pulmonary effect of beta-agonists).
No products indexed under this heading.

Bendroflumethiazide (The ECG changes and/or hypokalemia that may result from the administration of nonpotassium-sparing diuretics can be acutely worsened by beta-agonists, especially when the recommended dose of beta-agonist is exceeded).
No products indexed under this heading.

Betaxolol Hydrochloride (Beta-adrenergic blockers may produce severe bronchospasm in asthmatic patients, however, beta blockers do not block the pulmonary effect of beta-agonists). Products include:
- Betoptic S Ophthalmic Suspension 558

Bisoprolol Fumarate (Beta-adrenergic blockers may produce severe bronchospasm in asthmatic patients, however, beta blockers do not block the pulmonary effect of beta-agonists).
No products indexed under this heading.

Bumetanide (The ECG changes and/or hypokalemia that may result from the administration of nonpotassium-sparing diuretics can be acutely worsened by beta-agonists, especially when the recommended dose of beta-agonist is exceeded). Products include:
- Bumex Tablets 2746

Carteolol Hydrochloride (Beta-adrenergic blockers may produce severe bronchospasm in asthmatic patients, however, beta blockers do not block the pulmonary effect of beta-agonists). Products include:
- Carteolol Hydrochloride Ophthalmic Solution USP, 1% .... ⊙249

Chlorothiazide (The ECG changes and/or hypokalemia that may result from the administration of nonpotassium-sparing diuretics can be acutely worsened by beta-agonists, especially when the recommended dose of beta-agonist is exceeded). Products include:
- Diuril Oral Suspension 1954

Chlorothiazide Sodium (The ECG changes and/or hypokalemia that may result from the administration of nonpotassium-sparing diuretics can be acutely worsened by beta-agonists, especially when the recommended dose of beta-agonist is exceeded). Products include:
- Diuril Sodium Intravenous 2467

Clomipramine Hydrochloride (The action of salmeterol on the vascular system may be potentiated by tricyclic antidepressant).
No products indexed under this heading.

Desipramine Hydrochloride (The action of salmeterol on the vascular system may be potentiated by tricyclic antidepressant).
No products indexed under this heading.

Doxepin Hydrochloride (The action of salmeterol on the vascular system may be potentiated by tricyclic antidepressant).
No products indexed under this heading.

Esmolol Hydrochloride (Beta-adrenergic blockers may produce severe bronchospasm in asthmatic patients, however, beta blockers do not block the pulmonary effect of beta-agonists).
No products indexed under this heading.

Ethacrynic Acid (The ECG changes and/or hypokalemia that may result from the administration of nonpotassium-sparing diuretics can be acutely worsened by beta-agonists, especially when the recommended dose of beta-agonist is exceeded). Products include:
- Edecrin Tablets 1959

Furosemide (The ECG changes and/or hypokalemia that may result from the administration of nonpotassium-sparing diuretics can be acutely worsened by beta-agonists, especially when the recommended dose of beta-agonist is exceeded). Products include:
- Furosemide Tablets 2154

Hydrochlorothiazide (The ECG changes and/or hypokalemia that may result from the administration of nonpotassium-sparing diuretics can be acutely worsened by beta-agonists, especially when the recommended dose of beta-agonist is exceeded). Products include:

Aldoril Tablets **1910**
Atacand HCT **651**
Avalide Tablets **888**
Avalide Tablets **2874**
Benicar HCT Tablets **1044**
Diovan HCT Tablets **2196**
Dyazide Capsules **1423**
Hyzaar 50-12.5 Tablets **1990**
Hyzaar 100-12.5 Tablets **1990**
Hyzaar 100-25 Tablets **1990**
Lopressor HCT 50/25 Tablets **2241**
Lopressor HCT 100/25 Tablets **2241**
Lopressor HCT 100/50 Tablets **2241**
Lotensin HCT Tablets **2246**
Micardis HCT Tablets **856**
Moduretic Tablets **2028**
Prinzide Tablets **2056**
Teveten HCT Tablets **1737**
Timolide Tablets **2086**
Uniretic Tablets **3100**

Hydroflumethiazide (The ECG changes and/or hypokalemia that may result from the administration of nonpotassium-sparing diuretics can be acutely worsened by beta-agonists, especially when the recommended dose of beta-agonist is exceeded).
No products indexed under this heading.

Imipramine Hydrochloride (The action of salmeterol on the vascular system may be potentiated by tricyclic antidepressant).
No products indexed under this heading.

Imipramine Pamoate (The action of salmeterol on the vascular system may be potentiated by tricyclic antidepressant).
No products indexed under this heading.

Isocarboxazid (The action of salmeterol on the vascular system may be potentiated by MAO inhibitor).
No products indexed under this heading.

Labetalol Hydrochloride (Beta-adrenergic blockers may produce severe bronchospasm in asthmatic patients, however, beta blockers do not block the pulmonary effect of beta-agonists).
No products indexed under this heading.

Levobunolol Hydrochloride (Beta-adrenergic blockers may produce severe bronchospasm in asthmatic patients, however, beta blockers do not block the pulmonary effect of beta-agonists). Products include:

Betagan Ophthalmic Solution, USP .... ⊙**220**

Maprotiline Hydrochloride (The action of salmeterol on the vascular system may be potentiated by tricyclic antidepressant).
No products indexed under this heading.

Methyclothiazide (The ECG changes and/or hypokalemia that may result from the administration of nonpotassium-sparing diuretics can be acutely worsened by beta-agonists, especially when the recommended dose of beta-agonist is exceeded).
No products indexed under this heading.

Metipranolol Hydrochloride (Beta-adrenergic blockers may produce severe bronchospasm in asthmatic patients, however, beta blockers do not block the pulmonary effect of beta-agonists).
No products indexed under this heading.

Metoprolol Succinate (Beta-adrenergic blockers may produce severe bronchospasm in asthmatic patients, however, beta blockers do not block the pulmonary effect of beta-agonists). Products include:

Toprol-XL Tablets **668**

Metoprolol Tartrate (Beta-adrenergic blockers may produce severe bronchospasm in asthmatic patients, however, beta blockers do not block the pulmonary effect of beta-agonists). Products include:

Lopressor Injection **2238**
Lopressor Tablets **2238**
Lopressor HCT 50/25 Tablets **2241**
Lopressor HCT 100/25 Tablets **2241**
Lopressor HCT 100/50 Tablets **2241**

Moclobemide (The action of salmeterol on the vascular system may be potentiated by MAO inhibitor).
No products indexed under this heading.

Nadolol (Beta-adrenergic blockers may produce severe bronchospasm in asthmatic patients, however, beta blockers do not block the pulmonary effect of beta-agonists). Products include:

Nadolol Tablets **2159**

Nortriptyline Hydrochloride (The action of salmeterol on the vascular system may be potentiated by tricyclic antidepressant).
No products indexed under this heading.

Pargyline Hydrochloride (The action of salmeterol on the vascular system may be potentiated by MAO inhibitor).
No products indexed under this heading.

Penbutolol Sulfate (Beta-adrenergic blockers may produce severe bronchospasm in asthmatic patients, however, beta blockers do not block the pulmonary effect of beta-agonists).
No products indexed under this heading.

Phenelzine Sulfate (The action of salmeterol on the vascular system may be potentiated by MAO inhibitor).
No products indexed under this heading.

Pindolol (Beta-adrenergic blockers may produce severe bronchospasm in asthmatic patients, however, beta blockers do not block the pulmonary effect of beta-agonists).
No products indexed under this heading.

Polythiazide (The ECG changes and/or hypokalemia that may result from the administration of nonpotassium-sparing diuretics can be acutely worsened by beta-agonists, especially when the recommended dose of beta-agonist is exceeded).
No products indexed under this heading.

Procarbazine Hydrochloride (The action of salmeterol on the vascular system may be potentiated by MAO inhibitor). Products include:

Matulane Capsules **3191**

Propranolol Hydrochloride (Beta-adrenergic blockers may produce severe bronchospasm in asthmatic patients, however, beta blockers do not block the pulmonary effect of beta-agonists). Products include:

Inderal LA Long-Acting Capsules **3429**
InnoPran XL Capsules **2723**

Protriptyline Hydrochloride (The action of salmeterol on the vascular system may be potentiated by tricyclic antidepressant).
No products indexed under this heading.

Selegiline Hydrochloride (The action of salmeterol on the vascular system may be potentiated by MAO inhibitor). Products include:

Eldepryl Capsules **3208**
Zelapar Tablets **3372**

Sotalol Hydrochloride (Beta-adrenergic blockers may produce severe bronchospasm in asthmatic patients, however, beta blockers do not block the pulmonary effect of beta-agonists).
No products indexed under this heading.

Timolol Hemihydrate (Beta-adrenergic blockers may produce severe bronchospasm in asthmatic patients, however, beta blockers do not block the pulmonary effect of beta-agonists). Products include:

Betimol Ophthalmic Solution **3382**
Betimol Ophthalmic Solution .... ⊙**295**

Timolol Maleate (Beta-adrenergic blockers may produce severe bronchospasm in asthmatic patients, however, beta blockers do not block the pulmonary effect of beta-agonists). Products include:

Blocadren Tablets **1916**
Cosopt Sterile Ophthalmic Solution **1931**
Timolide Tablets **2086**
Timoptic Sterile Ophthalmic Solution **2088**
Timoptic in Ocudose **2091**
Timoptic-XE Sterile Ophthalmic Gel Forming Solution **2092**

Torsemide (The ECG changes and/or hypokalemia that may result from the administration of nonpotassium-sparing diuretics can be acutely worsened by beta-agonists, especially when the recommended dose of beta-agonist is exceeded). Products include:

Demadex Injection **2759**
Demadex Tablets **2759**

Tranylcypromine Sulfate (The action of salmeterol on the vascular system may be potentiated by MAO inhibitor). Products include:

Parnate Tablets **1527**

Trimipramine Maleate (The action of salmeterol on the vascular system may be potentiated by tricyclic antidepressant).
No products indexed under this heading.

SEROMYCIN CAPSULES

(Cycloserine) **1813**
May interact with antituberculosis drugs and certain other agents. Compounds in these categories include:

Aminosalicylic Acid (Co-administration has been associated with a few instances of vitamin B_{12} and/or folic acid deficiency, megaloblastic anemia, and sideroblastic anemia). Products include:

Paser Granules **1674**

p-Aminosalicylic Acid (Co-administration has been associated with a few instances of vitamin B_{12} and/or folic acid deficiency, megaloblastic anemia, and sideroblastic anemia).
No products indexed under this heading.

Ethambutol Hydrochloride (Co-administration has been associated with a few instances of vitamin B_{12} and/or folic acid deficiency, megaloblastic anemia, and sideroblastic anemia).
No products indexed under this heading.

Ethionamide (Co-administration has been reported to potentiate neurotoxic side effects). Products include:

Trecator Tablets **3487**

Isoniazid (Co-administration may result in increased incidence of CNS effects, such as dizziness or drowsiness).
No products indexed under this heading.

Pyrazinamide (Co-administration has been associated with a few instances of vitamin B_{12} and/or folic acid deficiency, megaloblastic anemia, and sideroblastic anemia).
No products indexed under this heading.

Rifampin (Co-administration has been associated with a few instances of vitamin B_{12} and/or folic acid deficiency, megaloblastic anemia, and sideroblastic anemia).
No products indexed under this heading.

Rifapentine (Co-administration has been associated with a few instances of vitamin B_{12} and/or folic acid deficiency, megaloblastic anemia, and sideroblastic anemia).
No products indexed under this heading.

Food Interactions

Alcohol (Concurrent use increases the possibility and risk of epileptic episodes).

SEROQUEL TABLETS

(Quetiapine Fumarate) **690**
May interact with antihypertensives, barbiturates, cytochrome p450 3a4 inhibitors (selected), dopamine agonists, glucocorticoids, phenytoin, and certain other agents. Compounds in these categories include:

Acebutolol Hydrochloride (Enhanced effects of certain antihypertensive agents).
No products indexed under this heading.

Acetazolamide (Co-administration with an inhibitor of CYP4503A may reduce oral clearance of quetiapine, resulting in an increase in maximum plasma concentration of quetiapine; dose adjustment of quetiapine will be necessary).
No products indexed under this heading.

Amiodarone Hydrochloride (Co-administration with an inhibitor of CYP4503A may reduce oral clearance of quetiapine, resulting in an increase in maximum plasma concentration of quetiapine; dose adjustment of quetiapine will be necessary).
No products indexed under this heading.

Amlodipine Besylate (Enhanced effects of certain antihypertensive agents). Products include:
Caduet Tablets ... 2508
Lotrel Capsules ... 2249
Norvasc Tablets ... 2545

Amprenavir (Co-administration with an inhibitor of CYP4503A may reduce oral clearance of quetiapine, resulting in an increase in maximum plasma concentration of quetiapine; dose adjustment of quetiapine will be necessary). Products include:
Agenerase Capsules ... 1327
Agenerase Oral Solution ... 1332

Anastrozole (Co-administration with an inhibitor of CYP4503A may reduce oral clearance of quetiapine, resulting in an increase in maximum plasma concentration of quetiapine; dose adjustment of quetiapine will be necessary). Products include:
Arimidex Tablets ... 673

Aprepitant (Co-administration with an inhibitor of CYP4503A may reduce oral clearance of quetiapine, resulting in an increase in maximum plasma concentration of quetiapine; dose adjustment of quetiapine will be necessary). Products include:
Emend Capsules ... 1963

Aprobarbital (Co-administration with hepatic enzyme inducers, such as barbiturates, may increase oral clearance).
No products indexed under this heading.

Atenolol (Enhanced effects of certain antihypertensive agents).
No products indexed under this heading.

Benazepril Hydrochloride (Enhanced effects of certain antihypertensive agents). Products include:
Lotensin Tablets ... 2243
Lotensin HCT Tablets ... 2246
Lotrel Capsules ... 2249

Bendroflumethiazide (Enhanced effects of certain antihypertensive agents).
No products indexed under this heading.

Betamethasone Acetate (Co-administration with hepatic enzyme inducers, such as glucocorticosteroids, may increase oral clearance).
No products indexed under this heading.

Betamethasone Sodium Phosphate (Co-administration with hepatic enzyme inducers, such as glucocorticosteroids, may increase oral clearance).
No products indexed under this heading.

Betaxolol Hydrochloride (Enhanced effects of certain antihypertensive agents). Products include:
Betoptic S Ophthalmic Suspension ... 558

Bisoprolol Fumarate (Enhanced effects of certain antihypertensive agents).
No products indexed under this heading.

Bromocriptine Mesylate (Quetiapine may antagonize the effects of dopamine agonists).
No products indexed under this heading.

Butabarbital (Co-administration with hepatic enzyme inducers, such as barbiturates, may increase oral clearance).
No products indexed under this heading.

Butalbital (Co-administration with hepatic enzyme inducers, such as barbiturates, may increase oral clearance).
No products indexed under this heading.

Candesartan Cilexetil (Enhanced effects of certain antihypertensive agents). Products include:
Atacand Tablets ... 649
Atacand HCT ... 651

Captopril (Enhanced effects of certain antihypertensive agents). Products include:
Captopril Tablets ... 2149

Carbamazepine (Co-administration with hepatic enzyme inducers, such as carbamazepine, may increase oral clearance). Products include:
Carbatrol Capsules ... 3171
Equetro Extended-Release Capsules ... 3180
Tegretol/Tegretol-XR ... 2295

Carteolol Hydrochloride (Enhanced effects of certain antihypertensive agents). Products include:
Carteolol Hydrochloride Ophthalmic Solution USP, 1% ... ⊙249

Chlorothiazide (Enhanced effects of certain antihypertensive agents). Products include:
Diuril Oral Suspension ... 1954

Chlorothiazide Sodium (Enhanced effects of certain antihypertensive agents). Products include:
Diuril Sodium Intravenous ... 2467

Chlorthalidone (Enhanced effects of certain antihypertensive agents). Products include:
Clorpres Tablets ... 2153

Cimetidine (Co-administration has resulted in a 20% decrease in the mean oral clearance of quetiapine). Products include:
Tagamet HB 200 Tablets ... ▣664

Cimetidine Hydrochloride (Co-administration with an inhibitor of CYP4503A may reduce oral clearance of quetiapine, resulting in an increase in maximum plasma concentration of quetiapine; dose adjustment of quetiapine will be necessary).
No products indexed under this heading.

Ciprofloxacin (Co-administration with an inhibitor of CYP4503A may reduce oral clearance of quetiapine, resulting in an increase in maximum plasma concentration of quetiapine; dose adjustment of quetiapine will be necessary). Products include:
Cipro Oral Suspension ... 2977
Cipro I.V. ... 2984
Cipro XR Tablets ... 2990
Ciprodex Otic Suspension ... 559

Clarithromycin (Co-administration with an inhibitor of CYP4503A may reduce oral clearance of quetiapine, resulting in an increase in maximum plasma concentration of quetiapine; dose adjustment of quetiapine will be necessary). Products include:
Biaxin/Biaxin XL ... 402
PREVPAC ... 3284

Clonidine (Enhanced effects of certain antihypertensive agents). Products include:
Catapres-TTS ... 844

Clonidine Hydrochloride (Enhanced effects of certain antihypertensive agents). Products include:
Catapres Tablets ... 843
Clorpres Tablets ... 2153

Clotrimazole (Co-administration with an inhibitor of CYP4503A may reduce oral clearance of quetiapine, resulting in an increase in maximum plasma concentration of quetiapine; dose adjustment of quetiapine will be necessary). Products include:
Desenex Athlete's Foot Cream ... ▣635
Lotrimin ... 3039
Lotrisone ... 3040

Cortisone Acetate (Co-administration with hepatic enzyme inducers, such as glucocorticosteroids, may increase oral clearance).
No products indexed under this heading.

Cyclosporine (Co-administration with an inhibitor of CYP4503A may reduce oral clearance of quetiapine, resulting in an increase in maximum plasma concentration of quetiapine; dose adjustment of quetiapine will be necessary). Products include:
Gengraf Capsules ... 459
Neoral Oral Solution ... 2259
Neoral Soft Gelatin Capsules ... 2259
Restasis Ophthalmic Emulsion ... 575
Sandimmune ... 2275

Dalfopristin (Co-administration with an inhibitor of CYP4503A may reduce oral clearance of quetiapine, resulting in an increase in maximum plasma concentration of quetiapine; dose adjustment of quetiapine will be necessary).
No products indexed under this heading.

Danazol (Co-administration with an inhibitor of CYP4503A may reduce oral clearance of quetiapine, resulting in an increase in maximum plasma concentration of quetiapine; dose adjustment of quetiapine will be necessary).
No products indexed under this heading.

Delavirdine Mesylate (Co-administration with an inhibitor of CYP4503A may reduce oral clearance of quetiapine, resulting in an increase in maximum plasma concentration of quetiapine; dose adjustment of quetiapine will be necessary). Products include:
Rescriptor Tablets ... 2551

Deserpidine (Enhanced effects of certain antihypertensive agents).
No products indexed under this heading.

Dexamethasone (Co-administration with hepatic enzyme inducers, such as glucocorticosteroids, may increase oral clearance). Products include:
Ciprodex Otic Suspension ... 559
Decadron Tablets ... 1951
TobraDex Ophthalmic Ointment ... 562
TobraDex Ophthalmic Suspension ... 563

Dexamethasone Acetate (Co-administration with hepatic enzyme inducers, such as glucocorticosteroids, may increase oral clearance).
No products indexed under this heading.

Dexamethasone Sodium Phosphate (Co-administration with hepatic enzyme inducers, such as glucocorticosteroids, may increase oral clearance).
No products indexed under this heading.

Diazoxide (Enhanced effects of certain antihypertensive agents). Products include:
Hyperstat I.V. ... 3017

Diltiazem Hydrochloride (Co-administration with an inhibitor of CYP4503A may reduce oral clearance of quetiapine, resulting in an increase in maximum plasma concentration of quetiapine; dose adjustment of quetiapine will be necessary). Products include:
Cardizem LA Extended Release Tablets ... 1728
Tiazac Capsules ... 1201

Diltiazem Maleate (Co-administration with an inhibitor of CYP4503A may reduce oral clearance of quetiapine, resulting in an increase in maximum plasma concentration of quetiapine; dose adjustment of quetiapine will be necessary).
No products indexed under this heading.

Divalproex Sodium (Co-administration of quetiapine (150 mg bid) and divalproex (500 mg bid) increased the mean maximum plasma concentration of quetiapine at steady state by 17% without affecting the extent of absorption or mean oral clearance. Co-administration also decreased the mean maximum concentration and extent of absorption of total and free valproic acid at steady state by 10% to 12% and increased mean oral clearance of total valproic acid by 11%). Products include:
Depakote Sprinkle Capsules ... 422
Depakote Tablets ... 427
Depakote ER Tablets ... 434

Dopamine Hydrochloride (Quetiapine may antagonize the effects of dopamine agonists).
No products indexed under this heading.

Doxazosin Mesylate (Enhanced effects of certain antihypertensive agents). Products include:
Cardura XL Tablets ... 2515

Efavirenz (Co-administration with an inhibitor of CYP4503A may reduce oral clearance of quetiapine, resulting in an increase in maximum plasma concentration of quetiapine; dose adjustment of quetiapine will be necessary). Products include:
Atripla Tablets ... 945
Sustiva Capsules ... 930
Sustiva Tablets ... 930

Enalapril Maleate (Enhanced effects of certain antihypertensive agents). Products include:
Vasotec I.V. Injection ... 2103

Enalaprilat (Enhanced effects of certain antihypertensive agents).
No products indexed under this heading.

Eprosartan Mesylate (Enhanced effects of certain antihypertensive agents). Products include:
Teveten Tablets ... 1735
Teveten HCT Tablets ... 1737

Erythromycin (Co-administration with an inhibitor of CYP4503A may reduce oral clearance of quetiapine, resulting in an increase in maximum plasma concentration of quetiapine; dose adjustment of quetiapine will be necessary). Products include:
Ery-Tab Tablets ... 449
Erythromycin Base Filmtab Tablets ... 455
Erythromycin Delayed-Release Capsules, USP ... 457

PCE Dispertab Tablets 515

Erythromycin Estolate (Co-administration with an inhibitor of CYP4503A may reduce oral clearance of quetiapine, resulting in an increase in maximum plasma concentration of quetiapine; dose adjustment of quetiapine will be necessary).

No products indexed under this heading.

Erythromycin Ethylsuccinate (Co-administration with an inhibitor of CYP4503A may reduce oral clearance of quetiapine, resulting in an increase in maximum plasma concentration of quetiapine; dose adjustment of quetiapine will be necessary). Products include:

E.E.S. 451
EryPed 447

Erythromycin Gluceptate (Co-administration with an inhibitor of CYP4503A may reduce oral clearance of quetiapine, resulting in an increase in maximum plasma concentration of quetiapine; dose adjustment of quetiapine will be necessary).

No products indexed under this heading.

Erythromycin Lactobionate (Co-administration with an inhibitor of CYP4503A may reduce oral clearance of quetiapine, resulting in an increase in maximum plasma concentration of quetiapine; dose adjustment of quetiapine will be necessary).

No products indexed under this heading.

Erythromycin Stearate (Co-administration with an inhibitor of CYP4503A may reduce oral clearance of quetiapine, resulting in an increase in maximum plasma concentration of quetiapine; dose adjustment of quetiapine will be necessary). Products include:

Erythrocin Stearate Filmtab Tablets 453

Esmolol Hydrochloride (Enhanced effects of certain antihypertensive agents).

No products indexed under this heading.

Esomeprazole Magnesium (Co-administration with an inhibitor of CYP4503A may reduce oral clearance of quetiapine, resulting in an increase in maximum plasma concentration of quetiapine; dose adjustment of quetiapine will be necessary). Products include:

Nexium Delayed-Release Capsules 655

Felodipine (Enhanced effects of certain antihypertensive agents).

No products indexed under this heading.

Fludrocortisone Acetate (Co-administration with hepatic enzyme inducers, such as glucocorticosteroids, may increase oral clearance).

No products indexed under this heading.

Fluoxetine Hydrochloride (Co-administration with an inhibitor of CYP4503A may reduce oral clearance of quetiapine, resulting in an increase in maximum plasma concentration of quetiapine; dose adjustment of quetiapine will be necessary). Products include:

Prozac Pulvules and Liquid 1801
Symbyax Capsules 1819

Fluvoxamine Maleate (Co-administration with an inhibitor of CYP4503A may reduce oral clearance of quetiapine, resulting in an increase in maximum plasma concentration of quetiapine; dose adjustment of quetiapine will be necessary).

No products indexed under this heading.

Fosamprenavir Calcium (Co-administration with an inhibitor of CYP4503A may reduce oral clearance of quetiapine, resulting in an increase in maximum plasma concentration of quetiapine; dose adjustment of quetiapine will be necessary). Products include:

Lexiva Tablets 1505

Fosinopril Sodium (Enhanced effects of certain antihypertensive agents).

No products indexed under this heading.

Fosphenytoin Sodium (Co-administration has resulted in increased mean oral clearance of quetiapine by 5-fold; increased dose of quetiapine may be required).

No products indexed under this heading.

Furosemide (Enhanced effects of certain antihypertensive agents). Products include:

Furosemide Tablets 2154

Guanabenz Acetate (Enhanced effects of certain antihypertensive agents).

No products indexed under this heading.

Guanethidine Monosulfate (Enhanced effects of certain antihypertensive agents).

No products indexed under this heading.

Hydralazine Hydrochloride (Enhanced effects of certain antihypertensive agents). Products include:

BiDil Tablets 2171

Hydrochlorothiazide (Enhanced effects of certain antihypertensive agents). Products include:

Aldoril Tablets 1910
Atacand HCT 651
Avalide Tablets 888
Avalide Tablets 2874
Benicar HCT Tablets 1044
Diovan HCT Tablets 2196
Dyazide Capsules 1423
Hyzaar 50-12.5 Tablets 1990
Hyzaar 100-12.5 Tablets 1990
Hyzaar 100-25 Tablets 1990
Lopressor HCT 50/25 Tablets 2241
Lopressor HCT 100/25 Tablets 2241
Lopressor HCT 100/50 Tablets 2241
Lotensin HCT Tablets 2246
Micardis HCT Tablets 856
Moduretic Tablets 2028
Prinzide Tablets 2056
Teveten HCT Tablets 1737
Timolide Tablets 2086
Uniretic Tablets 3100

Hydrocortisone (Co-administration with hepatic enzyme inducers, such as glucocorticosteroids, may increase oral clearance). Products include:

Colocort Rectal Suspension, USP (Retention) 100 mg/60 mL 2476
Hydrocortone Tablets 1989
Preparation H Hydrocortisone Cream 646

Hydrocortisone Acetate (Co-administration with hepatic enzyme inducers, such as glucocorticosteroids, may increase oral clearance). Products include:

Analpram-HC 1159
Pramosone 1161
ProctoFoam-HC 3099

Hydrocortisone Sodium Phosphate (Co-administration with hepatic enzyme inducers, such as glucocorticosteroids, may increase oral clearance).

No products indexed under this heading.

Hydrocortisone Sodium Succinate (Co-administration with hepatic enzyme inducers, such as glucocorticosteroids, may increase oral clearance).

No products indexed under this heading.

Hydroflumethiazide (Enhanced effects of certain antihypertensive agents).

No products indexed under this heading.

Indapamide (Enhanced effects of certain antihypertensive agents). Products include:

Indapamide Tablets 2156

Indinavir Sulfate (Co-administration with an inhibitor of CYP4503A may reduce oral clearance of quetiapine, resulting in an increase in maximum plasma concentration of quetiapine; dose adjustment of quetiapine will be necessary). Products include:

Crixivan Capsules 1940

Irbesartan (Enhanced effects of certain antihypertensive agents). Products include:

Avalide Tablets 888
Avalide Tablets 2874
Avapro Tablets 891
Avapro Tablets 2871

Isoniazid (Co-administration with an inhibitor of CYP4503A may reduce oral clearance of quetiapine, resulting in an increase in maximum plasma concentration of quetiapine; dose adjustment of quetiapine will be necessary).

No products indexed under this heading.

Isradipine (Enhanced effects of certain antihypertensive agents). Products include:

DynaCirc CR Tablets 2721

Ketoconazole (Co-administration of ketoconazole, a potent inhibitor of CYP4503A, reduced oral clearance of quetiapine by 84%, resulting in a 335% increase in maximum plasma concentration of quetiapine; dose adjustment of quetiapine will be necessary if it is used with ketoconazole). Products include:

Nizoral A-D Shampoo, 1% 1868

Labetalol Hydrochloride (Enhanced effects of certain antihypertensive agents).

No products indexed under this heading.

Levodopa (Quetiapine may antagonize the effects of levodopa). Products include:

Parcopa Orally Disintegrating Tablets 3097
Stalevo Tablets 2287

Lisinopril (Enhanced effects of certain antihypertensive agents). Products include:

Prinivil Tablets 2052
Prinzide Tablets 2056

Lopinavir (Co-administration with an inhibitor of CYP4503A may reduce oral clearance of quetiapine, resulting in an increase in maximum plasma concentration of quetiapine; dose adjustment of quetiapine will be necessary). Products include:

Kaletra 476

Loratadine (Co-administration with an inhibitor of CYP4503A may reduce oral clearance of quetiapine, resulting in an increase in maximum plasma concentration of quetiapine; dose adjustment of quetiapine will be necessary). Products include:

Alavert Allergy & Sinus D-12 Hour Tablets 771
Alavert 771
Children's Claritin Allergy Oral Solution 771
Claritin Non-Drowsy 24 Hour Tablets 772
Claritin Reditabs 24 Hour Non-Drowsy Tablets 772
Claritin-D Non-Drowsy 12 Hour Tablets 772
Claritin-D Non-Drowsy 24 Hour Tablets 772

Lorazepam (Co-administration has resulted in reduced (20%) mean oral clearance of lorazepam).

No products indexed under this heading.

Losartan Potassium (Enhanced effects of certain antihypertensive agents). Products include:

Cozaar Tablets 1935
Hyzaar 50-12.5 Tablets 1990
Hyzaar 100-12.5 Tablets 1990
Hyzaar 100-25 Tablets 1990

Mecamylamine Hydrochloride (Enhanced effects of certain antihypertensive agents).

No products indexed under this heading.

Mephobarbital (Co-administration with hepatic enzyme inducers, such as barbiturates, may increase oral clearance).

No products indexed under this heading.

Methyclothiazide (Enhanced effects of certain antihypertensive agents).

No products indexed under this heading.

Methyldopa (Enhanced effects of certain antihypertensive agents). Products include:

Aldoril Tablets 1910

Methyldopate Hydrochloride (Enhanced effects of certain antihypertensive agents).

No products indexed under this heading.

Methylprednisolone Acetate (Co-administration with hepatic enzyme inducers, such as glucocorticosteroids, may increase oral clearance). Products include:

Depo-Medrol Injectable Suspension 2617
Depo-Medrol Single-Dose Vial 2619

Methylprednisolone Sodium Succinate (Co-administration with hepatic enzyme inducers, such as glucocorticosteroids, may increase oral clearance).

No products indexed under this heading.

Metolazone (Enhanced effects of certain antihypertensive agents).

No products indexed under this heading.

Metoprolol Succinate (Enhanced effects of certain antihypertensive agents). Products include:

Toprol-XL Tablets 668

Metoprolol Tartrate (Enhanced effects of certain antihypertensive agents). Products include:

Metronidazole (Co-administration with an inhibitor of CYP4503A may reduce oral clearance of quetiapine, resulting in an increase in maximum plasma concentration of quetiapine; dose adjustment of quetiapine will be necessary). Products include:

Metronidazole Benzoate (Co-administration with an inhibitor of CYP4503A may reduce oral clearance of quetiapine, resulting in an increase in maximum plasma concentration of quetiapine; dose adjustment of quetiapine will be necessary).

No products indexed under this heading.

Metronidazole Hydrochloride (Co-administration with an inhibitor of CYP4503A may reduce oral clearance of quetiapine, resulting in an increase in maximum plasma concentration of quetiapine; dose adjustment of quetiapine will be necessary).

No products indexed under this heading.

Metyrosine (Enhanced effects of certain antihypertensive agents). Products include:

Mibefradil Dihydrochloride (Enhanced effects of certain antihypertensive agents).

No products indexed under this heading.

Miconazole (Co-administration with an inhibitor of CYP4503A may reduce oral clearance of quetiapine, resulting in an increase in maximum plasma concentration of quetiapine; dose adjustment of quetiapine will be necessary).

No products indexed under this heading.

Miconazole Nitrate (Co-administration with an inhibitor of CYP4503A may reduce oral clearance of quetiapine, resulting in an increase in maximum plasma concentration of quetiapine; dose adjustment of quetiapine will be necessary). Products include:

Minoxidil (Enhanced effects of certain antihypertensive agents). Products include:

Moexipril Hydrochloride (Enhanced effects of certain antihypertensive agents). Products include:

Nadolol (Enhanced effects of certain antihypertensive agents). Products include:

Nefazodone Hydrochloride (Co-administration with an inhibitor of CYP4503A may reduce oral clearance of quetiapine, resulting in an increase in maximum plasma concentration of quetiapine; dose adjustment of quetiapine will be necessary).

No products indexed under this heading.

Nelfinavir Mesylate (Co-administration with an inhibitor of CYP4503A may reduce oral clearance of quetiapine, resulting in an increase in maximum plasma concentration of quetiapine; dose adjustment of quetiapine will be necessary). Products include:

Nevirapine (Co-administration with an inhibitor of CYP4503A may reduce oral clearance of quetiapine, resulting in an increase in maximum plasma concentration of quetiapine; dose adjustment of quetiapine will be necessary). Products include:

Niacinamide (Co-administration with an inhibitor of CYP4503A may reduce oral clearance of quetiapine, resulting in an increase in maximum plasma concentration of quetiapine; dose adjustment of quetiapine will be necessary).

No products indexed under this heading.

Nicardipine Hydrochloride (Enhanced effects of certain antihypertensive agents). Products include:

Nicotinamide (Co-administration with an inhibitor of CYP4503A may reduce oral clearance of quetiapine, resulting in an increase in maximum plasma concentration of quetiapine; dose adjustment of quetiapine will be necessary). Products include:

Nifedipine (Co-administration with an inhibitor of CYP4503A may reduce oral clearance of quetiapine, resulting in an increase in maximum plasma concentration of quetiapine; dose adjustment of quetiapine will be necessary). Products include:

Nisoldipine (Enhanced effects of certain antihypertensive agents). Products include:

Nitroglycerin (Enhanced effects of certain antihypertensive agents). Products include:

Norfloxacin (Co-administration with an inhibitor of CYP4503A may reduce oral clearance of quetiapine, resulting in an increase in maximum plasma concentration of quetiapine; dose adjustment of quetiapine will be necessary). Products include:

Omeprazole (Co-administration with an inhibitor of CYP4503A may reduce oral clearance of quetiapine, resulting in an increase in maximum plasma concentration of quetiapine; dose adjustment of quetiapine will be necessary). Products include:

Paroxetine Hydrochloride (Co-administration with an inhibitor of CYP4503A may reduce oral clearance of quetiapine, resulting in an increase in maximum plasma concentration of quetiapine; dose adjustment of quetiapine will be necessary). Products include:

Penbutolol Sulfate (Enhanced effects of certain antihypertensive agents).

No products indexed under this heading.

Pentobarbital Sodium (Co-administration with hepatic enzyme inducers, such as barbiturates, may increase oral clearance). Products include:

Pergolide Mesylate (Quetiapine may antagonize the effects of dopamine agonists). Products include:

Perindopril Erbumine (Enhanced effects of certain antihypertensive agents). Products include:

Phenobarbital (Co-administration with hepatic enzyme inducers, such as barbiturates, may increase oral clearance). Products include:

Phenoxybenzamine Hydrochloride (Enhanced effects of certain antihypertensive agents). Products include:

Phentolamine Mesylate (Enhanced effects of certain antihypertensive agents).

No products indexed under this heading.

Phenytoin (Co-administration has resulted in increased mean oral clearance of quetiapine by 5-fold; increased dose of quetiapine may be required).

No products indexed under this heading.

Phenytoin Sodium (Co-administration has resulted in increased mean oral clearance of quetiapine by 5-fold; increased dose of quetiapine may be required). Products include:

Pindolol (Enhanced effects of certain antihypertensive agents).

No products indexed under this heading.

Polythiazide (Enhanced effects of certain antihypertensive agents).

No products indexed under this heading.

Pramipexole Dihydrochloride (Quetiapine may antagonize the effects of dopamine agonists). Products include:

Prazosin Hydrochloride (Enhanced effects of certain antihypertensive agents).

No products indexed under this heading.

Prednisolone Acetate (Co-administration with hepatic enzyme inducers, such as glucocorticosteroids, may increase oral clearance). Products include:

Prednisolone Sodium Phosphate (Co-administration with hepatic enzyme inducers, such as glucocorticosteroids, may increase oral clearance).

No products indexed under this heading.

Prednisolone Tebutate (Co-administration with hepatic enzyme inducers, such as glucocorticosteroids, may increase oral clearance).

No products indexed under this heading.

Prednisone (Co-administration with hepatic enzyme inducers, such as glucocorticosteroids, may increase oral clearance).

No products indexed under this heading.

Propoxyphene Hydrochloride (Co-administration with an inhibitor of CYP4503A may reduce oral clearance of quetiapine, resulting in an increase in maximum plasma concentration of quetiapine; dose adjustment of quetiapine will be necessary).

No products indexed under this heading.

Propoxyphene Napsylate (Co-administration with an inhibitor of CYP4503A may reduce oral clearance of quetiapine, resulting in an increase in maximum plasma concentration of quetiapine; dose adjustment of quetiapine will be necessary).

No products indexed under this heading.

Propranolol Hydrochloride (Enhanced effects of certain antihypertensive agents). Products include:

Quinapril Hydrochloride (Enhanced effects of certain antihypertensive agents).

No products indexed under this heading.

Quinidine (Co-administration with an inhibitor of CYP4503A may reduce oral clearance of quetiapine, resulting in an increase in maximum plasma concentration of quetiapine; dose adjustment of quetiapine will be necessary).

No products indexed under this heading.

Quinidine Hydrochloride (Co-administration with an inhibitor of CYP4503A may reduce oral clearance of quetiapine, resulting in an increase in maximum plasma concentration of quetiapine; dose adjustment of quetiapine will be necessary).

No products indexed under this heading.

Quinidine Polygalacturonate (Co-administration with an inhibitor of CYP4503A may reduce oral clearance of quetiapine, resulting in an increase in maximum plasma concentration of quetiapine; dose adjustment of quetiapine will be necessary).

No products indexed under this heading.

Quinidine Sulfate (Co-administration with an inhibitor of CYP4503A may reduce oral clearance of quetiapine, resulting in an increase in maximum plasma concentration of quetiapine; dose adjustment of quetiapine will be necessary).
No products indexed under this heading.

Quinine (Co-administration with an inhibitor of CYP4503A may reduce oral clearance of quetiapine, resulting in an increase in maximum plasma concentration of quetiapine; dose adjustment of quetiapine will be necessary).
No products indexed under this heading.

Quinine Sulfate (Co-administration with an inhibitor of CYP4503A may reduce oral clearance of quetiapine, resulting in an increase in maximum plasma concentration of quetiapine; dose adjustment of quetiapine will be necessary).
No products indexed under this heading.

Quinupristin (Co-administration with an inhibitor of CYP4503A may reduce oral clearance of quetiapine, resulting in an increase in maximum plasma concentration of quetiapine; dose adjustment of quetiapine will be necessary).
No products indexed under this heading.

Ramipril (Enhanced effects of certain antihypertensive agents). Products include:
Altace Capsules ... 1702

Ranitidine Bismuth Citrate (Co-administration with an inhibitor of CYP4503A may reduce oral clearance of quetiapine, resulting in an increase in maximum plasma concentration of quetiapine; dose adjustment of quetiapine will be necessary).
No products indexed under this heading.

Ranitidine Hydrochloride (Co-administration with an inhibitor of CYP4503A may reduce oral clearance of quetiapine, resulting in an increase in maximum plasma concentration of quetiapine; dose adjustment of quetiapine will be necessary). Products include:
Zantac ... 1624
Zantac Injection ... 1619
Zantac Injection Pharmacy Bulk Package ... 1622

Rauwolfia Serpentina (Enhanced effects of certain antihypertensive agents).
No products indexed under this heading.

Rescinnamine (Enhanced effects of certain antihypertensive agents).
No products indexed under this heading.

Reserpine (Enhanced effects of certain antihypertensive agents).
No products indexed under this heading.

Rifampin (Co-administration with hepatic enzyme inducers, such as rifampin, may increase oral clearance).
No products indexed under this heading.

Ritonavir (Co-administration with an inhibitor of CYP4503A may reduce oral clearance of quetiapine, resulting in an increase in maximum plasma concentration of quetiapine; dose adjustment of quetiapine will be necessary). Products include:
Kaletra ... 476
Norvir ... 503

Ropinirole Hydrochloride (Quetiapine may antagonize the effects of dopamine agonists). Products include:
Requip Tablets ... 1555

Saquinavir (Co-administration with an inhibitor of CYP4503A may reduce oral clearance of quetiapine, resulting in an increase in maximum plasma concentration of quetiapine; dose adjustment of quetiapine will be necessary).
No products indexed under this heading.

Saquinavir Mesylate (Co-administration with an inhibitor of CYP4503A may reduce oral clearance of quetiapine, resulting in an increase in maximum plasma concentration of quetiapine; dose adjustment of quetiapine will be necessary). Products include:
Invirase ... 2772

Secobarbital Sodium (Co-administration with hepatic enzyme inducers, such as barbiturates, may increase oral clearance).
No products indexed under this heading.

Sertraline Hydrochloride (Co-administration with an inhibitor of CYP4503A may reduce oral clearance of quetiapine, resulting in an increase in maximum plasma concentration of quetiapine; dose adjustment of quetiapine will be necessary). Products include:
Zoloft ... 2586

Sodium Nitroprusside (Enhanced effects of certain antihypertensive agents).
No products indexed under this heading.

Sotalol Hydrochloride (Enhanced effects of certain antihypertensive agents).
No products indexed under this heading.

Spirapril Hydrochloride (Enhanced effects of certain antihypertensive agents).
No products indexed under this heading.

Telmisartan (Enhanced effects of certain antihypertensive agents). Products include:
Micardis Tablets ... 854
Micardis HCT Tablets ... 856

Terazosin Hydrochloride (Enhanced effects of certain antihypertensive agents). Products include:
Hytrin Capsules ... 471

Thiamylal Sodium (Co-administration with hepatic enzyme inducers, such as barbiturates, may increase oral clearance).
No products indexed under this heading.

Thioridazine (Increases the oral clearance of quetiapine by 65%).
No products indexed under this heading.

Timolol Maleate (Enhanced effects of certain antihypertensive agents). Products include:
Blocadren Tablets ... 1916
Cosopt Sterile Ophthalmic Solution ... 1931
Timolide Tablets ... 2086
Timoptic Sterile Ophthalmic Solution ... 2088
Timoptic in Ocudose ... 2091
Timoptic-XE Sterile Ophthalmic Gel Forming Solution ... 2092

Torsemide (Enhanced effects of certain antihypertensive agents). Products include:
Demadex Injection ... 2759
Demadex Tablets ... 2759

Trandolapril (Enhanced effects of certain antihypertensive agents). Products include:
Mavik Tablets ... 486
Tarka Tablets ... 524

Triamcinolone (Co-administration with hepatic enzyme inducers, such as glucocorticosteroids, may increase oral clearance).
No products indexed under this heading.

Triamcinolone Acetonide (Co-administration with hepatic enzyme inducers, such as glucocorticosteroids, may increase oral clearance). Products include:
Azmacort Inhalation Aerosol ... 1726
Nasacort AQ Nasal Spray ... 2922

Triamcinolone Diacetate (Co-administration with hepatic enzyme inducers, such as glucocorticosteroids, may increase oral clearance).
No products indexed under this heading.

Triamcinolone Hexacetonide (Co-administration with hepatic enzyme inducers, such as glucocorticosteroids, may increase oral clearance).
No products indexed under this heading.

Trimethaphan Camsylate (Enhanced effects of certain antihypertensive agents).
No products indexed under this heading.

Troglitazone (Co-administration with an inhibitor of CYP4503A may reduce oral clearance of quetiapine, resulting in an increase in maximum plasma concentration of quetiapine; dose adjustment of quetiapine will be necessary).
No products indexed under this heading.

Troleandomycin (Co-administration with an inhibitor of CYP4503A may reduce oral clearance of quetiapine, resulting in an increase in maximum plasma concentration of quetiapine; dose adjustment of quetiapine will be necessary).
No products indexed under this heading.

Valproate Sodium (Co-administration with an inhibitor of CYP4503A may reduce oral clearance of quetiapine, resulting in an increase in maximum plasma concentration of quetiapine; dose adjustment of quetiapine will be necessary). Products include:
Depacon Injection ... 412

Valsartan (Enhanced effects of certain antihypertensive agents). Products include:
Diovan Tablets ... 2193
Diovan HCT Tablets ... 2196

Verapamil Hydrochloride (Co-administration with an inhibitor of CYP4503A may reduce oral clearance of quetiapine, resulting in an increase in maximum plasma concentration of quetiapine; dose adjustment of quetiapine will be necessary). Products include:
Covera-HS Tablets ... 3139
Tarka Tablets ... 524
Verelan PM Extended-Release Capsules, Controlled-Onset ... 3106

Voriconazole (Co-administration with an inhibitor of CYP4503A may reduce oral clearance of quetiapine, resulting in an increase in maximum plasma concentration of quetiapine; dose adjustment of quetiapine will be necessary). Products include:
VFEND I.V. ... 2564
VFEND Oral Suspension ... 2564
VFEND Tablets ... 2564

Zafirlukast (Co-administration with an inhibitor of CYP4503A may reduce oral clearance of quetiapine, resulting in an increase in maximum plasma concentration of quetiapine; dose adjustment of quetiapine will be necessary). Products include:
Accolate Tablets ... 671

Zileuton (Co-administration with an inhibitor of CYP4503A may reduce oral clearance of quetiapine, resulting in an increase in maximum plasma concentration of quetiapine; dose adjustment of quetiapine will be necessary). Products include:
Zyflo Tablets ... 1023

Food Interactions

Alcohol (The cognitive and motor effect of alcohol is potentiated; alcohol use should be avoided).

Food, unspecified (The bioavailability of quetiapine is marginally affected by administration with food, with Cmax and AUC values increased by 25% and 15%, respectively).

Grapefruit (Co-administration with an inhibitor of CYP4503A may reduce oral clearance of quetiapine, resulting in an increase in maximum plasma concentration of quetiapine; dose adjustment of quetiapine will be necessary).

Grapefruit Juice (Co-administration with an inhibitor of CYP4503A may reduce oral clearance of quetiapine, resulting in an increase in maximum plasma concentration of quetiapine; dose adjustment of quetiapine will be necessary).

SIMPLY SLEEP CAPLETS

(Diphenhydramine Hydrochloride) ... 1868
May interact with hypnotics and sedatives, tranquilizers, and certain other agents. Compounds in these categories include:

Alprazolam (Diphenhydramine is an antihistamine with sedative properties; concurrent use should be avoided). Products include:
Niravam Orally Disintegrating Tablets ... 3092

Buspirone Hydrochloride (Diphenhydramine is an antihistamine with sedative properties; concurrent use should be avoided).
No products indexed under this heading.

Chlordiazepoxide (Diphenhydramine is an antihistamine with sedative properties; concurrent use should be avoided).
No products indexed under this heading.

Chlordiazepoxide Hydrochloride (Diphenhydramine is an antihistamine with sedative properties; concurrent use should be avoided). Products include:
Librium Capsules ... 3347

Chlorpromazine (Diphenhydramine is an antihistamine with sedative properties; concurrent use should be avoided).
No products indexed under this heading.

Chlorpromazine Hydrochloride (Diphenhydramine is an antihistamine with sedative properties; concurrent use should be avoided).
No products indexed under this heading.

Chlorprothixene (Diphenhydramine is an antihistamine with sedative properties; concurrent use should be avoided).
No products indexed under this heading.

Chlorprothixene Hydrochloride (Diphenhydramine is an antihistamine with sedative properties; concurrent use should be avoided).
No products indexed under this heading.

Clorazepate Dipotassium (Diphenhydramine is an antihistamine with sedative properties; concurrent use should be avoided). Products include:
Tranxene 2474

Diazepam (Diphenhydramine is an antihistamine with sedative properties; concurrent use should be avoided). Products include:
Diastat Rectal Delivery System 3343
Valium Tablets 2819

Droperidol (Diphenhydramine is an antihistamine with sedative properties; concurrent use should be avoided).
No products indexed under this heading.

Estazolam (Diphenhydramine is an antihistamine with sedative properties; concurrent use should be avoided). Products include:
ProSom Tablets 517

Ethchlorvynol (Diphenhydramine is an antihistamine with sedative properties; concurrent use should be avoided).
No products indexed under this heading.

Ethinamate (Diphenhydramine is an antihistamine with sedative properties; concurrent use should be avoided).
No products indexed under this heading.

Fluphenazine Decanoate (Diphenhydramine is an antihistamine with sedative properties; concurrent use should be avoided).
No products indexed under this heading.

Fluphenazine Enanthate (Diphenhydramine is an antihistamine with sedative properties; concurrent use should be avoided).
No products indexed under this heading.

Fluphenazine Hydrochloride (Diphenhydramine is an antihistamine with sedative properties; concurrent use should be avoided).
No products indexed under this heading.

Flurazepam Hydrochloride (Diphenhydramine is an antihistamine with sedative properties; concurrent use should be avoided). Products include:
Dalmane Capsules 3342

Glutethimide (Diphenhydramine is an antihistamine with sedative properties; concurrent use should be avoided).
No products indexed under this heading.

Haloperidol (Diphenhydramine is an antihistamine with sedative properties; concurrent use should be avoided).
No products indexed under this heading.

Haloperidol Decanoate (Diphenhydramine is an antihistamine with sedative properties; concurrent use should be avoided).
No products indexed under this heading.

Hydroxyzine Hydrochloride (Diphenhydramine is an antihistamine with sedative properties; concurrent use should be avoided).
No products indexed under this heading.

Lorazepam (Diphenhydramine is an antihistamine with sedative properties; concurrent use should be avoided).
No products indexed under this heading.

Loxapine Hydrochloride (Diphenhydramine is an antihistamine with sedative properties; concurrent use should be avoided).
No products indexed under this heading.

Loxapine Succinate (Diphenhydramine is an antihistamine with sedative properties; concurrent use should be avoided).
No products indexed under this heading.

Meprobamate (Diphenhydramine is an antihistamine with sedative properties; concurrent use should be avoided).
No products indexed under this heading.

Mesoridazine Besylate (Diphenhydramine is an antihistamine with sedative properties; concurrent use should be avoided).
No products indexed under this heading.

Midazolam Hydrochloride (Diphenhydramine is an antihistamine with sedative properties; concurrent use should be avoided).
No products indexed under this heading.

Molindone Hydrochloride (Diphenhydramine is an antihistamine with sedative properties; concurrent use should be avoided). Products include:
Moban Tablets 1119

Oxazepam (Diphenhydramine is an antihistamine with sedative properties; concurrent use should be avoided).
No products indexed under this heading.

Perphenazine (Diphenhydramine is an antihistamine with sedative properties; concurrent use should be avoided).
No products indexed under this heading.

Prazepam (Diphenhydramine is an antihistamine with sedative properties; concurrent use should be avoided).
No products indexed under this heading.

Prochlorperazine (Diphenhydramine is an antihistamine with sedative properties; concurrent use should be avoided).
No products indexed under this heading.

Promethazine Hydrochloride (Diphenhydramine is an antihistamine with sedative properties; concurrent use should be avoided). Products include:
Phenergan Tablets and Suppositories 3440

Propofol (Diphenhydramine is an antihistamine with sedative properties; concurrent use should be avoided).
No products indexed under this heading.

Quazepam (Diphenhydramine is an antihistamine with sedative properties; concurrent use should be avoided).
No products indexed under this heading.

Ramelteon (Diphenhydramine is an antihistamine with sedative properties; concurrent use should be avoided). Products include:
Rozerem Tablets 3231

Secobarbital Sodium (Diphenhydramine is an antihistamine with sedative properties; concurrent use should be avoided).
No products indexed under this heading.

Temazepam (Diphenhydramine is an antihistamine with sedative properties; concurrent use should be avoided). Products include:
Restoril Capsules 1860

Thioridazine Hydrochloride (Diphenhydramine is an antihistamine with sedative properties; concurrent use should be avoided). Products include:
Thioridazine Hydrochloride Tablets 2163

Thiothixene (Diphenhydramine is an antihistamine with sedative properties; concurrent use should be avoided). Products include:
Thiothixene Capsules 2165

Triazolam (Diphenhydramine is an antihistamine with sedative properties; concurrent use should be avoided).
No products indexed under this heading.

Trifluoperazine Hydrochloride (Diphenhydramine is an antihistamine with sedative properties; concurrent use should be avoided).
No products indexed under this heading.

Zaleplon (Diphenhydramine is an antihistamine with sedative properties; concurrent use should be avoided). Products include:
Sonata Capsules 1717

Zolpidem Tartrate (Diphenhydramine is an antihistamine with sedative properties; concurrent use should be avoided). Products include:
Ambien Tablets 2851
Ambien CR Tablets 2855

Food Interactions

Alcohol (Diphenhydramine is an antihistamine with sedative properties; concurrent use with alcoholic beverages should be avoided).

SIMULECT FOR INJECTION

(Basiliximab) 2284
None cited in PDR database.

SINGULAIR TABLETS

(Montelukast Sodium) 2077
May interact with cytochrome p450 2c8 substrates (selected) and certain other agents. Compounds in these categories include:

Amiodarone Hydrochloride (Montelukast is a potent inhibitor of P450 2C8, but no in vivo drug interaction studies have been conducted between montelukast and cytochrome P450 2C8 substrates. Caution should be exercised when concomitantly administering a cytochrome P450 2C8 substrate).
No products indexed under this heading.

Amitriptyline Hydrochloride (Montelukast is a potent inhibitor of P450 2C8, but no in vivo drug interaction studies have been conducted between montelukast and cytochrome P450 2C8 substrates. Caution should be exercised when concomitantly administering a cytochrome P450 2C8 substrate).
No products indexed under this heading.

Amoxapine (Montelukast is a potent inhibitor of P450 2C8, but no in vivo drug interaction studies have been conducted between montelukast and cytochrome P450 2C8 substrates. Caution should be exercised when concomitantly administering a cytochrome P450 2C8 substrate).
No products indexed under this heading.

Benzphetamine Hydrochloride (Montelukast is a potent inhibitor of P450 2C8, but no in vivo drug interaction studies have been conducted between montelukast and cytochrome P450 2C8 substrates. Caution should be exercised when concomitantly administering a cytochrome P450 2C8 substrate).
No products indexed under this heading.

Carbamazepine (Montelukast is a potent inhibitor of P450 2C8, but no in vivo drug interaction studies have been conducted between montelukast and cytochrome P450 2C8 substrates. Caution should be exercised when concomitantly administering a cytochrome P450 2C8 substrate). Products include:
Carbatrol Capsules 3171
Equetro Extended-Release Capsules 3180
Tegretol/Tegretol-XR 2295

Clomipramine Hydrochloride (Montelukast is a potent inhibitor of P450 2C8, but no in vivo drug interaction studies have been conducted between montelukast and cytochrome P450 2C8 substrates. Caution should be exercised when concomitantly administering a cytochrome P450 2C8 substrate).
No products indexed under this heading.

Desipramine Hydrochloride (Montelukast is a potent inhibitor of P450 2C8, but no in vivo drug interaction studies have been conducted between montelukast and cytochrome P450 2C8 substrates. Caution should be exercised when concomitantly administering a cytochrome P450 2C8 substrate).
No products indexed under this heading.

Diazepam (Montelukast is a potent inhibitor of P450 2C8, but no in vivo drug interaction studies have been conducted between montelukast and cytochrome P450 2C8 substrates. Caution should be exercised when concomitantly administering a cytochrome P450 2C8 substrate). Products include:

Diclofenac Potassium (Montelukast is a potent inhibitor of P450 2C8, but no in vivo drug interaction studies have been conducted between montelukast and cytochrome P450 2C8 substrates. Caution should be exercised when concomitantly administering a cytochrome P450 2C8 substrate).

No products indexed under this heading.

Diclofenac Sodium (Montelukast is a potent inhibitor of P450 2C8, but no in vivo drug interaction studies have been conducted between montelukast and cytochrome P450 2C8 substrates. Caution should be exercised when concomitantly administering a cytochrome P450 2C8 substrate). Products include:

Docetaxel (Montelukast is a potent inhibitor of P450 2C8, but no in vivo drug interaction studies have been conducted between montelukast and cytochrome P450 2C8 substrates. Caution should be exercised when concomitantly administering a cytochrome P450 2C8 substrate). Products include:

Doxepin Hydrochloride (Montelukast is a potent inhibitor of P450 2C8, but no in vivo drug interaction studies have been conducted between montelukast and cytochrome P450 2C8 substrates. Caution should be exercised when concomitantly administering a cytochrome P450 2C8 substrate).

No products indexed under this heading.

Fluvastatin Sodium (Montelukast is a potent inhibitor of P450 2C8, but no in vivo drug interaction studies have been conducted between montelukast and cytochrome P450 2C8 substrates. Caution should be exercised when concomitantly administering a cytochrome P450 2C8 substrate). Products include:

Imipramine Hydrochloride (Montelukast is a potent inhibitor of P450 2C8, but no in vivo drug interaction studies have been conducted between montelukast and cytochrome P450 2C8 substrates. Caution should be exercised when concomitantly administering a cytochrome P450 2C8 substrate).

No products indexed under this heading.

Imipramine Pamoate (Montelukast is a potent inhibitor of P450 2C8, but no in vivo drug interaction studies have been conducted between montelukast and cytochrome P450 2C8 substrates. Caution should be exercised when concomitantly administering a cytochrome P450 2C8 substrate).

No products indexed under this heading.

Isotretinoin (Montelukast is a potent inhibitor of P450 2C8, but no in vivo drug interaction studies have been conducted between montelukast and cytochrome P450 2C8 substrates. Caution should be exercised when concomitantly administering a cytochrome P450 2C8 substrate). Products include:

Maprotiline Hydrochloride (Montelukast is a potent inhibitor of P450 2C8, but no in vivo drug interaction studies have been conducted between montelukast and cytochrome P450 2C8 substrates. Caution should be exercised when concomitantly administering a cytochrome P450 2C8 substrate).

No products indexed under this heading.

Mephobarbital (Montelukast is a potent inhibitor of P450 2C8, but no in vivo drug interaction studies have been conducted between montelukast and cytochrome P450 2C8 substrates. Caution should be exercised when concomitantly administering a cytochrome P450 2C8 substrate).

No products indexed under this heading.

Nortriptyline Hydrochloride (Montelukast is a potent inhibitor of P450 2C8, but no in vivo drug interaction studies have been conducted between montelukast and cytochrome P450 2C8 substrates. Caution should be exercised when concomitantly administering a cytochrome P450 2C8 substrate).

No products indexed under this heading.

Omeprazole (Montelukast is a potent inhibitor of P450 2C8, but no in vivo drug interaction studies have been conducted between montelukast and cytochrome P450 2C8 substrates. Caution should be exercised when concomitantly administering a cytochrome P450 2C8 substrate). Products include:

Paclitaxel (Montelukast is a potent inhibitor of P450 2C8, but no in vivo drug interaction studies have been conducted between montelukast and cytochrome P450 2C8 substrates. Caution should be exercised when concomitantly administering a cytochrome P450 2C8 substrate).

No products indexed under this heading.

Phenobarbital (Induces hepatic metabolism and decreases the AUC of montelukast approximately 40%; no dosage adjustment for Singulair is recommended). Products include:

Phenytoin (Montelukast is a potent inhibitor of P450 2C8, but no in vivo drug interaction studies have been conducted between montelukast and cytochrome P450 2C8 substrates. Caution should be exercised when concomitantly administering a cytochrome P450 2C8 substrate).

No products indexed under this heading.

Phenytoin Sodium (Montelukast is a potent inhibitor of P450 2C8, but no in vivo drug interaction studies have been conducted between montelukast and cytochrome P450 2C8 substrates. Caution should be exer-

cised when concomitantly administering a cytochrome P450 2C8 substrate). Products include:

Pioglitazone Hydrochloride (Montelukast is a potent inhibitor of P450 2C8, but no in vivo drug interaction studies have been conducted between montelukast and cytochrome P450 2C8 substrates. Caution should be exercised when concomitantly administering a cytochrome P450 2C8 substrate). Products include:

Protriptyline Hydrochloride (Montelukast is a potent inhibitor of P450 2C8, but no in vivo drug interaction studies have been conducted between montelukast and cytochrome P450 2C8 substrates. Caution should be exercised when concomitantly administering a cytochrome P450 2C8 substrate).

No products indexed under this heading.

Repaglinide (Montelukast is a potent inhibitor of P450 2C8, but no in vivo drug interaction studies have been conducted between montelukast and cytochrome P450 2C8 substrates. Caution should be exercised when concomitantly administering a cytochrome P450 2C8 substrate).

No products indexed under this heading.

Rifampin (Co-administration with CYP450 enzyme inducers, such as rifampin, may alter metabolism of montelukast; it is reasonable to employ appropriate clinical monitoring).

No products indexed under this heading.

Rosiglitazone Maleate (Montelukast is a potent inhibitor of P450 2C8, but no in vivo drug interaction studies have been conducted between montelukast and cytochrome P450 2C8 substrates. Caution should be exercised when concomitantly administering a cytochrome P450 2C8 substrate). Products include:

Rosiglitazone/Metformin (Montelukast is a potent inhibitor of P450 2C8, but no in vivo drug interaction studies have been conducted between montelukast and cytochrome P450 2C8 substrates. Caution should be exercised when concomitantly administering a cytochrome P450 2C8 substrate).

No products indexed under this heading.

Tolbutamide (Montelukast is a potent inhibitor of P450 2C8, but no in vivo drug interaction studies have been conducted between montelukast and cytochrome P450 2C8 substrates. Caution should be exercised when concomitantly administering a cytochrome P450 2C8 substrate).

No products indexed under this heading.

Tolbutamide Sodium (Montelukast is a potent inhibitor of P450 2C8, but no in vivo drug interaction studies have been conducted between montelukast and cytochrome P450 2C8 substrates. Caution should be exercised when concomitantly administering a cytochrome P450 2C8 substrate).

No products indexed under this heading.

Tretinoin (Montelukast is a potent inhibitor of P450 2C8, but no in vivo drug interaction studies have been conducted between montelukast and cytochrome P450 2C8 substrates. Caution should be exercised when concomitantly administering a cytochrome P450 2C8 substrate). Products include:

Trimipramine Maleate (Montelukast is a potent inhibitor of P450 2C8, but no in vivo drug interaction studies have been conducted between montelukast and cytochrome P450 2C8 substrates. Caution should be exercised when concomitantly administering a cytochrome P450 2C8 substrate).

No products indexed under this heading.

Verapamil Hydrochloride (Montelukast is a potent inhibitor of P450 2C8, but no in vivo drug interaction studies have been conducted between montelukast and cytochrome P450 2C8 substrates. Caution should be exercised when concomitantly administering a cytochrome P450 2C8 substrate). Products include:

Vitamin A (Montelukast is a potent inhibitor of P450 2C8, but no in vivo drug interaction studies have been conducted between montelukast and cytochrome P450 2C8 substrates. Caution should be exercised when concomitantly administering a cytochrome P450 2C8 substrate). Products include:

Vitamin A Acetate (Montelukast is a potent inhibitor of P450 2C8, but no in vivo drug interaction studies have been conducted between montelukast and cytochrome P450 2C8 substrates. Caution should be exercised when concomitantly administering a cytochrome P450 2C8 substrate).

No products indexed under this heading.

Warfarin Sodium (Montelukast is a potent inhibitor of P450 2C8, but no in vivo drug interaction studies have been conducted between montelukast and cytochrome P450 2C8 substrates. Caution should be exercised when concomitantly administering a cytochrome P450 2C8 substrate). Products include:

Zopiclone (Montelukast is a potent inhibitor of P450 2C8, but no in vivo drug interaction studies have been conducted between montelukast and cytochrome P450 2C8 substrates. Caution should be exercised when concomitantly administering a cytochrome P450 2C8 substrate).

No products indexed under this heading.

IMPORTANT NOTE: Always consult each drug listing in the patient's regimen for possible interactions.

SINGULAIR CHEWABLE TABLETS

(Montelukast Sodium) 2077
See Singulair Tablets

SINGULAIR ORAL GRANULES

(Montelukast Sodium) 2077
See Singulair Tablets

SKELAXIN TABLETS

(Metaxalone) 1716
May interact with barbiturates, central nervous system depressants, and certain other agents. Compounds in these categories include:

Alfentanil Hydrochloride (Skelaxin may enhance the effects of alcohol, barbiturates and other CNS depressants).
No products indexed under this heading.

Alprazolam (Skelaxin may enhance the effects of alcohol, barbiturates and other CNS depressants). Products include:
Niravam Orally Disintegrating Tablets 3092

Aprobarbital (Skelaxin may enhance the effects of alcohol, barbiturates and other CNS depressants).
No products indexed under this heading.

Buprenorphine Hydrochloride (Skelaxin may enhance the effects of alcohol, barbiturates and other CNS depressants). Products include:
Buprenex Injectable 2716
Suboxone Tablets 2717
Subutex Tablets 2717

Buspirone Hydrochloride (Skelaxin may enhance the effects of alcohol, barbiturates and other CNS depressants).
No products indexed under this heading.

Butabarbital (Skelaxin may enhance the effects of alcohol, barbiturates and other CNS depressants).
No products indexed under this heading.

Butalbital (Skelaxin may enhance the effects of alcohol, barbiturates and other CNS depressants).
No products indexed under this heading.

Chlordiazepoxide (Skelaxin may enhance the effects of alcohol, barbiturates and other CNS depressants).
No products indexed under this heading.

Chlordiazepoxide Hydrochloride (Skelaxin may enhance the effects of alcohol, barbiturates and other CNS depressants). Products include:
Librium Capsules 3347

Chlorpromazine (Skelaxin may enhance the effects of alcohol, barbiturates and other CNS depressants).
No products indexed under this heading.

Chlorpromazine Hydrochloride (Skelaxin may enhance the effects of alcohol, barbiturates and other CNS depressants).
No products indexed under this heading.

Chlorprothixene (Skelaxin may enhance the effects of alcohol, barbiturates and other CNS depressants).
No products indexed under this heading.

Chlorprothixene Hydrochloride (Skelaxin may enhance the effects of alcohol, barbiturates and other CNS depressants).
No products indexed under this heading.

Chlorprothixene Lactate (Skelaxin may enhance the effects of alcohol, barbiturates and other CNS depressants).
No products indexed under this heading.

Clorazepate Dipotassium (Skelaxin may enhance the effects of alcohol, barbiturates and other CNS depressants). Products include:
Tranxene 2474

Clozapine (Skelaxin may enhance the effects of alcohol, barbiturates and other CNS depressants). Products include:
Clozaril Tablets 2184
FazaClo Orally Disintegrating Tablets 551

Codeine Phosphate (Skelaxin may enhance the effects of alcohol, barbiturates and other CNS depressants). Products include:
Tylenol with Codeine Tablets 2391

Desflurane (Skelaxin may enhance the effects of alcohol, barbiturates and other CNS depressants).
No products indexed under this heading.

Dezocine (Skelaxin may enhance the effects of alcohol, barbiturates and other CNS depressants).
No products indexed under this heading.

Diazepam (Skelaxin may enhance the effects of alcohol, barbiturates and other CNS depressants). Products include:
Diastat Rectal Delivery System 3343
Valium Tablets 2819

Droperidol (Skelaxin may enhance the effects of alcohol, barbiturates and other CNS depressants).
No products indexed under this heading.

Enflurane (Skelaxin may enhance the effects of alcohol, barbiturates and other CNS depressants).
No products indexed under this heading.

Estazolam (Skelaxin may enhance the effects of alcohol, barbiturates and other CNS depressants). Products include:
ProSom Tablets 517

Ethanol (Skelaxin may enhance the effects of alcohol, barbiturates and other CNS depressants).
No products indexed under this heading.

Ethchlorvynol (Skelaxin may enhance the effects of alcohol, barbiturates and other CNS depressants).
No products indexed under this heading.

Ethinamate (Skelaxin may enhance the effects of alcohol, barbiturates and other CNS depressants).
No products indexed under this heading.

Ethyl Alcohol (Skelaxin may enhance the effects of alcohol, barbiturates and other CNS depressants).
No products indexed under this heading.

Fentanyl (Skelaxin may enhance the effects of alcohol, barbiturates and other CNS depressants). Products include:
Duragesic Transdermal System 2373
Ionsys Transdermal System 2379

Fentanyl Citrate (Skelaxin may enhance the effects of alcohol, barbiturates and other CNS depressants). Products include:
Actiq 979

Fluphenazine Decanoate (Skelaxin may enhance the effects of alcohol, barbiturates and other CNS depressants).
No products indexed under this heading.

Fluphenazine Enanthate (Skelaxin may enhance the effects of alcohol, barbiturates and other CNS depressants).
No products indexed under this heading.

Fluphenazine Hydrochloride (Skelaxin may enhance the effects of alcohol, barbiturates and other CNS depressants).
No products indexed under this heading.

Flurazepam Hydrochloride (Skelaxin may enhance the effects of alcohol, barbiturates and other CNS depressants). Products include:
Dalmane Capsules 3342

Glutethimide (Skelaxin may enhance the effects of alcohol, barbiturates and other CNS depressants).
No products indexed under this heading.

Haloperidol (Skelaxin may enhance the effects of alcohol, barbiturates and other CNS depressants).
No products indexed under this heading.

Haloperidol Decanoate (Skelaxin may enhance the effects of alcohol, barbiturates and other CNS depressants).
No products indexed under this heading.

Hydrocodone Bitartrate (Skelaxin may enhance the effects of alcohol, barbiturates and other CNS depressants). Products include:
Hycodan 1116
Hycotuss Expectorant Syrup 1117
Vicodin Tablets 535
Vicodin ES Tablets 536
Vicodin HP Tablets 538
Vicoprofen Tablets 539
Zydone Tablets 1139

Hydrocodone Polistirex (Skelaxin may enhance the effects of alcohol, barbiturates and other CNS depressants). Products include:
Tussionex Pennkinetic Extended-Release Suspension 3327

Hydromorphone Hydrochloride (Skelaxin may enhance the effects of alcohol, barbiturates and other CNS depressants). Products include:
Dilaudid 440
Dilaudid Non-Sterile Powder 440
Dilaudid Oral Liquid 445
Dilaudid Rectal Suppositories 440
Dilaudid Tablets 440
Dilaudid Tablets - 8 mg 445
Dilaudid-HP 442

Hydroxyzine Hydrochloride (Skelaxin may enhance the effects of alcohol, barbiturates and other CNS depressants).
No products indexed under this heading.

Isoflurane (Skelaxin may enhance the effects of alcohol, barbiturates and other CNS depressants).
No products indexed under this heading.

Ketamine Hydrochloride (Skelaxin may enhance the effects of alcohol, barbiturates and other CNS depressants).
No products indexed under this heading.

Levomethadyl Acetate Hydrochloride (Skelaxin may enhance the effects of alcohol, barbiturates and other CNS depressants).
No products indexed under this heading.

Levorphanol Tartrate (Skelaxin may enhance the effects of alcohol, barbiturates and other CNS depressants).
No products indexed under this heading.

Lorazepam (Skelaxin may enhance the effects of alcohol, barbiturates and other CNS depressants).
No products indexed under this heading.

Loxapine Hydrochloride (Skelaxin may enhance the effects of alcohol, barbiturates and other CNS depressants).
No products indexed under this heading.

Loxapine Succinate (Skelaxin may enhance the effects of alcohol, barbiturates and other CNS depressants).
No products indexed under this heading.

Meperidine Hydrochloride (Skelaxin may enhance the effects of alcohol, barbiturates and other CNS depressants).
No products indexed under this heading.

Mephobarbital (Skelaxin may enhance the effects of alcohol, barbiturates and other CNS depressants).
No products indexed under this heading.

Meprobamate (Skelaxin may enhance the effects of alcohol, barbiturates and other CNS depressants).
No products indexed under this heading.

Mesoridazine Besylate (Skelaxin may enhance the effects of alcohol, barbiturates and other CNS depressants).
No products indexed under this heading.

Methadone Hydrochloride (Skelaxin may enhance the effects of alcohol, barbiturates and other CNS depressants).
No products indexed under this heading.

Methohexital Sodium (Skelaxin may enhance the effects of alcohol, barbiturates and other CNS depressants).
No products indexed under this heading.

Methotrimeprazine (Skelaxin may enhance the effects of alcohol, barbiturates and other CNS depressants).
No products indexed under this heading.

Methoxyflurane (Skelaxin may enhance the effects of alcohol, barbiturates and other CNS depressants).
No products indexed under this heading.

Midazolam Hydrochloride (Skelaxin may enhance the effects of alcohol, barbiturates and other CNS depressants).
No products indexed under this heading.

Molindone Hydrochloride (Skelaxin may enhance the effects of alcohol, barbiturates and other CNS depressants). Products include:
Moban Tablets 1119

Morphine Sulfate (Skelaxin may enhance the effects of alcohol, barbiturates and other CNS depressants). Products include:
Avinza Capsules 1741
Kadian Capsules 577
MS Contin Tablets 2701

Olanzapine (Skelaxin may enhance the effects of alcohol, barbiturates and other CNS depressants). Products include:
Symbyax Capsules 1819
Zyprexa Tablets 1830
Zyprexa IntraMuscular 1830
Zyprexa ZYDIS Orally Disintegrating Tablets 1830

Oxazepam (Skelaxin may enhance the effects of alcohol, barbiturates and other CNS depressants).
No products indexed under this heading.

Oxycodone Hydrochloride (Skelaxin may enhance the effects of alcohol, barbiturates and other CNS depressants). Products include:
OxyContin Tablets 2703
OxyFast Oral Concentrate Solution 2708
OxyIR Capsules 2708
Percocet Tablets 1131
Percodan Tablets 1132

Pentobarbital Sodium (Skelaxin may enhance the effects of alcohol, barbiturates and other CNS depressants). Products include:
Nembutal Sodium Solution, USP 2470

Perphenazine (Skelaxin may enhance the effects of alcohol, barbiturates and other CNS depressants).
No products indexed under this heading.

Phenobarbital (Skelaxin may enhance the effects of alcohol, barbiturates and other CNS depressants). Products include:
Donnatal Extentabs 2493

Prazepam (Skelaxin may enhance the effects of alcohol, barbiturates and other CNS depressants).
No products indexed under this heading.

Prochlorperazine (Skelaxin may enhance the effects of alcohol, barbiturates and other CNS depressants).
No products indexed under this heading.

Promethazine Hydrochloride (Skelaxin may enhance the effects of alcohol, barbiturates and other CNS depressants). Products include:
Phenergan Tablets and Suppositories 3440

Propofol (Skelaxin may enhance the effects of alcohol, barbiturates and other CNS depressants).
No products indexed under this heading.

Propoxyphene Hydrochloride (Skelaxin may enhance the effects of alcohol, barbiturates and other CNS depressants).
No products indexed under this heading.

Propoxyphene Napsylate (Skelaxin may enhance the effects of alcohol, barbiturates and other CNS depressants).
No products indexed under this heading.

Quazepam (Skelaxin may enhance the effects of alcohol, barbiturates and other CNS depressants).
No products indexed under this heading.

Quetiapine Fumarate (Skelaxin may enhance the effects of alcohol, barbiturates and other CNS depressants). Products include:
Seroquel Tablets 690

Remifentanil Hydrochloride (Skelaxin may enhance the effects of alcohol, barbiturates and other CNS depressants).
No products indexed under this heading.

Risperidone (Skelaxin may enhance the effects of alcohol, barbiturates and other CNS depressants). Products include:
Risperdal 1676
Risperdal Consta Long-Acting Injection 1682
Risperdal M-Tab Orally Disintegrating Tablets 1676

Secobarbital Sodium (Skelaxin may enhance the effects of alcohol, barbiturates and other CNS depressants).
No products indexed under this heading.

Sevoflurane (Skelaxin may enhance the effects of alcohol, barbiturates and other CNS depressants). Products include:
Ultane Liquid for Inhalation 531

Sodium Oxybate (Skelaxin may enhance the effects of alcohol, barbiturates and other CNS depressants). Products include:
Xyrem Oral Solution 1688

Sufentanil Citrate (Skelaxin may enhance the effects of alcohol, barbiturates and other CNS depressants).
No products indexed under this heading.

Temazepam (Skelaxin may enhance the effects of alcohol, barbiturates and other CNS depressants). Products include:
Restoril Capsules 1860

Thiamylal Sodium (Skelaxin may enhance the effects of alcohol, barbiturates and other CNS depressants).
No products indexed under this heading.

Thioridazine Hydrochloride (Skelaxin may enhance the effects of alcohol, barbiturates and other CNS depressants). Products include:
Thioridazine Hydrochloride Tablets 2163

Thiothixene (Skelaxin may enhance the effects of alcohol, barbiturates and other CNS depressants). Products include:
Thiothixene Capsules 2165

Triazolam (Skelaxin may enhance the effects of alcohol, barbiturates and other CNS depressants).
No products indexed under this heading.

Trifluoperazine Hydrochloride (Skelaxin may enhance the effects of alcohol, barbiturates and other CNS depressants).
No products indexed under this heading.

Zaleplon (Skelaxin may enhance the effects of alcohol, barbiturates and other CNS depressants). Products include:
Sonata Capsules 1717

Ziprasidone Hydrochloride (Skelaxin may enhance the effects of alcohol, barbiturates and other CNS depressants). Products include:
Geodon Capsules 2529

Zolpidem Tartrate (Skelaxin may enhance the effects of alcohol, barbiturates and other CNS depressants). Products include:
Ambien Tablets 2851
Ambien CR Tablets 2855

Food Interactions

Alcohol (Skelaxin may enhance the effects of alcohol, barbiturates and other CNS depressants).

SLEEP-TITE CAPLETS

(Herbals, Multiple, Kava-Kava, Valeriana officinalis) 832
May interact with monoamine oxidase inhibitors and certain other agents. Compounds in these categories include:

Isocarboxazid (Concurrent use with monoamine oxidase inhibitors is not recommended).
No products indexed under this heading.

Moclobemide (Concurrent use with monoamine oxidase inhibitors is not recommended).
No products indexed under this heading.

Pargyline Hydrochloride (Concurrent use with monoamine oxidase inhibitors is not recommended).
No products indexed under this heading.

Phenelzine Sulfate (Concurrent use with monoamine oxidase inhibitors is not recommended).
No products indexed under this heading.

Procarbazine Hydrochloride (Concurrent use with monoamine oxidase inhibitors is not recommended). Products include:
Matulane Capsules 3191

Selegiline Hydrochloride (Concurrent use with monoamine oxidase inhibitors is not recommended). Products include:
Eldepryl Capsules 3208
Zelapar Tablets 3372

Tranylcypromine Sulfate (Concurrent use with monoamine oxidase inhibitors is not recommended). Products include:
Parnate Tablets 1527

Food Interactions

Alcohol (Concurrent use is not recommended).

SLOW FE IRON TABLETS

(Ferrous Sulfate) 818
May interact with tetracyclines and certain other agents. Compounds in these categories include:

Demeclocycline Hydrochloride (Absorption of oral tetracycline impaired).
No products indexed under this heading.

Doxycycline Calcium (Absorption of oral tetracycline impaired).
No products indexed under this heading.

Doxycycline Hyclate (Absorption of oral tetracycline impaired).
No products indexed under this heading.

Doxycycline Monohydrate (Absorption of oral tetracycline impaired). Products include:
Oracea Capsules 1000

Methacycline Hydrochloride (Absorption of oral tetracycline impaired).
No products indexed under this heading.

Minocycline Hydrochloride (Absorption of oral tetracycline impaired). Products include:
Solodyn Extended Release Tablets 1890

Oxytetracycline (Absorption of oral tetracycline impaired).
No products indexed under this heading.

Oxytetracycline Hydrochloride (Absorption of oral tetracycline impaired).
No products indexed under this heading.

Tetracycline Hydrochloride (Absorption of oral tetracycline impaired).
No products indexed under this heading.

SLOW FE WITH FOLIC ACID TABLETS

(Ferrous Sulfate, Folic Acid) 819
May interact with tetracyclines. Compounds in these categories include:

Demeclocycline Hydrochloride (Oral iron products interfere with oral absorption of tetracycline; do not take within two hours of each other).
No products indexed under this heading.

Doxycycline Calcium (Oral iron products interfere with oral absorption of tetracycline; do not take within two hours of each other).
No products indexed under this heading.

Doxycycline Hyclate (Oral iron products interfere with oral absorption of tetracycline; do not take within two hours of each other).
No products indexed under this heading.

Doxycycline Monohydrate (Oral iron products interfere with oral absorption of tetracycline; do not take within two hours of each other). Products include:
Oracea Capsules 1000

Methacycline Hydrochloride (Oral iron products interfere with oral absorption of tetracycline; do not take within two hours of each other).
No products indexed under this heading.

Minocycline Hydrochloride (Oral iron products interfere with oral absorption of tetracycline; do not take within two hours of each other). Products include:
Solodyn Extended Release Tablets 1890

Oxytetracycline Hydrochloride (Oral iron products interfere with oral absorption of tetracycline; do not take within two hours of each other).
No products indexed under this heading.

Tetracycline Hydrochloride (Oral iron products interfere with oral absorption of tetracycline; do not take within two hours of each other).
No products indexed under this heading.

SMILE'S PRID SALVE
(Homeopathic Formulations) .... ▣833
None cited in PDR database.

SOLODYN EXTENDED RELEASE TABLETS
(Minocycline Hydrochloride) 1890
May interact with antacids containing aluminum, calcium and magnesium, oral anticoagulants, iron containing oral preparations, oral contraceptives, penicillins, and certain other agents. Compounds in these categories include:

Aluminum Carbonate (Absorption of tetracyclines is impaired by antacids containing aluminum, calcium or magnesium).
No products indexed under this heading.

Aluminum Hydroxide (Absorption of tetracyclines is impaired by antacids containing aluminum, calcium or magnesium). Products include:
- Gaviscon Regular Strength Liquid .. ▣658
- Gaviscon Regular Strength Tablets.. ▣658
- Gaviscon Extra Strength Liquid ...... ▣658
- Gaviscon Extra Strength Tablets .... ▣658
- Maalox Regular Strength Antacid/Antigas Liquid................. 2175
- Maalox Max Maximum Strength Antacid/Anti-Gas Liquid................ 2176

5-Amino-Salicylic Acid (Since bacteriostatic drugs may interfere with bactericidal action of penicillin, it is advisable to avoid giving tetracycline-class drugs in conjunction with penicillin).
No products indexed under this heading.

Amoxicillin (Since bacteriostatic drugs may interfere with bactericidal action of penicillin, it is advisable to avoid giving tetracycline-class drugs in conjunction with penicillin). Products include:
- Amoxil Capsules 1343
- Amoxil Chewable Tablets 1343
- Amoxil Pediatric Drops for Oral Suspension 1343
- Amoxil Powder for Oral Suspension 1343
- Amoxil Tablets 1343
- Augmentin 1360
- Augmentin Tablets 1363
- Augmentin XR Extended-Release Tablets 1369
- Augmentin ES-600 Powder for Oral Suspension 1366
- PREVPAC 3284

Amoxicillin Trihydrate (Since bacteriostatic drugs may interfere with bactericidal action of penicillin, it is advisable to avoid giving tetracycline-class drugs in conjunction with penicillin).
No products indexed under this heading.

Ampicillin (Since bacteriostatic drugs may interfere with bactericidal action of penicillin, it is advisable to avoid giving tetracycline-class drugs in conjunction with penicillin).
No products indexed under this heading.

Ampicillin Sodium (Since bacteriostatic drugs may interfere with bactericidal action of penicillin, it is advisable to avoid giving tetracycline-class drugs in conjunction with penicillin).
No products indexed under this heading.

Ampicillin Trihydrate (Since bacteriostatic drugs may interfere with bactericidal action of penicillin, it is advisable to avoid giving tetracycline-class drugs in conjunction with penicillin).
No products indexed under this heading.

Anisindione (Because tetracyclines have been shown to depress plasma prothrombin activity, patients who are on anticoagulant therapy may require downward adjustment of their anticoagulant dosage). Products include:
- Miradon Tablets 3042

Azlocillin Sodium (Since bacteriostatic drugs may interfere with bactericidal action of penicillin, it is advisable to avoid giving tetracycline-class drugs in conjunction with penicillin).
No products indexed under this heading.

Bacampicillin Hydrochloride (Since bacteriostatic drugs may interfere with bactericidal action of penicillin, it is advisable to avoid giving tetracycline-class drugs in conjunction with penicillin).
No products indexed under this heading.

Carbenicillin Disodium (Since bacteriostatic drugs may interfere with bactericidal action of penicillin, it is advisable to avoid giving tetracycline-class drugs in conjunction with penicillin).
No products indexed under this heading.

Carbenicillin Indanyl Sodium (Since bacteriostatic drugs may interfere with bactericidal action of penicillin, it is advisable to avoid giving tetracycline-class drugs in conjunction with penicillin).
No products indexed under this heading.

Desogestrel (To avoid contraceptive failure, female patients are advised to use a second form of contraceptive during treatment with minocyline). Products include:
- Mircette Tablets 1066

Dicloxacillin Sodium (Since bacteriostatic drugs may interfere with bactericidal action of penicillin, it is advisable to avoid giving tetracycline-class drugs in conjunction with penicillin).
No products indexed under this heading.

Dicumarol (Because tetracyclines have been shown to depress plasma prothrombin activity, patients who are on anticoagulant therapy may require downward adjustment of their anticoagulant dosage).
No products indexed under this heading.

Ethinyl Estradiol (To avoid contraceptive failure, female patients are advised to use a second form of contraceptive during treatment with minocyline). Products include:
- Mircette Tablets 1066
- NuvaRing 2340
- Ortho-Cyclen/Ortho Tri-Cyclen 2429
- Ortho Evra Transdermal System 2417
- Ortho Tri-Cyclen Lo Tablets 2436
- Seasonique Tablets 1077
- Yasmin 28 Tablets 796
- Yaz Tablets 803

Ethynodiol Diacetate (To avoid contraceptive failure, female patients are advised to use a second form of contraceptive during treatment with minocyline).
No products indexed under this heading.

Ferrous Fumarate (Absorption of tetracyclines is impaired by iron-containing preparations).
No products indexed under this heading.

Ferrous Gluconate (Absorption of tetracyclines is impaired by iron-containing preparations).
No products indexed under this heading.

Ferrous Sulfate (Absorption of tetracyclines is impaired by iron-containing preparations). Products include:
- Slow Fe Iron Tablets .... ▣818
- Slow Fe with Folic Acid Tablets .... ▣819

Iron (Absorption of tetracyclines is impaired by iron-containing preparations).
No products indexed under this heading.

Levonorgestrel (To avoid contraceptive failure, female patients are advised to use a second form of contraceptive during treatment with minocyline). Products include:
- Climara Pro Transdermal System 776
- Mirena Intrauterine System 787
- Plan B Tablets 1076
- Seasonique Tablets 1077

Magaldrate (Absorption of tetracyclines is impaired by antacids containing aluminum, calcium or magnesium).
No products indexed under this heading.

Magnesium Hydroxide (Absorption of tetracyclines is impaired by antacids containing aluminum, calcium or magnesium). Products include:
- Maalox Regular Strength Antacid/Antigas Liquid................. 2175
- Maalox Max Maximum Strength Antacid/Anti-Gas Liquid................ 2176
- Pepcid Complete Chewable Tablets 1701

Magnesium Oxide (Absorption of tetracyclines is impaired by antacids containing aluminum, calcium or magnesium). Products include:
- Beelith Tablets 759
- PremCal Light, Regular, and Extra Strength Tablets................ ▣818

Mestranol (To avoid contraceptive failure, female patients are advised to use a second form of contraceptive during treatment with minocyline).
No products indexed under this heading.

Methoxyflurane (The concurrent use of tetracyclines and methoxyflurane has been reported to result in fatal renal toxicity).
No products indexed under this heading.

Mezlocillin Sodium (Since bacteriostatic drugs may interfere with bactericidal action of penicillin, it is advisable to avoid giving tetracycline-class drugs in conjunction with penicillin).
No products indexed under this heading.

Nafcillin Sodium (Since bacteriostatic drugs may interfere with bactericidal action of penicillin, it is advisable to avoid giving tetracycline-class drugs in conjunction with penicillin).
No products indexed under this heading.

Norethindrone (To avoid contraceptive failure, female patients are advised to use a second form of contraceptive during treatment with minocyline). Products include:
- Ortho Micronor Tablets 2426

Norethynodrel (To avoid contraceptive failure, female patients are advised to use a second form of contraceptive during treatment with minocyline).
No products indexed under this heading.

Norgestimate (To avoid contraceptive failure, female patients are advised to use a second form of contraceptive during treatment with minocyline). Products include:
- Ortho-Cyclen/Ortho Tri-Cyclen 2429
- Ortho Tri-Cyclen Lo Tablets 2436

Norgestrel (To avoid contraceptive failure, female patients are advised to use a second form of contraceptive during treatment with minocyline).
No products indexed under this heading.

Penicillin G Benzathine (Since bacteriostatic drugs may interfere with bactericidal action of penicillin, it is advisable to avoid giving tetracycline-class drugs in conjunction with penicillin). Products include:
- Bicillin C-R Injectable Suspension 1706

Penicillin G Potassium (Since bacteriostatic drugs may interfere with bactericidal action of penicillin, it is advisable to avoid giving tetracycline-class drugs in conjunction with penicillin).
No products indexed under this heading.

Penicillin G Procaine (Since bacteriostatic drugs may interfere with bactericidal action of penicillin, it is advisable to avoid giving tetracycline-class drugs in conjunction with penicillin). Products include:
- Bicillin C-R Injectable Suspension 1706

Penicillin G Sodium (Since bacteriostatic drugs may interfere with bactericidal action of penicillin, it is advisable to avoid giving tetracycline-class drugs in conjunction with penicillin).
No products indexed under this heading.

Penicillin V Potassium (Since bacteriostatic drugs may interfere with bactericidal action of penicillin, it is advisable to avoid giving tetracycline-class drugs in conjunction with penicillin).
No products indexed under this heading.

Polysaccharide Iron Complex (Absorption of tetracyclines is impaired by iron-containing preparations). Products include:
- Nu-Iron 150 Capsules 2127

Ticarcillin Disodium (Since bacteriostatic drugs may interfere with bactericidal action of penicillin, it is advisable to avoid giving tetracycline-class drugs in conjunction with penicillin). Products include:
- Timentin ADD-Vantage 1580

Timentin Injection Galaxy Container 1583
Timentin IV Infusion 1577
Timentin Pharmacy Bulk Package 1586

Warfarin Sodium (Because tetracyclines have been shown to depress plasma prothrombin activity, patients who are on anticoagulant therapy may require downward adjustment of their anticoagulant dosage). Products include:
Coumadin for Injection 898
Coumadin Tablets 898

SOLTAMOX ORAL SOLUTION

(Tamoxifen Citrate) 3527

May interact with oral anticoagulants, cytotoxic drugs, and certain other agents. Compounds in these categories include:

Aminoglutethimide (Plasma concentrations have been shown to be reduced when co-administered with aminoglutethimide).
No products indexed under this heading.

Anisindione (Concomitant administration of tamoxifen with coumarin type anticoagulants, a significant increase in anticoagulant effect may occur. Where such co-administration exists, careful monitoring of patient's prothrombin time is recommended). Products include:
Miradon Tablets 3042

Bleomycin Sulfate (There is an increased risk of thromboembolic events when cytotoxic agents are used in combination with tamoxifen).
No products indexed under this heading.

Cyclophosphamide (There is an increased risk of thromboembolic events when cytotoxic agents are used in combination with tamoxifen).
No products indexed under this heading.

Daunorubicin Hydrochloride (There is an increased risk of thromboembolic events occuring when cytotoxic agents are used in combination with tamoxifen).
No products indexed under this heading.

Dicumarol (Concomitant administration of tamoxifen with coumarin type anticoagulants, a significant increase in anticoagulant effect may occur. Where such co-administration exists, careful monitoring of patient's prothrombin time is recommended).
No products indexed under this heading.

Doxorubicin Hydrochloride (There is an increased risk of thromboembolic events occuring when cytotoxic agents are used in combination with tamoxifen).
No products indexed under this heading.

Epirubicin Hydrochloride (There is an increased risk of thromboembolic events occuring when cytotoxic agents are used in combination with tamoxifen).
No products indexed under this heading.

Fluorouracil (There is an increased risk of thromboembolic events occuring when cytotoxic agents are used in combination with tamoxifen). Products include:
Carac Cream, 0.5% 2879
Efudex 3363

Hydroxyurea (There is an increased risk of thromboembolic events occuring when cytotoxic agents are used in combination with tamoxifen).
No products indexed under this heading.

Letrozole (Tamoxifen reduced letrozole plasma concentrations by 37%). Products include:
Femara Tablets 2214

Methotrexate Sodium (There is an increased risk of thromboembolic events occuring when cytotoxic agents are used in combination with tamoxifen).
No products indexed under this heading.

Mitotane (There is an increased risk of thromboembolic events occuring when cytotoxic agents are used in combination with tamoxifen).
No products indexed under this heading.

Mitoxantrone Hydrochloride (There is an increased risk of thromboembolic events occuring when cytotoxic agents are used in combination with tamoxifen).
No products indexed under this heading.

Procarbazine Hydrochloride (There is an increased risk of thromboembolic events occuring when cytotoxic agents are used in combination with tamoxifen). Products include:
Matulane Capsules 3191

Rifampin (Plasma concentrations have been shown to be reduced when co-administered with rifampin).
No products indexed under this heading.

Vincristine Sulfate (There is an increased risk of thromboembolic events occuring when cytotoxic agents are used in combination with tamoxifen).
No products indexed under this heading.

Warfarin Sodium (Concomitant administration of tamoxifen with coumarin type anticoagulants, a significant increase in anticoagulant effect may occur. Where such co-administration exists, careful monitoring of patient's prothrombin time is recommended). Products include:
Coumadin for Injection 898
Coumadin Tablets 898

SOMAVERT INJECTION

(Pegvisomant) 2642

May interact with oral hypoglycemic agents, insulin, and narcotic analgesics. Compounds in these categories include:

Acarbose (Growth hormone opposes the effects of insulin on carbohydrate metabolism by decreasing insulin sensitivity; therefore, glucose tolerance may increase in some patients treated with pegvisomant. Acromegalic patients with diabetes mellitus being treated with insulin and/or oral hypoglycemic agents may require dose reductions of these therapeutic agents after initiation of therapy with pegvisomant; monitor and reduce dose when necessary). Products include:
Precose Tablets 751

Alfentanil Hydrochloride (In clinical studies, patients on opioids often needed higher serum pegvisomant concentrations to achieve appropriate IGF-I suppression compared with patients not receiving opioids).
No products indexed under this heading.

Buprenorphine Hydrochloride (In clinical studies, patients on opioids often needed higher serum pegvisomant concentrations to achieve appropriate IGF-I suppression compared with patients not receiving opioids). Products include:
Buprenex Injectable 2716
Suboxone Tablets 2717
Subutex Tablets 2717

Chlorpropamide (Growth hormone opposes the effects of insulin on carbohydrate metabolism by decreasing insulin sensitivity; therefore, glucose tolerance may increase in some patients treated with pegvisomant. Acromegalic patients with diabetes mellitus being treated with insulin and/or oral hypoglycemic agents may require dose reductions of these therapeutic agents after initiation of therapy with pegvisomant; monitor and reduce dose when necessary).
No products indexed under this heading.

Codeine Phosphate (In clinical studies, patients on opioids often needed higher serum pegvisomant concentrations to achieve appropriate IGF-I suppression compared with patients not receiving opioids). Products include:
Tylenol with Codeine Tablets 2391

Dezocine (In clinical studies, patients on opioids often needed higher serum pegvisomant concentrations to achieve appropriate IGF-I suppression compared with patients not receiving opioids).
No products indexed under this heading.

Fentanyl (In clinical studies, patients on opioids often needed higher serum pegvisomant concentrations to achieve appropriate IGF-I suppression compared with patients not receiving opioids). Products include:
Duragesic Transdermal System 2373
Ionsys Transdermal System 2379

Fentanyl Citrate (In clinical studies, patients on opioids often needed higher serum pegvisomant concentrations to achieve appropriate IGF-I suppression compared with patients not receiving opioids). Products include:
Actiq 979

Glimepiride (Growth hormone opposes the effects of insulin on carbohydrate metabolism by decreasing insulin sensitivity; therefore, glucose tolerance may increase in some patients treated with pegvisomant. Acromegalic patients with diabetes mellitus being treated with insulin and/or oral hypoglycemic agents may require dose reductions of these therapeutic agents after initiation of therapy with pegvisomant; monitor and reduce dose when necessary). Products include:
Avandaryl Tablets 1379
Duetact Tablets 3226

Glipizide (Growth hormone opposes the effects of insulin on carbohydrate metabolism by decreasing insulin sensitivity; therefore, glucose tolerance may increase in some patients treated with pegvisomant. Acromegalic patients with diabetes mellitus being treated with insulin and/or oral hypoglycemic agents may require dose reductions of these therapeutic agents after initiation of therapy with pegvisomant; monitor and reduce dose when necessary).
No products indexed under this heading.

Glyburide (Growth hormone opposes the effects of insulin on carbohydrate metabolism by decreasing insulin sensitivity; therefore, glucose tolerance may increase in some patients treated with pegvisomant. Acromegalic patients with diabetes mellitus being treated with insulin and/or oral hypoglycemic agents may require dose reductions of these therapeutic agents after initiation of therapy with pegvisomant; monitor and reduce dose when necessary).
No products indexed under this heading.

Hydrocodone Bitartrate (In clinical studies, patients on opioids often needed higher serum pegvisomant concentrations to achieve appropriate IGF-I suppression compared with patients not receiving opioids). Products include:
Hycodan 1116
Hycotuss Expectorant Syrup 1117
Vicodin Tablets 535
Vicodin ES Tablets 536
Vicodin HP Tablets 538
Vicoprofen Tablets 539
Zydone Tablets 1139

Hydrocodone Polistirex (In clinical studies, patients on opioids often needed higher serum pegvisomant concentrations to achieve appropriate IGF-I suppression compared with patients not receiving opioids). Products include:
Tussionex Pennkinetic Extended-Release Suspension 3327

Hydromorphone Hydrochloride (In clinical studies, patients on opioids often needed higher serum pegvisomant concentrations to achieve appropriate IGF-I suppression compared with patients not receiving opioids). Products include:
Dilaudid 440
Dilaudid Non-Sterile Powder 440
Dilaudid Oral Liquid 445
Dilaudid Rectal Suppositories 440
Dilaudid Tablets 440
Dilaudid Tablets - 8 mg 445
Dilaudid-HP 442

Insulin, Human, Zinc Suspension (Growth hormone opposes the effects of insulin on carbohydrate metabolism by decreasing insulin sensitivity; therefore, glucose tolerance may increase in some patients treated with pegvisomant. Acromegalic patients with diabetes mellitus being treated with insulin and/or oral hypoglycemic agents may require dose reductions of these therapeutic agents after initiation of therapy with pegvisomant; monitor and reduce dose when necessary). Products include:
Humulin L, 100 Units 1794
Humulin U, 100 Units 1800

Insulin, Human NPH (Growth hormone opposes the effects of insulin on carbohydrate metabolism by decreasing insulin sensitivity; therefore, glucose tolerance may increase in some patients treated with pegvisomant. Acromegalic patients with diabetes mellitus being treated with insulin and/or oral hypoglycemic agents may require dose reductions of these therapeutic agents after initiation of therapy with pegvisomant; monitor and reduce dose when necessary). Products include:

Insulin, Human Regular (Growth hormone opposes the effects of insulin on carbohydrate metabolism by decreasing insulin sensitivity; therefore, glucose tolerance may increase in some patients treated with pegvisomant. Acromegalic patients with diabetes mellitus being treated with insulin and/or oral hypoglycemic agents may require dose reductions of these therapeutic agents after initiation of therapy with pegvisomant; monitor and reduce dose when necessary). Products include:

Insulin, Human Regular and Human NPH Mixture (Growth hormone opposes the effects of insulin on carbohydrate metabolism by decreasing insulin sensitivity; therefore, glucose tolerance may increase in some patients treated with pegvisomant. Acromegalic patients with diabetes mellitus being treated with insulin and/or oral hypoglycemic agents may require dose reductions of these therapeutic agents after initiation of therapy with pegvisomant; monitor and reduce dose when necessary). Products include:

Insulin, NPH (Growth hormone opposes the effects of insulin on carbohydrate metabolism by decreasing insulin sensitivity; therefore, glucose tolerance may increase in some patients treated with pegvisomant. Acromegalic patients with diabetes mellitus being treated with insulin and/or oral hypoglycemic agents may require dose reductions of these therapeutic agents after initiation of therapy with pegvisomant; monitor and reduce dose when necessary).

No products indexed under this heading.

Insulin, Regular (Growth hormone opposes the effects of insulin on carbohydrate metabolism by decreasing insulin sensitivity; therefore, glucose tolerance may increase in some patients treated with pegvisomant. Acromegalic patients with diabetes mellitus being treated with insulin and/or oral hypoglycemic agents may require dose reductions of these therapeutic agents after initiation of therapy with pegvisomant; monitor and reduce dose when necessary).

No products indexed under this heading.

Insulin, Zinc Crystals (Growth hormone opposes the effects of insulin on carbohydrate metabolism by decreasing insulin sensitivity; therefore, glucose tolerance may increase in some patients treated with pegvisomant. Acromegalic patients with diabetes mellitus being treated with insulin and/or oral hypoglycemic agents may require dose

reductions of these therapeutic agents after initiation of therapy with pegvisomant; monitor and reduce dose when necessary).

No products indexed under this heading.

Insulin, Zinc Suspension (Growth hormone opposes the effects of insulin on carbohydrate metabolism by decreasing insulin sensitivity; therefore, glucose tolerance may increase in some patients treated with pegvisomant. Acromegalic patients with diabetes mellitus being treated with insulin and/or oral hypoglycemic agents may require dose reductions of these therapeutic agents after initiation of therapy with pegvisomant; monitor and reduce dose when necessary).

No products indexed under this heading.

Insulin Aspart, Human Regular (Growth hormone opposes the effects of insulin on carbohydrate metabolism by decreasing insulin sensitivity; therefore, glucose tolerance may increase in some patients treated with pegvisomant. Acromegalic patients with diabetes mellitus being treated with insulin and/or oral hypoglycemic agents may require dose reductions of these therapeutic agents after initiation of therapy with pegvisomant; monitor and reduce dose when necessary). Products include:

Insulin glargine (Growth hormone opposes the effects of insulin on carbohydrate metabolism by decreasing insulin sensitivity; therefore, glucose tolerance may increase in some patients treated with pegvisomant. Acromegalic patients with diabetes mellitus being treated with insulin and/or oral hypoglycemic agents may require dose reductions of these therapeutic agents after initiation of therapy with pegvisomant; monitor and reduce dose when necessary). Products include:

Insulin Lispro, Human (Growth hormone opposes the effects of insulin on carbohydrate metabolism by decreasing insulin sensitivity; therefore, glucose tolerance may increase in some patients treated with pegvisomant. Acromegalic patients with diabetes mellitus being treated with insulin and/or oral hypoglycemic agents may require dose reductions of these therapeutic agents after initiation of therapy with pegvisomant; monitor and reduce dose when necessary). Products include:

Insulin Lispro Protamine, Human (Growth hormone opposes the effects of insulin on carbohydrate metabolism by decreasing insulin sensitivity; therefore, glucose tolerance may increase in some patients treated with pegvisomant. Acromegalic patients with diabetes mellitus being treated with insulin and/or oral hypoglycemic agents may require dose reductions of these therapeutic agents after initiation of therapy with pegvisomant; monitor and reduce dose when necessary). Products include:

Levorphanol Tartrate (In clinical studies, patients on opioids often needed higher serum pegvisomant concentrations to achieve appropriate IGF-I suppression compared with patients not receiving opioids).

No products indexed under this heading.

Meperidine Hydrochloride (In clinical studies, patients on opioids often needed higher serum pegvisomant concentrations to achieve appropriate IGF-I suppression compared with patients not receiving opioids).

No products indexed under this heading.

Metformin Hydrochloride (Growth hormone opposes the effects of insulin on carbohydrate metabolism by decreasing insulin sensitivity; therefore, glucose tolerance may increase in some patients treated with pegvisomant. Acromegalic patients with diabetes mellitus being treated with insulin and/or oral hypoglycemic agents may require dose reductions of these therapeutic agents after initiation of therapy with pegvisomant; monitor and reduce dose when necessary). Products include:

Methadone Hydrochloride (In clinical studies, patients on opioids often needed higher serum pegvisomant concentrations to achieve appropriate IGF-I suppression compared with patients not receiving opioids).

No products indexed under this heading.

Miglitol (Growth hormone opposes the effects of insulin on carbohydrate metabolism by decreasing insulin sensitivity; therefore, glucose tolerance may increase in some patients treated with pegvisomant. Acromegalic patients with diabetes mellitus being treated with insulin and/or oral hypoglycemic agents may require dose reductions of these therapeutic agents after initiation of therapy with pegvisomant; monitor and reduce dose when necessary).

No products indexed under this heading.

Morphine Sulfate (In clinical studies, patients on opioids often needed higher serum pegvisomant concentrations to achieve appropriate IGF-I suppression compared with patients not receiving opioids). Products include:

Oxycodone Hydrochloride (In clinical studies, patients on opioids often needed higher serum pegvisomant concentrations to achieve appropriate IGF-I suppression compared with patients not receiving opioids). Products include:

Pioglitazone Hydrochloride (Growth hormone opposes the effects of insulin on carbohydrate

metabolism by decreasing insulin sensitivity; therefore, glucose tolerance may increase in some patients treated with pegvisomant. Acromegalic patients with diabetes mellitus being treated with insulin and/or oral hypoglycemic agents may require dose reductions of these therapeutic agents after initiation of therapy with pegvisomant; monitor and reduce dose when necessary). Products include:

Propoxyphene Hydrochloride (In clinical studies, patients on opioids often needed higher serum pegvisomant concentrations to achieve appropriate IGF-I suppression compared with patients not receiving opioids).

No products indexed under this heading.

Propoxyphene Napsylate (In clinical studies, patients on opioids often needed higher serum pegvisomant concentrations to achieve appropriate IGF-I suppression compared with patients not receiving opioids).

No products indexed under this heading.

Remifentanil Hydrochloride (In clinical studies, patients on opioids often needed higher serum pegvisomant concentrations to achieve appropriate IGF-I suppression compared with patients not receiving opioids).

No products indexed under this heading.

Repaglinide (Growth hormone opposes the effects of insulin on carbohydrate metabolism by decreasing insulin sensitivity; therefore, glucose tolerance may increase in some patients treated with pegvisomant. Acromegalic patients with diabetes mellitus being treated with insulin and/or oral hypoglycemic agents may require dose reductions of these therapeutic agents after initiation of therapy with pegvisomant; monitor and reduce dose when necessary).

No products indexed under this heading.

Rosiglitazone Maleate (Growth hormone opposes the effects of insulin on carbohydrate metabolism by decreasing insulin sensitivity; therefore, glucose tolerance may increase in some patients treated with pegvisomant. Acromegalic patients with diabetes mellitus being treated with insulin and/or oral hypoglycemic agents may require dose reductions of these therapeutic agents after initiation of therapy with pegvisomant; monitor and reduce dose when necessary). Products include:

Sufentanil Citrate (In clinical studies, patients on opioids often needed higher serum pegvisomant concentrations to achieve appropriate IGF-I suppression compared with patients not receiving opioids).

No products indexed under this heading.

Tolazamide (Growth hormone opposes the effects of insulin on carbohydrate metabolism by decreasing insulin sensitivity; therefore, glucose tolerance may

increase in some patients treated with pegvisomant. Acromegalic patients with diabetes mellitus being treated with insulin and/or oral hypoglycemic agents may require dose reductions of these therapeutic agents after initiation of therapy with pegvisomant; monitor and reduce dose when necessary).
No products indexed under this heading.

Tolbutamide (Growth hormone opposes the effects of insulin on carbohydrate metabolism by decreasing insulin sensitivity; therefore, glucose tolerance may increase in some patients treated with pegvisomant. Acromegalic patients with diabetes mellitus being treated with insulin and/or oral hypoglycemic agents may require dose reductions of these therapeutic agents after initiation of therapy with pegvisomant; monitor and reduce dose when necessary).
No products indexed under this heading.

Troglitazone (Growth hormone opposes the effects of insulin on carbohydrate metabolism by decreasing insulin sensitivity; therefore, glucose tolerance may increase in some patients treated with pegvisomant. Acromegalic patients with diabetes mellitus being treated with insulin and/or oral hypoglycemic agents may require dose reductions of these therapeutic agents after initiation of therapy with pegvisomant; monitor and reduce dose when necessary).
No products indexed under this heading.

SOMINEX ORIGINAL FORMULA TABLETS

(Diphenhydramine Hydrochloride) 616
May interact with hypnotics and sedatives, tranquilizers, and certain other agents. Compounds in these categories include:

Alprazolam (Concurrent use with tranquilizers is not recommended unless directed by a physician). Products include:
Niravam Orally Disintegrating Tablets 3092

Buspirone Hydrochloride (Concurrent use with tranquilizers is not recommended unless directed by a physician).
No products indexed under this heading.

Chlordiazepoxide (Concurrent use with tranquilizers is not recommended unless directed by a physician).
No products indexed under this heading.

Chlordiazepoxide Hydrochloride (Concurrent use with tranquilizers is not recommended unless directed by a physician). Products include:
Librium Capsules 3347

Chlorpromazine (Concurrent use with tranquilizers is not recommended unless directed by a physician).
No products indexed under this heading.

Chlorpromazine Hydrochloride (Concurrent use with tranquilizers is not recommended unless directed by a physician).
No products indexed under this heading.

Chlorprothixene (Concurrent use with tranquilizers is not recommended unless directed by a physician).
No products indexed under this heading.

Chlorprothixene Hydrochloride (Concurrent use with tranquilizers is not recommended unless directed by a physician).
No products indexed under this heading.

Clorazepate Dipotassium (Concurrent use with tranquilizers is not recommended unless directed by a physician). Products include:
Tranxene 2474

Diazepam (Concurrent use with tranquilizers is not recommended unless directed by a physician). Products include:
Diastat Rectal Delivery System 3343
Valium Tablets 2819

Droperidol (Concurrent use with tranquilizers is not recommended unless directed by a physician).
No products indexed under this heading.

Estazolam (Concurrent use with sedatives is not recommended unless directed by a physician). Products include:
ProSom Tablets 517

Ethchlorvynol (Concurrent use with sedatives is not recommended unless directed by a physician).
No products indexed under this heading.

Ethinamate (Concurrent use with sedatives is not recommended unless directed by a physician).
No products indexed under this heading.

Fluphenazine Decanoate (Concurrent use with tranquilizers is not recommended unless directed by a physician).
No products indexed under this heading.

Fluphenazine Enanthate (Concurrent use with tranquilizers is not recommended unless directed by a physician).
No products indexed under this heading.

Fluphenazine Hydrochloride (Concurrent use with tranquilizers is not recommended unless directed by a physician).
No products indexed under this heading.

Flurazepam Hydrochloride (Concurrent use with sedatives is not recommended unless directed by a physician). Products include:
Dalmane Capsules 3342

Glutethimide (Concurrent use with sedatives is not recommended unless directed by a physician).
No products indexed under this heading.

Haloperidol (Concurrent use with tranquilizers is not recommended unless directed by a physician).
No products indexed under this heading.

Haloperidol Decanoate (Concurrent use with tranquilizers is not recommended unless directed by a physician).
No products indexed under this heading.

Hydroxyzine Hydrochloride (Concurrent use with tranquilizers is not recommended unless directed by a physician).
No products indexed under this heading.

Lorazepam (Concurrent use with tranquilizers is not recommended unless directed by a physician).
No products indexed under this heading.

Loxapine Hydrochloride (Concurrent use with tranquilizers is not recommended unless directed by a physician).
No products indexed under this heading.

Loxapine Succinate (Concurrent use with tranquilizers is not recommended unless directed by a physician).
No products indexed under this heading.

Meprobamate (Concurrent use with tranquilizers is not recommended unless directed by a physician).
No products indexed under this heading.

Mesoridazine Besylate (Concurrent use with tranquilizers is not recommended unless directed by a physician).
No products indexed under this heading.

Midazolam Hydrochloride (Concurrent use with sedatives is not recommended unless directed by a physician).
No products indexed under this heading.

Molindone Hydrochloride (Concurrent use with tranquilizers is not recommended unless directed by a physician). Products include:
Moban Tablets 1119

Oxazepam (Concurrent use with tranquilizers is not recommended unless directed by a physician).
No products indexed under this heading.

Perphenazine (Concurrent use with tranquilizers is not recommended unless directed by a physician).
No products indexed under this heading.

Prazepam (Concurrent use with tranquilizers is not recommended unless directed by a physician).
No products indexed under this heading.

Prochlorperazine (Concurrent use with tranquilizers is not recommended unless directed by a physician).
No products indexed under this heading.

Promethazine Hydrochloride (Concurrent use with tranquilizers is not recommended unless directed by a physician). Products include:
Phenergan Tablets and Suppositories 3440

Propofol (Concurrent use with sedatives is not recommended unless directed by a physician).
No products indexed under this heading.

Quazepam (Concurrent use with sedatives is not recommended unless directed by a physician).
No products indexed under this heading.

Ramelteon (Concurrent use with sedatives is not recommended unless directed by a physician). Products include:
Rozerem Tablets 3231

Secobarbital Sodium (Concurrent use with sedatives is not recommended unless directed by a physician).
No products indexed under this heading.

Temazepam (Concurrent use with sedatives is not recommended unless directed by a physician). Products include:
Restoril Capsules 1860

Thioridazine Hydrochloride (Concurrent use with tranquilizers is not recommended unless directed by a physician). Products include:
Thioridazine Hydrochloride Tablets 2163

Thiothixene (Concurrent use with tranquilizers is not recommended unless directed by a physician). Products include:
Thiothixene Capsules 2165

Triazolam (Concurrent use with sedatives is not recommended unless directed by a physician).
No products indexed under this heading.

Trifluoperazine Hydrochloride (Concurrent use with tranquilizers is not recommended unless directed by a physician).
No products indexed under this heading.

Zaleplon (Concurrent use with sedatives is not recommended unless directed by a physician). Products include:
Sonata Capsules 1717

Zolpidem Tartrate (Concurrent use with sedatives is not recommended unless directed by a physician). Products include:
Ambien Tablets 2851
Ambien CR Tablets 2855

Food Interactions

Alcohol (Concurrent use of alcoholic beverages is not recommended).

SON FORMULA TABLETS

(Amino Acid Preparations) 1673
None cited in PDR database.

SONATA CAPSULES

(Zaleplon) 1717
May interact with antihistamines, central nervous system depressants, cytochrome p450 3a4 inducers (selected), cytochrome p450 3a4 inhibitors (selected), anticonvulsants, erythromycin, phenytoin, psychotropics, and certain other agents. Compounds in these categories include:

Acetazolamide (CYP3A4 inhibitors may decrease zaleplon's clearance, possibly increasing its concentration).
No products indexed under this heading.

Acrivastine (Concurrent use may produce additive CNS depressant effects).
No products indexed under this heading.

Alfentanil Hydrochloride (Concurrent use may produce additive CNS depressant effects).
No products indexed under this heading.

Allium sativum (CYP3A4 inhibitors may increase zaleplon's clearance, possibly decreasing its concentration).
No products indexed under this heading.

Alprazolam (Concurrent use may produce additive CNS depressant effects). Products include:
Niravam Orally Disintegrating Tablets ... 3092

Amiodarone Hydrochloride (CYP3A4 inhibitors may decrease zaleplon's clearance, possibly increasing its concentration).
No products indexed under this heading.

Amitriptyline Hydrochloride (Concurrent use may produce additive CNS depressant effects).
No products indexed under this heading.

Amoxapine (Concurrent use may produce additive CNS depressant effects).
No products indexed under this heading.

Amprenavir (CYP3A4 inhibitors may decrease zaleplon's clearance, possibly increasing its concentration). Products include:
Agenerase Capsules ... 1327
Agenerase Oral Solution ... 1332

Anastrozole (CYP3A4 inhibitors may decrease zaleplon's clearance, possibly increasing its concentration). Products include:
Arimidex Tablets ... 673

Aprepitant (CYP3A4 inhibitors may decrease zaleplon's clearance, possibly increasing its concentration). Products include:
Emend Capsules ... 1963

Aprobarbital (Concurrent use may produce additive CNS depressant effects).
No products indexed under this heading.

Astemizole (Concurrent use may produce additive CNS depressant effects).
No products indexed under this heading.

Azatadine Maleate (Concurrent use may produce additive CNS depressant effects).
No products indexed under this heading.

Betamethasone Acetate (CYP3A4 inhibitors may increase zaleplon's clearance, possibly decreasing its concentration).
No products indexed under this heading.

Betamethasone Sodium Phosphate (CYP3A4 inhibitors may increase zaleplon's clearance, possibly decreasing its concentration).
No products indexed under this heading.

Bromodiphenhydramine Hydrochloride (Concurrent use may produce additive CNS depressant effects).
No products indexed under this heading.

Brompheniramine Maleate (Concurrent use may produce additive CNS depressant effects). Products include:
Children's Dimetapp Cold & Allergy Elixir ... ▣730
Children's Dimetapp Cold & Allergy Chewable Tablets ... ▣730
Children's Dimetapp DM Cold & Cough Elixir ... ▣731

Buprenorphine Hydrochloride (Concurrent use may produce additive CNS depressant effects). Products include:
Buprenex Injectable ... 2716
Suboxone Tablets ... 2717
Subutex Tablets ... 2717

Buspirone Hydrochloride (Concurrent use may produce additive CNS depressant effects).
No products indexed under this heading.

Butabarbital (Concurrent use may produce additive CNS depressant effects).
No products indexed under this heading.

Butalbital (Concurrent use may produce additive CNS depressant effects).
No products indexed under this heading.

Carbamazepine (CYP3A4 is ordinarily a minor metabolizing enzyme of zaleplon, the co-administration of a potent inducer, such as carbamazepine, although not posing a safety concern, could lead to ineffectiveness of zaleplon; concurrent use with anticonvulsants may produce additive CNS depressant effects). Products include:
Carbatrol Capsules ... 3171
Equetro Extended-Release Capsules ... 3180
Tegretol/Tegretol-XR ... 2295

Cetirizine Hydrochloride (Concurrent use may produce additive CNS depressant effects). Products include:
Zyrtec Chewable Tablets ... 2594
Zyrtec ... 2594
Zyrtec-D 12 Hour Extended Release Tablets ... 2597

Chlordiazepoxide (Concurrent use may produce additive CNS depressant effects).
No products indexed under this heading.

Chlordiazepoxide Hydrochloride (Concurrent use may produce additive CNS depressant effects). Products include:
Librium Capsules ... 3347

Chlorpheniramine Maleate (Concurrent use may produce additive CNS depressant effects). Products include:
Advil Allergy Sinus Caplets ... ▣770
Advil Multi-Symptom Cold Caplets ... ▣770
BC Allergy Sinus Cold Powder ... ▣677
Comtrex Maximum Strength Cold & Cough Day/Night Caplets - Night Formulation ... ▣726
Comtrex Maximum Strength Day/Night Severe Cold & Sinus Caplets - Night Formulation ... ▣725
Contac Cold and Flu Maximum Strength Caplets ... ▣728
Contac Cold and Flu Day and Night Caplets (Night Formulation Only) ... ▣727
Children's Dimetapp Long Acting Cough Plus Cold Syrup ... ▣731
Robitussin Cough & Cold Long-Acting Liquid ... ▣735
Robitussin Cough & Allergy Syrup .. ▣736
Robitussin Cough & Cold Nighttime Liquid ... ▣736
Robitussin Cough, Cold & Flu Nighttime Liquid ... ▣738
Robitussin Pediatric Cough & Cold Long-Acting Liquid ... ▣735
Robitussin Pediatric Cough & Cold Nighttime Liquid ... ▣736
Triaminic Cold & Allergy Liquid ... ▣746
Triaminic Cough & Runny Nose Softchews ... ▣748
Children's Tylenol Plus Flu Oral Suspension ... ▣749
Tylenol Allergy Multi-Symptom Caplets with Cool Burst and Gelcaps ... 1872
Children's Tylenol Plus Cold Suspension Liquid ... 1879
Children's Tylenol Plus Cough & Runny Nose Suspension Liquid ... 1879
Children's Tylenol Plus Flu Suspension Liquid ... 1881
Children's Tylenol Plus Multi-Symptom Cold Suspension Liquid ... 1879
Tylenol Cold Head Congestion Nighttime Caplets with Cool Burst ... 1873
Tylenol Cold Multi-Symptom Nighttime Caplets with Cool Burst ... 1874
Tylenol Sinus Congestion & Pain Nighttime Caplets with Cool Burst ... 1876
Vicks 44M Cough, Cold & Flu Relief Liquid ... 2680
Pediatric Vicks 44m Cough & Cold Relief Liquid ... 2676
Children's Vicks NyQuil Cold/Cough Relief ... ▣756
Children's Vicks NyQuil Cold/Cough Relief Liquid ... 2680
Zicam Maximum Strength Flu Daytime ... ▣768

Chlorpheniramine Polistirex (Concurrent use may produce additive CNS depressant effects). Products include:
Tussionex Pennkinetic Extended-Release Suspension ... 3327

Chlorpheniramine Tannate (Concurrent use may produce additive CNS depressant effects).
No products indexed under this heading.

Chlorpromazine (Concurrent use may produce additive CNS depressant effects).
No products indexed under this heading.

Chlorpromazine Hydrochloride (Concurrent use may produce additive CNS depressant effects).
No products indexed under this heading.

Chlorprothixene (Concurrent use may produce additive CNS depressant effects).
No products indexed under this heading.

Chlorprothixene Hydrochloride (Concurrent use may produce additive CNS depressant effects).
No products indexed under this heading.

Chlorprothixene Lactate (Concurrent use may produce additive CNS depressant effects).
No products indexed under this heading.

Cimetidine (Co-administration has produced an 85% increase in the mean Cmax and AUC of zaleplon; an initial dose of 5 mg should be given to patients who are concomitantly being treated with cimetidine). Products include:
Tagamet HB 200 Tablets ... ▣664

Cimetidine Hydrochloride (Co-administration has produced an 85% increase in the mean Cmax and AUC of zaleplon; an initial dose of 5 mg should be given to patients who are concomitantly being treated with cimetidine).
No products indexed under this heading.

Ciprofloxacin (CYP3A4 inhibitors may decrease zaleplon's clearance, possibly increasing its concentration). Products include:
Cipro Oral Suspension ... 2977
Cipro I.V. ... 2984
Cipro XR Tablets ... 2990
Ciprodex Otic Suspension ... 559

Ciprofloxacin Hydrochloride (CYP3A4 inhibitors may increase zaleplon's clearance, possibly decreasing its concentration). Products include:
Ciloxan Ophthalmic Ointment ... 559
Ciloxan Ophthalmic Solution ... ⊙206
Cipro Tablets ... 2977
Proquin XR Tablets ... 1153

Cisplatin (CYP3A4 inhibitors may increase zaleplon's clearance, possibly decreasing its concentration).
No products indexed under this heading.

Clarithromycin (CYP3A4 inhibitors may decrease zaleplon's clearance, possibly increasing its concentration). Products include:
Biaxin/Biaxin XL ... 402
PREVPAC ... 3284

Clemastine Fumarate (Concurrent use may produce additive CNS depressant effects).
No products indexed under this heading.

Clorazepate Dipotassium (Concurrent use may produce additive CNS depressant effects). Products include:
Tranxene ... 2474

Clotrimazole (CYP3A4 inhibitors may decrease zaleplon's clearance, possibly increasing its concentration). Products include:
Desenex Athlete's Foot Cream ... ▣635
Lotrimin ... 3039
Lotrisone ... 3040

Clozapine (Concurrent use may produce additive CNS depressant effects). Products include:
Clozaril Tablets ... 2184
FazaClo Orally Disintegrating Tablets ... 551

Codeine Phosphate (Concurrent use may produce additive CNS depressant effects). Products include:
Tylenol with Codeine Tablets ... 2391

Cortisone Acetate (CYP3A4 inhibitors may increase zaleplon's clearance, possibly decreasing its concentration).
No products indexed under this heading.

Cyclosporine (CYP3A4 inhibitors may decrease zaleplon's clearance, possibly increasing its concentration). Products include:
Gengraf Capsules ... 459
Neoral Oral Solution ... 2259
Neoral Soft Gelatin Capsules ... 2259
Restasis Ophthalmic Emulsion ... 575
Sandimmune ... 2275

Cyproheptadine Hydrochloride (Concurrent use may produce additive CNS depressant effects).
No products indexed under this heading.

Dalfopristin (CYP3A4 inhibitors may decrease zaleplon's clearance, possibly increasing its concentration).
No products indexed under this heading.

Danazol (CYP3A4 inhibitors may decrease zaleplon's clearance, possibly increasing its concentration).
No products indexed under this heading.

Delavirdine Mesylate (CYP3A4 inhibitors may decrease zaleplon's clearance, possibly increasing its concentration). Products include:

Rescriptor Tablets 2551

Desflurane (Concurrent use may produce additive CNS depressant effects).
No products indexed under this heading.

Desipramine Hydrochloride (Concurrent use may produce additive CNS depressant effects).
No products indexed under this heading.

Dexamethasone (CYP3A4 inhibitors may increase zaleplon's clearance, possibly decreasing its concentration). Products include:
- Ciprodex Otic Suspension 559
- Decadron Tablets 1951
- TobraDex Ophthalmic Ointment 562
- TobraDex Ophthalmic Suspension 563

Dexamethasone Acetate (CYP3A4 inhibitors may increase zaleplon's clearance, possibly decreasing its concentration).
No products indexed under this heading.

Dexamethasone Sodium Phosphate (CYP3A4 inhibitors may increase zaleplon's clearance, possibly decreasing its concentration).
No products indexed under this heading.

Dexchlorpheniramine Maleate (Concurrent use may produce additive CNS depressant effects).
No products indexed under this heading.

Dezocine (Concurrent use may produce additive CNS depressant effects).
No products indexed under this heading.

Diazepam (Concurrent use may produce additive CNS depressant effects). Products include:
- Diastat Rectal Delivery System 3343
- Valium Tablets 2819

Diltiazem Hydrochloride (CYP3A4 inhibitors may decrease zaleplon's clearance, possibly increasing its concentration). Products include:
- Cardizem LA Extended Release Tablets 1728
- Tiazac Capsules 1201

Diltiazem Maleate (CYP3A4 inhibitors may decrease zaleplon's clearance, possibly increasing its concentration).
No products indexed under this heading.

Diphenhydramine Citrate (Concurrent use may produce additive CNS depressant effects). Products include:
- Advil PM Caplets 615
- Excedrin PM Caplets/Tablets/Geltabs 610
- Goody's PM Powder for Pain with Sleeplessness 612

Diphenhydramine Hydrochloride (Concurrent use may produce additive CNS depressant effects). Products include:
- Nytol QuickCaps Caplets 615
- Nytol QuickGels Softgels Maximum Strength 616
- Simply Sleep Caplets 1868
- Sominex Original Formula Tablets 616
- TheraFlu Warming Relief Nighttime Severe Cold 743
- TheraFlu Thin Strips Multi Symptom 744
- Triaminic Nighttime Cold & Cough Liquid 746
- Triaminic Thin Strips Cough & Runny Nose 749
- Extra Strength Tylenol PM Caplets, Vanilla Caplets, Geltabs, Gelcaps and Liquid 1875
- Tylenol Sore Throat Nighttime Liquid with Cool Burst 790
- Tylenol Allergy Multi-Symptom Nighttime Caplets with Cool Burst 1872
- Tylenol Severe Allergy Caplets 1872
- Children's Tylenol Plus Cold & Allergy Suspension Liquid 1878

Diphenylpyraline Hydrochloride (Concurrent use may produce additive CNS depressant effects).
No products indexed under this heading.

Divalproex Sodium (Concurrent use with anticonvulsants may produce additive CNS depressant effects). Products include:
- Depakote Sprinkle Capsules 422
- Depakote Tablets 427
- Depakote ER Tablets 434

Doxepin Hydrochloride (Concurrent use may produce additive CNS depressant effects).
No products indexed under this heading.

Doxorubicin Hydrochloride (CYP3A4 inhibitors may increase zaleplon's clearance, possibly decreasing its concentration).
No products indexed under this heading.

Droperidol (Concurrent use may produce additive CNS depressant effects).
No products indexed under this heading.

Efavirenz (CYP3A4 inhibitors may decrease zaleplon's clearance, possibly increasing its concentration). Products include:
- Atripla Tablets 945
- Sustiva Capsules 930
- Sustiva Tablets 930

Enflurane (Concurrent use may produce additive CNS depressant effects).
No products indexed under this heading.

Erythromycin (CYP3A4 is a minor metabolizing enzyme of zaleplon; the co-administration of a strong, selective CYP3A4 inhibitor (erythromycin) produced a 34% increase in zaleplon's plasma concentration. A routine dosage adjustment of zaleplon is not considered necessary). Products include:
- Ery-Tab Tablets 449
- Erythromycin Base Filmtab Tablets 455
- Erythromycin Delayed-Release Capsules, USP 457
- PCE Dispertab Tablets 515

Erythromycin Estolate (CYP3A4 is a minor metabolizing enzyme of zaleplon; the co-administration of a strong, selective CYP3A4 inhibitor (erythromycin) produced a 34% increase in zaleplon's plasma concentration. A routine dosage adjustment of zaleplon is not considered necessary).
No products indexed under this heading.

Erythromycin Ethylsuccinate (CYP3A4 is a minor metabolizing enzyme of zaleplon; the co-administration of a strong, selective CYP3A4 inhibitor (erythromycin) produced a 34% increase in zaleplon's plasma concentration. A routine dosage adjustment of zaleplon is not considered necessary). Products include:
- E.E.S. 451
- EryPed 447

Erythromycin Gluceptate (CYP3A4 is a minor metabolizing enzyme of zaleplon; the co-administration of a strong, selective CYP3A4 inhibitor (erythromycin) produced a 34% increase in zaleplon's plasma concentration. A routine dosage adjustment of zaleplon is not considered necessary).
No products indexed under this heading.

Erythromycin Lactobionate (CYP3A4 is a minor metabolizing enzyme of zaleplon; the co-administration of a strong, selective CYP3A4 inhibitor (erythromycin) produced a 34% increase in zaleplon's plasma concentration. A routine dosage adjustment of zaleplon is not considered necessary).
No products indexed under this heading.

Erythromycin Stearate (CYP3A4 is a minor metabolizing enzyme of zaleplon; the co-administration of a strong, selective CYP3A4 inhibitor (erythromycin) produced a 34% increase in zaleplon's plasma concentration. A routine dosage adjustment of zaleplon is not considered necessary). Products include:
- Erythrocin Stearate Filmtab Tablets 453

Esomeprazole Magnesium (CYP3A4 inhibitors may decrease zaleplon's clearance, possibly increasing its concentration). Products include:
- Nexium Delayed-Release Capsules 655

Estazolam (Concurrent use may produce additive CNS depressant effects). Products include:
- ProSom Tablets 517

Ethanol (Concurrent use may produce additive CNS depressant effects).
No products indexed under this heading.

Ethchlorvynol (Concurrent use may produce additive CNS depressant effects).
No products indexed under this heading.

Ethinamate (Concurrent use may produce additive CNS depressant effects).
No products indexed under this heading.

Ethosuximide (Concurrent use with anticonvulsants may produce additive CNS depressant effects).
No products indexed under this heading.

Ethotoin (Concurrent use with anticonvulsants may produce additive CNS depressant effects).
No products indexed under this heading.

Ethyl Alcohol (Concurrent use may produce additive CNS depressant effects).
No products indexed under this heading.

Felbamate (Concurrent use with anticonvulsants may produce additive CNS depressant effects).
No products indexed under this heading.

Fentanyl (Concurrent use may produce additive CNS depressant effects). Products include:
- Duragesic Transdermal System 2373
- Ionsys Transdermal System 2379

Fentanyl Citrate (Concurrent use may produce additive CNS depressant effects). Products include:
- Actiq 979

Fexofenadine Hydrochloride (Concurrent use may produce additive CNS depressant effects). Products include:
- Allegra 2844
- Allegra-D 12 Hour Extended-Release Tablets 2846
- Allegra-D 24 Hour Extended-Release Tablets 2849

Fluconazole (CYP3A4 inhibitors may decrease zaleplon's clearance, possibly increasing its concentration).
No products indexed under this heading.

Fludrocortisone Acetate (CYP3A4 inhibitors may increase zaleplon's clearance, possibly decreasing its concentration).
No products indexed under this heading.

Fluoxetine Hydrochloride (CYP3A4 inhibitors may decrease zaleplon's clearance, possibly increasing its concentration). Products include:
- Prozac Pulvules and Liquid 1801
- Symbyax Capsules 1819

Fluphenazine Decanoate (Concurrent use may produce additive CNS depressant effects).
No products indexed under this heading.

Fluphenazine Enanthate (Concurrent use may produce additive CNS depressant effects).
No products indexed under this heading.

Fluphenazine Hydrochloride (Concurrent use may produce additive CNS depressant effects).
No products indexed under this heading.

Flurazepam Hydrochloride (Concurrent use may produce additive CNS depressant effects). Products include:
- Dalmane Capsules 3342

Fluvoxamine Maleate (CYP3A4 inhibitors may decrease zaleplon's clearance, possibly increasing its concentration).
No products indexed under this heading.

Fosamprenavir Calcium (CYP3A4 inhibitors may decrease zaleplon's clearance, possibly increasing its concentration). Products include:
- Lexiva Tablets 1505

Fosphenytoin (Concurrent use with anticonvulsants may produce additive CNS depressant effects).
No products indexed under this heading.

Fosphenytoin Sodium (CYP3A4 is ordinarily a minor metabolizing enzyme of zaleplon, the co-administration of a potent inducer, such as phenytoin, although not posing a safety concern, could lead to ineffectiveness of zaleplon; concurrent use with anticonvulsants may produce additive CNS depressant effects).
No products indexed under this heading.

Gabapentin (Concurrent use with anticonvulsants may produce additive CNS depressant effects). Products include:
- Neurontin Capsules 2487
- Neurontin Oral Solution 2487
- Neurontin Tablets 2487

IMPORTANT NOTE: Always consult each drug listing in the patient's regimen for possible interactions.

Garlic Extract (CYP3A4 inhibitors may increase zaleplon's clearance, possibly decreasing its concentration).
No products indexed under this heading.

Garlic Oil (CYP3A4 inhibitors may increase zaleplon's clearance, possibly decreasing its concentration).
No products indexed under this heading.

Glutethimide (Concurrent use may produce additive CNS depressant effects).
No products indexed under this heading.

Haloperidol (Concurrent use may produce additive CNS depressant effects).
No products indexed under this heading.

Haloperidol Decanoate (Concurrent use may produce additive CNS depressant effects).
No products indexed under this heading.

Hydrocodone Bitartrate (Concurrent use may produce additive CNS depressant effects). Products include:
Hycodan 1116
Hycotuss Expectorant Syrup 1117
Vicodin Tablets 535
Vicodin ES Tablets 536
Vicodin HP Tablets 538
Vicoprofen Tablets 539
Zydone Tablets 1139

Hydrocodone Polistirex (Concurrent use may produce additive CNS depressant effects). Products include:
Tussionex Pennkinetic Extended-Release Suspension 3327

Hydrocortisone (CYP3A4 inhibitors may increase zaleplon's clearance, possibly decreasing its concentration). Products include:
Colocort Rectal Suspension, USP (Retention) 100 mg/60 mL 2476
Hydrocortone Tablets 1989
Preparation H Hydrocortisone Cream .... ▣ 646

Hydrocortisone Acetate (CYP3A4 inhibitors may increase zaleplon's clearance, possibly decreasing its concentration). Products include:
Analpram-HC 1159
Pramosone 1161
ProctoFoam-HC 3099

Hydrocortisone Butyrate (CYP3A4 inhibitors may increase zaleplon's clearance, possibly decreasing its concentration). Products include:
Locoid Lipocream Cream 1160

Hydrocortisone Cypionate (CYP3A4 inhibitors may increase zaleplon's clearance, possibly decreasing its concentration).
No products indexed under this heading.

Hydrocortisone Hemisuccinate (CYP3A4 inhibitors may increase zaleplon's clearance, possibly decreasing its concentration).
No products indexed under this heading.

Hydrocortisone Probutate (CYP3A4 inhibitors may increase zaleplon's clearance, possibly decreasing its concentration).
No products indexed under this heading.

Hydrocortisone Sodium Phosphate (CYP3A4 inhibitors may increase zaleplon's clearance, possibly decreasing its concentration).
No products indexed under this heading.

Hydrocortisone Sodium Succinate (CYP3A4 inhibitors may increase zaleplon's clearance, possibly decreasing its concentration).
No products indexed under this heading.

Hydrocortisone Valerate (CYP3A4 inhibitors may increase zaleplon's clearance, possibly decreasing its concentration).
No products indexed under this heading.

Hydromorphone Hydrochloride (Concurrent use may produce additive CNS depressant effects). Products include:
Dilaudid 440
Dilaudid Non-Sterile Powder 440
Dilaudid Oral Liquid 445
Dilaudid Rectal Suppositories 440
Dilaudid Tablets 440
Dilaudid Tablets - 8 mg 445
Dilaudid-HP 442

Hydroxyzine Hydrochloride (Concurrent use may produce additive CNS depressant effects).
No products indexed under this heading.

Hypericum (CYP3A4 inhibitors may increase zaleplon's clearance, possibly decreasing its concentration). Products include:
Satiete Tablets .... ▣ 832

Hypericum Perforatum (CYP3A4 inhibitors may increase zaleplon's clearance, possibly decreasing its concentration).
No products indexed under this heading.

Imipramine Hydrochloride (Concurrent use may produce additive CNS depressant effects).
No products indexed under this heading.

Imipramine Pamoate (Concurrent use may produce additive CNS depressant effects).
No products indexed under this heading.

Indinavir Sulfate (CYP3A4 inhibitors may decrease zaleplon's clearance, possibly increasing its concentration). Products include:
Crixivan Capsules 1940

Isocarboxazid (Concurrent use may produce additive CNS depressant effects).
No products indexed under this heading.

Isoflurane (Concurrent use may produce additive CNS depressant effects).
No products indexed under this heading.

Isoniazid (CYP3A4 inhibitors may decrease zaleplon's clearance, possibly increasing its concentration).
No products indexed under this heading.

Itraconazole (CYP3A4 inhibitors may decrease zaleplon's clearance, possibly increasing its concentration).
No products indexed under this heading.

Ketamine Hydrochloride (Concurrent use may produce additive CNS depressant effects).
No products indexed under this heading.

Ketoconazole (CYP3A4 inhibitors may decrease zaleplon's clearance, possibly increasing its concentration). Products include:
Nizoral A-D Shampoo, 1% 1868

Lamotrigine (Concurrent use with anticonvulsants may produce additive CNS depressant effects). Products include:
Lamictal 1481

Levetiracetam (Concurrent use with anticonvulsants may produce additive CNS depressant effects). Products include:
Keppra Injection 3320
Keppra Oral Solution 3314
Keppra Tablets 3314

Levomethadyl Acetate Hydrochloride (Concurrent use may produce additive CNS depressant effects).
No products indexed under this heading.

Levorphanol Tartrate (Concurrent use may produce additive CNS depressant effects).
No products indexed under this heading.

Lithium Carbonate (Concurrent use may produce additive CNS depressant effects). Products include:
Lithobid Tablets 1692

Lithium Citrate (Concurrent use may produce additive CNS depressant effects).
No products indexed under this heading.

Lopinavir (CYP3A4 inhibitors may decrease zaleplon's clearance, possibly increasing its concentration). Products include:
Kaletra 476

Loratadine (Concurrent use may produce additive CNS depressant effects). Products include:
Alavert Allergy & Sinus D-12 Hour Tablets .... ▣ 771
Alavert .... ▣ 771
Children's Claritin Allergy Oral Solution .... ▣ 771
Claritin Non-Drowsy 24 Hour Tablets .... ▣ 772
Claritin Reditabs 24 Hour Non-Drowsy Tablets .... ▣ 772
Claritin-D Non-Drowsy 12 Hour Tablets .... ▣ 772
Claritin-D Non-Drowsy 24 Hour Tablets .... ▣ 772

Lorazepam (Concurrent use may produce additive CNS depressant effects).
No products indexed under this heading.

Loxapine Hydrochloride (Concurrent use may produce additive CNS depressant effects).
No products indexed under this heading.

Loxapine Succinate (Concurrent use may produce additive CNS depressant effects).
No products indexed under this heading.

Maprotiline Hydrochloride (Concurrent use may produce additive CNS depressant effects).
No products indexed under this heading.

Meperidine Hydrochloride (Concurrent use may produce additive CNS depressant effects).
No products indexed under this heading.

Mephenytoin (Concurrent use with anticonvulsants may produce additive CNS depressant effects).
No products indexed under this heading.

Mephobarbital (Concurrent use may produce additive CNS depressant effects).
No products indexed under this heading.

Meprobamate (Concurrent use may produce additive CNS depressant effects).
No products indexed under this heading.

Mesoridazine Besylate (Concurrent use may produce additive CNS depressant effects).
No products indexed under this heading.

Methadone Hydrochloride (Concurrent use may produce additive CNS depressant effects).
No products indexed under this heading.

Methdilazine Hydrochloride (Concurrent use may produce additive CNS depressant effects).
No products indexed under this heading.

Methohexital Sodium (Concurrent use may produce additive CNS depressant effects).
No products indexed under this heading.

Methotrimeprazine (Concurrent use may produce additive CNS depressant effects).
No products indexed under this heading.

Methoxyflurane (Concurrent use may produce additive CNS depressant effects).
No products indexed under this heading.

Methsuximide (Concurrent use with anticonvulsants may produce additive CNS depressant effects).
No products indexed under this heading.

Methylprednisolone (CYP3A4 inhibitors may increase zaleplon's clearance, possibly decreasing its concentration).
No products indexed under this heading.

Methylprednisolone Acetate (CYP3A4 inhibitors may increase zaleplon's clearance, possibly decreasing its concentration). Products include:
Depo-Medrol Injectable Suspension 2617
Depo-Medrol Single-Dose Vial 2619

Methylprednisolone Sodium Succinate (CYP3A4 inhibitors may increase zaleplon's clearance, possibly decreasing its concentration).
No products indexed under this heading.

Metronidazole (CYP3A4 inhibitors may decrease zaleplon's clearance, possibly increasing its concentration). Products include:
Metrogel 1% 1211
MetroGel-Vaginal Gel 1855
Vandazole Vaginal Gel 3338

Metronidazole Benzoate (CYP3A4 inhibitors may decrease zaleplon's clearance, possibly increasing its concentration).
No products indexed under this heading.

Metronidazole Hydrochloride
(CYP3A4 inhibitors may decrease
zaleplon's clearance, possibly
increasing its concentration).
No products indexed under this
heading.

Miconazole (CYP3A4 inhibitors
may decrease zaleplon's clearance,
possibly increasing its
concentration).
No products indexed under this
heading.

Miconazole Nitrate (CYP3A4
inhibitors may decrease zaleplon's
clearance, possibly increasing its
concentration). Products include:
Desenex ▧635
Desenex Jock Itch Spray Powder ... ▧635

Midazolam Hydrochloride (Concurrent use may produce additive
CNS depressant effects).
No products indexed under this
heading.

Modafinil (CYP3A4 inhibitors may
increase zaleplon's clearance, possibly decreasing its concentration).
Products include:
Provigil Tablets 988

Molindone Hydrochloride (Concurrent use may produce additive
CNS depressant effects). Products
include:
Moban Tablets 1119

Morphine Sulfate (Concurrent use
may produce additive CNS depres-
sant effects). Products include:
Avinza Capsules 1741
Kadian Capsules 577
MS Contin Tablets 2701

Nefazodone Hydrochloride
(CYP3A4 inhibitors may decrease
zaleplon's clearance, possibly
increasing its concentration).
No products indexed under this
heading.

Nelfinavir Mesylate (CYP3A4
inhibitors may decrease zaleplon's
clearance, possibly increasing its
concentration). Products include:
Viracept 2577

Nevirapine (CYP3A4 inhibitors may
decrease zaleplon's clearance, pos-
sibly increasing its concentration).
Products include:
Viramune Oral Suspension 873
Viramune Tablets 873

Niacinamide (CYP3A4 inhibitors
may decrease zaleplon's clearance,
possibly increasing its
concentration).
No products indexed under this
heading.

Nicotinamide (CYP3A4 inhibitors
may decrease zaleplon's clearance,
possibly increasing its concentration). Products include:
Nicomide Tablets 1088

Nifedipine (CYP3A4 inhibitors may
decrease zaleplon's clearance, possibly increasing its concentration).
Products include:
Adalat CC Tablets 2964

Norfloxacin (CYP3A4 inhibitors
may decrease zaleplon's clearance,
possibly increasing its concentration). Products include:
Noroxin Tablets 2032

Nortriptyline Hydrochloride (Concurrent use may produce additive
CNS depressant effects).
No products indexed under this
heading.

Olanzapine (Concurrent use may
produce additive CNS depressant
effects). Products include:
Symbyax Capsules 1819

Zyprexa Tablets 1830
Zyprexa IntraMuscular 1830
Zyprexa ZYDIS Orally
Disintegrating Tablets 1830

Omeprazole (CYP3A4 inhibitors
may decrease zaleplon's clearance,
possibly increasing its concentration). Products include:
Zegerid Capsules 2958
Zegerid Powder for Oral Solution 2958

Oxazepam (Concurrent use may
produce additive CNS depressant
effects).
No products indexed under this
heading.

Oxcarbazepine (Concurrent use
with anticonvulsants may produce
additive CNS depressant effects).
Products include:
Trileptal Tablets 2300
Trileptal Oral Suspension 2300

Oxycodone Hydrochloride (Con-
current use may produce additive
CNS depressant effects). Products
include:
OxyContin Tablets 2703
OxyFast Oral Concentrate
Solution................................ 2708
OxyIR Capsules 2708
Percocet Tablets 1131
Percodan Tablets 1132

Paramethadione (Concurrent use
with anticonvulsants may produce
additive CNS depressant effects).
No products indexed under this
heading.

Paroxetine Hydrochloride
(CYP3A4 inhibitors may decrease
zaleplon's clearance, possibly
increasing its concentration).
Products include:
Paxil CR Controlled-Release
Tablets 1538
Paxil 1530

Pentobarbital Sodium (Concurrent use may produce additive CNS
depressant effects). Products
include:
Nembutal Sodium Solution, USP 2470

Perphenazine (Concurrent use
may produce additive CNS depressant effects).
No products indexed under this
heading.

Phenacemide (Concurrent use with
anticonvulsants may produce additive CNS depressant effects).
No products indexed under this
heading.

Phenelzine Sulfate (Concurrent
use may produce additive CNS
depressant effects).
No products indexed under this
heading.

Phenobarbital (CYP3A4 is ordinarily a minor metabolizing enzyme of
zaleplon, the co-administration of a
potent inducer, such as phenobarbital, although not posing a safety concern, could lead to ineffectiveness of
zaleplon; concurrent use with anticonvulsants may produce additive
CNS depressant effects). Products
include:
Donnatal Extentabs 2493

Phenobarbital Sodium (CYP3A4
inhibitors may increase zaleplon's
clearance, possibly decreasing its
concentration).
No products indexed under this
heading.

Phensuximide (Concurrent use
with anticonvulsants may produce
additive CNS depressant effects).
No products indexed under this
heading.

Phenytoin (CYP3A4 is ordinarily a
minor metabolizing enzyme of zaleplon, the co-administration of a
potent inducer, such as phenytoin,
although not posing a safety concern, could lead to ineffectiveness of
zaleplon; concurrent use with anticonvulsants may produce additive
CNS depressant effects).
No products indexed under this
heading.

Phenytoin Sodium (CYP3A4 is
ordinarily a minor metabolizing
enzyme of zaleplon, the co-
administration of a potent inducer,
such as phenytoin, although not posing a safety concern, could lead to
ineffectiveness of zaleplon; concurrent use with anticonvulsants may
produce additive CNS depressant
effects). Products include:
Phenytek Capsules 2160

Prazepam (Concurrent use may
produce additive CNS depressant
effects).
No products indexed under this
heading.

Prednisolone Acetate (CYP3A4
inhibitors may increase zaleplon's
clearance, possibly decreasing its
concentration). Products include:
Blephamide Ophthalmic Ointment 568
Blephamide Ophthalmic
Suspension 569
Poly-Pred Ophthalmic
Suspension ☉233
Pred Forte Ophthalmic
Suspension ☉235
Pred Mild Ophthalmic
Suspension ☉238
Pred-G Ophthalmic Ointment ☉237
Pred-G Ophthalmic Suspension ... ☉236

Prednisolone Sodium Phosphate
(CYP3A4 inhibitors may increase
zaleplon's clearance, possibly
decreasing its concentration).
No products indexed under this
heading.

Prednisolone Tebutate (CYP3A4
inhibitors may increase zaleplon's
clearance, possibly decreasing its
concentration).
No products indexed under this
heading.

Prednisone (CYP3A4 inhibitors may
increase zaleplon's clearance, possibly decreasing its concentration).
No products indexed under this
heading.

Primidone (Concurrent use with
anticonvulsants may produce additive CNS depressant effects).
No products indexed under this
heading.

Prochlorperazine (Concurrent use
may produce additive CNS depressant effects).
No products indexed under this
heading.

Promethazine Hydrochloride
(Co-administration of a single dose
of zaleplon and promethazine (10
and 25mg, respectively) resulted in
a 15% decrease in maximal plasma
concentrations of zalephon, but no
change in the area under the plasma
curve, however, the pharmacodynamics of co-administration of zalephon and promethazine have not
been evaluated. Caution should be
exercised when these 2 agents are
co-administered). Products include:
Phenergan Tablets and
Suppositories.......................... 3440

Propofol (Concurrent use may produce additive CNS depressant
effects).
No products indexed under this
heading.

Propoxyphene Hydrochloride
(Concurrent use may produce additive CNS depressant effects).
No products indexed under this
heading.

Propoxyphene Napsylate (Concurrent use may produce additive
CNS depressant effects).
No products indexed under this
heading.

Protriptyline Hydrochloride (Concurrent use may produce additive
CNS depressant effects).
No products indexed under this
heading.

Pyrilamine Maleate (Concurrent
use may produce additive CNS
depressant effects).
No products indexed under this
heading.

Pyrilamine Tannate (Concurrent
use may produce additive CNS
depressant effects).
No products indexed under this
heading.

Quazepam (Concurrent use may
produce additive CNS depressant
effects).
No products indexed under this
heading.

Quetiapine Fumarate (Concurrent
use may produce additive CNS
depressant effects). Products
include:
Seroquel Tablets 690

Quinidine (CYP3A4 inhibitors may
decrease zaleplon's clearance, possibly increasing its concentration).
No products indexed under this
heading.

Quinidine Hydrochloride (CYP3A4
inhibitors may decrease zaleplon's
clearance, possibly increasing its
concentration).
No products indexed under this
heading.

Quinidine Polygalacturonate
(CYP3A4 inhibitors may decrease
zaleplon's clearance, possibly
increasing its concentration).
No products indexed under this
heading.

Quinidine Sulfate (CYP3A4 inhibitors may decrease zaleplon's clearance, possibly increasing its
concentration).
No products indexed under this
heading.

Quinine (CYP3A4 inhibitors may
decrease zaleplon's clearance, possibly increasing its concentration).
No products indexed under this
heading.

Quinine Sulfate (CYP3A4 inhibitors
may decrease zaleplon's clearance,
possibly increasing its
concentration).
No products indexed under this
heading.

Quinupristin (CYP3A4 inhibitors
may decrease zaleplon's clearance,
possibly increasing its
concentration).
No products indexed under this
heading.

Ranitidine Bismuth Citrate
(CYP3A4 inhibitors may decrease
zaleplon's clearance, possibly
increasing its concentration).
No products indexed under this
heading.

IMPORTANT NOTE: Always consult each drug listing in the patient's regimen for possible interactions.

Ranitidine Hydrochloride (CYP3A4 inhibitors may decrease zaleplon's clearance, possibly increasing its concentration).
Products include:
Zantac 1624
Zantac Injection 1619
Zantac Injection Pharmacy Bulk Package 1622

Remifentanil Hydrochloride (Concurrent use may produce additive CNS depressant effects).
No products indexed under this heading.

Rifabutin (CYP3A4 inhibitors may increase zaleplon's clearance, possibly decreasing its concentration).
No products indexed under this heading.

Rifampicin (CYP3A4 inhibitors may increase zaleplon's clearance, possibly decreasing its concentration).
No products indexed under this heading.

Rifampin (The co-administration of a potent CYP3A4 enzyme inducer, although not posing a safety concern, could lead to ineffectiveness of zaleplon).
No products indexed under this heading.

Rifapentine (CYP3A4 inhibitors may increase zaleplon's clearance, possibly decreasing its concentration).
No products indexed under this heading.

Risperidone (Concurrent use may produce additive CNS depressant effects). Products include:
Risperdal 1676
Risperdal Consta Long-Acting Injection 1682
Risperdal M-Tab Orally Disintegrating Tablets 1676

Ritonavir (CYP3A4 inhibitors may decrease zaleplon's clearance, possibly increasing its concentration).
Products include:
Kaletra 476
Norvir 503

Saquinavir (CYP3A4 inhibitors may decrease zaleplon's clearance, possibly increasing its concentration).
No products indexed under this heading.

Saquinavir Mesylate (CYP3A4 inhibitors may decrease zaleplon's clearance, possibly increasing its concentration). Products include:
Invirase 2772

Secobarbital Sodium (Concurrent use may produce additive CNS depressant effects).
No products indexed under this heading.

Sertraline Hydrochloride (CYP3A4 inhibitors may decrease zaleplon's clearance, possibly increasing its concentration).
Products include:
Zoloft 2586

Sevoflurane (Concurrent use may produce additive CNS depressant effects). Products include:
Ultane Liquid for Inhalation 531

Sodium Oxybate (Concurrent use may produce additive CNS depressant effects). Products include:
Xyrem Oral Solution 1688

Sufentanil Citrate (Concurrent use may produce additive CNS depressant effects).
No products indexed under this heading.

Sulfinpyrazone (CYP3A4 inhibitors may increase zaleplon's clearance, possibly decreasing its concentration).
No products indexed under this heading.

Telithromycin (CYP3A4 inhibitors may decrease zaleplon's clearance, possibly increasing its concentration). Products include:
Ketek Tablets 2903

Temazepam (Concurrent use may produce additive CNS depressant effects). Products include:
Restoril Capsules 1860

Terfenadine (Concurrent use may produce additive CNS depressant effects).
No products indexed under this heading.

Theophylline (CYP3A4 inhibitors may increase zaleplon's clearance, possibly decreasing its concentration).
No products indexed under this heading.

Thiamylal Sodium (Concurrent use may produce additive CNS depressant effects).
No products indexed under this heading.

Thioridazine Hydrochloride (Co-administration has produced additive effects of decreased alertness and impaired psychomotor performance for 2 to 4 hours). Products include:
Thioridazine Hydrochloride Tablets 2163

Thiothixene (Concurrent use may produce additive CNS depressant effects). Products include:
Thiothixene Capsules 2165

Tiagabine Hydrochloride (Concurrent use with anticonvulsants may produce additive CNS depressant effects). Products include:
Gabitril Tablets 984

Topiramate (Concurrent use with anticonvulsants may produce additive CNS depressant effects).
Products include:
Topamax Sprinkle Capsules 2404
Topamax Tablets 2404

Tranylcypromine Sulfate (Concurrent use may produce additive CNS depressant effects). Products include:
Parnate Tablets 1527

Triamcinolone (CYP3A4 inhibitors may increase zaleplon's clearance, possibly decreasing its concentration).
No products indexed under this heading.

Triamcinolone Acetonide (CYP3A4 inhibitors may increase zaleplon's clearance, possibly decreasing its concentration).
Products include:
Azmacort Inhalation Aerosol 1726
Nasacort AQ Nasal Spray 2922

Triamcinolone Diacetate (CYP3A4 inhibitors may increase zaleplon's clearance, possibly decreasing its concentration).
No products indexed under this heading.

Triamcinolone Hexacetonide (CYP3A4 inhibitors may increase zaleplon's clearance, possibly decreasing its concentration).
No products indexed under this heading.

Triazolam (Concurrent use may produce additive CNS depressant effects).
No products indexed under this heading.

Trifluoperazine Hydrochloride (Concurrent use may produce additive CNS depressant effects).
No products indexed under this heading.

Trimeprazine Tartrate (Concurrent use may produce additive CNS depressant effects).
No products indexed under this heading.

Trimethadione (Concurrent use with anticonvulsants may produce additive CNS depressant effects).
No products indexed under this heading.

Trimipramine Maleate (Concurrent use may produce additive CNS depressant effects).
No products indexed under this heading.

Tripelennamine Hydrochloride (Concurrent use may produce additive CNS depressant effects).
No products indexed under this heading.

Triprolidine Hydrochloride (Concurrent use may produce additive CNS depressant effects).
No products indexed under this heading.

Troglitazone (CYP3A4 inhibitors may decrease zaleplon's clearance, possibly increasing its concentration).
No products indexed under this heading.

Troleandomycin (CYP3A4 inhibitors may decrease zaleplon's clearance, possibly increasing its concentration).
No products indexed under this heading.

Valproate Sodium (Concurrent use with anticonvulsants may produce additive CNS depressant effects).
Products include:
Depacon Injection 412

Valproic Acid (Concurrent use with anticonvulsants may produce additive CNS depressant effects).
Products include:
Depakene 417

Verapamil Hydrochloride (CYP3A4 inhibitors may decrease zaleplon's clearance, possibly increasing its concentration).
Products include:
Covera-HS Tablets 3139
Tarka Tablets 524
Verelan PM Extended-Release Capsules, Controlled-Onset 3106

Voriconazole (CYP3A4 inhibitors may decrease zaleplon's clearance, possibly increasing its concentration). Products include:
VFEND I.V. 2564
VFEND Oral Suspension 2564
VFEND Tablets 2564

Zafirlukast (CYP3A4 inhibitors may decrease zaleplon's clearance, possibly increasing its concentration).
Products include:
Accolate Tablets 671

Zileuton (CYP3A4 inhibitors may decrease zaleplon's clearance, possibly increasing its concentration).
Products include:
Zyflo Tablets 1023

Ziprasidone Hydrochloride (Concurrent use may produce additive CNS depressant effects). Products include:
Geodon Capsules 2529

Zolpidem Tartrate (Concurrent use may produce additive CNS depressant effects). Products include:
Ambien Tablets 2851
Ambien CR Tablets 2855

Zonisamide (Concurrent use with anticonvulsants may produce additive CNS depressant effects).
Products include:
Zonegran Capsules 1101

Food Interactions

Alcohol (Concurrent use may produce additive CNS depressant effects).

Food, unspecified (A high-fat/heavy meal prolongs the absorption of zaleplon compared to fasting state, delays tmax by approximately 2 hours and reduces Cmax approximately 35%; the effect of Sonata on sleep onset may be reduced if it is taken with or immediately after a high-fat/heavy meal).

Grapefruit (CYP3A4 inhibitors may decrease zaleplon's clearance, possibly increasing its concentration).

Grapefruit Juice (CYP3A4 inhibitors may decrease zaleplon's clearance, possibly increasing its concentration).

SORIATANE CAPSULES

(Acitretin) 1013

May interact with tetracyclines and certain other agents. Compounds in these categories include:

Demeclocycline Hydrochloride (Since both Soriatane and tetracyclines can cause increases in intracranial pressure, their combined use is contraindicated).
No products indexed under this heading.

Doxycycline Calcium (Since both Soriatane and tetracyclines can cause increases in intracranial pressure, their combined use is contraindicated).
No products indexed under this heading.

Doxycycline Hyclate (Since both Soriatane and tetracyclines can cause increases in intracranial pressure, their combined use is contraindicated).
No products indexed under this heading.

Doxycycline Monohydrate (Since both Soriatane and tetracyclines can cause increases in intracranial pressure, their combined use is contraindicated). Products include:
Oracea Capsules 1000

Glibenclamide (Acitretin treatment potentiated the blood glucose lowering affect of glibenclamide in 3 of the 7 male volunteers).
No products indexed under this heading.

Methacycline Hydrochloride (Since both Soriatane and tetracyclines can cause increases in intracranial pressure, their combined use is contraindicated).
No products indexed under this heading.

Methotrexate (An increased risk of hepatitis has been reported to result from combined use of methotrexate and etretinate).
No products indexed under this heading.

Minocycline Hydrochloride (Since both Soriatane and tetracy-

clines can cause increases in intracranial pressure, their combined use is contraindicated). Products include:
Solodyn Extended Release Tablets 1890
Oxytetracycline Hydrochloride (Since both Soriatane and tetracyclines can cause increases in intracranial pressure, their combined use is contraindicated).
No products indexed under this heading.
Phenytoin (If acitretin is given concurrently with phenytoin, the protein binding of phenytoin may be reduced).
No products indexed under this heading.
Tetracycline Hydrochloride (Since both Soriatane and tetracyclines can cause increases in intracranial pressure, their combined use is contraindicated).
No products indexed under this heading.
Vitamin A (Concomitant administration of vitamin A and/or other oral retinoids with acitretin must be avoided because of the risk of hypervitaminosis A). Products include:
Visutein Capsules 3329

Food Interactions

Alcohol (Clinical evidence has shown that etretinate can be formed with concurrent ingestion of acitretin and ethanol).

SPIRIVA HANDIHALER

(Tiotropium bromide) 869
May interact with anticholinergics and certain other agents. Compounds in these categories include:

Atropine Sulfate (Co-administration of tiotropium with other anticholinergic-containing drugs (e.g., ipratropium) has not been studied and is therefore not recommended). Products include:
Donnatal Extentabs 2493
Belladonna Alkaloids (Co-administration of tiotropium with other anticholinergic-containing drugs (e.g., ipratropium) has not been studied and is therefore not recommended). Products include:
Hyland's Teething Tablets 830
Benztropine Mesylate (Co-administration of tiotropium with other anticholinergic-containing drugs (e.g., ipratropium) has not been studied and is therefore not recommended).
No products indexed under this heading.
Biperiden Hydrochloride (Co-administration of tiotropium with other anticholinergic-containing drugs (e.g., ipratropium) has not been studied and is therefore not recommended).
No products indexed under this heading.
Cimetidine (Concomitant administration of cimetidine with tiotropium resulted in a 20% increase in the $AUC_{0\text{-}4h}$, a 28% increase in the renal clearance of tiotropium and no significant change in the Cmax and amount excreted in urine over 96 hours. Therefore, no clinically significant interaction occurred between tiotropium and cimetidine). Products include:
Tagamet HB 200 Tablets 664
Cimetidine Hydrochloride (Concomitant administration of cimetidine with tiotropium resulted in a 20% increase in the AUC0-4h, a 28% increase in the renal clearance of tiotropium and no significant change in the Cmax and amount excreted in urine over 96 hours. Therefore, no clinically significant interaction occurred between tiotropium and cimetidine).
No products indexed under this heading.
Clidinium Bromide (Co-administration of tiotropium with other anticholinergic-containing drugs (e.g., ipratropium) has not been studied and is therefore not recommended).
No products indexed under this heading.
Dicyclomine Hydrochloride (Co-administration of tiotropium with other anticholinergic-containing drugs (e.g., ipratropium) has not been studied and is therefore not recommended). Products include:
Bentyl Capsules 697
Bentyl Injection 697
Bentyl Syrup 697
Bentyl Tablets 697
Glycopyrrolate (Co-administration of tiotropium with other anticholinergic-containing drugs (e.g., ipratropium) has not been studied and is therefore not recommended).
No products indexed under this heading.
Hyoscyamine (Co-administration of tiotropium with other anticholinergic-containing drugs (e.g., ipratropium) has not been studied and is therefore not recommended).
No products indexed under this heading.
Hyoscyamine Sulfate (Co-administration of tiotropium with other anticholinergic-containing drugs (e.g., ipratropium) has not been studied and is therefore not recommended). Products include:
Donnatal Extentabs 2493
Prosed/DS Tablets 1157
Ipratropium Bromide (Co-administration of tiotropium with other anticholinergic-containing drugs (e.g., ipratropium) has not been studied and is therefore not recommended). Products include:
Atrovent Inhalation Solution 835
Atrovent HFA Inhalation Aerosol 841
Atrovent Nasal Spray 0.03% 837
Atrovent Nasal Spray 0.06% 839
Combivent Inhalation Aerosol 847
DuoNeb Inhalation Solution 1058
Mepenzolate Bromide (Co-administration of tiotropium with other anticholinergic-containing drugs (e.g., ipratropium) has not been studied and is therefore not recommended).
No products indexed under this heading.
Oxybutynin Chloride (Co-administration of tiotropium with other anticholinergic-containing drugs (e.g., ipratropium) has not been studied and is therefore not recommended). Products include:
Ditropan XL Extended-Release Tablets 2413
Procyclidine Hydrochloride (Co-administration of tiotropium with other anticholinergic-containing drugs (e.g., ipratropium) has not been studied and is therefore not recommended).
No products indexed under this heading.
Propantheline Bromide (Co-administration of tiotropium with other anticholinergic-containing drugs (e.g., ipratropium) has not been studied and is therefore not recommended).
No products indexed under this heading.
Scopolamine (Co-administration of tiotropium with other anticholinergic-containing drugs (e.g., ipratropium) has not been studied and is therefore not recommended). Products include:
Transderm Scōp Transdermal Therapeutic System 2177
Scopolamine Hydrobromide (Co-administration of tiotropium with other anticholinergic-containing drugs (e.g., ipratropium) has not been studied and is therefore not recommended). Products include:
Donnatal Extentabs 2493
Tolterodine Tartrate (Co-administration of tiotropium with other anticholinergic-containing drugs (e.g., ipratropium) has not been studied and is therefore not recommended). Products include:
Detrol Tablets 2628
Detrol LA Capsules 2631
Tridihexethyl Chloride (Co-administration of tiotropium with other anticholinergic-containing drugs (e.g., ipratropium) has not been studied and is therefore not recommended).
No products indexed under this heading.
Trihexyphenidyl Hydrochloride (Co-administration of tiotropium with other anticholinergic-containing drugs (e.g., ipratropium) has not been studied and is therefore not recommended).
No products indexed under this heading.

ST. JOSEPH 81 MG ASPIRIN CHEWABLE AND ENTERIC COATED TABLETS

(Aspirin) 1869
May interact with ACE inhibitors, beta blockers, anticoagulants, diuretics, oral hypoglycemic agents, non-steroidal anti-inflammatory agents, phenytoin, valproate, and certain other agents. Compounds in these categories include:

Acarbose (Moderate doses of aspirin may increase the effectiveness of oral hypoglycemic agents leading to hypoglycemia). Products include:
Precose Tablets 751
Acebutolol Hydrochloride (Decreased hypotensive effects of beta-blockers).
No products indexed under this heading.
Acetazolamide (Co-administration can lead to high serum concentrations of acetazolamide and its toxicity).
No products indexed under this heading.
Acetazolamide Sodium (Co-administration can lead to high serum concentrations of acetazolamide and its toxicity).
No products indexed under this heading.
Amiloride Hydrochloride (Diminished effectiveness of diuretics in patients with underlying renal or cardiovascular disease). Products include:
Midamor Tablets 2026
Moduretic Tablets 2028
Anisindione (Patients on anticoagulant therapy are at increased risk of bleeding). Products include:
Miradon Tablets 3042
Ardeparin Sodium (Patients on anticoagulant therapy are at increased risk of bleeding).
No products indexed under this heading.
Atenolol (Decreased hypotensive effects of beta-blockers).
No products indexed under this heading.
Benazepril Hydrochloride (Co-administration may result in diminished hyponatremic and hypotensive effects of ACE inhibitors). Products include:
Lotensin Tablets 2243
Lotensin HCT Tablets 2246
Lotrel Capsules 2249
Bendroflumethiazide (Diminished effectiveness of diuretics in patients with underlying renal or cardiovascular disease).
No products indexed under this heading.
Betaxolol Hydrochloride (Decreased hypotensive effects of beta-blockers). Products include:
Betoptic S Ophthalmic Suspension 558
Bisoprolol Fumarate (Decreased hypotensive effects of beta-blockers).
No products indexed under this heading.
Bumetanide (Diminished effectiveness of diuretics in patients with underlying renal or cardiovascular disease). Products include:
Bumex Tablets 2746
Captopril (Co-administration may result in diminished hyponatremic and hypotensive effects of ACE inhibitors). Products include:
Captopril Tablets 2149
Carteolol Hydrochloride (Decreased hypotensive effects of beta-blockers). Products include:
Carteolol Hydrochloride Ophthalmic Solution USP, 1% .... ⊙249
Celecoxib (Co-administration may increase bleeding or lead to decreased renal function). Products include:
Celebrex Capsules 3134
Chlorothiazide (Diminished effectiveness of diuretics in patients with underlying renal or cardiovascular disease). Products include:
Diuril Oral Suspension 1954
Chlorothiazide Sodium (Diminished effectiveness of diuretics in patients with underlying renal or cardiovascular disease). Products include:
Diuril Sodium Intravenous 2467

Chlorpropamide (Moderate doses of aspirin may increase the effectiveness of oral hypoglycemic agents leading to hypoglycemia).
No products indexed under this heading.

Chlorthalidone (Diminished effectiveness of diuretics in patients with underlying renal or cardiovascular disease). Products include:
Clorpres Tablets 2153

Dalteparin Sodium (Patients on anticoagulant therapy are at increased risk of bleeding). Products include:
Fragmin Injection 1097

Danaparoid Sodium (Patients on anticoagulant therapy are at increased risk of bleeding).
No products indexed under this heading.

Diclofenac Potassium (Co-administration may increase bleeding or lead to decreased renal function).
No products indexed under this heading.

Diclofenac Sodium (Co-administration may increase bleeding or lead to decreased renal function). Products include:
Arthrotec Tablets 3129
Voltaren Ophthalmic Solution 2309
Voltaren Tablets 2307
Voltaren-XR Tablets 2310

Dicumarol (Patients on anticoagulant therapy are at increased risk of bleeding).
No products indexed under this heading.

Divalproex Sodium (Salicylate can displace protein-bound valproic acid leading to an increase in serum valproic acid levels). Products include:
Depakote Sprinkle Capsules 422
Depakote Tablets 427
Depakote ER Tablets 434

Enalapril Maleate (Co-administration may result in diminished hyponatremic and hypotensive effects of ACE inhibitors). Products include:
Vasotec I.V. Injection 2103

Enalaprilat (Co-administration may result in diminished hyponatremic and hypotensive effects of ACE inhibitors).
No products indexed under this heading.

Enoxaparin Sodium (Patients on anticoagulant therapy are at increased risk of bleeding). Products include:
Lovenox Injection 2915

Esmolol Hydrochloride (Decreased hypotensive effects of beta-blockers).
No products indexed under this heading.

Ethacrynic Acid (Diminished effectiveness of diuretics in patients with underlying renal or cardiovascular disease). Products include:
Edecrin Tablets 1959

Etodolac (Co-administration may increase bleeding or lead to decreased renal function).
No products indexed under this heading.

Fenoprofen Calcium (Co-administration may increase bleeding or lead to decreased renal function). Products include:
Nalfon Capsules 2502

Flurbiprofen (Co-administration may increase bleeding or lead to decreased renal function).
No products indexed under this heading.

Fondaparinux Sodium (Patients on anticoagulant therapy are at increased risk of bleeding). Products include:
Arixtra Injection 1351

Fosinopril Sodium (Co-administration may result in diminished hyponatremic and hypotensive effects of ACE inhibitors).
No products indexed under this heading.

Fosphenytoin Sodium (Salicylate can displace protein-bound phenytoin leading to a decrease in the total concentration of phenytoin).
No products indexed under this heading.

Furosemide (Diminished effectiveness of diuretics in patients with underlying renal or cardiovascular disease). Products include:
Furosemide Tablets 2154

Glimepiride (Moderate doses of aspirin may increase the effectiveness of oral hypoglycemic agents leading to hypoglycemia). Products include:
Avandaryl Tablets 1379
Duetact Tablets 3226

Glipizide (Moderate doses of aspirin may increase the effectiveness of oral hypoglycemic agents leading to hypoglycemia).
No products indexed under this heading.

Glyburide (Moderate doses of aspirin may increase the effectiveness of oral hypoglycemic agents leading to hypoglycemia).
No products indexed under this heading.

Heparin Calcium (Patients on anticoagulant therapy are at increased risk of bleeding).
No products indexed under this heading.

Heparin Sodium (Aspirin can increase the anticoagulant activity of heparin increasing bleeding risk).
No products indexed under this heading.

Hydrochlorothiazide (Diminished effectiveness of diuretics in patients with underlying renal or cardiovascular disease). Products include:
Aldoril Tablets 1910
Atacand HCT 651
Avalide Tablets 888
Avalide Tablets 2874
Benicar HCT Tablets 1044
Diovan HCT Tablets 2196
Dyazide Capsules 1423
Hyzaar 50-12.5 Tablets 1990
Hyzaar 100-12.5 Tablets 1990
Hyzaar 100-25 Tablets 1990
Lopressor HCT 50/25 Tablets 2241
Lopressor HCT 100/25 Tablets 2241
Lopressor HCT 100/50 Tablets 2241
Lotensin HCT Tablets 2246
Micardis HCT Tablets 856
Moduretic Tablets 2028
Prinzide Tablets 2056
Teveten HCT Tablets 1737
Timolide Tablets 2086
Uniretic Tablets 3100

Hydroflumethiazide (Diminished effectiveness of diuretics in patients with underlying renal or cardiovascular disease).
No products indexed under this heading.

Ibuprofen (Co-administration may increase bleeding or lead to decreased renal function). Products include:
Advil Allergy Sinus Caplets .... ▣ 770
Advil .... ▣ 674
Children's Advil Oral Suspension .... ▣ 603
Children's Advil Chewable Tablets .... ▣ 603
Advil Cold & Sinus .... ▣ 723
Infants' Advil Concentrated Drops .... ▣ 604
Infants' Advil Concentrated Drops - White Grape (Dye-Free) .... ▣ 604
Junior Strength Advil Swallow Tablets .... ▣ 605
Advil Migraine Liquigels .... ▣ 608
Advil Multi-Symptom Cold Caplets .... ▣ 770
Advil PM Caplets .... ▣ 615
Motrin IB Tablets and Caplets 1866
Children's Motrin Oral Suspension 1867
Children's Motrin Non-Staining Dye-Free Oral Suspension 1867
Children's Motrin Cold Oral Suspension 1867
Infants' Motrin Concentrated Drops 1867
Infants' Motrin Non-Staining Dye-Free Concentrated Drops 1867
Junior Strength Motrin Caplets and Chewable Tablets 1867
Vicoprofen Tablets 539

Indapamide (Diminished effectiveness of diuretics in patients with underlying renal or cardiovascular disease). Products include:
Indapamide Tablets 2156

Indomethacin (Co-administration may increase bleeding or lead to decreased renal function). Products include:
Indocin 1995

Indomethacin Sodium Trihydrate (Co-administration may increase bleeding or lead to decreased renal function). Products include:
Indocin I.V. 2465

Ketoprofen (Co-administration may increase bleeding or lead to decreased renal function).
No products indexed under this heading.

Ketorolac Tromethamine (Co-administration may increase bleeding or lead to decreased renal function). Products include:
Acular Ophthalmic Solution 565
Acular LS Ophthalmic Solution 566

Labetalol Hydrochloride (Decreased hypotensive effects of beta-blockers).
No products indexed under this heading.

Levobunolol Hydrochloride (Decreased hypotensive effects of beta-blockers). Products include:
Betagan Ophthalmic Solution, USP .... ⊙ 220

Lisinopril (Co-administration may result in diminished hyponatremic and hypotensive effects of ACE inhibitors). Products include:
Prinivil Tablets 2052
Prinzide Tablets 2056

Low Molecular Weight Heparins (Patients on anticoagulant therapy are at increased risk of bleeding).
No products indexed under this heading.

Meclofenamate Sodium (Co-administration may increase bleeding or lead to decreased renal function).
No products indexed under this heading.

Mefenamic Acid (Co-administration may increase bleeding or lead to decreased renal function).
No products indexed under this heading.

Meloxicam (Co-administration may increase bleeding or lead to decreased renal function). Products include:
Mobic Oral Suspension 863
Mobic Tablets 863

Metformin Hydrochloride (Moderate doses of aspirin may increase the effectiveness of oral hypoglycemic agents leading to hypoglycemia). Products include:
ActoPlus Met Tablets 3214
Avandamet Tablets 1373
Fortamet Extended-Release Tablets 3115

Methotrexate Sodium (Salicylate can inhibit renal clearance of methotrexate leading to bone marrow toxicity, especially in the elderly or renal impaired).
No products indexed under this heading.

Methyclothiazide (Diminished effectiveness of diuretics in patients with underlying renal or cardiovascular disease).
No products indexed under this heading.

Metipranolol Hydrochloride (Decreased hypotensive effects of beta-blockers).
No products indexed under this heading.

Metolazone (Diminished effectiveness of diuretics in patients with underlying renal or cardiovascular disease).
No products indexed under this heading.

Metoprolol Succinate (Decreased hypotensive effects of beta-blockers). Products include:
Toprol-XL Tablets 668

Metoprolol Tartrate (Decreased hypotensive effects of beta-blockers). Products include:
Lopressor Injection 2238
Lopressor Tablets 2238
Lopressor HCT 50/25 Tablets 2241
Lopressor HCT 100/25 Tablets 2241
Lopressor HCT 100/50 Tablets 2241

Miglitol (Moderate doses of aspirin may increase the effectiveness of oral hypoglycemic agents leading to hypoglycemia).
No products indexed under this heading.

Moexipril Hydrochloride (Co-administration may result in diminished hyponatremic and hypotensive effects of ACE inhibitors). Products include:
Uniretic Tablets 3100
Univasc Tablets 3104

Nabumetone (Co-administration may increase bleeding or lead to decreased renal function).
No products indexed under this heading.

Nadolol (Decreased hypotensive effects of beta-blockers). Products include:
Nadolol Tablets 2159

Naproxen (Co-administration may increase bleeding or lead to decreased renal function). Products include:
EC-Naprosyn Delayed-Release Tablets 2761
Naprosyn Suspension 2761
Naprosyn Tablets 2761

Prevacid NapraPAC 3280

Naproxen Sodium (Co-administration may increase bleeding or lead to decreased renal function). Products include:
Aleve Caplets 742
Aleve Gelcaps 743
Aleve Tablets 743
Aleve Cold & Sinus Caplets 744
Anaprox Tablets 2761
Anaprox DS Tablets 2761

Oxaprozin (Co-administration may increase bleeding or lead to decreased renal function).
No products indexed under this heading.

Penbutolol Sulfate (Decreased hypotensive effects of beta-blockers).
No products indexed under this heading.

Perindopril Erbumine (Co-administration may result in diminished hyponatremic and hypotensive effects of ACE inhibitors). Products include:
Aceon Tablets (2 mg, 4 mg, 8 mg) 3194

Phenylbutazone (Co-administration may increase bleeding or lead to decreased renal function).
No products indexed under this heading.

Phenytoin (Salicylate can displace protein-bound phenytoin leading to a decrease in the total concentration of phenytoin).
No products indexed under this heading.

Phenytoin Sodium (Salicylate can displace protein-bound phenytoin leading to a decrease in the total concentration of phenytoin). Products include:
Phenytek Capsules 2160

Pindolol (Decreased hypotensive effects of beta-blockers).
No products indexed under this heading.

Pioglitazone Hydrochloride (Moderate doses of aspirin may increase the effectiveness of oral hypoglycemic agents leading to hypoglycemia). Products include:
ActoPlus Met Tablets 3214
Actos Tablets 3219
Duetact Tablets 3226

Piroxicam (Co-administration may increase bleeding or lead to decreased renal function).
No products indexed under this heading.

Polythiazide (Diminished effectiveness of diuretics in patients with underlying renal or cardiovascular disease).
No products indexed under this heading.

Probenecid (Salicylate antagonizes the uricosuric action of probenecid).
No products indexed under this heading.

Propranolol Hydrochloride (Decreased hypotensive effects of beta-blockers). Products include:
Inderal LA Long-Acting Capsules 3429
InnoPran XL Capsules 2723

Quinapril Hydrochloride (Co-administration may result in diminished hyponatremic and hypotensive effects of ACE inhibitors).
No products indexed under this heading.

Ramipril (Co-administration may result in diminished hyponatremic and hypotensive effects of ACE inhibitors). Products include:
Altace Capsules 1702

Repaglinide (Moderate doses of aspirin may increase the effectiveness of oral hypoglycemic agents leading to hypoglycemia).
No products indexed under this heading.

Rofecoxib (Co-administration may increase bleeding or lead to decreased renal function).
No products indexed under this heading.

Rosiglitazone Maleate (Moderate doses of aspirin may increase the effectiveness of oral hypoglycemic agents leading to hypoglycemia). Products include:
Avandamet Tablets 1373
Avandaryl Tablets 1379
Avandia Tablets 1384

Sotalol Hydrochloride (Decreased hypotensive effects of beta-blockers).
No products indexed under this heading.

Spirapril Hydrochloride (Co-administration may result in diminished hyponatremic and hypotensive effects of ACE inhibitors).
No products indexed under this heading.

Spironolactone (Diminished effectiveness of diuretics in patients with underlying renal or cardiovascular disease).
No products indexed under this heading.

Sulfinpyrazone (Salicylate antagonizes the uricosuric action of sulfinpyrazone).
No products indexed under this heading.

Sulindac (Co-administration may increase bleeding or lead to decreased renal function). Products include:
Clinoril Tablets 1924

Timolol Hemihydrate (Decreased hypotensive effects of beta-blockers). Products include:
Betimol Ophthalmic Solution 3382
Betimol Ophthalmic Solution .... ⊙ 295

Timolol Maleate (Decreased hypotensive effects of beta-blockers). Products include:
Blocadren Tablets 1916
Cosopt Sterile Ophthalmic Solution 1931
Timolide Tablets 2086
Timoptic Sterile Ophthalmic Solution 2088
Timoptic in Ocudose 2091
Timoptic-XE Sterile Ophthalmic Gel Forming Solution 2092

Tinzaparin Sodium (Patients on anticoagulant therapy are at increased risk of bleeding).
No products indexed under this heading.

Tolazamide (Moderate doses of aspirin may increase the effectiveness of oral hypoglycemic agents leading to hypoglycemia).
No products indexed under this heading.

Tolbutamide (Moderate doses of aspirin may increase the effectiveness of oral hypoglycemic agents leading to hypoglycemia).
No products indexed under this heading.

Tolmetin Sodium (Co-administration may increase bleeding or lead to decreased renal function).
No products indexed under this heading.

Torsemide (Diminished effectiveness of diuretics in patients with underlying renal or cardiovascular disease). Products include:
Demadex Injection 2759
Demadex Tablets 2759

Trandolapril (Co-administration may result in diminished hyponatremic and hypotensive effects of ACE inhibitors). Products include:
Mavik Tablets 486
Tarka Tablets 524

Triamterene (Diminished effectiveness of diuretics in patients with underlying renal or cardiovascular disease). Products include:
Dyazide Capsules 1423
Dyrenium Capsules 3400

Troglitazone (Moderate doses of aspirin may increase the effectiveness of oral hypoglycemic agents leading to hypoglycemia).
No products indexed under this heading.

Valdecoxib (Co-administration may increase bleeding or lead to decreased renal function).
No products indexed under this heading.

Valproate Sodium (Salicylate can displace protein-bound valproic acid leading to an increase in serum valproic acid levels). Products include:
Depacon Injection 412

Valproic Acid (Salicylate can displace protein-bound valproic acid leading to an increase in serum valproic acid levels). Products include:
Depakene 417

Warfarin Sodium (Aspirin can displace Warfarin from protein binding sites leading to prolongation of both the prothrombin time and the bleeding time). Products include:
Coumadin for Injection 898
Coumadin Tablets 898

Food Interactions

Alcohol (Chronic heavy alcohol users, 3 or more drinks per day, in combination with analgesic/antipyretic drug products containing aspirin increases the risk of adverse GI events, including stomach bleeding).

ST. JOSEPH 81 MG ASPIRIN

(Aspirin) 688

May interact with ACE inhibitors, aldosterone-inhibiting diuretic agents, beta blockers, anticoagulants, oral anticoagulants, diuretics, anticonvulsants, hydantoin anticonvulsants, oral hypoglycemic agents, loop diuretics, nonpotassium-sparing diuretics, non-steroidal anti-inflammatory agents, potassium-depleting diuretics, potassium sparing diuretics, and certain other agents. Compounds in these categories include:

Acarbose (Moderate doses of aspirin may increase the effectiveness of oral hypoglycemic drugs, leading to hypoglycemia). Products include:
Precose Tablets 751

Acebutolol Hydrochloride (The hypotensive effects of beta blockers may be diminished by the concomitant administration of aspirin due to inhibition of renal prostaglandins, leading to decreased renal blood flow and salt and fluid retention).
No products indexed under this heading.

Amiloride Hydrochloride (The effectiveness of diuretics in patients with underlying renal or cardiovascular disease may be diminished by the concomitant administration of aspirin due to inhibition of renal prostaglandins, leading to decreased renal blood flow, and salt and fluid retention). Products include:
Midamor Tablets 2026
Moduretic Tablets 2028

Anisindione (Patients on anticoagulant therapy are at increased risk for bleeding because of the drug-drug interaction and the effect on platelets). Products include:
Miradon Tablets 3042

Ardeparin Sodium (Patients on anticoagulant therapy are at increased risk for bleeding because of the drug-drug interaction and the effect on platelets).
No products indexed under this heading.

Atenolol (The hypotensive effects of beta blockers may be diminished by the concomitant administration of aspirin due to inhibition of renal prostaglandins, leading to decreased renal blood flow and salt and fluid retention).
No products indexed under this heading.

Benazepril Hydrochloride (The hyponatremic and hypotensive effects of ACE inhibitors may be diminished by the concomitant administration of aspirin due to its indirect effect on the renin-angiotensin conversion pathway). Products include:
Lotensin Tablets 2243
Lotensin HCT Tablets 2246
Lotrel Capsules 2249

Bendroflumethiazide (The effectiveness of diuretics in patients with underlying renal or cardiovascular disease may be diminished by the concomitant administration of aspirin due to inhibition of renal prostaglandins, leading to decreased renal blood flow, and salt and fluid retention).
No products indexed under this heading.

Betaxolol Hydrochloride (The hypotensive effects of beta blockers may be diminished by the concomitant administration of aspirin due to inhibition of renal prostaglandins, leading to decreased renal blood flow and salt and fluid retention). Products include:
Betoptic S Ophthalmic Suspension 558

Bisoprolol Fumarate (The hypotensive effects of beta blockers may be diminished by the concomitant administration of aspirin due to inhibition of renal prostaglandins, leading to decreased renal blood flow and salt and fluid retention).
No products indexed under this heading.

Bumetanide (The effectiveness of diuretics in patients with underlying renal or cardiovascular disease may be diminished by the concomitant administration of aspirin due to inhibition of renal prostaglandins, leading to decreased renal blood flow, and salt and fluid retention). Products include:
Bumex Tablets 2746

Captopril (The hyponatremic and hypotensive effects of ACE inhibitors may be diminished by the concomitant administration of aspirin due to

its indirect effect on the renin-angiotensin conversion pathway). Products include:
Captopril Tablets 2149

Carbamazepine (Salicylate can displace protein-bound phenytoin and valproic acid, leading to a decrease in the total concentration of phenytoin and an increase in serum valproic acid level). Products include:
Carbatrol Capsules 3171
Equetro Extended-Release Capsules.................................... 3180
Tegretol/Tegretol-XR 2295

Carteolol Hydrochloride (The hypotensive effects of beta blockers may be diminished by the concomitant administration of aspirin due to inhibition of renal prostaglandins, leading to decreased renal blood flow and salt and fluid retention). Products include:
Carteolol Hydrochloride Ophthalmic Solution USP, 1%....... ⊙249

Celecoxib (The concurrent use of aspirin with other NSAIDs should be avoided because this may increase bleeding or lead to decreased renal function). Products include:
Celebrex Capsules 3134

Chlorothiazide (The effectiveness of diuretics in patients with underlying renal or cardiovascular disease may be diminished by the concomitant administration of aspirin due to inhibition of renal prostaglandins, leading to decreased renal blood flow, and salt and fluid retention). Products include:
Diuril Oral Suspension 1954

Chlorothiazide Sodium (The effectiveness of diuretics in patients with underlying renal or cardiovascular disease may be diminished by the concomitant administration of aspirin due to inhibition of renal prostaglandins, leading to decreased renal blood flow, and salt and fluid retention). Products include:
Diuril Sodium Intravenous 2467

Chlorpropamide (Moderate doses of aspirin may increase the effectiveness of oral hypoglycemic drugs, leading to hypoglycemia).
No products indexed under this heading.

Chlorthalidone (The effectiveness of diuretics in patients with underlying renal or cardiovascular disease may be diminished by the concomitant administration of aspirin due to inhibition of renal prostaglandins, leading to decreased renal blood flow, and salt and fluid retention). Products include:
Clorpres Tablets 2153

Dalteparin Sodium (Patients on anticoagulant therapy are at increased risk for bleeding because of the drug-drug interaction and the effect on platelets). Products include:
Fragmin Injection 1097

Danaparoid Sodium (Patients on anticoagulant therapy are at increased risk for bleeding because of the drug-drug interaction and the effect on platelets).
No products indexed under this heading.

Diclofenac Potassium (The concurrent use of aspirin with other NSAIDs should be avoided because this may increase bleeding or lead to decreased renal function).
No products indexed under this heading.

Diclofenac Sodium (The concurrent use of aspirin with other NSAIDs should be avoided because this may increase bleeding or lead to decreased renal function). Products include:
Arthrotec Tablets 3129
Voltaren Ophthalmic Solution 2309
Voltaren Tablets 2307
Voltaren-XR Tablets 2310

Dicumarol (Patients on anticoagulant therapy are at increased risk for bleeding because of the drug-drug interaction and the effect on platelets).
No products indexed under this heading.

Divalproex Sodium (Salicylate can displace protein-bound phenytoin and valproic acid, leading to a decrease in the total concentration of phenytoin and an increase in serum valproic acid level). Products include:
Depakote Sprinkle Capsules 422
Depakote Tablets 427
Depakote ER Tablets 434

Enalapril Maleate (The hyponatremic and hypotensive effects of ACE inhibitors may be diminished by the concomitant administration of aspirin due to its indirect effect on the renin-angiotensin conversion pathway). Products include:
Vasotec I.V. Injection 2103

Enalaprilat (The hyponatremic and hypotensive effects of ACE inhibitors may be diminished by the concomitant administration of aspirin due to its indirect effect on the renin-angiotensin conversion pathway).
No products indexed under this heading.

Enoxaparin Sodium (Patients on anticoagulant therapy are at increased risk for bleeding because of the drug-drug interaction and the effect on platelets). Products include:
Lovenox Injection 2915

Esmolol Hydrochloride (The hypotensive effects of beta blockers may be diminished by the concomitant administration of aspirin due to inhibition of renal prostaglandins, leading to decreased renal blood flow and salt and fluid retention).
No products indexed under this heading.

Ethacrynic Acid (The effectiveness of diuretics in patients with underlying renal or cardiovascular disease may be diminished by the concomitant administration of aspirin due to inhibition of renal prostaglandins, leading to decreased renal blood flow, and salt and fluid retention). Products include:
Edecrin Tablets 1959

Ethosuximide (Salicylate can displace protein-bound phenytoin and valproic acid, leading to a decrease in the total concentration of phenytoin and an increase in serum valproic acid level).
No products indexed under this heading.

Ethotoin (Salicylate can displace protein-bound phenytoin and valproic acid, leading to a decrease in the total concentration of phenytoin and an increase in serum valproic acid level).
No products indexed under this heading.

Etodolac (The concurrent use of aspirin with other NSAIDs should be avoided because this may increase bleeding or lead to decreased renal function).
No products indexed under this heading.

Felbamate (Salicylate can displace protein-bound phenytoin and valproic acid, leading to a decrease in the total concentration of phenytoin and an increase in serum valproic acid level).
No products indexed under this heading.

Fenoprofen Calcium (The concurrent use of aspirin with other NSAIDs should be avoided because this may increase bleeding or lead to decreased renal function). Products include:
Nalfon Capsules 2502

Flurbiprofen (The concurrent use of aspirin with other NSAIDs should be avoided because this may increase bleeding or lead to decreased renal function).
No products indexed under this heading.

Fondaparinux Sodium (Patients on anticoagulant therapy are at increased risk for bleeding because of the drug-drug interaction and the effect on platelets). Products include:
Arixtra Injection 1351

Fosinopril Sodium (The hyponatremic and hypotensive effects of ACE inhibitors may be diminished by the concomitant administration of aspirin due to its indirect effect on the renin-angiotensin conversion pathway).
No products indexed under this heading.

Fosphenytoin (Salicylate can displace protein-bound phenytoin and valproic acid, leading to a decrease in the total concentration of phenytoin and an increase in serum valproic acid level).
No products indexed under this heading.

Fosphenytoin Sodium (Salicylate can displace protein-bound phenytoin and valproic acid, leading to a decrease in the total concentration of phenytoin and an increase in serum valproic acid level).
No products indexed under this heading.

Furosemide (The effectiveness of diuretics in patients with underlying renal or cardiovascular disease may be diminished by the concomitant administration of aspirin due to inhibition of renal prostaglandins, leading to decreased renal blood flow, and salt and fluid retention). Products include:
Furosemide Tablets 2154

Gabapentin (Salicylate can displace protein-bound phenytoin and valproic acid, leading to a decrease in the total concentration of phenytoin and an increase in serum valproic acid level). Products include:
Neurontin Capsules 2487
Neurontin Oral Solution 2487
Neurontin Tablets 2487

Glimepiride (Moderate doses of aspirin may increase the effectiveness of oral hypoglycemic drugs, leading to hypoglycemia). Products include:
Avandaryl Tablets 1379
Duetact Tablets 3226

Glipizide (Moderate doses of aspirin may increase the effectiveness of oral hypoglycemic drugs, leading to hypoglycemia).
No products indexed under this heading.

Glyburide (Moderate doses of aspirin may increase the effectiveness of oral hypoglycemic drugs, leading to hypoglycemia).
No products indexed under this heading.

Heparin Calcium (Patients on anticoagulant therapy are at increased risk for bleeding because of the drug-drug interaction and the effect on platelets. Aspirin can increase the anticoagulant activity of heparin, increasing bleeding risk).
No products indexed under this heading.

Heparin Sodium (Patients on anticoagulant therapy are at increased risk for bleeding because of the drug-drug interaction and the effect on platelets. Aspirin can increase the anticoagulant activity of heparin, increasing bleeding risk).
No products indexed under this heading.

Hydrochlorothiazide (The effectiveness of diuretics in patients with underlying renal or cardiovascular disease may be diminished by the concomitant administration of aspirin due to inhibition of renal prostaglandins, leading to decreased renal blood flow and salt and fluid retention). Products include:
Aldoril Tablets 1910
Atacand HCT 651
Avalide Tablets 888
Avalide Tablets 2874
Benicar HCT Tablets 1044
Diovan HCT Tablets 2196
Dyazide Capsules 1423
Hyzaar 50-12.5 Tablets 1990
Hyzaar 100-12.5 Tablets 1990
Hyzaar 100-25 Tablets 1990
Lopressor HCT 50/25 Tablets 2241
Lopressor HCT 100/25 Tablets 2241
Lopressor HCT 100/50 Tablets 2241
Lotensin HCT Tablets 2246
Micardis HCT Tablets 856
Moduretic Tablets 2028
Prinzide Tablets 2056
Teveten HCT Tablets 1737
Timolide Tablets 2086
Uniretic Tablets 3100

Hydroflumethiazide (The effectiveness of diuretics in patients with underlying renal or cardiovascular disease may be diminished by the concomitant administration of aspirin due to inhibition of renal prostaglandins, leading to decreased renal blood flow, and salt and fluid retention).
No products indexed under this heading.

Ibuprofen (The concurrent use of aspirin with other NSAIDs should be avoided because this may increase bleeding or lead to decreased renal function). Products include:
Advil Allergy Sinus Caplets .... ■770
Advil .... ■674
Children's Advil Oral Suspension .... ■603
Children's Advil Chewable Tablets .. ■603
Advil Cold & Sinus .... ■723
Infants' Advil Concentrated Drops .. ■604
Infants' Advil Concentrated Drops - White Grape (Dye-Free)............. ■604
Junior Strength Advil Swallow Tablets.. ■605
Advil Migraine Liquigels .... ■608
Advil Multi-Symptom Cold Caplets... ■770
Advil PM Caplets .... ■615

Indapamide (The effectiveness of diuretics in patients with underlying renal or cardiovascular disease may be diminished by the concomitant administration of aspirin due to inhibition of renal prostaglandins, leading to decreased renal blood flow, and salt and fluid retention). Products include:

Indomethacin (The concurrent use of aspirin with other NSAIDs should be avoided because this may increase bleeding or lead to decreased renal function). Products include:

Indomethacin Sodium Trihydrate (The concurrent use of aspirin with other NSAIDs should be avoided because this may increase bleeding or lead to decreased renal function). Products include:

Ketoprofen (The concurrent use of aspirin with other NSAIDs should be avoided because this may increase bleeding or lead to decreased renal function).
 No products indexed under this heading.

Ketorolac Tromethamine (The concurrent use of aspirin with other NSAIDs should be avoided because this may increase bleeding or lead to decreased renal function). Products include:

Labetalol Hydrochloride (The hypotensive effects of beta blockers may be diminished by the concomitant administration of aspirin due to inhibition of renal prostaglandins, leading to decreased renal blood flow and salt and fluid retention).
 No products indexed under this heading.

Lamotrigine (Salicylate can displace protein-bound phenytoin and valproic acid, leading to a decrease in the total concentration of phenytoin and an increase in serum valproic acid level). Products include:

Levetiracetam (Salicylate can displace protein-bound phenytoin and valproic acid, leading to a decrease in the total concentration of phenytoin and an increase in serum valproic acid level). Products include:

Levobunolol Hydrochloride (The hypotensive effects of beta blockers may be diminished by the concomitant administration of aspirin due to inhibition of renal prostaglandins, leading to decreased renal blood flow and salt and fluid retention). Products include:

Lisinopril (The hyponatremic and hypotensive effects of ACE inhibitors may be diminished by the concomitant administration of aspirin due to its indirect effect on the renin-angiotensin conversion pathway). Products include:

Low Molecular Weight Heparins (Patients on anticoagulant therapy are at increased risk for bleeding because of the drug-drug interaction and the effect on platelets).
 No products indexed under this heading.

Meclofenamate Sodium (The concurrent use of aspirin with other NSAIDs should be avoided because this may increase bleeding or lead to decreased renal function).
 No products indexed under this heading.

Mefenamic Acid (The concurrent use of aspirin with other NSAIDs should be avoided because this may increase bleeding or lead to decreased renal function).
 No products indexed under this heading.

Meloxicam (The concurrent use of aspirin with other NSAIDs should be avoided because this may increase bleeding or lead to decreased renal function). Products include:

Mephenytoin (Salicylate can displace protein-bound phenytoin and valproic acid, leading to a decrease in the total concentration of phenytoin and an increase in serum valproic acid level).
 No products indexed under this heading.

Metformin Hydrochloride (Moderate doses of aspirin may increase the effectiveness of oral hypoglycemic drugs, leading to hypoglycemia). Products include:

Methotrexate (Salicylate can inhibit renal clearance of methotrexate, leading to bone marrow toxicity, especially in the elderly and renally impaired).
 No products indexed under this heading.

Methsuximide (Salicylate can displace protein-bound phenytoin and valproic acid, leading to a decrease in the total concentration of phenytoin and an increase in serum valproic acid level).
 No products indexed under this heading.

Methyclothiazide (The effectiveness of diuretics in patients with underlying renal or cardiovascular disease may be diminished by the concomitant administration of aspirin due to inhibition of renal prostaglandins, leading to decreased renal blood flow, and salt and fluid retention).
 No products indexed under this heading.

Metipranolol Hydrochloride (The hypotensive effects of beta blockers may be diminished by the concomitant administration of aspirin due to inhibition of renal prostaglandins, leading to decreased renal blood flow and salt and fluid retention).
 No products indexed under this heading.

Metolazone (The effectiveness of diuretics in patients with underlying renal or cardiovascular disease may be diminished by the concomitant administration of aspirin due to inhibition of renal prostaglandins, leading to decreased renal blood flow, and salt and fluid retention).
 No products indexed under this heading.

Metoprolol Succinate (The hypotensive effects of beta blockers may be diminished by the concomitant administration of aspirin due to inhibition of renal prostaglandins, leading to decreased renal blood flow and salt and fluid retention). Products include:

Metoprolol Tartrate (The hypotensive effects of beta blockers may be diminished by the concomitant administration of aspirin due to inhibition of renal prostaglandins, leading to decreased renal blood flow and salt and fluid retention). Products include:

Miglitol (Moderate doses of aspirin may increase the effectiveness of oral hypoglycemic drugs, leading to hypoglycemia).
 No products indexed under this heading.

Moexipril Hydrochloride (The hyponatremic and hypotensive effects of ACE inhibitors may be diminished by the concomitant administration of aspirin due to its indirect effect on the renin-angiotensin conversion pathway). Products include:

Nabumetone (The concurrent use of aspirin with other NSAIDs should be avoided because this may increase bleeding or lead to decreased renal function).
 No products indexed under this heading.

Nadolol (The hypotensive effects of beta blockers may be diminished by the concomitant administration of aspirin due to inhibition of renal prostaglandins, leading to decreased renal blood flow and salt and fluid retention). Products include:

Naproxen (The concurrent use of aspirin with other NSAIDs should be avoided because this may increase bleeding or lead to decreased renal function). Products include:

Naproxen Sodium (The concurrent use of aspirin with other NSAIDs should be avoided because this may

increase bleeding or lead to decreased renal function). Products include:

Oxaprozin (The concurrent use of aspirin with other NSAIDs should be avoided because this may increase bleeding or lead to decreased renal function).
 No products indexed under this heading.

Oxcarbazepine (Salicylate can displace protein-bound phenytoin and valproic acid, leading to a decrease in the total concentration of phenytoin and an increase in serum valproic acid level). Products include:

Paramethadione (Salicylate can displace protein-bound phenytoin and valproic acid, leading to a decrease in the total concentration of phenytoin and an increase in serum valproic acid level).
 No products indexed under this heading.

Penbutolol Sulfate (The hypotensive effects of beta blockers may be diminished by the concomitant administration of aspirin due to inhibition of renal prostaglandins, leading to decreased renal blood flow and salt and fluid retention).
 No products indexed under this heading.

Perindopril Erbumine (The hyponatremic and hypotensive effects of ACE inhibitors may be diminished by the concomitant administration of aspirin due to its indirect effect on the renin-angiotensin conversion pathway). Products include:

Phenacemide (Salicylate can displace protein-bound phenytoin and valproic acid, leading to a decrease in the total concentration of phenytoin and an increase in serum valproic acid level).
 No products indexed under this heading.

Phenobarbital (Salicylate can displace protein-bound phenytoin and valproic acid, leading to a decrease in the total concentration of phenytoin and an increase in serum valproic acid level). Products include:

Phensuximide (Salicylate can displace protein-bound phenytoin and valproic acid, leading to a decrease in the total concentration of phenytoin and an increase in serum valproic acid level).
 No products indexed under this heading.

Phenylbutazone (The concurrent use of aspirin with other NSAIDs should be avoided because this may increase bleeding or lead to decreased renal function).
 No products indexed under this heading.

Phenytoin (Salicylate can displace protein-bound phenytoin and valproic acid, leading to a decrease in the total concentration of phenytoin and an increase in serum valproic acid level).
No products indexed under this heading.

Phenytoin Sodium (Salicylate can displace protein-bound phenytoin and valproic acid, leading to a decrease in the total concentration of phenytoin and an increase in serum valproic acid level). Products include:
Phenytek Capsules 2160

Pindolol (The hypotensive effects of beta blockers may be diminished by the concomitant administration of aspirin due to inhibition of renal prostaglandins, leading to decreased renal blood flow and salt and fluid retention).
No products indexed under this heading.

Pioglitazone Hydrochloride (Moderate doses of aspirin may increase the effectiveness of oral hypoglycemic drugs, leading to hypoglycemia).
Products include:
ActoPlus Met Tablets 3214
Actos Tablets 3219
Duetact Tablets 3226

Piroxicam (The concurrent use of aspirin with other NSAIDs should be avoided because this may increase bleeding or lead to decreased renal function).
No products indexed under this heading.

Polythiazide (The effectiveness of diuretics in patients with underlying renal or cardiovascular disease may be diminished by the concomitant administration of aspirin due to inhibition of renal prostaglandins, leading to decreased renal blood flow, and salt and fluid retention).
No products indexed under this heading.

Primidone (Salicylate can displace protein-bound phenytoin and valproic acid, leading to a decrease in the total concentration of phenytoin and an increase in serum valproic acid level).
No products indexed under this heading.

Probenecid (Salicylates antagonize the uricosuric action of uricosuric agents).
No products indexed under this heading.

Propranolol Hydrochloride (The hypotensive effects of beta blockers may be diminished by the concomitant administration of aspirin due to inhibition of renal prostaglandins, leading to decreased renal blood flow and salt and fluid retention).
Products include:
Inderal LA Long-Acting Capsules 3429
InnoPran XL Capsules 2723

Quinapril Hydrochloride (The hyponatremic and hypotensive effects of ACE inhibitors may be diminished by the concomitant administration of aspirin due to its indirect effect on the renin-angiotensin conversion pathway).
No products indexed under this heading.

Ramipril (The hyponatremic and hypotensive effects of ACE inhibitors may be diminished by the concomitant administration of aspirin due to its indirect effect on the renin-angiotensin conversion pathway).
Products include:
Altace Capsules 1702

Repaglinide (Moderate doses of aspirin may increase the effectiveness of oral hypoglycemic drugs, leading to hypoglycemia).
No products indexed under this heading.

Rofecoxib (The concurrent use of aspirin with other NSAIDs should be avoided because this may increase bleeding or lead to decreased renal function).
No products indexed under this heading.

Rosiglitazone Maleate (Moderate doses of aspirin may increase the effectiveness of oral hypoglycemic drugs, leading to hypoglycemia).
Products include:
Avandamet Tablets 1373
Avandaryl Tablets 1379
Avandia Tablets 1384

Sotalol Hydrochloride (The hypotensive effects of beta blockers may be diminished by the concomitant administration of aspirin due to inhibition of renal prostaglandins, leading to decreased renal blood flow and salt and fluid retention).
No products indexed under this heading.

Spirapril Hydrochloride (The hyponatremic and hypotensive effects of ACE inhibitors may be diminished by the concomitant administration of aspirin due to its indirect effect on the renin-angiotensin conversion pathway).
No products indexed under this heading.

Spironolactone (The effectiveness of diuretics in patients with underlying renal or cardiovascular disease may be diminished by the concomitant administration of aspirin due to inhibition of renal prostaglandins, leading to decreased renal blood flow, and salt and fluid retention).
No products indexed under this heading.

Sulfinpyrazone (Salicylates antagonize the uricosuric action of uricosuric agents).
No products indexed under this heading.

Sulindac (The concurrent use of aspirin with other NSAIDs should be avoided because this may increase bleeding or lead to decreased renal function). Products include:
Clinoril Tablets 1924

Tiagabine Hydrochloride (Salicylate can displace protein-bound phenytoin and valproic acid, leading to a decrease in the total concentration of phenytoin and an increase in serum valproic acid level). Products include:
Gabitril Tablets 984

Timolol Hemihydrate (The hypotensive effects of beta blockers may be diminished by the concomitant administration of aspirin due to inhibition of renal prostaglandins, leading to decreased renal blood flow and salt and fluid retention).
Products include:
Betimol Ophthalmic Solution 3382
Betimol Ophthalmic Solution .... ⊙295

Timolol Maleate (The hypotensive effects of beta blockers may be diminished by the concomitant administration of aspirin due to inhibition of renal prostaglandins, leading to decreased renal blood flow and salt and fluid retention).
Products include:
Blocadren Tablets 1916
Cosopt Sterile Ophthalmic Solution 1931
Timolide Tablets 2086
Timoptic Sterile Ophthalmic Solution 2088
Timoptic in Ocudose 2091
Timoptic-XE Sterile Ophthalmic Gel Forming Solution 2092

Tinzaparin Sodium (Patients on anticoagulant therapy are at increased risk for bleeding because of the drug-drug interaction and the effect on platelets).
No products indexed under this heading.

Tolazamide (Moderate doses of aspirin may increase the effectiveness of oral hypoglycemic drugs, leading to hypoglycemia).
No products indexed under this heading.

Tolbutamide (Moderate doses of aspirin may increase the effectiveness of oral hypoglycemic drugs, leading to hypoglycemia).
No products indexed under this heading.

Tolmetin Sodium (The concurrent use of aspirin with other NSAIDs should be avoided because this may increase bleeding or lead to decreased renal function).
No products indexed under this heading.

Topiramate (Salicylate can displace protein-bound phenytoin and valproic acid, leading to a decrease in the total concentration of phenytoin and an increase in serum valproic acid level). Products include:
Topamax Sprinkle Capsules 2404
Topamax Tablets 2404

Torsemide (The effectiveness of diuretics in patients with underlying renal or cardiovascular disease may be diminished by the concomitant administration of aspirin due to inhibition of renal prostaglandins, leading to decreased renal blood flow, and salt and fluid retention).
Products include:
Demadex Injection 2759
Demadex Tablets 2759

Trandolapril (The hyponatremic and hypotensive effects of ACE inhibitors may be diminished by the concomitant administration of aspirin due to its indirect effect on the renin-angiotensin conversion pathway).
Products include:
Mavik Tablets 486
Tarka Tablets 524

Triamterene (The effectiveness of diuretics in patients with underlying renal or cardiovascular disease may be diminished by the concomitant administration of aspirin due to inhibition of renal prostaglandins, leading to decreased renal blood flow, and salt and fluid retention).
Products include:
Dyazide Capsules 1423
Dyrenium Capsules 3400

Trimethadione (Salicylate can displace protein-bound phenytoin and valproic acid, leading to a decrease in the total concentration of phenytoin and an increase in serum valproic acid level).
No products indexed under this heading.

Troglitazone (Moderate doses of aspirin may increase the effectiveness of oral hypoglycemic drugs, leading to hypoglycemia).
No products indexed under this heading.

Valdecoxib (The concurrent use of aspirin with other NSAIDs should be avoided because this may increase bleeding or lead to decreased renal function).
No products indexed under this heading.

Valproate Sodium (Salicylate can displace protein-bound phenytoin and valproic acid, leading to a decrease in the total concentration of phenytoin and an increase in serum valproic acid level). Products include:
Depacon Injection 412

Valproic Acid (Salicylate can displace protein-bound phenytoin and valproic acid, leading to a decrease in the total concentration of phenytoin and an increase in serum valproic acid level). Products include:
Depakene 417

Warfarin Sodium (Patients on anticoagulant therapy are at increased risk for bleeding because of the drug-drug interaction and the effect on platelets. Aspirin can displace warfarin from protein binding sites, leading to prolongation of both prothrombin time and bleeding time).
Products include:
Coumadin for Injection 898
Coumadin Tablets 898

Zonisamide (Salicylate can displace protein-bound phenytoin and valproic acid, leading to a decrease in the total concentration of phenytoin and an increase in serum valproic acid level). Products include:
Zonegran Capsules 1101

Food Interactions

Alcohol (Consuming 3 or more alcoholic beverages can increase the risk of stomach bleeding).

STALEVO TABLETS

(Carbidopa, Entacapone, Levodopa)... 2287
May interact with antihypertensives, drugs metabolized by Catechol-O-methytransferase, dopamine D2 antagonists, iron containing oral preparations, monoamine oxidase inhibitors, tricyclic antidepressants, and certain other agents. Compounds in these categories include:

Acebutolol Hydrochloride (Symptomatic postural hypotension has occurred when carbidopa-levodopa was added to the treatment of a patient receiving antihypertensive drugs).
No products indexed under this heading.

Amitriptyline Hydrochloride (There have been rare reports of adverse reactions, including hypertension and dyskinesia, resulting from the concomitant use of tricylic antidepressants and carbidopa-levodopa).
No products indexed under this heading.

Amlodipine Besylate (Symptomatic postural hypotension has occurred when carbidopa-levodopa was added to the treatment of a patient receiving antihypertensive drugs).
Products include:
Caduet Tablets 2508

Lotrel Capsules 2249
Norvasc Tablets 2545

Amoxapine (There have been rare reports of adverse reactions, including hypertension and dyskinesia, resulting from the concomitant use of tricylic antidepressants and carbidopa-levodopa).
No products indexed under this heading.

Ampicillin (As most entacapone excretion is via the bile, caution should be exercised when drugs known to interfere with biliary excretion, glucuronidation, and intestinal beta-glucuronidase are given concurrently with entacapone).
No products indexed under this heading.

Ampicillin Sodium (As most entacapone excretion is via the bile, caution should be exercised when drugs known to interfere with biliary excretion, glucuronidation, and intestinal beta-glucuronidase are given concurrently with entacapone).
No products indexed under this heading.

Ampicillin Trihydrate (As most entacapone excretion is via the bile, caution should be exercised when drugs known to interfere with biliary excretion, glucuronidation, and intestinal beta-glucuronidase are given concurrently with entacapone).
No products indexed under this heading.

Apomorphine (Drugs known to be metabolized by COMT should be administered with caution in patients receiving entacapone regardless of the route of administration (including inhalation), as their interaction may result in increased heart rates, possibly arrhythmias, and excessive changes in blood pressure).
No products indexed under this heading.

Atenolol (Symptomatic postural hypotension has occurred when carbidopa-levodopa was added to the treatment of a patient receiving antihypertensive drugs).
No products indexed under this heading.

Bacampicillin Hydrochloride (As most entacapone excretion is via the bile, caution should be exercised when drugs known to interfere with biliary excretion, glucuronidation, and intestinal beta-glucuronidase are given concurrently with entacapone).
No products indexed under this heading.

Benazepril Hydrochloride (Symptomatic postural hypotension has occurred when carbidopa-levodopa was added to the treatment of a patient receiving antihypertensive drugs). Products include:
Lotensin Tablets 2243
Lotensin HCT Tablets 2246
Lotrel Capsules 2249

Bendroflumethiazide (Symptomatic postural hypotension has occurred when carbidopa-levodopa was added to the treatment of a patient receiving antihypertensive drugs).
No products indexed under this heading.

Betaxolol Hydrochloride (Symptomatic postural hypotension has occurred when carbidopa-levodopa was added to the treatment of a patient receiving antihypertensive drugs). Products include:
Betoptic S Ophthalmic Suspension.................................. 558

Bisoprolol Fumarate (Symptomatic postural hypotension has occurred when carbidopa-levodopa was added to the treatment of a patient receiving antihypertensive drugs).
No products indexed under this heading.

Bitolterol Mesylate (Drugs known to be metabolized by COMT should be administered with caution in patients receiving entacapone regardless of the route of administration (including inhalation), as their interaction may result in increased heart rates, possibly arrhythmias, and excessive changes in blood pressure).
No products indexed under this heading.

Candesartan Cilexetil (Symptomatic postural hypotension has occurred when carbidopa-levodopa was added to the treatment of a patient receiving antihypertensive drugs). Products include:
Atacand Tablets 649
Atacand HCT 651

Captopril (Symptomatic postural hypotension has occurred when carbidopa-levodopa was added to the treatment of a patient receiving antihypertensive drugs). Products include:
Captopril Tablets 2149

Carteolol Hydrochloride (Symptomatic postural hypotension has occurred when carbidopa-levodopa was added to the treatment of a patient receiving antihypertensive drugs). Products include:
Carteolol Hydrochloride Ophthalmic Solution USP, 1%....... ⊙249

Chloramphenicol (As most entacapone excretion is via the bile, caution should be exercised when drugs known to interfere with biliary excretion, glucuronidation, and intestinal beta-glucuronidase are given concurrently with entacapone).
No products indexed under this heading.

Chloramphenicol Palmitate (As most entacapone excretion is via the bile, caution should be exercised when drugs known to interfere with biliary excretion, glucuronidation, and intestinal beta-glucuronidase are given concurrently with entacapone).
No products indexed under this heading.

Chloramphenicol Sodium Succinate (As most entacapone excretion is via the bile, caution should be exercised when drugs known to interfere with biliary excretion, glucuronidation, and intestinal beta-glucuronidase are given concurrently with entacapone).
No products indexed under this heading.

Chlorothiazide (Symptomatic postural hypotension has occurred when carbidopa-levodopa was added to the treatment of a patient receiving antihypertensive drugs). Products include:
Diuril Oral Suspension 1954

Chlorothiazide Sodium (Symptomatic postural hypotension has occurred when carbidopa-levodopa was added to the treatment of a patient receiving antihypertensive drugs). Products include:
Diuril Sodium Intravenous 2467

Chlorpromazine (Dopamine D2 receptor antagonists may reduce the therapeutic effects of levodopa).
No products indexed under this heading.

Chlorpromazine Hydrochloride (Dopamine D2 receptor antagonists may reduce the therapeutic effects of levodopa).
No products indexed under this heading.

Chlorprothixene (Dopamine D2 receptor antagonists may reduce the therapeutic effects of levodopa).
No products indexed under this heading.

Chlorprothixene Hydrochloride (Dopamine D2 receptor antagonists may reduce the therapeutic effects of levodopa).
No products indexed under this heading.

Chlorthalidone (Symptomatic postural hypotension has occurred when carbidopa-levodopa was added to the treatment of a patient receiving antihypertensive drugs). Products include:
Clorpres Tablets 2153

Cholestyramine (As most entacapone excretion is via the bile, caution should be exercised when drugs known to interfere with biliary excretion, glucuronidation, and intestinal beta-glucuronidase are given concurrently with entacapone).
No products indexed under this heading.

Clomipramine Hydrochloride (There have been rare reports of adverse reactions, including hypertension and dyskinesia, resulting from the concomitant use of tricylic antidepressants and carbidopa-levodopa).
No products indexed under this heading.

Clonidine (Symptomatic postural hypotension has occurred when carbidopa-levodopa was added to the treatment of a patient receiving antihypertensive drugs). Products include:
Catapres-TTS 844

Clonidine Hydrochloride (Symptomatic postural hypotension has occurred when carbidopa-levodopa was added to the treatment of a patient receiving antihypertensive drugs). Products include:
Catapres Tablets 843
Clorpres Tablets 2153

Deserpidine (Symptomatic postural hypotension has occurred when carbidopa-levodopa was added to the treatment of a patient receiving antihypertensive drugs).
No products indexed under this heading.

Desipramine Hydrochloride (There have been rare reports of adverse reactions, including hypertension and dyskinesia, resulting from the concomitant use of tricylic antidepressants and carbidopa-levodopa).
No products indexed under this heading.

Diazoxide (Symptomatic postural hypotension has occurred when carbidopa-levodopa was added to the treatment of a patient receiving antihypertensive drugs). Products include:
Hyperstat I.V. 3017

Diltiazem Hydrochloride (Symptomatic postural hypotension has occurred when carbidopa-levodopa was added to the treatment of a patient receiving antihypertensive drugs). Products include:
Cardizem LA Extended Release Tablets 1728
Tiazac Capsules 1201

Dobutamine Hydrochloride (Drugs known to be metabolized by COMT should be administered with caution in patients receiving entacapone regardless of the route of administration (including inhalation), as their interaction may result in increased heart rates, possibly arrhythmias, and excessive changes in blood pressure).
No products indexed under this heading.

Dopamine Hydrochloride (Drugs known to be metabolized by COMT should be administered with caution in patients receiving entacapone regardless of the route of administration (including inhalation), as their interaction may result in increased heart rates, possibly arrhythmias, and excessive changes in blood pressure).
No products indexed under this heading.

Doxazosin Mesylate (Symptomatic postural hypotension has occurred when carbidopa-levodopa was added to the treatment of a patient receiving antihypertensive drugs). Products include:
Cardura XL Tablets 2515

Doxepin Hydrochloride (There have been rare reports of adverse reactions, including hypertension and dyskinesia, resulting from the concomitant use of tricylic antidepressants and carbidopa-levodopa).
No products indexed under this heading.

Enalapril Maleate (Symptomatic postural hypotension has occurred when carbidopa-levodopa was added to the treatment of a patient receiving antihypertensive drugs). Products include:
Vasotec I.V. Injection 2103

Enalaprilat (Symptomatic postural hypotension has occurred when carbidopa-levodopa was added to the treatment of a patient receiving antihypertensive drugs).
No products indexed under this heading.

Epinephrine (Drugs known to be metabolized by COMT should be administered with caution in patients receiving entacapone regardless of the route of administration (including inhalation), as their interaction may result in increased heart rates, possibly arrhythmias, and excessive changes in blood pressure). Products include:
EpiPen 1061
Primatene Mist .... ▣719
Twinject 0.15 3379
Twinject 0.3 3378

Epinephrine Bitartrate (Drugs known to be metabolized by COMT should be administered with caution in patients receiving entacapone regardless of the route of administration (including inhalation), as their interaction may result in increased heart rates, possibly arrhythmias, and excessive changes in blood pressure).
No products indexed under this heading.

Epinephrine Hydrochloride (Drugs known to be metabolized by COMT should be administered with caution in patients receiving entacapone regardless of the route of administration (including inhalation), as their interaction may result in increased heart rates, possibly arrhythmias, and excessive changes in blood pressure).
No products indexed under this heading.

Eprosartan Mesylate (Symptomatic postural hypotension has occurred when carbidopa-levodopa was added to the treatment of a patient receiving antihypertensive drugs).
Products include:
Teveten Tablets 1735
Teveten HCT Tablets 1737

Erythromycin (As most entacapone excretion is via the bile, caution should be exercised when drugs known to interfere with biliary excretion, glucuronidation, and intestinal beta-glucuronidase are given concurrently with entacapone). Products include:
Ery-Tab Tablets 449
Erythromycin Base Filmtab Tablets 455
Erythromycin Delayed-Release Capsules, USP 457
PCE Dispertab Tablets 515

Erythromycin Enteric Coated Tablets (As most entacapone excretion is via the bile, caution should be exercised when drugs known to interfere with biliary excretion, glucuronidation, and intestinal beta-glucuronidase are given concurrently with entacapone).
No products indexed under this heading.

Erythromycin Estolate (As most entacapone excretion is via the bile, caution should be exercised when drugs known to interfere with biliary excretion, glucuronidation, and intestinal beta-glucuronidase are given concurrently with entacapone).
No products indexed under this heading.

Erythromycin Ethylsuccinate (As most entacapone excretion is via the bile, caution should be exercised when drugs known to interfere with biliary excretion, glucuronidation, and intestinal beta-glucuronidase are given concurrently with entacapone).
Products include:
E.E.S. 451
EryPed 447

Erythromycin Gluceptate (As most entacapone excretion is via the bile, caution should be exercised when drugs known to interfere with biliary excretion, glucuronidation, and intestinal beta-glucuronidase are given concurrently with entacapone).
No products indexed under this heading.

Erythromycin Lactobionate (As most entacapone excretion is via the bile, caution should be exercised when drugs known to interfere with biliary excretion, glucuronidation, and intestinal beta-glucuronidase are given concurrently with entacapone).
No products indexed under this heading.

Erythromycin Stearate (As most entacapone excretion is via the bile, caution should be exercised when drugs known to interfere with biliary excretion, glucuronidation, and intestinal beta-glucuronidase are given concurrently with entacapone).
Products include:
Erythrocin Stearate Filmtab Tablets 453

Esmolol Hydrochloride (Symptomatic postural hypotension has occurred when carbidopa-levodopa was added to the treatment of a patient receiving antihypertensive drugs).
No products indexed under this heading.

Ethylpapaverine Hydrochloride (The beneficial effects of levodopa in Parkinson's disease have been reported to be reversed by papaverine).
No products indexed under this heading.

Felodipine (Symptomatic postural hypotension has occurred when carbidopa-levodopa was added to the treatment of a patient receiving antihypertensive drugs).
No products indexed under this heading.

Ferrous Fumarate (Iron salts may reduce the bioavailability of levodopa, carbidopa and entacapone).
No products indexed under this heading.

Ferrous Gluconate (Iron salts may reduce the bioavailability of levodopa, carbidopa and entacapone).
No products indexed under this heading.

Ferrous Sulfate (Iron salts may reduce the bioavailability of levodopa, carbidopa and entacapone). Products include:
Slow Fe Iron Tablets .... ▣818
Slow Fe with Folic Acid Tablets .... ▣819

Fluphenazine Decanoate (Dopamine D2 receptor antagonists may reduce the therapeutic effects of levodopa).
No products indexed under this heading.

Fluphenazine Enanthate (Dopamine D2 receptor antagonists may reduce the therapeutic effects of levodopa).
No products indexed under this heading.

Fluphenazine Hydrochloride (Dopamine D2 receptor antagonists may reduce the therapeutic effects of levodopa).
No products indexed under this heading.

Fosinopril Sodium (Symptomatic postural hypotension has occurred when carbidopa-levodopa was added to the treatment of a patient receiving antihypertensive drugs).
No products indexed under this heading.

Fosphenytoin (The beneficial effects of levodopa in Parkinson's disease have been reported to be reversed by phenytoin).
No products indexed under this heading.

Fosphenytoin Sodium (The beneficial effects of levodopa in Parkinson's disease have been reported to be reversed by phenytoin).
No products indexed under this heading.

Furosemide (Symptomatic postural hypotension has occurred when carbidopa-levodopa was added to the treatment of a patient receiving antihypertensive drugs). Products include:
Furosemide Tablets 2154

Guanabenz Acetate (Symptomatic postural hypotension has occurred when carbidopa-levodopa was added to the treatment of a patient receiving antihypertensive drugs).
No products indexed under this heading.

Guanethidine Monosulfate (Symptomatic postural hypotension has occurred when carbidopa-levodopa was added to the treatment of a patient receiving antihypertensive drugs).
No products indexed under this heading.

Haloperidol (Dopamine D2 receptor antagonists may reduce the therapeutic effects of levodopa).
No products indexed under this heading.

Haloperidol Decanoate (Dopamine D2 receptor antagonists may reduce the therapeutic effects of levodopa).
No products indexed under this heading.

Hydralazine Hydrochloride (Symptomatic postural hypotension has occurred when carbidopa-levodopa was added to the treatment of a patient receiving antihypertensive drugs). Products include:
BiDil Tablets 2171

Hydrochlorothiazide (Symptomatic postural hypotension has occurred when carbidopa-levodopa was added to the treatment of a patient receiving antihypertensive drugs).
Products include:
Aldoril Tablets 1910
Atacand HCT 651
Avalide Tablets 888
Avalide Tablets 2874
Benicar HCT Tablets 1044
Diovan HCT Tablets 2196
Dyazide Capsules 1423
Hyzaar 50-12.5 Tablets 1990
Hyzaar 100-12.5 Tablets 1990
Hyzaar 100-25 Tablets 1990
Lopressor HCT 50/25 Tablets 2241
Lopressor HCT 100/25 Tablets 2241
Lopressor HCT 100/50 Tablets 2241
Lotensin HCT Tablets 2246
Micardis HCT Tablets 856
Moduretic Tablets 2028
Prinzide Tablets 2056
Teveten HCT Tablets 1737
Timolide Tablets 2086
Uniretic Tablets 3100

Hydroflumethiazide (Symptomatic postural hypotension has occurred when carbidopa-levodopa was added to the treatment of a patient receiving antihypertensive drugs).
No products indexed under this heading.

Imipramine Hydrochloride (There have been rare reports of adverse reactions, including hypertension and dyskinesia, resulting from the concomitant use of tricylic antidepressants and carbidopa-levodopa).
No products indexed under this heading.

Imipramine Pamoate (There have been rare reports of adverse reactions, including hypertension and dyskinesia, resulting from the concomitant use of tricylic antidepressants and carbidopa-levodopa).
No products indexed under this heading.

Indapamide (Symptomatic postural hypotension has occurred when carbidopa-levodopa was added to the treatment of a patient receiving antihypertensive drugs). Products include:
Indapamide Tablets 2156

Irbesartan (Symptomatic postural hypotension has occurred when carbidopa-levodopa was added to the treatment of a patient receiving antihypertensive drugs). Products include:
Avalide Tablets 888
Avalide Tablets 2874
Avapro Tablets 891
Avapro Tablets 2871

Iron (Iron salts may reduce the bioavailability of levodopa, carbidopa and entacapone).
No products indexed under this heading.

Isocarboxazid (Nonselective monoamine oxidase (MAO) inhibitors are contraindicated for use with Stalevo).
No products indexed under this heading.

Isoetharine (Drugs known to be metabolized by COMT should be administered with caution in patients receiving entacapone regardless of the route of administration (including inhalation), as their interaction may result in increased heart rates, possibly arrhythmias, and excessive changes in blood pressure).
No products indexed under this heading.

Isoniazid (Isoniazid may reduce the therapeutic effects of levodopa).
No products indexed under this heading.

Isoproterenol Hydrochloride (Drugs known to be metabolized by COMT should be administered with caution in patients receiving entacapone regardless of the route of administration (including inhalation), as their interaction may result in increased heart rates, possibly arrhythmias, and excessive changes in blood pressure).
No products indexed under this heading.

Isoproterenol Sulfate (Drugs known to be metabolized by COMT should be administered with caution in patients receiving entacapone regardless of the route of administration (including inhalation), as their interaction may result in increased heart rates, possibly arrhythmias, and excessive changes in blood pressure).
No products indexed under this heading.

Isradipine (Symptomatic postural hypotension has occurred when carbidopa-levodopa was added to the treatment of a patient receiving antihypertensive drugs). Products include:
DynaCirc CR Tablets 2721

Labetalol Hydrochloride (Symptomatic postural hypotension has occurred when carbidopa-levodopa was added to the treatment of a patient receiving antihypertensive drugs).
No products indexed under this heading.

Lisinopril (Symptomatic postural hypotension has occurred when carbidopa-levodopa was added to the treatment of a patient receiving antihypertensive drugs). Products include:

Losartan Potassium (Symptomatic postural hypotension has occurred when carbidopa-levodopa was added to the treatment of a patient receiving antihypertensive drugs). Products include:

Loxapine Hydrochloride (Dopamine D2 receptor antagonists may reduce the therapeutic effects of levodopa).

No products indexed under this heading.

Loxapine Succinate (Dopamine D2 receptor antagonists may reduce the therapeutic effects of levodopa).

No products indexed under this heading.

Maprotiline Hydrochloride (There have been rare reports of adverse reactions, including hypertension and dyskinesia, resulting from the concomitant use of tricyclic antidepressants and carbidopa-levodopa).

No products indexed under this heading.

Mecamylamine Hydrochloride (Symptomatic postural hypotension has occurred when carbidopa-levodopa was added to the treatment of a patient receiving antihypertensive drugs).

No products indexed under this heading.

Mephenytoin (The beneficial effects of levodopa in Parkinson's disease have been reported to be reversed by phenytoin).

No products indexed under this heading.

Mesoridazine Besylate (Dopamine D2 receptor antagonists may reduce the therapeutic effects of levodopa).

No products indexed under this heading.

Methotrimeprazine (Dopamine D2 receptor antagonists may reduce the therapeutic effects of levodopa).

No products indexed under this heading.

Methyclothiazide (Symptomatic postural hypotension has occurred when carbidopa-levodopa was added to the treatment of a patient receiving antihypertensive drugs).

No products indexed under this heading.

Methyldopa (Drugs known to be metabolized by COMT should be administered with caution in patients receiving entacapone regardless of the route of administration (including inhalation), as their interaction may result in increased heart rates, possibly arrhythmias, and excessive changes in blood pressure). Products include:

Methyldopate Hydrochloride (Symptomatic postural hypotension has occurred when carbidopa-levodopa was added to the treatment of a patient receiving antihypertensive drugs).

No products indexed under this heading.

Metoclopramide Hydrochloride (Although metoclopramide may increase the bioavailability of levodopa by increasing gastric emptying, metoclopramide may also adversely affect disease control by its dopamine receptor antagonistic properties).

No products indexed under this heading.

Metolazone (Symptomatic postural hypotension has occurred when carbidopa-levodopa was added to the treatment of a patient receiving antihypertensive drugs).

No products indexed under this heading.

Metoprolol Succinate (Symptomatic postural hypotension has occurred when carbidopa-levodopa was added to the treatment of a patient receiving antihypertensive drugs). Products include:

Metoprolol Tartrate (Symptomatic postural hypotension has occurred when carbidopa-levodopa was added to the treatment of a patient receiving antihypertensive drugs). Products include:

Metyrosine (Symptomatic postural hypotension has occurred when carbidopa-levodopa was added to the treatment of a patient receiving antihypertensive drugs). Products include:

Mibefradil Dihydrochloride (Symptomatic postural hypotension has occurred when carbidopa-levodopa was added to the treatment of a patient receiving antihypertensive drugs).

No products indexed under this heading.

Minoxidil (Symptomatic postural hypotension has occurred when carbidopa-levodopa was added to the treatment of a patient receiving antihypertensive drugs). Products include:

Moclobemide (Nonselective monoamine oxidase (MAO) inhibitors are contraindicated for use with Stalevo).

No products indexed under this heading.

Moexipril Hydrochloride (Symptomatic postural hypotension has occurred when carbidopa-levodopa was added to the treatment of a patient receiving antihypertensive drugs). Products include:

Molindone Hydrochloride (Dopamine D2 receptor antagonists may reduce the therapeutic effects of levodopa). Products include:

Nadolol (Symptomatic postural hypotension has occurred when carbidopa-levodopa was added to

the treatment of a patient receiving antihypertensive drugs). Products include:

Nicardipine Hydrochloride (Symptomatic postural hypotension has occurred when carbidopa-levodopa was added to the treatment of a patient receiving antihypertensive drugs). Products include:

Nifedipine (Symptomatic postural hypotension has occurred when carbidopa-levodopa was added to the treatment of a patient receiving antihypertensive drugs). Products include:

Nisoldipine (Symptomatic postural hypotension has occurred when carbidopa-levodopa was added to the treatment of a patient receiving antihypertensive drugs). Products include:

Nitroglycerin (Symptomatic postural hypotension has occurred when carbidopa-levodopa was added to the treatment of a patient receiving antihypertensive drugs). Products include:

Norepinephrine Bitartrate (Drugs known to be metabolized by COMT should be administered with caution in patients receiving entacapone regardless of the route of administration (including inhalation), as their interaction may result in increased heart rates, possibly arrhythmias, and excessive changes in blood pressure).

No products indexed under this heading.

Nortriptyline Hydrochloride (There have been rare reports of adverse reactions, including hypertension and dyskinesia, resulting from the concomitant use of tricyclic antidepressants and carbidopa-levodopa).

No products indexed under this heading.

Papaverine (The beneficial effects of levodopa in Parkinson's disease have been reported to be reversed by papaverine).

No products indexed under this heading.

Papaverine Hydrochloride (The beneficial effects of levodopa in Parkinson's disease have been reported to be reversed by papaverine).

No products indexed under this heading.

Pargyline Hydrochloride (Nonselective monoamine oxidase (MAO) inhibitors are contraindicated for use with Stalevo).

No products indexed under this heading.

Penbutolol Sulfate (Symptomatic postural hypotension has occurred when carbidopa-levodopa was added to the treatment of a patient receiving antihypertensive drugs).

No products indexed under this heading.

Perindopril Erbumine (Symptomatic postural hypotension has occurred when carbidopa-levodopa was added to the treatment of a patient receiving antihypertensive drugs). Products include:

Perphenazine (Dopamine D2 receptor antagonists may reduce the therapeutic effects of levodopa).

No products indexed under this heading.

Phenelzine Sulfate (Nonselective monoamine oxidase (MAO) inhibitors are contraindicated for use with Stalevo).

No products indexed under this heading.

Phenoxybenzamine Hydrochloride (Symptomatic postural hypotension has occurred when carbidopa-levodopa was added to the treatment of a patient receiving antihypertensive drugs). Products include:

Phentolamine Mesylate (Symptomatic postural hypotension has occurred when carbidopa-levodopa was added to the treatment of a patient receiving antihypertensive drugs).

No products indexed under this heading.

Phenytoin (The beneficial effects of levodopa in Parkinson's disease have been reported to be reversed by phenytoin).

No products indexed under this heading.

Phenytoin Sodium (The beneficial effects of levodopa in Parkinson's disease have been reported to be reversed by phenytoin). Products include:

Pindolol (Symptomatic postural hypotension has occurred when carbidopa-levodopa was added to the treatment of a patient receiving antihypertensive drugs).

No products indexed under this heading.

Polysaccharide Iron Complex (Iron salts may reduce the bioavailability of levodopa, carbidopa and entacapone). Products include:

Polythiazide (Symptomatic postural hypotension has occurred when carbidopa-levodopa was added to the treatment of a patient receiving antihypertensive drugs).

No products indexed under this heading.

Prazosin Hydrochloride (Symptomatic postural hypotension has occurred when carbidopa-levodopa was added to the treatment of a patient receiving antihypertensive drugs).

No products indexed under this heading.

Probenecid (As most entacapone excretion is via the bile, caution should be exercised when drugs known to interfere with biliary excretion, glucuronidation, and intestinal beta-glucuronidase are given concurrently with entacapone).

No products indexed under this heading.

Procarbazine Hydrochloride (Nonselective monoamine oxidase (MAO) inhibitors are contraindicated for use with Stalevo). Products include:

IMPORTANT NOTE: Always consult each drug listing in the patient's regimen for possible interactions.

Prochlorperazine (Dopamine D2 receptor antagonists may reduce the therapeutic effects of levodopa).
No products indexed under this heading.

Promethazine Hydrochloride (Dopamine D2 receptor antagonists may reduce the therapeutic effects of levodopa). Products include:
Phenergan Tablets and Suppositories 3440

Propranolol Hydrochloride (Symptomatic postural hypotension has occurred when carbidopa-levodopa was added to the treatment of a patient receiving antihypertensive drugs). Products include:
Inderal LA Long-Acting Capsules 3429
InnoPran XL Capsules 2723

Protriptyline Hydrochloride (There have been rare reports of adverse reactions, including hypertension and dyskinesia, resulting from the concomitant use of tricylic antidepressants and carbidopa-levodopa).
No products indexed under this heading.

Quetiapine Fumarate (Dopamine D2 receptor antagonists may reduce the therapeutic effects of levodopa). Products include:
Seroquel Tablets 690

Quinapril Hydrochloride (Symptomatic postural hypotension has occurred when carbidopa-levodopa was added to the treatment of a patient receiving antihypertensive drugs).
No products indexed under this heading.

Ramipril (Symptomatic postural hypotension has occurred when carbidopa-levodopa was added to the treatment of a patient receiving antihypertensive drugs). Products include:
Altace Capsules 1702

Rauwolfia Serpentina (Symptomatic postural hypotension has occurred when carbidopa-levodopa was added to the treatment of a patient receiving antihypertensive drugs).
No products indexed under this heading.

Rescinnamine (Symptomatic postural hypotension has occurred when carbidopa-levodopa was added to the treatment of a patient receiving antihypertensive drugs).
No products indexed under this heading.

Reserpine (Symptomatic postural hypotension has occurred when carbidopa-levodopa was added to the treatment of a patient receiving antihypertensive drugs).
No products indexed under this heading.

Rifampicin (As most entacapone excretion is via the bile, caution should be exercised when drugs known to interfere with biliary excretion, glucuronidation, and intestinal beta-glucuronidase are given concurrently with entacapone).
No products indexed under this heading.

Risperidone (Dopamine D2 receptor antagonists may reduce the therapeutic effects of levodopa). Products include:
Risperdal 1676
Risperdal Consta Long-Acting Injection 1682
Risperdal M-Tab Orally Disintegrating Tablets 1676

Selegiline Hydrochloride (Nonselective monoamine oxidase (MAO) inhibitors are contraindicated for use with Stalevo). Products include:
Eldepryl Capsules 3208
Zelapar Tablets 3372

Sodium Nitroprusside (Symptomatic postural hypotension has occurred when carbidopa-levodopa was added to the treatment of a patient receiving antihypertensive drugs).
No products indexed under this heading.

Sotalol Hydrochloride (Symptomatic postural hypotension has occurred when carbidopa-levodopa was added to the treatment of a patient receiving antihypertensive drugs).
No products indexed under this heading.

Spirapril Hydrochloride (Symptomatic postural hypotension has occurred when carbidopa-levodopa was added to the treatment of a patient receiving antihypertensive drugs).
No products indexed under this heading.

Telmisartan (Symptomatic postural hypotension has occurred when carbidopa-levodopa was added to the treatment of a patient receiving antihypertensive drugs). Products include:
Micardis Tablets 854
Micardis HCT Tablets 856

Terazosin Hydrochloride (Symptomatic postural hypotension has occurred when carbidopa-levodopa was added to the treatment of a patient receiving antihypertensive drugs). Products include:
Hytrin Capsules 471

Thioridazine Hydrochloride (Dopamine D2 receptor antagonists may reduce the therapeutic effects of levodopa). Products include:
Thioridazine Hydrochloride Tablets 2163

Thiothixene (Dopamine D2 receptor antagonists may reduce the therapeutic effects of levodopa). Products include:
Thiothixene Capsules 2165

Timolol Maleate (Symptomatic postural hypotension has occurred when carbidopa-levodopa was added to the treatment of a patient receiving antihypertensive drugs). Products include:
Blocadren Tablets 1916
Cosopt Sterile Ophthalmic Solution 1931
Timolide Tablets 2086
Timoptic Sterile Ophthalmic Solution 2088
Timoptic in Ocudose 2091
Timoptic-XE Sterile Ophthalmic Gel Forming Solution 2092

Torsemide (Symptomatic postural hypotension has occurred when carbidopa-levodopa was added to the treatment of a patient receiving antihypertensive drugs). Products include:
Demadex Injection 2759
Demadex Tablets 2759

Trandolapril (Symptomatic postural hypotension has occurred when carbidopa-levodopa was added to the treatment of a patient receiving antihypertensive drugs). Products include:
Mavik Tablets 486
Tarka Tablets 524

Tranylcypromine Sulfate (Nonselective monoamine oxidase (MAO) inhibitors are contraindicated for use with Stalevo). Products include:
Parnate Tablets 1527

Trifluoperazine Hydrochloride (Dopamine D2 receptor antagonists may reduce the therapeutic effects of levodopa).
No products indexed under this heading.

Trimethaphan Camsylate (Symptomatic postural hypotension has occurred when carbidopa-levodopa was added to the treatment of a patient receiving antihypertensive drugs).
No products indexed under this heading.

Trimipramine Maleate (There have been rare reports of adverse reactions, including hypertension and dyskinesia, resulting from the concomitant use of tricylic antidepressants and carbidopa-levodopa).
No products indexed under this heading.

Valsartan (Symptomatic postural hypotension has occurred when carbidopa-levodopa was added to the treatment of a patient receiving antihypertensive drugs). Products include:
Diovan Tablets 2193
Diovan HCT Tablets 2196

Verapamil Hydrochloride (Symptomatic postural hypotension has occurred when carbidopa-levodopa was added to the treatment of a patient receiving antihypertensive drugs). Products include:
Covera-HS Tablets 3139
Tarka Tablets 524
Verelan PM Extended-Release Capsules, Controlled-Onset 3106

STARLIX TABLETS

(Nateglinide) 2292
May interact with beta blockers, corticosteroids, monoamine oxidase inhibitors, non-steroidal anti-inflammatory agents, salicylates, sympathomimetics, thiazides, thyroid preparations, and certain other agents. Compounds in these categories include:

Acebutolol Hydrochloride (The hypoglycemic action of nateglinide may be potentiated by non-selective beta-adrenergic-blocking agents).
No products indexed under this heading.

Albuterol (Co-administration with certain drugs, such as sympathomimetics, may reduce the hypoglycemic action of nateglinide and other oral antidiabetic drugs; when these drugs are administered to or withdrawn from patients receiving nateglinide, the patient should be observed closely for changes in glycemic control). Products include:
Proventil Inhalation Aerosol 3053

Albuterol Sulfate (Co-administration with certain drugs, such as sympathomimetics, may reduce the hypoglycemic action of nateglinide and other oral antidiabetic drugs; when these drugs are administered to or withdrawn from patients receiving nateglinide, the patient should be observed closely for changes in glycemic control). Products include:
AccuNeb Inhalation Solution 1055
Combivent Inhalation Aerosol 847
DuoNeb Inhalation Solution 1058
ProAir HFA Inhalation Aerosol 3300
Proventil Inhalation Solution 0.083% 3055
Proventil HFA Inhalation Aerosol 3056
Ventolin HFA Inhalation Aerosol 1600
VoSpire ER Tablets 1052

Aspirin (The hypoglycemic action of nateglinide may be potentiated by salicylates). Products include:
Aggrenox Capsules 822
Bayer Aspirin 744
BC Allergy Sinus Cold Powder .... ■677
BC Headache Powder .... ■677
Arthritis Strength BC Powder .... ■677
BC Sinus Cold Powder .... ■677
Excedrin Extra Strength Caplets/Tablets/Geltabs .... ■684
Excedrin Migraine Caplets/Tablets/Geltabs .... ■609
Goody's Body Pain Formula Powder .... ■684
Goody's Extra Strength Headache Powders .... ■611
Goody's Extra Strength Pain Relief Tablets .... ■685
Percodan Tablets 1132
St. Joseph 81 mg Aspirin Chewable and Enteric Coated Tablets 1869

Aspirin, Enteric Coated (The hypoglycemic action of nateglinide may be potentiated by salicylates).
No products indexed under this heading.

Aspirin Buffered (The hypoglycemic action of nateglinide may be potentiated by salicylates). Products include:
Bufferin Extra Strength Tablets .... ■678
Bufferin Regular Strength Tablets .... ■678

Atenolol (The hypoglycemic action of nateglinide may be potentiated by non-selective beta-adrenergic-blocking agents).
No products indexed under this heading.

Bendroflumethiazide (Co-administration with certain drugs, such as thiazides, may reduce the hypoglycemic action of nateglinide and other oral antidiabetic drugs; when these drugs are administered to or withdrawn from patients receiving nateglinide, the patient should be observed closely for changes in glycemic control).
No products indexed under this heading.

Betamethasone Acetate (Co-administration with certain drugs, such as corticosteroids, may reduce the hypoglycemic action of nateglinide and other oral antidiabetic drugs; when these drugs are administered to or withdrawn from patients receiving nateglinide, the patient should be observed closely for changes in glycemic control).
No products indexed under this heading.

Betamethasone Sodium Phosphate (Co-administration with certain drugs, such as corticosteroids, may reduce the hypoglycemic action of nateglinide and other oral antidiabetic drugs; when these drugs are administered to or withdrawn from patients receiving nateglinide, the patient should be observed closely for changes in glycemic control).
No products indexed under this heading.

Betaxolol Hydrochloride (The hypoglycemic action of nateglinide may be potentiated by non-selective beta-adrenergic-blocking agents). Products include:

Betoptic S Ophthalmic Suspension.................................. 558

Bisoprolol Fumarate (The hypoglycemic action of nateglinide may be potentiated by non-selective beta-adrenergic-blocking agents).

No products indexed under this heading.

Carteolol Hydrochloride (The hypoglycemic action of nateglinide may be potentiated by non-selective beta-adrenergic-blocking agents). Products include:

Carteolol Hydrochloride Ophthalmic Solution USP, 1%....... ⊙249

Celecoxib (The hypoglycemic action of nateglinide may be potentiated by non-steroidal anti-inflammatory agents). Products include:

Celebrex Capsules 3134

Chlorothiazide (Co-administration with certain drugs, such as thiazides, may reduce the hypoglycemic action of nateglinide and other oral antidiabetic drugs; when these drugs are administered to or withdrawn from patients receiving nateglinide, the patient should be observed closely for changes in glycemic control). Products include:

Diuril Oral Suspension 1954

Chlorothiazide Sodium (Co-administration with certain drugs, such as thiazides, may reduce the hypoglycemic action of nateglinide and other oral antidiabetic drugs; when these drugs are administered to or withdrawn from patients receiving nateglinide, the patient should be observed closely for changes in glycemic control). Products include:

Diuril Sodium Intravenous 2467

Choline Magnesium Trisalicylate (The hypoglycemic action of nateglinide may be potentiated by salicylates).

No products indexed under this heading.

Cortisone Acetate (Co-administration with certain drugs, such as corticosteroids, may reduce the hypoglycemic action of nateglinide and other oral antidiabetic drugs; when these drugs are administered to or withdrawn from patients receiving nateglinide, the patient should be observed closely for changes in glycemic control).

No products indexed under this heading.

Dexamethasone (Co-administration with certain drugs, such as corticosteroids, may reduce the hypoglycemic action of nateglinide and other oral antidiabetic drugs; when these drugs are administered to or withdrawn from patients receiving nateglinide, the patient should be observed closely for changes in glycemic control). Products include:

Ciprodex Otic Suspension 559
Decadron Tablets 1951
TobraDex Ophthalmic Ointment 562
TobraDex Ophthalmic Suspension ... 563

Dexamethasone Acetate (Co-administration with certain drugs, such as corticosteroids, may reduce the hypoglycemic action of nateglinide and other oral antidiabetic drugs; when these drugs are administered to or withdrawn from patients receiving nateglinide, the patient should be observed closely for changes in glycemic control).

No products indexed under this heading.

Dexamethasone Sodium Phosphate (Co-administration with certain drugs, such as corticosteroids, may reduce the hypoglycemic action of nateglinide and other oral antidiabetic drugs; when these drugs are administered to or withdrawn from patients receiving nateglinide, the patient should be observed closely for changes in glycemic control).

No products indexed under this heading.

Diclofenac Potassium (The hypoglycemic action of nateglinide may be potentiated by non-steroidal anti-inflammatory agents).

No products indexed under this heading.

Diclofenac Sodium (The hypoglycemic action of nateglinide may be potentiated by non-steroidal anti-inflammatory agents). Products include:

Arthrotec Tablets 3129
Voltaren Ophthalmic Solution 2309
Voltaren Tablets 2307
Voltaren-XR Tablets 2310

Diflunisal (The hypoglycemic action of nateglinide may be potentiated by salicylates). Products include:

Dolobid Tablets 1955

Dobutamine Hydrochloride (Co-administration with certain drugs, such as sympathomimetics, may reduce the hypoglycemic action of nateglinide and other oral antidiabetic drugs; when these drugs are administered to or withdrawn from patients receiving nateglinide, the patient should be observed closely for changes in glycemic control).

No products indexed under this heading.

Dopamine Hydrochloride (Co-administration with certain drugs, such as sympathomimetics, may reduce the hypoglycemic action of nateglinide and other oral antidiabetic drugs; when these drugs are administered to or withdrawn from patients receiving nateglinide, the patient should be observed closely for changes in glycemic control).

No products indexed under this heading.

Ephedrine Hydrochloride (Co-administration with certain drugs, such as sympathomimetics, may reduce the hypoglycemic action of nateglinide and other oral antidiabetic drugs; when these drugs are administered to or withdrawn from patients receiving nateglinide, the patient should be observed closely for changes in glycemic control).

No products indexed under this heading.

Ephedrine Sulfate (Co-administration with certain drugs, such as sympathomimetics, may reduce the hypoglycemic action of nateglinide and other oral antidiabetic drugs; when these drugs are administered to or withdrawn from patients receiving nateglinide, the patient should be observed closely for changes in glycemic control).

No products indexed under this heading.

Ephedrine Tannate (Co-administration with certain drugs, such as sympathomimetics, may reduce the hypoglycemic action of nateglinide and other oral antidiabetic drugs; when these drugs are administered to or withdrawn from patients receiving nateglinide, the patient should be observed closely for changes in glycemic control).

No products indexed under this heading.

Epinephrine (Co-administration with certain drugs, such as sympathomimetics, may reduce the hypoglycemic action of nateglinide and other oral antidiabetic drugs; when these drugs are administered to or withdrawn from patients receiving nateglinide, the patient should be observed closely for changes in glycemic control). Products include:

EpiPen 1061
Primatene Mist .... ▣719
Twinject 0.15 3379
Twinject 0.3 3378

Epinephrine Bitartrate (Co-administration with certain drugs, such as sympathomimetics, may reduce the hypoglycemic action of nateglinide and other oral antidiabetic drugs; when these drugs are administered to or withdrawn from patients receiving nateglinide, the patient should be observed closely for changes in glycemic control).

No products indexed under this heading.

Epinephrine Hydrochloride (Co-administration with certain drugs, such as sympathomimetics, may reduce the hypoglycemic action of nateglinide and other oral antidiabetic drugs; when these drugs are administered to or withdrawn from patients receiving nateglinide, the patient should be observed closely for changes in glycemic control).

No products indexed under this heading.

Esmolol Hydrochloride (The hypoglycemic action of nateglinide may be potentiated by non-selective beta-adrenergic-blocking agents).

No products indexed under this heading.

Etodolac (The hypoglycemic action of nateglinide may be potentiated by non-steroidal anti-inflammatory agents).

No products indexed under this heading.

Fenoprofen Calcium (The hypoglycemic action of nateglinide may be potentiated by non-steroidal anti-inflammatory agents). Products include:

Nalfon Capsules 2502

Fludrocortisone Acetate (Co-administration with certain drugs, such as corticosteroids, may reduce the hypoglycemic action of nateglinide and other oral antidiabetic drugs; when these drugs are administered to or withdrawn from patients receiving nateglinide, the patient should be observed closely for changes in glycemic control).

No products indexed under this heading.

Flurbiprofen (The hypoglycemic action of nateglinide may be potentiated by non-steroidal anti-inflammatory agents).

No products indexed under this heading.

Hydrochlorothiazide (Co-administration with certain drugs, such as thiazides, may reduce the hypoglycemic action of nateglinide and other oral antidiabetic drugs; when these drugs are administered to or withdrawn from patients receiving nateglinide, the patient should be observed closely for changes in glycemic control). Products include:

Aldoril Tablets 1910
Atacand HCT 651
Avalide Tablets 888
Avalide Tablets 2874
Benicar HCT Tablets 1044
Diovan HCT Tablets 2196
Dyazide Capsules 1423
Hyzaar 50-12.5 Tablets 1990
Hyzaar 100-12.5 Tablets 1990
Hyzaar 100-25 Tablets 1990
Lopressor HCT 50/25 Tablets 2241
Lopressor HCT 100/25 Tablets 2241
Lopressor HCT 100/50 Tablets 2241
Lotensin HCT Tablets 2246
Micardis HCT Tablets 856
Moduretic Tablets 2028
Prinzide Tablets 2056
Teveten HCT Tablets 1737
Timolide Tablets 2086
Uniretic Tablets 3100

Hydrocortisone (Co-administration with certain drugs, such as corticosteroids, may reduce the hypoglycemic action of nateglinide and other oral antidiabetic drugs; when these drugs are administered to or withdrawn from patients receiving nateglinide, the patient should be observed closely for changes in glycemic control). Products include:

Colocort Rectal Suspension, USP (Retention) 100 mg/60 mL........... 2476
Hydrocortone Tablets 1989
Preparation H Hydrocortisone Cream .... ▣646

Hydrocortisone Acetate (Co-administration with certain drugs, such as corticosteroids, may reduce the hypoglycemic action of nateglinide and other oral antidiabetic drugs; when these drugs are administered to or withdrawn from patients receiving nateglinide, the patient should be observed closely for changes in glycemic control). Products include:

Analpram-HC 1159
Pramosone 1161
ProctoFoam-HC 3099

Hydrocortisone Sodium Phosphate (Co-administration with certain drugs, such as corticosteroids, may reduce the hypoglycemic action of nateglinide and other oral antidiabetic drugs; when these drugs are administered to or withdrawn from patients receiving nateglinide, the patient should be observed closely for changes in glycemic control).

No products indexed under this heading.

Hydrocortisone Sodium Succinate (Co-administration with certain drugs, such as corticosteroids, may reduce the hypoglycemic action of nateglinide and other oral antidiabetic drugs; when these drugs are administered to or withdrawn from patients receiving nateglinide, the patient should be observed closely for changes in glycemic control).

No products indexed under this heading.

Hydroflumethiazide (Co-administration with certain drugs, such as thiazides, may reduce the hypoglycemic action of nateglinide and other oral antidiabetic drugs; when these drugs are administered to or withdrawn from patients receiving nateglinide, the patient should be observed closely for changes in glycemic control).
No products indexed under this heading.

Ibuprofen (The hypoglycemic action of nateglinide may be potentiated by non-steroidal anti-inflammatory agents). Products include:
- Advil Allergy Sinus Caplets .... ▣ 770
- Advil .... ▣ 674
- Children's Advil Oral Suspension .... ▣ 603
- Children's Advil Chewable Tablets .. ▣ 603
- Advil Cold & Sinus .... ▣ 723
- Infants' Advil Concentrated Drops .. ▣ 604
- Infants' Advil Concentrated Drops - White Grape (Dye-Free) .... ▣ 604
- Junior Strength Advil Swallow Tablets .... ▣ 605
- Advil Migraine Liquigels .... ▣ 608
- Advil Multi-Symptom Cold Caplets .... ▣ 770
- Advil PM Caplets .... ▣ 615
- Motrin IB Tablets and Caplets 1866
- Children's Motrin Oral Suspension ... 1867
- Children's Motrin Non-Staining Dye-Free Oral Suspension 1867
- Children's Motrin Cold Oral Suspension 1867
- Infants' Motrin Concentrated Drops 1867
- Infants' Motrin Non-Staining Dye-Free Concentrated Drops 1867
- Junior Strength Motrin Caplets and Chewable Tablets 1867
- Vicoprofen Tablets 539

Indomethacin (The hypoglycemic action of nateglinide may be potentiated by non-steroidal anti-inflammatory agents). Products include:
- Indocin 1995

Indomethacin Sodium Trihydrate (The hypoglycemic action of nateglinide may be potentiated by non-steroidal anti-inflammatory agents). Products include:
- Indocin I.V. 2465

Isocarboxazid (The hypoglycemic action of nateglinide may be potentiated by MAO inhibitors).
No products indexed under this heading.

Isoproterenol Hydrochloride (Co-administration with certain drugs, such as sympathomimetics, may reduce the hypoglycemic action of nateglinide and other oral antidiabetic drugs; when these drugs are administered to or withdrawn from patients receiving nateglinide, the patient should be observed closely for changes in glycemic control).
No products indexed under this heading.

Isoproterenol Sulfate (Co-administration with certain drugs, such as sympathomimetics, may reduce the hypoglycemic action of nateglinide and other oral antidiabetic drugs; when these drugs are administered to or withdrawn from patients receiving nateglinide, the patient should be observed closely for changes in glycemic control).
No products indexed under this heading.

Ketoprofen (The hypoglycemic action of nateglinide may be potentiated by non-steroidal anti-inflammatory agents).
No products indexed under this heading.

Ketorolac Tromethamine (The hypoglycemic action of nateglinide may be potentiated by non-steroidal anti-inflammatory agents). Products include:
- Acular Ophthalmic Solution 565
- Acular LS Ophthalmic Solution 566

Labetalol Hydrochloride (The hypoglycemic action of nateglinide may be potentiated by non-selective beta-adrenergic-blocking agents).
No products indexed under this heading.

Levalbuterol Hydrochloride (Co-administration with certain drugs, such as sympathomimetics, may reduce the hypoglycemic action of nateglinide and other oral antidiabetic drugs; when these drugs are administered to or withdrawn from patients receiving nateglinide, the patient should be observed closely for changes in glycemic control). Products include:
- Xopenex Inhalation Solution 3146
- Xopenex Inhalation Solution Concentrate 3150

Levobunolol Hydrochloride (The hypoglycemic action of nateglinide may be potentiated by non-selective beta-adrenergic-blocking agents). Products include:
- Betagan Ophthalmic Solution, USP .... ⊙ 220

Levothyroxine Sodium (Co-administration with certain drugs, such as thyroid products, may reduce the hypoglycemic action of nateglinide and other oral antidiabetic drugs; when these drugs are administered to or withdrawn from patients receiving nateglinide, the patient should be observed closely for changes in glycemic control). Products include:
- Levothroid Tablets 1186
- Levoxyl Tablets 1712
- Synthroid Tablets 520
- Westhroid Tablets 3403

Liothyronine Sodium (Co-administration with certain drugs, such as thyroid products, may reduce the hypoglycemic action of nateglinide and other oral antidiabetic drugs; when these drugs are administered to or withdrawn from patients receiving nateglinide, the patient should be observed closely for changes in glycemic control). Products include:
- Cytomel Tablets 1710
- Westhroid Tablets 3403

Liotrix (Co-administration with certain drugs, such as thyroid products, may reduce the hypoglycemic action of nateglinide and other oral antidiabetic drugs; when these drugs are administered to or withdrawn from patients receiving nateglinide, the patient should be observed closely for changes in glycemic control). Products include:
- Thyrolar Tablets 1199

Magnesium Salicylate (The hypoglycemic action of nateglinide may be potentiated by salicylates).
No products indexed under this heading.

Meclofenamate Sodium (The hypoglycemic action of nateglinide may be potentiated by non-steroidal anti-inflammatory agents).
No products indexed under this heading.

Mefenamic Acid (The hypoglycemic action of nateglinide may be potentiated by non-steroidal anti-inflammatory agents).
No products indexed under this heading.

Meloxicam (The hypoglycemic action of nateglinide may be potentiated by non-steroidal anti-inflammatory agents). Products include:
- Mobic Oral Suspension 863
- Mobic Tablets 863

Metaproterenol Sulfate (Co-administration with certain drugs, such as sympathomimetics, may reduce the hypoglycemic action of nateglinide and other oral antidiabetic drugs; when these drugs are administered to or withdrawn from patients receiving nateglinide, the patient should be observed closely for changes in glycemic control). Products include:
- Alupent Inhalation Aerosol 826

Metaraminol Bitartrate (Co-administration with certain drugs, such as sympathomimetics, may reduce the hypoglycemic action of nateglinide and other oral antidiabetic drugs; when these drugs are administered to or withdrawn from patients receiving nateglinide, the patient should be observed closely for changes in glycemic control).
No products indexed under this heading.

Methoxamine Hydrochloride (Co-administration with certain drugs, such as sympathomimetics, may reduce the hypoglycemic action of nateglinide and other oral antidiabetic drugs; when these drugs are administered to or withdrawn from patients receiving nateglinide, the patient should be observed closely for changes in glycemic control).
No products indexed under this heading.

Methyclothiazide (Co-administration with certain drugs, such as thiazides, may reduce the hypoglycemic action of nateglinide and other oral antidiabetic drugs; when these drugs are administered to or withdrawn from patients receiving nateglinide, the patient should be observed closely for changes in glycemic control).
No products indexed under this heading.

Methylprednisolone Acetate (Co-administration with certain drugs, such as corticosteroids, may reduce the hypoglycemic action of nateglinide and other oral antidiabetic drugs; when these drugs are administered to or withdrawn from patients receiving nateglinide, the patient should be observed closely for changes in glycemic control). Products include:
- Depo-Medrol Injectable Suspension 2617
- Depo-Medrol Single-Dose Vial 2619

Methylprednisolone Sodium Succinate (Co-administration with certain drugs, such as corticosteroids, may reduce the hypoglycemic action of nateglinide and other oral antidiabetic drugs; when these drugs are administered to or withdrawn from patients receiving nateglinide, the patient should be observed closely for changes in glycemic control).
No products indexed under this heading.

Metipranolol Hydrochloride (The hypoglycemic action of nateglinide may be potentiated by non-selective beta-adrenergic-blocking agents).
No products indexed under this heading.

Metoprolol Succinate (The hypoglycemic action of nateglinide may be potentiated by non-selective beta-adrenergic-blocking agents). Products include:
- Toprol-XL Tablets 668

Metoprolol Tartrate (The hypoglycemic action of nateglinide may be potentiated by non selective beta-adrenergic-blocking agents). Products include:
- Lopressor Injection 2238
- Lopressor Tablets 2238
- Lopressor HCT 50/25 Tablets 2241
- Lopressor HCT 100/25 Tablets 2241
- Lopressor HCT 100/50 Tablets 2241

Moclobemide (The hypoglycemic action of nateglinide may be potentiated by MAO inhibitors).
No products indexed under this heading.

Nabumetone (The hypoglycemic action of nateglinide may be potentiated by non-steroidal anti-inflammatory agents).
No products indexed under this heading.

Nadolol (The hypoglycemic action of nateglinide may be potentiated by non-selective beta-adrenergic-blocking agents). Products include:
- Nadolol Tablets 2159

Naproxen (The hypoglycemic action of nateglinide may be potentiated by non-steroidal anti-inflammatory agents). Products include:
- EC-Naprosyn Delayed-Release Tablets 2761
- Naprosyn Suspension 2761
- Naprosyn Tablets 2761
- Prevacid NapraPAC 3280

Naproxen Sodium (The hypoglycemic action of nateglinide may be potentiated by non-steroidal anti-inflammatory agents). Products include:
- Aleve Caplets 742
- Aleve Gelcaps 743
- Aleve Tablets 743
- Aleve Cold & Sinus Caplets 744
- Anaprox Tablets 2761
- Anaprox DS Tablets 2761

Norepinephrine Bitartrate (Co-administration with certain drugs, such as sympathomimetics, may reduce the hypoglycemic action of nateglinide and other oral antidiabetic drugs; when these drugs are administered to or withdrawn from patients receiving nateglinide, the patient should be observed closely for changes in glycemic control).
No products indexed under this heading.

Oxaprozin (The hypoglycemic action of nateglinide may be potentiated by non-steroidal anti-inflammatory agents).
No products indexed under this heading.

Pargyline Hydrochloride (The hypoglycemic action of nateglinide may be potentiated by MAO inhibitors).
No products indexed under this heading.

Penbutolol Sulfate (The hypoglycemic action of nateglinide may be potentiated by non-selective beta-adrenergic-blocking agents).
No products indexed under this heading.

(▣ Described in PDR For Nonprescription Drugs)

(⊙ Described in PDR For Ophthalmic Medicines™)

Phenelzine Sulfate (The hypoglycemic action of nateglinide may be potentiated by MAO inhibitors).
No products indexed under this heading.

Phenylbutazone (The hypoglycemic action of nateglinide may be potentiated by non-steroidal anti-inflammatory agents).
No products indexed under this heading.

Phenylephrine Bitartrate (Co-administration with certain drugs, such as sympathomimetics, may reduce the hypoglycemic action of nateglinide and other oral antidiabetic drugs; when these drugs are administered to or withdrawn from patients receiving nateglinide, the patient should be observed closely for changes in glycemic control).
No products indexed under this heading.

Phenylephrine Hydrochloride (Co-administration with certain drugs, such as sympathomimetics, may reduce the hypoglycemic action of nateglinide and other oral antidiabetic drugs; when these drugs are administered to or withdrawn from patients receiving nateglinide, the patient should be observed closely for changes in glycemic control). Products include:
- Comtrex Maximum Strength Non-Drowsy Cold & Cough Caplets 725
- Comtrex Maximum Strength Day/Night Severe Cold & Sinus Caplets - Day Formulation 725
- Comtrex Maximum Strength Day/Night Severe Cold & Sinus Caplets - Night Formulation 725
- Contac Cold and Flu Maximum Strength Caplets 728
- Contac Cold and Flu Day and Night Caplets (Day Formulation Only) 727
- Contac Cold and Flu Day and Night Caplets (Night Formulation Only) 727
- Contac Cold and Flu Non-Drowsy Caplets 728
- Contac-D Cold Non-Drowsy Tablets 729
- Children's Dimetapp Cold & Allergy Elixir 730
- Children's Dimetapp Cold & Allergy Chewable Tablets 730
- Children's Dimetapp DM Cold & Cough Elixir 731
- Toddler's Dimetapp Cold and Cough Drops 732
- Excedrin Sinus Headache Caplets/Tablets 610
- 4-Way Fast Acting Nasal Spray 775
- 4-Way Menthol Nasal Spray 775
- Preparation H Maximum Strength Cream 666
- Preparation H Cooling Gel 666
- Preparation H 666
- Refenesen PE Caplets 721
- Robitussin Cough & Allergy Syrup 736
- Robitussin Cough & Cold Nighttime Liquid 736
- Robitussin Cough, Cold & Flu Nighttime Liquid 738
- Robitussin Head & Chest Congestion PE Syrup 739
- Robitussin Pediatric Cough & Cold Nighttime Liquid 736
- TheraFlu Cold & Cough Hot Liquid 740
- TheraFlu Cold & Sore Throat Hot Liquid 741
- TheraFlu Flu & Sore Throat Hot Liquid 742
- TheraFlu Daytime Severe Cold Hot Liquid 742
- TheraFlu Nighttime Severe Cold Hot Liquid 740
- TheraFlu Warming Relief Daytime Severe Cold 743
- TheraFlu Warming Relief Nighttime Severe Cold 743
- Triaminic Chest & Nasal Congestion Liquid 746
- Triaminic Cold & Allergy Liquid 746
- Triaminic Daytime Cold & Cough Liquid 745
- Triaminic Nighttime Cold & Cough Liquid 746
- Triaminic Thin Strips Cold 748
- Triaminic Thin Strips Cold & Cough 778
- Triaminic Infant Thin Strips Decongestant 747
- Triaminic Infant Thin Strips Decongestant Plus Cough 747
- Children's Tylenol Plus Flu Oral Suspension 749
- Tylenol Cold Head Congestion Daytime Caplets with Cool Burst and Gelcaps 750
- Tylenol Cold Multi-Symptom Daytime Liquid 752
- Tylenol Cold Multi-Symptom Severe Daytime Liquid 752
- Concentrated Tylenol Infants' Drops Plus Cold & Cough 754
- Tylenol Allergy Multi-Symptom Caplets with Cool Burst and Gelcaps 1872
- Tylenol Allergy Multi-Symptom Nighttime Caplets with Cool Burst 1872
- Children's Tylenol Plus Cold Suspension Liquid 1879
- Children's Tylenol Plus Cold & Allergy Suspension Liquid 1878
- Children's Tylenol Plus Flu Suspension Liquid 1881
- Children's Tylenol Plus Multi-Symptom Cold Suspension Liquid 1879
- Tylenol Cold Head Congestion Daytime Caplets with Cool Burst 1873
- Tylenol Cold Head Congestion Nighttime Caplets with Cool Burst 1873
- Tylenol Cold Head Congestion Severe Caplets with Cool Burst 1873
- Tylenol Cold Multi-Symptom Daytime Caplets with Cool Burst and Gelcaps 1874
- Tylenol Cold Multi-Symptom Daytime Liquid with Citrus Burst 1874
- Tylenol Cold Multi-Symptom Nighttime Caplets with Cool Burst 1874
- Tylenol Cold Multi-Symptom Nighttime Liquid with Cool Burst 1874
- Tylenol Cold Multi-Symptom Severe Caplets with Cool Burst 1874
- Tylenol Cold Multi-Symptom Severe Daytime Liquid with Citrus Burst 1874
- Tylenol Sinus Congestion & Pain Daytime Caplets with Cool Burst and Gelcaps 1876
- Tylenol Sinus Congestion & Pain Nighttime Caplets with Cool Burst 1876
- Tylenol Sinus Congestion & Pain Severe Caplets with Cool Burst 1876
- Vicks 44D Cough & Head Congestion Relief Liquid 760
- Vicks DayQuil LiquiCaps/Liquid Multi-Symptom Cold/Flu Relief 761
- Zicam Cough Plus D Cough Spray 767

Phenylephrine Tannate (Co-administration with certain drugs, such as sympathomimetics, may reduce the hypoglycemic action of nateglinide and other oral antidiabetic drugs; when these drugs are administered to or withdrawn from patients receiving nateglinide, the patient should be observed closely for changes in glycemic control).
No products indexed under this heading.

Phenylpropanolamine Hydrochloride (Co-administration with certain drugs, such as sympathomimetics, may reduce the hypoglycemic action of nateglinide and other oral antidiabetic drugs; when these drugs are administered to or withdrawn from patients receiving nateglinide, the patient should be observed closely for changes in glycemic control).
No products indexed under this heading.

Pindolol (The hypoglycemic action of nateglinide may be potentiated by non-selective beta-adrenergic-blocking agents).
No products indexed under this heading.

Pirbuterol Acetate (Co-administration with certain drugs, such as sympathomimetics, may reduce the hypoglycemic action of nateglinide and other oral antidiabetic drugs; when these drugs are administered to or withdrawn from patients receiving nateglinide, the patient should be observed closely for changes in glycemic control). Products include:
- Maxair Autohaler 1852

Piroxicam (The hypoglycemic action of nateglinide may be potentiated by non-steroidal anti-inflammatory agents).
No products indexed under this heading.

Polythiazide (Co-administration with certain drugs, such as thiazides, may reduce the hypoglycemic action of nateglinide and other oral antidiabetic drugs; when these drugs are administered to or withdrawn from patients receiving nateglinide, the patient should be observed closely for changes in glycemic control).
No products indexed under this heading.

Prednisolone Acetate (Co-administration with certain drugs, such as corticosteroids, may reduce the hypoglycemic action of nateglinide and other oral antidiabetic drugs; when these drugs are administered to or withdrawn from patients receiving nateglinide, the patient should be observed closely for changes in glycemic control). Products include:
- Blephamide Ophthalmic Ointment 568
- Blephamide Ophthalmic Suspension 569
- Poly-Pred Ophthalmic Suspension .... ⊙233
- Pred Forte Ophthalmic Suspension .... ⊙235
- Pred Mild Ophthalmic Suspension .... ⊙238
- Pred-G Ophthalmic Ointment .... ⊙237
- Pred-G Ophthalmic Suspension .... ⊙236

Prednisolone Sodium Phosphate (Co-administration with certain drugs, such as corticosteroids, may reduce the hypoglycemic action of nateglinide and other oral antidiabetic drugs; when these drugs are administered to or withdrawn from patients receiving nateglinide, the patient should be observed closely for changes in glycemic control).
No products indexed under this heading.

Prednisolone Tebutate (Co-administration with certain drugs, such as corticosteroids, may reduce the hypoglycemic action of nateglinide and other oral antidiabetic drugs; when these drugs are administered to or withdrawn from patients receiving nateglinide, the patient should be observed closely for changes in glycemic control).
No products indexed under this heading.

Prednisone (Co-administration with certain drugs, such as corticosteroids, may reduce the hypoglycemic action of nateglinide and other oral antidiabetic drugs; when these drugs are administered to or withdrawn from patients receiving nateglinide, the patient should be observed closely for changes in glycemic control).
No products indexed under this heading.

Procarbazine Hydrochloride (The hypoglycemic action of nateglinide may be potentiated by MAO inhibitors). Products include:
- Matulane Capsules 3191

Propranolol Hydrochloride (The hypoglycemic action of nateglinide may be potentiated by non-selective beta-adrenergic-blocking agents). Products include:
- Inderal LA Long-Acting Capsules 3429
- InnoPran XL Capsules 2723

Pseudoephedrine Hydrochloride (Co-administration with certain drugs, such as sympathomimetics, may reduce the hypoglycemic action of nateglinide and other oral antidiabetic drugs; when these drugs are administered to or withdrawn from patients receiving nateglinide, the patient should be observed closely for changes in glycemic control). Products include:
- Advil Allergy Sinus Caplets 770
- Advil Cold & Sinus 723
- Advil Multi-Symptom Cold Caplets 770
- Aleve Cold & Sinus Caplets 744
- Allegra-D 12 Hour Extended-Release Tablets 2846
- Allegra-D 24 Hour Extended-Release Tablets 2849
- BC Cold Powder 677
- Comtrex Maximum Strength Cold & Cough Day/Night Caplets - Day Formulation 726
- Comtrex Maximum Strength Cold & Cough Day/Night Caplets - Night Formulation 726
- Children's Motrin Cold Oral Suspension 1867
- Mucinex D Extended-Release Bi-Layer Tablets 776
- Robitussin Cough & Cold CF Liquid 735
- Robitussin Cough & Cold Pediatric Drops 735
- Tylenol Sinus Congestion & Pain Nighttime Caplets with Cool Burst 778
- Tylenol Cold Severe Congestion Non-Drowsy Caplets with Cool Burst 1874
- Tylenol Sinus Severe Congestion Caplets with Cool Burst 1876
- Vicks 44D Cough & Head Congestion Relief Liquid 2679
- Vicks 44M Cough, Cold & Flu Relief Liquid 2680
- Vicks DayQuil Multi-Symptom Cold/Flu Relief LiquiCaps 2678
- Vicks DayQuil Multi-Symptom Cold/Flu Relief Liquid 2678
- Vicks NyQuil Multi-Symptom Cold/Flu Relief Liquid 2681
- Vicks NyQuil Multi-Symptom Cold/Flu Relief LiquiCaps 2681

Children's Vicks NyQuil Cold/Cough Relief Liquid 2680
Zyrtec-D 12 Hour Extended Release Tablets 2597

Pseudoephedrine Sulfate (Co-administration with certain drugs, such as sympathomimetics, may reduce the hypoglycemic action of nateglinide and other oral antidiabetic drugs; when these drugs are administered to or withdrawn from patients receiving nateglinide, the patient should be observed closely for changes in glycemic control). Products include:
Alavert Allergy & Sinus D-12 Hour Tablets .... ▣771
Clarinex-D 24-Hour Extended-Release Tablets 2998
Claritin-D Non-Drowsy 12 Hour Tablets .... ▣772
Claritin-D Non-Drowsy 24 Hour Tablets .... ▣772

Rofecoxib (The hypoglycemic action of nateglinide may be potentiated by non-steroidal anti-inflammatory agents).
No products indexed under this heading.

Salmeterol Xinafoate (Co-administration with certain drugs, such as sympathomimetics, may reduce the hypoglycemic action of nateglinide and other oral antidiabetic drugs; when these drugs are administered to or withdrawn from patients receiving nateglinide, the patient should be observed closely for changes in glycemic control). Products include:
Advair Diskus 100/50 1308
Advair Diskus 250/50 1308
Advair Diskus 500/50 1308
Advair HFA Inhalation Aerosol 1318
Serevent Diskus 1568

Salsalate (The hypoglycemic action of nateglinide may be potentiated by salicylates).
No products indexed under this heading.

Selegiline Hydrochloride (The hypoglycemic action of nateglinide may be potentiated by MAO inhibitors). Products include:
Eldepryl Capsules 3208
Zelapar Tablets 3372

Sotalol Hydrochloride (The hypoglycemic action of nateglinide may be potentiated by non-selective beta-adrenergic-blocking agents).
No products indexed under this heading.

Sulindac (The hypoglycemic action of nateglinide may be potentiated by non-steroidal anti-inflammatory agents). Products include:
Clinoril Tablets 1924

Terbutaline Sulfate (Co-administration with certain drugs, such as sympathomimetics, may reduce the hypoglycemic action of nateglinide and other oral antidiabetic drugs; when these drugs are administered to or withdrawn from patients receiving nateglinide, the patient should be observed closely for changes in glycemic control).
No products indexed under this heading.

Thyroglobulin (Co-administration with certain drugs, such as thyroid products, may reduce the hypoglycemic action of nateglinide and other oral antidiabetic drugs; when these drugs are administered to or withdrawn from patients receiving nateglinide, the patient should be observed closely for changes in glycemic control).
No products indexed under this heading.

Thyroid (Co-administration with certain drugs, such as thyroid products, may reduce the hypoglycemic action of nateglinide and other oral antidiabetic drugs; when these drugs are administered to or withdrawn from patients receiving nateglinide, the patient should be observed closely for changes in glycemic control).
No products indexed under this heading.

Thyroxine (Co-administration with certain drugs, such as thyroid products, may reduce the hypoglycemic action of nateglinide and other oral antidiabetic drugs; when these drugs are administered to or withdrawn from patients receiving nateglinide, the patient should be observed closely for changes in glycemic control).
No products indexed under this heading.

Thyroxine Sodium (Co-administration with certain drugs, such as thyroid products, may reduce the hypoglycemic action of nateglinide and other oral antidiabetic drugs; when these drugs are administered to or withdrawn from patients receiving nateglinide, the patient should be observed closely for changes in glycemic control).
No products indexed under this heading.

Timolol Hemihydrate (The hypoglycemic action of nateglinide may be potentiated by non-selective beta-adrenergic-blocking agents). Products include:
Betimol Ophthalmic Solution 3382
Betimol Ophthalmic Solution .... ⊙295

Timolol Maleate (The hypoglycemic action of nateglinide may be potentiated by non-selective beta-adrenergic-blocking agents). Products include:
Blocadren Tablets 1916
Cosopt Sterile Ophthalmic Solution 1931
Timolide Tablets 2086
Timoptic Sterile Ophthalmic Solution 2088
Timoptic in Ocudose 2091
Timoptic-XE Sterile Ophthalmic Gel Forming Solution 2092

Tolmetin Sodium (The hypoglycemic action of nateglinide may be potentiated by non-steroidal anti-inflammatory agents).
No products indexed under this heading.

Tranylcypromine Sulfate (The hypoglycemic action of nateglinide may be potentiated by MAO inhibitors). Products include:
Parnate Tablets 1527

Triamcinolone (Co-administration with certain drugs, such as corticosteroids, may reduce the hypoglycemic action of nateglinide and other oral antidiabetic drugs; when these drugs are administered to or withdrawn from patients receiving nateglinide, the patient should be observed closely for changes in glycemic control).
No products indexed under this heading.

Triamcinolone Acetonide (Co-administration with certain drugs, such as corticosteroids, may reduce the hypoglycemic action of nateglinide and other oral antidiabetic drugs; when these drugs are administered to or withdrawn from patients receiving nateglinide, the patient should be observed closely for changes in glycemic control). Products include:
Azmacort Inhalation Aerosol 1726
Nasacort AQ Nasal Spray 2922

Triamcinolone Diacetate (Co-administration with certain drugs, such as corticosteroids, may reduce the hypoglycemic action of nateglinide and other oral antidiabetic drugs; when these drugs are administered to or withdrawn from patients receiving nateglinide, the patient should be observed closely for changes in glycemic control).
No products indexed under this heading.

Triamcinolone Hexacetonide (Co-administration with certain drugs, such as corticosteroids, may reduce the hypoglycemic action of nateglinide and other oral antidiabetic drugs; when these drugs are administered to or withdrawn from patients receiving nateglinide, the patient should be observed closely for changes in glycemic control).
No products indexed under this heading.

Valdecoxib (The hypoglycemic action of nateglinide may be potentiated by non-steroidal anti-inflammatory agents).
No products indexed under this heading.

Food Interactions

Food, unspecified (Administration of nateglinide with liquid meal significantly reduces peak plasma levels).

STEPHAN CLARITY CAPSULES

(Amino Acid Preparations, Ginkgo biloba, Herbals with Vitamins) .... ▣819
None cited in PDR database.

STEPHAN ELASTICITY CAPSULES

(Amino Acid Preparations, Herbals with Vitamins & Minerals) .... ▣819
None cited in PDR database.

STEPHAN ELIXIR CAPSULES

(Amino Acid Preparations, Ginkgo biloba, Herbals with Vitamins & Minerals) .... ▣814
None cited in PDR database.

STEPHAN ESSENTIAL CAPSULES

(Amino Acid Preparations, Herbals with Vitamins & Minerals, Vitamins with Minerals) .... ▣820
None cited in PDR database.

STEPHAN FEMININE CAPSULES

(Amino Acid Preparations, Vitamins with Minerals) .... ▣833
None cited in PDR database.

STEPHAN FLEXIBILITY CAPSULES

(Amino Acid Preparations, Vitamins with Minerals) .... ▣820
None cited in PDR database.

STEPHAN LOVPIL CAPSULES

(Amino Acid Preparations, Herbals with Vitamins & Minerals) .... ▣820
None cited in PDR database.

STEPHAN MASCULINE CAPSULES

(Amino Acid Preparations, Herbals with Minerals) .... ▣821
None cited in PDR database.

STEPHAN PROTECTOR CAPSULES

(Amino Acid Preparations, Astragalus, Herbals, Multiple) .... ▣821
None cited in PDR database.

STEPHAN RELIEF CAPSULES

(Amino Acid Preparations, Herbals with Vitamins, Psyllium Preparations) .... ▣821
None cited in PDR database.

STEPHAN TRANQUILITY CAPSULES

(Amino Acid Preparations, Herbals with Vitamins & Minerals, Valeriana officinalis) .... ▣821
None cited in PDR database.

STRATTERA CAPSULES

(Atomoxetine Hydrochloride) 1814
May interact with beta-adrenergic stimulating agents, cytochrome p450 2d6 inhibitors (selected), monoamine oxidase inhibitors, vasopressors, and certain other agents. Compounds in these categories include:

Albuterol (Atomoxene HCl should be administered with caution to patients being treated with systematically-administered (oral or intravenous) albuterol (or other beta-2 agonists) because the action of albuterol on the cardiovascular system can be potentiated resulting in increases in heart rate and blood pressure). Products include:
Proventil Inhalation Aerosol 3053

Albuterol Sulfate (Atomoxene HCl should be administered with caution to patients being treated with systematically-administered (oral or intravenous) albuterol (or other beta-2 agonists) because the action of albuterol on the cardiovascular system can be potentiated resulting in increases in heart rate and blood pressure). Products include:
AccuNeb Inhalation Solution 1055
Combivent Inhalation Aerosol 847
DuoNeb Inhalation Solution 1058
ProAir HFA Inhalation Aerosol 3300
Proventil Inhalation Solution 0.083% 3055
Proventil HFA Inhalation Aerosol 3056
Ventolin HFA Inhalation Aerosol 1600
VoSpire ER Tablets 1052

Amiodarone Hydrochloride (CYP2D6 inhibitors increase atomexetine plasma levels; dosage adjustment of atomexetine when co-administered with CYP2D6 inhibitors may be necessary).
No products indexed under this heading.

Amitriptyline Hydrochloride (CYP2D6 inhibitors increase atomexetine plasma levels; dosage adjustment of atomexetine when co-administered with CYP2D6 inhibitors may be necessary).
No products indexed under this heading.

Amoxapine (CYP2D6 inhibitors increase atomexetine plasma levels; dosage adjustment of atomexetine when co-administered with CYP2D6 inhibitors may be necessary).
No products indexed under this heading.

Bitolterol Mesylate (Atomoxene HCl should be administered with caution to patients being treated with systematically-administered (oral or intravenous) albuterol (or other beta-2 agonists) because the action of albuterol on the cardiovascular system can be potentiated resulting in increases in heart rate and blood pressure).
No products indexed under this heading.

Bupropion Hydrochloride (CYP2D6 inhibitors increase atomexetine plasma levels; dosage adjustment of atomexetine when co-administered with CYP2D6 inhibitors may be necessary). Products include:
Wellbutrin Tablets **1603**
Wellbutrin SR Sustained-Release Tablets **1607**
Wellbutrin XL Extended-Release Tablets **1613**
Zyban Sustained-Release Tablets **1644**

Celecoxib (CYP2D6 inhibitors increase atomexetine plasma levels; dosage adjustment of atomexetine when co-administered with CYP2D6 inhibitors may be necessary). Products include:
Celebrex Capsules **3134**

Chloroquine Hydrochloride (CYP2D6 inhibitors increase atomexetine plasma levels; dosage adjustment of atomexetine when co-administered with CYP2D6 inhibitors may be necessary).
No products indexed under this heading.

Chloroquine Phosphate (CYP2D6 inhibitors increase atomexetine plasma levels; dosage adjustment of atomexetine when co-administered with CYP2D6 inhibitors may be necessary).
No products indexed under this heading.

Chlorpheniramine (CYP2D6 inhibitors increase atomexetine plasma levels; dosage adjustment of atomexetine when co-administered with CYP2D6 inhibitors may be necessary).
No products indexed under this heading.

Chlorpheniramine Maleate (CYP2D6 inhibitors increase atomexetine plasma levels; dosage adjustment of atomexetine when co-administered with CYP2D6 inhibitors may be necessary). Products include:
Advil Allergy Sinus Caplets **770**
Advil Multi-Symptom Cold Caplets **770**
BC Allergy Sinus Cold Powder **677**
Comtrex Maximum Strength Cold & Cough Day/Night Caplets - Night Formulation **726**
Comtrex Maximum Strength Day/Night Severe Cold & Sinus Caplets - Night Formulation **725**
Contac Cold and Flu Maximum Strength Caplets **728**
Contac Cold and Flu Day and Night Caplets (Night Formulation Only) **727**
Children's Dimetapp Long Acting Cough Plus Cold Syrup **731**
Robitussin Cough & Cold Long-Acting Liquid **735**
Robitussin Cough & Allergy Syrup .. **736**
Robitussin Cough & Cold Nighttime Liquid **736**
Robitussin Cough, Cold & Flu Nighttime Liquid **738**
Robitussin Pediatric Cough & Cold Long-Acting Liquid **735**
Robitussin Pediatric Cough & Cold Nighttime Liquid **736**
Triaminic Cold & Allergy Liquid **746**
Triaminic Cough & Runny Nose Softchews **748**
Children's Tylenol Plus Flu Oral Suspension **749**
Tylenol Allergy Multi-Symptom Caplets with Cool Burst and Gelcaps **1872**
Children's Tylenol Plus Cold Suspension Liquid **1879**
Children's Tylenol Plus Cough & Runny Nose Suspension Liquid **1879**
Children's Tylenol Plus Flu Suspension Liquid **1881**
Children's Tylenol Plus Multi-Symptom Cold Suspension Liquid **1879**
Tylenol Cold Head Congestion Nighttime Caplets with Cool Burst **1873**
Tylenol Cold Multi-Symptom Nighttime Caplets with Cool Burst **1874**
Tylenol Sinus Congestion & Pain Nighttime Caplets with Cool Burst **1876**
Vicks 44M Cough, Cold & Flu Relief Liquid **2680**
Pediatric Vicks 44m Cough & Cold Relief Liquid **2676**
Children's Vicks NyQuil Cold/Cough Relief **756**
Children's Vicks NyQuil Cold/Cough Relief Liquid **2680**
Zicam Maximum Strength Flu Daytime **768**

Chlorpheniramine Polistirex (CYP2D6 inhibitors increase atomexetine plasma levels; dosage adjustment of atomexetine when co-administered with CYP2D6 inhibitors may be necessary). Products include:
Tussionex Pennkinetic Extended-Release Suspension **3327**

Chlorpheniramine Tannate (CYP2D6 inhibitors increase atomexetine plasma levels; dosage adjustment of atomexetine when co-administered with CYP2D6 inhibitors may be necessary).
No products indexed under this heading.

Cimetidine (CYP2D6 inhibitors increase atomexetine plasma levels; dosage adjustment of atomexetine when co-administered with CYP2D6 inhibitors may be necessary). Products include:
Tagamet HB 200 Tablets **664**

Cimetidine Hydrochloride (CYP2D6 inhibitors increase atomexetine plasma levels; dosage adjustment of atomexetine when co-administered with CYP2D6 inhibitors may be necessary).
No products indexed under this heading.

Citalopram Hydrobromide (CYP2D6 inhibitors increase atomexetine plasma levels; dosage adjustment of atomexetine when co-administered with CYP2D6 inhibitors may be necessary). Products include:
Celexa **1176**

Clomipramine Hydrochloride (CYP2D6 inhibitors increase atomexetine plasma levels; dosage adjustment of atomexetine when co-administered with CYP2D6 inhibitors may be necessary).
No products indexed under this heading.

Cocaine Hydrochloride (CYP2D6 inhibitors increase atomexetine plasma levels; dosage adjustment of atomexetine when co-administered with CYP2D6 inhibitors may be necessary).
No products indexed under this heading.

Desipramine Hydrochloride (CYP2D6 inhibitors increase atomexetine plasma levels; dosage adjustment of atomexetine when co-administered with CYP2D6 inhibitors may be necessary).
No products indexed under this heading.

Diphenhydramine (CYP2D6 inhibitors increase atomexetine plasma levels; dosage adjustment of atomexetine when co-administered with CYP2D6 inhibitors may be necessary). Products include:
Tylenol Sore Throat Nighttime Liquid with Cool Burst **1877**

Diphenhydramine Hydrochloride (CYP2D6 inhibitors increase atomexetine plasma levels; dosage adjustment of atomexetine when co-administered with CYP2D6 inhibitors may be necessary). Products include:
Nytol QuickCaps Caplets **615**
Nytol QuickGels Softgels Maximum Strength **616**
Simply Sleep Caplets **1868**
Sominex Original Formula Tablets .. **616**
TheraFlu Warming Relief Nighttime Severe Cold **743**
TheraFlu Thin Strips Multi Symptom **744**
Triaminic Nighttime Cold & Cough Liquid **746**
Triaminic Thin Strips Cough & Runny Nose **749**
Extra Strength Tylenol PM Caplets, Vanilla Caplets, Geltabs, Gelcaps and Liquid **1875**
Tylenol Sore Throat Nighttime Liquid with Cool Burst **790**
Tylenol Allergy Multi-Symptom Nighttime Caplets with Cool Burst **1872**
Tylenol Severe Allergy Caplets **1872**
Children's Tylenol Plus Cold & Allergy Suspension Liquid **1878**

Dobutamine (Atomoxene HCl should be administered with caution to patients being treated with systematically-administered (oral or intravenous) albuterol (or other beta-2 agonists) because the action of albuterol on the cardiovascular system can be potentiated resulting in increases in heart rate and blood pressure).
No products indexed under this heading.

Dobutamine Hydrochloride (Atomoxene HCl should be administered with caution to patients being treated with systematically-administered (oral or intravenous) albuterol (or other beta-2 agonists) because the action of albuterol on the cardiovascular system can be potentiated resulting in increases in heart rate and blood pressure).
No products indexed under this heading.

Dopamine Hydrochloride (Because of the possible effects of blood pressure, atomoxetine hydrochloride should be used cautiously with pressor agents).
No products indexed under this heading.

Doxepin Hydrochloride (CYP2D6 inhibitors increase atomexetine plasma levels; dosage adjustment of atomexetine when co-administered with CYP2D6 inhibitors may be necessary).
No products indexed under this heading.

Ephedrine Hydrochloride (Atomoxene HCl should be administered with caution to patients being treated with systematically-administered (oral or intravenous) albuterol (or other beta-2 agonists) because the action of albuterol on the cardiovascular system can be potentiated resulting in increases in heart rate and blood pressure).
No products indexed under this heading.

Ephedrine Sulfate (Atomoxene HCl should be administered with caution to patients being treated with systematically-administered (oral or intravenous) albuterol (or other beta-2 agonists) because the action of albuterol on the cardiovascular system can be potentiated resulting in increases in heart rate and blood pressure).
No products indexed under this heading.

Ephedrine Tannate (Atomoxene HCl should be administered with caution to patients being treated with systematically-administered (oral or intravenous) albuterol (or other beta-2 agonists) because the action of albuterol on the cardiovascular system can be potentiated resulting in increases in heart rate and blood pressure).
No products indexed under this heading.

Epinephrine (Atomoxene HCl should be administered with caution to patients being treated with systematically-administered (oral or intravenous) albuterol (or other beta-2 agonists) because the action of albuterol on the cardiovascular system can be potentiated resulting in increases in heart rate and blood pressure). Products include:
EpiPen **1061**
Primatene Mist **719**
Twinject 0.15 .... **3379**
Twinject 0.3 .... **3378**

Epinephrine Bitartrate (Because of the possible effects of blood pressure, atomoxetine hydrochloride should be used cautiously with pressor agents).
No products indexed under this heading.

IMPORTANT NOTE: Always consult each drug listing in the patient's regimen for possible interactions.

Epinephrine Hydrochloride (Atomoxene HCl should be administered with caution to patients being treated with systematically-administered (oral or intravenous) albuterol (or other beta-2 agonists) because the action of albuterol on the cardiovascular system can be potentiated resulting in increases in heart rate and blood pressure).
No products indexed under this heading.

Escitalopram Oxalate (CYP2D6 inhibitors increase atomexetine plasma levels; dosage adjustment of atomexetine when co-administered with CYP2D6 inhibitors may be necessary). Products include:
Lexapro Oral Solution 1190
Lexapro Tablets 1190

Fluoxetine (CYP2D6 inhibitors increase atomexetine plasma levels; dosage adjustment of atomexetine when co-administered with CYP2D6 inhibitors may be necessary).
No products indexed under this heading.

Fluoxetine Hydrochloride (CYP2D6 inhibitors increase atomexetine plasma levels; dosage adjustment of atomoxetine when co-administered with CYP2D6 inhibitors may be necessary). Products include:
Prozac Pulvules and Liquid 1801
Symbyax Capsules 1819

Fluphenazine Decanoate (CYP2D6 inhibitors increase atomexetine plasma levels; dosage adjustment of atomexetine when co-administered with CYP2D6 inhibitors may be necessary).
No products indexed under this heading.

Fluphenazine Enanthate (CYP2D6 inhibitors increase atomexetine plasma levels; dosage adjustment of atomexetine when co-administered with CYP2D6 inhibitors may be necessary).
No products indexed under this heading.

Fluphenazine Hydrochloride (CYP2D6 inhibitors increase atomexetine plasma levels; dosage adjustment of atomexetine when co-administered with CYP2D6 inhibitors may be necessary).
No products indexed under this heading.

Fluvoxamine Maleate (CYP2D6 inhibitors increase atomexetine plasma levels; dosage adjustment of atomexetine when co-administered with CYP2D6 inhibitors may be necessary).
No products indexed under this heading.

Halofantrine Hydrochloride (CYP2D6 inhibitors increase atomexetine plasma levels; dosage adjustment of atomexetine when co-administered with CYP2D6 inhibitors may be necessary).
No products indexed under this heading.

Haloperidol (CYP2D6 inhibitors increase atomexetine plasma levels; dosage adjustment of atomexetine when co-administered with CYP2D6 inhibitors may be necessary).
No products indexed under this heading.

Haloperidol Decanoate (CYP2D6 inhibitors increase atomexetine plasma levels; dosage adjustment of atomexetine when co-administered with CYP2D6 inhibitors may be necessary).
No products indexed under this heading.

Hydroxychloroquine Sulfate (CYP2D6 inhibitors increase atomexetine plasma levels; dosage adjustment of atomexetine when co-administered with CYP2D6 inhibitors may be necessary).
No products indexed under this heading.

Imatinib Mesylate (CYP2D6 inhibitors increase atomexetine plasma levels; dosage adjustment of atomexetine when co-administered with CYP2D6 inhibitors may be necessary). Products include:
Gleevec Tablets 2227

Imipramine Hydrochloride (CYP2D6 inhibitors increase atomexetine plasma levels; dosage adjustment of atomexetine when co-administered with CYP2D6 inhibitors may be necessary).
No products indexed under this heading.

Imipramine Pamoate (CYP2D6 inhibitors increase atomexetine plasma levels; dosage adjustment of atomexetine when co-administered with CYP2D6 inhibitors may be necessary).
No products indexed under this heading.

Isocarboxazid (Concurrent use with MAOIs is contraindicated. Atomexetine should not be taken with MAOIs or within two weeks after discontinuing MAOI. Treatment with an MAOI should not be initiated within two weeks after discontinuing atomexetine).
No products indexed under this heading.

Isoetharine (Atomoxene HCl should be administered with caution to patients being treated with systematically-administered (oral or intravenous) albuterol (or other beta-2 agonists) because the action of albuterol on the cardiovascular system can be potentiated resulting in increases in heart rate and blood pressure).
No products indexed under this heading.

Isoproterenol Hydrochloride (Atomoxene HCl should be administered with caution to patients being treated with systematically-administered (oral or intravenous) albuterol (or other beta-2 agonists) because the action of albuterol on the cardiovascular system can be potentiated resulting in increases in heart rate and blood pressure).
No products indexed under this heading.

Isoproterenol Sulfate (Atomoxene HCl should be administered with caution to patients being treated with systematically-administered (oral or intravenous) albuterol (or other beta-2 agonists) because the action of albuterol on the cardiovascular system can be potentiated resulting in increases in heart rate and blood pressure).
No products indexed under this heading.

Levalbuterol Hydrochloride (Atomoxene HCl should be administered

with caution to patients being treated with systematically-administered (oral or intravenous) albuterol (or other beta-2 agonists) because the action of albuterol on the cardiovascular system can be potentiated resulting in increases in heart rate and blood pressure). Products include:
Xopenex Inhalation Solution 3146
Xopenex Inhalation Solution
Concentrate................................ 3150

Maprotiline Hydrochloride (CYP2D6 inhibitors increase atomexetine plasma levels; dosage adjustment of atomexetine when co-administered with CYP2D6 inhibitors may be necessary).
No products indexed under this heading.

Mephentermine Sulfate (Because of the possible effects of blood pressure, atomoxetine hydrochloride should be used cautiously with pressor agents).
No products indexed under this heading.

Metaproterenol Sulfate (Atomoxene HCl should be administered with caution to patients being treated with systematically-administered (oral or intravenous) albuterol (or other beta-2 agonists) because the action of albuterol on the cardiovascular system can be potentiated resulting in increases in heart rate and blood pressure). Products include:
Alupent Inhalation Aerosol 826

Metaraminol Bitartrate (Because of the possible effects of blood pressure, atomoxetine hydrochloride should be used cautiously with pressor agents).
No products indexed under this heading.

Methadone Hydrochloride (CYP2D6 inhibitors increase atomexetine plasma levels; dosage adjustment of atomexetine when co-administered with CYP2D6 inhibitors may be necessary).
No products indexed under this heading.

Methoxamine Hydrochloride (Because of the possible effects of blood pressure, atomoxetine hydrochloride should be used cautiously with pressor agents).
No products indexed under this heading.

Mibefradil Dihydrochloride (CYP2D6 inhibitors increase atomexetine plasma levels; dosage adjustment of atomexetine when co-administered with CYP2D6 inhibitors may be necessary).
No products indexed under this heading.

Midazolam Hydrochloride (Co-administration of atomexetine with midazolam, resulted in a 15% increase in AUC of midazolam).
No products indexed under this heading.

Moclobemide (Concurrent use with MAOIs is contraindicated. Atomexetine should not be taken with MAOIs or within two weeks after discontinuing MAOI. Treatment with an MAOI should not be initiated within two weeks after discontinuing atomexetine).
No products indexed under this heading.

Norepinephrine Bitartrate (Because of the possible effects of blood pressure, atomoxetine hydrochloride should be used cautiously with pressor agents).
No products indexed under this heading.

Nortriptyline Hydrochloride (CYP2D6 inhibitors increase atomexetine plasma levels; dosage adjustment of atomexetine when co-administered with CYP2D6 inhibitors may be necessary).
No products indexed under this heading.

Pargyline Hydrochloride (Concurrent use with MAOIs is contraindicated. Atomexetine should not be taken with MAOIs or within two weeks after discontinuing MAOI. Treatment with an MAOI should not be initiated within two weeks after discontinuing atomexetine).
No products indexed under this heading.

Paroxetine Hydrochloride (CYP2D6 inhibitors increase atomexetine plasma levels; dosage adjustment of atomexetine when co-administered with CYP2D6 inhibitors may be necessary). Products include:
Paxil CR Controlled-Release
Tablets... 1538
Paxil .. 1530

Perphenazine (CYP2D6 inhibitors increase atomexetine plasma levels; dosage adjustment of atomexetine when co-administered with CYP2D6 inhibitors may be necessary).
No products indexed under this heading.

Phenelzine Sulfate (Concurrent use with MAOIs is contraindicated. Atomexetine should not be taken with MAOIs or within two weeks after discontinuing MAOI. Treatment with an MAOI should not be initiated within two weeks after discontinuing atomexetine).
No products indexed under this heading.

Phenylephrine Hydrochloride (Because of the possible effects of blood pressure, atomoxetine hydrochloride should be used cautiously with pressor agents). Products include:
Comtrex Maximum Strength
Non-Drowsy Cold & Cough
Caplets.................................... ▣725
Comtrex Maximum Strength
Day/Night Severe Cold & Sinus
Caplets - Day Formulation ▣725
Comtrex Maximum Strength
Day/Night Severe Cold & Sinus
Caplets - Night Formulation......... ▣725
Contac Cold and Flu Maximum
Strength Caplets...................... ▣728
Contac Cold and Flu Day and
Night Caplets (Day Formulation
Only)....................................... ▣727
Contac Cold and Flu Day and
Night Caplets (Night
Formulation Only).................... ▣727
Contac Cold and Flu Non-Drowsy
Caplets.................................... ▣728
Contac-D Cold Non-Drowsy
Tablets.................................... ▣729
Children's Dimetapp Cold &
Allergy Elixir ▣730
Children's Dimetapp Cold &
Allergy Chewable Tablets............ ▣730
Children's Dimetapp DM Cold &
Cough Elixir ▣731
Toddler's Dimetapp Cold and
Cough Drops ▣732
Excedrin Sinus Headache
Caplets/Tablets......................... ▣610
4-Way Fast Acting Nasal Spray ▣775

4-Way Menthol Nasal Spray 775
Preparation H Maximum Strength Cream 666
Preparation H Cooling Gel 666
Preparation H 666
Refenesen PE Caplets 721
Robitussin Cough & Allergy Syrup .. 736
Robitussin Cough & Cold Nighttime Liquid 736
Robitussin Cough, Cold & Flu Nighttime Liquid 738
Robitussin Head & Chest Congestion PE Syrup 739
Robitussin Pediatric Cough & Cold Nighttime Liquid 736
TheraFlu Cold & Cough Hot Liquid 740
TheraFlu Cold & Sore Throat Hot Liquid 741
TheraFlu Flu & Sore Throat Hot Liquid 742
TheraFlu Daytime Severe Cold Hot Liquid 742
TheraFlu Nighttime Severe Cold Hot Liquid 740
TheraFlu Warming Relief Daytime Severe Cold 743
TheraFlu Warming Relief Nighttime Severe Cold 743
Triaminic Chest & Nasal Congestion Liquid 746
Triaminic Cold & Allergy Liquid 746
Triaminic Daytime Cold & Cough Liquid 745
Triaminic Nighttime Cold & Cough Liquid 746
Triaminic Thin Strips Cold 748
Triaminic Thin Strips Cold & Cough 778
Triaminic Infant Thin Strips Decongestant 747
Triaminic Infant Thin Strips Decongestant Plus Cough 747
Children's Tylenol Plus Flu Oral Suspension 749
Tylenol Cold Head Congestion Daytime Caplets with Cool Burst and Gelcaps 750
Tylenol Cold Multi-Symptom Daytime Liquid 752
Tylenol Cold Multi-Symptom Severe Daytime Liquid 752
Concentrated Tylenol Infants' Drops Plus Cold & Cough 754
Tylenol Allergy Multi-Symptom Caplets with Cool Burst and Gelcaps 1872
Tylenol Allergy Multi-Symptom Nighttime Caplets with Cool Burst 1872
Children's Tylenol Plus Cold Suspension Liquid 1879
Children's Tylenol Plus Cold & Allergy Suspension Liquid 1878
Children's Tylenol Plus Flu Suspension Liquid 1881
Children's Tylenol Plus Multi-Symptom Cold Suspension Liquid 1879
Tylenol Cold Head Congestion Daytime Caplets with Cool Burst 1873
Tylenol Cold Head Congestion Nighttime Caplets with Cool Burst 1873
Tylenol Cold Head Congestion Severe Caplets with Cool Burst..... 1873
Tylenol Cold Multi-Symptom Daytime Caplets with Cool Burst and Gelcaps 1874
Tylenol Cold Multi-Symptom Daytime Liquid with Citrus Burst... 1874
Tylenol Cold Multi-Symptom Nighttime Caplets with Cool Burst 1874
Tylenol Cold Multi-Symptom Nighttime Liquid with Cool Burst... 1874
Tylenol Cold Multi-Symptom Severe Caplets with Cool Burst..... 1874
Tylenol Cold Multi-Symptom Severe Daytime Liquid with Citrus Burst 1874
Tylenol Sinus Congestion & Pain Daytime Caplets with Cool Burst and Gelcaps 1876
Tylenol Sinus Congestion & Pain Nighttime Caplets with Cool Burst 1876
Tylenol Sinus Congestion & Pain Severe Caplets with Cool Burst..... 1876
Vicks 44D Cough & Head Congestion Relief Liquid............. 760
Vicks DayQuil LiquiCaps/Liquid Multi-Symptom Cold/Flu Relief..... 761
Zicam Cough Plus D Cough Spray... 767

Pirbuterol Acetate (Atomoxene HCl should be administered with caution to patients being treated with systematically-administered (oral or intravenous) albuterol (or other beta-2 agonists) because the action of albuterol on the cardiovascular system can be potentiated resulting in increases in heart rate and blood pressure). Products include:
Maxair Autohaler 1852

Procarbazine Hydrochloride (Concurrent use with MAOIs is contraindicated. Atomexetine should not be taken with MAOIs or within two weeks after discontinuing MAOI. Treatment with an MAOI should not be initiated within two weeks after discontinuing atomexetine). Products include:
Matulane Capsules 3191

Propafenone Hydrochloride (CYP2D6 inhibitors increase atomexetine plasma levels; dosage adjustment of atomexetine when co-administered with CYP2D6 inhibitors may be necessary). Products include:
Rythmol SR Capsules 2727

Propoxyphene Hydrochloride (CYP2D6 inhibitors increase atomexetine plasma levels; dosage adjustment of atomexetine when co-administered with CYP2D6 inhibitors may be necessary).
No products indexed under this heading.

Propoxyphene Napsylate (CYP2D6 inhibitors increase atomexetine plasma levels; dosage adjustment of atomexetine when co-administered with CYP2D6 inhibitors may be necessary).
No products indexed under this heading.

Protriptyline Hydrochloride (CYP2D6 inhibitors increase atomexetine plasma levels; dosage adjustment of atomexetine when co-administered with CYP2D6 inhibitors may be necessary).
No products indexed under this heading.

Quinacrine Hydrochloride (CYP2D6 inhibitors increase atomexetine plasma levels; dosage adjustment of atomexetine when co-administered with CYP2D6 inhibitors may be necessary).
No products indexed under this heading.

Quinidine (CYP2D6 inhibitors increase atomexetine plasma levels; dosage adjustment of atomexetine when co-administered with CYP2D6 inhibitors may be necessary).
No products indexed under this heading.

Quinidine Gluconate (CYP2D6 inhibitors increase atomexetine plasma levels; dosage adjustment of atomexetine when co-administered with CYP2D6 inhibitors may be necessary).
No products indexed under this heading.

Quinidine Hydrochloride (CYP2D6 inhibitors increase atomexetine plasma levels; dosage adjustment of atomexetine when co-administered with CYP2D6 inhibitors may be necessary).
No products indexed under this heading.

Quinidine Polygalacturonate (CYP2D6 inhibitors increase atomexetine plasma levels; dosage adjustment of atomexetine when co-administered with CYP2D6 inhibitors may be necessary).
No products indexed under this heading.

Quinidine Sulfate (CYP2D6 inhibitors increase atomexetine plasma levels; dosage adjustment of atomexetine when co-administered with CYP2D6 inhibitors may be necessary).
No products indexed under this heading.

Ranitidine Bismuth Citrate (CYP2D6 inhibitors increase atomexetine plasma levels; dosage adjustment of atomexetine when co-administered with CYP2D6 inhibitors may be necessary).
No products indexed under this heading.

Ranitidine Hydrochloride (CYP2D6 inhibitors increase atomexetine plasma levels; dosage adjustment of atomexetine when co-administered with CYP2D6 inhibitors may be necessary). Products include:
Zantac 1624
Zantac Injection 1619
Zantac Injection Pharmacy Bulk Package 1622

Ritonavir (CYP2D6 inhibitors increase atomexetine plasma levels; dosage adjustment of atomexetine when co-administered with CYP2D6 inhibitors may be necessary). Products include:
Kaletra 476
Norvir 503

Salmeterol Xinafoate (Atomoxene HCl should be administered with caution to patients being treated with systematically-administered (oral or intravenous) albuterol (or other beta-2 agonists) because the action of albuterol on the cardiovascular system can be potentiated resulting in increases in heart rate and blood pressure). Products include:
Advair Diskus 100/50 1308
Advair Diskus 250/50 1308
Advair Diskus 500/50 1308
Advair HFA Inhalation Aerosol 1318
Serevent Diskus 1568

Selegiline Hydrochloride (Concurrent use with MAOIs is contraindicated. Atomexetine should not be taken with MAOIs or within two weeks after discontinuing MAOI. Treatment with an MAOI should not be initiated within two weeks after discontinuing atomexetine). Products include:
Eldepryl Capsules 3208
Zelapar Tablets 3372

Sertraline Hydrochloride (CYP2D6 inhibitors increase atomexetine plasma levels; dosage adjustment of atomexetine when co-administered with CYP2D6 inhibitors may be necessary). Products include:
Zoloft 2586

Terbinafine Hydrochloride (CYP2D6 inhibitors increase atomexetine plasma levels; dosage adjustment of atomexetine when co-administered with CYP2D6 inhibitors may be necessary). Products include:
Lamisil Tablets 2232
Lamisil AT Creams (Athlete's Foot & Jock Itch)................................ 636

Terbutaline Sulfate (Atomoxene HCl should be administered with caution to patients being treated with systematically-administered (oral or intravenous) albuterol (or other beta-2 agonists) because the action of albuterol on the cardiovascular system can be potentiated resulting in increases in heart rate and blood pressure).
No products indexed under this heading.

Thioridazine Hydrochloride (CYP2D6 inhibitors increase atomexetine plasma levels; dosage adjustment of atomexetine when co-administered with CYP2D6 inhibitors may be necessary). Products include:
Thioridazine Hydrochloride Tablets 2163

Tranylcypromine Sulfate (Concurrent use with MAOIs is contraindicated. Atomexetine should not be taken with MAOIs or within two weeks after discontinuing MAOI. Treatment with an MAOI should not be initiated within two weeks after discontinuing atomexetine). Products include:
Parnate Tablets 1527

Trimipramine Maleate (CYP2D6 inhibitors increase atomexetine plasma levels; dosage adjustment of atomexetine when co-administered with CYP2D6 inhibitors may be necessary).
No products indexed under this heading.

STRIANT MUCOADHESIVE

(Testosterone) 1007
May interact with corticosteroids, insulin, and certain other agents. Compounds in these categories include:

ACTH (Concurrent administration of testosterone with ACTH or corticosteroids may enhance edema formation and should be administered cautiously, particularly in patients with cardiac or hepatic disease).
No products indexed under this heading.

Betamethasone Acetate (Concurrent administration of testosterone with ACTH or corticosteroids may enhance edema formation and should be administered cautiously, particularly in patients with cardiac or hepatic disease).
No products indexed under this heading.

Betamethasone Sodium Phosphate (Concurrent administration of testosterone with ACTH or corticosteroids may enhance edema formation and should be administered cautiously, particularly in patients with cardiac or hepatic disease).
No products indexed under this heading.

Cortisone Acetate (Concurrent administration of testosterone with ACTH or corticosteroids may enhance edema formation and should be administered cautiously, particularly in patients with cardiac or hepatic disease).
No products indexed under this heading.

Dexamethasone (Concurrent administration of testosterone with ACTH or corticosteroids may enhance edema formation and should be administered cautiously, particularly in patients with cardiac or hepatic disease). Products include:
Ciprodex Otic Suspension 559
Decadron Tablets 1951
TobraDex Ophthalmic Ointment 562
TobraDex Ophthalmic Suspension ... 563

Dexamethasone Acetate (Concurrent administration of testosterone with ACTH or corticosteroids may enhance edema formation and should be administered cautiously, particularly in patients with cardiac or hepatic disease).
No products indexed under this heading.

Dexamethasone Sodium Phosphate (Concurrent administration of testosterone with ACTH or corticosteroids may enhance edema formation and should be administered cautiously, particularly in patients with cardiac or hepatic disease).
No products indexed under this heading.

Fludrocortisone Acetate (Concurrent administration of testosterone with ACTH or corticosteroids may enhance edema formation and should be administered cautiously, particularly in patients with cardiac or hepatic disease).
No products indexed under this heading.

Hydrocortisone (Concurrent administration of testosterone with ACTH or corticosteroids may enhance edema formation and should be administered cautiously, particularly in patients with cardiac or hepatic disease). Products include:
Colocort Rectal Suspension, USP (Retention) 100 mg/60 mL........... 2476
Hydrocortone Tablets 1989
Preparation H Hydrocortisone Cream .... ▣646

Hydrocortisone Acetate (Concurrent administration of testosterone with ACTH or corticosteroids may enhance edema formation and should be administered cautiously, particularly in patients with cardiac or hepatic disease). Products include:
Analpram-HC 1159
Pramosone 1161
ProctoFoam-HC 3099

Hydrocortisone Sodium Phosphate (Concurrent administration of testosterone with ACTH or corticosteroids may enhance edema formation and should be administered cautiously, particularly in patients with cardiac or hepatic disease).
No products indexed under this heading.

Hydrocortisone Sodium Succinate (Concurrent administration of testosterone with ACTH or corticosteroids may enhance edema formation and should be administered cautiously, particularly in patients with cardiac or hepatic disease).
No products indexed under this heading.

Insulin, Human, Zinc Suspension (In diabetic patients, the metabolic effects of androgens may decrease blood glucose and, therefore, insulin requirements). Products include:
Humulin L, 100 Units 1794
Humulin U, 100 Units 1800

Insulin, Human NPH (In diabetic patients, the metabolic effects of androgens may decrease blood glucose and, therefore, insulin requirements). Products include:
Humulin N, 100 Units 1795
Humulin N Pen 1797

Insulin, Human Regular (In diabetic patients, the metabolic effects of androgens may decrease blood glucose and, therefore, insulin requirements). Products include:
Humulin R, 100 Units 1798

Insulin, Human Regular and Human NPH Mixture (In diabetic patients, the metabolic effects of androgens may decrease blood glucose and, therefore, insulin requirements). Products include:
Humulin 50/50, 100 Units 1791
Humulin 70/30 Pen 1793

Insulin, NPH (In diabetic patients, the metabolic effects of androgens may decrease blood glucose and, therefore, insulin requirements).
No products indexed under this heading.

Insulin, Regular (In diabetic patients, the metabolic effects of androgens may decrease blood glucose and, therefore, insulin requirements).
No products indexed under this heading.

Insulin, Zinc Crystals (In diabetic patients, the metabolic effects of androgens may decrease blood glucose and, therefore, insulin requirements).
No products indexed under this heading.

Insulin, Zinc Suspension (In diabetic patients, the metabolic effects of androgens may decrease blood glucose and, therefore, insulin requirements).
No products indexed under this heading.

Insulin Aspart, Human Regular (In diabetic patients, the metabolic effects of androgens may decrease blood glucose and, therefore, insulin requirements). Products include:
NovoLog Injection 2326

Insulin glargine (In diabetic patients, the metabolic effects of androgens may decrease blood glucose and, therefore, insulin requirements). Products include:
Lantus Injection 2909

Insulin Lispro, Human (In diabetic patients, the metabolic effects of androgens may decrease blood glucose and, therefore, insulin requirements). Products include:
Humalog-Pen 1781
Humalog Mix 50/50-Pen 1783
Humalog Mix 75/25-Pen 1785

Insulin Lispro Protamine, Human (In diabetic patients, the metabolic effects of androgens may decrease blood glucose and, therefore, insulin requirements). Products include:
Humalog Mix 50/50-Pen 1783
Humalog Mix 75/25-Pen 1785

Methylprednisolone Acetate (Concurrent administration of testosterone with ACTH or corticosteroids may enhance edema formation and should be administered cautiously, particularly in patients with cardiac or hepatic disease). Products include:
Depo-Medrol Injectable Suspension 2617
Depo-Medrol Single-Dose Vial 2619

Methylprednisolone Sodium Succinate (Concurrent administration of testosterone with ACTH or corticosteroids may enhance edema formation and should be administered cautiously, particularly in patients with cardiac or hepatic disease).
No products indexed under this heading.

Oxyphenbutazone (Concurrent administration of oxyphenbutazone and androgens may result in elevated serum levels of oxyphenbutazone).
No products indexed under this heading.

Prednisolone Acetate (Concurrent administration of testosterone with ACTH or corticosteroids may enhance edema formation and should be administered cautiously, particularly in patients with cardiac or hepatic disease). Products include:
Blephamide Ophthalmic Ointment 568
Blephamide Ophthalmic Suspension 569
Poly-Pred Ophthalmic Suspension .... ⊙233
Pred Forte Ophthalmic Suspension .... ⊙235
Pred Mild Ophthalmic Suspension .... ⊙238
Pred-G Ophthalmic Ointment .... ⊙237
Pred-G Ophthalmic Suspension ...... ⊙236

Prednisolone Sodium Phosphate (Concurrent administration of testosterone with ACTH or corticosteroids may enhance edema formation and should be administered cautiously, particularly in patients with cardiac or hepatic disease).
No products indexed under this heading.

Prednisolone Tebutate (Concurrent administration of testosterone with ACTH or corticosteroids may enhance edema formation and should be administered cautiously, particularly in patients with cardiac or hepatic disease).
No products indexed under this heading.

Prednisone (Concurrent administration of testosterone with ACTH or corticosteroids may enhance edema formation and should be administered cautiously, particularly in patients with cardiac or hepatic disease).
No products indexed under this heading.

Triamcinolone (Concurrent administration of testosterone with ACTH or corticosteroids may enhance edema formation and should be administered cautiously, particularly in patients with cardiac or hepatic disease).
No products indexed under this heading.

Triamcinolone Acetonide (Concurrent administration of testosterone with ACTH or corticosteroids may enhance edema formation and should be administered cautiously, particularly in patients with cardiac or hepatic disease). Products include:
Azmacort Inhalation Aerosol 1726
Nasacort AQ Nasal Spray 2922

Triamcinolone Diacetate (Concurrent administration of testosterone with ACTH or corticosteroids may enhance edema formation and should be administered cautiously, particularly in patients with cardiac or hepatic disease).
No products indexed under this heading.

Triamcinolone Hexacetonide (Concurrent administration of testosterone with ACTH or corticosteroids may enhance edema formation and should be administered cautiously, particularly in patients with cardiac or hepatic disease).
No products indexed under this heading.

STROMECTOL TABLETS

(Ivermectin) 2083
None cited in PDR database.

SUBOXONE TABLETS

(Buprenorphine Hydrochloride, Naloxone Hydrochloride).................... 2717
May interact with cytochrome p450 3a4 inhibitors (selected). Compounds in these categories include:

Acetazolamide (Buprenorphine is metabolized to norbuprenorphine by cytochrome CYP3A4. Because CYP3A4 inhibitors may increase plasma concentrations of buprenorphine, patients already on CYP3A4 inhibitors should have their dose of Subutex or Suboxone adjusted.).
No products indexed under this heading.

Amiodarone Hydrochloride (Buprenorphine is metabolized to norbuprenorphine by cytochrome CYP3A4. Because CYP3A4 inhibitors may increase plasma concentrations of buprenorphine, patients already on CYP3A4 inhibitors should have their dose of Subutex or Suboxone adjusted.).
No products indexed under this heading.

Amprenavir (Buprenorphine is metabolized to norbuprenorphine by cytochrome CYP3A4. Because CYP3A4 inhibitors may increase plasma concentrations of buprenorphine, patients already on CYP3A4 inhibitors should have their dose of Subutex or Suboxone adjusted). Products include:
Agenerase Capsules 1327
Agenerase Oral Solution 1332

Anastrozole (Buprenorphine is metabolized to norbuprenorphine by cytochrome CYP3A4. Because CYP3A4 inhibitors may increase plasma concentrations of buprenorphine, patients already on CYP3A4 inhibitors should have their dose of Subutex or Suboxone adjusted). Products include:
Arimidex Tablets 673

Aprepitant (Buprenorphine is metabolized to norbuprenorphine by cytochrome CYP3A4. Because CYP3A4 inhibitors may increase plasma concentrations of buprenorphine, patients already on CYP3A4 inhibitors should have their dose of Subutex or Subuxone adjusted). Products include:

Emend Capsules 1963

Cimetidine (Buprenorphine is metabolized to norbuprenorphine by cytochrome CYP3A4. Because CYP3A4 inhibitors may increase plasma concentrations of buprenorphine, patients already on CYP3A4 inhibitors should have their dose of Subutex or Subuxone adjusted). Products include:

Tagamet HB 200 Tablets 664

Cimetidine Hydrochloride (Buprenorphine is metabolized to norbuprenorphine by cytochrome CYP3A4. Because CYP3A4 inhibitors may increase plasma concentrations of buprenorphine, patients already on CYP3A4 inhibitors should have their dose of Subutex or Subuxone adjusted.).

No products indexed under this heading.

Ciprofloxacin (Buprenorphine is metabolized to norbuprenorphine by cytochrome CYP3A4. Because CYP3A4 inhibitors may increase plasma concentrations of buprenorphine, patients already on CYP3A4 inhibitors should have their dose of Subutex or Subuxone adjusted). Products include:

Cipro Oral Suspension 2977
Cipro I.V. 2984
Cipro XR Tablets 2990
Ciprodex Otic Suspension 559

Clarithromycin (Buprenorphine is metabolized to norbuprenorphine by cytochrome CYP3A4. Because CYP3A4 inhibitors may increase plasma concentrations of buprenorphine, patients already on CYP3A4 inhibitors should have their dose of Subutex or Subuxone adjusted). Products include:

Biaxin/Biaxin XL 402
PREVPAC 3284

Clotrimazole (Buprenorphine is metabolized to norbuprenorphine by cytochrome CYP3A4. Because CYP3A4 inhibitors may increase plasma concentrations of buprenorphine, patients already on CYP3A4 inhibitors should have their dose of Subutex or Subuxone adjusted). Products include:

Desenex Athlete's Foot Cream 635
Lotrimin 3039
Lotrisone 3040

Cyclosporine (Buprenorphine is metabolized to norbuprenorphine by cytochrome CYP3A4. Because CYP3A4 inhibitors may increase plasma concentrations of buprenorphine, patients already on CYP3A4 inhibitors should have their dose of Subutex or Subuxone adjusted). Products include:

Gengraf Capsules 459
Neoral Oral Solution 2259
Neoral Soft Gelatin Capsules 2259
Restasis Ophthalmic Emulsion 575
Sandimmune 2275

Dalfopristin (Buprenorphine is metabolized to norbuprenorphine by cytochrome CYP3A4. Because CYP3A4 inhibitors may increase plasma concentrations of buprenorphine, patients already on CYP3A4 inhibitors should have their dose of Subutex or Subuxone adjusted.).

No products indexed under this heading.

Danazol (Buprenorphine is metabolized to norbuprenorphine by cytochrome CYP3A4. Because CYP3A4 inhibitors may increase plasma concentrations of buprenorphine, patients already on CYP3A4 inhibitors should have their dose of Subutex or Subuxone adjusted.).

No products indexed under this heading.

Delavirdine Mesylate (Buprenorphine is metabolized to norbuprenorphine by cytochrome CYP3A4. Because CYP3A4 inhibitors may increase plasma concentrations of buprenorphine, patients already on CYP3A4 inhibitors should have their dose of Subutex or Subuxone adjusted). Products include:

Rescriptor Tablets 2551

Diltiazem Hydrochloride (Buprenorphine is metabolized to norbuprenorphine by cytochrome CYP3A4. Because CYP3A4 inhibitors may increase plasma concentrations of buprenorphine, patients already on CYP3A4 inhibitors should have their dose of Subutex or Subuxone adjusted). Products include:

Cardizem LA Extended Release Tablets 1728
Tiazac Capsules 1201

Diltiazem Maleate (Buprenorphine is metabolized to norbuprenorphine by cytochrome CYP3A4. Because CYP3A4 inhibitors may increase plasma concentrations of buprenorphine, patients already on CYP3A4 inhibitors should have their dose of Subutex or Subuxone adjusted.).

No products indexed under this heading.

Efavirenz (Buprenorphine is metabolized to norbuprenorphine by cytochrome CYP3A4. Because CYP3A4 inhibitors may increase plasma concentrations of buprenorphine, patients already on CYP3A4 inhibitors should have their dose of Subutex or Subuxone adjusted). Products include:

Atripla Tablets 945
Sustiva Capsules 930
Sustiva Tablets 930

Erythromycin (Buprenorphine is metabolized to norbuprenorphine by cytochrome CYP3A4. Because CYP3A4 inhibitors may increase plasma concentrations of buprenorphine, patients already on CYP3A4 inhibitors should have their dose of Subutex or Subuxone adjusted). Products include:

Ery-Tab Tablets 449
Erythromycin Base Filmtab Tablets 455
Erythromycin Delayed-Release Capsules, USP 457
PCE Dispertab Tablets 515

Erythromycin Estolate (Buprenorphine is metabolized to norbuprenorphine by cytochrome CYP3A4. Because CYP3A4 inhibitors may increase plasma concentrations of buprenorphine, patients already on CYP3A4 inhibitors should have their dose of Subutex or Subuxone adjusted.).

No products indexed under this heading.

Erythromycin Ethylsuccinate (Buprenorphine is metabolized to norbuprenorphine by cytochrome CYP3A4. Because CYP3A4 inhibitors may increase plasma concentrations of buprenorphine, patients already on CYP3A4 inhibitors should have their dose of Subutex or Subuxone adjusted). Products include:

E.E.S. 451
EryPed 447

Erythromycin Gluceptate (Buprenorphine is metabolized to norbuprenorphine by cytochrome CYP3A4. Because CYP3A4 inhibitors may increase plasma concentrations of buprenorphine, patients already on CYP3A4 inhibitors should have their dose of Subutex or Subuxone adjusted.).

No products indexed under this heading.

Erythromycin Lactobionate (Buprenorphine is metabolized to norbuprenorphine by cytochrome CYP3A4. Because CYP3A4 inhibitors may increase plasma concentrations of buprenorphine, patients already on CYP3A4 inhibitors should have their dose of Subutex or Subuxone adjusted.).

No products indexed under this heading.

Erythromycin Stearate (Buprenorphine is metabolized to norbuprenorphine by cytochrome CYP3A4. Because CYP3A4 inhibitors may increase plasma concentrations of buprenorphine, patients already on CYP3A4 inhibitors should have their dose of Subutex or Subuxone adjusted). Products include:

Erythrocin Stearate Filmtab Tablets 453

Esomeprazole Magnesium (Buprenorphine is metabolized to norbuprenorphine by cytochrome CYP3A4. Because CYP3A4 inhibitors may increase plasma concentrations of buprenorphine, patients already on CYP3A4 inhibitors should have their dose of Subutex or Subuxone adjusted). Products include:

Nexium Delayed-Release Capsules 655

Fluconazole (Buprenorphine is metabolized to norbuprenorphine by cytochrome CYP3A4. Because CYP3A4 inhibitors may increase plasma concentrations of buprenorphine, patients already on CYP3A4 inhibitors should have their dose of Subutex or Subuxone adjusted.).

No products indexed under this heading.

Fluoxetine Hydrochloride (Buprenorphine is metabolized to norbuprenorphine by cytochrome CYP3A4. Because CYP3A4 inhibitors may increase plasma concentrations of buprenorphine, patients already on CYP3A4 inhibitors should have their dose of Subutex or Subuxone adjusted). Products include:

Prozac Pulvules and Liquid 1801
Symbyax Capsules 1819

Fluvoxamine Maleate (Buprenorphine is metabolized to norbuprenorphine by cytochrome CYP3A4. Because CYP3A4 inhibitors may increase plasma concentrations of buprenorphine, patients already on CYP3A4 inhibitors should have their dose of Subutex or Subuxone adjusted.).

No products indexed under this heading.

Fosamprenavir Calcium (Buprenorphine is metabolized to norbuprenorphine by cytochrome CYP3A4. Because CYP3A4 inhibitors may increase plasma concentrations of buprenorphine, patients already on CYP3A4 inhibitors should have their dose of Subutex or Subuxone adjusted). Products include:

Lexiva Tablets 1505

Indinavir Sulfate (Buprenorphine is metabolized to norbuprenorphine by cytochrome CYP3A4. Because CYP3A4 inhibitors may increase plasma concentrations of buprenorphine, patients already on CYP3A4 inhibitors should have their dose of Subutex or Subuxone adjusted). Products include:

Crixivan Capsules 1940

Isoniazid (Buprenorphine is metabolized to norbuprenorphine by cytochrome CYP3A4. Because CYP3A4 inhibitors may increase plasma concentrations of buprenorphine, patients already on CYP3A4 inhibitors should have their dose of Subutex or Subuxone adjusted.).

No products indexed under this heading.

Itraconazole (Buprenorphine is metabolized to norbuprenorphine by cytochrome CYP3A4. Because CYP3A4 inhibitors may increase plasma concentrations of buprenorphine, patients already on CYP3A4 inhibitors should have their dose of Subutex or Subuxone adjusted.).

No products indexed under this heading.

Ketoconazole (Buprenorphine is metabolized to norbuprenorphine by cytochrome CYP3A4. Because CYP3A4 inhibitors may increase plasma concentrations of buprenorphine, patients already on CYP3A4 inhibitors should have their dose of Subutex or Subuxone adjusted). Products include:

Nizoral A-D Shampoo, 1% 1868

Lopinavir (Buprenorphine is metabolized to norbuprenorphine by cytochrome CYP3A4. Because CYP3A4 inhibitors may increase plasma concentrations of buprenorphine, patients already on CYP3A4 inhibitors should have their dose of Subutex or Subuxone adjusted). Products include:

Kaletra 476

Loratadine (Buprenorphine is metabolized to norbuprenorphine by cytochrome CYP3A4. Because CYP3A4 inhibitors may increase plasma concentrations of buprenorphine, patients already on CYP3A4 inhibitors should have their dose of Subutex or Subuxone adjusted). Products include:

Alavert Allergy & Sinus D-12 Hour Tablets 771
Alavert 771
Children's Claritin Allergy Oral Solution 771
Claritin Non-Drowsy 24 Hour Tablets 772
Claritin Reditabs 24 Hour Non-Drowsy Tablets 772
Claritin-D Non-Drowsy 12 Hour Tablets 772
Claritin-D Non-Drowsy 24 Hour Tablets 772

Metronidazole (Buprenorphine is metabolized to norbuprenorphine by cytochrome CYP3A4. Because CYP3A4 inhibitors may increase plasma concentrations of buprenorphine, patients already on CYP3A4 inhibitors should have their dose of Subutex or Subuxone adjusted). Products include:

Metrogel 1% 1211
MetroGel-Vaginal Gel 1855
Vandazole Vaginal Gel 3338

Metronidazole Benzoate
(Buprenorphine is metabolized to norbuprenorphine by cytochrome CYP3A4. Because CYP3A4 inhibitors may increase plasma concentrations of buprenorphine, patients already on CYP3A4 inhibitors should have their dose of Subutex or Suboxone adjusted.).
 No products indexed under this heading.

Metronidazole Hydrochloride
(Buprenorphine is metabolized to norbuprenorphine by cytochrome CYP3A4. Because CYP3A4 inhibitors may increase plasma concentrations of buprenorphine, patients already on CYP3A4 inhibitors should have their dose of Subutex or Suboxone adjusted.).
 No products indexed under this heading.

Miconazole (Buprenorphine is metabolized to norbuprenorphine by cytochrome CYP3A4. Because CYP3A4 inhibitors may increase plasma concentrations of buprenorphine, patients already on CYP3A4 inhibitors should have their dose of Subutex or Suboxone adjusted.).
 No products indexed under this heading.

Miconazole Nitrate (Buprenorphine is metabolized to norbuprenorphine by cytochrome CYP3A4. Because CYP3A4 inhibitors may increase plasma concentrations of buprenorphine, patients already on CYP3A4 inhibitors should have their dose of Subutex or Suboxone adjusted.). Products include:

Nefazodone Hydrochloride
(Buprenorphine is metabolized to norbuprenorphine by cytochrome CYP3A4. Because CYP3A4 inhibitors may increase plasma concentrations of buprenorphine, patients already on CYP3A4 inhibitors should have their dose of Subutex or Suboxone adjusted.).
 No products indexed under this heading.

Nelfinavir Mesylate (Buprenorphine is metabolized to norbuprenorphine by cytochrome CYP3A4. Because CYP3A4 inhibitors may increase plasma concentrations of buprenorphine, patients already on CYP3A4 inhibitors should have their dose of Subutex or Suboxone adjusted.). Products include:

Nevirapine (Buprenorphine is metabolized to norbuprenorphine by cytochrome CYP3A4. Because CYP3A4 inhibitors may increase plasma concentrations of buprenorphine, patients already on CYP3A4 inhibitors should have their dose of Subutex or Suboxone adjusted.). Products include:

Niacinamide (Buprenorphine is metabolized to norbuprenorphine by cytochrome CYP3A4. Because CYP3A4 inhibitors may increase plasma concentrations of buprenorphine, patients already on CYP3A4 inhibitors should have their dose of Subutex or Suboxone adjusted.).
 No products indexed under this heading.

Nicotinamide (Buprenorphine is metabolized to norbuprenorphine by

cytochrome CYP3A4. Because CYP3A4 inhibitors may increase plasma concentrations of buprenorphine, patients already on CYP3A4 inhibitors should have their dose of Subutex or Suboxone adjusted.). Products include:

Nifedipine (Buprenorphine is metabolized to norbuprenorphine by cytochrome CYP3A4. Because CYP3A4 inhibitors may increase plasma concentrations of buprenorphine, patients already on CYP3A4 inhibitors should have their dose of Subutex or Suboxone adjusted.). Products include:

Norfloxacin (Buprenorphine is metabolized to norbuprenorphine by cytochrome CYP3A4. Because CYP3A4 inhibitors may increase plasma concentrations of buprenorphine, patients already on CYP3A4 inhibitors should have their dose of Subutex or Suboxone adjusted.). Products include:

Omeprazole (Buprenorphine is metabolized to norbuprenorphine by cytochrome CYP3A4. Because CYP3A4 inhibitors may increase plasma concentrations of buprenorphine, patients already on CYP3A4 inhibitors should have their dose of Subutex or Suboxone adjusted.). Products include:

Paroxetine Hydrochloride
(Buprenorphine is metabolized to norbuprenorphine by cytochrome CYP3A4. Because CYP3A4 inhibitors may increase plasma concentrations of buprenorphine, patients already on CYP3A4 inhibitors should have their dose of Subutex or Suboxone adjusted.). Products include:

Propoxyphene Hydrochloride
(Buprenorphine is metabolized to norbuprenorphine by cytochrome CYP3A4. Because CYP3A4 inhibitors may increase plasma concentrations of buprenorphine, patients already on CYP3A4 inhibitors should have their dose of Subutex or Suboxone adjusted.).
 No products indexed under this heading.

Propoxyphene Napsylate
(Buprenorphine is metabolized to norbuprenorphine by cytochrome CYP3A4. Because CYP3A4 inhibitors may increase plasma concentrations of buprenorphine, patients already on CYP3A4 inhibitors should have their dose of Subutex or Suboxone adjusted.).
 No products indexed under this heading.

Quinidine (Buprenorphine is metabolized to norbuprenorphine by cytochrome CYP3A4. Because CYP3A4 inhibitors may increase plasma concentrations of buprenorphine, patients already on CYP3A4 inhibitors should have their dose of Subutex or Suboxone adjusted.).
 No products indexed under this heading.

Quinidine Hydrochloride
(Buprenorphine is metabolized to norbuprenorphine by cytochrome CYP3A4. Because CYP3A4 inhibitors may increase plasma concentrations of buprenorphine, patients already on CYP3A4 inhibitors should have their dose of Subutex or Suboxone adjusted.).
 No products indexed under this heading.

Quinidine Polygalacturonate
(Buprenorphine is metabolized to norbuprenorphine by cytochrome CYP3A4. Because CYP3A4 inhibitors may increase plasma concentrations of buprenorphine, patients already on CYP3A4 inhibitors should have their dose of Subutex or Suboxone adjusted.).
 No products indexed under this heading.

Quinidine Sulfate (Buprenorphine is metabolized to norbuprenorphine by cytochrome CYP3A4. Because CYP3A4 inhibitors may increase plasma concentrations of buprenorphine, patients already on CYP3A4 inhibitors should have their dose of Subutex or Suboxone adjusted.).
 No products indexed under this heading.

Quinine (Buprenorphine is metabolized to norbuprenorphine by cytochrome CYP3A4. Because CYP3A4 inhibitors may increase plasma concentrations of buprenorphine, patients already on CYP3A4 inhibitors should have their dose of Subutex or Suboxone adjusted.).
 No products indexed under this heading.

Quinine Sulfate (Buprenorphine is metabolized to norbuprenorphine by cytochrome CYP3A4. Because CYP3A4 inhibitors may increase plasma concentrations of buprenorphine, patients already on CYP3A4 inhibitors should have their dose of Subutex or Suboxone adjusted.).
 No products indexed under this heading.

Quinupristin (Buprenorphine is metabolized to norbuprenorphine by cytochrome CYP3A4. Because CYP3A4 inhibitors may increase plasma concentrations of buprenorphine, patients already on CYP3A4 inhibitors should have their dose of Subutex or Suboxone adjusted.).
 No products indexed under this heading.

Ranitidine Bismuth Citrate
(Buprenorphine is metabolized to norbuprenorphine by cytochrome CYP3A4. Because CYP3A4 inhibitors may increase plasma concentrations of buprenorphine, patients already on CYP3A4 inhibitors should have their dose of Subutex or Suboxone adjusted.).
 No products indexed under this heading.

Ranitidine Hydrochloride
(Buprenorphine is metabolized to norbuprenorphine by cytochrome CYP3A4. Because CYP3A4 inhibitors may increase plasma concentrations of buprenorphine, patients already on CYP3A4 inhibitors should have their dose of Subutex or Suboxone adjusted.). Products include:

Ritonavir (Buprenorphine is metabolized to norbuprenorphine by cytochrome CYP3A4. Because CYP3A4 inhibitors may increase plasma concentrations of buprenorphine, patients already on CYP3A4 inhibitors should have their dose of Subutex or Suboxone adjusted.). Products include:

Saquinavir (Buprenorphine is metabolized to norbuprenorphine by cytochrome CYP3A4. Because CYP3A4 inhibitors may increase plasma concentrations of buprenorphine, patients already on CYP3A4 inhibitors should have their dose of Subutex or Suboxone adjusted.).
 No products indexed under this heading.

Saquinavir Mesylate (Buprenorphine is metabolized to norbuprenorphine by cytochrome CYP3A4. Because CYP3A4 inhibitors may increase plasma concentrations of buprenorphine, patients already on CYP3A4 inhibitors should have their dose of Subutex or Suboxone adjusted.). Products include:

Sertraline Hydrochloride
(Buprenorphine is metabolized to norbuprenorphine by cytochrome CYP3A4. Because CYP3A4 inhibitors may increase plasma concentrations of buprenorphine, patients already on CYP3A4 inhibitors should have their dose of Subutex or Suboxone adjusted.). Products include:

Telithromycin (Buprenorphine is metabolized to norbuprenorphine by cytochrome CYP3A4. Because CYP3A4 inhibitors may increase plasma concentrations of buprenorphine, patients already on CYP3A4 inhibitors should have their dose of Subutex or Suboxone adjusted.). Products include:

Troglitazone (Buprenorphine is metabolized to norbuprenorphine by cytochrome CYP3A4. Because CYP3A4 inhibitors may increase plasma concentrations of buprenorphine, patients already on CYP3A4 inhibitors should have their dose of Subutex or Suboxone adjusted.).
 No products indexed under this heading.

Troleandomycin (Buprenorphine is metabolized to norbuprenorphine by cytochrome CYP3A4. Because CYP3A4 inhibitors may increase plasma concentrations of buprenorphine, patients already on CYP3A4 inhibitors should have their dose of Subutex or Suboxone adjusted.).
 No products indexed under this heading.

Valproate Sodium (Buprenorphine is metabolized to norbuprenorphine by cytochrome CYP3A4. Because CYP3A4 inhibitors may increase plasma concentrations of buprenorphine, patients already on CYP3A4 inhibitors should have their dose of Subutex or Suboxone adjusted.). Products include:

Verapamil Hydrochloride
(Buprenorphine is metabolized to norbuprenorphine by cytochrome CYP3A4. Because CYP3A4 inhibitors may increase plasma concentrations of buprenorphine, patients already

on CYP3A4 inhibitors should have their dose of Subutex or Subuxone adjusted). Products include:
- Covera-HS Tablets 3139
- Tarka Tablets 524
- Verelan PM Extended-Release Capsules, Controlled-Onset 3106

Voriconazole (Buprenorphine is metabolized to norbuprenorphine by cytochrome CYP3A4. Because CYP3A4 inhibitors may increase plasma concentrations of buprenorphine, patients already on CYP3A4 inhibitors should have their dose of Subutex or Subuxone adjusted). Products include:
- VFEND I.V. 2564
- VFEND Oral Suspension 2564
- VFEND Tablets 2564

Zafirlukast (Buprenorphine is metabolized to norbuprenorphine by cytochrome CYP3A4. Because CYP3A4 inhibitors may increase plasma concentrations of buprenorphine, patients already on CYP3A4 inhibitors should have their dose of Subutex or Subuxone adjusted). Products include:
- Accolate Tablets 671

Zileuton (Buprenorphine is metabolized to norbuprenorphine by cytochrome CYP3A4. Because CYP3A4 inhibitors may increase plasma concentrations of buprenorphine, patients already on CYP3A4 inhibitors should have their dose of Subutex or Subuxone adjusted). Products include:
- Zyflo Tablets 1023

Food Interactions

Grapefruit (Buprenorphine is metabolized to norbuprenorphine by cytochrome CYP3A4. Because CYP3A4 inhibitors may increase plasma concentrations of buprenorphine, patients already on CYP3A4 inhibitors should have their dose of Subutex or Subuxone adjusted).

Grapefruit Juice (Buprenorphine is metabolized to norbuprenorphine by cytochrome CYP3A4. Because CYP3A4 inhibitors may increase plasma concentrations of buprenorphine, patients already on CYP3A4 inhibitors should have their dose of Subutex or Subuxone adjusted).

SUBUTEX TABLETS

(Buprenorphine Hydrochloride) 2717

May interact with cytochrome p450 3a4 inhibitors (selected). Compounds in these categories include:

Acetazolamide (Buprenorphine is metabolized to norbuprenorphine by cytochrome CYP3A4. Because CYP3A4 inhibitors may increase plasma concentrations of buprenorphine, patients already on CYP3A4 inhibitors should have their dose of Subutex or Subuxone adjusted.).

No products indexed under this heading.

Amiodarone Hydrochloride (Buprenorphine is metabolized to norbuprenorphine by cytochrome CYP3A4. Because CYP3A4 inhibitors may increase plasma concentrations of buprenorphine, patients already on CYP3A4 inhibitors should have their dose of Subutex or Subuxone adjusted.).

No products indexed under this heading.

Amprenavir (Buprenorphine is metabolized to norbuprenorphine by cytochrome CYP3A4. Because CYP3A4 inhibitors may increase plasma concentrations of buprenorphine, patients already on CYP3A4 inhibitors should have their dose of Subutex or Subuxone adjusted). Products include:
- Agenerase Capsules 1327
- Agenerase Oral Solution 1332

Anastrozole (Buprenorphine is metabolized to norbuprenorphine by cytochrome CYP3A4. Because CYP3A4 inhibitors may increase plasma concentrations of buprenorphine, patients already on CYP3A4 inhibitors should have their dose of Subutex or Subuxone adjusted). Products include:
- Arimidex Tablets 673

Aprepitant (Buprenorphine is metabolized to norbuprenorphine by cytochrome CYP3A4. Because CYP3A4 inhibitors may increase plasma concentrations of buprenorphine, patients already on CYP3A4 inhibitors should have their dose of Subutex or Subuxone adjusted). Products include:
- Emend Capsules 1963

Cimetidine (Buprenorphine is metabolized to norbuprenorphine by cytochrome CYP3A4. Because CYP3A4 inhibitors may increase plasma concentrations of buprenorphine, patients already on CYP3A4 inhibitors should have their dose of Subutex or Subuxone adjusted). Products include:
- Tagamet HB 200 Tablets 664

Cimetidine Hydrochloride (Buprenorphine is metabolized to norbuprenorphine by cytochrome CYP3A4. Because CYP3A4 inhibitors may increase plasma concentrations of buprenorphine, patients already on CYP3A4 inhibitors should have their dose of Subutex or Subuxone adjusted.).

No products indexed under this heading.

Ciprofloxacin (Buprenorphine is metabolized to norbuprenorphine by cytochrome CYP3A4. Because CYP3A4 inhibitors may increase plasma concentrations of buprenorphine, patients already on CYP3A4 inhibitors should have their dose of Subutex or Subuxone adjusted). Products include:
- Cipro Oral Suspension 2977
- Cipro I.V. 2984
- Cipro XR Tablets 2990
- Ciprodex Otic Suspension 559

Clarithromycin (Buprenorphine is metabolized to norbuprenorphine by cytochrome CYP3A4. Because CYP3A4 inhibitors may increase plasma concentrations of buprenorphine, patients already on CYP3A4 inhibitors should have their dose of Subutex or Subuxone adjusted). Products include:
- Biaxin/Biaxin XL 402
- PREVPAC 3284

Clotrimazole (Buprenorphine is metabolized to norbuprenorphine by cytochrome CYP3A4. Because CYP3A4 inhibitors may increase plasma concentrations of buprenorphine, patients already on CYP3A4 inhibitors should have their dose of Subutex or Subuxone adjusted). Products include:
- Desenex Athlete's Foot Cream 635
- Lotrimin 3039
- Lotrisone 3040

Cyclosporine (Buprenorphine is metabolized to norbuprenorphine by cytochrome CYP3A4. Because CYP3A4 inhibitors may increase plasma concentrations of buprenorphine, patients already on CYP3A4 inhibitors should have their dose of Subutex or Subuxone adjusted). Products include:
- Gengraf Capsules 459
- Neoral Oral Solution 2259
- Neoral Soft Gelatin Capsules 2259
- Restasis Ophthalmic Emulsion 575
- Sandimmune 2275

Dalfopristin (Buprenorphine is metabolized to norbuprenorphine by cytochrome CYP3A4. Because CYP3A4 inhibitors may increase plasma concentrations of buprenorphine, patients already on CYP3A4 inhibitors should have their dose of Subutex or Subuxone adjusted.).

No products indexed under this heading.

Danazol (Buprenorphine is metabolized to norbuprenorphine by cytochrome CYP3A4. Because CYP3A4 inhibitors may increase plasma concentrations of buprenorphine, patients already on CYP3A4 inhibitors should have their dose of Subutex or Subuxone adjusted.).

No products indexed under this heading.

Delavirdine Mesylate (Buprenorphine is metabolized to norbuprenorphine by cytochrome CYP3A4. Because CYP3A4 inhibitors may increase plasma concentrations of buprenorphine, patients already on CYP3A4 inhibitors should have their dose of Subutex or Subuxone adjusted). Products include:
- Rescriptor Tablets 2551

Diltiazem Hydrochloride (Buprenorphine is metabolized to norbuprenorphine by cytochrome CYP3A4. Because CYP3A4 inhibitors may increase plasma concentrations of buprenorphine, patients already on CYP3A4 inhibitors should have their dose of Subutex or Subuxone adjusted). Products include:
- Cardizem LA Extended Release Tablets 1728
- Tiazac Capsules 1201

Diltiazem Maleate (Buprenorphine is metabolized to norbuprenorphine by cytochrome CYP3A4. Because CYP3A4 inhibitors may increase plasma concentrations of buprenorphine, patients already on CYP3A4 inhibitors should have their dose of Subutex or Subuxone adjusted.).

No products indexed under this heading.

Efavirenz (Buprenorphine is metabolized to norbuprenorphine by cytochrome CYP3A4. Because CYP3A4 inhibitors may increase plasma concentrations of buprenorphine, patients already on CYP3A4 inhibitors should have their dose of Subutex or Subuxone adjusted). Products include:
- Atripla Tablets 945
- Sustiva Capsules 930
- Sustiva Tablets 930

Erythromycin (Buprenorphine is metabolized to norbuprenorphine by cytochrome CYP3A4. Because CYP3A4 inhibitors may increase plasma concentrations of buprenorphine, patients already on CYP3A4 inhibitors should have their dose of Subutex or Subuxone adjusted). Products include:
- Ery-Tab Tablets 449
- Erythromycin Base Filmtab Tablets 455
- Erythromycin Delayed-Release Capsules, USP 457
- PCE Dispertab Tablets 515

Erythromycin Estolate (Buprenorphine is metabolized to norbuprenorphine by cytochrome CYP3A4. Because CYP3A4 inhibitors may increase plasma concentrations of buprenorphine, patients already on CYP3A4 inhibitors should have their dose of Subutex or Subuxone adjusted.).

No products indexed under this heading.

Erythromycin Ethylsuccinate (Buprenorphine is metabolized to norbuprenorphine by cytochrome CYP3A4. Because CYP3A4 inhibitors may increase plasma concentrations of buprenorphine, patients already on CYP3A4 inhibitors should have their dose of Subutex or Subuxone adjusted). Products include:
- E.E.S. 451
- EryPed 447

Erythromycin Gluceptate (Buprenorphine is metabolized to norbuprenorphine by cytochrome CYP3A4. Because CYP3A4 inhibitors may increase plasma concentrations of buprenorphine, patients already on CYP3A4 inhibitors should have their dose of Subutex or Subuxone adjusted.).

No products indexed under this heading.

Erythromycin Lactobionate (Buprenorphine is metabolized to norbuprenorphine by cytochrome CYP3A4. Because CYP3A4 inhibitors may increase plasma concentrations of buprenorphine, patients already on CYP3A4 inhibitors should have their dose of Subutex or Subuxone adjusted.).

No products indexed under this heading.

Erythromycin Stearate (Buprenorphine is metabolized to norbuprenorphine by cytochrome CYP3A4. Because CYP3A4 inhibitors may increase plasma concentrations of buprenorphine, patients already on CYP3A4 inhibitors should have their dose of Subutex or Subuxone adjusted). Products include:
- Erythrocin Stearate Filmtab Tablets 453

Esomeprazole Magnesium (Buprenorphine is metabolized to norbuprenorphine by cytochrome CYP3A4. Because CYP3A4 inhibitors may increase plasma concentrations of buprenorphine, patients already on CYP3A4 inhibitors should have their dose of Subutex or Subuxone adjusted). Products include:
- Nexium Delayed-Release Capsules 655

Fluconazole (Buprenorphine is metabolized to norbuprenorphine by cytochrome CYP3A4. Because CYP3A4 inhibitors may increase plasma concentrations of buprenorphine, patients already on CYP3A4 inhibitors should have their dose of Subutex or Subuxone adjusted.).

No products indexed under this heading.

Fluoxetine Hydrochloride (Buprenorphine is metabolized to norbuprenorphine by cytochrome CYP3A4. Because CYP3A4 inhibitors may increase plasma concentrations of buprenorphine, patients already on CYP3A4 inhibitors should have their dose of Subutex or Subuxone adjusted). Products include:
- Prozac Pulvules and Liquid 1801

Symbyax Capsules 1819

Fluvoxamine Maleate (Buprenorphine is metabolized to norbuprenorphine by cytochrome CYP3A4. Because CYP3A4 inhibitors may increase plasma concentrations of buprenorphine, patients already on CYP3A4 inhibitors should have their dose of Subutex or Suboxone adjusted.).

No products indexed under this heading.

Fosamprenavir Calcium (Buprenorphine is metabolized to norbuprenorphine by cytochrome CYP3A4. Because CYP3A4 inhibitors may increase plasma concentrations of buprenorphine, patients already on CYP3A4 inhibitors should have their dose of Subutex or Suboxone adjusted). Products include:

Lexiva Tablets 1505

Indinavir Sulfate (Buprenorphine is metabolized to norbuprenorphine by cytochrome CYP3A4. Because CYP3A4 inhibitors may increase plasma concentrations of buprenorphine, patients already on CYP3A4 inhibitors should have their dose of Subutex or Suboxone adjusted). Products include:

Crixivan Capsules 1940

Isoniazid (Buprenorphine is metabolized to norbuprenorphine by cytochrome CYP3A4. Because CYP3A4 inhibitors may increase plasma concentrations of buprenorphine, patients already on CYP3A4 inhibitors should have their dose of Subutex or Suboxone adjusted.).

No products indexed under this heading.

Itraconazole (Buprenorphine is metabolized to norbuprenorphine by cytochrome CYP3A4. Because CYP3A4 inhibitors may increase plasma concentrations of buprenorphine, patients already on CYP3A4 inhibitors should have their dose of Subutex or Suboxone adjusted.).

No products indexed under this heading.

Ketoconazole (Buprenorphine is metabolized to norbuprenorphine by cytochrome CYP3A4. Because CYP3A4 inhibitors may increase plasma concentrations of buprenorphine, patients already on CYP3A4 inhibitors should have their dose of Subutex or Suboxone adjusted). Products include:

Nizoral A-D Shampoo, 1% 1868

Lopinavir (Buprenorphine is metabolized to norbuprenorphine by cytochrome CYP3A4. Because CYP3A4 inhibitors may increase plasma concentrations of buprenorphine, patients already on CYP3A4 inhibitors should have their dose of Subutex or Suboxone adjusted). Products include:

Kaletra 476

Loratadine (Buprenorphine is metabolized to norbuprenorphine by cytochrome CYP3A4. Because CYP3A4 inhibitors may increase plasma concentrations of buprenorphine, patients already on CYP3A4 inhibitors should have their dose of Subutex or Suboxone adjusted). Products include:

Alavert Allergy & Sinus D-12 Hour Tablets .... ▣ 771

Alavert .... ▣ 771

Children's Claritin Allergy Oral Solution .... ▣ 771

Claritin Non-Drowsy 24 Hour Tablets .... ▣ 772

Claritin Reditabs 24 Hour Non-Drowsy Tablets .... ▣ 772

Claritin-D Non-Drowsy 12 Hour Tablets .... ▣ 772

Claritin-D Non-Drowsy 24 Hour Tablets .... ▣ 772

Metronidazole (Buprenorphine is metabolized to norbuprenorphine by cytochrome CYP3A4. Because CYP3A4 inhibitors may increase plasma concentrations of buprenorphine, patients already on CYP3A4 inhibitors should have their dose of Subutex or Suboxone adjusted). Products include:

Metrogel 1% 1211

MetroGel-Vaginal Gel 1855

Vandazole Vaginal Gel 3338

Metronidazole Benzoate (Buprenorphine is metabolized to norbuprenorphine by cytochrome CYP3A4. Because CYP3A4 inhibitors may increase plasma concentrations of buprenorphine, patients already on CYP3A4 inhibitors should have their dose of Subutex or Suboxone adjusted.).

No products indexed under this heading.

Metronidazole Hydrochloride (Buprenorphine is metabolized to norbuprenorphine by cytochrome CYP3A4. Because CYP3A4 inhibitors may increase plasma concentrations of buprenorphine, patients already on CYP3A4 inhibitors should have their dose of Subutex or Suboxone adjusted.).

No products indexed under this heading.

Miconazole (Buprenorphine is metabolized to norbuprenorphine by cytochrome CYP3A4. Because CYP3A4 inhibitors may increase plasma concentrations of buprenorphine, patients already on CYP3A4 inhibitors should have their dose of Subutex or Suboxone adjusted.).

No products indexed under this heading.

Miconazole Nitrate (Buprenorphine is metabolized to norbuprenorphine by cytochrome CYP3A4. Because CYP3A4 inhibitors may increase plasma concentrations of buprenorphine, patients already on CYP3A4 inhibitors should have their dose of Subutex or Suboxone adjusted). Products include:

Desenex .... ▣ 635

Desenex Jock Itch Spray Powder ... ▣ 635

Nefazodone Hydrochloride (Buprenorphine is metabolized to norbuprenorphine by cytochrome CYP3A4. Because CYP3A4 inhibitors may increase plasma concentrations of buprenorphine, patients already on CYP3A4 inhibitors should have their dose of Subutex or Suboxone adjusted.).

No products indexed under this heading.

Nelfinavir Mesylate (Buprenorphine is metabolized to norbuprenorphine by cytochrome CYP3A4. Because CYP3A4 inhibitors may increase plasma concentrations of buprenorphine, patients already on CYP3A4 inhibitors should have their dose of Subutex or Suboxone adjusted). Products include:

Viracept 2577

Nevirapine (Buprenorphine is metabolized to norbuprenorphine by cytochrome CYP3A4. Because CYP3A4 inhibitors may increase plasma concentrations of buprenorphine, patients already on CYP3A4 inhibitors should have their dose of Subutex or Suboxone adjusted). Products include:

Viramune Oral Suspension 873

Viramune Tablets 873

Niacinamide (Buprenorphine is metabolized to norbuprenorphine by cytochrome CYP3A4. Because CYP3A4 inhibitors may increase plasma concentrations of buprenorphine, patients already on CYP3A4 inhibitors should have their dose of Subutex or Suboxone adjusted.).

No products indexed under this heading.

Nicotinamide (Buprenorphine is metabolized to norbuprenorphine by cytochrome CYP3A4. Because CYP3A4 inhibitors may increase plasma concentrations of buprenorphine, patients already on CYP3A4 inhibitors should have their dose of Subutex or Suboxone adjusted). Products include:

Nicomide Tablets 1088

Nifedipine (Buprenorphine is metabolized to norbuprenorphine by cytochrome CYP3A4. Because CYP3A4 inhibitors may increase plasma concentrations of buprenorphine, patients already on CYP3A4 inhibitors should have their dose of Subutex or Suboxone adjusted). Products include:

Adalat CC Tablets 2964

Norfloxacin (Buprenorphine is metabolized to norbuprenorphine by cytochrome CYP3A4. Because CYP3A4 inhibitors may increase plasma concentrations of buprenorphine, patients already on CYP3A4 inhibitors should have their dose of Subutex or Suboxone adjusted). Products include:

Noroxin Tablets 2032

Omeprazole (Buprenorphine is metabolized to norbuprenorphine by cytochrome CYP3A4. Because CYP3A4 inhibitors may increase plasma concentrations of buprenorphine, patients already on CYP3A4 inhibitors should have their dose of Subutex or Suboxone adjusted). Products include:

Zegerid Capsules 2958

Zegerid Powder for Oral Solution 2958

Paroxetine Hydrochloride (Buprenorphine is metabolized to norbuprenorphine by cytochrome CYP3A4. Because CYP3A4 inhibitors may increase plasma concentrations of buprenorphine, patients already on CYP3A4 inhibitors should have their dose of Subutex or Suboxone adjusted). Products include:

Paxil CR Controlled-Release Tablets 1538

Paxil 1530

Propoxyphene Hydrochloride (Buprenorphine is metabolized to norbuprenorphine by cytochrome CYP3A4. Because CYP3A4 inhibitors may increase plasma concentrations of buprenorphine, patients already on CYP3A4 inhibitors should have their dose of Subutex or Suboxone adjusted.).

No products indexed under this heading.

Propoxyphene Napsylate (Buprenorphine is metabolized to norbuprenorphine by cytochrome CYP3A4. Because CYP3A4 inhibitors may increase plasma concentrations of buprenorphine, patients already on CYP3A4 inhibitors should have their dose of Subutex or Suboxone adjusted.).

No products indexed under this heading.

Quinidine (Buprenorphine is metabolized to norbuprenorphine by cytochrome CYP3A4. Because CYP3A4 inhibitors may increase plasma concentrations of buprenorphine, patients already on CYP3A4 inhibitors should have their dose of Subutex or Suboxone adjusted.).

No products indexed under this heading.

Quinidine Hydrochloride (Buprenorphine is metabolized to norbuprenorphine by cytochrome CYP3A4. Because CYP3A4 inhibitors may increase plasma concentrations of buprenorphine, patients already on CYP3A4 inhibitors should have their dose of Subutex or Suboxone adjusted.).

No products indexed under this heading.

Quinidine Polygalacturonate (Buprenorphine is metabolized to norbuprenorphine by cytochrome CYP3A4. Because CYP3A4 inhibitors may increase plasma concentrations of buprenorphine, patients already on CYP3A4 inhibitors should have their dose of Subutex or Suboxone adjusted.).

No products indexed under this heading.

Quinidine Sulfate (Buprenorphine is metabolized to norbuprenorphine by cytochrome CYP3A4. Because CYP3A4 inhibitors may increase plasma concentrations of buprenorphine, patients already on CYP3A4 inhibitors should have their dose of Subutex or Suboxone adjusted.).

No products indexed under this heading.

Quinine (Buprenorphine is metabolized to norbuprenorphine by cytochrome CYP3A4. Because CYP3A4 inhibitors may increase plasma concentrations of buprenorphine, patients already on CYP3A4 inhibitors should have their dose of Subutex or Suboxone adjusted.).

No products indexed under this heading.

Quinine Sulfate (Buprenorphine is metabolized to norbuprenorphine by cytochrome CYP3A4. Because CYP3A4 inhibitors may increase plasma concentrations of buprenorphine, patients already on CYP3A4 inhibitors should have their dose of Subutex or Suboxone adjusted.).

No products indexed under this heading.

Quinupristin (Buprenorphine is metabolized to norbuprenorphine by cytochrome CYP3A4. Because CYP3A4 inhibitors may increase plasma concentrations of buprenorphine, patients already on CYP3A4 inhibitors should have their dose of Subutex or Suboxone adjusted.).

No products indexed under this heading.

Ranitidine Bismuth Citrate (Buprenorphine is metabolized to norbuprenorphine by cytochrome CYP3A4. Because CYP3A4 inhibitors may increase plasma concentrations of buprenorphine, patients already on CYP3A4 inhibitors should have their dose of Subutex or Subuxone adjusted.).
No products indexed under this heading.

Ranitidine Hydrochloride (Buprenorphine is metabolized to norbuprenorphine by cytochrome CYP3A4. Because CYP3A4 inhibitors may increase plasma concentrations of buprenorphine, patients already on CYP3A4 inhibitors should have their dose of Subutex or Subuxone adjusted). Products include:
Zantac **1624**
Zantac Injection **1619**
Zantac Injection Pharmacy Bulk Package **1622**

Ritonavir (Buprenorphine is metabolized to norbuprenorphine by cytochrome CYP3A4. Because CYP3A4 inhibitors may increase plasma concentrations of buprenorphine, patients already on CYP3A4 inhibitors should have their dose of Subutex or Subuxone adjusted). Products include:
Kaletra **476**
Norvir **503**

Saquinavir (Buprenorphine is metabolized to norbuprenorphine by cytochrome CYP3A4. Because CYP3A4 inhibitors may increase plasma concentrations of buprenorphine, patients already on CYP3A4 inhibitors should have their dose of Subutex or Subuxone adjusted.).
No products indexed under this heading.

Saquinavir Mesylate (Buprenorphine is metabolized to norbuprenorphine by cytochrome CYP3A4. Because CYP3A4 inhibitors may increase plasma concentrations of buprenorphine, patients already on CYP3A4 inhibitors should have their dose of Subutex or Subuxone adjusted). Products include:
Invirase **2772**

Sertraline Hydrochloride (Buprenorphine is metabolized to norbuprenorphine by cytochrome CYP3A4. Because CYP3A4 inhibitors may increase plasma concentrations of buprenorphine, patients already on CYP3A4 inhibitors should have their dose of Subutex or Subuxone adjusted). Products include:
Zoloft **2586**

Telithromycin (Buprenorphine is metabolized to norbuprenorphine by cytochrome CYP3A4. Because CYP3A4 inhibitors may increase plasma concentrations of buprenorphine, patients already on CYP3A4 inhibitors should have their dose of Subutex or Subuxone adjusted). Products include:
Ketek Tablets **2903**

Troglitazone (Buprenorphine is metabolized to norbuprenorphine by cytochrome CYP3A4. Because CYP3A4 inhibitors may increase plasma concentrations of buprenorphine, patients already on CYP3A4 inhibitors should have their dose of Subutex or Subuxone adjusted.).
No products indexed under this heading.

Troleandomycin (Buprenorphine is metabolized to norbuprenorphine by cytochrome CYP3A4. Because CYP3A4 inhibitors may increase plasma concentrations of buprenorphine, patients already on CYP3A4 inhibitors should have their dose of Subutex or Subuxone adjusted.).
No products indexed under this heading.

Valproate Sodium (Buprenorphine is metabolized to norbuprenorphine by cytochrome CYP3A4. Because CYP3A4 inhibitors may increase plasma concentrations of buprenorphine, patients already on CYP3A4 inhibitors should have their dose of Subutex or Subuxone adjusted). Products include:
Depacon Injection **412**

Verapamil Hydrochloride (Buprenorphine is metabolized to norbuprenorphine by cytochrome CYP3A4. Because CYP3A4 inhibitors may increase plasma concentrations of buprenorphine, patients already on CYP3A4 inhibitors should have their dose of Subutex or Subuxone adjusted). Products include:
Covera-HS Tablets **3139**
Tarka Tablets **524**
Verelan PM Extended-Release Capsules, Controlled-Onset **3106**

Voriconazole (Buprenorphine is metabolized to norbuprenorphine by cytochrome CYP3A4. Because CYP3A4 inhibitors may increase plasma concentrations of buprenorphine, patients already on CYP3A4 inhibitors should have their dose of Subutex or Subuxone adjusted). Products include:
VFEND I.V. **2564**
VFEND Oral Suspension **2564**
VFEND Tablets **2564**

Zafirlukast (Buprenorphine is metabolized to norbuprenorphine by cytochrome CYP3A4. Because CYP3A4 inhibitors may increase plasma concentrations of buprenorphine, patients already on CYP3A4 inhibitors should have their dose of Subutex or Subuxone adjusted). Products include:
Accolate Tablets **671**

Zileuton (Buprenorphine is metabolized to norbuprenorphine by cytochrome CYP3A4. Because CYP3A4 inhibitors may increase plasma concentrations of buprenorphine, patients already on CYP3A4 inhibitors should have their dose of Subutex or Subuxone adjusted). Products include:
Zyflo Tablets **1023**

Food Interactions

Grapefruit (Buprenorphine is metabolized to norbuprenorphine by cytochrome CYP3A4. Because CYP3A4 inhibitors may increase plasma concentrations of buprenorphine, patients already on CYP3A4 inhibitors should have their dose of Subutex or Subuxone adjusted).

Grapefruit Juice (Buprenorphine is metabolized to norbuprenorphine by cytochrome CYP3A4. Because CYP3A4 inhibitors may increase plasma concentrations of buprenorphine, patients already on CYP3A4 inhibitors should have their dose of Subutex or Subuxone adjusted).

SULAR TABLETS

(Nisoldipine) **3122**
May interact with dexamethasone, phenytoin, quinidine, and certain other agents. Compounds in these categories include:

Atenolol (Greater blood pressure effect of Sular with concomitant use).
No products indexed under this heading.

Carbamazepine (Co-administration of nisoldipine with known CYP3A4 inducer, such as carbamazepine, should be avoided because of possible reduced nisoldipine plasma concentrations). Products include:
Carbatrol Capsules **3171**
Equetro Extended-Release Capsules **3180**
Tegretol/Tegretol-XR **2295**

Cimetidine (Concomitant use increases nisoldipine AUC and Cmax by 30% to 45%). Products include:
Tagamet HB 200 Tablets **664**

Cimetidine Hydrochloride (Concomitant use increases nisoldipine AUC and Cmax by 30% to 45%).
No products indexed under this heading.

Dexamethasone (Co-administration of nisoldipine with known CYP3A4 inducer, such as dexamethasone, should be avoided because of possible reduced nisoldipine plasma concentrations). Products include:
Ciprodex Otic Suspension **559**
Decadron Tablets **1951**
TobraDex Ophthalmic Ointment **562**
TobraDex Ophthalmic Suspension **563**

Dexamethasone Acetate (Co-administration of nisoldipine with known CYP3A4 inducer, such as dexamethasone, should be avoided because of possible reduced nisoldipine plasma concentrations).
No products indexed under this heading.

Dexamethasone Sodium Phosphate (Co-administration of nisoldipine with known CYP3A4 inducer, such as dexamethasone, should be avoided because of possible reduced nisoldipine plasma concentrations).
No products indexed under this heading.

Fosphenytoin Sodium (Co-administration in epileptic patients has resulted in reduced nisoldipine plasma concentrations to undetectable levels).
No products indexed under this heading.

Phenobarbital (Co-administration of nisoldipine with known CYP3A4 inducer, such as phenobarbital, should be avoided because of possible reduced nisoldipine plasma concentrations). Products include:
Donnatal Extentabs **2493**

Phenytoin (Co-administration in epileptic patients has resulted in reduced nisoldipine plasma concentrations to undetectable levels).
No products indexed under this heading.

Phenytoin Sodium (Co-administration in epileptic patients has resulted in reduced nisoldipine plasma concentrations to undetectable levels). Products include:
Phenytek Capsules **2160**

Propranolol Hydrochloride (Propanolol attenuates the heart rate increase following the administration of immediate-release nisoldipine). Products include:
Inderal LA Long-Acting Capsules **3429**
InnoPran XL Capsules **2723**

Quinidine (May decrease the bioavailability (AUC) of nisoldipine by 26%, but not the peak concentration; clinical significance is not known).
No products indexed under this heading.

Quinidine Gluconate (May decrease the bioavailability (AUC) of nisoldipine by 26%, but not the peak concentration; clinical significance is not known).
No products indexed under this heading.

Quinidine Hydrochloride (May decrease the bioavailability (AUC) of nisoldipine by 26%, but not the peak concentration; clinical significance is not known).
No products indexed under this heading.

Quinidine Polygalacturonate (May decrease the bioavailability (AUC) of nisoldipine by 26%, but not the peak concentration; clinical significance is not known).
No products indexed under this heading.

Quinidine Sulfate (May decrease the bioavailability (AUC) of nisoldipine by 26%, but not the peak concentration; clinical significance is not known).
No products indexed under this heading.

Ranitidine Hydrochloride (Concomitant use decreases AUC by 15% to 20%). Products include:
Zantac **1624**
Zantac Injection **1619**
Zantac Injection Pharmacy Bulk Package **1622**

Rifampin (Co-administration of nisoldipine with known CYP3A4 inducer, such as rifampin, should be avoided because of possible reduced nisoldipine plasma concentrations).
No products indexed under this heading.

Food Interactions

Diet, high-lipid (Food with a high fat content has a pronounced effect on the release of nisoldipine resulting in a significant increase in peak concentration (Cmax) by up to 300%; concomitant intake of high-fat meal should be avoided).

SULFAMYLON CREAM

(Mafenide Acetate) **2162**
None cited in PDR database.

SULFAMYLON FOR 5% TOPICAL SOLUTION

(Mafenide Acetate) **2162**
None cited in PDR database.

SUPRAX

(Cefixime) **1843**
May interact with oral anticoagulants and certain other agents. Compounds in these categories include:

Anisindione (Co-administration has resulted in increased prothrombin time, with or without clinical bleeding). Products include:
Miradon Tablets **3042**

Carbamazepine (Co-administration has resulted in elevated carbamazepine levels). Products include:

Carbatrol Capsules 3171
Equetro Extended-Release Capsules 3180
Tegretol/Tegretol-XR 2295

Dicumarol (Co-administration has resulted in increased prothrombin time, with or without clinical bleeding).
No products indexed under this heading.

Warfarin Sodium (Co-administration has resulted in increased prothrombin time, with or without clinical bleeding). Products include:
Coumadin for Injection 898
Coumadin Tablets 898

Food Interactions

Food, unspecified (Increases time to maximal absorption approximately 0.8 hour).

SURE2ENDURE TABLETS

(Glucosamine Hydrochloride, Herbals with Vitamins & Minerals) ...... ▣821
None cited in PDR database.

SUSTIVA CAPSULES

(Efavirenz) 930
May interact with central nervous system depressants, ergot-containing drugs, phenytoin, and certain other agents. Compounds in these categories include:

Alfentanil Hydrochloride (Potential for additive central nervous system effects when Sustiva is used concomitantly with other CNS depressants).
No products indexed under this heading.

Alprazolam (Potential for additive central nervous system effects when Sustiva is used concomitantly with other CNS depressants). Products include:
Niravam Orally Disintegrating Tablets 3092

Amprenavir (Efavirenz has the potential to decrease serum concentrations of amprenavir). Products include:
Agenerase Capsules 1327
Agenerase Oral Solution 1332

Aprobarbital (Potential for additive central nervous system effects when Sustiva is used concomitantly with other CNS depressants).
No products indexed under this heading.

Astemizole (Efavirenz has been shown *in vivo* to induce CYP3A4, other compounds that are substrates of CYP3A4, such as astemizole, may have decreased plasma concentrations when co-administered; *in vitro* efavirenz inhibits its 3A4, co-administration with the drugs primarily metabolized by this isoenzyme, such as astemizole, may result in altered plasma concentrations of astemizole; concurrent use should be avoided).
No products indexed under this heading.

Atazanavir (Co-administration has resulted in decreases in atazanavir Cmax (59%) and AUC (74%)).
No products indexed under this heading.

Azithromycin Dihydrate (Co-administration has resulted in increases in azithromycin Cmax (22%) with no change in AUC; no dosage adjustment is necessary).
No products indexed under this heading.

Buprenorphine Hydrochloride (Potential for additive central nervous system effects when Sustiva is used concomitantly with other CNS depressants). Products include:
Buprenex Injectable 2716
Suboxone Tablets 2717
Subutex Tablets 2717

Buspirone Hydrochloride (Potential for additive central nervous system effects when Sustiva is used concomitantly with other CNS depressants).
No products indexed under this heading.

Butabarbital (Potential for additive central nervous system effects when Sustiva is used concomitantly with other CNS depressants).
No products indexed under this heading.

Butalbital (Potential for additive central nervous system effects when Sustiva is used concomitantly with other CNS depressants).
No products indexed under this heading.

Carbamazepine (Potential for reduction in anticonvulsant and/or efavirenz plasma levels). Products include:
Carbatrol Capsules 3171
Equetro Extended-Release Capsules 3180
Tegretol/Tegretol-XR 2295

Chlordiazepoxide (Potential for additive central nervous system effects when Sustiva is used concomitantly with other CNS depressants).
No products indexed under this heading.

Chlordiazepoxide Hydrochloride (Potential for additive central nervous system effects when Sustiva is used concomitantly with other CNS depressants). Products include:
Librium Capsules 3347

Chlorpromazine (Potential for additive central nervous system effects when Sustiva is used concomitantly with other CNS depressants).
No products indexed under this heading.

Chlorpromazine Hydrochloride (Potential for additive central nervous system effects when Sustiva is used concomitantly with other CNS depressants).
No products indexed under this heading.

Chlorprothixene (Potential for additive central nervous system effects when Sustiva is used concomitantly with other CNS depressants).
No products indexed under this heading.

Chlorprothixene Hydrochloride (Potential for additive central nervous system effects when Sustiva is used concomitantly with other CNS depressants).
No products indexed under this heading.

Chlorprothixene Lactate (Potential for additive central nervous system effects when Sustiva is used concomitantly with other CNS depressants).
No products indexed under this heading.

Cisapride (Efavirenz has been shown *in vivo* to induce CYP3A4, other compounds that are substrates of CYP3A4, such as cisapride, may have decreased plasma concentrations when co-administered; *in vitro* efavirenz inhibits its 3A4, co-administration with the drugs primarily metabolized by this isoenzyme, such as cisapride, may result in altered plasma concentrations of cisapride; concurrent use should be avoided).
No products indexed under this heading.

Clarithromycin (Decreased plasma concentration of clarithromycin and increased 14-OH metabolite concentration; clinical significance is not known). Products include:
Biaxin/Biaxin XL 402
PREVPAC 3284

Clorazepate Dipotassium (Potential for additive central nervous system effects when Sustiva is used concomitantly with other CNS depressants). Products include:
Tranxene 2474

Clozapine (Potential for additive central nervous system effects when Sustiva is used concomitantly with other CNS depressants). Products include:
Clozaril Tablets 2184
FazaClo Orally Disintegrating Tablets 551

Codeine Phosphate (Potential for additive central nervous system effects when Sustiva is used concomitantly with other CNS depressants). Products include:
Tylenol with Codeine Tablets 2391

Desflurane (Potential for additive central nervous system effects when Sustiva is used concomitantly with other CNS depressants).
No products indexed under this heading.

Dezocine (Potential for additive central nervous system effects when Sustiva is used concomitantly with other CNS depressants).
No products indexed under this heading.

Diazepam (Potential for additive central nervous system effects when Sustiva is used concomitantly with other CNS depressants). Products include:
Diastat Rectal Delivery System 3343
Valium Tablets 2819

Dihydroergotamine Mesylate (Efavirenz has been shown *in vivo* to induce CYP3A4, other compounds that are substrates of CYP3A4, such as ergot derivatives, may have decreased plasma concentrations when co-administered; *in vitro* efavirenz inhibits 3A4, co-administration with the drugs primarily metabolized by this isoenzyme, such as ergot derivatives, may result in altered plasma concentrations of ergot derivatives; concurrent use should be avoided). Products include:
Migranal Nasal Spray 3348

Droperidol (Potential for additive central nervous system effects when Sustiva is used concomitantly with other CNS depressants).
No products indexed under this heading.

Enflurane (Potential for additive central nervous system effects when Sustiva is used concomitantly with other CNS depressants).
No products indexed under this heading.

Ergonovine Maleate (Efavirenz has been shown *in vivo* to induce CYP3A4, other compounds that are substrates of CYP3A4, such as ergot derivatives, may have decreased plasma concentrations when co-administered; *in vitro* efavirenz inhibits 3A4, co-administration with the drugs primarily metabolized by this isoenzyme, such as ergot derivatives, may result in altered plasma concentrations of ergot derivatives; concurrent use should be avoided).
No products indexed under this heading.

Ergotamine Tartrate (Efavirenz has been shown *in vivo* to induce CYP3A4, other compounds that are substrates of CYP3A4, such as ergot derivatives, may have decreased plasma concentrations when co-administered; *in vitro* efavirenz inhibits 3A4, co-administration with the drugs primarily metabolized by this isoenzyme, such as ergot derivatives, may result in altered plasma concentrations of ergot derivatives; concurrent use should be avoided).
No products indexed under this heading.

Estazolam (Potential for additive central nervous system effects when Sustiva is used concomitantly with other CNS depressants). Products include:
ProSom Tablets 517

Ethanol (Potential for additive central nervous system effects when Sustiva is used concomitantly with other CNS depressants).
No products indexed under this heading.

Ethchlorvynol (Potential for additive central nervous system effects when Sustiva is used concomitantly with other CNS depressants).
No products indexed under this heading.

Ethinamate (Potential for additive central nervous system effects when Sustiva is used concomitantly with other CNS depressants).
No products indexed under this heading.

Ethinyl Estradiol (Co-administration has resulted in increased AUC for ethinyl estradiol; there was no effect on efavirenz AUC or Cmax; clinical significance is unknown). Products include:
Mircette Tablets 1066
NuvaRing 2340
Ortho-Cyclen/Ortho Tri-Cyclen 2429
Ortho Evra Transdermal System 2417
Ortho Tri-Cyclen Lo Tablets 2436
Seasonique Tablets 1077
Yasmin 28 Tablets 796
Yaz Tablets 803

Ethyl Alcohol (Potential for additive central nervous system effects when Sustiva is used concomitantly with other CNS depressants).
No products indexed under this heading.

Fentanyl (Potential for additive central nervous system effects when Sustiva is used concomitantly with other CNS depressants). Products include:
Duragesic Transdermal System 2373
Ionsys Transdermal System 2379

Fentanyl Citrate (Potential for additive central nervous system effects when Sustiva is used concomitantly with other CNS depressants). Products include:
Actiq 979

Fluconazole (Co-administration has resulted in increase in 16% AUC for efavirenz; there was no change in fluconazole Cmax or AUC).

No products indexed under this heading.

Fluphenazine Decanoate (Potential for additive central nervous system effects when Sustiva is used concomitantly with other CNS depressants).

No products indexed under this heading.

Fluphenazine Enanthate (Potential for additive central nervous system effects when Sustiva is used concomitantly with other CNS depressants).

No products indexed under this heading.

Fluphenazine Hydrochloride (Potential for additive central nervous system effects when Sustiva is used concomitantly with other CNS depressants).

No products indexed under this heading.

Flurazepam Hydrochloride (Potential for additive central nervous system effects when Sustiva is used concomitantly with other CNS depressants). Products include:

Fosphenytoin Sodium (Potential for reduction in anticonvulsant and/ or efavirenz plasma levels).

No products indexed under this heading.

Glutethimide (Potential for additive central nervous system effects when Sustiva is used concomitantly with other CNS depressants).

No products indexed under this heading.

Haloperidol (Potential for additive central nervous system effects when Sustiva is used concomitantly with other CNS depressants).

No products indexed under this heading.

Haloperidol Decanoate (Potential for additive central nervous system effects when Sustiva is used concomitantly with other CNS depressants).

No products indexed under this heading.

Hydrocodone Bitartrate (Potential for additive central nervous system effects when Sustiva is used concomitantly with other CNS depressants). Products include:

Hydrocodone Polistirex (Potential for additive central nervous system effects when Sustiva is used concomitantly with other CNS depressants). Products include:

Hydromorphone Hydrochloride (Potential for additive central nervous system effects when Sustiva is used concomitantly with other CNS depressants). Products include:

Hydroxyzine Hydrochloride (Potential for additive central nervous system effects when Sustiva is used concomitantly with other CNS depressants).

No products indexed under this heading.

Hypericum (St. John's Wort is expected to substantially decrease plasma levels of efavirenz; concurrent use is not recommended). Products include:

Indinavir Sulfate (Decreased plasma concentration of indinavir; indinavir dose should be increased). Products include:

Isoflurane (Potential for additive central nervous system effects when Sustiva is used concomitantly with other CNS depressants).

No products indexed under this heading.

Itraconazole (Potential for decreased itraconazole concentrations).

No products indexed under this heading.

Ketamine Hydrochloride (Potential for additive central nervous system effects when Sustiva is used concomitantly with other CNS depressants).

No products indexed under this heading.

Ketoconazole (Potential for decreased ketoconazole concentrations). Products include:

Levomethadyl Acetate Hydrochloride (Potential for additive central nervous system effects when Sustiva is used concomitantly with other CNS depressants).

No products indexed under this heading.

Levorphanol Tartrate (Potential for additive central nervous system effects when Sustiva is used concomitantly with other CNS depressants).

No products indexed under this heading.

Lorazepam (Potential for additive central nervous system effects when Sustiva is used concomitantly with other CNS depressants).

No products indexed under this heading.

Loxapine Hydrochloride (Potential for additive central nervous system effects when Sustiva is used concomitantly with other CNS depressants).

No products indexed under this heading.

Loxapine Succinate (Potential for additive central nervous system effects when Sustiva is used concomitantly with other CNS depressants).

No products indexed under this heading.

Meperidine Hydrochloride (Potential for additive central nervous system effects when Sustiva is used concomitantly with other CNS depressants).

No products indexed under this heading.

Mephobarbital (Potential for additive central nervous system effects when Sustiva is used concomitantly with other CNS depressants).

No products indexed under this heading.

Meprobamate (Potential for additive central nervous system effects when Sustiva is used concomitantly with other CNS depressants).

No products indexed under this heading.

Mesoridazine Besylate (Potential for additive central nervous system effects when Sustiva is used concomitantly with other CNS depressants).

No products indexed under this heading.

Methadone Hydrochloride (Decreased plasma concentration of methadone; methadone dose may need to be increased).

No products indexed under this heading.

Methohexital Sodium (Potential for additive central nervous system effects when Sustiva is used concomitantly with other CNS depressants).

No products indexed under this heading.

Methotrimeprazine (Potential for additive central nervous system effects when Sustiva is used concomitantly with other CNS depressants).

No products indexed under this heading.

Methoxyflurane (Potential for additive central nervous system effects when Sustiva is used concomitantly with other CNS depressants).

No products indexed under this heading.

Methylergonovine Maleate (Efavirenz has been shown *in vivo* to induce CYP3A4, other compounds that are substrates of CYP3A4, such as ergot derivatives, may have decreased plasma concentrations when co-administered; *in vitro* efavirenz inhibits 3A4, co-administration with the drugs primarily metabolized by this isoenzyme, such as ergot derivatives, may result in altered plasma concentrations of ergot derivatives; concurrent use should be avoided).

No products indexed under this heading.

Methysergide Maleate (Efavirenz has been shown *in vivo* to induce CYP3A4, other compounds that are substrates of CYP3A4, such as ergot derivatives, may have decreased plasma concentrations when co-administered; *in vitro* efavirenz inhibits 3A4, co-administration with the drugs primarily metabolized by this isoenzyme, such as ergot derivatives, may result in altered plasma concentrations of ergot derivatives; concurrent use should be avoided).

No products indexed under this heading.

Midazolam Hydrochloride (Efavirenz has been shown *in vivo* to induce CYP3A4, other compounds that are substrates of CYP3A4, such as midazolam, may have decreased plasma concentrations when co-administered; *in vitro* efavirenz inhibits 3A4, co-administration with the drugs primarily metabolized by this isoenzyme, such as midazolam, may

result in altered plasma concentrations of midazolam; concurrent use should be avoided).

No products indexed under this heading.

Molindone Hydrochloride (Potential for additive central nervous system effects when Sustiva is used concomitantly with other CNS depressants). Products include:

Morphine Sulfate (Potential for additive central nervous system effects when Sustiva is used concomitantly with other CNS depressants). Products include:

Nelfinavir Mesylate (Co-administration in uninfected individuals has resulted in increases in AUC (20%) and Cmax (21%) for nelfinavir; no dose adjustment is necessary). Products include:

Olanzapine (Potential for additive central nervous system effects when Sustiva is used concomitantly with other CNS depressants). Products include:

Oxazepam (Potential for additive central nervous system effects when Sustiva is used concomitantly with other CNS depressants).

No products indexed under this heading.

Oxycodone Hydrochloride (Potential for additive central nervous system effects when Sustiva is used concomitantly with other CNS depressants). Products include:

Pentobarbital Sodium (Potential for additive central nervous system effects when Sustiva is used concomitantly with other CNS depressants). Products include:

Perphenazine (Potential for additive central nervous system effects when Sustiva is used concomitantly with other CNS depressants).

No products indexed under this heading.

Phenobarbital (Potential for reduction in anticonvulsant and/or efavirenz plasma levels). Products include:

Phenytoin (Potential for reduction in anticonvulsant and/or efavirenz plasma levels).

No products indexed under this heading.

Phenytoin Sodium (Potential for reduction in anticonvulsant and/or efavirenz plasma levels). Products include:

Prazepam (Potential for additive central nervous system effects when Sustiva is used concomitantly with other CNS depressants).

No products indexed under this heading.

Prochlorperazine (Potential for additive central nervous system effects when Sustiva is used concomitantly with other CNS depressants).
No products indexed under this heading.

Promethazine Hydrochloride (Potential for additive central nervous system effects when Sustiva is used concomitantly with other CNS depressants). Products include:
Phenergan Tablets and Suppositories 3440

Propofol (Potential for additive central nervous system effects when Sustiva is used concomitantly with other CNS depressants).
No products indexed under this heading.

Propoxyphene Hydrochloride (Potential for additive central nervous system effects when Sustiva is used concomitantly with other CNS depressants).
No products indexed under this heading.

Propoxyphene Napsylate (Potential for additive central nervous system effects when Sustiva is used concomitantly with other CNS depressants).
No products indexed under this heading.

Quazepam (Potential for additive central nervous system effects when Sustiva is used concomitantly with other CNS depressants).
No products indexed under this heading.

Quetiapine Fumarate (Potential for additive central nervous system effects when Sustiva is used concomitantly with other CNS depressants). Products include:
Seroquel Tablets 690

Remifentanil Hydrochloride (Potential for additive central nervous system effects when Sustiva is used concomitantly with other CNS depressants).
No products indexed under this heading.

Rifabutin (Decreased plasma concentration of rifabutin; rifabutin dose should be increased by 50%).
No products indexed under this heading.

Rifampin (Co-administration has resulted in decreased efavirenz plasma concentrations; clinical significance is unknown).
No products indexed under this heading.

Risperidone (Potential for additive central nervous system effects when Sustiva is used concomitantly with other CNS depressants). Products include:
Risperdal 1676
Risperdal Consta Long-Acting Injection 1682
Risperdal M-Tab Orally Disintegrating Tablets 1676

Ritonavir (Co-administration has resulted in increases in AUC for each drug by 20%; the combination was associated with a higher frequency of adverse clinical experiences including dizziness, nausea, paresthesia, and laboratory abnormalities (elevated liver enzymes)). Products include:
Kaletra 476
Norvir 503

Saquinavir (Co-administration with saquinavir soft gelatin capsule has resulted in decreases in AUC (62%) and Cmax (50%) for saquinavir; saquinavir should not be used as sole protease inhibitor in combination with Sustiva).
No products indexed under this heading.

Saquinavir Mesylate (Co-administration with saquinavir soft gelatin capsule has resulted in decreases in AUC (62%) and Cmax (50%) for saquinavir; saquinavir should not be used as sole protease inhibitor in combination with Sustiva). Products include:
Invirase 2772

Secobarbital Sodium (Potential for additive central nervous system effects when Sustiva is used concomitantly with other CNS depressants).
No products indexed under this heading.

Sevoflurane (Potential for additive central nervous system effects when Sustiva is used concomitantly with other CNS depressants). Products include:
Ultane Liquid for Inhalation 531

Sodium Oxybate (Potential for additive central nervous system effects when Sustiva is used concomitantly with other CNS depressants). Products include:
Xyrem Oral Solution 1688

Sufentanil Citrate (Potential for additive central nervous system effects when Sustiva is used concomitantly with other CNS depressants).
No products indexed under this heading.

Temazepam (Potential for additive central nervous system effects when Sustiva is used concomitantly with other CNS depressants). Products include:
Restoril Capsules 1860

Thiamylal Sodium (Potential for additive central nervous system effects when Sustiva is used concomitantly with other CNS depressants).
No products indexed under this heading.

Thioridazine Hydrochloride (Potential for additive central nervous system effects when Sustiva is used concomitantly with other CNS depressants). Products include:
Thioridazine Hydrochloride Tablets 2163

Thiothixene (Potential for additive central nervous system effects when Sustiva is used concomitantly with other CNS depressants). Products include:
Thiothixene Capsules 2165

Triazolam (Efavirenz has been shown *in vivo* to induce CYP3A4, other compounds that are substrates of CYP3A4, such as triazolam, may have decreased plasma concentrations when co-administered; *in vitro* efavirenz inhibits 3A4, co-administration with the drugs primarily metabolized by this isoenzyme, such as triazolam, may result in altered plasma concentrations of triazolam; concurrent use should be avoided).
No products indexed under this heading.

Trifluoperazine Hydrochloride (Potential for additive central nervous system effects when Sustiva is used concomitantly with other CNS depressants).
No products indexed under this heading.

Voriconazole (Co-administration has resulted in increases in voriconazole Cmax (38%) and AUC (44%); efavirenz will significantly decrease voriconazole concentration therefore co-administration is contraindicated). Products include:
VFEND I.V. 2564
VFEND Oral Suspension 2564
VFEND Tablets 2564

Warfarin Sodium (Co-administration may result in increased or decreased plasma concentrations and effects of warfarin). Products include:
Coumadin for Injection 898
Coumadin Tablets 898

Zaleplon (Potential for additive central nervous system effects when Sustiva is used concomitantly with other CNS depressants). Products include:
Sonata Capsules 1717

Ziprasidone Hydrochloride (Potential for additive central nervous system effects when Sustiva is used concomitantly with other CNS depressants). Products include:
Geodon Capsules 2529

Zolpidem Tartrate (Potential for additive central nervous system effects when Sustiva is used concomitantly with other CNS depressants). Products include:
Ambien Tablets 2851
Ambien CR Tablets 2855

Food Interactions

Alcohol (Potential for additive central nervous system effects when Sustiva is used concomitantly with alcohol).

Food, unspecified (High fat meal may increase the absorption of Sustiva and should be avoided; it can be taken with or without meals of normal composition).

SUSTIVA TABLETS

(Efavirenz) 930
See Sustiva Capsules

SUTENT CAPSULES

(Sunitinib malate) 2560
May interact with cytochrome p450 3a4 inducers (selected), cytochrome p450 3a4 inhibitors, potent, and certain other agents. Compounds in these categories include:

Allium sativum (Concurrent administration of sunitinib with CYP3A4 inducers (e.g., rifampin) may decrease plasma sunitinib concentrations. Dose increase of sunitinib to 87.5 mg daily should be considered with co-administration).
No products indexed under this heading.

Amprenavir (Concurrent administration of sunitinib with strong CYP3A4 inhibitors (e.g., ketoconazole) may increase sunitinib plasma concentrations. Dose reduction of sunitinib to 37.5 mg daily is recommended with co-administration). Products include:
Agenerase Capsules 1327
Agenerase Oral Solution 1332

Aprepitant (Concurrent administration of sunitinib with CYP3A4 inducers (e.g., rifampin) may decrease plasma sunitinib concentrations. Dose increase of sunitinib to 87.5 mg daily should be considered with co-administration). Products include:
Emend Capsules 1963

Atazanavir (Concurrent administration of sunitinib with strong CYP3A4 inhibitors (e.g., ketoconazole) may increase sunitinib plasma concentrations. Dose reduction of sunitinib to 37.5 mg daily is recommended with co-administration).
No products indexed under this heading.

Atazanavir sulfate (Concurrent administration of sunitinib with strong CYP3A4 inhibitors (e.g., ketoconazole) may increase sunitinib plasma concentrations. Dose reduction of sunitinib to 37.5 mg daily is recommended with co-administration). Products include:
Reyataz Capsules 921

Betamethasone Acetate (Concurrent administration of sunitinib with CYP3A4 inducers (e.g., rifampin) may decrease plasma sunitinib concentrations. Dose increase of sunitinib to 87.5 mg daily should be considered with co-administration).
No products indexed under this heading.

Betamethasone Sodium Phosphate (Concurrent administration of sunitinib with CYP3A4 inducers (e.g., rifampin) may decrease plasma sunitinib concentrations. Dose increase of sunitinib to 87.5 mg daily should be considered with co-administration).
No products indexed under this heading.

Carbamazepine (Concurrent administration of sunitinib with CYP3A4 inducers (e.g., rifampin) may decrease plasma sunitinib concentrations. Dose increase of sunitinib to 87.5 mg daily should be considered with co-administration). Products include:
Carbatrol Capsules 3171
Equetro Extended-Release Capsules 3180
Tegretol/Tegretol-XR 2295

Ciprofloxacin Hydrochloride (Concurrent administration of sunitinib with CYP3A4 inducers (e.g., rifampin) may decrease plasma sunitinib concentrations. Dose increase of sunitinib to 87.5 mg daily should be considered with co-administration). Products include:
Ciloxan Ophthalmic Ointment 559
Ciloxan Ophthalmic Solution .... ⊙206
Cipro Tablets 2977
Proquin XR Tablets 1153

Cisplatin (Concurrent administration of sunitinib with CYP3A4 inducers (e.g., rifampin) may decrease plasma sunitinib concentrations. Dose increase of sunitinib to 87.5 mg daily should be considered with co-administration).
No products indexed under this heading.

Clarithromycin (Concurrent administration of sunitinib with strong CYP3A4 inhibitors (e.g., ketoconazole) may increase sunitinib plasma concentrations. Dose reduction of sunitinib to 37.5 mg daily is recommended with co-administration). Products include:
Biaxin/Biaxin XL 402
PREVPAC 3284

Cortisone Acetate (Concurrent administration of sunitinib with CYP3A4 inducers (e.g., rifampin) may decrease plasma sunitinib concentrations. Dose increase of sunitinib to 87.5 mg daily should be considered with co-administration).
No products indexed under this heading.

Dexamethasone (Concurrent administration of sunitinib with CYP3A4 inducers (e.g., rifampin) may decrease plasma sunitinib concentrations. Dose increase of sunitinib to 87.5 mg daily should be considered with co-administration). Products include:
- Ciprodex Otic Suspension 559
- Decadron Tablets 1951
- TobraDex Ophthalmic Ointment 562
- TobraDex Ophthalmic Suspension ... 563

Dexamethasone Acetate (Concurrent administration of sunitinib with CYP3A4 inducers (e.g., rifampin) may decrease plasma sunitinib concentrations. Dose increase of sunitinib to 87.5 mg daily should be considered with co-administration).
No products indexed under this heading.

Dexamethasone Sodium Phosphate (Concurrent administration of sunitinib with CYP3A4 inducers (e.g., rifampin) may decrease plasma sunitinib concentrations. Dose increase of sunitinib to 87.5 mg daily should be considered with co-administration).
No products indexed under this heading.

Doxorubicin Hydrochloride (Concurrent administration of sunitinib with CYP3A4 inducers (e.g., rifampin) may decrease plasma sunitinib concentrations. Dose increase of sunitinib to 87.5 mg daily should be considered with co-administration).
No products indexed under this heading.

Efavirenz (Concurrent administration of sunitinib with CYP3A4 inducers (e.g., rifampin) may decrease plasma sunitinib concentrations. Dose increase of sunitinib to 87.5 mg daily should be considered with co-administration). Products include:
- Atripla Tablets 945
- Sustiva Capsules 930
- Sustiva Tablets 930

Ethosuximide (Concurrent administration of sunitinib with CYP3A4 inducers (e.g., rifampin) may decrease plasma sunitinib concentrations. Dose increase of sunitinib to 87.5 mg daily should be considered with co-administration).
No products indexed under this heading.

Felbamate (Concurrent administration of sunitinib with CYP3A4 inducers (e.g., rifampin) may decrease plasma sunitinib concentrations. Dose increase of sunitinib to 87.5 mg daily should be considered with co-administration).
No products indexed under this heading.

Fludrocortisone Acetate (Concurrent administration of sunitinib with CYP3A4 inducers (e.g., rifampin) may decrease plasma sunitinib concentrations. Dose increase of sunitinib to 87.5 mg daily should be considered with co-administration).
No products indexed under this heading.

Fosamprenavir Calcium (Concurrent administration of sunitinib with strong CYP3A4 inhibitors (e.g., ketoconazole) may increase sunitinib plasma concentrations. Dose reduction of sunitinib to 37.5 mg daily is recommended with co-administration). Products include:
- Lexiva Tablets 1505

Fosphenytoin Sodium (Concurrent administration of sunitinib with CYP3A4 inducers (e.g., rifampin) may decrease plasma sunitinib concentrations. Dose increase of sunitinib to 87.5 mg daily should be considered with co-administration).
No products indexed under this heading.

Garlic Extract (Concurrent administration of sunitinib with CYP3A4 inducers (e.g., rifampin) may decrease plasma sunitinib concentrations. Dose increase of sunitinib to 87.5 mg daily should be considered with co-administration).
No products indexed under this heading.

Garlic Oil (Concurrent administration of sunitinib with CYP3A4 inducers (e.g., rifampin) may decrease plasma sunitinib concentrations. Dose increase of sunitinib to 87.5 mg daily should be considered with co-administration).
No products indexed under this heading.

Hydrocortisone (Concurrent administration of sunitinib with CYP3A4 inducers (e.g., rifampin) may decrease plasma sunitinib concentrations. Dose increase of sunitinib to 87.5 mg daily should be considered with co-administration). Products include:
- Colocort Rectal Suspension, USP (Retention) 100 mg/60 mL........... 2476
- Hydrocortone Tablets 1989
- Preparation H Hydrocortisone Cream 646

Hydrocortisone Acetate (Concurrent administration of sunitinib with CYP3A4 inducers (e.g., rifampin) may decrease plasma sunitinib concentrations. Dose increase of sunitinib to 87.5 mg daily should be considered with co-administration). Products include:
- Analpram-HC 1159
- Pramosone 1161
- ProctoFoam-HC 3099

Hydrocortisone Butyrate (Concurrent administration of sunitinib with CYP3A4 inducers (e.g., rifampin) may decrease plasma sunitinib concentrations. Dose increase of sunitinib to 87.5 mg daily should be considered with co-administration). Products include:
- Locoid Lipocream Cream 1160

Hydrocortisone Cypionate (Concurrent administration of sunitinib with CYP3A4 inducers (e.g., rifampin) may decrease plasma sunitinib concentrations. Dose increase of sunitinib to 87.5 mg daily should be considered with co-administration).
No products indexed under this heading.

Hydrocortisone Hemisuccinate (Concurrent administration of sunitinib with CYP3A4 inducers (e.g., rifampin) may decrease plasma sunitinib concentrations. Dose increase of sunitinib to 87.5 mg daily should be considered with co-administration).
No products indexed under this heading.

Hydrocortisone Probutate (Concurrent administration of sunitinib with CYP3A4 inducers (e.g., rifampin) may decrease plasma sunitinib concentrations. Dose increase of sunitinib to 87.5 mg daily should be considered with co-administration).
No products indexed under this heading.

Hydrocortisone Sodium Phosphate (Concurrent administration of sunitinib with CYP3A4 inducers (e.g., rifampin) may decrease plasma sunitinib concentrations. Dose increase of sunitinib to 87.5 mg daily should be considered with co-administration).
No products indexed under this heading.

Hydrocortisone Sodium Succinate (Concurrent administration of sunitinib with CYP3A4 inducers (e.g., rifampin) may decrease plasma sunitinib concentrations. Dose increase of sunitinib to 87.5 mg daily should be considered with co-administration).
No products indexed under this heading.

Hydrocortisone Valerate (Concurrent administration of sunitinib with CYP3A4 inducers (e.g., rifampin) may decrease plasma sunitinib concentrations. Dose increase of sunitinib to 87.5 mg daily should be considered with co-administration).
No products indexed under this heading.

Hypericum (Co-administration of St. John's wort with sunitinib may decrease plasma concentrations of sunitinib unpredictably. Avoid concurrent administration of St. John's wort with sunitinib). Products include:
- Satiete Tablets 832

Hypericum Perforatum (Co-administration of St. John's wort with sunitinib may decrease plasma concentrations of sunitinib unpredictably. Avoid concurrent administration of St. John's wort with sunitinib).
No products indexed under this heading.

Indinavir Sulfate (Concurrent administration of sunitinib with strong CYP3A4 inhibitors (e.g., ketoconazole) may increase sunitinib plasma concentrations. Dose reduction of sunitinib to 37.5 mg daily is recommended with co-administration). Products include:
- Crixivan Capsules 1940

Itraconazole (Concurrent administration of sunitinib with strong CYP3A4 inhibitors (e.g., ketoconazole) may increase sunitinib plasma concentrations. Dose reduction of sunitinib to 37.5 mg daily is recommended with co-administration).
No products indexed under this heading.

Ketoconazole (Concurrent administration of sunitinib with strong CYP3A4 inhibitors (e.g., ketoconazole) may increase sunitinib plasma concentrations. Dose reduction of sunitinib to 37.5 mg daily is recommended with co-administration). Products include:
- Nizoral A-D Shampoo, 1% 1868

Lopinavir (Concurrent administration of sunitinib with strong CYP3A4 inhibitors (e.g., ketoconazole) may increase sunitinib plasma concentrations. Dose reduction of sunitinib to 37.5 mg daily is recommended with co-administration). Products include:
- Kaletra 476

Mephenytoin (Concurrent administration of sunitinib with CYP3A4 inducers (e.g., rifampin) may decrease plasma sunitinib concentrations. Dose increase of sunitinib to 87.5 mg daily should be considered with co-administration).
No products indexed under this heading.

Methsuximide (Concurrent administration of sunitinib with CYP3A4 inducers (e.g., rifampin) may decrease plasma sunitinib concentrations. Dose increase of sunitinib to 87.5 mg daily should be considered with co-administration).
No products indexed under this heading.

Methylprednisolone (Concurrent administration of sunitinib with CYP3A4 inducers (e.g., rifampin) may decrease plasma sunitinib concentrations. Dose increase of sunitinib to 87.5 mg daily should be considered with co-administration).
No products indexed under this heading.

Methylprednisolone Acetate (Concurrent administration of sunitinib with CYP3A4 inducers (e.g., rifampin) may decrease plasma sunitinib concentrations. Dose increase of sunitinib to 87.5 mg daily should be considered with co-administration). Products include:
- Depo-Medrol Injectable Suspension 2617
- Depo-Medrol Single-Dose Vial 2619

Methylprednisolone Sodium Succinate (Concurrent administration of sunitinib with CYP3A4 inducers (e.g., rifampin) may decrease plasma sunitinib concentrations. Dose increase of sunitinib to 87.5 mg daily should be considered with co-administration).
No products indexed under this heading.

Modafinil (Concurrent administration of sunitinib with CYP3A4 inducers (e.g., rifampin) may decrease plasma sunitinib concentrations. Dose increase of sunitinib to 87.5 mg daily should be considered with co-administration). Products include:
- Provigil Tablets 988

Nefazodone Hydrochloride (Concurrent administration of sunitinib with strong CYP3A4 inhibitors (e.g., ketoconazole) may increase sunitinib plasma concentrations. Dose reduction of sunitinib to 37.5 mg daily is recommended with co-administration).
No products indexed under this heading.

Nelfinavir Mesylate (Concurrent administration of sunitinib with strong CYP3A4 inhibitors (e.g., ketoconazole) may increase sunitinib plasma concentrations. Dose reduction of sunitinib to 37.5 mg daily is recommended with co-administration). Products include:
- Viracept 2577

Nevirapine (Concurrent administration of sunitinib with CYP3A4 inducers (e.g., rifampin) may decrease plasma sunitinib concentrations. Dose increase of sunitinib to 87.5 mg daily should be considered with co-administration). Products include:

Viramune Oral Suspension 873
Viramune Tablets 873

Oxcarbazepine (Concurrent administration of sunitinib with CYP3A4 inducers (e.g., rifampin) may decrease plasma sunitinib concentrations. Dose increase of sunitinib to 87.5 mg daily should be considered with co-administration).
Products include:
Trileptal Tablets 2300
Trileptal Oral Suspension 2300

Phenobarbital (Concurrent administration of sunitinib with CYP3A4 inducers (e.g., rifampin) may decrease plasma sunitinib concentrations. Dose increase of sunitinib to 87.5 mg daily should be considered with co-administration).
Products include:
Donnatal Extentabs 2493

Phenobarbital Sodium (Concurrent administration of sunitinib with CYP3A4 inducers (e.g., rifampin) may decrease plasma sunitinib concentrations. Dose increase of sunitinib to 87.5 mg daily should be considered with co-administration).
No products indexed under this heading.

Phenytoin (Concurrent administration of sunitinib with CYP3A4 inducers (e.g., rifampin) may decrease plasma sunitinib concentrations. Dose increase of sunitinib to 87.5 mg daily should be considered with co-administration).
No products indexed under this heading.

Phenytoin Sodium (Concurrent administration of sunitinib with CYP3A4 inducers (e.g., rifampin) may decrease plasma sunitinib concentrations. Dose increase of sunitinib to 87.5 mg daily should be considered with co-administration).
Products include:
Phenytek Capsules 2160

Prednisolone Acetate (Concurrent administration of sunitinib with CYP3A4 inducers (e.g., rifampin) may decrease plasma sunitinib concentrations. Dose increase of sunitinib to 87.5 mg daily should be considered with co-administration).
Products include:
Blephamide Ophthalmic Ointment 568
Blephamide Ophthalmic Suspension 569
Poly-Pred Ophthalmic Suspension .... ⊙233
Pred Forte Ophthalmic Suspension .... ⊙235
Pred Mild Ophthalmic Suspension .... ⊙238
Pred-G Ophthalmic Ointment .... ⊙237
Pred-G Ophthalmic Suspension ...... ⊙236

Prednisolone Sodium Phosphate (Concurrent administration of sunitinib with CYP3A4 inducers (e.g., rifampin) may decrease plasma sunitinib concentrations. Dose increase of sunitinib to 87.5 mg daily should be considered with co-administration).
No products indexed under this heading.

Prednisolone Tebutate (Concurrent administration of sunitinib with CYP3A4 inducers (e.g., rifampin) may decrease plasma sunitinib concentrations. Dose increase of sunitinib to 87.5 mg daily should be considered with co-administration).
No products indexed under this heading.

Prednisone (Concurrent administration of sunitinib with CYP3A4 inducers (e.g., rifampin) may decrease plasma sunitinib concentrations. Dose increase of sunitinib to 87.5 mg daily should be considered with co-administration).
No products indexed under this heading.

Primidone (Concurrent administration of sunitinib with CYP3A4 inducers (e.g., rifampin) may decrease plasma sunitinib concentrations. Dose increase of sunitinib to 87.5 mg daily should be considered with co-administration).
No products indexed under this heading.

Rifabutin (Concurrent administration of sunitinib with CYP3A4 inducers (e.g., rifampin) may decrease plasma sunitinib concentrations. Dose increase of sunitinib to 87.5 mg daily should be considered with co-administration).
No products indexed under this heading.

Rifampicin (Concurrent administration of sunitinib with CYP3A4 inducers (e.g., rifampin) may decrease plasma sunitinib concentrations. Dose increase of sunitinib to 87.5 mg daily should be considered with co-administration).
No products indexed under this heading.

Rifampin (Concurrent administration of sunitinib with CYP3A4 inducers (e.g., rifampin) may decrease plasma sunitinib concentrations. Dose increase of sunitinib to 87.5 mg daily should be considered with co-administration).
No products indexed under this heading.

Rifapentine (Concurrent administration of sunitinib with CYP3A4 inducers (e.g., rifampin) may decrease plasma sunitinib concentrations. Dose increase of sunitinib to 87.5 mg daily should be considered with co-administration).
No products indexed under this heading.

Ritonavir (Concurrent administration of sunitinib with strong CYP3A4 inhibitors (e.g., ketoconazole) may increase sunitinib plasma concentrations. Dose reduction of sunitinib to 37.5 mg daily is recommended with co-administration). Products include:
Kaletra 476
Norvir 503

Saquinavir (Concurrent administration of sunitinib with strong CYP3A4 inhibitors (e.g., ketoconazole) may increase sunitinib plasma concentrations. Dose reduction of sunitinib to 37.5 mg daily is recommended with co-administration).
No products indexed under this heading.

Saquinavir Mesylate (Concurrent administration of sunitinib with strong CYP3A4 inhibitors (e.g., ketoconazole) may increase sunitinib plasma concentrations. Dose reduction of sunitinib to 37.5 mg daily is recommended with co-administration). Products include:
Invirase 2772

Sulfinpyrazone (Concurrent administration of sunitinib with CYP3A4 inducers (e.g., rifampin) may decrease plasma sunitinib concentrations. Dose increase of sunitinib to 87.5 mg daily should be considered with co-administration).
No products indexed under this heading.

Telithromycin (Concurrent administration of sunitinib with strong CYP3A4 inhibitors (e.g., ketoconazole) may increase sunitinib plasma concentrations. Dose reduction of sunitinib to 37.5 mg daily is recommended with co-administration).
Products include:
Ketek Tablets 2903

Theophylline (Concurrent administration of sunitinib with CYP3A4 inducers (e.g., rifampin) may decrease plasma sunitinib concentrations. Dose increase of sunitinib to 87.5 mg daily should be considered with co-administration).
No products indexed under this heading.

Triamcinolone (Concurrent administration of sunitinib with CYP3A4 inducers (e.g., rifampin) may decrease plasma sunitinib concentrations. Dose increase of sunitinib to 87.5 mg daily should be considered with co-administration).
No products indexed under this heading.

Triamcinolone Acetonide (Concurrent administration of sunitinib with CYP3A4 inducers (e.g., rifampin) may decrease plasma sunitinib concentrations. Dose increase of sunitinib to 87.5 mg daily should be considered with co-administration). Products include:
Azmacort Inhalation Aerosol 1726
Nasacort AQ Nasal Spray 2922

Triamcinolone Diacetate (Concurrent administration of sunitinib with CYP3A4 inducers (e.g., rifampin) may decrease plasma sunitinib concentrations. Dose increase of sunitinib to 87.5 mg daily should be considered with co-administration).
No products indexed under this heading.

Triamcinolone Hexacetonide (Concurrent administration of sunitinib with CYP3A4 inducers (e.g., rifampin) may decrease plasma sunitinib concentrations. Dose increase of sunitinib to 87.5 mg daily should be considered with co-administration).
No products indexed under this heading.

Troglitazone (Concurrent administration of sunitinib with CYP3A4 inducers (e.g., rifampin) may decrease plasma sunitinib concentrations. Dose increase of sunitinib to 87.5 mg daily should be considered with co-administration).
No products indexed under this heading.

Troleandomycin (Concurrent administration of sunitinib with strong CYP3A4 inhibitors (e.g., ketoconazole) may increase sunitinib plasma concentrations. Dose reduction of sunitinib to 37.5 mg daily is recommended with co-administration).
No products indexed under this heading.

Voriconazole (Concurrent administration of sunitinib with strong CYP3A4 inhibitors (e.g., ketoconazole) may increase sunitinib plasma concentrations. Dose reduction of sunitinib to 37.5 mg daily is recommended with co-administration).
Products include:
VFEND I.V. 2564
VFEND Oral Suspension 2564
VFEND Tablets 2564

Food Interactions

Grapefruit (Grapefruit may increase plasma concentrations of sunitinib malate).

Grapefruit Juice (Grapefruit may increase plasma concentrations of sunitinib maleate).

SYMBICORT 80/4.5 INHALATION AEROSOL

(Budesonide, Formoterol fumarate dihydrate).. 3511
May interact with beta blockers, cytochrome p450 3a4 inhibitors (selected), diuretics, monoamine oxidase inhibitors, tricyclic antidepressants, and certain other agents. Compounds in these categories include:

Acebutolol Hydrochloride (Beta-blockers (including eye drops) may not only block the pulmonary effect of beta-agonists (e.g., formoterol- a component of Symbicort), but may produce severe bronchospasm in asthma patients).
No products indexed under this heading.

Acetazolamide (Concomitant administration of CYP3A4 inhibitors (e.g., itraconazole, clarithromycin, erythromycin, etc.) may inhibit the metabolism of, and increase the systemic exposure to, budesonide. Caution should be exercised with co-administration of Symbicort with potent CYP3A4 inhibitors).
No products indexed under this heading.

Amiloride Hydrochloride (The ECG changes and/or hypokalemia that may result from the administration of nonpotassium-sparing diuretics (e.g., loop or thiazide diuretics) can be acutely worsened by beta-agonists, especially when the recommended dose of the beta-agonist is exceeded. Caution is advised with co-administration of Symbicort with nonpotassium-sparing diuretics).
Products include:
Midamor Tablets 2026
Moduretic Tablets 2028

Amiodarone Hydrochloride (Concomitant administration of CYP3A4 inhibitors (e.g., itraconazole, clarithromycin, erythromycin, etc.) may inhibit the metabolism of, and increase the systemic exposure to, budesonide. Caution should be exercised with co-administration of Symbicort with potent CYP3A4 inhibitors).
No products indexed under this heading.

Amitriptyline Hydrochloride (Symbicort should be administered with caution to patients treated with TCAs, or within 2 weeks of discontinuation of TCAs, since these agents may potentiate formoterol action on the vascular system).
No products indexed under this heading.

Amoxapine (Symbicort should be administered with caution to patients treated with TCAs, or within 2 weeks of discontinuation of TCAs, since these agents may potentiate formoterol action on the vascular system).
No products indexed under this heading.

Amprenavir (Concomitant administration of CYP3A4 inhibitors (e.g., itraconazole, clarithromycin, erythromycin, etc.) may inhibit the metabolism of, and increase the systemic exposure to, budesonide. Caution should be exercised with co-administration of Symbicort with potent CYP3A4 inhibitors). Products include:
Agenerase Capsules **1327**
Agenerase Oral Solution **1332**

Anastrozole (Concomitant administration of CYP3A4 inhibitors (e.g., itraconazole, clarithromycin, erythromycin, etc.) may inhibit the metabolism of, and increase the systemic exposure to, budesonide. Caution should be exercised with co-administration of Symbicort with potent CYP3A4 inhibitors). Products include:
Arimidex Tablets **673**

Aprepitant (Concomitant administration of CYP3A4 inhibitors (e.g., itraconazole, clarithromycin, erythromycin, etc.) may inhibit the metabolism of, and increase the systemic exposure to, budesonide. Caution should be exercised with co-administration of Symbicort with potent CYP3A4 inhibitors). Products include:
Emend Capsules **1963**

Atenolol (Beta-blockers (including eye drops) may not only block the pulmonary effect of beta-agonists (e.g., formoterol- a component of Symbicort), but may produce severe bronchospasm in asthma patients).
No products indexed under this heading.

Bendroflumethiazide (The ECG changes and/or hypokalemia that may result from the administration of nonpotassium-sparing diuretics (e.g., loop or thiazide diuretics) can be acutely worsened by beta-agonists, especially when the recommended dose of the beta-agonist is exceeded. Caution is advised with co-administration of Symbicort with nonpotassium-sparing diuretics).
No products indexed under this heading.

Betaxolol Hydrochloride (Beta-blockers (including eye drops) may not only block the pulmonary effect of beta-agonists (e.g., formoterol- a component of Symbicort), but may produce severe bronchospasm in asthma patients). Products include:
Betoptic S Ophthalmic Suspension................................ **558**

Bisoprolol Fumarate (Beta-blockers (including eye drops) may not only block the pulmonary effect of beta-agonists (e.g., formoterol- a component of Symbicort), but may produce severe bronchospasm in asthma patients).
No products indexed under this heading.

Bumetanide (The ECG changes and/or hypokalemia that may result from the administration of nonpotassium-sparing diuretics (e.g., loop or thiazide diuretics) can be acutely worsened by beta-agonists, especially when the recommended dose of the beta-agonist is exceeded. Caution is advised with co-administration of Symbicort with nonpotassium-sparing diuretics). Products include:
Bumex Tablets **2746**

Carteolol Hydrochloride (Beta-blockers (including eye drops) may not only block the pulmonary effect of beta-agonists (e.g., formoterol- a component of Symbicort), but may produce severe bronchospasm in asthma patients). Products include:
Carteolol Hydrochloride Ophthalmic Solution USP, 1%...... ⊙**249**

Chlorothiazide (The ECG changes and/or hypokalemia that may result from the administration of nonpotassium-sparing diuretics (e.g., loop or thiazide diuretics) can be acutely worsened by beta-agonists, especially when the recommended dose of the beta-agonist is exceeded. Caution is advised with co-administration of Symbicort with nonpotassium-sparing diuretics). Products include:
Diuril Oral Suspension **1954**

Chlorothiazide Sodium (The ECG changes and/or hypokalemia that may result from the administration of nonpotassium-sparing diuretics (e.g., loop or thiazide diuretics) can be acutely worsened by beta-agonists, especially when the recommended dose of the beta-agonist is exceeded. Caution is advised with co-administration of Symbicort with nonpotassium-sparing diuretics). Products include:
Diuril Sodium Intravenous **2467**

Chlorthalidone (The ECG changes and/or hypokalemia that may result from the administration of nonpotassium-sparing diuretics (e.g., loop or thiazide diuretics) can be acutely worsened by beta-agonists, especially when the recommended dose of the beta-agonist is exceeded. Caution is advised with co-administration of Symbicort with nonpotassium-sparing diuretics). Products include:
Clorpres Tablets **2153**

Cimetidine (Concomitant administration of CYP3A4 inhibitors (e.g., itraconazole, clarithromycin, erythromycin, etc.) may inhibit the metabolism of, and increase the systemic exposure to, budesonide. Caution should be exercised with co-administration of Symbicort with potent CYP3A4 inhibitors). Products include:
Tagamet HB 200 Tablets .... ▣**664**

Cimetidine Hydrochloride (Concomitant administration of CYP3A4 inhibitors (e.g., itraconazole, clarithromycin, erythromycin, etc.) may inhibit the metabolism of, and increase the systemic exposure to, budesonide. Caution should be exercised with co-administration of Symbicort with potent CYP3A4 inhibitors).
No products indexed under this heading.

Ciprofloxacin (Concomitant administration of CYP3A4 inhibitors (e.g., itraconazole, clarithromycin, erythromycin, etc.) may inhibit the metabolism of, and increase the systemic exposure to, budesonide. Caution should be exercised with co-administration of Symbicort with potent CYP3A4 inhibitors). Products include:
Cipro Oral Suspension **2977**
Cipro I.V. **2984**
Cipro XR Tablets **2990**
Ciprodex Otic Suspension **559**

Clarithromycin (Concomitant administration of CYP3A4 inhibitors (e.g., itraconazole, clarithromycin, erythromycin, etc.) may inhibit the metabolism of, and increase the systemic exposure to, budesonide. Caution should be exercised with co-administration of Symbicort with potent CYP3A4 inhibitors). Products include:
Biaxin/Biaxin XL **402**
PREVPAC **3284**

Clomipramine Hydrochloride (Symbicort should be administered with caution to patients treated with TCAs, or within 2 weeks of discontinuation of TCAs, since these agents may potentiate formoterol action on the vascular system).
No products indexed under this heading.

Clotrimazole (Concomitant administration of CYP3A4 inhibitors (e.g., itraconazole, clarithromycin, erythromycin, etc.) may inhibit the metabolism of, and increase the systemic exposure to, budesonide. Caution should be exercised with co-administration of Symbicort with potent CYP3A4 inhibitors). Products include:
Desenex Athlete's Foot Cream .... ▣**635**
Lotrimin **3039**
Lotrisone **3040**

Cyclosporine (Concomitant administration of CYP3A4 inhibitors (e.g., itraconazole, clarithromycin, erythromycin, etc.) may inhibit the metabolism of, and increase the systemic exposure to, budesonide. Caution should be exercised with co-administration of Symbicort with potent CYP3A4 inhibitors). Products include:
Gengraf Capsules **459**
Neoral Oral Solution **2259**
Neoral Soft Gelatin Capsules **2259**
Restasis Ophthalmic Emulsion **575**
Sandimmune **2275**

Dalfopristin (Concomitant administration of CYP3A4 inhibitors (e.g., itraconazole, clarithromycin, erythromycin, etc.) may inhibit the metabolism of, and increase the systemic exposure to, budesonide. Caution should be exercised with co-administration of Symbicort with potent CYP3A4 inhibitors).
No products indexed under this heading.

Danazol (Concomitant administration of CYP3A4 inhibitors (e.g., itraconazole, clarithromycin, erythromycin, etc.) may inhibit the metabolism of, and increase the systemic exposure to, budesonide. Caution should be exercised with co-administration of Symbicort with potent CYP3A4 inhibitors).
No products indexed under this heading.

Delavirdine Mesylate (Concomitant administration of CYP3A4 inhibitors (e.g., itraconazole, clarithromycin, erythromycin, etc.) may inhibit the metabolism of, and increase the systemic exposure to, budesonide. Caution should be exercised with co-administration of Symbicort with potent CYP3A4 inhibitors). Products include:
Rescriptor Tablets **2551**

Desipramine Hydrochloride (Symbicort should be administered with caution to patients treated with TCAs, or within 2 weeks of discontinuation of TCAs, since these agents may potentiate formoterol action on the vascular system).
No products indexed under this heading.

Diltiazem Hydrochloride (Concomitant administration of CYP3A4 inhibitors (e.g., itraconazole, clarithromycin, erythromycin, etc.) may inhibit the metabolism of, and increase the systemic exposure to, budesonide. Caution should be exercised with co-administration of Symbicort with potent CYP3A4 inhibitors). Products include:
Cardizem LA Extended Release Tablets **1728**
Tiazac Capsules **1201**

Diltiazem Maleate (Concomitant administration of CYP3A4 inhibitors (e.g., itraconazole, clarithromycin, erythromycin, etc.) may inhibit the metabolism of, and increase the systemic exposure to, budesonide. Caution should be exercised with co-administration of Symbicort with potent CYP3A4 inhibitors).
No products indexed under this heading.

Doxepin Hydrochloride (Symbicort should be administered with caution to patients treated with TCAs, or within 2 weeks of discontinuation of TCAs, since these agents may potentiate formoterol action on the vascular system).
No products indexed under this heading.

Efavirenz (Concomitant administration of CYP3A4 inhibitors (e.g., itraconazole, clarithromycin, erythromycin, etc.) may inhibit the metabolism of, and increase the systemic exposure to, budesonide. Caution should be exercised with co-administration of Symbicort with potent CYP3A4 inhibitors). Products include:
Atripla Tablets **945**
Sustiva Capsules **930**
Sustiva Tablets **930**

Erythromycin (Concomitant administration of CYP3A4 inhibitors (e.g., itraconazole, clarithromycin, erythromycin, etc.) may inhibit the metabolism of, and increase the systemic exposure to, budesonide. Caution should be exercised with co-administration of Symbicort with potent CYP3A4 inhibitors). Products include:
Ery-Tab Tablets **449**
Erythromycin Base Filmtab Tablets **455**
Erythromycin Delayed-Release Capsules, USP............................. **457**
PCE Dispertab Tablets **515**

Erythromycin Estolate (Concomitant administration of CYP3A4 inhibitors (e.g., itraconazole, clarithromycin, erythromycin, etc.) may inhibit the metabolism of, and increase the systemic exposure to, budesonide. Caution should be exercised with co-administration of Symbicort with potent CYP3A4 inhibitors).
No products indexed under this heading.

Erythromycin Ethylsuccinate (Concomitant administration of CYP3A4 inhibitors (e.g., itraconazole, clarithromycin, erythromycin, etc.) may inhibit the metabolism of, and increase the systemic exposure to, budesonide. Caution should be exercised with co-administration of Symbicort with potent CYP3A4 inhibitors). Products include:

Erythromycin Gluceptate (Concomitant administration of CYP3A4 inhibitors (e.g., itraconazole, clarithromycin, erythromycin, etc.) may inhibit the metabolism of, and increase the systemic exposure to, budesonide. Caution should be exercised with co-administration of Symbicort with potent CYP3A4 inhibitors).

No products indexed under this heading.

Erythromycin Lactobionate (Concomitant administration of CYP3A4 inhibitors (e.g., itraconazole, clarithromycin, erythromycin, etc.) may inhibit the metabolism of, and increase the systemic exposure to, budesonide. Caution should be exercised with co-administration of Symbicort with potent CYP3A4 inhibitors).

No products indexed under this heading.

Erythromycin Stearate (Concomitant administration of CYP3A4 inhibitors (e.g., itraconazole, clarithromycin, erythromycin, etc.) may inhibit the metabolism of, and increase the systemic exposure to, budesonide. Caution should be exercised with co-administration of Symbicort with potent CYP3A4 inhibitors). Products include:

Esmolol Hydrochloride (Beta-blockers (including eye drops) may not only block the pulmonary effect of beta-agonists (e.g., formoterol- a component of Symbicort), but may produce severe bronchospasm in asthma patients).

No products indexed under this heading.

Esomeprazole Magnesium (Concomitant administration of CYP3A4 inhibitors (e.g., itraconazole, clarithromycin, erythromycin, etc.) may inhibit the metabolism of, and increase the systemic exposure to, budesonide. Caution should be exercised with co-administration of Symbicort with potent CYP3A4 inhibitors). Products include:

Ethacrynic Acid (The ECG changes and/or hypokalemia that may result from the administration of nonpotassium-sparing diuretics (e.g., loop or thiazide diuretics) can be acutely worsened by beta-agonists, especially when the recommended dose of the beta-agonist is exceeded. Caution is advised with co-administration of Symbicort with nonpotassium-sparing diuretics). Products include:

Fluconazole (Concomitant administration of CYP3A4 inhibitors (e.g., itraconazole, clarithromycin, erythromycin, etc.) may inhibit the metabolism of, and increase the systemic exposure to, budesonide. Caution should be exercised with co-administration of Symbicort with potent CYP3A4 inhibitors).

No products indexed under this heading.

Fluoxetine Hydrochloride (Concomitant administration of CYP3A4

inhibitors (e.g., itraconazole, clarithromycin, erythromycin, etc.) may inhibit the metabolism of, and increase the systemic exposure to, budesonide. Caution should be exercised with co-administration of Symbicort with potent CYP3A4 inhibitors). Products include:

Fluvoxamine Maleate (Concomitant administration of CYP3A4 inhibitors (e.g., itraconazole, clarithromycin, erythromycin, etc.) may inhibit the metabolism of, and increase the systemic exposure to, budesonide. Caution should be exercised with co-administration of Symbicort with potent CYP3A4 inhibitors).

No products indexed under this heading.

Fosamprenavir Calcium (Concomitant administration of CYP3A4 inhibitors (e.g., itraconazole, clarithromycin, erythromycin, etc.) may inhibit the metabolism of, and increase the systemic exposure to, budesonide. Caution should be exercised with co-administration of Symbicort with potent CYP3A4 inhibitors). Products include:

Furosemide (The ECG changes and/or hypokalemia that may result from the administration of nonpotassium-sparing diuretics (e.g., loop or thiazide diuretics) can be acutely worsened by beta-agonists, especially when the recommended dose of the beta-agonist is exceeded. Caution is advised with co-administration of Symbicort with nonpotassium-sparing diuretics). Products include:

Hydrochlorothiazide (The ECG changes and/or hypokalemia that may result from the administration of nonpotassium-sparing diuretics (e.g., loop or thiazide diuretics) can be acutely worsened by beta-agonists, especially when the recommended dose of the beta-agonist is exceeded. Caution is advised with co-administration of Symbicort with nonpotassium-sparing diuretics). Products include:

Hydroflumethiazide (The ECG changes and/or hypokalemia that may result from the administration of nonpotassium-sparing diuretics (e.g., loop or thiazide diuretics) can be acutely worsened by beta-agonists, especially when the recommended dose of the beta-agonist is exceeded. Caution is advised with co-administration of Symbicort with nonpotassium-sparing diuretics).

No products indexed under this heading.

Imipramine Hydrochloride (Symbicort should be administered with caution to patients treated with TCAs, or within 2 weeks of discontinuation of TCAs, since these agents may potentiate formoterol action on the vascular system).

No products indexed under this heading.

Imipramine Pamoate (Symbicort should be administered with caution to patients treated with TCAs, or within 2 weeks of discontinuation of TCAs, since these agents may potentiate formoterol action on the vascular system).

No products indexed under this heading.

Indapamide (The ECG changes and/or hypokalemia that may result from the administration of nonpotassium-sparing diuretics (e.g., loop or thiazide diuretics) can be acutely worsened by beta-agonists, especially when the recommended dose of the beta-agonist is exceeded. Caution is advised with co-administration of Symbicort with nonpotassium-sparing diuretics). Products include:

Indinavir Sulfate (Concomitant administration of CYP3A4 inhibitors (e.g., itraconazole, clarithromycin, erythromycin, etc.) may inhibit the metabolism of, and increase the systemic exposure to, budesonide. Caution should be exercised with co-administration of Symbicort with potent CYP3A4 inhibitors). Products include:

Isocarboxazid (Symbicort should be administered with caution to patients treated with MAOIs, or within 2 weeks of discontinuation of MAOIs, since these agents may potentiate formoterol action on the vascular system).

No products indexed under this heading.

Isoniazid (Concomitant administration of CYP3A4 inhibitors (e.g., itraconazole, clarithromycin, erythromycin, etc.) may inhibit the metabolism of, and increase the systemic exposure to, budesonide. Caution should be exercised with co-administration of Symbicort with potent CYP3A4 inhibitors).

No products indexed under this heading.

Itraconazole (Concomitant administration of CYP3A4 inhibitors (e.g., itraconazole, clarithromycin, erythromycin, etc.) may inhibit the metabolism of, and increase the systemic exposure to, budesonide. Caution should be exercised with co-administration of Symbicort with potent CYP3A4 inhibitors).

No products indexed under this heading.

Ketoconazole (Co-administration of ketoconazole and Symbicort increases the mean plasma concentration of orally administered budesonide. Caution should be excercised when considering co-administration of Symbicort with long-term ketoconazole). Products include:

Labetalol Hydrochloride (Beta-blockers (including eye drops) may not only block the pulmonary effect of beta-agonists (e.g., formoterol- a component of Symbicort), but may produce severe bronchospasm in asthma patients).

No products indexed under this heading.

Levobunolol Hydrochloride (Beta-blockers (including eye drops) may not only block the pulmonary effect of beta-agonists (e.g., formoterol- a component of Symbicort), but may produce severe bronchospasm in asthma patients). Products include:

Lopinavir (Concomitant administration of CYP3A4 inhibitors (e.g., itraconazole, clarithromycin, erythromycin, etc.) may inhibit the metabolism of, and increase the systemic exposure to, budesonide. Caution should be exercised with co-administration of Symbicort with potent CYP3A4 inhibitors). Products include:

Loratadine (Concomitant administration of CYP3A4 inhibitors (e.g., itraconazole, clarithromycin, erythromycin, etc.) may inhibit the metabolism of, and increase the systemic exposure to, budesonide. Caution should be exercised with co-administration of Symbicort with potent CYP3A4 inhibitors). Products include:

Maprotiline Hydrochloride (Symbicort should be administered with caution to patients treated with TCAs, or within 2 weeks of discontinuation of TCAs, since these agents may potentiate formoterol action on the vascular system).

No products indexed under this heading.

Methyclothiazide (The ECG changes and/or hypokalemia that may result from the administration of nonpotassium-sparing diuretics (e.g., loop or thiazide diuretics) can be acutely worsened by beta-agonists, especially when the recommended dose of the beta-agonist is exceeded. Caution is advised with co-administration of Symbicort with nonpotassium-sparing diuretics).

No products indexed under this heading.

Metipranolol Hydrochloride (Beta-blockers (including eye drops) may not only block the pulmonary effect of beta-agonists (e.g., formoterol- a component of Symbicort), but may produce severe bronchospasm in asthma patients).

No products indexed under this heading.

Metolazone (The ECG changes and/or hypokalemia that may result from the administration of nonpotassium-sparing diuretics (e.g., loop or thiazide diuretics) can be acutely worsened by beta-agonists, especially when the recommended dose of the beta-agonist is exceeded. Caution is advised with co-administration of Symbicort with nonpotassium-sparing diuretics).
No products indexed under this heading.

Metoprolol Succinate (Beta-blockers (including eye drops) may not only block the pulmonary effect of beta-agonists (e.g., formoterol- a component of Symbicort), but may produce severe bronchospasm in asthma patients). Products include:
Toprol-XL Tablets 668

Metoprolol Tartrate (Beta-blockers (including eye drops) may not only block the pulmonary effect of beta-agonists (e.g., formoterol- a component of Symbicort), but may produce severe bronchospasm in asthma patients). Products include:
Lopressor Injection 2238
Lopressor Tablets 2238
Lopressor HCT 50/25 Tablets 2241
Lopressor HCT 100/25 Tablets 2241
Lopressor HCT 100/50 Tablets 2241

Metronidazole (Concomitant administration of CYP3A4 inhibitors (e.g., itraconazole, clarithromycin, erythromycin, etc.) may inhibit the metabolism of, and increase the systemic exposure to, budesonide. Caution should be exercised with co-administration of Symbicort with potent CYP3A4 inhibitors). Products include:
Metrogel 1% 1211
MetroGel-Vaginal Gel 1855
Vandazole Vaginal Gel 3338

Metronidazole Benzoate (Concomitant administration of CYP3A4 inhibitors (e.g., itraconazole, clarithromycin, erythromycin, etc.) may inhibit the metabolism of, and increase the systemic exposure to, budesonide. Caution should be exercised with co-administration of Symbicort with potent CYP3A4 inhibitors).
No products indexed under this heading.

Metronidazole Hydrochloride (Concomitant administration of CYP3A4 inhibitors (e.g., itraconazole, clarithromycin, erythromycin, etc.) may inhibit the metabolism of, and increase the systemic exposure to, budesonide. Caution should be exercised with co-administration of Symbicort with potent CYP3A4 inhibitors).
No products indexed under this heading.

Miconazole (Concomitant administration of CYP3A4 inhibitors (e.g., itraconazole, clarithromycin, erythromycin, etc.) may inhibit the metabolism of, and increase the systemic exposure to, budesonide. Caution should be exercised with co-administration of Symbicort with potent CYP3A4 inhibitors).
No products indexed under this heading.

Miconazole Nitrate (Concomitant administration of CYP3A4 inhibitors (e.g., itraconazole, clarithromycin, erythromycin, etc.) may inhibit the metabolism of, and increase the systemic exposure to, budesonide. Caution should be exercised with co-administration of Symbicort with potent CYP3A4 inhibitors). Products include:
Desenex 635
Desenex Jock Itch Spray Powder 635

Moclobemide (Symbicort should be administered with caution to patients treated with MAOIs, or within 2 weeks of discontinuation of MAOIs, since these agents may potentiate formoterol action on the vascular system).
No products indexed under this heading.

Nadolol (Beta-blockers (including eye drops) may not only block the pulmonary effect of beta-agonists (e.g., formoterol- a component of Symbicort), but may produce severe bronchospasm in asthma patients). Products include:
Nadolol Tablets 2159

Nefazodone Hydrochloride (Concomitant administration of CYP3A4 inhibitors (e.g., itraconazole, clarithromycin, erythromycin, etc.) may inhibit the metabolism of, and increase the systemic exposure to, budesonide. Caution should be exercised with co-administration of Symbicort with potent CYP3A4 inhibitors).
No products indexed under this heading.

Nelfinavir Mesylate (Concomitant administration of CYP3A4 inhibitors (e.g., itraconazole, clarithromycin, erythromycin, etc.) may inhibit the metabolism of, and increase the systemic exposure to, budesonide. Caution should be exercised with co-administration of Symbicort with potent CYP3A4 inhibitors). Products include:
Viracept 2577

Nevirapine (Concomitant administration of CYP3A4 inhibitors (e.g., itraconazole, clarithromycin, erythromycin, etc.) may inhibit the metabolism of, and increase the systemic exposure to, budesonide. Caution should be exercised with co-administration of Symbicort with potent CYP3A4 inhibitors). Products include:
Viramune Oral Suspension 873
Viramune Tablets 873

Niacinamide (Concomitant administration of CYP3A4 inhibitors (e.g., itraconazole, clarithromycin, erythromycin, etc.) may inhibit the metabolism of, and increase the systemic exposure to, budesonide. Caution should be exercised with co-administration of Symbicort with potent CYP3A4 inhibitors).
No products indexed under this heading.

Nicotinamide (Concomitant administration of CYP3A4 inhibitors (e.g., itraconazole, clarithromycin, erythromycin, etc.) may inhibit the metabolism of, and increase the systemic exposure to, budesonide. Caution should be exercised with co-administration of Symbicort with potent CYP3A4 inhibitors). Products include:
Nicomide Tablets 1088

Nifedipine (Concomitant administration of CYP3A4 inhibitors (e.g., itraconazole, clarithromycin, erythromycin, etc.) may inhibit the metabolism of, and increase the systemic exposure to, budesonide. Caution should be exercised with co-administration of Symbicort with potent CYP3A4 inhibitors). Products include:
Adalat CC Tablets 2964

Norfloxacin (Concomitant administration of CYP3A4 inhibitors (e.g., itraconazole, clarithromycin, erythromycin, etc.) may inhibit the metabolism of, and increase the systemic exposure to, budesonide. Caution should be exercised with co-administration of Symbicort with potent CYP3A4 inhibitors). Products include:
Noroxin Tablets 2032

Nortriptyline Hydrochloride (Symbicort should be administered with caution to patients treated with TCAs, or within 2 weeks of discontinuation of TCAs, since these agents may potentiate formoterol action on the vascular system).
No products indexed under this heading.

Omeprazole (Concomitant administration of CYP3A4 inhibitors (e.g., itraconazole, clarithromycin, erythromycin, etc.) may inhibit the metabolism of, and increase the systemic exposure to, budesonide. Caution should be exercised with co-administration of Symbicort with potent CYP3A4 inhibitors). Products include:
Zegerid Capsules 2958
Zegerid Powder for Oral Solution 2958

Pargyline Hydrochloride (Symbicort should be administered with caution to patients treated with MAOIs, or within 2 weeks of discontinuation of MAOIs, since these agents may potentiate formoterol action on the vascular system).
No products indexed under this heading.

Paroxetine Hydrochloride (Concomitant administration of CYP3A4 inhibitors (e.g., itraconazole, clarithromycin, erythromycin, etc.) may inhibit the metabolism of, and increase the systemic exposure to, budesonide. Caution should be exercised with co-administration of Symbicort with potent CYP3A4 inhibitors). Products include:
Paxil CR Controlled-Release Tablets 1538
Paxil 1530

Penbutolol Sulfate (Beta-blockers (including eye drops) may not only block the pulmonary effect of beta-agonists (e.g., formoterol- a component of Symbicort), but may produce severe bronchospasm in asthma patients).
No products indexed under this heading.

Phenelzine Sulfate (Symbicort should be administered with caution to patients treated with MAOIs, or within 2 weeks of discontinuation of MAOIs, since these agents may potentiate formoterol action on the vascular system).
No products indexed under this heading.

Pindolol (Beta-blockers (including eye drops) may not only block the pulmonary effect of beta-agonists (e.g., formoterol- a component of Symbicort), but may produce severe bronchospasm in asthma patients).
No products indexed under this heading.

Polythiazide (The ECG changes and/or hypokalemia that may result from the administration of nonpotassium-sparing diuretics (e.g., loop or thiazide diuretics) can be acutely worsened by beta-agonists, especially when the recommended dose of the beta-agonist is exceeded. Caution is advised with co-administration of Symbicort with nonpotassium-sparing diuretics).
No products indexed under this heading.

Procarbazine Hydrochloride (Symbicort should be administered with caution to patients treated with MAOIs, or within 2 weeks of discontinuation of MAOIs, since these agents may potentiate formoterol action on the vascular system). Products include:
Matulane Capsules 3191

Propoxyphene Hydrochloride (Concomitant administration of CYP3A4 inhibitors (e.g., itraconazole, clarithromycin, erythromycin, etc.) may inhibit the metabolism of, and increase the systemic exposure to, budesonide. Caution should be exercised with co-administration of Symbicort with potent CYP3A4 inhibitors).
No products indexed under this heading.

Propoxyphene Napsylate (Concomitant administration of CYP3A4 inhibitors (e.g., itraconazole, clarithromycin, erythromycin, etc.) may inhibit the metabolism of, and increase the systemic exposure to, budesonide. Caution should be exercised with co-administration of Symbicort with potent CYP3A4 inhibitors).
No products indexed under this heading.

Propranolol Hydrochloride (Beta-blockers (including eye drops) may not only block the pulmonary effect of beta-agonists (e.g., formoterol- a component of Symbicort), but may produce severe bronchospasm in asthma patients). Products include:
Inderal LA Long-Acting Capsules 3429
InnoPran XL Capsules 2723

Protriptyline Hydrochloride (Symbicort should be administered with caution to patients treated with TCAs, or within 2 weeks of discontinuation of TCAs, since these agents may potentiate formoterol action on the vascular system).
No products indexed under this heading.

Quinidine (Concomitant administration of CYP3A4 inhibitors (e.g., itraconazole, clarithromycin, erythromycin, etc.) may inhibit the metabolism of, and increase the systemic exposure to, budesonide. Caution should be exercised with co-administration of Symbicort with potent CYP3A4 inhibitors).
No products indexed under this heading.

Quinidine Hydrochloride (Concomitant administration of CYP3A4 inhibitors (e.g., itraconazole, clarithromycin, erythromycin, etc.) may inhibit the metabolism of, and increase the systemic exposure to, budesonide. Caution should be exercised with co-administration of Symbicort with potent CYP3A4 inhibitors).
No products indexed under this heading.

Quinidine Polygalacturonate (Concomitant administration of CYP3A4 inhibitors (e.g., itraconazole, clarithromycin, erythromycin, etc.) may inhibit the metabolism of, and increase the systemic exposure to, budesonide. Caution should be exercised with co-administration of Symbicort with potent CYP3A4 inhibitors).
No products indexed under this heading.

Quinidine Sulfate (Concomitant administration of CYP3A4 inhibitors (e.g., itraconazole, clarithromycin, erythromycin, etc.) may inhibit the metabolism of, and increase the systemic exposure to, budesonide. Caution should be exercised with co-administration of Symbicort with potent CYP3A4 inhibitors).
No products indexed under this heading.

Quinine (Concomitant administration of CYP3A4 inhibitors (e.g., itraconazole, clarithromycin, erythromycin, etc.) may inhibit the metabolism of, and increase the systemic exposure to, budesonide. Caution should be exercised with co-administration of Symbicort with potent CYP3A4 inhibitors).
No products indexed under this heading.

Quinine Sulfate (Concomitant administration of CYP3A4 inhibitors (e.g., itraconazole, clarithromycin, erythromycin, etc.) may inhibit the metabolism of, and increase the systemic exposure to, budesonide. Caution should be exercised with co-administration of Symbicort with potent CYP3A4 inhibitors).
No products indexed under this heading.

Quinupristin (Concomitant administration of CYP3A4 inhibitors (e.g., itraconazole, clarithromycin, erythromycin, etc.) may inhibit the metabolism of, and increase the systemic exposure to, budesonide. Caution should be exercised with co-administration of Symbicort with potent CYP3A4 inhibitors).
No products indexed under this heading.

Ranitidine Bismuth Citrate (Concomitant administration of CYP3A4 inhibitors (e.g., itraconazole, clarithromycin, erythromycin, etc.) may inhibit the metabolism of, and increase the systemic exposure to, budesonide. Caution should be exercised with co-administration of Symbicort with potent CYP3A4 inhibitors).
No products indexed under this heading.

Ranitidine Hydrochloride (Concomitant administration of CYP3A4 inhibitors (e.g., itraconazole, clarithromycin, erythromycin, etc.) may inhibit the metabolism of, and increase the systemic exposure to, budesonide. Caution should be exercised with co-administration of Symbicort with potent CYP3A4 inhibitors). Products include:
Zantac 1624
Zantac Injection 1619
Zantac Injection Pharmacy Bulk Package 1622

Ritonavir (Concomitant administration of CYP3A4 inhibitors (e.g., itraconazole, clarithromycin, erythromycin, etc.) may inhibit the metabolism of, and increase the systemic exposure to, budesonide. Caution should be exercised with co-administration of Symbicort with potent CYP3A4 inhibitors). Products include:
Kaletra 476
Norvir 503

Saquinavir (Concomitant administration of CYP3A4 inhibitors (e.g., itraconazole, clarithromycin, erythromycin, etc.) may inhibit the metabolism of, and increase the systemic exposure to, budesonide. Caution should be exercised with co-administration of Symbicort with potent CYP3A4 inhibitors).
No products indexed under this heading.

Saquinavir Mesylate (Concomitant administration of CYP3A4 inhibitors (e.g., itraconazole, clarithromycin, erythromycin, etc.) may inhibit the metabolism of, and increase the systemic exposure to, budesonide. Caution should be exercised with co-administration of Symbicort with potent CYP3A4 inhibitors). Products include:
Invirase 2772

Selegiline Hydrochloride (Symbicort should be administered with caution to patients treated with MAOIs, or within 2 weeks of discontinuation of MAOIs, since these agents may potentiate formoterol action on the vascular system). Products include:
Eldepryl Capsules 3208
Zelapar Tablets 3372

Sertraline Hydrochloride (Concomitant administration of CYP3A4 inhibitors (e.g., itraconazole, clarithromycin, erythromycin, etc.) may inhibit the metabolism of, and increase the systemic exposure to, budesonide. Caution should be exercised with co-administration of Symbicort with potent CYP3A4 inhibitors). Products include:
Zoloft 2586

Sotalol Hydrochloride (Beta-blockers (including eye drops) may not only block the pulmonary effect of beta-agonists (e.g., formoterol- a component of Symbicort), but may produce severe bronchospasm in asthma patients).
No products indexed under this heading.

Spironolactone (The ECG changes and/or hypokalemia that may result from the administration of nonpotassium-sparing diuretics (e.g., loop or thiazide diuretics) can be acutely worsened by beta-agonists, especially when the recommended dose of the beta-agonist is exceeded. Caution is advised with co-administration of Symbicort with nonpotassium-sparing diuretics).
No products indexed under this heading.

Telithromycin (Concomitant administration of CYP3A4 inhibitors (e.g., itraconazole, clarithromycin, erythromycin, etc.) may inhibit the metabolism of, and increase the systemic exposure to, budesonide. Caution should be exercised with co-administration of Symbicort with potent CYP3A4 inhibitors). Products include:
Ketek Tablets 2903

Timolol Hemihydrate (Beta-blockers (including eye drops) may not only block the pulmonary effect of beta-agonists (e.g., formoterol- a component of Symbicort), but may produce severe bronchospasm in asthma patients). Products include:
Betimol Ophthalmic Solution 3382
Betimol Ophthalmic Solution .... ⊙295

Timolol Maleate (Beta-blockers (including eye drops) may not only block the pulmonary effect of beta-agonists (e.g., formoterol- a component of Symbicort), but may produce severe bronchospasm in asthma patients). Products include:
Blocadren Tablets 1916
Cosopt Sterile Ophthalmic Solution 1931
Timolide Tablets 2086
Timoptic Sterile Ophthalmic Solution 2088
Timoptic in Ocudose 2091
Timoptic-XE Sterile Ophthalmic Gel Forming Solution 2092

Torsemide (The ECG changes and/or hypokalemia that may result from the administration of nonpotassium-sparing diuretics (e.g., loop or thiazide diuretics) can be acutely worsened by beta-agonists, especially when the recommended dose of the beta-agonist is exceeded. Caution is advised with co-administration of Symbicort with nonpotassium-sparing diuretics). Products include:
Demadex Injection 2759
Demadex Tablets 2759

Tranylcypromine Sulfate (Symbicort should be administered with caution to patients treated with MAOIs, or within 2 weeks of discontinuation of MAOIs, since these agents may potentiate formoterol action on the vascular system). Products include:
Parnate Tablets 1527

Triamterene (The ECG changes and/or hypokalemia that may result from the administration of nonpotassium-sparing diuretics (e.g., loop or thiazide diuretics) can be acutely worsened by beta-agonists, especially when the recommended dose of the beta-agonist is exceeded. Caution is advised with co-administration of Symbicort with nonpotassium-sparing diuretics). Products include:
Dyazide Capsules 1423
Dyrenium Capsules 3400

Trimipramine Maleate (Symbicort should be administered with caution to patients treated with TCAs, or within 2 weeks of discontinuation of TCAs, since these agents may potentiate formoterol action on the vascular system).
No products indexed under this heading.

Troglitazone (Concomitant administration of CYP3A4 inhibitors (e.g., itraconazole, clarithromycin, erythromycin, etc.) may inhibit the metabolism of, and increase the systemic exposure to, budesonide. Caution should be exercised with co-administration of Symbicort with potent CYP3A4 inhibitors).
No products indexed under this heading.

Troleandomycin (Concomitant administration of CYP3A4 inhibitors (e.g., itraconazole, clarithromycin, erythromycin, etc.) may inhibit the metabolism of, and increase the systemic exposure to, budesonide. Caution should be exercised with co-administration of Symbicort with potent CYP3A4 inhibitors).
No products indexed under this heading.

Valproate Sodium (Concomitant administration of CYP3A4 inhibitors (e.g., itraconazole, clarithromycin, erythromycin, etc.) may inhibit the metabolism of, and increase the systemic exposure to, budesonide. Caution should be exercised with co-administration of Symbicort with potent CYP3A4 inhibitors). Products include:
Depacon Injection 412

Verapamil Hydrochloride (Concomitant administration of CYP3A4 inhibitors (e.g., itraconazole, clarithromycin, erythromycin, etc.) may inhibit the metabolism of, and increase the systemic exposure to, budesonide. Caution should be exercised with co-administration of Symbicort with potent CYP3A4 inhibitors). Products include:
Covera-HS Tablets 3139
Tarka Tablets 524
Verelan PM Extended-Release Capsules, Controlled-Onset 3106

Voriconazole (Concomitant administration of CYP3A4 inhibitors (e.g., itraconazole, clarithromycin, erythromycin, etc.) may inhibit the metabolism of, and increase the systemic exposure to, budesonide. Caution should be exercised with co-administration of Symbicort with potent CYP3A4 inhibitors). Products include:
VFEND I.V. 2564
VFEND Oral Suspension 2564
VFEND Tablets 2564

Zafirlukast (Concomitant administration of CYP3A4 inhibitors (e.g., itraconazole, clarithromycin, erythromycin, etc.) may inhibit the metabolism of, and increase the systemic exposure to, budesonide. Caution should be exercised with co-administration of Symbicort with potent CYP3A4 inhibitors). Products include:
Accolate Tablets 671

Zileuton (Concomitant administration of CYP3A4 inhibitors (e.g., itraconazole, clarithromycin, erythromycin, etc.) may inhibit the metabolism of, and increase the systemic exposure to, budesonide. Caution should be exercised with co-administration of Symbicort with potent CYP3A4 inhibitors). Products include:
Zyflo Tablets 1023

Food Interactions

Grapefruit (Concomitant administration of CYP3A4 inhibitors (e.g., itraconazole, clarithromycin, erythromycin, etc.) may inhibit the metabolism of, and increase the systemic exposure to, budesonide. Caution should be exercised with co-administration of Symbicort with potent CYP3A4 inhibitors).

Grapefruit Juice (Concomitant administration of CYP3A4 inhibitors (e.g., itraconazole, clarithromycin, erythromycin, etc.) may inhibit the metabolism of, and increase the systemic exposure to, budesonide. Caution should be exercised with co-administration of Symbicort with potent CYP3A4 inhibitors).

SYMBICORT 160/4.5 INHALATION AEROSOL

(Budesonide, Formoterol fumarate dihydrate) 3511
See Symbicort 80/4.5 Inhalation Aerosol

SYMBYAX CAPSULES
(Fluoxetine Hydrochloride, Olanzapine) 1819
May interact with antihypertensives, cytochrome p450 1a2 inducers (selected), cytochrome p450 2d6 substrates (selected), dopamine agonists, monoamine oxidase inhibitors, non-steroidal anti-inflammatory agents, phenytoin, highly protein bound drugs (selected), tricyclic antidepressants, and certain other agents. Compounds in these categories include:

5-hydroxytryptophan (Five patients receiving fluoxetine in combination with tryptophan experienced adverse reactions, including agitation, restlessness, and gastrointestinal distress).
No products indexed under this heading.

Acebutolol Hydrochloride (Because of the potential for olanzapine to induce hypotension, Symbyax may enhance the effects of certain antihypertensive agents).
No products indexed under this heading.

Alprazolam (Co-administration of alprazolam and fluoxetine resulted in increased alprazolam plasma concentrations and in further psychomotor performance decrement due to increased alprazolam levels). Products include:
Niravam Orally Disintegrating Tablets 3092

Amiodarone Hydrochloride (Because fluoxetine is tightly bound to plasma protein, the administration of fluoxetine to a patient taking another drug that is tightly bound to protein may cause a shift in plasma concentrations potentially resulting in an adverse effect. Conversely, adverse effects may result from displacement of protein-bound fluoxetine by other tightly bound drugs).
No products indexed under this heading.

Amitriptyline Hydrochloride (In two fluoxetine studies, previously stable plasma levels of imipramine and desipramine have increased >2- to 10-fold when fluoxetine has been administered in combination. This influence may persist for three weeks or longer after fluoxetine is discontinued. Thus, the dose of TCA may need to be reduced and plasma TCA concentrations may need to be monitored temporarily when Symbyax is co-administered or has been recently discontinued).
No products indexed under this heading.

Amlodipine Besylate (Because of the potential for olanzapine to induce hypotension, Symbyax may enhance the effects of certain antihypertensive agents). Products include:
Caduet Tablets 2508
Lotrel Capsules 2249
Norvasc Tablets 2545

Amoxapine (In two fluoxetine studies, previously stable plasma levels of imipramine and desipramine have increased >2- to 10-fold when fluoxetine has been administered in combination. This influence may persist for three weeks or longer after fluoxetine is discontinued. Thus, the dose of TCA may need to be reduced and plasma TCA concentrations may need to be monitored temporarily when Symbyax is co-administered or has been recently discontinued).
No products indexed under this heading.

Amphetamine Aspartate (Fluoxetine, like other agents that are metabolized by CYP2D6, inhibits the activity of this isoenzyme. Therapy with medications that are predominately metabolized by the CYP2D6 system and have a relatively narrow therapeutic index should be initiated at the low end of the dose range if the patient is receiving fluoxetine concurrently or has taken it in the previous five weeks. If fluoxetine is added to the treatment regimen of a patient already receiving a drug metabolized by CYP2D6, the need for a decreased dose of the original medication should be considered). Products include:
Adderall Tablets 3164
Adderall XR Capsules 3166

Amphetamine Aspartate Monohydrate (Fluoxetine, like other agents that are metabolized by CYP2D6, inhibits the activity of this isoenzyme. Therapy with medications that are predominately metabolized by the CYP2D6 system and have a relatively narrow therapeutic index should be initiated at the low end of the dose range if the patient is receiving fluoxetine concurrently or has taken it in the previous five weeks. If fluoxetine is added to the treatment regimen of a patient already receiving a drug metabolized by CYP2D6, the need for a decreased dose of the original medication should be considered).
No products indexed under this heading.

Amphetamine Sulfate (Fluoxetine, like other agents that are metabolized by CYP2D6, inhibits the activity of this isoenzyme. Therapy with medications that are predominately metabolized by the CYP2D6 system and have a relatively narrow therapeutic index should be initiated at the low end of the dose range if the patient is receiving fluoxetine concurrently or has taken it in the previous five weeks. If fluoxetine is added to the treatment regimen of a patient already receiving a drug metabolized by CYP2D6, the need for a decreased dose of the original medication should be considered). Products include:
Adderall Tablets 3164
Adderall XR Capsules 3166

Aspirin (Serotonin release by platelets plays an important role in hemostasis. Studies have demonstrated an association between the use of psychotropic drugs that interfere with serotonin reuptake and the occurrence of upper gastrointestinal bleeding. These studies have also shown that concurrent use of aspirin potentiated the risk of bleeding. Therefore, patients should be cautioned about the use of aspirin concurrently with Symbyax). Products include:
Aggrenox Capsules 822
Bayer Aspirin 744
BC Allergy Sinus Cold Powder 677
BC Headache Powder 677
Arthritis Strength BC Powder 677
BC Sinus Cold Powder 677
Excedrin Extra Strength Caplets/Tablets/Geltabs 684
Excedrin Migraine Caplets/Tablets/Geltabs 609
Goody's Body Pain Formula Powder 684
Goody's Extra Strength Headache Powders 611
Goody's Extra Strength Pain Relief Tablets 685
Percodan Tablets 1132
St. Joseph 81 mg Aspirin Chewable and Enteric Coated Tablets 1869

Aspirin, Enteric Coated (Serotonin release by platelets plays an important role in hemostasis. Studies have demonstrated an association between the use of psychotropic drugs that interfere with serotonin reuptake and the occurrence of upper gastrointestinal bleeding. These studies have also shown that concurrent use of aspirin potentiated the risk of bleeding. Therefore, patients should be cautioned about the use of aspirin concurrently with Symbyax).
No products indexed under this heading.

Aspirin Buffered (Serotonin release by platelets plays an important role in hemostasis. Studies have demonstrated an association between the use of psychotropic drugs that interfere with serotonin reuptake and the occurrence of upper gastrointestinal bleeding. These studies have also shown that concurrent use of aspirin potentiated the risk of bleeding. Therefore, patients should be cautioned about the use of aspirin concurrently with Symbyax). Products include:
Bufferin Extra Strength Tablets 678
Bufferin Regular Strength Tablets 678

Atenolol (Because of the potential for olanzapine to induce hypotension, Symbyax may enhance the effects of certain antihypertensive agents).
No products indexed under this heading.

Atomoxetine Hydrochloride (Fluoxetine, like other agents that are metabolized by CYP2D6, inhibits the activity of this isoenzyme. Therapy with medications that are predominately metabolized by the CYP2D6 system and have a relatively narrow therapeutic index should be initiated at the low end of the dose range if the patient is receiving fluoxetine concurrently or has taken it in the previous five weeks. If fluoxetine is added to the treatment regimen of a patient already receiving a drug metabolized by CYP2D6, the need for a decreased dose of the original medication should be considered). Products include:
Strattera Capsules 1814

Atovaquone (Because fluoxetine is tightly bound to plasma protein, the administration of fluoxetine to a patient taking another drug that is tightly bound to protein may cause a shift in plasma concentrations potentially resulting in an adverse effect. Conversely, adverse effects may result from displacement of protein-bound fluoxetine by other tightly bound drugs). Products include:
Malarone Pediatric Tablets 1517
Malarone Tablets 1517
Mepron Suspension 1521

Benazepril Hydrochloride (Because of the potential for olanzapine to induce hypotension, Symbyax may enhance the effects of certain antihypertensive agents). Products include:
Lotensin Tablets 2243
Lotensin HCT Tablets 2246
Lotrel Capsules 2249

Bendroflumethiazide (Because of the potential for olanzapine to induce hypotension, Symbyax may enhance the effects of certain antihypertensive agents).
No products indexed under this heading.

Betaxolol Hydrochloride (Because of the potential for olanzapine to induce hypotension, Symbyax may enhance the effects of certain antihypertensive agents). Products include:
Betoptic S Ophthalmic Suspension 558

Bisoprolol Fumarate (Because of the potential for olanzapine to induce hypotension, Symbyax may enhance the effects of certain antihypertensive agents).
No products indexed under this heading.

Bromocriptine Mesylate (The olanzapine component of Symbyax may antagonize the effects of levodopa and dopamine agonists).
No products indexed under this heading.

Candesartan Cilexetil (Because of the potential for olanzapine to induce hypotension, Symbyax may enhance the effects of certain antihypertensive agents). Products include:
Atacand Tablets 649
Atacand HCT 651

Captopril (Because of the potential for olanzapine to induce hypotension, Symbyax may enhance the effects of certain antihypertensive agents). Products include:
Captopril Tablets 2149

Carbamazepine (Carbamazepine therapy (200mg bid) causes an approximate 50% increase in the clearance of olanzapine; higher daily doses of carbamazepine may cause an even greater increase in olanzapine clearance. Patients on stable dose of carbamazepine have developed elevated plasma anticonvulsant concentrations and clinical anticonvulsant toxicity following initiation of concomitant fluoxetine treatment). Products include:
Carbatrol Capsules 3171
Equetro Extended-Release Capsules 3180
Tegretol/Tegretol-XR 2295

Carteolol Hydrochloride (Because of the potential for olanzapine to induce hypotension, Symbyax may enhance the effects of certain antihypertensive agents). Products include:
Carteolol Hydrochloride Ophthalmic Solution USP, 1% .... ⊙249

Carvedilol (Fluoxetine, like other agents that are metabolized by CYP2D6, inhibits the activity of this isoenzyme. Therapy with medications that are predominately metabolized by the CYP2D6 system and have a relatively narrow therapeutic index should be initiated at the low end of the dose range if the patient is receiving fluoxetine concurrently or has taken it in the previous five weeks. If fluoxetine is added to the treatment regimen of a patient already receiving a drug metabolized by CYP2D6, the need for a decreased dose of the original medication should be considered). Products include:
Coreg Tablets 1414

Cefonicid Sodium (Because fluoxetine is tightly bound to plasma protein, the administration of fluoxetine to a patient taking another drug that is tightly bound to protein may cause a shift in plasma concentrations potentially resulting in an adverse effect. Conversely, adverse effects may result from displacement of protein-bound fluoxetine by other tightly bound drugs).
No products indexed under this heading.

Celecoxib (Serotonin release by platelets plays an important role in hemostasis. Studies have demonstrated an association between the use of psychotropic drugs that interfere with serotonin reuptake and the occurrence of upper gastrointestinal bleeding. These studies have also shown that concurrent use of an NSAID potentiated the risk of bleeding. Therefore, patients should be cautioned about the use of NSAIDs concurrently with Symbyax).
Products include:
Celebrex Capsules 3134

Cevimeline Hydrochloride (Fluoxetine, like other agents that are metabolized by CYP2D6, inhibits the activity of this isoenzyme. Therapy with medications that are predominately metabolized by the CYP2D6 system and have a relatively narrow therapeutic index should be initiated at the low end of the dose range if the patient is receiving fluoxetine concurrently or has taken it in the previous five weeks. If fluoxetine is added to the treatment regimen of a patient already receiving a drug metabolized by CYP2D6, the need for a decreased dose of the original medication should be considered).
Products include:
Evoxac Capsules 1047

Chlordiazepoxide (Because fluoxetine is tightly bound to plasma protein, the administration of fluoxetine to a patient taking another drug that is tightly bound to protein may cause a shift in plasma concentrations potentially resulting in an adverse effect. Conversely, adverse effects may result from displacement of protein-bound fluoxetine by other tightly bound drugs).
No products indexed under this heading.

Chlordiazepoxide Hydrochloride (Because fluoxetine is tightly bound to plasma protein, the administration of fluoxetine to a patient taking another drug that is tightly bound to protein may cause a shift in plasma concentrations potentially resulting in an adverse effect. Conversely, adverse effects may result from displacement of protein-bound fluoxetine by other tightly bound drugs).
Products include:
Librium Capsules 3347

Chlorothiazide (Because of the potential for olanzapine to induce hypotension, Symbyax may enhance the effects of certain antihypertensive agents). Products include:
Diuril Oral Suspension 1954

Chlorothiazide Sodium (Because of the potential for olanzapine to induce hypotension, Symbyax may enhance the effects of certain antihypertensive agents). Products include:
Diuril Sodium Intravenous 2467

Chlorpromazine (Fluoxetine, like other agents that are metabolized by CYP2D6, inhibits the activity of this isoenzyme. Therapy with medications that are predominately metabolized by the CYP2D6 system and have a relatively narrow therapeutic index should be initiated at the low end of the dose range if the patient is receiving fluoxetine concurrently or has taken it in the previous five weeks. If fluoxetine is added to the treatment regimen of a patient already receiving a drug metabolized by CYP2D6, the need for a decreased dose of the original medication should be considered).
No products indexed under this heading.

Chlorpromazine Hydrochloride (Fluoxetine, like other agents that are metabolized by CYP2D6, inhibits the activity of this isoenzyme. Therapy with medications that are predominately metabolized by the CYP2D6 system and have a relatively narrow therapeutic index should be initiated at the low end of the dose range if the patient is receiving fluoxetine concurrently or has taken it in the previous five weeks. If fluoxetine is added to the treatment regimen of a patient already receiving a drug metabolized by CYP2D6, the need for a decreased dose of the original medication should be considered).
No products indexed under this heading.

Chlorpropamide (Fluoxetine, like other agents that are metabolized by CYP2D6, inhibits the activity of this isoenzyme. Therapy with medications that are predominately metabolized by the CYP2D6 system and have a relatively narrow therapeutic index should be initiated at the low end of the dose range if the patient is receiving fluoxetine concurrently or has taken it in the previous five weeks. If fluoxetine is added to the treatment regimen of a patient already receiving a drug metabolized by CYP2D6, the need for a decreased dose of the original medication should be considered).
No products indexed under this heading.

Chlorthalidone (Because of the potential for olanzapine to induce hypotension, Symbyax may enhance the effects of certain antihypertensive agents). Products include:
Clorpres Tablets 2153

Citalopram Hydrobromide (Agents that induce CYP1A2 or glucuronyl transferase enzymes may cause an increase in olanzapine concentration). Products include:
Celexa 1176

Clomipramine Hydrochloride (In two fluoxetine studies, previously stable plasma levels of imipramine and desipramine have increased >2- to 10-fold when fluoxetine has been administered in combination. This influence may persist for three weeks or longer after fluoxetine is discontinued. Thus, the dose of TCA may need to be reduced and plasma TCA concentrations may need to be monitored temporarily when Symbyax is co-administered or has been recently discontinued).
No products indexed under this heading.

Clonidine (Because of the potential for olanzapine to induce hypotension, Symbyax may enhance the effects of certain antihypertensive agents). Products include:
Catapres-TTS 844

Clonidine Hydrochloride (Because of the potential for olanzapine to induce hypotension, Symbyax may enhance the effects of certain antihypertensive agents). Products include:
Catapres Tablets 843
Clorpres Tablets 2153

Clozapine (Elevation of blood levels of clozapine has been observed in patients receiving concomitant fluoxetine). Products include:
Clozaril Tablets 2184
FazaClo Orally Disintegrating Tablets 551

Codeine Phosphate (Fluoxetine, like other agents that are metabolized by CYP2D6, inhibits the activity of this isoenzyme. Therapy with medications that are predominately metabolized by the CYP2D6 system and have a relatively narrow therapeutic index should be initiated at the low end of the dose range if the patient is receiving fluoxetine concurrently or has taken it in the previous five weeks. If fluoxetine is added to the treatment regimen of a patient already receiving a drug metabolized by CYP2D6, the need for a decreased dose of the original medication should be considered).
Products include:
Tylenol with Codeine Tablets 2391

Codeine Sulfate (Fluoxetine, like other agents that are metabolized by CYP2D6, inhibits the activity of this isoenzyme. Therapy with medications that are predominately metabolized by the CYP2D6 system and have a relatively narrow therapeutic index should be initiated at the low end of the dose range if the patient is receiving fluoxetine concurrently or has taken it in the previous five weeks. If fluoxetine is added to the treatment regimen of a patient already receiving a drug metabolized by CYP2D6, the need for a decreased dose of the original medication should be considered).
No products indexed under this heading.

Cyclobenzaprine Hydrochloride (Fluoxetine, like other agents that are metabolized by CYP2D6, inhibits the activity of this isoenzyme. Therapy with medications that are predominately metabolized by the CYP2D6 system and have a relatively narrow therapeutic index should be initiated at the low end of the dose range if the patient is receiving fluoxetine concurrently or has taken it in the previous five weeks. If fluoxetine is added to the treatment regimen of a patient already receiving a drug metabolized by CYP2D6, the need for a decreased dose of the original medication should be considered).
No products indexed under this heading.

Cyclosporine (Because fluoxetine is tightly bound to plasma protein, the administration of fluoxetine to a patient taking another drug that is tightly bound to protein may cause a shift in plasma concentrations potentially resulting in an adverse effect. Conversely, adverse effects may result from displacement of protein-bound fluoxetine by other tightly bound drugs). Products include:
Gengraf Capsules 459
Neoral Oral Solution 2259
Neoral Soft Gelatin Capsules 2259
Restasis Ophthalmic Emulsion 575
Sandimmune 2275

Deserpidine (Because of the potential for olanzapine to induce hypotension, Symbyax may enhance the effects of certain antihypertensive agents).
No products indexed under this heading.

Desipramine Hydrochloride (In two fluoxetine studies, previously stable plasma levels of imipramine and desipramine have increased >2- to 10-fold when fluoxetine has been administered in combination. This influence may persist for three weeks or longer after fluoxetine is discontinued. Thus, the dose of TCA may need to be reduced and plasma TCA concentrations may need to be monitored temporarily when Symbyax is co-administered or has been recently discontinued).
No products indexed under this heading.

Dexfenfluramine Hydrochloride (Fluoxetine, like other agents that are metabolized by CYP2D6, inhibits the activity of this isoenzyme. Therapy with medications that are predominately metabolized by the CYP2D6 system and have a relatively narrow therapeutic index should be initiated at the low end of the dose range if the patient is receiving fluoxetine concurrently or has taken it in the previous five weeks. If fluoxetine is added to the treatment regimen of a patient already receiving a drug metabolized by CYP2D6, the need for a decreased dose of the original medication should be considered).
No products indexed under this heading.

Dextromethorphan Hydrobromide (Fluoxetine, like other agents that are metabolized by CYP2D6, inhibits the activity of this isoenzyme. Therapy with medications that are predominately metabolized by the CYP2D6 system and have a relatively narrow therapeutic index should be initiated at the low end of the dose range if the patient is receiving fluoxetine concurrently or has taken it in the previous five weeks. If fluoxetine is added to the treatment regimen of a patient already receiving a drug metabolized by CYP2D6, the need for a decreased dose of the original medication should be considered).
Products include:
Comtrex Maximum Strength Cold & Cough Day/Night Caplets - Day Formulation .... ■ 726
Comtrex Maximum Strength Cold & Cough Day/Night Caplets - Night Formulation .... ■ 726
Comtrex Maximum Strength Non-Drowsy Cold & Cough Caplets .... ■ 725
Children's Dimetapp DM Cold & Cough Elixir .... ■ 731
Children's Dimetapp Long Acting Cough Plus Cold Syrup .... ■ 731
Toddler's Dimetapp Cold and Cough Drops .... ■ 732
Mucinex DM Extended-Release Bi-Layer Tablets .... ■ 720
Refenesen DM Caplets .... ■ 721
Robitussin Cough & Cold CF Liquid .... ■ 735
Robitussin Cough & Cold Long-Acting Liquid .... ■ 735
Robitussin Cough & Allergy Syrup .. ■ 736
Robitussin Cough & Cold Nighttime Liquid .... ■ 736
Robitussin Cough & Cold Pediatric Drops .... ■ 735

Robitussin Cough, Cold & Flu Nighttime Liquid 738
Robitussin Cough & Congestion Liquid 738
Robitussin Cough Gels Long-Acting 737
Robitussin Cough Long Acting Liquid 739
Robitussin Cough DM Syrup 738
Robitussin Cough DM Infant Drops 738
Robitussin Pediatric Cough Long Acting Liquid 739
Robitussin Pediatric Cough & Cold Long-Acting Liquid 735
Robitussin Pediatric Cough & Cold Nighttime Liquid 736
Robitussin Sugar Free Cough 738
TheraFlu Cold & Cough Hot Liquid 740
TheraFlu Warming Relief Daytime Severe Cold 743
TheraFlu Thin Strips Long Acting Cough 744
Triaminic Daytime Cold & Cough Liquid 745
Triaminic Cough & Sore Throat Liquid 747
Triaminic Cough & Runny Nose Softchews 748
Triaminic Thin Strips Cold & Cough 778
Triaminic Infant Thin Strips Decongestant Plus Cough 747
Children's Tylenol Plus Flu Oral Suspension 749
Tylenol Cold Head Congestion Daytime Caplets with Cool Burst and Gelcaps 750
Tylenol Cold Multi-Symptom Daytime Liquid 752
Tylenol Cold Multi-Symptom Severe Daytime Liquid 752
Concentrated Tylenol Infants' Drops Plus Cold & Cough 754
Children's Tylenol Plus Cough & Runny Nose Suspension Liquid 1879
Children's Tylenol Plus Cough & Sore Throat Suspension Liquid 1879
Children's Tylenol Plus Flu Suspension Liquid 1881
Children's Tylenol Plus Multi-Symptom Cold Suspension Liquid 1879
Tylenol Cold Severe Congestion Non-Drowsy Caplets with Cool Burst 1874
Tylenol Cold Head Congestion Daytime Caplets with Cool Burst 1873
Tylenol Cold Head Congestion Nighttime Caplets with Cool Burst 1873
Tylenol Cold Head Congestion Severe Caplets with Cool Burst 1873
Tylenol Cold Multi-Symptom Daytime Caplets with Cool Burst and Gelcaps 1874
Tylenol Cold Multi-Symptom Daytime Liquid with Citrus Burst 1874
Tylenol Cold Multi-Symptom Nighttime Caplets with Cool Burst 1874
Tylenol Cold Multi-Symptom Nighttime Liquid with Cool Burst 1874
Tylenol Cold Multi-Symptom Severe Caplets with Cool Burst 1874
Tylenol Cold Multi-Symptom Severe Daytime Liquid with Citrus Burst 1874
Tylenol Cough & Sore Throat Daytime Liquid with Cool Burst 1877
Tylenol Cough & Sore Throat Nighttime Liquid with Cool Burst 1877
Concentrated Tylenol Infants' Drops Plus Cold and Cough 1879
Vicks 44 Cough Relief Liquid 2679
Vicks 44D Cough & Head Congestion Relief Liquid 2679
Vicks 44E Cough & Chest Congestion Relief Liquid 2679
Pediatric Vicks 44e Cough & Chest Congestion Relief Liquid 2676
Vicks 44M Cough, Cold & Flu Relief Liquid 2680
Pediatric Vicks 44m Cough & Cold Relief Liquid 2676
Vicks DayQuil LiquiCaps/Liquid Multi-Symptom Cold/Flu Relief 761
Vicks DayQuil Multi-Symptom Cold/Flu Relief LiquiCaps 2678
Vicks DayQuil Multi-Symptom Cold/Flu Relief Liquid 2678
Vicks NyQuil Multi-Symptom Cold/Flu Relief Liquid 2681
Children's Vicks NyQuil Cold/Cough Relief 756
Vicks NyQuil Multi-Symptom Cold/Flu Relief LiquiCaps 2681
Vicks NyQuil LiquiCaps/Liquid Multi-Symptom Cold/Flu Relief 763
Vicks NyQuil Cough Liquid 2680
Children's Vicks NyQuil Cold/Cough Relief Liquid 2680
Zicam Cough Max Nighttime Cough Spray 767
Zicam Cough Max Cough Spray 767
Zicam Cough Max Cough Melts 767
Zicam Cough Plus D Cough Spray 767
Zicam Cough Relief Cough Spray 767
Zicam Maximum Strength Flu Daytime 768
Zicam Maximum Strength Flu Nighttime 768

Dextromethorphan Polistirex (Fluoxetine, like other agents that are metabolized by CYP2D6, inhibits the activity of this isoenzyme. Therapy with medications that are predominately metabolized by the CYP2D6 system and have a relatively narrow therapeutic index should be initiated at the low end of the dose range if the patient is receiving fluoxetine concurrently or has taken it in the previous five weeks. If fluoxetine is added to the treatment regimen of a patient already receiving a drug metabolized by CYP2D6, the need for a decreased dose of the original medication should be considered). Products include:
Delsym Extended-Release Suspension 12 Hour Cough Suppressant 611

Diazepam (The co-administration of diazepam with olanzapine may potentiate the orthostatic hypotension observed with olanzapine). Products include:
Diastat Rectal Delivery System 3343
Valium Tablets 2819

Diazoxide (Because of the potential for olanzapine to induce hypotension, Symbyax may enhance the effects of certain antihypertensive agents). Products include:
Hyperstat I.V. 3017

Diclofenac Potassium (Serotonin release by platelets plays an important role in hemostasis. Studies have demonstrated an association between the use of psychotropic drugs that interfere with serotonin reuptake and the occurrence of upper gastrointestinal bleeding. These studies have also shown that concurrent use of an NSAID potentiated the risk of bleeding. Therefore, patients should be cautioned about the use of NSAIDs concurrently with Symbyax).
No products indexed under this heading.

Diclofenac Sodium (Serotonin release by platelets plays an important role in hemostasis. Studies have demonstrated an association between the use of psychotropic drugs that interfere with serotonin reuptake and the occurrence of upper gastrointestinal bleeding. These studies have also shown that concurrent use of an NSAID potentiated the risk of bleeding. Therefore, patients should be cautioned about the use of NSAIDs concurrently with Symbyax). Products include:
Arthrotec Tablets 3129
Voltaren Ophthalmic Solution 2309
Voltaren Tablets 2307
Voltaren-XR Tablets 2310

Diltiazem Hydrochloride (Because of the potential for olanzapine to induce hypotension, Symbyax may enhance the effects of certain antihypertensive agents). Products include:
Cardizem LA Extended Release Tablets 1728
Tiazac Capsules 1201

Diltiazem Maleate (Agents that induce CYP1A2 or glucuronyl transferase enzymes may cause an increase in olanzapine concentration).
No products indexed under this heading.

Dipyridamole (Because fluoxetine is tightly bound to plasma protein, the administration of fluoxetine to a patient taking another drug that is tightly bound to protein may cause a shift in plasma concentrations potentially resulting in an adverse effect. Conversely, adverse effects may result from displacement of protein-bound fluoxetine by other tightly bound drugs). Products include:
Aggrenox Capsules 822
Persantine Tablets 868

Dolasetron Mesylate (Fluoxetine, like other agents that are metabolized by CYP2D6, inhibits the activity of this isoenzyme. Therapy with medications that are predominately metabolized by the CYP2D6 system and have a relatively narrow therapeutic index should be initiated at the low end of the dose range if the patient is receiving fluoxetine concurrently or has taken it in the previous five weeks. If fluoxetine is added to the treatment regimen of a patient already receiving a drug metabolized by CYP2D6, the need for a decreased dose of the original medication should be considered). Products include:
Anzemet Injection 2859
Anzemet Tablets 2862

Donepezil Hydrochloride (Fluoxetine, like other agents that are metabolized by CYP2D6, inhibits the activity of this isoenzyme. Therapy with medications that are predominately metabolized by the CYP2D6 system and have a relatively narrow therapeutic index should be initiated at the low end of the dose range if the patient is receiving fluoxetine concurrently or has taken it in the previous five weeks. If fluoxetine is added to the treatment regimen of a patient already receiving a drug metabolized by CYP2D6, the need for a decreased dose of the original medication should be considered). Products include:
Aricept Tablets 1094
Aricept ODT Tablets 1094

Dopamine Hydrochloride (The olanzapine component of Symbyax may antagonize the effects of levodopa and dopamine agonists).
No products indexed under this heading.

Doxazosin Mesylate (Because of the potential for olanzapine to induce hypotension, Symbyax may enhance the effects of certain antihypertensive agents). Products include:
Cardura XL Tablets 2515

Doxepin Hydrochloride (In two fluoxetine studies, previously stable plasma levels of imipramine and desipramine have increased >2- to 10-fold when fluoxetine has been administered in combination. This influence may persist for three weeks or longer after fluoxetine is discontinued. Thus, the dose of TCA may need to be reduced and plasma TCA concentrations may need to be monitored temporarily when Symbyax is co-administered or has been recently discontinued).
No products indexed under this heading.

Enalapril Maleate (Because of the potential for olanzapine to induce hypotension, Symbyax may enhance the effects of certain antihypertensive agents). Products include:
Vasotec I.V. Injection 2103

Enalaprilat (Because of the potential for olanzapine to induce hypotension, Symbyax may enhance the effects of certain antihypertensive agents).
No products indexed under this heading.

Encainide Hydrochloride (Fluoxetine, like other agents that are metabolized by CYP2D6, inhibits the activity of this isoenzyme. Therapy with medications that are predominately metabolized by the CYP2D6 system and have a relatively narrow therapeutic index should be initiated at the low end of the dose range if the patient is receiving fluoxetine concurrently or has taken it in the previous five weeks. If fluoxetine is added to the treatment regimen of a patient already receiving a drug metabolized by CYP2D6, the need for a decreased dose of the original medication should be considered).
No products indexed under this heading.

Eprosartan Mesylate (Because of the potential for olanzapine to induce hypotension, Symbyax may enhance the effects of certain antihypertensive agents). Products include:
Teveten Tablets 1735
Teveten HCT Tablets 1737

Erythromycin (Agents that induce CYP1A2 or glucuronyl transferase enzymes may cause an increase in olanzapine concentration). Products include:
Ery-Tab Tablets 449
Erythromycin Base Filmtab Tablets 455
Erythromycin Delayed-Release Capsules, USP 457
PCE Dispertab Tablets 515

Erythromycin Estolate (Agents that induce CYP1A2 or glucuronyl transferase enzymes may cause an increase in olanzapine concentration).
No products indexed under this heading.

Erythromycin Ethylsuccinate (Agents that induce CYP1A2 or glucuronyl transferase enzymes may cause an increase in olanzapine concentration). Products include:
E.E.S. 451
EryPed 447

Erythromycin Gluceptate (Agents that induce CYP1A2 or glucuronyl transferase enzymes may cause an increase in olanzapine concentration).
No products indexed under this heading.

IMPORTANT NOTE: Always consult each drug listing in the patient's regimen for possible interactions.

Erythromycin Lactobionate (Agents that induce CYP1A2 or glucuronyl transferase enzymes may cause an increase in olanzapine concentration).
No products indexed under this heading.

Erythromycin Stearate (Agents that induce CYP1A2 or glucuronyl transferase enzymes may cause an increase in olanzapine concentration). Products include:
Erythrocin Stearate Filmtab Tablets ... 453

Esmolol Hydrochloride (Because of the potential for olanzapine to induce hypotension, Symbyax may enhance the effects of certain antihypertensive agents).
No products indexed under this heading.

Etodolac (Serotonin release by platelets plays an important role in hemostasis. Studies have demonstrated an association between the use of psychotropic drugs that interfere with serotonin reuptake and the occurrence of upper gastrointestinal bleeding. These studies have also shown that concurrent use of an NSAID potentiated the risk of bleeding. Therefore, patients should be cautioned about the use of NSAIDs concurrently with Symbyax).
No products indexed under this heading.

Felodipine (Because of the potential for olanzapine to induce hypotension, Symbyax may enhance the effects of certain antihypertensive agents).
No products indexed under this heading.

Fenoprofen Calcium (Serotonin release by platelets plays an important role in hemostasis. Studies have demonstrated an association between the use of psychotropic drugs that interfere with serotonin reuptake and the occurrence of upper gastrointestinal bleeding. These studies have also shown that concurrent use of an NSAID potentiated the risk of bleeding. Therefore, patients should be cautioned about the use of NSAIDs concurrently with Symbyax). Products include:
Nalfon Capsules ... 2502

Fentanyl (Fluoxetine, like other agents that are metabolized by CYP2D6, inhibits the activity of this isoenzyme. Therapy with medications that are predominately metabolized by the CYP2D6 system and have a relatively narrow therapeutic index should be initiated at the low end of the dose range if the patient is receiving fluoxetine concurrently or has taken it in the previous five weeks. If fluoxetine is added to the treatment regimen of a patient already receiving a drug metabolized by CYP2D6, the need for a decreased dose of the original medication should be considered). Products include:
Duragesic Transdermal System ... 2373
Ionsys Transdermal System ... 2379

Fentanyl Citrate (Fluoxetine, like other agents that are metabolized by CYP2D6, inhibits the activity of this isoenzyme. Therapy with medications that are predominately metabolized by the CYP2D6 system and have a relatively narrow therapeutic index should be initiated at the low end of the dose range if the patient is receiving fluoxetine concurrently or has taken it in the previous five weeks. If fluoxetine is added to the treatment regimen of a patient already receiving a drug metabolized by CYP2D6, the need for a decreased dose of the original medication should be considered). Products include:
Actiq ... 979

Flecainide Acetate (Fluoxetine, like other agents that are metabolized by CYP2D6, inhibits the activity of this isoenzyme. Therapy with medications that are predominately metabolized by the CYP2D6 system and have a relatively narrow therapeutic index should be initiated at the low end of the dose range if the patient is receiving fluoxetine concurrently or has taken it in the previous five weeks. If fluoxetine is added to the treatment regimen of a patient already receiving a drug metabolized by CYP2D6, the need for a decreased dose of the original medication should be considered). Products include:
Tambocor Tablets ... 1856

Fluoxetine (Fluoxetine, like other agents that are metabolized by CYP2D6, inhibits the activity of this isoenzyme. Therapy with medications that are predominately metabolized by the CYP2D6 system and have a relatively narrow therapeutic index should be initiated at the low end of the dose range if the patient is receiving fluoxetine concurrently or has taken it in the previous five weeks. If fluoxetine is added to the treatment regimen of a patient already receiving a drug metabolized by CYP2D6, the need for a decreased dose of the original medication should be considered).
No products indexed under this heading.

Fluphenazine Decanoate (Fluoxetine, like other agents that are metabolized by CYP2D6, inhibits the activity of this isoenzyme. Therapy with medications that are predominately metabolized by the CYP2D6 system and have a relatively narrow therapeutic index should be initiated at the low end of the dose range if the patient is receiving fluoxetine concurrently or has taken it in the previous five weeks. If fluoxetine is added to the treatment regimen of a patient already receiving a drug metabolized by CYP2D6, the need for a decreased dose of the original medication should be considered).
No products indexed under this heading.

Fluphenazine Enanthate (Fluoxetine, like other agents that are metabolized by CYP2D6, inhibits the activity of this isoenzyme. Therapy with medications that are predominately metabolized by the CYP2D6 system and have a relatively narrow therapeutic index should be initiated at the low end of the dose range if the patient is receiving fluoxetine concurrently or has taken it in the previous five weeks. If fluoxetine is added to the treatment regimen of a patient already receiving a drug metabolized by CYP2D6, the need for a decreased dose of the original medication should be considered).
No products indexed under this heading.

Fluphenazine Hydrochloride (Fluoxetine, like other agents that are metabolized by CYP2D6, inhibits the activity of this isoenzyme. Therapy with medications that are predominately metabolized by the CYP2D6 system and have a relatively narrow therapeutic index should be initiated at the low end of the dose range if the patient is receiving fluoxetine concurrently or has taken it in the previous five weeks. If fluoxetine is added to the treatment regimen of a patient already receiving a drug metabolized by CYP2D6, the need for a decreased dose of the original medication should be considered).
No products indexed under this heading.

Flurazepam Hydrochloride (Because fluoxetine is tightly bound to plasma protein, the administration of fluoxetine to a patient taking another drug that is tightly bound to protein may cause a shift in plasma concentrations potentially resulting in an adverse effect. Conversely, adverse effects may result from displacement of protein-bound fluoxetine by other tightly bound drugs). Products include:
Dalmane Capsules ... 3342

Flurbiprofen (Serotonin release by platelets plays an important role in hemostasis. Studies have demonstrated an association between the use of psychotropic drugs that interfere with serotonin reuptake and the occurrence of upper gastrointestinal bleeding. These studies have also shown that concurrent use of an NSAID potentiated the risk of bleeding. Therefore, patients should be cautioned about the use of NSAIDs concurrently with Symbyax).
No products indexed under this heading.

Fluvoxamine (Fluvoxamine, a CYP1A2 inhibitor, decreases the clearance of olanzapine. This results in a mean increase in olanzapine Cmax and AUC following fluvoxamine administration. Lower doses of the olanzapine component of Symbyax should be considered in patients receiving concomitant treatment with fluvoxamine).
No products indexed under this heading.

Fluvoxamine Maleate (Fluvoxamine, a CYP1A2 inhibitor, decreases the clearance of olanzapine. This results in a mean increase in olanzapine Cmax and AUC following fluvoxamine administration. Lower doses of the olanzapine component of Symbyax should be considered in patients receiving concomitant treatment with fluvoxamine).
No products indexed under this heading.

Formoterol Fumarate (Fluoxetine, like other agents that are metabolized by CYP2D6, inhibits the activity of this isoenzyme. Therapy with medications that are predominately metabolized by the CYP2D6 system and have a relatively narrow therapeutic index should be initiated at the low end of the dose range if the patient is receiving fluoxetine concurrently or has taken it in the previous five weeks. If fluoxetine is added to the treatment regimen of a patient already receiving a drug metabolized by CYP2D6, the need for a decreased dose of the original medication should be considered). Products include:
Foradil Aerolizer ... 3010

Fosinopril Sodium (Because of the potential for olanzapine to induce hypotension, Symbyax may enhance the effects of certain antihypertensive agents).
No products indexed under this heading.

Fosphenytoin Sodium (Patients on stable doses of phenytoin have developed elevated plasma levels of phenytoin with clinical pheytoin toxicity following initiation of concomitant fluoxetine).
No products indexed under this heading.

Furosemide (Because of the potential for olanzapine to induce hypotension, Symbyax may enhance the effects of certain antihypertensive agents). Products include:
Furosemide Tablets ... 2154

Galantamine Hydrobromide (Fluoxetine, like other agents that are metabolized by CYP2D6, inhibits the activity of this isoenzyme. Therapy with medications that are predominately metabolized by the CYP2D6 system and have a relatively narrow therapeutic index should be initiated at the low end of the dose range if the patient is receiving fluoxetine concurrently or has taken it in the previous five weeks. If fluoxetine is added to the treatment regimen of a patient already receiving a drug metabolized by CYP2D6, the need for a decreased dose of the original medication should be considered). Products include:
Razadyne ... 2399
Razadyne ER Extended-Release Capsules ... 2399

Glipizide (Because fluoxetine is tightly bound to plasma protein, the administration of fluoxetine to a patient taking another drug that is tightly bound to protein may cause a shift in plasma concentrations potentially resulting in an adverse effect. Conversely, adverse effects may result from displacement of protein-bound fluoxetine by other tightly bound drugs).
No products indexed under this heading.

Guanabenz Acetate (Because of the potential for olanzapine to induce hypotension, Symbyax may enhance the effects of certain antihypertensive agents).
No products indexed under this heading.

Guanethidine Monosulfate (Because of the potential for olanzapine to induce hypotension, Symbyax may enhance the effects of certain antihypertensive agents).
No products indexed under this heading.

Haloperidol (Elevation of blood levels of haloperidol has been observed in patients receiving concomitant fluoxetine).
No products indexed under this heading.

Haloperidol Decanoate (Elevation of blood levels of haloperidol has been observed in patients receiving concomitant fluoxetine).
No products indexed under this heading.

Haloperidol Lactate (Elevation of blood levels of haloperidol have been observed in patients receiving concomitant fluoxetine).
No products indexed under this heading.

Hydralazine Hydrochloride (Because of the potential for olanzapine to induce hypotension, Symbyax may enhance the effects of certain antihypertensive agents).
Products include:
BiDil Tablets 2171

Hydrochlorothiazide (Because of the potential for olanzapine to induce hypotension, Symbyax may enhance the effects of certain antihypertensive agents). Products include:
Aldoril Tablets 1910
Atacand HCT 651
Avalide Tablets 888
Avalide Tablets 2874
Benicar HCT Tablets 1044
Diovan HCT Tablets 2196
Dyazide Capsules 1423
Hyzaar 50-12.5 Tablets 1990
Hyzaar 100-12.5 Tablets 1990
Hyzaar 100-25 Tablets 1990
Lopressor HCT 50/25 Tablets 2241
Lopressor HCT 100/25 Tablets 2241
Lopressor HCT 100/50 Tablets 2241
Lotensin HCT Tablets 2246
Micardis HCT Tablets 856
Moduretic Tablets 2028
Prinzide Tablets 2056
Teveten HCT Tablets 1737
Timolide Tablets 2086
Uniretic Tablets 3100

Hydrocodone Bitartrate (Fluoxetine, like other agents that are metabolized by CYP2D6, inhibits the activity of this isoenzyme. Therapy with medications that are predominately metabolized by the CYP2D6 system and have a relatively narrow therapeutic index should be initiated at the low end of the dose range if the patient is receiving fluoxetine concurrently or has taken it in the previous five weeks. If fluoxetine is added to the treatment regimen of a patient already receiving a drug metabolized by CYP2D6, the need for a decreased dose of the original medication should be considered).
Products include:
Hycodan 1116
Hycotuss Expectorant Syrup 1117
Vicodin Tablets 535
Vicodin ES Tablets 536
Vicodin HP Tablets 538
Vicoprofen Tablets 539
Zydone Tablets 1139

Hydroflumethiazide (Because of the potential for olanzapine to induce hypotension, Symbyax may enhance the effects of certain antihypertensive agents).
No products indexed under this heading.

Hypericum (Agents that induce CYP1A2 or glucuronyl transferase enzymes may cause an increase in olanzapine concentration). Products include:
Satiete Tablets 832

Ibuprofen (Serotonin release by platelets plays an important role in hemostasis. Studies have demonstrated an association between the use of psychotropic drugs that interfere with serotonin reuptake and the occurrence of upper gastrointestinal bleeding. These studies have also shown that concurrent use of an NSAID potentiated the risk of bleeding. Therefore, patients should be cautioned about the use of NSAIDs concurrently with Symbyax).
Products include:
Advil Allergy Sinus Caplets 770
Advil 674
Children's Advil Oral Suspension 603
Children's Advil Chewable Tablets 603
Advil Cold & Sinus 723
Infants' Advil Concentrated Drops 604
Infants' Advil Concentrated Drops - White Grape (Dye-Free) 604
Junior Strength Advil Swallow Tablets 605
Advil Migraine Liquigels 608
Advil Multi-Symptom Cold Caplets 770
Advil PM Caplets 615
Motrin IB Tablets and Caplets 1866
Children's Motrin Oral Suspension 1867
Children's Motrin Non-Staining Dye-Free Oral Suspension 1867
Children's Motrin Cold Oral Suspension 1867
Infants' Motrin Concentrated Drops 1867
Infants' Motrin Non-Staining Dye-Free Concentrated Drops 1867
Junior Strength Motrin Caplets and Chewable Tablets 1867
Vicoprofen Tablets 539

Imipramine Hydrochloride (In two fluoxetine studies, previously stable plasma levels of imipramine and desipramine have increased >2- to 10-fold when fluoxetine has been administered in combination. This influence may persist for three weeks or longer after fluoxetine is discontinued. Thus, the dose of TCA may need to be reduced and plasma TCA concentrations may need to be monitored temporarily when Symbyax is co-administered or has been recently discontinued).
No products indexed under this heading.

Imipramine Pamoate (In two fluoxetine studies, previously stable plasma levels of imipramine and desipramine have increased >2- to 10-fold when fluoxetine has been administered in combination. This influence may persist for three weeks or longer after fluoxetine is discontinued. Thus, the dose of TCA may need to be reduced and plasma TCA concentrations may need to be monitored temporarily when Symbyax is co-administered or has been recently discontinued).
No products indexed under this heading.

Indapamide (Because of the potential for olanzapine to induce hypotension, Symbyax may enhance the effects of certain antihypertensive agents). Products include:
Indapamide Tablets 2156

Indomethacin (Serotonin release by platelets plays an important role in hemostasis. Studies have demonstrated an association between the use of psychotropic drugs that interfere with serotonin reuptake and the occurrence of upper gastrointestinal bleeding. These studies have also shown that concurrent use of an NSAID potentiated the risk of bleeding. Therefore, patients should be cautioned about the use of NSAIDs concurrently with Symbyax).
Products include:
Indocin 1995

Indomethacin Sodium Trihydrate (Serotonin release by platelets plays an important role in hemostasis. Studies have demonstrated an association between the use of psychotropic drugs that interfere with serotonin reuptake and the occurrence of upper gastrointestinal bleeding. These studies have also shown that concurrent use of an NSAID potentiated the risk of bleeding. Therefore, patients should be cautioned about the use of NSAIDs concurrently with Symbyax).
Products include:
Indocin I.V. 2465

Indoramin Hydrochloride (Fluoxetine, like other agents that are metabolized by CYP2D6, inhibits the activity of this isoenzyme. Therapy with medications that are predominately metabolized by the CYP2D6 system and have a relatively narrow therapeutic index should be initiated at the low end of the dose range if the patient is receiving fluoxetine concurrently or has taken it in the previous five weeks. If fluoxetine is added to the treatment regimen of a patient already receiving a drug metabolized by CYP2D6, the need for a decreased dose of the original medication should be considered).
No products indexed under this heading.

Insulin (Agents that induce CYP1A2 or glucuronyl transferase enzymes may cause an increase in olanzapine concentration).
No products indexed under this heading.

Irbesartan (Because of the potential for olanzapine to induce hypotension, Symbyax may enhance the effects of certain antihypertensive agents). Products include:
Avalide Tablets 888
Avalide Tablets 2874
Avapro Tablets 891
Avapro Tablets 2871

Isocarboxazid (Concomitant use in patients taking MAO inhibitors is contraindicated. There have been reports of serious, sometimes fatal, reactions in patients receiving, or who have recently discontinued, fluoxetine and are then started on an MAO inhibitor. Therefore, Symbyax should not be used in combination with, or within a minimum of 14 days of discontinuing, MAO inhibitors).
No products indexed under this heading.

Isradipine (Because of the potential for olanzapine to induce hypotension, Symbyax may enhance the effects of certain antihypertensive agents). Products include:
DynaCirc CR Tablets 2721

Ketoprofen (Serotonin release by platelets plays an important role in hemostasis. Studies have demonstrated an association between the use of psychotropic drugs that interfere with serotonin reuptake and the occurrence of upper gastrointestinal bleeding. These studies have also shown that concurrent use of an NSAID potentiated the risk of bleeding. Therefore, patients should be cautioned about the use of NSAIDs concurrently with Symbyax).
No products indexed under this heading.

Ketorolac Tromethamine (Serotonin release by platelets plays an important role in hemostasis. Studies have demonstrated an association between the use of psychotropic drugs that interfere with serotonin reuptake and the occurrence of upper gastrointestinal bleeding. These studies have also shown that concurrent use of an NSAID potentiated the risk of bleeding. Therefore, patients should be cautioned about the use of NSAIDs concurrently with Symbyax). Products include:
Acular Ophthalmic Solution 565
Acular LS Ophthalmic Solution 566

Labetalol Hydrochloride (Because of the potential for olanzapine to induce hypotension, Symbyax may enhance the effects of certain antihypertensive agents).
No products indexed under this heading.

Lansoprazole (Agents that induce CYP1A2 or glucuronyl transferase enzymes may cause an increase in olanzapine concentration). Products include:
Prevacid Delayed-Release Capsules 3271
Prevacid for Delayed-Release Oral Suspension 3271
Prevacid SoluTab Delayed-Release Orally Disintegrating Tablets 3271
Prevacid I.V. for Injection 3277
Prevacid NapraPAC 3280
PREVPAC 3284

Levodopa (The olanzapine component of Symbyax may antagonize the effects of levodopa and dopamine agonists). Products include:
Parcopa Orally Disintegrating Tablets 3097
Stalevo Tablets 2287

Lidocaine (Fluoxetine, like other agents that are metabolized by CYP2D6, inhibits the activity of this isoenzyme. Therapy with medications that are predominately metabolized by the CYP2D6 system and have a relatively narrow therapeutic index should be initiated at the low end of the dose range if the patient is receiving fluoxetine concurrently or has taken it in the previous five weeks. If fluoxetine is added to the treatment regimen of a patient already receiving a drug metabolized by CYP2D6, the need for a decreased dose of the original medication should be considered).
Products include:
Lidoderm Patch 1118
Synera Topical Patch 1137

Lidocaine Hydrochloride (Fluoxetine, like other agents that are metabolized by CYP2D6, inhibits the activity of this isoenzyme. Therapy with medications that are predominately metabolized by the CYP2D6 system and have a relatively narrow therapeutic index should be initiated at the low end of the dose range if the patient is receiving fluoxetine concurrently or has taken it in the previous five weeks. If fluoxetine is added to the treatment regimen of a patient already receiving a drug metabolized by CYP2D6, the need for a decreased dose of the original medication should be considered).
No products indexed under this heading.

Lisinopril (Because of the potential for olanzapine to induce hypotension, Symbyax may enhance the effects of certain antihypertensive agents). Products include:
Prinivil Tablets 2052
Prinzide Tablets 2056

Lithium (There have been reports of both increased and decreased lithium levels when lithium was used concomitantly with fluoxetine. Cases of lithium toxicity and increased serotonergic effects have been reported. Lithium levels should be monitored in patients taking Symbyax concomitantly with lithium).
No products indexed under this heading.

Lithium Carbonate (There have been reports of both increased and decreased lithium levels when lithium

was used concomitantly with fluoxetine. Cases of lithium toxicity and increased serotonergic effects have been reported. Lithium levels should be monitored in patients taking Symbyax concomitantly with lithium). Products include:

Lithobid Tablets 1692

Lithium Citrate (There have been reports of both increased and decreased lithium levels when lithium was used concomitantly with fluoxetine. Cases of lithium toxicity and increased serotonergic effects have been reported. Lithium levels should be monitored in patients taking Symbyax concomitantly with lithium).

No products indexed under this heading.

Losartan Potassium (Because of the potential for olanzapine to induce hypotension, Symbyax may enhance the effects of certain antihypertensive agents). Products include:

Cozaar Tablets 1935
Hyzaar 50-12.5 Tablets 1990
Hyzaar 100-12.5 Tablets 1990
Hyzaar 100-25 Tablets 1990

Maprotiline Hydrochloride (In two fluoxetine studies, previously stable plasma levels of imipramine and desipramine have increased >2- to 10-fold when fluoxetine has been administered in combination. This influence may persist for three weeks or longer after fluoxetine is discontinued. Thus, the dose of TCA may need to be reduced and plasma TCA concentrations may need to be monitored temporarily when Symbyax is co-administered or has been recently discontinued).

No products indexed under this heading.

Mecamylamine Hydrochloride (Because of the potential for olanzapine to induce hypotension, Symbyax may enhance the effects of certain antihypertensive agents).

No products indexed under this heading.

Meclofenamate Sodium (Serotonin release by platelets plays an important role in hemostasis. Studies have demonstrated an association between the use of psychotropic drugs that interfere with serotonin reuptake and the occurrence of upper gastrointestinal bleeding. These studies have also shown that concurrent use of an NSAID potentiated the risk of bleeding. Therefore, patients should be cautioned about the use of NSAIDs concurrently with Symbyax).

No products indexed under this heading.

Mefenamic Acid (Serotonin release by platelets plays an important role in hemostasis. Studies have demonstrated an association between the use of psychotropic drugs that interfere with serotonin reuptake and the occurrence of upper gastrointestinal bleeding. These studies have also shown that concurrent use of an NSAID potentiated the risk of bleeding. Therefore, patients should be cautioned about the use of NSAIDs concurrently with Symbyax).

No products indexed under this heading.

Meloxicam (Serotonin release by platelets plays an important role in hemostasis. Studies have demonstrated an association between the use of psychotropic drugs that inter-

fere with serotonin reuptake and the occurrence of upper gastrointestinal bleeding. These studies have also shown that concurrent use of an NSAID potentiated the risk of bleeding. Therefore, patients should be cautioned about the use of NSAIDs concurrently with Symbyax). Products include:

Mobic Oral Suspension 863
Mobic Tablets 863

Meperidine Hydrochloride (Fluoxetine, like other agents that are metabolized by CYP2D6, inhibits the activity of this isoenzyme. Therapy with medications that are predominately metabolized by the CYP2D6 system and have a relatively narrow therapeutic index should be initiated at the low end of the dose range if the patient is receiving fluoxetine concurrently or has taken it in the previous five weeks. If fluoxetine is added to the treatment regimen of a patient already receiving a drug metabolized by CYP2D6, the need for a decreased dose of the original medication should be considered).

No products indexed under this heading.

Methadone Hydrochloride (Fluoxetine, like other agents that are metabolized by CYP2D6, inhibits the activity of this isoenzyme. Therapy with medications that are predominately metabolized by the CYP2D6 system and have a relatively narrow therapeutic index should be initiated at the low end of the dose range if the patient is receiving fluoxetine concurrently or has taken it in the previous five weeks. If fluoxetine is added to the treatment regimen of a patient already receiving a drug metabolized by CYP2D6, the need for a decreased dose of the original medication should be considered).

No products indexed under this heading.

Methamphetamine Hydrochloride (Fluoxetine, like other agents that are metabolized by CYP2D6, inhibits the activity of this isoenzyme. Therapy with medications that are predominately metabolized by the CYP2D6 system and have a relatively narrow therapeutic index should be initiated at the low end of the dose range if the patient is receiving fluoxetine concurrently or has taken it in the previous five weeks. If fluoxetine is added to the treatment regimen of a patient already receiving a drug metabolized by CYP2D6, the need for a decreased dose of the original medication should be considered). Products include:

Desoxyn Tablets, USP 2462

Methyclothiazide (Because of the potential for olanzapine to induce hypotension, Symbyax may enhance the effects of certain antihypertensive agents).

No products indexed under this heading.

Methyldopa (Because of the potential for olanzapine to induce hypotension, Symbyax may enhance the effects of certain antihypertensive agents). Products include:

Aldoril Tablets 1910

Methyldopate Hydrochloride (Because of the potential for olanzapine to induce hypotension, Symbyax may enhance the effects of certain antihypertensive agents).

No products indexed under this heading.

Metolazone (Because of the potential for olanzapine to induce hypotension, Symbyax may enhance the effects of certain antihypertensive agents).

No products indexed under this heading.

Metoprolol Succinate (Because of the potential for olanzapine to induce hypotension, Symbyax may enhance the effects of certain antihypertensive agents). Products include:

Toprol-XL Tablets 668

Metoprolol Tartrate (Because of the potential for olanzapine to induce hypotension, Symbyax may enhance the effects of certain antihypertensive agents). Products include:

Lopressor Injection 2238
Lopressor Tablets 2238
Lopressor HCT 50/25 Tablets 2241
Lopressor HCT 100/25 Tablets 2241
Lopressor HCT 100/50 Tablets 2241

Metyrosine (Because of the potential for olanzapine to induce hypotension, Symbyax may enhance the effects of certain antihypertensive agents). Products include:

Demser Capsules 1953

Mexiletine Hydrochloride (Fluoxetine, like other agents that are metabolized by CYP2D6, inhibits the activity of this isoenzyme. Therapy with medications that are predominately metabolized by the CYP2D6 system and have a relatively narrow therapeutic index should be initiated at the low end of the dose range if the patient is receiving fluoxetine concurrently or has taken it in the previous five weeks. If fluoxetine is added to the treatment regimen of a patient already receiving a drug metabolized by CYP2D6, the need for a decreased dose of the original medication should be considered).

No products indexed under this heading.

Mibefradil Dihydrochloride (Because of the potential for olanzapine to induce hypotension, Symbyax may enhance the effects of certain antihypertensive agents).

No products indexed under this heading.

Midazolam Hydrochloride (Because fluoxetine is tightly bound to plasma protein, the administration of fluoxetine to a patient taking another drug that is tightly bound to protein may cause a shift in plasma concentrations potentially resulting in an adverse effect. Conversely, adverse effects may result from displacement of protein-bound fluoxetine by other tightly bound drugs).

No products indexed under this heading.

Minoxidil (Because of the potential for olanzapine to induce hypotension, Symbyax may enhance the effects of certain antihypertensive agents). Products include:

Men's Rogaine Extra Strength Hair Regrowth Treatment Topical Solution, Ocean Rush Scent and Original Unscented ▣◪633
Men's Rogaine Foam Hair Regrowth Treatment ▣◪633
Women's Rogaine Hair Regrowth Treatment Topical Solution, Spring Bloom Scent and Original Unscented ▣◪634

Mirtazapine (Fluoxetine, like other agents that are metabolized by CYP2D6, inhibits the activity of this isoenzyme. Therapy with medications that are predominately metabo-

lized by the CYP2D6 system and have a relatively narrow therapeutic index should be initiated at the low end of the dose range if the patient is receiving fluoxetine concurrently or has taken it in the previous five weeks. If fluoxetine is added to the treatment regimen of a patient already receiving a drug metabolized by CYP2D6, the need for a decreased dose of the original medication should be considered).

No products indexed under this heading.

Moclobemide (Concomitant use in patients taking MAO inhibitors is contraindicated. There have been reports of serious, sometimes fatal, reactions in patients receiving, or who have recently discontinued, fluoxetine and are then started on an MAO inhibitor. Therefore, Symbyax should not be used in combination with, or within a minimum of 14 days of discontinuing, MAO inhibitors).

No products indexed under this heading.

Moexipril Hydrochloride (Because of the potential for olanzapine to induce hypotension, Symbyax may enhance the effects of certain antihypertensive agents). Products include:

Uniretic Tablets 3100
Univasc Tablets 3104

Morphine Sulfate (Fluoxetine, like other agents that are metabolized by CYP2D6, inhibits the activity of this isoenzyme. Therapy with medications that are predominately metabolized by the CYP2D6 system and have a relatively narrow therapeutic index should be initiated at the low end of the dose range if the patient is receiving fluoxetine concurrently or has taken it in the previous five weeks. If fluoxetine is added to the treatment regimen of a patient already receiving a drug metabolized by CYP2D6, the need for a decreased dose of the original medication should be considered). Products include:

Avinza Capsules 1741
Kadian Capsules 577
MS Contin Tablets 2701

Nabumetone (Serotonin release by platelets plays an important role in hemostasis. Studies have demonstrated an association between the use of psychotropic drugs that interfere with serotonin reuptake and the occurrence of upper gastrointestinal bleeding. These studies have also shown that concurrent use of an NSAID potentiated the risk of bleeding. Therefore, patients should be cautioned about the use of NSAIDs concurrently with Symbyax).

No products indexed under this heading.

Nadolol (Because of the potential for olanzapine to induce hypotension, Symbyax may enhance the effects of certain antihypertensive agents). Products include:

Nadolol Tablets 2159

Nafcillin Sodium (Agents that induce CYP1A2 or glucuronyl transferase enzymes may cause an increase in olanzapine concentration).

No products indexed under this heading.

Naproxen (Serotonin release by platelets plays an important role in hemostasis. Studies have demonstrated an association between the

use of psychotropic drugs that interfere with serotonin reuptake and the occurrence of upper gastrointestinal bleeding. These studies have also shown that concurrent use of an NSAID potentiated the risk of bleeding. Therefore, patients should be cautioned about the use of NSAIDs concurrently with Symbyax).
Products include:
- EC-Naprosyn Delayed-Release Tablets 2761
- Naprosyn Suspension 2761
- Naprosyn Tablets 2761
- Prevacid NapraPAC 3280

Naproxen Sodium (Serotonin release by platelets plays an important role in hemostasis. Studies have demonstrated an association between the use of psychotropic drugs that interfere with serotonin reuptake and the occurrence of upper gastrointestinal bleeding. These studies have also shown that concurrent use of an NSAID potentiated the risk of bleeding. Therefore, patients should be cautioned about the use of NSAIDs concurrently with Symbyax). Products include:
- Aleve Caplets 742
- Aleve Gelcaps 743
- Aleve Tablets 743
- Aleve Cold & Sinus Caplets 744
- Anaprox Tablets 2761
- Anaprox DS Tablets 2761

Nelfinavir Mesylate (Fluoxetine, like other agents that are metabolized by CYP2D6, inhibits the activity of this isoenzyme. Therapy with medications that are predominately metabolized by the CYP2D6 system and have a relatively narrow therapeutic index should be initiated at the low end of the dose range if the patient is receiving fluoxetine concurrently or has taken it in the previous five weeks. If fluoxetine is added to the treatment regimen of a patient already receiving a drug metabolized by CYP2D6, the need for a decreased dose of the original medication should be considered).
Products include:
- Viracept 2577

Nicardipine Hydrochloride (Because of the potential for olanzapine to induce hypotension, Symbyax may enhance the effects of certain antihypertensive agents).
Products include:
- Cardene I.V. 2497

Nicotine (Agents that induce CYP1A2 or glucuronyl transferase enzymes may cause an increase in olanzapine concentration). Products include:
- NicoDerm CQ Clear Patch 622

Nicotine Polacrilex (Agents that induce CYP1A2 or glucuronyl transferase enzymes may cause an increase in olanzapine concentration).
No products indexed under this heading.

Nicotine Salicylate (Agents that induce CYP1A2 or glucuronyl transferase enzymes may cause an increase in olanzapine concentration).
No products indexed under this heading.

Nicotine Sulfate (Agents that induce CYP1A2 or glucuronyl transferase enzymes may cause an increase in olanzapine concentration).
No products indexed under this heading.

Nifedipine (Because of the potential for olanzapine to induce hypotension, Symbyax may enhance the effects of certain antihypertensive agents). Products include:
- Adalat CC Tablets 2964

Nisoldipine (Because of the potential for olanzapine to induce hypotension, Symbyax may enhance the effects of certain antihypertensive agents). Products include:
- Sular Tablets 3122

Nitroglycerin (Because of the potential for olanzapine to induce hypotension, Symbyax may enhance the effects of certain antihypertensive agents). Products include:
- Nitro-Dur Transdermal Infusion System 3046
- Nitrolingual Pumpspray 3120

Nortriptyline Hydrochloride (In two fluoxetine studies, previously stable plasma levels of imipramine and desipramine have increased >2- to 10-fold when fluoxetine has been administered in combination. This influence may persist for three weeks or longer after fluoxetine is discontinued. Thus, the dose of TCA may need to be reduced and plasma TCA concentrations may need to be monitored temporarily when Symbyax is co-administered or has been recently discontinued).
No products indexed under this heading.

Omeprazole (Fluoxetine, like other agents that are metabolized by CYP2D6, inhibits the activity of this isoenzyme. Therapy with medications that are predominately metabolized by the CYP2D6 system and have a relatively narrow therapeutic index should be initiated at the low end of the dose range if the patient is receiving fluoxetine concurrently or has taken it in the previous five weeks. If fluoxetine is added to the treatment regimen of a patient already receiving a drug metabolized by CYP2D6, the need for a decreased dose of the original medication should be considered).
Products include:
- Zegerid Capsules 2958
- Zegerid Powder for Oral Solution 2958

Ondansetron (Fluoxetine, like other agents that are metabolized by CYP2D6, inhibits the activity of this isoenzyme. Therapy with medications that are predominately metabolized by the CYP2D6 system and have a relatively narrow therapeutic index should be initiated at the low end of the dose range if the patient is receiving fluoxetine concurrently or has taken it in the previous five weeks. If fluoxetine is added to the treatment regimen of a patient already receiving a drug metabolized by CYP2D6, the need for a decreased dose of the original medication should be considered).
Products include:
- Zofran ODT Orally Disintegrating Tablets 1639

Ondansetron Hydrochloride (Fluoxetine, like other agents that are metabolized by CYP2D6, inhibits the activity of this isoenzyme. Therapy with medications that are predominately metabolized by the CYP2D6 system and have a relatively narrow therapeutic index should be initiated at the low end of the dose range if the patient is receiving fluoxetine concurrently or has taken it in the previous five weeks. If fluoxetine is added to the treatment regimen of a patient already receiving a drug metabolized by CYP2D6, the need for a decreased dose of the original medication should be considered).
Products include:
- Zofran Injection 1634
- Zofran 1639

Oxaprozin (Serotonin release by platelets plays an important role in hemostasis. Studies have demonstrated an association between the use of psychotropic drugs that interfere with serotonin reuptake and the occurrence of upper gastrointestinal bleeding. These studies have also shown that concurrent use of an NSAID potentiated the risk of bleeding. Therefore, patients should be cautioned about the use of NSAIDs concurrently with Symbyax).
No products indexed under this heading.

Oxazepam (Because fluoxetine is tightly bound to plasma protein, the administration of fluoxetine to a patient taking another drug that is tightly bound to protein may cause a shift in plasma concentrations potentially resulting in an adverse effect. Conversely, adverse effects may result from displacement of protein-bound fluoxetine by other tightly bound drugs).
No products indexed under this heading.

Oxycodone Hydrochloride (Fluoxetine, like other agents that are metabolized by CYP2D6, inhibits the activity of this isoenzyme. Therapy with medications that are predominately metabolized by the CYP2D6 system and have a relatively narrow therapeutic index should be initiated at the low end of the dose range if the patient is receiving fluoxetine concurrently or has taken it in the previous five weeks. If fluoxetine is added to the treatment regimen of a patient already receiving a drug metabolized by CYP2D6, the need for a decreased dose of the original medication should be considered).
Products include:
- OxyContin Tablets 2703
- OxyFast Oral Concentrate Solution 2708
- OxyIR Capsules 2708
- Percocet Tablets 1131
- Percodan Tablets 1132

Paclitaxel (Fluoxetine, like other agents that are metabolized by CYP2D6, inhibits the activity of this isoenzyme. Therapy with medications that are predominately metabolized by the CYP2D6 system and have a relatively narrow therapeutic index should be initiated at the low end of the dose range if the patient is receiving fluoxetine concurrently or has taken it in the previous five weeks. If fluoxetine is added to the treatment regimen of a patient already receiving a drug metabolized by CYP2D6, the need for a decreased dose of the original medication should be considered).
No products indexed under this heading.

Pargyline Hydrochloride (Concomitant use in patients taking MAO inhibitors is contraindicated. There have been reports of serious, sometimes fatal, reactions in patients receiving, or who have recently discontinued, fluoxetine and are then started on an MAO inhibitor. Therefore, Symbyax should not be used in combination with, or within a minimum of 14 days of discontinuing, MAO inhibitors).
No products indexed under this heading.

Paroxetine Hydrochloride (Fluoxetine, like other agents that are metabolized by CYP2D6, inhibits the activity of this isoenzyme. Therapy with medications that are predominately metabolized by the CYP2D6 system and have a relatively narrow therapeutic index should be initiated at the low end of the dose range if the patient is receiving fluoxetine concurrently or has taken it in the previous five weeks. If fluoxetine is added to the treatment regimen of a patient already receiving a drug metabolized by CYP2D6, the need for a decreased dose of the original medication should be considered).
Products include:
- Paxil CR Controlled-Release Tablets 1538
- Paxil 1530

Penbutolol Sulfate (Because of the potential for olanzapine to induce hypotension, Symbyax may enhance the effects of certain antihypertensive agents).
No products indexed under this heading.

Pergolide Mesylate (The olanzapine component of Symbyax may antagonize the effects of levodopa and dopamine agonists). Products include:
- Permax Tablets 3356

Perindopril Erbumine (Because of the potential for olanzapine to induce hypotension, Symbyax may enhance the effects of certain antihypertensive agents). Products include:
- Aceon Tablets (2 mg, 4 mg, 8 mg) 3194

Phenelzine Sulfate (Concomitant use in patients taking MAO inhibitors is contraindicated. There have been reports of serious, sometimes fatal, reactions in patients receiving, or who have recently discontinued, fluoxetine and are then started on an MAO inhibitor. Therefore, Symbyax should not be used in combination with, or within a minimum of 14 days of discontinuing, MAO inhibitors).
No products indexed under this heading.

Phenobarbital (Agents that induce CYP1A2 or glucuronyl transferase enzymes may cause an increase in olanzapine concentration). Products include:
- Donnatal Extentabs 2493

Phenoxybenzamine Hydrochloride (Because of the potential for olanzapine to induce hypotension, Symbyax may enhance the effects of certain antihypertensive agents).
Products include:
- Dibenzyline Capsules 3399

Phentolamine Mesylate (Because of the potential for olanzapine to induce hypotension, Symbyax may enhance the effects of certain antihypertensive agents).
No products indexed under this heading.

Phenylbutazone (Serotonin release by platelets plays an important role in hemostasis. Studies have demonstrated an association between the use of psychotropic drugs that interfere with serotonin reuptake and the occurrence of upper gastrointestinal bleeding. These studies have also shown that

concurrent use of an NSAID potentiated the risk of bleeding. Therefore, patients should be cautioned about the use of NSAIDs concurrently with Symbyax).
No products indexed under this heading.

Phenytoin (Patients on stable doses of phenytoin have developed elevated plasma levels of phenytoin with clinical pheytoin toxicity following initiation of concomitant fluoxetine).
No products indexed under this heading.

Phenytoin Sodium (Patients on stable doses of phenytoin have developed elevated plasma levels of phenytoin with clinical pheytoin toxicity following initiation of concomitant fluoxetine). Products include:
Phenytek Capsules 2160

Pimozide (Concomitant use in patients taking pimozide is contraindicated).
No products indexed under this heading.

Pindolol (Because of the potential for olanzapine to induce hypotension, Symbyax may enhance the effects of certain antihypertensive agents).
No products indexed under this heading.

Piroxicam (Serotonin release by platelets plays an important role in hemostasis. Studies have demonstrated an association between the use of psychotropic drugs that interfere with serotonin reuptake and the occurrence of upper gastrointestinal bleeding. These studies have also shown that concurrent use of an NSAID potentiated the risk of bleeding. Therefore, patients should be cautioned about the use of NSAIDs concurrently with Symbyax).
No products indexed under this heading.

Polythiazide (Because of the potential for olanzapine to induce hypotension, Symbyax may enhance the effects of certain antihypertensive agents).
No products indexed under this heading.

Pramipexole Dihydrochloride (The olanzapine component of Symbyax may antagonize the effects of levodopa and dopamine agonists). Products include:
Mirapex Tablets 859

Prazosin Hydrochloride (Because of the potential for olanzapine to induce hypotension, Symbyax may enhance the effects of certain antihypertensive agents).
No products indexed under this heading.

Primidone (Agents that induce CYP1A2 or glucuronyl transferase enzymes may cause an increase in olanzapine concentration).
No products indexed under this heading.

Procarbazine Hydrochloride (Concomitant use in patients taking MAO inhibitors is contraindicated. There have been reports of serious, sometimes fatal, reactions in patients receiving, or who have recently discontinued, fluoxetine and are then started on an MAO inhibitor. Therefore, Symbyax should not be used in combination with, or within a minimum of 14 days of discontinuing, MAO inhibitors). Products include:
Matulane Capsules 3191

Propafenone Hydrochloride (Fluoxetine, like other agents that are metabolized by CYP2D6, inhibits the activity of this isoenzyme. Therapy with medications that are predominately metabolized by the CYP2D6 system and have a relatively narrow therapeutic index should be initiated at the low end of the dose range if the patient is receiving fluoxetine concurrently or has taken it in the previous five weeks. If fluoxetine is added to the treatment regimen of a patient already receiving a drug metabolized by CYP2D6, the need for a decreased dose of the original medication should be considered). Products include:
Rythmol SR Capsules 2727

Propoxyphene Hydrochloride (Fluoxetine, like other agents that are metabolized by CYP2D6, inhibits the activity of this isoenzyme. Therapy with medications that are predominately metabolized by the CYP2D6 system and have a relatively narrow therapeutic index should be initiated at the low end of the dose range if the patient is receiving fluoxetine concurrently or has taken it in the previous five weeks. If fluoxetine is added to the treatment regimen of a patient already receiving a drug metabolized by CYP2D6, the need for a decreased dose of the original medication should be considered).
No products indexed under this heading.

Propoxyphene Napsylate (Fluoxetine, like other agents that are metabolized by CYP2D6, inhibits the activity of this isoenzyme. Therapy with medications that are predominately metabolized by the CYP2D6 system and have a relatively narrow therapeutic index should be initiated at the low end of the dose range if the patient is receiving fluoxetine concurrently or has taken it in the previous five weeks. If fluoxetine is added to the treatment regimen of a patient already receiving a drug metabolized by CYP2D6, the need for a decreased dose of the original medication should be considered).
No products indexed under this heading.

Propranolol Hydrochloride (Because of the potential for olanzapine to induce hypotension, Symbyax may enhance the effects of certain antihypertensive agents). Products include:
Inderal LA Long-Acting Capsules 3429
InnoPran XL Capsules 2723

Protriptyline Hydrochloride (In two fluoxetine studies, previously stable plasma levels of imipramine and desipramine have increased >2- to 10-fold when fluoxetine has been administered in combination. This influence may persist for three weeks or longer after fluoxetine is discontinued. Thus, the dose of TCA may need to be reduced and plasma TCA concentrations may need to be monitored temporarily when Symbyax is co-administered or has been recently discontinued).
No products indexed under this heading.

Quetiapine Fumarate (Fluoxetine, like other agents that are metabolized by CYP2D6, inhibits the activity of this isoenzyme. Therapy with medications that are predominately metabolized by the CYP2D6 system and have a relatively narrow therapeutic index should be initiated at the low end of the dose range if the patient is receiving fluoxetine concurrently or has taken it in the previous five weeks. If fluoxetine is added to the treatment regimen of a patient already receiving a drug metabolized by CYP2D6, the need for a decreased dose of the original medication should be considered). Products include:
Seroquel Tablets 690

Quinapril Hydrochloride (Because of the potential for olanzapine to induce hypotension, Symbyax may enhance the effects of certain antihypertensive agents).
No products indexed under this heading.

Quinidine Gluconate (Fluoxetine, like other agents that are metabolized by CYP2D6, inhibits the activity of this isoenzyme. Therapy with medications that are predominately metabolized by the CYP2D6 system and have a relatively narrow therapeutic index should be initiated at the low end of the dose range if the patient is receiving fluoxetine concurrently or has taken it in the previous five weeks. If fluoxetine is added to the treatment regimen of a patient already receiving a drug metabolized by CYP2D6, the need for a decreased dose of the original medication should be considered).
No products indexed under this heading.

Quinidine Hydrochloride (Fluoxetine, like other agents that are metabolized by CYP2D6, inhibits the activity of this isoenzyme. Therapy with medications that are predominately metabolized by the CYP2D6 system and have a relatively narrow therapeutic index should be initiated at the low end of the dose range if the patient is receiving fluoxetine concurrently or has taken it in the previous five weeks. If fluoxetine is added to the treatment regimen of a patient already receiving a drug metabolized by CYP2D6, the need for a decreased dose of the original medication should be considered).
No products indexed under this heading.

Quinidine Polygalacturonate (Fluoxetine, like other agents that are metabolized by CYP2D6, inhibits the activity of this isoenzyme. Therapy with medications that are predominately metabolized by the CYP2D6 system and have a relatively narrow therapeutic index should be initiated at the low end of the dose range if the patient is receiving fluoxetine concurrently or has taken it in the previous five weeks. If fluoxetine is added to the treatment regimen of a patient already receiving a drug metabolized by CYP2D6, the need for a decreased dose of the original medication should be considered).
No products indexed under this heading.

Quinidine Sulfate (Fluoxetine, like other agents that are metabolized by CYP2D6, inhibits the activity of this isoenzyme. Therapy with medications that are predominately metabolized by the CYP2D6 system and have a relatively narrow therapeutic index should be initiated at the low end of the dose range if the patient is receiving fluoxetine concurrently or has taken it in the previous five weeks. If fluoxetine is added to the treatment regimen of a patient already receiving a drug metabolized by CYP2D6, the need for a decreased dose of the original medication should be considered).
No products indexed under this heading.

Ramipril (Because of the potential for olanzapine to induce hypotension, Symbyax may enhance the effects of certain antihypertensive agents). Products include:
Altace Capsules 1702

Rauwolfia Serpentina (Because of the potential for olanzapine to induce hypotension, Symbyax may enhance the effects of certain antihypertensive agents).
No products indexed under this heading.

Rescinnamine (Because of the potential for olanzapine to induce hypotension, Symbyax may enhance the effects of certain antihypertensive agents).
No products indexed under this heading.

Reserpine (Because of the potential for olanzapine to induce hypotension, Symbyax may enhance the effects of certain antihypertensive agents).
No products indexed under this heading.

Rifampicin (Agents that induce CYP1A2 or glucuronyl transferase enzymes may cause an increase in olanzapine concentration).
No products indexed under this heading.

Rifampin (Agents that induce CYP1A2 or glucuronyl transferase enzymes may cause an increase in olanzapine concentration).
No products indexed under this heading.

Risperidone (Fluoxetine, like other agents that are metabolized by CYP2D6, inhibits the activity of this isoenzyme. Therapy with medications that are predominately metabolized by the CYP2D6 system and have a relatively narrow therapeutic index should be initiated at the low end of the dose range if the patient is receiving fluoxetine concurrently or has taken it in the previous five weeks. If fluoxetine is added to the treatment regimen of a patient already receiving a drug metabolized by CYP2D6, the need for a decreased dose of the original medication should be considered). Products include:
Risperdal 1676
Risperdal Consta Long-Acting Injection 1682
Risperdal M-Tab Orally Disintegrating Tablets 1676

Ritonavir (Fluoxetine, like other agents that are metabolized by CYP2D6, inhibits the activity of this isoenzyme. Therapy with medications that are predominately metabolized by the CYP2D6 system and have a relatively narrow therapeutic index should be initiated at the low end of the dose range if the patient is receiving fluoxetine concurrently or has taken it in the previous five weeks. If fluoxetine is added to the treatment regimen of a patient already receiving a drug metabolized by CYP2D6, the need for a decreased dose of the original medication should be considered). Products include:

- Kaletra 476
- Norvir 503

Rofecoxib (Serotonin release by platelets plays an important role in hemostasis. Studies have demonstrated an association between the use of psychotropic drugs that interfere with serotonin reuptake and the occurrence of upper gastrointestinal bleeding. These studies have also shown that concurrent use of an NSAID potentiated the risk of bleeding. Therefore, patients should be cautioned about the use of NSAIDs concurrently with Symbyax).

No products indexed under this heading.

Ropinirole Hydrochloride (The olanzapine component of Symbyax may antagonize the effects of levodopa and dopamine agonists). Products include:

- Requip Tablets 1555

Selegiline Hydrochloride (Concomitant use in patients taking MAO inhibitors is contraindicated. There have been reports of serious, sometimes fatal, reactions in patients receiving, or who have recently discontinued, fluoxetine and are then started on an MAO inhibitor. Therefore, Symbyax should not be used in combination with, or within a minimum of 14 days of discontinuing, MAO inhibitors). Products include:

- Eldepryl Capsules 3208
- Zelapar Tablets 3372

Sodium Nitroprusside (Because of the potential for olanzapine to induce hypotension, Symbyax may enhance the effects of certain antihypertensive agents).

No products indexed under this heading.

Sotalol Hydrochloride (Because of the potential for olanzapine to induce hypotension, Symbyax may enhance the effects of certain antihypertensive agents).

No products indexed under this heading.

Spirapril Hydrochloride (Because of the potential for olanzapine to induce hypotension, Symbyax may enhance the effects of certain antihypertensive agents).

No products indexed under this heading.

Sulindac (Serotonin release by platelets plays an important role in hemostasis. Studies have demonstrated an association between the use of psychotropic drugs that interfere with serotonin reuptake and the occurrence of upper gastrointestinal bleeding. These studies have also shown that concurrent use of an NSAID potentiated the risk of bleeding. Therefore, patients should be cautioned about the use of NSAIDs concurrently with Symbyax). Products include:

- Clinoril Tablets 1924

Sumatriptan (There have been rare postmarketing reports describing patients with weakness, hyperreflexia, and incoordination following the use of an SSRI and sumatriptan. If concomitant treatment with sumatriptan and an SSRI is clinically warranted, appropriate observation of the patient is advised). Products include:

- Imitrex Nasal Spray 1467

Sumatriptan Succinate (There have been rare postmarketing reports describing patients with weakness, hyperreflexia, and incoordination following the use of an SSRI and sumatriptan. If concomitant treatment with sumatriptan and an SSRI is clinically warranted, appropriate observation of the patient is advised). Products include:

- Imitrex Injection 1463
- Imitrex Tablets 1471

Tamoxifen Citrate (Fluoxetine, like other agents that are metabolized by CYP2D6, inhibits the activity of this isoenzyme. Therapy with medications that are predominately metabolized by the CYP2D6 system and have a relatively narrow therapeutic index should be initiated at the low end of the dose range if the patient is receiving fluoxetine concurrently or has taken it in the previous five weeks. If fluoxetine is added to the treatment regimen of a patient already receiving a drug metabolized by CYP2D6, the need for a decreased dose of the original medication should be considered). Products include:

- Soltamox Oral Solution 3527

Telmisartan (Because of the potential for olanzapine to induce hypotension, Symbyax may enhance the effects of certain antihypertensive agents). Products include:

- Micardis Tablets 854
- Micardis HCT Tablets 856

Temazepam (Because fluoxetine is tightly bound to plasma protein, the administration of fluoxetine to a patient taking another drug that is tightly bound to protein may cause a shift in plasma concentrations potentially resulting in an adverse effect. Conversely, adverse effects may result from displacement of protein-bound fluoxetine by other tightly bound drugs). Products include:

- Restoril Capsules 1860

Teniposide (Fluoxetine, like other agents that are metabolized by CYP2D6, inhibits the activity of this isoenzyme. Therapy with medications that are predominately metabolized by the CYP2D6 system and have a relatively narrow therapeutic index should be initiated at the low end of the dose range if the patient is receiving fluoxetine concurrently or has taken it in the previous five weeks. If fluoxetine is added to the treatment regimen of a patient already receiving a drug metabolized by CYP2D6, the need for a decreased dose of the original medication should be considered).

No products indexed under this heading.

Terazosin Hydrochloride (Because of the potential for olanzapine to induce hypotension, Symbyax may enhance the effects of certain antihypertensive agents). Products include:

- Hytrin Capsules 471

Testosterone (Fluoxetine, like other agents that are metabolized by CYP2D6, inhibits the activity of this isoenzyme. Therapy with medications that are predominately metabolized by the CYP2D6 system and have a relatively narrow therapeutic index should be initiated at the low end of the dose range if the patient is receiving fluoxetine concurrently or has taken it in the previous five weeks. If fluoxetine is added to the treatment regimen of a patient already receiving a drug metabolized by CYP2D6, the need for a decreased dose of the original medication should be considered). Products include:

- AndroGel 3329
- Striant Mucoadhesive 1007
- Testim 1% Gel 695

Testosterone Cypionate (Fluoxetine, like other agents that are metabolized by CYP2D6, inhibits the activity of this isoenzyme. Therapy with medications that are predominately metabolized by the CYP2D6 system and have a relatively narrow therapeutic index should be initiated at the low end of the dose range if the patient is receiving fluoxetine concurrently or has taken it in the previous five weeks. If fluoxetine is added to the treatment regimen of a patient already receiving a drug metabolized by CYP2D6, the need for a decreased dose of the original medication should be considered).

No products indexed under this heading.

Testosterone Enanthate (Fluoxetine, like other agents that are metabolized by CYP2D6, inhibits the activity of this isoenzyme. Therapy with medications that are predominately metabolized by the CYP2D6 system and have a relatively narrow therapeutic index should be initiated at the low end of the dose range if the patient is receiving fluoxetine concurrently or has taken it in the previous five weeks. If fluoxetine is added to the treatment regimen of a patient already receiving a drug metabolized by CYP2D6, the need for a decreased dose of the original medication should be considered).

No products indexed under this heading.

Testosterone Propionate (Fluoxetine, like other agents that are metabolized by CYP2D6, inhibits the activity of this isoenzyme. Therapy with medications that are predominately metabolized by the CYP2D6 system and have a relatively narrow therapeutic index should be initiated at the low end of the dose range if the patient is receiving fluoxetine concurrently or has taken it in the previous five weeks. If fluoxetine is added to the treatment regimen of a patient already receiving a drug metabolized by CYP2D6, the need for a decreased dose of the original medication should be considered).

No products indexed under this heading.

Thioridazine (Concomitant use in patients taking Thioridazine is contraindicated. Thioridazine should not be administered with Symbyax or administered within a minimum of 5 weeks after discontinuation of Symbyax).

No products indexed under this heading.

Thioridazine Hydrochloride (Concomitant use in patients taking Thioridazine is contraindicated. Thioridazine should not be administered with Symbyax or administered within a minimum of 5 weeks after discontinuation of Symbyax). Products include:

- Thioridazine Hydrochloride Tablets 2163

Timolol Maleate (Because of the potential for olanzapine to induce hypotension, Symbyax may enhance the effects of certain antihypertensive agents). Products include:

- Blocadren Tablets 1916
- Cosopt Sterile Ophthalmic Solution 1931
- Timolide Tablets 2086
- Timoptic Sterile Ophthalmic Solution 2088
- Timoptic in Ocudose 2091
- Timoptic-XE Sterile Ophthalmic Gel Forming Solution 2092

Tobacco (Agents that induce CYP1A2 or glucuronyl transferase enzymes may cause an increase in olanzapine concentration).

No products indexed under this heading.

Tolbutamide (Because fluoxetine is tightly bound to plasma protein, the administration of fluoxetine to a patient taking another drug that is tightly bound to protein may cause a shift in plasma concentrations potentially resulting in an adverse effect. Conversely, adverse effects may result from displacement of protein-bound fluoxetine by other tightly bound drugs).

No products indexed under this heading.

Tolmetin Sodium (Serotonin release by platelets plays an important role in hemostasis. Studies have demonstrated an association between the use of psychotropic drugs that interfere with serotonin reuptake and the occurrence of upper gastrointestinal bleeding. These studies have also shown that concurrent use of an NSAID potentiated the risk of bleeding. Therefore, patients should be cautioned about the use of NSAIDs concurrently with Symbyax).

No products indexed under this heading.

Tolterodine Tartrate (Fluoxetine, like other agents that are metabolized by CYP2D6, inhibits the activity of this isoenzyme. Therapy with medications that are predominately metabolized by the CYP2D6 system and have a relatively narrow therapeutic index should be initiated at the low end of the dose range if the patient is receiving fluoxetine concurrently or has taken it in the previous five weeks. If fluoxetine is added to the treatment regimen of a patient already receiving a drug metabolized by CYP2D6, the need for a decreased dose of the original medication should be considered). Products include:

- Detrol Tablets 2628
- Detrol LA Capsules 2631

Torsemide (Because of the potential for olanzapine to induce hypotension, Symbyax may enhance the effects of certain antihypertensive agents). Products include:

- Demadex Injection 2759
- Demadex Tablets 2759

Tramadol Hydrochloride (Fluoxetine, like other agents that are metabolized by CYP2D6, inhibits the activity of this isoenzyme. Therapy with medications that are predominately metabolized by the CYP2D6 system and have a relatively narrow therapeutic index should be initiated at the low end of the dose range if the patient is receiving fluoxetine concurrently or has taken it in the previous five weeks. If fluoxetine is added to the treatment regimen of a patient already receiving a drug metabolized by CYP2D6, the need for a decreased dose of the original medication should be considered). Products include:

Ultram ER Tablets 2392

Trandolapril (Because of the potential for olanzapine to induce hypotension, Symbyax may enhance the effects of certain antihypertensive agents). Products include:

Mavik Tablets 486
Tarka Tablets 524

Tranylcypromine Sulfate (Concomitant use in patients taking MAO inhibitors is contraindicated. There have been reports of serious, sometimes fatal, reactions in patients receiving, or who have recently discontinued, fluoxetine and are then started on an MAO inhibitor. Therefore, Symbyax should not be used in combination with, or within a minimum of 14 days of discontinuing, MAO inhibitors). Products include:

Parnate Tablets 1527

Trazodone Hydrochloride (Fluoxetine, like other agents that are metabolized by CYP2D6, inhibits the activity of this isoenzyme. Therapy with medications that are predominately metabolized by the CYP2D6 system and have a relatively narrow therapeutic index should be initiated at the low end of the dose range if the patient is receiving fluoxetine concurrently or has taken it in the previous five weeks. If fluoxetine is added to the treatment regimen of a patient already receiving a drug metabolized by CYP2D6, the need for a decreased dose of the original medication should be considered).

No products indexed under this heading.

Triazolam (Fluoxetine, like other agents that are metabolized by CYP2D6, inhibits the activity of this isoenzyme. Therapy with medications that are predominately metabolized by the CYP2D6 system and have a relatively narrow therapeutic index should be initiated at the low end of the dose range if the patient is receiving fluoxetine concurrently or has taken it in the previous five weeks. If fluoxetine is added to the treatment regimen of a patient already receiving a drug metabolized by CYP2D6, the need for a decreased dose of the original medication should be considered).

No products indexed under this heading.

Trimethaphan Camsylate (Because of the potential for olanzapine to induce hypotension, Symbyax may enhance the effects of certain antihypertensive agents).

No products indexed under this heading.

Trimipramine Maleate (In two fluoxetine studies, previously stable plasma levels of imipramine and desipramine have increased >2- to 10-fold when fluoxetine has been administered in combination. This influence may persist for three weeks or longer after fluoxetine is discontinued. Thus, the dose of TCA may need to be reduced and plasma TCA concentrations may need to be monitored temporarily when Symbyax is co-administered or has been recently discontinued).

No products indexed under this heading.

L-Tryptophan (Five patients receiving fluoxetine in combination with tryptophan experienced adverse reactions, including agitation, restlessness, and gastrointestinal distress). Products include:

L-Tryptophan Capsules 2145

Valdecoxib (Serotonin release by platelets plays an important role in hemostasis. Studies have demonstrated an association between the use of psychotropic drugs that interfere with serotonin reuptake and the occurrence of upper gastrointestinal bleeding. These studies have also shown that concurrent use of an NSAID potentiated the risk of bleeding. Therefore, patients should be cautioned about the use of NSAIDs concurrently with Symbyax).

No products indexed under this heading.

Valsartan (Because of the potential for olanzapine to induce hypotension, Symbyax may enhance the effects of certain antihypertensive agents). Products include:

Diovan Tablets 2193
Diovan HCT Tablets 2196

Venlafaxine Hydrochloride (Fluoxetine, like other agents that are metabolized by CYP2D6, inhibits the activity of this isoenzyme. Therapy with medications that are predominately metabolized by the CYP2D6 system and have a relatively narrow therapeutic index should be initiated at the low end of the dose range if the patient is receiving fluoxetine concurrently or has taken it in the previous five weeks. If fluoxetine is added to the treatment regimen of a patient already receiving a drug metabolized by CYP2D6, the need for a decreased dose of the original medication should be considered). Products include:

Effexor Tablets 3411
Effexor XR Capsules 3417

Verapamil Hydrochloride (Because of the potential for olanzapine to induce hypotension, Symbyax may enhance the effects of certain antihypertensive agents). Products include:

Covera-HS Tablets 3139
Tarka Tablets 524
Verelan PM Extended-Release Capsules, Controlled-Onset 3106

Vinblastine Sulfate (Fluoxetine, like other agents that are metabolized by CYP2D6, inhibits the activity of this isoenzyme. Therapy with medications that are predominately metabolized by the CYP2D6 system and have a relatively narrow therapeutic index should be initiated at the low end of the dose range if the patient is receiving fluoxetine concurrently or has taken it in the previous five weeks. If fluoxetine is added to the treatment regimen of a patient already receiving a drug metabolized by CYP2D6, the need for a decreased dose of the original medication should be considered).

No products indexed under this heading.

Warfarin Sodium (Altered anticoagulant effects, including increased bleeding, have been reported when fluoxetine is co-administered with warfarin. Patients receiving warfarin therapy should receive careful coagulation monitoring when Symbyax is initiated or stopped). Products include:

Coumadin for Injection 898
Coumadin Tablets 898

Zonisamide (Fluoxetine, like other agents that are metabolized by CYP2D6, inhibits the activity of this isoenzyme. Therapy with medications that are predominately metabolized by the CYP2D6 system and have a relatively narrow therapeutic index should be initiated at the low end of the dose range if the patient is receiving fluoxetine concurrently or has taken it in the previous five weeks. If fluoxetine is added to the treatment regimen of a patient already receiving a drug metabolized by CYP2D6, the need for a decreased dose of the original medication should be considered). Products include:

Zonegran Capsules 1101

Food Interactions

Alcohol (Alcohol may potentiate the orthostatic effect of olanzapine, increasing the risk of orthostatic hypotension. Therefore, patients should be advised to avoid alcohol while taking Symbyax).

Broccoli (Agents that induce CYP1A2 or glucuronyl transferase enzymes may cause an increase in olanzapine concentration).

Brussel Sprouts (Agents that induce CYP1A2 or glucuronyl transferase enzymes may cause an increase in olanzapine concentration).

Charbroiled Food (Agents that induce CYP1A2 or glucuronyl transferase enzymes may cause an increase in olanzapine concentration).

SYMLIN INJECTION

(Pramlintide Acetate) 613

May interact with ACE inhibitors, anticholinergics, fibrates, drugs affecting gastrointestinal motility, oral hypoglycemic agents, insulin, monoamine oxidase inhibitors, salicylates, sulfonylureas, and certain other agents. Compounds in these categories include:

Acarbose (Due to its effects on gastric emptying, pramlintide acetate therapy should not be considered for patients taking agents that slow the intestinal absorption of nutrients (eg, alpha-glucosidase inhibitors)). Products include:

Precose Tablets 751

Albuterol (Due to its effects on gastric emptying, pramlintide acetate therapy should not be considered for patients taking drugs that alter gastrointestinal motility and agents that slow the intestinal absorption of nutrients). Products include:

Proventil Inhalation Aerosol 3053

Albuterol Sulfate (Due to its effects on gastric emptying, pramlintide acetate therapy should not be considered for patients taking drugs that alter gastrointestinal motility and agents that slow the intestinal absorption of nutrients). Products include:

AccuNeb Inhalation Solution 1055
Combivent Inhalation Aerosol 847
DuoNeb Inhalation Solution 1058
ProAir HFA Inhalation Aerosol 3300
Proventil Inhalation Solution 0.083% 3055
Proventil HFA Inhalation Aerosol 3056
Ventolin HFA Inhalation Aerosol 1600
VoSpire ER Tablets 1052

Alfentanil Hydrochloride (Due to its effects on gastric emptying, pramlintide acetate therapy should not be considered for patients taking drugs that alter gastrointestinal motility and agents that slow the intestinal absorption of nutrients).

No products indexed under this heading.

Amitriptyline Hydrochloride (Due to its effects on gastric emptying, pramlintide acetate therapy should not be considered for patients taking drugs that alter gastrointestinal motility and agents that slow the intestinal absorption of nutrients).

No products indexed under this heading.

Amlodipine Besylate (Due to its effects on gastric emptying, pramlintide acetate therapy should not be considered for patients taking drugs that alter gastrointestinal motility and agents that slow the intestinal absorption of nutrients). Products include:

Caduet Tablets 2508
Lotrel Capsules 2249
Norvasc Tablets 2545

Amoxapine (Due to its effects on gastric emptying, pramlintide acetate therapy should not be considered for patients taking drugs that alter gastrointestinal motility and agents that slow the intestinal absorption of nutrients).

No products indexed under this heading.

Anti-infectives, oral, unspecified (Pramlintide acetate has the potential to delay the absorption of concomitantly administered oral medications. When the rapid onset of a concomitant orally administered agent is a critical determinant of effectiveness, the agent should be administered at least 1 hr prior to or 2 hrs after pramlintide acetate injection).

No products indexed under this heading.

Aspirin (May increase the blood glucose-lowering effect and susceptibility to hypoglycemia, which may necessitate further insulin dose adjustments and particularly close monitoring of blood glucose). Products include:

Aggrenox Capsules 822
Bayer Aspirin 744
BC Allergy Sinus Cold Powder .... ▣677
BC Headache Powder .... ▣677
Arthritis Strength BC Powder .... ▣677
BC Sinus Cold Powder .... ▣677
Excedrin Extra Strength Caplets/Tablets/Geltabs .... ▣684
Excedrin Migraine Caplets/Tablets/Geltabs .... ▣609
Goody's Body Pain Formula Powder .... ▣684
Goody's Extra Strength Headache Powders .... ▣611
Goody's Extra Strength Pain Relief Tablets .... ▣685
Percodan Tablets 1132
St. Joseph 81 mg Aspirin Chewable and Enteric Coated Tablets 1869

Aspirin, Enteric Coated (May increase the blood glucose-lowering effect and susceptibility to hypoglycemia, which may necessitate further insulin dose adjustments and particularly close monitoring of blood glucose).

No products indexed under this heading.

Aspirin Buffered (May increase the blood glucose-lowering effect and

susceptibility to hypoglycemia, which may necessitate further insulin dose adjustments and particularly close monitoring of blood glucose).
Products include:
Bufferin Extra Strength Tablets 678
Bufferin Regular Strength Tablets ... 678

Astemizole (Due to its effects on gastric emptying, pramlintide acetate therapy should not be considered for patients taking drugs that alter gastrointestinal motility and agents that slow the intestinal absorption of nutrients).
No products indexed under this heading.

Atropine Sulfate (Due to its effects on gastric emptying, pramlintide acetate therapy should not be considered for patients taking drugs that alter gastrointestinal motility and agents that slow the intestinal absorption of nutrients). Products include:
Donnatal Extentabs 2493

Azatadine Maleate (Due to its effects on gastric emptying, pramlintide acetate therapy should not be considered for patients taking drugs that alter gastrointestinal motility and agents that slow the intestinal absorption of nutrients).
No products indexed under this heading.

Belladonna Alkaloids (Due to its effects on gastric emptying, pramlintide acetate therapy should not be considered for patients taking drugs that alter gastrointestinal motility and agents that slow the intestinal absorption of nutrients). Products include:
Hyland's Teething Tablets 830

Benazepril Hydrochloride (May increase the blood glucose-lowering effect and susceptibility to hypoglycemia, which may necessitate further insulin dose adjustments and particularly close monitoring of blood glucose). Products include:
Lotensin Tablets 2243
Lotensin HCT Tablets 2246
Lotrel Capsules 2249

Benztropine Mesylate (Due to its effects on gastric emptying, pramlintide acetate therapy should not be considered for patients taking drugs that alter gastrointestinal motility and agents that slow the intestinal absorption of nutrients).
No products indexed under this heading.

Bepridil Hydrochloride (Due to its effects on gastric emptying, pramlintide acetate therapy should not be considered for patients taking drugs that alter gastrointestinal motility and agents that slow the intestinal absorption of nutrients).
No products indexed under this heading.

Bethanechol Chloride (Due to its effects on gastric emptying, pramlintide acetate therapy should not be considered for patients taking drugs that alter gastrointestinal motility and agents that slow the intestinal absorption of nutrients).
No products indexed under this heading.

Biperiden Hydrochloride (Due to its effects on gastric emptying, pramlintide acetate therapy should not be considered for patients taking drugs that alter gastrointestinal motility and agents that slow the intestinal absorption of nutrients).
No products indexed under this heading.

Bitolterol Mesylate (Due to its effects on gastric emptying, pramlintide acetate therapy should not be considered for patients taking drugs that alter gastrointestinal motility and agents that slow the intestinal absorption of nutrients).
No products indexed under this heading.

Bromocriptine Mesylate (Due to its effects on gastric emptying, pramlintide acetate therapy should not be considered for patients taking drugs that alter gastrointestinal motility and agents that slow the intestinal absorption of nutrients).
No products indexed under this heading.

Bromodiphenhydramine Hydrochloride (Due to its effects on gastric emptying, pramlintide acetate therapy should not be considered for patients taking drugs that alter gastrointestinal motility and agents that slow the intestinal absorption of nutrients).
No products indexed under this heading.

Brompheniramine Maleate (Due to its effects on gastric emptying, pramlintide acetate therapy should not be considered for patients taking drugs that alter gastrointestinal motility and agents that slow the intestinal absorption of nutrients).
Products include:
Children's Dimetapp Cold & Allergy Elixir 730
Children's Dimetapp Cold & Allergy Chewable Tablets............ 730
Children's Dimetapp DM Cold & Cough Elixir 731

Buprenorphine Hydrochloride (Due to its effects on gastric emptying, pramlintide acetate therapy should not be considered for patients taking drugs that alter gastrointestinal motility and agents that slow the intestinal absorption of nutrients). Products include:
Buprenex Injectable 2716
Suboxone Tablets 2717
Subutex Tablets 2717

Captopril (May increase the blood glucose-lowering effect and susceptibility to hypoglycemia, which may necessitate further insulin dose adjustments and particularly close monitoring of blood glucose).
Products include:
Captopril Tablets 2149

Cevimeline Hydrochloride (Due to its effects on gastric emptying, pramlintide acetate therapy should not be considered for patients taking drugs that alter gastrointestinal motility and agents that slow the intestinal absorption of nutrients).
Products include:
Evoxac Capsules 1047

Chlorpheniramine Maleate (Due to its effects on gastric emptying, pramlintide acetate therapy should not be considered for patients taking drugs that alter gastrointestinal motility and agents that slow the intestinal absorption of nutrients).
Products include:
Advil Allergy Sinus Caplets 770
Advil Multi-Symptom Cold Caplets 770
BC Allergy Sinus Cold Powder 677
Comtrex Maximum Strength Cold & Cough Day/Night Caplets - Night Formulation 726
Comtrex Maximum Strength Day/Night Severe Cold & Sinus Caplets - Night Formulation 725
Contac Cold and Flu Maximum Strength Caplets........................ 728
Contac Cold and Flu Day and Night Caplets (Night Formulation Only)....................... 727
Children's Dimetapp Long Acting Cough Plus Cold Syrup............... 731
Robitussin Cough & Cold Long-Acting Liquid 735
Robitussin Cough & Allergy Syrup .. 736
Robitussin Cough & Cold Nighttime Liquid......................... 736
Robitussin Cough, Cold & Flu Nighttime Liquid......................... 738
Robitussin Pediatric Cough & Cold Long-Acting Liquid.............. 735
Robitussin Pediatric Cough & Cold Nighttime Liquid................. 736
Triaminic Cold & Allergy Liquid 746
Triaminic Cough & Runny Nose Softchews 748
Children's Tylenol Plus Flu Oral Suspension... 749
Tylenol Allergy Multi-Symptom Caplets with Cool Burst and Gelcaps 1872
Children's Tylenol Plus Cold Suspension Liquid 1879
Children's Tylenol Plus Cough & Runny Nose Suspension Liquid 1879
Children's Tylenol Plus Flu Suspension Liquid 1881
Children's Tylenol Plus Multi-Symptom Cold Suspension Liquid 1879
Tylenol Cold Head Congestion Nighttime Caplets with Cool Burst... 1873
Tylenol Cold Multi-Symptom Nighttime Caplets with Cool Burst... 1874
Tylenol Sinus Congestion & Pain Nighttime Caplets with Cool Burst... 1876
Vicks 44M Cough, Cold & Flu Relief Liquid................................. 2680
Pediatric Vicks 44m Cough & Cold Relief Liquid.......................... 2676
Children's Vicks NyQuil Cold/Cough Relief........................ 756
Children's Vicks NyQuil Cold/Cough Relief Liquid 2680
Zicam Maximum Strength Flu Daytime 768

Chlorpheniramine Polistirex (Due to its effects on gastric emptying, pramlintide acetate therapy should not be considered for patients taking drugs that alter gastrointestinal motility and agents that slow the intestinal absorption of nutrients).
Products include:
Tussionex Pennkinetic Extended-Release Suspension 3327

Chlorpheniramine Tannate (Due to its effects on gastric emptying, pramlintide acetate therapy should not be considered for patients taking drugs that alter gastrointestinal motility and agents that slow the intestinal absorption of nutrients).
No products indexed under this heading.

Chlorpropamide (May increase the blood glucose-lowering effect and susceptibility to hypoglycemia, which may necessitate further insulin dose adjustments and particularly close monitoring of blood glucose).
No products indexed under this heading.

Choline Magnesium Trisalicylate (May increase the blood glucose-lowering effect and susceptibility to hypoglycemia, which may necessitate further insulin dose adjustments and particularly close monitoring of blood glucose).
No products indexed under this heading.

Cisapride (Due to its effects on gastric emptying, pramlintide acetate therapy should not be considered for patients taking drugs that alter gastrointestinal motility and agents that slow the intestinal absorption of nutrients).
No products indexed under this heading.

Clemastine Fumarate (Due to its effects on gastric emptying, pramlintide acetate therapy should not be considered for patients taking drugs that alter gastrointestinal motility and agents that slow the intestinal absorption of nutrients).
No products indexed under this heading.

Clidinium Bromide (Due to its effects on gastric emptying, pramlintide acetate therapy should not be considered for patients taking drugs that alter gastrointestinal motility and agents that slow the intestinal absorption of nutrients).
No products indexed under this heading.

Clofibrate (May increase the blood glucose-lowering effect and susceptibility to hypoglycemia, which may necessitate further insulin dose adjustments and particularly close monitoring of blood glucose).
No products indexed under this heading.

Clomipramine Hydrochloride (Due to its effects on gastric emptying, pramlintide acetate therapy should not be considered for patients taking drugs that alter gastrointestinal motility and agents that slow the intestinal absorption of nutrients).
No products indexed under this heading.

Codeine Phosphate (Due to its effects on gastric emptying, pramlintide acetate therapy should not be considered for patients taking drugs that alter gastrointestinal motility and agents that slow the intestinal absorption of nutrients). Products include:
Tylenol with Codeine Tablets 2391

Cyproheptadine Hydrochloride (Due to its effects on gastric emptying, pramlintide acetate therapy should not be considered for patients taking drugs that alter gastrointestinal motility and agents that slow the intestinal absorption of nutrients).
No products indexed under this heading.

Desipramine Hydrochloride (Due to its effects on gastric emptying, pramlintide acetate therapy should not be considered for patients taking drugs that alter gastrointestinal motility and agents that slow the intestinal absorption of nutrients).
No products indexed under this heading.

Dexchlorpheniramine Maleate (Due to its effects on gastric emptying, pramlintide acetate therapy should not be considered for patients taking drugs that alter gastrointestinal motility and agents that slow the intestinal absorption of nutrients).
No products indexed under this heading.

Dezocine (Due to its effects on gastric emptying, pramlintide acetate therapy should not be considered for patients taking drugs that alter gastrointestinal motility and agents that slow the intestinal absorption of nutrients).
No products indexed under this heading.

Dicyclomine Hydrochloride (Due to its effects on gastric emptying, pramlintide acetate therapy should not be considered for patients taking drugs that alter gastrointestinal motility and agents that slow the intestinal absorption of nutrients). Products include:
Bentyl Capsules 697
Bentyl Injection 697
Bentyl Syrup 697
Bentyl Tablets 697

Diflunisal (May increase the blood glucose-lowering effect and susceptibility to hypoglycemia, which may necessitate further insulin dose adjustments and particularly close monitoring of blood glucose). Products include:
Dolobid Tablets 1955

Diltiazem Hydrochloride (Due to its effects on gastric emptying, pramlintide acetate therapy should not be considered for patients taking drugs that alter gastrointestinal motility and agents that slow the intestinal absorption of nutrients). Products include:
Cardizem LA Extended Release Tablets 1728
Tiazac Capsules 1201

Diphenhydramine Citrate (Due to its effects on gastric emptying, pramlintide acetate therapy should not be considered for patients taking drugs that alter gastrointestinal motility and agents that slow the intestinal absorption of nutrients). Products include:
Advil PM Caplets .... ■615
Excedrin PM Caplets/Tablets/Geltabs .... ■610
Goody's PM Powder for Pain with Sleeplessness .... ■612

Diphenhydramine Hydrochloride (Due to its effects on gastric emptying, pramlintide acetate therapy should not be considered for patients taking drugs that alter gastrointestinal motility and agents that slow the intestinal absorption of nutrients). Products include:
Nytol QuickCaps Caplets .... ■615
Nytol QuickGels Softgels Maximum Strength .... ■616
Simply Sleep Caplets 1868
Sominex Original Formula Tablets .. ■616
TheraFlu Warming Relief Nighttime Severe Cold .... ■743
TheraFlu Thin Strips Multi Symptom .... ■744
Triaminic Nighttime Cold & Cough Liquid .... ■746
Triaminic Thin Strips Cough & Runny Nose .... ■749
Extra Strength Tylenol PM Caplets, Vanilla Caplets, Geltabs, Gelcaps and Liquid 1875
Tylenol Sore Throat Nighttime Liquid with Cool Burst .... ■790
Tylenol Allergy Multi-Symptom Nighttime Caplets with Cool Burst 1872
Tylenol Severe Allergy Caplets 1872
Children's Tylenol Plus Cold & Allergy Suspension Liquid 1878

Diphenylpyraline Hydrochloride (Due to its effects on gastric emptying, pramlintide acetate therapy should not be considered for patients taking drugs that alter gastrointestinal motility and agents that slow the intestinal absorption of nutrients).
No products indexed under this heading.

Disopyramide (May increase the blood glucose-lowering effect and susceptibility to hypoglycemia, which may necessitate further insulin dose adjustments and particularly close monitoring of blood glucose).
No products indexed under this heading.

Disopyramide Phosphate (May increase the blood glucose-lowering effect and susceptibility to hypoglycemia, which may necessitate further insulin dose adjustments and particularly close monitoring of blood glucose).
No products indexed under this heading.

Dobutamine (Due to its effects on gastric emptying, pramlintide acetate therapy should not be considered for patients taking drugs that alter gastrointestinal motility and agents that slow the intestinal absorption of nutrients).
No products indexed under this heading.

Dobutamine Hydrochloride (Due to its effects on gastric emptying, pramlintide acetate therapy should not be considered for patients taking drugs that alter gastrointestinal motility and agents that slow the intestinal absorption of nutrients).
No products indexed under this heading.

Domperidone (Due to its effects on gastric emptying, pramlintide acetate therapy should not be considered for patients taking drugs that alter gastrointestinal motility and agents that slow the intestinal absorption of nutrients).
No products indexed under this heading.

Donepezil Hydrochloride (Due to its effects on gastric emptying, pramlintide acetate therapy should not be considered for patients taking drugs that alter gastrointestinal motility and agents that slow the intestinal absorption of nutrients). Products include:
Aricept Tablets 1094
Aricept ODT Tablets 1094

Dopamine Hydrochloride (Due to its effects on gastric emptying, pramlintide acetate therapy should not be considered for patients taking drugs that alter gastrointestinal motility and agents that slow the intestinal absorption of nutrients).
No products indexed under this heading.

Doxepin Hydrochloride (Due to its effects on gastric emptying, pramlintide acetate therapy should not be considered for patients taking drugs that alter gastrointestinal motility and agents that slow the intestinal absorption of nutrients).
No products indexed under this heading.

Edrophonium Chloride (Due to its effects on gastric emptying, pramlintide acetate therapy should not be considered for patients taking drugs that alter gastrointestinal motility and agents that slow the intestinal absorption of nutrients).
No products indexed under this heading.

Enalapril Maleate (May increase the blood glucose-lowering effect and susceptibility to hypoglycemia, which may necessitate further insulin dose adjustments and particularly close monitoring of blood glucose). Products include:
Vasotec I.V. Injection 2103

Enalaprilat (May increase the blood glucose-lowering effect and susceptibility to hypoglycemia, which may necessitate further insulin dose adjustments and particularly close monitoring of blood glucose).
No products indexed under this heading.

Ephedrine Hydrochloride (Due to its effects on gastric emptying, pramlintide acetate therapy should not be considered for patients taking drugs that alter gastrointestinal motility and agents that slow the intestinal absorption of nutrients).
No products indexed under this heading.

Ephedrine Sulfate (Due to its effects on gastric emptying, pramlintide acetate therapy should not be considered for patients taking drugs that alter gastrointestinal motility and agents that slow the intestinal absorption of nutrients).
No products indexed under this heading.

Ephedrine Tannate (Due to its effects on gastric emptying, pramlintide acetate therapy should not be considered for patients taking drugs that alter gastrointestinal motility and agents that slow the intestinal absorption of nutrients).
No products indexed under this heading.

Epinephrine (Due to its effects on gastric emptying, pramlintide acetate therapy should not be considered for patients taking drugs that alter gastrointestinal motility and agents that slow the intestinal absorption of nutrients). Products include:
EpiPen 1061
Primatene Mist .... ■719
Twinject 0.15 3379
Twinject 0.3 3378

Epinephrine Hydrochloride (Due to its effects on gastric emptying, pramlintide acetate therapy should not be considered for patients taking drugs that alter gastrointestinal motility and agents that slow the intestinal absorption of nutrients).
No products indexed under this heading.

Erythromycin (Due to its effects on gastric emptying, pramlintide acetate therapy should not be considered for patients taking drugs that alter gastrointestinal motility and agents that slow the intestinal absorption of nutrients). Products include:
Ery-Tab Tablets 449
Erythromycin Base Filmtab Tablets 455
Erythromycin Delayed-Release Capsules, USP 457
PCE Dispertab Tablets 515

Erythromycin Estolate (Due to its effects on gastric emptying, pramlintide acetate therapy should not be considered for patients taking drugs that alter gastrointestinal motility and agents that slow the intestinal absorption of nutrients).
No products indexed under this heading.

Erythromycin Ethylsuccinate (Due to its effects on gastric emptying, pramlintide acetate therapy should not be considered for patients taking drugs that alter gastrointestinal motility and agents that slow the intestinal absorption of nutrients). Products include:
E.E.S. 451
EryPed 447

Erythromycin Gluceptate (Due to its effects on gastric emptying, pramlintide acetate therapy should not be considered for patients taking drugs that alter gastrointestinal motility and agents that slow the intestinal absorption of nutrients).
No products indexed under this heading.

Erythromycin Stearate (Due to its effects on gastric emptying, pramlintide acetate therapy should not be considered for patients taking drugs that alter gastrointestinal motility and agents that slow the intestinal absorption of nutrients). Products include:
Erythrocin Stearate Filmtab Tablets 453

Felodipine (Due to its effects on gastric emptying, pramlintide acetate therapy should not be considered for patients taking drugs that alter gastrointestinal motility and agents that slow the intestinal absorption of nutrients).
No products indexed under this heading.

Fenofibrate (May increase the blood glucose-lowering effect and susceptibility to hypoglycemia, which may necessitate further insulin dose adjustments and particularly close monitoring of blood glucose). Products include:
Lofibra Tablets 1219
Lofibra Capsules 1216
Tricor Tablets 527
Triglide Tablets 3123

Fentanyl (Due to its effects on gastric emptying, pramlintide acetate therapy should not be considered for patients taking drugs that alter gastrointestinal motility and agents that slow the intestinal absorption of nutrients). Products include:
Duragesic Transdermal System 2373
Ionsys Transdermal System 2379

Fentanyl Citrate (Due to its effects on gastric emptying, pramlintide acetate therapy should not be considered for patients taking drugs that alter gastrointestinal motility and agents that slow the intestinal absorption of nutrients). Products include:
Actiq 979

Fluoxetine (May increase the blood glucose-lowering effect and susceptibility to hypoglycemia, which may necessitate further insulin dose adjustments and particularly close monitoring of blood glucose).
No products indexed under this heading.

Fluoxetine Hydrochloride (May increase the blood glucose-lowering effect and susceptibility to hypoglycemia, which may necessitate further insulin dose adjustments and particularly close monitoring of blood glucose). Products include:

Fosinopril Sodium (May increase the blood glucose-lowering effect and susceptibility to hypoglycemia, which may necessitate further insulin dose adjustments and particularly close monitoring of blood glucose).

No products indexed under this heading.

Galantamine Hydrobromide (Due to its effects on gastric emptying, pramlintide acetate therapy should not be considered for patients taking drugs that alter gastrointestinal motility and agents that slow the intestinal absorption of nutrients). Products include:

Gemfibrozil (May increase the blood glucose-lowering effect and susceptibility to hypoglycemia, which may necessitate further insulin dose adjustments and particularly close monitoring of blood glucose).

No products indexed under this heading.

Glimepiride (May increase the blood glucose-lowering effect and susceptibility to hypoglycemia, which may necessitate further insulin dose adjustments and particularly close monitoring of blood glucose). Products include:

Glipizide (May increase the blood glucose-lowering effect and susceptibility to hypoglycemia, which may necessitate further insulin dose adjustments and particularly close monitoring of blood glucose).

No products indexed under this heading.

Glyburide (May increase the blood glucose-lowering effect and susceptibility to hypoglycemia, which may necessitate further insulin dose adjustments and particularly close monitoring of blood glucose).

No products indexed under this heading.

Glycopyrrolate (Due to its effects on gastric emptying, pramlintide acetate therapy should not be considered for patients taking drugs that alter gastrointestinal motility and agents that slow the intestinal absorption of nutrients).

No products indexed under this heading.

Hydrocodone Bitartrate (Due to its effects on gastric emptying, pramlintide acetate therapy should not be considered for patients taking drugs that alter gastrointestinal motility and agents that slow the intestinal absorption of nutrients). Products include:

Hydrocodone Polistirex (Due to its effects on gastric emptying, pramlintide acetate therapy should not be considered for patients taking drugs that alter gastrointestinal

motility and agents that slow the intestinal absorption of nutrients). Products include:

Hydromorphone Hydrochloride (Due to its effects on gastric emptying, pramlintide acetate therapy should not be considered for patients taking drugs that alter gastrointestinal motility and agents that slow the intestinal absorption of nutrients). Products include:

Hyoscyamine (Due to its effects on gastric emptying, pramlintide acetate therapy should not be considered for patients taking drugs that alter gastrointestinal motility and agents that slow the intestinal absorption of nutrients).

No products indexed under this heading.

Hyoscyamine Sulfate (Due to its effects on gastric emptying, pramlintide acetate therapy should not be considered for patients taking drugs that alter gastrointestinal motility and agents that slow the intestinal absorption of nutrients). Products include:

Imipramine Hydrochloride (Due to its effects on gastric emptying, pramlintide acetate therapy should not be considered for patients taking drugs that alter gastrointestinal motility and agents that slow the intestinal absorption of nutrients).

No products indexed under this heading.

Imipramine Pamoate (Due to its effects on gastric emptying, pramlintide acetate therapy should not be considered for patients taking drugs that alter gastrointestinal motility and agents that slow the intestinal absorption of nutrients).

No products indexed under this heading.

Insulin, Human, Zinc Suspension (The addition of any antihyperglycemic agent, such as pramlintide acetate, to an existing regimen of one or more anti-hyperglycemic agents (eg, insulin) may necessitate further insulin dose adjustments and particularly close monitoring of blood glucose). Products include:

Insulin, Human NPH (The addition of any antihyperglycemic agent, such as pramlintide acetate, to an existing regimen of one or more anti-hyperglycemic agents (eg, insulin) may necessitate further insulin dose adjustments and particularly close monitoring of blood glucose). Products include:

Insulin, Human Regular (The addition of any antihyperglycemic agent, such as pramlintide acetate, to an existing regimen of one or more anti-hyperglycemic agents (eg, insulin) may necessitate further insulin dose adjustments and particularly close monitoring of blood glucose). Products include:

Insulin, Human Regular and Human NPH Mixture (The addition of any antihyperglycemic agent, such as pramlintide acetate, to an existing regimen of one or more anti-hyperglycemic agents (eg, insulin) may necessitate further insulin dose adjustments and particularly close monitoring of blood glucose). Products include:

Insulin, NPH (The addition of any antihyperglycemic agent, such as pramlintide acetate, to an existing regimen of one or more anti-hyperglycemic agents (eg, insulin) may necessitate further insulin dose adjustments and particularly close monitoring of blood glucose).

No products indexed under this heading.

Insulin, Regular (The addition of any antihyperglycemic agent, such as pramlintide acetate, to an existing regimen of one or more anti-hyperglycemic agents (eg, insulin) may necessitate further insulin dose adjustments and particularly close monitoring of blood glucose).

No products indexed under this heading.

Insulin, Zinc Crystals (The addition of any antihyperglycemic agent, such as pramlintide acetate, to an existing regimen of one or more anti-hyperglycemic agents (eg, insulin) may necessitate further insulin dose adjustments and particularly close monitoring of blood glucose).

No products indexed under this heading.

Insulin, Zinc Suspension (The addition of any antihyperglycemic agent, such as pramlintide acetate, to an existing regimen of one or more anti-hyperglycemic agents (eg, insulin) may necessitate further insulin dose adjustments and particularly close monitoring of blood glucose).

No products indexed under this heading.

Insulin Aspart, Human Regular (The addition of any antihyperglycemic agent, such as pramlintide acetate, to an existing regimen of one or more anti-hyperglycemic agents (eg, insulin) may necessitate further insulin dose adjustments and particularly close monitoring of blood glucose). Products include:

Insulin glargine (The addition of any antihyperglycemic agent, such as pramlintide acetate, to an existing regimen of one or more anti-hyperglycemic agents (eg, insulin) may necessitate further insulin dose adjustments and particularly close monitoring of blood glucose). Products include:

Insulin Lispro, Human (The addition of any antihyperglycemic agent, such as pramlintide acetate, to an existing regimen of one or more anti-hyperglycemic agents (eg, insulin) may necessitate further insulin dose adjustments and particularly close monitoring of blood glucose). Products include:

Insulin Lispro Protamine, Human (The addition of any antihyperglyce-

mic agent, such as pramlintide acetate, to an existing regimen of one or more anti-hyperglycemic agents (eg, insulin) may necessitate further insulin dose adjustments and particularly close monitoring of blood glucose). Products include:

Ipratropium Bromide (Due to its effects on gastric emptying, pramlintide acetate therapy should not be considered for patients taking drugs that alter gastrointestinal motility and agents that slow the intestinal absorption of nutrients). Products include:

Isocarboxazid (May increase the blood glucose-lowering effect and susceptibility to hypoglycemia, which may necessitate further insulin dose adjustments and particularly close monitoring of blood glucose).

No products indexed under this heading.

Isoetharine (Due to its effects on gastric emptying, pramlintide acetate therapy should not be considered for patients taking drugs that alter gastrointestinal motility and agents that slow the intestinal absorption of nutrients).

No products indexed under this heading.

Isoproterenol Hydrochloride (Due to its effects on gastric emptying, pramlintide acetate therapy should not be considered for patients taking drugs that alter gastrointestinal motility and agents that slow the intestinal absorption of nutrients).

No products indexed under this heading.

Isoproterenol Sulfate (Due to its effects on gastric emptying, pramlintide acetate therapy should not be considered for patients taking drugs that alter gastrointestinal motility and agents that slow the intestinal absorption of nutrients).

No products indexed under this heading.

Isradipine (Due to its effects on gastric emptying, pramlintide acetate therapy should not be considered for patients taking drugs that alter gastrointestinal motility and agents that slow the intestinal absorption of nutrients). Products include:

Levalbuterol Hydrochloride (Due to its effects on gastric emptying, pramlintide acetate therapy should not be considered for patients taking drugs that alter gastrointestinal motility and agents that slow the intestinal absorption of nutrients). Products include:

Levorphanol Tartrate (Due to its effects on gastric emptying, pramlintide acetate therapy should not be considered for patients taking drugs that alter gastrointestinal motility and agents that slow the intestinal absorption of nutrients).

No products indexed under this heading.

Lisinopril (May increase the blood glucose-lowering effect and susceptibility to hypoglycemia, which may necessitate further insulin dose adjustments and particularly close monitoring of blood glucose). Products include:

Prinivil Tablets **2052**
Prinzide Tablets **2056**

Magnesium Salicylate (May increase the blood glucose-lowering effect and susceptibility to hypoglycemia, which may necessitate further insulin dose adjustments and particularly close monitoring of blood glucose).

No products indexed under this heading.

Maprotiline Hydrochloride (Due to its effects on gastric emptying, pramlintide acetate therapy should not be considered for patients taking drugs that alter gastrointestinal motility and agents that slow the intestinal absorption of nutrients).

No products indexed under this heading.

Mepenzolate Bromide (Due to its effects on gastric emptying, pramlintide acetate therapy should not be considered for patients taking drugs that alter gastrointestinal motility and agents that slow the intestinal absorption of nutrients).

No products indexed under this heading.

Meperidine Hydrochloride (Due to its effects on gastric emptying, pramlintide acetate therapy should not be considered for patients taking drugs that alter gastrointestinal motility and agents that slow the intestinal absorption of nutrients).

No products indexed under this heading.

Metaproterenol Sulfate (Due to its effects on gastric emptying, pramlintide acetate therapy should not be considered for patients taking drugs that alter gastrointestinal motility and agents that slow the intestinal absorption of nutrients). Products include:

Alupent Inhalation Aerosol **826**

Metformin Hydrochloride (May increase the blood glucose-lowering effect and susceptibility to hypoglycemia, which may necessitate further insulin dose adjustments and particularly close monitoring of blood glucose). Products include:

ActoPlus Met Tablets **3214**
Avandamet Tablets **1373**
Fortamet Extended-Release Tablets **3115**

Methadone Hydrochloride (Due to its effects on gastric emptying, pramlintide acetate therapy should not be considered for patients taking drugs that alter gastrointestinal motility and agents that slow the intestinal absorption of nutrients).

No products indexed under this heading.

Methdilazine Hydrochloride (Due to its effects on gastric emptying, pramlintide acetate therapy should not be considered for patients taking drugs that alter gastrointestinal motility and agents that slow the intestinal absorption of nutrients).

No products indexed under this heading.

Metoclopramide Hydrochloride (Due to its effects on gastric emptying, pramlintide acetate therapy should not be considered for patients taking drugs that alter gastrointestinal motility and agents that slow the intestinal absorption of nutrients).

No products indexed under this heading.

Mibefradil Dihydrochloride (Due to its effects on gastric emptying, pramlintide acetate therapy should not be considered for patients taking drugs that alter gastrointestinal motility and agents that slow the intestinal absorption of nutrients).

No products indexed under this heading.

Miglitol (Due to its effects on gastric emptying, pramlintide acetate therapy should not be considered for patients taking drugs that slow the intestinal absorption of nutrients (eg, alpha-glucosidase inhibitors)).

No products indexed under this heading.

Moclobemide (May increase the blood glucose-lowering effect and susceptibility to hypoglycemia, which may necessitate further insulin dose adjustments and particularly close monitoring of blood glucose).

No products indexed under this heading.

Moexipril Hydrochloride (May increase the blood glucose-lowering effect and susceptibility to hypoglycemia, which may necessitate further insulin dose adjustments and particularly close monitoring of blood glucose). Products include:

Uniretic Tablets **3100**
Univasc Tablets **3104**

Morphine Sulfate (Due to its effects on gastric emptying, pramlintide acetate therapy should not be considered for patients taking drugs that alter gastrointestinal motility and agents that slow the intestinal absorption of nutrients). Products include:

Avinza Capsules **1741**
Kadian Capsules **577**
MS Contin Tablets **2701**

Neostigmine Bromide (Due to its effects on gastric emptying, pramlintide acetate therapy should not be considered for patients taking drugs that alter gastrointestinal motility and agents that slow the intestinal absorption of nutrients).

No products indexed under this heading.

Neostigmine Methylsulfate (Due to its effects on gastric emptying, pramlintide acetate therapy should not be considered for patients taking drugs that alter gastrointestinal motility and agents that slow the intestinal absorption of nutrients).

No products indexed under this heading.

Nicardipine Hydrochloride (Due to its effects on gastric emptying, pramlintide acetate therapy should not be considered for patients taking drugs that alter gastrointestinal motility and agents that slow the intestinal absorption of nutrients). Products include:

Cardene I.V. **2497**

Nifedipine (Due to its effects on gastric emptying, pramlintide acetate therapy should not be considered for patients taking drugs that alter gastrointestinal motility and agents that slow the intestinal absorption of nutrients). Products include:

Adalat CC Tablets **2964**

Nimodipine (Due to its effects on gastric emptying, pramlintide acetate therapy should not be considered for patients taking drugs that alter gastrointestinal motility and agents that slow the intestinal absorption of nutrients). Products include:

Nimotop Capsules **749**

Nisoldipine (Due to its effects on gastric emptying, pramlintide acetate therapy should not be considered for patients taking drugs that alter gastrointestinal motility and agents that slow the intestinal absorption of nutrients). Products include:

Sular Tablets **3122**

Nortriptyline Hydrochloride (Due to its effects on gastric emptying, pramlintide acetate therapy should not be considered for patients taking drugs that alter gastrointestinal motility and agents that slow the intestinal absorption of nutrients).

No products indexed under this heading.

Octreotide Acetate (Due to its effects on gastric emptying, pramlintide acetate therapy should not be considered for patients taking drugs that alter gastrointestinal motility and agents that slow the intestinal absorption of nutrients). Products include:

Sandostatin Injection **2278**
Sandostatin LAR Depot **2280**

Oral Medications, unspecified (Pramlintide has the potential to delay the absorption of co-administered oral medications. When the rapid onset of a concomitant orally administered agent is a critical determinant of effectiveness (such as analgesics), the agent should be administered at least 1 hour prior to or 2 hours after pramlintide injection).

No products indexed under this heading.

Oxybutynin Chloride (Due to its effects on gastric emptying, pramlintide acetate therapy should not be considered for patients taking drugs that alter gastrointestinal motility and agents that slow the intestinal absorption of nutrients). Products include:

Ditropan XL Extended-Release Tablets **2413**

Oxycodone Hydrochloride (Due to its effects on gastric emptying, pramlintide acetate therapy should not be considered for patients taking drugs that alter gastrointestinal motility and agents that slow the intestinal absorption of nutrients). Products include:

OxyContin Tablets **2703**
OxyFast Oral Concentrate Solution **2708**
OxyIR Capsules **2708**
Percocet Tablets **1131**
Percodan Tablets **1132**

Oxyphenonium Bromide (Due to its effects on gastric emptying, pramlintide acetate therapy should not be considered for patients taking drugs that alter gastrointestinal motility and agents that slow the intestinal absorption of nutrients).

No products indexed under this heading.

Pargyline Hydrochloride (May increase the blood glucose-lowering effect and susceptibility to hypoglycemia, which may necessitate further insulin dose adjustments and particularly close monitoring of blood glucose).

No products indexed under this heading.

Pentoxifylline (May increase the blood glucose-lowering effect and susceptibility to hypoglycemia, which may necessitate further insulin dose adjustments and particularly close monitoring of blood glucose).

No products indexed under this heading.

Pergolide Mesylate (Due to its effects on gastric emptying, pramlintide acetate therapy should not be considered for patients taking drugs that alter gastrointestinal motility and agents that slow the intestinal absorption of nutrients). Products include:

Permax Tablets **3356**

Perindopril Erbumine (May increase the blood glucose-lowering effect and susceptibility to hypoglycemia, which may necessitate further insulin dose adjustments and particularly close monitoring of blood glucose). Products include:

Aceon Tablets (2 mg, 4 mg, 8 mg) **3194**

Phenelzine Sulfate (May increase the blood glucose-lowering effect and susceptibility to hypoglycemia, which may necessitate further insulin dose adjustments and particularly close monitoring of blood glucose).

No products indexed under this heading.

Pioglitazone Hydrochloride (May increase the blood glucose-lowering effect and susceptibility to hypoglycemia, which may necessitate further insulin dose adjustments and particularly close monitoring of blood glucose). Products include:

ActoPlus Met Tablets **3214**
Actos Tablets **3219**
Duetact Tablets **3226**

Pirbuterol Acetate (Due to its effects on gastric emptying, pramlintide acetate therapy should not be considered for patients taking drugs that alter gastrointestinal motility and agents that slow the intestinal absorption of nutrients). Products include:

Maxair Autohaler **1852**

Pramipexole Dihydrochloride (Due to its effects on gastric emptying, pramlintide acetate therapy should not be considered for patients taking drugs that alter gastrointestinal motility and agents that slow the intestinal absorption of nutrients). Products include:

Mirapex Tablets **859**

Procainamide Hydrochloride (Due to its effects on gastric emptying, pramlintide acetate therapy should not be considered for patients taking drugs that alter gastrointestinal motility and agents that slow the intestinal absorption of nutrients).

No products indexed under this heading.

Procarbazine Hydrochloride (May increase the blood glucose-lowering effect and susceptibility to hypoglycemia, which may necessitate further insulin dose adjustments and particularly close monitoring of blood glucose). Products include:

Procyclidine Hydrochloride (Due to its effects on gastric emptying, pramlintide acetate therapy should not be considered for patients taking drugs that alter gastrointestinal motility and agents that slow the intestinal absorption of nutrients).

No products indexed under this heading.

Promethazine Hydrochloride (Due to its effects on gastric emptying, pramlintide acetate therapy should not be considered for patients taking drugs that alter gastrointestinal motility and agents that slow the intestinal absorption of nutrients). Products include:

Propantheline Bromide (Due to its effects on gastric emptying, pramlintide acetate therapy should not be considered for patients taking drugs that alter gastrointestinal motility and agents that slow the intestinal absorption of nutrients).

No products indexed under this heading.

Propoxyphene Hydrochloride (May increase the blood glucose-lowering effect and susceptibility to hypoglycemia, which may necessitate further insulin dose adjustments and particularly close monitoring of blood glucose).

No products indexed under this heading.

Propoxyphene Napsylate (May increase the blood glucose-lowering effect and susceptibility to hypoglycemia, which may necessitate further insulin dose adjustments and particularly close monitoring of blood glucose).

No products indexed under this heading.

Protriptyline Hydrochloride (Due to its effects on gastric emptying, pramlintide acetate therapy should not be considered for patients taking drugs that alter gastrointestinal motility and agents that slow the intestinal absorption of nutrients).

No products indexed under this heading.

Pyridostigmine Bromide (Due to its effects on gastric emptying, pramlintide acetate therapy should not be considered for patients taking drugs that alter gastrointestinal motility and agents that slow the intestinal absorption of nutrients).

No products indexed under this heading.

Pyrilamine Maleate (Due to its effects on gastric emptying, pramlintide acetate therapy should not be considered for patients taking drugs that alter gastrointestinal motility and agents that slow the intestinal absorption of nutrients).

No products indexed under this heading.

Pyrilamine Tannate (Due to its effects on gastric emptying, pramlintide acetate therapy should not be considered for patients taking drugs that alter gastrointestinal motility and agents that slow the intestinal absorption of nutrients).

No products indexed under this heading.

Quinapril Hydrochloride (May increase the blood glucose-lowering effect and susceptibility to hypoglycemia, which may necessitate further insulin dose adjustments and particularly close monitoring of blood glucose).

No products indexed under this heading.

Quinidine Gluconate (Due to its effects on gastric emptying, pramlintide acetate therapy should not be considered for patients taking drugs that alter gastrointestinal motility and agents that slow the intestinal absorption of nutrients).

No products indexed under this heading.

Quinidine Polygalacturonate (Due to its effects on gastric emptying, pramlintide acetate therapy should not be considered for patients taking drugs that alter gastrointestinal motility and agents that slow the intestinal absorption of nutrients).

No products indexed under this heading.

Quinidine Sulfate (Due to its effects on gastric emptying, pramlintide acetate therapy should not be considered for patients taking drugs that alter gastrointestinal motility and agents that slow the intestinal absorption of nutrients).

No products indexed under this heading.

Ramipril (May increase the blood glucose-lowering effect and susceptibility to hypoglycemia, which may necessitate further insulin dose adjustments and particularly close monitoring of blood glucose). Products include:

Remifentanil Hydrochloride (Due to its effects on gastric emptying, pramlintide acetate therapy should not be considered for patients taking drugs that alter gastrointestinal motility and agents that slow the intestinal absorption of nutrients).

No products indexed under this heading.

Repaglinide (May increase the blood glucose-lowering effect and susceptibility to hypoglycemia, which may necessitate further insulin dose adjustments and particularly close monitoring of blood glucose).

No products indexed under this heading.

Rivastigmine Tartrate (Due to its effects on gastric emptying, pramlintide acetate therapy should not be considered for patients taking drugs that alter gastrointestinal motility and agents that slow the intestinal absorption of nutrients). Products include:

Ropinirole Hydrochloride (Due to its effects on gastric emptying, pramlintide acetate therapy should not be considered for patients taking drugs that alter gastrointestinal motility and agents that slow the intestinal absorption of nutrients). Products include:

Rosiglitazone Maleate (May increase the blood glucose-lowering effect and susceptibility to hypoglycemia, which may necessitate fur-

ther insulin dose adjustments and particularly close monitoring of blood glucose). Products include:

Salmeterol Xinafoate (Due to its effects on gastric emptying, pramlintide acetate therapy should not be considered for patients taking drugs that alter gastrointestinal motility and agents that slow the intestinal absorption of nutrients). Products include:

Salsalate (May increase the blood glucose-lowering effect and susceptibility to hypoglycemia, which may necessitate further insulin dose adjustments and particularly close monitoring of blood glucose).

No products indexed under this heading.

Scopolamine (Due to its effects on gastric emptying, pramlintide acetate therapy should not be considered for patients taking drugs that alter gastrointestinal motility and agents that slow the intestinal absorption of nutrients). Products include:

Scopolamine Hydrobromide (Due to its effects on gastric emptying, pramlintide acetate therapy should not be considered for patients taking drugs that alter gastrointestinal motility and agents that slow the intestinal absorption of nutrients). Products include:

Selegiline Hydrochloride (May increase the blood glucose-lowering effect and susceptibility to hypoglycemia, which may necessitate further insulin dose adjustments and particularly close monitoring of blood glucose). Products include:

Spirapril Hydrochloride (May increase the blood glucose-lowering effect and susceptibility to hypoglycemia, which may necessitate further insulin dose adjustments and particularly close monitoring of blood glucose).

No products indexed under this heading.

Sucralfate (Due to its effects on gastric emptying, pramlintide acetate therapy should not be considered for patients taking drugs that alter gastrointestinal motility and agents that slow the intestinal absorption of nutrients). Products include:

Sufentanil Citrate (Due to its effects on gastric emptying, pramlintide acetate therapy should not be considered for patients taking drugs that alter gastrointestinal motility and agents that slow the intestinal absorption of nutrients).

No products indexed under this heading.

Sulfamethoxazole (May increase the blood glucose-lowering effect and susceptibility to hypoglycemia, which may necessitate further insulin dose adjustments and particularly close monitoring of blood glucose).

No products indexed under this heading.

Sulfisoxazole Acetyl (May increase the blood glucose-lowering effect and susceptibility to hypoglycemia, which may necessitate further insulin dose adjustments and particularly close monitoring of blood glucose).

No products indexed under this heading.

Sulfisoxazole Diolamine (May increase the blood glucose-lowering effect and susceptibility to hypoglycemia, which may necessitate further insulin dose adjustments and particularly close monitoring of blood glucose).

No products indexed under this heading.

Tacrine Hydrochloride (Due to its effects on gastric emptying, pramlintide acetate therapy should not be considered for patients taking drugs that alter gastrointestinal motility and agents that slow the intestinal absorption of nutrients).

No products indexed under this heading.

Terbutaline Sulfate (Due to its effects on gastric emptying, pramlintide acetate therapy should not be considered for patients taking drugs that alter gastrointestinal motility and agents that slow the intestinal absorption of nutrients).

No products indexed under this heading.

Tolazamide (May increase the blood glucose-lowering effect and susceptibility to hypoglycemia, which may necessitate further insulin dose adjustments and particularly close monitoring of blood glucose).

No products indexed under this heading.

Tolbutamide (May increase the blood glucose-lowering effect and susceptibility to hypoglycemia, which may necessitate further insulin dose adjustments and particularly close monitoring of blood glucose).

No products indexed under this heading.

Tolterodine Tartrate (Due to its effects on gastric emptying, pramlintide acetate therapy should not be considered for patients taking drugs that alter gastrointestinal motility and agents that slow the intestinal absorption of nutrients). Products include:

Trandolapril (May increase the blood glucose-lowering effect and susceptibility to hypoglycemia, which may necessitate further insulin dose adjustments and particularly close monitoring of blood glucose). Products include:

Tranylcypromine Sulfate (May increase the blood glucose-lowering effect and susceptibility to hypoglycemia, which may necessitate further insulin dose adjustments and particularly close monitoring of blood glucose). Products include:

IMPORTANT NOTE: Always consult each drug listing in the patient's regimen for possible interactions.

Tridihexethyl Chloride (Due to its effects on gastric emptying, pramlintide acetate therapy should not be considered for patients taking drugs that alter gastrointestinal motility and agents that slow the intestinal absorption of nutrients).
No products indexed under this heading.

Trihexyphenidyl Hydrochloride (Due to its effects on gastric emptying, pramlintide acetate therapy should not be considered for patients taking drugs that alter gastrointestinal motility and agents that slow the intestinal absorption of nutrients).
No products indexed under this heading.

Trimeprazine Tartrate (Due to its effects on gastric emptying, pramlintide acetate therapy should not be considered for patients taking drugs that alter gastrointestinal motility and agents that slow the intestinal absorption of nutrients).
No products indexed under this heading.

Trimipramine Maleate (Due to its effects on gastric emptying, pramlintide acetate therapy should not be considered for patients taking drugs that alter gastrointestinal motility and agents that slow the intestinal absorption of nutrients).
No products indexed under this heading.

Tripelennamine Hydrochloride (Due to its effects on gastric emptying, pramlintide acetate therapy should not be considered for patients taking drugs that alter gastrointestinal motility and agents that slow the intestinal absorption of nutrients).
No products indexed under this heading.

Triprolidine Hydrochloride (Due to its effects on gastric emptying, pramlintide acetate therapy should not be considered for patients taking drugs that alter gastrointestinal motility and agents that slow the intestinal absorption of nutrients).
No products indexed under this heading.

Troglitazone (May increase the blood glucose-lowering effect and susceptibility to hypoglycemia, which may necessitate further insulin dose adjustments and particularly close monitoring of blood glucose).
No products indexed under this heading.

Verapamil Hydrochloride (Due to its effects on gastric emptying, pramlintide acetate therapy should not be considered for patients taking drugs that alter gastrointestinal motility and agents that slow the intestinal absorption of nutrients). Products include:
Covera-HS Tablets 3139
Tarka Tablets 524
Verelan PM Extended-Release Capsules, Controlled-Onset 3106

SYMMETREL TABLETS
(Amantadine Hydrochloride) 1135
May interact with anticholinergics, central nervous system stimulants, quinidine, and certain other agents. Compounds in these categories include:

Amphetamine Resins (Co-administration with central nervous system stimulants requires careful observation).
No products indexed under this heading.

Atropine Sulfate (Agents with anticholinergic properties may potentiate the anticholinergic-like side effects of amantadine). Products include:
Donnatal Extentabs 2493

Belladonna Alkaloids (Agents with anticholinergic properties may potentiate the anticholinergic-like side effects of amantadine). Products include:
Hyland's Teething Tablets .... ▣830

Benztropine Mesylate (Agents with anticholinergic properties may potentiate the anticholinergic-like side effects of amantadine).
No products indexed under this heading.

Biperiden Hydrochloride (Agents with anticholinergic properties may potentiate the anticholinergic-like side effects of amantadine).
No products indexed under this heading.

Clidinium Bromide (Agents with anticholinergic properties may potentiate the anticholinergic-like side effects of amantadine).
No products indexed under this heading.

Dextroamphetamine Sulfate (Co-administration with central nervous system stimulants requires careful observation). Products include:
Adderall Tablets 3164
Adderall XR Capsules 3166
Dexedrine 1420
DextroStat Tablets 3179

Dicyclomine Hydrochloride (Agents with anticholinergic properties may potentiate the anticholinergic-like side effects of amantadine). Products include:
Bentyl Capsules 697
Bentyl Injection 697
Bentyl Syrup 697
Bentyl Tablets 697

Glycopyrrolate (Agents with anticholinergic properties may potentiate the anticholinergic-like side effects of amantadine).
No products indexed under this heading.

Hydrochlorothiazide (Co-administration with triamterene-hydrochlorothiazide capsules has resulted in a higher plasma amantadine concentration in a patient with Parkinsonism; it is not known which components of triamterene-hydrochlorothiazide capsules contributed to this interaction). Products include:
Aldoril Tablets 1910
Atacand HCT 651
Avalide Tablets 888
Avalide Tablets 2874
Benicar HCT Tablets 1044
Diovan HCT Tablets 2196
Dyazide Capsules 1423
Hyzaar 50-12.5 Tablets 1990
Hyzaar 100-12.5 Tablets 1990
Hyzaar 100-25 Tablets 1990
Lopressor HCT 50/25 Tablets 2241
Lopressor HCT 100/25 Tablets 2241
Lopressor HCT 100/50 Tablets 2241
Lotensin HCT Tablets 2246
Micardis HCT Tablets 856
Moduretic Tablets 2028
Prinzide Tablets 2056
Teveten HCT Tablets 1737
Timolide Tablets 2086
Uniretic Tablets 3100

Hyoscyamine (Agents with anticholinergic properties may potentiate the anticholinergic-like side effects of amantadine).
No products indexed under this heading.

Hyoscyamine Sulfate (Agents with anticholinergic properties may potentiate the anticholinergic-like side effects of amantadine). Products include:
Donnatal Extentabs 2493
Prosed/DS Tablets 1157

Ipratropium Bromide (Agents with anticholinergic properties may potentiate the anticholinergic-like side effects of amantadine). Products include:
Atrovent Inhalation Solution 835
Atrovent HFA Inhalation Aerosol 841
Atrovent Nasal Spray 0.03% 837
Atrovent Nasal Spray 0.06% 839
Combivent Inhalation Aerosol 847
DuoNeb Inhalation Solution 1058

Mepenzolate Bromide (Agents with anticholinergic properties may potentiate the anticholinergic-like side effects of amantadine).
No products indexed under this heading.

Methamphetamine Hydrochloride (Co-administration with central nervous system stimulants requires careful observation). Products include:
Desoxyn Tablets, USP 2462

Methylphenidate (Co-administration with central nervous system stimulants requires careful observation). Products include:
Daytrana Transdermal Patch 3174

Methylphenidate Hydrochloride (Co-administration with central nervous system stimulants requires careful observation). Products include:
Concertá Extended-Release Tablets 1881
Metadate CD Capsules 3323
Ritalin Hydrochloride Tablets 2269
Ritalin LA Capsules 2271
Ritalin-SR Tablets 2269

Oxybutynin Chloride (Agents with anticholinergic properties may potentiate the anticholinergic-like side effects of amantadine). Products include:
Ditropan XL Extended-Release Tablets 2413

Pemoline (Co-administration with central nervous system stimulants requires careful observation).
No products indexed under this heading.

Procyclidine Hydrochloride (Agents with anticholinergic properties may potentiate the anticholinergic-like side effects of amantadine).
No products indexed under this heading.

Propantheline Bromide (Agents with anticholinergic properties may potentiate the anticholinergic-like side effects of amantadine).
No products indexed under this heading.

Quinidine (Co-administration of quinidine with amantadine has been shown to reduce the renal clearance of amantadine by about 30%).
No products indexed under this heading.

Quinidine Gluconate (Co-administration of quinidine with amantadine has been shown to reduce the renal clearance of amantadine by about 30%).
No products indexed under this heading.

Quinidine Hydrochloride (Co-administration of quinidine with amantadine has been shown to reduce the renal clearance of amantadine by about 30%).
No products indexed under this heading.

Quinidine Polygalacturonate (Co-administration of quinidine with amantadine has been shown to reduce the renal clearance of amantadine by about 30%).
No products indexed under this heading.

Quinidine Sulfate (Co-administration of quinidine with amantadine has been shown to reduce the renal clearance of amantadine by about 30%).
No products indexed under this heading.

Quinine (Co-administration of quinine with amantadine has been shown to reduce the renal clearance of amantadine).
No products indexed under this heading.

Scopolamine (Agents with anticholinergic properties may potentiate the anticholinergic-like side effects of amantadine). Products include:
Transderm Scōp Transdermal Therapeutic System 2177

Scopolamine Hydrobromide (Agents with anticholinergic properties may potentiate the anticholinergic-like side effects of amantadine). Products include:
Donnatal Extentabs 2493

Thioridazine Hydrochloride (Co-administration has been reported to worsen the tremor in elderly patients with Parkinson's disease). Products include:
Thioridazine Hydrochloride Tablets 2163

Tolterodine Tartrate (Agents with anticholinergic properties may potentiate the anticholinergic-like side effects of amantadine). Products include:
Detrol Tablets 2628
Detrol LA Capsules 2631

Triamterene (Co-administration with triamterene-hydrochlorothiazide capsules has resulted in a higher plasma amantadine concentration in a patient with Parkinsonism; it is not known which components of triamterene-hydrochlorothiazide capsules contributed to this interaction). Products include:
Dyazide Capsules 1423
Dyrenium Capsules 3400

Tridihexethyl Chloride (Agents with anticholinergic properties may potentiate the anticholinergic-like side effects of amantadine).
No products indexed under this heading.

Trihexyphenidyl Hydrochloride (Agents with anticholinergic properties may potentiate the anticholinergic-like side effects of amantadine).
No products indexed under this heading.

Food Interactions

Alcohol (May increase the potential for CNS effects such as dizziness, confusion, light-headedness and orthostatic hypotension; avoid excessive alcohol usage).

SYNAGIS INTRAMUSCULAR POWDER

(Palivizumab) 1897
None cited in PDR database.

SYNAGIS INTRAMUSCULAR SOLUTION

(Palivizumab) 1897
None cited in PDR database.

SYNERA TOPICAL PATCH

(Lidocaine, Tetracaine) 1137
May interact with antiarrhythmics, local anesthetics, and para-aminobenzoic acid based local anesthetics. Compounds in these categories include:

Acebutolol Hydrochloride (Synera should be used with caution in patients receiving Class I antiarrythmic drugs (such as tocainamide and mexiletine) since the systemic toxic effects are thought to be additive and potentially synergistic with lidocaine and tetracaine).
No products indexed under this heading.

Adenosine (Synera should be used with caution in patients receiving Class I antiarrythmic drugs (such as tocainamide and mexiletine) since the systemic toxic effects are thought to be additive and potentially synergistic with lidocaine and tetracaine). Products include:
Adenocard Injection 617
Adenoscan 619

Amiodarone Hydrochloride (Synera should be used with caution in patients receiving Class I antiarrythmic drugs (such as tocainamide and mexiletine) since the systemic toxic effects are thought to be additive and potentially synergistic with lidocaine and tetracaine).
No products indexed under this heading.

Bretylium Tosylate (Synera should be used with caution in patients receiving Class I antiarrythmic drugs (such as tocainamide and mexiletine) since the systemic toxic effects are thought to be additive and potentially synergistic with lidocaine and tetracaine).
No products indexed under this heading.

Bupivacaine Hydrochloride (When Synera is used concomitantly with other products containing local anesthetic agents, the amount absorbed from all formulations should be considered since the systemic toxic effects are thought to be additive and potentially synergistic with lidocaine and tetracaine).
No products indexed under this heading.

Chloroprocaine Hydrochloride (When Synera is used concomitantly with other products containing local anesthetic agents, the amount absorbed from all formulations should be considered since the systemic toxic effects are thought to be additive and potentially synergistic with lidocaine and tetracaine).
No products indexed under this heading.

Disopyramide Phosphate (Synera should be used with caution in patients receiving Class I antiarrythmic drugs (such as tocainamide and mexiletine) since the systemic toxic effects are thought to be additive and potentially synergistic with lidocaine and tetracaine).
No products indexed under this heading.

Dofetilide (Synera should be used with caution in patients receiving Class I antiarrythmic drugs (such as tocainamide and mexiletine) since the systemic toxic effects are thought to be additive and potentially synergistic with lidocaine and tetracaine).
No products indexed under this heading.

Etidocaine Hydrochloride (When Synera is used concomitantly with other products containing local anesthetic agents, the amount absorbed from all formulations should be considered since the systemic toxic effects are thought to be additive and potentially synergistic with lidocaine and tetracaine).
No products indexed under this heading.

Flecainide Acetate (Synera should be used with caution in patients receiving Class I antiarrythmic drugs (such as tocainamide and mexiletine) since the systemic toxic effects are thought to be additive and potentially synergistic with lidocaine and tetracaine). Products include:
Tambocor Tablets 1856

Levobupivacaine Hydrochloride (When Synera is used concomitantly with other products containing local anesthetic agents, the amount absorbed from all formulations should be considered since the systemic toxic effects are thought to be additive and potentially synergistic with lidocaine and tetracaine).
No products indexed under this heading.

Lidocaine Hydrochloride (Synera should be used with caution in patients receiving Class I antiarrythmic drugs (such as tocainamide and mexiletine) since the systemic toxic effects are thought to be additive and potentially synergistic with lidocaine and tetracaine).
No products indexed under this heading.

Mepivacaine Hydrochloride (When Synera is used concomitantly with other products containing local anesthetic agents, the amount absorbed from all formulations should be considered since the systemic toxic effects are thought to be additive and potentially synergistic with lidocaine and tetracaine).
No products indexed under this heading.

Mexiletine Hydrochloride (Synera should be used with caution in patients receiving Class I antiarrythmic drugs (such as tocainamide and mexiletine) since the systemic toxic effects are thought to be additive and potentially synergistic with lidocaine and tetracaine).
No products indexed under this heading.

Moricizine Hydrochloride (Synera should be used with caution in patients receiving Class I antiarrythmic drugs (such as tocainamide and mexiletine) since the systemic toxic effects are thought to be additive and potentially synergistic with lidocaine and tetracaine).
No products indexed under this heading.

Procainamide Hydrochloride (Synera should be used with caution in patients receiving Class I antiarrythmic drugs (such as tocainamide and mexiletine) since the systemic toxic effects are thought to be additive and potentially synergistic with lidocaine and tetracaine).
No products indexed under this heading.

Procaine Hydrochloride (Synera is contraindicated in patients with a para-aminobenzoic acid (PABA) hypersensitivity).
No products indexed under this heading.

Propafenone Hydrochloride (Synera should be used with caution in patients receiving Class I antiarrythmic drugs (such as tocainamide and mexiletine) since the systemic toxic effects are thought to be additive and potentially synergistic with lidocaine and tetracaine). Products include:
Rythmol SR Capsules 2727

Propranolol Hydrochloride (Synera should be used with caution in patients receiving Class I antiarrythmic drugs (such as tocainamide and mexiletine) since the systemic toxic effects are thought to be additive and potentially synergistic with lidocaine and tetracaine). Products include:
Inderal LA Long-Acting Capsules 3429
InnoPran XL Capsules 2723

Quinidine Gluconate (Synera should be used with caution in patients receiving Class I antiarrythmic drugs (such as tocainamide and mexiletine) since the systemic toxic effects are thought to be additive and potentially synergistic with lidocaine and tetracaine).
No products indexed under this heading.

Quinidine Polygalacturonate (Synera should be used with caution in patients receiving Class I antiarrythmic drugs (such as tocainamide and mexiletine) since the systemic toxic effects are thought to be additive and potentially synergistic with lidocaine and tetracaine).
No products indexed under this heading.

Quinidine Sulfate (Synera should be used with caution in patients receiving Class I antiarrythmic drugs (such as tocainamide and mexiletine) since the systemic toxic effects are thought to be additive and potentially synergistic with lidocaine and tetracaine).
No products indexed under this heading.

Sotalol Hydrochloride (Synera should be used with caution in patients receiving Class I antiarrythmic drugs (such as tocainamide and mexiletine) since the systemic toxic effects are thought to be additive and potentially synergistic with lidocaine and tetracaine).
No products indexed under this heading.

Tetracaine Hydrochloride (Synera is contraindicated in patients with a para-aminobenzoic acid (PABA) hypersensitivity). Products include:
Cetacaine Topical Anesthetic 999

Tocainide Hydrochloride (Synera should be used with caution in patients receiving Class I antiarrythmic drugs (such as tocainamide and mexiletine) since the systemic toxic effects are thought to be additive and potentially synergistic with lidocaine and tetracaine).
No products indexed under this heading.

Verapamil Hydrochloride (Synera should be used with caution in patients receiving Class I antiarrythmic drugs (such as tocainamide and mexiletine) since the systemic toxic effects are thought to be additive and potentially synergistic with lidocaine and tetracaine). Products include:
Covera-HS Tablets 3139
Tarka Tablets 524
Verelan PM Extended-Release Capsules, Controlled-Onset........... 3106

SYNERGYDEFENSE CAPSULES

(Herbals, Multiple) 833
None cited in PDR database.

SYNTHROID TABLETS

(Levothyroxine Sodium) 520
May interact with androgens, antithyroid agents, beta blockers, oral anticoagulants, cytokines, dopamine agonists, estrogens, glucocorticoids, cardiac glycosides, hepatic microsomal enzyme inducers, oral hypoglycemic agents, insulin, lithium preparations, phenytoin, radiographic iodinated contrast media, salicylates, sulfonamides, sulfonylureas, sympathomimetics, thiazides, tricyclic antidepressants, xanthines, and certain other agents. Compounds in these categories include:

Acarbose (Requirements of oral antidiabetic agents may be reduced in hypothyroid patients with diabetes and may be subsequently increased with initiation of thyroid hormone therapy). Products include:
Precose Tablets 751

Acebutolol Hydrochloride (Alters thyroid hormone or TSH levels; actions of some beta blockers may be impaired when hypothyroid patients become euthyroid).
No products indexed under this heading.

Albuterol (Possible increased risk of coronary insufficiency in patients with coronary artery disease). Products include:
Proventil Inhalation Aerosol 3053

Albuterol Sulfate (Possible increased risk of coronary insufficiency in patients with coronary artery disease). Products include:
AccuNeb Inhalation Solution 1055
Combivent Inhalation Aerosol 847
DuoNeb Inhalation Solution 1058
ProAir HFA Inhalation Aerosol 3300

Proventil Inhalation Solution 0.083% 3055
Proventil HFA Inhalation Aerosol 3056
Ventolin HFA Inhalation Aerosol 1600
VoSpire ER Tablets 1052

Aldesleukin (Cytokines have been reported to induce both hyperthyroidism or hypothyroidism; dosage adjustment may be necessary). Products include:
Proleukin for Injection 2266

Aluminum Hydroxide (Binds and decreases absorption of levothyroxine sodium from the gastrointestinal tract). Products include:
Gaviscon Regular Strength Liquid .. ▣658
Gaviscon Regular Strength Tablets .... ▣658
Gaviscon Extra Strength Liquid .... ▣658
Gaviscon Extra Strength Tablets .... ▣658
Maalox Regular Strength Antacid/Antigas Liquid 2175
Maalox Max Maximum Strength Antacid/Anti-Gas Liquid 2176

Aminoglutethimide (Alters thyroid hormone or TSH levels).
No products indexed under this heading.

Aminophylline (Theophylline clearance may be decreased in hypothyroid patients and return toward normal when euthyroid state is achieved).
No products indexed under this heading.

p-Aminosalicylic Acid (Alters thyroid hormone or TSH levels).
No products indexed under this heading.

Amiodarone Hydrochloride (Amiodarone therapy alone can cause hypothyroidism or hyperthyroidism).
No products indexed under this heading.

Amitriptyline Hydrochloride (Concurrent use may increase the therapeutic and toxic effects of both drugs; onset of action of tricyclics may be accelerated).
No products indexed under this heading.

Amoxapine (Concurrent use may increase the therapeutic and toxic effects of both drugs; onset of action of tricyclics may be accelerated).
No products indexed under this heading.

Anisindione (The hypoprothrombinemic effect of anticoagulants may be potentiated). Products include:
Miradon Tablets 3042

Asparaginase (May inhibit levothyroxine sodium binding to serum proteins or alter the concentrations of serum proteins). Products include:
Elspar for Injection 2463
Elspar for Injection 1960

Aspirin (May inhibit levothyroxine sodium binding to serum proteins or alter the concentrations of serum proteins). Products include:
Aggrenox Capsules 822
Bayer Aspirin 744
BC Allergy Sinus Cold Powder .... ▣677
BC Headache Powder .... ▣677
Arthritis Strength BC Powder .... ▣677
BC Sinus Cold Powder .... ▣677
Excedrin Extra Strength Caplets/Tablets/Geltabs .... ▣684
Excedrin Migraine Caplets/Tablets/Geltabs .... ▣609
Goody's Body Pain Formula Powder .... ▣684
Goody's Extra Strength Headache Powders .... ▣611
Goody's Extra Strength Pain Relief Tablets .... ▣685
Percodan Tablets 1132
St. Joseph 81 mg Aspirin Chewable and Enteric Coated Tablets 1869

Aspirin, Enteric Coated (May inhibit levothyroxine sodium binding to serum proteins or alter the concentrations of serum proteins).
No products indexed under this heading.

Aspirin Buffered (May inhibit levothyroxine sodium binding to serum proteins or alter the concentrations of serum proteins). Products include:
Bufferin Extra Strength Tablets .... ▣678
Bufferin Regular Strength Tablets .... ▣678

Atenolol (Alters thyroid hormone or TSH levels; actions of some beta blockers may be impaired when hypothyroid patients become euthyroid).
No products indexed under this heading.

Bendroflumethiazide (Alters thyroid hormone or TSH levels).
No products indexed under this heading.

Betamethasone Acetate (May inhibit levothyroxine sodium binding to serum proteins or alter the concentrations of serum proteins).
No products indexed under this heading.

Betamethasone Sodium Phosphate (May inhibit levothyroxine sodium binding to serum proteins or alter the concentrations of serum proteins).
No products indexed under this heading.

Betaxolol Hydrochloride (Alters thyroid hormone or TSH levels; actions of some beta blockers may be impaired when hypothyroid patients become euthyroid). Products include:
Betoptic S Ophthalmic Suspension 558

Bisoprolol Fumarate (Alters thyroid hormone or TSH levels; actions of some beta blockers may be impaired when hypothyroid patients become euthyroid).
No products indexed under this heading.

Bromocriptine Mesylate (Alters thyroid hormone or TSH levels).
No products indexed under this heading.

Carbamazepine (Alters thyroid hormone or TSH levels). Products include:
Carbatrol Capsules 3171
Equetro Extended-Release Capsules 3180
Tegretol/Tegretol-XR 2295

Carteolol Hydrochloride (Alters thyroid hormone or TSH levels; actions of some beta blockers may be impaired when hypothyroid patients become euthyroid). Products include:
Carteolol Hydrochloride Ophthalmic Solution USP, 1% .... ⊙249

Chloral Hydrate (Alters thyroid hormone or TSH levels).
No products indexed under this heading.

Chlorothiazide (Alters thyroid hormone or TSH levels). Products include:
Diuril Oral Suspension 1954

Chlorothiazide Sodium (Alters thyroid hormone or TSH levels). Products include:
Diuril Sodium Intravenous 2467

Chlorotrianisene (Estrogens or estrogen-containing compounds may inhibit levothyroxine sodium binding to serum proteins or alter the concentrations of serum proteins).
No products indexed under this heading.

Chlorpropamide (Alters thyroid hormone or TSH levels; requirements of oral antidiabetic agents may be reduced in hypothyroid patients with diabetes and may be subsequently increased with initiation of thyroid hormone therapy).
No products indexed under this heading.

Cholestyramine (Binds and decreases absorption of levothyroxine sodium from the gastrointestinal tract).
No products indexed under this heading.

Choline Magnesium Trisalicylate (May inhibit levothyroxine sodium binding to serum proteins or alter the concentrations of serum proteins).
No products indexed under this heading.

Clofibrate (May inhibit levothyroxine sodium binding to serum proteins or alter the concentrations of serum proteins).
No products indexed under this heading.

Clomipramine Hydrochloride (Concurrent use may increase the therapeutic and toxic effects of both drugs; onset of action of tricyclics may be accelerated).
No products indexed under this heading.

Colestipol Hydrochloride (Binds and decreases absorption of levothyroxine sodium from the gastrointestinal tract).
No products indexed under this heading.

Cortisone Acetate (May inhibit levothyroxine sodium binding to serum proteins or alter the concentrations of serum proteins).
No products indexed under this heading.

Desipramine Hydrochloride (Concurrent use may increase the therapeutic and toxic effects of both drugs; onset of action of tricyclics may be accelerated).
No products indexed under this heading.

Deslanoside (Therapeutic effects of digitalis glycosides may be reduced; serum digitalis levels may be decreased in hyperthyroidism or when a hypothyroid patient becomes euthyroid).
No products indexed under this heading.

Dexamethasone (May inhibit levothyroxine sodium binding to serum proteins or alter the concentrations of serum proteins). Products include:
Ciprodex Otic Suspension 559
Decadron Tablets 1951
TobraDex Ophthalmic Ointment 562
TobraDex Ophthalmic Suspension ... 563

Dexamethasone Acetate (May inhibit levothyroxine sodium binding to serum proteins or alter the concentrations of serum proteins).
No products indexed under this heading.

Dexamethasone Sodium Phosphate (May inhibit levothyroxine sodium binding to serum proteins or alter the concentrations of serum proteins).
No products indexed under this heading.

Diatrizoate Meglumine (Alters thyroid hormone or TSH levels).
No products indexed under this heading.

Diatrizoate Sodium (Alters thyroid hormone or TSH levels).
No products indexed under this heading.

Diazepam (Alters thyroid hormone or TSH levels). Products include:
Diastat Rectal Delivery System 3343
Valium Tablets 2819

Dicumarol (The hypoprothrombinemic effect of anticoagulants may be potentiated).
No products indexed under this heading.

Dienestrol (Estrogens or estrogen-containing compounds may inhibit levothyroxine sodium binding to serum proteins or alter the concentrations of serum proteins).
No products indexed under this heading.

Diethylstilbestrol (Estrogens or estrogen-containing compounds may inhibit levothyroxine sodium binding to serum proteins or alter the concentrations of serum proteins).
No products indexed under this heading.

Diflunisal (May inhibit levothyroxine sodium binding to serum proteins or alter the concentrations of serum proteins). Products include:
Dolobid Tablets 1955

Digitalis Glycoside Preparations (Therapeutic effects of digitalis glycosides may be reduced; serum digitalis levels may be decreased in hyperthyroidism or when a hypothyroid patient becomes euthyroid).
No products indexed under this heading.

Digitoxin (Therapeutic effects of digitalis glycosides may be reduced; serum digitalis levels may be decreased in hyperthyroidism or when a hypothyroid patient becomes euthyroid).
No products indexed under this heading.

Digoxin (Therapeutic effects of digitalis glycosides may be reduced; serum digitalis levels may be decreased in hyperthyroidism or when a hypothyroid patient becomes euthyroid). Products include:
Lanoxicaps Capsules 1490
Lanoxin Injection 1494
Lanoxin Injection Pediatric 1497
Lanoxin Tablets 1500

Dobutamine Hydrochloride (Possible increased risk of coronary insufficiency in patients with coronary artery disease).
No products indexed under this heading.

Dopamine Hydrochloride (Alters thyroid hormone or TSH levels).
No products indexed under this heading.

Doxepin Hydrochloride (Concurrent use may increase the therapeutic and toxic effects of both drugs; onset of action of tricyclics may be accelerated).
No products indexed under this heading.

Dyphylline (Theophylline clearance may be decreased in hypothyroid patients and return toward normal when euthyroid state is achieved).
No products indexed under this heading.

Ephedrine Hydrochloride (Possible increased risk of coronary insufficiency in patients with coronary artery disease).
No products indexed under this heading.

Ephedrine Sulfate (Possible increased risk of coronary insufficiency in patients with coronary artery disease).
No products indexed under this heading.

Ephedrine Tannate (Possible increased risk of coronary insufficiency in patients with coronary artery disease).
No products indexed under this heading.

Epinephrine (Possible increased risk of coronary insufficiency in patients with coronary artery disease). Products include:
EpiPen **1061**
Primatene Mist **719**
Twinject 0.15 .... **3379**
Twinject 0.3 .... **3378**

Epinephrine Bitartrate (Possible increased risk of coronary insufficiency in patients with coronary artery disease).
No products indexed under this heading.

Epinephrine Hydrochloride (Possible increased risk of coronary insufficiency in patients with coronary artery disease).
No products indexed under this heading.

Esmolol Hydrochloride (Alters thyroid hormone or TSH levels; actions of some beta blockers may be impaired when hypothyroid patients become euthyroid).
No products indexed under this heading.

Estradiol (Estrogens or estrogen-containing compounds may inhibit levothyroxine sodium binding to serum proteins or alter the concentrations of serum proteins). Products include:
Angeliq Tablets **762**
Climara Transdermal System **771**
Climara Pro Transdermal System **776**
Estrasorb Topical Emulsion **1147**
Estring Vaginal Ring **2635**
Menostar Transdermal System **782**
Vagifem Tablets **2334**

Estrogens, Conjugated (Estrogens or estrogen-containing compounds may inhibit levothyroxine sodium binding to serum proteins or alter the concentrations of serum proteins). Products include:
Premarin Intravenous **3442**
Premarin Tablets **3446**
Premarin Vaginal Cream **3452**
Premphase Tablets **3456**
Prempro Tablets **3456**

Estrogens, Esterified (Estrogens or estrogen-containing compounds may inhibit levothyroxine sodium binding to serum proteins or alter the concentrations of serum proteins). Products include:
Estratest Tablets **3199**
Estratest H.S. Tablets **3199**

Estropipate (Estrogens or estrogen-containing compounds may inhibit levothyroxine sodium binding to serum proteins or alter the concentrations of serum proteins).
No products indexed under this heading.

Ethanol (Alters thyroid hormone or TSH levels).
No products indexed under this heading.

Ethinyl Estradiol (Estrogens or estrogen-containing compounds may inhibit levothyroxine sodium binding to serum proteins or alter the concentrations of serum proteins). Products include:
Mircette Tablets **1066**
NuvaRing **2340**
Ortho-Cyclen/Ortho Tri-Cyclen **2429**
Ortho Evra Transdermal System **2417**
Ortho Tri-Cyclen Lo Tablets **2436**
Seasonique Tablets **1077**
Yasmin 28 Tablets **796**
Yaz Tablets **803**

Ethiodized Oil (Alters thyroid hormone or TSH levels).
No products indexed under this heading.

Ethionamide (Alters thyroid hormone or TSH levels). Products include:
Trecator Tablets **3487**

Ferrous Sulfate (Binds and decreases absorption of levothyroxine sodium from the gastrointestinal tract). Products include:
Slow Fe Iron Tablets **818**
Slow Fe with Folic Acid Tablets **819**

Fludrocortisone Acetate (May inhibit levothyroxine sodium binding to serum proteins or alter the concentrations of serum proteins).
No products indexed under this heading.

Fluorouracil (May inhibit levothyroxine sodium binding to serum proteins or alter the concentrations of serum proteins). Products include:
Carac Cream, 0.5% **2879**
Efudex **3363**

Fluoxymesterone (May inhibit levothyroxine sodium binding to serum proteins or alter the concentrations of serum proteins; alters TSH or thyroid hormone levels). Products include:
Androxy Tablets **3335**

Fosphenytoin Sodium (Alters thyroid hormone or TSH levels).
No products indexed under this heading.

Furosemide (May inhibit levothyroxine sodium binding to serum proteins or alter the concentrations of serum proteins). Products include:
Furosemide Tablets **2154**

Gadopentetate Dimeglumine (Alters thyroid hormone or TSH levels).
No products indexed under this heading.

Glimepiride (Alters thyroid hormone or TSH levels; requirements of oral antidiabetic agents may be reduced in hypothyroid patients with diabetes and may be subsequently increased with initiation of thyroid hormone therapy). Products include:
Avandaryl Tablets **1379**
Duetact Tablets **3226**

Glipizide (Alters thyroid hormone or TSH levels; requirements of oral antidiabetic agents may be reduced in hypothyroid patients with diabetes and may be subsequently increased with initiation of thyroid hormone therapy).
No products indexed under this heading.

Glyburide (Alters thyroid hormone or TSH levels; requirements of oral antidiabetic agents may be reduced in hypothyroid patients with diabetes and may be subsequently increased with initiation of thyroid hormone therapy).
No products indexed under this heading.

Heparin Sodium (Alters thyroid hormone or TSH levels).
No products indexed under this heading.

Hydrochlorothiazide (Alters thyroid hormone or TSH levels). Products include:
Aldoril Tablets **1910**
Atacand HCT **651**
Avalide Tablets **888**
Avalide Tablets **2874**
Benicar HCT Tablets **1044**
Diovan HCT Tablets **2196**
Dyazide Capsules **1423**
Hyzaar 50-12.5 Tablets **1990**
Hyzaar 100-12.5 Tablets **1990**
Hyzaar 100-25 Tablets **1990**
Lopressor HCT 50/25 Tablets **2241**
Lopressor HCT 100/25 Tablets **2241**
Lopressor HCT 100/50 Tablets **2241**
Lotensin HCT Tablets **2246**
Micardis HCT Tablets **856**
Moduretic Tablets **2028**
Prinzide Tablets **2056**
Teveten HCT Tablets **1737**
Timolide Tablets **2086**
Uniretic Tablets **3100**

Hydrocortisone (May inhibit levothyroxine sodium binding to serum proteins or alter the concentrations of serum proteins). Products include:
Colocort Rectal Suspension, USP (Retention) 100 mg/60 mL **2476**
Hydrocortone Tablets **1989**
Preparation H Hydrocortisone Cream **646**

Hydrocortisone Acetate (May inhibit levothyroxine sodium binding to serum proteins or alter the concentrations of serum proteins). Products include:
Analpram-HC **1159**
Pramosone **1161**
ProctoFoam-HC **3099**

Hydrocortisone Sodium Phosphate (May inhibit levothyroxine sodium binding to serum proteins or alter the concentrations of serum proteins).
No products indexed under this heading.

Hydrocortisone Sodium Succinate (May inhibit levothyroxine sodium binding to serum proteins or alter the concentrations of serum proteins).
No products indexed under this heading.

Hydroflumethiazide (Alters thyroid hormone or TSH levels).
No products indexed under this heading.

Imipramine Hydrochloride (Concurrent use may increase the therapeutic and toxic effects of both drugs; onset of action of tricyclics may be accelerated).
No products indexed under this heading.

Imipramine Pamoate (Concurrent use may increase the therapeutic and toxic effects of both drugs; onset of action of tricyclics may be accelerated).
No products indexed under this heading.

Insulin, Human, Zinc Suspension (Requirements of insulin may be reduced in hypothyroid patients with diabetes and may be subsequently increased with initiation of thyroid hormone therapy). Products include:
Humulin L, 100 Units **1794**
Humulin U, 100 Units **1800**

Insulin, Human NPH (Requirements of insulin may be reduced in hypothyroid patients with diabetes and may be subsequently increased with initiation of thyroid hormone therapy). Products include:
Humulin N, 100 Units **1795**
Humulin N Pen **1797**

Insulin, Human Regular (Requirements of insulin may be reduced in hypothyroid patients with diabetes and may be subsequently increased with initiation of thyroid hormone therapy). Products include:
Humulin R, 100 Units **1798**

Insulin, Human Regular and Human NPH Mixture (Requirements of insulin may be reduced in hypothyroid patients with diabetes and may be subsequently increased with initiation of thyroid hormone therapy). Products include:
Humulin 50/50, 100 Units **1791**
Humulin 70/30 Pen **1793**

Insulin, NPH (Requirements of insulin may be reduced in hypothyroid patients with diabetes and may be subsequently increased with initiation of thyroid hormone therapy).
No products indexed under this heading.

Insulin, Regular (Requirements of insulin may be reduced in hypothyroid patients with diabetes and may be subsequently increased with initiation of thyroid hormone therapy).
No products indexed under this heading.

Insulin, Zinc Crystals (Requirements of insulin may be reduced in hypothyroid patients with diabetes and may be subsequently increased with initiation of thyroid hormone therapy).
No products indexed under this heading.

Insulin, Zinc Suspension (Requirements of insulin may be reduced in hypothyroid patients with diabetes and may be subsequently increased with initiation of thyroid hormone therapy).
No products indexed under this heading.

Insulin Aspart, Human Regular (Requirements of insulin may be reduced in hypothyroid patients with diabetes and may be subsequently increased with initiation of thyroid hormone therapy). Products include:
NovoLog Injection **2326**

Insulin glargine (Requirements of insulin may be reduced in hypothyroid patients with diabetes and may be subsequently increased with initiation of thyroid hormone therapy). Products include:
Lantus Injection **2909**

Insulin Lispro, Human (Requirements of insulin may be reduced in hypothyroid patients with diabetes and may be subsequently increased with initiation of thyroid hormone therapy). Products include:

- Humalog-Pen ... 1781
- Humalog Mix 50/50-Pen ... 1783
- Humalog Mix 75/25-Pen ... 1785

Insulin Lispro Protamine, Human (Requirements of insulin may be reduced in hypothyroid patients with diabetes and may be subsequently increased with initiation of thyroid hormone therapy). Products include:

- Humalog Mix 50/50-Pen ... 1783
- Humalog Mix 75/25-Pen ... 1785

Interferon alfa-2a, Recombinant (Cytokines have been reported to induce both hyperthyroidism or hypothyroidism; dosage adjustment may be necessary).

No products indexed under this heading.

Interferon alfa-2b, Recombinant (Cytokines have been reported to induce both hyperthyroidism or hypothyroidism; dosage adjustment may be necessary). Products include:

- Intron A for Injection ... 3024
- Rebetron Combination Therapy ... 3063

Interferon alfa-N3 (Human Leukocyte Derived) (Cytokines have been reported to induce both hyperthyroidism or hypothyroidism; dosage adjustment may be necessary). Products include:

- Alferon N Injection ... 1665

Interferon Beta-1b (Cytokines have been reported to induce both hyperthyroidism or hypothyroidism; dosage adjustment may be necessary). Products include:

- Betaseron for SC Injection ... 767

Interferon Gamma-1B (Cytokines have been reported to induce both hyperthyroidism or hypothyroidism; dosage adjustment may be necessary). Products include:

- Actimmune ... 1671

Iodamide Meglumine (Alters thyroid hormone or TSH levels).

No products indexed under this heading.

Iodinated Glycerol (Alters thyroid hormone or TSH levels).

No products indexed under this heading.

Iodine, radiolabeled (Uptake of radiolabeled ions may be decreased).

No products indexed under this heading.

Iohexol (Alters thyroid hormone or TSH levels).

No products indexed under this heading.

Iopamidol (Alters thyroid hormone or TSH levels).

No products indexed under this heading.

Iopanoic Acid (Alters thyroid hormone or TSH levels).

No products indexed under this heading.

Iothalamate Meglumine (Alters thyroid hormone or TSH levels).

No products indexed under this heading.

Ioxaglate Meglumine (Alters thyroid hormone or TSH levels).

No products indexed under this heading.

Ioxaglate Sodium (Alters thyroid hormone or TSH levels).

No products indexed under this heading.

Isoproterenol Hydrochloride (Possible increased risk of coronary insufficiency in patients with coronary artery disease).

No products indexed under this heading.

Isoproterenol Sulfate (Possible increased risk of coronary insufficiency in patients with coronary artery disease).

No products indexed under this heading.

Ketamine Hydrochloride (Coadministration produces marked hypertension and tachycardia).

No products indexed under this heading.

Labetalol Hydrochloride (Alters thyroid hormone or TSH levels; actions of some beta blockers may be impaired when hypothyroid patients become euthyroid).

No products indexed under this heading.

Levalbuterol Hydrochloride (Possible increased risk of coronary insufficiency in patients with coronary artery disease). Products include:

- Xopenex Inhalation Solution ... 3146
- Xopenex Inhalation Solution Concentrate ... 3150

Levobunolol Hydrochloride (Alters thyroid hormone or TSH levels; actions of some beta blockers may be impaired when hypothyroid patients become euthyroid). Products include:

- Betagan Ophthalmic Solution, USP ... ⊙220

Levodopa (Alters thyroid hormone or TSH levels). Products include:

- Parcopa Orally Disintegrating Tablets ... 3097
- Stalevo Tablets ... 2287

Lithium (Blocks the TSH-mediated release of T4 and T3; thyroid function should be carefully monitored during lithium initiation, stablization, and maintenence; if hypothyroidism occurs during lithium treatment, a higher than usual Synthroid dose may be required).

No products indexed under this heading.

Lithium Carbonate (Blocks the TSH-mediated release of T4 and T3; thyroid function should therefore be carefully monitored during lithium initiation, stablization, and maintenence; if hypothyroidism occurs during lithium treatment, a higher than usual Synthroid dose may be required). Products include:

- Lithobid Tablets ... 1692

Lithium Citrate (Blocks the TSH-mediated release of T4 and T3; thyroid function should therefore be carefully monitored during lithium initiation, stablization, and maintenence; if hypothyroidism occurs during lithium treatment, a higher than usual Synthroid dose may be required).

No products indexed under this heading.

Lovastatin (Alters thyroid hormone or TSH levels). Products include:

- Advicor Tablets ... 1722
- Altoprev Extended-Release Tablets ... 3109
- Mevacor Tablets ... 2021

Magnesium Salicylate (May inhibit levothyroxine sodium binding to serum proteins or alter the concentrations of serum proteins).

No products indexed under this heading.

Maprotiline Hydrochloride (Risk of cardiac arrhythmias may increase).

No products indexed under this heading.

Meclofenamate Sodium (Meclofenamic acid may inhibit levothyroxine sodium binding to serum proteins or alter the concentrations of serum proteins).

No products indexed under this heading.

Mefenamic Acid (May inhibit levothyroxine sodium binding to serum proteins or alter the concentrations of serum proteins).

No products indexed under this heading.

Mercaptopurine (Alters thyroid hormone or TSH levels).

No products indexed under this heading.

Metaproterenol Sulfate (Possible increased risk of coronary insufficiency in patients with coronary artery disease). Products include:

- Alupent Inhalation Aerosol ... 826

Metaraminol Bitartrate (Possible increased risk of coronary insufficiency in patients with coronary artery disease).

No products indexed under this heading.

Metformin Hydrochloride (Requirements of oral antidiabetic agents may be reduced in hypothyroid patients with diabetes and may be subsequently increased with initiation of thyroid hormone therapy). Products include:

- ActoPlus Met Tablets ... 3214
- Avandamet Tablets ... 1373
- Fortamet Extended-Release Tablets ... 3115

Methadone Hydrochloride (May inhibit levothyroxine sodium binding to serum proteins or alter the concentrations of serum proteins).

No products indexed under this heading.

Methimazole (Alters thyroid hormone or TSH levels).

No products indexed under this heading.

Methoxamine Hydrochloride (Possible increased risk of coronary insufficiency in patients with coronary artery disease).

No products indexed under this heading.

Methyclothiazide (Alters thyroid hormone or TSH levels).

No products indexed under this heading.

Methylprednisolone Acetate (May inhibit levothyroxine sodium binding to serum proteins or alter the concentrations of serum proteins). Products include:

- Depo-Medrol Injectable Suspension ... 2617
- Depo-Medrol Single-Dose Vial ... 2619

Methylprednisolone Sodium Succinate (May inhibit levothyroxine sodium binding to serum proteins or alter the concentrations of serum proteins).

No products indexed under this heading.

Methyltestosterone (May inhibit levothyroxine sodium binding to serum proteins or alter the concentrations of serum proteins; alters TSH or thyroid hormone levels). Products include:

- Estratest Tablets ... 3199
- Estratest H.S. Tablets ... 3199

Metipranolol Hydrochloride (Alters thyroid hormone or TSH levels; actions of some beta blockers may be impaired when hypothyroid patients become euthyroid).

No products indexed under this heading.

Metoclopramide Hydrochloride (Alters thyroid hormone or TSH levels).

No products indexed under this heading.

Metoprolol Succinate (Alters thyroid hormone or TSH levels; actions of some beta blockers may be impaired when hypothyroid patients become euthyroid). Products include:

- Toprol-XL Tablets ... 668

Metoprolol Tartrate (Alters thyroid hormone or TSH levels; actions of some beta blockers may be impaired when hypothyroid patients become euthyroid). Products include:

- Lopressor Injection ... 2238
- Lopressor Tablets ... 2238
- Lopressor HCT 50/25 Tablets ... 2241
- Lopressor HCT 100/25 Tablets ... 2241
- Lopressor HCT 100/50 Tablets ... 2241

Miglitol (Requirements of oral antidiabetic agents may be reduced in hypothyroid patients with diabetes and may be subsequently increased with initiation of thyroid hormone therapy).

No products indexed under this heading.

Mitotane (Alters thyroid hormone or TSH levels).

No products indexed under this heading.

Nadolol (Alters thyroid hormone or TSH levels; actions of some beta blockers may be impaired when hypothyroid patients become euthyroid). Products include:

- Nadolol Tablets ... 2159

Norepinephrine Bitartrate (Possible increased risk of coronary insufficiency in patients with coronary artery disease).

No products indexed under this heading.

Nortriptyline Hydrochloride (Concurrent use may increase the therapeutic and toxic effects of both drugs; onset of action of tricyclics may be accelerated).

No products indexed under this heading.

Octreotide Acetate (Alters thyroid hormone or TSH levels). Products include:

- Sandostatin Injection ... 2278
- Sandostatin LAR Depot ... 2280

Oxandrolone (May inhibit levothyroxine sodium binding to serum proteins or alter the concentrations of serum proteins; alters TSH or thyroid hormone levels). Products include:

- Oxandrin Tablets ... 2962

Oxymetholone (May inhibit levothyroxine sodium binding to serum proteins or alter the concentrations of serum proteins; alters TSH or thyroid hormone levels).

No products indexed under this heading.

IMPORTANT NOTE: Always consult each drug listing in the patient's regimen for possible interactions.

Repaglinide (Requirements of oral antidiabetic agents may be reduced in hypothyroid patients with diabetes and may be subsequently increased with initiation of thyroid hormone therapy).
No products indexed under this heading.

Resorcinol (Alters thyroid hormone or TSH levels).
No products indexed under this heading.

Rifampin (Alters thyroid hormone or TSH levels).
No products indexed under this heading.

Rifapentine (Alters thyroid hormone or TSH levels).
No products indexed under this heading.

Ropinirole Hydrochloride (Alters thyroid hormone or TSH levels). Products include:
Requip Tablets **1555**

Rosiglitazone Maleate (Requirements of oral antidiabetic agents may be reduced in hypothyroid patients with diabetes and may be subsequently increased with initiation of thyroid hormone therapy). Products include:
Avandamet Tablets **1373**
Avandaryl Tablets **1379**
Avandia Tablets **1384**

Salmeterol Xinafoate (Possible increased risk of coronary insufficiency in patients with coronary artery disease). Products include:
Advair Diskus 100/50 .... **1308**
Advair Diskus 250/50 .... **1308**
Advair Diskus 500/50 .... **1308**
Advair HFA Inhalation Aerosol **1318**
Serevent Diskus **1568**

Salsalate (May inhibit levothyroxine sodium binding to serum proteins or alter the concentrations of serum proteins).
No products indexed under this heading.

Sodium Iodide I 123 (Uptake of radiolabeled ions may be decreased).
No products indexed under this heading.

Sodium Iodide I 131 (Uptake of radiolabeled ions may be decreased).
No products indexed under this heading.

Sodium Nitroprusside (Alters thyroid hormone or TSH levels).
No products indexed under this heading.

Sodium Pertechnetate (Alters thyroid hormone or TSH levels).
No products indexed under this heading.

Sodium Polystyrene Sulfonate (Binds and decreases absorption of levothyroxine sodium from the gastrointestinal tract).
No products indexed under this heading.

Somatrem (Excessive concurrent use of thyroid hormone may accelerate epiphyseal closure; untreated hypothyroidism may interfere with the growth response to somatrem).
No products indexed under this heading.

Somatropin (Excessive concurrent use of thyroid hormone may accelerate epiphyseal closure; untreated hypothyroidism may interfere with the growth response to somatrem). Products include:
Genotropin Lyophilized Powder **2638**
Humatrope Vials and Cartridges **1787**
Norditropin Cartridges **2323**
Nutropin for Injection **1239**
Nutropin AQ Injection **1243**
Nutropin AQ Pen **1243**
Nutropin AQ Pen Cartridge **1243**

Sotalol Hydrochloride (Alters thyroid hormone or TSH levels; actions of some beta blockers may be impaired when hypothyroid patients become euthyroid).
No products indexed under this heading.

Stanozolol (May inhibit levothyroxine sodium binding to serum proteins or alter the concentrations of serum proteins; alters TSH or thyroid hormone levels).
No products indexed under this heading.

Sucralfate (Binds and decreases absorption of levothyroxine sodium from the gastrointestinal tract). Products include:
Carafate Suspension **701**
Carafate Tablets **701**

Sulfacytine (Alters thyroid hormone or TSH levels).
No products indexed under this heading.

Sulfamethizole (Alters thyroid hormone or TSH levels).
No products indexed under this heading.

Sulfamethoxazole (Alters thyroid hormone or TSH levels).
No products indexed under this heading.

Sulfasalazine (Alters thyroid hormone or TSH levels).
No products indexed under this heading.

Sulfinpyrazone (Alters thyroid hormone or TSH levels).
No products indexed under this heading.

Sulfisoxazole Acetyl (Alters thyroid hormone or TSH levels).
No products indexed under this heading.

Sulfisoxazole Diolamine (Alters thyroid hormone or TSH levels).
No products indexed under this heading.

Tamoxifen Citrate (May inhibit levothyroxine sodium binding to serum proteins or alter the concentrations of serum proteins). Products include:
Soltamox Oral Solution **3527**

Terbutaline Sulfate (Possible increased risk of coronary insufficiency in patients with coronary artery disease).
No products indexed under this heading.

Theophylline (Theophylline clearance may be decreased in hypothyroid patients and return toward normal when euthyroid state is achieved).
No products indexed under this heading.

Theophylline Anhydrous (Theophylline clearance may be decreased in hypothyroid patients and return toward normal when euthyroid state is achieved). Products include:
Uniphyl Tablets **2710**

Theophylline Calcium Salicylate (Theophylline clearance may be decreased in hypothyroid patients and return toward normal when euthyroid state is achieved).
No products indexed under this heading.

Theophylline Dihydroxypropyl (Glyceryl) (Theophylline clearance may be decreased in hypothyroid patients and return toward normal when euthyroid state is achieved).
No products indexed under this heading.

Theophylline Ethylenediamine (Theophylline clearance may be decreased in hypothyroid patients and return toward normal when euthyroid state is achieved).
No products indexed under this heading.

Theophylline Sodium Glycinate (Theophylline clearance may be decreased in hypothyroid patients and return toward normal when euthyroid state is achieved).
No products indexed under this heading.

Timolol Hemihydrate (Alters thyroid hormone or TSH levels; actions of some beta blockers may be impaired when hypothyroid patients become euthyroid). Products include:
Betimol Ophthalmic Solution **3382**
Betimol Ophthalmic Solution .... ⊙ **295**

Timolol Maleate (Alters thyroid hormone or TSH levels; actions of some beta blockers may be impaired when hypothyroid patients become euthyroid). Products include:
Blocadren Tablets **1916**
Cosopt Sterile Ophthalmic Solution **1931**
Timolide Tablets **2086**
Timoptic Sterile Ophthalmic Solution **2088**
Timoptic in Ocudose **2091**
Timoptic-XE Sterile Ophthalmic Gel Forming Solution **2092**

Tolazamide (Alters thyroid hormone or TSH levels; requirements of oral antidiabetic agents may be reduced in hypothyroid patients with diabetes and may be subsequently increased with initiation of thyroid hormone therapy).
No products indexed under this heading.

Tolbutamide (Alters thyroid hormone or TSH levels; requirements of oral antidiabetic agents may be reduced in hypothyroid patients with diabetes and may be subsequently increased with initiation of thyroid hormone therapy).
No products indexed under this heading.

Triamcinolone (May inhibit levothyroxine sodium binding to serum proteins or alter the concentrations of serum proteins).
No products indexed under this heading.

Triamcinolone Acetonide (May inhibit levothyroxine sodium binding to serum proteins or alter the concentrations of serum proteins). Products include:
Azmacort Inhalation Aerosol **1726**
Nasacort AQ Nasal Spray **2922**

Triamcinolone Diacetate (May inhibit levothyroxine sodium binding to serum proteins or alter the concentrations of serum proteins).
No products indexed under this heading.

Triamcinolone Hexacetonide (May inhibit levothyroxine sodium binding to serum proteins or alter the concentrations of serum proteins).
No products indexed under this heading.

Trimipramine Maleate (Concurrent use may increase the therapeutic and toxic effects of both drugs; onset of action of tricyclics may be accelerated).
No products indexed under this heading.

Troglitazone (Requirements of oral antidiabetic agents may be reduced in hypothyroid patients with diabetes and may be subsequently increased with initiation of thyroid hormone therapy).
No products indexed under this heading.

Tyropanoate Sodium (Alters thyroid hormone or TSH levels).
No products indexed under this heading.

Warfarin Sodium (The hypoprothrombinemic effect of anticoagulants may be potentiated). Products include:
Coumadin for Injection **898**
Coumadin Tablets **898**

Food Interactions

Soybean Formula, Children's (Binds and decreases absorption of levothyroxine sodium from the gastrointestinal tract).

SYPRINE CAPSULES

(Trientine Hydrochloride) **2085**
None cited in PDR database.

SYSTANE LUBRICANT EYE DROPS

(Polyethylene Glycol, Propylene Glycol) **562**
None cited in PDR database.

TABLOID TABLETS

(Thioguanine) **1575**
May interact with cytotoxic drugs, drugs that inhibit thiopurine methyltransferase (TPMT), and certain other agents. Compounds in these categories include:

Bleomycin Sulfate (Combination therapy may produce hepatic disease).
No products indexed under this heading.

Busulfan (Potential for esophageal varices associated with abnormal liver function tests). Products include:
I.V. Busulfex **2493**
Myleran Tablets **1525**

Cyclophosphamide (Combination therapy may produce hepatic disease).
No products indexed under this heading.

Daunorubicin Hydrochloride (Combination therapy may produce hepatic disease).
No products indexed under this heading.

Doxorubicin Hydrochloride (Combination therapy may produce hepatic disease).
No products indexed under this heading.

Epirubicin Hydrochloride (Combination therapy may produce hepatic disease).
No products indexed under this heading.

Fluorouracil (Combination therapy may produce hepatic disease). Products include:
Carac Cream, 0.5% 2879
Efudex 3363

Hydroxyurea (Combination therapy may produce hepatic disease).
No products indexed under this heading.

Mercaptopurine (Complete cross-resistance).
No products indexed under this heading.

Mesalamine (Individuals with inherited deficiency of the enzyme TPMT are unusually sensitive to the myelosuppressive effects of mercaptopurine and are prone to developing rapid bone marrow suppression; co-administration with drugs that inhibit TPMT could exacerbate this toxicity). Products include:
Asacol Delayed-Release Tablets 2692
Canasa Rectal Suppositories 699
Pentasa Capsules 3185

Mesalazine (Individuals with inherited deficiency of the enzyme TPMT are unusually sensitive to the myelosuppressive effects of mercaptopurine and are prone to developing rapid bone marrow suppression; co-administration with drugs that inhibit TPMT could exacerbate this toxicity).
No products indexed under this heading.

Methotrexate Sodium (Combination therapy may produce hepatic disease).
No products indexed under this heading.

Mitotane (Combination therapy may produce hepatic disease).
No products indexed under this heading.

Mitoxantrone Hydrochloride (Combination therapy may produce hepatic disease).
No products indexed under this heading.

Olsalazine Sodium (Individuals with inherited deficiency of the enzyme TPMT are unusually sensitive to the myelosuppressive effects of mercaptopurine and are prone to developing rapid bone marrow suppression; co-administration with drugs that inhibit TPMT could exacerbate this toxicity).
No products indexed under this heading.

Procarbazine Hydrochloride (Combination therapy may produce hepatic disease). Products include:
Matulane Capsules 3191

Sulphasalazine (Individuals with inherited deficiency of the enzyme TPMT are unusually sensitive to the myelosuppressive effects of mercaptopurine and are prone to developing rapid bone marrow suppression; co-administration with drugs that inhibit TPMT could exacerbate this toxicity).
No products indexed under this heading.

Tamoxifen Citrate (Combination therapy may produce hepatic disease). Products include:
Soltamox Oral Solution 3527

Vincristine Sulfate (Combination therapy may produce hepatic disease).
No products indexed under this heading.

TAGAMET HB 200 TABLETS

(Cimetidine) 664
May interact with dihydropyridine calcium channel blockers, xanthines, and certain other agents. Compounds in these categories include:

Aminophylline (Increased AUC of theophylline by 14% and peak levels by 15% when used concurrently at the maximum recommended OTC dose level; clinically significant pharmacokinetic interactions have been reported at prescription doses).
No products indexed under this heading.

Amlodipine Besylate (Clinically significant pharmacokinetic interactions have been reported with concurrent use at prescription doses of cimetidine; patients are advised to consult their physician). Products include:
Caduet Tablets 2508
Lotrel Capsules 2249
Norvasc Tablets 2545

Dyphylline (Increased AUC of theophylline by 14% and peak levels by 15% when used concurrently at the maximum recommended OTC dose level; clinically significant pharmacokinetic interactions have been reported at prescription doses).
No products indexed under this heading.

Felodipine (Clinically significant pharmacokinetic interactions have been reported with concurrent use at prescription doses of cimetidine; patients are advised to consult their physician).
No products indexed under this heading.

Isradipine (Clinically significant pharmacokinetic interactions have been reported with concurrent use at prescription doses of cimetidine; patients are advised to consult their physician). Products include:
DynaCirc CR Tablets 2721

Nicardipine Hydrochloride (Clinically significant pharmacokinetic interactions have been reported with concurrent use at prescription doses of cimetidine; patients are advised to consult their physician). Products include:
Cardene I.V. 2497

Nifedipine (Clinically significant pharmacokinetic interactions have been reported with concurrent use at prescription doses of cimetidine; patients are advised to consult their physician). Products include:
Adalat CC Tablets 2964

Nimodipine (Clinically significant pharmacokinetic interactions have been reported with concurrent use at prescription doses of cimetidine; patients are advised to consult their physician). Products include:
Nimotop Capsules 749

Phenytoin (Clinically significant pharmacokinetic interactions have been reported with concurrent use at prescription doses of cimetidine; patients are advised to consult their physician).
No products indexed under this heading.

Phenytoin Sodium (Clinically significant pharmacokinetic interactions have been reported with concurrent use at prescription doses of cimetidine; patients are advised to consult their physician). Products include:
Phenytek Capsules 2160

Theophylline (Increased AUC of theophylline by 14% and peak levels by 15% when used concurrently at the maximum recommended OTC dose level; clinically significant pharmacokinetic interactions have been reported at prescription doses).
No products indexed under this heading.

Theophylline Anhydrous (Increased AUC of theophylline by 14% and peak levels by 15% when used concurrently at the maximum recommended OTC dose level; clinically significant pharmacokinetic interactions have been reported at prescription doses). Products include:
Uniphyl Tablets 2710

Theophylline Calcium Salicylate (Increased AUC of theophylline by 14% and peak levels by 15% when used concurrently at the maximum recommended OTC dose level; clinically significant pharmacokinetic interactions have been reported at prescription doses).
No products indexed under this heading.

Theophylline Dihydroxypropyl (Glyceryl) (Increased AUC of theophylline by 14% and peak levels by 15% when used concurrently at the maximum recommended OTC dose level; clinically significant pharmacokinetic interactions have been reported at prescription doses).
No products indexed under this heading.

Theophylline Ethylenediamine (Increased AUC of theophylline by 14% and peak levels by 15% when used concurrently at the maximum recommended OTC dose level; clinically significant pharmacokinetic interactions have been reported at prescription doses).
No products indexed under this heading.

Theophylline Sodium Glycinate (Increased AUC of theophylline by 14% and peak levels by 15% when used concurrently at the maximum recommended OTC dose level; clinically significant pharmacokinetic interactions have been reported at prescription doses).
No products indexed under this heading.

Triazolam (Potential for increased AUC of triazolam by 26-28% and increased peak levels by 11-23%).
No products indexed under this heading.

Warfarin Sodium (Clinically significant pharmacokinetic interactions have been reported with concurrent use at prescription doses of cimetidine; patients are advised to consult their physician). Products include:
Coumadin for Injection 898
Coumadin Tablets 898

TAHITIAN NONI LEAF SERUM SOOTHING GEL

(Herbal Medicines, unspecified) 833
None cited in PDR database.

TAHITIAN NONI LIQUID

(Dietary Supplement) 834
None cited in PDR database.

TAHITIAN NONI SEED OIL

(Herbal Medicines, unspecified) 834
None cited in PDR database.

TAMBOCOR TABLETS

(Flecainide Acetate) 1856
May interact with beta blockers, phenytoin, quinidine, and certain other agents. Compounds in these categories include:

Acebutolol Hydrochloride (Co-administration of flecainide with beta adrenergic blocking agents may result in possible additive negative inotropic effects; combined therapy has not resulted in adverse effects).
No products indexed under this heading.

Amiodarone Hydrochloride (When amiodarone is added to flecainide therapy, plasma flecainide levels may increase two-fold or more in some patients, if flecainide dosage is not reduced).
No products indexed under this heading.

Atenolol (Co-administration of flecainide with beta adrenergic blocking agents may result in possible additive negative inotropic effects; combined therapy has not resulted in adverse effects).
No products indexed under this heading.

Betaxolol Hydrochloride (Co-administration of flecainide with beta adrenergic blocking agents may result in possible additive negative inotropic effects; combined therapy has not resulted in adverse effects). Products include:
Betoptic S Ophthalmic Suspension 558

Bisoprolol Fumarate (Co-administration of flecainide with beta adrenergic blocking agents may result in possible additive negative inotropic effects; combined therapy has not resulted in adverse effects).
No products indexed under this heading.

Carbamazepine (Limited data in patients receiving known enzyme inducers, such as carbamazepine, indicate only a 30% increase in the rate of flecainide elimination). Products include:
Carbatrol Capsules 3171
Equetro Extended-Release Capsules 3180
Tegretol/Tegretol-XR 2295

Carteolol Hydrochloride (Co-administration of flecainide with beta adrenergic blocking agents may result in possible additive negative inotropic effects; combined therapy has not resulted in adverse effects). Products include:
Carteolol Hydrochloride Ophthalmic Solution USP, 1% .... ⊙249

Cimetidine (Increases plasma levels by about 30% and half-life by about 10%). Products include:
Tagamet HB 200 Tablets 664

Cimetidine Hydrochloride (Increases plasma levels by about 30% and half-life by about 10%).
No products indexed under this heading.

Digoxin (Co-administration in individuals stabilized on a maintenance dose of digoxin has resulted in increased plasma digoxin levels by 13% to 19% at six hours postdose). Products include:
- Lanoxicaps Capsules 1490
- Lanoxin Injection 1494
- Lanoxin Injection Pediatric 1497
- Lanoxin Tablets 1500

Disopyramide Phosphate (Co-administration is not recommended because both drugs have negative inotropic properties).
No products indexed under this heading.

Esmolol Hydrochloride (Co-administration of flecainide with beta adrenergic blocking agents may result in possible additive negative inotropic effects; combined therapy has not resulted in adverse effects).
No products indexed under this heading.

Fosphenytoin Sodium (Limited data in patients receiving known enzyme inducers, such as phenytoin, indicate only a 30% increase in the rate of flecainide elimination).
No products indexed under this heading.

Labetalol Hydrochloride (Co-administration of flecainide with beta adrenergic blocking agents may result in possible additive negative inotropic effects; combined therapy has not resulted in adverse effects).
No products indexed under this heading.

Levobunolol Hydrochloride (Co-administration of flecainide with beta adrenergic blocking agents may result in possible additive negative inotropic effects; combined therapy has not resulted in adverse effects). Products include:
- Betagan Ophthalmic Solution, USP... ⊙220

Metipranolol Hydrochloride (Co-administration of flecainide with beta adrenergic blocking agents may result in possible additive negative inotropic effects; combined therapy has not resulted in adverse effects).
No products indexed under this heading.

Metoprolol Succinate (Co-administration of flecainide with beta adrenergic blocking agents may result in possible additive negative inotropic effects; combined therapy has not resulted in adverse effects). Products include:
- Toprol-XL Tablets 668

Metoprolol Tartrate (Co-administration of flecainide with beta adrenergic blocking agents may result in possible additive negative inotropic effects; combined therapy has not resulted in adverse effects). Products include:
- Lopressor Injection 2238
- Lopressor Tablets 2238
- Lopressor HCT 50/25 Tablets 2241
- Lopressor HCT 100/25 Tablets 2241
- Lopressor HCT 100/50 Tablets 2241

Nadolol (Co-administration of flecainide with beta adrenergic blocking agents may result in possible additive negative inotropic effects; combined therapy has not resulted in adverse effects). Products include:
- Nadolol Tablets 2159

Penbutolol Sulfate (Co-administration of flecainide with beta adrenergic blocking agents may result in possible additive negative inotropic effects; combined therapy has not resulted in adverse effects).
No products indexed under this heading.

Phenobarbital (Limited data in patients receiving known enzyme inducers, such as phenobarbital, indicate only a 30% increase in the rate of flecainide elimination). Products include:
- Donnatal Extentabs 2493

Phenytoin (Limited data in patients receiving known enzyme inducers, such as phenytoin, indicate only a 30% increase in the rate of flecainide elimination).
No products indexed under this heading.

Phenytoin Sodium (Limited data in patients receiving known enzyme inducers, such as phenytoin, indicate only a 30% increase in the rate of flecainide elimination). Products include:
- Phenytek Capsules 2160

Pindolol (Co-administration of flecainide with beta adrenergic blocking agents may result in possible additive negative inotropic effects; combined therapy has not resulted in adverse effects).
No products indexed under this heading.

Propranolol Hydrochloride (Co-administration has resulted in increased flecainide and propranolol levels by about 20% and 30% respectively; concurrent use in this study has resulted in additive negative inotropic effects). Products include:
- Inderal LA Long-Acting Capsules 3429
- InnoPran XL Capsules 2723

Quinidine (Drugs that inhibit cytochrome P4502D6, such as quinidine, might increase the plasma-concentrations of flecainide in patients who are on chronic flecainide therapy).
No products indexed under this heading.

Quinidine Gluconate (Drugs that inhibit cytochrome P4502D6, such as quinidine, might increase the plasma-concentrations of flecainide in patients who are on chronic flecainide therapy).
No products indexed under this heading.

Quinidine Hydrochloride (Drugs that inhibit cytochrome P4502D6, such as quinidine, might increase the plasma-concentrations of flecainide in patients who are on chronic flecainide therapy).
No products indexed under this heading.

Quinidine Polygalacturonate (Drugs that inhibit cytochrome P4502D6, such as quinidine, might increase the plasma-concentrations of flecainide in patients who are on chronic flecainide therapy).
No products indexed under this heading.

Quinidine Sulfate (Drugs that inhibit cytochrome P4502D6, such as quinidine, might increase the plasma-concentrations of flecainide in patients who are on chronic flecainide therapy).
No products indexed under this heading.

Sotalol Hydrochloride (Co-administration of flecainide with beta adrenergic blocking agents may result in possible additive negative inotropic effects; combined therapy has not resulted in adverse effects).
No products indexed under this heading.

Timolol Hemihydrate (Co-administration of flecainide with beta adrenergic blocking agents may result in possible additive negative inotropic effects; combined therapy has not resulted in adverse effects). Products include:
- Betimol Ophthalmic Solution 3382
- Betimol Ophthalmic Solution .... ⊙295

Timolol Maleate (Co-administration of flecainide with beta adrenergic blocking agents may result in possible additive negative inotropic effects; combined therapy has not resulted in adverse effects). Products include:
- Blocadren Tablets 1916
- Cosopt Sterile Ophthalmic Solution.. 1931
- Timolide Tablets 2086
- Timoptic Sterile Ophthalmic Solution.. 2088
- Timoptic in Ocudose 2091
- Timoptic-XE Sterile Ophthalmic Gel Forming Solution 2092

Verapamil Hydrochloride (Co-administration is not recommended because both drugs have negative inotropic properties). Products include:
- Covera-HS Tablets 3139
- Tarka Tablets 524
- Verelan PM Extended-Release Capsules, Controlled-Onset.......... 3106

Food Interactions

Dairy products (Milk may inhibit absorption in infants; a reduction in Tambocor dosage should be considered when milk is removed from the diet of infants).

TAMIFLU CAPSULES

(Oseltamivir Phosphate) 2807
May interact with:

Probenecid (Co-administration with probenecid results in an approximate two-fold increase in exposure to oseltamivir due to a decrease in active anionic tubular secretion in the kidneys; no dose adjustments are required due to the safety margin of oseltamivir).
No products indexed under this heading.

TAMIFLU ORAL SUSPENSION

(Oseltamivir Phosphate) 2807
See Tamiflu Capsules

TARCEVA TABLETS

(Erlotinib) 1259
May interact with cytochrome p450 3a4 inducers (selected), cytochrome p450 3a4 inhibitors (selected), and certain other agents. Compounds in these categories include:

Acetazolamide (Caution when administering or taking erlotinib with strong CYP3A4 inhibitors such as atazanavir, clarithromycin, indinavir, itraconazole, nefazodone, nelfinavir, ritonavir, saquinavir, telithromycin, troleandomycin, and voriconazole).
No products indexed under this heading.

Allium sativum (Pre-treatment with the CYP3A4 inducer rifampicin decreased erlotinib AUC by about 2/3. Alternate treatments lacking CYP3A4 inducing activity should be considered. If an alternative treatment is unavailable, an erlotinib dose greater than 150 mg should be considered. If the erlotinib dose is adjusted upward, the dose will need to be reduced upon discontinuation of rifampicin or otehr CYP3A4 inducers).
No products indexed under this heading.

Amiodarone Hydrochloride (Caution when administering or taking erlotinib with strong CYP3A4 inhibitors such as atazanavir, clarithromycin, indinavir, itraconazole, nefazodone, nelfinavir, ritonavir, saquinavir, telithromycin, troleandomycin, and voriconazole).
No products indexed under this heading.

Amprenavir (Caution when administering or taking erlotinib with strong CYP3A4 inhibitors such as atazanavir, clarithromycin, indinavir, itraconazole, nefazodone, nelfinavir, ritonavir, saquinavir, telithromycin, troleandomycin, and voriconazole). Products include:
- Agenerase Capsules 1327
- Agenerase Oral Solution 1332

Anastrozole (Caution when administering or taking erlotinib with strong CYP3A4 inhibitors such as atazanavir, clarithromycin, indinavir, itraconazole, nefazodone, nelfinavir, ritonavir, saquinavir, telithromycin, troleandomycin, and voriconazole). Products include:
- Arimidex Tablets 673

Aprepitant (Caution when administering or taking erlotinib with strong CYP3A4 inhibitors such as atazanavir, clarithromycin, indinavir, itraconazole, nefazodone, nelfinavir, ritonavir, saquinavir, telithromycin, troleandomycin, and voriconazole). Products include:
- Emend Capsules 1963

Atazanavir (Co-treatment with the potent CYP3A4 inhibitor ketoconazole increases erlotinib AUC by 2/3. Caution should be used when administering or taking erlotinib with ketoconazole and other strong CYP3A4 inhibitors such as atazanavir).
No products indexed under this heading.

Atazanavir sulfate (Co-treatment with the potent CYP3A4 inhibitor ketoconazole increases erlotinib AUC by 2/3. Caution should be used when administering or taking erlotinib with ketoconazole and other strong CYP3A4 inhibitors such as atazanavir). Products include:

Reyataz Capsules 921

Betamethasone Acetate (Pre-treatment with the CYP3A4 inducer rifampicin decreased erlotinib AUC by about 2/3. Alternate treatments lacking CYP3A4 inducing activity should be considered. If an alternative treatment is unavailable, an erlotinib dose greater than 150 mg should be considered. If the erlotinib dose is adjusted upward, the dose will need to be reduced upon discontinuation of rifampicin or otehr CYP3A4 inducers).

No products indexed under this heading.

Betamethasone Sodium Phosphate (Pre-treatment with the CYP3A4 inducer rifampicin decreased erlotinib AUC by about 2/3. Alternate treatments lacking CYP3A4 inducing activity should be considered. If an alternative treatment is unavailable, an erlotinib dose greater than 150 mg should be considered. If the erlotinib dose is adjusted upward, the dose will need to be reduced upon discontinuation of rifampicin or otehr CYP3A4 inducers).

No products indexed under this heading.

Carbamazepine (Pre-treatment with the CYP3A4 inducer rifampicin decreased erlotinib AUC by about 2/3. Alternate treatments lacking CYP3A4 inducing activity should be considered. If an alternative treatment is unavailable, an erlotinib dose greater than 150 mg should be considered. If the erlotinib dose is adjusted upward, the dose will need to be reduced upon discontinuation of rifampicin or otehr CYP3A4 inducers). Products include:

Carbatrol Capsules 3171
Equetro Extended-Release Capsules 3180
Tegretol/Tegretol-XR 2295

Cimetidine (Caution when administering or taking erlotinib with strong CYP3A4 inhibitors such as atazanavir, clarithromycin, indinavir, itraconazole, nefazodone, nelfinavir, ritonavir, saquinavir, telithromycin, troleandomycin, and voriconazole). Products include:

Tagamet HB 200 Tablets 664

Cimetidine Hydrochloride (Caution when administering or taking erlotinib with strong CYP3A4 inhibitors such as atazanavir, clarithromycin, indinavir, itraconazole, nefazodone, nelfinavir, ritonavir, saquinavir, telithromycin, troleandomycin, and voriconazole).

No products indexed under this heading.

Ciprofloxacin (Caution when administering or taking erlotinib with strong CYP3A4 inhibitors such as atazanavir, clarithromycin, indinavir, itraconazole, nefazodone, nelfinavir, ritonavir, saquinavir, telithromycin, troleandomycin, and voriconazole). Products include:

Cipro Oral Suspension 2977
Cipro I.V. 2984
Cipro XR Tablets 2990
Ciprodex Otic Suspension 559

Ciprofloxacin Hydrochloride (Pre-treatment with the CYP3A4 inducer rifampicin decreased erlotinib AUC by about 2/3. Alternate treatments lacking CYP3A4 inducing activity should be considered. If an alternative treatment is unavailable, an erlotinib dose greater than 150 mg should be considered. If the erlotinib dose is adjusted upward, the dose will need to be reduced upon discontinuation of rifampicin or otehr CYP3A4 inducers). Products include:

Ciloxan Ophthalmic Ointment 559
Ciloxan Ophthalmic Solution .... ⊙206
Cipro Tablets 2977
Proquin XR Tablets 1153

Cisplatin (Pre-treatment with the CYP3A4 inducer rifampicin decreased erlotinib AUC by about 2/3. Alternate treatments lacking CYP3A4 inducing activity should be considered. If an alternative treatment is unavailable, an erlotinib dose greater than 150 mg should be considered. If the erlotinib dose is adjusted upward, the dose will need to be reduced upon discontinuation of rifampicin or otehr CYP3A4 inducers).

No products indexed under this heading.

Clarithromycin (Co-treatment with the potent CYP3A4 inhibitor ketoconazole increases erlotinib AUC by 2/3. Caution should be used when administering or taking erlotinib with ketoconazole and other strong CYP3A4 inhibitors such as clarithromycin). Products include:

Biaxin/Biaxin XL 402
PREVPAC 3284

Clotrimazole (Caution when administering or taking erlotinib with strong CYP3A4 inhibitors such as atazanavir, clarithromycin, indinavir, itraconazole, nefazodone, nelfinavir, ritonavir, saquinavir, telithromycin, troleandomycin, and voriconazole). Products include:

Desenex Athlete's Foot Cream 635
Lotrimin 3039
Lotrisone 3040

Cortisone Acetate (Pre-treatment with the CYP3A4 inducer rifampicin decreased erlotinib AUC by about 2/3. Alternate treatments lacking CYP3A4 inducing activity should be considered. If an alternative treatment is unavailable, an erlotinib dose greater than 150 mg should be considered. If the erlotinib dose is adjusted upward, the dose will need to be reduced upon discontinuation of rifampicin or otehr CYP3A4 inducers).

No products indexed under this heading.

Cyclosporine (Caution when administering or taking erlotinib with strong CYP3A4 inhibitors such as atazanavir, clarithromycin, indinavir, itraconazole, nefazodone, nelfinavir, ritonavir, saquinavir, telithromycin, troleandomycin, and voriconazole). Products include:

Gengraf Capsules 459
Neoral Oral Solution 2259
Neoral Soft Gelatin Capsules 2259
Restasis Ophthalmic Emulsion 575
Sandimmune 2275

Dalfopristin (Caution when administering or taking erlotinib with strong CYP3A4 inhibitors such as atazanavir, clarithromycin, indinavir, itraconazole, nefazodone, nelfinavir, ritonavir, saquinavir, telithromycin, troleandomycin, and voriconazole).

No products indexed under this heading.

Danazol (Caution when administering or taking erlotinib with strong CYP3A4 inhibitors such as atazanavir, clarithromycin, indinavir, itraconazole, nefazodone, nelfinavir, ritonavir, saquinavir, telithromycin, troleandomycin, and voriconazole).

No products indexed under this heading.

Delavirdine Mesylate (Caution when administering or taking erlotinib with strong CYP3A4 inhibitors such as atazanavir, clarithromycin, indinavir, itraconazole, nefazodone, nelfinavir, ritonavir, saquinavir, telithromycin, troleandomycin, and voriconazole). Products include:

Rescriptor Tablets 2551

Dexamethasone (Pre-treatment with the CYP3A4 inducer rifampicin decreased erlotinib AUC by about 2/3. Alternate treatments lacking CYP3A4 inducing activity should be considered. If an alternative treatment is unavailable, an erlotinib dose greater than 150 mg should be considered. If the erlotinib dose is adjusted upward, the dose will need to be reduced upon discontinuation of rifampicin or otehr CYP3A4 inducers). Products include:

Ciprodex Otic Suspension 559
Decadron Tablets 1951
TobraDex Ophthalmic Ointment 562
TobraDex Ophthalmic Suspension ... 563

Dexamethasone Acetate (Pre-treatment with the CYP3A4 inducer rifampicin decreased erlotinib AUC by about 2/3. Alternate treatments lacking CYP3A4 inducing activity should be considered. If an alternative treatment is unavailable, an erlotinib dose greater than 150 mg should be considered. If the erlotinib dose is adjusted upward, the dose will need to be reduced upon discontinuation of rifampicin or otehr CYP3A4 inducers).

No products indexed under this heading.

Dexamethasone Sodium Phosphate (Pre-treatment with the CYP3A4 inducer rifampicin decreased erlotinib AUC by about 2/3. Alternate treatments lacking CYP3A4 inducing activity should be considered. If an alternative treatment is unavailable, an erlotinib dose greater than 150 mg should be considered. If the erlotinib dose is adjusted upward, the dose will need to be reduced upon discontinuation of rifampicin or otehr CYP3A4 inducers).

No products indexed under this heading.

Diltiazem Hydrochloride (Caution when administering or taking erlotinib with strong CYP3A4 inhibitors such as atazanavir, clarithromycin, indinavir, itraconazole, nefazodone, nelfinavir, ritonavir, saquinavir, telithromycin, troleandomycin, and voriconazole). Products include:

Cardizem LA Extended Release Tablets 1728
Tiazac Capsules 1201

Diltiazem Maleate (Caution when administering or taking erlotinib with strong CYP3A4 inhibitors such as atazanavir, clarithromycin, indinavir, itraconazole, nefazodone, nelfinavir, ritonavir, saquinavir, telithromycin, troleandomycin, and voriconazole).

No products indexed under this heading.

Doxorubicin Hydrochloride (Pre-treatment with the CYP3A4 inducer rifampicin decreased erlotinib AUC by about 2/3. Alternate treatments lacking CYP3A4 inducing activity should be considered. If an alternative treatment is unavailable, an erlotinib dose greater than 150 mg should be considered. If the erlotinib dose is adjusted upward, the dose will need to be reduced upon discontinuation of rifampicin or otehr CYP3A4 inducers).

No products indexed under this heading.

Efavirenz (Caution when administering or taking erlotinib with strong CYP3A4 inhibitors such as atazanavir, clarithromycin, indinavir, itraconazole, nefazodone, nelfinavir, ritonavir, saquinavir, telithromycin, troleandomycin, and voriconazole). Products include:

Atripla Tablets 945
Sustiva Capsules 930
Sustiva Tablets 930

Erythromycin (Caution when administering or taking erlotinib with strong CYP3A4 inhibitors such as atazanavir, clarithromycin, indinavir, itraconazole, nefazodone, nelfinavir, ritonavir, saquinavir, telithromycin, troleandomycin, and voriconazole). Products include:

Ery-Tab Tablets 449
Erythromycin Base Filmtab Tablets 455
Erythromycin Delayed-Release Capsules, USP 457
PCE Dispertab Tablets 515

Erythromycin Estolate (Caution when administering or taking erlotinib with strong CYP3A4 inhibitors such as atazanavir, clarithromycin, indinavir, itraconazole, nefazodone, nelfinavir, ritonavir, saquinavir, telithromycin, troleandomycin, and voriconazole).

No products indexed under this heading.

Erythromycin Ethylsuccinate (Caution when administering or taking erlotinib with strong CYP3A4 inhibitors such as atazanavir, clarithromycin, indinavir, itraconazole, nefazodone, nelfinavir, ritonavir, saquinavir, telithromycin, troleandomycin, and voriconazole). Products include:

E.E.S. 451
EryPed 447

Erythromycin Gluceptate (Caution when administering or taking erlotinib with strong CYP3A4 inhibitors such as atazanavir, clarithromycin, indinavir, itraconazole, nefazodone, nelfinavir, ritonavir, saquinavir, telithromycin, troleandomycin, and voriconazole).

No products indexed under this heading.

Erythromycin Lactobionate (Caution when administering or taking erlotinib with strong CYP3A4 inhibitors such as atazanavir, clarithromycin, indinavir, itraconazole, nefazodone, nelfinavir, ritonavir, saquinavir, telithromycin, troleandomycin, and voriconazole).

No products indexed under this heading.

Erythromycin Stearate (Caution when administering or taking erlotinib with strong CYP3A4 inhibitors such as atazanavir, clarithromycin, indinavir, itraconazole, nefazodone, nelfinavir, ritonavir, saquinavir, telithromycin, troleandomycin, and voriconazole). Products include:

Erythrocin Stearate Filmtab Tablets 453

Esomeprazole Magnesium (Caution when administering or taking erlotinib with strong CYP3A4 inhibitors such as atazanavir, clarithromycin, indinavir, itraconazole, nefazodone, nelfinavir, ritonavir, saquinavir, telithromycin, troleandomycin, and voriconazole). Products include:

Nexium Delayed-Release Capsules 655

Ethosuximide (Pre-treatment with the CYP3A4 inducer rifampicin decreased erlotinib AUC by about 2/3. Alternate treatments lacking CYP3A4 inducing activity should be considered. If an alternative treatment is unavailable, an erlotinib dose greater than 150 mg should be considered. If the erlotinib dose is adjusted upward, the dose will need to be reduced upon discontinuation of rifampicin or otehr CYP3A4 inducers).

No products indexed under this heading.

Felbamate (Pre-treatment with the CYP3A4 inducer rifampicin decreased erlotinib AUC by about 2/3. Alternate treatments lacking CYP3A4 inducing activity should be considered. If an alternative treatment is unavailable, an erlotinib dose greater than 150 mg should be considered. If the erlotinib dose is adjusted upward, the dose will need to be reduced upon discontinuation of rifampicin or otehr CYP3A4 inducers).

No products indexed under this heading.

Fluconazole (Caution when administering or taking erlotinib with strong CYP3A4 inhibitors such as atazanavir, clarithromycin, indinavir, itraconazole, nefazodone, nelfinavir, ritonavir, saquinavir, telithromycin, troleandomycin, and voriconazole).

No products indexed under this heading.

Fludrocortisone Acetate (Pre-treatment with the CYP3A4 inducer rifampicin decreased erlotinib AUC by about 2/3. Alternate treatments lacking CYP3A4 inducing activity should be considered. If an alternative treatment is unavailable, an erlotinib dose greater than 150 mg should be considered. If the erlotinib dose is adjusted upward, the dose will need to be reduced upon discontinuation of rifampicin or otehr CYP3A4 inducers).

No products indexed under this heading.

Fluoxetine Hydrochloride (Caution when administering or taking erlotinib with strong CYP3A4 inhibitors such as atazanavir, clarithromycin, indinavir, itraconazole, nefazodone, nelfinavir, ritonavir, saquinavir, telithromycin, troleandomycin, and voriconazole). Products include:

Prozac Pulvules and Liquid 1801
Symbyax Capsules 1819

Fluvoxamine Maleate (Caution when administering or taking erlotinib with strong CYP3A4 inhibitors such as atazanavir, clarithromycin, indinavir, itraconazole, nefazodone, nelfinavir, ritonavir, saquinavir, telithromycin, troleandomycin, and voriconazole).

No products indexed under this heading.

Fosamprenavir Calcium (Caution when administering or taking erlotinib with strong CYP3A4 inhibitors such as atazanavir, clarithromycin, indinavir, itraconazole, nefazodone, nelfinavir, ritonavir, saquinavir, telithromycin, troleandomycin, and voriconazole). Products include:

Lexiva Tablets 1505

Fosphenytoin Sodium (Pre-treatment with the CYP3A4 inducer rifampicin decreased erlotinib AUC by about 2/3. Alternate treatments lacking CYP3A4 inducing activity should be considered. If an alternative treatment is unavailable, an erlotinib dose greater than 150 mg should be considered. If the erlotinib dose is adjusted upward, the dose will need to be reduced upon discontinuation of rifampicin or otehr CYP3A4 inducers).

No products indexed under this heading.

Garlic Extract (Pre-treatment with the CYP3A4 inducer rifampicin decreased erlotinib AUC by about 2/3. Alternate treatments lacking CYP3A4 inducing activity should be considered. If an alternative treatment is unavailable, an erlotinib dose greater than 150 mg should be considered. If the erlotinib dose is adjusted upward, the dose will need to be reduced upon discontinuation of rifampicin or otehr CYP3A4 inducers).

No products indexed under this heading.

Garlic Oil (Pre-treatment with the CYP3A4 inducer rifampicin decreased erlotinib AUC by about 2/3. Alternate treatments lacking CYP3A4 inducing activity should be considered. If an alternative treatment is unavailable, an erlotinib dose greater than 150 mg should be considered. If the erlotinib dose is adjusted upward, the dose will need to be reduced upon discontinuation of rifampicin or otehr CYP3A4 inducers).

No products indexed under this heading.

Hydrocortisone (Pre-treatment with the CYP3A4 inducer rifampicin decreased erlotinib AUC by about 2/3. Alternate treatments lacking CYP3A4 inducing activity should be considered. If an alternative treatment is unavailable, an erlotinib dose greater than 150 mg should be considered. If the erlotinib dose is adjusted upward, the dose will need to be reduced upon discontinuation of rifampicin or otehr CYP3A4 inducers). Products include:

Colocort Rectal Suspension, USP (Retention) 100 mg/60 mL.......... 2476
Hydrocortone Tablets 1989
Preparation H Hydrocortisone Cream .... ◙ 646

Hydrocortisone Acetate (Pre-treatment with the CYP3A4 inducer rifampicin decreased erlotinib AUC by about 2/3. Alternate treatments lacking CYP3A4 inducing activity should be considered. If an alternative treatment is unavailable, an erlotinib dose greater than 150 mg should be considered. If the erlotinib dose is adjusted upward, the dose will need to be reduced upon discontinuation of rifampicin or otehr CYP3A4 inducers). Products include:

Analpram-HC 1159
Pramosone 1161
ProctoFoam-HC 3099

Hydrocortisone Butyrate (Pre-treatment with the CYP3A4 inducer rifampicin decreased erlotinib AUC by about 2/3. Alternate treatments lacking CYP3A4 inducing activity should be considered. If an alternative treatment is unavailable, an erlotinib dose greater than 150 mg should be considered. If the erlotinib dose is adjusted upward, the dose will need to be reduced upon discontinuation of rifampicin or otehr CYP3A4 inducers). Products include:

Locoid Lipocream Cream 1160

Hydrocortisone Cypionate (Pre-treatment with the CYP3A4 inducer rifampicin decreased erlotinib AUC by about 2/3. Alternate treatments lacking CYP3A4 inducing activity should be considered. If an alternative treatment is unavailable, an erlotinib dose greater than 150 mg should be considered. If the erlotinib dose is adjusted upward, the dose will need to be reduced upon discontinuation of rifampicin or otehr CYP3A4 inducers).

No products indexed under this heading.

Hydrocortisone Hemisuccinate (Pre-treatment with the CYP3A4 inducer rifampicin decreased erlotinib AUC by about 2/3. Alternate treatments lacking CYP3A4 inducing activity should be considered. If an alternative treatment is unavailable, an erlotinib dose greater than 150 mg should be considered. If the erlotinib dose is adjusted upward, the dose will need to be reduced upon discontinuation of rifampicin or otehr CYP3A4 inducers).

No products indexed under this heading.

Hydrocortisone Probutate (Pre-treatment with the CYP3A4 inducer rifampicin decreased erlotinib AUC by about 2/3. Alternate treatments lacking CYP3A4 inducing activity should be considered. If an alternative treatment is unavailable, an erlotinib dose greater than 150 mg should be considered. If the erlotinib dose is adjusted upward, the dose will need to be reduced upon discontinuation of rifampicin or otehr CYP3A4 inducers).

No products indexed under this heading.

Hydrocortisone Sodium Phosphate (Pre-treatment with the CYP3A4 inducer rifampicin decreased erlotinib AUC by about 2/3. Alternate treatments lacking CYP3A4 inducing activity should be considered. If an alternative treatment is unavailable, an erlotinib dose greater than 150 mg should be considered. If the erlotinib dose is adjusted upward, the dose will need to be reduced upon discontinuation of rifampicin or otehr CYP3A4 inducers).

No products indexed under this heading.

Hydrocortisone Sodium Succinate (Pre-treatment with the CYP3A4 inducer rifampicin decreased erlotinib AUC by about 2/3. Alternate treatments lacking CYP3A4 inducing activity should be considered. If an alternative treatment is unavailable, an erlotinib dose greater than 150 mg should be considered. If the erlotinib dose is adjusted upward, the dose will need to be reduced upon discontinuation of rifampicin or otehr CYP3A4 inducers).

No products indexed under this heading.

Hydrocortisone Valerate (Pre-treatment with the CYP3A4 inducer rifampicin decreased erlotinib AUC by about 2/3. Alternate treatments lacking CYP3A4 inducing activity should be considered. If an alternative treatment is unavailable, an erlotinib dose greater than 150 mg should be considered. If the erlotinib dose is adjusted upward, the dose will need to be reduced upon discontinuation of rifampicin or otehr CYP3A4 inducers).

No products indexed under this heading.

Hypericum (Pre-treatment with the CYP3A4 inducer rifampicin decreased erlotinib AUC by about 2/3. Alternate treatments lacking CYP3A4 inducing activity should be considered. If an alternative treatment is unavailable, an erlotinib dose greater than 150 mg should be considered. If the erlotinib dose is adjusted upward, the dose will need to be reduced upon discontinuation of rifampicin or otehr CYP3A4 inducers). Products include:

Satiete Tablets .... ◙ 832

Hypericum Perforatum (Pre-treatment with the CYP3A4 inducer rifampicin decreased erlotinib AUC by about 2/3. Alternate treatments lacking CYP3A4 inducing activity should be considered. If an alternative treatment is unavailable, an erlotinib dose greater than 150 mg should be considered. If the erlotinib dose is adjusted upward, the dose will need to be reduced upon discontinuation of rifampicin or otehr CYP3A4 inducers).

No products indexed under this heading.

Indinavir Sulfate (Co-treatment with the potent CYP3A4 inhibitor ketoconazole increases erlotinib AUC by 2/3. Caution should be used when administering or taking erlotinib with ketoconazole and other strong CYP3A4 inhibitors such as indinavir). Products include:

Crixivan Capsules 1940

Isoniazid (Caution when administering or taking erlotinib with strong CYP3A4 inhibitors such as atazanavir, clarithromycin, indinavir, itraconazole, nefazodone, nelfinavir, ritonavir, saquinavir, telithromycin, troleandomycin, and voriconazole).

No products indexed under this heading.

Itraconazole (Co-treatment with the potent CYP3A4 inhibitor ketoconazole increases erlotinib AUC by 2/3. Caution should be used when administering or taking erlotinib with ketoconazole and other strong CYP3A4 inhibitors such as itraconazole).

No products indexed under this heading.

Ketoconazole (Co-treatment with the potent CYP3A4 inhibitor ketoconazole increases erlotinib AUC by 2/3. Caution should be used when administering or taking erlotinib with ketoconazole and other strong CYP3A4 inhibitors). Products include:

Nizoral A-D Shampoo, 1% 1868

Lopinavir (Caution when administering or taking erlotinib with strong CYP3A4 inhibitors such as atazanavir, clarithromycin, indinavir, itraconazole, nefazodone, nelfinavir, ritonavir, saquinavir, telithromycin, troleandomycin, and voriconazole). Products include:

Kaletra ... 476

Loratadine (Caution when administering or taking erlotinib with strong CYP3A4 inhibitors such as atazanavir, clarithromycin, indinavir, itraconazole, nefazodone, nelfinavir, ritonavir, saquinavir, telithromycin, troleandomycin, and voriconazole). Products include:

Alavert Allergy & Sinus D-12 Hour Tablets ... ▣771
Alavert ... ▣771
Children's Claritin Allergy Oral Solution ... ▣771
Claritin Non-Drowsy 24 Hour Tablets ... ▣772
Claritin Reditabs 24 Hour Non-Drowsy Tablets ... ▣772
Claritin-D Non-Drowsy 12 Hour Tablets ... ▣772
Claritin-D Non-Drowsy 24 Hour Tablets ... ▣772

Mephenytoin (Pre-treatment with the CYP3A4 inducer rifampicin decreased erlotinib AUC by about 2/3. Alternate treatments lacking CYP3A4 inducing activity should be considered. If an alternative treatment is unavailable, an erlotinib dose greater than 150 mg should be considered. If the erlotinib dose is adjusted upward, the dose will need to be reduced upon discontinuation of rifampicin or otehr CYP3A4 inducers).

No products indexed under this heading.

Methsuximide (Pre-treatment with the CYP3A4 inducer rifampicin decreased erlotinib AUC by about 2/3. Alternate treatments lacking CYP3A4 inducing activity should be considered. If an alternative treatment is unavailable, an erlotinib dose greater than 150 mg should be considered. If the erlotinib dose is adjusted upward, the dose will need to be reduced upon discontinuation of rifampicin or otehr CYP3A4 inducers).

No products indexed under this heading.

Methylprednisolone (Pre-treatment with the CYP3A4 inducer rifampicin decreased erlotinib AUC by about 2/3. Alternate treatments lacking CYP3A4 inducing activity should be considered. If an alternative treatment is unavailable, an erlotinib dose greater than 150 mg should be considered. If the erlotinib dose is adjusted upward, the dose will need to be reduced upon discontinuation of rifampicin or otehr CYP3A4 inducers).

No products indexed under this heading.

Methylprednisolone Acetate (Pre-treatment with the CYP3A4 inducer rifampicin decreased erlotinib AUC by about 2/3. Alternate treatments lacking CYP3A4 inducing activity should be considered. If an alternative treatment is unavailable, an erlotinib dose greater than 150 mg should be considered. If the erlotinib dose is adjusted upward, the dose will need to be reduced upon discontinuation of rifampicin or otehr CYP3A4 inducers). Products include:

Depo-Medrol Injectable Suspension ... 2617
Depo-Medrol Single-Dose Vial ... 2619

Methylprednisolone Sodium Succinate (Pre-treatment with the CYP3A4 inducer rifampicin decreased erlotinib AUC by about 2/3. Alternate treatments lacking CYP3A4 inducing activity should be considered. If an alternative treatment is unavailable, an erlotinib dose greater than 150 mg should be considered. If the erlotinib dose is adjusted upward, the dose will need to be reduced upon discontinuation of rifampicin or otehr CYP3A4 inducers).

No products indexed under this heading.

Metronidazole (Caution when administering or taking erlotinib with strong CYP3A4 inhibitors such as atazanavir, clarithromycin, indinavir, itraconazole, nefazodone, nelfinavir, ritonavir, saquinavir, telithromycin, troleandomycin, and voriconazole). Products include:

Metrogel 1% ... 1211
MetroGel-Vaginal Gel ... 1855
Vandazole Vaginal Gel ... 3338

Metronidazole Benzoate (Caution when administering or taking erlotinib with strong CYP3A4 inhibitors such as atazanavir, clarithromycin, indinavir, itraconazole, nefazodone, nelfinavir, ritonavir, saquinavir, telithromycin, troleandomycin, and voriconazole).

No products indexed under this heading.

Metronidazole Hydrochloride (Caution when administering or taking erlotinib with strong CYP3A4 inhibitors such as atazanavir, clarithromycin, indinavir, itraconazole, nefazodone, nelfinavir, ritonavir, saquinavir, telithromycin, troleandomycin, and voriconazole).

No products indexed under this heading.

Miconazole (Caution when administering or taking erlotinib with strong CYP3A4 inhibitors such as atazanavir, clarithromycin, indinavir, itraconazole, nefazodone, nelfinavir, ritonavir, saquinavir, telithromycin, troleandomycin, and voriconazole).

No products indexed under this heading.

Miconazole Nitrate (Caution when administering or taking erlotinib with strong CYP3A4 inhibitors such as atazanavir, clarithromycin, indinavir, itraconazole, nefazodone, nelfinavir, ritonavir, saquinavir, telithromycin, troleandomycin, and voriconazole). Products include:

Desenex ... ▣635
Desenex Jock Itch Spray Powder ... ▣635

Modafinil (Pre-treatment with the CYP3A4 inducer rifampicin decreased erlotinib AUC by about 2/3. Alternate treatments lacking CYP3A4 inducing activity should be considered. If an alternative treatment is unavailable, an erlotinib dose greater than 150 mg should be considered. If the erlotinib dose is adjusted upward, the dose will need to be reduced upon discontinuation of rifampicin or otehr CYP3A4 inducers). Products include:

Provigil Tablets ... 988

Nefazodone Hydrochloride (Co-treatment with the potent CYP3A4 inhibitor ketoconazole increases erlotinib AUC by 2/3. Caution should be used when administering or taking erlotinib with ketoconazole and other strong CYP3A4 inhibitors such as nefazodone).

No products indexed under this heading.

Nelfinavir Mesylate (Co-treatment with the potent CYP3A4 inhibitor ketoconazole increases erlotinib AUC by 2/3. Caution should be used when administering or taking erlotinib with ketoconazole and other strong CYP3A4 inhibitors such as nelfinavir). Products include:

Viracept ... 2577

Nevirapine (Caution when administering or taking erlotinib with strong CYP3A4 inhibitors such as atazanavir, clarithromycin, indinavir, itraconazole, nefazodone, nelfinavir, ritonavir, saquinavir, telithromycin, troleandomycin, and voriconazole). Products include:

Viramune Oral Suspension ... 873
Viramune Tablets ... 873

Niacinamide (Caution when administering or taking erlotinib with strong CYP3A4 inhibitors such as atazanavir, clarithromycin, indinavir, itraconazole, nefazodone, nelfinavir, ritonavir, saquinavir, telithromycin, troleandomycin, and voriconazole).

No products indexed under this heading.

Nicotinamide (Caution when administering or taking erlotinib with strong CYP3A4 inhibitors such as atazanavir, clarithromycin, indinavir, itraconazole, nefazodone, nelfinavir, ritonavir, saquinavir, telithromycin, troleandomycin, and voriconazole). Products include:

Nicomide Tablets ... 1088

Nifedipine (Caution when administering or taking erlotinib with strong CYP3A4 inhibitors such as atazanavir, clarithromycin, indinavir, itraconazole, nefazodone, nelfinavir, ritonavir, saquinavir, telithromycin, troleandomycin, and voriconazole). Products include:

Adalat CC Tablets ... 2964

Norfloxacin (Caution when administering or taking erlotinib with strong CYP3A4 inhibitors such as atazanavir, clarithromycin, indinavir, itraconazole, nefazodone, nelfinavir, ritonavir, saquinavir, telithromycin, troleandomycin, and voriconazole). Products include:

Noroxin Tablets ... 2032

Omeprazole (Caution when administering or taking erlotinib with strong CYP3A4 inhibitors such as atazanavir, clarithromycin, indinavir, itraconazole, nefazodone, nelfinavir, ritonavir, saquinavir, telithromycin, troleandomycin, and voriconazole). Products include:

Zegerid Capsules ... 2958
Zegerid Powder for Oral Solution ... 2958

Oxcarbazepine (Pre-treatment with the CYP3A4 inducer rifampicin decreased erlotinib AUC by about 2/3. Alternate treatments lacking CYP3A4 inducing activity should be considered. If an alternative treatment is unavailable, an erlotinib dose greater than 150 mg should be considered. If the erlotinib dose is adjusted upward, the dose will need to be reduced upon discontinuation of rifampicin or otehr CYP3A4 inducers). Products include:

Trileptal Tablets ... 2300
Trileptal Oral Suspension ... 2300

Paroxetine Hydrochloride (Caution when administering or taking erlotinib with strong CYP3A4 inhibitors such as atazanavir, clarithromycin, indinavir, itraconazole, nefazodone, nelfinavir, ritonavir, saquinavir, telithromycin, troleandomycin, and voriconazole). Products include:

Paxil CR Controlled-Release Tablets ... 1538
Paxil ... 1530

Phenobarbital (Pre-treatment with the CYP3A4 inducer rifampicin decreased erlotinib AUC by about 2/3. Alternate treatments lacking CYP3A4 inducing activity should be considered. If an alternative treatment is unavailable, an erlotinib dose greater than 150 mg should be considered. If the erlotinib dose is adjusted upward, the dose will need to be reduced upon discontinuation of rifampicin or otehr CYP3A4 inducers). Products include:

Donnatal Extentabs ... 2493

Phenobarbital Sodium (Pre-treatment with the CYP3A4 inducer rifampicin decreased erlotinib AUC by about 2/3. Alternate treatments lacking CYP3A4 inducing activity should be considered. If an alternative treatment is unavailable, an erlotinib dose greater than 150 mg should be considered. If the erlotinib dose is adjusted upward, the dose will need to be reduced upon discontinuation of rifampicin or otehr CYP3A4 inducers).

No products indexed under this heading.

Phenytoin (Pre-treatment with the CYP3A4 inducer rifampicin decreased erlotinib AUC by about 2/3. Alternate treatments lacking CYP3A4 inducing activity should be considered. If an alternative treatment is unavailable, an erlotinib dose greater than 150 mg should be considered. If the erlotinib dose is adjusted upward, the dose will need to be reduced upon discontinuation of rifampicin or otehr CYP3A4 inducers).

No products indexed under this heading.

Phenytoin Sodium (Pre-treatment with the CYP3A4 inducer rifampicin decreased erlotinib AUC by about 2/3. Alternate treatments lacking CYP3A4 inducing activity should be considered. If an alternative treatment is unavailable, an erlotinib dose greater than 150 mg should be considered. If the erlotinib dose is adjusted upward, the dose will need to be reduced upon discontinuation of rifampicin or otehr CYP3A4 inducers). Products include:

Phenytek Capsules ... 2160

Prednisolone Acetate (Pre-treatment with the CYP3A4 inducer rifampicin decreased erlotinib AUC by about 2/3. Alternate treatments lacking CYP3A4 inducing activity should be considered. If an alternative treatment is unavailable, an erlotinib dose greater than 150 mg should be considered. If the erlotinib dose is adjusted upward, the dose will need to be reduced upon discontinuation of rifampicin or otehr CYP3A4 inducers). Products include:

Blephamide Ophthalmic Ointment ... 568
Blephamide Ophthalmic Suspension ... 569
Poly-Pred Ophthalmic Suspension ... ⊙233
Pred Forte Ophthalmic Suspension ... ⊙235
Pred Mild Ophthalmic Suspension ... ⊙238
Pred-G Ophthalmic Ointment ... ⊙237
Pred-G Ophthalmic Suspension ... ⊙236

Prednisolone Sodium Phosphate (Pre-treatment with the CYP3A4 inducer rifampicin decreased erlotinib AUC by about 2/3. Alternate treatments lacking CYP3A4 inducing activity should be considered. If an alternative treatment is unavailable, an erlotinib dose greater than 150 mg should be considered. If the erlotinib dose is adjusted upward, the dose will need to be reduced upon discontinuation of rifampicin or otehr CYP3A4 inducers).
No products indexed under this heading.

Prednisolone Tebutate (Pre-treatment with the CYP3A4 inducer rifampicin decreased erlotinib AUC by about 2/3. Alternate treatments lacking CYP3A4 inducing activity should be considered. If an alternative treatment is unavailable, an erlotinib dose greater than 150 mg should be considered. If the erlotinib dose is adjusted upward, the dose will need to be reduced upon discontinuation of rifampicin or otehr CYP3A4 inducers).
No products indexed under this heading.

Prednisone (Pre-treatment with the CYP3A4 inducer rifampicin decreased erlotinib AUC by about 2/3. Alternate treatments lacking CYP3A4 inducing activity should be considered. If an alternative treatment is unavailable, an erlotinib dose greater than 150 mg should be considered. If the erlotinib dose is adjusted upward, the dose will need to be reduced upon discontinuation of rifampicin or otehr CYP3A4 inducers).
No products indexed under this heading.

Primidone (Pre-treatment with the CYP3A4 inducer rifampicin decreased erlotinib AUC by about 2/3. Alternate treatments lacking CYP3A4 inducing activity should be considered. If an alternative treatment is unavailable, an erlotinib dose greater than 150 mg should be considered. If the erlotinib dose is adjusted upward, the dose will need to be reduced upon discontinuation of rifampicin or otehr CYP3A4 inducers).
No products indexed under this heading.

Propoxyphene Hydrochloride (Caution when administering or taking erlotinib with strong CYP3A4 inhibitors such as atazanavir, clarithromycin, indinavir, itraconazole, nefazodone, nelfinavir, ritonavir, saquinavir, telithromycin, troleandomycin, and voriconazole).
No products indexed under this heading.

Propoxyphene Napsylate (Caution when administering or taking erlotinib with strong CYP3A4 inhibitors such as atazanavir, clarithromycin, indinavir, itraconazole, nefazodone, nelfinavir, ritonavir, saquinavir, telithromycin, troleandomycin, and voriconazole).
No products indexed under this heading.

Quinidine (Caution when administering or taking erlotinib with strong CYP3A4 inhibitors such as atazanavir, clarithromycin, indinavir, itraconazole, nefazodone, nelfinavir, ritonavir, saquinavir, telithromycin, troleandomycin, and voriconazole).
No products indexed under this heading.

Quinidine Hydrochloride (Caution when administering or taking erlotinib with strong CYP3A4 inhibitors such as atazanavir, clarithromycin, indinavir, itraconazole, nefazodone, nelfinavir, ritonavir, saquinavir, telithromycin, troleandomycin, and voriconazole).
No products indexed under this heading.

Quinidine Polygalacturonate (Caution when administering or taking erlotinib with strong CYP3A4 inhibitors such as atazanavir, clarithromycin, indinavir, itraconazole, nefazodone, nelfinavir, ritonavir, saquinavir, telithromycin, troleandomycin, and voriconazole).
No products indexed under this heading.

Quinidine Sulfate (Caution when administering or taking erlotinib with strong CYP3A4 inhibitors such as atazanavir, clarithromycin, indinavir, itraconazole, nefazodone, nelfinavir, ritonavir, saquinavir, telithromycin, troleandomycin, and voriconazole).
No products indexed under this heading.

Quinine (Caution when administering or taking erlotinib with strong CYP3A4 inhibitors such as atazanavir, clarithromycin, indinavir, itraconazole, nefazodone, nelfinavir, ritonavir, saquinavir, telithromycin, troleandomycin, and voriconazole).
No products indexed under this heading.

Quinine Sulfate (Caution when administering or taking erlotinib with strong CYP3A4 inhibitors such as atazanavir, clarithromycin, indinavir, itraconazole, nefazodone, nelfinavir, ritonavir, saquinavir, telithromycin, troleandomycin, and voriconazole).
No products indexed under this heading.

Quinupristin (Caution when administering or taking erlotinib with strong CYP3A4 inhibitors such as atazanavir, clarithromycin, indinavir, itraconazole, nefazodone, nelfinavir, ritonavir, saquinavir, telithromycin, troleandomycin, and voriconazole).
No products indexed under this heading.

Ranitidine Bismuth Citrate (Caution when administering or taking erlotinib with strong CYP3A4 inhibitors such as atazanavir, clarithromycin, indinavir, itraconazole, nefazodone, nelfinavir, ritonavir, saquinavir, telithromycin, troleandomycin, and voriconazole).
No products indexed under this heading.

Ranitidine Hydrochloride (Caution when administering or taking erlotinib with strong CYP3A4 inhibitors such as atazanavir, clarithromycin, indinavir, itraconazole, nefazodone, nelfinavir, ritonavir, saquinavir, telithromycin, troleandomycin, and voriconazole). Products include:
Zantac 1624
Zantac Injection 1619
Zantac Injection Pharmacy Bulk Package 1622

Rifabutin (Pre-treatment with the CYP3A4 inducer rifampicin decreased erlotinib AUC by about 2/3. Alternate treatments lacking CYP3A4 inducing activity should be considered. If an alternative treatment is unavailable, an erlotinib dose greater than 150 mg should be considered. If the erlotinib dose is adjusted upward, the dose will need to be reduced upon discontinuation of rifampicin or otehr CYP3A4 inducers).
No products indexed under this heading.

Rifampicin (Pre-treatment with the CYP3A4 inducer rifampicin decreased erlotinib AUC by about 2/3. Alternate treatments lacking CYP3A4 inducing activity should be considered. If an alternative treatment is unavailable, an erlotinib dose greater than 150 mg should be considered. If the erlotinib dose is adjusted upward, the dose will need to be reduced upon discontinuation of rifampicin or otehr CYP3A4 inducers).
No products indexed under this heading.

Rifampin (Pre-treatment with the CYP3A4 inducer rifampicin decreased erlotinib AUC by about 2/3. Alternate treatments lacking CYP3A4 inducing activity should be considered. If an alternative treatment is unavailable, an erlotinib dose greater than 150 mg should be considered. If the erlotinib dose is adjusted upward, the dose will need to be reduced upon discontinuation of rifampicin or otehr CYP3A4 inducers).
No products indexed under this heading.

Rifapentine (Pre-treatment with the CYP3A4 inducer rifampicin decreased erlotinib AUC by about 2/3. Alternate treatments lacking CYP3A4 inducing activity should be considered. If an alternative treatment is unavailable, an erlotinib dose greater than 150 mg should be considered. If the erlotinib dose is adjusted upward, the dose will need to be reduced upon discontinuation of rifampicin or otehr CYP3A4 inducers).
No products indexed under this heading.

Ritonavir (Co-treatment with the potent CYP3A4 inhibitor ketoconazole increases erlotinib AUC by 2/3. Caution should be used when administering or taking erlotinib with ketoconazole and other strong CYP3A4 inhibitors such as ritonavir). Products include:
Kaletra 476
Norvir 503

Saquinavir (Co-treatment with the potent CYP3A4 inhibitor ketoconazole increases erlotinib AUC by 2/3. Caution should be used when administering or taking erlotinib with ketoconazole and other strong CYP3A4 inhibitors such as saquinavir).
No products indexed under this heading.

Saquinavir Mesylate (Co-treatment with the potent CYP3A4 inhibitor ketoconazole increases erlotinib AUC by 2/3. Caution should be used when administering or taking erlotinib with ketoconazole and other strong CYP3A4 inhibitors such as saquinavir). Products include:
Invirase 2772

Sertraline Hydrochloride (Caution when administering or taking erlotinib with strong CYP3A4 inhibitors such as atazanavir, clarithromycin, indinavir, itraconazole, nefazodone, nelfinavir, ritonavir, saquinavir, telithromycin, troleandomycin, and voriconazole). Products include:
Zoloft 2586

Sulfinpyrazone (Pre-treatment with the CYP3A4 inducer rifampicin decreased erlotinib AUC by about 2/3. Alternate treatments lacking CYP3A4 inducing activity should be considered. If an alternative treatment is unavailable, an erlotinib dose greater than 150 mg should be considered. If the erlotinib dose is adjusted upward, the dose will need to be reduced upon discontinuation of rifampicin or otehr CYP3A4 inducers).
No products indexed under this heading.

Telithromycin (Co-treatment with the potent CYP3A4 inhibitor ketoconazole increases erlotinib AUC by 2/3. Caution should be used when administering or taking erlotinib with ketoconazole and other strong CYP3A4 inhibitors such as telithromycin). Products include:
Ketek Tablets 2903

Theophylline (Pre-treatment with the CYP3A4 inducer rifampicin decreased erlotinib AUC by about 2/3. Alternate treatments lacking CYP3A4 inducing activity should be considered. If an alternative treatment is unavailable, an erlotinib dose greater than 150 mg should be considered. If the erlotinib dose is adjusted upward, the dose will need to be reduced upon discontinuation of rifampicin or otehr CYP3A4 inducers).
No products indexed under this heading.

Triamcinolone (Pre-treatment with the CYP3A4 inducer rifampicin decreased erlotinib AUC by about 2/3. Alternate treatments lacking CYP3A4 inducing activity should be considered. If an alternative treatment is unavailable, an erlotinib dose greater than 150 mg should be considered. If the erlotinib dose is adjusted upward, the dose will need to be reduced upon discontinuation of rifampicin or otehr CYP3A4 inducers).
No products indexed under this heading.

Triamcinolone Acetonide (Pre-treatment with the CYP3A4 inducer rifampicin decreased erlotinib AUC by about 2/3. Alternate treatments lacking CYP3A4 inducing activity should be considered. If an alternative treatment is unavailable, an erlotinib dose greater than 150 mg should be considered. If the erlotinib dose is adjusted upward, the dose will need to be reduced upon discontinuation of rifampicin or otehr CYP3A4 inducers). Products include:
Azmacort Inhalation Aerosol 1726
Nasacort AQ Nasal Spray 2922

Triamcinolone Diacetate (Pre-treatment with the CYP3A4 inducer rifampicin decreased erlotinib AUC by about 2/3. Alternate treatments lacking CYP3A4 inducing activity should be considered. If an alternative treatment is unavailable, an erlotinib dose greater than 150 mg should be considered. If the erlotinib dose is adjusted upward, the dose will need to be reduced upon discontinuation of rifampicin or otehr CYP3A4 inducers).
No products indexed under this heading.

Triamcinolone Hexacetonide (Pre-treatment with the CYP3A4 inducer rifampicin decreased erlo-

tinib AUC by about 2/3. Alternate treatments lacking CYP3A4 inducing activity should be considered. If an alternative treatment is unavailable, an erlotinib dose greater than 150 mg should be considered. If the erlotinib dose is adjusted upward, the dose will need to be reduced upon discontinuation of rifampicin or otehr CYP3A4 inducers).
No products indexed under this heading.

Troglitazone (Caution when administering or taking erlotinib with strong CYP3A4 inhibitors such as atazanavir, clarithromycin, indinavir, itraconazole, nefazodone, nelfinavir, ritonavir, saquinavir, telithromycin, troleandomycin, and voriconazole).
No products indexed under this heading.

Troleandomycin (Co-treatment with the potent CYP3A4 inhibitor ketoconazole increases erlotinib AUC by 2/3. Caution should be used when administering or taking erlotinib with ketoconazole and other strong CYP3A4 inhibitors such as troleandomycin).
No products indexed under this heading.

Valproate Sodium (Caution when administering or taking erlotinib with strong CYP3A4 inhibitors such as atazanavir, clarithromycin, indinavir, itraconazole, nefazodone, nelfinavir, ritonavir, saquinavir, telithromycin, troleandomycin, and voriconazole). Products include:
Depacon Injection 412

Verapamil Hydrochloride (Caution when administering or taking erlotinib with strong CYP3A4 inhibitors such as atazanavir, clarithromycin, indinavir, itraconazole, nefazodone, nelfinavir, ritonavir, saquinavir, telithromycin, troleandomycin, and voriconazole). Products include:
Covera-HS Tablets 3139
Tarka Tablets 524
Verelan PM Extended-Release Capsules, Controlled-Onset 3106

Voriconazole (Co-treatment with the potent CYP3A4 inhibitor ketoconazole increases erlotinib AUC by 2/3. Caution should be used when administering or taking erlotinib with ketoconazole and other strong CYP3A4 inhibitors such as voriconazole). Products include:
VFEND I.V. 2564
VFEND Oral Suspension 2564
VFEND Tablets 2564

Zafirlukast (Caution when administering or taking erlotinib with strong CYP3A4 inhibitors such as atazanavir, clarithromycin, indinavir, itraconazole, nefazodone, nelfinavir, ritonavir, saquinavir, telithromycin, troleandomycin, and voriconazole). Products include:
Accolate Tablets 671

Zileuton (Caution when administering or taking erlotinib with strong CYP3A4 inhibitors such as atazanavir, clarithromycin, indinavir, itraconazole, nefazodone, nelfinavir, ritonavir, saquinavir, telithromycin, troleandomycin, and voriconazole). Products include:
Zyflo Tablets 1023

Food Interactions

Grapefruit (Caution when administering or taking erlotinib with strong CYP3A4 inhibitors such as atazanavir, clarithromycin, indinavir, itraconazole, nefazodone, nelfinavir, ritonavir, saquinavir, telithromycin, troleandomycin, and voriconazole).

Grapefruit Juice (Caution when administering or taking erlotinib with strong CYP3A4 inhibitors such as atazanavir, clarithromycin, indinavir, itraconazole, nefazodone, nelfinavir, ritonavir, saquinavir, telithromycin, troleandomycin, and voriconazole).

TARCEVA TABLETS

(Erlotinib) 2444
May interact with cytochrome p450 3a4 inducers (selected), cytochrome p450 3a4 inhibitors (selected), and certain other agents. Compounds in these categories include:

Acetazolamide (Caution when administering or taking erlotinib with strong CYP3A4 inhibitors such as atazanavir, clarithromycin, indinavir, itraconazole, nefazodone, nelfinavir, ritonavir, saquinavir, telithromycin, troleandomycin, and voriconazole).
No products indexed under this heading.

Allium sativum (Pre-treatment with the CYP3A4 inducer rifampicin decreased erlotinib AUC by about 2/3. Alternate treatments lacking CYP3A4 inducing activity should be considered. If an alternative treatment is unavailable, an erlotinib dose greater than 150 mg should be considered. If the erlotinib dose is adjusted upward, the dose will need to be reduced upon discontinuation of rifampicin or otehr CYP3A4 inducers).
No products indexed under this heading.

Amiodarone Hydrochloride (Caution when administering or taking erlotinib with strong CYP3A4 inhibitors such as atazanavir, clarithromycin, indinavir, itraconazole, nefazodone, nelfinavir, ritonavir, saquinavir, telithromycin, troleandomycin, and voriconazole).
No products indexed under this heading.

Amprenavir (Caution when administering or taking erlotinib with strong CYP3A4 inhibitors such as atazanavir, clarithromycin, indinavir, itraconazole, nefazodone, nelfinavir, ritonavir, saquinavir, telithromycin, troleandomycin, and voriconazole). Products include:
Agenerase Capsules 1327
Agenerase Oral Solution 1332

Anastrozole (Caution when administering or taking erlotinib with strong CYP3A4 inhibitors such as atazanavir, clarithromycin, indinavir, itraconazole, nefazodone, nelfinavir, ritonavir, saquinavir, telithromycin, troleandomycin, and voriconazole). Products include:
Arimidex Tablets 673

Aprepitant (Caution when administering or taking erlotinib with strong CYP3A4 inhibitors such as atazanavir, clarithromycin, indinavir, itraconazole, nefazodone, nelfinavir, ritonavir, saquinavir, telithromycin, troleandomycin, and voriconazole). Products include:
Emend Capsules 1963

Atazanavir (Co-treatment with the potent CYP3A4 inhibitor ketoconazole increases erlotinib AUC by 2/3. Caution should be used when administering or taking erlotinib with ketoconazole and other strong CYP3A4 inhibitors such as atazanavir).
No products indexed under this heading.

Atazanavir sulfate (Co-treatment with the potent CYP3A4 inhibitor ketoconazole increases erlotinib AUC by 2/3. Caution should be used when administering or taking erlotinib with ketoconazole and other strong CYP3A4 inhibitors such as atazanavir). Products include:
Reyataz Capsules 921

Betamethasone Acetate (Pre-treatment with the CYP3A4 inducer rifampicin decreased erlotinib AUC by about 2/3. Alternate treatments lacking CYP3A4 inducing activity should be considered. If an alternative treatment is unavailable, an erlotinib dose greater than 150 mg should be considered. If the erlotinib dose is adjusted upward, the dose will need to be reduced upon discontinuation of rifampicin or otehr CYP3A4 inducers).
No products indexed under this heading.

Betamethasone Sodium Phosphate (Pre-treatment with the CYP3A4 inducer rifampicin decreased erlotinib AUC by about 2/3. Alternate treatments lacking CYP3A4 inducing activity should be considered. If an alternative treatment is unavailable, an erlotinib dose greater than 150 mg should be considered. If the erlotinib dose is adjusted upward, the dose will need to be reduced upon discontinuation of rifampicin or otehr CYP3A4 inducers).
No products indexed under this heading.

Carbamazepine (Pre-treatment with the CYP3A4 inducer rifampicin decreased erlotinib AUC by about 2/3. Alternate treatments lacking CYP3A4 inducing activity should be considered. If an alternative treatment is unavailable, an erlotinib dose greater than 150 mg should be considered. If the erlotinib dose is adjusted upward, the dose will need to be reduced upon discontinuation of rifampicin or otehr CYP3A4 inducers). Products include:
Carbatrol Capsules 3171
Equetro Extended-Release Capsules 3180
Tegretol/Tegretol-XR 2295

Cimetidine (Caution when administering or taking erlotinib with strong CYP3A4 inhibitors such as atazanavir, clarithromycin, indinavir, itraconazole, nefazodone, nelfinavir, ritonavir, saquinavir, telithromycin, troleandomycin, and voriconazole). Products include:
Tagamet HB 200 Tablets .... ▣ 664

Cimetidine Hydrochloride (Caution when administering or taking erlotinib with strong CYP3A4 inhibitors such as atazanavir, clarithromycin, indinavir, itraconazole, nefazodone, nelfinavir, ritonavir, saquinavir, telithromycin, troleandomycin, and voriconazole).
No products indexed under this heading.

Ciprofloxacin (Caution when administering or taking erlotinib with strong CYP3A4 inhibitors such as atazanavir, clarithromycin, indinavir, itraconazole, nefazodone, nelfinavir, ritonavir, saquinavir, telithromycin, troleandomycin, and voriconazole). Products include:
Cipro Oral Suspension 2977
Cipro I.V. 2984
Cipro XR Tablets 2990
Ciprodex Otic Suspension 559

Ciprofloxacin Hydrochloride (Pre-treatment with the CYP3A4 inducer rifampicin decreased erlotinib AUC by about 2/3. Alternate treatments lacking CYP3A4 inducing activity should be considered. If an alternative treatment is unavailable, an erlotinib dose greater than 150 mg should be considered. If the erlotinib dose is adjusted upward, the dose will need to be reduced upon discontinuation of rifampicin or otehr CYP3A4 inducers). Products include:
Ciloxan Ophthalmic Ointment 559
Ciloxan Ophthalmic Solution .... ⊙ 206
Cipro Tablets 2977
Proquin XR Tablets 1153

Cisplatin (Pre-treatment with the CYP3A4 inducer rifampicin decreased erlotinib AUC by about 2/3. Alternate treatments lacking CYP3A4 inducing activity should be considered. If an alternative treatment is unavailable, an erlotinib dose greater than 150 mg should be considered. If the erlotinib dose is adjusted upward, the dose will need to be reduced upon discontinuation of rifampicin or otehr CYP3A4 inducers).
No products indexed under this heading.

Clarithromycin (Co-treatment with the potent CYP3A4 inhibitor ketoconazole increases erlotinib AUC by 2/3. Caution should be used when administering or taking erlotinib with ketoconazole and other strong CYP3A4 inhibitors such as clarithromycin). Products include:
Biaxin/Biaxin XL 402
PREVPAC 3284

Clotrimazole (Caution when administering or taking erlotinib with strong CYP3A4 inhibitors such as atazanavir, clarithromycin, indinavir, itraconazole, nefazodone, nelfinavir, ritonavir, saquinavir, telithromycin, troleandomycin, and voriconazole). Products include:
Desenex Athlete's Foot Cream .... ▣ 635
Lotrimin 3039
Lotrisone 3040

Cortisone Acetate (Pre-treatment with the CYP3A4 inducer rifampicin decreased erlotinib AUC by about 2/3. Alternate treatments lacking CYP3A4 inducing activity should be considered. If an alternative treatment is unavailable, an erlotinib dose greater than 150 mg should be considered. If the erlotinib dose is adjusted upward, the dose will need to be reduced upon discontinuation of rifampicin or otehr CYP3A4 inducers).
No products indexed under this heading.

Cyclosporine (Caution when administering or taking erlotinib with strong CYP3A4 inhibitors such as atazanavir, clarithromycin, indinavir, itraconazole, nefazodone, nelfinavir, ritonavir, saquinavir, telithromycin, troleandomycin, and voriconazole). Products include:
Gengraf Capsules 459
Neoral Oral Solution 2259

Hydrocortone Tablets 1989
Preparation H Hydrocortisone Cream 646

Hydrocortisone Acetate (Pre-treatment with the CYP3A4 inducer rifampicin decreased erlotinib AUC by about 2/3. Alternate treatments lacking CYP3A4 inducing activity should be considered. If an alternative treatment is unavailable, an erlotinib dose greater than 150 mg should be considered. If the erlotinib dose is adjusted upward, the dose will need to be reduced upon discontinuation of rifampicin or otehr CYP3A4 inducers). Products include:
Analpram-HC 1159
Pramosone 1161
ProctoFoam-HC 3099

Hydrocortisone Butyrate (Pre-treatment with the CYP3A4 inducer rifampicin decreased erlotinib AUC by about 2/3. Alternate treatments lacking CYP3A4 inducing activity should be considered. If an alternative treatment is unavailable, an erlotinib dose greater than 150 mg should be considered. If the erlotinib dose is adjusted upward, the dose will need to be reduced upon discontinuation of rifampicin or otehr CYP3A4 inducers). Products include:
Locoid Lipocream Cream 1160

Hydrocortisone Cypionate (Pre-treatment with the CYP3A4 inducer rifampicin decreased erlotinib AUC by about 2/3. Alternate treatments lacking CYP3A4 inducing activity should be considered. If an alternative treatment is unavailable, an erlotinib dose greater than 150 mg should be considered. If the erlotinib dose is adjusted upward, the dose will need to be reduced upon discontinuation of rifampicin or otehr CYP3A4 inducers).
No products indexed under this heading.

Hydrocortisone Hemisuccinate (Pre-treatment with the CYP3A4 inducer rifampicin decreased erlotinib AUC by about 2/3. Alternate treatments lacking CYP3A4 inducing activity should be considered. If an alternative treatment is unavailable, an erlotinib dose greater than 150 mg should be considered. If the erlotinib dose is adjusted upward, the dose will need to be reduced upon discontinuation of rifampicin or otehr CYP3A4 inducers).
No products indexed under this heading.

Hydrocortisone Probutate (Pre-treatment with the CYP3A4 inducer rifampicin decreased erlotinib AUC by about 2/3. Alternate treatments lacking CYP3A4 inducing activity should be considered. If an alternative treatment is unavailable, an erlotinib dose greater than 150 mg should be considered. If the erlotinib dose is adjusted upward, the dose will need to be reduced upon discontinuation of rifampicin or otehr CYP3A4 inducers).
No products indexed under this heading.

Hydrocortisone Sodium Phosphate (Pre-treatment with the CYP3A4 inducer rifampicin decreased erlotinib AUC by about 2/3. Alternate treatments lacking CYP3A4 inducing activity should be considered. If an alternative treatment is unavailable, an erlotinib dose greater than 150 mg should be considered. If the erlotinib dose is adjusted upward, the dose will need to be reduced upon discontinuation of rifampicin or otehr CYP3A4 inducers).
No products indexed under this heading.

Hydrocortisone Sodium Succinate (Pre-treatment with the CYP3A4 inducer rifampicin decreased erlotinib AUC by about 2/3. Alternate treatments lacking CYP3A4 inducing activity should be considered. If an alternative treatment is unavailable, an erlotinib dose greater than 150 mg should be considered. If the erlotinib dose is adjusted upward, the dose will need to be reduced upon discontinuation of rifampicin or otehr CYP3A4 inducers).
No products indexed under this heading.

Hydrocortisone Valerate (Pre-treatment with the CYP3A4 inducer rifampicin decreased erlotinib AUC by about 2/3. Alternate treatments lacking CYP3A4 inducing activity should be considered. If an alternative treatment is unavailable, an erlotinib dose greater than 150 mg should be considered. If the erlotinib dose is adjusted upward, the dose will need to be reduced upon discontinuation of rifampicin or otehr CYP3A4 inducers).
No products indexed under this heading.

Hypericum (Pre-treatment with the CYP3A4 inducer rifampicin decreased erlotinib AUC by about 2/3. Alternate treatments lacking CYP3A4 inducing activity should be considered. If an alternative treatment is unavailable, an erlotinib dose greater than 150 mg should be considered. If the erlotinib dose is adjusted upward, the dose will need to be reduced upon discontinuation of rifampicin or otehr CYP3A4 inducers). Products include:
Satiete Tablets 832

Hypericum Perforatum (Pre-treatment with the CYP3A4 inducer rifampicin decreased erlotinib AUC by about 2/3. Alternate treatments lacking CYP3A4 inducing activity should be considered. If an alternative treatment is unavailable, an erlotinib dose greater than 150 mg should be considered. If the erlotinib dose is adjusted upward, the dose will need to be reduced upon discontinuation of rifampicin or otehr CYP3A4 inducers).
No products indexed under this heading.

Indinavir Sulfate (Co-treatment with the potent CYP3A4 inhibitor ketoconazole increases erlotinib AUC by 2/3. Caution should be used when administering or taking erlotinib with ketoconazole and other strong CYP3A4 inhibitors such as indinavir). Products include:
Crixivan Capsules 1940

Isoniazid (Caution when administering or taking erlotinib with strong CYP3A4 inhibitors such as atazanavir, clarithromycin, indinavir, itraconazole, nefazodone, nelfinavir, ritonavir, saquinavir, telithromycin, troleandomycin, and voriconazole).
No products indexed under this heading.

Itraconazole (Co-treatment with the potent CYP3A4 inhibitor ketoconazole increases erlotinib AUC by 2/3. Caution should be used when administering or taking erlotinib with ketoconazole and other strong CYP3A4 inhibitors such as itraconazole).
No products indexed under this heading.

Ketoconazole (Co-treatment with the potent CYP3A4 inhibitor ketoconazole increases erlotinib AUC by 2/3. Caution should be used when administering or taking erlotinib with ketoconazole and other strong CYP3A4 inhibitors). Products include:
Nizoral A-D Shampoo, 1% 1868

Lopinavir (Caution when administering or taking erlotinib with strong CYP3A4 inhibitors such as atazanavir, clarithromycin, indinavir, itraconazole, nefazodone, nelfinavir, ritonavir, saquinavir, telithromycin, troleandomycin, and voriconazole). Products include:
Kaletra 476

Loratadine (Caution when administering or taking erlotinib with strong CYP3A4 inhibitors such as atazanavir, clarithromycin, indinavir, itraconazole, nefazodone, nelfinavir, ritonavir, saquinavir, telithromycin, troleandomycin, and voriconazole). Products include:
Alavert Allergy & Sinus D-12 Hour Tablets 771
Alavert 771
Children's Claritin Allergy Oral Solution 771
Claritin Non-Drowsy 24 Hour Tablets 772
Claritin Reditabs 24 Hour Non-Drowsy Tablets 772
Claritin-D Non-Drowsy 12 Hour Tablets 772
Claritin-D Non-Drowsy 24 Hour Tablets 772

Mephenytoin (Pre-treatment with the CYP3A4 inducer rifampicin decreased erlotinib AUC by about 2/3. Alternate treatments lacking CYP3A4 inducing activity should be considered. If an alternative treatment is unavailable, an erlotinib dose greater than 150 mg should be considered. If the erlotinib dose is adjusted upward, the dose will need to be reduced upon discontinuation of rifampicin or otehr CYP3A4 inducers).
No products indexed under this heading.

Methsuximide (Pre-treatment with the CYP3A4 inducer rifampicin decreased erlotinib AUC by about 2/3. Alternate treatments lacking CYP3A4 inducing activity should be considered. If an alternative treatment is unavailable, an erlotinib dose greater than 150 mg should be considered. If the erlotinib dose is adjusted upward, the dose will need to be reduced upon discontinuation of rifampicin or otehr CYP3A4 inducers).
No products indexed under this heading.

Methylprednisolone (Pre-treatment with the CYP3A4 inducer rifampicin decreased erlotinib AUC by about 2/3. Alternate treatments lacking CYP3A4 inducing activity should be considered. If an alternative treatment is unavailable, an erlotinib dose greater than 150 mg should be considered. If the erlotinib dose is adjusted upward, the dose will need to be reduced upon discontinuation of rifampicin or otehr CYP3A4 inducers).
No products indexed under this heading.

Methylprednisolone Acetate (Pre-treatment with the CYP3A4 inducer rifampicin decreased erlotinib AUC by about 2/3. Alternate treatments lacking CYP3A4 inducing activity should be considered. If an alternative treatment is unavailable, an erlotinib dose greater than 150 mg should be considered. If the erlotinib dose is adjusted upward, the dose will need to be reduced upon discontinuation of rifampicin or otehr CYP3A4 inducers). Products include:
Depo-Medrol Injectable Suspension 2617
Depo-Medrol Single-Dose Vial 2619

Methylprednisolone Sodium Succinate (Pre-treatment with the CYP3A4 inducer rifampicin decreased erlotinib AUC by about 2/3. Alternate treatments lacking CYP3A4 inducing activity should be considered. If an alternative treatment is unavailable, an erlotinib dose greater than 150 mg should be considered. If the erlotinib dose is adjusted upward, the dose will need to be reduced upon discontinuation of rifampicin or otehr CYP3A4 inducers).
No products indexed under this heading.

Metronidazole (Caution when administering or taking erlotinib with strong CYP3A4 inhibitors such as atazanavir, clarithromycin, indinavir, itraconazole, nefazodone, nelfinavir, ritonavir, saquinavir, telithromycin, troleandomycin, and voriconazole). Products include:
Metrogel 1% 1211
MetroGel-Vaginal Gel 1855
Vandazole Vaginal Gel 3338

Metronidazole Benzoate (Caution when administering or taking erlotinib with strong CYP3A4 inhibitors such as atazanavir, clarithromycin, indinavir, itraconazole, nefazodone, nelfinavir, ritonavir, saquinavir, telithromycin, troleandomycin, and voriconazole).
No products indexed under this heading.

Metronidazole Hydrochloride (Caution when administering or taking erlotinib with strong CYP3A4 inhibitors such as atazanavir, clarithromycin, indinavir, itraconazole, nefazodone, nelfinavir, ritonavir, saquinavir, telithromycin, troleandomycin, and voriconazole).
No products indexed under this heading.

Miconazole (Caution when administering or taking erlotinib with strong CYP3A4 inhibitors such as atazanavir, clarithromycin, indinavir, itraconazole, nefazodone, nelfinavir, ritonavir, saquinavir, telithromycin, troleandomycin, and voriconazole).
No products indexed under this heading.

Miconazole Nitrate (Caution when administering or taking erlotinib with strong CYP3A4 inhibitors such as atazanavir, clarithromycin, indinavir, itraconazole, nefazodone, nelfinavir, ritonavir, saquinavir, telithromycin, troleandomycin, and voriconazole). Products include:
Desenex 635
Desenex Jock Itch Spray Powder ... 635

Modafinil (Pre-treatment with the CYP3A4 inducer rifampicin decreased erlotinib AUC by about 2/3. Alternate treatments lacking CYP3A4 inducing activity should be considered. If an alternative treatment is unavailable, an erlotinib dose greater than 150 mg should be considered. If the erlotinib dose is adjusted upward, the dose will need to be reduced upon discontinuation of rifampicin or otehr CYP3A4 inducers). Products include:

Provigil Tablets 988

Nefazodone Hydrochloride (Co-treatment with the potent CYP3A4 inhibitor ketoconazole increases erlotinib AUC by 2/3. Caution should be used when administering or taking erlotinib with ketoconazole and other strong CYP3A4 inhibitors such as nefazodone).

No products indexed under this heading.

Nelfinavir Mesylate (Co-treatment with the potent CYP3A4 inhibitor ketoconazole increases erlotinib AUC by 2/3. Caution should be used when administering or taking erlotinib with ketoconazole and other strong CYP3A4 inhibitors such as nelfinavir). Products include:

Viracept 2577

Nevirapine (Caution when administering or taking erlotinib with strong CYP3A4 inhibitors such as atazanavir, clarithromycin, indinavir, itraconazole, nefazodone, nelfinavir, ritonavir, saquinavir, telithromycin, troleandomycin, and voriconazole). Products include:

Viramune Oral Suspension 873
Viramune Tablets 873

Niacinamide (Caution when administering or taking erlotinib with strong CYP3A4 inhibitors such as atazanavir, clarithromycin, indinavir, itraconazole, nefazodone, nelfinavir, ritonavir, saquinavir, telithromycin, troleandomycin, and voriconazole).

No products indexed under this heading.

Nicotinamide (Caution when administering or taking erlotinib with strong CYP3A4 inhibitors such as atazanavir, clarithromycin, indinavir, itraconazole, nefazodone, nelfinavir, ritonavir, saquinavir, telithromycin, troleandomycin, and voriconazole). Products include:

Nicomide Tablets 1088

Nifedipine (Caution when administering or taking erlotinib with strong CYP3A4 inhibitors such as atazanavir, clarithromycin, indinavir, itraconazole, nefazodone, nelfinavir, ritonavir, saquinavir, telithromycin, troleandomycin, and voriconazole). Products include:

Adalat CC Tablets 2964

Norfloxacin (Caution when administering or taking erlotinib with strong CYP3A4 inhibitors such as atazanavir, clarithromycin, indinavir, itraconazole, nefazodone, nelfinavir, ritonavir, saquinavir, telithromycin, troleandomycin, and voriconazole). Products include:

Noroxin Tablets 2032

Omeprazole (Caution when administering or taking erlotinib with strong CYP3A4 inhibitors such as atazanavir, clarithromycin, indinavir, itraconazole, nefazodone, nelfinavir, ritonavir, saquinavir, telithromycin, troleandomycin, and voriconazole). Products include:

Zegerid Capsules 2958
Zegerid Powder for Oral Solution 2958

Oxcarbazepine (Pre-treatment with the CYP3A4 inducer rifampicin decreased erlotinib AUC by about 2/3. Alternate treatments lacking CYP3A4 inducing activity should be considered. If an alternative treatment is unavailable, an erlotinib dose greater than 150 mg should be considered. If the erlotinib dose is adjusted upward, the dose will need to be reduced upon discontinuation of rifampicin or otehr CYP3A4 inducers). Products include:

Trileptal Tablets 2300
Trileptal Oral Suspension 2300

Paroxetine Hydrochloride (Caution when administering or taking erlotinib with strong CYP3A4 inhibitors such as atazanavir, clarithromycin, indinavir, itraconazole, nefazodone, nelfinavir, ritonavir, saquinavir, telithromycin, troleandomycin, and voriconazole). Products include:

Paxil CR Controlled-Release Tablets 1538
Paxil 1530

Phenobarbital (Pre-treatment with the CYP3A4 inducer rifampicin decreased erlotinib AUC by about 2/3. Alternate treatments lacking CYP3A4 inducing activity should be considered. If an alternative treatment is unavailable, an erlotinib dose greater than 150 mg should be considered. If the erlotinib dose is adjusted upward, the dose will need to be reduced upon discontinuation of rifampicin or otehr CYP3A4 inducers). Products include:

Donnatal Extentabs 2493

Phenobarbital Sodium (Pre-treatment with the CYP3A4 inducer rifampicin decreased erlotinib AUC by about 2/3. Alternate treatments lacking CYP3A4 inducing activity should be considered. If an alternative treatment is unavailable, an erlotinib dose greater than 150 mg should be considered. If the erlotinib dose is adjusted upward, the dose will need to be reduced upon discontinuation of rifampicin or otehr CYP3A4 inducers).

No products indexed under this heading.

Phenytoin (Pre-treatment with the CYP3A4 inducer rifampicin decreased erlotinib AUC by about 2/3. Alternate treatments lacking CYP3A4 inducing activity should be considered. If an alternative treatment is unavailable, an erlotinib dose greater than 150 mg should be considered. If the erlotinib dose is adjusted upward, the dose will need to be reduced upon discontinuation of rifampicin or otehr CYP3A4 inducers).

No products indexed under this heading.

Phenytoin Sodium (Pre-treatment with the CYP3A4 inducer rifampicin decreased erlotinib AUC by about 2/3. Alternate treatments lacking CYP3A4 inducing activity should be considered. If an alternative treatment is unavailable, an erlotinib dose greater than 150 mg should be considered. If the erlotinib dose is adjusted upward, the dose will need to be reduced upon discontinuation of rifampicin or otehr CYP3A4 inducers). Products include:

Phenytek Capsules 2160

Prednisolone Acetate (Pre-treatment with the CYP3A4 inducer rifampicin decreased erlotinib AUC by about 2/3. Alternate treatments lacking CYP3A4 inducing activity should be considered. If an alternative treatment is unavailable, an erlotinib dose greater than 150 mg should be considered. If the erlotinib dose is adjusted upward, the dose will need to be reduced upon discontinuation of rifampicin or otehr CYP3A4 inducers). Products include:

Blephamide Ophthalmic Ointment 568
Blephamide Ophthalmic Suspension 569
Poly-Pred Ophthalmic Suspension ⊙233
Pred Forte Ophthalmic Suspension ⊙235
Pred Mild Ophthalmic Suspension ⊙238
Pred-G Ophthalmic Ointment ⊙237
Pred-G Ophthalmic Suspension ⊙236

Prednisolone Sodium Phosphate (Pre-treatment with the CYP3A4 inducer rifampicin decreased erlotinib AUC by about 2/3. Alternate treatments lacking CYP3A4 inducing activity should be considered. If an alternative treatment is unavailable, an erlotinib dose greater than 150 mg should be considered. If the erlotinib dose is adjusted upward, the dose will need to be reduced upon discontinuation of rifampicin or otehr CYP3A4 inducers).

No products indexed under this heading.

Prednisolone Tebutate (Pre-treatment with the CYP3A4 inducer rifampicin decreased erlotinib AUC by about 2/3. Alternate treatments lacking CYP3A4 inducing activity should be considered. If an alternative treatment is unavailable, an erlotinib dose greater than 150 mg should be considered. If the erlotinib dose is adjusted upward, the dose will need to be reduced upon discontinuation of rifampicin or otehr CYP3A4 inducers).

No products indexed under this heading.

Prednisone (Pre-treatment with the CYP3A4 inducer rifampicin decreased erlotinib AUC by about 2/3. Alternate treatments lacking CYP3A4 inducing activity should be considered. If an alternative treatment is unavailable, an erlotinib dose greater than 150 mg should be considered. If the erlotinib dose is adjusted upward, the dose will need to be reduced upon discontinuation of rifampicin or otehr CYP3A4 inducers).

No products indexed under this heading.

Primidone (Pre-treatment with the CYP3A4 inducer rifampicin decreased erlotinib AUC by about 2/3. Alternate treatments lacking CYP3A4 inducing activity should be considered. If an alternative treatment is unavailable, an erlotinib dose greater than 150 mg should be considered. If the erlotinib dose is adjusted upward, the dose will need to be reduced upon discontinuation of rifampicin or otehr CYP3A4 inducers).

No products indexed under this heading.

Propoxyphene Hydrochloride (Caution when administering or taking erlotinib with strong CYP3A4 inhibitors such as atazanavir, clarithromycin, indinavir, itraconazole, nefazodone, nelfinavir, ritonavir, saquinavir, telithromycin, troleandomycin, and voriconazole).

No products indexed under this heading.

Propoxyphene Napsylate (Caution when administering or taking erlotinib with strong CYP3A4 inhibitors such as atazanavir, clarithromycin, indinavir, itraconazole, nefazodone, nelfinavir, ritonavir, saquinavir, telithromycin, troleandomycin, and voriconazole).

No products indexed under this heading.

Quinidine (Caution when administering or taking erlotinib with strong CYP3A4 inhibitors such as atazanavir, clarithromycin, indinavir, itraconazole, nefazodone, nelfinavir, ritonavir, saquinavir, telithromycin, troleandomycin, and voriconazole).

No products indexed under this heading.

Quinidine Hydrochloride (Caution when administering or taking erlotinib with strong CYP3A4 inhibitors such as atazanavir, clarithromycin, indinavir, itraconazole, nefazodone, nelfinavir, ritonavir, saquinavir, telithromycin, troleandomycin, and voriconazole).

No products indexed under this heading.

Quinidine Polygalacturonate (Caution when administering or taking erlotinib with strong CYP3A4 inhibitors such as atazanavir, clarithromycin, indinavir, itraconazole, nefazodone, nelfinavir, ritonavir, saquinavir, telithromycin, troleandomycin, and voriconazole).

No products indexed under this heading.

Quinidine Sulfate (Caution when administering or taking erlotinib with strong CYP3A4 inhibitors such as atazanavir, clarithromycin, indinavir, itraconazole, nefazodone, nelfinavir, ritonavir, saquinavir, telithromycin, troleandomycin, and voriconazole).

No products indexed under this heading.

Quinine (Caution when administering or taking erlotinib with strong CYP3A4 inhibitors such as atazanavir, clarithromycin, indinavir, itraconazole, nefazodone, nelfinavir, ritonavir, saquinavir, telithromycin, troleandomycin, and voriconazole).

No products indexed under this heading.

Quinine Sulfate (Caution when administering or taking erlotinib with strong CYP3A4 inhibitors such as atazanavir, clarithromycin, indinavir, itraconazole, nefazodone, nelfinavir, ritonavir, saquinavir, telithromycin, troleandomycin, and voriconazole).

No products indexed under this heading.

Quinupristin (Caution when administering or taking erlotinib with strong CYP3A4 inhibitors such as atazanavir, clarithromycin, indinavir, itraconazole, nefazodone, nelfinavir, ritonavir, saquinavir, telithromycin, troleandomycin, and voriconazole).

No products indexed under this heading.

Ranitidine Bismuth Citrate (Caution when administering or taking erlotinib with strong CYP3A4 inhibitors such as atazanavir, clarithromycin, indinavir, itraconazole, nefazodone, nelfinavir, ritonavir, saquinavir, telithromycin, troleandomycin, and voriconazole).
No products indexed under this heading.

Ranitidine Hydrochloride (Caution when administering or taking erlotinib with strong CYP3A4 inhibitors such as atazanavir, clarithromycin, indinavir, itraconazole, nefazodone, nelfinavir, ritonavir, saquinavir, telithromycin, troleandomycin, and voriconazole). Products include:
Zantac **1624**
Zantac Injection **1619**
Zantac Injection Pharmacy Bulk Package **1622**

Rifabutin (Pre-treatment with the CYP3A4 inducer rifampicin decreased erlotinib AUC by about 2/3. Alternate treatments lacking CYP3A4 inducing activity should be considered. If an alternative treatment is unavailable, an erlotinib dose greater than 150 mg should be considered. If the erlotinib dose is adjusted upward, the dose will need to be reduced upon discontinuation of rifampicin or otehr CYP3A4 inducers).
No products indexed under this heading.

Rifampicin (Pre-treatment with the CYP3A4 inducer rifampicin decreased erlotinib AUC by about 2/3. Alternate treatments lacking CYP3A4 inducing activity should be considered. If an alternative treatment is unavailable, an erlotinib dose greater than 150 mg should be considered. If the erlotinib dose is adjusted upward, the dose will need to be reduced upon discontinuation of rifampicin or otehr CYP3A4 inducers).
No products indexed under this heading.

Rifampin (Pre-treatment with the CYP3A4 inducer rifampicin decreased erlotinib AUC by about 2/3. Alternate treatments lacking CYP3A4 inducing activity should be considered. If an alternative treatment is unavailable, an erlotinib dose greater than 150 mg should be considered. If the erlotinib dose is adjusted upward, the dose will need to be reduced upon discontinuation of rifampicin or otehr CYP3A4 inducers).
No products indexed under this heading.

Rifapentine (Pre-treatment with the CYP3A4 inducer rifampicin decreased erlotinib AUC by about 2/3. Alternate treatments lacking CYP3A4 inducing activity should be considered. If an alternative treatment is unavailable, an erlotinib dose greater than 150 mg should be considered. If the erlotinib dose is adjusted upward, the dose will need to be reduced upon discontinuation of rifampicin or otehr CYP3A4 inducers).
No products indexed under this heading.

Ritonavir (Co-treatment with the potent CYP3A4 inhibitor ketoconazole increases erlotinib AUC by 2/3. Caution should be used when administering or taking erlotinib with ketoconazole and other strong CYP3A4 inhibitors such as ritonavir). Products include:
Kaletra **476**
Norvir **503**

Saquinavir (Co-treatment with the potent CYP3A4 inhibitor ketoconazole increases erlotinib AUC by 2/3. Caution should be used when administering or taking erlotinib with ketoconazole and other strong CYP3A4 inhibitors such as saquinavir).
No products indexed under this heading.

Saquinavir Mesylate (Co-treatment with the potent CYP3A4 inhibitor ketoconazole increases erlotinib AUC by 2/3. Caution should be used when administering or taking erlotinib with ketoconazole and other strong CYP3A4 inhibitors such as saquinavir). Products include:
Invirase **2772**

Sertraline Hydrochloride (Caution when administering or taking erlotinib with strong CYP3A4 inhibitors such as atazanavir, clarithromycin, indinavir, itraconazole, nefazodone, nelfinavir, ritonavir, saquinavir, telithromycin, troleandomycin, and voriconazole). Products include:
Zoloft **2586**

Sulfinpyrazone (Pre-treatment with the CYP3A4 inducer rifampicin decreased erlotinib AUC by about 2/3. Alternate treatments lacking CYP3A4 inducing activity should be considered. If an alternative treatment is unavailable, an erlotinib dose greater than 150 mg should be considered. If the erlotinib dose is adjusted upward, the dose will need to be reduced upon discontinuation of rifampicin or otehr CYP3A4 inducers).
No products indexed under this heading.

Telithromycin (Co-treatment with the potent CYP3A4 inhibitor ketoconazole increases erlotinib AUC by 2/3. Caution should be used when administering or taking erlotinib with ketoconazole and other strong CYP3A4 inhibitors such as telithromycin). Products include:
Ketek Tablets **2903**

Theophylline (Pre-treatment with the CYP3A4 inducer rifampicin decreased erlotinib AUC by about 2/3. Alternate treatments lacking CYP3A4 inducing activity should be considered. If an alternative treatment is unavailable, an erlotinib dose greater than 150 mg should be considered. If the erlotinib dose is adjusted upward, the dose will need to be reduced upon discontinuation of rifampicin or otehr CYP3A4 inducers).
No products indexed under this heading.

Triamcinolone (Pre-treatment with the CYP3A4 inducer rifampicin decreased erlotinib AUC by about 2/3. Alternate treatments lacking CYP3A4 inducing activity should be considered. If an alternative treatment is unavailable, an erlotinib dose greater than 150 mg should be considered. If the erlotinib dose is adjusted upward, the dose will need to be reduced upon discontinuation of rifampicin or otehr CYP3A4 inducers).
No products indexed under this heading.

Triamcinolone Acetonide (Pre-treatment with the CYP3A4 inducer rifampicin decreased erlotinib AUC by about 2/3. Alternate treatments lacking CYP3A4 inducing activity should be considered. If an alternative treatment is unavailable, an erlotinib dose greater than 150 mg should be considered. If the erlotinib dose is adjusted upward, the dose will need to be reduced upon discontinuation of rifampicin or otehr CYP3A4 inducers). Products include:
Azmacort Inhalation Aerosol **1726**
Nasacort AQ Nasal Spray **2922**

Triamcinolone Diacetate (Pre-treatment with the CYP3A4 inducer rifampicin decreased erlotinib AUC by about 2/3. Alternate treatments lacking CYP3A4 inducing activity should be considered. If an alternative treatment is unavailable, an erlotinib dose greater than 150 mg should be considered. If the erlotinib dose is adjusted upward, the dose will need to be reduced upon discontinuation of rifampicin or otehr CYP3A4 inducers).
No products indexed under this heading.

Triamcinolone Hexacetonide (Pre-treatment with the CYP3A4 inducer rifampicin decreased erlotinib AUC by about 2/3. Alternate treatments lacking CYP3A4 inducing activity should be considered. If an alternative treatment is unavailable, an erlotinib dose greater than 150 mg should be considered. If the erlotinib dose is adjusted upward, the dose will need to be reduced upon discontinuation of rifampicin or otehr CYP3A4 inducers).
No products indexed under this heading.

Troglitazone (Caution when administering or taking erlotinib with strong CYP3A4 inhibitors such as atazanavir, clarithromycin, indinavir, itraconazole, nefazodone, nelfinavir, ritonavir, saquinavir, telithromycin, troleandomycin, and voriconazole).
No products indexed under this heading.

Troleandomycin (Co-treatment with the potent CYP3A4 inhibitor ketoconazole increases erlotinib AUC by 2/3. Caution should be used when administering or taking erlotinib with ketoconazole and other strong CYP3A4 inhibitors such as troleandomycin).
No products indexed under this heading.

Valproate Sodium (Caution when administering or taking erlotinib with strong CYP3A4 inhibitors such as atazanavir, clarithromycin, indinavir, itraconazole, nefazodone, nelfinavir, ritonavir, saquinavir, telithromycin, troleandomycin, and voriconazole). Products include:
Depacon Injection **412**

Verapamil Hydrochloride (Caution when administering or taking erlotinib with strong CYP3A4 inhibitors such as atazanavir, clarithromycin, indinavir, itraconazole, nefazodone, nelfinavir, ritonavir, saquinavir, telithromycin, troleandomycin, and voriconazole). Products include:
Covera-HS Tablets **3139**
Tarka Tablets **524**
Verelan PM Extended-Release Capsules, Controlled-Onset **3106**

Voriconazole (Co-treatment with the potent CYP3A4 inhibitor ketoconazole increases erlotinib AUC by 2/3. Caution should be used when administering or taking erlotinib with ketoconazole and other strong CYP3A4 inhibitors such as voriconazole). Products include:
VFEND I.V. **2564**
VFEND Oral Suspension **2564**
VFEND Tablets **2564**

Zafirlukast (Caution when administering or taking erlotinib with strong CYP3A4 inhibitors such as atazanavir, clarithromycin, indinavir, itraconazole, nefazodone, nelfinavir, ritonavir, saquinavir, telithromycin, troleandomycin, and voriconazole). Products include:
Accolate Tablets **671**

Zileuton (Caution when administering or taking erlotinib with strong CYP3A4 inhibitors such as atazanavir, clarithromycin, indinavir, itraconazole, nefazodone, nelfinavir, ritonavir, saquinavir, telithromycin, troleandomycin, and voriconazole). Products include:
Zyflo Tablets **1023**

Food Interactions

Grapefruit (Caution when administering or taking erlotinib with strong CYP3A4 inhibitors such as atazanavir, clarithromycin, indinavir, itraconazole, nefazodone, nelfinavir, ritonavir, saquinavir, telithromycin, troleandomycin, and voriconazole).

Grapefruit Juice (Caution when administering or taking erlotinib with strong CYP3A4 inhibitors such as atazanavir, clarithromycin, indinavir, itraconazole, nefazodone, nelfinavir, ritonavir, saquinavir, telithromycin, troleandomycin, and voriconazole).

TARGRETIN CAPSULES

(Bexarotene) **1747**
May interact with erythromycin, oral hypoglycemic agents, insulin, oral contraceptives, phenytoin, protease inhibitors, and certain other agents. Compounds in these categories include:

Acarbose (Bexarotene could enhance the action of hypoglycemic agents resulting in hypoglycemia). Products include:
Precose Tablets **751**

Amiodarone Hydrochloride (Bexarotene is metabolized by CYP4503A4; co-administration with inhibitors of CYP4503A4, such as amiodarone, would be expected to lead to an increase in plasma bexarotene concentrations).
No products indexed under this heading.

Amprenavir (Bexarotene is metabolized by CYP4503A4; co-administration with inhibitors of CYP4503A4, such as protease inhibitors, would be expected to lead to an increase in plasma bexarotene concentrations). Products include:
Agenerase Capsules **1327**
Agenerase Oral Solution **1332**

Carbamazepine (Bexarotene is metabolized by CYP4503A4; co-administration with inducers of CYP4503A4, such as carbamazepine, may cause a reduction in plasma bexarotene concentrations). Products include:
Carbatrol Capsules **3171**
Equetro Extended-Release Capsules **3180**
Tegretol/Tegretol-XR **2295**

Chlorpropamide (Bexarotene could enhance the action of hypoglycemic agents resulting in hypoglycemia).
No products indexed under this heading.

Desogestrel (Bexarotene may theoretically increase the rate of metabolism and reduce plasma concentrations of other substrates metabolized by CYP4503A4, including hormonal contraceptives; it is strongly recommended that two reliable forms of contraception be used concurrently, one of which should be non-hormonal). Products include:
Mircette Tablets 1066

Erythromycin (Bexarotene is metabolized by CYP4503A4; co-administration with inhibitors of CYP4503A4, such as erythromycin, would be expected to lead to an increase in plasma bexarotene concentrations). Products include:
Ery-Tab Tablets 449
Erythromycin Base Filmtab Tablets 455
Erythromycin Delayed-Release Capsules, USP 457
PCE Dispertab Tablets 515

Erythromycin Estolate (Bexarotene is metabolized by CYP4503A4; co-administration with inhibitors of CYP4503A4, such as erythromycin, would be expected to lead to an increase in plasma bexarotene concentrations).
No products indexed under this heading.

Erythromycin Ethylsuccinate (Bexarotene is metabolized by CYP4503A4; co-administration with inhibitors of CYP4503A4, such as erythromycin, would be expected to lead to an increase in plasma bexarotene concentrations). Products include:
E.E.S. 451
EryPed 447

Erythromycin Gluceptate (Bexarotene is metabolized by CYP4503A4; co-administration with inhibitors of CYP4503A4, such as erythromycin, would be expected to lead to an increase in plasma bexarotene concentrations).
No products indexed under this heading.

Erythromycin Lactobionate (Bexarotene is metabolized by CYP4503A4; co-administration with inhibitors of CYP4503A4, such as erythromycin, would be expected to lead to an increase in plasma bexarotene concentrations).
No products indexed under this heading.

Erythromycin Stearate (Bexarotene is metabolized by CYP4503A4; co-administration with inhibitors of CYP4503A4, such as erythromycin, would be expected to lead to an increase in plasma bexarotene concentrations). Products include:
Erythrocin Stearate Filmtab Tablets 453

Ethinyl Estradiol (Bexarotene may theoretically increase the rate of metabolism and reduce plasma concentrations of other substrates metabolized by CYP4503A4, including hormonal contraceptives; it is strongly recommended that two reliable forms of contraception be used concurrently, one of which should be non-hormonal). Products include:
Mircette Tablets 1066
NuvaRing 2340
Ortho-Cyclen/Ortho Tri-Cyclen 2429
Ortho Evra Transdermal System 2417
Ortho Tri-Cyclen Lo Tablets 2436
Seasonique Tablets 1077
Yasmin 28 Tablets 796
Yaz Tablets 803

Ethynodiol Diacetate (Bexarotene may theoretically increase the rate of metabolism and reduce plasma concentrations of other substrates metabolized by CYP4503A4, including hormonal contraceptives; it is strongly recommended that two reliable forms of contraception be used concurrently, one of which should be non-hormonal).
No products indexed under this heading.

Fosphenytoin Sodium (Bexarotene is metabolized by CYP4503A4; co-administration with inducers of CYP4503A4, such as phenytoin, may cause a reduction in plasma bexarotene concentrations).
No products indexed under this heading.

Gemfibrozil (Co-administration has resulted in substantial increases in plasma bexarotene concentrations; concomitant administration is not recommended).
No products indexed under this heading.

Glimepiride (Bexarotene could enhance the action of hypoglycemic agents resulting in hypoglycemia). Products include:
Avandaryl Tablets 1379
Duetact Tablets 3226

Glipizide (Bexarotene could enhance the action of hypoglycemic agents resulting in hypoglycemia).
No products indexed under this heading.

Glyburide (Bexarotene could enhance the action of hypoglycemic agents resulting in hypoglycemia).
No products indexed under this heading.

Hypericum (Bexarotene is metabolized by CYP4503A4; co-administration with inducers of CYP4503A4, such as St. John's Wort, may cause a reduction in plasma bexarotene concentrations). Products include:
Satiete Tablets .... ▣832

Indinavir Sulfate (Bexarotene is metabolized by CYP4503A4; co-administration with inhibitors of CYP4503A4, such as protease inhibitors, would be expected to lead to an increase in plasma bexarotene concentrations). Products include:
Crixivan Capsules 1940

Insulin, Human, Zinc Suspension (Bexarotene could enhance the action of insulin resulting in hypoglycemia). Products include:
Humulin L, 100 Units 1794
Humulin U, 100 Units 1800

Insulin, Human NPH (Bexarotene could enhance the action of insulin resulting in hypoglycemia). Products include:
Humulin N, 100 Units 1795
Humulin N Pen 1797

Insulin, Human Regular (Bexarotene could enhance the action of insulin resulting in hypoglycemia). Products include:
Humulin R, 100 Units 1798

Insulin, Human Regular and Human NPH Mixture (Bexarotene could enhance the action of insulin resulting in hypoglycemia). Products include:
Humulin 50/50, 100 Units 1791
Humulin 70/30 Pen 1793

Insulin, NPH (Bexarotene could enhance the action of insulin resulting in hypoglycemia).
No products indexed under this heading.

Insulin, Regular (Bexarotene could enhance the action of insulin resulting in hypoglycemia).
No products indexed under this heading.

Insulin, Zinc Crystals (Bexarotene could enhance the action of insulin resulting in hypoglycemia).
No products indexed under this heading.

Insulin, Zinc Suspension (Bexarotene could enhance the action of insulin resulting in hypoglycemia).
No products indexed under this heading.

Insulin Aspart, Human Regular (Bexarotene could enhance the action of insulin resulting in hypoglycemia). Products include:
NovoLog Injection 2326

Insulin glargine (Bexarotene could enhance the action of insulin resulting in hypoglycemia). Products include:
Lantus Injection 2909

Insulin Lispro, Human (Bexarotene could enhance the action of insulin resulting in hypoglycemia). Products include:
Humalog-Pen 1781
Humalog Mix 50/50-Pen 1783
Humalog Mix 75/25-Pen 1785

Insulin Lispro Protamine, Human (Bexarotene could enhance the action of insulin resulting in hypoglycemia). Products include:
Humalog Mix 50/50-Pen 1783
Humalog Mix 75/25-Pen 1785

Itraconazole (Bexarotene is metabolized by CYP4503A4; co-administration with inhibitors of CYP4503A4, such as itraconazole, would be expected to lead to an increase in plasma bexarotene concentrations).
No products indexed under this heading.

Ketoconazole (Bexarotene is metabolized by CYP4503A4; co-administration with inhibitors of CYP4503A4, such as ketoconazole, would be expected to lead to an increase in plasma concentrations). Products include:
Nizoral A-D Shampoo, 1% 1868

Levonorgestrel (Bexarotene may theoretically increase the rate of metabolism and reduce plasma concentrations of other substrates metabolized by CYP4503A4, including hormonal contraceptives; it is strongly recommended that two reliable forms of contraception be used concurrently, one of which should be non-hormonal). Products include:
Climara Pro Transdermal System 776
Mirena Intrauterine System 787
Plan B Tablets 1076
Seasonique Tablets 1077

Lopinavir (Bexarotene is metabolized by CYP4503A4; co-administration with inhibitors of CYP4503A4, such as protease inhibitors, would be expected to lead to an increase in plasma bexarotene concentrations). Products include:
Kaletra 476

Mestranol (Bexarotene may theoretically increase the rate of metabolism and reduce plasma concentrations of other substrates metabolized by CYP4503A4, including hormonal contraceptives; it is strongly recommended that two reliable forms of contraception be used concurrently, one of which should be non-hormonal).
No products indexed under this heading.

Metformin Hydrochloride (Bexarotene could enhance the action of hypoglycemic agents resulting in hypoglycemia). Products include:
ActoPlus Met Tablets 3214
Avandamet Tablets 1373
Fortamet Extended-Release Tablets 3115

Miglitol (Bexarotene could enhance the action of hypoglycemic agents resulting in hypoglycemia).
No products indexed under this heading.

Nefazodone Hydrochloride (Bexarotene is metabolized by CYP4503A4; co-administration with inhibitors of CYP4503A4, such as nefazodone, would be expected to lead to an increase in plasma bexarotene concentrations).
No products indexed under this heading.

Nelfinavir Mesylate (Bexarotene is metabolized by CYP4503A4; co-administration with inhibitors of CYP4503A4, such as protease inhibitors, would be expected to lead to an increase in plasma bexarotene concentrations). Products include:
Viracept 2577

Norethindrone (Bexarotene may theoretically increase the rate of metabolism and reduce plasma concentrations of other substrates metabolized by CYP4503A4, including hormonal contraceptives; it is strongly recommended that two reliable forms of contraception be used concurrently, one of which should be non-hormonal). Products include:
Ortho Micronor Tablets 2426

Norethynodrel (Bexarotene may theoretically increase the rate of metabolism and reduce plasma concentrations of other substrates metabolized by CYP4503A4, including hormonal contraceptives; it is strongly recommended that two reliable forms of contraception be used concurrently, one of which should be non-hormonal).
No products indexed under this heading.

Norgestimate (Bexarotene may theoretically increase the rate of metabolism and reduce plasma concentrations of other substrates metabolized by CYP4503A4, including hormonal contraceptives; it is strongly recommended that two reliable forms of contraception be used concurrently, one of which should be non-hormonal). Products include:
Ortho-Cyclen/Ortho Tri-Cyclen 2429
Ortho Tri-Cyclen Lo Tablets 2436

Norgestrel (Bexarotene may theoretically increase the rate of metabolism and reduce plasma concentrations of other substrates metabolized by CYP4503A4, including hormonal contraceptives; it is strongly recommended that two reliable forms of contraception be used concurrently, one of which should be non-hormonal).
No products indexed under this heading.

Phenobarbital (Bexarotene is metabolized by CYP4503A4; co-administration with inducers of CYP4503A4, such as phenobarbital, may cause a reduction in plasma bexarotene concentrations).
Products include:
Donnatal Extentabs **2493**

Phenytoin (Bexarotene is metabolized by CYP4503A4; co-administration with inducers of CYP4503A4, such as phenytoin, may cause a reduction in plasma bexarotene concentrations).
No products indexed under this heading.

Phenytoin Sodium (Bexarotene is metabolized by CYP4503A4; co-administration with inducers of CYP4503A4, such as phenytoin, may cause a reduction in plasma bexarotene concentrations).
Products include:
Phenytek Capsules **2160**

Pioglitazone Hydrochloride (Bexarotene could enhance the action of hypoglycemic agents resulting in hypoglycemia). Products include:
ActoPlus Met Tablets **3214**
Actos Tablets **3219**
Duetact Tablets **3226**

Repaglinide (Bexarotene could enhance the action of hypoglycemic agents resulting in hypoglycemia).
No products indexed under this heading.

Rifampin (Bexarotene is metabolized by CYP4503A4; co-administration with inducers of CYP4503A4, such as rifampin, may cause a reduction in plasma bexarotene concentrations).
No products indexed under this heading.

Ritonavir (Bexarotene is metabolized by CYP4503A4; co-administration with inhibitors of CYP4503A4, such as protease inhibitors, would be expected to lead to an increase in plasma bexarotene concentrations). Products include:
Kaletra **476**
Norvir **503**

Rosiglitazone Maleate (Bexarotene could enhance the action of hypoglycemic agents resulting in hypoglycemia). Products include:
Avandamet Tablets **1373**
Avandaryl Tablets **1379**
Avandia Tablets **1384**

Saquinavir (Bexarotene is metabolized by CYP4503A4; co-administration with inhibitors of CYP4503A4, such as protease inhibitors, would be expected to lead to an increase in plasma bexarotene concentrations).
No products indexed under this heading.

Saquinavir Mesylate (Bexarotene is metabolized by CYP4503A4; co-administration with inhibitors of CYP4503A4, such as protease inhibitors, would be expected to lead to an increase in plasma bexarotene concentrations). Products include:
Invirase **2772**

Tamoxifen Citrate (Co-administration has resulted in a modest decrease in plasma concentrations of tamoxifen). Products include:
Soltamox Oral Solution **3527**

Tolazamide (Bexarotene could enhance the action of hypoglycemic agents resulting in hypoglycemia).
No products indexed under this heading.

Tolbutamide (Bexarotene could enhance the action of hypoglycemic agents resulting in hypoglycemia).
No products indexed under this heading.

Troglitazone (Bexarotene could enhance the action of hypoglycemic agents resulting in hypoglycemia).
No products indexed under this heading.

Vitamin A (Potential for additive toxic effects because of the relationship of bexarotene to vitamin A; patients should be advised to limit their vitamin A intake). Products include:
Visutein Capsules **3329**

Food Interactions

Food, unspecified (Co-administration with a fat-containing meal has resulted in higher plasma bexarotene AUC and Cmax values; because safety and efficacy data are based upon administration with food, it is recommended that Targretin capsules be administered with or immediately following a meal).

Grapefruit Juice (Bexarotene is metabolized by CYP403A4; co-administration with inhibitors of CYP4503A4, such as grapefruit juice, would be expected to lead to an increase in plasma bexarotene concentrations).

TARKA TABLETS

(Trandolapril, Verapamil Hydrochloride)........................ **524**
May interact with beta blockers, diuretics, cardiac glycosides, inhalant anesthetics, lithium preparations, neuromuscular blocking agents, potassium preparations, potassium sparing diuretics, quinidine, xanthines, and certain other agents. Compounds in these categories include:

Acebutolol Hydrochloride (Co-administration of beta blockers and verapamil may result in additive effects on heart rate, atrioventricular conduction, and/or cardiac contractility).
No products indexed under this heading.

Amiloride Hydrochloride (Increased risk of hyperkalemia; patients on diuretics, especially those on recently instituted diuretic therapy, may occasionally experience an excessive reduction of blood pressure after initiation of therapy with Tarka). Products include:
Midamor Tablets **2026**
Moduretic Tablets **2028**

Aminophylline (Verapamil may inhibit the clearance and increase the plasma levels of theophylline).
No products indexed under this heading.

Atenolol (Co-administration of beta blockers and verapamil may result in additive effects on heart rate, atrioventricular conduction, and/or cardiac contractility).
No products indexed under this heading.

Atracurium Besylate (Verapamil may potentiate the activity of neuromuscular blocking agents).
No products indexed under this heading.

Bendroflumethiazide (Patients on diuretics, especially those on recently instituted diuretic therapy, may occasionally experience an excessive reduction of blood pressure after initiation of therapy with Tarka).
No products indexed under this heading.

Betaxolol Hydrochloride (Co-administration of beta blockers and verapamil may result in additive effects on heart rate, atrioventricular conduction, and/or cardiac contractility). Products include:
Betoptic S Ophthalmic Suspension........................ **558**

Bisoprolol Fumarate (Co-administration of beta blockers and verapamil may result in additive effects on heart rate, atrioventricular conduction, and/or cardiac contractility).
No products indexed under this heading.

Bumetanide (Patients on diuretics, especially those on recently instituted diuretic therapy, may occasionally experience an excessive reduction of blood pressure after initiation of therapy with Tarka). Products include:
Bumex Tablets **2746**

Carbamazepine (Combined therapy of verapamil and carbamazepine may increase carbamazepine concentrations resulting in side effects such as diplopia, ataxia, and headache). Products include:
Carbatrol Capsules **3171**
Equetro Extended-Release Capsules........................ **3180**
Tegretol/Tegretol-XR **2295**

Carteolol Hydrochloride (Co-administration of beta blockers and verapamil may result in additive effects on heart rate, atrioventricular conduction, and/or cardiac contractility). Products include:
Carteolol Hydrochloride Ophthalmic Solution USP, 1%....... ⊙ **249**

Chlorothiazide (Patients on diuretics, especially those on recently instituted diuretic therapy, may occasionally experience an excessive reduction of blood pressure after initiation of therapy with Tarka).
Products include:
Diuril Oral Suspension **1954**

Chlorothiazide Sodium (Patients on diuretics, especially those on recently instituted diuretic therapy, may occasionally experience an excessive reduction of blood pressure after initiation of therapy with Tarka). Products include:
Diuril Sodium Intravenous **2467**

Chlorthalidone (Patients on diuretics, especially those on recently instituted diuretic therapy, may occasionally experience an excessive reduction of blood pressure after initiation of therapy with Tarka).
Products include:
Clorpres Tablets **2153**

Cimetidine (Variable results on clearance have been obtained in acute studies during concomitant therapy; clearance of verapamil may be reduced or unchanged). Products include:
Tagamet HB 200 Tablets .... ▣ **664**

Cimetidine Hydrochloride (Variable results on clearance have been obtained in acute studies during concomitant therapy; clearance of verapamil may be reduced or unchanged).
No products indexed under this heading.

Cisatracurium Besylate (Verapamil may potentiate the activity of neuromuscular blocking agents).
Products include:
Nimbex Injection **498**

Cyclosporine (Increased serum levels of cyclosporine). Products include:
Gengraf Capsules **459**
Neoral Oral Solution **2259**
Neoral Soft Gelatin Capsules **2259**
Restasis Ophthalmic Emulsion **575**
Sandimmune **2275**

Desflurane (Potential for excessive cardiovascular depression).
No products indexed under this heading.

Deslanoside (Chronic verapamil therapy can increase serum digoxin levels by 50% to 75% during the first week, and this can result in digoxin toxicity; patient should be carefully monitored to avoid over- or under-digitalization).
No products indexed under this heading.

Digitalis Glycoside Preparations (Chronic verapamil therapy can increase serum digoxin levels by 50% to 75% during the first week, and this can result in digoxin toxicity; patient should be carefully monitored to avoid over- or under-digitalization).
No products indexed under this heading.

Digitoxin (Chronic verapamil therapy can increase serum digoxin levels by 50% to 75% during the first week, and this can result in digoxin toxicity; patient should be carefully monitored to avoid over- or under-digitalization).
No products indexed under this heading.

Digoxin (Chronic verapamil therapy can increase serum digoxin levels by 50% to 75% during the first week, and this can result in digoxin toxicity; patient should be carefully monitored to avoid over- or under-digitalization).
Products include:
Lanoxicaps Capsules **1490**
Lanoxin Injection **1494**
Lanoxin Injection Pediatric **1497**
Lanoxin Tablets **1500**

Doxacurium Chloride (Verapamil may potentiate the activity of neuromuscular blocking agents).
No products indexed under this heading.

Dyphylline (Verapamil may inhibit the clearance and increase the plasma levels of theophylline).
No products indexed under this heading.

Enflurane (Potential for excessive cardiovascular depression).
No products indexed under this heading.

Esmolol Hydrochloride (Co-administration of beta blockers and verapamil may result in additive effects on heart rate, atrioventricular conduction, and/or cardiac contractility).
No products indexed under this heading.

Ethacrynic Acid (Patients on diuretics, especially those on recently instituted diuretic therapy, may occasionally experience an excessive reduction of blood pressure after initiation of therapy with Tarka). Products include:

Edecrin Tablets 1959

Flecainide Acetate (Concomitant use may result in additive effects on myocardial contractility, AV conduction and repolarization; concurrent use of flecainide and verapamil may result in additive inotropic effect and prolongation of atrioventricular conduction). Products include:

Tambocor Tablets 1856

Furosemide (Patients on diuretics, especially those on recently instituted diuretic therapy, may occasionally experience an excessive reduction of blood pressure after initiation of therapy with Tarka). Products include:

Furosemide Tablets 2154

Halothane (Potential for excessive cardiovascular depression).

No products indexed under this heading.

Hydrochlorothiazide (Patients on diuretics, especially those on recently instituted diuretic therapy, may occasionally experience an excessive reduction of blood pressure after initiation of therapy with Tarka). Products include:

Aldoril Tablets 1910
Atacand HCT 651
Avalide Tablets 888
Avalide Tablets 2874
Benicar HCT Tablets 1044
Diovan HCT Tablets 2196
Dyazide Capsules 1423
Hyzaar 50-12.5 Tablets 1990
Hyzaar 100-12.5 Tablets 1990
Hyzaar 100-25 Tablets 1990
Lopressor HCT 50/25 Tablets 2241
Lopressor HCT 100/25 Tablets 2241
Lopressor HCT 100/50 Tablets 2241
Lotensin HCT Tablets 2246
Micardis HCT Tablets 856
Moduretic Tablets 2028
Prinzide Tablets 2056
Teveten HCT Tablets 1737
Timolide Tablets 2086
Uniretic Tablets 3100

Hydroflumethiazide (Patients on diuretics, especially those on recently instituted diuretic therapy, may occasionally experience an excessive reduction of blood pressure after initiation of therapy with Tarka).

No products indexed under this heading.

Indapamide (Patients on diuretics, especially those on recently instituted diuretic therapy, may occasionally experience an excessive reduction of blood pressure after initiation of therapy with Tarka). Products include:

Indapamide Tablets 2156

Isoflurane (Potential for excessive cardiovascular depression).

No products indexed under this heading.

Labetalol Hydrochloride (Co-administration of beta blockers and verapamil may result in additive effects on heart rate, atrioventricular conduction, and/or cardiac contractility).

No products indexed under this heading.

Levobunolol Hydrochloride (Co-administration of beta blockers and verapamil may result in additive effects on heart rate, atrioventricular conduction, and/or cardiac contractility). Products include:

Betagan Ophthalmic Solution, USP.. ⊙220

Lithium (Co-administration results in increased sensitivity to the effects of lithium (neurotoxicity) with either no change or increase in serum lithium levels; increased lithium levels have been reported in patients receiving lithium and ACE inhibitor).

No products indexed under this heading.

Lithium Carbonate (Co-administration results in increased sensitivity to the effects of lithium (neurotoxicity) with either no change or increase in serum lithium levels; increased lithium levels have been reported in patients receiving lithium and ACE inhibitor). Products include:

Lithobid Tablets 1692

Lithium Citrate (Co-administration results in increased sensitivity to the effects of lithium (neurotoxicity) with either no change or increase in serum lithium levels; increased lithium levels have been reported in patients receiving lithium and ACE inhibitor).

No products indexed under this heading.

Methoxyflurane (Potential for excessive cardiovascular depression).

No products indexed under this heading.

Methyclothiazide (Patients on diuretics, especially those on recently instituted diuretic therapy, may occasionally experience an excessive reduction of blood pressure after initiation of therapy with Tarka).

No products indexed under this heading.

Metipranolol Hydrochloride (Co-administration of beta blockers and verapamil may result in additive effects on heart rate, atrioventricular conduction, and/or cardiac contractility).

No products indexed under this heading.

Metocurine Iodide (Verapamil may potentiate the activity of neuromuscular blocking agents).

No products indexed under this heading.

Metolazone (Patients on diuretics, especially those on recently instituted diuretic therapy, may occasionally experience an excessive reduction of blood pressure after initiation of therapy with Tarka).

No products indexed under this heading.

Metoprolol Succinate (Co-administration of beta blockers and verapamil may result in additive effects on heart rate, atrioventricular conduction, and/or cardiac contractility). Products include:

Toprol-XL Tablets 668

Metoprolol Tartrate (Co-administration of beta blockers and verapamil may result in additive effects on heart rate, atrioventricular conduction, and/or cardiac contractility). Products include:

Lopressor Injection 2238
Lopressor Tablets 2238
Lopressor HCT 50/25 Tablets 2241
Lopressor HCT 100/25 Tablets 2241
Lopressor HCT 100/50 Tablets 2241

Mivacurium Chloride (Verapamil may potentiate the activity of neuromuscular blocking agents). Products include:

Mivacron Injection 493

Nadolol (Co-administration of beta blockers and verapamil may result in additive effects on heart rate, atrioventricular conduction, and/or cardiac contractility). Products include:

Nadolol Tablets 2159

Pancuronium Bromide (Verapamil may potentiate the activity of neuromuscular blocking agents).

No products indexed under this heading.

Penbutolol Sulfate (Co-administration of beta blockers and verapamil may result in additive effects on heart rate, atrioventricular conduction, and/or cardiac contractility).

No products indexed under this heading.

Phenobarbital (May increase verapamil clearance). Products include:

Donnatal Extentabs 2493

Pindolol (Co-administration of beta blockers and verapamil may result in additive effects on heart rate, atrioventricular conduction, and/or cardiac contractility).

No products indexed under this heading.

Polythiazide (Patients on diuretics, especially those on recently instituted diuretic therapy, may occasionally experience an excessive reduction of blood pressure after initiation of therapy with Tarka).

No products indexed under this heading.

Potassium Acid Phosphate (Increased risk of hyperkalemia). Products include:

K-Phos Original (Sodium Free) Tablets 760

Potassium Bicarbonate (Increased risk of hyperkalemia).

No products indexed under this heading.

Potassium Chloride (Increased risk of hyperkalemia). Products include:

Colyte with Flavor Packs for Oral Solution.. 3088
HalfLytely and Bisacodyl Tablets Bowel Prep Kit with Flavors Packs.. 881
K-Dur Extended-Relase Tablets 3033
K-Lor Oral Solution 474
K-Tab Tablets 475
MoviPrep Oral Solution 2839
TriLyte with Flavor Packs for Oral Solution.. 3100

Potassium Citrate (Increased risk of hyperkalemia). Products include:

Urocit-K Tablets 2144

Potassium Gluconate (Increased risk of hyperkalemia).

No products indexed under this heading.

Potassium Phosphate (Increased risk of hyperkalemia). Products include:

K-Phos Neutral Tablets 760

Propranolol Hydrochloride (Co-administration of beta blockers and verapamil may result in additive effects on heart rate, atrioventricular conduction, and/or cardiac contractility). Products include:

Inderal LA Long-Acting Capsules 3429
InnoPran XL Capsules 2723

Quinidine (Concomitant use of verapamil and quinidine has resulted in significant hypotension and/or increased quinidine levels during verapamil therapy).

No products indexed under this heading.

Quinidine Gluconate (Concomitant use of verapamil and quinidine has resulted in significant hypotension and/or increased quinidine levels during verapamil therapy).

No products indexed under this heading.

Quinidine Hydrochloride (Concomitant use of verapamil and quinidine has resulted in significant hypotension and/or increased quinidine levels during verapamil therapy).

No products indexed under this heading.

Quinidine Polygalacturonate (Concomitant use of verapamil and quinidine has resulted in significant hypotension and/or increased quinidine levels during verapamil therapy).

No products indexed under this heading.

Quinidine Sulfate (Concomitant use of verapamil and quinidine has resulted in significant hypotension and/or increased quinidine levels during verapamil therapy).

No products indexed under this heading.

Rapacuronium Bromide (Verapamil may potentiate the activity of neuromuscular blocking agents).

No products indexed under this heading.

Rifampin (May markedly reduce oral verapamil bioavailability).

No products indexed under this heading.

Rocuronium Bromide (Verapamil may potentiate the activity of neuromuscular blocking agents). Products include:

Zemuron Injection 2346

Sotalol Hydrochloride (Co-administration of beta blockers and verapamil may result in additive effects on heart rate, atrioventricular conduction, and/or cardiac contractility).

No products indexed under this heading.

Spironolactone (Increased risk of hyperkalemia; patients on diuretics, especially those on recently instituted diuretic therapy, may occasionally experience an excessive reduction of blood pressure after initiation of therapy with Tarka).

No products indexed under this heading.

Succinylcholine Chloride (Verapamil may potentiate the activity of neuromuscular blocking agents).

No products indexed under this heading.

Theophylline (Verapamil may inhibit the clearance and increase the plasma levels of theophylline).

No products indexed under this heading.

Theophylline Anhydrous (Verapamil may inhibit the clearance and increase the plasma levels of theophylline). Products include:

Uniphyl Tablets 2710

Theophylline Calcium Salicylate (Verapamil may inhibit the clearance and increase the plasma levels of theophylline).

No products indexed under this heading.

Theophylline Dihydroxypropyl (Glyceryl) (Verapamil may inhibit the clearance and increase the plasma levels of theophylline).
No products indexed under this heading.

Theophylline Ethylenediamine (Verapamil may inhibit the clearance and increase the plasma levels of theophylline).
No products indexed under this heading.

Theophylline Sodium Glycinate (Verapamil may inhibit the clearance and increase the plasma levels of theophylline).
No products indexed under this heading.

Timolol Hemihydrate (Concomitant use of timolol eye drops and verapamil has resulted in asymptomatic bradycardia with wandering atrial pacemaker). Products include:
Betimol Ophthalmic Solution 3382
Betimol Ophthalmic Solution .... ⊙295

Timolol Maleate (Concomitant use of timolol eye drops and verapamil has resulted in asymptomatic bradycardia with wandering atrial pacemaker). Products include:
Blocadren Tablets 1916
Cosopt Sterile Ophthalmic Solution.. 1931
Timolide Tablets 2086
Timoptic Sterile Ophthalmic Solution.. 2088
Timoptic in Ocudose 2091
Timoptic-XE Sterile Ophthalmic Gel Forming Solution................... 2092

Torsemide (Patients on diuretics, especially those on recently instituted diuretic therapy, may occasionally experience an excessive reduction of blood pressure after initiation of therapy with Tarka). Products include:
Demadex Injection 2759
Demadex Tablets 2759

Triamterene (Increased risk of hyperkalemia; patients on diuretics, especially those on recently instituted diuretic therapy, may occasionally experience an excessive reduction of blood pressure after initiation of therapy with Tarka). Products include:
Dyazide Capsules 1423
Dyrenium Capsules 3400

Vecuronium Bromide (Verapamil may potentiate the activity of neuromuscular blocking agents).
No products indexed under this heading.

Food Interactions

Food, unspecified (Co-administration with food decreases verapamil bioavailability and the time to peak plasma concentration is delayed; bioavailability of trandolapril is not altered; Tarka should be administered with food).

TASMAR TABLETS
(Tolcapone) 3358
May interact with central nervous system depressants, nonselective MAO inhibitors, and certain other agents. Compounds in these categories include:

Alfentanil Hydrochloride (Possible additive sedative effects when used in combination with CNS depressants).
No products indexed under this heading.

Alprazolam (Possible additive sedative effects when used in combination with CNS depressants). Products include:
Niravam Orally Disintegrating Tablets.. 3092

Apomorphine (Tolcapone may influence the pharmacokinetics of drugs metabolized by COMT; dosage adjustments should be considered when co-administered).
No products indexed under this heading.

Aprobarbital (Possible additive sedative effects when used in combination with CNS depressants).
No products indexed under this heading.

Buprenorphine Hydrochloride (Possible additive sedative effects when used in combination with CNS depressants). Products include:
Buprenex Injectable 2716
Suboxone Tablets 2717
Subutex Tablets 2717

Buspirone Hydrochloride (Possible additive sedative effects when used in combination with CNS depressants).
No products indexed under this heading.

Butabarbital (Possible additive sedative effects when used in combination with CNS depressants).
No products indexed under this heading.

Butalbital (Possible additive sedative effects when used in combination with CNS depressants).
No products indexed under this heading.

Chlordiazepoxide (Possible additive sedative effects when used in combination with CNS depressants).
No products indexed under this heading.

Chlordiazepoxide Hydrochloride (Possible additive sedative effects when used in combination with CNS depressants). Products include:
Librium Capsules 3347

Chlorpromazine (Possible additive sedative effects when used in combination with CNS depressants).
No products indexed under this heading.

Chlorpromazine Hydrochloride (Possible additive sedative effects when used in combination with CNS depressants).
No products indexed under this heading.

Chlorprothixene (Possible additive sedative effects when used in combination with CNS depressants).
No products indexed under this heading.

Chlorprothixene Hydrochloride (Possible additive sedative effects when used in combination with CNS depressants).
No products indexed under this heading.

Chlorprothixene Lactate (Possible additive sedative effects when used in combination with CNS depressants).
No products indexed under this heading.

Clorazepate Dipotassium (Possible additive sedative effects when used in combination with CNS depressants). Products include:
Tranxene 2474

Clozapine (Possible additive sedative effects when used in combination with CNS depressants). Products include:
Clozaril Tablets 2184
FazaClo Orally Disintegrating Tablets... 551

Codeine Phosphate (Possible additive sedative effects when used in combination with CNS depressants). Products include:
Tylenol with Codeine Tablets 2391

Desflurane (Possible additive sedative effects when used in combination with CNS depressants).
No products indexed under this heading.

Desipramine Hydrochloride (Co-administration of tolcapone with levodopa/carbidopa and desipramine has resulted in slight increase in frequency of adverse events; caution should be exercised when co-administered).
No products indexed under this heading.

Dezocine (Possible additive sedative effects when used in combination with CNS depressants).
No products indexed under this heading.

Diazepam (Possible additive sedative effects when used in combination with CNS depressants). Products include:
Diastat Rectal Delivery System 3343
Valium Tablets 2819

Dobutamine Hydrochloride (Tolcapone may influence the pharmacokinetics of drugs metabolized by COMT; dosage adjustments should be considered when co-administered).
No products indexed under this heading.

Droperidol (Possible additive sedative effects when used in combination with CNS depressants).
No products indexed under this heading.

Enflurane (Possible additive sedative effects when used in combination with CNS depressants).
No products indexed under this heading.

Estazolam (Possible additive sedative effects when used in combination with CNS depressants). Products include:
ProSom Tablets 517

Ethanol (Possible additive sedative effects when used in combination with CNS depressants).
No products indexed under this heading.

Ethchlorvynol (Possible additive sedative effects when used in combination with CNS depressants).
No products indexed under this heading.

Ethinamate (Possible additive sedative effects when used in combination with CNS depressants).
No products indexed under this heading.

Ethyl Alcohol (Possible additive sedative effects when used in combination with CNS depressants).
No products indexed under this heading.

Fentanyl (Possible additive sedative effects when used in combination with CNS depressants). Products include:
Duragesic Transdermal System 2373
Ionsys Transdermal System 2379

Fentanyl Citrate (Possible additive sedative effects when used in combination with CNS depressants). Products include:
Actiq 979

Fluphenazine Decanoate (Possible additive sedative effects when used in combination with CNS depressants).
No products indexed under this heading.

Fluphenazine Enanthate (Possible additive sedative effects when used in combination with CNS depressants).
No products indexed under this heading.

Fluphenazine Hydrochloride (Possible additive sedative effects when used in combination with CNS depressants).
No products indexed under this heading.

Flurazepam Hydrochloride (Possible additive sedative effects when used in combination with CNS depressants). Products include:
Dalmane Capsules 3342

Glutethimide (Possible additive sedative effects when used in combination with CNS depressants).
No products indexed under this heading.

Haloperidol (Possible additive sedative effects when used in combination with CNS depressants).
No products indexed under this heading.

Haloperidol Decanoate (Possible additive sedative effects when used in combination with CNS depressants).
No products indexed under this heading.

Hydrocodone Bitartrate (Possible additive sedative effects when used in combination with CNS depressants). Products include:
Hycodan 1116
Hycotuss Expectorant Syrup 1117
Vicodin Tablets 535
Vicodin ES Tablets 536
Vicodin HP Tablets 538
Vicoprofen Tablets 539
Zydone Tablets 1139

Hydrocodone Polistirex (Possible additive sedative effects when used in combination with CNS depressants). Products include:
Tussionex Pennkinetic Extended-Release Suspension...... 3327

Hydromorphone Hydrochloride (Possible additive sedative effects when used in combination with CNS depressants). Products include:
Dilaudid 440
Dilaudid Non-Sterile Powder 440
Dilaudid Oral Liquid 445
Dilaudid Rectal Suppositories 440
Dilaudid Tablets 440
Dilaudid Tablets - 8 mg 445
Dilaudid-HP 442

Hydroxyzine Hydrochloride (Possible additive sedative effects when used in combination with CNS depressants).
No products indexed under this heading.

Isocarboxazid (The combination, in theory, of tolcapone and nonselective MAO inhibitor may result in inhibition of the majority of the pathways responsible for normal catecholamine metabolism; patients should ordinarily not be treated concomitantly).
No products indexed under this heading.

Isoflurane (Possible additive sedative effects when used in combination with CNS depressants).
No products indexed under this heading.

Isoproterenol Hydrochloride (Tolcapone may influence the pharmacokinetics of drugs metabolized by COMT; dosage adjustments should be considered when co-administered).
No products indexed under this heading.

Ketamine Hydrochloride (Possible additive sedative effects when used in combination with CNS depressants).
No products indexed under this heading.

Levodopa (Tolcapone enhances levodopa bioavailability and, therefore, may increase the occurence of orthostatic hypotension; tolcapone may potentiate the dopaminergic side effects of levodopa and may cause and/or exacerbate preexisting dyskinesia). Products include:
Parcopa Orally Disintegrating Tablets 3097
Stalevo Tablets 2287

Levomethadyl Acetate Hydrochloride (Possible additive sedative effects when used in combination with CNS depressants).
No products indexed under this heading.

Levorphanol Tartrate (Possible additive sedative effects when used in combination with CNS depressants).
No products indexed under this heading.

Lorazepam (Possible additive sedative effects when used in combination with CNS depressants).
No products indexed under this heading.

Loxapine Hydrochloride (Possible additive sedative effects when used in combination with CNS depressants).
No products indexed under this heading.

Loxapine Succinate (Possible additive sedative effects when used in combination with CNS depressants).
No products indexed under this heading.

Meperidine Hydrochloride (Possible additive sedative effects when used in combination with CNS depressants).
No products indexed under this heading.

Mephobarbital (Possible additive sedative effects when used in combination with CNS depressants).
No products indexed under this heading.

Meprobamate (Possible additive sedative effects when used in combination with CNS depressants).
No products indexed under this heading.

Mesoridazine Besylate (Possible additive sedative effects when used in combination with CNS depressants).
No products indexed under this heading.

Methadone Hydrochloride (Possible additive sedative effects when used in combination with CNS depressants).
No products indexed under this heading.

Methohexital Sodium (Possible additive sedative effects when used in combination with CNS depressants).
No products indexed under this heading.

Methotrimeprazine (Possible additive sedative effects when used in combination with CNS depressants).
No products indexed under this heading.

Methoxyflurane (Possible additive sedative effects when used in combination with CNS depressants).
No products indexed under this heading.

Methyldopa (Tolcapone may influence the pharmacokinetics of drugs metabolized by COMT; dosage adjustments should be considered when co-administered). Products include:
Aldoril Tablets 1910

Midazolam Hydrochloride (Possible additive sedative effects when used in combination with CNS depressants).
No products indexed under this heading.

Molindone Hydrochloride (Possible additive sedative effects when used in combination with CNS depressants). Products include:
Moban Tablets 1119

Morphine Sulfate (Possible additive sedative effects when used in combination with CNS depressants). Products include:
Avinza Capsules 1741
Kadian Capsules 577
MS Contin Tablets 2701

Olanzapine (Possible additive sedative effects when used in combination with CNS depressants). Products include:
Symbyax Capsules 1819
Zyprexa Tablets 1830
Zyprexa IntraMuscular 1830
Zyprexa ZYDIS Orally Disintegrating Tablets.................. 1830

Oxazepam (Possible additive sedative effects when used in combination with CNS depressants).
No products indexed under this heading.

Oxycodone Hydrochloride (Possible additive sedative effects when used in combination with CNS depressants). Products include:
OxyContin Tablets 2703
OxyFast Oral Concentrate Solution 2708
OxyIR Capsules 2708
Percocet Tablets 1131
Percodan Tablets 1132

Pargyline Hydrochloride (The combination, in theory, of tolcapone and non-selective MAO inhibitor may result in inhibition of the majority of the pathways responsible for normal catecholamine metabolism; patients should ordinarily not be treated concomitantly).
No products indexed under this heading.

Pentobarbital Sodium (Possible additive sedative effects when used in combination with CNS depressants). Products include:
Nembutal Sodium Solution, USP 2470

Perphenazine (Possible additive sedative effects when used in combination with CNS depressants).
No products indexed under this heading.

Phenelzine Sulfate (The combination, in theory, of tolcapone and non-selective MAO inhibitor may result in inhibition of the majority of the pathways responsible for normal catecholamine metabolism; patients should ordinarily not be treated concomitantly).
No products indexed under this heading.

Phenobarbital (Possible additive sedative effects when used in combination with CNS depressants). Products include:
Donnatal Extentabs 2493

Prazepam (Possible additive sedative effects when used in combination with CNS depressants).
No products indexed under this heading.

Procarbazine Hydrochloride (The combination, in theory, of tolcapone and non-selective MAO inhibitor may result in inhibition of the majority of the pathways responsible for normal catecholamine metabolism; patients should ordinarily not be treated concomitantly). Products include:
Matulane Capsules 3191

Prochlorperazine (Possible additive sedative effects when used in combination with CNS depressants).
No products indexed under this heading.

Promethazine Hydrochloride (Possible additive sedative effects when used in combination with CNS depressants). Products include:
Phenergan Tablets and Suppositories............................... 3440

Propofol (Possible additive sedative effects when used in combination with CNS depressants).
No products indexed under this heading.

Propoxyphene Hydrochloride (Possible additive sedative effects when used in combination with CNS depressants).
No products indexed under this heading.

Propoxyphene Napsylate (Possible additive sedative effects when used in combination with CNS depressants).
No products indexed under this heading.

Quazepam (Possible additive sedative effects when used in combination with CNS depressants).
No products indexed under this heading.

Quetiapine Fumarate (Possible additive sedative effects when used in combination with CNS depressants). Products include:
Seroquel Tablets 690

Remifentanil Hydrochloride (Possible additive sedative effects when used in combination with CNS depressants).
No products indexed under this heading.

Risperidone (Possible additive sedative effects when used in combination with CNS depressants). Products include:
Risperdal 1676
Risperdal Consta Long-Acting Injection 1682
Risperdal M-Tab Orally Disintegrating Tablets.................. 1676

Secobarbital Sodium (Possible additive sedative effects when used in combination with CNS depressants).
No products indexed under this heading.

Sevoflurane (Possible additive sedative effects when used in combination with CNS depressants).
Products include:
Ultane Liquid for Inhalation 531

Sufentanil Citrate (Possible additive sedative effects when used in combination with CNS depressants).
No products indexed under this heading.

Temazepam (Possible additive sedative effects when used in combination with CNS depressants).
Products include:
Restoril Capsules 1860

Thiamylal Sodium (Possible additive sedative effects when used in combination with CNS depressants).
No products indexed under this heading.

Thioridazine Hydrochloride (Possible additive sedative effects when used in combination with CNS depressants). Products include:
Thioridazine Hydrochloride Tablets.. 2163

Thiothixene (Possible additive sedative effects when used in combination with CNS depressants).
Products include:
Thiothixene Capsules 2165

Tranylcypromine Sulfate (The combination, in theory, of tolcapone and non-selective MAO inhibitor may result in inhibition of the majority of the pathways responsible for normal catecholamine metabolism; patients should ordinarily not be treated concomitantly). Products include:
Parnate Tablets 1527

Triazolam (Possible additive sedative effects when used in combination with CNS depressants).
No products indexed under this heading.

Trifluoperazine Hydrochloride (Possible additive sedative effects when used in combination with CNS depressants).
No products indexed under this heading.

Zaleplon (Possible additive sedative effects when used in combination with CNS depressants). Products include:
Sonata Capsules 1717

Ziprasidone Hydrochloride (Possible additive sedative effects when used in combination with CNS depressants). Products include:
Geodon Capsules 2529

Zolpidem Tartrate (Possible additive sedative effects when used in combination with CNS depressants). Products include:
Ambien Tablets 2851
Ambien CR Tablets 2855

Food Interactions

Alcohol (Possible additive sedative effects when used in combination with CNS depressants, such as alcohol).

Food, unspecified (Food given within 1 hour before and 2 hours after dosing of tolcapone decreases the relative bioavailability by 10% to 20%; Tasmar may be taken with or without food).

TAXOTERE INJECTION CONCENTRATE

(Docetaxel) 2932

May interact with cytochrome p450 3a4 inhibitors (selected). Compounds in these categories include:

Acetazolamide (Metabolism of docetaxel may be inhibited by co-administration with CYP3A4 inhibitors, thereby leading to substantial increases in docetaxel blood concentrations).

No products indexed under this heading.

Amiodarone Hydrochloride (Metabolism of docetaxel may be inhibited by co-administration with CYP3A4 inhibitors, thereby leading to substantial increases in docetaxel blood concentrations).

No products indexed under this heading.

Amprenavir (Metabolism of docetaxel may be inhibited by co-administration with CYP3A4 inhibitors, thereby leading to substantial increases in docetaxel blood concentrations). Products include:

- Agenerase Capsules 1327
- Agenerase Oral Solution 1332

Anastrozole (Metabolism of docetaxel may be inhibited by co-administration with CYP3A4 inhibitors, thereby leading to substantial increases in docetaxel blood concentrations). Products include:

- Arimidex Tablets 673

Aprepitant (Metabolism of docetaxel may be inhibited by co-administration with CYP3A4 inhibitors, thereby leading to substantial increases in docetaxel blood concentrations). Products include:

- Emend Capsules 1963

Cimetidine (Metabolism of docetaxel may be inhibited by co-administration with CYP3A4 inhibitors, thereby leading to substantial increases in docetaxel blood concentrations). Products include:

- Tagamet HB 200 Tablets 664

Cimetidine Hydrochloride (Metabolism of docetaxel may be inhibited by co-administration with CYP3A4 inhibitors, thereby leading to substantial increases in docetaxel blood concentrations).

No products indexed under this heading.

Ciprofloxacin (Metabolism of docetaxel may be inhibited by co-administration with CYP3A4 inhibitors, thereby leading to substantial increases in docetaxel blood concentrations). Products include:

- Cipro Oral Suspension 2977
- Cipro I.V. 2984
- Cipro XR Tablets 2990
- Ciprodex Otic Suspension 559

Clarithromycin (Metabolism of docetaxel may be inhibited by co-administration with CYP3A4 inhibitors, thereby leading to substantial increases in docetaxel blood concentrations). Products include:

- Biaxin/Biaxin XL 402
- PREVPAC 3284

Clotrimazole (Metabolism of docetaxel may be inhibited by co-administration with CYP3A4 inhibitors, thereby leading to substantial increases in docetaxel blood concentrations). Products include:

- Desenex Athlete's Foot Cream 635
- Lotrimin 3039
- Lotrisone 3040

Cyclosporine (Metabolism of docetaxel may be inhibited by co-administration with CYP3A4 inhibitors, thereby leading to substantial increases in docetaxel blood concentrations). Products include:

- Gengraf Capsules 459
- Neoral Oral Solution 2259
- Neoral Soft Gelatin Capsules 2259
- Restasis Ophthalmic Emulsion 575
- Sandimmune 2275

Dalfopristin (Metabolism of docetaxel may be inhibited by co-administration with CYP3A4 inhibitors, thereby leading to substantial increases in docetaxel blood concentrations).

No products indexed under this heading.

Danazol (Metabolism of docetaxel may be inhibited by co-administration with CYP3A4 inhibitors, thereby leading to substantial increases in docetaxel blood concentrations).

No products indexed under this heading.

Delavirdine Mesylate (Metabolism of docetaxel may be inhibited by co-administration with CYP3A4 inhibitors, thereby leading to substantial increases in docetaxel blood concentrations). Products include:

- Rescriptor Tablets 2551

Diltiazem Hydrochloride (Metabolism of docetaxel may be inhibited by co-administration with CYP3A4 inhibitors, thereby leading to substantial increases in docetaxel blood concentrations). Products include:

- Cardizem LA Extended Release Tablets 1728
- Tiazac Capsules 1201

Diltiazem Maleate (Metabolism of docetaxel may be inhibited by co-administration with CYP3A4 inhibitors, thereby leading to substantial increases in docetaxel blood concentrations).

No products indexed under this heading.

Efavirenz (Metabolism of docetaxel may be inhibited by co-administration with CYP3A4 inhibitors, thereby leading to substantial increases in docetaxel blood concentrations). Products include:

- Atripla Tablets 945
- Sustiva Capsules 930
- Sustiva Tablets 930

Erythromycin (Metabolism of docetaxel may be inhibited by co-administration with CYP3A4 inhibitors, thereby leading to substantial increases in docetaxel blood concentrations). Products include:

- Ery-Tab Tablets 449
- Erythromycin Base Filmtab Tablets 455
- Erythromycin Delayed-Release Capsules, USP 457
- PCE Dispertab Tablets 515

Erythromycin Estolate (Metabolism of docetaxel may be inhibited by co-administration with CYP3A4 inhibitors, thereby leading to substantial increases in docetaxel blood concentrations).

No products indexed under this heading.

Erythromycin Ethylsuccinate (Metabolism of docetaxel may be inhibited by co-administration with CYP3A4 inhibitors, thereby leading to substantial increases in docetaxel blood concentrations). Products include:

- E.E.S. 451
- EryPed 447

Erythromycin Gluceptate (Metabolism of docetaxel may be inhibited by co-administration with CYP3A4 inhibitors, thereby leading to substantial increases in docetaxel blood concentrations).

No products indexed under this heading.

Erythromycin Lactobionate (Metabolism of docetaxel may be inhibited by co-administration with CYP3A4 inhibitors, thereby leading to substantial increases in docetaxel blood concentrations).

No products indexed under this heading.

Erythromycin Stearate (Metabolism of docetaxel may be inhibited by co-administration with CYP3A4 inhibitors, thereby leading to substantial increases in docetaxel blood concentrations). Products include:

- Erythrocin Stearate Filmtab Tablets 453

Esomeprazole Magnesium (Metabolism of docetaxel may be inhibited by co-administration with CYP3A4 inhibitors, thereby leading to substantial increases in docetaxel blood concentrations). Products include:

- Nexium Delayed-Release Capsules 655

Fluconazole (Metabolism of docetaxel may be inhibited by co-administration with CYP3A4 inhibitors, thereby leading to substantial increases in docetaxel blood concentrations).

No products indexed under this heading.

Fluoxetine Hydrochloride (Metabolism of docetaxel may be inhibited by co-administration with CYP3A4 inhibitors, thereby leading to substantial increases in docetaxel blood concentrations). Products include:

- Prozac Pulvules and Liquid 1801
- Symbyax Capsules 1819

Fluvoxamine Maleate (Metabolism of docetaxel may be inhibited by co-administration with CYP3A4 inhibitors, thereby leading to substantial increases in docetaxel blood concentrations).

No products indexed under this heading.

Fosamprenavir Calcium (Metabolism of docetaxel may be inhibited by co-administration with CYP3A4 inhibitors, thereby leading to substantial increases in docetaxel blood concentrations). Products include:

- Lexiva Tablets 1505

Indinavir Sulfate (Metabolism of docetaxel may be inhibited by co-administration with CYP3A4 inhibitors, thereby leading to substantial increases in docetaxel blood concentrations). Products include:

- Crixivan Capsules 1940

Isoniazid (Metabolism of docetaxel may be inhibited by co-administration with CYP3A4 inhibitors, thereby leading to substantial increases in docetaxel blood concentrations).

No products indexed under this heading.

Itraconazole (Metabolism of docetaxel may be inhibited by co-administration with CYP3A4 inhibitors, thereby leading to substantial increases in docetaxel blood concentrations).

No products indexed under this heading.

Ketoconazole (Metabolism of docetaxel may be inhibited by co-administration with CYP3A4 inhibitors, thereby leading to substantial increases in docetaxel blood concentrations). Products include:

- Nizoral A-D Shampoo, 1% 1868

Lopinavir (Metabolism of docetaxel may be inhibited by co-administration with CYP3A4 inhibitors, thereby leading to substantial increases in docetaxel blood concentrations). Products include:

- Kaletra 476

Loratadine (Metabolism of docetaxel may be inhibited by co-administration with CYP3A4 inhibitors, thereby leading to substantial increases in docetaxel blood concentrations). Products include:

- Alavert Allergy & Sinus D-12 Hour Tablets 771
- Alavert 771
- Children's Claritin Allergy Oral Solution 771
- Claritin Non-Drowsy 24 Hour Tablets 772
- Claritin Reditabs 24 Hour Non-Drowsy Tablets 772
- Claritin-D Non-Drowsy 12 Hour Tablets 772
- Claritin-D Non-Drowsy 24 Hour Tablets 772

Metronidazole (Metabolism of docetaxel may be inhibited by co-administration with CYP3A4 inhibitors, thereby leading to substantial increases in docetaxel blood concentrations). Products include:

- Metrogel 1% 1211
- MetroGel-Vaginal Gel 1855
- Vandazole Vaginal Gel 3338

Metronidazole Benzoate (Metabolism of docetaxel may be inhibited by co-administration with CYP3A4 inhibitors, thereby leading to substantial increases in docetaxel blood concentrations).

No products indexed under this heading.

Metronidazole Hydrochloride (Metabolism of docetaxel may be inhibited by co-administration with CYP3A4 inhibitors, thereby leading to substantial increases in docetaxel blood concentrations).

No products indexed under this heading.

Miconazole (Metabolism of docetaxel may be inhibited by co-administration with CYP3A4 inhibitors, thereby leading to substantial increases in docetaxel blood concentrations).

No products indexed under this heading.

Miconazole Nitrate (Metabolism of docetaxel may be inhibited by co-administration with CYP3A4 inhibitors, thereby leading to substantial increases in docetaxel blood concentrations). Products include:

- Desenex 635
- Desenex Jock Itch Spray Powder 635

Nefazodone Hydrochloride (Metabolism of docetaxel may be inhibited by co-administration with CYP3A4 inhibitors, thereby leading to substantial increases in docetaxel blood concentrations).
No products indexed under this heading.

Nelfinavir Mesylate (Metabolism of docetaxel may be inhibited by co-administration with CYP3A4 inhibitors, thereby leading to substantial increases in docetaxel blood concentrations). Products include:
Viracept 2577

Nevirapine (Metabolism of docetaxel may be inhibited by co-administration with CYP3A4 inhibitors, thereby leading to substantial increases in docetaxel blood concentrations). Products include:
Viramune Oral Suspension 873
Viramune Tablets 873

Niacinamide (Metabolism of docetaxel may be inhibited by co-administration with CYP3A4 inhibitors, thereby leading to substantial increases in docetaxel blood concentrations).
No products indexed under this heading.

Nicotinamide (Metabolism of docetaxel may be inhibited by co-administration with CYP3A4 inhibitors, thereby leading to substantial increases in docetaxel blood concentrations). Products include:
Nicomide Tablets 1088

Nifedipine (Metabolism of docetaxel may be inhibited by co-administration with CYP3A4 inhibitors, thereby leading to substantial increases in docetaxel blood concentrations). Products include:
Adalat CC Tablets 2964

Norfloxacin (Metabolism of docetaxel may be inhibited by co-administration with CYP3A4 inhibitors, thereby leading to substantial increases in docetaxel blood concentrations). Products include:
Noroxin Tablets 2032

Omeprazole (Metabolism of docetaxel may be inhibited by co-administration with CYP3A4 inhibitors, thereby leading to substantial increases in docetaxel blood concentrations). Products include:
Zegerid Capsules 2958
Zegerid Powder for Oral Solution 2958

Paroxetine Hydrochloride (Metabolism of docetaxel may be inhibited by co-administration with CYP3A4 inhibitors, thereby leading to substantial increases in docetaxel blood concentrations). Products include:
Paxil CR Controlled-Release Tablets 1538
Paxil 1530

Propoxyphene Hydrochloride (Metabolism of docetaxel may be inhibited by co-administration with CYP3A4 inhibitors, thereby leading to substantial increases in docetaxel blood concentrations).
No products indexed under this heading.

Propoxyphene Napsylate (Metabolism of docetaxel may be inhibited by co-administration with CYP3A4 inhibitors, thereby leading to substantial increases in docetaxel blood concentrations).
No products indexed under this heading.

Quinidine (Metabolism of docetaxel may be inhibited by co-administration with CYP3A4 inhibitors, thereby leading to substantial increases in docetaxel blood concentrations).
No products indexed under this heading.

Quinidine Hydrochloride (Metabolism of docetaxel may be inhibited by co-administration with CYP3A4 inhibitors, thereby leading to substantial increases in docetaxel blood concentrations).
No products indexed under this heading.

Quinidine Polygalacturonate (Metabolism of docetaxel may be inhibited by co-administration with CYP3A4 inhibitors, thereby leading to substantial increases in docetaxel blood concentrations).
No products indexed under this heading.

Quinidine Sulfate (Metabolism of docetaxel may be inhibited by co-administration with CYP3A4 inhibitors, thereby leading to substantial increases in docetaxel blood concentrations).
No products indexed under this heading.

Quinine (Metabolism of docetaxel may be inhibited by co-administration with CYP3A4 inhibitors, thereby leading to substantial increases in docetaxel blood concentrations).
No products indexed under this heading.

Quinine Sulfate (Metabolism of docetaxel may be inhibited by co-administration with CYP3A4 inhibitors, thereby leading to substantial increases in docetaxel blood concentrations).
No products indexed under this heading.

Quinupristin (Metabolism of docetaxel may be inhibited by co-administration with CYP3A4 inhibitors, thereby leading to substantial increases in docetaxel blood concentrations).
No products indexed under this heading.

Ranitidine Bismuth Citrate (Metabolism of docetaxel may be inhibited by co-administration with CYP3A4 inhibitors, thereby leading to substantial increases in docetaxel blood concentrations).
No products indexed under this heading.

Ranitidine Hydrochloride (Metabolism of docetaxel may be inhibited by co-administration with CYP3A4 inhibitors, thereby leading to substantial increases in docetaxel blood concentrations). Products include:
Zantac 1624
Zantac Injection 1619
Zantac Injection Pharmacy Bulk Package 1622

Ritonavir (Metabolism of docetaxel may be inhibited by co-administration with CYP3A4 inhibitors, thereby leading to substantial increases in docetaxel blood concentrations). Products include:
Kaletra 476
Norvir 503

Saquinavir (Metabolism of docetaxel may be inhibited by co-administration with CYP3A4 inhibitors, thereby leading to substantial increases in docetaxel blood concentrations).
No products indexed under this heading.

Saquinavir Mesylate (Metabolism of docetaxel may be inhibited by co-administration with CYP3A4 inhibitors, thereby leading to substantial increases in docetaxel blood concentrations). Products include:
Invirase 2772

Sertraline Hydrochloride (Metabolism of docetaxel may be inhibited by co-administration with CYP3A4 inhibitors, thereby leading to substantial increases in docetaxel blood concentrations). Products include:
Zoloft 2586

Telithromycin (Metabolism of docetaxel may be inhibited by co-administration with CYP3A4 inhibitors, thereby leading to substantial increases in docetaxel blood concentrations). Products include:
Ketek Tablets 2903

Troglitazone (Metabolism of docetaxel may be inhibited by co-administration with CYP3A4 inhibitors, thereby leading to substantial increases in docetaxel blood concentrations).
No products indexed under this heading.

Troleandomycin (Metabolism of docetaxel may be inhibited by co-administration with CYP3A4 inhibitors, thereby leading to substantial increases in docetaxel blood concentrations).
No products indexed under this heading.

Valproate Sodium (Metabolism of docetaxel may be inhibited by co-administration with CYP3A4 inhibitors, thereby leading to substantial increases in docetaxel blood concentrations). Products include:
Depacon Injection 412

Verapamil Hydrochloride (Metabolism of docetaxel may be inhibited by co-administration with CYP3A4 inhibitors, thereby leading to substantial increases in docetaxel blood concentrations). Products include:
Covera-HS Tablets 3139
Tarka Tablets 524
Verelan PM Extended-Release Capsules, Controlled-Onset 3106

Voriconazole (Metabolism of docetaxel may be inhibited by co-administration with CYP3A4 inhibitors, thereby leading to substantial increases in docetaxel blood concentrations). Products include:
VFEND I.V. 2564
VFEND Oral Suspension 2564
VFEND Tablets 2564

Zafirlukast (Metabolism of docetaxel may be inhibited by co-administration with CYP3A4 inhibitors, thereby leading to substantial increases in docetaxel blood concentrations). Products include:
Accolate Tablets 671

Zileuton (Metabolism of docetaxel may be inhibited by co-administration with CYP3A4 inhibitors, thereby leading to substantial increases in docetaxel blood concentrations). Products include:
Zyflo Tablets 1023

Food Interactions

Grapefruit (Metabolism of docetaxel may be inhibited by co-administration with CYP3A4 inhibitors, thereby leading to substantial increases in docetaxel blood concentrations).

Grapefruit Juice (Metabolism of docetaxel may be inhibited by co-administration with CYP3A4 inhibitors, thereby leading to substantial increases in docetaxel blood concentrations).

TĒGREEN 97 CAPSULES

(Camellia sinensis) 2672
May interact with oral anticoagulants. Compounds in these categories include:

Anisindione (Concurrent use with anticoagulants requires consultation with a physician). Products include:
Miradon Tablets 3042

Dicumarol (Concurrent use with anticoagulants requires consultation with a physician).
No products indexed under this heading.

Warfarin Sodium (Concurrent use with anticoagulants requires consultation with a physician). Products include:
Coumadin for Injection 898
Coumadin Tablets 898

TEGRETOL SUSPENSION

(Carbamazepine) 2295
See Tegretol-XR Tablets

TEGRETOL TABLETS

(Carbamazepine) 2295
See Tegretol-XR Tablets

TEGRETOL CHEWABLE TABLETS

(Carbamazepine) 2295
See Tegretol-XR Tablets

TEGRETOL-XR TABLETS

(Carbamazepine) 2295
May interact with calcium channel blockers, corticosteroids, doxycycline, anticonvulsants, erythromycin, lithium preparations, macrolide antibiotics, monoamine oxidase inhibitors, oral contraceptives, phenytoin, protease inhibitors, tricyclic antidepressants, valproate, xanthines, and certain other agents. Compounds in these categories include:

Acetaminophen (Carbamazepine induces hepatic CYP activity; carbamazepine causes, or would be expected to cause, decreased levels of acetaminophen). Products include:
Comtrex Maximum Strength Cold & Cough Day/Night Caplets - Day Formulation .... ■ 726
Comtrex Maximum Strength Cold & Cough Day/Night Caplets - Night Formulation .... ■ 726
Comtrex Maximum Strength Non-Drowsy Cold & Cough Caplets .... ■ 725
Comtrex Maximum Strength Day/Night Severe Cold & Sinus Caplets - Day Formulation .... ■ 725
Comtrex Maximum Strength Day/Night Severe Cold & Sinus Caplets - Night Formulation .... ■ 725
Contac Cold and Flu Maximum Strength Caplets .... ■ 728
Contac Cold and Flu Day and Night Caplets (Day Formulation Only) .... ■ 727
Contac Cold and Flu Day and Night Caplets (Night Formulation Only) .... ■ 727
Contac Cold and Flu Non-Drowsy Caplets .... ■ 728

Excedrin Extra Strength Caplets/Tablets/Geltabs............ 684
Excedrin Migraine Caplets/Tablets/Geltabs............ 609
Excedrin PM Caplets/Tablets/Geltabs............ 610
Excedrin Sinus Headache Caplets/Tablets............ 610
Excedrin Tension Headache Caplets/Tablets/Geltabs............ 611
Goody's Body Pain Formula Powder............ 684
Goody's Extra Strength Headache Powders............ 611
Goody's Extra Strength Pain Relief Tablets............ 685
Goody's PM Powder for Pain with Sleeplessness............ 612
Percocet Tablets............ 1131
Robitussin Cough, Cold & Flu Nighttime Liquid............ 738
TheraFlu Cold & Sore Throat Hot Liquid............ 741
TheraFlu Flu & Chest Congestion Hot Liquid............ 741
TheraFlu Flu & Sore Throat Hot Liquid............ 742
TheraFlu Daytime Severe Cold Hot Liquid............ 742
TheraFlu Nighttime Severe Cold Hot Liquid............ 740
TheraFlu Warming Relief Daytime Severe Cold............ 743
TheraFlu Warming Relief Nighttime Severe Cold............ 743
Triaminic Cough & Sore Throat Liquid............ 747
Regular Strength Tylenol Tablets............ 1870
Children's Tylenol with Flavor Creator............ 679
Children's Tylenol Plus Flu Oral Suspension............ 749
Tylenol Cold Head Congestion Daytime Caplets with Cool Burst and Gelcaps............ 750
Tylenol Cold Multi-Symptom Daytime Liquid............ 752
Tylenol Cold Multi-Symptom Severe Daytime Liquid............ 752
Tylenol 8 Hour Extended Release Caplets............ 1870
Tylenol............ 1870
Extra Strength Tylenol PM Caplets, Vanilla Caplets, Geltabs, Gelcaps and Liquid............ 1875
Extra Strength Tylenol Rapid Release Gels............ 1870
Concentrated Tylenol Infants' Drops Plus Cold & Cough............ 754
Tylenol with Codeine Tablets............ 2391
Tylenol Allergy Multi-Symptom Caplets with Cool Burst and Gelcaps............ 1872
Tylenol Allergy Multi-Symptom Nighttime Caplets with Cool Burst............ 1872
Tylenol Severe Allergy Caplets............ 1872
Tylenol Arthritis Pain Extended Release Caplets and Geltabs............ 1870
Tylenol Chest Congestion Caplets with Cool Burst............ 1872
Tylenol Chest Congestion Liquid with Cool Burst............ 1872
Children's Tylenol Suspension Liquid and Meltaways............ 1878
Children's Tylenol Plus Cold Suspension Liquid............ 1879
Children's Tylenol Plus Cold & Allergy Suspension Liquid............ 1878
Children's Tylenol Plus Cough & Runny Nose Suspension Liquid............ 1879
Children's Tylenol Plus Cough & Sore Throat Suspension Liquid............ 1879
Children's Tylenol Suspension with Flavor Creator............ 1878
Children's Tylenol Plus Flu Suspension Liquid............ 1881
Children's Tylenol Plus Multi-Symptom Cold Suspension Liquid............ 1879
Tylenol Cold Severe Congestion Non-Drowsy Caplets with Cool Burst............ 1874
Tylenol Cold Head Congestion Daytime Caplets with Cool Burst............ 1873
Tylenol Cold Head Congestion Nighttime Caplets with Cool Burst............ 1873
Tylenol Cold Head Congestion Severe Caplets with Cool Burst............ 1873
Tylenol Cold Multi-Symptom Daytime Caplets with Cool Burst and Gelcaps............ 1874
Tylenol Cold Multi-Symptom Daytime Liquid with Citrus Burst............ 1874
Tylenol Cold Multi-Symptom Nighttime Caplets with Cool Burst............ 1874
Tylenol Cold Multi-Symptom Nighttime Liquid with Cool Burst............ 1874
Tylenol Cold Multi-Symptom Severe Caplets with Cool Burst............ 1874
Tylenol Cold Multi-Symptom Severe Daytime Liquid with Citrus Burst............ 1874
Tylenol Cough & Sore Throat Daytime Liquid with Cool Burst............ 1877
Tylenol Cough & Sore Throat Nighttime Liquid with Cool Burst............ 1877
Concentrated Tylenol Infants' Drops............ 1878
Concentrated Tylenol Infants' Drops Plus Cold............ 1879
Concentrated Tylenol Infants' Drops Plus Cold and Cough............ 1879
Jr. Tylenol Meltaways............ 1878
Tylenol Sinus Severe Congestion Caplets with Cool Burst............ 1876
Tylenol Sinus Congestion & Pain Daytime Caplets with Cool Burst and Gelcaps............ 1876
Tylenol Sinus Congestion & Pain Nighttime Caplets with Cool Burst............ 1876
Tylenol Sinus Congestion & Pain Severe Caplets with Cool Burst............ 1876
Tylenol Sore Throat Daytime Liquid with Cool Burst............ 1877
Tylenol Sore Throat Nighttime Liquid with Cool Burst............ 1877
Women's Tylenol Menstrual Relief Caplets............ 1877
Vicks 44M Cough, Cold & Flu Relief Liquid............ 2680
Vicks DayQuil LiquiCaps/Liquid Multi-Symptom Cold/Flu Relief............ 761
Vicks DayQuil Multi-Symptom Cold/Flu Relief LiquiCaps............ 2678
Vicks DayQuil Multi-Symptom Cold/Flu Relief Liquid............ 2678
Vicks NyQuil Multi-Symptom Cold/Flu Relief Liquid............ 2681
Vicks NyQuil Multi-Symptom Cold/Flu Relief LiquiCaps............ 2681
Vicks NyQuil LiquiCaps/Liquid Multi-Symptom Cold/Flu Relief............ 763
Vicodin Tablets............ 535
Vicodin ES Tablets............ 536
Vicodin HP Tablets............ 538
Zicam Maximum Strength Flu Daytime............ 768
Zicam Maximum Strength Flu Nighttime............ 768
Zydone Tablets............ 1139

Alprazolam (Carbamazepine induces hepatic CYP activity; carbamazepine causes, or would be expected to cause, decreased levels of alprazolam). Products include:
Niravam Orally Disintegrating Tablets............ 3092

Aminophylline (Co-administration with CYP3A4 inducers, such as theophylline, has been shown, or that would be expected, to decrease carbamazepine plasma levels; carbamazepine induces hepatic CYP activity; carbamazepine causes, or would be expected to cause decreased levels of theophylline).
No products indexed under this heading.

Amitriptyline Hydrochloride (Since carbamazepine induces hepatic CYP activity, carbamazepine may cause decreased levels of tricyclic antidepressants).
No products indexed under this heading.

Amlodipine Besylate (Since carbamazepine induces hepatic CYP activity, carbamazepine may cause decreased levels of the dihydropyridine calcium channel blockers). Products include:
Caduet Tablets............ 2508
Lotrel Capsules............ 2249
Norvasc Tablets............ 2545

Amoxapine (Since carbamazepine induces hepatic CYP activity, carbamazepine may cause decreased levels of tricyclic antidepressants).
No products indexed under this heading.

Amprenavir (Since carbamazepine induces hepatic CYP activity, carbamazepine may cause decreased levels of protease inhibitors). Products include:
Agenerase Capsules............ 1327
Agenerase Oral Solution............ 1332

Azithromycin Dihydrate (Co-administration with CYP3A4 inhibitors, such as macrolides, inhibits carbamazepine metabolism and has been shown, or would be expected to increase carbamazepine plasma levels).
No products indexed under this heading.

Bepridil Hydrochloride (Since carbamazepine induces hepatic CYP activity, carbamazepine may cause decreased levels of the dihydropyridine calcium channel blockers).
No products indexed under this heading.

Betamethasone Acetate (Since carbamazepine induces hepatic CYP activity, carbamazepine may cause decreased levels of corticosteroids).
No products indexed under this heading.

Betamethasone Sodium Phosphate (Since carbamazepine induces hepatic CYP activity, carbamazepine may cause decreased levels of corticosteroids).
No products indexed under this heading.

Chlorpromazine Hydrochloride (Concurrent use of Thorazine solution and Tegretol Suspension has resulted in an orange rubbery precipitate in stool; Tegretol Suspension should not be administered simultaneously with other liquid medications).
No products indexed under this heading.

Cimetidine (Co-administration with CYP3A4 inhibitors, such as cimetidine, inhibits carbamazepine metabolism and has been shown, or would be expected to increase carbamazepine plasma levels). Products include:
Tagamet HB 200 Tablets............ 664

Cimetidine Hydrochloride (Co-administration with CYP3A4 inhibitors, such as cimetidine inhibits carbamazepine metabolism and has been shown, or would be expected to increase carbamazepine plasma levels).
No products indexed under this heading.

Cisplatin (Co-administration with CYP3A4 inducers, such as cisplatin, has been shown, or that would be expected, to decrease carbamazepine plasma levels).
No products indexed under this heading.

Clarithromycin (Co-administration with CYP3A4 inhibitors, such as macrolides, inhibits carbamazepine metabolism and has been shown, or would be expected to increase carbamazepine plasma levels). Products include:
Biaxin/Biaxin XL............ 402
PREVPAC............ 3284

Clomipramine Hydrochloride (Carbamazepine increases clomipramine plasma levels).
No products indexed under this heading.

Clonazepam (Carbamazepine induces hepatic CYP activity; carbamazepine causes, or would be expected to cause, decreased levels of clonazepam; combination therapy with other anticonvulsant drugs has resulted in alterations in thyroid function). Products include:
Klonopin............ 2778

Clozapine (Carbamazepine induces hepatic CYP activity: carbamazepine causes, or would be expected to cause decreased levels of clozapine). Products include:
Clozaril Tablets............ 2184
FazaClo Orally Disintegrating Tablets............ 551

Cortisone Acetate (Since carbamazepine induces hepatic CYP activity, carbamazepine may cause decreased levels of corticosteroids).
No products indexed under this heading.

Cyclosporine (Since carbamazepine induces hepatic CYP activity, carbamazepine may cause decreased levels of cyclosporine). Products include:
Gengraf Capsules............ 459
Neoral Oral Solution............ 2259
Neoral Soft Gelatin Capsules............ 2259
Restasis Ophthalmic Emulsion............ 575
Sandimmune............ 2275

Danazol (Co-administration with CYP3A4 inhibitors, such as danazol, inhibits carbamazepine metabolism and has been shown, or would be expected to increase carbamazepine plasma levels).
No products indexed under this heading.

Desipramine Hydrochloride (Since carbamazepine induces hepatic CYP activity, carbamazepine may cause decreased levels of tricyclic antidepressants).
No products indexed under this heading.

Desogestrel (Carbamazepine induces hepatic CYP activity; carbamazepine causes, or would be expected to cause, decreased levels of oral contraceptives; breakthrough bleeding has been reported among patients receiving concomitant oral and subdermal contraceptives and their reliability may be adversely affected). Products include:
Mircette Tablets............ 1066

Dexamethasone (Since carbamazepine induces hepatic CYP activity, carbamazepine may cause decreased levels of corticosteroids). Products include:
Ciprodex Otic Suspension............ 559
Decadron Tablets............ 1951
TobraDex Ophthalmic Ointment............ 562
TobraDex Ophthalmic Suspension............ 563

Dexamethasone Acetate (Since carbamazepine induces hepatic CYP activity, carbamazepine may cause decreased levels of corticosteroids).
No products indexed under this heading.

Dexamethasone Sodium Phosphate (Since carbamazepine induces hepatic CYP activity, carbamazepine may cause decreased levels of corticosteroids).

No products indexed under this heading.

Dicumarol (Carbamazepine induces hepatic CYP activity; carbamazepine causes, or would be expected to cause, decreased levels of dicumarol).

No products indexed under this heading.

Diltiazem Hydrochloride (Co-administration with CYP3A4 inhibitors, such as diltiazem, inhibits carbamazepine metabolism and has been shown, or would be expected to increase carbamazepine plasma levels). Products include:

Cardizem LA Extended Release Tablets............................. 1728
Tiazac Capsules 1201

Dirithromycin (Co-administration with CYP3A4 inhibitors, such as macrolides, inhibits carbamazepine metabolism and has been shown, or would be expected to increase carbamazepine plasma levels).

No products indexed under this heading.

Divalproex Sodium (Co-administration with CYP3A4 inhibitors, such as valproate, inhibits carbamazepine metabolism and has been shown, or would be expected to increase carbamazepine (active 10, 11-epoxide) plasma levels; carbamazepine causes, or would be expected to cause, decreased levels of valproate; combination therapy with other anticonvulsant drugs has resulted in alterations in thyroid function). Products include:

Depakote Sprinkle Capsules 422
Depakote Tablets 427
Depakote ER Tablets 434

Doxepin Hydrochloride (Since carbamazepine induces hepatic CYP activity, carbamazepine may cause decreased levels of tricyclic antidepressants).

No products indexed under this heading.

Doxorubicin Hydrochloride (Co-administration with CYP3A4 inducers, such as doxorubicin, has been shown, or that would be expected, to decrease carbamazepine plasma levels).

No products indexed under this heading.

Doxycycline Calcium (Carbamazepine induces hepatic CYP activity; carbamazepine causes, or would be expected to cause, decreased levels of doxycycline).

No products indexed under this heading.

Doxycycline Hyclate (Carbamazepine induces hepatic CYP activity; carbamazepine causes, or would be expected to cause, decreased levels of doxycycline).

No products indexed under this heading.

Doxycycline Monohydrate (Carbamazepine induces hepatic CYP activity; carbamazepine causes, or would be expected to cause, decreased levels of doxycycline). Products include:

Oracea Capsules 1000

Dyphylline (Co-administration with CYP3A4 inducers, such as theophylline, has been shown, or that would be expected, to decrease carbamazepine plasma levels; carbamazepine induces hepatic CYP activity; carbamazepine causes, or would be expected to cause decreased levels of theophylline).

No products indexed under this heading.

Erythromycin (Co-administration with CYP3A4 inhibitors, such as erythromycin, inhibits carbamazepine metabolism and has been shown, or would be expected to increase carbamazepine plasma levels). Products include:

Ery-Tab Tablets 449
Erythromycin Base Filmtab Tablets ... 455
Erythromycin Delayed-Release Capsules, USP 457
PCE Dispertab Tablets 515

Erythromycin Estolate (Co-administration with CYP3A4 inhibitors, such as erythromycin, inhibits carbamazepine metabolism and has been shown, or would be expected to increase carbamazepine plasma levels).

No products indexed under this heading.

Erythromycin Ethylsuccinate (Co-administration with CYP3A4 inhibitors, such as erythromycin, inhibits carbamazepine metabolism and has been shown, or would be expected to increase carbamazepine plasma levels). Products include:

E.E.S. ... 451
EryPed ... 447

Erythromycin Gluceptate (Co-administration with CYP3A4 inhibitors, such as erythromycin, inhibits carbamazepine metabolism and has been shown, or would be expected to increase carbamazepine plasma levels).

No products indexed under this heading.

Erythromycin Lactobionate (Co-administration with CYP3A4 inhibitors, such as erythromycin, inhibits carbamazepine metabolism and has been shown, or would be expected to increase carbamazepine plasma levels).

No products indexed under this heading.

Erythromycin Stearate (Co-administration with CYP3A4 inhibitors, such as erythromycin, inhibits carbamazepine metabolism and has been shown, or would be expected to increase carbamazepine plasma levels). Products include:

Erythrocin Stearate Filmtab Tablets ... 453

Ethinyl Estradiol (Carbamazepine induces hepatic CYP activity; carbamazepine causes, or would be expected to cause, decreased levels of oral contraceptives; breakthrough bleeding has been reported among patients receiving concomitant oral and subdermal contraceptives and their reliability may be adversely affected). Products include:

Mircette Tablets 1066
NuvaRing 2340
Ortho-Cyclen/Ortho Tri-Cyclen 2429
Ortho Evra Transdermal System 2417
Ortho Tri-Cyclen Lo Tablets 2436
Seasonique Tablets 1077
Yasmin 28 Tablets 796
Yaz Tablets 803

Ethosuximide (Carbamazepine induces hepatic CYP activity; carbamazepine causes, or would be expected to cause, decreased levels of ethosuximide; combination therapy with other anticonvulsant drugs has resulted in alterations in thyroid function).

No products indexed under this heading.

Ethotoin (Combination therapy with other anticonvulsant drugs has resulted in alterations in thyroid function. Since carbamazepine induces hepatic CYP activity, carbamazepine may cause decreased levels of zonisamide).

No products indexed under this heading.

Ethynodiol Diacetate (Carbamazepine induces hepatic CYP activity; carbamazepine causes, or would be expected to cause, decreased levels of oral contraceptives; breakthrough bleeding has been reported among patients receiving concomitant oral and subdermal contraceptives and their reliability may be adversely affected).

No products indexed under this heading.

Felbamate (Co-administration with CYP3A4 inducers, such as felbamate, has been shown, or that would be expected, to decrease carbamazepine and increased levels of the 10, 11-epoxide plasma levels; combination therapy with other anticonvulsant drugs has resulted in alterations in thyroid function).

No products indexed under this heading.

Felodipine (Since carbamazepine induces hepatic CYP activity, carbamazepine may cause decreased levels of the dihydropyridine calcium channel blockers).

No products indexed under this heading.

Fludrocortisone Acetate (Since carbamazepine induces hepatic CYP activity, carbamazepine may cause decreased levels of corticosteroids).

No products indexed under this heading.

Fluoxetine Hydrochloride (Co-administration with CYP3A4 inhibitors, such as fluoxetine, inhibits carbamazepine metabolism and has been shown, or would be expected to increase carbamazepine plasma levels). Products include:

Prozac Pulvules and Liquid 1801
Symbyax Capsules 1819

Fosphenytoin (Combination therapy with other anticonvulsant drugs has resulted in alterations in thyroid function. Since carbamazepine induces hepatic CYP activity, carbamazepine may cause decreased levels of zonisamide).

No products indexed under this heading.

Fosphenytoin Sodium (Co-administration with CYP3A4 inducers, such as phenytoin, has been shown, or that would be expected, to decrease carbamazepine plasma levels; carbamazepine increases phenytoin plasma levels; carbamazepine induces hepatic CYP activity; carbamazepine causes, or would be expected to cause, decreased levels of phenytoin; combination therapy with other anticonvulsant drugs has resulted in alterations in thyroid

function).

No products indexed under this heading.

Gabapentin (Combination therapy with other anticonvulsant drugs has resulted in alterations in thyroid function. Since carbamazepine induces hepatic CYP activity, carbamazepine may cause decreased levels of zonisamide). Products include:

Neurontin Capsules 2487
Neurontin Oral Solution 2487
Neurontin Tablets 2487

Haloperidol (Carbamazepine induces hepatic CYP activity; carbamazepine causes, or would be expected to cause, decreased levels of haloperidol).

No products indexed under this heading.

Haloperidol Decanoate (Carbamazepine induces hepatic CYP activity; carbamazepine causes, or would be expected to cause, decreased levels of haloperidol).

No products indexed under this heading.

Hydrocortisone (Since carbamazepine induces hepatic CYP activity, carbamazepine may cause decreased levels of corticosteroids). Products include:

Colocort Rectal Suspension, USP (Retention) 100 mg/60 mL........... 2476
Hydrocortone Tablets 1989
Preparation H Hydrocortisone Cream ... ▣646

Hydrocortisone Acetate (Since carbamazepine induces hepatic CYP activity, carbamazepine may cause decreased levels of corticosteroids). Products include:

Analpram-HC 1159
Pramosone 1161
ProctoFoam-HC 3099

Hydrocortisone Sodium Phosphate (Since carbamazepine induces hepatic CYP activity, carbamazepine may cause decreased levels of corticosteroids).

No products indexed under this heading.

Hydrocortisone Sodium Succinate (Since carbamazepine induces hepatic CYP activity, carbamazepine may cause decreased levels of corticosteroids).

No products indexed under this heading.

Imipramine Hydrochloride (Since carbamazepine induces hepatic CYP activity, carbamazepine may cause decreased levels of tricyclic antidepressants).

No products indexed under this heading.

Imipramine Pamoate (Since carbamazepine induces hepatic CYP activity, carbamazepine may cause decreased levels of tricyclic antidepressants).

No products indexed under this heading.

Indinavir Sulfate (Since carbamazepine induces hepatic CYP activity, carbamazepine may cause decreased levels of protease inhibitors). Products include:

Crixivan Capsules 1940

Isocarboxazid (Because of the relationship of carbamazepine to other tricyclic compounds, on theoretical grounds, co-administration with MAO inhibitors is contraindicated).

No products indexed under this heading.

Isoniazid (Co-administration with CYP3A4 inhibitors, such as isoniazid, inhibits carbamazepine metabolism and has been shown, or would be expected to increase carbamazepine plasma levels).
No products indexed under this heading.

Isradipine (Since carbamazepine induces hepatic CYP activity, carbamazepine may cause decreased levels of the dihydropyridine calcium channel blockers). Products include:
DynaCirc CR Tablets 2721

Itraconazole (Co-administration with CYP3A4 inhibitors, such as itraconazole, inhibits carbamazepine metabolism and has been shown, or would be expected to increase carbamazepine plasma levels. Since carbamazepine induces hepatic CYP activity, carbamazepine may cause decreased levels of itraconazole).
No products indexed under this heading.

Ketoconazole (Co-administration with CYP3A4 inhibitors, such as ketoconazole, inhibits carbamazepine metabolism and has been shown, or would be expected to increase carbamazepine plasma levels). Products include:
Nizoral A-D Shampoo, 1% 1868

Lamotrigine (Carbamazepine induces hepatic CYP activity; carbamazepine causes, or would be expected to cause, decreased levels of lamotrigine; combination therapy with other anticonvulsant drugs has resulted in alterations in thyroid function). Products include:
Lamictal 1481

Levetiracetam (Combination therapy with other anticonvulsant drugs has resulted in alterations in thyroid function. Since carbamazepine induces hepatic CYP activity, carbamazepine may cause decreased levels of zonisamide). Products include:
Keppra Injection 3320
Keppra Oral Solution 3314
Keppra Tablets 3314

Levonorgestrel (Carbamazepine induces hepatic CYP activity; carbamazepine causes, or would be expected to cause, decreased levels of oral contraceptives; breakthrough bleeding has been reported among patients receiving concomitant oral and subdermal contraceptives and their reliability may be adversely affected). Products include:
Climara Pro Transdermal System 776
Mirena Intrauterine System 787
Plan B Tablets 1076
Seasonique Tablets 1077

Levothyroxine Sodium (Since carbamazepine induces hepatic CYP activity, carbamazepine may cause decreased levels of levothyroxine). Products include:
Levothroid Tablets 1186
Levoxyl Tablets 1712
Synthroid Tablets 520
Westhroid Tablets 3403

Lithium (Co-administration may increase the risk of nuerotoxic side effects).
No products indexed under this heading.

Lithium Carbonate (Co-administration may increase the risk of nuerotoxic side effects). Products include:
Lithobid Tablets 1692

Lithium Citrate (Co-administration may increase the risk of nuerotoxic side effects).
No products indexed under this heading.

Lopinavir (Since carbamazepine induces hepatic CYP activity, carbamazepine may cause decreased levels of protease inhibitors). Products include:
Kaletra 476

Loratadine (Co-administration with CYP3A4 inhibitors, such as loratadine, inhibits carbamazepine metabolism and has been shown, or would be expected to increase carbamazepine plasma levels). Products include:
Alavert Allergy & Sinus D-12 Hour Tablets 771
Alavert 771
Children's Claritin Allergy Oral Solution 771
Claritin Non-Drowsy 24 Hour Tablets 772
Claritin Reditabs 24 Hour Non-Drowsy Tablets 772
Claritin-D Non-Drowsy 12 Hour Tablets 772
Claritin-D Non-Drowsy 24 Hour Tablets 772

Maprotiline Hydrochloride (Since carbamazepine induces hepatic CYP activity, carbamazepine may cause decreased levels of tricyclic antidepressants).
No products indexed under this heading.

Mephenytoin (Combination therapy with other anticonvulsant drugs has resulted in alterations in thyroid function. Since carbamazepine induces hepatic CYP activity, carbamazepine may cause decreased levels of zonisamide).
No products indexed under this heading.

Mestranol (Carbamazepine induces hepatic CYP activity; carbamazepine causes, or would be expected to cause, decreased levels of oral contraceptives; breakthrough bleeding has been reported among patients receiving concomitant oral and subdermal contraceptives and their reliability may be adversely affected).
No products indexed under this heading.

Methadone Hydrochloride (Since carbamazepine induces hepatic CYP activity, carbamazepine may cause decreased levels of methadone).
No products indexed under this heading.

Methsuximide (Carbamazepine induces hepatic CYP activity; carbamazepine causes, or would be expected to cause, decreased levels of methsuximide; combination therapy with other anticonvulsant drugs has resulted in alterations in thyroid function).
No products indexed under this heading.

Methylprednisolone Acetate (Since carbamazepine induces hepatic CYP activity, carbamazepine may cause decreased levels of corticosteroids). Products include:
Depo-Medrol Injectable Suspension 2617
Depo-Medrol Single-Dose Vial 2619

Methylprednisolone Sodium Succinate (Since carbamazepine induces hepatic CYP activity, carbamazepine may cause decreased levels of corticosteroids).
No products indexed under this heading.

Mibefradil Dihydrochloride (Since carbamazepine induces hepatic CYP activity, carbamazepine may cause decreased levels of the dihydropyridine calcium channel blockers).
No products indexed under this heading.

Midazolam Hydrochloride (Since carbamazepine induces hepatic CYP activity, carbamazepine may cause decreased levels of midazolam).
No products indexed under this heading.

Moclobemide (Because of the relationship of carbamazepine to other tricyclic compounds, on theoretical grounds, co-administration with MAO inhibitors is contraindicated).
No products indexed under this heading.

Nelfinavir Mesylate (Since carbamazepine induces hepatic CYP activity, carbamazepine may cause decreased levels of protease inhibitors). Products include:
Viracept 2577

Niacinamide (Co-administration with CYP3A4 inhibitors, such as niacinamide, inhibits carbamazepine metabolism and has been shown, or would be expected to increase carbamazepine plasma levels).
No products indexed under this heading.

Nicardipine Hydrochloride (Since carbamazepine induces hepatic CYP activity, carbamazepine may cause decreased levels of the dihydropyridine calcium channel blockers). Products include:
Cardene I.V. 2497

Nicotinamide (Co-administration with CYP3A4 inhibitors, such as nicotinamide, inhibits carbamazepine metabolism and has been shown, or would be expected to increase carbamazepine plasma levels). Products include:
Nicomide Tablets 1088

Nifedipine (Since carbamazepine induces hepatic CYP activity, carbamazepine may cause decreased levels of the dihydropyridine calcium channel blockers). Products include:
Adalat CC Tablets 2964

Nimodipine (Since carbamazepine induces hepatic CYP activity, carbamazepine may cause decreased levels of the dihydropyridine calcium channel blockers). Products include:
Nimotop Capsules 749

Nisoldipine (Since carbamazepine induces hepatic CYP activity, carbamazepine may cause decreased levels of the dihydropyridine calcium channel blockers). Products include:
Sular Tablets 3122

Norethindrone (Carbamazepine induces hepatic CYP activity; carbamazepine causes, or would be expected to cause, decreased levels of oral contraceptives; breakthrough bleeding has been reported among patients receiving concomitant oral and subdermal contraceptives and their reliability may be adversely affected). Products include:
Ortho Micronor Tablets 2426

Norethynodrel (Carbamazepine induces hepatic CYP activity; carbamazepine causes, or would be expected to cause, decreased levels of oral contraceptives; breakthrough bleeding has been reported among patients receiving concomitant oral and subdermal contraceptives and their reliability may be adversely affected).
No products indexed under this heading.

Norgestimate (Carbamazepine induces hepatic CYP activity; carbamazepine causes, or would be expected to cause, decreased levels of oral contraceptives; breakthrough bleeding has been reported among patients receiving concomitant oral and subdermal contraceptives and their reliability may be adversely affected). Products include:
Ortho-Cyclen/Ortho Tri-Cyclen 2429
Ortho Tri-Cyclen Lo Tablets 2436

Norgestrel (Carbamazepine induces hepatic CYP activity; carbamazepine causes, or would be expected to cause, decreased levels of oral contraceptives; breakthrough bleeding has been reported among patients receiving concomitant oral and subdermal contraceptives and their reliability may be adversely affected).
No products indexed under this heading.

Nortriptyline Hydrochloride (Since carbamazepine induces hepatic CYP activity, carbamazepine may cause decreased levels of tricyclic antidepressants).
No products indexed under this heading.

Olanzapine (Since carbamazepine induces hepatic CYP activity, carbamazepine may cause decreased levels of olanzapine). Products include:
Symbyax Capsules 1819
Zyprexa Tablets 1830
Zyprexa IntraMuscular 1830
Zyprexa ZYDIS Orally Disintegrating Tablets 1830

Oxcarbazepine (Combination therapy with other anticonvulsant drugs has resulted in alterations in thyroid function. Since carbamazepine induces hepatic CYP activity, carbamazepine may cause decreased levels of oxcarbazepine). Products include:
Trileptal Tablets 2300
Trileptal Oral Suspension 2300

Paramethadione (Combination therapy with other anticonvulsant drugs has resulted in alterations in thyroid function. Since carbamazepine induces hepatic CYP activity, carbamazepine may cause decreased levels of zonisamide).
No products indexed under this heading.

Pargyline Hydrochloride (Because of the relationship of carbamazepine to other tricyclic compounds, on theoretical grounds, co-administration with MAO inhibitors is contraindicated).
No products indexed under this heading.

Phenacemide (Combination therapy with other anticonvulsant drugs has resulted in alterations in thyroid function. Since carbamazepine induces hepatic CYP activity, carbamazepine may cause decreased levels of zonisamide).
No products indexed under this heading.

Phenelzine Sulfate (Because of the relationship of carbamazepine to other tricyclic compounds, on theoretical grounds, co-administration with MAO inhibitors is contraindicated).
No products indexed under this heading.

Phenobarbital (Co-administration with CYP3A4 inducers, such as phenobarbital, has been shown, or that would be expected, to decrease carbamazepine plasma levels; carbamezepine increases phenobarbital plasma levels; combination therapy with other anticonvulsant drugs has resulted in alterations of thyroid function). Products include:
Donnatal Extentabs 2493

Phensuximide (Carbamazepine induces hepatic CYP activity; carbamazepine causes, or would be expected to cause, decreased levels of phensuximide; combination therapy with other anticonvulsant drugs has resulted in alterations in thyroid function).
No products indexed under this heading.

Phenytoin (Co-administration with CYP3A4 inducers, such as phenytoin, has been shown, or that would be expected, to decrease carbamazepine plasma levels; carbamazepine increases phenytoin plasma levels; carbamazepine induces hepatic CYP activity; carbamazepine causes, or would be expected to cause, decreased levels of phenytoin; combination therapy with other anticonvulsant drugs has resulted in alterations in thyroid function).
No products indexed under this heading.

Phenytoin Sodium (Co-administration with CYP3A4 inducers, such as phenytoin, has been shown, or that would be expected, to decrease carbamazepine plasma levels; carbamazepine increases phenytoin plasma levels; carbamazepine induces hepatic CYP activity; carbamazepine causes, or would be expected to cause, decreased levels of phenytoin; combination therapy with other anticonvulsant drugs has resulted in alterations in thyroid function). Products include:
Phenytek Capsules 2160

Praziquantel (Since carbamazepine induces hepatic CYP activity, carbamazepine may cause decreased levels of praziquantel). Products include:
Biltricide Tablets 2976

Prednisolone Acetate (Since carbamazepine induces hepatic CYP activity, carbamazepine may cause decreased levels of corticosteroids). Products include:
Blephamide Ophthalmic Ointment 568
Blephamide Ophthalmic Suspension 569
Poly-Pred Ophthalmic Suspension .... ⊙233
Pred Forte Ophthalmic Suspension .... ⊙235
Pred Mild Ophthalmic Suspension .... ⊙238
Pred-G Ophthalmic Ointment .... ⊙237
Pred-G Ophthalmic Suspension .... ⊙236

Prednisolone Sodium Phosphate (Since carbamazepine induces hepatic CYP activity, carbamazepine may cause decreased levels of corticosteroids).
No products indexed under this heading.

Prednisolone Tebutate (Since carbamazepine induces hepatic CYP activity, carbamazepine may cause decreased levels of corticosteroids).
No products indexed under this heading.

Prednisone (Since carbamazepine induces hepatic CYP activity, carbamazepine may cause decreased levels of corticosteroids).
No products indexed under this heading.

Primidone (Co-administration with CYP3A4 inducers, such as primidone, has been shown, or that would be expected, to decrease carbamazepine plasma levels; carbamazepine increases primidone plasma levels; combination therapy with other anticonvulsant drugs has resulted in alterations in thyroid function).
No products indexed under this heading.

Procarbazine Hydrochloride (Because of the relationship of carbamazepine to other tricyclic compounds, on theoretical grounds, co-administration with MAO inhibitors is contraindicated). Products include:
Matulane Capsules 3191

Propoxyphene Hydrochloride (Co-administration with CYP3A4 inhibitors, such as propoxyphene, inhibits carbamazepine metabolism and has been shown, or would be expected to increase carbamazepine plasma levels).
No products indexed under this heading.

Propoxyphene Napsylate (Co-administration with CYP3A4 inhibitors, such as propoxyphene, inhibits carbamazepine metabolism and has been shown, or would be expected to increase carbamazepine plasma levels).
No products indexed under this heading.

Protriptyline Hydrochloride (Since carbamazepine induces hepatic CYP activity, carbamazepine may cause decreased levels of tricyclic antidepressants).
No products indexed under this heading.

Rifampin (Co-administration with CYP3A4 inducers, such as rifampin, has been shown, or that would be expected, to decrease carbamazepine plasma levels).
No products indexed under this heading.

Risperidone (Since carbamazepine induces hepatic CYP activity, carbamazepine may cause decreased levels of risperidone). Products include:
Risperdal 1676
Risperdal Consta Long-Acting Injection 1682
Risperdal M-Tab Orally Disintegrating Tablets 1676

Ritonavir (Since carbamazepine induces hepatic CYP activity, carbamazepine may cause decreased levels of protease inhibitors). Products include:
Kaletra 476
Norvir 503

Saquinavir (Since carbamazepine induces hepatic CYP activity, carbamazepine may cause decreased levels of protease inhibitors).
No products indexed under this heading.

Saquinavir Mesylate (Since carbamazepine induces hepatic CYP activity, carbamazepine may cause decreased levels of protease inhibitors). Products include:
Invirase 2772

Selegiline Hydrochloride (Because of the relationship of carbamazepine to other tricyclic compounds, on theoretical grounds, co-administration with MAO inhibitors is contraindicated). Products include:
Eldepryl Capsules 3208
Zelapar Tablets 3372

Terfenadine (Co-administration with CYP3A4 inhibitors, such as terfenadine, inhibits carbamazepine metabolism and has been shown, or would be expected to increase carbamazepine plasma levels).
No products indexed under this heading.

Theophylline (Co-administration with CYP3A4 inducers, such as theophylline, has been shown, or that would be expected, to decrease carbamazepine plasma levels; carbamazepine induces hepatic CYP activity; carbamazepine causes, or would be expected to cause decreased levels of theophylline).
No products indexed under this heading.

Theophylline Anhydrous (Co-administration with CYP3A4 inducers, such as theophylline, has been shown, or that would be expected, to decrease carbamazepine plasma levels; carbamazepine induces hepatic CYP activity; carbamazepine causes, or would be expected to cause decreased levels of theophylline). Products include:
Uniphyl Tablets 2710

Theophylline Calcium Salicylate (Co-administration with CYP3A4 inducers, such as theophylline, has been shown, or that would be expected, to decrease carbamazepine plasma levels; carbamazepine induces hepatic CYP activity; carbamazepine causes, or would be expected to cause decreased levels of theophylline).
No products indexed under this heading.

Theophylline Dihydroxypropyl (Glyceryl) (Co-administration with CYP3A4 inducers, such as theophylline, has been shown, or that would be expected, to decrease carbamazepine plasma levels; carbamazepine induces hepatic CYP activity; carbamazepine causes, or would be expected to cause decreased levels of theophylline).
No products indexed under this heading.

Theophylline Ethylenediamine (Co-administration with CYP3A4 inducers, such as theophylline, has been shown, or that would be expected, to decrease carbamazepine plasma levels; carbamazepine induces hepatic CYP activity; carbamazepine causes, or would be expected to cause decreased levels of theophylline).
No products indexed under this heading.

Theophylline Sodium Glycinate (Co-administration with CYP3A4 inducers, such as theophylline, has been shown, or that would be expected, to decrease carbamazepine plasma levels; carbamazepine induces hepatic CYP activity; carbamazepine causes, or would be expected to cause decreased levels of theophylline).
No products indexed under this heading.

Thioridazine Hydrochloride (Concurrent use of Mellaril Solution and Tegretol Suspension has resulted in an orange rubbery precipitate in stool; Tegretol Suspension should not be administered simultaneously with other liquid medications). Products include:
Thioridazine Hydrochloride Tablets 2163

Tiagabine Hydrochloride (Carbamazepine induces hepatic CYP activity; carbamazepine causes, or would be expected to cause, decreased levels of tiagabine; combination therapy with other anticonvulsant drugs has resulted in alterations in thyroid function). Products include:
Gabitril Tablets 984

Topiramate (Carbamazepine induces hepatic CYP activity; carbamazepine causes, or would be expected to cause, decreased levels of topiramate; combination therapy with other anticonvulsant drugs has resulted in alterations in thyroid function). Products include:
Topamax Sprinkle Capsules 2404
Topamax Tablets 2404

Tramadol Hydrochloride (Since carbamazepine induces hepatic CYP activity, carbamazepine may cause decreased levels of tramadol). Products include:
Ultram ER Tablets 2392

Tranylcypromine Sulfate (Because of the relationship of carbamazepine to other tricyclic compounds, on theoretical grounds, co-administration with MAO inhibitors is contraindicated). Products include:
Parnate Tablets 1527

Triamcinolone (Since carbamazepine induces hepatic CYP activity, carbamazepine may cause decreased levels of corticosteroids).
No products indexed under this heading.

Triamcinolone Acetonide (Since carbamazepine induces hepatic CYP activity, carbamazepine may cause decreased levels of corticosteroids). Products include:
Azmacort Inhalation Aerosol 1726
Nasacort AQ Nasal Spray 2922

Triamcinolone Diacetate (Since carbamazepine induces hepatic CYP activity, carbamazepine may cause decreased levels of corticosteroids).
No products indexed under this heading.

Triamcinolone Hexacetonide (Since carbamazepine induces hepatic CYP activity, carbamazepine may cause decreased levels of corticosteroids).
No products indexed under this heading.

Trimethadione (Combination therapy with other anticonvulsant drugs has resulted in alterations in thyroid function. Since carbamazepine induces hepatic CYP activity, carbamazepine may cause decreased levels of zonisamide).
No products indexed under this heading.

Trimipramine Maleate (Since carbamazepine induces hepatic CYP activity, carbamazepine may cause decreased levels of tricyclic antidepressants).
No products indexed under this heading.

Troleandomycin (Co-administration with CYP3A4 inhibitors, such as macrolides, inhibits carbamazepine metabolism and has been shown, or would be expected to increase carbamazepine plasma levels).
No products indexed under this heading.

Valproate Sodium (Co-administration with CYP3A4 inhibitors, such as valproate, inhibits carbamazepine metabolism and has been shown, or would be expected to increase carbamazepine (active 10, 11-epoxide) plasma levels; carbamazepine causes, or would be expected to cause, decreased levels of valproate; combination therapy with other anticonvulsant drugs has resulted in alterations in thyroid function). Products include:
Depacon Injection 412

Valproic Acid (Co-administration with CYP3A4 inhibitors, such as valproate, inhibits carbamazepine metabolism and has been shown, or would be expected to increase carbamazepine (active 10, 11-epoxide) plasma levels; carbamazepine causes, or would be expected to cause, decreased levels of valproate; combination therapy with other anticonvulsant drugs has resulted in alterations in thyroid function). Products include:
Depakene 417

Verapamil Hydrochloride (Co-administration with CYP3A4 inhibitors, such as verapamil, inhibits carbamazepine metabolism and has been shown, or would be expected to increase carbamazepine plasma levels). Products include:
Covera-HS Tablets 3139
Tarka Tablets 524
Verelan PM Extended-Release Capsules, Controlled-Onset 3106

Warfarin Sodium (Carbamazepine induces hepatic CYP activity; carbamazepine causes, or would be expected to cause, decreased levels of warfarin). Products include:
Coumadin for Injection 898
Coumadin Tablets 898

Zonisamide (Combination therapy with other anticonvulsant drugs has resulted in alterations in thyroid function. Since carbamazepine induces hepatic CYP activity, carbamazepine may cause decreased levels of zonisamide). Products include:
Zonegran Capsules 1101

TEMODAR CAPSULES

(Temozolomide) 3073
May interact with valproate and certain other agents. Compounds in these categories include:

Divalproex Sodium (Co-administration with valproic acid decreases oral clearance of temozolomide by about 5%; the clinical implication of this effect is not known). Products include:
Depakote Sprinkle Capsules 422
Depakote Tablets 427
Depakote ER Tablets 434

Valproate Sodium (Co-administration with valproic acid decreases oral clearance of temozolomide by about 5%; the clinical implication of this effect is not known). Products include:
Depacon Injection 412

Valproic Acid (Co-administration with valproic acid decreases oral clearance of temozolomide by about 5%; the clinical implication of this effect is not known). Products include:
Depakene 417

Food Interactions

Food, unspecified (Co-administration with a modified high-fat breakfast has resulted in decrease in mean plasma concentration and AUC by 32% and 9%, respectively, and 2-fold increase in Tmax).

TEMOVATE CREAM

(Clobetasol Propionate) 2668
None cited in PDR database.

TEMOVATE GEL

(Clobetasol Propionate) 2669
None cited in PDR database.

TEMOVATE OINTMENT

(Clobetasol Propionate) 2668
None cited in PDR database.

TEMOVATE SCALP APPLICATION

(Clobetasol Propionate) 2670
None cited in PDR database.

TEMOVATE E EMOLLIENT

(Clobetasol Propionate) 2671
None cited in PDR database.

TEQUIN INJECTION

(Gatifloxacin) 938
See Tequin Tablets

TEQUIN INJECTION IN 5% DEXTROSE

(Gatifloxacin) 938
See Tequin Tablets

TEQUIN TABLETS

(Gatifloxacin) 938
May interact with corticosteroids, erythromycin, oral hypoglycemic agents, insulin, iron containing oral preparations, magnesium-containing antacids, non-steroidal anti-inflammatory agents, psychotropics, quinidine, tricyclic antidepressants, and certain other agents. Compounds in these categories include:

Acarbose (During the postmarketing period, co-administration has resulted in hypoglycemic episodes, in some cases severe). Products include:
Precose Tablets 751

Alprazolam (Gatifloxacin may have the potential to prolong the QTc interval; co-administration with drugs known to prolong QT interval should be avoided). Products include:
Niravam Orally Disintegrating Tablets 3092

Aluminum Hydroxide (Systemic exposure to Tequin Tablets is reduced by co-administration of Tequin Tablets with antacids containing aluminum salts; Tequin Tablets can be administered 4 hours before the administration of antacids). Products include:
Gaviscon Regular Strength Liquid 658
Gaviscon Regular Strength Tablets 658
Gaviscon Extra Strength Liquid 658
Gaviscon Extra Strength Tablets 658
Maalox Regular Strength Antacid/Antigas Liquid 2175
Maalox Max Maximum Strength Antacid/Anti-Gas Liquid 2176

Amiodarone Hydrochloride (Gatifloxacin may have the potential to prolong the QTc interval; co-administration with drugs known to prolong QT interval should be avoided).
No products indexed under this heading.

Amitriptyline Hydrochloride (Gatifloxacin may have the potential to prolong the QTc interval; co-administration with drugs known to prolong QT interval should be avoided).
No products indexed under this heading.

Amoxapine (Gatifloxacin may have the potential to prolong the QTc interval; co-administration with drugs known to prolong QT interval should be avoided).
No products indexed under this heading.

Arsenic Trioxide (Gatifloxacin may have the potential to prolong the QTc interval; co-administration with drugs known to prolong QT interval should be avoided). Products include:
Trisenox Injection 993

Betamethasone Acetate (Post-marketing surveillance reports indicate that this risk may be increased in patients receiving concomitant corticosteroids, especially the elderly).
No products indexed under this heading.

Betamethasone Sodium Phosphate (Post-marketing surveillance reports indicate that this risk may be increased in patients receiving concomitant corticosteroids, especially the elderly).
No products indexed under this heading.

Buspirone Hydrochloride (Gatifloxacin may have the potential to prolong the QTc interval; co-administration with drugs known to prolong QT interval should be avoided).
No products indexed under this heading.

Celecoxib (Co-administration of non-steroidal anti-inflammatory agents with quinolones may increase the risks of CNS stimulation and convulsions; these events have not been observed with gatifloxacin in preclinical and clinical trials). Products include:
Celebrex Capsules 3134

Chlordiazepoxide (Gatifloxacin may have the potential to prolong the QTc interval; co-administration with drugs known to prolong QT interval should be avoided).
No products indexed under this heading.

Chlordiazepoxide Hydrochloride (Gatifloxacin may have the potential to prolong the QTc interval; co-administration with drugs known to prolong QT interval should be avoided). Products include:
Librium Capsules 3347

Chlorpromazine (Gatifloxacin may have the potential to prolong the QTc interval; co-administration with drugs known to prolong QT interval should be avoided).
No products indexed under this heading.

Chlorpromazine Hydrochloride (Gatifloxacin may have the potential to prolong the QTc interval; co-administration with drugs known to prolong QT interval should be avoided).
No products indexed under this heading.

Chlorpropamide (During the post-marketing period, co-administration has resulted in hypoglycemic episodes, in some cases severe).
No products indexed under this heading.

Chlorprothixene (Gatifloxacin may have the potential to prolong the QTc interval; co-administration with drugs known to prolong QT interval should be avoided).
No products indexed under this heading.

Chlorprothixene Hydrochloride (Gatifloxacin may have the potential to prolong the QTc interval; co-administration with drugs known to prolong QT interval should be avoided).
No products indexed under this heading.

Cisapride (Gatifloxacin may have the potential to prolong the QTc interval; co-administration with drugs known to prolong QT interval should be avoided).
No products indexed under this heading.

Clomipramine Hydrochloride (Gatifloxacin may have the potential to prolong the QTc interval; co-administration with drugs known to prolong QT interval should be avoided).
No products indexed under this heading.

Clorazepate Dipotassium (Gatifloxacin may have the potential to prolong the QTc interval; co-administration with drugs known to prolong QT interval should be avoided). Products include:
Tranxene 2474

Clozapine (Gatifloxacin may have the potential to prolong the QTc interval; co-administration with drugs known to prolong QT interval should be avoided). Products include:
Clozaril Tablets 2184
FazaClo Orally Disintegrating Tablets 551

Cortisone Acetate (Post-marketing surveillance reports indicate that this risk may be increased in patients receiving concomitant corticosteroids, especially the elderly).
No products indexed under this heading.

Desipramine Hydrochloride (Gatifloxacin may have the potential to prolong the QTc interval; co-administration with drugs known to prolong QT interval should be avoided).
No products indexed under this heading.

Dexamethasone (Post-marketing surveillance reports indicate that this risk may be increased in patients receiving concomitant corticosteroids, especially the elderly). Products include:

- Ciprodex Otic Suspension 559
- Decadron Tablets 1951
- TobraDex Ophthalmic Ointment 562
- TobraDex Ophthalmic Suspension ... 563

Dexamethasone Acetate (Post-marketing surveillance reports indicate that this risk may be increased in patients receiving concomitant corticosteroids, especially the elderly).

No products indexed under this heading.

Dexamethasone Sodium Phosphate (Post-marketing surveillance reports indicate that this risk may be increased in patients receiving concomitant corticosteroids, especially the elderly).

No products indexed under this heading.

Diazepam (Gatifloxacin may have the potential to prolong the QTc interval; co-administration with drugs known to prolong QT interval should be avoided). Products include:

- Diastat Rectal Delivery System 3343
- Valium Tablets 2819

Diclofenac Potassium (Co-administration of non-steroidal anti-inflammatory agents with quinolones may increase the risks of CNS stimulation and convulsions; these events have not been observed with gatifloxacin in pre-clinical and clinical trials).

No products indexed under this heading.

Diclofenac Sodium (Co-administration of non-steroidal anti-inflammatory agents with quinolones may increase the risks of CNS stimulation and convulsions; these events have not been observed with gatifloxacin in pre-clinical and clinical trials). Products include:

- Arthrotec Tablets 3129
- Voltaren Ophthalmic Solution 2309
- Voltaren Tablets 2307
- Voltaren-XR Tablets 2310

Digoxin (Co-administration has resulted in modest increases in Cmax and AUC of digoxin; although dose adjustments for digoxin are not warranted with initiation of gatifloxacin treatment; patients taking digoxin should be monitored for signs and symptoms of toxicity). Products include:

- Lanoxicaps Capsules 1490
- Lanoxin Injection 1494
- Lanoxin Injection Pediatric 1497
- Lanoxin Tablets 1500

Doxepin Hydrochloride (Gatifloxacin may have the potential to prolong the QTc interval; co-administration with drugs known to prolong QT interval should be avoided).

No products indexed under this heading.

Droperidol (Gatifloxacin may have the potential to prolong the QTc interval; co-administration with drugs known to prolong QT interval should be avoided).

No products indexed under this heading.

Erythromycin (Gatifloxacin may have the potential to prolong the QTc interval; co-administration with drugs known to prolong QT interval should be avoided). Products include:

- Ery-Tab Tablets 449
- Erythromycin Base Filmtab Tablets 455
- Erythromycin Delayed-Release Capsules, USP 457
- PCE Dispertab Tablets 515

Erythromycin Estolate (Gatifloxacin may have the potential to prolong the QTc interval; co-administration with drugs known to prolong QT interval should be avoided).

No products indexed under this heading.

Erythromycin Ethylsuccinate (Gatifloxacin may have the potential to prolong the QTc interval; co-administration with drugs known to prolong QT interval should be avoided). Products include:

- E.E.S. 451
- EryPed 447

Erythromycin Gluceptate (Gatifloxacin may have the potential to prolong the QTc interval; co-administration with drugs known to prolong QT interval should be avoided).

No products indexed under this heading.

Erythromycin Lactobionate (Gatifloxacin may have the potential to prolong the QTc interval; co-administration with drugs known to prolong QT interval should be avoided).

No products indexed under this heading.

Erythromycin Stearate (Gatifloxacin may have the potential to prolong the QTc interval; co-administration with drugs known to prolong QT interval should be avoided). Products include:

- Erythrocin Stearate Filmtab Tablets 453

Etodolac (Co-administration of non-steroidal anti-inflammatory agents with quinolones may increase the risks of CNS stimulation and convulsions; these events have not been observed with gatifloxacin in pre-clinical and clinical trials).

No products indexed under this heading.

Fenoprofen Calcium (Co-administration of non-steroidal anti-inflammatory agents with quinolones may increase the risks of CNS stimulation and convulsions; these events have not been observed with gatifloxacin in pre-clinical and clinical trials). Products include:

- Nalfon Capsules 2502

Ferrous Fumarate (Systemic exposure to gatifloxacin is reduced by co-administration of gatifloxacin with iron-containing products; Tequin can be administered 4 hours before the administration of iron-containing products).

No products indexed under this heading.

Ferrous Gluconate (Systemic exposure to gatifloxacin is reduced by co-administration of gatifloxacin with iron-containing products; Tequin can be administered 4 hours before the administration of iron-containing products).

No products indexed under this heading.

Ferrous Sulfate (Systemic exposure to Tequin Tablets is reduced by co-administration of Tequin Tablets with ferrous sulfate; Tequin Tablets can be administered 4 hours before the administration of iron-containing products). Products include:

- Slow Fe Iron Tablets .... ■ 818
- Slow Fe with Folic Acid Tablets .... ■ 819

Fludrocortisone Acetate (Post-marketing surveillance reports indicate that this risk may be increased in patients receiving concomitant corticosteroids, especially the elderly).

No products indexed under this heading.

Fluphenazine Decanoate (Gatifloxacin may have the potential to prolong the QTc interval; co-administration with drugs known to prolong QT interval should be avoided).

No products indexed under this heading.

Fluphenazine Enanthate (Gatifloxacin may have the potential to prolong the QTc interval; co-administration with drugs known to prolong QT interval should be avoided).

No products indexed under this heading.

Fluphenazine Hydrochloride (Gatifloxacin may have the potential to prolong the QTc interval; co-administration with drugs known to prolong QT interval should be avoided).

No products indexed under this heading.

Flurbiprofen (Co-administration of non-steroidal anti-inflammatory agents with quinolones may increase the risks of CNS stimulation and convulsions; these events have not been observed with gatifloxacin in pre-clinical and clinical trials).

No products indexed under this heading.

Glimepiride (During the postmarketing period, co-administration has resulted in hypoglycemic episodes, in some cases severe). Products include:

- Avandaryl Tablets 1379
- Duetact Tablets 3226

Glipizide (During the postmarketing period, co-administration has resulted in hypoglycemic episodes, in some cases severe).

No products indexed under this heading.

Glyburide (During the postmarketing period, co-administration has resulted in hypoglycemic episodes, in some cases severe).

No products indexed under this heading.

Haloperidol (Gatifloxacin may have the potential to prolong the QTc interval; co-administration with drugs known to prolong QT interval should be avoided).

No products indexed under this heading.

Haloperidol Decanoate (Gatifloxacin may have the potential to prolong the QTc interval; co-administration with drugs known to prolong QT interval should be avoided).

No products indexed under this heading.

Hydrocortisone (Post-marketing surveillance reports indicate that this risk may be increased in patients receiving concomitant corticosteroids, especially the elderly). Products include:

- Colocort Rectal Suspension, USP (Retention) 100 mg/60 mL 2476
- Hydrocortone Tablets 1989
- Preparation H Hydrocortisone Cream .... ■ 646

Hydrocortisone Acetate (Post-marketing surveillance reports indicate that this risk may be increased in patients receiving concomitant corticosteroids, especially the elderly). Products include:

- Analpram-HC 1159
- Pramosone 1161
- ProctoFoam-HC 3099

Hydrocortisone Sodium Phosphate (Post-marketing surveillance reports indicate that this risk may be increased in patients receiving concomitant corticosteroids, especially the elderly).

No products indexed under this heading.

Hydrocortisone Sodium Succinate (Post-marketing surveillance reports indicate that this risk may be increased in patients receiving concomitant corticosteroids, especially the elderly).

No products indexed under this heading.

Hydroxyzine Hydrochloride (Gatifloxacin may have the potential to prolong the QTc interval; co-administration with drugs known to prolong QT interval should be avoided).

No products indexed under this heading.

Ibuprofen (Co-administration of non-steroidal anti-inflammatory agents with quinolones may increase the risks of CNS stimulation and convulsions; these events have not been observed with gatifloxacin in pre-clinical and clinical trials). Products include:

- Advil Allergy Sinus Caplets .... ■ 770
- Advil .... ■ 674
- Children's Advil Oral Suspension .... ■ 603
- Children's Advil Chewable Tablets .. ■ 603
- Advil Cold & Sinus .... ■ 723
- Infants' Advil Concentrated Drops .. ■ 604
- Infants' Advil Concentrated Drops - White Grape (Dye-Free) .... ■ 604
- Junior Strength Advil Swallow Tablets .... ■ 605
- Advil Migraine Liquigels .... ■ 608
- Advil Multi-Symptom Cold Caplets .... ■ 770
- Advil PM Caplets .... ■ 615
- Motrin IB Tablets and Caplets 1866
- Children's Motrin Oral Suspension ... 1867
- Children's Motrin Non-Staining Dye-Free Oral Suspension 1867
- Children's Motrin Cold Oral Suspension 1867
- Infants' Motrin Concentrated Drops 1867
- Infants' Motrin Non-Staining Dye-Free Concentrated Drops 1867
- Junior Strength Motrin Caplets and Chewable Tablets 1867
- Vicoprofen Tablets 539

Imipramine Hydrochloride (Gatifloxacin may have the potential to prolong the QTc interval; co-administration with drugs known to prolong QT interval should be avoided).

No products indexed under this heading.

Imipramine Pamoate (Gatifloxacin may have the potential to prolong the QTc interval; co-administration with drugs known to prolong QT interval should be avoided).

No products indexed under this heading.

Indomethacin (Co-administration of non-steroidal anti-inflammatory agents with quinolones may increase the risks of CNS stimulation and convulsions; these events have not been observed with gatifloxacin in pre-clinical and clinical trials). Products include:

Indocin 1995

Indomethacin Sodium Trihydrate (Co-administration of non-steroidal anti-inflammatory agents with quinolones may increase the risks of CNS stimulation and convulsions; these events have not been observed with gatifloxacin in pre-clinical and clinical trials). Products include:

Indocin I.V. 2465

Insulin, Human, Zinc Suspension (As with other quinolones, disturbances of blood glucose, including symptomatic hyper- and hypoglycemia have been reported, usually in diabetic patients receiving insulin). Products include:

Humulin L, 100 Units 1794
Humulin U, 100 Units 1800

Insulin, Human NPH (As with other quinolones, disturbances of blood glucose, including symptomatic hyper- and hypoglycemia have been reported, usually in diabetic patients receiving insulin). Products include:

Humulin N, 100 Units 1795
Humulin N Pen 1797

Insulin, Human Regular (As with other quinolones, disturbances of blood glucose, including symptomatic hyper- and hypoglycemia have been reported, usually in diabetic patients receiving insulin). Products include:

Humulin R, 100 Units 1798

Insulin, Human Regular and Human NPH Mixture (As with other quinolones, disturbances of blood glucose, including symptomatic hyper- and hypoglycemia have been reported, usually in diabetic patients receiving insulin). Products include:

Humulin 50/50, 100 Units 1791
Humulin 70/30 Pen 1793

Insulin, NPH (As with other quinolones, disturbances of blood glucose, including symptomatic hyper- and hypoglycemia have been reported, usually in diabetic patients receiving insulin).

No products indexed under this heading.

Insulin, Regular (As with other quinolones, disturbances of blood glucose, including symptomatic hyper- and hypoglycemia have been reported, usually in diabetic patients receiving insulin).

No products indexed under this heading.

Insulin, Zinc Crystals (As with other quinolones, disturbances of blood glucose, including symptomatic hyper- and hypoglycemia have been reported, usually in diabetic patients receiving insulin).

No products indexed under this heading.

Insulin, Zinc Suspension (As with other quinolones, disturbances of blood glucose, including symptomatic hyper- and hypoglycemia have been reported, usually in diabetic patients receiving insulin).

No products indexed under this heading.

Insulin Aspart, Human Regular (As with other quinolones, disturbances of blood glucose, including symptomatic hyper- and hypoglycemia have been reported, usually in diabetic patients receiving insulin). Products include:

NovoLog Injection 2326

Insulin glargine (As with other quinolones, disturbances of blood glucose, including symptomatic hyper- and hypoglycemia have been reported, usually in diabetic patients receiving insulin). Products include:

Lantus Injection 2909

Insulin Lispro, Human (As with other quinolones, disturbances of blood glucose, including symptomatic hyper- and hypoglycemia have been reported, usually in diabetic patients receiving insulin). Products include:

Humalog-Pen 1781
Humalog Mix 50/50-Pen 1783
Humalog Mix 75/25-Pen 1785

Insulin Lispro Protamine, Human (As with other quinolones, disturbances of blood glucose, including symptomatic hyper- and hypoglycemia have been reported, usually in diabetic patients receiving insulin). Products include:

Humalog Mix 50/50-Pen 1783
Humalog Mix 75/25-Pen 1785

Iron (Systemic exposure to gatifloxacin is reduced by co-administration of gatifloxacin with iron-containing products; Tequin can be administered 4 hours before the administration of iron-containing products).

No products indexed under this heading.

Isocarboxazid (Gatifloxacin may have the potential to prolong the QTc interval; co-administration with drugs known to prolong QT interval should be avoided).

No products indexed under this heading.

Ketoprofen (Co-administration of non-steroidal anti-inflammatory agents with quinolones may increase the risks of CNS stimulation and convulsions; these events have not been observed with gatifloxacin in pre-clinical and clinical trials).

No products indexed under this heading.

Ketorolac Tromethamine (Co-administration of non-steroidal anti-inflammatory agents with quinolones may increase the risks of CNS stimulation and convulsions; these events have not been observed with gatifloxacin in pre-clinical and clinical trials). Products include:

Acular Ophthalmic Solution 565
Acular LS Ophthalmic Solution 566

Lithium Carbonate (Gatifloxacin may have the potential to prolong the QTc interval; co-administration with drugs known to prolong QT interval should be avoided). Products include:

Lithobid Tablets 1692

Lithium Citrate (Gatifloxacin may have the potential to prolong the QTc interval; co-administration with drugs known to prolong QT interval should be avoided).

No products indexed under this heading.

Lorazepam (Gatifloxacin may have the potential to prolong the QTc interval; co-administration with drugs known to prolong QT interval should be avoided).

No products indexed under this heading.

Loxapine Hydrochloride (Gatifloxacin may have the potential to prolong the QTc interval; co-administration with drugs known to prolong QT interval should be avoided).

No products indexed under this heading.

Loxapine Succinate (Gatifloxacin may have the potential to prolong the QTc interval; co-administration with drugs known to prolong QT interval should be avoided).

No products indexed under this heading.

Magaldrate (Systemic exposure to Tequin Tablets is reduced by co-administration of Tequin Tablets with antacids containing magnesium salts; Tequin Tablets can be administered 4 hours before the administration of antacids).

No products indexed under this heading.

Magnesium Carbonate (Systemic exposure to gatifloxacin is reduced by concomitant administration of gatifloxacin and antacids containing magnesium). Products include:

Gaviscon Regular Strength Liquid .. ▣658
Gaviscon Extra Strength Liquid ...... ▣658
Gaviscon Extra Strength Tablets .... ▣658

Magnesium Hydroxide (Systemic exposure to Tequin Tablets is reduced by co-administration of Tequin Tablets with antacids containing magnesium salts; Tequin Tablets can be administered 4 hours before the administration of antacids). Products include:

Maalox Regular Strength Antacid/Antigas Liquid 2175
Maalox Max Maximum Strength Antacid/Anti-Gas Liquid 2176
Pepcid Complete Chewable Tablets 1701

Magnesium Oxide (Systemic exposure to Tequin Tablets is reduced by co-administration of Tequin Tablets with antacids containing magnesium salts; Tequin Tablets can be administered 4 hours before the administration of antacids). Products include:

Beelith Tablets 759
PremCal Light, Regular, and Extra Strength Tablets .... ▣818

Magnesium Trisilicate (Systemic exposure to gatifloxacin is reduced by concomitant administration of gatifloxacin and antacids containing magnesium). Products include:

Gaviscon Regular Strength Tablets .... ▣658

Maprotiline Hydrochloride (Gatifloxacin may have the potential to prolong the QTc interval; co-administration with drugs known to prolong QT interval should be avoided).

No products indexed under this heading.

Meclofenamate Sodium (Co-administration of non-steroidal anti-inflammatory agents with quinolones may increase the risks of CNS stimulation and convulsions; these events have not been observed with gatifloxacin in pre-clinical and clinical trials).

No products indexed under this heading.

Mefenamic Acid (Co-administration of non-steroidal anti-inflammatory agents with quinolones may increase the risks of CNS stimulation and convulsions; these events have not been observed with gatifloxacin in pre-clinical and clinical trials).

No products indexed under this heading.

Meloxicam (Co-administration of non-steroidal anti-inflammatory agents with quinolones may increase the risks of CNS stimulation and convulsions; these events have not been observed with gatifloxacin in pre-clinical and clinical trials). Products include:

Mobic Oral Suspension 863
Mobic Tablets 863

Meprobamate (Gatifloxacin may have the potential to prolong the QTc interval; co-administration with drugs known to prolong QT interval should be avoided).

No products indexed under this heading.

Mesoridazine Besylate (Gatifloxacin may have the potential to prolong the QTc interval; co-administration with drugs known to prolong QT interval should be avoided).

No products indexed under this heading.

Metformin Hydrochloride (During the postmarketing period, co-administration has resulted in hypoglycemic episodes, in some cases severe). Products include:

ActoPlus Met Tablets 3214
Avandamet Tablets 1373
Fortamet Extended-Release Tablets 3115

Methylprednisolone Acetate (Post-marketing surveillance reports indicate that this risk may be increased in patients receiving concomitant corticosteroids, especially the elderly). Products include:

Depo-Medrol Injectable Suspension 2617
Depo-Medrol Single-Dose Vial 2619

Methylprednisolone Sodium Succinate (Post-marketing surveillance reports indicate that this risk may be increased in patients receiving concomitant corticosteroids, especially the elderly).

No products indexed under this heading.

Midazolam Hydrochloride (Gatifloxacin may have the potential to prolong the QTc interval; co-administration with drugs known to prolong QT interval should be avoided).

No products indexed under this heading.

Miglitol (During the postmarketing period, co-administration has resulted in hypoglycemic episodes, in some cases severe).

No products indexed under this heading.

Molindone Hydrochloride (Gatifloxacin may have the potential to prolong the QTc interval; co-administration with drugs known to prolong QT interval should be avoided). Products include:

Moban Tablets 1119

Multivitamins (Systemic exposure to gatifloxacin is reduced by concomitant administration of gatifloxacin and ferrous sulfate. Gatifloxacin can be administered 4 hours before the administration of dietary supplements containing zinc, magnesium, or iron (such as multivitamins)).
No products indexed under this heading.

Nabumetone (Co-administration of non-steroidal anti-inflammatory agents with quinolones may increase the risks of CNS stimulation and convulsions; these events have not been observed with gatifloxacin in pre-clinical and clinical trials).
No products indexed under this heading.

Naproxen (Co-administration of non-steroidal anti-inflammatory agents with quinolones may increase the risks of CNS stimulation and convulsions; these events have not been observed with gatifloxacin in pre-clinical and clinical trials). Products include:
EC-Naprosyn Delayed-Release Tablets 2761
Naprosyn Suspension 2761
Naprosyn Tablets 2761
Prevacid NapraPAC 3280

Naproxen Sodium (Co-administration of non-steroidal anti-inflammatory agents with quinolones may increase the risks of CNS stimulation and convulsions; these events have not been observed with gatifloxacin in pre-clinical and clinical trials). Products include:
Aleve Caplets 742
Aleve Gelcaps 743
Aleve Tablets 743
Aleve Cold & Sinus Caplets 744
Anaprox Tablets 2761
Anaprox DS Tablets 2761

Nortriptyline Hydrochloride (Gatifloxacin may have the potential to prolong the QTc interval; co-administration with drugs known to prolong QT interval should be avoided).
No products indexed under this heading.

Olanzapine (Gatifloxacin may have the potential to prolong the QTc interval; co-administration with drugs known to prolong QT interval should be avoided). Products include:
Symbyax Capsules 1819
Zyprexa Tablets 1830
Zyprexa IntraMuscular 1830
Zyprexa ZYDIS Orally Disintegrating Tablets 1830

Oxaprozin (Co-administration of non-steroidal anti-inflammatory agents with quinolones may increase the risks of CNS stimulation and convulsions; these events have not been observed with gatifloxacin in pre-clinical and clinical trials).
No products indexed under this heading.

Oxazepam (Gatifloxacin may have the potential to prolong the QTc interval; co-administration with drugs known to prolong QT interval should be avoided).
No products indexed under this heading.

Perphenazine (Gatifloxacin may have the potential to prolong the QTc interval; co-administration with drugs known to prolong QT interval should be avoided).
No products indexed under this heading.

Phenelzine Sulfate (Gatifloxacin may have the potential to prolong the QTc interval; co-administration with drugs known to prolong QT interval should be avoided).
No products indexed under this heading.

Phenylbutazone (Co-administration of non-steroidal anti-inflammatory agents with quinolones may increase the risks of CNS stimulation and convulsions; these events have not been observed with gatifloxacin in pre-clinical and clinical trials).
No products indexed under this heading.

Pimozide (Gatifloxacin may have the potential to prolong the QTc interval; co-administration with drugs known to prolong QT interval should be avoided).
No products indexed under this heading.

Pioglitazone Hydrochloride (During the postmarketing period, co-administration has resulted in hypoglycemic episodes, in some cases severe). Products include:
ActoPlus Met Tablets 3214
Actos Tablets 3219
Duetact Tablets 3226

Piroxicam (Co-administration of non-steroidal anti-inflammatory agents with quinolones may increase the risks of CNS stimulation and convulsions; these events have not been observed with gatifloxacin in pre-clinical and clinical trials).
No products indexed under this heading.

Polysaccharide Iron Complex (Systemic exposure to gatifloxacin is reduced by co-administration of gatifloxacin with iron-containing products; Tequin can be administered 4 hours before the administration of iron-containing products). Products include:
Nu-Iron 150 Capsules 2127

Prazepam (Gatifloxacin may have the potential to prolong the QTc interval; co-administration with drugs known to prolong QT interval should be avoided).
No products indexed under this heading.

Prednisolone Acetate (Post-marketing surveillance reports indicate that this risk may be increased in patients receiving concomitant corticosteroids, especially the elderly). Products include:
Blephamide Ophthalmic Ointment 568
Blephamide Ophthalmic Suspension 569
Poly-Pred Ophthalmic Suspension .... ⊙233
Pred Forte Ophthalmic Suspension .... ⊙235
Pred Mild Ophthalmic Suspension .... ⊙238
Pred-G Ophthalmic Ointment .... ⊙237
Pred-G Ophthalmic Suspension .... ⊙236

Prednisolone Sodium Phosphate (Post-marketing surveillance reports indicate that this risk may be increased in patients receiving concomitant corticosteroids, especially the elderly).
No products indexed under this heading.

Prednisolone Tebutate (Post-marketing surveillance reports indicate that this risk may be increased in patients receiving concomitant corticosteroids, especially the elderly).
No products indexed under this heading.

Prednisone (Post-marketing surveillance reports indicate that this risk may be increased in patients receiving concomitant corticosteroids, especially the elderly).
No products indexed under this heading.

Probenecid (Systemic exposure to gatifloxacin is increased following co-administration of gatifloxacin with probenecid resulting in a 42% increase in AUC and a 44% longer half-life of gatifloxacin).
No products indexed under this heading.

Procainamide Hydrochloride (Gatifloxacin may have the potential to prolong the QTc interval; co-administration with drugs known to prolong QT interval should be avoided).
No products indexed under this heading.

Prochlorperazine (Gatifloxacin may have the potential to prolong the QTc interval; co-administration with drugs known to prolong QT interval should be avoided).
No products indexed under this heading.

Promethazine Hydrochloride (Gatifloxacin may have the potential to prolong the QTc interval; co-administration with drugs known to prolong QT interval should be avoided). Products include:
Phenergan Tablets and Suppositories 3440

Protriptyline Hydrochloride (Gatifloxacin may have the potential to prolong the QTc interval; co-administration with drugs known to prolong QT interval should be avoided).
No products indexed under this heading.

Quetiapine Fumarate (Gatifloxacin may have the potential to prolong the QTc interval; co-administration with drugs known to prolong QT interval should be avoided). Products include:
Seroquel Tablets 690

Quinidine (Gatifloxacin may have the potential to prolong the QTc interval; co-administration with drugs known to prolong QT interval should be avoided).
No products indexed under this heading.

Quinidine Gluconate (Gatifloxacin may have the potential to prolong the QTc interval; co-administration with drugs known to prolong QT interval should be avoided).
No products indexed under this heading.

Quinidine Hydrochloride (Gatifloxacin may have the potential to prolong the QTc interval; co-administration with drugs known to prolong QT interval should be avoided).
No products indexed under this heading.

Quinidine Polygalacturonate (Gatifloxacin may have the potential to prolong the QTc interval; co-administration with drugs known to prolong QT interval should be avoided).
No products indexed under this heading.

Quinidine Sulfate (Gatifloxacin may have the potential to prolong the QTc interval; co-administration with drugs known to prolong QT interval should be avoided).
No products indexed under this heading.

Repaglinide (During the postmarketing period, co-administration has resulted in hypoglycemic episodes, in some cases severe).
No products indexed under this heading.

Risperidone (Gatifloxacin may have the potential to prolong the QTc interval; co-administration with drugs known to prolong QT interval should be avoided). Products include:
Risperdal 1676
Risperdal Consta Long-Acting Injection 1682
Risperdal M-Tab Orally Disintegrating Tablets 1676

Rofecoxib (Co-administration of non-steroidal anti-inflammatory agents with quinolones may increase the risks of CNS stimulation and convulsions; these events have not been observed with gatifloxacin in pre-clinical and clinical trials).
No products indexed under this heading.

Rosiglitazone Maleate (During the postmarketing period, co-administration has resulted in hypoglycemic episodes, in some cases severe). Products include:
Avandamet Tablets 1373
Avandaryl Tablets 1379
Avandia Tablets 1384

Sotalol Hydrochloride (Gatifloxacin may have the potential to prolong the QTc interval; co-administration with drugs known to prolong QT interval should be avoided).
No products indexed under this heading.

Sulindac (Co-administration of non-steroidal anti-inflammatory agents with quinolones may increase the risks of CNS stimulation and convulsions; these events have not been observed with gatifloxacin in pre-clinical and clinical trials). Products include:
Clinoril Tablets 1924

Thioridazine Hydrochloride (Gatifloxacin may have the potential to prolong the QTc interval; co-administration with drugs known to prolong QT interval should be avoided). Products include:
Thioridazine Hydrochloride Tablets 2163

Thiothixene (Gatifloxacin may have the potential to prolong the QTc interval; co-administration with drugs known to prolong QT interval should be avoided). Products include:
Thiothixene Capsules 2165

Tolazamide (During the postmarketing period, co-administration has resulted in hypoglycemic episodes, in some cases severe).
No products indexed under this heading.

Tolbutamide (During the postmarketing period, co-administration has resulted in hypoglycemic episodes, in some cases severe).
No products indexed under this heading.

Tolmetin Sodium (Co-administration of non-steroidal anti-inflammatory agents with quinolones may increase the risks of CNS stimulation and convulsions; these events have not been observed with gatifloxacin in pre-clinical and clinical trials).
No products indexed under this heading.

Tranylcypromine Sulfate (Gatifloxacin may have the potential to prolong the QTc interval; co-administration with drugs known to prolong QT interval should be avoided). Products include:
Parnate Tablets 1527

Triamcinolone (Post-marketing surveillance reports indicate that this risk may be increased in patients receiving concomitant corticosteroids, especially the elderly).
No products indexed under this heading.

Triamcinolone Acetonide (Post-marketing surveillance reports indicate that this risk may be increased in patients receiving concomitant corticosteroids, especially the elderly). Products include:
Azmacort Inhalation Aerosol 1726
Nasacort AQ Nasal Spray 2922

Triamcinolone Diacetate (Post-marketing surveillance reports indicate that this risk may be increased in patients receiving concomitant corticosteroids, especially the elderly).
No products indexed under this heading.

Triamcinolone Hexacetonide (Post-marketing surveillance reports indicate that this risk may be increased in patients receiving concomitant corticosteroids, especially the elderly).
No products indexed under this heading.

Trifluoperazine Hydrochloride (Gatifloxacin may have the potential to prolong the QTc interval; co-administration with drugs known to prolong QT interval should be avoided).
No products indexed under this heading.

Trimipramine Maleate (Gatifloxacin may have the potential to prolong the QTc interval; co-administration with drugs known to prolong QT interval should be avoided).
No products indexed under this heading.

Troglitazone (During the postmarketing period, co-administration has resulted in hypoglycemic episodes, in some cases severe).
No products indexed under this heading.

Valdecoxib (Co-administration of non-steroidal anti-inflammatory agents with quinolones may increase the risks of CNS stimulation and convulsions; these events have not been observed with gatifloxacin in pre-clinical and clinical trials).
No products indexed under this heading.

Zinc-Containing Multivitamins (Systemic exposure to gatifloxacin is reduced by concomitant administration of gatifloxacin and ferrous sulfate. Gatifloxacin can be administered 4 hours before the administration of dietary supplements containing zinc, magnesium, or iron (such as multivitamins)).
No products indexed under this heading.

Zinc Sulfate (Gatifloxacin can be administered 4 hours before the administration of zinc-containing supplements). Products include:
Visine A.C. Seasonal Itching and Redness Relief Drops .... ⊙ 289
Zinc-220 Capsules 580

Ziprasidone Hydrochloride (Gatifloxacin may have the potential to prolong the QTc interval; co-administration with drugs known to prolong QT interval should be avoided). Products include:
Geodon Capsules 2529

TESSALON CAPSULES

(Benzonatate) 1199
None cited in PDR database.

TESSALON PERLES

(Benzonatate) 1199
None cited in PDR database.

TESTIM 1% GEL

(Testosterone) 695
May interact with corticosteroids, insulin, and certain other agents. Compounds in these categories include:

ACTH (Co-administration of testoterone with ACTH may enhance edema formation).
No products indexed under this heading.

Betamethasone Acetate (Co-administration of testosterone with corticosteroids may enhance edema formation).
No products indexed under this heading.

Betamethasone Sodium Phosphate (Co-administration of testosterone with corticosteroids may enhance edema formation).
No products indexed under this heading.

Cortisone Acetate (Co-administration of testosterone with corticosteroids may enhance edema formation).
No products indexed under this heading.

Dexamethasone (Co-administration of testosterone with corticosteroids may enhance edema formation). Products include:
Ciprodex Otic Suspension 559
Decadron Tablets 1951
TobraDex Ophthalmic Ointment 562
TobraDex Ophthalmic Suspension ... 563

Dexamethasone Acetate (Co-administration of testosterone with corticosteroids may enhance edema formation).
No products indexed under this heading.

Dexamethasone Sodium Phosphate (Co-administration of testosterone with corticosteroids may enhance edema formation).
No products indexed under this heading.

Fludrocortisone Acetate (Co-administration of testosterone with corticosteroids may enhance edema formation).
No products indexed under this heading.

Hydrocortisone (Co-administration of testosterone with corticosteroids may enhance edema formation). Products include:
Colocort Rectal Suspension, USP (Retention) 100 mg/60 mL........... 2476
Hydrocortone Tablets 1989
Preparation H Hydrocortisone Cream .... ▣ 646

Hydrocortisone Acetate (Co-administration of testosterone with corticosteroids may enhance edema formation). Products include:
Analpram-HC 1159
Pramosone 1161
ProctoFoam-HC 3099

Hydrocortisone Sodium Phosphate (Co-administration of testosterone with corticosteroids may enhance edema formation).
No products indexed under this heading.

Hydrocortisone Sodium Succinate (Co-administration of testosterone with corticosteroids may enhance edema formation).
No products indexed under this heading.

Insulin, Human, Zinc Suspension (In diabetic patients, the metabolic effects of androgens may decrease blood glucose and, therefore, insulin requirements). Products include:
Humulin L, 100 Units 1794
Humulin U, 100 Units 1800

Insulin, Human NPH (In diabetic patients, the metabolic effects of androgens may decrease blood glucose and, therefore, insulin requirements). Products include:
Humulin N, 100 Units 1795
Humulin N Pen 1797

Insulin, Human Regular (In diabetic patients, the metabolic effects of androgens may decrease blood glucose and, therefore, insulin requirements). Products include:
Humulin R, 100 Units 1798

Insulin, Human Regular and Human NPH Mixture (In diabetic patients, the metabolic effects of androgens may decrease blood glucose and, therefore, insulin requirements). Products include:
Humulin 50/50, 100 Units 1791
Humulin 70/30 Pen 1793

Insulin, NPH (In diabetic patients, the metabolic effects of androgens may decrease blood glucose and, therefore, insulin requirements).
No products indexed under this heading.

Insulin, Regular (In diabetic patients, the metabolic effects of androgens may decrease blood glucose and, therefore, insulin requirements).
No products indexed under this heading.

Insulin, Zinc Crystals (In diabetic patients, the metabolic effects of androgens may decrease blood glucose and, therefore, insulin requirements).
No products indexed under this heading.

Insulin, Zinc Suspension (In diabetic patients, the metabolic effects of androgens may decrease blood glucose and, therefore, insulin requirements).
No products indexed under this heading.

Insulin Aspart, Human Regular (In diabetic patients, the metabolic effects of androgens may decrease blood glucose and, therefore, insulin requirements). Products include:
NovoLog Injection 2326

Insulin glargine (In diabetic patients, the metabolic effects of androgens may decrease blood glucose and, therefore, insulin requirements). Products include:
Lantus Injection 2909

Insulin Lispro, Human (In diabetic patients, the metabolic effects of androgens may decrease blood glucose and, therefore, insulin requirements). Products include:
Humalog-Pen 1781
Humalog Mix 50/50-Pen 1783
Humalog Mix 75/25-Pen 1785

Insulin Lispro Protamine, Human (In diabetic patients, the metabolic effects of androgens may decrease blood glucose and, therefore, insulin requirements). Products include:
Humalog Mix 50/50-Pen 1783
Humalog Mix 75/25-Pen 1785

Methylprednisolone Acetate (Co-administration of testosterone with corticosteroids may enhance edema formation). Products include:
Depo-Medrol Injectable Suspension 2617
Depo-Medrol Single-Dose Vial 2619

Methylprednisolone Sodium Succinate (Co-administration of testosterone with corticosteroids may enhance edema formation).
No products indexed under this heading.

Oxyphenbutazone (Co-administration of androgens and oxyphenbutazone may result in elevated serum levels of oxyphenbutazone).
No products indexed under this heading.

Prednisolone Acetate (Co-administration of testosterone with corticosteroids may enhance edema formation). Products include:
Blephamide Ophthalmic Ointment 568
Blephamide Ophthalmic Suspension.................................. 569
Poly-Pred Ophthalmic Suspension .... ⊙ 233
Pred Forte Ophthalmic Suspension .... ⊙ 235
Pred Mild Ophthalmic Suspension .... ⊙ 238
Pred-G Ophthalmic Ointment .... ⊙ 237
Pred-G Ophthalmic Suspension ...... ⊙ 236

Prednisolone Sodium Phosphate (Co-administration of testosterone with corticosteroids may enhance edema formation).
No products indexed under this heading.

Prednisolone Tebutate (Co-administration of testosterone with corticosteroids may enhance edema formation).
No products indexed under this heading.

Prednisone (Co-administration of testosterone with corticosteroids may enhance edema formation).
No products indexed under this heading.

Propranolol Hydrochloride (Co-administration of injectable testosterone cypionate has resulted in an increased clearance of propranolol). Products include:

Inderal LA Long-Acting Capsules 3429
InnoPran XL Capsules 2723

Triamcinolone (Co-administration of testosterone with corticosteroids may enhance edema formation).

No products indexed under this heading.

Triamcinolone Acetonide (Co-administration of testosterone with corticosteroids may enhance edema formation). Products include:

Azmacort Inhalation Aerosol 1726
Nasacort AQ Nasal Spray 2922

Triamcinolone Diacetate (Co-administration of testosterone with corticosteroids may enhance edema formation).

No products indexed under this heading.

Triamcinolone Hexacetonide (Co-administration of testosterone with corticosteroids may enhance edema formation).

No products indexed under this heading.

TEVETEN TABLETS

(Eprosartan Mesylate) 1735

Food Interactions

Food, unspecified (Co-administration with food delays absorption and causes variable changes in Cmax and AUC values which do not appear clinically important).

TEVETEN HCT TABLETS

(Eprosartan Mesylate, Hydrochlorothiazide).......................... 1737

May interact with antihypertensives, barbiturates, corticosteroids, cardiac glycosides, oral hypoglycemic agents, insulin, lithium preparations, narcotic analgesics, nondepolarizing neuromuscular blocking agents, nonsteroidal anti-inflammatory agents, potassium preparations, potassium sparing diuretics, and certain other agents. Compounds in these categories include:

Acarbose (Hyperglycemia may occur with thiazide diuretics; oral hypoglycemic dosage may need to be adjusted). Products include:

Precose Tablets 751

Acebutolol Hydrochloride (Co-administration of thiazides with other antihypertensive agents may lead to additive effects or potentiation).

No products indexed under this heading.

ACTH (Intensifies the electrolyte balance, particularly hypokalemia).

No products indexed under this heading.

Alfentanil Hydrochloride (Narcotics may potentiate orthostatic hypotension).

No products indexed under this heading.

Amiloride Hydrochloride (Concomitant use of potassium sparing diuretics with eprosartan may lead to hyperkalemia). Products include:

Midamor Tablets 2026
Moduretic Tablets 2028

Amlodipine Besylate (Co-administration of thiazides with other antihypertensive agents may lead to additive effects or potentiation). Products include:

Caduet Tablets 2508
Lotrel Capsules 2249
Norvasc Tablets 2545

Aprobarbital (Barbiturates may potentiate orthostatic hypotension).

No products indexed under this heading.

Atenolol (Co-administration of thiazides with other antihypertensive agents may lead to additive effects or potentiation).

No products indexed under this heading.

Atracurium Besylate (Possible increased responsiveness to muscle relaxants).

No products indexed under this heading.

Benazepril Hydrochloride (Co-administration of thiazides with other antihypertensive agents may lead to additive effects or potentiation). Products include:

Lotensin Tablets 2243
Lotensin HCT Tablets 2246
Lotrel Capsules 2249

Bendroflumethiazide (Co-administration of thiazides with other antihypertensive agents may lead to additive effects or potentiation).

No products indexed under this heading.

Betamethasone Acetate (Corticosteroids intensify the electrolyte imbalance, particularly hypokalemia).

No products indexed under this heading.

Betamethasone Sodium Phosphate (Corticosteroids intensify the electrolyte imbalance, particularly hypokalemia).

No products indexed under this heading.

Betaxolol Hydrochloride (Co-administration of thiazides with other antihypertensive agents may lead to additive effects or potentiation). Products include:

Betoptic S Ophthalmic Suspension................................. 558

Bisoprolol Fumarate (Co-administration of thiazides with other antihypertensive agents may lead to additive effects or potentiation).

No products indexed under this heading.

Buprenorphine Hydrochloride (Narcotics may potentiate orthostatic hypotension). Products include:

Buprenex Injectable 2716
Suboxone Tablets 2717
Subutex Tablets 2717

Butabarbital (Barbiturates may potentiate orthostatic hypotension).

No products indexed under this heading.

Butalbital (Barbiturates may potentiate orthostatic hypotension).

No products indexed under this heading.

Candesartan Cilexetil (Co-administration of thiazides with other antihypertensive agents may lead to additive effects or potentiation). Products include:

Atacand Tablets 649
Atacand HCT 651

Captopril (Co-administration of thiazides with other antihypertensive agents may lead to additive effects or potentiation). Products include:

Captopril Tablets 2149

Carteolol Hydrochloride (Co-administration of thiazides with other antihypertensive agents may lead to additive effects or potentiation). Products include:

Carteolol Hydrochloride Ophthalmic Solution USP, 1%....... ⊙ 249

Celecoxib (Nonsteroidal anti-inflammatory agents can reduce the natriuretic, diuretic, and antihypertensive effects). Products include:

Celebrex Capsules 3134

Chlorothiazide (Co-administration of thiazides with other antihypertensive agents may lead to additive effects or potentiation). Products include:

Diuril Oral Suspension 1954

Chlorothiazide Sodium (Co-administration of thiazides with other antihypertensive agents may lead to additive effects or potentiation). Products include:

Diuril Sodium Intravenous 2467

Chlorpropamide (Hyperglycemia may occur with thiazide diuretics; oral hypoglycemic dosage may need to be adjusted).

No products indexed under this heading.

Chlorthalidone (Co-administration of thiazides with other antihypertensive agents may lead to additive effects or potentiation). Products include:

Clorpres Tablets 2153

Cholestyramine (Binds hydrochlorothiazide and reduces its absorption from gastrointestinal tract by 85%).

No products indexed under this heading.

Cisatracurium Besylate (Possible increased responsiveness to muscle relaxants). Products include:

Nimbex Injection 498

Clonidine (Co-administration of thiazides with other antihypertensive agents may lead to additive effects or potentiation). Products include:

Catapres-TTS 844

Clonidine Hydrochloride (Co-administration of thiazides with other antihypertensive agents may lead to additive effects or potentiation). Products include:

Catapres Tablets 843
Clorpres Tablets 2153

Codeine Phosphate (Narcotics may potentiate orthostatic hypotension). Products include:

Tylenol with Codeine Tablets 2391

Colestipol Hydrochloride (Binds hydrochlorothiazide and reduces its absorption from gastrointestinal tract by 43%).

No products indexed under this heading.

Cortisone Acetate (Corticosteroids intensify the electrolyte imbalance, particularly hypokalemia).

No products indexed under this heading.

Deserpidine (Co-administration of thiazides with other antihypertensive agents may lead to additive effects or potentiation).

No products indexed under this heading.

Deslanoside (Thiazide-induced hypokalemia may cause cardiac arrhythmias and may also sensitize or exaggerate response of the heart to the toxic effects of digitalis).

No products indexed under this heading.

Dexamethasone (Corticosteroids intensify the electrolyte imbalance, particularly hypokalemia). Products include:

Ciprodex Otic Suspension 559
Decadron Tablets 1951
TobraDex Ophthalmic Ointment 562
TobraDex Ophthalmic Suspension ... 563

Dexamethasone Acetate (Corticosteroids intensify the electrolyte imbalance, particularly hypokalemia).

No products indexed under this heading.

Dexamethasone Sodium Phosphate (Corticosteroids intensify the electrolyte imbalance, particularly hypokalemia).

No products indexed under this heading.

Dezocine (Narcotics may potentiate orthostatic hypotension).

No products indexed under this heading.

Diazoxide (Co-administration of thiazides with other antihypertensive agents may lead to additive effects or potentiation). Products include:

Hyperstat I.V. 3017

Diclofenac Potassium (Nonsteroidal anti-inflammatory agents can reduce the natriuretic, diuretic, and antihypertensive effects).

No products indexed under this heading.

Diclofenac Sodium (Nonsteroidal anti-inflammatory agents can reduce the natriuretic, diuretic, and antihypertensive effects). Products include:

Arthrotec Tablets 3129
Voltaren Ophthalmic Solution 2309
Voltaren Tablets 2307
Voltaren-XR Tablets 2310

Digitalis Glycoside Preparations (Thiazide-induced hypokalemia may cause cardiac arrhythmias and may also sensitize or exaggerate response of the heart to the toxic effects of digitalis).

No products indexed under this heading.

Digitoxin (Thiazide-induced hypokalemia may cause cardiac arrhythmias and may also sensitize or exaggerate response of the heart to the toxic effects of digitalis).

No products indexed under this heading.

Digoxin (Thiazide-induced hypokalemia may cause cardiac arrhythmias and may also sensitize or exaggerate response of the heart to the toxic effects of digitalis). Products include:

Lanoxicaps Capsules 1490
Lanoxin Injection 1494
Lanoxin Injection Pediatric 1497
Lanoxin Tablets 1500

Diltiazem Hydrochloride (Co-administration of thiazides with other antihypertensive agents may lead to additive effects or potentiation). Products include:

Cardizem LA Extended Release Tablets 1728
Tiazac Capsules 1201

Doxazosin Mesylate (Co-administration of thiazides with other antihypertensive agents may lead to additive effects or potentiation). Products include:

Cardura XL Tablets 2515

Enalapril Maleate (Co-administration of thiazides with other antihypertensive agents may lead to additive effects or potentiation). Products include:

Vasotec I.V. Injection 2103

Enalaprilat (Co-administration of thiazides with other antihypertensive agents may lead to additive effects or potentiation).
No products indexed under this heading.

Esmolol Hydrochloride (Co-administration of thiazides with other antihypertensive agents may lead to additive effects or potentiation).
No products indexed under this heading.

Etodolac (Nonsteroidal anti-inflammatory agents can reduce the natriuretic, diuretic, and antihypertensive effects).
No products indexed under this heading.

Felodipine (Co-administration of thiazides with other antihypertensive agents may lead to additive effects or potentiation).
No products indexed under this heading.

Fenoprofen Calcium (Nonsteroidal anti-inflammatory agents can reduce the natriuretic, diuretic, and antihypertensive effects). Products include:
Nalfon Capsules **2502**

Fentanyl (Narcotics may potentiate orthostatic hypotension). Products include:
Duragesic Transdermal System **2373**
Ionsys Transdermal System **2379**

Fentanyl Citrate (Narcotics may potentiate orthostatic hypotension). Products include:
Actiq **979**

Fludrocortisone Acetate (Corticosteroids intensify the electrolyte imbalance, particularly hypokalemia).
No products indexed under this heading.

Flurbiprofen (Nonsteroidal anti-inflammatory agents can reduce the natriuretic, diuretic, and antihypertensive effects).
No products indexed under this heading.

Fosinopril Sodium (Co-administration of thiazides with other antihypertensive agents may lead to additive effects or potentiation).
No products indexed under this heading.

Furosemide (Co-administration of thiazides with other antihypertensive agents may lead to additive effects or potentiation). Products include:
Furosemide Tablets **2154**

Glimepiride (Hyperglycemia may occur with thiazide diuretics; oral hypoglycemic dosage may need to be adjusted). Products include:
Avandaryl Tablets **1379**
Duetact Tablets **3226**

Glipizide (Hyperglycemia may occur with thiazide diuretics; oral hypoglycemic dosage may need to be adjusted).
No products indexed under this heading.

Glyburide (Hyperglycemia may occur with thiazide diuretics; oral hypoglycemic dosage may need to be adjusted).
No products indexed under this heading.

Guanabenz Acetate (Co-administration of thiazides with other antihypertensive agents may lead to additive effects or potentiation).
No products indexed under this heading.

Guanethidine Monosulfate (Co-administration of thiazides with other antihypertensive agents may lead to additive effects or potentiation).
No products indexed under this heading.

Hydralazine Hydrochloride (Co-administration of thiazides with other antihypertensive agents may lead to additive effects or potentiation). Products include:
BiDil Tablets **2171**

Hydrocodone Bitartrate (Narcotics may potentiate orthostatic hypotension). Products include:
Hycodan **1116**
Hycotuss Expectorant Syrup **1117**
Vicodin Tablets **535**
Vicodin ES Tablets **536**
Vicodin HP Tablets **538**
Vicoprofen Tablets **539**
Zydone Tablets **1139**

Hydrocodone Polistirex (Narcotics may potentiate orthostatic hypotension). Products include:
Tussionex Pennkinetic Extended-Release Suspension **3327**

Hydrocortisone (Corticosteroids intensify the electrolyte imbalance, particularly hypokalemia). Products include:
Colocort Rectal Suspension, USP (Retention) 100 mg/60 mL **2476**
Hydrocortone Tablets **1989**
Preparation H Hydrocortisone Cream **646**

Hydrocortisone Acetate (Corticosteroids intensify the electrolyte imbalance, particularly hypokalemia). Products include:
Analpram-HC **1159**
Pramosone **1161**
ProctoFoam-HC **3099**

Hydrocortisone Sodium Phosphate (Corticosteroids intensify the electrolyte imbalance, particularly hypokalemia).
No products indexed under this heading.

Hydrocortisone Sodium Succinate (Corticosteroids intensify the electrolyte imbalance, particularly hypokalemia).
No products indexed under this heading.

Hydroflumethiazide (Co-administration of thiazides with other antihypertensive agents may lead to additive effects or potentiation).
No products indexed under this heading.

Hydromorphone Hydrochloride (Narcotics may potentiate orthostatic hypotension). Products include:
Dilaudid **440**
Dilaudid Non-Sterile Powder **440**
Dilaudid Oral Liquid **445**
Dilaudid Rectal Suppositories **440**
Dilaudid Tablets **440**
Dilaudid Tablets - 8 mg **445**
Dilaudid-HP **442**

Ibuprofen (Nonsteroidal anti-inflammatory agents can reduce the natriuretic, diuretic, and antihypertensive effects). Products include:
Advil Allergy Sinus Caplets **770**
Advil **674**
Children's Advil Oral Suspension **603**
Children's Advil Chewable Tablets **603**
Advil Cold & Sinus **723**
Infants' Advil Concentrated Drops **604**
Infants' Advil Concentrated Drops - White Grape (Dye-Free) **604**
Junior Strength Advil Swallow Tablets **605**
Advil Migraine Liquigels **608**
Advil Multi-Symptom Cold Caplets **770**
Advil PM Caplets **615**
Motrin IB Tablets and Caplets **1866**
Children's Motrin Oral Suspension **1867**
Children's Motrin Non-Staining Dye-Free Oral Suspension **1867**
Children's Motrin Cold Oral Suspension **1867**
Infants' Motrin Concentrated Drops **1867**
Infants' Motrin Non-Staining Dye-Free Concentrated Drops **1867**
Junior Strength Motrin Caplets and Chewable Tablets **1867**
Vicoprofen Tablets **539**

Indapamide (Co-administration of thiazides with other antihypertensive agents may lead to additive effects or potentiation). Products include:
Indapamide Tablets **2156**

Indomethacin (Nonsteroidal anti-inflammatory agents can reduce the natriuretic, diuretic, and antihypertensive effects). Products include:
Indocin **1995**

Indomethacin Sodium Trihydrate (Nonsteroidal anti-inflammatory agents can reduce the natriuretic, diuretic, and antihypertensive effects). Products include:
Indocin I.V. **2465**

Insulin, Human, Zinc Suspension (Hyperglycemia may occur with thiazide diuretics; insulin dosage may need to be adjusted). Products include:
Humulin L, 100 Units **1794**
Humulin U, 100 Units **1800**

Insulin, Human NPH (Hyperglycemia may occur with thiazide diuretics; insulin dosage may need to be adjusted). Products include:
Humulin N, 100 Units **1795**
Humulin N Pen **1797**

Insulin, Human Regular (Hyperglycemia may occur with thiazide diuretics; insulin dosage may need to be adjusted). Products include:
Humulin R, 100 Units **1798**

Insulin, Human Regular and Human NPH Mixture (Hyperglycemia may occur with thiazide diuretics; insulin dosage may need to be adjusted). Products include:
Humulin 50/50, 100 Units **1791**
Humulin 70/30 Pen **1793**

Insulin, NPH (Hyperglycemia may occur with thiazide diuretics; insulin dosage may need to be adjusted).
No products indexed under this heading.

Insulin, Regular (Hyperglycemia may occur with thiazide diuretics; insulin dosage may need to be adjusted).
No products indexed under this heading.

Insulin, Zinc Crystals (Hyperglycemia may occur with thiazide diuretics; insulin dosage may need to be adjusted).
No products indexed under this heading.

Insulin, Zinc Suspension (Hyperglycemia may occur with thiazide diuretics; insulin dosage may need to be adjusted).
No products indexed under this heading.

Insulin Aspart, Human Regular (Hyperglycemia may occur with thiazide diuretics; insulin dosage may need to be adjusted). Products include:
NovoLog Injection **2326**

Insulin glargine (Hyperglycemia may occur with thiazide diuretics; insulin dosage may need to be adjusted). Products include:
Lantus Injection **2909**

Insulin Lispro, Human (Hyperglycemia may occur with thiazide diuretics; insulin dosage may need to be adjusted). Products include:
Humalog-Pen **1781**
Humalog Mix 50/50-Pen **1783**
Humalog Mix 75/25-Pen **1785**

Insulin Lispro Protamine, Human (Hyperglycemia may occur with thiazide diuretics; insulin dosage may need to be adjusted). Products include:
Humalog Mix 50/50-Pen **1783**
Humalog Mix 75/25-Pen **1785**

Irbesartan (Co-administration of thiazides with other antihypertensive agents may lead to additive effects or potentiation). Products include:
Avalide Tablets **888**
Avalide Tablets **2874**
Avapro Tablets **891**
Avapro Tablets **2871**

Isradipine (Co-administration of thiazides with other antihypertensive agents may lead to additive effects or potentiation). Products include:
DynaCirc CR Tablets **2721**

Ketoprofen (Nonsteroidal anti-inflammatory agents can reduce the natriuretic, diuretic, and antihypertensive effects).
No products indexed under this heading.

Ketorolac Tromethamine (Nonsteroidal anti-inflammatory agents can reduce the natriuretic, diuretic, and antihypertensive effects). Products include:
Acular Ophthalmic Solution **565**
Acular LS Ophthalmic Solution **566**

Labetalol Hydrochloride (Co-administration of thiazides with other antihypertensive agents may lead to additive effects or potentiation).
No products indexed under this heading.

Levorphanol Tartrate (Narcotics may potentiate orthostatic hypotension).
No products indexed under this heading.

Lisinopril (Co-administration of thiazides with other antihypertensive agents may lead to additive effects or potentiation). Products include:
Prinivil Tablets **2052**
Prinzide Tablets **2056**

Lithium (Diuretics reduce the renal clearance of lithium and add a high risk of lithium toxicity).
No products indexed under this heading.

Lithium Carbonate (Diuretics reduce the renal clearance of lithium and add a high risk of lithium toxicity). Products include:
Lithobid Tablets **1692**

Lithium Citrate (Diuretics reduce the renal clearance of lithium and add a high risk of lithium toxicity).
No products indexed under this heading.

Losartan Potassium (Co-administration of thiazides with other antihypertensive agents may lead to additive effects or potentiation). Products include:
Cozaar Tablets **1935**
Hyzaar 50-12.5 Tablets **1990**
Hyzaar 100-12.5 Tablets **1990**
Hyzaar 100-25 Tablets **1990**

Mecamylamine Hydrochloride (Co-administration of thiazides with other antihypertensive agents may lead to additive effects or potentiation).
No products indexed under this heading.

Meclofenamate Sodium (Nonsteroidal anti-inflammatory agents can reduce the natriuretic, diuretic, and antihypertensive effects).
No products indexed under this heading.

Mefenamic Acid (Nonsteroidal anti-inflammatory agents can reduce the natriuretic, diuretic, and antihypertensive effects).
No products indexed under this heading.

Meloxicam (Nonsteroidal anti-inflammatory agents can reduce the natriuretic, diuretic, and antihypertensive effects). Products include:
Mobic Oral Suspension 863
Mobic Tablets 863

Meperidine Hydrochloride (Narcotics may potentiate orthostatic hypotension).
No products indexed under this heading.

Mephobarbital (Barbiturates may potentiate orthostatic hypotension).
No products indexed under this heading.

Metformin Hydrochloride (Hyperglycemia may occur with thiazide diuretics; oral hypoglycemic dosage may need to be adjusted). Products include:
ActoPlus Met Tablets 3214
Avandamet Tablets 1373
Fortamet Extended-Release Tablets 3115

Methadone Hydrochloride (Narcotics may potentiate orthostatic hypotension).
No products indexed under this heading.

Methyclothiazide (Co-administration of thiazides with other antihypertensive agents may lead to additive effects or potentiation).
No products indexed under this heading.

Methyldopa (Co-administration of thiazides with other antihypertensive agents may lead to additive effects or potentiation). Products include:
Aldoril Tablets 1910

Methyldopate Hydrochloride (Co-administration of thiazides with other antihypertensive agents may lead to additive effects or potentiation).
No products indexed under this heading.

Methylprednisolone Acetate (Corticosteroids intensify the electrolyte imbalance, particularly hypokalemia). Products include:
Depo-Medrol Injectable Suspension 2617
Depo-Medrol Single-Dose Vial 2619

Methylprednisolone Sodium Succinate (Corticosteroids intensify the electrolyte imbalance, particularly hypokalemia).
No products indexed under this heading.

Metocurine Iodide (Possible increased responsiveness to muscle relaxants).
No products indexed under this heading.

Metolazone (Co-administration of thiazides with other antihypertensive agents may lead to additive effects or potentiation).
No products indexed under this heading.

Metoprolol Succinate (Co-administration of thiazides with other antihypertensive agents may lead to additive effects or potentiation). Products include:
Toprol-XL Tablets 668

Metoprolol Tartrate (Co-administration of thiazides with other antihypertensive agents may lead to additive effects or potentiation). Products include:
Lopressor Injection 2238
Lopressor Tablets 2238
Lopressor HCT 50/25 Tablets 2241
Lopressor HCT 100/25 Tablets 2241
Lopressor HCT 100/50 Tablets 2241

Metyrosine (Co-administration of thiazides with other antihypertensive agents may lead to additive effects or potentiation). Products include:
Demser Capsules 1953

Mibefradil Dihydrochloride (Co-administration of thiazides with other antihypertensive agents may lead to additive effects or potentiation).
No products indexed under this heading.

Miglitol (Hyperglycemia may occur with thiazide diuretics; oral hypoglycemic dosage may need to be adjusted).
No products indexed under this heading.

Minoxidil (Co-administration of thiazides with other antihypertensive agents may lead to additive effects or potentiation). Products include:
Men's Rogaine Extra Strength Hair Regrowth Treatment Topical Solution, Ocean Rush Scent and Original Unscented .... ▣633
Men's Rogaine Foam Hair Regrowth Treatment .... ▣633
Women's Rogaine Hair Regrowth Treatment Topical Solution, Spring Bloom Scent and Original Unscented .... ▣634

Mivacurium Chloride (Possible increased responsiveness to muscle relaxants). Products include:
Mivacron Injection 493

Moexipril Hydrochloride (Co-administration of thiazides with other antihypertensive agents may lead to additive effects or potentiation). Products include:
Uniretic Tablets 3100
Univasc Tablets 3104

Morphine Sulfate (Narcotics may potentiate orthostatic hypotension). Products include:
Avinza Capsules 1741
Kadian Capsules 577
MS Contin Tablets 2701

Nabumetone (Nonsteroidal anti-inflammatory agents can reduce the natriuretic, diuretic, and antihypertensive effects).
No products indexed under this heading.

Nadolol (Co-administration of thiazides with other antihypertensive agents may lead to additive effects or potentiation). Products include:
Nadolol Tablets 2159

Naproxen (Nonsteroidal anti-inflammatory agents can reduce the natriuretic, diuretic, and antihypertensive effects). Products include:
EC-Naprosyn Delayed-Release Tablets 2761
Naprosyn Suspension 2761
Naprosyn Tablets 2761
Prevacid NapraPAC 3280

Naproxen Sodium (Nonsteroidal anti-inflammatory agents can reduce the natriuretic, diuretic, and antihypertensive effects). Products include:
Aleve Caplets 742
Aleve Gelcaps 743
Aleve Tablets 743
Aleve Cold & Sinus Caplets 744
Anaprox Tablets 2761
Anaprox DS Tablets 2761

Nicardipine Hydrochloride (Co-administration of thiazides with other antihypertensive agents may lead to additive effects or potentiation). Products include:
Cardene I.V. 2497

Nifedipine (Co-administration of thiazides with other antihypertensive agents may lead to additive effects or potentiation). Products include:
Adalat CC Tablets 2964

Nisoldipine (Co-administration of thiazides with other antihypertensive agents may lead to additive effects or potentiation). Products include:
Sular Tablets 3122

Nitroglycerin (Co-administration of thiazides with other antihypertensive agents may lead to additive effects or potentiation). Products include:
Nitro-Dur Transdermal Infusion System 3046
Nitrolingual Pumpspray 3120

Norepinephrine Bitartrate (Possible decreased response to pressor amines).
No products indexed under this heading.

Oxaprozin (Nonsteroidal anti-inflammatory agents can reduce the natriuretic, diuretic, and antihypertensive effects).
No products indexed under this heading.

Oxycodone Hydrochloride (Narcotics may potentiate orthostatic hypotension). Products include:
OxyContin Tablets 2703
OxyFast Oral Concentrate Solution 2708
OxyIR Capsules 2708
Percocet Tablets 1131
Percodan Tablets 1132

Pancuronium Bromide (Possible increased responsiveness to muscle relaxants).
No products indexed under this heading.

Penbutolol Sulfate (Co-administration of thiazides with other antihypertensive agents may lead to additive effects or potentiation).
No products indexed under this heading.

Pentobarbital Sodium (Barbiturates may potentiate orthostatic hypotension). Products include:
Nembutal Sodium Solution, USP 2470

Perindopril Erbumine (Co-administration of thiazides with other antihypertensive agents may lead to additive effects or potentiation). Products include:
Aceon Tablets (2 mg, 4 mg, 8 mg) 3194

Phenobarbital (Barbiturates may potentiate orthostatic hypotension). Products include:
Donnatal Extentabs 2493

Phenoxybenzamine Hydrochloride (Co-administration of thiazides with other antihypertensive agents may lead to additive effects or potentiation). Products include:
Dibenzyline Capsules 3399

Phentolamine Mesylate (Co-administration of thiazides with other antihypertensive agents may lead to additive effects or potentiation).
No products indexed under this heading.

Phenylbutazone (Nonsteroidal anti-inflammatory agents can reduce the natriuretic, diuretic, and antihypertensive effects).
No products indexed under this heading.

Pindolol (Co-administration of thiazides with other antihypertensive agents may lead to additive effects or potentiation).
No products indexed under this heading.

Pioglitazone Hydrochloride (Hyperglycemia may occur with thiazide diuretics; oral hypoglycemic dosage may need to be adjusted). Products include:
ActoPlus Met Tablets 3214
Actos Tablets 3219
Duetact Tablets 3226

Piroxicam (Nonsteroidal anti-inflammatory agents can reduce the natriuretic, diuretic, and antihypertensive effects).
No products indexed under this heading.

Polythiazide (Co-administration of thiazides with other antihypertensive agents may lead to additive effects or potentiation).
No products indexed under this heading.

Potassium Acid Phosphate (Concomitant use of potassium supplements with eprosartan may lead to hyperkalemia). Products include:
K-Phos Original (Sodium Free) Tablets 760

Potassium Bicarbonate (Concomitant use of potassium supplements with eprosartan may lead to hyperkalemia).
No products indexed under this heading.

Potassium Chloride (Concomitant use of potassium supplements with eprosartan may lead to hyperkalemia). Products include:
Colyte with Flavor Packs for Oral Solution 3088
HalfLytely and Bisacodyl Tablets Bowel Prep Kit with Flavors Packs 881
K-Dur Extended-Relase Tablets 3033
K-Lor Oral Solution 474
K-Tab Tablets 475
MoviPrep Oral Solution 2839
TriLyte with Flavor Packs for Oral Solution 3100

Potassium Citrate (Concomitant use of potassium supplements with eprosartan may lead to hyperkalemia). Products include:
Urocit-K Tablets 2144

Potassium Gluconate (Concomitant use of potassium supplements with eprosartan may lead to hyperkalemia).
No products indexed under this heading.

Potassium Phosphate (Concomitant use of potassium supplements with eprosartan may lead to hyperkalemia). Products include:
K-Phos Neutral Tablets 760

Prazosin Hydrochloride (Co-administration of thiazides with other antihypertensive agents may lead to additive effects or potentiation).
No products indexed under this heading.

Prednisolone Acetate (Corticosteroids intensify the electrolyte imbalance, particularly hypokalemia). Products include:
Blephamide Ophthalmic Ointment 568
Blephamide Ophthalmic Suspension 569
Poly-Pred Ophthalmic Suspension .... ⊙233
Pred Forte Ophthalmic Suspension .... ⊙235
Pred Mild Ophthalmic Suspension .... ⊙238
Pred-G Ophthalmic Ointment .... ⊙237
Pred-G Ophthalmic Suspension .... ⊙236

Prednisolone Sodium Phosphate (Corticosteroids intensify the electrolyte imbalance, particularly hypokalemia).
No products indexed under this heading.

Prednisolone Tebutate (Corticosteroids intensify the electrolyte imbalance, particularly hypokalemia).
No products indexed under this heading.

Prednisone (Corticosteroids intensify the electrolyte imbalance, particularly hypokalemia).
No products indexed under this heading.

Propoxyphene Hydrochloride (Narcotics may potentiate orthostatic hypotension).
No products indexed under this heading.

Propoxyphene Napsylate (Narcotics may potentiate orthostatic hypotension).
No products indexed under this heading.

Propranolol Hydrochloride (Co-administration of thiazides with other antihypertensive agents may lead to additive effects or potentiation). Products include:
Inderal LA Long-Acting Capsules 3429
InnoPran XL Capsules 2723

Quinapril Hydrochloride (Co-administration of thiazides with other antihypertensive agents may lead to additive effects or potentiation).
No products indexed under this heading.

Ramipril (Co-administration of thiazides with other antihypertensive agents may lead to additive effects or potentiation). Products include:
Altace Capsules 1702

Rapacuronium Bromide (Possible increased responsiveness to muscle relaxants).
No products indexed under this heading.

Rauwolfia Serpentina (Co-administration of thiazides with other antihypertensive agents may lead to additive effects or potentiation).
No products indexed under this heading.

Remifentanil Hydrochloride (Narcotics may potentiate orthostatic hypotension).
No products indexed under this heading.

Repaglinide (Hyperglycemia may occur with thiazide diuretics; oral hypoglycemic dosage may need to be adjusted).
No products indexed under this heading.

Rescinnamine (Co-administration of thiazides with other antihypertensive agents may lead to additive effects or potentiation).
No products indexed under this heading.

Reserpine (Co-administration of thiazides with other antihypertensive agents may lead to additive effects or potentiation).
No products indexed under this heading.

Rocuronium Bromide (Possible increased responsiveness to muscle relaxants). Products include:
Zemuron Injection 2346

Rofecoxib (Nonsteroidal anti-inflammatory agents can reduce the natriuretic, diuretic, and antihypertensive effects).
No products indexed under this heading.

Rosiglitazone Maleate (Hyperglycemia may occur with thiazide diuretics; oral hypoglycemic dosage may need to be adjusted). Products include:
Avandamet Tablets 1373
Avandaryl Tablets 1379
Avandia Tablets 1384

Secobarbital Sodium (Barbiturates may potentiate orthostatic hypotension).
No products indexed under this heading.

Sodium Nitroprusside (Co-administration of thiazides with other antihypertensive agents may lead to additive effects or potentiation).
No products indexed under this heading.

Sotalol Hydrochloride (Co-administration of thiazides with other antihypertensive agents may lead to additive effects or potentiation).
No products indexed under this heading.

Spirapril Hydrochloride (Co-administration of thiazides with other antihypertensive agents may lead to additive effects or potentiation).
No products indexed under this heading.

Spironolactone (Concomitant use of potassium sparing diuretics with eprosartan may lead to hyperkalemia).
No products indexed under this heading.

Sufentanil Citrate (Narcotics may potentiate orthostatic hypotension).
No products indexed under this heading.

Sulindac (Nonsteroidal anti-inflammatory agents can reduce the natriuretic, diuretic, and antihypertensive effects). Products include:
Clinoril Tablets 1924

Telmisartan (Co-administration of thiazides with other antihypertensive agents may lead to additive effects or potentiation). Products include:
Micardis Tablets 854
Micardis HCT Tablets 856

Terazosin Hydrochloride (Co-administration of thiazides with other antihypertensive agents may lead to additive effects or potentiation). Products include:
Hytrin Capsules 471

Thiamylal Sodium (Barbiturates may potentiate orthostatic hypotension).
No products indexed under this heading.

Timolol Maleate (Co-administration of thiazides with other antihypertensive agents may lead to additive effects or potentiation). Products include:
Blocadren Tablets 1916
Cosopt Sterile Ophthalmic Solution 1931
Timolide Tablets 2086
Timoptic Sterile Ophthalmic Solution 2088
Timoptic in Ocudose 2091
Timoptic-XE Sterile Ophthalmic Gel Forming Solution 2092

Tolazamide (Hyperglycemia may occur with thiazide diuretics; oral hypoglycemic dosage may need to be adjusted).
No products indexed under this heading.

Tolbutamide (Hyperglycemia may occur with thiazide diuretics; oral hypoglycemic dosage may need to be adjusted).
No products indexed under this heading.

Tolmetin Sodium (Nonsteroidal anti-inflammatory agents can reduce the natriuretic, diuretic, and antihypertensive effects).
No products indexed under this heading.

Torsemide (Co-administration of thiazides with other antihypertensive agents may lead to additive effects or potentiation). Products include:
Demadex Injection 2759
Demadex Tablets 2759

Trandolapril (Co-administration of thiazides with other antihypertensive agents may lead to additive effects or potentiation). Products include:
Mavik Tablets 486
Tarka Tablets 524

Triamcinolone (Corticosteroids intensify the electrolyte imbalance, particularly hypokalemia).
No products indexed under this heading.

Triamcinolone Acetonide (Corticosteroids intensify the electrolyte imbalance, particularly hypokalemia). Products include:
Azmacort Inhalation Aerosol 1726
Nasacort AQ Nasal Spray 2922

Triamcinolone Diacetate (Corticosteroids intensify the electrolyte imbalance, particularly hypokalemia).
No products indexed under this heading.

Triamcinolone Hexacetonide (Corticosteroids intensify the electrolyte imbalance, particularly hypokalemia).
No products indexed under this heading.

Triamterene (Concomitant use of potassium sparing diuretics with eprosartan may lead to hyperkalemia). Products include:
Dyazide Capsules 1423
Dyrenium Capsules 3400

Trimethaphan Camsylate (Co-administration of thiazides with other antihypertensive agents may lead to additive effects or potentiation).
No products indexed under this heading.

Troglitazone (Hyperglycemia may occur with thiazide diuretics; oral hypoglycemic dosage may need to be adjusted).
No products indexed under this heading.

Tubocurarine Chloride (Possible increased responsiveness to muscle relaxant).
No products indexed under this heading.

Valdecoxib (Nonsteroidal anti-inflammatory agents can reduce the natriuretic, diuretic, and antihypertensive effects).
No products indexed under this heading.

Valsartan (Co-administration of thiazides with other antihypertensive agents may lead to additive effects or potentiation). Products include:
Diovan Tablets 2193
Diovan HCT Tablets 2196

Vecuronium Bromide (Possible increased responsiveness to muscle relaxants).
No products indexed under this heading.

Verapamil Hydrochloride (Co-administration of thiazides with other antihypertensive agents may lead to additive effects or potentiation). Products include:
Covera-HS Tablets 3139
Tarka Tablets 524
Verelan PM Extended-Release Capsules, Controlled-Onset 3106

Food Interactions

Alcohol (May potentiate orthostatic hypotension).

TEV-TROPIN FOR INJECTION

(Somatropin (rDNA Origin)) 1222
May interact with glucocorticoids. Compounds in these categories include:

Betamethasone Acetate (Glucocorticoid therapy may inhibit the growth-promoting effect of human growth hormone. Patients with co-existing ACTH deficiency should have their glucocorticoid replacement dose carefully adjusted to avoid an inhibitory effect on growth).
No products indexed under this heading.

Betamethasone Sodium Phosphate (Glucocorticoid therapy may inhibit the growth-promoting effect of human growth hormone. Patients with co-existing ACTH deficiency should have their glucocorticoid replacement dose carefully adjusted to avoid an inhibitory effect on growth).
No products indexed under this heading.

Cortisone Acetate (Glucocorticoid therapy may inhibit the growth-promoting effect of human growth hormone. Patients with co-existing ACTH deficiency should have their glucocorticoid replacement dose carefully adjusted to avoid an inhibitory effect on growth).
No products indexed under this heading.

Dexamethasone (Glucocorticoid therapy may inhibit the growth-promoting effect of human growth hormone. Patients with co-existing ACTH deficiency should have their glucocorticoid replacement dose carefully adjusted to avoid an inhibitory effect on growth). Products include:
Ciprodex Otic Suspension 559
Decadron Tablets 1951
TobraDex Ophthalmic Ointment 562
TobraDex Ophthalmic Suspension 563

Dexamethasone Acetate (Glucocorticoid therapy may inhibit the growth-promoting effect of human growth hormone. Patients with co-existing ACTH deficiency should have their glucocorticoid replacement dose carefully adjusted to avoid an inhibitory effect on growth).
No products indexed under this heading.

Dexamethasone Sodium Phosphate (Glucocorticoid therapy may inhibit the growth-promoting effect of human growth hormone. Patients with co-existing ACTH deficiency should have their glucocorticoid replacement dose carefully adjusted to avoid an inhibitory effect on growth).
No products indexed under this heading.

Fludrocortisone Acetate (Glucocorticoid therapy may inhibit the growth-promoting effect of human growth hormone. Patients with co-existing ACTH deficiency should have their glucocorticoid replacement dose carefully adjusted to avoid an inhibitory effect on growth).
No products indexed under this heading.

Hydrocortisone (Glucocorticoid therapy may inhibit the growth-promoting effect of human growth hormone. Patients with co-existing ACTH deficiency should have their glucocorticoid replacement dose carefully adjusted to avoid an inhibitory effect on growth). Products include:

Colocort Rectal Suspension, USP (Retention) 100 mg/60 mL **2476**
Hydrocortone Tablets **1989**
Preparation H Hydrocortisone Cream .... ▣**646**

Hydrocortisone Acetate (Glucocorticoid therapy may inhibit the growth-promoting effect of human growth hormone. Patients with co-existing ACTH deficiency should have their glucocorticoid replacement dose carefully adjusted to avoid an inhibitory effect on growth). Products include:

Analpram-HC **1159**
Pramosone **1161**
ProctoFoam-HC **3099**

Hydrocortisone Sodium Phosphate (Glucocorticoid therapy may inhibit the growth-promoting effect of human growth hormone. Patients with co-existing ACTH deficiency should have their glucocorticoid replacement dose carefully adjusted to avoid an inhibitory effect on growth).
No products indexed under this heading.

Hydrocortisone Sodium Succinate (Glucocorticoid therapy may inhibit the growth-promoting effect of human growth hormone. Patients with co-existing ACTH deficiency should have their glucocorticoid replacement dose carefully adjusted to avoid an inhibitory effect on growth).
No products indexed under this heading.

Methylprednisolone Acetate (Glucocorticoid therapy may inhibit the growth-promoting effect of human growth hormone. Patients with co-existing ACTH deficiency should have their glucocorticoid replacement dose carefully adjusted to avoid an inhibitory effect on growth). Products include:

Depo-Medrol Injectable Suspension **2617**
Depo-Medrol Single-Dose Vial **2619**

Methylprednisolone Sodium Succinate (Glucocorticoid therapy may inhibit the growth-promoting effect of human growth hormone. Patients with co-existing ACTH deficiency should have their glucocorticoid replacement dose carefully adjusted to avoid an inhibitory effect on growth).
No products indexed under this heading.

Prednisolone Acetate (Glucocorticoid therapy may inhibit the growth-promoting effect of human growth hormone. Patients with co-existing ACTH deficiency should have their glucocorticoid replacement dose carefully adjusted to avoid an inhibitory effect on growth). Products include:

Blephamide Ophthalmic Ointment **568**
Blephamide Ophthalmic Suspension **569**
Poly-Pred Ophthalmic Suspension .... ⊙**233**
Pred Forte Ophthalmic Suspension .... ⊙**235**
Pred Mild Ophthalmic Suspension .... ⊙**238**
Pred-G Ophthalmic Ointment .... ⊙**237**
Pred-G Ophthalmic Suspension .... ⊙**236**

Prednisolone Sodium Phosphate (Glucocorticoid therapy may inhibit the growth-promoting effect of human growth hormone. Patients with co-existing ACTH deficiency should have their glucocorticoid replacement dose carefully adjusted to avoid an inhibitory effect on growth).
No products indexed under this heading.

Prednisolone Tebutate (Glucocorticoid therapy may inhibit the growth-promoting effect of human growth hormone. Patients with co-existing ACTH deficiency should have their glucocorticoid replacement dose carefully adjusted to avoid an inhibitory effect on growth).
No products indexed under this heading.

Prednisone (Glucocorticoid therapy may inhibit the growth-promoting effect of human growth hormone. Patients with co-existing ACTH deficiency should have their glucocorticoid replacement dose carefully adjusted to avoid an inhibitory effect on growth).
No products indexed under this heading.

Triamcinolone (Glucocorticoid therapy may inhibit the growth-promoting effect of human growth hormone. Patients with co-existing ACTH deficiency should have their glucocorticoid replacement dose carefully adjusted to avoid an inhibitory effect on growth).
No products indexed under this heading.

Triamcinolone Acetonide (Glucocorticoid therapy may inhibit the growth-promoting effect of human growth hormone. Patients with co-existing ACTH deficiency should have their glucocorticoid replacement dose carefully adjusted to avoid an inhibitory effect on growth). Products include:

Azmacort Inhalation Aerosol **1726**
Nasacort AQ Nasal Spray **2922**

Triamcinolone Diacetate (Glucocorticoid therapy may inhibit the growth-promoting effect of human growth hormone. Patients with co-existing ACTH deficiency should have their glucocorticoid replacement dose carefully adjusted to avoid an inhibitory effect on growth).
No products indexed under this heading.

Triamcinolone Hexacetonide (Glucocorticoid therapy may inhibit the growth-promoting effect of human growth hormone. Patients with co-existing ACTH deficiency should have their glucocorticoid replacement dose carefully adjusted to avoid an inhibitory effect on growth).
No products indexed under this heading.

THALOMID CAPSULES

(Thalidomide) **965**

May interact with barbiturates, drugs that may exacerbate peripheral neuropathy (selected), phenytoin, protease inhibitors, and certain other agents. Compounds in these categories include:

Amprenavir (Concomitant use of HIV-protease inhibitors with hormonal contraceptives may reduce the effectiveness of contraception; women requiring treatment with HIV-protease inhibitors must use two other highly effective methods of contraception or abstain from heterosexual sexual intercourse during treatment with thalidomide). Products include:

Agenerase Capsules **1327**
Agenerase Oral Solution **1332**

Aprobarbital (Thalidomide has been reported to enhance the sedative activity of barbiturates).
No products indexed under this heading.

Butabarbital (Thalidomide has been reported to enhance the sedative activity of barbiturates).
No products indexed under this heading.

Butalbital (Thalidomide has been reported to enhance the sedative activity of barbiturates).
No products indexed under this heading.

Carbamazepine (Concomitant use of carbamazepine with hormonal contraceptives may reduce the effectiveness of contraception; women requiring treatment with carbamazepine must use two other highly effective methods of contraception or abstain from heterosexual sexual intercourse during treatment with thalidomide). Products include:

Carbatrol Capsules **3171**
Equetro Extended-Release Capsules **3180**
Tegretol/Tegretol-XR **2295**

Carboplatin (Peripheral neuropathy is a common, potentially severe, side effect of treatment with thalidomide; therefore, concomitant use of drugs known to be associated with peripheral neuropathy should be undertaken with caution).
No products indexed under this heading.

Chlorpromazine (Thalidomide has been reported to enhance the sedative activity of chlorpromazine).
No products indexed under this heading.

Chlorpromazine Hydrochloride (Thalidomide has been reported to enhance the sedative activity of chlorpromazine).
No products indexed under this heading.

Didanosine (Peripheral neuropathy is a common, potentially severe, side effect of treatment with thalidomide; therefore, concomitant use of drugs known to be associated with peripheral neuropathy should be undertaken with caution).
No products indexed under this heading.

Fosphenytoin Sodium (Concomitant use of phenytoin with hormonal contraceptives may reduce the effectiveness of contraception; women requiring treatment with phenytoin must use two other highly effective methods of contraception or abstain from heterosexual sexual intercourse during treatment with thalidomide).
No products indexed under this heading.

Griseofulvin (Concomitant use of griseofulvin with hormonal contraceptives may reduce the effectiveness of contraception; women requiring treatment with griseofulvin must use two other highly effective methods of contraception or abstain from heterosexual sexual intercourse during treatment with thalidomide). Products include:

Gris-PEG Tablets **2502**

Indinavir Sulfate (Concomitant use of HIV-protease inhibitors with hormonal contraceptives may reduce the effectiveness of contraception; women requiring treatment with HIV-protease inhibitors must use two other highly effective methods of contraception or abstain from heterosexual sexual intercourse during treatment with thalidomide). Products include:

Crixivan Capsules **1940**

Isoniazid (Peripheral neuropathy is a common, potentially severe, side effect of treatment with thalidomide; therefore, concomitant use of drugs known to be associated with peripheral neuropathy should be undertaken with caution).
No products indexed under this heading.

Lopinavir (Concomitant use of HIV-protease inhibitors with hormonal contraceptives may reduce the effectiveness of contraception; women requiring treatment with HIV-protease inhibitors must use two other highly effective methods of contraception or abstain from heterosexual sexual intercourse during treatment with thalidomide). Products include:

Kaletra **476**

Mephobarbital (Thalidomide has been reported to enhance the sedative activity of barbiturates).
No products indexed under this heading.

Nelfinavir Mesylate (Concomitant use of HIV-protease inhibitors with hormonal contraceptives may reduce the effectiveness of contraception; women requiring treatment with HIV-protease inhibitors must use two other highly effective methods of contraception or abstain from heterosexual sexual intercourse during treatment with thalidomide). Products include:

Viracept .. 2577

Paclitaxel (Peripheral neuropathy is a common, potentially severe, side effect of treatment with thalidomide; therefore, concomitant use of drugs known to be associated with peripheral neuropathy should be undertaken with caution).
No products indexed under this heading.

Pentobarbital Sodium (Thalidomide has been reported to enhance the sedative activity of barbiturates). Products include:
Nembutal Sodium Solution, USP 2470

Phenobarbital (Thalidomide has been reported to enhance the sedative activity of barbiturates). Products include:
Donnatal Extentabs 2493

Phenytoin (Concomitant use of phenytoin with hormonal contraceptives may reduce the effectiveness of contraception; women requiring treatment with phenytoin must use two other highly effective methods of contraception or abstain from heterosexual sexual intercourse during treatment with thalidomide).
No products indexed under this heading.

Phenytoin Sodium (Concomitant use of phenytoin with hormonal contraceptives may reduce the effectiveness of contraception; women requiring treatment with phenytoin must use two other highly effective methods of contraception or abstain from heterosexual sexual intercourse during treatment with thalidomide). Products include:
Phenytek Capsules 2160

Reserpine (Thalidomide has been reported to enhance the sedative activity of reserpine).
No products indexed under this heading.

Rifabutin (Concomitant use of rifabutin with hormonal contraceptives may reduce the effectiveness of contraception; women requiring treatment with rifabutin must use two other highly effective methods of contraception or abstain from heterosexual sexual intercourse during treatment with thalidomide).
No products indexed under this heading.

Rifampin (Concomitant use of rifampin with hormonal contraceptives may reduce the effectiveness of contraception; women requiring treatment with rifampin must use two other highly effective methods of contraception or abstain from heterosexual sexual intercourse during treatment with thalidomide).
No products indexed under this heading.

Ritonavir (Concomitant use of HIV-protease inhibitors with hormonal contraceptives may reduce the effectiveness of contraception; women requiring treatment with HIV-protease inhibitors must use two other highly effective methods of contraception or abstain from heterosexual sexual intercourse during treatment with thalidomide). Products include:
Kaletra .. 476
Norvir ... 503

Saquinavir (Concomitant use of HIV-protease inhibitors with hormonal contraceptives may reduce the effectiveness of contraception; women requiring treatment with HIV-protease inhibitors must use two other highly effective methods of contraception or abstain from heterosexual sexual intercourse during treatment with thalidomide).
No products indexed under this heading.

Saquinavir Mesylate (Concomitant use of HIV-protease inhibitors with hormonal contraceptives may reduce the effectiveness of contraception; women requiring treatment with HIV-protease inhibitors must use two other highly effective methods of contraception or abstain from heterosexual sexual intercourse during treatment with thalidomide). Products include:
Invirase ... 2772

Secobarbital Sodium (Thalidomide has been reported to enhance the sedative activity of barbiturates).
No products indexed under this heading.

Stavudine (Peripheral neuropathy is a common, potentially severe, side effect of treatment with thalidomide; therefore, concomitant use of drugs known to be associated with peripheral neuropathy should be undertaken with caution).
No products indexed under this heading.

Thiamylal Sodium (Thalidomide has been reported to enhance the sedative activity of barbiturates).
No products indexed under this heading.

Zalcitabine (Peripheral neuropathy is a common, potentially severe, side effect of treatment with thalidomide; therefore, concomitant use of drugs known to be associated with peripheral neuropathy should be undertaken with caution).
No products indexed under this heading.

Food Interactions

Alcohol (Thalidomide has been reported to enhance the sedative activity of alcohol).

Food, unspecified (Co-administration of Thalomid with a high fat meal causes minor changes in the observed AUC and Cmax values; however, it causes an increase in Tmax to approximately 6 hours).

THERAFLU COLD & COUGH HOT LIQUID

(Dextromethorphan Hydrobromide, Pheniramine Maleate, Phenylephrine Hydrochloride) ▣ 740
May interact with hypnotics and sedatives, monoamine oxidase inhibitors, tranquilizers, and certain other agents. Compounds in these categories include:

Alprazolam (Concurrent use with tranquilizers may increase drowsiness; use caution when co-administering). Products include:
Niravam Orally Disintegrating Tablets ... 3092

Buspirone Hydrochloride (Concurrent use with tranquilizers may increase drowsiness; use caution when co-administering).
No products indexed under this heading.

Chlordiazepoxide (Concurrent use with tranquilizers may increase drowsiness; use caution when co-administering).
No products indexed under this heading.

Chlordiazepoxide Hydrochloride (Concurrent use with tranquilizers may increase drowsiness; use caution when co-administering). Products include:
Librium Capsules 3347

Chlorpromazine (Concurrent use with tranquilizers may increase drowsiness; use caution when co-administering).
No products indexed under this heading.

Chlorpromazine Hydrochloride (Concurrent use with tranquilizers may increase drowsiness; use caution when co-administering).
No products indexed under this heading.

Chlorprothixene (Concurrent use with tranquilizers may increase drowsiness; use caution when co-administering).
No products indexed under this heading.

Chlorprothixene Hydrochloride (Concurrent use with tranquilizers may increase drowsiness; use caution when co-administering).
No products indexed under this heading.

Clorazepate Dipotassium (Concurrent use with tranquilizers may increase drowsiness; use caution when co-administering). Products include:
Tranxene ... 2474

Diazepam (Concurrent use with tranquilizers may increase drowsiness; use caution when co-administering). Products include:
Diastat Rectal Delivery System 3343
Valium Tablets 2819

Droperidol (Concurrent use with tranquilizers may increase drowsiness; use caution when co-administering).
No products indexed under this heading.

Estazolam (Concurrent use with sedatives may increase drowsiness; use caution when co-administering). Products include:
ProSom Tablets 517

Ethchlorvynol (Concurrent use with sedatives may increase drowsiness; use caution when co-administering).
No products indexed under this heading.

Ethinamate (Concurrent use with sedatives may increase drowsiness; use caution when co-administering).
No products indexed under this heading.

Fluphenazine Decanoate (Concurrent use with tranquilizers may increase drowsiness; use caution when co-administering).
No products indexed under this heading.

Fluphenazine Enanthate (Concurrent use with tranquilizers may increase drowsiness; use caution when co-administering).
No products indexed under this heading.

Fluphenazine Hydrochloride (Concurrent use with tranquilizers may increase drowsiness; use caution when co-administering).
No products indexed under this heading.

Flurazepam Hydrochloride (Concurrent use with sedatives may increase drowsiness; use caution when co-administering). Products include:
Dalmane Capsules 3342

Glutethimide (Concurrent use with sedatives may increase drowsiness; use caution when co-administering).
No products indexed under this heading.

Haloperidol (Concurrent use with tranquilizers may increase drowsiness; use caution when co-administering).
No products indexed under this heading.

Haloperidol Decanoate (Concurrent use with tranquilizers may increase drowsiness; use caution when co-administering).
No products indexed under this heading.

Hydroxyzine Hydrochloride (Concurrent use with tranquilizers may increase drowsiness; use caution when co-administering).
No products indexed under this heading.

Isocarboxazid (Do not use while taking, or for two weeks after stopping, MAO inhibitors).
No products indexed under this heading.

Lorazepam (Concurrent use with sedatives may increase drowsiness; use caution when co-administering).
No products indexed under this heading.

Loxapine Hydrochloride (Concurrent use with tranquilizers may increase drowsiness; use caution when co-administering).
No products indexed under this heading.

Loxapine Succinate (Concurrent use with tranquilizers may increase drowsiness; use caution when co-administering).
No products indexed under this heading.

Meprobamate (Concurrent use with tranquilizers may increase drowsiness; use caution when co-administering).
No products indexed under this heading.

Mesoridazine Besylate (Concurrent use with tranquilizers may increase drowsiness; use caution when co-administering).
No products indexed under this heading.

Midazolam Hydrochloride (Concurrent use with sedatives may increase drowsiness; use caution when co-administering).
No products indexed under this heading.

Moclobemide (Do not use while taking, or for two weeks after stopping, MAO inhibitors).
No products indexed under this heading.

Molindone Hydrochloride (Concurrent use with tranquilizers may increase drowsiness; use caution when co-administering). Products include:
Moban Tablets 1119

Oxazepam (Concurrent use with tranquilizers may increase drowsiness; use caution when co-administering).
No products indexed under this heading.

IMPORTANT NOTE: Always consult each drug listing in the patient's regimen for possible interactions.

Pargyline Hydrochloride (Do not use while taking, or for two weeks after stopping, MAO inhibitors).
No products indexed under this heading.

Perphenazine (Concurrent use with tranquilizers may increase drowsiness; use caution when co-administering).
No products indexed under this heading.

Phenelzine Sulfate (Do not use while taking, or for two weeks after stopping, MAO inhibitors).
No products indexed under this heading.

Prazepam (Concurrent use with tranquilizers may increase drowsiness; use caution when co-administering).
No products indexed under this heading.

Procarbazine Hydrochloride (Do not use while taking, or for two weeks after stopping, MAO inhibitors). Products include:
Matulane Capsules **3191**

Prochlorperazine (Concurrent use with tranquilizers may increase drowsiness; use caution when co-administering).
No products indexed under this heading.

Promethazine Hydrochloride (Concurrent use with tranquilizers may increase drowsiness; use caution when co-administering). Products include:
Phenergan Tablets and Suppositories **3440**

Propofol (Concurrent use with sedatives may increase drowsiness; use caution when co-administering).
No products indexed under this heading.

Quazepam (Concurrent use with sedatives may increase drowsiness; use caution when co-administering).
No products indexed under this heading.

Ramelteon (Concurrent use with sedatives may increase drowsiness; use caution when co-administering). Products include:
Rozerem Tablets **3231**

Secobarbital Sodium (Concurrent use with sedatives may increase drowsiness; use caution when co-administering).
No products indexed under this heading.

Selegiline Hydrochloride (Do not use while taking, or for two weeks after stopping, MAO inhibitors). Products include:
Eldepryl Capsules **3208**
Zelapar Tablets **3372**

Temazepam (Concurrent use with sedatives may increase drowsiness; use caution when co-administering). Products include:
Restoril Capsules **1860**

Thioridazine Hydrochloride (Concurrent use with tranquilizers may increase drowsiness; use caution when co-administering). Products include:
Thioridazine Hydrochloride Tablets **2163**

Thiothixene (Concurrent use with tranquilizers may increase drowsiness; use caution when co-administering). Products include:
Thiothixene Capsules **2165**

Tranylcypromine Sulfate (Do not use while taking, or for two weeks after stopping, MAO inhibitors). Products include:
Parnate Tablets **1527**

Triazolam (Concurrent use with sedatives may increase drowsiness; use caution when co-administering).
No products indexed under this heading.

Trifluoperazine Hydrochloride (Concurrent use with tranquilizers may increase drowsiness; use caution when co-administering).
No products indexed under this heading.

Zaleplon (Concurrent use with sedatives may increase drowsiness; use caution when co-administering). Products include:
Sonata Capsules **1717**

Zolpidem Tartrate (Concurrent use with sedatives may increase drowsiness; use caution when co-administering). Products include:
Ambien Tablets **2851**
Ambien CR Tablets **2855**

Food Interactions

Alcohol (Concurrent use may increase drowsiness; avoid alcoholic drinks).

THERAFLU COLD & SORE THROAT HOT LIQUID

(Acetaminophen, Pheniramine Maleate, Phenylephrine Hydrochloride)................................... **741**
May interact with hypnotics and sedatives, monoamine oxidase inhibitors, tranquilizers, and certain other agents. Compounds in these categories include:

Alprazolam (Concurrent use with tranquilizers may increase drowsiness; use caution when co-administering). Products include:
Niravam Orally Disintegrating Tablets **3092**

Buspirone Hydrochloride (Concurrent use with tranquilizers may increase drowsiness; use caution when co-administering).
No products indexed under this heading.

Chlordiazepoxide (Concurrent use with tranquilizers may increase drowsiness; use caution when co-administering).
No products indexed under this heading.

Chlordiazepoxide Hydrochloride (Concurrent use with tranquilizers may increase drowsiness; use caution when co-administering). Products include:
Librium Capsules **3347**

Chlorpromazine (Concurrent use with tranquilizers may increase drowsiness; use caution when co-administering).
No products indexed under this heading.

Chlorpromazine Hydrochloride (Concurrent use with tranquilizers may increase drowsiness; use caution when co-administering).
No products indexed under this heading.

Chlorprothixene (Concurrent use with tranquilizers may increase drowsiness; use caution when co-administering).
No products indexed under this heading.

Chlorprothixene Hydrochloride (Concurrent use with tranquilizers may increase drowsiness; use caution when co-administering).
No products indexed under this heading.

Clorazepate Dipotassium (Concurrent use with tranquilizers may increase drowsiness; use caution when co-administering). Products include:
Tranxene **2474**

Diazepam (Concurrent use with tranquilizers may increase drowsiness; use caution when co-administering). Products include:
Diastat Rectal Delivery System **3343**
Valium Tablets **2819**

Droperidol (Concurrent use with tranquilizers may increase drowsiness; use caution when co-administering).
No products indexed under this heading.

Estazolam (Concurrent use with sedatives may increase drowsiness; use caution when co-administering). Products include:
ProSom Tablets **517**

Ethchlorvynol (Concurrent use with sedatives may increase drowsiness; use caution when co-administering).
No products indexed under this heading.

Ethinamate (Concurrent use with sedatives may increase drowsiness; use caution when co-administering).
No products indexed under this heading.

Fluphenazine Decanoate (Concurrent use with tranquilizers may increase drowsiness; use caution when co-administering).
No products indexed under this heading.

Fluphenazine Enanthate (Concurrent use with tranquilizers may increase drowsiness; use caution when co-administering).
No products indexed under this heading.

Fluphenazine Hydrochloride (Concurrent use with tranquilizers may increase drowsiness; use caution when co-administering).
No products indexed under this heading.

Flurazepam Hydrochloride (Concurrent use with sedatives may increase drowsiness; use caution when co-administering). Products include:
Dalmane Capsules **3342**

Glutethimide (Concurrent use with sedatives may increase drowsiness; use caution when co-administering).
No products indexed under this heading.

Haloperidol (Concurrent use with tranquilizers may increase drowsiness; use caution when co-administering).
No products indexed under this heading.

Haloperidol Decanoate (Concurrent use with tranquilizers may increase drowsiness; use caution when co-administering).
No products indexed under this heading.

Hydroxyzine Hydrochloride (Concurrent use with tranquilizers may increase drowsiness; use caution when co-administering).
No products indexed under this heading.

Isocarboxazid (Do not use while taking, or for two weeks after stopping, MAO inhibitors).
No products indexed under this heading.

Lorazepam (Concurrent use with sedatives may increase drowsiness; use caution when co-administering).
No products indexed under this heading.

Loxapine Hydrochloride (Concurrent use with tranquilizers may increase drowsiness; use caution when co-administering).
No products indexed under this heading.

Loxapine Succinate (Concurrent use with tranquilizers may increase drowsiness; use caution when co-administering).
No products indexed under this heading.

Meprobamate (Concurrent use with tranquilizers may increase drowsiness; use caution when co-administering).
No products indexed under this heading.

Mesoridazine Besylate (Concurrent use with tranquilizers may increase drowsiness; use caution when co-administering).
No products indexed under this heading.

Midazolam Hydrochloride (Concurrent use with sedatives may increase drowsiness; use caution when co-administering).
No products indexed under this heading.

Moclobemide (Do not use while taking, or for two weeks after stopping, MAO inhibitors).
No products indexed under this heading.

Molindone Hydrochloride (Concurrent use with tranquilizers may increase drowsiness; use caution when co-administering). Products include:
Moban Tablets **1119**

Oxazepam (Concurrent use with tranquilizers may increase drowsiness; use caution when co-administering).
No products indexed under this heading.

Pargyline Hydrochloride (Do not use while taking, or for two weeks after stopping, MAO inhibitors).
No products indexed under this heading.

Perphenazine (Concurrent use with tranquilizers may increase drowsiness; use caution when co-administering).
No products indexed under this heading.

Phenelzine Sulfate (Do not use while taking, or for two weeks after stopping, MAO inhibitors).
No products indexed under this heading.

Prazepam (Concurrent use with tranquilizers may increase drowsiness; use caution when co-administering).
No products indexed under this heading.

Procarbazine Hydrochloride (Do not use while taking, or for two weeks after stopping, MAO inhibitors). Products include:
Matulane Capsules **3191**

Prochlorperazine (Concurrent use with tranquilizers may increase drowsiness; use caution when co-administering).
> No products indexed under this heading.

Promethazine Hydrochloride (Concurrent use with tranquilizers may increase drowsiness; use caution when co-administering). Products include:
> Phenergan Tablets and Suppositories 3440

Propofol (Concurrent use with sedatives may increase drowsiness; use caution when co-administering).
> No products indexed under this heading.

Quazepam (Concurrent use with sedatives may increase drowsiness; use caution when co-administering).
> No products indexed under this heading.

Ramelteon (Concurrent use with sedatives may increase drowsiness; use caution when co-administering). Products include:
> Rozerem Tablets 3231

Secobarbital Sodium (Concurrent use with sedatives may increase drowsiness; use caution when co-administering).
> No products indexed under this heading.

Selegiline Hydrochloride (Do not use while taking, or for two weeks after stopping, MAO inhibitors). Products include:
> Eldepryl Capsules 3208
> Zelapar Tablets 3372

Temazepam (Concurrent use with sedatives may increase drowsiness; use caution when co-administering). Products include:
> Restoril Capsules 1860

Thioridazine Hydrochloride (Concurrent use with tranquilizers may increase drowsiness; use caution when co-administering). Products include:
> Thioridazine Hydrochloride Tablets 2163

Thiothixene (Concurrent use with tranquilizers may increase drowsiness; use caution when co-administering). Products include:
> Thiothixene Capsules 2165

Tranylcypromine Sulfate (Do not use while taking, or for two weeks after stopping, MAO inhibitors). Products include:
> Parnate Tablets 1527

Triazolam (Concurrent use with sedatives may increase drowsiness; use caution when co-administering).
> No products indexed under this heading.

Trifluoperazine Hydrochloride (Concurrent use with tranquilizers may increase drowsiness; use caution when co-administering).
> No products indexed under this heading.

Zaleplon (Concurrent use with sedatives may increase drowsiness; use caution when co-administering). Products include:
> Sonata Capsules 1717

Zolpidem Tartrate (Concurrent use with sedatives may increase drowsiness; use caution when co-administering). Products include:
> Ambien Tablets 2851
> Ambien CR Tablets 2855

Food Interactions

Alcohol (Concurrent use may increase drowsiness; avoid alcoholic drinks).

THERAFLU FLU & CHEST CONGESTION HOT LIQUID
(Acetaminophen, Guaifenesin) ▣741

Food Interactions

Alcohol (Avoid alcoholic drinks).

THERAFLU FLU & SORE THROAT HOT LIQUID
(Acetaminophen, Pheniramine Maleate, Phenylephrine Hydrochloride) ▣742
May interact with hypnotics and sedatives, monoamine oxidase inhibitors, tranquilizers, and certain other agents. Compounds in these categories include:

Alprazolam (Concurrent use with tranquilizers may increase drowsiness; use caution when co-administering). Products include:
> Niravam Orally Disintegrating Tablets 3092

Buspirone Hydrochloride (Concurrent use with tranquilizers may increase drowsiness; use caution when co-administering).
> No products indexed under this heading.

Chlordiazepoxide (Concurrent use with tranquilizers may increase drowsiness; use caution when co-administering).
> No products indexed under this heading.

Chlordiazepoxide Hydrochloride (Concurrent use with tranquilizers may increase drowsiness; use caution when co-administering). Products include:
> Librium Capsules 3347

Chlorpromazine (Concurrent use with tranquilizers may increase drowsiness; use caution when co-administering).
> No products indexed under this heading.

Chlorpromazine Hydrochloride (Concurrent use with tranquilizers may increase drowsiness; use caution when co-administering).
> No products indexed under this heading.

Chlorprothixene (Concurrent use with tranquilizers may increase drowsiness; use caution when co-administering).
> No products indexed under this heading.

Chlorprothixene Hydrochloride (Concurrent use with tranquilizers may increase drowsiness; use caution when co-administering).
> No products indexed under this heading.

Clorazepate Dipotassium (Concurrent use with tranquilizers may increase drowsiness; use caution when co-administering). Products include:
> Tranxene 2474

Diazepam (Concurrent use with tranquilizers may increase drowsiness; use caution when co-administering). Products include:
> Diastat Rectal Delivery System 3343
> Valium Tablets 2819

Droperidol (Concurrent use with tranquilizers may increase drowsiness; use caution when co-administering).
> No products indexed under this heading.

Estazolam (Concurrent use with sedatives may increase drowsiness; use caution when co-administering). Products include:
> ProSom Tablets 517

Ethchlorvynol (Concurrent use with sedatives may increase drowsiness; use caution when co-administering).
> No products indexed under this heading.

Ethinamate (Concurrent use with sedatives may increase drowsiness; use caution when co-administering).
> No products indexed under this heading.

Fluphenazine Decanoate (Concurrent use with tranquilizers may increase drowsiness; use caution when co-administering).
> No products indexed under this heading.

Fluphenazine Enanthate (Concurrent use with tranquilizers may increase drowsiness; use caution when co-administering).
> No products indexed under this heading.

Fluphenazine Hydrochloride (Concurrent use with tranquilizers may increase drowsiness; use caution when co-administering).
> No products indexed under this heading.

Flurazepam Hydrochloride (Concurrent use with sedatives may increase drowsiness; use caution when co-administering). Products include:
> Dalmane Capsules 3342

Glutethimide (Concurrent use with sedatives may increase drowsiness; use caution when co-administering).
> No products indexed under this heading.

Haloperidol (Concurrent use with tranquilizers may increase drowsiness; use caution when co-administering).
> No products indexed under this heading.

Haloperidol Decanoate (Concurrent use with tranquilizers may increase drowsiness; use caution when co-administering).
> No products indexed under this heading.

Hydroxyzine Hydrochloride (Concurrent use with tranquilizers may increase drowsiness; use caution when co-administering).
> No products indexed under this heading.

Isocarboxazid (Do not use while taking, or for two weeks after stopping, MAO inhibitors).
> No products indexed under this heading.

Lorazepam (Concurrent use with sedatives may increase drowsiness; use caution when co-administering).
> No products indexed under this heading.

Loxapine Hydrochloride (Concurrent use with tranquilizers may increase drowsiness; use caution when co-administering).
> No products indexed under this heading.

Loxapine Succinate (Concurrent use with tranquilizers may increase drowsiness; use caution when co-administering).
> No products indexed under this heading.

Meprobamate (Concurrent use with tranquilizers may increase drowsiness; use caution when co-administering).
> No products indexed under this heading.

Mesoridazine Besylate (Concurrent use with tranquilizers may increase drowsiness; use caution when co-administering).
> No products indexed under this heading.

Midazolam Hydrochloride (Concurrent use with sedatives may increase drowsiness; use caution when co-administering).
> No products indexed under this heading.

Moclobemide (Do not use while taking, or for two weeks after stopping, MAO inhibitors).
> No products indexed under this heading.

Molindone Hydrochloride (Concurrent use with tranquilizers may increase drowsiness; use caution when co-administering). Products include:
> Moban Tablets 1119

Oxazepam (Concurrent use with tranquilizers may increase drowsiness; use caution when co-administering).
> No products indexed under this heading.

Pargyline Hydrochloride (Do not use while taking, or for two weeks after stopping, MAO inhibitors).
> No products indexed under this heading.

Perphenazine (Concurrent use with tranquilizers may increase drowsiness; use caution when co-administering).
> No products indexed under this heading.

Phenelzine Sulfate (Do not use while taking, or for two weeks after stopping, MAO inhibitors).
> No products indexed under this heading.

Prazepam (Concurrent use with tranquilizers may increase drowsiness; use caution when co-administering).
> No products indexed under this heading.

Procarbazine Hydrochloride (Do not use while taking, or for two weeks after stopping, MAO inhibitors). Products include:
> Matulane Capsules 3191

Prochlorperazine (Concurrent use with tranquilizers may increase drowsiness; use caution when co-administering).
> No products indexed under this heading.

Promethazine Hydrochloride (Concurrent use with tranquilizers may increase drowsiness; use caution when co-administering). Products include:
> Phenergan Tablets and Suppositories 3440

Propofol (Concurrent use with sedatives may increase drowsiness; use caution when co-administering).
> No products indexed under this heading.

IMPORTANT NOTE: Always consult each drug listing in the patient's regimen for possible interactions.

Quazepam (Concurrent use with sedatives may increase drowsiness; use caution when co-administering).
No products indexed under this heading.

Ramelteon (Concurrent use with sedatives may increase drowsiness; use caution when co-administering). Products include:
Rozerem Tablets 3231

Secobarbital Sodium (Concurrent use with sedatives may increase drowsiness; use caution when co-administering).
No products indexed under this heading.

Selegiline Hydrochloride (Do not use while taking, or for two weeks after stopping, MAO inhibitors). Products include:
Eldepryl Capsules 3208
Zelapar Tablets 3372

Temazepam (Concurrent use with sedatives may increase drowsiness; use caution when co-administering). Products include:
Restoril Capsules 1860

Thioridazine Hydrochloride (Concurrent use with tranquilizers may increase drowsiness; use caution when co-administering). Products include:
Thioridazine Hydrochloride Tablets 2163

Thiothixene (Concurrent use with tranquilizers may increase drowsiness; use caution when co-administering). Products include:
Thiothixene Capsules 2165

Tranylcypromine Sulfate (Do not use while taking, or for two weeks after stopping, MAO inhibitors). Products include:
Parnate Tablets 1527

Triazolam (Concurrent use with sedatives may increase drowsiness; use caution when co-administering).
No products indexed under this heading.

Trifluoperazine Hydrochloride (Concurrent use with tranquilizers may increase drowsiness; use caution when co-administering).
No products indexed under this heading.

Zaleplon (Concurrent use with sedatives may increase drowsiness; use caution when co-administering). Products include:
Sonata Capsules 1717

Zolpidem Tartrate (Concurrent use with sedatives may increase drowsiness; use caution when co-administering). Products include:
Ambien Tablets 2851
Ambien CR Tablets 2855

Food Interactions

Alcohol (Concurrent use may increase drowsiness; avoid alcoholic drinks).

THERAFLU DAYTIME SEVERE COLD HOT LIQUID

(Acetaminophen, Phenylephrine Hydrochloride).................................. ▣742
May interact with monoamine oxidase inhibitors and certain other agents. Compounds in these categories include:

Isocarboxazid (Concurrent and/or sequential use with MAO inhibitors is not recommended).
No products indexed under this heading.

Moclobemide (Concurrent and/or sequential use with MAO inhibitors is not recommended).
No products indexed under this heading.

Pargyline Hydrochloride (Concurrent and/or sequential use with MAO inhibitors is not recommended).
No products indexed under this heading.

Phenelzine Sulfate (Concurrent and/or sequential use with MAO inhibitors is not recommended).
No products indexed under this heading.

Procarbazine Hydrochloride (Concurrent and/or sequential use with MAO inhibitors is not recommended). Products include:
Matulane Capsules 3191

Selegiline Hydrochloride (Concurrent and/or sequential use with MAO inhibitors is not recommended). Products include:
Eldepryl Capsules 3208
Zelapar Tablets 3372

Tranylcypromine Sulfate (Concurrent and/or sequential use with MAO inhibitors is not recommended). Products include:
Parnate Tablets 1527

Food Interactions

Alcohol (Chronic heavy alcohol users, 3 or more drinks per day, should consult their physicians for advice on when and how they should take pain relievers/fever reducers, including acetaminophen; may increase the drowsiness effect).

THERAFLU NIGHTTIME SEVERE COLD HOT LIQUID

(Acetaminophen, Pheniramine Maleate, Phenylephrine Hydrochloride)................................ ▣740
May interact with hypnotics and sedatives, monoamine oxidase inhibitors, tranquilizers, and certain other agents. Compounds in these categories include:

Alprazolam (Concurrent use with tranquilizers may increase drowsiness; use caution when co-administering). Products include:
Niravam Orally Disintegrating Tablets 3092

Buspirone Hydrochloride (Concurrent use with tranquilizers may increase drowsiness; use caution when co-administering).
No products indexed under this heading.

Chlordiazepoxide (Concurrent use with tranquilizers may increase drowsiness; use caution when co-administering).
No products indexed under this heading.

Chlordiazepoxide Hydrochloride (Concurrent use with tranquilizers may increase drowsiness; use caution when co-administering). Products include:
Librium Capsules 3347

Chlorpromazine (Concurrent use with tranquilizers may increase drowsiness; use caution when co-administering).
No products indexed under this heading.

Chlorpromazine Hydrochloride (Concurrent use with tranquilizers may increase drowsiness; use caution when co-administering).
No products indexed under this heading.

Chlorprothixene (Concurrent use with tranquilizers may increase drowsiness; use caution when co-administering).
No products indexed under this heading.

Chlorprothixene Hydrochloride (Concurrent use with tranquilizers may increase drowsiness; use caution when co-administering).
No products indexed under this heading.

Clorazepate Dipotassium (Concurrent use with tranquilizers may increase drowsiness; use caution when co-administering). Products include:
Tranxene 2474

Diazepam (Concurrent use with tranquilizers may increase drowsiness; use caution when co-administering). Products include:
Diastat Rectal Delivery System 3343
Valium Tablets 2819

Droperidol (Concurrent use with tranquilizers may increase drowsiness; use caution when co-administering).
No products indexed under this heading.

Estazolam (Concurrent use with sedatives may increase drowsiness; use caution when co-administering). Products include:
ProSom Tablets 517

Ethchlorvynol (Concurrent use with sedatives may increase drowsiness; use caution when co-administering).
No products indexed under this heading.

Ethinamate (Concurrent use with sedatives may increase drowsiness; use caution when co-administering).
No products indexed under this heading.

Fluphenazine Decanoate (Concurrent use with tranquilizers may increase drowsiness; use caution when co-administering).
No products indexed under this heading.

Fluphenazine Enanthate (Concurrent use with tranquilizers may increase drowsiness; use caution when co-administering).
No products indexed under this heading.

Fluphenazine Hydrochloride (Concurrent use with tranquilizers may increase drowsiness; use caution when co-administering).
No products indexed under this heading.

Flurazepam Hydrochloride (Concurrent use with sedatives may increase drowsiness; use caution when co-administering). Products include:
Dalmane Capsules 3342

Glutethimide (Concurrent use with sedatives may increase drowsiness; use caution when co-administering).
No products indexed under this heading.

Haloperidol (Concurrent use with tranquilizers may increase drowsiness; use caution when co-administering).
No products indexed under this heading.

Haloperidol Decanoate (Concurrent use with tranquilizers may increase drowsiness; use caution when co-administering).
No products indexed under this heading.

Hydroxyzine Hydrochloride (Concurrent use with tranquilizers may increase drowsiness; use caution when co-administering).
No products indexed under this heading.

Isocarboxazid (Do not use while taking, or for two weeks after stopping, MAO inhibitors).
No products indexed under this heading.

Lorazepam (Concurrent use with sedatives may increase drowsiness; use caution when co-administering).
No products indexed under this heading.

Loxapine Hydrochloride (Concurrent use with tranquilizers may increase drowsiness; use caution when co-administering).
No products indexed under this heading.

Loxapine Succinate (Concurrent use with tranquilizers may increase drowsiness; use caution when co-administering).
No products indexed under this heading.

Meprobamate (Concurrent use with tranquilizers may increase drowsiness; use caution when co-administering).
No products indexed under this heading.

Mesoridazine Besylate (Concurrent use with tranquilizers may increase drowsiness; use caution when co-administering).
No products indexed under this heading.

Midazolam Hydrochloride (Concurrent use with sedatives may increase drowsiness; use caution when co-administering).
No products indexed under this heading.

Moclobemide (Do not use while taking, or for two weeks after stopping, MAO inhibitors).
No products indexed under this heading.

Molindone Hydrochloride (Concurrent use with tranquilizers may increase drowsiness; use caution when co-administering). Products include:
Moban Tablets 1119

Oxazepam (Concurrent use with tranquilizers may increase drowsiness; use caution when co-administering).
No products indexed under this heading.

Pargyline Hydrochloride (Do not use while taking, or for two weeks after stopping, MAO inhibitors).
No products indexed under this heading.

Perphenazine (Concurrent use with tranquilizers may increase drowsiness; use caution when co-administering).
No products indexed under this heading.

Phenelzine Sulfate (Do not use while taking, or for two weeks after stopping, MAO inhibitors).
No products indexed under this heading.

Prazepam (Concurrent use with tranquilizers may increase drowsiness; use caution when co-administering).
No products indexed under this heading.

Procarbazine Hydrochloride (Do not use while taking, or for two weeks after stopping, MAO inhibitors). Products include:
Matulane Capsules 3191

Prochlorperazine (Concurrent use with tranquilizers may increase drowsiness; use caution when co-administering).
No products indexed under this heading.

Promethazine Hydrochloride (Concurrent use with tranquilizers may increase drowsiness; use caution when co-administering). Products include:
Phenergan Tablets and Suppositories 3440

Propofol (Concurrent use with sedatives may increase drowsiness; use caution when co-administering).
No products indexed under this heading.

Quazepam (Concurrent use with sedatives may increase drowsiness; use caution when co-administering).
No products indexed under this heading.

Ramelteon (Concurrent use with sedatives may increase drowsiness; use caution when co-administering). Products include:
Rozerem Tablets 3231

Secobarbital Sodium (Concurrent use with sedatives may increase drowsiness; use caution when co-administering).
No products indexed under this heading.

Selegiline Hydrochloride (Do not use while taking, or for two weeks after stopping, MAO inhibitors). Products include:
Eldepryl Capsules 3208
Zelapar Tablets 3372

Temazepam (Concurrent use with sedatives may increase drowsiness; use caution when co-administering). Products include:
Restoril Capsules 1860

Thioridazine Hydrochloride (Concurrent use with tranquilizers may increase drowsiness; use caution when co-administering). Products include:
Thioridazine Hydrochloride Tablets 2163

Thiothixene (Concurrent use with tranquilizers may increase drowsiness; use caution when co-administering). Products include:
Thiothixene Capsules 2165

Tranylcypromine Sulfate (Do not use while taking, or for two weeks after stopping, MAO inhibitors). Products include:
Parnate Tablets 1527

Triazolam (Concurrent use with sedatives may increase drowsiness; use caution when co-administering).
No products indexed under this heading.

Trifluoperazine Hydrochloride (Concurrent use with tranquilizers may increase drowsiness; use caution when co-administering).
No products indexed under this heading.

Zaleplon (Concurrent use with sedatives may increase drowsiness; use caution when co-administering). Products include:
Sonata Capsules 1717

Zolpidem Tartrate (Concurrent use with sedatives may increase drowsiness; use caution when co-administering). Products include:
Ambien Tablets 2851
Ambien CR Tablets 2855

Food Interactions

Alcohol (Concurrent use may increase drowsiness; avoid alcoholic drinks).

THERAFLU WARMING RELIEF DAYTIME SEVERE COLD

(Acetaminophen, Dextromethorphan Hydrobromide, Phenylephrine Hydrochloride)............ 743
May interact with monoamine oxidase inhibitors and certain agents. Compounds in these categories include:

Isocarboxazid (Concurrent or sequential use with MAO inhibitors is not recommended).
No products indexed under this heading.

Moclobemide (Concurrent or sequential use with MAO inhibitors is not recommended).
No products indexed under this heading.

Pargyline Hydrochloride (Concurrent or sequential use with MAO inhibitors is not recommended).
No products indexed under this heading.

Phenelzine Sulfate (Concurrent or sequential use with MAO inhibitors is not recommended).
No products indexed under this heading.

Procarbazine Hydrochloride (Concurrent or sequential use with MAO inhibitors is not recommended). Products include:
Matulane Capsules 3191

Selegiline Hydrochloride (Concurrent or sequential use with MAO inhibitors is not recommended). Products include:
Eldepryl Capsules 3208
Zelapar Tablets 3372

Tranylcypromine Sulfate (Concurrent or sequential use with MAO inhibitors is not recommended). Products include:
Parnate Tablets 1527

Food Interactions

Alcohol (Consuming 3 or more alcoholic beverages with this product may cause hepatotoxicity).

THERAFLU WARMING RELIEF NIGHTTIME SEVERE COLD

(Acetaminophen, Diphenhydramine Hydrochloride, Phenylephrine Hydrochloride)............ 743
May interact with hypnotics and sedatives, monoamine oxidase inhibitors, tranquilizers, and certain other agents. Compounds in these categories include:

Alprazolam (May increase drowsiness effect). Products include:
Niravam Orally Disintegrating Tablets 3092

Buspirone Hydrochloride (May increase drowsiness effect).
No products indexed under this heading.

Chlordiazepoxide (May increase drowsiness effect).
No products indexed under this heading.

Chlordiazepoxide Hydrochloride (May increase drowsiness effect). Products include:
Librium Capsules 3347

Chlorpromazine (May increase drowsiness effect).
No products indexed under this heading.

Chlorpromazine Hydrochloride (May increase drowsiness effect).
No products indexed under this heading.

Chlorprothixene (May increase drowsiness effect).
No products indexed under this heading.

Chlorprothixene Hydrochloride (May increase drowsiness effect).
No products indexed under this heading.

Clorazepate Dipotassium (May increase drowsiness effect). Products include:
Tranxene 2474

Diazepam (May increase drowsiness effect). Products include:
Diastat Rectal Delivery System 3343
Valium Tablets 2819

Droperidol (May increase drowsiness effect).
No products indexed under this heading.

Estazolam (May increase drowsiness effect). Products include:
ProSom Tablets 517

Ethchlorvynol (May increase drowsiness effect).
No products indexed under this heading.

Ethinamate (May increase drowsiness effect).
No products indexed under this heading.

Fluphenazine Decanoate (May increase drowsiness effect).
No products indexed under this heading.

Fluphenazine Enanthate (May increase drowsiness effect).
No products indexed under this heading.

Fluphenazine Hydrochloride (May increase drowsiness effect).
No products indexed under this heading.

Flurazepam Hydrochloride (May increase drowsiness effect). Products include:
Dalmane Capsules 3342

Glutethimide (May increase drowsiness effect).
No products indexed under this heading.

Haloperidol (May increase drowsiness effect).
No products indexed under this heading.

Haloperidol Decanoate (May increase drowsiness effect).
No products indexed under this heading.

Hydroxyzine Hydrochloride (May increase drowsiness effect).
No products indexed under this heading.

Isocarboxazid (Concurrent or sequential use of MAO inhibitors is not recommended).
No products indexed under this heading.

Lorazepam (May increase drowsiness effect).
No products indexed under this heading.

Loxapine Hydrochloride (May increase drowsiness effect).
No products indexed under this heading.

Loxapine Succinate (May increase drowsiness effect).
No products indexed under this heading.

Meprobamate (May increase drowsiness effect).
No products indexed under this heading.

Mesoridazine Besylate (May increase drowsiness effect).
No products indexed under this heading.

Midazolam Hydrochloride (May increase drowsiness effect).
No products indexed under this heading.

Moclobemide (Concurrent or sequential use of MAO inhibitors is not recommended).
No products indexed under this heading.

Molindone Hydrochloride (May increase drowsiness effect). Products include:
Moban Tablets 1119

Oxazepam (May increase drowsiness effect).
No products indexed under this heading.

Pargyline Hydrochloride (Concurrent or sequential use of MAO inhibitors is not recommended).
No products indexed under this heading.

Perphenazine (May increase drowsiness effect).
No products indexed under this heading.

Phenelzine Sulfate (Concurrent or sequential use of MAO inhibitors is not recommended).
No products indexed under this heading.

Prazepam (May increase drowsiness effect).
No products indexed under this heading.

Procarbazine Hydrochloride (Concurrent or sequential use of MAO inhibitors is not recommended). Products include:
Matulane Capsules 3191

Prochlorperazine (May increase drowsiness effect).
No products indexed under this heading.

Promethazine Hydrochloride (May increase drowsiness effect). Products include:
Phenergan Tablets and Suppositories 3440

Propofol (May increase drowsiness effect).
No products indexed under this heading.

Quazepam (May increase drowsiness effect).
No products indexed under this heading.

Ramelteon (May increase drowsiness effect). Products include:
Rozerem Tablets 3231

Secobarbital Sodium (May increase drowsiness effect).
No products indexed under this heading.

Selegiline Hydrochloride (Concurrent or sequential use of MAO inhibitors is not recommended). Products include:
Eldepryl Capsules 3208
Zelapar Tablets 3372

Temazepam (May increase drowsiness effect). Products include:
Restoril Capsules 1860

Thioridazine Hydrochloride (May increase drowsiness effect). Products include:
Thioridazine Hydrochloride Tablets 2163

Thiothixene (May increase drowsiness effect). Products include:
Thiothixene Capsules 2165

Tranylcypromine Sulfate (Concurrent or sequential use of MAO inhibitors is not recommended). Products include:
Parnate Tablets 1527

Triazolam (May increase drowsiness effect).
No products indexed under this heading.

Trifluoperazine Hydrochloride (May increase drowsiness effect).
No products indexed under this heading.

Zaleplon (May increase drowsiness effect). Products include:
Sonata Capsules 1717

Zolpidem Tartrate (May increase drowsiness effect). Products include:
Ambien Tablets 2851
Ambien CR Tablets 2855

Food Interactions

Alcohol (Consuming 3 or more alcoholic beverages with this product may cause hepatotoxicity).

THERAFLU THIN STRIPS LONG ACTING COUGH

(Dextromethorphan Hydrobromide) .... ▣744
May interact with monoamine oxidase inhibitors. Compounds in these categories include:

Isocarboxazid (Do not use concurrently with, or for two weeks after stopping, MAO Inhibitors).
No products indexed under this heading.

Moclobemide (Do not use concurrently with, or for two weeks after stopping, MAO Inhibitors).
No products indexed under this heading.

Pargyline Hydrochloride (Do not use concurrently with, or for two weeks after stopping, MAO Inhibitors).
No products indexed under this heading.

Phenelzine Sulfate (Do not use concurrently with, or for two weeks after stopping, MAO Inhibitors).
No products indexed under this heading.

Procarbazine Hydrochloride (Do not use concurrently with, or for two weeks after stopping, MAO Inhibitors). Products include:
Matulane Capsules 3191

Selegiline Hydrochloride (Do not use concurrently with, or for two weeks after stopping, MAO Inhibitors). Products include:
Eldepryl Capsules 3208
Zelapar Tablets 3372

Tranylcypromine Sulfate (Do not use concurrently with, or for two weeks after stopping, MAO Inhibitors). Products include:
Parnate Tablets 1527

THERAFLU THIN STRIPS MULTI SYMPTOM

(Diphenhydramine Hydrochloride) ..... ▣744
May interact with hypnotics and sedatives, tranquilizers, and certain other agents. Compounds in these categories include:

Alprazolam (Co-administration with tranquilizers may increase drowsiness). Products include:
Niravam Orally Disintegrating Tablets 3092

Buspirone Hydrochloride (Co-administration with tranquilizers may increase drowsiness).
No products indexed under this heading.

Chlordiazepoxide (Co-administration with tranquilizers may increase drowsiness).
No products indexed under this heading.

Chlordiazepoxide Hydrochloride (Co-administration with tranquilizers may increase drowsiness). Products include:
Librium Capsules 3347

Chlorpromazine (Co-administration with tranquilizers may increase drowsiness).
No products indexed under this heading.

Chlorpromazine Hydrochloride (Co-administration with tranquilizers may increase drowsiness).
No products indexed under this heading.

Chlorprothixene (Co-administration with tranquilizers may increase drowsiness).
No products indexed under this heading.

Chlorprothixene Hydrochloride (Co-administration with tranquilizers may increase drowsiness).
No products indexed under this heading.

Clorazepate Dipotassium (Co-administration with tranquilizers may increase drowsiness). Products include:
Tranxene 2474

Diazepam (Co-administration with tranquilizers may increase drowsiness). Products include:
Diastat Rectal Delivery System 3343
Valium Tablets 2819

Droperidol (Co-administration with tranquilizers may increase drowsiness).
No products indexed under this heading.

Estazolam (Co-administration with sedatives may increase drowsiness). Products include:
ProSom Tablets 517

Ethchlorvynol (Co-administration with sedatives may increase drowsiness).
No products indexed under this heading.

Ethinamate (Co-administration with sedatives may increase drowsiness).
No products indexed under this heading.

Fluphenazine Decanoate (Co-administration with tranquilizers may increase drowsiness).
No products indexed under this heading.

Fluphenazine Enanthate (Co-administration with tranquilizers may increase drowsiness).
No products indexed under this heading.

Fluphenazine Hydrochloride (Co-administration with tranquilizers may increase drowsiness).
No products indexed under this heading.

Flurazepam Hydrochloride (Co-administration with sedatives may increase drowsiness). Products include:
Dalmane Capsules 3342

Glutethimide (Co-administration with sedatives may increase drowsiness).
No products indexed under this heading.

Haloperidol (Co-administration with tranquilizers may increase drowsiness).
No products indexed under this heading.

Haloperidol Decanoate (Co-administration with tranquilizers may increase drowsiness).
No products indexed under this heading.

Hydroxyzine Hydrochloride (Co-administration with tranquilizers may increase drowsiness).
No products indexed under this heading.

Lorazepam (Co-administration with sedatives may increase drowsiness).
No products indexed under this heading.

Loxapine Hydrochloride (Co-administration with tranquilizers may increase drowsiness).
No products indexed under this heading.

Loxapine Succinate (Co-administration with tranquilizers may increase drowsiness).
No products indexed under this heading.

Meprobamate (Co-administration with tranquilizers may increase drowsiness).
No products indexed under this heading.

Mesoridazine Besylate (Co-administration with tranquilizers may increase drowsiness).
No products indexed under this heading.

Midazolam Hydrochloride (Co-administration with sedatives may increase drowsiness).
No products indexed under this heading.

Molindone Hydrochloride (Co-administration with tranquilizers may increase drowsiness). Products include:
Moban Tablets 1119

Oxazepam (Co-administration with tranquilizers may increase drowsiness).
No products indexed under this heading.

Perphenazine (Co-administration with tranquilizers may increase drowsiness).
No products indexed under this heading.

Prazepam (Co-administration with tranquilizers may increase drowsiness).
No products indexed under this heading.

Prochlorperazine (Co-administration with tranquilizers may increase drowsiness).
No products indexed under this heading.

Promethazine Hydrochloride (Co-administration with tranquilizers may increase drowsiness). Products include:
Phenergan Tablets and Suppositories 3440

Propofol (Co-administration with sedatives may increase drowsiness).
No products indexed under this heading.

Quazepam (Co-administration with sedatives may increase drowsiness).
No products indexed under this heading.

Ramelteon (Co-administration with sedatives may increase drowsiness). Products include:
Rozerem Tablets 3231

Secobarbital Sodium (Co-administration with sedatives may increase drowsiness).
No products indexed under this heading.

Temazepam (Co-administration with sedatives may increase drowsiness). Products include:
Restoril Capsules 1860

Thioridazine Hydrochloride (Co-administration with tranquilizers may increase drowsiness). Products include:
Thioridazine Hydrochloride Tablets 2163

Thiothixene (Co-administration with tranquilizers may increase drowsiness). Products include:
Thiothixene Capsules 2165

Triazolam (Co-administration with sedatives may increase drowsiness).
No products indexed under this heading.

Trifluoperazine Hydrochloride (Co-administration with tranquilizers may increase drowsiness).
No products indexed under this heading.

Zaleplon (Co-administration with sedatives may increase drowsiness). Products include:
Sonata Capsules 1717

Zolpidem Tartrate (Co-administration with sedatives may increase drowsiness). Products include:
Ambien Tablets 2851
Ambien CR Tablets 2855

Food Interactions

Alcohol (Co-administration with alcohol may increase drowsiness).

THERA-GESIC CREME

(Menthol, Methyl Salicylate) 2141
None cited in PDR database.

THERMACARE HEAT WRAPS

(Device) 2677
None cited in PDR database.

THIOLA TABLETS

(Tiopronin) 2141
None cited in PDR database.

THIORIDAZINE HYDROCHLORIDE TABLETS
(Thioridazine Hydrochloride) **2163**
May interact with central nervous system depressants, erythromycin, potassium-depleting diuretics, quinidine, and certain other agents. Compounds in these categories include:

Alfentanil Hydrochloride (Thioridazine is capable of potentiating CNS depressants).
No products indexed under this heading.

Alprazolam (Thioridazine is capable of potentiating CNS depressants). Products include:
Niravam Orally Disintegrating Tablets **3092**

Amiodarone Hydrochloride (Thioridazine has been shown to prolong QTc interval in a dose-related manner; drugs with this potential have been associated with Torsade de pointes-type arrhythmias and sudden death; co-administration with other drugs that are known to prolong QTc interval is contraindicated).
No products indexed under this heading.

Aprobarbital (Thioridazine is capable of potentiating CNS depressants).
No products indexed under this heading.

Arsenic Trioxide (Thioridazine has been shown to prolong QTc interval in a dose-related manner; drugs with this potential have been associated with torsade de pointes-type arrhythmias and sudden death; co-administration with other drugs that are known to prolong QTc interval is contraindicated). Products include:
Trisenox Injection **993**

Atropine Sulfate (Thioridazine is capable of potentiating atropine). Products include:
Donnatal Extentabs **2493**

Bendroflumethiazide (Hypokalemia may result from diuretic therapy and this may increase the risk of QT prolongation and arrhythmias; co-administration may increase the risk of serious, potentially fatal, cardiac arrhythmias).
No products indexed under this heading.

Bepridil Hydrochloride (Thioridazine has been shown to prolong QTc interval in a dose-related manner; drugs with this potential have been associated with torsade de pointes-type arrhythmias and sudden death; co-administration with other drugs that are known to prolong QTc interval is contraindicated).
No products indexed under this heading.

Bumetanide (Hypokalemia may result from diuretic therapy and this may increase the risk of QT prolongation and arrhythmias; co-administration may increase the risk of serious, potentially fatal, cardiac arrhythmias). Products include:
Bumex Tablets **2746**

Buprenorphine Hydrochloride (Thioridazine is capable of potentiating CNS depressants). Products include:
Buprenex Injectable **2716**
Suboxone Tablets **2717**
Subutex Tablets **2717**

Buspirone Hydrochloride (Thioridazine is capable of potentiating CNS depressants).
No products indexed under this heading.

Butabarbital (Thioridazine is capable of potentiating CNS depressants).
No products indexed under this heading.

Butalbital (Thioridazine is capable of potentiating CNS depressants).
No products indexed under this heading.

Chlordiazepoxide (Thioridazine is capable of potentiating CNS depressants).
No products indexed under this heading.

Chlordiazepoxide Hydrochloride (Thioridazine is capable of potentiating CNS depressants). Products include:
Librium Capsules **3347**

Chlorothiazide (Hypokalemia may result from diuretic therapy and this may increase the risk of QT prolongation and arrhythmias; co-administration may increase the risk of serious, potentially fatal, cardiac arrhythmias). Products include:
Diuril Oral Suspension **1954**

Chlorothiazide Sodium (Hypokalemia may result from diuretic therapy and this may increase the risk of QT prolongation and arrhythmias; co-administration may increase the risk of serious, potentially fatal, cardiac arrhythmias). Products include:
Diuril Sodium Intravenous **2467**

Chlorpromazine (Thioridazine is capable of potentiating CNS depressants).
No products indexed under this heading.

Chlorpromazine Hydrochloride (Thioridazine is capable of potentiating CNS depressants).
No products indexed under this heading.

Chlorprothixene (Thioridazine is capable of potentiating CNS depressants).
No products indexed under this heading.

Chlorprothixene Hydrochloride (Thioridazine is capable of potentiating CNS depressants).
No products indexed under this heading.

Chlorprothixene Lactate (Thioridazine is capable of potentiating CNS depressants).
No products indexed under this heading.

Clorazepate Dipotassium (Thioridazine is capable of potentiating CNS depressants). Products include:
Tranxene **2474**

Clozapine (Thioridazine is capable of potentiating CNS depressants). Products include:
Clozaril Tablets **2184**
FazaClo Orally Disintegrating Tablets **551**

Codeine Phosphate (Thioridazine is capable of potentiating CNS depressants). Products include:
Tylenol with Codeine Tablets **2391**

Desflurane (Thioridazine is capable of potentiating CNS depressants).
No products indexed under this heading.

Desipramine Hydrochloride (Thioridazine has been shown to prolong QTc interval in a dose-related manner; drugs with this potential have been associated with torsade de pointes-type arrhythmias and sudden death; co-administration with other drugs that are known to prolong QTc interval is contraindicated).
No products indexed under this heading.

Dezocine (Thioridazine is capable of potentiating CNS depressants).
No products indexed under this heading.

Diazepam (Thioridazine is capable of potentiating CNS depressants). Products include:
Diastat Rectal Delivery System **3343**
Valium Tablets **2819**

Disopyramide Phosphate (Thioridazine has been shown to prolong QTc interval in a dose-related manner; drugs with this potential have been associated with torsade de pointes-type arrhythmias and sudden death; co-administration with other drugs that are known to prolong QTc interval is contraindicated).
No products indexed under this heading.

Dofetilide (Thioridazine has been shown to prolong QTc interval in a dose-related manner; drugs with this potential have been associated with Torsade de pointes-type arrhythmias and sudden death; co-administration with other drugs that are known to prolong QTc interval is contraindicated).
No products indexed under this heading.

Dolasetron Mesylate (Thioridazine has been shown to prolong QTc interval in a dose-related manner; drugs with this potential have been associated with Torsade de pointes-type arrhythmias and sudden death; co-administration with other drugs that are known to prolong QTc interval is contraindicated). Products include:
Anzemet Injection **2859**
Anzemet Tablets **2862**

Droperidol (Thioridazine has been shown to prolong QTc interval in a dose-related manner; drugs with this potential have been associated with torsade de pointes-type arrhythmias and sudden death; co-administration with other drugs that are known to prolong QTc interval is contraindicated).
No products indexed under this heading.

Enflurane (Thioridazine is capable of potentiating CNS depressants).
No products indexed under this heading.

Epinephrine (Thioridazine causes orthostatic hypotension, especially in female patients; use of epinephrine should be avoided in view of the fact that phenothiazines may induce a reversed epinephrine effect). Products include:
EpiPen **1061**
Primatene Mist **719**
Twinject 0.15 .... **3379**
Twinject 0.3 .... **3378**

Epinephrine Hydrochloride (Thioridazine causes orthostatic hypotension, especially in female patients; use of epinephrine should be avoided in view of the fact that phenothiazines may induce a reversed epinephrine effect).
No products indexed under this heading.

Erythromycin (Thioridazine has been shown to prolong QTc interval in a dose-related manner; drugs with this potential have been associated with torsade de pointes-type arrhythmias and sudden death; co-administration with other drugs that are known to prolong QTc interval is contraindicated). Products include:
Ery-Tab Tablets **449**
Erythromycin Base Filmtab Tablets **455**
Erythromycin Delayed-Release Capsules, USP **457**
PCE Dispertab Tablets **515**

Erythromycin Estolate (Thioridazine has been shown to prolong QTc interval in a dose-related manner; drugs with this potential have been associated with torsade de pointes-type arrhythmias and sudden death; co-administration with other drugs that are known to prolong QTc interval is contraindicated).
No products indexed under this heading.

Erythromycin Ethylsuccinate (Thioridazine has been shown to prolong QTc interval in a dose-related manner; drugs with this potential have been associated with torsade de pointes-type arrhythmias and sudden death; co-administration with other drugs that are known to prolong QTc interval is contraindicated). Products include:
E.E.S. **451**
EryPed **447**

Erythromycin Gluceptate (Thioridazine has been shown to prolong QTc interval in a dose-related manner; drugs with this potential have been associated with torsade de pointes-type arrhythmias and sudden death; co-administration with other drugs that are known to prolong QTc interval is contraindicated).
No products indexed under this heading.

Erythromycin Lactobionate (Thioridazine has been shown to prolong QTc interval in a dose-related manner; drugs with this potential have been associated with torsade de pointes-type arrhythmias and sudden death; co-administration with other drugs that are known to prolong QTc interval is contraindicated).
No products indexed under this heading.

Erythromycin Stearate (Thioridazine has been shown to prolong QTc interval in a dose-related manner; drugs with this potential have been associated with torsade de pointes-type arrhythmias and sudden death; co-administration with other drugs that are known to prolong QTc interval is contraindicated). Products include:
Erythrocin Stearate Filmtab Tablets **453**

Estazolam (Thioridazine is capable of potentiating CNS depressants). Products include:
ProSom Tablets **517**

Ethacrynic Acid (Hypokalemia may result from diuretic therapy and this may increase the risk of QT prolongation and arrhythmias; co-administration may increase the risk of serious, potentially fatal, cardiac arrhythmias). Products include:

Edecrin Tablets 1959

Ethanol (Thioridazine is capable of potentiating CNS depressants).

No products indexed under this heading.

Ethchlorvynol (Thioridazine is capable of potentiating CNS depressants).

No products indexed under this heading.

Ethinamate (Thioridazine is capable of potentiating CNS depressants).

No products indexed under this heading.

Ethyl Alcohol (Thioridazine is capable of potentiating CNS depressants).

No products indexed under this heading.

Fentanyl (Thioridazine is capable of potentiating CNS depressants). Products include:

Duragesic Transdermal System 2373
Ionsys Transdermal System 2379

Fentanyl Citrate (Thioridazine is capable of potentiating CNS depressants). Products include:

Actiq ... 979

Flecainide Acetate (Thioridazine has been shown to prolong QTc interval in a dose-related manner; drugs with this potential have been associated with Torsade de pointes-type arrhythmias and sudden death; co-administration with other drugs that are known to prolong QTc interval is contraindicated). Products include:

Tambocor Tablets 1856

Fluoxetine Hydrochloride (Co-administration with drugs that inhibit CYP450 2D6 isoenzyme will appreciably inhibit metabolism of thioridazine and resulting elevated levels of thioridazine would be expected to augment the prolongation of QTc interval and may increase the risk of serious, potentially fatal, cardiac arrhythmias; concurrent use is contraindicated). Products include:

Prozac Pulvules and Liquid 1801
Symbyax Capsules 1819

Fluphenazine Decanoate (Thioridazine is capable of potentiating CNS depressants).

No products indexed under this heading.

Fluphenazine Enanthate (Thioridazine is capable of potentiating CNS depressants).

No products indexed under this heading.

Fluphenazine Hydrochloride (Thioridazine is capable of potentiating CNS depressants).

No products indexed under this heading.

Flurazepam Hydrochloride (Thioridazine is capable of potentiating CNS depressants). Products include:

Dalmane Capsules 3342

Fluvoxamine Maleate (Co-administration with drugs that inhibit CYP450 2D6 isoenzyme will appreciably inhibit metabolism of thioridazine and resulting elevated levels of thioridazine would be expected to augment the prolongation of QTc interval and may increase the risk of serious, potentially fatal, cardiac arrhythmias; concurrent use is contraindicated).

No products indexed under this heading.

Furosemide (Hypokalemia may result from diuretic therapy and this may increase the risk of QT prolongation and arrhythmias; co-administration may increase the risk of serious, potentially fatal, cardiac arrhythmias). Products include:

Furosemide Tablets 2154

Gatifloxacin (Thioridazine has been shown to prolong QTc interval in a dose-related manner; drugs with this potential have been associated with torsade de pointes-type arrhythmias and sudden death; co-administration with other drugs that are known to prolong QTc interval is contraindicated). Products include:

Tequin Injection 938
Tequin Injection in 5% Dextrose 938
Tequin Tablets 938
Zymar Ophthalmic Solution 575

Glutethimide (Thioridazine is capable of potentiating CNS depressants).

No products indexed under this heading.

Halofantrine (Thioridazine has been shown to prolong QTc interval in a dose-related manner; drugs with this potential have been associated with Torsade de pointes-type arrhythmias and sudden death; co-administration with other drugs that are known to prolong QTc interval is contraindicated).

No products indexed under this heading.

Haloperidol (Thioridazine is capable of potentiating CNS depressants).

No products indexed under this heading.

Haloperidol Decanoate (Thioridazine is capable of potentiating CNS depressants).

No products indexed under this heading.

Hydrochlorothiazide (Hypokalemia may result from diuretic therapy and this may increase the risk of QT prolongation and arrhythmias; co-administration may increase the risk of serious, potentially fatal, cardiac arrhythmias). Products include:

Aldoril Tablets 1910
Atacand HCT 651
Avalide Tablets 888
Avalide Tablets 2874
Benicar HCT Tablets 1044
Diovan HCT Tablets 2196
Dyazide Capsules 1423
Hyzaar 50-12.5 Tablets 1990
Hyzaar 100-12.5 Tablets 1990
Hyzaar 100-25 Tablets 1990
Lopressor HCT 50/25 Tablets 2241
Lopressor HCT 100/25 Tablets 2241
Lopressor HCT 100/50 Tablets 2241
Lotensin HCT Tablets 2246
Micardis HCT Tablets 856
Moduretic Tablets 2028
Prinzide Tablets 2056
Teveten HCT Tablets 1737
Timolide Tablets 2086
Uniretic Tablets 3100

Hydrocodone Bitartrate (Thioridazine is capable of potentiating CNS depressants). Products include:

Hycodan 1116
Hycotuss Expectorant Syrup 1117
Vicodin Tablets 535
Vicodin ES Tablets 536
Vicodin HP Tablets 538
Vicoprofen Tablets 539
Zydone Tablets 1139

Hydrocodone Polistirex (Thioridazine is capable of potentiating CNS depressants). Products include:

Tussionex Pennkinetic
Extended-Release Suspension 3327

Hydroflumethiazide (Hypokalemia may result from diuretic therapy and this may increase the risk of QT prolongation and arrhythmias; co-administration may increase the risk of serious, potentially fatal, cardiac arrhythmias).

No products indexed under this heading.

Hydromorphone Hydrochloride (Thioridazine is capable of potentiating CNS depressants). Products include:

Dilaudid 440
Dilaudid Non-Sterile Powder 440
Dilaudid Oral Liquid 445
Dilaudid Rectal Suppositories 440
Dilaudid Tablets 440
Dilaudid Tablets - 8 mg 445
Dilaudid-HP 442

Hydroxyzine Hydrochloride (Thioridazine is capable of potentiating CNS depressants).

No products indexed under this heading.

Ibutilide Fumarate (Thioridazine has been shown to prolong QTc interval in a dose-related manner; drugs with this potential have been associated with torsade de pointes-type arrhythmias and sudden death; co-administration with other drugs that are known to prolong QTc interval is contraindicated).

No products indexed under this heading.

Isoflurane (Thioridazine is capable of potentiating CNS depressants).

No products indexed under this heading.

Ketamine Hydrochloride (Thioridazine is capable of potentiating CNS depressants).

No products indexed under this heading.

Levomethadyl Acetate Hydrochloride (Thioridazine has been shown to prolong QTc interval in a dose-related manner; drugs with this potential have been associated with torsade de pointes-type arrhythmias and sudden death; co-administration with other drugs that are known to prolong QTc interval is contraindicated).

No products indexed under this heading.

Levorphanol Tartrate (Thioridazine is capable of potentiating CNS depressants).

No products indexed under this heading.

Lorazepam (Thioridazine is capable of potentiating CNS depressants).

No products indexed under this heading.

Loxapine Hydrochloride (Thioridazine is capable of potentiating CNS depressants).

No products indexed under this heading.

Loxapine Succinate (Thioridazine is capable of potentiating CNS depressants).

No products indexed under this heading.

Mefloquine Hydrochloride (Thioridazine has been shown to prolong QTc interval in a dose-related manner; drugs with this potential have been associated with Torsade de pointes-type arrhythmias and sudden death; co-administration with other drugs that are known to prolong QTc interval is contraindicated). Products include:

Lariam Tablets 2786

Meperidine Hydrochloride (Thioridazine is capable of potentiating CNS depressants).

No products indexed under this heading.

Mephobarbital (Thioridazine is capable of potentiating CNS depressants).

No products indexed under this heading.

Meprobamate (Thioridazine is capable of potentiating CNS depressants).

No products indexed under this heading.

Mesoridazine Besylate (Thioridazine is capable of potentiating CNS depressants).

No products indexed under this heading.

Methadone Hydrochloride (Thioridazine is capable of potentiating CNS depressants).

No products indexed under this heading.

Methohexital Sodium (Thioridazine is capable of potentiating CNS depressants).

No products indexed under this heading.

Methotrimeprazine (Thioridazine is capable of potentiating CNS depressants).

No products indexed under this heading.

Methoxyflurane (Thioridazine is capable of potentiating CNS depressants).

No products indexed under this heading.

Methyclothiazide (Hypokalemia may result from diuretic therapy and this may increase the risk of QT prolongation and arrhythmias; co-administration may increase the risk of serious, potentially fatal, cardiac arrhythmias).

No products indexed under this heading.

Midazolam Hydrochloride (Thioridazine is capable of potentiating CNS depressants).

No products indexed under this heading.

Molindone Hydrochloride (Thioridazine is capable of potentiating CNS depressants). Products include:

Moban Tablets 1119

Morphine Sulfate (Thioridazine is capable of potentiating CNS depressants). Products include:

Avinza Capsules 1741
Kadian Capsules 577
MS Contin Tablets 2701

Moxifloxacin Hydrochloride (Thioridazine has been shown to prolong QTc interval in a dose-related manner; drugs with this potential have been associated with torsade de pointes-type arrhythmias and sudden death; co-administration with other drugs that are known to prolong QTc interval is contraindicated). Products include:

Olanzapine (Thioridazine is capable of potentiating CNS depressants). Products include:

Oxazepam (Thioridazine is capable of potentiating CNS depressants).
No products indexed under this heading.

Oxycodone Hydrochloride (Thioridazine is capable of potentiating CNS depressants). Products include:

Paroxetine Hydrochloride (Co-administration with drugs that inhibit CYP450 2D6 isoenzyme will appreciably inhibit metabolism of thioridazine and resulting elevated levels of thioridazine would be expected to augment the prolongation of QTc interval and may increase the risk of serious, potentially fatal, cardiac arrhythmias; concurrent use is contraindicated). Products include:

Pentamidine Isethionate (Thioridazine has been shown to prolong QTc interval in a dose-related manner; drugs with this potential have been associated with torsade de pointes-type arrhythmias and sudden death; co-administration with other drugs that are known to prolong QTc interval is contraindicated).
No products indexed under this heading.

Pentobarbital Sodium (Thioridazine is capable of potentiating CNS depressants). Products include:
Nembutal Sodium Solution, USP 2470

Perphenazine (Thioridazine is capable of potentiating CNS depressants).
No products indexed under this heading.

Phenobarbital (Thioridazine is capable of potentiating CNS depressants). Products include:
Donnatal Extentabs 2493

Pimozide (Thioridazine has been shown to prolong QTc interval in a dose-related manner; drugs with this potential have been associated with torsade de pointes-type arrhythmias and sudden death; co-administration with other drugs that are known to prolong QTc interval is contraindicated).
No products indexed under this heading.

Pindolol (Co-administration with drugs that inhibit CYP450 2D6 isoenzyme will appreciably inhibit metabolism of thioridazine and resulting elevated levels of thioridazine would be expected to augment the prolongation of QTc interval and may increase the risk of serious, potentially fatal, cardiac arrhythmias; concurrent use is contraindicated).
No products indexed under this heading.

Polythiazide (Hypokalemia may result from diuretic therapy and this may increase the risk of QT prolongation and arrhythmias; co-administration may increase the risk of serious, potentially fatal, cardiac arrhythmias).
No products indexed under this heading.

Prazepam (Thioridazine is capable of potentiating CNS depressants).
No products indexed under this heading.

Procainamide Hydrochloride (Thioridazine has been shown to prolong QTc interval in a dose-related manner; drugs with this potential have been associated with torsade de pointes-type arrhythmias and sudden death; co-administration with other drugs that are known to prolong QTc interval is contraindicated).
No products indexed under this heading.

Prochlorperazine (Thioridazine is capable of potentiating CNS depressants).
No products indexed under this heading.

Promethazine Hydrochloride (Thioridazine is capable of potentiating CNS depressants). Products include:
Phenergan Tablets and
 Suppositories 3440

Propofol (Thioridazine is capable of potentiating CNS depressants).
No products indexed under this heading.

Propoxyphene Hydrochloride (Thioridazine is capable of potentiating CNS depressants).
No products indexed under this heading.

Propoxyphene Napsylate (Thioridazine is capable of potentiating CNS depressants).
No products indexed under this heading.

Propranolol Hydrochloride (Co-administration with drugs that inhibit CYP450 2D6 isoenzyme will appreciably inhibit metabolism of thioridazine and resulting elevated levels of thioridazine would be expected to augment the prolongation of QTc interval and may increase the risk of serious, potentially fatal, cardiac arrhythmias; concurrent use is contraindicated). Products include:

Quazepam (Thioridazine is capable of potentiating CNS depressants).
No products indexed under this heading.

Quetiapine Fumarate (Thioridazine is capable of potentiating CNS depressants). Products include:
Seroquel Tablets 690

Quinidine (Thioridazine has been shown to prolong QTc interval in a dose-related manner; drugs with this potential have been associated with torsade de pointes-type arrhythmias and sudden death; co-administration with other drugs that are known to prolong QTc interval is contraindicated).
No products indexed under this heading.

Quinidine Gluconate (Thioridazine has been shown to prolong QTc interval in a dose-related manner; drugs with this potential have been associated with torsade de pointes-type arrhythmias and sudden death; co-administration with other drugs that are known to prolong QTc interval is contraindicated).
No products indexed under this heading.

Quinidine Hydrochloride (Thioridazine has been shown to prolong QTc interval in a dose-related manner; drugs with this potential have been associated with torsade de pointes-type arrhythmias and sudden death; co-administration with other drugs that are known to prolong QTc interval is contraindicated).
No products indexed under this heading.

Quinidine Polygalacturonate (Thioridazine has been shown to prolong QTc interval in a dose-related manner; drugs with this potential have been associated with torsade de pointes-type arrhythmias and sudden death; co-administration with other drugs that are known to prolong QTc interval is contraindicated).
No products indexed under this heading.

Quinidine Sulfate (Thioridazine has been shown to prolong QTc interval in a dose-related manner; drugs with this potential have been associated with torsade de pointes-type arrhythmias and sudden death; co-administration with other drugs that are known to prolong QTc interval is contraindicated).
No products indexed under this heading.

Remifentanil Hydrochloride (Thioridazine is capable of potentiating CNS depressants).
No products indexed under this heading.

Risperidone (Thioridazine is capable of potentiating CNS depressants). Products include:

Secobarbital Sodium (Thioridazine is capable of potentiating CNS depressants).
No products indexed under this heading.

Sevoflurane (Thioridazine is capable of potentiating CNS depressants). Products include:
Ultane Liquid for Inhalation 531

Sotalol Hydrochloride (Thioridazine has been shown to prolong QTc interval in a dose-related manner; drugs with this potential have been associated with torsade de pointes-type arrhythmias and sudden death; co-administration with other drugs that are known to prolong QTc interval is contraindicated).
No products indexed under this heading.

Sparfloxacin (Thioridazine has been shown to prolong QTc interval in a dose-related manner; drugs with this potential have been associated with torsade de pointes-type arrhythmias and sudden death; co-administration with other drugs that are known to prolong QTc interval is contraindicated).
No products indexed under this heading.

Sufentanil Citrate (Thioridazine is capable of potentiating CNS depressants).
No products indexed under this heading.

Tacrolimus (Thioridazine has been shown to prolong QTc interval in a dose-related manner; drugs with this potential have been associated with torsade de pointes-type arrhythmias and sudden death; co-administration with other drugs that are known to prolong QTc interval is contraindicated). Products include:

Temazepam (Thioridazine is capable of potentiating CNS depressants). Products include:
Restoril Capsules 1860

Thiamylal Sodium (Thioridazine is capable of potentiating CNS depressants).
No products indexed under this heading.

Thiothixene (Thioridazine is capable of potentiating CNS depressants). Products include:
Thiothixene Capsules 2165

Torsemide (Hypokalemia may result from diuretic therapy and this may increase the risk of QT prolongation and arrhythmias; co-administration may increase the risk of serious, potentially fatal, cardiac arrhythmias). Products include:

Triazolam (Thioridazine is capable of potentiating CNS depressants).
No products indexed under this heading.

Trifluoperazine Hydrochloride (Thioridazine is capable of potentiating CNS depressants).
No products indexed under this heading.

Zaleplon (Thioridazine is capable of potentiating CNS depressants). Products include:
Sonata Capsules 1717

Ziprasidone Hydrochloride (Thioridazine has been shown to prolong QTc interval in a dose-related manner; drugs with this potential have been associated with torsade de pointes-type arrhythmias and sudden death; co-administration with other drugs that are known to prolong QTc interval is contraindicated). Products include:
Geodon Capsules 2529

Ziprasidone Mesylate (Thioridazine has been shown to prolong QTc interval in a dose-related manner; drugs with this potential have been associated with torsade de pointes-type arrhythmias and sudden death; co-administration with other drugs that are known to prolong QTc interval is contraindicated). Products include:
Geodon for Injection 2529

Zolpidem Tartrate (Thioridazine is capable of potentiating CNS depressants). Products include:

Food Interactions

Alcohol (Thioridazine is capable of potentiating CNS depressants).

IMPORTANT NOTE: Always consult each drug listing in the patient's regimen for possible interactions.

THIOTHIXENE CAPSULES
(Thiothixene) 2165
May interact with belladona products, central nervous system depressants, and certain other agents. Compounds in these categories include:

Alfentanil Hydrochloride (Possible additive effects which may include hypotension).
No products indexed under this heading.

Alprazolam (Possible additive effects which may include hypotension). Products include:
Niravam Orally Disintegrating Tablets 3092

Aprobarbital (Possible additive effects which may include hypotension).
No products indexed under this heading.

Atropine Sulfate (Thiothixene exhibits weak anticholinergic properties; concurrent use with atropine or related drugs requires caution). Products include:
Donnatal Extentabs 2493

Belladonna Alkaloids (Thiothixene exhibits weak anticholinergic properties; concurrent use with atropine or related drugs requires caution). Products include:
Hyland's Teething Tablets .... ▣ 830

Buprenorphine Hydrochloride (Possible additive effects which may include hypotension). Products include:
Buprenex Injectable 2716
Suboxone Tablets 2717
Subutex Tablets 2717

Buspirone Hydrochloride (Possible additive effects which may include hypotension).
No products indexed under this heading.

Butabarbital (Possible additive effects which may include hypotension).
No products indexed under this heading.

Butalbital (Possible additive effects which may include hypotension).
No products indexed under this heading.

Chlordiazepoxide (Possible additive effects which may include hypotension).
No products indexed under this heading.

Chlordiazepoxide Hydrochloride (Possible additive effects which may include hypotension). Products include:
Librium Capsules 3347

Chlorpromazine (Possible additive effects which may include hypotension).
No products indexed under this heading.

Chlorpromazine Hydrochloride (Possible additive effects which may include hypotension).
No products indexed under this heading.

Chlorprothixene (Possible additive effects which may include hypotension).
No products indexed under this heading.

Chlorprothixene Hydrochloride (Possible additive effects which may include hypotension).
No products indexed under this heading.

Chlorprothixene Lactate (Possible additive effects which may include hypotension).
No products indexed under this heading.

Clorazepate Dipotassium (Possible additive effects which may include hypotension). Products include:
Tranxene 2474

Clozapine (Possible additive effects which may include hypotension). Products include:
Clozaril Tablets 2184
FazaClo Orally Disintegrating Tablets 551

Codeine Phosphate (Possible additive effects which may include hypotension). Products include:
Tylenol with Codeine Tablets 2391

Desflurane (Possible additive effects which may include hypotension).
No products indexed under this heading.

Dezocine (Possible additive effects which may include hypotension).
No products indexed under this heading.

Diazepam (Possible additive effects which may include hypotension). Products include:
Diastat Rectal Delivery System 3343
Valium Tablets 2819

Droperidol (Possible additive effects which may include hypotension).
No products indexed under this heading.

Enflurane (Possible additive effects which may include hypotension).
No products indexed under this heading.

Estazolam (Possible additive effects which may include hypotension). Products include:
ProSom Tablets 517

Ethanol (Possible additive effects which may include hypotension).
No products indexed under this heading.

Ethchlorvynol (Possible additive effects which may include hypotension).
No products indexed under this heading.

Ethinamate (Possible additive effects which may include hypotension).
No products indexed under this heading.

Ethyl Alcohol (Possible additive effects which may include hypotension).
No products indexed under this heading.

Fentanyl (Possible additive effects which may include hypotension). Products include:
Duragesic Transdermal System 2373
Ionsys Transdermal System 2379

Fentanyl Citrate (Possible additive effects which may include hypotension). Products include:
Actiq 979

Fluphenazine Decanoate (Possible additive effects which may include hypotension).
No products indexed under this heading.

Fluphenazine Enanthate (Possible additive effects which may include hypotension).
No products indexed under this heading.

Fluphenazine Hydrochloride (Possible additive effects which may include hypotension).
No products indexed under this heading.

Flurazepam Hydrochloride (Possible additive effects which may include hypotension). Products include:
Dalmane Capsules 3342

Glutethimide (Possible additive effects which may include hypotension).
No products indexed under this heading.

Haloperidol (Possible additive effects which may include hypotension).
No products indexed under this heading.

Haloperidol Decanoate (Possible additive effects which may include hypotension).
No products indexed under this heading.

Hydrocodone Bitartrate (Possible additive effects which may include hypotension). Products include:
Hycodan 1116
Hycotuss Expectorant Syrup 1117
Vicodin Tablets 535
Vicodin ES Tablets 536
Vicodin HP Tablets 538
Vicoprofen Tablets 539
Zydone Tablets 1139

Hydrocodone Polistirex (Possible additive effects which may include hypotension). Products include:
Tussionex Pennkinetic Extended-Release Suspension 3327

Hydromorphone Hydrochloride (Possible additive effects which may include hypotension). Products include:
Dilaudid 440
Dilaudid Non-Sterile Powder 440
Dilaudid Oral Liquid 445
Dilaudid Rectal Suppositories 440
Dilaudid Tablets 440
Dilaudid Tablets - 8 mg 445
Dilaudid-HP 442

Hydroxyzine Hydrochloride (Possible additive effects which may include hypotension).
No products indexed under this heading.

Hyoscyamine (Thiothixene exhibits weak anticholinergic properties; concurrent use with atropine or related drugs requires caution).
No products indexed under this heading.

Hyoscyamine Sulfate (Thiothixene exhibits weak anticholinergic properties; concurrent use with atropine or related drugs requires caution). Products include:
Donnatal Extentabs 2493
Prosed/DS Tablets 1157

Isoflurane (Possible additive effects which may include hypotension).
No products indexed under this heading.

Ketamine Hydrochloride (Possible additive effects which may include hypotension).
No products indexed under this heading.

Levomethadyl Acetate Hydrochloride (Possible additive effects which may include hypotension).
No products indexed under this heading.

Levorphanol Tartrate (Possible additive effects which may include hypotension).
No products indexed under this heading.

Lorazepam (Possible additive effects which may include hypotension).
No products indexed under this heading.

Loxapine Hydrochloride (Possible additive effects which may include hypotension).
No products indexed under this heading.

Loxapine Succinate (Possible additive effects which may include hypotension).
No products indexed under this heading.

Meperidine Hydrochloride (Possible additive effects which may include hypotension).
No products indexed under this heading.

Mephobarbital (Possible additive effects which may include hypotension).
No products indexed under this heading.

Meprobamate (Possible additive effects which may include hypotension).
No products indexed under this heading.

Mesoridazine Besylate (Possible additive effects which may include hypotension).
No products indexed under this heading.

Methadone Hydrochloride (Possible additive effects which may include hypotension).
No products indexed under this heading.

Methohexital Sodium (Possible additive effects which may include hypotension).
No products indexed under this heading.

Methotrimeprazine (Possible additive effects which may include hypotension).
No products indexed under this heading.

Methoxyflurane (Possible additive effects which may include hypotension).
No products indexed under this heading.

Midazolam Hydrochloride (Possible additive effects which may include hypotension).
No products indexed under this heading.

Molindone Hydrochloride (Possible additive effects which may include hypotension). Products include:
Moban Tablets 1119

Morphine Sulfate (Possible additive effects which may include hypotension). Products include:
Avinza Capsules 1741
Kadian Capsules 577
MS Contin Tablets 2701

Olanzapine (Possible additive effects which may include hypotension). Products include:
Symbyax Capsules 1819
Zyprexa Tablets 1830
Zyprexa IntraMuscular 1830
Zyprexa ZYDIS Orally Disintegrating Tablets 1830

Oxazepam (Possible additive effects which may include hypotension).
No products indexed under this heading.

Oxycodone Hydrochloride (Possible additive effects which may include hypotension). Products include:
OxyContin Tablets 2703
OxyFast Oral Concentrate Solution 2708
OxyIR Capsules 2708
Percocet Tablets 1131
Percodan Tablets 1132

Pentobarbital Sodium (Possible additive effects which may include hypotension). Products include:
Nembutal Sodium Solution, USP 2470

Perphenazine (Possible additive effects which may include hypotension).
No products indexed under this heading.

Phenobarbital (Possible additive effects which may include hypotension). Products include:
Donnatal Extentabs 2493

Prazepam (Possible additive effects which may include hypotension).
No products indexed under this heading.

Prochlorperazine (Possible additive effects which may include hypotension).
No products indexed under this heading.

Promethazine Hydrochloride (Possible additive effects which may include hypotension). Products include:
Phenergan Tablets and Suppositories 3440

Propofol (Possible additive effects which may include hypotension).
No products indexed under this heading.

Propoxyphene Hydrochloride (Possible additive effects which may include hypotension).
No products indexed under this heading.

Propoxyphene Napsylate (Possible additive effects which may include hypotension).
No products indexed under this heading.

Quazepam (Possible additive effects which may include hypotension).
No products indexed under this heading.

Quetiapine Fumarate (Possible additive effects which may include hypotension). Products include:
Seroquel Tablets 690

Remifentanil Hydrochloride (Possible additive effects which may include hypotension).
No products indexed under this heading.

Risperidone (Possible additive effects which may include hypotension). Products include:
Risperdal 1676
Risperdal Consta Long-Acting Injection 1682
Risperdal M-Tab Orally Disintegrating Tablets 1676

Scopolamine (Thiothixene exhibits weak anticholinergic properties; concurrent use with atropine or related drugs requires caution). Products include:
Transderm Scōp Transdermal Therapeutic System 2177

Scopolamine Hydrobromide (Thiothixene exhibits weak anticholinergic properties; concurrent use with atropine or related drugs requires caution). Products include:
Donnatal Extentabs 2493

Secobarbital Sodium (Possible additive effects which may include hypotension).
No products indexed under this heading.

Sevoflurane (Possible additive effects which may include hypotension). Products include:
Ultane Liquid for Inhalation 531

Sufentanil Citrate (Possible additive effects which may include hypotension).
No products indexed under this heading.

Temazepam (Possible additive effects which may include hypotension). Products include:
Restoril Capsules 1860

Thiamylal Sodium (Possible additive effects which may include hypotension).
No products indexed under this heading.

Thioridazine Hydrochloride (Possible additive effects which may include hypotension). Products include:
Thioridazine Hydrochloride Tablets 2163

Triazolam (Possible additive effects which may include hypotension).
No products indexed under this heading.

Trifluoperazine Hydrochloride (Possible additive effects which may include hypotension).
No products indexed under this heading.

Zaleplon (Possible additive effects which may include hypotension). Products include:
Sonata Capsules 1717

Ziprasidone Hydrochloride (Possible additive effects which may include hypotension). Products include:
Geodon Capsules 2529

Zolpidem Tartrate (Possible additive effects which may include hypotension). Products include:
Ambien Tablets 2851
Ambien CR Tablets 2855

Food Interactions

Alcohol (Possible additive effects which may include hypotension).

THROMBATE III

(Antithrombin III) 3257
May interact with:

Heparin Sodium (The anticoagulant effect of heparin is enhanced by concurrent treatment with antithrombin III; reduced dosage of heparin may be required).
No products indexed under this heading.

THYMOGLOBULIN FOR INTRAVENOUS INFUSION

(Anti-thymocyte Globulin) 1284
May interact with immunosuppressive agents and certain other agents. Compounds in these categories include:

Azathioprine (Co-administration with standard immunosuppressive regimen may predispose patients to over-immunosuppression; decrease in maintenance immunosuppression therapy during the period of antibody therapy may be needed).
No products indexed under this heading.

Basiliximab (Co-administration with standard immunosuppressive regimen may predispose patients to over-immunosuppression; decrease in maintenance immunosuppression therapy during the period of antibody therapy may be needed). Products include:
Simulect for Injection 2284

Cyclosporine (Co-administration with standard immunosuppressive regimen may predispose patients to over-immunosuppression; decrease in maintenance immunosuppression therapy during the period of antibody therapy may be needed). Products include:
Gengraf Capsules 459
Neoral Oral Solution 2259
Neoral Soft Gelatin Capsules 2259
Restasis Ophthalmic Emulsion 575
Sandimmune 2275

Globulin, immune (rabbit) (Thymoglobulin can stimulate the production of antibodies which cross-react with rabbit immune globulin).
No products indexed under this heading.

Muromonab-CD3 (Co-administration with standard immunosuppressive regimen may predispose patients to over-immunosuppression; decrease in maintenance immunosuppression therapy during the period of antibody therapy may be needed). Products include:
Orthoclone OKT3 Sterile Solution 2360

Mycophenolate Mofetil (Co-administration with standard immunosuppressive regimen may predispose patients to over-immunosuppression; decrease in maintenance immunosuppression therapy during the period of antibody therapy may be needed). Products include:
CellCept Capsules 2747
CellCept Oral Suspension 2747
CellCept Tablets 2747

Sirolimus (Co-administration with standard immunosuppressive regimen may predispose patients to over-immunosuppression; decrease in maintenance immunosuppression therapy during the period of antibody therapy may be needed). Products include:
Rapamune Oral Solution and Tablets 3475

Tacrolimus (Co-administration with standard immunosuppressive regimen may predispose patients to over-immunosuppression; decrease in maintenance immunosuppression therapy during the period of antibody therapy may be needed). Products include:
Prograf Capsules and Injection 632
Protopic Ointment 638

THYROGEN FOR INJECTION

(Thyrotropin alfa) 1286
None cited in PDR database.

THYROLAR TABLETS

(Liotrix) 1199
May interact with oral anticoagulants, estrogens, oral hypoglycemic agents, insulin, oral contraceptives, and certain other agents. Compounds in these categories include:

Acarbose (Initiating thyroid replacement therapy may cause increases in roal hypoglycemic requirements. The effects seen are poorly understood and depend upon a variety of factors such as dose and type of thyroid preparations and endocrine status of the patient. Patients receiving oral hypoglycemics should be closely watched during initiation of thyroid replacement therapy). Products include:
Precose Tablets 751

Anisindione (Thyroid hormones appear to increase catabolism of vitamin K-dependent clotting factors. If oral anticoagulants are also being given, compensatory increases in clotting factor synthesis are impaired. Patients stabilized on oral anticoagulants who are found to require thyroid replacement therapy should be watched very closely when thyroid is started. If a patient is truly hypothyroid, it is likely that a reduction in anticoagulant dosage will be required. No special precautions appear to be necessary when oral anticoagulant therapy is begun in a patient already stabilized on maintenance thyroid replacement therapy). Products include:
Miradon Tablets 3042

Chlorotrianisene (Estrogens tend to increase serum thyroxine-binding globulin (TBg). In a patient with a nonfunctioning thyroid gland who is receiving thyroid replacement therapy, free levothyroxine may be decreased when estrogens are started, thus increasing thyroid requirements. However, if the patient's thyroid gland has sufficient function, the decreased free thyroxine will result in a compensatory increase in thyroxine output by the thyroid. Therefore, patients without a functioning thyroid gland who are on thyroid replacement therapy may need to increase their thyroid dose if estrogens or estrogen-containing oral contraceptives are given).
No products indexed under this heading.

Chlorpropamide (Initiating thyroid replacement therapy may cause increases in roal hypoglycemic requirements. The effects seen are poorly understood and depend upon a variety of factors such as dose and type of thyroid preparations and endocrine status of the patient. Patients receiving oral hypoglycemics should be closely watched during initiation of thyroid replacement therapy).
No products indexed under this heading.

Cholestyramine (Cholestyramine binds both T4 and T3 in the intesting thus impairing absorption of these thyroid hormones. In vitro studues indicate that the binding is not easily removed. Therefore, 4-5 hours should elapse between the administration of cholestyramine and thyroid hormones).

No products indexed under this heading.

Colestipol (Colestipol binds both T4 and T3 in the intesting thus impairing absorption of these thyroid hormones. In vitro studues indicate that the binding is not easily removed. Therefore, 4-5 hours should elapse between the administration of colestipol and thyroid hormones).

No products indexed under this heading.

Colestipol Hydrochloride (Colestipol binds both T4 and T3 in the intesting thus impairing absorption of these thyroid hormones. In vitro studies indicate that the binding is not easily removed. Therefore, 4-5 hours should elapse between the administration of colestipol and thyroid hormones).

No products indexed under this heading.

Desogestrel (Estrogens tend to increase serum thyroxine-binding globulin (TBg). In a patient with a nonfunctioning thyroid gland who is receiving thyroid replacement therapy, free levothyroxine may be decreased when estrogens are started, thus increasing thyroid requirements. However, if the patient's thyroid gland has sufficient function, the decreased free thyroxine will result in a compensatory increase in thyroxine output by the thyroid. Therefore, patients without a functioning thyroid gland who are on thyroid replacement therapy may need to increase their thyroid dose if estrogens or estrogen-containing oral contraceptives are given). Products include:

Mircette Tablets 1066

Dicumarol (Thyroid hormones appear to increase catabolism of vitamin K-dependent clotting factors. If oral anticoagulants are also being given, compensatory increases in clotting factor synthesis are impaired. Patients stabilized on oral anticoagulants who are found to require thyroid replacement therapy should be watched very closely when thyroid is started. If a patient is truly hypothyroid, it is likely that a reduction in anticoagulant dosage will be required. No special precautions appear to be necessary when oral anticoagulant therapy is begun in a patient already stabilized on maintenance thyroid replacement therapy).

No products indexed under this heading.

Dienestrol (Estrogens tend to increase serum thyroxine-binding globulin (TBg). In a patient with a nonfunctioning thyroid gland who is receiving thyroid replacement therapy, free levothyroxine may be decreased when estrogens are started, thus increasing thyroid requirements. However, if the patient's thyroid gland has sufficient function, the decreased free thyroxine will result in a compensatory increase in thyroxine output by the thyroid. Therefore, patients without a functioning

thyroid gland who are on thyroid replacement therapy may need to increase their thyroid dose if estrogens or estrogen-containing oral contraceptives are given).

No products indexed under this heading.

Diethylstilbestrol (Estrogens tend to increase serum thyroxine-binding globulin (TBg). In a patient with a nonfunctioning thyroid gland who is receiving thyroid replacement therapy, free levothyroxine may be decreased when estrogens are started, thus increasing thyroid requirements. However, if the patient's thyroid gland has sufficient function, the decreased free thyroxine will result in a compensatory increase in thyroxine output by the thyroid. Therefore, patients without a functioning thyroid gland who are on thyroid replacement therapy may need to increase their thyroid dose if estrogens or estrogen-containing oral contraceptives are given).

No products indexed under this heading.

Estradiol (Estrogens tend to increase serum thyroxine-binding globulin (TBg). In a patient with a nonfunctioning thyroid gland who is receiving thyroid replacement therapy, free levothyroxine may be decreased when estrogens are started, thus increasing thyroid requirements. However, if the patient's thyroid gland has sufficient function, the decreased free thyroxine will result in a compensatory increase in thyroxine output by the thyroid. Therefore, patients without a functioning thyroid gland who are on thyroid replacement therapy may need to increase their thyroid dose if estrogens or estrogen-containing oral contraceptives are given). Products include:

Angeliq Tablets 762
Climara Transdermal System 771
Climara Pro Transdermal System 776
Estrasorb Topical Emulsion 1147
Estring Vaginal Ring 2635
Menostar Transdermal System 782
Vagifem Tablets 2334

Estrogens, Conjugated (Estrogens tend to increase serum thyroxine-binding globulin (TBg). In a patient with a nonfunctioning thyroid gland who is receiving thyroid replacement therapy, free levothyroxine may be decreased when estrogens are started, thus increasing thyroid requirements. However, if the patient's thyroid gland has sufficient function, the decreased free thyroxine will result in a compensatory increase in thyroxine output by the thyroid. Therefore, patients without a functioning thyroid gland who are on thyroid replacement therapy may need to increase their thyroid dose if estrogens or estrogen-containing oral contraceptives are given). Products include:

Premarin Intravenous 3442
Premarin Tablets 3446
Premarin Vaginal Cream 3452
Premphase Tablets 3456
Prempro Tablets 3456

Estrogens, Esterified (Estrogens tend to increase serum thyroxine-binding globulin (TBg). In a patient with a nonfunctioning thyroid gland who is receiving thyroid replacement therapy, free levothyroxine may be decreased when estrogens are started, thus increasing thyroid require-

ments. However, if the patient's thyroid gland has sufficient function, the decreased free thyroxine will result in a compensatory increase in thyroxine output by the thyroid. Therefore, patients without a functioning thyroid gland who are on thyroid replacement therapy may need to increase their thyroid dose if estrogens or estrogen-containing oral contraceptives are given). Products include:

Estratest Tablets 3199
Estratest H.S. Tablets 3199

Estropipate (Estrogens tend to increase serum thyroxine-binding globulin (TBg). In a patient with a nonfunctioning thyroid gland who is receiving thyroid replacement therapy, free levothyroxine may be decreased when estrogens are started, thus increasing thyroid requirements. However, if the patient's thyroid gland has sufficient function, the decreased free thyroxine will result in a compensatory increase in thyroxine output by the thyroid. Therefore, patients without a functioning thyroid gland who are on thyroid replacement therapy may need to increase their thyroid dose if estrogens or estrogen-containing oral contraceptives are given).

No products indexed under this heading.

Ethinyl Estradiol (Estrogens tend to increase serum thyroxine-binding globulin (TBg). In a patient with a nonfunctioning thyroid gland who is receiving thyroid replacement therapy, free levothyroxine may be decreased when estrogens are started, thus increasing thyroid requirements. However, if the patient's thyroid gland has sufficient function, the decreased free thyroxine will result in a compensatory increase in thyroxine output by the thyroid. Therefore, patients without a functioning thyroid gland who are on thyroid replacement therapy may need to increase their thyroid dose if estrogens or estrogen-containing oral contraceptives are given). Products include:

Mircette Tablets 1066
NuvaRing 2340
Ortho-Cyclen/Ortho Tri-Cyclen 2429
Ortho Evra Transdermal System 2417
Ortho Tri-Cyclen Lo Tablets 2436
Seasonique Tablets 1077
Yasmin 28 Tablets 796
Yaz Tablets 803

Ethynodiol Diacetate (Estrogens tend to increase serum thyroxine-binding globulin (TBg). In a patient with a nonfunctioning thyroid gland who is receiving thyroid replacement therapy, free levothyroxine may be decreased when estrogens are started, thus increasing thyroid requirements. However, if the patient's thyroid gland has sufficient function, the decreased free thyroxine will result in a compensatory increase in thyroxine output by the thyroid. Therefore, patients without a functioning thyroid gland who are on thyroid replacement therapy may need to increase their thyroid dose if estrogens or estrogen-containing oral contraceptives are given).

No products indexed under this heading.

Glimepiride (Initiating thyroid replacement therapy may cause increases in roal hypoglycemic requirements. The effects seen are poorly understood and depend upon

a variety of factors such as dose and type of thyroid preparations and endocrine status of the patient. Patients receiving oral hypoglycemics should be closely watched during initiation of thyroid replacement therapy). Products include:

Avandaryl Tablets 1379
Duetact Tablets 3226

Glipizide (Initiating thyroid replacement therapy may cause increases in roal hypoglycemic requirements. The effects seen are poorly understood and depend upon a variety of factors such as dose and type of thyroid preparations and endocrine status of the patient. Patients receiving oral hypoglycemics should be closely watched during initiation of thyroid replacement therapy).

No products indexed under this heading.

Glyburide (Initiating thyroid replacement therapy may cause increases in roal hypoglycemic requirements. The effects seen are poorly understood and depend upon a variety of factors such as dose and type of thyroid preparations and endocrine status of the patient. Patients receiving oral hypoglycemics should be closely watched during initiation of thyroid replacement therapy).

No products indexed under this heading.

Insulin, Human, Zinc Suspension (Initiating thyroid replacement therapy may cause increases in requirements. The effects seen are poorly understood and depend upon a variety of factors such as dose and type of thyroid preparations and endocrine status of the patient. Patients receiving insulin should be closely watched during initiation of thyroid replacement therapy). Products include:

Humulin L, 100 Units 1794
Humulin U, 100 Units 1800

Insulin, Human NPH (Initiating thyroid replacement therapy may cause increases in requirements. The effects seen are poorly understood and depend upon a variety of factors such as dose and type of thyroid preparations and endocrine status of the patient. Patients receiving insulin should be closely watched during initiation of thyroid replacement therapy). Products include:

Humulin N, 100 Units 1795
Humulin N Pen 1797

Insulin, Human Regular (Initiating thyroid replacement therapy may cause increases in requirements. The effects seen are poorly understood and depend upon a variety of factors such as dose and type of thyroid preparations and endocrine status of the patient. Patients receiving insulin should be closely watched during initiation of thyroid replacement therapy). Products include:

Humulin R, 100 Units 1798

Insulin, Human Regular and Human NPH Mixture (Initiating thyroid replacement therapy may cause increases in requirements. The effects seen are poorly understood and depend upon a variety of factors such as dose and type of thyroid preparations and endocrine status of the patient. Patients receiving insulin should be closely watched during initiation of thyroid replacement therapy). Products include:

Humulin 50/50, 100 Units 1791
Humulin 70/30 Pen 1793

Insulin, NPH (Initiating thyroid replacement therapy may cause increases in requirements. The effects seen are poorly understood and depend upon a variety of factors such as dose and type of thyroid preparations and endocrine status of the patient. Patients receiving insulin should be closely watched during initiation of thyroid replacement therapy).

No products indexed under this heading.

Insulin, Regular (Initiating thyroid replacement therapy may cause increases in requirements. The effects seen are poorly understood and depend upon a variety of factors such as dose and type of thyroid preparations and endocrine status of the patient. Patients receiving insulin should be closely watched during initiation of thyroid replacement therapy).

No products indexed under this heading.

Insulin, Zinc Crystals (Initiating thyroid replacement therapy may cause increases in requirements. The effects seen are poorly understood and depend upon a variety of factors such as dose and type of thyroid preparations and endocrine status of the patient. Patients receiving insulin should be closely watched during initiation of thyroid replacement therapy).

No products indexed under this heading.

Insulin, Zinc Suspension (Initiating thyroid replacement therapy may cause increases in requirements. The effects seen are poorly understood and depend upon a variety of factors such as dose and type of thyroid preparations and endocrine status of the patient. Patients receiving insulin should be closely watched during initiation of thyroid replacement therapy).

No products indexed under this heading.

Insulin Aspart, Human Regular (Initiating thyroid replacement therapy may cause increases in requirements. The effects seen are poorly understood and depend upon a variety of factors such as dose and type of thyroid preparations and endocrine status of the patient. Patients receiving insulin should be closely watched during initiation of thyroid replacement therapy). Products include:

NovoLog Injection 2326

Insulin glargine (Initiating thyroid replacement therapy may cause increases in requirements. The effects seen are poorly understood and depend upon a variety of factors such as dose and type of thyroid preparations and endocrine status of the patient. Patients receiving insulin should be closely watched during initiation of thyroid replacement therapy). Products include:

Lantus Injection 2909

Insulin Lispro, Human (Initiating thyroid replacement therapy may cause increases in requirements. The effects seen are poorly understood and depend upon a variety of factors such as dose and type of thyroid preparations and endocrine status of the patient. Patients receiv-

ing insulin should be closely watched during initiation of thyroid replacement therapy). Products include:

Humalog-Pen 1781
Humalog Mix 50/50-Pen 1783
Humalog Mix 75/25-Pen 1785

Insulin Lispro Protamine, Human (Initiating thyroid replacement therapy may cause increases in requirements. The effects seen are poorly understood and depend upon a variety of factors such as dose and type of thyroid preparations and endocrine status of the patient. Patients receiving insulin should be closely watched during initiation of thyroid replacement therapy). Products include:

Humalog Mix 50/50-Pen 1783
Humalog Mix 75/25-Pen 1785

Levonorgestrel (Estrogens tend to increase serum thyroxine-binding globulin (TBg). In a patient with a nonfunctioning thyroid gland who is receiving thyroid replacement therapy, free levothyroxine may be decreased when estrogens are started, thus increasing thyroid requirements. However, if the patient's thyroid gland has sufficient function, the decreased free thyroxine will result in a compensatory increase in thyroxine output by the thyroid. Therefore, patients without a functioning thyroid gland who are on thyroid replacement therapy may need to increase their thyroid dose if estrogens or estrogen-containing oral contraceptives are given). Products include:

Climara Pro Transdermal System 776
Mirena Intrauterine System 787
Plan B Tablets 1076
Seasonique Tablets 1077

Mestranol (Estrogens tend to increase serum thyroxine-binding globulin (TBg). In a patient with a nonfunctioning thyroid gland who is receiving thyroid replacement therapy, free levothyroxine may be decreased when estrogens are started, thus increasing thyroid requirements. However, if the patient's thyroid gland has sufficient function, the decreased free thyroxine will result in a compensatory increase in thyroxine output by the thyroid. Therefore, patients without a functioning thyroid gland who are on thyroid replacement therapy may need to increase their thyroid dose if estrogens or estrogen-containing oral contraceptives are given).

No products indexed under this heading.

Metformin Hydrochloride (Initiating thyroid replacement therapy may cause increases in roal hypoglycemic requirements. The effects seen are poorly understood and depend upon a variety of factors such as dose and type of thyroid preparations and endocrine status of the patient. Patients receiving oral hypoglycemics should be closely watched during initiation of thyroid replacement therapy). Products include:

ActoPlus Met Tablets 3214
Avandamet Tablets 1373
Fortamet Extended-Release Tablets ... 3115

Miglitol (Initiating thyroid replacement therapy may cause increases in roal hypoglycemic requirements. The effects seen are poorly understood and depend upon a variety of factors such as dose and type of thyroid preparations and endocrine status of the patient. Patients receiving oral hypoglycemics should be closely watched during initiation of thyroid replacement therapy).

No products indexed under this heading.

Norethindrone (Estrogens tend to increase serum thyroxine-binding globulin (TBg). In a patient with a nonfunctioning thyroid gland who is receiving thyroid replacement therapy, free levothyroxine may be decreased when estrogens are started, thus increasing thyroid requirements. However, if the patient's thyroid gland has sufficient function, the decreased free thyroxine will result in a compensatory increase in thyroxine output by the thyroid. Therefore, patients without a functioning thyroid gland who are on thyroid replacement therapy may need to increase their thyroid dose if estrogens or estrogen-containing oral contraceptives are given). Products include:

Ortho Micronor Tablets 2426

Norethynodrel (Estrogens tend to increase serum thyroxine-binding globulin (TBg). In a patient with a nonfunctioning thyroid gland who is receiving thyroid replacement therapy, free levothyroxine may be decreased when estrogens are started, thus increasing thyroid requirements. However, if the patient's thyroid gland has sufficient function, the decreased free thyroxine will result in a compensatory increase in thyroxine output by the thyroid. Therefore, patients without a functioning thyroid gland who are on thyroid replacement therapy may need to increase their thyroid dose if estrogens or estrogen-containing oral contraceptives are given).

No products indexed under this heading.

Norgestimate (Estrogens tend to increase serum thyroxine-binding globulin (TBg). In a patient with a nonfunctioning thyroid gland who is receiving thyroid replacement therapy, free levothyroxine may be decreased when estrogens are started, thus increasing thyroid requirements. However, if the patient's thyroid gland has sufficient function, the decreased free thyroxine will result in a compensatory increase in thyroxine output by the thyroid. Therefore, patients without a functioning thyroid gland who are on thyroid replacement therapy may need to increase their thyroid dose if estrogens or estrogen-containing oral contraceptives are given). Products include:

Ortho-Cyclen/Ortho Tri-Cyclen 2429
Ortho Tri-Cyclen Lo Tablets 2436

Norgestrel (Estrogens tend to increase serum thyroxine-binding globulin (TBg). In a patient with a nonfunctioning thyroid gland who is receiving thyroid replacement therapy, free levothyroxine may be decreased when estrogens are started, thus increasing thyroid requirements. However, if the patient's thyroid gland has sufficient function, the

decreased free thyroxine will result in a compensatory increase in thyroxine output by the thyroid. Therefore, patients without a functioning thyroid gland who are on thyroid replacement therapy may need to increase their thyroid dose if estrogens or estrogen-containing oral contraceptives are given).

No products indexed under this heading.

Pioglitazone Hydrochloride (Initiating thyroid replacement therapy may cause increases in roal hypoglycemic requirements. The effects seen are poorly understood and depend upon a variety of factors such as dose and type of thyroid preparations and endocrine status of the patient. Patients receiving oral hypoglycemics should be closely watched during initiation of thyroid replacement therapy). Products include:

ActoPlus Met Tablets 3214
Actos Tablets 3219
Duetact Tablets 3226

Polyestradiol Phosphate (Estrogens tend to increase serum thyroxine-binding globulin (TBg). In a patient with a nonfunctioning thyroid gland who is receiving thyroid replacement therapy, free levothyroxine may be decreased when estrogens are started, thus increasing thyroid requirements. However, if the patient's thyroid gland has sufficient function, the decreased free thyroxine will result in a compensatory increase in thyroxine output by the thyroid. Therefore, patients without a functioning thyroid gland who are on thyroid replacement therapy may need to increase their thyroid dose if estrogens or estrogen-containing oral contraceptives are given).

No products indexed under this heading.

Quinestrol (Estrogens tend to increase serum thyroxine-binding globulin (TBg). In a patient with a nonfunctioning thyroid gland who is receiving thyroid replacement therapy, free levothyroxine may be decreased when estrogens are started, thus increasing thyroid requirements. However, if the patient's thyroid gland has sufficient function, the decreased free thyroxine will result in a compensatory increase in thyroxine output by the thyroid. Therefore, patients without a functioning thyroid gland who are on thyroid replacement therapy may need to increase their thyroid dose if estrogens or estrogen-containing oral contraceptives are given).

No products indexed under this heading.

Repaglinide (Initiating thyroid replacement therapy may cause increases in roal hypoglycemic requirements. The effects seen are poorly understood and depend upon a variety of factors such as dose and type of thyroid preparations and endocrine status of the patient. Patients receiving oral hypoglycemics should be closely watched during initiation of thyroid replacement therapy).

No products indexed under this heading.

Rosiglitazone Maleate (Initiating thyroid replacement therapy may cause increases in roal hypoglycemic requirements. The effects seen are poorly understood and depend upon a variety of factors such as dose and type of thyroid preparations and endocrine status of the patient. Patients receiving oral hypoglycemics should be closely watched during initiation of thyroid replacement therapy). Products include:

Avandamet Tablets 1373
Avandaryl Tablets 1379
Avandia Tablets 1384

Tolazamide (Initiating thyroid replacement therapy may cause increases in roal hypoglycemic requirements. The effects seen are poorly understood and depend upon a variety of factors such as dose and type of thyroid preparations and endocrine status of the patient. Patients receiving oral hypoglycemics should be closely watched during initiation of thyroid replacement therapy).
No products indexed under this heading.

Tolbutamide (Initiating thyroid replacement therapy may cause increases in roal hypoglycemic requirements. The effects seen are poorly understood and depend upon a variety of factors such as dose and type of thyroid preparations and endocrine status of the patient. Patients receiving oral hypoglycemics should be closely watched during initiation of thyroid replacement therapy).
No products indexed under this heading.

Troglitazone (Initiating thyroid replacement therapy may cause increases in roal hypoglycemic requirements. The effects seen are poorly understood and depend upon a variety of factors such as dose and type of thyroid preparations and endocrine status of the patient. Patients receiving oral hypoglycemics should be closely watched during initiation of thyroid replacement therapy).
No products indexed under this heading.

Warfarin Sodium (Thyroid hormones appear to increase catabolism of vitamin K-dependent clotting factors. If oral anticoagulants are also being given, compensatory increases in clotting factor synthesis are impaired. Patients stabilized on oral anticoagulants who are found to require thyroid replacement therapy should be watched very closely when thyroid is started. If a patient is truly hypothyroid, it is likely that a reduction in anticoagulant dosage will be required. No special precautions appear to be necessary when oral anticoagulant therapy is begun in a patient already stabilized on maintenance thyroid replacement therapy). Products include:

Coumadin for Injection 898
Coumadin Tablets 898

TIAZAC CAPSULES

(Diltiazem Hydrochloride) 1201
May interact with anesthetics, beta blockers, erythromycin, cardiac glycosides, phenytoin, and certain other agents. Compounds in these categories include:

Acebutolol Hydrochloride (Concomitant use of diltiazem with beta blockers may result in additive effects on cardiac conduction).
No products indexed under this heading.

Alfentanil Hydrochloride (Calcium channel blockers potentiate the depression of cardiac contractility, conductivity, and automaticity as well as vascular dilation associated with anesthetics).
No products indexed under this heading.

Amiodarone Hydrochloride (Agents known to affect cardiac contractility, such as amiodarone, may produce additive inhibition of cardiac conduction leading to increased risk of AV block).
No products indexed under this heading.

Atenolol (Concomitant use of diltiazem with beta blockers may result in additive effects on cardiac conduction).
No products indexed under this heading.

Betaxolol Hydrochloride (Concomitant use of diltiazem with beta blockers may result in additive effects on cardiac conduction). Products include:

Betoptic S Ophthalmic Suspension 558

Bisoprolol Fumarate (Concomitant use of diltiazem with beta blockers may result in additive effects on cardiac conduction).
No products indexed under this heading.

Carbamazepine (Co-administration has resulted in increased serum levels of carbamazepine resulting in toxicity in some patients). Products include:

Carbatrol Capsules 3171
Equetro Extended-Release Capsules 3180
Tegretol/Tegretol-XR 2295

Carteolol Hydrochloride (Concomitant use of diltiazem with beta blockers may result in additive effects on cardiac conduction). Products include:

Carteolol Hydrochloride Ophthalmic Solution USP, 1% .... ⊙ 249

Cimetidine (Co-administration has resulted in inhibition of hepatic cytochrome P450 by cimetidine producing significant increase in peak diltiazem plasma levels and AUC; am adjustment in diltiazem dosage may be warranted). Products include:

Tagamet HB 200 Tablets .... ▣ 664

Cimetidine Hydrochloride (Co-administration has resulted in inhibition of hepatic cytochrome P450 by cimetidine producing significant increase in peak diltiazem plasma levels and AUC; am adjustment in diltiazem dosage may be warranted).
No products indexed under this heading.

Cyclosporine (Diltiazem inhibits cytochrome P450 3A enzyme and co-administration may result in increased cyclosporine concentrations; a reduction in cyclosporine dose may be required, especially in renal and cardiac transplant recipients). Products include:

Gengraf Capsules 459
Neoral Oral Solution 2259
Neoral Soft Gelatin Capsules 2259
Restasis Ophthalmic Emulsion 575
Sandimmune 2275

Deslanoside (Concomitant use of diltiazem with digitalis may result in additive effects on cardiac conduction).
No products indexed under this heading.

Digitalis Glycoside Preparations (Concomitant use of diltiazem with digitalis may result in additive effects on cardiac conduction).
No products indexed under this heading.

Digitoxin (Concomitant use of diltiazem with digitalis may result in additive effects on cardiac conduction).
No products indexed under this heading.

Digoxin (Co-administration has resulted in increased plasma digoxin concentrations in some patients; concomitant use of diltiazem with digitalis may result in additive effects on cardiac conduction). Products include:

Lanoxicaps Capsules 1490
Lanoxin Injection 1494
Lanoxin Injection Pediatric 1497
Lanoxin Tablets 1500

Enflurane (Calcium channel blockers potentiate the depression of cardiac contractility, conductivity, and automaticity as well as vascular dilation associated with anesthetics).
No products indexed under this heading.

Erythromycin (Diltiazem is both a substrate and inhibitor of the CYP4503A4; co-administration with inhibitors of this enzyme system, such as erythromycin, may have significant impact on the side effect profile of diltiazem). Products include:

Ery-Tab Tablets 449
Erythromycin Base Filmtab Tablets 455
Erythromycin Delayed-Release Capsules, USP 457
PCE Dispertab Tablets 515

Erythromycin Estolate (Diltiazem is both a substrate and inhibitor of the CYP4503A4; co-administration with inhibitors of this enzyme system, such as erythromycin, may have significant impact on the side effect profile of diltiazem).
No products indexed under this heading.

Erythromycin Ethylsuccinate (Diltiazem is both a substrate and inhibitor of the CYP4503A4; co-administration with inhibitors of this enzyme system, such as erythromycin, may have significant impact on the side effect profile of diltiazem). Products include:

E.E.S. 451
EryPed 447

Erythromycin Gluceptate (Diltiazem is both a substrate and inhibitor of the CYP4503A4; co-administration with inhibitors of this enzyme system, such as erythromycin, may have significant impact on the side effect profile of diltiazem).
No products indexed under this heading.

Erythromycin Lactobionate (Diltiazem is both a substrate and inhibitor of the CYP4503A4; co-administration with inhibitors of this enzyme system, such as erythromycin, may have significant impact on the side effect profile of diltiazem).
No products indexed under this heading.

Erythromycin Stearate (Diltiazem is both a substrate and inhibitor of the CYP4503A4; co-administration with inhibitors of this enzyme system, such as erythromycin, may have significant impact on the side effect profile of diltiazem). Products include:

Erythrocin Stearate Filmtab Tablets 453

Esmolol Hydrochloride (Concomitant use of diltiazem with beta blockers may result in additive effects on cardiac conduction).
No products indexed under this heading.

Fentanyl Citrate (Calcium channel blockers potentiate the depression of cardiac contractility, conductivity, and automaticity as well as vascular dilation associated with anesthetics). Products include:

Actiq 979

Fluoxetine Hydrochloride (Diltiazem undergoes biotransformation by cytochrome P450 mixed funciton oxidase; co-administration with other agents which follow the same route of biotransformation may result in competitve inhibition of metabolism). Products include:

Prozac Pulvules and Liquid 1801
Symbyax Capsules 1819

Fluvoxamine Maleate (Diltiazem undergoes biotransformation by cytochrome P450 mixed funciton oxidase; co-administration with other agents which follow the same route of biotransformation may result in competitve inhibition of metabolism).
No products indexed under this heading.

Fosphenytoin Sodium (Diltiazem is both a substrate and inhibitor of the CYP4503A4; co-administration with inducers of this enzyme system, such as phenytoin, may have significant impact on the efficacy of diltiazem).
No products indexed under this heading.

Halothane (Calcium channel blockers potentiate the depression of cardiac contractility, conductivity, and automaticity as well as vascular dilation associated with anesthetics).
No products indexed under this heading.

Isoflurane (Calcium channel blockers potentiate the depression of cardiac contractility, conductivity, and automaticity as well as vascular dilation associated with anesthetics).
No products indexed under this heading.

Ketamine Hydrochloride (Calcium channel blockers potentiate the depression of cardiac contractility, conductivity, and automaticity as well as vascular dilation associated with anesthetics).
No products indexed under this heading.

Ketoconazole (Diltiazem is both a substrate and inhibitor of the CYP4503A4; co-administration with inhibitors of this enzyme system, such as ketoconazole, may have significant impact on the side effect profile of diltiazem). Products include:

Nizoral A-D Shampoo, 1% 1868

Labetalol Hydrochloride (Concomitant use of diltiazem with beta blockers may result in additive effects on cardiac conduction).
No products indexed under this heading.

Levobunolol Hydrochloride (Concomitant use of diltiazem with beta blockers may result in additive effects on cardiac conduction). Products include:
Betagan Ophthalmic Solution, USP ⊙ 220

Lovastatin (Co-administration has resulted in a 3-4 times increase in mean lovastatin AUC and Cmax). Products include:
Advicor Tablets 1722
Altoprev Extended-Release Tablets 3109
Mevacor Tablets 2021

Methohexital Sodium (Calcium channel blockers potentiate the depression of cardiac contractility, conductivity, and automaticity as well as vascular dilation associated with anesthetics).
No products indexed under this heading.

Metipranolol Hydrochloride (Concomitant use of diltiazem with beta blockers may result in additive effects on cardiac conduction).
No products indexed under this heading.

Metoprolol Succinate (Concomitant use of diltiazem with beta blockers may result in additive effects on cardiac conduction). Products include:
Toprol-XL Tablets 668

Metoprolol Tartrate (Concomitant use of diltiazem with beta blockers may result in additive effects on cardiac conduction). Products include:
Lopressor Injection 2238
Lopressor Tablets 2238
Lopressor HCT 50/25 Tablets 2241
Lopressor HCT 100/25 Tablets 2241
Lopressor HCT 100/50 Tablets 2241

Midazolam Hydrochloride (Co-administration has resulted in increased AUC of midazolam by 3-4 fold and the Cmax by 2-fold; the elimination half-life of midazolam also increased during co-administration).
No products indexed under this heading.

Nadolol (Concomitant use of diltiazem with beta blockers may result in additive effects on cardiac conduction). Products include:
Nadolol Tablets 2159

Penbutolol Sulfate (Concomitant use of diltiazem with beta blockers may result in additive effects on cardiac conduction).
No products indexed under this heading.

Phenobarbital (Diltiazem is both a substrate and inhibitor of the CYP4503A4; co-administration with inducers of this enzyme system, such as phenobarbital, may have significant impact on the efficacy of diltiazem). Products include:
Donnatal Extentabs 2493

Phenytoin (Diltiazem is both a substrate and inhibitor of the CYP4503A4; co-administration with inducers of this enzyme system, such as phenytoin, may have significant impact on the efficacy of diltiazem).
No products indexed under this heading.

Phenytoin Sodium (Diltiazem is both a substrate and inhibitor of the CYP4503A4; co-administration with inducers of this enzyme system, such as phenytoin, may have significant impact on the efficacy of diltiazem). Products include:
Phenytek Capsules 2160

Pindolol (Concomitant use of diltiazem with beta blockers may result in additive effects on cardiac conduction).
No products indexed under this heading.

Propofol (Calcium channel blockers potentiate the depression of cardiac contractility, conductivity, and automaticity as well as vascular dilation associated with anesthetics).
No products indexed under this heading.

Propranolol Hydrochloride (Concomitant use of diltiazem with propranolol resulted in increased propranolol levels and bioavailability of propanolol was increased by approximately 50%; Concurrent therapy of diltiazem with beta blockers may result in additive effects on cardiac conduction). Products include:
Inderal LA Long-Acting Capsules 3429
InnoPran XL Capsules 2723

Ranitidine Hydrochloride (Co-administration produces smaller, nonsignificant increase in diltiazem plasma levels). Products include:
Zantac 1624
Zantac Injection 1619
Zantac Injection Pharmacy Bulk Package 1622

Remifentanil Hydrochloride (Calcium channel blockers potentiate the depression of cardiac contractility, conductivity, and automaticity as well as vascular dilation associated with anesthetics).
No products indexed under this heading.

Rifampin (Co-administration has resulted in lowered diltiazem plasma concentrations to undetectable levels; co-administration should be avoided).
No products indexed under this heading.

Ritonavir (Diltiazem is both a substrate and inhibitor of the CYP4503A4; co-administration with inhibitors of this enzyme system, such as ritonavir, may have significant impact on the side effect profile of diltiazem). Products include:
Kaletra 476
Norvir 503

Sotalol Hydrochloride (Concomitant use of diltiazem with beta blockers may result in additive effects on cardiac conduction).
No products indexed under this heading.

Sufentanil Citrate (Calcium channel blockers potentiate the depression of cardiac contractility, conductivity, and automaticity as well as vascular dilation associated with anesthetics).
No products indexed under this heading.

Thiamylal Sodium (Calcium channel blockers potentiate the depression of cardiac contractility, conductivity, and automaticity as well as vascular dilation associated with anesthetics).
No products indexed under this heading.

Timolol Hemihydrate (Concomitant use of diltiazem with beta blockers may result in additive effects on cardiac conduction). Products include:
Betimol Ophthalmic Solution 3382
Betimol Ophthalmic Solution ⊙ 295

Timolol Maleate (Concomitant use of diltiazem with beta blockers may result in additive effects on cardiac conduction). Products include:
Blocadren Tablets 1916
Cosopt Sterile Ophthalmic Solution 1931
Timolide Tablets 2086
Timoptic Sterile Ophthalmic Solution 2088
Timoptic in Ocudose 2091
Timoptic-XE Sterile Ophthalmic Gel Forming Solution 2092

Triazolam (Co-administration has resulted in increased AUC of triazolam by 3-4 fold and the Cmax by 2-fold; the elimination half-life of triazolam also increased during co-administration).
No products indexed under this heading.

TICLID TABLETS

(Ticlopidine Hydrochloride) 2810

May interact with antacids, anticoagulants, non-steroidal anti-inflammatory agents, phenytoin, xanthines, and certain other agents. Compounds in these categories include:

Aluminum Carbonate (18% decrease in plasma levels of ticlopidine when administered after antacids).
No products indexed under this heading.

Aluminum Hydroxide (18% decrease in plasma levels of ticlopidine when administered after antacids). Products include:
Gaviscon Regular Strength Liquid ▣ 658
Gaviscon Regular Strength Tablets ▣ 658
Gaviscon Extra Strength Liquid ▣ 658
Gaviscon Extra Strength Tablets ▣ 658
Maalox Regular Strength Antacid/Antigas Liquid 2175
Maalox Max Maximum Strength Antacid/Anti-Gas Liquid 2176

Aminophylline (Co-administration may result in significant increase in the theophylline elimination half-life and a comparable reduction in total plasma clearance of theophylline).
No products indexed under this heading.

Anisindione (The tolerance and safety of co-administration has not been established; anticoagulant should be discontinued prior to Ticlid administration). Products include:
Miradon Tablets 3042

Ardeparin Sodium (The tolerance and safety of co-administration has not been established; anticoagulant should be discontinued prior to Ticlid administration).
No products indexed under this heading.

Aspirin (Ticlopidine potentiates the effect of aspirin on collagen-induced platelet aggregation; concurrent use is not recommended). Products include:
Aggrenox Capsules 822
Bayer Aspirin 744
BC Allergy Sinus Cold Powder ▣ 677
BC Headache Powder ▣ 677
Arthritis Strength BC Powder ▣ 677
BC Sinus Cold Powder ▣ 677
Excedrin Extra Strength Caplets/Tablets/Geltabs ▣ 684
Excedrin Migraine Caplets/Tablets/Geltabs ▣ 609
Goody's Body Pain Formula Powder ▣ 684
Goody's Extra Strength Headache Powders ▣ 611
Goody's Extra Strength Pain Relief Tablets ▣ 685
Percodan Tablets 1132
St. Joseph 81 mg Aspirin Chewable and Enteric Coated Tablets 1869

Celecoxib (Ticlopidine potentiates the effect of NSAIDS on platelet aggregation). Products include:
Celebrex Capsules 3134

Cimetidine (Chronic administration of cimetidine reduces the clearance of a single dose of ticlopidine by 50%). Products include:
Tagamet HB 200 Tablets ▣ 664

Cimetidine Hydrochloride (Chronic administration of cimetidine reduces the clearance of a single dose of ticlopidine by 50%).
No products indexed under this heading.

Dalteparin Sodium (The tolerance and safety of co-administration has not been established; anticoagulant should be discontinued prior to Ticlid administration). Products include:
Fragmin Injection 1097

Danaparoid Sodium (The tolerance and safety of co-administration has not been established; anticoagulant should be discontinued prior to Ticlid administration).
No products indexed under this heading.

Diclofenac Potassium (Ticlopidine potentiates the effect of NSAIDS on platelet aggregation).
No products indexed under this heading.

Diclofenac Sodium (Ticlopidine potentiates the effect of NSAIDS on platelet aggregation). Products include:
Arthrotec Tablets 3129
Voltaren Ophthalmic Solution 2309
Voltaren Tablets 2307
Voltaren-XR Tablets 2310

Dicumarol (The tolerance and safety of co-administration has not been established; anticoagulant should be discontinued prior to Ticlid administration).
No products indexed under this heading.

Digoxin (Co-administration resulted in slight decrease in digoxin plasma levels; little or no change in efficacy of digoxin). Products include:
Lanoxicaps Capsules 1490
Lanoxin Injection 1494
Lanoxin Injection Pediatric 1497
Lanoxin Tablets 1500

Dyphylline (Co-administration may result in significant increase in the theophylline elimination half-life and a comparable reduction in total plasma clearance of theophylline).
No products indexed under this heading.

Enoxaparin Sodium (The tolerance and safety of co-administration has not been established; anticoagulant should be discontinued prior to Ticlid administration). Products include:
Lovenox Injection 2915

Etodolac (Ticlopidine potentiates the effect of NSAIDS on platelet aggregation).
No products indexed under this heading.

Fenoprofen Calcium (Ticlopidine potentiates the effect of NSAIDS on platelet aggregation). Products include:
Nalfon Capsules 2502

Flurbiprofen (Ticlopidine potentiates the effect of NSAIDS on platelet aggregation).
No products indexed under this heading.

Fondaparinux Sodium (The tolerance and safety of co-administration has not been established; anticoagulant should be discontinued prior to Ticlid administration). Products include:
Arixtra Injection 1351

Fosphenytoin Sodium (Co-administration has resulted in several cases of elevated phenytoin plasma levels with associated somnolence and lethargy; caution is advised).
No products indexed under this heading.

Heparin Calcium (The tolerance and safety of co-administration has not been established; anticoagulant should be discontinued prior to Ticlid administration).
No products indexed under this heading.

Heparin Sodium (The tolerance and safety of co-administration has not been established; anticoagulant should be discontinued prior to Ticlid administration).
No products indexed under this heading.

Ibuprofen (Ticlopidine potentiates the effect of NSAIDS on platelet aggregation). Products include:
Advil Allergy Sinus Caplets .... ▣770
Advil .... ▣674
Children's Advil Oral Suspension .... ▣603
Children's Advil Chewable Tablets .. ▣603
Advil Cold & Sinus .... ▣723
Infants' Advil Concentrated Drops .. ▣604
Infants' Advil Concentrated Drops - White Grape (Dye-Free)............. ▣604
Junior Strength Advil Swallow Tablets.. ▣605
Advil Migraine Liquigels .... ▣608
Advil Multi-Symptom Cold Caplets... ▣770
Advil PM Caplets .... ▣615
Motrin IB Tablets and Caplets 1866
Children's Motrin Oral Suspension ... 1867
Children's Motrin Non-Staining Dye-Free Oral Suspension............ 1867
Children's Motrin Cold Oral Suspension 1867
Infants' Motrin Concentrated Drops... 1867
Infants' Motrin Non-Staining Dye-Free Concentrated Drops....... 1867
Junior Strength Motrin Caplets and Chewable Tablets.................. 1867
Vicoprofen Tablets 539

Indomethacin (Ticlopidine potentiates the effect of NSAIDS on platelet aggregation). Products include:
Indocin 1995

Indomethacin Sodium Trihydrate (Ticlopidine potentiates the effect of NSAIDS on platelet aggregation). Products include:
Indocin I.V. 2465

Ketoprofen (Ticlopidine potentiates the effect of NSAIDS on platelet aggregation).
No products indexed under this heading.

Ketorolac Tromethamine (Ticlopidine potentiates the effect of NSAIDS on platelet aggregation). Products include:
Acular Ophthalmic Solution 565
Acular LS Ophthalmic Solution 566

Low Molecular Weight Heparins (The tolerance and safety of co-administration has not been established; anticoagulant should be discontinued prior to Ticlid administration).
No products indexed under this heading.

Magaldrate (18% decrease in plasma levels of ticlopidine when administered after antacids).
No products indexed under this heading.

Magnesium Hydroxide (18% decrease in plasma levels of ticlopidine when administered after antacids). Products include:
Maalox Regular Strength Antacid/Antigas Liquid................. 2175
Maalox Max Maximum Strength Antacid/Anti-Gas Liquid................ 2176
Pepcid Complete Chewable Tablets.. 1701

Magnesium Oxide (18% decrease in plasma levels of ticlopidine when administered after antacids). Products include:
Beelith Tablets 759
PremCal Light, Regular, and Extra Strength Tablets................ ▣818

Meclofenamate Sodium (Ticlopidine potentiates the effect of NSAIDS on platelet aggregation).
No products indexed under this heading.

Mefenamic Acid (Ticlopidine potentiates the effect of NSAIDS on platelet aggregation).
No products indexed under this heading.

Meloxicam (Ticlopidine potentiates the effect of NSAIDS on platelet aggregation). Products include:
Mobic Oral Suspension 863
Mobic Tablets 863

Nabumetone (Ticlopidine potentiates the effect of NSAIDS on platelet aggregation).
No products indexed under this heading.

Naproxen (Ticlopidine potentiates the effect of NSAIDS on platelet aggregation). Products include:
EC-Naprosyn Delayed-Release Tablets.. 2761
Naprosyn Suspension 2761
Naprosyn Tablets 2761
Prevacid NapraPAC 3280

Naproxen Sodium (Ticlopidine potentiates the effect of NSAIDS on platelet aggregation). Products include:
Aleve Caplets 742
Aleve Gelcaps 743
Aleve Tablets 743
Aleve Cold & Sinus Caplets 744
Anaprox Tablets 2761
Anaprox DS Tablets 2761

Oxaprozin (Ticlopidine potentiates the effect of NSAIDS on platelet aggregation).
No products indexed under this heading.

Phenylbutazone (Ticlopidine potentiates the effect of NSAIDS on platelet aggregation).
No products indexed under this heading.

Phenytoin (Co-administration has resulted in several cases of elevated phenytoin plasma levels with associated somnolence and lethargy; caution is advised).
No products indexed under this heading.

Phenytoin Sodium (Co-administration has resulted in several cases of elevated phenytoin plasma levels with associated somnolence and lethargy; caution is advised). Products include:
Phenytek Capsules 2160

Piroxicam (Ticlopidine potentiates the effect of NSAIDS on platelet aggregation).
No products indexed under this heading.

Propranolol Hydrochloride (Exercise caution if co-administered; *in vitro* studies indicate no alteration of plasma protein binding of propranolol). Products include:
Inderal LA Long-Acting Capsules 3429
InnoPran XL Capsules 2723

Rofecoxib (Ticlopidine potentiates the effect of NSAIDS on platelet aggregation).
No products indexed under this heading.

Sodium Bicarbonate (18% decrease in plasma levels of ticlopidine when administered after antacids). Products include:
Colyte with Flavor Packs for Oral Solution.. 3088
HalfLytely and Bisacodyl Tablets Bowel Prep Kit with Flavors Packs... 881
TriLyte with Flavor Packs for Oral Solution.. 3100

Sulindac (Ticlopidine potentiates the effect of NSAIDS on platelet aggregation). Products include:
Clinoril Tablets 1924

Theophylline (Co-administration may result in significant increase in the theophylline elimination half-life and a comparable reduction in total plasma clearance of theophylline).
No products indexed under this heading.

Theophylline Anhydrous (Co-administration may result in significant increase in the theophylline elimination half-life and a comparable reduction in total plasma clearance of theophylline). Products include:
Uniphyl Tablets 2710

Theophylline Calcium Salicylate (Co-administration may result in significant increase in the theophylline elimination half-life and a comparable reduction in total plasma clearance of theophylline).
No products indexed under this heading.

Theophylline Dihydroxypropyl (Glyceryl) (Co-administration may result in significant increase in the theophylline elimination half-life and a comparable reduction in total plasma clearance of theophylline).
No products indexed under this heading.

Theophylline Ethylenediamine (Co-administration may result in significant increase in the theophylline elimination half-life and a comparable reduction in total plasma clearance of theophylline).
No products indexed under this heading.

Theophylline Sodium Glycinate (Co-administration may result in significant increase in the theophylline elimination half-life and a comparable reduction in total plasma clearance of theophylline).
No products indexed under this heading.

Tinzaparin Sodium (The tolerance and safety of co-administration has not been established; anticoagulant should be discontinued prior to Ticlid administration).
No products indexed under this heading.

Tolmetin Sodium (Ticlopidine potentiates the effect of NSAIDS on platelet aggregation).
No products indexed under this heading.

Valdecoxib (Ticlopidine potentiates the effect of NSAIDS on platelet aggregation).
No products indexed under this heading.

Warfarin Sodium (The tolerance and safety of co-administration has not been established; anticoagulant should be discontinued prior to Ticlid administration). Products include:
Coumadin for Injection 898
Coumadin Tablets 898

Food Interactions

Meal, unspecified (Administration after meals results in a 20% increase in the AUC of ticlopidine).

TIMENTIN ADD-VANTAGE

(Clavulanate Potassium, Ticarcillin Disodium)... 1580
See Timentin IV Infusion

TIMENTIN INJECTION GALAXY CONTAINER

(Clavulanate Potassium, Ticarcillin Disodium)... 1583
See Timentin IV Infusion

TIMENTIN IV INFUSION

(Clavulanate Potassium, Ticarcillin Disodium)... 1577
May interact with aminoglycosides and certain other agents. Compounds in these categories include:

Amikacin Sulfate (The mixing of Timentin with an aminoglycoside in solutions for parental administration can result in substantial inactivation of the aminoglycoside).
No products indexed under this heading.

Gentamicin Sulfate (The mixing of Timentin with an aminoglycoside in solutions for parental administration can result in substantial inactivation of the aminoglycoside). Products include:
Garamycin Injectable 3014
Pred-G Ophthalmic Ointment .... ⊙237
Pred-G Ophthalmic Suspension ...... ⊙236

Kanamycin Sulfate (The mixing of Timentin with an aminoglycoside in solutions for parental administration can result in substantial inactivation of the aminoglycoside).
No products indexed under this heading.

Probenecid (Interferes with the renal tubular secretion of ticarcillin, thereby increasing serum concentrations and prolonged serum half-life of the antibiotic).
No products indexed under this heading.

Streptomycin Sulfate (The mixing of Timentin with an aminoglycoside in solutions for parental administration can result in substantial inactivation of the aminoglycoside).
No products indexed under this heading.

Tobramycin (The mixing of Timentin with an aminoglycoside in solutions for parental administration can result in substantial inactivation of the aminoglycoside). Products include:

TOBI Solution for Inhalation 2298
TobraDex Ophthalmic Ointment 562
TobraDex Ophthalmic Suspension ... 563
Zylet Ophthalmic Suspension .... ⊙259

Tobramycin Sulfate (The mixing of Timentin with an aminoglycoside in solutions for parental administration can result in substantial inactivation of the aminoglycoside).

No products indexed under this heading.

TIMENTIN PHARMACY BULK PACKAGE

(Clavulanate Potassium, Ticarcillin Disodium).. 1586

See Timentin IV Infusion

TIMOLIDE TABLETS

(Hydrochlorothiazide, Timolol Maleate)... 2086

May interact with antihypertensives, catecholamine depleting drugs, calcium channel blockers, cardiac glycosides, oral hypoglycemic agents, insulin, lithium preparations, non-steroidal anti-inflammatory agents, quinidine, and certain other agents. Compounds in these categories include:

Acarbose (Beta-blockers may mask the signs and symptoms of hypoglycemia). Products include:

Precose Tablets 751

Acebutolol Hydrochloride (Timolide may potentiate the action of other antihypertensive agents used concomitantly).

No products indexed under this heading.

Amlodipine Besylate (Hypotension, AV conduction disturbances, and left ventricular failure have been reported in some patients receiving beta-adrenergic blocking agents when an oral calcium antagonist was added to the treatment regimen). Products include:

Caduet Tablets 2508
Lotrel Capsules 2249
Norvasc Tablets 2545

Atenolol (Timolide may potentiate the action of other antihypertensive agents used concomitantly).

No products indexed under this heading.

Benazepril Hydrochloride (Timolide may potentiate the action of other antihypertensive agents used concomitantly). Products include:

Lotensin Tablets 2243
Lotensin HCT Tablets 2246
Lotrel Capsules 2249

Bendroflumethiazide (Timolide may potentiate the action of other antihypertensive agents used concomitantly).

No products indexed under this heading.

Bepridil Hydrochloride (Hypotension, AV conduction disturbances, and left ventricular failure have been reported in some patients receiving beta-adrenergic blocking agents when an oral calcium antagonist was added to the treatment regimen).

No products indexed under this heading.

Betaxolol Hydrochloride (Timolide may potentiate the action of other antihypertensive agents used concomitantly). Products include:

Betoptic S Ophthalmic Suspension.................................. 558

Bisoprolol Fumarate (Timolide may potentiate the action of other antihypertensive agents used concomitantly).

No products indexed under this heading.

Candesartan Cilexetil (Timolide may potentiate the action of other antihypertensive agents used concomitantly). Products include:

Atacand Tablets 649
Atacand HCT 651

Captopril (Timolide may potentiate the action of other antihypertensive agents used concomitantly). Products include:

Captopril Tablets 2149

Carteolol Hydrochloride (Timolide may potentiate the action of other antihypertensive agents used concomitantly). Products include:

Carteolol Hydrochloride Ophthalmic Solution USP, 1%....... ⊙249

Celecoxib (NSAIDs reduce the diuretic, natriuretic, and antihypertensive effects of Timolide). Products include:

Celebrex Capsules 3134

Chlorothiazide (Timolide may potentiate the action of other antihypertensive agents used concomitantly). Products include:

Diuril Oral Suspension 1954

Chlorothiazide Sodium (Timolide may potentiate the action of other antihypertensive agents used concomitantly). Products include:

Diuril Sodium Intravenous 2467

Chlorpropamide (Beta-blockers may mask the signs and symptoms of hypoglycemia).

No products indexed under this heading.

Chlorthalidone (Timolide may potentiate the action of other antihypertensive agents used concomitantly). Products include:

Clorpres Tablets 2153

Cholestyramine (Cholestyramine resin has potential of binding hydrochlorothiazide and reducing its absorption from the GI tract by up to 85%).

No products indexed under this heading.

Clonidine (Beta adrenergic blocking agents may exacerbate the rebound hypertension which can follow the withdrawal of clonidine). Products include:

Catapres-TTS 844

Clonidine Hydrochloride (Beta adrenergic blocking agents may exacerbate the rebound hypertension which can follow the withdrawal of clonidine). Products include:

Catapres Tablets 843
Clorpres Tablets 2153

Colestipol Hydrochloride (Colestipol resin has potential of binding hydrochlorothiazide and reducing its absorption from the GI tract by up to 43%).

No products indexed under this heading.

Deserpidine (Close observation of the patient is recommended when Timolide is administered to patients receiving catecholamine-depleting drugs such as reserpine, because of possible additive effects and the production of hypotension and/or marked bradycardia, which may produce vertigo, syncope, or postural hypotension).

No products indexed under this heading.

Deslanoside (The concomitant use of beta-adrenergic blocking agents with digitalis and either diltiazem or verapamil may have additive effects in prolonging AV conduction time. Hypokalemia may develop during thiazide therapy and may cause cardiac arrhythmia and may also sensitize or exaggerate the response of the heart to the toxic effects of digitalis (e.g., increased ventricular irritability)).

No products indexed under this heading.

Diazoxide (Timolide may potentiate the action of other antihypertensive agents used concomitantly). Products include:

Hyperstat I.V. 3017

Diclofenac Potassium (NSAIDs reduce the diuretic, natriuretic, and antihypertensive effects of Timolide).

No products indexed under this heading.

Diclofenac Sodium (NSAIDs reduce the diuretic, natriuretic, and antihypertensive effects of Timolide). Products include:

Arthrotec Tablets 3129
Voltaren Ophthalmic Solution 2309
Voltaren Tablets 2307
Voltaren-XR Tablets 2310

Digitalis Glycoside Preparations (The concomitant use of beta-adrenergic blocking agents with digitalis and either diltiazem or verapamil may have additive effects in prolonging AV conduction time. Hypokalemia may develop during thiazide therapy and may cause cardiac arrhythmia and may also sensitize or exaggerate the response of the heart to the toxic effects of digitalis (e.g., increased ventricular irritability)).

No products indexed under this heading.

Digitoxin (The concomitant use of beta-adrenergic blocking agents with digitalis and either diltiazem or verapamil may have additive effects in prolonging AV conduction time. Hypokalemia may develop during thiazide therapy and may cause cardiac arrhythmia and may also sensitize or exaggerate the response of the heart to the toxic effects of digitalis (e.g., increased ventricular irritability)).

No products indexed under this heading.

Digoxin (The concomitant use of beta-adrenergic blocking agents with digitalis and either diltiazem or verapamil may have additive effects in prolonging AV conduction time. Hypokalemia may develop during thiazide therapy and may cause cardiac arrhythmia and may also sensitize or exaggerate the response of the heart to the toxic effects of digitalis (e.g., increased ventricular irritability)). Products include:

Lanoxicaps Capsules 1490
Lanoxin Injection 1494
Lanoxin Injection Pediatric 1497
Lanoxin Tablets 1500

Diltiazem Hydrochloride (Left ventricular failure and AV conduction disturbances). Products include:

Cardizem LA Extended Release Tablets 1728
Tiazac Capsules 1201

Doxazosin Mesylate (Timolide may potentiate the action of other antihypertensive agents used concomitantly). Products include:

Cardura XL Tablets 2515

Enalapril Maleate (Timolide may potentiate the action of other antihypertensive agents used concomitantly). Products include:

Vasotec I.V. Injection 2103

Enalaprilat (Timolide may potentiate the action of other antihypertensive agents used concomitantly).

No products indexed under this heading.

Eprosartan Mesylate (Timolide may potentiate the action of other antihypertensive agents used concomitantly). Products include:

Teveten Tablets 1735
Teveten HCT Tablets 1737

Esmolol Hydrochloride (Timolide may potentiate the action of other antihypertensive agents used concomitantly).

No products indexed under this heading.

Etodolac (NSAIDs reduce the diuretic, natriuretic, and antihypertensive effects of Timolide).

No products indexed under this heading.

Felodipine (Hypotension, AV conduction disturbances, and left ventricular failure have been reported in some patients receiving beta-adrenergic blocking agents when an oral calcium antagonist was added to the treatment regimen).

No products indexed under this heading.

Fenoprofen Calcium (NSAIDs reduce the diuretic, natriuretic, and antihypertensive effects of Timolide). Products include:

Nalfon Capsules 2502

Flurbiprofen (NSAIDs reduce the diuretic, natriuretic, and antihypertensive effects of Timolide).

No products indexed under this heading.

Fosinopril Sodium (Timolide may potentiate the action of other antihypertensive agents used concomitantly).

No products indexed under this heading.

Furosemide (Timolide may potentiate the action of other antihypertensive agents used concomitantly). Products include:

Furosemide Tablets 2154

Glimepiride (Beta-blockers may mask the signs and symptoms of hypoglycemia). Products include:

Avandaryl Tablets 1379
Duetact Tablets 3226

Glipizide (Beta-blockers may mask the signs and symptoms of hypoglycemia).

No products indexed under this heading.

Glyburide (Beta-blockers may mask the signs and symptoms of hypoglycemia).

No products indexed under this heading.

Guanabenz Acetate (Timolide may potentiate the action of other antihypertensive agents used concomitantly).
No products indexed under this heading.

Guanethidine Monosulfate (Close observation of the patient is recommended when Timolide is administered to patients receiving catecholamine-depleting drugs such as reserpine, because of possible additive effects and the production of hypotension and/or marked bradycardia, which may produce vertigo, syncope, or postural hypotension).
No products indexed under this heading.

Hydralazine Hydrochloride (Timolide may potentiate the action of other antihypertensive agents used concomitantly). Products include:
BiDil Tablets 2171

Hydroflumethiazide (Timolide may potentiate the action of other antihypertensive agents used concomitantly).
No products indexed under this heading.

Ibuprofen (NSAIDs reduce the diuretic, natriuretic, and antihypertensive effects of Timolide). Products include:
Advil Allergy Sinus Caplets .... ▣770
Advil .... ▣674
Children's Advil Oral Suspension .... ▣603
Children's Advil Chewable Tablets .. ▣603
Advil Cold & Sinus .... ▣723
Infants' Advil Concentrated Drops .. ▣604
Infants' Advil Concentrated Drops - White Grape (Dye-Free)............. ▣604
Junior Strength Advil Swallow Tablets... ▣605
Advil Migraine Liquigels .... ▣608
Advil Multi-Symptom Cold Caplets.. ▣770
Advil PM Caplets .... ▣615
Motrin IB Tablets and Caplets 1866
Children's Motrin Oral Suspension ... 1867
Children's Motrin Non-Staining Dye-Free Oral Suspension............ 1867
Children's Motrin Cold Oral Suspension 1867
Infants' Motrin Concentrated Drops.. 1867
Infants' Motrin Non-Staining Dye-Free Concentrated Drops...... 1867
Junior Strength Motrin Caplets and Chewable Tablets.................. 1867
Vicoprofen Tablets 539

Indapamide (Timolide may potentiate the action of other antihypertensive agents used concomitantly). Products include:
Indapamide Tablets 2156

Indomethacin (NSAIDs reduce the diuretic, natriuretic, and antihypertensive effects of Timolide). Products include:
Indocin 1995

Indomethacin Sodium Trihydrate (NSAIDs reduce the diuretic, natriuretic, and antihypertensive effects of Timolide). Products include:
Indocin I.V. 2465

Insulin, Human, Zinc Suspension (Beta-blockers may mask the signs and symptoms of acute hypoglycemia. Insulin requirements may be altered). Products include:
Humulin L, 100 Units 1794
Humulin U, 100 Units 1800

Insulin, Human NPH (Beta-blockers may mask the signs and symptoms of acute hypoglycemia. Insulin requirements may be altered). Products include:
Humulin N, 100 Units 1795
Humulin N Pen 1797

Insulin, Human Regular (Beta-blockers may mask the signs and symptoms of acute hypoglycemia. Insulin requirements may be altered). Products include:
Humulin R, 100 Units 1798

Insulin, Human Regular and Human NPH Mixture (Beta-blockers may mask the signs and symptoms of acute hypoglycemia. Insulin requirements may be altered). Products include:
Humulin 50/50, 100 Units 1791
Humulin 70/30 Pen 1793

Insulin, NPH (Beta-blockers may mask the signs and symptoms of acute hypoglycemia. Insulin requirements may be altered.).
No products indexed under this heading.

Insulin, Regular (Beta-blockers may mask the signs and symptoms of acute hypoglycemia. Insulin requirements may be altered.).
No products indexed under this heading.

Insulin, Zinc Crystals (Beta-blockers may mask the signs and symptoms of acute hypoglycemia. Insulin requirements may be altered.).
No products indexed under this heading.

Insulin, Zinc Suspension (Beta-blockers may mask the signs and symptoms of acute hypoglycemia. Insulin requirements may be altered.).
No products indexed under this heading.

Insulin Aspart, Human Regular (Beta-blockers may mask the signs and symptoms of acute hypoglycemia. Insulin requirements may be altered). Products include:
NovoLog Injection 2326

Insulin glargine (Beta-blockers may mask the signs and symptoms of acute hypoglycemia. Insulin requirements may be altered). Products include:
Lantus Injection 2909

Insulin Lispro, Human (Beta-blockers may mask the signs and symptoms of acute hypoglycemia. Insulin requirements may be altered). Products include:
Humalog-Pen 1781
Humalog Mix 50/50-Pen 1783
Humalog Mix 75/25-Pen 1785

Insulin Lispro Protamine, Human (Beta-blockers may mask the signs and symptoms of acute hypoglycemia. Insulin requirements may be altered). Products include:
Humalog Mix 50/50-Pen 1783
Humalog Mix 75/25-Pen 1785

Irbesartan (Timolide may potentiate the action of other antihypertensive agents used concomitantly). Products include:
Avalide Tablets 888
Avalide Tablets 2874
Avapro Tablets 891
Avapro Tablets 2871

Isradipine (Hypotension, AV conduction disturbances, and left ventricular failure have been reported in some patients receiving beta-adrenergic blocking agents when an oral calcium antagonist was added to the treatment regimen). Products include:
DynaCirc CR Tablets 2721

Ketoprofen (NSAIDs reduce the diuretic, natriuretic, and antihypertensive effects of Timolide).
No products indexed under this heading.

Ketorolac Tromethamine (NSAIDs reduce the diuretic, natriuretic, and antihypertensive effects of Timolide). Products include:
Acular Ophthalmic Solution 565
Acular LS Ophthalmic Solution 566

Labetalol Hydrochloride (Timolide may potentiate the action of other antihypertensive agents used concomitantly).
No products indexed under this heading.

Lisinopril (Timolide may potentiate the action of other antihypertensive agents used concomitantly). Products include:
Prinivil Tablets 2052
Prinzide Tablets 2056

Lithium (Lithium generally should not be given with diuretics because they reduce its renal clearance and add a high risk of lithium toxicity).
No products indexed under this heading.

Lithium Carbonate (Lithium generally should not be given with diuretics because they reduce its renal clearance and add a high risk of lithium toxicity). Products include:
Lithobid Tablets 1692

Lithium Citrate (Lithium generally should not be given with diuretics because they reduce its renal clearance and add a high risk of lithium toxicity).
No products indexed under this heading.

Losartan Potassium (Timolide may potentiate the action of other antihypertensive agents used concomitantly). Products include:
Cozaar Tablets 1935
Hyzaar 50-12.5 Tablets 1990
Hyzaar 100-12.5 Tablets 1990
Hyzaar 100-25 Tablets 1990

Mecamylamine Hydrochloride (Timolide may potentiate the action of other antihypertensive agents used concomitantly).
No products indexed under this heading.

Meclofenamate Sodium (NSAIDs reduce the diuretic, natriuretic, and antihypertensive effects of Timolide).
No products indexed under this heading.

Mefenamic Acid (NSAIDs reduce the diuretic, natriuretic, and antihypertensive effects of Timolide).
No products indexed under this heading.

Meloxicam (NSAIDs reduce the diuretic, natriuretic, and antihypertensive effects of Timolide). Products include:
Mobic Oral Suspension 863
Mobic Tablets 863

Metformin Hydrochloride (Beta-blockers may mask the signs and symptoms of hypoglycemia). Products include:
ActoPlus Met Tablets 3214
Avandamet Tablets 1373
Fortamet Extended-Release Tablets 3115

Methyclothiazide (Timolide may potentiate the action of other antihypertensive agents used concomitantly).
No products indexed under this heading.

Methyldopa (Timolide may potentiate the action of other antihypertensive agents used concomitantly). Products include:
Aldoril Tablets 1910

Methyldopate Hydrochloride (Timolide may potentiate the action of other antihypertensive agents used concomitantly).
No products indexed under this heading.

Metolazone (Timolide may potentiate the action of other antihypertensive agents used concomitantly).
No products indexed under this heading.

Metoprolol Succinate (Timolide may potentiate the action of other antihypertensive agents used concomitantly). Products include:
Toprol-XL Tablets 668

Metoprolol Tartrate (Timolide may potentiate the action of other antihypertensive agents used concomitantly). Products include:
Lopressor Injection 2238
Lopressor Tablets 2238
Lopressor HCT 50/25 Tablets 2241
Lopressor HCT 100/25 Tablets 2241
Lopressor HCT 100/50 Tablets 2241

Metyrosine (Timolide may potentiate the action of other antihypertensive agents used concomitantly). Products include:
Demser Capsules 1953

Mibefradil Dihydrochloride (Hypotension, AV conduction disturbances, and left ventricular failure have been reported in some patients receiving beta-adrenergic blocking agents when an oral calcium antagonist was added to the treatment regimen).
No products indexed under this heading.

Miglitol (Beta-blockers may mask the signs and symptoms of hypoglycemia).
No products indexed under this heading.

Minoxidil (Timolide may potentiate the action of other antihypertensive agents used concomitantly). Products include:
Men's Rogaine Extra Strength Hair Regrowth Treatment Topical Solution, Ocean Rush Scent and Original Unscented ..... ▣633
Men's Rogaine Foam Hair Regrowth Treatment.................... ▣633
Women's Rogaine Hair Regrowth Treatment Topical Solution, Spring Bloom Scent and Original Unscented...................... ▣634

Moexipril Hydrochloride (Timolide may potentiate the action of other antihypertensive agents used concomitantly). Products include:
Uniretic Tablets 3100
Univasc Tablets 3104

Nabumetone (NSAIDs reduce the diuretic, natriuretic, and antihypertensive effects of Timolide).
No products indexed under this heading.

Nadolol (Timolide may potentiate the action of other antihypertensive agents used concomitantly). Products include:
Nadolol Tablets 2159

TIMOPTIC STERILE OPHTHALMIC SOLUTION
See Timoptic in Ocudose

TIMOPTIC IN OCUDOSE
May interact with beta blockers, catecholamine depleting drugs, calcium channel blockers, cardiac glycosides, oral hypoglycemic agents, insulin, quinidine, and certain other agents. Compounds in these categories include:

IMPORTANT NOTE: Always consult each drug listing in the patient's regimen for possible interactions.

Acebutolol Hydrochloride (Concurrent use with systemic beta blocker may have additive effects of beta blockade, both systemic and on intraocular pressure).
No products indexed under this heading.

Amlodipine Besylate (Possible atrioventricular conduction disturbances, left ventricular failure, or hypotension when used concurrently). Products include:
- Caduet Tablets 2508
- Lotrel Capsules 2249
- Norvasc Tablets 2545

Atenolol (Concurrent use with systemic beta blocker may have additive effects of beta blockade, both systemic and on intraocular pressure).
No products indexed under this heading.

Bepridil Hydrochloride (Possible atrioventricular conduction disturbances, left ventricular failure, or hypotension when used concurrently).
No products indexed under this heading.

Betaxolol Hydrochloride (Concurrent use with systemic beta blocker may have additive effects of beta blockade, both systemic and on intraocular pressure; concurrent use of two topical beta blockers is not recommended). Products include:
- Betoptic S Ophthalmic Suspension 558

Bisoprolol Fumarate (Concurrent use with systemic beta blocker may have additive effects of beta blockade, both systemic and on intraocular pressure).
No products indexed under this heading.

Carteolol Hydrochloride (Concurrent use with systemic beta blocker may have additive effects of beta blockade, both systemic and on intraocular pressure; concurrent use of two topical beta blockers is not recommended). Products include:
- Carteolol Hydrochloride Ophthalmic Solution USP, 1% .... ⊙ 249

Chlorpropamide (Beta blocking agents, usually systemic, may mask the sign and symptoms of acute hypoglycemia).
No products indexed under this heading.

Clonidine (Oral beta-adrenergic blocking agents may exacerbate the rebound hypertension which can follow the withdrawal of clonidine; there have been no reports of exacerbation of rebound hypertension with ophthalmic timolol). Products include:
- Catapres-TTS 844

Clonidine Hydrochloride (Oral beta-adrenergic blocking agents may exacerbate the rebound hypertension which can follow the withdrawal of clonidine; there have been no reports of exacerbation of rebound hypertension with ophthalmic timolol). Products include:
- Catapres Tablets 843
- Clorpres Tablets 2153

Deserpidine (Possible additive effects and the production of hypotension and/or bradycardia).
No products indexed under this heading.

Deslanoside (Co-administration with digitalis and calcium antagonists may have additive effects in prolonging atrioventricular conduction time).
No products indexed under this heading.

Digitalis Glycoside Preparations (Co-administration with digitalis and calcium antagonists may have additive effects in prolonging atrioventricular conduction time).
No products indexed under this heading.

Digitoxin (Co-administration with digitalis and calcium antagonists may have additive effects in prolonging atrioventricular conduction time).
No products indexed under this heading.

Digoxin (Co-administration with digitalis and calcium antagonists may have additive effects in prolonging atrioventricular conduction time). Products include:
- Lanoxicaps Capsules 1490
- Lanoxin Injection 1494
- Lanoxin Injection Pediatric 1497
- Lanoxin Tablets 1500

Diltiazem Hydrochloride (Possible atrioventricular conduction disturbances, left ventricular failure, or hypotension when used concurrently). Products include:
- Cardizem LA Extended Release Tablets 1728
- Tiazac Capsules 1201

Epinephrine (Patients with a history of atopy or anaphylactic reactions to a variety of allergens may be unresponsive to the usual dose of injectable epinephrine used to treat allergic reactions). Products include:
- EpiPen 1061
- Primatene Mist .... ■ 719
- Twinject 0.15 3379
- Twinject 0.3 3378

Epinephrine Bitartrate (Patients with a history of atopy or anaphylactic reactions to a variety of allergens may be unresponsive to the usual dose of injectable epinephrine used to treat allergic reactions).
No products indexed under this heading.

Esmolol Hydrochloride (Concurrent use with systemic beta blocker may have additive effects of beta blockade, both systemic and on intraocular pressure).
No products indexed under this heading.

Felodipine (Possible atrioventricular conduction disturbances, left ventricular failure, or hypotension when used concurrently).
No products indexed under this heading.

Glimepiride (Beta blocking agents, usually systemic, may mask the sign and symptoms of acute hypoglycemia). Products include:
- Avandaryl Tablets 1379
- Duetact Tablets 3226

Glipizide (Beta blocking agents, usually systemic, may mask the sign and symptoms of acute hypoglycemia).
No products indexed under this heading.

Glyburide (Beta blocking agents, usually systemic, may mask the sign and symptoms of acute hypoglycemia).
No products indexed under this heading.

Guanethidine Monosulfate (Possible additive effects and the production of hypotension and/or bradycardia).
No products indexed under this heading.

Insulin, Human, Zinc Suspension (Beta blocking agents, usually systemic, may mask the sign and symptoms of acute hypoglycemia). Products include:
- Humulin L, 100 Units 1794
- Humulin U, 100 Units 1800

Insulin, Human NPH (Beta blocking agents, usually systemic, may mask the sign and symptoms of acute hypoglycemia). Products include:
- Humulin N, 100 Units 1795
- Humulin N Pen 1797

Insulin, Human Regular (Beta blocking agents, usually systemic, may mask the sign and symptoms of acute hypoglycemia). Products include:
- Humulin R, 100 Units 1798

Insulin, Human Regular and Human NPH Mixture (Beta blocking agents, usually systemic, may mask the sign and symptoms of acute hypoglycemia). Products include:
- Humulin 50/50, 100 Units 1791
- Humulin 70/30 Pen 1793

Insulin, NPH (Beta blocking agents, usually systemic, may mask the sign and symptoms of acute hypoglycemia).
No products indexed under this heading.

Insulin, Regular (Beta blocking agents, usually systemic, may mask the sign and symptoms of acute hypoglycemia).
No products indexed under this heading.

Insulin, Zinc Crystals (Beta blocking agents, usually systemic, may mask the sign and symptoms of acute hypoglycemia).
No products indexed under this heading.

Insulin, Zinc Suspension (Beta blocking agents, usually systemic, may mask the sign and symptoms of acute hypoglycemia).
No products indexed under this heading.

Insulin Aspart, Human Regular (Beta blocking agents, usually systemic, may mask the sign and symptoms of acute hypoglycemia). Products include:
- NovoLog Injection 2326

Insulin glargine (Beta blocking agents, usually systemic, may mask the sign and symptoms of acute hypoglycemia). Products include:
- Lantus Injection 2909

Insulin Lispro, Human (Beta blocking agents, usually systemic, may mask the sign and symptoms of acute hypoglycemia). Products include:
- Humalog-Pen 1781
- Humalog Mix 50/50-Pen 1783
- Humalog Mix 75/25-Pen 1785

Insulin Lispro Protamine, Human (Beta blocking agents, usually systemic, may mask the sign and symptoms of acute hypoglycemia). Products include:
- Humalog Mix 50/50-Pen 1783
- Humalog Mix 75/25-Pen 1785

Isradipine (Possible atrioventricular conduction disturbances, left ventricular failure, or hypotension when used concurrently). Products include:
- DynaCirc CR Tablets 2721

Labetalol Hydrochloride (Concurrent use with systemic beta blocker may have additive effects of beta blockade, both systemic and on intraocular pressure).
No products indexed under this heading.

Levobunolol Hydrochloride (Concurrent use of two topical beta blockers is not recommended). Products include:
- Betagan Ophthalmic Solution, USP .... ⊙ 220

Metformin Hydrochloride (Beta blocking agents, usually systemic, may mask the sign and symptoms of acute hypoglycemia). Products include:
- ActoPlus Met Tablets 3214
- Avandamet Tablets 1373
- Fortamet Extended-Release Tablets 3115

Metipranolol Hydrochloride (Concurrent use of two topical beta blockers is not recommended).
No products indexed under this heading.

Metoprolol Succinate (Concurrent use with systemic beta blocker may have additive effects of beta blockade, both systemic and on intraocular pressure). Products include:
- Toprol-XL Tablets 668

Metoprolol Tartrate (Concurrent use with systemic beta blocker may have additive effects of beta blockade, both systemic and on intraocular pressure). Products include:
- Lopressor Injection 2238
- Lopressor Tablets 2238
- Lopressor HCT 50/25 Tablets 2241
- Lopressor HCT 100/25 Tablets 2241
- Lopressor HCT 100/50 Tablets 2241

Mibefradil Dihydrochloride (Possible atrioventricular conduction disturbances, left ventricular failure, or hypotension when used concurrently).
No products indexed under this heading.

Miglitol (Beta blocking agents, usually systemic, may mask the sign and symptoms of acute hypoglycemia).
No products indexed under this heading.

Nadolol (Concurrent use with systemic beta blocker may have additive effects of beta blockade, both systemic and on intraocular pressure). Products include:
- Nadolol Tablets 2159

Nicardipine Hydrochloride (Possible atrioventricular conduction disturbances, left ventricular failure, or hypotension when used concurrently). Products include:
- Cardene I.V. 2497

Nifedipine (Possible atrioventricular conduction disturbances, left ventricular failure, or hypotension when used concurrently). Products include:
- Adalat CC Tablets 2964

Nimodipine (Possible atrioventricular conduction disturbances, left ventricular failure, or hypotension when used concurrently). Products include:
- Nimotop Capsules 749

Nisoldipine (Possible atrioventricular conduction disturbances, left ven-

tricular failure, or hypotension when used concurrently). Products include:
Sular Tablets 3122

Penbutolol Sulfate (Concurrent use with systemic beta blocker may have additive effects of beta blockade, both systemic and on intraocular pressure).
No products indexed under this heading.

Pindolol (Concurrent use with systemic beta blocker may have additive effects of beta blockade, both systemic and on intraocular pressure).
No products indexed under this heading.

Pioglitazone Hydrochloride (Beta blocking agents, usually systemic, may mask the sign and symptoms of acute hypoglycemia). Products include:
ActoPlus Met Tablets 3214
Actos Tablets 3219
Duetact Tablets 3226

Propranolol Hydrochloride (Concurrent use with systemic beta blocker may have additive effects of beta blockade, both systemic and on intraocular pressure). Products include:
Inderal LA Long-Acting Capsules 3429
InnoPran XL Capsules 2723

Quinidine (Co-administration has resulted in potentiated systemic beta-blockade, e.g., decreased heart rate).
No products indexed under this heading.

Quinidine Gluconate (Co-administration has resulted in potentiated systemic beta-blockade, e.g., decreased heart rate).
No products indexed under this heading.

Quinidine Hydrochloride (Co-administration has resulted in potentiated systemic beta-blockade, e.g., decreased heart rate).
No products indexed under this heading.

Quinidine Polygalacturonate (Co-administration has resulted in potentiated systemic beta-blockade, e.g., decreased heart rate).
No products indexed under this heading.

Quinidine Sulfate (Co-administration has resulted in potentiated systemic beta-blockade, e.g., decreased heart rate).
No products indexed under this heading.

Rauwolfia Serpentina (Possible additive effects and the production of hypotension and/or bradycardia).
No products indexed under this heading.

Repaglinide (Beta blocking agents, usually systemic, may mask the sign and symptoms of acute hypoglycemia).
No products indexed under this heading.

Rescinnamine (Possible additive effects and the production of hypotension and/or bradycardia).
No products indexed under this heading.

Reserpine (Possible additive effects and the production of hypotension and/or bradycardia).
No products indexed under this heading.

Rosiglitazone Maleate (Beta blocking agents, usually systemic, may mask the sign and symptoms of acute hypoglycemia). Products include:
Avandamet Tablets 1373
Avandaryl Tablets 1379
Avandia Tablets 1384

Sotalol Hydrochloride (Concurrent use with systemic beta blocker may have additive effects of beta blockade, both systemic and on intraocular pressure).
No products indexed under this heading.

Timolol Hemihydrate (Concurrent use of two topical beta blockers is not recommended). Products include:
Betimol Ophthalmic Solution 3382
Betimol Ophthalmic Solution .... ⊙295

Tolazamide (Beta blocking agents, usually systemic, may mask the sign and symptoms of acute hypoglycemia).
No products indexed under this heading.

Tolbutamide (Beta blocking agents, usually systemic, may mask the sign and symptoms of acute hypoglycemia).
No products indexed under this heading.

Troglitazone (Beta blocking agents, usually systemic, may mask the sign and symptoms of acute hypoglycemia).
No products indexed under this heading.

Verapamil Hydrochloride (Possible atrioventricular conduction disturbances, left ventricular failure, or hypotension when used concurrently). Products include:
Covera-HS Tablets 3139
Tarka Tablets 524
Verelan PM Extended-Release Capsules, Controlled-Onset........... 3106

TIMOPTIC-XE STERILE OPHTHALMIC GEL FORMING SOLUTION

(Timolol Maleate) 2092
See Timoptic in Ocudose

TINDAMAX TABLETS

(Tinidazole) 2142
May interact with oral anticoagulants, lithium preparations, and phenytoin. Compounds in these categories include:

Anisindione (May enhance the effect of warfarin and other coumarin anticoagulants resulting in a prolongation of prothrombin time. The dosage of oral anticoagulants may need to be adjusted during co-administration and up to 8 days after tinidazole discontinuation). Products include:
Miradon Tablets 3042

Cholestyramine (It is advisable to separate dosing of cholestyramine and tinidazole to minimize any potential effect on the oral bioavailability of tinidazole).
No products indexed under this heading.

Cimetidine (Co-administration with drugs that inhibit the activity of liver microsomal enzymes, such as cimetidine, may prolong the half-life and decrease the plasma clearance of tinidazole, increasing the plasma level of tinidazole). Products include:
Tagamet HB 200 Tablets .... ▣664

Cimetidine Hydrochloride (Co-administration with drugs that inhibit the activity of liver microsomal enzymes, such as cimetidine, may prolong the half-life and decrease the plasma clearance of tinidazole, increasing the plasma level of tinidazole).
No products indexed under this heading.

Cyclosporine (Metronidazole has the potential to increase the levels of cyclosporine. During tinidazole co-administration, the patient should be monitored for signs of calcineurin-inhibitor associated toxicities). Products include:
Gengraf Capsules 459
Neoral Oral Solution 2259
Neoral Soft Gelatin Capsules 2259
Restasis Ophthalmic Emulsion 575
Sandimmune 2275

Dicumarol (May enhance the effect of warfarin and other coumarin anticoagulants resulting in a prolongation of prothrombin time. The dosage of oral anticoagulants may need to be adjusted during co-administration and up to 8 days after tinidazole discontinuation).
No products indexed under this heading.

Disulfiram (Psychotic reactions have been reported in alcoholic patients using metronidazole and disulfiram concurrently. Though no similar reactions have been reported with tinidazole, tinidazole should not be given to patients who have taken disulfiram within the last two weeks).
No products indexed under this heading.

Ethanol (Alcoholic beverages and preparations containing ethanol should be avoided during tinidazole therapy and for three days afterward because abdominal cramps, nausea, vomiting, headaches and flushing may occur).
No products indexed under this heading.

Fluorouracil (Metronidazole was shown to decrease the clearance of fluorouracil, resulting in side-effects without an increase in therapeutic benefits. If the concomitant use of tinidazole and fluorouracil cannot be avoided, the patient should be monitored for fluorouracil-associated toxicities). Products include:
Carac Cream, 0.5% 2879
Efudex 3363

Fosphenytoin Sodium (Concomitant administration of oral metronidazole and IV phenytoin was reported to result in prolongation of the half-life and reduction in the clearance of phenytoin. This may occur with tinidazole. Phenytoin and fosphenytoin may accelerate the elimination of tinidazole, decreasing the plasma level of tinidazole).
No products indexed under this heading.

Ketoconazole (Co-administration with drugs that inhibit the activity of liver microsomal enzymes, such as ketoconazole, may prolong the half-life and decrease the plasma clearance of tinidazole, increasing the plasma level of tinidazole). Products include:
Nizoral A-D Shampoo, 1% 1868

Lithium (Consideration should be given to measuring serum lithium creatinine levels after several days of simultaneous lithium and tinidazole treatment to detect potential lithium intoxication).
No products indexed under this heading.

Lithium Carbonate (Consideration should be given to measuring serum lithium creatinine levels after several days of simultaneous lithium and tinidazole treatment to detect potential lithium intoxication). Products include:
Lithobid Tablets 1692

Lithium Citrate (Consideration should be given to measuring serum lithium creatinine levels after several days of simultaneous lithium and tinidazole treatment to detect potential lithium intoxication).
No products indexed under this heading.

Oxytetracycline (Oxytetracycline was reported to antagonize the therapeutic effect of metronidazole and may potentially have the same effect on tinidazole).
No products indexed under this heading.

Oxytetracycline Hydrochloride (Oxytetracycline was reported to antagonize the therapeutic effect of metronidazole and may potentially have the same effect on tinidazole).
No products indexed under this heading.

Phenobarbital (Co-administration with drugs that induce liver microsomal enzymes, such as phenobarbital, may accelerate the elimination of tinidazole, decreasing the plasma level of tinidazole). Products include:
Donnatal Extentabs 2493

Phenobarbital Sodium (Co-administration with drugs that induce liver microsomal enzymes, such as phenobarbital, may accelerate the elimination of tinidazole, decreasing the plasma level of tinidazole).
No products indexed under this heading.

Phenytoin (Concomitant administration of oral metronidazole and IV phenytoin was reported to result in prolongation of the half-life and reduction in the clearance of phenytoin. This may occur with tinidazole. Phenytoin and fosphenytoin may accelerate the elimination of tinidazole, decreasing the plasma level of tinidazole).
No products indexed under this heading.

Phenytoin Sodium (Concomitant administration of oral metronidazole and IV phenytoin was reported to result in prolongation of the half-life and reduction in the clearance of phenytoin. This may occur with tinidazole. Phenytoin and fosphenytoin may accelerate the elimination of tinidazole, decreasing the plasma level of tinidazole). Products include:
Phenytek Capsules 2160

Propylene Glycol (Preparations containing propylene glycol should be avoided during tinidazole therapy and for three days afterward because abdominal cramps, nausea, vomiting, headaches and flushing may occur). Products include:
Systane Lubricant Eye Drops 562

Propylene Glycol-containing Solutions (Preparations containing propylene glycol should be avoided during tinidazole therapy and for three days afterward because abdominal cramps, nausea, vomiting, headaches and flushing may occur).
No products indexed under this heading.

Rifampin (Co-administration with drugs that induce liver microsomal enzymes, such as rifampin, may accelerate the elimination of tinidazole, decreasing the plasma level of tinidazole).
No products indexed under this heading.

Tacrolimus (Metronidazole has the potential to increase the levels of tacrolimus. During tinidazole co-administration, the patient should be monitored for signs of calcineurin-inhibitor associated toxins). Products include:
Prograf Capsules and Injection 632
Protopic Ointment 638

Warfarin Sodium (May enhance the effect of warfarin and other coumarin anticoagulants resulting in a prolongation of prothrombin time. The dosage of oral anticoagulants may need to be adjusted during co-administration and up to 8 days after tinidazole discontinuation). Products include:
Coumadin for Injection 898
Coumadin Tablets 898

Food Interactions

Alcohol (Alcoholic beverages should be avoided during tinidazole therapy and for three days afterward because abdominal cramps, nausea, vomiting, headaches and flushing may occur).

TNKASE I.V.

(Tenecteplase) 1264
May interact with vitamin K antagonists and certain other agents. Compounds in these categories include:

Abciximab (Drugs that alter platelet function, such as abciximab, may increase the risk of bleeding if administered prior to or after tenecteplase therapy). Products include:
ReoPro Vials 1809

Aspirin (Drugs that alter platelet function, such as aspirin, may increase the risk of bleeding if administered prior to or after tenecteplase therapy). Products include:
Aggrenox Capsules 822
Bayer Aspirin 744
BC Allergy Sinus Cold Powder .... ▣677
BC Headache Powder .... ▣677
Arthritis Strength BC Powder .... ▣677
BC Sinus Cold Powder .... ▣677
Excedrin Extra Strength Caplets/Tablets/Geltabs .... ▣684
Excedrin Migraine Caplets/Tablets/Geltabs .... ▣609
Goody's Body Pain Formula Powder .... ▣684
Goody's Extra Strength Headache Powders .... ▣611
Goody's Extra Strength Pain Relief Tablets .... ▣685
Percodan Tablets 1132
St. Joseph 81 mg Aspirin Chewable and Enteric Coated Tablets 1869

Clopidogrel Bisulfate (Drugs that alter platelet function, such as clopidogrel, may increase the risk of bleeding if administered prior to or after tenecteplase therapy). Products include:
Plavix Tablets 917
Plavix Tablets 2926

Dicumarol (Co-administration increases the risk of bleeding).
No products indexed under this heading.

Dipyridamole (Drugs that alter platelet function, such as dipyridamole, may increase the risk of bleeding if administered prior to or after tenecteplase therapy). Products include:
Aggrenox Capsules 822
Persantine Tablets 868

Epitifibatide (Drugs that alter platelet function, such as epitifibatide, may increase the risk of bleeding if administered prior to or after tenecteplase therapy).
No products indexed under this heading.

Ticlopidine Hydrochloride (Drugs that alter platelet function, such as ticlopidine, may increase the risk of bleeding if administered prior to or after tenecteplase therapy). Products include:
Ticlid Tablets 2810

Tirofiban Hydrochloride (Drugs that alter platelet function, such as tirofiban, may increase the risk of bleeding if administered prior to or after tenecteplase therapy). Products include:
Aggrastat 1907

Warfarin Sodium (Co-administration increases the risk of bleeding). Products include:
Coumadin for Injection 898
Coumadin Tablets 898

TOBI SOLUTION FOR INHALATION

(Tobramycin) 2298
May interact with aminoglycosides and certain other agents. Compounds in these categories include:

Amikacin Sulfate (Co-administration in some patients receiving TOBI and extensive previous or concomitant parenteral aminoglycosides has resulted in hearing loss; potential for increased risk of neurotoxicity and/or ototoxicity).
No products indexed under this heading.

Ethacrynic Acid (Some diuretics, such as ethacrynic acid, can enhance aminoglycoside toxicity by altering antibiotic concentrations in serum and tissue; TOBI should not be administered with ethacrynic acid). Products include:
Edecrin Tablets 1959

Furosemide (Some diuretics, such as furosemide, can enhance aminoglycoside toxicity by altering antibiotic concentrations in serum and tissue; TOBI should not be administered with furosemide). Products include:
Furosemide Tablets 2154

Gentamicin Sulfate (Co-administration in some patients receiving TOBI and extensive previous or concomitant parenteral aminoglycosides has resulted in hearing loss; potential for increased risk of neurotoxicity and/or ototoxicity). Products include:
Garamycin Injectable 3014
Pred-G Ophthalmic Ointment .... ⊙237
Pred-G Ophthalmic Suspension ...... ⊙236

Kanamycin Sulfate (Co-administration in some patients receiving TOBI and extensive previous or concomitant parenteral aminoglycosides has resulted in hearing loss; potential for increased risk of neurotoxicity and/or ototoxicity).
No products indexed under this heading.

Mannitol (Some diuretics, such as mannitol, can enhance aminoglycoside toxicity by altering antibiotic concentrations in serum and tissue; TOBI should not be administered with mannitol).
No products indexed under this heading.

Streptomycin Sulfate (Co-administration in some patients receiving TOBI and extensive previous or concomitant parenteral aminoglycosides has resulted in hearing loss; potential for increased risk of neurotoxicity and/or ototoxicity).
No products indexed under this heading.

Tobramycin Sulfate (Co-administration in some patients receiving TOBI and extensive previous or concomitant parenteral aminoglycosides has resulted in hearing loss; potential for increased risk of neurotoxicity and/or ototoxicity).
No products indexed under this heading.

Urea (Some diuretics, such as systemic urea, can enhance aminoglycoside toxicity by altering antibiotic concentrations in serum and tissue; TOBI should not be administered with urea). Products include:
Accuzyme Debriding Ointment 1662
Accuzyme SE Spray Emulsion 1662
Panafil Ointment 1663
Panafil SE Spray Emulsion 1663

TOBRADEX OPHTHALMIC OINTMENT

(Dexamethasone, Tobramycin) 562
May interact with aminoglycosides. Compounds in these categories include:

Amikacin Sulfate (Monitor the total serum concentration if administered with systemic aminoglycoside).
No products indexed under this heading.

Gentamicin Sulfate (Monitor the total serum concentration if administered with systemic aminoglycoside). Products include:
Garamycin Injectable 3014
Pred-G Ophthalmic Ointment .... ⊙237
Pred-G Ophthalmic Suspension ...... ⊙236

Kanamycin Sulfate (Monitor the total serum concentration if administered with systemic aminoglycoside).
No products indexed under this heading.

Streptomycin Sulfate (Monitor the total serum concentration if administered with systemic aminoglycoside).
No products indexed under this heading.

Tobramycin Sulfate (Monitor the total serum concentration if administered with systemic aminoglycoside).
No products indexed under this heading.

TOBRADEX OPHTHALMIC SUSPENSION

(Dexamethasone, Tobramycin) 563
See TobraDex Ophthalmic Ointment

TOPAMAX SPRINKLE CAPSULES

(Topiramate) 2404
See Topamax Tablets

TOPAMAX TABLETS

(Topiramate) 2404
May interact with carbonic anhydrase inhibitors, central nervous system depressants, lithium preparations, oral contraceptives, phenytoin, valproate, and certain other agents. Compounds in these categories include:

Acetazolamide (Co-administration of topiramate with carbonic anhydrase inhibitors may create a physiological environment that increases the risk of kidney stone formation; concurrent use should be avoided).
No products indexed under this heading.

Alfentanil Hydrochloride (Potential for increased CNS depression).
No products indexed under this heading.

Alprazolam (Potential for increased CNS depression). Products include:
Niravam Orally Disintegrating Tablets 3092

Amitriptyline Hydrochloride (There was a 12% increase in AUC and Cmax for amitriptyline (25mg per day) in 18 normal subjects receiving 200mg/day of topiramate. Some subjects may experience a large increase in amitriptyline concentration in the presence of topiramate and any adjustments in amitriptyline dose should be made according to the patient's clinical response and not on the basis of plasma levels).
No products indexed under this heading.

Aprobarbital (Potential for increased CNS depression).
No products indexed under this heading.

Buprenorphine Hydrochloride (Potential for increased CNS depression). Products include:
Buprenex Injectable 2716
Suboxone Tablets 2717
Subutex Tablets 2717

Buspirone Hydrochloride (Potential for increased CNS depression).
No products indexed under this heading.

Butabarbital (Potential for increased CNS depression).
No products indexed under this heading.

Butalbital (Potential for increased CNS depression).
No products indexed under this heading.

Carbamazepine (Co-administration has resulted in 40% decrease in topiramate concentration and no change in carbamazepine concentration). Products include:
Carbatrol Capsules 3171
Equetro Extended-Release Capsules 3180
Tegretol/Tegretol-XR 2295

Chlordiazepoxide (Potential for increased CNS depression).
No products indexed under this heading.

Chlordiazepoxide Hydrochloride (Potential for increased CNS depression). Products include:
Librium Capsules 3347

Chlorpromazine (Potential for increased CNS depression).
No products indexed under this heading.

Chlorpromazine Hydrochloride (Potential for increased CNS depression).
No products indexed under this heading.

Chlorprothixene (Potential for increased CNS depression).
No products indexed under this heading.

Chlorprothixene Hydrochloride (Potential for increased CNS depression).
No products indexed under this heading.

Chlorprothixene Lactate (Potential for increased CNS depression).
No products indexed under this heading.

Clorazepate Dipotassium (Potential for increased CNS depression). Products include:
Tranxene ... 2474

Clozapine (Potential for increased CNS depression). Products include:
Clozaril Tablets ... 2184
FazaClo Orally Disintegrating Tablets ... 551

Codeine Phosphate (Potential for increased CNS depression). Products include:
Tylenol with Codeine Tablets ... 2391

Desflurane (Potential for increased CNS depression).
No products indexed under this heading.

Desogestrel (The possibility of decreased contraceptive efficacy and increased breakthrough bleeding should be considered in patients taking combination oral contraceptive products with topiramate). Products include:
Mircette Tablets ... 1066

Dezocine (Potential for increased CNS depression).
No products indexed under this heading.

Diazepam (Potential for increased CNS depression). Products include:
Diastat Rectal Delivery System ... 3343
Valium Tablets ... 2819

Dichlorphenamide (Co-administration of topiramate with carbonic anhydrase inhibitors may create a physiological environment that increases the risk of kidney stone formation; concurrent use should be avoided). Products include:
Daranide Tablets ... 1950

Digoxin (Co-administration has resulted in decreased serum digoxin AUC by 12%; clinical significance of this interaction is unknown). Products include:
Lanoxicaps Capsules ... 1490
Lanoxin Injection ... 1494
Lanoxin Injection Pediatric ... 1497
Lanoxin Tablets ... 1500

Divalproex Sodium (Co-administration resulted in an 11% decrease in valproic acid concentration and a 14% decrease in topiramate concentration. Concomitant administration of topiramate and valproic acid has been associated with hyperammonemia, with or without encephalopathy, in patients who have tolerated either drug alone). Products include:
Depakote Sprinkle Capsules ... 422
Depakote Tablets ... 427
Depakote ER Tablets ... 434

Dorzolamide Hydrochloride (Co-administration of topiramate with carbonic anhydrase inhibitors may create a physiological environment that increases the risk of kidney stone formation; concurrent use should be avoided). Products include:
Cosopt Sterile Ophthalmic Solution ... 1931
Trusopt Sterile Ophthalmic Solution ... 2095

Droperidol (Potential for increased CNS depression).
No products indexed under this heading.

Enflurane (Potential for increased CNS depression).
No products indexed under this heading.

Estazolam (Potential for increased CNS depression). Products include:
ProSom Tablets ... 517

Ethanol (Potential for increased CNS depression).
No products indexed under this heading.

Ethchlorvynol (Potential for increased CNS depression).
No products indexed under this heading.

Ethinamate (Potential for increased CNS depression).
No products indexed under this heading.

Ethinyl Estradiol (The possibility of decreased contraceptive efficacy and increased breakthrough bleeding should be considered in patients taking combination oral contraceptive products with topiramate). Products include:
Mircette Tablets ... 1066
NuvaRing ... 2340
Ortho-Cyclen/Ortho Tri-Cyclen ... 2429
Ortho Evra Transdermal System ... 2417
Ortho Tri-Cyclen Lo Tablets ... 2436
Seasonique Tablets ... 1077
Yasmin 28 Tablets ... 796
Yaz Tablets ... 803

Ethyl Alcohol (Potential for increased CNS depression).
No products indexed under this heading.

Ethynodiol Diacetate (The possibility of decreased contraceptive efficacy and increased breakthrough bleeding should be considered in patients taking combination oral contraceptive products with topiramate).
No products indexed under this heading.

Fentanyl (Potential for increased CNS depression). Products include:
Duragesic Transdermal System ... 2373
Ionsys Transdermal System ... 2379

Fentanyl Citrate (Potential for increased CNS depression). Products include:
Actiq ... 979

Fluphenazine Decanoate (Potential for increased CNS depression).
No products indexed under this heading.

Fluphenazine Enanthate (Potential for increased CNS depression).
No products indexed under this heading.

Fluphenazine Hydrochloride (Potential for increased CNS depression).
No products indexed under this heading.

Flurazepam Hydrochloride (Potential for increased CNS depression). Products include:
Dalmane Capsules ... 3342

Fosphenytoin Sodium (Co-administration has resulted in 48% decrease in topiramate concentration and no change or 25% increase in phenytoin concentration).
No products indexed under this heading.

Glutethimide (Potential for increased CNS depression).
No products indexed under this heading.

Haloperidol (Potential for increased CNS depression).
No products indexed under this heading.

Haloperidol Decanoate (Potential for increased CNS depression).
No products indexed under this heading.

Hydrochlorothiazide (A study done in healthy volunteers indicated that topiramate Cmax increased by 27% and AUC increased by 29% when HCTZ was added to topiramate. The addition of HCTZ to topiramate therapy may require an adjustment of the topiramate dose. The steady state pharmacokinetics of HCTZ were not significantly influenced by the concomitant administration of topiramate. Clinical laboratory results indicated decreases in serum potassium after topiramate of HCTZ administration, which were greater when HCTZ and topiramate were administered in combination). Products include:
Aldoril Tablets ... 1910
Atacand HCT ... 651
Avalide Tablets ... 888
Avalide Tablets ... 2874
Benicar HCT Tablets ... 1044
Diovan HCT Tablets ... 2196
Dyazide Capsules ... 1423
Hyzaar 50-12.5 Tablets ... 1990
Hyzaar 100-12.5 Tablets ... 1990
Hyzaar 100-25 Tablets ... 1990
Lopressor HCT 50/25 Tablets ... 2241
Lopressor HCT 100/25 Tablets ... 2241
Lopressor HCT 100/50 Tablets ... 2241
Lotensin HCT Tablets ... 2246
Micardis HCT Tablets ... 856
Moduretic Tablets ... 2028
Prinzide Tablets ... 2056
Teveten HCT Tablets ... 1737
Timolide Tablets ... 2086
Uniretic Tablets ... 3100

Hydrochlorothiazide Hydrochloride (A study done in healthy volunteers indicated that topiramate Cmax increased by 27% and AUC increased by 29% when HCTZ was added to topiramate. The addition of HCTZ to topiramate therapy may require an adjustment of the topiramate dose. The steady state pharmacokinetics of HCTZ were not significantly influenced by the concomitant administration of topiramate. Clinical laboratory results indicated decreases in serum potassium after topiramate of HCTZ administration, which were greater when HCTZ and topiramate were administered in combination).
No products indexed under this heading.

Hydrocodone Bitartrate (Potential for increased CNS depression). Products include:
Hycodan ... 1116
Hycotuss Expectorant Syrup ... 1117
Vicodin Tablets ... 535
Vicodin ES Tablets ... 536
Vicodin HP Tablets ... 538
Vicoprofen Tablets ... 539
Zydone Tablets ... 1139

Hydrocodone Polistirex (Potential for increased CNS depression). Products include:
Tussionex Pennkinetic Extended-Release Suspension ... 3327

Hydromorphone Hydrochloride (Potential for increased CNS depression). Products include:
Dilaudid ... 440
Dilaudid Non-Sterile Powder ... 440
Dilaudid Oral Liquid ... 445
Dilaudid Rectal Suppositories ... 440
Dilaudid Tablets ... 440
Dilaudid Tablets - 8 mg ... 445
Dilaudid-HP ... 442

Hydroxyzine Hydrochloride (Potential for increased CNS depression).
No products indexed under this heading.

Isoflurane (Potential for increased CNS depression).
No products indexed under this heading.

Ketamine Hydrochloride (Potential for increased CNS depression).
No products indexed under this heading.

Levomethadyl Acetate Hydrochloride (Potential for increased CNS depression).
No products indexed under this heading.

Levonorgestrel (The possibility of decreased contraceptive efficacy and increased breakthrough bleeding should be considered in patients taking combination oral contraceptive products with topiramate). Products include:
Climara Pro Transdermal System ... 776
Mirena Intrauterine System ... 787
Plan B Tablets ... 1076
Seasonique Tablets ... 1077

Levorphanol Tartrate (Potential for increased CNS depression).
No products indexed under this heading.

Lithium (Multiple dosing of topiramate 100mg every 12 hours has decreased the AUC and Cmax of lithium (300mg every 8 hrs) by 20%).
No products indexed under this heading.

Lithium Carbonate (Multiple dosing of topiramate 100mg every 12 hours has decreased the AUC and Cmax of lithium (300mg every 8 hrs) by 20%). Products include:
Lithobid Tablets ... 1692

Lithium Citrate (Multiple dosing of topiramate 100mg every 12 hours has decreased the AUC and Cmax of lithium (300mg every 8 hrs) by 20%).
No products indexed under this heading.

Lorazepam (Potential for increased CNS depression).
No products indexed under this heading.

Loxapine Hydrochloride (Potential for increased CNS depression).
No products indexed under this heading.

Loxapine Succinate (Potential for increased CNS depression).
No products indexed under this heading.

Meperidine Hydrochloride (Potential for increased CNS depression).
No products indexed under this heading.

Mephobarbital (Potential for increased CNS depression).
No products indexed under this heading.

Meprobamate (Potential for increased CNS depression).
No products indexed under this heading.

Mesoridazine Besylate (Potential for increased CNS depression).
No products indexed under this heading.

Mestranol (The possibility of decreased contraceptive efficacy and increased breakthrough bleeding should be considered in patients taking combination oral contraceptive products with topiramate).
No products indexed under this heading.

Metformin (Co-administration has resulted in increased metformin mean AUC and Cmax and decreased CL/F; oral plasma clearance of Topiramate appears to be reduced with co-administration; clinical significance of these findings is unclear).
No products indexed under this heading.

Methadone Hydrochloride (Potential for increased CNS depression).
No products indexed under this heading.

Methazolamide (Co-administration of topiramate with carbonic anhydrase inhibitors may create a physiological environment that increases the risk of kidney stone formation; concurrent use should be avoided).
No products indexed under this heading.

Methohexital Sodium (Potential for increased CNS depression).
No products indexed under this heading.

Methotrimeprazine (Potential for increased CNS depression).
No products indexed under this heading.

Methoxyflurane (Potential for increased CNS depression).
No products indexed under this heading.

Midazolam Hydrochloride (Potential for increased CNS depression).
No products indexed under this heading.

Molindone Hydrochloride (Potential for increased CNS depression).
Products include:
Moban Tablets ... 1119

Morphine Sulfate (Potential for increased CNS depression).
Products include:
Avinza Capsules ... 1741
Kadian Capsules ... 577
MS Contin Tablets ... 2701

Norethindrone (The possibility of decreased contraceptive efficacy and increased breakthrough bleeding should be considered in patients taking combination oral contraceptive products with topiramate).
Products include:
Ortho Micronor Tablets ... 2426

Norethynodrel (The possibility of decreased contraceptive efficacy and increased breakthrough bleeding should be considered in patients taking combination oral contraceptive products with topiramate).
No products indexed under this heading.

Norgestimate (The possibility of decreased contraceptive efficacy and increased breakthrough bleeding should be considered in patients taking combination oral contraceptive products with topiramate).
Products include:
Ortho-Cyclen/Ortho Tri-Cyclen ... 2429
Ortho Tri-Cyclen Lo Tablets ... 2436

Norgestrel (The possibility of decreased contraceptive efficacy and increased breakthrough bleeding should be considered in patients taking combination oral contraceptive products with topiramate).
No products indexed under this heading.

Olanzapine (Potential for increased CNS depression). Products include:
Symbyax Capsules ... 1819
Zyprexa Tablets ... 1830
Zyprexa IntraMuscular ... 1830
Zyprexa ZYDIS Orally Disintegrating Tablets ... 1830

Oxazepam (Potential for increased CNS depression).
No products indexed under this heading.

Oxycodone Hydrochloride (Potential for increased CNS depression). Products include:
OxyContin Tablets ... 2703
OxyFast Oral Concentrate Solution ... 2708
OxyIR Capsules ... 2708
Percocet Tablets ... 1131
Percodan Tablets ... 1132

Pentobarbital Sodium (Potential for increased CNS depression).
Products include:
Nembutal Sodium Solution, USP ... 2470

Perphenazine (Potential for increased CNS depression).
No products indexed under this heading.

Phenobarbital (Potential for increased CNS depression).
Products include:
Donnatal Extentabs ... 2493

Phenytoin (Co-administration has resulted in 48% decrease in topiramate concentration and no change or 25% increase in phenytoin concentration).
No products indexed under this heading.

Phenytoin Sodium (Co-administration has resulted in 48% decrease in topiramate concentration and no change or 25% increase in phenytoin concentration).
Products include:
Phenytek Capsules ... 2160

Pioglitazone Hydrochloride (When topiramate is added to pioglitazone therapy or pioglitazone is added to topiramate therapy, careful attention should be given to the routine monitoring of patients for adequate control of their diabetic disease status). Products include:
ActoPlus Met Tablets ... 3214
Actos Tablets ... 3219
Duetact Tablets ... 3226

Prazepam (Potential for increased CNS depression).
No products indexed under this heading.

Prochlorperazine (Potential for increased CNS depression).
No products indexed under this heading.

Promethazine Hydrochloride (Potential for increased CNS depression). Products include:
Phenergan Tablets and Suppositories ... 3440

Propofol (Potential for increased CNS depression).
No products indexed under this heading.

Propoxyphene Hydrochloride (Potential for increased CNS depression).
No products indexed under this heading.

Propoxyphene Napsylate (Potential for increased CNS depression).
No products indexed under this heading.

Quazepam (Potential for increased CNS depression).
No products indexed under this heading.

Quetiapine Fumarate (Potential for increased CNS depression).
Products include:
Seroquel Tablets ... 690

Remifentanil Hydrochloride (Potential for increased CNS depression).
No products indexed under this heading.

Risperidone (There was a 25% decrease in exposure to risperidone (2mg single dose) in 12 healthy volunteers receiving 200mg/day of topiramate. Therefore, patients receiving risperidone in combination with topiramate should be closely monitored for clinical response).
Products include:
Risperdal ... 1676
Risperdal Consta Long-Acting Injection ... 1682
Risperdal M-Tab Orally Disintegrating Tablets ... 1676

Secobarbital Sodium (Potential for increased CNS depression).
No products indexed under this heading.

Sevoflurane (Potential for increased CNS depression).
Products include:
Ultane Liquid for Inhalation ... 531

Sodium Oxybate (Potential for increased CNS depression).
Products include:
Xyrem Oral Solution ... 1688

Sufentanil Citrate (Potential for increased CNS depression).
No products indexed under this heading.

Temazepam (Potential for increased CNS depression).
Products include:
Restoril Capsules ... 1860

Thiamylal Sodium (Potential for increased CNS depression).
No products indexed under this heading.

Thioridazine Hydrochloride (Potential for increased CNS depression). Products include:
Thioridazine Hydrochloride Tablets ... 2163

Thiothixene (Potential for increased CNS depression). Products include:
Thiothixene Capsules ... 2165

Torsemide (Co-administration of topiramate with carbonic anhydrase inhibitors may create a physiological environment that increases the risk of kidney stone formation; concurrent use should be avoided).
Products include:
Demadex Injection ... 2759
Demadex Tablets ... 2759

Triazolam (Potential for increased CNS depression).
No products indexed under this heading.

Trifluoperazine Hydrochloride (Potential for increased CNS depression).
No products indexed under this heading.

Valproate Sodium (Co-administration resulted in an 11% decrease in valproic acid concentration and a 14% decrease in topiramate concentration. Concomitant administration of topiramate and valproic acid has been associated with hyperammonemia, with or without encephalopathy, in patients who have tolerated either drug alone).
Products include:
Depacon Injection ... 412

Valproic Acid (Co-administration resulted in an 11% decrease in valproic acid concentration and a 14% decrease in topiramate concentration. Concomitant administration of topiramate and valproic acid has been associated with hyperammonemia, with or without encephalopathy, in patients who have tolerated either drug alone). Products include:
Depakene ... 417

Zaleplon (Potential for increased CNS depression). Products include:
Sonata Capsules ... 1717

Ziprasidone Hydrochloride (Potential for increased CNS depression). Products include:
Geodon Capsules ... 2529

Zolpidem Tartrate (Potential for increased CNS depression).
Products include:
Ambien Tablets ... 2851
Ambien CR Tablets ... 2855

Food Interactions

Alcohol (Potential for increased CNS depression).

TOPROL-XL TABLETS
(Metoprolol Succinate) ... 668
May interact with catecholamine depleting drugs and cytochrome p450 2d6 inhibitors (selected). Compounds in these categories include:

Amiodarone Hydrochloride (Co-administration of metoprolol with drugs that inhibit CYP2D6, such as quinidine, is likely to increase metoprolol concentration; this increase in plasma concentration would decrease the cardioselectivity of metoprolol).
No products indexed under this heading.

Amitriptyline Hydrochloride (Co-administration of metoprolol with drugs that inhibit CYP2D6, such as quinidine, is likely to increase metoprolol concentration; this increase in plasma concentration would decrease the cardioselectivity of metoprolol).
No products indexed under this heading.

Amoxapine (Co-administration of metoprolol with drugs that inhibit CYP2D6, such as quinidine, is likely to increase metoprolol concentration; this increase in plasma concentration would decrease the cardioselectivity of metoprolol).
No products indexed under this heading.

Bupropion Hydrochloride (Co-administration of metoprolol with drugs that inhibit CYP2D6, such as quinidine, is likely to increase metoprolol concentration; this increase in plasma concentration would decrease the cardioselectivity of metoprolol). Products include:

Wellbutrin Tablets 1603
Wellbutrin SR Sustained-Release Tablets 1607
Wellbutrin XL Extended-Release Tablets 1613
Zyban Sustained-Release Tablets 1644

Celecoxib (Co-administration of metoprolol with drugs that inhibit CYP2D6, such as quinidine, is likely to increase metoprolol concentration; this increase in plasma concentration would decrease the cardioselectivity of metoprolol). Products include:

Celebrex Capsules 3134

Chloroquine Hydrochloride (Co-administration of metoprolol with drugs that inhibit CYP2D6, such as quinidine, is likely to increase metoprolol concentration; this increase in plasma concentration would decrease the cardioselectivity of metoprolol).

No products indexed under this heading.

Chloroquine Phosphate (Co-administration of metoprolol with drugs that inhibit CYP2D6, such as quinidine, is likely to increase metoprolol concentration; this increase in plasma concentration would decrease the cardioselectivity of metoprolol).

No products indexed under this heading.

Chlorpheniramine (Co-administration of metoprolol with drugs that inhibit CYP2D6, such as quinidine, is likely to increase metoprolol concentration; this increase in plasma concentration would decrease the cardioselectivity of metoprolol).

No products indexed under this heading.

Chlorpheniramine Maleate (Co-administration of metoprolol with drugs that inhibit CYP2D6, such as quinidine, is likely to increase metoprolol concentration; this increase in plasma concentration would decrease the cardioselectivity of metoprolol). Products include:

Advil Allergy Sinus Caplets 770
Advil Multi-Symptom Cold Caplets 770
BC Allergy Sinus Cold Powder 677
Comtrex Maximum Strength Cold & Cough Day/Night Caplets - Night Formulation 726
Comtrex Maximum Strength Day/Night Severe Cold & Sinus Caplets - Night Formulation 725
Contac Cold and Flu Maximum Strength Caplets 728
Contac Cold and Flu Day and Night Caplets (Night Formulation Only) 727
Children's Dimetapp Long Acting Cough Plus Cold Syrup 731
Robitussin Cough & Cold Long-Acting Liquid 735
Robitussin Cough & Allergy Syrup .. 736
Robitussin Cough & Cold Nighttime Liquid 736
Robitussin Cough, Cold & Flu Nighttime Liquid 738
Robitussin Pediatric Cough & Cold Long-Acting Liquid 735
Robitussin Pediatric Cough & Cold Nighttime Liquid 736
Triaminic Cold & Allergy Liquid 746
Triaminic Cough & Runny Nose Softchews 748
Children's Tylenol Plus Flu Oral Suspension 749
Tylenol Allergy Multi-Symptom Caplets with Cool Burst and Gelcaps 1872
Children's Tylenol Plus Cold Suspension Liquid 1879
Children's Tylenol Plus Cough & Runny Nose Suspension Liquid 1879
Children's Tylenol Plus Flu Suspension Liquid 1881
Children's Tylenol Plus Multi-Symptom Cold Suspension Liquid 1879
Tylenol Cold Head Congestion Nighttime Caplets with Cool Burst 1873
Tylenol Cold Multi-Symptom Nighttime Caplets with Cool Burst 1874
Tylenol Sinus Congestion & Pain Nighttime Caplets with Cool Burst 1876
Vicks 44M Cough, Cold & Flu Relief Liquid 2680
Pediatric Vicks 44m Cough & Cold Relief Liquid 2676
Children's Vicks NyQuil Cold/Cough Relief 756
Children's Vicks NyQuil Cold/Cough Relief Liquid 2680
Zicam Maximum Strength Flu Daytime 768

Chlorpheniramine Polistirex (Co-administration of metoprolol with drugs that inhibit CYP2D6, such as quinidine, is likely to increase metoprolol concentration; this increase in plasma concentration would decrease the cardioselectivity of metoprolol). Products include:

Tussionex Pennkinetic Extended-Release Suspension 3327

Chlorpheniramine Tannate (Co-administration of metoprolol with drugs that inhibit CYP2D6, such as quinidine, is likely to increase metoprolol concentration; this increase in plasma concentration would decrease the cardioselectivity of metoprolol).

No products indexed under this heading.

Cimetidine (Co-administration of metoprolol with drugs that inhibit CYP2D6, such as quinidine, is likely to increase metoprolol concentration; this increase in plasma concentration would decrease the cardioselectivity of metoprolol). Products include:

Tagamet HB 200 Tablets 664

Cimetidine Hydrochloride (Co-administration of metoprolol with drugs that inhibit CYP2D6, such as quinidine, is likely to increase metoprolol concentration; this increase in plasma concentration would decrease the cardioselectivity of metoprolol).

No products indexed under this heading.

Citalopram Hydrobromide (Co-administration of metoprolol with drugs that inhibit CYP2D6, such as quinidine, is likely to increase metoprolol concentration; this increase in plasma concentration would decrease the cardioselectivity of metoprolol). Products include:

Celexa 1176

Clomipramine Hydrochloride (Co-administration of metoprolol with drugs that inhibit CYP2D6, such as quinidine, is likely to increase metoprolol concentration; this increase in plasma concentration would decrease the cardioselectivity of metoprolol).

No products indexed under this heading.

Clonidine (Beta-blockers may exacerbate the rebound hypertension which can follow the withdrawal of clonidine. If co-administered, withdraw beta-blockers several days before the gradual withdrawal of clonidine. If replacing clonidine by beta-blocker therapy, delay start of beta-blockers for several days after clonidine administration has stopped). Products include:

Catapres-TTS 844

Cocaine Hydrochloride (Co-administration of metoprolol with drugs that inhibit CYP2D6, such as quinidine, is likely to increase metoprolol concentration; this increase in plasma concentration would decrease the cardioselectivity of metoprolol).

No products indexed under this heading.

Deserpidine (Catecholamine-depleting drugs may have an additive effect when given with beta-blocking agents; monitor closely for signs of hypotension or marked bradycardia).

No products indexed under this heading.

Desipramine Hydrochloride (Co-administration of metoprolol with drugs that inhibit CYP2D6, such as quinidine, is likely to increase metoprolol concentration; this increase in plasma concentration would decrease the cardioselectivity of metoprolol).

No products indexed under this heading.

Diltiazem Hydrochloride (Because of significant inotropic and chronotropic effects in patients treated with beta-blockers and calcium-channel blockers of the diltiazem type, caution should be exercised in patients treated with these agents concomitantly). Products include:

Cardizem LA Extended Release Tablets 1728
Tiazac Capsules 1201

Diphenhydramine (Co-administration of metoprolol with drugs that inhibit CYP2D6, such as quinidine, is likely to increase metoprolol concentration; this increase in plasma concentration would decrease the cardioselectivity of metoprolol). Products include:

Tylenol Sore Throat Nighttime Liquid with Cool Burst 1877

Diphenhydramine Hydrochloride (Co-administration of metoprolol with drugs that inhibit CYP2D6, such as quinidine, is likely to increase metoprolol concentration; this increase in plasma concentration would decrease the cardioselectivity of metoprolol). Products include:

Nytol QuickCaps Caplets 615
Nytol QuickGels Softgels Maximum Strength........................ 616
Simply Sleep Caplets 1868
Sominex Original Formula Tablets .. 616
TheraFlu Warming Relief Nighttime Severe Cold.............. 743
TheraFlu Thin Strips Multi Symptom................................... 744
Triaminic Nighttime Cold & Cough Liquid.......................... 746
Triaminic Thin Strips Cough & Runny Nose 749
Extra Strength Tylenol PM Caplets, Vanilla Caplets, Geltabs, Gelcaps and Liquid......... 1875
Tylenol Sore Throat Nighttime Liquid with Cool Burst 790
Tylenol Allergy Multi-Symptom Nighttime Caplets with Cool Burst 1872
Tylenol Severe Allergy Caplets 1872
Children's Tylenol Plus Cold & Allergy Suspension Liquid 1878

Doxepin Hydrochloride (Co-administration of metoprolol with drugs that inhibit CYP2D6, such as quinidine, is likely to increase metoprolol concentration; this increase in plasma concentration would decrease the cardioselectivity of metoprolol).

No products indexed under this heading.

Epinephrine Hydrochloride (Potential unresponsiveness to the usual dose of epinephrine to treat allergic reactions in certain patients).

No products indexed under this heading.

Escitalopram Oxalate (Co-administration of metoprolol with drugs that inhibit CYP2D6, such as quinidine, is likely to increase metoprolol concentration; this increase in plasma concentration would decrease the cardioselectivity of metoprolol). Products include:

Lexapro Oral Solution 1190
Lexapro Tablets 1190

Fluoxetine (Co-administration of metoprolol with drugs that inhibit CYP2D6, such as quinidine, is likely to increase metoprolol concentration; this increase in plasma concentration would decrease the cardioselectivity of metoprolol).

No products indexed under this heading.

Fluoxetine Hydrochloride (Co-administration with drugs that inhibit CYP2D6, such as fluoxetine, are likely to increase metoprolol concentrations; these increases in plasma concentration would decrease the cardioselectivity of metoprolol). Products include:

Prozac Pulvules and Liquid 1801
Symbyax Capsules 1819

Fluphenazine Decanoate (Co-administration of metoprolol with drugs that inhibit CYP2D6, such as quinidine, is likely to increase metoprolol concentration; this increase in plasma concentration would decrease the cardioselectivity of metoprolol).

No products indexed under this heading.

Fluphenazine Enanthate (Co-administration of metoprolol with drugs that inhibit CYP2D6, such as quinidine, is likely to increase metoprolol concentration; this increase in plasma concentration would decrease the cardioselectivity of metoprolol).

No products indexed under this heading.

Fluphenazine Hydrochloride (Co-administration of metoprolol with drugs that inhibit CYP2D6, such as quinidine, is likely to increase metoprolol concentration; this increase in plasma concentration would decrease the cardioselectivity of metoprolol).

No products indexed under this heading.

Fluvoxamine Maleate (Co-administration of metoprolol with drugs that inhibit CYP2D6, such as quinidine, is likely to increase metoprolol concentration; this increase in plasma concentration would decrease the cardioselectivity of metoprolol).

No products indexed under this heading.

Guanethidine Monosulfate (Catecholamine-depleting drugs may have an additive effect when given with beta-blocking agents; monitor closely for signs of hypotension or marked bradycardia).
No products indexed under this heading.

Halofantrine Hydrochloride (Co-administration of metoprolol with drugs that inhibit CYP2D6, such as quinidine, is likely to increase metoprolol concentration; this increase in plasma concentration would decrease the cardioselectivity of metoprolol).
No products indexed under this heading.

Haloperidol (Co-administration of metoprolol with drugs that inhibit CYP2D6, such as quinidine, is likely to increase metoprolol concentration; this increase in plasma concentration would decrease the cardioselectivity of metoprolol).
No products indexed under this heading.

Haloperidol Decanoate (Co-administration of metoprolol with drugs that inhibit CYP2D6, such as quinidine, is likely to increase metoprolol concentration; this increase in plasma concentration would decrease the cardioselectivity of metoprolol).
No products indexed under this heading.

Hydroxychloroquine Sulfate (Co-administration of metoprolol with drugs that inhibit CYP2D6, such as quinidine, is likely to increase metoprolol concentration; this increase in plasma concentration would decrease the cardioselectivity of metoprolol).
No products indexed under this heading.

Imatinib Mesylate (Co-administration of metoprolol with drugs that inhibit CYP2D6, such as quinidine, is likely to increase metoprolol concentration; this increase in plasma concentration would decrease the cardioselectivity of metoprolol). Products include:
Gleevec Tablets 2227

Imipramine Hydrochloride (Co-administration of metoprolol with drugs that inhibit CYP2D6, such as quinidine, is likely to increase metoprolol concentration; this increase in plasma concentration would decrease the cardioselectivity of metoprolol).
No products indexed under this heading.

Imipramine Pamoate (Co-administration of metoprolol with drugs that inhibit CYP2D6, such as quinidine, is likely to increase metoprolol concentration; this increase in plasma concentration would decrease the cardioselectivity of metoprolol).
No products indexed under this heading.

Isocarboxazid (Catecholamine-depleting drugs may have an additive effect when given with beta-blocking agents; monitor closely for signs of hypotension or marked bradycardia).
No products indexed under this heading.

Maprotiline Hydrochloride (Co-administration of metoprolol with drugs that inhibit CYP2D6, such as quinidine, is likely to increase metoprolol concentration; this increase in plasma concentration would decrease the cardioselectivity of metoprolol).
No products indexed under this heading.

Methadone Hydrochloride (Co-administration of metoprolol with drugs that inhibit CYP2D6, such as quinidine, is likely to increase metoprolol concentration; this increase in plasma concentration would decrease the cardioselectivity of metoprolol).
No products indexed under this heading.

Mibefradil Dihydrochloride (Co-administration of metoprolol with drugs that inhibit CYP2D6, such as quinidine, is likely to increase metoprolol concentration; this increase in plasma concentration would decrease the cardioselectivity of metoprolol).
No products indexed under this heading.

Moclobemide (Catecholamine-depleting drugs may have an additive effect when given with beta-blocking agents; monitor closely for signs of hypotension or marked bradycardia).
No products indexed under this heading.

Nortriptyline Hydrochloride (Co-administration of metoprolol with drugs that inhibit CYP2D6, such as quinidine, is likely to increase metoprolol concentration; this increase in plasma concentration would decrease the cardioselectivity of metoprolol).
No products indexed under this heading.

Pargyline Hydrochloride (Catecholamine-depleting drugs may have an additive effect when given with beta-blocking agents; monitor closely for signs of hypotension or marked bradycardia).
No products indexed under this heading.

Paroxetine Hydrochloride (Co-administration with drugs that inhibit CYP2D6, such as paroxetine, are likely to increase metoprolol concentrations; these increases in plasma concentration would decrease the cardioselectivity of metoprolol). Products include:
Paxil CR Controlled-Release Tablets 1538
Paxil 1530

Perphenazine (Co-administration of metoprolol with drugs that inhibit CYP2D6, such as quinidine, is likely to increase metoprolol concentration; this increase in plasma concentration would decrease the cardioselectivity of metoprolol).
No products indexed under this heading.

Phenelzine Sulfate (Catecholamine-depleting drugs may have an additive effect when given with beta-blocking agents; monitor closely for signs of hypotension or marked bradycardia).
No products indexed under this heading.

Procarbazine Hydrochloride (Catecholamine-depleting drugs may have an additive effect when given with beta-blocking agents; monitor closely for signs of hypotension or marked bradycardia). Products include:
Matulane Capsules 3191

Propafenone Hydrochloride (Co-administration with drugs that inhibit CYP2D6, such as propafenone, are likely to increase metoprolol concentrations; these increases in plasma concentration would decrease the cardioselectivity of metoprolol). Products include:
Rythmol SR Capsules 2727

Propoxyphene Hydrochloride (Co-administration of metoprolol with drugs that inhibit CYP2D6, such as quinidine, is likely to increase metoprolol concentration; this increase in plasma concentration would decrease the cardioselectivity of metoprolol).
No products indexed under this heading.

Propoxyphene Napsylate (Co-administration of metoprolol with drugs that inhibit CYP2D6, such as quinidine, is likely to increase metoprolol concentration; this increase in plasma concentration would decrease the cardioselectivity of metoprolol).
No products indexed under this heading.

Protriptyline Hydrochloride (Co-administration of metoprolol with drugs that inhibit CYP2D6, such as quinidine, is likely to increase metoprolol concentration; this increase in plasma concentration would decrease the cardioselectivity of metoprolol).
No products indexed under this heading.

Quinacrine Hydrochloride (Co-administration of metoprolol with drugs that inhibit CYP2D6, such as quinidine, is likely to increase metoprolol concentration; this increase in plasma concentration would decrease the cardioselectivity of metoprolol).
No products indexed under this heading.

Quinidine Gluconate (Co-administration of metoprolol with drugs that inhibit CYP2D6, such as quinidine, is likely to increase metoprolol concentration; this increase in plasma concentration would decrease the cardioselectivity of metoprolol).
No products indexed under this heading.

Quinidine Hydrochloride (Co-administration of metoprolol with drugs that inhibit CYP2D6, such as quinidine, is likely to increase metoprolol concentration; this increase in plasma concentration would decrease the cardioselectivity of metoprolol).
No products indexed under this heading.

Quinidine Polygalacturonate (Co-administration of metoprolol with drugs that inhibit CYP2D6, such as quinidine, is likely to increase metoprolol concentration; this increase in plasma concentration would decrease the cardioselectivity of metoprolol).
No products indexed under this heading.

Quinidine Sulfate (Co-administration of metoprolol with drugs that inhibit CYP2D6, such as quinidine, is likely to increase metoprolol concentration; this increase in plasma concentration would decrease the cardioselectivity of metoprolol).
No products indexed under this heading.

Ranitidine Bismuth Citrate (Co-administration of metoprolol with drugs that inhibit CYP2D6, such as quinidine, is likely to increase metoprolol concentration; this increase in plasma concentration would decrease the cardioselectivity of metoprolol).
No products indexed under this heading.

Ranitidine Hydrochloride (Co-administration of metoprolol with drugs that inhibit CYP2D6, such as quinidine, is likely to increase metoprolol concentration; this increase in plasma concentration would decrease the cardioselectivity of metoprolol). Products include:
Zantac 1624
Zantac Injection 1619
Zantac Injection Pharmacy Bulk Package.. 1622

Rauwolfia Serpentina (Catecholamine-depleting drugs may have an additive effect when given with beta-blocking agents; monitor closely for signs of hypotension or marked bradycardia).
No products indexed under this heading.

Rescinnamine (Catecholamine-depleting drugs may have an additive effect when given with beta-blocking agents; monitor closely for signs of hypotension or marked bradycardia).
No products indexed under this heading.

Reserpine (Catecholamine-depleting drugs may have an additive effect when given with beta-blocking agents; monitor closely for signs of hypotension or marked bradycardia).
No products indexed under this heading.

Ritonavir (Co-administration of metoprolol with drugs that inhibit CYP2D6, such as quinidine, is likely to increase metoprolol concentration; this increase in plasma concentration would decrease the cardioselectivity of metoprolol). Products include:
Kaletra 476
Norvir 503

Selegiline Hydrochloride (Catecholamine-depleting drugs may have an additive effect when given with beta-blocking agents; monitor closely for signs of hypotension or marked bradycardia). Products include:
Eldepryl Capsules 3208
Zelapar Tablets 3372

Sertraline Hydrochloride (Co-administration of metoprolol with drugs that inhibit CYP2D6, such as quinidine, is likely to increase metoprolol concentration; this increase in plasma concentration would decrease the cardioselectivity of metoprolol). Products include:
Zoloft 2586

Terbinafine Hydrochloride (Co-administration of metoprolol with drugs that inhibit CYP2D6, such as quinidine, is likely to increase metoprolol concentration; this increase in plasma concentration would decrease the cardioselectivity of metoprolol). Products include:

Lamisil Tablets 2232
Lamisil AT Creams (Athlete's Foot & Jock Itch) 636

Thioridazine Hydrochloride (Co-administration of metoprolol with drugs that inhibit CYP2D6, such as quinidine, is likely to increase metoprolol concentration; this increase in plasma concentration would decrease the cardioselectivity of metoprolol). Products include:

Thioridazine Hydrochloride Tablets 2163

Tranylcypromine Sulfate (Catecholamine-depleting drugs may have an additive effect when given with beta-blocking agents; monitor closely for signs of hypotension or marked bradycardia). Products include:

Parnate Tablets 1527

Trimipramine Maleate (Co-administration of metoprolol with drugs that inhibit CYP2D6, such as quinidine, is likely to increase metoprolol concentration; this increase in plasma concentration would decrease the cardioselectivity of metoprolol).

No products indexed under this heading.

Verapamil Hydrochloride (Because of significant inotropic and chronotropic effects in patients treated with beta-blockers and calcium-channel blockers of the verapamil type, caution should be exercised in patients treated with these agents concomitantly). Products include:

Covera-HS Tablets 3139
Tarka Tablets 524
Verelan PM Extended-Release Capsules, Controlled-Onset 3106

TRACLEER TABLETS

(Bosentan) 545

May interact with cytochrome p450 2c9 inhibitors (selected), cytochrome p450 3a4 inhibitors (selected), oral contraceptives, and certain other agents. Compounds in these categories include:

Acetazolamide (Co-administration of both a CYP2C9 inhibitor and a CYP3A4 inhibitor with bosentan will likely lead to large increases in plasma concentrations of bosentan and is not recommended).

No products indexed under this heading.

Amiodarone Hydrochloride (Co-administration of both a CYP2C9 inhibitor and a CYP3A4 inhibitor with bosentan will likely lead to large increases in plasma concentrations of bosentan and is not recommended).

No products indexed under this heading.

Amprenavir (Co-administration of both a CYP2C9 inhibitor and a CYP3A4 inhibitor with bosentan will likely lead to large increases in plasma concentrations of bosentan and is not recommended). Products include:

Agenerase Capsules 1327
Agenerase Oral Solution 1332

Anastrozole (Co-administration of both a CYP2C9 inhibitor and a CYP3A4 inhibitor with bosentan will likely lead to large increases in plasma concentrations of bosentan and is not recommended). Products include:

Arimidex Tablets 673

Aprepitant (Co-administration of both a CYP2C9 inhibitor and a CYP3A4 inhibitor with bosentan will likely lead to large increases in plasma concentrations of bosentan and is not recommended). Products include:

Emend Capsules 1963

Atorvastatin Calcium (Bosentan is expected to reduce plasma concentrations of statins that have significant metabolism by CYP3A4, such as atorvastatin). Products include:

Caduet Tablets 2508
Lipitor Tablets 2483

Bendroflumethiazide (Co-administration of both a CYP2C9 inhibitor and a CYP3A4 inhibitor with bosentan will likely lead to large increases in plasma concentrations of bosentan and is not recommended).

No products indexed under this heading.

Chloramphenicol (Co-administration of both a CYP2C9 inhibitor and a CYP3A4 inhibitor with bosentan will likely lead to large increases in plasma concentrations of bosentan and is not recommended).

No products indexed under this heading.

Chlorothiazide (Co-administration of both a CYP2C9 inhibitor and a CYP3A4 inhibitor with bosentan will likely lead to large increases in plasma concentrations of bosentan and is not recommended). Products include:

Diuril Oral Suspension 1954

Chlorothiazide Sodium (Co-administration of both a CYP2C9 inhibitor and a CYP3A4 inhibitor with bosentan will likely lead to large increases in plasma concentrations of bosentan and is not recommended). Products include:

Diuril Sodium Intravenous 2467

Chlorpropamide (Co-administration of both a CYP2C9 inhibitor and a CYP3A4 inhibitor with bosentan will likely lead to large increases in plasma concentrations of bosentan and is not recommended).

No products indexed under this heading.

Cimetidine (Co-administration of both a CYP2C9 inhibitor and a CYP3A4 inhibitor with bosentan will likely lead to large increases in plasma concentrations of bosentan and is not recommended). Products include:

Tagamet HB 200 Tablets 664

Cimetidine Hydrochloride (Co-administration of both a CYP2C9 inhibitor and a CYP3A4 inhibitor with bosentan will likely lead to large increases in plasma concentrations of bosentan and is not recommended).

No products indexed under this heading.

Ciprofloxacin (Co-administration of both a CYP2C9 inhibitor and a CYP3A4 inhibitor with bosentan will likely lead to large increases in plasma concentrations of bosentan and is not recommended). Products include:

Cipro Oral Suspension 2977
Cipro I.V. 2984
Cipro XR Tablets 2990
Ciprodex Otic Suspension 559

Clarithromycin (Co-administration of both a CYP2C9 inhibitor and a CYP3A4 inhibitor with bosentan will likely lead to large increases in plasma concentrations of bosentan and is not recommended). Products include:

Biaxin/Biaxin XL 402
PREVPAC 3284

Clopidogrel Hydrogen Sulfate (Co-administration of both a CYP2C9 inhibitor and a CYP3A4 inhibitor with bosentan will likely lead to large increases in plasma concentrations of bosentan and is not recommended).

No products indexed under this heading.

Clotrimazole (Co-administration of both a CYP2C9 inhibitor and a CYP3A4 inhibitor with bosentan will likely lead to large increases in plasma concentrations of bosentan and is not recommended). Products include:

Desenex Athlete's Foot Cream 635
Lotrimin 3039
Lotrisone 3040

Cyclosporine (Co-administration has resulted in markedly increased plasma concentrations of bosentan; concurrent use is contraindicated). Products include:

Gengraf Capsules 459
Neoral Oral Solution 2259
Neoral Soft Gelatin Capsules 2259
Restasis Ophthalmic Emulsion 575
Sandimmune 2275

Dalfopristin (Co-administration of both a CYP2C9 inhibitor and a CYP3A4 inhibitor with bosentan will likely lead to large increases in plasma concentrations of bosentan and is not recommended).

No products indexed under this heading.

Danazol (Co-administration of both a CYP2C9 inhibitor and a CYP3A4 inhibitor with bosentan will likely lead to large increases in plasma concentrations of bosentan and is not recommended).

No products indexed under this heading.

Delavirdine Mesylate (Co-administration of both a CYP2C9 inhibitor and a CYP3A4 inhibitor with bosentan will likely lead to large increases in plasma concentrations of bosentan and is not recommended). Products include:

Rescriptor Tablets 2551

Desogestrel (Co-administration increases the possibility of failure of contraception. Women should practice additional methods of contraception). Products include:

Mircette Tablets 1066

Diclofenac Potassium (Co-administration of both a CYP2C9 inhibitor and a CYP3A4 inhibitor with bosentan will likely lead to large increases in plasma concentrations of bosentan and is not recommended).

No products indexed under this heading.

Diclofenac Sodium (Co-administration of both a CYP2C9 inhibitor and a CYP3A4 inhibitor with bosentan will likely lead to large increases in plasma concentrations of bosentan and is not recommended). Products include:

Arthrotec Tablets 3129
Voltaren Ophthalmic Solution 2309
Voltaren Tablets 2307
Voltaren-XR Tablets 2310

Diltiazem Hydrochloride (Co-administration of both a CYP2C9 inhibitor and a CYP3A4 inhibitor with bosentan will likely lead to large increases in plasma concentrations of bosentan and is not recommended). Products include:

Cardizem LA Extended Release Tablets 1728
Tiazac Capsules 1201

Diltiazem Maleate (Co-administration of both a CYP2C9 inhibitor and a CYP3A4 inhibitor with bosentan will likely lead to large increases in plasma concentrations of bosentan and is not recommended).

No products indexed under this heading.

Disulfiram (Co-administration of both a CYP2C9 inhibitor and a CYP3A4 inhibitor with bosentan will likely lead to large increases in plasma concentrations of bosentan and is not recommended).

No products indexed under this heading.

Efavirenz (Co-administration of both a CYP2C9 inhibitor and a CYP3A4 inhibitor with bosentan will likely lead to large increases in plasma concentrations of bosentan and is not recommended). Products include:

Atripla Tablets 945
Sustiva Capsules 930
Sustiva Tablets 930

Erythromycin (Co-administration of both a CYP2C9 inhibitor and a CYP3A4 inhibitor with bosentan will likely lead to large increases in plasma concentrations of bosentan and is not recommended). Products include:

Ery-Tab Tablets 449
Erythromycin Base Filmtab Tablets 455
Erythromycin Delayed-Release Capsules, USP 457
PCE Dispertab Tablets 515

Erythromycin Estolate (Co-administration of both a CYP2C9 inhibitor and a CYP3A4 inhibitor with bosentan will likely lead to large increases in plasma concentrations of bosentan and is not recommended).

No products indexed under this heading.

Erythromycin Ethylsuccinate (Co-administration of both a CYP2C9 inhibitor and a CYP3A4 inhibitor with bosentan will likely lead to large increases in plasma concentrations of bosentan and is not recommended). Products include:

E.E.S. 451
EryPed 447

Erythromycin Gluceptate (Co-administration of both a CYP2C9 inhibitor and a CYP3A4 inhibitor with bosentan will likely lead to large increases in plasma concentrations of bosentan and is not recommended).

No products indexed under this heading.

Erythromycin Lactobionate (Co-administration of both a CYP2C9 inhibitor and a CYP3A4 inhibitor with bosentan will likely lead to large increases in plasma concentrations of bosentan and is not recommended).
No products indexed under this heading.

Erythromycin Stearate (Co-administration of both a CYP2C9 inhibitor and a CYP3A4 inhibitor with bosentan will likely lead to large increases in plasma concentrations of bosentan and is not recommended). Products include:
Erythrocin Stearate Filmtab Tablets 453

Esomeprazole Magnesium (Co-administration of both a CYP2C9 inhibitor and a CYP3A4 inhibitor with bosentan will likely lead to large increases in plasma concentrations of bosentan and is not recommended). Products include:
Nexium Delayed-Release Capsules 655

Ethinyl Estradiol (Co-administration increases the possibility of failure of contraception. Women should practice additional methods of contraception). Products include:
Mircette Tablets 1066
NuvaRing 2340
Ortho-Cyclen/Ortho Tri-Cyclen 2429
Ortho Evra Transdermal System 2417
Ortho Tri-Cyclen Lo Tablets 2436
Seasonique Tablets 1077
Yasmin 28 Tablets 796
Yaz Tablets 803

Ethynodiol Diacetate (Co-administration increases the possibility of failure of contraception. Women should practice additional methods of contraception).
No products indexed under this heading.

Fenofibrate (Co-administration of both a CYP2C9 inhibitor and a CYP3A4 inhibitor with bosentan will likely lead to large increases in plasma concentrations of bosentan and is not recommended). Products include:
Lofibra Tablets 1219
Lofibra Capsules 1216
Tricor Tablets 527
Triglide Tablets 3123

Fluconazole (Co-administration of both a CYP2C9 inhibitor and a CYP3A4 inhibitor with bosentan will likely lead to large increases in plasma concentrations of bosentan and is not recommended).
No products indexed under this heading.

Fluorouracil (Co-administration of both a CYP2C9 inhibitor and a CYP3A4 inhibitor with bosentan will likely lead to large increases in plasma concentrations of bosentan and is not recommended). Products include:
Carac Cream, 0.5% 2879
Efudex 3363

Fluoxetine Hydrochloride (Co-administration of both a CYP2C9 inhibitor and a CYP3A4 inhibitor with bosentan will likely lead to large increases in plasma concentrations of bosentan and is not recommended). Products include:
Prozac Pulvules and Liquid 1801
Symbyax Capsules 1819

Flurbiprofen (Co-administration of both a CYP2C9 inhibitor and a CYP3A4 inhibitor with bosentan will likely lead to large increases in plasma concentrations of bosentan and is not recommended).
No products indexed under this heading.

Flurbiprofen Sodium (Co-administration of both a CYP2C9 inhibitor and a CYP3A4 inhibitor with bosentan will likely lead to large increases in plasma concentrations of bosentan and is not recommended). Products include:
Ocufen Ophthalmic Solution .... ⊙ 232

Fluvastatin Sodium (Co-administration of both a CYP2C9 inhibitor and a CYP3A4 inhibitor with bosentan will likely lead to large increases in plasma concentrations of bosentan and is not recommended). Products include:
Lescol Capsules 2233
Lescol XL Tablets 2233

Fluvoxamine Maleate (Co-administration of both a CYP2C9 inhibitor and a CYP3A4 inhibitor with bosentan will likely lead to large increases in plasma concentrations of bosentan and is not recommended).
No products indexed under this heading.

Fosamprenavir Calcium (Co-administration of both a CYP2C9 inhibitor and a CYP3A4 inhibitor with bosentan will likely lead to large increases in plasma concentrations of bosentan and is not recommended). Products include:
Lexiva Tablets 1505

Gemfibrozil (Co-administration of both a CYP2C9 inhibitor and a CYP3A4 inhibitor with bosentan will likely lead to large increases in plasma concentrations of bosentan and is not recommended).
No products indexed under this heading.

Glipizide (Co-administration of both a CYP2C9 inhibitor and a CYP3A4 inhibitor with bosentan will likely lead to large increases in plasma concentrations of bosentan and is not recommended).
No products indexed under this heading.

Glyburide (Co-administration increases the risk of liver enzyme elevation; concurrent use is contraindicated).
No products indexed under this heading.

Hydrochlorothiazide (Co-administration of both a CYP2C9 inhibitor and a CYP3A4 inhibitor with bosentan will likely lead to large increases in plasma concentrations of bosentan and is not recommended). Products include:
Aldoril Tablets 1910
Atacand HCT 651
Avalide Tablets 888
Avalide Tablets 2874
Benicar HCT Tablets 1044
Diovan HCT Tablets 2196
Dyazide Capsules 1423
Hyzaar 50-12.5 Tablets 1990
Hyzaar 100-12.5 Tablets 1990
Hyzaar 100-25 Tablets 1990
Lopressor HCT 50/25 Tablets 2241
Lopressor HCT 100/25 Tablets 2241
Lopressor HCT 100/50 Tablets 2241
Lotensin HCT Tablets 2246
Micardis HCT Tablets 856
Moduretic Tablets 2028
Prinzide Tablets 2056
Teveten HCT Tablets 1737
Timolide Tablets 2086
Uniretic Tablets 3100

Hydroflumethiazide (Co-administration of both a CYP2C9 inhibitor and a CYP3A4 inhibitor with bosentan will likely lead to large increases in plasma concentrations of bosentan and is not recommended).
No products indexed under this heading.

Imatinib Mesylate (Co-administration of both a CYP2C9 inhibitor and a CYP3A4 inhibitor with bosentan will likely lead to large increases in plasma concentrations of bosentan and is not recommended). Products include:
Gleevec Tablets 2227

Indinavir Sulfate (Co-administration of both a CYP2C9 inhibitor and a CYP3A4 inhibitor with bosentan will likely lead to large increases in plasma concentrations of bosentan and is not recommended). Products include:
Crixivan Capsules 1940

Isoniazid (Co-administration of both a CYP2C9 inhibitor and a CYP3A4 inhibitor with bosentan will likely lead to large increases in plasma concentrations of bosentan and is not recommended).
No products indexed under this heading.

Itraconazole (Co-administration of both a CYP2C9 inhibitor and a CYP3A4 inhibitor with bosentan will likely lead to large increases in plasma concentrations of bosentan and is not recommended).
No products indexed under this heading.

Ketoconazole (Co-administration increases the plasma concentrations of bosentan by approximately two-fold). Products include:
Nizoral A-D Shampoo, 1% 1868

Ketoprofen (Co-administration of both a CYP2C9 inhibitor and a CYP3A4 inhibitor with bosentan will likely lead to large increases in plasma concentrations of bosentan and is not recommended).
No products indexed under this heading.

Leflunomide (Co-administration of both a CYP2C9 inhibitor and a CYP3A4 inhibitor with bosentan will likely lead to large increases in plasma concentrations of bosentan and is not recommended).
No products indexed under this heading.

Levonorgestrel (Co-administration increases the possibility of failure of contraception. Women should practice additional methods of contraception). Products include:
Climara Pro Transdermal System 776
Mirena Intrauterine System 787
Plan B Tablets 1076
Seasonique Tablets 1077

Lopinavir (Co-administration of both a CYP2C9 inhibitor and a CYP3A4 inhibitor with bosentan will likely lead to large increases in plasma concentrations of bosentan and is not recommended). Products include:
Kaletra 476

Loratadine (Co-administration of both a CYP2C9 inhibitor and a CYP3A4 inhibitor with bosentan will likely lead to large increases in plasma concentrations of bosentan and is not recommended). Products include:
Alavert Allergy & Sinus D-12 Hour Tablets .... ■ 771
Alavert .... ■ 771
Children's Claritin Allergy Oral Solution .... ■ 771
Claritin Non-Drowsy 24 Hour Tablets .... ■ 772
Claritin Reditabs 24 Hour Non-Drowsy Tablets .... ■ 772
Claritin-D Non-Drowsy 12 Hour Tablets .... ■ 772
Claritin-D Non-Drowsy 24 Hour Tablets .... ■ 772

Lovastatin (Bosentan is expected to reduce plasma concentrations of statins that have significant metabolism by CYP3A4, such as lovastatin). Products include:
Advicor Tablets 1722
Altoprev Extended-Release Tablets 3109
Mevacor Tablets 2021

Mestranol (Co-administration increases the possibility of failure of contraception. Women should practice additional methods of contraception).
No products indexed under this heading.

Methyclothiazide (Co-administration of both a CYP2C9 inhibitor and a CYP3A4 inhibitor with bosentan will likely lead to large increases in plasma concentrations of bosentan and is not recommended).
No products indexed under this heading.

Metronidazole (Co-administration of both a CYP2C9 inhibitor and a CYP3A4 inhibitor with bosentan will likely lead to large increases in plasma concentrations of bosentan and is not recommended). Products include:
Metrogel 1% 1211
MetroGel-Vaginal Gel 1855
Vandazole Vaginal Gel 3338

Metronidazole Benzoate (Co-administration of both a CYP2C9 inhibitor and a CYP3A4 inhibitor with bosentan will likely lead to large increases in plasma concentrations of bosentan and is not recommended).
No products indexed under this heading.

Metronidazole Hydrochloride (Co-administration of both a CYP2C9 inhibitor and a CYP3A4 inhibitor with bosentan will likely lead to large increases in plasma concentrations of bosentan and is not recommended).
No products indexed under this heading.

Miconazole (Co-administration of both a CYP2C9 inhibitor and a CYP3A4 inhibitor with bosentan will likely lead to large increases in plasma concentrations of bosentan and is not recommended).
No products indexed under this heading.

Miconazole Nitrate (Co-administration of both a CYP2C9 inhibitor and a CYP3A4 inhibitor with bosentan will likely lead to large increases in plasma concentrations of bosentan and is not recommended). Products include:
Desenex .... ■ 635
Desenex Jock Itch Spray Powder .... ■ 635

Modafinil (Co-administration of both a CYP2C9 inhibitor and a CYP3A4

inhibitor with bosentan will likely lead to large increases in plasma concentrations of bosentan and is not recommended). Products include:

Nefazodone Hydrochloride (Co-administration of both a CYP2C9 inhibitor and a CYP3A4 inhibitor with bosentan will likely lead to large increases in plasma concentrations of bosentan and is not recommended).
No products indexed under this heading.

Nelfinavir Mesylate (Co-administration of both a CYP2C9 inhibitor and a CYP3A4 inhibitor with bosentan will likely lead to large increases in plasma concentrations of bosentan and is not recommended). Products include:

Nevirapine (Co-administration of both a CYP2C9 inhibitor and a CYP3A4 inhibitor with bosentan will likely lead to large increases in plasma concentrations of bosentan and is not recommended). Products include:

Niacinamide (Co-administration of both a CYP2C9 inhibitor and a CYP3A4 inhibitor with bosentan will likely lead to large increases in plasma concentrations of bosentan and is not recommended).
No products indexed under this heading.

Nicotinamide (Co-administration of both a CYP2C9 inhibitor and a CYP3A4 inhibitor with bosentan will likely lead to large increases in plasma concentrations of bosentan and is not recommended). Products include:

Nifedipine (Co-administration of both a CYP2C9 inhibitor and a CYP3A4 inhibitor with bosentan will likely lead to large increases in plasma concentrations of bosentan and is not recommended). Products include:

Norethindrone (Co-administration increases the possibility of failure of contraception. Women should practice additional methods of contraception). Products include:

Norethynodrel (Co-administration increases the possibility of failure of contraception. Women should practice additional methods of contraception).
No products indexed under this heading.

Norfloxacin (Co-administration of both a CYP2C9 inhibitor and a CYP3A4 inhibitor with bosentan will likely lead to large increases in plasma concentrations of bosentan and is not recommended). Products include:

Norgestimate (Co-administration increases the possibility of failure of contraception. Women should practice additional methods of contraception). Products include:

Norgestrel (Co-administration increases the possibility of failure of contraception. Women should practice additional methods of contraception).
No products indexed under this heading.

Omeprazole (Co-administration of both a CYP2C9 inhibitor and a CYP3A4 inhibitor with bosentan will likely lead to large increases in plasma concentrations of bosentan and is not recommended). Products include:

Oxiconazole Nitrate (Co-administration of both a CYP2C9 inhibitor and a CYP3A4 inhibitor with bosentan will likely lead to large increases in plasma concentrations of bosentan and is not recommended). Products include:

Paroxetine Hydrochloride (Co-administration of both a CYP2C9 inhibitor and a CYP3A4 inhibitor with bosentan will likely lead to large increases in plasma concentrations of bosentan and is not recommended). Products include:

Phenylbutazone (Co-administration of both a CYP2C9 inhibitor and a CYP3A4 inhibitor with bosentan will likely lead to large increases in plasma concentrations of bosentan and is not recommended).
No products indexed under this heading.

Polythiazide (Co-administration of both a CYP2C9 inhibitor and a CYP3A4 inhibitor with bosentan will likely lead to large increases in plasma concentrations of bosentan and is not recommended).
No products indexed under this heading.

Propoxyphene Hydrochloride (Co-administration of both a CYP2C9 inhibitor and a CYP3A4 inhibitor with bosentan will likely lead to large increases in plasma concentrations of bosentan and is not recommended).
No products indexed under this heading.

Propoxyphene Napsylate (Co-administration of both a CYP2C9 inhibitor and a CYP3A4 inhibitor with bosentan will likely lead to large increases in plasma concentrations of bosentan and is not recommended).
No products indexed under this heading.

Quinidine (Co-administration of both a CYP2C9 inhibitor and a CYP3A4 inhibitor with bosentan will likely lead to large increases in plasma concentrations of bosentan and is not recommended).
No products indexed under this heading.

Quinidine Hydrochloride (Co-administration of both a CYP2C9 inhibitor and a CYP3A4 inhibitor with bosentan will likely lead to large increases in plasma concentrations of bosentan and is not recommended).
No products indexed under this heading.

Quinidine Polygalacturonate (Co-administration of both a CYP2C9 inhibitor and a CYP3A4 inhibitor with bosentan will likely lead to large increases in plasma concentrations of bosentan and is not recommended).
No products indexed under this heading.

Quinidine Sulfate (Co-administration of both a CYP2C9 inhibitor and a CYP3A4 inhibitor with bosentan will likely lead to large increases in plasma concentrations of bosentan and is not recommended).
No products indexed under this heading.

Quinine (Co-administration of both a CYP2C9 inhibitor and a CYP3A4 inhibitor with bosentan will likely lead to large increases in plasma concentrations of bosentan and is not recommended).
No products indexed under this heading.

Quinine Sulfate (Co-administration of both a CYP2C9 inhibitor and a CYP3A4 inhibitor with bosentan will likely lead to large increases in plasma concentrations of bosentan and is not recommended).
No products indexed under this heading.

Quinupristin (Co-administration of both a CYP2C9 inhibitor and a CYP3A4 inhibitor with bosentan will likely lead to large increases in plasma concentrations of bosentan and is not recommended).
No products indexed under this heading.

Ranitidine Bismuth Citrate (Co-administration of both a CYP2C9 inhibitor and a CYP3A4 inhibitor with bosentan will likely lead to large increases in plasma concentrations of bosentan and is not recommended).
No products indexed under this heading.

Ranitidine Hydrochloride (Co-administration of both a CYP2C9 inhibitor and a CYP3A4 inhibitor with bosentan will likely lead to large increases in plasma concentrations of bosentan and is not recommended). Products include:

Ritonavir (Co-administration of both a CYP2C9 inhibitor and a CYP3A4 inhibitor with bosentan will likely lead to large increases in plasma concentrations of bosentan and is not recommended). Products include:

Saquinavir (Co-administration of both a CYP2C9 inhibitor and a CYP3A4 inhibitor with bosentan will likely lead to large increases in plasma concentrations of bosentan and is not recommended).
No products indexed under this heading.

Saquinavir Mesylate (Co-administration of both a CYP2C9 inhibitor and a CYP3A4 inhibitor with bosentan will likely lead to large increases in plasma concentrations of bosentan and is not recommended). Products include:

Sertraline Hydrochloride (Co-administration of both a CYP2C9 inhibitor and a CYP3A4 inhibitor with bosentan will likely lead to large increases in plasma concentrations of bosentan and is not recommended). Products include:

Simvastatin (Co-administration decreases plasma concentrations of simvastatin and its active metabolite by 50%). Products include:

Sulfacytine (Co-administration of both a CYP2C9 inhibitor and a CYP3A4 inhibitor with bosentan will likely lead to large increases in plasma concentrations of bosentan and is not recommended).
No products indexed under this heading.

Sulfamethizole (Co-administration of both a CYP2C9 inhibitor and a CYP3A4 inhibitor with bosentan will likely lead to large increases in plasma concentrations of bosentan and is not recommended).
No products indexed under this heading.

Sulfamethoxazole (Co-administration of both a CYP2C9 inhibitor and a CYP3A4 inhibitor with bosentan will likely lead to large increases in plasma concentrations of bosentan and is not recommended).
No products indexed under this heading.

Sulfasalazine (Co-administration of both a CYP2C9 inhibitor and a CYP3A4 inhibitor with bosentan will likely lead to large increases in plasma concentrations of bosentan and is not recommended).
No products indexed under this heading.

Sulfinpyrazone (Co-administration of both a CYP2C9 inhibitor and a CYP3A4 inhibitor with bosentan will likely lead to large increases in plasma concentrations of bosentan and is not recommended).
No products indexed under this heading.

Sulfisoxazole Acetyl (Co-administration of both a CYP2C9 inhibitor and a CYP3A4 inhibitor with bosentan will likely lead to large increases in plasma concentrations of bosentan and is not recommended).
No products indexed under this heading.

Sulfisoxazole Diolamine (Co-administration of both a CYP2C9 inhibitor and a CYP3A4 inhibitor with bosentan will likely lead to large increases in plasma concentrations of bosentan and is not recommended).
No products indexed under this heading.

Tacrolimus (Caution should be exercised if tacrolimus and bosentan are used together). Products include:

IMPORTANT NOTE: Always consult each drug listing in the patient's regimen for possible interactions.

Telithromycin (Co-administration of both a CYP2C9 inhibitor and a CYP3A4 inhibitor with bosentan will likely lead to large increases in plasma concentrations of bosentan and is not recommended). Products include:
Ketek Tablets **2903**

Terconazole (Co-administration of both a CYP2C9 inhibitor and a CYP3A4 inhibitor with bosentan will likely lead to large increases in plasma concentrations of bosentan and is not recommended).
No products indexed under this heading.

Ticlopidine Hydrochloride (Co-administration of both a CYP2C9 inhibitor and a CYP3A4 inhibitor with bosentan will likely lead to large increases in plasma concentrations of bosentan and is not recommended). Products include:
Ticlid Tablets **2810**

Tolazamide (Co-administration of both a CYP2C9 inhibitor and a CYP3A4 inhibitor with bosentan will likely lead to large increases in plasma concentrations of bosentan and is not recommended).
No products indexed under this heading.

Tolbutamide (Co-administration of both a CYP2C9 inhibitor and a CYP3A4 inhibitor with bosentan will likely lead to large increases in plasma concentrations of bosentan and is not recommended).
No products indexed under this heading.

Tolbutamide Sodium (Co-administration of both a CYP2C9 inhibitor and a CYP3A4 inhibitor with bosentan will likely lead to large increases in plasma concentrations of bosentan and is not recommended).
No products indexed under this heading.

Troglitazone (Co-administration of both a CYP2C9 inhibitor and a CYP3A4 inhibitor with bosentan will likely lead to large increases in plasma concentrations of bosentan and is not recommended).
No products indexed under this heading.

Troleandomycin (Co-administration of both a CYP2C9 inhibitor and a CYP3A4 inhibitor with bosentan will likely lead to large increases in plasma concentrations of bosentan and is not recommended).
No products indexed under this heading.

Valproate Sodium (Co-administration of both a CYP2C9 inhibitor and a CYP3A4 inhibitor with bosentan will likely lead to large increases in plasma concentrations of bosentan and is not recommended). Products include:
Depacon Injection **412**

Verapamil Hydrochloride (Co-administration of both a CYP2C9 inhibitor and a CYP3A4 inhibitor with bosentan will likely lead to large increases in plasma concentrations of bosentan and is not recommended). Products include:
Covera-HS Tablets **3139**
Tarka Tablets **524**
Verelan PM Extended-Release Capsules, Controlled-Onset **3106**

Voriconazole (Co-administration of both a CYP2C9 inhibitor and a CYP3A4 inhibitor with bosentan will likely lead to large increases in plasma concentrations of bosentan and is not recommended). Products include:
VFEND I.V. **2564**
VFEND Oral Suspension **2564**
VFEND Tablets **2564**

Zafirlukast (Co-administration of both a CYP2C9 inhibitor and a CYP3A4 inhibitor with bosentan will likely lead to large increases in plasma concentrations of bosentan and is not recommended). Products include:
Accolate Tablets **671**

Zileuton (Co-administration of both a CYP2C9 inhibitor and a CYP3A4 inhibitor with bosentan will likely lead to large increases in plasma concentrations of bosentan and is not recommended). Products include:
Zyflo Tablets **1023**

Food Interactions

Grapefruit (Co-administration of both a CYP2C9 inhibitor and a CYP3A4 inhibitor with bosentan will likely lead to large increases in plasma concentrations of bosentan and is not recommended).

Grapefruit Juice (Co-administration of both a CYP2C9 inhibitor and a CYP3A4 inhibitor with bosentan will likely lead to large increases in plasma concentrations of bosentan and is not recommended).

TRANSDERM SCOP TRANSDERMAL THERAPEUTIC SYSTEM

(Scopolamine) **2177**
May interact with anticholinergics, antihistamines, central nervous system depressants, hypnotics and sedatives, muscle relaxants, tranquilizers, tricyclic antidepressants, and certain other agents. Compounds in these categories include:

Acrivastine (Antihistamines have anticholinergic properties and co-administration may result in additive effects).
No products indexed under this heading.

Alfentanil Hydrochloride (Scopolamine is an anticholinergic agent and causes certain CNS effects, such as drowsiness and dizziness, and hence it should be used with care in patients on concomitant therapy).
No products indexed under this heading.

Alprazolam (Scopolamine is an anticholinergic agent and causes certain CNS effects, such as drowsiness and dizziness, and hence it should be used with care in patients on concomitant therapy). Products include:
Niravam Orally Disintegrating Tablets **3092**

Amitriptyline Hydrochloride (Tricyclic antidepressants have anticholinergic properties and co-administration may result in additive effects).
No products indexed under this heading.

Amoxapine (Tricyclic antidepressants have anticholinergic properties and co-administration may result in additive effects).
No products indexed under this heading.

Aprobarbital (Scopolamine is an anticholinergic agent and causes certain CNS effects, such as drowsiness and dizziness, and hence it should be used with care in patients on concomitant therapy).
No products indexed under this heading.

Astemizole (Antihistamines have anticholinergic properties and co-administration may result in additive effects).
No products indexed under this heading.

Atracurium Besylate (Co-administration may result in addititve anticholinergic effects).
No products indexed under this heading.

Atropine Sulfate (Co-administration may result in additive anticholinergic effects). Products include:
Donnatal Extentabs **2493**

Azatadine Maleate (Antihistamines have anticholinergic properties and co-administration may result in additive effects).
No products indexed under this heading.

Baclofen (Co-administration may result in addititve anticholinergic effects).
No products indexed under this heading.

Belladonna Alkaloids (Co-administration may result in additive anticholinergic effects). Products include:
Hyland's Teething Tablets .... ▣**830**

Benztropine Mesylate (Co-administration may result in additive anticholinergic effects).
No products indexed under this heading.

Biperiden Hydrochloride (Co-administration may result in additive anticholinergic effects).
No products indexed under this heading.

Bromodiphenhydramine Hydrochloride (Antihistamines have anticholinergic properties and co-administration may result in additive effects).
No products indexed under this heading.

Brompheniramine Maleate (Antihistamines have anticholinergic properties and co-administration may result in additive effects). Products include:
Children's Dimetapp Cold & Allergy Elixir .... ▣**730**
Children's Dimetapp Cold & Allergy Chewable Tablets .... ▣**730**
Children's Dimetapp DM Cold & Cough Elixir .... ▣**731**

Buprenorphine Hydrochloride (Scopolamine is an anticholinergic agent and causes certain CNS effects, such as drowsiness and dizziness, and hence it should be used with care in patients on concomitant therapy). Products include:
Buprenex Injectable **2716**
Suboxone Tablets **2717**
Subutex Tablets **2717**

Buspirone Hydrochloride (Scopolamine is an anticholinergic agent and causes certain CNS effects, such as drowsiness and dizziness, and hence it should be used with care in patients on concomitant therapy).
No products indexed under this heading.

Butabarbital (Scopolamine is an anticholinergic agent and causes certain CNS effects, such as drowsiness and dizziness, and hence it should be used with care in patients on concomitant therapy).
No products indexed under this heading.

Butalbital (Scopolamine is an anticholinergic agent and causes certain CNS effects, such as drowsiness and dizziness, and hence it should be used with care in patients on concomitant therapy).
No products indexed under this heading.

Carisoprodol (Co-administration may result in addititve anticholinergic effects).
No products indexed under this heading.

Cetirizine Hydrochloride (Antihistamines have anticholinergic properties and co-administration may result in additive effects). Products include:
Zyrtec Chewable Tablets **2594**
Zyrtec **2594**
Zyrtec-D 12 Hour Extended Release Tablets **2597**

Chlordiazepoxide (Scopolamine is an anticholinergic agent and causes certain CNS effects, such as drowsiness and dizziness, and hence it should be used with care in patients on concomitant therapy).
No products indexed under this heading.

Chlordiazepoxide Hydrochloride (Scopolamine is an anticholinergic agent and causes certain CNS effects, such as drowsiness and dizziness, and hence it should be used with care in patients on concomitant therapy). Products include:
Librium Capsules **3347**

Chlorpheniramine Maleate (Antihistamines have anticholinergic properties and co-administration may result in additive effects). Products include:
Advil Allergy Sinus Caplets .... ▣**770**
Advil Multi-Symptom Cold Caplets .... ▣**770**
BC Allergy Sinus Cold Powder .... ▣**677**
Comtrex Maximum Strength Cold & Cough Day/Night Caplets - Night Formulation .... ▣**726**
Comtrex Maximum Strength Day/Night Severe Cold & Sinus Caplets - Night Formulation .... ▣**725**
Contac Cold and Flu Maximum Strength Caplets .... ▣**728**
Contac Cold and Flu Day and Night Caplets (Night Formulation Only) .... ▣**727**
Children's Dimetapp Long Acting Cough Plus Cold Syrup .... ▣**731**
Robitussin Cough & Cold Long-Acting Liquid .... ▣**735**
Robitussin Cough & Allergy Syrup .. ▣**736**
Robitussin Cough & Cold Nighttime Liquid .... ▣**736**
Robitussin Cough, Cold & Flu Nighttime Liquid .... ▣**738**
Robitussin Pediatric Cough & Cold Long-Acting Liquid .... ▣**735**
Robitussin Pediatric Cough & Cold Nighttime Liquid .... ▣**736**
Triaminic Cold & Allergy Liquid .... ▣**746**
Triaminic Cough & Runny Nose Softchews .... ▣**748**
Children's Tylenol Plus Flu Oral Suspension .... ▣**749**
Tylenol Allergy Multi-Symptom Caplets with Cool Burst and Gelcaps **1872**
Children's Tylenol Plus Cold Suspension Liquid **1879**
Children's Tylenol Plus Cough & Runny Nose Suspension Liquid **1879**

Children's Tylenol Plus Flu Suspension Liquid 1881
Children's Tylenol Plus Multi-Symptom Cold Suspension Liquid 1879
Tylenol Cold Head Congestion Nighttime Caplets with Cool Burst 1873
Tylenol Cold Multi-Symptom Nighttime Caplets with Cool Burst 1874
Tylenol Sinus Congestion & Pain Nighttime Caplets with Cool Burst 1876
Vicks 44M Cough, Cold & Flu Relief Liquid 2680
Pediatric Vicks 44m Cough & Cold Relief Liquid 2676
Children's Vicks NyQuil Cold/Cough Relief 756
Children's Vicks NyQuil Cold/Cough Relief Liquid 2680
Zicam Maximum Strength Flu Daytime 768

Chlorpheniramine Polistirex (Antihistamines have anticholinergic properties and co-administration may result in additive effects). Products include:
Tussionex Pennkinetic Extended-Release Suspension 3327

Chlorpheniramine Tannate (Antihistamines have anticholinergic properties and co-administration may result in additive effects).
No products indexed under this heading.

Chlorpromazine (Scopolamine is an anticholinergic agent and causes certain CNS effects, such as drowsiness and dizziness, and hence it should be used with care in patients on concomitant therapy).
No products indexed under this heading.

Chlorpromazine Hydrochloride (Scopolamine is an anticholinergic agent and causes certain CNS effects, such as drowsiness and dizziness, and hence it should be used with care in patients on concomitant therapy).
No products indexed under this heading.

Chlorprothixene (Scopolamine is an anticholinergic agent and causes certain CNS effects, such as drowsiness and dizziness, and hence it should be used with care in patients on concomitant therapy).
No products indexed under this heading.

Chlorprothixene Hydrochloride (Scopolamine is an anticholinergic agent and causes certain CNS effects, such as drowsiness and dizziness, and hence it should be used with care in patients on concomitant therapy).
No products indexed under this heading.

Chlorprothixene Lactate (Scopolamine is an anticholinergic agent and causes certain CNS effects, such as drowsiness and dizziness, and hence it should be used with care in patients on concomitant therapy).
No products indexed under this heading.

Chlorzoxazone (Co-administration may result in addititve anticholinergic effects).
No products indexed under this heading.

Cisatracurium Besylate (Co-administration may result in addititve anticholinergic effects). Products include:
Nimbex Injection 498

Clemastine Fumarate (Antihistamines have anticholinergic properties and co-administration may result in additive effects).
No products indexed under this heading.

Clidinium Bromide (Co-administration may result in additive anticholinergic effects).
No products indexed under this heading.

Clomipramine Hydrochloride (Tricyclic antidepressants have anticholinergic properties and co-administration may result in additive effects).
No products indexed under this heading.

Clorazepate Dipotassium (Scopolamine is an anticholinergic agent and causes certain CNS effects, such as drowsiness and dizziness, and hence it should be used with care in patients on concomitant therapy). Products include:
Tranxene 2474

Clozapine (Scopolamine is an anticholinergic agent and causes certain CNS effects, such as drowsiness and dizziness, and hence it should be used with care in patients on concomitant therapy). Products include:
Clozaril Tablets 2184
FazaClo Orally Disintegrating Tablets 551

Codeine Phosphate (Scopolamine is an anticholinergic agent and causes certain CNS effects, such as drowsiness and dizziness, and hence it should be used with care in patients on concomitant therapy). Products include:
Tylenol with Codeine Tablets 2391

Cyclobenzaprine Hydrochloride (Co-administration may result in addititve anticholinergic effects).
No products indexed under this heading.

Cyproheptadine Hydrochloride (Antihistamines have anticholinergic properties and co-administration may result in additive effects).
No products indexed under this heading.

Dantrolene Sodium (Co-administration may result in addititve anticholinergic effects). Products include:
Dantrium Capsules 2694
Dantrium Intravenous 2695

Desflurane (Scopolamine is an anticholinergic agent and causes certain CNS effects, such as drowsiness and dizziness, and hence it should be used with care in patients on concomitant therapy).
No products indexed under this heading.

Desipramine Hydrochloride (Tricyclic antidepressants have anticholinergic properties and co-administration may result in additive effects).
No products indexed under this heading.

Dexchlorpheniramine Maleate (Antihistamines have anticholinergic properties and co-administration may result in additive effects).
No products indexed under this heading.

Dezocine (Scopolamine is an anticholinergic agent and causes certain CNS effects, such as drowsiness and dizziness, and hence it should be used with care in patients on concomitant therapy).
No products indexed under this heading.

Diazepam (Scopolamine is an anticholinergic agent and causes certain CNS effects, such as drowsiness and dizziness, and hence it should be used with care in patients on concomitant therapy). Products include:
Diastat Rectal Delivery System 3343
Valium Tablets 2819

Dicyclomine Hydrochloride (Co-administration may result in additive anticholinergic effects). Products include:
Bentyl Capsules 697
Bentyl Injection 697
Bentyl Syrup 697
Bentyl Tablets 697

Diphenhydramine Citrate (Antihistamines have anticholinergic properties and co-administration may result in additive effects). Products include:
Advil PM Caplets 615
Excedrin PM Caplets/Tablets/Geltabs 610
Goody's PM Powder for Pain with Sleeplessness 612

Diphenhydramine Hydrochloride (Antihistamines have anticholinergic properties and co-administration may result in additive effects). Products include:
Nytol QuickCaps Caplets 615
Nytol QuickGels Softgels Maximum Strength 616
Simply Sleep Caplets 1868
Sominex Original Formula Tablets .. 616
TheraFlu Warming Relief Nighttime Severe Cold 743
TheraFlu Thin Strips Multi Symptom 744
Triaminic Nighttime Cold & Cough Liquid 746
Triaminic Thin Strips Cough & Runny Nose 749
Extra Strength Tylenol PM Caplets, Vanilla Caplets, Geltabs, Gelcaps and Liquid 1875
Tylenol Sore Throat Nighttime Liquid with Cool Burst 790
Tylenol Allergy Multi-Symptom Nighttime Caplets with Cool Burst 1872
Tylenol Severe Allergy Caplets 1872
Children's Tylenol Plus Cold & Allergy Suspension Liquid 1878

Diphenylpyraline Hydrochloride (Antihistamines have anticholinergic properties and co-administration may result in additive effects).
No products indexed under this heading.

Doxacurium Chloride (Co-administration may result in addititve anticholinergic effects).
No products indexed under this heading.

Doxepin Hydrochloride (Tricyclic antidepressants have anticholinergic properties and co-administration may result in additive effects).
No products indexed under this heading.

Droperidol (Scopolamine is an anticholinergic agent and causes certain CNS effects, such as drowsiness and dizziness, and hence it should be used with care in patients on concomitant therapy).
No products indexed under this heading.

Enflurane (Scopolamine is an anticholinergic agent and causes certain CNS effects, such as drowsiness and dizziness, and hence it should be used with care in patients on concomitant therapy).
No products indexed under this heading.

Estazolam (Scopolamine is an anticholinergic agent and causes certain CNS effects, such as drowsiness and dizziness, and hence it should be used with care in patients on concomitant therapy). Products include:
ProSom Tablets 517

Ethanol (Scopolamine is an anticholinergic agent and causes certain CNS effects, such as drowsiness and dizziness, and hence it should be used with care in patients on concomitant therapy).
No products indexed under this heading.

Ethchlorvynol (Scopolamine is an anticholinergic agent and causes certain CNS effects, such as drowsiness and dizziness, and hence it should be used with care in patients on concomitant therapy).
No products indexed under this heading.

Ethinamate (Scopolamine is an anticholinergic agent and causes certain CNS effects, such as drowsiness and dizziness, and hence it should be used with care in patients on concomitant therapy).
No products indexed under this heading.

Ethyl Alcohol (Scopolamine is an anticholinergic agent and causes certain CNS effects, such as drowsiness and dizziness, and hence it should be used with care in patients on concomitant therapy).
No products indexed under this heading.

Fentanyl (Scopolamine is an anticholinergic agent and causes certain CNS effects, such as drowsiness and dizziness, and hence it should be used with care in patients on concomitant therapy). Products include:
Duragesic Transdermal System 2373
Ionsys Transdermal System 2379

Fentanyl Citrate (Scopolamine is an anticholinergic agent and causes certain CNS effects, such as drowsiness and dizziness, and hence it should be used with care in patients on concomitant therapy). Products include:
Actiq 979

Fexofenadine Hydrochloride (Antihistamines have anticholinergic properties and co-administration may result in additive effects). Products include:
Allegra 2844
Allegra-D 12 Hour Extended-Release Tablets 2846
Allegra-D 24 Hour Extended-Release Tablets 2849

Fluphenazine Decanoate (Scopolamine is an anticholinergic agent and causes certain CNS effects, such as drowsiness and dizziness, and hence it should be used with care in patients on concomitant therapy).
No products indexed under this heading.

Fluphenazine Enanthate (Scopolamine is an anticholinergic agent and causes certain CNS effects, such as drowsiness and dizziness, and hence it should be used with care in patients on concomitant therapy).

No products indexed under this heading.

Fluphenazine Hydrochloride (Scopolamine is an anticholinergic agent and causes certain CNS effects, such as drowsiness and dizziness, and hence it should be used with care in patients on concomitant therapy).

No products indexed under this heading.

Flurazepam Hydrochloride (Scopolamine is an anticholinergic agent and causes certain CNS effects, such as drowsiness and dizziness, and hence it should be used with care in patients on concomitant therapy). Products include:

Dalmane Capsules 3342

Glutethimide (Scopolamine is an anticholinergic agent and causes certain CNS effects, such as drowsiness and dizziness, and hence it should be used with care in patients on concomitant therapy).

No products indexed under this heading.

Glycopyrrolate (Co-administration may result in additive anticholinergic effects).

No products indexed under this heading.

Haloperidol (Scopolamine is an anticholinergic agent and causes certain CNS effects, such as drowsiness and dizziness, and hence it should be used with care in patients on concomitant therapy).

No products indexed under this heading.

Haloperidol Decanoate (Scopolamine is an anticholinergic agent and causes certain CNS effects, such as drowsiness and dizziness, and hence it should be used with care in patients on concomitant therapy).

No products indexed under this heading.

Hydrocodone Bitartrate (Scopolamine is an anticholinergic agent and causes certain CNS effects, such as drowsiness and dizziness, and hence it should be used with care in patients on concomitant therapy). Products include:

Hycodan 1116
Hycotuss Expectorant Syrup 1117
Vicodin Tablets 535
Vicodin ES Tablets 536
Vicodin HP Tablets 538
Vicoprofen Tablets 539
Zydone Tablets 1139

Hydrocodone Polistirex (Scopolamine is an anticholinergic agent and causes certain CNS effects, such as drowsiness and dizziness, and hence it should be used with care in patients on concomitant therapy). Products include:

Tussionex Pennkinetic
Extended-Release Suspension 3327

Hydromorphone Hydrochloride (Scopolamine is an anticholinergic agent and causes certain CNS effects, such as drowsiness and dizziness, and hence it should be used with care in patients on concomitant therapy). Products include:

Dilaudid 440
Dilaudid Non-Sterile Powder 440
Dilaudid Oral Liquid 445

Dilaudid Rectal Suppositories 440
Dilaudid Tablets 440
Dilaudid Tablets - 8 mg 445
Dilaudid-HP 442

Hydroxyzine Hydrochloride (Scopolamine is an anticholinergic agent and causes certain CNS effects, such as drowsiness and dizziness, and hence it should be used with care in patients on concomitant therapy).

No products indexed under this heading.

Hyoscyamine (Co-administration may result in additive anticholinergic effects).

No products indexed under this heading.

Hyoscyamine Sulfate (Co-administration may result in additive anticholinergic effects). Products include:

Donnatal Extentabs 2493
Prosed/DS Tablets 1157

Imipramine Hydrochloride (Tricyclic antidepressants have anticholinergic properties and co-administration may result in additive effects).

No products indexed under this heading.

Imipramine Pamoate (Tricyclic antidepressants have anticholinergic properties and co-administration may result in additive effects).

No products indexed under this heading.

Ipratropium Bromide (Co-administration may result in additive anticholinergic effects). Products include:

Atrovent Inhalation Solution 835
Atrovent HFA Inhalation Aerosol 841
Atrovent Nasal Spray 0.03% 837
Atrovent Nasal Spray 0.06% 839
Combivent Inhalation Aerosol 847
DuoNeb Inhalation Solution 1058

Isoflurane (Scopolamine is an anticholinergic agent and causes certain CNS effects, such as drowsiness and dizziness, and hence it should be used with care in patients on concomitant therapy).

No products indexed under this heading.

Ketamine Hydrochloride (Scopolamine is an anticholinergic agent and causes certain CNS effects, such as drowsiness and dizziness, and hence it should be used with care in patients on concomitant therapy).

No products indexed under this heading.

Levomethadyl Acetate Hydrochloride (Scopolamine is an anticholinergic agent and causes certain CNS effects, such as drowsiness and dizziness, and hence it should be used with care in patients on concomitant therapy).

No products indexed under this heading.

Levorphanol Tartrate (Scopolamine is an anticholinergic agent and causes certain CNS effects, such as drowsiness and dizziness, and hence it should be used with care in patients on concomitant therapy).

No products indexed under this heading.

Loratadine (Antihistamines have anticholinergic properties and co-administration may result in additive effects). Products include:

Alavert Allergy & Sinus D-12 Hour
Tablets 🔲771
Alavert 🔲771

Children's Claritin Allergy Oral
Solution 🔲771
Claritin Non-Drowsy 24 Hour
Tablets 🔲772
Claritin Reditabs 24 Hour
Non-Drowsy Tablets 🔲772
Claritin-D Non-Drowsy 12 Hour
Tablets 🔲772
Claritin-D Non-Drowsy 24 Hour
Tablets 🔲772

Lorazepam (Scopolamine is an anticholinergic agent and causes certain CNS effects, such as drowsiness and dizziness, and hence it should be used with care in patients on concomitant therapy).

No products indexed under this heading.

Loxapine Hydrochloride (Scopolamine is an anticholinergic agent and causes certain CNS effects, such as drowsiness and dizziness, and hence it should be used with care in patients on concomitant therapy).

No products indexed under this heading.

Loxapine Succinate (Scopolamine is an anticholinergic agent and causes certain CNS effects, such as drowsiness and dizziness, and hence it should be used with care in patients on concomitant therapy).

No products indexed under this heading.

Maprotiline Hydrochloride (Tricyclic antidepressants have anticholinergic properties and co-administration may result in additive effects).

No products indexed under this heading.

Meclizine Hydrochloride (Antihistamines have anticholinergic properties and co-administration may result in additive effects).

No products indexed under this heading.

Mepenzolate Bromide (Co-administration may result in additive anticholinergic effects).

No products indexed under this heading.

Meperidine Hydrochloride (Scopolamine is an anticholinergic agent and causes certain CNS effects, such as drowsiness and dizziness, and hence it should be used with care in patients on concomitant therapy).

No products indexed under this heading.

Mephobarbital (Scopolamine is an anticholinergic agent and causes certain CNS effects, such as drowsiness and dizziness, and hence it should be used with care in patients on concomitant therapy).

No products indexed under this heading.

Meprobamate (Scopolamine is an anticholinergic agent and causes certain CNS effects, such as drowsiness and dizziness, and hence it should be used with care in patients on concomitant therapy).

No products indexed under this heading.

Mesoridazine Besylate (Scopolamine is an anticholinergic agent and causes certain CNS effects, such as drowsiness and dizziness, and hence it should be used with care in patients on concomitant therapy).

No products indexed under this heading.

Metaxalone (Co-administration may result in additive anticholinergic effects). Products include:

Skelaxin Tablets 1716

Methadone Hydrochloride (Scopolamine is an anticholinergic agent and causes certain CNS effects, such as drowsiness and dizziness, and hence it should be used with care in patients on concomitant therapy).

No products indexed under this heading.

Methdilazine Hydrochloride (Antihistamines have anticholinergic properties and co-administration may result in additive effects).

No products indexed under this heading.

Methocarbamol (Co-administration may result in additive anticholinergic effects).

No products indexed under this heading.

Methohexital Sodium (Scopolamine is an anticholinergic agent and causes certain CNS effects, such as drowsiness and dizziness, and hence it should be used with care in patients on concomitant therapy).

No products indexed under this heading.

Methotrimeprazine (Scopolamine is an anticholinergic agent and causes certain CNS effects, such as drowsiness and dizziness, and hence it should be used with care in patients on concomitant therapy).

No products indexed under this heading.

Methoxyflurane (Scopolamine is an anticholinergic agent and causes certain CNS effects, such as drowsiness and dizziness, and hence it should be used with care in patients on concomitant therapy).

No products indexed under this heading.

Midazolam Hydrochloride (Scopolamine is an anticholinergic agent and causes certain CNS effects, such as drowsiness and dizziness, and hence it should be used with care in patients on concomitant therapy).

No products indexed under this heading.

Mivacurium Chloride (Co-administration may result in additive anticholinergic effects). Products include:

Mivacron Injection 493

Molindone Hydrochloride (Scopolamine is an anticholinergic agent and causes certain CNS effects, such as drowsiness and dizziness, and hence it should be used with care in patients on concomitant therapy). Products include:

Moban Tablets 1119

Morphine Sulfate (Scopolamine is an anticholinergic agent and causes certain CNS effects, such as drowsiness and dizziness, and hence it should be used with care in patients on concomitant therapy). Products include:

Avinza Capsules 1741
Kadian Capsules 577
MS Contin Tablets 2701

Nortriptyline Hydrochloride (Tricyclic antidepressants have anticholinergic properties and co-administration may result in additive effects).

No products indexed under this heading.

Olanzapine (Scopolamine is an anticholinergic agent and causes certain CNS effects, such as drowsiness and dizziness, and hence it should be used with care in patients on concomitant therapy). Products include:

Oral Medications, unspecified (The absorption of oral medications may be decreased during the concurrent use of scopolamine because of decreased gastric motility and delayed gastric emptying).

No products indexed under this heading.

Orphenadrine Citrate (Co-administration may result in additive anticholinergic effects). Products include:

Oxazepam (Scopolamine is an anticholinergic agent and causes certain CNS effects, such as drowsiness and dizziness, and hence it should be used with care in patients on concomitant therapy).

No products indexed under this heading.

Oxybutynin Chloride (Co-administration may result in additive anticholinergic effects). Products include:

Oxycodone Hydrochloride (Scopolamine is an anticholinergic agent and causes certain CNS effects, such as drowsiness and dizziness, and hence it should be used with care in patients on concomitant therapy). Products include:

Pancuronium Bromide (Co-administration may result in additive anticholinergic effects).

No products indexed under this heading.

Pentobarbital Sodium (Scopolamine is an anticholinergic agent and causes certain CNS effects, such as drowsiness and dizziness, and hence it should be used with care in patients on concomitant therapy). Products include:

Perphenazine (Scopolamine is an anticholinergic agent and causes certain CNS effects, such as drowsiness and dizziness, and hence it should be used with care in patients on concomitant therapy).

No products indexed under this heading.

Phenobarbital (Scopolamine is an anticholinergic agent and causes certain CNS effects, such as drowsiness and dizziness, and hence it should be used with care in patients on concomitant therapy). Products include:

Prazepam (Scopolamine is an anticholinergic agent and causes certain CNS effects, such as drowsiness and dizziness, and hence it should be used with care in patients on concomitant therapy).

No products indexed under this heading.

Prochlorperazine (Scopolamine is an anticholinergic agent and causes certain CNS effects, such as drowsiness and dizziness, and hence it should be used with care in patients on concomitant therapy).

No products indexed under this heading.

Procyclidine Hydrochloride (Co-administration may result in additive anticholinergic effects).

No products indexed under this heading.

Promethazine Hydrochloride (Antihistamines have anticholinergic properties and co-administration may result in additive effects). Products include:

Propantheline Bromide (Co-administration may result in additive anticholinergic effects).

No products indexed under this heading.

Propofol (Scopolamine is an anticholinergic agent and causes certain CNS effects, such as drowsiness and dizziness, and hence it should be used with care in patients on concomitant therapy).

No products indexed under this heading.

Propoxyphene Hydrochloride (Scopolamine is an anticholinergic agent and causes certain CNS effects, such as drowsiness and dizziness, and hence it should be used with care in patients on concomitant therapy).

No products indexed under this heading.

Propoxyphene Napsylate (Scopolamine is an anticholinergic agent and causes certain CNS effects, such as drowsiness and dizziness, and hence it should be used with care in patients on concomitant therapy).

No products indexed under this heading.

Protriptyline Hydrochloride (Tricyclic antidepressants have anticholinergic properties and co-administration may result in additive effects).

No products indexed under this heading.

Pyrilamine Maleate (Antihistamines have anticholinergic properties and co-administration may result in additive effects).

No products indexed under this heading.

Pyrilamine Tannate (Antihistamines have anticholinergic properties and co-administration may result in additive effects).

No products indexed under this heading.

Quazepam (Scopolamine is an anticholinergic agent and causes certain CNS effects, such as drowsiness and dizziness, and hence it should be used with care in patients on concomitant therapy).

No products indexed under this heading.

Quetiapine Fumarate (Scopolamine is an anticholinergic agent and causes certain CNS effects, such as drowsiness and dizziness, and hence it should be used with care in patients on concomitant therapy). Products include:

Ramelteon (Scopolamine is an anticholinergic agent and causes certain CNS effects, such as drowsiness and dizziness, and hence it should be used with care in patients on concomitant therapy). Products include:

Rapacuronium Bromide (Co-administration may result in additive anticholinergic effects).

No products indexed under this heading.

Remifentanil Hydrochloride (Scopolamine is an anticholinergic agent and causes certain CNS effects, such as drowsiness and dizziness, and hence it should be used with care in patients on concomitant therapy).

No products indexed under this heading.

Risperidone (Scopolamine is an anticholinergic agent and causes certain CNS effects, such as drowsiness and dizziness, and hence it should be used with care in patients on concomitant therapy). Products include:

Rocuronium Bromide (Co-administration may result in additive anticholinergic effects). Products include:

Scopolamine Hydrobromide (Co-administration may result in additive anticholinergic effects). Products include:

Secobarbital Sodium (Scopolamine is an anticholinergic agent and causes certain CNS effects, such as drowsiness and dizziness, and hence it should be used with care in patients on concomitant therapy).

No products indexed under this heading.

Sevoflurane (Scopolamine is an anticholinergic agent and causes certain CNS effects, such as drowsiness and dizziness, and hence it should be used with care in patients on concomitant therapy). Products include:

Sodium Oxybate (Scopolamine is an anticholinergic agent and causes certain CNS effects, such as drowsiness and dizziness, and hence it should be used with care in patients on concomitant therapy). Products include:

Succinylcholine Chloride (Co-administration may result in additive anticholinergic effects).

No products indexed under this heading.

Sufentanil Citrate (Scopolamine is an anticholinergic agent and causes certain CNS effects, such as drowsiness and dizziness, and hence it should be used with care in patients on concomitant therapy).

No products indexed under this heading.

Temazepam (Scopolamine is an anticholinergic agent and causes certain CNS effects, such as drowsiness and dizziness, and hence it should be used with care in patients on concomitant therapy). Products include:

Terfenadine (Antihistamines have anticholinergic properties and co-administration may result in additive effects).

No products indexed under this heading.

Thiamylal Sodium (Scopolamine is an anticholinergic agent and causes certain CNS effects, such as drowsiness and dizziness, and hence it should be used with care in patients on concomitant therapy).

No products indexed under this heading.

Thioridazine Hydrochloride (Scopolamine is an anticholinergic agent and causes certain CNS effects, such as drowsiness and dizziness, and hence it should be used with care in patients on concomitant therapy). Products include:

Thiothixene (Scopolamine is an anticholinergic agent and causes certain CNS effects, such as drowsiness and dizziness, and hence it should be used with care in patients on concomitant therapy). Products include:

Tolterodine Tartrate (Co-administration may result in additive anticholinergic effects). Products include:

Triazolam (Scopolamine is an anticholinergic agent and causes certain CNS effects, such as drowsiness and dizziness, and hence it should be used with care in patients on concomitant therapy).

No products indexed under this heading.

Tridihexethyl Chloride (Co-administration may result in additive anticholinergic effects).

No products indexed under this heading.

Trifluoperazine Hydrochloride (Scopolamine is an anticholinergic agent and causes certain CNS effects, such as drowsiness and dizziness, and hence it should be used with care in patients on concomitant therapy).

No products indexed under this heading.

Trimeprazine Tartrate (Antihistamines have anticholinergic properties and co-administration may result in additive effects).

No products indexed under this heading.

Trimipramine Maleate (Tricyclic antidepressants have anticholinergic properties and co-administration may result in additive effects).
No products indexed under this heading.

Tripelennamine Hydrochloride (Antihistamines have anticholinergic properties and co-administration may result in additive effects).
No products indexed under this heading.

Triprolidine Hydrochloride (Antihistamines have anticholinergic properties and co-administration may result in additive effects).
No products indexed under this heading.

Vecuronium Bromide (Co-administration may result in addititve anticholinergic effects).
No products indexed under this heading.

Zaleplon (Scopolamine is an anticholinergic agent and causes certain CNS effects, such as drowsiness and dizziness, and hence it should be used with care in patients on concomitant therapy). Products include:
Sonata Capsules **1717**

Ziprasidone Hydrochloride (Scopolamine is an anticholinergic agent and causes certain CNS effects, such as drowsiness and dizziness, and hence it should be used with care in patients on concomitant therapy). Products include:
Geodon Capsules **2529**

Zolpidem Tartrate (Scopolamine is an anticholinergic agent and causes certain CNS effects, such as drowsiness and dizziness, and hence it should be used with care in patients on concomitant therapy). Products include:
Ambien Tablets **2851**
Ambien CR Tablets **2855**

Food Interactions

Alcohol (Scopolamine is an anticholinergic agent and causes certain CNS effects, such as drowsiness and dizziness, and hence it should be used with care in patients on concomitant therapy).

4LIFE TRANSFER FACTOR PLUS ADVANCED FORMULA

(Amino Acid Preparations) .... ■**835**
None cited in PDR database.

TRANXENE T-TAB TABLETS

(Clorazepate Dipotassium) **2474**
May interact with barbiturates, central nervous system depressants, antidepressant drugs, hypnotics and sedatives, monoamine oxidase inhibitors, narcotic analgesics, phenothiazines, and certain other agents. Compounds in these categories include:

Alfentanil Hydrochloride (Actions of benzodiazepines may be potentiated).
No products indexed under this heading.

Alprazolam (Actions of benzodiazepines may be potentiated). Products include:
Niravam Orally Disintegrating Tablets **3092**

Amitriptyline Hydrochloride (Actions of benzodiazepines may be potentiated).
No products indexed under this heading.

Amoxapine (Actions of benzodiazepines may be potentiated).
No products indexed under this heading.

Aprobarbital (Actions of benzodiazepines may be potentiated).
No products indexed under this heading.

Buprenorphine Hydrochloride (Actions of benzodiazepines may be potentiated). Products include:
Buprenex Injectable **2716**
Suboxone Tablets **2717**
Subutex Tablets **2717**

Bupropion Hydrochloride (Actions of benzodiazepines may be potentiated). Products include:
Wellbutrin Tablets **1603**
Wellbutrin SR Sustained-Release Tablets **1607**
Wellbutrin XL Extended-Release Tablets **1613**
Zyban Sustained-Release Tablets **1644**

Buspirone Hydrochloride (Actions of benzodiazepines may be potentiated).
No products indexed under this heading.

Butabarbital (Actions of benzodiazepines may be potentiated).
No products indexed under this heading.

Butalbital (Actions of benzodiazepines may be potentiated).
No products indexed under this heading.

Chlordiazepoxide (Actions of benzodiazepines may be potentiated).
No products indexed under this heading.

Chlordiazepoxide Hydrochloride (Actions of benzodiazepines may be potentiated). Products include:
Librium Capsules **3347**

Chlorpromazine (Actions of benzodiazepines may be potentiated).
No products indexed under this heading.

Chlorpromazine Hydrochloride (Actions of benzodiazepines may be potentiated).
No products indexed under this heading.

Chlorprothixene (Actions of benzodiazepines may be potentiated).
No products indexed under this heading.

Chlorprothixene Hydrochloride (Actions of benzodiazepines may be potentiated).
No products indexed under this heading.

Chlorprothixene Lactate (Actions of benzodiazepines may be potentiated).
No products indexed under this heading.

Citalopram Hydrobromide (Actions of benzodiazepines may be potentiated). Products include:
Celexa **1176**

Clozapine (Actions of benzodiazepines may be potentiated). Products include:
Clozaril Tablets **2184**
FazaClo Orally Disintegrating Tablets **551**

Codeine Phosphate (Actions of benzodiazepines may be potentiated). Products include:
Tylenol with Codeine Tablets **2391**

Desflurane (Actions of benzodiazepines may be potentiated).
No products indexed under this heading.

Desipramine Hydrochloride (Actions of benzodiazepines may be potentiated).
No products indexed under this heading.

Dezocine (Actions of benzodiazepines may be potentiated).
No products indexed under this heading.

Diazepam (Actions of benzodiazepines may be potentiated). Products include:
Diastat Rectal Delivery System **3343**
Valium Tablets **2819**

Doxepin Hydrochloride (Actions of benzodiazepines may be potentiated).
No products indexed under this heading.

Droperidol (Actions of benzodiazepines may be potentiated).
No products indexed under this heading.

Enflurane (Actions of benzodiazepines may be potentiated).
No products indexed under this heading.

Estazolam (Actions of benzodiazepines may be potentiated; increased sedation with concurrent use). Products include:
ProSom Tablets **517**

Ethanol (Actions of benzodiazepines may be potentiated).
No products indexed under this heading.

Ethchlorvynol (Actions of benzodiazepines may be potentiated; increased sedation with concurrent use).
No products indexed under this heading.

Ethinamate (Actions of benzodiazepines may be potentiated; increased sedation with concurrent use).
No products indexed under this heading.

Ethyl Alcohol (Actions of benzodiazepines may be potentiated).
No products indexed under this heading.

Fentanyl (Actions of benzodiazepines may be potentiated). Products include:
Duragesic Transdermal System **2373**
Ionsys Transdermal System **2379**

Fentanyl Citrate (Actions of benzodiazepines may be potentiated). Products include:
Actiq **979**

Fluoxetine Hydrochloride (Actions of benzodiazepines may be potentiated). Products include:
Prozac Pulvules and Liquid **1801**
Symbyax Capsules **1819**

Fluphenazine Decanoate (Actions of benzodiazepines may be potentiated).
No products indexed under this heading.

Fluphenazine Enanthate (Actions of benzodiazepines may be potentiated).
No products indexed under this heading.

Fluphenazine Hydrochloride (Actions of benzodiazepines may be potentiated).
No products indexed under this heading.

Flurazepam Hydrochloride (Actions of benzodiazepines may be potentiated; increased sedation with concurrent use). Products include:
Dalmane Capsules **3342**

Glutethimide (Actions of benzodiazepines may be potentiated; increased sedation with concurrent use).
No products indexed under this heading.

Haloperidol (Actions of benzodiazepines may be potentiated).
No products indexed under this heading.

Haloperidol Decanoate (Actions of benzodiazepines may be potentiated).
No products indexed under this heading.

Hydrocodone Bitartrate (Actions of benzodiazepines may be potentiated). Products include:
Hycodan **1116**
Hycotuss Expectorant Syrup **1117**
Vicodin Tablets **535**
Vicodin ES Tablets **536**
Vicodin HP Tablets **538**
Vicoprofen Tablets **539**
Zydone Tablets **1139**

Hydrocodone Polistirex (Actions of benzodiazepines may be potentiated). Products include:
Tussionex Pennkinetic Extended-Release Suspension **3327**

Hydromorphone Hydrochloride (Actions of benzodiazepines may be potentiated). Products include:
Dilaudid **440**
Dilaudid Non-Sterile Powder **440**
Dilaudid Oral Liquid **445**
Dilaudid Rectal Suppositories **440**
Dilaudid Tablets **440**
Dilaudid Tablets - 8 mg **445**
Dilaudid-HP **442**

Hydroxyzine Hydrochloride (Actions of benzodiazepines may be potentiated).
No products indexed under this heading.

Imipramine Hydrochloride (Actions of benzodiazepines may be potentiated).
No products indexed under this heading.

Imipramine Pamoate (Actions of benzodiazepines may be potentiated).
No products indexed under this heading.

Isocarboxazid (Actions of benzodiazepines may be potentiated).
No products indexed under this heading.

Isoflurane (Actions of benzodiazepines may be potentiated).
No products indexed under this heading.

Ketamine Hydrochloride (Actions of benzodiazepines may be potentiated).
No products indexed under this heading.

Levomethadyl Acetate Hydrochloride (Actions of benzodiazepines may be potentiated).
No products indexed under this heading.

Levorphanol Tartrate (Actions of benzodiazepines may be potentiated).
No products indexed under this heading.

Lorazepam (Actions of benzodiazepines may be potentiated; increased sedation with concurrent use).
No products indexed under this heading.

Loxapine Hydrochloride (Actions of benzodiazepines may be potentiated).
No products indexed under this heading.

Loxapine Succinate (Actions of benzodiazepines may be potentiated).
No products indexed under this heading.

Maprotiline Hydrochloride (Actions of benzodiazepines may be potentiated).
No products indexed under this heading.

Meperidine Hydrochloride (Actions of benzodiazepines may be potentiated).
No products indexed under this heading.

Mephobarbital (Actions of benzodiazepines may be potentiated).
No products indexed under this heading.

Meprobamate (Actions of benzodiazepines may be potentiated).
No products indexed under this heading.

Mesoridazine Besylate (Actions of benzodiazepines may be potentiated).
No products indexed under this heading.

Methadone Hydrochloride (Actions of benzodiazepines may be potentiated).
No products indexed under this heading.

Methohexital Sodium (Actions of benzodiazepines may be potentiated).
No products indexed under this heading.

Methotrimeprazine (Actions of benzodiazepines may be potentiated).
No products indexed under this heading.

Methoxyflurane (Actions of benzodiazepines may be potentiated).
No products indexed under this heading.

Midazolam Hydrochloride (Actions of benzodiazepines may be potentiated; increased sedation with concurrent use).
No products indexed under this heading.

Mirtazapine (Actions of benzodiazepines may be potentiated).
No products indexed under this heading.

Moclobemide (Actions of benzodiazepines may be potentiated).
No products indexed under this heading.

Molindone Hydrochloride (Actions of benzodiazepines may be potentiated). Products include:
Moban Tablets **1119**

Morphine Sulfate (Actions of benzodiazepines may be potentiated).
Products include:
Avinza Capsules **1741**
Kadian Capsules **577**
MS Contin Tablets **2701**

Nefazodone Hydrochloride (Actions of benzodiazepines may be potentiated).
No products indexed under this heading.

Nortriptyline Hydrochloride (Actions of benzodiazepines may be potentiated).
No products indexed under this heading.

Olanzapine (Actions of benzodiazepines may be potentiated).
Products include:
Symbyax Capsules **1819**
Zyprexa Tablets **1830**
Zyprexa IntraMuscular **1830**
Zyprexa ZYDIS Orally Disintegrating Tablets **1830**

Oxazepam (Actions of benzodiazepines may be potentiated).
No products indexed under this heading.

Oxycodone Hydrochloride (Actions of benzodiazepines may be potentiated). Products include:
OxyContin Tablets **2703**
OxyFast Oral Concentrate Solution **2708**
OxyIR Capsules **2708**
Percocet Tablets **1131**
Percodan Tablets **1132**

Pargyline Hydrochloride (Actions of benzodiazepines may be potentiated).
No products indexed under this heading.

Paroxetine Hydrochloride (Actions of benzodiazepines may be potentiated). Products include:
Paxil CR Controlled-Release Tablets **1538**
Paxil **1530**

Pentobarbital Sodium (Actions of benzodiazepines may be potentiated). Products include:
Nembutal Sodium Solution, USP **2470**

Perphenazine (Actions of benzodiazepines may be potentiated).
No products indexed under this heading.

Phenelzine Sulfate (Actions of benzodiazepines may be potentiated).
No products indexed under this heading.

Phenobarbital (Actions of benzodiazepines may be potentiated).
Products include:
Donnatal Extentabs **2493**

Prazepam (Actions of benzodiazepines may be potentiated).
No products indexed under this heading.

Procarbazine Hydrochloride (Actions of benzodiazepines may be potentiated). Products include:
Matulane Capsules **3191**

Prochlorperazine (Actions of benzodiazepines may be potentiated).
No products indexed under this heading.

Promethazine Hydrochloride (Actions of benzodiazepines may be potentiated). Products include:
Phenergan Tablets and Suppositories **3440**

Propofol (Actions of benzodiazepines may be potentiated; increased sedation with concurrent use).
No products indexed under this heading.

Propoxyphene Hydrochloride (Actions of benzodiazepines may be potentiated).
No products indexed under this heading.

Propoxyphene Napsylate (Actions of benzodiazepines may be potentiated).
No products indexed under this heading.

Protriptyline Hydrochloride (Actions of benzodiazepines may be potentiated).
No products indexed under this heading.

Quazepam (Actions of benzodiazepines may be potentiated; increased sedation with concurrent use).
No products indexed under this heading.

Quetiapine Fumarate (Actions of benzodiazepines may be potentiated). Products include:
Seroquel Tablets **690**

Ramelteon (Actions of benzodiazepines may be potentiated; increased sedation with concurrent use). Products include:
Rozerem Tablets **3231**

Remifentanil Hydrochloride (Actions of benzodiazepines may be potentiated).
No products indexed under this heading.

Risperidone (Actions of benzodiazepines may be potentiated).
Products include:
Risperdal **1676**
Risperdal Consta Long-Acting Injection **1682**
Risperdal M-Tab Orally Disintegrating Tablets **1676**

Secobarbital Sodium (Actions of benzodiazepines may be potentiated).
No products indexed under this heading.

Selegiline Hydrochloride (Actions of benzodiazepines may be potentiated). Products include:
Eldepryl Capsules **3208**
Zelapar Tablets **3372**

Sertraline Hydrochloride (Actions of benzodiazepines may be potentiated). Products include:
Zoloft **2586**

Sevoflurane (Actions of benzodiazepines may be potentiated).
Products include:
Ultane Liquid for Inhalation **531**

Sufentanil Citrate (Actions of benzodiazepines may be potentiated).
No products indexed under this heading.

Temazepam (Actions of benzodiazepines may be potentiated; increased sedation with concurrent use). Products include:
Restoril Capsules **1860**

Thiamylal Sodium (Actions of benzodiazepines may be potentiated).
No products indexed under this heading.

Thioridazine Hydrochloride (Actions of benzodiazepines may be potentiated). Products include:
Thioridazine Hydrochloride Tablets **2163**

Thiothixene (Actions of benzodiazepines may be potentiated).
Products include:
Thiothixene Capsules **2165**

Tranylcypromine Sulfate (Actions of benzodiazepines may be potentiated). Products include:
Parnate Tablets **1527**

Trazodone Hydrochloride (Actions of benzodiazepines may be potentiated).
No products indexed under this heading.

Triazolam (Actions of benzodiazepines may be potentiated; increased sedation with concurrent use).
No products indexed under this heading.

Trifluoperazine Hydrochloride (Actions of benzodiazepines may be potentiated).
No products indexed under this heading.

Trimipramine Maleate (Actions of benzodiazepines may be potentiated).
No products indexed under this heading.

Venlafaxine Hydrochloride (Actions of benzodiazepines may be potentiated). Products include:
Effexor Tablets **3411**
Effexor XR Capsules **3417**

Zaleplon (Actions of benzodiazepines may be potentiated).
Products include:
Sonata Capsules **1717**

Ziprasidone Hydrochloride (Actions of benzodiazepines may be potentiated). Products include:
Geodon Capsules **2529**

Zolpidem Tartrate (Actions of benzodiazepines may be potentiated; increased sedation with concurrent use). Products include:
Ambien Tablets **2851**
Ambien CR Tablets **2855**

Food Interactions

Alcohol (Actions of benzodiazepines may be potentiated; prolonged sleeping time).

TRANXENE-SD TABLETS

(Clorazepate Dipotassium) **2474**
May interact with:

See (Tranxene T-TAB Tablets).
No products indexed under this heading.

TRANXENE-SD HALF STRENGTH TABLETS

(Clorazepate Dipotassium) **2474**
May interact with:

See (Tranxene T-TAB Tablets).
No products indexed under this heading.

TRASYLOL INJECTION

(Aprotinin) **754**
May interact with fibrinolytic agents and certain other agents. Compounds in these categories include:

Alteplase (Aprotinin may inhibit the effects of fibrinolytic agents).
Products include:
Activase I.V. **1223**
Cathflo Activase **1231**

Anistreplase (Aprotinin may inhibit the effects of fibrinolytic agents).
No products indexed under this heading.

Captopril (Aprotinin may block the acute hypotensive effects of captopril). Products include:
Captopril Tablets **2149**

Heparin Sodium (Aprotinin, in the presence of heparin, has been found to prolong the activated clotting time (ACT) as measured by surface activation methods).
No products indexed under this heading.

Streptokinase (Aprotinin may inhibit the effects of fibrinolytic agents).
No products indexed under this heading.

Urokinase (Aprotinin may inhibit the effects of fibrinolytic agents).
No products indexed under this heading.

TRAUMEEL INJECTION SOLUTION
(Homeopathic Formulations) 1664
None cited in PDR database.

TRAVATAN OPHTHALMIC SOLUTION
(Travoprost) 563
None cited in PDR database.

TRECATOR TABLETS
(Ethionamide) 3487
May interact with antituberculosis drugs and certain other agents. Compounds in these categories include:

Aminosalicylic Acid (Ethionamide may potentiate the adverse effects of other antituberculous drugs administered concomitantly). Products include:
Paser Granules 1674

p-Aminosalicylic Acid (Ethionamide may potentiate the adverse effects of other antituberculous drugs administered concomitantly).
No products indexed under this heading.

Cycloserine (Ethionamide may potentiate the adverse effects of other antituberculous drugs administered concomitantly. In particular, convulsions have been reported when ethionamide is administered with cycloserine and special care should be taken when the treatment regimen includes both of these drugs). Products include:
Seromycin Capsules 1813

Ethambutol Hydrochloride (Ethionamide may potentiate the adverse effects of other antituberculous drugs administered concomitantly).
No products indexed under this heading.

Ethanol (Excessive ethanol ingestion should be avoided because a psychotic reaction has been reported).
No products indexed under this heading.

Isoniazid (Ethionamide has been found to temporarily raise serum concentrations of isoniazid).
No products indexed under this heading.

Pyrazinamide (Ethionamide may potentiate the adverse effects of other antituberculous drugs administered concomitantly).
No products indexed under this heading.

Rifampin (Ethionamide may potentiate the adverse effects of other antituberculous drugs administered concomitantly).
No products indexed under this heading.

Rifapentine (Ethionamide may potentiate the adverse effects of other antituberculous drugs administered concomitantly).
No products indexed under this heading.

Food Interactions

Alcohol (Excessive ethanol ingestion should be avoided because a psychotic reaction has been reported).

TRELSTAR DEPOT
(Triptorelin Pamoate) 3394
May interact with drugs which may cause hyperprolactinemia and certain other agents. Compounds in these categories include:

Alprazolam (Hyperprolactinemic drugs should not be prescribed concomitantly with triptorelin, since hyperprolactinemia reduces the number of pituitary GnRH receptors). Products include:
Niravam Orally Disintegrating Tablets 3092

Chlorpromazine (Hyperprolactinemic drugs should not be prescribed concomitantly with triptorelin, since hyperprolactinemia reduces the number of pituitary GnRH receptors).
No products indexed under this heading.

Chlorpromazine Hydrochloride (Hyperprolactinemic drugs should not be prescribed concomitantly with triptorelin, since hyperprolactinemia reduces the number of pituitary GnRH receptors).
No products indexed under this heading.

Chlorprothixene (Hyperprolactinemic drugs should not be prescribed concomitantly with triptorelin, since hyperprolactinemia reduces the number of pituitary GnRH receptors).
No products indexed under this heading.

Chlorprothixene Hydrochloride (Hyperprolactinemic drugs should not be prescribed concomitantly with triptorelin, since hyperprolactinemia reduces the number of pituitary GnRH receptors).
No products indexed under this heading.

Fluoxetine Hydrochloride (Hyperprolactinemic drugs should not be prescribed concomitantly with triptorelin, since hyperprolactinemia reduces the number of pituitary GnRH receptors). Products include:
Prozac Pulvules and Liquid 1801
Symbyax Capsules 1819

Fluphenazine Decanoate (Hyperprolactinemic drugs should not be prescribed concomitantly with triptorelin, since hyperprolactinemia reduces the number of pituitary GnRH receptors).
No products indexed under this heading.

Fluphenazine Enanthate (Hyperprolactinemic drugs should not be prescribed concomitantly with triptorelin, since hyperprolactinemia reduces the number of pituitary GnRH receptors).
No products indexed under this heading.

Fluphenazine Hydrochloride (Hyperprolactinemic drugs should not be prescribed concomitantly with triptorelin, since hyperprolactinemia reduces the number of pituitary GnRH receptors).
No products indexed under this heading.

Haloperidol (Hyperprolactinemic drugs should not be prescribed concomitantly with triptorelin, since hyperprolactinemia reduces the number of pituitary GnRH receptors).
No products indexed under this heading.

Haloperidol Decanoate (Hyperprolactinemic drugs should not be prescribed concomitantly with triptorelin, since hyperprolactinemia reduces the number of pituitary GnRH receptors).
No products indexed under this heading.

Loxapine Hydrochloride (Hyperprolactinemic drugs should not be prescribed concomitantly with triptorelin, since hyperprolactinemia reduces the number of pituitary GnRH receptors).
No products indexed under this heading.

Loxapine Succinate (Hyperprolactinemic drugs should not be prescribed concomitantly with triptorelin, since hyperprolactinemia reduces the number of pituitary GnRH receptors).
No products indexed under this heading.

Mesoridazine Besylate (Hyperprolactinemic drugs should not be prescribed concomitantly with triptorelin, since hyperprolactinemia reduces the number of pituitary GnRH receptors).
No products indexed under this heading.

Methotrimeprazine (Hyperprolactinemic drugs should not be prescribed concomitantly with triptorelin, since hyperprolactinemia reduces the number of pituitary GnRH receptors).
No products indexed under this heading.

Methyldopa (Hyperprolactinemic drugs should not be prescribed concomitantly with triptorelin, since hyperprolactinemia reduces the number of pituitary GnRH receptors). Products include:
Aldoril Tablets 1910

Metoclopramide Hydrochloride (Hyperprolactinemic drugs should not be prescribed concomitantly with triptorelin, since hyperprolactinemia reduces the number of pituitary GnRH receptors).
No products indexed under this heading.

Molindone Hydrochloride (Hyperprolactinemic drugs should not be prescribed concomitantly with triptorelin, since hyperprolactinemia reduces the number of pituitary GnRH receptors). Products include:
Moban Tablets 1119

Olanzapine (Hyperprolactinemic drugs should not be prescribed concomitantly with triptorelin, since hyperprolactinemia reduces the number of pituitary GnRH receptors). Products include:
Symbyax Capsules 1819
Zyprexa Tablets 1830
Zyprexa IntraMuscular 1830
Zyprexa ZYDIS Orally Disintegrating Tablets 1830

Perphenazine (Hyperprolactinemic drugs should not be prescribed concomitantly with triptorelin, since hyperprolactinemia reduces the number of pituitary GnRH receptors).
No products indexed under this heading.

Prochlorperazine (Hyperprolactinemic drugs should not be prescribed concomitantly with triptorelin, since hyperprolactinemia reduces the number of pituitary GnRH receptors).
No products indexed under this heading.

Promethazine Hydrochloride (Hyperprolactinemic drugs should not be prescribed concomitantly with triptorelin, since hyperprolactinemia reduces the number of pituitary GnRH receptors). Products include:
Phenergan Tablets and Suppositories 3440

Quetiapine Fumarate (Hyperprolactinemic drugs should not be prescribed concomitantly with triptorelin, since hyperprolactinemia reduces the number of pituitary GnRH receptors). Products include:
Seroquel Tablets 690

Risperidone (Hyperprolactinemic drugs should not be prescribed concomitantly with triptorelin, since hyperprolactinemia reduces the number of pituitary GnRH receptors). Products include:
Risperdal 1676
Risperdal Consta Long-Acting Injection 1682
Risperdal M-Tab Orally Disintegrating Tablets 1676

Sertraline Hydrochloride (Hyperprolactinemic drugs should not be prescribed concomitantly with triptorelin, since hyperprolactinemia reduces the number of pituitary GnRH receptors). Products include:
Zoloft 2586

Thioridazine Hydrochloride (Hyperprolactinemic drugs should not be prescribed concomitantly with triptorelin, since hyperprolactinemia reduces the number of pituitary GnRH receptors). Products include:
Thioridazine Hydrochloride Tablets 2163

Thiothixene (Hyperprolactinemic drugs should not be prescribed concomitantly with triptorelin, since hyperprolactinemia reduces the number of pituitary GnRH receptors). Products include:
Thiothixene Capsules 2165

Trifluoperazine Hydrochloride (Hyperprolactinemic drugs should not be prescribed concomitantly with triptorelin, since hyperprolactinemia reduces the number of pituitary GnRH receptors).
No products indexed under this heading.

Verapamil Hydrochloride (Hyperprolactinemic drugs should not be prescribed concomitantly with triptorelin, since hyperprolactinemia reduces the number of pituitary GnRH receptors). Products include:
Covera-HS Tablets 3139
Tarka Tablets 524
Verelan PM Extended-Release Capsules, Controlled-Onset........... 3106

Ziprasidone Hydrochloride (Hyperprolactinemic drugs should not be prescribed concomitantly with triptorelin, since hyperprolactinemia reduces the number of pituitary GnRH receptors). Products include:
Geodon Capsules 2529

Ziprasidone Mesylate (Hyperprolactinemic drugs should not be prescribed concomitantly with triptorelin, since hyperprolactinemia reduces the number of pituitary GnRH receptors). Products include:
Geodon for Injection 2529

TRELSTAR LA SUSPENSION
(Triptorelin Pamoate) 3397
May interact with drugs which may cause hyperprolactinemia and certain other agents. Compounds in these categories include:

Alprazolam (Hyperprolactinemic drugs should not be prescribed concomitantly with triptorelin pamoate since hyperprolactinemia reduces the number of pituitary GnRH receptors). Products include:

Chlorpromazine (Hyperprolactine-mic drugs should not be prescribed concomitantly with triptorelin pamoate since hyperprolactinemia reduces the number of pituitary GnRH receptors).
No products indexed under this heading.

Chlorpromazine Hydrochloride (Hyperprolactinemic drugs should not be prescribed concomitantly with triptorelin pamoate since hyperprolactinemia reduces the number of pituitary GnRH receptors).
No products indexed under this heading.

Chlorprothixene (Hyperprolactine-mic drugs should not be prescribed concomitantly with triptorelin pamoate since hyperprolactinemia reduces the number of pituitary GnRH receptors).
No products indexed under this heading.

Chlorprothixene Hydrochloride (Hyperprolactinemic drugs should not be prescribed concomitantly with triptorelin pamoate since hyperprolactinemia reduces the number of pituitary GnRH receptors).
No products indexed under this heading.

Fluoxetine Hydrochloride (Hyperprolactinemic drugs should not be prescribed concomitantly with triptorelin pamoate since hyperprolactinemia reduces the number of pituitary GnRH receptors). Products include:

Fluphenazine Decanoate (Hyperprolactinemic drugs should not be prescribed concomitantly with triptorelin pamoate since hyperprolactinemia reduces the number of pituitary GnRH receptors).
No products indexed under this heading.

Fluphenazine Enanthate (Hyperprolactinemic drugs should not be prescribed concomitantly with triptorelin pamoate since hyperprolactinemia reduces the number of pituitary GnRH receptors).
No products indexed under this heading.

Fluphenazine Hydrochloride (Hyperprolactinemic drugs should not be prescribed concomitantly with triptorelin pamoate since hyperprolactinemia reduces the number of pituitary GnRH receptors).
No products indexed under this heading.

Haloperidol (Hyperprolactinemic drugs should not be prescribed concomitantly with triptorelin pamoate since hyperprolactinemia reduces the number of pituitary GnRH receptors).
No products indexed under this heading.

Haloperidol Decanoate (Hyperprolactinemic drugs should not be prescribed concomitantly with triptorelin pamoate since hyperprolactinemia reduces the number of pituitary GnRH receptors).
No products indexed under this heading.

Loxapine Hydrochloride (Hyperprolactinemic drugs should not be prescribed concomitantly with triptorelin pamoate since hyperprolactinemia reduces the number of pituitary GnRH receptors).
No products indexed under this heading.

Loxapine Succinate (Hyperprolactinemic drugs should not be prescribed concomitantly with triptorelin pamoate since hyperprolactinemia reduces the number of pituitary GnRH receptors).
No products indexed under this heading.

Mesoridazine Besylate (Hyperprolactinemic drugs should not be prescribed concomitantly with triptorelin pamoate since hyperprolactinemia reduces the number of pituitary GnRH receptors).
No products indexed under this heading.

Methotrimeprazine (Hyperprolactinemic drugs should not be prescribed concomitantly with triptorelin pamoate since hyperprolactinemia reduces the number of pituitary GnRH receptors).
No products indexed under this heading.

Methyldopa (Hyperprolactinemic drugs should not be prescribed concomitantly with triptorelin pamoate since hyperprolactinemia reduces the number of pituitary GnRH receptors). Products include:

Metoclopramide Hydrochloride (Hyperprolactinemic drugs should not be prescribed concomitantly with triptorelin pamoate since hyperprolactinemia reduces the number of pituitary GnRH receptors).
No products indexed under this heading.

Molindone Hydrochloride (Hyperprolactinemic drugs should not be prescribed concomitantly with triptorelin pamoate since hyperprolactinemia reduces the number of pituitary GnRH receptors). Products include:

Olanzapine (Hyperprolactinemic drugs should not be prescribed concomitantly with triptorelin pamoate since hyperprolactinemia reduces the number of pituitary GnRH receptors). Products include:

Perphenazine (Hyperprolactinemic drugs should not be prescribed concomitantly with triptorelin pamoate since hyperprolactinemia reduces the number of pituitary GnRH receptors).
No products indexed under this heading.

Prochlorperazine (Hyperprolactinemic drugs should not be prescribed concomitantly with triptorelin pamoate since hyperprolactinemia reduces the number of pituitary GnRH receptors).
No products indexed under this heading.

Promethazine Hydrochloride (Hyperprolactinemic drugs should not be prescribed concomitantly with triptorelin pamoate since hyperpro-

lactinemia reduces the number of pituitary GnRH receptors). Products include:

Quetiapine Fumarate (Hyperprolactinemic drugs should not be prescribed concomitantly with triptorelin pamoate since hyperprolactinemia reduces the number of pituitary GnRH receptors). Products include:

Risperidone (Hyperprolactinemic drugs should not be prescribed concomitantly with triptorelin pamoate since hyperprolactinemia reduces the number of pituitary GnRH receptors). Products include:

Sertraline Hydrochloride (Hyperprolactinemic drugs should not be prescribed concomitantly with triptorelin pamoate since hyperprolactinemia reduces the number of pituitary GnRH receptors). Products include:

Thioridazine Hydrochloride (Hyperprolactinemic drugs should not be prescribed concomitantly with triptorelin pamoate since hyperprolactinemia reduces the number of pituitary GnRH receptors). Products include:

Thiothixene (Hyperprolactinemic drugs should not be prescribed concomitantly with triptorelin pamoate since hyperprolactinemia reduces the number of pituitary GnRH receptors). Products include:

Trifluoperazine Hydrochloride (Hyperprolactinemic drugs should not be prescribed concomitantly with triptorelin pamoate since hyperprolactinemia reduces the number of pituitary GnRH receptors).
No products indexed under this heading.

Verapamil Hydrochloride (Hyperprolactinemic drugs should not be prescribed concomitantly with triptorelin pamoate since hyperprolactinemia reduces the number of pituitary GnRH receptors). Products include:

Ziprasidone Hydrochloride (Hyperprolactinemic drugs should not be prescribed concomitantly with triptorelin pamoate since hyperprolactinemia reduces the number of pituitary GnRH receptors). Products include:

Ziprasidone Mesylate (Hyperprolactinemic drugs should not be prescribed concomitantly with triptorelin pamoate since hyperprolactinemia reduces the number of pituitary GnRH receptors). Products include:

TRIAMINIC CHEST & NASAL CONGESTION LIQUID

(Guaifenesin, Phenylephrine Hydrochloride)................................ 746
May interact with monoamine oxidase inhibitors. Compounds in these categories include:

Isocarboxazid (Concurrent and/or sequential use with MAO inhibitors is not recommended).
No products indexed under this heading.

Moclobemide (Concurrent and/or sequential use with MAO inhibitors is not recommended).
No products indexed under this heading.

Pargyline Hydrochloride (Concurrent and/or sequential use with MAO inhibitors is not recommended).
No products indexed under this heading.

Phenelzine Sulfate (Concurrent and/or sequential use with MAO inhibitors is not recommended).
No products indexed under this heading.

Procarbazine Hydrochloride (Concurrent and/or sequential use with MAO inhibitors is not recommended). Products include:

Selegiline Hydrochloride (Concurrent and/or sequential use with MAO inhibitors is not recommended). Products include:

Tranylcypromine Sulfate (Concurrent and/or sequential use with MAO inhibitors is not recommended). Products include:

TRIAMINIC COLD & ALLERGY LIQUID

(Chlorpheniramine Maleate, Phenylephrine Hydrochloride)........... 746
May interact with:

See (Triaminic Night Time Cough & Cold Liquid).
No products indexed under this heading.

TRIAMINIC DAYTIME COLD & COUGH LIQUID

(Dextromethorphan Hydrobromide, Phenylephrine Hydrochloride)................................ 745
May interact with monoamine oxidase inhibitors. Compounds in these categories include:

Isocarboxazid (Concurrent and/or sequential use with MAO inhibitors is not recommended).
No products indexed under this heading.

Moclobemide (Concurrent and/or sequential use with MAO inhibitors is not recommended).
No products indexed under this heading.

Pargyline Hydrochloride (Concurrent and/or sequential use with MAO inhibitors is not recommended).
No products indexed under this heading.

Phenelzine Sulfate (Concurrent and/or sequential use with MAO inhibitors is not recommended).
No products indexed under this heading.

IMPORTANT NOTE: Always consult each drug listing in the patient's regimen for possible interactions.

Procarbazine Hydrochloride (Concurrent and/or sequential use with MAO inhibitors is not recommended). Products include:
Matulane Capsules 3191

Selegiline Hydrochloride (Concurrent and/or sequential use with MAO inhibitors is not recommended). Products include:
Eldepryl Capsules 3208
Zelapar Tablets 3372

Tranylcypromine Sulfate (Concurrent and/or sequential use with MAO inhibitors is not recommended). Products include:
Parnate Tablets 1527

TRIAMINIC NIGHTTIME COLD & COUGH LIQUID
(Diphenhydramine Hydrochloride, Phenylephrine Hydrochloride)............ 746
May interact with hypnotics and sedatives, monoamine oxidase inhibitors, tranquilizers, and certain other agents. Compounds in these categories include:

Alprazolam (May increase drowsiness effect). Products include:
Niravam Orally Disintegrating Tablets.. 3092

Buspirone Hydrochloride (May increase drowsiness effect).
No products indexed under this heading.

Chlordiazepoxide (May increase drowsiness effect).
No products indexed under this heading.

Chlordiazepoxide Hydrochloride (May increase drowsiness effect). Products include:
Librium Capsules 3347

Chlorpromazine (May increase drowsiness effect).
No products indexed under this heading.

Chlorpromazine Hydrochloride (May increase drowsiness effect).
No products indexed under this heading.

Chlorprothixene (May increase drowsiness effect).
No products indexed under this heading.

Chlorprothixene Hydrochloride (May increase drowsiness effect).
No products indexed under this heading.

Clorazepate Dipotassium (May increase drowsiness effect). Products include:
Tranxene 2474

Diazepam (May increase drowsiness effect). Products include:
Diastat Rectal Delivery System 3343
Valium Tablets 2819

Droperidol (May increase drowsiness effect).
No products indexed under this heading.

Estazolam (May increase drowsiness effect). Products include:
ProSom Tablets 517

Ethchlorvynol (May increase drowsiness effect).
No products indexed under this heading.

Ethinamate (May increase drowsiness effect).
No products indexed under this heading.

Fluphenazine Decanoate (May increase drowsiness effect).
No products indexed under this heading.

Fluphenazine Enanthate (May increase drowsiness effect).
No products indexed under this heading.

Fluphenazine Hydrochloride (May increase drowsiness effect).
No products indexed under this heading.

Flurazepam Hydrochloride (May increase drowsiness effect). Products include:
Dalmane Capsules 3342

Glutethimide (May increase drowsiness effect).
No products indexed under this heading.

Haloperidol (May increase drowsiness effect).
No products indexed under this heading.

Haloperidol Decanoate (May increase drowsiness effect).
No products indexed under this heading.

Hydroxyzine Hydrochloride (May increase drowsiness effect).
No products indexed under this heading.

Isocarboxazid (Concurrent and/or sequential use with MAO inhibitors is not recommended).
No products indexed under this heading.

Lorazepam (May increase drowsiness effect).
No products indexed under this heading.

Loxapine Hydrochloride (May increase drowsiness effect).
No products indexed under this heading.

Loxapine Succinate (May increase drowsiness effect).
No products indexed under this heading.

Meprobamate (May increase drowsiness effect).
No products indexed under this heading.

Mesoridazine Besylate (May increase drowsiness effect).
No products indexed under this heading.

Midazolam Hydrochloride (May increase drowsiness effect).
No products indexed under this heading.

Moclobemide (Concurrent and/or sequential use with MAO inhibitors is not recommended).
No products indexed under this heading.

Molindone Hydrochloride (May increase drowsiness effect). Products include:
Moban Tablets 1119

Oxazepam (May increase drowsiness effect).
No products indexed under this heading.

Pargyline Hydrochloride (Concurrent and/or sequential use with MAO inhibitors is not recommended).
No products indexed under this heading.

Perphenazine (May increase drowsiness effect).
No products indexed under this heading.

Phenelzine Sulfate (Concurrent and/or sequential use with MAO inhibitors is not recommended).
No products indexed under this heading.

Prazepam (May increase drowsiness effect).
No products indexed under this heading.

Procarbazine Hydrochloride (Concurrent and/or sequential use with MAO inhibitors is not recommended). Products include:
Matulane Capsules 3191

Prochlorperazine (May increase drowsiness effect).
No products indexed under this heading.

Promethazine Hydrochloride (May increase drowsiness effect). Products include:
Phenergan Tablets and Suppositories.............................. 3440

Propofol (May increase drowsiness effect).
No products indexed under this heading.

Quazepam (May increase drowsiness effect).
No products indexed under this heading.

Ramelteon (May increase drowsiness effect). Products include:
Rozerem Tablets 3231

Secobarbital Sodium (May increase drowsiness effect).
No products indexed under this heading.

Selegiline Hydrochloride (Concurrent and/or sequential use with MAO inhibitors is not recommended). Products include:
Eldepryl Capsules 3208
Zelapar Tablets 3372

Temazepam (May increase drowsiness effect). Products include:
Restoril Capsules 1860

Thioridazine Hydrochloride (May increase drowsiness effect). Products include:
Thioridazine Hydrochloride Tablets 2163

Thiothixene (May increase drowsiness effect). Products include:
Thiothixene Capsules 2165

Tranylcypromine Sulfate (Concurrent and/or sequential use with MAO inhibitors is not recommended). Products include:
Parnate Tablets 1527

Triazolam (May increase drowsiness effect).
No products indexed under this heading.

Trifluoperazine Hydrochloride (May increase drowsiness effect).
No products indexed under this heading.

Zaleplon (May increase drowsiness effect). Products include:
Sonata Capsules 1717

Zolpidem Tartrate (May increase drowsiness effect). Products include:
Ambien Tablets 2851
Ambien CR Tablets 2855

Food Interactions

Alcohol (Concomitant consumption of alcohol may cause liver damage).

TRIAMINIC COUGH & SORE THROAT LIQUID
(Acetaminophen, Dextromethorphan Hydrobromide)..... 747
May interact with monoamine oxidase inhibitors. Compounds in these categories include:

Isocarboxazid (Concurrent and/or sequential use with MAO inhibitors is not recommended).
No products indexed under this heading.

Moclobemide (Concurrent and/or sequential use with MAO inhibitors is not recommended).
No products indexed under this heading.

Pargyline Hydrochloride (Concurrent and/or sequential use with MAO inhibitors is not recommended).
No products indexed under this heading.

Phenelzine Sulfate (Concurrent and/or sequential use with MAO inhibitors is not recommended).
No products indexed under this heading.

Procarbazine Hydrochloride (Concurrent and/or sequential use with MAO inhibitors is not recommended). Products include:
Matulane Capsules 3191

Selegiline Hydrochloride (Concurrent and/or sequential use with MAO inhibitors is not recommended). Products include:
Eldepryl Capsules 3208
Zelapar Tablets 3372

Tranylcypromine Sulfate (Concurrent and/or sequential use with MAO inhibitors is not recommended). Products include:
Parnate Tablets 1527

TRIAMINIC COUGH & RUNNY NOSE SOFTCHEWS
(Chlorpheniramine Maleate, Dextromethorphan Hydrobromide).... 748
May interact with hypnotics and sedatives, monoamine oxidase inhibitors, tranquilizers, and certain other agents. Compounds in these categories include:

Alprazolam (May increase drowsiness effect). Products include:
Niravam Orally Disintegrating Tablets.. 3092

Buspirone Hydrochloride (May increase drowsiness effect).
No products indexed under this heading.

Chlordiazepoxide (May increase drowsiness effect).
No products indexed under this heading.

Chlordiazepoxide Hydrochloride (May increase drowsiness effect). Products include:
Librium Capsules 3347

Chlorpromazine (May increase drowsiness effect).
No products indexed under this heading.

Chlorpromazine Hydrochloride (May increase drowsiness effect).
No products indexed under this heading.

Chlorprothixene (May increase drowsiness effect).
No products indexed under this heading.

Chlorprothixene Hydrochloride (May increase drowsiness effect).
No products indexed under this heading.

Clorazepate Dipotassium (May increase drowsiness effect). Products include:
Tranxene 2474

Diazepam (May increase drowsiness effect). Products include:
Diastat Rectal Delivery System 3343
Valium Tablets 2819

Droperidol (May increase drowsiness effect).
No products indexed under this heading.

Estazolam (May increase drowsiness effect). Products include:
ProSom Tablets 517

Ethchlorvynol (May increase drowsiness effect).
No products indexed under this heading.

Ethinamate (May increase drowsiness effect).
No products indexed under this heading.

Fluphenazine Decanoate (May increase drowsiness effect).
No products indexed under this heading.

Fluphenazine Enanthate (May increase drowsiness effect).
No products indexed under this heading.

Fluphenazine Hydrochloride (May increase drowsiness effect).
No products indexed under this heading.

Flurazepam Hydrochloride (May increase drowsiness effect). Products include:
Dalmane Capsules 3342

Glutethimide (May increase drowsiness effect).
No products indexed under this heading.

Haloperidol (May increase drowsiness effect).
No products indexed under this heading.

Haloperidol Decanoate (May increase drowsiness effect).
No products indexed under this heading.

Hydroxyzine Hydrochloride (May increase drowsiness effect).
No products indexed under this heading.

Isocarboxazid (Concurrent and/or sequential use with MAO inhibitors is not recommended).
No products indexed under this heading.

Lorazepam (May increase drowsiness effect).
No products indexed under this heading.

Loxapine Hydrochloride (May increase drowsiness effect).
No products indexed under this heading.

Loxapine Succinate (May increase drowsiness effect).
No products indexed under this heading.

Meprobamate (May increase drowsiness effect).
No products indexed under this heading.

Mesoridazine Besylate (May increase drowsiness effect).
No products indexed under this heading.

Midazolam Hydrochloride (May increase drowsiness effect).
No products indexed under this heading.

Moclobemide (Concurrent and/or sequential use with MAO inhibitors is not recommended).
No products indexed under this heading.

Molindone Hydrochloride (May increase drowsiness effect). Products include:
Moban Tablets 1119

Oxazepam (May increase drowsiness effect).
No products indexed under this heading.

Pargyline Hydrochloride (Concurrent and/or sequential use with MAO inhibitors is not recommended).
No products indexed under this heading.

Perphenazine (May increase drowsiness effect).
No products indexed under this heading.

Phenelzine Sulfate (Concurrent and/or sequential use with MAO inhibitors is not recommended).
No products indexed under this heading.

Prazepam (May increase drowsiness effect).
No products indexed under this heading.

Procarbazine Hydrochloride (Concurrent and/or sequential use with MAO inhibitors is not recommended). Products include:
Matulane Capsules 3191

Prochlorperazine (May increase drowsiness effect).
No products indexed under this heading.

Promethazine Hydrochloride (May increase drowsiness effect). Products include:
Phenergan Tablets and Suppositories 3440

Propofol (May increase drowsiness effect).
No products indexed under this heading.

Quazepam (May increase drowsiness effect).
No products indexed under this heading.

Ramelteon (May increase drowsiness effect). Products include:
Rozerem Tablets 3231

Secobarbital Sodium (May increase drowsiness effect).
No products indexed under this heading.

Selegiline Hydrochloride (Concurrent and/or sequential use with MAO inhibitors is not recommended). Products include:
Eldepryl Capsules 3208
Zelapar Tablets 3372

Temazepam (May increase drowsiness effect). Products include:
Restoril Capsules 1860

Thioridazine Hydrochloride (May increase drowsiness effect). Products include:
Thioridazine Hydrochloride Tablets 2163

Thiothixene (May increase drowsiness effect). Products include:
Thiothixene Capsules 2165

Tranylcypromine Sulfate (Concurrent and/or sequential use with MAO inhibitors is not recommended). Products include:
Parnate Tablets 1527

Triazolam (May increase drowsiness effect).
No products indexed under this heading.

Trifluoperazine Hydrochloride (May increase drowsiness effect).
No products indexed under this heading.

Zaleplon (May increase drowsiness effect). Products include:
Sonata Capsules 1717

Zolpidem Tartrate (May increase drowsiness effect). Products include:
Ambien Tablets 2851
Ambien CR Tablets 2855

Food Interactions

Alcohol (May increase drowsiness effect).

TRIAMINIC THIN STRIPS COLD

(Phenylephrine Hydrochloride) 748
May interact with monoamine oxidase inhibitors. Compounds in these categories include:

Isocarboxazid (Concurrent and/or sequential use with MAO inhibitors is not recommended).
No products indexed under this heading.

Moclobemide (Concurrent and/or sequential use with MAO inhibitors is not recommended).
No products indexed under this heading.

Pargyline Hydrochloride (Concurrent and/or sequential use with MAO inhibitors is not recommended).
No products indexed under this heading.

Phenelzine Sulfate (Concurrent and/or sequential use with MAO inhibitors is not recommended).
No products indexed under this heading.

Procarbazine Hydrochloride (Concurrent and/or sequential use with MAO inhibitors is not recommended). Products include:
Matulane Capsules 3191

Selegiline Hydrochloride (Concurrent and/or sequential use with MAO inhibitors is not recommended). Products include:
Eldepryl Capsules 3208
Zelapar Tablets 3372

Tranylcypromine Sulfate (Concurrent and/or sequential use with MAO inhibitors is not recommended). Products include:
Parnate Tablets 1527

TRIAMINIC THIN STRIPS COLD & COUGH

(Dextromethorphan Hydrobromide, Phenylephrine Hydrochloride) 778
May interact with monoamine oxidase inhibitors. Compounds in these categories include:

Isocarboxazid (Concurrent and/or sequential use with MAO inhibitors is not recommended).
No products indexed under this heading.

Moclobemide (Concurrent and/or sequential use with MAO inhibitors is not recommended).
No products indexed under this heading.

Pargyline Hydrochloride (Concurrent and/or sequential use with MAO inhibitors is not recommended).
No products indexed under this heading.

Phenelzine Sulfate (Concurrent and/or sequential use with MAO inhibitors is not recommended).
No products indexed under this heading.

Procarbazine Hydrochloride (Concurrent and/or sequential use with MAO inhibitors is not recommended). Products include:
Matulane Capsules 3191

Selegiline Hydrochloride (Concurrent and/or sequential use with MAO inhibitors is not recommended). Products include:
Eldepryl Capsules 3208
Zelapar Tablets 3372

Tranylcypromine Sulfate (Concurrent and/or sequential use with MAO inhibitors is not recommended). Products include:
Parnate Tablets 1527

TRIAMINIC THIN STRIPS COUGH & RUNNY NOSE

(Diphenhydramine Hydrochloride) 749
May interact with hypnotics and sedatives and tranquilizers. Compounds in these categories include:

Alprazolam (Tranquilizers may increase the drowsiness effect). Products include:
Niravam Orally Disintegrating Tablets 3092

Buspirone Hydrochloride (Tranquilizers may increase the drowsiness effect).
No products indexed under this heading.

Chlordiazepoxide (Tranquilizers may increase the drowsiness effect).
No products indexed under this heading.

Chlordiazepoxide Hydrochloride (Tranquilizers may increase the drowsiness effect). Products include:
Librium Capsules 3347

Chlorpromazine (Tranquilizers may increase the drowsiness effect).
No products indexed under this heading.

Chlorpromazine Hydrochloride (Tranquilizers may increase the drowsiness effect).
No products indexed under this heading.

Chlorprothixene (Tranquilizers may increase the drowsiness effect).
No products indexed under this heading.

Chlorprothixene Hydrochloride (Tranquilizers may increase the drowsiness effect).
No products indexed under this heading.

Clorazepate Dipotassium (Tranquilizers may increase the drowsiness effect). Products include:
Tranxene 2474

Diazepam (Tranquilizers may increase the drowsiness effect). Products include:
Diastat Rectal Delivery System 3343
Valium Tablets 2819

Droperidol (Tranquilizers may increase the drowsiness effect).
No products indexed under this heading.

Estazolam (Sedatives may increase the drowsiness effect). Products include:
ProSom Tablets 517

Ethchlorvynol (Sedatives may increase the drowsiness effect).
No products indexed under this heading.

Ethinamate (Sedatives may increase the drowsiness effect).
No products indexed under this heading.

Fluphenazine Decanoate (Tranquilizers may increase the drowsiness effect).
No products indexed under this heading.

Fluphenazine Enanthate (Tranquilizers may increase the drowsiness effect).
No products indexed under this heading.

Fluphenazine Hydrochloride (Tranquilizers may increase the drowsiness effect).
No products indexed under this heading.

Flurazepam Hydrochloride (Sedatives may increase the drowsiness effect). Products include:
Dalmane Capsules 3342

Glutethimide (Sedatives may increase the drowsiness effect).
No products indexed under this heading.

Haloperidol (Tranquilizers may increase the drowsiness effect).
No products indexed under this heading.

Haloperidol Decanoate (Tranquilizers may increase the drowsiness effect).
No products indexed under this heading.

Hydroxyzine Hydrochloride (Tranquilizers may increase the drowsiness effect).
No products indexed under this heading.

Lorazepam (Sedatives may increase the drowsiness effect).
No products indexed under this heading.

Loxapine Hydrochloride (Tranquilizers may increase the drowsiness effect).
No products indexed under this heading.

Loxapine Succinate (Tranquilizers may increase the drowsiness effect).
No products indexed under this heading.

Meprobamate (Tranquilizers may increase the drowsiness effect).
No products indexed under this heading.

Mesoridazine Besylate (Tranquilizers may increase the drowsiness effect).
No products indexed under this heading.

Midazolam Hydrochloride (Sedatives may increase the drowsiness effect).
No products indexed under this heading.

Molindone Hydrochloride (Tranquilizers may increase the drowsiness effect). Products include:
Moban Tablets 1119

Oxazepam (Tranquilizers may increase the drowsiness effect).
No products indexed under this heading.

Perphenazine (Tranquilizers may increase the drowsiness effect).
No products indexed under this heading.

Prazepam (Tranquilizers may increase the drowsiness effect).
No products indexed under this heading.

Prochlorperazine (Tranquilizers may increase the drowsiness effect).
No products indexed under this heading.

Promethazine Hydrochloride (Tranquilizers may increase the drowsiness effect). Products include:
Phenergan Tablets and Suppositories 3440

Propofol (Sedatives may increase the drowsiness effect).
No products indexed under this heading.

Quazepam (Sedatives may increase the drowsiness effect).
No products indexed under this heading.

Ramelteon (Sedatives may increase the drowsiness effect). Products include:
Rozerem Tablets 3231

Secobarbital Sodium (Sedatives may increase the drowsiness effect).
No products indexed under this heading.

Temazepam (Sedatives may increase the drowsiness effect). Products include:
Restoril Capsules 1860

Thioridazine Hydrochloride (Tranquilizers may increase the drowsiness effect). Products include:
Thioridazine Hydrochloride Tablets 2163

Thiothixene (Tranquilizers may increase the drowsiness effect). Products include:
Thiothixene Capsules 2165

Triazolam (Sedatives may increase the drowsiness effect).
No products indexed under this heading.

Trifluoperazine Hydrochloride (Tranquilizers may increase the drowsiness effect).
No products indexed under this heading.

Zaleplon (Sedatives may increase the drowsiness effect). Products include:
Sonata Capsules 1717

Zolpidem Tartrate (Sedatives may increase the drowsiness effect). Products include:
Ambien Tablets 2851
Ambien CR Tablets 2855

TRIAMINIC INFANT THIN STRIPS DECONGESTANT

(Phenylephrine Hydrochloride) .... ▣747
May interact with monoamine oxidase inhibitors. Compounds in these categories include:

Isocarboxazid (Concurrent and/or sequential use with MAO inhibitors is not recommended).
No products indexed under this heading.

Moclobemide (Concurrent and/or sequential use with MAO inhibitors is not recommended).
No products indexed under this heading.

Pargyline Hydrochloride (Concurrent and/or sequential use with MAO inhibitors is not recommended).
No products indexed under this heading.

Phenelzine Sulfate (Concurrent and/or sequential use with MAO inhibitors is not recommended).
No products indexed under this heading.

Procarbazine Hydrochloride (Concurrent and/or sequential use with MAO inhibitors is not recommended). Products include:
Matulane Capsules 3191

Selegiline Hydrochloride (Concurrent and/or sequential use with MAO inhibitors is not recommended). Products include:
Eldepryl Capsules 3208
Zelapar Tablets 3372

Tranylcypromine Sulfate (Concurrent and/or sequential use with MAO inhibitors is not recommended). Products include:
Parnate Tablets 1527

TRIAMINIC INFANT THIN STRIPS DECONGESTANT PLUS COUGH

(Dextromethorphan Hydrobromide, Phenylephrine Hydrochloride) .... ▣747
May interact with monoamine oxidase inhibitors. Compounds in these categories include:

Isocarboxazid (Concurrent and/or sequential use with MAO inhibitors is not recommended).
No products indexed under this heading.

Moclobemide (Concurrent and/or sequential use with MAO inhibitors is not recommended).
No products indexed under this heading.

Pargyline Hydrochloride (Concurrent and/or sequential use with MAO inhibitors is not recommended).
No products indexed under this heading.

Phenelzine Sulfate (Concurrent and/or sequential use with MAO inhibitors is not recommended).
No products indexed under this heading.

Procarbazine Hydrochloride (Concurrent and/or sequential use with MAO inhibitors is not recommended). Products include:
Matulane Capsules 3191

Selegiline Hydrochloride (Concurrent and/or sequential use with MAO inhibitors is not recommended). Products include:
Eldepryl Capsules 3208
Zelapar Tablets 3372

Tranylcypromine Sulfate (Concurrent and/or sequential use with MAO inhibitors is not recommended). Products include:
Parnate Tablets 1527

TRIAZ CLEANSER

(Benzoyl Peroxide) 1892
None cited in PDR database.

TRIAZ GEL

(Benzoyl Peroxide) 1892
None cited in PDR database.

TRIAZ PADS

(Benzoyl Peroxide) 1892
None cited in PDR database.

TRICOR TABLETS

(Fenofibrate) 527
May interact with bile acid sequestering agents, oral anticoagulants, HMG-CoA reductase inhibitors, immunosuppressive agents, nephrotoxic agents, and certain other agents. Compounds in these categories include:

Abacavir Sulfate (The benefits and risks of using fenofibrate tablets with immunosuppressants and other potentially nephrotoxic agents should be carefully considered and the lowest effective dose employed). Products include:
Epzicom Tablets 1436
Trizivir Tablets 1589
Ziagen 1626

Acyclovir (The benefits and risks of using fenofibrate tablets with immunosuppressants and other potentially nephrotoxic agents should be carefully considered and the lowest effective dose employed). Products include:
Zovirax 1643
Zovirax Cream 820
Zovirax Ointment 821

Acyclovir Sodium (The benefits and risks of using fenofibrate tablets with immunosuppressants and other potentially nephrotoxic agents should be carefully considered and the lowest effective dose employed).
No products indexed under this heading.

Alatrofloxacin Mesylate (The benefits and risks of using fenofibrate tablets with immunosuppressants and other potentially nephrotoxic agents should be carefully considered and the lowest effective dose employed).
No products indexed under this heading.

Aldesleukin (The benefits and risks of using fenofibrate tablets with immunosuppressants and other potentially nephrotoxic agents should be carefully considered and the lowest effective dose employed). Products include:
Proleukin for Injection 2266

Amikacin Sulfate (The benefits and risks of using fenofibrate tablets with immunosuppressants and other potentially nephrotoxic agents should be carefully considered and the lowest effective dose employed).
No products indexed under this heading.

Amoxicillin (The benefits and risks of using fenofibrate tablets with immunosuppressants and other potentially nephrotoxic agents should be carefully considered and the lowest effective dose employed). Products include:
Amoxil Capsules 1343
Amoxil Chewable Tablets 1343
Amoxil Pediatric Drops for Oral Suspension 1343
Amoxil Powder for Oral Suspension 1343
Amoxil Tablets 1343
Augmentin 1360
Augmentin Tablets 1363
Augmentin XR Extended-Release Tablets 1369
Augmentin ES-600 Powder for Oral Suspension 1366
PREVPAC 3284

Amoxicillin Trihydrate (The benefits and risks of using fenofibrate tablets with immunosuppressants and other potentially nephrotoxic agents should be carefully considered and the lowest effective dose employed).
No products indexed under this heading.

Amphotericin B (The benefits and risks of using fenofibrate tablets with immunosuppressants and other potentially nephrotoxic agents should be carefully considered and the lowest effective dose employed).
No products indexed under this heading.

Amphotericin B, liposomal (The benefits and risks of using fenofibrate tablets with immunosuppressants and other potentially nephrotoxic agents should be carefully considered and the lowest effective dose employed). Products include:

AmBisome for Injection 620

Amphotericin B Cholesteryl Sulfate (The benefits and risks of using fenofibrate tablets with immunosuppressants and other potentially nephrotoxic agents should be carefully considered and the lowest effective dose employed).

No products indexed under this heading.

Amphotericin B Lipid Complex (The benefits and risks of using fenofibrate tablets with immunosuppressants and other potentially nephrotoxic agents should be carefully considered and the lowest effective dose employed). Products include:

Abelcet Injection 1141

Ampicillin (The benefits and risks of using fenofibrate tablets with immunosuppressants and other potentially nephrotoxic agents should be carefully considered and the lowest effective dose employed).

No products indexed under this heading.

Ampicillin Sodium (The benefits and risks of using fenofibrate tablets with immunosuppressants and other potentially nephrotoxic agents should be carefully considered and the lowest effective dose employed).

No products indexed under this heading.

Ampicillin Trihydrate (The benefits and risks of using fenofibrate tablets with immunosuppressants and other potentially nephrotoxic agents should be carefully considered and the lowest effective dose employed).

No products indexed under this heading.

Amprenavir (The benefits and risks of using fenofibrate tablets with immunosuppressants and other potentially nephrotoxic agents should be carefully considered and the lowest effective dose employed). Products include:

Agenerase Capsules 1327
Agenerase Oral Solution 1332

Anisindione (Caution should be exercised when anticoagulants are given in conjunction with fenofibrate because of the potentiation of coumarin-type anticoagulants in prolonging the PT/INR. The dosage of the anticoagulant should be reduced to maintain the PT/INR at the desired level to prevent bleeding complications. Frequent PT/INR determinations are advisable until it has been definitely determined that the PT/INR has stabilized). Products include:

Miradon Tablets 3042

Aspirin (The benefits and risks of using fenofibrate tablets with immunosuppressants and other potentially nephrotoxic agents should be carefully considered and the lowest effective dose employed). Products include:

Aggrenox Capsules 822
Bayer Aspirin 744
BC Allergy Sinus Cold Powder 677
BC Headache Powder 677
Arthritis Strength BC Powder 677
BC Sinus Cold Powder 677
Excedrin Extra Strength Caplets/Tablets/Geltabs 684
Excedrin Migraine Caplets/Tablets/Geltabs 609
Goody's Body Pain Formula Powder 684
Goody's Extra Strength Headache Powders 611
Goody's Extra Strength Pain Relief Tablets 685
Percodan Tablets 1132
St. Joseph 81 mg Aspirin Chewable and Enteric Coated Tablets 1869

Atazanavir (The benefits and risks of using fenofibrate tablets with immunosuppressants and other potentially nephrotoxic agents should be carefully considered and the lowest effective dose employed).

No products indexed under this heading.

Atorvastatin Calcium (Co-administration of fibric acid derivatives and HMG-CoA reductase inhibitors has been associated with rhabdomyolysis, markedly elevated creatine kinase levels and myoglobulinuria, leading in a high proportion of cases to acute renal failure; the combined use should be avoided unless the benefit of further alterations in lipid levels is likely to outweigh the increased risk of this combination). Products include:

Caduet Tablets 2508
Lipitor Tablets 2483

Azathioprine (The benefits and risks of using fenofibrate tablets with immunosuppressants and other potentially nephrotoxic agents should be carefully considered and the lowest effective dose employed).

No products indexed under this heading.

Azithromycin Dihydrate (The benefits and risks of using fenofibrate tablets with immunosuppressants and other potentially nephrotoxic agents should be carefully considered and the lowest effective dose employed).

No products indexed under this heading.

Azlocillin Sodium (The benefits and risks of using fenofibrate tablets with immunosuppressants and other potentially nephrotoxic agents should be carefully considered and the lowest effective dose employed).

No products indexed under this heading.

Aztreonam (The benefits and risks of using fenofibrate tablets with immunosuppressants and other potentially nephrotoxic agents should be carefully considered and the lowest effective dose employed).

No products indexed under this heading.

Bacampicillin Hydrochloride (The benefits and risks of using fenofibrate tablets with immunosuppressants and other potentially nephrotoxic agents should be carefully considered and the lowest effective dose employed).

No products indexed under this heading.

Balsalazide Disodium (The benefits and risks of using fenofibrate tablets with immunosuppressants and other potentially nephrotoxic agents should be carefully considered and the lowest effective dose employed). Products include:

Colazal Capsules 2838

Basiliximab (The benefits and risks of using fenofibrate tablets with immunosuppressants and other potentially nephrotoxic agents should be carefully considered and the lowest effective dose employed). Products include:

Simulect for Injection 2284

Benazepril Hydrochloride (The benefits and risks of using fenofibrate tablets with immunosuppressants and other potentially nephrotoxic agents should be carefully considered and the lowest effective dose employed). Products include:

Lotensin Tablets 2243
Lotensin HCT Tablets 2246
Lotrel Capsules 2249

Bendroflumethiazide (The benefits and risks of using fenofibrate tablets with immunosuppressants and other potentially nephrotoxic agents should be carefully considered and the lowest effective dose employed).

No products indexed under this heading.

Caffeine (The benefits and risks of using fenofibrate tablets with immunosuppressants and other potentially nephrotoxic agents should be carefully considered and the lowest effective dose employed). Products include:

BC Headache Powder 677
Arthritis Strength BC Powder 677
Excedrin Extra Strength Caplets/Tablets/Geltabs 684
Excedrin Migraine Caplets/Tablets/Geltabs 609
Excedrin Tension Headache Caplets/Tablets/Geltabs 611
Goody's Extra Strength Headache Powders 611
Goody's Extra Strength Pain Relief Tablets 685
Vivarin 602
Winrgy Dietary Supplement 823

Captopril (The benefits and risks of using fenofibrate tablets with immunosuppressants and other potentially nephrotoxic agents should be carefully considered and the lowest effective dose employed). Products include:

Captopril Tablets 2149

Carbenicillin Disodium (The benefits and risks of using fenofibrate tablets with immunosuppressants and other potentially nephrotoxic agents should be carefully considered and the lowest effective dose employed).

No products indexed under this heading.

Carbenicillin Indanyl Sodium (The benefits and risks of using fenofibrate tablets with immunosuppressants and other potentially nephrotoxic agents should be carefully considered and the lowest effective dose employed).

No products indexed under this heading.

Carboplatin (The benefits and risks of using fenofibrate tablets with immunosuppressants and other potentially nephrotoxic agents should be carefully considered and the lowest effective dose employed).

No products indexed under this heading.

Carmustine (BCNU) (The benefits and risks of using fenofibrate tablets with immunosuppressants and other potentially nephrotoxic agents should be carefully considered and the lowest effective dose employed).

No products indexed under this heading.

Cefaclor (The benefits and risks of using fenofibrate tablets with immunosuppressants and other potentially nephrotoxic agents should be carefully considered and the lowest effective dose employed).

No products indexed under this heading.

Cefadroxil (The benefits and risks of using fenofibrate tablets with immunosuppressants and other potentially nephrotoxic agents should be carefully considered and the lowest effective dose employed).

No products indexed under this heading.

Cefamandole Nafate (The benefits and risks of using fenofibrate tablets with immunosuppressants and other potentially nephrotoxic agents should be carefully considered and the lowest effective dose employed).

No products indexed under this heading.

Cefazolin Sodium (The benefits and risks of using fenofibrate tablets with immunosuppressants and other potentially nephrotoxic agents should be carefully considered and the lowest effective dose employed).

No products indexed under this heading.

Cefdinir (The benefits and risks of using fenofibrate tablets with immunosuppressants and other potentially nephrotoxic agents should be carefully considered and the lowest effective dose employed). Products include:

Omnicef Capsules 511
Omnicef for Oral Suspension 511

Cefepime Hydrochloride (The benefits and risks of using fenofibrate tablets with immunosuppressants and other potentially nephrotoxic agents should be carefully considered and the lowest effective dose employed). Products include:

Maxipime for Injection 1105

Cefixime (The benefits and risks of using fenofibrate tablets with immunosuppressants and other potentially nephrotoxic agents should be carefully considered and the lowest effective dose employed). Products include:

Suprax 1843

Cefmetazole Sodium (The benefits and risks of using fenofibrate tablets with immunosuppressants and other potentially nephrotoxic agents should be carefully considered and the lowest effective dose employed).

No products indexed under this heading.

Cefonicid Sodium (The benefits and risks of using fenofibrate tablets with immunosuppressants and other potentially nephrotoxic agents should be carefully considered and the lowest effective dose employed).

No products indexed under this heading.

Cefoperazone Sodium (The benefits and risks of using fenofibrate tablets with immunosuppressants and other potentially nephrotoxic agents should be carefully considered and the lowest effective dose employed).

No products indexed under this heading.

Ceforanide (The benefits and risks of using fenofibrate tablets with immunosuppressants and other potentially nephrotoxic agents should be carefully considered and the lowest effective dose employed).
No products indexed under this heading.

Cefotaxime Sodium (The benefits and risks of using fenofibrate tablets with immunosuppressants and other potentially nephrotoxic agents should be carefully considered and the lowest effective dose employed).
No products indexed under this heading.

Cefotetan (The benefits and risks of using fenofibrate tablets with immunosuppressants and other potentially nephrotoxic agents should be carefully considered and the lowest effective dose employed).
No products indexed under this heading.

Cefoxitin Sodium (The benefits and risks of using fenofibrate tablets with immunosuppressants and other potentially nephrotoxic agents should be carefully considered and the lowest effective dose employed).
Products include:
Mefoxin for Injection 2012
Mefoxin Premixed Intravenous Solution.. 2016

Cefpodoxime Proxetil (The benefits and risks of using fenofibrate tablets with immunosuppressants and other potentially nephrotoxic agents should be carefully considered and the lowest effective dose employed). Products include:
Vantin Tablets and Oral Suspension 2645

Cefprozil (The benefits and risks of using fenofibrate tablets with immunosuppressants and other potentially nephrotoxic agents should be carefully considered and the lowest effective dose employed).
No products indexed under this heading.

Ceftazidime (The benefits and risks of using fenofibrate tablets with immunosuppressants and other potentially nephrotoxic agents should be carefully considered and the lowest effective dose employed).
Products include:
Fortaz 1453

Ceftizoxime Sodium (The benefits and risks of using fenofibrate tablets with immunosuppressants and other potentially nephrotoxic agents should be carefully considered and the lowest effective dose employed).
No products indexed under this heading.

Ceftriaxone Sodium (The benefits and risks of using fenofibrate tablets with immunosuppressants and other potentially nephrotoxic agents should be carefully considered and the lowest effective dose employed).
Products include:
Rocephin Injectable Vials, ADD-Vantage, Galaxy, Bulk............ 2800

Cefuroxime Axetil (The benefits and risks of using fenofibrate tablets with immunosuppressants and other potentially nephrotoxic agents should be carefully considered and the lowest effective dose employed).
Products include:
Ceftin 1407

Cefuroxime Sodium (The benefits and risks of using fenofibrate tablets with immunosuppressants and other potentially nephrotoxic agents should be carefully considered and the lowest effective dose employed).
No products indexed under this heading.

Celecoxib (The benefits and risks of using fenofibrate tablets with immunosuppressants and other potentially nephrotoxic agents should be carefully considered and the lowest effective dose employed).
Products include:
Celebrex Capsules 3134

Cephalexin (The benefits and risks of using fenofibrate tablets with immunosuppressants and other potentially nephrotoxic agents should be carefully considered and the lowest effective dose employed).
Products include:
Keflex Capsules 549

Cephalothin Sodium (The benefits and risks of using fenofibrate tablets with immunosuppressants and other potentially nephrotoxic agents should be carefully considered and the lowest effective dose employed).
No products indexed under this heading.

Cephapirin Sodium (The benefits and risks of using fenofibrate tablets with immunosuppressants and other potentially nephrotoxic agents should be carefully considered and the lowest effective dose employed).
No products indexed under this heading.

Cephradine (The benefits and risks of using fenofibrate tablets with immunosuppressants and other potentially nephrotoxic agents should be carefully considered and the lowest effective dose employed).
No products indexed under this heading.

Cerivastatin Sodium (Co-administration of fibric acid derivatives and HMG-CoA reductase inhibitors has been associated with rhabdomyolysis, markedly elevated creatine kinase levels and myoglobulinuria, leading in a high proportion of cases to acute renal failure; the combined use should be avoided unless the benefit of further alterations in lipid levels is likely to outweigh the increased risk of this combination).
No products indexed under this heading.

Chlorothiazide (The benefits and risks of using fenofibrate tablets with immunosuppressants and other potentially nephrotoxic agents should be carefully considered and the lowest effective dose employed).
Products include:
Diuril Oral Suspension 1954

Chlorothiazide Sodium (The benefits and risks of using fenofibrate tablets with immunosuppressants and other potentially nephrotoxic agents should be carefully considered and the lowest effective dose employed). Products include:
Diuril Sodium Intravenous 2467

Chlorpropamide (The benefits and risks of using fenofibrate tablets with immunosuppressants and other potentially nephrotoxic agents should be carefully considered and the lowest effective dose employed).
No products indexed under this heading.

Cholestyramine (Bile acid sequestrants may bind fenofibrate; fenofibrate should be taken at least 1 hours before or 4-6 hours after a bile acid binding resin to avoid impeding its absorption).
No products indexed under this heading.

Cidofovir (The benefits and risks of using fenofibrate tablets with immunosuppressants and other potentially nephrotoxic agents should be carefully considered and the lowest effective dose employed).
No products indexed under this heading.

Cilastatin Sodium (The benefits and risks of using fenofibrate tablets with immunosuppressants and other potentially nephrotoxic agents should be carefully considered and the lowest effective dose employed).
Products include:
Primaxin I.M. 2045
Primaxin I.V. 2048

Cimetidine (The benefits and risks of using fenofibrate tablets with immunosuppressants and other potentially nephrotoxic agents should be carefully considered and the lowest effective dose employed).
Products include:
Tagamet HB 200 Tablets .... ◘664

Cimetidine Hydrochloride (The benefits and risks of using fenofibrate tablets with immunosuppressants and other potentially nephrotoxic agents should be carefully considered and the lowest effective dose employed).
No products indexed under this heading.

Cisplatin (The benefits and risks of using fenofibrate tablets with immunosuppressants and other potentially nephrotoxic agents should be carefully considered and the lowest effective dose employed).
No products indexed under this heading.

Cladribine (The benefits and risks of using fenofibrate tablets with immunosuppressants and other potentially nephrotoxic agents should be carefully considered and the lowest effective dose employed).
Products include:
Leustatin Injection 2357

Clozapine (The benefits and risks of using fenofibrate tablets with immunosuppressants and other potentially nephrotoxic agents should be carefully considered and the lowest effective dose employed).
Products include:
Clozaril Tablets 2184
FazaClo Orally Disintegrating Tablets 551

Colesevelam Hydrochloride (Bile acid sequestrants may bind fenofibrate; fenofibrate should be taken at least 1 hours before or 4-6 hours after a bile acid binding resin to avoid impeding its absorption).
Products include:
WelChol Tablets 1050

Colestipol Hydrochloride (Bile acid sequestrants may bind fenofibrate; fenofibrate should be taken at least 1 hours before or 4-6 hours after a bile acid binding resin to avoid impeding its absorption).
No products indexed under this heading.

Colistimethate Sodium (The benefits and risks of using fenofibrate tablets with immunosuppressants and other potentially nephrotoxic agents should be carefully considered and the lowest effective dose employed).
No products indexed under this heading.

Colistin Sulfate (The benefits and risks of using fenofibrate tablets with immunosuppressants and other potentially nephrotoxic agents should be carefully considered and the lowest effective dose employed).
No products indexed under this heading.

Cyclophosphamide (The benefits and risks of using fenofibrate tablets with immunosuppressants and other potentially nephrotoxic agents should be carefully considered and the lowest effective dose employed).
No products indexed under this heading.

Cyclosporine (Because Cyclosporine can produce nephrotoxicity with decreases in creatinine clearance and rises in serum creatinine, and because renal excretion is the primary elimination route of fibrate drugs including fenofibrate, there is a risk that an interactionwill lead to deterioration. The benefits and risks of using fenofibrate tablets with immunosuppressants and other potentially nephrotoxic agents should be carefully considered and the lowest effective dose employed). Products include:
Gengraf Capsules 459
Neoral Oral Solution 2259
Neoral Soft Gelatin Capsules 2259
Restasis Ophthalmic Emulsion 575
Sandimmune 2275

Cytarabine (The benefits and risks of using fenofibrate tablets with immunosuppressants and other potentially nephrotoxic agents should be carefully considered and the lowest effective dose employed).
No products indexed under this heading.

Cytarabine Liposome (The benefits and risks of using fenofibrate tablets with immunosuppressants and other potentially nephrotoxic agents should be carefully considered and the lowest effective dose employed). Products include:
DepoCyt Injection 1143

Delavirdine Mesylate (The benefits and risks of using fenofibrate tablets with immunosuppressants and other potentially nephrotoxic agents should be carefully considered and the lowest effective dose employed). Products include:
Rescriptor Tablets 2551

Diatrizoate Meglumine (The benefits and risks of using fenofibrate tablets with immunosuppressants and other potentially nephrotoxic agents should be carefully considered and the lowest effective dose employed).
No products indexed under this heading.

Diatrizoate Sodium (The benefits and risks of using fenofibrate tablets with immunosuppressants and other potentially nephrotoxic agents should be carefully considered and the lowest effective dose employed).
No products indexed under this heading.

Diclofenac Potassium (The benefits and risks of using fenofibrate tablets with immunosuppressants and other potentially nephrotoxic agents should be carefully considered and the lowest effective dose employed).

 No products indexed under this heading.

Diclofenac Sodium (The benefits and risks of using fenofibrate tablets with immunosuppressants and other potentially nephrotoxic agents should be carefully considered and the lowest effective dose employed). Products include:

Arthrotec Tablets	3129
Voltaren Ophthalmic Solution	2309
Voltaren Tablets	2307
Voltaren-XR Tablets	2310

Dicloxacillin Sodium (The benefits and risks of using fenofibrate tablets with immunosuppressants and other potentially nephrotoxic agents should be carefully considered and the lowest effective dose employed).

 No products indexed under this heading.

Dicumarol (Caution should be exercised when anticoagulants are given in conjunction with fenofibrate because of the potentiation of coumarin-type anticoagulants in prolonging the PT/INR. The dosage of the anticoagulant should be reduced to maintain the PT/INR at the desired level to prevent bleeding complications. Frequent PT/INR determinations are advisable until it has been definitely determined that the PT/INR has stabilized).

 No products indexed under this heading.

Didanosine (The benefits and risks of using fenofibrate tablets with immunosuppressants and other potentially nephrotoxic agents should be carefully considered and the lowest effective dose employed).

 No products indexed under this heading.

Efavirenz (The benefits and risks of using fenofibrate tablets with immunosuppressants and other potentially nephrotoxic agents should be carefully considered and the lowest effective dose employed). Products include:

Atripla Tablets	945
Sustiva Capsules	930
Sustiva Tablets	930

Emtricitabine (The benefits and risks of using fenofibrate tablets with immunosuppressants and other potentially nephrotoxic agents should be carefully considered and the lowest effective dose employed). Products include:

Atripla Tablets	945
Emtriva Capsules	1287
Emtriva Oral Solution	1287
Truvada Tablets	1296

Enalapril Maleate (The benefits and risks of using fenofibrate tablets with immunosuppressants and other potentially nephrotoxic agents should be carefully considered and the lowest effective dose employed). Products include:

Vasotec I.V. Injection	2103

Enalaprilat (The benefits and risks of using fenofibrate tablets with immunosuppressants and other potentially nephrotoxic agents should be carefully considered and the lowest effective dose employed).

 No products indexed under this heading.

Enfuvirtide (The benefits and risks of using fenofibrate tablets with immunosuppressants and other potentially nephrotoxic agents should be carefully considered and the lowest effective dose employed). Products include:

Fuzeon Injection	2767

Ethiodized Oil (The benefits and risks of using fenofibrate tablets with immunosuppressants and other potentially nephrotoxic agents should be carefully considered and the lowest effective dose employed).

 No products indexed under this heading.

Etodolac (The benefits and risks of using fenofibrate tablets with immunosuppressants and other potentially nephrotoxic agents should be carefully considered and the lowest effective dose employed).

 No products indexed under this heading.

Fenoprofen Calcium (The benefits and risks of using fenofibrate tablets with immunosuppressants and other potentially nephrotoxic agents should be carefully considered and the lowest effective dose employed). Products include:

Nalfon Capsules	2502

Filgrastim (The benefits and risks of using fenofibrate tablets with immunosuppressants and other potentially nephrotoxic agents should be carefully considered and the lowest effective dose employed). Products include:

Neupogen for Injection	603

Fluorouracil (The benefits and risks of using fenofibrate tablets with immunosuppressants and other potentially nephrotoxic agents should be carefully considered and the lowest effective dose employed). Products include:

Carac Cream, 0.5%	2879
Efudex	3363

Flurbiprofen (The benefits and risks of using fenofibrate tablets with immunosuppressants and other potentially nephrotoxic agents should be carefully considered and the lowest effective dose employed).

 No products indexed under this heading.

Fluvastatin Sodium (Coadministration of fibric acid derivatives and HMG-CoA reductase inhibitors has been associated with rhabdomyolysis, markedly elevated creatine kinase levels and myoglobulinuria, leading in a high proportion of cases to acute renal failure; the combined use should be avoided unless the benefit of further alterations in lipid levels is likely to outweigh the increased risk of this combination). Products include:

Lescol Capsules	2233
Lescol XL Tablets	2233

Foscarnet Sodium (The benefits and risks of using fenofibrate tablets with immunosuppressants and other potentially nephrotoxic agents should be carefully considered and the lowest effective dose employed).

 No products indexed under this heading.

Fosinopril Sodium (The benefits and risks of using fenofibrate tablets with immunosuppressants and other potentially nephrotoxic agents should be carefully considered and the lowest effective dose employed).

 No products indexed under this heading.

Furosemide (The benefits and risks of using fenofibrate tablets with immunosuppressants and other potentially nephrotoxic agents should be carefully considered and the lowest effective dose employed). Products include:

Furosemide Tablets	2154

Gadopentetate Dimeglumine (The benefits and risks of using fenofibrate tablets with immunosuppressants and other potentially nephrotoxic agents should be carefully considered and the lowest effective dose employed).

 No products indexed under this heading.

Gentamicin (The benefits and risks of using fenofibrate tablets with immunosuppressants and other potentially nephrotoxic agents should be carefully considered and the lowest effective dose employed).

 No products indexed under this heading.

Gentamicin Sulfate (The benefits and risks of using fenofibrate tablets with immunosuppressants and other potentially nephrotoxic agents should be carefully considered and the lowest effective dose employed). Products include:

Garamycin Injectable	3014
Pred-G Ophthalmic Ointment	⊙237
Pred-G Ophthalmic Suspension	⊙236

Glipizide (The benefits and risks of using fenofibrate tablets with immunosuppressants and other potentially nephrotoxic agents should be carefully considered and the lowest effective dose employed).

 No products indexed under this heading.

Globulin, Immune (Human) (The benefits and risks of using fenofibrate tablets with immunosuppressants and other potentially nephrotoxic agents should be carefully considered and the lowest effective dose employed). Products include:

Flebogamma 5%, Immune Globulin Intravenous (Human)	1658
GamaSTAN	3234

Glyburide (The benefits and risks of using fenofibrate tablets with immunosuppressants and other potentially nephrotoxic agents should be carefully considered and the lowest effective dose employed).

 No products indexed under this heading.

Gold Therapy (The benefits and risks of using fenofibrate tablets with immunosuppressants and other potentially nephrotoxic agents should be carefully considered and the lowest effective dose employed).

 No products indexed under this heading.

HMG-CoA Reductase Inhibitors (The benefits and risks of using fenofibrate tablets with immunosuppressants and other potentially nephrotoxic agents should be carefully considered and the lowest effective dose employed).

 No products indexed under this heading.

Hydrochlorothiazide (The benefits and risks of using fenofibrate tablets with immunosuppressants and other potentially nephrotoxic agents should be carefully considered and the lowest effective dose employed). Products include:

Aldoril Tablets	1910
Atacand HCT	651
Avalide Tablets	888
Avalide Tablets	2874
Benicar HCT Tablets	1044
Diovan HCT Tablets	2196
Dyazide Capsules	1423
Hyzaar 50-12.5 Tablets	1990
Hyzaar 100-12.5 Tablets	1990
Hyzaar 100-25 Tablets	1990
Lopressor HCT 50/25 Tablets	2241
Lopressor HCT 100/25 Tablets	2241
Lopressor HCT 100/50 Tablets	2241
Lotensin HCT Tablets	2246
Micardis HCT Tablets	856
Moduretic Tablets	2028
Prinzide Tablets	2056
Teveten HCT Tablets	1737
Timolide Tablets	2086
Uniretic Tablets	3100

Hydroflumethiazide (The benefits and risks of using fenofibrate tablets with immunosuppressants and other potentially nephrotoxic agents should be carefully considered and the lowest effective dose employed).

 No products indexed under this heading.

Ibuprofen (The benefits and risks of using fenofibrate tablets with immunosuppressants and other potentially nephrotoxic agents should be carefully considered and the lowest effective dose employed). Products include:

Advil Allergy Sinus Caplets	▣770
Advil	▣674
Children's Advil Oral Suspension	▣603
Children's Advil Chewable Tablets	▣603
Advil Cold & Sinus	▣723
Infants' Advil Concentrated Drops	▣604
Infants' Advil Concentrated Drops - White Grape (Dye-Free)	▣604
Junior Strength Advil Swallow Tablets	▣605
Advil Migraine Liquigels	▣608
Advil Multi-Symptom Cold Caplets	▣770
Advil PM Caplets	▣615
Motrin IB Tablets and Caplets	1866
Children's Motrin Oral Suspension	1867
Children's Motrin Non-Staining Dye-Free Oral Suspension	1867
Children's Motrin Cold Oral Suspension	1867
Infants' Motrin Concentrated Drops	1867
Infants' Motrin Non-Staining Dye-Free Concentrated Drops	1867
Junior Strength Motrin Caplets and Chewable Tablets	1867
Vicoprofen Tablets	539

Idarubicin Hydrochloride (The benefits and risks of using fenofibrate tablets with immunosuppressants and other potentially nephrotoxic agents should be carefully considered and the lowest effective dose employed).

 No products indexed under this heading.

IMPORTANT NOTE: Always consult each drug listing in the patient's regimen for possible interactions.

Ifosfamide (The benefits and risks of using fenofibrate tablets with immunosuppressants and other potentially nephrotoxic agents should be carefully considered and the lowest effective dose employed). No products indexed under this heading.

Imipenem (The benefits and risks of using fenofibrate tablets with immunosuppressants and other potentially nephrotoxic agents should be carefully considered and the lowest effective dose employed). Products include:

Primaxin I.M. 2045
Primaxin I.V. 2048

Immune Globulin Intravenous (Human) (The benefits and risks of using fenofibrate tablets with immunosuppressants and other potentially nephrotoxic agents should be carefully considered and the lowest effective dose employed). Products include:

Carimune NF 3499
Gammagard Liquid 721
Gammagard S/D 724
Gamunex Immune Globulin I.V., 10% ... 3235

Indinavir Sulfate (The benefits and risks of using fenofibrate tablets with immunosuppressants and other potentially nephrotoxic agents should be carefully considered and the lowest effective dose employed). Products include:

Crixivan Capsules 1940

Indomethacin (The benefits and risks of using fenofibrate tablets with immunosuppressants and other potentially nephrotoxic agents should be carefully considered and the lowest effective dose employed). Products include:

Indocin ... 1995

Indomethacin Sodium Trihydrate (The benefits and risks of using fenofibrate tablets with immunosuppressants and other potentially nephrotoxic agents should be carefully considered and the lowest effective dose employed). Products include:

Indocin I.V. 2465

Interferon Beta-1b (The benefits and risks of using fenofibrate tablets with immunosuppressants and other potentially nephrotoxic agents should be carefully considered and the lowest effective dose employed). Products include:

Betaseron for SC Injection 767

Interleukin-2 (The benefits and risks of using fenofibrate tablets with immunosuppressants and other potentially nephrotoxic agents should be carefully considered and the lowest effective dose employed). No products indexed under this heading.

Iodamide Meglumine (The benefits and risks of using fenofibrate tablets with immunosuppressants and other potentially nephrotoxic agents should be carefully considered and the lowest effective dose employed). No products indexed under this heading.

Iohexol (The benefits and risks of using fenofibrate tablets with immunosuppressants and other potentially nephrotoxic agents should be carefully considered and the lowest effective dose employed). No products indexed under this heading.

Iopamidol (The benefits and risks of using fenofibrate tablets with immunosuppressants and other potentially nephrotoxic agents should be carefully considered and the lowest effective dose employed). No products indexed under this heading.

Iopanoic Acid (The benefits and risks of using fenofibrate tablets with immunosuppressants and other potentially nephrotoxic agents should be carefully considered and the lowest effective dose employed). No products indexed under this heading.

Iothalamate Meglumine (The benefits and risks of using fenofibrate tablets with immunosuppressants and other potentially nephrotoxic agents should be carefully considered and the lowest effective dose employed). No products indexed under this heading.

Ioxaglate Meglumine (The benefits and risks of using fenofibrate tablets with immunosuppressants and other potentially nephrotoxic agents should be carefully considered and the lowest effective dose employed). No products indexed under this heading.

Ioxaglate Sodium (The benefits and risks of using fenofibrate tablets with immunosuppressants and other potentially nephrotoxic agents should be carefully considered and the lowest effective dose employed). No products indexed under this heading.

Kanamycin Sulfate (The benefits and risks of using fenofibrate tablets with immunosuppressants and other potentially nephrotoxic agents should be carefully considered and the lowest effective dose employed). No products indexed under this heading.

Ketoprofen (The benefits and risks of using fenofibrate tablets with immunosuppressants and other potentially nephrotoxic agents should be carefully considered and the lowest effective dose employed). No products indexed under this heading.

Ketorolac Tromethamine (The benefits and risks of using fenofibrate tablets with immunosuppressants and other potentially nephrotoxic agents should be carefully considered and the lowest effective dose employed). Products include:

Acular Ophthalmic Solution 565
Acular LS Ophthalmic Solution 566

Lamium album (The benefits and risks of using fenofibrate tablets with immunosuppressants and other potentially nephrotoxic agents should be carefully considered and the lowest effective dose employed). No products indexed under this heading.

Lisinopril (The benefits and risks of using fenofibrate tablets with immunosuppressants and other potentially nephrotoxic agents should be carefully considered and the lowest effective dose employed). Products include:

Prinivil Tablets 2052
Prinzide Tablets 2056

Lithium (The benefits and risks of using fenofibrate tablets with immunosuppressants and other potentially nephrotoxic agents should be carefully considered and the lowest effective dose employed). No products indexed under this heading.

Lithium Carbonate (The benefits and risks of using fenofibrate tablets with immunosuppressants and other potentially nephrotoxic agents should be carefully considered and the lowest effective dose employed). Products include:

Lithobid Tablets 1692

Lithium Citrate (The benefits and risks of using fenofibrate tablets with immunosuppressants and other potentially nephrotoxic agents should be carefully considered and the lowest effective dose employed). No products indexed under this heading.

Lopinavir (The benefits and risks of using fenofibrate tablets with immunosuppressants and other potentially nephrotoxic agents should be carefully considered and the lowest effective dose employed). Products include:

Kaletra ... 476

Loracarbef (The benefits and risks of using fenofibrate tablets with immunosuppressants and other potentially nephrotoxic agents should be carefully considered and the lowest effective dose employed). No products indexed under this heading.

Lovastatin (Co-administration of fibric acid derivatives and HMG-CoA reductase inhibitors has been associated with rhabdomyolysis, markedly elevated creatine kinase levels and myoglobulinuria, leading in a high proportion of cases to acute renal failure; the combined use should be avoided unless the benefit of further alterations in lipid levels is likely to outweigh the increased risk of this combination). Products include:

Advicor Tablets 1722
Altoprev Extended-Release Tablets .. 3109
Mevacor Tablets 2021

Meclofenamate Sodium (The benefits and risks of using fenofibrate tablets with immunosuppressants and other potentially nephrotoxic agents should be carefully considered and the lowest effective dose employed). No products indexed under this heading.

Mefenamic Acid (The benefits and risks of using fenofibrate tablets with immunosuppressants and other potentially nephrotoxic agents should be carefully considered and the lowest effective dose employed). No products indexed under this heading.

Meloxicam (The benefits and risks of using fenofibrate tablets with immunosuppressants and other potentially nephrotoxic agents should be carefully considered and the lowest effective dose employed). Products include:

Mobic Oral Suspension 863
Mobic Tablets 863

Melphalan Hydrochloride (The benefits and risks of using fenofibrate tablets with immunosuppressants and other potentially nephro-

toxic agents should be carefully considered and the lowest effective dose employed). Products include:

Alkeran for Injection 955

Mesalamine (The benefits and risks of using fenofibrate tablets with immunosuppressants and other potentially nephrotoxic agents should be carefully considered and the lowest effective dose employed). Products include:

Asacol Delayed-Release Tablets 2692
Canasa Rectal Suppositories 699
Pentasa Capsules 3185

Methimazole (The benefits and risks of using fenofibrate tablets with immunosuppressants and other potentially nephrotoxic agents should be carefully considered and the lowest effective dose employed). No products indexed under this heading.

Methotrexate (The benefits and risks of using fenofibrate tablets with immunosuppressants and other potentially nephrotoxic agents should be carefully considered and the lowest effective dose employed). No products indexed under this heading.

Methotrexate Sodium (The benefits and risks of using fenofibrate tablets with immunosuppressants and other potentially nephrotoxic agents should be carefully considered and the lowest effective dose employed). No products indexed under this heading.

Methyclothiazide (The benefits and risks of using fenofibrate tablets with immunosuppressants and other potentially nephrotoxic agents should be carefully considered and the lowest effective dose employed). No products indexed under this heading.

Mezlocillin Sodium (The benefits and risks of using fenofibrate tablets with immunosuppressants and other potentially nephrotoxic agents should be carefully considered and the lowest effective dose employed). No products indexed under this heading.

Minocycline Hydrochloride (The benefits and risks of using fenofibrate tablets with immunosuppressants and other potentially nephrotoxic agents should be carefully considered and the lowest effective dose employed). Products include:

Solodyn Extended Release Tablets .. 1890

Mitomycin (Mitomycin-C) (The benefits and risks of using fenofibrate tablets with immunosuppressants and other potentially nephrotoxic agents should be carefully considered and the lowest effective dose employed). No products indexed under this heading.

Moexipril Hydrochloride (The benefits and risks of using fenofibrate tablets with immunosuppressants and other potentially nephrotoxic agents should be carefully considered and the lowest effective dose employed). Products include:

Uniretic Tablets 3100
Univasc Tablets 3104

Muromonab-CD3 (The benefits and risks of using fenofibrate tablets with immunosuppressants and other potentially nephrotoxic agents should be carefully considered and the lowest effective dose employed). Products include:

Orthoclone OKT3 Sterile Solution 2360

Mycophenolate Mofetil (The benefits and risks of using fenofibrate tablets with immunosuppressants and other potentially nephrotoxic agents should be carefully considered and the lowest effective dose employed). Products include:

CellCept Capsules 2747
CellCept Oral Suspension 2747
CellCept Tablets 2747

Nabumetone (The benefits and risks of using fenofibrate tablets with immunosuppressants and other potentially nephrotoxic agents should be carefully considered and the lowest effective dose employed).

No products indexed under this heading.

Nafcillin Sodium (The benefits and risks of using fenofibrate tablets with immunosuppressants and other potentially nephrotoxic agents should be carefully considered and the lowest effective dose employed).

No products indexed under this heading.

Naproxen (The benefits and risks of using fenofibrate tablets with immunosuppressants and other potentially nephrotoxic agents should be carefully considered and the lowest effective dose employed). Products include:

EC-Naprosyn Delayed-Release Tablets 2761
Naprosyn Suspension 2761
Naprosyn Tablets 2761
Prevacid NapraPAC 3280

Naproxen Sodium (The benefits and risks of using fenofibrate tablets with immunosuppressants and other potentially nephrotoxic agents should be carefully considered and the lowest effective dose employed). Products include:

Aleve Caplets 742
Aleve Gelcaps 743
Aleve Tablets 743
Aleve Cold & Sinus Caplets 744
Anaprox Tablets 2761
Anaprox DS Tablets 2761

Nelfinavir Mesylate (The benefits and risks of using fenofibrate tablets with immunosuppressants and other potentially nephrotoxic agents should be carefully considered and the lowest effective dose employed). Products include:

Viracept 2577

Neomycin (The benefits and risks of using fenofibrate tablets with immunosuppressants and other potentially nephrotoxic agents should be carefully considered and the lowest effective dose employed). Products include:

Neosporin Antibiotic Ointment 643
Neosporin + Pain Relief Antibiotic Cream and Ointment (Maximum Strength).................... 643

Neomycin, oral (The benefits and risks of using fenofibrate tablets with immunosuppressants and other potentially nephrotoxic agents should be carefully considered and the lowest effective dose employed).

No products indexed under this heading.

Neomycin Sulfate (The benefits and risks of using fenofibrate tablets with immunosuppressants and other potentially nephrotoxic agents should be carefully considered and the lowest effective dose employed). Products include:

Neosporin Ophthalmic Solution Sterile .... ⊙265
Poly-Pred Ophthalmic Suspension .... ⊙233

Nevirapine (The benefits and risks of using fenofibrate tablets with immunosuppressants and other potentially nephrotoxic agents should be carefully considered and the lowest effective dose employed). Products include:

Viramune Oral Suspension 873
Viramune Tablets 873

Norfloxacin (The benefits and risks of using fenofibrate tablets with immunosuppressants and other potentially nephrotoxic agents should be carefully considered and the lowest effective dose employed). Products include:

Noroxin Tablets 2032

Olsalazine Sodium (The benefits and risks of using fenofibrate tablets with immunosuppressants and other potentially nephrotoxic agents should be carefully considered and the lowest effective dose employed).

No products indexed under this heading.

Omeprazole (The benefits and risks of using fenofibrate tablets with immunosuppressants and other potentially nephrotoxic agents should be carefully considered and the lowest effective dose employed). Products include:

Zegerid Capsules 2958
Zegerid Powder for Oral Solution 2958

Oxaprozin (The benefits and risks of using fenofibrate tablets with immunosuppressants and other potentially nephrotoxic agents should be carefully considered and the lowest effective dose employed).

No products indexed under this heading.

Pamidronate Disodium (The benefits and risks of using fenofibrate tablets with immunosuppressants and other potentially nephrotoxic agents should be carefully considered and the lowest effective dose employed). Products include:

Aredia for Injection 2179

Paroxetine Hydrochloride (The benefits and risks of using fenofibrate tablets with immunosuppressants and other potentially nephrotoxic agents should be carefully considered and the lowest effective dose employed). Products include:

Paxil CR Controlled-Release Tablets 1538
Paxil 1530

Penicillamine (The benefits and risks of using fenofibrate tablets with immunosuppressants and other potentially nephrotoxic agents should be carefully considered and the lowest effective dose employed). Products include:

Cuprimine Capsules 1947

Penicillin G Benzathine (The benefits and risks of using fenofibrate tablets with immunosuppressants and other potentially nephrotoxic agents should be carefully considered and the lowest effective dose employed). Products include:

Bicillin C-R Injectable Suspension 1706

Penicillin G Potassium (The benefits and risks of using fenofibrate tablets with immunosuppressants and other potentially nephrotoxic agents should be carefully considered and the lowest effective dose employed).

No products indexed under this heading.

Penicillin G Procaine (The benefits and risks of using fenofibrate tablets with immunosuppressants and other potentially nephrotoxic agents should be carefully considered and the lowest effective dose employed). Products include:

Bicillin C-R Injectable Suspension 1706

Penicillin G Sodium (The benefits and risks of using fenofibrate tablets with immunosuppressants and other potentially nephrotoxic agents should be carefully considered and the lowest effective dose employed).

No products indexed under this heading.

Penicillin V Potassium (The benefits and risks of using fenofibrate tablets with immunosuppressants and other potentially nephrotoxic agents should be carefully considered and the lowest effective dose employed).

No products indexed under this heading.

Pentamidine Isethionate (The benefits and risks of using fenofibrate tablets with immunosuppressants and other potentially nephrotoxic agents should be carefully considered and the lowest effective dose employed).

No products indexed under this heading.

Perindopril Erbumine (The benefits and risks of using fenofibrate tablets with immunosuppressants and other potentially nephrotoxic agents should be carefully considered and the lowest effective dose employed). Products include:

Aceon Tablets (2 mg, 4 mg, 8 mg).. 3194

Phenylbutazone (The benefits and risks of using fenofibrate tablets with immunosuppressants and other potentially nephrotoxic agents should be carefully considered and the lowest effective dose employed).

No products indexed under this heading.

Piroxicam (The benefits and risks of using fenofibrate tablets with immunosuppressants and other potentially nephrotoxic agents should be carefully considered and the lowest effective dose employed).

No products indexed under this heading.

Plicamycin (The benefits and risks of using fenofibrate tablets with immunosuppressants and other potentially nephrotoxic agents should be carefully considered and the lowest effective dose employed).

No products indexed under this heading.

Polymyxin (The benefits and risks of using fenofibrate tablets with immunosuppressants and other potentially nephrotoxic agents should be carefully considered and the lowest effective dose employed).

No products indexed under this heading.

Polymyxin B Sulfate (The benefits and risks of using fenofibrate tablets with immunosuppressants and other potentially nephrotoxic agents should be carefully considered and the lowest effective dose employed). Products include:

Neosporin Antibiotic Ointment 643
Neosporin Ophthalmic Solution Sterile .... ⊙265
Neosporin + Pain Relief Antibiotic Cream and Ointment (Maximum Strength).................... 643
Poly-Pred Ophthalmic Suspension .... ⊙233
Polysporin First Aid Antibiotic Ointment...................................... 643
Polytrim Ophthalmic Solution 574

Polythiazide (The benefits and risks of using fenofibrate tablets with immunosuppressants and other potentially nephrotoxic agents should be carefully considered and the lowest effective dose employed).

No products indexed under this heading.

Pravastatin Sodium (Co-administration of fibric acid derivatives and HMG-CoA reductase inhibitors has been associated with rhabdomyolysis, markedly elevated creatine kinase levels and myoglobulinuria, leading in a high proportion of cases to acute renal failure; the combined use should be avoided unless the benefit of further alterations in lipid levels is likely to outweigh the increased risk of this combination).

No products indexed under this heading.

Probenecid (The benefits and risks of using fenofibrate tablets with immunosuppressants and other potentially nephrotoxic agents should be carefully considered and the lowest effective dose employed).

No products indexed under this heading.

Quinapril Hydrochloride (The benefits and risks of using fenofibrate tablets with immunosuppressants and other potentially nephrotoxic agents should be carefully considered and the lowest effective dose employed).

No products indexed under this heading.

Rabeprazole Sodium (The benefits and risks of using fenofibrate tablets with immunosuppressants and other potentially nephrotoxic agents should be carefully considered and the lowest effective dose employed). Products include:

Aciphex Tablets 1090

Ramipril (The benefits and risks of using fenofibrate tablets with immunosuppressants and other potentially nephrotoxic agents should be carefully considered and the lowest effective dose employed). Products include:

Altace Capsules 1702

Rifampin (The benefits and risks of using fenofibrate tablets with immunosuppressants and other potentially nephrotoxic agents should be carefully considered and the lowest effective dose employed).

No products indexed under this heading.

Riluzole (The benefits and risks of using fenofibrate tablets with immunosuppressants and other potentially nephrotoxic agents should be carefully considered and the lowest effective dose employed). Products include:

Rilutek Tablets 2930

Ritonavir (The benefits and risks of using fenofibrate tablets with immunosuppressants and other potentially nephrotoxic agents should be carefully considered and the lowest effective dose employed). Products include:

Kaletra ... 476
Norvir ... 503

Rofecoxib (The benefits and risks of using fenofibrate tablets with immunosuppressants and other potentially nephrotoxic agents should be carefully considered and the lowest effective dose employed).

No products indexed under this heading.

Saquinavir (The benefits and risks of using fenofibrate tablets with immunosuppressants and other potentially nephrotoxic agents should be carefully considered and the lowest effective dose employed).

No products indexed under this heading.

Sibutramine Hydrochloride Monohydrate (The benefits and risks of using fenofibrate tablets with immunosuppressants and other potentially nephrotoxic agents should be carefully considered and the lowest effective dose employed). Products include:

Meridia Capsules ... 489

Simvastatin (Co-administration of fibric acid derivatives and HMG-CoA reductase inhibitors has been associated with rhabdomyolysis, markedly elevated creatine kinase levels and myoglobulinuria, leading in a high proportion of cases to acute renal failure; the combined use should be avoided unless the benefit of further alterations in lipid levels is likely to outweigh the increased risk of this combination). Products include:

Vytorin 10/10 Tablets ... 2114
Vytorin 10/10 Tablets ... 3077
Vytorin 10/20 Tablets ... 2114
Vytorin 10/20 Tablets ... 3077
Vytorin 10/40 Tablets ... 2114
Vytorin 10/40 Tablets ... 3077
Vytorin 10/80 Tablets ... 2114
Vytorin 10/80 Tablets ... 3077
Zocor Tablets ... 2105

Sirolimus (The benefits and risks of using fenofibrate tablets with immunosuppressants and other potentially nephrotoxic agents should be carefully considered and the lowest effective dose employed). Products include:

Rapamune Oral Solution and Tablets ... 3475

Spirapril Hydrochloride (The benefits and risks of using fenofibrate tablets with immunosuppressants and other potentially nephrotoxic agents should be carefully considered and the lowest effective dose employed).

No products indexed under this heading.

Stavudine (The benefits and risks of using fenofibrate tablets with immunosuppressants and other potentially nephrotoxic agents should be carefully considered and the lowest effective dose employed).

No products indexed under this heading.

Streptomycin Sulfate (The benefits and risks of using fenofibrate tablets with immunosuppressants and other potentially nephrotoxic agents should be carefully considered and the lowest effective dose employed).

No products indexed under this heading.

Streptozocin (The benefits and risks of using fenofibrate tablets with immunosuppressants and other potentially nephrotoxic agents should be carefully considered and the lowest effective dose employed).

No products indexed under this heading.

Sulfacytine (The benefits and risks of using fenofibrate tablets with immunosuppressants and other potentially nephrotoxic agents should be carefully considered and the lowest effective dose employed).

No products indexed under this heading.

Sulfamethizole (The benefits and risks of using fenofibrate tablets with immunosuppressants and other potentially nephrotoxic agents should be carefully considered and the lowest effective dose employed).

No products indexed under this heading.

Sulfamethoxazole (The benefits and risks of using fenofibrate tablets with immunosuppressants and other potentially nephrotoxic agents should be carefully considered and the lowest effective dose employed).

No products indexed under this heading.

Sulfasalazine (The benefits and risks of using fenofibrate tablets with immunosuppressants and other potentially nephrotoxic agents should be carefully considered and the lowest effective dose employed).

No products indexed under this heading.

Sulfinpyrazone (The benefits and risks of using fenofibrate tablets with immunosuppressants and other potentially nephrotoxic agents should be carefully considered and the lowest effective dose employed).

No products indexed under this heading.

Sulfisoxazole Acetyl (The benefits and risks of using fenofibrate tablets with immunosuppressants and other potentially nephrotoxic agents should be carefully considered and the lowest effective dose employed).

No products indexed under this heading.

Sulfisoxazole Diolamine (The benefits and risks of using fenofibrate tablets with immunosuppressants and other potentially nephrotoxic agents should be carefully considered and the lowest effective dose employed).

No products indexed under this heading.

Sulindac (The benefits and risks of using fenofibrate tablets with immunosuppressants and other potentially nephrotoxic agents should be carefully considered and the lowest effective dose employed). Products include:

Clinoril Tablets ... 1924

Tacrolimus (The benefits and risks of using fenofibrate tablets with immunosuppressants and other potentially nephrotoxic agents should be carefully considered and the lowest effective dose employed). Products include:

Prograf Capsules and Injection ... 632
Protopic Ointment ... 638

Tenofovir Disoproxil Fumarate (The benefits and risks of using fenofibrate tablets with immunosuppressants and other potentially nephrotoxic agents should be carefully considered and the lowest effective dose employed). Products include:

Atripla Tablets ... 945
Truvada Tablets ... 1296
Viread Tablets ... 1301

Thioguanine (The benefits and risks of using fenofibrate tablets with immunosuppressants and other potentially nephrotoxic agents should be carefully considered and the lowest effective dose employed). Products include:

Tabloid Tablets ... 1575

Ticarcillin Disodium (The benefits and risks of using fenofibrate tablets with immunosuppressants and other potentially nephrotoxic agents should be carefully considered and the lowest effective dose employed). Products include:

Timentin ADD-Vantage ... 1580
Timentin Injection Galaxy Container ... 1583
Timentin IV Infusion ... 1577
Timentin Pharmacy Bulk Package ... 1586

Tobramycin (The benefits and risks of using fenofibrate tablets with immunosuppressants and other potentially nephrotoxic agents should be carefully considered and the lowest effective dose employed). Products include:

TOBI Solution for Inhalation ... 2298
TobraDex Ophthalmic Ointment ... 562
TobraDex Ophthalmic Suspension ... 563
Zylet Ophthalmic Suspension ... ⊙259

Tobramycin Sulfate (The benefits and risks of using fenofibrate tablets with immunosuppressants and other potentially nephrotoxic agents should be carefully considered and the lowest effective dose employed).

No products indexed under this heading.

Tolazamide (The benefits and risks of using fenofibrate tablets with immunosuppressants and other potentially nephrotoxic agents should be carefully considered and the lowest effective dose employed).

No products indexed under this heading.

Tolbutamide (The benefits and risks of using fenofibrate tablets with immunosuppressants and other potentially nephrotoxic agents should be carefully considered and the lowest effective dose employed).

No products indexed under this heading.

Tolmetin Sodium (The benefits and risks of using fenofibrate tablets with immunosuppressants and other potentially nephrotoxic agents should be carefully considered and the lowest effective dose employed).

No products indexed under this heading.

Trandolapril (The benefits and risks of using fenofibrate tablets with immunosuppressants and other potentially nephrotoxic agents should be carefully considered and the lowest effective dose employed). Products include:

Mavik Tablets ... 486
Tarka Tablets ... 524

Triamterene (The benefits and risks of using fenofibrate tablets with immunosuppressants and other potentially nephrotoxic agents should be carefully considered and the lowest effective dose employed). Products include:

Dyazide Capsules ... 1423
Dyrenium Capsules ... 3400

Trimethadione (The benefits and risks of using fenofibrate tablets with immunosuppressants and other potentially nephrotoxic agents should be carefully considered and the lowest effective dose employed).

No products indexed under this heading.

Trovafloxacin Mesylate (The benefits and risks of using fenofibrate tablets with immunosuppressants and other potentially nephrotoxic agents should be carefully considered and the lowest effective dose employed).

No products indexed under this heading.

Tyropanoate Sodium (The benefits and risks of using fenofibrate tablets with immunosuppressants and other potentially nephrotoxic agents should be carefully considered and the lowest effective dose employed).

No products indexed under this heading.

Valacyclovir Hydrochloride (The benefits and risks of using fenofibrate tablets with immunosuppressants and other potentially nephrotoxic agents should be carefully considered and the lowest effective dose employed). Products include:

Valtrex Caplets ... 1597

Valdecoxib (The benefits and risks of using fenofibrate tablets with immunosuppressants and other potentially nephrotoxic agents should be carefully considered and the lowest effective dose employed).

No products indexed under this heading.

Vancomycin Hydrochloride (The benefits and risks of using fenofibrate tablets with immunosuppressants and other potentially nephrotoxic agents should be carefully considered and the lowest effective dose employed). Products include:

Vancocin HCl Capsules, USP ... 3380

Voriconazole (The benefits and risks of using fenofibrate tablets with immunosuppressants and other potentially nephrotoxic agents should be carefully considered and the lowest effective dose employed). Products include:

VFEND I.V. ... 2564
VFEND Oral Suspension ... 2564
VFEND Tablets ... 2564

Warfarin Sodium (Caution should be exercised when anticoagulants are given in conjunction with fenofibrate because of the potentiation of coumarin-type anticoagulants in prolonging the PT/INR. The dosage of the anticoagulant should be reduced to maintain the PT/INR at the desired level to prevent bleeding complications. Frequent PT/INR determinations are advisable until it has been definitely determined that the PT/INR has stabilized). Products include:

Coumadin for Injection ... 898
Coumadin Tablets ... 898

Zalcitabine (The benefits and risks of using fenofibrate tablets with immunosuppressants and other potentially nephrotoxic agents should be carefully considered and the lowest effective dose employed).

No products indexed under this heading.

Zidovudine (The benefits and risks of using fenofibrate tablets with immunosuppressants and other potentially nephrotoxic agents should be carefully considered and the lowest effective dose employed). Products include:

Zoledronic acid (The benefits and risks of using fenofibrate tablets with immunosuppressants and other potentially nephrotoxic agents should be carefully considered and the lowest effective dose employed). Products include:

Food Interactions

Food, unspecified (The absorption of fenofibrate is increased when administered with food; Tricor should be given with meals).

TRIGLIDE TABLETS

May interact with bile acid sequestering agents, oral anticoagulants, cytochrome p450 2c19 substrates (selected), cytochrome p450 2c9 substrates (selected), HMG-CoA reductase inhibitors, immunosuppressive agents, nephrotoxic agents, and certain other agents. Compounds in these categories include:

Abacavir Sulfate (The benefits and risks of using fenofibrate with immunosuppressants and other potentially nephrotoxic agents should be carefully considered, and the lowest effective dose employed). Products include:

Acarbose (Fenofibrates are mild-moderate inhibitors of CYP2C9 at therapeutic concentrations). Products include:

Acyclovir (The benefits and risks of using fenofibrate with immunosuppressants and other potentially nephrotoxic agents should be carefully considered, and the lowest effective dose employed). Products include:

Acyclovir Sodium (The benefits and risks of using fenofibrate with immunosuppressants and other potentially nephrotoxic agents should be carefully considered, and the lowest effective dose employed).
No products indexed under this heading.

Alatrofloxacin Mesylate (The benefits and risks of using fenofibrate with immunosuppressants and other potentially nephrotoxic agents should be carefully considered, and the lowest effective dose employed).
No products indexed under this heading.

Aldesleukin (The benefits and risks of using fenofibrate with immunosuppressants and other potentially nephrotoxic agents should be carefully considered, and the lowest effective dose employed). Products include:

Amikacin Sulfate (The benefits and risks of using fenofibrate with immunosuppressants and other potentially nephrotoxic agents should be carefully considered, and the lowest effective dose employed).
No products indexed under this heading.

Amitriptyline Hydrochloride (Fenofibrates are mild-moderate inhibitors of CYP2C9 at therapeutic concentrations).
No products indexed under this heading.

Amoxapine (Fenofibrates are weak inhibitors of CYP2C19 at therapeutic concentrations).
No products indexed under this heading.

Amoxicillin (The benefits and risks of using fenofibrate with immunosuppressants and other potentially nephrotoxic agents should be carefully considered, and the lowest effective dose employed). Products include:

Amoxicillin Trihydrate (The benefits and risks of using fenofibrate with immunosuppressants and other potentially nephrotoxic agents should be carefully considered, and the lowest effective dose employed).
No products indexed under this heading.

Amphotericin B (The benefits and risks of using fenofibrate with immunosuppressants and other potentially nephrotoxic agents should be carefully considered, and the lowest effective dose employed).
No products indexed under this heading.

Amphotericin B, liposomal (The benefits and risks of using fenofibrate with immunosuppressants and other potentially nephrotoxic agents should be carefully considered, and the lowest effective dose employed). Products include:

Amphotericin B Cholesteryl Sulfate (The benefits and risks of using fenofibrate with immunosuppressants and other potentially nephrotoxic agents should be carefully considered, and the lowest effective dose employed).
No products indexed under this heading.

Amphotericin B Lipid Complex (The benefits and risks of using fenofibrate with immunosuppressants and other potentially nephrotoxic agents should be carefully considered, and the lowest effective dose employed). Products include:

Ampicillin (The benefits and risks of using fenofibrate with immunosuppressants and other potentially nephrotoxic agents should be carefully considered, and the lowest effective dose employed).
No products indexed under this heading.

Ampicillin Sodium (The benefits and risks of using fenofibrate with immunosuppressants and other potentially nephrotoxic agents should be carefully considered, and the lowest effective dose employed).
No products indexed under this heading.

Ampicillin Trihydrate (The benefits and risks of using fenofibrate with immunosuppressants and other potentially nephrotoxic agents should be carefully considered, and the lowest effective dose employed).
No products indexed under this heading.

Amprenavir (The benefits and risks of using fenofibrate with immunosuppressants and other potentially nephrotoxic agents should be carefully considered, and the lowest effective dose employed). Products include:

Anisindione (Caution should be exercised when anticoagulants are given in conjunction with fenofibrate because of the potentiation of coumarin-type anticoagulants in prolonging the prothrombin time/INR. The dosage of the anticoagulant should be reduced to maintain the prothrombin time/INR at the desired level to prevent bleeding complications. Frequent prothrombin time/INR determinations are advisably until it has been definitely determined that the prothrombin time/INR has stabilized). Products include:

Aspirin (The benefits and risks of using fenofibrate with immunosuppressants and other potentially nephrotoxic agents should be carefully considered, and the lowest effective dose employed). Products include:

Atazanavir (The benefits and risks of using fenofibrate with immunosuppressants and other potentially nephrotoxic agents should be carefully considered, and the lowest effective dose employed).
No products indexed under this heading.

Atorvastatin Calcium (The combined use of fenofibrates and HMG-CoA reductase inhibitors should be avoided unless the benefit of further alterations in lipid levels is likely to outweigh the increased risk of this drug combination. The combined use of fibric acid derivatives and HMG-CoA reductase inhibitors has been associated, in the absence of a marked pharmacokinetic interaction, in numerous case reports, with rhabdomyolysis, markedly elevated creatine kinase (CK) levels and myoglobinuria, leading in a high proportion of cases to acute renal failure). Products include:

Azathioprine (The benefits and risks of using fenofibrate with immunosuppressants and other potentially nephrotoxic agents should be carefully considered, and the lowest effective dose employed).
No products indexed under this heading.

Azithromycin Dihydrate (The benefits and risks of using fenofibrate with immunosuppressants and other potentially nephrotoxic agents should be carefully considered, and the lowest effective dose employed).
No products indexed under this heading.

Azlocillin Sodium (The benefits and risks of using fenofibrate with immunosuppressants and other potentially nephrotoxic agents should be carefully considered, and the lowest effective dose employed).
No products indexed under this heading.

Aztreonam (The benefits and risks of using fenofibrate with immunosuppressants and other potentially nephrotoxic agents should be carefully considered, and the lowest effective dose employed).
No products indexed under this heading.

Bacampicillin Hydrochloride (The benefits and risks of using fenofibrate with immunosuppressants and other potentially nephrotoxic agents should be carefully considered, and the lowest effective dose employed).
No products indexed under this heading.

Balsalazide Disodium (The benefits and risks of using fenofibrate with immunosuppressants and other potentially nephrotoxic agents should be carefully considered, and the lowest effective dose employed). Products include:

Basiliximab (The benefits and risks of using fenofibrate with immunosuppressants and other potentially nephrotoxic agents should be carefully considered, and the lowest effective dose employed). Products include:

Benazepril Hydrochloride (The benefits and risks of using fenofibrate with immunosuppressants and other potentially nephrotoxic agents should be carefully considered, and the lowest effective dose employed). Products include:

Bendroflumethiazide (The benefits and risks of using fenofibrate with immunosuppressants and other potentially nephrotoxic agents should be carefully considered, and the lowest effective dose employed).
No products indexed under this heading.

Caffeine (The benefits and risks of using fenofibrate with immunosuppressants and other potentially nephrotoxic agents should be carefully considered, and the lowest effective dose employed). Products include:

IMPORTANT NOTE: Always consult each drug listing in the patient's regimen for possible interactions.

Excedrin Tension Headache Caplets/Tablets/Geltabs .... ▣ 611
Goody's Extra Strength Headache Powders .... ▣ 611
Goody's Extra Strength Pain Relief Tablets .... ▣ 685
Vivarin .... ▣ 602
Winrgy Dietary Supplement .... ▣ 823

Candesartan Cilexetil (Fenofibrates are mild-moderate inhibitors of CYP2C9 at therapeutic concentrations). Products include:
Atacand Tablets 649
Atacand HCT 651

Captopril (The benefits and risks of using fenofibrate with immunosuppressants and other potentially nephrotoxic agents should be carefully considered, and the lowest effective dose employed). Products include:
Captopril Tablets 2149

Carbenicillin Disodium (The benefits and risks of using fenofibrate with immunosuppressants and other potentially nephrotoxic agents should be carefully considered, and the lowest effective dose employed).
No products indexed under this heading.

Carbenicillin Indanyl Sodium (The benefits and risks of using fenofibrate with immunosuppressants and other potentially nephrotoxic agents should be carefully considered, and the lowest effective dose employed).
No products indexed under this heading.

Carboplatin (The benefits and risks of using fenofibrate with immunosuppressants and other potentially nephrotoxic agents should be carefully considered, and the lowest effective dose employed).
No products indexed under this heading.

Carisoprodol (Fenofibrates are weak inhibitors of CYP2C19 at therapeutic concentrations).
No products indexed under this heading.

Carmustine (BCNU) (The benefits and risks of using fenofibrate with immunosuppressants and other potentially nephrotoxic agents should be carefully considered, and the lowest effective dose employed).
No products indexed under this heading.

Carvedilol (Fenofibrates are mild-moderate inhibitors of CYP2C9 at therapeutic concentrations). Products include:
Coreg Tablets 1414

Cefaclor (The benefits and risks of using fenofibrate with immunosuppressants and other potentially nephrotoxic agents should be carefully considered, and the lowest effective dose employed).
No products indexed under this heading.

Cefadroxil (The benefits and risks of using fenofibrate with immunosuppressants and other potentially nephrotoxic agents should be carefully considered, and the lowest effective dose employed).
No products indexed under this heading.

Cefamandole Nafate (The benefits and risks of using fenofibrate with immunosuppressants and other potentially nephrotoxic agents should be carefully considered, and the lowest effective dose employed).
No products indexed under this heading.

Cefazolin Sodium (The benefits and risks of using fenofibrate with immunosuppressants and other potentially nephrotoxic agents should be carefully considered, and the lowest effective dose employed).
No products indexed under this heading.

Cefdinir (The benefits and risks of using fenofibrate with immunosuppressants and other potentially nephrotoxic agents should be carefully considered, and the lowest effective dose employed). Products include:
Omnicef Capsules 511
Omnicef for Oral Suspension 511

Cefepime Hydrochloride (The benefits and risks of using fenofibrate with immunosuppressants and other potentially nephrotoxic agents should be carefully considered, and the lowest effective dose employed). Products include:
Maxipime for Injection 1105

Cefixime (The benefits and risks of using fenofibrate with immunosuppressants and other potentially nephrotoxic agents should be carefully considered, and the lowest effective dose employed). Products include:
Suprax 1843

Cefmetazole Sodium (The benefits and risks of using fenofibrate with immunosuppressants and other potentially nephrotoxic agents should be carefully considered, and the lowest effective dose employed).
No products indexed under this heading.

Cefonicid Sodium (The benefits and risks of using fenofibrate with immunosuppressants and other potentially nephrotoxic agents should be carefully considered, and the lowest effective dose employed).
No products indexed under this heading.

Cefoperazone Sodium (The benefits and risks of using fenofibrate with immunosuppressants and other potentially nephrotoxic agents should be carefully considered, and the lowest effective dose employed).
No products indexed under this heading.

Ceforanide (The benefits and risks of using fenofibrate with immunosuppressants and other potentially nephrotoxic agents should be carefully considered, and the lowest effective dose employed).
No products indexed under this heading.

Cefotaxime Sodium (The benefits and risks of using fenofibrate with immunosuppressants and other potentially nephrotoxic agents should be carefully considered, and the lowest effective dose employed).
No products indexed under this heading.

Cefotetan (The benefits and risks of using fenofibrate with immunosuppressants and other potentially nephrotoxic agents should be carefully considered, and the lowest effective dose employed).
No products indexed under this heading.

Cefoxitin Sodium (The benefits and risks of using fenofibrate with immunosuppressants and other potentially nephrotoxic agents should be carefully considered, and the lowest effective dose employed). Products include:
Mefoxin for Injection 2012
Mefoxin Premixed Intravenous Solution 2016

Cefpodoxime Proxetil (The benefits and risks of using fenofibrate with immunosuppressants and other potentially nephrotoxic agents should be carefully considered, and the lowest effective dose employed). Products include:
Vantin Tablets and Oral Suspension 2645

Cefprozil (The benefits and risks of using fenofibrate with immunosuppressants and other potentially nephrotoxic agents should be carefully considered, and the lowest effective dose employed).
No products indexed under this heading.

Ceftazidime (The benefits and risks of using fenofibrate with immunosuppressants and other potentially nephrotoxic agents should be carefully considered, and the lowest effective dose employed). Products include:
Fortaz 1453

Ceftizoxime Sodium (The benefits and risks of using fenofibrate with immunosuppressants and other potentially nephrotoxic agents should be carefully considered, and the lowest effective dose employed).
No products indexed under this heading.

Ceftriaxone Sodium (The benefits and risks of using fenofibrate with immunosuppressants and other potentially nephrotoxic agents should be carefully considered, and the lowest effective dose employed). Products include:
Rocephin Injectable Vials, ADD-Vantage, Galaxy, Bulk........... 2800

Cefuroxime Axetil (The benefits and risks of using fenofibrate with immunosuppressants and other potentially nephrotoxic agents should be carefully considered, and the lowest effective dose employed). Products include:
Ceftin 1407

Cefuroxime Sodium (The benefits and risks of using fenofibrate with immunosuppressants and other potentially nephrotoxic agents should be carefully considered, and the lowest effective dose employed).
No products indexed under this heading.

Celecoxib (Fenofibrates are mild-moderate inhibitors of CYP2C9 at therapeutic concentrations). Products include:
Celebrex Capsules 3134

Cephalexin (The benefits and risks of using fenofibrate with immunosuppressants and other potentially nephrotoxic agents should be carefully considered, and the lowest effective dose employed). Products include:
Keflex Capsules 549

Cephalothin Sodium (The benefits and risks of using fenofibrate with immunosuppressants and other potentially nephrotoxic agents should be carefully considered, and the lowest effective dose employed).
No products indexed under this heading.

Cephapirin Sodium (The benefits and risks of using fenofibrate with immunosuppressants and other potentially nephrotoxic agents should be carefully considered, and the lowest effective dose employed).
No products indexed under this heading.

Cephradine (The benefits and risks of using fenofibrate with immunosuppressants and other potentially nephrotoxic agents should be carefully considered, and the lowest effective dose employed).
No products indexed under this heading.

Cerivastatin Sodium (The combined use of fenofibrates and HMG-CoA reductase inhibitors should be avoided unless the benefit of further alterations in lipid levels is likely to outweigh the increased risk of this drug combination. The combined use of fibric acid derivatives and HMG-CoA reductase inhibitors has been associated, in the absence of a marked pharmacokinetic interaction, in numerous case reports, with rhabdomyolysis, markedly elevated creatine kinase (CK) levels and myoglobinuria, leading in a high proportion of cases to acute renal failure).
No products indexed under this heading.

Chlorothiazide (The benefits and risks of using fenofibrate with immunosuppressants and other potentially nephrotoxic agents should be carefully considered, and the lowest effective dose employed). Products include:
Diuril Oral Suspension 1954

Chlorothiazide Sodium (The benefits and risks of using fenofibrate with immunosuppressants and other potentially nephrotoxic agents should be carefully considered, and the lowest effective dose employed). Products include:
Diuril Sodium Intravenous 2467

Chlorpropamide (Fenofibrates are mild-moderate inhibitors of CYP2C9 at therapeutic concentrations).
No products indexed under this heading.

Cholestyramine (Bile acid sequestrants have been shown to bind to other drugs given concurrently. Therefore, fenofibrates should be taken at least 1 hour before, or 4-6 hours after a bile acid binding resin to avoid impeding its absorption).
No products indexed under this heading.

Cidofovir (The benefits and risks of using fenofibrate with immunosuppressants and other potentially nephrotoxic agents should be carefully considered, and the lowest effective dose employed).
No products indexed under this heading.

Cilastatin Sodium (The benefits and risks of using fenofibrate with immunosuppressants and other potentially nephrotoxic agents should be carefully considered, and the lowest effective dose employed). Products include:
Primaxin I.M. 2045
Primaxin I.V. 2048

Cilostazol (Fenofibrates are weak inhibitors of CYP2C19 at therapeutic concentrations). Products include:
Pletal Tablets 2455

Cimetidine (The benefits and risks of using fenofibrate with immunosuppressants and other potentially nephrotoxic agents should be carefully considered, and the lowest effective dose employed). Products include:
Tagamet HB 200 Tablets .... ▣ 664

Cimetidine Hydrochloride (The benefits and risks of using fenofibrate with immunosuppressants and other potentially nephrotoxic agents should be carefully considered, and the lowest effective dose employed).
No products indexed under this heading.

Cisplatin (The benefits and risks of using fenofibrate with immunosuppressants and other potentially nephrotoxic agents should be carefully considered, and the lowest effective dose employed).
No products indexed under this heading.

Citalopram Hydrobromide (Fenofibrates are weak inhibitors of CYP2C19 at therapeutic concentrations). Products include:
Celexa ... 1176

Cladribine (The benefits and risks of using fenofibrate with immunosuppressants and other potentially nephrotoxic agents should be carefully considered, and the lowest effective dose employed). Products include:
Leustatin Injection ... 2357

Clomipramine Hydrochloride (Fenofibrates are mild-moderate inhibitors of CYP2C9 at therapeutic concentrations).
No products indexed under this heading.

Clozapine (The benefits and risks of using fenofibrate with immunosuppressants and other potentially nephrotoxic agents should be carefully considered, and the lowest effective dose employed). Products include:
Clozaril Tablets ... 2184
FazaClo Orally Disintegrating Tablets ... 551

Colesevelam Hydrochloride (Bile acid sequestrants have been shown to bind to other drugs given concurrently. Therefore, fenofibrates should be taken at least 1 hour before, or 4-6 hours after a bile acid binding resin to avoid impeding its absorption). Products include:
WelChol Tablets ... 1050

Colestipol Hydrochloride (Bile acid sequestrants have been shown to bind to other drugs given concurrently. Therefore, fenofibrates should be taken at least 1 hour before, or 4-6 hours after a bile acid binding resin to avoid impeding its absorption).
No products indexed under this heading.

Colistimethate Sodium (The benefits and risks of using fenofibrate with immunosuppressants and other potentially nephrotoxic agents should be carefully considered, and the lowest effective dose employed).
No products indexed under this heading.

Colistin Sulfate (The benefits and risks of using fenofibrate with immunosuppressants and other potentially nephrotoxic agents should be carefully considered, and the lowest effective dose employed).
No products indexed under this heading.

Cyclophosphamide (Fenofibrates are weak inhibitors of CYP2C19 at therapeutic concentrations).
No products indexed under this heading.

Cyclosporine (Because cyclosporine can produce nephrotoxicity with decreases in creatinine clearance and rises in serum creatinine, and because renal excretion is the primary elimination route of fibrate drugs including fenofibrate, there is a risk that an interaction will lead to deterioration). Products include:
Gengraf Capsules ... 459
Neoral Oral Solution ... 2259
Neoral Soft Gelatin Capsules ... 2259
Restasis Ophthalmic Emulsion ... 575
Sandimmune ... 2275

Cytarabine (The benefits and risks of using fenofibrate with immunosuppressants and other potentially nephrotoxic agents should be carefully considered, and the lowest effective dose employed).
No products indexed under this heading.

Cytarabine Liposome (The benefits and risks of using fenofibrate with immunosuppressants and other potentially nephrotoxic agents should be carefully considered, and the lowest effective dose employed). Products include:
DepoCyt Injection ... 1143

Delavirdine Mesylate (The benefits and risks of using fenofibrate with immunosuppressants and other potentially nephrotoxic agents should be carefully considered, and the lowest effective dose employed). Products include:
Rescriptor Tablets ... 2551

Desipramine Hydrochloride (Fenofibrates are weak inhibitors of CYP2C19 at therapeutic concentrations).
No products indexed under this heading.

Desogestrel (Fenofibrates are mild-moderate inhibitors of CYP2C9 at therapeutic concentrations). Products include:
Mircette Tablets ... 1066

Dextromethorphan (Fenofibrates are mild-moderate inhibitors of CYP2C9 at therapeutic concentrations).
No products indexed under this heading.

Dextromethorphan Hydrobromide (Fenofibrates are weak inhibitors of CYP2C19 at therapeutic concentrations). Products include:
Comtrex Maximum Strength Cold & Cough Day/Night Caplets - Day Formulation ... 726
Comtrex Maximum Strength Cold & Cough Day/Night Caplets - Night Formulation ... 726
Comtrex Maximum Strength Non-Drowsy Cold & Cough Caplets ... 725
Children's Dimetapp DM Cold & Cough Elixir ... 731
Children's Dimetapp Long Acting Cough Plus Cold Syrup ... 731
Toddler's Dimetapp Cold and Cough Drops ... 732
Mucinex DM Extended-Release Bi-Layer Tablets ... 720
Refenesen DM Caplets ... 721
Robitussin Cough & Cold CF Liquid ... 735
Robitussin Cough & Cold Long-Acting Liquid ... 735
Robitussin Cough & Allergy Syrup ... 736
Robitussin Cough & Cold Nighttime Liquid ... 736
Robitussin Cough & Cold Pediatric Drops ... 735
Robitussin Cough, Cold & Flu Nighttime Liquid ... 738
Robitussin Cough & Congestion Liquid ... 738
Robitussin Cough Gels Long-Acting ... 737
Robitussin Cough Long Acting Liquid ... 739
Robitussin Cough DM Syrup ... 738
Robitussin Cough DM Infant Drops ... 738
Robitussin Pediatric Cough Long Acting Liquid ... 739
Robitussin Pediatric Cough & Cold Long-Acting Liquid ... 735
Robitussin Pediatric Cough & Cold Nighttime Liquid ... 736
Robitussin Sugar Free Cough ... 738
TheraFlu Cold & Cough Hot Liquid ... 740
TheraFlu Warming Relief Daytime Severe Cold ... 743
TheraFlu Thin Strips Long Acting Cough ... 744
Triaminic Daytime Cold & Cough Liquid ... 745
Triaminic Cough & Sore Throat Liquid ... 747
Triaminic Cough & Runny Nose Softchews ... 748
Triaminic Thin Strips Cold & Cough ... 778
Triaminic Infant Thin Strips Decongestant Plus Cough ... 747
Children's Tylenol Plus Flu Oral Suspension ... 749
Tylenol Cold Head Congestion Daytime Caplets with Cool Burst and Gelcaps ... 750
Tylenol Cold Multi-Symptom Daytime Liquid ... 752
Tylenol Cold Multi-Symptom Severe Daytime Liquid ... 752
Concentrated Tylenol Infants' Drops Plus Cold & Cough ... 754
Children's Tylenol Plus Cough & Runny Nose Suspension Liquid ... 1879
Children's Tylenol Plus Cough & Sore Throat Suspension Liquid ... 1879
Children's Tylenol Plus Flu Suspension Liquid ... 1881
Children's Tylenol Plus Multi-Symptom Cold Suspension Liquid ... 1879
Tylenol Cold Severe Congestion Non-Drowsy Caplets with Cool Burst ... 1874
Tylenol Cold Head Congestion Daytime Caplets with Cool Burst ... 1873
Tylenol Cold Head Congestion Nighttime Caplets with Cool Burst ... 1873
Tylenol Cold Head Congestion Severe Caplets with Cool Burst ... 1873
Tylenol Cold Multi-Symptom Daytime Caplets with Cool Burst and Gelcaps ... 1874
Tylenol Cold Multi-Symptom Daytime Liquid with Citrus Burst ... 1874
Tylenol Cold Multi-Symptom Nighttime Caplets with Cool Burst ... 1874
Tylenol Cold Multi-Symptom Nighttime Liquid with Cool Burst ... 1874
Tylenol Cold Multi-Symptom Severe Caplets with Cool Burst ... 1874
Tylenol Cold Multi-Symptom Severe Daytime Liquid with Citrus Burst ... 1874
Tylenol Cough & Sore Throat Daytime Liquid with Cool Burst ... 1877
Tylenol Cough & Sore Throat Nighttime Liquid with Cool Burst ... 1877
Concentrated Tylenol Infants' Drops Plus Cold and Cough ... 1879
Vicks 44 Cough Relief Liquid ... 2679
Vicks 44D Cough & Head Congestion Relief Liquid ... 2679
Vicks 44E Cough & Chest Congestion Relief Liquid ... 2679
Pediatric Vicks 44e Cough & Chest Congestion Relief Liquid ... 2676
Vicks 44M Cough, Cold & Flu Relief Liquid ... 2680
Pediatric Vicks 44m Cough & Cold Relief Liquid ... 2676
Vicks DayQuil LiquiCaps/Liquid Multi-Symptom Cold/Flu Relief ... 761
Vicks DayQuil Multi-Symptom Cold/Flu Relief LiquiCaps ... 2678
Vicks DayQuil Multi-Symptom Cold/Flu Relief Liquid ... 2678
Vicks NyQuil Multi-Symptom Cold/Flu Relief Liquid ... 2681
Children's Vicks NyQuil Cold/Cough Relief ... 756
Vicks NyQuil Multi-Symptom Cold/Flu Relief LiquiCaps ... 2681
Vicks NyQuil LiquiCaps/Liquid Multi-Symptom Cold/Flu Relief ... 763
Vicks NyQuil Cough Liquid ... 2680
Children's Vicks NyQuil Cold/Cough Relief Liquid ... 2680
Zicam Cough Max Nighttime Cough Spray ... 767
Zicam Cough Max Cough Spray ... 767
Zicam Cough Max Cough Melts ... 767
Zicam Cough Plus D Cough Spray ... 767
Zicam Cough Relief Cough Spray ... 767
Zicam Maximum Strength Flu Daytime ... 768
Zicam Maximum Strength Flu Nighttime ... 768

Diatrizoate Meglumine (The benefits and risks of using fenofibrate with immunosuppressants and other potentially nephrotoxic agents should be carefully considered, and the lowest effective dose employed).
No products indexed under this heading.

Diatrizoate Sodium (The benefits and risks of using fenofibrate with immunosuppressants and other potentially nephrotoxic agents should be carefully considered, and the lowest effective dose employed).
No products indexed under this heading.

Diazepam (Fenofibrates are mild-moderate inhibitors of CYP2C9 at therapeutic concentrations). Products include:
Diastat Rectal Delivery System ... 3343
Valium Tablets ... 2819

Diclofenac Potassium (Fenofibrates are mild-moderate inhibitors of CYP2C9 at therapeutic concentrations).
No products indexed under this heading.

Diclofenac Sodium (Fenofibrates are mild-moderate inhibitors of CYP2C9 at therapeutic concentrations). Products include:
Arthrotec Tablets ... 3129
Voltaren Ophthalmic Solution ... 2309
Voltaren Tablets ... 2307
Voltaren-XR Tablets ... 2310

Dicloxacillin Sodium (The benefits and risks of using fenofibrate with immunosuppressants and other potentially nephrotoxic agents should be carefully considered, and the lowest effective dose employed).
No products indexed under this heading.

Dicumarol (Caution should be exercised when anticoagulants are given in conjunction with fenofibrate because of the potentiation of coumarin-type anticoagulants in prolonging the prothrombin time/INR. The dosage of the anticoagulant should be reduced to maintain the prothrombin time/INR at the desired level to prevent bleeding complications. Frequent prothrombin time/INR determinations are advisably until it has been definitely determined that the prothrombin time/INR has stabilized).
No products indexed under this heading.

Didanosine (The benefits and risks of using fenofibrate with immunosuppressants and other potentially nephrotoxic agents should be carefully considered, and the lowest effective dose employed).
No products indexed under this heading.

IMPORTANT NOTE: Always consult each drug listing in the patient's regimen for possible interactions.

Divalproex Sodium (Fenofibrates are weak inhibitors of CYP2C19 at therapeutic concentrations). Products include:
- Depakote Sprinkle Capsules 422
- Depakote Tablets 427
- Depakote ER Tablets 434

Doxepin Hydrochloride (Fenofibrates are weak inhibitors of CYP2C19 at therapeutic concentrations).
No products indexed under this heading.

Dronabinol (Fenofibrates are mild-moderate inhibitors of CYP2C9 at therapeutic concentrations). Products include:
- Marinol Capsules 3333

Efavirenz (The benefits and risks of using fenofibrate with immunosuppressants and other potentially nephrotoxic agents should be carefully considered, and the lowest effective dose employed). Products include:
- Atripla Tablets 945
- Sustiva Capsules 930
- Sustiva Tablets 930

Emtricitabine (The benefits and risks of using fenofibrate with immunosuppressants and other potentially nephrotoxic agents should be carefully considered, and the lowest effective dose employed). Products include:
- Atripla Tablets 945
- Emtriva Capsules 1287
- Emtriva Oral Solution 1287
- Truvada Tablets 1296

Enalapril Maleate (The benefits and risks of using fenofibrate with immunosuppressants and other potentially nephrotoxic agents should be carefully considered, and the lowest effective dose employed). Products include:
- Vasotec I.V. Injection 2103

Enalaprilat (The benefits and risks of using fenofibrate with immunosuppressants and other potentially nephrotoxic agents should be carefully considered, and the lowest effective dose employed).
No products indexed under this heading.

Enfuvirtide (The benefits and risks of using fenofibrate with immunosuppressants and other potentially nephrotoxic agents should be carefully considered, and the lowest effective dose employed). Products include:
- Fuzeon Injection 2767

Eprosartan Mesylate (Fenofibrates are mild-moderate inhibitors of CYP2C9 at therapeutic concentrations). Products include:
- Teveten Tablets 1735
- Teveten HCT Tablets 1737

Esomeprazole Magnesium (Fenofibrates are weak inhibitors of CYP2C19 at therapeutic concentrations). Products include:
- Nexium Delayed-Release Capsules 655

Ethiodized Oil (The benefits and risks of using fenofibrate with immunosuppressants and other potentially nephrotoxic agents should be carefully considered, and the lowest effective dose employed).
No products indexed under this heading.

Ethosuximide (Fenofibrates are weak inhibitors of CYP2C19 at therapeutic concentrations).
No products indexed under this heading.

Ethotoin (Fenofibrates are weak inhibitors of CYP2C19 at therapeutic concentrations).
No products indexed under this heading.

Etodolac (Fenofibrates are mild-moderate inhibitors of CYP2C9 at therapeutic concentrations).
No products indexed under this heading.

Felbamate (Fenofibrates are weak inhibitors of CYP2C19 at therapeutic concentrations).
No products indexed under this heading.

Fenoprofen Calcium (Fenofibrates are mild-moderate inhibitors of CYP2C9 at therapeutic concentrations). Products include:
- Nalfon Capsules 2502

Filgrastim (The benefits and risks of using fenofibrate with immunosuppressants and other potentially nephrotoxic agents should be carefully considered, and the lowest effective dose employed). Products include:
- Neupogen for Injection 603

Fluorouracil (The benefits and risks of using fenofibrate with immunosuppressants and other potentially nephrotoxic agents should be carefully considered, and the lowest effective dose employed). Products include:
- Carac Cream, 0.5% 2879
- Efudex 3363

Fluoxetine Hydrochloride (Fenofibrates are mild-moderate inhibitors of CYP2C9 at therapeutic concentrations). Products include:
- Prozac Pulvules and Liquid 1801
- Symbyax Capsules 1819

Flurbiprofen (Fenofibrates are mild-moderate inhibitors of CYP2C9 at therapeutic concentrations).
No products indexed under this heading.

Flurbiprofen Sodium (Fenofibrates are mild-moderate inhibitors of CYP2C9 at therapeutic concentrations). Products include:
- Ocufen Ophthalmic Solution .... ⊙ 232

Fluvastatin Sodium (The combined use of fenofibrates and HMG-CoA reductase inhibitors should be avoided unless the benefit of further alterations in lipid levels is likely to outweigh the increased risk of this drug combination. The combined use of fibric acid derivatives and HMG-CoA reductase inhibitors has been associated, in the absence of a marked pharmacokinetic interaction, in numerous case reports, with rhabdomyolysis, markedly elevated creatine kinase (CK) levels and myoglobinuria, leading in a high proportion of cases to acute renal failure). Products include:
- Lescol Capsules 2233
- Lescol XL Tablets 2233

Formoterol Fumarate (Fenofibrates are weak inhibitors of CYP2C19 at therapeutic concentrations). Products include:
- Foradil Aerolizer 3010

Foscarnet Sodium (The benefits and risks of using fenofibrate with immunosuppressants and other potentially nephrotoxic agents should be carefully considered, and the lowest effective dose employed).
No products indexed under this heading.

Fosinopril Sodium (The benefits and risks of using fenofibrate with immunosuppressants and other potentially nephrotoxic agents should be carefully considered, and the lowest effective dose employed).
No products indexed under this heading.

Fosphenytoin (Fenofibrates are weak inhibitors of CYP2C19 at therapeutic concentrations).
No products indexed under this heading.

Fosphenytoin Sodium (Fenofibrates are weak inhibitors of CYP2C19 at therapeutic concentrations).
No products indexed under this heading.

Furosemide (The benefits and risks of using fenofibrate with immunosuppressants and other potentially nephrotoxic agents should be carefully considered, and the lowest effective dose employed). Products include:
- Furosemide Tablets 2154

Gabapentin (Fenofibrates are weak inhibitors of CYP2C19 at therapeutic concentrations). Products include:
- Neurontin Capsules 2487
- Neurontin Oral Solution 2487
- Neurontin Tablets 2487

Gadopentetate Dimeglumine (The benefits and risks of using fenofibrate with immunosuppressants and other potentially nephrotoxic agents should be carefully considered, and the lowest effective dose employed).
No products indexed under this heading.

Gentamicin (The benefits and risks of using fenofibrate with immunosuppressants and other potentially nephrotoxic agents should be carefully considered, and the lowest effective dose employed).
No products indexed under this heading.

Gentamicin Sulfate (The benefits and risks of using fenofibrate with immunosuppressants and other potentially nephrotoxic agents should be carefully considered, and the lowest effective dose employed). Products include:
- Garamycin Injectable 3014
- Pred-G Ophthalmic Ointment .... ⊙ 237
- Pred-G Ophthalmic Suspension .... ⊙ 236

Glimepiride (Fenofibrates are mild-moderate inhibitors of CYP2C9 at therapeutic concentrations). Products include:
- Avandaryl Tablets 1379
- Duetact Tablets 3226

Glipizide (Fenofibrates are mild-moderate inhibitors of CYP2C9 at therapeutic concentrations).
No products indexed under this heading.

Globulin, Immune (Human) (The benefits and risks of using fenofibrate with immunosuppressants and other potentially nephrotoxic agents should be carefully considered, and the lowest effective dose employed). Products include:
- Flebogamma 5%, Immune Globulin Intravenous (Human) 1658
- GamaSTAN 3234

Glyburide (The benefits and risks of using fenofibrate with immunosuppressants and other potentially nephrotoxic agents should be carefully considered, and the lowest effective dose employed).
No products indexed under this heading.

Gold Therapy (The benefits and risks of using fenofibrate with immunosuppressants and other potentially nephrotoxic agents should be carefully considered, and the lowest effective dose employed).
No products indexed under this heading.

HMG-CoA Reductase Inhibitors (The benefits and risks of using fenofibrate with immunosuppressants and other potentially nephrotoxic agents should be carefully considered, and the lowest effective dose employed).
No products indexed under this heading.

Hydrochlorothiazide (The benefits and risks of using fenofibrate with immunosuppressants and other potentially nephrotoxic agents should be carefully considered, and the lowest effective dose employed). Products include:
- Aldoril Tablets 1910
- Atacand HCT 651
- Avalide Tablets 888
- Avalide Tablets 2874
- Benicar HCT Tablets 1044
- Diovan HCT Tablets 2196
- Dyazide Capsules 1423
- Hyzaar 50-12.5 Tablets 1990
- Hyzaar 100-12.5 Tablets 1990
- Hyzaar 100-25 Tablets 1990
- Lopressor HCT 50/25 Tablets 2241
- Lopressor HCT 100/25 Tablets 2241
- Lopressor HCT 100/50 Tablets 2241
- Lotensin HCT Tablets 2246
- Micardis HCT Tablets 856
- Moduretic Tablets 2028
- Prinzide Tablets 2056
- Teveten HCT Tablets 1737
- Timolide Tablets 2086
- Uniretic Tablets 3100

Hydroflumethiazide (The benefits and risks of using fenofibrate with immunosuppressants and other potentially nephrotoxic agents should be carefully considered, and the lowest effective dose employed).
No products indexed under this heading.

Ibuprofen (Fenofibrates are mild-moderate inhibitors of CYP2C9 at therapeutic concentrations). Products include:
- Advil Allergy Sinus Caplets .... ▣ 770
- Advil .... ▣ 674
- Children's Advil Oral Suspension .... ▣ 603
- Children's Advil Chewable Tablets .... ▣ 603
- Advil Cold & Sinus .... ▣ 723
- Infants' Advil Concentrated Drops .... ▣ 604
- Infants' Advil Concentrated Drops - White Grape (Dye-Free) .... ▣ 604
- Junior Strength Advil Swallow Tablets .... ▣ 605
- Advil Migraine Liquigels .... ▣ 608
- Advil Multi-Symptom Cold Caplets .... ▣ 770
- Advil PM Caplets .... ▣ 615
- Motrin IB Tablets and Caplets 1866
- Children's Motrin Oral Suspension 1867
- Children's Motrin Non-Staining Dye-Free Oral Suspension 1867
- Children's Motrin Cold Oral Suspension 1867
- Infants' Motrin Concentrated Drops 1867
- Infants' Motrin Non-Staining Dye-Free Concentrated Drops 1867
- Junior Strength Motrin Caplets and Chewable Tablets 1867
- Vicoprofen Tablets 539

Idarubicin Hydrochloride (The benefits and risks of using fenofibrate with immunosuppressants and other potentially nephrotoxic agents should be carefully considered, and the lowest effective dose employed).
No products indexed under this heading.

Ifosfamide (The benefits and risks of using fenofibrate with immunosuppressants and other potentially nephrotoxic agents should be carefully considered, and the lowest effective dose employed).
No products indexed under this heading.

Imipenem (The benefits and risks of using fenofibrate with immunosuppressants and other potentially nephrotoxic agents should be carefully considered, and the lowest effective dose employed). Products include:
Primaxin I.M. 2045
Primaxin I.V. 2048

Imipramine Hydrochloride (Fenofibrates are mild-moderate inhibitors of CYP2C9 at therapeutic concentrations).
No products indexed under this heading.

Imipramine Pamoate (Fenofibrates are weak inhibitors of CYP2C19 at therapeutic concentrations).
No products indexed under this heading.

Immune Globulin Intravenous (Human) (The benefits and risks of using fenofibrate with immunosuppressants and other potentially nephrotoxic agents should be carefully considered, and the lowest effective dose employed). Products include:
Carimune NF 3499
Gammagard Liquid 721
Gammagard S/D 724
Gamunex Immune Globulin I.V., 10% 3235

Indinavir Sulfate (The benefits and risks of using fenofibrate with immunosuppressants and other potentially nephrotoxic agents should be carefully considered, and the lowest effective dose employed). Products include:
Crixivan Capsules 1940

Indomethacin (Fenofibrates are mild-moderate inhibitors of CYP2C9 at therapeutic concentrations). Products include:
Indocin 1995

Indomethacin Sodium Trihydrate (Fenofibrates are mild-moderate inhibitors of CYP2C9 at therapeutic concentrations). Products include:
Indocin I.V. 2465

Interferon Beta-1b (The benefits and risks of using fenofibrate with immunosuppressants and other potentially nephrotoxic agents should be carefully considered, and the lowest effective dose employed). Products include:
Betaseron for SC Injection 767

Interleuken-2 (The benefits and risks of using fenofibrate with immunosuppressants and other potentially nephrotoxic agents should be carefully considered, and the lowest effective dose employed).
No products indexed under this heading.

Iodamide Meglumine (The benefits and risks of using fenofibrate with immunosuppressants and other potentially nephrotoxic agents should be carefully considered, and the lowest effective dose employed).
No products indexed under this heading.

Iohexol (The benefits and risks of using fenofibrate with immunosuppressants and other potentially nephrotoxic agents should be carefully considered, and the lowest effective dose employed).
No products indexed under this heading.

Iopamidol (The benefits and risks of using fenofibrate with immunosuppressants and other potentially nephrotoxic agents should be carefully considered, and the lowest effective dose employed).
No products indexed under this heading.

Iopanoic Acid (The benefits and risks of using fenofibrate with immunosuppressants and other potentially nephrotoxic agents should be carefully considered, and the lowest effective dose employed).
No products indexed under this heading.

Iothalamate Meglumine (The benefits and risks of using fenofibrate with immunosuppressants and other potentially nephrotoxic agents should be carefully considered, and the lowest effective dose employed).
No products indexed under this heading.

Ioxaglate Meglumine (The benefits and risks of using fenofibrate with immunosuppressants and other potentially nephrotoxic agents should be carefully considered, and the lowest effective dose employed).
No products indexed under this heading.

Ioxaglate Sodium (The benefits and risks of using fenofibrate with immunosuppressants and other potentially nephrotoxic agents should be carefully considered, and the lowest effective dose employed).
No products indexed under this heading.

Irbesartan (Fenofibrates are mild-moderate inhibitors of CYP2C9 at therapeutic concentrations). Products include:
Avalide Tablets 888
Avalide Tablets 2874
Avapro Tablets 891
Avapro Tablets 2871

Kanamycin Sulfate (The benefits and risks of using fenofibrate with immunosuppressants and other potentially nephrotoxic agents should be carefully considered, and the lowest effective dose employed).
No products indexed under this heading.

Ketoprofen (Fenofibrates are mild-moderate inhibitors of CYP2C9 at therapeutic concentrations).
No products indexed under this heading.

Ketorolac Tromethamine (Fenofibrates are mild-moderate inhibitors of CYP2C9 at therapeutic concentrations). Products include:
Acular Ophthalmic Solution 565
Acular LS Ophthalmic Solution 566

Lamium album (The benefits and risks of using fenofibrate with immunosuppressants and other potentially nephrotoxic agents should be carefully considered, and the lowest effective dose employed).
No products indexed under this heading.

Lamotrigine (Fenofibrates are weak inhibitors of CYP2C19 at therapeutic concentrations). Products include:
Lamictal 1481

Lansoprazole (Fenofibrates are mild-moderate inhibitors of CYP2C9 at therapeutic concentrations). Products include:
Prevacid Delayed-Release Capsules 3271
Prevacid for Delayed-Release Oral Suspension 3271
Prevacid SoluTab Delayed-Release Orally Disintegrating Tablets 3271
Prevacid I.V. for Injection 3277
Prevacid NapraPAC 3280
PREVPAC 3284

Levetiracetam (Fenofibrates are weak inhibitors of CYP2C19 at therapeutic concentrations). Products include:
Keppra Injection 3320
Keppra Oral Solution 3314
Keppra Tablets 3314

Lisinopril (The benefits and risks of using fenofibrate with immunosuppressants and other potentially nephrotoxic agents should be carefully considered, and the lowest effective dose employed). Products include:
Prinivil Tablets 2052
Prinzide Tablets 2056

Lithium (The benefits and risks of using fenofibrate with immunosuppressants and other potentially nephrotoxic agents should be carefully considered, and the lowest effective dose employed).
No products indexed under this heading.

Lithium Carbonate (The benefits and risks of using fenofibrate with immunosuppressants and other potentially nephrotoxic agents should be carefully considered, and the lowest effective dose employed). Products include:
Lithobid Tablets 1692

Lithium Citrate (The benefits and risks of using fenofibrate with immunosuppressants and other potentially nephrotoxic agents should be carefully considered, and the lowest effective dose employed).
No products indexed under this heading.

Lopinavir (The benefits and risks of using fenofibrate with immunosuppressants and other potentially nephrotoxic agents should be carefully considered, and the lowest effective dose employed). Products include:
Kaletra 476

Loracarbef (The benefits and risks of using fenofibrate with immunosuppressants and other potentially nephrotoxic agents should be carefully considered, and the lowest effective dose employed).
No products indexed under this heading.

Losartan Potassium (Fenofibrates are mild-moderate inhibitors of CYP2C9 at therapeutic concentrations). Products include:
Cozaar Tablets 1935
Hyzaar 50-12.5 Tablets 1990
Hyzaar 100-12.5 Tablets 1990
Hyzaar 100-25 Tablets 1990

Lovastatin (The combined use of fenofibrates and HMG-CoA reductase inhibitors should be avoided unless the benefit of further alterations in lipid levels is likely to outweigh the increased risk of this drug combination. The combined use of fibric acid derivatives and HMG-CoA reductase inhibitors has been associated, in the absence of a marked pharmacokinetic interaction, in numerous case reports, with rhabdomyolysis, markedly elevated creatine kinase (CK) levels and myoglobinuria, leading in a high proportion of cases to acute renal failure). Products include:
Advicor Tablets 1722
Altoprev Extended-Release Tablets 3109
Mevacor Tablets 2021

Maprotiline Hydrochloride (Fenofibrates are weak inhibitors of CYP2C19 at therapeutic concentrations).
No products indexed under this heading.

Meclofenamate Sodium (Fenofibrates are mild-moderate inhibitors of CYP2C9 at therapeutic concentrations).
No products indexed under this heading.

Mefenamic Acid (Fenofibrates are mild-moderate inhibitors of CYP2C9 at therapeutic concentrations).
No products indexed under this heading.

Meloxicam (Fenofibrates are mild-moderate inhibitors of CYP2C9 at therapeutic concentrations). Products include:
Mobic Oral Suspension 863
Mobic Tablets 863

Melphalan Hydrochloride (The benefits and risks of using fenofibrate with immunosuppressants and other potentially nephrotoxic agents should be carefully considered, and the lowest effective dose employed). Products include:
Alkeran for Injection 955

Mephenytoin (Fenofibrates are weak inhibitors of CYP2C19 at therapeutic concentrations).
No products indexed under this heading.

Mephobarbital (Fenofibrates are weak inhibitors of CYP2C19 at therapeutic concentrations).
No products indexed under this heading.

Meprobamate (Fenofibrates are weak inhibitors of CYP2C19 at therapeutic concentrations).
No products indexed under this heading.

Mesalamine (The benefits and risks of using fenofibrate with immunosuppressants and other potentially nephrotoxic agents should be carefully considered, and the lowest effective dose employed). Products include:
Asacol Delayed-Release Tablets 2692
Canasa Rectal Suppositories 699
Pentasa Capsules 3185

Metformin Hydrochloride (Fenofibrates are mild-moderate inhibitors of CYP2C9 at therapeutic concentrations). Products include:
ActoPlus Met Tablets 3214
Avandamet Tablets 1373
Fortamet Extended-Release Tablets 3115

Methimazole (The benefits and risks of using fenofibrate with immunosuppressants and other potentially nephrotoxic agents should be carefully considered, and the lowest effective dose employed).

No products indexed under this heading.

Methotrexate (The benefits and risks of using fenofibrate with immunosuppressants and other potentially nephrotoxic agents should be carefully considered, and the lowest effective dose employed).

No products indexed under this heading.

Methotrexate Sodium (The benefits and risks of using fenofibrate with immunosuppressants and other potentially nephrotoxic agents should be carefully considered, and the lowest effective dose employed).

No products indexed under this heading.

Methsuximide (Fenofibrates are weak inhibitors of CYP2C19 at therapeutic concentrations).

No products indexed under this heading.

Methyclothiazide (The benefits and risks of using fenofibrate with immunosuppressants and other potentially nephrotoxic agents should be carefully considered, and the lowest effective dose employed).

No products indexed under this heading.

Mezlocillin Sodium (The benefits and risks of using fenofibrate with immunosuppressants and other potentially nephrotoxic agents should be carefully considered, and the lowest effective dose employed).

No products indexed under this heading.

Midazolam Hydrochloride (Fenofibrates are weak inhibitors of CYP2C19 at therapeutic concentrations).

No products indexed under this heading.

Miglitol (Fenofibrates are mild-moderate inhibitors of CYP2C9 at therapeutic concentrations).

No products indexed under this heading.

Minocycline Hydrochloride (The benefits and risks of using fenofibrate with immunosuppressants and other potentially nephrotoxic agents should be carefully considered, and the lowest effective dose employed). Products include:

Mirtazapine (Fenofibrates are mild-moderate inhibitors of CYP2C9 at therapeutic concentrations).

No products indexed under this heading.

Mitomycin (Mitomycin-C) (The benefits and risks of using fenofibrate with immunosuppressants and other potentially nephrotoxic agents should be carefully considered, and the lowest effective dose employed).

No products indexed under this heading.

Moexipril Hydrochloride (The benefits and risks of using fenofibrate with immunosuppressants and other potentially nephrotoxic agents should be carefully considered, and the lowest effective dose employed). Products include:

Montelukast Sodium (Fenofibrates are mild-moderate inhibitors of CYP2C9 at therapeutic concentrations). Products include:

Muromonab-CD3 (The benefits and risks of using fenofibrate with immunosuppressants and other potentially nephrotoxic agents should be carefully considered, and the lowest effective dose employed). Products include:

Mycophenolate Mofetil (The benefits and risks of using fenofibrate with immunosuppressants and other potentially nephrotoxic agents should be carefully considered, and the lowest effective dose employed). Products include:

Nabumetone (Fenofibrates are mild-moderate inhibitors of CYP2C9 at therapeutic concentrations).

No products indexed under this heading.

Nafcillin Sodium (The benefits and risks of using fenofibrate with immunosuppressants and other potentially nephrotoxic agents should be carefully considered, and the lowest effective dose employed).

No products indexed under this heading.

Naproxen (Fenofibrates are mild-moderate inhibitors of CYP2C9 at therapeutic concentrations). Products include:

Naproxen Sodium (Fenofibrates are mild-moderate inhibitors of CYP2C9 at therapeutic concentrations). Products include:

Nateglinide (Fenofibrates are mild-moderate inhibitors of CYP2C9 at therapeutic concentrations). Products include:

Nelfinavir Mesylate (Fenofibrates are weak inhibitors of CYP2C19 at therapeutic concentrations). Products include:

Neomycin (The benefits and risks of using fenofibrate with immunosuppressants and other potentially nephrotoxic agents should be carefully considered, and the lowest effective dose employed). Products include:

Neomycin, oral (The benefits and risks of using fenofibrate with immunosuppressants and other potentially nephrotoxic agents should be carefully considered, and the lowest effective dose employed).

No products indexed under this heading.

Neomycin Sulfate (The benefits and risks of using fenofibrate with immunosuppressants and other potentially nephrotoxic agents

should be carefully considered, and the lowest effective dose employed). Products include:

Nevirapine (The benefits and risks of using fenofibrate with immunosuppressants and other potentially nephrotoxic agents should be carefully considered, and the lowest effective dose employed). Products include:

Nilutamide (Fenofibrates are weak inhibitors of CYP2C19 at therapeutic concentrations).

No products indexed under this heading.

Norfloxacin (The benefits and risks of using fenofibrate with immunosuppressants and other potentially nephrotoxic agents should be carefully considered, and the lowest effective dose employed). Products include:

Nortriptyline Hydrochloride (Fenofibrates are weak inhibitors of CYP2C19 at therapeutic concentrations).

No products indexed under this heading.

Olsalazine Sodium (The benefits and risks of using fenofibrate with immunosuppressants and other potentially nephrotoxic agents should be carefully considered, and the lowest effective dose employed).

No products indexed under this heading.

Omeprazole (Fenofibrates are mild-moderate inhibitors of CYP2C9 at therapeutic concentrations). Products include:

Oxaprozin (Fenofibrates are mild-moderate inhibitors of CYP2C9 at therapeutic concentrations).

No products indexed under this heading.

Oxcarbazepine (Fenofibrates are weak inhibitors of CYP2C19 at therapeutic concentrations). Products include:

Pamidronate Disodium (The benefits and risks of using fenofibrate with immunosuppressants and other potentially nephrotoxic agents should be carefully considered, and the lowest effective dose employed). Products include:

Pantoprazole Sodium (Fenofibrates are weak inhibitors of CYP2C19 at therapeutic concentrations). Products include:

Paramethadione (Fenofibrates are weak inhibitors of CYP2C19 at therapeutic concentrations).

No products indexed under this heading.

Paroxetine Hydrochloride (The benefits and risks of using fenofibrate with immunosuppressants and other potentially nephrotoxic agents should be carefully considered, and the lowest effective dose employed). Products include:

Penicillamine (The benefits and risks of using fenofibrate with immunosuppressants and other potentially nephrotoxic agents should be carefully considered, and the lowest effective dose employed). Products include:

Penicillin G Benzathine (The benefits and risks of using fenofibrate with immunosuppressants and other potentially nephrotoxic agents should be carefully considered, and the lowest effective dose employed). Products include:

Penicillin G Potassium (The benefits and risks of using fenofibrate with immunosuppressants and other potentially nephrotoxic agents should be carefully considered, and the lowest effective dose employed).

No products indexed under this heading.

Penicillin G Procaine (The benefits and risks of using fenofibrate with immunosuppressants and other potentially nephrotoxic agents should be carefully considered, and the lowest effective dose employed). Products include:

Penicillin G Sodium (The benefits and risks of using fenofibrate with immunosuppressants and other potentially nephrotoxic agents should be carefully considered, and the lowest effective dose employed).

No products indexed under this heading.

Penicillin V Potassium (The benefits and risks of using fenofibrate with immunosuppressants and other potentially nephrotoxic agents should be carefully considered, and the lowest effective dose employed).

No products indexed under this heading.

Pentamidine Isethionate (Fenofibrates are weak inhibitors of CYP2C19 at therapeutic concentrations).

No products indexed under this heading.

Perindopril Erbumine (The benefits and risks of using fenofibrate with immunosuppressants and other potentially nephrotoxic agents should be carefully considered, and the lowest effective dose employed). Products include:

Phenacemide (Fenofibrates are weak inhibitors of CYP2C19 at therapeutic concentrations).

No products indexed under this heading.

Phenobarbital (Fenofibrates are weak inhibitors of CYP2C19 at therapeutic concentrations). Products include:

Phenobarbital Sodium (Fenofibrates are weak inhibitors of CYP2C19 at therapeutic concentrations).

No products indexed under this heading.

Phensuximide (Fenofibrates are weak inhibitors of CYP2C19 at therapeutic concentrations).

No products indexed under this heading.

(▣ Described in PDR For Nonprescription Drugs) (⊙ Described in PDR For Ophthalmic Medicines™)

Phenylbutazone (Fenofibrates are mild-moderate inhibitors of CYP2C9 at therapeutic concentrations).
No products indexed under this heading.

Phenytoin (Fenofibrates are weak inhibitors of CYP2C19 at therapeutic concentrations).
No products indexed under this heading.

Phenytoin Sodium (Fenofibrates are mild-moderate inhibitors of CYP2C9 at therapeutic concentrations). Products include:
Phenytek Capsules 2160

Pioglitazone Hydrochloride (Fenofibrates are mild-moderate inhibitors of CYP2C9 at therapeutic concentrations). Products include:
ActoPlus Met Tablets 3214
Actos Tablets 3219
Duetact Tablets 3226

Piroxicam (Fenofibrates are mild-moderate inhibitors of CYP2C9 at therapeutic concentrations).
No products indexed under this heading.

Plicamycin (The benefits and risks of using fenofibrate with immunosuppressants and other potentially nephrotoxic agents should be carefully considered, and the lowest effective dose employed).
No products indexed under this heading.

Polymyxin (The benefits and risks of using fenofibrate with immunosuppressants and other potentially nephrotoxic agents should be carefully considered, and the lowest effective dose employed).
No products indexed under this heading.

Polymyxin B Sulfate (The benefits and risks of using fenofibrate with immunosuppressants and other potentially nephrotoxic agents should be carefully considered, and the lowest effective dose employed). Products include:
Neosporin Antibiotic Ointment .... ▣643
Neosporin Ophthalmic Solution Sterile .... ⊙265
Neosporin + Pain Relief Antibiotic Cream and Ointment (Maximum Strength) .... ▣643
Poly-Pred Ophthalmic Suspension .... ⊙233
Polysporin First Aid Antibiotic Ointment .... ▣643
Polytrim Ophthalmic Solution 574

Polythiazide (The benefits and risks of using fenofibrate with immunosuppressants and other potentially nephrotoxic agents should be carefully considered, and the lowest effective dose employed).
No products indexed under this heading.

Pravastatin Sodium (The combined use of fenofibrates and HMG-CoA reductase inhibitors should be avoided unless the benefit of further alterations in lipid levels is likely to outweigh the increased risk of this drug combination. The combined use of fibric acid derivatives and HMG-CoA reductase inhibitors has been associated, in the absence of a marked pharmacokinetic interaction, in numerous case reports, with rhabdomyolysis, markedly elevated creatine kinase (CK) levels and myoglobinuria, leading in a high proportion of cases to acute renal failure).
No products indexed under this heading.

Primidone (Fenofibrates are weak inhibitors of CYP2C19 at therapeutic concentrations).
No products indexed under this heading.

Probenecid (The benefits and risks of using fenofibrate with immunosuppressants and other potentially nephrotoxic agents should be carefully considered, and the lowest effective dose employed).
No products indexed under this heading.

Progesterone (Fenofibrates are weak inhibitors of CYP2C19 at therapeutic concentrations). Products include:
Prochieve 4% Gel 1003
Prochieve 8% Gel 1003
Prometrium Capsules (100 mg, 200 mg) 3203

Proguanil Hydrochloride (Fenofibrates are weak inhibitors of CYP2C19 at therapeutic concentrations). Products include:
Malarone Pediatric Tablets 1517
Malarone Tablets 1517

Propranolol Hydrochloride (Fenofibrates are weak inhibitors of CYP2C19 at therapeutic concentrations). Products include:
Inderal LA Long-Acting Capsules 3429
InnoPran XL Capsules 2723

Protriptyline Hydrochloride (Fenofibrates are weak inhibitors of CYP2C19 at therapeutic concentrations).
No products indexed under this heading.

Quinapril Hydrochloride (The benefits and risks of using fenofibrate with immunosuppressants and other potentially nephrotoxic agents should be carefully considered, and the lowest effective dose employed).
No products indexed under this heading.

Rabeprazole Sodium (Fenofibrates are weak inhibitors of CYP2C19 at therapeutic concentrations). Products include:
Aciphex Tablets 1090

Ramipril (The benefits and risks of using fenofibrate with immunosuppressants and other potentially nephrotoxic agents should be carefully considered, and the lowest effective dose employed). Products include:
Altace Capsules 1702

Repaglinide (Fenofibrates are mild-moderate inhibitors of CYP2C9 at therapeutic concentrations).
No products indexed under this heading.

Rifampin (The benefits and risks of using fenofibrate with immunosuppressants and other potentially nephrotoxic agents should be carefully considered, and the lowest effective dose employed).
No products indexed under this heading.

Riluzole (The benefits and risks of using fenofibrate with immunosuppressants and other potentially nephrotoxic agents should be carefully considered, and the lowest effective dose employed). Products include:
Rilutek Tablets 2930

Ritonavir (The benefits and risks of using fenofibrate with immunosuppressants and other potentially nephrotoxic agents should be carefully considered, and the lowest effective dose employed). Products include:
Kaletra 476
Norvir 503

Rofecoxib (Fenofibrates are mild-moderate inhibitors of CYP2C9 at therapeutic concentrations).
No products indexed under this heading.

Rosiglitazone Maleate (Fenofibrates are mild-moderate inhibitors of CYP2C9 at therapeutic concentrations). Products include:
Avandamet Tablets 1373
Avandaryl Tablets 1379
Avandia Tablets 1384

Saquinavir (The benefits and risks of using fenofibrate with immunosuppressants and other potentially nephrotoxic agents should be carefully considered, and the lowest effective dose employed).
No products indexed under this heading.

Sertraline Hydrochloride (Fenofibrates are weak inhibitors of CYP2C19 at therapeutic concentrations). Products include:
Zoloft 2586

Sibutramine Hydrochloride Monohydrate (The benefits and risks of using fenofibrate with immunosuppressants and other potentially nephrotoxic agents should be carefully considered, and the lowest effective dose employed). Products include:
Meridia Capsules 489

Sildenafil Citrate (Fenofibrates are mild-moderate inhibitors of CYP2C9 at therapeutic concentrations). Products include:
Revatio Tablets 2557
Viagra Tablets 2573

Simvastatin (The combined use of fenofibrates and HMG-CoA reductase inhibitors should be avoided unless the benefit of further alterations in lipid levels is likely to outweigh the increased risk of this drug combination. The combined use of fibric acid derivatives and HMG-CoA reductase inhibitors has been associated, in the absence of a marked pharmacokinetic interaction, in numerous case reports, with rhabdomyolysis, markedly elevated creatine kinase (CK) levels and myoglobinuria, leading in a high proportion of cases to acute renal failure). Products include:
Vytorin 10/10 Tablets 2114
Vytorin 10/10 Tablets 3077
Vytorin 10/20 Tablets 2114
Vytorin 10/20 Tablets 3077
Vytorin 10/40 Tablets 2114
Vytorin 10/40 Tablets 3077
Vytorin 10/80 Tablets 2114
Vytorin 10/80 Tablets 3077
Zocor Tablets 2105

Sirolimus (The benefits and risks of using fenofibrate with immunosuppressants and other potentially nephrotoxic agents should be carefully considered, and the lowest effective dose employed). Products include:
Rapamune Oral Solution and Tablets 3475

Spirapril Hydrochloride (The benefits and risks of using fenofibrate with immunosuppressants and other potentially nephrotoxic agents should be carefully considered, and the lowest effective dose employed).
No products indexed under this heading.

Stavudine (The benefits and risks of using fenofibrate with immunosuppressants and other potentially nephrotoxic agents should be carefully considered, and the lowest effective dose employed).
No products indexed under this heading.

Streptomycin Sulfate (The benefits and risks of using fenofibrate with immunosuppressants and other potentially nephrotoxic agents should be carefully considered, and the lowest effective dose employed).
No products indexed under this heading.

Streptozocin (The benefits and risks of using fenofibrate with immunosuppressants and other potentially nephrotoxic agents should be carefully considered, and the lowest effective dose employed).
No products indexed under this heading.

Sulfacytine (The benefits and risks of using fenofibrate with immunosuppressants and other potentially nephrotoxic agents should be carefully considered, and the lowest effective dose employed).
No products indexed under this heading.

Sulfamethizole (The benefits and risks of using fenofibrate with immunosuppressants and other potentially nephrotoxic agents should be carefully considered, and the lowest effective dose employed).
No products indexed under this heading.

Sulfamethoxazole (Fenofibrates are mild-moderate inhibitors of CYP2C9 at therapeutic concentrations).
No products indexed under this heading.

Sulfasalazine (The benefits and risks of using fenofibrate with immunosuppressants and other potentially nephrotoxic agents should be carefully considered, and the lowest effective dose employed).
No products indexed under this heading.

Sulfinpyrazone (The benefits and risks of using fenofibrate with immunosuppressants and other potentially nephrotoxic agents should be carefully considered, and the lowest effective dose employed).
No products indexed under this heading.

Sulfisoxazole Acetyl (The benefits and risks of using fenofibrate with immunosuppressants and other potentially nephrotoxic agents should be carefully considered, and the lowest effective dose employed).
No products indexed under this heading.

Sulfisoxazole Diolamine (The benefits and risks of using fenofibrate with immunosuppressants and other potentially nephrotoxic agents should be carefully considered, and the lowest effective dose employed).
No products indexed under this heading.

Sulindac (Fenofibrates are mild-moderate inhibitors of CYP2C9 at therapeutic concentrations). Products include:
Clinoril Tablets 1924

Suprofen (Fenofibrates are mild-moderate inhibitors of CYP2C9 at therapeutic concentrations).
No products indexed under this heading.

Tacrolimus (The benefits and risks of using fenofibrate with immunosuppressants and other potentially nephrotoxic agents should be carefully considered, and the lowest effective dose employed). Products include:
Prograf Capsules and Injection 632
Protopic Ointment 638

Tamoxifen Citrate (Fenofibrates are mild-moderate inhibitors of CYP2C9 at therapeutic concentrations). Products include:
Soltamox Oral Solution 3527

Telmisartan (Fenofibrates are mild-moderate inhibitors of CYP2C9 at therapeutic concentrations). Products include:
Micardis Tablets 854
Micardis HCT Tablets 856

Teniposide (Fenofibrates are weak inhibitors of CYP2C19 at therapeutic concentrations).
No products indexed under this heading.

Tenofovir Disoproxil Fumarate (The benefits and risks of using fenofibrate with immunosuppressants and other potentially nephrotoxic agents should be carefully considered, and the lowest effective dose employed). Products include:
Atripla Tablets 945
Truvada Tablets 1296
Viread Tablets 1301

Thioguanine (The benefits and risks of using fenofibrate with immunosuppressants and other potentially nephrotoxic agents should be carefully considered, and the lowest effective dose employed). Products include:
Tabloid Tablets 1575

Thioridazine (Fenofibrates are weak inhibitors of CYP2C19 at therapeutic concentrations).
No products indexed under this heading.

Thioridazine Hydrochloride (Fenofibrates are weak inhibitors of CYP2C19 at therapeutic concentrations). Products include:
Thioridazine Hydrochloride Tablets 2163

Tiagabine Hydrochloride (Fenofibrates are weak inhibitors of CYP2C19 at therapeutic concentrations). Products include:
Gabitril Tablets 984

Ticarcillin Disodium (The benefits and risks of using fenofibrate with immunosuppressants and other potentially nephrotoxic agents should be carefully considered, and the lowest effective dose employed). Products include:
Timentin ADD-Vantage 1580
Timentin Injection Galaxy Container 1583
Timentin IV Infusion 1577
Timentin Pharmacy Bulk Package 1586

Tobramycin (The benefits and risks of using fenofibrate with immunosuppressants and other potentially nephrotoxic agents should be carefully considered, and the lowest effective dose employed). Products include:
TOBI Solution for Inhalation 2298
TobraDex Ophthalmic Ointment 562
TobraDex Ophthalmic Suspension ... 563
Zylet Ophthalmic Suspension .... ⊙259

Tobramycin Sulfate (The benefits and risks of using fenofibrate with immunosuppressants and other potentially nephrotoxic agents should be carefully considered, and the lowest effective dose employed).
No products indexed under this heading.

Tolazamide (Fenofibrates are mild-moderate inhibitors of CYP2C9 at therapeutic concentrations).
No products indexed under this heading.

Tolbutamide (Fenofibrates are mild-moderate inhibitors of CYP2C9 at therapeutic concentrations).
No products indexed under this heading.

Tolbutamide Sodium (Fenofibrates are mild-moderate inhibitors of CYP2C9 at therapeutic concentrations).
No products indexed under this heading.

Tolmetin Sodium (Fenofibrates are mild-moderate inhibitors of CYP2C9 at therapeutic concentrations).
No products indexed under this heading.

Topiramate (Fenofibrates are weak inhibitors of CYP2C19 at therapeutic concentrations). Products include:
Topamax Sprinkle Capsules 2404
Topamax Tablets 2404

Torsemide (Fenofibrates are mild-moderate inhibitors of CYP2C9 at therapeutic concentrations). Products include:
Demadex Injection 2759
Demadex Tablets 2759

Trandolapril (The benefits and risks of using fenofibrate with immunosuppressants and other potentially nephrotoxic agents should be carefully considered, and the lowest effective dose employed). Products include:
Mavik Tablets 486
Tarka Tablets 524

Triamterene (The benefits and risks of using fenofibrate with immunosuppressants and other potentially nephrotoxic agents should be carefully considered, and the lowest effective dose employed). Products include:
Dyazide Capsules 1423
Dyrenium Capsules 3400

Trimethadione (Fenofibrates are weak inhibitors of CYP2C19 at therapeutic concentrations).
No products indexed under this heading.

Trimipramine Maleate (Fenofibrates are weak inhibitors of CYP2C19 at therapeutic concentrations).
No products indexed under this heading.

Troglitazone (Fenofibrates are mild-moderate inhibitors of CYP2C9 at therapeutic concentrations).
No products indexed under this heading.

Trovafloxacin Mesylate (The benefits and risks of using fenofibrate with immunosuppressants and other potentially nephrotoxic agents should be carefully considered, and the lowest effective dose employed).
No products indexed under this heading.

Tyropanoate Sodium (The benefits and risks of using fenofibrate with immunosuppressants and other potentially nephrotoxic agents should be carefully considered, and the lowest effective dose employed).
No products indexed under this heading.

Valacyclovir Hydrochloride (The benefits and risks of using fenofibrate with immunosuppressants and other potentially nephrotoxic agents should be carefully considered, and the lowest effective dose employed). Products include:
Valtrex Caplets 1597

Valdecoxib (Fenofibrates are mild-moderate inhibitors of CYP2C9 at therapeutic concentrations).
No products indexed under this heading.

Valproate Sodium (Fenofibrates are weak inhibitors of CYP2C19 at therapeutic concentrations). Products include:
Depacon Injection 412

Valproic Acid (Fenofibrates are weak inhibitors of CYP2C19 at therapeutic concentrations). Products include:
Depakene 417

Valsartan (Fenofibrates are mild-moderate inhibitors of CYP2C9 at therapeutic concentrations). Products include:
Diovan Tablets 2193
Diovan HCT Tablets 2196

Vancomycin Hydrochloride (The benefits and risks of using fenofibrate with immunosuppressants and other potentially nephrotoxic agents should be carefully considered, and the lowest effective dose employed). Products include:
Vancocin HCl Capsules, USP 3380

Verapamil Hydrochloride (Fenofibrates are mild-moderate inhibitors of CYP2C9 at therapeutic concentrations). Products include:
Covera-HS Tablets 3139
Tarka Tablets 524
Verelan PM Extended-Release Capsules, Controlled-Onset........... 3106

Voriconazole (Fenofibrates are mild-moderate inhibitors of CYP2C9 at therapeutic concentrations). Products include:
VFEND I.V. 2564
VFEND Oral Suspension 2564
VFEND Tablets 2564

Warfarin Sodium (Caution should be exercised when anticoagulants are given in conjunction with fenofibrate because of the potentiation of coumarin-type anticoagulants in prolonging the prothrombin time/INR. The dosage of the anticoagulant should be reduced to maintain the prothrombin time/INR at the desired level to prevent bleeding complications. Frequent prothrombin time/INR determinations are advisably until it has been definitely determined that the prothrombin time/INR has stabilized). Products include:
Coumadin for Injection 898
Coumadin Tablets 898

Zafirlukast (Fenofibrates are mild-moderate inhibitors of CYP2C9 at therapeutic concentrations). Products include:
Accolate Tablets 671

Zalcitabine (The benefits and risks of using fenofibrate with immunosuppressants and other potentially nephrotoxic agents should be carefully considered, and the lowest effective dose employed).
No products indexed under this heading.

Zidovudine (The benefits and risks of using fenofibrate with immunosuppressants and other potentially nephrotoxic agents should be carefully considered, and the lowest effective dose employed). Products include:
Combivir Tablets 1411
Retrovir 1560
Retrovir IV Infusion 1564
Trizivir Tablets 1589

Zileuton (Fenofibrates are mild-moderate inhibitors of CYP2C9 at therapeutic concentrations). Products include:
Zyflo Tablets 1023

Zoledronic acid (The benefits and risks of using fenofibrate with immunosuppressants and other potentially nephrotoxic agents should be carefully considered, and the lowest effective dose employed). Products include:
Zometa for Intravenous Infusion 2315

Zonisamide (Fenofibrates are weak inhibitors of CYP2C19 at therapeutic concentrations). Products include:
Zonegran Capsules 1101

TRILEPTAL TABLETS

(Oxcarbazepine) 2300
May interact with dihydropyridine calcium channel blockers, oral contraceptives, phenytoin, valproate, and certain other agents. Compounds in these categories include:

Amlodipine Besylate (Oxcarbazepine and MHD induce a subgroup of the CYP4503A family responsible for the metabolism of dihydropyridine calcium channel antagonists, resulting in a lower plasma concentration of these drugs). Products include:
Caduet Tablets 2508
Lotrel Capsules 2249
Norvasc Tablets 2545

Carbamazepine (Co-administration with carbamazepine decreases the plasma levels of MHD (29% to 40%)). Products include:
Carbatrol Capsules 3171
Equetro Extended-Release Capsules 3180
Tegretol/Tegretol-XR 2295

Desogestrel (Concurrent use of oxcarbazepine with hormonal contraceptives may render these contraceptives less effective). Products include:
Mircette Tablets 1066

Divalproex Sodium (Co-administration decreases MHD concentration by 18%). Products include:
Depakote Sprinkle Capsules 422
Depakote Tablets 427
Depakote ER Tablets 434

Ethinyl Estradiol (Co-administration with an oral contraceptive containing ethinyl estradiol and levonorgestrel results in the decreased mean AUC value of EE by 48% to 52%, therefore, concurrent use of Trileptal with hormonal contraceptives may render these contraceptives less effective; studies with other oral or implant contraceptives have not been studied). Products include:

Mircette Tablets 1066
NuvaRing 2340
Ortho-Cyclen/Ortho Tri-Cyclen 2429
Ortho Evra Transdermal System 2417
Ortho Tri-Cyclen Lo Tablets 2436
Seasonique Tablets 1077
Yasmin 28 Tablets 796
Yaz Tablets 803

Ethynodiol Diacetate (Concurrent use of oxcarbazepine with hormonal contraceptives may render these contraceptives less effective).
No products indexed under this heading.

Felodipine (Repeated co-administration of Trileptal lowers felodipine AUC by 28%).
No products indexed under this heading.

Fosphenytoin Sodium (Co-administration increases the plasma phenytoin levels by up to 40%; phenytoin decreases the plasma levels of its active metabolite monohydroxy metabolite (MHD); a decrease in the dose of phenytoin may be required).
No products indexed under this heading.

Isradipine (Oxcarbazepine and MHD induce a subgroup of the CYP4503A family responsible for the metabolism of dihydropyridine calcium channel antagonists, resulting in a lower plasma concentration of these drugs). Products include:
DynaCirc CR Tablets 2721

Levonorgestrel (Co-administration with an oral contraceptive containing ethinyl estradiol and levonorgestrel results in the decreased mean AUC value of EE by 48% to 52%, therefore, concurrent use of Trileptal with hormonal contraceptives may render these contraceptives less effective; studies with other oral or implant contraceptives have not been studied). Products include:
Climara Pro Transdermal System 776
Mirena Intrauterine System 787
Plan B Tablets 1076
Seasonique Tablets 1077

Mestranol (Concurrent use of oxcarbazepine with hormonal contraceptives may render these contraceptives less effective).
No products indexed under this heading.

Nicardipine Hydrochloride (Oxcarbazepine and MHD induce a subgroup of the CYP4503A family responsible for the metabolism of dihydropyridine calcium channel antagonists, resulting in a lower plasma concentration of these drugs). Products include:
Cardene I.V. 2497

Nifedipine (Oxcarbazepine and MHD induce a subgroup of the CYP4503A family responsible for the metabolism of dihydropyridine calcium channel antagonists, resulting in a lower plasma concentration of these drugs). Products include:
Adalat CC Tablets 2964

Nimodipine (Oxcarbazepine and MHD induce a subgroup of the CYP4503A family responsible for the metabolism of dihydropyridine calcium channel antagonists, resulting in a lower plasma concentration of these drugs). Products include:
Nimotop Capsules 749

Norethindrone (Concurrent use of oxcarbazepine with hormonal contraceptives may render these contraceptives less effective). Products include:
Ortho Micronor Tablets 2426

Norethynodrel (Concurrent use of oxcarbazepine with hormonal contraceptives may render these contraceptives less effective).
No products indexed under this heading.

Norgestimate (Concurrent use of oxcarbazepine with hormonal contraceptives may render these contraceptives less effective). Products include:
Ortho-Cyclen/Ortho Tri-Cyclen 2429
Ortho Tri-Cyclen Lo Tablets 2436

Norgestrel (Concurrent use of oxcarbazepine with hormonal contraceptives may render these contraceptives less effective).
No products indexed under this heading.

Phenobarbital (Co-administration with phenobarbital decreases the plasma levels of MHD (29% to 40%); concurrent use increases the phenobarbital level by approximately 15%). Products include:
Donnatal Extentabs 2493

Phenytoin (Co-administration increases the plasma phenytoin levels by up to 40%; phenytoin decreases the plasma levels of its active metabolite monohydroxy metabolite (MHD); a decrease in the dose of phenytoin may be required).
No products indexed under this heading.

Phenytoin Sodium (Co-administration increases the plasma phenytoin levels by up to 40%; phenytoin decreases the plasma levels of its active metabolite monohydroxy metabolite (MHD); a decrease in the dose of phenytoin may be required). Products include:
Phenytek Capsules 2160

Valproate Sodium (Co-administration decreases MHD concentration by 18%). Products include:
Depacon Injection 412

Valproic Acid (Co-administration decreases MHD concentration by 18%). Products include:
Depakene 417

Verapamil Hydrochloride (Produces a decrease of 20% of the plasma levels of MHD). Products include:
Covera-HS Tablets 3139
Tarka Tablets 524
Verelan PM Extended-Release Capsules, Controlled-Onset........... 3106

Food Interactions

Alcohol (Oxcarbazepine causes dizziness and somnolence, concurrent use with alcohol could result in possible additive sedative effect).

TRILEPTAL ORAL SUSPENSION

(Oxcarbazepine) 2300

See Trileptal Tablets

TRI-LUMA CREAM

(Fluocinolone Acetonide, Hydroquinone, Tretinoin).................... 1213

May interact with drugs known to be photosensitizers and certain other agents. Compounds in these categories include:

Acetazolamide (Patients should be cautioned on concomitant use of medications that are known to be photosensitizing).
No products indexed under this heading.

Acitretin (Patients should be cautioned on concomitant use of medications that are known to be photosensitizing). Products include:
Soriatane Capsules 1013

Alatrofloxacin Mesylate (Patients should be cautioned on concomitant use of medications that are known to be photosensitizing).
No products indexed under this heading.

Anthralin (Patients should be cautioned on concomitant use of medications that are known to be photosensitizing). Products include:
Psoriatec Cream 1089

Bendroflumethiazide (Patients should be cautioned on concomitant use of medications that are known to be photosensitizing).
No products indexed under this heading.

Chlorothiazide (Patients should be cautioned on concomitant use of medications that are known to be photosensitizing). Products include:
Diuril Oral Suspension 1954

Chlorothiazide Sodium (Patients should be cautioned on concomitant use of medications that are known to be photosensitizing). Products include:
Diuril Sodium Intravenous 2467

Chlorpromazine (Patients should be cautioned on concomitant use of medications that are known to be photosensitizing).
No products indexed under this heading.

Chlorpromazine Hydrochloride (Patients should be cautioned on concomitant use of medications that are known to be photosensitizing).
No products indexed under this heading.

Chlorpropamide (Patients should be cautioned on concomitant use of medications that are known to be photosensitizing).
No products indexed under this heading.

Ciprofloxacin (Patients should be cautioned on concomitant use of medications that are known to be photosensitizing). Products include:
Cipro Oral Suspension 2977
Cipro I.V. 2984
Cipro XR Tablets 2990
Ciprodex Otic Suspension 559

Ciprofloxacin Hydrochloride (Patients should be cautioned on concomitant use of medications that are known to be photosensitizing). Products include:
Ciloxan Ophthalmic Ointment 559
Ciloxan Ophthalmic Solution .... ⊙206
Cipro Tablets 2977
Proquin XR Tablets 1153

Coal Tar (Patients should be cautioned on concomitant use of medications that are known to be photosensitizing).
No products indexed under this heading.

Demeclocycline Hydrochloride (Patients should be cautioned on concomitant use of medications that are known to be photosensitizing).
No products indexed under this heading.

Doxycycline Calcium (Patients should be cautioned on concomitant use of medications that are known to be photosensitizing).
No products indexed under this heading.

Doxycycline Hyclate (Patients should be cautioned on concomitant use of medications that are known to be photosensitizing).
No products indexed under this heading.

Doxycycline Monohydrate (Patients should be cautioned on concomitant use of medications that are known to be photosensitizing). Products include:
Oracea Capsules 1000

Enoxacin (Patients should be cautioned on concomitant use of medications that are known to be photosensitizing).
No products indexed under this heading.

Fluphenazine Decanoate (Patients should be cautioned on concomitant use of medications that are known to be photosensitizing).
No products indexed under this heading.

Fluphenazine Enanthate (Patients should be cautioned on concomitant use of medications that are known to be photosensitizing).
No products indexed under this heading.

Fluphenazine Hydrochloride (Patients should be cautioned on concomitant use of medications that are known to be photosensitizing).
No products indexed under this heading.

Furosemide (Patients should be cautioned on concomitant use of medications that are known to be photosensitizing). Products include:
Furosemide Tablets 2154

Glipizide (Patients should be cautioned on concomitant use of medications that are known to be photosensitizing).
No products indexed under this heading.

Glyburide (Patients should be cautioned on concomitant use of medications that are known to be photosensitizing).
No products indexed under this heading.

Grepafloxacin Hydrochloride (Patients should be cautioned on concomitant use of medications that are known to be photosensitizing).
No products indexed under this heading.

Griseofulvin (Patients should be cautioned on concomitant use of medications that are known to be photosensitizing). Products include:
Gris-PEG Tablets 2502

Hydrochlorothiazide (Patients should be cautioned on concomitant use of medications that are known to be photosensitizing). Products include:
Aldoril Tablets 1910
Atacand HCT 651
Avalide Tablets 888
Avalide Tablets 2874
Benicar HCT Tablets 1044
Diovan HCT Tablets 2196
Dyazide Capsules 1423
Hyzaar 50-12.5 Tablets 1990
Hyzaar 100-12.5 Tablets 1990
Hyzaar 100-25 Tablets 1990
Lopressor HCT 50/25 Tablets 2241
Lopressor HCT 100/25 Tablets 2241
Lopressor HCT 100/50 Tablets 2241
Lotensin HCT Tablets 2246
Micardis HCT Tablets 856
Moduretic Tablets 2028
Prinzide Tablets 2056
Teveten HCT Tablets 1737

Timolide Tablets 2086
Uniretic Tablets 3100

Hydroflumethiazide (Patients should be cautioned on concomitant use of medications that are known to be photosensitizing).
No products indexed under this heading.

Lomefloxacin Hydrochloride (Patients should be cautioned on concomitant use of medications that are known to be photosensitizing).
No products indexed under this heading.

Mesoridazine Besylate (Patients should be cautioned on concomitant use of medications that are known to be photosensitizing).
No products indexed under this heading.

Metabromsalan (Patients should be cautioned on concomitant use of medications that are known to be photosensitizing).
No products indexed under this heading.

Methacycline Hydrochloride (Patients should be cautioned on concomitant use of medications that are known to be photosensitizing).
No products indexed under this heading.

Methotrimeprazine (Patients should be cautioned on concomitant use of medications that are known to be photosensitizing).
No products indexed under this heading.

Methyclothiazide (Patients should be cautioned on concomitant use of medications that are known to be photosensitizing).
No products indexed under this heading.

Minocycline Hydrochloride (Patients should be cautioned on concomitant use of medications that are known to be photosensitizing). Products include:

Solodyn Extended Release Tablets 1890

Nalidixic Acid (Patients should be cautioned on concomitant use of medications that are known to be photosensitizing).
No products indexed under this heading.

Norfloxacin (Patients should be cautioned on concomitant use of medications that are known to be photosensitizing). Products include:

Noroxin Tablets 2032

Ofloxacin (Patients should be cautioned on concomitant use of medications that are known to be photosensitizing). Products include:

Floxin Otic Solution 1049

Oxytetracycline Hydrochloride (Patients should be cautioned on concomitant use of medications that are known to be photosensitizing).
No products indexed under this heading.

Perphenazine (Patients should be cautioned on concomitant use of medications that are known to be photosensitizing).
No products indexed under this heading.

Polythiazide (Patients should be cautioned on concomitant use of medications that are known to be photosensitizing).
No products indexed under this heading.

Prochlorperazine (Patients should be cautioned on concomitant use of medications that are known to be photosensitizing).
No products indexed under this heading.

Promethazine Hydrochloride (Patients should be cautioned on concomitant use of medications that are known to be photosensitizing). Products include:

Phenergan Tablets and Suppositories 3440

Salicylic Acid (Patients should avoid products containing keratolytic agents).
No products indexed under this heading.

Sulfamethizole (Patients should be cautioned on concomitant use of medications that are known to be photosensitizing).
No products indexed under this heading.

Sulfamethoxazole (Patients should be cautioned on concomitant use of medications that are known to be photosensitizing).
No products indexed under this heading.

Sulfasalazine (Patients should be cautioned on concomitant use of medications that are known to be photosensitizing).
No products indexed under this heading.

Sulfinpyrazone (Patients should be cautioned on concomitant use of medications that are known to be photosensitizing).
No products indexed under this heading.

Sulfisoxazole Acetyl (Patients should be cautioned on concomitant use of medications that are known to be photosensitizing).
No products indexed under this heading.

Sulfisoxazole Diolamine (Patients should be cautioned on concomitant use of medications that are known to be photosensitizing).
No products indexed under this heading.

Tetrachlorosalicylanilide (Patients should be cautioned on concomitant use of medications that are known to be photosensitizing).
No products indexed under this heading.

Tetracycline Hydrochloride (Patients should be cautioned on concomitant use of medications that are known to be photosensitizing).
No products indexed under this heading.

Thioridazine Hydrochloride (Patients should be cautioned on concomitant use of medications that are known to be photosensitizing). Products include:

Thioridazine Hydrochloride Tablets 2163

Tolazamide (Patients should be cautioned on concomitant use of medications that are known to be photosensitizing).
No products indexed under this heading.

Tolbutamide (Patients should be cautioned on concomitant use of medications that are known to be photosensitizing).
No products indexed under this heading.

Trifluoperazine Hydrochloride (Patients should be cautioned on concomitant use of medications that are known to be photosensitizing).
No products indexed under this heading.

Trovafloxacin Mesylate (Patients should be cautioned on concomitant use of medications that are known to be photosensitizing).
No products indexed under this heading.

Food Interactions

Alcohol (Patients should avoid topical products containing high alcohol concentrations).

TRILYTE WITH FLAVOR PACKS FOR ORAL SOLUTION

(PEG-3350, Potassium Chloride, Sodium Bicarbonate, Sodium Chloride)............................ 3100
May interact with:

Oral Medications, unspecified (Oral medication administered within one hour of the start of administration of TriLyte with flavor packs may be flushed from the gastrointestinal tract and not absorbed).
No products indexed under this heading.

TRISENOX INJECTION

(Arsenic Trioxide) 993
May interact with potassium-depleting diuretics, quinidine, and certain other agents. Compounds in these categories include:

Amiodarone Hydrochloride (Arsenic trioxide can cause QT interval prolongation and complete AV block; QT prolongation can lead to torsade de pointes-type ventricular arrhythmias, which can be fatal; co-administration with other drugs that can prolong the QT interval, such as certain anti-arrhythmics, increases the risk and extent of QT prolongation).
No products indexed under this heading.

Amphotericin B (Arsenic trioxide can cause QT interval prolongation and complete AV block; QT prolongation can lead to torsade de pointes-type ventricular arrhythmias, which can be fatal; co-administration with other drugs that can prolong the QT interval, such as amphotericin B, increases the risk and extent of QT prolongation).
No products indexed under this heading.

Bendroflumethiazide (Arsenic trioxide can cause QT interval prolongation and complete AV block; QT prolongation can lead to torsade de pointes-type ventricular arrhythmias, which can be fatal; co-administration with other drugs that cause hypokalemia or hypomagnesemia resulting in prolongation of the QT interval, such as potassium-wasting diuretics, increases the risk and extent of QT prolongation).
No products indexed under this heading.

Bumetanide (Arsenic trioxide can cause QT interval prolongation and complete AV block; QT prolongation can lead to torsade de pointes-type ventricular arrhythmias, which can be fatal; co-administration with other drugs that cause hypokalemia or hypomagnesemia resulting in prolongation of the QT interval, such as potassium-wasting diuretics, increases the risk and extent of QT prolongation). Products include:

Bumex Tablets 2746

Chlorothiazide (Arsenic trioxide can cause QT interval prolongation and complete AV block; QT prolongation can lead to torsade de pointes-type ventricular arrhythmias, which can be fatal; co-administration with other drugs that cause hypokalemia or hypomagnesemia resulting in prolongation of the QT interval, such as potassium-wasting diuretics, increases the risk and extent of QT prolongation). Products include:

Diuril Oral Suspension 1954

Chlorothiazide Sodium (Arsenic trioxide can cause QT interval prolongation and complete AV block; QT prolongation can lead to torsade de pointes-type ventricular arrhythmias, which can be fatal; co-administration with other drugs that cause hypokalemia or hypomagnesemia resulting in prolongation of the QT interval, such as potassium-wasting diuretics, increases the risk and extent of QT prolongation). Products include:

Diuril Sodium Intravenous 2467

Ethacrynic Acid (Arsenic trioxide can cause QT interval prolongation and complete AV block; QT prolongation can lead to torsade de pointes-type ventricular arrhythmias, which can be fatal; co-administration with other drugs that cause hypokalemia or hypomagnesemia resulting in prolongation of the QT interval, such as potassium-wasting diuretics, increases the risk and extent of QT prolongation). Products include:

Edecrin Tablets 1959

Furosemide (Arsenic trioxide can cause QT interval prolongation and complete AV block; QT prolongation can lead to torsade de pointes-type ventricular arrhythmias, which can be fatal; co-administration with other drugs that cause hypokalemia or hypomagnesemia resulting in prolongation of the QT interval, such as potassium-wasting diuretics, increases the risk and extent of QT prolongation). Products include:

Furosemide Tablets 2154

Hydrochlorothiazide (Arsenic trioxide can cause QT interval prolongation and complete AV block; QT prolongation can lead to torsade de pointes-type ventricular arrhythmias, which can be fatal; co-administration with other drugs that cause hypokalemia or hypomagnesemia resulting in prolongation of the QT interval, such as potassium-wasting diuretics, increases the risk and extent of QT prolongation). Products include:

Aldoril Tablets 1910
Atacand HCT 651
Avalide Tablets 888
Avalide Tablets 2874
Benicar HCT Tablets 1044
Diovan HCT Tablets 2196
Dyazide Capsules 1423
Hyzaar 50-12.5 Tablets 1990
Hyzaar 100-12.5 Tablets 1990
Hyzaar 100-25 Tablets 1990
Lopressor HCT 50/25 Tablets 2241
Lopressor HCT 100/25 Tablets 2241
Lopressor HCT 100/50 Tablets 2241
Lotensin HCT Tablets 2246
Micardis HCT Tablets 856
Moduretic Tablets 2028
Prinzide Tablets 2056
Teveten HCT Tablets 1737
Timolide Tablets 2086

Uniretic Tablets 3100

Hydroflumethiazide (Arsenic trioxide can cause QT interval prolongation and complete AV block; QT prolongation can lead to torsade de pointes-type ventricular arrhythmias, which can be fatal; co-administration with other drugs that cause hypokalemia or hypomagnesemia resulting in prolongation of the QT interval, such as potassium-wasting diuretics, increases the risk and extent of QT prolongation).
No products indexed under this heading.

Methyclothiazide (Arsenic trioxide can cause QT interval prolongation and complete AV block; QT prolongation can lead to torsade de pointes-type ventricular arrhythmias, which can be fatal; co-administration with other drugs that cause hypokalemia or hypomagnesemia resulting in prolongation of the QT interval, such as potassium-wasting diuretics, increases the risk and extent of QT prolongation).
No products indexed under this heading.

Polythiazide (Arsenic trioxide can cause QT interval prolongation and complete AV block; QT prolongation can lead to torsade de pointes-type ventricular arrhythmias, which can be fatal; co-administration with other drugs that cause hypokalemia or hypomagnesemia resulting in prolongation of the QT interval, such as potassium-wasting diuretics, increases the risk and extent of QT prolongation).
No products indexed under this heading.

Procainamide Hydrochloride (Arsenic trioxide can cause QT interval prolongation and complete AV block; QT prolongation can lead to torsade de pointes-type ventricular arrhythmias, which can be fatal; co-administration with other drugs that can prolong the QT interval, such as certain antiarrhythmics, increases the risk and extent of QT prolongation).
No products indexed under this heading.

Quinidine (Arsenic trioxide can cause QT interval prolongation and complete AV block; QT prolongation can lead to torsade de pointes-type ventricular arrhythmias, which can be fatal; co-administration with other drugs that can prolong the QT interval, such as certain anti-arrhythmic quinidine, increases the risk and extent of QT prolongation).
No products indexed under this heading.

Quinidine Gluconate (Arsenic trioxide can cause QT interval prolongation and complete AV block; QT prolongation can lead to torsade de pointes-type ventricular arrhythmias, which can be fatal; co-administration with other drugs that can prolong the QT interval, such as certain anti-arrhythmic quinidine, increases the risk and extent of QT prolongation).
No products indexed under this heading.

Quinidine Hydrochloride (Arsenic trioxide can cause QT interval prolongation and complete AV block; QT prolongation can lead to torsade de pointes-type ventricular arrhythmias, which can be fatal; co-administration with other drugs that can prolong the QT interval, such as certain anti-arrhythmic quinidine, increases the risk and extent of QT prolongation).
No products indexed under this heading.

Quinidine Polygalacturonate (Arsenic trioxide can cause QT interval prolongation and complete AV block; QT prolongation can lead to torsade de pointes-type ventricular arrhythmias, which can be fatal; co-administration with other drugs that can prolong the QT interval, such as certain anti-arrhythmic quinidine, increases the risk and extent of QT prolongation).
No products indexed under this heading.

Quinidine Sulfate (Arsenic trioxide can cause QT interval prolongation and complete AV block; QT prolongation can lead to torsade de pointes-type ventricular arrhythmias, which can be fatal; co-administration with other drugs that can prolong the QT interval, such as certain anti-arrhythmic quinidine, increases the risk and extent of QT prolongation).
No products indexed under this heading.

Sotalol Hydrochloride (Arsenic trioxide can cause QT interval prolongation and complete AV block; QT prolongation can lead to torsade de pointes-type ventricular arrhythmias, which can be fatal; co-administration with other drugs that can prolong the QT interval, such as certain anti-arrhythmics, increases the risk and extent of QT prolongation).
No products indexed under this heading.

Thioridazine Hydrochloride (Arsenic trioxide can cause QT interval prolongation and complete AV block; QT prolongation can lead to torsade de pointes-type ventricular arrhythmias, which can be fatal; co-administration with other drugs that can prolong the QT interval, such as thioridazine, increases the risk and extent of QT prolongation). Products include:
Thioridazine Hydrochloride Tablets 2163

Torsemide (Arsenic trioxide can cause QT interval prolongation and complete AV block; QT prolongation can lead to torsade de pointes-type ventricular arrhythmias, which can be fatal; co-administration with other drugs that cause hypokalemia or hypomagnesemia resulting in prolongation of the QT interval, such as potassium-wasting diuretics, increases the risk and extent of QT prolongation). Products include:
Demadex Injection 2759
Demadex Tablets 2759

TRIZIVIR TABLETS

(Abacavir Sulfate, Lamivudine, Zidovudine).. 1589

May interact with cytotoxic drugs, valproate, and certain other agents. Compounds in these categories include:

Atovaquone (Co-administration may alter zidovudine blood concentrations; routine dose modification is not warranted). Products include:
Malarone Pediatric Tablets 1517
Malarone Tablets 1517
Mepron Suspension 1521

Bleomycin Sulfate (Co-administration with cytotoxic agents may increase the hematologic toxicity of zidovudine).
No products indexed under this heading.

Cyclophosphamide (Co-administration with cytotoxic agents may increase the hematologic toxicity of zidovudine).
No products indexed under this heading.

Daunorubicin Hydrochloride (Co-administration with cytotoxic agents may increase the hematologic toxicity of zidovudine).
No products indexed under this heading.

Divalproex Sodium (Co-administration may alter zidovudine blood concentrations; routine dose modification is not warranted). Products include:
Depakote Sprinkle Capsules 422
Depakote Tablets 427
Depakote ER Tablets 434

Doxorubicin Hydrochloride (Co-administration with cytotoxic agents may increase the hematologic toxicity of zidovudine).
No products indexed under this heading.

Emtricitabine (Trizivir should not be administered concomitantly with emtricitabine). Products include:
Atripla Tablets 945
Emtriva Capsules 1287
Emtriva Oral Solution 1287
Truvada Tablets 1296

Epirubicin Hydrochloride (Co-administration with cytotoxic agents may increase the hematologic toxicity of zidovudine).
No products indexed under this heading.

Fluconazole (Co-administration may alter zidovudine blood concentrations; routine dose modification is not warranted).
No products indexed under this heading.

Fluorouracil (Co-administration with cytotoxic agents may increase the hematologic toxicity of zidovudine). Products include:
Carac Cream, 0.5% 2879
Efudex 3363

Ganciclovir (Co-administration may increase the hematologic toxicity of zidovudine).
No products indexed under this heading.

Ganciclovir Sodium (Co-administration may increase the hematologic toxicity of zidovudine).
No products indexed under this heading.

Hydroxyurea (Co-administration with cytotoxic agents may increase the hematologic toxicity of zidovudine).
No products indexed under this heading.

Interferon alfa-2a, Recombinant (Hepatic decompensation (some fatal) has occurred in HIV/HCV co-infected patients receiving combination antiretroviral for HIV and interferon alfa and ribavirin. Patients receiving interferon alfa with or without ribavirin and Trizivir should be closely monitored for treatment-associated toxicities, especially hepatic decompensation, neutropenia and anemia. Discontinuation of Trizivir should be considered as medically appropriate. Dose reduction or discontinuation of interferon, alfa, ribavirin or both should also be considered if worsening clinical toxicities are observed, including hepatic decompensation (e.g., Childs Pugh greater than 6)).
No products indexed under this heading.

Interferon alfa-N3 (Human Leukocyte Derived) (Hepatic decompensation (some fatal) has occurred in HIV/HCV co-infected patients receiving combination antiretroviral for HIV and interferon alfa and ribavirin. Patients receiving interferon alfa with or without ribavirin and Trizivir should be closely monitored for treatment-associated toxicities, especially hepatic decompensation, neutropenia and anemia. Discontinuation of Trizivir should be considered as medically appropriate. Dose reduction or discontinuation of interferon, alfa, ribavirin or both should also be considered if worsening clinical toxicities are observed, including hepatic decompensation (e.g., Childs Pugh greater than 6)). Products include:
Alferon N Injection 1665

Methadone Hydrochloride (Co-administration may alter zidovudine blood concentrations; routine dose modification is not warranted).
No products indexed under this heading.

Methotrexate Sodium (Co-administration with cytotoxic agents may increase the hematologic toxicity of zidovudine).
No products indexed under this heading.

Mitotane (Co-administration with cytotoxic agents may increase the hematologic toxicity of zidovudine).
No products indexed under this heading.

Mitoxantrone Hydrochloride (Co-administration with cytotoxic agents may increase the hematologic toxicity of zidovudine).
No products indexed under this heading.

Nelfinavir Mesylate (Co-administration may alter lamivudine and zidovudine blood concentrations; routine dose modification is not warranted). Products include:
Viracept 2577

Probenecid (Co-administration may alter zidovudine blood concentrations; routine dose modification is not warranted).
No products indexed under this heading.

Procarbazine Hydrochloride (Co-administration with cytotoxic agents may increase the hematologic toxicity of zidovudine). Products include:
Matulane Capsules 3191

Ribavirin (Co-administration of zidovudine with ribavirin should be avoided since an antagonistic relationship has been demonstrated in vitro). Products include:
Copegus Tablets 2754
Rebetol 3058
Rebetron Combination Therapy 3063
Ribavirin, USP Capsules 3068
Virazole for Inhalation Solution 3370

Ritonavir (Co-administration may alter zidovudine blood concentrations; routine dose modification is not warranted). Products include:

Kaletra 476
Norvir 503

Stavudine (Co-administration of zidovudine with stavudine should be avoided since an antagonistic relationship has been demonstrated in vitro).
No products indexed under this heading.

Sulfamethoxazole (Co-administration with trimethoprim/sulfamethoxazole may alter lamivudine blood concentrations; routine dose modification is not warranted).
No products indexed under this heading.

Tamoxifen Citrate (Co-administration with cytotoxic agents may increase the hematologic toxicity of zidovudine). Products include:
Soltamox Oral Solution 3527

Trimethoprim (Co-administration with trimethoprim/sulfamethoxazole may alter lamivudine blood concentrations; routine dose modification is not warranted).
No products indexed under this heading.

Valproate Sodium (Co-administration may alter zidovudine blood concentrations; routine dose modification is not warranted).
Products include:
Depacon Injection 412

Valproic Acid (Co-administration may alter zidovudine blood concentrations; routine dose modification is not warranted). Products include:
Depakene 417

Vincristine Sulfate (Co-administration with cytotoxic agents may increase the hematologic toxicity of zidovudine).
No products indexed under this heading.

Zalacitabine (Lamivudine and zalcitabine may inhibit the intracellular phosphorylation of one another; co-administration is not recommended).
No products indexed under this heading.

Food Interactions

Alcohol (Concurrent use decreases the elimination of abacavir causing an increase in overall exposure).

TRUSOPT STERILE OPHTHALMIC SOLUTION

(Dorzolamide Hydrochloride) 2095
May interact with carbonic anhydrase inhibitors and certain other agents. Compounds in these categories include:

Acetazolamide (Potential for an additive effect on the known systemic effects of carbonic anhydrase inhibition in patients receiving a systemic carbonic anhydrase inhibitor and Trusopt).
No products indexed under this heading.

Acetazolamide Sodium (Potential for an additive effect on the known systemic effects of carbonic anhydrase inhibition in patients receiving a systemic carbonic anhydrase inhibitor and Trusopt).
No products indexed under this heading.

Aspirin (Potential for acid-base and electrolyte disturbances with concomitant use; these disturbances have been reported with oral agent and have not been reported during clinical trials with Trusopt). Products include:
Aggrenox Capsules 822
Bayer Aspirin 744
BC Allergy Sinus Cold Powder .... ■677
BC Headache Powder .... ■677
Arthritis Strength BC Powder .... ■677
BC Sinus Cold Powder .... ■677
Excedrin Extra Strength Caplets/Tablets/Geltabs .... ■684
Excedrin Migraine Caplets/Tablets/Geltabs .... ■609
Goody's Body Pain Formula Powder .... ■684
Goody's Extra Strength Headache Powders .... ■611
Goody's Extra Strength Pain Relief Tablets .... ■685
Percodan Tablets 1132
St. Joseph 81 mg Aspirin Chewable and Enteric Coated Tablets 1869

Dichlorphenamide (Potential for an additive effect on the known systemic carbonic anhydrase inhibition in patients receiving a systemic carbonic anhydrase inhibitor and Trusopt). Products include:
Daranide Tablets 1950

Methazolamide (Potential for an additive effect on the known systemic effects of carbonic anhydrase inhibition in patients receiving a systemic carbonic anhydrase inhibitor and Trusopt).
No products indexed under this heading.

TRUVADA TABLETS

(Emtricitabine, Tenofovir Disoproxil Fumarate)... 1296
May interact with cationic drugs that are eliminated by renal tubular and certain other agents. Compounds in these categories include:

Acyclovir (Since emtricitabine and tenofovir are primarily eliminated by the kidneys, co-administration of Truvada with drugs that reduce renal function or compete for active tubular secretion, may increase serum concentrations of emtricitabine, tenofovir, and/or other renally eliminated drugs, such as acyclovir).
Products include:
Zovirax 1643
Zovirax Cream 820
Zovirax Ointment 821

Acyclovir Sodium (Since emtricitabine and tenofovir are primarily eliminated by the kidneys, co-administration of Truvada with drugs that reduce renal function or compete for active tubular secretion, may increase serum concentrations of emtricitabine, tenofovir, and/or other renally eliminated drugs, such as acyclovir).
No products indexed under this heading.

Adefovir dipivoxil (Since emtricitabine and tenofovir are primarily eliminated by the kidneys, co-administration of Truvada with drugs that reduce renal function or compete for active tubular secretion, may increase serum concentrations of emtricitabine, tenofovir, and/or other renally eliminated drugs, such as adefovir dipivoxil). Products include:
Hepsera Tablets 1292

Amiloride Hydrochloride (Co-administration of Truvada with drugs that are eliminated by active tubular secretion, may increase concentrations of emtricitabine, tenofovir, and/or the co-administered drug).
Products include:
Midamor Tablets 2026
Moduretic Tablets 2028

Atazanavir (Atazanavir and lopinavir/ritonavir have been shown to increase tenofovir concentrations. Patients receiving atazanavir and lopinavir/ritonavir and Truvada should be monitored for Truvada-associated adverse events. Truvada should be discontinued in patients who develop Truvada-associated adverse events. Tenofovir decreases the AUC and Cmin of atazanavir. When co-administered with Truvada, it is recommended that atazanavir 300 mg is given with ritonavir 100 mg. Atazanavir without ritonavir should not be co-administered with Truvada).
No products indexed under this heading.

Atazanavir sulfate (Atazanavir and lopinavir/ritonavir have been shown to increase tenofovir concentrations. Patients receiving atazanavir and lopinavir/ritonavir and Truvada should be monitored for Truvada-associated adverse events. Truvada should be discontinued in patients who develop Truvada-associated adverse events. Tenofovir decreases the AUC and Cmin of atazanavir. When co-administered with Truvada, it is recommended that atazanavir 300 mg is given with ritonavir 100 mg. Atazanavir without ritonavir should not be co-administered with Truvada). Products include:
Reyataz Capsules 921

Cidofovir (Since emtricitabine and tenofovir are primarily eliminated by the kidneys, co-administration of Truvada with drugs that reduce renal function or compete for active tubular secretion, may increase serum concentrations of emtricitabine, tenofovir, and/or other renally eliminated drugs, such as cidofovir).
No products indexed under this heading.

Didanosine (When tenofovir disoproxil fumarate was administered with didanosine, the Cmax and AUC of didanosine, administered as either the buffered or enteric-coated formulation, increased significantly. Higher didanosine concentrations could potentiate didanosine-associated adverse events. Co-administration of Truvada and didanosine should be undertaken with caution, and patients receiving this combination should be monitored closely for didanosine-associated adverse events. Didanosine should be discontinued in patients who develop didanosine-associated adverse events).
No products indexed under this heading.

Digoxin (Co-administration of Truvada with drugs that are eliminated by active tubular secretion, may increase concentrations of emtricitabine, tenofovir, and/or the co-administered drug). Products include:
Lanoxicaps Capsules 1490
Lanoxin Injection 1494
Lanoxin Injection Pediatric 1497
Lanoxin Tablets 1500

Ganciclovir (Since emtricitabine and tenofovir are primarily eliminated by the kidneys, co-administration of Truvada with drugs that reduce renal function or compete for active tubular secretion, may increase serum concentrations of emtricitabine, tenofovir, and/or other renally eliminated drugs, such as ganciclovir).
No products indexed under this heading.

Ganciclovir Sodium (Since emtricitabine and tenofovir are primarily eliminated by the kidneys, co-administration of Truvada with drugs that reduce renal function or compete for active tubular secretion, may increase serum concentrations of emtricitabine, tenofovir, and/or other renally eliminated drugs, such as ganciclovir).
No products indexed under this heading.

Lamivudine (Due to similarities between emtricitabine and lamivudine, Truvada should not be co-administered with other drugs containing lamivudine). Products include:
Combivir Tablets 1411
Epivir 1427
Epivir-HBV 1432
Epzicom Tablets 1436
Trizivir Tablets 1589

Lopinavir (Atazanavir and lopinavir/ritonavir have been shown to increase tenofovir concentrations. Patients receiving atazanavir and lopinavir/ritonavir and Truvada should be monitored for Truvada-associated adverse events. Truvada should be discontinued in patients who develop Truvada-associated adverse events). Products include:
Kaletra 476

Morphine Sulfate (Co-administration of Truvada with drugs that are eliminated by active tubular secretion, may increase concentrations of emtricitabine, tenofovir, and/or the co-administered drug).
Products include:
Avinza Capsules 1741
Kadian Capsules 577
MS Contin Tablets 2701

Procainamide Hydrochloride (Co-administration of Truvada with drugs that are eliminated by active tubular secretion, may increase concentrations of emtricitabine, tenofovir, and/or the co-administered drug).
No products indexed under this heading.

Quinidine Gluconate (Co-administration of Truvada with drugs that are eliminated by active tubular secretion, may increase concentrations of emtricitabine, tenofovir, and/or the co-administered drug).
No products indexed under this heading.

Quinidine Polygalacturonate (Co-administration of Truvada with drugs that are eliminated by active tubular secretion, may increase concentrations of emtricitabine, tenofovir, and/or the co-administered drug).
No products indexed under this heading.

Quinidine Sulfate (Co-administration of Truvada with drugs that are eliminated by active tubular secretion, may increase concentrations of emtricitabine, tenofovir, and/or the co-administered drug).
No products indexed under this heading.

Quinine Sulfate (Co-administration of Truvada with drugs that are eliminated by active tubular secretion, may increase concentrations of emtricitabine, tenofovir, and/or the co-administered drug).
No products indexed under this heading.

Ranitidine Hydrochloride (Co-administration of Truvada with drugs that are eliminated by active tubular

secretion, may increase concentrations of emtricitabine, tenofovir, and/or the co-administered drug). Products include:
- Zantac 1624
- Zantac Injection 1619
- Zantac Injection Pharmacy Bulk Package 1622

Ritonavir (Coadministration of tenofovir and ritonavir resulted in 23% increase in Cmin). Products include:
- Kaletra 476
- Norvir 503

Saquinavir (Coadministration of tenofovir and saquinavir resulted in a 22% increase in Cmax).
No products indexed under this heading.

Triamterene (Co-administration of Truvada with drugs that are eliminated by active tubular secretion, may increase concentrations of emtricitabine, tenofovir, and/or the co-administered drug). Products include:
- Dyazide Capsules 1423
- Dyrenium Capsules 3400

Trimethoprim (Co-administration of Truvada with drugs that are eliminated by active tubular secretion, may increase concentrations of emtricitabine, tenofovir, and/or the co-administered drug).
No products indexed under this heading.

Trimethoprim Sulfate (Co-administration of Truvada with drugs that are eliminated by active tubular secretion, may increase concentrations of emtricitabine, tenofovir, and/or the co-administered drug). Products include:
- Polytrim Ophthalmic Solution 574

Valacyclovir Hydrochloride (Since emtricitabine and tenofovir are primarily eliminated by the kidneys, co-administration of Truvada with drugs that reduce renal function or compete for active tubular secretion, may increase serum concentrations of emtricitabine, tenofovir, and/or other renally eliminated drugs, such as valacyclovir). Products include:
- Valtrex Caplets 1597

Valganciclovir Hydrochloride (Since emtricitabine and tenofovir are primarily eliminated by the kidneys, co-administration of Truvada with drugs that reduce renal function or compete for active tubular secretion, may increase serum concentrations of emtricitabine, tenofovir, and/or other renally eliminated drugs, such as valganciclovir). Products include:
- Valcyte Tablets 2813

Vancomycin Hydrochloride (Co-administration of Truvada with drugs that are eliminated by active tubular secretion, may increase concentrations of emtricitabine, tenofovir, and/or the co-administered drug). Products include:
- Vancocin HCl Capsules, USP 3380

Zidovudine (Coadministration of 200 mg of emtricitabine and 300 mg of zidovudine over a one week period resulted in a 17% increase in Cmax and a 13% increase in AUC). Products include:
- Combivir Tablets 1411
- Retrovir 1560
- Retrovir IV Infusion 1564
- Trizivir Tablets 1589

TUMS E-X ANTACID/ CALCIUM TABLETS

(Calcium Carbonate) 664
See Tums Regular Antacid/Calcium Tablets

TUMS E-X SUGAR FREE ANTACID/CALCIUM TABLETS

(Calcium Carbonate) 664
See Tums Regular Antacid/Calcium Tablets

TUMS REGULAR ANTACID/ CALCIUM TABLETS

(Calcium Carbonate) 664
May interact with:

Prescription Drugs, unspecified (Antacids may interact with certain unspecified prescription drugs).
No products indexed under this heading.

TUMS ULTRA ANTACID/ CALCIUM TABLETS

(Calcium Carbonate) 664
See Tums Regular Antacid/Calcium Tablets

TUSSIONEX PENNKINETIC EXTENDED-RELEASE SUSPENSION

(Chlorpheniramine Polistirex, Hydrocodone Polistirex) 3327
May interact with anticholinergics, antihistamines, central nervous system depressants, monoamine oxidase inhibitors, tricyclic antidepressants, and certain other agents. Compounds in these categories include:

Acrivastine (Combined therapy may result in additive CNS depression).
No products indexed under this heading.

Alfentanil Hydrochloride (Combined therapy may result in additive CNS depression).
No products indexed under this heading.

Alprazolam (Combined therapy may result in additive CNS depression). Products include:
- Niravam Orally Disintegrating Tablets 3092

Amitriptyline Hydrochloride (Co-administration of hydrocodone with MAO inhibitors may increase the effect of tricyclic antidepressant or hydrocodone).
No products indexed under this heading.

Amoxapine (Co-administration of hydrocodone with MAO inhibitors may increase the effect of tricyclic antidepressant or hydrocodone).
No products indexed under this heading.

Aprobarbital (Combined therapy may result in additive CNS depression).
No products indexed under this heading.

Astemizole (Combined therapy may result in additive CNS depression).
No products indexed under this heading.

Atropine Sulfate (Concurrent use of other anticholinergic agents with hydrocodone may produce paralytic ileus). Products include:
- Donnatal Extentabs 2493

Azatadine Maleate (Combined therapy may result in additive CNS depression).
No products indexed under this heading.

Belladonna Alkaloids (Concurrent use of other anticholinergic agents with hydrocodone may produce paralytic ileus). Products include:
- Hyland's Teething Tablets 830

Benztropine Mesylate (Concurrent use of other anticholinergic agents with hydrocodone may produce paralytic ileus).
No products indexed under this heading.

Biperiden Hydrochloride (Concurrent use of other anticholinergic agents with hydrocodone may produce paralytic ileus).
No products indexed under this heading.

Bromodiphenhydramine Hydrochloride (Combined therapy may result in additive CNS depression).
No products indexed under this heading.

Brompheniramine Maleate (Combined therapy may result in additive CNS depression). Products include:
- Children's Dimetapp Cold & Allergy Elixir 730
- Children's Dimetapp Cold & Allergy Chewable Tablets 730
- Children's Dimetapp DM Cold & Cough Elixir 731

Buprenorphine Hydrochloride (Combined therapy may result in additive CNS depression). Products include:
- Buprenex Injectable 2716
- Suboxone Tablets 2717
- Subutex Tablets 2717

Buspirone Hydrochloride (Combined therapy may result in additive CNS depression).
No products indexed under this heading.

Butabarbital (Combined therapy may result in additive CNS depression).
No products indexed under this heading.

Butalbital (Combined therapy may result in additive CNS depression).
No products indexed under this heading.

Cetirizine Hydrochloride (Combined therapy may result in additive CNS depression). Products include:
- Zyrtec Chewable Tablets 2594
- Zyrtec 2594
- Zyrtec-D 12 Hour Extended Release Tablets 2597

Chlordiazepoxide (Combined therapy may result in additive CNS depression).
No products indexed under this heading.

Chlordiazepoxide Hydrochloride (Combined therapy may result in additive CNS depression). Products include:
- Librium Capsules 3347

Chlorpheniramine Maleate (Combined therapy may result in additive CNS depression). Products include:
- Advil Allergy Sinus Caplets 770
- Advil Multi-Symptom Cold Caplets 770
- BC Allergy Sinus Cold Powder 677
- Comtrex Maximum Strength Cold & Cough Day/Night Caplets - Night Formulation 726
- Comtrex Maximum Strength Day/Night Severe Cold & Sinus Caplets - Night Formulation 725
- Contac Cold and Flu Maximum Strength Caplets 728
- Contac Cold and Flu Day and Night Caplets (Night Formulation Only) 727
- Children's Dimetapp Long Acting Cough Plus Cold Syrup 731
- Robitussin Cough & Cold Long-Acting Liquid 735
- Robitussin Cough & Allergy Syrup 736
- Robitussin Cough & Cold Nighttime Liquid 736
- Robitussin Cough, Cold & Flu Nighttime Liquid 738
- Robitussin Pediatric Cough & Cold Long-Acting Liquid 735
- Robitussin Pediatric Cough & Cold Nighttime Liquid 736
- Triaminic Cold & Allergy Liquid 746
- Triaminic Cough & Runny Nose Softchews 748
- Children's Tylenol Plus Flu Oral Suspension 749
- Tylenol Allergy Multi-Symptom Caplets with Cool Burst and Gelcaps 1872
- Children's Tylenol Plus Cold Suspension Liquid 1879
- Children's Tylenol Plus Cough & Runny Nose Suspension Liquid 1879
- Children's Tylenol Plus Flu Suspension Liquid 1881
- Children's Tylenol Plus Multi-Symptom Cold Suspension Liquid 1879
- Tylenol Cold Head Congestion Nighttime Caplets with Cool Burst 1873
- Tylenol Cold Multi-Symptom Nighttime Caplets with Cool Burst 1874
- Tylenol Sinus Congestion & Pain Nighttime Caplets with Cool Burst 1876
- Vicks 44M Cough, Cold & Flu Relief Liquid 2680
- Pediatric Vicks 44m Cough & Cold Relief Liquid 2676
- Children's Vicks NyQuil Cold/Cough Relief 756
- Children's Vicks NyQuil Cold/Cough Relief Liquid 2680
- Zicam Maximum Strength Flu Daytime 768

Chlorpheniramine Tannate (Combined therapy may result in additive CNS depression).
No products indexed under this heading.

Chlorpromazine (Combined therapy may result in additive CNS depression).
No products indexed under this heading.

Chlorpromazine Hydrochloride (Combined therapy may result in additive CNS depression).
No products indexed under this heading.

Chlorprothixene (Combined therapy may result in additive CNS depression).
No products indexed under this heading.

Chlorprothixene Hydrochloride (Combined therapy may result in additive CNS depression).
No products indexed under this heading.

Chlorprothixene Lactate (Combined therapy may result in additive CNS depression).
No products indexed under this heading.

Clemastine Fumarate (Combined therapy may result in additive CNS depression).
No products indexed under this heading.

Clidinium Bromide (Concurrent use of other anticholinergic agents with hydrocodone may produce paralytic ileus).

No products indexed under this heading.

Clomipramine Hydrochloride (Co-administration of hydrocodone with MAO inhibitors may increase the effect of tricyclic antidepressant or hydrocodone).

No products indexed under this heading.

Clorazepate Dipotassium (Combined therapy may result in additive CNS depression). Products include:

Tranxene 2474

Clozapine (Combined therapy may result in additive CNS depression). Products include:

Clozaril Tablets 2184
FazaClo Orally Disintegrating Tablets 551

Codeine Phosphate (Combined therapy may result in additive CNS depression). Products include:

Tylenol with Codeine Tablets 2391

Cyproheptadine Hydrochloride (Combined therapy may result in additive CNS depression).

No products indexed under this heading.

Desflurane (Combined therapy may result in additive CNS depression).

No products indexed under this heading.

Desipramine Hydrochloride (Co-administration of hydrocodone with MAO inhibitors may increase the effect of tricyclic antidepressant or hydrocodone).

No products indexed under this heading.

Dexchlorpheniramine Maleate (Combined therapy may result in additive CNS depression).

No products indexed under this heading.

Dezocine (Combined therapy may result in additive CNS depression).

No products indexed under this heading.

Diazepam (Combined therapy may result in additive CNS depression). Products include:

Diastat Rectal Delivery System 3343
Valium Tablets 2819

Dicyclomine Hydrochloride (Concurrent use of other anticholinergic agents with hydrocodone may produce paralytic ileus). Products include:

Bentyl Capsules 697
Bentyl Injection 697
Bentyl Syrup 697
Bentyl Tablets 697

Diphenhydramine Citrate (Combined therapy may result in additive CNS depression). Products include:

Advil PM Caplets ▪□615
Excedrin PM Caplets/Tablets/Geltabs ▪□610
Goody's PM Powder for Pain with Sleeplessness ▪□612

Diphenhydramine Hydrochloride (Combined therapy may result in additive CNS depression). Products include:

Nytol QuickCaps Caplets ▪□615
Nytol QuickGels Softgels Maximum Strength ▪□616
Simply Sleep Caplets 1868
Sominex Original Formula Tablets .. ▪□616
TheraFlu Warming Relief Nighttime Severe Cold ▪□743
TheraFlu Thin Strips Multi Symptom ▪□744

Triaminic Nighttime Cold & Cough Liquid ▪□746
Triaminic Thin Strips Cough & Runny Nose ▪□749
Extra Strength Tylenol PM Caplets, Vanilla Caplets, Geltabs, Gelcaps and Liquid......... 1875
Tylenol Sore Throat Nighttime Liquid with Cool Burst ▪□790
Tylenol Allergy Multi-Symptom Nighttime Caplets with Cool Burst 1872
Tylenol Severe Allergy Caplets 1872
Children's Tylenol Plus Cold & Allergy Suspension Liquid 1878

Diphenylpyraline Hydrochloride (Combined therapy may result in additive CNS depression).

No products indexed under this heading.

Doxepin Hydrochloride (Co-administration of hydrocodone with MAO inhibitors may increase the effect of tricyclic antidepressant or hydrocodone).

No products indexed under this heading.

Droperidol (Combined therapy may result in additive CNS depression).

No products indexed under this heading.

Enflurane (Combined therapy may result in additive CNS depression).

No products indexed under this heading.

Estazolam (Combined therapy may result in additive CNS depression). Products include:

ProSom Tablets 517

Ethanol (Combined therapy may result in additive CNS depression).

No products indexed under this heading.

Ethchlorvynol (Combined therapy may result in additive CNS depression).

No products indexed under this heading.

Ethinamate (Combined therapy may result in additive CNS depression).

No products indexed under this heading.

Ethyl Alcohol (Combined therapy may result in additive CNS depression).

No products indexed under this heading.

Fentanyl (Combined therapy may result in additive CNS depression). Products include:

Duragesic Transdermal System 2373
Ionsys Transdermal System 2379

Fentanyl Citrate (Combined therapy may result in additive CNS depression). Products include:

Actiq 979

Fexofenadine Hydrochloride (Combined therapy may result in additive CNS depression). Products include:

Allegra 2844
Allegra-D 12 Hour Extended-Release Tablets 2846
Allegra-D 24 Hour Extended-Release Tablets 2849

Fluphenazine Decanoate (Combined therapy may result in additive CNS depression).

No products indexed under this heading.

Fluphenazine Enanthate (Combined therapy may result in additive CNS depression).

No products indexed under this heading.

Fluphenazine Hydrochloride (Combined therapy may result in additive CNS depression).

No products indexed under this heading.

Flurazepam Hydrochloride (Combined therapy may result in additive CNS depression). Products include:

Dalmane Capsules 3342

Glutethimide (Combined therapy may result in additive CNS depression).

No products indexed under this heading.

Glycopyrrolate (Concurrent use of other anticholinergic agents with hydrocodone may produce paralytic ileus).

No products indexed under this heading.

Haloperidol (Combined therapy may result in additive CNS depression).

No products indexed under this heading.

Haloperidol Decanoate (Combined therapy may result in additive CNS depression).

No products indexed under this heading.

Hydrocodone Bitartrate (Combined therapy may result in additive CNS depression). Products include:

Hycodan 1116
Hycotuss Expectorant Syrup 1117
Vicodin Tablets 535
Vicodin ES Tablets 536
Vicodin HP Tablets 538
Vicoprofen Tablets 539
Zydone Tablets 1139

Hydromorphone Hydrochloride (Combined therapy may result in additive CNS depression). Products include:

Dilaudid 440
Dilaudid Non-Sterile Powder 440
Dilaudid Oral Liquid 445
Dilaudid Rectal Suppositories 440
Dilaudid Tablets 440
Dilaudid Tablets - 8 mg 445
Dilaudid-HP 442

Hydroxyzine Hydrochloride (Combined therapy may result in additive CNS depression).

No products indexed under this heading.

Hyoscyamine (Concurrent use of other anticholinergic agents with hydrocodone may produce paralytic ileus).

No products indexed under this heading.

Hyoscyamine Sulfate (Concurrent use of other anticholinergic agents with hydrocodone may produce paralytic ileus). Products include:

Donnatal Extentabs 2493
Prosed/DS Tablets 1157

Imipramine Hydrochloride (Co-administration of hydrocodone with MAO inhibitors may increase the effect of tricyclic antidepressant or hydrocodone).

No products indexed under this heading.

Imipramine Pamoate (Co-administration of hydrocodone with MAO inhibitors may increase the effect of tricyclic antidepressant or hydrocodone).

No products indexed under this heading.

Ipratropium Bromide (Concurrent use of other anticholinergic agents with hydrocodone may produce paralytic ileus). Products include:

Atrovent Inhalation Solution 835
Atrovent HFA Inhalation Aerosol 841
Atrovent Nasal Spray 0.03% 837
Atrovent Nasal Spray 0.06% 839
Combivent Inhalation Aerosol 847
DuoNeb Inhalation Solution 1058

Isocarboxazid (Co-administration of hydrocodone with MAO inhibitors may increase the effect of MAOI or hydrocodone).

No products indexed under this heading.

Isoflurane (Combined therapy may result in additive CNS depression).

No products indexed under this heading.

Ketamine Hydrochloride (Combined therapy may result in additive CNS depression).

No products indexed under this heading.

Levomethadyl Acetate Hydrochloride (Combined therapy may result in additive CNS depression).

No products indexed under this heading.

Levorphanol Tartrate (Combined therapy may result in additive CNS depression).

No products indexed under this heading.

Loratadine (Combined therapy may result in additive CNS depression). Products include:

Alavert Allergy & Sinus D-12 Hour Tablets ▪□771
Alavert ▪□771
Children's Claritin Allergy Oral Solution ▪□771
Claritin Non-Drowsy 24 Hour Tablets ▪□772
Claritin Reditabs 24 Hour Non-Drowsy Tablets ▪□772
Claritin-D Non-Drowsy 12 Hour Tablets ▪□772
Claritin-D Non-Drowsy 24 Hour Tablets ▪□772

Lorazepam (Combined therapy may result in additive CNS depression).

No products indexed under this heading.

Loxapine Hydrochloride (Combined therapy may result in additive CNS depression).

No products indexed under this heading.

Loxapine Succinate (Combined therapy may result in additive CNS depression).

No products indexed under this heading.

Maprotiline Hydrochloride (Co-administration of hydrocodone with MAO inhibitors may increase the effect of tricyclic antidepressant or hydrocodone).

No products indexed under this heading.

Mepenzolate Bromide (Concurrent use of other anticholinergic agents with hydrocodone may produce paralytic ileus).

No products indexed under this heading.

Meperidine Hydrochloride (Combined therapy may result in additive CNS depression).

No products indexed under this heading.

Mephobarbital (Combined therapy may result in additive CNS depression).

No products indexed under this heading.

Meprobamate (Combined therapy may result in additive CNS depression).
　No products indexed under this heading.

Mesoridazine Besylate (Combined therapy may result in additive CNS depression).
　No products indexed under this heading.

Methadone Hydrochloride (Combined therapy may result in additive CNS depression).
　No products indexed under this heading.

Methdilazine Hydrochloride (Combined therapy may result in additive CNS depression).
　No products indexed under this heading.

Methohexital Sodium (Combined therapy may result in additive CNS depression).
　No products indexed under this heading.

Methotrimeprazine (Combined therapy may result in additive CNS depression).
　No products indexed under this heading.

Methoxyflurane (Combined therapy may result in additive CNS depression).
　No products indexed under this heading.

Midazolam Hydrochloride (Combined therapy may result in additive CNS depression).
　No products indexed under this heading.

Moclobemide (Co-administration of hydrocodone with MAO inhibitors may increase the effect of MAOI or hydrocodone).
　No products indexed under this heading.

Molindone Hydrochloride (Combined therapy may result in additive CNS depression). Products include:
　Moban Tablets 1119

Morphine Sulfate (Combined therapy may result in additive CNS depression). Products include:
　Avinza Capsules 1741
　Kadian Capsules 577
　MS Contin Tablets 2701

Nortriptyline Hydrochloride (Co-administration of hydrocodone with MAO inhibitors may increase the effect of tricyclic antidepressant or hydrocodone).
　No products indexed under this heading.

Olanzapine (Combined therapy may result in additive CNS depression). Products include:
　Symbyax Capsules 1819
　Zyprexa Tablets 1830
　Zyprexa IntraMuscular 1830
　Zyprexa ZYDIS Orally
　　Disintegrating Tablets................... 1830

Oxazepam (Combined therapy may result in additive CNS depression).
　No products indexed under this heading.

Oxybutynin Chloride (Concurrent use of other anticholinergic agents with hydrocodone may produce paralytic ileus). Products include:
　Ditropan XL Extended-Release
　　Tablets... 2413

Oxycodone Hydrochloride (Combined therapy may result in additive CNS depression). Products include:
　OxyContin Tablets 2703

OxyFast Oral Concentrate
　Solution...................................... 2708
OxyIR Capsules 2708
Percocet Tablets 1131
Percodan Tablets 1132

Pargyline Hydrochloride (Co-administration of hydrocodone with MAO inhibitors may increase the effect of MAOI or hydrocodone).
　No products indexed under this heading.

Pentobarbital Sodium (Combined therapy may result in additive CNS depression). Products include:
　Nembutal Sodium Solution, USP 2470

Perphenazine (Combined therapy may result in additive CNS depression).
　No products indexed under this heading.

Phenelzine Sulfate (Co-administration of hydrocodone with MAO inhibitors may increase the effect of MAOI or hydrocodone).
　No products indexed under this heading.

Phenobarbital (Combined therapy may result in additive CNS depression). Products include:
　Donnatal Extentabs 2493

Prazepam (Combined therapy may result in additive CNS depression).
　No products indexed under this heading.

Procarbazine Hydrochloride (Co-administration of hydrocodone with MAO inhibitors may increase the effect of MAOI or hydrocodone). Products include:
　Matulane Capsules 3191

Prochlorperazine (Combined therapy may result in additive CNS depression).
　No products indexed under this heading.

Procyclidine Hydrochloride (Concurrent use of other anticholinergic agents with hydrocodone may produce paralytic ileus).
　No products indexed under this heading.

Promethazine Hydrochloride (Combined therapy may result in additive CNS depression). Products include:
　Phenergan Tablets and
　　Suppositories.............................. 3440

Propantheline Bromide (Concurrent use of other anticholinergic agents with hydrocodone may produce paralytic ileus).
　No products indexed under this heading.

Propofol (Combined therapy may result in additive CNS depression).
　No products indexed under this heading.

Propoxyphene Hydrochloride (Combined therapy may result in additive CNS depression).
　No products indexed under this heading.

Propoxyphene Napsylate (Combined therapy may result in additive CNS depression).
　No products indexed under this heading.

Protriptyline Hydrochloride (Co-administration of hydrocodone with MAO inhibitors may increase the effect of tricyclic antidepressant or hydrocodone).
　No products indexed under this heading.

Pyrilamine Maleate (Combined therapy may result in additive CNS depression).
　No products indexed under this heading.

Pyrilamine Tannate (Combined therapy may result in additive CNS depression).
　No products indexed under this heading.

Quazepam (Combined therapy may result in additive CNS depression).
　No products indexed under this heading.

Quetiapine Fumarate (Combined therapy may result in additive CNS depression). Products include:
　Seroquel Tablets 690

Remifentanil Hydrochloride (Combined therapy may result in additive CNS depression).
　No products indexed under this heading.

Risperidone (Combined therapy may result in additive CNS depression). Products include:
　Risperdal .. 1676
　Risperdal Consta Long-Acting
　　Injection 1682
　Risperdal M-Tab Orally
　　Disintegrating Tablets.................. 1676

Scopolamine (Concurrent use of other anticholinergic agents with hydrocodone may produce paralytic ileus). Products include:
　Transderm Scōp Transdermal
　　Therapeutic System 2177

Scopolamine Hydrobromide (Concurrent use of other anticholinergic agents with hydrocodone may produce paralytic ileus). Products include:
　Donnatal Extentabs 2493

Secobarbital Sodium (Combined therapy may result in additive CNS depression).
　No products indexed under this heading.

Selegiline Hydrochloride (Co-administration of hydrocodone with MAO inhibitors may increase the effect of MAOI or hydrocodone). Products include:
　Eldepryl Capsules 3208
　Zelapar Tablets 3372

Sevoflurane (Combined therapy may result in additive CNS depression). Products include:
　Ultane Liquid for Inhalation 531

Sodium Oxybate (Combined therapy may result in additive CNS depression). Products include:
　Xyrem Oral Solution 1688

Sufentanil Citrate (Combined therapy may result in additive CNS depression).
　No products indexed under this heading.

Temazepam (Combined therapy may result in additive CNS depression). Products include:
　Restoril Capsules 1860

Terfenadine (Combined therapy may result in additive CNS depression).
　No products indexed under this heading.

Thiamylal Sodium (Combined therapy may result in additive CNS depression).
　No products indexed under this heading.

Thioridazine Hydrochloride (Combined therapy may result in additive CNS depression). Products include:

Thioridazine Hydrochloride
　Tablets ... 2163

Thiothixene (Combined therapy may result in additive CNS depression). Products include:
　Thiothixene Capsules 2165

Tolterodine Tartrate (Concurrent use of other anticholinergic agents with hydrocodone may produce paralytic ileus). Products include:
　Detrol Tablets 2628
　Detrol LA Capsules 2631

Tranylcypromine Sulfate (Co-administration of hydrocodone with MAO inhibitors may increase the effect of MAOI or hydrocodone). Products include:
　Parnate Tablets 1527

Triazolam (Combined therapy may result in additive CNS depression).
　No products indexed under this heading.

Tridihexethyl Chloride (Concurrent use of other anticholinergic agents with hydrocodone may produce paralytic ileus).
　No products indexed under this heading.

Trifluoperazine Hydrochloride (Combined therapy may result in additive CNS depression).
　No products indexed under this heading.

Trihexyphenidyl Hydrochloride (Concurrent use of other anticholinergic agents with hydrocodone may produce paralytic ileus).
　No products indexed under this heading.

Trimeprazine Tartrate (Combined therapy may result in additive CNS depression).
　No products indexed under this heading.

Trimipramine Maleate (Co-administration of hydrocodone with MAO inhibitors may increase the effect of tricyclic antidepressant or hydrocodone).
　No products indexed under this heading.

Tripelennamine Hydrochloride (Combined therapy may result in additive CNS depression).
　No products indexed under this heading.

Triprolidine Hydrochloride (Combined therapy may result in additive CNS depression).
　No products indexed under this heading.

Zaleplon (Combined therapy may result in additive CNS depression). Products include:
　Sonata Capsules 1717

Ziprasidone Hydrochloride (Combined therapy may result in additive CNS depression). Products include:
　Geodon Capsules 2529

Zolpidem Tartrate (Combined therapy may result in additive CNS depression). Products include:
　Ambien Tablets 2851
　Ambien CR Tablets 2855

Food Interactions

Alcohol (Combined use may result in additive CNS depression).

TWINJECT 0.3
(Epinephrine) 3378
See Twinject 0.15

IMPORTANT NOTE: Always consult each drug listing in the patient's regimen for possible interactions.

TWINJECT 0.15
(Epinephrine) 3379
May interact with alpha adrenergic blockers, beta blockers, diuretics, ergot-containing drugs, cardiac glycosides, monoamine oxidase inhibitors, phenothiazines, tricyclic antidepressants, and certain other agents. Compounds in these categories include:

Acebutolol Hydrochloride (The cardiostimulating and bronchodilating effects of epinephrine are antagonized by beta-adrenergic blocking drugs).
No products indexed under this heading.

Amiloride Hydrochloride (Patients who receive epinephrine while concomitantly taking diuretics should be observed carefully for the development of cardiac arrhythmias). Products include:
Midamor Tablets 2026
Moduretic Tablets 2028

Amitriptyline Hydrochloride (The effects of epinephrine may be potentiated by tricyclic antidepressants).
No products indexed under this heading.

Amoxapine (The effects of epinephrine may be potentiated by tricyclic antidepressants).
No products indexed under this heading.

Atenolol (The cardiostimulating and bronchodilating effects of epinephrine are antagonized by beta-adrenergic blocking drugs).
No products indexed under this heading.

Bendroflumethiazide (Patients who receive epinephrine while concomitantly taking diuretics should be observed carefully for the development of cardiac arrhythmias).
No products indexed under this heading.

Betaxolol Hydrochloride (The cardiostimulating and bronchodilating effects of epinephrine are antagonized by beta-adrenergic blocking drugs). Products include:
Betoptic S Ophthalmic Suspension 558

Bisoprolol Fumarate (The cardiostimulating and bronchodilating effects of epinephrine are antagonized by beta-adrenergic blocking drugs).
No products indexed under this heading.

Bumetanide (Patients who receive epinephrine while concomitantly taking diuretics should be observed carefully for the development of cardiac arrhythmias). Products include:
Bumex Tablets 2746

Carteolol Hydrochloride (The cardiostimulating and bronchodilating effects of epinephrine are antagonized by beta-adrenergic blocking drugs). Products include:
Carteolol Hydrochloride Ophthalmic Solution USP, 1% .... ⊙249

Chlorothiazide (Patients who receive epinephrine while concomitantly taking diuretics should be observed carefully for the development of cardiac arrhythmias). Products include:
Diuril Oral Suspension 1954

Chlorothiazide Sodium (Patients who receive epinephrine while concomitantly taking diuretics should be observed carefully for the development of cardiac arrhythmias). Products include:
Diuril Sodium Intravenous 2467

Chlorpheniramine (The effects of epinephrine may be potentiated by certain antihistamines, notably chlorpheniramine).
No products indexed under this heading.

Chlorpheniramine Maleate (The effects of epinephrine may be potentiated by certain antihistamines, notably chlorpheniramine). Products include:
Advil Allergy Sinus Caplets .... ▣770
Advil Multi-Symptom Cold Caplets .... ▣770
BC Allergy Sinus Cold Powder .... ▣677
Comtrex Maximum Strength Cold & Cough Day/Night Caplets - Night Formulation .... ▣726
Comtrex Maximum Strength Day/Night Severe Cold & Sinus Caplets - Night Formulation .... ▣725
Contac Cold and Flu Maximum Strength Caplets .... ▣728
Contac Cold and Flu Day and Night Caplets (Night Formulation Only) .... ▣727
Children's Dimetapp Long Acting Cough Plus Cold Syrup .... ▣731
Robitussin Cough & Cold Long-Acting Liquid .... ▣735
Robitussin Cough & Allergy Syrup .. ▣736
Robitussin Cough & Cold Nighttime Liquid .... ▣736
Robitussin Cough, Cold & Flu Nighttime Liquid .... ▣738
Robitussin Pediatric Cough & Cold Long-Acting Liquid .... ▣735
Robitussin Pediatric Cough & Cold Nighttime Liquid .... ▣736
Triaminic Cold & Allergy Liquid .... ▣746
Triaminic Cough & Runny Nose Softchews .... ▣748
Children's Tylenol Plus Flu Oral Suspension .... ▣749
Tylenol Allergy Multi-Symptom Caplets with Cool Burst and Gelcaps 1872
Children's Tylenol Plus Cold Suspension Liquid 1879
Children's Tylenol Plus Cough & Runny Nose Suspension Liquid 1879
Children's Tylenol Plus Flu Suspension Liquid 1881
Children's Tylenol Plus Multi-Symptom Cold Suspension Liquid 1879
Tylenol Cold Head Congestion Nighttime Caplets with Cool Burst 1873
Tylenol Cold Multi-Symptom Nighttime Caplets with Cool Burst 1874
Tylenol Sinus Congestion & Pain Nighttime Caplets with Cool Burst 1876
Vicks 44M Cough, Cold & Flu Relief Liquid 2680
Pediatric Vicks 44m Cough & Cold Relief Liquid 2676
Children's Vicks NyQuil Cold/Cough Relief .... ▣756
Children's Vicks NyQuil Cold/Cough Relief Liquid 2680
Zicam Maximum Strength Flu Daytime .... ▣768

Chlorpheniramine Polistirex (The effects of epinephrine may be potentiated by certain antihistamines, notably chlorpheniramine). Products include:
Tussionex Pennkinetic Extended-Release Suspension 3327

Chlorpheniramine Preparations (The effects of epinephrine may be potentiated by certain antihistamines, notably chlorpheniramine).
No products indexed under this heading.

Chlorpheniramine Tannate (The effects of epinephrine may be potentiated by certain antihistamines, notably chlorpheniramine).
No products indexed under this heading.

Chlorpromazine (Phenothiazines may reverse the pressor effects of epinephrine).
No products indexed under this heading.

Chlorpromazine Hydrochloride (Phenothiazines may reverse the pressor effects of epinephrine).
No products indexed under this heading.

Chlorthalidone (Patients who receive epinephrine while concomitantly taking diuretics should be observed carefully for the development of cardiac arrhythmias). Products include:
Clorpres Tablets 2153

Clomipramine Hydrochloride (The effects of epinephrine may be potentiated by tricyclic antidepressants).
No products indexed under this heading.

Desipramine Hydrochloride (The effects of epinephrine may be potentiated by tricyclic antidepressants).
No products indexed under this heading.

Deslanoside (Patients who receive epinephrine while concomitantly takng cardiac glycosides should be observed carefully for the development of cardiac arrhythmias).
No products indexed under this heading.

Digitalis Glycoside Preparations (Patients who receive epinephrine while concomitantly takng cardiac glycosides should be observed carefully for the development of cardiac arrhythmias).
No products indexed under this heading.

Digitoxin (Patients who receive epinephrine while concomitantly takng cardiac glycosides should be observed carefully for the development of cardiac arrhythmias).
No products indexed under this heading.

Digoxin (Patients who receive epinephrine while concomitantly takng cardiac glycosides should be observed carefully for the development of cardiac arrhythmias). Products include:
Lanoxicaps Capsules 1490
Lanoxin Injection 1494
Lanoxin Injection Pediatric 1497
Lanoxin Tablets 1500

Dihydroergotamine Mesylate (Ergot alkaloids may reverse the pressor effects of epinephrine). Products include:
Migranal Nasal Spray 3348

Diphenhydramine (The effects of epinephrine may be potentiated by certain antihistamines, notably diphenhydramine). Products include:
Tylenol Sore Throat Nighttime Liquid with Cool Burst 1877

Diphenhydramine Citrate (The effects of epinephrine may be potentiated by certain antihistamines, notably diphenhydramine). Products include:
Advil PM Caplets .... ▣615
Excedrin PM Caplets/Tablets/Geltabs .... ▣610
Goody's PM Powder for Pain with Sleeplessness .... ▣612

Diphenhydramine Hydrochloride (The effects of epinephrine may be potentiated by certain antihistamines, notably diphenhydramine). Products include:
Nytol QuickCaps Caplets .... ▣615
Nytol QuickGels Softgels Maximum Strength .... ▣616
Simply Sleep Caplets 1868
Sominex Original Formula Tablets .. ▣616
TheraFlu Warming Relief Nighttime Severe Cold .... ▣743
TheraFlu Thin Strips Multi Symptom .... ▣744
Triaminic Nighttime Cold & Cough Liquid .... ▣746
Triaminic Thin Strips Cough & Runny Nose .... ▣749
Extra Strength Tylenol PM Caplets, Vanilla Caplets, Geltabs, Gelcaps and Liquid 1875
Tylenol Sore Throat Nighttime Liquid with Cool Burst .... ▣790
Tylenol Allergy Multi-Symptom Nighttime Caplets with Cool Burst 1872
Tylenol Severe Allergy Caplets 1872
Children's Tylenol Plus Cold & Allergy Suspension Liquid 1878

Doxazosin Mesylate (The vasoconstricting and hypertensive effects of epinephrine are antagonized by alpha-adrenergic blocking drugs). Products include:
Cardura XL Tablets 2515

Doxepin Hydrochloride (The effects of epinephrine may be potentiated by tricyclic antidepressants).
No products indexed under this heading.

Ergonovine Maleate (Ergot alkaloids may reverse the pressor effects of epinephrine).
No products indexed under this heading.

Ergotamine Tartrate (Ergot alkaloids may reverse the pressor effects of epinephrine).
No products indexed under this heading.

Esmolol Hydrochloride (The cardiostimulating and bronchodilating effects of epinephrine are antagonized by beta-adrenergic blocking drugs).
No products indexed under this heading.

Ethacrynic Acid (Patients who receive epinephrine while concomitantly taking diuretics should be observed carefully for the development of cardiac arrhythmias). Products include:
Edecrin Tablets 1959

Fluphenazine Decanoate (Phenothiazines may reverse the pressor effects of epinephrine).
No products indexed under this heading.

Fluphenazine Enanthate (Phenothiazines may reverse the pressor effects of epinephrine).
No products indexed under this heading.

Fluphenazine Hydrochloride (Phenothiazines may reverse the pressor effects of epinephrine).
No products indexed under this heading.

Furosemide (Patients who receive epinephrine while concomitantly taking diuretics should be observed carefully for the development of cardiac arrhythmias). Products include:
Furosemide Tablets 2154

Hydrochlorothiazide (Patients who receive epinepherine while concomitantly taking diuretics should be observed carefully for the development of cardiac arrhythmias). Products include:

- Aldoril Tablets 1910
- Atacand HCT 651
- Avalide Tablets 888
- Avalide Tablets 2874
- Benicar HCT Tablets 1044
- Diovan HCT Tablets 2196
- Dyazide Capsules 1423
- Hyzaar 50-12.5 Tablets 1990
- Hyzaar 100-12.5 Tablets 1990
- Hyzaar 100-25 Tablets 1990
- Lopressor HCT 50/25 Tablets 2241
- Lopressor HCT 100/25 Tablets 2241
- Lopressor HCT 100/50 Tablets 2241
- Lotensin HCT Tablets 2246
- Micardis HCT Tablets 856
- Moduretic Tablets 2028
- Prinzide Tablets 2056
- Teveten HCT Tablets 1737
- Timolide Tablets 2086
- Uniretic Tablets 3100

Hydroflumethiazide (Patients who receive epinepherine while concomitantly taking diuretics should be observed carefully for the development of cardiac arrhythmias).

No products indexed under this heading.

Imipramine Hydrochloride (The effects of epinepherine may be potentiated by tricyclic antidepressants).

No products indexed under this heading.

Imipramine Pamoate (The effects of epinepherine may be potentiated by tricyclic antidepressants).

No products indexed under this heading.

Indapamide (Patients who receive epinepherine while concomitantly taking diuretics should be observed carefully for the development of cardiac arrhythmias). Products include:

- Indapamide Tablets 2156

Isocarboxazid (The effects of epinepherine may be potentiated by monoamine oxidase inhibitors).

No products indexed under this heading.

Labetalol Hydrochloride (The cardiostimulating and bronchodilating effects of epinepherine are antagonized by beta-adrenergic blocking drugs).

No products indexed under this heading.

Levobunolol Hydrochloride (The cardiostimulating and bronchodilating effects of epinepherine are antagonized by beta-adrenergic blocking drugs). Products include:

- Betagan Ophthalmic Solution, USP .... ⊙ 220

Levothyroxine Sodium (The effects of epinepherine may be potentiated by certain sodium levothyroxine). Products include:

- Levothroid Tablets 1186
- Levoxyl Tablets 1712
- Synthroid Tablets 520
- Westhroid Tablets 3403

Maprotiline Hydrochloride (The effects of epinepherine may be potentiated by tricyclic antidepressants).

No products indexed under this heading.

Mesoridazine Besylate (Phenothiazines may reverse the pressor effects of epinepherine).

No products indexed under this heading.

Methotrimeprazine (Phenothiazines may reverse the pressor effects of epinepherine).

No products indexed under this heading.

Methyclothiazide (Patients who receive epinepherine while concomitantly taking diuretics should be observed carefully for the development of cardiac arrhythmias).

No products indexed under this heading.

Methylergonovine Maleate (Ergot alkaloids may reverse the pressor effects of epinepherine).

No products indexed under this heading.

Methysergide Maleate (Ergot alkaloids may reverse the pressor effects of epinepherine).

No products indexed under this heading.

Metipranolol Hydrochloride (The cardiostimulating and bronchodilating effects of epinepherine are antagonized by beta-adrenergic blocking drugs).

No products indexed under this heading.

Metolazone (Patients who receive epinepherine while concomitantly taking diuretics should be observed carefully for the development of cardiac arrhythmias).

No products indexed under this heading.

Metoprolol Succinate (The cardiostimulating and bronchodilating effects of epinepherine are antagonized by beta-adrenergic blocking drugs). Products include:

- Toprol-XL Tablets 668

Metoprolol Tartrate (The cardiostimulating and bronchodilating effects of epinepherine are antagonized by beta-adrenergic blocking drugs). Products include:

- Lopressor Injection 2238
- Lopressor Tablets 2238
- Lopressor HCT 50/25 Tablets 2241
- Lopressor HCT 100/25 Tablets 2241
- Lopressor HCT 100/50 Tablets 2241

Moclobemide (The effects of epinepherine may be potentiated by monoamine oxidase inhibitors).

No products indexed under this heading.

Nadolol (The cardiostimulating and bronchodilating effects of epinepherine are antagonized by beta-adrenergic blocking drugs). Products include:

- Nadolol Tablets 2159

Nortriptyline Hydrochloride (The effects of epinepherine may be potentiated by tricyclic antidepressants).

No products indexed under this heading.

Pargyline Hydrochloride (The effects of epinepherine may be potentiated by monoamine oxidase inhibitors).

No products indexed under this heading.

Penbutolol Sulfate (The cardiostimulating and bronchodilating effects of epinepherine are antagonized by beta-adrenergic blocking drugs).

No products indexed under this heading.

Perphenazine (Phenothiazines may reverse the pressor effects of epinepherine).

No products indexed under this heading.

Phenelzine Sulfate (The effects of epinepherine may be potentiated by monoamine oxidase inhibitors).

No products indexed under this heading.

Pindolol (The cardiostimulating and bronchodilating effects of epinepherine are antagonized by beta-adrenergic blocking drugs).

No products indexed under this heading.

Polythiazide (Patients who receive epinepherine while concomitantly taking diuretics should be observed carefully for the development of cardiac arrhythmias).

No products indexed under this heading.

Prazosin Hydrochloride (The vasoconstricting and hypertensive effects of epinepherine are antagonized by alpha-adrenergic blocking drugs).

No products indexed under this heading.

Procarbazine Hydrochloride (The effects of epinepherine may be potentiated by monoamine oxidase inhibitors). Products include:

- Matulane Capsules 3191

Prochlorperazine (Phenothiazines may reverse the pressor effects of epinepherine).

No products indexed under this heading.

Promethazine Hydrochloride (Phenothiazines may reverse the pressor effects of epinepherine). Products include:

- Phenergan Tablets and Suppositories 3440

Propranolol Hydrochloride (The cardiostimulating and bronchodilating effects of epinepherine are antagonized by beta-adrenergic blocking drugs). Products include:

- Inderal LA Long-Acting Capsules 3429
- InnoPran XL Capsules 2723

Protriptyline Hydrochloride (The effects of epinepherine may be potentiated by tricyclic antidepressants).

No products indexed under this heading.

Selegiline Hydrochloride (The effects of epinepherine may be potentiated by monoamine oxidase inhibitors). Products include:

- Eldepryl Capsules 3208
- Zelapar Tablets 3372

Sotalol Hydrochloride (The cardiostimulating and bronchodilating effects of epinepherine are antagonized by beta-adrenergic blocking drugs).

No products indexed under this heading.

Spironolactone (Patients who receive epinepherine while concomitantly taking diuretics should be observed carefully for the development of cardiac arrhythmias).

No products indexed under this heading.

Tamsulosin Hydrochloride (The vasoconstricting and hypertensive effects of epinepherine are antagonized by alpha-adrenergic blocking drugs). Products include:

- Flomax Capsules 850

Terazosin Hydrochloride (The vasoconstricting and hypertensive effects of epinepherine are antagonized by alpha-adrenergic blocking drugs). Products include:

- Hytrin Capsules 471

Thioridazine Hydrochloride (Phenothiazines may reverse the pressor effects of epinepherine). Products include:

- Thioridazine Hydrochloride Tablets 2163

Timolol Hemihydrate (The cardiostimulating and bronchodilating effects of epinepherine are antagonized by beta-adrenergic blocking drugs). Products include:

- Betimol Ophthalmic Solution 3382
- Betimol Ophthalmic Solution .... ⊙ 295

Timolol Maleate (The cardiostimulating and bronchodilating effects of epinepherine are antagonized by beta-adrenergic blocking drugs). Products include:

- Blocadren Tablets 1916
- Cosopt Sterile Ophthalmic Solution 1931
- Timolide Tablets 2086
- Timoptic Sterile Ophthalmic Solution 2088
- Timoptic in Ocudose 2091
- Timoptic-XE Sterile Ophthalmic Gel Forming Solution 2092

Torsemide (Patients who receive epinepherine while concomitantly taking diuretics should be observed carefully for the development of cardiac arrhythmias). Products include:

- Demadex Injection 2759
- Demadex Tablets 2759

Tranylcypromine Sulfate (The effects of epinepherine may be potentiated by monoamine oxidase inhibitors). Products include:

- Parnate Tablets 1527

Triamterene (Patients who receive epinepherine while concomitantly taking diuretics should be observed carefully for the development of cardiac arrhythmias). Products include:

- Dyazide Capsules 1423
- Dyrenium Capsules 3400

Trifluoperazine Hydrochloride (Phenothiazines may reverse the pressor effects of epinepherine).

No products indexed under this heading.

Trimipramine Maleate (The effects of epinepherine may be potentiated by tricyclic antidepressants).

No products indexed under this heading.

Tripelennamine Hydrochloride (The effects of epinepherine may be potentiated by certain antihistamines, notably tripelennamine).

No products indexed under this heading.

TWINRIX VACCINE

(Hepatitis A Vaccine, Inactivated, Hepatitis B Vaccine, Recombinant) 1595

None cited in PDR database.

TYGACIL FOR INJECTION

(Tigecycline) 3488

May interact with oral contraceptives and certain other agents. Compounds in these categories include:

Desogestrel (Concurrent use of antibacterial drugs with oral contraceptives may render oral contraceptives less effective). Products include:

- Mircette Tablets 1066

Ethinyl Estradiol (Concurrent use of antibacterial drugs with oral contraceptives may render oral contraceptives less effective). Products include:

- Mircette Tablets 1066
- NuvaRing 2340

Ortho-Cyclen/Ortho Tri-Cyclen 2429
Ortho Evra Transdermal System 2417
Ortho Tri-Cyclen Lo Tablets 2436
Seasonique Tablets 1077
Yasmin 28 Tablets 796
Yaz Tablets 803

Ethynodiol Diacetate (Concurrent use of antibacterial drugs with oral contraceptives may render oral contraceptives less effective).
No products indexed under this heading.

Levonorgestrel (Concurrent use of antibacterial drugs with oral contraceptives may render oral contraceptives less effective). Products include:
Climara Pro Transdermal System 776
Mirena Intrauterine System 787
Plan B Tablets 1076
Seasonique Tablets 1077

Mestranol (Concurrent use of antibacterial drugs with oral contraceptives may render oral contraceptives less effective).
No products indexed under this heading.

Norethindrone (Concurrent use of antibacterial drugs with oral contraceptives may render oral contraceptives less effective). Products include:
Ortho Micronor Tablets 2426

Norethynodrel (Concurrent use of antibacterial drugs with oral contraceptives may render oral contraceptives less effective).
No products indexed under this heading.

Norgestimate (Concurrent use of antibacterial drugs with oral contraceptives may render oral contraceptives less effective). Products include:
Ortho-Cyclen/Ortho Tri-Cyclen 2429
Ortho Tri-Cyclen Lo Tablets 2436

Norgestrel (Concurrent use of antibacterial drugs with oral contraceptives may render oral contraceptives less effective).
No products indexed under this heading.

Warfarin Sodium (Prothrombin time or other suitable anticoagulation test should be monitored if tigecycline is administered with warfarin). Products include:
Coumadin for Injection 898
Coumadin Tablets 898

REGULAR STRENGTH TYLENOL TABLETS
(Acetaminophen) 1870

Food Interactions

Alcohol (Chronic heavy alcohol users, 3 or more drinks per day, should consult their physicians for advice on when and how they should take pain relievers including acetaminophen).

TYLENOL 8 HOUR EXTENDED RELEASE CAPLETS
(Acetaminophen) .... ▣695

Food Interactions

Alcohol (Chronic heavy alcohol users, 3 or more drinks per day, should consult their physicians for advice on when and how they should take pain relievers including acetaminophen).

TYLENOL CHEST CONGESTION CAPLETS WITH COOL BURST
(Acetaminophen, Guaifenesin) .... ▣722

Food Interactions

Alcohol (Consuming 3 or more alcoholic beverages with this product may cause hepatotoxicity).

TYLENOL CHEST CONGESTION LIQUID WITH COOL BURST
(Acetaminophen, Guaifenesin) .... ▣722
See Tylenol Chest Congestion Caplets with Cool Burst

CHILDREN'S TYLENOL WITH FLAVOR CREATOR
(Acetaminophen) .... ▣679
None cited in PDR database.

CHILDREN'S TYLENOL PLUS COUGH & RUNNY NOSE SUSPENSION LIQUID
(Acetaminophen, Chlorpheniramine Maleate, Dextromethorphan Hydrobromide).... ▣754
May interact with hypnotics and sedatives, monoamine oxidase inhibitors, and tranquilizers. Compounds in these categories include:

Alprazolam (Concurrent use may increase drowsiness effect). Products include:
Niravam Orally Disintegrating Tablets 3092

Buspirone Hydrochloride (Concurrent use may increase drowsiness effect).
No products indexed under this heading.

Chlordiazepoxide (Concurrent use may increase drowsiness effect).
No products indexed under this heading.

Chlordiazepoxide Hydrochloride (Concurrent use may increase drowsiness effect). Products include:
Librium Capsules 3347

Chlorpromazine (Concurrent use may increase drowsiness effect).
No products indexed under this heading.

Chlorpromazine Hydrochloride (Concurrent use may increase drowsiness effect).
No products indexed under this heading.

Chlorprothixene (Concurrent use may increase drowsiness effect).
No products indexed under this heading.

Chlorprothixene Hydrochloride (Concurrent use may increase drowsiness effect).
No products indexed under this heading.

Clorazepate Dipotassium (Concurrent use may increase drowsiness effect). Products include:
Tranxene 2474

Diazepam (Concurrent use may increase drowsiness effect). Products include:
Diastat Rectal Delivery System 3343
Valium Tablets 2819

Droperidol (Concurrent use may increase drowsiness effect).
No products indexed under this heading.

Estazolam (Concurrent use may increase drowsiness effect). Products include:
ProSom Tablets 517

Ethchlorvynol (Concurrent use may increase drowsiness effect).
No products indexed under this heading.

Ethinamate (Concurrent use may increase drowsiness effect).
No products indexed under this heading.

Fluphenazine Decanoate (Concurrent use may increase drowsiness effect).
No products indexed under this heading.

Fluphenazine Enanthate (Concurrent use may increase drowsiness effect).
No products indexed under this heading.

Fluphenazine Hydrochloride (Concurrent use may increase drowsiness effect).
No products indexed under this heading.

Flurazepam Hydrochloride (Concurrent use may increase drowsiness effect). Products include:
Dalmane Capsules 3342

Glutethimide (Concurrent use may increase drowsiness effect).
No products indexed under this heading.

Haloperidol (Concurrent use may increase drowsiness effect).
No products indexed under this heading.

Haloperidol Decanoate (Concurrent use may increase drowsiness effect).
No products indexed under this heading.

Hydroxyzine Hydrochloride (Concurrent use may increase drowsiness effect).
No products indexed under this heading.

Isocarboxazid (Do not use while taking, or 2 weeks after stopping, MAO inhibitors).
No products indexed under this heading.

Lorazepam (Concurrent use may increase drowsiness effect).
No products indexed under this heading.

Loxapine Hydrochloride (Concurrent use may increase drowsiness effect).
No products indexed under this heading.

Loxapine Succinate (Concurrent use may increase drowsiness effect).
No products indexed under this heading.

Meprobamate (Concurrent use may increase drowsiness effect).
No products indexed under this heading.

Mesoridazine Besylate (Concurrent use may increase drowsiness effect).
No products indexed under this heading.

Midazolam Hydrochloride (Concurrent use may increase drowsiness effect).
No products indexed under this heading.

Moclobemide (Do not use while taking, or 2 weeks after stopping, MAO inhibitors).
No products indexed under this heading.

Molindone Hydrochloride (Concurrent use may increase drowsiness effect). Products include:
Moban Tablets 1119

Oxazepam (Concurrent use may increase drowsiness effect).
No products indexed under this heading.

Pargyline Hydrochloride (Do not use while taking, or 2 weeks after stopping, MAO inhibitors).
No products indexed under this heading.

Perphenazine (Concurrent use may increase drowsiness effect).
No products indexed under this heading.

Phenelzine Sulfate (Do not use while taking, or 2 weeks after stopping, MAO inhibitors).
No products indexed under this heading.

Prazepam (Concurrent use may increase drowsiness effect).
No products indexed under this heading.

Procarbazine Hydrochloride (Do not use while taking, or 2 weeks after stopping, MAO inhibitors). Products include:
Matulane Capsules 3191

Prochlorperazine (Concurrent use may increase drowsiness effect).
No products indexed under this heading.

Promethazine Hydrochloride (Concurrent use may increase drowsiness effect). Products include:
Phenergan Tablets and Suppositories.............................. 3440

Propofol (Concurrent use may increase drowsiness effect).
No products indexed under this heading.

Quazepam (Concurrent use may increase drowsiness effect).
No products indexed under this heading.

Ramelteon (Concurrent use may increase drowsiness effect). Products include:
Rozerem Tablets 3231

Secobarbital Sodium (Concurrent use may increase drowsiness effect).
No products indexed under this heading.

Selegiline Hydrochloride (Do not use while taking, or 2 weeks after stopping, MAO inhibitors). Products include:
Eldepryl Capsules 3208
Zelapar Tablets 3372

Temazepam (Concurrent use may increase drowsiness effect). Products include:
Restoril Capsules 1860

Thioridazine Hydrochloride (Concurrent use may increase drowsiness effect). Products include:
Thioridazine Hydrochloride Tablets 2163

Thiothixene (Concurrent use may increase drowsiness effect). Products include:
Thiothixene Capsules 2165

Tranylcypromine Sulfate (Do not use while taking, or 2 weeks after stopping, MAO inhibitors). Products include:
Parnate Tablets 1527

Triazolam (Concurrent use may increase drowsiness effect).
No products indexed under this heading.

Trifluoperazine Hydrochloride (Concurrent use may increase drowsiness effect).
No products indexed under this heading.

Zaleplon (Concurrent use may increase drowsiness effect). Products include:
Sonata Capsules 1717

Zolpidem Tartrate (Concurrent use may increase drowsiness effect). Products include:
Ambien Tablets 2851
Ambien CR Tablets 2855

CHILDREN'S TYLENOL PLUS COUGH & SORE THROAT SUSPENSION LIQUID

(Acetaminophen, Dextromethorphan Hydrobromide).... ▣ 754
May interact with monoamine oxidase inhibitors. Compounds in these categories include:

Isocarbazid (Do not use while taking, or 2 weeks after stopping, MAO inhibitors).
No products indexed under this heading.

Moclobemide (Do not use while taking, or 2 weeks after stopping, MAO inhibitors).
No products indexed under this heading.

Pargyline Hydrochloride (Do not use while taking, or 2 weeks after stopping, MAO inhibitors).
No products indexed under this heading.

Phenelzine Sulfate (Do not use while taking, or 2 weeks after stopping, MAO inhibitors).
No products indexed under this heading.

Procarbazine Hydrochloride (Do not use while taking, or 2 weeks after stopping, MAO inhibitors). Products include:
Matulane Capsules 3191

Selegiline Hydrochloride (Do not use while taking, or 2 weeks after stopping, MAO inhibitors). Products include:
Eldepryl Capsules 3208
Zelapar Tablets 3372

Tranylcypromine Sulfate (Do not use while taking, or 2 weeks after stopping, MAO inhibitors). Products include:
Parnate Tablets 1527

CHILDREN'S TYLENOL PLUS COLD SUSPENSION LIQUID

(Acetaminophen, Chlorpheniramine Maleate, Phenylephrine Hydrochloride)........... ▣ 754
May interact with hypnotics and sedatives, monoamine oxidase inhibitors, tranquilizers, and certain other agents. Compounds in these categories include:

Alprazolam (Concurrent use may increase the drowsiness effect). Products include:
Niravam Orally Disintegrating Tablets ... 3092

Buspirone Hydrochloride (Concurrent use may increase the drowsiness effect).
No products indexed under this heading.

Chlordiazepoxide (Concurrent use may increase the drowsiness effect).
No products indexed under this heading.

Chlordiazepoxide Hydrochloride (Concurrent use may increase the drowsiness effect). Products include:

Librium Capsules 3347

Chlorpromazine (Concurrent use may increase the drowsiness effect).
No products indexed under this heading.

Chlorpromazine Hydrochloride (Concurrent use may increase the drowsiness effect).
No products indexed under this heading.

Chlorprothixene (Concurrent use may increase the drowsiness effect).
No products indexed under this heading.

Chlorprothixene Hydrochloride (Concurrent use may increase the drowsiness effect).
No products indexed under this heading.

Clorazepate Dipotassium (Concurrent use may increase the drowsiness effect). Products include:
Tranxene .. 2474

Diazepam (Concurrent use may increase the drowsiness effect). Products include:
Diastat Rectal Delivery System 3343
Valium Tablets 2819

Droperidol (Concurrent use may increase the drowsiness effect).
No products indexed under this heading.

Estazolam (Concurrent use may increase the drowsiness effect). Products include:
ProSom Tablets 517

Ethchlorvynol (Concurrent use may increase the drowsiness effect).
No products indexed under this heading.

Ethinamate (Concurrent use may increase the drowsiness effect).
No products indexed under this heading.

Fluphenazine Decanoate (Concurrent use may increase the drowsiness effect).
No products indexed under this heading.

Fluphenazine Enanthate (Concurrent use may increase the drowsiness effect).
No products indexed under this heading.

Fluphenazine Hydrochloride (Concurrent use may increase the drowsiness effect).
No products indexed under this heading.

Flurazepam Hydrochloride (Concurrent use may increase the drowsiness effect). Products include:
Dalmane Capsules 3342

Glutethimide (Concurrent use may increase the drowsiness effect).
No products indexed under this heading.

Haloperidol (Concurrent use may increase the drowsiness effect).
No products indexed under this heading.

Haloperidol Decanoate (Concurrent use may increase the drowsiness effect).
No products indexed under this heading.

Hydroxyzine Hydrochloride (Concurrent use may increase the drowsiness effect).
No products indexed under this heading.

Isocarboxazid (Avoid concurrent use while taking, or for up to 2 weeks after stopping, MAO inhibitors).
No products indexed under this heading.

Lorazepam (Concurrent use may increase the drowsiness effect).
No products indexed under this heading.

Loxapine Hydrochloride (Concurrent use may increase the drowsiness effect).
No products indexed under this heading.

Loxapine Succinate (Concurrent use may increase the drowsiness effect).
No products indexed under this heading.

Meprobamate (Concurrent use may increase the drowsiness effect).
No products indexed under this heading.

Mesoridazine Besylate (Concurrent use may increase the drowsiness effect).
No products indexed under this heading.

Midazolam Hydrochloride (Concurrent use may increase the drowsiness effect).
No products indexed under this heading.

Moclobemide (Avoid concurrent use while taking, or for up to 2 weeks after stopping, MAO inhibitors).
No products indexed under this heading.

Molindone Hydrochloride (Concurrent use may increase the drowsiness effect). Products include:
Moban Tablets 1119

Oxazepam (Concurrent use may increase the drowsiness effect).
No products indexed under this heading.

Pargyline Hydrochloride (Avoid concurrent use while taking, or for up to 2 weeks after stopping, MAO inhibitors).
No products indexed under this heading.

Perphenazine (Concurrent use may increase the drowsiness effect).
No products indexed under this heading.

Phenelzine Sulfate (Avoid concurrent use while taking, or for up to 2 weeks after stopping, MAO inhibitors).
No products indexed under this heading.

Prazepam (Concurrent use may increase the drowsiness effect).
No products indexed under this heading.

Procarbazine Hydrochloride (Avoid concurrent use while taking, or for up to 2 weeks after stopping, MAO inhibitors). Products include:
Matulane Capsules 3191

Prochlorperazine (Concurrent use may increase the drowsiness effect).
No products indexed under this heading.

Promethazine Hydrochloride (Concurrent use may increase the drowsiness effect). Products include:
Phenergan Tablets and Suppositories 3440

Propofol (Concurrent use may increase the drowsiness effect).
No products indexed under this heading.

Quazepam (Concurrent use may increase the drowsiness effect).
No products indexed under this heading.

Ramelteon (Concurrent use may increase the drowsiness effect). Products include:
Rozerem Tablets 3231

Secobarbital Sodium (Concurrent use may increase the drowsiness effect).
No products indexed under this heading.

Selegiline Hydrochloride (Avoid concurrent use while taking, or up to 2 weeks after stopping, MAO inhibitors). Products include:
Eldepryl Capsules 3208
Zelapar Tablets 3372

Temazepam (Concurrent use may increase the drowsiness effect). Products include:
Restoril Capsules 1860

Thioridazine Hydrochloride (Concurrent use may increase the drowsiness effect). Products include:
Thioridazine Hydrochloride Tablets 2163

Thiothixene (Concurrent use may increase the drowsiness effect). Products include:
Thiothixene Capsules 2165

Tranylcypromine Sulfate (Avoid concurrent use while taking, or for up to 2 weeks after stopping, MAO inhibitors). Products include:
Parnate Tablets 1527

Triazolam (Concurrent use may increase the drowsiness effect).
No products indexed under this heading.

Trifluoperazine Hydrochloride (Concurrent use may increase the drowsiness effect).
No products indexed under this heading.

Zaleplon (Concurrent use may increase the drowsiness effect). Products include:
Sonata Capsules 1717

Zolpidem Tartrate (Concurrent use may increase the drowsiness effect). Products include:
Ambien Tablets 2851
Ambien CR Tablets 2855

CHILDREN'S TYLENOL PLUS MULTI-SYMPTOM COLD SUSPENSION LIQUID

(Acetaminophen, Chlorpheniramine Maleate, Dextromethorphan Hydrobromide, Phenylephrine Hydrochloride)........... ▣ 754
See Children's Tylenol Plus Cold Suspension Liquid

CHILDREN'S TYLENOL PLUS COLD & ALLERGY ORAL SUSPENSION

(Acetaminophen, Diphenhydramine Hydrochloride, Phenylephrine Hydrochloride)........... ▣ 716
May interact with hypnotics and sedatives, monoamine oxidase inhibitors, tranquilizers, and certain other agents. Compounds in these categories include:

Alprazolam (Concurrent use of tranquilizers may increase the drowsiness effect). Products include:
Niravam Orally Disintegrating Tablets ... 3092

IMPORTANT NOTE: Always consult each drug listing in the patient's regimen for possible interactions.

Buspirone Hydrochloride (Concurrent use of tranquilizers may increase the drowsiness effect).
 No products indexed under this heading.

Chlordiazepoxide (Concurrent use of tranquilizers may increase the drowsiness effect).
 No products indexed under this heading.

Chlordiazepoxide Hydrochloride (Concurrent use of tranquilizers may increase the drowsiness effect). Products include:
 Librium Capsules 3347

Chlorpromazine (Concurrent use of tranquilizers may increase the drowsiness effect).
 No products indexed under this heading.

Chlorpromazine Hydrochloride (Concurrent use of tranquilizers may increase the drowsiness effect).
 No products indexed under this heading.

Chlorprothixene (Concurrent use of tranquilizers may increase the drowsiness effect).
 No products indexed under this heading.

Chlorprothixene Hydrochloride (Concurrent use of tranquilizers may increase the drowsiness effect).
 No products indexed under this heading.

Clorazepate Dipotassium (Concurrent use of tranquilizers may increase the drowsiness effect). Products include:
 Tranxene 2474

Diazepam (Concurrent use of tranquilizers may increase the drowsiness effect). Products include:
 Diastat Rectal Delivery System 3343
 Valium Tablets 2819

Diphenhydramine (Concurrent use with other products containing diphenhydramine is not recommended). Products include:
 Tylenol Sore Throat Nighttime Liquid with Cool Burst 1877

Diphenhydramine Citrate (Concurrent use with other products containing diphenhydramine is not recommended). Products include:
 Advil PM Caplets ▣615
 Excedrin PM Caplets/Tablets/Geltabs............. ▣610
 Goody's PM Powder for Pain with Sleeplessness ▣612

Droperidol (Concurrent use of tranquilizers may increase the drowsiness effect).
 No products indexed under this heading.

Estazolam (Concurrent use of sedatives may increase drowsiness effect). Products include:
 ProSom Tablets 517

Ethchlorvynol (Concurrent use of sedatives may increase drowsiness effect).
 No products indexed under this heading.

Ethinamate (Concurrent use of sedatives may increase drowsiness effect).
 No products indexed under this heading.

Fluphenazine Decanoate (Concurrent use of tranquilizers may increase the drowsiness effect).
 No products indexed under this heading.

Fluphenazine Enanthate (Concurrent use of tranquilizers may increase the drowsiness effect).
 No products indexed under this heading.

Fluphenazine Hydrochloride (Concurrent use of tranquilizers may increase the drowsiness effect).
 No products indexed under this heading.

Flurazepam Hydrochloride (Concurrent use of sedatives may increase drowsiness effect). Products include:
 Dalmane Capsules 3342

Glutethimide (Concurrent use of sedatives may increase drowsiness effect).
 No products indexed under this heading.

Haloperidol (Concurrent use of tranquilizers may increase the drowsiness effect).
 No products indexed under this heading.

Haloperidol Decanoate (Concurrent use of tranquilizers may increase the drowsiness effect).
 No products indexed under this heading.

Hydroxyzine Hydrochloride (Concurrent use of tranquilizers may increase the drowsiness effect).
 No products indexed under this heading.

Isocarboxazid (Avoid concurrent use while taking, or for up to 2 weeks after stopping, MAO inhibitors).
 No products indexed under this heading.

Lorazepam (Concurrent use of sedatives may increase drowsiness effect).
 No products indexed under this heading.

Loxapine Hydrochloride (Concurrent use of tranquilizers may increase the drowsiness effect).
 No products indexed under this heading.

Loxapine Succinate (Concurrent use of tranquilizers may increase the drowsiness effect).
 No products indexed under this heading.

Meprobamate (Concurrent use of tranquilizers may increase the drowsiness effect).
 No products indexed under this heading.

Mesoridazine Besylate (Concurrent use of tranquilizers may increase the drowsiness effect).
 No products indexed under this heading.

Midazolam Hydrochloride (Concurrent use of sedatives may increase drowsiness effect).
 No products indexed under this heading.

Moclobemide (Avoid concurrent use while taking, or for up to 2 weeks after stopping, MAO inhibitors).
 No products indexed under this heading.

Molindone Hydrochloride (Concurrent use of tranquilizers may increase the drowsiness effect). Products include:
 Moban Tablets 1119

Oxazepam (Concurrent use of tranquilizers may increase the drowsiness effect).
 No products indexed under this heading.

Pargyline Hydrochloride (Avoid concurrent use while taking, or for up to 2 weeks after stopping, MAO inhibitors).
 No products indexed under this heading.

Perphenazine (Concurrent use of tranquilizers may increase the drowsiness effect).
 No products indexed under this heading.

Phenelzine Sulfate (Avoid concurrent use while taking, or for up to 2 weeks after stopping, MAO inhibitors).
 No products indexed under this heading.

Prazepam (Concurrent use of tranquilizers may increase the drowsiness effect).
 No products indexed under this heading.

Procarbazine Hydrochloride (Avoid concurrent use while taking, or for up to 2 weeks after stopping, MAO inhibitors). Products include:
 Matulane Capsules 3191

Prochlorperazine (Concurrent use of tranquilizers may increase the drowsiness effect).
 No products indexed under this heading.

Promethazine Hydrochloride (Concurrent use of tranquilizers may increase the drowsiness effect). Products include:
 Phenergan Tablets and Suppositories............................... 3440

Propofol (Concurrent use of sedatives may increase drowsiness effect).
 No products indexed under this heading.

Quazepam (Concurrent use of sedatives may increase drowsiness effect).
 No products indexed under this heading.

Ramelteon (Concurrent use of sedatives may increase drowsiness effect). Products include:
 Rozerem Tablets 3231

Secobarbital Sodium (Concurrent use of sedatives may increase drowsiness effect).
 No products indexed under this heading.

Selegiline Hydrochloride (Avoid concurrent use while taking, or for up to 2 weeks after stopping, MAO inhibitors). Products include:
 Eldepryl Capsules 3208
 Zelapar Tablets 3372

Temazepam (Concurrent use of sedatives may increase drowsiness effect). Products include:
 Restoril Capsules 1860

Thioridazine Hydrochloride (Concurrent use of tranquilizers may increase the drowsiness effect). Products include:
 Thioridazine Hydrochloride Tablets .. 2163

Thiothixene (Concurrent use of tranquilizers may increase the drowsiness effect). Products include:
 Thiothixene Capsules 2165

Tranylcypromine Sulfate (Avoid concurrent use while taking, or for up to 2 weeks after stopping, MAO inhibitors).

 Parnate Tablets 1527

Triazolam (Concurrent use of sedatives may increase drowsiness effect).
 No products indexed under this heading.

Trifluoperazine Hydrochloride (Concurrent use of tranquilizers may increase the drowsiness effect).
 No products indexed under this heading.

Zaleplon (Concurrent use of sedatives may increase drowsiness effect). Products include:
 Sonata Capsules 1717

Zolpidem Tartrate (Concurrent use of sedatives may increase drowsiness effect). Products include:
 Ambien Tablets 2851
 Ambien CR Tablets 2855

CHILDREN'S TYLENOL PLUS FLU ORAL SUSPENSION

(Acetaminophen, Chlorpheniramine Maleate, Dextromethorphan Hydrobromide, Phenylephrine Hydrochloride)............ ▣749
May interact with hypnotics and sedatives, monoamine oxidase inhibitors, and tranquilizers. Compounds in these categories include:

Alprazolam (Concurrent use of tranquilizers may increase the drowsiness effect). Products include:
 Niravam Orally Disintegrating Tablets ... 3092

Buspirone Hydrochloride (Concurrent use of tranquilizers may increase the drowsiness effect).
 No products indexed under this heading.

Chlordiazepoxide (Concurrent use of tranquilizers may increase the drowsiness effect).
 No products indexed under this heading.

Chlordiazepoxide Hydrochloride (Concurrent use of tranquilizers may increase the drowsiness effect). Products include:
 Librium Capsules 3347

Chlorpromazine (Concurrent use of tranquilizers may increase the drowsiness effect).
 No products indexed under this heading.

Chlorpromazine Hydrochloride (Concurrent use of tranquilizers may increase the drowsiness effect).
 No products indexed under this heading.

Chlorprothixene (Concurrent use of tranquilizers may increase the drowsiness effect).
 No products indexed under this heading.

Chlorprothixene Hydrochloride (Concurrent use of tranquilizers may increase the drowsiness effect).
 No products indexed under this heading.

Clorazepate Dipotassium (Concurrent use of tranquilizers may increase the drowsiness effect). Products include:
 Tranxene .. 2474

Diazepam (Concurrent use of tranquilizers may increase the drowsiness effect). Products include:
 Diastat Rectal Delivery System 3343
 Valium Tablets 2819

Droperidol (Concurrent use of tranquilizers may increase the drowsiness effect).

No products indexed under this heading.

Estazolam (Concurrent use of sedatives may increase the drowsiness effect). Products include:

Ethchlorvynol (Concurrent use of sedatives may increase the drowsiness effect).

No products indexed under this heading.

Ethinamate (Concurrent use of sedatives may increase the drowsiness effect).

No products indexed under this heading.

Fluphenazine Decanoate (Concurrent use of tranquilizers may increase the drowsiness effect).

No products indexed under this heading.

Fluphenazine Enanthate (Concurrent use of tranquilizers may increase the drowsiness effect).

No products indexed under this heading.

Fluphenazine Hydrochloride (Concurrent use of tranquilizers may increase the drowsiness effect).

No products indexed under this heading.

Flurazepam Hydrochloride (Concurrent use of sedatives may increase the drowsiness effect). Products include:

Glutethimide (Concurrent use of sedatives may increase the drowsiness effect).

No products indexed under this heading.

Haloperidol (Concurrent use of tranquilizers may increase the drowsiness effect).

No products indexed under this heading.

Haloperidol Decanoate (Concurrent use of tranquilizers may increase the drowsiness effect).

No products indexed under this heading.

Hydroxyzine Hydrochloride (Concurrent use of tranquilizers may increase the drowsiness effect).

No products indexed under this heading.

Isocarboxazid (Avoid concurrent use while taking, or for up to 2 weeks after stopping, MAO inhibitors).

No products indexed under this heading.

Lorazepam (Concurrent use of sedatives may increase the drowsiness effect).

No products indexed under this heading.

Midazolam Hydrochloride (Concurrent use of sedatives may increase the drowsiness effect).

No products indexed under this heading.

Moclobemide (Avoid concurrent use while taking, or for up to 2 weeks after stopping, MAO inhibitors).

No products indexed under this heading.

Pargyline Hydrochloride (Avoid concurrent use while taking, or for up to 2 weeks after stopping, MAO inhibitors).

No products indexed under this heading.

Phenelzine Sulfate (Avoid concurrent use while taking, or for up to 2 weeks after stopping, MAO inhibitors).

No products indexed under this heading.

Procarbazine Hydrochloride (Avoid concurrent use while taking, or for up to 2 weeks after stopping, MAO inhibitors). Products include:

Propofol (Concurrent use of sedatives may increase the drowsiness effect).

No products indexed under this heading.

Quazepam (Concurrent use of sedatives may increase the drowsiness effect).

No products indexed under this heading.

Ramelteon (Concurrent use of sedatives may increase the drowsiness effect). Products include:

Secobarbital Sodium (Concurrent use of sedatives may increase the drowsiness effect).

No products indexed under this heading.

Selegiline Hydrochloride (Avoid concurrent use while taking, or for up to 2 weeks after stopping, MAO inhibitors). Products include:

Temazepam (Concurrent use of sedatives may increase the drowsiness effect). Products include:

Tranylcypromine Sulfate (Avoid concurrent use while taking, or for up to 2 weeks after stopping, MAO inhibitors). Products include:

Triazolam (Concurrent use of sedatives may increase the drowsiness effect).

No products indexed under this heading.

Zaleplon (Concurrent use of sedatives may increase the drowsiness effect). Products include:

Zolpidem Tartrate (Concurrent use of sedatives may increase the drowsiness effect). Products include:

TYLENOL COLD HEAD CONGESTION DAYTIME CAPLETS WITH COOL BURST AND GELCAPS

(Acetaminophen, Dextromethorphan Hydrobromide, Phenylephrine Hydrochloride)........... ▣750 May interact with monoamine oxidase inhibitors and certain other agents. Compounds in these categories include:

Isocarboxazid (Do not use while taking, or for 2 weeks after stopping, MAOI drugs).

No products indexed under this heading.

Moclobemide (Do not use while taking, or for 2 weeks after stopping, MAOI drugs).

No products indexed under this heading.

Pargyline Hydrochloride (Do not use while taking, or for 2 weeks after stopping, MAOI drugs).

No products indexed under this heading.

Phenelzine Sulfate (Do not use while taking, or for 2 weeks after stopping, MAOI drugs).

No products indexed under this heading.

Procarbazine Hydrochloride (Do not use while taking, or for 2 weeks after stopping, MAOI drugs). Products include:

Selegiline Hydrochloride (Do not use while taking, or for 2 weeks after stopping, MAOI drugs). Products include:

Tranylcypromine Sulfate (Do not use while taking, or for 2 weeks after stopping, MAOI drugs). Products include:

Food Interactions

Alcohol (Concomitant consumption of alcohol may cause liver damage).

TYLENOL COLD HEAD CONGESTION NIGHTTIME CAPLETS WITH COOL BURST

(Acetaminophen, Chlorpheniramine Maleate, Dextromethorphan Hydrobromide, Phenylephrine Hydrochloride)........... ▣750 May interact with hypnotics and sedatives, monoamine oxidase inhibitors, tranquilizers, and certain other agents. Compounds in these categories include:

Alprazolam (May increase drowsiness effect). Products include:

Buspirone Hydrochloride (May increase drowsiness effect).

No products indexed under this heading.

Chlordiazepoxide (May increase drowsiness effect).

No products indexed under this heading.

Chlordiazepoxide Hydrochloride (May increase drowsiness effect). Products include:

Chlorpromazine (May increase drowsiness effect).

No products indexed under this heading.

Chlorpromazine Hydrochloride (May increase drowsiness effect).

No products indexed under this heading.

Chlorprothixene (May increase drowsiness effect).

No products indexed under this heading.

Chlorprothixene Hydrochloride (May increase drowsiness effect).

No products indexed under this heading.

Clorazepate Dipotassium (May increase drowsiness effect). Products include:

Diazepam (May increase drowsiness effect). Products include:

Droperidol (May increase drowsiness effect).

No products indexed under this heading.

Estazolam (May increase drowsiness effect). Products include:

Ethchlorvynol (May increase drowsiness effect).

No products indexed under this heading.

Ethinamate (May increase drowsiness effect).

No products indexed under this heading.

Fluphenazine Decanoate (May increase drowsiness effect).

No products indexed under this heading.

Fluphenazine Enanthate (May increase drowsiness effect).

No products indexed under this heading.

Fluphenazine Hydrochloride (May increase drowsiness effect).

No products indexed under this heading.

Flurazepam Hydrochloride (May increase drowsiness effect). Products include:

Glutethimide (May increase drowsiness effect).

No products indexed under this heading.

Haloperidol (May increase drowsiness effect).

No products indexed under this heading.

Haloperidol Decanoate (May increase drowsiness effect).

No products indexed under this heading.

Hydroxyzine Hydrochloride (May increase drowsiness effect).

No products indexed under this heading.

Isocarboxazid (Concurrent and/or sequential use with MAO inhibitors is not recommended).

No products indexed under this heading.

Lorazepam (May increase drowsiness effect).

No products indexed under this heading.

Loxapine Hydrochloride (May increase drowsiness effect).

No products indexed under this heading.

Loxapine Succinate (May increase drowsiness effect).

No products indexed under this heading.

Meprobamate (May increase drowsiness effect).

No products indexed under this heading.

Mesoridazine Besylate (May increase drowsiness effect).

No products indexed under this heading.

Midazolam Hydrochloride (May increase drowsiness effect).

No products indexed under this heading.

Moclobemide (Concurrent and/or sequential use with MAO inhibitors is not recommended).

No products indexed under this heading.

Molindone Hydrochloride (May increase drowsiness effect). Products include:
 Moban Tablets 1119

Oxazepam (May increase drowsiness effect).
 No products indexed under this heading.

Pargyline Hydrochloride (Concurrent and/or sequential use with MAO inhibitors is not recommended).
 No products indexed under this heading.

Perphenazine (May increase drowsiness effect).
 No products indexed under this heading.

Phenelzine Sulfate (Concurrent and/or sequential use with MAO inhibitors is not recommended).
 No products indexed under this heading.

Prazepam (May increase drowsiness effect).
 No products indexed under this heading.

Procarbazine Hydrochloride (Concurrent and/or sequential use with MAO inhibitors is not recommended). Products include:
 Matulane Capsules 3191

Prochlorperazine (May increase drowsiness effect).
 No products indexed under this heading.

Promethazine Hydrochloride (May increase drowsiness effect). Products include:
 Phenergan Tablets and Suppositories 3440

Propofol (May increase drowsiness effect).
 No products indexed under this heading.

Quazepam (May increase drowsiness effect).
 No products indexed under this heading.

Ramelteon (May increase drowsiness effect). Products include:
 Rozerem Tablets 3231

Secobarbital Sodium (May increase drowsiness effect).
 No products indexed under this heading.

Selegiline Hydrochloride (Concurrent and/or sequential use with MAO inhibitors is not recommended). Products include:
 Eldepryl Capsules 3208
 Zelapar Tablets 3372

Temazepam (May increase drowsiness effect). Products include:
 Restoril Capsules 1860

Thioridazine Hydrochloride (May increase drowsiness effect). Products include:
 Thioridazine Hydrochloride Tablets .. 2163

Thiothixene (May increase drowsiness effect). Products include:
 Thiothixene Capsules 2165

Tranylcypromine Sulfate (Concurrent and/or sequential use with MAO inhibitors is not recommended). Products include:
 Parnate Tablets 1527

Triazolam (May increase drowsiness effect).
 No products indexed under this heading.

Trifluoperazine Hydrochloride (May increase drowsiness effect).
 No products indexed under this heading.

Zaleplon (May increase drowsiness effect). Products include:
 Sonata Capsules 1717

Zolpidem Tartrate (May increase drowsiness effect). Products include:
 Ambien Tablets 2851
 Ambien CR Tablets 2855

Food Interactions

Alcohol (Concomitant consumption of alcohol may cause liver damage).

TYLENOL COLD HEAD CONGESTION SEVERE CAPLETS WITH COOL BURST

(Acetaminophen, Dextromethorphan Hydrobromide, Guaifenesin, Phenylephrine Hydrochloride) ⏺▣ 750
May interact with hypnotics and sedatives, monoamine oxidase inhibitors, tranquilizers, and certain other agents. Compounds in these categories include:

Alprazolam (May increase drowsiness effect). Products include:
 Niravam Orally Disintegrating Tablets .. 3092

Buspirone Hydrochloride (May increase drowsiness effect).
 No products indexed under this heading.

Chlordiazepoxide (May increase drowsiness effect).
 No products indexed under this heading.

Chlordiazepoxide Hydrochloride (May increase drowsiness effect). Products include:
 Librium Capsules 3347

Chlorpromazine (May increase drowsiness effect).
 No products indexed under this heading.

Chlorpromazine Hydrochloride (May increase drowsiness effect).
 No products indexed under this heading.

Chlorprothixene (May increase drowsiness effect).
 No products indexed under this heading.

Chlorprothixene Hydrochloride (May increase drowsiness effect).
 No products indexed under this heading.

Clorazepate Dipotassium (May increase drowsiness effect). Products include:
 Tranxene 2474

Diazepam (May increase drowsiness effect). Products include:
 Diastat Rectal Delivery System 3343
 Valium Tablets 2819

Droperidol (May increase drowsiness effect).
 No products indexed under this heading.

Estazolam (May increase drowsiness effect). Products include:
 ProSom Tablets 517

Ethchlorvynol (May increase drowsiness effect).
 No products indexed under this heading.

Ethinamate (May increase drowsiness effect).
 No products indexed under this heading.

Fluphenazine Decanoate (May increase drowsiness effect).
 No products indexed under this heading.

Fluphenazine Enanthate (May increase drowsiness effect).
 No products indexed under this heading.

Fluphenazine Hydrochloride (May increase drowsiness effect).
 No products indexed under this heading.

Flurazepam Hydrochloride (May increase drowsiness effect). Products include:
 Dalmane Capsules 3342

Glutethimide (May increase drowsiness effect).
 No products indexed under this heading.

Haloperidol (May increase drowsiness effect).
 No products indexed under this heading.

Haloperidol Decanoate (May increase drowsiness effect).
 No products indexed under this heading.

Hydroxyzine Hydrochloride (May increase drowsiness effect).
 No products indexed under this heading.

Isocarboxazid (Concurrent and/or sequential use with MAO inhibitors is not recommended).
 No products indexed under this heading.

Lorazepam (May increase drowsiness effect).
 No products indexed under this heading.

Loxapine Hydrochloride (May increase drowsiness effect).
 No products indexed under this heading.

Loxapine Succinate (May increase drowsiness effect).
 No products indexed under this heading.

Meprobamate (May increase drowsiness effect).
 No products indexed under this heading.

Mesoridazine Besylate (May increase drowsiness effect).
 No products indexed under this heading.

Midazolam Hydrochloride (May increase drowsiness effect).
 No products indexed under this heading.

Moclobemide (Concurrent and/or sequential use with MAO inhibitors is not recommended).
 No products indexed under this heading.

Molindone Hydrochloride (May increase drowsiness effect). Products include:
 Moban Tablets 1119

Oxazepam (May increase drowsiness effect).
 No products indexed under this heading.

Pargyline Hydrochloride (Concurrent and/or sequential use with MAO inhibitors is not recommended).
 No products indexed under this heading.

Perphenazine (May increase drowsiness effect).
 No products indexed under this heading.

Phenelzine Sulfate (Concurrent and/or sequential use with MAO inhibitors is not recommended).
 No products indexed under this heading.

Prazepam (May increase drowsiness effect).
 No products indexed under this heading.

Procarbazine Hydrochloride (Concurrent and/or sequential use with MAO inhibitors is not recommended). Products include:
 Matulane Capsules 3191

Prochlorperazine (May increase drowsiness effect).
 No products indexed under this heading.

Promethazine Hydrochloride (May increase drowsiness effect). Products include:
 Phenergan Tablets and Suppositories 3440

Propofol (May increase drowsiness effect).
 No products indexed under this heading.

Quazepam (May increase drowsiness effect).
 No products indexed under this heading.

Ramelteon (May increase drowsiness effect). Products include:
 Rozerem Tablets 3231

Secobarbital Sodium (May increase drowsiness effect).
 No products indexed under this heading.

Selegiline Hydrochloride (Concurrent and/or sequential use with MAO inhibitors is not recommended). Products include:
 Eldepryl Capsules 3208
 Zelapar Tablets 3372

Temazepam (May increase drowsiness effect). Products include:
 Restoril Capsules 1860

Thioridazine Hydrochloride (May increase drowsiness effect). Products include:
 Thioridazine Hydrochloride Tablets .. 2163

Thiothixene (May increase drowsiness effect). Products include:
 Thiothixene Capsules 2165

Tranylcypromine Sulfate (Concurrent and/or sequential use with MAO inhibitors is not recommended). Products include:
 Parnate Tablets 1527

Triazolam (May increase drowsiness effect).
 No products indexed under this heading.

Trifluoperazine Hydrochloride (May increase drowsiness effect).
 No products indexed under this heading.

Zaleplon (May increase drowsiness effect). Products include:
 Sonata Capsules 1717

Zolpidem Tartrate (May increase drowsiness effect). Products include:
 Ambien Tablets 2851
 Ambien CR Tablets 2855

Food Interactions

Alcohol (Concomitant consumption of alcohol with acetaminophen may cause liver damage; alcohol may increase drowsiness effect).

TYLENOL COLD MULTI-SYMPTOM DAYTIME CAPLETS WITH COOL BURST AND GELCAPS

(Acetaminophen, Dextromethorphan Hydrobromide, Phenylephrine Hydrochloride) 752

May interact with monoamine oxidase inhibitors and certain other agents. Compounds in these categories include:

Isocarboxazid (Do not use while taking, or for 2 weeks after stopping, MAOI drugs).
No products indexed under this heading.

Moclobemide (Do not use while taking, or for 2 weeks after stopping, MAOI drugs).
No products indexed under this heading.

Pargyline Hydrochloride (Do not use while taking, or for 2 weeks after stopping, MAOI drugs).
No products indexed under this heading.

Phenelzine Sulfate (Do not use while taking, or for 2 weeks after stopping, MAOI drugs).
No products indexed under this heading.

Procarbazine Hydrochloride (Do not use while taking, or for 2 weeks after stopping, MAOI drugs). Products include:
Matulane Capsules 3191

Selegiline Hydrochloride (Do not use while taking, or for 2 weeks after stopping, MAOI drugs). Products include:
Eldepryl Capsules 3208
Zelapar Tablets 3372

Tranylcypromine Sulfate (Do not use while taking, or for 2 weeks after stopping, MAOI drugs). Products include:
Parnate Tablets 1527

Food Interactions

Alcohol (Concomitant consumption of alcohol may cause liver damage).

TYLENOL COLD MULTI-SYMPTOM DAYTIME LIQUID

(Acetaminophen, Dextromethorphan Hydrobromide, Phenylephrine Hydrochloride) 752

May interact with monoamine oxidase inhibitors and certain other agents. Compounds in these categories include:

Isocarboxazid (Do not use while taking, or 2 weeks after stopping, MAO inhibitors).
No products indexed under this heading.

Moclobemide (Do not use while taking, or 2 weeks after stopping, MAO inhibitors).
No products indexed under this heading.

Pargyline Hydrochloride (Do not use while taking, or 2 weeks after stopping, MAO inhibitors).
No products indexed under this heading.

Phenelzine Sulfate (Do not use while taking, or 2 weeks after stopping, MAO inhibitors).
No products indexed under this heading.

Procarbazine Hydrochloride (Do not use while taking, or 2 weeks after stopping, MAO inhibitors). Products include:
Matulane Capsules 3191

Selegiline Hydrochloride (Do not use while taking, or 2 weeks after stopping, MAO inhibitors). Products include:
Eldepryl Capsules 3208
Zelapar Tablets 3372

Tranylcypromine Sulfate (Do not use while taking, or 2 weeks after stopping, MAO inhibitors). Products include:
Parnate Tablets 1527

Food Interactions

Alcohol (Chronic heavy alcohol users, 3 or more drinks per day, should consult their physicians for advice on when and how they should take pain relievers including acetaminophen).

TYLENOL COLD MULTI-SYMPTOM NIGHTTIME LIQUID WITH COOL BURST

(Acetaminophen, Dextromethorphan Hydrobromide, Doxylamine Succinate, Phenylephrine Hydrochloride) 752

May interact with hypnotics and sedatives, monoamine oxidase inhibitors, tranquilizers, and certain other agents. Compounds in these categories include:

Alprazolam (May increase drowsiness effect). Products include:
Niravam Orally Disintegrating Tablets 3092

Buspirone Hydrochloride (May increase drowsiness effect).
No products indexed under this heading.

Chlordiazepoxide (May increase drowsiness effect).
No products indexed under this heading.

Chlordiazepoxide Hydrochloride (May increase drowsiness effect). Products include:
Librium Capsules 3347

Chlorpromazine (May increase drowsiness effect).
No products indexed under this heading.

Chlorpromazine Hydrochloride (May increase drowsiness effect).
No products indexed under this heading.

Chlorprothixene (May increase drowsiness effect).
No products indexed under this heading.

Chlorprothixene Hydrochloride (May increase drowsiness effect).
No products indexed under this heading.

Clorazepate Dipotassium (May increase drowsiness effect). Products include:
Tranxene 2474

Diazepam (May increase drowsiness effect). Products include:
Diastat Rectal Delivery System 3343
Valium Tablets 2819

Droperidol (May increase drowsiness effect).
No products indexed under this heading.

Estazolam (May increase drowsiness effect). Products include:
ProSom Tablets 517

Ethchlorvynol (May increase drowsiness effect).
No products indexed under this heading.

Ethinamate (May increase drowsiness effect).
No products indexed under this heading.

Fluphenazine Decanoate (May increase drowsiness effect).
No products indexed under this heading.

Fluphenazine Enanthate (May increase drowsiness effect).
No products indexed under this heading.

Fluphenazine Hydrochloride (May increase drowsiness effect).
No products indexed under this heading.

Flurazepam Hydrochloride (May increase drowsiness effect). Products include:
Dalmane Capsules 3342

Glutethimide (May increase drowsiness effect).
No products indexed under this heading.

Haloperidol (May increase drowsiness effect).
No products indexed under this heading.

Haloperidol Decanoate (May increase drowsiness effect).
No products indexed under this heading.

Hydroxyzine Hydrochloride (May increase drowsiness effect).
No products indexed under this heading.

Isocarboxazid (Concurrent and/or sequential use with MAO inhibitors is not recommended).
No products indexed under this heading.

Lorazepam (May increase drowsiness effect).
No products indexed under this heading.

Loxapine Hydrochloride (May increase drowsiness effect).
No products indexed under this heading.

Loxapine Succinate (May increase drowsiness effect).
No products indexed under this heading.

Meprobamate (May increase drowsiness effect).
No products indexed under this heading.

Mesoridazine Besylate (May increase drowsiness effect).
No products indexed under this heading.

Midazolam Hydrochloride (May increase drowsiness effect).
No products indexed under this heading.

Moclobemide (Concurrent and/or sequential use with MAO inhibitors is not recommended).
No products indexed under this heading.

Molindone Hydrochloride (May increase drowsiness effect). Products include:
Moban Tablets 1119

Oxazepam (May increase drowsiness effect).
No products indexed under this heading.

Pargyline Hydrochloride (Concurrent and/or sequential use with MAO inhibitors is not recommended).
No products indexed under this heading.

Perphenazine (May increase drowsiness effect).
No products indexed under this heading.

Phenelzine Sulfate (Concurrent and/or sequential use with MAO inhibitors is not recommended).
No products indexed under this heading.

Prazepam (May increase drowsiness effect).
No products indexed under this heading.

Procarbazine Hydrochloride (Concurrent and/or sequential use with MAO inhibitors is not recommended). Products include:
Matulane Capsules 3191

Prochlorperazine (May increase drowsiness effect).
No products indexed under this heading.

Promethazine Hydrochloride (May increase drowsiness effect). Products include:
Phenergan Tablets and Suppositories 3440

Propofol (May increase drowsiness effect).
No products indexed under this heading.

Quazepam (May increase drowsiness effect).
No products indexed under this heading.

Ramelteon (May increase drowsiness effect). Products include:
Rozerem Tablets 3231

Secobarbital Sodium (May increase drowsiness effect).
No products indexed under this heading.

Selegiline Hydrochloride (Concurrent and/or sequential use with MAO inhibitors is not recommended). Products include:
Eldepryl Capsules 3208
Zelapar Tablets 3372

Temazepam (May increase drowsiness effect). Products include:
Restoril Capsules 1860

Thioridazine Hydrochloride (May increase drowsiness effect). Products include:
Thioridazine Hydrochloride Tablets 2163

Thiothixene (May increase drowsiness effect). Products include:
Thiothixene Capsules 2165

Tranylcypromine Sulfate (Concurrent and/or sequential use with MAO inhibitors is not recommended). Products include:
Parnate Tablets 1527

Triazolam (May increase drowsiness effect).
No products indexed under this heading.

Trifluoperazine Hydrochloride (May increase drowsiness effect).
No products indexed under this heading.

Zaleplon (May increase drowsiness effect). Products include:
Sonata Capsules 1717

Zolpidem Tartrate (May increase drowsiness effect). Products include:
Ambien Tablets 2851
Ambien CR Tablets 2855

Food Interactions

Alcohol (Concomitant consumption of alcohol may cause liver damage).

TYLENOL COLD MULTI-SYMPTOM SEVERE CAPLETS WITH COOL BURST
(Acetaminophen, Dextromethorphan Hydrobromide, Guaifenesin, Phenylephrine Hydrochloride) .... ■ 752
May interact with monoamine oxidase inhibitors and certain other agents. Compounds in these categories include:

Isocarboxazid (Do not use while taking, or 2 weeks after stopping, MAO inhibitors).
No products indexed under this heading.

Moclobemide (Do not use while taking, or 2 weeks after stopping, MAO inhibitors).
No products indexed under this heading.

Pargyline Hydrochloride (Do not use while taking, or 2 weeks after stopping, MAO inhibitors).
No products indexed under this heading.

Phenelzine Sulfate (Do not use while taking, or 2 weeks after stopping, MAO inhibitors).
No products indexed under this heading.

Procarbazine Hydrochloride (Do not use while taking, or 2 weeks after stopping, MAO inhibitors). Products include:
Matulane Capsules 3191

Selegiline Hydrochloride (Do not use while taking, or 2 weeks after stopping, MAO inhibitors). Products include:
Eldepryl Capsules 3208
Zelapar Tablets 3372

Tranylcypromine Sulfate (Do not use while taking, or 2 weeks after stopping, MAO inhibitors). Products include:
Parnate Tablets 1527

Food Interactions

Alcohol (Chronic heavy alcohol users, 3 or more drinks per day, should consult their physicians for advice on when and how they should take pain relievers including acetaminophen).

TYLENOL COLD MULTI-SYMPTOM SEVERE DAYTIME LIQUID
(Acetaminophen, Dextromethorphan Hydrobromide, Guaifenesin, Phenylephrine Hydrochloride) .... ■ 752
May interact with monoamine oxidase inhibitors and certain other agents. Compounds in these categories include:

Isocarboxazid (Do not use while taking, or for 2 weeks after stopping, MAOI drugs).
No products indexed under this heading.

Moclobemide (Do not use while taking, or for 2 weeks after stopping, MAOI drugs).
No products indexed under this heading.

Pargyline Hydrochloride (Do not use while taking, or for 2 weeks after stopping, MAOI drugs).
No products indexed under this heading.

Phenelzine Sulfate (Do not use while taking, or for 2 weeks after stopping, MAOI drugs).
No products indexed under this heading.

Procarbazine Hydrochloride (Do not use while taking, or for 2 weeks after stopping, MAOI drugs). Products include:
Matulane Capsules 3191

Selegiline Hydrochloride (Do not use while taking, or for 2 weeks after stopping, MAOI drugs). Products include:
Eldepryl Capsules 3208
Zelapar Tablets 3372

Tranylcypromine Sulfate (Do not use while taking, or for 2 weeks after stopping, MAOI drugs). Products include:
Parnate Tablets 1527

Food Interactions

Alcohol (Concomitant consumption of alcohol may cause liver damage).

TYLENOL COUGH & SORE THROAT DAYTIME LIQUID WITH COOL BURST
(Acetaminophen, Dextromethorphan Hydrobromide) .... ■ 790
May interact with monoamine oxidase inhibitors and certain other agents. Compounds in these categories include:

Isocarboxazid (Concurrent and/or sequential use with MAO inhibitors is not recommended).
No products indexed under this heading.

Moclobemide (Concurrent and/or sequential use with MAO inhibitors is not recommended).
No products indexed under this heading.

Pargyline Hydrochloride (Concurrent and/or sequential use with MAO inhibitors is not recommended).
No products indexed under this heading.

Phenelzine Sulfate (Concurrent and/or sequential use with MAO inhibitors is not recommended).
No products indexed under this heading.

Procarbazine Hydrochloride (Concurrent and/or sequential use with MAO inhibitors is not recommended). Products include:
Matulane Capsules 3191

Selegiline Hydrochloride (Concurrent and/or sequential use with MAO inhibitors is not recommended). Products include:
Eldepryl Capsules 3208
Zelapar Tablets 3372

Tranylcypromine Sulfate (Concurrent and/or sequential use with MAO inhibitors is not recommended). Products include:
Parnate Tablets 1527

Food Interactions

Alcohol (Concomitant consumption of alcohol may cause liver damage).

TYLENOL COUGH & SORE THROAT NIGHTTIME LIQUID WITH COOL BURST
(Acetaminophen, Dextromethorphan Hydrobromide, Doxylamine Succinate) .... ■ 790
May interact with hypnotics and sedatives, monoamine oxidase inhibitors, tranquilizers, and certain other agents. Compounds in these categories include:

Alprazolam (Co-administration with tranquilizers may increase drowsiness). Products include:
Niravam Orally Disintegrating Tablets 3092

Buspirone Hydrochloride (Co-administration with tranquilizers may increase drowsiness).
No products indexed under this heading.

Chlordiazepoxide (Co-administration with tranquilizers may increase drowsiness).
No products indexed under this heading.

Chlordiazepoxide Hydrochloride (Co-administration with tranquilizers may increase drowsiness). Products include:
Librium Capsules 3347

Chlorpromazine (Co-administration with tranquilizers may increase drowsiness).
No products indexed under this heading.

Chlorpromazine Hydrochloride (Co-administration with tranquilizers may increase drowsiness).
No products indexed under this heading.

Chlorprothixene (Co-administration with tranquilizers may increase drowsiness).
No products indexed under this heading.

Chlorprothixene Hydrochloride (Co-administration with tranquilizers may increase drowsiness).
No products indexed under this heading.

Clorazepate Dipotassium (Co-administration with tranquilizers may increase drowsiness). Products include:
Tranxene 2474

Diazepam (Co-administration with tranquilizers may increase drowsiness). Products include:
Diastat Rectal Delivery System 3343
Valium Tablets 2819

Droperidol (Co-administration with tranquilizers may increase drowsiness).
No products indexed under this heading.

Estazolam (Co-administration with sedatives may increase drowsiness). Products include:
ProSom Tablets 517

Ethchlorvynol (Co-administration with sedatives may increase drowsiness).
No products indexed under this heading.

Ethinamate (Co-administration with sedatives may increase drowsiness).
No products indexed under this heading.

Fluphenazine Decanoate (Co-administration with tranquilizers may increase drowsiness).
No products indexed under this heading.

Fluphenazine Enanthate (Co-administration with tranquilizers may increase drowsiness).
No products indexed under this heading.

Fluphenazine Hydrochloride (Co-administration with tranquilizers may increase drowsiness).
No products indexed under this heading.

Flurazepam Hydrochloride (Co-administration with sedatives may increase drowsiness). Products include:
Dalmane Capsules 3342

Glutethimide (Co-administration with sedatives may increase drowsiness).
No products indexed under this heading.

Haloperidol (Co-administration with tranquilizers may increase drowsiness).
No products indexed under this heading.

Haloperidol Decanoate (Co-administration with tranquilizers may increase drowsiness).
No products indexed under this heading.

Hydroxyzine Hydrochloride (Co-administration with tranquilizers may increase drowsiness).
No products indexed under this heading.

Isocarboxazid (Concurrent and/or sequential use with MAO inhibitors is not recommended).
No products indexed under this heading.

Lorazepam (Co-administration with sedatives may increase drowsiness).
No products indexed under this heading.

Loxapine Hydrochloride (Co-administration with tranquilizers may increase drowsiness).
No products indexed under this heading.

Loxapine Succinate (Co-administration with tranquilizers may increase drowsiness).
No products indexed under this heading.

Meprobamate (Co-administration with tranquilizers may increase drowsiness).
No products indexed under this heading.

Mesoridazine Besylate (Co-administration with tranquilizers may increase drowsiness).
No products indexed under this heading.

Midazolam Hydrochloride (Co-administration with sedatives may increase drowsiness).
No products indexed under this heading.

Moclobemide (Concurrent and/or sequential use with MAO inhibitors is not recommended).
No products indexed under this heading.

Molindone Hydrochloride (Co-administration with tranquilizers may increase drowsiness). Products include:
Moban Tablets 1119

Oxazepam (Co-administration with tranquilizers may increase drowsiness).
No products indexed under this heading.

Pargyline Hydrochloride (Concurrent and/or sequential use with MAO inhibitors is not recommended).
No products indexed under this heading.

Perphenazine (Co-administration with tranquilizers may increase drowsiness).
No products indexed under this heading.

Phenelzine Sulfate (Concurrent and/or sequential use with MAO inhibitors is not recommended).
No products indexed under this heading.

Prazepam (Co-administration with tranquilizers may increase drowsiness).
No products indexed under this heading.

Procarbazine Hydrochloride (Concurrent and/or sequential use with MAO inhibitors is not recommended). Products include:
Matulane Capsules ... 3191

Prochlorperazine (Co-administration with tranquilizers may increase drowsiness).
No products indexed under this heading.

Promethazine Hydrochloride (Co-administration with tranquilizers may increase drowsiness). Products include:
Phenergan Tablets and Suppositories ... 3440

Propofol (Co-administration with sedatives may increase drowsiness).
No products indexed under this heading.

Quazepam (Co-administration with sedatives may increase drowsiness).
No products indexed under this heading.

Ramelteon (Co-administration with sedatives may increase drowsiness). Products include:
Rozerem Tablets ... 3231

Secobarbital Sodium (Co-administration with sedatives may increase drowsiness).
No products indexed under this heading.

Selegiline Hydrochloride (Concurrent and/or sequential use with MAO inhibitors is not recommended). Products include:
Eldepryl Capsules ... 3208
Zelapar Tablets ... 3372

Temazepam (Co-administration with sedatives may increase drowsiness). Products include:
Restoril Capsules ... 1860

Thioridazine Hydrochloride (Co-administration with tranquilizers may increase drowsiness). Products include:
Thioridazine Hydrochloride Tablets ... 2163

Thiothixene (Co-administration with tranquilizers may increase drowsiness). Products include:
Thiothixene Capsules ... 2165

Tranylcypromine Sulfate (Concurrent and/or sequential use with MAO inhibitors is not recommended). Products include:
Parnate Tablets ... 1527

Triazolam (Co-administration with sedatives may increase drowsiness).
No products indexed under this heading.

Trifluoperazine Hydrochloride (Co-administration with tranquilizers may increase drowsiness).
No products indexed under this heading.

Zaleplon (Co-administration with sedatives may increase drowsiness). Products include:
Sonata Capsules ... 1717

Zolpidem Tartrate (Co-administration with sedatives may increase drowsiness). Products include:
Ambien Tablets ... 2851
Ambien CR Tablets ... 2855

Food Interactions

Alcohol (Concomitant consumption of alcohol may cause liver damage).

TYLENOL 8 HOUR EXTENDED RELEASE CAPLETS

(Acetaminophen) ... 1870
See Regular Strength Tylenol Tablets

EXTRA STRENGTH TYLENOL CAPLETS, COOL CAPLETS, GO TABS AND EZ TABS

(Acetaminophen) ... 1870
See Regular Strength Tylenol Tablets

EXTRA STRENGTH TYLENOL ADULT RAPID BLAST LIQUID

(Acetaminophen) ... 1870
See Regular Strength Tylenol Tablets

EXTRA STRENGTH TYLENOL PM CAPLETS, VANILLA CAPLETS, GELTABS, GELCAPS AND LIQUID

(Acetaminophen, Diphenhydramine Hydrochloride) ... 1875
May interact with tranquilizers and certain other agents. Compounds in these categories include:

Alprazolam (Concurrent use may increase the drowsiness effect). Products include:
Niravam Orally Disintegrating Tablets ... 3092

Buspirone Hydrochloride (Concurrent use may increase the drowsiness effect).
No products indexed under this heading.

Chlordiazepoxide (Concurrent use may increase the drowsiness effect).
No products indexed under this heading.

Chlordiazepoxide Hydrochloride (Concurrent use may increase the drowsiness effect). Products include:
Librium Capsules ... 3347

Chlorpromazine (Concurrent use may increase the drowsiness effect).
No products indexed under this heading.

Chlorpromazine Hydrochloride (Concurrent use may increase the drowsiness effect).
No products indexed under this heading.

Chlorprothixene (Concurrent use may increase the drowsiness effect).
No products indexed under this heading.

Chlorprothixene Hydrochloride (Concurrent use may increase the drowsiness effect).
No products indexed under this heading.

Clorazepate Dipotassium (Concurrent use may increase the drowsiness effect). Products include:
Tranxene ... 2474

Diazepam (Concurrent use may increase the drowsiness effect). Products include:
Diastat Rectal Delivery System ... 3343
Valium Tablets ... 2819

Droperidol (Concurrent use may increase the drowsiness effect).
No products indexed under this heading.

Estazolam (Concurrent use may increase the drowsiness effect). Products include:
ProSom Tablets ... 517

Ethchlorvynol (Concurrent use may increase the drowsiness effect).
No products indexed under this heading.

Ethinamate (Concurrent use may increase the drowsiness effect).
No products indexed under this heading.

Fluphenazine Decanoate (Concurrent use may increase the drowsiness effect).
No products indexed under this heading.

Fluphenazine Enanthate (Concurrent use may increase the drowsiness effect).
No products indexed under this heading.

Fluphenazine Hydrochloride (Concurrent use may increase the drowsiness effect).
No products indexed under this heading.

Flurazepam Hydrochloride (Concurrent use may increase the drowsiness effect). Products include:
Dalmane Capsules ... 3342

Glutethimide (Concurrent use may increase the drowsiness effect).
No products indexed under this heading.

Haloperidol (Concurrent use may increase the drowsiness effect).
No products indexed under this heading.

Haloperidol Decanoate (Concurrent use may increase the drowsiness effect).
No products indexed under this heading.

Hydroxyzine Hydrochloride (Concurrent use may increase the drowsiness effect).
No products indexed under this heading.

Lorazepam (Concurrent use may increase the drowsiness effect).
No products indexed under this heading.

Loxapine Hydrochloride (Concurrent use may increase the drowsiness effect).
No products indexed under this heading.

Loxapine Succinate (Concurrent use may increase the drowsiness effect).
No products indexed under this heading.

Meprobamate (Concurrent use may increase the drowsiness effect).
No products indexed under this heading.

Mesoridazine Besylate (Concurrent use may increase the drowsiness effect).
No products indexed under this heading.

Midazolam Hydrochloride (Concurrent use may increase the drowsiness effect).
No products indexed under this heading.

Molindone Hydrochloride (Concurrent use may increase the drowsiness effect). Products include:
Moban Tablets ... 1119

Oxazepam (Concurrent use may increase the drowsiness effect).
No products indexed under this heading.

Perphenazine (Concurrent use may increase the drowsiness effect).
No products indexed under this heading.

Prazepam (Concurrent use may increase the drowsiness effect).
No products indexed under this heading.

Prochlorperazine (Concurrent use may increase the drowsiness effect).
No products indexed under this heading.

Promethazine Hydrochloride (Concurrent use may increase the drowsiness effect). Products include:
Phenergan Tablets and Suppositories ... 3440

Propofol (Concurrent use may increase the drowsiness effect).
No products indexed under this heading.

Quazepam (Concurrent use may increase the drowsiness effect).
No products indexed under this heading.

Ramelteon (Concurrent use may increase the drowsiness effect). Products include:
Rozerem Tablets ... 3231

Secobarbital Sodium (Concurrent use may increase the drowsiness effect).
No products indexed under this heading.

Temazepam (Concurrent use may increase the drowsiness effect). Products include:
Restoril Capsules ... 1860

Thioridazine Hydrochloride (Concurrent use may increase the drowsiness effect). Products include:
Thioridazine Hydrochloride Tablets ... 2163

Thiothixene (Concurrent use may increase the drowsiness effect). Products include:
Thiothixene Capsules ... 2165

Triazolam (Concurrent use may increase the drowsiness effect).
No products indexed under this heading.

Trifluoperazine Hydrochloride (Concurrent use may increase the drowsiness effect).
No products indexed under this heading.

Zaleplon (Concurrent use may increase the drowsiness effect). Products include:
Sonata Capsules ... 1717

Zolpidem Tartrate (Concurrent use may increase the drowsiness effect). Products include:
Ambien Tablets ... 2851
Ambien CR Tablets ... 2855

Food Interactions

Alcohol (Concurrent use may increase drowsiness effect; chronic heavy alcohol abusers, 3 or more drinks per day, may be at increased risk of liver toxicity from excessive acetaminophen use).

EXTRA STRENGTH TYLENOL RAPID RELEASE GELS

(Acetaminophen) 1870

See Regular Strength Tylenol Tablets

CONCENTRATED TYLENOL INFANTS' DROPS PLUS COLD & COUGH

(Acetaminophen, Dextromethorphan Hydrobromide, Phenylephrine Hydrochloride)............ ◘754

May interact with monoamine oxidase inhibitors. Compounds in these categories include:

Isocarboxazid (Avoid concurrent use while taking, or for up to 2 weeks after stopping, MAO inhibitors).
No products indexed under this heading.

Moclobemide (Avoid concurrent use while taking, or for up to 2 weeks after stopping, MAO inhibitors).
No products indexed under this heading.

Pargyline Hydrochloride (Avoid concurrent use while taking, or for up to 2 weeks after stopping, MAO inhibitors).
No products indexed under this heading.

Phenelzine Sulfate (Avoid concurrent use while taking, or for up to 2 weeks after stopping, MAO inhibitors).
No products indexed under this heading.

Procarbazine Hydrochloride (Avoid concurrent use while taking, or for up to 2 weeks after stopping, MAO inhibitors). Products include:
Matulane Capsules 3191

Selegiline Hydrochloride (Avoid concurrent use while taking, or for up to 2 weeks after stopping, MAO inhibitors). Products include:
Eldepryl Capsules 3208
Zelapar Tablets 3372

Tranylcypromine Sulfate (Avoid concurrent use while taking, or for up to 2 weeks after stopping, MAO inhibitors). Products include:
Parnate Tablets 1527

TYLENOL SINUS SEVERE CONGESTION CAPLETS WITH COOL BURST

(Acetaminophen, Guaifenesin, Pseudoephedrine Hydrochloride)....... ◘778

May interact with monoamine oxidase inhibitors and certain other agents. Compounds in these categories include:

Isocarboxazid (Do not use while taking, or 2 weeks after stopping, MAO inhibitors).
No products indexed under this heading.

Moclobemide (Do not use while taking, or 2 weeks after stopping, MAO inhibitors).
No products indexed under this heading.

Pargyline Hydrochloride (Do not use while taking, or 2 weeks after stopping, MAO inhibitors).
No products indexed under this heading.

Phenelzine Sulfate (Do not use while taking, or 2 weeks after stopping, MAO inhibitors).
No products indexed under this heading.

Procarbazine Hydrochloride (Do not use while taking, or 2 weeks after stopping, MAO inhibitors). Products include:
Matulane Capsules 3191

Selegiline Hydrochloride (Do not use while taking, or 2 weeks after stopping, MAO inhibitors). Products include:
Eldepryl Capsules 3208
Zelapar Tablets 3372

Tranylcypromine Sulfate (Do not use while taking, or 2 weeks after stopping, MAO inhibitors). Products include:
Parnate Tablets 1527

Food Interactions

Alcohol (Chronic heavy alcohol users, 3 or more drinks per day, should consult their physicians for advice on when and how they should take pain relievers including acetaminophen).

TYLENOL SINUS CONGESTION & PAIN NIGHTTIME CAPLETS WITH COOL BURST

(Acetaminophen, Doxylamine Succinate, Pseudoephedrine Hydrochloride)................................ ◘778

TYLENOL SORE THROAT DAYTIME LIQUID WITH COOL BURST

(Acetaminophen) .... ◘790

Food Interactions

Alcohol (Concomitant consumption of alcohol may cause liver damage).

TYLENOL SORE THROAT NIGHTTIME LIQUID WITH COOL BURST

(Acetaminophen, Diphenhydramine Hydrochloride)....... ◘790

May interact with hypnotics and sedatives, tranquilizers, and certain other agents. Compounds in these categories include:

Alprazolam (May increase drowsiness effect). Products include:
Niravam Orally Disintegrating Tablets 3092

Buspirone Hydrochloride (May increase drowsiness effect).
No products indexed under this heading.

Chlordiazepoxide (May increase drowsiness effect).
No products indexed under this heading.

Chlordiazepoxide Hydrochloride (May increase drowsiness effect). Products include:
Librium Capsules 3347

Chlorpromazine (May increase drowsiness effect).
No products indexed under this heading.

Chlorpromazine Hydrochloride (May increase drowsiness effect).
No products indexed under this heading.

Chlorprothixene (May increase drowsiness effect).
No products indexed under this heading.

Chlorprothixene Hydrochloride (May increase drowsiness effect).
No products indexed under this heading.

Clorazepate Dipotassium (May increase drowsiness effect). Products include:
Tranxene 2474

Diazepam (May increase drowsiness effect). Products include:
Diastat Rectal Delivery System 3343
Valium Tablets 2819

Droperidol (May increase drowsiness effect).
No products indexed under this heading.

Estazolam (May increase drowsiness effect). Products include:
ProSom Tablets 517

Ethchlorvynol (May increase drowsiness effect).
No products indexed under this heading.

Ethinamate (May increase drowsiness effect).
No products indexed under this heading.

Fluphenazine Decanoate (May increase drowsiness effect).
No products indexed under this heading.

Fluphenazine Enanthate (May increase drowsiness effect).
No products indexed under this heading.

Fluphenazine Hydrochloride (May increase drowsiness effect).
No products indexed under this heading.

Flurazepam Hydrochloride (May increase drowsiness effect). Products include:
Dalmane Capsules 3342

Glutethimide (May increase drowsiness effect).
No products indexed under this heading.

Haloperidol (May increase drowsiness effect).
No products indexed under this heading.

Haloperidol Decanoate (May increase drowsiness effect).
No products indexed under this heading.

Hydroxyzine Hydrochloride (May increase drowsiness effect).
No products indexed under this heading.

Lorazepam (May increase drowsiness effect).
No products indexed under this heading.

Loxapine Hydrochloride (May increase drowsiness effect).
No products indexed under this heading.

Loxapine Succinate (May increase drowsiness effect).
No products indexed under this heading.

Meprobamate (May increase drowsiness effect).
No products indexed under this heading.

Mesoridazine Besylate (May increase drowsiness effect).
No products indexed under this heading.

Midazolam Hydrochloride (May increase drowsiness effect).
No products indexed under this heading.

Molindone Hydrochloride (May increase drowsiness effect). Products include:
Moban Tablets 1119

Oxazepam (May increase drowsiness effect).
No products indexed under this heading.

Perphenazine (May increase drowsiness effect).
No products indexed under this heading.

Prazepam (May increase drowsiness effect).
No products indexed under this heading.

Prochlorperazine (May increase drowsiness effect).
No products indexed under this heading.

Promethazine Hydrochloride (May increase drowsiness effect). Products include:
Phenergan Tablets and Suppositories.............................. 3440

Propofol (May increase drowsiness effect).
No products indexed under this heading.

Quazepam (May increase drowsiness effect).
No products indexed under this heading.

Ramelteon (May increase drowsiness effect). Products include:
Rozerem Tablets 3231

Secobarbital Sodium (May increase drowsiness effect).
No products indexed under this heading.

Temazepam (May increase drowsiness effect). Products include:
Restoril Capsules 1860

Thioridazine Hydrochloride (May increase drowsiness effect). Products include:
Thioridazine Hydrochloride Tablets 2163

Thiothixene (May increase drowsiness effect). Products include:
Thiothixene Capsules 2165

Triazolam (May increase drowsiness effect).
No products indexed under this heading.

Trifluoperazine Hydrochloride (May increase drowsiness effect).
No products indexed under this heading.

Zaleplon (May increase drowsiness effect). Products include:
Sonata Capsules 1717

Zolpidem Tartrate (May increase drowsiness effect). Products include:
Ambien Tablets 2851
Ambien CR Tablets 2855

Food Interactions

Alcohol (Concomitant consumption of alcohol with acetaminophen may cause liver damage; alcohol may increase drowsiness effect).

TYLENOL WITH CODEINE TABLETS

(Acetaminophen, Codeine Phosphate).. 2391

May interact with anticholinergics and central nervous system depressants. Compounds in these categories include:

Alfentanil Hydrochloride (Coadministration with other CNS depressants may exhibit an additive CNS depression).
No products indexed under this heading.

Alprazolam (Co-administration with other CNS depressants may exhibit an additive CNS depression). Products include:
Niravam Orally Disintegrating Tablets 3092

Aprobarbital (Co-administration with other CNS depressants may exhibit an additive CNS depression).
No products indexed under this heading.

Atropine Sulfate (Co-administration of codeine with anticholinergics may produce paralytic ileus). Products include:
Donnatal Extentabs 2493

Belladonna Alkaloids (Co-administration of codeine with anticholinergics may produce paralytic ileus). Products include:
Hyland's Teething Tablets 830

Benztropine Mesylate (Co-administration of codeine with anticholinergics may produce paralytic ileus).
No products indexed under this heading.

Biperiden Hydrochloride (Co-administration of codeine with anticholinergics may produce paralytic ileus).
No products indexed under this heading.

Buprenorphine Hydrochloride (Co-administration with other CNS depressants may exhibit an additive CNS depression). Products include:
Buprenex Injectable 2716
Suboxone Tablets 2717
Subutex Tablets 2717

Buspirone Hydrochloride (Co-administration with other CNS depressants may exhibit an additive CNS depression).
No products indexed under this heading.

Butabarbital (Co-administration with other CNS depressants may exhibit an additive CNS depression).
No products indexed under this heading.

Butalbital (Co-administration with other CNS depressants may exhibit an additive CNS depression).
No products indexed under this heading.

Chlordiazepoxide (Co-administration with other CNS depressants may exhibit an additive CNS depression).
No products indexed under this heading.

Chlordiazepoxide Hydrochloride (Co-administration with other CNS depressants may exhibit an additive CNS depression). Products include:
Librium Capsules 3347

Chlorpromazine (Co-administration with other CNS depressants may exhibit an additive CNS depression).
No products indexed under this heading.

Chlorpromazine Hydrochloride (Co-administration with other CNS depressants may exhibit an additive CNS depression).
No products indexed under this heading.

Chlorprothixene (Co-administration with other CNS depressants may exhibit an additive CNS depression).
No products indexed under this heading.

Chlorprothixene Hydrochloride (Co-administration with other CNS depressants may exhibit an additive CNS depression).
No products indexed under this heading.

Chlorprothixene Lactate (Co-administration with other CNS depressants may exhibit an additive CNS depression).
No products indexed under this heading.

Clidinium Bromide (Co-administration of codeine with anticholinergics may produce paralytic ileus).
No products indexed under this heading.

Clorazepate Dipotassium (Co-administration with other CNS depressants may exhibit an additive CNS depression). Products include:
Tranxene 2474

Clozapine (Co-administration with other CNS depressants may exhibit an additive CNS depression). Products include:
Clozaril Tablets 2184
FazaClo Orally Disintegrating Tablets 551

Desflurane (Co-administration with other CNS depressants may exhibit an additive CNS depression).
No products indexed under this heading.

Dezocine (Co-administration with other CNS depressants may exhibit an additive CNS depression).
No products indexed under this heading.

Diazepam (Co-administration with other CNS depressants may exhibit an additive CNS depression). Products include:
Diastat Rectal Delivery System 3343
Valium Tablets 2819

Dicyclomine Hydrochloride (Co-administration of codeine with anticholinergics may produce paralytic ileus). Products include:
Bentyl Capsules 697
Bentyl Injection 697
Bentyl Syrup 697
Bentyl Tablets 697

Droperidol (Co-administration with other CNS depressants may exhibit an additive CNS depression).
No products indexed under this heading.

Enflurane (Co-administration with other CNS depressants may exhibit an additive CNS depression).
No products indexed under this heading.

Estazolam (Co-administration with other CNS depressants may exhibit an additive CNS depression). Products include:
ProSom Tablets 517

Ethanol (Co-administration with other CNS depressants may exhibit an additive CNS depression).
No products indexed under this heading.

Ethchlorvynol (Co-administration with other CNS depressants may exhibit an additive CNS depression).
No products indexed under this heading.

Ethinamate (Co-administration with other CNS depressants may exhibit an additive CNS depression).
No products indexed under this heading.

Ethyl Alcohol (Co-administration with other CNS depressants may exhibit an additive CNS depression).
No products indexed under this heading.

Fentanyl (Co-administration with other CNS depressants may exhibit an additive CNS depression). Products include:
Duragesic Transdermal System 2373
Ionsys Transdermal System 2379

Fentanyl Citrate (Co-administration with other CNS depressants may exhibit an additive CNS depression). Products include:
Actiq 979

Fluphenazine Decanoate (Co-administration with other CNS depressants may exhibit an additive CNS depression).
No products indexed under this heading.

Fluphenazine Enanthate (Co-administration with other CNS depressants may exhibit an additive CNS depression).
No products indexed under this heading.

Fluphenazine Hydrochloride (Co-administration with other CNS depressants may exhibit an additive CNS depression).
No products indexed under this heading.

Flurazepam Hydrochloride (Co-administration with other CNS depressants may exhibit an additive CNS depression). Products include:
Dalmane Capsules 3342

Glutethimide (Co-administration with other CNS depressants may exhibit an additive CNS depression).
No products indexed under this heading.

Glycopyrrolate (Co-administration of codeine with anticholinergics may produce paralytic ileus).
No products indexed under this heading.

Haloperidol (Co-administration with other CNS depressants may exhibit an additive CNS depression).
No products indexed under this heading.

Haloperidol Decanoate (Co-administration with other CNS depressants may exhibit an additive CNS depression).
No products indexed under this heading.

Hydrocodone Bitartrate (Co-administration with other CNS depressants may exhibit an additive CNS depression). Products include:
Hycodan 1116
Hycotuss Expectorant Syrup 1117
Vicodin Tablets 535
Vicodin ES Tablets 536
Vicodin HP Tablets 538
Vicoprofen Tablets 539
Zydone Tablets 1139

Hydrocodone Polistirex (Co-administration with other CNS depressants may exhibit an additive CNS depression). Products include:
Tussionex Pennkinetic Extended-Release Suspension 3327

Hydromorphone Hydrochloride (Co-administration with other CNS depressants may exhibit an additive CNS depression). Products include:
Dilaudid 440
Dilaudid Non-Sterile Powder 440
Dilaudid Oral Liquid 445
Dilaudid Rectal Suppositories 440
Dilaudid Tablets 440
Dilaudid Tablets - 8 mg 445
Dilaudid-HP 442

Hydroxyzine Hydrochloride (Co-administration with other CNS depressants may exhibit an additive CNS depression).
No products indexed under this heading.

Hyoscyamine (Co-administration of codeine with anticholinergics may produce paralytic ileus).
No products indexed under this heading.

Hyoscyamine Sulfate (Co-administration of codeine with anticholinergics may produce paralytic ileus). Products include:
Donnatal Extentabs 2493
Prosed/DS Tablets 1157

Ipratropium Bromide (Co-administration of codeine with anticholinergics may produce paralytic ileus). Products include:
Atrovent Inhalation Solution 835
Atrovent HFA Inhalation Aerosol 841
Atrovent Nasal Spray 0.03% 837
Atrovent Nasal Spray 0.06% 839
Combivent Inhalation Aerosol 847
DuoNeb Inhalation Solution 1058

Isoflurane (Co-administration with other CNS depressants may exhibit an additive CNS depression).
No products indexed under this heading.

Ketamine Hydrochloride (Co-administration with other CNS depressants may exhibit an additive CNS depression).
No products indexed under this heading.

Levomethadyl Acetate Hydrochloride (Co-administration with other CNS depressants may exhibit an additive CNS depression).
No products indexed under this heading.

Levorphanol Tartrate (Co-administration with other CNS depressants may exhibit an additive CNS depression).
No products indexed under this heading.

Lorazepam (Co-administration with other CNS depressants may exhibit an additive CNS depression).
No products indexed under this heading.

Loxapine Hydrochloride (Co-administration with other CNS depressants may exhibit an additive CNS depression).
No products indexed under this heading.

Loxapine Succinate (Co-administration with other CNS depressants may exhibit an additive CNS depression).
No products indexed under this heading.

Mepenzolate Bromide (Co-administration of codeine with anticholinergics may produce paralytic ileus).
No products indexed under this heading.

Meperidine Hydrochloride (Co-administration with other CNS depressants may exhibit an additive CNS depression).
No products indexed under this heading.

Mephobarbital (Co-administration with other CNS depressants may exhibit an additive CNS depression).
No products indexed under this heading.

IMPORTANT NOTE: Always consult each drug listing in the patient's regimen for possible interactions.

Meprobamate (Co-administration with other CNS depressants may exhibit an additive CNS depression).
No products indexed under this heading.

Mesoridazine Besylate (Co-administration with other CNS depressants may exhibit an additive CNS depression).
No products indexed under this heading.

Methadone Hydrochloride (Co-administration with other CNS depressants may exhibit an additive CNS depression).
No products indexed under this heading.

Methohexital Sodium (Co-administration with other CNS depressants may exhibit an additive CNS depression).
No products indexed under this heading.

Methotrimeprazine (Co-administration with other CNS depressants may exhibit an additive CNS depression).
No products indexed under this heading.

Methoxyflurane (Co-administration with other CNS depressants may exhibit an additive CNS depression).
No products indexed under this heading.

Midazolam Hydrochloride (Co-administration with other CNS depressants may exhibit an additive CNS depression).
No products indexed under this heading.

Molindone Hydrochloride (Co-administration with other CNS depressants may exhibit an additive CNS depression). Products include:
Moban Tablets ... 1119

Morphine Sulfate (Co-administration with other CNS depressants may exhibit an additive CNS depression). Products include:
Avinza Capsules ... 1741
Kadian Capsules ... 577
MS Contin Tablets ... 2701

Olanzapine (Co-administration with other CNS depressants may exhibit an additive CNS depression). Products include:
Symbyax Capsules ... 1819
Zyprexa Tablets ... 1830
Zyprexa IntraMuscular ... 1830
Zyprexa ZYDIS Orally Disintegrating Tablets ... 1830

Oxazepam (Co-administration with other CNS depressants may exhibit an additive CNS depression).
No products indexed under this heading.

Oxybutynin Chloride (Co-administration of codeine with anticholinergics may produce paralytic ileus). Products include:
Ditropan XL Extended-Release Tablets ... 2413

Oxycodone Hydrochloride (Co-administration with other CNS depressants may exhibit an additive CNS depression). Products include:
OxyContin Tablets ... 2703
OxyFast Oral Concentrate Solution ... 2708
OxyIR Capsules ... 2708
Percocet Tablets ... 1131
Percodan Tablets ... 1132

Pentobarbital Sodium (Co-administration with other CNS depressants may exhibit an additive CNS depression). Products include:
Nembutal Sodium Solution, USP ... 2470

Perphenazine (Co-administration with other CNS depressants may exhibit an additive CNS depression).
No products indexed under this heading.

Phenobarbital (Co-administration with other CNS depressants may exhibit an additive CNS depression). Products include:
Donnatal Extentabs ... 2493

Prazepam (Co-administration with other CNS depressants may exhibit an additive CNS depression).
No products indexed under this heading.

Prochlorperazine (Co-administration with other CNS depressants may exhibit an additive CNS depression).
No products indexed under this heading.

Procyclidine Hydrochloride (Co-administration of codeine with anticholinergics may produce paralytic ileus).
No products indexed under this heading.

Promethazine Hydrochloride (Co-administration with other CNS depressants may exhibit an additive CNS depression). Products include:
Phenergan Tablets and Suppositories ... 3440

Propantheline Bromide (Co-administration of codeine with anticholinergics may produce paralytic ileus).
No products indexed under this heading.

Propofol (Co-administration with other CNS depressants may exhibit an additive CNS depression).
No products indexed under this heading.

Propoxyphene Hydrochloride (Co-administration with other CNS depressants may exhibit an additive CNS depression).
No products indexed under this heading.

Propoxyphene Napsylate (Co-administration with other CNS depressants may exhibit an additive CNS depression).
No products indexed under this heading.

Quazepam (Co-administration with other CNS depressants may exhibit an additive CNS depression).
No products indexed under this heading.

Quetiapine Fumarate (Co-administration with other CNS depressants may exhibit an additive CNS depression). Products include:
Seroquel Tablets ... 690

Remifentanil Hydrochloride (Co-administration with other CNS depressants may exhibit an additive CNS depression).
No products indexed under this heading.

Risperidone (Co-administration with other CNS depressants may exhibit an additive CNS depression). Products include:
Risperdal ... 1676
Risperdal Consta Long-Acting Injection ... 1682
Risperdal M-Tab Orally Disintegrating Tablets ... 1676

Scopolamine (Co-administration of codeine with anticholinergics may produce paralytic ileus). Products include:
Transderm Scōp Transdermal Therapeutic System ... 2177

Scopolamine Hydrobromide (Co-administration of codeine with anticholinergics may produce paralytic ileus). Products include:
Donnatal Extentabs ... 2493

Secobarbital Sodium (Co-administration with other CNS depressants may exhibit an additive CNS depression).
No products indexed under this heading.

Sevoflurane (Co-administration with other CNS depressants may exhibit an additive CNS depression). Products include:
Ultane Liquid for Inhalation ... 531

Sodium Oxybate (Co-administration with other CNS depressants may exhibit an additive CNS depression). Products include:
Xyrem Oral Solution ... 1688

Sufentanil Citrate (Co-administration with other CNS depressants may exhibit an additive CNS depression).
No products indexed under this heading.

Temazepam (Co-administration with other CNS depressants may exhibit an additive CNS depression). Products include:
Restoril Capsules ... 1860

Thiamylal Sodium (Co-administration with other CNS depressants may exhibit an additive CNS depression).
No products indexed under this heading.

Thioridazine Hydrochloride (Co-administration with other CNS depressants may exhibit an additive CNS depression). Products include:
Thioridazine Hydrochloride Tablets ... 2163

Thiothixene (Co-administration with other CNS depressants may exhibit an additive CNS depression). Products include:
Thiothixene Capsules ... 2165

Tolterodine Tartrate (Co-administration of codeine with anticholinergics may produce paralytic ileus). Products include:
Detrol Tablets ... 2628
Detrol LA Capsules ... 2631

Triazolam (Co-administration with other CNS depressants may exhibit an additive CNS depression).
No products indexed under this heading.

Tridihexethyl Chloride (Co-administration of codeine with anticholinergics may produce paralytic ileus).
No products indexed under this heading.

Trifluoperazine Hydrochloride (Co-administration with other CNS depressants may exhibit an additive CNS depression).
No products indexed under this heading.

Trihexyphenidyl Hydrochloride (Co-administration of codeine with anticholinergics may produce paralytic ileus).
No products indexed under this heading.

Zaleplon (Co-administration with other CNS depressants may exhibit an additive CNS depression). Products include:
Sonata Capsules ... 1717

Ziprasidone Hydrochloride (Co-administration with other CNS depressants may exhibit an additive CNS depression). Products include:
Geodon Capsules ... 2529

Zolpidem Tartrate (Co-administration with other CNS depressants may exhibit an additive CNS depression). Products include:
Ambien Tablets ... 2851
Ambien CR Tablets ... 2855

Food Interactions

Alcohol (Concurrent use with other CNS depressants may exhibit an additive CNS depression).

WOMEN'S TYLENOL MENSTRUAL RELIEF CAPLETS
(Acetaminophen, Pamabrom) ... 803

TYLENOL ALLERGY MULTI-SYMPTOM CAPLETS WITH COOL BURST AND GELCAPS
(Acetaminophen, Chlorpheniramine Maleate, Phenylephrine Hydrochloride) ... 1872
See Tylenol Severe Allergy Caplets

TYLENOL ALLERGY MULTI-SYMPTOM NIGHTTIME CAPLETS WITH COOL BURST
(Acetaminophen, Diphenhydramine Hydrochloride, Phenylephrine Hydrochloride) ... 1872
See Tylenol Severe Allergy Caplets

TYLENOL SEVERE ALLERGY CAPLETS
(Acetaminophen, Diphenhydramine Hydrochloride) ... 1872
May interact with hypnotics and sedatives, monoamine oxidase inhibitors, tranquilizers, and certain other agents. Compounds in these categories include:

Alprazolam (Concurrent use may increase drowsiness). Products include:
Niravam Orally Disintegrating Tablets ... 3092

Buspirone Hydrochloride (Concurrent use may increase drowsiness).
No products indexed under this heading.

Chlordiazepoxide (Concurrent use may increase drowsiness).
No products indexed under this heading.

Chlordiazepoxide Hydrochloride (Concurrent use may increase drowsiness). Products include:
Librium Capsules ... 3347

Chlorpromazine (Concurrent use may increase drowsiness).
No products indexed under this heading.

Chlorpromazine Hydrochloride (Concurrent use may increase drowsiness).
No products indexed under this heading.

Chlorprothixene (Concurrent use may increase drowsiness).
No products indexed under this heading.

Chlorprothixene Hydrochloride (Concurrent use may increase drowsiness).
No products indexed under this heading.

Clorazepate Dipotassium (Concurrent use may increase drowsiness). Products include:
Tranxene 2474

Diazepam (Concurrent use may increase drowsiness). Products include:
Diastat Rectal Delivery System 3343
Valium Tablets 2819

Droperidol (Concurrent use may increase drowsiness).
No products indexed under this heading.

Estazolam (Concurrent use may increase drowsiness effect). Products include:
ProSom Tablets 517

Ethchlorvynol (Concurrent use may increase drowsiness effect).
No products indexed under this heading.

Ethinamate (Concurrent use may increase drowsiness effect).
No products indexed under this heading.

Fluphenazine Decanoate (Concurrent use may increase drowsiness).
No products indexed under this heading.

Fluphenazine Enanthate (Concurrent use may increase drowsiness).
No products indexed under this heading.

Fluphenazine Hydrochloride (Concurrent use may increase drowsiness).
No products indexed under this heading.

Flurazepam Hydrochloride (Concurrent use may increase drowsiness effect). Products include:
Dalmane Capsules 3342

Glutethimide (Concurrent use may increase drowsiness effect).
No products indexed under this heading.

Haloperidol (Concurrent use may increase drowsiness).
No products indexed under this heading.

Haloperidol Decanoate (Concurrent use may increase drowsiness).
No products indexed under this heading.

Hydroxyzine Hydrochloride (Concurrent use may increase drowsiness).
No products indexed under this heading.

Isocarboxazid (Concurrent and/or sequential use with MAO inhibitors is not recommended).
No products indexed under this heading.

Lorazepam (Concurrent use may increase drowsiness effect).
No products indexed under this heading.

Loxapine Hydrochloride (Concurrent use may increase drowsiness).
No products indexed under this heading.

Loxapine Succinate (Concurrent use may increase drowsiness).
No products indexed under this heading.

Meprobamate (Concurrent use may increase drowsiness).
No products indexed under this heading.

Mesoridazine Besylate (Concurrent use may increase drowsiness).
No products indexed under this heading.

Midazolam Hydrochloride (Concurrent use may increase drowsiness effect).
No products indexed under this heading.

Moclobemide (Concurrent and/or sequential use with MAO inhibitors is not recommended).
No products indexed under this heading.

Molindone Hydrochloride (Concurrent use may increase drowsiness). Products include:
Moban Tablets 1119

Oxazepam (Concurrent use may increase drowsiness).
No products indexed under this heading.

Pargyline Hydrochloride (Concurrent and/or sequential use with MAO inhibitors is not recommended).
No products indexed under this heading.

Perphenazine (Concurrent use may increase drowsiness).
No products indexed under this heading.

Phenelzine Sulfate (Concurrent and/or sequential use with MAO inhibitors is not recommended).
No products indexed under this heading.

Prazepam (Concurrent use may increase drowsiness).
No products indexed under this heading.

Procarbazine Hydrochloride (Concurrent and/or sequential use with MAO inhibitors is not recommended). Products include:
Matulane Capsules 3191

Prochlorperazine (Concurrent use may increase drowsiness).
No products indexed under this heading.

Promethazine Hydrochloride (Concurrent use may increase drowsiness). Products include:
Phenergan Tablets and Suppositories 3440

Propofol (Concurrent use may increase drowsiness effect).
No products indexed under this heading.

Quazepam (Concurrent use may increase drowsiness effect).
No products indexed under this heading.

Ramelteon (Concurrent use may increase drowsiness effect). Products include:
Rozerem Tablets 3231

Secobarbital Sodium (Concurrent use may increase drowsiness effect).
No products indexed under this heading.

Selegiline Hydrochloride (Concurrent and/or sequential use with MAO inhibitors is not recommended). Products include:
Eldepryl Capsules 3208
Zelapar Tablets 3372

Temazepam (Concurrent use may increase drowsiness effect). Products include:
Restoril Capsules 1860

Thioridazine Hydrochloride (Concurrent use may increase drowsiness). Products include:
Thioridazine Hydrochloride Tablets 2163

Thiothixene (Concurrent use may increase drowsiness). Products include:
Thiothixene Capsules 2165

Tranylcypromine Sulfate (Concurrent and/or sequential use with MAO inhibitors is not recommended). Products include:
Parnate Tablets 1527

Triazolam (Concurrent use may increase drowsiness effect).
No products indexed under this heading.

Trifluoperazine Hydrochloride (Concurrent use may increase drowsiness).
No products indexed under this heading.

Zaleplon (Concurrent use may increase drowsiness effect). Products include:
Sonata Capsules 1717

Zolpidem Tartrate (Concurrent use may increase drowsiness effect). Products include:
Ambien Tablets 2851
Ambien CR Tablets 2855

Food Interactions

Alcohol (Concurrent use may increase drowsiness effect; chronic heavy alcohol abusers, 3 or more drinks per day, may be at increased risk of liver toxicity from excessive acetaminophen use).

TYLENOL ARTHRITIS PAIN EXTENDED RELEASE CAPLETS AND GELTABS

(Acetaminophen) 1870
See Regular Strength Tylenol Tablets

TYLENOL CHEST CONGESTION CAPLETS WITH COOL BURST

(Acetaminophen, Guaifenesin) 1872

Food Interactions

Alcohol (Concurrent use may increase drowsiness effect; chronic heavy alcohol abusers, 3 or more drinks per day, may be at increased risk of liver toxicity from excessive acetaminophen use).

TYLENOL CHEST CONGESTION LIQUID WITH COOL BURST

(Acetaminophen, Guaifenesin) 1872
See Tylenol Chest Congestion Caplets with Cool Burst

CHILDREN'S TYLENOL SUSPENSION LIQUID AND MELTAWAYS

(Acetaminophen) 1878
None cited in PDR database.

CHILDREN'S TYLENOL PLUS COLD SUSPENSION LIQUID

(Acetaminophen, Chlorpheniramine Maleate, Phenylephrine Hydrochloride) 1879
May interact with hypnotics and sedatives, monoamine oxidase inhibitors, and tranquilizers. Compounds in these categories include:

Alprazolam (Concurrent use may increase drowiness effect). Products include:
Niravam Orally Disintegrating Tablets 3092

Buspirone Hydrochloride (Concurrent use may increase drowiness effect).
No products indexed under this heading.

Chlordiazepoxide (Concurrent use may increase drowiness effect).
No products indexed under this heading.

Chlordiazepoxide Hydrochloride (Concurrent use may increase drowiness effect). Products include:
Librium Capsules 3347

Chlorpromazine (Concurrent use may increase drowiness effect).
No products indexed under this heading.

Chlorpromazine Hydrochloride (Concurrent use may increase drowiness effect).
No products indexed under this heading.

Chlorprothixene (Concurrent use may increase drowiness effect).
No products indexed under this heading.

Chlorprothixene Hydrochloride (Concurrent use may increase drowiness effect).
No products indexed under this heading.

Clorazepate Dipotassium (Concurrent use may increase drowiness effect). Products include:
Tranxene 2474

Diazepam (Concurrent use may increase drowiness effect). Products include:
Diastat Rectal Delivery System 3343
Valium Tablets 2819

Droperidol (Concurrent use may increase drowiness effect).
No products indexed under this heading.

Estazolam (Concurrent use may increase drowsiness effect). Products include:
ProSom Tablets 517

Ethchlorvynol (Concurrent use may increase drowsiness effect).
No products indexed under this heading.

Ethinamate (Concurrent use may increase drowsiness effect).
No products indexed under this heading.

Fluphenazine Decanoate (Concurrent use may increase drowiness effect).
No products indexed under this heading.

Fluphenazine Enanthate (Concurrent use may increase drowiness effect).
No products indexed under this heading.

Fluphenazine Hydrochloride (Concurrent use may increase drowiness effect).
No products indexed under this heading.

Flurazepam Hydrochloride (Concurrent use may increase drowsiness effect). Products include:
Dalmane Capsules 3342

Glutethimide (Concurrent use may increase drowsiness effect).
No products indexed under this heading.

Haloperidol (Concurrent use may increase drowiness effect).
No products indexed under this heading.

Haloperidol Decanoate (Concurrent use may increase drowiness effect).
No products indexed under this heading.

Hydroxyzine Hydrochloride (Concurrent use may increase drowsiness effect).

 No products indexed under this heading.

Isocarboxazid (Concurrent and/or sequential use with MAO inhibitors is not recommended).

 No products indexed under this heading.

Lorazepam (Concurrent use may increase drowsiness effect).

 No products indexed under this heading.

Midazolam Hydrochloride (Concurrent use may increase drowsiness effect).

 No products indexed under this heading.

Moclobemide (Concurrent and/or sequential use with MAO inhibitors is not recommended).

 No products indexed under this heading.

Pargyline Hydrochloride (Concurrent and/or sequential use with MAO inhibitors is not recommended).

 No products indexed under this heading.

Phenelzine Sulfate (Concurrent and/or sequential use with MAO inhibitors is not recommended).

 No products indexed under this heading.

Procarbazine Hydrochloride (Concurrent and/or sequential use with MAO inhibitors is not recommended). Products include:

 Matulane Capsules 3191

Propofol (Concurrent use may increase drowsiness effect).

 No products indexed under this heading.

Quazepam (Concurrent use may increase drowsiness effect).

 No products indexed under this heading.

Ramelteon (Concurrent use may increase drowsiness effect). Products include:

 Rozerem Tablets 3231

Secobarbital Sodium (Concurrent use may increase drowsiness effect).

 No products indexed under this heading.

Selegiline Hydrochloride (Concurrent and/or sequential use with MAO inhibitors is not recommended). Products include:

 Eldepryl Capsules 3208
 Zelapar Tablets 3372

Temazepam (Concurrent use may increase drowsiness effect). Products include:

 Restoril Capsules 1860

Tranylcypromine Sulfate (Concurrent and/or sequential use with MAO inhibitors is not recommended). Products include:

 Parnate Tablets 1527

Triazolam (Concurrent use may increase drowsiness effect).

 No products indexed under this heading.

Zaleplon (Concurrent use may increase drowsiness effect). Products include:

 Sonata Capsules 1717

Zolpidem Tartrate (Concurrent use may increase drowsiness effect). Products include:

 Ambien Tablets 2851
 Ambien CR Tablets 2855

CHILDREN'S TYLENOL PLUS COLD & ALLERGY SUSPENSION LIQUID

(Acetaminophen, Diphenhydramine Hydrochloride, Phenylephrine Hydrochloride)..................................... 1878

May interact with hypnotics and sedatives, monoamine oxidase inhibitors, and tranquilizers. Compounds in these categories include:

Alprazolam (Concurrent use may increase drowsiness). Products include:

 Niravam Orally Disintegrating Tablets.. 3092

Buspirone Hydrochloride (Concurrent use may increase drowsiness).

 No products indexed under this heading.

Chlordiazepoxide (Concurrent use may increase drowsiness).

 No products indexed under this heading.

Chlordiazepoxide Hydrochloride (Concurrent use may increase drowsiness). Products include:

 Librium Capsules 3347

Chlorpromazine (Concurrent use may increase drowsiness).

 No products indexed under this heading.

Chlorpromazine Hydrochloride (Concurrent use may increase drowsiness).

 No products indexed under this heading.

Chlorprothixene (Concurrent use may increase drowsiness).

 No products indexed under this heading.

Chlorprothixene Hydrochloride (Concurrent use may increase drowsiness).

 No products indexed under this heading.

Clorazepate Dipotassium (Concurrent use may increase drowsiness). Products include:

 Tranxene ... 2474

Diazepam (Concurrent use may increase drowsiness). Products include:

 Diastat Rectal Delivery System 3343
 Valium Tablets 2819

Droperidol (Concurrent use may increase drowsiness).

 No products indexed under this heading.

Estazolam (Concurrent use may increase drowsiness effect). Products include:

 ProSom Tablets 517

Ethchlorvynol (Concurrent use may increase drowsiness effect).

 No products indexed under this heading.

Ethinamate (Concurrent use may increase drowsiness effect).

 No products indexed under this heading.

Fluphenazine Decanoate (Concurrent use may increase drowsiness).

 No products indexed under this heading.

Fluphenazine Enanthate (Concurrent use may increase drowsiness).

 No products indexed under this heading.

Fluphenazine Hydrochloride (Concurrent use may increase drowsiness).

 No products indexed under this heading.

Flurazepam Hydrochloride (Concurrent use may increase drowsiness effect). Products include:

 Dalmane Capsules 3342

Glutethimide (Concurrent use may increase drowsiness effect).

 No products indexed under this heading.

Haloperidol (Concurrent use may increase drowsiness).

 No products indexed under this heading.

Haloperidol Decanoate (Concurrent use may increase drowsiness).

 No products indexed under this heading.

Hydroxyzine Hydrochloride (Concurrent use may increase drowsiness).

 No products indexed under this heading.

Isocarboxazid (Concurrent and/or sequential use with MAO inhibitors is not recommended).

 No products indexed under this heading.

Lorazepam (Concurrent use may increase drowsiness effect).

 No products indexed under this heading.

Loxapine Hydrochloride (Concurrent use may increase drowsiness).

 No products indexed under this heading.

Loxapine Succinate (Concurrent use may increase drowsiness).

 No products indexed under this heading.

Meprobamate (Concurrent use may increase drowsiness).

 No products indexed under this heading.

Mesoridazine Besylate (Concurrent use may increase drowsiness).

 No products indexed under this heading.

Midazolam Hydrochloride (Concurrent use may increase drowsiness effect).

 No products indexed under this heading.

Moclobemide (Concurrent and/or sequential use with MAO inhibitors is not recommended).

 No products indexed under this heading.

Molindone Hydrochloride (Concurrent use may increase drowsiness). Products include:

 Moban Tablets 1119

Oxazepam (Concurrent use may increase drowsiness).

 No products indexed under this heading.

Pargyline Hydrochloride (Concurrent and/or sequential use with MAO inhibitors is not recommended).

 No products indexed under this heading.

Perphenazine (Concurrent use may increase drowsiness).

 No products indexed under this heading.

Phenelzine Sulfate (Concurrent and/or sequential use with MAO inhibitors is not recommended).

 No products indexed under this heading.

Prazepam (Concurrent use may increase drowsiness).

 No products indexed under this heading.

Procarbazine Hydrochloride (Concurrent and/or sequential use with MAO inhibitors is not recommended). Products include:

 Matulane Capsules 3191

Prochlorperazine (Concurrent use may increase drowsiness).

 No products indexed under this heading.

Promethazine Hydrochloride (Concurrent use may increase drowsiness). Products include:

 Phenergan Tablets and Suppositories............................... 3440

Propofol (Concurrent use may increase drowsiness effect).

 No products indexed under this heading.

Quazepam (Concurrent use may increase drowsiness effect).

 No products indexed under this heading.

Ramelteon (Concurrent use may increase drowsiness effect). Products include:

 Rozerem Tablets 3231

Secobarbital Sodium (Concurrent use may increase drowsiness effect).

 No products indexed under this heading.

Selegiline Hydrochloride (Concurrent and/or sequential use with MAO inhibitors is not recommended). Products include:

 Eldepryl Capsules 3208
 Zelapar Tablets 3372

Temazepam (Concurrent use may increase drowsiness effect). Products include:

 Restoril Capsules 1860

Thioridazine Hydrochloride (Concurrent use may increase drowsiness). Products include:

 Thioridazine Hydrochloride Tablets... 2163

Thiothixene (Concurrent use may increase drowsiness). Products include:

 Thiothixene Capsules 2165

Tranylcypromine Sulfate (Concurrent and/or sequential use with MAO inhibitors is not recommended). Products include:

 Parnate Tablets 1527

Triazolam (Concurrent use may increase drowsiness effect).

 No products indexed under this heading.

Trifluoperazine Hydrochloride (Concurrent use may increase drowsiness).

 No products indexed under this heading.

Zaleplon (Concurrent use may increase drowsiness effect). Products include:

 Sonata Capsules 1717

Zolpidem Tartrate (Concurrent use may increase drowsiness effect). Products include:

 Ambien Tablets 2851
 Ambien CR Tablets 2855

(▨ Described in PDR For Nonprescription Drugs) (☉ Described in PDR For Ophthalmic Medicines™)

CHILDREN'S TYLENOL PLUS COUGH & RUNNY NOSE SUSPENSION LIQUID

(Acetaminophen, Chlorpheniramine Maleate, Dextromethorphan Hydrobromide) 1879

May interact with hypnotics and sedatives, monoamine oxidase inhibitors, and tranquilizers. Compounds in these categories include:

Alprazolam (Concurrent use may increase drowsiness effect). Products include:
Niravam Orally Disintegrating Tablets .. 3092

Buspirone Hydrochloride (Concurrent use may increase drowsiness effect).
No products indexed under this heading.

Chlordiazepoxide (Concurrent use may increase drowsiness effect).
No products indexed under this heading.

Chlordiazepoxide Hydrochloride (Concurrent use may increase drowsiness effect). Products include:
Librium Capsules 3347

Chlorpromazine (Concurrent use may increase drowsiness effect).
No products indexed under this heading.

Chlorpromazine Hydrochloride (Concurrent use may increase drowsiness effect).
No products indexed under this heading.

Chlorprothixene (Concurrent use may increase drowsiness effect).
No products indexed under this heading.

Chlorprothixene Hydrochloride (Concurrent use may increase drowsiness effect).
No products indexed under this heading.

Clorazepate Dipotassium (Concurrent use may increase drowsiness effect). Products include:
Tranxene .. 2474

Diazepam (Concurrent use may increase drowsiness effect). Products include:
Diastat Rectal Delivery System 3343
Valium Tablets 2819

Droperidol (Concurrent use may increase drowsiness effect).
No products indexed under this heading.

Estazolam (Concurrent use may increase drowsiness effect). Products include:
ProSom Tablets 517

Ethchlorvynol (Concurrent use may increase drowsiness effect).
No products indexed under this heading.

Ethinamate (Concurrent use may increase drowsiness effect).
No products indexed under this heading.

Fluphenazine Decanoate (Concurrent use may increase drowsiness effect).
No products indexed under this heading.

Fluphenazine Enanthate (Concurrent use may increase drowsiness effect).
No products indexed under this heading.

Fluphenazine Hydrochloride (Concurrent use may increase drowsiness effect).
No products indexed under this heading.

Flurazepam Hydrochloride (Concurrent use may increase drowsiness effect). Products include:
Dalmane Capsules 3342

Glutethimide (Concurrent use may increase drowsiness effect).
No products indexed under this heading.

Haloperidol (Concurrent use may increase drowsiness effect).
No products indexed under this heading.

Haloperidol Decanoate (Concurrent use may increase drowsiness effect).
No products indexed under this heading.

Hydroxyzine Hydrochloride (Concurrent use may increase drowsiness effect).
No products indexed under this heading.

Isocarboxazid (Concurrent and/or sequential use with MAO inhibitors is not recommended).
No products indexed under this heading.

Lorazepam (Concurrent use may increase drowsiness effect).
No products indexed under this heading.

Midazolam Hydrochloride (Concurrent use may increase drowsiness effect).
No products indexed under this heading.

Moclobemide (Concurrent and/or sequential use with MAO inhibitors is not recommended).
No products indexed under this heading.

Pargyline Hydrochloride (Concurrent and/or sequential use with MAO inhibitors is not recommended).
No products indexed under this heading.

Phenelzine Sulfate (Concurrent and/or sequential use with MAO inhibitors is not recommended).
No products indexed under this heading.

Procarbazine Hydrochloride (Concurrent and/or sequential use with MAO inhibitors is not recommended). Products include:
Matulane Capsules 3191

Propofol (Concurrent use may increase drowsiness effect).
No products indexed under this heading.

Quazepam (Concurrent use may increase drowsiness effect).
No products indexed under this heading.

Ramelteon (Concurrent use may increase drowsiness effect). Products include:
Rozerem Tablets 3231

Secobarbital Sodium (Concurrent use may increase drowsiness effect).
No products indexed under this heading.

Selegiline Hydrochloride (Concurrent and/or sequential use with MAO inhibitors is not recommended). Products include:
Eldepryl Capsules 3208
Zelapar Tablets 3372

Temazepam (Concurrent use may increase drowsiness effect). Products include:
Restoril Capsules 1860

Tranylcypromine Sulfate (Concurrent and/or sequential use with MAO inhibitors is not recommended). Products include:
Parnate Tablets 1527

Triazolam (Concurrent use may increase drowsiness effect).
No products indexed under this heading.

Zaleplon (Concurrent use may increase drowsiness effect). Products include:
Sonata Capsules 1717

Zolpidem Tartrate (Concurrent use may increase drowsiness effect). Products include:
Ambien Tablets 2851
Ambien CR Tablets 2855

CHILDREN'S TYLENOL PLUS COUGH & SORE THROAT SUSPENSION LIQUID

(Acetaminophen, Dextromethorphan Hydrobromide) 1879

May interact with monoamine oxidase inhibitors. Compounds in these categories include:

Isocarboxazid (Concurrent and/or sequential use with MAO inhibitors is not recommended).
No products indexed under this heading.

Moclobemide (Concurrent and/or sequential use with MAO inhibitors is not recommended).
No products indexed under this heading.

Pargyline Hydrochloride (Concurrent and/or sequential use with MAO inhibitors is not recommended).
No products indexed under this heading.

Phenelzine Sulfate (Concurrent and/or sequential use with MAO inhibitors is not recommended).
No products indexed under this heading.

Procarbazine Hydrochloride (Concurrent and/or sequential use with MAO inhibitors is not recommended). Products include:
Matulane Capsules 3191

Selegiline Hydrochloride (Concurrent and/or sequential use with MAO inhibitors is not recommended). Products include:
Eldepryl Capsules 3208
Zelapar Tablets 3372

Tranylcypromine Sulfate (Concurrent and/or sequential use with MAO inhibitors is not recommended). Products include:
Parnate Tablets 1527

CHILDREN'S TYLENOL SUSPENSION WITH FLAVOR CREATOR

(Acetaminophen) 1878
None cited in PDR database.

CHILDREN'S TYLENOL PLUS FLU SUSPENSION LIQUID

(Acetaminophen, Chlorpheniramine Maleate, Dextromethorphan Hydrobromide, Phenylephrine Hydrochloride) 1881

May interact with hypnotics and sedatives, monoamine oxidase inhibitors, tranquilizers, and certain other agents. Compounds in these categories include:

Alprazolam (Concurrent use may increase the drowsiness effect). Products include:
Niravam Orally Disintegrating Tablets .. 3092

Buspirone Hydrochloride (Concurrent use may increase the drowsiness effect).
No products indexed under this heading.

Chlordiazepoxide (Concurrent use may increase the drowsiness effect).
No products indexed under this heading.

Chlordiazepoxide Hydrochloride (Concurrent use may increase the drowsiness effect). Products include:
Librium Capsules 3347

Chlorpromazine (Concurrent use may increase the drowsiness effect).
No products indexed under this heading.

Chlorpromazine Hydrochloride (Concurrent use may increase the drowsiness effect).
No products indexed under this heading.

Chlorprothixene (Concurrent use may increase the drowsiness effect).
No products indexed under this heading.

Chlorprothixene Hydrochloride (Concurrent use may increase the drowsiness effect).
No products indexed under this heading.

Clorazepate Dipotassium (Concurrent use may increase the drowsiness effect). Products include:
Tranxene .. 2474

Diazepam (Concurrent use may increase the drowsiness effect). Products include:
Diastat Rectal Delivery System 3343
Valium Tablets 2819

Droperidol (Concurrent use may increase the drowsiness effect).
No products indexed under this heading.

Estazolam (Concurrent use may increase the drowsiness effect). Products include:
ProSom Tablets 517

Ethchlorvynol (Concurrent use may increase the drowsiness effect).
No products indexed under this heading.

Ethinamate (Concurrent use may increase the drowsiness effect).
No products indexed under this heading.

Fluphenazine Decanoate (Concurrent use may increase the drowsiness effect).
No products indexed under this heading.

Fluphenazine Enanthate (Concurrent use may increase the drowsiness effect).
No products indexed under this heading.

IMPORTANT NOTE: Always consult each drug listing in the patient's regimen for possible interactions.

Fluphenazine Hydrochloride (Concurrent use may increase the drowsiness effect).
 No products indexed under this heading.

Flurazepam Hydrochloride (Concurrent use may increase the drowsiness effect). Products include:
 Dalmane Capsules 3342

Glutethimide (Concurrent use may increase the drowsiness effect).
 No products indexed under this heading.

Haloperidol (Concurrent use may increase the drowsiness effect).
 No products indexed under this heading.

Haloperidol Decanoate (Concurrent use may increase the drowsiness effect).
 No products indexed under this heading.

Hydroxyzine Hydrochloride (Concurrent use may increase the drowsiness effect).
 No products indexed under this heading.

Isocarboxazid (Concurrent and/or sequential use with MAO inhibitors is not recommended).
 No products indexed under this heading.

Lorazepam (Concurrent use may increase the drowsiness effect).
 No products indexed under this heading.

Loxapine Hydrochloride (Concurrent use may increase the drowsiness effect).
 No products indexed under this heading.

Loxapine Succinate (Concurrent use may increase the drowsiness effect).
 No products indexed under this heading.

Meprobamate (Concurrent use may increase the drowsiness effect).
 No products indexed under this heading.

Mesoridazine Besylate (Concurrent use may increase the drowsiness effect).
 No products indexed under this heading.

Midazolam Hydrochloride (Concurrent use may increase the drowsiness effect).
 No products indexed under this heading.

Moclobemide (Concurrent and/or sequential use with MAO inhibitors is not recommended).
 No products indexed under this heading.

Molindone Hydrochloride (Concurrent use may increase the drowsiness effect). Products include:
 Moban Tablets 1119

Oxazepam (Concurrent use may increase the drowsiness effect).
 No products indexed under this heading.

Pargyline Hydrochloride (Concurrent and/or sequential use with MAO inhibitors is not recommended).
 No products indexed under this heading.

Perphenazine (Concurrent use may increase the drowsiness effect).
 No products indexed under this heading.

Phenelzine Sulfate (Concurrent and/or sequential use with MAO inhibitors is not recommended).
 No products indexed under this heading.

Prazepam (Concurrent use may increase the drowsiness effect).
 No products indexed under this heading.

Procarbazine Hydrochloride (Concurrent and/or sequential use with MAO inhibitors is not recommended). Products include:
 Matulane Capsules 3191

Prochlorperazine (Concurrent use may increase the drowsiness effect).
 No products indexed under this heading.

Promethazine Hydrochloride (Concurrent use may increase the drowsiness effect). Products include:
 Phenergan Tablets and Suppositories............................... 3440

Propofol (Concurrent use may increase the drowsiness effect).
 No products indexed under this heading.

Quazepam (Concurrent use may increase the drowsiness effect).
 No products indexed under this heading.

Ramelteon (Concurrent use may increase the drowsiness effect). Products include:
 Rozerem Tablets 3231

Secobarbital Sodium (Concurrent use may increase the drowsiness effect).
 No products indexed under this heading.

Selegiline Hydrochloride (Concurrent and/or sequential use with MAO inhibitors is not recommended). Products include:
 Eldepryl Capsules 3208
 Zelapar Tablets 3372

Temazepam (Concurrent use may increase the drowsiness effect). Products include:
 Restoril Capsules 1860

Thioridazine Hydrochloride (Concurrent use may increase the drowsiness effect). Products include:
 Thioridazine Hydrochloride Tablets 2163

Thiothixene (Concurrent use may increase the drowsiness effect). Products include:
 Thiothixene Capsules 2165

Tranylcypromine Sulfate (Concurrent and/or sequential use with MAO inhibitors is not recommended). Products include:
 Parnate Tablets 1527

Triazolam (Concurrent use may increase the drowsiness effect).
 No products indexed under this heading.

Trifluoperazine Hydrochloride (Concurrent use may increase the drowsiness effect).
 No products indexed under this heading.

Zaleplon (Concurrent use may increase the drowsiness effect). Products include:
 Sonata Capsules 1717

Zolpidem Tartrate (Concurrent use may increase the drowsiness effect). Products include:
 Ambien Tablets 2851
 Ambien CR Tablets 2855

CHILDREN'S TYLENOL PLUS MULTI-SYMPTOM COLD SUSPENSION LIQUID

(Acetaminophen, Chlorpheniramine Maleate, Dextromethorphan Hydrobromide, Phenylephrine Hydrochloride)..................... 1879
See Children's Tylenol Plus Cold Suspension Liquid

TYLENOL COLD SEVERE CONGESTION NON-DROWSY CAPLETS WITH COOL BURST

(Acetaminophen, Dextromethorphan Hydrobromide, Guaifenesin, Pseudoephedrine Hydrochloride)..................... 1874
May interact with monoamine oxidase inhibitors and certain other agents. Compounds in these categories include:

Isocarboxazid (Concurrent and/or sequential use with MAO inhibitors is not recommended).
 No products indexed under this heading.

Moclobemide (Concurrent and/or sequential use with MAO inhibitors is not recommended).
 No products indexed under this heading.

Pargyline Hydrochloride (Concurrent and/or sequential use with MAO inhibitors is not recommended).
 No products indexed under this heading.

Phenelzine Sulfate (Concurrent and/or sequential use with MAO inhibitors is not recommended).
 No products indexed under this heading.

Procarbazine Hydrochloride (Concurrent and/or sequential use with MAO inhibitors is not recommended). Products include:
 Matulane Capsules 3191

Selegiline Hydrochloride (Concurrent and/or sequential use with MAO inhibitors is not recommended). Products include:
 Eldepryl Capsules 3208
 Zelapar Tablets 3372

Tranylcypromine Sulfate (Concurrent and/or sequential use with MAO inhibitors is not recommended). Products include:
 Parnate Tablets 1527

Food Interactions

Alcohol (Chronic heavy alcohol abusers, 3 or more drinks per day, may be at increased risk of liver toxicity from acetaminophen use).

TYLENOL COLD HEAD CONGESTION DAYTIME CAPLETS WITH COOL BURST

(Acetaminophen, Dextromethorphan Hydrobromide, Phenylephrine Hydrochloride)............ 1873
May interact with monoamine oxidase inhibitors and certain other agents. Compounds in these categories include:

Isocarboxazid (Concurrent and/or sequential use with MAO inhibitors is not recommended).
 No products indexed under this heading.

Moclobemide (Concurrent and/or sequential use with MAO inhibitors is not recommended).
 No products indexed under this heading.

Pargyline Hydrochloride (Concurrent and/or sequential use with MAO inhibitors is not recommended).
 No products indexed under this heading.

Phenelzine Sulfate (Concurrent and/or sequential use with MAO inhibitors is not recommended).
 No products indexed under this heading.

Procarbazine Hydrochloride (Concurrent and/or sequential use with MAO inhibitors is not recommended). Products include:
 Matulane Capsules 3191

Selegiline Hydrochloride (Concurrent and/or sequential use with MAO inhibitors is not recommended). Products include:
 Eldepryl Capsules 3208
 Zelapar Tablets 3372

Tranylcypromine Sulfate (Concurrent and/or sequential use with MAO inhibitors is not recommended). Products include:
 Parnate Tablets 1527

Food Interactions

Alcohol (Concurrent use may increase drowsiness effect; chronic heavy alcohol abusers, 3 or more drinks per day, may be at increased risk of liver toxicity from excessive acetaminophen use).

TYLENOL COLD HEAD CONGESTION NIGHTTIME CAPLETS WITH COOL BURST

(Acetaminophen, Chlorpheniramine Maleate, Dextromethorphan Hydrobromide, Phenylephrine Hydrochloride)..................... 1873
May interact with hypnotics and sedatives, monoamine oxidase inhibitors, tranquilizers, and certain other agents. Compounds in these categories include:

Alprazolam (Concurrent use may increase drowsiness). Products include:
 Niravam Orally Disintegrating Tablets 3092

Buspirone Hydrochloride (Concurrent use may increase drowsiness).
 No products indexed under this heading.

Chlordiazepoxide (Concurrent use may increase drowsiness).
 No products indexed under this heading.

Chlordiazepoxide Hydrochloride (Concurrent use may increase drowsiness). Products include:
 Librium Capsules 3347

Chlorpromazine (Concurrent use may increase drowsiness).
 No products indexed under this heading.

Chlorpromazine Hydrochloride (Concurrent use may increase drowsiness).
 No products indexed under this heading.

Chlorprothixene (Concurrent use may increase drowsiness).
 No products indexed under this heading.

Chlorprothixene Hydrochloride (Concurrent use may increase drowsiness).
 No products indexed under this heading.

Clorazepate Dipotassium (Concurrent use may increase drowsiness). Products include:
 Tranxene 2474

Diazepam (Concurrent use may increase drowsiness). Products include:
 Diastat Rectal Delivery System 3343
 Valium Tablets 2819

Droperidol (Concurrent use may increase drowsiness).
 No products indexed under this heading.

Estazolam (Concurrent use may increase drowsiness effect). Products include:
 ProSom Tablets 517

Ethchlorvynol (Concurrent use may increase drowsiness effect).
 No products indexed under this heading.

Ethinamate (Concurrent use may increase drowsiness effect).
 No products indexed under this heading.

Fluphenazine Decanoate (Concurrent use may increase drowsiness).
 No products indexed under this heading.

Fluphenazine Enanthate (Concurrent use may increase drowsiness).
 No products indexed under this heading.

Fluphenazine Hydrochloride (Concurrent use may increase drowsiness).
 No products indexed under this heading.

Flurazepam Hydrochloride (Concurrent use may increase drowsiness effect). Products include:
 Dalmane Capsules 3342

Glutethimide (Concurrent use may increase drowsiness effect).
 No products indexed under this heading.

Haloperidol (Concurrent use may increase drowsiness).
 No products indexed under this heading.

Haloperidol Decanoate (Concurrent use may increase drowsiness).
 No products indexed under this heading.

Hydroxyzine Hydrochloride (Concurrent use may increase drowsiness).
 No products indexed under this heading.

Isocarboxazid (Concurrent and/or sequential use with MAO inhibitors is not recommended).
 No products indexed under this heading.

Lorazepam (Concurrent use may increase drowsiness effect).
 No products indexed under this heading.

Loxapine Hydrochloride (Concurrent use may increase drowsiness).
 No products indexed under this heading.

Loxapine Succinate (Concurrent use may increase drowsiness).
 No products indexed under this heading.

Meprobamate (Concurrent use may increase drowsiness).
 No products indexed under this heading.

Mesoridazine Besylate (Concurrent use may increase drowsiness).
 No products indexed under this heading.

Midazolam Hydrochloride (Concurrent use may increase drowsiness effect).
 No products indexed under this heading.

Moclobemide (Concurrent and/or sequential use with MAO inhibitors is not recommended).
 No products indexed under this heading.

Molindone Hydrochloride (Concurrent use may increase drowsiness). Products include:
 Moban Tablets 1119

Oxazepam (Concurrent use may increase drowsiness).
 No products indexed under this heading.

Pargyline Hydrochloride (Concurrent and/or sequential use with MAO inhibitors is not recommended).
 No products indexed under this heading.

Perphenazine (Concurrent use may increase drowsiness).
 No products indexed under this heading.

Phenelzine Sulfate (Concurrent and/or sequential use with MAO inhibitors is not recommended).
 No products indexed under this heading.

Prazepam (Concurrent use may increase drowsiness).
 No products indexed under this heading.

Procarbazine Hydrochloride (Concurrent and/or sequential use with MAO inhibitors is not recommended). Products include:
 Matulane Capsules 3191

Prochlorperazine (Concurrent use may increase drowsiness).
 No products indexed under this heading.

Promethazine Hydrochloride (Concurrent use may increase drowsiness). Products include:
 Phenergan Tablets and Suppositories.............................. 3440

Propofol (Concurrent use may increase drowsiness effect).
 No products indexed under this heading.

Quazepam (Concurrent use may increase drowsiness effect).
 No products indexed under this heading.

Ramelteon (Concurrent use may increase drowsiness effect). Products include:
 Rozerem Tablets 3231

Secobarbital Sodium (Concurrent use may increase drowsiness effect).
 No products indexed under this heading.

Selegiline Hydrochloride (Concurrent and/or sequential use with MAO inhibitors is not recommended). Products include:
 Eldepryl Capsules 3208
 Zelapar Tablets 3372

Temazepam (Concurrent use may increase drowsiness effect). Products include:
 Restoril Capsules 1860

Thioridazine Hydrochloride (Concurrent use may increase drowsiness). Products include:

Thioridazine Hydrochloride Tablets .. 2163

Thiothixene (Concurrent use may increase drowsiness). Products include:
 Thiothixene Capsules 2165

Tranylcypromine Sulfate (Concurrent and/or sequential use with MAO inhibitors is not recommended). Products include:
 Parnate Tablets 1527

Triazolam (Concurrent use may increase drowsiness effect).
 No products indexed under this heading.

Trifluoperazine Hydrochloride (Concurrent use may increase drowsiness).
 No products indexed under this heading.

Zaleplon (Concurrent use may increase drowsiness effect). Products include:
 Sonata Capsules 1717

Zolpidem Tartrate (Concurrent use may increase drowsiness effect). Products include:
 Ambien Tablets 2851
 Ambien CR Tablets 2855

Food Interactions

Alcohol (Concurrent use may increase drowsiness effect; chronic heavy alcohol abusers, 3 or more drinks per day, may be at increased risk of liver toxicity from excessive acetaminophen use).

TYLENOL COLD HEAD CONGESTION SEVERE CAPLETS WITH COOL BURST

(Acetaminophen, Dextromethorphan Hydrobromide, Guaifenesin, Phenylephrine Hydrochloride)................................. 1873
See Tylenol Cold Head Congestion Daytime Caplets with Cool Burst

TYLENOL COLD MULTI-SYMPTOM DAYTIME CAPLETS WITH COOL BURST AND GELCAPS

(Acetaminophen, Dextromethorphan Hydrobromide, Phenylephrine Hydrochloride)............. 1874
May interact with monoamine oxidase inhibitors and certain other agents. Compounds in these categories include:

Isocarboxazid (Concurrent and/or sequential use with MAO inhibitors is not recommended).
 No products indexed under this heading.

Moclobemide (Concurrent and/or sequential use with MAO inhibitors is not recommended).
 No products indexed under this heading.

Pargyline Hydrochloride (Concurrent and/or sequential use with MAO inhibitors is not recommended).
 No products indexed under this heading.

Phenelzine Sulfate (Concurrent and/or sequential use with MAO inhibitors is not recommended).
 No products indexed under this heading.

Procarbazine Hydrochloride (Concurrent and/or sequential use with MAO inhibitors is not recommended). Products include:
 Matulane Capsules 3191

Selegiline Hydrochloride (Concurrent and/or sequential use with MAO inhibitors is not recommended). Products include:
 Eldepryl Capsules 3208
 Zelapar Tablets 3372

Tranylcypromine Sulfate (Concurrent and/or sequential use with MAO inhibitors is not recommended). Products include:
 Parnate Tablets 1527

Food Interactions

Alcohol (Consumption of 3 or more alcoholic drinks every day, need to ask your doctor whether you should take acetaminophen; may be at increased risk of liver toxicity from acetaminophen use).

TYLENOL COLD MULTI-SYMPTOM DAYTIME LIQUID WITH CITRUS BURST

(Acetaminophen, Dextromethorphan Hydrobromide, Phenylephrine Hydrochloride)............. 1874
See Tylenol Cold Multi-Symptom Daytime Caplets with Cool Burst and Gelcaps

TYLENOL COLD MULTI-SYMPTOM NIGHTTIME CAPLETS WITH COOL BURST

(Acetaminophen, Chlorpheniramine Maleate, Dextromethorphan Hydrobromide, Phenylephrine Hydrochloride)................................. 1874
See Tylenol Cold Multi-Symptom Daytime Caplets with Cool Burst and Gelcaps

TYLENOL COLD MULTI-SYMPTOM NIGHTTIME LIQUID WITH COOL BURST

(Acetaminophen, Dextromethorphan Hydrobromide, Doxylamine Succinate, Phenylephrine Hydrochloride)............. 1874
See Tylenol Cold Multi-Symptom Daytime Caplets with Cool Burst and Gelcaps

TYLENOL COLD MULTI-SYMPTOM SEVERE CAPLETS WITH COOL BURST

(Acetaminophen, Dextromethorphan Hydrobromide, Guaifenesin, Phenylephrine Hydrochloride)................................. 1874
See Tylenol Cold Multi-Symptom Daytime Caplets with Cool Burst and Gelcaps

TYLENOL COLD MULTI-SYMPTOM SEVERE DAYTIME LIQUID WITH CITRUS BURST

(Acetaminophen, Dextromethorphan Hydrobromide, Guaifenesin, Phenylephrine Hydrochloride)................................. 1874
See Tylenol Cold Multi-Symptom Daytime Caplets with Cool Burst and Gelcaps

IMPORTANT NOTE: Always consult each drug listing in the patient's regimen for possible interactions.

TYLENOL COUGH & SORE THROAT DAYTIME LIQUID WITH COOL BURST

(Acetaminophen, Dextromethorphan Hydrobromide)...... **1877**
May interact with monoamine oxidase inhibitors and certain other agents. Compounds in these categories include:

Isocarboxazid (Avoid use with, or for two weeks after stopping, MAOI drugs).
No products indexed under this heading.

Moclobemide (Avoid use with, or for two weeks after stopping, MAOI drugs).
No products indexed under this heading.

Pargyline Hydrochloride (Avoid use with, or for two weeks after stopping, MAOI drugs).
No products indexed under this heading.

Phenelzine Sulfate (Avoid use with, or for two weeks after stopping, MAOI drugs).
No products indexed under this heading.

Procarbazine Hydrochloride (Avoid use with, or for two weeks after stopping, MAOI drugs). Products include:
Matulane Capsules **3191**

Seleglline Hydrochloride (Avoid use with, or for two weeks after stopping, MAOI drugs). Products include:
Eldepryl Capsules **3208**
Zelapar Tablets **3372**

Tranylcypromine Sulfate (Avoid use with, or for two weeks after stopping, MAOI drugs). Products include:
Parnate Tablets **1527**

Food Interactions

Alcohol (Consumption of 3 or more alcoholic drinks everyday, need to ask your doctor whether you should take acetaminophen; may be at increased risk of liver toxicity from acetaminophen use).

TYLENOL COUGH & SORE THROAT NIGHTTIME LIQUID WITH COOL BURST

(Acetaminophen, Dextromethorphan Hydrobromide, Doxylamine Succinate)........................ **1877**
See Tylenol Sore Throat Nighttime Liquid with Cool Burst

CONCENTRATED TYLENOL INFANTS' DROPS

(Acetaminophen) **1878**
None cited in PDR database.

CONCENTRATED TYLENOL INFANTS' DROPS PLUS COLD

(Acetaminophen) **1879**
See Concentrated Tylenol Infants' Drops Plus Cold and Cough

CONCENTRATED TYLENOL INFANTS' DROPS PLUS COLD AND COUGH

(Acetaminophen, Dextromethorphan Hydrobromide)...... **1879**
May interact with monoamine oxidase inhibitors. Compounds in these categories include:

Isocarboxazid (Concurrent and/or sequential use with MAO inhibitors is not recommended).
No products indexed under this heading.

Moclobemide (Concurrent and/or sequential use with MAO inhibitors is not recommended).
No products indexed under this heading.

Pargyline Hydrochloride (Concurrent and/or sequential use with MAO inhibitors is not recommended).
No products indexed under this heading.

Phenelzine Sulfate (Concurrent and/or sequential use with MAO inhibitors is not recommended).
No products indexed under this heading.

Procarbazine Hydrochloride (Concurrent and/or sequential use with MAO inhibitors is not recommended). Products include:
Matulane Capsules **3191**

Seleglline Hydrochloride (Concurrent and/or sequential use with MAO inhibitors is not recommended). Products include:
Eldepryl Capsules **3208**
Zelapar Tablets **3372**

Tranylcypromine Sulfate (Concurrent and/or sequential use with MAO inhibitors is not recommended). Products include:
Parnate Tablets **1527**

JR. TYLENOL MELTAWAYS

(Acetaminophen) **1878**
None cited in PDR database.

TYLENOL SINUS SEVERE CONGESTION CAPLETS WITH COOL BURST

(Acetaminophen, Guaifenesin, Pseudoephedrine Hydrochloride)........ **1876**
May interact with monoamine oxidase inhibitors and certain other agents. Compounds in these categories include:

Isocarboxazid (Concurrent and/or sequential use with MAO inhibitors is not recommended).
No products indexed under this heading.

Moclobemide (Concurrent and/or sequential use with MAO inhibitors is not recommended).
No products indexed under this heading.

Pargyline Hydrochloride (Concurrent and/or sequential use with MAO inhibitors is not recommended).
No products indexed under this heading.

Phenelzine Sulfate (Concurrent and/or sequential use with MAO inhibitors is not recommended).
No products indexed under this heading.

Procarbazine Hydrochloride (Concurrent and/or sequential use with MAO inhibitors is not recommended). Products include:
Matulane Capsules **3191**

Selegiline Hydrochloride (Concurrent and/or sequential use with MAO inhibitors is not recommended).
Products include:
Eldepryl Capsules **3208**
Zelapar Tablets **3372**

Tranylcypromine Sulfate (Concurrent and/or sequential use with MAO inhibitors is not recommended).
Products include:
Parnate Tablets **1527**

Food Interactions

Alcohol (Concurrent use may increase drowsiness effect; chronic heavy alcohol abusers, 3 or more drinks per day, may be at increased risk of liver toxicity from excessive accetaminophen use).

TYLENOL SINUS CONGESTION & PAIN DAYTIME CAPLETS WITH COOL BURST AND GELCAPS

(Acetaminophen, Phenylephrine Hydrochloride).................................... **1876**
May interact with monoamine oxidase inhibitors and certain other agents. Compounds in these categories include:

Isocarboxazid (Concurrent and/or sequential use with MAO inhibitors is not recommended).
No products indexed under this heading.

Moclobemide (Concurrent and/or sequential use with MAO inhibitors is not recommended).
No products indexed under this heading.

Pargyline Hydrochloride (Concurrent and/or sequential use with MAO inhibitors is not recommended).
No products indexed under this heading.

Phenelzine Sulfate (Concurrent and/or sequential use with MAO inhibitors is not recommended).
No products indexed under this heading.

Procarbazine Hydrochloride (Concurrent and/or sequential use with MAO inhibitors is not recommended). Products include:
Matulane Capsules **3191**

Selegiline Hydrochloride (Concurrent and/or sequential use with MAO inhibitors is not recommended).
Products include:
Eldepryl Capsules **3208**
Zelapar Tablets **3372**

Tranylcypromine Sulfate (Concurrent and/or sequential use with MAO inhibitors is not recommended).
Products include:
Parnate Tablets **1527**

Food Interactions

Alcohol (Concurrent use may increase drowsiness effect; chronic heavy alcohol abusers, 3 or more drinks per day, may be at increased risk of liver toxicity from excessive acetaminophen use).

TYLENOL SINUS CONGESTION & PAIN NIGHTTIME CAPLETS WITH COOL BURST

(Acetaminophen, Chlorpheniramine Maleate, Phenylephrine Hydrochloride).................................... **1876**
May interact with hypnotics and sedatives, monoamine oxidase inhibitors, tranquilizers, and certain other agents. Compounds in these categories include:

Alprazolam (May increase drowsiness effect). Products include:

Niravam Orally Disintegrating Tablets .. **3092**
Buspirone Hydrochloride (May increase drowsiness effect).
No products indexed under this heading.

Chlordiazepoxide (May increase drowsiness effect).
No products indexed under this heading.

Chlordiazepoxide Hydrochloride (May increase drowsiness effect).
Products include:
Librium Capsules **3347**

Chlorpromazine (May increase drowsiness effect).
No products indexed under this heading.

Chlorpromazine Hydrochloride (May increase drowsiness effect).
No products indexed under this heading.

Chlorprothixene (May increase drowsiness effect).
No products indexed under this heading.

Chlorprothixene Hydrochloride (May increase drowsiness effect).
No products indexed under this heading.

Clorazepate Dipotassium (May increase drowsiness effect).
Products include:
Tranxene .. **2474**

Diazepam (May increase drowsiness effect). Products include:
Diastat Rectal Delivery System **3343**
Valium Tablets **2819**

Droperidol (May increase drowsiness effect).
No products indexed under this heading.

Estazolam (May increase drowsiness effect). Products include:
ProSom Tablets **517**

Ethchlorvynol (May increase drowsiness effect).
No products indexed under this heading.

Ethinamate (May increase drowsiness effect).
No products indexed under this heading.

Fluphenazine Decanoate (May increase drowsiness effect).
No products indexed under this heading.

Fluphenazine Enanthate (May increase drowsiness effect).
No products indexed under this heading.

Fluphenazine Hydrochloride (May increase drowsiness effect).
No products indexed under this heading.

Flurazepam Hydrochloride (May increase drowsiness effect).
Products include:
Dalmane Capsules **3342**

Glutethimide (May increase drowsiness effect).
No products indexed under this heading.

Haloperidol (May increase drowsiness effect).
No products indexed under this heading.

Haloperidol Decanoate (May increase drowsiness effect).
No products indexed under this heading.

Hydroxyzine Hydrochloride (May increase drowsiness effect).
No products indexed under this heading.

Isocarboxazid (Concurrent and/or sequential use with MAO inhibitors is not recommended).
No products indexed under this heading.

Lorazepam (May increase drowsiness effect).
No products indexed under this heading.

Loxapine Hydrochloride (May increase drowsiness effect).
No products indexed under this heading.

Loxapine Succinate (May increase drowsiness effect).
No products indexed under this heading.

Meprobamate (May increase drowsiness effect).
No products indexed under this heading.

Mesoridazine Besylate (May increase drowsiness effect).
No products indexed under this heading.

Midazolam Hydrochloride (May increase drowsiness effect).
No products indexed under this heading.

Moclobemide (Concurrent and/or sequential use with MAO inhibitors is not recommended).
No products indexed under this heading.

Molindone Hydrochloride (May increase drowsiness effect). Products include:
Moban Tablets **1119**

Oxazepam (May increase drowsiness effect).
No products indexed under this heading.

Pargyline Hydrochloride (Concurrent and/or sequential use with MAO inhibitors is not recommended).
No products indexed under this heading.

Perphenazine (May increase drowsiness effect).
No products indexed under this heading.

Phenelzine Sulfate (Concurrent and/or sequential use with MAO inhibitors is not recommended).
No products indexed under this heading.

Prazepam (May increase drowsiness effect).
No products indexed under this heading.

Procarbazine Hydrochloride (Concurrent and/or sequential use with MAO inhibitors is not recommended). Products include:
Matulane Capsules **3191**

Prochlorperazine (May increase drowsiness effect).
No products indexed under this heading.

Promethazine Hydrochloride (May increase drowsiness effect). Products include:
Phenergan Tablets and Suppositories **3440**

Propofol (May increase drowsiness effect).
No products indexed under this heading.

Quazepam (May increase drowsiness effect).
No products indexed under this heading.

Ramelteon (May increase drowsiness effect). Products include:
Rozerem Tablets **3231**

Secobarbital Sodium (May increase drowsiness effect).
No products indexed under this heading.

Selegiline Hydrochloride (Concurrent and/or sequential use with MAO inhibitors is not recommended). Products include:
Eldepryl Capsules **3208**
Zelapar Tablets **3372**

Temazepam (May increase drowsiness effect). Products include:
Restoril Capsules **1860**

Thioridazine Hydrochloride (May increase drowsiness effect). Products include:
Thioridazine Hydrochloride Tablets **2163**

Thiothixene (May increase drowsiness effect). Products include:
Thiothixene Capsules **2165**

Tranylcypromine Sulfate (Concurrent and/or sequential use with MAO inhibitors is not recommended). Products include:
Parnate Tablets **1527**

Triazolam (May increase drowsiness effect).
No products indexed under this heading.

Trifluoperazine Hydrochloride (May increase drowsiness effect).
No products indexed under this heading.

Zaleplon (May increase drowsiness effect). Products include:
Sonata Capsules **1717**

Zolpidem Tartrate (May increase drowsiness effect). Products include:
Ambien Tablets **2851**
Ambien CR Tablets **2855**

Food Interactions

Alcohol (May increase drowsiness effect).

TYLENOL SINUS CONGESTION & PAIN SEVERE CAPLETS WITH COOL BURST

(Acetaminophen, Guaifenesin, Phenylephrine Hydrochloride) **1876**
May interact with monoamine oxidase inhibitors and certain other agents. Compounds in these categories include:

Isocarboxazid (Concurrent and/or sequential use with MAO inhibitors is not recommended).
No products indexed under this heading.

Moclobemide (Concurrent and/or sequential use with MAO inhibitors is not recommended).
No products indexed under this heading.

Pargyline Hydrochloride (Concurrent and/or sequential use with MAO inhibitors is not recommended).
No products indexed under this heading.

Phenelzine Sulfate (Concurrent and/or sequential use with MAO inhibitors is not recommended).
No products indexed under this heading.

Procarbazine Hydrochloride (Concurrent and/or sequential use with MAO inhibitors is not recommended). Products include:
Matulane Capsules **3191**

Selegiline Hydrochloride (Concurrent and/or sequential use with MAO inhibitors is not recommended). Products include:
Eldepryl Capsules **3208**
Zelapar Tablets **3372**

Tranylcypromine Sulfate (Concurrent and/or sequential use with MAO inhibitors is not recommended). Products include:
Parnate Tablets **1527**

Food Interactions

Alcohol (Avoid concurrent use; chronic heavy alcohol abusers, 3 or more drinks per day, may be at increased risk of liver toxicity from acetaminophen use).

TYLENOL SORE THROAT DAYTIME LIQUID WITH COOL BURST

(Acetaminophen) **1877**
See Tylenol Cough & Sore Throat Daytime Liquid with Cool Burst

TYLENOL SORE THROAT NIGHTTIME LIQUID WITH COOL BURST

(Acetaminophen, Diphenhydramine).............................. **1877**
May interact with hypnotics and sedatives, monoamine oxidase inhibitors, tranquilizers, and certain other agents. Compounds in these categories include:

Alprazolam (Concurrent use may cause drowsiness effect). Products include:
Niravam Orally Disintegrating Tablets **3092**

Buspirone Hydrochloride (Concurrent use may cause drowsiness effect).
No products indexed under this heading.

Chlordiazepoxide (Concurrent use may cause drowsiness effect).
No products indexed under this heading.

Chlordiazepoxide Hydrochloride (Concurrent use may cause drowsiness effect). Products include:
Librium Capsules **3347**

Chlorpromazine (Concurrent use may cause drowsiness effect).
No products indexed under this heading.

Chlorpromazine Hydrochloride (Concurrent use may cause drowsiness effect).
No products indexed under this heading.

Chlorprothixene (Concurrent use may cause drowsiness effect).
No products indexed under this heading.

Chlorprothixene Hydrochloride (Concurrent use may cause drowsiness effect).
No products indexed under this heading.

Clorazepate Dipotassium (Concurrent use may cause drowsiness effect). Products include:
Tranxene **2474**

Diazepam (Concurrent use may cause drowsiness effect). Products include:
Diastat Rectal Delivery System **3343**
Valium Tablets **2819**

Diphenhydramine Hydrochloride (Do not use with any other product containing diphenhydramine, even one used on skin). Products include:
Nytol QuickCaps Caplets **615**
Nytol QuickGels Softgels Maximum Strength..................... **616**
Simply Sleep Caplets **1868**
Sominex Original Formula Tablets .. **616**
TheraFlu Warming Relief Nighttime Severe Cold **743**
TheraFlu Thin Strips Multi Symptom.................................. **744**
Triaminic Nighttime Cold & Cough Liquid.............................. **746**
Triaminic Thin Strips Cough & Runny Nose **749**
Extra Strength Tylenol PM Caplets, Vanilla Caplets, Geltabs, Gelcaps and Liquid.......... **1875**
Tylenol Sore Throat Nighttime Liquid with Cool Burst................ **790**
Tylenol Allergy Multi-Symptom Nighttime Caplets with Cool Burst.. **1872**
Tylenol Severe Allergy Caplets **1872**
Children's Tylenol Plus Cold & Allergy Suspension Liquid............ **1878**

Droperidol (Concurrent use may cause drowsiness effect).
No products indexed under this heading.

Estazolam (Concurrent use may increase drowsiness effect). Products include:
ProSom Tablets **517**

Ethchlorvynol (Concurrent use may increase drowsiness effect).
No products indexed under this heading.

Ethinamate (Concurrent use may increase drowsiness effect).
No products indexed under this heading.

Fluphenazine Decanoate (Concurrent use may cause drowsiness effect).
No products indexed under this heading.

Fluphenazine Enanthate (Concurrent use may cause drowsiness effect).
No products indexed under this heading.

Fluphenazine Hydrochloride (Concurrent use may cause drowsiness effect).
No products indexed under this heading.

Flurazepam Hydrochloride (Concurrent use may increase drowsiness effect). Products include:
Dalmane Capsules **3342**

Glutethimide (Concurrent use may increase drowsiness effect).
No products indexed under this heading.

Haloperidol (Concurrent use may cause drowsiness effect).
No products indexed under this heading.

Haloperidol Decanoate (Concurrent use may cause drowsiness effect).
No products indexed under this heading.

Hydroxyzine Hydrochloride (Concurrent use may cause drowsiness effect).
No products indexed under this heading.

Isocarboxazid (Concurrent and/or sequential use with MAO inhibitors is not recommended).
No products indexed under this heading.

Lorazepam (Concurrent use may increase drowsiness effect).
No products indexed under this heading.

Midazolam Hydrochloride (Concurrent use may increase drowsiness effect).
No products indexed under this heading.

Moclobemide (Concurrent and/or sequential use with MAO inhibitors is not recommended).
No products indexed under this heading.

Pargyline Hydrochloride (Concurrent and/or sequential use with MAO inhibitors is not recommended).
No products indexed under this heading.

Phenelzine Sulfate (Concurrent and/or sequential use with MAO inhibitors is not recommended).
No products indexed under this heading.

Procarbazine Hydrochloride (Concurrent and/or sequential use with MAO inhibitors is not recommended). Products include:
Matulane Capsules **3191**

Propofol (Concurrent use may increase drowsiness effect).
No products indexed under this heading.

Quazepam (Concurrent use may increase drowsiness effect).
No products indexed under this heading.

Ramelteon (Concurrent use may increase drowsiness effect).
Products include:
Rozerem Tablets **3231**

Secobarbital Sodium (Concurrent use may increase drowsiness effect).
No products indexed under this heading.

Selegiline Hydrochloride (Concurrent and/or sequential use with MAO inhibitors is not recommended).
Products include:
Eldepryl Capsules **3208**
Zelapar Tablets **3372**

Temazepam (Concurrent use may increase drowsiness effect).
Products include:
Restoril Capsules **1860**

Tranylcypromine Sulfate (Concurrent and/or sequential use with MAO inhibitors is not recommended).
Products include:
Parnate Tablets **1527**

Triazolam (Concurrent use may increase drowsiness effect).
No products indexed under this heading.

Zaleplon (Concurrent use may increase drowsiness effect).
Products include:
Sonata Capsules **1717**

Zolpidem Tartrate (Concurrent use may increase drowsiness effect).
Products include:
Ambien Tablets **2851**
Ambien CR Tablets **2855**

Food Interactions

Alcohol (Concurrent use may increase drowsiness effect; chronic heavy alcohol abusers, 3 or more drinks perday, may be at increased risk of liver toxicity from excessive acetaminophen use).

WOMEN'S TYLENOL MENSTRUAL RELIEF CAPLETS

(Acetaminophen, Pamabrom) **1877**

Food Interactions

Alcohol (Chronic heavy alcohol users, 3 or more drinks per day, should consult their physicians for advice on when and how they should take pain relievers, including acetaminophen).

ULTANE LIQUID FOR INHALATION

(Sevoflurane) **531**

May interact with benzodiazepines, narcotic analgesics, nondepolarizing neuromuscular blocking agents, and certain other agents. Compounds in these categories include:

Alfentanil Hydrochloride (Benzodiazepines would be expected to decrease the MAC of sevoflurane in the same manner as with other inhalational anesthetics. Sevoflurane administration is compatible with benzodiazepines and opioids as commonly used in surgical practice).
No products indexed under this heading.

Alprazolam (Benzodiazepines would be expected to decrease the MAC of sevoflurane in the same manner as with other inhalational anesthetics. Sevoflurane administration is compatible with benzodiazepines and opioids as commonly used in surgical practice). Products include:
Niravam Orally Disintegrating Tablets **3092**

Atracurium Besylate (Sevoflurane increases both the intensity and duration of neuromuscular blockade induced by non-depolarizing muscle relaxants. When used to supplement alfentanil-nitrous oxide anesthesia, sevoflurane and isoflurane equally potentiate neuromuscular block induced with pancuronium, vecuronium or atracurium. Among available non-depolarizing agents, only vecuronium, pancuronium and atracurium interactions have been studied during sevoflurane anesthesia. In the absence of specific guidelines: 1) For endotracheal intubation, do not reduce the dose of non-depolarizing muscle relaxants. 2) During maintenance of anesthesia, the required dose of non-depolarizing muscle relaxants is likely to be reduced compared to that during nitrous oxide/opioid anesthesia).
No products indexed under this heading.

Buprenorphine Hydrochloride (Benzodiazepines would be expected to decrease the MAC of sevoflurane in the same manner as with other inhalational anesthetics. Sevoflurane administration is compatible with benzodiazepines and opioids as commonly used in surgical practice).
Products include:
Buprenex Injectable **2716**
Suboxone Tablets **2717**
Subutex Tablets **2717**

Chlordiazepoxide (Benzodiazepines would be expected to decrease the MAC of sevoflurane in the same manner as with other inhalational anesthetics. Sevoflurane administration is compatible with benzodiazepines and opioids as commonly used in surgical practice).
No products indexed under this heading.

Chlordiazepoxide Hydrochloride (Benzodiazepines would be expected to decrease the MAC of sevoflurane in the same manner as with other inhalational anesthetics. Sevoflurane administration is compatible with benzodiazepines and opioids as commonly used in surgical practice).
Products include:
Librium Capsules **3347**

Cisatracurium Besylate (Sevoflurane increases both the intensity and duration of neuromuscular blockade induced by non-depolarizing muscle relaxants. When used to supplement alfentanil-nitrous oxide anesthesia, sevoflurane and isoflurane equally potentiate neuromuscular block induced with pancuronium, vecuronium or atracurium. Among available non-depolarizing agents, only vecuronium, pancuronium and atracurium interactions have been studied during sevoflurane anesthesia. In the absence of specific guidelines: 1) For endotracheal intubation, do not reduce the dose of non-depolarizing muscle relaxants. 2) During maintenance of anesthesia, the required dose of non-depolarizing muscle relaxants is likely to be reduced compared to that during nitrous oxide/opioid anesthesia). Products include:
Nimbex Injection **498**

Clorazepate Dipotassium (Benzodiazepines would be expected to decrease the MAC of sevoflurane in the same manner as with other inhalational anesthetics. Sevoflurane administration is compatible with benzodiazepines and opioids as commonly used in surgical practice).
Products include:
Tranxene **2474**

Codeine Phosphate (Benzodiazepines would be expected to decrease the MAC of sevoflurane in the same manner as with other inhalational anesthetics. Sevoflurane administration is compatible with benzodiazepines and opioids as commonly used in surgical practice).
Products include:
Tylenol with Codeine Tablets **2391**

Dezocine (Benzodiazepines would be expected to decrease the MAC of sevoflurane in the same manner as with other inhalational anesthetics. Sevoflurane administration is compatible with benzodiazepines and opioids as commonly used in surgical practice).
No products indexed under this heading.

Diazepam (Benzodiazepines would be expected to decrease the MAC of sevoflurane in the same manner as with other inhalational anesthetics. Sevoflurane administration is compatible with benzodiazepines and opioids as commonly used in surgical practice). Products include:
Diastat Rectal Delivery System **3343**
Valium Tablets **2819**

Estazolam (Benzodiazepines would be expected to decrease the MAC of sevoflurane in the same manner as with other inhalational anesthetics. Sevoflurane administration is compatible with benzodiazepines and opioids as commonly used in surgical practice). Products include:
ProSom Tablets **517**

Fentanyl (Benzodiazepines would be expected to decrease the MAC of sevoflurane in the same manner as with other inhalational anesthetics. Sevoflurane administration is compatible with benzodiazepines and opioids as commonly used in surgical practice). Products include:
Duragesic Transdermal System **2373**
Ionsys Transdermal System **2379**

Fentanyl Citrate (Benzodiazepines would be expected to decrease the MAC of sevoflurane in the same manner as with other inhalational anesthetics. Sevoflurane administration is compatible with benzodiazepines and opioids as commonly used in surgical practice). Products include:
Actiq **979**

Flurazepam Hydrochloride (Benzodiazepines would be expected to decrease the MAC of sevoflurane in the same manner as with other inhalational anesthetics. Sevoflurane administration is compatible with benzodiazepines and opioids as commonly used in surgical practice).
Products include:
Dalmane Capsules **3342**

Halazepam (Benzodiazepines would be expected to decrease the MAC of sevoflurane in the same manner as with other inhalational anesthetics. Sevoflurane administration is compatible with benzodiazepines and opioids as commonly used in surgical practice).
No products indexed under this heading.

Hydrocodone Bitartrate (Benzodiazepines would be expected to decrease the MAC of sevoflurane in the same manner as with other inhalational anesthetics. Sevoflurane administration is compatible with benzodiazepines and opioids as commonly used in surgical practice).
Products include:
Hycodan **1116**
Hycotuss Expectorant Syrup **1117**
Vicodin Tablets **535**
Vicodin ES Tablets **536**
Vicodin HP Tablets **538**
Vicoprofen Tablets **539**
Zydone Tablets **1139**

Hydrocodone Polistirex (Benzodiazepines would be expected to decrease the MAC of sevoflurane in the same manner as with other inhalational anesthetics. Sevoflurane administration is compatible with benzodiazepines and opioids as commonly used in surgical practice).
Products include:
Tussionex Pennkinetic Extended-Release Suspension...... **3327**

Hydromorphone Hydrochloride (Benzodiazepines would be expected to decrease the MAC of sevoflurane in the same manner as with other inhalational anesthetics. Sevoflurane administration is compatible with benzodiazepines and opioids as commonly used in surgical practice).
Products include:
Dilaudid **440**
Dilaudid Non-Sterile Powder **440**
Dilaudid Oral Liquid **445**
Dilaudid Rectal Suppositories **440**
Dilaudid Tablets **440**
Dilaudid Tablets - 8 mg **445**
Dilaudid-HP **442**

Levorphanol Tartrate (Benzodiazepines would be expected to decrease the MAC of sevoflurane in the same manner as with other inhalational anesthetics. Sevoflurane administration is compatible with benzodiazepines and opioids as commonly used in surgical practice).
No products indexed under this heading.

Lorazepam (Benzodiazepines would be expected to decrease the MAC of sevoflurane in the same manner as with other inhalational anesthetics. Sevoflurane administration is compatible with benzodiazepines and opioids as commonly used in surgical practice).
No products indexed under this heading.

Meperidine Hydrochloride (Benzodiazepines would be expected to decrease the MAC of sevoflurane in the same manner as with other inhalational anesthetics. Sevoflurane administration is compatible with benzodiazepines and opioids as commonly used in surgical practice).
No products indexed under this heading.

Methadone Hydrochloride (Benzodiazepines would be expected to decrease the MAC of sevoflurane in the same manner as with other inhalational anesthetics. Sevoflurane administration is compatible with benzodiazepines and opioids as commonly used in surgical practice).
No products indexed under this heading.

Metocurine Iodide (Sevoflurane increases both the intensity and duration of neuromuscular blockade induced by non-depolarizing muscle relaxants. When used to supplement alfentanil-nitrous oxide anesthesia, sevoflurane and isoflurane equally potentiate neuromuscular block induced with pancuronium, vecuronium or atracurium. Among available non-depolarizing agents, only vecuronium, pancuronium and atracurium interactions have been studied during sevoflurane anesthesia. In the absence of specific guidelines: 1) For endotracheal intubation, do not reduce the dose of non-depolarizing muscle relaxants. 2) During maintenance of anesthesia, the required dose of non-depolarizing muscle relaxants is likely to be reduced compared to that during nitrous oxide/opioid anesthesia).
No products indexed under this heading.

Midazolam Hydrochloride (Benzodiazepines would be expected to decrease the MAC of sevoflurane in the same manner as with other inhalational anesthetics. Sevoflurane administration is compatible with benzodiazepines and opioids as commonly used in surgical practice).
No products indexed under this heading.

Mivacurium Chloride (Sevoflurane increases both the intensity and duration of neuromuscular blockade induced by non-depolarizing muscle relaxants. When used to supplement alfentanil-nitrous oxide anesthesia, sevoflurane and isoflurane equally potentiate neuromuscular block induced with pancuronium, vecuronium or atracurium. Among available non-depolarizing agents, only vecuronium, pancuronium and atracurium interactions have been studied during sevoflurane anesthesia. In the absence of specific guidelines: 1) For endotracheal intubation, do not reduce the dose of non-depolarizing muscle relaxants. 2) During maintenance of anesthesia, the required dose of non-depolarizing muscle relaxants is likely to be reduced compared to that during nitrous oxide/opioid anesthesia). Products include:
Mivacron Injection 493

Morphine Sulfate (Benzodiazepines would be expected to decrease the MAC of sevoflurane in the same manner as with other inhalational anesthetics. Sevoflurane administration is compatible with benzodiazepines and opioids as commonly used in surgical practice). Products include:
Avinza Capsules 1741
Kadian Capsules 577
MS Contin Tablets 2701

Nitrous Oxide (As with other halogenated volatile anesthetics, the anesthetic requirement for sevoflurane is decreased when administered in combination with nitrous oxide. Using 50% nitrous oxide, the MAC equivalent dose requirement is reduced approximately 50% in adults and approximately 25% in pediatrics patients).
No products indexed under this heading.

Oxazepam (Benzodiazepines would be expected to decrease the MAC of sevoflurane in the same manner as with other inhalational anesthetics. Sevoflurane administration is compatible with benzodiazepines and opioids as commonly used in surgical practice).
No products indexed under this heading.

Oxycodone Hydrochloride (Benzodiazepines would be expected to decrease the MAC of sevoflurane in the same manner as with other inhalational anesthetics. Sevoflurane administration is compatible with benzodiazepines and opioids as commonly used in surgical practice). Products include:
OxyContin Tablets 2703
OxyFast Oral Concentrate Solution 2708
OxyIR Capsules 2708
Percocet Tablets 1131
Percodan Tablets 1132

Pancuronium Bromide (Sevoflurane increases both the intensity and duration of neuromuscular blockade induced by non-depolarizing muscle relaxants. When used to supplement alfentanil-nitrous oxide anesthesia, sevoflurane and isoflurane equally potentiate neuromuscular block induced with pancuronium, vecuronium or atracurium. Among available non-depolarizing agents, only vecuronium, pancuronium and atracurium interactions have been studied during sevoflurane anesthesia. In the absence of specific guidelines: 1) For endotracheal intubation, do not reduce the dose of non-depolarizing muscle relaxants. 2) During maintenance of anesthesia, the required dose of non-depolarizing muscle relaxants is likely to be reduced compared to that during nitrous oxide/opioid anesthesia).
No products indexed under this heading.

Prazepam (Benzodiazepines would be expected to decrease the MAC of sevoflurane in the same manner as with other inhalational anesthetics. Sevoflurane administration is compatible with benzodiazepines and opioids as commonly used in surgical practice).
No products indexed under this heading.

Propoxyphene Hydrochloride (Benzodiazepines would be expected to decrease the MAC of sevoflurane in the same manner as with other inhalational anesthetics. Sevoflurane administration is compatible with benzodiazepines and opioids as commonly used in surgical practice).
No products indexed under this heading.

Propoxyphene Napsylate (Benzodiazepines would be expected to decrease the MAC of sevoflurane in the same manner as with other inhalational anesthetics. Sevoflurane administration is compatible with benzodiazepines and opioids as commonly used in surgical practice).
No products indexed under this heading.

Quazepam (Benzodiazepines would be expected to decrease the MAC of sevoflurane in the same manner as with other inhalational anesthetics. Sevoflurane administration is compatible with benzodiazepines and opioids as commonly used in surgical practice).
No products indexed under this heading.

Rapacuronium Bromide (Sevoflurane increases both the intensity and duration of neuromuscular blockade induced by non-depolarizing muscle relaxants. When used to supplement alfentanil-nitrous oxide anesthesia, sevoflurane and isoflurane equally potentiate neuromuscular block induced with pancuronium, vecuronium or atracurium. Among available non-depolarizing agents, only vecuronium, pancuronium and atracurium interactions have been studied during sevoflurane anesthesia. In the absence of specific guidelines: 1) For endotracheal intubation, do not reduce the dose of non-depolarizing muscle relaxants. 2) During maintenance of anesthesia, the required dose of non-depolarizing muscle relaxants is likely to be reduced compared to that during nitrous oxide/opioid anesthesia).
No products indexed under this heading.

Remifentanil Hydrochloride (Benzodiazepines would be expected to decrease the MAC of sevoflurane in the same manner as with other inhalational anesthetics. Sevoflurane administration is compatible with benzodiazepines and opioids as commonly used in surgical practice).
No products indexed under this heading.

Rocuronium Bromide (Sevoflurane increases both the intensity and duration of neuromuscular blockade induced by non-depolarizing muscle relaxants. When used to supplement alfentanil-nitrous oxide anesthesia, sevoflurane and isoflurane equally potentiate neuromuscular block induced with pancuronium, vecuronium or atracurium. Among available non-depolarizing agents, only vecuronium, pancuronium and atracurium interactions have been studied during sevoflurane anesthesia. In the absence of specific guidelines: 1) For endotracheal intubation, do not reduce the dose of non-depolarizing muscle relaxants. 2) During maintenance of anesthesia, the required dose of non-depolarizing muscle relaxants is likely to be reduced compared to that during nitrous oxide/opioid anesthesia). Products include:
Zemuron Injection 2346

Sufentanil Citrate (Benzodiazepines would be expected to decrease the MAC of sevoflurane in the same manner as with other inhalational anesthetics. Sevoflurane administration is compatible with benzodiazepines and opioids as commonly used in surgical practice).
No products indexed under this heading.

Temazepam (Benzodiazepines would be expected to decrease the MAC of sevoflurane in the same manner as with other inhalational anesthetics. Sevoflurane administration is compatible with benzodiazepines and opioids as commonly used in surgical practice). Products include:
Restoril Capsules 1860

Triazolam (Benzodiazepines would be expected to decrease the MAC of sevoflurane in the same manner as with other inhalational anesthetics. Sevoflurane administration is compatible with benzodiazepines and opioids as commonly used in surgical practice).
No products indexed under this heading.

Vecuronium Bromide (Sevoflurane increases both the intensity and duration of neuromuscular blockade induced by non-depolarizing muscle relaxants. When used to supplement alfentanil-nitrous oxide anesthesia, sevoflurane and isoflurane equally potentiate neuromuscular block induced with pancuronium, vecuronium or atracurium. Among available non-depolarizing agents, only vecuronium, pancuronium and atracurium interactions have been studied during sevoflurane anesthesia. In the absence of specific guidelines: 1) For endotracheal intubation, do not reduce the dose of non-depolarizing muscle relaxants. 2) During maintenance of anesthesia, the required dose of non-depolarizing muscle relaxants is likely to be reduced compared to that during nitrous oxide/opioid anesthesia).
No products indexed under this heading.

ULTRAM ER TABLETS

(Tramadol Hydrochloride) 2392
May interact with anesthetics, central nervous system depressants, cytochrome p450 2d6 inhibitors (selected), cytochrome p450 3a4 inducers (selected), cytochrome p450 3a4 inhibitors (selected), hypnotics and sedatives, monoamine oxidase inhibitors, narcotic analgesics, antipsychotic agents, phenothiazines, psychotropics, quinidine, selective serotonin reuptake inhibitors, tranquilizers, tricyclic antidepressants, and certain other agents. Compounds in these categories include:

Acetazolamide (Administration of CYP3A4 inhibitors, such as ketoconazole and erythromycin, with tramadol hydrochloride may effect the meatbolism of tramadol leading to altered tramadol exposure).
No products indexed under this heading.

Alfentanil Hydrochloride (Tramadol hydrochloride is contraindicated in acute intoxication with narcotics, opioids, and centrally-acting analgesics. Concomitant use of tramadol increases the seizure risk in patients taking opioids. Tramadol hydrochloride should be used with caution and in reduced dosages when adminis-

tered to patients receiving CNS depressants, such as opioids or narcotics. Tramadol hydrochloride increases the risk of CNS and respiratory depression. Tramadol may be expected to have additive effects when used in conjunction with other opioids).
No products indexed under this heading.

Allium sativum (Administration of CYP3A4 inducers, such as rifampin or St. John's Wort, with tramadol hydrochloride may effect the meatbolism of tramadol leading to altered tramadol exposure).
No products indexed under this heading.

Alprazolam (Tramadol hydrochloride is contraindicated in acute intoxication with psychotropic drugs). Products include:
Niravam Orally Disintegrating Tablets 3092

Amiodarone Hydrochloride (In vitro drug interaction studies in human liver microsomes indicate that concomitant administration with inhibitors of CYP2D6 could result in some inhibition of the metabolism of tramadol).
No products indexed under this heading.

Amitriptyline Hydrochloride (Tramadol hydrochloride is contraindicated in acute intoxication with psychotropic drugs).
No products indexed under this heading.

Amoxapine (Tramadol hydrochloride is contraindicated in acute intoxication with psychotropic drugs).
No products indexed under this heading.

Amprenavir (Administration of CYP3A4 inhibitors, such as ketoconazole and erythromycin, with tramadol hydrochloride may effect the meatbolism of tramadol leading to altered tramadol exposure). Products include:
Agenerase Capsules 1327
Agenerase Oral Solution 1332

Anastrozole (Administration of CYP3A4 inhibitors, such as ketoconazole and erythromycin, with tramadol hydrochloride may effect the meatbolism of tramadol leading to altered tramadol exposure). Products include:
Arimidex Tablets 673

Aprepitant (Administration of CYP3A4 inhibitors, such as ketoconazole and erythromycin, with tramadol hydrochloride may effect the meatbolism of tramadol leading to altered tramadol exposure). Products include:
Emend Capsules 1963

Aprobarbital (Tramadol hydrochloride should be used with caution and in reduced dosages when administered to patients receiving CNS depressants, such as alcohol, opioids, anesthetic agents, narcotics, phenothiazines, tranquilizers, or sedative hypnotics. Tramadol hydrochloride increases the risk of CNS and respiratory depression).
No products indexed under this heading.

Aripiprazole (Administration of tramadol may increase the seizure risk in patients taking neuroleptics or other drugs that reduce the seizure threshold). Products include:
Abilify Oral Solution 882
Abilify Oral Solution 2450
Abilify Discmelt Orally Disintegrating Tablets 882
Abilify Discmelt Orally Disintegrating Tablets 2450
Abilify Tablets 882
Abilify Tablets 2450

Betamethasone Acetate (Administration of CYP3A4 inducers, such as rifampin or St. John's Wort, with tramadol hydrochloride may effect the meatbolism of tramadol leading to altered tramadol exposure).
No products indexed under this heading.

Betamethasone Sodium Phosphate (Administration of CYP3A4 inducers, such as rifampin or St. John's Wort, with tramadol hydrochloride may effect the meatbolism of tramadol leading to altered tramadol exposure).
No products indexed under this heading.

Buprenorphine Hydrochloride (Tramadol hydrochloride is contraindicated in acute intoxication with narcotics, opioids, and centrally-acting analgesics. Concomitant use of tramadol increases the seizure risk in patients taking opioids. Tramadol hydrochloride should be used with caution and in reduced dosages when administered to patients receiving CNS depressants, such as opioids or narcotics. Tramadol hydrochloride increases the risk of CNS and respiratory depression. Tramadol may be expected to have additive effects when used in conjunction with other opioids). Products include:
Buprenex Injectable 2716
Suboxone Tablets 2717
Subutex Tablets 2717

Bupropion Hydrochloride (In vitro drug interaction studies in human liver microsomes indicate that concomitant administration with inhibitors of CYP2D6 could result in some inhibition of the metabolism of tramadol). Products include:
Wellbutrin Tablets 1603
Wellbutrin SR Sustained-Release Tablets 1607
Wellbutrin XL Extended-Release Tablets 1613
Zyban Sustained-Release Tablets 1644

Buspirone Hydrochloride (Tramadol hydrochloride is contraindicated in acute intoxication with psychotropic drugs).
No products indexed under this heading.

Butabarbital (Tramadol hydrochloride should be used with caution and in reduced dosages when administered to patients receiving CNS depressants, such as alcohol, opioids, anesthetic agents, narcotics, phenothiazines, tranquilizers, or sedative hypnotics. Tramadol hydrochloride increases the risk of CNS and respiratory depression).
No products indexed under this heading.

Butalbital (Tramadol hydrochloride should be used with caution and in reduced dosages when administered to patients receiving CNS depressants, such as alcohol, opioids, anesthetic agents, narcotics, phenothiazines, tranquilizers, or sedative hypnotics. Tramadol hydrochloride increases the risk of CNS and respiratory depression).
No products indexed under this heading.

Carbamazepine (Patients taking carbamazepine, a CYP3A4 inducer, may have a significantly reduced analgesic effect of tramadol. Because carbamazepine increases tramadol metabolism and because of the seizure risk associated with tramadol, concomitant administration of tramadol hydrochloride and carbamazepine is not recommended). Products include:
Carbatrol Capsules 3171
Equetro Extended-Release Capsules 3180
Tegretol/Tegretol-XR 2295

Celecoxib (In vitro drug interaction studies in human liver microsomes indicate that concomitant administration with inhibitors of CYP2D6 could result in some inhibition of the metabolism of tramadol). Products include:
Celebrex Capsules 3134

Chlordiazepoxide (Tramadol hydrochloride is contraindicated in acute intoxication with psychotropic drugs).
No products indexed under this heading.

Chlordiazepoxide Hydrochloride (Tramadol hydrochloride is contraindicated in acute intoxication with psychotropic drugs). Products include:
Librium Capsules 3347

Chloroquine Hydrochloride (In vitro drug interaction studies in human liver microsomes indicate that concomitant administration with inhibitors of CYP2D6 could result in some inhibition of the metabolism of tramadol).
No products indexed under this heading.

Chloroquine Phosphate (In vitro drug interaction studies in human liver microsomes indicate that concomitant administration with inhibitors of CYP2D6 could result in some inhibition of the metabolism of tramadol).
No products indexed under this heading.

Chlorpheniramine (In vitro drug interaction studies in human liver microsomes indicate that concomitant administration with inhibitors of CYP2D6 could result in some inhibition of the metabolism of tramadol).
No products indexed under this heading.

Chlorpheniramine Maleate (In vitro drug interaction studies in human liver microsomes indicate that concomitant administration with inhibitors of CYP2D6 could result in some inhibition of the metabolism of tramadol). Products include:
Advil Allergy Sinus Caplets .... ▣770
Advil Multi-Symptom Cold Caplets .... ▣770
BC Allergy Sinus Cold Powder .... ▣677
Comtrex Maximum Strength Cold & Cough Day/Night Caplets - Night Formulation .... ▣726
Comtrex Maximum Strength Day/Night Severe Cold & Sinus Caplets - Night Formulation .... ▣725
Contac Cold and Flu Maximum Strength Caplets .... ▣728
Contac Cold and Flu Day and Night Caplets (Night Formulation Only) .... ▣727
Children's Dimetapp Long Acting Cough Plus Cold Syrup .... ▣731
Robitussin Cough & Cold Long-Acting Liquid .... ▣735
Robitussin Cough & Allergy Syrup .... ▣736
Robitussin Cough & Cold Nighttime Liquid .... ▣736
Robitussin Cough, Cold & Flu Nighttime Liquid .... ▣738
Robitussin Pediatric Cough & Cold Long-Acting Liquid .... ▣735
Robitussin Pediatric Cough & Cold Nighttime Liquid .... ▣736
Triaminic Cold & Allergy Liquid .... ▣746
Triaminic Cough & Runny Nose Softchews .... ▣748
Children's Tylenol Plus Flu Oral Suspension .... ▣749
Tylenol Allergy Multi-Symptom Caplets with Cool Burst and Gelcaps 1872
Children's Tylenol Plus Cold Suspension Liquid 1879
Children's Tylenol Plus Cough & Runny Nose Suspension Liquid 1879
Children's Tylenol Plus Flu Suspension Liquid 1881
Children's Tylenol Plus Multi-Symptom Cold Suspension Liquid 1879
Tylenol Cold Head Congestion Nighttime Caplets with Cool Burst 1873
Tylenol Cold Multi-Symptom Nighttime Caplets with Cool Burst 1874
Tylenol Sinus Congestion & Pain Nighttime Caplets with Cool Burst 1876
Vicks 44M Cough, Cold & Flu Relief Liquid 2680
Pediatric Vicks 44m Cough & Cold Relief Liquid 2676
Children's Vicks NyQuil Cold/Cough Relief .... ▣756
Children's Vicks NyQuil Cold/Cough Relief Liquid 2680
Zicam Maximum Strength Flu Daytime .... ▣768

Chlorpheniramine Polistirex (In vitro drug interaction studies in human liver microsomes indicate that concomitant administration with inhibitors of CYP2D6 could result in some inhibition of the metabolism of tramadol). Products include:
Tussionex Pennkinetic Extended-Release Suspension 3327

Chlorpheniramine Tannate (In vitro drug interaction studies in human liver microsomes indicate that concomitant administration with inhibitors of CYP2D6 could result in some inhibition of the metabolism of tramadol).
No products indexed under this heading.

Chlorpromazine (Tramadol hydrochloride is contraindicated in acute intoxication with psychotropic drugs).
No products indexed under this heading.

Chlorpromazine Hydrochloride (Tramadol hydrochloride is contraindicated in acute intoxication with psychotropic drugs).
No products indexed under this heading.

Chlorprothixene (Tramadol hydrochloride is contraindicated in acute intoxication with psychotropic drugs).
No products indexed under this heading.

Chlorprothixene Hydrochloride (Tramadol hydrochloride is contraindicated in acute intoxication with psychotropic drugs).
No products indexed under this heading.

Chlorprothixene Lactate (Tramadol hydrochloride should be used with caution and in reduced dosages when administered to patients receiving CNS depressants, such as alcohol, opioids, anesthetic agents, narcotics, phenothiazines, tranquilizers, or sedative hypnotics. Tramadol hydrochloride increases the risk of CNS and respiratory depression).
No products indexed under this heading.

Cimetidine (In vitro drug interaction studies in human liver microsomes indicate that concomitant administration with inhibitors of CYP2D6 could result in some inhibition of the metabolism of tramadol). Products include:
Tagamet HB 200 Tablets 664

Cimetidine Hydrochloride (In vitro drug interaction studies in human liver microsomes indicate that concomitant administration with inhibitors of CYP2D6 could result in some inhibition of the metabolism of tramadol).
No products indexed under this heading.

Ciprofloxacin (Administration of CYP3A4 inhibitors, such as ketoconazole and erythromycin, with tramadol hydrochloride may effect the meatbolism of tramadol leading to altered tramadol exposure).
Products include:
Cipro Oral Suspension 2977
Cipro I.V. 2984
Cipro XR Tablets 2990
Ciprodex Otic Suspension 559

Ciprofloxacin Hydrochloride (Administration of CYP3A4 inducers, such as rifampin or St. John's Wort, with tramadol hydrochloride may effect the meatbolism of tramadol leading to altered tramadol exposure). Products include:
Ciloxan Ophthalmic Ointment 559
Ciloxan Ophthalmic Solution .... ⊙ 206
Cipro Tablets 2977
Proquin XR Tablets 1153

Cisplatin (Administration of CYP3A4 inducers, such as rifampin or St. John's Wort, with tramadol hydrochloride may effect the meatbolism of tramadol leading to altered tramadol exposure).
No products indexed under this heading.

Citalopram Hydrobromide (Concomitant use of tramadol increases the seizure risk in patients taking selective serotonin re-uptake inhibitors. Concomitant use of tramadol with SSRIs increases the risk of adverse events, including seizure and serotonin syndrome). Products include:
Celexa 1176

Clarithromycin (Administration of CYP3A4 inhibitors, such as ketoconazole and erythromycin, with tramadol hydrochloride may effect the meatbolism of tramadol leading to altered tramadol exposure).
Products include:
Biaxin/Biaxin XL 402
PREVPAC 3284

Clomipramine Hydrochloride (Concomitant use of tramadol increases the seizure risk in patients taking tricyclic antidepressants).
No products indexed under this heading.

Clorazepate Dipotassium (Tramadol hydrochloride is contraindicated in acute intoxication with psychotropic drugs). Products include:
Tranxene 2474

Clotrimazole (Administration of CYP3A4 inhibitors, such as ketoconazole and erythromycin, with tramadol hydrochloride may effect the meatbolism of tramadol leading to altered tramadol exposure).
Products include:
Desenex Athlete's Foot Cream 635
Lotrimin 3039
Lotrisone 3040

Clozapine (Tramadol hydrochloride is contraindicated in acute intoxication with psychotropic drugs).
Products include:
Clozaril Tablets 2184
FazaClo Orally Disintegrating Tablets 551

Cocaine Hydrochloride (In vitro drug interaction studies in human liver microsomes indicate that concomitant administration with inhibitors of CYP2D6 could result in some inhibition of the metabolism of tramadol).
No products indexed under this heading.

Codeine Phosphate (Tramadol hydrochloride is contraindicated in acute intoxication with narcotics, opioids, and centrally-acting analgesics. Concomitant use of tramadol increases the seizure risk in patients taking opioids. Tramadol hydrochloride should be used with caution and in reduced dosages when administered to patients receiving CNS depressants, such as opioids or narcotics. Tramadol hydrochloride increases the risk of CNS and respiratory depression. Tramadol may be expected to have additive effects when used in conjunction with other opioids). Products include:
Tylenol with Codeine Tablets 2391

Cortisone Acetate (Administration of CYP3A4 inducers, such as rifampin or St. John's Wort, with tramadol hydrochloride may effect the meatbolism of tramadol leading to altered tramadol exposure).
No products indexed under this heading.

Cyclobenzaprine (Concomitant use of tramadol increases the seizure risk in patients taking tricyclic compounds, such as cyclobenzaprine).
No products indexed under this heading.

Cyclobenzaprine Hydrochloride (Concomitant use of tramadol increases the seizure risk in patients taking tricyclic compounds, such as cyclobenzaprine).
No products indexed under this heading.

Cyclosporine (Administration of CYP3A4 inhibitors, such as ketoconazole and erythromycin, with tramadol hydrochloride may effect the meatbolism of tramadol leading to altered tramadol exposure).
Products include:
Gengraf Capsules 459
Neoral Oral Solution 2259
Neoral Soft Gelatin Capsules 2259
Restasis Ophthalmic Emulsion 575
Sandimmune 2275

Dalfopristin (Administration of CYP3A4 inhibitors, such as ketoconazole and erythromycin, with tramadol hydrochloride may effect the meatbolism of tramadol leading to altered tramadol exposure).
No products indexed under this heading.

Danazol (Administration of CYP3A4 inhibitors, such as ketoconazole and erythromycin, with tramadol hydrochloride may effect the meatbolism of tramadol leading to altered tramadol exposure).
No products indexed under this heading.

Delavirdine Mesylate (Administration of CYP3A4 inhibitors, such as ketoconazole and erythromycin, with tramadol hydrochloride may effect the meatbolism of tramadol leading to altered tramadol exposure).
Products include:
Rescriptor Tablets 2551

Desflurane (Tramadol hydrochloride should be used with caution and in reduced dosages when administered to patients receiving CNS depressants, such as alcohol, opioids, anesthetic agents, narcotics, phenothiazines, tranquilizers, or sedative hypnotics. Tramadol hydrochloride increases the risk of CNS and respiratory depression).
No products indexed under this heading.

Desipramine Hydrochloride (Tramadol hydrochloride is contraindicated in acute intoxication with psychotropic drugs).
No products indexed under this heading.

Dexamethasone (Administration of CYP3A4 inducers, such as rifampin or St. John's Wort, with tramadol hydrochloride may effect the meatbolism of tramadol leading to altered tramadol exposure). Products include:
Ciprodex Otic Suspension 559
Decadron Tablets 1951
TobraDex Ophthalmic Ointment 562
TobraDex Ophthalmic Suspension ... 563

Dexamethasone Acetate (Administration of CYP3A4 inducers, such as rifampin or St. John's Wort, with tramadol hydrochloride may effect the meatbolism of tramadol leading to altered tramadol exposure).
No products indexed under this heading.

Dexamethasone Sodium Phosphate (Administration of CYP3A4 inducers, such as rifampin or St. John's Wort, with tramadol hydrochloride may effect the meatbolism of tramadol leading to altered tramadol exposure).
No products indexed under this heading.

Dezocine (Tramadol hydrochloride is contraindicated in acute intoxication with narcotics, opioids, and centrally-acting analgesics. Concomitant use of tramadol increases the seizure risk in patients taking opioids. Tramadol hydrochloride should be used with caution and in reduced dosages when administered to patients receiving CNS depressants, such as opioids or narcotics. Tramadol hydrochloride increases the risk of CNS and respiratory depression. Tramadol may be expected to have additive effects when used in conjunction with other opioids).
No products indexed under this heading.

Diazepam (Tramadol hydrochloride is contraindicated in acute intoxication with psychotropic drugs).
Products include:
Diastat Rectal Delivery System 3343
Valium Tablets 2819

Digoxin (Post-marketing surveillance of tramadol has revealed rare reports of digoxin toxicity). Products include:
Lanoxicaps Capsules 1490
Lanoxin Injection 1494
Lanoxin Injection Pediatric 1497
Lanoxin Tablets 1500

Diltiazem Hydrochloride (Administration of CYP3A4 inhibitors, such as ketoconazole and erythromycin, with tramadol hydrochloride may effect the meatbolism of tramadol leading to altered tramadol exposure). Products include:
Cardizem LA Extended Release Tablets 1728
Tiazac Capsules 1201

Diltiazem Maleate (Administration of CYP3A4 inhibitors, such as ketoconazole and erythromycin, with tramadol hydrochloride may effect the meatbolism of tramadol leading to altered tramadol exposure).
No products indexed under this heading.

Diphenhydramine (In vitro drug interaction studies in human liver microsomes indicate that concomitant administration with inhibitors of CYP2D6 could result in some inhibition of the metabolism of tramadol).
Products include:
Tylenol Sore Throat Nighttime Liquid with Cool Burst.................. 1877

Diphenhydramine Hydrochloride (In vitro drug interaction studies in human liver microsomes indicate that concomitant administration with inhibitors of CYP2D6 could result in some inhibition of the metabolism of tramadol). Products include:
Nytol QuickCaps Caplets 615
Nytol QuickGels Softgels Maximum Strength...................... 616
Simply Sleep Caplets 1868
Sominex Original Formula Tablets .. 616
TheraFlu Warming Relief Nighttime Severe Cold 743
TheraFlu Thin Strips Multi Symptom.................................. 744
Triaminic Nighttime Cold & Cough Liquid................................ 746
Triaminic Thin Strips Cough & Runny Nose 749
Extra Strength Tylenol PM Caplets, Vanilla Caplets, Geltabs, Gelcaps and Liquid.......... 1875
Tylenol Sore Throat Nighttime Liquid with Cool Burst 790
Tylenol Allergy Multi-Symptom Nighttime Caplets with Cool Burst... 1872
Tylenol Severe Allergy Caplets 1872
Children's Tylenol Plus Cold & Allergy Suspension Liquid............ 1878

Doxepin Hydrochloride (Tramadol hydrochloride is contraindicated in acute intoxication with psychotropic drugs).
No products indexed under this heading.

Doxorubicin Hydrochloride (Administration of CYP3A4 inducers, such as rifampin or St. John's Wort, with tramadol hydrochloride may effect the meatbolism of tramadol leading to altered tramadol exposure).
No products indexed under this heading.

Droperidol (Tramadol hydrochloride is contraindicated in acute intoxication with psychotropic drugs).
No products indexed under this heading.

Efavirenz (Administration of CYP3A4 inhibitors, such as ketoconazole and erythromycin, with tramadol hydrochloride may effect the meatbolism of tramadol leading to altered tramadol exposure). Products include:

Enflurane (Tramadol hydrochloride should be used with caution and in reduced dosages when administered to patients receiving CNS depressants, such as alcohol, opioids, anesthetic agents, narcotics, phenothiazines, tranquilizers, or sedative hypnotics. Tramadol hydrochloride increases the risk of CNS and respiratory depression).

No products indexed under this heading.

Erythromycin (Administration of CYP3A4 inhibitors, such as ketoconazole and erythromycin, with tramadol hydrochloride may effect the meatbolism of tramadol leading to altered tramadol exposure). Products include:

Erythromycin Estolate (Administration of CYP3A4 inhibitors, such as ketoconazole and erythromycin, with tramadol hydrochloride may effect the meatbolism of tramadol leading to altered tramadol exposure).

No products indexed under this heading.

Erythromycin Ethylsuccinate (Administration of CYP3A4 inhibitors, such as ketoconazole and erythromycin, with tramadol hydrochloride may effect the meatbolism of tramadol leading to altered tramadol exposure). Products include:

Erythromycin Gluceptate (Administration of CYP3A4 inhibitors, such as ketoconazole and erythromycin, with tramadol hydrochloride may effect the meatbolism of tramadol leading to altered tramadol exposure).

No products indexed under this heading.

Erythromycin Lactobionate (Administration of CYP3A4 inhibitors, such as ketoconazole and erythromycin, with tramadol hydrochloride may effect the meatbolism of tramadol leading to altered tramadol exposure).

No products indexed under this heading.

Erythromycin Stearate (Administration of CYP3A4 inhibitors, such as ketoconazole and erythromycin, with tramadol hydrochloride may effect the meatbolism of tramadol leading to altered tramadol exposure). Products include:

Escitalopram Oxalate (Concomitant use of tramadol increases the seizure risk in patients taking selective serotonin re-uptake inhibitors. Concomitant use of tramadol with SSRIs increases the risk of adverse events, including seizure and serotonin syndrome). Products include:

Esomeprazole Magnesium (Administration of CYP3A4 inhibitors, such as ketoconazole and erythro-

mycin, with tramadol hydrochloride may effect the meatbolism of tramadol leading to altered tramadol exposure). Products include:

Estazolam (Tramadol hydrochloride is contraindicated in acute intoxication with hypnotics. Tramadol hydrochloride should be used with caution and in reduced dosages when administered to patients receiving CNS depressants, such as sedative hypnotics. Tramadol hydrochloride increases the risk of CNS and respiratory depression). Products include:

Ethanol (Tramadol hydrochloride should be used with caution and in reduced dosages when administered to patients receiving CNS depressants, such as alcohol, opioids, anesthetic agents, narcotics, phenothiazines, tranquilizers, or sedative hypnotics. Tramadol hydrochloride increases the risk of CNS and respiratory depression).

No products indexed under this heading.

Ethchlorvynol (Tramadol hydrochloride is contraindicated in acute intoxication with hypnotics. Tramadol hydrochloride should be used with caution and in reduced dosages when administered to patients receiving CNS depressants, such as sedative hypnotics. Tramadol hydrochloride increases the risk of CNS and respiratory depression).

No products indexed under this heading.

Ethinamate (Tramadol hydrochloride is contraindicated in acute intoxication with hypnotics. Tramadol hydrochloride should be used with caution and in reduced dosages when administered to patients receiving CNS depressants, such as sedative hypnotics. Tramadol hydrochloride increases the risk of CNS and respiratory depression).

No products indexed under this heading.

Ethosuximide (Administration of CYP3A4 inducers, such as rifampin or St. John's Wort, with tramadol hydrochloride may effect the meatbolism of tramadol leading to altered tramadol exposure).

No products indexed under this heading.

Ethyl Alcohol (Tramadol hydrochloride should be used with caution and in reduced dosages when administered to patients receiving CNS depressants, such as alcohol, opioids, anesthetic agents, narcotics, phenothiazines, tranquilizers, or sedative hypnotics. Tramadol hydrochloride increases the risk of CNS and respiratory depression).

No products indexed under this heading.

Felbamate (Administration of CYP3A4 inducers, such as rifampin or St. John's Wort, with tramadol hydrochloride may effect the meatbolism of tramadol leading to altered tramadol exposure).

No products indexed under this heading.

Fentanyl (Tramadol hydrochloride is contraindicated in acute intoxication with narcotics, opioids, and centrally-acting analgesics. Concomitant use of tramadol increases the seizure risk in patients taking opioids. Tra-

madol hydrochloride should be used with caution and in reduced dosages when administered to patients receiving CNS depressants, such as opioids or narcotics. Tramadol hydrochloride increases the risk of CNS and respiratory depression. Tramadol may be expected to have additive effects when used in conjunction with other opioids). Products include:

Fentanyl Citrate (Tramadol hydrochloride is contraindicated in acute intoxication with narcotics, opioids, and centrally-acting analgesics. Concomitant use of tramadol increases the seizure risk in patients taking opioids. Tramadol hydrochloride should be used with caution and in reduced dosages when administered to patients receiving CNS depressants, such as opioids or narcotics. Tramadol hydrochloride increases the risk of CNS and respiratory depression. Tramadol may be expected to have additive effects when used in conjunction with other opioids). Products include:

Fluconazole (Administration of CYP3A4 inhibitors, such as ketoconazole and erythromycin, with tramadol hydrochloride may effect the meatbolism of tramadol leading to altered tramadol exposure).

No products indexed under this heading.

Fludrocortisone Acetate (Administration of CYP3A4 inducers, such as rifampin or St. John's Wort, with tramadol hydrochloride may effect the meatbolism of tramadol leading to altered tramadol exposure).

No products indexed under this heading.

Fluoxetine (In vitro drug interaction studies in human liver microsomes indicate that concomitant administration with inhibitors of CYP2D6 could result in some inhibition of the metabolism of tramadol).

No products indexed under this heading.

Fluoxetine Hydrochloride (Concomitant use of tramadol increases the seizure risk in patients taking selective serotonin re-uptake inhibitors. Concomitant use of tramadol with SSRIs increases the risk of adverse events, including seizure and serotonin syndrome). Products include:

Fluphenazine Decanoate (Tramadol hydrochloride is contraindicated in acute intoxication with psychotropic drugs).

No products indexed under this heading.

Fluphenazine Enanthate (Tramadol hydrochloride is contraindicated in acute intoxication with psychotropic drugs).

No products indexed under this heading.

Fluphenazine Hydrochloride (Tramadol hydrochloride is contraindicated in acute intoxication with psychotropic drugs).

No products indexed under this heading.

Flurazepam Hydrochloride (Tramadol hydrochloride is contraindicated in acute intoxication with hyp-

notics. Tramadol hydrochloride should be used with caution and in reduced dosages when administered to patients receiving CNS depressants, such as sedative hypnotics. Tramadol hydrochloride increases the risk of CNS and respiratory depression). Products include:

Fluvoxamine Maleate (Concomitant use of tramadol increases the seizure risk in patients taking selective serotonin re-uptake inhibitors. Concomitant use of tramadol with SSRIs increases the risk of adverse events, including seizure and serotonin syndrome).

No products indexed under this heading.

Fosamprenavir Calcium (Administration of CYP3A4 inhibitors, such as ketoconazole and erythromycin, with tramadol hydrochloride may effect the meatbolism of tramadol leading to altered tramadol exposure). Products include:

Fosphenytoin Sodium (Administration of CYP3A4 inducers, such as rifampin or St. John's Wort, with tramadol hydrochloride may effect the meatbolism of tramadol leading to altered tramadol exposure).

No products indexed under this heading.

Garlic Extract (Administration of CYP3A4 inducers, such as rifampin or St. John's Wort, with tramadol hydrochloride may effect the meatbolism of tramadol leading to altered tramadol exposure).

No products indexed under this heading.

Garlic Oil (Administration of CYP3A4 inducers, such as rifampin or St. John's Wort, with tramadol hydrochloride may effect the meatbolism of tramadol leading to altered tramadol exposure).

No products indexed under this heading.

Glutethimide (Tramadol hydrochloride is contraindicated in acute intoxication with hypnotics. Tramadol hydrochloride should be used with caution and in reduced dosages when administered to patients receiving CNS depressants, such as sedative hypnotics. Tramadol hydrochloride increases the risk of CNS and respiratory depression).

No products indexed under this heading.

Halofantrine Hydrochloride (In vitro drug interaction studies in human liver microsomes indicate that concomitant administration with inhibitors of CYP2D6 could result in some inhibition of the metabolism of tramadol).

No products indexed under this heading.

Haloperidol (Tramadol hydrochloride is contraindicated in acute intoxication with psychotropic drugs).

No products indexed under this heading.

Haloperidol Decanoate (Tramadol hydrochloride is contraindicated in acute intoxication with psychotropic drugs).

No products indexed under this heading.

Halothane (Tramadol hydrochloride should be used with caution and in reduced dosages when administered to patients receiving CNS depressants, such as anesthetic agents. Tramadol hydrochloride increases the risk of CNS and respiratory depression).
No products indexed under this heading.

Hydrocodone Bitartrate (Tramadol hydrochloride is contraindicated in acute intoxication with narcotics, opioids, and centrally-acting analgesics. Concomitant use of tramadol increases the seizure risk in patients taking opioids. Tramadol hydrochloride should be used with caution and in reduced dosages when administered to patients receiving CNS depressants, such as opioids or narcotics. Tramadol hydrochloride increases the risk of CNS and respiratory depression. Tramadol may be expected to have additive effects when used in conjunction with other opioids). Products include:
Hycodan 1116
Hycotuss Expectorant Syrup 1117
Vicodin Tablets 535
Vicodin ES Tablets 536
Vicodin HP Tablets 538
Vicoprofen Tablets 539
Zydone Tablets 1139

Hydrocodone Polistirex (Tramadol hydrochloride is contraindicated in acute intoxication with narcotics, opioids, and centrally-acting analgesics. Concomitant use of tramadol increases the seizure risk in patients taking opioids. Tramadol hydrochloride should be used with caution and in reduced dosages when administered to patients receiving CNS depressants, such as opioids or narcotics. Tramadol hydrochloride increases the risk of CNS and respiratory depression. Tramadol may be expected to have additive effects when used in conjunction with other opioids). Products include:
Tussionex Pennkinetic Extended-Release Suspension 3327

Hydrocortisone (Administration of CYP3A4 inducers, such as rifampin or St. John's Wort, with tramadol hydrochloride may effect the meatbolism of tramadol leading to altered tramadol exposure). Products include:
Colocort Rectal Suspension, USP (Retention) 100 mg/60 mL 2476
Hydrocortone Tablets 1989
Preparation H Hydrocortisone Cream 646

Hydrocortisone Acetate (Administration of CYP3A4 inducers, such as rifampin or St. John's Wort, with tramadol hydrochloride may effect the meatbolism of tramadol leading to altered tramadol exposure). Products include:
Analpram-HC 1159
Pramosone 1161
ProctoFoam-HC 3099

Hydrocortisone Butyrate (Administration of CYP3A4 inducers, such as rifampin or St. John's Wort, with tramadol hydrochloride may effect the meatbolism of tramadol leading to altered tramadol exposure). Products include:
Locoid Lipocream Cream 1160

Hydrocortisone Cypionate (Administration of CYP3A4 inducers, such as rifampin or St. John's Wort, with tramadol hydrochloride may effect the meatbolism of tramadol leading to altered tramadol exposure).
No products indexed under this heading.

Hydrocortisone Hemisuccinate (Administration of CYP3A4 inducers, such as rifampin or St. John's Wort, with tramadol hydrochloride may effect the meatbolism of tramadol leading to altered tramadol exposure).
No products indexed under this heading.

Hydrocortisone Probutate (Administration of CYP3A4 inducers, such as rifampin or St. John's Wort, with tramadol hydrochloride may effect the meatbolism of tramadol leading to altered tramadol exposure).
No products indexed under this heading.

Hydrocortisone Sodium Phosphate (Administration of CYP3A4 inducers, such as rifampin or St. John's Wort, with tramadol hydrochloride may effect the meatbolism of tramadol leading to altered tramadol exposure).
No products indexed under this heading.

Hydrocortisone Sodium Succinate (Administration of CYP3A4 inducers, such as rifampin or St. John's Wort, with tramadol hydrochloride may effect the meatbolism of tramadol leading to altered tramadol exposure).
No products indexed under this heading.

Hydrocortisone Valerate (Administration of CYP3A4 inducers, such as rifampin or St. John's Wort, with tramadol hydrochloride may effect the meatbolism of tramadol leading to altered tramadol exposure).
No products indexed under this heading.

Hydromorphone Hydrochloride (Tramadol hydrochloride is contraindicated in acute intoxication with narcotics, opioids, and centrally-acting analgesics. Concomitant use of tramadol increases the seizure risk in patients taking opioids. Tramadol hydrochloride should be used with caution and in reduced dosages when administered to patients receiving CNS depressants, such as opioids or narcotics. Tramadol hydrochloride increases the risk of CNS and respiratory depression. Tramadol may be expected to have additive effects when used in conjunction with other opioids). Products include:
Dilaudid 440
Dilaudid Non-Sterile Powder 440
Dilaudid Oral Liquid 445
Dilaudid Rectal Suppositories 440
Dilaudid Tablets 440
Dilaudid Tablets - 8 mg 445
Dilaudid-HP 442

Hydroxychloroquine Sulfate (In vitro drug interaction studies in human liver microsomes indicate that concomitant administration with inhibitors of CYP2D6 could result in some inhibition of the metabolism of tramadol).
No products indexed under this heading.

Hydroxyzine Hydrochloride (Tramadol hydrochloride is contraindicated in acute intoxication with psychotropic drugs).
No products indexed under this heading.

Hypericum (Administration of CYP3A4 inducers, such as rifampin or St. John's Wort, with tramadol hydrochloride may effect the meatbolism of tramadol leading to altered tramadol exposure). Products include:
Satiete Tablets 832

Hypericum Perforatum (Administration of CYP3A4 inducers, such as rifampin or St. John's Wort, with tramadol hydrochloride may effect the meatbolism of tramadol leading to altered tramadol exposure).
No products indexed under this heading.

Imatinib Mesylate (In vitro drug interaction studies in human liver microsomes indicate that concomitant administration with inhibitors of CYP2D6 could result in some inhibition of the metabolism of tramadol). Products include:
Gleevec Tablets 2227

Imipramine Hydrochloride (Tramadol hydrochloride is contraindicated in acute intoxication with psychotropic drugs).
No products indexed under this heading.

Imipramine Pamoate (Tramadol hydrochloride is contraindicated in acute intoxication with psychotropic drugs).
No products indexed under this heading.

Indinavir Sulfate (Administration of CYP3A4 inhibitors, such as ketoconazole and erythromycin, with tramadol hydrochloride may effect the meatbolism of tramadol leading to altered tramadol exposure). Products include:
Crixivan Capsules 1940

Isocarboxazid (Tramadol hydrochloride is contraindicated in acute intoxication with psychotropic drugs).
No products indexed under this heading.

Isoflurane (Tramadol hydrochloride should be used with caution and in reduced dosages when administered to patients receiving CNS depressants, such as alcohol, opioids, anesthetic agents, narcotics, phenothiazines, tranquilizers, or sedative hypnotics. Tramadol hydrochloride increases the risk of CNS and respiratory depression).
No products indexed under this heading.

Isoniazid (Administration of CYP3A4 inhibitors, such as ketoconazole and erythromycin, with tramadol hydrochloride may effect the meatbolism of tramadol leading to altered tramadol exposure).
No products indexed under this heading.

Itraconazole (Administration of CYP3A4 inhibitors, such as ketoconazole and erythromycin, with tramadol hydrochloride may effect the meatbolism of tramadol leading to altered tramadol exposure).
No products indexed under this heading.

Ketamine Hydrochloride (Tramadol hydrochloride should be used with caution and in reduced dosages when administered to patients receiving CNS depressants, such as alcohol, opioids, anesthetic agents, narcotics, phenothiazines, tranquilizers, or sedative hypnotics. Tramadol hydrochloride increases the risk of CNS and respiratory depression).
No products indexed under this heading.

Ketoconazole (Administration of CYP3A4 inhibitors, such as ketoconazole and erythromycin, with tramadol hydrochloride may effect the meatbolism of tramadol leading to altered tramadol exposure). Products include:
Nizoral A-D Shampoo, 1% 1868

Levomethadyl Acetate Hydrochloride (Tramadol hydrochloride should be used with caution and in reduced dosages when administered to patients receiving CNS depressants, such as alcohol, opioids, anesthetic agents, narcotics, phenothiazines, tranquilizers, or sedative hypnotics. Tramadol hydrochloride increases the risk of CNS and respiratory depression).
No products indexed under this heading.

Levorphanol Tartrate (Tramadol hydrochloride is contraindicated in acute intoxication with narcotics, opioids, and centrally-acting analgesics. Concomitant use of tramadol increases the seizure risk in patients taking opioids. Tramadol hydrochloride should be used with caution and in reduced dosages when administered to patients receiving CNS depressants, such as opioids or narcotics. Tramadol hydrochloride increases the risk of CNS and respiratory depression. Tramadol may be expected to have additive effects when used in conjunction with other opioids).
No products indexed under this heading.

Lithium Carbonate (Tramadol hydrochloride is contraindicated in acute intoxication with psychotropic drugs). Products include:
Lithobid Tablets 1692

Lithium Citrate (Tramadol hydrochloride is contraindicated in acute intoxication with psychotropic drugs).
No products indexed under this heading.

Lopinavir (Administration of CYP3A4 inhibitors, such as ketoconazole and erythromycin, with tramadol hydrochloride may effect the meatbolism of tramadol leading to altered tramadol exposure). Products include:
Kaletra 476

Loratadine (Administration of CYP3A4 inhibitors, such as ketoconazole and erythromycin, with tramadol hydrochloride may effect the meatbolism of tramadol leading to altered tramadol exposure). Products include:
Alavert Allergy & Sinus D-12 Hour Tablets 771
Alavert 771
Children's Claritin Allergy Oral Solution 771
Claritin Non-Drowsy 24 Hour Tablets 772
Claritin Reditabs 24 Hour Non-Drowsy Tablets 772

Lorazepam (Tramadol hydrochloride is contraindicated in acute intoxication with hypnotics. Tramadol hydrochloride should be used with caution and in reduced dosages when administered to patients receiving CNS depressants, such as sedative hypnotics. Tramadol hydrochloride increases the risk of CNS and respiratory depression).
No products indexed under this heading.

Loxapine Hydrochloride (Tramadol hydrochloride is contraindicated in acute intoxication with psychotropic drugs).
No products indexed under this heading.

Loxapine Succinate (Tramadol hydrochloride is contraindicated in acute intoxication with psychotropic drugs).
No products indexed under this heading.

Maprotiline Hydrochloride (Tramadol hydrochloride is contraindicated in acute intoxication with psychotropic drugs).
No products indexed under this heading.

Meperidine Hydrochloride (Tramadol hydrochloride is contraindicated in acute intoxication with narcotics, opioids, and centrally-acting analgesics. Concomitant use of tramadol increases the seizure risk in patients taking opioids. Tramadol hydrochloride should be used with caution and in reduced dosages when administered to patients receiving CNS depressants, such as opioids or narcotics. Tramadol hydrochloride increases the risk of CNS and respiratory depression. Tramadol may be expected to have additive effects when used in conjunction with other opioids).
No products indexed under this heading.

Mephenytoin (Administration of CYP3A4 inducers, such as rifampin or St. John's Wort, with tramadol hydrochloride may effect the meatbolism of tramadol leading to altered tramadol exposure).
No products indexed under this heading.

Mephobarbital (Tramadol hydrochloride should be used with caution and in reduced dosages when administered to patients receiving CNS depressants, such as alcohol, opioids, anesthetic agents, narcotics, phenothiazines, tranquilizers, or sedative hypnotics. Tramadol hydrochloride increases the risk of CNS and respiratory depression).
No products indexed under this heading.

Meprobamate (Tramadol hydrochloride is contraindicated in acute intoxication with psychotropic drugs).
No products indexed under this heading.

Mesoridazine Besylate (Tramadol hydrochloride is contraindicated in acute intoxication with psychotropic drugs).
No products indexed under this heading.

Methadone Hydrochloride (Tramadol hydrochloride is contraindi-

cated in acute intoxication with narcotics, opioids, and centrally-acting analgesics. Concomitant use of tramadol increases the seizure risk in patients taking opioids. Tramadol hydrochloride should be used with caution and in reduced dosages when administered to patients receiving CNS depressants, such as opioids or narcotics. Tramadol hydrochloride increases the risk of CNS and respiratory depression. Tramadol may be expected to have additive effects when used in conjunction with other opioids).
No products indexed under this heading.

Methohexital Sodium (Tramadol hydrochloride should be used with caution and in reduced dosages when administered to patients receiving CNS depressants, such as alcohol, opioids, anesthetic agents, narcotics, phenothiazines, tranquilizers, or sedative hypnotics. Tramadol hydrochloride increases the risk of CNS and respiratory depression).
No products indexed under this heading.

Methotrimeprazine (Administration of tramadol may increase the seizure risk in patients taking neuroleptics or other drugs that reduce the seizure threshold).
No products indexed under this heading.

Methoxyflurane (Tramadol hydrochloride should be used with caution and in reduced dosages when administered to patients receiving CNS depressants, such as alcohol, opioids, anesthetic agents, narcotics, phenothiazines, tranquilizers, or sedative hypnotics. Tramadol hydrochloride increases the risk of CNS and respiratory depression).
No products indexed under this heading.

Methsuximide (Administration of CYP3A4 inducers, such as rifampin or St. John's Wort, with tramadol hydrochloride may effect the meatbolism of tramadol leading to altered tramadol exposure).
No products indexed under this heading.

Methylprednisolone (Administration of CYP3A4 inducers, such as rifampin or St. John's Wort, with tramadol hydrochloride may effect the meatbolism of tramadol leading to altered tramadol exposure).
No products indexed under this heading.

Methylprednisolone Acetate (Administration of CYP3A4 inducers, such as rifampin or St. John's Wort, with tramadol hydrochloride may effect the meatbolism of tramadol leading to altered tramadol exposure). Products include:

Methylprednisolone Sodium Succinate (Administration of CYP3A4 inducers, such as rifampin or St. John's Wort, with tramadol hydrochloride may effect the meatbolism of tramadol leading to altered tramadol exposure).
No products indexed under this heading.

Metronidazole (Administration of CYP3A4 inhibitors, such as ketoconazole and erythromycin, with tramadol hydrochloride may effect

the meatbolism of tramadol leading to altered tramadol exposure). Products include:

Metronidazole Benzoate (Administration of CYP3A4 inhibitors, such as ketoconazole and erythromycin, with tramadol hydrochloride may effect the meatbolism of tramadol leading to altered tramadol exposure).
No products indexed under this heading.

Metronidazole Hydrochloride (Administration of CYP3A4 inhibitors, such as ketoconazole and erythromycin, with tramadol hydrochloride may effect the meatbolism of tramadol leading to altered tramadol exposure).
No products indexed under this heading.

Mibefradil Dihydrochloride (In vitro drug interaction studies in human liver microsomes indicate that concomitant administration with inhibitors of CYP2D6 could result in some inhibition of the metabolism of tramadol).
No products indexed under this heading.

Miconazole (Administration of CYP3A4 inhibitors, such as ketoconazole and erythromycin, with tramadol hydrochloride may effect the meatbolism of tramadol leading to altered tramadol exposure).
No products indexed under this heading.

Miconazole Nitrate (Administration of CYP3A4 inhibitors, such as ketoconazole and erythromycin, with tramadol hydrochloride may effect the meatbolism of tramadol leading to altered tramadol exposure). Products include:

Midazolam Hydrochloride (Tramadol hydrochloride is contraindicated in acute intoxication with hypnotics. Tramadol hydrochloride should be used with caution and in reduced dosages when administered to patients receiving CNS depressants, such as sedative hypnotics. Tramadol hydrochloride increases the risk of CNS and respiratory depression).
No products indexed under this heading.

Moclobemide (Administration of tramadol may increase the seizure risk in patients taking monoamine oxidase inhibitors or other drugs that reduce the seizure threshold. Use tramadol with great caution in patients taking MAO inhibitors. Concomitant use of tramadol with MAO inhibitors increases the risk of adverse events, including seizure and serotonin syndrome).
No products indexed under this heading.

Modafinil (Administration of CYP3A4 inducers, such as rifampin or St. John's Wort, with tramadol hydrochloride may effect the meatbolism of tramadol leading to altered tramadol exposure). Products include:

Molindone Hydrochloride (Tramadol hydrochloride is contraindicated in acute intoxication with psychotropic drugs). Products include:

Morphine Sulfate (Tramadol hydrochloride is contraindicated in acute intoxication with narcotics, opioids, and centrally-acting analgesics. Concomitant use of tramadol increases the seizure risk in patients taking opioids. Tramadol hydrochloride should be used with caution and in reduced dosages when administered to patients receiving CNS depressants, such as opioids or narcotics. Tramadol hydrochloride increases the risk of CNS and respiratory depression. Tramadol may be expected to have additive effects when used in conjunction with other opioids). Products include:

Nefazodone Hydrochloride (Administration of CYP3A4 inhibitors, such as ketoconazole and erythromycin, with tramadol hydrochloride may effect the meatbolism of tramadol leading to altered tramadol exposure).
No products indexed under this heading.

Nelfinavir Mesylate (Administration of CYP3A4 inhibitors, such as ketoconazole and erythromycin, with tramadol hydrochloride may effect the meatbolism of tramadol leading to altered tramadol exposure). Products include:

Nevirapine (Administration of CYP3A4 inhibitors, such as ketoconazole and erythromycin, with tramadol hydrochloride may effect the meatbolism of tramadol leading to altered tramadol exposure). Products include:

Niacinamide (Administration of CYP3A4 inhibitors, such as ketoconazole and erythromycin, with tramadol hydrochloride may effect the meatbolism of tramadol leading to altered tramadol exposure).
No products indexed under this heading.

Nicotinamide (Administration of CYP3A4 inhibitors, such as ketoconazole and erythromycin, with tramadol hydrochloride may effect the meatbolism of tramadol leading to altered tramadol exposure). Products include:

Nifedipine (Administration of CYP3A4 inhibitors, such as ketoconazole and erythromycin, with tramadol hydrochloride may effect the meatbolism of tramadol leading to altered tramadol exposure). Products include:

Norfloxacin (Administration of CYP3A4 inhibitors, such as ketoconazole and erythromycin, with tramadol hydrochloride may effect the meatbolism of tramadol leading to altered tramadol exposure). Products include:

Nortriptyline Hydrochloride (Tramadol hydrochloride is contraindicated in acute intoxication with psychotropic drugs).
No products indexed under this heading.

Olanzapine (Tramadol hydrochloride is contraindicated in acute intoxication with psychotropic drugs).
Products include:
Symbyax Capsules 1819
Zyprexa Tablets 1830
Zyprexa IntraMuscular 1830
Zyprexa ZYDIS Orally Disintegrating Tablets 1830

Omeprazole (Administration of CYP3A4 inhibitors, such as ketoconazole and erythromycin, with tramadol hydrochloride may effect the meatbolism of tramadol leading to altered tramadol exposure).
Products include:
Zegerid Capsules 2958
Zegerid Powder for Oral Solution 2958

Oxazepam (Tramadol hydrochloride is contraindicated in acute intoxication with psychotropic drugs).
No products indexed under this heading.

Oxcarbazepine (Administration of CYP3A4 inducers, such as rifampin or St. John's Wort, with tramadol hydrochloride may effect the meatbolism of tramadol leading to altered tramadol exposure). Products include:
Trileptal Tablets 2300
Trileptal Oral Suspension 2300

Oxycodone Hydrochloride (Tramadol hydrochloride is contraindicated in acute intoxication with narcotics, opioids, and centrally-acting analgesics. Concomitant use of tramadol increases the seizure risk in patients taking opioids. Tramadol hydrochloride should be used with caution and in reduced dosages when administered to patients receiving CNS depressants, such as opioids or narcotics. Tramadol hydrochloride increases the risk of CNS and respiratory depression. Tramadol may be expected to have additive effects when used in conjunction with other opioids).
Products include:
OxyContin Tablets 2703
OxyFast Oral Concentrate Solution 2708
OxyIR Capsules 2708
Percocet Tablets 1131
Percodan Tablets 1132

Pargyline Hydrochloride (Administration of tramadol may increase the seizure risk in patients taking monoamine oxidase inhibitors or other drugs that reduce the seizure threshold. Use tramadol with great caution in patients taking MAO inhibitors. Concomitant use of tramadol withMAO inhibitors increases the risk of adverse events, including seizure and serotonin syndrome).
No products indexed under this heading.

Paroxetine Hydrochloride (Concomitant use of tramadol increases the seizure risk in patients taking selective serotonin re-uptake inhibitors. Concomitant use of tramadol with SSRIs increases the risk of adverse events, including seizure and serotonin syndrome). Products include:
Paxil CR Controlled-Release Tablets 1538
Paxil 1530

Pentobarbital Sodium (Tramadol hydrochloride should be used with caution and in reduced dosages when administered to patients receiving CNS depressants, such as alcohol, opioids, anesthetic agents, narcotics, phenothiazines, tranquilizers, or sedative hypnotics. Tramadol hydrochloride increases the risk of CNS and respiratory depression).
Products include:
Nembutal Sodium Solution, USP 2470

Perphenazine (Tramadol hydrochloride is contraindicated in acute intoxication with psychotropic drugs).
No products indexed under this heading.

Phenelzine Sulfate (Tramadol hydrochloride is contraindicated in acute intoxication with psychotropic drugs).
No products indexed under this heading.

Phenobarbital (Tramadol hydrochloride should be used with caution and in reduced dosages when administered to patients receiving CNS depressants, such as alcohol, opioids, anesthetic agents, narcotics, phenothiazines, tranquilizers, or sedative hypnotics. Tramadol hydrochloride increases the risk of CNS and respiratory depression). Products include:
Donnatal Extentabs 2493

Phenobarbital Sodium (Administration of CYP3A4 inducers, such as rifampin or St. John's Wort, with tramadol hydrochloride may effect the meatbolism of tramadol leading to altered tramadol exposure).
No products indexed under this heading.

Phenytoin (Administration of CYP3A4 inducers, such as rifampin or St. John's Wort, with tramadol hydrochloride may effect the meatbolism of tramadol leading to altered tramadol exposure).
No products indexed under this heading.

Phenytoin Sodium (Administration of CYP3A4 inducers, such as rifampin or St. John's Wort, with tramadol hydrochloride may effect the meatbolism of tramadol leading to altered tramadol exposure).
Products include:
Phenytek Capsules 2160

Pimozide (Administration of tramadol may increase the seizure risk in patients taking neuroleptics or other drugs that reduce the seizure threshold).
No products indexed under this heading.

Prazepam (Tramadol hydrochloride is contraindicated in acute intoxication with psychotropic drugs).
No products indexed under this heading.

Prednisolone Acetate (Administration of CYP3A4 inducers, such as rifampin or St. John's Wort, with tramadol hydrochloride may effect the meatbolism of tramadol leading to altered tramadol exposure).
Products include:
Blephamide Ophthalmic Ointment 568
Blephamide Ophthalmic Suspension 569
Poly-Pred Ophthalmic Suspension .... ⊙ 233
Pred Forte Ophthalmic Suspension .... ⊙ 235
Pred Mild Ophthalmic Suspension .... ⊙ 238
Pred-G Ophthalmic Ointment .... ⊙ 237
Pred-G Ophthalmic Suspension .... ⊙ 236

Prednisolone Sodium Phosphate (Administration of CYP3A4 inducers, such as rifampin or St. John's Wort, with tramadol hydrochloride may effect the meatbolism of tramadol leading to altered tramadol exposure).
No products indexed under this heading.

Prednisolone Tebutate (Administration of CYP3A4 inducers, such as rifampin or St. John's Wort, with tramadol hydrochloride may effect the meatbolism of tramadol leading to altered tramadol exposure).
No products indexed under this heading.

Prednisone (Administration of CYP3A4 inducers, such as rifampin or St. John's Wort, with tramadol hydrochloride may effect the meatbolism of tramadol leading to altered tramadol exposure).
No products indexed under this heading.

Primidone (Administration of CYP3A4 inducers, such as rifampin or St. John's Wort, with tramadol hydrochloride may effect the meatbolism of tramadol leading to altered tramadol exposure).
No products indexed under this heading.

Procarbazine Hydrochloride (Administration of tramadol may increase the seizure risk in patients taking monoamine oxidase inhibitors or other drugs that reduce the seizure threshold. Use tramadol with great caution in patients taking MAO inhibitors. Concomitant use of tramadol withMAO inhibitors increases the risk of adverse events, including seizure and serotonin syndrome).
Products include:
Matulane Capsules 3191

Prochlorperazine (Tramadol hydrochloride is contraindicated in acute intoxication with psychotropic drugs).
No products indexed under this heading.

Promethazine (Concomitant use of tramadol increases the seizure risk in patients taking tricyclic compounds, such as promethazine).
No products indexed under this heading.

Promethazine Hydrochloride (Concomitant use of tramadol increases the seizure risk in patients taking tricyclic compounds, such as promethazine). Products include:
Phenergan Tablets and Suppositories 3440

Propafenone Hydrochloride (In vitro drug interaction studies in human liver microsomes indicate that concomitant administration with inhibitors of CYP2D6 could result in some inhibition of the metabolism of tramadol). Products include:
Rythmol SR Capsules 2727

Propofol (Tramadol hydrochloride is contraindicated in acute intoxication with hypnotics. Tramadol hydrochloride should be used with caution and in reduced dosages when administered to patients receiving CNS depressants, such as sedative hypnotics. Tramadol hydrochloride increases the risk of CNS and respiratory depression).
No products indexed under this heading.

Propoxyphene Hydrochloride (Tramadol hydrochloride is contraindicated in acute intoxication with narcotics, opioids, and centrally-acting analgesics. Concomitant use of tramadol increases the seizure risk in patients taking opioids. Tramadol hydrochloride should be used with caution and in reduced dosages when administered to patients receiving CNS depressants, such as opioids or narcotics. Tramadol hydrochloride increases the risk of CNS and respiratory depression. Tramadol may be expected to have additive effects when used in conjunction with other opioids).
No products indexed under this heading.

Propoxyphene Napsylate (Tramadol hydrochloride is contraindicated in acute intoxication with narcotics, opioids, and centrally-acting analgesics. Concomitant use of tramadol increases the seizure risk in patients taking opioids. Tramadol hydrochloride should be used with caution and in reduced dosages when administered to patients receiving CNS depressants, such as opioids or narcotics. Tramadol hydrochloride increases the risk of CNS and respiratory depression. Tramadol may be expected to have additive effects when used in conjunction with other opioids).
No products indexed under this heading.

Protriptyline Hydrochloride (Tramadol hydrochloride is contraindicated in acute intoxication with psychotropic drugs).
No products indexed under this heading.

Quazepam (Tramadol hydrochloride is contraindicated in acute intoxication with hypnotics. Tramadol hydrochloride should be used with caution and in reduced dosages when administered to patients receiving CNS depressants, such as sedative hypnotics. Tramadol hydrochloride increases the risk of CNS and respiratory depression).
No products indexed under this heading.

Quetiapine Fumarate (Tramadol hydrochloride is contraindicated in acute intoxication with psychotropic drugs). Products include:
Seroquel Tablets 690

Quinacrine Hydrochloride (In vitro drug interaction studies in human liver microsomes indicate that concomitant administration with inhibitors of CYP2D6 could result in some inhibition of the metabolism of tramadol).
No products indexed under this heading.

Quinidine (Administration of CYP3A4 inhibitors, such as ketoconazole and erythromycin, with tramadol hydrochloride may effect the meatbolism of tramadol leading to altered tramadol exposure).
No products indexed under this heading.

Quinidine Gluconate (In vitro drug interaction studies in human liver microsomes indicate that concomitant administration with inhibitors of CYP2D6 could result in some inhibition of the metabolism of tramadol).
No products indexed under this heading.

Quinidine Hydrochloride (In vitro drug interaction studies in human liver microsomes indicate that concomitant administration with inhibitors of CYP2D6 could result in some inhibition of the metabolism of tramadol).
No products indexed under this heading.

Quinidine Polygalacturonate (In vitro drug interaction studies in human liver microsomes indicate that concomitant administration with inhibitors of CYP2D6 could result in some inhibition of the metabolism of tramadol).
No products indexed under this heading.

Quinidine Sulfate (In vitro drug interaction studies in human liver microsomes indicate that concomitant administration with inhibitors of CYP2D6 could result in some inhibition of the metabolism of tramadol).
No products indexed under this heading.

Quinine (Administration of CYP3A4 inhibitors, such as ketoconazole and erythromycin, with tramadol hydrochloride may effect the meatbolism of tramadol leading to altered tramadol exposure).
No products indexed under this heading.

Quinine Sulfate (Administration of CYP3A4 inhibitors, such as ketoconazole and erythromycin, with tramadol hydrochloride may effect the meatbolism of tramadol leading to altered tramadol exposure).
No products indexed under this heading.

Quinupristin (Administration of CYP3A4 inhibitors, such as ketoconazole and erythromycin, with tramadol hydrochloride may effect the meatbolism of tramadol leading to altered tramadol exposure).
No products indexed under this heading.

Ramelteon (Tramadol hydrochloride is contraindicated in acute intoxication with hypnotics. Tramadol hydrochloride should be used with caution and in reduced dosages when administered to patients receiving CNS depressants, such as sedative hypnotics. Tramadol hydrochloride increases the risk of CNS and respiratory depression).
Products include:
Rozerem Tablets 3231

Ranitidine Bismuth Citrate (In vitro drug interaction studies in human liver microsomes indicate that concomitant administration with inhibitors of CYP2D6 could result in some inhibition of the metabolism of tramadol).
No products indexed under this heading.

Ranitidine Hydrochloride (In vitro drug interaction studies in human liver microsomes indicate that concomitant administration with inhibitors of CYP2D6 could result in some inhibition of the metabolism of tramadol). Products include:
Zantac 1624
Zantac Injection 1619
Zantac Injection Pharmacy Bulk Package 1622

Remifentanil Hydrochloride (Tramadol hydrochloride is contraindicated in acute intoxication with narcotics, opioids, and centrally-acting analgesics. Concomitant use of tramadol increases the seizure risk in patients taking opioids. Tramadol hydrochloride should be used with caution and in reduced dosages when administered to patients receiving CNS depressants, such as opioids or narcotics. Tramadol hydrochloride increases the risk of CNS and respiratory depression. Tramadol may be expected to have additive effects when used in conjunction with other opioids).
No products indexed under this heading.

Rifabutin (Administration of CYP3A4 inducers, such as rifampin or St. John's Wort, with tramadol hydrochloride may effect the metabolism of tramadol leading to altered tramadol exposure).
No products indexed under this heading.

Rifampicin (Administration of CYP3A4 inducers, such as rifampin or St. John's Wort, with tramadol hydrochloride may effect the metabolism of tramadol leading to altered tramadol exposure).
No products indexed under this heading.

Rifampin (Administration of CYP3A4 inducers, such as rifampin or St. John's Wort, with tramadol hydrochloride may effect the metabolism of tramadol leading to altered tramadol exposure).
No products indexed under this heading.

Rifapentine (Administration of CYP3A4 inducers, such as rifampin or St. John's Wort, with tramadol hydrochloride may effect the metabolism of tramadol leading to altered tramadol exposure).
No products indexed under this heading.

Risperidone (Tramadol hydrochloride is contraindicated in acute intoxication with psychotropic drugs). Products include:
Risperdal 1676
Risperdal Consta Long-Acting Injection 1682
Risperdal M-Tab Orally Disintegrating Tablets 1676

Ritonavir (In vitro drug interaction studies in human liver microsomes indicate that concomitant administration with inhibitors of CYP2D6 could result in some inhibition of the metabolism of tramadol). Products include:
Kaletra 476
Norvir 503

Saquinavir (Administration of CYP3A4 inhibitors, such as ketoconazole and erythromycin, with tramadol hydrochloride may effect the meatbolism of tramadol leading to altered tramadol exposure).
No products indexed under this heading.

Saquinavir Mesylate (Administration of CYP3A4 inhibitors, such as ketoconazole and erythromycin, with tramadol hydrochloride may effect the meatbolism of tramadol leading to altered tramadol exposure).
Products include:
Invirase 2772

Secobarbital Sodium (Tramadol hydrochloride is contraindicated in acute intoxication with hypnotics. Tramadol hydrochloride should be used with caution and in reduced dosages when administered to patients receiving CNS depressants, such as sedative hypnotics. Tramadol hydrochloride increases the risk of CNS and respiratory depression).
No products indexed under this heading.

Selegiline Hydrochloride (Administration of tramadol may increase the seizure risk in patients taking monoamine oxidase inhibitors or other drugs that reduce the seizure threshold. Use tramadol with great caution in patients taking MAO inhibitors. Concomitant use of tramadol withMAO inhibitors increases the risk of adverse events, including seizure and serotonin syndrome). Products include:
Eldepryl Capsules 3208
Zelapar Tablets 3372

Sertraline Hydrochloride (Concomitant use of tramadol increases the seizure risk in patients taking selective serotonin re-uptake inhibitors. Concomitant use of tramadol with SSRIs increases the risk of adverse events, including seizure and serotonin syndrome). Products include:
Zoloft 2586

Sevoflurane (Tramadol hydrochloride should be used with caution and in reduced dosages when administered to patients receiving CNS depressants, such as alcohol, opioids, anesthetic agents, narcotics, phenothiazines, tranquilizers, or sedative hypnotics. Tramadol hydrochloride increases the risk of CNS and respiratory depression). Products include:
Ultane Liquid for Inhalation 531

Sodium Oxybate (Tramadol hydrochloride should be used with caution and in reduced dosages when administered to patients receiving CNS depressants, such as alcohol, opioids, anesthetic agents, narcotics, phenothiazines, tranquilizers, or sedative hypnotics. Tramadol hydrochloride increases the risk of CNS and respiratory depression). Products include:
Xyrem Oral Solution 1688

Sufentanil Citrate (Tramadol hydrochloride is contraindicated in acute intoxication with narcotics, opioids, and centrally-acting analgesics. Concomitant use of tramadol increases the seizure risk in patients taking opioids. Tramadol hydrochloride should be used with caution and in reduced dosages when administered to patients receiving CNS depressants, such as opioids or narcotics. Tramadol hydrochloride increases the risk of CNS and respiratory depression. Tramadol may be expected to have additive effects when used in conjunction with other opioids).
No products indexed under this heading.

Sulfinpyrazone (Administration of CYP3A4 inducers, such as rifampin or St. John's Wort, with tramadol hydrochloride may effect the metabolism of tramadol leading to altered tramadol exposure).
No products indexed under this heading.

Telithromycin (Administration of CYP3A4 inhibitors, such as ketoconazole and erythromycin, with tramadol hydrochloride may effect the meatbolism of tramadol leading to altered tramadol exposure). Products include:
Ketek Tablets 2903

Temazepam (Tramadol hydrochloride is contraindicated in acute intoxication with hypnotics. Tramadol hydrochloride should be used with caution and in reduced dosages when administered to patients receiving CNS depressants, such as sedative hypnotics. Tramadol hydrochloride increases the risk of CNS and respiratory depression). Products include:
Restoril Capsules 1860

Terbinafine Hydrochloride (In vitro drug interaction studies in human liver microsomes indicate that concomitant administration with inhibitors of CYP2D6 could result in some inhibition of the metabolism of tramadol). Products include:
Lamisil Tablets 2232
Lamisil AT Creams (Athlete's Foot & Jock Itch) .... ◘636

Theophylline (Administration of CYP3A4 inducers, such as rifampin or St. John's Wort, with tramadol hydrochloride may effect the metabolism of tramadol leading to altered tramadol exposure).
No products indexed under this heading.

Thiamylal Sodium (Tramadol hydrochloride should be used with caution and in reduced dosages when administered to patients receiving CNS depressants, such as alcohol, opioids, anesthetic agents, narcotics, phenothiazines, tranquilizers, or sedative hypnotics. Tramadol hydrochloride increases the risk of CNS and respiratory depression).
No products indexed under this heading.

Thioridazine Hydrochloride (Tramadol hydrochloride is contraindicated in acute intoxication with psychotropic drugs). Products include:
Thioridazine Hydrochloride Tablets 2163

Thiothixene (Tramadol hydrochloride is contraindicated in acute intoxication with psychotropic drugs). Products include:
Thiothixene Capsules 2165

Tranylcypromine Sulfate (Tramadol hydrochloride is contraindicated in acute intoxication with psychotropic drugs). Products include:
Parnate Tablets 1527

Triamcinolone (Administration of CYP3A4 inducers, such as rifampin or St. John's Wort, with tramadol hydrochloride may effect the metabolism of tramadol leading to altered tramadol exposure).
No products indexed under this heading.

Triamcinolone Acetonide (Administration of CYP3A4 inducers, such as rifampin or St. John's Wort, with tramadol hydrochloride may effect the metabolism of tramadol leading to altered tramadol exposure). Products include:
Azmacort Inhalation Aerosol 1726
Nasacort AQ Nasal Spray 2922

Triamcinolone Diacetate (Administration of CYP3A4 inducers, such as rifampin or St. John's Wort, with tramadol hydrochloride may effect the meatbolism of tramadol leading to altered tramadol exposure).
No products indexed under this heading.

Triamcinolone Hexacetonide (Administration of CYP3A4 inducers, such as rifampin or St. John's Wort, with tramadol hydrochloride may effect the meatbolism of tramadol leading to altered tramadol exposure).
No products indexed under this heading.

Triazolam (Tramadol hydrochloride is contraindicated in acute intoxication with hypnotics. Tramadol hydrochloride should be used with caution and in reduced dosages when administered to patients receiving CNS depressants, such as sedative hypnotics. Tramadol hydrochloride increases the risk of CNS and respiratory depression).
No products indexed under this heading.

Trifluoperazine Hydrochloride (Tramadol hydrochloride is contraindicated in acute intoxication with psychotropic drugs).
No products indexed under this heading.

Trimipramine Maleate (Tramadol hydrochloride is contraindicated in acute intoxication with psychotropic drugs).
No products indexed under this heading.

Troglitazone (Administration of CYP3A4 inhibitors, such as ketoconazole and erythromycin, with tramadol hydrochloride may effect the meatbolism of tramadol leading to altered tramadol exposure).
No products indexed under this heading.

Troleandomycin (Administration of CYP3A4 inhibitors, such as ketoconazole and erythromycin, with tramadol hydrochloride may effect the meatbolism of tramadol leading to altered tramadol exposure).
No products indexed under this heading.

Valproate Sodium (Administration of CYP3A4 inhibitors, such as ketoconazole and erythromycin, with tramadol hydrochloride may effect the meatbolism of tramadol leading to altered tramadol exposure). Products include:
Depacon Injection 412

Verapamil Hydrochloride (Administration of CYP3A4 inhibitors, such as ketoconazole and erythromycin, with tramadol hydrochloride may effect the meatbolism of tramadol leading to altered tramadol exposure). Products include:
Covera-HS Tablets 3139
Tarka Tablets 524
Verelan PM Extended-Release Capsules, Controlled-Onset 3106

Voriconazole (Administration of CYP3A4 inhibitors, such as ketoconazole and erythromycin, with tramadol hydrochloride may effect the meatbolism of tramadol leading to altered tramadol exposure). Products include:
VFEND I.V. 2564
VFEND Oral Suspension 2564
VFEND Tablets 2564

Warfarin Sodium (Post-marketing surveillance of tramadol has revealed rare reports of alteration of warfarin effect, including elevation of prothrombin times). Products include:
Coumadin for Injection 898
Coumadin Tablets 898

Zafirlukast (Administration of CYP3A4 inhibitors, such as ketoconazole and erythromycin, with tramadol hydrochloride may effect the meatbolism of tramadol leading to altered tramadol exposure). Products include:
Accolate Tablets 671

Zaleplon (Tramadol hydrochloride is contraindicated in acute intoxication with hypnotics. Tramadol hydrochloride should be used with caution and in reduced dosages when administered to patients receiving CNS depressants, such as sedative hypnotics. Tramadol hydrochloride increases the risk of CNS and respiratory depression). Products include:
Sonata Capsules 1717

Zileuton (Administration of CYP3A4 inhibitors, such as ketoconazole and erythromycin, with tramadol hydrochloride may effect the meatbolism of tramadol leading to altered tramadol exposure). Products include:
Zyflo Tablets 1023

Ziprasidone Hydrochloride (Tramadol hydrochloride is contraindicated in acute intoxication with psychotropic drugs). Products include:
Geodon Capsules 2529

Zolpidem Tartrate (Tramadol hydrochloride is contraindicated in acute intoxication with hypnotics. Tramadol hydrochloride should be used with caution and in reduced dosages when administered to patients receiving CNS depressants, such as sedative hypnotics. Tramadol hydrochloride increases the risk of CNS and respiratory depression). Products include:
Ambien Tablets 2851
Ambien CR Tablets 2855

Food Interactions

Alcohol (Tramadol hydrochloride is contraindicated in acute intoxication with alcohol. Tramadol hydrochloride should be used with caution and in reduced dosages when administered to patients receiving CNS depressants, such as alcohol. Tramadol may be expected to have additive effects when used in conjunction with alcohol).

Grapefruit (Administration of CYP3A4 inhibitors, such as ketoconazole and erythromycin, with tramadol hydrochloride may effect the meatbolism of tramadol leading to altered tramadol exposure).

Grapefruit Juice (Administration of CYP3A4 inhibitors, such as ketoconazole and erythromycin, with tramadol hydrochloride may effect the meatbolism of tramadol leading to altered tramadol exposure).

ULTRASE CAPSULES
(Pancrelipase) 708

Food Interactions

Food having a pH greater than 5.5 (Can dissolve the protective coating resulting in early release of enzymes, irritation of oral mucosa, and/or loss of enzyme activity).

ULTRASE MT CAPSULES
(Pancrelipase) 709

Food Interactions

Food having a pH greater than 5.5 (Can dissolve the protective enteric shell).

UNIPHYL TABLETS
(Theophylline Anhydrous) 2710
May interact with erythromycin, lithium preparations, and certain other agents. Compounds in these categories include:

Adenosine (Theophylline blocks adenosine receptors; higher doses of adenosine may be required to achieve desired effect). Products include:
Adenocard Injection 617
Adenoscan 619

Allopurinol (Decreases theophylline clearance at allopurinol doses greater than or equal to 600 mg/day).
No products indexed under this heading.

Aminoglutethimide (Increases theophylline clearance by induction of microsomal enzyme).
No products indexed under this heading.

Carbamazepine (Increases theophylline clearance by induction of microsomal enzyme). Products include:
Carbatrol Capsules 3171
Equetro Extended-Release Capsules 3180
Tegretol/Tegretol-XR 2295

Cimetidine (Decreases theophylline clearance by inhibiting cytochrome P450 1A2). Products include:
Tagamet HB 200 Tablets .... ▣664

Cimetidine Hydrochloride (Decreases theophylline clearance by inhibiting cytochrome P450 1A2).
No products indexed under this heading.

Ciprofloxacin (Decreases theophylline clearance by inhibiting cytochrome P450 1A2). Products include:
Cipro Oral Suspension 2977
Cipro I.V. 2984
Cipro XR Tablets 2990
Ciprodex Otic Suspension 559

Ciprofloxacin Hydrochloride (Decreases theophylline clearance by inhibiting cytochrome P450 1A2). Products include:
Ciloxan Ophthalmic Ointment 559
Ciloxan Ophthalmic Solution .... ⊙206
Cipro Tablets 2977
Proquin XR Tablets 1153

Clarithromycin (Decreases theophylline clearance by inhibiting cytochrome P450 3A3). Products include:
Biaxin/Biaxin XL 402
PREVPAC 3284

Diazepam (Benzodiazepines increase CNS concentrations of adenosine, a potent CNS depressant, while theophylline blocks adenosine receptors; larger diazepam doses may be required to produce desired level of sedation; discontinuation of theophylline without reduction of diazepam dose may result in respiratory depression). Products include:
Diastat Rectal Delivery System 3343
Valium Tablets 2819

Disulfiram (Decreases theophylline clearance by inhibiting hydroxylation and demethylation).
No products indexed under this heading.

Enoxacin (Decreases theophylline clearance by inhibiting cytochrome P450 1A2).
No products indexed under this heading.

Ephedrine Hydrochloride (Co-administration results in synergistic CNS effects resulting in increased frequency of nausea, nervousness, and insomnia).
No products indexed under this heading.

Ephedrine Sulfate (Co-administration results in synergistic CNS effects resulting in increased frequency of nausea, nervousness, and insomnia).
No products indexed under this heading.

Ephedrine Tannate (Co-administration results in synergistic CNS effects resulting in increased frequency of nausea, nervousness, and insomnia).
No products indexed under this heading.

Erythromycin (Erythromycin metabolite decreases theophylline clearance by inhibiting cytochrome P450 3A3; decreased erythromycin steady-state serum concentrations). Products include:
Ery-Tab Tablets 449
Erythromycin Base Filmtab Tablets 455
Erythromycin Delayed-Release Capsules, USP 457
PCE Dispertab Tablets 515

Erythromycin Estolate (Erythromycin metabolite decreases theophylline clearance by inhibiting cytochrome P450 3A3; decreased erythromycin steady-state serum concentrations).
No products indexed under this heading.

Erythromycin Ethylsuccinate (Erythromycin metabolite decreases theophylline clearance by inhibiting cytochrome P450 3A3; decreased erythromycin steady-state serum concentrations). Products include:
E.E.S. 451
EryPed 447

Erythromycin Gluceptate (Erythromycin metabolite decreases theophylline clearance by inhibiting cytochrome P450 3A3; decreased erythromycin steady-state serum concentrations).
No products indexed under this heading.

Erythromycin Lactobionate (Erythromycin metabolite decreases theophylline clearance by inhibiting cytochrome P450 3A3; decreased erythromycin steady-state serum concentrations).
No products indexed under this heading.

Erythromycin Stearate (Erythromycin metabolite decreases theophylline clearance by inhibiting cytochrome P450 3A3; decreased erythromycin steady-state serum concentrations). Products include:
Erythrocin Stearate Filmtab Tablets 453

Ethinyl Estradiol (Estrogen containing oral contraceptives decreases theophylline clearance in dose dependent fashion). Products include:
Mircette Tablets 1066
NuvaRing 2340
Ortho-Cyclen/Ortho Tri-Cyclen 2429
Ortho Evra Transdermal System 2417

Ortho Tri-Cyclen Lo Tablets 2436
Seasonique Tablets 1077
Yasmin 28 Tablets 796
Yaz Tablets 803

Flurazepam Hydrochloride (Benzodiazepines increase CNS concentrations of adenosine, a potent CNS depressant, while theophylline blocks adenosine receptors; larger flurazepam doses may be required to produce desired level of sedation; discontinuation of theophylline without reduction of flurazepam dose may result in respiratory depression). Products include:
Dalmane Capsules 3342

Fluvoxamine Maleate (Decreases theophylline clearance by inhibiting cytochrome P450 1A2).
No products indexed under this heading.

Halothane (Halothane sensitizes the myocardium to catecholamines; theophylline increases release of endogenous catecholamines resulting in increased risk of ventricular arrhythmias).
No products indexed under this heading.

Hypericum (Increases theophylline clearance; higher doses of theophylline may be required to achieve desired effect; stopping St. John's Wort may result in theophylline toxicity). Products include:
Satiete Tablets .... ◘832

Interferon alfa-2a, Recombinant (Decreases theophylline clearance).
No products indexed under this heading.

Isoproterenol Hydrochloride (Co-administration with intravenous isoproterenol decreases theophylline clearance).
No products indexed under this heading.

Ketamine Hydrochloride (May lower theophylline seizure threshold).
No products indexed under this heading.

Lithium (Theophylline increases renal lithium clearance; increase in lithium dose may be required to achieve a therapeutic serum concentration).
No products indexed under this heading.

Lithium Carbonate (Theophylline increases renal lithium clearance; increase in lithium dose may be required to achieve a therapeutic serum concentration). Products include:
Lithobid Tablets 1692

Lithium Citrate (Theophylline increases renal lithium clearance; increase in lithium dose may be required to achieve a therapeutic serum concentration).
No products indexed under this heading.

Lorazepam (Benzodiazepines increase CNS concentrations of adenosine, a potent CNS depressant, while theophylline blocks adenosine receptors; larger lorazepam doses may be required to produce desired level of sedation; discontinuation of theophylline without reduction of lorazepam dose may result in respiratory depression).
No products indexed under this heading.

Mestranol (Estrogen containing oral contraceptives decreases theophylline clearance in dose dependent fashion).
No products indexed under this heading.

Methotrexate Sodium (Decreases theophylline clearance).
No products indexed under this heading.

Mexiletine Hydrochloride (Decreases theophylline clearance by inhibiting hydroxylation and demethylation).
No products indexed under this heading.

Midazolam Hydrochloride (Benzodiazepines increase CNS concentrations of adenosine, a potent CNS depressant, while theophylline blocks adenosine receptors; larger midazolam doses may be required to produce desired level of sedation; discontinuation of theophylline without reduction of midazolam dose may result in respiratory depression).
No products indexed under this heading.

Moricizine Hydrochloride (Increases theophylline clearance).
No products indexed under this heading.

Pancuronium Bromide (Theophylline may antagonize non-depolarizing neuromuscular blocking effects; possibly due to phosphodiesterase inhibition; larger pancuronium doses may be required to achieve neuromuscular blockade).
No products indexed under this heading.

Pentoxifylline (Decreases theophylline clearance).
No products indexed under this heading.

Phenobarbital (Increases theophylline clearance by induction of microsomal enzyme). Products include:
Donnatal Extentabs 2493

Phenytoin (Phenytoin increases theophylline clearance by increasing microsomal enzyme activity; theophylline decreases phenytoin absorption).
No products indexed under this heading.

Phenytoin Sodium (Phenytoin increases theophylline clearance by increasing microsomal enzyme activity; theophylline decreases phenytoin absorption). Products include:
Phenytek Capsules 2160

Propafenone Hydrochloride (Decreases theophylline clearance). Products include:
Rythmol SR Capsules 2727

Propranolol Hydrochloride (Decreases theophylline clearance by inhibiting cytochrome P450 1A2). Products include:
Inderal LA Long-Acting Capsules 3429
InnoPran XL Capsules 2723

Rifampin (Increases theophylline clearance by increasing cytochrome P450 1A2 and 3A3 activity).
No products indexed under this heading.

Sulfinpyrazone (Increases theophylline clearance by increasing demethylation and hydroxylation; decreases renal clearance of theophylline).
No products indexed under this heading.

Tacrine Hydrochloride (Decreases theophylline clearance by inhibiting cytochrome P450 1A2 and also increases renal clearance of theophylline).
No products indexed under this heading.

Thiabendazole (Decreases theophylline clearance). Products include:
Mintezol 2027

Ticlopidine Hydrochloride (Decreases theophylline clearance). Products include:
Ticlid Tablets 2810

Troleandomycin (Decreases theophylline clearance by inhibiting cytochrome P450 3A3).
No products indexed under this heading.

Verapamil Hydrochloride (Decreases theophylline clearance by inhibiting hydroxylation and demethylation). Products include:
Covera-HS Tablets 3139
Tarka Tablets 524
Verelan PM Extended-Release Capsules, Controlled-Onset........... 3106

Food Interactions

Alcohol (Concurrent use with a single dose of alcohol (3mL/kg of whiskey) decreases theophylline clearance for up to 24 hours).

Diet, high-lipid (Co-administration with a standardized high-fat meal results in increased peak plasma concentration and bioavailability; however, a precipitous increase in the rate and extent of absorption was not evident; the dosing should be ideally administered consistently either with or without food).

UNIRETIC TABLETS

(Hydrochlorothiazide, Moexipril Hydrochloride)................................. 3100
May interact with barbiturates, beta blockers, corticosteroids, oral hypoglycemic agents, insulin, lithium preparations, narcotic analgesics, non-steroidal anti-inflammatory agents, potassium preparations, potassium sparing diuretics, and certain other agents. Compounds in these categories include:

Acarbose (Thiazide diuretic may reduce glucose tolerance; concomitant use may require dosage adjustment of oral hypoglycemic agents). Products include:
Precose Tablets 751

Acebutolol Hydrochloride (ACE inhibitors have less than additive effects with beta-adrenergic blockers, presumably because both work by inhibiting the renin-angiotension system).
No products indexed under this heading.

ACTH (Concomitant use of thiazides with ACTH may intensify electrolyte depletion, particularly hypokalemia).
No products indexed under this heading.

Alfentanil Hydrochloride (Co-administration of narcotics with thiazide diuretics may result in potentiation of orthostatic hypotension).
No products indexed under this heading.

Amiloride Hydrochloride (Potassium-sparing diuretics can increase the risk of hyperkalemia). Products include:
Midamor Tablets 2026
Moduretic Tablets 2028

Aprobarbital (Co-administration of barbiturate with thiazide diuretics may result in potentiation of orthostatic hypotension).
No products indexed under this heading.

Atenolol (ACE inhibitors have less than additive effects with beta-adrenergic blockers, presumably because both work by inhibiting the renin-angiotension system).
No products indexed under this heading.

Betamethasone Acetate (Concomitant use of thiazides with corticosteroids may intensify electrolyte depletion, particularly hypokalemia).
No products indexed under this heading.

Betamethasone Sodium Phosphate (Concomitant use of thiazides with corticosteroids may intensify electrolyte depletion, particularly hypokalemia).
No products indexed under this heading.

Betaxolol Hydrochloride (ACE inhibitors have less than additive effects with beta-adrenergic blockers, presumably because both work by inhibiting the renin-angiotension system). Products include:
Betoptic S Ophthalmic Suspension.................................. 558

Bisoprolol Fumarate (ACE inhibitors have less than additive effects with beta-adrenergic blockers, presumably because both work by inhibiting the renin-angiotension system).
No products indexed under this heading.

Buprenorphine Hydrochloride (Co-administration of narcotics with thiazide diuretics may result in potentiation of orthostatic hypotension). Products include:
Buprenex Injectable 2716
Suboxone Tablets 2717
Subutex Tablets 2717

Butabarbital (Co-administration of barbiturate with thiazide diuretics may result in potentiation of orthostatic hypotension).
No products indexed under this heading.

Butalbital (Co-administration of barbiturate with thiazide diuretics may result in potentiation of orthostatic hypotension).
No products indexed under this heading.

Carteolol Hydrochloride (ACE inhibitors have less than additive effects with beta-adrenergic blockers, presumably because both work by inhibiting the renin-angiotension system). Products include:
Carteolol Hydrochloride Ophthalmic Solution USP, 1%....... ⊙249

Celecoxib (NSAIDs can reduce the diuretic, natriuretic, and antihypertensive effects of thiazides). Products include:
Celebrex Capsules 3134

Chlorpropamide (Thiazide diuretic may reduce glucose tolerance; concomitant use may require dosage adjustment of oral hypoglycemic agents).
No products indexed under this heading.

Cholestyramine (Absorption of hydrochlorothiazide is impaired in the presence of anionic exchange resins; binds the hydrochlorothiazide and reduces its absorption from GI tract by up to 85%).
No products indexed under this heading.

Codeine Phosphate (Co-administration of narcotics with thiazide diuretics may result in potentiation of orthostatic hypotension). Products include:
Tylenol with Codeine Tablets 2391

Colestipol Hydrochloride (Absorption of hydrochlorothiazide is impaired in the presence of anionic exchange resins; binds the hydrochlorothiazide and reduces its absorption from GI tract by up to 43%).
No products indexed under this heading.

Cortisone Acetate (Concomitant use of thiazides with corticosteroids may intensify electrolyte depletion, particularly hypokalemia).
No products indexed under this heading.

Dexamethasone (Concomitant use of thiazides with corticosteroids may intensify electrolyte depletion, particularly hypokalemia). Products include:
Ciprodex Otic Suspension 559
Decadron Tablets 1951
TobraDex Ophthalmic Ointment 562
TobraDex Ophthalmic Suspension 563

Dexamethasone Acetate (Concomitant use of thiazides with corticosteroids may intensify electrolyte depletion, particularly hypokalemia).
No products indexed under this heading.

Dexamethasone Sodium Phosphate (Concomitant use of thiazides with corticosteroids may intensify electrolyte depletion, particularly hypokalemia).
No products indexed under this heading.

Dezocine (Co-administration of narcotics with thiazide diuretics may result in potentiation of orthostatic hypotension).
No products indexed under this heading.

Diclofenac Potassium (NSAIDs can reduce the diuretic, natriuretic, and antihypertensive effects of thiazides).
No products indexed under this heading.

Diclofenac Sodium (NSAIDs can reduce the diuretic, natriuretic, and antihypertensive effects of thiazides). Products include:
Arthrotec Tablets 3129
Voltaren Ophthalmic Solution 2309
Voltaren Tablets 2307
Voltaren-XR Tablets 2310

Esmolol Hydrochloride (ACE inhibitors have less than additive effects with beta-adrenergic blockers, presumably because both work by inhibiting the renin-angiotension system).
No products indexed under this heading.

Etodolac (NSAIDs can reduce the diuretic, natriuretic, and antihypertensive effects of thiazides).
No products indexed under this heading.

Fenoprofen Calcium (NSAIDs can reduce the diuretic, natriuretic, and antihypertensive effects of thiazides). Products include:
Nalfon Capsules 2502

Fentanyl (Co-administration of narcotics with thiazide diuretics may result in potentiation of orthostatic hypotension). Products include:
Duragesic Transdermal System 2373
Ionsys Transdermal System 2379

Fentanyl Citrate (Co-administration of narcotics with thiazide diuretics may result in potentiation of orthostatic hypotension). Products include:
Actiq 979

Fludrocortisone Acetate (Concomitant use of thiazides with corticosteroids may intensify electrolyte depletion, particularly hypokalemia).
No products indexed under this heading.

Flurbiprofen (NSAIDs can reduce the diuretic, natriuretic, and antihypertensive effects of thiazides).
No products indexed under this heading.

Glimepiride (Thiazide diuretic may reduce glucose tolerance; concomitant use may require dosage adjustment of oral hypoglycemic agents). Products include:
Avandaryl Tablets 1379
Duetact Tablets 3226

Glipizide (Thiazide diuretic may reduce glucose tolerance; concomitant use may require dosage adjustment of oral hypoglycemic agents).
No products indexed under this heading.

Glyburide (Thiazide diuretic may reduce glucose tolerance; concomitant use may require dosage adjustment of oral hypoglycemic agents).
No products indexed under this heading.

Guanabenz Acetate (Co-administration increases the absorption of hydrochlorothiazide).
No products indexed under this heading.

Hydrocodone Bitartrate (Co-administration of narcotics with thiazide diuretics may result in potentiation of orthostatic hypotension). Products include:
Hycodan 1116
Hycotuss Expectorant Syrup 1117
Vicodin Tablets 535
Vicodin ES Tablets 536
Vicodin HP Tablets 538
Vicoprofen Tablets 539
Zydone Tablets 1139

Hydrocodone Polistirex (Co-administration of narcotics with thiazide diuretics may result in potentiation of orthostatic hypotension). Products include:
Tussionex Pennkinetic Extended-Release Suspension 3327

Hydrocortisone (Concomitant use of thiazides with corticosteroids may intensify electrolyte depletion, particularly hypokalemia). Products include:
Colocort Rectal Suspension, USP (Retention) 100 mg/60 mL........... 2476
Hydrocortone Tablets 1989
Preparation H Hydrocortisone Cream .... ▣646

Hydrocortisone Acetate (Concomitant use of thiazides with corticosteroids may intensify electrolyte depletion, particularly hypokalemia). Products include:
Analpram-HC 1159
Pramosone 1161
ProctoFoam-HC 3099

Hydrocortisone Sodium Phosphate (Concomitant use of thiazides with corticosteroids may intensify electrolyte depletion, particularly hypokalemia).
No products indexed under this heading.

Hydrocortisone Sodium Succinate (Concomitant use of thiazides with corticosteroids may intensify electrolyte depletion, particularly hypokalemia).
No products indexed under this heading.

Hydromorphone Hydrochloride (Co-administration of narcotics with thiazide diuretics may result in potentiation of orthostatic hypotension). Products include:
Dilaudid 440
Dilaudid Non-Sterile Powder 440
Dilaudid Oral Liquid 445
Dilaudid Rectal Suppositories 440
Dilaudid Tablets 440
Dilaudid Tablets - 8 mg 445
Dilaudid-HP 442

Ibuprofen (NSAIDs can reduce the diuretic, natriuretic, and antihypertensive effects of thiazides). Products include:
Advil Allergy Sinus Caplets .... ▣770
Advil .... ▣674
Children's Advil Oral Suspension .... ▣603
Children's Advil Chewable Tablets .. ▣603
Advil Cold & Sinus .... ▣723
Infants' Advil Concentrated Drops .. ▣604
Infants' Advil Concentrated Drops - White Grape (Dye-Free)............. ▣604
Junior Strength Advil Swallow Tablets.. ▣605
Advil Migraine Liquigels .... ▣608
Advil Multi-Symptom Cold Caplets.. ▣770
Advil PM Caplets .... ▣615
Motrin IB Tablets and Caplets 1866
Children's Motrin Oral Suspension ... 1867
Children's Motrin Non-Staining Dye-Free Oral Suspension............ 1867
Children's Motrin Cold Oral Suspension 1867
Infants' Motrin Concentrated Drops.. 1867
Infants' Motrin Non-Staining Dye-Free Concentrated Drops....... 1867
Junior Strength Motrin Caplets and Chewable Tablets.................. 1867
Vicoprofen Tablets 539

Indomethacin (NSAIDs can reduce the diuretic, natriuretic, and antihypertensive effects of thiazides). Products include:
Indocin 1995

Indomethacin Sodium Trihydrate (NSAIDs can reduce the diuretic, natriuretic, and antihypertensive effects of thiazides). Products include:
Indocin I.V. 2465

Insulin, Human, Zinc Suspension (Thiazide diuretic may reduce glucose tolerance; concomitant use may require dosage adjustment of insulin). Products include:
Humulin L, 100 Units 1794
Humulin U, 100 Units 1800

Insulin, Human NPH (Thiazide diuretic may reduce glucose tolerance; concomitant use may require dosage adjustment of insulin). Products include:
Humulin N, 100 Units 1795
Humulin N Pen 1797

Insulin, Human Regular (Thiazide diuretic may reduce glucose tolerance; concomitant use may require dosage adjustment of insulin). Products include:
Humulin R, 100 Units 1798

Insulin, Human Regular and Human NPH Mixture (Thiazide diuretic may reduce glucose tolerance; concomitant use may require dosage adjustment of insulin). Products include:
Humulin 50/50, 100 Units 1791
Humulin 70/30 Pen 1793

Insulin, NPH (Thiazide diuretic may reduce glucose tolerance; concomitant use may require dosage adjustment of insulin).
No products indexed under this heading.

Insulin, Regular (Thiazide diuretic may reduce glucose tolerance; concomitant use may require dosage adjustment of insulin).
No products indexed under this heading.

Insulin, Zinc Crystals (Thiazide diuretic may reduce glucose tolerance; concomitant use may require dosage adjustment of insulin).
No products indexed under this heading.

Insulin, Zinc Suspension (Thiazide diuretic may reduce glucose tolerance; concomitant use may require dosage adjustment of insulin).
No products indexed under this heading.

Insulin Aspart, Human Regular (Thiazide diuretic may reduce glucose tolerance; concomitant use may require dosage adjustment of insulin). Products include:
NovoLog Injection 2326

Insulin glargine (Thiazide diuretic may reduce glucose tolerance; concomitant use may require dosage adjustment of insulin). Products include:
Lantus Injection 2909

Insulin Lispro, Human (Thiazide diuretic may reduce glucose tolerance; concomitant use may require dosage adjustment of insulin). Products include:
Humalog-Pen 1781
Humalog Mix 50/50-Pen 1783
Humalog Mix 75/25-Pen 1785

Insulin Lispro Protamine, Human (Thiazide diuretic may reduce glucose tolerance; concomitant use may require dosage adjustment of insulin). Products include:
Humalog Mix 50/50-Pen 1783
Humalog Mix 75/25-Pen 1785

Ketoprofen (NSAIDs can reduce the diuretic, natriuretic, and antihypertensive effects of thiazides).
No products indexed under this heading.

Ketorolac Tromethamine (NSAIDs can reduce the diuretic, natriuretic, and antihypertensive effects of thiazides). Products include:
Acular Ophthalmic Solution 565
Acular LS Ophthalmic Solution 566

Labetalol Hydrochloride (ACE inhibitors have less than additive effects with beta-adrenergic blockers, presumably because both work by inhibiting the renin-angiotension system).
No products indexed under this heading.

Levobunolol Hydrochloride (ACE inhibitors have less than additive effects with beta-adrenergic blockers, presumably because both work by inhibiting the renin-angiotension system). Products include:
Betagan Ophthalmic Solution, USP... ⊙220

Levorphanol Tartrate (Co-administration of narcotics with thiazide diuretics may result in potentiation of orthostatic hypotension).
No products indexed under this heading.

Lithium (Co-administration of ACE inhibitors and lithium has resulted in increased serum lithium levels and symptoms of lithium toxicity).
No products indexed under this heading.

Lithium Carbonate (Co-administration of ACE inhibitors and lithium has resulted in increased serum lithium levels and symptoms of lithium toxicity). Products include:
Lithobid Tablets 1692

Lithium Citrate (Co-administration of ACE inhibitors and lithium has resulted in increased serum lithium levels and symptoms of lithium toxicity).
No products indexed under this heading.

Meclofenamate Sodium (NSAIDs can reduce the diuretic, natriuretic, and antihypertensive effects of thiazides).
No products indexed under this heading.

Mefenamic Acid (NSAIDs can reduce the diuretic, natriuretic, and antihypertensive effects of thiazides).
No products indexed under this heading.

Meloxicam (NSAIDs can reduce the diuretic, natriuretic, and antihypertensive effects of thiazides). Products include:
Mobic Oral Suspension 863
Mobic Tablets 863

Meperidine Hydrochloride (Co-administration of narcotics with thiazide diuretics may result in potentiation of orthostatic hypotension).
No products indexed under this heading.

Mephobarbital (Co-administration of barbiturate with thiazide diuretics may result in potentiation of orthostatic hypotension).
No products indexed under this heading.

Metformin Hydrochloride (Thiazide diuretic may reduce glucose tolerance; concomitant use may require dosage adjustment of oral hypoglycemic agents). Products include:
ActoPlus Met Tablets 3214
Avandamet Tablets 1373
Fortamet Extended-Release Tablets 3115

Methadone Hydrochloride (Co-administration of narcotics with thiazide diuretics may result in potentiation of orthostatic hypotension).
No products indexed under this heading.

Methylprednisolone Acetate (Concomitant use of thiazides with corticosteroids may intensify electrolyte depletion, particularly hypokalemia). Products include:
Depo-Medrol Injectable Suspension 2617
Depo-Medrol Single-Dose Vial 2619

Methylprednisolone Sodium Succinate (Concomitant use of thiazides with corticosteroids may intensify electrolyte depletion, particularly hypokalemia).
No products indexed under this heading.

Metipranolol Hydrochloride (ACE inhibitors have less than additive effects with beta-adrenergic blockers, presumably because both work by inhibiting the renin-angiotensin system).
No products indexed under this heading.

Metoprolol Succinate (ACE inhibitors have less than additive effects with beta-adrenergic blockers, presumably because both work by inhibiting the renin-angiotensin system). Products include:
Toprol-XL Tablets 668

Metoprolol Tartrate (ACE inhibitors have less than additive effects with beta-adrenergic blockers, presumably because both work by inhibiting the renin-angiotensin system). Products include:
Lopressor Injection 2238
Lopressor Tablets 2238
Lopressor HCT 50/25 Tablets 2241
Lopressor HCT 100/25 Tablets 2241
Lopressor HCT 100/50 Tablets 2241

Miglitol (Thiazide diuretic may reduce glucose tolerance; concomitant use may require dosage adjustment of oral hypoglycemic agents).
No products indexed under this heading.

Morphine Sulfate (Co-administration of narcotics with thiazide diuretics may result in potentiation of orthostatic hypotension). Products include:
Avinza Capsules 1741
Kadian Capsules 577
MS Contin Tablets 2701

Nabumetone (NSAIDs can reduce the diuretic, natriuretic, and antihypertensive effects of thiazides).
No products indexed under this heading.

Nadolol (ACE inhibitors have less than additive effects with beta-adrenergic blockers, presumably because both work by inhibiting the renin-angiotensin system). Products include:
Nadolol Tablets 2159

Naproxen (NSAIDs can reduce the diuretic, natriuretic, and antihypertensive effects of thiazides). Products include:
EC-Naprosyn Delayed-Release Tablets 2761
Naprosyn Suspension 2761
Naprosyn Tablets 2761
Prevacid NapraPAC 3280

Naproxen Sodium (NSAIDs can reduce the diuretic, natriuretic, and antihypertensive effects of thiazides). Products include:
Aleve Caplets 742
Aleve Gelcaps 743
Aleve Cold & Sinus Caplets 744
Anaprox Tablets 2761
Anaprox DS Tablets 2761

Norepinephrine Bitartrate (Thiazide diuretics may decrease arterial responsiveness to pressor amines).
No products indexed under this heading.

Oxaprozin (NSAIDs can reduce the diuretic, natriuretic, and antihypertensive effects of thiazides).
No products indexed under this heading.

Oxycodone Hydrochloride (Co-administration of narcotics with thiazide diuretics may result in potentiation of orthostatic hypotension). Products include:
OxyContin Tablets 2703
OxyFast Oral Concentrate Solution 2708
OxyIR Capsules 2708
Percocet Tablets 1131
Percodan Tablets 1132

Penbutolol Sulfate (ACE inhibitors have less than additive effects with beta-adrenergic blockers, presumably because both work by inhibiting the renin-angiotensin system).
No products indexed under this heading.

Pentobarbital Sodium (Co-administration of barbiturate with thiazide diuretics may result in potentiation of orthostatic hypotension). Products include:
Nembutal Sodium Solution, USP 2470

Phenobarbital (Co-administration of barbiturate with thiazide diuretics may result in potentiation of orthostatic hypotension). Products include:
Donnatal Extentabs 2493

Phenylbutazone (NSAIDs can reduce the diuretic, natriuretic, and antihypertensive effects of thiazides).
No products indexed under this heading.

Pindolol (ACE inhibitors have less than additive effects with beta-adrenergic blockers, presumably because both work by inhibiting the renin-angiotensin system).
No products indexed under this heading.

Pioglitazone Hydrochloride (Thiazide diuretic may reduce glucose tolerance; concomitant use may require dosage adjustment of oral hypoglycemic agents). Products include:
ActoPlus Met Tablets 3214
Actos Tablets 3219
Duetact Tablets 3226

Piroxicam (NSAIDs can reduce the diuretic, natriuretic, and antihypertensive effects of thiazides).
No products indexed under this heading.

Potassium Acid Phosphate (Potassium supplements can increase the risk of hyperkalemia). Products include:
K-Phos Original (Sodium Free) Tablets 760

Potassium Bicarbonate (Potassium supplements can increase the risk of hyperkalemia).
No products indexed under this heading.

Potassium Chloride (Potassium supplements can increase the risk of hyperkalemia). Products include:
Colyte with Flavor Packs for Oral Solution 3088
HalfLytely and Bisacodyl Tablets Bowel Prep Kit with Flavors Packs 881
K-Dur Extended-Relase Tablets 3033
K-Lor Oral Solution 474
K-Tab Tablets 475
MoviPrep Oral Solution 2839
TriLyte with Flavor Packs for Oral Solution 3100

Potassium Citrate (Potassium supplements can increase the risk of hyperkalemia). Products include:
Urocit-K Tablets 2144

Potassium Gluconate (Potassium supplements can increase the risk of hyperkalemia).
No products indexed under this heading.

Potassium Phosphate (Potassium supplements can increase the risk of hyperkalemia). Products include:
K-Phos Neutral Tablets 760

Prednisolone Acetate (Concomitant use of thiazides with corticosteroids may intensify electrolyte depletion, particularly hypokalemia). Products include:
Blephamide Ophthalmic Ointment 568
Blephamide Ophthalmic Suspension 569
Poly-Pred Ophthalmic Suspension .... ⊙233
Pred Forte Ophthalmic Suspension .... ⊙235
Pred Mild Ophthalmic Suspension .... ⊙238
Pred-G Ophthalmic Ointment .... ⊙237
Pred-G Ophthalmic Suspension ...... ⊙236

Prednisolone Sodium Phosphate (Concomitant use of thiazides with corticosteroids may intensify electrolyte depletion, particularly hypokalemia).
No products indexed under this heading.

Prednisolone Tebutate (Concomitant use of thiazides with corticosteroids may intensify electrolyte depletion, particularly hypokalemia).
No products indexed under this heading.

Prednisone (Concomitant use of thiazides with corticosteroids may intensify electrolyte depletion, particularly hypokalemia).
No products indexed under this heading.

Propantheline Bromide (Co-administration increases the absorption of hydrochlorothiazide).
No products indexed under this heading.

Propoxyphene Hydrochloride (Co-administration of narcotics with thiazide diuretics may result in potentiation of orthostatic hypotension).
No products indexed under this heading.

Propoxyphene Napsylate (Co-administration of narcotics with thiazide diuretics may result in potentiation of orthostatic hypotension).
No products indexed under this heading.

Propranolol Hydrochloride (ACE inhibitors have less than additive effects with beta-adrenergic blockers, presumably because both work by inhibiting the renin-angiotensin system). Products include:
Inderal LA Long-Acting Capsules 3429
InnoPran XL Capsules 2723

Remifentanil Hydrochloride (Co-administration of narcotics with thiazide diuretics may result in potentiation of orthostatic hypotension).
No products indexed under this heading.

Repaglinide (Thiazide diuretic may reduce glucose tolerance; concomitant use may require dosage adjustment of oral hypoglycemic agents).
No products indexed under this heading.

Rofecoxib (NSAIDs can reduce the diuretic, natriuretic, and antihypertensive effects of thiazides).
No products indexed under this heading.

Rosiglitazone Maleate (Thiazide diuretic may reduce glucose tolerance; concomitant use may require dosage adjustment of oral hypoglycemic agents). Products include:
Avandamet Tablets 1373
Avandaryl Tablets 1379
Avandia Tablets 1384

Secobarbital Sodium (Co-administration of barbiturate with thiazide diuretics may result in potentiation of orthostatic hypotension).
No products indexed under this heading.

Sotalol Hydrochloride (ACE inhibitors have less than additive effects with beta-adrenergic blockers, presumably because both work by inhibiting the renin-angiotension system).
No products indexed under this heading.

Spironolactone (Potassium-sparing diuretics can increase the risk of hyperkalemia).
No products indexed under this heading.

Sufentanil Citrate (Co-administration of narcotics with thiazide diuretics may result in potentiation of orthostatic hypotension).
No products indexed under this heading.

Sulindac (NSAIDs can reduce the diuretic, natriuretic, and antihypertensive effects of thiazides).
Products include:
Clinoril Tablets 1924

Thiamylal Sodium (Co-administration of barbiturate with thiazide diuretics may result in potentiation of orthostatic hypotension).
No products indexed under this heading.

Timolol Hemihydrate (ACE inhibitors have less than additive effects with beta-adrenergic blockers, presumably because both work by inhibiting the renin-angiotension system).
Products include:
Betimol Ophthalmic Solution 3382
Betimol Ophthalmic Solution .... ⊙295

Timolol Maleate (ACE inhibitors have less than additive effects with beta-adrenergic blockers, presumably because both work by inhibiting the renin-angiotension system).
Products include:
Blocadren Tablets 1916
Cosopt Sterile Ophthalmic Solution 1931
Timolide Tablets 2086
Timoptic Sterile Ophthalmic Solution 2088
Timoptic in Ocudose 2091
Timoptic-XE Sterile Ophthalmic Gel Forming Solution 2092

Tolazamide (Thiazide diuretic may reduce glucose tolerance; concomitant use may require dosage adjustment of oral hypoglycemic agents).
No products indexed under this heading.

Tolbutamide (Thiazide diuretic may reduce glucose tolerance; concomitant use may require dosage adjustment of oral hypoglycemic agents).
No products indexed under this heading.

Tolmetin Sodium (NSAIDs can reduce the diuretic, natriuretic, and antihypertensive effects of thiazides).
No products indexed under this heading.

Triamcinolone (Concomitant use of thiazides with corticosteroids may intensify electrolyte depletion, particularly hypokalemia).
No products indexed under this heading.

Triamcinolone Acetonide (Concomitant use of thiazides with corticosteroids may intensify electrolyte depletion, particularly hypokalemia).
Products include:
Azmacort Inhalation Aerosol 1726
Nasacort AQ Nasal Spray 2922

Triamcinolone Diacetate (Concomitant use of thiazides with corticosteroids may intensify electrolyte depletion, particularly hypokalemia).
No products indexed under this heading.

Triamcinolone Hexacetonide (Concomitant use of thiazides with corticosteroids may intensify electrolyte depletion, particularly hypokalemia).
No products indexed under this heading.

Triamterene (Potassium-sparing diuretics can increase the risk of hyperkalemia). Products include:
Dyazide Capsules 1423
Dyrenium Capsules 3400

Troglitazone (Thiazide diuretic may reduce glucose tolerance; concomitant use may require dosage adjustment of oral hypoglycemic agents).
No products indexed under this heading.

Tubocurarine Chloride (Thiazide diuretics may increase the responsiveness to tubocurarine).
No products indexed under this heading.

Valdecoxib (NSAIDs can reduce the diuretic, natriuretic, and antihypertensive effects of thiazides).
No products indexed under this heading.

Food Interactions

Alcohol (Co-administration of alcohol with thiazide diuretics may result in potentiation of orthostatic hypotension).

Food, unspecified (Bioavailability varies with formulation and food intake which reduces Cmax and AUC of moexiprilat by about 70% and 40% respectively after ingestion of low-fat breakfast or by 80% and 50% respectively after the ingestion of a high-fat breakfast; patients should be advised to take Uniretic one hour before a meal).

UNIVASC TABLETS

(Moexipril Hydrochloride) 3104
May interact with diuretics, lithium preparations, potassium preparations, potassium sparing diuretics, and certain other agents. Compounds in these categories include:

Amiloride Hydrochloride (Co-administration can increase the risk of hyperkalemia; therefore, potassium-sparing diuretics should be given with caution, and serum potassium should be monitored).
Products include:
Midamor Tablets 2026
Moduretic Tablets 2028

Bendroflumethiazide (Co-administration may result in excessive reductions in blood pressure. This can be minimized by discontinuing diuretic therapy for several days or cautiously increasing salt intake before initiating with moexipril. If this is not possible, the starting dose of moexipril should be reduced).
No products indexed under this heading.

Bumetanide (Co-administration may result in excessive reductions in blood pressure. This can be minimized by discontinuing diuretic therapy for several days or cautiously increasing salt intake before initiating with moexipril. If this is not possible, the starting dose of moexipril should be reduced). Products include:
Bumex Tablets 2746

Chlorothiazide (Co-administration may result in excessive reductions in blood pressure. This can be minimized by discontinuing diuretic therapy for several days or cautiously increasing salt intake before initiating with moexipril. If this is not possible, the starting dose of moexipril should be reduced). Products include:
Diuril Oral Suspension 1954

Chlorothiazide Sodium (Co-administration may result in excessive reductions in blood pressure. This can be minimized by discontinuing diuretic therapy for several days or cautiously increasing salt intake before initiating with moexipril. If this is not possible, the starting dose of moexipril should be reduced).
Products include:
Diuril Sodium Intravenous 2467

Chlorthalidone (Co-administration may result in excessive reductions in blood pressure. This can be minimized by discontinuing diuretic therapy for several days or cautiously increasing salt intake before initiating with moexipril. If this is not possible, the starting dose of moexipril should be reduced). Products include:
Clorpres Tablets 2153

Ethacrynic Acid (Co-administration may result in excessive reductions in blood pressure. This can be minimized by discontinuing diuretic therapy for several days or cautiously increasing salt intake before initiating with moexipril. If this is not possible, the starting dose of moexipril should be reduced). Products include:
Edecrin Tablets 1959

Furosemide (Co-administration may result in excessive reductions in blood pressure. This can be minimized by discontinuing diuretic therapy for several days or cautiously increasing salt intake before initiating with moexipril. If this is not possible, the starting dose of moexipril should be reduced). Products include:
Furosemide Tablets 2154

Hydrochlorothiazide (Co-administration may result in excessive reductions in blood pressure. This can be minimized by discontinuing diuretic therapy for several days or cautiously increasing salt intake before initiating with moexipril. If this is not possible, the starting dose of moexipril should be reduced).
Products include:
Aldoril Tablets 1910
Atacand HCT 651
Avalide Tablets 888
Avalide Tablets 2874
Benicar HCT Tablets 1044
Diovan HCT Tablets 2196
Dyazide Capsules 1423
Hyzaar 50-12.5 Tablets 1990
Hyzaar 100-12.5 Tablets 1990
Hyzaar 100-25 Tablets 1990
Lopressor HCT 50/25 Tablets 2241
Lopressor HCT 100/25 Tablets 2241
Lopressor HCT 100/50 Tablets 2241
Lotensin HCT Tablets 2246
Micardis HCT Tablets 856
Moduretic Tablets 2028
Prinzide Tablets 2056
Teveten HCT Tablets 1737
Timolide Tablets 2086
Uniretic Tablets 3100

Hydroflumethiazide (Co-administration may result in excessive reductions in blood pressure. This can be minimized by discontinuing diuretic therapy for several days or cautiously increasing salt intake before initiating with moexipril. If this is not possible, the starting dose of moexipril should be reduced).
No products indexed under this heading.

Indapamide (Co-administration may result in excessive reductions in blood pressure. This can be minimized by discontinuing diuretic therapy for several days or cautiously increasing salt intake before initiating with moexipril. If this is not possible, the starting dose of moexipril should be reduced). Products include:
Indapamide Tablets 2156

Lithium (Increased serum lithium levels and symptoms of lithium toxicity have been reported during concomitant use. Lithium should be co-administered with caution, and frequent monitoring of serum lithium levels is recommended).
No products indexed under this heading.

Lithium Carbonate (Increased serum lithium levels and symptoms of lithium toxicity have been reported during concomitant use. Lithium should be co-administered with caution, and frequent monitoring of serum lithium levels is recommended).
Products include:
Lithobid Tablets 1692

Lithium Citrate (Increased serum lithium levels and symptoms of lithium toxicity have been reported during concomitant use. Lithium should be co-administered with caution, and frequent monitoring of serum lithium levels is recommended).
No products indexed under this heading.

Methyclothiazide (Co-administration may result in excessive reductions in blood pressure. This can be minimized by discontinuing diuretic therapy for several days or cautiously increasing salt intake before initiating with moexipril. If this is not possible, the starting dose of moexipril should be reduced).
No products indexed under this heading.

Metolazone (Co-administration may result in excessive reductions in blood pressure. This can be minimized by discontinuing diuretic therapy for several days or cautiously increasing salt intake before initiating with moexipril. If this is not possible, the starting dose of moexipril should be reduced).
No products indexed under this heading.

Polythiazide (Co-administration may result in excessive reductions in blood pressure. This can be minimized by discontinuing diuretic therapy for several days or cautiously increasing salt intake before initiating with moexipril. If this is not possible, the starting dose of moexipril should be reduced).
No products indexed under this heading.

Potassium Acid Phosphate (Co-administration can increase the risk of hyperkalemia; therefore, potassium supplements should be given with caution, and serum potassium should be monitored). Products include:

K-Phos Original (Sodium Free) Tablets 760

Potassium Bicarbonate (Co-administration can increase the risk of hyperkalemia; therefore, potassium supplements should be given with caution, and serum potassium should be monitored).

No products indexed under this heading.

Potassium Chloride (Co-administration can increase the risk of hyperkalemia; therefore, potassium supplements should be given with caution, and serum potassium should be monitored). Products include:

Colyte with Flavor Packs for Oral Solution 3088
HalfLytely and Bisacodyl Tablets Bowel Prep Kit with Flavors Packs 881
K-Dur Extended-Relase Tablets 3033
K-Lor Oral Solution 474
K-Tab Tablets 475
MoviPrep Oral Solution 2839
TriLyte with Flavor Packs for Oral Solution 3100

Potassium Citrate (Co-administration can increase the risk of hyperkalemia; therefore, potassium supplements should be given with caution, and serum potassium should be monitored). Products include:

Urocit-K Tablets 2144

Potassium Gluconate (Co-administration can increase the risk of hyperkalemia; therefore, potassium supplements should be given with caution, and serum potassium should be monitored).

No products indexed under this heading.

Potassium Phosphate (Co-administration can increase the risk of hyperkalemia; therefore, potassium supplements should be given with caution, and serum potassium should be monitored). Products include:

K-Phos Neutral Tablets 760

Spironolactone (Co-administration can increase the risk of hyperkalemia; therefore, potassium-sparing diuretics should be given with caution, and serum potassium should be monitored).

No products indexed under this heading.

Torsemide (Co-administration may result in excessive reductions in blood pressure. This can be minimized by discontinuing diuretic therapy for several days or cautiously increasing salt intake before initiating with moexipril. If this is not possible, the starting dose of moexipril should be reduced). Products include:

Demadex Injection 2759
Demadex Tablets 2759

Triamterene (Co-administration can increase the risk of hyperkalemia; therefore, potassium-sparing diuretics should be given with caution, and serum potassium should be monitored). Products include:

Dyazide Capsules 1423
Dyrenium Capsules 3400

Food Interactions

Food, unspecified (Food reduces Cmax and AUC by about 70% and 40% respectively after ingestion of a low-fat breakfast or by 80% and 50% respectively after the ingestion of high-fat breakfast).

UROCIT-K TABLETS

(Potassium Citrate) 2144

May interact with anticholinergics and potassium sparing diuretics. Compounds in these categories include:

Amiloride Hydrochloride (Co-administration can produce severe hyperkalemia; concurrent use should be avoided). Products include:

Midamor Tablets 2026
Moduretic Tablets 2028

Atropine Sulfate (Co-administration with drugs that slow gastrointestinal transit time, such as anticholinergics, can be expected to increase the gastrointestinal irritation produced by potassium salts; concurrent use is contraindicated). Products include:

Donnatal Extentabs 2493

Belladonna Alkaloids (Co-administration with drugs that slow gastrointestinal transit time, such as anticholinergics, can be expected to increase the gastrointestinal irritation produced by potassium salts; concurrent use is contraindicated). Products include:

Hyland's Teething Tablets ..... ▣830

Benztropine Mesylate (Co-administration with drugs that slow gastrointestinal transit time, such as anticholinergics, can be expected to increase the gastrointestinal irritation produced by potassium salts; concurrent use is contraindicated).

No products indexed under this heading.

Biperiden Hydrochloride (Co-administration with drugs that slow gastrointestinal transit time, such as anticholinergics, can be expected to increase the gastrointestinal irritation produced by potassium salts; concurrent use is contraindicated).

No products indexed under this heading.

Clidinium Bromide (Co-administration with drugs that slow gastrointestinal transit time, such as anticholinergics, can be expected to increase the gastrointestinal irritation produced by potassium salts; concurrent use is contraindicated).

No products indexed under this heading.

Dicyclomine Hydrochloride (Co-administration with drugs that slow gastrointestinal transit time, such as anticholinergics, can be expected to increase the gastrointestinal irritation produced by potassium salts; concurrent use is contraindicated). Products include:

Bentyl Capsules 697
Bentyl Injection 697
Bentyl Syrup 697
Bentyl Tablets 697

Glycopyrrolate (Co-administration with drugs that slow gastrointestinal transit time, such as anticholinergics, can be expected to increase the gastrointestinal irritation produced by potassium salts; concurrent use is contraindicated).

No products indexed under this heading.

Hyoscyamine (Co-administration with drugs that slow gastrointestinal transit time, such as anticholinergics, can be expected to increase the gastrointestinal irritation produced by potassium salts; concurrent use is contraindicated).

No products indexed under this heading.

Hyoscyamine Sulfate (Co-administration with drugs that slow gastrointestinal transit time, such as anticholinergics, can be expected to increase the gastrointestinal irritation produced by potassium salts; concurrent use is contraindicated). Products include:

Donnatal Extentabs 2493
Prosed/DS Tablets 1157

Ipratropium Bromide (Co-administration with drugs that slow gastrointestinal transit time, such as anticholinergics, can be expected to increase the gastrointestinal irritation produced by potassium salts; concurrent use is contraindicated). Products include:

Atrovent Inhalation Solution 835
Atrovent HFA Inhalation Aerosol 841
Atrovent Nasal Spray 0.03% 837
Atrovent Nasal Spray 0.06% 839
Combivent Inhalation Aerosol 847
DuoNeb Inhalation Solution 1058

Mepenzolate Bromide (Co-administration with drugs that slow gastrointestinal transit time, such as anticholinergics, can be expected to increase the gastrointestinal irritation produced by potassium salts; concurrent use is contraindicated).

No products indexed under this heading.

Oxybutynin Chloride (Co-administration with drugs that slow gastrointestinal transit time, such as anticholinergics, can be expected to increase the gastrointestinal irritation produced by potassium salts; concurrent use is contraindicated). Products include:

Ditropan XL Extended-Release Tablets 2413

Procyclidine Hydrochloride (Co-administration with drugs that slow gastrointestinal transit time, such as anticholinergics, can be expected to increase the gastrointestinal irritation produced by potassium salts; concurrent use is contraindicated).

No products indexed under this heading.

Propantheline Bromide (Co-administration with drugs that slow gastrointestinal transit time, such as anticholinergics, can be expected to increase the gastrointestinal irritation produced by potassium salts; concurrent use is contraindicated).

No products indexed under this heading.

Scopolamine (Co-administration with drugs that slow gastrointestinal transit time, such as anticholinergics, can be expected to increase the gastrointestinal irritation produced by potassium salts; concurrent use is contraindicated). Products include:

Transderm Scōp Transdermal Therapeutic System 2177

Scopolamine Hydrobromide (Co-administration with drugs that slow gastrointestinal transit time, such as anticholinergics, can be expected to increase the gastrointestinal irritation produced by potassium salts; concurrent use is contraindicated). Products include:

Donnatal Extentabs 2493

Spironolactone (Co-administration can produce severe hyperkalemia; concurrent use should be avoided).

No products indexed under this heading.

Tolterodine Tartrate (Co-administration with drugs that slow gastrointestinal transit time, such as anticholinergics, can be expected to increase the gastrointestinal irritation produced by potassium salts; concurrent use is contraindicated). Products include:

Detrol Tablets 2628
Detrol LA Capsules 2631

Triamterene (Co-administration can produce severe hyperkalemia; concurrent use should be avoided). Products include:

Dyazide Capsules 1423
Dyrenium Capsules 3400

Tridihexethyl Chloride (Co-administration with drugs that slow gastrointestinal transit time, such as anticholinergics, can be expected to increase the gastrointestinal irritation produced by potassium salts; concurrent use is contraindicated).

No products indexed under this heading.

Trihexyphenidyl Hydrochloride (Co-administration with drugs that slow gastrointestinal transit time, such as anticholinergics, can be expected to increase the gastrointestinal irritation produced by potassium salts; concurrent use is contraindicated).

No products indexed under this heading.

UROQID-ACID NO. 2 TABLETS

(Methenamine Mandelate, Sodium Acid Phosphate) 760

May interact with:

Acetazolamide (Reduces the effectiveness of methenamine by causing urine to become alkaline).

No products indexed under this heading.

ACTH (Concurrent use with sodium phosphate may result in hypernatremia).

No products indexed under this heading.

Aluminum Carbonate (Reduces the effectiveness of methenamine by causing urine to become alkaline).

No products indexed under this heading.

Aluminum Hydroxide (Reduces the effectiveness of methenamine by causing urine to become alkaline). Products include:

Gaviscon Regular Strength Liquid ..... ▣658
Gaviscon Regular Strength Tablets ..... ▣658
Gaviscon Extra Strength Liquid ..... ▣658
Gaviscon Extra Strength Tablets ..... ▣658
Maalox Regular Strength Antacid/Antigas Liquid 2175
Maalox Max Maximum Strength Antacid/Anti-Gas Liquid 2176

Aspirin (Concurrent use may lead to increased serum salicylate levels since excretion of salicylates is reduced in acidic urine). Products include:

Aggrenox Capsules 822
Bayer Aspirin 744
BC Allergy Sinus Cold Powder ..... ▣677
BC Headache Powder ..... ▣677
Arthritis Strength BC Powder ..... ▣677
BC Sinus Cold Powder ..... ▣677

- Excedrin Extra Strength Caplets/Tablets/Geltabs 684
- Excedrin Migraine Caplets/Tablets/Geltabs 609
- Goody's Body Pain Formula Powder 684
- Goody's Extra Strength Headache Powders 611
- Goody's Extra Strength Pain Relief Tablets 685
- Percodan Tablets 1132
- St. Joseph 81 mg Aspirin Chewable and Enteric Coated Tablets 1869

Bendroflumethiazide (Reduces the effectiveness of methenamine by causing urine to become alkaline).
No products indexed under this heading.

Betamethasone Acetate (Concurrent use with sodium phosphate may result in hypernatremia).
No products indexed under this heading.

Betamethasone Sodium Phosphate (Concurrent use with sodium phosphate may result in hypernatremia).
No products indexed under this heading.

Chlorothiazide (Reduces the effectiveness of methenamine by causing urine to become alkaline). Products include:
- Diuril Oral Suspension 1954

Chlorothiazide Sodium (Reduces the effectiveness of methenamine by causing urine to become alkaline). Products include:
- Diuril Sodium Intravenous 2467

Choline Magnesium Trisalicylate (Concurrent use may lead to increased serum salicylate levels since excretion of salicylates is reduced in acidic urine).
No products indexed under this heading.

Cortisone Acetate (Concurrent use with sodium phosphate may result in hypernatremia).
No products indexed under this heading.

Deserpidine (Concurrent use with sodium phosphate may result in hypernatremia).
No products indexed under this heading.

Desoxycorticosterone Acetate (Concurrent use with sodium phosphate may result in hypernatremia).
No products indexed under this heading.

Desoxycorticosterone Pivalate (Concurrent use with sodium phosphate may result in hypernatremia).
No products indexed under this heading.

Dexamethasone (Concurrent use with sodium phosphate may result in hypernatremia). Products include:
- Ciprodex Otic Suspension 559
- Decadron Tablets 1951
- TobraDex Ophthalmic Ointment 562
- TobraDex Ophthalmic Suspension ... 563

Dexamethasone Acetate (Concurrent use with sodium phosphate may result in hypernatremia).
No products indexed under this heading.

Dexamethasone Sodium Phosphate (Concurrent use with sodium phosphate may result in hypernatremia).
No products indexed under this heading.

Diazoxide (Concurrant use with sodium phosphate may result in hypernatremia). Products include:
- Hyperstat I.V. 3017

Dichlorphenamide (Reduces the effectiveness of methenamine by causing urine to become alkaline). Products include:
- Daranide Tablets 1950

Diflunisal (Concurrent use may lead to increased serum salicylate levels since excretion of salicylates is reduced in acidic urine). Products include:
- Dolobid Tablets 1955

Fludrocortisone Acetate (Concurrent use with sodium phosphate may result in hypernatremia).
No products indexed under this heading.

Guanethidine Monosulfate (Concurrent use with sodium phosphate may result in hypernatremia).
No products indexed under this heading.

Hydralazine Hydrochloride (Concurrent use with sodium phosphate may result in hypernatremia). Products include:
- BiDil Tablets 2171

Hydrochlorothiazide (Reduces the effectiveness of methenamine by causing urine to become alkaline). Products include:
- Aldoril Tablets 1910
- Atacand HCT 651
- Avalide Tablets 888
- Avalide Tablets 2874
- Benicar HCT Tablets 1044
- Diovan HCT Tablets 2196
- Dyazide Capsules 1423
- Hyzaar 50-12.5 Tablets 1990
- Hyzaar 100-12.5 Tablets 1990
- Hyzaar 100-25 Tablets 1990
- Lopressor HCT 50/25 Tablets 2241
- Lopressor HCT 100/25 Tablets 2241
- Lopressor HCT 100/50 Tablets 2241
- Lotensin HCT Tablets 2246
- Micardis HCT Tablets 856
- Moduretic Tablets 2028
- Prinzide Tablets 2056
- Teveten HCT Tablets 1737
- Timolide Tablets 2086
- Uniretic Tablets 3100

Hydrocortisone (Concurrent use with sodium phosphate may result in hypernatremia). Products include:
- Colocort Rectal Suspension, USP (Retention) 100 mg/60 mL 2476
- Hydrocortone Tablets 1989
- Preparation H Hydrocortisone Cream 646

Hydrocortisone Acetate (Concurrent use with sodium phosphate may result in hypernatremia). Products include:
- Analpram-HC 1159
- Pramosone 1161
- ProctoFoam-HC 3099

Hydrocortisone Sodium Phosphate (Concurrent use with sodium phosphate may result in hypernatremia).
No products indexed under this heading.

Hydrocortisone Sodium Succinate (Concurrent use with sodium phosphate may result in hypernatremia).
No products indexed under this heading.

Hydroflumethiazide (Reduces the effectiveness of methenamine by causing urine to become alkaline).
No products indexed under this heading.

Magaldrate (Reduces the effectiveness of methenamine by causing urine to become alkaline).
No products indexed under this heading.

Magnesium Hydroxide (Reduces the effectiveness of methenamine by causing urine to become alkaline). Products include:
- Maalox Regular Strength Antacid/Antigas Liquid 2175
- Maalox Max Maximum Strength Antacid/Anti-Gas Liquid 2176
- Pepcid Complete Chewable Tablets 1701

Magnesium Oxide (Reduces the effectiveness of methenamine by causing urine to become alkaline). Products include:
- Beelith Tablets 759
- PremCal Light, Regular, and Extra Strength Tablets 818

Magnesium Salicylate (Concurrent use may lead to increased serum salicylate levels since excretion of salicylates is reduced in acidic urine).
No products indexed under this heading.

Methazolamide (Reduces the effectiveness of methenamine by causing urine to become alkaline).
No products indexed under this heading.

Methyclothiazide (Reduces the effectiveness of methenamine by causing urine to become alkaline).
No products indexed under this heading.

Methyldopa (Concurrent use with sodium phosphate may result in hypernatremia). Products include:
- Aldoril Tablets 1910

Methylprednisolone Acetate (Concurrent use with sodium phosphate may result in hypernatremia). Products include:
- Depo-Medrol Injectable Suspension 2617
- Depo-Medrol Single-Dose Vial 2619

Methylprednisolone Sodium Succinate (Concurrent use with sodium phosphate may result in hypernatremia).
No products indexed under this heading.

Polythiazide (Reduces the effectiveness of methenamine by causing urine to become alkaline).
No products indexed under this heading.

Potassium Citrate (Reduces the effectiveness of methenamine by causing urine to become alkaline). Products include:
- Urocit-K Tablets 2144

Prednisolone Acetate (Concurrent use with sodium phosphate may result in hypernatremia). Products include:
- Blephamide Ophthalmic Ointment 568
- Blephamide Ophthalmic Suspension 569
- Poly-Pred Ophthalmic Suspension .... ⊙233
- Pred Forte Ophthalmic Suspension .... ⊙235
- Pred Mild Ophthalmic Suspension .... ⊙238
- Pred-G Ophthalmic Ointment .... ⊙237
- Pred-G Ophthalmic Suspension ...... ⊙236

Prednisolone Sodium Phosphate (Concurrent use with sodium phosphate may result in hypernatremia).
No products indexed under this heading.

Prednisolone Tebutate (Concurrent use with sodium phosphate may result in hypernatremia).
No products indexed under this heading.

Prednisone (Concurrent use with sodium phosphate may result in hypernatremia).
No products indexed under this heading.

Rauwolfia Serpentina (Concurrent use with sodium phosphate may result in hypernatremia).
No products indexed under this heading.

Rescinnamine (Concurrent use with sodium phosphate may result in hypernatremia).
No products indexed under this heading.

Reserpine (Concurrent use with sodium phosphate may result in hypernatremia).
No products indexed under this heading.

Salsalate (Concurrent use may lead to increased serum salicylate levels since excretion of salicylates is reduced in acidic urine).
No products indexed under this heading.

Sodium Bicarbonate (Reduces the effectiveness of methenamine by causing urine to become alkaline). Products include:
- Colyte with Flavor Packs for Oral Solution 3088
- HalfLytely and Bisacodyl Tablets Bowel Prep Kit with Flavors Packs 881
- TriLyte with Flavor Packs for Oral Solution 3100

Sodium Citrate (Reduces the effectiveness of methenamine by causing urine to become alkaline).
No products indexed under this heading.

Sulfamethizole (Concurrent use with sulfamethizole and formaldehyde forms an insoluble precipitate in acid urine and increases the risk of crystaluria).
No products indexed under this heading.

Triamcinolone (Concurrent use with sodium phosphate may result in hypernatremia).
No products indexed under this heading.

Triamcinolone Acetonide (Concurrent use with sodium phosphate may result in hypernatremia). Products include:
- Azmacort Inhalation Aerosol 1726
- Nasacort AQ Nasal Spray 2922

Triamcinolone Diacetate (Concurrent use with sodium phosphate may result in hypernatremia).
No products indexed under this heading.

Triamcinolone Hexacetonide (Concurrent use with sodium phosphate may result in hypernatremia).
No products indexed under this heading.

UROXATRAL TABLETS

(Alfuzosin Hydrochloride) 2943

May interact with alpha adrenergic blockers and cytochrome p450 3a4 inhibitors (selected). Compounds in these categories include:

Acetazolamide (Uroxatral should not be co-administered with potent CYP3A4 inhibitors such as ketoconazole, itraconazole, and ritonavir, since alfuzosin blood levels are increased).
No products indexed under this heading.

Amiodarone Hydrochloride
(Uroxatral should not be co-administered with potent CYP3A4 inhibitors such as ketoconazole, itraconazole, and ritonavir, since alfuzosin blood levels are increased).
 No products indexed under this heading.

Amprenavir (Uroxatral should not be co-administered with potent CYP3A4 inhibitors such as ketoconazole, itraconazole, and ritonavir, since alfuzosin blood levels are increased). Products include:
Agenerase Capsules 1327
Agenerase Oral Solution 1332

Anastrozole (Uroxatral should not be co-administered with potent CYP3A4 inhibitors such as ketoconazole, itraconazole, and ritonavir, since alfuzosin blood levels are increased). Products include:
Arimidex Tablets 673

Aprepitant (Uroxatral should not be co-administered with potent CYP3A4 inhibitors such as ketoconazole, itraconazole, and ritonavir, since alfuzosin blood levels are increased). Products include:
Emend Capsules 1963

Cimetidine (Uroxatral should not be co-administered with potent CYP3A4 inhibitors such as ketoconazole, itraconazole, and ritonavir, since alfuzosin blood levels are increased). Products include:
Tagamet HB 200 Tablets ▣664

Cimetidine Hydrochloride (Uroxatral should not be co-administered with potent CYP3A4 inhibitors such as ketoconazole, itraconazole, and ritonavir, since alfuzosin blood levels are increased).
 No products indexed under this heading.

Ciprofloxacin (Uroxatral should not be co-administered with potent CYP3A4 inhibitors such as ketoconazole, itraconazole, and ritonavir, since alfuzosin blood levels are increased). Products include:
Cipro Oral Suspension 2977
Cipro I.V. ... 2984
Cipro XR Tablets 2990
Ciprodex Otic Suspension 559

Clarithromycin (Uroxatral should not be co-administered with potent CYP3A4 inhibitors such as ketoconazole, itraconazole, and ritonavir, since alfuzosin blood levels are increased). Products include:
Biaxin/Biaxin XL 402
PREVPAC 3284

Clotrimazole (Uroxatral should not be co-administered with potent CYP3A4 inhibitors such as ketoconazole, itraconazole, and ritonavir, since alfuzosin blood levels are increased). Products include:
Desenex Athlete's Foot Cream ▣635
Lotrimin ... 3039
Lotrisone ... 3040

Cyclosporine (Uroxatral should not be co-administered with potent CYP3A4 inhibitors such as ketoconazole, itraconazole, and ritonavir, since alfuzosin blood levels are increased). Products include:
Gengraf Capsules 459
Neoral Oral Solution 2259
Neoral Soft Gelatin Capsules 2259
Restasis Ophthalmic Emulsion 575
Sandimmune 2275

Dalfopristin (Uroxatral should not be co-administered with potent CYP3A4 inhibitors such as ketoconazole, itraconazole, and ritonavir, since alfuzosin blood levels are increased).
 No products indexed under this heading.

Danazol (Uroxatral should not be co-administered with potent CYP3A4 inhibitors such as ketoconazole, itraconazole, and ritonavir, since alfuzosin blood levels are increased).
 No products indexed under this heading.

Delavirdine Mesylate (Uroxatral should not be co-administered with potent CYP3A4 inhibitors such as ketoconazole, itraconazole, and ritonavir, since alfuzosin blood levels are increased). Products include:
Rescriptor Tablets 2551

Diltiazem Hydrochloride (Uroxatral should not be co-administered with potent CYP3A4 inhibitors such as ketoconazole, itraconazole, and ritonavir, since alfuzosin blood levels are increased). Products include:
Cardizem LA Extended Release Tablets ... 1728
Tiazac Capsules 1201

Diltiazem Maleate (Uroxatral should not be co-administered with potent CYP3A4 inhibitors such as ketoconazole, itraconazole, and ritonavir, since alfuzosin blood levels are increased).
 No products indexed under this heading.

Doxazosin Mesylate (Interactions may be expected; uroxatral should not be used in combination with other alpha-blockers). Products include:
Cardura XL Tablets 2515

Efavirenz (Uroxatral should not be co-administered with potent CYP3A4 inhibitors such as ketoconazole, itraconazole, and ritonavir, since alfuzosin blood levels are increased). Products include:
Atripla Tablets 945
Sustiva Capsules 930
Sustiva Tablets 930

Erythromycin (Uroxatral should not be co-administered with potent CYP3A4 inhibitors such as ketoconazole, itraconazole, and ritonavir, since alfuzosin blood levels are increased). Products include:
Ery-Tab Tablets 449
Erythromycin Base Filmtab Tablets .. 455
Erythromycin Delayed-Release Capsules, USP 457
PCE Dispertab Tablets 515

Erythromycin Estolate (Uroxatral should not be co-administered with potent CYP3A4 inhibitors such as ketoconazole, itraconazole, and ritonavir, since alfuzosin blood levels are increased).
 No products indexed under this heading.

Erythromycin Ethylsuccinate (Uroxatral should not be co-administered with potent CYP3A4 inhibitors such as ketoconazole, itraconazole, and ritonavir, since alfuzosin blood levels are increased). Products include:
E.E.S. .. 451
EryPed ... 447

Erythromycin Gluceptate (Uroxatral should not be co-administered with potent CYP3A4 inhibitors such as ketoconazole, itraconazole, and ritonavir, since alfuzosin blood levels are increased).
 No products indexed under this heading.

Erythromycin Lactobionate (Uroxatral should not be co-administered with potent CYP3A4 inhibitors such as ketoconazole, itraconazole, and ritonavir, since alfuzosin blood levels are increased).
 No products indexed under this heading.

Erythromycin Stearate (Uroxatral should not be co-administered with potent CYP3A4 inhibitors such as ketoconazole, itraconazole, and ritonavir, since alfuzosin blood levels are increased). Products include:
Erythrocin Stearate Filmtab Tablets .. 453

Esomeprazole Magnesium (Uroxatral should not be co-administered with potent CYP3A4 inhibitors such as ketoconazole, itraconazole, and ritonavir, since alfuzosin blood levels are increased). Products include:
Nexium Delayed-Release Capsules 655

Fluconazole (Uroxatral should not be co-administered with potent CYP3A4 inhibitors such as ketoconazole, itraconazole, and ritonavir, since alfuzosin blood levels are increased).
 No products indexed under this heading.

Fluoxetine Hydrochloride (Uroxatral should not be co-administered with potent CYP3A4 inhibitors such as ketoconazole, itraconazole, and ritonavir, since alfuzosin blood levels are increased). Products include:
Prozac Pulvules and Liquid 1801
Symbyax Capsules 1819

Fluvoxamine Maleate (Uroxatral should not be co-administered with potent CYP3A4 inhibitors such as ketoconazole, itraconazole, and ritonavir, since alfuzosin blood levels are increased).
 No products indexed under this heading.

Fosamprenavir Calcium (Uroxatral should not be co-administered with potent CYP3A4 inhibitors such as ketoconazole, itraconazole, and ritonavir, since alfuzosin blood levels are increased). Products include:
Lexiva Tablets 1505

Indinavir Sulfate (Uroxatral should not be co-administered with potent CYP3A4 inhibitors such as ketoconazole, itraconazole, and ritonavir, since alfuzosin blood levels are increased). Products include:
Crixivan Capsules 1940

Isoniazid (Uroxatral should not be co-administered with potent CYP3A4 inhibitors such as ketoconazole, itraconazole, and ritonavir, since alfuzosin blood levels are increased).
 No products indexed under this heading.

Itraconazole (Uroxatral should not be co-administered with potent CYP3A4 inhibitors such as ketoconazole, itraconazole, and ritonavir, since alfuzosin blood levels are increased).
 No products indexed under this heading.

Ketoconazole (Uroxatral should not be co-administered with potent CYP3A4 inhibitors such as ketoconazole, itraconazole, and ritonavir, since alfuzosin blood levels are increased). Products include:
Nizoral A-D Shampoo, 1% 1868

Lopinavir (Uroxatral should not be co-administered with potent CYP3A4 inhibitors such as ketoconazole, itraconazole, and ritonavir, since alfuzosin blood levels are increased). Products include:
Kaletra ... 476

Loratadine (Uroxatral should not be co-administered with potent CYP3A4 inhibitors such as ketoconazole, itraconazole, and ritonavir, since alfuzosin blood levels are increased). Products include:
Alavert Allergy & Sinus D-12 Hour Tablets .. ▣771
Alavert .. ▣771
Children's Claritin Allergy Oral Solution .. ▣771
Claritin Non-Drowsy 24 Hour Tablets .. ▣772
Claritin Reditabs 24 Hour Non-Drowsy Tablets ▣772
Claritin-D Non-Drowsy 12 Hour Tablets .. ▣772
Claritin-D Non-Drowsy 24 Hour Tablets .. ▣772

Metronidazole (Uroxatral should not be co-administered with potent CYP3A4 inhibitors such as ketoconazole, itraconazole, and ritonavir, since alfuzosin blood levels are increased). Products include:
Metrogel 1% 1211
MetroGel-Vaginal Gel 1855
Vandazole Vaginal Gel 3338

Metronidazole Benzoate (Uroxatral should not be co-administered with potent CYP3A4 inhibitors such as ketoconazole, itraconazole, and ritonavir, since alfuzosin blood levels are increased).
 No products indexed under this heading.

Metronidazole Hydrochloride (Uroxatral should not be co-administered with potent CYP3A4 inhibitors such as ketoconazole, itraconazole, and ritonavir, since alfuzosin blood levels are increased).
 No products indexed under this heading.

Miconazole (Uroxatral should not be co-administered with potent CYP3A4 inhibitors such as ketoconazole, itraconazole, and ritonavir, since alfuzosin blood levels are increased).
 No products indexed under this heading.

Miconazole Nitrate (Uroxatral should not be co-administered with potent CYP3A4 inhibitors such as ketoconazole, itraconazole, and ritonavir, since alfuzosin blood levels are increased). Products include:
Desenex .. ▣635
Desenex Jock Itch Spray Powder ... ▣635

Nefazodone Hydrochloride (Uroxatral should not be co-administered with potent CYP3A4 inhibitors such as ketoconazole, itraconazole, and ritonavir, since alfuzosin blood levels are increased).
 No products indexed under this heading.

Nelfinavir Mesylate (Uroxatral should not be co-administered with potent CYP3A4 inhibitors such as ketoconazole, itraconazole, and ritonavir, since alfuzosin blood levels are increased). Products include:

Viracept ... 2577

Nevirapine (Uroxatral should not be co-administered with potent CYP3A4 inhibitors such as ketoconazole, itraconazole, and ritonavir, since alfuzosin blood levels are increased). Products include:
Viramune Oral Suspension 873
Viramune Tablets 873

Niacinamide (Uroxatral should not be co-administered with potent CYP3A4 inhibitors such as ketoconazole, itraconazole, and ritonavir, since alfuzosin blood levels are increased).
No products indexed under this heading.

Nicotinamide (Uroxatral should not be co-administered with potent CYP3A4 inhibitors such as ketoconazole, itraconazole, and ritonavir, since alfuzosin blood levels are increased). Products include:
Nicomide Tablets 1088

Nifedipine (Uroxatral should not be co-administered with potent CYP3A4 inhibitors such as ketoconazole, itraconazole, and ritonavir, since alfuzosin blood levels are increased). Products include:
Adalat CC Tablets 2964

Norfloxacin (Uroxatral should not be co-administered with potent CYP3A4 inhibitors such as ketoconazole, itraconazole, and ritonavir, since alfuzosin blood levels are increased). Products include:
Noroxin Tablets 2032

Omeprazole (Uroxatral should not be co-administered with potent CYP3A4 inhibitors such as ketoconazole, itraconazole, and ritonavir, since alfuzosin blood levels are increased). Products include:
Zegerid Capsules 2958
Zegerid Powder for Oral Solution 2958

Paroxetine Hydrochloride (Uroxatral should not be co-administered with potent CYP3A4 inhibitors such as ketoconazole, itraconazole, and ritonavir, since alfuzosin blood levels are increased). Products include:
Paxil CR Controlled-Release Tablets .. 1538
Paxil ... 1530

Prazosin Hydrochloride (Interactions may be expected; uroxatral should not be used in combination with other alpha-blockers).
No products indexed under this heading.

Propoxyphene Hydrochloride (Uroxatral should not be co-administered with potent CYP3A4 inhibitors such as ketoconazole, itraconazole, and ritonavir, since alfuzosin blood levels are increased).
No products indexed under this heading.

Propoxyphene Napsylate (Uroxatral should not be co-administered with potent CYP3A4 inhibitors such as ketoconazole, itraconazole, and ritonavir, since alfuzosin blood levels are increased).
No products indexed under this heading.

Quinidine (Uroxatral should not be co-administered with potent CYP3A4 inhibitors such as ketoconazole, itraconazole, and ritonavir, since alfuzosin blood levels are increased).
No products indexed under this heading.

Quinidine Hydrochloride (Uroxatral should not be co-administered with potent CYP3A4 inhibitors such as ketoconazole, itraconazole, and ritonavir, since alfuzosin blood levels are increased).
No products indexed under this heading.

Quinidine Polygalacturonate (Uroxatral should not be co-administered with potent CYP3A4 inhibitors such as ketoconazole, itraconazole, and ritonavir, since alfuzosin blood levels are increased).
No products indexed under this heading.

Quinidine Sulfate (Uroxatral should not be co-administered with potent CYP3A4 inhibitors such as ketoconazole, itraconazole, and ritonavir, since alfuzosin blood levels are increased).
No products indexed under this heading.

Quinine (Uroxatral should not be co-administered with potent CYP3A4 inhibitors such as ketoconazole, itraconazole, and ritonavir, since alfuzosin blood levels are increased).
No products indexed under this heading.

Quinine Sulfate (Uroxatral should not be co-administered with potent CYP3A4 inhibitors such as ketoconazole, itraconazole, and ritonavir, since alfuzosin blood levels are increased).
No products indexed under this heading.

Quinupristin (Uroxatral should not be co-administered with potent CYP3A4 inhibitors such as ketoconazole, itraconazole, and ritonavir, since alfuzosin blood levels are increased).
No products indexed under this heading.

Ranitidine Bismuth Citrate (Uroxatral should not be co-administered with potent CYP3A4 inhibitors such as ketoconazole, itraconazole, and ritonavir, since alfuzosin blood levels are increased).
No products indexed under this heading.

Ranitidine Hydrochloride (Uroxatral should not be co-administered with potent CYP3A4 inhibitors such as ketoconazole, itraconazole, and ritonavir, since alfuzosin blood levels are increased). Products include:
Zantac ... 1624
Zantac Injection 1619
Zantac Injection Pharmacy Bulk Package 1622

Ritonavir (Uroxatral should not be co-administered with potent CYP3A4 inhibitors such as ketoconazole, itraconazole, and ritonavir, since alfuzosin blood levels are increased). Products include:
Kaletra ... 476
Norvir ... 503

Saquinavir (Uroxatral should not be co-administered with potent CYP3A4 inhibitors such as ketoconazole, itraconazole, and ritonavir, since alfuzosin blood levels are increased).
No products indexed under this heading.

Saquinavir Mesylate (Uroxatral should not be co-administered with potent CYP3A4 inhibitors such as ketoconazole, itraconazole, and ritonavir, since alfuzosin blood levels are increased). Products include:
Invirase 2772

Sertraline Hydrochloride (Uroxatral should not be co-administered with potent CYP3A4 inhibitors such as ketoconazole, itraconazole, and ritonavir, since alfuzosin blood levels are increased). Products include:
Zoloft ... 2586

Tamsulosin Hydrochloride (Interactions may be expected; uroxatral should not be used in combination with other alpha-blockers). Products include:
Flomax Capsules 850

Telithromycin (Uroxatral should not be co-administered with potent CYP3A4 inhibitors such as ketoconazole, itraconazole, and ritonavir, since alfuzosin blood levels are increased). Products include:
Ketek Tablets 2903

Terazosin Hydrochloride (Interactions may be expected; uroxatral should not be used in combination with other alpha-blockers). Products include:
Hytrin Capsules 471

Troglitazone (Uroxatral should not be co-administered with potent CYP3A4 inhibitors such as ketoconazole, itraconazole, and ritonavir, since alfuzosin blood levels are increased).
No products indexed under this heading.

Troleandomycin (Uroxatral should not be co-administered with potent CYP3A4 inhibitors such as ketoconazole, itraconazole, and ritonavir, since alfuzosin blood levels are increased).
No products indexed under this heading.

Valproate Sodium (Uroxatral should not be co-administered with potent CYP3A4 inhibitors such as ketoconazole, itraconazole, and ritonavir, since alfuzosin blood levels are increased). Products include:
Depacon Injection 412

Verapamil Hydrochloride (Uroxatral should not be co-administered with potent CYP3A4 inhibitors such as ketoconazole, itraconazole, and ritonavir, since alfuzosin blood levels are increased). Products include:
Covera-HS Tablets 3139
Tarka Tablets 524
Verelan PM Extended-Release Capsules, Controlled-Onset.......... 3106

Voriconazole (Uroxatral should not be co-administered with potent CYP3A4 inhibitors such as ketoconazole, itraconazole, and ritonavir, since alfuzosin blood levels are increased). Products include:
VFEND I.V. 2564
VFEND Oral Suspension 2564
VFEND Tablets 2564

Zafirlukast (Uroxatral should not be co-administered with potent CYP3A4 inhibitors such as ketoconazole, itraconazole, and ritonavir, since alfuzosin blood levels are increased). Products include:
Accolate Tablets 671

Zileuton (Uroxatral should not be co-administered with potent CYP3A4 inhibitors such as ketoconazole, itraconazole, and ritonavir, since alfuzosin blood levels are increased). Products include:
Zyflo Tablets 1023

Food Interactions

Grapefruit (Uroxatral should not be co-administered with potent CYP3A4 inhibitors such as ketoconazole, itraconazole, and ritonavir, since alfuzosin blood levels are increased).

Grapefruit Juice (Uroxatral should not be co-administered with potent CYP3A4 inhibitors such as ketoconazole, itraconazole, and ritonavir, since alfuzosin blood levels are increased).

URSO 250 TABLETS
(Ursodiol) 710
May interact with bile acid sequestering agents, estrogens, lipid-lowering drugs, oral contraceptives, and certain other agents. Compounds in these categories include:

Aluminum Hydroxide (Aluminum-based antacids have been shown to adsorb bile acid in vitro and may be expected to interfere with ursodiol in the same manner as the bile acid sequestering agents). Products include:
Gaviscon Regular Strength Liquid .. ☜658
Gaviscon Regular Strength Tablets.................................... ☜658
Gaviscon Extra Strength Liquid ☜658
Gaviscon Extra Strength Tablets ☜658
Maalox Regular Strength Antacid/Antigas Liquid.................. 2175
Maalox Max Maximum Strength Antacid/Anti-Gas Liquid................ 2176

Atorvastatin Calcium (Lipid-lowering drugs increase hepatic cholesterol secretion and encourage cholesterol gallstone formation and hence may counteract the effectiveness of ursodiol). Products include:
Caduet Tablets 2508
Lipitor Tablets 2483

Cerivastatin Sodium (Lipid-lowering drugs increase hepatic cholesterol secretion and encourage cholesterol gallstone formation and hence may counteract the effectiveness of ursodiol).
No products indexed under this heading.

Chlorotrianisene (Estrogens and oral contraceptives increase hepatic cholesterol excretion and encourage cholesterol gallstone formation and hence may counteract the effectiveness of ursodiol).
No products indexed under this heading.

Cholestyramine (Lipid-lowering drugs increase hepatic cholesterol secretion and encourage cholesterol gallstone formation and hence may counteract the effectiveness of ursodiol).
No products indexed under this heading.

Clofibrate (Lipid-lowering drugs increase hepatic cholesterol secretion and encourage cholesterol gallstone formation and hence may counteract the effectiveness of ursodiol).
No products indexed under this heading.

Colesevelam Hydrochloride (Bile sequestering agents may interfere with the action of ursodiol by reducing its absorption). Products include:
WelChol Tablets 1050

Colestipol Hydrochloride (Lipid-lowering drugs increase hepatic cholesterol secretion and encourage cholesterol gallstone formation and hence may counteract the effectiveness of ursodiol).
No products indexed under this heading.

Desogestrel (Estrogens and oral contraceptives increase hepatic cholesterol secretion and encourage cholesterol gallstone formation and hence may counteract the effectiveness of ursodiol). Products include:
- Mircette Tablets 1066

Dienestrol (Estrogens and oral contraceptives increase hepatic cholesterol excretion and encourage cholesterol gallstone formation and hence may counteract the effectiveness of ursodiol).
No products indexed under this heading.

Diethylstilbestrol (Estrogens and oral contraceptives increase hepatic cholesterol excretion and encourage cholesterol gallstone formation and hence may counteract the effectiveness of ursodiol).
No products indexed under this heading.

Estradiol (Estrogens and oral contraceptives increase hepatic cholesterol excretion and encourage cholesterol gallstone formation and hence may counteract the effectiveness of ursodiol). Products include:
- Angeliq Tablets 762
- Climara Transdermal System 771
- Climara Pro Transdermal System 776
- Estrasorb Topical Emulsion 1147
- Estring Vaginal Ring 2635
- Menostar Transdermal System 782
- Vagifem Tablets 2334

Estrogens, Conjugated (Estrogens and oral contraceptives increase hepatic cholesterol excretion and encourage cholesterol gallstone formation and hence may counteract the effectiveness of ursodiol). Products include:
- Premarin Intravenous 3442
- Premarin Tablets 3446
- Premarin Vaginal Cream 3452
- Premphase Tablets 3456
- Prempro Tablets 3456

Estrogens, Esterified (Estrogens and oral contraceptives increase hepatic cholesterol excretion and encourage cholesterol gallstone formation and hence may counteract the effectiveness of ursodiol).
Products include:
- Estratest Tablets 3199
- Estratest H.S. Tablets 3199

Estropipate (Estrogens and oral contraceptives increase hepatic cholesterol excretion and encourage cholesterol gallstone formation and hence may counteract the effectiveness of ursodiol).
No products indexed under this heading.

Ethinyl Estradiol (Estrogens and oral contraceptives increase hepatic cholesterol secretion and encourage cholesterol gallstone formation and hence may counteract the effectiveness of ursodiol). Products include:
- Mircette Tablets 1066
- NuvaRing 2340
- Ortho-Cyclen/Ortho Tri-Cyclen 2429
- Ortho Evra Transdermal System 2417
- Ortho Tri-Cyclen Lo Tablets 2436
- Seasonique Tablets 1077
- Yasmin 28 Tablets 796
- Yaz Tablets 803

Ethynodiol Diacetate (Estrogens and oral contraceptives increase hepatic cholesterol secretion and encourage cholesterol gallstone formation and hence may counteract the effectiveness of ursodiol).
No products indexed under this heading.

Fenofibrate (Lipid-lowering drugs increase hepatic cholesterol secretion and encourage cholesterol gallstone formation and hence may counteract the effectiveness of ursodiol). Products include:
- Lofibra Tablets 1219
- Lofibra Capsules 1216
- Tricor Tablets 527
- Triglide Tablets 3123

Fluvastatin Sodium (Lipid-lowering drugs increase hepatic cholesterol secretion and encourage cholesterol gallstone formation and hence may counteract the effectiveness of ursodiol). Products include:
- Lescol Capsules 2233
- Lescol XL Tablets 2233

Gemfibrozil (Lipid-lowering drugs increase hepatic cholesterol secretion and encourage cholesterol gallstone formation and hence may counteract the effectiveness of ursodiol).
No products indexed under this heading.

Levonorgestrel (Estrogens and oral contraceptives increase hepatic cholesterol secretion and encourage cholesterol gallstone formation and hence may counteract the effectiveness of ursodiol). Products include:
- Climara Pro Transdermal System 776
- Mirena Intrauterine System 787
- Plan B Tablets 1076
- Seasonique Tablets 1077

Lovastatin (Lipid-lowering drugs increase hepatic cholesterol secretion and encourage cholesterol gallstone formation and hence may counteract the effectiveness of ursodiol). Products include:
- Advicor Tablets 1722
- Altoprev Extended-Release Tablets 3109
- Mevacor Tablets 2021

Mestranol (Estrogens and oral contraceptives increase hepatic cholesterol secretion and encourage cholesterol gallstone formation and hence may counteract the effectiveness of ursodiol).
No products indexed under this heading.

Norethindrone (Estrogens and oral contraceptives increase hepatic cholesterol secretion and encourage cholesterol gallstone formation and hence may counteract the effectiveness of ursodiol). Products include:
- Ortho Micronor Tablets 2426

Norethynodrel (Estrogens and oral contraceptives increase hepatic cholesterol secretion and encourage cholesterol gallstone formation and hence may counteract the effectiveness of ursodiol).
No products indexed under this heading.

Norgestimate (Estrogens and oral contraceptives increase hepatic cholesterol secretion and encourage cholesterol gallstone formation and hence may counteract the effectiveness of ursodiol). Products include:
- Ortho-Cyclen/Ortho Tri-Cyclen 2429
- Ortho Tri-Cyclen Lo Tablets 2436

Norgestrel (Estrogens and oral contraceptives increase hepatic cholesterol secretion and encourage cholesterol gallstone formation and hence may counteract the effectiveness of ursodiol).
No products indexed under this heading.

Polyestradiol Phosphate (Estrogens and oral contraceptives increase hepatic cholesterol excretion and encourage cholesterol gallstone formation and hence may counteract the effectiveness of ursodiol).
No products indexed under this heading.

Pravastatin Sodium (Lipid-lowering drugs increase hepatic cholesterol secretion and encourage cholesterol gallstone formation and hence may counteract the effectiveness of ursodiol).
No products indexed under this heading.

Probucol (Lipid-lowering drugs increase hepatic cholesterol secretion and encourage cholesterol gallstone formation and hence may counteract the effectiveness of ursodiol).
No products indexed under this heading.

Quinestrol (Estrogens and oral contraceptives increase hepatic cholesterol excretion and encourage cholesterol gallstone formation and hence may counteract the effectiveness of ursodiol).
No products indexed under this heading.

Simvastatin (Lipid-lowering drugs increase hepatic cholesterol secretion and encourage cholesterol gallstone formation and hence may counteract the effectiveness of ursodiol). Products include:
- Vytorin 10/10 Tablets 2114
- Vytorin 10/10 Tablets 3077
- Vytorin 10/20 Tablets 2114
- Vytorin 10/20 Tablets 3077
- Vytorin 10/40 Tablets 2114
- Vytorin 10/40 Tablets 3077
- Vytorin 10/80 Tablets 2114
- Vytorin 10/80 Tablets 3077
- Zocor Tablets 2105

URSO FORTE TABLETS

(Ursodiol) 710
See Urso 250 Tablets

VAGIFEM TABLETS

(Estradiol) 2334
None cited in PDR database.

VAGISTAT-1

(Tioconazole) .... ▣804
May interact with:

Petrolatum-containing vaginal lubricants (Concomitant use is not advised).
No products indexed under this heading.

Precoital Douche (Concomitant use is not advised).
No products indexed under this heading.

Vaginal Diaphragm & Apparatus (Diaphragms may be damaged and fail to prevent pregnancy or sexually transmitted disease).
No products indexed under this heading.

Vaginally administered preparations, unspecified (Concomitant use is not advised).
No products indexed under this heading.

VALCYTE TABLETS

(Valganciclovir Hydrochloride) 2813
May interact with:

Didanosine (Valganciclovir is extensively converted to ganciclovir; co-administration of ganciclovir with didanosine has resulted in decreased AUC of ganciclovir and increased AUC of didanosine; patients should be monitored for didanosine toxicity).
No products indexed under this heading.

Mycophenolate Mofetil (Valganciclovir is extensively converted to ganciclovir; co-administration of ganciclovir with mycophenolate in patients with normal renal function has not resulted in any effect on PK parameters, however, patients with renal impairment should be monitored carefully as levels of metabolites or both drugs may increase). Products include:
- CellCept Capsules 2747
- CellCept Oral Suspension 2747
- CellCept Tablets 2747

Probenecid (Valganciclovir is extensively converted to ganciclovir; co-administration of ganciclovir with probenecid results in increase in AUC of ganciclovir and decrease in ganciclovir renal cleareance; patients on concomitant therapy should be monitored for evidence of ganciclovir toxicity).
No products indexed under this heading.

Trimethoprim (Valganciclovir is extensively converted to ganciclovir; co-administration of ganciclovir with trimethoprim has resulted in decreased renal clearance and increased half-life of ganciclovir and an increase in Cmax of trimethoprim; effects of this interaction are not likely to be clinically significant).
No products indexed under this heading.

Zalcitabine (Valganciclovir is extensively converted to ganciclovir; co-administration of ganciclovir with zalcitabine has resulted in increased AUC of ganciclovir; effects of this interaction are not likely to be clinically significant).
No products indexed under this heading.

Zidovudine (Valganciclovir is extensively converted to ganciclovir; co-administration of ganciclovir with zidovudine has resulted in decreased AUC of ganciclovir and increased AUC of zidovudine; zidovudine and valganciclovir each have the potential to cause neutropenia and anemia; some patients may not tolerate concomitant therapy at full dosage).
Products include:
- Combivir Tablets 1411
- Retrovir 1560
- Retrovir IV Infusion 1564
- Trizivir Tablets 1589

Food Interactions

Food, unspecified (Co-administration with high fat meals has resulted in increased steady-state ganciclovir AUC and Cmax without any prolongation in time to peak plasma concentrations; Valcyte should be administered with food).

VALIUM TABLETS

(Diazepam) 2819

May interact with barbiturates, central nervous system depressants, antidepressant drugs, anticonvulsants, monoamine oxidase inhibitors, narcotic analgesics, phenothiazines, and certain other agents. Compounds in these categories include:

Alfentanil Hydrochloride (May potentiate the actions of diazepam).
No products indexed under this heading.

Alprazolam (May potentiate the actions of diazepam). Products include:
Niravam Orally Disintegrating Tablets 3092

Amitriptyline Hydrochloride (May potentiate the actions of diazepam).
No products indexed under this heading.

Amoxapine (May potentiate the actions of diazepam).
No products indexed under this heading.

Aprobarbital (May potentiate the actions of diazepam).
No products indexed under this heading.

Buprenorphine Hydrochloride (May potentiate the actions of diazepam). Products include:
Buprenex Injectable 2716
Suboxone Tablets 2717
Subutex Tablets 2717

Bupropion Hydrochloride (May potentiate the actions of diazepam). Products include:
Wellbutrin Tablets 1603
Wellbutrin SR Sustained-Release Tablets 1607
Wellbutrin XL Extended-Release Tablets 1613
Zyban Sustained-Release Tablets 1644

Buspirone Hydrochloride (May potentiate the actions of diazepam).
No products indexed under this heading.

Butabarbital (May potentiate the actions of diazepam).
No products indexed under this heading.

Butalbital (May potentiate the actions of diazepam).
No products indexed under this heading.

Carbamazepine (Co-administration of diazepam as an adjunct in treating convulsive disorders results in possibility of an increase in the frequency and/or severity of grand mal seizures which may require an increase in the dosage of standard anticonvulsant agent). Products include:
Carbatrol Capsules 3171
Equetro Extended-Release Capsules 3180
Tegretol/Tegretol-XR 2295

Chlordiazepoxide (May potentiate the actions of diazepam).
No products indexed under this heading.

Chlordiazepoxide Hydrochloride (May potentiate the actions of diazepam). Products include:
Librium Capsules 3347

Chlorpromazine (May potentiate the actions of diazepam).
No products indexed under this heading.

Chlorpromazine Hydrochloride (May potentiate the actions of diazepam).
No products indexed under this heading.

Chlorprothixene (May potentiate the actions of diazepam).
No products indexed under this heading.

Chlorprothixene Hydrochloride (May potentiate the actions of diazepam).
No products indexed under this heading.

Chlorprothixene Lactate (May potentiate the actions of diazepam).
No products indexed under this heading.

Cimetidine (Co-administration delays diazepam clearance; clinical significance of this interaction is unclear). Products include:
Tagamet HB 200 Tablets 664

Cimetidine Hydrochloride (Co-administration delays diazepam clearance; clinical significance of this interaction is unclear).
No products indexed under this heading.

Citalopram Hydrobromide (May potentiate the actions of diazepam). Products include:
Celexa 1176

Clonazepam (Co-administration of diazepam as an adjunct in treating convulsive disorders results in possibility of an increase in the frequency and/or severity of grand mal seizures which may require an increase in the dosage of standard anticonvulsant agent; may potentiate the CNS depression caused by diazepam). Products include:
Klonopin 2778

Clorazepate Dipotassium (May potentiate the actions of diazepam). Products include:
Tranxene 2474

Clozapine (May potentiate the actions of diazepam). Products include:
Clozaril Tablets 2184
FazaClo Orally Disintegrating Tablets 551

Codeine Phosphate (May potentiate the actions of diazepam). Products include:
Tylenol with Codeine Tablets 2391

Desflurane (May potentiate the actions of diazepam).
No products indexed under this heading.

Desipramine Hydrochloride (May potentiate the actions of diazepam).
No products indexed under this heading.

Dezocine (May potentiate the actions of diazepam).
No products indexed under this heading.

Divalproex Sodium (Co-administration of diazepam as an adjunct in treating convulsive disorders results in possibility of an increase in the frequency and/or severity of grand mal seizures which may require an increase in the dosage of standard anticonvulsant agent). Products include:
Depakote Sprinkle Capsules 422
Depakote Tablets 427
Depakote ER Tablets 434

Doxepin Hydrochloride (May potentiate the actions of diazepam).
No products indexed under this heading.

Droperidol (May potentiate the actions of diazepam).
No products indexed under this heading.

Enflurane (May potentiate the actions of diazepam).
No products indexed under this heading.

Estazolam (May potentiate the actions of diazepam). Products include:
ProSom Tablets 517

Ethanol (May potentiate the actions of diazepam).
No products indexed under this heading.

Ethchlorvynol (May potentiate the actions of diazepam).
No products indexed under this heading.

Ethinamate (May potentiate the actions of diazepam).
No products indexed under this heading.

Ethosuximide (Co-administration of diazepam as an adjunct in treating convulsive disorders results in possibility of an increase in the frequency and/or severity of grand mal seizures which may require an increase in the dosage of standard anticonvulsant agent).
No products indexed under this heading.

Ethotoin (Co-administration of diazepam as an adjunct in treating convulsive disorders results in possibility of an increase in the frequency and/or severity of grand mal seizures which may require an increase in the dosage of standard anticonvulsant agent).
No products indexed under this heading.

Ethyl Alcohol (May potentiate the actions of diazepam).
No products indexed under this heading.

Felbamate (Co-administration of diazepam as an adjunct in treating convulsive disorders results in possibility of an increase in the frequency and/or severity of grand mal seizures which may require an increase in the dosage of standard anticonvulsant agent).
No products indexed under this heading.

Fentanyl (May potentiate the actions of diazepam). Products include:
Duragesic Transdermal System 2373
Ionsys Transdermal System 2379

Fentanyl Citrate (May potentiate the actions of diazepam). Products include:
Actiq 979

Fluoxetine Hydrochloride (May potentiate the actions of diazepam). Products include:
Prozac Pulvules and Liquid 1801
Symbyax Capsules 1819

Fluphenazine Decanoate (May potentiate the actions of diazepam).
No products indexed under this heading.

Fluphenazine Enanthate (May potentiate the actions of diazepam).
No products indexed under this heading.

Fluphenazine Hydrochloride (May potentiate the actions of diazepam).
No products indexed under this heading.

Flurazepam Hydrochloride (May potentiate the actions of diazepam). Products include:
Dalmane Capsules 3342

Fosphenytoin (Co-administration of diazepam as an adjunct in treating convulsive disorders results in possibility of an increase in the frequency and/or severity of grand mal seizures which may require an increase in the dosage of standard anticonvulsant agent).
No products indexed under this heading.

Fosphenytoin Sodium (Co-administration of diazepam as an adjunct in treating convulsive disorders results in possibility of an increase in the frequency and/or severity of grand mal seizures which may require an increase in the dosage of standard anticonvulsant agent).
No products indexed under this heading.

Gabapentin (Co-administration of diazepam as an adjunct in treating convulsive disorders results in possibility of an increase in the frequency and/or severity of grand mal seizures which may require an increase in the dosage of standard anticonvulsant agent). Products include:
Neurontin Capsules 2487
Neurontin Oral Solution 2487
Neurontin Tablets 2487

Glutethimide (May potentiate the actions of diazepam).
No products indexed under this heading.

Haloperidol (May potentiate the actions of diazepam).
No products indexed under this heading.

Haloperidol Decanoate (May potentiate the actions of diazepam).
No products indexed under this heading.

Hydrocodone Bitartrate (May potentiate the actions of diazepam). Products include:
Hycodan 1116
Hycotuss Expectorant Syrup 1117
Vicodin Tablets 535
Vicodin ES Tablets 536
Vicodin HP Tablets 538
Vicoprofen Tablets 539
Zydone Tablets 1139

Hydrocodone Polistirex (May potentiate the actions of diazepam). Products include:
Tussionex Pennkinetic Extended-Release Suspension 3327

Hydromorphone Hydrochloride (May potentiate the actions of diazepam). Products include:
Dilaudid 440
Dilaudid Non-Sterile Powder 440
Dilaudid Oral Liquid 445
Dilaudid Rectal Suppositories 440
Dilaudid Tablets 440
Dilaudid Tablets - 8 mg 445
Dilaudid-HP 442

Hydroxyzine Hydrochloride (May potentiate the actions of diazepam).
No products indexed under this heading.

Imipramine Hydrochloride (May potentiate the actions of diazepam).
No products indexed under this heading.

Imipramine Pamoate (May potentiate the actions of diazepam).
No products indexed under this heading.

Isocarboxazid (May potentiate the actions of diazepam).
No products indexed under this heading.

Isoflurane (May potentiate the actions of diazepam).
No products indexed under this heading.

Ketamine Hydrochloride (May potentiate the actions of diazepam).
No products indexed under this heading.

Lamotrigine (Co-administration of diazepam as an adjunct in treating convulsive disorders results in possibility of an increase in the frequency and/or severity of grand mal seizures which may require an increase in the dosage of standard anticonvulsant agent). Products include:
Lamictal 1481

Levetiracetam (Co-administration of diazepam as an adjunct in treating convulsive disorders results in possibility of an increase in the frequency and/or severity of grand mal seizures which may require an increase in the dosage of standard anticonvulsant agent). Products include:
Keppra Injection 3320
Keppra Oral Solution 3314
Keppra Tablets 3314

Levomethadyl Acetate Hydrochloride (May potentiate the actions of diazepam).
No products indexed under this heading.

Levorphanol Tartrate (May potentiate the actions of diazepam).
No products indexed under this heading.

Lorazepam (May potentiate the actions of diazepam).
No products indexed under this heading.

Loxapine Hydrochloride (May potentiate the actions of diazepam).
No products indexed under this heading.

Loxapine Succinate (May potentiate the actions of diazepam).
No products indexed under this heading.

Maprotiline Hydrochloride (May potentiate the actions of diazepam).
No products indexed under this heading.

Meperidine Hydrochloride (May potentiate the actions of diazepam).
No products indexed under this heading.

Mephenytoin (Co-administration of diazepam as an adjunct in treating convulsive disorders results in possibility of an increase in the frequency and/or severity of grand mal seizures which may require an increase in the dosage of standard anticonvulsant agent).
No products indexed under this heading.

Mephobarbital (May potentiate the actions of diazepam).
No products indexed under this heading.

Meprobamate (May potentiate the actions of diazepam).
No products indexed under this heading.

Mesoridazine Besylate (May potentiate the actions of diazepam).
No products indexed under this heading.

Methadone Hydrochloride (May potentiate the actions of diazepam).
No products indexed under this heading.

Methohexital Sodium (May potentiate the actions of diazepam).
No products indexed under this heading.

Methotrimeprazine (May potentiate the actions of diazepam).
No products indexed under this heading.

Methoxyflurane (May potentiate the actions of diazepam).
No products indexed under this heading.

Methsuximide (Co-administration of diazepam as an adjunct in treating convulsive disorders results in possibility of an increase in the frequency and/or severity of grand mal seizures which may require an increase in the dosage of standard anticonvulsant agent).
No products indexed under this heading.

Midazolam Hydrochloride (May potentiate the actions of diazepam).
No products indexed under this heading.

Mirtazapine (May potentiate the actions of diazepam).
No products indexed under this heading.

Moclobemide (May potentiate the actions of diazepam).
No products indexed under this heading.

Molindone Hydrochloride (May potentiate the actions of diazepam). Products include:
Moban Tablets 1119

Morphine Sulfate (May potentiate the actions of diazepam). Products include:
Avinza Capsules 1741
Kadian Capsules 577
MS Contin Tablets 2701

Nefazodone Hydrochloride (May potentiate the actions of diazepam).
No products indexed under this heading.

Nortriptyline Hydrochloride (May potentiate the actions of diazepam).
No products indexed under this heading.

Olanzapine (May potentiate the actions of diazepam). Products include:
Symbyax Capsules 1819
Zyprexa Tablets 1830
Zyprexa IntraMuscular 1830
Zyprexa ZYDIS Orally Disintegrating Tablets 1830

Oxazepam (May potentiate the actions of diazepam).
No products indexed under this heading.

Oxcarbazepine (Co-administration of diazepam as an adjunct in treating convulsive disorders results in possibility of an increase in the frequency and/or severity of grand mal seizures which may require an increase in the dosage of standard anticonvulsant agent). Products include:
Trileptal Tablets 2300
Trileptal Oral Suspension 2300

Oxycodone Hydrochloride (May potentiate the actions of diazepam). Products include:
OxyContin Tablets 2703
OxyFast Oral Concentrate Solution 2708
OxyIR Capsules 2708
Percocet Tablets 1131
Percodan Tablets 1132

Paramethadione (Co-administration of diazepam as an adjunct in treating convulsive disorders results in possibility of an increase in the frequency and/or severity of grand mal seizures which may require an increase in the dosage of standard anticonvulsant agent).
No products indexed under this heading.

Pargyline Hydrochloride (May potentiate the actions of diazepam).
No products indexed under this heading.

Paroxetine Hydrochloride (May potentiate the actions of diazepam). Products include:
Paxil CR Controlled-Release Tablets 1538
Paxil 1530

Pentobarbital Sodium (May potentiate the actions of diazepam). Products include:
Nembutal Sodium Solution, USP 2470

Perphenazine (May potentiate the actions of diazepam).
No products indexed under this heading.

Phenacemide (Co-administration of diazepam as an adjunct in treating convulsive disorders results in possibility of an increase in the frequency and/or severity of grand mal seizures which may require an increase in the dosage of standard anticonvulsant agent).
No products indexed under this heading.

Phenelzine Sulfate (May potentiate the actions of diazepam).
No products indexed under this heading.

Phenobarbital (Co-administration of diazepam as an adjunct in treating convulsive disorders results in possibility of an increase in the frequency and/or severity of grand mal seizures which may require an increase in the dosage of standard anticonvulsant agent; may potentiate the CNS depression caused by diazepam). Products include:
Donnatal Extentabs 2493

Phensuximide (Co-administration of diazepam as an adjunct in treating convulsive disorders results in possibility of an increase in the frequency and/or severity of grand mal seizures which may require an increase in the dosage of standard anticonvulsant agent).
No products indexed under this heading.

Phenytoin (Co-administration of diazepam as an adjunct in treating convulsive disorders results in possibility of an increase in the frequency and/or severity of grand mal seizures which may require an increase in the dosage of standard anticonvulsant agent).
No products indexed under this heading.

Phenytoin Sodium (Co-administration of diazepam as an adjunct in treating convulsive disorders results in possibility of an increase in the frequency and/or severity of grand mal seizures which may require an increase in the dosage of standard anticonvulsant agent). Products include:
Phenytek Capsules 2160

Prazepam (May potentiate the actions of diazepam).
No products indexed under this heading.

Primidone (Co-administration of diazepam as an adjunct in treating convulsive disorders results in possibility of an increase in the frequency and/or severity of grand mal seizures which may require an increase in the dosage of standard anticonvulsant agent).
No products indexed under this heading.

Procarbazine Hydrochloride (May potentiate the actions of diazepam). Products include:
Matulane Capsules 3191

Prochlorperazine (May potentiate the actions of diazepam).
No products indexed under this heading.

Promethazine Hydrochloride (May potentiate the actions of diazepam). Products include:
Phenergan Tablets and Suppositories 3440

Propofol (May potentiate the actions of diazepam).
No products indexed under this heading.

Propoxyphene Hydrochloride (May potentiate the actions of diazepam).
No products indexed under this heading.

Propoxyphene Napsylate (May potentiate the actions of diazepam).
No products indexed under this heading.

Protriptyline Hydrochloride (May potentiate the actions of diazepam).
No products indexed under this heading.

Quazepam (May potentiate the actions of diazepam).
No products indexed under this heading.

Quetiapine Fumarate (May potentiate the actions of diazepam). Products include:
Seroquel Tablets 690

Remifentanil Hydrochloride (May potentiate the actions of diazepam).
No products indexed under this heading.

Risperidone (May potentiate the actions of diazepam). Products include:
Risperdal 1676
Risperdal Consta Long-Acting Injection 1682
Risperdal M-Tab Orally Disintegrating Tablets 1676

Secobarbital Sodium (May potentiate the actions of diazepam).
No products indexed under this heading.

Selegiline Hydrochloride (May potentiate the actions of diazepam). Products include:
Eldepryl Capsules 3208
Zelapar Tablets 3372

Sertraline Hydrochloride (May potentiate the actions of diazepam). Products include:
Zoloft 2586

Sevoflurane (May potentiate the actions of diazepam). Products include:
Ultane Liquid for Inhalation 531

Sufentanil Citrate (May potentiate the actions of diazepam).
No products indexed under this heading.

Temazepam (May potentiate the actions of diazepam). Products include:
Restoril Capsules **1860**

Thiamylal Sodium (May potentiate the actions of diazepam).
No products indexed under this heading.

Thioridazine Hydrochloride (May potentiate the actions of diazepam). Products include:
Thioridazine Hydrochloride Tablets **2163**

Thiothixene (May potentiate the actions of diazepam). Products include:
Thiothixene Capsules **2165**

Tiagabine Hydrochloride (Co-administration of diazepam as an adjunct in treating convulsive disorders results in possibility of an increase in the frequency and/or severity of grand mal seizures which may require an increase in the dosage of standard anticonvulsant agent). Products include:
Gabitril Tablets **984**

Topiramate (Co-administration of diazepam as an adjunct in treating convulsive disorders results in possibility of an increase in the frequency and/or severity of grand mal seizures which may require an increase in the dosage of standard anticonvulsant agent). Products include:
Topamax Sprinkle Capsules **2404**
Topamax Tablets **2404**

Tranylcypromine Sulfate (May potentiate the actions of diazepam). Products include:
Parnate Tablets **1527**

Trazodone Hydrochloride (May potentiate the actions of diazepam).
No products indexed under this heading.

Triazolam (May potentiate the actions of diazepam).
No products indexed under this heading.

Trifluoperazine Hydrochloride (May potentiate the actions of diazepam).
No products indexed under this heading.

Trimethadione (Co-administration of diazepam as an adjunct in treating convulsive disorders results in possibility of an increase in the frequency and/or severity of grand mal seizures which may require an increase in the dosage of standard anticonvulsant agent).
No products indexed under this heading.

Trimipramine Maleate (May potentiate the actions of diazepam).
No products indexed under this heading.

Valproate Sodium (Co-administration of diazepam as an adjunct in treating convulsive disorders results in possibility of an increase in the frequency and/or severity of grand mal seizures which may require an increase in the dosage of standard anticonvulsant agent). Products include:
Depacon Injection **412**

Valproic Acid (Co-administration of diazepam as an adjunct in treating convulsive disorders results in possibility of an increase in the frequency and/or severity of grand mal seizures which may require an increase in the dosage of standard anticonvulsant agent). Products include:
Depakene **417**

Venlafaxine Hydrochloride (May potentiate the actions of diazepam). Products include:
Effexor Tablets **3411**
Effexor XR Capsules **3417**

Zaleplon (May potentiate the actions of diazepam). Products include:
Sonata Capsules **1717**

Ziprasidone Hydrochloride (May potentiate the actions of diazepam). Products include:
Geodon Capsules **2529**

Zolpidem Tartrate (May potentiate the actions of diazepam). Products include:
Ambien Tablets **2851**
Ambien CR Tablets **2855**

Zonisamide (Co-administration of diazepam as an adjunct in treating convulsive disorders results in possibility of an increase in the frequency and/or severity of grand mal seizures which may require an increase in the dosage of standard anticonvulsant agent). Products include:
Zonegran Capsules **1101**

Food Interactions

Alcohol (May potentiate the actions of diazepam).

VALTREX CAPLETS

(Valacyclovir Hydrochloride) **1597**
May interact with:

Cimetidine (Co-administration reduces renal clearance of acyclovir causing an increase in acyclovir AUC and Cmax). Products include:
Tagamet HB 200 Tablets .... ▣**664**

Cimetidine Hydrochloride (Co-administration reduces renal clearance of acyclovir causing an increase in acyclovir AUC and Cmax).
No products indexed under this heading.

Probenecid (Co-administration reduces renal clearance of acyclovir causing an increase in acyclovir AUC and Cmax).
No products indexed under this heading.

VANCOCIN HCL CAPSULES, USP

(Vancomycin Hydrochloride) **3380**
May interact with aminoglycosides, anesthetics, and certain other agents. Compounds in these categories include:

Alfentanil Hydrochloride (Co-administration with anesthetic agents has been associated with erythema and histamine-like flushing in children).
No products indexed under this heading.

Amikacin Sulfate (Concurrent and/or sequential use may result in increased potential for neurotoxicity and/or nephrotoxicity).
No products indexed under this heading.

Amphotericin B (Concurrent and/or sequential use may result in increased potential for neurotoxicity and/or nephrotoxicity).
No products indexed under this heading.

Bacitracin Zinc (Concurrent and/or sequential use may result in increased potential for neurotoxicity and/or nephrotoxicity).
No products indexed under this heading.

Cisplatin (Concurrent and/or sequential use may result in increased potential for neurotoxicity and/or nephrotoxicity).
No products indexed under this heading.

Colistin Sulfate (Concurrent and/or sequential use may result in increased potential for neurotoxicity and/or nephrotoxicity).
No products indexed under this heading.

Enflurane (Co-administration with anesthetic agents has been associated with erythema and histamine-like flushing in children).
No products indexed under this heading.

Fentanyl Citrate (Co-administration with anesthetic agents has been associated with erythema and histamine-like flushing in children). Products include:
Actiq **979**

Gentamicin Sulfate (Concurrent and/or sequential use may result in increased potential for neurotoxicity and/or nephrotoxicity). Products include:
Garamycin Injectable **3014**
Pred-G Ophthalmic Ointment .... ⊙**237**
Pred-G Ophthalmic Suspension ...... ⊙**236**

Halothane (Co-administration with anesthetic agents has been associated with erythema and histamine-like flushing in children).
No products indexed under this heading.

Isoflurane (Co-administration with anesthetic agents has been associated with erythema and histamine-like flushing in children).
No products indexed under this heading.

Kanamycin Sulfate (Concurrent and/or sequential use may result in increased potential for neurotoxicity and/or nephrotoxicity).
No products indexed under this heading.

Ketamine Hydrochloride (Co-administration with anesthetic agents has been associated with erythema and histamine-like flushing in children).
No products indexed under this heading.

Methohexital Sodium (Co-administration with anesthetic agents has been associated with erythema and histamine-like flushing in children).
No products indexed under this heading.

Midazolam Hydrochloride (Co-administration with anesthetic agents has been associated with erythema and histamine-like flushing in children).
No products indexed under this heading.

Polymyxin B Sulfate (Concurrent and/or sequential use may result in increased potential for neurotoxicity and/or nephrotoxicity). Products include:
Neosporin Antibiotic Ointment .... ▣**643**
Neosporin Ophthalmic Solution Sterile .... ⊙**265**
Neosporin + Pain Relief Antibiotic Cream and Ointment (Maximum Strength).................. ▣**643**
Poly-Pred Ophthalmic Suspension .... ⊙**233**
Polysporin First Aid Antibiotic Ointment.................................. ▣**643**
Polytrim Ophthalmic Solution **574**

Propofol (Co-administration with anesthetic agents has been associated with erythema and histamine-like flushing in children).
No products indexed under this heading.

Remifentanil Hydrochloride (Co-administration with anesthetic agents has been associated with erythema and histamine-like flushing in children).
No products indexed under this heading.

Streptomycin Sulfate (Concurrent and/or sequential use may result in increased potential for neurotoxicity and/or nephrotoxicity).
No products indexed under this heading.

Sufentanil Citrate (Co-administration with anesthetic agents has been associated with erythema and histamine-like flushing in children).
No products indexed under this heading.

Thiamylal Sodium (Co-administration with anesthetic agents has been associated with erythema and histamine-like flushing in children).
No products indexed under this heading.

Tobramycin (Concurrent and/or sequential use may result in increased potential for neurotoxicity and/or nephrotoxicity). Products include:
TOBI Solution for Inhalation **2298**
TobraDex Ophthalmic Ointment **562**
TobraDex Ophthalmic Suspension ... **563**
Zylet Ophthalmic Suspension .... ⊙**259**

Tobramycin Sulfate (Concurrent and/or sequential use may result in increased potential for neurotoxicity and/or nephrotoxicity).
No products indexed under this heading.

Viomycin (Concurrent and/or sequential use may result in increased potential for neurotoxicity and/or nephrotoxicity).
No products indexed under this heading.

VANDAZOLE VAGINAL GEL

(Metronidazole) **3338**
May interact with oral anticoagulants, lithium preparations, and certain other agents. Compounds in these categories include:

Anisindione (Oral metronidazole has been reported to potentiate the anticoagulant effect of warfarin and other coumarin anticoagulants, resulting in a prolongation of prothrombin time. The possible drug interaction should be considered when metronidazole vaginal gelis prescribed for patients on this type of anticoagulant therapy). Products include:
Miradon Tablets **3042**

Dicumarol (Oral metronidazole has been reported to potentiate the anticoagulant effect of warfarin and other coumarin anticoagulants, resulting in a prolongation of prothrombin time. The possible drug interaction should be considered when metronidazole vaginal gelis prescribed for patients on this type of anticoagulant therapy).
No products indexed under this heading.

Disulfiram (Metronidazole vaginal gel should not be administered to patients who have taken disulfiram within the last two weeks).
No products indexed under this heading.

Lithium (In patients stabilized on relatively high doses of lithium, short-term oral metronidazole therapy has been associated with elevation of serum lithium levels and, in a few cases, signs of lithium toxicity).
No products indexed under this heading.

Lithium Carbonate (In patients stabilized on relatively high doses of lithium, short-term oral metronidazole therapy has been associated with elevation of serum lithium levels and, in a few cases, signs of lithium toxicity). Products include:
Lithobid Tablets 1692

Lithium Citrate (In patients stabilized on relatively high doses of lithium, short-term oral metronidazole therapy has been associated with elevation of serum lithium levels and, in a few cases, signs of lithium toxicity).
No products indexed under this heading.

Petrolatum-containing vaginal lubricants (The patient should be instructed not to engage in vaginal intercourse, or use other vaginal products during treatment).
No products indexed under this heading.

Vaginal Diaphragm & Apparatus (The patient should be instructed not to engage in vaginal intercourse, or use other vaginal products during treatment).
No products indexed under this heading.

Vaginally administered preparations, unspecified (The patient should be instructed not to engage in vaginal intercourse, or use other vaginal products during treatment).
No products indexed under this heading.

Warfarin Sodium (Oral metronidazole has been reported to potentiate the anticoagulant effect of warfarin and other coumarin anticoagulants, resulting in a prolongation of prothrombin time. The possible drug interaction should be considered when metronidazole vaginal gelis prescribed for patients on this type of anticoagulant therapy). Products include:
Coumadin for Injection 898
Coumadin Tablets 898

Food Interactions

Alcohol (The patient should be cautioned about drinking alcohol while being treated with metronidazole vaginal gel).

VANOS CREAM

(Fluocinonide) 1893
None cited in PDR database.

VANTAS

(Histrelin Acetate) 3375
None cited in PDR database.

VANTIN TABLETS AND ORAL SUSPENSION

(Cefpodoxime Proxetil) 2645
May interact with aminoglycosides, antacids, anticholinergics, histamine H2-receptor antagonists, and certain other agents. Compounds in these categories include:

Aluminum Carbonate (High doses of antacids reduces peak plasma levels by 24% and the extent of absorption by 27%; the rate of absorption is not altered).
No products indexed under this heading.

Aluminum Hydroxide (High doses of antacids reduces peak plasma levels by 24% and the extent of absorption by 27%; the rate of absorption is not altered). Products include:
Gaviscon Regular Strength Liquid .. ▣ 658
Gaviscon Regular Strength Tablets...................................... ▣ 658
Gaviscon Extra Strength Liquid ...... ▣ 658
Gaviscon Extra Strength Tablets .... ▣ 658
Maalox Regular Strength Antacid/Antigas Liquid................. 2175
Maalox Max Maximum Strength Antacid/Anti-Gas Liquid................ 2176

Amikacin Sulfate (Close monitoring of renal function is required when co-administered with compounds of known nephrotoxicity potential, such as aminoglycosides).
No products indexed under this heading.

Atropine Sulfate (Oral anti-cholinergics delay peak plasma levels but do not affect the extent of absorption). Products include:
Donnatal Extentabs 2493

Belladonna Alkaloids (Oral anti-cholinergics delay peak plasma levels but do not affect the extent of absorption). Products include:
Hyland's Teething Tablets .... ▣ 830

Benztropine Mesylate (Oral anti-cholinergics delay peak plasma levels but do not affect the extent of absorption).
No products indexed under this heading.

Biperiden Hydrochloride (Oral anti-cholinergics delay peak plasma levels but do not affect the extent of absorption).
No products indexed under this heading.

Cimetidine (High doses of H_2 blockers reduces peak plasma levels by 42% and the extent of absorption by 32%; the rate of absorption is not altered). Products include:
Tagamet HB 200 Tablets .... ▣ 664

Cimetidine Hydrochloride (High doses of H_2 blockers reduces peak plasma levels by 42% and the extent of absorption by 32%; the rate of absorption is not altered).
No products indexed under this heading.

Clidinium Bromide (Oral anti-cholinergics delay peak plasma levels but do not affect the extent of absorption).
No products indexed under this heading.

Dicyclomine Hydrochloride (Oral anti-cholinergics delay peak plasma levels but do not affect the extent of absorption). Products include:
Bentyl Capsules 697
Bentyl Injection 697
Bentyl Syrup 697
Bentyl Tablets 697

Famotidine (High doses of H_2 blockers reduces peak plasma levels by 42% and the extent of absorption by 32%; the rate of absorption is not altered). Products include:
Pepcid Injection 2040
Pepcid 2038
Pepcid AC Gelcaps 1701
Pepcid AC Tablets 1701
Maximum Strength Pepcid AC Tablets 1701
Pepcid Complete Chewable Tablets 1701

Gentamicin Sulfate (Close monitoring of renal function is required when co-administered with compounds of known nephrotoxicity potential, such as aminoglycosides). Products include:
Garamycin Injectable 3014
Pred-G Ophthalmic Ointment .... ⊙ 237
Pred-G Ophthalmic Suspension ...... ⊙ 236

Glycopyrrolate (Oral anti-cholinergics delay peak plasma levels but do not affect the extent of absorption).
No products indexed under this heading.

Hyoscyamine (Oral anti-cholinergics delay peak plasma levels but do not affect the extent of absorption).
No products indexed under this heading.

Hyoscyamine Sulfate (Oral anti-cholinergics delay peak plasma levels but do not affect the extent of absorption). Products include:
Donnatal Extentabs 2493
Prosed/DS Tablets 1157

Ipratropium Bromide (Oral anti-cholinergics delay peak plasma levels but do not affect the extent of absorption). Products include:
Atrovent Inhalation Solution 835
Atrovent HFA Inhalation Aerosol 841
Atrovent Nasal Spray 0.03% 837
Atrovent Nasal Spray 0.06% 839
Combivent Inhalation Aerosol 847
DuoNeb Inhalation Solution 1058

Kanamycin Sulfate (Close monitoring of renal function is required when co-administered with compounds of known nephrotoxicity potential, such as aminoglycosides).
No products indexed under this heading.

Magaldrate (High doses of antacids reduces peak plasma levels by 24% and the extent of absorption by 27%; the rate of absorption is not altered).
No products indexed under this heading.

Magnesium Hydroxide (High doses of antacids reduces peak plasma levels by 24% and the extent of absorption by 27%; the rate of absorption is not altered). Products include:
Maalox Regular Strength Antacid/Antigas Liquid................. 2175
Maalox Max Maximum Strength Antacid/Anti-Gas Liquid................ 2176
Pepcid Complete Chewable Tablets 1701

Magnesium Oxide (High doses of antacids reduces peak plasma levels by 24% and the extent of absorption by 27%; the rate of absorption is not altered). Products include:
Beelith Tablets 759
PremCal Light, Regular, and Extra Strength Tablets................. ▣ 818

Mepenzolate Bromide (Oral anti-cholinergics delay peak plasma levels but do not affect the extent of absorption).
No products indexed under this heading.

Nephrotoxic Drugs (Close monitoring of renal function is required when co-administered with compounds of known nephrotoxicity potential).
No products indexed under this heading.

Nizatidine (High doses of H_2 blockers reduces peak plasma levels by 42% and the extent of absorption by 32%; the rate of absorption is not altered). Products include:
Axid Oral Solution 879

Oxybutynin Chloride (Oral anti-cholinergics delay peak plasma levels but do not affect the extent of absorption). Products include:
Ditropan XL Extended-Release Tablets 2413

Probenecid (Renal excretion of cefpodoxime is inhibited by probenecid and resulting in an approximately 31% increase in AUC and 20% increase in peak plasma levels).
No products indexed under this heading.

Procyclidine Hydrochloride (Oral anti-cholinergics delay peak plasma levels but do not affect the extent of absorption).
No products indexed under this heading.

Propantheline Bromide (Oral anti-cholinergics delay peak plasma levels but do not affect the extent of absorption).
No products indexed under this heading.

Ranitidine Bismuth Citrate (High doses of H_2 blockers reduces peak plasma levels by 42% and the extent of absorption by 32%; the rate of absorption is not altered).
No products indexed under this heading.

Ranitidine Hydrochloride (High doses of H_2 blockers reduces peak plasma levels by 42% and the extent of absorption by 32%; the rate of absorption is not altered). Products include:
Zantac 1624
Zantac Injection 1619
Zantac Injection Pharmacy Bulk Package 1622

Scopolamine (Oral anti-cholinergics delay peak plasma levels but do not affect the extent of absorption). Products include:
Transderm Scōp Transdermal Therapeutic System 2177

Scopolamine Hydrobromide (Oral anti-cholinergics delay peak plasma levels but do not affect the extent of absorption). Products include:
Donnatal Extentabs 2493

Sodium Bicarbonate (High doses of antacids reduces peak plasma levels by 24% and the extent of absorption by 27%; the rate of absorption is not altered). Products include:
Colyte with Flavor Packs for Oral Solution 3088
HalfLytely and Bisacodyl Tablets Bowel Prep Kit with Flavors Packs 881
TriLyte with Flavor Packs for Oral Solution 3100

tions of co-administered drugs that are primarily metabolized by CYP3A4). Products include:

Actiq ... 979

Fluconazole (Conivaptan is a substrate of CYP3A4. Co-administration of conivaptan with CYP3A4 inhibitors could lead to an increase in conivaptan concentrations. Concomitant use of conivaptan with potent CYP3A4 inhibitors is contraindicated).

No products indexed under this heading.

Fluoxetine Hydrochloride (Conivaptan is a substrate of CYP3A4. Co-administration of conivaptan with CYP3A4 inhibitors could lead to an increase in conivaptan concentrations. Concomitant use of conivaptan with potent CYP3A4 inhibitors is contraindicated). Products include:

Prozac Pulvules and Liquid ... 1801
Symbyax Capsules ... 1819

Fluvoxamine Maleate (Conivaptan is a substrate of CYP3A4. Co-administration of conivaptan with CYP3A4 inhibitors could lead to an increase in conivaptan concentrations. Concomitant use of conivaptan with potent CYP3A4 inhibitors is contraindicated).

No products indexed under this heading.

Fosamprenavir Calcium (Conivaptan is a substrate of CYP3A4. Co-administration of conivaptan with CYP3A4 inhibitors could lead to an increase in conivaptan concentrations. Concomitant use of conivaptan with potent CYP3A4 inhibitors is contraindicated). Products include:

Lexiva Tablets ... 1505

Haloperidol (Conivaptan is a potent inhibitor of CYP3A4. Conivaptan may increase plasma concentrations of co-administered drugs that are primarily metabolized by CYP3A4).

No products indexed under this heading.

Haloperidol Decanoate (Conivaptan is a potent inhibitor of CYP3A4. Conivaptan may increase plasma concentrations of co-administered drugs that are primarily metabolized by CYP3A4).

No products indexed under this heading.

Haloperidol Lactate (Conivaptan is a potent inhibitor of CYP3A4. Conivaptan may increase plasma concentrations of co-administered drugs that are primarily metabolized by CYP3A4).

No products indexed under this heading.

Indinavir Sulfate (Conivaptan is a substrate of CYP3A4. Co-administration of conivaptan with CYP3A4 inhibitors could lead to an increase in conivaptan concentrations. Concomitant use of conivaptan with potent CYP3A4 inhibitors is contraindicated). Products include:

Crixivan Capsules ... 1940

Isoniazid (Conivaptan is a substrate of CYP3A4. Co-administration of conivaptan with CYP3A4 inhibitors could lead to an increase in conivaptan concentrations. Concomitant use of conivaptan with potent CYP3A4 inhibitors is contraindicated).

No products indexed under this heading.

Isradipine (Conivaptan is a potent inhibitor of CYP3A4. Conivaptan may increase plasma concentrations of co-administered drugs that are primarily metabolized by CYP3A4). Products include:

DynaCirc CR Tablets ... 2721

Itraconazole (Conivaptan is a substrate of CYP3A4. Co-administration of conivaptan with CYP3A4 inhibitors could lead to an increase in conivaptan concentrations. Concomitant use of conivaptan with potent CYP3A4 inhibitors is contraindicated).

No products indexed under this heading.

Ketoconazole (Conivaptan is a substrate of CYP3A4. Co-administration of conivaptan with CYP3A4 inhibitors could lead to an increase in conivaptan concentrations. Concomitant use of conivaptan with potent CYP3A4 inhibitors is contraindicated). Products include:

Nizoral A-D Shampoo, 1% ... 1868

Levonorgestrel (Conivaptan is a potent inhibitor of CYP3A4. Conivaptan may increase plasma concentrations of co-administered drugs that are primarily metabolized by CYP3A4). Products include:

Climara Pro Transdermal System ... 776
Mirena Intrauterine System ... 787
Plan B Tablets ... 1076
Seasonique Tablets ... 1077

Lidocaine (Conivaptan is a potent inhibitor of CYP3A4. Conivaptan may increase plasma concentrations of co-administered drugs that are primarily metabolized by CYP3A4). Products include:

Lidoderm Patch ... 1118
Synera Topical Patch ... 1137

Lidocaine Hydrochloride (Conivaptan is a potent inhibitor of CYP3A4. Conivaptan may increase plasma concentrations of co-administered drugs that are primarily metabolized by CYP3A4).

No products indexed under this heading.

Lopinavir (Conivaptan is a substrate of CYP3A4. Co-administration of conivaptan with CYP3A4 inhibitors could lead to an increase in conivaptan concentrations. Concomitant use of conivaptan with potent CYP3A4 inhibitors is contraindicated). Products include:

Kaletra ... 476

Loratadine (Conivaptan is a substrate of CYP3A4. Co-administration of conivaptan with CYP3A4 inhibitors could lead to an increase in conivaptan concentrations. Concomitant use of conivaptan with potent CYP3A4 inhibitors is contraindicated). Products include:

Alavert Allergy & Sinus D-12 Hour Tablets ... 771
Alavert ... 771
Children's Claritin Allergy Oral Solution ... 771
Claritin Non-Drowsy 24 Hour Tablets ... 772
Claritin Reditabs 24 Hour Non-Drowsy Tablets ... 772
Claritin-D Non-Drowsy 12 Hour Tablets ... 772
Claritin-D Non-Drowsy 24 Hour Tablets ... 772

Lovastatin (Conivaptan is a potent inhibitor of CYP3A4. Conivaptan may increase plasma concentrations of co-administered drugs that are primarily metabolized by CYP3A4). Products include:

Advicor Tablets ... 1722
Altoprev Extended-Release Tablets ... 3109
Mevacor Tablets ... 2021

Mestranol (Conivaptan is a potent inhibitor of CYP3A4. Conivaptan may increase plasma concentrations of co-administered drugs that are primarily metabolized by CYP3A4).

No products indexed under this heading.

Methadone Hydrochloride (Conivaptan is a potent inhibitor of CYP3A4. Conivaptan may increase plasma concentrations of co-administered drugs that are primarily metabolized by CYP3A4).

No products indexed under this heading.

Metronidazole (Conivaptan is a substrate of CYP3A4. Co-administration of conivaptan with CYP3A4 inhibitors could lead to an increase in conivaptan concentrations. Concomitant use of conivaptan with potent CYP3A4 inhibitors is contraindicated). Products include:

Metrogel 1% ... 1211
MetroGel-Vaginal Gel ... 1855
Vandazole Vaginal Gel ... 3338

Metronidazole Benzoate (Conivaptan is a substrate of CYP3A4. Co-administration of conivaptan with CYP3A4 inhibitors could lead to an increase in conivaptan concentrations. Concomitant use of conivaptan with potent CYP3A4 inhibitors is contraindicated).

No products indexed under this heading.

Metronidazole Hydrochloride (Conivaptan is a substrate of CYP3A4. Co-administration of conivaptan with CYP3A4 inhibitors could lead to an increase in conivaptan concentrations. Concomitant use of conivaptan with potent CYP3A4 inhibitors is contraindicated).

No products indexed under this heading.

Miconazole (Conivaptan is a substrate of CYP3A4. Co-administration of conivaptan with CYP3A4 inhibitors could lead to an increase in conivaptan concentrations. Concomitant use of conivaptan with potent CYP3A4 inhibitors is contraindicated).

No products indexed under this heading.

Miconazole Nitrate (Conivaptan is a substrate of CYP3A4. Co-administration of conivaptan with CYP3A4 inhibitors could lead to an increase in conivaptan concentrations. Concomitant use of conivaptan with potent CYP3A4 inhibitors is contraindicated). Products include:

Desenex ... 635
Desenex Jock Itch Spray Powder ... 635

Midazolam Hydrochloride (Conivaptan is a potent inhibitor of CYP3A4. Conivaptan may increase plasma concentrations of co-administered drugs that are primarily metabolized by CYP3A4).

No products indexed under this heading.

Nefazodone Hydrochloride (Conivaptan is a substrate of CYP3A4. Co-administration of conivaptan with CYP3A4 inhibitors could lead to an increase in conivaptan concentrations. Concomitant use of conivaptan with potent CYP3A4 inhibitors is contraindicated).

No products indexed under this heading.

Nelfinavir Mesylate (Conivaptan is a substrate of CYP3A4. Co-administration of conivaptan with CYP3A4 inhibitors could lead to an increase in conivaptan concentrations. Concomitant use of conivaptan with potent CYP3A4 inhibitors is contraindicated). Products include:

Viracept ... 2577

Nevirapine (Conivaptan is a substrate of CYP3A4. Co-administration of conivaptan with CYP3A4 inhibitors could lead to an increase in conivaptan concentrations. Concomitant use of conivaptan with potent CYP3A4 inhibitors is contraindicated). Products include:

Viramune Oral Suspension ... 873
Viramune Tablets ... 873

Niacinamide (Conivaptan is a substrate of CYP3A4. Co-administration of conivaptan with CYP3A4 inhibitors could lead to an increase in conivaptan concentrations. Concomitant use of conivaptan with potent CYP3A4 inhibitors is contraindicated).

No products indexed under this heading.

Nicardipine Hydrochloride (Conivaptan is a potent inhibitor of CYP3A4. Conivaptan may increase plasma concentrations of co-administered drugs that are primarily metabolized by CYP3A4). Products include:

Cardene I.V. ... 2497

Nicotinamide (Conivaptan is a substrate of CYP3A4. Co-administration of conivaptan with CYP3A4 inhibitors could lead to an increase in conivaptan concentrations. Concomitant use of conivaptan with potent CYP3A4 inhibitors is contraindicated). Products include:

Nicomide Tablets ... 1088

Nifedipine (Conivaptan is a substrate of CYP3A4. Co-administration of conivaptan with CYP3A4 inhibitors could lead to an increase in conivaptan concentrations. Concomitant use of conivaptan with potent CYP3A4 inhibitors is contraindicated). Products include:

Adalat CC Tablets ... 2964

Nimodipine (Conivaptan is a potent inhibitor of CYP3A4. Conivaptan may increase plasma concentrations of co-administered drugs that are primarily metabolized by CYP3A4). Products include:

Nimotop Capsules ... 749

Nisoldipine (Conivaptan is a potent inhibitor of CYP3A4. Conivaptan may increase plasma concentrations of co-administered drugs that are primarily metabolized by CYP3A4). Products include:

Sular Tablets ... 3122

Nitrendipine (Conivaptan is a potent inhibitor of CYP3A4. Conivaptan may increase plasma concentrations of co-administered drugs that are primarily metabolized by CYP3A4).

No products indexed under this heading.

Norethindrone (Conivaptan is a potent inhibitor of CYP3A4. Conivaptan may increase plasma concentrations of co-administered drugs that are primarily metabolized by CYP3A4). Products include:

Ortho Micronor Tablets ... 2426

Norethindrone Acetate (Conivaptan is a potent inhibitor of CYP3A4. Conivaptan may increase plasma concentrations of co-administered drugs that are primarily metabolized by CYP3A4).

No products indexed under this heading.

Norfloxacin (Conivaptan is a substrate of CYP3A4. Co-administration of conivaptan with CYP3A4 inhibitors could lead to an increase in conivaptan concentrations. Concomitant use of conivaptan with potent CYP3A4 inhibitors is contraindicated). Products include:
Noroxin Tablets 2032

Norgestrel (Conivaptan is a potent inhibitor of CYP3A4. Conivaptan may increase plasma concentrations of co-administered drugs that are primarily metabolized by CYP3A4).
No products indexed under this heading.

Omeprazole (Conivaptan is a substrate of CYP3A4. Co-administration of conivaptan with CYP3A4 inhibitors could lead to an increase in conivaptan concentrations. Concomitant use of conivaptan with potent CYP3A4 inhibitors is contraindicated). Products include:
Zegerid Capsules 2958
Zegerid Powder for Oral Solution 2958

Ondansetron (Conivaptan is a potent inhibitor of CYP3A4. Conivaptan may increase plasma concentrations of co-administered drugs that are primarily metabolized by CYP3A4). Products include:
Zofran ODT Orally Disintegrating Tablets 1639

Ondansetron Hydrochloride (Conivaptan is a potent inhibitor of CYP3A4. Conivaptan may increase plasma concentrations of co-administered drugs that are primarily metabolized by CYP3A4). Products include:
Zofran Injection 1634
Zofran 1639

Paclitaxel (Conivaptan is a potent inhibitor of CYP3A4. Conivaptan may increase plasma concentrations of co-administered drugs that are primarily metabolized by CYP3A4).
No products indexed under this heading.

Paroxetine Hydrochloride (Conivaptan is a substrate of CYP3A4. Co-administration of conivaptan with CYP3A4 inhibitors could lead to an increase in conivaptan concentrations. Concomitant use of conivaptan with potent CYP3A4 inhibitors is contraindicated). Products include:
Paxil CR Controlled-Release Tablets 1538
Paxil 1530

Pimozide (Conivaptan is a potent inhibitor of CYP3A4. Conivaptan may increase plasma concentrations of co-administered drugs that are primarily metabolized by CYP3A4).
No products indexed under this heading.

Polyestradiol Phosphate (Conivaptan is a potent inhibitor of CYP3A4. Conivaptan may increase plasma concentrations of co-administered drugs that are primarily metabolized by CYP3A4).
No products indexed under this heading.

Propoxyphene Hydrochloride (Conivaptan is a substrate of CYP3A4. Co-administration of conivaptan with CYP3A4 inhibitors could lead to an increase in conivaptan concentrations. Concomitant use of conivaptan with potent CYP3A4 inhibitors is contraindicated).
No products indexed under this heading.

Propoxyphene Napsylate (Conivaptan is a substrate of CYP3A4. Co-administration of conivaptan with CYP3A4 inhibitors could lead to an increase in conivaptan concentrations. Concomitant use of conivaptan with potent CYP3A4 inhibitors is contraindicated).
No products indexed under this heading.

Quinidine (Conivaptan is a substrate of CYP3A4. Co-administration of conivaptan with CYP3A4 inhibitors could lead to an increase in conivaptan concentrations. Concomitant use of conivaptan with potent CYP3A4 inhibitors is contraindicated).
No products indexed under this heading.

Quinidine Gluconate (Conivaptan is a potent inhibitor of CYP3A4. Conivaptan may increase plasma concentrations of co-administered drugs that are primarily metabolized by CYP3A4).
No products indexed under this heading.

Quinidine Hydrochloride (Conivaptan is a substrate of CYP3A4. Co-administration of conivaptan with CYP3A4 inhibitors could lead to an increase in conivaptan concentrations. Concomitant use of conivaptan with potent CYP3A4 inhibitors is contraindicated).
No products indexed under this heading.

Quinidine Polygalacturonate (Conivaptan is a substrate of CYP3A4. Co-administration of conivaptan with CYP3A4 inhibitors could lead to an increase in conivaptan concentrations. Concomitant use of conivaptan with potent CYP3A4 inhibitors is contraindicated).
No products indexed under this heading.

Quinidine Sulfate (Conivaptan is a substrate of CYP3A4. Co-administration of conivaptan with CYP3A4 inhibitors could lead to an increase in conivaptan concentrations. Concomitant use of conivaptan with potent CYP3A4 inhibitors is contraindicated).
No products indexed under this heading.

Quinine (Conivaptan is a substrate of CYP3A4. Co-administration of conivaptan with CYP3A4 inhibitors could lead to an increase in conivaptan concentrations. Concomitant use of conivaptan with potent CYP3A4 inhibitors is contraindicated).
No products indexed under this heading.

Quinine Sulfate (Conivaptan is a substrate of CYP3A4. Co-administration of conivaptan with CYP3A4 inhibitors could lead to an increase in conivaptan concentrations. Concomitant use of conivaptan with potent CYP3A4 inhibitors is contraindicated).
No products indexed under this heading.

Quinupristin (Conivaptan is a substrate of CYP3A4. Co-administration of conivaptan with CYP3A4 inhibitors could lead to an increase in conivaptan concentrations. Concomitant use of conivaptan with potent CYP3A4 inhibitors is contraindicated).
No products indexed under this heading.

Ranitidine Bismuth Citrate (Conivaptan is a substrate of CYP3A4. Co-administration of conivaptan with CYP3A4 inhibitors could lead to an increase in conivaptan concentrations. Concomitant use of conivaptan with potent CYP3A4 inhibitors is contraindicated).
No products indexed under this heading.

Ranitidine Hydrochloride (Conivaptan is a substrate of CYP3A4. Co-administration of conivaptan with CYP3A4 inhibitors could lead to an increase in conivaptan concentrations. Concomitant use of conivaptan with potent CYP3A4 inhibitors is contraindicated). Products include:
Zantac 1624
Zantac Injection 1619
Zantac Injection Pharmacy Bulk Package 1622

Rifabutin (Conivaptan is a potent inhibitor of CYP3A4. Conivaptan may increase plasma concentrations of co-administered drugs that are primarily metabolized by CYP3A4).
No products indexed under this heading.

Ritonavir (Conivaptan is a substrate of CYP3A4. Co-administration of conivaptan with CYP3A4 inhibitors could lead to an increase in conivaptan concentrations. Concomitant use of conivaptan with potent CYP3A4 inhibitors is contraindicated). Products include:
Kaletra 476
Norvir 503

Saquinavir (Conivaptan is a substrate of CYP3A4. Co-administration of conivaptan with CYP3A4 inhibitors could lead to an increase in conivaptan concentrations. Concomitant use of conivaptan with potent CYP3A4 inhibitors is contraindicated).
No products indexed under this heading.

Saquinavir Mesylate (Conivaptan is a substrate of CYP3A4. Co-administration of conivaptan with CYP3A4 inhibitors could lead to an increase in conivaptan concentrations. Concomitant use of conivaptan with potent CYP3A4 inhibitors is contraindicated). Products include:
Invirase 2772

Sertraline Hydrochloride (Conivaptan is a substrate of CYP3A4. Co-administration of conivaptan with CYP3A4 inhibitors could lead to an increase in conivaptan concentrations. Concomitant use of conivaptan with potent CYP3A4 inhibitors is contraindicated). Products include:
Zoloft 2586

Sildenafil Citrate (Conivaptan is a potent inhibitor of CYP3A4. Conivaptan may increase plasma concentrations of co-administered drugs that are primarily metabolized by CYP3A4). Products include:
Revatio Tablets 2557
Viagra Tablets 2573

Simvastatin (Conivaptan is a potent inhibitor of CYP3A4. Conivaptan may increase plasma concentrations of co-administered drugs that are primarily metabolized by CYP3A4). Products include:
Vytorin 10/10 Tablets 2114
Vytorin 10/10 Tablets 3077
Vytorin 10/20 Tablets 2114
Vytorin 10/20 Tablets 3077
Vytorin 10/40 Tablets 2114
Vytorin 10/40 Tablets 3077
Vytorin 10/80 Tablets 2114
Vytorin 10/80 Tablets 3077
Zocor Tablets 2105

Sirolimus (Conivaptan is a potent inhibitor of CYP3A4. Conivaptan may increase plasma concentrations of co-administered drugs that are primarily metabolized by CYP3A4). Products include:
Rapamune Oral Solution and Tablets 3475

Tacrolimus (Conivaptan is a potent inhibitor of CYP3A4. Conivaptan may increase plasma concentrations of co-administered drugs that are primarily metabolized by CYP3A4). Products include:
Prograf Capsules and Injection 632
Protopic Ointment 638

Tamoxifen Citrate (Conivaptan is a potent inhibitor of CYP3A4. Conivaptan may increase plasma concentrations of co-administered drugs that are primarily metabolized by CYP3A4). Products include:
Soltamox Oral Solution 3527

Telithromycin (Conivaptan is a substrate of CYP3A4. Co-administration of conivaptan with CYP3A4 inhibitors could lead to an increase in conivaptan concentrations. Concomitant use of conivaptan with potent CYP3A4 inhibitors is contraindicated). Products include:
Ketek Tablets 2903

Tiagabine Hydrochloride (Conivaptan is a potent inhibitor of CYP3A4. Conivaptan may increase plasma concentrations of co-administered drugs that are primarily metabolized by CYP3A4). Products include:
Gabitril Tablets 984

Tolterodine Tartrate (Conivaptan is a potent inhibitor of CYP3A4. Conivaptan may increase plasma concentrations of co-administered drugs that are primarily metabolized by CYP3A4). Products include:
Detrol Tablets 2628
Detrol LA Capsules 2631

Trazodone Hydrochloride (Conivaptan is a potent inhibitor of CYP3A4. Conivaptan may increase plasma concentrations of co-administered drugs that are primarily metabolized by CYP3A4).
No products indexed under this heading.

Triazolam (Conivaptan is a potent inhibitor of CYP3A4. Conivaptan may increase plasma concentrations of co-administered drugs that are primarily metabolized by CYP3A4).
No products indexed under this heading.

Troglitazone (Conivaptan is a substrate of CYP3A4. Co-administration of conivaptan with CYP3A4 inhibitors could lead to an increase in conivaptan concentrations. Concomitant use of conivaptan with potent CYP3A4 inhibitors is contraindicated).
No products indexed under this heading.

Troleandomycin (Conivaptan is a substrate of CYP3A4. Co-administration of conivaptan with CYP3A4 inhibitors could lead to an increase in conivaptan concentrations. Concomitant use of conivaptan with potent CYP3A4 inhibitors is contraindicated).
No products indexed under this heading.

Valproate Sodium (Conivaptan is a substrate of CYP3A4. Co-

administration of conivaptan with CYP3A4 inhibitors could lead to an increase in conivaptan concentrations. Concomitant use of conivaptan with potent CYP3A4 inhibitors is contraindicated). Products include:
- Depacon Injection 412

Verapamil Hydrochloride (Conivaptan is a substrate of CYP3A4. Co-administration of conivaptan with CYP3A4 inhibitors could lead to an increase in conivaptan concentrations. Concomitant use of conivaptan with potent CYP3A4 inhibitors is contraindicated). Products include:
- Covera-HS Tablets 3139
- Tarka Tablets 524
- Verelan PM Extended-Release Capsules, Controlled-Onset.......... 3106

Vinblastine Sulfate (Conivaptan is a potent inhibitor of CYP3A4. Conivaptan may increase plasma concentrations of co-administered drugs that are primarily metabolized by CYP3A4).
No products indexed under this heading.

Vincristine Sulfate (Conivaptan is a potent inhibitor of CYP3A4. Conivaptan may increase plasma concentrations of co-administered drugs that are primarily metabolized by CYP3A4).
No products indexed under this heading.

Voriconazole (Conivaptan is a substrate of CYP3A4. Co-administration of conivaptan with CYP3A4 inhibitors could lead to an increase in conivaptan concentrations. Concomitant use of conivaptan with potent CYP3A4 inhibitors is contraindicated). Products include:
- VFEND I.V. 2564
- VFEND Oral Suspension 2564
- VFEND Tablets 2564

Warfarin Sodium (Conivaptan is a potent inhibitor of CYP3A4. Conivaptan may increase plasma concentrations of co-administered drugs that are primarily metabolized by CYP3A4). Products include:
- Coumadin for Injection 898
- Coumadin Tablets 898

Zafirlukast (Conivaptan is a substrate of CYP3A4. Co-administration of conivaptan with CYP3A4 inhibitors could lead to an increase in conivaptan concentrations. Concomitant use of conivaptan with potent CYP3A4 inhibitors is contraindicated). Products include:
- Accolate Tablets 671

Zileuton (Conivaptan is a substrate of CYP3A4. Co-administration of conivaptan with CYP3A4 inhibitors could lead to an increase in conivaptan concentrations. Concomitant use of conivaptan with potent CYP3A4 inhibitors is contraindicated). Products include:
- Zyflo Tablets 1023

Food Interactions

Grapefruit (Conivaptan is a substrate of CYP3A4. Co-administration of conivaptan with CYP3A4 inhibitors could lead to an increase in conivaptan concentrations. Concomitant use of conivaptan with potent CYP3A4 inhibitors is contraindicated).

Grapefruit Juice (Conivaptan is a substrate of CYP3A4. Co-administration of conivaptan with CYP3A4 inhibitors could lead to an increase in conivaptan concentrations. Concomitant use of conivaptan with potent CYP3A4 inhibitors is contraindicated).

VAQTA

(Hepatitis A Vaccine, Inactivated) 2097

May interact with typhoid vaccine and certain other agents. Compounds in these categories include:

Typhoid Vaccine (Co-administration of Vaqta, typhoid and yellow fever vaccines has resulted in reduced GMTs for hepatitis A compared to Vaqta alone; however, following the receipt of the booster dose of Vaqta the GMTs for hepatits A in these two groups were observed to be comparable).
No products indexed under this heading.

Typhoid Vaccine Live Oral TY21a (Co-administration of Vaqta, typhoid and yellow fever vaccines has resulted in reduced GMTs for hepatitis A compared to Vaqta alone; however, following the receipt of the booster dose of Vaqta the GMTs for hepatits A in these two groups were observed to be comparable). Products include:
- Vivotif 819

Typhoid Vi Polysaccharide Vaccine (Co-administration of Vaqta, typhoid and yellow fever vaccines has resulted in reduced GMTs for hepatitis A compared to Vaqta alone; however, following the receipt of the booster dose of Vaqta the GMTs for hepatits A in these two groups were observed to be comparable).
No products indexed under this heading.

Yellow Fever Vaccine (Co-administration of Vaqta, typhoid and yellow fever vaccines has resulted in reduced GMTs for hepatitis A compared to Vaqta alone; however, following the receipt of the booster dose of Vaqta the GMTs for hepatitis A in these two groups were observed to be comparable).
No products indexed under this heading.

VARIVAX

(Varicella Virus Vaccine Live) 2100

May interact with corticosteroids, salicylates, and certain other agents. Compounds in these categories include:

Aspirin (Vaccine recipients should avoid use of salicylates for 6 weeks after vaccination with Varivax because of the potential for Reye's syndrome). Products include:
- Aggrenox Capsules 822
- Bayer Aspirin 744
- BC Allergy Sinus Cold Powder 677
- BC Headache Powder 677
- Arthritis Strength BC Powder 677
- BC Sinus Cold Powder 677
- Excedrin Extra Strength Caplets/Tablets/Geltabs.......... 684
- Excedrin Migraine Caplets/Tablets/Geltabs.......... 609
- Goody's Body Pain Formula Powder.......... 684
- Goody's Extra Strength Headache Powders.......... 611
- Goody's Extra Strength Pain Relief Tablets.......... 685
- Percodan Tablets 1132
- St. Joseph 81 mg Aspirin Chewable and Enteric Coated Tablets.......... 1869

Aspirin, Enteric Coated (Vaccine recipients should avoid use of salicylates for 6 weeks after vaccination with Varivax because of the potential for Reye's syndrome).
No products indexed under this heading.

Aspirin Buffered (Vaccine recipients should avoid use of salicylates for 6 weeks after vaccination with Varivax because of the potential for Reye's syndrome). Products include:
- Bufferin Extra Strength Tablets 678
- Bufferin Regular Strength Tablets 678

Azathioprine (Concurrent use in individuals who are on immunosuppressant drugs can result in greater susceptibility to infections; co-administration is contraindicated).
No products indexed under this heading.

Betamethasone Acetate (Co-administration in individuals on immunosuppressant doses of corticosteroids can result in more extensive vaccine-associated rash or disseminated disease).
No products indexed under this heading.

Betamethasone Sodium Phosphate (Co-administration in individuals on immunosuppressant doses of corticosteroids can result in more extensive vaccine-associated rash or disseminated disease).
No products indexed under this heading.

Choline Magnesium Trisalicylate (Vaccine recipients should avoid use of salicylates for 6 weeks after vaccination with Varivax because of the potential for Reye's syndrome).
No products indexed under this heading.

Cortisone Acetate (Co-administration in individuals on immunosuppressant doses of corticosteroids can result in more extensive vaccine-associated rash or disseminated disease).
No products indexed under this heading.

Cyclosporine (Concurrent use in individuals who are on immunosuppressant drugs can result in greater susceptibility to infections; co-administration is contraindicated). Products include:
- Gengraf Capsules 459
- Neoral Oral Solution 2259
- Neoral Soft Gelatin Capsules 2259
- Restasis Ophthalmic Emulsion 575
- Sandimmune 2275

Dexamethasone (Co-administration in individuals on immunosuppressant doses of corticosteroids can result in more extensive vaccine-associated rash or disseminated disease). Products include:
- Ciprodex Otic Suspension 559
- Decadron Tablets 1951
- TobraDex Ophthalmic Ointment 562
- TobraDex Ophthalmic Suspension 563

Dexamethasone Acetate (Co-administration in individuals on immunosuppressant doses of corticosteroids can result in more extensive vaccine-associated rash or disseminated disease).
No products indexed under this heading.

Dexamethasone Sodium Phosphate (Co-administration in individuals on immunosuppressant doses of corticosteroids can result in more extensive vaccine-associated rash or disseminated disease).
No products indexed under this heading.

Diflunisal (Vaccine recipients should avoid use of salicylates for 6 weeks after vaccination with Varivax because of the potential for Reye's syndrome). Products include:
- Dolobid Tablets 1955

Fludrocortisone Acetate (Co-administration in individuals on immunosuppressant doses of corticosteroids can result in more extensive vaccine-associated rash or disseminated disease).
No products indexed under this heading.

Globulin, Immune (Human) (Vaccination should be deferred for at least 5 months following immune globulin administration; following administration of Varivax, immune globulin should not be given for 2 months). Products include:
- Flebogamma 5%, Immune Globulin Intravenous (Human).......... 1658
- GamaSTAN 3234

Hydrocortisone (Co-administration in individuals on immunosuppressant doses of corticosteroids can result in more extensive vaccine-associated rash or disseminated disease). Products include:
- Colocort Rectal Suspension, USP (Retention) 100 mg/60 mL.......... 2476
- Hydrocortone Tablets 1989
- Preparation H Hydrocortisone Cream 646

Hydrocortisone Acetate (Co-administration in individuals on immunosuppressant doses of corticosteroids can result in more extensive vaccine-associated rash or disseminated disease). Products include:
- Analpram-HC 1159
- Pramosone 1161
- ProctoFoam-HC 3099

Hydrocortisone Sodium Phosphate (Co-administration in individuals on immunosuppressant doses of corticosteroids can result in more extensive vaccine-associated rash or disseminated disease).
No products indexed under this heading.

Hydrocortisone Sodium Succinate (Co-administration in individuals on immunosuppressant doses of corticosteroids can result in more extensive vaccine-associated rash or disseminated disease).
No products indexed under this heading.

Magnesium Salicylate (Vaccine recipients should avoid use of salicylates for 6 weeks after vaccination with Varivax because of the potential for Reye's syndrome).
No products indexed under this heading.

Methylprednisolone Acetate (Co-administration in individuals on immunosuppressant doses of corticosteroids can result in more extensive vaccine-associated rash or disseminated disease). Products include:
- Depo-Medrol Injectable Suspension 2617
- Depo-Medrol Single-Dose Vial 2619

Methylprednisolone Sodium Succinate (Co-administration in individuals on immunosuppressant doses of corticosteroids can result in more extensive vaccine-associated rash or disseminated disease).
No products indexed under this heading.

Muromonab-CD3 (Concurrent use in individuals who are on immunosuppressant drugs can result in greater susceptibility to infections; co-administration is contraindicated). Products include:
Orthoclone OKT3 Sterile Solution 2360

Mycophenolate Mofetil (Concurrent use in individuals who are on immunosuppressant drugs can result in greater susceptibility to infections; co-administration is contraindicated). Products include:
CellCept Capsules 2747
CellCept Oral Suspension 2747
CellCept Tablets 2747

Prednisolone Acetate (Co-administration in individuals on immunosuppressant doses of corticosteroids can result in more extensive vaccine-associated rash or disseminated disease). Products include:
Blephamide Ophthalmic Ointment 568
Blephamide Ophthalmic Suspension.................................. 569
Poly-Pred Ophthalmic Suspension .... ⊙233
Pred Forte Ophthalmic Suspension .... ⊙235
Pred Mild Ophthalmic Suspension .... ⊙238
Pred-G Ophthalmic Ointment .... ⊙237
Pred-G Ophthalmic Suspension ...... ⊙236

Prednisolone Sodium Phosphate (Co-administration in individuals on immunosuppressant doses of corticosteroids can result in more extensive vaccine-associated rash or disseminated disease).
No products indexed under this heading.

Prednisolone Tebutate (Co-administration in individuals on immunosuppressant doses of corticosteroids can result in more extensive vaccine-associated rash or disseminated disease).
No products indexed under this heading.

Prednisone (Co-administration in individuals on immunosuppressant doses of corticosteroids can result in more extensive vaccine-associated rash or disseminated disease).
No products indexed under this heading.

Salsalate (Vaccine recipients should avoid use of salicylates for 6 weeks after vaccination with Varivax because of the potential for Reye's syndrome).
No products indexed under this heading.

Tacrolimus (Concurrent use in individuals who are on immunosuppressant drugs can result in greater susceptibility to infections; co-administration is contraindicated). Products include:
Prograf Capsules and Injection 632
Protopic Ointment 638

Triamcinolone (Co-administration in individuals on immunosuppressant doses of corticosteroids can result in more extensive vaccine-associated rash or disseminated disease).
No products indexed under this heading.

Triamcinolone Acetonide (Co-administration in individuals on immunosuppressant doses of corticosteroids can result in more extensive vaccine-associated rash or disseminated disease). Products include:
Azmacort Inhalation Aerosol 1726
Nasacort AQ Nasal Spray 2922

Triamcinolone Diacetate (Co-administration in individuals on immunosuppressant doses of corticosteroids can result in more extensive vaccine-associated rash or disseminated disease).
No products indexed under this heading.

Triamcinolone Hexacetonide (Co-administration in individuals on immunosuppressant doses of corticosteroids can result in more extensive vaccine-associated rash or disseminated disease).
No products indexed under this heading.

VASOTEC I.V. INJECTION

(Enalapril Maleate) 2103
May interact with diuretics, lithium preparations, non-steroidal anti-inflammatory agents, potassium preparations, and potassium sparing diuretics. Compounds in these categories include:

Amiloride Hydrochloride (Enalapril attenuates diuretic-induced potassium loss; concomitant use can lead to hyperkalemia; frequent monitoring of serum potassium is recommended if used concurrently; co-administration can result in excessive hypotension). Products include:
Midamor Tablets 2026
Moduretic Tablets 2028

Bendroflumethiazide (Co-administration of enalapril in patients on diuretics, especially those in whom diuretic therapy was recently instituted, may occasionally experience excessive hypotension; antihypertensive effects of enalapril are augmented by antihypertensive agents that cause renin release).
No products indexed under this heading.

Bumetanide (Co-administration of enalapril in patients on diuretics, especially those in whom diuretic therapy was recently instituted, may occasionally experience excessive hypotension; antihypertensive effects of enalapril are augmented by antihypertensive agents that cause renin release). Products include:
Bumex Tablets 2746

Celecoxib (Co-administration with NSAIDs may diminish the antihypertensive effect of ACE inhibitors; potential for further deterioration of renal function in patients with compromised renal function when used concurrently). Products include:
Celebrex Capsules 3134

Chlorothiazide (Co-administration of enalapril in patients on diuretics, especially those in whom diuretic therapy was recently instituted, may occasionally experience excessive hypotension; antihypertensive effects of enalapril are augmented by antihypertensive agents that cause renin release). Products include:
Diuril Oral Suspension 1954

Chlorothiazide Sodium (Co-administration of enalapril in patients on diuretics, especially those in whom diuretic therapy was recently instituted, may occasionally experience excessive hypotension; antihypertensive effects of enalapril are augmented by antihypertensive agents that cause renin release). Products include:
Diuril Sodium Intravenous 2467

Chlorthalidone (Co-administration of enalapril in patients on diuretics, especially those in whom diuretic therapy was recently instituted, may occasionally experience excessive hypotension; antihypertensive effects of enalapril are augmented by antihypertensive agents that cause renin release). Products include:
Clorpres Tablets 2153

Diclofenac Potassium (Co-administration with NSAIDs may diminish the antihypertensive effect of ACE inhibitors; potential for further deterioration of renal function in patients with compromised renal function when used concurrently).
No products indexed under this heading.

Diclofenac Sodium (Co-administration with NSAIDs may diminish the antihypertensive effect of ACE inhibitors; potential for further deterioration of renal function in patients with compromised renal function when used concurrently). Products include:
Arthrotec Tablets 3129
Voltaren Ophthalmic Solution 2309
Voltaren Tablets 2307
Voltaren-XR Tablets 2310

Ethacrynic Acid (Co-administration of enalapril in patients on diuretics, especially those in whom diuretic therapy was recently instituted, may occasionally experience excessive hypotension; antihypertensive effects of enalapril are augmented by antihypertensive agents that cause renin release). Products include:
Edecrin Tablets 1959

Etodolac (Co-administration with NSAIDs may diminish the antihypertensive effect of ACE inhibitors; potential for further deterioration of renal function in patients with compromised renal function when used concurrently).
No products indexed under this heading.

Fenoprofen Calcium (Co-administration with NSAIDs may diminish the antihypertensive effect of ACE inhibitors; potential for further deterioration of renal function in patients with compromised renal function when used concurrently). Products include:
Nalfon Capsules 2502

Flurbiprofen (Co-administration with NSAIDs may diminish the antihypertensive effect of ACE inhibitors; potential for further deterioration of renal function in patients with compromised renal function when used concurrently).
No products indexed under this heading.

Furosemide (Co-administration of enalapril in patients on diuretics, especially those in whom diuretic therapy was recently instituted, may occasionally experience excessive hypotension; antihypertensive effects of enalapril are augmented by antihypertensive agents that cause renin release). Products include:
Furosemide Tablets 2154

Hydrochlorothiazide (Co-administration of enalapril in patients on diuretics, especially those in whom diuretic therapy was recently instituted, may occasionally experience excessive hypotension; antihypertensive effects of enalapril are augmented by antihypertensive agents that cause renin release). Products include:
Aldoril Tablets 1910
Atacand HCT 651
Avalide Tablets 888
Avalide Tablets 2874
Benicar HCT Tablets 1044
Diovan HCT Tablets 2196
Dyazide Capsules 1423
Hyzaar 50-12.5 Tablets 1990
Hyzaar 100-12.5 Tablets 1990
Hyzaar 100-25 Tablets 1990
Lopressor HCT 50/25 Tablets 2241
Lopressor HCT 100/25 Tablets 2241
Lopressor HCT 100/50 Tablets 2241
Lotensin HCT Tablets 2246
Micardis HCT Tablets 856
Moduretic Tablets 2028
Prinzide Tablets 2056
Teveten HCT Tablets 1737
Timolide Tablets 2086
Uniretic Tablets 3100

Hydroflumethiazide (Co-administration of enalapril in patients on diuretics, especially those in whom diuretic therapy was recently instituted, may occasionally experience excessive hypotension; antihypertensive effects of enalapril are augmented by antihypertensive agents that cause renin release).
No products indexed under this heading.

Ibuprofen (Co-administration with NSAIDs may diminish the antihypertensive effect of ACE inhibitors; potential for further deterioration of renal function in patients with compromised renal function when used concurrently). Products include:
Advil Allergy Sinus Caplets .... ▣770
Advil .... ▣674
Children's Advil Oral Suspension .... ▣603
Children's Advil Chewable Tablets .. ▣603
Advil Cold & Sinus .... ▣723
Infants' Advil Concentrated Drops .. ▣604
Infants' Advil Concentrated Drops - White Grape (Dye-Free).............. ▣604
Junior Strength Advil Swallow Tablets.. ▣605
Advil Migraine Liquigels .... ▣608
Advil Multi-Symptom Cold Caplets.. ▣770
Advil PM Caplets .... ▣615
Motrin IB Tablets and Caplets 1866
Children's Motrin Oral Suspension ... 1867
Children's Motrin Non-Staining Dye-Free Oral Suspension............ 1867
Children's Motrin Cold Oral Suspension 1867
Infants' Motrin Concentrated Drops.. 1867
Infants' Motrin Non-Staining Dye-Free Concentrated Drops....... 1867
Junior Strength Motrin Caplets and Chewable Tablets.................. 1867
Vicoprofen Tablets 539

Indapamide (Co-administration of enalapril in patients on diuretics, especially those in whom diuretic therapy was recently instituted, may occasionally experience excessive hypotension; antihypertensive effects of enalapril are augmented by antihypertensive agents that cause renin release). Products include:

Indomethacin (Co-administration with NSAIDs may diminish the antihypertensive effect of ACE inhibitors; potential for further deterioration of renal function in patients with compromised renal function when used concurrently). Products include:

Indomethacin Sodium Trihydrate (Co-administration with NSAIDs may diminish the antihypertensive effect of ACE inhibitors; potential for further deterioration of renal function in patients with compromised renal function when used concurrently). Products include:

Ketoprofen (Co-administration with NSAIDs may diminish the antihypertensive effect of ACE inhibitors; potential for further deterioration of renal function in patients with compromised renal function when used concurrently).
No products indexed under this heading.

Ketorolac Tromethamine (Co-administration with NSAIDs may diminish the antihypertensive effect of ACE inhibitors; potential for further deterioration of renal function in patients with compromised renal function when used concurrently). Products include:

Lithium (Co-administration of lithium with drugs that cause elimination of sodium, including ACE inhibitors, can lead to lithium toxicity).
No products indexed under this heading.

Lithium Carbonate (Co-administration of lithium with drugs that cause elimination of sodium, including ACE inhibitors, can lead to lithium toxicity). Products include:

Lithium Citrate (Co-administration of lithium with drugs that cause elimination of sodium, including ACE inhibitors, can lead to lithium toxicity).
No products indexed under this heading.

Meclofenamate Sodium (Co-administration with NSAIDs may diminish the antihypertensive effect of ACE inhibitors; potential for further deterioration of renal function in patients with compromised renal function when used concurrently).
No products indexed under this heading.

Mefenamic Acid (Co-administration with NSAIDs may diminish the antihypertensive effect of ACE inhibitors; potential for further deterioration of renal function in patients with compromised renal function when used concurrently).
No products indexed under this heading.

Meloxicam (Co-administration with NSAIDs may diminish the antihypertensive effect of ACE inhibitors; potential for further deterioration of renal function in patients with compromised renal function when used concurrently). Products include:

Methyclothiazide (Co-administration of enalapril in patients on diuretics, especially those in whom diuretic therapy was recently instituted, may occasionally experience excessive hypotension; antihypertensive effects of enalapril are augmented by antihypertensive agents that cause renin release).
No products indexed under this heading.

Metolazone (Co-administration of enalapril in patients on diuretics, especially those in whom diuretic therapy was recently instituted, may occasionally experience excessive hypotension; antihypertensive effects of enalapril are augmented by antihypertensive agents that cause renin release).
No products indexed under this heading.

Nabumetone (Co-administration with NSAIDs may diminish the antihypertensive effect of ACE inhibitors; potential for further deterioration of renal function in patients with compromised renal function when used concurrently).
No products indexed under this heading.

Naproxen (Co-administration with NSAIDs may diminish the antihypertensive effect of ACE inhibitors; potential for further deterioration of renal function in patients with compromised renal function when used concurrently). Products include:

Naproxen Sodium (Co-administration with NSAIDs may diminish the antihypertensive effect of ACE inhibitors; potential for further deterioration of renal function in patients with compromised renal function when used concurrently). Products include:

Oxaprozin (Co-administration with NSAIDs may diminish the antihypertensive effect of ACE inhibitors; potential for further deterioration of renal function in patients with compromised renal function when used concurrently).
No products indexed under this heading.

Phenylbutazone (Co-administration with NSAIDs may diminish the antihypertensive effect of ACE inhibitors; potential for further deterioration of renal function in patients with compromised renal function when used concurrently).
No products indexed under this heading.

Piroxicam (Co-administration with NSAIDs may diminish the antihypertensive effect of ACE inhibitors; potential for further deterioration of renal function in patients with compromised renal function when used concurrently).
No products indexed under this heading.

Polythiazide (Co-administration of enalapril in patients on diuretics, especially those in whom diuretic therapy was recently instituted, may occasionally experience excessive hypotension; antihypertensive effects of enalapril are augmented by antihypertensive agents that cause renin release).
No products indexed under this heading.

Potassium Acid Phosphate (Concomitant use of potassium-containing salt substitute or potassium supplements can lead to hyperkalemia; frequent monitoring of serum potassium is recommended if used concurrently). Products include:

Potassium Bicarbonate (Concomitant use of potassium-containing salt substitute or potassium supplements can lead to hyperkalemia; frequent monitoring of serum potassium is recommended if used concurrently).
No products indexed under this heading.

Potassium Chloride (Concomitant use of potassium-containing salt substitute or potassium supplements can lead to hyperkalemia; frequent monitoring of serum potassium is recommended if used concurrently). Products include:

Potassium Citrate (Concomitant use of potassium-containing salt substitute or potassium supplements can lead to hyperkalemia; frequent monitoring of serum potassium is recommended if used concurrently). Products include:

Potassium Gluconate (Concomitant use of potassium-containing salt substitute or potassium supplements can lead to hyperkalemia; frequent monitoring of serum potassium is recommended if used concurrently).
No products indexed under this heading.

Potassium Phosphate (Concomitant use of potassium-containing salt substitute or potassium supplements can lead to hyperkalemia; frequent monitoring of serum potassium is recommended if used concurrently). Products include:

Rofecoxib (Co-administration with NSAIDs may diminish the antihypertensive effect of ACE inhibitors; potential for further deterioration of renal function in patients with compromised renal function when used concurrently).
No products indexed under this heading.

Spironolactone (Enalapril attenuates diuretic-induced potassium loss; concomitant use can lead to hyperkalemia; frequent monitoring of serum potassium is recommended if used concurrently; co-administration can result in excessive hypotension).
No products indexed under this heading.

Sulindac (Co-administration with NSAIDs may diminish the antihypertensive effect of ACE inhibitors; potential for further deterioration of renal function in patients with compromised renal function when used concurrently). Products include:

Tolmetin Sodium (Co-administration with NSAIDs may diminish the antihypertensive effect of ACE inhibitors; potential for further deterioration of renal function in patients with compromised renal function when used concurrently).
No products indexed under this heading.

Torsemide (Co-administration of enalapril in patients on diuretics, especially those in whom diuretic therapy was recently instituted, may occasionally experience excessive hypotension; antihypertensive effects of enalapril are augmented by antihypertensive agents that cause renin release). Products include:

Triamterene (Enalapril attenuates diuretic-induced potassium loss; concomitant use can lead to hyperkalemia; frequent monitoring of serum potassium is recommended if used concurrently; co-administration can result in excessive hypotension). Products include:

Valdecoxib (Co-administration with NSAIDs may diminish the antihypertensive effect of ACE inhibitors; potential for further deterioration of renal function in patients with compromised renal function when used concurrently).
No products indexed under this heading.

VELCADE FOR INJECTION

May interact with cytochrome p450 2c19 substrates (selected), cytochrome p450 3a4 inducers (selected), cytochrome p450 3a4 inhibitors (selected), and oral hypoglycemic agents. Compounds in these categories include:

Acarbose (Patients on oral antidiabetic agents receiving bortezomib treatment may require close monitoring of their blood glucose levels and adjustment of the dose of their antidiabetic medication; during clinical trials, hypoglycemia and hyperglycemia were reported in diabetic patients receiving oral hypoglycemics). Products include:

Acetazolamide (Patients who are concomitantly receiving Velcade and drugs that are inhibitors or inducers of cytochrome P450 3A4 should be closely monitored for either toxicities or reduced efficacy).
No products indexed under this heading.

Allium sativum (Patients who are concomitantly receiving Velcade and drugs that are inhibitors or inducers of cytochrome P450 3A4 should be closely monitored for either toxicities or reduced efficacy).
No products indexed under this heading.

Amiodarone Hydrochloride (Patients who are concomitantly receiving Velcade and drugs that are inhibitors or inducers of cytochrome P450 3A4 should be closely monitored for either toxicities or reduced efficacy).
No products indexed under this heading.

Amitriptyline Hydrochloride (Bortezomib may inhibit 2C19 activity and increase exposure to drugs that are substrates for this enzyme).
No products indexed under this heading.

Amoxapine (Bortezomib may inhibit 2C19 activity and increase exposure to drugs that are substrates for this enzyme).
No products indexed under this heading.

Amprenavir (Patients who are concomitantly receiving Velcade and drugs that are inhibitors or inducers of cytochrome P450 3A4 should be closely monitored for either toxicities or reduced efficacy). Products include:
Agenerase Capsules **1327**
Agenerase Oral Solution **1332**

Anastrozole (Patients who are concomitantly receiving Velcade and drugs that are inhibitors or inducers of cytochrome P450 3A4 should be closely monitored for either toxicities or reduced efficacy). Products include:
Arimidex Tablets **673**

Aprepitant (Patients who are concomitantly receiving Velcade and drugs that are inhibitors or inducers of cytochrome P450 3A4 should be closely monitored for either toxicities or reduced efficacy). Products include:
Emend Capsules **1963**

Betamethasone Acetate (Patients who are concomitantly receiving Velcade and drugs that are inhibitors or inducers of cytochrome P450 3A4 should be closely monitored for either toxicities or reduced efficacy).
No products indexed under this heading.

Betamethasone Sodium Phosphate (Patients who are concomitantly receiving Velcade and drugs that are inhibitors or inducers of cytochrome P450 3A4 should be closely monitored for either toxicities or reduced efficacy).
No products indexed under this heading.

Carbamazepine (Patients who are concomitantly receiving Velcade and drugs that are inhibitors or inducers of cytochrome P450 3A4 should be closely monitored for either toxicities or reduced efficacy). Products include:
Carbatrol Capsules **3171**
Equetro Extended-Release Capsules **3180**
Tegretol/Tegretol-XR **2295**

Carisoprodol (Bortezomib may inhibit 2C19 activity and increase exposure to drugs that are substrates for this enzyme).
No products indexed under this heading.

Chlorpropamide (Patients on oral antidiabetic agents receiving bortezomib treatment may require close monitoring of their blood glucose levels and adjustment of the dose of their antidiabetic medication; during clinical trials, hypoglycemia and hyperglycemia were reported in diabetic patients receiving oral hypoglycemics).
No products indexed under this heading.

Cilostazol (Bortezomib may inhibit 2C19 activity and increase exposure to drugs that are substrates for this enzyme). Products include:
Pletal Tablets **2455**

Cimetidine (Patients who are concomitantly receiving Velcade and drugs that are inhibitors or inducers of cytochrome P450 3A4 should be closely monitored for either toxicities or reduced efficacy). Products include:
Tagamet HB 200 Tablets .... ▣**664**

Cimetidine Hydrochloride (Patients who are concomitantly receiving Velcade and drugs that are inhibitors or inducers of cytochrome P450 3A4 should be closely monitored for either toxicities or reduced efficacy).
No products indexed under this heading.

Ciprofloxacin (Patients who are concomitantly receiving Velcade and drugs that are inhibitors or inducers of cytochrome P450 3A4 should be closely monitored for either toxicities or reduced efficacy). Products include:
Cipro Oral Suspension **2977**
Cipro I.V. **2984**
Cipro XR Tablets **2990**
Ciprodex Otic Suspension **559**

Ciprofloxacin Hydrochloride (Patients who are concomitantly receiving Velcade and drugs that are inhibitors or inducers of cytochrome P450 3A4 should be closely monitored for either toxicities or reduced efficacy). Products include:
Ciloxan Ophthalmic Ointment **559**
Ciloxan Ophthalmic Solution .... ⊙**206**
Cipro Tablets **2977**
Proquin XR Tablets **1153**

Cisplatin (Patients who are concomitantly receiving Velcade and drugs that are inhibitors or inducers of cytochrome P450 3A4 should be closely monitored for either toxicities or reduced efficacy).
No products indexed under this heading.

Citalopram Hydrobromide (Bortezomib may inhibit 2C19 activity and increase exposure to drugs that are substrates for this enzyme). Products include:
Celexa **1176**

Clarithromycin (Patients who are concomitantly receiving Velcade and drugs that are inhibitors or inducers of cytochrome P450 3A4 should be closely monitored for either toxicities or reduced efficacy). Products include:
Biaxin/Biaxin XL **402**
PREVPAC **3284**

Clomipramine Hydrochloride (Bortezomib may inhibit 2C19 activity and increase exposure to drugs that are substrates for this enzyme).
No products indexed under this heading.

Clotrimazole (Patients who are concomitantly receiving Velcade and drugs that are inhibitors or inducers of cytochrome P450 3A4 should be closely monitored for either toxicities or reduced efficacy). Products include:
Desenex Athlete's Foot Cream .... ▣**635**
Lotrimin **3039**
Lotrisone **3040**

Cortisone Acetate (Patients who are concomitantly receiving Velcade and drugs that are inhibitors or inducers of cytochrome P450 3A4 should be closely monitored for either toxicities or reduced efficacy).
No products indexed under this heading.

Cyclophosphamide (Bortezomib may inhibit 2C19 activity and increase exposure to drugs that are substrates for this enzyme).
No products indexed under this heading.

Cyclosporine (Patients who are concomitantly receiving Velcade and drugs that are inhibitors or inducers of cytochrome P450 3A4 should be closely monitored for either toxicities or reduced efficacy). Products include:
Gengraf Capsules **459**
Neoral Oral Solution **2259**
Neoral Soft Gelatin Capsules **2259**
Restasis Ophthalmic Emulsion **575**
Sandimmune **2275**

Dalfopristin (Patients who are concomitantly receiving Velcade and drugs that are inhibitors or inducers of cytochrome P450 3A4 should be closely monitored for either toxicities or reduced efficacy).
No products indexed under this heading.

Danazol (Patients who are concomitantly receiving Velcade and drugs that are inhibitors or inducers of cytochrome P450 3A4 should be closely monitored for either toxicities or reduced efficacy).
No products indexed under this heading.

Delavirdine Mesylate (Patients who are concomitantly receiving Velcade and drugs that are inhibitors or inducers of cytochrome P450 3A4 should be closely monitored for either toxicities or reduced efficacy). Products include:
Rescriptor Tablets **2551**

Desipramine Hydrochloride (Bortezomib may inhibit 2C19 activity and increase exposure to drugs that are substrates for this enzyme).
No products indexed under this heading.

Dexamethasone (Patients who are concomitantly receiving Velcade and drugs that are inhibitors or inducers of cytochrome P450 3A4 should be closely monitored for either toxicities or reduced efficacy). Products include:
Ciprodex Otic Suspension **559**
Decadron Tablets **1951**
TobraDex Ophthalmic Ointment **562**
TobraDex Ophthalmic Suspension **563**

Dexamethasone Acetate (Patients who are concomitantly receiving Velcade and drugs that are inhibitors or inducers of cytochrome P450 3A4 should be closely monitored for either toxicities or reduced efficacy).
No products indexed under this heading.

Dexamethasone Sodium Phosphate (Patients who are concomitantly receiving Velcade and drugs that are inhibitors or inducers of cytochrome P450 3A4 should be closely monitored for either toxicities or reduced efficacy).
No products indexed under this heading.

Dextromethorphan (Bortezomib may inhibit 2C19 activity and increase exposure to drugs that are substrates for this enzyme).
No products indexed under this heading.

Dextromethorphan Hydrobromide (Bortezomib may inhibit 2C19 activity and increase exposure to drugs that are substrates for this enzyme). Products include:
Comtrex Maximum Strength Cold & Cough Day/Night Caplets - Day Formulation .... ▣**726**
Comtrex Maximum Strength Cold & Cough Day/Night Caplets - Night Formulation .... ▣**726**
Comtrex Maximum Strength Non-Drowsy Cold & Cough Caplets .... ▣**725**
Children's Dimetapp DM Cold & Cough Elixir .... ▣**731**
Children's Dimetapp Long Acting Cough Plus Cold Syrup .... ▣**731**
Toddler's Dimetapp Cold and Cough Drops .... ▣**732**
Mucinex DM Extended-Release Bi-Layer Tablets .... ▣**720**
Refenesen DM Caplets .... ▣**721**
Robitussin Cough & Cold CF Liquid .... ▣**735**
Robitussin Cough & Cold Long-Acting Liquid .... ▣**735**
Robitussin Cough & Allergy Syrup .. ▣**736**
Robitussin Cough & Cold Nighttime Liquid .... ▣**736**
Robitussin Cough & Cold Pediatric Drops .... ▣**735**
Robitussin Cough, Cold & Flu Nighttime Liquid .... ▣**738**
Robitussin Cough & Congestion Liquid .... ▣**738**
Robitussin Cough Gels Long-Acting .... ▣**737**
Robitussin Cough Long Acting Liquid .... ▣**739**
Robitussin Cough DM Syrup .... ▣**738**
Robitussin Cough DM Infant Drops .... ▣**738**
Robitussin Pediatric Cough Long Acting Liquid .... ▣**739**
Robitussin Pediatric Cough & Cold Long-Acting Liquid .... ▣**735**
Robitussin Pediatric Cough & Cold Nighttime Liquid .... ▣**736**
Robitussin Sugar Free Cough .... ▣**738**
TheraFlu Cold & Cough Hot Liquid .... ▣**740**
TheraFlu Warming Relief Daytime Severe Cold .... ▣**743**
TheraFlu Thin Strips Long Acting Cough .... ▣**744**
Triaminic Daytime Cold & Cough Liquid .... ▣**745**
Triaminic Cough & Sore Throat Liquid .... ▣**747**
Triaminic Cough & Runny Nose Softchews .... ▣**748**
Triaminic Thin Strips Cold & Cough .... ▣**778**
Triaminic Infant Thin Strips Decongestant Plus Cough .... ▣**747**
Children's Tylenol Plus Flu Oral Suspension .... ▣**749**

Diazepam (Bortezomib may inhibit 2C19 activity and increase exposure to drugs that are substrates for this enzyme). Products include:

Diltiazem Hydrochloride (Patients who are concomitantly receiving Vel-

cade and drugs that are inhibitors or inducers of cytochrome P450 3A4 should be closely monitored for either toxicities or reduced efficacy). Products include:

Diltiazem Maleate (Patients who are concomitantly receiving Velcade and drugs that are inhibitors or inducers of cytochrome P450 3A4 should be closely monitored for either toxicities or reduced efficacy).
No products indexed under this heading.

Divalproex Sodium (Bortezomib may inhibit 2C19 activity and increase exposure to drugs that are substrates for this enzyme). Products include:

Doxepin Hydrochloride (Bortezomib may inhibit 2C19 activity and increase exposure to drugs that are substrates for this enzyme).
No products indexed under this heading.

Doxorubicin Hydrochloride (Patients who are concomitantly receiving Velcade and drugs that are inhibitors or inducers of cytochrome P450 3A4 should be closely monitored for either toxicities or reduced efficacy).
No products indexed under this heading.

Efavirenz (Patients who are concomitantly receiving Velcade and drugs that are inhibitors or inducers of cytochrome P450 3A4 should be closely monitored for either toxicities or reduced efficacy). Products include:

Erythromycin (Patients who are concomitantly receiving Velcade and drugs that are inhibitors or inducers of cytochrome P450 3A4 should be closely monitored for either toxicities or reduced efficacy). Products include:

Erythromycin Estolate (Patients who are concomitantly receiving Velcade and drugs that are inhibitors or inducers of cytochrome P450 3A4 should be closely monitored for either toxicities or reduced efficacy).
No products indexed under this heading.

Erythromycin Ethylsuccinate (Patients who are concomitantly receiving Velcade and drugs that are inhibitors or inducers of cytochrome P450 3A4 should be closely monitored for either toxicities or reduced efficacy). Products include:

Erythromycin Gluceptate (Patients who are concomitantly receiving Velcade and drugs that are inhibitors or inducers of cytochrome P450 3A4 should be closely monitored for either toxicities or reduced efficacy).
No products indexed under this heading.

Erythromycin Lactobionate (Patients who are concomitantly receiving Velcade and drugs that are inhibitors or inducers of cytochrome P450 3A4 should be closely monitored for either toxicities or reduced efficacy).
No products indexed under this heading.

Erythromycin Stearate (Patients who are concomitantly receiving Velcade and drugs that are inhibitors or inducers of cytochrome P450 3A4 should be closely monitored for either toxicities or reduced efficacy). Products include:

Esomeprazole Magnesium (Patients who are concomitantly receiving Velcade and drugs that are inhibitors or inducers of cytochrome P450 3A4 should be closely monitored for either toxicities or reduced efficacy). Products include:

Ethosuximide (Patients who are concomitantly receiving Velcade and drugs that are inhibitors or inducers of cytochrome P450 3A4 should be closely monitored for either toxicities or reduced efficacy).
No products indexed under this heading.

Ethotoin (Bortezomib may inhibit 2C19 activity and increase exposure to drugs that are substrates for this enzyme).
No products indexed under this heading.

Felbamate (Patients who are concomitantly receiving Velcade and drugs that are inhibitors or inducers of cytochrome P450 3A4 should be closely monitored for either toxicities or reduced efficacy).
No products indexed under this heading.

Fluconazole (Patients who are concomitantly receiving Velcade and drugs that are inhibitors or inducers of cytochrome P450 3A4 should be closely monitored for either toxicities or reduced efficacy).
No products indexed under this heading.

Fludrocortisone Acetate (Patients who are concomitantly receiving Velcade and drugs that are inhibitors or inducers of cytochrome P450 3A4 should be closely monitored for either toxicities or reduced efficacy).
No products indexed under this heading.

Fluoxetine Hydrochloride (Patients who are concomitantly receiving Velcade and drugs that are inhibitors or inducers of cytochrome P450 3A4 should be closely monitored for either toxicities or reduced efficacy). Products include:

Fluvoxamine Maleate (Patients who are concomitantly receiving Velcade and drugs that are inhibitors or inducers of cytochrome P450 3A4 should be closely monitored for either toxicities or reduced efficacy).
No products indexed under this heading.

Formoterol Fumarate (Bortezomib may inhibit 2C19 activity and increase exposure to drugs that are substrates for this enzyme).
Products include:

Fosamprenavir Calcium (Patients who are concomitantly receiving Velcade and drugs that are inhibitors or inducers of cytochrome P450 3A4 should be closely monitored for either toxicities or reduced efficacy). Products include:

Fosphenytoin (Bortezomib may inhibit 2C19 activity and increase exposure to drugs that are substrates for this enzyme).
No products indexed under this heading.

Fosphenytoin Sodium (Patients who are concomitantly receiving Velcade and drugs that are inhibitors or inducers of cytochrome P450 3A4 should be closely monitored for either toxicities or reduced efficacy).
No products indexed under this heading.

Gabapentin (Bortezomib may inhibit 2C19 activity and increase exposure to drugs that are substrates for this enzyme). Products include:

Garlic Extract (Patients who are concomitantly receiving Velcade and drugs that are inhibitors or inducers of cytochrome P450 3A4 should be closely monitored for either toxicities or reduced efficacy).
No products indexed under this heading.

Garlic Oil (Patients who are concomitantly receiving Velcade and drugs that are inhibitors or inducers of cytochrome P450 3A4 should be closely monitored for either toxicities or reduced efficacy).
No products indexed under this heading.

Glimepiride (Patients on oral antidiabetic agents receiving bortezomib treatment may require close monitoring of their blood glucose levels and adjustment of the dose of their antidiabetic medication; during clinical trials, hypoglycemia and hyperglycemia were reported in diabetic patients receiving oral hypoglycemics). Products include:

Glipizide (Patients on oral antidiabetic agents receiving bortezomib treatment may require close monitoring of their blood glucose levels and adjustment of the dose of their antidiabetic medication; during clinical trials, hypoglycemia and hyperglycemia were reported in diabetic patients receiving oral hypoglycemics).
No products indexed under this heading.

Glyburide (Patients on oral antidiabetic agents receiving bortezomib treatment may require close monitoring of their blood glucose levels and adjustment of the dose of their antidiabetic medication; during clinical trials, hypoglycemia and hyperglycemia were reported in diabetic patients receiving oral hypoglycemics).
No products indexed under this heading.

Hydrocortisone (Patients who are concomitantly receiving Velcade and drugs that are inhibitors or inducers of cytochrome P450 3A4 should be

closely monitored for either toxicities or reduced efficacy). Products include:
Colocort Rectal Suspension, USP (Retention) 100 mg/60 mL 2476
Hydrocortone Tablets 1989
Preparation H Hydrocortisone Cream .... ▣646

Hydrocortisone Acetate (Patients who are concomitantly receiving Velcade and drugs that are inhibitors or inducers of cytochrome P450 3A4 should be closely monitored for either toxicities or reduced efficacy). Products include:
Analpram-HC 1159
Pramosone 1161
ProctoFoam-HC 3099

Hydrocortisone Butyrate (Patients who are concomitantly receiving Velcade and drugs that are inhibitors or inducers of cytochrome P450 3A4 should be closely monitored for either toxicities or reduced efficacy). Products include:
Locoid Lipocream Cream 1160

Hydrocortisone Cypionate (Patients who are concomitantly receiving Velcade and drugs that are inhibitors or inducers of cytochrome P450 3A4 should be closely monitored for either toxicities or reduced efficacy).
No products indexed under this heading.

Hydrocortisone Hemisuccinate (Patients who are concomitantly receiving Velcade and drugs that are inhibitors or inducers of cytochrome P450 3A4 should be closely monitored for either toxicities or reduced efficacy).
No products indexed under this heading.

Hydrocortisone Probutate (Patients who are concomitantly receiving Velcade and drugs that are inhibitors or inducers of cytochrome P450 3A4 should be closely monitored for either toxicities or reduced efficacy).
No products indexed under this heading.

Hydrocortisone Sodium Phosphate (Patients who are concomitantly receiving Velcade and drugs that are inhibitors or inducers of cytochrome P450 3A4 should be closely monitored for either toxicities or reduced efficacy).
No products indexed under this heading.

Hydrocortisone Sodium Succinate (Patients who are concomitantly receiving Velcade and drugs that are inhibitors or inducers of cytochrome P450 3A4 should be closely monitored for either toxicities or reduced efficacy).
No products indexed under this heading.

Hydrocortisone Valerate (Patients who are concomitantly receiving Velcade and drugs that are inhibitors or inducers of cytochrome P450 3A4 should be closely monitored for either toxicities or reduced efficacy).
No products indexed under this heading.

Hypericum (Patients who are concomitantly receiving Velcade and drugs that are inhibitors or inducers of cytochrome P450 3A4 should be closely monitored for either toxicities or reduced efficacy). Products include:
Satiete Tablets .... ▣832

Hypericum Perforatum (Patients who are concomitantly receiving Velcade and drugs that are inhibitors or inducers of cytochrome P450 3A4 should be closely monitored for either toxicities or reduced efficacy).
No products indexed under this heading.

Imipramine Hydrochloride (Bortezomib may inhibit 2C19 activity and increase exposure to drugs that are substrates for this enzyme).
No products indexed under this heading.

Imipramine Pamoate (Bortezomib may inhibit 2C19 activity and increase exposure to drugs that are substrates for this enzyme).
No products indexed under this heading.

Indinavir Sulfate (Patients who are concomitantly receiving Velcade and drugs that are inhibitors or inducers of cytochrome P450 3A4 should be closely monitored for either toxicities or reduced efficacy). Products include:
Crixivan Capsules 1940

Indomethacin (Bortezomib may inhibit 2C19 activity and increase exposure to drugs that are substrates for this enzyme). Products include:
Indocin 1995

Indomethacin Sodium Trihydrate (Bortezomib may inhibit 2C19 activity and increase exposure to drugs that are substrates for this enzyme). Products include:
Indocin I.V. 2465

Isoniazid (Patients who are concomitantly receiving Velcade and drugs that are inhibitors or inducers of cytochrome P450 3A4 should be closely monitored for either toxicities or reduced efficacy).
No products indexed under this heading.

Itraconazole (Patients who are concomitantly receiving Velcade and drugs that are inhibitors or inducers of cytochrome P450 3A4 should be closely monitored for either toxicities or reduced efficacy).
No products indexed under this heading.

Ketoconazole (Patients who are concomitantly receiving Velcade and drugs that are inhibitors or inducers of cytochrome P450 3A4 should be closely monitored for either toxicities or reduced efficacy). Products include:
Nizoral A-D Shampoo, 1% 1868

Lamotrigine (Bortezomib may inhibit 2C19 activity and increase exposure to drugs that are substrates for this enzyme). Products include:
Lamictal 1481

Lansoprazole (Bortezomib may inhibit 2C19 activity and increase exposure to drugs that are substrates for this enzyme). Products include:
Prevacid Delayed-Release Capsules 3271
Prevacid for Delayed-Release Oral Suspension 3271
Prevacid SoluTab Delayed-Release Orally Disintegrating Tablets 3271
Prevacid I.V. for Injection 3277
Prevacid NapraPAC 3280
PREVPAC 3284

Levetiracetam (Bortezomib may inhibit 2C19 activity and increase exposure to drugs that are substrates for this enzyme). Products include:
Keppra Injection 3320
Keppra Oral Solution 3314
Keppra Tablets 3314

Lopinavir (Patients who are concomitantly receiving Velcade and drugs that are inhibitors or inducers of cytochrome P450 3A4 should be closely monitored for either toxicities or reduced efficacy). Products include:
Kaletra 476

Loratadine (Patients who are concomitantly receiving Velcade and drugs that are inhibitors or inducers of cytochrome P450 3A4 should be closely monitored for either toxicities or reduced efficacy). Products include:
Alavert Allergy & Sinus D-12 Hour Tablets .... ▣771
Alavert .... ▣771
Children's Claritin Allergy Oral Solution .... ▣771
Claritin Non-Drowsy 24 Hour Tablets .... ▣772
Claritin Reditabs 24 Hour Non-Drowsy Tablets .... ▣772
Claritin-D Non-Drowsy 12 Hour Tablets .... ▣772
Claritin-D Non-Drowsy 24 Hour Tablets .... ▣772

Maprotiline Hydrochloride (Bortezomib may inhibit 2C19 activity and increase exposure to drugs that are substrates for this enzyme).
No products indexed under this heading.

Mephenytoin (Patients who are concomitantly receiving Velcade and drugs that are inhibitors or inducers of cytochrome P450 3A4 should be closely monitored for either toxicities or reduced efficacy).
No products indexed under this heading.

Mephobarbital (Bortezomib may inhibit 2C19 activity and increase exposure to drugs that are substrates for this enzyme).
No products indexed under this heading.

Meprobamate (Bortezomib may inhibit 2C19 activity and increase exposure to drugs that are substrates for this enzyme).
No products indexed under this heading.

Metformin Hydrochloride (Patients on oral antidiabetic agents receiving bortezomib treatment may require close monitoring of their blood glucose levels and adjustment of the dose of their antidiabetic medication; during clinical trials, hypoglycemia and hyperglycemia were reported in diabetic patients receiving oral hypoglycemics). Products include:
ActoPlus Met Tablets 3214
Avandamet Tablets 1373
Fortamet Extended-Release Tablets 3115

Methsuximide (Patients who are concomitantly receiving Velcade and drugs that are inhibitors or inducers of cytochrome P450 3A4 should be closely monitored for either toxicities or reduced efficacy).
No products indexed under this heading.

Methylprednisolone (Patients who are concomitantly receiving Velcade and drugs that are inhibitors or inducers of cytochrome P450 3A4 should be closely monitored for either toxicities or reduced efficacy).
No products indexed under this heading.

Methylprednisolone Acetate (Patients who are concomitantly receiving Velcade and drugs that are inhibitors or inducers of cytochrome P450 3A4 should be closely monitored for either toxicities or reduced efficacy). Products include:
Depo-Medrol Injectable Suspension 2617
Depo-Medrol Single-Dose Vial 2619

Methylprednisolone Sodium Succinate (Patients who are concomitantly receiving Velcade and drugs that are inhibitors or inducers of cytochrome P450 3A4 should be closely monitored for either toxicities or reduced efficacy).
No products indexed under this heading.

Metronidazole (Patients who are concomitantly receiving Velcade and drugs that are inhibitors or inducers of cytochrome P450 3A4 should be closely monitored for either toxicities or reduced efficacy). Products include:
Metrogel 1% 1211
MetroGel-Vaginal Gel 1855
Vandazole Vaginal Gel 3338

Metronidazole Benzoate (Patients who are concomitantly receiving Velcade and drugs that are inhibitors or inducers of cytochrome P450 3A4 should be closely monitored for either toxicities or reduced efficacy).
No products indexed under this heading.

Metronidazole Hydrochloride (Patients who are concomitantly receiving Velcade and drugs that are inhibitors or inducers of cytochrome P450 3A4 should be closely monitored for either toxicities or reduced efficacy).
No products indexed under this heading.

Miconazole (Patients who are concomitantly receiving Velcade and drugs that are inhibitors or inducers of cytochrome P450 3A4 should be closely monitored for either toxicities or reduced efficacy).
No products indexed under this heading.

Miconazole Nitrate (Patients who are concomitantly receiving Velcade and drugs that are inhibitors or inducers of cytochrome P450 3A4 should be closely monitored for either toxicities or reduced efficacy). Products include:
Desenex .... ▣635
Desenex Jock Itch Spray Powder .... ▣635

Midazolam Hydrochloride (Bortezomib may inhibit 2C19 activity and increase exposure to drugs that are substrates for this enzyme).
No products indexed under this heading.

Miglitol (Patients on oral antidiabetic agents receiving bortezomib treatment may require close monitoring of their blood glucose levels and adjustment of the dose of their antidiabetic medication; during clinical trials, hypoglycemia and hyperglycemia were reported in diabetic patients receiving oral hypoglycemics).
No products indexed under this heading.

Modafinil (Patients who are concomitantly receiving Velcade and drugs that are inhibitors or inducers of cytochrome P450 3A4 should be closely monitored for either toxicities or reduced efficacy). Products include:

Nefazodone Hydrochloride (Patients who are concomitantly receiving Velcade and drugs that are inhibitors or inducers of cytochrome P450 3A4 should be closely monitored for either toxicities or reduced efficacy).
No products indexed under this heading.

Nelfinavir Mesylate (Patients who are concomitantly receiving Velcade and drugs that are inhibitors or inducers of cytochrome P450 3A4 should be closely monitored for either toxicities or reduced efficacy). Products include:

Nevirapine (Patients who are concomitantly receiving Velcade and drugs that are inhibitors or inducers of cytochrome P450 3A4 should be closely monitored for either toxicities or reduced efficacy). Products include:

Niacinamide (Patients who are concomitantly receiving Velcade and drugs that are inhibitors or inducers of cytochrome P450 3A4 should be closely monitored for either toxicities or reduced efficacy).
No products indexed under this heading.

Nicotinamide (Patients who are concomitantly receiving Velcade and drugs that are inhibitors or inducers of cytochrome P450 3A4 should be closely monitored for either toxicities or reduced efficacy). Products include:

Nifedipine (Patients who are concomitantly receiving Velcade and drugs that are inhibitors or inducers of cytochrome P450 3A4 should be closely monitored for either toxicities or reduced efficacy). Products include:

Nilutamide (Bortezomib may inhibit 2C19 activity and increase exposure to drugs that are substrates for this enzyme).
No products indexed under this heading.

Norfloxacin (Patients who are concomitantly receiving Velcade and drugs that are inhibitors or inducers of cytochrome P450 3A4 should be closely monitored for either toxicities or reduced efficacy). Products include:

Nortriptyline Hydrochloride (Bortezomib may inhibit 2C19 activity and increase exposure to drugs that are substrates for this enzyme).
No products indexed under this heading.

Omeprazole (Patients who are concomitantly receiving Velcade and drugs that are inhibitors or inducers of cytochrome P450 3A4 should be closely monitored for either toxicities or reduced efficacy). Products include:

Oxcarbazepine (Patients who are concomitantly receiving Velcade and drugs that are inhibitors or inducers of cytochrome P450 3A4 should be closely monitored for either toxicities or reduced efficacy). Products include:

Pantoprazole Sodium (Bortezomib may inhibit 2C19 activity and increase exposure to drugs that are substrates for this enzyme). Products include:

Paramethadione (Bortezomib may inhibit 2C19 activity and increase exposure to drugs that are substrates for this enzyme).
No products indexed under this heading.

Paroxetine Hydrochloride (Patients who are concomitantly receiving Velcade and drugs that are inhibitors or inducers of cytochrome P450 3A4 should be closely monitored for either toxicities or reduced efficacy). Products include:

Pentamidine Isethionate (Bortezomib may inhibit 2C19 activity and increase exposure to drugs that are substrates for this enzyme).
No products indexed under this heading.

Phenacemide (Bortezomib may inhibit 2C19 activity and increase exposure to drugs that are substrates for this enzyme).
No products indexed under this heading.

Phenobarbital (Patients who are concomitantly receiving Velcade and drugs that are inhibitors or inducers of cytochrome P450 3A4 should be closely monitored for either toxicities or reduced efficacy). Products include:

Phenobarbital Sodium (Patients who are concomitantly receiving Velcade and drugs that are inhibitors or inducers of cytochrome P450 3A4 should be closely monitored for either toxicities or reduced efficacy).
No products indexed under this heading.

Phensuximide (Bortezomib may inhibit 2C19 activity and increase exposure to drugs that are substrates for this enzyme).
No products indexed under this heading.

Phenytoin (Patients who are concomitantly receiving Velcade and drugs that are inhibitors or inducers of cytochrome P450 3A4 should be closely monitored for either toxicities or reduced efficacy).
No products indexed under this heading.

Phenytoin Sodium (Patients who are concomitantly receiving Velcade and drugs that are inhibitors or inducers of cytochrome P450 3A4 should be closely monitored for either toxicities or reduced efficacy). Products include:

Pioglitazone Hydrochloride (Patients on oral antidiabetic agents receiving bortezomib treatment may require close monitoring of their blood glucose levels and adjustment of the dose of their antidiabetic medication; during clinical trials, hypoglycemia and hyperglycemia were reported in diabetic patients receiving oral hypoglycemics). Products include:

Prednisolone Acetate (Patients who are concomitantly receiving Velcade and drugs that are inhibitors or inducers of cytochrome P450 3A4 should be closely monitored for either toxicities or reduced efficacy). Products include:

Prednisolone Sodium Phosphate (Patients who are concomitantly receiving Velcade and drugs that are inhibitors or inducers of cytochrome P450 3A4 should be closely monitored for either toxicities or reduced efficacy).
No products indexed under this heading.

Prednisolone Tebutate (Patients who are concomitantly receiving Velcade and drugs that are inhibitors or inducers of cytochrome P450 3A4 should be closely monitored for either toxicities or reduced efficacy).
No products indexed under this heading.

Prednisone (Patients who are concomitantly receiving Velcade and drugs that are inhibitors or inducers of cytochrome P450 3A4 should be closely monitored for either toxicities or reduced efficacy).
No products indexed under this heading.

Primidone (Patients who are concomitantly receiving Velcade and drugs that are inhibitors or inducers of cytochrome P450 3A4 should be closely monitored for either toxicities or reduced efficacy).
No products indexed under this heading.

Progesterone (Bortezomib may inhibit 2C19 activity and increase exposure to drugs that are substrates for this enzyme). Products include:

Proguanil Hydrochloride (Bortezomib may inhibit 2C19 activity and increase exposure to drugs that are substrates for this enzyme). Products include:

Propoxyphene Hydrochloride (Patients who are concomitantly receiving Velcade and drugs that are inhibitors or inducers of cytochrome P450 3A4 should be closely monitored for either toxicities or reduced efficacy).
No products indexed under this heading.

Propoxyphene Napsylate (Patients who are concomitantly receiving Velcade and drugs that are inhibitors or inducers of cytochrome P450 3A4 should be closely monitored for either toxicities or reduced efficacy).
No products indexed under this heading.

Propranolol Hydrochloride (Bortezomib may inhibit 2C19 activity and increase exposure to drugs that are substrates for this enzyme). Products include:

Protriptyline Hydrochloride (Bortezomib may inhibit 2C19 activity and increase exposure to drugs that are substrates for this enzyme).
No products indexed under this heading.

Quinidine (Patients who are concomitantly receiving Velcade and drugs that are inhibitors or inducers of cytochrome P450 3A4 should be closely monitored for either toxicities or reduced efficacy).
No products indexed under this heading.

Quinidine Hydrochloride (Patients who are concomitantly receiving Velcade and drugs that are inhibitors or inducers of cytochrome P450 3A4 should be closely monitored for either toxicities or reduced efficacy).
No products indexed under this heading.

Quinidine Polygalacturonate (Patients who are concomitantly receiving Velcade and drugs that are inhibitors or inducers of cytochrome P450 3A4 should be closely monitored for either toxicities or reduced efficacy).
No products indexed under this heading.

Quinidine Sulfate (Patients who are concomitantly receiving Velcade and drugs that are inhibitors or inducers of cytochrome P450 3A4 should be closely monitored for either toxicities or reduced efficacy).
No products indexed under this heading.

Quinine (Patients who are concomitantly receiving Velcade and drugs that are inhibitors or inducers of cytochrome P450 3A4 should be closely monitored for either toxicities or reduced efficacy).
No products indexed under this heading.

IMPORTANT NOTE: Always consult each drug listing in the patient's regimen for possible interactions.

Quinine Sulfate (Patients who are concomitantly receiving Velcade and drugs that are inhibitors or inducers of cytochrome P450 3A4 should be closely monitored for either toxicities or reduced efficacy).

No products indexed under this heading.

Quinupristin (Patients who are concomitantly receiving Velcade and drugs that are inhibitors or inducers of cytochrome P450 3A4 should be closely monitored for either toxicities or reduced efficacy).

No products indexed under this heading.

Rabeprazole Sodium (Bortezomib may inhibit 2C19 activity and increase exposure to drugs that are substrates for this enzyme). Products include:

Aciphex Tablets 1090

Ranitidine Bismuth Citrate (Patients who are concomitantly receiving Velcade and drugs that are inhibitors or inducers of cytochrome P450 3A4 should be closely monitored for either toxicities or reduced efficacy).

No products indexed under this heading.

Ranitidine Hydrochloride (Patients who are concomitantly receiving Velcade and drugs that are inhibitors or inducers of cytochrome P450 3A4 should be closely monitored for either toxicities or reduced efficacy). Products include:

Zantac **1624**
Zantac Injection **1619**
Zantac Injection Pharmacy Bulk
Package **1622**

Repaglinide (Patients on oral antidiabetic agents receiving bortezomib treatment may require close monitoring of their blood glucose levels and adjustment of the dose of their antidiabetic medication; during clinical trials, hypoglycemia and hyperglycemia were reported in diabetic patients receiving oral hypoglycemics).

No products indexed under this heading.

Rifabutin (Patients who are concomitantly receiving Velcade and drugs that are inhibitors or inducers of cytochrome P450 3A4 should be closely monitored for either toxicities or reduced efficacy).

No products indexed under this heading.

Rifampicin (Patients who are concomitantly receiving Velcade and drugs that are inhibitors or inducers of cytochrome P450 3A4 should be closely monitored for either toxicities or reduced efficacy).

No products indexed under this heading.

Rifampin (Patients who are concomitantly receiving Velcade and drugs that are inhibitors or inducers of cytochrome P450 3A4 should be closely monitored for either toxicities or reduced efficacy).

No products indexed under this heading.

Rifapentine (Patients who are concomitantly receiving Velcade and drugs that are inhibitors or inducers of cytochrome P450 3A4 should be closely monitored for either toxicities or reduced efficacy).

No products indexed under this heading.

Ritonavir (Patients who are concomitantly receiving Velcade and drugs that are inhibitors or inducers of cytochrome P450 3A4 should be closely monitored for either toxicities or reduced efficacy). Products include:

Kaletra 476
Norvir .. 503

Rosiglitazone Maleate (Patients on oral antidiabetic agents receiving bortezomib treatment may require close monitoring of their blood glucose levels and adjustment of the dose of their antidiabetic medication; during clinical trials, hypoglycemia and hyperglycemia were reported in diabetic patients receiving oral hypoglycemics). Products include:

Avandamet Tablets **1373**
Avandaryl Tablets **1379**
Avandia Tablets **1384**

Saquinavir (Patients who are concomitantly receiving Velcade and drugs that are inhibitors or inducers of cytochrome P450 3A4 should be closely monitored for either toxicities or reduced efficacy).

No products indexed under this heading.

Saquinavir Mesylate (Patients who are concomitantly receiving Velcade and drugs that are inhibitors or inducers of cytochrome P450 3A4 should be closely monitored for either toxicities or reduced efficacy). Products include:

Invirase **2772**

Sertraline Hydrochloride (Patients who are concomitantly receiving Velcade and drugs that are inhibitors or inducers of cytochrome P450 3A4 should be closely monitored for either toxicities or reduced efficacy). Products include:

Zoloft .. **2586**

Sulfinpyrazone (Patients who are concomitantly receiving Velcade and drugs that are inhibitors or inducers of cytochrome P450 3A4 should be closely monitored for either toxicities or reduced efficacy).

No products indexed under this heading.

Telithromycin (Patients who are concomitantly receiving Velcade and drugs that are inhibitors or inducers of cytochrome P450 3A4 should be closely monitored for either toxicities or reduced efficacy). Products include:

Ketek Tablets **2903**

Teniposide (Bortezomib may inhibit 2C19 activity and increase exposure to drugs that are substrates for this enzyme).

No products indexed under this heading.

Theophylline (Patients who are concomitantly receiving Velcade and drugs that are inhibitors or inducers of cytochrome P450 3A4 should be closely monitored for either toxicities or reduced efficacy).

No products indexed under this heading.

Thioridazine (Bortezomib may inhibit 2C19 activity and increase exposure to drugs that are substrates for this enzyme).

No products indexed under this heading.

Thioridazine Hydrochloride (Bortezomib may inhibit 2C19 activity and increase exposure to drugs that are substrates for this enzyme). Products include:

Thioridazine Hydrochloride
Tablets 2163

Tiagabine Hydrochloride (Bortezomib may inhibit 2C19 activity and increase exposure to drugs that are substrates for this enzyme). Products include:

Gabitril Tablets 984

Tolazamide (Patients on oral antidiabetic agents receiving bortezomib treatment may require close monitoring of their blood glucose levels and adjustment of the dose of their antidiabetic medication; during clinical trials, hypoglycemia and hyperglycemia were reported in diabetic patients receiving oral hypoglycemics).

No products indexed under this heading.

Tolbutamide (Bortezomib may inhibit 2C19 activity and increase exposure to drugs that are substrates for this enzyme).

No products indexed under this heading.

Tolbutamide Sodium (Bortezomib may inhibit 2C19 activity and increase exposure to drugs that are substrates for this enzyme).

No products indexed under this heading.

Topiramate (Bortezomib may inhibit 2C19 activity and increase exposure to drugs that are substrates for this enzyme). Products include:

Topamax Sprinkle Capsules **2404**
Topamax Tablets **2404**

Triamcinolone (Patients who are concomitantly receiving Velcade and drugs that are inhibitors or inducers of cytochrome P450 3A4 should be closely monitored for either toxicities or reduced efficacy).

No products indexed under this heading.

Triamcinolone Acetonide (Patients who are concomitantly receiving Velcade and drugs that are inhibitors or inducers of cytochrome P450 3A4 should be closely monitored for either toxicities or reduced efficacy). Products include:

Azmacort Inhalation Aerosol **1726**
Nasacort AQ Nasal Spray **2922**

Triamcinolone Diacetate (Patients who are concomitantly receiving Velcade and drugs that are inhibitors or inducers of cytochrome P450 3A4 should be closely monitored for either toxicities or reduced efficacy).

No products indexed under this heading.

Triamcinolone Hexacetonide (Patients who are concomitantly receiving Velcade and drugs that are inhibitors or inducers of cytochrome P450 3A4 should be closely monitored for either toxicities or reduced efficacy).

No products indexed under this heading.

Trimethadione (Bortezomib may inhibit 2C19 activity and increase exposure to drugs that are substrates for this enzyme).

No products indexed under this heading.

Trimipramine Maleate (Bortezomib may inhibit 2C19 activity and increase exposure to drugs that are substrates for this enzyme).

No products indexed under this heading.

Troglitazone (Patients who are concomitantly receiving Velcade and drugs that are inhibitors or inducers of cytochrome P450 3A4 should be closely monitored for either toxicities or reduced efficacy).

No products indexed under this heading.

Troleandomycin (Patients who are concomitantly receiving Velcade and drugs that are inhibitors or inducers of cytochrome P450 3A4 should be closely monitored for either toxicities or reduced efficacy).

No products indexed under this heading.

Valproate Sodium (Patients who are concomitantly receiving Velcade and drugs that are inhibitors or inducers of cytochrome P450 3A4 should be closely monitored for either toxicities or reduced efficacy). Products include:

Depacon Injection 412

Valproic Acid (Bortezomib may inhibit 2C19 activity and increase exposure to drugs that are substrates for this enzyme). Products include:

Depakene 417

Verapamil Hydrochloride (Patients who are concomitantly receiving Velcade and drugs that are inhibitors or inducers of cytochrome P450 3A4 should be closely monitored for either toxicities or reduced efficacy). Products include:

Covera-HS Tablets 3139
Tarka Tablets 524
Verelan PM Extended-Release
Capsules, Controlled-Onset........... 3106

Voriconazole (Patients who are concomitantly receiving Velcade and drugs that are inhibitors or inducers of cytochrome P450 3A4 should be closely monitored for either toxicities or reduced efficacy). Products include:

VFEND I.V. 2564
VFEND Oral Suspension 2564
VFEND Tablets 2564

Warfarin Sodium (Bortezomib may inhibit 2C19 activity and increase exposure to drugs that are substrates for this enzyme). Products include:

Coumadin for Injection 898
Coumadin Tablets 898

Zafirlukast (Patients who are concomitantly receiving Velcade and drugs that are inhibitors or inducers of cytochrome P450 3A4 should be closely monitored for either toxicities or reduced efficacy). Products include:

Accolate Tablets 671

Zileuton (Patients who are concomitantly receiving Velcade and drugs that are inhibitors or inducers of cytochrome P450 3A4 should be closely monitored for either toxicities or reduced efficacy). Products include:

Zyflo Tablets 1023

Zonisamide (Bortezomib may inhibit 2C19 activity and increase exposure to drugs that are substrates for this enzyme). Products include:

Zonegran Capsules 1101

Food Interactions

Grapefruit (Patients who are concomitantly receiving Velcade and drugs that are inhibitors or inducers of cytochrome P450 3A4 should be closely monitored for either toxicities or reduced efficacy).

Grapefruit Juice (Patients who are concomitantly receiving Velcade and drugs that are inhibitors or inducers of cytochrome P450 3A4 should be closely monitored for either toxicities or reduced efficacy).

VEMMA NUTRITION PROGRAM - ESSENTIAL MINERALS

(Minerals, Multiple) 835
None cited in PDR database.

VEMMA NUTRITION PROGRAM - MANGOSTEEN PLUS

(Aloe vera, Folic Acid, Herbals with Vitamins, Phytonutrients, Vitamins, Multiple).. 835
None cited in PDR database.

VENTAVIS INHALATION SOLUTION

(Iloprost) 1020
May interact with antihypertensives, anticoagulants, and vasodilators. Compounds in these categories include:

Acebutolol Hydrochloride (Iloprost has the potential to increase the hypotensive effect of vasodilators and antihypertensive agents).
No products indexed under this heading.

Amlodipine Besylate (Iloprost has the potential to increase the hypotensive effect of vasodilators and antihypertensive agents). Products include:
Caduet Tablets 2508
Lotrel Capsules 2249
Norvasc Tablets 2545

Amyl Nitrite (Iloprost has the potential to increase the hypotensive effect of vasodilators and antihypertensive agents).
No products indexed under this heading.

Anisindione (Since iloprost inhibits platelet function, there is a potential for increased risk of bleeding, particularly in patients maintained on anticoagulants). Products include:
Miradon Tablets 3042

Ardeparin Sodium (Since iloprost inhibits platelet function, there is a potential for increased risk of bleeding, particularly in patients maintained on anticoagulants).
No products indexed under this heading.

Atenolol (Iloprost has the potential to increase the hypotensive effect of vasodilators and antihypertensive agents).
No products indexed under this heading.

Benazepril Hydrochloride (Iloprost has the potential to increase the hypotensive effect of vasodilators and antihypertensive agents). Products include:
Lotensin Tablets 2243
Lotensin HCT Tablets 2246
Lotrel Capsules 2249

Bendroflumethiazide (Iloprost has the potential to increase the hypotensive effect of vasodilators and antihypertensive agents).
No products indexed under this heading.

Betaxolol Hydrochloride (Iloprost has the potential to increase the hypotensive effect of vasodilators and antihypertensive agents). Products include:
Betoptic S Ophthalmic Suspension................................. 558

Bisoprolol Fumarate (Iloprost has the potential to increase the hypotensive effect of vasodilators and antihypertensive agents).
No products indexed under this heading.

Candesartan Cilexetil (Iloprost has the potential to increase the hypotensive effect of vasodilators and antihypertensive agents). Products include:
Atacand Tablets 649
Atacand HCT 651

Captopril (Iloprost has the potential to increase the hypotensive effect of vasodilators and antihypertensive agents). Products include:
Captopril Tablets 2149

Carteolol Hydrochloride (Iloprost has the potential to increase the hypotensive effect of vasodilators and antihypertensive agents). Products include:
Carteolol Hydrochloride Ophthalmic Solution USP, 1%....... ⊙249

Chlorothiazide (Iloprost has the potential to increase the hypotensive effect of vasodilators and antihypertensive agents). Products include:
Diuril Oral Suspension 1954

Chlorothiazide Sodium (Iloprost has the potential to increase the hypotensive effect of vasodilators and antihypertensive agents). Products include:
Diuril Sodium Intravenous 2467

Chlorthalidone (Iloprost has the potential to increase the hypotensive effect of vasodilators and antihypertensive agents). Products include:
Clorpres Tablets 2153

Clonidine (Iloprost has the potential to increase the hypotensive effect of vasodilators and antihypertensive agents). Products include:
Catapres-TTS 844

Clonidine Hydrochloride (Iloprost has the potential to increase the hypotensive effect of vasodilators and antihypertensive agents). Products include:
Catapres Tablets 843
Clorpres Tablets 2153

Dalteparin Sodium (Since iloprost inhibits platelet function, there is a potential for increased risk of bleeding, particularly in patients maintained on anticoagulants). Products include:
Fragmin Injection 1097

Danaparoid Sodium (Since iloprost inhibits platelet function, there is a potential for increased risk of bleeding, particularly in patients maintained on anticoagulants).
No products indexed under this heading.

Deserpidine (Iloprost has the potential to increase the hypotensive effect of vasodilators and antihypertensive agents).
No products indexed under this heading.

Diazoxide (Iloprost has the potential to increase the hypotensive effect of vasodilators and antihypertensive agents). Products include:
Hyperstat I.V. 3017

Dicumarol (Since iloprost inhibits platelet function, there is a potential for increased risk of bleeding, particularly in patients maintained on anticoagulants).
No products indexed under this heading.

Diltiazem Hydrochloride (Iloprost has the potential to increase the hypotensive effect of vasodilators and antihypertensive agents). Products include:
Cardizem LA Extended Release Tablets 1728
Tiazac Capsules 1201

Doxazosin Mesylate (Iloprost has the potential to increase the hypotensive effect of vasodilators and antihypertensive agents). Products include:
Cardura XL Tablets 2515

Enalapril Maleate (Iloprost has the potential to increase the hypotensive effect of vasodilators and antihypertensive agents). Products include:
Vasotec I.V. Injection 2103

Enalaprilat (Iloprost has the potential to increase the hypotensive effect of vasodilators and antihypertensive agents).
No products indexed under this heading.

Enoxaparin Sodium (Since iloprost inhibits platelet function, there is a potential for increased risk of bleeding, particularly in patients maintained on anticoagulants). Products include:
Lovenox Injection 2915

Epoprostenol Sodium (Iloprost has the potential to increase the hypotensive effect of vasodilators and antihypertensive agents).
No products indexed under this heading.

Eprosartan Mesylate (Iloprost has the potential to increase the hypotensive effect of vasodilators and antihypertensive agents). Products include:
Teveten Tablets 1735
Teveten HCT Tablets 1737

Esmolol Hydrochloride (Iloprost has the potential to increase the hypotensive effect of vasodilators and antihypertensive agents).
No products indexed under this heading.

Ethaverine Hydrochloride (Iloprost has the potential to increase the hypotensive effect of vasodilators and antihypertensive agents).
No products indexed under this heading.

Felodipine (Iloprost has the potential to increase the hypotensive effect of vasodilators and antihypertensive agents).
No products indexed under this heading.

Fondaparinux Sodium (Since iloprost inhibits platelet function, there is a potential for increased risk of bleeding, particularly in patients maintained on anticoagulants). Products include:
Arixtra Injection 1351

Fosinopril Sodium (Iloprost has the potential to increase the hypotensive effect of vasodilators and antihypertensive agents).
No products indexed under this heading.

Furosemide (Iloprost has the potential to increase the hypotensive effect of vasodilators and antihypertensive agents). Products include:
Furosemide Tablets 2154

Guanabenz Acetate (Iloprost has the potential to increase the hypotensive effect of vasodilators and antihypertensive agents).
No products indexed under this heading.

Guanethidine Monosulfate (Iloprost has the potential to increase the hypotensive effect of vasodilators and antihypertensive agents).
No products indexed under this heading.

Heparin Calcium (Since iloprost inhibits platelet function, there is a potential for increased risk of bleeding, particularly in patients maintained on anticoagulants).
No products indexed under this heading.

Heparin Sodium (Since iloprost inhibits platelet function, there is a potential for increased risk of bleeding, particularly in patients maintained on anticoagulants).
No products indexed under this heading.

Hydralazine Hydrochloride (Iloprost has the potential to increase the hypotensive effect of vasodilators and antihypertensive agents). Products include:
BiDil Tablets 2171

Hydrochlorothiazide (Iloprost has the potential to increase the hypotensive effect of vasodilators and antihypertensive agents). Products include:
Aldoril Tablets 1910
Atacand HCT 651
Avalide Tablets 888
Avalide Tablets 2874
Benicar HCT Tablets 1044
Diovan HCT Tablets 2196
Dyazide Capsules 1423
Hyzaar 50-12.5 Tablets 1990
Hyzaar 100-12.5 Tablets 1990
Hyzaar 100-25 Tablets 1990
Lopressor HCT 50/25 Tablets 2241
Lopressor HCT 100/25 Tablets 2241
Lopressor HCT 100/50 Tablets 2241
Lotensin HCT Tablets 2246
Micardis HCT Tablets 856
Moduretic Tablets 2028
Prinzide Tablets 2056
Teveten HCT Tablets 1737
Timolide Tablets 2086
Uniretic Tablets 3100

Hydroflumethiazide (Iloprost has the potential to increase the hypotensive effect of vasodilators and antihypertensive agents).
No products indexed under this heading.

Indapamide (Iloprost has the potential to increase the hypotensive effect of vasodilators and antihypertensive agents). Products include:
Indapamide Tablets 2156

Irbesartan (Iloprost has the potential to increase the hypotensive effect of vasodilators and antihypertensive agents). Products include:
Avalide Tablets 888
Avalide Tablets 2874
Avapro Tablets 891
Avapro Tablets 2871

Isosorbide Dinitrate (Iloprost has the potential to increase the hypotensive effect of vasodilators and antihypertensive agents). Products include:
BiDil Tablets 2171

Isosorbide Mononitrate (Iloprost has the potential to increase the hypotensive effect of vasodilators and antihypertensive agents). Products include:
Imdur Tablets 3018

Isoxsuprine Hydrochloride (Iloprost has the potential to increase the hypotensive effect of vasodilators and antihypertensive agents).
No products indexed under this heading.

IMPORTANT NOTE: Always consult each drug listing in the patient's regimen for possible interactions.

Isradipine (Iloprost has the potential to increase the hypotensive effect of vasodilators and antihypertensive agents). Products include:
- DynaCirc CR Tablets ... 2721

Labetalol Hydrochloride (Iloprost has the potential to increase the hypotensive effect of vasodilators and antihypertensive agents).
- No products indexed under this heading.

Lisinopril (Iloprost has the potential to increase the hypotensive effect of vasodilators and antihypertensive agents). Products include:
- Prinivil Tablets ... 2052
- Prinzide Tablets ... 2056

Losartan Potassium (Iloprost has the potential to increase the hypotensive effect of vasodilators and antihypertensive agents). Products include:
- Cozaar Tablets ... 1935
- Hyzaar 50-12.5 Tablets ... 1990
- Hyzaar 100-12.5 Tablets ... 1990
- Hyzaar 100-25 Tablets ... 1990

Low Molecular Weight Heparins (Since iloprost inhibits platelet function, there is a potential for increased risk of bleeding, particularly in patients maintained on anticoagulants).
- No products indexed under this heading.

Mecamylamine Hydrochloride (Iloprost has the potential to increase the hypotensive effect of vasodilators and antihypertensive agents).
- No products indexed under this heading.

Methyclothiazide (Iloprost has the potential to increase the hypotensive effect of vasodilators and antihypertensive agents).
- No products indexed under this heading.

Methyldopa (Iloprost has the potential to increase the hypotensive effect of vasodilators and antihypertensive agents). Products include:
- Aldoril Tablets ... 1910

Methyldopate Hydrochloride (Iloprost has the potential to increase the hypotensive effect of vasodilators and antihypertensive agents).
- No products indexed under this heading.

Metolazone (Iloprost has the potential to increase the hypotensive effect of vasodilators and antihypertensive agents).
- No products indexed under this heading.

Metoprolol Succinate (Iloprost has the potential to increase the hypotensive effect of vasodilators and antihypertensive agents). Products include:
- Toprol-XL Tablets ... 668

Metoprolol Tartrate (Iloprost has the potential to increase the hypotensive effect of vasodilators and antihypertensive agents). Products include:
- Lopressor Injection ... 2238
- Lopressor Tablets ... 2238
- Lopressor HCT 50/25 Tablets ... 2241
- Lopressor HCT 100/25 Tablets ... 2241
- Lopressor HCT 100/50 Tablets ... 2241

Metyrosine (Iloprost has the potential to increase the hypotensive effect of vasodilators and antihypertensive agents). Products include:
- Demser Capsules ... 1953

Mibefradil Dihydrochloride (Iloprost has the potential to increase the hypotensive effect of vasodilators and antihypertensive agents).
- No products indexed under this heading.

Minoxidil (Iloprost has the potential to increase the hypotensive effect of vasodilators and antihypertensive agents). Products include:
- Men's Rogaine Extra Strength Hair Regrowth Treatment Topical Solution, Ocean Rush Scent and Original Unscented ... ▣633
- Men's Rogaine Foam Hair Regrowth Treatment ... ▣633
- Women's Rogaine Hair Regrowth Treatment Topical Solution, Spring Bloom Scent and Original Unscented ... ▣634

Moexipril Hydrochloride (Iloprost has the potential to increase the hypotensive effect of vasodilators and antihypertensive agents). Products include:
- Uniretic Tablets ... 3100
- Univasc Tablets ... 3104

Nadolol (Iloprost has the potential to increase the hypotensive effect of vasodilators and antihypertensive agents). Products include:
- Nadolol Tablets ... 2159

Nicardipine Hydrochloride (Iloprost has the potential to increase the hypotensive effect of vasodilators and antihypertensive agents). Products include:
- Cardene I.V. ... 2497

Nifedipine (Iloprost has the potential to increase the hypotensive effect of vasodilators and antihypertensive agents). Products include:
- Adalat CC Tablets ... 2964

Nisoldipine (Iloprost has the potential to increase the hypotensive effect of vasodilators and antihypertensive agents). Products include:
- Sular Tablets ... 3122

Nitroglycerin (Iloprost has the potential to increase the hypotensive effect of vasodilators and antihypertensive agents). Products include:
- Nitro-Dur Transdermal Infusion System ... 3046
- Nitrolingual Pumpspray ... 3120

Nitroglycerin, long-acting formulations (Iloprost has the potential to increase the hypotensive effect of vasodilators and antihypertensive agents).
- No products indexed under this heading.

Nitroglycerin Intravenous (Iloprost has the potential to increase the hypotensive effect of vasodilators and antihypertensive agents).
- No products indexed under this heading.

Papaverine (Iloprost has the potential to increase the hypotensive effect of vasodilators and antihypertensive agents).
- No products indexed under this heading.

Papaverine Hydrochloride (Iloprost has the potential to increase the hypotensive effect of vasodilators and antihypertensive agents).
- No products indexed under this heading.

Penbutolol Sulfate (Iloprost has the potential to increase the hypotensive effect of vasodilators and antihypertensive agents).
- No products indexed under this heading.

Perindopril Erbumine (Iloprost has the potential to increase the hypotensive effect of vasodilators and antihypertensive agents). Products include:
- Aceon Tablets (2 mg, 4 mg, 8 mg) ... 3194

Phenoxybenzamine Hydrochloride (Iloprost has the potential to increase the hypotensive effect of vasodilators and antihypertensive agents). Products include:
- Dibenzyline Capsules ... 3399

Phentolamine Mesylate (Iloprost has the potential to increase the hypotensive effect of vasodilators and antihypertensive agents).
- No products indexed under this heading.

Pindolol (Iloprost has the potential to increase the hypotensive effect of vasodilators and antihypertensive agents).
- No products indexed under this heading.

Polythiazide (Iloprost has the potential to increase the hypotensive effect of vasodilators and antihypertensive agents).
- No products indexed under this heading.

Prazosin Hydrochloride (Iloprost has the potential to increase the hypotensive effect of vasodilators and antihypertensive agents).
- No products indexed under this heading.

Propranolol Hydrochloride (Iloprost has the potential to increase the hypotensive effect of vasodilators and antihypertensive agents). Products include:
- Inderal LA Long-Acting Capsules ... 3429
- InnoPran XL Capsules ... 2723

Quinapril Hydrochloride (Iloprost has the potential to increase the hypotensive effect of vasodilators and antihypertensive agents).
- No products indexed under this heading.

Ramipril (Iloprost has the potential to increase the hypotensive effect of vasodilators and antihypertensive agents). Products include:
- Altace Capsules ... 1702

Rauwolfia Serpentina (Iloprost has the potential to increase the hypotensive effect of vasodilators and antihypertensive agents).
- No products indexed under this heading.

Rescinnamine (Iloprost has the potential to increase the hypotensive effect of vasodilators and antihypertensive agents).
- No products indexed under this heading.

Reserpine (Iloprost has the potential to increase the hypotensive effect of vasodilators and antihypertensive agents).
- No products indexed under this heading.

Sodium Nitroprusside (Iloprost has the potential to increase the hypotensive effect of vasodilators and antihypertensive agents).
- No products indexed under this heading.

Sotalol Hydrochloride (Iloprost has the potential to increase the hypotensive effect of vasodilators and antihypertensive agents).
- No products indexed under this heading.

Spirapril Hydrochloride (Iloprost has the potential to increase the hypotensive effect of vasodilators and antihypertensive agents).
- No products indexed under this heading.

Telmisartan (Iloprost has the potential to increase the hypotensive effect of vasodilators and antihypertensive agents). Products include:
- Micardis Tablets ... 854
- Micardis HCT Tablets ... 856

Terazosin Hydrochloride (Iloprost has the potential to increase the hypotensive effect of vasodilators and antihypertensive agents). Products include:
- Hytrin Capsules ... 471

Timolol Maleate (Iloprost has the potential to increase the hypotensive effect of vasodilators and antihypertensive agents). Products include:
- Blocadren Tablets ... 1916
- Cosopt Sterile Ophthalmic Solution ... 1931
- Timolide Tablets ... 2086
- Timoptic Sterile Ophthalmic Solution ... 2088
- Timoptic in Ocudose ... 2091
- Timoptic-XE Sterile Ophthalmic Gel Forming Solution ... 2092

Tinzaparin Sodium (Since iloprost inhibits platelet function, there is a potential for increased risk of bleeding, particularly in patients maintained on anticoagulants).
- No products indexed under this heading.

Tolazoline Hydrochloride (Iloprost has the potential to increase the hypotensive effect of vasodilators and antihypertensive agents).
- No products indexed under this heading.

Torsemide (Iloprost has the potential to increase the hypotensive effect of vasodilators and antihypertensive agents). Products include:
- Demadex Injection ... 2759
- Demadex Tablets ... 2759

Trandolapril (Iloprost has the potential to increase the hypotensive effect of vasodilators and antihypertensive agents). Products include:
- Mavik Tablets ... 486
- Tarka Tablets ... 524

Trimethaphan Camsylate (Iloprost has the potential to increase the hypotensive effect of vasodilators and antihypertensive agents).
- No products indexed under this heading.

Valsartan (Iloprost has the potential to increase the hypotensive effect of vasodilators and antihypertensive agents). Products include:
- Diovan Tablets ... 2193
- Diovan HCT Tablets ... 2196

Verapamil Hydrochloride (Iloprost has the potential to increase the hypotensive effect of vasodilators and antihypertensive agents). Products include:
- Covera-HS Tablets ... 3139
- Tarka Tablets ... 524
- Verelan PM Extended-Release Capsules, Controlled-Onset ... 3106

Warfarin Sodium (Since iloprost inhibits platelet function, there is a potential for increased risk of bleeding, particularly in patients maintained on anticoagulants). Products include:
- Coumadin for Injection ... 898
- Coumadin Tablets ... 898

Food Interactions

Alcohol (Iloprost has the potential to increase the hypotensive effect of vasodilators and antihypertensive agents).

VENTOLIN HFA INHALATION AEROSOL

(Albuterol Sulfate) 1600

May interact with monoamine oxidase inhibitors, nonpotassium-sparing diuretics, sympathomimetic bronchodilators, sympathomimetics, tricyclic antidepressants, and certain other agents. Compounds in these categories include:

Albuterol (Co-administration with other short-acting sympathomimetic aerosol bronchodilators should not be used concomitantly with albuterol). Products include:
- Proventil Inhalation Aerosol 3053

Amitriptyline Hydrochloride (Co-administration with tricyclic antidepressants may potentiate action of albuterol on the vascular system).
No products indexed under this heading.

Amoxapine (Co-administration with tricyclic antidepressants may potentiate action of albuterol on the vascular system).
No products indexed under this heading.

Bendroflumethiazide (The ECG changes and/or hypokalemia that may result from the adminstration of nonpotassium-sparing diuretics can be acutely worsened by beta-agonists, especially when the recommended dose of beta-agonist is exceeded).
No products indexed under this heading.

Bitolterol Mesylate (Co-administration with other short-acting sympathomimetic aerosol bronchodilators should not be used concomitantly with albuterol).
No products indexed under this heading.

Bumetanide (The ECG changes and/or hypokalemia that may result from the adminstration of nonpotassium-sparing diuretics can be acutely worsened by beta-agonists, especially when the recommended dose of beta-agonist is exceeded). Products include:
- Bumex Tablets 2746

Chlorothiazide (The ECG changes and/or hypokalemia that may result from the adminstration of nonpotassium-sparing diuretics can be acutely worsened by beta-agonists, especially when the recommended dose of beta-agonist is exceeded). Products include:
- Diuril Oral Suspension 1954

Chlorothiazide Sodium (The ECG changes and/or hypokalemia that may result from the adminstration of nonpotassium-sparing diuretics can be acutely worsened by beta-agonists, especially when the recommended dose of beta-agonist is exceeded). Products include:
- Diuril Sodium Intravenous 2467

Clomipramine Hydrochloride (Co-administration with tricyclic antidepressants may potentiate action of albuterol on the vascular system).
No products indexed under this heading.

Desipramine Hydrochloride (Co-administration with tricyclic antidepressants may potentiate action of albuterol on the vascular system).
No products indexed under this heading.

Digoxin (Co-administration of intravenous and oral administration of albuterol to volunteers who had received digoxin for 10 days has resulted in mean decrease in digoxin levels; the clinical significance of this finding is unknown). Products include:
- Lanoxicaps Capsules 1490
- Lanoxin Injection 1494
- Lanoxin Injection Pediatric 1497
- Lanoxin Tablets 1500

Dobutamine Hydrochloride (Co-administration with other adrenergic agents may result in deleterious cardiovascular events).
No products indexed under this heading.

Dopamine Hydrochloride (Co-administration with other adrenergic agents may result in deleterious cardiovascular events).
No products indexed under this heading.

Doxepin Hydrochloride (Co-administration with tricyclic antidepressants may potentiate action of albuterol on the vascular system).
No products indexed under this heading.

Ephedrine Hydrochloride (Co-administration with other short-acting sympathomimetic aerosol bronchodilators should not be used concomitantly with albuterol).
No products indexed under this heading.

Ephedrine Sulfate (Co-administration with other short-acting sympathomimetic aerosol bronchodilators should not be used concomitantly with albuterol).
No products indexed under this heading.

Ephedrine Tannate (Co-administration with other short-acting sympathomimetic aerosol bronchodilators should not be used concomitantly with albuterol).
No products indexed under this heading.

Epinephrine (Co-administration with other short-acting sympathomimetic aerosol bronchodilators should not be used concomitantly with albuterol). Products include:
- EpiPen 1061
- Primatene Mist 719
- Twinject 0.15 3379
- Twinject 0.3 3378

Epinephrine Bitartrate (Co-administration with other adrenergic agents may result in deleterious cardiovascular events).
No products indexed under this heading.

Epinephrine Hydrochloride (Co-administration with other short-acting sympathomimetic aerosol bronchodilators should not be used concomitantly with albuterol).
No products indexed under this heading.

Ethacrynic Acid (The ECG changes and/or hypokalemia that may result from the adminstration of nonpotassium-sparing diuretics can be acutely worsened by beta-agonists, especially when the recommended dose of beta-agonist is exceeded). Products include:
- Edecrin Tablets 1959

Furosemide (The ECG changes and/or hypokalemia that may result from the adminstration of nonpotassium-sparing diuretics can be acutely worsened by beta-agonists, especially when the recommended dose of beta-agonist is exceeded). Products include:
- Furosemide Tablets 2154

Hydrochlorothiazide (The ECG changes and/or hypokalemia that may result from the adminstration of nonpotassium-sparing diuretics can be acutely worsened by beta-agonists, especially when the recommended dose of beta-agonist is exceeded). Products include:
- Aldoril Tablets 1910
- Atacand HCT 651
- Avalide Tablets 888
- Avalide Tablets 2874
- Benicar HCT Tablets 1044
- Diovan HCT Tablets 2196
- Dyazide Capsules 1423
- Hyzaar 50-12.5 Tablets 1990
- Hyzaar 100-12.5 Tablets 1990
- Hyzaar 100-25 Tablets 1990
- Lopressor HCT 50/25 Tablets 2241
- Lopressor HCT 100/25 Tablets 2241
- Lopressor HCT 100/50 Tablets 2241
- Lotensin HCT Tablets 2246
- Micardis HCT Tablets 856
- Moduretic Tablets 2028
- Prinzide Tablets 2056
- Teveten HCT Tablets 1737
- Timolide Tablets 2086
- Uniretic Tablets 3100

Hydroflumethiazide (The ECG changes and/or hypokalemia that may result from the adminstration of nonpotassium-sparing diuretics can be acutely worsened by beta-agonists, especially when the recommended dose of beta-agonist is exceeded).
No products indexed under this heading.

Imipramine Hydrochloride (Co-administration with tricyclic antidepressants may potentiate action of albuterol on the vascular system).
No products indexed under this heading.

Imipramine Pamoate (Co-administration with tricyclic antidepressants may potentiate action of albuterol on the vascular system).
No products indexed under this heading.

Isocarboxazid (Co-administration with MAO inhibitors may potentiate action of albuterol on the vascular system).
No products indexed under this heading.

Isoetharine (Co-administration with other short-acting sympathomimetic aerosol bronchodilators should not be used concomitantly with albuterol).
No products indexed under this heading.

Isoproterenol Hydrochloride (Co-administration with other short-acting sympathomimetic aerosol bronchodilators should not be used concomitantly with albuterol).
No products indexed under this heading.

Isoproterenol Sulfate (Co-administration with other short-acting sympathomimetic aerosol bronchodilators should not be used concomitantly with albuterol).
No products indexed under this heading.

Levalbuterol Hydrochloride (Co-administration with other short-acting sympathomimetic aerosol bronchodilators should not be used concomitantly with albuterol). Products include:
- Xopenex Inhalation Solution 3146
- Xopenex Inhalation Solution Concentrate 3150

Maprotiline Hydrochloride (Co-administration with tricyclic antidepressants may potentiate action of albuterol on the vascular system).
No products indexed under this heading.

Metaproterenol Sulfate (Co-administration with other short-acting sympathomimetic aerosol bronchodilators should not be used concomitantly with albuterol). Products include:
- Alupent Inhalation Aerosol 826

Metaraminol Bitartrate (Co-administration with other adrenergic agents may result in deleterious cardiovascular events).
No products indexed under this heading.

Methoxamine Hydrochloride (Co-administration with other adrenergic agents may result in deleterious cardiovascular events).
No products indexed under this heading.

Methyclothiazide (The ECG changes and/or hypokalemia that may result from the adminstration of nonpotassium-sparing diuretics can be acutely worsened by beta-agonists, especially when the recommended dose of beta-agonist is exceeded).
No products indexed under this heading.

Moclobemide (Co-administration with MAO inhibitors may potentiate action of albuterol on the vascular system).
No products indexed under this heading.

Norepinephrine Bitartrate (Co-administration with other adrenergic agents may result in deleterious cardiovascular events).
No products indexed under this heading.

Nortriptyline Hydrochloride (Co-administration with tricyclic antidepressants may potentiate action of albuterol on the vascular system).
No products indexed under this heading.

Pargyline Hydrochloride (Co-administration with MAO inhibitors may potentiate action of albuterol on the vascular system).
No products indexed under this heading.

Phenelzine Sulfate (Co-administration with MAO inhibitors may potentiate action of albuterol on the vascular system).
No products indexed under this heading.

Phenylephrine Bitartrate (Co-administration with other adrenergic agents may result in deleterious cardiovascular events).
No products indexed under this heading.

Phenylephrine Hydrochloride (Co-administration with other adrenergic agents may result in deleterious cardiovascular events). Products include:
- Comtrex Maximum Strength Non-Drowsy Cold & Cough Caplets 725

Phenylephrine Tannate (Co-administration with other adrenergic agents may result in deleterious cardiovascular events).

No products indexed under this heading.

Phenylpropanolamine Hydrochloride (Co-administration with other adrenergic agents may result in deleterious cardiovascular events).

No products indexed under this heading.

Pirbuterol Acetate (Co-administration with other short-acting sympathomimetic aerosol bronchodilators should not be used concomitantly with albuterol). Products include:

Polythiazide (The ECG changes and/or hypokalemia that may result from the adminstration of nonpotassium-sparing diuretics can be acutely worsened by beta-agonists, especially when the recommended dose of beta-agonist is exceeded).

No products indexed under this heading.

Procarbazine Hydrochloride (Co-administration with MAO inhibitors may potentiate action of albuterol on the vascular system). Products include:

Protriptyline Hydrochloride (Co-administration with tricyclic antidepressants may potentiate action of albuterol on the vascular system).

No products indexed under this heading.

Pseudoephedrine Hydrochloride (Co-administration with other adrenergic agents may result in deleterious cardiovascular events). Products include:

Pseudoephedrine Sulfate (Co-administration with other adrenergic agents may result in deleterious cardiovascular events). Products include:

Salmeterol Xinafoate (Co-administration with other short-acting sympathomimetic aerosol bronchodilators should not be used concomitantly with albuterol). Products include:

Selegiline Hydrochloride (Co-administration with MAO inhibitors may potentiate action of albuterol on the vascular system). Products include:

Terbutaline Sulfate (Co-administration with other short-acting sympathomimetic aerosol bronchodilators should not be used concomitantly with albuterol).

No products indexed under this heading.

Torsemide (The ECG changes and/or hypokalemia that may result from the adminstration of nonpotassium-sparing diuretics can be acutely worsened by beta-agonists, especially when the recommended dose of beta-agonist is exceeded). Products include:

Tranylcypromine Sulfate (Co-administration with MAO inhibitors may potentiate action of albuterol on the vascular system). Products include:

Trimipramine Maleate (Co-administration with tricyclic antidepressants may potentiate action of albuterol on the vascular system).

No products indexed under this heading.

VERELAN PM EXTENDED-RELEASE CAPSULES, CONTROLLED-ONSET

(Verapamil Hydrochloride) 3106

May interact with ACE inhibitors, antihypertensives, beta blockers, cytochrome p450 3a4 inducers (selected), cytochrome p450 3a4 inhibitors (selected), diuretics, cardiac glycosides, inhalant anesthetics, lithium preparations, neuromuscular blocking agents, quinidine, theophyllines, vasodilators, and certain other agents. Compounds in these categories include:

Acebutolol Hydrochloride (Concomitant therapy with beta-adrenergic blockers and verapamil may result in additive negative effects on heart rate, A-V conduction, and/or cardiac contractility; excessive bradycardia and A-V block have been reported with concurrent use in hypertensive patients. This combination should be used only with caution and close monitoring).

No products indexed under this heading.

Acetazolamide (Clinically significant interactions have been reported with inhibitors of cytochrome P450 3A4 causing elevation of plasma levels of verapamil).

No products indexed under this heading.

Allium sativum (Clinically significant interactions have been reported with inducers of cytochrome P450 3A4 causing a lowering of plasma levels of verapamil).

No products indexed under this heading.

Amiloride Hydrochloride (Co-administration with oral antihypertensive agents (eg, diuretics) will usually have an additive effect on lowering blood pressure). Products include:

Amiodarone Hydrochloride (Clinically significant interactions have been reported with inhibitors of cytochrome P450 3A4 causing elevation of plasma levels of verapamil).

No products indexed under this heading.

Amlodipine Besylate (Co-administration with oral antihypertensive agents will usually have an additive effect on lowering blood pressure). Products include:

Amprenavir (Clinically significant interactions have been reported with inhibitors of cytochrome P450 3A4 causing elevation of plasma levels of verapamil). Products include:

Amyl Nitrite (Co-administration with oral antihypertensive agents (eg, vasodilators) will usually have an additive effect on lowering blood pressure).
No products indexed under this heading.

Anastrozole (Clinically significant interactions have been reported with inhibitors of cytochrome P450 3A4 causing elevation of plasma levels of verapamil). Products include:
Arimidex Tablets 673

Aprepitant (Clinically significant interactions have been reported with inducers of cytochrome P450 3A4 causing a lowering of plasma levels of verapamil). Products include:
Emend Capsules 1963

Aspirin (Co-administration, in a few reported cases, has led to increased bleeding times greater than those observed with aspirin alone).
Products include:
Aggrenox Capsules 822
Bayer Aspirin 744
BC Allergy Sinus Cold Powder .... ▣677
BC Headache Powder .... ▣677
Arthritis Strength BC Powder .... ▣677
BC Sinus Cold Powder .... ▣677
Excedrin Extra Strength Caplets/Tablets/Geltabs .... ▣684
Excedrin Migraine Caplets/Tablets/Geltabs .... ▣609
Goody's Body Pain Formula Powder .... ▣684
Goody's Extra Strength Headache Powders .... ▣611
Goody's Extra Strength Pain Relief Tablets .... ▣685
Percodan Tablets 1132
St. Joseph 81 mg Aspirin Chewable and Enteric Coated Tablets 1869

Aspirin, Enteric Coated (Co-administration, in a few reported cases, has led to increased bleeding times greater than those observed with aspirin alone).
No products indexed under this heading.

Aspirin Buffered (Co-administration, in a few reported cases, has led to increased bleeding times greater than those observed with aspirin alone). Products include:
Bufferin Extra Strength Tablets .... ▣678
Bufferin Regular Strength Tablets .... ▣678

Atenolol (Concomitant therapy with beta-adrenergic blockers and verapamil may result in additive negative effects on heart rate, A-V conduction, and/or cardiac contractility; excessive bradycardia and A-V block have been reported with concurrent use in hypertensive patients. This combination should be used only with caution and close monitoring).
No products indexed under this heading.

Atracurium Besylate (Clinical data and animal studies suggest that verapamil may potentiate the activity of neuromuscular blocking agents (curare-like and depolarizing). It may be necessary to decrease the dose of verapamil and/or the dose of the neuromuscular blocking agent when the drugs are used concomitantly).
No products indexed under this heading.

Benazepril Hydrochloride (Co-administration with oral antihypertensive agents will usually have an additive effect on lowering blood pressure). Products include:
Lotensin Tablets 2243
Lotensin HCT Tablets 2246
Lotrel Capsules 2249

Bendroflumethiazide (Co-administration with oral antihypertensive agents will usually have an additive effect on lowering blood pressure).
No products indexed under this heading.

Betamethasone Acetate (Clinically significant interactions have been reported with inducers of cytochrome P450 3A4 causing a lowering of plasma levels of verapamil).
No products indexed under this heading.

Betamethasone Sodium Phosphate (Clinically significant interactions have been reported with inducers of cytochrome P450 3A4 causing a lowering of plasma levels of verapamil).
No products indexed under this heading.

Betaxolol Hydrochloride (Concomitant therapy with beta-adrenergic blockers and verapamil may result in additive negative effects on heart rate, A-V conduction, and/or cardiac contractility; excessive bradycardia and A-V block have been reported with concurrent use in hypertensive patients. This combination should be used only with caution and close monitoring). Products include:
Betoptic S Ophthalmic Suspension 558

Bisoprolol Fumarate (Concomitant therapy with beta-adrenergic blockers and verapamil may result in additive negative effects on heart rate, A-V conduction, and/or cardiac contractility; excessive bradycardia and A-V block have been reported with concurrent use in hypertensive patients. This combination should be used only with caution and close monitoring).
No products indexed under this heading.

Bumetanide (Co-administration with oral antihypertensive agents (eg, diuretics) will usually have an additive effect on lowering blood pressure). Products include:
Bumex Tablets 2746

Candesartan Cilexetil (Co-administration with oral antihypertensive agents will usually have an additive effect on lowering blood pressure). Products include:
Atacand Tablets 649
Atacand HCT 651

Captopril (Co-administration with oral antihypertensive agents will usually have an additive effect on lowering blood pressure). Products include:
Captopril Tablets 2149

Carbamazepine (Verapamil therapy may increase carbamazepine concentrations during combined therapy resulting in side effects such as diplopia, headache, ataxia, or dizziness). Products include:
Carbatrol Capsules 3171
Equetro Extended-Release Capsules 3180
Tegretol/Tegretol-XR 2295

Carteolol Hydrochloride (Concomitant therapy with beta-adrenergic blockers and verapamil may result in additive negative effects on heart rate, A-V conduction, and/or cardiac contractility; excessive bradycardia and A-V block have been reported with concurrent use in hypertensive patients. This combination should be used only with caution and close monitoring). Products include:
Carteolol Hydrochloride Ophthalmic Solution USP, 1% .... ⊙249

Chlorothiazide (Co-administration with oral antihypertensive agents will usually have an additive effect on lowering blood pressure). Products include:
Diuril Oral Suspension 1954

Chlorothiazide Sodium (Co-administration with oral antihypertensive agents will usually have an additive effect on lowering blood pressure). Products include:
Diuril Sodium Intravenous 2467

Chlorthalidone (Co-administration with oral antihypertensive agents will usually have an additive effect on lowering blood pressure). Products include:
Clorpres Tablets 2153

Cimetidine (The interaction between cimetidine and chronically administered verapamil has not been studied. Variable results on clearance have been obtained in acute studies of healthy volunteers; clearance of verapamil was either reduced or unchanged). Products include:
Tagamet HB 200 Tablets .... ▣664

Cimetidine Hydrochloride (The interaction between cimetidine and chronically administered verapamil has not been studied. Variable results on clearance have been obtained in acute studies of healthy volunteers; clearance of verapamil was either reduced or unchanged).
No products indexed under this heading.

Ciprofloxacin (Clinically significant interactions have been reported with inhibitors of cytochrome P450 3A4 causing elevation of plasma levels of verapamil). Products include:
Cipro Oral Suspension 2977
Cipro I.V. 2984
Cipro XR Tablets 2990
Ciprodex Otic Suspension 559

Ciprofloxacin Hydrochloride (Clinically significant interactions have been reported with inducers of cytochrome P450 3A4 causing a lowering of plasma levels of verapamil). Products include:
Ciloxan Ophthalmic Ointment 559
Ciloxan Ophthalmic Solution .... ⊙206
Cipro Tablets 2977
Proquin XR Tablets 1153

Cisatracurium Besylate (Clinical data and animal studies suggest that verapamil may potentiate the activity of neuromuscular blocking agents (curare-like and depolarizing). It may be necessary to decrease the dose of verapamil and/or the dose of the neuromuscular blocking agent when the drugs are used concomitantly). Products include:
Nimbex Injection 498

Cisplatin (Clinically significant interactions have been reported with inducers of cytochrome P450 3A4 causing a lowering of plasma levels of verapamil).
No products indexed under this heading.

Clarithromycin (Clinically significant interactions have been reported with inhibitors of cytochrome P450 3A4 causing elevation of plasma levels of verapamil). Products include:
Biaxin/Biaxin XL 402
PREVPAC 3284

Clonidine (Co-administration with oral antihypertensive agents will usually have an additive effect on lowering blood pressure). Products include:
Catapres-TTS 844

Clonidine Hydrochloride (Co-administration with oral antihypertensive agents will usually have an additive effect on lowering blood pressure). Products include:
Catapres Tablets 843
Clorpres Tablets 2153

Clotrimazole (Clinically significant interactions have been reported with inhibitors of cytochrome P450 3A4 causing elevation of plasma levels of verapamil). Products include:
Desenex Athlete's Foot Cream .... ▣635
Lotrimin 3039
Lotrisone 3040

Cortisone Acetate (Clinically significant interactions have been reported with inducers of cytochrome P450 3A4 causing a lowering of plasma levels of verapamil).
No products indexed under this heading.

Cyclosporine (Verapamil therapy may increase serum levels of cyclosporine). Products include:
Gengraf Capsules 459
Neoral Oral Solution 2259
Neoral Soft Gelatin Capsules 2259
Restasis Ophthalmic Emulsion 575
Sandimmune 2275

Dalfopristin (Clinically significant interactions have been reported with inhibitors of cytochrome P450 3A4 causing elevation of plasma levels of verapamil).
No products indexed under this heading.

Danazol (Clinically significant interactions have been reported with inhibitors of cytochrome P450 3A4 causing elevation of plasma levels of verapamil).
No products indexed under this heading.

Delavirdine Mesylate (Clinically significant interactions have been reported with inhibitors of cytochrome P450 3A4 causing elevation of plasma levels of verapamil).
Products include:
Rescriptor Tablets 2551

Deserpidine (Co-administration with oral antihypertensive agents will usually have an additive effect on lowering blood pressure).
No products indexed under this heading.

Desflurane (When used concomitantly, inhalation anesthetics and calcium antagonists, such as verapamil, should each be titrated carefully to avoid excessive cardiovascular depression).
No products indexed under this heading.

Deslanoside (Chronic verapamil treatment can increase serum digoxin levels by 50% to 70% during the first week of therapy and this may result in digitalis toxicity. The influence of verapamil on digoxin kinetics is magnified in hepatic cirrhosis patients).
No products indexed under this heading.

Dexamethasone (Clinically significant interactions have been reported with inducers of cytochrome P450

3A4 causing a lowering of plasma levels of verapamil). Products include:

Ciprodex Otic Suspension 559
Decadron Tablets 1951
TobraDex Ophthalmic Ointment 562
TobraDex Ophthalmic Suspension ... 563

Dexamethasone Acetate (Clinically significant interactions have been reported with inducers of cytochrome P450 3A4 causing a lowering of plasma levels of verapamil).
No products indexed under this heading.

Dexamethasone Sodium Phosphate (Clinically significant interactions have been reported with inducers of cytochrome P450 3A4 causing a lowering of plasma levels of verapamil).
No products indexed under this heading.

Diazoxide (Co-administration with oral antihypertensive agents will usually have an additive effect on lowering blood pressure). Products include:

Hyperstat I.V. 3017

Digitalis Glycoside Preparations (Chronic verapamil treatment can increase serum digoxin levels by 50% to 70% during the first week of therapy and this may result in digitalis toxicity.The influence of verapamil on digoxin kinetics is magnified in hepatic cirrhosis patients).
No products indexed under this heading.

Digitoxin (Chronic verapamil treatment can increase serum digoxin levels by 50% to 70% during the first week of therapy and this may result in digitalis toxicity.The influence of verapamil on digoxin kinetics is magnified in hepatic cirrhosis patients).
No products indexed under this heading.

Digoxin (Chronic verapamil treatment can increase serum digoxin levels by 50% to 70% during the first week of therapy and this may result in digitalis toxicity.The influence of verapamil on digoxin kinetics is magnified in hepatic cirrhosis patients). Products include:

Lanoxicaps Capsules 1490
Lanoxin Injection 1494
Lanoxin Injection Pediatric 1497
Lanoxin Tablets 1500

Diltiazem Hydrochloride (Co-administration with oral antihypertensive agents will usually have an additive effect on lowering blood pressure). Products include:

Cardizem LA Extended Release Tablets 1728
Tiazac Capsules 1201

Diltiazem Maleate (Clinically significant interactions have been reported with inhibitors of cytochrome P450 3A4 causing elevation of plasma levels of verapamil).
No products indexed under this heading.

Disopyramide (Disopyramide should not be administered within 48 hours before, or 24 hours after, verapamil administration).
No products indexed under this heading.

Disopyramide Phosphate (Disopyramide should not be administered within 48 hours before or 24 hours after verapamil administration).
No products indexed under this heading.

Doxacurium Chloride (Clinical data and animal studies suggest that verapamil may potentiate the activity of neuromuscular blocking agents (curare-like and depolarizing). It may be necessary to decrease the dose of verapamil and/or the dose of the neuromuscular blocking agent when the drugs are used concomitantly).
No products indexed under this heading.

Doxazosin Mesylate (Concomitant use of agents that attenuate alpha-adrenergic function, such as doxazosin, may result in excessive reduction in blood pressure). Products include:

Cardura XL Tablets 2515

Doxorubicin Hydrochloride (Verapamil can increase the efficacy of doxorubicin both in tissue culture systems and in patients. It raises the serum doxorubicin levels).
No products indexed under this heading.

Doxorubicin Hydrochloride Liposome (Verapamil can increase the efficacy of doxorubicin both in tissue culture systems and in patients. It raises the serum doxorubicin levels). Products include:

Doxil Injection 2351

Efavirenz (Clinically significant interactions have been reported with inducers of cytochrome P450 3A4 causing a lowering of plasma levels of verapamil). Products include:

Atripla Tablets 945
Sustiva Capsules 930
Sustiva Tablets 930

Enalapril Maleate (Co-administration with oral antihypertensive agents will usually have an additive effect on lowering blood pressure). Products include:

Vasotec I.V. Injection 2103

Enalaprilat (Co-administration with oral antihypertensive agents will usually have an additive effect on lowering blood pressure).
No products indexed under this heading.

Enflurane (When used concomitantly, inhalation anesthetics and calcium antagonists, such as verapamil, should each be titrated carefully to avoid excessive cardiovascular depression).
No products indexed under this heading.

Epoprostenol Sodium (Co-administration with oral antihypertensive agents (eg, vasodilators) will usually have an additive effect on lowering blood pressure).
No products indexed under this heading.

Eprosartan Mesylate (Co-administration with oral antihypertensive agents will usually have an additive effect on lowering blood pressure). Products include:

Teveten Tablets 1735
Teveten HCT Tablets 1737

Erythromycin (Clinically significant interactions have been reported with inhibitors of cytochrome P450 3A4 causing elevation of plasma levels of verapamil). Products include:

Ery-Tab Tablets 449
Erythromycin Base Filmtab Tablets 455
Erythromycin Delayed-Release Capsules, USP 457
PCE Dispertab Tablets 515

Erythromycin Estolate (Clinically significant interactions have been reported with inhibitors of cytochrome P450 3A4 causing elevation of plasma levels of verapamil).
No products indexed under this heading.

Erythromycin Ethylsuccinate (Clinically significant interactions have been reported with inhibitors of cytochrome P450 3A4 causing elevation of plasma levels of verapamil). Products include:

E.E.S. 451
EryPed 447

Erythromycin Gluceptate (Clinically significant interactions have been reported with inhibitors of cytochrome P450 3A4 causing elevation of plasma levels of verapamil).
No products indexed under this heading.

Erythromycin Lactobionate (Clinically significant interactions have been reported with inhibitors of cytochrome P450 3A4 causing elevation of plasma levels of verapamil).
No products indexed under this heading.

Erythromycin Stearate (Clinically significant interactions have been reported with inhibitors of cytochrome P450 3A4 causing elevation of plasma levels of verapamil). Products include:

Erythrocin Stearate Filmtab Tablets 453

Esmolol Hydrochloride (Concomitant therapy with beta-adrenergic blockers and verapamil may result in additive negative effects on heart rate, A-V conduction, and/or cardiac contractility; excessive bradycardia and A-V block have been reported with concurrent use in hypertensive patients.This combination should be used only with caution and close monitoring).
No products indexed under this heading.

Esomeprazole Magnesium (Clinically significant interactions have been reported with inhibitors of cytochrome P450 3A4 causing elevation of plasma levels of verapamil). Products include:

Nexium Delayed-Release Capsules 655

Ethacrynic Acid (Co-administration with oral antihypertensive agents (eg, diuretics) will usually have an additive effect on lowering blood pressure). Products include:

Edecrin Tablets 1959

Ethaverine Hydrochloride (Co-administration with oral antihypertensive agents (eg, vasodilators) will usually have an additive effect on lowering blood pressure).
No products indexed under this heading.

Ethosuximide (Clinically significant interactions have been reported with inducers of cytochrome P450 3A4 causing a lowering of plasma levels of verapamil).
No products indexed under this heading.

Felbamate (Clinically significant interactions have been reported with inducers of cytochrome P450 3A4 causing a lowering of plasma levels of verapamil).
No products indexed under this heading.

Felodipine (Co-administration with oral antihypertensive agents will usually have an additive effect on lowering blood pressure).
No products indexed under this heading.

Flecainide Acetate (Concomitant administration of flecainide and verapamil may have additive effects on myocardial contractility, A-V conduction, and repolarization). Products include:

Tambocor Tablets 1856

Fluconazole (Clinically significant interactions have been reported with inhibitors of cytochrome P450 3A4 causing elevation of plasma levels of verapamil).
No products indexed under this heading.

Fludrocortisone Acetate (Clinically significant interactions have been reported with inducers of cytochrome P450 3A4 causing a lowering of plasma levels of verapamil).
No products indexed under this heading.

Fluoxetine Hydrochloride (Clinically significant interactions have been reported with inhibitors of cytochrome P450 3A4 causing elevation of plasma levels of verapamil). Products include:

Prozac Pulvules and Liquid 1801
Symbyax Capsules 1819

Fluvoxamine Maleate (Clinically significant interactions have been reported with inhibitors of cytochrome P450 3A4 causing elevation of plasma levels of verapamil).
No products indexed under this heading.

Fosamprenavir Calcium (Clinically significant interactions have been reported with inhibitors of cytochrome P450 3A4 causing elevation of plasma levels of verapamil). Products include:

Lexiva Tablets 1505

Fosinopril Sodium (Co-administration with oral antihypertensive agents will usually have an additive effect on lowering blood pressure).
No products indexed under this heading.

Fosphenytoin Sodium (Clinically significant interactions have been reported with inducers of cytochrome P450 3A4 causing a lowering of plasma levels of verapamil).
No products indexed under this heading.

Furosemide (Co-administration with oral antihypertensive agents will usually have an additive effect on lowering blood pressure). Products include:

Furosemide Tablets 2154

Garlic Extract (Clinically significant interactions have been reported with inducers of cytochrome P450 3A4 causing a lowering of plasma levels of verapamil).
No products indexed under this heading.

Garlic Oil (Clinically significant interactions have been reported with inducers of cytochrome P450 3A4 causing a lowering of plasma levels of verapamil).
No products indexed under this heading.

Guanabenz Acetate (Co-administration with oral antihypertensive agents will usually have an additive effect on lowering blood pressure).
No products indexed under this heading.

Guanethidine Monosulfate (Co-administration with oral antihypertensive agents will usually have an additive effect on lowering blood pressure).
No products indexed under this heading.

Halothane (When used concomitantly, inhalation anesthetics and calcium antagonists, such as verapamil, should each be titrated carefully to avoid excessive cardiovascular depression).
No products indexed under this heading.

Hydralazine Hydrochloride (Co-administration with oral antihypertensive agents will usually have an additive effect on lowering blood pressure). Products include:
BiDil Tablets 2171

Hydrochlorothiazide (Co-administration with oral antihypertensive agents will usually have an additive effect on lowering blood pressure). Products include:
Aldoril Tablets 1910
Atacand HCT 651
Avalide Tablets 888
Avalide Tablets 2874
Benicar HCT Tablets 1044
Diovan HCT Tablets 2196
Dyazide Capsules 1423
Hyzaar 50-12.5 Tablets 1990
Hyzaar 100-12.5 Tablets 1990
Hyzaar 100-25 Tablets 1990
Lopressor HCT 50/25 Tablets 2241
Lopressor HCT 100/25 Tablets 2241
Lopressor HCT 100/50 Tablets 2241
Lotensin HCT Tablets 2246
Micardis HCT Tablets 856
Moduretic Tablets 2028
Prinzide Tablets 2056
Teveten HCT Tablets 1737
Timolide Tablets 2086
Uniretic Tablets 3100

Hydrocortisone (Clinically significant interactions have been reported with inducers of cytochrome P450 3A4 causing a lowering of plasma levels of verapamil). Products include:
Colocort Rectal Suspension, USP (Retention) 100 mg/60 mL 2476
Hydrocortone Tablets 1989
Preparation H Hydrocortisone Cream 646

Hydrocortisone Acetate (Clinically significant interactions have been reported with inducers of cytochrome P450 3A4 causing a lowering of plasma levels of verapamil). Products include:
Analpram-HC 1159
Pramosone 1161
ProctoFoam-HC 3099

Hydrocortisone Butyrate (Clinically significant interactions have been reported with inducers of cytochrome P450 3A4 causing a lowering of plasma levels of verapamil). Products include:
Locoid Lipocream Cream 1160

Hydrocortisone Cypionate (Clinically significant interactions have been reported with inducers of cytochrome P450 3A4 causing a lowering of plasma levels of verapamil).
No products indexed under this heading.

Hydrocortisone Hemisuccinate (Clinically significant interactions have been reported with inducers of cytochrome P450 3A4 causing a lowering of plasma levels of verapamil).
No products indexed under this heading.

Hydrocortisone Probutate (Clinically significant interactions have been reported with inducers of cytochrome P450 3A4 causing a lowering of plasma levels of verapamil).
No products indexed under this heading.

Hydrocortisone Sodium Phosphate (Clinically significant interactions have been reported with inducers of cytochrome P450 3A4 causing a lowering of plasma levels of verapamil).
No products indexed under this heading.

Hydrocortisone Sodium Succinate (Clinically significant interactions have been reported with inducers of cytochrome P450 3A4 causing a lowering of plasma levels of verapamil).
No products indexed under this heading.

Hydrocortisone Valerate (Clinically significant interactions have been reported with inducers of cytochrome P450 3A4 causing a lowering of plasma levels of verapamil).
No products indexed under this heading.

Hydroflumethiazide (Co-administration with oral antihypertensive agents will usually have an additive effect on lowering blood pressure).
No products indexed under this heading.

Hypericum (Clinically significant interactions have been reported with inducers of cytochrome P450 3A4 causing a lowering of plasma levels of verapamil). Products include:
Satiete Tablets 832

Hypericum Perforatum (Clinically significant interactions have been reported with inducers of cytochrome P450 3A4 causing a lowering of plasma levels of verapamil).
No products indexed under this heading.

Indapamide (Co-administration with oral antihypertensive agents will usually have an additive effect on lowering blood pressure). Products include:
Indapamide Tablets 2156

Indinavir Sulfate (Clinically significant interactions have been reported with inhibitors of cytochrome P450 3A4 causing elevation of plasma levels of verapamil). Products include:
Crixivan Capsules 1940

Irbesartan (Co-administration with oral antihypertensive agents will usually have an additive effect on lowering blood pressure). Products include:
Avalide Tablets 888
Avalide Tablets 2874
Avapro Tablets 891
Avapro Tablets 2871

Isoflurane (When used concomitantly, inhalation anesthetics and calcium antagonists, such as verapamil, should each be titrated carefully to avoid excessive cardiovascular depression).
No products indexed under this heading.

Isoniazid (Clinically significant interactions have been reported with inhibitors of cytochrome P450 3A4 causing elevation of plasma levels of verapamil).
No products indexed under this heading.

Isosorbide Dinitrate (Co-administration with oral antihypertensive agents (eg, vasodilators) will usually have an additive effect on lowering blood pressure). Products include:
BiDil Tablets 2171

Isosorbide Mononitrate (Co-administration with oral antihypertensive agents (eg, vasodilators) will usually have an additive effect on lowering blood pressure). Products include:
Imdur Tablets 3018

Isoxsuprine Hydrochloride (Co-administration with oral antihypertensive agents (eg, vasodilators) will usually have an additive effect on lowering blood pressure).
No products indexed under this heading.

Isradipine (Co-administration with oral antihypertensive agents will usually have an additive effect on lowering blood pressure). Products include:
DynaCirc CR Tablets 2721

Itraconazole (Clinically significant interactions have been reported with inhibitors of cytochrome P450 3A4 causing elevation of plasma levels of verapamil).
No products indexed under this heading.

Ketoconazole (Clinically significant interactions have been reported with inhibitors of cytochrome P450 3A4 causing elevation of plasma levels of verapamil). Products include:
Nizoral A-D Shampoo, 1% 1868

Labetalol Hydrochloride (Concomitant therapy with beta-adrenergic blockers and verapamil may result in additive negative effects on heart rate, A-V conduction, and/or cardiac contractility; excessive bradycardia and A-V block have been reported with concurrent use in hypertensive patients.This combination should be used only with caution and close monitoring).
No products indexed under this heading.

Levobunolol Hydrochloride (Concomitant therapy with beta-adrenergic blockers and verapamil may result in additive negative effects on heart rate, A-V conduction, and/or cardiac contractility; excessive bradycardia and A-V block have been reported with concurrent use in hypertensive patients.This combination should be used only with caution and close monitoring). Products include:
Betagan Ophthalmic Solution, USP .... ⊙220

Lisinopril (Co-administration with oral antihypertensive agents will usually have an additive effect on lowering blood pressure). Products include:
Prinivil Tablets 2052
Prinzide Tablets 2056

Lithium (Increased sensitivity to the effects of lithium (neurotoxicity) has been reported during concomitant verapamil-lithium therapy with either no change or an increase in serum lithium levels. However, the addition of verapamil has also resulted in the lowering of serum lithium levels in patients receiving chronic stable oral lithium. Patients receiving both drugs must be monitored carefully).
No products indexed under this heading.

Lithium Carbonate (Increased sensitivity to the effects of lithium (neurotoxicity) has been reported during concomitant verapamil-lithium therapy with either no change or an increase in serum lithium levels. However, the addition of verapamil has also resulted in the lowering of serum lithium levels in patients receiving chronic stable oral lithium. Patients receiving both drugs must be monitored carefully). Products include:
Lithobid Tablets 1692

Lithium Citrate (Increased sensitivity to the effects of lithium (neurotoxicity) has been reported during concomitant verapamil-lithium therapy with either no change or an increase in serum lithium levels. However, the addition of verapamil has also resulted in the lowering of serum lithium levels in patients receiving chronic stable oral lithium. Patients receiving both drugs must be monitored carefully).
No products indexed under this heading.

Lopinavir (Clinically significant interactions have been reported with inhibitors of cytochrome P450 3A4 causing elevation of plasma levels of verapamil). Products include:
Kaletra 476

Loratadine (Clinically significant interactions have been reported with inhibitors of cytochrome P450 3A4 causing elevation of plasma levels of verapamil). Products include:
Alavert Allergy & Sinus D-12 Hour Tablets 771
Alavert 771
Children's Claritin Allergy Oral Solution 771
Claritin Non-Drowsy 24 Hour Tablets 772
Claritin Reditabs 24 Hour Non-Drowsy Tablets 772
Claritin-D Non-Drowsy 12 Hour Tablets 772
Claritin-D Non-Drowsy 24 Hour Tablets 772

Losartan Potassium (Co-administration with oral antihypertensive agents will usually have an additive effect on lowering blood pressure). Products include:
Cozaar Tablets 1935
Hyzaar 50-12.5 Tablets 1990
Hyzaar 100-12.5 Tablets 1990
Hyzaar 100-25 Tablets 1990

Mecamylamine Hydrochloride (Co-administration with oral antihypertensive agents will usually have an additive effect on lowering blood pressure).
No products indexed under this heading.

Mephenytoin (Clinically significant interactions have been reported with inducers of cytochrome P450 3A4 causing a lowering of plasma levels of verapamil).
No products indexed under this heading.

Methoxyflurane (When used concomitantly, inhalation anesthetics and calcium antagonists, such as verapamil, should each be titrated carefully to avoid excessive cardiovascular depression).
No products indexed under this heading.

Methsuximide (Clinically significant interactions have been reported with inducers of cytochrome P450 3A4 causing a lowering of plasma levels of verapamil).
No products indexed under this heading.

Methyclothiazide (Co-administration with oral antihypertensive agents will usually have an additive effect on lowering blood pressure).
No products indexed under this heading.

Methyldopa (Co-administration with oral antihypertensive agents will usually have an additive effect on lowering blood pressure). Products include:
Aldoril Tablets 1910

Methyldopate Hydrochloride (Co-administration with oral antihypertensive agents will usually have an additive effect on lowering blood pressure).
No products indexed under this heading.

Methylprednisolone (Clinically significant interactions have been reported with inducers of cytochrome P450 3A4 causing a lowering of plasma levels of verapamil).
No products indexed under this heading.

Methylprednisolone Acetate (Clinically significant interactions have been reported with inducers of cytochrome P450 3A4 causing a lowering of plasma levels of verapamil). Products include:
Depo-Medrol Injectable
Suspension 2617
Depo-Medrol Single-Dose Vial 2619

Methylprednisolone Sodium Succinate (Clinically significant interactions have been reported with inducers of cytochrome P450 3A4 causing a lowering of plasma levels of verapamil).
No products indexed under this heading.

Metipranolol Hydrochloride (Concomitant therapy with beta-adrenergic blockers and verapamil may result in additive negative effects on heart rate, A-V conduction, and/or cardiac contractility; excessive bradycardia and A-V block have been reported with concurrent use in hypertensive patients. This combination should be used only with caution and close monitoring).
No products indexed under this heading.

Metocurine Iodide (Clinical data and animal studies suggest that verapamil may potentiate the activity of neuromuscular blocking agents (curare-like and depolarizing). It may be necessary to decrease the dose of verapamil and/or the dose of the neuromuscular blocking agent when the drugs are used concomitantly).
No products indexed under this heading.

Metolazone (Co-administration with oral antihypertensive agents will usually have an additive effect on lowering blood pressure).
No products indexed under this heading.

Metoprolol Succinate (Co-administration has resulted in a decrease in metoprolol clearance; concomitant therapy may result in additive negative effects on heart rate, A-V conduction, and/or cardiac contractility; excessive bradycardia and A-V block have been reported with concurrent use in hypertensive patients). Products include:
Toprol-XL Tablets 668

Metoprolol Tartrate (Co-administration has resulted in a decrease in metoprolol clearance; concomitant therapy may result in additive negative effects on heart rate, A-V conduction, and/or cardiac contractility; excessive bradycardia and A-V block have been reported with concurrent use in hypertensive patients). Products include:
Lopressor Injection 2238
Lopressor Tablets 2238
Lopressor HCT 50/25 Tablets 2241
Lopressor HCT 100/25 Tablets 2241
Lopressor HCT 100/50 Tablets 2241

Metronidazole (Clinically significant interactions have been reported with inhibitors of cytochrome P450 3A4 causing elevation of plasma levels of verapamil). Products include:
Metrogel 1% 1211
MetroGel-Vaginal Gel 1855
Vandazole Vaginal Gel 3338

Metronidazole Benzoate (Clinically significant interactions have been reported with inhibitors of cytochrome P450 3A4 causing elevation of plasma levels of verapamil).
No products indexed under this heading.

Metronidazole Hydrochloride (Clinically significant interactions have been reported with inhibitors of cytochrome P450 3A4 causing elevation of plasma levels of verapamil).
No products indexed under this heading.

Metyrosine (Co-administration with oral antihypertensive agents will usually have an additive effect on lowering blood pressure). Products include:
Demser Capsules 1953

Mibefradil Dihydrochloride (Co-administration with oral antihypertensive agents will usually have an additive effect on lowering blood pressure).
No products indexed under this heading.

Miconazole (Clinically significant interactions have been reported with inhibitors of cytochrome P450 3A4 causing elevation of plasma levels of verapamil).
No products indexed under this heading.

Miconazole Nitrate (Clinically significant interactions have been

reported with inhibitors of cytochrome P450 3A4 causing elevation of plasma levels of verapamil). Products include:
Desenex .. 🔲635
Desenex Jock Itch Spray Powder ... 🔲635

Minoxidil (Co-administration with oral antihypertensive agents will usually have an additive effect on lowering blood pressure). Products include:
Men's Rogaine Extra Strength
Hair Regrowth Treatment
Topical Solution, Ocean Rush
Scent and Original Unscented 🔲633
Men's Rogaine Foam Hair
Regrowth Treatment 🔲633
Women's Rogaine Hair Regrowth
Treatment Topical Solution,
Spring Bloom Scent and
Original Unscented 🔲634

Mivacurium Chloride (Clinical data and animal studies suggest that verapamil may potentiate the activity of neuromuscular blocking agents (curare-like and depolarizing). It may be necessary to decrease the dose of verapamil and/or the dose of the neuromuscular blocking agent when the drugs are used concomitantly). Products include:
Mivacron Injection 493

Modafinil (Clinically significant interactions have been reported with inducers of cytochrome P450 3A4 causing a lowering of plasma levels of verapamil). Products include:
Provigil Tablets 988

Moexipril Hydrochloride (Co-administration with oral antihypertensive agents will usually have an additive effect on lowering blood pressure). Products include:
Uniretic Tablets 3100
Univasc Tablets 3104

Nadolol (Concomitant therapy with beta-adrenergic blockers and verapamil may result in additive negative effects on heart rate, A-V conduction, and/or cardiac contractility; excessive bradycardia and A-V block have been reported with concurrent use in hypertensive patients. This combination should be used only with caution and close monitoring). Products include:
Nadolol Tablets 2159

Nefazodone Hydrochloride (Clinically significant interactions have been reported with inhibitors of cytochrome P450 3A4 causing elevation of plasma levels of verapamil).
No products indexed under this heading.

Nelfinavir Mesylate (Clinically significant interactions have been reported with inhibitors of cytochrome P450 3A4 causing elevation of plasma levels of verapamil). Products include:
Viracept .. 2577

Nevirapine (Clinically significant interactions have been reported with inducers of cytochrome P450 3A4 causing a lowering of plasma levels of verapamil). Products include:
Viramune Oral Suspension 873
Viramune Tablets 873

Niacinamide (Clinically significant interactions have been reported with inhibitors of cytochrome P450 3A4 causing elevation of plasma levels of verapamil).
No products indexed under this heading.

Nicardipine Hydrochloride (Co-administration with oral antihyperten-

sive agents will usually have an additive effect on lowering blood pressure). Products include:
Cardene I.V. 2497

Nicotinamide (Clinically significant interactions have been reported with inhibitors of cytochrome P450 3A4 causing elevation of plasma levels of verapamil). Products include:
Nicomide Tablets 1088

Nifedipine (Co-administration with oral antihypertensive agents will usually have an additive effect on lowering blood pressure). Products include:
Adalat CC Tablets 2964

Nisoldipine (Co-administration with oral antihypertensive agents will usually have an additive effect on lowering blood pressure). Products include:
Sular Tablets 3122

Nitroglycerin (Verapamil has been given concomitantly with short- and long-acting nitrates without any undesirable drug interactions. The pharmacologic profile of both drugs and the clinical experience suggest beneficial interactions). Products include:
Nitro-Dur Transdermal Infusion
System 3046
Nitrolingual Pumpspray 3120

Nitroglycerin, long-acting formulations (Co-administration with oral antihypertensive agents (eg, vasodilators) will usually have an additive effect on lowering blood pressure).
No products indexed under this heading.

Nitroglycerin Intravenous (Co-administration with oral antihypertensive agents (eg, vasodilators) will usually have an additive effect on lowering blood pressure).
No products indexed under this heading.

Norfloxacin (Clinically significant interactions have been reported with inhibitors of cytochrome P450 3A4 causing elevation of plasma levels of verapamil). Products include:
Noroxin Tablets 2032

Omeprazole (Clinically significant interactions have been reported with inhibitors of cytochrome P450 3A4 causing elevation of plasma levels of verapamil). Products include:
Zegerid Capsules 2958
Zegerid Powder for Oral Solution 2958

Oxcarbazepine (Clinically significant interactions have been reported with inducers of cytochrome P450 3A4 causing a lowering of plasma levels of verapamil). Products include:
Trileptal Tablets 2300
Trileptal Oral Suspension 2300

Paclitaxel (Concomitant administration of R-verapamil can decrease the clearance of paclitaxel).
No products indexed under this heading.

Paclitaxel, protein-bound (Concomitant administration of verapamil can decrease the clearance of paclitaxel).
No products indexed under this heading.

Pancuronium Bromide (Clinical data and animal studies suggest that verapamil may potentiate the activity of neuromuscular blocking agents (curare-like and depolarizing). It may be necessary to decrease the dose of verapamil and/or the dose of the neuromuscular blocking agent when the drugs are used concomitantly).
No products indexed under this heading.

Papaverine (Co-administration with oral antihypertensive agents (eg, vasodilators) will usually have an additive effect on lowering blood pressure).
No products indexed under this heading.

Papaverine Hydrochloride (Co-administration with oral antihypertensive agents (eg, vasodilators) will usually have an additive effect on lowering blood pressure).
No products indexed under this heading.

Paroxetine Hydrochloride (Clinically significant interactions have been reported with inhibitors of cytochrome P450 3A4 causing elevation of plasma levels of verapamil). Products include:
Paxil CR Controlled-Release Tablets **1538**
Paxil **1530**

Penbutolol Sulfate (Concomitant therapy with beta-adrenergic blockers and verapamil may result in additive negative effects on heart rate, A-V conduction, and/or cardiac contractility; excessive bradycardia and A-V block have been reported with concurrent use in hypertensive patients.This combination should be used only with caution and close monitoring).
No products indexed under this heading.

Perindopril Erbumine (Co-administration with oral antihypertensive agents will usually have an additive effect on lowering blood pressure). Products include:
Aceon Tablets (2 mg, 4 mg, 8 mg) **3194**

Phenobarbital (Combined therapy with phenobarbital may increase verapamil clearance). Products include:
Donnatal Extentabs **2493**

Phenobarbital Sodium (Clinically significant interactions have been reported with inducers of cytochrome P450 3A4 causing a lowering of plasma levels of verapamil).
No products indexed under this heading.

Phenoxybenzamine Hydrochloride (Co-administration with oral antihypertensive agents will usually have an additive effect on lowering blood pressure). Products include:
Dibenzyline Capsules **3399**

Phentolamine Mesylate (Co-administration with oral antihypertensive agents will usually have an additive effect on lowering blood pressure).
No products indexed under this heading.

Phenytoin (Clinically significant interactions have been reported with inducers of cytochrome P450 3A4 causing a lowering of plasma levels of verapamil).
No products indexed under this heading.

Phenytoin Sodium (Clinically significant interactions have been reported with inducers of cytochrome P450 3A4 causing a lowering of plasma levels of verapamil).
Products include:
Phenytek Capsules **2160**

Pindolol (Concomitant therapy with beta-adrenergic blockers and verapamil may result in additive negative effects on heart rate, A-V conduction, and/or cardiac contractility; excessive bradycardia and A-V block have been reported with concurrent use in hypertensive patients.This combination should be used only with caution and close monitoring).
No products indexed under this heading.

Polythiazide (Co-administration with oral antihypertensive agents will usually have an additive effect on lowering blood pressure).
No products indexed under this heading.

Prazosin Hydrochloride (Concomitant use of agents that attenuate alpha-adrenergic function, such as prazosin, may result in excessive reduction in blood pressure).
No products indexed under this heading.

Prednisolone Acetate (Clinically significant interactions have been reported with inducers of cytochrome P450 3A4 causing a lowering of plasma levels of verapamil).
Products include:
Blephamide Ophthalmic Ointment **568**
Blephamide Ophthalmic Suspension **569**
Poly-Pred Ophthalmic Suspension .... **⊙233**
Pred Forte Ophthalmic Suspension .... **⊙235**
Pred Mild Ophthalmic Suspension .... **⊙238**
Pred-G Ophthalmic Ointment .... **⊙237**
Pred-G Ophthalmic Suspension .... **⊙236**

Prednisolone Sodium Phosphate (Clinically significant interactions have been reported with inducers of cytochrome P450 3A4 causing a lowering of plasma levels of verapamil).
No products indexed under this heading.

Prednisolone Tebutate (Clinically significant interactions have been reported with inducers of cytochrome P450 3A4 causing a lowering of plasma levels of verapamil).
No products indexed under this heading.

Prednisone (Clinically significant interactions have been reported with inducers of cytochrome P450 3A4 causing a lowering of plasma levels of verapamil).
No products indexed under this heading.

Primidone (Clinically significant interactions have been reported with inducers of cytochrome P450 3A4 causing a lowering of plasma levels of verapamil).
No products indexed under this heading.

Propoxyphene Hydrochloride (Clinically significant interactions have been reported with inhibitors of cytochrome P450 3A4 causing elevation of plasma levels of verapamil).
No products indexed under this heading.

Propoxyphene Napsylate (Clinically significant interactions have been reported with inhibitors of cytochrome P450 3A4 causing elevation of plasma levels of verapamil).
No products indexed under this heading.

Propranolol Hydrochloride (Concomitant therapy with beta-adrenergic blockers and verapamil may result in additive negative effects on heart rate, A-V conduction, and/or cardiac contractility; excessive bradycardia and A-V block have been reported with concurrent use in hypertensive patients.This combination should be used only with caution and close monitoring). Products include:
Inderal LA Long-Acting Capsules **3429**
InnoPran XL Capsules **2723**

Quinapril Hydrochloride (Co-administration with oral antihypertensive agents will usually have an additive effect on lowering blood pressure).
No products indexed under this heading.

Quinidine (In a small number of patients with hypertrophic cardiomyopathy, co-administration has resulted in significant hypotension; combined use in these patients should probably be avoided).
No products indexed under this heading.

Quinidine Gluconate (In a small number of patients with hypertrophic cardiomyopathy, co-administration has resulted in significant hypotension; combined use in these patients should probably be avoided).
No products indexed under this heading.

Quinidine Hydrochloride (In a small number of patients with hypertrophic cardiomyopathy, co-administration has resulted in significant hypotension; combined use in these patients should probably be avoided).
No products indexed under this heading.

Quinidine Polygalacturonate (In a small number of patients with hypertrophic cardiomyopathy, co-administration has resulted in significant hypotension; combined use in these patients should probably be avoided).
No products indexed under this heading.

Quinidine Sulfate (In a small number of patients with hypertrophic cardiomyopathy, co-administration has resulted in significant hypotension; combined use in these patients should probably be avoided).
No products indexed under this heading.

Quinine (Clinically significant interactions have been reported with inhibitors of cytochrome P450 3A4 causing elevation of plasma levels of verapamil).
No products indexed under this heading.

Quinine Sulfate (Clinically significant interactions have been reported with inhibitors of cytochrome P450 3A4 causing elevation of plasma levels of verapamil).
No products indexed under this heading.

Quinupristin (Clinically significant interactions have been reported with inhibitors of cytochrome P450 3A4 causing elevation of plasma levels of verapamil).
No products indexed under this heading.

Ramipril (Co-administration with oral antihypertensive agents will usually have an additive effect on lowering blood pressure). Products include:
Altace Capsules **1702**

Ranitidine Bismuth Citrate (Clinically significant interactions have been reported with inhibitors of cytochrome P450 3A4 causing elevation of plasma levels of verapamil).
No products indexed under this heading.

Ranitidine Hydrochloride (Clinically significant interactions have been reported with inhibitors of cytochrome P450 3A4 causing elevation of plasma levels of verapamil).
Products include:
Zantac **1624**
Zantac Injection **1619**
Zantac Injection Pharmacy Bulk Package **1622**

Rapacuronium Bromide (Clinical data and animal studies suggest that verapamil may potentiate the activity of neuromuscular blocking agents (curare-like and depolarizing). It may be necessary to decrease the dose of verapamil and/or the dose of the neuromuscular blocking agent when the drugs are used concomitantly).
No products indexed under this heading.

Rauwolfia Serpentina (Co-administration with oral antihypertensive agents will usually have an additive effect on lowering blood pressure).
No products indexed under this heading.

Rescinnamine (Co-administration with oral antihypertensive agents will usually have an additive effect on lowering blood pressure).
No products indexed under this heading.

Reserpine (Co-administration with oral antihypertensive agents will usually have an additive effect on lowering blood pressure).
No products indexed under this heading.

Rifabutin (Clinically significant interactions have been reported with inducers of cytochrome P450 3A4 causing a lowering of plasma levels of verapamil).
No products indexed under this heading.

Rifampicin (Clinically significant interactions have been reported with inducers of cytochrome P450 3A4 causing a lowering of plasma levels of verapamil).
No products indexed under this heading.

Rifampin (Combined therapy with rifampin may markedly reduce oral verapamil bioavailability).
No products indexed under this heading.

Rifapentine (Clinically significant interactions have been reported with inducers of cytochrome P450 3A4 causing a lowering of plasma levels of verapamil).
No products indexed under this heading.

Ritonavir (Clinically significant interactions have been reported with inhibitors of cytochrome P450 3A4 causing elevation of plasma levels of verapamil). Products include:
Kaletra ... 476
Norvir ... 503

Rocuronium Bromide (Clinical data and animal studies suggest that verapamil may potentiate the activity of neuromuscular blocking agents (curare-like and depolarizing). It may be necessary to decrease the dose of verapamil and/or the dose of the neuromuscular blocking agent when the drugs are used concomitantly). Products include:
Zemuron Injection ... 2346

Saquinavir (Clinically significant interactions have been reported with inhibitors of cytochrome P450 3A4 causing elevation of plasma levels of verapamil).
No products indexed under this heading.

Saquinavir Mesylate (Clinically significant interactions have been reported with inhibitors of cytochrome P450 3A4 causing elevation of plasma levels of verapamil). Products include:
Invirase ... 2772

Sertraline Hydrochloride (Clinically significant interactions have been reported with inhibitors of cytochrome P450 3A4 causing elevation of plasma levels of verapamil). Products include:
Zoloft ... 2586

Sodium Nitroprusside (Co-administration with oral antihypertensive agents will usually have an additive effect on lowering blood pressure).
No products indexed under this heading.

Sotalol Hydrochloride (Concomitant therapy with beta-adrenergic blockers and verapamil may result in additive negative effects on heart rate, A-V conduction, and/or cardiac contractility; excessive bradycardia and A-V block have been reported with concurrent use in hypertensive patients.This combination should be used only with caution and close monitoring).
No products indexed under this heading.

Spirapril Hydrochloride (Co-administration with oral antihypertensive agents will usually have an additive effect on lowering blood pressure).
No products indexed under this heading.

Spironolactone (Co-administration with oral antihypertensive agents (eg, diuretics) will usually have an additive effect on lowering blood pressure).
No products indexed under this heading.

Succinylcholine Chloride (Clinical data and animal studies suggest that verapamil may potentiate the activity of neuromuscular blocking agents (curare-like and depolarizing). It may be necessary to decrease the dose of verapamil and/or the dose of the neuromuscular blocking agent when the drugs are used concomitantly).
No products indexed under this heading.

Sulfinpyrazone (Clinically significant interactions have been reported with inducers of cytochrome P450 3A4 causing a lowering of plasma levels of verapamil).
No products indexed under this heading.

Telithromycin (Clinically significant interactions have been reported with inhibitors of cytochrome P450 3A4 causing elevation of plasma levels of verapamil). Products include:
Ketek Tablets ... 2903

Telmisartan (Co-administration with oral antihypertensive agents will usually have an additive effect on lowering blood pressure). Products include:
Micardis Tablets ... 854
Micardis HCT Tablets ... 856

Terazosin Hydrochloride (Concomitant use of agents that attenuate alpha-adrenergic function, such as terazosin, may result in excessive reduction in blood pressure). Products include:
Hytrin Capsules ... 471

Theophylline (Clinically significant interactions have been reported with inducers of cytochrome P450 3A4 causing a lowering of plasma levels of verapamil).
No products indexed under this heading.

Theophylline Anhydrous (Verapamil may inhibit the clearance and increase the plasma levels of theophylline). Products include:
Uniphyl Tablets ... 2710

Theophylline Calcium Salicylate (Verapamil may inhibit the clearance and increase the plasma levels of theophylline).
No products indexed under this heading.

Theophylline Dihydroxypropyl (Glyceryl) (Verapamil may inhibit the clearance and increase the plasma levels of theophylline).
No products indexed under this heading.

Theophylline Ethylenediamine (Verapamil may inhibit the clearance and increase the plasma levels of theophylline).
No products indexed under this heading.

Theophylline Sodium Glycinate (Verapamil may inhibit the clearance and increase the plasma levels of theophylline).
No products indexed under this heading.

Timolol Hemihydrate (Co-administration of oral verapamil and timolol eye drops has resulted in asymptomatic bradycardia with a wandering atrial pacemaker). Products include:
Betimol Ophthalmic Solution ... 3382
Betimol Ophthalmic Solution ... ⊙ 295

Timolol Maleate (Co-administration of oral verapamil and timolol eye drops has resulted in asymptomatic bradycardia with a wandering atrial pacemaker; concomitant therapy may result in additive negative effects on heart rate, A-V conduction, and/or cardiac contractility;excessive bradycardia and A-V block have been reported with concurrent use in hypertensive patients). Products include:
Blocadren Tablets ... 1916
Cosopt Sterile Ophthalmic Solution ... 1931
Timolide Tablets ... 2086
Timoptic Sterile Ophthalmic Solution ... 2088
Timoptic in Ocudose ... 2091
Timoptic-XE Sterile Ophthalmic Gel Forming Solution ... 2092

Tolazoline Hydrochloride (Co-administration with oral antihypertensive agents (eg, vasodilators) will usually have an additive effect on lowering blood pressure).
No products indexed under this heading.

Torsemide (Co-administration with oral antihypertensive agents will usually have an additive effect on lowering blood pressure). Products include:
Demadex Injection ... 2759
Demadex Tablets ... 2759

Trandolapril (Co-administration with oral antihypertensive agents will usually have an additive effect on lowering blood pressure). Products include:
Mavik Tablets ... 486
Tarka Tablets ... 524

Triamcinolone (Clinically significant interactions have been reported with inducers of cytochrome P450 3A4 causing a lowering of plasma levels of verapamil).
No products indexed under this heading.

Triamcinolone Acetonide (Clinically significant interactions have been reported with inducers of cytochrome P450 3A4 causing a lowering of plasma levels of verapamil). Products include:
Azmacort Inhalation Aerosol ... 1726
Nasacort AQ Nasal Spray ... 2922

Triamcinolone Diacetate (Clinically significant interactions have been reported with inducers of cytochrome P450 3A4 causing a lowering of plasma levels of verapamil).
No products indexed under this heading.

Triamcinolone Hexacetonide (Clinically significant interactions have been reported with inducers of cytochrome P450 3A4 causing a lowering of plasma levels of verapamil).
No products indexed under this heading.

Triamterene (Co-administration with oral antihypertensive agents (eg, diuretics) will usually have an additive effect on lowering blood pressure). Products include:
Dyazide Capsules ... 1423
Dyrenium Capsules ... 3400

Trimethaphan Camsylate (Co-administration with oral antihypertensive agents will usually have an additive effect on lowering blood pressure).
No products indexed under this heading.

Troglitazone (Clinically significant interactions have been reported with inducers of cytochrome P450 3A4 causing a lowering of plasma levels of verapamil).
No products indexed under this heading.

Troleandomycin (Clinically significant interactions have been reported with inhibitors of cytochrome P450 3A4 causing elevation of plasma levels of verapamil).
No products indexed under this heading.

Tubocurarine Chloride (Verapamil may potentiate the activity of neuromuscular blocking drugs).
No products indexed under this heading.

Valproate Sodium (Clinically significant interactions have been reported with inhibitors of cytochrome P450 3A4 causing elevation of plasma levels of verapamil). Products include:
Depacon Injection ... 412

Valsartan (Co-administration with oral antihypertensive agents will usually have an additive effect on lowering blood pressure). Products include:
Diovan Tablets ... 2193
Diovan HCT Tablets ... 2196

Vecuronium Bromide (Clinical data and animal studies suggest that verapamil may potentiate the activity of neuromuscular blocking agents (curare-like and depolarizing). It may be necessary to decrease the dose of verapamil and/or the dose of the neuromuscular blocking agent when the drugs are used concomitantly).
No products indexed under this heading.

Voriconazole (Clinically significant interactions have been reported with inhibitors of cytochrome P450 3A4 causing elevation of plasma levels of verapamil). Products include:
VFEND I.V. ... 2564
VFEND Oral Suspension ... 2564
VFEND Tablets ... 2564

Zafirlukast (Clinically significant interactions have been reported with inhibitors of cytochrome P450 3A4 causing elevation of plasma levels of verapamil). Products include:
Accolate Tablets ... 671

Zileuton (Clinically significant interactions have been reported with inhibitors of cytochrome P450 3A4 causing elevation of plasma levels of verapamil). Products include:
Zyflo Tablets ... 1023

Food Interactions

Alcohol (Verapamil has been found to significantly inhibit ethanol elimination resulting in elevated blood ethanol concentration that may prolong the intoxicating effects of alcohol).

Grapefruit (Grapefruit juice may significantly increase concentrations of verapamil).

Grapefruit Juice (Grapefruit juice may significantly increase concentrations of verapamil).

VESANOID CAPSULES

(Tretinoin) ... 2820

May interact with cytochrome p450 3a4 inducers (selected), cytochrome p450 3a4 inhibitors (selected), erythromycin, glucocorticoids, tetracyclines, and certain other agents. Compounds in these categories include:

Acetazolamide (Tretinoin is metaboized by the hepatic P450 system; therefore, there is a potential for alteration of pharmacokinetic parameters in patients administered concomitant medications that are also inducers of this system. To date, there is no data to suggestthat co-use with these medications increases or decreases either efficacy or toxicity of tretinoin).
No products indexed under this heading.

Allium sativum (Tretinoin is metaboized by the hepatic P450 system; therefore, there is a potential for alteration of pharmacokinetic parameters in patients administered concomitant medications that are also inducers of this system. To date, there is no data to suggestthat co-use with these medications increases or decreases either efficacy or toxicity of tretinoin).

No products indexed under this heading.

Aminocaproic Acid (Cases of fatal thrombotic complications have been reported rarely in patients concomitantly treated with tretinoin and anti-fibrinolytic agents. Therefore, caution should be exercised when administering tretinoin concomitantly with these agents).

No products indexed under this heading.

Amiodarone Hydrochloride (Tretinoin is metabolized by the hepatic P450 system; therefore, there is a potential for alteration of pharmacokinetic parameters in patients administered concomitant medications that are also inducers of this system. To date, there is no data to suggest-that co-use with these medications increases or decreases either efficacy or toxicity of tretinoin).

No products indexed under this heading.

Amprenavir (Tretinoin is metaboized by the hepatic P450 system; therefore, there is a potential for alteration of pharmacokinetic parameters in patients administered concomitant medications that are also inducers of this system. To date, there is no data to suggestthat co-use with these medications increases or decreases either efficacy or toxicity of tretinoin). Products include:

Agenerase Capsules 1327
Agenerase Oral Solution 1332

Anastrozole (Tretinoin is metabolized by the hepatic P450 system; therefore, there is a potential for alteration of pharmacokinetic parameters in patients administered concomitant medications that are also inducers of this system. To date, there is no data to suggestthat co-use with these medications increases or decreases either efficacy or toxicity of tretinoin). Products include:

Arimidex Tablets 673

Aprepitant (Tretinoin is metaboized by the hepatic P450 system; therefore, there is a potential for alteration of pharmacokinetic parameters in patients administered concomitant medications that are also inducers of this system. To date, there is no data to suggestthat co-use with these medications increases or decreases either efficacy or toxicity of tretinoin). Products include:

Emend Capsules 1963

Aprotinin (Cases of fatal thrombotic complications have been reported rarely in patients concomitantly treated with tretinoin and anti-fibrinolytic agents. Therefore, caution should be exercised when administering tretinoin concomitantly with these agents). Products include:

Trasylol Injection 754

Betamethasone Acetate (Potential for alteration of pharmacokinetic parameters in patients on concomitant drugs that are inducers of hepatic CYP enzymes).

No products indexed under this heading.

Betamethasone Sodium Phosphate (Potential for alteration of pharmacokinetic parameters in patients on concomitant drugs that are inducers of hepatic CYP enzymes).

No products indexed under this heading.

Carbamazepine (Tretinoin is metabolized by the hepatic P450 system; therefore, there is a potential for alteration of pharmacokinetic parameters in patients administered concomitant medications that are also inducers of this system. To date, there is no data to suggestthat co-use with these medications increases or decreases either efficacy or toxicity of tretinoin). Products include:

Carbatrol Capsules 3171
Equetro Extended-Release
 Capsules.................................... 3180
Tegretol/Tegretol-XR 2295

Cimetidine (Potential for alteration of pharmacokinetic parameters in patients on concomitant drugs that inhibit hepatic CYP enzymes). Products include:

Tagamet HB 200 Tablets ▣▣664

Cimetidine Hydrochloride (Potential for alteration of pharmacokinetic parameters in patients on concomitant drugs that inhibit hepatic CYP enzymes).

No products indexed under this heading.

Ciprofloxacin (Tretinoin is metaboized by the hepatic P450 system; therefore, there is a potential for alteration of pharmacokinetic parameters in patients administered concomitant medications that are also inducers of this system. To date, there is no data to suggestthat co-use with these medications increases or decreases either efficacy or toxicity of tretinoin). Products include:

Cipro Oral Suspension 2977
Cipro I.V. 2984
Cipro XR Tablets 2990
Ciprodex Otic Suspension 559

Ciprofloxacin Hydrochloride (Tretinoin is metaboized by the hepatic P450 system; therefore, there is a potential for alteration of pharmacokinetic parameters in patients administered concomitant medications that are also inducers of this system. To date, there is no data to suggestthat co-use with these medications increases or decreases either efficacy or toxicity of tretinoin). Products include:

Ciloxan Ophthalmic Ointment 559
Ciloxan Ophthalmic Solution ⊙206
Cipro Tablets 2977
Proquin XR Tablets 1153

Cisplatin (Tretinoin is metabolized by the hepatic P450 system; therefore, there is a potential for alteration of pharmacokinetic parameters in patients administered concomitant medications that are also inducers of this system. To date, there is no data to suggestthat co-use with these medications increases or decreases either efficacy or toxicity of tretinoin).

No products indexed under this heading.

Clarithromycin (Tretinoin is metabolized by the hepatic P450 system; therefore, there is a potential for alteration of pharmacokinetic parameters in patients administered concomitant medications that are also inducers of this system. To date, there is no data to suggestthat co-use with these medications increases or decreases either efficacy or toxicity of tretinoin). Products include:

Biaxin/Biaxin XL 402
PREVPAC 3284

Clotrimazole (Tretinoin is metabolized by the hepatic P450 system; therefore, there is a potential for alteration of pharmacokinetic parameters in patients administered concomitant medications that are also inducers of this system. To date, there is no data to suggestthat co-use with these medications increases or decreases either efficacy or toxicity of tretinoin). Products include:

Desenex Athlete's Foot Cream ▣▣635
Lotrimin .. 3039
Lotrisone 3040

Cortisone Acetate (Potential for alteration of pharmacokinetic parameters in patients on concomitant drugs that are inducers of hepatic CYP enzymes).

No products indexed under this heading.

Cyclosporine (Potential for alteration of pharmacokinetic parameters in patients on concomitant drugs that inhibit hepatic CYP enzymes). Products include:

Gengraf Capsules 459
Neoral Oral Solution 2259
Neoral Soft Gelatin Capsules 2259
Restasis Ophthalmic Emulsion 575
Sandimmune 2275

Dalfopristin (Tretinoin is metabolized by the hepatic P450 system; therefore, there is a potential for alteration of pharmacokinetic parameters in patients administered concomitant medications that are also inducers of this system. To date, there is no data to suggestthat co-use with these medications increases or decreases either efficacy or toxicity of tretinoin).

No products indexed under this heading.

Danazol (Tretinoin is metabolized by the hepatic P450 system; therefore, there is a potential for alteration of pharmacokinetic parameters in patients administered concomitant medications that are also inducers of this system. To date, there is no data to suggestthat co-use with these medications increases or decreases either efficacy or toxicity of tretinoin).

No products indexed under this heading.

Delavirdine Mesylate (Tretinoin is metabolized by the hepatic P450 system; therefore, there is a potential for alteration of pharmacokinetic parameters in patients administered concomitant medications that are also inducers of this system. To date, there is no data to suggestthat co-use with these medications increases or decreases either efficacy or toxicity of tretinoin). Products include:

Rescriptor Tablets, 2551

Demeclocycline Hydrochloride (Tretinoin may cause pseudotumor cerebri/intracranial hypertension. Concomitant administration of tretinoin and agents known to cause pseudotumor cerebri/intracranial hypertension as well might increase the risk of this condition).

No products indexed under this heading.

Dexamethasone (Potential for alteration of pharmacokinetic parameters in patients on concomitant drugs that are inducers of hepatic CYP enzymes). Products include:

Ciprodex Otic Suspension 559
Decadron Tablets 1951
TobraDex Ophthalmic Ointment 562
TobraDex Ophthalmic Suspension ... 563

Dexamethasone Acetate (Potential for alteration of pharmacokinetic parameters in patients on concomitant drugs that are inducers of hepatic CYP enzymes).

No products indexed under this heading.

Dexamethasone Sodium Phosphate (Potential for alteration of pharmacokinetic parameters in patients on concomitant drugs that are inducers of hepatic CYP enzymes).

No products indexed under this heading.

Diltiazem Hydrochloride (Potential for alteration of pharmacokinetic parameters in patients on concomitant drugs that inhibit hepatic CYP enzymes). Products include:

Cardizem LA Extended Release
 Tablets 1728
Tiazac Capsules 1201

Diltiazem Maleate (Tretinoin is metaboized by the hepatic P450 system; therefore, there is a potential for alteration of pharmacokinetic parameters in patients administered concomitant medications that are also inducers of this system. To date, there is no data to suggestthat co-use with these medications increases or decreases either efficacy or toxicity of tretinoin).

No products indexed under this heading.

Doxorubicin Hydrochloride (Tretinoin is metabolized by the hepatic P450 system; therefore, there is a potential for alteration of pharmacokinetic parameters in patients administered concomitant medications that are also inducers of this system. To date, there is no data to suggest-that co-use with these medications increases or decreases either efficacy or toxicity of tretinoin).

No products indexed under this heading.

Doxycycline Calcium (Tretinoin may cause pseudotumor cerebri/intracranial hypertension. Concomitant administration of tretinoin and agents known to cause pseudotumor cerebri/intracranial hypertension as well might increase the risk of this condition).

No products indexed under this heading.

Doxycycline Hyclate (Tretinoin may cause pseudotumor cerebri/intracranial hypertension. Concomitant administration of tretinoin and agents known to cause pseudotumor cerebri/intracranial hypertension as well might increase the risk of this condition).

No products indexed under this heading.

Doxycycline Monohydrate (Tretinoin may cause pseudotumor cerebri/intracranial hypertension. Concomitant administration of tretinoin and agents known to cause pseudotumor cerebri/intracranial hypertension as well might increase the risk of this condition). Products include:

Oracea Capsules 1000

Efavirenz (Tretinoin is metaboized by the hepatic P450 system; therefore, there is a potential for alteration of pharmacokinetic parameters in patients administered concomitant medications that are also inducers of this system. To date, there is no data to suggestthat co-use with these medications increases or decreases either efficacy or toxicity of tretinoin). Products include:

Atripla Tablets 945
Sustiva Capsules 930
Sustiva Tablets 930

Erythromycin (Potential for alteration of pharmacokinetic parameters in patients on concomitant drugs that inhibit hepatic CYP enzymes). Products include:

Ery-Tab Tablets 449
Erythromycin Base Filmtab Tablets 455
Erythromycin Delayed-Release Capsules, USP 457
PCE Dispertab Tablets 515

Erythromycin Estolate (Potential for alteration of pharmacokinetic parameters in patients on concomitant drugs that inhibit hepatic CYP enzymes).

No products indexed under this heading.

Erythromycin Ethylsuccinate (Potential for alteration of pharmacokinetic parameters in patients on concomitant drugs that inhibit hepatic CYP enzymes). Products include:

E.E.S. 451
EryPed 447

Erythromycin Gluceptate (Potential for alteration of pharmacokinetic parameters in patients on concomitant drugs that inhibit hepatic CYP enzymes).

No products indexed under this heading.

Erythromycin Lactobionate (Potential for alteration of pharmacokinetic parameters in patients on concomitant drugs that inhibit hepatic CYP enzymes).

No products indexed under this heading.

Erythromycin Stearate (Potential for alteration of pharmacokinetic parameters in patients on concomitant drugs that inhibit hepatic CYP enzymes). Products include:

Erythrocin Stearate Filmtab Tablets 453

Esomeprazole Magnesium (Tretinoin is metaboized by the hepatic P450 system; therefore, there is a potential for alteration of pharmacokinetic parameters in patients administered concomitant medications that are also inducers of this system. To date, there is no data to suggest that co-use with these medications increases or decreases either efficacy or toxicity of tretinoin). Products include:

Nexium Delayed-Release Capsules 655

Ethosuximide (Tretinoin is metaboized by the hepatic P450 system; therefore, there is a potential for alteration of pharmacokinetic parameters in patients administered concomitant medications that are also inducers of this system. To date, there is no data to suggestthat co-use with these medications increases or decreases either efficacy or toxicity of tretinoin).

No products indexed under this heading.

Felbamate (Tretinoin is metaboized by the hepatic P450 system; therefore, there is a potential for alteration of pharmacokinetic parameters in patients administered concomitant medications that are also inducers of this system. To date, there is no data to suggestthat co-use with these medications increases or decreases either efficacy or toxicity of tretinoin).

No products indexed under this heading.

Fluconazole (Tretinoin is metaboized by the hepatic P450 system; therefore, there is a potential for alteration of pharmacokinetic parameters in patients administered concomitant medications that are also inducers of this system. To date, there is no data to suggestthat co-use with these medications increases or decreases either efficacy or toxicity of tretinoin).

No products indexed under this heading.

Fludrocortisone Acetate (Potential for alteration of pharmacokinetic parameters in patients on concomitant drugs that are inducers of hepatic CYP enzymes).

No products indexed under this heading.

Fluoxetine Hydrochloride (Tretinoin is metaboized by the hepatic P450 system; therefore, there is a potential for alteration of pharmacokinetic parameters in patients administered concomitant medications that are also inducers of this system. To date, there is no data to suggest that co-use with these medications increases or decreases either efficacy or toxicity of tretinoin). Products include:

Prozac Pulvules and Liquid 1801
Symbyax Capsules 1819

Fluvoxamine Maleate (Tretinoin is metaboized by the hepatic P450 system; therefore, there is a potential for alteration of pharmacokinetic parameters in patients administered concomitant medications that are also inducers of this system. To date, there is no data to suggestthat co-use with these medications increases or decreases either efficacy or toxicity of tretinoin).

No products indexed under this heading.

Fosamprenavir Calcium (Tretinoin is metaboized by the hepatic P450 system; therefore, there is a potential for alteration of pharmacokinetic parameters in patients administered concomitant medications that are also inducers of this system. To date, there is no data to suggestthat co-use with these medications increases or decreases either efficacy or toxicity of tretinoin). Products include:

Lexiva Tablets 1505

Fosphenytoin Sodium (Tretinoin is metaboized by the hepatic P450 system; therefore, there is a potential for alteration of pharmacokinetic parameters in patients administered concomitant medications that are also inducers of this system. To date, there is no data to suggestthat co-use with these medications increases or decreases either efficacy or toxicity of tretinoin).

No products indexed under this heading.

Garlic Extract (Tretinoin is metaboized by the hepatic P450 system; therefore, there is a potential for alteration of pharmacokinetic parameters in patients administered concomitant medications that are also inducers of this system. To date, there is no data to suggestthat co-use with these medications increases or decreases either efficacy or toxicity of tretinoin).

No products indexed under this heading.

Garlic Oil (Tretinoin is metaboized by the hepatic P450 system; therefore, there is a potential for alteration of pharmacokinetic parameters in patients administered concomitant medications that are also inducers of this system. To date, there is no data to suggestthat co-use with these medications increases or decreases either efficacy or toxicity of tretinoin).

No products indexed under this heading.

Hydrocortisone (Potential for alteration of pharmacokinetic parameters in patients on concomitant drugs that are inducers of hepatic CYP enzymes). Products include:

Colocort Rectal Suspension, USP (Retention) 100 mg/60 mL 2476
Hydrocortone Tablets 1989
Preparation H Hydrocortisone Cream .... ■646

Hydrocortisone Acetate (Potential for alteration of pharmacokinetic parameters in patients on concomitant drugs that are inducers of hepatic CYP enzymes). Products include:

Analpram-HC 1159
Pramosone 1161
ProctoFoam-HC 3099

Hydrocortisone Butyrate (Tretinoin is metaboized by the hepatic P450 system; therefore, there is a potential for alteration of pharmacokinetic parameters in patients administered concomitant medications that are also inducers of this system. To date, there is no data to suggest that co-use with these medications increases or decreases either efficacy or toxicity of tretinoin). Products include:

Locoid Lipocream Cream 1160

Hydrocortisone Cypionate (Tretinoin is metaboized by the hepatic P450 system; therefore, there is a potential for alteration of pharmacokinetic parameters in patients administered concomitant medications that are also inducers of this system. To date, there is no data to suggest that co-use with these medications increases or decreases either efficacy or toxicity of tretinoin).

No products indexed under this heading.

Hydrocortisone Hemisuccinate (Tretinoin is metaboized by the hepatic P450 system; therefore, there is a potential for alteration of pharmacokinetic parameters in patients administered concomitant medications that are also inducers of this system. To date, there is no data to suggestthat co-use with these medications increases or decreases either efficacy or toxicity of tretinoin).

No products indexed under this heading.

Hydrocortisone Probutate (Tretinoin is metaboized by the hepatic P450 system; therefore, there is a potential for alteration of pharmacokinetic parameters in patients administered concomitant medications that are also inducers of this system. To date, there is no data to suggest that co-use with these medications increases or decreases either efficacy or toxicity of tretinoin).

No products indexed under this heading.

Hydrocortisone Sodium Phosphate (Potential for alteration of pharmacokinetic parameters in patients on concomitant drugs that are inducers of hepatic CYP enzymes).

No products indexed under this heading.

Hydrocortisone Sodium Succinate (Potential for alteration of pharmacokinetic parameters in patients on concomitant drugs that are inducers of hepatic CYP enzymes).

No products indexed under this heading.

Hydrocortisone Valerate (Tretinoin is metaboized by the hepatic P450 system; therefore, there is a potential for alteration of pharmacokinetic parameters in patients administered concomitant medications that are also inducers of this system. To date, there is no data to suggest that co-use with these medications increases or decreases either efficacy or toxicity of tretinoin).

No products indexed under this heading.

Hypericum (Tretinoin is metaboized by the hepatic P450 system; therefore, there is a potential for alteration of pharmacokinetic parameters in patients administered concomitant medications that are also inducers of this system. To date, there is no data to suggestthat co-use with these medications increases or decreases either efficacy or toxicity of tretinoin). Products include:

Satiete Tablets .... ■832

Hypericum Perforatum (Tretinoin is metaboized by the hepatic P450 system; therefore, there is a potential for alteration of pharmacokinetic parameters in patients administered concomitant medications that are also inducers of this system. To date, there is no data to suggestthat co-use with these medications increases or decreases either efficacy or toxicity of tretinoin).

No products indexed under this heading.

Indinavir Sulfate (Tretinoin is metaboized by the hepatic P450 system; therefore, there is a potential for alteration of pharmacokinetic parameters in patients administered concomitant medications that are also inducers of this system. To date, there is no data to suggestthat co-use with these medications increases or decreases either efficacy or toxicity of tretinoin). Products include:

Crixivan Capsules 1940

Isoniazid (Tretinoin is metaboized by the hepatic P450 system; therefore, there is a potential for alteration of pharmacokinetic parameters in patients administered concomitant medications that are also inducers of this system. To date, there is no data to suggestthat co-use with these medications increases or decreases either efficacy or toxicity of tretinoin).

No products indexed under this heading.

Itraconazole (Tretinoin is metaboized by the hepatic P450 system; therefore, there is a potential for alteration of pharmacokinetic parameters in patients administered concomitant medications that are also inducers of this system. To date, there is no data to suggestthat co-use with these medications increases or decreases either efficacy or toxicity of tretinoin).

No products indexed under this heading.

Ketoconazole (Potential for alteration of pharmacokinetic parameters in patients on concomitant drugs that inhibit hepatic CYP enzymes). Products include:

Nizoral A-D Shampoo, 1% 1868

Lopinavir (Tretinoin is metaboized by the hepatic P450 system; therefore, there is a potential for alteration of pharmacokinetic parameters in patients administered concomitant medications that are also inducers of this system. To date, there is no data to suggestthat co-use with these medications increases or decreases either efficacy or toxicity of tretinoin). Products include:

Kaletra 476

Loratadine (Tretinoin is metaboized by the hepatic P450 system; therefore, there is a potential for alteration of pharmacokinetic parameters in patients administered concomitant medications that are also inducers of this system. To date, there is no data to suggestthat co-use with these medications increases or decreases either efficacy or toxicity of tretinoin). Products include:

Alavert Allergy & Sinus D-12 Hour Tablets 771
Alavert 771
Children's Claritin Allergy Oral Solution 771
Claritin Non-Drowsy 24 Hour Tablets 772
Claritin Reditabs 24 Hour Non-Drowsy Tablets 772
Claritin-D Non-Drowsy 12 Hour Tablets 772
Claritin-D Non-Drowsy 24 Hour Tablets 772

Mephenytoin (Tretinoin is metaboized by the hepatic P450 system; therefore, there is a potential for alteration of pharmacokinetic parameters in patients administered concomitant medications that are also inducers of this system. To date, there is no data to suggestthat co-use with these medications increases or decreases either efficacy or toxicity of tretinoin).

No products indexed under this heading.

Methacycline Hydrochloride (Tretinoin may cause pseudotumor cerebri/intracranial hypertension. Concomitant administration of tretinoin and agents known to cause pseudotumor cerebri/intracranial hypertension as well might increase the risk of this condition).

No products indexed under this heading.

Methsuximide (Tretinoin is metaboized by the hepatic P450 system; therefore, there is a potential for alteration of pharmacokinetic parameters in patients administered concomitant medications that are also inducers of this system. To date, there is no data to suggestthat co-use with these medications increases or decreases either efficacy or toxicity of tretinoin).

No products indexed under this heading.

Methylprednisolone (Tretinoin is metaboized by the hepatic P450 system; therefore, there is a potential for alteration of pharmacokinetic parameters in patients administered concomitant medications that are also inducers of this system. To date, there is no data to suggestthat co-use with these medications increases or decreases either efficacy or toxicity of tretinoin).

No products indexed under this heading.

Methylprednisolone Acetate (Potential for alteration of pharmacokinetic parameters in patients on concomitant drugs that are inducers of hepatic CYP enzymes). Products include:

Depo-Medrol Injectable Suspension 2617
Depo-Medrol Single-Dose Vial 2619

Methylprednisolone Sodium Succinate (Potential for alteration of pharmacokinetic parameters in patients on concomitant drugs that are inducers of hepatic CYP enzymes).

No products indexed under this heading.

Metronidazole (Tretinoin is metaboized by the hepatic P450 system; therefore, there is a potential for alteration of pharmacokinetic parameters in patients administered concomitant medications that are also inducers of this system. To date, there is no data to suggestthat co-use with these medications increases or decreases either efficacy or toxicity of tretinoin). Products include:

Metrogel 1% 1211
MetroGel-Vaginal Gel 1855
Vandazole Vaginal Gel 3338

Metronidazole Benzoate (Tretinoin is metaboized by the hepatic P450 system; therefore, there is a potential for alteration of pharmacokinetic parameters in patients administered concomitant medications that are also inducers of this system. To date, there is no data to suggest-that co-use with these medications increases or decreases either efficacy or toxicity of tretinoin).

No products indexed under this heading.

Metronidazole Hydrochloride (Tretinoin is metaboized by the hepatic P450 system; therefore, there is a potential for alteration of pharmacokinetic parameters in patients administered concomitant medications that are also inducers of this system. To date, there is no data to suggestthat co-use with these medications increases or decreases either efficacy or toxicity of tretinoin).

No products indexed under this heading.

Miconazole (Tretinoin is metaboized by the hepatic P450 system; therefore, there is a potential for alteration of pharmacokinetic parameters in patients administered concomitant medications that are also inducers of this system. To date, there is no data to suggestthat co-use with these medications increases or decreases either efficacy or toxicity of tretinoin).

No products indexed under this heading.

Miconazole Nitrate (Tretinoin is metaboized by the hepatic P450 system; therefore, there is a potential for alteration of pharmacokinetic parameters in patients administered concomitant medications that are also inducers of this system. To date, there is no data to suggestthat co-use with these medications increases or decreases either efficacy or toxicity of tretinoin). Products include:

Desenex 635
Desenex Jock Itch Spray Powder ... 635

Minocycline Hydrochloride (Tretinoin may cause pseudotumor cerebri/intracranial hypertension. Concomitant administration of tretinoin and agents known to cause pseudotumor cerebri/intracranial hypertension as well might increase the risk of this condition). Products include:

Solodyn Extended Release Tablets 1890

Modafinil (Tretinoin is metaboized by the hepatic P450 system; therefore, there is a potential for alteration of pharmacokinetic parameters in patients administered concomitant medications that are also inducers of this system. To date, there is no data to suggestthat co-use with these medications increases or decreases either efficacy or toxicity of tretinoin). Products include:

Provigil Tablets 988

Nefazodone Hydrochloride (Tretinoin is metaboized by the hepatic P450 system; therefore, there is a potential for alteration of pharmacokinetic parameters in patients administered concomitant medications that are also inducers of this system. To date, there is no data to suggest-that co-use with these medications increases or decreases either efficacy or toxicity of tretinoin).

No products indexed under this heading.

Nelfinavir Mesylate (Tretinoin is metaboized by the hepatic P450 system; therefore, there is a potential for alteration of pharmacokinetic parameters in patients administered concomitant medications that are also inducers of this system. To date, there is no data to suggestthat co-use with these medications increases or decreases either efficacy or toxicity of tretinoin). Products include:

Viracept 2577

Nevirapine (Tretinoin is metaboized by the hepatic P450 system; therefore, there is a potential for alteration of pharmacokinetic parameters in patients administered concomitant medications that are also inducers of this system. To date, there is no data to suggestthat co-use with these medications increases or decreases either efficacy or toxicity of tretinoin). Products include:

Viramune Oral Suspension 873
Viramune Tablets 873

Niacinamide (Tretinoin is metaboized by the hepatic P450 system; therefore, there is a potential for alteration of pharmacokinetic parameters in patients administered concomitant medications that are also inducers of this system. To date, there is no data to suggestthat co-use with these medications increases or decreases either efficacy or toxicity of tretinoin).

No products indexed under this heading.

Nicotinamide (Tretinoin is metaboized by the hepatic P450 system; therefore, there is a potential for alteration of pharmacokinetic parameters in patients administered concomitant medications that are also inducers of this system. To date, there is no data to suggestthat co-use with these medications increases or decreases either efficacy or toxicity of tretinoin). Products include:

Nicomide Tablets 1088

Nifedipine (Tretinoin is metaboized by the hepatic P450 system; therefore, there is a potential for alteration of pharmacokinetic parameters in patients administered concomitant medications that are also inducers of this system. To date, there is no data to suggestthat co-use with these medications increases or decreases either efficacy or toxicity of tretinoin). Products include:

Adalat CC Tablets 2964

Norfloxacin (Tretinoin is metaboized by the hepatic P450 system; therefore, there is a potential for alteration of pharmacokinetic parameters in patients administered concomitant medications that are also inducers of this system. To date, there is no data to suggestthat co-use with these medications increases or decreases either efficacy or toxicity of tretinoin). Products include:

Noroxin Tablets 2032

Omeprazole (Tretinoin is metaboized by the hepatic P450 system; therefore, there is a potential for alteration of pharmacokinetic parameters in patients administered concomitant medications that are also inducers of this system. To date, there is no data to suggestthat co-use with these medications increases or decreases either efficacy or toxicity of tretinoin). Products include:

Zegerid Capsules 2958
Zegerid Powder for Oral Solution 2958

Oxcarbazepine (Tretinoin is metaboized by the hepatic P450 system; therefore, there is a potential for alteration of pharmacokinetic parameters in patients administered concomitant medications that are also inducers of this system. To date, there is no data to suggestthat co-use with these medications increases or decreases either efficacy or toxicity of tretinoin). Products include:

Trileptal Tablets 2300
Trileptal Oral Suspension 2300

Oxytetracycline Hydrochloride
(Tretinoin may cause pseudotumor cerebri/intracranial hypertension. Concomitant administration of tretinoin and agents known to cause pseudotumor cerebri/intracranial hypertension as well might increase the risk of this condition).

No products indexed under this heading.

Paroxetine Hydrochloride (Tretinoin is metaboized by the hepatic P450 system; therefore, there is a potential for alteration of pharmacokinetic parameters in patients administered concomitant medications that are also inducers of this system. To date, there is no data to suggestthat co-use with these medications increases or decreases either efficacy or toxicity of tretinoin). Products include:

Paxil CR Controlled-Release
Tablets .. 1538
Paxil ... 1530

Pentobarbital Sodium (Potential for alteration of pharmacokinetic parameters in patients on concomitant drugs that are inducers of hepatic CYP enzymes). Products include:

Nembutal Sodium Solution, USP 2470

Phenobarbital (Potential for alteration of pharmacokinetic parameters in patients on concomitant drugs that are inducers of hepatic CYP enzymes). Products include:

Donnatal Extentabs 2493

Phenobarbital Sodium (Tretinoin is metaboized by the hepatic P450 system; therefore, there is a potential for alteration of pharmacokinetic parameters in patients administered concomitant medications that are also inducers of this system. To date, there is no data to suggestthat co-use with these medications increases or decreases either efficacy or toxicity of tretinoin).

No products indexed under this heading.

Phenytoin (Tretinoin is metaboized by the hepatic P450 system; therefore, there is a potential for alteration of pharmacokinetic parameters in patients administered concomitant medications that are also inducers of this system. To date, there is no data to suggestthat co-use with these medications increases or decreases either efficacy or toxicity of tretinoin).

No products indexed under this heading.

Phenytoin Sodium (Tretinoin is metaboized by the hepatic P450 system; therefore, there is a potential for alteration of pharmacokinetic parameters in patients administered concomitant medications that are also inducers of this system. To date, there is no data to suggestthat co-use with these medications increases or decreases either efficacy or toxicity of tretinoin). Products include:

Phenytek Capsules 2160

Prednisolone Acetate (Potential for alteration of pharmacokinetic parameters in patients on concomi-

tant drugs that are inducers of hepatic CYP enzymes). Products include:

Blephamide Ophthalmic Ointment 568
Blephamide Ophthalmic
Suspension 569
Poly-Pred Ophthalmic
Suspension ⊙233
Pred Forte Ophthalmic
Suspension ⊙235
Pred Mild Ophthalmic
Suspension ⊙238
Pred-G Ophthalmic Ointment ⊙237
Pred-G Ophthalmic Suspension ⊙236

Prednisolone Sodium Phosphate
(Potential for alteration of pharmacokinetic parameters in patients on concomitant drugs that are inducers of hepatic CYP enzymes).

No products indexed under this heading.

Prednisolone Tebutate (Potential for alteration of pharmacokinetic parameters in patients on concomitant drugs that are inducers of hepatic CYP enzymes).

No products indexed under this heading.

Prednisone (Potential for alteration of pharmacokinetic parameters in patients on concomitant drugs that are inducers of hepatic CYP enzymes).

No products indexed under this heading.

Primidone (Tretinoin is metaboized by the hepatic P450 system; therefore, there is a potential for alteration of pharmacokinetic parameters in patients administered concomitant medications that are also inducers of this system. To date, there is no data to suggestthat co-use with these medications increases or decreases either efficacy or toxicity of tretinoin).

No products indexed under this heading.

Propoxyphene Hydrochloride
(Tretinoin is metaboized by the hepatic P450 system; therefore, there is a potential for alteration of pharmacokinetic parameters in patients administered concomitant medications that are also inducers of this system. To date, there is no data to suggestthat co-use with these medications increases or decreases either efficacy or toxicity of tretinoin).

No products indexed under this heading.

Propoxyphene Napsylate (Tretinoin is metaboized by the hepatic P450 system; therefore, there is a potential for alteration of pharmacokinetic parameters in patients administered concomitant medications that are also inducers of this system. To date, there is no data to suggestthat co-use with these medications increases or decreases either efficacy or toxicity of tretinoin).

No products indexed under this heading.

Quinidine (Tretinoin is metaboized by the hepatic P450 system; therefore, there is a potential for alteration of pharmacokinetic parameters in patients administered concomitant medications that are also inducers of this system. To date, there is no data to suggestthat co-use with these medications increases or decreases either efficacy or toxicity of tretinoin).

No products indexed under this heading.

Quinidine Hydrochloride (Tretinoin is metaboized by the hepatic P450 system; therefore, there is a potential for alteration of pharmacokinetic parameters in patients administered concomitant medications that are also inducers of this system. To date, there is no data to suggestthat co-use with these medications increases or decreases either efficacy or toxicity of tretinoin).

No products indexed under this heading.

Quinidine Polygalacturonate
(Tretinoin is metaboized by the hepatic P450 system; therefore, there is a potential for alteration of pharmacokinetic parameters in patients administered concomitant medications that are also inducers of this system. To date, there is no data to suggestthat co-use with these medications increases or decreases either efficacy or toxicity of tretinoin).

No products indexed under this heading.

Quinidine Sulfate (Tretinoin is metaboized by the hepatic P450 system; therefore, there is a potential for alteration of pharmacokinetic parameters in patients administered concomitant medications that are also inducers of this system. To date, there is no data to suggestthat co-use with these medications increases or decreases either efficacy or toxicity of tretinoin).

No products indexed under this heading.

Quinine (Tretinoin is metaboized by the hepatic P450 system; therefore, there is a potential for alteration of pharmacokinetic parameters in patients administered concomitant medications that are also inducers of this system. To date, there is no data to suggestthat co-use with these medications increases or decreases either efficacy or toxicity of tretinoin).

No products indexed under this heading.

Quinine Sulfate (Tretinoin is metaboized by the hepatic P450 system; therefore, there is a potential for alteration of pharmacokinetic parameters in patients administered concomitant medications that are also inducers of this system. To date, there is no data to suggestthat co-use with these medications increases or decreases either efficacy or toxicity of tretinoin).

No products indexed under this heading.

Quinupristin (Tretinoin is metaboized by the hepatic P450 system; therefore, there is a potential for alteration of pharmacokinetic parameters in patients administered concomitant medications that are also inducers of this system. To date, there is no data to suggestthat co-use with these medications increases or decreases either efficacy or toxicity of tretinoin).

No products indexed under this heading.

Ranitidine Bismuth Citrate (Tretinoin is metaboized by the hepatic P450 system; therefore, there is a potential for alteration of pharmacokinetic parameters in patients administered concomitant medications that are also inducers of this system. To date, there is no data to suggestthat co-use with these medications increases or decreases either efficacy or toxicity of tretinoin).

No products indexed under this heading.

Ranitidine Hydrochloride (Tretinoin is metaboized by the hepatic P450 system; therefore, there is a potential for alteration of pharmacokinetic parameters in patients administered concomitant medications that are also inducers of this system. To date, there is no data to suggestthat co-use with these medications increases or decreases either efficacy or toxicity of tretinoin). Products include:

Zantac .. 1624
Zantac Injection 1619
Zantac Injection Pharmacy Bulk
Package... 1622

Rifabutin (Tretinoin is metaboized by the hepatic P450 system; therefore, there is a potential for alteration of pharmacokinetic parameters in patients administered concomitant medications that are also inducers of this system. To date, there is no data to suggestthat co-use with these medications increases or decreases either efficacy or toxicity of tretinoin).

No products indexed under this heading.

Rifampicin (Tretinoin is metaboized by the hepatic P450 system; therefore, there is a potential for alteration of pharmacokinetic parameters in patients administered concomitant medications that are also inducers of this system. To date, there is no data to suggestthat co-use with these medications increases or decreases either efficacy or toxicity of tretinoin).

No products indexed under this heading.

Rifampin (Potential for alteration of pharmacokinetic parameters in patients on concomitant drugs that are inducers of hepatic CYP enzymes).

No products indexed under this heading.

Rifapentine (Tretinoin is metaboized by the hepatic P450 system; therefore, there is a potential for alteration of pharmacokinetic parameters in patients administered concomitant medications that are also inducers of this system. To date, there is no data to suggestthat co-use with these medications increases or decreases either efficacy or toxicity of tretinoin).

No products indexed under this heading.

Ritonavir (Tretinoin is metaboized by the hepatic P450 system; therefore, there is a potential for alteration of pharmacokinetic parameters in patients administered concomitant medications that are also inducers of this system. To date, there is no data to suggestthat co-use with these medications increases or decreases either efficacy or toxicity of tretinoin). Products include:

Kaletra ... 476

Norvir 503

Saquinavir (Tretinoin is metaboized by the hepatic P450 system; therefore, there is a potential for alteration of pharmacokinetic parameters in patients administered concomitant medications that are also inducers of this system. To date, there is no data to suggestthat co-use with these medications increases or decreases either efficacy or toxicity of tretinoin).

No products indexed under this heading.

Saquinavir Mesylate (Tretinoin is metaboized by the hepatic P450 system; therefore, there is a potential for alteration of pharmacokinetic parameters in patients administered concomitant medications that are also inducers of this system. To date, there is no data to suggestthat co-use with these medications increases or decreases either efficacy or toxicity of tretinoin). Products include:

Invirase 2772

Sertraline Hydrochloride (Tretinoin is metaboized by the hepatic P450 system; therefore, there is a potential for alteration of pharmacokinetic parameters in patients administered concomitant medications that are also inducers of this system. To date, there is no data to suggest that co-use with these medications increases or decreases either efficacy or toxicity of tretinoin). Products include:

Zoloft 2586

Sulfinpyrazone (Tretinoin is metaboized by the hepatic P450 system; therefore, there is a potential for alteration of pharmacokinetic parameters in patients administered concomitant medications that are also inducers of this system. To date, there is no data to suggestthat co-use with these medications increases or decreases either efficacy or toxicity of tretinoin).

No products indexed under this heading.

Telithromycin (Tretinoin is metaboized by the hepatic P450 system; therefore, there is a potential for alteration of pharmacokinetic parameters in patients administered concomitant medications that are also inducers of this system. To date, there is no data to suggestthat co-use with these medications increases or decreases either efficacy or toxicity of tretinoin). Products include:

Ketek Tablets 2903

Tetracycline Hydrochloride (Tretinoin may cause pseudotumor cerebri/intracranial hypertension. Concomitant administration of tretinoin and agents known to cause pseudotumor cerebri/intracranial hypertension as well might increase the risk of this condition).

No products indexed under this heading.

Theophylline (Tretinoin is metaboized by the hepatic P450 system; therefore, there is a potential for alteration of pharmacokinetic parameters in patients administered concomitant medications that are also inducers of this system. To date, there is no data to suggestthat co-use with these medications increases or decreases either efficacy or toxicity of tretinoin).

No products indexed under this heading.

Tranexamic Acid (Cases of fatal thrombotic complications have been reported rarely in patients concomitantly treated with tretinoin and antifibrinolytic agents. Therefore, caution should be exercised when administering tretinoin concomitantly with these agents).

No products indexed under this heading.

Triamcinolone (Potential for alteration of pharmacokinetic parameters in patients on concomitant drugs that are inducers of hepatic CYP enzymes).

No products indexed under this heading.

Triamcinolone Acetonide (Potential for alteration of pharmacokinetic parameters in patients on concomitant drugs that are inducers of hepatic CYP enzymes). Products include:

Azmacort Inhalation Aerosol 1726
Nasacort AQ Nasal Spray 2922

Triamcinolone Diacetate (Potential for alteration of pharmacokinetic parameters in patients on concomitant drugs that are inducers of hepatic CYP enzymes).

No products indexed under this heading.

Triamcinolone Hexacetonide (Potential for alteration of pharmacokinetic parameters in patients on concomitant drugs that are inducers of hepatic CYP enzymes).

No products indexed under this heading.

Troglitazone (Tretinoin is metaboized by the hepatic P450 system; therefore, there is a potential for alteration of pharmacokinetic parameters in patients administered concomitant medications that are also inducers of this system. To date, there is no data to suggestthat co-use with these medications increases or decreases either efficacy or toxicity of tretinoin).

No products indexed under this heading.

Troleandomycin (Tretinoin is metaboized by the hepatic P450 system; therefore, there is a potential for alteration of pharmacokinetic parameters in patients administered concomitant medications that are also inducers of this system. To date, there is no data to suggestthat co-use with these medications increases or decreases either efficacy or toxicity of tretinoin).

No products indexed under this heading.

Valproate Sodium (Tretinoin is metaboized by the hepatic P450 system; therefore, there is a potential for alteration of pharmacokinetic parameters in patients administered concomitant medications that are also inducers of this system. To date, there is no data to suggestthat co-use with these medications increases or decreases either efficacy or toxicity of tretinoin). Products include:

Depacon Injection 412

Verapamil Hydrochloride (Potential for alteration of pharmacokinetic parameters in patients on concomitant drugs that inhibit hepatic CYP enzymes). Products include:

Covera-HS Tablets 3139
Tarka Tablets 524
Verelan PM Extended-Release Capsules, Controlled-Onset.......... 3106

Vitamin A (Vesanoid must not be administered in combination with vitamin A because of symptoms of hypervitaminosis A could be aggravated). Products include:

Visutein Capsules 3329

Voriconazole (Tretinoin is metaboized by the hepatic P450 system; therefore, there is a potential for alteration of pharmacokinetic parameters in patients administered concomitant medications that are also inducers of this system. To date, there is no data to suggestthat co-use with these medications increases or decreases either efficacy or toxicity of tretinoin). Products include:

VFEND I.V. 2564
VFEND Oral Suspension 2564
VFEND Tablets 2564

Zafirlukast (Tretinoin is metaboized by the hepatic P450 system; therefore, there is a potential for alteration of pharmacokinetic parameters in patients administered concomitant medications that are also inducers of this system. To date, there is no data to suggestthat co-use with these medications increases or decreases either efficacy or toxicity of tretinoin). Products include:

Accolate Tablets 671

Zileuton (Tretinoin is metaboized by the hepatic P450 system; therefore, there is a potential for alteration of pharmacokinetic parameters in patients administered concomitant medications that are also inducers of this system. To date, there is no data to suggestthat co-use with these medications increases or decreases either efficacy or toxicity of tretinoin). Products include:

Zyflo Tablets 1023

Food Interactions

Food, unspecified (The absorption of retinoids as a class has been shown to be enhanced when taken with food).

Grapefruit (Tretinoin is metaboized by the hepatic P450 system; therefore, there is a potential for alteration of pharmacokinetic parameters in patients administered concomitant medications that are also inducers of this system. To date, there is no data to suggestthat co-use with these medications increases or decreases either efficacy or toxicity of tretinoin).

Grapefruit Juice (Tretinoin is metaboized by the hepatic P450 system; therefore, there is a potential for alteration of pharmacokinetic parameters in patients administered concomitant medications that are also inducers of this system. To date, there is no data to suggestthat co-use with these medications increases or decreases either efficacy or toxicity of tretinoin).

VESICARE TABLETS

(Solifenacin Succinate) 646

May interact with cytochrome p450 3a4 inhibitors, potent and drugs that prolong the QT interval. Compounds in these categories include:

Amiodarone Hydrochloride (In a study of the effect of solifenacin on the QT interval in 76 healthy women, the QT prolonging effect appered less with solifenacin 10 mg than with 30 mg (three times the maximum recommended dose), and the effect of solifenacin 30 mg did not appear as large as that of the positive control moxifloxacin at its therapeutic dose. This observation should be considered in clinical decisions to prescribe solifenacin succinate for patients with a known history of QT prolongation or patients who are taking medications known to prolong the QT interval).

No products indexed under this heading.

Amitriptyline Hydrochloride (In a study of the effect of solifenacin on the QT interval in 76 healthy women, the QT prolonging effect appered less with solifenacin 10 mg than with 30 mg (three times the maximum recommended dose), and the effect of solifenacin 30 mg did not appear as large as that of the positive control moxifloxacin at its therapeutic dose. This observation should be considered in clinical decisions to prescribe solifenacin succinate for patients with a known history of QT prolongation or patients who are taking medications known to prolong the QT interval).

No products indexed under this heading.

Amoxapine (In a study of the effect of solifenacin on the QT interval in 76 healthy women, the QT prolonging effect appered less with solifenacin 10 mg than with 30 mg (three times the maximum recommended dose), and the effect of solifenacin 30 mg did not appear as large as that of the positive control moxifloxacin at its therapeutic dose. This observation should be considered in clinical decisions to prescribe solifenacin succinate for patients with a known history of QT prolongation or patients who are taking medications known to prolong the QT interval).

No products indexed under this heading.

Amprenavir (Do not exceed a 5 mg daily dose of solifenacin succinate when administered with therapeutic doses of ketoconazole or other potent CYP3A4 inhibitors). Products include:

Agenerase Capsules 1327
Agenerase Oral Solution 1332

Astemizole (In a study of the effect of solifenacin on the QT interval in 76 healthy women, the QT prolonging effect appered less with solifenacin 10 mg than with 30 mg (three times the maximum recommended dose), and the effect of solifenacin 30 mg did not appear as large as that of the positive control moxifloxacin at its therapeutic dose. This observation should be considered in clinical decisions to prescribe solifenacin succinate for patients with a known history of QT prolongation or patients who are taking medications known to prolong the QT interval).

No products indexed under this heading.

Atazanavir (Do not exceed a 5 mg daily dose of solifenacin succinate when administered with therapeutic doses of ketoconazole or other potent CYP3A4 inhibitors).

No products indexed under this heading.

Atazanavir sulfate (Do not exceed a 5 mg daily dose of solifenacin succinate when administered with therapeutic doses of ketoconazole or other potent CYP3A4 inhibitors). Products include:

Reyataz Capsules 921

Bretylium Tosylate (In a study of the effect of solifenacin on the QT interval in 76 healthy women, the QT prolonging effect appered less with solifenacin 10 mg than with 30 mg (three times the maximum recommended dose), and the effect of solifenacin 30 mg did not appear as large as that of the positive control moxifloxacin at its therapeutic dose. This observation should be considered in clinical decisions to prescribe solifenacin succinate for patients with a known history of QT prolongation or patients who are taking medications known to prolong the QT interval).

No products indexed under this heading.

Chlorpromazine (In a study of the effect of solifenacin on the QT interval in 76 healthy women, the QT prolonging effect appered less with solifenacin 10 mg than with 30 mg (three times the maximum recommended dose), and the effect of solifenacin 30 mg did not appear as large as that of the positive control moxifloxacin at its therapeutic dose. This observation should be considered in clinical decisions to prescribe solifenacin succinate for patients with a known history of QT prolongation or patients who are taking medications known to prolong the QT interval).

No products indexed under this heading.

Chlorpromazine Hydrochloride (In a study of the effect of solifenacin on the QT interval in 76 healthy women, the QT prolonging effect appered less with solifenacin 10 mg than with 30 mg (three times the maximum recommended dose), and the effect of solifenacin 30 mg did not appear as large as that of the positive control moxifloxacin at its therapeutic dose. This observation should be considered in clinical decisions to prescribe solifenacin succinate for patients with a known history of QT prolongation or patients who are taking medications known to prolong the QT interval).

No products indexed under this heading.

Clarithromycin (Do not exceed a 5 mg daily dose of solifenacin succinate when administered with therapeutic doses of ketoconazole or other potent CYP3A4 inhibitors). Products include:

Biaxin/Biaxin XL 402
PREVPAC 3284

Clomipramine Hydrochloride (In a study of the effect of solifenacin on the QT interval in 76 healthy women, the QT prolonging effect appered less with solifenacin 10 mg than with 30 mg (three times the maximum recommended dose), and the effect of solifenacin 30 mg did not appear as large as that of the positive control moxifloxacin at its therapeutic dose. This observation should be considered in clinical decisions to prescribe solifenacin succinate for patients with a known history of QT prolongation or patients who are taking medications known to prolong the QT interval).

No products indexed under this heading.

Desipramine Hydrochloride (In a study of the effect of solifenacin on the QT interval in 76 healthy women, the QT prolonging effect appered less with solifenacin 10 mg than with 30 mg (three times the maximum recommended dose), and the effect of solifenacin 30 mg did not appear as large as that of the positive control moxifloxacin at its therapeutic dose. This observation should be considered in clinical decisions to prescribe solifenacin succinate for patients with a known history of QT prolongation or patients who are taking medications known to prolong the QT interval).

No products indexed under this heading.

Disopyramide Phosphate (In a study of the effect of solifenacin on the QT interval in 76 healthy women, the QT prolonging effect appered less with solifenacin 10 mg than with 30 mg (three times the maximum recommended dose), and the effect of solifenacin 30 mg did not appear as large as that of the positive control moxifloxacin at its therapeutic dose. This observation should be considered in clinical decisions to prescribe solifenacin succinate for patients with a known history of QT prolongation or patients who are taking medications known to prolong the QT interval).

No products indexed under this heading.

Dofetilide (In a study of the effect of solifenacin on the QT interval in 76 healthy women, the QT prolonging effect appered less with solifenacin 10 mg than with 30 mg (three times the maximum recommended dose), and the effect of solifenacin 30 mg did not appear as large as that of the positive control moxifloxacin at its therapeutic dose. This observation should be considered in clinical decisions to prescribe solifenacin succinate for patients with a known history of QT prolongation or patients who are taking medications known to prolong the QT interval).

No products indexed under this heading.

Doxepin Hydrochloride (In a study of the effect of solifenacin on the QT interval in 76 healthy women, the QT prolonging effect appered less with solifenacin 10 mg than with 30 mg (three times the maximum recommended dose), and the effect of solifenacin 30 mg did not appear as large as that of the positive control moxifloxacin at its therapeutic dose. This observation should be considered in clinical decisions to prescribe solifenacin succinate for patients with a known history of QT prolongation or patients who are taking medications known to prolong the QT interval).

No products indexed under this heading.

Flecainide Acetate (In a study of the effect of solifenacin on the QT interval in 76 healthy women, the QT prolonging effect appered less with solifenacin 10 mg than with 30 mg (three times the maximum recommended dose), and the effect of solifenacin 30 mg did not appear as large as that of the positive control moxifloxacin at its therapeutic dose. This observation should be considered in clinical decisions to prescribe solifenacin succinate for patients with a known history of QT prolongation or patients who are taking medications known to prolong the QT interval). Products include:

Tambocor Tablets 1856

Fluphenazine Decanoate (In a study of the effect of solifenacin on the QT interval in 76 healthy women, the QT prolonging effect appered less with solifenacin 10 mg than with 30 mg (three times the maximum recommended dose), and the effect of solifenacin 30 mg did not appear as large as that of the positive control moxifloxacin at its therapeutic dose. This observation should be considered in clinical decisions to prescribe solifenacin succinate for patients with a known history of QT prolongation or patients who are taking medications known to prolong the QT interval).

No products indexed under this heading.

Fluphenazine Enanthate (In a study of the effect of solifenacin on the QT interval in 76 healthy women, the QT prolonging effect appered less with solifenacin 10 mg than with 30 mg (three times the maximum recommended dose), and the effect of solifenacin 30 mg did not appear as large as that of the positive control moxifloxacin at its therapeutic dose. This observation should be considered in clinical decisions to prescribe solifenacin succinate for patients with a known history of QT prolongation or patients who are taking medications known to prolong the QT interval).

No products indexed under this heading.

Fluphenazine Hydrochloride (In a study of the effect of solifenacin on the QT interval in 76 healthy women, the QT prolonging effect appered less with solifenacin 10 mg than with 30 mg (three times the maximum recommended dose), and the effect of solifenacin 30 mg did not appear as large as that of the positive control moxifloxacin at its therapeutic dose. This observation should be considered in clinical decisions to prescribe solifenacin succinate for patients with a known history of QT prolongation or patients who are taking medications known to prolong the QT interval).

No products indexed under this heading.

Fosamprenavir Calcium (Do not exceed a 5 mg daily dose of solifenacin succinate when administered with therapeutic doses of ketoconazole or other potent CYP3A4 inhibitors). Products include:

Lexiva Tablets 1505

Imipramine Hydrochloride (In a study of the effect of solifenacin on the QT interval in 76 healthy women, the QT prolonging effect appered less with solifenacin 10 mg than with 30 mg (three times the maximum recommended dose), and the effect of solifenacin 30 mg did not appear as large as that of the positive control moxifloxacin at its therapeutic dose. This observation should be considered in clinical decisions to prescribe solifenacin succinate for patients with a known history of QT prolongation or patients who are taking medications known to prolong the QT interval).

No products indexed under this heading.

Imipramine Pamoate (In a study of the effect of solifenacin on the QT interval in 76 healthy women, the QT prolonging effect appered less with solifenacin 10 mg than with 30 mg (three times the maximum recommended dose), and the effect of solifenacin 30 mg did not appear as large as that of the positive control moxifloxacin at its therapeutic dose. This observation should be considered in clinical decisions to prescribe solifenacin succinate for patients with a known history of QT prolongation or patients who are taking medications known to prolong the QT interval).

No products indexed under this heading.

Indinavir Sulfate (Do not exceed a 5 mg daily dose of solifenacin succinate when administered with therapeutic doses of ketoconazole or other potent CYP3A4 inhibitors). Products include:

Crixivan Capsules 1940

Itraconazole (Do not exceed a 5 mg daily dose of solifenacin succinate when administered with therapeutic doses of ketoconazole or other potent CYP3A4 inhibitors).

No products indexed under this heading.

Ketoconazole (Do not exceed a 5 mg daily dose of solifenacin succinate when administered with therapeutic doses of ketoconazole or other potent CYP3A4 inhibitors). Products include:

Nizoral A-D Shampoo, 1% 1868

Lidocaine Hydrochloride (In a study of the effect of solifenacin on the QT interval in 76 healthy women, the QT prolonging effect appered less with solifenacin 10 mg than with 30 mg (three times the maximum recommended dose), and the effect of solifenacin 30 mg did not appear as large as that of the positive control moxifloxacin at its therapeutic dose. This observation should be considered in clinical decisions to prescribe solifenacin succinate for patients with a known history of QT prolongation or patients who are taking medications known to prolong the QT interval).

No products indexed under this heading.

Lopinavir (Do not exceed a 5 mg daily dose of solifenacin succinate when administered with therapeutic doses of ketoconazole or other potent CYP3A4 inhibitors). Products include:

Kaletra 476

Maprotiline Hydrochloride (In a study of the effect of solifenacin on the QT interval in 76 healthy women, the QT prolonging effect appered less with solifenacin 10 mg than with 30 mg (three times the maximum recommended dose), and the effect of solifenacin 30 mg did not appear as large as that of the positive control moxifloxacin at its therapeutic dose. This observation should be considered in clinical decisions to prescribe solifenacin succinate for patients with a known history of QT prolongation or patients who are taking medications known to prolong the QT interval).

No products indexed under this heading.

Mesoridazine Besylate (In a study of the effect of solifenacin on the QT interval in 76 healthy women, the QT prolonging effect appered less with solifenacin 10 mg than with 30 mg (three times the maximum recommended dose), and the effect of solifenacin 30 mg did not appear as large as that of the positive control moxifloxacin at its therapeutic dose. This observation should be considered in clinical decisions to prescribe solifenacin succinate for patients with a known history of QT prolongation or patients who are taking medications known to prolong the QT interval).

No products indexed under this heading.

Mexiletine Hydrochloride (In a study of the effect of solifenacin on the QT interval in 76 healthy women, the QT prolonging effect appered less with solifenacin 10 mg than with 30 mg (three times the maximum recommended dose), and the effect of solifenacin 30 mg did not appear as large as that of the positive control moxifloxacin at its therapeutic dose. This observation should be considered in clinical decisions to prescribe solifenacin succinate for patients with a known history of QT prolongation or patients who are taking medications known to prolong the QT interval).

No products indexed under this heading.

Nefazodone Hydrochloride (Do not exceed a 5 mg daily dose of solifenacin succinate when administered with therapeutic doses of ketoconazole or other potent CYP3A4 inhibitors).

No products indexed under this heading.

Nelfinavir Mesylate (Do not exceed a 5 mg daily dose of solifenacin succinate when administered with therapeutic doses of ketoconazole or other potent CYP3A4 inhibitors). Products include:

Nortriptyline Hydrochloride (In a study of the effect of solifenacin on the QT interval in 76 healthy women, the QT prolonging effect appered less with solifenacin 10 mg than with 30 mg (three times the maximum recommended dose), and the effect of solifenacin 30 mg did not appear as large as that of the positive control moxifloxacin at its therapeutic dose. This observation should be considered in clinical decisions to prescribe solifenacin succinate for patients with a known history of QT prolongation or patients who are taking medications known to prolong the QT interval).

No products indexed under this heading.

Perphenazine (In a study of the effect of solifenacin on the QT interval in 76 healthy women, the QT prolonging effect appered less with solifenacin 10 mg than with 30 mg (three times the maximum recommended dose), and the effect of solifenacin 30 mg did not appear as large as that of the positive control moxifloxacin at its therapeutic dose. This observation should be considered in clinical decisions to prescribe solifenacin succinate for patients with a known history of QT prolongation or patients who are taking medications known to prolong the QT interval).

No products indexed under this heading.

Procainamide Hydrochloride (In a study of the effect of solifenacin on the QT interval in 76 healthy women, the QT prolonging effect appered less with solifenacin 10 mg than with

30 mg (three times the maximum recommended dose), and the effect of solifenacin 30 mg did not appear as large as that of the positive control moxifloxacin at its therapeutic dose. This observation should be considered in clinical decisions to prescribe solifenacin succinate for patients with a known history of QT prolongation or patients who are taking medications known to prolong the QT interval).

No products indexed under this heading.

Prochlorperazine (In a study of the effect of solifenacin on the QT interval in 76 healthy women, the QT prolonging effect appered less with solifenacin 10 mg than with 30 mg (three times the maximum recommended dose), and the effect of solifenacin 30 mg did not appear as large as that of the positive control moxifloxacin at its therapeutic dose. This observation should be considered in clinical decisions to prescribe solifenacin succinate for patients with a known history of QT prolongation or patients who are taking medications known to prolong the QT interval).

No products indexed under this heading.

Promethazine Hydrochloride (In a study of the effect of solifenacin on the QT interval in 76 healthy women, the QT prolonging effect appered less with solifenacin 10 mg than with 30 mg (three times the maximum recommended dose), and the effect of solifenacin 30 mg did not appear as large as that of the positive control moxifloxacin at its therapeutic dose. This observation should be considered in clinical decisions to prescribe solifenacin succinate for patients with a known history of QT prolongation or patients who are taking medications known to prolong the QT interval). Products include:

Propafenone Hydrochloride (In a study of the effect of solifenacin on the QT interval in 76 healthy women, the QT prolonging effect appered less with solifenacin 10 mg than with 30 mg (three times the maximum recommended dose), and the effect of solifenacin 30 mg did not appear as large as that of the positive control moxifloxacin at its therapeutic dose. This observation should be considered in clinical decisions to prescribe solifenacin succinate for patients with a known history of QT prolongation or patients who are taking medications known to prolong the QT interval). Products include:

Protriptyline Hydrochloride (In a study of the effect of solifenacin on the QT interval in 76 healthy women, the QT prolonging effect appered less with solifenacin 10 mg than with 30 mg (three times the maximum recommended dose), and the effect of solifenacin 30 mg did not appear as large as that of the positive control moxifloxacin at its therapeutic dose. This observation should be considered in clinical decisions to prescribe solifenacin succinate for patients with a known history of QT prolongation or patients who are taking medications known to prolong

the QT interval).

No products indexed under this heading.

Quinidine Gluconate (In a study of the effect of solifenacin on the QT interval in 76 healthy women, the QT prolonging effect appered less with solifenacin 10 mg than with 30 mg (three times the maximum recommended dose), and the effect of solifenacin 30 mg did not appear as large as that of the positive control moxifloxacin at its therapeutic dose. This observation should be considered in clinical decisions to prescribe solifenacin succinate for patients with a known history of QT prolongation or patients who are taking medications known to prolong the QT interval).

No products indexed under this heading.

Quinidine Polygalacturonate (In a study of the effect of solifenacin on the QT interval in 76 healthy women, the QT prolonging effect appered less with solifenacin 10 mg than with 30 mg (three times the maximum recommended dose), and the effect of solifenacin 30 mg did not appear as large as that of the positive control moxifloxacin at its therapeutic dose. This observation should be considered in clinical decisions to prescribe solifenacin succinate for patients with a known history of QT prolongation or patients who are taking medications known to prolong the QT interval).

No products indexed under this heading.

Quinidine Sulfate (In a study of the effect of solifenacin on the QT interval in 76 healthy women, the QT prolonging effect appered less with solifenacin 10 mg than with 30 mg (three times the maximum recommended dose), and the effect of solifenacin 30 mg did not appear as large as that of the positive control moxifloxacin at its therapeutic dose. This observation should be considered in clinical decisions to prescribe solifenacin succinate for patients with a known history of QT prolongation or patients who are taking medications known to prolong the QT interval).

No products indexed under this heading.

Ritonavir (Do not exceed a 5 mg daily dose of solifenacin succinate when administered with therapeutic doses of ketoconazole or other potent CYP3A4 inhibitors). Products include:

Saquinavir (Do not exceed a 5 mg daily dose of solifenacin succinate when administered with therapeutic doses of ketoconazole or other potent CYP3A4 inhibitors).

No products indexed under this heading.

Saquinavir Mesylate (Do not exceed a 5 mg daily dose of solifenacin succinate when administered with therapeutic doses of ketoconazole or other potent CYP3A4 inhibitors). Products include:

Telithromycin (Do not exceed a 5 mg daily dose of solifenacin succinate when administered with thera-

peutic doses of ketoconazole or other potent CYP3A4 inhibitors). Products include:

Thioridazine Hydrochloride (In a study of the effect of solifenacin on the QT interval in 76 healthy women, the QT prolonging effect appered less with solifenacin 10 mg than with 30 mg (three times the maximum recommended dose), and the effect of solifenacin 30 mg did not appear as large as that of the positive control moxifloxacin at its therapeutic dose. This observation should be considered in clinical decisions to prescribe solifenacin succinate for patients with a known history of QT prolongation or patients who are taking medications known to prolong the QT interval). Products include:

Tocainide Hydrochloride (In a study of the effect of solifenacin on the QT interval in 76 healthy women, the QT prolonging effect appered less with solifenacin 10 mg than with 30 mg (three times the maximum recommended dose), and the effect of solifenacin 30 mg did not appear as large as that of the positive control moxifloxacin at its therapeutic dose. This observation should be considered in clinical decisions to prescribe solifenacin succinate for patients with a known history of QT prolongation or patients who are taking medications known to prolong the QT interval).

No products indexed under this heading.

Trifluoperazine Hydrochloride (In a study of the effect of solifenacin on the QT interval in 76 healthy women, the QT prolonging effect appered less with solifenacin 10 mg than with 30 mg (three times the maximum recommended dose), and the effect of solifenacin 30 mg did not appear as large as that of the positive control moxifloxacin at its therapeutic dose. This observation should be considered in clinical decisions to prescribe solifenacin succinate for patients with a known history of QT prolongation or patients who are taking medications known to prolong the QT interval).

No products indexed under this heading.

Trimipramine Maleate (In a study of the effect of solifenacin on the QT interval in 76 healthy women, the QT prolonging effect appered less with solifenacin 10 mg than with 30 mg (three times the maximum recommended dose), and the effect of solifenacin 30 mg did not appear as large as that of the positive control moxifloxacin at its therapeutic dose. This observation should be considered in clinical decisions to prescribe solifenacin succinate for patients with a known history of QT prolongation or patients who are taking medications known to prolong the QT interval).

No products indexed under this heading.

Troleandomycin (Do not exceed a 5 mg daily dose of solifenacin succinate when administered with therapeutic doses of ketoconazole or other potent CYP3A4 inhibitors).

No products indexed under this heading.

Voriconazole (Do not exceed a 5 mg daily dose of solifenacin succinate when administered with therapeutic doses of ketoconazole or other potent CYP3A4 inhibitors). Products include:
VFEND I.V. 2564
VFEND Oral Suspension 2564
VFEND Tablets 2564

Ziprasidone Hydrochloride (In a study of the effect of solifenacin on the QT interval in 76 healthy women, the QT prolonging effect appered less with solifenacin 10 mg than with 30 mg (three times the maximum recommended dose), and the effect of solifenacin 30 mg did not appear as large as that of the positive control moxifloxacin at its therapeutic dose. This observation should be considered in clinical decisions to prescribe solifenacin succinate for patients with a known history of QT prolongation or patients who are taking medications known to prolong the QT interval). Products include:
Geodon Capsules 2529

VFEND I.V.
(Voriconazole) 2564
See VFEND Tablets

VFEND ORAL SUSPENSION
(Voriconazole) 2564
See VFEND Tablets

VFEND TABLETS
(Voriconazole) 2564
May interact with barbiturates, benzodiazepine that are metabolized by CYP3A4, calcium channel blockers that are metabolized by CYP3A4, oral anticoagulants, cytochrome p450 2c19 inducers (selected), cytochrome p450 2c19 inhibitors (selected), cytochrome p450 2c9 inducers (selected), cytochrome p450 2c9 inhibitors (selected), cytochrome p450 3a4 inducers (selected), cytochrome p450 3a4 inhibitors (selected), ergot-containing drugs, Non-nucleoside reverse transcriptase inhibtors, oral contraceptives, phenytoin, prednisolone, proton pump inhibitor, quinidine, statins that are metabolized by CYP3A4, sulfonylureas that are substrate of CYP2C9, vinca alkaloids, and certain other agents. Compounds in these categories include:

Acetazolamide (CYP3A4 inhibitors may increase voriconazole systemic exposure (plasma concentrations)).
No products indexed under this heading.

Allium sativum (CYP3A4 inducers may decrease voriconazole systemic exposure (plasma concentrations)).
No products indexed under this heading.

Alprazolam (Co-administration may increase plasma concentrations of benzodiazepines that are metabolized by CYP3A4). Products include:
Niravam Orally Disintegrating Tablets 3092

Amiodarone Hydrochloride (CYP2C9 inhibitors may increase voriconazole systemic exposure (plasma concentrations)).
No products indexed under this heading.

Amlodipine Besylate (Co-administration may increase plasma concentrations of calcium channel blockers that are metabolized by CYP3A4). Products include:
Caduet Tablets 2508
Lotrel Capsules 2249
Norvasc Tablets 2545

Amprenavir (Voriconazole may inhibit the metabolism of amprenavir; amprenavir may inhibit the metabolism of voriconazole). Products include:
Agenerase Capsules 1327
Agenerase Oral Solution 1332

Anastrozole (CYP2C9 inhibitors may increase voriconazole systemic exposure (plasma concentrations)). Products include:
Arimidex Tablets 673

Anisindione (Co-administration may increase prothrombin time). Products include:
Miradon Tablets 3042

Aprepitant (CYP2C9 inducers may decrease voriconazole systemic exposure (plasma concentrations)). Products include:
Emend Capsules 1963

Aprobarbital (Long-acting barbiturates are likely to significantly decrease plasma voriconazole concentrations. Co-administration of voriconazole with long-acting barbiturates is contraindicated).
No products indexed under this heading.

Astemizole (Co-administration with a CYP3A4 substrate, such as astemizole, may result in inhibition of the metabolism of astemizole; increased plasma concentrations of astemizole can lead to QT prolongation and rare occurrence of torsade de pointes; co-administration is contraindicated).
No products indexed under this heading.

Atorvastatin Calcium (Co-administration may increase plasma concentrations of statins that are metabolized by CYP3A4). Products include:
Caduet Tablets 2508
Lipitor Tablets 2483

Bendroflumethiazide (CYP2C9 inhibitors may increase voriconazole systemic exposure (plasma concentrations)).
No products indexed under this heading.

Betamethasone Acetate (CYP3A4 inducers may decrease voriconazole systemic exposure (plasma concentrations)).
No products indexed under this heading.

Betamethasone Sodium Phosphate (CYP3A4 inducers may decrease voriconazole systemic exposure (plasma concentrations)).
No products indexed under this heading.

Butabarbital (Long-acting barbiturates are likely to significantly decrease plasma voriconazole concentrations. Co-administration of voriconazole with long-acting barbiturates is contraindicated).
No products indexed under this heading.

Butalbital (Long-acting barbiturates are likely to significantly decrease plasma voriconazole concentrations. Co-administration of voriconazole with long-acting barbiturates is contraindicated).
No products indexed under this heading.

Carbamazepine (Co-administration with potent inducer of CYP450, such as carbamazepine, is likely to significantly decrease plasma voriconazole concentrations; co-administration is contraindicated). Products include:
Carbatrol Capsules 3171
Equetro Extended-Release Capsules 3180
Tegretol/Tegretol-XR 2295

Chloramphenicol (CYP2C9 inhibitors may increase voriconazole systemic exposure (plasma concentrations)).
No products indexed under this heading.

Chlorothiazide (CYP2C9 inhibitors may increase voriconazole systemic exposure (plasma concentrations)). Products include:
Diuril Oral Suspension 1954

Chlorothiazide Sodium (CYP2C9 inhibitors may increase voriconazole systemic exposure (plasma concentrations)). Products include:
Diuril Sodium Intravenous 2467

Chlorpropamide (CYP2C9 inhibitors may increase voriconazole systemic exposure (plasma concentrations)).
No products indexed under this heading.

Cimetidine (Increases voriconazole steady state Cmax and AUC by an average of 18% and 23%, respectively; no dosage adjustment required). Products include:
Tagamet HB 200 Tablets .... ■ 664

Cimetidine Hydrochloride (Increases voriconazole steady state Cmax and AUC by an average of 18% and 23%, respectively; no dosage adjustment required).
No products indexed under this heading.

Ciprofloxacin (CYP3A4 inhibitors may increase voriconazole systemic exposure (plasma concentrations)). Products include:
Cipro Oral Suspension 2977
Cipro I.V. 2984
Cipro XR Tablets 2990
Ciprodex Otic Suspension 559

Ciprofloxacin Hydrochloride (CYP3A4 inducers may decrease voriconazole systemic exposure (plasma concentrations)). Products include:
Ciloxan Ophthalmic Ointment 559
Ciloxan Ophthalmic Solution .... ⊙ 206
Cipro Tablets 2977
Proquin XR Tablets 1153

Cisapride (Co-administration with a CYP3A4 substrate, such as cisapride, may result in inhibition of the metabolism of cisapride; increased plasma concentrations of cisapride can lead to QT prolongation and rare occurrence of torsade de pointes; co-administration is contraindicated).
No products indexed under this heading.

Cisplatin (CYP3A4 inducers may decrease voriconazole systemic exposure (plasma concentrations)).
No products indexed under this heading.

Citalopram Hydrobromide (CYP2C19 inhibitors may increase voriconazole systemic exposure (plasma concentrations)). Products include:
Celexa 1176

Clarithromycin (CYP3A4 inhibitors may increase voriconazole systemic exposure (plasma concentrations)). Products include:
Biaxin/Biaxin XL 402
PREVPAC 3284

Clopidogrel Hydrogen Sulfate (CYP2C9 inhibitors may increase voriconazole systemic exposure (plasma concentrations)).
No products indexed under this heading.

Clotrimazole (CYP2C9 inhibitors may increase voriconazole systemic exposure (plasma concentrations)). Products include:
Desenex Athlete's Foot Cream .... ■ 635
Lotrimin 3039
Lotrisone 3040

Cortisone Acetate (CYP3A4 inducers may decrease voriconazole systemic exposure (plasma concentrations)).
No products indexed under this heading.

Cyclosporine (Co-administration results in increased exposure to cyclosporine; it is recommended that the cyclosporine dose be reduced by one-half when initiating the therapy; close and frequent monitoring of cyclosporine levels is recommended when voriconazole is discontinued). Products include:
Gengraf Capsules 459
Neoral Oral Solution 2259
Neoral Soft Gelatin Capsules 2259
Restasis Ophthalmic Emulsion 575
Sandimmune 2275

Dalfopristin (CYP3A4 inhibitors may increase voriconazole systemic exposure (plasma concentrations)).
No products indexed under this heading.

Danazol (CYP3A4 inhibitors may increase voriconazole systemic exposure (plasma concentrations)).
No products indexed under this heading.

Delavirdine Mesylate (May inhibit the metabolism of voriconazole; voriconazole may inhibit the metabolism of delavirdine). Products include:
Rescriptor Tablets 2551

Desogestrel (Co-administration with oral contraceptives containing ethinyl estradiol and norethindrone may increase drug plasma levels of ethinyl estradiol, norethindrone, and voriconazole. Monitoring for adverse events related to oral contraceptives is recommended during co-administration). Products include:
Mircette Tablets 1066

Dexamethasone (CYP2C9 inducers may decrease voriconazole systemic exposure (plasma concentrations)). Products include:
Ciprodex Otic Suspension 559
Decadron Tablets 1951
TobraDex Ophthalmic Ointment 562
TobraDex Ophthalmic Suspension ... 563

Dexamethasone Acetate (CYP3A4 inducers may decrease voriconazole systemic exposure (plasma concentrations)).
No products indexed under this heading.

Dexamethasone Sodium Phosphate (CYP3A4 inducers may decrease voriconazole systemic exposure (plasma concentrations)).
No products indexed under this heading.

Diazepam (Co-administration may increase plasma concentrations of benzodiazepines that are metabolized by CYP3A4). Products include:
Diastat Rectal Delivery System 3343
Valium Tablets 2819

Diclofenac Potassium (CYP2C9 inhibitors may increase voriconazole systemic exposure (plasma concentrations)).
No products indexed under this heading.

Diclofenac Sodium (CYP2C9 inhibitors may increase voriconazole systemic exposure (plasma concentrations)). Products include:
Arthrotec Tablets 3129
Voltaren Ophthalmic Solution 2309
Voltaren Tablets 2307
Voltaren-XR Tablets 2310

Dicumarol (Co-administration may increase prothrombin time).
No products indexed under this heading.

Dihydroergotamine Mesylate (Co-administration may result in increased plasma concentrations of ergot alkaloids and this can lead to ergotism; co-administration is contraindicated). Products include:
Migranal Nasal Spray 3348

Diltiazem Hydrochloride (Co-administration may increase plasma concentrations of calcium channel blockers that are metabolized by CYP3A4). Products include:
Cardizem LA Extended Release Tablets 1728
Tiazac Capsules 1201

Diltiazem Maleate (CYP3A4 inhibitors may increase voriconazole systemic exposure (plasma concentrations)).
No products indexed under this heading.

Disulfiram (CYP2C9 inhibitors may increase voriconazole systemic exposure (plasma concentrations)).
No products indexed under this heading.

Doxorubicin Hydrochloride (CYP3A4 inducers may decrease voriconazole systemic exposure (plasma concentrations)).
No products indexed under this heading.

Efavirenz (May inhibit the metabolism of voriconazole; the metabolism of voriconazole may be induced by efavirenz. Co-administration is contraindicated). Products include:
Atripla Tablets 945
Sustiva Capsules 930
Sustiva Tablets 930

Ergonovine Maleate (Co-administration may result in increased plasma concentrations of ergot alkaloids and this can lead to ergotism; co-administration is contraindicated).
No products indexed under this heading.

Ergotamine Tartrate (Co-administration may result in increased plasma concentrations of ergot alkaloids and this can lead to ergotism; co-administration is contraindicated).
No products indexed under this heading.

Erythromycin (CYP3A4 inhibitors may increase voriconazole systemic exposure (plasma concentrations)). Products include:
Ery-Tab Tablets 449
Erythromycin Base Filmtab Tablets 455
Erythromycin Delayed-Release Capsules, USP 457
PCE Dispertab Tablets 515

Erythromycin Estolate (CYP3A4 inhibitors may increase voriconazole systemic exposure (plasma concentrations)).
No products indexed under this heading.

Erythromycin Ethylsuccinate (CYP3A4 inhibitors may increase voriconazole systemic exposure (plasma concentrations)). Products include:
E.E.S. 451
EryPed 447

Erythromycin Gluceptate (CYP3A4 inhibitors may increase voriconazole systemic exposure (plasma concentrations)).
No products indexed under this heading.

Erythromycin Lactobionate (CYP3A4 inhibitors may increase voriconazole systemic exposure (plasma concentrations)).
No products indexed under this heading.

Erythromycin Stearate (CYP3A4 inhibitors may increase voriconazole systemic exposure (plasma concentrations)). Products include:
Erythrocin Stearate Filmtab Tablets 453

Esomeprazole Magnesium (The metabolism of other proton pump inhibitors may also be inhibited by voriconazole and may result in increased plasma concentrations of other proton pump inhibitors). Products include:
Nexium Delayed-Release Capsules 655

Ethinyl Estradiol (Co-administration with oral contraceptives containing ethinyl estradiol and norethindrone may increase drug plasma levels of ethinyl estradiol, norethindrone, and voriconazole. Monitoring for adverse events related to oral contraceptives is recommended during co-administration). Products include:
Mircette Tablets 1066
NuvaRing 2340
Ortho-Cyclen/Ortho Tri-Cyclen 2429
Ortho Evra Transdermal System 2417
Ortho Tri-Cyclen Lo Tablets 2436
Seasonique Tablets 1077
Yasmin 28 Tablets 796
Yaz Tablets 803

Ethosuximide (CYP3A4 inducers may decrease voriconazole systemic exposure (plasma concentrations)).
No products indexed under this heading.

Ethynodiol Diacetate (Co-administration with oral contraceptives containing ethinyl estradiol and norethindrone may increase drug plasma levels of ethinyl estradiol, norethindrone, and voriconazole. Monitoring for adverse events related to oral contraceptives is recommended during co-administration).
No products indexed under this heading.

Felbamate (CYP2C19 inhibitors may increase voriconazole systemic exposure (plasma concentrations)).
No products indexed under this heading.

Felodipine (Co-administration may increase plasma concentrations of calcium channel blockers that are metabolized by CYP3A4).
No products indexed under this heading.

Fenofibrate (CYP2C9 inhibitors may increase voriconazole systemic exposure (plasma concentrations)). Products include:
Lofibra Tablets 1219
Lofibra Capsules 1216
Tricor Tablets 527
Triglide Tablets 3123

Fluconazole (CYP2C9 inhibitors may increase voriconazole systemic exposure (plasma concentrations)).
No products indexed under this heading.

Fludrocortisone Acetate (CYP3A4 inducers may decrease voriconazole systemic exposure (plasma concentrations)).
No products indexed under this heading.

Fluorouracil (CYP2C9 inhibitors may increase voriconazole systemic exposure (plasma concentrations)). Products include:
Carac Cream, 0.5% 2879
Efudex 3363

Fluoxetine (CYP2C19 inhibitors may increase voriconazole systemic exposure (plasma concentrations)).
No products indexed under this heading.

Fluoxetine Hydrochloride (CYP2C19 inhibitors may increase voriconazole systemic exposure (plasma concentrations)). Products include:
Prozac Pulvules and Liquid 1801
Symbyax Capsules 1819

Flurbiprofen (CYP2C9 inhibitors may increase voriconazole systemic exposure (plasma concentrations)).
No products indexed under this heading.

Flurbiprofen Sodium (CYP2C9 inhibitors may increase voriconazole systemic exposure (plasma concentrations)). Products include:
Ocufen Ophthalmic Solution .... ⊙ 232

Fluvastatin Sodium (CYP2C19 inhibitors may increase voriconazole systemic exposure (plasma concentrations)). Products include:
Lescol Capsules 2233
Lescol XL Tablets 2233

Fluvoxamine (CYP2C19 inhibitors may increase voriconazole systemic exposure (plasma concentrations)).
No products indexed under this heading.

Fluvoxamine Maleate (CYP2C19 inhibitors may increase voriconazole systemic exposure (plasma concentrations)).
No products indexed under this heading.

Fosamprenavir Calcium (CYP3A4 inhibitors may increase voriconazole systemic exposure (plasma concentrations)). Products include:
Lexiva Tablets 1505

Fosphenytoin Sodium (Co-administration results in decreased steady-state Cmax and AUC of orally administered voriconazole and increased steady-state Cmax and AUC of phenytoin; frequent monitoring of plasma phenytoin levels and related adverse events is recommended).
No products indexed under this heading.

Garlic Extract (CYP3A4 inducers may decrease voriconazole systemic exposure (plasma concentrations)).
No products indexed under this heading.

Garlic Oil (CYP3A4 inducers may decrease voriconazole systemic exposure (plasma concentrations)).
No products indexed under this heading.

Gemfibrozil (CYP2C9 inhibitors may increase voriconazole systemic exposure (plasma concentrations)).
No products indexed under this heading.

Glipizide (Co-administration may increase plasma concentrations of sulfonylureas that are metabolized by CYP2C9 and, therefore, cause hypoglycemia).
No products indexed under this heading.

Glyburide (Co-administration may increase plasma concentrations of sulfonylureas that are metabolized by CYP2C9 and, therefore, cause hypoglycemia).
No products indexed under this heading.

Hydrochlorothiazide (CYP2C9 inhibitors may increase voriconazole systemic exposure (plasma concentrations)). Products include:
Aldoril Tablets 1910
Atacand HCT 651
Avalide Tablets 888
Avalide Tablets 2874
Benicar HCT Tablets 1044
Diovan HCT Tablets 2196
Dyazide Capsules 1423
Hyzaar 50-12.5 Tablets 1990
Hyzaar 100-12.5 Tablets 1990
Hyzaar 100-25 Tablets 1990
Lopressor HCT 50/25 Tablets 2241
Lopressor HCT 100/25 Tablets 2241
Lopressor HCT 100/50 Tablets 2241
Lotensin HCT Tablets 2246
Micardis HCT Tablets 856
Moduretic Tablets 2028
Prinzide Tablets 2056
Teveten HCT Tablets 1737
Timolide Tablets 2086
Uniretic Tablets 3100

Hydrocortisone (CYP3A4 inducers may decrease voriconazole systemic exposure (plasma concentrations)). Products include:
Colocort Rectal Suspension, USP (Retention) 100 mg/60 mL 2476
Hydrocortone Tablets 1989
Preparation H Hydrocortisone Cream 646

Hydrocortisone Acetate (CYP3A4 inducers may decrease voriconazole systemic exposure (plasma concentrations)). Products include:
Analpram-HC 1159
Pramosone 1161
ProctoFoam-HC 3099

Hydrocortisone Butyrate (CYP3A4 inducers may decrease voriconazole systemic exposure (plasma concentrations)). Products include:
Locoid Lipocream Cream 1160

Hydrocortisone Cypionate (CYP3A4 inducers may decrease voriconazole systemic exposure (plasma concentrations)).
No products indexed under this heading.

Hydrocortisone Hemisuccinate (CYP3A4 inducers may decrease voriconazole systemic exposure (plasma concentrations)).
No products indexed under this heading.

Hydrocortisone Probutate (CYP3A4 inducers may decrease voriconazole systemic exposure (plasma concentrations)).
No products indexed under this heading.

Hydrocortisone Sodium Phosphate (CYP3A4 inducers may decrease voriconazole systemic exposure (plasma concentrations)).
No products indexed under this heading.

Hydrocortisone Sodium Succinate (CYP3A4 inducers may decrease voriconazole systemic exposure (plasma concentrations)).
No products indexed under this heading.

Hydrocortisone Valerate (CYP3A4 inducers may decrease voriconazole systemic exposure (plasma concentrations)).
No products indexed under this heading.

Hydroflumethiazide (CYP2C9 inhibitors may increase voriconazole systemic exposure (plasma concentrations)).
No products indexed under this heading.

Hypericum (CYP3A4 inducers may decrease voriconazole systemic exposure (plasma concentrations)). Products include:
Satiete Tablets .... ▣832

Hypericum Perforatum (CYP3A4 inducers may decrease voriconazole systemic exposure (plasma concentrations)).
No products indexed under this heading.

Imatinib Mesylate (CYP2C9 inhibitors may increase voriconazole systemic exposure (plasma concentrations)). Products include:
Gleevec Tablets 2227

Indinavir Sulfate (CYP3A4 inhibitors may increase voriconazole systemic exposure (plasma concentrations)). Products include:
Crixivan Capsules 1940

Indomethacin (CYP2C19 inhibitors may increase voriconazole systemic exposure (plasma concentrations)). Products include:
Indocin 1995

Indomethacin Sodium Trihydrate (CYP2C19 inhibitors may increase voriconazole systemic exposure (plasma concentrations)). Products include:
Indocin I.V. 2465

Isoniazid (CYP2C19 inhibitors may increase voriconazole systemic exposure (plasma concentrations)).
No products indexed under this heading.

Itraconazole (CYP2C9 inhibitors may increase voriconazole systemic exposure (plasma concentrations)).
No products indexed under this heading.

Ketoconazole (CYP2C19 inhibitors may increase voriconazole systemic exposure (plasma concentrations)). Products include:
Nizoral A-D Shampoo, 1% 1868

Ketoprofen (CYP2C9 inhibitors may increase voriconazole systemic exposure (plasma concentrations)).
No products indexed under this heading.

Lansoprazole (The metabolism of other proton pump inhibitors may also be inhibited by voriconazole and may result in increased plasma concentrations of other proton pump inhibitors). Products include:
Prevacid Delayed-Release Capsules 3271
Prevacid for Delayed-Release Oral Suspension 3271
Prevacid SoluTab Delayed-Release Orally Disintegrating Tablets 3271
Prevacid I.V. for Injection 3277
Prevacid NapraPAC 3280
PREVPAC 3284

Leflunomide (CYP2C9 inhibitors may increase voriconazole systemic exposure (plasma concentrations)).
No products indexed under this heading.

Letrozole (CYP2C19 inhibitors may increase voriconazole systemic exposure (plasma concentrations)). Products include:
Femara Tablets 2214

Levonorgestrel (Co-administration with oral contraceptives containing ethinyl estradiol and norethindrone may increase drug plasma levels of ethinyl estradiol, norethindrone, and voriconazole. Monitoring for adverse events related to oral contraceptives is recommended during co-administration). Products include:
Climara Pro Transdermal System 776
Mirena Intrauterine System 787
Plan B Tablets 1076
Seasonique Tablets 1077

Lopinavir (CYP3A4 inhibitors may increase voriconazole systemic exposure (plasma concentrations)). Products include:
Kaletra 476

Loratadine (CYP3A4 inhibitors may increase voriconazole systemic exposure (plasma concentrations)). Products include:
Alavert Allergy & Sinus D-12 Hour Tablets .... ▣771
Alavert .... ▣771
Children's Claritin Allergy Oral Solution .... ▣771
Claritin Non-Drowsy 24 Hour Tablets .... ▣772
Claritin Reditabs 24 Hour Non-Drowsy Tablets .... ▣772
Claritin-D Non-Drowsy 12 Hour Tablets .... ▣772
Claritin-D Non-Drowsy 24 Hour Tablets .... ▣772

Lovastatin (Co-administration may increase plasma concentrations of statins that are metabolized by CYP3A4). Products include:
Advicor Tablets 1722
Altoprev Extended-Release Tablets 3109
Mevacor Tablets 2021

Mephenytoin (CYP3A4 inducers may decrease voriconazole systemic exposure (plasma concentrations)).
No products indexed under this heading.

Mephobarbital (Co-administration with potent inducer of CYP450, such as long-acting barbiturates- mephobarbital, is likely to significantly decrease plasma voriconazole concentrations; co-administration is contraindicated).
No products indexed under this heading.

Mestranol (Co-administration with oral contraceptives containing ethinyl estradiol and norethindrone may increase drug plasma levels of ethinyl estradiol, norethindrone, and voriconazole. Monitoring for adverse events related to oral contraceptives is recommended during co-administration).
No products indexed under this heading.

Methadone Hydrochloride (Increased plasma concentrations of methadone have been associated with toxicity, including QT prolongation. Frequent monitoring for adverse events and toxicity related to methadone is recommended during co-administration. Dose reduction of methadone may be needed).
No products indexed under this heading.

Methsuximide (CYP3A4 inducers may decrease voriconazole systemic exposure (plasma concentrations)).
No products indexed under this heading.

Methyclothiazide (CYP2C9 inhibitors may increase voriconazole systemic exposure (plasma concentrations)).
No products indexed under this heading.

Methylergonovine Maleate (Co-administration may result in increased plasma concentrations of ergot alkaloids and this can lead to ergotism; co-administration is contraindicated).
No products indexed under this heading.

Methylprednisolone (CYP3A4 inducers may decrease voriconazole systemic exposure (plasma concentrations)).
No products indexed under this heading.

Methylprednisolone Acetate (CYP3A4 inducers may decrease voriconazole systemic exposure (plasma concentrations)). Products include:
Depo-Medrol Injectable Suspension 2617
Depo-Medrol Single-Dose Vial 2619

Methylprednisolone Sodium Succinate (CYP3A4 inducers may decrease voriconazole systemic exposure (plasma concentrations)).
No products indexed under this heading.

Methysergide Maleate (Co-administration may result in increased plasma concentrations of ergot alkaloids and this can lead to ergotism; co-administration is contraindicated).
No products indexed under this heading.

Metronidazole (CYP2C9 inhibitors may increase voriconazole systemic exposure (plasma concentrations)). Products include:
Metrogel 1% 1211
MetroGel-Vaginal Gel 1855
Vandazole Vaginal Gel 3338

Metronidazole Benzoate (CYP2C9 inhibitors may increase voriconazole systemic exposure (plasma concentrations)).
No products indexed under this heading.

Metronidazole Hydrochloride (CYP2C9 inhibitors may increase voriconazole systemic exposure (plasma concentrations)).
No products indexed under this heading.

Miconazole (CYP2C9 inhibitors may increase voriconazole systemic exposure (plasma concentrations)).
No products indexed under this heading.

Miconazole Nitrate (CYP3A4 inhibitors may increase voriconazole systemic exposure (plasma concentrations)). Products include:
Desenex .... ▣635
Desenex Jock Itch Spray Powder .... ▣635

Midazolam Hydrochloride (Co-administration may increase plasma concentrations of benzodiazepines that are metabolized by CYP3A4).
No products indexed under this heading.

Modafinil (CYP2C19 inhibitors may increase voriconazole systemic exposure (plasma concentrations)). Products include:
Provigil Tablets 988

Nefazodone Hydrochloride (CYP3A4 inhibitors may increase voriconazole systemic exposure (plasma concentrations)).
No products indexed under this heading.

Nelfinavir Mesylate (Voriconazole may inhibit the metabolism of nelfinavir). Products include:
Viracept 2577

Nevirapine (The metabolism of voriconazole may be induced by nevirapine). Products include:
Viramune Oral Suspension 873
Viramune Tablets 873

Niacinamide (CYP3A4 inhibitors may increase voriconazole systemic exposure (plasma concentrations)).
No products indexed under this heading.

Nicotinamide (CYP3A4 inhibitors may increase voriconazole systemic exposure (plasma concentrations)). Products include:
Nicomide Tablets 1088

Nifedipine (Co-administration may increase plasma concentrations of calcium channel blockers that are metabolized by CYP3A4). Products include:
Adalat CC Tablets 2964

Nisoldipine (Co-administration may increase plasma concentrations of calcium channel blockers that are metabolized by CYP3A4). Products include:
Sular Tablets 3122

Norethindrone (Co-administration with oral contraceptives containing ethinyl estradiol and norethindrone may increase drug plasma levels of ethinyl estradiol, norethindrone, and voriconazole. Monitoring for adverse events related to oral contraceptives is recommended during co-administration). Products include:
Ortho Micronor Tablets 2426

Norethindrone Acetate (CYP2C19 inducers may decrease voriconazole systemic exposure (plasma concentrations)).
No products indexed under this heading.

Norethynodrel (Co-administration with oral contraceptives containing ethinyl estradiol and norethindrone may increase drug plasma levels of ethinyl estradiol, norethindrone, and voriconazole. Monitoring for adverse events related to oral contraceptives is recommended during co-administration).
No products indexed under this heading.

Norfloxacin (CYP3A4 inhibitors may increase voriconazole systemic exposure (plasma concentrations)). Products include:
Noroxin Tablets 2032

Norgestimate (Co-administration with oral contraceptives containing ethinyl estradiol and norethindrone may increase drug plasma levels of ethinyl estradiol, norethindrone, and voriconazole. Monitoring for adverse events related to oral contraceptives is recommended during co-administration). Products include:

Ortho-Cyclen/Ortho Tri-Cyclen 2429
Ortho Tri-Cyclen Lo Tablets 2436

Norgestrel (Co-administration with oral contraceptives containing ethinyl estradiol and norethindrone may increase drug plasma levels of ethinyl estradiol, norethindrone, and voriconazole. Monitoring for adverse events related to oral contraceptives is recommended during co-administration).
No products indexed under this heading.

Omeprazole (Co-administration results in a significant increase in omeprazole plasma exposure; when initiating therapy with VFEND in patients already receiving omeprazole doses of 40 mg or greater, reduce the omeprazole dose by one-half). Products include:

Zegerid Capsules 2958
Zegerid Powder for Oral Solution 2958

Oxcarbazepine (CYP2C19 inhibitors may increase voriconazole systemic exposure (plasma concentrations)). Products include:

Trileptal Tablets 2300
Trileptal Oral Suspension 2300

Oxiconazole Nitrate (CYP2C9 inhibitors may increase voriconazole systemic exposure (plasma concentrations)). Products include:

Oxistat 2667

Pantoprazole Sodium (The metabolism of other proton pump inhibitors may also be inhibited by voriconazole and may result in increased plasma concentrations of other proton pump inhibitors). Products include:

Protonix I.V. 3472
Protonix Tablets 3469

Paroxetine Hydrochloride (CYP2C19 inhibitors may increase voriconazole systemic exposure (plasma concentrations)). Products include:

Paxil CR Controlled-Release Tablets 1538
Paxil 1530

Pentobarbital Sodium (Long-acting barbiturates are likely to significantly decrease plasma voriconazole concentrations. Co-administration of voriconazole with long-acting barbiturates is contraindicated). Products include:

Nembutal Sodium Solution, USP 2470

Phenobarbital (Co-administration with potent inducer of CYP450, such as long-acting barbiturates- phenobarbital, are likely to significantly decrease plasma voriconazole concentrations; co-administration is contraindicated). Products include:

Donnatal Extentabs 2493

Phenobarbital Sodium (CYP2C19 inducers may decrease voriconazole systemic exposure (plasma concentrations)).
No products indexed under this heading.

Phenylbutazone (CYP2C9 inhibitors may increase voriconazole systemic exposure (plasma concentrations)).
No products indexed under this heading.

Phenytoin (Co-administration results in decreased steady-state Cmax and AUC of orally administered voriconazole and increased steady-state Cmax and AUC of phenytoin; frequent monitoring of plasma phenytoin levels and related adverse events is recommended).
No products indexed under this heading.

Phenytoin Sodium (Co-administration results in decreased steady-state Cmax and AUC of orally administered voriconazole and increased steady-state Cmax and AUC of phenytoin; frequent monitoring of plasma phenytoin levels and related adverse events is recommended). Products include:

Phenytek Capsules 2160

Pimozide (Co-administration with a CYP3A4 substrate, such as pimozide, may result in inhibition of the metabolism of pimozide; increased plasma concentrations of pimozide can lead to QT prolongation and rare occurrence of torsade de pointes; co-administration is contraindicated).
No products indexed under this heading.

Polythiazide (CYP2C9 inhibitors may increase voriconazole systemic exposure (plasma concentrations)).
No products indexed under this heading.

Prednisolone (Increased Cmax and AUC of prednisolone by 11% and 34%, respectively; no dosage adjustments of prednisolone are needed).
No products indexed under this heading.

Prednisolone Acetate (Increased Cmax and AUC of prednisolone by 11% and 34%, respectively; no dosage adjustments of prednisolone are needed). Products include:

Blephamide Ophthalmic Ointment 568
Blephamide Ophthalmic Suspension.................................. 569
Poly-Pred Ophthalmic Suspension .... ⊙233
Pred Forte Ophthalmic Suspension .... ⊙235
Pred Mild Ophthalmic Suspension .... ⊙238
Pred-G Ophthalmic Ointment .... ⊙237
Pred-G Ophthalmic Suspension ...... ⊙236

Prednisolone Sodium Phosphate (Increased Cmax and AUC of prednisolone by 11% and 34%, respectively; no dosage adjustments of prednisolone are needed).
No products indexed under this heading.

Prednisolone Tebutate (Increased Cmax and AUC of prednisolone by 11% and 34%, respectively; no dosage adjustments of prednisolone are needed).
No products indexed under this heading.

Prednisone (CYP2C19 inducers may decrease voriconazole systemic exposure (plasma concentrations)).
No products indexed under this heading.

Primidone (CYP2C9 inducers may decrease voriconazole systemic exposure (plasma concentrations)).
No products indexed under this heading.

Propoxyphene Hydrochloride (CYP3A4 inhibitors may increase voriconazole systemic exposure (plasma concentrations)).
No products indexed under this heading.

Propoxyphene Napsylate (CYP3A4 inhibitors may increase voriconazole systemic exposure (plasma concentrations)).
No products indexed under this heading.

Quinidine (Co-administration with a CYP3A4 substrate, such as quinidine, may result in inhibition of the metabolism of quinidine; increased plasma concentrations of quinidine can lead to QT prolongation and rare occurrence of torsade de pointes; co-administration is contraindicated).
No products indexed under this heading.

Quinidine Gluconate (Co-administration with a CYP3A4 substrate, such as quinidine, may result in inhibition of the metabolism of quinidine; increased plasma concentrations of quinidine can lead to QT prolongation and rare occurrence of torsade de pointes; co-administration is contraindicated).
No products indexed under this heading.

Quinidine Hydrochloride (Co-administration with a CYP3A4 substrate, such as quinidine, may result in inhibition of the metabolism of quinidine; increased plasma concentrations of quinidine can lead to QT prolongation and rare occurrence of torsade de pointes; co-administration is contraindicated).
No products indexed under this heading.

Quinidine Polygalacturonate (Co-administration with a CYP3A4 substrate, such as quinidine, may result in inhibition of the metabolism of quinidine; increased plasma concentrations of quinidine can lead to QT prolongation and rare occurrence of torsade de pointes; co-administration is contraindicated).
No products indexed under this heading.

Quinidine Sulfate (Co-administration with a CYP3A4 substrate, such as quinidine, may result in inhibition of the metabolism of quinidine; increased plasma concentrations of quinidine can lead to QT prolongation and rare occurrence of torsade de pointes; co-administration is contraindicated).
No products indexed under this heading.

Quinine (CYP3A4 inhibitors may increase voriconazole systemic exposure (plasma concentrations)).
No products indexed under this heading.

Quinine Sulfate (CYP3A4 inhibitors may increase voriconazole systemic exposure (plasma concentrations)).
No products indexed under this heading.

Quinupristin (CYP3A4 inhibitors may increase voriconazole systemic exposure (plasma concentrations)).
No products indexed under this heading.

Rabeprazole Sodium (The metabolism of other proton pump inhibitors may also be inhibited by voriconazole and may result in increased plasma concentrations of other proton pump inhibitors). Products include:

Aciphex Tablets 1090

Ranitidine Bismuth Citrate (CYP3A4 inhibitors may increase voriconazole systemic exposure (plasma concentrations)).
No products indexed under this heading.

Ranitidine Hydrochloride (CYP3A4 inhibitors may increase voriconazole systemic exposure (plasma concentrations)). Products include:

Zantac 1624
Zantac Injection 1619
Zantac Injection Pharmacy Bulk Package 1622

Rifabutin (Co-administration results in a significant increase in rifabutin plasma exposure; co-administration is contraindicated).
No products indexed under this heading.

Rifampicin (CYP3A4 inducers may decrease voriconazole systemic exposure (plasma concentrations)).
No products indexed under this heading.

Rifampin (Co-administration with a potent inducer of CYP450, such as rifampin, can significantly reduce the systemic exposure; doubling the dose of voriconazole does not restore adequate exposure to voriconazole; co-administration is contraindicated).
No products indexed under this heading.

Rifapentine (CYP2C9 inducers may decrease voriconazole systemic exposure (plasma concentrations)).
No products indexed under this heading.

Ritonavir (Co-administration of voriconazole with high-dose ritonavir (400 mg q12h) is contraindicated because ritonavir (400 mg q12h) significantly decreases plasma concentrations in healthy subjects. Co-administration of voriconazole and low-dose ritonavir (100 mg q12h) should be avoided unless an assessment of the benefit-risk to the patient justifies the use of voriconazole). Products include:

Kaletra 476
Norvir 503

Saquinavir (Voriconazole may inhibit the metabolism of saquinavir; saquinavir may inhibit the metabolism of voriconazole).
No products indexed under this heading.

Saquinavir Mesylate (Voriconazole may inhibit the metabolism of saquinavir; saquinavir may inhibit the metabolism of voriconazole). Products include:

Invirase 2772

Secobarbital Sodium (Long-acting barbiturates are likely to significantly decrease plasma voriconazole concentrations. Co-administration of voriconazole with long-acting barbiturates is contraindicated).
No products indexed under this heading.

Sertraline Hydrochloride (CYP2C19 inhibitors may increase voriconazole systemic exposure (plasma concentrations)). Products include:

Zoloft 2586

Simvastatin (Co-administration may increase plasma concentrations of statins that are metabolized by CYP3A4). Products include:
- Vytorin 10/10 Tablets 2114
- Vytorin 10/10 Tablets 3077
- Vytorin 10/20 Tablets 2114
- Vytorin 10/20 Tablets 3077
- Vytorin 10/40 Tablets 2114
- Vytorin 10/40 Tablets 3077
- Vytorin 10/80 Tablets 2114
- Vytorin 10/80 Tablets 3077
- Zocor Tablets 2105

Sirolimus (Co-administration with a CYP3A4 substrate, such as sirolimus, can significantly increase the systemic exposure of sirolimus; co-administration is contraindicated). Products include:
- Rapamune Oral Solution and Tablets 3475

Sulfacytine (CYP2C9 inhibitors may increase voriconazole systemic exposure (plasma concentrations)).
No products indexed under this heading.

Sulfamethizole (CYP2C9 inhibitors may increase voriconazole systemic exposure (plasma concentrations)).
No products indexed under this heading.

Sulfamethoxazole (CYP2C9 inhibitors may increase voriconazole systemic exposure (plasma concentrations)).
No products indexed under this heading.

Sulfaphenazole (CYP2C19 inhibitors may increase voriconazole systemic exposure (plasma concentrations)).
No products indexed under this heading.

Sulfasalazine (CYP2C9 inhibitors may increase voriconazole systemic exposure (plasma concentrations)).
No products indexed under this heading.

Sulfinpyrazone (CYP2C9 inhibitors may increase voriconazole systemic exposure (plasma concentrations)).
No products indexed under this heading.

Sulfisoxazole Acetyl (CYP2C9 inhibitors may increase voriconazole systemic exposure (plasma concentrations)).
No products indexed under this heading.

Sulfisoxazole Diolamine (CYP2C9 inhibitors may increase voriconazole systemic exposure (plasma concentrations)).
No products indexed under this heading.

Tacrolimus (Co-administration results in increased exposure to tacrolimus; it is recommended that the tacrolimus dose be reduced by one-half when initiating the therapy; close and frequent monitoring of tacrolimus levels is recommended when voriconazole is discontinued). Products include:
- Prograf Capsules and Injection 632
- Protopic Ointment 638

Telithromycin (CYP3A4 inhibitors may increase voriconazole systemic exposure (plasma concentrations)). Products include:
- Ketek Tablets 2903

Telmisartan (CYP2C19 inhibitors may increase voriconazole systemic exposure (plasma concentrations)). Products include:
- Micardis Tablets 854
- Micardis HCT Tablets 856

Terconazole (CYP2C9 inhibitors may increase voriconazole systemic exposure (plasma concentrations)).
No products indexed under this heading.

Terfenadine (Co-administration with a CYP3A4 substrate, such as terfenadine, may result in inhibition of the metabolism of terfenadine; increased plasma concentrations of terfenadine can lead to QT prolongation and rare occurrence of torsade de pointes; co-administration is contraindicated).
No products indexed under this heading.

Theophylline (CYP3A4 inducers may decrease voriconazole systemic exposure (plasma concentrations)).
No products indexed under this heading.

Thiamylal Sodium (Long-acting barbiturates are likely to significantly decrease plasma voriconazole concentrations. Co-administration of voriconazole with long-acting barbiturates is contraindicated).
No products indexed under this heading.

Ticlopidine Hydrochloride (CYP2C19 inhibitors may increase voriconazole systemic exposure (plasma concentrations)). Products include:
- Ticlid Tablets 2810

Tolazamide (CYP2C9 inhibitors may increase voriconazole systemic exposure (plasma concentrations)).
No products indexed under this heading.

Tolbutamide (Co-administration may increase plasma concentrations of sulfonylureas that are metabolized by CYP2C9 and, therefore, cause hypoglycemia).
No products indexed under this heading.

Tolbutamide Sodium (CYP2C19 inhibitors may increase voriconazole systemic exposure (plasma concentrations)).
No products indexed under this heading.

Topiramate (CYP2C19 inhibitors may increase voriconazole systemic exposure (plasma concentrations)). Products include:
- Topamax Sprinkle Capsules 2404
- Topamax Tablets 2404

Triamcinolone (CYP3A4 inducers may decrease voriconazole systemic exposure (plasma concentrations)).
No products indexed under this heading.

Triamcinolone Acetonide (CYP3A4 inducers may decrease voriconazole systemic exposure (plasma concentrations)). Products include:
- Azmacort Inhalation Aerosol 1726
- Nasacort AQ Nasal Spray 2922

Triamcinolone Diacetate (CYP3A4 inducers may decrease voriconazole systemic exposure (plasma concentrations)).
No products indexed under this heading.

Triamcinolone Hexacetonide (CYP3A4 inducers may decrease voriconazole systemic exposure (plasma concentrations)).
No products indexed under this heading.

Triazolam (Co-administration may increase plasma concentrations of benzodiazepines that are metabolized by CYP3A4).
No products indexed under this heading.

Troglitazone (CYP2C9 inhibitors may increase voriconazole systemic exposure (plasma concentrations)).
No products indexed under this heading.

Troleandomycin (CYP3A4 inhibitors may increase voriconazole systemic exposure (plasma concentrations)).
No products indexed under this heading.

Valproate Sodium (CYP3A4 inhibitors may increase voriconazole systemic exposure (plasma concentrations)). Products include:
- Depacon Injection 412

Verapamil Hydrochloride (Co-administration may increase plasma concentrations of calcium channel blockers that are metabolized by CYP3A4). Products include:
- Covera-HS Tablets 3139
- Tarka Tablets 524
- Verelan PM Extended-Release Capsules, Controlled-Onset 3106

Vinblastine Sulfate (Co-administration may increase plasma concentrations of vinca alkaloids and lead to neurotoxicity).
No products indexed under this heading.

Vincristine Sulfate (Co-administration may increase plasma concentrations of vinca alkaloids and lead to neurotoxicity).
No products indexed under this heading.

Vinorelbine Tartrate (Co-administration may increase plasma concentrations of vinca alkaloids and lead to neurotoxicity).
No products indexed under this heading.

Warfarin Sodium (Co-administration significantly increases maximum prothrombin time by 2-times). Products include:
- Coumadin for Injection 898
- Coumadin Tablets 898

Zafirlukast (CYP2C9 inhibitors may increase voriconazole systemic exposure (plasma concentrations)). Products include:
- Accolate Tablets 671

Zileuton (CYP3A4 inhibitors may increase voriconazole systemic exposure (plasma concentrations)). Products include:
- Zyflo Tablets 1023

Food Interactions

Food, unspecified (When multiple doses of voriconazole are administered with high fat meals, the mean Cmax and AUC are reduced; VFEND tablets should be taken at least one hour before or one hour following a meal).

Grapefruit (CYP3A4 inhibitors may increase voriconazole systemic exposure (plasma concentrations)).

Grapefruit Juice (CYP3A4 inhibitors may increase voriconazole systemic exposure (plasma concentrations)).

VIADUR IMPLANT

(Leuprolide Acetate) 757
None cited in PDR database.

VIAGRA TABLETS

(Sildenafil Citrate) 2573
May interact with alpha adrenergic blockers, nonspecific beta-blockers, erythromycin, loop diuretics, nitrates and nitrites, protease inhibitors, potassium sparing diuretics, and certain other agents. Compounds in these categories include:

Alprostadil (The safety and efficacy of combinations of Viagra with other treatments for erectile dysfunction have not been studied; therefore, the use of such combinations is not recommended). Products include:
- Caverject Impulse Injection 2612
- Edex Injection 3089

Amiloride Hydrochloride (The AUC of the active metabolite, N-desmethyl sildenafil, was increased 62% by potassium-sparing diuretics; these effects on the metabolite are not expected to be of clinical consequence). Products include:
- Midamor Tablets 2026
- Moduretic Tablets 2028

Amlodipine Besylate (Co-administration in hypertensive patients has resulted in mean additional reduction on supine blood pressure by 8 mmHg systolic and 7 mmHg diastolic). Products include:
- Caduet Tablets 2508
- Lotrel Capsules 2249
- Norvasc Tablets 2545

Amprenavir (Although the interaction between other protease inhibitors and sildenafil has not been studied, their concomitant use is expected to increase sildenafil levels). Products include:
- Agenerase Capsules 1327
- Agenerase Oral Solution 1332

Amyl Nitrite (Viagra has been shown to potentiate the hypotensive effects of nitrates, and its administration to patients who are using organic nitrates, either regularly and/or intermittently, in any form is therefore contraindicated).
No products indexed under this heading.

Bumetanide (The AUC of the active metabolite, N-desmethyl sildenafil, was increased 62% by loop diuretics; these effects on the metabolite are not expected to be of clinical consequence). Products include:
- Bumex Tablets 2746

Cimetidine (Co-administration of sildenafil with non-specific CYP inhibitors, such as cimetidine, has caused a 56% increase in plasma sildenafil concentrations; potential for reduction in sildenafil clearance). Products include:
- Tagamet HB 200 Tablets .... ▣664

Cimetidine Hydrochloride (Co-administration of sildenafil with non-specific CYP inhibitors, such as cimetidine, has caused a 56% increase in plasma sildenafil concentrations; potential for reduction in sildenafil clearance).
No products indexed under this heading.

Doxazosin Mesylate (Simultaneous administration of sildenafil citrate doses above 25mg and an alpha-blocker may lead to symptomatic hypotension in some patients. Therefore, Viagra doses above 25mg should not be taken within four hours of taking alpha-blockers). Products include:
- Cardura XL Tablets 2515

Erythrityl Tetranitrate (Viagra has been shown to potentiate the hypotensive effects of nitrates, and its administration to patients who are using organic nitrates, either regularly and/or intermittently, in any form is therefore contraindicated).
No products indexed under this heading.

Erythromycin (Co-administration of sildenafil with a specific CYP3A4 inhibitor, such as erythromycin, at steady state has resulted in a 182% increase in sildenafil systemic exposure; potential for reduction in sildenafil clearance). Products include:
Ery-Tab Tablets 449
Erythromycin Base Filmtab Tablets 455
Erythromycin Delayed-Release Capsules, USP 457
PCE Dispertab Tablets 515

Erythromycin Estolate (Co-administration of sildenafil with a specific CYP3A4 inhibitor, such as erythromycin, at steady state has resulted in a 182% increase in sildenafil systemic exposure; potential for reduction in sildenafil clearance).
No products indexed under this heading.

Erythromycin Ethylsuccinate (Co-administration of sildenafil with a specific CYP3A4 inhibitor, such as erythromycin, at steady state has resulted in a 182% increase in sildenafil systemic exposure; potential for reduction in sildenafil clearance). Products include:
E.E.S. 451
EryPed 447

Erythromycin Gluceptate (Co-administration of sildenafil with a specific CYP3A4 inhibitor, such as erythromycin, at steady state has resulted in a 182% increase in sildenafil systemic exposure; potential for reduction in sildenafil clearance).
No products indexed under this heading.

Erythromycin Lactobionate (Co-administration of sildenafil with a specific CYP3A4 inhibitor, such as erythromycin, at steady state has resulted in a 182% increase in sildenafil systemic exposure; potential for reduction in sildenafil clearance).
No products indexed under this heading.

Erythromycin Stearate (Co-administration of sildenafil with a specific CYP3A4 inhibitor, such as erythromycin, at steady state has resulted in a 182% increase in sildenafil systemic exposure; potential for reduction in sildenafil clearance). Products include:
Erythrocin Stearate Filmtab Tablets 453

Ethacrynic Acid (The AUC of the active metabolite, N-desmethyl sildenafil, was increased 62% by loop diuretics; these effects on the metabolite are not expected to be of clinical consequence). Products include:
Edecrin Tablets 1959

Furosemide (The AUC of the active metabolite, N-desmethyl sildenafil, was increased 62% by loop diuretics; these effects on the metabolite are not expected to be of clinical consequence). Products include:
Furosemide Tablets 2154

Indinavir Sulfate (Although the interaction between other protease inhibitors and sildenafil has not been studied, their concomitant use is expected to increase sildenafil levels). Products include:
Crixivan Capsules 1940

Isosorbide Dinitrate (Viagra has been shown to potentiate the hypotensive effects of nitrates, and its administration to patients who are using organic nitrates, either regularly and/or intermittently, in any form is therefore contraindicated). Products include:
BiDil Tablets 2171

Isosorbide Mononitrate (Viagra has been shown to potentiate the hypotensive effects of nitrates, and its administration to patients who are using organic nitrates, either regularly and/or intermittently, in any form is therefore contraindicated). Products include:
Imdur Tablets 3018

Itraconazole (Co-administration of sildenafil with a stronger CYP3A4 inhibitor, such as itraconazole, would be expected to have a greater effect on the increase in sildenafil systemic exposure and a reduction in sildenafil clearance).
No products indexed under this heading.

Ketoconazole (Co-administration of sildenafil with a stronger CYP3A4 inhibitor, such as ketoconazole, would be expected to have a greater effect on the increase in sildenafil systemic exposure and a reduction in sildenafil clearance). Products include:
Nizoral A-D Shampoo, 1% 1868

Labetalol Hydrochloride (Co-administration with nonspecific beta-blockers has resulted in the AUC of the active metabolite, N-desmethyl sildenafil by 102%; these effects on the metabolite are not expected to be of clinical consequences).
No products indexed under this heading.

Lopinavir (Although the interaction between other protease inhibitors and sildenafil has not been studied, their concomitant use is expected to increase sildenafil levels). Products include:
Kaletra 476

Nadolol (Co-administration with nonspecific beta-blockers has resulted in the AUC of the active metabolite, N-desmethyl sildenafil by 102%; these effects on the metabolite are not expected to be of clinical consequences). Products include:
Nadolol Tablets 2159

Nelfinavir Mesylate (Although the interaction between other protease inhibitors and sildenafil has not been studied, their concomitant use is expected to increase sildenafil levels). Products include:
Viracept 2577

Nitroglycerin (Viagra has been shown to potentiate the hypotensive effects of nitrates, and its administration to patients who are using organic nitrates, either regularly and/or intermittently, in any form is therefore contraindicated). Products include:
Nitro-Dur Transdermal Infusion System 3046
Nitrolingual Pumpspray 3120

Pentaerythritol Tetranitrate (Viagra has been shown to potentiate the hypotensive effects of nitrates, and its administration to patients who are using organic nitrates, either regularly and/or intermittently, in any form is therefore contraindicated).
No products indexed under this heading.

Pindolol (Co-administration with nonspecific beta-blockers has resulted in the AUC of the active metabolite, N-desmethyl sildenafil by 102%; these effects on the metabolite are not expected to be of clinical consequences).
No products indexed under this heading.

Prazosin Hydrochloride (Simultaneous administration of sildenafil citrate doses above 25mg and an alpha-blocker may lead to symptomatic hypotension in some patients. Therefore, Viagra doses above 25mg should not be taken within four hours of taking alpha-blockers).
No products indexed under this heading.

Propranolol Hydrochloride (Co-administration with nonspecific beta-blockers has resulted in the AUC of the active metabolite, N-desmethyl sildenafil by 102%; these effects on the metabolite are not expected to be of clinical consequences). Products include:
Inderal LA Long-Acting Capsules 3429
InnoPran XL Capsules 2723

Rifampin (Co-administration of sildenafil with CYP3A4 inducers, such as rifampin, would be expected to result in decreased plasma levels of sildenafil).
No products indexed under this heading.

Ritonavir (Co-administration of ritonavir substantially increases serum concentrations of sildenafil, 11-fold increase in AUC; visual disturbances have occurred more commonly at higher systemic levels of sildenafil; decreased blood pressure, syncope, and prolonged erection have been reported in some healthy subjects exposed to high doses of sildenafil; a decrease in sildenafil dosage is recommended). Products include:
Kaletra 476
Norvir 503

Saquinavir (Co-administration of HIV protease inhibitor saquinavir, CYP3A4 inhibitor, at steady-state has resulted in a 140% increase in sildenafil Cmax and a 210% increase in sildenafil plasma AUC).
No products indexed under this heading.

Saquinavir Mesylate (Although the interaction between other protease inhibitors and sildenafil has not been studied, their concomitant use is expected to increase sildenafil levels). Products include:
Invirase 2772

Spironolactone (The AUC of the active metabolite, N-desmethyl sildenafil, was increased 62% by potassium-sparing diuretics; these effects on the metabolite are not expected to be of clinical consequence).
No products indexed under this heading.

Tamsulosin Hydrochloride (Simultaneous administration of sildenafil citrate doses above 25mg and an alpha-blocker may lead to symptomatic hypotension in some patients. Therefore, Viagra doses above 25mg should not be taken within four hours of taking alpha-blockers). Products include:
Flomax Capsules 850

Terazosin Hydrochloride (Simultaneous administration of sildenafil citrate doses above 25mg and an alpha-blocker may lead to symptomatic hypotension in some patients. Therefore, Viagra doses above 25mg should not be taken within four hours of taking alpha-blockers). Products include:
Hytrin Capsules 471

Timolol Maleate (Co-administration with nonspecific beta-blockers has resulted in the AUC of the active metabolite, N-desmethyl sildenafil by 102%; these effects on the metabolite are not expected to be of clinical consequences). Products include:
Blocadren Tablets 1916
Cosopt Sterile Ophthalmic Solution 1931
Timolide Tablets 2086
Timoptic Sterile Ophthalmic Solution 2088
Timoptic in Ocudose 2091
Timoptic-XE Sterile Ophthalmic Gel Forming Solution 2092

Torsemide (The AUC of the active metabolite, N-desmethyl sildenafil, was increased 62% by loop diuretics; these effects on the metabolite are not expected to be of clinical consequence). Products include:
Demadex Injection 2759
Demadex Tablets 2759

Triamterene (The AUC of the active metabolite, N-desmethyl sildenafil, was increased 62% by potassium-sparing diuretics; these effects on the metabolite are not expected to be of clinical consequence). Products include:
Dyazide Capsules 1423
Dyrenium Capsules 3400

Food Interactions

Food, unspecified (When Viagra is taken with a high fat meal, the rate of absorption is reduced with a mean delay in Tmax of 60 minutes and a mean reduction in Cmax of 29%).

VIBE LIQUID MULTI-NUTRIENT SUPPLEMENT

(Herbals with Vitamins & Minerals, Vitamins with Minerals) 822
May interact with:

Vitamin A (Concurrent use with other Vitamin A supplements is not recommended). Products include:
Visutein Capsules 3329

VICKS 44 COUGH RELIEF LIQUID

(Dextromethorphan Hydrobromide) ... 2679
See Vicks 44E Cough & Chest Congestion Relief Liquid

VICKS 44D COUGH & HEAD CONGESTION RELIEF LIQUID

(Dextromethorphan Hydrobromide, Pseudoephedrine Hydrochloride) 2679
See Vicks 44E Cough & Chest Congestion Relief Liquid

VICKS 44E COUGH & CHEST CONGESTION RELIEF LIQUID
(Dextromethorphan Hydrobromide, Guaifenesin) 2679
May interact with monoamine oxidase inhibitors. Compounds in these categories include:

Isocarboxazid (Concurrent and/or sequential use with MAO inhibitors is not recommended).
No products indexed under this heading.

Moclobemide (Concurrent and/or sequential use with MAO inhibitors is not recommended).
No products indexed under this heading.

Pargyline Hydrochloride (Concurrent and/or sequential use with MAO inhibitors is not recommended).
No products indexed under this heading.

Phenelzine Sulfate (Concurrent and/or sequential use with MAO inhibitors is not recommended).
No products indexed under this heading.

Procarbazine Hydrochloride (Concurrent and/or sequential use with MAO inhibitors is not recommended). Products include:
Matulane Capsules 3191

Selegiline Hydrochloride (Concurrent and/or sequential use with MAO inhibitors is not recommended). Products include:
Eldepryl Capsules 3208
Zelapar Tablets 3372

Tranylcypromine Sulfate (Concurrent and/or sequential use with MAO inhibitors is not recommended). Products include:
Parnate Tablets 1527

PEDIATRIC VICKS 44E COUGH & CHEST CONGESTION RELIEF LIQUID
(Dextromethorphan Hydrobromide, Guaifenesin) 2676
See Vicks 44E Cough & Chest Congestion Relief Liquid

VICKS 44M COUGH, COLD & FLU RELIEF LIQUID
(Acetaminophen, Chlorpheniramine Maleate, Dextromethorphan Hydrobromide, Pseudoephedrine Hydrochloride) 2680
May interact with hypnotics and sedatives, monoamine oxidase inhibitors, tranquilizers, and certain other agents. Compounds in these categories include:

Alprazolam (May increase drowsiness effect). Products include:
Niravam Orally Disintegrating Tablets 3092

Buspirone Hydrochloride (May increase drowsiness effect).
No products indexed under this heading.

Chlordiazepoxide (May increase drowsiness effect).
No products indexed under this heading.

Chlordiazepoxide Hydrochloride (May increase drowsiness effect). Products include:
Librium Capsules 3347

Chlorpromazine (May increase drowsiness effect).
No products indexed under this heading.

Chlorpromazine Hydrochloride (May increase drowsiness effect).
No products indexed under this heading.

Chlorprothixene (May increase drowsiness effect).
No products indexed under this heading.

Chlorprothixene Hydrochloride (May increase drowsiness effect).
No products indexed under this heading.

Clorazepate Dipotassium (May increase drowsiness effect). Products include:
Tranxene 2474

Diazepam (May increase drowsiness effect). Products include:
Diastat Rectal Delivery System 3343
Valium Tablets 2819

Droperidol (May increase drowsiness effect).
No products indexed under this heading.

Estazolam (May increase drowsiness effect). Products include:
ProSom Tablets 517

Ethchlorvynol (May increase drowsiness effect).
No products indexed under this heading.

Ethinamate (May increase drowsiness effect).
No products indexed under this heading.

Fluphenazine Decanoate (May increase drowsiness effect).
No products indexed under this heading.

Fluphenazine Enanthate (May increase drowsiness effect).
No products indexed under this heading.

Fluphenazine Hydrochloride (May increase drowsiness effect).
No products indexed under this heading.

Flurazepam Hydrochloride (May increase drowsiness effect). Products include:
Dalmane Capsules 3342

Glutethimide (May increase drowsiness effect).
No products indexed under this heading.

Haloperidol (May increase drowsiness effect).
No products indexed under this heading.

Haloperidol Decanoate (May increase drowsiness effect).
No products indexed under this heading.

Hydroxyzine Hydrochloride (May increase drowsiness effect).
No products indexed under this heading.

Isocarboxazid (Concurrent and/or sequential use with MAO inhibitors is not recommended).
No products indexed under this heading.

Lorazepam (May increase drowsiness effect).
No products indexed under this heading.

Loxapine Hydrochloride (May increase drowsiness effect).
No products indexed under this heading.

Loxapine Succinate (May increase drowsiness effect).
No products indexed under this heading.

Meprobamate (May increase drowsiness effect).
No products indexed under this heading.

Mesoridazine Besylate (May increase drowsiness effect).
No products indexed under this heading.

Midazolam Hydrochloride (May increase drowsiness effect).
No products indexed under this heading.

Moclobemide (Concurrent and/or sequential use with MAO inhibitors is not recommended).
No products indexed under this heading.

Molindone Hydrochloride (May increase drowsiness effect). Products include:
Moban Tablets 1119

Oxazepam (May increase drowsiness effect).
No products indexed under this heading.

Pargyline Hydrochloride (Concurrent and/or sequential use with MAO inhibitors is not recommended).
No products indexed under this heading.

Perphenazine (May increase drowsiness effect).
No products indexed under this heading.

Phenelzine Sulfate (Concurrent and/or sequential use with MAO inhibitors is not recommended).
No products indexed under this heading.

Prazepam (May increase drowsiness effect).
No products indexed under this heading.

Procarbazine Hydrochloride (Concurrent and/or sequential use with MAO inhibitors is not recommended). Products include:
Matulane Capsules 3191

Prochlorperazine (May increase drowsiness effect).
No products indexed under this heading.

Promethazine Hydrochloride (May increase drowsiness effect). Products include:
Phenergan Tablets and Suppositories 3440

Propofol (May increase drowsiness effect).
No products indexed under this heading.

Quazepam (May increase drowsiness effect).
No products indexed under this heading.

Ramelteon (May increase drowsiness effect). Products include:
Rozerem Tablets 3231

Secobarbital Sodium (May increase drowsiness effect).
No products indexed under this heading.

Selegiline Hydrochloride (Concurrent and/or sequential use with MAO inhibitors is not recommended). Products include:
Eldepryl Capsules 3208
Zelapar Tablets 3372

Temazepam (May increase drowsiness effect). Products include:
Restoril Capsules 1860

Thioridazine Hydrochloride (May increase drowsiness effect). Products include:
Thioridazine Hydrochloride Tablets 2163

Thiothixene (May increase drowsiness effect). Products include:
Thiothixene Capsules 2165

Tranylcypromine Sulfate (Concurrent and/or sequential use with MAO inhibitors is not recommended). Products include:
Parnate Tablets 1527

Triazolam (May increase drowsiness effect).
No products indexed under this heading.

Trifluoperazine Hydrochloride (May increase drowsiness effect).
No products indexed under this heading.

Zaleplon (May increase drowsiness effect). Products include:
Sonata Capsules 1717

Zolpidem Tartrate (May increase drowsiness effect). Products include:
Ambien Tablets 2851
Ambien CR Tablets 2855

Food Interactions

Alcohol (May increase drowsiness effect; patients consuming 3 or more alcoholic drinks per day should consult their physician for advice on when and how they should take this medication).

VICKS 44D COUGH & HEAD CONGESTION RELIEF LIQUID
(Dextromethorphan Hydrobromide, Phenylephrine Hydrochloride) .... ▣ 760
May interact with monoamine oxidase inhibitors. Compounds in these categories include:

Isocarboxazid (Concurrent and/or sequential use with MAO inhibitors is not recommended).
No products indexed under this heading.

Moclobemide (Concurrent and/or sequential use with MAO inhibitors is not recommended).
No products indexed under this heading.

Pargyline Hydrochloride (Concurrent and/or sequential use with MAO inhibitors is not recommended).
No products indexed under this heading.

Phenelzine Sulfate (Concurrent and/or sequential use with MAO inhibitors is not recommended).
No products indexed under this heading.

Procarbazine Hydrochloride (Concurrent and/or sequential use with MAO inhibitors is not recommended). Products include:
Matulane Capsules 3191

Selegiline Hydrochloride (Concurrent and/or sequential use with MAO inhibitors is not recommended). Products include:
Eldepryl Capsules 3208
Zelapar Tablets 3372

Tranylcypromine Sulfate (Concurrent and/or sequential use with MAO inhibitors is not recommended). Products include:
Parnate Tablets 1527

VICKS 44E COUGH & CHEST CONGESTION RELIEF LIQUID
(Dextromethorphan Hydrobromide, Guaifenesin) .... ▣ 760

VICKS 44M COUGH, COLD & FLU RELIEF LIQUID
(Acetaminophen, Chlorpheniramine Maleate, Dextromethorphan Hydrobromide).... 760
May interact with hypnotics and sedatives, monoamine oxidase inhibitors, tranquilizers, and certain other agents. Compounds in these categories include:

Alprazolam (May increase drowsiness effect). Products include:
Niravam Orally Disintegrating Tablets 3092

Buspirone Hydrochloride (May increase drowsiness effect).
No products indexed under this heading.

Chlordiazepoxide (May increase drowsiness effect).
No products indexed under this heading.

Chlordiazepoxide Hydrochloride (May increase drowsiness effect). Products include:
Librium Capsules 3347

Chlorpromazine (May increase drowsiness effect).
No products indexed under this heading.

Chlorpromazine Hydrochloride (May increase drowsiness effect).
No products indexed under this heading.

Chlorprothixene (May increase drowsiness effect).
No products indexed under this heading.

Chlorprothixene Hydrochloride (May increase drowsiness effect).
No products indexed under this heading.

Clorazepate Dipotassium (May increase drowsiness effect). Products include:
Tranxene 2474

Diazepam (May increase drowsiness effect). Products include:
Diastat Rectal Delivery System 3343
Valium Tablets 2819

Droperidol (May increase drowsiness effect).
No products indexed under this heading.

Estazolam (May increase drowsiness effect). Products include:
ProSom Tablets 517

Ethchlorvynol (May increase drowsiness effect).
No products indexed under this heading.

Ethinamate (May increase drowsiness effect).
No products indexed under this heading.

Fluphenazine Decanoate (May increase drowsiness effect).
No products indexed under this heading.

Fluphenazine Enanthate (May increase drowsiness effect).
No products indexed under this heading.

Fluphenazine Hydrochloride (May increase drowsiness effect).
No products indexed under this heading.

Flurazepam Hydrochloride (May increase drowsiness effect). Products include:
Dalmane Capsules 3342

Glutethimide (May increase drowsiness effect).
No products indexed under this heading.

Haloperidol (May increase drowsiness effect).
No products indexed under this heading.

Haloperidol Decanoate (May increase drowsiness effect).
No products indexed under this heading.

Hydroxyzine Hydrochloride (May increase drowsiness effect).
No products indexed under this heading.

Isocarboxazid (Concurrent and/or sequential use with MAO inhibitors is not recommended).
No products indexed under this heading.

Lorazepam (May increase drowsiness effect).
No products indexed under this heading.

Loxapine Hydrochloride (May increase drowsiness effect).
No products indexed under this heading.

Loxapine Succinate (May increase drowsiness effect).
No products indexed under this heading.

Meprobamate (May increase drowsiness effect).
No products indexed under this heading.

Mesoridazine Besylate (May increase drowsiness effect).
No products indexed under this heading.

Midazolam Hydrochloride (May increase drowsiness effect).
No products indexed under this heading.

Moclobemide (Concurrent and/or sequential use with MAO inhibitors is not recommended).
No products indexed under this heading.

Molindone Hydrochloride (May increase drowsiness effect). Products include:
Moban Tablets 1119

Oxazepam (May increase drowsiness effect).
No products indexed under this heading.

Pargyline Hydrochloride (Concurrent and/or sequential use with MAO inhibitors is not recommended).
No products indexed under this heading.

Perphenazine (May increase drowsiness effect).
No products indexed under this heading.

Phenelzine Sulfate (Concurrent and/or sequential use with MAO inhibitors is not recommended).
No products indexed under this heading.

Prazepam (May increase drowsiness effect).
No products indexed under this heading.

Procarbazine Hydrochloride (Concurrent and/or sequential use with MAO inhibitors is not recommended). Products include:
Matulane Capsules 3191

Prochlorperazine (May increase drowsiness effect).
No products indexed under this heading.

Promethazine Hydrochloride (May increase drowsiness effect). Products include:
Phenergan Tablets and Suppositories 3440

Propofol (May increase drowsiness effect).
No products indexed under this heading.

Quazepam (May increase drowsiness effect).
No products indexed under this heading.

Ramelteon (May increase drowsiness effect). Products include:
Rozerem Tablets 3231

Secobarbital Sodium (May increase drowsiness effect).
No products indexed under this heading.

Selegiline Hydrochloride (Concurrent and/or sequential use with MAO inhibitors is not recommended). Products include:
Eldepryl Capsules 3208
Zelapar Tablets 3372

Temazepam (May increase drowsiness effect). Products include:
Restoril Capsules 1860

Thioridazine Hydrochloride (May increase drowsiness effect). Products include:
Thioridazine Hydrochloride Tablets 2163

Thiothixene (May increase drowsiness effect). Products include:
Thiothixene Capsules 2165

Tranylcypromine Sulfate (Concurrent and/or sequential use with MAO inhibitors is not recommended). Products include:
Parnate Tablets 1527

Triazolam (May increase drowsiness effect).
No products indexed under this heading.

Trifluoperazine Hydrochloride (May increase drowsiness effect).
No products indexed under this heading.

Zaleplon (May increase drowsiness effect). Products include:
Sonata Capsules 1717

Zolpidem Tartrate (May increase drowsiness effect). Products include:
Ambien Tablets 2851
Ambien CR Tablets 2855

Food Interactions

Alcohol (Concomitant consumption of alcohol may cause liver damage).

PEDIATRIC VICKS 44M COUGH & COLD RELIEF LIQUID
(Chlorpheniramine Maleate, Dextromethorphan Hydrobromide)...... 2676
May interact with hypnotics and sedatives, monoamine oxidase inhibitors, tranquilizers, and certain other agents. Compounds in these categories include:

Alprazolam (May increase drowsiness effect). Products include:
Niravam Orally Disintegrating Tablets 3092

Buspirone Hydrochloride (May increase drowsiness effect).
No products indexed under this heading.

Chlordiazepoxide (May increase drowsiness effect).
No products indexed under this heading.

Chlordiazepoxide Hydrochloride (May increase drowsiness effect). Products include:
Librium Capsules 3347

Chlorpromazine (May increase drowsiness effect).
No products indexed under this heading.

Chlorpromazine Hydrochloride (May increase drowsiness effect).
No products indexed under this heading.

Chlorprothixene (May increase drowsiness effect).
No products indexed under this heading.

Chlorprothixene Hydrochloride (May increase drowsiness effect).
No products indexed under this heading.

Clorazepate Dipotassium (May increase drowsiness effect). Products include:
Tranxene 2474

Diazepam (May increase drowsiness effect). Products include:
Diastat Rectal Delivery System 3343
Valium Tablets 2819

Droperidol (May increase drowsiness effect).
No products indexed under this heading.

Estazolam (May increase drowsiness effect). Products include:
ProSom Tablets 517

Ethchlorvynol (May increase drowsiness effect).
No products indexed under this heading.

Ethinamate (May increase drowsiness effect).
No products indexed under this heading.

Fluphenazine Decanoate (May increase drowsiness effect).
No products indexed under this heading.

Fluphenazine Enanthate (May increase drowsiness effect).
No products indexed under this heading.

Fluphenazine Hydrochloride (May increase drowsiness effect).
No products indexed under this heading.

Flurazepam Hydrochloride (May increase drowsiness effect). Products include:
Dalmane Capsules 3342

Glutethimide (May increase drowsiness effect).
No products indexed under this heading.

Haloperidol (May increase drowsiness effect).
No products indexed under this heading.

Haloperidol Decanoate (May increase drowsiness effect).
No products indexed under this heading.

Hydroxyzine Hydrochloride (May increase drowsiness effect).
No products indexed under this heading.

Isocarboxazid (Concurrent and/or sequential use with MAO inhibitors is not recommended).
No products indexed under this heading.

Lorazepam (May increase drowsiness effect).
No products indexed under this heading.

Loxapine Hydrochloride (May increase drowsiness effect).
No products indexed under this heading.

Loxapine Succinate (May increase drowsiness effect).
No products indexed under this heading.

Meprobamate (May increase drowsiness effect).
No products indexed under this heading.

Mesoridazine Besylate (May increase drowsiness effect).
No products indexed under this heading.

Midazolam Hydrochloride (May increase drowsiness effect).
No products indexed under this heading.

Moclobemide (Concurrent and/or sequential use with MAO inhibitors is not recommended).
No products indexed under this heading.

Molindone Hydrochloride (May increase drowsiness effect). Products include:
Moban Tablets ... 1119

Oxazepam (May increase drowsiness effect).
No products indexed under this heading.

Pargyline Hydrochloride (Concurrent and/or sequential use with MAO inhibitors is not recommended).
No products indexed under this heading.

Perphenazine (May increase drowsiness effect).
No products indexed under this heading.

Phenelzine Sulfate (Concurrent and/or sequential use with MAO inhibitors is not recommended).
No products indexed under this heading.

Prazepam (May increase drowsiness effect).
No products indexed under this heading.

Procarbazine Hydrochloride (Concurrent and/or sequential use with MAO inhibitors is not recommended). Products include:
Matulane Capsules ... 3191

Prochlorperazine (May increase drowsiness effect).
No products indexed under this heading.

Promethazine Hydrochloride (May increase drowsiness effect). Products include:
Phenergan Tablets and Suppositories ... 3440

Propofol (May increase drowsiness effect).
No products indexed under this heading.

Quazepam (May increase drowsiness effect).
No products indexed under this heading.

Ramelteon (May increase drowsiness effect). Products include:
Rozerem Tablets ... 3231

Secobarbital Sodium (May increase drowsiness effect).
No products indexed under this heading.

Selegiline Hydrochloride (Concurrent and/or sequential use with MAO inhibitors is not recommended). Products include:
Eldepryl Capsules ... 3208
Zelapar Tablets ... 3372

Temazepam (May increase drowsiness effect). Products include:
Restoril Capsules ... 1860

Thioridazine Hydrochloride (May increase drowsiness effect). Products include:
Thioridazine Hydrochloride Tablets ... 2163

Thiothixene (May increase drowsiness effect). Products include:
Thiothixene Capsules ... 2165

Tranylcypromine Sulfate (Concurrent and/or sequential use with MAO inhibitors is not recommended). Products include:
Parnate Tablets ... 1527

Triazolam (May increase drowsiness effect).
No products indexed under this heading.

Trifluoperazine Hydrochloride (May increase drowsiness effect).
No products indexed under this heading.

Zaleplon (May increase drowsiness effect). Products include:
Sonata Capsules ... 1717

Zolpidem Tartrate (May increase drowsiness effect). Products include:
Ambien Tablets ... 2851
Ambien CR Tablets ... 2855

Food Interactions

Alcohol (May increase drowsiness effect).

VICKS DAYQUIL LIQUICAPS/LIQUID MULTI-SYMPTOM COLD

(Acetaminophen, Dextromethorphan Hydrobromide, Phenylephrine Hydrochloride) ... 761
May interact with monoamine oxidase inhibitors and certain other agents. Compounds in these categories include:

Isocarboxazid (Concurrent and/or sequential use with MAO inhibitors is not recommended).
No products indexed under this heading.

Moclobemide (Concurrent and/or sequential use with MAO inhibitors is not recommended).
No products indexed under this heading.

Pargyline Hydrochloride (Concurrent and/or sequential use with MAO inhibitors is not recommended).
No products indexed under this heading.

Phenelzine Sulfate (Concurrent and/or sequential use with MAO inhibitors is not recommended).
No products indexed under this heading.

Procarbazine Hydrochloride (Concurrent and/or sequential use with MAO inhibitors is not recommended). Products include:
Matulane Capsules ... 3191

Selegiline Hydrochloride (Concurrent and/or sequential use with MAO inhibitors is not recommended). Products include:
Eldepryl Capsules ... 3208
Zelapar Tablets ... 3372

Tranylcypromine Sulfate (Concurrent and/or sequential use with MAO inhibitors is not recommended). Products include:
Parnate Tablets ... 1527

Food Interactions

Alcohol (Concomitant consumption of alcohol may cause liver damage).

VICKS COUGH DROPS, MENTHOL & CHERRY FLAVORS

(Menthol) ... 2678
None cited in PDR database.

VICKS DAYQUIL MULTI-SYMPTOM COLD

(Acetaminophen, Dextromethorphan Hydrobromide, Pseudoephedrine Hydrochloride) ... 2678
See Vicks DayQuil Multi-Symptom Cold/Flu Relief LiquiCaps

VICKS DAYQUIL MULTI-SYMPTOM COLD LIQUICAPS

(Acetaminophen, Dextromethorphan Hydrobromide, Pseudoephedrine Hydrochloride) ... 2678
May interact with monoamine oxidase inhibitors and certain other agents. Compounds in these categories include:

Isocarboxazid (Concurrent and/or sequential use with MAO inhibitors is not recommended).
No products indexed under this heading.

Moclobemide (Concurrent and/or sequential use with MAO inhibitors is not recommended).
No products indexed under this heading.

Pargyline Hydrochloride (Concurrent and/or sequential use with MAO inhibitors is not recommended).
No products indexed under this heading.

Phenelzine Sulfate (Concurrent and/or sequential use with MAO inhibitors is not recommended).
No products indexed under this heading.

Procarbazine Hydrochloride (Concurrent and/or sequential use with MAO inhibitors is not recommended). Products include:
Matulane Capsules ... 3191

Selegiline Hydrochloride (Concurrent and/or sequential use with MAO inhibitors is not recommended). Products include:
Eldepryl Capsules ... 3208
Zelapar Tablets ... 3372

Tranylcypromine Sulfate (Concurrent and/or sequential use with MAO inhibitors is not recommended). Products include:
Parnate Tablets ... 1527

Food Interactions

Alcohol (Patients consuming 3 or more alcoholic drinks per day should consult their physician for advice on when and how they should take this medication).

VICKS NYQUIL/ MULTI-SYMPTOM COLD LIQUID

(Acetaminophen, Dextromethorphan Hydrobromide, Doxylamine Succinate, Pseudoephedrine Hydrochloride) ... 2681
See Vicks NyQuil Multi-Symptom Cold/Flu Relief LiquiCaps

CHILDREN'S VICKS NYQUIL COLD/COUGH RELIEF

(Chlorpheniramine Maleate, Dextromethorphan Hydrobromide) ... 756
May interact with hypnotics and sedatives, monoamine oxidase inhibitors, tranquilizers, and certain other agents. Compounds in these categories include:

Alprazolam (May increase drowsiness effect). Products include:
Niravam Orally Disintegrating Tablets ... 3092

Buspirone Hydrochloride (May increase drowsiness effect).
No products indexed under this heading.

Chlordiazepoxide (May increase drowsiness effect).
No products indexed under this heading.

Chlordiazepoxide Hydrochloride (May increase drowsiness effect). Products include:
Librium Capsules ... 3347

Chlorpromazine (May increase drowsiness effect).
No products indexed under this heading.

Chlorpromazine Hydrochloride (May increase drowsiness effect).
No products indexed under this heading.

Chlorprothixene (May increase drowsiness effect).
No products indexed under this heading.

Chlorprothixene Hydrochloride (May increase drowsiness effect).
No products indexed under this heading.

Clorazepate Dipotassium (May increase drowsiness effect). Products include:
Tranxene ... 2474

Diazepam (May increase drowsiness effect). Products include:
Diastat Rectal Delivery System ... 3343
Valium Tablets ... 2819

Droperidol (May increase drowsiness effect).
No products indexed under this heading.

Estazolam (May increase drowsiness effect). Products include:
ProSom Tablets ... 517

Ethchlorvynol (May increase drowsiness effect).
No products indexed under this heading.

Ethinamate (May increase drowsiness effect).
No products indexed under this heading.

Fluphenazine Decanoate (May increase drowsiness effect).
No products indexed under this heading.

Fluphenazine Enanthate (May increase drowsiness effect).
No products indexed under this heading.

Fluphenazine Hydrochloride (May increase drowsiness effect).
No products indexed under this heading.

Flurazepam Hydrochloride (May increase drowsiness effect). Products include:
Dalmane Capsules ... 3342

Glutethimide (May increase drowsiness effect).
No products indexed under this heading.

Haloperidol (May increase drowsiness effect).
No products indexed under this heading.

Haloperidol Decanoate (May increase drowsiness effect).
No products indexed under this heading.

Hydroxyzine Hydrochloride (May increase drowsiness effect).
No products indexed under this heading.

Isocarboxazid (Concurrent and/or sequential use with MAO inhibitors is not recommended).

No products indexed under this heading.

Lorazepam (May increase drowsiness effect).

No products indexed under this heading.

Loxapine Hydrochloride (May increase drowsiness effect).

No products indexed under this heading.

Loxapine Succinate (May increase drowsiness effect).

No products indexed under this heading.

Meprobamate (May increase drowsiness effect).

No products indexed under this heading.

Mesoridazine Besylate (May increase drowsiness effect).

No products indexed under this heading.

Midazolam Hydrochloride (May increase drowsiness effect).

No products indexed under this heading.

Moclobemide (Concurrent and/or sequential use with MAO inhibitors is not recommended).

No products indexed under this heading.

Molindone Hydrochloride (May increase drowsiness effect).
Products include:
Moban Tablets 1119

Oxazepam (May increase drowsiness effect).

No products indexed under this heading.

Pargyline Hydrochloride (Concurrent and/or sequential use with MAO inhibitors is not recommended).

No products indexed under this heading.

Perphenazine (May increase drowsiness effect).

No products indexed under this heading.

Phenelzine Sulfate (Concurrent and/or sequential use with MAO inhibitors is not recommended).

No products indexed under this heading.

Prazepam (May increase drowsiness effect).

No products indexed under this heading.

Procarbazine Hydrochloride (Concurrent and/or sequential use with MAO inhibitors is not recommended). Products include:
Matulane Capsules 3191

Prochlorperazine (May increase drowsiness effect).

No products indexed under this heading.

Promethazine Hydrochloride (May increase drowsiness effect).
Products include:
Phenergan Tablets and
Suppositories............................. 3440

Propofol (May increase drowsiness effect).

No products indexed under this heading.

Quazepam (May increase drowsiness effect).

No products indexed under this heading.

Ramelteon (May increase drowsiness effect). Products include:

Rozerem Tablets 3231

Secobarbital Sodium (May increase drowsiness effect).

No products indexed under this heading.

Selegiline Hydrochloride (Concurrent and/or sequential use with MAO inhibitors is not recommended). Products include:
Eldepryl Capsules 3208
Zelapar Tablets 3372

Temazepam (May increase drowsiness effect). Products include:
Restoril Capsules 1860

Thioridazine Hydrochloride (May increase drowsiness effect).
Products include:
Thioridazine Hydrochloride
Tablets .. 2163

Thiothixene (May increase drowsiness effect). Products include:
Thiothixene Capsules 2165

Tranylcypromine Sulfate (Concurrent and/or sequential use with MAO inhibitors is not recommended). Products include:
Parnate Tablets 1527

Triazolam (May increase drowsiness effect).

No products indexed under this heading.

Trifluoperazine Hydrochloride (May increase drowsiness effect).

No products indexed under this heading.

Zaleplon (May increase drowsiness effect). Products include:
Sonata Capsules 1717

Zolpidem Tartrate (May increase drowsiness effect). Products include:
Ambien Tablets 2851
Ambien CR Tablets 2855

Food Interactions

Alcohol (Concomitant consumption of alcohol may cause liver damage).

VICKS NYQUIL MULTI-SYMPTOM COLD LIQUICAPS

(Acetaminophen, Dextromethorphan Hydrobromide, Doxylamine Succinate, Pseudoephedrine Hydrochloride)........ 2681
May interact with hypnotics and sedatives, monoamine oxidase inhibitors, tranquilizers, and certain other agents. Compounds in these categories include:

Alprazolam (May increase drowsiness effect). Products include:
Niravam Orally Disintegrating
Tablets .. 3092

Buspirone Hydrochloride (May increase drowsiness effect).

No products indexed under this heading.

Chlordiazepoxide (May increase drowsiness effect).

No products indexed under this heading.

Chlordiazepoxide Hydrochloride (May increase drowsiness effect).
Products include:
Librium Capsules 3347

Chlorpromazine (May increase drowsiness effect).

No products indexed under this heading.

Chlorpromazine Hydrochloride (May increase drowsiness effect).

No products indexed under this heading.

Chlorprothixene (May increase drowsiness effect).

No products indexed under this heading.

Chlorprothixene Hydrochloride (May increase drowsiness effect).

No products indexed under this heading.

Clorazepate Dipotassium (May increase drowsiness effect). Products include:
Tranxene 2474

Diazepam (May increase drowsiness effect). Products include:
Diastat Rectal Delivery System 3343
Valium Tablets 2819

Droperidol (May increase drowsiness effect).

No products indexed under this heading.

Estazolam (May increase drowsiness effect). Products include:
ProSom Tablets 517

Ethchlorvynol (May increase drowsiness effect).

No products indexed under this heading.

Ethinamate (May increase drowsiness effect).

No products indexed under this heading.

Fluphenazine Decanoate (May increase drowsiness effect).

No products indexed under this heading.

Fluphenazine Enanthate (May increase drowsiness effect).

No products indexed under this heading.

Fluphenazine Hydrochloride (May increase drowsiness effect).

No products indexed under this heading.

Flurazepam Hydrochloride (May increase drowsiness effect).
Products include:
Dalmane Capsules 3342

Glutethimide (May increase drowsiness effect).

No products indexed under this heading.

Haloperidol (May increase drowsiness effect).

No products indexed under this heading.

Haloperidol Decanoate (May increase drowsiness effect).

No products indexed under this heading.

Hydroxyzine Hydrochloride (May increase drowsiness effect).

No products indexed under this heading.

Isocarboxazid (Concurrent and/or sequential use with MAO inhibitors is not recommended).

No products indexed under this heading.

Lorazepam (May increase drowsiness effect).

No products indexed under this heading.

Loxapine Hydrochloride (May increase drowsiness effect).

No products indexed under this heading.

Loxapine Succinate (May increase drowsiness effect).

No products indexed under this heading.

Meprobamate (May increase drowsiness effect).

No products indexed under this heading.

Mesoridazine Besylate (May increase drowsiness effect).

No products indexed under this heading.

Midazolam Hydrochloride (May increase drowsiness effect).

No products indexed under this heading.

Moclobemide (Concurrent and/or sequential use with MAO inhibitors is not recommended).

No products indexed under this heading.

Molindone Hydrochloride (May increase drowsiness effect).
Products include:
Moban Tablets................................ 1119

Oxazepam (May increase drowsiness effect).

No products indexed under this heading.

Pargyline Hydrochloride (Concurrent and/or sequential use with MAO inhibitors is not recommended).

No products indexed under this heading.

Perphenazine (May increase drowsiness effect).

No products indexed under this heading.

Phenelzine Sulfate (Concurrent and/or sequential use with MAO inhibitors is not recommended).

No products indexed under this heading.

Prazepam (May increase drowsiness effect).

No products indexed under this heading.

Procarbazine Hydrochloride (Concurrent and/or sequential use with MAO inhibitors is not recommended). Products include:
Matulane Capsules 3191

Prochlorperazine (May increase drowsiness effect).

No products indexed under this heading.

Promethazine Hydrochloride (May increase drowsiness effect).
Products include:
Phenergan Tablets and
Suppositories............................. 3440

Propofol (May increase drowsiness effect).

No products indexed under this heading.

Quazepam (May increase drowsiness effect).

No products indexed under this heading.

Ramelteon (May increase drowsiness effect). Products include:
Rozerem Tablets 3231

Secobarbital Sodium (May increase drowsiness effect).

No products indexed under this heading.

Selegiline Hydrochloride (Concurrent and/or sequential use with MAO inhibitors is not recommended). Products include:
Eldepryl Capsules 3208
Zelapar Tablets 3372

Temazepam (May increase drowsiness effect). Products include:
Restoril Capsules 1860

Thioridazine Hydrochloride (May increase drowsiness effect).
Products include:
Thioridazine Hydrochloride
Tablets .. 2163

Thiothixene (May increase drowsiness effect). Products include:
Thiothixene Capsules 2165

Tranylcypromine Sulfate (Concurrent and/or sequential use with MAO inhibitors is not recommended). Products include:

IMPORTANT NOTE: Always consult each drug listing in the patient's regimen for possible interactions.

Parnate Tablets 1527

Triazolam (May increase drowsiness effect).
No products indexed under this heading.

Trifluoperazine Hydrochloride (May increase drowsiness effect).
No products indexed under this heading.

Zaleplon (May increase drowsiness effect). Products include:
Sonata Capsules 1717

Zolpidem Tartrate (May increase drowsiness effect). Products include:
Ambien Tablets 2851
Ambien CR Tablets 2855

Food Interactions

Alcohol (May increase drowsiness effect; patients consuming 3 or more alcoholic drinks per day should consult their physician for advice on when and how they should take this medication).

VICKS NYQUIL LIQUICAPS/LIQUID MULTI-SYMPTOM COLD/FLU RELIEF

(Acetaminophen, Dextromethorphan Hydrobromide, Doxylamine Succinate).................... ▣ 763
May interact with hypnotics and sedatives, monoamine oxidase inhibitors, tranquilizers, and certain other agents. Compounds in these categories include:

Alprazolam (May increase drowsiness effect). Products include:
Niravam Orally Disintegrating Tablets 3092

Buspirone Hydrochloride (May increase drowsiness effect).
No products indexed under this heading.

Chlordiazepoxide (May increase drowsiness effect).
No products indexed under this heading.

Chlordiazepoxide Hydrochloride (May increase drowsiness effect). Products include:
Librium Capsules 3347

Chlorpromazine (May increase drowsiness effect).
No products indexed under this heading.

Chlorpromazine Hydrochloride (May increase drowsiness effect).
No products indexed under this heading.

Chlorprothixene (May increase drowsiness effect).
No products indexed under this heading.

Chlorprothixene Hydrochloride (May increase drowsiness effect).
No products indexed under this heading.

Clorazepate Dipotassium (May increase drowsiness effect). Products include:
Tranxene 2474

Diazepam (May increase drowsiness effect). Products include:
Diastat Rectal Delivery System 3343
Valium Tablets 2819

Droperidol (May increase drowsiness effect).
No products indexed under this heading.

Estazolam (May increase drowsiness effect). Products include:
ProSom Tablets 517

Ethchlorvynol (May increase drowsiness effect).
No products indexed under this heading.

Ethinamate (May increase drowsiness effect).
No products indexed under this heading.

Fluphenazine Decanoate (May increase drowsiness effect).
No products indexed under this heading.

Fluphenazine Enanthate (May increase drowsiness effect).
No products indexed under this heading.

Fluphenazine Hydrochloride (May increase drowsiness effect).
No products indexed under this heading.

Flurazepam Hydrochloride (May increase drowsiness effect). Products include:
Dalmane Capsules 3342

Glutethimide (May increase drowsiness effect).
No products indexed under this heading.

Haloperidol (May increase drowsiness effect).
No products indexed under this heading.

Haloperidol Decanoate (May increase drowsiness effect).
No products indexed under this heading.

Hydroxyzine Hydrochloride (May increase drowsiness effect).
No products indexed under this heading.

Isocarboxazid (Do not use while taking, or for 2 weeks after stopping, MAO inhibitors).
No products indexed under this heading.

Lorazepam (May increase drowsiness effect).
No products indexed under this heading.

Loxapine Hydrochloride (May increase drowsiness effect).
No products indexed under this heading.

Loxapine Succinate (May increase drowsiness effect).
No products indexed under this heading.

Meprobamate (May increase drowsiness effect).
No products indexed under this heading.

Mesoridazine Besylate (May increase drowsiness effect).
No products indexed under this heading.

Midazolam Hydrochloride (May increase drowsiness effect).
No products indexed under this heading.

Moclobemide (Do not use while taking, or for 2 weeks after stopping, MAO inhibitors).
No products indexed under this heading.

Molindone Hydrochloride (May increase drowsiness effect). Products include:
Moban Tablets 1119

Oxazepam (May increase drowsiness effect).
No products indexed under this heading.

Pargyline Hydrochloride (Do not use while taking, or for 2 weeks after stopping, MAO inhibitors).
No products indexed under this heading.

Perphenazine (May increase drowsiness effect).
No products indexed under this heading.

Phenelzine Sulfate (Do not use while taking, or for 2 weeks after stopping, MAO inhibitors).
No products indexed under this heading.

Prazepam (May increase drowsiness effect).
No products indexed under this heading.

Procarbazine Hydrochloride (Do not use while taking, or for 2 weeks after stopping, MAO inhibitors). Products include:
Matulane Capsules 3191

Prochlorperazine (May increase drowsiness effect).
No products indexed under this heading.

Promethazine Hydrochloride (May increase drowsiness effect). Products include:
Phenergan Tablets and Suppositories 3440

Propofol (May increase drowsiness effect).
No products indexed under this heading.

Quazepam (May increase drowsiness effect).
No products indexed under this heading.

Ramelteon (May increase drowsiness effect). Products include:
Rozerem Tablets 3231

Secobarbital Sodium (May increase drowsiness effect).
No products indexed under this heading.

Selegiline Hydrochloride (Do not use while taking, or for 2 weeks after stopping, MAO inhibitors). Products include:
Eldepryl Capsules 3208
Zelapar Tablets 3372

Temazepam (May increase drowsiness effect). Products include:
Restoril Capsules 1860

Thioridazine Hydrochloride (May increase drowsiness effect). Products include:
Thioridazine Hydrochloride Tablets 2163

Thiothixene (May increase drowsiness effect). Products include:
Thiothixene Capsules 2165

Tranylcypromine Sulfate (Do not use while taking, or for 2 weeks after stopping, MAO inhibitors). Products include:
Parnate Tablets 1527

Triazolam (May increase drowsiness effect).
No products indexed under this heading.

Trifluoperazine Hydrochloride (May increase drowsiness effect).
No products indexed under this heading.

Zaleplon (May increase drowsiness effect). Products include:
Sonata Capsules 1717

Zolpidem Tartrate (May increase drowsiness effect). Products include:
Ambien Tablets 2851
Ambien CR Tablets 2855

Food Interactions

Alcohol (Chronic heavy alcohol users, 3 or more drinks per day, are at increased risk of liver toxicity from excessive acetaminophen use; alcohol increases drowsiness effect and concurrent use of alcoholic beverages should be avoided).

VICKS NYQUIL COUGH LIQUID

(Dextromethorphan Hydrobromide, Doxylamine Succinate)....................... 2680
See Vicks NyQuil Multi-Symptom Cold/Flu Relief LiquiCaps

CHILDREN'S VICKS NYQUIL COLD/COUGH RELIEF LIQUID

(Chlorpheniramine Maleate, Dextromethorphan Hydrobromide, Pseudoephedrine Hydrochloride)........ 2680
May interact with hypnotics and sedatives, monoamine oxidase inhibitors, tranquilizers, and certain other agents. Compounds in these categories include:

Alprazolam (May increase drowsiness effect). Products include:
Niravam Orally Disintegrating Tablets 3092

Buspirone Hydrochloride (May increase drowsiness effect).
No products indexed under this heading.

Chlordiazepoxide (May increase drowsiness effect).
No products indexed under this heading.

Chlordiazepoxide Hydrochloride (May increase drowsiness effect). Products include:
Librium Capsules 3347

Chlorpromazine (May increase drowsiness effect).
No products indexed under this heading.

Chlorpromazine Hydrochloride (May increase drowsiness effect).
No products indexed under this heading.

Chlorprothixene (May increase drowsiness effect).
No products indexed under this heading.

Chlorprothixene Hydrochloride (May increase drowsiness effect).
No products indexed under this heading.

Clorazepate Dipotassium (May increase drowsiness effect). Products include:
Tranxene 2474

Diazepam (May increase drowsiness effect). Products include:
Diastat Rectal Delivery System 3343
Valium Tablets 2819

Droperidol (May increase drowsiness effect).
No products indexed under this heading.

Estazolam (May increase drowsiness effect). Products include:
ProSom Tablets 517

Ethchlorvynol (May increase drowsiness effect).
No products indexed under this heading.

Ethinamate (May increase drowsiness effect).
No products indexed under this heading.

Fluphenazine Decanoate (May increase drowsiness effect).
No products indexed under this heading.

Fluphenazine Enanthate (May increase drowsiness effect).
No products indexed under this heading.

Fluphenazine Hydrochloride (May increase drowsiness effect).
No products indexed under this heading.

Flurazepam Hydrochloride (May increase drowsiness effect). Products include:
Dalmane Capsules **3342**

Glutethimide (May increase drowsiness effect).
No products indexed under this heading.

Haloperidol (May increase drowsiness effect).
No products indexed under this heading.

Haloperidol Decanoate (May increase drowsiness effect).
No products indexed under this heading.

Hydroxyzine Hydrochloride (May increase drowsiness effect).
No products indexed under this heading.

Isocarboxazid (Concurrent and/or sequential use with MAO inhibitors is not recommended).
No products indexed under this heading.

Lorazepam (May increase drowsiness effect).
No products indexed under this heading.

Loxapine Hydrochloride (May increase drowsiness effect).
No products indexed under this heading.

Loxapine Succinate (May increase drowsiness effect).
No products indexed under this heading.

Meprobamate (May increase drowsiness effect).
No products indexed under this heading.

Mesoridazine Besylate (May increase drowsiness effect).
No products indexed under this heading.

Midazolam Hydrochloride (May increase drowsiness effect).
No products indexed under this heading.

Moclobemide (Concurrent and/or sequential use with MAO inhibitors is not recommended).
No products indexed under this heading.

Molindone Hydrochloride (May increase drowsiness effect). Products include:
Moban Tablets **1119**

Oxazepam (May increase drowsiness effect).
No products indexed under this heading.

Pargyline Hydrochloride (Concurrent and/or sequential use with MAO inhibitors is not recommended).
No products indexed under this heading.

Perphenazine (May increase drowsiness effect).
No products indexed under this heading.

Phenelzine Sulfate (Concurrent and/or sequential use with MAO inhibitors is not recommended).
No products indexed under this heading.

Prazepam (May increase drowsiness effect).
No products indexed under this heading.

Procarbazine Hydrochloride (Concurrent and/or sequential use with MAO inhibitors is not recommended). Products include:
Matulane Capsules **3191**

Prochlorperazine (May increase drowsiness effect).
No products indexed under this heading.

Promethazine Hydrochloride (May increase drowsiness effect). Products include:
Phenergan Tablets and Suppositories.............................. **3440**

Propofol (May increase drowsiness effect).
No products indexed under this heading.

Quazepam (May increase drowsiness effect).
No products indexed under this heading.

Ramelteon (May increase drowsiness effect). Products include:
Rozerem Tablets **3231**

Secobarbital Sodium (May increase drowsiness effect).
No products indexed under this heading.

Selegiline Hydrochloride (Concurrent and/or sequential use with MAO inhibitors is not recommended). Products include:
Eldepryl Capsules **3208**
Zelapar Tablets **3372**

Temazepam (May increase drowsiness effect). Products include:
Restoril Capsules **1860**

Thioridazine Hydrochloride (May increase drowsiness effect). Products include:
Thioridazine Hydrochloride Tablets **2163**

Thiothixene (May increase drowsiness effect). Products include:
Thiothixene Capsules **2165**

Tranylcypromine Sulfate (Concurrent and/or sequential use with MAO inhibitors is not recommended). Products include:
Parnate Tablets **1527**

Triazolam (May increase drowsiness effect).
No products indexed under this heading.

Trifluoperazine Hydrochloride (May increase drowsiness effect).
No products indexed under this heading.

Zaleplon (May increase drowsiness effect). Products include:
Sonata Capsules **1717**

Zolpidem Tartrate (May increase drowsiness effect). Products include:
Ambien Tablets **2851**
Ambien CR Tablets **2855**

Food Interactions

Alcohol (May increase drowsiness effect).

VICKS SINEX NASAL SPRAY AND ULTRA FINE MIST FOR SINUS RELIEF

(Oxymetazoline Hydrochloride) **2681**
None cited in PDR database.

VICKS SINEX 12-HOUR NASAL SPRAY AND ULTRA FINE MIST FOR SINUS RELIEF

(Oxymetazoline Hydrochloride) **2681**
None cited in PDR database.

VICKS VAPOR INHALER

(Levmetamfetamine) **2682**
None cited in PDR database.

VICKS VAPORUB CREAM

(Camphor, Menthol) **2682**
None cited in PDR database.

VICKS VAPORUB OINTMENT

(Camphor, Eucalyptus, Oil of, Menthol).. **2682**
None cited in PDR database.

VICKS VAPOSTEAM

(Camphor) **2682**
None cited in PDR database.

VICODIN TABLETS

(Acetaminophen, Hydrocodone Bitartrate)... **535**
May interact with antihistamines, central nervous system depressants, monoamine oxidase inhibitors, narcotic analgesics, tricyclic antidepressants, and certain other agents. Compounds in these categories include:

Acrivastine (May exhibit an additive CNS depression).
No products indexed under this heading.

Alfentanil Hydrochloride (May exhibit an additive CNS depression).
No products indexed under this heading.

Alprazolam (May exhibit an additive CNS depression). Products include:
Niravam Orally Disintegrating Tablets **3092**

Amitriptyline Hydrochloride (Co-administration may increase the effect of either antidepressant or hydrocodone).
No products indexed under this heading.

Amoxapine (Co-administration may increase the effect of either antidepressant or hydrocodone).
No products indexed under this heading.

Aprobarbital (May exhibit an additive CNS depression).
No products indexed under this heading.

Astemizole (May exhibit an additive CNS depression).
No products indexed under this heading.

Azatadine Maleate (May exhibit an additive CNS depression).
No products indexed under this heading.

Bromodiphenhydramine Hydrochloride (May exhibit an additive CNS depression).
No products indexed under this heading.

Brompheniramine Maleate (May exhibit an additive CNS depression). Products include:
Children's Dimetapp Cold & Allergy Elixir **730**
Children's Dimetapp Cold & Allergy Chewable Tablets............. **730**
Children's Dimetapp DM Cold & Cough Elixir **731**

Buprenorphine Hydrochloride (May exhibit an additive CNS depression). Products include:
Buprenex Injectable **2716**
Suboxone Tablets **2717**
Subutex Tablets **2717**

Buspirone Hydrochloride (May exhibit an additive CNS depression).
No products indexed under this heading.

Butabarbital (May exhibit an additive CNS depression).
No products indexed under this heading.

Butalbital (May exhibit an additive CNS depression).
No products indexed under this heading.

Cetirizine Hydrochloride (May exhibit an additive CNS depression). Products include:
Zyrtec Chewable Tablets **2594**
Zyrtec **2594**
Zyrtec-D 12 Hour Extended Release Tablets.......................... **2597**

Chlordiazepoxide (May exhibit an additive CNS depression).
No products indexed under this heading.

Chlordiazepoxide Hydrochloride (May exhibit an additive CNS depression). Products include:
Librium Capsules **3347**

Chlorpheniramine Maleate (May exhibit an additive CNS depression). Products include:
Advil Allergy Sinus Caplets **770**
Advil Multi-Symptom Cold Caplets.. **770**
BC Allergy Sinus Cold Powder **677**
Comtrex Maximum Strength Cold & Cough Day/Night Caplets - Night Formulation **726**
Comtrex Maximum Strength Day/Night Severe Cold & Sinus Caplets - Night Formulation......... **725**
Contac Cold and Flu Maximum Strength Caplets........................ **728**
Contac Cold and Flu Day and Night Caplets (Night Formulation Only)...................... **727**
Children's Dimetapp Long Acting Cough Plus Cold Syrup............... **731**
Robitussin Cough & Cold Long-Acting Liquid **735**
Robitussin Cough & Allergy Syrup .. **736**
Robitussin Cough & Cold Nighttime Liquid.......................... **736**
Robitussin Cough, Cold & Flu Nighttime Liquid.......................... **738**
Robitussin Pediatric Cough & Cold Long-Acting Liquid.............. **735**
Robitussin Pediatric Cough & Cold Nighttime Liquid.................. **736**
Triaminic Cold & Allergy Liquid **746**
Triaminic Cough & Runny Nose Softchews **748**
Children's Tylenol Plus Flu Oral Suspension................................ **749**
Tylenol Allergy Multi-Symptom Caplets with Cool Burst and Gelcaps.. **1872**
Children's Tylenol Plus Cold Suspension Liquid **1879**
Children's Tylenol Plus Cough & Runny Nose Suspension Liquid..... **1879**
Children's Tylenol Plus Flu Suspension Liquid **1881**
Children's Tylenol Plus Multi-Symptom Cold Suspension Liquid **1879**
Tylenol Cold Head Congestion Nighttime Caplets with Cool Burst.. **1873**
Tylenol Cold Multi-Symptom Nighttime Caplets with Cool Burst.. **1874**
Tylenol Sinus Congestion & Pain Nighttime Caplets with Cool Burst.. **1876**
Vicks 44M Cough, Cold & Flu Relief Liquid................................ **2680**
Pediatric Vicks 44m Cough & Cold Relief Liquid........................ **2676**
Children's Vicks NyQuil Cold/Cough Relief........................ **756**
Children's Vicks NyQuil Cold/Cough Relief Liquid **2680**
Zicam Maximum Strength Flu Daytime.. **768**

Chlorpheniramine Polistirex (May exhibit an additive CNS depression). Products include:
Tussionex Pennkinetic Extended-Release Suspension 3327

Chlorpheniramine Tannate (May exhibit an additive CNS depression).
No products indexed under this heading.

Chlorpromazine (May exhibit an additive CNS depression).
No products indexed under this heading.

Chlorpromazine Hydrochloride (May exhibit an additive CNS depression).
No products indexed under this heading.

Chlorprothixene (May exhibit an additive CNS depression).
No products indexed under this heading.

Chlorprothixene Hydrochloride (May exhibit an additive CNS depression).
No products indexed under this heading.

Chlorprothixene Lactate (May exhibit an additive CNS depression).
No products indexed under this heading.

Clemastine Fumarate (May exhibit an additive CNS depression).
No products indexed under this heading.

Clomipramine Hydrochloride (Co-administration may increase the effect of either antidepressant or hydrocodone).
No products indexed under this heading.

Clorazepate Dipotassium (May exhibit an additive CNS depression). Products include:
Tranxene 2474

Clozapine (May exhibit an additive CNS depression). Products include:
Clozaril Tablets 2184
FazaClo Orally Disintegrating Tablets 551

Codeine Phosphate (May exhibit an additive CNS depression). Products include:
Tylenol with Codeine Tablets 2391

Cyproheptadine Hydrochloride (May exhibit an additive CNS depression).
No products indexed under this heading.

Desflurane (May exhibit an additive CNS depression).
No products indexed under this heading.

Desipramine Hydrochloride (Co-administration may increase the effect of either antidepressant or hydrocodone).
No products indexed under this heading.

Dexchlorpheniramine Maleate (May exhibit an additive CNS depression).
No products indexed under this heading.

Dezocine (May exhibit an additive CNS depression).
No products indexed under this heading.

Diazepam (May exhibit an additive CNS depression). Products include:
Diastat Rectal Delivery System 3343
Valium Tablets 2819

Diphenhydramine Citrate (May exhibit an additive CNS depression). Products include:
Advil PM Caplets .... ■615
Excedrin PM Caplets/Tablets/Geltabs .... ■610
Goody's PM Powder for Pain with Sleeplessness .... ■612

Diphenhydramine Hydrochloride (May exhibit an additive CNS depression). Products include:
Nytol QuickCaps Caplets .... ■615
Nytol QuickGels Softgels Maximum Strength...................... ■616
Simply Sleep Caplets 1868
Sominex Original Formula Tablets .. ■616
TheraFlu Warming Relief Nighttime Severe Cold............... ■743
TheraFlu Thin Strips Multi Symptom.................................... ■744
Triaminic Nighttime Cold & Cough Liquid............................. ■746
Triaminic Thin Strips Cough & Runny Nose .... ■749
Extra Strength Tylenol PM Caplets, Vanilla Caplets, Geltabs, Gelcaps and Liquid......... 1875
Tylenol Sore Throat Nighttime Liquid with Cool Burst................ ■790
Tylenol Allergy Multi-Symptom Nighttime Caplets with Cool Burst.. 1872
Tylenol Severe Allergy Caplets 1872
Children's Tylenol Plus Cold & Allergy Suspension Liquid............ 1878

Diphenylpyraline Hydrochloride (May exhibit an additive CNS depression).
No products indexed under this heading.

Doxepin Hydrochloride (Co-administration may increase the effect of either antidepressant or hydrocodone).
No products indexed under this heading.

Droperidol (May exhibit an additive CNS depression).
No products indexed under this heading.

Enflurane (May exhibit an additive CNS depression).
No products indexed under this heading.

Estazolam (May exhibit an additive CNS depression). Products include:
ProSom Tablets 517

Ethanol (May exhibit an additive CNS depression).
No products indexed under this heading.

Ethchlorvynol (May exhibit an additive CNS depression).
No products indexed under this heading.

Ethinamate (May exhibit an additive CNS depression).
No products indexed under this heading.

Ethyl Alcohol (May exhibit an additive CNS depression).
No products indexed under this heading.

Fentanyl (May exhibit an additive CNS depression). Products include:
Duragesic Transdermal System....... 2373
Ionsys Transdermal System 2379

Fentanyl Citrate (May exhibit an additive CNS depression). Products include:
Actiq 979

Fexofenadine Hydrochloride (May exhibit an additive CNS depression). Products include:
Allegra 2844
Allegra-D 12 Hour Extended-Release Tablets............ 2846
Allegra-D 24 Hour Extended-Release Tablets............ 2849

Fluphenazine Decanoate (May exhibit an additive CNS depression).
No products indexed under this heading.

Fluphenazine Enanthate (May exhibit an additive CNS depression).
No products indexed under this heading.

Fluphenazine Hydrochloride (May exhibit an additive CNS depression).
No products indexed under this heading.

Flurazepam Hydrochloride (May exhibit an additive CNS depression). Products include:
Dalmane Capsules 3342

Glutethimide (May exhibit an additive CNS depression).
No products indexed under this heading.

Haloperidol (May exhibit an additive CNS depression).
No products indexed under this heading.

Haloperidol Decanoate (May exhibit an additive CNS depression).
No products indexed under this heading.

Hydrocodone Polistirex (May exhibit an additive CNS depression). Products include:
Tussionex Pennkinetic Extended-Release Suspension...... 3327

Hydromorphone Hydrochloride (May exhibit an additive CNS depression). Products include:
Dilaudid 440
Dilaudid Non-Sterile Powder 440
Dilaudid Oral Liquid 445
Dilaudid Rectal Suppositories 440
Dilaudid Tablets 440
Dilaudid Tablets - 8 mg 445
Dilaudid-HP 442

Hydroxyzine Hydrochloride (May exhibit an additive CNS depression).
No products indexed under this heading.

Imipramine Hydrochloride (Co-administration may increase the effect of either antidepressant or hydrocodone).
No products indexed under this heading.

Imipramine Pamoate (Co-administration may increase the effect of either antidepressant or hydrocodone).
No products indexed under this heading.

Isocarboxazid (Co-administration may increase the effect of either the MAO inhibitor or hydrocodone).
No products indexed under this heading.

Isoflurane (May exhibit an additive CNS depression).
No products indexed under this heading.

Ketamine Hydrochloride (May exhibit an additive CNS depression).
No products indexed under this heading.

Levomethadyl Acetate Hydrochloride (May exhibit an additive CNS depression).
No products indexed under this heading.

Levorphanol Tartrate (May exhibit an additive CNS depression).
No products indexed under this heading.

Loratadine (May exhibit an additive CNS depression). Products include:
Alavert Allergy & Sinus D-12 Hour Tablets.. ■771
Alavert .... ■771
Children's Claritin Allergy Oral Solution .... ■771
Claritin Non-Drowsy 24 Hour Tablets.. ■772
Claritin Reditabs 24 Hour Non-Drowsy Tablets .... ■772
Claritin-D Non-Drowsy 12 Hour Tablets.. ■772
Claritin-D Non-Drowsy 24 Hour Tablets.. ■772

Lorazepam (May exhibit an additive CNS depression).
No products indexed under this heading.

Loxapine Hydrochloride (May exhibit an additive CNS depression).
No products indexed under this heading.

Loxapine Succinate (May exhibit an additive CNS depression).
No products indexed under this heading.

Maprotiline Hydrochloride (Co-administration may increase the effect of either antidepressant or hydrocodone).
No products indexed under this heading.

Meperidine Hydrochloride (May exhibit an additive CNS depression).
No products indexed under this heading.

Mephobarbital (May exhibit an additive CNS depression).
No products indexed under this heading.

Meprobamate (May exhibit an additive CNS depression).
No products indexed under this heading.

Mesoridazine Besylate (May exhibit an additive CNS depression).
No products indexed under this heading.

Methadone Hydrochloride (May exhibit an additive CNS depression).
No products indexed under this heading.

Methdilazine Hydrochloride (May exhibit an additive CNS depression).
No products indexed under this heading.

Methohexital Sodium (May exhibit an additive CNS depression).
No products indexed under this heading.

Methotrimeprazine (May exhibit an additive CNS depression).
No products indexed under this heading.

Methoxyflurane (May exhibit an additive CNS depression).
No products indexed under this heading.

Midazolam Hydrochloride (May exhibit an additive CNS depression).
No products indexed under this heading.

Moclobemide (Co-administration may increase the effect of either the MAO inhibitor or hydrocodone).
No products indexed under this heading.

Molindone Hydrochloride (May exhibit an additive CNS depression). Products include:
Moban Tablets 1119

Morphine Sulfate (May exhibit an additive CNS depression). Products include:
Avinza Capsules 1741
Kadian Capsules 577
MS Contin Tablets 2701

Nortriptyline Hydrochloride (Co-administration may increase the effect of either antidepressant or hydrocodone).
No products indexed under this heading.

Olanzapine (May exhibit an additive CNS depression). Products include:
Symbyax Capsules 1819
Zyprexa Tablets 1830
Zyprexa IntraMuscular 1830
Zyprexa ZYDIS Orally Disintegrating Tablets 1830

Oxazepam (May exhibit an additive CNS depression).
No products indexed under this heading.

Oxycodone Hydrochloride (May exhibit an additive CNS depression). Products include:
OxyContin Tablets 2703
OxyFast Oral Concentrate Solution 2708
OxyIR Capsules 2708
Percocet Tablets 1131
Percodan Tablets 1132

Pargyline Hydrochloride (Co-administration may increase the effect of either the MAO inhibitor or hydrocodone).
No products indexed under this heading.

Pentobarbital Sodium (May exhibit an additive CNS depression). Products include:
Nembutal Sodium Solution, USP 2470

Perphenazine (May exhibit an additive CNS depression).
No products indexed under this heading.

Phenelzine Sulfate (Co-administration may increase the effect of either the MAO inhibitor or hydrocodone).
No products indexed under this heading.

Phenobarbital (May exhibit an additive CNS depression). Products include:
Donnatal Extentabs 2493

Prazepam (May exhibit an additive CNS depression).
No products indexed under this heading.

Procarbazine Hydrochloride (Co-administration may increase the effect of either the MAO inhibitor or hydrocodone). Products include:
Matulane Capsules 3191

Prochlorperazine (May exhibit an additive CNS depression).
No products indexed under this heading.

Promethazine Hydrochloride (May exhibit an additive CNS depression). Products include:
Phenergan Tablets and Suppositories 3440

Propofol (May exhibit an additive CNS depression).
No products indexed under this heading.

Propoxyphene Hydrochloride (May exhibit an additive CNS depression).
No products indexed under this heading.

Propoxyphene Napsylate (May exhibit an additive CNS depression).
No products indexed under this heading.

Protriptyline Hydrochloride (Co-administration may increase the effect of either antidepressant or hydrocodone).
No products indexed under this heading.

Pyrilamine Maleate (May exhibit an additive CNS depression).
No products indexed under this heading.

Pyrilamine Tannate (May exhibit an additive CNS depression).
No products indexed under this heading.

Quazepam (May exhibit an additive CNS depression).
No products indexed under this heading.

Quetiapine Fumarate (May exhibit an additive CNS depression). Products include:
Seroquel Tablets 690

Remifentanil Hydrochloride (May exhibit an additive CNS depression).
No products indexed under this heading.

Risperidone (May exhibit an additive CNS depression). Products include:
Risperdal 1676
Risperdal Consta Long-Acting Injection 1682
Risperdal M-Tab Orally Disintegrating Tablets 1676

Secobarbital Sodium (May exhibit an additive CNS depression).
No products indexed under this heading.

Selegiline Hydrochloride (Co-administration may increase the effect of either the MAO inhibitor or hydrocodone). Products include:
Eldepryl Capsules 3208
Zelapar Tablets 3372

Sevoflurane (May exhibit an additive CNS depression). Products include:
Ultane Liquid for Inhalation 531

Sufentanil Citrate (May exhibit an additive CNS depression).
No products indexed under this heading.

Temazepam (May exhibit an additive CNS depression). Products include:
Restoril Capsules 1860

Terfenadine (May exhibit an additive CNS depression).
No products indexed under this heading.

Thiamylal Sodium (May exhibit an additive CNS depression).
No products indexed under this heading.

Thioridazine Hydrochloride (May exhibit an additive CNS depression). Products include:
Thioridazine Hydrochloride Tablets 2163

Thiothixene (May exhibit an additive CNS depression). Products include:
Thiothixene Capsules 2165

Tranylcypromine Sulfate (Co-administration may increase the effect of either the MAO inhibitor or hydrocodone). Products include:
Parnate Tablets 1527

Triazolam (May exhibit an additive CNS depression).
No products indexed under this heading.

Trifluoperazine Hydrochloride (May exhibit an additive CNS depression).
No products indexed under this heading.

Trimeprazine Tartrate (May exhibit an additive CNS depression).
No products indexed under this heading.

Trimipramine Maleate (Co-administration may increase the effect of either antidepressant or hydrocodone).
No products indexed under this heading.

Tripelennamine Hydrochloride (May exhibit an additive CNS depression).
No products indexed under this heading.

Triprolidine Hydrochloride (May exhibit an additive CNS depression).
No products indexed under this heading.

Zaleplon (May exhibit an additive CNS depression). Products include:
Sonata Capsules 1717

Ziprasidone Hydrochloride (May exhibit an additive CNS depression). Products include:
Geodon Capsules 2529

Zolpidem Tartrate (May exhibit an additive CNS depression). Products include:
Ambien Tablets 2851
Ambien CR Tablets 2855

Food Interactions

Alcohol (May exhibit an additive CNS depression).

VICODIN ES TABLETS

(Acetaminophen, Hydrocodone Bitartrate) 536
May interact with anticholinergics, central nervous system depressants, narcotic analgesics, psychotropics, tranquilizers, tricyclic antidepressants, and certain other agents. Compounds in these categories include:

Alfentanil Hydrochloride (Additive CNS depression; the dose of one or both agents should be reduced).
No products indexed under this heading.

Alprazolam (Additive CNS depression; the dose of one or both agents should be reduced). Products include:
Niravam Orally Disintegrating Tablets 3092

Amitriptyline Hydrochloride (Concurrent use of tricyclic antidepressants and hydrocodone preparations may increase the effect of either the antidepressant or hydrocodone).
No products indexed under this heading.

Amoxapine (Concurrent use of tricyclic antidepressants and hydrocodone preparations may increase the effect of either the antidepressant or hydrocodone).
No products indexed under this heading.

Aprobarbital (Additive CNS depression; the dose of one or both agents should be reduced).
No products indexed under this heading.

Atropine Sulfate (May produce paralytic ileus). Products include:
Donnatal Extentabs 2493

Belladonna Alkaloids (May produce paralytic ileus). Products include:
Hyland's Teething Tablets 830

Benztropine Mesylate (May produce paralytic ileus).
No products indexed under this heading.

Biperiden Hydrochloride (May produce paralytic ileus).
No products indexed under this heading.

Buprenorphine Hydrochloride (Additive CNS depression; the dose of one or both agents should be reduced). Products include:
Buprenex Injectable 2716
Suboxone Tablets 2717
Subutex Tablets 2717

Buspirone Hydrochloride (Additive CNS depression; the dose of one or both agents should be reduced).
No products indexed under this heading.

Butabarbital (Additive CNS depression; the dose of one or both agents should be reduced).
No products indexed under this heading.

Butalbital (Additive CNS depression; the dose of one or both agents should be reduced).
No products indexed under this heading.

Chlordiazepoxide (Additive CNS depression; the dose of one or both agents should be reduced).
No products indexed under this heading.

Chlordiazepoxide Hydrochloride (Additive CNS depression; the dose of one or both agents should be reduced). Products include:
Librium Capsules 3347

Chlorpromazine (Additive CNS depression; the dose of one or both agents should be reduced).
No products indexed under this heading.

Chlorpromazine Hydrochloride (Additive CNS depression; the dose of one or both agents should be reduced).
No products indexed under this heading.

Chlorprothixene (Additive CNS depression; the dose of one or both agents should be reduced).
No products indexed under this heading.

Chlorprothixene Hydrochloride (Additive CNS depression; the dose of one or both agents should be reduced).
No products indexed under this heading.

Chlorprothixene Lactate (Additive CNS depression; the dose of one or both agents should be reduced).
No products indexed under this heading.

Clidinium Bromide (May produce paralytic ileus).
No products indexed under this heading.

Clomipramine Hydrochloride (Concurrent use of tricyclic antidepressants and hydrocodone preparations may increase the effect of either the antidepressant or hydrocodone).
No products indexed under this heading.

Clorazepate Dipotassium (Additive CNS depression; the dose of one or both agents should be reduced). Products include:
Tranxene 2474

Clozapine (Additive CNS depression; the dose of one or both agents should be reduced). Products include:
Clozaril Tablets 2184
FazaClo Orally Disintegrating Tablets 551

Codeine Phosphate (Additive CNS depression; the dose of one or both agents should be reduced). Products include:

Desflurane (Additive CNS depression; the dose of one or both agents should be reduced).

No products indexed under this heading.

Desipramine Hydrochloride (Concurrent use of tricyclic antidepressants and hydrocodone preparations may increase the effect of either the antidepressant or hydrocodone).

No products indexed under this heading.

Dezocine (Additive CNS depression; the dose of one or both agents should be reduced).

No products indexed under this heading.

Diazepam (Additive CNS depression; the dose of one or both agents should be reduced). Products include:

Dicyclomine Hydrochloride (May produce paralytic ileus). Products include:

Doxepin Hydrochloride (Concurrent use of tricyclic antidepressants and hydrocodone preparations may increase the effect of either the antidepressant or hydrocodone).

No products indexed under this heading.

Droperidol (Additive CNS depression; the dose of one or both agents should be reduced).

No products indexed under this heading.

Enflurane (Additive CNS depression; the dose of one or both agents should be reduced).

No products indexed under this heading.

Estazolam (Additive CNS depression; the dose of one or both agents should be reduced). Products include:

Ethanol (Additive CNS depression; the dose of one or both agents should be reduced).

No products indexed under this heading.

Ethchlorvynol (Additive CNS depression; the dose of one or both agents should be reduced).

No products indexed under this heading.

Ethinamate (Additive CNS depression; the dose of one or both agents should be reduced).

No products indexed under this heading.

Ethyl Alcohol (Additive CNS depression; the dose of one or both agents should be reduced).

No products indexed under this heading.

Fentanyl (Additive CNS depression; the dose of one or both agents should be reduced). Products include:

Fentanyl Citrate (Additive CNS depression; the dose of one or both agents should be reduced). Products include:

Fluphenazine Decanoate (Additive CNS depression; the dose of one or both agents should be reduced).

No products indexed under this heading.

Fluphenazine Enanthate (Additive CNS depression; the dose of one or both agents should be reduced).

No products indexed under this heading.

Fluphenazine Hydrochloride (Additive CNS depression; the dose of one or both agents should be reduced).

No products indexed under this heading.

Flurazepam Hydrochloride (Additive CNS depression; the dose of one or both agents should be reduced). Products include:

Glutethimide (Additive CNS depression; the dose of one or both agents should be reduced).

No products indexed under this heading.

Glycopyrrolate (May produce paralytic ileus).

No products indexed under this heading.

Haloperidol (Additive CNS depression; the dose of one or both agents should be reduced).

No products indexed under this heading.

Haloperidol Decanoate (Additive CNS depression; the dose of one or both agents should be reduced).

No products indexed under this heading.

Hydrocodone Polistirex (Additive CNS depression; the dose of one or both agents should be reduced). Products include:

Hydromorphone Hydrochloride (Additive CNS depression; the dose of one or both agents should be reduced). Products include:

Hydroxyzine Hydrochloride (Additive CNS depression; the dose of one or both agents should be reduced).

No products indexed under this heading.

Hyoscyamine (May produce paralytic ileus).

No products indexed under this heading.

Hyoscyamine Sulfate (May produce paralytic ileus). Products include:

Imipramine Hydrochloride (Concurrent use of tricyclic antidepressants and hydrocodone preparations may increase the effect of either the antidepressant or hydrocodone).

No products indexed under this heading.

Imipramine Pamoate (Concurrent use of tricyclic antidepressants and hydrocodone preparations may increase the effect of either the antidepressant or hydrocodone).

No products indexed under this heading.

Ipratropium Bromide (May produce paralytic ileus). Products include:

Isocarboxazid (Concurrent use of MAO inhibitor and hydrocodone preparations may increase the effect of either the MAO inhibitor or hydrocodone).

No products indexed under this heading.

Isoflurane (Additive CNS depression; the dose of one or both agents should be reduced).

No products indexed under this heading.

Ketamine Hydrochloride (Additive CNS depression; the dose of one or both agents should be reduced).

No products indexed under this heading.

Levomethadyl Acetate Hydrochloride (Additive CNS depression; the dose of one or both agents should be reduced).

No products indexed under this heading.

Levorphanol Tartrate (Additive CNS depression; the dose of one or both agents should be reduced).

No products indexed under this heading.

Lithium Carbonate (Additive CNS depression; the dose of one or both agents should be reduced). Products include:

Lithium Citrate (Additive CNS depression; the dose of one or both agents should be reduced).

No products indexed under this heading.

Lorazepam (Additive CNS depression; the dose of one or both agents should be reduced).

No products indexed under this heading.

Loxapine Hydrochloride (Additive CNS depression; the dose of one or both agents should be reduced).

No products indexed under this heading.

Loxapine Succinate (Additive CNS depression; the dose of one or both agents should be reduced).

No products indexed under this heading.

Maprotiline Hydrochloride (Concurrent use of tricyclic antidepressants and hydrocodone preparations may increase the effect of either the antidepressant or hydrocodone).

No products indexed under this heading.

Mepenzolate Bromide (May produce paralytic ileus).

No products indexed under this heading.

Meperidine Hydrochloride (Additive CNS depression; the dose of one or both agents should be reduced).

No products indexed under this heading.

Mephobarbital (Additive CNS depression; the dose of one or both agents should be reduced).

No products indexed under this heading.

Meprobamate (Additive CNS depression; the dose of one or both agents should be reduced).

No products indexed under this heading.

Mesoridazine Besylate (Additive CNS depression; the dose of one or both agents should be reduced).

No products indexed under this heading.

Methadone Hydrochloride (Additive CNS depression; the dose of one or both agents should be reduced).

No products indexed under this heading.

Methohexital Sodium (Additive CNS depression; the dose of one or both agents should be reduced).

No products indexed under this heading.

Methotrimeprazine (Additive CNS depression; the dose of one or both agents should be reduced).

No products indexed under this heading.

Methoxyflurane (Additive CNS depression; the dose of one or both agents should be reduced).

No products indexed under this heading.

Midazolam Hydrochloride (Additive CNS depression; the dose of one or both agents should be reduced).

No products indexed under this heading.

Molindone Hydrochloride (Additive CNS depression; the dose of one or both agents should be reduced). Products include:

Morphine Sulfate (Additive CNS depression; the dose of one or both agents should be reduced). Products include:

Nortriptyline Hydrochloride (Concurrent use of tricyclic antidepressants and hydrocodone preparations may increase the effect of either the antidepressant or hydrocodone).

No products indexed under this heading.

Olanzapine (Additive CNS depression; the dose of one or both agents should be reduced). Products include:

Oxazepam (Additive CNS depression; the dose of one or both agents should be reduced).

No products indexed under this heading.

Oxybutynin Chloride (May produce paralytic ileus). Products include:

Oxycodone Hydrochloride (Additive CNS depression; the dose of one or both agents should be reduced). Products include:

OxyFast Oral Concentrate Solution 2708
OxyIR Capsules 2708
Percocet Tablets 1131
Percodan Tablets 1132

Pentobarbital Sodium (Additive CNS depression; the dose of one or both agents should be reduced). Products include:
Nembutal Sodium Solution, USP 2470

Perphenazine (Additive CNS depression; the dose of one or both agents should be reduced).
No products indexed under this heading.

Phenelzine Sulfate (Concurrent use of MAO inhibitor and hydrocodone preparations may increase the effect of either the MAO inhibitor or hydrocodone).
No products indexed under this heading.

Phenobarbital (Additive CNS depression; the dose of one or both agents should be reduced). Products include:
Donnatal Extentabs 2493

Prazepam (Additive CNS depression; the dose of one or both agents should be reduced).
No products indexed under this heading.

Prochlorperazine (Additive CNS depression; the dose of one or both agents should be reduced).
No products indexed under this heading.

Procyclidine Hydrochloride (May produce paralytic ileus).
No products indexed under this heading.

Promethazine Hydrochloride (Additive CNS depression; the dose of one or both agents should be reduced). Products include:
Phenergan Tablets and Suppositories 3440

Propantheline Bromide (May produce paralytic ileus).
No products indexed under this heading.

Propofol (Additive CNS depression; the dose of one or both agents should be reduced).
No products indexed under this heading.

Propoxyphene Hydrochloride (Additive CNS depression; the dose of one or both agents should be reduced).
No products indexed under this heading.

Propoxyphene Napsylate (Additive CNS depression; the dose of one or both agents should be reduced).
No products indexed under this heading.

Protriptyline Hydrochloride (Concurrent use of tricyclic antidepressants and hydrocodone preparations may increase the effect of either the antidepressant or hydrocodone).
No products indexed under this heading.

Quazepam (Additive CNS depression; the dose of one or both agents should be reduced).
No products indexed under this heading.

Quetiapine Fumarate (Additive CNS depression; the dose of one or both agents should be reduced). Products include:
Seroquel Tablets 690

Remifentanil Hydrochloride (Additive CNS depression; the dose of one or both agents should be reduced).
No products indexed under this heading.

Risperidone (Additive CNS depression; the dose of one or both agents should be reduced). Products include:
Risperdal 1676
Risperdal Consta Long-Acting Injection 1682
Risperdal M-Tab Orally Disintegrating Tablets 1676

Scopolamine (May produce paralytic ileus). Products include:
Transderm Scōp Transdermal Therapeutic System 2177

Scopolamine Hydrobromide (May produce paralytic ileus). Products include:
Donnatal Extentabs 2493

Secobarbital Sodium (Additive CNS depression; the dose of one or both agents should be reduced).
No products indexed under this heading.

Selegiline Hydrochloride (Concurrent use of MAO inhibitor and hydrocodone preparations may increase the effect of either the MAO inhibitor or hydrocodone). Products include:
Eldepryl Capsules 3208
Zelapar Tablets 3372

Sevoflurane (Additive CNS depression; the dose of one or both agents should be reduced). Products include:
Ultane Liquid for Inhalation 531

Sufentanil Citrate (Additive CNS depression; the dose of one or both agents should be reduced).
No products indexed under this heading.

Temazepam (Additive CNS depression; the dose of one or both agents should be reduced). Products include:
Restoril Capsules 1860

Thiamylal Sodium (Additive CNS depression; the dose of one or both agents should be reduced).
No products indexed under this heading.

Thioridazine Hydrochloride (Additive CNS depression; the dose of one or both agents should be reduced). Products include:
Thioridazine Hydrochloride Tablets 2163

Thiothixene (Additive CNS depression; the dose of one or both agents should be reduced). Products include:
Thiothixene Capsules 2165

Tolterodine Tartrate (May produce paralytic ileus). Products include:
Detrol Tablets 2628
Detrol LA Capsules 2631

Tranylcypromine Sulfate (Concurrent use of MAO inhibitor and hydrocodone preparations may increase the effect of either the MAO inhibitor or hydrocodone). Products include:
Parnate Tablets 1527

Triazolam (Additive CNS depression; the dose of one or both agents should be reduced).
No products indexed under this heading.

Tridihexethyl Chloride (May produce paralytic ileus).
No products indexed under this heading.

Trifluoperazine Hydrochloride (Additive CNS depression; the dose of one or both agents should be reduced).
No products indexed under this heading.

Trihexyphenidyl Hydrochloride (May produce paralytic ileus).
No products indexed under this heading.

Trimipramine Maleate (Concurrent use of tricyclic antidepressants and hydrocodone preparations may increase the effect of either the antidepressant or hydrocodone).
No products indexed under this heading.

Zaleplon (Additive CNS depression; the dose of one or both agents should be reduced). Products include:
Sonata Capsules 1717

Ziprasidone Hydrochloride (Additive CNS depression; the dose of one or both agents should be reduced). Products include:
Geodon Capsules 2529

Zolpidem Tartrate (Additive CNS depression; the dose of one or both agents should be reduced). Products include:
Ambien Tablets 2851
Ambien CR Tablets 2855

Food Interactions

Alcohol (Additive CNS depression).

VICODIN HP TABLETS

(Acetaminophen, Hydrocodone Bitartrate) 538

May interact with antihistamines, central nervous system depressants, monoamine oxidase inhibitors, narcotic analgesics, tranquilizers, tricyclic antidepressants, and certain other agents. Compounds in these categories include:

Acrivastine (Co-administration may result in an additive CNS depression).
No products indexed under this heading.

Alfentanil Hydrochloride (Co-administration may result in an additive CNS depression).
No products indexed under this heading.

Alprazolam (Co-administration may result in an additive CNS depression). Products include:
Niravam Orally Disintegrating Tablets 3092

Amitriptyline Hydrochloride (Co-administration with tricyclic antidepressants may increase the effect of either hydrocodone or the tricyclic antidepressant).
No products indexed under this heading.

Amoxapine (Co-administration with tricyclic antidepressants may increase the effect of either hydrocodone or the tricyclic antidepressant).
No products indexed under this heading.

Aprobarbital (Co-administration may result in an additive CNS depression).
No products indexed under this heading.

Astemizole (Co-administration may result in an additive CNS depression).
No products indexed under this heading.

Azatadine Maleate (Co-administration may result in an additive CNS depression).
No products indexed under this heading.

Bromodiphenhydramine Hydrochloride (Co-administration may result in an additive CNS depression).
No products indexed under this heading.

Brompheniramine Maleate (Co-administration may result in an additive CNS depression). Products include:
Children's Dimetapp Cold & Allergy Elixir 730
Children's Dimetapp Cold & Allergy Chewable Tablets 730
Children's Dimetapp DM Cold & Cough Elixir 731

Buprenorphine Hydrochloride (Co-administration may result in an additive CNS depression). Products include:
Buprenex Injectable 2716
Suboxone Tablets 2717
Subutex Tablets 2717

Buspirone Hydrochloride (Co-administration may result in an additive CNS depression).
No products indexed under this heading.

Butabarbital (Co-administration may result in an additive CNS depression).
No products indexed under this heading.

Butalbital (Co-administration may result in an additive CNS depression).
No products indexed under this heading.

Cetirizine Hydrochloride (Co-administration may result in an additive CNS depression). Products include:
Zyrtec Chewable Tablets 2594
Zyrtec 2594
Zyrtec-D 12 Hour Extended Release Tablets 2597

Chlordiazepoxide (Co-administration may result in an additive CNS depression).
No products indexed under this heading.

Chlordiazepoxide Hydrochloride (Co-administration may result in an additive CNS depression). Products include:
Librium Capsules 3347

Chlorpheniramine Maleate (Co-administration may result in an additive CNS depression). Products include:
Advil Allergy Sinus Caplets 770
Advil Multi-Symptom Cold Caplets 770
BC Allergy Sinus Cold Powder 677
Comtrex Maximum Strength Cold & Cough Day/Night Caplets - Night Formulation 726
Comtrex Maximum Strength Day/Night Severe Cold & Sinus Caplets - Night Formulation 725
Contac Cold and Flu Maximum Strength Caplets 728
Contac Cold and Flu Day and Night Caplets (Night Formulation Only) 727
Children's Dimetapp Long Acting Cough Plus Cold Syrup 731
Robitussin Cough & Cold Long-Acting Liquid 735
Robitussin Cough & Allergy Syrup 736
Robitussin Cough & Cold Nighttime Liquid 736
Robitussin Cough, Cold & Flu Nighttime Liquid 738

Chlorpheniramine Polistirex (Co-administration may result in an additive CNS depression). Products include:
 Tussionex Pennkinetic
 Extended-Release Suspension...... 3327

Chlorpheniramine Tannate (Co-administration may result in an additive CNS depression).
 No products indexed under this heading.

Chlorpromazine (Co-administration may result in an additive CNS depression).
 No products indexed under this heading.

Chlorpromazine Hydrochloride (Co-administration may result in an additive CNS depression).
 No products indexed under this heading.

Chlorprothixene (Co-administration may result in an additive CNS depression).
 No products indexed under this heading.

Chlorprothixene Hydrochloride (Co-administration may result in an additive CNS depression).
 No products indexed under this heading.

Chlorprothixene Lactate (Co-administration may result in an additive CNS depression).
 No products indexed under this heading.

Clemastine Fumarate (Co-administration may result in an additive CNS depression).
 No products indexed under this heading.

Clomipramine Hydrochloride (Co-administration with tricyclic antidepressants may increase the effect of either hydrocodone or the tricyclic antidepressant).
 No products indexed under this heading.

Clorazepate Dipotassium (Co-administration may result in an additive CNS depression). Products include:
 Tranxene 2474

Clozapine (Co-administration may result in an additive CNS depression). Products include:
 Clozaril Tablets 2184
 FazaClo Orally Disintegrating
 Tablets 551

Codeine Phosphate (Co-administration may result in an additive CNS depression). Products include:
 Tylenol with Codeine Tablets 2391

Cyproheptadine Hydrochloride (Co-administration may result in an additive CNS depression).
 No products indexed under this heading.

Desflurane (Co-administration may result in an additive CNS depression).
 No products indexed under this heading.

Desipramine Hydrochloride (Co-administration with tricyclic antidepressants may increase the effect of either hydrocodone or the tricyclic antidepressant).
 No products indexed under this heading.

Dexchlorpheniramine Maleate (Co-administration may result in an additive CNS depression).
 No products indexed under this heading.

Dezocine (Co-administration may result in an additive CNS depression).
 No products indexed under this heading.

Diazepam (Co-administration may result in an additive CNS depression). Products include:
 Diastat Rectal Delivery System 3343
 Valium Tablets 2819

Diphenhydramine Citrate (Co-administration may result in an additive CNS depression). Products include:
 Advil PM Caplets ▣615
 Excedrin PM
 Caplets/Tablets/Geltabs............. ▣610
 Goody's PM Powder for Pain with
 Sleeplessness ▣612

Diphenhydramine Hydrochloride (Co-administration may result in an additive CNS depression). Products include:
 Nytol QuickCaps Caplets ▣615
 Nytol QuickGels Softgels
 Maximum Strength.................... ▣616
 Simply Sleep Caplets 1868
 Sominex Original Formula Tablets .. ▣616
 TheraFlu Warming Relief
 Nighttime Severe Cold............... ▣743
 TheraFlu Thin Strips Multi
 Symptom................................. ▣744
 Triaminic Nighttime Cold &
 Cough Liquid............................. ▣746
 Triaminic Thin Strips Cough &
 Runny Nose ▣749
 Extra Strength Tylenol PM
 Caplets, Vanilla Caplets,
 Geltabs, Gelcaps and Liquid........ 1875
 Tylenol Sore Throat Nighttime
 Liquid with Cool Burst ▣790
 Tylenol Allergy Multi-Symptom
 Nighttime Caplets with Cool
 Burst.. 1872
 Tylenol Severe Allergy Caplets 1872
 Children's Tylenol Plus Cold &
 Allergy Suspension Liquid 1878

Diphenylpyraline Hydrochloride (Co-administration may result in an additive CNS depression).
 No products indexed under this heading.

Doxepin Hydrochloride (Co-administration with tricyclic antidepressants may increase the effect of either hydrocodone or the tricyclic antidepressant).
 No products indexed under this heading.

Droperidol (Co-administration may result in an additive CNS depression).
 No products indexed under this heading.

Enflurane (Co-administration may result in an additive CNS depression).
 No products indexed under this heading.

Estazolam (Co-administration may result in an additive CNS depression). Products include:
 ProSom Tablets 517

Ethanol (Co-administration may result in an additive CNS depression).
 No products indexed under this heading.

Ethchlorvynol (Co-administration may result in an additive CNS depression).
 No products indexed under this heading.

Ethinamate (Co-administration may result in an additive CNS depression).
 No products indexed under this heading.

Ethyl Alcohol (Co-administration may result in an additive CNS depression).
 No products indexed under this heading.

Fentanyl (Co-administration may result in an additive CNS depression). Products include:
 Duragesic Transdermal System 2373
 Ionsys Transdermal System 2379

Fentanyl Citrate (Co-administration may result in an additive CNS depression). Products include:
 Actiq ... 979

Fexofenadine Hydrochloride (Co-administration may result in an additive CNS depression). Products include:
 Allegra ... 2844
 Allegra-D 12 Hour
 Extended-Release Tablets............. 2846
 Allegra-D 24 Hour
 Extended-Release Tablets............. 2849

Fluphenazine Decanoate (Co-administration may result in an additive CNS depression).
 No products indexed under this heading.

Fluphenazine Enanthate (Co-administration may result in an additive CNS depression).
 No products indexed under this heading.

Fluphenazine Hydrochloride (Co-administration may result in an additive CNS depression).
 No products indexed under this heading.

Flurazepam Hydrochloride (Co-administration may result in an additive CNS depression). Products include:
 Dalmane Capsules 3342

Glutethimide (Co-administration may result in an additive CNS depression).
 No products indexed under this heading.

Haloperidol (Co-administration may result in an additive CNS depression).
 No products indexed under this heading.

Haloperidol Decanoate (Co-administration may result in an additive CNS depression).
 No products indexed under this heading.

Hydrocodone Polistirex (Co-administration may result in an additive CNS depression). Products include:
 Tussionex Pennkinetic
 Extended-Release Suspension...... 3327

Hydromorphone Hydrochloride (Co-administration may result in an additive CNS depression). Products include:
 Dilaudid 440
 Dilaudid Non-Sterile Powder 440
 Dilaudid Oral Liquid 445
 Dilaudid Rectal Suppositories 440
 Dilaudid Tablets 440
 Dilaudid Tablets - 8 mg 445
 Dilaudid-HP 442

Hydroxyzine Hydrochloride (Co-administration may result in an additive CNS depression).
 No products indexed under this heading.

Imipramine Hydrochloride (Co-administration with tricyclic antidepressants may increase the effect of either hydrocodone or the tricyclic antidepressant).
 No products indexed under this heading.

Imipramine Pamoate (Co-administration with tricyclic antidepressants may increase the effect of either hydrocodone or the tricyclic antidepressant).
 No products indexed under this heading.

Isocarboxazid (Co-administration with an MAO inhibitor may increase the effect of either hydrocodone or the MAO inhibitor).
 No products indexed under this heading.

Isoflurane (Co-administration may result in an additive CNS depression).
 No products indexed under this heading.

Ketamine Hydrochloride (Co-administration may result in an additive CNS depression).
 No products indexed under this heading.

Levomethadyl Acetate Hydrochloride (Co-administration may result in an additive CNS depression).
 No products indexed under this heading.

Levorphanol Tartrate (Co-administration may result in an additive CNS depression).
 No products indexed under this heading.

Loratadine (Co-administration may result in an additive CNS depression). Products include:
 Alavert Allergy & Sinus D-12 Hour
 Tablets....................................... ▣771
 Alavert ... ▣771
 Children's Claritin Allergy Oral
 Solution..................................... ▣771

Claritin Non-Drowsy 24 Hour Tablets....................................... 772
Claritin Reditabs 24 Hour Non-Drowsy Tablets.................... 772
Claritin-D Non-Drowsy 12 Hour Tablets....................................... 772
Claritin-D Non-Drowsy 24 Hour Tablets....................................... 772

Lorazepam (Co-administration may result in an additive CNS depression).
No products indexed under this heading.

Loxapine Hydrochloride (Co-administration may result in an additive CNS depression).
No products indexed under this heading.

Loxapine Succinate (Co-administration may result in an additive CNS depression).
No products indexed under this heading.

Maprotiline Hydrochloride (Co-administration with tricyclic antidepressants may increase the effect of either hydrocodone or the tricyclic antidepressant).
No products indexed under this heading.

Meperidine Hydrochloride (Co-administration may result in an additive CNS depression).
No products indexed under this heading.

Mephobarbital (Co-administration may result in an additive CNS depression).
No products indexed under this heading.

Meprobamate (Co-administration may result in an additive CNS depression).
No products indexed under this heading.

Mesoridazine Besylate (Co-administration may result in an additive CNS depression).
No products indexed under this heading.

Methadone Hydrochloride (Co-administration may result in an additive CNS depression).
No products indexed under this heading.

Methdilazine Hydrochloride (Co-administration may result in an additive CNS depression).
No products indexed under this heading.

Methohexital Sodium (Co-administration may result in an additive CNS depression).
No products indexed under this heading.

Methotrimeprazine (Co-administration may result in an additive CNS depression).
No products indexed under this heading.

Methoxyflurane (Co-administration may result in an additive CNS depression).
No products indexed under this heading.

Midazolam Hydrochloride (Co-administration may result in an additive CNS depression).
No products indexed under this heading.

Moclobemide (Co-administration with an MAO inhibitor may increase the effect of either hydrocodone or the MAO inhibitor).
No products indexed under this heading.

Molindone Hydrochloride (Co-administration may result in an additive CNS depression). Products include:
Moban Tablets 1119

Morphine Sulfate (Co-administration may result in an additive CNS depression). Products include:
Avinza Capsules 1741
Kadian Capsules 577
MS Contin Tablets 2701

Nortriptyline Hydrochloride (Co-administration with tricyclic antidepressants may increase the effect of either hydrocodone or the tricyclic antidepressant).
No products indexed under this heading.

Olanzapine (Co-administration may result in an additive CNS depression). Products include:
Symbyax Capsules 1819
Zyprexa Tablets 1830
Zyprexa IntraMuscular 1830
Zyprexa ZYDIS Orally Disintegrating Tablets.................. 1830

Oxazepam (Co-administration may result in an additive CNS depression).
No products indexed under this heading.

Oxycodone Hydrochloride (Co-administration may result in an additive CNS depression). Products include:
OxyContin Tablets 2703
OxyFast Oral Concentrate Solution....................................... 2708
OxyIR Capsules 2708
Percocet Tablets 1131
Percodan Tablets 1132

Pargyline Hydrochloride (Co-administration with an MAO inhibitor may increase the effect of either hydrocodone or the MAO inhibitor).
No products indexed under this heading.

Pentobarbital Sodium (Co-administration may result in an additive CNS depression). Products include:
Nembutal Sodium Solution, USP...... 2470

Perphenazine (Co-administration may result in an additive CNS depression).
No products indexed under this heading.

Phenelzine Sulfate (Co-administration with an MAO inhibitor may increase the effect of either hydrocodone or the MAO inhibitor).
No products indexed under this heading.

Phenobarbital (Co-administration may result in an additive CNS depression). Products include:
Donnatal Extentabs 2493

Prazepam (Co-administration may result in an additive CNS depression).
No products indexed under this heading.

Procarbazine Hydrochloride (Co-administration with an MAO inhibitor may increase the effect of either hydrocodone or the MAO inhibitor). Products include:
Matulane Capsules 3191

Prochlorperazine (Co-administration may result in an additive CNS depression).
No products indexed under this heading.

Promethazine Hydrochloride (Co-administration may result in an additive CNS depression). Products include:
Phenergan Tablets and Suppositories 3440

Propofol (Co-administration may result in an additive CNS depression).
No products indexed under this heading.

Propoxyphene Hydrochloride (Co-administration may result in an additive CNS depression).
No products indexed under this heading.

Propoxyphene Napsylate (Co-administration may result in an additive CNS depression).
No products indexed under this heading.

Protriptyline Hydrochloride (Co-administration with tricyclic antidepressants may increase the effect of either hydrocodone or the tricyclic antidepressant).
No products indexed under this heading.

Pyrilamine Maleate (Co-administration may result in an additive CNS depression).
No products indexed under this heading.

Pyrilamine Tannate (Co-administration may result in an additive CNS depression).
No products indexed under this heading.

Quazepam (Co-administration may result in an additive CNS depression).
No products indexed under this heading.

Quetiapine Fumarate (Co-administration may result in an additive CNS depression). Products include:
Seroquel Tablets 690

Remifentanil Hydrochloride (Co-administration may result in an additive CNS depression).
No products indexed under this heading.

Risperidone (Co-administration may result in an additive CNS depression). Products include:
Risperdal 1676
Risperdal Consta Long-Acting Injection 1682
Risperdal M-Tab Orally Disintegrating Tablets.................. 1676

Secobarbital Sodium (Co-administration may result in an additive CNS depression).
No products indexed under this heading.

Selegiline Hydrochloride (Co-administration with an MAO inhibitor may increase the effect of either hydrocodone or the MAO inhibitor). Products include:
Eldepryl Capsules 3208
Zelapar Tablets 3372

Sevoflurane (Co-administration may result in an additive CNS depression). Products include:
Ultane Liquid for Inhalation 531

Sufentanil Citrate (Co-administration may result in an additive CNS depression).
No products indexed under this heading.

Temazepam (Co-administration may result in an additive CNS depression). Products include:
Restoril Capsules 1860

Terfenadine (Co-administration may result in an additive CNS depression).
No products indexed under this heading.

Thiamylal Sodium (Co-administration may result in an additive CNS depression).
No products indexed under this heading.

Thioridazine Hydrochloride (Co-administration may result in an additive CNS depression). Products include:
Thioridazine Hydrochloride Tablets 2163

Thiothixene (Co-administration may result in an additive CNS depression). Products include:
Thiothixene Capsules 2165

Tranylcypromine Sulfate (Co-administration with an MAO inhibitor may increase the effect of either hydrocodone or the MAO inhibitor). Products include:
Parnate Tablets 1527

Triazolam (Co-administration may result in an additive CNS depression).
No products indexed under this heading.

Trifluoperazine Hydrochloride (Co-administration may result in an additive CNS depression).
No products indexed under this heading.

Trimeprazine Tartrate (Co-administration may result in an additive CNS depression).
No products indexed under this heading.

Trimipramine Maleate (Co-administration with tricyclic antidepressants may increase the effect of either hydrocodone or the tricyclic antidepressant).
No products indexed under this heading.

Tripelennamine Hydrochloride (Co-administration may result in an additive CNS depression).
No products indexed under this heading.

Triprolidine Hydrochloride (Co-administration may result in an additive CNS depression).
No products indexed under this heading.

Zaleplon (Co-administration may result in an additive CNS depression). Products include:
Sonata Capsules 1717

Ziprasidone Hydrochloride (Co-administration may result in an additive CNS depression). Products include:
Geodon Capsules 2529

Zolpidem Tartrate (Co-administration may result in an additive CNS depression). Products include:
Ambien Tablets 2851
Ambien CR Tablets 2855

Food Interactions

Alcohol (Concurrent use results in an additive CNS depression).

VICOPROFEN TABLETS
(Hydrocodone Bitartrate, Ibuprofen) 539
May interact with ACE inhibitors, anticholinergics, central nervous system depressants, lithium preparations, monoamine oxidase inhibitors, thiazides, tricyclic antidepressants, and certain other agents. Compounds in these categories include:

Alfentanil Hydrochloride (May exhibit additive CNS depression).
No products indexed under this heading.

Alprazolam (May exhibit additive CNS depression). Products include:
Niravam Orally Disintegrating Tablets 3092

Amitriptyline Hydrochloride (Co-administration of tricyclic antidepressants with hydrocodone preparations may increase the effect of either the antidepressant or hydrocodone).
No products indexed under this heading.

Amoxapine (Co-administration of tricyclic antidepressants with hydrocodone preparations may increase the effect of either the antidepressant or hydrocodone).
No products indexed under this heading.

Aprobarbital (May exhibit additive CNS depression).
No products indexed under this heading.

Aspirin (Co-administration of Vicoprofen and aspirin may increase the risk of adverse effects; concurrent use should be avoided). Products include:
Aggrenox Capsules 822
Bayer Aspirin 744
BC Allergy Sinus Cold Powder .... ■677
BC Headache Powder .... ■677
Arthritis Strength BC Powder .... ■677
BC Sinus Cold Powder .... ■677
Excedrin Extra Strength Caplets/Tablets/Geltabs .... ■684
Excedrin Migraine Caplets/Tablets/Geltabs .... ■609
Goody's Body Pain Formula Powder .... ■684
Goody's Extra Strength Headache Powders .... ■611
Goody's Extra Strength Pain Relief Tablets .... ■685
Percodan Tablets 1132
St. Joseph 81 mg Aspirin Chewable and Enteric Coated Tablets 1869

Aspirin, Enteric Coated (Co-administration of Vicoprofen and aspirin may increase the risk of adverse effects; concurrent use should be avoided).
No products indexed under this heading.

Aspirin Buffered (Co-administration of Vicoprofen and aspirin may increase the risk of adverse effects; concurrent use should be avoided). Products include:
Bufferin Extra Strength Tablets .... ■678
Bufferin Regular Strength Tablets .... ■678

Atropine Sulfate (Concurrent use of anticholinergics with hydrocodone preparations may produce paralytic ileus). Products include:
Donnatal Extentabs 2493

Belladonna Alkaloids (Concurrent use of anticholinergics with hydrocodone preparations may produce paralytic ileus). Products include:
Hyland's Teething Tablets .... ■830

Benazepril Hydrochloride (NSAIDs may diminish the antihypertensive effect of ACE inhibitors). Products include:
Lotensin Tablets 2243
Lotensin HCT Tablets 2246
Lotrel Capsules 2249

Bendroflumethiazide (Ibuprofen has been shown to reduce the natriuretic effect of thiazides in some patients).
No products indexed under this heading.

Benztropine Mesylate (Concurrent use of anticholinergics with hydrocodone preparations may produce paralytic ileus).
No products indexed under this heading.

Biperiden Hydrochloride (Concurrent use of anticholinergics with hydrocodone preparations may produce paralytic ileus).
No products indexed under this heading.

Buprenorphine Hydrochloride (May exhibit additive CNS depression). Products include:
Buprenex Injectable 2716
Suboxone Tablets 2717
Subutex Tablets 2717

Buspirone Hydrochloride (May exhibit additive CNS depression).
No products indexed under this heading.

Butabarbital (May exhibit additive CNS depression).
No products indexed under this heading.

Butalbital (May exhibit additive CNS depression).
No products indexed under this heading.

Captopril (NSAIDs may diminish the antihypertensive effect of ACE inhibitors). Products include:
Captopril Tablets 2149

Chlordiazepoxide (May exhibit additive CNS depression).
No products indexed under this heading.

Chlordiazepoxide Hydrochloride (May exhibit additive CNS depression). Products include:
Librium Capsules 3347

Chlorothiazide (Ibuprofen has been shown to reduce the natriuretic effect of thiazides in some patients). Products include:
Diuril Oral Suspension 1954

Chlorothiazide Sodium (Ibuprofen has been shown to reduce the natriuretic effect of thiazides in some patients). Products include:
Diuril Sodium Intravenous 2467

Chlorpromazine (May exhibit additive CNS depression).
No products indexed under this heading.

Chlorpromazine Hydrochloride (May exhibit additive CNS depression).
No products indexed under this heading.

Chlorprothixene (May exhibit additive CNS depression).
No products indexed under this heading.

Chlorprothixene Hydrochloride (May exhibit additive CNS depression).
No products indexed under this heading.

Chlorprothixene Lactate (May exhibit additive CNS depression).
No products indexed under this heading.

Clidinium Bromide (Concurrent use of anticholinergics with hydrocodone preparations may produce paralytic ileus).
No products indexed under this heading.

Clomipramine Hydrochloride (Co-administration of tricyclic antidepressants with hydrocodone preparations may increase the effect of either the antidepressant or hydrocodone).
No products indexed under this heading.

Clorazepate Dipotassium (May exhibit additive CNS depression). Products include:
Tranxene 2474

Clozapine (May exhibit additive CNS depression). Products include:
Clozaril Tablets 2184
FazaClo Orally Disintegrating Tablets 551

Codeine Phosphate (May exhibit additive CNS depression). Products include:
Tylenol with Codeine Tablets 2391

Desflurane (May exhibit additive CNS depression).
No products indexed under this heading.

Desipramine Hydrochloride (Co-administration of tricyclic antidepressants with hydrocodone preparations may increase the effect of either the antidepressant or hydrocodone).
No products indexed under this heading.

Dezocine (May exhibit additive CNS depression).
No products indexed under this heading.

Diazepam (May exhibit additive CNS depression). Products include:
Diastat Rectal Delivery System 3343
Valium Tablets 2819

Dicyclomine Hydrochloride (Concurrent use of anticholinergics with hydrocodone preparations may produce paralytic ileus). Products include:
Bentyl Capsules 697
Bentyl Injection 697
Bentyl Syrup 697
Bentyl Tablets 697

Doxepin Hydrochloride (Co-administration of tricyclic antidepressants with hydrocodone preparations may increase the effect of either the antidepressant or hydrocodone).
No products indexed under this heading.

Droperidol (May exhibit additive CNS depression).
No products indexed under this heading.

Enalapril Maleate (NSAIDs may diminish the antihypertensive effect of ACE inhibitors). Products include:
Vasotec I.V. Injection 2103

Enalaprilat (NSAIDs may diminish the antihypertensive effect of ACE inhibitors).
No products indexed under this heading.

Enflurane (May exhibit additive CNS depression).
No products indexed under this heading.

Estazolam (May exhibit additive CNS depression). Products include:
ProSom Tablets 517

Ethanol (May exhibit additive CNS depression).
No products indexed under this heading.

Ethchlorvynol (May exhibit additive CNS depression).
No products indexed under this heading.

Ethinamate (May exhibit additive CNS depression).
No products indexed under this heading.

Ethyl Alcohol (May exhibit additive CNS depression).
No products indexed under this heading.

Fentanyl (May exhibit additive CNS depression). Products include:
Duragesic Transdermal System 2373
Ionsys Transdermal System 2379

Fentanyl Citrate (May exhibit additive CNS depression). Products include:
Actiq 979

Fluphenazine Decanoate (May exhibit additive CNS depression).
No products indexed under this heading.

Fluphenazine Enanthate (May exhibit additive CNS depression).
No products indexed under this heading.

Fluphenazine Hydrochloride (May exhibit additive CNS depression).
No products indexed under this heading.

Flurazepam Hydrochloride (May exhibit additive CNS depression). Products include:
Dalmane Capsules 3342

Fosinopril Sodium (NSAIDs may diminish the antihypertensive effect of ACE inhibitors).
No products indexed under this heading.

Furosemide (Ibuprofen has been shown to reduce the natriuretic effect of furosemide). Products include:
Furosemide Tablets 2154

Glutethimide (May exhibit additive CNS depression).
No products indexed under this heading.

Glycopyrrolate (Concurrent use of anticholinergics with hydrocodone preparations may produce paralytic ileus).
No products indexed under this heading.

Haloperidol (May exhibit additive CNS depression).
No products indexed under this heading.

Haloperidol Decanoate (May exhibit additive CNS depression).
No products indexed under this heading.

Hydrochlorothiazide (Ibuprofen has been shown to reduce the natriuretic effect of thiazides in some patients). Products include:
Aldoril Tablets 1910
Atacand HCT 651
Avalide Tablets 888
Avalide Tablets 2874
Benicar HCT Tablets 1044
Diovan HCT Tablets 2196
Dyazide Capsules 1423
Hyzaar 50-12.5 Tablets 1990
Hyzaar 100-12.5 Tablets 1990
Hyzaar 100-25 Tablets 1990
Lopressor HCT 50/25 Tablets 2241

Hydrocodone Polistirex (May exhibit additive CNS depression). Products include:

Hydroflumethiazide (Ibuprofen has been shown to reduce the natriuretic effect of thiazides in some patients).

No products indexed under this heading.

Hydromorphone Hydrochloride (May exhibit additive CNS depression). Products include:

Hydroxyzine Hydrochloride (May exhibit additive CNS depression).

No products indexed under this heading.

Hyoscyamine (Concurrent use of anticholinergics with hydrocodone preparations may produce paralytic ileus).

No products indexed under this heading.

Hyoscyamine Sulfate (Concurrent use of anticholinergics with hydrocodone preparations may produce paralytic ileus). Products include:

Imipramine Hydrochloride (Co-administration of tricyclic antidepressants with hydrocodone preparations may increase the effect of either the antidepressant or hydrocodone).

No products indexed under this heading.

Imipramine Pamoate (Co-administration of tricyclic antidepressants with hydrocodone preparations may increase the effect of either the antidepressant or hydrocodone).

No products indexed under this heading.

Ipratropium Bromide (Concurrent use of anticholinergics with hydrocodone preparations may produce paralytic ileus). Products include:

Isocarboxazid (Co-administration of MAO inhibitors with hydrocodone preparations may increase the effect of either the MAO inhibitors or hydrocodone).

No products indexed under this heading.

Isoflurane (May exhibit additive CNS depression).

No products indexed under this heading.

Ketamine Hydrochloride (May exhibit additive CNS depression).

No products indexed under this heading.

Levomethadyl Acetate Hydrochloride (May exhibit additive CNS depression).

No products indexed under this heading.

Levorphanol Tartrate (May exhibit additive CNS depression).

No products indexed under this heading.

Lisinopril (NSAIDs may diminish the antihypertensive effect of ACE inhibitors). Products include:

Lithium (Ibuprofen has been shown to elevate plasma lithium concentration and reduce renal clearance).

No products indexed under this heading.

Lithium Carbonate (Ibuprofen has been shown to elevate plasma lithium concentration and reduce renal clearance). Products include:

Lithium Citrate (Ibuprofen has been shown to elevate plasma lithium concentration and reduce renal clearance).

No products indexed under this heading.

Lorazepam (May exhibit additive CNS depression).

No products indexed under this heading.

Loxapine Hydrochloride (May exhibit additive CNS depression).

No products indexed under this heading.

Loxapine Succinate (May exhibit additive CNS depression).

No products indexed under this heading.

Maprotiline Hydrochloride (Co-administration of tricyclic antidepressants with hydrocodone preparations may increase the effect of either the antidepressant or hydrocodone).

No products indexed under this heading.

Mepenzolate Bromide (Concurrent use of anticholinergics with hydrocodone preparations may produce paralytic ileus).

No products indexed under this heading.

Meperidine Hydrochloride (May exhibit additive CNS depression).

No products indexed under this heading.

Mephobarbital (May exhibit additive CNS depression).

No products indexed under this heading.

Meprobamate (May exhibit additive CNS depression).

No products indexed under this heading.

Mesoridazine Besylate (May exhibit additive CNS depression).

No products indexed under this heading.

Methadone Hydrochloride (May exhibit additive CNS depression).

No products indexed under this heading.

Methohexital Sodium (May exhibit additive CNS depression).

No products indexed under this heading.

Methotrexate Sodium (Ibuprofen, in animal studies, has been reported to competitively inhibit methotrexate accumulation; this could lead to enhanced toxicity of methotrexate).

No products indexed under this heading.

Methotrimeprazine (May exhibit additive CNS depression).

No products indexed under this heading.

Methoxyflurane (May exhibit additive CNS depression).

No products indexed under this heading.

Methyclothiazide (Ibuprofen has been shown to reduce the natriuretic effect of thiazides in some patients).

No products indexed under this heading.

Midazolam Hydrochloride (May exhibit additive CNS depression).

No products indexed under this heading.

Moclobemide (Co-administration of MAO inhibitors with hydrocodone preparations may increase the effect of either the MAO inhibitors or hydrocodone).

No products indexed under this heading.

Moexipril Hydrochloride (NSAIDs may diminish the antihypertensive effect of ACE inhibitors). Products include:

Molindone Hydrochloride (May exhibit additive CNS depression). Products include:

Morphine Sulfate (May exhibit additive CNS depression). Products include:

Nortriptyline Hydrochloride (Co-administration of tricyclic antidepressants with hydrocodone preparations may increase the effect of either the antidepressant or hydrocodone).

No products indexed under this heading.

Olanzapine (May exhibit additive CNS depression). Products include:

Oxazepam (May exhibit additive CNS depression).

No products indexed under this heading.

Oxybutynin Chloride (Concurrent use of anticholinergics with hydrocodone preparations may produce paralytic ileus). Products include:

Oxycodone Hydrochloride (May exhibit additive CNS depression). Products include:

Pargyline Hydrochloride (Co-administration of MAO inhibitors with hydrocodone preparations may increase the effect of either the MAO inhibitors or hydrocodone).

No products indexed under this heading.

Pentobarbital Sodium (May exhibit additive CNS depression). Products include:

Perindopril Erbumine (NSAIDs may diminish the antihypertensive effect of ACE inhibitors). Products include:

Perphenazine (May exhibit additive CNS depression).

No products indexed under this heading.

Phenelzine Sulfate (Co-administration of MAO inhibitors with hydrocodone preparations may increase the effect of either the MAO inhibitors or hydrocodone).

No products indexed under this heading.

Phenobarbital (May exhibit additive CNS depression). Products include:

Polythiazide (Ibuprofen has been shown to reduce the natriuretic effect of thiazides in some patients).

No products indexed under this heading.

Prazepam (May exhibit additive CNS depression).

No products indexed under this heading.

Procarbazine Hydrochloride (Co-administration of MAO inhibitors with hydrocodone preparations may increase the effect of either the MAO inhibitors or hydrocodone). Products include:

Prochlorperazine (May exhibit additive CNS depression).

No products indexed under this heading.

Procyclidine Hydrochloride (Concurrent use of anticholinergics with hydrocodone preparations may produce paralytic ileus).

No products indexed under this heading.

Promethazine Hydrochloride (May exhibit additive CNS depression). Products include:

Propantheline Bromide (Concurrent use of anticholinergics with hydrocodone preparations may produce paralytic ileus).

No products indexed under this heading.

Propofol (May exhibit additive CNS depression).

No products indexed under this heading.

Propoxyphene Hydrochloride (May exhibit additive CNS depression).

No products indexed under this heading.

Propoxyphene Napsylate (May exhibit additive CNS depression).

No products indexed under this heading.

Protriptyline Hydrochloride (Co-administration of tricyclic antidepressants with hydrocodone preparations may increase the effect of either the antidepressant or hydrocodone).

No products indexed under this heading.

Quazepam (May exhibit additive CNS depression).

No products indexed under this heading.

Quetiapine Fumarate (May exhibit additive CNS depression). Products include:

Quinapril Hydrochloride (NSAIDs may diminish the antihypertensive effect of ACE inhibitors).
No products indexed under this heading.

Ramipril (NSAIDs may diminish the antihypertensive effect of ACE inhibitors). Products include:
Altace Capsules 1702

Remifentanil Hydrochloride (May exhibit additive CNS depression).
No products indexed under this heading.

Risperidone (May exhibit additive CNS depression). Products include:
Risperdal 1676
Risperdal Consta Long-Acting Injection 1682
Risperdal M-Tab Orally Disintegrating Tablets.................. 1676

Scopolamine (Concurrent use of anticholinergics with hydrocodone preparations may produce paralytic ileus). Products include:
Transderm Scōp Transdermal Therapeutic System 2177

Scopolamine Hydrobromide (Concurrent use of anticholinergics with hydrocodone preparations may produce paralytic ileus). Products include:
Donnatal Extentabs 2493

Secobarbital Sodium (May exhibit additive CNS depression).
No products indexed under this heading.

Selegiline Hydrochloride (Co-administration of MAO inhibitors with hydrocodone preparations may increase the effect of either the MAO inhibitors or hydrocodone). Products include:
Eldepryl Capsules 3208
Zelapar Tablets 3372

Sevoflurane (May exhibit additive CNS depression). Products include:
Ultane Liquid for Inhalation 531

Spirapril Hydrochloride (NSAIDs may diminish the antihypertensive effect of ACE inhibitors).
No products indexed under this heading.

Sufentanil Citrate (May exhibit additive CNS depression).
No products indexed under this heading.

Temazepam (May exhibit additive CNS depression). Products include:
Restoril Capsules 1860

Thiamylal Sodium (May exhibit additive CNS depression).
No products indexed under this heading.

Thioridazine Hydrochloride (May exhibit additive CNS depression). Products include:
Thioridazine Hydrochloride Tablets.. 2163

Thiothixene (May exhibit additive CNS depression). Products include:
Thiothixene Capsules 2165

Tolterodine Tartrate (Concurrent use of anticholinergics with hydrocodone preparations may produce paralytic ileus). Products include:
Detrol Tablets 2628
Detrol LA Capsules 2631

Trandolapril (NSAIDs may diminish the antihypertensive effect of ACE inhibitors). Products include:
Mavik Tablets 486
Tarka Tablets 524

Tranylcypromine Sulfate (Co-administration of MAO inhibitors with hydrocodone preparations may increase the effect of either the MAO inhibitors or hydrocodone). Products include:
Parnate Tablets 1527

Triazolam (May exhibit additive CNS depression).
No products indexed under this heading.

Tridihexethyl Chloride (Concurrent use of anticholinergics with hydrocodone preparations may produce paralytic ileus).
No products indexed under this heading.

Trifluoperazine Hydrochloride (May exhibit additive CNS depression).
No products indexed under this heading.

Trihexyphenidyl Hydrochloride (Concurrent use of anticholinergics with hydrocodone preparations may produce paralytic ileus).
No products indexed under this heading.

Trimipramine Maleate (Co-administration of tricyclic antidepressants with hydrocodone preparations may increase the effect of either the antidepressant or hydrocodone).
No products indexed under this heading.

Warfarin Sodium (The effects of warfarin and NSAIDs on GI bleeding are synergistic). Products include:
Coumadin for Injection 898
Coumadin Tablets 898

Zaleplon (May exhibit additive CNS depression). Products include:
Sonata Capsules 1717

Ziprasidone Hydrochloride (May exhibit additive CNS depression). Products include:
Geodon Capsules 2529

Zolpidem Tartrate (May exhibit additive CNS depression). Products include:
Ambien Tablets 2851
Ambien CR Tablets 2855

Food Interactions

Alcohol (May exhibit additive CNS depression).

VIGAMOX OPHTHALMIC SOLUTION

(Moxifloxacin Hydrochloride) 564
None cited in PDR database.

VIOKASE POWDER

(Pancrelipase) 711
None cited in PDR database.

VIOKASE TABLETS

(Pancrelipase) 711
None cited in PDR database.

VIRACEPT ORAL POWDER

(Nelfinavir Mesylate) 2577
See Viracept Tablets

VIRACEPT TABLETS

(Nelfinavir Mesylate) 2577
May interact with cytochrome p450 2c19 inducers (selected), cytochrome p450 2c19 inhibitors (selected), cytochrome p450 3a inducers (selected), cytochrome p450 3a inhibitors (selected), dihydropyridine calcium channel blockers, ergot-containing drugs, oral contraceptives, phenytoin, quinidine, statins that are metabolized by CYP3A4, and certain other agents. Compounds in these categories include:

Allium sativum (Nelfinavir is metabolized by CYP3A and CYP2C19; co-administration of Viracept and drugs that induce CYP3A or CYP2C19 may decrease nelfinavir plasma concentrations and reduce its therapeutic effect).
No products indexed under this heading.

Amiodarone Hydrochloride (Nelfinavir is an inhibitor of CYP3A and co-administration with drugs primarily metabolized by CYP3A, such as amiodarone, could result in competition for CYP3A by nelfinavir; contraindicated due to potential for serious and/or life-threatening reactions, such as cardiac arrhythmias).
No products indexed under this heading.

Amlodipine Besylate (Nelfinavir is an inhibitor of CYP450 3A enzymes which are responsible for the metabolism of dihydropyridine calcium channel blockers; co-administration may result in increased plasma concentrations of these calcium channel blockers). Products include:
Caduet Tablets 2508
Lotrel Capsules 2249
Norvasc Tablets 2545

Amprenavir (Nelfinavir is metabolized by CYP3A and CYP2C19; co-administration of Viracept and drugs that inhibit CYP3A or CYP2C19 may increase nelfinavir plasma concentrations). Products include:
Agenerase Capsules 1327
Agenerase Oral Solution 1332

Aprepitant (Nelfinavir is metabolized by CYP3A and CYP2C19; co-administration of Viracept and drugs that induce CYP3A or CYP2C19 may decrease nelfinavir plasma concentrations and reduce its therapeutic effect). Products include:
Emend Capsules 1963

Atorvastatin Calcium (Nelfinavir is an inhibitor of CYP3A and co-administration with drugs primarily metabolized by CYP3A could increase the risk of myopathy including rhabdomyolysis). Products include:
Caduet Tablets 2508
Lipitor Tablets 2483

Azithromycin Dihydrate (Co-administrations results in increases in azithromycin plasma concentrations).
No products indexed under this heading.

Carbamazepine (May decrease nelfinavir plasma concentrations; Viracept may not be effective due to decreased nelfinavir plasma concentrations in patients taking carbamazepine). Products include:
Carbatrol Capsules 3171
Equetro Extended-Release Capsules..................................... 3180
Tegretol/Tegretol-XR 2295

Cerivastatin Sodium (Nelfinavir is an inhibitor of CYP3A and co-administration with drugs primarily metabolized by CYP3A, such as cerivastatin, could increase the risk of myopathy including rhabdomyolysis).
No products indexed under this heading.

Cimetidine (Nelfinavir is metabolized by CYP3A and CYP2C19; co-administration of Viracept and drugs that inhibit CYP3A or CYP2C19 may increase nelfinavir plasma concentrations). Products include:
Tagamet HB 200 Tablets .... ▣664

Cimetidine Hydrochloride (Nelfinavir is metabolized by CYP3A and CYP2C19; co-administration of Viracept and drugs that inhibit CYP3A or CYP2C19 may increase nelfinavir plasma concentrations).
No products indexed under this heading.

Ciprofloxacin (Nelfinavir is metabolized by CYP3A and CYP2C19; co-administration of Viracept and drugs that inhibit CYP3A or CYP2C19 may increase nelfinavir plasma concentrations). Products include:
Cipro Oral Suspension 2977
Cipro I.V. 2984
Cipro XR Tablets 2990
Ciprodex Otic Suspension 559

Ciprofloxacin Hydrochloride (Nelfinavir is metabolized by CYP3A and CYP2C19; co-administration of Viracept and drugs that inhibit CYP3A or CYP2C19 may increase nelfinavir plasma concentrations). Products include:
Ciloxan Ophthalmic Ointment........... 559
Ciloxan Ophthalmic Solution .... ⊙206
Cipro Tablets 2977
Proquin XR Tablets 1153

Cisapride (Nelfinavir is an inhibitor of CYP3A and co-administration with drugs primarily metabolized by CYP3A, such as cisapride, could affect hepatic metabolism of cisapride and create the potential for serious and/or life-threatening adverse events; concurrent use is contraindicated).
No products indexed under this heading.

Citalopram Hydrobromide (Nelfinavir is metabolized by CYP3A and CYP2C19; co-administration of Viracept and drugs that inhibit CYP3A or CYP2C19 may increase nelfinavir plasma concentrations). Products include:
Celexa 1176

Clarithromycin (Nelfinavir is metabolized by CYP3A and CYP2C19; co-administration of Viracept and drugs that inhibit CYP3A or CYP2C19 may increase nelfinavir plasma concentrations). Products include:
Biaxin/Biaxin XL 402
PREVPAC 3284

Cyclosporine (Nelfinavir is an inhibitor of CYP450 3A enzymes which are responsible for the metabolism of immunosuppressants, such as cyclosporine; co-administration may result in increased plasma concentrations of immunosuppressants). Products include:
Gengraf Capsules 459
Neoral Oral Solution 2259
Neoral Soft Gelatin Capsules 2259
Restasis Ophthalmic Emulsion 575
Sandimmune 2275

Delavirdine Mesylate (Co-administration results in increases in nelfinavir plasma concentrations and decreases in delavirdine plasma concentrations; appropriate doses for these combinations, with respect to safety and efficacy, have not been established). Products include:
- Rescriptor Tablets 2551

Desogestrel (Nelfinavir is metabolized by CYP3A and CYP2C19; co-administration of Viracept and drugs that inhibit CYP3A or CYP2C19 may increase nelfinavir plasma concentrations). Products include:
- Mircette Tablets 1066

Dexamethasone (Nelfinavir is metabolized by CYP3A and CYP2C19; co-administration of Viracept and drugs that induce CYP3A or CYP2C19 may decrease nelfinavir plasma concentrations and reduce its therapeutic effect). Products include:
- Ciprodex Otic Suspension 559
- Decadron Tablets 1951
- TobraDex Ophthalmic Ointment 562
- TobraDex Ophthalmic Suspension ... 563

Didanosine (Co-administration with didanosine indicates no change in AUC or Cmax of nelfinavir; however, it is recommended that didanosine be administered on an empty stomach; therefore, nelfinavir should be administered with food one hour after or more than 2 hours before didanosine).
- No products indexed under this heading.

Dihydroergotamine Mesylate (Nelfinavir is an inhibitor of CYP3A and co-administration with drugs primarily metabolized by CYP3A, such as ergot derivatives, could result in competition for CYP3A by nelfinavir; inhibition of the metabolism of ergot derivatives could create a potential for serious cardiac arrhythmias or prolong adverse events; contraindicated due to potential for serious and/or life-threatening reactions, such as acute ergot toxicity characterized by peripheral vasospasm and ischemia of the extremities and other tissues). Products include:
- Migranal Nasal Spray 3348

Diltiazem Hydrochloride (Nelfinavir is metabolized by CYP3A and CYP2C19; co-administration of Viracept and drugs that inhibit CYP3A or CYP2C19 may increase nelfinavir plasma concentrations). Products include:
- Cardizem LA Extended Release Tablets 1728
- Tiazac Capsules 1201

Diltiazem Maleate (Nelfinavir is metabolized by CYP3A and CYP2C19; co-administration of Viracept and drugs that inhibit CYP3A or CYP2C19 may increase nelfinavir plasma concentrations).
- No products indexed under this heading.

Efavirenz (Nelfinavir is metabolized by CYP3A and CYP2C19; co-administration of Viracept and drugs that inhibit CYP3A or CYP2C19 may increase nelfinavir plasma concentrations). Products include:
- Atripla Tablets 945
- Sustiva Capsules 930
- Sustiva Tablets 930

Ergonovine Maleate (Nelfinavir is an inhibitor of CYP3A and co-administration with drugs primarily metabolized by CYP3A, such as ergot derivatives, could result in competition for CYP3A by nelfinavir; inhibition of the metabolism of ergot derivatives could create a potential for serious cardiac arrhythmias or prolong adverse events; contraindicated due to potential for serious and/or life-threatening reactions, such as acute ergot toxicity characterized by peripheral vasospasm and ischemia of the extremities and other tissues).
- No products indexed under this heading.

Ergotamine Tartrate (Nelfinavir is an inhibitor of CYP3A and co-administration with drugs primarily metabolized by CYP3A, such as ergot derivatives, could result in competition for CYP3A by nelfinavir; inhibition of the metabolism of ergot derivatives could create a potential for serious cardiac arrhythmias or prolong adverse events; contraindicated due to potential for serious and/or life-threatening reactions, such as acute ergot toxicity characterized by peripheral vasospasm and ischemia of the extremities and other tissues).
- No products indexed under this heading.

Erythromycin (Nelfinavir is metabolized by CYP3A and CYP2C19; co-administration of Viracept and drugs that inhibit CYP3A or CYP2C19 may increase nelfinavir plasma concentrations). Products include:
- Ery-Tab Tablets 449
- Erythromycin Base Filmtab Tablets 455
- Erythromycin Delayed-Release Capsules, USP 457
- PCE Dispertab Tablets 515

Ethinyl Estradiol (Co-administration with oral contraceptives containing ethinyl estradiol results in decreased ethinyl estradiol plasma concentrations; alternative or additional contraceptive measures should be used when oral contraceptives and Viracept are co-administered). Products include:
- Mircette Tablets 1066
- NuvaRing 2340
- Ortho-Cyclen/Ortho Tri-Cyclen 2429
- Ortho Evra Transdermal System 2417
- Ortho Tri-Cyclen Lo Tablets 2436
- Seasonique Tablets 1077
- Yasmin 28 Tablets 796
- Yaz Tablets 803

Ethosuximide (Nelfinavir is metabolized by CYP3A and CYP2C19; co-administration of Viracept and drugs that induce CYP3A or CYP2C19 may decrease nelfinavir plasma concentrations and reduce its therapeutic effect).
- No products indexed under this heading.

Ethynodiol Diacetate (Nelfinavir is metabolized by CYP3A and CYP2C19; co-administration of Viracept and drugs that inhibit CYP3A or CYP2C19 may increase nelfinavir plasma concentrations).
- No products indexed under this heading.

Felbamate (Nelfinavir is metabolized by CYP3A and CYP2C19; co-administration of Viracept and drugs that inhibit CYP3A or CYP2C19 may increase nelfinavir plasma concentrations).
- No products indexed under this heading.

Felodipine (Nelfinavir is an inhibitor of CYP450 3A enzymes which are responsible for the metabolism of dihydropyridine calcium channel blockers; co-administration may result in increased plasma concentrations of these calcium channel blockers).
- No products indexed under this heading.

Fluconazole (Nelfinavir is metabolized by CYP3A and CYP2C19; co-administration of Viracept and drugs that inhibit CYP3A or CYP2C19 may increase nelfinavir plasma concentrations).
- No products indexed under this heading.

Fluoxetine (Nelfinavir is metabolized by CYP3A and CYP2C19; co-administration of Viracept and drugs that inhibit CYP3A or CYP2C19 may increase nelfinavir plasma concentrations).
- No products indexed under this heading.

Fluoxetine Hydrochloride (Nelfinavir is metabolized by CYP3A and CYP2C19; co-administration of Viracept and drugs that inhibit CYP3A or CYP2C19 may increase nelfinavir plasma concentrations). Products include:
- Prozac Pulvules and Liquid 1801
- Symbyax Capsules 1819

Fluticasone Propionate (Concomitant use of fluticasone propionate and nelfinavir may increase plasma concentrations of fluticasone propionate. Use with caution. Consider alternatives to fluticasone propionate, particularly for long-term use). Products include:
- Advair Diskus 100/50 1308
- Advair Diskus 250/50 1308
- Advair Diskus 500/50 1308
- Advair HFA Inhalation Aerosol 1318
- Cutivate Cream 2662
- Cutivate Lotion 0.05% 2664
- Cutivate Ointment 2665
- Flonase Nasal Spray 1440
- Flovent Diskus 1443

Fluticasone Propionate HFA (Concomitant use of fluticasone propionate and nelfinavir may increase plasma concentrations of fluticasone propionate. Use with caution. Consider alternatives to fluticasone propionate, particularly for long-term use). Products include:
- Flovent HFA 1447

Fluvastatin Sodium (Nelfinavir is metabolized by CYP3A and CYP2C19; co-administration of Viracept and drugs that inhibit CYP3A or CYP2C19 may increase nelfinavir plasma concentrations). Products include:
- Lescol Capsules 2233
- Lescol XL Tablets 2233

Fluvoxamine (Nelfinavir is metabolized by CYP3A and CYP2C19; co-administration of Viracept and drugs that inhibit CYP3A or CYP2C19 may increase nelfinavir plasma concentrations).
- No products indexed under this heading.

Fluvoxamine Maleate (Nelfinavir is metabolized by CYP3A and CYP2C19; co-administration of Viracept and drugs that inhibit CYP3A or CYP2C19 may increase nelfinavir plasma concentrations).
- No products indexed under this heading.

Fosphenytoin Sodium (Nelfinavir may decrease phenytoin levels. Phenytoin plasma/serum concentrations should be monitored; phenytoin dose may require adjustment to compensate for altered phenytoin concentration. Phenytoin may also decrease Cmin of nelfinavir).
- No products indexed under this heading.

Hypericum (Concomitant use of St. John's Wort or products containing St. John's Wort and nelfinavir is expected to substantially decrease protease inhibitor concentrations and may result in sub-optimal levels of nelfinavir and lead to loss of virologic response and possible resistance to nelfinavir or other co-administered antiretroviral agents). Products include:
- Satiete Tablets 832

Indinavir Sulfate (Co-administration results in increases in both nelfinavir and indinavir plasma concentrations; appropriate doses for this combination, with respect to safety and efficacy, have not been established). Products include:
- Crixivan Capsules 1940

Indomethacin (Nelfinavir is metabolized by CYP3A and CYP2C19; co-administration of Viracept and drugs that inhibit CYP3A or CYP2C19 may increase nelfinavir plasma concentrations). Products include:
- Indocin 1995

Indomethacin Sodium Trihydrate (Nelfinavir is metabolized by CYP3A and CYP2C19; co-administration of Viracept and drugs that inhibit CYP3A or CYP2C19 may increase nelfinavir plasma concentrations). Products include:
- Indocin I.V. 2465

Isoniazid (Nelfinavir is metabolized by CYP3A and CYP2C19; co-administration of Viracept and drugs that inhibit CYP3A or CYP2C19 may increase nelfinavir plasma concentrations).
- No products indexed under this heading.

Isradipine (Nelfinavir is an inhibitor of CYP450 3A enzymes which are responsible for the metabolism of dihydropyridine calcium channel blockers; co-administration may result in increased plasma concentrations of these calcium channel blockers). Products include:
- DynaCirc CR Tablets 2721

Itraconazole (Nelfinavir is metabolized by CYP3A and CYP2C19; co-administration of Viracept and drugs that inhibit CYP3A or CYP2C19 may increase nelfinavir plasma concentrations).
- No products indexed under this heading.

Ketoconazole (Nelfinavir is metabolized by CYP3A and CYP2C19; co-administration of Viracept and drugs that inhibit CYP3A or CYP2C19 may increase nelfinavir plasma concentrations). Products include:
- Nizoral A-D Shampoo, 1% 1868

Lamivudine (Nelfinavir increases lamivudine's AUC and Cmax by 10% and 31%, respectively). Products include:
- Combivir Tablets 1411
- Epivir 1427
- Epivir-HBV 1432
- Epzicom Tablets 1436
- Trizivir Tablets 1589

Lansoprazole (Nelfinavir is metabolized by CYP3A and CYP2C19; co-administration of Viracept and drugs that inhibit CYP3A or CYP2C19 may increase nelfinavir plasma concentrations). Products include:

Letrozole (Nelfinavir is metabolized by CYP3A and CYP2C19; co-administration of Viracept and drugs that inhibit CYP3A or CYP2C19 may increase nelfinavir plasma concentrations). Products include:

Levonorgestrel (Nelfinavir is metabolized by CYP3A and CYP2C19; co-administration of Viracept and drugs that inhibit CYP3A or CYP2C19 may increase nelfinavir plasma concentrations). Products include:

Lopinavir (Nelfinavir is metabolized by CYP3A and CYP2C19; co-administration of Viracept and drugs that inhibit CYP3A or CYP2C19 may increase nelfinavir plasma concentrations). Products include:

Lovastatin (Nelfinavir is an inhibitor of CYP3A and co-administration with drugs primarily metabolized by CYP3A could increase the risk of myopathy including rhabdomyolysis. Products include:

Mestranol (Nelfinavir is metabolized by CYP3A and CYP2C19; co-administration of Viracept and drugs that inhibit CYP3A or CYP2C19 may increase nelfinavir plasma concentrations).

No products indexed under this heading.

Methadone Hydrochloride (Co-administration with methadone results in a decrease in methadone plasma concentrations; dosage of methadone may need to be increased).

No products indexed under this heading.

Methylergonovine Maleate (Nelfinavir is an inhibitor of CYP3A and co-administration with drugs primarily metabolized by CYP3A, such as ergot derivatives, could result in competition for CYP3A by nelfinavir; inhibition of the metabolism of ergot derivatives could create a potential for serious cardiac arrhythmias or prolong adverse events; contraindicated due to potential for serious and/or life-threatening reactions, such as acute ergot toxicity characterized by peripheral vasospasm and ischemia of the extremities and other tissues).

No products indexed under this heading.

Methysergide Maleate (Nelfinavir is an inhibitor of CYP3A and co-administration with drugs primarily metabolized by CYP3A, such as ergot derivatives, could result in competition for CYP3A by nelfinavir; inhibition of the metabolism of ergot derivatives could create a potential for serious cardiac arrhythmias or prolong adverse events; contraindicated due to potential for serious and/or life-threatening reactions, such as acute ergot toxicity characterized by peripheral vasospasm and ischemia of the extremities and other tissues).

No products indexed under this heading.

Metronidazole (Nelfinavir is metabolized by CYP3A and CYP2C19; co-administration of Viracept and drugs that inhibit CYP3A or CYP2C19 may increase nelfinavir plasma concentrations). Products include:

Metronidazole Benzoate (Nelfinavir is metabolized by CYP3A and CYP2C19; co-administration of Viracept and drugs that inhibit CYP3A or CYP2C19 may increase nelfinavir plasma concentrations).

No products indexed under this heading.

Metronidazole Hydrochloride (Nelfinavir is metabolized by CYP3A and CYP2C19; co-administration of Viracept and drugs that inhibit CYP3A or CYP2C19 may increase nelfinavir plasma concentrations).

No products indexed under this heading.

Miconazole (Nelfinavir is metabolized by CYP3A and CYP2C19; co-administration of Viracept and drugs that inhibit CYP3A or CYP2C19 may increase nelfinavir plasma concentrations).

No products indexed under this heading.

Midazolam Hydrochloride (Nelfinavir is an inhibitor of CYP3A and co-administration with drugs primarily metabolized by CYP3A, such as midazolam, could affect hepatic metabolism of midazolam; contraindicated due to potential for serious and/or life-threatening reactions, such as prolonged or increased sedation or respiratory depression).

No products indexed under this heading.

Modafinil (Nelfinavir is metabolized by CYP3A and CYP2C19; co-administration of Viracept and drugs that inhibit CYP3A or CYP2C19 may increase nelfinavir plasma concentrations). Products include:

Nefazodone Hydrochloride (Nelfinavir is metabolized by CYP3A and CYP2C19; co-administration of Viracept and drugs that inhibit CYP3A or CYP2C19 may increase nelfinavir plasma concentrations).

No products indexed under this heading.

Nevirapine (Nelfinavir is metabolized by CYP3A and CYP2C19; co-administration of Viracept and drugs that induce CYP3A or CYP2C19 may decrease nelfinavir plasma concentrations and reduce its therapeutic effect). Products include:

Nicardipine Hydrochloride (Nelfinavir is an inhibitor of CYP450 3A enzymes which are responsible for the metabolism of dihydropyridine calcium channel blockers; co-administration may result in increased plasma concentrations of these calcium channel blockers). Products include:

Nifedipine (Nelfinavir is an inhibitor of CYP450 3A enzymes which are responsible for the metabolism of dihydropyridine calcium channel blockers; co-administration may result in increased plasma concentrations of these calcium channel blockers). Products include:

Nimodipine (Nelfinavir is an inhibitor of CYP450 3A enzymes which are responsible for the metabolism of dihydropyridine calcium channel blockers; co-administration may result in increased plasma concentrations of these calcium channel blockers). Products include:

Norethindrone (Co-administration with oral contraceptives containing norethindrone results in decreased norethindrone AUC by approximately 18%; alternative or additional contraceptive measures should be used when oral contraceptives and Viracept are co-administered). Products include:

Norethindrone Acetate (Co-administration with oral contraceptives containing norethindrone results in decreased norethindrone AUC by approximately 18%; alternative or additional contraceptive measures should be used when oral contraceptives and Viracept are co-administered).

No products indexed under this heading.

Norethynodrel (Nelfinavir is metabolized by CYP3A and CYP2C19; co-administration of Viracept and drugs that inhibit CYP3A or CYP2C19 may increase nelfinavir plasma concentrations).

No products indexed under this heading.

Norfloxacin (Nelfinavir is metabolized by CYP3A and CYP2C19; co-administration of Viracept and drugs that inhibit CYP3A or CYP2C19 may increase nelfinavir plasma concentrations). Products include:

Norgestimate (Nelfinavir is metabolized by CYP3A and CYP2C19; co-administration of Viracept and drugs that inhibit CYP3A or CYP2C19 may increase nelfinavir plasma concentrations). Products include:

Norgestrel (Nelfinavir is metabolized by CYP3A and CYP2C19; co-administration of Viracept and drugs that inhibit CYP3A or CYP2C19 may increase nelfinavir plasma concentrations).

No products indexed under this heading.

Omeprazole (Co-administration may lead to a decrease in nelfinavir concentrations that may lead to a loss of virologic response and possible resistance to nelfinavir). Products include:

Omeprazole magnesium (Co-administration may lead to a decrease in nelfinavir concentrations that may lead to a loss of virologic response and possible resistance to nelfinavir). Products include:

Oxcarbazepine (Nelfinavir is metabolized by CYP3A and CYP2C19; co-administration of Viracept and drugs that inhibit CYP3A or CYP2C19 may increase nelfinavir plasma concentrations). Products include:

Paroxetine Hydrochloride (Nelfinavir is metabolized by CYP3A and CYP2C19; co-administration of Viracept and drugs that inhibit CYP3A or CYP2C19 may increase nelfinavir plasma concentrations). Products include:

Phenobarbital (May decrease nelfinavir plasma concentrations; Viracept may not be effective due to decreased nelfinavir plasma concentrations in patients taking phenobarbital). Products include:

Phenobarbital Sodium (Nelfinavir is metabolized by CYP3A and CYP2C19; co-administration of Viracept and drugs that induce CYP3A or CYP2C19 may decrease nelfinavir plasma concentrations and reduce its therapeutic effect).

No products indexed under this heading.

Phenytoin (Nelfinavir may decrease phenytoin levels. Phenytoin plasma/serum concentrations should be monitored; phenytoin dose may require adjustment to compensate for altered phenytoin concentration. Phenytoin may also decrease Cmin of nelfinavir).

No products indexed under this heading.

Phenytoin Sodium (Nelfinavir may decrease phenytoin levels. Phenytoin plasma/serum concentrations should be monitored; phenytoin dose may require adjustment to compensate for altered phenytoin concentration. Phenytoin may also decrease Cmin of nelfinavir). Products include:

Pimozide (Concurrent use with nelfinavir is contraindicted due to potential for serious and/or life-threatening reactions, such as cardiac arrhythmias).

No products indexed under this heading.

Prednisone (Nelfinavir is metabolized by CYP3A and CYP2C19; co-administration of Viracept and drugs that induce CYP3A or CYP2C19 may decrease nelfinavir plasma concentrations and reduce its therapeutic effect).

No products indexed under this heading.

Quinidine (Nelfinavir is an inhibitor of CYP3A and co-administration with drugs primarily metabolized by CYP3A, such as quinidine, could result in competition for CYP3A by nelfinavir; contraindicated due to potential for serious and/or life-threatening reactions, such as cardiac arrhythmias).

No products indexed under this heading.

Quinidine Gluconate (Nelfinavir is an inhibitor of CYP3A and co-administration with drugs primarily metabolized by CYP3A, such as quinidine, could result in competition for CYP3A by nelfinavir; contraindicated due to potential for serious and/or life-threatening reactions, such as cardiac arrhythmias).
No products indexed under this heading.

Quinidine Hydrochloride (Nelfinavir is an inhibitor of CYP3A and co-administration with drugs primarily metabolized by CYP3A, such as quinidine, could result in competition for CYP3A by nelfinavir; contraindicated due to potential for serious and/or life-threatening reactions, such as cardiac arrhythmias).
No products indexed under this heading.

Quinidine Polygalacturonate (Nelfinavir is an inhibitor of CYP3A and co-administration with drugs primarily metabolized by CYP3A, such as quinidine, could result in competition for CYP3A by nelfinavir; contraindicated due to potential for serious and/or life-threatening reactions, such as cardiac arrhythmias).
No products indexed under this heading.

Quinidine Sulfate (Nelfinavir is an inhibitor of CYP3A and co-administration with drugs primarily metabolized by CYP3A, such as quinidine, could result in competition for CYP3A by nelfinavir; contraindicated due to potential for serious and/or life-threatening reactions, such as cardiac arrhythmias).
No products indexed under this heading.

Quinine (Nelfinavir is metabolized by CYP3A and CYP2C19; co-administration of Viracept and drugs that inhibit CYP3A or CYP2C19 may increase nelfinavir plasma concentrations).
No products indexed under this heading.

Quinine Sulfate (Nelfinavir is metabolized by CYP3A and CYP2C19; co-administration of Viracept and drugs that inhibit CYP3A or CYP2C19 may increase nelfinavir plasma concentrations).
No products indexed under this heading.

Rifabutin (It is recommended that the dose of rifabutin be reduced to one-half the usual dose when administered with nelfinavir; co-administration results in no change or a decrease in nelfinavir plasma concentrations (depending upon dosage) and increases in rifabutin plasma concentrations).
No products indexed under this heading.

Rifampicin (Nelfinavir is metabolized by CYP3A and CYP2C19; co-administration of Viracept and drugs that induce CYP3A or CYP2C19 may decrease nelfinavir plasma concentrations and reduce its therapeutic effect).
No products indexed under this heading.

Rifampin (Co-administration with rifampin results in decreased nelfinavir AUC and Cmax; may lead to loss of virologic response and possible resistance to nelfinavir or other co-administered antiretroviral agents).
No products indexed under this heading.

Rifapentine (Nelfinavir is metabolized by CYP3A and CYP2C19; co-administration of Viracept and drugs that induce CYP3A or CYP2C19 may decrease nelfinavir plasma concentrations and reduce its therapeutic effect).
No products indexed under this heading.

Ritonavir (Co-administration results in increased nelfinavir plasma concentrations; appropriate doses for this combination, with respect to safety and efficacy, have not been established). Products include:
Kaletra 476
Norvir 503

Saquinavir (Co-administration results in increase in saquinavir plasma concentrations; appropriate doses for this combination, with respect to safety and efficacy, have not been established).
No products indexed under this heading.

Saquinavir Mesylate (Co-administration results in increase in saquinavir plasma concentrations; appropriate doses for this combination, with respect to safety and efficacy, have not been established). Products include:
Invirase 2772

Sertraline Hydrochloride (Nelfinavir is metabolized by CYP3A and CYP2C19; co-administration of Viracept and drugs that inhibit CYP3A or CYP2C19 may increase nelfinavir plasma concentrations). Products include:
Zoloft 2586

Sildenafil Citrate (Co-administration of a protease inhibitor with sildenafil is expected to substantially increase sildenafil concentrations and may result in an increase in sildenafil-associated adverse events, including hypotension, visual changes, and priapism; sildenafil should not exceed a maximum single dose of 25 mg in a 48 hour period when administered in patients receiving protease inhibitors). Products include:
Revatio Tablets 2557
Viagra Tablets 2573

Simvastatin (Nelfinavir is an inhibitor of CYP3A and co-administration with drugs primarily metabolized by CYP3A could increase the risk of myopathy including rhabdomyolysis). Products include:
Vytorin 10/10 Tablets 2114
Vytorin 10/10 Tablets 3077
Vytorin 10/20 Tablets 2114
Vytorin 10/20 Tablets 3077
Vytorin 10/40 Tablets 2114
Vytorin 10/40 Tablets 3077
Vytorin 10/80 Tablets 2114
Vytorin 10/80 Tablets 3077
Zocor Tablets 2105

Sirolimus (Nelfinavir is an inhibitor of CYP450 3A enzymes which are responsible for the metabolism of immunosuppressants, such as sirolimus; co-administration may result in increased plasma concentrations of immunosuppressants). Products include:
Rapamune Oral Solution and Tablets 3475

Sulfaphenazole (Nelfinavir is metabolized by CYP3A and CYP2C19; co-administration of Viracept and drugs that inhibit CYP3A or CYP2C19 may increase nelfinavir plasma concentrations).
No products indexed under this heading.

Tacrolimus (Nelfinavir is an inhibitor of CYP450 3A enzymes which are responsible for the metabolism of immunosuppressants, such as tacrolimus; co-administration may result in increased plasma concentrations of immunosuppressants). Products include:
Prograf Capsules and Injection 632
Protopic Ointment 638

Telmisartan (Nelfinavir is metabolized by CYP3A and CYP2C19; co-administration of Viracept and drugs that inhibit CYP3A or CYP2C19 may increase nelfinavir plasma concentrations). Products include:
Micardis Tablets 854
Micardis HCT Tablets 856

Ticlopidine Hydrochloride (Nelfinavir is metabolized by CYP3A and CYP2C19; co-administration of Viracept and drugs that inhibit CYP3A or CYP2C19 may increase nelfinavir plasma concentrations). Products include:
Ticlid Tablets 2810

Tolbutamide (Nelfinavir is metabolized by CYP3A and CYP2C19; co-administration of Viracept and drugs that inhibit CYP3A or CYP2C19 may increase nelfinavir plasma concentrations).
No products indexed under this heading.

Tolbutamide Sodium (Nelfinavir is metabolized by CYP3A and CYP2C19; co-administration of Viracept and drugs that inhibit CYP3A or CYP2C19 may increase nelfinavir plasma concentrations).
No products indexed under this heading.

Topiramate (Nelfinavir is metabolized by CYP3A and CYP2C19; co-administration of Viracept and drugs that inhibit CYP3A or CYP2C19 may increase nelfinavir plasma concentrations). Products include:
Topamax Sprinkle Capsules 2404
Topamax Tablets 2404

Trazodone Hydrochloride (Concomitant use of trazodone and nelfinavir mesylate may increase plasma concentrations of trazodone. Adverse events of nausea, dizziness, hypotension, and syncope have been observed following co-administration of trazodone and ritonavir. If trazodone is used with a CYP3A4 inhibitor, such as nelfinavir mesylate, the combination should be used with caution and a lower dose of trazodone should be considered).
No products indexed under this heading.

Triazolam (Nelfinavir is an inhibitor of CYP3A and co-administration with drugs primarily metabolized by CYP3A, such as triazolam, could affect hepatic metabolism of triazolam; contraindicated due to potential for serious and/or life-threatening reactions, such as prolonged or increased sedation or respiratory depression).
No products indexed under this heading.

Troleandomycin (Nelfinavir is metabolized by CYP3A and CYP2C19; co-administration of Viracept and drugs that inhibit CYP3A or CYP2C19 may increase nelfinavir plasma concentrations).
No products indexed under this heading.

Venlafaxine Hydrochloride (Nelfinavir is metabolized by CYP3A and CYP2C19; co-administration of Viracept and drugs that inhibit CYP3A or CYP2C19 may increase nelfinavir plasma concentrations). Products include:
Effexor Tablets 3411
Effexor XR Capsules 3417

Verapamil Hydrochloride (Nelfinavir is metabolized by CYP3A and CYP2C19; co-administration of Viracept and drugs that inhibit CYP3A or CYP2C19 may increase nelfinavir plasma concentrations). Products include:
Covera-HS Tablets 3139
Tarka Tablets 524
Verelan PM Extended-Release Capsules, Controlled-Onset 3106

Voriconazole (Nelfinavir is metabolized by CYP3A and CYP2C19; co-administration of Viracept and drugs that inhibit CYP3A or CYP2C19 may increase nelfinavir plasma concentrations). Products include:
VFEND I.V. 2564
VFEND Oral Suspension 2564
VFEND Tablets 2564

Zafirlukast (Nelfinavir is metabolized by CYP3A and CYP2C19; co-administration of Viracept and drugs that inhibit CYP3A or CYP2C19 may increase nelfinavir plasma concentrations). Products include:
Accolate Tablets 671

Zidovudine (Nelfinavir decreases zidovudine's AUC and Cmax by 35% and 31%, respectively). Products include:
Combivir Tablets 1411
Retrovir 1560
Retrovir IV Infusion 1564
Trizivir Tablets 1589

Zileuton (Nelfinavir is metabolized by CYP3A and CYP2C19; co-administration of Viracept and drugs that inhibit CYP3A or CYP2C19 may increase nelfinavir plasma concentrations). Products include:
Zyflo Tablets 1023

Food Interactions

Food, unspecified (Maximum plasma concentrations and AUC were 2- to 3-fold higher under fed conditions compared to fasting; Viracept should be taken with a meal or light snack).

Grapefruit (Nelfinavir is metabolized by CYP3A and CYP2C19; co-administration of Viracept and drugs that inhibit CYP3A or CYP2C19 may increase nelfinavir plasma concentrations).

VIRAMUNE ORAL SUSPENSION

(Nevirapine) 873
See Viramune Tablets

VIRAMUNE TABLETS

(Nevirapine) 873

May interact with antiarrhythmics, azole antifungals, calcium channel blockers, antineoplastics, anticoagulants, anticonvulsants, ergot-containing drugs, drugs affecting gastrointestinal motility, immunosuppressive agents, narcotic analgesics, oral contraceptives, and certain other agents. Compounds in these categories include:

Acebutolol Hydrochloride (Plasma concentrations of antiarrhythmics may be decreased by co-administration with nevirapine. Dose adjustment of co-administered drug may be needed due to possible decrease in clinical effect.).
No products indexed under this heading.

Adenosine (Plasma concentrations of antiarrhythmics may be decreased by co-administration with nevirapine. Dose adjustment of co-administered drug may be needed due to possible decrease in clinical effect). Products include:
Adenocard Injection 617
Adenoscan 619

Albuterol (Plasma concentrations of GI motility agents may be decreased by co-administration with nevirapine. Dose adjustment of co-administered drug may be needed due to possible decrease in clinical effect). Products include:
Proventil Inhalation Aerosol 3053

Albuterol Sulfate (Plasma concentrations of GI motility agents may be decreased by co-administration with nevirapine. Dose adjustment of co-administered drug may be needed due to possible decrease in clinical effect). Products include:
AccuNeb Inhalation Solution 1055
Combivent Inhalation Aerosol 847
DuoNeb Inhalation Solution 1058
ProAir HFA Inhalation Aerosol 3300
Proventil Inhalation Solution 0.083% 3055
Proventil HFA Inhalation Aerosol 3056
Ventolin HFA Inhalation Aerosol 1600
VoSpire ER Tablets 1052

Alfentanil Hydrochloride (Plasma concentrations of GI motility agents may be decreased by co-administration with nevirapine. Dose adjustment of co-administered drug may be needed due to possible decrease in clinical effect.).
No products indexed under this heading.

Altretamine (Plasma concentrations of cancer chemotherapeutic agents may be decreased by co-administration with nevirapine. Dose adjustment of co-administered drug may be needed due to possible decrease in clinical effect.).
No products indexed under this heading.

Amiodarone Hydrochloride (Plasma concentrations of antiarrhythmics may be decreased by co-administration with nevirapine. Dose adjustment of co-administered drug may be needed due to possible decrease in clinical effect.).
No products indexed under this heading.

Amitriptyline Hydrochloride (Plasma concentrations of GI motility agents may be decreased by co-administration with nevirapine. Dose adjustment of co-administered drug may be needed due to possible decrease in clinical effect.).
No products indexed under this heading.

Amlodipine Besylate (Plasma concentrations of calcium channel blockers may be decreased by co-administration with nevirapine. Dose adjustment of co-administered drug may be needed due to possible decrease in clinical effect). Products include:
Caduet Tablets 2508
Lotrel Capsules 2249
Norvasc Tablets 2545

Amoxapine (Plasma concentrations of GI motility agents may be decreased by co-administration with nevirapine. Dose adjustment of co-administered drug may be needed due to possible decrease in clinical effect.).
No products indexed under this heading.

Anastrozole (Plasma concentrations of cancer chemotherapeutic agents may be decreased by co-administration with nevirapine. Dose adjustment of co-administered drug may be needed due to possible decrease in clinical effect). Products include:
Arimidex Tablets 673

Anisindione (Plasma concentrations of antithrombotics may be increased by co-administration with nevirapine. Dose adjustment of co-administered drug may be needed due to possible decrease in clinical effect). Products include:
Miradon Tablets 3042

Ardeparin Sodium (Plasma concentrations of antithrombotics may be increased by co-administration with nevirapine. Dose adjustment of co-administered drug may be needed due to possible decrease in clinical effect.).
No products indexed under this heading.

Asparaginase (Plasma concentrations of cancer chemotherapeutic agents may be decreased by co-administration with nevirapine. Dose adjustment of co-administered drug may be needed due to possible decrease in clinical effect). Products include:
Elspar for Injection 2463
Elspar for Injection 1960

Astemizole (Plasma concentrations of GI motility agents may be decreased by co-administration with nevirapine. Dose adjustment of co-administered drug may be needed due to possible decrease in clinical effect.).
No products indexed under this heading.

Atropine Sulfate (Plasma concentrations of GI motility agents may be decreased by co-administration with nevirapine. Dose adjustment of co-administered drug may be needed due to possible decrease in clinical effect). Products include:
Donnatal Extentabs 2493

Azatadine Maleate (Plasma concentrations of GI motility agents may be decreased by co-administration with nevirapine. Dose adjustment of co-administered drug may be needed due to possible decrease in clinical effect.).
No products indexed under this heading.

Azathioprine (Plasma concentrations of immunosuppressants may be decreased by co-administration with nevirapine. Dose adjustment of co-administered drug may be needed due to possible decrease in clinical effect.).
No products indexed under this heading.

Basiliximab (Plasma concentrations of immunosuppressants may be decreased by co-administration with nevirapine. Dose adjustment of co-administered drug may be needed due to possible decrease in clinical effect). Products include:
Simulect for Injection 2284

Belladonna Alkaloids (Plasma concentrations of GI motility agents may be decreased by co-administration with nevirapine. Dose adjustment of co-administered drug may be needed due to possible decrease in clinical effect). Products include:
Hyland's Teething Tablets .... ◼◻830

Benztropine Mesylate (Plasma concentrations of GI motility agents may be decreased by co-administration with nevirapine. Dose adjustment of co-administered drug may be needed due to possible decrease in clinical effect.).
No products indexed under this heading.

Bepridil Hydrochloride (Plasma concentrations of calcium channel blockers may be decreased by co-administration with nevirapine. Dose adjustment of co-administered drug may be needed due to possible decrease in clinical effect.).
No products indexed under this heading.

Bethanechol Chloride (Plasma concentrations of GI motility agents may be decreased by co-administration with nevirapine. Dose adjustment of co-administered drug may be needed due to possible decrease in clinical effect.).
No products indexed under this heading.

Bicalutamide (Plasma concentrations of cancer chemotherapeutic agents may be decreased by co-administration with nevirapine. Dose adjustment of co-administered drug may be needed due to possible decrease in clinical effect.).
No products indexed under this heading.

Biperiden Hydrochloride (Plasma concentrations of GI motility agents may be decreased by co-administration with nevirapine. Dose adjustment of co-administered drug may be needed due to possible decrease in clinical effect.).
No products indexed under this heading.

Bitolterol Mesylate (Plasma concentrations of GI motility agents may be decreased by co-administration with nevirapine. Dose adjustment of co-administered drug may be needed due to possible decrease in clinical effect.).
No products indexed under this heading.

Bleomycin Sulfate (Plasma concentrations of cancer chemotherapeutic agents may be decreased by co-administration with nevirapine. Dose adjustment of co-administered drug may be needed due to possible decrease in clinical effect.).
No products indexed under this heading.

Bretylium Tosylate (Plasma concentrations of antiarrhythmics may be decreased by co-administration with nevirapine. Dose adjustment of co-administered drug may be needed due to possible decrease in clinical effect.).
No products indexed under this heading.

Bromocriptine Mesylate (Plasma concentrations of GI motility agents may be decreased by co-administration with nevirapine. Dose adjustment of co-administered drug may be needed due to possible decrease in clinical effect.).
No products indexed under this heading.

Bromodiphenhydramine Hydrochloride (Plasma concentrations of GI motility agents may be decreased by co-administration with nevirapine. Dose adjustment of co-administered drug may be needed due to possible decrease in clinical effect.).
No products indexed under this heading.

Brompheniramine Maleate (Plasma concentrations of GI motility agents may be decreased by co-administration with nevirapine. Dose adjustment of co-administered drug may be needed due to possible decrease in clinical effect). Products include:
Children's Dimetapp Cold & Allergy Elixir .... ◼◻730
Children's Dimetapp Cold & Allergy Chewable Tablets .... ◼◻730
Children's Dimetapp DM Cold & Cough Elixir .... ◼◻731

Buprenorphine Hydrochloride (Plasma concentrations of GI motility agents may be decreased by co-administration with nevirapine. Dose adjustment of co-administered drug may be needed due to possible decrease in clinical effect). Products include:
Buprenex Injectable 2716
Suboxone Tablets 2717
Subutex Tablets 2717

Busulfan (Plasma concentrations of cancer chemotherapeutic agents may be decreased by co-administration with nevirapine. Dose adjustment of co-administered drug may be needed due to possible decrease in clinical effect). Products include:
I.V. Busulfex 2493
Myleran Tablets 1525

Carbamazepine (Plasma concentrations of anticonvulsants may be decreased by co-administration with nevirapine. Dose adjustment of co-administered drug may be needed due to possible decrease in clinical effect). Products include:

Carbatrol Capsules 3171
Equetro Extended-Release Capsules 3180
Tegretol/Tegretol-XR 2295

Carboplatin (Plasma concentrations of cancer chemotherapeutic agents may be decreased by co-administration with nevirapine. Dose adjustment of co-administered drug may be needed due to possible decrease in clinical effect.).
No products indexed under this heading.

Carmustine (BCNU) (Plasma concentrations of cancer chemotherapeutic agents may be decreased by co-administration with nevirapine. Dose adjustment of co-administered drug may be needed due to possible decrease in clinical effect.).
No products indexed under this heading.

Cevimeline Hydrochloride (Plasma concentrations of GI motility agents may be decreased by co-administration with nevirapine. Dose adjustment of co-administered drug may be needed due to possible decrease in clinical effect). Products include:
Evoxac Capsules 1047

Chlorambucil (Plasma concentrations of cancer chemotherapeutic agents may be decreased by co-administration with nevirapine. Dose adjustment of co-administered drug may be needed due to possible decrease in clinical effect). Products include:
Leukeran Tablets 1504

Chlorpheniramine Maleate (Plasma concentrations of GI motility agents may be decreased by co-administration with nevirapine. Dose adjustment of co-administered drug may be needed due to possible decrease in clinical effect). Products include:
Advil Allergy Sinus Caplets 770
Advil Multi-Symptom Cold Caplets 770
BC Allergy Sinus Cold Powder 677
Comtrex Maximum Strength Cold & Cough Day/Night Caplets - Night Formulation 726
Comtrex Maximum Strength Day/Night Severe Cold & Sinus Caplets - Night Formulation 725
Contac Cold and Flu Maximum Strength Caplets 728
Contac Cold and Flu Day and Night Caplets (Night Formulation Only) 727
Children's Dimetapp Long Acting Cough Plus Cold Syrup 731
Robitussin Cough & Cold Long-Acting Liquid 735
Robitussin Cough & Allergy Syrup 736
Robitussin Cough & Cold Nighttime Liquid 736
Robitussin Cough, Cold & Flu Nighttime Liquid 738
Robitussin Pediatric Cough & Cold Long-Acting Liquid 735
Robitussin Pediatric Cough & Cold Nighttime Liquid 736
Triaminic Cold & Allergy Liquid 746
Triaminic Cough & Runny Nose Softchews 748
Children's Tylenol Plus Flu Oral Suspension 749
Tylenol Allergy Multi-Symptom Caplets with Cool Burst and Gelcaps 1872
Children's Tylenol Plus Cold Suspension Liquid 1879
Children's Tylenol Plus Cough & Runny Nose Suspension Liquid 1879
Children's Tylenol Plus Flu Suspension Liquid 1881
Children's Tylenol Plus Multi-Symptom Cold Suspension Liquid 1879
Tylenol Cold Head Congestion Nighttime Caplets with Cool Burst 1873
Tylenol Cold Multi-Symptom Nighttime Caplets with Cool Burst 1874
Tylenol Sinus Congestion & Pain Nighttime Caplets with Cool Burst 1876
Vicks 44M Cough, Cold & Flu Relief Liquid 2680
Pediatric Vicks 44m Cough & Cold Relief Liquid 2676
Children's Vicks NyQuil Cold/Cough Relief 756
Children's Vicks NyQuil Cold/Cough Relief Liquid 2680
Zicam Maximum Strength Flu Daytime 768

Chlorpheniramine Polistirex (Plasma concentrations of GI motility agents may be decreased by co-administration with nevirapine. Dose adjustment of co-administered drug may be needed due to possible decrease in clinical effect). Products include:
Tussionex Pennkinetic Extended-Release Suspension 3327

Chlorpheniramine Tannate (Plasma concentrations of GI motility agents may be decreased by co-administration with nevirapine. Dose adjustment of co-administered drug may be needed due to possible decrease in clinical effect.).
No products indexed under this heading.

Cisapride (Plasma concentrations of GI motility agents may be decreased by co-administration with nevirapine. Dose adjustment of co-administered drug may be needed due to possible decrease in clinical effect.).
No products indexed under this heading.

Cisplatin (Plasma concentrations of cancer chemotherapeutic agents may be decreased by co-administration with nevirapine. Dose adjustment of co-administered drug may be needed due to possible decrease in clinical effect.).
No products indexed under this heading.

Clarithromycin (Clarithromycin exposure was significantly decreased by nevirapine; however, 14-OH-metabolite concentrations were increased. Because clarithromycin active metabolite has reduced activity against Mycobacterium Avium-Intracellulare Complex, overall activity against this pathogen may be altered. Alternatives to clarithromycin, such as azithromycin, should be considered). Products include:
Biaxin/Biaxin XL 402
PREVPAC 3284

Clemastine Fumarate (Plasma concentrations of GI motility agents may be decreased by co-administration with nevirapine. Dose adjustment of co-administered drug may be needed due to possible decrease in clinical effect.).
No products indexed under this heading.

Clidinium Bromide (Plasma concentrations of GI motility agents may be decreased by co-administration with nevirapine. Dose adjustment of co-administered drug may be needed due to possible decrease in clinical effect.).
No products indexed under this heading.

Clomipramine Hydrochloride (Plasma concentrations of GI motility agents may be decreased by co-administration with nevirapine. Dose adjustment of co-administered drug may be needed due to possible decrease in clinical effect.).
No products indexed under this heading.

Clotrimazole (Plasma concentrations of antifungals may be decreased by co-administration with nevirapine. Dose adjustment of co-administered drug may be needed due to possible decrease in clinical effect). Products include:
Desenex Athlete's Foot Cream 635
Lotrimin 3039
Lotrisone 3040

Codeine Phosphate (Plasma concentrations of GI motility agents may be decreased by co-administration with nevirapine. Dose adjustment of co-administered drug may be needed due to possible decrease in clinical effect). Products include:
Tylenol with Codeine Tablets 2391

Cyclophosphamide (Plasma concentrations of cancer chemotherapeutic agents may be decreased by co-administration with nevirapine. Dose adjustment of co-administered drug may be needed due to possible decrease in clinical effect.).
No products indexed under this heading.

Cyclosporine (Plasma concentrations of immunosuppressants may be decreased by co-administration with nevirapine. Dose adjustment of co-administered drug may be needed due to possible decrease in clinical effect). Products include:
Gengraf Capsules 459
Neoral Oral Solution 2259
Neoral Soft Gelatin Capsules 2259
Restasis Ophthalmic Emulsion 575
Sandimmune 2275

Cyproheptadine Hydrochloride (Plasma concentrations of GI motility agents may be decreased by co-administration with nevirapine. Dose adjustment of co-administered drug may be needed due to possible decrease in clinical effect.).
No products indexed under this heading.

Dacarbazine (Plasma concentrations of cancer chemotherapeutic agents may be decreased by co-administration with nevirapine. Dose adjustment of co-administered drug may be needed due to possible decrease in clinical effect.).
No products indexed under this heading.

Dalteparin Sodium (Plasma concentrations of antithrombotics may be increased by co-administration with nevirapine. Dose adjustment of co-administered drug may be needed due to possible decrease in clinical effect). Products include:
Fragmin Injection 1097

Danaparoid Sodium (Plasma concentrations of antithrombotics may be increased by co-administration with nevirapine. Dose adjustment of co-administered drug may be needed due to possible decrease in clinical effect.).
No products indexed under this heading.

Daunorubicin Citrate (Plasma concentrations of cancer chemotherapeutic agents may be decreased by co-administration with nevirapine. Dose adjustment of co-administered drug may be needed due to possible decrease in clinical effect.).
No products indexed under this heading.

Daunorubicin Hydrochloride (Plasma concentrations of cancer chemotherapeutic agents may be decreased by co-administration with nevirapine. Dose adjustment of co-administered drug may be needed due to possible decrease in clinical effect.).
No products indexed under this heading.

Denileukin Diftitox (Plasma concentrations of cancer chemotherapeutic agents may be decreased by co-administration with nevirapine. Dose adjustment of co-administered drug may be needed due to possible decrease in clinical effect). Products include:
Ontak Vials 1745

Desipramine Hydrochloride (Plasma concentrations of GI motility agents may be decreased by co-administration with nevirapine. Dose adjustment of co-administered drug may be needed due to possible decrease in clinical effect.).
No products indexed under this heading.

Desogestrel (Oral contraceptives and other hormonal methods of birth control should not be used as the sole method of contraception in women taking nevirapine, may lower plasma levels of these medications. An alternative or additional method of contraception is recommended). Products include:
Mircette Tablets 1066

Dexchlorpheniramine Maleate (Plasma concentrations of GI motility agents may be decreased by co-administration with nevirapine. Dose adjustment of co-administered drug may be needed due to possible decrease in clinical effect.).
No products indexed under this heading.

Dezocine (Plasma concentrations of GI motility agents may be decreased by co-administration with nevirapine. Dose adjustment of co-administered drug may be needed due to possible decrease in clinical effect.).
No products indexed under this heading.

Dicumarol (Plasma concentrations of antithrombotics may be increased by co-administration with nevirapine. Dose adjustment of co-administered drug may be needed due to possible decrease in clinical effect.).
No products indexed under this heading.

Dicyclomine Hydrochloride (Plasma concentrations of GI motility agents may be decreased by co-administration with nevirapine. Dose adjustment of co-administered drug may be needed due to possible decrease in clinical effect). Products include:
Bentyl Capsules 697
Bentyl Injection 697
Bentyl Syrup 697
Bentyl Tablets 697

Dihydroergotamine Mesylate (Plasma concentrations of ergot alkaloids may be decreased by co-administration with nevirapine. Dose adjustment of co-administered drug may be needed due to possible decrease in clinical effect). Products include:

Migranal Nasal Spray 3348

Diltiazem Hydrochloride (Plasma concentrations of calcium channel blockers may be decreased by co-administration with nevirapine. Dose adjustment of co-administered drug may be needed due to possible decrease in clinical effect). Products include:

Cardizem LA Extended Release Tablets 1728
Tiazac Capsules 1201

Diphenhydramine Citrate (Plasma concentrations of GI motility agents may be decreased by co-administration with nevirapine. Dose adjustment of co-administered drug may be needed due to possible decrease in clinical effect). Products include:

Advil PM Caplets .... ▣615
Excedrin PM Caplets/Tablets/Geltabs .... ▣610
Goody's PM Powder for Pain with Sleeplessness .... ▣612

Diphenhydramine Hydrochloride (Plasma concentrations of GI motility agents may be decreased by co-administration with nevirapine. Dose adjustment of co-administered drug may be needed due to possible decrease in clinical effect). Products include:

Nytol QuickCaps Caplets .... ▣615
Nytol QuickGels Softgels Maximum Strength .... ▣616
Simply Sleep Caplets 1868
Sominex Original Formula Tablets .. ▣616
TheraFlu Warming Relief Nighttime Severe Cold .... ▣743
TheraFlu Thin Strips Multi Symptom .... ▣744
Triaminic Nighttime Cold & Cough Liquid .... ▣746
Triaminic Thin Strips Cough & Runny Nose .... ▣749
Extra Strength Tylenol PM Caplets, Vanilla Caplets, Geltabs, Gelcaps and Liquid 1875
Tylenol Sore Throat Nighttime Liquid with Cool Burst .... ▣790
Tylenol Allergy Multi-Symptom Nighttime Caplets with Cool Burst 1872
Tylenol Severe Allergy Caplets 1872
Children's Tylenol Plus Cold & Allergy Suspension Liquid 1878

Diphenylpyraline Hydrochloride (Plasma concentrations of GI motility agents may be decreased by co-administration with nevirapine. Dose adjustment of co-administered drug may be needed due to possible decrease in clinical effect.).

No products indexed under this heading.

Disopyramide Phosphate (Plasma concentrations of antiarrhythmics may be decreased by co-administration with nevirapine. Dose adjustment of co-administered drug may be needed due to possible decrease in clinical effect.).

No products indexed under this heading.

Divalproex Sodium (Plasma concentrations of anticonvulsants may be decreased by co-administration with nevirapine. Dose adjustment of co-administered drug may be needed due to possible decrease in clinical effect). Products include:

Depakote Sprinkle Capsules 422
Depakote Tablets 427
Depakote ER Tablets 434

Dobutamine (Plasma concentrations of GI motility agents may be decreased by co-administration with nevirapine. Dose adjustment of co-administered drug may be needed due to possible decrease in clinical effect.).

No products indexed under this heading.

Dobutamine Hydrochloride (Plasma concentrations of GI motility agents may be decreased by co-administration with nevirapine. Dose adjustment of co-administered drug may be needed due to possible decrease in clinical effect.).

No products indexed under this heading.

Docetaxel (Plasma concentrations of cancer chemotherapeutic agents may be decreased by co-administration with nevirapine. Dose adjustment of co-administered drug may be needed due to possible decrease in clinical effect). Products include:

Taxotere Injection Concentrate 2932

Dofetilide (Plasma concentrations of antiarrhythmics may be decreased by co-administration with nevirapine. Dose adjustment of co-administered drug may be needed due to possible decrease in clinical effect.).

No products indexed under this heading.

Domperidone (Plasma concentrations of GI motility agents may be decreased by co-administration with nevirapine. Dose adjustment of co-administered drug may be needed due to possible decrease in clinical effect.).

No products indexed under this heading.

Donepezil Hydrochloride (Plasma concentrations of GI motility agents may be decreased by co-administration with nevirapine. Dose adjustment of co-administered drug may be needed due to possible decrease in clinical effect). Products include:

Aricept Tablets 1094
Aricept ODT Tablets 1094

Dopamine Hydrochloride (Plasma concentrations of GI motility agents may be decreased by co-administration with nevirapine. Dose adjustment of co-administered drug may be needed due to possible decrease in clinical effect.).

No products indexed under this heading.

Doxepin Hydrochloride (Plasma concentrations of GI motility agents may be decreased by co-administration with nevirapine. Dose adjustment of co-administered drug may be needed due to possible decrease in clinical effect.).

No products indexed under this heading.

Doxorubicin Hydrochloride (Plasma concentrations of cancer chemotherapeutic agents may be decreased by co-administration with nevirapine. Dose adjustment of co-administered drug may be needed due to possible decrease in clinical effect.).

No products indexed under this heading.

Edrophonium Chloride (Plasma concentrations of GI motility agents may be decreased by co-administration with nevirapine. Dose adjustment of co-administered drug may be needed due to possible decrease in clinical effect.).

No products indexed under this heading.

Efavirenz (Efavirenz plasma concentration levels are decreased when used concomitantly with nevirapine. Appropriate doses for this combination are not established). Products include:

Atripla Tablets 945
Sustiva Capsules 930
Sustiva Tablets 930

Enoxaparin Sodium (Plasma concentrations of antithrombotics may be increased by co-administration with nevirapine. Dose adjustment of co-administered drug may be needed due to possible decrease in clinical effect). Products include:

Lovenox Injection 2915

Ephedrine Hydrochloride (Plasma concentrations of GI motility agents may be decreased by co-administration with nevirapine. Dose adjustment of co-administered drug may be needed due to possible decrease in clinical effect.).

No products indexed under this heading.

Ephedrine Sulfate (Plasma concentrations of GI motility agents may be decreased by co-administration with nevirapine. Dose adjustment of co-administered drug may be needed due to possible decrease in clinical effect.).

No products indexed under this heading.

Ephedrine Tannate (Plasma concentrations of GI motility agents may be decreased by co-administration with nevirapine. Dose adjustment of co-administered drug may be needed due to possible decrease in clinical effect.).

No products indexed under this heading.

Epinephrine (Plasma concentrations of GI motility agents may be decreased by co-administration with nevirapine. Dose adjustment of co-administered drug may be needed due to possible decrease in clinical effect). Products include:

EpiPen 1061
Primatene Mist .... ▣719
Twinject 0.15 3379
Twinject 0.3 3378

Epinephrine Hydrochloride (Plasma concentrations of GI motility agents may be decreased by co-administration with nevirapine. Dose adjustment of co-administered drug may be needed due to possible decrease in clinical effect.).

No products indexed under this heading.

Epirubicin Hydrochloride (Plasma concentrations of cancer chemotherapeutic agents may be decreased by co-administration with nevirapine. Dose adjustment of co-administered drug may be needed due to possible decrease in clinical effect.).

No products indexed under this heading.

Ergonovine Maleate (Plasma concentrations of ergot alkaloids may be decreased by co-administration with nevirapine. Dose adjustment of co-administered drug may be needed due to possible decrease in clinical effect.).

No products indexed under this heading.

Ergotamine Tartrate (Plasma concentrations of ergot alkaloids may be decreased by co-administration with nevirapine. Dose adjustment of co-administered drug may be needed due to possible decrease in clinical effect.).

No products indexed under this heading.

Erythromycin (Plasma concentrations of GI motility agents may be decreased by co-administration with nevirapine. Dose adjustment of co-administered drug may be needed due to possible decrease in clinical effect). Products include:

Ery-Tab Tablets 449
Erythromycin Base Filmtab Tablets 455
Erythromycin Delayed-Release Capsules, USP 457
PCE Dispertab Tablets 515

Erythromycin Estolate (Plasma concentrations of GI motility agents may be decreased by co-administration with nevirapine. Dose adjustment of co-administered drug may be needed due to possible decrease in clinical effect.).

No products indexed under this heading.

Erythromycin Ethylsuccinate (Plasma concentrations of GI motility agents may be decreased by co-administration with nevirapine. Dose adjustment of co-administered drug may be needed due to possible decrease in clinical effect). Products include:

E.E.S. 451
EryPed 447

Erythromycin Gluceptate (Plasma concentrations of GI motility agents may be decreased by co-administration with nevirapine. Dose adjustment of co-administered drug may be needed due to possible decrease in clinical effect.).

No products indexed under this heading.

Erythromycin Stearate (Plasma concentrations of GI motility agents may be decreased by co-administration with nevirapine. Dose adjustment of co-administered drug may be needed due to possible decrease in clinical effect). Products include:

Erythrocin Stearate Filmtab Tablets 453

Estramustine Phosphate Sodium (Plasma concentrations of cancer chemotherapeutic agents may be decreased by co-administration with nevirapine. Dose adjustment of co-administered drug may be needed due to possible decrease in clinical effect). Products include:

Emcyt Capsules 2634

Ethinyl Estradiol (When ethinyl estradiol and Viramune are co-administered, the AUC for ethinyl estradiol is decreased by 20%). Products include:

Mircette Tablets 1066
NuvaRing 2340
Ortho-Cyclen/Ortho Tri-Cyclen 2429
Ortho Evra Transdermal System 2417
Ortho Tri-Cyclen Lo Tablets 2436

Seasonique Tablets 1077
Yasmin 28 Tablets 796
Yaz Tablets 803

Ethosuximide (Plasma concentrations of anticonvulsants may be decreased by co-administration with nevirapine. Dose adjustment of co-administered drug may be needed due to possible decrease in clinical effect.).
No products indexed under this heading.

Ethotoin (Plasma concentrations of anticonvulsants may be decreased by co-administration with nevirapine. Dose adjustment of co-administered drug may be needed due to possible decrease in clinical effect.).
No products indexed under this heading.

Ethynodiol Diacetate (Oral contraceptives and other hormonal methods of birth control should not be used as the sole method of contraception in women taking nevirapine, may lower plasma levels of these medications. An alternative or additional method of contraception is recommended.).
No products indexed under this heading.

Etoposide (Plasma concentrations of cancer chemotherapeutic agents may be decreased by co-administration with nevirapine. Dose adjustment of co-administered drug may be needed due to possible decrease in clinical effect.).
No products indexed under this heading.

Exemestane (Plasma concentrations of cancer chemotherapeutic agents may be decreased by co-administration with nevirapine. Dose adjustment of co-administered drug may be needed due to possible decrease in clinical effect). Products include:
Aromasin Tablets 2600

Felbamate (Plasma concentrations of anticonvulsants may be decreased by co-administration with nevirapine. Dose adjustment of co-administered drug may be needed due to possible decrease in clinical effect.).
No products indexed under this heading.

Felodipine (Plasma concentrations of calcium channel blockers may be decreased by co-administration with nevirapine. Dose adjustment of co-administered drug may be needed due to possible decrease in clinical effect.).
No products indexed under this heading.

Fentanyl (Plasma concentrations of GI motility agents may be decreased by co-administration with nevirapine. Dose adjustment of co-administered drug may be needed due to possible decrease in clinical effect). Products include:
Duragesic Transdermal System 2373
Ionsys Transdermal System 2379

Fentanyl Citrate (Plasma concentrations of GI motility agents may be decreased by co-administration with nevirapine. Dose adjustment of co-administered drug may be needed due to possible decrease in clinical effect). Products include:
Actiq 979

Flecainide Acetate (Plasma concentrations of antiarrhythmics may be decreased by co-administration with nevirapine. Dose adjustment of co-administered drug may be needed due to possible decrease in clinical effect). Products include:
Tambocor Tablets 1856

Floxuridine (Plasma concentrations of cancer chemotherapeutic agents may be decreased by co-administration with nevirapine. Dose adjustment of co-administered drug may be needed due to possible decrease in clinical effect.).
No products indexed under this heading.

Fluconazole (Administration of fluconazole resulted in an approximate 100% increase in nevirapine exposure, based on a comparison to historic data. Because of the risk of increased exposure to nevirapine, caution should be used in concomitant administration, and patients should be monitored closely for nevirapine associated adverse events.).
No products indexed under this heading.

Fluorouracil (Plasma concentrations of cancer chemotherapeutic agents may be decreased by co-administration with nevirapine. Dose adjustment of co-administered drug may be needed due to possible decrease in clinical effect). Products include:
Carac Cream, 0.5% 2879
Efudex 3363

Flutamide (Plasma concentrations of cancer chemotherapeutic agents may be decreased by co-administration with nevirapine. Dose adjustment of co-administered drug may be needed due to possible decrease in clinical effect). Products include:
Eulexin Capsules 3009

Fondaparinux Sodium (Plasma concentrations of antithrombotics may be increased by co-administration with nevirapine. Dose adjustment of co-administered drug may be needed due to possible decrease in clinical effect). Products include:
Arixtra Injection 1351

Fosphenytoin (Plasma concentrations of anticonvulsants may be decreased by co-administration with nevirapine. Dose adjustment of co-administered drug may be needed due to possible decrease in clinical effect.).
No products indexed under this heading.

Fosphenytoin Sodium (Plasma concentrations of anticonvulsants may be decreased by co-administration with nevirapine. Dose adjustment of co-administered drug may be needed due to possible decrease in clinical effect.).
No products indexed under this heading.

Gabapentin (Plasma concentrations of anticonvulsants may be decreased by co-administration with nevirapine. Dose adjustment of co-administered drug may be needed due to possible decrease in clinical effect). Products include:
Neurontin Capsules 2487
Neurontin Oral Solution 2487
Neurontin Tablets 2487

Galantamine Hydrobromide (Plasma concentrations of GI motility agents may be decreased by co-administration with nevirapine. Dose adjustment of co-administered drug may be needed due to possible decrease in clinical effect). Products include:
Razadyne 2399
Razadyne ER Extended-Release Capsules 2399

Gemcitabine Hydrochloride (Plasma concentrations of cancer chemotherapeutic agents may be decreased by co-administration with nevirapine. Dose adjustment of co-administered drug may be needed due to possible decrease in clinical effect). Products include:
Gemzar for Injection 1771

Glycopyrrolate (Plasma concentrations of GI motility agents may be decreased by co-administration with nevirapine. Dose adjustment of co-administered drug may be needed due to possible decrease in clinical effect.).
No products indexed under this heading.

Heparin Calcium (Plasma concentrations of antithrombotics may be increased by co-administration with nevirapine. Dose adjustment of co-administered drug may be needed due to possible decrease in clinical effect.).
No products indexed under this heading.

Heparin Sodium (Plasma concentrations of antithrombotics may be increased by co-administration with nevirapine. Dose adjustment of co-administered drug may be needed due to possible decrease in clinical effect.).
No products indexed under this heading.

Hydrocodone Bitartrate (Plasma concentrations of GI motility agents may be decreased by co-administration with nevirapine. Dose adjustment of co-administered drug may be needed due to possible decrease in clinical effect). Products include:
Hycodan 1116
Hycotuss Expectorant Syrup 1117
Vicodin Tablets 535
Vicodin ES Tablets 536
Vicodin HP Tablets 538
Vicoprofen Tablets 539
Zydone Tablets 1139

Hydrocodone Polistirex (Plasma concentrations of GI motility agents may be decreased by co-administration with nevirapine. Dose adjustment of co-administered drug may be needed due to possible decrease in clinical effect). Products include:
Tussionex Pennkinetic Extended-Release Suspension 3327

Hydromorphone Hydrochloride (Plasma concentrations of GI motility agents may be decreased by co-administration with nevirapine. Dose adjustment of co-administered drug may be needed due to possible decrease in clinical effect). Products include:
Dilaudid 440
Dilaudid Non-Sterile Powder 440
Dilaudid Oral Liquid 445
Dilaudid Rectal Suppositories 440
Dilaudid Tablets 440
Dilaudid Tablets - 8 mg 445
Dilaudid-HP 442

Hydroxyurea (Plasma concentrations of cancer chemotherapeutic agents may be decreased by co-administration with nevirapine. Dose adjustment of co-administered drug may be needed due to possible decrease in clinical effect.).
No products indexed under this heading.

Hyoscyamine (Plasma concentrations of GI motility agents may be decreased by co-administration with nevirapine. Dose adjustment of co-administered drug may be needed due to possible decrease in clinical effect.).
No products indexed under this heading.

Hyoscyamine Sulfate (Plasma concentrations of GI motility agents may be decreased by co-administration with nevirapine. Dose adjustment of co-administered drug may be needed due to possible decrease in clinical effect). Products include:
Donnatal Extentabs 2493
Prosed/DS Tablets 1157

Idarubicin Hydrochloride (Plasma concentrations of cancer chemotherapeutic agents may be decreased by co-administration with nevirapine. Dose adjustment of co-administered drug may be needed due to possible decrease in clinical effect.).
No products indexed under this heading.

Ifosfamide (Plasma concentrations of cancer chemotherapeutic agents may be decreased by co-administration with nevirapine. Dose adjustment of co-administered drug may be needed due to possible decrease in clinical effect.).
No products indexed under this heading.

Imipramine Hydrochloride (Plasma concentrations of GI motility agents may be decreased by co-administration with nevirapine. Dose adjustment of co-administered drug may be needed due to possible decrease in clinical effect.).
No products indexed under this heading.

Imipramine Pamoate (Plasma concentrations of GI motility agents may be decreased by co-administration with nevirapine. Dose adjustment of co-administered drug may be needed due to possible decrease in clinical effect.).
No products indexed under this heading.

Indinavir Sulfate (Appropriate doses for this combination are not established, but an increase in the dosage of indinavir may be required). Products include:
Crixivan Capsules 1940

Interferon alfa-2a, Recombinant (Plasma concentrations of cancer chemotherapeutic agents may be decreased by co-administration with nevirapine. Dose adjustment of co-administered drug may be needed due to possible decrease in clinical effect.).
No products indexed under this heading.

Interferon alfa-2b, Recombinant (Plasma concentrations of cancer chemotherapeutic agents may be decreased by co-administration with nevirapine. Dose adjustment of co-administered drug may be needed due to possible decrease in clinical effect). Products include:

Ipratropium Bromide (Plasma concentrations of GI motility agents may be decreased by co-administration with nevirapine. Dose adjustment of co-administered drug may be needed due to possible decrease in clinical effect). Products include:

Irinotecan Hydrochloride (Plasma concentrations of cancer chemotherapeutic agents may be decreased by co-administration with nevirapine. Dose adjustment of co-administered drug may be needed due to possible decrease in clinical effect). Products include:

Isoetharine (Plasma concentrations of GI motility agents may be decreased by co-administration with nevirapine. Dose adjustment of co-administered drug may be needed due to possible decrease in clinical effect.).

No products indexed under this heading.

Isoproterenol Hydrochloride (Plasma concentrations of GI motility agents may be decreased by co-administration with nevirapine. Dose adjustment of co-administered drug may be needed due to possible decrease in clinical effect.).

No products indexed under this heading.

Isoproterenol Sulfate (Plasma concentrations of GI motility agents may be decreased by co-administration with nevirapine. Dose adjustment of co-administered drug may be needed due to possible decrease in clinical effect.).

No products indexed under this heading.

Isradipine (Plasma concentrations of calcium channel blockers may be decreased by co-administration with nevirapine. Dose adjustment of co-administered drug may be needed due to possible decrease in clinical effect). Products include:

Itraconazole (Plasma concentrations of antifungals may be decreased by co-administration with nevirapine. Dose adjustment of co-administered drug may be needed due to possible decrease in clinical effect.).

No products indexed under this heading.

Ketoconazole (Nevirapine and ketoconazole should not be administered concomitantly because decreases in ketoconazole plasma concentrations may reduce the efficacy of the drug). Products include:

Lamotrigine (Plasma concentrations of anticonvulsants may be decreased by co-administration with nevirapine. Dose adjustment of co-administered drug may be needed due to possible decrease in clinical effect). Products include:

Levalbuterol Hydrochloride (Plasma concentrations of GI motility agents may be decreased by co-administration with nevirapine. Dose adjustment of co-administered drug may be needed due to possible decrease in clinical effect). Products include:

Levamisole Hydrochloride (Plasma concentrations of cancer chemotherapeutic agents may be decreased by co-administration with nevirapine. Dose adjustment of co-administered drug may be needed due to possible decrease in clinical effect.).

No products indexed under this heading.

Levetiracetam (Plasma concentrations of anticonvulsants may be decreased by co-administration with nevirapine. Dose adjustment of co-administered drug may be needed due to possible decrease in clinical effect). Products include:

Levonorgestrel (Oral contraceptives and other hormonal methods of birth control should not be used as the sole method of contraception in women taking nevirapine, may lower plasma levels of these medications. An alternative or additional method of contraception is recommended). Products include:

Levorphanol Tartrate (Plasma concentrations of GI motility agents may be decreased by co-administration with nevirapine. Dose adjustment of co-administered drug may be needed due to possible decrease in clinical effect.).

No products indexed under this heading.

Lidocaine Hydrochloride (Plasma concentrations of antiarrhythmics may be decreased by co-administration with nevirapine. Dose adjustment of co-administered drug may be needed due to possible decrease in clinical effect.).

No products indexed under this heading.

Lomustine (CCNU) (Plasma concentrations of cancer chemotherapeutic agents may be decreased by co-administration with nevirapine. Dose adjustment of co-administered drug may be needed due to possible decrease in clinical effect.).

No products indexed under this heading.

Lopinavir (A dose increase of lopinavir/ritonavir to 533/133 mg twice daily with food is recommended in combination with nevirapine). Products include:

Low Molecular Weight Heparins (Plasma concentrations of antithrombotics may be increased by co-administration with nevirapine. Dose adjustment of co-administered drug may be needed due to possible decrease in clinical effect.).

No products indexed under this heading.

Maprotiline Hydrochloride (Plasma concentrations of GI motility agents may be decreased by co-administration with nevirapine. Dose adjustment of co-administered drug may be needed due to possible decrease in clinical effect.).

No products indexed under this heading.

Mechlorethamine Hydrochloride (Plasma concentrations of cancer chemotherapeutic agents may be decreased by co-administration with nevirapine. Dose adjustment of co-administered drug may be needed due to possible decrease in clinical effect). Products include:

Megestrol Acetate (Plasma concentrations of cancer chemotherapeutic agents may be decreased by co-administration with nevirapine. Dose adjustment of co-administered drug may be needed due to possible decrease in clinical effect). Products include:

Melphalan (Plasma concentrations of cancer chemotherapeutic agents may be decreased by co-administration with nevirapine. Dose adjustment of co-administered drug may be needed due to possible decrease in clinical effect). Products include:

Mepenzolate Bromide (Plasma concentrations of GI motility agents may be decreased by co-administration with nevirapine. Dose adjustment of co-administered drug may be needed due to possible decrease in clinical effect.).

No products indexed under this heading.

Meperidine Hydrochloride (Plasma concentrations of GI motility agents may be decreased by co-administration with nevirapine. Dose adjustment of co-administered drug may be needed due to possible decrease in clinical effect.).

No products indexed under this heading.

Mephenytoin (Plasma concentrations of anticonvulsants may be decreased by co-administration with nevirapine. Dose adjustment of co-administered drug may be needed due to possible decrease in clinical effect.).

No products indexed under this heading.

Mercaptopurine (Plasma concentrations of cancer chemotherapeutic agents may be decreased by co-administration with nevirapine. Dose adjustment of co-administered drug may be needed due to possible decrease in clinical effect.).

No products indexed under this heading.

Mestranol (Oral contraceptives and other hormonal methods of birth control should not be used as the sole method of contraception in women taking nevirapine, may lower plasma levels of these medications. An alternative or additional method of contraception is recommended.).

No products indexed under this heading.

Metaproterenol Sulfate (Plasma concentrations of GI motility agents may be decreased by co-administration with nevirapine. Dose adjustment of co-administered drug

may be needed due to possible decrease in clinical effect). Products include:

Methadone Hydrochloride (Methadone levels may be decreased; increased dosages may be required to prevent symptoms of opiate withdrawal. Methadone maintained patients beginning nevirapine therapy should be monitored for evidence of withdrawal and methadone dose should be adjusted accordingly.).

No products indexed under this heading.

Methdilazine Hydrochloride (Plasma concentrations of GI motility agents may be decreased by co-administration with nevirapine. Dose adjustment of co-administered drug may be needed due to possible decrease in clinical effect.).

No products indexed under this heading.

Methotrexate Sodium (Plasma concentrations of cancer chemotherapeutic agents may be decreased by co-administration with nevirapine. Dose adjustment of co-administered drug may be needed due to possible decrease in clinical effect.).

No products indexed under this heading.

Methsuximide (Plasma concentrations of anticonvulsants may be decreased by co-administration with nevirapine. Dose adjustment of co-administered drug may be needed due to possible decrease in clinical effect.).

No products indexed under this heading.

Methylergonovine Maleate (Plasma concentrations of ergot alkaloids may be decreased by co-administration with nevirapine. Dose adjustment of co-administered drug may be needed due to possible decrease in clinical effect.).

No products indexed under this heading.

Methysergide Maleate (Plasma concentrations of ergot alkaloids may be decreased by co-administration with nevirapine. Dose adjustment of co-administered drug may be needed due to possible decrease in clinical effect.).

No products indexed under this heading.

Metoclopramide Hydrochloride (Plasma concentrations of GI motility agents may be decreased by co-administration with nevirapine. Dose adjustment of co-administered drug may be needed due to possible decrease in clinical effect.).

No products indexed under this heading.

Mexiletine Hydrochloride (Plasma concentrations of antiarrhythmics may be decreased by co-administration with nevirapine. Dose adjustment of co-administered drug may be needed due to possible decrease in clinical effect.).

No products indexed under this heading.

Mibefradil Dihydrochloride (Plasma concentrations of calcium channel blockers may be decreased by co-administration with nevirapine. Dose adjustment of co-administered drug may be needed due to possible decrease in clinical effect.).

No products indexed under this heading.

Miconazole (Plasma concentrations of antifungals may be decreased by co-administration with nevirapine. Dose adjustment of co-administered drug may be needed due to possible decrease in clinical effect.).
No products indexed under this heading.

Mitomycin (Mitomycin-C) (Plasma concentrations of cancer chemotherapeutic agents may be decreased by co-administration with nevirapine. Dose adjustment of co-administered drug may be needed due to possible decrease in clinical effect.).
No products indexed under this heading.

Mitotane (Plasma concentrations of cancer chemotherapeutic agents may be decreased by co-administration with nevirapine. Dose adjustment of co-administered drug may be needed due to possible decrease in clinical effect.).
No products indexed under this heading.

Mitoxantrone Hydrochloride (Plasma concentrations of cancer chemotherapeutic agents may be decreased by co-administration with nevirapine. Dose adjustment of co-administered drug may be needed due to possible decrease in clinical effect.).
No products indexed under this heading.

Moricizine Hydrochloride (Plasma concentrations of antiarrhythmics may be decreased by co-administration with nevirapine. Dose adjustment of co-administered drug may be needed due to possible decrease in clinical effect.).
No products indexed under this heading.

Morphine Sulfate (Plasma concentrations of GI motility agents may be decreased by co-administration with nevirapine. Dose adjustment of co-administered drug may be needed due to possible decrease in clinical effect). Products include:
Avinza Capsules 1741
Kadian Capsules 577
MS Contin Tablets 2701

Muromonab-CD3 (Plasma concentrations of immunosuppressants may be decreased by co-administration with nevirapine. Dose adjustment of co-administered drug may be needed due to possible decrease in clinical effect). Products include:
Orthoclone OKT3 Sterile Solution 2360

Mycophenolate Mofetil (Plasma concentrations of immunosuppressants may be decreased by co-administration with nevirapine. Dose adjustment of co-administered drug may be needed due to possible decrease in clinical effect). Products include:
CellCept Capsules 2747
CellCept Oral Suspension 2747
CellCept Tablets 2747

Nelfinavir Mesylate (When nelfinavir and Viramune are co-administered, the plasma concentrations of nelfinavir and the nelfinavir-M8 metabolite are decreased. The appropriate dose for nelfinavir in combination with nevirapine, with respect to safety and efficacy, has not been established). Products include:
Viracept 2577

Neostigmine Bromide (Plasma concentrations of GI motility agents may be decreased by co-administration with nevirapine. Dose adjustment of co-administered drug may be needed due to possible decrease in clinical effect.).
No products indexed under this heading.

Neostigmine Methylsulfate (Plasma concentrations of GI motility agents may be decreased by co-administration with nevirapine. Dose adjustment of co-administered drug may be needed due to possible decrease in clinical effect.).
No products indexed under this heading.

Nicardipine Hydrochloride (Plasma concentrations of calcium channel blockers may be decreased by co-administration with nevirapine. Dose adjustment of co-administered drug may be needed due to possible decrease in clinical effect). Products include:
Cardene I.V. 2497

Nifedipine (Plasma concentrations of calcium channel blockers may be decreased by co-administration with nevirapine. Dose adjustment of co-administered drug may be needed due to possible decrease in clinical effect). Products include:
Adalat CC Tablets 2964

Nimodipine (Plasma concentrations of calcium channel blockers may be decreased by co-administration with nevirapine. Dose adjustment of co-administered drug may be needed due to possible decrease in clinical effect). Products include:
Nimotop Capsules 749

Nisoldipine (Plasma concentrations of calcium channel blockers may be decreased by co-administration with nevirapine. Dose adjustment of co-administered drug may be needed due to possible decrease in clinical effect). Products include:
Sular Tablets 3122

Norethindrone (When norethindrone and Viramune are co-administered, the AUC and Cmax for norethindrone are decreased by 19% and 16%, respectively). Products include:
Ortho Micronor Tablets 2426

Norethynodrel (Oral contraceptives and other hormonal methods of birth control should not be used as the sole method of contraception in women taking nevirapine, may lower plasma levels of these medications. An alternative or additional method of contraception is recommended.).
No products indexed under this heading.

Norgestimate (Oral contraceptives and other hormonal methods of birth control should not be used as the sole method of contraception in women taking nevirapine, may lower plasma levels of these medications. An alternative or additional method of contraception is recommended). Products include:
Ortho-Cyclen/Ortho Tri-Cyclen 2429
Ortho Tri-Cyclen Lo Tablets 2436

Norgestrel (Oral contraceptives and other hormonal methods of birth control should not be used as the sole method of contraception in women taking nevirapine, may lower plasma levels of these medications. An alternative or additional method of contraception is recommended.).
No products indexed under this heading.

Nortriptyline Hydrochloride (Plasma concentrations of GI motility agents may be decreased by co-administration with nevirapine. Dose adjustment of co-administered drug may be needed due to possible decrease in clinical effect.).
No products indexed under this heading.

Octreotide Acetate (Plasma concentrations of GI motility agents may be decreased by co-administration with nevirapine. Dose adjustment of co-administered drug may be needed due to possible decrease in clinical effect). Products include:
Sandostatin Injection 2278
Sandostatin LAR Depot 2280

Oxaliplatin (Plasma concentrations of cancer chemotherapeutic agents may be decreased by co-administration with nevirapine. Dose adjustment of co-administered drug may be needed due to possible decrease in clinical effect). Products include:
Eloxatin for Injection 2892

Oxcarbazepine (Plasma concentrations of anticonvulsants may be decreased by co-administration with nevirapine. Dose adjustment of co-administered drug may be needed due to possible decrease in clinical effect). Products include:
Trileptal Tablets 2300
Trileptal Oral Suspension 2300

Oxiconazole Nitrate (Plasma concentrations of antifungals may be decreased by co-administration with nevirapine. Dose adjustment of co-administered drug may be needed due to possible decrease in clinical effect). Products include:
Oxistat 2667

Oxybutynin Chloride (Plasma concentrations of GI motility agents may be decreased by co-administration with nevirapine. Dose adjustment of co-administered drug may be needed due to possible decrease in clinical effect). Products include:
Ditropan XL Extended-Release Tablets 2413

Oxycodone Hydrochloride (Plasma concentrations of GI motility agents may be decreased by co-administration with nevirapine. Dose adjustment of co-administered drug may be needed due to possible decrease in clinical effect). Products include:
OxyContin Tablets 2703
OxyFast Oral Concentrate Solution 2708
OxyIR Capsules 2708
Percocet Tablets 1131
Percodan Tablets 1132

Oxyphenonium Bromide (Plasma concentrations of GI motility agents may be decreased by co-administration with nevirapine. Dose adjustment of co-administered drug may be needed due to possible decrease in clinical effect.).
No products indexed under this heading.

Paclitaxel (Plasma concentrations of cancer chemotherapeutic agents may be decreased by co-administration with nevirapine. Dose adjustment of co-administered drug may be needed due to possible decrease in clinical effect.).
No products indexed under this heading.

Paramethadione (Plasma concentrations of anticonvulsants may be decreased by co-administration with nevirapine. Dose adjustment of co-administered drug may be needed due to possible decrease in clinical effect.).
No products indexed under this heading.

Pergolide Mesylate (Plasma concentrations of GI motility agents may be decreased by co-administration with nevirapine. Dose adjustment of co-administered drug may be needed due to possible decrease in clinical effect). Products include:
Permax Tablets 3356

Phenacemide (Plasma concentrations of anticonvulsants may be decreased by co-administration with nevirapine. Dose adjustment of co-administered drug may be needed due to possible decrease in clinical effect.).
No products indexed under this heading.

Phenobarbital (Plasma concentrations of anticonvulsants may be decreased by co-administration with nevirapine. Dose adjustment of co-administered drug may be needed due to possible decrease in clinical effect). Products include:
Donnatal Extentabs 2493

Phensuximide (Plasma concentrations of anticonvulsants may be decreased by co-administration with nevirapine. Dose adjustment of co-administered drug may be needed due to possible decrease in clinical effect.).
No products indexed under this heading.

Phenytoin (Plasma concentrations of anticonvulsants may be decreased by co-administration with nevirapine. Dose adjustment of co-administered drug may be needed due to possible decrease in clinical effect.).
No products indexed under this heading.

Phenytoin Sodium (Plasma concentrations of anticonvulsants may be decreased by co-administration with nevirapine. Dose adjustment of co-administered drug may be needed due to possible decrease in clinical effect). Products include:
Phenytek Capsules 2160

Pirbuterol Acetate (Plasma concentrations of GI motility agents may be decreased by co-administration with nevirapine. Dose adjustment of co-administered drug may be needed due to possible decrease in clinical effect). Products include:
Maxair Autohaler 1852

Pramipexole Dihydrochloride (Plasma concentrations of GI motility agents may be decreased by co-administration with nevirapine. Dose adjustment of co-administered drug may be needed due to possible decrease in clinical effect). Products include:
Mirapex Tablets 859

Primidone (Plasma concentrations of anticonvulsants may be decreased by co-administration with nevirapine. Dose adjustment of co-administered drug may be needed due to possible decrease in clinical effect.).
 No products indexed under this heading.

Procainamide Hydrochloride (Plasma concentrations of antiarrhythmics may be decreased by co-administration with nevirapine. Dose adjustment of co-administered drug may be needed due to possible decrease in clinical effect.).
 No products indexed under this heading.

Procarbazine Hydrochloride (Plasma concentrations of cancer chemotherapeutic agents may be decreased by co-administration with nevirapine. Dose adjustment of co-administered drug may be needed due to possible decrease in clinical effect). Products include:
 Matulane Capsules **3191**

Procyclidine Hydrochloride (Plasma concentrations of GI motility agents may be decreased by co-administration with nevirapine. Dose adjustment of co-administered drug may be needed due to possible decrease in clinical effect.).
 No products indexed under this heading.

Promethazine Hydrochloride (Plasma concentrations of GI motility agents may be decreased by co-administration with nevirapine. Dose adjustment of co-administered drug may be needed due to possible decrease in clinical effect). Products include:
 Phenergan Tablets and Suppositories................................. **3440**

Propafenone Hydrochloride (Plasma concentrations of antiarrhythmics may be decreased by co-administration with nevirapine. Dose adjustment of co-administered drug may be needed due to possible decrease in clinical effect). Products include:
 Rythmol SR Capsules **2727**

Propantheline Bromide (Plasma concentrations of GI motility agents may be decreased by co-administration with nevirapine. Dose adjustment of co-administered drug may be needed due to possible decrease in clinical effect.).
 No products indexed under this heading.

Propoxyphene Hydrochloride (Plasma concentrations of GI motility agents may be decreased by co-administration with nevirapine. Dose adjustment of co-administered drug may be needed due to possible decrease in clinical effect.).
 No products indexed under this heading.

Propoxyphene Napsylate (Plasma concentrations of GI motility agents may be decreased by co-administration with nevirapine. Dose adjustment of co-administered drug may be needed due to possible decrease in clinical effect.).
 No products indexed under this heading.

Propranolol Hydrochloride (Plasma concentrations of antiarrhythmics may be decreased by co-administration with nevirapine. Dose adjustment of co-administered drug

may be needed due to possible decrease in clinical effect). Products include:
 Inderal LA Long-Acting Capsules **3429**
 InnoPran XL Capsules **2723**

Protriptyline Hydrochloride (Plasma concentrations of GI motility agents may be decreased by co-administration with nevirapine. Dose adjustment of co-administered drug may be needed due to possible decrease in clinical effect.).
 No products indexed under this heading.

Pyridostigmine Bromide (Plasma concentrations of GI motility agents may be decreased by co-administration with nevirapine. Dose adjustment of co-administered drug may be needed due to possible decrease in clinical effect.).
 No products indexed under this heading.

Pyrilamine Maleate (Plasma concentrations of GI motility agents may be decreased by co-administration with nevirapine. Dose adjustment of co-administered drug may be needed due to possible decrease in clinical effect.).
 No products indexed under this heading.

Pyrilamine Tannate (Plasma concentrations of GI motility agents may be decreased by co-administration with nevirapine. Dose adjustment of co-administered drug may be needed due to possible decrease in clinical effect.).
 No products indexed under this heading.

Quinidine Gluconate (Plasma concentrations of antiarrhythmics may be decreased by co-administration with nevirapine. Dose adjustment of co-administered drug may be needed due to possible decrease in clinical effect.).
 No products indexed under this heading.

Quinidine Polygalacturonate (Plasma concentrations of antiarrhythmics may be decreased by co-administration with nevirapine. Dose adjustment of co-administered drug may be needed due to possible decrease in clinical effect.).
 No products indexed under this heading.

Quinidine Sulfate (Plasma concentrations of antiarrhythmics may be decreased by co-administration with nevirapine. Dose adjustment of co-administered drug may be needed due to possible decrease in clinical effect.).
 No products indexed under this heading.

Remifentanil Hydrochloride (Plasma concentrations of GI motility agents may be decreased by co-administration with nevirapine. Dose adjustment of co-administered drug may be needed due to possible decrease in clinical effect.).
 No products indexed under this heading.

Rifabutin (Rifabutin and its metabolite concentrations were moderately increased. Due to high intersubject variability, however, some patients may experience large increases in rifabutin exposure and may be at higher risk for rifabutin toxicity. Therefore, caution should be used in concomitant administration.).
 No products indexed under this heading.

Rifampin (Nevirapine and rifampin should not be administered concomitantly because decreases in nevirapine plasma concentrations may reduce the efficacy of the drug. Physicians needing to treat patients co-infected with tuberculosis and using a nevirapine containing regimen may use rifabutin instead.).
 No products indexed under this heading.

Rivastigmine Tartrate (Plasma concentrations of GI motility agents may be decreased by co-administration with nevirapine. Dose adjustment of co-administered drug may be needed due to possible decrease in clinical effect). Products include:
 Exelon Capsules **2206**
 Exelon Oral Solution **2206**

Ropinirole Hydrochloride (Plasma concentrations of GI motility agents may be decreased by co-administration with nevirapine. Dose adjustment of co-administered drug may be needed due to possible decrease in clinical effect). Products include:
 Requip Tablets **1555**

Salmeterol Xinafoate (Plasma concentrations of GI motility agents may be decreased by co-administration with nevirapine. Dose adjustment of co-administered drug may be needed due to possible decrease in clinical effect). Products include:
 Advair Diskus 100/50 **1308**
 Advair Diskus 250/50 **1308**
 Advair Diskus 500/50 **1308**
 Advair HFA Inhalation Aerosol **1318**
 Serevent Diskus **1568**

Saquinavir (Saquinavir concentrations may be decreased when used concomitantly with nevirapine. Appropriate doses for this combination are not established, but an increase in the dosage of saquinavir may be required.).
 No products indexed under this heading.

Scopolamine (Plasma concentrations of GI motility agents may be decreased by co-administration with nevirapine. Dose adjustment of co-administered drug may be needed due to possible decrease in clinical effect). Products include:
 Transderm Scōp Transdermal Therapeutic System **2177**

Scopolamine Hydrobromide (Plasma concentrations of GI motility agents may be decreased by co-administration with nevirapine. Dose adjustment of co-administered drug may be needed due to possible decrease in clinical effect). Products include:
 Donnatal Extentabs **2493**

Sirolimus (Plasma concentrations of immunosuppressants may be decreased by co-administration with nevirapine. Dose adjustment of co-administered drug may be needed due to possible decrease in clinical effect). Products include:
 Rapamune Oral Solution and Tablets **3475**

Sotalol Hydrochloride (Plasma concentrations of antiarrhythmics may be decreased by co-administration with nevirapine. Dose adjustment of co-administered drug may be needed due to possible decrease in clinical effect.).
 No products indexed under this heading.

Streptozocin (Plasma concentrations of cancer chemotherapeutic agents may be decreased by co-administration with nevirapine. Dose adjustment of co-administered drug may be needed due to possible decrease in clinical effect.).
 No products indexed under this heading.

Sucralfate (Plasma concentrations of GI motility agents may be decreased by co-administration with nevirapine. Dose adjustment of co-administered drug may be needed due to possible decrease in clinical effect). Products include:
 Carafate Suspension **701**
 Carafate Tablets **701**

Sufentanil Citrate (Plasma concentrations of GI motility agents may be decreased by co-administration with nevirapine. Dose adjustment of co-administered drug may be needed due to possible decrease in clinical effect.).
 No products indexed under this heading.

Tacrine Hydrochloride (Plasma concentrations of GI motility agents may be decreased by co-administration with nevirapine. Dose adjustment of co-administered drug may be needed due to possible decrease in clinical effect.).
 No products indexed under this heading.

Tacrolimus (Plasma concentrations of immunosuppressants may be decreased by co-administration with nevirapine. Dose adjustment of co-administered drug may be needed due to possible decrease in clinical effect). Products include:
 Prograf Capsules and Injection **632**
 Protopic Ointment **638**

Tamoxifen Citrate (Plasma concentrations of cancer chemotherapeutic agents may be decreased by co-administration with nevirapine. Dose adjustment of co-administered drug may be needed due to possible decrease in clinical effect). Products include:
 Soltamox Oral Solution **3527**

Teniposide (Plasma concentrations of cancer chemotherapeutic agents may be decreased by co-administration with nevirapine. Dose adjustment of co-administered drug may be needed due to possible decrease in clinical effect.).
 No products indexed under this heading.

Terbutaline Sulfate (Plasma concentrations of GI motility agents may be decreased by co-administration with nevirapine. Dose adjustment of co-administered drug may be needed due to possible decrease in clinical effect.).
 No products indexed under this heading.

Terconazole (Plasma concentrations of antifungals may be decreased by co-administration with nevirapine. Dose adjustment of co-administered drug may be needed due to possible decrease in clinical effect.).
 No products indexed under this heading.

Thioguanine (Plasma concentrations of cancer chemotherapeutic agents may be decreased by co-administration with nevirapine. Dose adjustment of co-administered drug may be needed due to possible decrease in clinical effect). Products include:

Thiotepa (Plasma concentrations of cancer chemotherapeutic agents may be decreased by co-administration with nevirapine. Dose adjustment of co-administered drug may be needed due to possible decrease in clinical effect.).

No products indexed under this heading.

Tiagabine Hydrochloride (Plasma concentrations of anticonvulsants may be decreased by co-administration with nevirapine. Dose adjustment of co-administered drug may be needed due to possible decrease in clinical effect). Products include:

Tinzaparin Sodium (Plasma concentrations of antithrombotics may be increased by co-administration with nevirapine. Dose adjustment of co-administered drug may be needed due to possible decrease in clinical effect.).

No products indexed under this heading.

Tocainide Hydrochloride (Plasma concentrations of antiarrhythmics may be decreased by co-administration with nevirapine. Dose adjustment of co-administered drug may be needed due to possible decrease in clinical effect.).

No products indexed under this heading.

Tolterodine Tartrate (Plasma concentrations of GI motility agents may be decreased by co-administration with nevirapine. Dose adjustment of co-administered drug may be needed due to possible decrease in clinical effect). Products include:

Topiramate (Plasma concentrations of anticonvulsants may be decreased by co-administration with nevirapine. Dose adjustment of co-administered drug may be needed due to possible decrease in clinical effect). Products include:

Topotecan Hydrochloride (Plasma concentrations of cancer chemotherapeutic agents may be decreased by co-administration with nevirapine. Dose adjustment of co-administered drug may be needed due to possible decrease in clinical effect). Products include:

Toremifene Citrate (Plasma concentrations of cancer chemotherapeutic agents may be decreased by co-administration with nevirapine. Dose adjustment of co-administered drug may be needed due to possible decrease in clinical effect.).

No products indexed under this heading.

Tridihexethyl Chloride (Plasma concentrations of GI motility agents may be decreased by co-administration with nevirapine. Dose adjustment of co-administered drug may be needed due to possible decrease in clinical effect.).

No products indexed under this heading.

Trihexyphenidyl Hydrochloride (Plasma concentrations of GI motility agents may be decreased by co-administration with nevirapine. Dose adjustment of co-administered drug may be needed due to possible decrease in clinical effect.).

No products indexed under this heading.

Trimeprazine Tartrate (Plasma concentrations of GI motility agents may be decreased by co-administration with nevirapine. Dose adjustment of co-administered drug may be needed due to possible decrease in clinical effect.).

No products indexed under this heading.

Trimethadione (Plasma concentrations of anticonvulsants may be decreased by co-administration with nevirapine. Dose adjustment of co-administered drug may be needed due to possible decrease in clinical effect.).

No products indexed under this heading.

Trimipramine Maleate (Plasma concentrations of GI motility agents may be decreased by co-administration with nevirapine. Dose adjustment of co-administered drug may be needed due to possible decrease in clinical effect.).

No products indexed under this heading.

Tripelennamine Hydrochloride (Plasma concentrations of GI motility agents may be decreased by co-administration with nevirapine. Dose adjustment of co-administered drug may be needed due to possible decrease in clinical effect.).

No products indexed under this heading.

Triprolidine Hydrochloride (Plasma concentrations of GI motility agents may be decreased by co-administration with nevirapine. Dose adjustment of co-administered drug may be needed due to possible decrease in clinical effect.).

No products indexed under this heading.

Valproate Sodium (Plasma concentrations of anticonvulsants may be decreased by co-administration with nevirapine. Dose adjustment of co-administered drug may be needed due to possible decrease in clinical effect). Products include:

Valproic Acid (Plasma concentrations of anticonvulsants may be decreased by co-administration with nevirapine. Dose adjustment of co-administered drug may be needed due to possible decrease in clinical effect). Products include:

Valrubicin (Plasma concentrations of cancer chemotherapeutic agents may be decreased by co-administration with nevirapine. Dose adjustment of co-administered drug may be needed due to possible decrease in clinical effect.).

No products indexed under this heading.

Verapamil Hydrochloride (Plasma concentrations of antiarrhythmics may be decreased by co-administration with nevirapine. Dose adjustment of co-administered drug may be needed due to possible decrease in clinical effect). Products include:

Vincristine Sulfate (Plasma concentrations of cancer chemotherapeutic agents may be decreased by co-administration with nevirapine. Dose adjustment of co-administered drug may be needed due to possible decrease in clinical effect.).

No products indexed under this heading.

Vinorelbine Tartrate (Plasma concentrations of cancer chemotherapeutic agents may be decreased by co-administration with nevirapine. Dose adjustment of co-administered drug may be needed due to possible decrease in clinical effect.).

No products indexed under this heading.

Warfarin Sodium (Plasma concentrations of antithrombotics may be increased by co-administration with nevirapine. Dose adjustment of co-administered drug may be needed due to possible decrease in clinical effect). Products include:

Zidovudine (When zidovudine and Viramune are co-administered the AUC and Cmax for zidovudine are decreased by 28% and 30%, respectively). Products include:

Zonisamide (Plasma concentrations of anticonvulsants may be decreased by co-administration with nevirapine. Dose adjustment of co-administered drug may be needed due to possible decrease in clinical effect). Products include:

VIRAZOLE FOR INHALATION SOLUTION

None cited in PDR database.

VIREAD TABLETS

May interact with:

Acyclovir (Co-administration with drugs that reduce renal function or compete for active tubular secretion may increase serum concentrations of tenofovir and/or increase the concentrations of other renally eliminated drugs, such as acyclovir). Products include:

Acyclovir Sodium (Co-administration with drugs that reduce renal function or compete for active tubular secretion may increase serum concentrations of tenofovir and/or increase the concentrations of other renally eliminated drugs, such as acyclovir).

No products indexed under this heading.

Atazanavir (Tenofovir decreases the AUC and Cmin of atazanavir. When co-administered with tenofovir, it is recommended that atazanavir 300mg is given with ritonavir 100mg. Atazanavir without ritonavir should not be co-administered with tenofovir. Atazanavir may increase the Cmax, AUC and Cmin of tenofovir).

No products indexed under this heading.

Atazanavir sulfate (Tenofovir decreases the AUC and Cmin of atazanavir. When co-administered with tenofovir, it is recommended that atazanavir 300mg is given with ritonavir 100mg. Atazanavir without ritonavir should not be co-administered with tenofovir. Atazanavir may increase the Cmax, AUC and Cmin of tenofovir). Products include:

Cidofovir (Co-administration with drugs that reduce renal function or compete for active tubular secretion may increase serum concentrations of tenofovir and/or increase the concentrations of other renally eliminated drugs, such as cidofovir).

No products indexed under this heading.

Didanosine (Co-administration results in increased AUC and Cmax of didanosine and could potentiate didanosine-associated adverse events. Discontinue didanosine if didanosine-associated adverse events develop).

No products indexed under this heading.

Ganciclovir (Co-administration with drugs that reduce renal function or compete for active tubular secretion may increase serum concentrations of tenofovir and/or increase the concentrations of other renally eliminated drugs, such as ganciclovir).

No products indexed under this heading.

Indinavir Sulfate (Co-administration of tenofovir with indinavir has resulted in increased Cmax tenofovir and decreased Cmax for indinavir). Products include:

Lamivudine (Co-administration of tenofovir with lamivudine has resulted in decreased Cmax for lamivudine). Products include:

Lopinavir (Co-administration of tenofovir with lopinavir has resulted in increased Cmax, AUC, and Cmin for tenofovir and decreased AUC, Cmax, and Cmin for lopinavir). Products include:

Ritonavir (Coadministration of tenofovir and ritonavir resulted in a 23% increase in Cmin). Products include:

Saquinavir (Coadministration of tenofovir and saquinavir resulted in a 22% increse in Cmax).

No products indexed under this heading.

Valacyclovir Hydrochloride (Co-administration with drugs that reduce renal function or compete for active tubular secretion may

increase serum concentrations of tenofovir and/or increase the concentrations of other renally eliminated drugs, such as valacyclovir). Products include:
Valtrex Caplets 1597

Valganciclovir Hydrochloride (Co-administration with drugs that reduce renal function or compete for active tubular secretion may increase serum concentrations of tenofovir and/or increase the concentrations of other renally eliminated drugs, such as valganciclovir). Products include:
Valcyte Tablets 2813

Food Interactions

Food, unspecified (Increases the bioavailability and delays the time to tenofovir Cmax; Viread should be taken with a meal).

VIROPTIC OPHTHALMIC SOLUTION
(Trifluridine) ⊙266
None cited in PDR database.

VISINE ORIGINAL EYE DROPS
(Tetrahydrozoline Hydrochloride) ⊙290
None cited in PDR database.

VISINE A.C. SEASONAL ITCHING AND REDNESS RELIEF DROPS
(Tetrahydrozoline Hydrochloride, Zinc Sulfate) ⊙289
None cited in PDR database.

ADVANCED RELIEF VISINE EYE DROPS
(Dextran 70, Polyethylene Glycol, Povidone, Tetrahydrozoline Hydrochloride) ⊙288
None cited in PDR database.

VISINE FOR CONTACTS REWETTING DROPS
(Glycerin, Hydroxypropyl Methylcellulose) ⊙289
None cited in PDR database.

VISINE L.R. LONG LASTING EYE DROPS
(Oxymetazoline Hydrochloride) ⊙290
None cited in PDR database.

VISINE TEARS EYE DROPS
(Glycerin, Hypromellose, Polyethylene Glycol) ⊙290
None cited in PDR database.

VISINE PURE TEARS EYE DROPS SINGLE DROP DISPENSER
(Glycerin, Hypromellose, Polyethylene Glycol) ⊙291
None cited in PDR database.

VISINE PURE TEARS PORTABLES
(Glycerin, Hypromellose, Polyethylene Glycol) ⊙291
None cited in PDR database.

VISINE-A EYE ALLERGY RELIEF EYE DROPS
(Naphazoline Hydrochloride, Pheniramine Maleate) ⊙289
None cited in PDR database.

VISUDYNE FOR INJECTION
(Verteporfin) 2305
May interact with calcium channel blockers, anticoagulants, phenothiazines, sulfonamides, sulfonylureas, tetracyclines, thiazides, and certain other agents. Compounds in these categories include:

Amlodipine Besylate (Co-administration with calcium channel blockers could enhance the rate of verteporfin's uptake by the vascular endothelium). Products include:
Caduet Tablets 2508
Lotrel Capsules 2249
Norvasc Tablets 2545

Anisindione (Co-administration with drugs that decrease clotting would be expected to decrease verteporfin activity). Products include:
Miradon Tablets 3042

Ardeparin Sodium (Co-administration with drugs that decrease clotting would be expected to decrease verteporfin activity).
No products indexed under this heading.

Aspirin (Co-administration with drugs that decrease platelet aggregation would be expected to decrease verteporfin activity). Products include:
Aggrenox Capsules 822
Bayer Aspirin 744
BC Allergy Sinus Cold Powder ▣677
BC Headache Powder ▣677
Arthritis Strength BC Powder ▣677
BC Sinus Cold Powder ▣677
Excedrin Extra Strength Caplets/Tablets/Geltabs ▣684
Excedrin Migraine Caplets/Tablets/Geltabs ▣609
Goody's Body Pain Formula Powder ▣684
Goody's Extra Strength Headache Powders ▣611
Goody's Extra Strength Pain Relief Tablets ▣685
Percodan Tablets 1132
St. Joseph 81 mg Aspirin Chewable and Enteric Coated Tablets 1869

Bendroflumethiazide (Co-administration with other photosensitizing agents, such as thiazide diuretics, could increase the potential for skin photosensitivity reactions).
No products indexed under this heading.

Bepridil Hydrochloride (Co-administration with calcium channel blockers could enhance the rate of verteporfin's uptake by the vascular endothelium).
No products indexed under this heading.

Chlorothiazide (Co-administration with other photosensitizing agents, such as thiazide diuretics, could increase the potential for skin photosensitivity reactions). Products include:
Diuril Oral Suspension 1954

Chlorothiazide Sodium (Co-administration with other photosensitizing agents, such as thiazide diuretics, could increase the potential for skin photosensitivity reactions). Products include:
Diuril Sodium Intravenous 2467

Chlorpromazine (Co-administration with other photosensitizing agents, such as phenothiazines, could increase the potential for skin photosensitivity reactions).
No products indexed under this heading.

Chlorpromazine Hydrochloride (Co-administration with other photosensitizing agents, such as phenothiazines, could increase the potential for skin photosensitivity reactions).
No products indexed under this heading.

Chlorpropamide (Co-administration with other photosensitizing agents, such as sulfonylurea hypoglycemic agents, could increase the potential for skin photosensitivity reactions).
No products indexed under this heading.

Clopidogrel Bisulfate (Co-administration with drugs that decrease platelet aggregation would be expected to decrease verteporfin activity). Products include:
Plavix Tablets 917
Plavix Tablets 2926

Dalteparin Sodium (Co-administration with drugs that decrease clotting would be expected to decrease verteporfin activity). Products include:
Fragmin Injection 1097

Danaparoid Sodium (Co-administration with drugs that decrease clotting would be expected to decrease verteporfin activity).
No products indexed under this heading.

Demeclocycline Hydrochloride (Co-administration with other photosensitizing agents, such as tetracyclines, could increase the potential for skin photosensitivity reactions).
No products indexed under this heading.

Dicumarol (Co-administration with drugs that decrease clotting would be expected to decrease verteporfin activity).
No products indexed under this heading.

Diltiazem Hydrochloride (Co-administration with calcium channel blockers could enhance the rate of verteporfin's uptake by the vascular endothelium). Products include:
Cardizem LA Extended Release Tablets 1728
Tiazac Capsules 1201

Dimethyl Sulfoxide (Co-administration with compounds that quench active oxygen species or scavenge radicals, such as dimethyl sulfoxide, would be expected to decrease verteporfin activity).
No products indexed under this heading.

Dipyridamole (Co-administration with drugs that decrease platelet aggregation would be expected to decrease verteporfin activity). Products include:
Aggrenox Capsules 822
Persantine Tablets 868

Doxycycline Calcium (Co-administration with other photosensitizing agents, such as tetracyclines, could increase the potential for skin photosensitivity reactions).
No products indexed under this heading.

Doxycycline Hyclate (Co-administration with other photosensitizing agents, such as tetracyclines, could increase the potential for skin photosensitivity reactions).
No products indexed under this heading.

Doxycycline Monohydrate (Co-administration with other photosensitizing agents, such as tetracyclines,

could increase the potential for skin photosensitivity reactions). Products include:
Oracea Capsules 1000

Enoxaparin Sodium (Co-administration with drugs that decrease clotting would be expected to decrease verteporfin activity). Products include:
Lovenox Injection 2915

Felodipine (Co-administration with calcium channel blockers could enhance the rate of verteporfin's uptake by the vascular endothelium).
No products indexed under this heading.

Fluphenazine Decanoate (Co-administration with other photosensitizing agents, such as phenothiazines, could increase the potential for skin photosensitivity reactions).
No products indexed under this heading.

Fluphenazine Enanthate (Co-administration with other photosensitizing agents, such as phenothiazines, could increase the potential for skin photosensitivity reactions).
No products indexed under this heading.

Fluphenazine Hydrochloride (Co-administration with other photosensitizing agents, such as phenothiazines, could increase the potential for skin photosensitivity reactions).
No products indexed under this heading.

Fondaparinux Sodium (Co-administration with drugs that decrease clotting would be expected to decrease verteporfin activity). Products include:
Arixtra Injection 1351

Glimepiride (Co-administration with other photosensitizing agents, such as sulfonylurea hypoglycemic agents, could increase the potential for skin photosensitivity reactions). Products include:
Avandaryl Tablets 1379
Duetact Tablets 3226

Glipizide (Co-administration with other photosensitizing agents, such as sulfonylurea hypoglycemic agents, could increase the potential for skin photosensitivity reactions).
No products indexed under this heading.

Glyburide (Co-administration with other photosensitizing agents, such as sulfonylurea hypoglycemic agents, could increase the potential for skin photosensitivity reactions).
No products indexed under this heading.

Griseofulvin (Co-administration with other photosensitizing agents, such as griseofulvin, could increase the potential for skin photosensitivity reactions). Products include:
Gris-PEG Tablets 2502

Heparin Calcium (Co-administration with drugs that decrease clotting would be expected to decrease verteporfin activity).
No products indexed under this heading.

Heparin Sodium (Co-administration with drugs that decrease clotting would be expected to decrease verteporfin activity).
No products indexed under this heading.

Hydrochlorothiazide (Co-administration with other photosensitizing agents, such as thiazide diuretics, could increase the potential for skin photosensitivity reactions). Products include:

Aldoril Tablets 1910
Atacand HCT 651
Avalide Tablets 888
Avalide Tablets 2874
Benicar HCT Tablets 1044
Diovan HCT Tablets 2196
Dyazide Capsules 1423
Hyzaar 50-12.5 Tablets 1990
Hyzaar 100-12.5 Tablets 1990
Hyzaar 100-25 Tablets 1990
Lopressor HCT 50/25 Tablets 2241
Lopressor HCT 100/25 Tablets 2241
Lopressor HCT 100/50 Tablets 2241
Lotensin HCT Tablets 2246
Micardis HCT Tablets 856
Moduretic Tablets 2028
Prinzide Tablets 2056
Teveten HCT Tablets 1737
Timolide Tablets 2086
Uniretic Tablets 3100

Hydroflumethiazide (Co-administration with other photosensitizing agents, such as thiazide diuretics, could increase the potential for skin photosensitivity reactions).
No products indexed under this heading.

Isradipine (Co-administration with calcium channel blockers could enhance the rate of verteporfin's uptake by the vascular endothelium). Products include:

DynaCirc CR Tablets 2721

Low Molecular Weight Heparins (Co-administration with drugs that decrease clotting would be expected to decrease verteporfin activity).
No products indexed under this heading.

Mannitol (Co-administration with compounds that quench active oxygen species or scavenge radicals, such as mannitol, would be expected to decrease verteporfin activity).
No products indexed under this heading.

Mesoridazine Besylate (Co-administration with other photosensitizing agents, such as phenothiazines, could increase the potential for skin photosensitivity reactions).
No products indexed under this heading.

Methacycline Hydrochloride (Co-administration with other photosensitizing agents, such as tetracyclines, could increase the potential for skin photosensitivity reactions).
No products indexed under this heading.

Methotrimeprazine (Co-administration with other photosensitizing agents, such as phenothiazines, could increase the potential for skin photosensitivity reactions).
No products indexed under this heading.

Methyclothiazide (Co-administration with other photosensitizing agents, such as thiazide diuretics, could increase the potential for skin photosensitivity reactions).
No products indexed under this heading.

Mibefradil Dihydrochloride (Co-administration with calcium channel blockers could enhance the rate of verteporfin's uptake by the vascular endothelium).
No products indexed under this heading.

Minocycline Hydrochloride (Co-administration with other photosensitizing agents, such as tetracyclines, could increase the potential for skin photosensitivity reactions). Products include:

Solodyn Extended Release Tablets 1890

Nicardipine Hydrochloride (Co-administration with calcium channel blockers could enhance the rate of verteporfin's uptake by the vascular endothelium). Products include:

Cardene I.V. 2497

Nifedipine (Co-administration with calcium channel blockers could enhance the rate of verteporfin's uptake by the vascular endothelium). Products include:

Adalat CC Tablets 2964

Nimodipine (Co-administration with calcium channel blockers could enhance the rate of verteporfin's uptake by the vascular endothelium). Products include:

Nimotop Capsules 749

Nisoldipine (Co-administration with calcium channel blockers could enhance the rate of verteporfin's uptake by the vascular endothelium). Products include:

Sular Tablets 3122

Oxytetracycline Hydrochloride (Co-administration with other photosensitizing agents, such as tetracyclines, could increase the potential for skin photosensitivity reactions).
No products indexed under this heading.

Perphenazine (Co-administration with other photosensitizing agents, such as phenothiazines, could increase the potential for skin photosensitivity reactions).
No products indexed under this heading.

Polymyxin B Sulfate (Co-administration with polymyxin B could enhance the rate of verteporfin's uptake by the vascular endothelium). Products include:

Neosporin Antibiotic Ointment .... ▣ 643
Neosporin Ophthalmic Solution Sterile .... ⊙ 265
Neosporin + Pain Relief Antibiotic Cream and Ointment (Maximum Strength).................... ▣ 643
Poly-Pred Ophthalmic Suspension .... ⊙ 233
Polysporin First Aid Antibiotic Ointment.................................... ▣ 643
Polytrim Ophthalmic Solution 574

Polythiazide (Co-administration with other photosensitizing agents, such as thiazide diuretics, could increase the potential for skin photosensitivity reactions).
No products indexed under this heading.

Prochlorperazine (Co-administration with other photosensitizing agents, such as phenothiazines, could increase the potential for skin photosensitivity reactions).
No products indexed under this heading.

Promethazine Hydrochloride (Co-administration with other photosensitizing agents, such as phenothiazines, could increase the potential for skin photosensitivity reactions). Products include:

Phenergan Tablets and Suppositories.............................. 3440

Sulfacytine (Co-administration with other photosensitizing agents, such as sulfonamides, could increase the potential for skin photosensitivity reactions).
No products indexed under this heading.

Sulfamethizole (Co-administration with other photosensitizing agents, such as sulfonamides, could increase the potential for skin photosensitivity reactions).
No products indexed under this heading.

Sulfamethoxazole (Co-administration with other photosensitizing agents, such as sulfonamides, could increase the potential for skin photosensitivity reactions).
No products indexed under this heading.

Sulfasalazine (Co-administration with other photosensitizing agents, such as sulfonamides, could increase the potential for skin photosensitivity reactions).
No products indexed under this heading.

Sulfinpyrazone (Co-administration with other photosensitizing agents, such as sulfonamides, could increase the potential for skin photosensitivity reactions).
No products indexed under this heading.

Sulfisoxazole Acetyl (Co-administration with other photosensitizing agents, such as sulfonamides, could increase the potential for skin photosensitivity reactions).
No products indexed under this heading.

Sulfisoxazole Diolamine (Co-administration with other photosensitizing agents, such as sulfonamides, could increase the potential for skin photosensitivity reactions).
No products indexed under this heading.

Tetracycline Hydrochloride (Co-administration with other photosensitizing agents, such as tetracyclines, could increase the potential for skin photosensitivity reactions).
No products indexed under this heading.

Thioridazine Hydrochloride (Co-administration with other photosensitizing agents, such as phenothiazines, could increase the potential for skin photosensitivity reactions). Products include:

Thioridazine Hydrochloride Tablets 2163

Tinzaparin Sodium (Co-administration with drugs that decrease clotting would be expected to decrease verteporfin activity).
No products indexed under this heading.

Tolazamide (Co-administration with other photosensitizing agents, such as sulfonylurea hypoglycemic agents, could increase the potential for skin photosensitivity reactions).
No products indexed under this heading.

Tolbutamide (Co-administration with other photosensitizing agents, such as sulfonylurea hypoglycemic agents, could increase the potential for skin photosensitivity reactions).
No products indexed under this heading.

Trifluoperazine Hydrochloride (Co-administration with other photosensitizing agents, such as phenothiazines, could increase the potential for skin photosensitivity reactions).
No products indexed under this heading.

Verapamil Hydrochloride (Co-administration with calcium channel blockers could enhance the rate of verteporfin's uptake by the vascular endothelium). Products include:

Covera-HS Tablets 3139
Tarka Tablets 524
Verelan PM Extended-Release Capsules, Controlled-Onset........... 3106

Warfarin Sodium (Co-administration with drugs that decrease clotting would be expected to decrease verteporfin activity). Products include:

Coumadin for Injection 898
Coumadin Tablets 898

Food Interactions

Alcohol (Co-administration with compounds that quench active oxygen species or scavenge radicals, such as ethanol, would be expected to decrease verteporfin activity).

VISUTEIN CAPSULES

(Acetylcysteine, Carotenoids, Lutein, Vitamin A, Vitamin B_2, Zinc)...... 3329
None cited in PDR database.

VIVA LUBRICATING EYE DROPS

(Polysorbate 80) .... ⊙ 293
None cited in PDR database.

VIVAGLOBIN

(Immune Globulin Subcutaneous (Human)).. 3506
May interact with vaccines, live. Compounds in these categories include:

BCG Vaccine (Immunoglobulin administration can transiently impair the efficacy of live attenuated virus vaccines).
No products indexed under this heading.

Measles, Mumps, Rubella and Varicella Virus Vaccine Live (Immunoglobulin administration can transiently impair the efficacy of live attenuated virus vaccines). Products include:

ProQuad 2064

Measles, Mumps & Rubella Virus Vaccine, Live (Immunoglobulin administration can transiently impair the efficacy of live attenuated virus vaccines). Products include:

M-M-R II 2006

Measles & Rubella Virus Vaccine Live (Immunoglobulin administration can transiently impair the efficacy of live attenuated virus vaccines).
No products indexed under this heading.

Measles Virus Vaccine Live (Immunoglobulin administration can transiently impair the efficacy of live attenuated virus vaccines). Products include:

Attenuvax 1914

Mumps Virus Vaccine, Live (Immunoglobulin administration can transiently impair the efficacy of live attenuated virus vaccines). Products include:

Mumpsvax 2031

Poliovirus Vaccine, Live, Oral, Trivalent, Types 1,2,3 (Sabin) (Immunoglobulin administration can transiently impair the efficacy of live attenuated virus vaccines).
No products indexed under this heading.

Rotavirus Vaccine, Live, Oral, Tetravalent (Immunoglobulin administration can transiently impair the efficacy of live attenuated virus vaccines).
No products indexed under this heading.

Rubella & Mumps Virus Vaccine Live (Immunoglobulin administration can transiently impair the efficacy of live attenuated virus vaccines).
No products indexed under this heading.

Rubella Virus Vaccine Live (Immunoglobulin administration can transiently impair the efficacy of live attenuated virus vaccines). Products include:
Meruvax II 2019

Smallpox Vaccine (Immunoglobulin administration can transiently impair the efficacy of live attenuated virus vaccines).
No products indexed under this heading.

Typhoid Vaccine (Immunoglobulin administration can transiently impair the efficacy of live attenuated virus vaccines).
No products indexed under this heading.

Varicella Virus Vaccine Live (Immunoglobulin administration can transiently impair the efficacy of live attenuated virus vaccines). Products include:
Varivax 2100

Yellow Fever Vaccine (Immunoglobulin administration can transiently impair the efficacy of live attenuated virus vaccines).
No products indexed under this heading.

VIVARIN CAPLETS

(Caffeine) .... ▣602
May interact with:

Beverages, containing medications (Concurrent use may cause nervousness, irritability, sleeplessness, and occasionally, rapid heartbeat).
No products indexed under this heading.

Caffeine-containing medications (Concurrent use may cause nervousness, irritability, sleeplessness, and occasionally, rapid heartbeat).
No products indexed under this heading.

Food, containing medications (Concurrent use may cause nervousness, irritability, sleeplessness, and occasionally, rapid heartbeat).
No products indexed under this heading.

VIVARIN TABLETS

(Caffeine) .... ▣602
See Vivarin Caplets

VIVITROL

(Naltrexone) 995
May interact with narcotic analgesics and certain other agents. Compounds in these categories include:

Alfentanil Hydrochloride (Naltrexone is contraindicated in patients receiving opioid analgesics).
No products indexed under this heading.

Buprenorphine Hydrochloride (Naltrexone is contraindicated in patients receiving opioid analgesics). Products include:
Buprenex Injectable 2716
Suboxone Tablets 2717
Subutex Tablets 2717

Codeine Phosphate (Naltrexone is contraindicated in patients receiving opioid analgesics). Products include:
Tylenol with Codeine Tablets 2391

Dezocine (Naltrexone is contraindicated in patients receiving opioid analgesics).
No products indexed under this heading.

Fentanyl (Naltrexone is contraindicated in patients receiving opioid analgesics). Products include:
Duragesic Transdermal System 2373
Ionsys Transdermal System 2379

Fentanyl Citrate (Naltrexone is contraindicated in patients receiving opioid analgesics). Products include:
Actiq 979

Hydrocodone Bitartrate (Naltrexone is contraindicated in patients receiving opioid analgesics). Products include:
Hycodan 1116
Hycotuss Expectorant Syrup 1117
Vicodin Tablets 535
Vicodin ES Tablets 536
Vicodin HP Tablets 538
Vicoprofen Tablets 539
Zydone Tablets 1139

Hydrocodone Polistirex (Naltrexone is contraindicated in patients receiving opioid analgesics). Products include:
Tussionex Pennkinetic Extended-Release Suspension 3327

Hydromorphone Hydrochloride (Naltrexone is contraindicated in patients receiving opioid analgesics). Products include:
Dilaudid 440
Dilaudid Non-Sterile Powder 440
Dilaudid Oral Liquid 445
Dilaudid Rectal Suppositories 440
Dilaudid Tablets 440
Dilaudid Tablets - 8 mg 445
Dilaudid-HP 442

Levorphanol Tartrate (Naltrexone is contraindicated in patients receiving opioid analgesics).
No products indexed under this heading.

Meperidine Hydrochloride (Naltrexone is contraindicated in patients receiving opioid analgesics).
No products indexed under this heading.

Methadone Hydrochloride (Naltrexone is contraindicated in patients receiving opioid analgesics).
No products indexed under this heading.

Morphine Sulfate (Naltrexone is contraindicated in patients receiving opioid analgesics). Products include:
Avinza Capsules 1741
Kadian Capsules 577
MS Contin Tablets 2701

Opioid Analgesics (Naltrexone is contraindicated in patients receiving opioid analgesics).
No products indexed under this heading.

Opium Preparations (Naltrexone antagonizes the effects of opioid containing medicines, such as cough and cold remedies, antidiarrheal preparations and opioid analgesics).
No products indexed under this heading.

Oxycodone Hydrochloride (Naltrexone is contraindicated in patients receiving opioid analgesics). Products include:
OxyContin Tablets 2703
OxyFast Oral Concentrate Solution 2708
OxyIR Capsules 2708
Percocet Tablets 1131
Percodan Tablets 1132

Propoxyphene Hydrochloride (Naltrexone is contraindicated in patients receiving opioid analgesics).
No products indexed under this heading.

Propoxyphene Napsylate (Naltrexone is contraindicated in patients receiving opioid analgesics).
No products indexed under this heading.

Remifentanil Hydrochloride (Naltrexone is contraindicated in patients receiving opioid analgesics).
No products indexed under this heading.

Sufentanil Citrate (Naltrexone is contraindicated in patients receiving opioid analgesics).
No products indexed under this heading.

VIVOTIF

(Typhoid Vaccine Live Oral TY21a) 819
May interact with:

Chloroquine Phosphate (Several antimalarials, such as chloroquine, possess antibacterial activity which may interfere with the immune response rate; in one study, concomitant treatment did not result in significant reduction in the immune response, therefore, these drugs can be administered together).
No products indexed under this heading.

Mefloquine Hydrochloride (Several antimalarials, such as mefloquine, possess antibacterial activity which may interfere with the immune response rate; in one study, concomitant treatment did not result in significant reduction in the immune response, therefore, these drugs can be administered together). Products include:
Lariam Tablets 2786

Proguanil (The simultaneous administration of proguanil results in a significant decrease in the immune response rate).
No products indexed under this heading.

VOLTAREN OPHTHALMIC SOLUTION

(Diclofenac Sodium) 2309
May interact with anticoagulants and corticosteroids. Compounds in these categories include:

Anisindione (It is recommended that diclofenac ophthalmic suspension be used with caution in patients who are receiving other medications which may prolong bleeding time). Products include:
Miradon Tablets 3042

Ardeparin Sodium (It is recommended that diclofenac ophthalmic suspension be used with caution in patients who are receiving other medications which may prolong bleeding time).
No products indexed under this heading.

Betamethasone Acetate (All topical nonsteroidal anti-inflammatory drugs (NSAIDs) may slow or delay healing. Topical corticosteroids are also known to slow or delay healing. Concomitant use of topical NSAIDs and topical steroids may increase the potential for healing problems).
No products indexed under this heading.

Betamethasone Sodium Phosphate (All topical nonsteroidal anti-inflammatory drugs (NSAIDs) may slow or delay healing. Topical corticosteroids are also known to slow or delay healing. Concomitant use of topical NSAIDs and topical steroids may increase the potential for healing problems).
No products indexed under this heading.

Cortisone Acetate (All topical nonsteroidal anti-inflammatory drugs (NSAIDs) may slow or delay healing. Topical corticosteroids are also known to slow or delay healing. Concomitant use of topical NSAIDs and topical steroids may increase the potential for healing problems).
No products indexed under this heading.

Dalteparin Sodium (It is recommended that diclofenac ophthalmic suspension be used with caution in patients who are receiving other medications which may prolong bleeding time). Products include:
Fragmin Injection 1097

Danaparoid Sodium (It is recommended that diclofenac ophthalmic suspension be used with caution in patients who are receiving other medications which may prolong bleeding time).
No products indexed under this heading.

Dexamethasone (All topical nonsteroidal anti-inflammatory drugs (NSAIDs) may slow or delay healing. Topical corticosteroids are also known to slow or delay healing. Concomitant use of topical NSAIDs and topical steroids may increase the potential for healing problems). Products include:
Ciprodex Otic Suspension 559
Decadron Tablets 1951
TobraDex Ophthalmic Ointment 562
TobraDex Ophthalmic Suspension ... 563

Dexamethasone Acetate (All topical nonsteroidal anti-inflammatory drugs (NSAIDs) may slow or delay healing. Topical corticosteroids are also known to slow or delay healing. Concomitant use of topical NSAIDs and topical steroids may increase the potential for healing problems).
No products indexed under this heading.

Dexamethasone Sodium Phosphate (All topical nonsteroidal anti-inflammatory drugs (NSAIDs) may slow or delay healing. Topical corticosteroids are also known to slow or delay healing. Concomitant use of topical NSAIDs and topical steroids may increase the potential for healing problems).
No products indexed under this heading.

Dicumarol (It is recommended that diclofenac ophthalmic suspension be used with caution in patients who are receiving other medications which may prolong bleeding time).
No products indexed under this heading.

Enoxaparin Sodium (It is recommended that diclofenac ophthalmic suspension be used with caution in patients who are receiving other medications which may prolong bleeding time). Products include:

Lovenox Injection 2915

Fludrocortisone Acetate (All topical nonsteroidal anti-inflammatory drugs (NSAIDs) may slow or delay healing. Topical corticosteroids are also known to slow or delay healing. Concomitant use of topical NSAIDs and topical steroids may increase the potential for healing problems).

No products indexed under this heading.

Fondaparinux Sodium (It is recommended that diclofenac ophthalmic suspension be used with caution in patients who are receiving other medications which may prolong bleeding time). Products include:

Arixtra Injection 1351

Heparin Calcium (It is recommended that diclofenac ophthalmic suspension be used with caution in patients who are receiving other medications which may prolong bleeding time).

No products indexed under this heading.

Heparin Sodium (It is recommended that diclofenac ophthalmic suspension be used with caution in patients who are receiving other medications which may prolong bleeding time).

No products indexed under this heading.

Hydrocortisone (All topical nonsteroidal anti-inflammatory drugs (NSAIDs) may slow or delay healing. Topical corticosteroids are also known to slow or delay healing. Concomitant use of topical NSAIDs and topical steroids may increase the potential for healing problems). Products include:

Colocort Rectal Suspension, USP (Retention) 100 mg/60 mL 2476
Hydrocortone Tablets 1989
Preparation H Hydrocortisone Cream .... ▣646

Hydrocortisone Acetate (All topical nonsteroidal anti-inflammatory drugs (NSAIDs) may slow or delay healing. Topical corticosteroids are also known to slow or delay healing. Concomitant use of topical NSAIDs and topical steroids may increase the potential for healing problems). Products include:

Analpram-HC 1159
Pramosone 1161
ProctoFoam-HC 3099

Hydrocortisone Sodium Phosphate (All topical nonsteroidal anti-inflammatory drugs (NSAIDs) may slow or delay healing. Topical corticosteroids are also known to slow or delay healing. Concomitant use of topical NSAIDs and topical steroids may increase the potential for healing problems).

No products indexed under this heading.

Hydrocortisone Sodium Succinate (All topical nonsteroidal anti-inflammatory drugs (NSAIDs) may slow or delay healing. Topical corticosteroids are also known to slow or delay healing. Concomitant use of topical NSAIDs and topical steroids may increase the potential for healing problems).

No products indexed under this heading.

Low Molecular Weight Heparins (It is recommended that diclofenac ophthalmic suspension be used with caution in patients who are receiving other medications which may prolong bleeding time).

No products indexed under this heading.

Methylprednisolone Acetate (All topical nonsteroidal anti-inflammatory drugs (NSAIDs) may slow or delay healing. Topical corticosteroids are also known to slow or delay healing. Concomitant use of topical NSAIDs and topical steroids may increase the potential for healing problems). Products include:

Depo-Medrol Injectable Suspension 2617
Depo-Medrol Single-Dose Vial 2619

Methylprednisolone Sodium Succinate (All topical nonsteroidal anti-inflammatory drugs (NSAIDs) may slow or delay healing. Topical corticosteroids are also known to slow or delay healing. Concomitant use of topical NSAIDs and topical steroids may increase the potential for healing problems).

No products indexed under this heading.

Prednisolone Acetate (All topical nonsteroidal anti-inflammatory drugs (NSAIDs) may slow or delay healing. Topical corticosteroids are also known to slow or delay healing. Concomitant use of topical NSAIDs and topical steroids may increase the potential for healing problems). Products include:

Blephamide Ophthalmic Ointment 568
Blephamide Ophthalmic Suspension 569
Poly-Pred Ophthalmic Suspension .... ⊙233
Pred Forte Ophthalmic Suspension .... ⊙235
Pred Mild Ophthalmic Suspension .... ⊙238
Pred-G Ophthalmic Ointment .... ⊙237
Pred-G Ophthalmic Suspension .... ⊙236

Prednisolone Sodium Phosphate (All topical nonsteroidal anti-inflammatory drugs (NSAIDs) may slow or delay healing. Topical corticosteroids are also known to slow or delay healing. Concomitant use of topical NSAIDs and topical steroids may increase the potential for healing problems).

No products indexed under this heading.

Prednisolone Tebutate (All topical nonsteroidal anti-inflammatory drugs (NSAIDs) may slow or delay healing. Topical corticosteroids are also known to slow or delay healing. Concomitant use of topical NSAIDs and topical steroids may increase the potential for healing problems).

No products indexed under this heading.

Prednisone (All topical nonsteroidal anti-inflammatory drugs (NSAIDs) may slow or delay healing. Topical corticosteroids are also known to slow or delay healing. Concomitant use of topical NSAIDs and topical steroids may increase the potential for healing problems).

No products indexed under this heading.

Tinzaparin Sodium (It is recommended that diclofenac ophthalmic suspension be used with caution in patients who are receiving other medications which may prolong bleeding time).

No products indexed under this heading.

Triamcinolone (All topical nonsteroidal anti-inflammatory drugs (NSAIDs) may slow or delay healing. Topical corticosteroids are also known to slow or delay healing. Concomitant use of topical NSAIDs and topical steroids may increase the potential for healing problems).

No products indexed under this heading.

Triamcinolone Acetonide (All topical nonsteroidal anti-inflammatory drugs (NSAIDs) may slow or delay healing. Topical corticosteroids are also known to slow or delay healing. Concomitant use of topical NSAIDs and topical steroids may increase the potential for healing problems). Products include:

Azmacort Inhalation Aerosol 1726
Nasacort AQ Nasal Spray 2922

Triamcinolone Diacetate (All topical nonsteroidal anti-inflammatory drugs (NSAIDs) may slow or delay healing. Topical corticosteroids are also known to slow or delay healing. Concomitant use of topical NSAIDs and topical steroids may increase the potential for healing problems).

No products indexed under this heading.

Triamcinolone Hexacetonide (All topical nonsteroidal anti-inflammatory drugs (NSAIDs) may slow or delay healing. Topical corticosteroids are also known to slow or delay healing. Concomitant use of topical NSAIDs and topical steroids may increase the potential for healing problems).

No products indexed under this heading.

Warfarin Sodium (It is recommended that diclofenac ophthalmic suspension be used with caution in patients who are receiving other medications which may prolong bleeding time). Products include:

Coumadin for Injection 898
Coumadin Tablets 898

VOLTAREN TABLETS

(Diclofenac Sodium) 2307

May interact with ACE inhibitors, lithium preparations, thiazides, and certain other agents. Compounds in these categories include:

Aspirin (When diclofenac is administered with aspirin, its protein binding is reduced; the clinical significance of this interaction is not known). Products include:

Aggrenox Capsules 822
Bayer Aspirin 744
BC Allergy Sinus Cold Powder .... ▣677
BC Headache Powder .... ▣677
Arthritis Strength BC Powder .... ▣677
BC Sinus Cold Powder .... ▣677
Excedrin Extra Strength Caplets/Tablets/Geltabs .... ▣684
Excedrin Migraine Caplets/Tablets/Geltabs .... ▣609
Goody's Body Pain Formula Powder .... ▣684
Goody's Extra Strength Headache Powders .... ▣611
Goody's Extra Strength Pain Relief Tablets .... ▣685
Percodan Tablets 1132
St. Joseph 81 mg Aspirin Chewable and Enteric Coated Tablets 1869

Benazepril Hydrochloride (Reports suggest that NSAIDs may diminish the antihypertensive effect of ACE inhibitors; this interaction should be given consideration in patients taking NSAIDs concomitantly with ACE inhibitors). Products include:

Lotensin Tablets 2243
Lotensin HCT Tablets 2246
Lotrel Capsules 2249

Bendroflumethiazide (Studies have shown that diclofenac can reduce the natriuretic effect of furosemide and thiazides in some patients; during concomitant therapy with NSAIDs, the patient should be observed closely for signs of renal failure, as well as to assure diuretic efficacy).

No products indexed under this heading.

Captopril (Reports suggest that NSAIDs may diminish the antihypertensive effect of ACE inhibitors; this interaction should be given consideration in patients taking NSAIDs concomitantly with ACE inhibitors). Products include:

Captopril Tablets 2149

Chlorothiazide (Studies have shown that diclofenac can reduce the natriuretic effect of furosemide and thiazides in some patients; during concomitant therapy with NSAIDs, the patient should be observed closely for signs of renal failure, as well as to assure diuretic efficacy). Products include:

Diuril Oral Suspension 1954

Chlorothiazide Sodium (Studies have shown that diclofenac can reduce the natriuretic effect of furosemide and thiazides in some patients; during concomitant therapy with NSAIDs, the patient should be observed closely for signs of renal failure, as well as to assure diuretic efficacy). Products include:

Diuril Sodium Intravenous 2467

Cyclosporine (Diclofenac may affect renal prostaglandins and increase the toxicity of certain drugs; concomitant therapy with diclofenac may increase cyclosporine's nephrotoxicity; caution should be used when administered concomitantly with cyclosporine). Products include:

Gengraf Capsules 459
Neoral Oral Solution 2259
Neoral Soft Gelatin Capsules 2259
Restasis Ophthalmic Emulsion 575
Sandimmune 2275

Enalapril Maleate (Reports suggest that NSAIDs may diminish the antihypertensive effect of ACE inhibitors; this interaction should be given consideration in patients taking NSAIDs concomitantly with ACE inhibitors). Products include:

Vasotec I.V. Injection 2103

Enalaprilat (Reports suggest that NSAIDs may diminish the antihypertensive effect of ACE inhibitors; this interaction should be given consideration in patients taking NSAIDs concomitantly with ACE inhibitors).

No products indexed under this heading.

Fosinopril Sodium (Reports suggest that NSAIDs may diminish the antihypertensive effect of ACE inhibitors; this interaction should be given consideration in patients taking NSAIDs concomitantly with ACE inhibitors).
No products indexed under this heading.

Furosemide (Studies have shown that diclofenac can reduce the natriuretic effect of furosemide and thiazides in some patients; during concomitant therapy with NSAIDs, the patient should be observed closely for signs of renal failure, as well as to assure diuretic efficacy). Products include:
Furosemide Tablets 2154

Hydrochlorothiazide (Studies have shown that diclofenac can reduce the natriuretic effect of furosemide and thiazides in some patients; during concomitant therapy with NSAIDs, the patient should be observed closely for signs of renal failure, as well as to assure diuretic efficacy). Products include:
Aldoril Tablets 1910
Atacand HCT 651
Avalide Tablets 888
Avalide Tablets 2874
Benicar HCT Tablets 1044
Diovan HCT Tablets 2196
Dyazide Capsules 1423
Hyzaar 50-12.5 Tablets 1990
Hyzaar 100-12.5 Tablets 1990
Hyzaar 100-25 Tablets 1990
Lopressor HCT 50/25 Tablets 2241
Lopressor HCT 100/25 Tablets 2241
Lopressor HCT 100/50 Tablets 2241
Lotensin HCT Tablets 2246
Micardis HCT Tablets 856
Moduretic Tablets 2028
Prinzide Tablets 2056
Teveten HCT Tablets 1737
Timolide Tablets 2086
Uniretic Tablets 3100

Hydroflumethiazide (Studies have shown that diclofenac can reduce the natriuretic effect of furosemide and thiazides in some patients; during concomitant therapy with NSAIDs, the patient should be observed closely for signs of renal failure, as well as to assure diuretic efficacy).
No products indexed under this heading.

Lisinopril (Reports suggest that NSAIDs may diminish the antihypertensive effect of ACE inhibitors; this interaction should be given consideration in patients taking NSAIDs concomitantly with ACE inhibitors). Products include:
Prinivil Tablets 2052
Prinzide Tablets 2056

Lithium (NSAIDs have produced an elevation of plasma lithium levels and a reduction in renal lithium clearance; these effects have been attributed to inhibition of renal prostaglandin synthesis by the NSAID; monitor for signs of lithium toxicity).
No products indexed under this heading.

Lithium Carbonate (NSAIDs have produced an elevation of plasma lithium levels and a reduction in renal lithium clearance; these effects have been attributed to inhibition of renal prostaglandin synthesis by the NSAID; monitor for signs of lithium toxicity). Products include:
Lithobid Tablets 1692

Lithium Citrate (NSAIDs have produced an elevation of plasma lithium levels and a reduction in renal lithium clearance; these effects have been attributed to inhibition of renal prostaglandin synthesis by the NSAID; monitor for signs of lithium toxicity).
No products indexed under this heading.

Methotrexate Sodium (NSAIDs have been reported to competitively inhibit methotrexate accumulation in animal studies; this may indicate that they could enhance the toxicity of methotrexate; caution should be given when NSAIDs are administered concomitantly with methotrexate).
No products indexed under this heading.

Methyclothiazide (Studies have shown that diclofenac can reduce the natriuretic effect of furosemide and thiazides in some patients; during concomitant therapy with NSAIDs, the patient should be observed closely for signs of renal failure, as well as to assure diuretic efficacy).
No products indexed under this heading.

Moexipril Hydrochloride (Reports suggest that NSAIDs may diminish the antihypertensive effect of ACE inhibitors; this interaction should be given consideration in patients taking NSAIDs concomitantly with ACE inhibitors). Products include:
Uniretic Tablets 3100
Univasc Tablets 3104

Perindopril Erbumine (Reports suggest that NSAIDs may diminish the antihypertensive effect of ACE inhibitors; this interaction should be given consideration in patients taking NSAIDs concomitantly with ACE inhibitors). Products include:
Aceon Tablets (2 mg, 4 mg, 8 mg) 3194

Polythiazide (Studies have shown that diclofenac can reduce the natriuretic effect of furosemide and thiazides in some patients; during concomitant therapy with NSAIDs, the patient should be observed closely for signs of renal failure, as well as to assure diuretic efficacy).
No products indexed under this heading.

Quinapril Hydrochloride (Reports suggest that NSAIDs may diminish the antihypertensive effect of ACE inhibitors; this interaction should be given consideration in patients taking NSAIDs concomitantly with ACE inhibitors).
No products indexed under this heading.

Ramipril (Reports suggest that NSAIDs may diminish the antihypertensive effect of ACE inhibitors; this interaction should be given consideration in patients taking NSAIDs concomitantly with ACE inhibitors). Products include:
Altace Capsules 1702

Spirapril Hydrochloride (Reports suggest that NSAIDs may diminish the antihypertensive effect of ACE inhibitors; this interaction should be given consideration in patients taking NSAIDs concomitantly with ACE inhibitors).
No products indexed under this heading.

Trandolapril (Reports suggest that NSAIDs may diminish the antihypertensive effect of ACE inhibitors; this interaction should be given consideration in patients taking NSAIDs concomitantly with ACE inhibitors). Products include:
Mavik Tablets 486
Tarka Tablets 524

Warfarin Sodium (The effects of warfarin and NSAIDs on GI bleeding are synergistic, such that users of both drugs together have a risk of serious GI bleeding higher than users of either drug alone). Products include:
Coumadin for Injection 898
Coumadin Tablets 898

VOLTAREN-XR TABLETS

(Diclofenac Sodium) 2310
See Voltaren Tablets

VOSPIRE ER TABLETS

(Albuterol Sulfate) 1052
May interact with beta blockers, loop diuretics, monoamine oxidase inhibitors, nonpotassium-sparing diuretics, sympathomimetics, sympathomimetic aerosol bronchodilators, thiazides, tricyclic antidepressants, and certain other agents. Compounds in these categories include:

Acebutolol Hydrochloride (Beta-adrenergic receptor blocking agents not only block the pulmonary effect of beta-agonists, such as albuterol extended-release tablets, but may produce severe bronchospasm in asthmatic patients. Therefore, patients with asthma should not normally be treated with beta-blockers. However, under certain circumstances, e.g., as prophylaxis after myocardial infarction, there may be no acceptable alternatives to the use of beta-adrenergic blocking agents in patients with asthma. In this setting, cardio-selective beta-blockers could be considered, although they should be administered with caution).
No products indexed under this heading.

Albuterol (The concomitant use of albuterol extended-release tablets and other oral sympathomimetic agents is not recommended since such combined use may lead to deleterious cardiovascular effects. This recommendation does not preclude the judicious use of an aerosol bronchodilator of the adrenergic stimulant type in patients receiving albuterol extended-release tablets. Such concomitant use, however, should be individualized and not given on a routine basis. If regular co-administration is required, then alternative therapy should be considered). Products include:
Proventil Inhalation Aerosol 3053

Amitriptyline Hydrochloride (Albuterol should be administered with extreme caution to patients being treated with tricyclic antidepressants or within two weeks of discontinuation of such agents, because the action of albuterol on the vascular system may be potentiated).
No products indexed under this heading.

Amoxapine (Albuterol should be administered with extreme caution to patients being treated with tricyclic antidepressants or within two weeks of discontinuation of such agents, because the action of albuterol on the vascular system may be potentiated).
No products indexed under this heading.

Atenolol (Beta-adrenergic receptor blocking agents not only block the pulmonary effect of beta-agonists, such as albuterol extended-release tablets, but may produce severe bronchospasm in asthmatic patients. Therefore, patients with asthma should not normally be treated with beta-blockers. However, under certain circumstances, e.g., as prophylaxis after myocardial infarction, there may be no acceptable alternatives to the use of beta-adrenergic blocking agents in patients with asthma. In this setting, cardio-selective beta-blockers could be considered, although they should be administered with caution).
No products indexed under this heading.

Bendroflumethiazide (The ECG changse and/or hypokalemia that may result from the administration of nonpotassium-sparing diuretics (such as thiazide diuretics) can be acutely worsened by beta-agonists, especially when the recommended dose of the beta-agonist is exceeded. Although the clinical significance of these effects is not known, caution is advised in the co-administration of beta-agonists with nonpotassium-sparing diuretics).
No products indexed under this heading.

Betaxolol Hydrochloride (Beta-adrenergic receptor blocking agents not only block the pulmonary effect of beta-agonists, such as albuterol extended-release tablets, but may produce severe bronchospasm in asthmatic patients. Therefore, patients with asthma should not normally be treated with beta-blockers. However, under certain circumstances, e.g., as prophylaxis after myocardial infarction, there may be no acceptable alternatives to the use of beta-adrenergic blocking agents in patients with asthma. In this setting, cardio-selective beta-blockers could be considered, although they should be administered with caution). Products include:
Betoptic S Ophthalmic Suspension 558

Bisoprolol Fumarate (Beta-adrenergic receptor blocking agents not only block the pulmonary effect of beta-agonists, such as albuterol extended-release tablets, but may produce severe bronchospasm in asthmatic patients. Therefore, patients with asthma should not normally be treated with beta-blockers. However, under certain circumstances, e.g., as prophylaxis after myocardial infarction, there may be no acceptable alternatives to the use of beta-adrenergic blocking agents in patients with asthma. In this setting, cardio-selective beta-blockers could be considered, although they should be administered with caution).
No products indexed under this heading.

Bitolterol Mesylate (The concomitant use of albuterol extended-

release tablets and other oral sympathomimetic agents is not recommended since such combined use may lead to deleterious cardiovascular effects. This recommendation does not preclude the judicious use of an aerosol bronchodilator of the adrenergic stimulant type in patients receiving albuterol extended-release tablets. Such concomitant use, however, should be individualized and not given on a routine basis. If regular coadministration is required, then alternative therapy should be considered).
No products indexed under this heading.

Bumetanide (The ECG changes and/or hypokalemia that may result from the administration of nonpotassium-sparing diuretics (such as loop diuretics) can be acutely worsened by beta-agonists, especially when the recommended dose of the beta-agonist is exceeded. Although the clinical significance of these effects is not known, caution is advised in the coadministration of beta-agonists with nonpotassium-sparing diuretics).
Products include:
Bumex Tablets **2746**

Carteolol Hydrochloride (Beta-adrenergic receptor blocking agents not only block the pulmonary effect of beta-agonists, such as albuterol extended-release tablets, but may produce severe bronchospasm in asthmatic patients. Therefore, patients with asthma should not normally be treated with beta-blockers. However, under certain circumstances, e.g., as prophylaxis after myocardial infarction, there may be no acceptable alternatives to the use of beta-adrenergic blocking agents in patients with asthma. In this setting, cardio-selective beta-blockers could be considered, although they should be administered with caution).
Products include:
Carteolol Hydrochloride Ophthalmic Solution USP, 1%........ ⊙**249**

Chlorothiazide (The ECG changse and/or hypokalemia that may result from the administration of nonpotassium-sparing diuretics (such as thiazide diuretics) can be acutely worsened by beta-agonists, especially when the recommended dose of the beta-agonist is exceeded. Although the clinical significance of these effects is not known, caution is advised in the coadministration of beta-agonists with nonpotassium-sparing diuretics).
Products include:
Diuril Oral Suspension **1954**

Chlorothiazide Sodium (The ECG changse and/or hypokalemia that may result from the administration of nonpotassium-sparing diuretics (such as thiazide diuretics) can be acutely worsened by beta-agonists, especially when the recommended dose of the beta-agonist is exceeded. Although the clinical significance of these effects is not known, caution is advised in the coadministration of beta-agonists with nonpotassium-sparing diuretics).
Products include:
Diuril Sodium Intravenous **2467**

Clomipramine Hydrochloride (Albuterol should be administered with extreme caution to patients being treated with tricyclic antidepressants or within two weeks of discontinuation of such agents, because the action of albuterol on the vascular system may be potentiated).
No products indexed under this heading.

Desipramine Hydrochloride (Albuterol should be administered with extreme caution to patients being treated with tricyclic antidepressants or within two weeks of discontinuation of such agents, because the action of albuterol on the vascular system may be potentiated).
No products indexed under this heading.

Digoxin (Mean decreases of 16% to 22% in serum digoxin levels were demonstrated after single dose intravenous and oral administration of albuterol, respectively, to normal volunteers who had received digoxin for 10 days. It would be prudent to carefully evaluatethe serum digoxin levels in patients who are currently receiving digoxin and albuterol).
Products include:
Lanoxicaps Capsules **1490**
Lanoxin Injection **1494**
Lanoxin Injection Pediatric **1497**
Lanoxin Tablets **1500**

Doxepin Hydrochloride (Albuterol should be administered with extreme caution to patients being treated with tricyclic antidepressants or within two weeks of discontinuation of such agents, because the action of albuterol on the vascular system may be potentiated).
No products indexed under this heading.

Esmolol Hydrochloride (Beta-adrenergic receptor blocking agents not only block the pulmonary effect of beta-agonists, such as albuterol extended-release tablets, but may produce severe bronchospasm in asthmatic patients. Therefore, patients with asthma should not normally be treated with beta-blockers. However, under certain circumstances, e.g., as prophylaxis after myocardial infarction, there may be no acceptable alternatives to the use of beta-adrenergic blocking agents in patients with asthma. In this setting, cardio-selective beta-blockers could be considered, although they should be administered with caution).
No products indexed under this heading.

Ethacrynic Acid (The ECG changes and/or hypokalemia that may result from the administration of nonpotassium-sparing diuretics (such as loop diuretics) can be acutely worsened by beta-agonists, especially when the recommended dose of the beta-agonist is exceeded. Although the clinical significance of these effects is not known, caution is advised in the coadministration of beta-agonists with nonpotassium-sparing diuretics).
Products include:
Edecrin Tablets **1959**

Furosemide (The ECG changes and/or hypokalemia that may result from the administration of nonpotassium-sparing diuretics (such as loop diuretics) can be acutely worsened by beta-agonists, especially when the recommended dose of the beta-agonist is exceeded. Although the clinical significance of these effects is not known, caution is advised in the coadministration of beta-agonists with nonpotassium-sparing diuretics).
Products include:
Furosemide Tablets **2154**

Hydrochlorothiazide (The ECG changse and/or hypokalemia that may result from the administration of nonpotassium-sparing diuretics (such as thiazide diuretics) can be acutely worsened by beta-agonists, especially when the recommended dose of the beta-agonist is exceeded. Although the clinical significance of these effects is not known, caution is advised in the coadministration of beta-agonists with nonpotassium-sparing diuretics).
Products include:
Aldoril Tablets **1910**
Atacand HCT **651**
Avalide Tablets **888**
Avalide Tablets **2874**
Benicar HCT Tablets **1044**
Diovan HCT Tablets **2196**
Dyazide Capsules **1423**
Hyzaar 50-12.5 Tablets **1990**
Hyzaar 100-12.5 Tablets **1990**
Hyzaar 100-25 Tablets **1990**
Lopressor HCT 50/25 Tablets **2241**
Lopressor HCT 100/25 Tablets **2241**
Lopressor HCT 100/50 Tablets **2241**
Lotensin HCT Tablets **2246**
Micardis HCT Tablets **856**
Moduretic Tablets **2028**
Prinzide Tablets **2056**
Teveten HCT Tablets **1737**
Timolide Tablets **2086**
Uniretic Tablets **3100**

Hydroflumethiazide (The ECG changse and/or hypokalemia that may result from the administration of nonpotassium-sparing diuretics (such as thiazide diuretics) can be acutely worsened by beta-agonists, especially when the recommended dose of the beta-agonist is exceeded. Although the clinical significance of these effects is not known, caution is advised in the coadministration of beta-agonists with nonpotassium-sparing diuretics).
No products indexed under this heading.

Imipramine Hydrochloride (Albuterol should be administered with extreme caution to patients being treated with tricyclic antidepressants or within two weeks of discontinuation of such agents, because the action of albuterol on the vascular system may be potentiated).
No products indexed under this heading.

Imipramine Pamoate (Albuterol should be administered with extreme caution to patients being treated with tricyclic antidepressants or within two weeks of discontinuation of such agents, because the action of albuterol on the vascular system may be potentiated).
No products indexed under this heading.

Isocarboxazid (Albuterol should be administered with extreme caution to patients being treated with monoamine oxidase inhibitors or within two weeks of discontinuation of such agents, because the action of albuterol on the vascular system may be potentiated).
No products indexed under this heading.

Isoetharine (The concomitant use of albuterol extended-release tablets and other oral sympathomimetic agents is not recommended since such combined use may lead to deleterious cardiovascular effects. This recommendation does not preclude the judicious use of an aerosol bronchodilator of the adrenergic stimulant type in patients receiving albuterol extended-release tablets. Such concomitant use, however, should be individualized and not given on a routine basis. If regular coadministration is required, then alternative therapy should be considered).
No products indexed under this heading.

Isoproterenol Hydrochloride (The concomitant use of albuterol extended-release tablets and other oral sympathomimetic agents is not recommended since such combined use may lead to deleterious cardiovascular effects. This recommendation does not preclude the judicious use of an aerosol bronchodilator of the adrenergic stimulant type in patients receiving albuterol extended-release tablets. Such concomitant use, however, should be individualized and not given on a routine basis. If regular coadministration is required, then alternative therapy should be considered).
No products indexed under this heading.

Labetalol Hydrochloride (Beta-adrenergic receptor blocking agents not only block the pulmonary effect of beta-agonists, such as albuterol extended-release tablets, but may produce severe bronchospasm in asthmatic patients. Therefore, patients with asthma should not normally be treated with beta-blockers. However, under certain circumstances, e.g., as prophylaxis after myocardial infarction, there may be no acceptable alternatives to the use of beta-adrenergic blocking agents in patients with asthma. In this setting, cardio-selective beta-blockers could be considered, although they should be administered with caution).
No products indexed under this heading.

Levalbuterol Hydrochloride (The concomitant use of albuterol extended-release tablets and other oral sympathomimetic agents is not recommended since such combined use may lead to deleterious cardiovascular effects. This recommendation does not preclude the judicious use of an aerosol bronchodilator of the adrenergic stimulant type in patients receiving albuterol extended-release tablets. Such concomitant use, however, should be individualized and not given on a routine basis. If regular coadministration is required, then alternative therapy should be considered). Products include:
Xopenex Inhalation Solution **3146**
Xopenex Inhalation Solution Concentrate **3150**

Levobunolol Hydrochloride (Beta-adrenergic receptor blocking agents not only block the pulmonary effect of beta-agonists, such as albuterol extended-release tablets, but may produce severe bronchospasm in asthmatic patients. Therefore, patients with asthma should not normally be treated with beta-blockers. However, under certain circumstances, e.g., as prophylaxis after myocardial infarction, there may be no acceptable alternatives to the use of beta-adrenergic blocking agents in patients with asthma. In this setting, cardio-selective beta-blockers could be considered, although they should be administered with caution). Products include:

Betagan Ophthalmic Solution, USP .... ⊙220

Maprotiline Hydrochloride (Albuterol should be administered with extreme caution to patients being treated with tricyclic antidepressants or within two weeks of discontinuation of such agents, because the action of albuterol on the vascular system may be potentiated).

No products indexed under this heading.

Metaproterenol Sulfate (The concomitant use of albuterol extended-release tablets and other oral sympathomimetic agents is not recommended since such combined use may lead to deleterious cardiovascular effects. This recommendation does not preclude the judicious use of an aerosol bronchodilator of the adrenergic stimulant type in patients receiving albuterol extended-release tablets. Such concomitant use, however, should be individualized and not given on a routine basis. If regular co-administration is required, then alternative therapy should be considered). Products include:

Alupent Inhalation Aerosol 826

Methyclothiazide (The ECG change and/or hypokalemia that may result from the administration of nonpotassium-sparing diuretics (such as thiazide diuretics) can be acutely worsened by beta-agonists, especially when the recommended dose of the beta-agonist is exceeded. Although the clinical significance of these effects is not known, caution is advised in the co-administration of beta-agonists with nonpotassium-sparing diuretics).

No products indexed under this heading.

Metipranolol Hydrochloride (Beta-adrenergic receptor blocking agents not only block the pulmonary effect of beta-agonists, such as albuterol extended-release tablets, but may produce severe bronchospasm in asthmatic patients. Therefore, patients with asthma should not normally be treated with beta-blockers. However, under certain circumstances, e.g., as prophylaxis after myocardial infarction, there may be no acceptable alternatives to the use of beta-adrenergic blocking agents in patients with asthma. In this setting, cardio-selective beta-blockers could be considered, although they should be administered with caution).

No products indexed under this heading.

Metoprolol Succinate (Beta-adrenergic receptor blocking agents not only block the pulmonary effect of beta-agonists, such as albuterol extended-release tablets, but may produce severe bronchospasm in asthmatic patients. Therefore, patients with asthma should not normally be treated with beta-blockers. However, under certain circumstances, e.g., as prophylaxis after myocardial infarction, there may be no acceptable alternatives to the use of beta-adrenergic blocking agents in patients with asthma. In this setting, cardio-selective beta-blockers could be considered, although they should be administered with caution). Products include:

Toprol-XL Tablets 668

Metoprolol Tartrate (Beta-adrenergic receptor blocking agents not only block the pulmonary effect of beta-agonists, such as albuterol extended-release tablets, but may produce severe bronchospasm in asthmatic patients. Therefore, patients with asthma should not normally be treated with beta-blockers. However, under certain circumstances, e.g., as prophylaxis after myocardial infarction, there may be no acceptable alternatives to the use of beta-adrenergic blocking agents in patients with asthma. In this setting, cardio-selective beta-blockers could be considered, although they should be administered with caution). Products include:

Lopressor Injection 2238
Lopressor Tablets 2238
Lopressor HCT 50/25 Tablets 2241
Lopressor HCT 100/25 Tablets 2241
Lopressor HCT 100/50 Tablets 2241

Moclobemide (Albuterol should be administered with extreme caution to patients being treated with monoamine oxidase inhibitors or within two weeks of discontinuation of such agents, because the action of albuterol on the vascular system may be potentiated).

No products indexed under this heading.

Nadolol (Beta-adrenergic receptor blocking agents not only block the pulmonary effect of beta-agonists, such as albuterol extended-release tablets, but may produce severe bronchospasm in asthmatic patients. Therefore, patients with asthma should not normally be treated with beta-blockers. However, under certain circumstances, e.g., as prophylaxis after myocardial infarction, there may be no acceptable alternatives to the use of beta-adrenergic blocking agents in patients with asthma. In this setting, cardio-selective beta-blockers could be considered, although they should be administered with caution). Products include:

Nadolol Tablets 2159

Nortriptyline Hydrochloride (Albuterol should be administered with extreme caution to patients being treated with tricyclic antidepressants or within two weeks of discontinuation of such agents, because the action of albuterol on the vascular system may be potentiated).

No products indexed under this heading.

Pargyline Hydrochloride (Albuterol should be administered with extreme caution to patients being treated with monoamine oxidase inhibitors or within two weeks of discontinuation of such agents, because the action of albuterol on the vascular system may be potentiated).

No products indexed under this heading.

Penbutolol Sulfate (Beta-adrenergic receptor blocking agents not only block the pulmonary effect of beta-agonists, such as albuterol extended-release tablets, but may produce severe bronchospasm in asthmatic patients. Therefore, patients with asthma should not normally be treated with beta-blockers. However, under certain circumstances, e.g., as prophylaxis after myocardial infarction, there may be no acceptable alternatives to the use of beta-adrenergic blocking agents in patients with asthma. In this setting, cardio-selective beta-blockers could be considered, although they should be administered with caution).

No products indexed under this heading.

Phenelzine Sulfate (Albuterol should be administered with extreme caution to patients being treated with monoamine oxidase inhibitors or within two weeks of discontinuation of such agents, because the action of albuterol on the vascular system may be potentiated).

No products indexed under this heading.

Pindolol (Beta-adrenergic receptor blocking agents not only block the pulmonary effect of beta-agonists, such as albuterol extended-release tablets, but may produce severe bronchospasm in asthmatic patients. Therefore, patients with asthma should not normally be treated with beta-blockers. However, under certain circumstances, e.g., as prophylaxis after myocardial infarction, there may be no acceptable alternatives to the use of beta-adrenergic blocking agents in patients with asthma. In this setting, cardio-selective beta-blockers could be considered, although they should be administered with caution).

No products indexed under this heading.

Pirbuterol Acetate (The concomitant use of albuterol extended-release tablets and other oral sympathomimetic agents is not recommended since such combined use may lead to deleterious cardiovascular effects. This recommendation does not preclude the judicious use of an aerosol bronchodilator of the adrenergic stimulant type in patients receiving albuterol extended-release tablets. Such concomitant use, however, should be individualized and not given on a routine basis. If regular co-administration is required, then alternative therapy should be considered). Products include:

Maxair Autohaler 1852

Polythiazide (The ECG changse and/or hypokalemia that may result from the administration of nonpotassium-sparing diuretics (such as thiazide diuretics) can be acutely worsened by beta-agonists, especially when the recommended dose of the beta-agonist is exceeded. Although the clinical significance of these effects is not known, caution is advised in the co-administration of beta-agonists with nonpotassium-sparing diuretics).

No products indexed under this heading.

Procarbazine Hydrochloride (Albuterol should be administered with extreme caution to patients being treated with monoamine oxidase inhibitors or within two weeks of discontinuation of such agents, because the action of albuterol on the vascular system may be potentiated). Products include:

Matulane Capsules 3191

Propranolol Hydrochloride (Beta-adrenergic receptor blocking agents not only block the pulmonary effect of beta-agonists, such as albuterol extended-release tablets, but may produce severe bronchospasm in asthmatic patients. Therefore, patients with asthma should not normally be treated with beta-blockers. However, under certain circumstances, e.g., as prophylaxis after myocardial infarction, there may be no acceptable alternatives to the use of beta-adrenergic blocking agents in patients with asthma. In this setting, cardio-selective beta-blockers could be considered, although they should be administered with caution). Products include:

Inderal LA Long-Acting Capsules 3429
InnoPran XL Capsules 2723

Protriptyline Hydrochloride (Albuterol should be administered with extreme caution to patients being treated with tricyclic antidepressants or within two weeks of discontinuation of such agents, because the action of albuterol on the vascular system may be potentiated).

No products indexed under this heading.

Salmeterol Xinafoate (The concomitant use of albuterol extended-release tablets and other oral sympathomimetic agents is not recommended since such combined use may lead to deleterious cardiovascular effects. This recommendation does not preclude the judicious use of an aerosol bronchodilator of the adrenergic stimulant type in patients receiving albuterol extended-release tablets. Such concomitant use, however, should be individualized and not given on a routine basis. If regular co-administration is required, then alternative therapy should be considered). Products include:

Advair Diskus 100/50 1308
Advair Diskus 250/50 1308
Advair Diskus 500/50 1308
Advair HFA Inhalation Aerosol 1318
Serevent Diskus 1568

Selegiline Hydrochloride (Albuterol should be administered with extreme caution to patients being treated with monoamine oxidase inhibitors or within two weeks of discontinuation of such agents, because the action of albuterol on the vascular system may be potentiated). Products include:

Eldepryl Capsules 3208
Zelapar Tablets 3372

Sotalol Hydrochloride (Beta-adrenergic receptor blocking agents not only block the pulmonary effect of beta-agonists, such as albuterol extended-release tablets, but may produce severe bronchospasm in asthmatic patients. Therefore, patients with asthma should not normally be treated with beta-blockers. However, under certain circumstances, e.g., as prophylaxis after myocardial infarction, there may be no acceptable alternatives to the use of beta-adrenergic blocking agents in patients with asthma. In this setting, cardio-selective beta-blockers could be considered, although they should be administered with caution).

No products indexed under this heading.

Terbutaline Sulfate (The concomitant use of albuterol extended-release tablets and other oral sympathomimetic agents is not recommended since such combined use may lead to deleterious cardiovascular effects. This recommendation does not preclude the judicious use of an aerosol bronchodilator of the adrenergic stimulant type in patients receiving albuterol extended-release tablets. Such concomitant use, however, should be individualized and not given on a routine basis. If regular co-administration is required, then alternative therapy should be considered).

No products indexed under this heading.

Timolol Hemihydrate (Beta-adrenergic receptor blocking agents not only block the pulmonary effect of beta-agonists, such as albuterol extended-release tablets, but may produce severe bronchospasm in asthmatic patients. Therefore, patients with asthma should not normally be treated with beta-blockers. However, under certain circumstances, e.g., as prophylaxis after myocardial infarction, there may be no acceptable alternatives to the use of beta-adrenergic blocking agents in patients with asthma. In this setting, cardio-selective beta-blockers could be considered, although they should be administered with caution). Products include:

Betimol Ophthalmic Solution 3382
Betimol Ophthalmic Solution .... ⊙295

Timolol Maleate (Beta-adrenergic receptor blocking agents not only block the pulmonary effect of beta-agonists, such as albuterol extended-release tablets, but may produce severe bronchospasm in asthmatic patients. Therefore, patients with asthma should not normally be treated with beta-blockers. However, under certain circumstances, e.g., as prophylaxis after myocardial infarction, there may be no acceptable alternatives to the use of beta-adrenergic blocking agents in patients with asthma. In this setting, cardio-selective beta-blockers could be considered, although they should be administered with caution). Products include:

Blocadren Tablets 1916
Cosopt Sterile Ophthalmic Solution 1931
Timolide Tablets 2086
Timoptic Sterile Ophthalmic Solution 2088
Timoptic in Ocudose 2091
Timoptic-XE Sterile Ophthalmic Gel Forming Solution 2092

Torsemide (The ECG changes and/or hypokalemia that may result from the administration of nonpotassium-sparing diuretics (such as loop diuretics) can be acutely worsened by beta-agonists, especially when the recommended dose of the beta-agonist is exceeded. Although the clinical significance of these effects is not known, caution is advised in the co-administration of beta-agonists with nonpotassium-sparing diuretics). Products include:

Demadex Injection 2759
Demadex Tablets 2759

Tranylcypromine Sulfate (Albuterol should be administered with extreme caution to patients being treated with monoamine oxidase inhibitors or within two weeks of discontinuation of such agents, because the action of albuterol on the vascular system may be potentiated). Products include:

Parnate Tablets 1527

Trimipramine Maleate (Albuterol should be administered with extreme caution to patients being treated with tricyclic antidepressants or within two weeks of discontinuation of such agents, because the action of albuterol on the vascular system may be potentiated).

No products indexed under this heading.

VYTORIN 10/10 TABLETS

(Ezetimibe, Simvastatin) 2114

May interact with oral anticoagulants, cytochrome p450 3a4 inhibitors, potent, erythromycin, fibrates, protease inhibitors, and certain other agents. Compounds in these categories include:

Amiodarone Hydrochloride (The dose of Vytorin should not exceed 10/20 mg daily in patients receiving concomitant medication with amiodarone. The combined use of Vytorin at doses higher than 10/20 mg daily with amiodarone should be avoided unless the clinical benefit is likely to outweigh the increased risk of myopathy).

No products indexed under this heading.

Amprenavir (Simvastatin is a substrate of cytochrome P450 3A4 (CYP3A4). When simvastatin is used with potent inhibitors of CYP3A4, elevated plasma levels of HMG-CoA reductase inhibitory activity can increase the risk of myopathy and rhabdomyolysis, particulary with higher doses of simvastatin. The use of Vytorin concomitantly with potent CYP3A4 inhibitors, such as erythromycin, should be avoided). Products include:

Agenerase Capsules 1327
Agenerase Oral Solution 1332

Anisindione (Simvastatin modestly potentiated the effect of coumarin anticoagulants; monitor prothrombin time during co-administration). Products include:

Miradon Tablets 3042

Atazanavir (Simvastatin is a substrate of cytochrome P450 3A4 (CYP3A4). When simvastatin is used with potent inhibitors of CYP3A4, elevated plasma levels of HMG-CoA reductase inhibitory activity can increase the risk of myopathy and rhabdomyolysis, particulary with higher doses of simvastatin. Concomitant use should be avoided unless the benefits of combined therapy outweigh the increased risk. If treatment with potent CYP3A4 inhibitors is unavoidable, therapy with Vytorin should be suspended during the course of treatment).

No products indexed under this heading.

Atazanavir sulfate (Simvastatin is a substrate of cytochrome P450 3A4 (CYP3A4). When simvastatin is used with potent inhibitors of CYP3A4, elevated plasma levels of HMG-CoA reductase inhibitory activity can increase the risk of myopathy and rhabdomyolysis, particulary with higher doses of simvastatin. Concomitant use should be avoided unless the benefits of combined therapy outweigh the increased risk. If treatment with potent CYP3A4 inhibitors is unavoidable, therapy with Vytorin should be suspended during the course of treatment). Products include:

Reyataz Capsules 921

Cholestyramine (Co-administration decreased the mean AUC of total ezetimibe by approximately 55%; therefore, the incremental LDL-C reduction due to adding ezetimibe/simvastatin to cholestyramine may be reduced).

No products indexed under this heading.

Clarithromycin (Simvastatin is a substrate of cytochrome P450 3A4 (CYP3A4). When simvastatin is used with potent inhibitors of CYP3A4, elevated plasma levels of HMG-CoA reductase inhibitory activity can increase the risk of myopathy and rhabdomyolysis, particulary with higher doses of simvastatin. The use of Vytorin concomitantly with potent CYP3A4 inhibitors, such as clarithromycin, should be avoided). Products include:

Biaxin/Biaxin XL 402
PREVPAC 3284

Clofibrate (The safety and effectiveness of ezetimibe administered with fibrates have not been established. There is an increased risk of myopathy when simvastatin is used concomitantly with fibrates. Therefore, the concomitant use of Vytorin and fibrates should be avoided).

No products indexed under this heading.

Cyclosporine (The dose of Vytorin should not exceed 10/10 mg daily in patients receiving concomitant medication with cyclosporine. The benefits of the use of Vytorin in patients receiving cyclosporine should be carefully weighed against the risks of this combination). Products include:

Gengraf Capsules 459
Neoral Oral Solution 2259
Neoral Soft Gelatin Capsules 2259
Restasis Ophthalmic Emulsion 575
Sandimmune 2275

Danazol (The dose of Vytorin should not exceed 10/10 mg daily in patients receiving concomitant medication with danazol. The benefits of the use of Vytorin in patients receiving danazol should be carefully weighed against the risks of this combination).

No products indexed under this heading.

Dicumarol (Simvastatin modestly potentiated the effect of coumarin anticoagulants; monitor prothrombin time during co-administration).

No products indexed under this heading.

Digoxin (Co-administration resulted in a slight elevation (less than 0.3 ng/mL) in plasma digoxin concentrations). Products include:

Lanoxicaps Capsules 1490
Lanoxin Injection 1494
Lanoxin Injection Pediatric 1497
Lanoxin Tablets 1500

Erythromycin (Simvastatin is a substrate of cytochrome P450 3A4 (CYP3A4). When simvastatin is used with potent inhibitors of CYP3A4, elevated plasma levels of HMG-CoA reductase inhibitory activity can increase the risk of myopathy and rhabdomyolysis, particulary with higher doses of simvastatin. The use of Vytorin concomitantly with potent CYP3A4 inhibitors, such as erythromycin, should be avoided). Products include:

Ery-Tab Tablets 449
Erythromycin Base Filmtab Tablets 455
Erythromycin Delayed-Release Capsules, USP 457
PCE Dispertab Tablets 515

Erythromycin Estolate (Simvastatin is a substrate of cytochrome P450 3A4 (CYP3A4). When simvastatin is used with potent inhibitors of CYP3A4, elevated plasma levels of HMG-CoA reductase inhibitory activity can increase the risk of myopathy and rhabdomyolysis, particulary with higher doses of simvastatin. The use of Vytorin concomitantly with potent CYP3A4 inhibitors, such as erythromycin, should be avoided).

No products indexed under this heading.

Erythromycin Ethylsuccinate (Simvastatin is a substrate of cytochrome P450 3A4 (CYP3A4). When simvastatin is used with potent inhibitors of CYP3A4, elevated plasma levels of HMG-CoA reductase inhibitory activity can increase the risk of myopathy and rhabdomyolysis, particulary with higher doses of simvastatin. The use of Vytorin concomitantly with potent CYP3A4 inhibitors, such as erythromycin, should be avoided). Products include:

E.E.S. 451
EryPed 447

Erythromycin Gluceptate (Simvastatin is a substrate of cytochrome P450 3A4 (CYP3A4). When simvastatin is used with potent inhibitors of CYP3A4, elevated plasma levels of HMG-CoA reductase inhibitory activity can increase the risk of myopathy and rhabdomyolysis, particulary with higher doses of simvastatin. The use of Vytorin concomitantly with potent CYP3A4 inhibitors, such as erythromycin, should be avoided).

No products indexed under this heading.

Erythromycin Lactobionate (Simvastatin is a substrate of cytochrome P450 3A4 (CYP3A4). When simvastatin is used with potent inhibitors of CYP3A4, elevated plasma levels of HMG-CoA reductase inhibitory activity can increase the risk of myopathy and rhabdomyolysis, particulary with higher doses of simvastatin. The use of Vytorin concomitantly with potent CYP3A4 inhibitors, such as erythromycin, should be avoided).

No products indexed under this heading.

Erythromycin Stearate (Simvastatin is a substrate of cytochrome P450 3A4 (CYP3A4). When simvastatin is used with potent inhibitors of CYP3A4, elevated plasma levels of HMG-CoA reductase inhibitory activity can increase the risk of myopathy and rhabdomyolysis, particulary with higher doses of simvastatin. The use of Vytorin concomitantly with potent CYP3A4 inhibitors, such as erythromycin, should be avoided). Products include:

Erythrocin Stearate Filmtab Tablets 453

Fenofibrate (The safety and effectiveness of ezetimibe administered with fibrates have not been estab-

IMPORTANT NOTE: Always consult each drug listing in the patient's regimen for possible interactions.

lished. There is an increased risk of myopathy when simvastatin is used concomitantly with fibrates. Therefore, the concomitant use of Vytorin and fibrates should be avoided). Products include:

Lofibra Tablets ... 1219
Lofibra Capsules ... 1216
Tricor Tablets ... 527
Triglide Tablets ... 3123

Fosamprenavir Calcium (Simvastatin is a substrate of cytochrome P450 3A4 (CYP3A4). When simvastatin is used with potent inhibitors of CYP3A4, elevated plasma levels of HMG-CoA reductase inhibitory activity can increase the risk of myopathy and rhabdomyolysis, particulary with higher doses of simvastatin. Concomitant use should be avoided unless the benefits of combined therapy outweigh the increased risk. If treatment with potent CYP3A4 inhibitors is unavoidable, therapy with Vytorin should be suspended during the course of treatment). Products include:

Lexiva Tablets ... 1505

Gemfibrozil (There is an increased risk of myopathy when simvastatin is used concomitantly with fibrates (especially gemfibrozil). The combined use of simvastatin with gemfibrozil should be avoided, uless the benefits are likely to outweigh the increased risks of this drug combination. The dose of simvastatin should not exceed 10 mg daily in patients receiving concomitant medication with gemfibrozil. Therefore, although not recommended, if Vytorin is used in combination with gemfibrozil, the dose should not exceed 10/10 mg daily).

No products indexed under this heading.

Indinavir Sulfate (Simvastatin is a substrate of cytochrome P450 3A4 (CYP3A4). When simvastatin is used with potent inhibitors of CYP3A4, elevated plasma levels of HMG-CoA reductase inhibitory activity can increase the risk of myopathy and rhabdomyolysis, particulary with higher doses of simvastatin. The use of Vytorin concomitantly with potent CYP3A4 inhibitors, such as erythromycin, should be avoided). Products include:

Crixivan Capsules ... 1940

Itraconazole (Simvastatin is a substrate of cytochrome P450 3A4 (CYP3A4). When simvastatin is used with potent inhibitors of CYP3A4, elevated plasma levels of HMG-CoA reductase inhibitory activity can increase the risk of myopathy and rhabdomyolysis, particulary with higher doses of simvastatin. The use of Vytorin concomitantly with potent CYP3A4 inhibitors, such as itraconazole, should be avoided).

No products indexed under this heading.

Ketoconazole (Simvastatin is a substrate of cytochrome P450 3A4 (CYP3A4). When simvastatin is used with potent inhibitors of CYP3A4, elevated plasma levels of HMG-CoA reductase inhibitory activity can increase the risk of myopathy and rhabdomyolysis, particulary with higher doses of simvastatin. The use of Vytorin concomitantly with potent CYP3A4 inhibitors, such as ketoconazole, should be avoided). Products include:

Nizoral A-D Shampoo, 1% ... 1868

Lopinavir (Simvastatin is a substrate of cytochrome P450 3A4 (CYP3A4). When simvastatin is used with potent inhibitors of CYP3A4, elevated plasma levels of HMG-CoA reductase inhibitory activity can increase the risk of myopathy and rhabdomyolysis, particulary with higher doses of simvastatin. The use of Vytorin concomitantly with potent CYP3A4 inhibitors, such as erythromycin, should be avoided). Products include:

Kaletra ... 476

Nefazodone Hydrochloride (Simvastatin is a substrate of cytochrome P450 3A4 (CYP3A4). When simvastatin is used with potent inhibitors of CYP3A4, elevated plasma levels of HMG-CoA reductase inhibitory activity can increase the risk of myopathy and rhabdomyolysis, particulary with higher doses of simvastatin. The use of Vytorin concomitantly with potent CYP3A4 inhibitors, such as nefazodone, should be avoided).

No products indexed under this heading.

Nelfinavir Mesylate (Simvastatin is a substrate of cytochrome P450 3A4 (CYP3A4). When simvastatin is used with potent inhibitors of CYP3A4, elevated plasma levels of HMG-CoA reductase inhibitory activity can increase the risk of myopathy and rhabdomyolysis, particulary with higher doses of simvastatin. The use of Vytorin concomitantly with potent CYP3A4 inhibitors, such as erythromycin, should be avoided). Products include:

Viracept ... 2577

Niacin (Caution should be used when prescribing lipid-lowering doses (>=1 gm/day) of niacin with Vytorin, as niacin can cause myopathy when given alone. The benefit of further alterations in lipid levels by the combined use of Vytorin with niacin should be carefully weighed against the potential risks of this drug combination). Products include:

Advicor Tablets ... 1722
Niaspan Extended-Release Tablets ... 1730

Niacinamide (Caution should be used when prescribing lipid-lowering doses (≤1 gm/day) of niacin with Vytorin, as niacin can cause myopathy when given alone. The benefit of further alterations in lipid levels by the combined use of Vytorin with niacin should be carefully weighed against the potential risks of this drug combination).

No products indexed under this heading.

Niacinamide Hydroiodide (Caution should be used when prescribing lipid-lowering doses (≤1 gm/day) of niacin with Vytorin, as niacin can cause myopathy when given alone. The benefit of further alterations in lipid levels by the combined use of Vytorin with niacin should be carefully weighed against the potential risks of this drug combination).

No products indexed under this heading.

Ritonavir (Simvastatin is a substrate of cytochrome P450 3A4 (CYP3A4). When simvastatin is used with potent inhibitors of CYP3A4, elevated plasma levels of HMG-CoA reductase inhibitory activity can increase the risk of myopathy and rhabdomyolysis, particulary with higher doses of simvastatin. The use of Vytorin concomitantly with potent CYP3A4 inhibitors, such as erythromycin, should be avoided). Products include:

Kaletra ... 476
Norvir ... 503

Saquinavir (Simvastatin is a substrate of cytochrome P450 3A4 (CYP3A4). When simvastatin is used with potent inhibitors of CYP3A4, elevated plasma levels of HMG-CoA reductase inhibitory activity can increase the risk of myopathy and rhabdomyolysis, particulary with higher doses of simvastatin. The use of Vytorin concomitantly with potent CYP3A4 inhibitors, such as erythromycin, should be avoided).

No products indexed under this heading.

Saquinavir Mesylate (Simvastatin is a substrate of cytochrome P450 3A4 (CYP3A4). When simvastatin is used with potent inhibitors of CYP3A4, elevated plasma levels of HMG-CoA reductase inhibitory activity can increase the risk of myopathy and rhabdomyolysis, particulary with higher doses of simvastatin. The use of Vytorin concomitantly with potent CYP3A4 inhibitors, such as erythromycin, should be avoided). Products include:

Invirase ... 2772

Telithromycin (Simvastatin is a substrate of cytochrome P450 3A4 (CYP3A4). When simvastatin is used with potent inhibitors of CYP3A4, elevated plasma levels of HMG-CoA reductase inhibitory activity can increase the risk of myopathy and rhabdomyolysis, particulary with higher doses of simvastatin. The use of Vytorin concomitantly with potent CYP3A4 inhibitors, such as telithromycin, should be avoided). Products include:

Ketek Tablets ... 2903

Troleandomycin (Simvastatin is a substrate of cytochrome P450 3A4 (CYP3A4). When simvastatin is used with potent inhibitors of CYP3A4, elevated plasma levels of HMG-CoA reductase inhibitory activity can increase the risk of myopathy and rhabdomyolysis, particulary with higher doses of simvastatin. Concomitant use should be avoided unless the benefits of combined therapy outweigh the increased risk. If treatment with potent CYP3A4 inhibitors is unavoidable, therapy with Vytorin should be suspended during the course of treatment).

No products indexed under this heading.

Verapamil Hydrochloride (The dose of Vytorin should not exceed 10/20 mg daily in patients receiving concomitant medication with verapamil. The combined use of Vytorin at doses higher than 10/20 mg daily with verapamil should be avoided unless the clinical benefit is likely to outweigh the increased risk of myopathy). Products include:

Covera-HS Tablets ... 3139
Tarka Tablets ... 524
Verelan PM Extended-Release Capsules, Controlled-Onset ... 3106

Voriconazole (Simvastatin is a substrate of cytochrome P450 3A4 (CYP3A4). When simvastatin is used with potent inhibitors of CYP3A4, elevated plasma levels of HMG-CoA reductase inhibitory activity can increase the risk of myopathy and rhabdomyolysis, particulary with higher doses of simvastatin. Concomitant use should be avoided unless the benefits of combined therapy outweigh the increased risk. If treatment with potent CYP3A4 inhibitors is unavoidable, therapy with Vytorin should be suspended during the course of treatment). Products include:

VFEND I.V. ... 2564
VFEND Oral Suspension ... 2564
VFEND Tablets ... 2564

Warfarin Sodium (Simvastatin modestly potentiated the effect of coumarin anticoagulants; monitor prothrombin time during co-administration). Products include:

Coumadin for Injection ... 898
Coumadin Tablets ... 898

Food Interactions

Grapefruit (Concomitant use of Vytorin and large quantities of grapefruit juice should be avoided).

Grapefruit Juice (Concomitant use of Vytorin and large quantities of grapefruit juice should be avoided).

VYTORIN 10/10 TABLETS

(Ezetimibe, Simvastatin) ... 3077

May interact with oral anticoagulants, erythromycin, fibrates, protease inhibitors, and certain other agents. Compounds in these categories include:

Amiodarone Hydrochloride (Co-administration increases the risk of myopathy/rhabdomyolysis; caution should be exercised and the dose of ezetimibe/simvastatin should not exceed 10/20 mg).

No products indexed under this heading.

Amprenavir (Co-administration with potent CYP3A4 inhibitors, such as HIV protease inhibitors, increases the risk of myopathy/rhabdomyolysis; concurrent use should be avoided). Products include:

Agenerase Capsules ... 1327
Agenerase Oral Solution ... 1332

Anisindione (Simvastatin modestly potentiated the effect of coumarin anticoagulants). Products include:

Miradon Tablets ... 3042

Cholestyramine (Co-administration decreased the mean AUC of total ezetimibe by approximately 55%; therefore, the incremental LDL-C reduction due to adding ezetimibe/simvastatin to cholestyramine may be reduced).

No products indexed under this heading.

Clarithromycin (Co-administration with potent CYP3A4 inhibitors, such as clarithromycin, increases the risk of myopathy/rhabdomyolysis; the dose of ezetimibe/simvastatin should not exceed 10/10 mg). Products include:

Biaxin/Biaxin XL ... 402
PREVPAC ... 3284

Clofibrate (Co-administration with other lipid-lowering drugs that can cause myopathy when given alone, such as fibrates, increases the risk of myopathy/rhabdomyolysis; concurrent use should be avoided).

No products indexed under this heading.

Cyclosporine (Co-administration with potent CYP3A4 inhibitors, such as cyclosporine, increases the risk

of myopathy/rhabdomyolysis; the dose of ezetimibe/simvastatin should not exceed 10/10 mg).
Products include:
Gengraf Capsules 459
Neoral Oral Solution 2259
Neoral Soft Gelatin Capsules 2259
Restasis Ophthalmic Emulsion 575
Sandimmune 2275

Dicumarol (Simvastatin modestly potentiated the effect of coumarin anticoagulants).
No products indexed under this heading.

Digoxin (Co-administration resulted in a slight elevation (less than 0.3 ng/mL) in plasma digoxin concentrations). Products include:
Lanoxicaps Capsules 1490
Lanoxin Injection 1494
Lanoxin Injection Pediatric 1497
Lanoxin Tablets 1500

Erythromycin (Co-administration with potent CYP3A4 inhibitors, such as erythromycin, increases the risk of myopathy/rhabdomyolysis; concurrent use should be avoided).
Products include:
Ery-Tab Tablets 449
Erythromycin Base Filmtab Tablets 455
Erythromycin Delayed-Release Capsules, USP 457
PCE Dispertab Tablets 515

Erythromycin Estolate (Co-administration with potent CYP3A4 inhibitors, such as erythromycin, increases the risk of myopathy/rhabdomyolysis; concurrent use should be avoided).
No products indexed under this heading.

Erythromycin Ethylsuccinate (Co-administration with potent CYP3A4 inhibitors, such as erythromycin, increases the risk of myopathy/rhabdomyolysis; concurrent use should be avoided).
Products include:
E.E.S. 451
EryPed 447

Erythromycin Gluceptate (Co-administration with potent CYP3A4 inhibitors, such as erythromycin, increases the risk of myopathy/rhabdomyolysis; concurrent use should be avoided).
No products indexed under this heading.

Erythromycin Lactobionate (Co-administration with potent CYP3A4 inhibitors, such as erythromycin, increases the risk of myopathy/rhabdomyolysis; concurrent use should be avoided).
No products indexed under this heading.

Erythromycin Stearate (Co-administration with potent CYP3A4 inhibitors, such as erythromycin, increases the risk of myopathy/rhabdomyolysis; concurrent use should be avoided). Products include:
Erythrocin Stearate Filmtab Tablets 453

Fenofibrate (Co-administration with fibrates increases the risk of myopathy/rhabdomyolysis; concurrent use should be avoided. In a pharmacokinetic study, fenofibrate increased total ezetimibe concentrations by 1.5-fold). Products include:
Lofibra Tablets 1219
Lofibra Capsules 1216
Tricor Tablets 527
Triglide Tablets 3123

Gemfibrozil (Co-administration with gemfibrozil increases the risk of myopathy/rhabdomyolysis. In a pharmacokinetic study, gemfibrozil increased total ezetimibe concentrations by 1.7-fold).
No products indexed under this heading.

Indinavir Sulfate (Co-administration with potent CYP3A4 inhibitors, such as HIV protease inhibitors, increases the risk of myopathy/rhabdomyolysis; concurrent use should be avoided).
Products include:
Crixivan Capsules 1940

Itraconazole (Co-administration with potent CYP3A4 inhibitors, such as itraconazole, increases the risk of myopathy/rhabdomyolysis; concurrent use should be avoided).
No products indexed under this heading.

Ketoconazole (Co-administration with potent CYP3A4 inhibitors, such as ketoconazole, increases the risk of myopathy/rhabdomyolysis; concurrent use should be avoided).
Products include:
Nizoral A-D Shampoo, 1% 1868

Lopinavir (Co-administration with potent CYP3A4 inhibitors, such as HIV protease inhibitors, increases the risk of myopathy/rhabdomyolysis; concurrent use should be avoided). Products include:
Kaletra 476

Nefazodone Hydrochloride (Co-administration with potent CYP3A4 inhibitors, such as nefazodone, increases the risk of myopathy/rhabdomyolysis; concurrent use should be avoided).
No products indexed under this heading.

Nelfinavir Mesylate (Co-administration with potent CYP3A4 inhibitors, such as HIV protease inhibitors, increases the risk of myopathy/rhabdomyolysis; concurrent use should be avoided).
Products include:
Viracept 2577

Niacin (Caution with greater than or equal to 1 gram per day of niacin with ezetimibe/simvastatin as niacin can cause myopathy when given alone). Products include:
Advicor Tablets 1722
Niaspan Extended-Release Tablets 1730

Ritonavir (Co-administration with potent CYP3A4 inhibitors, such as HIV protease inhibitors, increases the risk of myopathy/rhabdomyolysis; concurrent use should be avoided). Products include:
Kaletra 476
Norvir 503

Saquinavir (Co-administration with potent CYP3A4 inhibitors, such as HIV protease inhibitors, increases the risk of myopathy/rhabdomyolysis; concurrent use should be avoided).
No products indexed under this heading.

Saquinavir Mesylate (Co-administration with potent CYP3A4 inhibitors, such as HIV protease inhibitors, increases the risk of myopathy/rhabdomyolysis; concurrent use should be avoided).
Products include:
Invirase 2772

Verapamil Hydrochloride (Co-administration increases the risk of myopathy/rhabdomyolysis; caution should be exercised and the dose of ezetimibe/simvastatin should not exceed 10/20 mg). Products include:
Covera-HS Tablets 3139
Tarka Tablets 524
Verelan PM Extended-Release Capsules, Controlled-Onset 3106

Warfarin Sodium (Simvastatin modestly potentiated the effect of coumarin anticoagulants). Products include:
Coumadin for Injection 898
Coumadin Tablets 898

Food Interactions

Grapefruit Juice (Co-administration with potent CYP3A4 inhibitors, such as large quantities of grapefruit juice (greater than 1 quart daily), increases the risk of myopathy/rhabdomyolysis; concurrent use should be avoided).

VYTORIN 10/20 TABLETS
(Ezetimibe, Simvastatin) 2114
See Vytorin 10/10 Tablets

VYTORIN 10/20 TABLETS
(Ezetimibe, Simvastatin) 3077
See Vytorin 10/10 Tablets

VYTORIN 10/40 TABLETS
(Ezetimibe, Simvastatin) 2114
See Vytorin 10/10 Tablets

VYTORIN 10/40 TABLETS
(Ezetimibe, Simvastatin) 3077
See Vytorin 10/10 Tablets

VYTORIN 10/80 TABLETS
(Ezetimibe, Simvastatin) 2114
See Vytorin 10/10 Tablets

VYTORIN 10/80 TABLETS
(Ezetimibe, Simvastatin) 3077
See Vytorin 10/10 Tablets

WELCHOL TABLETS
(Colesevelam Hydrochloride) 1050
May interact with:

Verapamil Hydrochloride (Co-administration of sustained-release verapamil with colesevelam results in decreased Cmax and AUC of sustained-release verapamil by approximately 31% and 11%, respectively; because of high variability in the bioavailability of verapamil, the clinical significance of this finding is unclear). Products include:
Covera-HS Tablets 3139
Tarka Tablets 524
Verelan PM Extended-Release Capsules, Controlled-Onset 3106

WELLBUTRIN TABLETS
(Bupropion Hydrochloride) 1603
See Wellbutrin SR Sustained-Release Tablets

WELLBUTRIN SR SUSTAINED-RELEASE TABLETS
(Bupropion Hydrochloride) 1607
May interact with benzodiazepines, corticosteroids, cytochrome p450 2d6 substrates (selected), antidepressant drugs, monoamine oxidase inhibitors, antipsychotic agents, phenytoin, drugs which lower seizure threshold, xanthines, and certain other agents. Compounds in these categories include:

Alprazolam (Bupropion is associated with a dose-related risk of seizures; excessive use of benzodiazepine sedatives is associated with increased risk of seizures; bupropion is contraindicated in patients undergoing abrupt discontinuation of benzodiazepine sedatives). Products include:
Niravam Orally Disintegrating Tablets 3092

Amantadine Hydrochloride (Limited clinical data suggest higher incidence of adverse experiences with co-administration; use small initial dose and gradually increase doses).
Products include:
Symmetrel Tablets 1135

Aminophylline (Bupropion is associated with a dose-related risk of seizures; co-administration with drugs that lower seizure threshold may increase the risk of seizures with bupropion; concurrent use should be undertaken with extreme caution).
No products indexed under this heading.

Amitriptyline Hydrochloride (Bupropion is associated with a dose-related risk of seizures; co-administration with drugs that lower seizure threshold may increase the risk of seizure with bupropion; concurrent use should be undertaken with extreme caution).
No products indexed under this heading.

Amoxapine (Bupropion is associated with a dose-related risk of seizures; co-administration with drugs that lower seizure threshold may increase the risk of seizure with bupropion; concurrent use should be undertaken with extreme caution).
No products indexed under this heading.

Amphetamine Aspartate (Co-administration of bupropion with drugs that are metabolized by the CYP2D6 isoenzyme should be approached with caution and should be initiated at the lower end of the dose range of the concomitant medication. If bupropion is added to the treatment regimen of a patient already receiving a drug metabolized by CYP2D6, the need to decrease the dose of the original medication should be considered, particularly for those concomitant medications with a narrow therapeutic index).
Products include:
Adderall Tablets 3164
Adderall XR Capsules 3166

Amphetamine Aspartate Monohydrate (Co-administration of bupropion with drugs that are metabolized by the CYP2D6 isoenzyme should be approached with caution and should be initiated at the lower end of the dose range of the concomitant medication. If bupropion is added to the treatment regimen of a patient already receiving a drug metabolized by CYP2D6, the need to decrease the dose of the original medication should be considered, particularly for those concomitant medications with a narrow therapeutic index).
No products indexed under this heading.

Amphetamine Sulfate (Co-administration of bupropion with drugs that are metabolized by the CYP2D6 isoenzyme should be approached with caution and should be initiated at the lower end of the dose range of the concomitant medication. If bupropion is added to the treatment regimen of a patient already receiving a drug metabolized by CYP2D6, the need to decrease the dose of the original medication should be considered, particularly for those concomitant medications with a narrow therapeutic index). Products include:

Adderall Tablets 3164
Adderall XR Capsules 3166

Aripiprazole (Concurrent administration of bupropion and agents that lower seizure threshold (e.g., antipsychotics) should be undertaken only with extreme caution. Low initial dosing and gradual dose increases should be employed). Products include:

Abilify Oral Solution 882
Abilify Oral Solution 2450
Abilify Discmelt Orally Disintegrating Tablets 882
Abilify Discmelt Orally Disintegrating Tablets 2450
Abilify Tablets 882
Abilify Tablets 2450

Atomoxetine Hydrochloride (Co-administration of bupropion with drugs that are metabolized by the CYP2D6 isoenzyme should be approached with caution and should be initiated at the lower end of the dose range of the concomitant medication. If bupropion is added to the treatment regimen of a patient already receiving a drug metabolized by CYP2D6, the need to decrease the dose of the original medication should be considered, particularly for those concomitant medications with a narrow therapeutic index). Products include:

Strattera Capsules 1814

Betamethasone Acetate (Bupropion is associated with a dose-related risk of seizures; co-administration with drugs that lower seizure threshold, such as systemic steroids, may increase the risk of seizure with bupropion).

No products indexed under this heading.

Betamethasone Sodium Phosphate (Bupropion is associated with a dose-related risk of seizures; co-administration with drugs that lower seizure threshold, such as systemic steroids, may increase the risk of seizure with bupropion).

No products indexed under this heading.

Bisoprolol Fumarate (Co-administration of bupropion with drugs that are metabolized by the CYP2D6 isoenzyme should be approached with caution and should be initiated at the lower end of the dose range of the concomitant medication. If bupropion is added to the treatment regimen of a patient already receiving a drug metabolized by CYP2D6, the need to decrease the dose of the original medication should be considered, particularly for those concomitant medications with a narrow therapeutic index).

No products indexed under this heading.

Bupropion (Patients should be made aware that both formulations of Wellbutrin contain the same active moiety found in Zyban, an aid to smoking cessation; combination is contraindicated).

No products indexed under this heading.

Captopril (Co-administration of bupropion with drugs that are metabolized by the CYP2D6 isoenzyme should be approached with caution and should be initiated at the lower end of the dose range of the concomitant medication. If bupropion is added to the treatment regimen of a patient already receiving a drug metabolized by CYP2D6, the need to decrease the dose of the original medication should be considered, particularly for those concomitant medications with a narrow therapeutic index). Products include:

Captopril Tablets 2149

Carbamazepine (May induce the metabolism of bupropion). Products include:

Carbatrol Capsules 3171
Equetro Extended-Release Capsules 3180
Tegretol/Tegretol-XR 2295

Carvedilol (Co-administration of bupropion with drugs that are metabolized by the CYP2D6 isoenzyme should be approached with caution and should be initiated at the lower end of the dose range of the concomitant medication. If bupropion is added to the treatment regimen of a patient already receiving a drug metabolized by CYP2D6, the need to decrease the dose of the original medication should be considered, particularly for those concomitant medications with a narrow therapeutic index). Products include:

Coreg Tablets 1414

Cevimeline Hydrochloride (Co-administration of bupropion with drugs that are metabolized by the CYP2D6 isoenzyme should be approached with caution and should be initiated at the lower end of the dose range of the concomitant medication. If bupropion is added to the treatment regimen of a patient already receiving a drug metabolized by CYP2D6, the need to decrease the dose of the original medication should be considered, particularly for those concomitant medications with a narrow therapeutic index). Products include:

Evoxac Capsules 1047

Chlordiazepoxide (Bupropion is associated with a dose-related risk of seizures; excessive use of benzodiazepine sedatives is associated with increased risk of seizures; bupropion is contraindicated in patients undergoing abrupt discontinuation of benzodiazepine sedatives).

No products indexed under this heading.

Chlordiazepoxide Hydrochloride (Bupropion is associated with a dose-related risk of seizures; excessive use of benzodiazepine sedatives is associated with increased risk of seizures; bupropion is contraindicated in patients undergoing abrupt discontinuation of benzodiazepine sedatives). Products include:

Librium Capsules 3347

Chlorpromazine (Bupropion is associated with a dose-related risk of seizures; co-administration with drugs that lower seizure threshold may increase the risk of seizure with bupropion; concurrent use should be undertaken with extreme caution).

No products indexed under this heading.

Chlorpromazine Hydrochloride (Bupropion is associated with a dose-related risk of seizures; co-administration with drugs that lower seizure threshold may increase the risk of seizure with bupropion; concurrent use should be undertaken with extreme caution).

No products indexed under this heading.

Chlorpropamide (Co-administration of bupropion with drugs that are metabolized by the CYP2D6 isoenzyme should be approached with caution and should be initiated at the lower end of the dose range of the concomitant medication. If bupropion is added to the treatment regimen of a patient already receiving a drug metabolized by CYP2D6, the need to decrease the dose of the original medication should be considered, particularly for those concomitant medications with a narrow therapeutic index).

No products indexed under this heading.

Chlorprothixene (Concurrent administration of bupropion and agents that lower seizure threshold (e.g., antipsychotics) should be undertaken only with extreme caution. Low initial dosing and gradual dose increases should be employed).

No products indexed under this heading.

Chlorprothixene Hydrochloride (Concurrent administration of bupropion and agents that lower seizure threshold (e.g., antipsychotics) should be undertaken only with extreme caution. Low initial dosing and gradual dose increases should be employed).

No products indexed under this heading.

Cimetidine (May inhibit the metabolism of bupropion). Products include:

Tagamet HB 200 Tablets .... ▣ 664

Cimetidine Hydrochloride (May induce the metabolism of bupropion).

No products indexed under this heading.

Citalopram Hydrobromide (Concurrent administration of bupropion and agents that lower seizure threshold (e.g., other antidepressants) should be undertaken only with extreme caution. Low initial dosing and gradual dose increases should be employed). Products include:

Celexa 1176

Clomipramine Hydrochloride (Co-administration of bupropion with drugs that are metabolized by the CYP2D6 isoenzyme should be approached with caution and should be initiated at the lower end of the dose range of the concomitant medication. If bupropion is added to the treatment regimen of a patient already receiving a drug metabolized by CYP2D6, the need to decrease the dose of the original medication should be considered, particularly for those concomitant medications with a narrow therapeutic index).

No products indexed under this heading.

Clorazepate Dipotassium (Bupropion is associated with a dose-related risk of seizures; excessive use of benzodiazepine sedatives is associated with increased risk of seizures; bupropion is contraindicated in patients undergoing abrupt discontinuation of benzodiazepine sedatives). Products include:

Tranxene 2474

Clozapine (Co-administration of bupropion with drugs that are metabolized by the CYP2D6 isoenzyme should be approached with caution and should be initiated at the lower end of the dose range of the concomitant medication. If bupropion is added to the treatment regimen of a patient already receiving a drug metabolized by CYP2D6, the need to decrease the dose of the original medication should be considered, particularly for those concomitant medications with a narrow therapeutic index). Products include:

Clozaril Tablets 2184
FazaClo Orally Disintegrating Tablets 551

Codeine Phosphate (Co-administration of bupropion with drugs that are metabolized by the CYP2D6 isoenzyme should be approached with caution and should be initiated at the lower end of the dose range of the concomitant medication. If bupropion is added to the treatment regimen of a patient already receiving a drug metabolized by CYP2D6, the need to decrease the dose of the original medication should be considered, particularly for those concomitant medications with a narrow therapeutic index). Products include:

Tylenol with Codeine Tablets 2391

Codeine Sulfate (Co-administration of bupropion with drugs that are metabolized by the CYP2D6 isoenzyme should be approached with caution and should be initiated at the lower end of the dose range of the concomitant medication. If bupropion is added to the treatment regimen of a patient already receiving a drug metabolized by CYP2D6, the need to decrease the dose of the original medication should be considered, particularly for those concomitant medications with a narrow therapeutic index).

No products indexed under this heading.

Cortisone Acetate (Bupropion is associated with a dose-related risk of seizures; co-administration with drugs that lower seizure threshold, such as systemic steroids, may increase the risk of seizure with bupropion).

No products indexed under this heading.

Cyclobenzaprine Hydrochloride (Co-administration of bupropion with drugs that are metabolized by the CYP2D6 isoenzyme should be approached with caution and should be initiated at the lower end of the dose range of the concomitant medication. If bupropion is added to the treatment regimen of a patient already receiving a drug metabolized by CYP2D6, the need to decrease the dose of the original medication should be considered, particularly for those concomitant medications with a narrow therapeutic index).

No products indexed under this heading.

Cyclophosphamide (Bupropion is primarily metabolized, based on in vitro studies, to the morpholinol metabolite by cytochrome P450IIB6 isoenzyme; therefore, the potential exists for a drug interaction with agents that affect the cytochrome P450IIB6 metabolism, such as cyclophosphamide).
No products indexed under this heading.

Desipramine Hydrochloride (Co-administration of bupropion with drugs that are metabolized by the CYP2D6 isoenzyme, including desipramine, should be approached with caution and should be initiated at the lower end of the dose range of the concomitant medication. If bupropion is added to the treatment regimen of a patient already receiving a drug metabolized by CYP2D6, the need to decrease the dose of the original medication should be considered, particularly for those concomitant medications with a narrow therapeutic index).
No products indexed under this heading.

Dexamethasone (Bupropion is associated with a dose-related risk of seizures; co-administration with drugs that lower seizure threshold, such as systemic steroids, may increase the risk of seizure with bupropion). Products include:
Ciprodex Otic Suspension 559
Decadron Tablets 1951
TobraDex Ophthalmic Ointment 562
TobraDex Ophthalmic Suspension ... 563

Dexamethasone Acetate (Bupropion is associated with a dose-related risk of seizures; co-administration with drugs that lower seizure threshold, such as systemic steroids, may increase the risk of seizure with bupropion).
No products indexed under this heading.

Dexamethasone Sodium Phosphate (Bupropion is associated with a dose-related risk of seizures; co-administration with drugs that lower seizure threshold, such as systemic steroids, may increase the risk of seizure with bupropion).
No products indexed under this heading.

Dexfenfluramine Hydrochloride (Co-administration of bupropion with drugs that are metabolized by the CYP2D6 isoenzyme should be approached with caution and should be initiated at the lower end of the dose range of the concomitant medication. If bupropion is added to the treatment regimen of a patient already receiving a drug metabolized by CYP2D6, the need to decrease the dose of the original medication should be considered, particularly for those concomitant medications with a narrow therapeutic index).
No products indexed under this heading.

Dextromethorphan Hydrobromide (Co-administration of bupropion with drugs that are metabolized by the CYP2D6 isoenzyme should be approached with caution and should be initiated at the lower end of the dose range of the concomitant medication. If bupropion is added to the treatment regimen of a patient already receiving a drug metabolized by CYP2D6, the need to decrease the dose of the original medication should be considered, particularly for those concomitant medications with a narrow therapeutic index). Products include:
Comtrex Maximum Strength Cold & Cough Day/Night Caplets - Day Formulation .... ■ 726
Comtrex Maximum Strength Cold & Cough Day/Night Caplets - Night Formulation .... ■ 726
Comtrex Maximum Strength Non-Drowsy Cold & Cough Caplets .... ■ 725
Children's Dimetapp DM Cold & Cough Elixir .... ■ 731
Children's Dimetapp Long Acting Cough Plus Cold Syrup .... ■ 731
Toddler's Dimetapp Cold and Cough Drops .... ■ 732
Mucinex DM Extended-Release Bi-Layer Tablets .... ■ 720
Refenesen DM Caplets .... ■ 721
Robitussin Cough & Cold CF Liquid .... ■ 735
Robitussin Cough & Cold Long-Acting Liquid .... ■ 735
Robitussin Cough & Allergy Syrup .. ■ 736
Robitussin Cough & Cold Nighttime Liquid .... ■ 736
Robitussin Cough & Cold Pediatric Drops .... ■ 735
Robitussin Cough, Cold & Flu Nighttime Liquid .... ■ 738
Robitussin Cough & Congestion Liquid .... ■ 738
Robitussin Cough Gels Long-Acting .... ■ 737
Robitussin Cough Long Acting Liquid .... ■ 739
Robitussin Cough DM Syrup .... ■ 738
Robitussin Cough DM Infant Drops .... ■ 738
Robitussin Pediatric Cough Long Acting Liquid .... ■ 739
Robitussin Pediatric Cough & Cold Long-Acting Liquid .... ■ 735
Robitussin Pediatric Cough & Cold Nighttime Liquid .... ■ 736
Robitussin Sugar Free Cough .... ■ 738
TheraFlu Cold & Cough Hot Liquid .... ■ 740
TheraFlu Warming Relief Daytime Severe Cold .... ■ 743
TheraFlu Thin Strips Long Acting Cough .... ■ 744
Triaminic Daytime Cold & Cough Liquid .... ■ 745
Triaminic Cough & Sore Throat Liquid .... ■ 747
Triaminic Cough & Runny Nose Softchews .... ■ 748
Triaminic Thin Strips Cold & Cough .... ■ 778
Triaminic Infant Thin Strips Decongestant Plus Cough .... ■ 747
Children's Tylenol Plus Flu Oral Suspension .... ■ 749
Tylenol Cold Head Congestion Daytime Caplets with Cool Burst and Gelcaps .... ■ 750
Tylenol Cold Multi-Symptom Daytime Liquid .... ■ 752
Tylenol Cold Multi-Symptom Severe Daytime Liquid .... ■ 752
Concentrated Tylenol Infants' Drops Plus Cold & Cough .... ■ 754
Children's Tylenol Plus Cough & Runny Nose Suspension Liquid 1879
Children's Tylenol Plus Cough & Sore Throat Suspension Liquid 1879
Children's Tylenol Plus Flu Suspension Liquid 1881
Children's Tylenol Plus Multi-Symptom Cold Suspension Liquid 1879
Tylenol Cold Severe Congestion Non-Drowsy Caplets with Cool Burst 1874
Tylenol Cold Head Congestion Daytime Caplets with Cool Burst 1873
Tylenol Cold Head Congestion Nighttime Caplets with Cool Burst 1873
Tylenol Cold Head Congestion Severe Caplets with Cool Burst..... 1873
Tylenol Cold Multi-Symptom Daytime Caplets with Cool Burst and Gelcaps 1874
Tylenol Cold Multi-Symptom Daytime Liquid with Citrus Burst... 1874
Tylenol Cold Multi-Symptom Nighttime Caplets with Cool Burst 1874
Tylenol Cold Multi-Symptom Nighttime Liquid with Cool Burst... 1874
Tylenol Cold Multi-Symptom Severe Caplets with Cool Burst..... 1874
Tylenol Cold Multi-Symptom Severe Daytime Liquid with Citrus Burst 1874
Tylenol Cough & Sore Throat Daytime Liquid with Cool Burst...... 1877
Tylenol Cough & Sore Throat Nighttime Liquid with Cool Burst... 1877
Concentrated Tylenol Infants' Drops Plus Cold and Cough 1879
Vicks 44 Cough Relief Liquid 2679
Vicks 44D Cough & Head Congestion Relief Liquid 2679
Vicks 44E Cough & Chest Congestion Relief Liquid 2679
Pediatric Vicks 44e Cough & Chest Congestion Relief Liquid...... 2676
Vicks 44M Cough, Cold & Flu Relief Liquid 2680
Pediatric Vicks 44m Cough & Cold Relief Liquid 2676
Vicks DayQuil LiquiCaps/Liquid Multi-Symptom Cold/Flu Relief..... ■ 761
Vicks DayQuil Multi-Symptom Cold/Flu Relief LiquiCaps 2678
Vicks DayQuil Multi-Symptom Cold/Flu Relief Liquid 2678
Vicks NyQuil Multi-Symptom Cold/Flu Relief Liquid 2681
Children's Vicks NyQuil Cold/Cough Relief .... ■ 756
Vicks NyQuil Multi-Symptom Cold/Flu Relief LiquiCaps 2681
Vicks NyQuil LiquiCaps/Liquid Multi-Symptom Cold/Flu Relief..... ■ 763
Vicks NyQuil Cough Liquid 2680
Children's Vicks NyQuil Cold/Cough Relief Liquid 2680
Zicam Cough Max Nighttime Cough Spray .... ■ 767
Zicam Cough Max Cough Spray ..... ■ 767
Zicam Cough Max Cough Melts ...... ■ 767
Zicam Cough Plus D Cough Spray .... ■ 767
Zicam Cough Relief Cough Spray ... ■ 767
Zicam Maximum Strength Flu Daytime .... ■ 768
Zicam Maximum Strength Flu Nighttime .... ■ 768

Dextromethorphan Polistirex (Co-administration of bupropion with drugs that are metabolized by the CYP2D6 isoenzyme should be approached with caution and should be initiated at the lower end of the dose range of the concomitant medication. If bupropion is added to the treatment regimen of a patient already receiving a drug metabolized by CYP2D6, the need to decrease the dose of the original medication should be considered, particularly for those concomitant medications with a narrow therapeutic index). Products include:
Delsym Extended-Release Suspension 12 Hour Cough Suppressant .... ■ 611

Diazepam (Bupropion is associated with a dose-related risk of seizures; excessive use of benzodiazepine sedatives is associated with increased risk of seizures; bupropion is contraindicated in patients undergoing abrupt discontinuation of benzodiazepine sedatives). Products include:
Diastat Rectal Delivery System 3343
Valium Tablets 2819

Dolasetron Mesylate (Co-administration of bupropion with drugs that are metabolized by the CYP2D6 isoenzyme should be approached with caution and should be initiated at the lower end of the dose range of the concomitant medication. If bupropion is added to the treatment regimen of a patient already receiving a drug metabolized by CYP2D6, the need to decrease the dose of the original medication should be considered, particularly for those concomitant medications with a narrow therapeutic index). Products include:
Anzemet Injection 2859
Anzemet Tablets 2862

Donepezil Hydrochloride (Co-administration of bupropion with drugs that are metabolized by the CYP2D6 isoenzyme should be approached with caution and should be initiated at the lower end of the dose range of the concomitant medication. If bupropion is added to the treatment regimen of a patient already receiving a drug metabolized by CYP2D6, the need to decrease the dose of the original medication should be considered, particularly for those concomitant medications with a narrow therapeutic index). Products include:
Aricept Tablets 1094
Aricept ODT Tablets 1094

Doxepin Hydrochloride (Bupropion is associated with a dose-related risk of seizures; co-administration with drugs that lower seizure threshold may increase the risk of seizure with bupropion; concurrent use should be undertaken with extreme caution).
No products indexed under this heading.

Dyphylline (Bupropion is associated with a dose-related risk of seizures; co-administration with drugs that lower seizure threshold may increase the risk of seizures with bupropion; concurrent use should be undertaken with extreme caution).
No products indexed under this heading.

Encainide Hydrochloride (Co-administration of bupropion with drugs that are metabolized by the CYP2D6 isoenzyme should be approached with caution and should be initiated at the lower end of the dose range of the concomitant medication. If bupropion is added to the treatment regimen of a patient already receiving a drug metabolized by CYP2D6, the need to decrease the dose of the original medication should be considered, particularly for those concomitant medications with a narrow therapeutic index).
No products indexed under this heading.

Escitalopram Oxalate (Concurrent administration of bupropion and agents that lower seizure threshold (e.g., other antidepressants) should be undertaken only with extreme caution. Low initial dosing and gradual dose increases should be employed). Products include:
Lexapro Oral Solution 1190
Lexapro Tablets 1190

Estazolam (Bupropion is associated with a dose-related risk of seizures; excessive use of benzodiazepine sedatives is associated with increased risk of seizures; bupropion is contraindicated in patients undergoing abrupt discontinuation of benzodiazepine sedatives). Products include:
ProSom Tablets 517

Fentanyl (Co-administration of bupropion with drugs that are metabolized by the CYP2D6 isoenzyme should be approached with caution and should be initiated at the lower end of the dose range of the concomitant medication. If bupropion is added to the treatment regimen of a patient already receiving a drug metabolized by CYP2D6, the need to decrease the dose of the original medication should be considered, particularly for those concomitant medications with a narrow therapeutic index). Products include:

Duragesic Transdermal System 2373
Ionsys Transdermal System 2379

Fentanyl Citrate (Co-administration of bupropion with drugs that are metabolized by the CYP2D6 isoenzyme should be approached with caution and should be initiated at the lower end of the dose range of the concomitant medication. If bupropion is added to the treatment regimen of a patient already receiving a drug metabolized by CYP2D6, the need to decrease the dose of the original medication should be considered, particularly for those concomitant medications with a narrow therapeutic index). Products include:

Actiq 979

Flecainide Acetate (Co-administration of bupropion with drugs that are metabolized by the CYP2D6 isoenzyme, including flecainide, should be approached with caution and should be initiated at the lower end of the dose range of the concomitant medication. If bupropion is added to the treatment regimen of a patient already receiving a drug metabolized by CYP2D6, the need to decrease the dose of the original medication should be considered, particularly for those concomitant medications with a narrow therapeutic index). Products include:

Tambocor Tablets 1856

Fludrocortisone Acetate (Bupropion is associated with a dose-related risk of seizures; co-administration with drugs that lower seizure threshold, such as systemic steroids, may increase the risk of seizure with bupropion).

No products indexed under this heading.

Fluoxetine (Co-administration of bupropion with drugs that are metabolized by the CYP2D6 isoenzyme, including fluoxetine, should be approached with caution and should be initiated at the lower end of the dose range of the concomitant medication. If bupropion is added to the treatment regimen of a patient already receiving a drug metabolized by CYP2D6, the need to decrease the dose of the original medication should be considered, particularly for those concomitant medications with a narrow therapeutic index).

No products indexed under this heading.

Fluoxetine Hydrochloride (Co-administration of bupropion with drugs that are metabolized by the CYP2D6 isoenzyme, including fluoxetine, should be approached with caution and should be initiated at the lower end of the dose range of the concomitant medication. If bupropion is added to the treatment regimen of a patient already receiving a drug metabolized by CYP2D6, the need to decrease the dose of the original medication should be consid-

ered, particularly for those concomitant medications with a narrow therapeutic index). Products include:

Prozac Pulvules and Liquid 1801
Symbyax Capsules 1819

Fluphenazine Decanoate (Bupropion is associated with a dose-related risk of seizures; co-administration with drugs that lower seizure threshold may increase the risk of seizure with bupropion; concurrent use should be undertaken with extreme caution).

No products indexed under this heading.

Fluphenazine Enanthate (Bupropion is associated with a dose-related risk of seizures; co-administration with drugs that lower seizure threshold may increase the risk of seizure with bupropion; concurrent use should be undertaken with extreme caution).

No products indexed under this heading.

Fluphenazine Hydrochloride (Bupropion is associated with a dose-related risk of seizures; co-administration with drugs that lower seizure threshold may increase the risk of seizure with bupropion; concurrent use should be undertaken with extreme caution).

No products indexed under this heading.

Flurazepam Hydrochloride (Bupropion is associated with a dose-related risk of seizures; excessive use of benzodiazepine sedatives is associated with increased risk of seizures; bupropion is contraindicated in patients undergoing abrupt discontinuation of benzodiazepine sedatives). Products include:

Dalmane Capsules 3342

Fluvoxamine Maleate (Co-administration of bupropion with drugs that are metabolized by the CYP2D6 isoenzyme should be approached with caution and should be initiated at the lower end of the dose range of the concomitant medication. If bupropion is added to the treatment regimen of a patient already receiving a drug metabolized by CYP2D6, the need to decrease the dose of the original medication should be considered, particularly for those concomitant medications with a narrow therapeutic index).

No products indexed under this heading.

Formoterol Fumarate (Co-administration of bupropion with drugs that are metabolized by the CYP2D6 isoenzyme should be approached with caution and should be initiated at the lower end of the dose range of the concomitant medication. If bupropion is added to the treatment regimen of a patient already receiving a drug metabolized by CYP2D6, the need to decrease the dose of the original medication should be considered, particularly for those concomitant medications with a narrow therapeutic index). Products include:

Foradil Aerolizer 3010

Fosphenytoin Sodium (May induce the metabolism of bupropion).

No products indexed under this heading.

Galantamine Hydrobromide (Co-administration of bupropion with drugs that are metabolized by the CYP2D6 isoenzyme should be

approached with caution and should be initiated at the lower end of the dose range of the concomitant medication. If bupropion is added to the treatment regimen of a patient already receiving a drug metabolized by CYP2D6, the need to decrease the dose of the original medication should be considered, particularly for those concomitant medications with a narrow therapeutic index). Products include:

Razadyne 2399
Razadyne ER Extended-Release
Capsules 2399

Halazepam (Bupropion is associated with a dose-related risk of seizures; excessive use of benzodiazepine sedatives is associated with increased risk of seizures; bupropion is contraindicated in patients undergoing abrupt discontinuation of benzodiazepine sedatives).

No products indexed under this heading.

Haloperidol (Co-administration of bupropion with drugs that are metabolized by the CYP2D6 isoenzyme, including haloperidol, should be approached with caution and should be initiated at the lower end of the dose range of the concomitant medication. If bupropion is added to the treatment regimen of a patient already receiving a drug metabolized by CYP2D6, the need to decrease the dose of the original medication should be considered, particularly for those concomitant medications with a narrow therapeutic index).

No products indexed under this heading.

Haloperidol Decanoate (Co-administration of bupropion with drugs that are metabolized by the CYP2D6 isoenzyme, including haloperidol, should be approached with caution and should be initiated at the lower end of the dose range of the concomitant medication. If bupropion is added to the treatment regimen of a patient already receiving a drug metabolized by CYP2D6, the need to decrease the dose of the original medication should be considered, particularly for those concomitant medications with a narrow therapeutic index).

No products indexed under this heading.

Haloperidol Lactate (Co-administration of bupropion with drugs that are metabolized by the CYP2D6 isoenzyme, including haloperidol, should be approached with caution and should be initiated at the lower end of the dose range of the concomitant medication. If bupropion is added to the treatment regimen of a patient already receiving a drug metabolized by CYP2D6, the need to decrease the dose of the original medication should be considered, particularly for those concomitant medications with a narrow therapeutic index).

No products indexed under this heading.

Hydrocodone Bitartrate (Co-administration of bupropion with drugs that are metabolized by the CYP2D6 isoenzyme should be approached with caution and should be initiated at the lower end of the concomitant medication. If bupropion is added to the treatment regimen of a patient already receiving a drug metabolized

by CYP2D6, the need to decrease the dose of the original medication should be considered, particularly for those concomitant medications with a narrow therapeutic index). Products include:

Hycodan 1116
Hycotuss Expectorant Syrup 1117
Vicodin Tablets 535
Vicodin ES Tablets 536
Vicodin HP Tablets 538
Vicoprofen Tablets 539
Zydone Tablets 1139

Hydrocortisone (Bupropion is associated with a dose-related risk of seizures; co-administration with drugs that lower seizure threshold, such as systemic steroids, may increase the risk of seizure with bupropion). Products include:

Colocort Rectal Suspension, USP
(Retention) 100 mg/60 mL........... 2476
Hydrocortone Tablets 1989
Preparation H Hydrocortisone
Cream ▣◻646

Hydrocortisone Acetate (Bupropion is associated with a dose-related risk of seizures; co-administration with drugs that lower seizure threshold, such as systemic steroids, may increase the risk of seizure with bupropion). Products include:

Analpram-HC 1159
Pramosone 1161
ProctoFoam-HC 3099

Hydrocortisone Sodium Phosphate (Bupropion is associated with a dose-related risk of seizures; co-administration with drugs that lower seizure threshold, such as systemic steroids, may increase the risk of seizure with bupropion).

No products indexed under this heading.

Hydrocortisone Sodium Succinate (Bupropion is associated with a dose-related risk of seizures; co-administration with drugs that lower seizure threshold, such as systemic steroids, may increase the risk of seizure with bupropion).

No products indexed under this heading.

Imipramine Hydrochloride (Co-administration of bupropion with drugs that are metabolized by the CYP2D6 isoenzyme, including imipramine, should be approached with caution and should be initiated at the lower end of the dose range of the concomitant medication. If bupropion is added to the treatment regimen of a patient already receiving a drug metabolized by CYP2D6, the need to decrease the dose of the original medication should be considered, particularly for those concomitant medications with a narrow therapeutic index).

No products indexed under this heading.

Imipramine Pamoate (Co-administration of bupropion with drugs that are metabolized by the CYP2D6 isoenzyme, including imipramine, should be approached with caution and should be initiated at the lower end of the dose range of the concomitant medication. If bupropion is added to the treatment regimen of a patient already receiving a drug metabolized by CYP2D6, the need to decrease the dose of the original medication should be considered, particularly for those concomitant medications with a narrow therapeutic index).

No products indexed under this heading.

Indoramin Hydrochloride (Co-administration of bupropion with drugs that are metabolized by the CYP2D6 isoenzyme should be approached with caution and should be initiated at the lower end of the dose range of the concomitant medication. If bupropion is added to the treatment regimen of a patient already receiving a drug metabolized by CYP2D6, the need to decrease the dose of the original medication should be considered, particularly for those concomitant medications with a narrow therapeutic index).

No products indexed under this heading.

Isocarboxazid (Concurrent and/or sequential use with MAO inhibitors is contraindicated).

No products indexed under this heading.

Labetalol Hydrochloride (Co-administration of bupropion with drugs that are metabolized by the CYP2D6 isoenzyme should be approached with caution and should be initiated at the lower end of the dose range of the concomitant medication. If bupropion is added to the treatment regimen of a patient already receiving a drug metabolized by CYP2D6, the need to decrease the dose of the original medication should be considered, particularly for those concomitant medications with a narrow therapeutic index).

No products indexed under this heading.

Levodopa (Limited clinical data suggest higher incidence of adverse experiences with co-administration; use small initial dose and gradually increase doses). Products include:

Lidocaine (Co-administration of bupropion with drugs that are metabolized by the CYP2D6 isoenzyme should be approached with caution and should be initiated at the lower end of the dose range of the concomitant medication. If bupropion is added to the treatment regimen of a patient already receiving a drug metabolized by CYP2D6, the need to decrease the dose of the original medication should be considered, particularly for those concomitant medications with a narrow therapeutic index). Products include:

Lidocaine Hydrochloride (Co-administration of bupropion with drugs that are metabolized by the CYP2D6 isoenzyme should be approached with caution and should be initiated at the lower end of the dose range of the concomitant medication. If bupropion is added to the treatment regimen of a patient already receiving a drug metabolized by CYP2D6, the need to decrease the dose of the original medication should be considered, particularly for those concomitant medications with a narrow therapeutic index).

No products indexed under this heading.

Lithium Carbonate (Concurrent administration of bupropion and agents that lower seizure threshold (e.g., antipsychotics) should be

undertaken only with extreme caution. Low initial dosing and gradual dose increases should be employed). Products include:

Lithium Citrate (Concurrent administration of bupropion and agents that lower seizure threshold (e.g., antipsychotics) should be undertaken only with extreme caution. Low initial dosing and gradual dose increases should be employed).

No products indexed under this heading.

Lorazepam (Bupropion is associated with a dose-related risk of seizures; excessive use of benzodiazepine sedatives is associated with increased risk of seizures; bupropion is contraindicated in patients undergoing abrupt discontinuation of benzodiazepine sedatives).

No products indexed under this heading.

Loxapine Hydrochloride (Concurrent administration of bupropion and agents that lower seizure threshold (e.g., antipsychotics) should be undertaken only with extreme caution. Low initial dosing and gradual dose increases should be employed).

No products indexed under this heading.

Loxapine Succinate (Concurrent administration of bupropion and agents that lower seizure threshold (e.g., antipsychotics) should be undertaken only with extreme caution. Low initial dosing and gradual dose increases should be employed).

No products indexed under this heading.

Maprotiline Hydrochloride (Bupropion is associated with a dose-related risk of seizures; co-administration with drugs that lower seizure threshold may increase the risk of seizure with bupropion; concurrent use should be undertaken with extreme caution).

No products indexed under this heading.

Meperidine Hydrochloride (Co-administration of bupropion with drugs that are metabolized by the CYP2D6 isoenzyme should be approached with caution and should be initiated at the lower end of the dose range of the concomitant medication. If bupropion is added to the treatment regimen of a patient already receiving a drug metabolized by CYP2D6, the need to decrease the dose of the original medication should be considered, particularly for those concomitant medications with a narrow therapeutic index).

No products indexed under this heading.

Mesoridazine Besylate (Bupropion is associated with a dose-related risk of seizures; co-administration with drugs that lower seizure threshold may increase the risk of seizure with bupropion; concurrent use should be undertaken with extreme caution).

No products indexed under this heading.

Methadone Hydrochloride (Co-administration of bupropion with drugs that are metabolized by the CYP2D6 isoenzyme should be approached with caution and should be initiated at the lower end of the

dose range of the concomitant medication. If bupropion is added to the treatment regimen of a patient already receiving a drug metabolized by CYP2D6, the need to decrease the dose of the original medication should be considered, particularly for those concomitant medications with a narrow therapeutic index).

No products indexed under this heading.

Methamphetamine Hydrochloride (Co-administration of bupropion with drugs that are metabolized by the CYP2D6 isoenzyme should be approached with caution and should be initiated at the lower end of the dose range of the concomitant medication. If bupropion is added to the treatment regimen of a patient already receiving a drug metabolized by CYP2D6, the need to decrease the dose of the original medication should be considered, particularly for those concomitant medications with a narrow therapeutic index). Products include:

Methotrimeprazine (Concurrent administration of bupropion and agents that lower seizure threshold (e.g., antipsychotics) should be undertaken only with extreme caution. Low initial dosing and gradual dose increases should be employed).

No products indexed under this heading.

Methylprednisolone Acetate (Bupropion is associated with a dose-related risk of seizures; co-administration with drugs that lower seizure threshold, such as systemic steroids, may increase the risk of seizure with bupropion). Products include:

Methylprednisolone Sodium Succinate (Bupropion is associated with a dose-related risk of seizures; co-administration with drugs that lower seizure threshold, such as systemic steroids, may increase the risk of seizure with bupropion).

No products indexed under this heading.

Metoprolol Succinate (Co-administration of bupropion with drugs that are metabolized by the CYP2D6 isoenzyme, including metoprolol, should be approached with caution and should be initiated at the lower end of the dose range of the concomitant medication. If bupropion is added to the treatment regimen of a patient already receiving a drug metabolized by CYP2D6, the need to decrease the dose of the original medication should be considered, particularly for those concomitant medications with a narrow therapeutic index). Products include:

Metoprolol Tartrate (Co-administration of bupropion with drugs that are metabolized by the CYP2D6 isoenzyme, including metoprolol, should be approached with caution and should be initiated at the lower end of the dose range of the concomitant medication. If bupropion is added to the treatment regimen of a patient already receiving a drug metabolized by CYP2D6, the need to decrease the dose of the original medication should be consid-

ered, particularly for those concomitant medications with a narrow therapeutic index). Products include:

Mexiletine Hydrochloride (Co-administration of bupropion with drugs that are metabolized by the CYP2D6 isoenzyme should be approached with caution and should be initiated at the lower end of the dose range of the concomitant medication. If bupropion is added to the treatment regimen of a patient already receiving a drug metabolized by CYP2D6, the need to decrease the dose of the original medication should be considered, particularly for those concomitant medications with a narrow therapeutic index).

No products indexed under this heading.

Midazolam Hydrochloride (Bupropion is associated with a dose-related risk of seizures; excessive use of benzodiazepine sedatives is associated with increased risk of seizures; bupropion is contraindicated in patients undergoing abrupt discontinuation of benzodiazepine sedatives).

No products indexed under this heading.

Mirtazapine (Co-administration of bupropion with drugs that are metabolized by the CYP2D6 isoenzyme should be approached with caution and should be initiated at the lower end of the dose range of the concomitant medication. If bupropion is added to the treatment regimen of a patient already receiving a drug metabolized by CYP2D6, the need to decrease the dose of the original medication should be considered, particularly for those concomitant medications with a narrow therapeutic index).

No products indexed under this heading.

Moclobemide (Concurrent and/or sequential use with MAO inhibitors is contraindicated).

No products indexed under this heading.

Molindone Hydrochloride (Concurrent administration of bupropion and agents that lower seizure threshold (e.g., antipsychotics) should be undertaken only with extreme caution. Low initial dosing and gradual dose increases should be employed). Products include:

Morphine Sulfate (Co-administration of bupropion with drugs that are metabolized by the CYP2D6 isoenzyme should be approached with caution and should be initiated at the lower end of the dose range of the concomitant medication. If bupropion is added to the treatment regimen of a patient already receiving a drug metabolized by CYP2D6, the need to decrease the dose of the original medication should be considered, particularly for those concomitant medications with a narrow therapeutic index). Products include:

IMPORTANT NOTE: Always consult each drug listing in the patient's regimen for possible interactions.

Nefazodone Hydrochloride (Concurrent administration of bupropion and agents that lower seizure threshold (e.g., other antidepressants) should be undertaken only with extreme caution. Low initial dosing and gradual dose increases should be employed).
No products indexed under this heading.

Nelfinavir Mesylate (Co-administration of bupropion with drugs that are metabolized by the CYP2D6 isoenzyme should be approached with caution and should be initiated at the lower end of the dose range of the concomitant medication. If bupropion is added to the treatment regimen of a patient already receiving a drug metabolized by CYP2D6, the need to decrease the dose of the original medication should be considered, particularly for those concomitant medications with a narrow therapeutic index). Products include:
Viracept **2577**

Nicotine (Co-administration has resulted in a higher incidence of treatment-emergent hypertension). Products include:
NicoDerm CQ Clear Patch .... ■**622**

Nortriptyline Hydrochloride (Co-administration of bupropion with drugs that are metabolized by the CYP2D6 isoenzyme, including nortriptyline, should be approached with caution and should be initiated at the lower end of the dose range of the concomitant medication. If bupropion is added to the treatment regimen of a patient already receiving a drug metabolized by CYP2D6, the need to decrease the dose of the original medication should be considered, particularly for those concomitant medications with a narrow therapeutic index).
No products indexed under this heading.

Olanzapine (Co-administration of bupropion with drugs that are metabolized by the CYP2D6 isoenzyme should be approached with caution and should be initiated at the lower end of the dose range of the concomitant medication. If bupropion is added to the treatment regimen of a patient already receiving a drug metabolized by CYP2D6, the need to decrease the dose of the original medication should be considered, particularly for those concomitant medications with a narrow therapeutic index). Products include:
Symbyax Capsules **1819**
Zyprexa Tablets **1830**
Zyprexa IntraMuscular **1830**
Zyprexa ZYDIS Orally Disintegrating Tablets **1830**

Omeprazole (Co-administration of bupropion with drugs that are metabolized by the CYP2D6 isoenzyme should be approached with caution and should be initiated at the lower end of the dose range of the concomitant medication. If bupropion is added to the treatment regimen of a patient already receiving a drug metabolized by CYP2D6, the need to decrease the dose of the original medication should be considered, particularly for those concomitant medications with a narrow therapeutic index). Products include:
Zegerid Capsules **2958**
Zegerid Powder for Oral Solution **2958**

Ondansetron (Co-administration of bupropion with drugs that are metabolized by the CYP2D6 isoenzyme should be approached with caution and should be initiated at the lower end of the dose range of the concomitant medication. If bupropion is added to the treatment regimen of a patient already receiving a drug metabolized by CYP2D6, the need to decrease the dose of the original medication should be considered, particularly for those concomitant medications with a narrow therapeutic index). Products include:
Zofran ODT Orally Disintegrating Tablets **1639**

Ondansetron Hydrochloride (Co-administration of bupropion with drugs that are metabolized by the CYP2D6 isoenzyme should be approached with caution and should be initiated at the lower end of the dose range of the concomitant medication. If bupropion is added to the treatment regimen of a patient already receiving a drug metabolized by CYP2D6, the need to decrease the dose of the original medication should be considered, particularly for those concomitant medications with a narrow therapeutic index). Products include:
Zofran Injection **1634**
Zofran **1639**

Orphenadrine Citrate (Bupropion is primarily metabolized, based on in vitro studies, to hydroxybupropion by cytochrome P450IIB6 isoenzyme; therefore, the potential exists for a drug interaction with agents that affect the cytochrome P450IIB6 metabolism, such as orphenadrine). Products include:
Norflex Injection **1856**

Oxazepam (Bupropion is associated with a dose-related risk of seizures; excessive use of benzodiazepine sedatives is associated with increased risk of seizures; bupropion is contraindicated in patients undergoing abrupt discontinuation of benzodiazepine sedatives).
No products indexed under this heading.

Oxycodone Hydrochloride (Co-administration of bupropion with drugs that are metabolized by the CYP2D6 isoenzyme should be approached with caution and should be initiated at the lower end of the dose range of the concomitant medication. If bupropion is added to the treatment regimen of a patient already receiving a drug metabolized by CYP2D6, the need to decrease the dose of the original medication should be considered, particularly for those concomitant medications with a narrow therapeutic index). Products include:
OxyContin Tablets **2703**
OxyFast Oral Concentrate Solution **2708**
OxyIR Capsules **2708**
Percocet Tablets **1131**
Percodan Tablets **1132**

Paclitaxel (Co-administration of bupropion with drugs that are metabolized by the CYP2D6 isoenzyme should be approached with caution and should be initiated at the lower end of the dose range of the concomitant medication. If bupropion is added to the treatment regimen of a patient already receiving a drug metabolized by CYP2D6, the need to decrease the dose of the original medication should be considered, particularly for those concomitant medications with a narrow therapeutic index).
No products indexed under this heading.

Pargyline Hydrochloride (Concurrent and/or sequential use with MAO inhibitors is contraindicated).
No products indexed under this heading.

Paroxetine Hydrochloride (Co-administration of bupropion with drugs that are metabolized by the CYP2D6 isoenzyme, including paroxetine, should be approached with caution and should be initiated at the lower end of the dose range of the concomitant medication. If bupropion is added to the treatment regimen of a patient already receiving a drug metabolized by CYP2D6, the need to decrease the dose of the original medication should be considered, particularly for those concomitant medications with a narrow therapeutic index). Products include:
Paxil CR Controlled-Release Tablets **1538**
Paxil **1530**

Perphenazine (Bupropion is associated with a dose-related risk of seizures; co-administration with drugs that lower seizure threshold may increase the risk of seizure with bupropion; concurrent use should be undertaken with extreme caution).
No products indexed under this heading.

Phenelzine Sulfate (Concurrent and/or sequential use with MAO inhibitors is contraindicated; acute toxicity of bupropion is enhanced by phenelzine in animal models).
No products indexed under this heading.

Phenobarbital (May induce the metabolism of bupropion). Products include:
Donnatal Extentabs **2493**

Phenytoin (May induce the metabolism of bupropion).
No products indexed under this heading.

Phenytoin Sodium (May induce the metabolism of bupropion). Products include:
Phenytek Capsules **2160**

Pimozide (Concurrent administration of bupropion and agents that lower seizure threshold (e.g., antipsychotics) should be undertaken only with extreme caution. Low initial dosing and gradual dose increases should be employed).
No products indexed under this heading.

Pindolol (Co-administration of bupropion with drugs that are metabolized by the CYP2D6 isoenzyme should be approached with caution and should be initiated at the lower end of the dose range of the concomitant medication. If bupropion is added to the treatment regimen of a patient already receiving a drug metabolized by CYP2D6, the need to decrease the dose of the original medication should be considered, particularly for those concomitant medications with a narrow therapeutic index).
No products indexed under this heading.

Prazepam (Bupropion is associated with a dose-related risk of seizures; excessive use of benzodiazepine sedatives is associated with increased risk of seizures; bupropion is contraindicated in patients undergoing abrupt discontinuation of benzodiazepine sedatives).
No products indexed under this heading.

Prednisolone Acetate (Bupropion is associated with a dose-related risk of seizures; co-administration with drugs that lower seizure threshold, such as systemic steroids, may increase the risk of seizure with bupropion). Products include:
Blephamide Ophthalmic Ointment **568**
Blephamide Ophthalmic Suspension **569**
Poly-Pred Ophthalmic Suspension .... ⊙**233**
Pred Forte Ophthalmic Suspension .... ⊙**235**
Pred Mild Ophthalmic Suspension .... ⊙**238**
Pred-G Ophthalmic Ointment .... ⊙**237**
Pred-G Ophthalmic Suspension .... ⊙**236**

Prednisolone Sodium Phosphate (Bupropion is associated with a dose-related risk of seizures; co-administration with drugs that lower seizure threshold, such as systemic steroids, may increase the risk of seizure with bupropion).
No products indexed under this heading.

Prednisolone Tebutate (Bupropion is associated with a dose-related risk of seizures; co-administration with drugs that lower seizure threshold, such as systemic steroids, may increase the risk of seizure with bupropion).
No products indexed under this heading.

Prednisone (Bupropion is associated with a dose-related risk of seizures; co-administration with drugs that lower seizure threshold, such as systemic steroids, may increase the risk of seizure with bupropion).
No products indexed under this heading.

Procarbazine Hydrochloride (Concurrent and/or sequential use with MAO inhibitors is contraindicated). Products include:
Matulane Capsules **3191**

Prochlorperazine (Bupropion is associated with a dose-related risk of seizures; co-administration with drugs that lower seizure threshold may increase the risk of seizure with bupropion; concurrent use should be undertaken with extreme caution).
No products indexed under this heading.

Promethazine Hydrochloride (Bupropion is associated with a dose-related risk of seizures; co-administration with drugs that lower seizure threshold may increase the risk of seizure with bupropion; concurrent use should be undertaken with extreme caution). Products include:
Phenergan Tablets and Suppositories **3440**

Propafenone Hydrochloride (Co-administration of bupropion with drugs that are metabolized by the CYP2D6 isoenzyme, including propafenone, should be approached with caution and should be initiated at the lower end of the dose range of the concomitant medication. If bupropion is added to the treatment regimen of a patient already receiving a drug metabolized by CYP2D6, the need to decrease the dose of the original medication should be considered, particularly for those concomitant medications with a narrow therapeutic index). Products include:

Rythmol SR Capsules 2727

Propoxyphene Hydrochloride

(Co-administration of bupropion with drugs that are metabolized by the CYP2D6 isoenzyme should be approached with caution and should be initiated at the lower end of the dose range of the concomitant medication. If bupropion is added to the treatment regimen of a patient already receiving a drug metabolized by CYP2D6, the need to decrease the dose of the original medication should be considered, particularly for those concomitant medications with a narrow therapeutic index).

No products indexed under this heading.

Propoxyphene Napsylate

(Co-administration of bupropion with drugs that are metabolized by the CYP2D6 isoenzyme should be approached with caution and should be initiated at the lower end of the dose range of the concomitant medication. If bupropion is added to the treatment regimen of a patient already receiving a drug metabolized by CYP2D6, the need to decrease the dose of the original medication should be considered, particularly for those concomitant medications with a narrow therapeutic index).

No products indexed under this heading.

Propranolol Hydrochloride

(Co-administration of bupropion with drugs that are metabolized by the CYP2D6 isoenzyme should be approached with caution and should be initiated at the lower end of the dose range of the concomitant medication. If bupropion is added to the treatment regimen of a patient already receiving a drug metabolized by CYP2D6, the need to decrease the dose of the original medication should be considered, particularly for those concomitant medications with a narrow therapeutic index). Products include:

Inderal LA Long-Acting Capsules 3429
InnoPran XL Capsules 2723

Protriptyline Hydrochloride

(Bupropion is associated with a dose-related risk of seizures; co-administration with drugs that lower seizure threshold may increase the risk of seizure with bupropion; concurrent use should be undertaken with extreme caution).

No products indexed under this heading.

Quazepam

(Bupropion is associated with a dose-related risk of seizures; excessive use of benzodiazepine sedatives is associated with increased risk of seizures; bupropion is contraindicated in patients undergoing abrupt discontinuation of benzodiazepine sedatives).

No products indexed under this heading.

Quetiapine Fumarate

(Co-administration of bupropion with drugs that are metabolized by the CYP2D6 isoenzyme should be approached with caution and should be initiated at the lower end of the dose range of the concomitant medication. If bupropion is added to the

treatment regimen of a patient already receiving a drug metabolized by CYP2D6, the need to decrease the dose of the original medication should be considered, particularly for those concomitant medications with a narrow therapeutic index). Products include:

Seroquel Tablets 690

Quinidine Gluconate

(Co-administration of bupropion with drugs that are metabolized by the CYP2D6 isoenzyme should be approached with caution and should be initiated at the lower end of the dose range of the concomitant medication. If bupropion is added to the treatment regimen of a patient already receiving a drug metabolized by CYP2D6, the need to decrease the dose of the original medication should be considered, particularly for those concomitant medications with a narrow therapeutic index).

No products indexed under this heading.

Quinidine Hydrochloride

(Co-administration of bupropion with drugs that are metabolized by the CYP2D6 isoenzyme should be approached with caution and should be initiated at the lower end of the dose range of the concomitant medication. If bupropion is added to the treatment regimen of a patient already receiving a drug metabolized by CYP2D6, the need to decrease the dose of the original medication should be considered, particularly for those concomitant medications with a narrow therapeutic index).

No products indexed under this heading.

Quinidine Polygalacturonate

(Co-administration of bupropion with drugs that are metabolized by the CYP2D6 isoenzyme should be approached with caution and should be initiated at the lower end of the dose range of the concomitant medication. If bupropion is added to the treatment regimen of a patient already receiving a drug metabolized by CYP2D6, the need to decrease the dose of the original medication should be considered, particularly for those concomitant medications with a narrow therapeutic index).

No products indexed under this heading.

Quinidine Sulfate

(Co-administration of bupropion with drugs that are metabolized by the CYP2D6 isoenzyme should be approached with caution and should be initiated at the lower end of the dose range of the concomitant medication. If bupropion is added to the treatment regimen of a patient already receiving a drug metabolized by CYP2D6, the need to decrease the dose of the original medication should be considered, particularly for those concomitant medications with a narrow therapeutic index).

No products indexed under this heading.

Risperidone

(Co-administration of bupropion with drugs that are metabolized by the CYP2D6 isoenzyme, including risperidone, should be approached with caution and should be initiated at the lower end of the dose range of the concomitant medication. If bupropion is added to the treatment regimen of a patient already receiving a drug metabolized by CYP2D6, the need to decrease

the dose of the original medication should be considered, particularly for those concomitant medications with a narrow therapeutic index). Products include:

Risperdal ... 1676
Risperdal Consta Long-Acting
 Injection 1682
Risperdal M-Tab Orally
 Disintegrating Tablets.................. 1676

Ritonavir

(Co-administration of bupropion with drugs that are metabolized by the CYP2D6 isoenzyme should be approached with caution and should be initiated at the lower end of the dose range of the concomitant medication. If bupropion is added to the treatment regimen of a patient already receiving a drug metabolized by CYP2D6, the need to decrease the dose of the original medication should be considered, particularly for those concomitant medications with a narrow therapeutic index). Products include:

Kaletra 476
Norvir 503

Selegiline Hydrochloride

(Concurrent and/or sequential use with MAO inhibitors is contraindicated). Products include:

Eldepryl Capsules 3208
Zelapar Tablets 3372

Sertraline Hydrochloride

(Co-administration of bupropion with drugs that are metabolized by the CYP2D6 isoenzyme, including sertraline, should be approached with caution and should be initiated at the lower end of the dose range of the concomitant medication. If bupropion is added to the treatment regimen of a patient already receiving a drug metabolized by CYP2D6, the need to decrease the dose of the original medication should be considered, particularly for those concomitant medications with a narrow therapeutic index). Products include:

Zoloft ... 2586

Tamoxifen Citrate

(Co-administration of bupropion with drugs that are metabolized by the CYP2D6 isoenzyme should be approached with caution and should be initiated at the lower end of the dose range of the concomitant medication. If bupropion is added to the treatment regimen of a patient already receiving a drug metabolized by CYP2D6, the need to decrease the dose of the original medication should be considered, particularly for those concomitant medications with a narrow therapeutic index). Products include:

Soltamox Oral Solution 3527

Temazepam

(Bupropion is associated with a dose-related risk of seizures; excessive use of benzodiazepine sedatives is associated with increased risk of seizures; bupropion is contraindicated in patients undergoing abrupt discontinuation of benzodiazepine sedatives). Products include:

Restoril Capsules 1860

Teniposide

(Co-administration of bupropion with drugs that are metabolized by the CYP2D6 isoenzyme should be approached with caution and should be initiated at the lower end of the dose range of the concomitant medication. If bupropion is added to the treatment regimen of a patient already receiving a drug metabolized by CYP2D6, the need to decrease the dose of the original

medication should be considered, particularly for those concomitant medications with a narrow therapeutic index).

No products indexed under this heading.

Testosterone

(Co-administration of bupropion with drugs that are metabolized by the CYP2D6 isoenzyme should be approached with caution and should be initiated at the lower end of the dose range of the concomitant medication. If bupropion is added to the treatment regimen of a patient already receiving a drug metabolized by CYP2D6, the need to decrease the dose of the original medication should be considered, particularly for those concomitant medications with a narrow therapeutic index). Products include:

AndroGel 3329
Striant Mucoadhesive 1007
Testim 1% Gel 695

Testosterone Cypionate

(Co-administration of bupropion with drugs that are metabolized by the CYP2D6 isoenzyme should be approached with caution and should be initiated at the lower end of the dose range of the concomitant medication. If bupropion is added to the treatment regimen of a patient already receiving a drug metabolized by CYP2D6, the need to decrease the dose of the original medication should be considered, particularly for those concomitant medications with a narrow therapeutic index).

No products indexed under this heading.

Testosterone Enanthate

(Co-administration of bupropion with drugs that are metabolized by the CYP2D6 isoenzyme should be approached with caution and should be initiated at the lower end of the dose range of the concomitant medication. If bupropion is added to the treatment regimen of a patient already receiving a drug metabolized by CYP2D6, the need to decrease the dose of the original medication should be considered, particularly for those concomitant medications with a narrow therapeutic index).

No products indexed under this heading.

Testosterone Propionate

(Co-administration of bupropion with drugs that are metabolized by the CYP2D6 isoenzyme should be approached with caution and should be initiated at the lower end of the dose range of the concomitant medication. If bupropion is added to the treatment regimen of a patient already receiving a drug metabolized by CYP2D6, the need to decrease the dose of the original medication should be considered, particularly for those concomitant medications with a narrow therapeutic index).

No products indexed under this heading.

Theophylline

(Bupropion is associated with a dose-related risk of seizures; co-administration with drugs that lower seizure threshold may increase the risk of seizures with bupropion; concurrent use should be undertaken with extreme caution).

No products indexed under this heading.

Theophylline Anhydrous

(Bupropion is associated with a dose-related risk of seizures; co-administration with drugs that lower

IMPORTANT NOTE: Always consult each drug listing in the patient's regimen for possible interactions.

seizure threshold may increase the risk of seizures with bupropion; concurrent use should be undertaken with extreme caution). Products include:

Uniphyl Tablets 2710

Theophylline Calcium Salicylate (Bupropion is associated with a dose-related risk of seizures; co-administration with drugs that lower seizure threshold may increase the risk of seizures with bupropion; concurrent use should be undertaken with extreme caution).

No products indexed under this heading.

Theophylline Dihydroxypropyl (Glyceryl) (Bupropion is associated with a dose-related risk of seizures; co-administration with drugs that lower seizure threshold may increase the risk of seizures with bupropion; concurrent use should be undertaken with extreme caution).

No products indexed under this heading.

Theophylline Ethylenediamine (Bupropion is associated with a dose-related risk of seizures; co-administration with drugs that lower seizure threshold may increase the risk of seizures with bupropion; concurrent use should be undertaken with extreme caution).

No products indexed under this heading.

Theophylline Sodium Glycinate (Bupropion is associated with a dose-related risk of seizures; co-administration with drugs that lower seizure threshold may increase the risk of seizures with bupropion; concurrent use should be undertaken with extreme caution).

No products indexed under this heading.

Thioridazine (Co-administration of bupropion with drugs that are metabolized by the CYP2D6 isoenzyme, including thioridazine, should be approached with caution and should be initiated at the lower end of the dose range of the concomitant medication. If bupropion is added to the treatment regimen of a patient already receiving a drug metabolized by CYP2D6, the need to decrease the dose of the original medication should be considered, particularly for those concomitant medications with a narrow therapeutic index).

No products indexed under this heading.

Thioridazine Hydrochloride (Co-administration of bupropion with drugs that are metabolized by the CYP2D6 isoenzyme, including thioridazine, should be approached with caution and should be initiated at the lower end of the dose range of the concomitant medication. If bupropion is added to the treatment regimen of a patient already receiving a drug metabolized by CYP2D6, the need to decrease the dose of the original medication should be considered, particularly for those concomitant medications with a narrow therapeutic index). Products include:

Thioridazine Hydrochloride Tablets 2163

Thiotepa (Bupropion is primarily metabolized, based on in vitro studies, to hydroxybupropion by cytochrome P450IIB6 isoenzyme; therefore, the potential exists for a drug interaction with agents that affect the cytochrome P450IIB6 metabolism, such as thiotepa).

No products indexed under this heading.

Thiothixene (Concurrent administration of bupropion and agents that lower seizure threshold (e.g., antipsychotics) should be undertaken only with extreme caution. Low initial dosing and gradual dose increases should be employed). Products include:

Thiothixene Capsules 2165

Timolol Maleate (Co-administration of bupropion with drugs that are metabolized by the CYP2D6 isoenzyme should be approached with caution and should be initiated at the lower end of the dose range of the concomitant medication. If bupropion is added to the treatment regimen of a patient already receiving a drug metabolized by CYP2D6, the need to decrease the dose of the original medication should be considered, particularly for those concomitant medications with a narrow therapeutic index). Products include:

Blocadren Tablets 1916
Cosopt Sterile Ophthalmic Solution 1931
Timolide Tablets 2086
Timoptic Sterile Ophthalmic Solution 2088
Timoptic in Ocudose 2091
Timoptic-XE Sterile Ophthalmic Gel Forming Solution 2092

Tolterodine Tartrate (Co-administration of bupropion with drugs that are metabolized by the CYP2D6 isoenzyme should be approached with caution and should be initiated at the lower end of the dose range of the concomitant medication. If bupropion is added to the treatment regimen of a patient already receiving a drug metabolized by CYP2D6, the need to decrease the dose of the original medication should be considered, particularly for those concomitant medications with a narrow therapeutic index). Products include:

Detrol Tablets 2628
Detrol LA Capsules 2631

Tramadol Hydrochloride (Co-administration of bupropion with drugs that are metabolized by the CYP2D6 isoenzyme should be approached with caution and should be initiated at the lower end of the dose range of the concomitant medication. If bupropion is added to the treatment regimen of a patient already receiving a drug metabolized by CYP2D6, the need to decrease the dose of the original medication should be considered, particularly for those concomitant medications with a narrow therapeutic index). Products include:

Ultram ER Tablets 2392

Tranylcypromine Sulfate (Concurrent and/or sequential use with MAO inhibitors is contraindicated). Products include:

Parnate Tablets 1527

Trazodone Hydrochloride (Bupropion is associated with a dose-related risk of seizures; co-administration with drugs that lower seizure threshold may increase the risk of seizure with bupropion; concurrent use should be undertaken with extreme caution).

No products indexed under this heading.

Triamcinolone (Bupropion is associated with a dose-related risk of seizures; co-administration with drugs that lower seizure threshold, such as systemic steroids, may increase the risk of seizure with bupropion).

No products indexed under this heading.

Triamcinolone Acetonide (Bupropion is associated with a dose-related risk of seizures; co-administration with drugs that lower seizure threshold, such as systemic steroids, may increase the risk of seizure with bupropion). Products include:

Azmacort Inhalation Aerosol 1726
Nasacort AQ Nasal Spray 2922

Triamcinolone Diacetate (Bupropion is associated with a dose-related risk of seizures; co-administration with drugs that lower seizure threshold, such as systemic steroids, may increase the risk of seizure with bupropion).

No products indexed under this heading.

Triamcinolone Hexacetonide (Bupropion is associated with a dose-related risk of seizures; co-administration with drugs that lower seizure threshold, such as systemic steroids, may increase the risk of seizure with bupropion).

No products indexed under this heading.

Triazolam (Bupropion is associated with a dose-related risk of seizures; excessive use of benzodiazepine sedatives is associated with increased risk of seizures; bupropion is contraindicated in patients undergoing abrupt discontinuation of benzodiazepine sedatives).

No products indexed under this heading.

Trifluoperazine Hydrochloride (Bupropion is associated with a dose-related risk of seizures; co-administration with drugs that lower seizure threshold may increase the risk of seizure with bupropion; concurrent use should be undertaken with extreme caution).

No products indexed under this heading.

Trimipramine Maleate (Bupropion is associated with a dose-related risk of seizures; co-administration with drugs that lower seizure threshold may increase the risk of seizure with bupropion; concurrent use should be undertaken with extreme caution).

No products indexed under this heading.

Venlafaxine Hydrochloride (Co-administration of bupropion with drugs that are metabolized by the CYP2D6 isoenzyme should be approached with caution and should be initiated at the lower end of the dose range of the concomitant medication. If bupropion is added to the treatment regimen of a patient already receiving a drug metabolized by CYP2D6, the need to decrease the dose of the original medication should be considered, particularly for those concomitant medications with a narrow therapeutic index). Products include:

Effexor Tablets 3411
Effexor XR Capsules 3417

Vinblastine Sulfate (Co-administration of bupropion with drugs that are metabolized by the CYP2D6 isoenzyme should be approached with caution and should be initiated at the lower end of the dose range of the concomitant medication. If bupropion is added to the treatment regimen of a patient already receiving a drug metabolized by CYP2D6, the need to decrease the dose of the original medication should be considered, particularly for those concomitant medications with a narrow therapeutic index).

No products indexed under this heading.

Warfarin Sodium (Altered PT and/or INR, infrequently associated with hemorrhagic or thrombotic complications, were observed when bupropion was co-administered with warfarin). Products include:

Coumadin for Injection 898
Coumadin Tablets 898

Ziprasidone Hydrochloride (Concurrent administration of bupropion and agents that lower seizure threshold (e.g., antipsychotics) should be undertaken only with extreme caution. Low initial dosing and gradual dose increases should be employed). Products include:

Geodon Capsules 2529

Zonisamide (Co-administration of bupropion with drugs that are metabolized by the CYP2D6 isoenzyme should be approached with caution and should be initiated at the lower end of the dose range of the concomitant medication. If bupropion is added to the treatment regimen of a patient already receiving a drug metabolized by CYP2D6, the need to decrease the dose of the original medication should be considered, particularly for those concomitant medications with a narrow therapeutic index). Products include:

Zonegran Capsules 1101

Food Interactions

Alcohol (Bupropion hydrochloride is contraindicated in patients undergoing abrupt discontinuation of alcohol. The consumption of alcohol during treatment with bupropion hydrochloride should be minimized or avoided).

Food, unspecified (Food increases Cmax and AUC of bupropion by 11% and 17%, respectively; no clinically significant food effect).

WELLBUTRIN XL EXTENDED-RELEASE TABLETS

(Bupropion Hydrochloride) 1613

See Wellbutrin SR Sustained-Release Tablets

WESTHROID TABLETS

(Levothyroxine Sodium, Liothyronine Sodium) 3403

May interact with androgens, corticosteroids, oral anticoagulants, estrogens, oral hypoglycemic agents, insulin, oral contraceptives, salicylates, and certain other agents. Compounds in these categories include:

Acarbose (Initiating thyroid replacement therapy may cause increases in insulin or oral hypoglycemic requirements). Products include:

Precose Tablets 751

Anisindione (Thyroid hormones appear to increase catabolism of vitamin K-dependent clotting factors. If oral anticoagulants are also being given, compensatory increases in clotting factor synthesis are impaired). Products include:

Miradon Tablets 3042

Aspirin (Preparations containing salicylates are known to interfere with laboratory tests performed in patients on thyroid hormone therapy). Products include:

Aggrenox Capsules 822
Bayer Aspirin 744
BC Allergy Sinus Cold Powder .... ■677
BC Headache Powder .... ■677
Arthritis Strength BC Powder .... ■677
BC Sinus Cold Powder .... ■677
Excedrin Extra Strength Caplets/Tablets/Geltabs .... ■684
Excedrin Migraine Caplets/Tablets/Geltabs .... ■609
Goody's Body Pain Formula Powder .... ■684
Goody's Extra Strength Headache Powders .... ■611
Goody's Extra Strength Pain Relief Tablets .... ■685
Percodan Tablets 1132
St. Joseph 81 mg Aspirin Chewable and Enteric Coated Tablets 1869

Aspirin, Enteric Coated (Preparations containing salicylates are known to interfere with laboratory tests performed in patients on thyroid hormone therapy).

No products indexed under this heading.

Aspirin Buffered (Preparations containing salicylates are known to interfere with laboratory tests performed in patients on thyroid hormone therapy). Products include:

Bufferin Extra Strength Tablets ...... ■678
Bufferin Regular Strength Tablets ... ■678

Betamethasone Acetate (Corticosteroids are known to interfere with laboratory tests performed in patients on thyroid hormone therapy).

No products indexed under this heading.

Betamethasone Sodium Phosphate (Corticosteroids are known to interfere with laboratory tests performed in patients on thyroid hormone therapy).

No products indexed under this heading.

Chlorotrianisene (Patients without a functioning thyroid gland who are on thyroid replacement therapy may need to increase their thyroid dose if estrogens are given. Estrogens are also known to interfere with laboratory tests performed in patients on thyroid hormone therapy).

No products indexed under this heading.

Chlorpropamide (Initiating thyroid replacement therapy may cause increases in insulin or oral hypoglycemic requirements).

No products indexed under this heading.

Cholestyramine (Cholestyramine binds both levothyroxine and liothyronine in the intestine, thus impairing absorption of these thyroid hormones. Four to five hours should elapse between administration of cholestyramine and thyroid hormones).

No products indexed under this heading.

Choline Magnesium Trisalicylate (Preparations containing salicylates are known to interfere with laboratory tests performed in patients on thyroid hormone therapy).

No products indexed under this heading.

Colestipol (Colestipol binds both levothyroxine and liothyronine in the intestine, thus impairing absorption of these thyroid hormones. Four to five hours should elapse between administration of colestipol and thyroid hormones).

No products indexed under this heading.

Colestipol Hydrochloride (Colestipol binds both levothyroxine and liothyronine in the intestine, thus impairing absorption of these thyroid hormones. Four to five hours should elapse between administration of colestipol and thyroid hormones).

No products indexed under this heading.

Cortisone Acetate (Corticosteroids are known to interfere with laboratory tests performed in patients on thyroid hormone therapy).

No products indexed under this heading.

Desogestrel (Patients without a functioning thyroid gland who are on thyroid replacement therapy may need to increase their thyroid dose if estrogens are given. Estrogens containing oral contraceptives are also known to interfere with laboratory tests performed in patients on thyroid hormone therapy). Products include:

Mircette Tablets 1066

Dexamethasone (Corticosteroids are known to interfere with laboratory tests performed in patients on thyroid hormone therapy). Products include:

Ciprodex Otic Suspension 559
Decadron Tablets 1951
TobraDex Ophthalmic Ointment 562
TobraDex Ophthalmic Suspension ... 563

Dexamethasone Acetate (Corticosteroids are known to interfere with laboratory tests performed in patients on thyroid hormone therapy).

No products indexed under this heading.

Dexamethasone Sodium Phosphate (Corticosteroids are known to interfere with laboratory tests performed in patients on thyroid hormone therapy).

No products indexed under this heading.

Dicumarol (Thyroid hormones appear to increase catabolism of vitamin K-dependent clotting factors. If oral anticoagulants are also being given, compensatory increases in clotting factor synthesis are impaired).

No products indexed under this heading.

Dienestrol (Patients without a functioning thyroid gland who are on thyroid replacement therapy may need to increase their thyroid dose if estrogens are given. Estrogens are also known to interfere with laboratory tests performed in patients on thyroid hormone therapy).

No products indexed under this heading.

Diethylstilbestrol (Patients without a functioning thyroid gland who are on thyroid replacement therapy may need to increase their thyroid dose if estrogens are given. Estrogens are also known to interfere with laboratory tests performed in patients on thyroid hormone therapy).

No products indexed under this heading.

Diflunisal (Preparations containing salicylates are known to interfere with laboratory tests performed in patients on thyroid hormone therapy). Products include:

Dolobid Tablets 1955

Estradiol (Patients without a functioning thyroid gland who are on thyroid replacement therapy may need to increase their thyroid dose if estrogens are given. Estrogens are also known to interfere with laboratory tests performed in patients on thyroid hormone therapy). Products include:

Angeliq Tablets 762
Climara Transdermal System 771
Climara Pro Transdermal System 776
Estrasorb Topical Emulsion 1147
Estring Vaginal Ring 2635
Menostar Transdermal System 782
Vagifem Tablets 2334

Estrogens, Conjugated (Patients without a functioning thyroid gland who are on thyroid replacement therapy may need to increase their thyroid dose if estrogens are given. Estrogens are also known to interfere with laboratory tests performed in patients on thyroid hormone therapy). Products include:

Premarin Intravenous 3442
Premarin Tablets 3446
Premarin Vaginal Cream 3452
Premphase Tablets 3456
Prempro Tablets 3456

Estrogens, Esterified (Patients without a functioning thyroid gland who are on thyroid replacement therapy may need to increase their thyroid dose if estrogens are given. Estrogens are also known to interfere with laboratory tests performed in patients on thyroid hormone therapy). Products include:

Estratest Tablets 3199
Estratest H.S. Tablets 3199

Estropipate (Patients without a functioning thyroid gland who are on thyroid replacement therapy may need to increase their thyroid dose if estrogens are given. Estrogens are also known to interfere with laboratory tests performed in patients on thyroid hormone therapy).

No products indexed under this heading.

Ethinyl Estradiol (Patients without a functioning thyroid gland who are on thyroid replacement therapy may need to increase their thyroid dose if estrogens are given. Estrogens are also known to interfere with laboratory tests performed in patients on thyroid hormone therapy). Products include:

Mircette Tablets 1066
NuvaRing 2340
Ortho-Cyclen/Ortho Tri-Cyclen 2429
Ortho Evra Transdermal System 2417
Ortho Tri-Cyclen Lo Tablets 2436
Seasonique Tablets 1077
Yasmin 28 Tablets 796
Yaz Tablets 803

Ethynodiol Diacetate (Patients without a functioning thyroid gland who are on thyroid replacement therapy may need to increase their thyroid dose if estrogens are given. Estrogens containing oral contraceptives are also known to interfere with laboratory tests performed in patients on thyroid hormone therapy).

No products indexed under this heading.

Fludrocortisone Acetate (Corticosteroids are known to interfere with laboratory tests performed in patients on thyroid hormone therapy).

No products indexed under this heading.

Fluoxymesterone (Androgens are known to interfere with laboratory tests performed in patients on thyroid hormone therapy). Products include:

Androxy Tablets 3335

Glimepiride (Initiating thyroid replacement therapy may cause increases in insulin or oral hypoglycemic requirements). Products include:

Avandaryl Tablets 1379
Duetact Tablets 3226

Glipizide (Initiating thyroid replacement therapy may cause increases in insulin or oral hypoglycemic requirements).

No products indexed under this heading.

Glyburide (Initiating thyroid replacement therapy may cause increases in insulin or oral hypoglycemic requirements).

No products indexed under this heading.

Hydrocortisone (Corticosteroids are known to interfere with laboratory tests performed in patients on thyroid hormone therapy). Products include:

Colocort Rectal Suspension, USP (Retention) 100 mg/60 mL.......... 2476
Hydrocortone Tablets 1989
Preparation H Hydrocortisone Cream .... ■646

Hydrocortisone Acetate (Corticosteroids are known to interfere with laboratory tests performed in patients on thyroid hormone therapy). Products include:

Analpram-HC 1159
Pramosone 1161
ProctoFoam-HC 3099

Hydrocortisone Sodium Phosphate (Corticosteroids are known to interfere with laboratory tests performed in patients on thyroid hormone therapy).

No products indexed under this heading.

Hydrocortisone Sodium Succinate (Corticosteroids are known to interfere with laboratory tests performed in patients on thyroid hormone therapy).

No products indexed under this heading.

Insulin, Human, Zinc Suspension (Initiating thyroid replacement therapy may cause increases in insulin or oral hypoglycemic requirements). Products include:

Humulin L, 100 Units 1794
Humulin U, 100 Units 1800

Insulin, Human NPH (Initiating thyroid replacement therapy may cause

increases in insulin or oral hypoglycemic requirements). Products
include:

Humulin N, 100 Units 1795
Humulin N Pen 1797

Insulin, Human Regular (Initiating
thyroid replacement therapy may
cause increases in insulin or oral
hypoglycemic requirements).
Products include:

Humulin R, 100 Units 1798

**Insulin, Human Regular and
Human NPH Mixture** (Initiating
thyroid replacement therapy may
cause increases in insulin or oral
hypoglycemic requirements).
Products include:

Humulin 50/50, 100 Units 1791
Humulin 70/30 Pen 1793

Insulin, NPH (Initiating thyroid
replacement therapy may cause
increases in insulin or oral hypoglycemic requirements).

No products indexed under this
heading.

Insulin, Regular (Initiating thyroid
replacement therapy may cause
increases in insulin or oral hypoglycemic requirements).

No products indexed under this
heading.

Insulin, Zinc Crystals (Initiating
thyroid replacement therapy may
cause increases in insulin or oral
hypoglycemic requirements).

No products indexed under this
heading.

Insulin, Zinc Suspension (Initiating
thyroid replacement therapy may
cause increases in insulin or oral
hypoglycemic requirements).

No products indexed under this
heading.

Insulin Aspart, Human Regular
(Initiating thyroid replacement therapy may cause increases in insulin or
oral hypoglycemic requirements).
Products include:

NovoLog Injection 2326

Insulin glargine (Initiating thyroid
replacement therapy may cause
increases in insulin or oral hypoglycemic requirements). Products
include:

Lantus Injection 2909

Insulin Lispro, Human (Initiating
thyroid replacement therapy may
cause increases in insulin or oral
hypoglycemic requirements).
Products include:

Humalog-Pen 1781
Humalog Mix 50/50-Pen 1783
Humalog Mix 75/25-Pen 1785

Insulin Lispro Protamine, Human
(Initiating thyroid replacement therapy may cause increases in insulin or
oral hypoglycemic requirements).
Products include:

Humalog Mix 50/50-Pen 1783
Humalog Mix 75/25-Pen 1785

Iodine Preparations (Iodine-
containing preparations are known
to interfere with laboratory tests performed in patients on thyroid hormone therapy).

No products indexed under this
heading.

Levonorgestrel (Patients without a
functioning thyroid gland who are on
thyroid replacement therapy may
need to increase their thyroid dose if
estrogens are given. Estrogens containing oral contraceptives are also
known to interfere with laboratory
tests performed in patients on thyroid hormone therapy). Products
include:

Climara Pro Transdermal System 776
Mirena Intrauterine System 787
Plan B Tablets 1076
Seasonique Tablets 1077

Magnesium Salicylate (Preparations containing salicylates are
known to interfere with laboratory
tests performed in patients on thyroid hormone therapy).

No products indexed under this
heading.

Mestranol (Patients without a functioning thyroid gland who are on thyroid replacement therapy may need
to increase their thyroid dose if
estrogens are given. Estrogens containing oral contraceptives are also
known to interfere with laboratory
tests performed in patients on thyroid hormone therapy).

No products indexed under this
heading.

Metformin Hydrochloride (Initiating thyroid replacement therapy may
cause increases in insulin or oral
hypoglycemic requirements).
Products include:

ActoPlus Met Tablets 3214
Avandamet Tablets 1373
Fortamet Extended-Release
Tablets ... 3115

Methylprednisolone Acetate
(Corticosteroids are known to interfere with laboratory tests performed
in patients on thyroid hormone therapy). Products include:

Depo-Medrol Injectable
Suspension 2617
Depo-Medrol Single-Dose Vial 2619

**Methylprednisolone Sodium
Succinate** (Corticosteroids are
known to interfere with laboratory
tests performed in patients on thyroid hormone therapy).

No products indexed under this
heading.

Methyltestosterone (Androgens
are known to interfere with laboratory tests performed in patients on
thyroid hormone therapy). Products
include:

Estratest Tablets 3199
Estratest H.S. Tablets 3199

Miglitol (Initiating thyroid replacement therapy may cause increases
in insulin or oral hypoglycemic
requirements).

No products indexed under this
heading.

Norethindrone (Patients without a
functioning thyroid gland who are on
thyroid replacement therapy may
need to increase their thyroid dose if
estrogens are given. Estrogens containing oral contraceptives are also
known to interfere with laboratory
tests performed in patients on thyroid hormone therapy). Products
include:

Ortho Micronor Tablets 2426

Norethynodrel (Patients without a
functioning thyroid gland who are on
thyroid replacement therapy may
need to increase their thyroid dose if
estrogens are given. Estrogens containing oral contraceptives are also
known to interfere with laboratory
tests performed in patients on thyroid hormone therapy).

No products indexed under this
heading.

Norgestimate (Patients without a
functioning thyroid gland who are on
thyroid replacement therapy may
need to increase their thyroid dose if
estrogens are given. Estrogens containing oral contraceptives are also
known to interfere with laboratory

tests performed in patients on thyroid hormone therapy). Products
include:

Ortho-Cyclen/Ortho Tri-Cyclen 2429
Ortho Tri-Cyclen Lo Tablets 2436

Norgestrel (Patients without a functioning thyroid gland who are on thyroid replacement therapy may need
to increase their thyroid dose if
estrogens are given. Estrogens containing oral contraceptives are also
known to interfere with laboratory
tests performed in patients on thyroid hormone therapy).

No products indexed under this
heading.

Oxandrolone (Androgens are
known to interfere with laboratory
tests performed in patients on thyroid hormone therapy). Products
include:

Oxandrin Tablets 2962

Oxymetholone (Androgens are
known to interfere with laboratory
tests performed in patients on thyroid hormone therapy).

No products indexed under this
heading.

Pioglitazone Hydrochloride (Initiating thyroid replacement therapy
may cause increases in insulin or
oral hypoglycemic requirements).
Products include:

ActoPlus Met Tablets 3214
Actos Tablets 3219
Duetact Tablets 3226

Polyestradiol Phosphate (Patients
without a functioning thyroid gland
who are on thyroid replacement therapy may need to increase their thyroid dose if estrogens are given.
Estrogens are also known to interfere with laboratory tests performed
in patients on thyroid hormone
therapy).

No products indexed under this
heading.

Prednisolone Acetate (Corticosteroids are known to interfere with
laboratory tests performed in
patients on thyroid hormone therapy). Products include:

Blephamide Ophthalmic Ointment 568
Blephamide Ophthalmic
Suspension 569
Poly-Pred Ophthalmic
Suspension ⊙233
Pred Forte Ophthalmic
Suspension ⊙235
Pred Mild Ophthalmic
Suspension ⊙238
Pred-G Ophthalmic Ointment ⊙237
Pred-G Ophthalmic Suspension ⊙236

Prednisolone Sodium Phosphate
(Corticosteroids are known to interfere with laboratory tests performed
in patients on thyroid hormone
therapy).

No products indexed under this
heading.

Prednisolone Tebutate (Corticosteroids are known to interfere with
laboratory tests performed in
patients on thyroid hormone
therapy).

No products indexed under this
heading.

Prednisone (Corticosteroids are
known to interfere with laboratory
tests performed in patients on thyroid hormone therapy).

No products indexed under this
heading.

Quinestrol (Patients without a functioning thyroid gland who are on thyroid replacement therapy may need
to increase their thyroid dose if
estrogens are given. Estrogens are
also known to interfere with labora-
ry tests performed in patients on
thyroid hormone therapy).

No products indexed under this
heading.

Repaglinide (Initiating thyroid
replacement therapy may cause
increases in insulin or oral hypoglycemic requirements).

No products indexed under this
heading.

Rosiglitazone Maleate (Initiating
thyroid replacement therapy may
cause increases in insulin or oral
hypoglycemic requirements).
Products include:

Avandamet Tablets 1373
Avandaryl Tablets 1379
Avandia Tablets 1384

Salsalate (Preparations containing
salicylates are known to interfere
with laboratory tests performed in
patients on thyroid hormone
therapy).

No products indexed under this
heading.

Stanozolol (Androgens are known
to interfere with laboratory tests performed in patients on thyroid hormone therapy).

No products indexed under this
heading.

Tolazamide (Initiating thyroid
replacement therapy may cause
increases in insulin or oral hypoglycemic requirements).

No products indexed under this
heading.

Tolbutamide (Initiating thyroid
replacement therapy may cause
increases in insulin or oral hypoglycemic requirements).

No products indexed under this
heading.

Triamcinolone (Corticosteroids are
known to interfere with laboratory
tests performed in patients on thyroid hormone therapy).

No products indexed under this
heading.

Triamcinolone Acetonide (Corticosteroids are known to interfere
with laboratory tests performed in
patients on thyroid hormone therapy). Products include:

Azmacort Inhalation Aerosol 1726
Nasacort AQ Nasal Spray 2922

Triamcinolone Diacetate (Corticosteroids are known to interfere
with laboratory tests performed in
patients on thyroid hormone
therapy).

No products indexed under this
heading.

Triamcinolone Hexacetonide
(Corticosteroids are known to interfere with laboratory tests performed
in patients on thyroid hormone
therapy).

No products indexed under this
heading.

Troglitazone (Initiating thyroid
replacement therapy may cause
increases in insulin or oral hypoglycemic requirements).

No products indexed under this
heading.

Warfarin Sodium (Thyroid hormones appear to increase catabolism of vitamin K-dependent clotting
factors. If oral anticoagulants are

also being given, compensatory increases in clotting factor synthesis are impaired). Products include:
Coumadin for Injection 898
Coumadin Tablets 898

WINOMEG3COMPLEX CAPSULES
(Docosahexaenoic Acid (DHA), EPA (Eicosapentaenoic Acid), Omega-3-acid ethyl esters, Omega-3 Acids, Omega-B Acids)............................ ▣
None cited in PDR database.

WINRGY DIETARY SUPPLEMENT
(Amino Acid Preparations, Caffeine, Vitamins with Minerals)........ ▣823
May interact with:

Aluminum Carbonate (Concomitant use with aluminum-containing antacids should be avoided).
No products indexed under this heading.

Aluminum Hydroxide (Concomitant use with aluminum-containing antacids should be avoided).
Products include:
Gaviscon Regular Strength Liquid .. ▣658
Gaviscon Regular Strength Tablets.. ▣658
Gaviscon Extra Strength Liquid ...... ▣658
Gaviscon Extra Strength Tablets .... ▣658
Maalox Regular Strength Antacid/Antigas Liquid.................. 2175
Maalox Max Maximum Strength Antacid/Anti-Gas Liquid................. 2176

WINRHO SDF
(Rh_0 (D) Immune Globulin (Human)) 732
May interact with vaccines, live. Compounds in these categories include:

BCG Vaccine (Other antibodies contained in WinRho SDF may interfere with the response to live virus vaccines such as measles, mumps, polio or rubella. Therefore, immunization with live vaccines should not be given within 3 months after WinRho SDF administration).
No products indexed under this heading.

Measles, Mumps, Rubella and Varicella Virus Vaccine Live (Other antibodies contained in WinRho SDF may interfere with the response to live virus vaccines such as measles, mumps, polio or rubella. Therefore, immunization with live vaccines should not be given within 3 months after WinRho SDF administration).
Products include:
ProQuad 2064

Measles, Mumps & Rubella Virus Vaccine, Live (Other antibodies contained in WinRho SDF may interfere with the response to live virus vaccines such as measles, mumps, polio or rubella. Therefore, immunization with live vaccines should not be given within 3 months after WinRho SDF administration).
Products include:
M-M-R II 2006

Measles & Rubella Virus Vaccine Live (Other antibodies contained in WinRho SDF may interfere with the response to live virus vaccines such as measles, mumps, polio or rubella. Therefore, immunization with live vaccines should not be given within 3 months after WinRho SDF administration).
No products indexed under this heading.

Measles Virus Vaccine Live (Other antibodies contained in WinRho SDF may interfere with the response to live virus vaccines such as measles, mumps, polio or rubella. Therefore, immunization with live vaccines should not be given within 3 months after WinRho SDF administration).
Products include:
Attenuvax 1914

Mumps Virus Vaccine, Live (Other antibodies contained in WinRho SDF may interfere with the response to live virus vaccines such as measles, mumps, polio or rubella. Therefore, immunization with live vaccines should not be given within 3 months after WinRho SDF administration).
Products include:
Mumpsvax 2031

Poliovirus Vaccine, Live, Oral, Trivalent, Types 1,2,3 (Sabin) (Other antibodies contained in WinRho SDF may interfere with the response to live virus vaccines such as measles, mumps, polio or rubella. Therefore, immunization with live vaccines should not be given within 3 months after WinRho SDF administration).
No products indexed under this heading.

Rotavirus Vaccine, Live, Oral, Tetravalent (Other antibodies contained in WinRho SDF may interfere with the response to live virus vaccines such as measles, mumps, polio or rubella. Therefore, immunization with live vaccines should not be given within 3 months after WinRho SDF administration).
No products indexed under this heading.

Rubella & Mumps Virus Vaccine Live (Other antibodies contained in WinRho SDF may interfere with the response to live virus vaccines such as measles, mumps, polio or rubella. Therefore, immunization with live vaccines should not be given within 3 months after WinRho SDF administration).
No products indexed under this heading.

Rubella Virus Vaccine Live (Other antibodies contained in WinRho SDF may interfere with the response to live virus vaccines such as measles, mumps, polio or rubella. Therefore, immunization with live vaccines should not be given within 3 months after WinRho SDF administration).
Products include:
Meruvax II 2019

Smallpox Vaccine (Other antibodies contained in WinRho SDF may interfere with the response to live virus vaccines such as measles, mumps, polio or rubella. Therefore, immunization with live vaccines should not be given within 3 months after WinRho SDF administration).
No products indexed under this heading.

Typhoid Vaccine (Other antibodies contained in WinRho SDF may interfere with the response to live virus vaccines such as measles, mumps, polio or rubella. Therefore, immunization with live vaccines should not be given within 3 months after WinRho SDF administration).
No products indexed under this heading.

Varicella Virus Vaccine Live (Other antibodies contained in WinRho SDF may interfere with the response to live virus vaccines such as measles, mumps, polio or rubella. Therefore, immunization with live vaccines should not be given within 3 months after WinRho SDF administration).
Products include:
Varivax 2100

Yellow Fever Vaccine (Other antibodies contained in WinRho SDF may interfere with the response to live virus vaccines such as measles, mumps, polio or rubella. Therefore, immunization with live vaccines should not be given within 3 months after WinRho SDF administration).
No products indexed under this heading.

WOBENZYM TABLETS
(Dietary Supplement) 1862
May interact with oral anticoagulants. Compounds in these categories include:

Anisindione (The use of Wobenzym should be graduated when taken in conjunction with anticoagulants).
Products include:
Miradon Tablets 3042

Dicumarol (The use of Wobenzym should be graduated when taken in conjunction with anticoagulants).
No products indexed under this heading.

Warfarin Sodium (The use of Wobenzym should be graduated when taken in conjunction with anticoagulants). Products include:
Coumadin for Injection 898
Coumadin Tablets 898

XALATAN STERILE OPHTHALMIC SOLUTION
(Latanoprost) 2649
May interact with:

Thimerosal (In vitro studies have shown that precipitation occurs when eye drops containing thimerosal are mixed with Xalatan; administer with an interval of at least five minutes between applications).
No products indexed under this heading.

XALATAN OPHTHALMIC SOLUTION
(Latanoprost) .... ⊙291

XELODA TABLETS
(Capecitabine) 2822
May interact with oral anticoagulants, phenytoin, and certain other agents. Compounds in these categories include:

Aluminum Hydroxide (Co-administration of capecitabine with aluminum hydroxide- and magnesium hydroxide-containing antacids has resulted in a small increase in plasma concentrations of capecitabine and one metabolite (5'DFCR)).
Products include:
Gaviscon Regular Strength Liquid .. ▣658
Gaviscon Regular Strength Tablets.. ▣658
Gaviscon Extra Strength Liquid ...... ▣658
Gaviscon Extra Strength Tablets .... ▣658
Maalox Regular Strength Antacid/Antigas Liquid.................. 2175
Maalox Max Maximum Strength Antacid/Anti-Gas Liquid................. 2176

Anisindione (Co-administration has resulted in altered coagulation parameters and/or bleeding).
Products include:
Miradon Tablets 3042

Dicumarol (Co-administration has resulted in altered coagulation parameters and/or bleeding).
No products indexed under this heading.

Fosphenytoin Sodium (Co-administration has resulted in toxicity associated with elevated phenytoin levels).
No products indexed under this heading.

Leucovorin Calcium (The concentrations of 5-fluorouracil, capecitabine is a prodrug and it is converted to 5-FU, is increased and its toxicity may be enhanced by leucovorin; deaths from severe enterocolitis, diarrhea, and dehydration have been reported in elderly patients receiving fluorouracil and leucovorin).
No products indexed under this heading.

Magnesium Hydroxide (Co-administration of capecitabine with aluminum hydroxide- and magnesium hydroxide-containing antacids has resulted in a small increase in plasma concentrations of capecitabine and one metabolite (5'DFCR)).
Products include:
Maalox Regular Strength Antacid/Antigas Liquid................. 2175
Maalox Max Maximum Strength Antacid/Anti-Gas Liquid................. 2176
Pepcid Complete Chewable Tablets 1701

Phenytoin (Co-administration has resulted in toxicity associated with elevated phenytoin levels).
No products indexed under this heading.

Phenytoin Sodium (Co-administration has resulted in toxicity associated with elevated phenytoin levels). Products include:
Phenytek Capsules 2160

Warfarin Sodium (Co-administration has resulted in altered coagulation parameters and/or bleeding). Products include:
Coumadin for Injection 898
Coumadin Tablets 898

Food Interactions

Food, unspecified (Reduces both rate and extent of absorption of capecitabine and delays Tmax of both parent and 5-FU).

XENADERM OINTMENT
(Balsam Peru, Castor Oil, Trypsin) 1664
None cited in PDR database.

XENICAL CAPSULES
(Orlistat) 2831
May interact with:

Beta-Carotene (Orlistat has been shown to reduce the absorption of some fat soluble vitamins; the vitamin supplement should be taken once a day at least 2 hours before or after the administration of orlistat).
No products indexed under this heading.

Cyclosporine (Co-administration has resulted in reduction in cyclosporine plasma levels; concurrent use is not recommended; if used concurrently, cyclosporine should be taken at least 2 hours before or after Xenical). Products include:
Gengraf Capsules 459
Neoral Oral Solution 2259
Neoral Soft Gelatin Capsules 2259
Restasis Ophthalmic Emulsion 575
Sandimmune 2275

Pravastatin Sodium (Co-administration results in additive lipid lowering effect of pravastatin; modest increases in pravastatin plasma concentrations were observed during co-administration).
No products indexed under this heading.

Vitamin A (Orlistat has been shown to reduce the absorption of some fat soluble vitamins; the vitamin supplement should be taken once a day at least 2 hours before or after the administration of orlistat). Products include:
- Visutein Capsules ... 3329

Vitamin D (Orlistat has been shown to reduce the absorption of some fat soluble vitamins; the vitamin supplement should be taken once a day at least 2 hours before or after the administration of orlistat). Products include:
- Active Calcium Tablets ... 3339
- Caltrate 600 PLUS ... ▣809
- Caltrate 600 + D Tablets ... ▣809
- D-Cal Chewable Caplets ... ▣812
- Os-Cal 250 + D Tablets ... ▣817
- Os-Cal 500 + D Tablets ... ▣817

Vitamin E (Orlistat has been shown to reduce the absorption of some fat soluble vitamins; the vitamin supplement should be taken once a day at least 2 hours before or after the administration of orlistat). Products include:
- Bausch & Lomb Ocuvite Adult Eye Vitamin and Mineral Supplement Soft Gels ... ▣706
- Bausch & Lomb Ocuvite Adult 50+ Eye Vitamin and Mineral Supplement Soft Gels ... ▣706
- MarineOmega Softgel Capsules ... 2672
- Ocuvite Adult Vitamin and Mineral Supplement ... ⊙253
- Ocuvite Adult 50+ Vitamin and Mineral Supplement ... ⊙253

Vitamin K_1 (Absorption of vitamin K may be decreased). Products include:
- Mephyton Tablets ... 2018

Warfarin Sodium (Vitamin K absorption may be decreased with orlistat; patients on chronic stable doses of warfarin who are prescribed orlistat should be monitored closely for changes in coagulation parameters). Products include:
- Coumadin for Injection ... 898
- Coumadin Tablets ... 898

Food Interactions

Food, unspecified (Gastrointestinal events may increase when orlistat is taken with a diet high in fat).

XERAC AC SOLUTION

(Aluminum Chloride) ... 2507
None cited in PDR database.

XIFAXAN TABLETS

(Rifaximin) ... 2842
None cited in PDR database.

XIGRIS POWDER FOR INTRAVENOUS INFUSION

(Drotrecogin alfa (activated)) ... 1828
May interact with oral anticoagulants, glycoprotein (GP) IIb/IIIa inhibitors, platelet inhibitors, thrombolytics, and certain other agents. Compounds in these categories include:

Abciximab (Bleeding is the most common serious adverse effect associated with drotrecogin alfa therapy; recent administration (within 7 days) of glycoprotein IIb/IIIa therapy increases the risk of bleeding). Products include:
- ReoPro Vials ... 1809

Alteplase (Bleeding is the most common serious adverse effect associated with drotrecogin alfa therapy; recent administration (within 3 days) of thrombolytic therapy increases the risk of bleeding). Products include:
- Activase I.V. ... 1223
- Cathflo Activase ... 1231

Anisindione (Bleeding is the most common serious adverse effect associated with drotrecogin alfa therapy; recent administration (within 7 days) of oral anticoagulant therapy increases the risk of bleeding). Products include:
- Miradon Tablets ... 3042

Anistreplase (Bleeding is the most common serious adverse effect associated with drotrecogin alfa therapy; recent administration (within 3 days) of thrombolytic therapy increases the risk of bleeding).
No products indexed under this heading.

Aspirin (Bleeding is the most common serious adverse effect associated with drotrecogin alfa therapy; recent administration (within 7 days) of more than 650mg per day of aspirin or other platelet inhibitors increases the risk of bleeding). Products include:
- Aggrenox Capsules ... 822
- Bayer Aspirin ... 744
- BC Allergy Sinus Cold Powder ... ▣677
- BC Headache Powder ... ▣677
- Arthritis Strength BC Powder ... ▣677
- BC Sinus Cold Powder ... ▣677
- Excedrin Extra Strength Caplets/Tablets/Geltabs ... ▣684
- Excedrin Migraine Caplets/Tablets/Geltabs ... ▣609
- Goody's Body Pain Formula Powder ... ▣684
- Goody's Extra Strength Headache Powders ... ▣611
- Goody's Extra Strength Pain Relief Tablets ... ▣685
- Percodan Tablets ... 1132
- St. Joseph 81 mg Aspirin Chewable and Enteric Coated Tablets ... 1869

Aspirin, Enteric Coated (Bleeding is the most common serious adverse effect associated with drotrecogin alfa therapy; recent administration (within 7 days) of more than 650mg per day of aspirin or other platelet inhibitors increases the risk of bleeding).
No products indexed under this heading.

Aspirin Buffered (Bleeding is the most common serious adverse effect associated with drotrecogin alfa therapy; recent administration (within 7 days) of more than 650mg per day of aspirin or other platelet inhibitors increases the risk of bleeding). Products include:
- Bufferin Extra Strength Tablets ... ▣678
- Bufferin Regular Strength Tablets ... ▣678

Azlocillin Sodium (Bleeding is the most common serious adverse effect associated with drotrecogin alfa therapy; recent administration (within 7 days) of more than 650mg per day of aspirin or other platelet inhibitors increases the risk of bleeding).
No products indexed under this heading.

Carbenicillin Indanyl Sodium (Bleeding is the most common serious adverse effect associated with drotrecogin alfa therapy; recent administration (within 7 days) of more than 650mg per day of aspirin or other platelet inhibitors increases the risk of bleeding).
No products indexed under this heading.

Choline Magnesium Trisalicylate (Bleeding is the most common serious adverse effect associated with drotrecogin alfa therapy; recent administration (within 7 days) of more than 650mg per day of aspirin or other platelet inhibitors increases the risk of bleeding).
No products indexed under this heading.

Clopidogrel Bisulfate (Bleeding is the most common serious adverse effect associated with drotrecogin alfa therapy; recent administration (within 7 days) of more than 650mg per day of aspirin or other platelet inhibitors increases the risk of bleeding). Products include:
- Plavix Tablets ... 917
- Plavix Tablets ... 2926

Diclofenac Potassium (Bleeding is the most common serious adverse effect associated with drotrecogin alfa therapy; recent administration (within 7 days) of more than 650mg per day of aspirin or other platelet inhibitors increases the risk of bleeding).
No products indexed under this heading.

Diclofenac Sodium (Bleeding is the most common serious adverse effect associated with drotrecogin alfa therapy; recent administration (within 7 days) of more than 650mg per day of aspirin or other platelet inhibitors increases the risk of bleeding). Products include:
- Arthrotec Tablets ... 3129
- Voltaren Ophthalmic Solution ... 2309
- Voltaren Tablets ... 2307
- Voltaren-XR Tablets ... 2310

Dicumarol (Bleeding is the most common serious adverse effect associated with drotrecogin alfa therapy; recent administration (within 7 days) of oral anticoagulant therapy increases the risk of bleeding).
No products indexed under this heading.

Diflunisal (Bleeding is the most common serious adverse effect associated with drotrecogin alfa therapy; recent administration (within 7 days) of more than 650mg per day of aspirin or other platelet inhibitors increases the risk of bleeding). Products include:
- Dolobid Tablets ... 1955

Dipyridamole (Bleeding is the most common serious adverse effect associated with drotrecogin alfa therapy; recent administration (within 7 days) of more than 650mg per day of aspirin or other platelet inhibitors increases the risk of bleeding). Products include:
- Aggrenox Capsules ... 822
- Persantine Tablets ... 868

Eptifibatide (Bleeding is the most common serious adverse effect associated with drotrecogin alfa therapy; recent administration (within 7 days) of glycoprotein IIb/IIIa therapy increases the risk of bleeding). Products include:
- Integrilin Injection ... 3020

Fenoprofen Calcium (Bleeding is the most common serious adverse effect associated with drotrecogin alfa therapy; recent administration (within 7 days) of more than 650mg per day of aspirin or other platelet inhibitors increases the risk of bleeding). Products include:
- Nalfon Capsules ... 2502

Flurbiprofen (Bleeding is the most common serious adverse effect associated with drotrecogin alfa therapy; recent administration (within 7 days) of more than 650mg per day of aspirin or other platelet inhibitors increases the risk of bleeding).
No products indexed under this heading.

Heparin Sodium (Bleeding is the most common serious adverse effect associated with drotrecogin alfa therapy; concurrent therapeutic dosing of heparin used to treat an active thrombotic or embolic event increases the risk of bleeding; low dose heparin does not appear to affect safety).
No products indexed under this heading.

Ibuprofen (Bleeding is the most common serious adverse effect associated with drotrecogin alfa therapy; recent administration (within 7 days) of more than 650mg per day of aspirin or other platelet inhibitors increases the risk of bleeding). Products include:
- Advil Allergy Sinus Caplets ... ▣770
- Advil ... ▣674
- Children's Advil Oral Suspension ... ▣603
- Children's Advil Chewable Tablets ... ▣603
- Advil Cold & Sinus ... ▣723
- Infants' Advil Concentrated Drops ... ▣604
- Infants' Advil Concentrated Drops - White Grape (Dye-Free) ... ▣604
- Junior Strength Advil Swallow Tablets ... ▣605
- Advil Migraine Liquigels ... ▣608
- Advil Multi-Symptom Cold Caplets ... ▣770
- Advil PM Caplets ... ▣615
- Motrin IB Tablets and Caplets ... 1866
- Children's Motrin Oral Suspension ... 1867
- Children's Motrin Non-Staining Dye-Free Oral Suspension ... 1867
- Children's Motrin Cold Oral Suspension ... 1867
- Infants' Motrin Concentrated Drops ... 1867
- Infants' Motrin Non-Staining Dye-Free Concentrated Drops ... 1867
- Junior Strength Motrin Caplets and Chewable Tablets ... 1867
- Vicoprofen Tablets ... 539

Indomethacin (Bleeding is the most common serious adverse effect associated with drotrecogin alfa therapy; recent administration (within 7 days) of more than 650mg per day of aspirin or other platelet inhibitors increases the risk of bleeding). Products include:
- Indocin ... 1995

Indomethacin Sodium Trihydrate (Bleeding is the most common serious adverse effect associated with drotrecogin alfa therapy; recent administration (within 7 days) of more than 650mg per day of aspirin or other platelet inhibitors increases the risk of bleeding). Products include:
- Indocin I.V. ... 2465

Ketoprofen (Bleeding is the most common serious adverse effect associated with drotrecogin alfa therapy; recent administration (within 7 days) of more than 650mg per day of aspirin or other platelet inhibitors increases the risk of bleeding).
No products indexed under this heading.

Magnesium Salicylate (Bleeding is the most common serious adverse effect associated with drotrecogin alfa therapy; recent administration (within 7 days) of more than 650mg per day of aspirin or other platelet inhibitors increases the risk of bleeding).
No products indexed under this heading.

Meclofenamate Sodium (Bleeding is the most common serious adverse effect associated with drotrecogin alfa therapy; recent administration (within 7 days) of more than 650mg per day of aspirin or other platelet inhibitors increases the risk of bleeding).
No products indexed under this heading.

Mefenamic Acid (Bleeding is the most common serious adverse effect associated with drotrecogin alfa therapy; recent administration (within 7 days) of more than 650mg per day of aspirin or other platelet inhibitors increases the risk of bleeding).
No products indexed under this heading.

Mezlocillin Sodium (Bleeding is the most common serious adverse effect associated with drotrecogin alfa therapy; recent administration (within 7 days) of more than 650mg per day of aspirin or other platelet inhibitors increases the risk of bleeding).
No products indexed under this heading.

Nafcillin Sodium (Bleeding is the most common serious adverse effect associated with drotrecogin alfa therapy; recent administration (within 7 days) of more than 650mg per day of aspirin or other platelet inhibitors increases the risk of bleeding).
No products indexed under this heading.

Naproxen (Bleeding is the most common serious adverse effect associated with drotrecogin alfa therapy; recent administration (within 7 days) of more than 650mg per day of aspirin or other platelet inhibitors increases the risk of bleeding). Products include:
EC-Naprosyn Delayed-Release Tablets 2761
Naprosyn Suspension 2761
Naprosyn Tablets 2761
Prevacid NapraPAC 3280

Naproxen Sodium (Bleeding is the most common serious adverse effect associated with drotrecogin alfa therapy; recent administration (within 7 days) of more than 650mg per day of aspirin or other platelet inhibitors increases the risk of bleeding). Products include:
Aleve Caplets 742
Aleve Gelcaps 743
Aleve Tablets 743
Aleve Cold & Sinus Caplets 744
Anaprox Tablets 2761
Anaprox DS Tablets 2761

Penicillin G Benzathine (Bleeding is the most common serious adverse effect associated with drotrecogin alfa therapy; recent administration (within 7 days) of more than 650mg per day of aspirin or other platelet inhibitors increases the risk of bleeding). Products include:
Bicillin C-R Injectable Suspension 1706

Penicillin G Procaine (Bleeding is the most common serious adverse effect associated with drotrecogin alfa therapy; recent administration (within 7 days) of more than 650mg per day of aspirin or other platelet inhibitors increases the risk of bleeding). Products include:
Bicillin C-R Injectable Suspension 1706

Phenylbutazone (Bleeding is the most common serious adverse effect associated with drotrecogin alfa therapy; recent administration (within 7 days) of more than 650mg per day of aspirin or other platelet inhibitors increases the risk of bleeding).
No products indexed under this heading.

Piroxicam (Bleeding is the most common serious adverse effect associated with drotrecogin alfa therapy; recent administration (within 7 days) of more than 650mg per day of aspirin or other platelet inhibitors increases the risk of bleeding).
No products indexed under this heading.

Reteplase (Bleeding is the most common serious adverse effect associated with drotrecogin alfa therapy; recent administration (within 3 days) of thrombolytic therapy increases the risk of bleeding). Products include:
Retavase 2499

Salsalate (Bleeding is the most common serious adverse effect associated with drotrecogin alfa therapy; recent administration (within 7 days) of more than 650mg per day of aspirin or other platelet inhibitors increases the risk of bleeding).
No products indexed under this heading.

Streptokinase (Bleeding is the most common serious adverse effect associated with drotrecogin alfa therapy; recent administration (within 3 days) of thrombolytic therapy increases the risk of bleeding).
No products indexed under this heading.

Sulindac (Bleeding is the most common serious adverse effect associated with drotrecogin alfa therapy; recent administration (within 7 days) of more than 650mg per day of aspirin or other platelet inhibitors increases the risk of bleeding). Products include:
Clinoril Tablets 1924

Ticarcillin Disodium (Bleeding is the most common serious adverse effect associated with drotrecogin alfa therapy; recent administration (within 7 days) of more than 650mg per day of aspirin or other platelet inhibitors increases the risk of bleeding). Products include:
Timentin ADD-Vantage 1580
Timentin Injection Galaxy Container 1583
Timentin IV Infusion 1577
Timentin Pharmacy Bulk Package 1586

Ticlopidine Hydrochloride (Bleeding is the most common serious adverse effect associated with drotrecogin alfa therapy; recent administration (within 7 days) of more than 650mg per day of aspirin or other platelet inhibitors increases the risk of bleeding). Products include:
Ticlid Tablets 2810

Tirofiban Hydrochloride (Bleeding is the most common serious adverse effect associated with drotrecogin alfa therapy; recent administration (within 7 days) of glycoprotein IIb/IIIa therapy increases the risk of bleeding). Products include:
Aggrastat 1907

Tolmetin Sodium (Bleeding is the most common serious adverse effect associated with drotrecogin alfa therapy; recent administration (within 7 days) of more than 650mg per day of aspirin or other platelet inhibitors increases the risk of bleeding).
No products indexed under this heading.

Urokinase (Bleeding is the most common serious adverse effect associated with drotrecogin alfa therapy; recent administration (within 3 days) of thrombolytic therapy increases the risk of bleeding).
No products indexed under this heading.

Warfarin Sodium (Bleeding is the most common serious adverse effect associated with drotrecogin alfa therapy; recent administration (within 7 days) of oral anticoagulant therapy increases the risk of bleeding). Products include:
Coumadin for Injection 898
Coumadin Tablets 898

XOLAIR

(Omalizumab) 1266
None cited in PDR database.

XOPENEX INHALATION SOLUTION

(Levalbuterol Hydrochloride) 3146
May interact with beta blockers, monoamine oxidase inhibitors, potassium-depleting diuretics, sympathomimetic aerosol bronchodilators, tricyclic antidepressants, and certain other agents. Compounds in these categories include:

Acebutolol Hydrochloride (Beta-adrenergic receptor blocking agents block the pulmonary effect of beta agonist and may produce severe bronchospasm in asthmatic patients).
No products indexed under this heading.

Albuterol (Potential for deleterious cardiovascular effects with concomitant use). Products include:
Proventil Inhalation Aerosol 3053

Amitriptyline Hydrochloride (Action of levalbuterol on the vascular system may be potentiated).
No products indexed under this heading.

Amoxapine (Action of levalbuterol on the vascular system may be potentiated).
No products indexed under this heading.

Atenolol (Beta-adrenergic receptor blocking agents block the pulmonary effect of beta agonist and may produce severe bronchospasm in asthmatic patients).
No products indexed under this heading.

Bendroflumethiazide (The ECG changes and/or hypokalemia that may result from the administration of non-potassium sparing diuretics can be acutely worsened by beta-agonists).
No products indexed under this heading.

Betaxolol Hydrochloride (Beta-adrenergic receptor blocking agents block the pulmonary effect of beta agonist and may produce severe bronchospasm in asthmatic patients). Products include:
Betoptic S Ophthalmic Suspension 558

Bisoprolol Fumarate (Beta-adrenergic receptor blocking agents block the pulmonary effect of beta agonist and may produce severe bronchospasm in asthmatic patients).
No products indexed under this heading.

Bitolterol Mesylate (Potential for deleterious cardiovascular effects with concomitant use).
No products indexed under this heading.

Bumetanide (The ECG changes and/or hypokalemia that may result from the administration of non-potassium sparing diuretics can be acutely worsened by beta-agonists). Products include:
Bumex Tablets 2746

Carteolol Hydrochloride (Beta-adrenergic receptor blocking agents block the pulmonary effect of beta agonist and may produce severe bronchospasm in asthmatic patients). Products include:
Carteolol Hydrochloride Ophthalmic Solution USP, 1%....... ⊙249

Chlorothiazide (The ECG changes and/or hypokalemia that may result from the administration of non-potassium sparing diuretics can be acutely worsened by beta-agonists). Products include:
Diuril Oral Suspension 1954

Chlorothiazide Sodium (The ECG changes and/or hypokalemia that may result from the administration of non-potassium sparing diuretics can be acutely worsened by beta-agonists). Products include:
Diuril Sodium Intravenous 2467

Clomipramine Hydrochloride (Action of levalbuterol on the vascular system may be potentiated).
No products indexed under this heading.

Desipramine Hydrochloride (Action of levalbuterol on the vascular system may be potentiated).
No products indexed under this heading.

Digoxin (Mean decreases of 16% and 22% in serum digoxin levels were demonstrated after the single-dose intravenous and oral administration of racemic albuterol, respectively; clinical significance of this finding is unclear). Products include:
Lanoxicaps Capsules 1490
Lanoxin Injection 1494
Lanoxin Injection Pediatric 1497
Lanoxin Tablets 1500

Doxepin Hydrochloride (Action of levalbuterol on the vascular system may be potentiated).
No products indexed under this heading.

Esmolol Hydrochloride (Beta-adrenergic receptor blocking agents block the pulmonary effect of beta agonist and may produce severe bronchospasm in asthmatic patients).
No products indexed under this heading.

Ethacrynic Acid (The ECG changes and/or hypokalemia that may result from the administration of non-potassium sparing diuretics can be acutely worsened by beta-agonists). Products include:
Edecrin Tablets 1959

Furosemide (The ECG changes and/or hypokalemia that may result from the administration of non-potassium sparing diuretics can be acutely worsened by beta-agonists). Products include:
Furosemide Tablets 2154

Hydrochlorothiazide (The ECG changes and/or hypokalemia that may result from the administration of non-potassium sparing diuretics can be acutely worsened by beta-agonists). Products include:
Aldoril Tablets 1910
Atacand HCT 651
Avalide Tablets 888
Avalide Tablets 2874
Benicar HCT Tablets 1044
Diovan HCT Tablets 2196
Dyazide Capsules 1423
Hyzaar 50-12.5 Tablets 1990
Hyzaar 100-12.5 Tablets 1990
Hyzaar 100-25 Tablets 1990
Lopressor HCT 50/25 Tablets 2241
Lopressor HCT 100/25 Tablets 2241
Lopressor HCT 100/50 Tablets 2241
Lotensin HCT Tablets 2246
Micardis HCT Tablets 856
Moduretic Tablets 2028
Prinzide Tablets 2056
Teveten HCT Tablets 1737
Timolide Tablets 2086
Uniretic Tablets 3100

Hydroflumethiazide (The ECG changes and/or hypokalemia that may result from the administration of non-potassium sparing diuretics can be acutely worsened by beta-agonists).
No products indexed under this heading.

Imipramine Hydrochloride (Action of levalbuterol on the vascular system may be potentiated).
No products indexed under this heading.

Imipramine Pamoate (Action of levalbuterol on the vascular system may be potentiated).
No products indexed under this heading.

Isocarboxazid (Action of levalbuterol on the vascular system may be potentiated).
No products indexed under this heading.

Isoetharine (Potential for deleterious cardiovascular effects with concomitant use).
No products indexed under this heading.

Isoproterenol Hydrochloride (Potential for deleterious cardiovascular effects with concomitant use).
No products indexed under this heading.

Labetalol Hydrochloride (Beta-adrenergic receptor blocking agents block the pulmonary effect of beta agonist and may produce severe bronchospasm in asthmatic patients).
No products indexed under this heading.

Levobunolol Hydrochloride (Beta-adrenergic receptor blocking agents block the pulmonary effect of beta agonist and may produce severe bronchospasm in asthmatic patients). Products include:
Betagan Ophthalmic Solution, USP .... ⊙220

Maprotiline Hydrochloride (Action of levalbuterol on the vascular system may be potentiated).
No products indexed under this heading.

Metaproterenol Sulfate (Potential for deleterious cardiovascular effects with concomitant use). Products include:
Alupent Inhalation Aerosol 826

Methyclothiazide (The ECG changes and/or hypokalemia that may result from the administration of non-potassium sparing diuretics can be acutely worsened by beta-agonists).
No products indexed under this heading.

Metipranolol Hydrochloride (Beta-adrenergic receptor blocking agents block the pulmonary effect of beta agonist and may produce severe bronchospasm in asthmatic patients).
No products indexed under this heading.

Metoprolol Succinate (Beta-adrenergic receptor blocking agents block the pulmonary effect of beta agonist and may produce severe bronchospasm in asthmatic patients). Products include:
Toprol-XL Tablets 668

Metoprolol Tartrate (Beta-adrenergic receptor blocking agents block the pulmonary effect of beta agonist and may produce severe bronchospasm in asthmatic patients). Products include:
Lopressor Injection 2238
Lopressor Tablets 2238
Lopressor HCT 50/25 Tablets 2241
Lopressor HCT 100/25 Tablets 2241
Lopressor HCT 100/50 Tablets 2241

Moclobemide (Action of levalbuterol on the vascular system may be potentiated).
No products indexed under this heading.

Nadolol (Beta-adrenergic receptor blocking agents block the pulmonary effect of beta agonist and may produce severe bronchospasm in asthmatic patients). Products include:
Nadolol Tablets 2159

Nortriptyline Hydrochloride (Action of levalbuterol on the vascular system may be potentiated).
No products indexed under this heading.

Pargyline Hydrochloride (Action of levalbuterol on the vascular system may be potentiated).
No products indexed under this heading.

Penbutolol Sulfate (Beta-adrenergic receptor blocking agents block the pulmonary effect of beta agonist and may produce severe bronchospasm in asthmatic patients).
No products indexed under this heading.

Phenelzine Sulfate (Action of levalbuterol on the vascular system may be potentiated).
No products indexed under this heading.

Pindolol (Beta-adrenergic receptor blocking agents block the pulmonary effect of beta agonist and may produce severe bronchospasm in asthmatic patients).
No products indexed under this heading.

Pirbuterol Acetate (Potential for deleterious cardiovascular effects with concomitant use). Products include:
Maxair Autohaler 1852

Polythiazide (The ECG changes and/or hypokalemia that may result from the administration of non-potassium sparing diuretics can be acutely worsened by beta-agonists).
No products indexed under this heading.

Procarbazine Hydrochloride (Action of levalbuterol on the vascular system may be potentiated). Products include:
Matulane Capsules 3191

Propranolol Hydrochloride (Beta-adrenergic receptor blocking agents block the pulmonary effect of beta agonist and may produce severe bronchospasm in asthmatic patients). Products include:
Inderal LA Long-Acting Capsules 3429
InnoPran XL Capsules 2723

Protriptyline Hydrochloride (Action of levalbuterol on the vascular system may be potentiated).
No products indexed under this heading.

Salmeterol Xinafoate (Potential for deleterious cardiovascular effects with concomitant use). Products include:
Advair Diskus 100/50 1308
Advair Diskus 250/50 1308
Advair Diskus 500/50 1308
Advair HFA Inhalation Aerosol 1318
Serevent Diskus 1568

Selegiline Hydrochloride (Action of levalbuterol on the vascular system may be potentiated). Products include:
Eldepryl Capsules 3208
Zelapar Tablets 3372

Sotalol Hydrochloride (Beta-adrenergic receptor blocking agents block the pulmonary effect of beta agonist and may produce severe bronchospasm in asthmatic patients).
No products indexed under this heading.

Terbutaline Sulfate (Potential for deleterious cardiovascular effects with concomitant use).
No products indexed under this heading.

Timolol Hemihydrate (Beta-adrenergic receptor blocking agents block the pulmonary effect of beta agonist and may produce severe bronchospasm in asthmatic patients). Products include:
Betimol Ophthalmic Solution 3382
Betimol Ophthalmic Solution .... ⊙295

Timolol Maleate (Beta-adrenergic receptor blocking agents block the pulmonary effect of beta agonist and may produce severe bronchospasm in asthmatic patients). Products include:
Blocadren Tablets 1916
Cosopt Sterile Ophthalmic Solution 1931
Timolide Tablets 2086
Timoptic Sterile Ophthalmic Solution 2088
Timoptic in Ocudose 2091
Timoptic-XE Sterile Ophthalmic Gel Forming Solution 2092

Torsemide (The ECG changes and/or hypokalemia that may result from the administration of non-potassium sparing diuretics can be acutely worsened by beta-agonists). Products include:
Demadex Injection 2759
Demadex Tablets 2759

Tranylcypromine Sulfate (Action of levalbuterol on the vascular system may be potentiated). Products include:
Parnate Tablets 1527

Trimipramine Maleate (Action of levalbuterol on the vascular system may be potentiated).
No products indexed under this heading.

XOPENEX INHALATION SOLUTION CONCENTRATE

(Levalbuterol Hydrochloride) 3150
See Xopenex Inhalation Solution

XOPENEX HFA INHALATION AEROSOL

(Levalbuterol Tartrate) 3154
See Xopenex Inhalation Solution

XYREM ORAL SOLUTION

(Sodium Oxybate) 1688
May interact with central nervous system depressants, hypnotics and sedatives, and certain other agents. Compounds in these categories include:

Alfentanil Hydrochloride (Sodium oxybate should not be used in combination with other CNS depressants).
No products indexed under this heading.

Alprazolam (Sodium oxybate should not be used in combination with other CNS depressants). Products include:
Niravam Orally Disintegrating Tablets 3092

Aprobarbital (Sodium oxybate should not be used in combination with other CNS depressants).
No products indexed under this heading.

Buprenorphine Hydrochloride (Sodium oxybate should not be used in combination with other CNS depressants). Products include:
Buprenex Injectable 2716
Suboxone Tablets 2717
Subutex Tablets 2717

Buspirone Hydrochloride (Sodium oxybate should not be used in combination with other CNS depressants).
No products indexed under this heading.

Butabarbital (Sodium oxybate should not be used in combination with other CNS depressants).
No products indexed under this heading.

Butalbital (Sodium oxybate should not be used in combination with other CNS depressants).
No products indexed under this heading.

Chlordiazepoxide (Sodium oxybate should not be used in combination with other CNS depressants).
No products indexed under this heading.

Chlordiazepoxide Hydrochloride (Sodium oxybate should not be used in combination with other CNS depressants). Products include:
Librium Capsules 3347

Chlorpromazine (Sodium oxybate should not be used in combination with other CNS depressants).
No products indexed under this heading.

Chlorpromazine Hydrochloride (Sodium oxybate should not be used in combination with other CNS depressants).
No products indexed under this heading.

Chlorprothixene (Sodium oxybate should not be used in combination with other CNS depressants).
No products indexed under this heading.

Chlorprothixene Hydrochloride (Sodium oxybate should not be used in combination with other CNS depressants).
No products indexed under this heading.

Chlorprothixene Lactate (Sodium oxybate should not be used in combination with other CNS depressants).
No products indexed under this heading.

Clorazepate Dipotassium (Sodium oxybate should not be used in combination with other CNS depressants). Products include:
Tranxene .. 2474

Clozapine (Sodium oxybate should not be used in combination with other CNS depressants). Products include:
Clozaril Tablets 2184
FazaClo Orally Disintegrating Tablets .. 551

Codeine Phosphate (Sodium oxybate should not be used in combination with other CNS depressants). Products include:
Tylenol with Codeine Tablets 2391

Desflurane (Sodium oxybate should not be used in combination with other CNS depressants).
No products indexed under this heading.

Dezocine (Sodium oxybate should not be used in combination with other CNS depressants).
No products indexed under this heading.

Diazepam (Sodium oxybate should not be used in combination with other CNS depressants). Products include:
Diastat Rectal Delivery System 3343
Valium Tablets 2819

Droperidol (Sodium oxybate should not be used in combination with other CNS depressants).
No products indexed under this heading.

Enflurane (Sodium oxybate should not be used in combination with other CNS depressants).
No products indexed under this heading.

Estazolam (Sodium oxybate is contraindicated in patients being treated with sedative hypnotic agents). Products include:
ProSom Tablets 517

Ethanol (Sodium oxybate should not be used in combination with other CNS depressants).
No products indexed under this heading.

Ethchlorvynol (Sodium oxybate is contraindicated in patients being treated with sedative hypnotic agents).
No products indexed under this heading.

Ethinamate (Sodium oxybate is contraindicated in patients being treated with sedative hypnotic agents).
No products indexed under this heading.

Ethyl Alcohol (Sodium oxybate should not be used in combination with other CNS depressants).
No products indexed under this heading.

Fentanyl (Sodium oxybate should not be used in combination with other CNS depressants). Products include:
Duragesic Transdermal System 2373
Ionsys Transdermal System 2379

Fentanyl Citrate (Sodium oxybate should not be used in combination with other CNS depressants). Products include:
Actiq .. 979

Fluphenazine Decanoate (Sodium oxybate should not be used in combination with other CNS depressants).
No products indexed under this heading.

Fluphenazine Enanthate (Sodium oxybate should not be used in combination with other CNS depressants).
No products indexed under this heading.

Fluphenazine Hydrochloride (Sodium oxybate should not be used in combination with other CNS depressants).
No products indexed under this heading.

Flurazepam Hydrochloride (Sodium oxybate is contraindicated in patients being treated with sedative hypnotic agents). Products include:
Dalmane Capsules 3342

Glutethimide (Sodium oxybate is contraindicated in patients being treated with sedative hypnotic agents).
No products indexed under this heading.

Haloperidol (Sodium oxybate should not be used in combination with other CNS depressants).
No products indexed under this heading.

Haloperidol Decanoate (Sodium oxybate should not be used in combination with other CNS depressants).
No products indexed under this heading.

Hydrocodone Bitartrate (Sodium oxybate should not be used in combination with other CNS depressants). Products include:
Hycodan ... 1116
Hycotuss Expectorant Syrup 1117
Vicodin Tablets 535
Vicodin ES Tablets 536
Vicodin HP Tablets 538
Vicoprofen Tablets 539
Zydone Tablets 1139

Hydrocodone Polistirex (Sodium oxybate should not be used in combination with other CNS depressants). Products include:
Tussionex Pennkinetic Extended-Release Suspension 3327

Hydromorphone Hydrochloride (Sodium oxybate should not be used in combination with other CNS depressants). Products include:
Dilaudid ... 440
Dilaudid Non-Sterile Powder 440
Dilaudid Oral Liquid 445
Dilaudid Rectal Suppositories 440
Dilaudid Tablets 440
Dilaudid Tablets - 8 mg 445
Dilaudid-HP 442

Hydroxyzine Hydrochloride (Sodium oxybate should not be used in combination with other CNS depressants).
No products indexed under this heading.

Isoflurane (Sodium oxybate should not be used in combination with other CNS depressants).
No products indexed under this heading.

Ketamine Hydrochloride (Sodium oxybate should not be used in combination with other CNS depressants).
No products indexed under this heading.

Levomethadyl Acetate Hydrochloride (Sodium oxybate should not be used in combination with other CNS depressants).
No products indexed under this heading.

Levorphanol Tartrate (Sodium oxybate should not be used in combination with other CNS depressants).
No products indexed under this heading.

Lorazepam (Sodium oxybate is contraindicated in patients being treated with sedative hypnotic agents).
No products indexed under this heading.

Loxapine Hydrochloride (Sodium oxybate should not be used in combination with other CNS depressants).
No products indexed under this heading.

Loxapine Succinate (Sodium oxybate should not be used in combination with other CNS depressants).
No products indexed under this heading.

Meperidine Hydrochloride (Sodium oxybate should not be used in combination with other CNS depressants).
No products indexed under this heading.

Mephobarbital (Sodium oxybate should not be used in combination with other CNS depressants).
No products indexed under this heading.

Meprobamate (Sodium oxybate should not be used in combination with other CNS depressants).
No products indexed under this heading.

Mesoridazine Besylate (Sodium oxybate should not be used in combination with other CNS depressants).
No products indexed under this heading.

Methadone Hydrochloride (Sodium oxybate should not be used in combination with other CNS depressants).
No products indexed under this heading.

Methohexital Sodium (Sodium oxybate should not be used in combination with other CNS depressants).
No products indexed under this heading.

Methotrimeprazine (Sodium oxybate should not be used in combination with other CNS depressants).
No products indexed under this heading.

Methoxyflurane (Sodium oxybate should not be used in combination with other CNS depressants).
No products indexed under this heading.

Midazolam Hydrochloride (Sodium oxybate is contraindicated in patients being treated with sedative hypnotic agents).
No products indexed under this heading.

Molindone Hydrochloride (Sodium oxybate should not be used in combination with other CNS depressants). Products include:
Moban Tablets 1119

Morphine Sulfate (Sodium oxybate should not be used in combination with other CNS depressants). Products include:
Avinza Capsules 1741
Kadian Capsules 577
MS Contin Tablets 2701

Olanzapine (Sodium oxybate should not be used in combination with other CNS depressants). Products include:
Symbyax Capsules 1819
Zyprexa Tablets 1830
Zyprexa IntraMuscular 1830
Zyprexa ZYDIS Orally Disintegrating Tablets.................. 1830

Oxazepam (Sodium oxybate should not be used in combination with other CNS depressants).
No products indexed under this heading.

Oxycodone Hydrochloride (Sodium oxybate should not be used in combination with other CNS depressants). Products include:
OxyContin Tablets 2703
OxyFast Oral Concentrate Solution 2708
OxyIR Capsules 2708
Percocet Tablets 1131
Percodan Tablets 1132

Pentobarbital Sodium (Sodium oxybate should not be used in combination with other CNS depressants). Products include:
Nembutal Sodium Solution, USP 2470

Perphenazine (Sodium oxybate should not be used in combination with other CNS depressants).
No products indexed under this heading.

Phenobarbital (Sodium oxybate should not be used in combination with other CNS depressants). Products include:
Donnatal Extentabs 2493

Prazepam (Sodium oxybate should not be used in combination with other CNS depressants).
No products indexed under this heading.

Prochlorperazine (Sodium oxybate should not be used in combination with other CNS depressants).
No products indexed under this heading.

Promethazine Hydrochloride (Sodium oxybate should not be used in combination with other CNS depressants). Products include:

IMPORTANT NOTE: Always consult each drug listing in the patient's regimen for possible interactions.

Food Interactions

Alcohol (The combined use of alcohol with sodium oxybate may result in potentiation of the central nervous system-depressant effects of sodium oxybate and alcohol).

YASMIN 28 TABLETS

(Drospirenone, Ethinyl Estradiol)........ 796
May interact with ACE inhibitors, aldosterone-inhibiting diuretic agents, angiotensin-II receptor antagonists, non-steroidal anti-inflammatory agents, phenytoin, prednisolone, potassium sparing diuretics, tetracyclines, xanthines, and certain other agents. Compounds in these categories include:

Amiloride Hydrochloride (Yasmin has the potential to cause hyperkalemia in high-risk patients; co-administration with other drugs that have the potential to increase serum potassium, such as potassium-sparing diuretics, may increase this risk further). Products include:

Aminophylline (Co-administration of products containing ethinyl estradiol may inhibit the metabolism of other compounds, such as theophylline, resulting in increased plasma concentrations of theophylline).
No products indexed under this heading.

Ampicillin (Pregnancy while taking oral contraceptives has been reported when oral contraceptives were administered with ampicillin; clinical pharmacokinetic studies have not demonstrated any consistent effect of antibiotics (other than rifampin) on plasma concentrations of synthetic steroids).
No products indexed under this heading.

Ampicillin Sodium (Pregnancy while taking oral contraceptives has been reported when oral contraceptives were administered with ampicillin; clinical pharmacokinetic studies have not demonstrated any consistent effect of antibiotics (other than rifampin) on plasma concentrations of synthetic steroids).
No products indexed under this heading.

(▣ Described in PDR For Nonprescription Drugs) (☉ Described in PDR For Ophthalmic Medicines™)

Atorvastatin Calcium (Co-administration of atorvastatin and an oral contraceptive increased AUC values for ethinyl estradiol by approximately 20%). Products include:

Caduet Tablets 2508
Lipitor Tablets 2483

Benazepril Hydrochloride (Yasmin has the potential to cause hyperkalemia in high-risk patients; co-administration with other drugs that have the potential to increase serum potassium, such as ACE inhibitors, may increase this risk further). Products include:

Lotensin Tablets 2243
Lotensin HCT Tablets 2246
Lotrel Capsules 2249

Candesartan Cilexetil (Yasmin has the potential to cause hyperkalemia in high-risk patients; co-administration with other drugs that have the potential to increase serum potassium, such as angiotensin-II receptor antagonists, may increase this risk further). Products include:

Atacand Tablets 649
Atacand HCT 651

Captopril (Yasmin has the potential to cause hyperkalemia in high-risk patients; co-administration with other drugs that have the potential to increase serum potassium, such as ACE inhibitors, may increase this risk further). Products include:

Captopril Tablets 2149

Carbamazepine (Co-administration results in increased metabolism of ethinyl estradiol and/or some progestins which could result in a reduction of contraceptive effectiveness). Products include:

Carbatrol Capsules 3171
Equetro Extended-Release Capsules 3180
Tegretol/Tegretol-XR 2295

Celecoxib (Yasmin has the potential to cause hyperkalemia in high-risk patients; co-administration with other drugs that have the potential to increase serum potassium, such as NSAIDs, may increase this risk further). Products include:

Celebrex Capsules 3134

Clofibrate (Co-administration of products containing ethinyl estradiol may increase clearance of clofibric acid).

No products indexed under this heading.

Cyclosporine (Co-administration of products containing ethinyl estradiol may inhibit the metabolism of other compounds, such as cyclosporine, resulting in increased plasma concentrations of cyclosporine). Products include:

Gengraf Capsules 459
Neoral Oral Solution 2259
Neoral Soft Gelatin Capsules 2259
Restasis Ophthalmic Emulsion 575
Sandimmune 2275

Demeclocycline Hydrochloride (Pregnancy while taking oral contraceptives has been reported when oral contraceptives were administered with tetracyclines; clinical pharmacokinetic studies have not demonstrated any consistent effect of antibiotics (other than rifampin) on plasma concentrations of synthetic steroids).

No products indexed under this heading.

Diclofenac Potassium (Yasmin has the potential to cause hyperkalemia in high-risk patients; co-administration with other drugs that have the potential to increase serum potassium, such as NSAIDs, may increase this risk further).

No products indexed under this heading.

Diclofenac Sodium (Yasmin has the potential to cause hyperkalemia in high-risk patients; co-administration with other drugs that have the potential to increase serum potassium, such as NSAIDs, may increase this risk further). Products include:

Arthrotec Tablets 3129
Voltaren Ophthalmic Solution 2309
Voltaren Tablets 2307
Voltaren-XR Tablets 2310

Doxycycline Calcium (Pregnancy while taking oral contraceptives has been reported when oral contraceptives were administered with tetracyclines; clinical pharmacokinetic studies have not demonstrated any consistent effect of antibiotics (other than rifampin) on plasma concentrations of synthetic steroids).

No products indexed under this heading.

Doxycycline Hyclate (Pregnancy while taking oral contraceptives has been reported when oral contraceptives were administered with tetracyclines; clinical pharmacokinetic studies have not demonstrated any consistent effect of antibiotics (other than rifampin) on plasma concentrations of synthetic steroids).

No products indexed under this heading.

Doxycycline Monohydrate (Pregnancy while taking oral contraceptives has been reported when oral contraceptives were administered with tetracyclines; clinical pharmacokinetic studies have not demonstrated any consistent effect of antibiotics (other than rifampin) on plasma concentrations of synthetic steroids). Products include:

Oracea Capsules 1000

Dyphylline (Co-administration of products containing ethinyl estradiol may inhibit the metabolism of other compounds, such as theophylline, resulting in increased plasma concentrations of theophylline).

No products indexed under this heading.

Enalapril Maleate (Yasmin has the potential to cause hyperkalemia in high-risk patients; co-administration with other drugs that have the potential to increase serum potassium, such as ACE inhibitors, may increase this risk further). Products include:

Vasotec I.V. Injection 2103

Enalaprilat (Yasmin has the potential to cause hyperkalemia in high-risk patients; co-administration with other drugs that have the potential to increase serum potassium, such as ACE inhibitors, may increase this risk further).

No products indexed under this heading.

Eprosartan Mesylate (Yasmin has the potential to cause hyperkalemia in high-risk patients; co-administration with other drugs that have the potential to increase serum potassium, such as angiotensin-II receptor antagonists, may increase this risk further). Products include:

Teveten Tablets 1735
Teveten HCT Tablets 1737

Etodolac (Yasmin has the potential to cause hyperkalemia in high-risk patients; co-administration with other drugs that have the potential to increase serum potassium, such as NSAIDs, may increase this risk further).

No products indexed under this heading.

Fenoprofen Calcium (Yasmin has the potential to cause hyperkalemia in high-risk patients; co-administration with other drugs that have the potential to increase serum potassium, such as NSAIDs, may increase this risk further). Products include:

Nalfon Capsules 2502

Flurbiprofen (Yasmin has the potential to cause hyperkalemia in high-risk patients; co-administration with other drugs that have the potential to increase serum potassium, such as NSAIDs, may increase this risk further).

No products indexed under this heading.

Fosinopril Sodium (Yasmin has the potential to cause hyperkalemia in high-risk patients; co-administration with other drugs that have the potential to increase serum potassium, such as ACE inhibitors, may increase this risk further).

No products indexed under this heading.

Fosphenytoin Sodium (Co-administration results in increased metabolism of ethinyl estradiol and/or some progestins which could result in a reduction of contraceptive effectiveness).

No products indexed under this heading.

Griseofulvin (Pregnancy while taking oral contraceptives has been reported when oral contraceptives were administered with griseofulvin; clinical pharmacokinetic studies have not demonstrated any consistent effect of antibiotics (other than rifampin) on plasma concentrations of synthetic steroids). Products include:

Gris-PEG Tablets 2502

Heparin Sodium (Yasmin has the potential to cause hyperkalemia in high-risk patients; co-administration with other drugs that have the potential to increase serum potassium, such as heparin, may increase this risk further).

No products indexed under this heading.

Hypericum (Herbal products containing St. John's Wort may induce hepatic enzyme and p-glycoprotein transport and may reduce the effectiveness of oral contraceptives and emergency contraceptive pills; potential for breakthrough bleeding). Products include:

Satiete Tablets 832

Ibuprofen (Yasmin has the potential to cause hyperkalemia in high-risk patients; co-administration with other drugs that have the potential to increase serum potassium, such as NSAIDs, may increase this risk further). Products include:

Advil Allergy Sinus Caplets 770
Advil 674
Children's Advil Oral Suspension 603
Children's Advil Chewable Tablets 603
Advil Cold & Sinus 723
Infants' Advil Concentrated Drops 604
Infants' Advil Concentrated Drops - White Grape (Dye-Free) 604
Junior Strength Advil Swallow Tablets 605
Advil Migraine Liquigels 608
Advil Multi-Symptom Cold Caplets 770
Advil PM Caplets 615
Motrin IB Tablets and Caplets 1866
Children's Motrin Oral Suspension 1867
Children's Motrin Non-Staining Dye-Free Oral Suspension 1867
Children's Motrin Cold Oral Suspension 1867
Infants' Motrin Concentrated Drops 1867
Infants' Motrin Non-Staining Dye-Free Concentrated Drops 1867
Junior Strength Motrin Caplets and Chewable Tablets 1867
Vicoprofen Tablets 539

Indomethacin (Yasmin has the potential to cause hyperkalemia in high-risk patients; co-administration with other drugs that have the potential to increase serum potassium, such as NSAIDs, may increase this risk further). Products include:

Indocin 1995

Indomethacin Sodium Trihydrate (Yasmin has the potential to cause hyperkalemia in high-risk patients; co-administration with other drugs that have the potential to increase serum potassium, such as NSAIDs, may increase this risk further). Products include:

Indocin I.V. 2465

Irbesartan (Yasmin has the potential to cause hyperkalemia in high-risk patients; co-administration with other drugs that have the potential to increase serum potassium, such as angiotensin-II receptor antagonists, may increase this risk further). Products include:

Avalide Tablets 888
Avalide Tablets 2874
Avapro Tablets 891
Avapro Tablets 2871

Ketoprofen (Yasmin has the potential to cause hyperkalemia in high-risk patients; co-administration with other drugs that have the potential to increase serum potassium, such as NSAIDs, may increase this risk further).

No products indexed under this heading.

Ketorolac Tromethamine (Yasmin has the potential to cause hyperkalemia in high-risk patients; co-administration with other drugs that have the potential to increase serum potassium, such as NSAIDs, may increase this risk further). Products include:

Acular Ophthalmic Solution 565
Acular LS Ophthalmic Solution 566

Lisinopril (Yasmin has the potential to cause hyperkalemia in high-risk patients; co-administration with other drugs that have the potential to increase serum potassium, such as ACE inhibitors, may increase this risk further). Products include:

Prinivil Tablets 2052
Prinzide Tablets 2056

Losartan Potassium (Yasmin has the potential to cause hyperkalemia in high-risk patients; co-administration with other drugs that have the potential to increase serum potassium, such as angiotensin-II receptor antagonists, may increase this risk further). Products include:

Cozaar Tablets 1935
Hyzaar 50-12.5 Tablets 1990
Hyzaar 100-12.5 Tablets 1990

Theophylline Ethylenediamine (Co-administration of products containing ethinyl estradiol may inhibit the metabolism of other compounds, such as theophylline, resulting in increased plasma concentrations of theophylline).
No products indexed under this heading.

Theophylline Sodium Glycinate (Co-administration of products containing ethinyl estradiol may inhibit the metabolism of other compounds, such as theophylline, resulting in increased plasma concentrations of theophylline).
No products indexed under this heading.

Tolmetin Sodium (Yasmin has the potential to cause hyperkalemia in high-risk patients; co-administration with other drugs that have the potential to increase serum potassium, such as NSAIDs, may increase this risk further).
No products indexed under this heading.

Trandolapril (Yasmin has the potential to cause hyperkalemia in high-risk patients; co-administration with other drugs that have the potential to increase serum potassium, such as ACE inhibitors, may increase this risk further). Products include:
Mavik Tablets 486
Tarka Tablets 524

Triamterene (Yasmin has the potential to cause hyperkalemia in high-risk patients; co-administration with other drugs that have the potential to increase serum potassium, such as potassium-sparing diuretics, may increase this risk further).
Products include:
Dyazide Capsules 1423
Dyrenium Capsules 3400

Valdecoxib (Yasmin has the potential to cause hyperkalemia in high-risk patients; co-administration with other drugs that have the potential to increase serum potassium, such as NSAIDs, may increase this risk further).
No products indexed under this heading.

Valsartan (Yasmin has the potential to cause hyperkalemia in high-risk patients; co-administration with other drugs that have the potential to increase serum potassium, such as angiotensin-II receptor antagonists, may increase this risk further).
Products include:
Diovan Tablets 2193
Diovan HCT Tablets 2196

Vitamin C (May increase plasma levels of ethinyl estradiol possibly by inhibition of conjugation). Products include:
Bausch & Lomb Ocuvite Adult Eye Vitamin and Mineral Supplement Soft Gels 706
Bausch & Lomb Ocuvite Adult 50+ Eye Vitamin and Mineral Supplement Soft Gels 706
Ocuvite Adult Vitamin and Mineral Supplement 253
Ocuvite Adult 50+ Vitamin and Mineral Supplement 253
Peridin-C Vitamin C Supplement 818

YAZ TABLETS

(Drospirenone, Ethinyl Estradiol) 803
May interact with ACE inhibitors, aldosterone-inhibiting diuretic agents, angiotensin-II receptor antagonists, anticonvulsants, non-steroidal anti-inflammatory agents, potassium preparations, prednisolone, potassium sparing diuretics, tetracyclines, theophyllines, and certain other agents. Compounds in these categories include:

Acetaminophen (Ascorbic acid and acetaminophen may increase plasma concentrations of some synthetic estrogens, possibly by inhibition of conjugation. Decreased plasma concentrations of acetaminophen have been noted when administered with oral contraceptives). Products include:
Comtrex Maximum Strength Cold & Cough Day/Night Caplets - Day Formulation 726
Comtrex Maximum Strength Cold & Cough Day/Night Caplets - Night Formulation 726
Comtrex Maximum Strength Non-Drowsy Cold & Cough Caplets 725
Comtrex Maximum Strength Day/Night Severe Cold & Sinus Caplets - Day Formulation 725
Comtrex Maximum Strength Day/Night Severe Cold & Sinus Caplets - Night Formulation 725
Contac Cold and Flu Maximum Strength Caplets 728
Contac Cold and Flu Day and Night Caplets (Day Formulation Only) 727
Contac Cold and Flu Day and Night Caplets (Night Formulation Only) 727
Contac Cold and Flu Non-Drowsy Caplets 728
Excedrin Extra Strength Caplets/Tablets/Geltabs 684
Excedrin Migraine Caplets/Tablets/Geltabs 609
Excedrin PM Caplets/Tablets/Geltabs 610
Excedrin Sinus Headache Caplets/Tablets 610
Excedrin Tension Headache Caplets/Tablets/Geltabs 611
Goody's Body Pain Formula Powder 684
Goody's Extra Strength Headache Powders 611
Goody's Extra Strength Pain Relief Tablets 685
Goody's PM Powder for Pain with Sleeplessness 612
Percocet Tablets 1131
Robitussin Cough, Cold & Flu Nighttime Liquid 738
TheraFlu Cold & Sore Throat Hot Liquid 741
TheraFlu Flu & Chest Congestion Hot Liquid 741
TheraFlu Flu & Sore Throat Hot Liquid 742
TheraFlu Daytime Severe Cold Hot Liquid 742
TheraFlu Nighttime Severe Cold Hot Liquid 740
TheraFlu Warming Relief Daytime Severe Cold 743
TheraFlu Warming Relief Nighttime Severe Cold 743
Triaminic Cough & Sore Throat Liquid 747
Regular Strength Tylenol Tablets 1870
Children's Tylenol with Flavor Creator 679
Children's Tylenol Plus Flu Oral Suspension 749
Tylenol Cold Head Congestion Daytime Caplets with Cool Burst and Gelcaps 750
Tylenol Cold Multi-Symptom Daytime Liquid 752
Tylenol Cold Multi-Symptom Severe Daytime Liquid 752
Tylenol 8 Hour Extended Release Caplets 1870
Tylenol 1870
Extra Strength Tylenol PM Caplets, Vanilla Caplets, Geltabs, Gelcaps and Liquid 1875
Extra Strength Tylenol Rapid Release Gels 1870
Concentrated Tylenol Infants' Drops Plus Cold & Cough 754
Tylenol with Codeine Tablets 2391
Tylenol Allergy Multi-Symptom Caplets with Cool Burst and Gelcaps 1872
Tylenol Allergy Multi-Symptom Nighttime Caplets with Cool Burst 1872
Tylenol Severe Allergy Caplets 1872
Tylenol Arthritis Pain Extended Release Caplets and Geltabs 1870
Tylenol Chest Congestion Caplets with Cool Burst 1872
Tylenol Chest Congestion Liquid with Cool Burst 1872
Children's Tylenol Suspension Liquid and Meltaways 1878
Children's Tylenol Plus Cold Suspension Liquid 1879
Children's Tylenol Plus Cold & Allergy Suspension Liquid 1878
Children's Tylenol Plus Cough & Runny Nose Suspension Liquid 1879
Children's Tylenol Plus Cough & Sore Throat Suspension Liquid 1879
Children's Tylenol Suspension with Flavor Creator 1878
Children's Tylenol Plus Flu Suspension Liquid 1881
Children's Tylenol Plus Multi-Symptom Cold Suspension Liquid 1879
Tylenol Cold Severe Congestion Non-Drowsy Caplets with Cool Burst 1874
Tylenol Cold Head Congestion Daytime Caplets with Cool Burst 1873
Tylenol Cold Head Congestion Nighttime Caplets with Cool Burst 1873
Tylenol Cold Head Congestion Severe Caplets with Cool Burst 1873
Tylenol Cold Multi-Symptom Daytime Caplets with Cool Burst and Gelcaps 1874
Tylenol Cold Multi-Symptom Daytime Liquid with Citrus Burst 1874
Tylenol Cold Multi-Symptom Nighttime Caplets with Cool Burst 1874
Tylenol Cold Multi-Symptom Nighttime Liquid with Cool Burst 1874
Tylenol Cold Multi-Symptom Severe Caplets with Cool Burst 1874
Tylenol Cold Multi-Symptom Severe Daytime Liquid with Citrus Burst 1874
Tylenol Cough & Sore Throat Daytime Liquid with Cool Burst 1877
Tylenol Cough & Sore Throat Nighttime Liquid with Cool Burst 1877
Concentrated Tylenol Infants' Drops 1878
Concentrated Tylenol Infants' Drops Plus Cold 1879
Concentrated Tylenol Infants' Drops Plus Cold and Cough 1879
Jr. Tylenol Meltaways 1878
Tylenol Sinus Severe Congestion Caplets with Cool Burst 1876
Tylenol Sinus Congestion & Pain Daytime Caplets with Cool Burst and Gelcaps 1876
Tylenol Sinus Congestion & Pain Nighttime Caplets with Cool Burst 1876
Tylenol Sinus Congestion & Pain Severe Caplets with Cool Burst 1876
Tylenol Sore Throat Daytime Liquid with Cool Burst 1877
Tylenol Sore Throat Nighttime Liquid with Cool Burst 1877
Women's Tylenol Menstrual Relief Caplets 1877
Vicks 44M Cough, Cold & Flu Relief Liquid 2680
Vicks DayQuil LiquiCaps/Liquid Multi-Symptom Cold/Flu Relief 761
Vicks DayQuil Multi-Symptom Cold/Flu Relief LiquiCaps 2678
Vicks DayQuil Multi-Symptom Cold/Flu Relief Liquid 2678
Vicks NyQuil Multi-Symptom Cold/Flu Relief Liquid 2681
Vicks NyQuil Multi-Symptom Cold/Flu Relief LiquiCaps 2681
Vicks NyQuil LiquiCaps/Liquid Multi-Symptom Cold/Flu Relief 763
Vicodin Tablets 535
Vicodin ES Tablets 536
Vicodin HP Tablets 538
Zicam Maximum Strength Flu Daytime 768
Zicam Maximum Strength Flu Nighttime 768
Zydone Tablets 1139

Amiloride Hydrochloride (YAZ has the potential to cause hyperkalemia in high-risk patients; co-administration with other drugs that have the potential to increase serum potassium, such as potassium-sparing diuretics, may increase the risk further). Products include:
Midamor Tablets 2026
Moduretic Tablets 2028

Ampicillin (Pregnancy while taking combined hormonal contraceptives has been reported when the combined hormonal contraceptives were administered with antimicrobials such as ampicillin).
No products indexed under this heading.

Ampicillin Sodium (Pregnancy while taking combined hormonal contraceptives has been reported when the combined hormonal contraceptives were administered with antimicrobials such as ampicillin).
No products indexed under this heading.

Ampicillin Trihydrate (Pregnancy while taking combined hormonal contraceptives has been reported when the combined hormonal contraceptives were administered with antimicrobials such as ampicillin).
No products indexed under this heading.

Ascorbic Acid (Ascorbic acid and acetaminophen may increase plasma concentrations of some synthetic estrogens, possibly by inhibition of conjugation). Products include:
MoviPrep Oral Solution 2839

Atorvastatin Calcium (Co-administration of atorvastatin and an oral contraceptive increased AUC values for norethindrone and ethinyl estradiol by approximately 30% and 20%, respectively). Products include:
Caduet Tablets 2508
Lipitor Tablets 2483

Benazepril Hydrochloride (YAZ has the potential to cause hyperkalemia in high-risk patients; co-administration with other drugs that have the potential to increase serum potassium, such as ACE inhibitors, may increase the risk further).
Products include:
Lotensin Tablets 2243
Lotensin HCT Tablets 2246
Lotrel Capsules 2249

Candesartan Cilexetil (YAZ has the potential to cause hyperkalemia in high-risk patients; co-administration with other drugs that have the potential to increase serum potassium, such as angiotensin-II receptor antagonists, may increase the risk further). Products include:
Atacand Tablets 649
Atacand HCT 651

Captopril (YAZ has the potential to cause hyperkalemia in high-risk patients; co-administration with other drugs that have the potential to increase serum potassium, such as ACE inhibitors, may increase the risk further). Products include:
Captopril Tablets 2149

Carbamazepine (Co-administration results in increased metabolism of ethinyl estradiol and/or some progestins which could result in a reduction of contraceptive effectiveness). Products include:
Carbatrol Capsules 3171
Equetro Extended-Release Capsules 3180
Tegretol/Tegretol-XR 2295

IMPORTANT NOTE: Always consult each drug listing in the patient's regimen for possible interactions.

Celecoxib (YAZ has the potential to cause hyperkalemia in high-risk patients; co-administration with other drugs that have the potential to increase serum potassium, such as NSAIDs, may increase the risk further). Products include:
Celebrex Capsules 3134

Clofibrate (Co-administration of products containing ethinyl estradiol may increase clearance of clofibric acid).
No products indexed under this heading.

Clofibric Acid (Increased clearance of clofibric acid has been noted when administered with oral contraceptives).
No products indexed under this heading.

Cyclosporine (Increased plasma concentrations of cyclosporine have been reported with concomitant administration of oral contraceptives). Products include:
Gengraf Capsules 459
Neoral Oral Solution 2259
Neoral Soft Gelatin Capsules 2259
Restasis Ophthalmic Emulsion 575
Sandimmune 2275

Demeclocycline Hydrochloride (Pregnancy while taking combined hormonal contraceptives has been reported when the combined hormonal contraceptives were administered with antimicrobials such as tetracycline).
No products indexed under this heading.

Diclofenac Potassium (YAZ has the potential to cause hyperkalemia in high-risk patients; co-administration with other drugs that have the potential to increase serum potassium, such as NSAIDs, may increase the risk further).
No products indexed under this heading.

Diclofenac Sodium (YAZ has the potential to cause hyperkalemia in high-risk patients; co-administration with other drugs that have the potential to increase serum potassium, such as NSAIDs, may increase the risk further). Products include:
Arthrotec Tablets 3129
Voltaren Ophthalmic Solution 2309
Voltaren Tablets 2307
Voltaren-XR Tablets 2310

Divalproex Sodium (Anticonvulsants have been shown to increase the metabolism of ethinyl estradiol and/or some progestins, which could result in a reduction of contraceptive effectiveness). Products include:
Depakote Sprinkle Capsules 422
Depakote Tablets 427
Depakote ER Tablets 434

Doxycycline Calcium (Pregnancy while taking combined hormonal contraceptives has been reported when the combined hormonal contraceptives were administered with antimicrobials such as tetracycline).
No products indexed under this heading.

Doxycycline Hyclate (Pregnancy while taking combined hormonal contraceptives has been reported when the combined hormonal contraceptives were administered with antimicrobials such as tetracycline).
No products indexed under this heading.

Doxycycline Monohydrate (Pregnancy while taking combined hormonal contraceptives has been reported when the combined hormonal contraceptives were administered with antimicrobials such as tetracycline). Products include:
Oracea Capsules 1000

Enalapril Maleate (YAZ has the potential to cause hyperkalemia in high-risk patients; co-administration with other drugs that have the potential to increase serum potassium, such as ACE inhibitors, may increase the risk further). Products include:
Vasotec I.V. Injection 2103

Enalaprilat (YAZ has the potential to cause hyperkalemia in high-risk patients; co-administration with other drugs that have the potential to increase serum potassium, such as ACE inhibitors, may increase the risk further).
No products indexed under this heading.

Eprosartan Mesylate (YAZ has the potential to cause hyperkalemia in high-risk patients; co-administration with other drugs that have the potential to increase serum potassium, such as angiotensin-II receptor antagonists, may increase the risk further). Products include:
Teveten Tablets 1735
Teveten HCT Tablets 1737

Ethosuximide (Anticonvulsants have been shown to increase the metabolism of ethinyl estradiol and/or some progestins, which could result in a reduction of contraceptive effectiveness).
No products indexed under this heading.

Ethotoin (Anticonvulsants have been shown to increase the metabolism of ethinyl estradiol and/or some progestins, which could result in a reduction of contraceptive effectiveness).
No products indexed under this heading.

Etodolac (YAZ has the potential to cause hyperkalemia in high-risk patients; co-administration with other drugs that have the potential to increase serum potassium, such as NSAIDs, may increase the risk further).
No products indexed under this heading.

Felbamate (Anticonvulsants have been shown to increase the metabolism of ethinyl estradiol and/or some progestins, which could result in a reduction of contraceptive effectiveness).
No products indexed under this heading.

Fenoprofen Calcium (YAZ has the potential to cause hyperkalemia in high-risk patients; co-administration with other drugs that have the potential to increase serum potassium, such as NSAIDs, may increase the risk further). Products include:
Nalfon Capsules 2502

Flurbiprofen (YAZ has the potential to cause hyperkalemia in high-risk patients; co-administration with other drugs that have the potential to increase serum potassium, such as NSAIDs, may increase the risk further).
No products indexed under this heading.

Fosinopril Sodium (YAZ has the potential to cause hyperkalemia in high-risk patients; co-administration with other drugs that have the potential to increase serum potassium, such as ACE inhibitors, may increase the risk further).
No products indexed under this heading.

Fosphenytoin (Anticonvulsants have been shown to increase the metabolism of ethinyl estradiol and/or some progestins, which could result in a reduction of contraceptive effectiveness).
No products indexed under this heading.

Gabapentin (Anticonvulsants have been shown to increase the metabolism of ethinyl estradiol and/or some progestins, which could result in a reduction of contraceptive effectiveness). Products include:
Neurontin Capsules 2487
Neurontin Oral Solution 2487
Neurontin Tablets 2487

Griseofulvin (Pregnancy while taking combined hormonal contraceptives has been reported when the combined hormonal contraceptives were administered with antimicrobials such as griseofulvin). Products include:
Gris-PEG Tablets 2502

Heparin Calcium (YAZ has the potential to cause hyperkalemia in high-risk patients; co-administration with other drugs that have the potential to increase serum potassium, such as heparin, may increase the risk further).
No products indexed under this heading.

Heparin Sodium (YAZ has the potential to cause hyperkalemia in high-risk patients; co-administration with other drugs that have the potential to increase serum potassium, such as heparin, may increase the risk further).
No products indexed under this heading.

Hypericum (Herbal products containing St. John's Wort may induce hepatic enzyme and p-glycoprotein transporter and may reduce the effectiveness of oral contraceptives and emergency contraceptive pills. This may also result in breakthrough bleeding). Products include:
Satiete Tablets .... ■ 832

Hypericum Perforatum (Herbal products containing St. John's Wort may induce hepatic enzyme and p-glycoprotein transporter and may reduce the effectiveness of oral contraceptives and emergency contraceptive pills. This may also result in breakthrough bleeding).
No products indexed under this heading.

Ibuprofen (YAZ has the potential to cause hyperkalemia in high-risk patients; co-administration with other drugs that have the potential to increase serum potassium, such as NSAIDs, may increase the risk further). Products include:
Advil Allergy Sinus Caplets .... ■ 770
Advil .... ■ 674
Children's Advil Oral Suspension .... ■ 603
Children's Advil Chewable Tablets .... ■ 603
Advil Cold & Sinus .... ■ 723
Infants' Advil Concentrated Drops .... ■ 604
Infants' Advil Concentrated Drops - White Grape (Dye-Free) .... ■ 604
Junior Strength Advil Swallow Tablets .... ■ 605
Advil Migraine Liquigels .... ■ 608
Advil Multi-Symptom Cold Caplets .... ■ 770
Advil PM Caplets .... ■ 615
Motrin IB Tablets and Caplets 1866
Children's Motrin Oral Suspension 1867
Children's Motrin Non-Staining Dye-Free Oral Suspension 1867
Children's Motrin Cold Oral Suspension 1867
Infants' Motrin Concentrated Drops 1867
Infants' Motrin Non-Staining Dye-Free Concentrated Drops 1867
Junior Strength Motrin Caplets and Chewable Tablets 1867
Vicoprofen Tablets 539

Indomethacin (YAZ has the potential to cause hyperkalemia in high-risk patients; co-administration with other drugs that have the potential to increase serum potassium, such as NSAIDs, may increase the risk further). Products include:
Indocin 1995

Indomethacin Sodium Trihydrate (YAZ has the potential to cause hyperkalemia in high-risk patients; co-administration with other drugs that have the potential to increase serum potassium, such as NSAIDs, may increase the risk further). Products include:
Indocin I.V. 2465

Irbesartan (YAZ has the potential to cause hyperkalemia in high-risk patients; co-administration with other drugs that have the potential to increase serum potassium, such as angiotensin-II receptor antagonists, may increase the risk further). Products include:
Avalide Tablets 888
Avalide Tablets 2874
Avapro Tablets 891
Avapro Tablets 2871

Ketoprofen (YAZ has the potential to cause hyperkalemia in high-risk patients; co-administration with other drugs that have the potential to increase serum potassium, such as NSAIDs, may increase the risk further).
No products indexed under this heading.

Ketorolac Tromethamine (YAZ has the potential to cause hyperkalemia in high-risk patients; co-administration with other drugs that have the potential to increase serum potassium, such as NSAIDs, may increase the risk further). Products include:
Acular Ophthalmic Solution 565
Acular LS Ophthalmic Solution 566

Lamotrigine (Anticonvulsants have been shown to increase the metabolism of ethinyl estradiol and/or some progestins, which could result in a reduction of contraceptive effectiveness). Products include:
Lamictal 1481

Levetiracetam (Anticonvulsants have been shown to increase the metabolism of ethinyl estradiol and/or some progestins, which could result in a reduction of contraceptive effectiveness). Products include:
Keppra Injection 3320
Keppra Oral Solution 3314
Keppra Tablets 3314

Lisinopril (YAZ has the potential to cause hyperkalemia in high-risk patients; co-administration with other drugs that have the potential to increase serum potassium, such as ACE inhibitors, may increase the risk further). Products include:
Prinivil Tablets 2052

Prinzide Tablets 2056

Losartan Potassium (YAZ has the potential to cause hyperkalemia in high-risk patients; co-administration with other drugs that have the potential to increase serum potassium, such as angiotensin-II receptor antagonists, may increase the risk further). Products include:

Cozaar Tablets 1935
Hyzaar 50-12.5 Tablets 1990
Hyzaar 100-12.5 Tablets 1990
Hyzaar 100-25 Tablets 1990

Low Molecular Weight Heparins (YAZ has the potential to cause hyperkalemia in high-risk patients; co-administration with other drugs that have the potential to increase serum potassium, such as heparin, may increase the risk further).

No products indexed under this heading.

Meclofenamate Sodium (YAZ has the potential to cause hyperkalemia in high-risk patients; co-administration with other drugs that have the potential to increase serum potassium, such as NSAIDs, may increase the risk further).

No products indexed under this heading.

Mefenamic Acid (YAZ has the potential to cause hyperkalemia in high-risk patients; co-administration with other drugs that have the potential to increase serum potassium, such as NSAIDs, may increase the risk further).

No products indexed under this heading.

Meloxicam (YAZ has the potential to cause hyperkalemia in high-risk patients; co-administration with other drugs that have the potential to increase serum potassium, such as NSAIDs, may increase the risk further). Products include:

Mobic Oral Suspension 863
Mobic Tablets 863

Mephenytoin (Anticonvulsants have been shown to increase the metabolism of ethinyl estradiol and/or some progestins, which could result in a reduction of contraceptive effectiveness).

No products indexed under this heading.

Methacycline Hydrochloride (Pregnancy while taking combined hormonal contraceptives has been reported when the combined hormonal contraceptives were administered with antimicrobials such as tetracycline).

No products indexed under this heading.

Methsuximide (Anticonvulsants have been shown to increase the metabolism of ethinyl estradiol and/or some progestins, which could result in a reduction of contraceptive effectiveness).

No products indexed under this heading.

Minocycline Hydrochloride (Pregnancy while taking combined hormonal contraceptives has been reported when the combined hormonal contraceptives were administered with antimicrobials such as tetracycline). Products include:

Solodyn Extended Release Tablets 1890

Moexipril Hydrochloride (YAZ has the potential to cause hyperkalemia in high-risk patients; co-administration with other drugs that have the potential to increase serum potassium, such as ACE inhibitors, may increase the risk further). Products include:

Uniretic Tablets 3100
Univasc Tablets 3104

Morphine Sulfate (Increased clearance of morphine has been noted when administered with oral contraceptives). Products include:

Avinza Capsules 1741
Kadian Capsules 577
MS Contin Tablets 2701

Morphine sulfate, liposomal (Increased clearance of morphine has been noted when administered with oral contraceptives). Products include:

DepoDur Extended-Release Injection 1110

Nabumetone (YAZ has the potential to cause hyperkalemia in high-risk patients; co-administration with other drugs that have the potential to increase serum potassium, such as NSAIDs, may increase the risk further).

No products indexed under this heading.

Naproxen (YAZ has the potential to cause hyperkalemia in high-risk patients; co-administration with other drugs that have the potential to increase serum potassium, such as NSAIDs, may increase the risk further). Products include:

EC-Naprosyn Delayed-Release Tablets 2761
Naprosyn Suspension 2761
Naprosyn Tablets 2761
Prevacid NapraPAC 3280

Naproxen Sodium (YAZ has the potential to cause hyperkalemia in high-risk patients; co-administration with other drugs that have the potential to increase serum potassium, such as NSAIDs, may increase the risk further). Products include:

Aleve Caplets 742
Aleve Gelcaps 743
Aleve Tablets 743
Aleve Cold & Sinus Caplets 744
Anaprox Tablets 2761
Anaprox DS Tablets 2761

Oxaprozin (YAZ has the potential to cause hyperkalemia in high-risk patients; co-administration with other drugs that have the potential to increase serum potassium, such as NSAIDs, may increase the risk further).

No products indexed under this heading.

Oxcarbazepine (Anticonvulsants have been shown to increase the metabolism of ethinyl estradiol and/or some progestins, which could result in a reduction of contraceptive effectiveness). Products include:

Trileptal Tablets 2300
Trileptal Oral Suspension 2300

Oxytetracycline Hydrochloride (Pregnancy while taking combined hormonal contraceptives has been reported when the combined hormonal contraceptives were administered with antimicrobials such as tetracycline).

No products indexed under this heading.

Paramethadione (Anticonvulsants have been shown to increase the metabolism of ethinyl estradiol and/or some progestins, which could result in a reduction of contraceptive effectiveness).

No products indexed under this heading.

Perindopril Erbumine (YAZ has the potential to cause hyperkalemia in high-risk patients; co-administration with other drugs that have the potential to increase serum potassium, such as ACE inhibitors, may increase the risk further). Products include:

Aceon Tablets (2 mg, 4 mg, 8 mg) 3194

Phenacemide (Anticonvulsants have been shown to increase the metabolism of ethinyl estradiol and/or some progestins, which could result in a reduction of contraceptive effectiveness).

No products indexed under this heading.

Phenobarbital (Co-administration results in increased metabolism of ethinyl estradiol and/or some progestins which could result in a reduction of contraceptive effectiveness). Products include:

Donnatal Extentabs 2493

Phensuximide (Anticonvulsants have been shown to increase the metabolism of ethinyl estradiol and/or some progestins, which could result in a reduction of contraceptive effectiveness).

No products indexed under this heading.

Phenylbutazone (A reduction in contraceptive effectiveness and an increased incidence of menstrual irregularities has been suggested with phenylbutazone).

No products indexed under this heading.

Piroxicam (YAZ has the potential to cause hyperkalemia in high-risk patients; co-administration with other drugs that have the potential to increase serum potassium, such as NSAIDs, may increase the risk further).

No products indexed under this heading.

Potassium Acid Phosphate (YAZ has the potential to cause hyperkalemia in high-risk patients; co-administration with other drugs that have the potential to increase serum potassium, such as potassium supplementation, may increase the risk further). Products include:

K-Phos Original (Sodium Free) Tablets 760

Potassium Bicarbonate (YAZ has the potential to cause hyperkalemia in high-risk patients; co-administration with other drugs that have the potential to increase serum potassium, such as potassium supplementation, may increase the risk further).

No products indexed under this heading.

Potassium Chloride (YAZ has the potential to cause hyperkalemia in high-risk patients; co-administration with other drugs that have the potential to increase serum potassium, such as potassium supplementation, may increase the risk further). Products include:

Colyte with Flavor Packs for Oral Solution 3088
HalfLytely and Bisacodyl Tablets Bowel Prep Kit with Flavors Packs 881
K-Dur Extended-Relase Tablets 3033
K-Lor Oral Solution 474
K-Tab Tablets 475
MoviPrep Oral Solution 2839
TriLyte with Flavor Packs for Oral Solution 3100

Potassium Citrate (YAZ has the potential to cause hyperkalemia in high-risk patients; co-administration with other drugs that have the potential to increase serum potassium, such as potassium supplementation, may increase the risk further). Products include:

Urocit-K Tablets 2144

Potassium Gluconate (YAZ has the potential to cause hyperkalemia in high-risk patients; co-administration with other drugs that have the potential to increase serum potassium, such as potassium supplementation, may increase the risk further).

No products indexed under this heading.

Potassium Phosphate (YAZ has the potential to cause hyperkalemia in high-risk patients; co-administration with other drugs that have the potential to increase serum potassium, such as potassium supplementation, may increase the risk further). Products include:

K-Phos Neutral Tablets 760

Prednisolone (Increased plasma concentrations of prednisolone have been reported with concomitant administration of oral contraceptives).

No products indexed under this heading.

Prednisolone Acetate (Increased plasma concentrations of prednisolone have been reported with concomitant administration of oral contraceptives). Products include:

Blephamide Ophthalmic Ointment 568
Blephamide Ophthalmic Suspension 569
Poly-Pred Ophthalmic Suspension .... ⊙233
Pred Forte Ophthalmic Suspension .... ⊙235
Pred Mild Ophthalmic Suspension .... ⊙238
Pred-G Ophthalmic Ointment .... ⊙237
Pred-G Ophthalmic Suspension ...... ⊙236

Prednisolone Sodium Phosphate (Increased plasma concentrations of prednisolone have been reported with concomitant administration of oral contraceptives).

No products indexed under this heading.

Prednisolone Tebutate (Increased plasma concentrations of prednisolone have been reported with concomitant administration of oral contraceptives).

No products indexed under this heading.

Primidone (Anticonvulsants have been shown to increase the metabolism of ethinyl estradiol and/or some progestins, which could result in a reduction of contraceptive effectiveness).

No products indexed under this heading.

Quinapril Hydrochloride (YAZ has the potential to cause hyperkalemia in high-risk patients; co-administration with other drugs that have the potential to increase serum potassium, such as ACE inhibitors, may increase the risk further).

No products indexed under this heading.

Ramipril (YAZ has the potential to cause hyperkalemia in high-risk patients; co-administration with other drugs that have the potential to

increase serum potassium, such as ACE inhibitors, may increase the risk further). Products include:
Altace Capsules 1702

Rifampin (Co-administration results in increased metabolism of ethinyl estradiol precipitating a reduction in contraceptive effectiveness and an increase in menstrual irregularities).
No products indexed under this heading.

Rofecoxib (YAZ has the potential to cause hyperkalemia in high-risk patients; co-administration with other drugs that have the potential to increase serum potassium, such as NSAIDs, may increase the risk further).
No products indexed under this heading.

Salicylic Acid (Increased clearance of salicylic acid has been noted when administered with oral contraceptives).
No products indexed under this heading.

Spirapril Hydrochloride (YAZ has the potential to cause hyperkalemia in high-risk patients; co-administration with other drugs that have the potential to increase serum potassium, such as ACE inhibitors, may increase the risk further).
No products indexed under this heading.

Spironolactone (YAZ has the potential to cause hyperkalemia in high-risk patients; co-administration with other drugs that have the potential to increase serum potassium, such as aldosterone antagonists, may increase the risk further).
No products indexed under this heading.

Sulindac (YAZ has the potential to cause hyperkalemia in high-risk patients; co-administration with other drugs that have the potential to increase serum potassium, such as NSAIDs, may increase the risk further). Products include:
Clinoril Tablets 1924

Telmisartan (YAZ has the potential to cause hyperkalemia in high-risk patients; co-administration with other drugs that have the potential to increase serum potassium, such as angiotensin-II receptor antagonists, may increase the risk further).
Products include:
Micardis Tablets 854
Micardis HCT Tablets 856

Temazepam (Increased clearance of temazepam has been noted when administered with oral contraceptives). Products include:
Restoril Capsules 1860

Tetracycline Hydrochloride (Pregnancy while taking combined hormonal contraceptives has been reported when the combined hormonal contraceptives were administered with antimicrobials such as tetracycline).
No products indexed under this heading.

Theophylline (Increased plasma concentrations of theophylline have been reported with concomitant administration of oral contraceptives).
No products indexed under this heading.

Theophylline Anhydrous (Increased plasma concentrations of theophylline have been reported with concomitant administration of oral contraceptives). Products include:
Uniphyl Tablets 2710

Theophylline Calcium Salicylate (Increased plasma concentrations of theophylline have been reported with concomitant administration of oral contraceptives).
No products indexed under this heading.

Theophylline Dihydroxypropyl (Glyceryl) (Increased plasma concentrations of theophylline have been reported with concomitant administration of oral contraceptives).
No products indexed under this heading.

Theophylline Ethylenediamine (Increased plasma concentrations of theophylline have been reported with concomitant administration of oral contraceptives).
No products indexed under this heading.

Theophylline Sodium Glycinate (Increased plasma concentrations of theophylline have been reported with concomitant administration of oral contraceptives).
No products indexed under this heading.

Tiagabine Hydrochloride (Anticonvulsants have been shown to increase the metabolism of ethinyl estradiol and/or some progestins, which could result in a reduction of contraceptive effectiveness).
Products include:
Gabitril Tablets 984

Tolmetin Sodium (YAZ has the potential to cause hyperkalemia in high-risk patients; co-administration with other drugs that have the potential to increase serum potassium, such as NSAIDs, may increase the risk further).
No products indexed under this heading.

Topiramate (Anticonvulsants have been shown to increase the metabolism of ethinyl estradiol and/or some progestins, which could result in a reduction of contraceptive effectiveness). Products include:
Topamax Sprinkle Capsules 2404
Topamax Tablets 2404

Trandolapril (YAZ has the potential to cause hyperkalemia in high-risk patients; co-administration with other drugs that have the potential to increase serum potassium, such as ACE inhibitors, may increase the risk further). Products include:
Mavik Tablets 486
Tarka Tablets 524

Triamterene (YAZ has the potential to cause hyperkalemia in high-risk patients; co-administration with other drugs that have the potential to increase serum potassium, such as potassium-sparing diuretics, may increase the risk further). Products include:
Dyazide Capsules 1423
Dyrenium Capsules 3400

Trimethadione (Anticonvulsants have been shown to increase the metabolism of ethinyl estradiol and/or some progestins, which could result in a reduction of contraceptive effectiveness).
No products indexed under this heading.

Valdecoxib (YAZ has the potential to cause hyperkalemia in high-risk patients; co-administration with other drugs that have the potential to increase serum potassium, such as NSAIDs, may increase the risk further).
No products indexed under this heading.

Valproate Sodium (Anticonvulsants have been shown to increase the metabolism of ethinyl estradiol and/or some progestins, which could result in a reduction of contraceptive effectiveness). Products include:
Depacon Injection 412

Valproic Acid (Anticonvulsants have been shown to increase the metabolism of ethinyl estradiol and/or some progestins, which could result in a reduction of contraceptive effectiveness). Products include:
Depakene 417

Valsartan (YAZ has the potential to cause hyperkalemia in high-risk patients; co-administration with other drugs that have the potential to increase serum potassium, such as angiotensin-II receptor antagonists, may increase the risk further).
Products include:
Diovan Tablets 2193
Diovan HCT Tablets 2196

Vitamin C (May increase plasma levels of ethinyl estradiol possibly by inhibition of conjugation). Products include:
Bausch & Lomb Ocuvite Adult Eye Vitamin and Mineral Supplement Soft Gels .... ▣706
Bausch & Lomb Ocuvite Adult 50+ Eye Vitamin and Mineral Supplement Soft Gels .... ▣706
Ocuvite Adult Vitamin and Mineral Supplement .... ⊙253
Ocuvite Adult 50+ Vitamin and Mineral Supplement .... ⊙253
Peridin-C Vitamin C Supplement ..... ▣818

Zonisamide (Anticonvulsants have been shown to increase the metabolism of ethinyl estradiol and/or some progestins, which could result in a reduction of contraceptive effectiveness). Products include:
Zonegran Capsules 1101

ZANTAC 25 EFFERDOSE TABLETS
(Ranitidine Hydrochloride) 1624
See Zantac 150 Tablets

ZANTAC 150 EFFERDOSE TABLETS
(Ranitidine Hydrochloride) 1624
See Zantac 150 Tablets

ZANTAC INJECTION
(Ranitidine Hydrochloride) 1619
See Zantac 150 Tablets

ZANTAC INJECTION PHARMACY BULK PACKAGE
(Ranitidine Hydrochloride) 1622
May interact with:

Triazolam (Ranitidine, similar to other agents that lower gastric acidity, has been shown to increase the absorption of triazolam resulting in increased plasma concentrations on average 14% to 28%; the clinical significance of this finding is unknown).
No products indexed under this heading.

Warfarin Sodium (Potential for increased or decreased prothrombin time; doses of ranitidine up to 400 mg per day had no effect on prothrombin time or warfarin clearance). Products include:
Coumadin for Injection 898
Coumadin Tablets 898

ZANTAC INJECTION PREMIXED
(Ranitidine Hydrochloride) 1619
See Zantac 150 Tablets

ZANTAC SYRUP
(Ranitidine Hydrochloride) 1624
See Zantac 150 Tablets

ZANTAC 150 TABLETS
(Ranitidine Hydrochloride) 1624
May interact with:

Triazolam (Ranitidine, similar to other agents that lower gastric acidity, has been shown to increase the absorption of triazolam resulting in increased plasma concentrations on average 14% to 28%; the clinical significance of this finding is unknown).
No products indexed under this heading.

Warfarin Sodium (Potential for increased or decreased prothrombin time; doses of ranitidine up to 400 mg per day had no effect on prothrombin time or warfarin clearance). Products include:
Coumadin for Injection 898
Coumadin Tablets 898

ZANTAC 300 TABLETS
(Ranitidine Hydrochloride) 1624
See Zantac 150 Tablets

ZAVITA LIQUID HERBAL SUPPLEMENT
(Herbals, Multiple) .... ▣823
None cited in PDR database.

ZEEL SOLUTION
(Arnica montana, Herbals, Multiple, Sulfur) 1665
None cited in PDR database.

ZEGERID CAPSULES
(Omeprazole) 2958
See Zegerid Powder for Oral Solution

ZEGERID POWDER FOR ORAL SOLUTION
(Omeprazole) 2958
May interact with benzodiazepines, iron containing oral preparations, phenytoin, and certain other agents. Compounds in these categories include:

Alprazolam (Potential for metabolism interaction via cytochrome P450 system). Products include:
Niravam Orally Disintegrating Tablets 3092

Atazanavir (Co-administration of omeprazole and atazanavir has been reported to reduce the plasma levels of atazanavir).
No products indexed under this heading.

Atazanavir sulfate (Co-administration of omeprazole and atazanavir has been reported to reduce the plasma levels of atazanavir). Products include:
Reyataz Capsules 921

Bacampicillin Hydrochloride (Omeprazole may interfere with gastric absorption of drugs, such as ampicillin esters, where gastric pH is an important determinant of their bioavailability).
No products indexed under this heading.

Chlordiazepoxide (Potential for metabolism interaction via cytochrome P450 system).
No products indexed under this heading.

Chlordiazepoxide Hydrochloride (Potential for metabolism interaction via cytochrome P450 system). Products include:
Librium Capsules 3347

Clarithromycin (Co-administration may result in increases in plasma levels of omeprazole, clarithromycin, and 14-hydroxy-clarithromycin). Products include:
Biaxin/Biaxin XL 402
PREVPAC 3284

Clorazepate Dipotassium (Potential for metabolism interaction via cytochrome P450 system). Products include:
Tranxene 2474

Cyclosporine (Potential for metabolism interaction via cytochrome P450 system). Products include:
Gengraf Capsules 459
Neoral Oral Solution 2259
Neoral Soft Gelatin Capsules 2259
Restasis Ophthalmic Emulsion 575
Sandimmune 2275

Diazepam (Potential for metabolism interaction via cytochrome P450 system; prolonged elimination of diazepam). Products include:
Diastat Rectal Delivery System 3343
Valium Tablets 2819

Disulfiram (Potential for metabolism interaction via cytochrome P450 system).
No products indexed under this heading.

Estazolam (Potential for metabolism interaction via cytochrome P450 system). Products include:
ProSom Tablets 517

Ferrous Fumarate (Omeprazole may interfere with gastric absorption of drugs, such as iron salts, where gastric pH is an important determinant of their bioavailability).
No products indexed under this heading.

Ferrous Gluconate (Omeprazole may interfere with gastric absorption of drugs, such as iron salts, where gastric pH is an important determinant of their bioavailability).
No products indexed under this heading.

Ferrous Sulfate (Omeprazole may interfere with gastric absorption of drugs, such as iron salts, where gastric pH is an important determinant of their bioavailability). Products include:
Slow Fe Iron Tablets 818
Slow Fe with Folic Acid Tablets 819

Flurazepam Hydrochloride (Potential for metabolism interaction via cytochrome P450 system). Products include:
Dalmane Capsules 3342

Fosphenytoin Sodium (Prolonged elimination of phenytoin).
No products indexed under this heading.

Halazepam (Potential for metabolism interaction via cytochrome P450 system).
No products indexed under this heading.

Iron (Omeprazole may interfere with gastric absorption of drugs, such as iron salts, where gastric pH is an important determinant of their bioavailability).
No products indexed under this heading.

Ketoconazole (Omeprazole may interfere with gastric absorption of drugs, such as ketoconazole, where gastric pH is an important determinant of their bioavailability). Products include:
Nizoral A-D Shampoo, 1% 1868

Lorazepam (Potential for metabolism interaction via cytochrome P450 system).
No products indexed under this heading.

Midazolam Hydrochloride (Potential for metabolism interaction via cytochrome P450 system).
No products indexed under this heading.

Oxazepam (Potential for metabolism interaction via cytochrome P450 system).
No products indexed under this heading.

Phenytoin (Prolonged elimination of phenytoin).
No products indexed under this heading.

Phenytoin Sodium (Prolonged elimination of phenytoin). Products include:
Phenytek Capsules 2160

Polysaccharide Iron Complex (Omeprazole may interfere with gastric absorption of drugs, such as iron salts, where gastric pH is an important determinant of their bioavailability). Products include:
Nu-Iron 150 Capsules 2127

Prazepam (Potential for metabolism interaction via cytochrome P450 system).
No products indexed under this heading.

Quazepam (Potential for metabolism interaction via cytochrome P450 system).
No products indexed under this heading.

Tacrolimus (Co-administration of omeprazole and tacrolimus may increase the serum levels of tacrolimus). Products include:
Prograf Capsules and Injection 632
Protopic Ointment 638

Temazepam (Potential for metabolism interaction via cytochrome P450 system). Products include:
Restoril Capsules 1860

Triazolam (Potential for metabolism interaction via cytochrome P450 system).
No products indexed under this heading.

Warfarin Sodium (Prolonged elimination of warfarin, and reports of increased INR and prothrombin time with concurrent use). Products include:
Coumadin for Injection 898
Coumadin Tablets 898

ZELAPAR TABLETS

(Selegiline Hydrochloride) 3372
May interact with cytochrome p450 3a4 inducers (selected), tricyclic antidepressants, and certain other agents. Compounds in these categories include:

Allium sativum (Drugs that induce CYP3A4 should be used with caution).
No products indexed under this heading.

Amitriptyline Hydrochloride (Severe CNS toxicity associated with hyperpyrexia and death has been reported with the combination of tricyclic antidepressants and non-selective MAOIs or a selective MAO-B inhibitor).
No products indexed under this heading.

Amoxapine (Severe CNS toxicity associated with hyperpyrexia and death has been reported with the combination of tricyclic antidepressants and non-selective MAOIs or a selective MAO-B inhibitor).
No products indexed under this heading.

Aprepitant (Drugs that induce CYP3A4 should be used with caution). Products include:
Emend Capsules 1963

Betamethasone Acetate (Drugs that induce CYP3A4 should be used with caution).
No products indexed under this heading.

Betamethasone Sodium Phosphate (Drugs that induce CYP3A4 should be used with caution).
No products indexed under this heading.

Carbamazepine (Drugs that induce CYP3A4 should be used with caution). Products include:
Carbatrol Capsules 3171
Equetro Extended-Release Capsules 3180
Tegretol/Tegretol-XR 2295

Carbidopa (Selegiline hydrochloride may potentiate the dopaminergic side effects of carbidopa and may cause or exacerbate preexisting dyskinesia). Products include:
Parcopa Orally Disintegrating Tablets 3097
Stalevo Tablets 2287

Ciprofloxacin Hydrochloride (Drugs that induce CYP3A4 should be used with caution). Products include:
Ciloxan Ophthalmic Ointment 559
Ciloxan Ophthalmic Solution .... ⊙206
Cipro Tablets 2977
Proquin XR Tablets 1153

Cisplatin (Drugs that induce CYP3A4 should be used with caution).
No products indexed under this heading.

Clomipramine Hydrochloride (Severe CNS toxicity associated with hyperpyrexia and death has been reported with the combination of tricyclic antidepressants and non-selective MAOIs or a selective MAO-B inhibitor).
No products indexed under this heading.

Cortisone Acetate (Drugs that induce CYP3A4 should be used with caution).
No products indexed under this heading.

Desipramine Hydrochloride (Severe CNS toxicity associated with hyperpyrexia and death has been reported with the combination of tricyclic antidepressants and non-selective MAOIs or a selective MAO-B inhibitor).
No products indexed under this heading.

Dexamethasone (Drugs that induce CYP3A4 should be used with caution). Products include:
Ciprodex Otic Suspension 559
Decadron Tablets 1951
TobraDex Ophthalmic Ointment 562
TobraDex Ophthalmic Suspension 563

Dexamethasone Acetate (Drugs that induce CYP3A4 should be used with caution).
No products indexed under this heading.

Dexamethasone Sodium Phosphate (Drugs that induce CYP3A4 should be used with caution).
No products indexed under this heading.

Dextromethorphan (Selegiline hydrochloride should not be used with the antitussive agent dextromethorphan. The combination of MAO inhibitors and dextromethorphan has been reported to cause brief episodes of psychosis or bizarre behavior).
No products indexed under this heading.

Doxepin Hydrochloride (Severe CNS toxicity associated with hyperpyrexia and death has been reported with the combination of tricyclic antidepressants and non-selective MAOIs or a selective MAO-B inhibitor).
No products indexed under this heading.

Doxorubicin Hydrochloride (Drugs that induce CYP3A4 should be used with caution).
No products indexed under this heading.

Efavirenz (Drugs that induce CYP3A4 should be used with caution). Products include:
Atripla Tablets 945
Sustiva Capsules 930
Sustiva Tablets 930

Ephedrine Hydrochloride (One case of hypertensive crisis has been reported in a patient taking the recommended dose of swallowed selegiline and ephedrine, a sympathomimetic medication).
No products indexed under this heading.

Ephedrine Sulfate (One case of hypertensive crisis has been reported in a patient taking the recommended dose of swallowed selegiline and ephedrine, a sympathomimetic medication).
No products indexed under this heading.

Ephedrine Tannate (One case of hypertensive crisis has been reported in a patient taking the recommended dose of swallowed selegiline and ephedrine, a sympathomimetic medication).
No products indexed under this heading.

Ethosuximide (Drugs that induce CYP3A4 should be used with caution).
No products indexed under this heading.

Felbamate (Drugs that induce CYP3A4 should be used with caution).
No products indexed under this heading.

Fludrocortisone Acetate (Drugs that induce CYP3A4 should be used with caution).
No products indexed under this heading.

Fluoxetine (Serious, sometimes fatal, reactions with signs and symptoms including hyperthermia, rigidity, myoclonus, autonomic instability with rapid vital sign fluctuation, and mental status changes progressing to extreme agitation, delirium, and coma have been reported in patients receiving a combination of selective serotonin reuptake inhibitors including fluoxetine and non-selective MAOIs or the selective MAO-B inhibitor selegiline).
No products indexed under this heading.

Fluvoxamine (Serious, sometimes fatal, reactions with signs and symptoms including hyperthermia, rigidity, myoclonus, autonomic instability with rapid vital sign fluctuation, and mental status changes progressing to extreme agitation, delirium, and coma have been reported in patients receiving a combination of selective serotonin reuptake inhibitors including fluvoxamine and non-selective MAOIs or the selective MAO-B inhibitor selegiline).
No products indexed under this heading.

Fosphenytoin Sodium (Drugs that induce CYP3A4 should be used with caution).
No products indexed under this heading.

Garlic Extract (Drugs that induce CYP3A4 should be used with caution).
No products indexed under this heading.

Garlic Oil (Drugs that induce CYP3A4 should be used with caution).
No products indexed under this heading.

Hydrocortisone (Drugs that induce CYP3A4 should be used with caution). Products include:
Colocort Rectal Suspension, USP (Retention) 100 mg/60 mL **2476**
Hydrocortone Tablets **1989**
Preparation H Hydrocortisone Cream .... ▣ **646**

Hydrocortisone Acetate (Drugs that induce CYP3A4 should be used with caution). Products include:
Analpram-HC **1159**
Pramosone **1161**
ProctoFoam-HC **3099**

Hydrocortisone Butyrate (Drugs that induce CYP3A4 should be used with caution). Products include:
Locoid Lipocream Cream **1160**

Hydrocortisone Cypionate (Drugs that induce CYP3A4 should be used with caution).
No products indexed under this heading.

Hydrocortisone Hemisuccinate (Drugs that induce CYP3A4 should be used with caution).
No products indexed under this heading.

Hydrocortisone Probutate (Drugs that induce CYP3A4 should be used with caution).
No products indexed under this heading.

Hydrocortisone Sodium Phosphate (Drugs that induce CYP3A4 should be used with caution).
No products indexed under this heading.

Hydrocortisone Sodium Succinate (Drugs that induce CYP3A4 should be used with caution).
No products indexed under this heading.

Hydrocortisone Valerate (Drugs that induce CYP3A4 should be used with caution).
No products indexed under this heading.

Hypericum (Drugs that induce CYP3A4 should be used with caution). Products include:
Satiete Tablets .... ▣ **832**

Hypericum Perforatum (Drugs that induce CYP3A4 should be used with caution).
No products indexed under this heading.

Imipramine Hydrochloride (Severe CNS toxicity associated with hyperpyrexia and death has been reported with the combination of tricyclic antidepressants and non-selective MAOIs or a selective MAO-B inhibitor).
No products indexed under this heading.

Imipramine Pamoate (Severe CNS toxicity associated with hyperpyrexia and death has been reported with the combination of tricyclic antidepressants and non-selective MAOIs or a selective MAO-B inhibitor).
No products indexed under this heading.

Levodopa (Selegiline hydrochloride may potentiate the dopaminergic side effects of levodopa and may cause or exacerbate preexisting dyskinesia). Products include:
Parcopa Orally Disintegrating Tablets **3097**
Stalevo Tablets **2287**

Maprotiline Hydrochloride (Severe CNS toxicity associated with hyperpyrexia and death has been reported with the combination of tricyclic antidepressants and non-selective MAOIs or a selective MAO-B inhibitor).
No products indexed under this heading.

Meperidine Hydrochloride (Selegiline hydrochloride is contraindicated for use with meperidine. Serious reactions have been precipitated with concomitant use of meperidine and MAO inhibitors including selective MAO-B inhibitors. At least 14 days should elapse between discontinuation of selegiline hydrochloride and inititation of treatment with meperidine).
No products indexed under this heading.

Mephenytoin (Drugs that induce CYP3A4 should be used with caution).
No products indexed under this heading.

Methadone Hydrochloride (Selegiline hydrochloride should not be administered with methadone. Serious reactions have been precipitated with concomitant use of analgesics and MAO inhibitors including selective MAO-B inhibitors. At least 14 days should elapse between discontinuation of selegiline hydrochloride and inititation of treatment with methadone).
No products indexed under this heading.

Methsuximide (Drugs that induce CYP3A4 should be used with caution).
No products indexed under this heading.

Methylprednisolone (Drugs that induce CYP3A4 should be used with caution).
No products indexed under this heading.

Methylprednisolone Acetate (Drugs that induce CYP3A4 should be used with caution). Products include:
Depo-Medrol Injectable Suspension **2617**
Depo-Medrol Single-Dose Vial **2619**

Methylprednisolone Sodium Succinate (Drugs that induce CYP3A4 should be used with caution).
No products indexed under this heading.

Modafinil (Drugs that induce CYP3A4 should be used with caution). Products include:
Provigil Tablets **988**

Nevirapine (Drugs that induce CYP3A4 should be used with caution). Products include:
Viramune Oral Suspension **873**
Viramune Tablets **873**

Nortriptyline Hydrochloride (Severe CNS toxicity associated with hyperpyrexia and death has been reported with the combination of tricyclic antidepressants and non-selective MAOIs or a selective MAO-B inhibitor).
No products indexed under this heading.

Oxcarbazepine (Drugs that induce CYP3A4 should be used with caution). Products include:
Trileptal Tablets **2300**
Trileptal Oral Suspension **2300**

Paroxetine Hydrochloride (Serious, sometimes fatal, reactions with signs and symptoms including hyperthermia, rigidity, myoclonus, autonomic instability with rapid vital sign fluctuation, and mental status changes progressing to extreme agitation, delirium, and coma have been reported in patients receiving a combination of selective serotonin reuptake inhibitors including paroxetine and non-selective MAOIs or the selective MAO-B inhibitor selegiline). Products include:
Paxil CR Controlled-Release Tablets **1538**
Paxil **1530**

Phenobarbital (Drugs that induce CYP3A4 should be used with caution). Products include:
Donnatal Extentabs **2493**

Phenobarbital Sodium (Drugs that induce CYP3A4 should be used with caution).
No products indexed under this heading.

Phenytoin (Drugs that induce CYP3A4 should be used with caution).
No products indexed under this heading.

Phenytoin Sodium (Drugs that induce CYP3A4 should be used with caution). Products include:
Phenytek Capsules **2160**

Prednisolone Acetate (Drugs that induce CYP3A4 should be used with caution). Products include:
Blephamide Ophthalmic Ointment **568**
Blephamide Ophthalmic Suspension.................................. **569**
Poly-Pred Ophthalmic Suspension .... ⊙ **233**
Pred Forte Ophthalmic Suspension .... ⊙ **235**
Pred Mild Ophthalmic Suspension .... ⊙ **238**
Pred-G Ophthalmic Ointment .... ⊙ **237**
Pred-G Ophthalmic Suspension ...... ⊙ **236**

Prednisolone Sodium Phosphate (Drugs that induce CYP3A4 should be used with caution).
No products indexed under this heading.

Prednisolone Tebutate (Drugs that induce CYP3A4 should be used with caution).
No products indexed under this heading.

Prednisone (Drugs that induce CYP3A4 should be used with caution).
No products indexed under this heading.

Primidone (Drugs that induce CYP3A4 should be used with caution).
No products indexed under this heading.

Propoxyphene Hydrochloride (Selegiline hydrochloride should not be administered with propoxyphene. Serious reactions have been precipitated with concomitant use of analgesics and MAO inhibitors including selective MAO-B inhibitors. At least 14 days should elapse between discontinuation of selegiline hydrochloride and inititation of treatment with propoxyphene).
No products indexed under this heading.

Protriptyline Hydrochloride (Severe CNS toxicity associated with hyperpyrexia and death has been reported with the combination of tricyclic antidepressants and non-selective MAOIs or a selective MAO-B inhibitor).
No products indexed under this heading.

Rifabutin (Drugs that induce CYP3A4 should be used with caution).
No products indexed under this heading.

Rifampicin (Drugs that induce CYP3A4 should be used with caution).
No products indexed under this heading.

Rifampin (Drugs that induce CYP3A4 should be used with caution).
No products indexed under this heading.

Rifapentine (Drugs that induce CYP3A4 should be used with caution).
No products indexed under this heading.

Sertraline Hydrochloride (Serious, sometimes fatal, reactions with signs and symptoms including hyperthermia, rigidity, myoclonus, autonomic instability with rapid vital sign fluctuation, and mental status changes progressing to extreme agitation, delirium, and coma have been reported in patients receiving a combination of selective serotonin reuptake inhibitors including sertraline and non-selective MAOIs or the selective MAO-B inhibitor selegiline). Products include:

Zoloft **2586**

Sulfinpyrazone (Drugs that induce CYP3A4 should be used with caution).

No products indexed under this heading.

Theophylline (Drugs that induce CYP3A4 should be used with caution).

No products indexed under this heading.

Tramadol Hydrochloride (Selegiline hydrochloride should not be administered with tramadol. Serious reactions have been precipitated with concomitant use of analgesics and MAO inhibitors including selective MAO-B inhibitors. At least 14 days should elapse between discontinuation of selegiline hydrochloride and inititation of treatment with tramadol). Products include:

Ultram ER Tablets **2392**

Triamcinolone (Drugs that induce CYP3A4 should be used with caution).

No products indexed under this heading.

Triamcinolone Acetonide (Drugs that induce CYP3A4 should be used with caution). Products include:

Azmacort Inhalation Aerosol **1726**
Nasacort AQ Nasal Spray **2922**

Triamcinolone Diacetate (Drugs that induce CYP3A4 should be used with caution).

No products indexed under this heading.

Triamcinolone Hexacetonide (Drugs that induce CYP3A4 should be used with caution).

No products indexed under this heading.

Trimipramine Maleate (Severe CNS toxicity associated with hyperpyrexia and death has been reported with the combination of tricyclic antidepressants and non-selective MAOIs or a selective MAO-B inhibitor).

No products indexed under this heading.

Troglitazone (Drugs that induce CYP3A4 should be used with caution).

No products indexed under this heading.

Venlafaxine Hydrochloride (Serious, sometimes fatal, reactions with signs and symptoms including hyperthermia, rigidity, myoclonus, autonomic instability with rapid vital sign fluctuation, and mental status changes progressing to extreme agitation, delirium, and coma have been reported in patients receiving a combination of selective serotonin-norepinephrine reuptake inhibitors including venlafaxine and non-selective MAOIs or the selective MAO-B inhibitor selegiline). Products include:

Effexor Tablets **3411**
Effexor XR Capsules **3417**

ZELNORM TABLETS

(Tegaserod maleate) **2312**
May interact with:

Digoxin (Reduced peak plasma concentrations of digoxin by approximately 15%; this reduction in bioavailability is not considered clinically relevant). Products include:

Lanoxicaps Capsules **1490**
Lanoxin Injection **1494**
Lanoxin Injection Pediatric **1497**
Lanoxin Tablets **1500**

Food Interactions

Food, unspecified (Reduces the bioavailability of tegaserod; Zelnorm should be taken before meals).

ZEMAIRA

(Alpha$_1$-Proteinase Inhibitor (Human)).............................. **3509**
None cited in PDR database.

ZEMPLAR CAPSULES

(Paricalcitol) **541**
May interact with cytochrome p450 3a4 inhibitors, potent and certain other agents. Compounds in these categories include:

Amprenavir (A study has demonstrated that ketoconazole approximately doubled paricalcitol AUC. Since paricalcitol is partially metabolized by CYP3A and ketoconazole is known to be a strong inhibitor of cytochrome P450 3A enzyme, care should be taken while dosing paricalcitol with ketoconazole and other strong P450 3A inhibitors. Dose adjustment of paricalcitol capsules may be required and iPTH and serum calcium concentrations should be closely monitored if a patient initiates or discontinues therapy with a strong CYP3A4 inhibitor, such as ketoconazole). Products include:

Agenerase Capsules **1327**
Agenerase Oral Solution **1332**

Atazanavir (A study has demonstrated that ketoconazole approximately doubled paricalcitol AUC. Since paricalcitol is partially metabolized by CYP3A and ketoconazole is known to be a strong inhibitor of cytochrome P450 3A enzyme, care should be taken while dosing paricalcitol with ketoconazole and other strong P450 3A inhibitors. Dose adjustment of paricalcitol capsules may be required and iPTH and serum calcium concentrations should be closely monitored if a patient initiates or discontinues therapy with a strong CYP3A4 inhibitor, such as ketoconazole).

No products indexed under this heading.

Atazanavir sulfate (A study has demonstrated that ketoconazole approximately doubled paricalcitol AUC. Since paricalcitol is partially metabolized by CYP3A and ketoconazole is known to be a strong inhibitor of cytochrome P450 3A enzyme, care should be taken while dosing paricalcitol with ketoconazole and other strong P450 3A inhibitors. Dose adjustment of paricalcitol capsules may be required and iPTH and serum calcium concentrations should be closely monitored if a patient initiates or discontinues therapy with a strong CYP3A4 inhibitor, such as ketoconazole). Products include:

Reyataz Capsules **921**

Cholestyramine (Drugs that impair intestinal absorption of fat-soluble vitamins, such as cholestyramine, may interfere with the absorption of paricalcitol).

No products indexed under this heading.

Clarithromycin (A study has demonstrated that ketoconazole approximately doubled paricalcitol AUC. Since paricalcitol is partially metabolized by CYP3A and ketoconazole is known to be a strong inhibitor of cytochrome P450 3A enzyme, care should be taken while dosing paricalcitol with ketoconazole and other strong P450 3A inhibitors. Dose adjustment of paricalcitol capsules may be required and iPTH and serum calcium concentrations should be closely monitored if a patient initiates or discontinues therapy with a strong CYP3A4 inhibitor, such as ketoconazole). Products include:

Biaxin/Biaxin XL **402**
PREVPAC **3284**

Fosamprenavir Calcium (A study has demonstrated that ketoconazole approximately doubled paricalcitol AUC. Since paricalcitol is partially metabolized by CYP3A and ketoconazole is known to be a strong inhibitor of cytochrome P450 3A enzyme, care should be taken while dosing paricalcitol with ketoconazole and other strong P450 3A inhibitors. Dose adjustment of paricalcitol capsules may be required and iPTH and serum calcium concentrations should be closely monitored if a patient initiates or discontinues therapy with a strong CYP3A4 inhibitor, such as ketoconazole). Products include:

Lexiva Tablets **1505**

Indinavir Sulfate (A study has demonstrated that ketoconazole approximately doubled paricalcitol AUC. Since paricalcitol is partially metabolized by CYP3A and ketoconazole is known to be a strong inhibitor of cytochrome P450 3A enzyme, care should be taken while dosing paricalcitol with ketoconazole and other strong P450 3A inhibitors. Dose adjustment of paricalcitol capsules may be required and iPTH and serum calcium concentrations should be closely monitored if a patient initiates or discontinues therapy with a strong CYP3A4 inhibitor, such as ketoconazole). Products include:

Crixivan Capsules **1940**

Itraconazole (A study has demonstrated that ketoconazole approximately doubled paricalcitol AUC. Since paricalcitol is partially metabolized by CYP3A and ketoconazole is known to be a strong inhibitor of cytochrome P450 3A enzyme, care should be taken while dosing paricalcitol with ketoconazole and other strong P450 3A inhibitors. Dose adjustment of paricalcitol capsules may be required and iPTH and serum calcium concentrations should be closely monitored if a patient initiates or discontinues therapy with a strong CYP3A4 inhibitor, such as ketoconazole).

No products indexed under this heading.

Ketoconazole (A study has demonstrated that ketoconazole approximately doubled paricalcitol AUC. Since paricalcitol is partially metabolized by CYP3A and ketoconazole is known to be a strong inhibitor of cytochrome P450 3A enzyme, care should be taken while dosing paricalcitol with ketoconazole and other strong P450 3A inhibitors. Dose adjustment of paricalcitol capsules may be required and iPTH and serum calcium concentrations should be closely monitored if a patient initiates or discontinues therapy with a strong CYP3A4 inhibitor, such as ketoconazole). Products include:

Nizoral A-D Shampoo, 1% **1868**

Lopinavir (A study has demonstrated that ketoconazole approximately doubled paricalcitol AUC. Since paricalcitol is partially metabolized by CYP3A and ketoconazole is known to be a strong inhibitor of cytochrome P450 3A enzyme, care should be taken while dosing paricalcitol with ketoconazole and other strong P450 3A inhibitors. Dose adjustment of paricalcitol capsules may be required and iPTH and serum calcium concentrations should be closely monitored if a patient initiates or discontinues therapy with a strong CYP3A4 inhibitor, such as ketoconazole). Products include:

Kaletra **476**

Nefazodone Hydrochloride (A study has demonstrated that ketoconazole approximately doubled paricalcitol AUC. Since paricalcitol is partially metabolized by CYP3A and ketoconazole is known to be a strong inhibitor of cytochrome P450 3A enzyme, care should be taken while dosing paricalcitol with ketoconazole and other strong P450 3A inhibitors. Dose adjustment of paricalcitol capsules may be required and iPTH and serum calcium concentrations should be closely monitored if a patient initiates or discontinues therapy with a strong CYP3A4 inhibitor, such as ketoconazole).

No products indexed under this heading.

Nelfinavir Mesylate (A study has demonstrated that ketoconazole approximately doubled paricalcitol AUC. Since paricalcitol is partially metabolized by CYP3A and ketoconazole is known to be a strong inhibitor of cytochrome P450 3A enzyme, care should be taken while dosing paricalcitol with ketoconazole and other strong P450 3A inhibitors. Dose adjustment of paricalcitol capsules may be required and iPTH and serum calcium concentrations should be closely monitored if a patient initiates or discontinues therapy with a strong CYP3A4 inhibitor, such as ketoconazole). Products include:

Viracept **2577**

Ritonavir (A study has demonstrated that ketoconazole approximately doubled paricalcitol AUC. Since paricalcitol is partially metabolized by CYP3A and ketoconazole is known to be a strong inhibitor of cytochrome P450 3A enzyme, care should be taken while dosing paricalcitol with ketoconazole and other strong P450 3A inhibitors. Dose adjustment of paricalcitol capsules may be required and iPTH and serum calcium concentrations should be closely monitored if a patient initiates or discontinues therapy with a strong CYP3A4 inhibitor, such as ketoconazole). Products include:

Kaletra **476**
Norvir **503**

IMPORTANT NOTE: Always consult each drug listing in the patient's regimen for possible interactions.

Saquinavir (A study has demonstrated that ketoconazole approximately doubled paricalcitol AUC. Since paricalcitol is partially metabolized by CYP3A and ketoconazole is known to be a strong inhibitor of cytochrome P450 3A enzyme, care should be taken while dosing paricalcitol with ketoconazole and other strong P450 3A inhibitors. Dose adjustment of paricalcitol capsules may be required and iPTH and serum calcium concentrations should be closely monitored if a patient initiates or discontinues therapy with a strong CYP3A4 inhibitor, such as ketoconazole).
No products indexed under this heading.

Saquinavir Mesylate (A study has demonstrated that ketoconazole approximately doubled paricalcitol AUC. Since paricalcitol is partially metabolized by CYP3A and ketoconazole is known to be a strong inhibitor of cytochrome P450 3A enzyme, care should be taken while dosing paricalcitol with ketoconazole and other strong P450 3A inhibitors. Dose adjustment of paricalcitol capsules may be required and iPTH and serum calcium concentrations should be closely monitored if a patient initiates or discontinues therapy with a strong CYP3A4 inhibitor, such as ketoconazole). Products include:
Invirase 2772

Telithromycin (A study has demonstrated that ketoconazole approximately doubled paricalcitol AUC. Since paricalcitol is partially metabolized by CYP3A and ketoconazole is known to be a strong inhibitor of cytochrome P450 3A enzyme, care should be taken while dosing paricalcitol with ketoconazole and other strong P450 3A inhibitors. Dose adjustment of paricalcitol capsules may be required and iPTH and serum calcium concentrations should be closely monitored if a patient initiates or discontinues therapy with a strong CYP3A4 inhibitor, such as ketoconazole). Products include:
Ketek Tablets 2903

Troleandomycin (A study has demonstrated that ketoconazole approximately doubled paricalcitol AUC. Since paricalcitol is partially metabolized by CYP3A and ketoconazole is known to be a strong inhibitor of cytochrome P450 3A enzyme, care should be taken while dosing paricalcitol with ketoconazole and other strong P450 3A inhibitors. Dose adjustment of paricalcitol capsules may be required and iPTH and serum calcium concentrations should be closely monitored if a patient initiates or discontinues therapy with a strong CYP3A4 inhibitor, such as ketoconazole).
No products indexed under this heading.

Voriconazole (A study has demonstrated that ketoconazole approximately doubled paricalcitol AUC. Since paricalcitol is partially metabolized by CYP3A and ketoconazole is known to be a strong inhibitor of cytochrome P450 3A enzyme, care should be taken while dosing paricalcitol with ketoconazole and other strong P450 3A inhibitors. Dose adjustment of paricalcitol capsules may be required and iPTH and serum calcium concentrations should be closely monitored if a patient initiates or discontinues therapy with a strong CYP3A4 inhibitor, such as ketoconazole). Products include:
VFEND I.V. 2564
VFEND Oral Suspension 2564
VFEND Tablets 2564

ZEMPLAR INJECTION

(Paricalcitol) 543
May interact with cardiac glycosides and certain other agents. Compounds in these categories include:

Atazanavir (Care should be taken while dosing paricalcitol with ketoconazole and other strong P450 3A inhibitiors including atazanavir, clarithromycin, indinavir, itraconazole, nefazodone, nelfinavir, ritonavir, saquinavir, telithromycin, or voriconazole due to a doubling of paricalcitol AUC and an increased mean half life when co-administered with these agents).
No products indexed under this heading.

Atazanavir sulfate (Care should be taken while dosing paricalcitol with ketoconazole and other strong P450 3A inhibitiors including atazanavir, clarithromycin, indinavir, itraconazole, nefazodone, nelfinavir, ritonavir, saquinavir, telithromycin, or voriconazole due to a doubling of paricalcitol AUC and an increased mean half life when co-administered with these agents). Products include:
Reyataz Capsules 921

Calcitriol (Vitamin D-related compounds should not be taken concomitantly with paricalcitol). Products include:
Calcijex Injection 411
Rocaltrol Capsules 2798
Rocaltrol Oral Solution 2798

Clarithromycin (Care should be taken while dosing paricalcitol with ketoconazole and other strong P450 3A inhibitiors including atazanavir, clarithromycin, indinavir, itraconazole, nefazodone, nelfinavir, ritonavir, saquinavir, telithromycin, or voriconazole due to a doubling of paricalcitol AUC and an increased mean half life when co-administered with these agents). Products include:
Biaxin/Biaxin XL 402
PREVPAC 3284

Deslanoside (Digitalis toxicity is potentiated by hypercalcemia of any cause, so caution should be applied when digitalis compounds are prescribed concomitantly with paricalcitol).
No products indexed under this heading.

Digitalis Glycoside Preparations (Digitalis toxicity is potentiated by hypercalcemia of any cause, so caution should be applied when digitalis compounds are prescribed concomitantly with paricalcitol).
No products indexed under this heading.

Digitoxin (Digitalis toxicity is potentiated by hypercalcemia of any cause, so caution should be applied when digitalis compounds are prescribed concomitantly with paricalcitol).
No products indexed under this heading.

Digoxin (Digitalis toxicity is potentiated by hypercalcemia of any cause, so caution should be applied when digitalis compounds are prescribed concomitantly with paricalcitol). Products include:
Lanoxicaps Capsules 1490
Lanoxin Injection 1494
Lanoxin Injection Pediatric 1497
Lanoxin Tablets 1500

Indinavir Sulfate (Care should be taken while dosing paricalcitol with ketoconazole and other strong P450 3A inhibitiors including atazanavir, clarithromycin, indinavir, itraconazole, nefazodone, nelfinavir, ritonavir, saquinavir, telithromycin, or voriconazole due to a doubling of paricalcitol AUC and an increased mean half life when co-administered with these agents). Products include:
Crixivan Capsules 1940

Itraconazole (Care should be taken while dosing paricalcitol with ketoconazole and other strong P450 3A inhibitiors including atazanavir, clarithromycin, indinavir, itraconazole, nefazodone, nelfinavir, ritonavir, saquinavir, telithromycin, or voriconazole due to a doubling of paricalcitol AUC and an increased mean half life when co-administered with these agents).
No products indexed under this heading.

Ketoconazole (Care should be taken while dosing paricalcitol with ketoconazole and other strong P450 3A inhibitiors including atazanavir, clarithromycin, indinavir, itraconazole, nefazodone, nelfinavir, ritonavir, saquinavir, telithromycin, or voriconazole due to a doubling of paricalcitol AUC and an increased mean half life when co-administered with these agents). Products include:
Nizoral A-D Shampoo, 1% 1868

Nefazodone Hydrochloride (Care should be taken while dosing paricalcitol with ketoconazole and other strong P450 3A inhibitiors including atazanavir, clarithromycin, indinavir, itraconazole, nefazodone, nelfinavir, ritonavir, saquinavir, telithromycin, or voriconazole due to a doubling of paricalcitol AUC and an increased mean half life when co-administered with these agents).
No products indexed under this heading.

Nelfinavir Mesylate (Care should be taken while dosing paricalcitol with ketoconazole and other strong P450 3A inhibitiors including atazanavir, clarithromycin, indinavir, itraconazole, nefazodone, nelfinavir, ritonavir, saquinavir, telithromycin, or voriconazole due to a doubling of paricalcitol AUC and an increased mean half life when co-administered with these agents). Products include:
Viracept 2577

Potassium Acid Phosphate (Phosphate compounds should not be taken concomitantly with paricalcitol). Products include:
K-Phos Original (Sodium Free) Tablets 760

Potassium Phosphate (Phosphate compounds should not be taken concomitantly with paricalcitol). Products include:
K-Phos Neutral Tablets 760

Ritonavir (Care should be taken while dosing paricalcitol with ketoconazole and other strong P450 3A inhibitiors including atazanavir, clarithromycin, indinavir, itraconazole, nefazodone, nelfinavir, ritonavir, saquinavir, telithromycin, or voriconazole due to a doubling of paricalcitol AUC and an increased mean half life when co-administered with these agents). Products include:
Kaletra 476
Norvir 503

Saquinavir (Care should be taken while dosing paricalcitol with ketoconazole and other strong P450 3A inhibitiors including atazanavir, clarithromycin, indinavir, itraconazole, nefazodone, nelfinavir, ritonavir, saquinavir, telithromycin, or voriconazole due to a doubling of paricalcitol AUC and an increased mean half life when co-administered with these agents).
No products indexed under this heading.

Saquinavir Mesylate (Care should be taken while dosing paricalcitol with ketoconazole and other strong P450 3A inhibitiors including atazanavir, clarithromycin, indinavir, itraconazole, nefazodone, nelfinavir, ritonavir, saquinavir, telithromycin, or voriconazole due to a doubling of paricalcitol AUC and an increased mean half life when co-administered with these agents). Products include:
Invirase 2772

Telithromycin (Care should be taken while dosing paricalcitol with ketoconazole and other strong P450 3A inhibitiors including atazanavir, clarithromycin, indinavir, itraconazole, nefazodone, nelfinavir, ritonavir, saquinavir, telithromycin, or voriconazole due to a doubling of paricalcitol AUC and an increased mean half life when co-administered with these agents). Products include:
Ketek Tablets 2903

Voriconazole (Care should be taken while dosing paricalcitol with ketoconazole and other strong P450 3A inhibitiors including atazanavir, clarithromycin, indinavir, itraconazole, nefazodone, nelfinavir, ritonavir, saquinavir, telithromycin, or voriconazole due to a doubling of paricalcitol AUC and an increased mean half life when co-administered with these agents). Products include:
VFEND I.V. 2564
VFEND Oral Suspension 2564
VFEND Tablets 2564

ZEMURON INJECTION

(Rocuronium Bromide) 2346
May interact with aminoglycosides, anticonvulsants, inhalant anesthetics, tetracyclines, and certain other agents. Compounds in these categories include:

Amikacin Sulfate (Possible prolongation of neuromuscular blockade).
No products indexed under this heading.

Bacitracin (Possible prolongation of neuromuscular blockade). Products include:
Neosporin Antibiotic Ointment .... ▣643
Polysporin First Aid Antibiotic Ointment .... ▣643

Carbamazepine (Potential for apparent resistance to the effects of rocuronium in the form of diminished magnitude of neuromuscular blockade). Products include:
Carbatrol Capsules 3171
Equetro Extended-Release Capsules 3180
Tegretol/Tegretol-XR 2295

Colistimethate Sodium (Possible prolongation of neuromuscular blockade).
No products indexed under this heading.

Colistin Sulfate (Possible prolongation of neuromuscular blockade).
No products indexed under this heading.

Demeclocycline Hydrochloride (Possible prolongation of neuromuscular blockade).
No products indexed under this heading.

Desflurane (Possible enhanced activity of neuromuscular blocking agent).
No products indexed under this heading.

Divalproex Sodium (Potential for apparent resistance to the effects of rocuronium in the form of diminished magnitude of neuromuscular blockade). Products include:
Depakote Sprinkle Capsules 422
Depakote Tablets 427
Depakote ER Tablets 434

Doxycycline Calcium (Possible prolongation of neuromuscular blockade).
No products indexed under this heading.

Doxycycline Hyclate (Possible prolongation of neuromuscular blockade).
No products indexed under this heading.

Doxycycline Monohydrate (Possible prolongation of neuromuscular blockade). Products include:
Oracea Capsules 1000

Enflurane (Possible enhanced activity of neuromuscular blocking agent; may prolong the duration of action).
No products indexed under this heading.

Ethosuximide (Potential for apparent resistance to the effects of rocuronium in the form of diminished magnitude of neuromuscular blockade).
No products indexed under this heading.

Ethotoin (Potential for apparent resistance to the effects of rocuronium in the form of diminished magnitude of neuromuscular blockade).
No products indexed under this heading.

Felbamate (Potential for apparent resistance to the effects of rocuronium in the form of diminished magnitude of neuromuscular blockade).
No products indexed under this heading.

Fosphenytoin (Potential for apparent resistance to the effects of rocuronium in the form of diminished magnitude of neuromuscular blockade).
No products indexed under this heading.

Fosphenytoin Sodium (Potential for apparent resistance to the effects of rocuronium in the form of diminished magnitude of neuromuscular blockade).
No products indexed under this heading.

Gabapentin (Potential for apparent resistance to the effects of rocuronium in the form of diminished magnitude of neuromuscular blockade). Products include:
Neurontin Capsules 2487
Neurontin Oral Solution 2487
Neurontin Tablets 2487

Gentamicin Sulfate (Possible prolongation of neuromuscular blockade). Products include:
Garamycin Injectable 3014
Pred-G Ophthalmic Ointment .... ⊙237
Pred-G Ophthalmic Suspension .... ⊙236

Halothane (Possible enhanced activity of neuromuscular blocking agent).
No products indexed under this heading.

Isoflurane (Possible enhanced activity of neuromuscular blocking agent; may prolong the duration of action).
No products indexed under this heading.

Kanamycin Sulfate (Possible prolongation of neuromuscular blockade).
No products indexed under this heading.

Lamotrigine (Potential for apparent resistance to the effects of rocuronium in the form of diminished magnitude of neuromuscular blockade). Products include:
Lamictal 1481

Levetiracetam (Potential for apparent resistance to the effects of rocuronium in the form of diminished magnitude of neuromuscular blockade). Products include:
Keppra Injection 3320
Keppra Oral Solution 3314
Keppra Tablets 3314

Lithium Carbonate (May increase the duration of neuromuscular block). Products include:
Lithobid Tablets 1692

Lithium Citrate (May increase the duration of neuromuscular block).
No products indexed under this heading.

Magnesium Sulfate Injection (May enhance the neuromuscular blockade).
No products indexed under this heading.

Mephenytoin (Potential for apparent resistance to the effects of rocuronium in the form of diminished magnitude of neuromuscular blockade).
No products indexed under this heading.

Methacycline Hydrochloride (Possible prolongation of neuromuscular blockade).
No products indexed under this heading.

Methoxyflurane (Possible enhanced activity of neuromuscular blocking agent).
No products indexed under this heading.

Methsuximide (Potential for apparent resistance to the effects of rocuronium in the form of diminished magnitude of neuromuscular blockade).
No products indexed under this heading.

Minocycline Hydrochloride (Possible prolongation of neuromuscular blockade). Products include:
Solodyn Extended Release Tablets 1890

Oxcarbazepine (Potential for apparent resistance to the effects of rocuronium in the form of diminished magnitude of neuromuscular blockade). Products include:
Trileptal Tablets 2300
Trileptal Oral Suspension 2300

Oxytetracycline Hydrochloride (Possible prolongation of neuromuscular blockade).
No products indexed under this heading.

Paramethadione (Potential for apparent resistance to the effects of rocuronium in the form of diminished magnitude of neuromuscular blockade).
No products indexed under this heading.

Phenacemide (Potential for apparent resistance to the effects of rocuronium in the form of diminished magnitude of neuromuscular blockade).
No products indexed under this heading.

Phenobarbital (Potential for apparent resistance to the effects of rocuronium in the form of diminished magnitude of neuromuscular blockade). Products include:
Donnatal Extentabs 2493

Phensuximide (Potential for apparent resistance to the effects of rocuronium in the form of diminished magnitude of neuromuscular blockade).
No products indexed under this heading.

Phenytoin (Potential for apparent resistance to the effects of rocuronium in the form of diminished magnitude of neuromuscular blockade).
No products indexed under this heading.

Phenytoin Sodium (Potential for apparent resistance to the effects of rocuronium in the form of diminished magnitude of neuromuscular blockade). Products include:
Phenytek Capsules 2160

Polymyxin B Sulfate (Possible prolongation of neuromuscular blockade). Products include:
Neosporin Antibiotic Ointment .... ▣643
Neosporin Ophthalmic Solution Sterile .... ⊙265
Neosporin + Pain Relief Antibiotic Cream and Ointment (Maximum Strength) .... ▣643
Poly-Pred Ophthalmic Suspension .... ⊙233
Polysporin First Aid Antibiotic Ointment .... ▣643
Polytrim Ophthalmic Solution 574

Primidone (Potential for apparent resistance to the effects of rocuronium in the form of diminished magnitude of neuromuscular blockade).
No products indexed under this heading.

Procainamide Hydrochloride (May increase the duration of neuromuscular block).
No products indexed under this heading.

Quinidine Gluconate (Possible recurrent paralysis; increased duration of neuromusclar block).
No products indexed under this heading.

Quinidine Polygalacturonate (Possible recurrent paralysis; increased duration of neuromusclar block).
No products indexed under this heading.

Quinidine Sulfate (Possible recurrent paralysis; increased duration of neuromusclar block).
No products indexed under this heading.

Streptomycin Sulfate (Possible prolongation of neuromuscular blockade).
No products indexed under this heading.

Succinylcholine Chloride (Rocuronium should not be given until recovery from succinylcholine has been observed).
No products indexed under this heading.

Tetracycline Hydrochloride (Possible prolongation of neuromuscular blockade).
No products indexed under this heading.

Tiagabine Hydrochloride (Potential for apparent resistance to the effects of rocuronium in the form of diminished magnitude of neuromuscular blockade). Products include:
Gabitril Tablets 984

Tobramycin (Possible prolongation of neuromuscular blockade). Products include:
TOBI Solution for Inhalation 2298
TobraDex Ophthalmic Ointment 562
TobraDex Ophthalmic Suspension 563
Zylet Ophthalmic Suspension .... ⊙259

Tobramycin Sulfate (Possible prolongation of neuromuscular blockade).
No products indexed under this heading.

Topiramate (Potential for apparent resistance to the effects of rocuronium in the form of diminished magnitude of neuromuscular blockade). Products include:
Topamax Sprinkle Capsules 2404
Topamax Tablets 2404

Trimethadione (Potential for apparent resistance to the effects of rocuronium in the form of diminished magnitude of neuromuscular blockade).
No products indexed under this heading.

Valproate Sodium (Potential for apparent resistance to the effects of rocuronium in the form of diminished magnitude of neuromuscular blockade). Products include:
Depacon Injection 412

Valproic Acid (Potential for apparent resistance to the effects of rocuronium in the form of diminished magnitude of neuromuscular blockade). Products include:
Depakene 417

Vancomycin Hydrochloride (Possible prolongation of neuromuscular blockade). Products include:
Vancocin HCl Capsules, USP 3380

Zonisamide (Potential for apparent resistance to the effects of rocuronium in the form of diminished magnitude of neuromuscular blockade). Products include:
Zonegran Capsules 1101

ZETIA TABLETS

(Ezetimibe) 2120
May interact with antacids, fibrates, and certain other agents. Compounds in these categories include:

Aluminum Carbonate (Coadministration had no significant effect on the oral bioavailability of total ezetimibe, ezetimibe-glucuronide, or ezetimibe based on AUC values. The Cmax value of total ezetimibe was decreased by 30%).
No products indexed under this heading.

Aluminum Hydroxide (Coadministration had no significant effect on the oral bioavailability of total ezetimibe, ezetimibe-glucuronide, or ezetimibe based on

AUC values. The Cmax value of total ezetimibe was decreased by 30%). Products include:

Gaviscon Regular Strength Liquid .. ■ 658
Gaviscon Regular Strength Tablets .... ■ 658
Gaviscon Extra Strength Liquid ...... ■ 658
Gaviscon Extra Strength Tablets .... ■ 658
Maalox Regular Strength Antacid/Antigas Liquid 2175
Maalox Max Maximum Strength Antacid/Anti-Gas Liquid 2176

Cholestyramine (Co-administration of cholestyramine decreased the mean AUC values of total ezetimibe and ezetimibe approximately 55% and 80%, respectively. The incremental LDL-C reduction due to adding ezetimibe to cholestyramine may be reduced by this interaction).

No products indexed under this heading.

Clofibrate (The safety and effectiveness of ezetimibe administered with fibrates other than fenofibrate has not been studied. Fibrates may increase cholesterol excretion into the bile leading to cholelithiasis. If cholelithiasis is suspected in a patient receivingezetimibe and fenofibrate, gallbladder studies are indicated and alternative lipid-lowering therapy should be considered. Co-administration of ezetimibe with fibrates other than fenofibrate is not recommended).

No products indexed under this heading.

Cyclosporine (Caution should be exercised when initiating ezetimibe in patients treated with cyclosporine due to increased exposure to ezetimibe. This exposure may be greater in patients with severe renal insufficiency). Products include:

Gengraf Capsules 459
Neoral Oral Solution 2259
Neoral Soft Gelatin Capsules 2259
Restasis Ophthalmic Emulsion 575
Sandimmune 2275

Fenofibrate (Co-administration of fenofibrate increased the mean Cmax and AUC values of total ezetimibe approximately 64% and 48%, respectively). Products include:

Lofibra Tablets 1219
Lofibra Capsules 1216
Tricor Tablets 527
Triglide Tablets 3123

Gemfibrozil (Co-administration increased total ezetimibe by approximately 1.7-fold).

No products indexed under this heading.

Magaldrate (Co-administration had no significant effect on the oral bioavailability of total ezetimibe, ezetimibe-glucuronide, or ezetimibe based on AUC values. The Cmax value of total ezetimibe was decreased by 30%).

No products indexed under this heading.

Magnesium Hydroxide (Co-administration had no significant effect on the oral bioavailability of total ezetimibe, ezetimibe-glucuronide, or ezetimibe based on AUC values. The Cmax value of total ezetimibe was decreased by 30%). Products include:

Maalox Regular Strength Antacid/Antigas Liquid 2175
Maalox Max Maximum Strength Antacid/Anti-Gas Liquid 2176
Pepcid Complete Chewable Tablets 1701

Magnesium Oxide (Co-administration had no significant effect on the oral bioavailability of total ezetimibe, ezetimibe-glucuronide, or ezetimibe based on AUC values. The Cmax value of total ezetimibe was decreased by 30%). Products include:

Beelith Tablets 759
PremCal Light, Regular, and Extra Strength Tablets .... ■ 818

Sodium Bicarbonate (Co-administration had no significant effect on the oral bioavailability of total ezetimibe, ezetimibe-glucuronide, or ezetimibe based on AUC values. The Cmax value of total ezetimibe was decreased by 30%). Products include:

Colyte with Flavor Packs for Oral Solution 3088
HalfLytely and Bisacodyl Tablets Bowel Prep Kit with Flavors Packs 881
TriLyte with Flavor Packs for Oral Solution 3100

Warfarin Sodium (There have been post-marketing reports of increased INR in patients who had ezetimibe added to warfarin. Most of these patients were also on other medications). Products include:

Coumadin for Injection 898
Coumadin Tablets 898

ZETIA TABLETS

(Ezetimibe) 3083

May interact with antacids, fibrates, HMG-CoA reductase inhibitors, and certain other agents. Compounds in these categories include:

Aluminum Carbonate (Co-administration had no significant effect on the oral bioavailability of total ezetimibe, ezetimibe-glucuronide, or ezetimibe based on AUC values. The Cmax value of total ezetimibe was decreased by 30%).

No products indexed under this heading.

Aluminum Hydroxide (Co-administration had no significant effect on the oral bioavailability of total ezetimibe, ezetimibe-glucuronide, or ezetimibe based on AUC values. The Cmax value of total ezetimibe was decreased by 30%). Products include:

Gaviscon Regular Strength Liquid .. ■ 658
Gaviscon Regular Strength Tablets .... ■ 658
Gaviscon Extra Strength Liquid ...... ■ 658
Gaviscon Extra Strength Tablets .... ■ 658
Maalox Regular Strength Antacid/Antigas Liquid 2175
Maalox Max Maximum Strength Antacid/Anti-Gas Liquid 2176

Atorvastatin Calcium (In controlled clinical studies of ezetimbe initiated concurrently with an HMG-CoA reductase inhibitor, the incidence of consecutive elevations (greater than or equal to 3 x ULN) in serum transaminases was 1.3% for patients treated with ezetimbe administered with HMG-CoA reductase inhibitors and 0.4% for patients treated with HMG-CoA reductase inhibitors alone. When ezetimbe is co-administered with an HMG-CoA reductase inhibitor, liver function tests should be performed at initiation of therapy and according to the recommendations of the HMG-CoA reductase inhibitor. The combination of ezetimbe with a HMG-CoA inhibitor is contraindicated in patients with active liver disease or unexplained persistent elevations in serum transaminases). Products include:

Caduet Tablets 2508
Lipitor Tablets 2483

Cerivastatin Sodium (In controlled clinical studies of ezetimbe initiated concurrently with an HMG-CoA reductase inhibitor, the incidence of consecutive elevations (greater than or equal to 3 x ULN) in serum transaminases was 1.3% for patients treated with ezetimbe administered with HMG-CoA reductase inhibitors and 0.4% for patients treated with HMG-CoA reductase inhibitors alone. When ezetimbe is co-administered with an HMG-CoA reductase inhibitor, liver function tests should be performed at initiation of therapy and according to the recommendations of the HMG-CoA reductase inhibitor. The combination of ezetimbe with a HMG-CoA inhibitor is contraindicated in patients with active liver disease or unexplained persistent elevations in serum transaminases).

No products indexed under this heading.

Cholestyramine (Co-administration decreased the mean AUC of total ezetimibe by approximately 55%. Incremental LDL-C reduction may be reduced).

No products indexed under this heading.

Clofibrate (The safety and effectiveness of ezetimbe administration with fibrates has not been established. Co-administration of ezetimbe with fibrates is not recommended until use in patients is studied).

No products indexed under this heading.

Cyclosporine (Caution should be exercised when initiating ezetimibe in patients treated with cyclosporine due to increased exposure to ezetimibe. This exposure may be greater in patients with severe renal insufficiency). Products include:

Gengraf Capsules 459
Neoral Oral Solution 2259
Neoral Soft Gelatin Capsules 2259
Restasis Ophthalmic Emulsion 575
Sandimmune 2275

Fenofibrate (Co-administration increased total ezetimbe concentrations by approximately 1.5-fold. Concurrent use of fibrates is not recommended). Products include:

Lofibra Tablets 1219
Lofibra Capsules 1216
Tricor Tablets 527
Triglide Tablets 3123

Fluvastatin Sodium (In controlled clinical studies of ezetimbe initiated concurrently with an HMG-CoA reductase inhibitor, the incidence of consecutive elevations (greater than or equal to 3 x ULN) in serum transaminases was 1.3% for patients treated with ezetimbe administered with HMG-CoA reductase inhibitors and 0.4% for patients treated with HMG-CoA reductase inhibitors alone. When ezetimbe is co-administered with an HMG-CoA reductase inhibitor, liver function tests should be performed at initiation of therapy and according to the recommendations of the HMG-CoA reductase inhibitor. The combination of ezetimbe with a HMG-CoA inhibitor is contraindicated in patients with active liver disease or unexplained persistent elevations in serum transaminases). Products include:

Lescol Capsules 2233
Lescol XL Tablets 2233

Gemfibrozil (Co-administration increased total ezetimbe concentrations by approximately 1.7-fold).

No products indexed under this heading.

Lovastatin (In controlled clinical studies of ezetimbe initiated concurrently with an HMG-CoA reductase inhibitor, the incidence of consecutive elevations (greater than or equal to 3 x ULN) in serum transaminases was 1.3% for patients treated with ezetimbe administered with HMG-CoA reductase inhibitors and 0.4% for patients treated with HMG-CoA reductase inhibitors alone. When ezetimbe is co-administered with an HMG-CoA reductase inhibitor, liver function tests should be performed at initiation of therapy and according to the recommendations of the HMG-CoA reductase inhibitor. The combination of ezetimbe with a HMG-CoA inhibitor is contraindicated in patients with active liver disease or unexplained persistent elevations in serum transaminases). Products include:

Advicor Tablets 1722
Altoprev Extended-Release Tablets 3109
Mevacor Tablets 2021

Magaldrate (Co-administration had no significant effect on the oral bioavailability of total ezetimibe, ezetimibe-glucuronide, or ezetimibe based on AUC values. The Cmax value of total ezetimibe was decreased by 30%).

No products indexed under this heading.

Magnesium Hydroxide (Co-administration had no significant effect on the oral bioavailability of total ezetimibe, ezetimibe-glucuronide, or ezetimibe based on AUC values. The Cmax value of total ezetimibe was decreased by 30%). Products include:

Maalox Regular Strength Antacid/Antigas Liquid 2175
Maalox Max Maximum Strength Antacid/Anti-Gas Liquid 2176
Pepcid Complete Chewable Tablets 1701

Magnesium Oxide (Co-administration had no significant effect on the oral bioavailability of total ezetimibe, ezetimibe-glucuronide, or ezetimibe based on AUC values. The Cmax value of total ezetimibe was decreased by 30%). Products include:

Beelith Tablets 759
PremCal Light, Regular, and Extra Strength Tablets .... ■ 818

Pravastatin Sodium (In controlled clinical studies of ezetimibe initiated concurrently with an HMG-CoA reductase inhibitor, the incidence of consecutive elevations (greater than or equal to 3 x ULN) in serum transaminases was 1.3% for patients treated with ezetimbe administered with HMG-CoA reductase inhibitors and 0.4% for patients treated with HMG-CoA reductase inhibitors alone. When ezetimbe is co-administered with an HMG-CoA reductase inhibitor, liver function tests should be performed at initiation of therapy and according to the recommendations of the HMG-CoA reductase inhibitor. The combination of ezetimbe with a HMG-CoA inhibitor is contraindicated in patients with active liver disease or unexplained persistent elevations

in serum transaminases).
No products indexed under this heading.

Simvastatin (In controlled clinical studies of ezetimbe initiated concurrently with an HMG-CoA reductase inhibitor, the incidence of consecutive elevations (greater than or equal to 3 x ULN) in serum transaminases was 1.3% for patients treated with ezetimbe administered with HMG-CoA reductase inhibitors and 0.4% for patients treated with HMG-CoA reductase inhibitors alone. When ezetimbe is co-administered with an HMG-CoA reductase inhibitor, liver function tests should be performed at initiation of therapy and according to the recommendations of the HMG-CoA reductase inhibitor. The combination of ezetimbe with a HMG-CoA inhibitor is contraindicated in patients with active liver disease or unexplained persistent elevations in serum transaminases). Products include:
Vytorin 10/10 Tablets 2114
Vytorin 10/10 Tablets 3077
Vytorin 10/20 Tablets 2114
Vytorin 10/20 Tablets 3077
Vytorin 10/40 Tablets 2114
Vytorin 10/40 Tablets 3077
Vytorin 10/80 Tablets 2114
Vytorin 10/80 Tablets 3077
Zocor Tablets 2105

Sodium Bicarbonate (Co-administration had no significant effect on the oral bioavailability of total ezetimibe, ezetimibe-glucuronide, or ezetimibe based on AUC values. The Cmax value of total ezetimibe was decreased by 30%). Products include:
Colyte with Flavor Packs for Oral Solution 3088
HalfLytely and Bisacodyl Tablets Bowel Prep Kit with Flavors Packs 881
TriLyte with Flavor Packs for Oral Solution 3100

Warfarin Sodium (It has been reported that patients who had ezetimibe added to warfarin have had an increased International Normalized Ratio (INR). Most of these patients were also on other medications). Products include:
Coumadin for Injection 898
Coumadin Tablets 898

ZIAGEN ORAL SOLUTION
(Abacavir Sulfate) 1626
See Ziagen Tablets

ZIAGEN TABLETS
(Abacavir Sulfate) 1626
May interact with:

Lamivudine (Ziagen should not be co-administered with Epzicom or Trizivir). Products include:
Combivir Tablets 1411
Epivir 1427
Epivir-HBV 1432
Epzicom Tablets 1436
Trizivir Tablets 1589

Methadone Hydrochloride (Co-administration in patients on methadone-maintenance therapy has resulted in increased methadone clearance by 22%. This alteration will not result in a methadone dose modification in the majority of patients; however, an increased methadone dose may be required in a small number of patients).
No products indexed under this heading.

Food Interactions

Alcohol (Decreases the elimination of abacavir causing an increase in overall exposure).

ZICAM ALLERGY RELIEF
(Galphimia Glauca, Histanium Hydrochloricum, Luffa operculata, Sulfur) 774
None cited in PDR database.

ZICAM COLD REMEDY CHEWABLES
(Zincum Aceticum, Zincum Gluconicum) 766
None cited in PDR database.

ZICAM COLD REMEDY CHEWCAPS
(Zincum Aceticum, Zincum Gluconicum) 766
None cited in PDR database.

ZICAM COLD REMEDY GEL SWABS
(Zincum Gluconicum) 766
None cited in PDR database.

ZICAM COLD REMEDY NASAL GEL
(Zincum Gluconicum) 766
None cited in PDR database.

ZICAM COLD REMEDY ORAL MIST
(Zincum Aceticum, Zincum Gluconicum) 766
None cited in PDR database.

ZICAM COLD REMEDY RAPIDMELTS
(Zincum Aceticum, Zincum Gluconicum) 766
None cited in PDR database.

ZICAM COLD REMEDY RAPIDMELTS WITH VITAMIN C
(Zincum Aceticum, Zincum Gluconicum) 766
None cited in PDR database.

ZICAM COLD REMEDY SWABS KIDS SIZE
(Zincum Gluconicum) 766
None cited in PDR database.

ZICAM COUGH MAX NIGHTTIME COUGH SPRAY
(Dextromethorphan Hydrobromide) 767
May interact with monoamine oxidase inhibitors. Compounds in these categories include:

Isocarboxazid (Avoid concurrent use while taking, or for up to 2 weeks after stopping MAO inhibitors).
No products indexed under this heading.

Moclobemide (Avoid concurrent use while taking, or for up to 2 weeks after stopping MAO inhibitors).
No products indexed under this heading.

Pargyline Hydrochloride (Avoid concurrent use while taking, or for up to 2 weeks after stopping MAO inhibitors).
No products indexed under this heading.

Phenelzine Sulfate (Avoid concurrent use while taking, or for up to 2 weeks after stopping MAO inhibitors).
No products indexed under this heading.

Procarbazine Hydrochloride (Avoid concurrent use while taking, or for up to 2 weeks after stopping MAO inhibitors). Products include:
Matulane Capsules 3191

Selegiline Hydrochloride (Avoid concurrent use while taking, or for up to 2 weeks after stopping MAO inhibitors). Products include:
Eldepryl Capsules 3208
Zelapar Tablets 3372

Tranylcypromine Sulfate (Avoid concurrent use while taking, or for up to 2 weeks after stopping MAO inhibitors). Products include:
Parnate Tablets 1527

ZICAM COUGH MAX COUGH SPRAY
(Dextromethorphan Hydrobromide) 767
May interact with monoamine oxidase inhibitors. Compounds in these categories include:

Isocarboxazid (Avoid concurrent use while taking, or for up to 2 weeks after stopping MAO inhibitors).
No products indexed under this heading.

Moclobemide (Avoid concurrent use while taking, or for up to 2 weeks after stopping MAO inhibitors).
No products indexed under this heading.

Pargyline Hydrochloride (Avoid concurrent use while taking, or for up to 2 weeks after stopping MAO inhibitors).
No products indexed under this heading.

Phenelzine Sulfate (Avoid concurrent use while taking, or for up to 2 weeks after stopping MAO inhibitors).
No products indexed under this heading.

Procarbazine Hydrochloride (Avoid concurrent use while taking, or for up to 2 weeks after stopping MAO inhibitors). Products include:
Matulane Capsules 3191

Selegiline Hydrochloride (Avoid concurrent use while taking, or for up to 2 weeks after stopping MAO inhibitors). Products include:
Eldepryl Capsules 3208
Zelapar Tablets 3372

Tranylcypromine Sulfate (Avoid concurrent use while taking, or for up to 2 weeks after stopping MAO inhibitors). Products include:
Parnate Tablets 1527

ZICAM COUGH MAX COUGH MELTS
(Dextromethorphan Hydrobromide) 767
May interact with monoamine oxidase inhibitors. Compounds in these categories include:

Isocarboxazid (Avoid concurrent use while taking, or for up to 2 weeks after stopping MAO inhibitors).
No products indexed under this heading.

Moclobemide (Avoid concurrent use while taking, or for up to 2 weeks after stopping MAO inhibitors).
No products indexed under this heading.

Pargyline Hydrochloride (Avoid concurrent use while taking, or for up to 2 weeks after stopping MAO inhibitors).
No products indexed under this heading.

Phenelzine Sulfate (Avoid concurrent use while taking, or for up to 2 weeks after stopping MAO inhibitors).
No products indexed under this heading.

Procarbazine Hydrochloride (Avoid concurrent use while taking, or for up to 2 weeks after stopping MAO inhibitors). Products include:
Matulane Capsules 3191

Selegiline Hydrochloride (Avoid concurrent use while taking, or for up to 2 weeks after stopping MAO inhibitors). Products include:
Eldepryl Capsules 3208
Zelapar Tablets 3372

Tranylcypromine Sulfate (Avoid concurrent use while taking, or for up to 2 weeks after stopping MAO inhibitors). Products include:
Parnate Tablets 1527

ZICAM COUGH PLUS D COUGH SPRAY
(Dextromethorphan Hydrobromide, Phenylephrine Hydrochloride) 767
May interact with monoamine oxidase inhibitors. Compounds in these categories include:

Isocarboxazid (Avoid concurrent use while taking, or for up to 2 weeks after stopping MAO inhibitors).
No products indexed under this heading.

Moclobemide (Avoid concurrent use while taking, or for up to 2 weeks after stopping MAO inhibitors).
No products indexed under this heading.

Pargyline Hydrochloride (Avoid concurrent use while taking, or for up to 2 weeks after stopping MAO inhibitors).
No products indexed under this heading.

Phenelzine Sulfate (Avoid concurrent use while taking, or for up to 2 weeks after stopping MAO inhibitors).
No products indexed under this heading.

Procarbazine Hydrochloride (Avoid concurrent use while taking, or for up to 2 weeks after stopping MAO inhibitors). Products include:
Matulane Capsules 3191

Selegiline Hydrochloride (Avoid concurrent use while taking, or for up to 2 weeks after stopping MAO inhibitors). Products include:
Eldepryl Capsules 3208
Zelapar Tablets 3372

Tranylcypromine Sulfate (Avoid concurrent use while taking, or for up to 2 weeks after stopping MAO inhibitors). Products include:
Parnate Tablets 1527

ZICAM COUGH RELIEF COUGH SPRAY
(Dextromethorphan Hydrobromide)................................ ▣767
May interact with monoamine oxidase inhibitors. Compounds in these categories include:

Isocarboxazid (Avoid concurrent use while taking, or for up to 2 weeks after stopping MAO inhibitors).
No products indexed under this heading.

Moclobemide (Avoid concurrent use while taking, or for up to 2 weeks after stopping MAO inhibitors).
No products indexed under this heading.

Pargyline Hydrochloride (Avoid concurrent use while taking, or for up to 2 weeks after stopping MAO inhibitors).
No products indexed under this heading.

Phenelzine Sulfate (Avoid concurrent use while taking, or for up to 2 weeks after stopping MAO inhibitors).
No products indexed under this heading.

Procarbazine Hydrochloride (Avoid concurrent use while taking, or for up to 2 weeks after stopping MAO inhibitors). Products include:
Matulane Capsules 3191

Selegiline Hydrochloride (Avoid concurrent use while taking, or for up to 2 weeks after stopping MAO inhibitors). Products include:
Eldepryl Capsules 3208
Zelapar Tablets 3372

Tranylcypromine Sulfate (Avoid concurrent use while taking, or for up to 2 weeks after stopping MAO inhibitors). Products include:
Parnate Tablets 1527

ZICAM EXTREME CONGESTION RELIEF
(Oxymetazoline Hydrochloride) .... ▣767
None cited in PDR database.

ZICAM MAXIMUM STRENGTH FLU DAYTIME
(Acetaminophen, Chlorpheniramine Maleate, Dextromethorphan Hydrobromide).... ▣768
May interact with hypnotics and sedatives, monoamine oxidase inhibitors, tranquilizers, and certain other agents. Compounds in these categories include:

Alprazolam (Concurrent use may increase drowsiness). Products include:
Niravam Orally Disintegrating Tablets.. 3092

Buspirone Hydrochloride (Concurrent use may increase drowsiness).
No products indexed under this heading.

Chlordiazepoxide (Concurrent use may increase drowsiness).
No products indexed under this heading.

Chlordiazepoxide Hydrochloride (Concurrent use may increase drowsiness). Products include:
Librium Capsules 3347

Chlorpromazine (Concurrent use may increase drowsiness).
No products indexed under this heading.

Chlorpromazine Hydrochloride (Concurrent use may increase drowsiness).
No products indexed under this heading.

Chlorprothixene (Concurrent use may increase drowsiness).
No products indexed under this heading.

Chlorprothixene Hydrochloride (Concurrent use may increase drowsiness).
No products indexed under this heading.

Clorazepate Dipotassium (Concurrent use may increase drowsiness). Products include:
Tranxene 2474

Diazepam (Concurrent use may increase drowsiness). Products include:
Diastat Rectal Delivery System 3343
Valium Tablets 2819

Droperidol (Concurrent use may increase drowsiness).
No products indexed under this heading.

Estazolam (Concurrent use may increase drowsiness). Products include:
ProSom Tablets 517

Ethchlorvynol (Concurrent use may increase drowsiness).
No products indexed under this heading.

Ethinamate (Concurrent use may increase drowsiness).
No products indexed under this heading.

Fluphenazine Decanoate (Concurrent use may increase drowsiness).
No products indexed under this heading.

Fluphenazine Enanthate (Concurrent use may increase drowsiness).
No products indexed under this heading.

Fluphenazine Hydrochloride (Concurrent use may increase drowsiness).
No products indexed under this heading.

Flurazepam Hydrochloride (Concurrent use may increase drowsiness). Products include:
Dalmane Capsules 3342

Glutethimide (Concurrent use may increase drowsiness).
No products indexed under this heading.

Haloperidol (Concurrent use may increase drowsiness).
No products indexed under this heading.

Haloperidol Decanoate (Concurrent use may increase drowsiness).
No products indexed under this heading.

Hydroxyzine Hydrochloride (Concurrent use may increase drowsiness).
No products indexed under this heading.

Isocarboxazid (Do not use while taking, or 2 weeks after stopping, MAO inhibitors).
No products indexed under this heading.

Lorazepam (Concurrent use may increase drowsiness).
No products indexed under this heading.

Loxapine Hydrochloride (Concurrent use may increase drowsiness).
No products indexed under this heading.

Loxapine Succinate (Concurrent use may increase drowsiness).
No products indexed under this heading.

Meprobamate (Concurrent use may increase drowsiness).
No products indexed under this heading.

Mesoridazine Besylate (Concurrent use may increase drowsiness).
No products indexed under this heading.

Midazolam Hydrochloride (Concurrent use may increase drowsiness).
No products indexed under this heading.

Moclobemide (Do not use while taking, or 2 weeks after stopping, MAO inhibitors).
No products indexed under this heading.

Molindone Hydrochloride (Concurrent use may increase drowsiness). Products include:
Moban Tablets 1119

Oxazepam (Concurrent use may increase drowsiness).
No products indexed under this heading.

Pargyline Hydrochloride (Do not use while taking, or 2 weeks after stopping, MAO inhibitors).
No products indexed under this heading.

Perphenazine (Concurrent use may increase drowsiness).
No products indexed under this heading.

Phenelzine Sulfate (Do not use while taking, or 2 weeks after stopping, MAO inhibitors).
No products indexed under this heading.

Prazepam (Concurrent use may increase drowsiness).
No products indexed under this heading.

Procarbazine Hydrochloride (Do not use while taking, or 2 weeks after stopping, MAO inhibitors). Products include:
Matulane Capsules 3191

Prochlorperazine (Concurrent use may increase drowsiness).
No products indexed under this heading.

Promethazine Hydrochloride (Concurrent use may increase drowsiness). Products include:
Phenergan Tablets and Suppositories.............................. 3440

Propofol (Concurrent use may increase drowsiness).
No products indexed under this heading.

Quazepam (Concurrent use may increase drowsiness).
No products indexed under this heading.

Ramelteon (Concurrent use may increase drowsiness). Products include:
Rozerem Tablets 3231

Secobarbital Sodium (Concurrent use may increase drowsiness).
No products indexed under this heading.

Selegiline Hydrochloride (Do not use while taking, or 2 weeks after stopping, MAO inhibitors). Products include:
Eldepryl Capsules 3208
Zelapar Tablets 3372

Temazepam (Concurrent use may increase drowsiness). Products include:
Restoril Capsules 1860

Thioridazine Hydrochloride (Concurrent use may increase drowsiness). Products include:
Thioridazine Hydrochloride Tablets 2163

Thiothixene (Concurrent use may increase drowsiness). Products include:
Thiothixene Capsules 2165

Tranylcypromine Sulfate (Do not use while taking, or 2 weeks after stopping, MAO inhibitors). Products include:
Parnate Tablets 1527

Triazolam (Concurrent use may increase drowsiness).
No products indexed under this heading.

Trifluoperazine Hydrochloride (Concurrent use may increase drowsiness).
No products indexed under this heading.

Zaleplon (Concurrent use may increase drowsiness). Products include:
Sonata Capsules 1717

Zolpidem Tartrate (Concurrent use may increase drowsiness). Products include:
Ambien Tablets 2851
Ambien CR Tablets 2855

Food Interactions

Alcohol (Concurrent use may increase drowsiness; avoid alcoholic beverages).

ZICAM MAXIMUM STRENGTH FLU NIGHTTIME
(Acetaminophen, Dextromethorphan Hydrobromide, Doxylamine Succinate)..................... ▣768
May interact with hypnotics and sedatives, monoamine oxidase inhibitors, tranquilizers, and certain other agents. Compounds in these categories include:

Alprazolam (Concurrent use may increase drowsiness). Products include:
Niravam Orally Disintegrating Tablets.. 3092

Buspirone Hydrochloride (Concurrent use may increase drowsiness).
No products indexed under this heading.

Chlordiazepoxide (Concurrent use may increase drowsiness).
No products indexed under this heading.

Chlordiazepoxide Hydrochloride (Concurrent use may increase drowsiness). Products include:
Librium Capsules 3347

Chlorpromazine (Concurrent use may increase drowsiness).
No products indexed under this heading.

Chlorpromazine Hydrochloride (Concurrent use may increase drowsiness).
No products indexed under this heading.

Chlorprothixene (Concurrent use may increase drowsiness).
No products indexed under this heading.

Chlorprothixene Hydrochloride (Concurrent use may increase drowsiness).
No products indexed under this heading.

Clorazepate Dipotassium (Concurrent use may increase drowsiness). Products include:
Tranxene 2474

Diazepam (Concurrent use may increase drowsiness). Products include:
Diastat Rectal Delivery System 3343
Valium Tablets 2819

Droperidol (Concurrent use may increase drowsiness).
No products indexed under this heading.

Estazolam (Concurrent use may increase drowsiness). Products include:
ProSom Tablets 517

Ethchlorvynol (Concurrent use may increase drowsiness).
No products indexed under this heading.

Ethinamate (Concurrent use may increase drowsiness).
No products indexed under this heading.

Fluphenazine Decanoate (Concurrent use may increase drowsiness).
No products indexed under this heading.

Fluphenazine Enanthate (Concurrent use may increase drowsiness).
No products indexed under this heading.

Fluphenazine Hydrochloride (Concurrent use may increase drowsiness).
No products indexed under this heading.

Flurazepam Hydrochloride (Concurrent use may increase drowsiness). Products include:
Dalmane Capsules 3342

Glutethimide (Concurrent use may increase drowsiness).
No products indexed under this heading.

Haloperidol (Concurrent use may increase drowsiness).
No products indexed under this heading.

Haloperidol Decanoate (Concurrent use may increase drowsiness).
No products indexed under this heading.

Hydroxyzine Hydrochloride (Concurrent use may increase drowsiness).
No products indexed under this heading.

Isocarboxazid (Do not use while taking, or 2 weeks after stopping, MAO inhibitors).
No products indexed under this heading.

Lorazepam (Concurrent use may increase drowsiness).
No products indexed under this heading.

Loxapine Hydrochloride (Concurrent use may increase drowsiness).
No products indexed under this heading.

Loxapine Succinate (Concurrent use may increase drowsiness).
No products indexed under this heading.

Meprobamate (Concurrent use may increase drowsiness).
No products indexed under this heading.

Mesoridazine Besylate (Concurrent use may increase drowsiness).
No products indexed under this heading.

Midazolam Hydrochloride (Concurrent use may increase drowsiness).
No products indexed under this heading.

Moclobemide (Do not use while taking, or 2 weeks after stopping, MAO inhibitors).
No products indexed under this heading.

Molindone Hydrochloride (Concurrent use may increase drowsiness). Products include:
Moban Tablets 1119

Oxazepam (Concurrent use may increase drowsiness).
No products indexed under this heading.

Pargyline Hydrochloride (Do not use while taking, or 2 weeks after stopping, MAO inhibitors).
No products indexed under this heading.

Perphenazine (Concurrent use may increase drowsiness).
No products indexed under this heading.

Phenelzine Sulfate (Do not use while taking, or 2 weeks after stopping, MAO inhibitors).
No products indexed under this heading.

Prazepam (Concurrent use may increase drowsiness).
No products indexed under this heading.

Procarbazine Hydrochloride (Do not use while taking, or 2 weeks after stopping, MAO inhibitors). Products include:
Matulane Capsules 3191

Prochlorperazine (Concurrent use may increase drowsiness).
No products indexed under this heading.

Promethazine Hydrochloride (Concurrent use may increase drowsiness). Products include:
Phenergan Tablets and Suppositories 3440

Propofol (Concurrent use may increase drowsiness).
No products indexed under this heading.

Quazepam (Concurrent use may increase drowsiness).
No products indexed under this heading.

Ramelteon (Concurrent use may increase drowsiness). Products include:
Rozerem Tablets 3231

Secobarbital Sodium (Concurrent use may increase drowsiness).
No products indexed under this heading.

Selegiline Hydrochloride (Do not use while taking, or 2 weeks after stopping, MAO inhibitors). Products include:
Eldepryl Capsules 3208
Zelapar Tablets 3372

Temazepam (Concurrent use may increase drowsiness). Products include:
Restoril Capsules 1860

Thioridazine Hydrochloride (Concurrent use may increase drowsiness). Products include:
Thioridazine Hydrochloride Tablets 2163

Thiothixene (Concurrent use may increase drowsiness). Products include:
Thiothixene Capsules 2165

Tranylcypromine Sulfate (Do not use while taking, or 2 weeks after stopping, MAO inhibitors). Products include:
Parnate Tablets 1527

Triazolam (Concurrent use may increase drowsiness).
No products indexed under this heading.

Trifluoperazine Hydrochloride (Concurrent use may increase drowsiness).
No products indexed under this heading.

Zaleplon (Concurrent use may increase drowsiness). Products include:
Sonata Capsules 1717

Zolpidem Tartrate (Concurrent use may increase drowsiness). Products include:
Ambien Tablets 2851
Ambien CR Tablets 2855

Food Interactions

Alcohol (Concurrent use may increase drowsiness; avoid alcoholic beverages).

ZICAM INTENSE SINUS RELIEF

(Oxymetazoline Hydrochloride) .... ▣767
None cited in PDR database.

ZINACEF FOR INJECTION

(Cefuroxime) 1631
See Zinacef Injection

ZINACEF INJECTION

(Cefuroxime) 1631
May interact with aminoglycosides, oral anticoagulants, and certain other agents. Compounds in these categories include:

Amikacin Sulfate (Concomitant administration may produce nephrotoxicity).
No products indexed under this heading.

Anisindione (Cephalosporins may be associated with a fall in prothrombin activity; those at risk include patients stabilized on anticoagulants). Products include:
Miradon Tablets 3042

Dicumarol (Cephalosporins may be associated with a fall in prothrombin activity; those at risk include patients stabilized on anticoagulants).
No products indexed under this heading.

Gentamicin Sulfate (Concomitant administration may produce nephrotoxicity). Products include:
Garamycin Injectable 3014
Pred-G Ophthalmic Ointment .... ⊙237
Pred-G Ophthalmic Suspension ...... ⊙236

Kanamycin Sulfate (Concomitant administration may produce nephrotoxicity).
No products indexed under this heading.

Probenecid (Concurrent administration of probenecid decreases renal clearance and increases peak serum levels of cefuroxime).
No products indexed under this heading.

Streptomycin Sulfate (Concomitant administration may produce nephrotoxicity).
No products indexed under this heading.

Tobramycin (Concomitant administration may produce nephrotoxicity). Products include:
TOBI Solution for Inhalation 2298
TobraDex Ophthalmic Ointment 562
TobraDex Ophthalmic Suspension ... 563
Zylet Ophthalmic Suspension .... ⊙259

Tobramycin Sulfate (Concomitant administration may produce nephrotoxicity).
No products indexed under this heading.

Warfarin Sodium (Cephalosporins may be associated with a fall in prothrombin activity; those at risk include patients stabilized on anticoagulants). Products include:
Coumadin for Injection 898
Coumadin Tablets 898

ZINC-220 CAPSULES

(Zinc Sulfate) 580
None cited in PDR database.

ZINECARD FOR INJECTION

(Dexrazoxane) 2650
May interact with antineoplastics and certain other agents. Compounds in these categories include:

Altretamine (Dexrazoxane may add to the myelosuppression caused by chemotherapeutic agents).
No products indexed under this heading.

Anastrozole (Dexrazoxane may add to the myelosuppression caused by chemotherapeutic agents). Products include:
Arimidex Tablets 673

Asparaginase (Dexrazoxane may add to the myelosuppression caused by chemotherapeutic agents). Products include:
Elspar for Injection 2463
Elspar for Injection 1960

Bicalutamide (Dexrazoxane may add to the myelosuppression caused by chemotherapeutic agents).
No products indexed under this heading.

Bleomycin Sulfate (Dexrazoxane may add to the myelosuppression caused by chemotherapeutic agents).
No products indexed under this heading.

Busulfan (Dexrazoxane may add to the myelosuppression caused by chemotherapeutic agents). Products include:
I.V. Busulfex 2493
Myleran Tablets 1525

Carboplatin (Dexrazoxane may add to the myelosuppression caused by chemotherapeutic agents).
No products indexed under this heading.

Carmustine (BCNU) (Dexrazoxane may add to the myelosuppression caused by chemotherapeutic agents).
No products indexed under this heading.

Chlorambucil (Dexrazoxane may add to the myelosuppression caused by chemotherapeutic agents). Products include:
Leukeran Tablets 1504

Cisplatin (Dexrazoxane may add to the myelosuppression caused by chemotherapeutic agents).
No products indexed under this heading.

Cyclophosphamide (Use of dexrazoxane concurrently with the initiation of fluorouracil, doxorubicin and cyclophosphamide (FAC) therapy may interfere with the antitumor efficacy of the regimen).
No products indexed under this heading.

Dacarbazine (Dexrazoxane may add to the myelosuppression caused by chemotherapeutic agents).
No products indexed under this heading.

Daunorubicin Citrate (Use of dexrazoxane concurrently with the initiation of fluorouracil, doxorubicin and cyclophosphamide (FAC) therapy may interfere with the antitumor efficacy of the regimen).
No products indexed under this heading.

Daunorubicin Hydrochloride (Dexrazoxane may add to the myelosuppression caused by chemotherapeutic agents).
No products indexed under this heading.

Denileukin Diftitox (Dexrazoxane may add to the myelosuppression caused by chemotherapeutic agents). Products include:
Ontak Vials 1745

Docetaxel (Dexrazoxane may add to the myelosuppression caused by chemotherapeutic agents). Products include:
Taxotere Injection Concentrate 2932

Doxorubicin Hydrochloride (Use of dexrazoxane concurrently with the initiation of fluorouracil, doxorubicin and cyclophosphamide (FAC) therapy may interfere with the antitumor efficacy of the regimen).
No products indexed under this heading.

Epirubicin Hydrochloride (Dexrazoxane may add to the myelosuppression caused by chemotherapeutic agents).
No products indexed under this heading.

Estramustine Phosphate Sodium (Dexrazoxane may add to the myelosuppression caused by chemotherapeutic agents). Products include:
Emcyt Capsules 2634

Etoposide (Dexrazoxane may add to the myelosuppression caused by chemotherapeutic agents).
No products indexed under this heading.

Exemestane (Dexrazoxane may add to the myelosuppression caused by chemotherapeutic agents). Products include:
Aromasin Tablets 2600

Floxuridine (Dexrazoxane may add to the myelosuppression caused by chemotherapeutic agents).
No products indexed under this heading.

Fluorouracil (Use of dexrazoxane concurrently with the initiation of fluorouracil, doxorubicin and cyclophosphamide (FAC) therapy may interfere with the antitumor efficacy of the regimen). Products include:
Carac Cream, 0.5% 2879
Efudex 3363

Flutamide (Dexrazoxane may add to the myelosuppression caused by chemotherapeutic agents). Products include:
Eulexin Capsules 3009

Gemcitabine Hydrochloride (Dexrazoxane may add to the myelosuppression caused by chemotherapeutic agents). Products include:
Gemzar for Injection 1771

Hydroxyurea (Dexrazoxane may add to the myelosuppression caused by chemotherapeutic agents).
No products indexed under this heading.

Idarubicin Hydrochloride (Dexrazoxane may add to the myelosuppression caused by chemotherapeutic agents).
No products indexed under this heading.

Ifosfamide (Dexrazoxane may add to the myelosuppression caused by chemotherapeutic agents).
No products indexed under this heading.

Interferon alfa-2a, Recombinant (Dexrazoxane may add to the myelosuppression caused by chemotherapeutic agents).
No products indexed under this heading.

Interferon alfa-2b, Recombinant (Dexrazoxane may add to the myelosuppression caused by chemotherapeutic agents). Products include:
Intron A for Injection 3024
Rebetron Combination Therapy 3063

Irinotecan Hydrochloride (Dexrazoxane may add to the myelosuppression caused by chemotherapeutic agents). Products include:
Camptosar Injection 2604

Levamisole Hydrochloride (Dexrazoxane may add to the myelosuppression caused by chemotherapeutic agents).
No products indexed under this heading.

Lomustine (CCNU) (Dexrazoxane may add to the myelosuppression caused by chemotherapeutic agents).
No products indexed under this heading.

Mechlorethamine Hydrochloride (Dexrazoxane may add to the myelosuppression caused by chemotherapeutic agents). Products include:
Mustargen for Injection 2468

Megestrol Acetate (Dexrazoxane may add to the myelosuppression caused by chemotherapeutic agents). Products include:
Megace ES Oral Suspension 2481

Melphalan (Dexrazoxane may add to the myelosuppression caused by chemotherapeutic agents). Products include:
Alkeran Tablets 956

Mercaptopurine (Dexrazoxane may add to the myelosuppression caused by chemotherapeutic agents).
No products indexed under this heading.

Methotrexate Sodium (Dexrazoxane may add to the myelosuppression caused by chemotherapeutic agents).
No products indexed under this heading.

Mitomycin (Mitomycin-C) (Dexrazoxane may add to the myelosuppression caused by chemotherapeutic agents).
No products indexed under this heading.

Mitotane (Dexrazoxane may add to the myelosuppression caused by chemotherapeutic agents).
No products indexed under this heading.

Mitoxantrone Hydrochloride (Dexrazoxane may add to the myelosuppression caused by chemotherapeutic agents).
No products indexed under this heading.

Paclitaxel (Dexrazoxane may add to the myelosuppression caused by chemotherapeutic agents).
No products indexed under this heading.

Procarbazine Hydrochloride (Dexrazoxane may add to the myelosuppression caused by chemotherapeutic agents). Products include:
Matulane Capsules 3191

Streptozocin (Dexrazoxane may add to the myelosuppression caused by chemotherapeutic agents).
No products indexed under this heading.

Tamoxifen Citrate (Dexrazoxane may add to the myelosuppression caused by chemotherapeutic agents). Products include:
Soltamox Oral Solution 3527

Teniposide (Dexrazoxane may add to the myelosuppression caused by chemotherapeutic agents).
No products indexed under this heading.

Thioguanine (Dexrazoxane may add to the myelosuppression caused by chemotherapeutic agents). Products include:
Tabloid Tablets 1575

Thiotepa (Dexrazoxane may add to the myelosuppression caused by chemotherapeutic agents).
No products indexed under this heading.

Topotecan Hydrochloride (Dexrazoxane may add to the myelosuppression caused by chemotherapeutic agents). Products include:
Hycamtin for Injection 1458

Toremifene Citrate (Dexrazoxane may add to the myelosuppression caused by chemotherapeutic agents).
No products indexed under this heading.

Valrubicin (Dexrazoxane may add to the myelosuppression caused by chemotherapeutic agents).
No products indexed under this heading.

Vincristine Sulfate (Dexrazoxane may add to the myelosuppression caused by chemotherapeutic agents).
No products indexed under this heading.

Vinorelbine Tartrate (Dexrazoxane may add to the myelosuppression caused by chemotherapeutic agents).
No products indexed under this heading.

ZMAX FOR ORAL SUSPENSION

(Azithromycin) 2583
May interact with phenytoin and certain other agents. Compounds in these categories include:

Cyclosporine (Carefully monitor cyclosporine concentrations when used concomitantly with azithromycin). Products include:
Gengraf Capsules 459
Neoral Oral Solution 2259
Neoral Soft Gelatin Capsules 2259
Restasis Ophthalmic Emulsion 575
Sandimmune 2275

Digoxin (Caution is advised since macrolide antibiotics elevate digoxin serum levels). Products include:
Lanoxicaps Capsules 1490
Lanoxin Injection 1494
Lanoxin Injection Pediatric 1497
Lanoxin Tablets 1500

Dihydroergotamine Mesylate (Carefully monitor patients taking dihydroergotamine and azithromycin concomitantly, due to acute ergot toxicity characterized by severe peripheral vasospams and dysesthesia). Products include:
Migranal Nasal Spray 3348

Ergotamine Tartrate (Carefully monitor patients taking ergotamine and azithromycin concomitantly, due to acute ergot toxicity characterized by severe peripheral vasospams and dysesthesia).
No products indexed under this heading.

Fosphenytoin Sodium (Carefully monitor phenytoin concentrations when used concomitantly with azithromycin).
No products indexed under this heading.

Hexobarbital (Carefully monitor hexobarbital concentrations when used concomitantly with azithromycin).
No products indexed under this heading.

Nelfinavir Mesylate (Co-administration of nelfinavir at steady-state with a single dose of azithromycin (2 x 600 mg tablets) results in increased azithromycin serum concentrations. Although a dose adjustment of azithromycin is not recommended when administered in combination with nelfinavir, close monitoring for known side effects of azithromycin, such as liver enzyme abnormalties and hearing impairment, is warranted). Products include:
Viracept 2577

Phenytoin (Carefully monitor phenytoin concentrations when used concomitantly with azithromycin).
No products indexed under this heading.

Phenytoin Sodium (Carefully monitor phenytoin concentrations when used concomitantly with azithromycin). Products include:
Phenytek Capsules 2160

Warfarin Sodium (Azithromycin did not affect the prothrombin time response to a single dose of warfarin. However, prudent medical practice dictates careful monitoring of prothrombin time in all patients treated with azithromycin and warfarin concomitantly. Concurrent use of macrolides and warfarin in clinical practice has been associated with increased anticoagulant effects). Products include:

Coumadin for Injection 898
Coumadin Tablets 898

ZOCOR TABLETS
(Simvastatin) 2105
May interact with azole antifungals, oral anticoagulants, cytochrome p450 3a inhibitors (selected), erythromycin, fibrates, protease inhibitors, and certain other agents. Compounds in these categories include:

Amiodarone Hydrochloride (Co-administration has resulted in myopathy, especially in patients on a higher dose of simvastatin; the dose of simvastatin should not exceed 20 mg daily in patients on concomitant amiodarone).
No products indexed under this heading.

Amprenavir (Description: Potent inhibators of CYP3A4 can raise the plasma levels of HMG-CoA reductase inhibitory activity and increase the risk of myopathy and rhabdomyolysis, particulary with higher doses of simvastin). Products include:
Agenerase Capsules 1327
Agenerase Oral Solution 1332

Anisindione (Simvastatin modestly potentiates the effect of coumarin anticoagulants; the prothrombin time is increased from baseline). Products include:
Miradon Tablets 3042

Aprepitant (Description: Potent inhibators of CYP3A4 can raise the plasma levels of HMG-CoA reductase inhibitory activity and increase the risk of myopathy and rhabdomyolysis, particulary with higher doses of simvastin). Products include:
Emend Capsules 1963

Cimetidine (Description: Potent inhibators of CYP3A4 can raise the plasma levels of HMG-CoA reductase inhibitory activity and increase the risk of myopathy and rhabdomyolysis, particulary with higher doses of simvastin). Products include:
Tagamet HB 200 Tablets 664

Cimetidine Hydrochloride (Description: Potent inhibators of CYP3A4 can raise the plasma levels of HMG-CoA reductase inhibitory activity and increase the risk of myopathy and rhabdomyolysis, particulary with higher doses of simvastin).
No products indexed under this heading.

Ciprofloxacin (Description: Potent inhibators of CYP3A4 can raise the plasma levels of HMG-CoA reductase inhibitory activity and increase the risk of myopathy and rhabdomyolysis, particulary with higher doses of simvastin). Products include:
Cipro Oral Suspension 2977
Cipro I.V. 2984
Cipro XR Tablets 2990
Ciprodex Otic Suspension 559

Ciprofloxacin Hydrochloride (Description: Potent inhibators of CYP3A4 can raise the plasma levels of HMG-CoA reductase inhibitory activity and increase the risk of myopathy and rhabdomyolysis, particulary with higher doses of simvastin). Products include:
Ciloxan Ophthalmic Ointment 559
Ciloxan Ophthalmic Solution .... ⊙ 206
Cipro Tablets 2977
Proquin XR Tablets 1153

Clarithromycin (Simvastatin is metabolized by CYP3A4; co-administration with potent inhibitors of CYP3A4, such as clarithromycin increases the risk of myopathy by reducing the elimination of simvastatin; concurrent use should be avoided). Products include:
Biaxin/Biaxin XL 402
PREVPAC 3284

Clofibrate (The incidence and severity of myopathy are increased by co-administration of HMG-CoA reductase inhibitors with drugs that cause myopathy when given alone, such as fibrates. In patients on concomitant fibrates, the dose of simvastatin should generally not exceed 10 mg/day).
No products indexed under this heading.

Clotrimazole (The risk of myopathy appears to be increased by high levels of HMG-CoA reductase inhibitory activity and the drugs that share the same metabolic pathways as simvastatin, such as antifungal azoles, can raise the plasma levels of simvastatin and may increase the risk of myopathy). Products include:
Desenex Athlete's Foot Cream 635
Lotrimin 3039
Lotrisone 3040

Cyclosporine (The risk of myopathy appears to be increased by high levels of HMG-CoA reductase inhibitory activity and the drugs that share the same metabolic pathways as simvastatin, such as cyclosporine, can raise the plasma levels of simvastatin and may increase the risk of myopathy; in patients on concomitant cyclosporine, the dose of simvastatin should begin with 5 mg/day and not exceed 10 mg/day). Products include:
Gengraf Capsules 459
Neoral Oral Solution 2259
Neoral Soft Gelatin Capsules 2259
Restasis Ophthalmic Emulsion 575
Sandimmune 2275

Danazol (The risk of myopathy/rhabdomyolysis is increased by concomitant administration of danazol, particularly with higher doses of simvastatin. The does of simvastatin should not exceed 10 mg daily in patients receiving concomitant medication with danazol).
No products indexed under this heading.

Delavirdine Mesylate (Description: Potent inhibators of CYP3A4 can raise the plasma levels of HMG-CoA reductase inhibitory activity and increase the risk of myopathy and rhabdomyolysis, particulary with higher doses of simvastin). Products include:
Rescriptor Tablets 2551

Dicumarol (Simvastatin modestly potentiates the effect of coumarin anticoagulants; the prothrombin time is increased from baseline).
No products indexed under this heading.

Digoxin (Slight elevation in digoxin plasma levels; patients taking digoxin should be monitored appropriately when simvastatin is initiated). Products include:
Lanoxicaps Capsules 1490
Lanoxin Injection 1494
Lanoxin Injection Pediatric 1497
Lanoxin Tablets 1500

Diltiazem Hydrochloride (Description: Potent inhibators of CYP3A4 can raise the plasma levels of HMG-CoA reductase inhibitory activity and increase the risk of myopathy and rhabdomyolysis, particulary with higher doses of simvastin). Products include:
Cardizem LA Extended Release Tablets 1728
Tiazac Capsules 1201

Diltiazem Maleate (Description: Potent inhibators of CYP3A4 can raise the plasma levels of HMG-CoA reductase inhibitory activity and increase the risk of myopathy and rhabdomyolysis, particulary with higher doses of simvastin).
No products indexed under this heading.

Efavirenz (Description: Potent inhibators of CYP3A4 can raise the plasma levels of HMG-CoA reductase inhibitory activity and increase the risk of myopathy and rhabdomyolysis, particulary with higher doses of simvastin). Products include:
Atripla Tablets 945
Sustiva Capsules 930
Sustiva Tablets 930

Erythromycin (Simvastatin is metabolized by CYP3A4; co-administration with potent inhibitors of CYP3A4, such as erythromycin, increases the risk of myopathy by reducing the elimination of simvastatin; concurrent use should be avoided). Products include:
Ery-Tab Tablets 449
Erythromycin Base Filmtab Tablets 455
Erythromycin Delayed-Release Capsules, USP 457
PCE Dispertab Tablets 515

Erythromycin Estolate (Simvastatin is metabolized by CYP3A4; co-administration with potent inhibitors of CYP3A4, such as erythromycin, increases the risk of myopathy by reducing the elimination of simvastatin; concurrent use should be avoided).
No products indexed under this heading.

Erythromycin Ethylsuccinate (Simvastatin is metabolized by CYP3A4; co-administration with potent inhibitors of CYP3A4, such as erythromycin, increases the risk of myopathy by reducing the elimination of simvastatin; concurrent use should be avoided). Products include:
E.E.S. 451
EryPed 447

Erythromycin Gluceptate (Simvastatin is metabolized by CYP3A4; co-administration with potent inhibitors of CYP3A4, such as erythromycin, increases the risk of myopathy by reducing the elimination of simvastatin; concurrent use should be avoided).
No products indexed under this heading.

Erythromycin Lactobionate (Simvastatin is metabolized by CYP3A4; co-administration with potent inhibitors of CYP3A4, such as erythromycin, increases the risk of myopathy by reducing the elimination of simvastatin; concurrent use should be avoided).
No products indexed under this heading.

Erythromycin Stearate (Simvastatin is metabolized by CYP3A4; co-administration with potent inhibitors of CYP3A4, such as erythromycin, increases the risk of myopathy by reducing the elimination of simvastatin; concurrent use should be avoided). Products include:
Erythrocin Stearate Filmtab Tablets 453

Fenofibrate (The incidence and severity of myopathy are increased by co-administration of HMG-CoA reductase inhibitors with drugs that cause myopathy when given alone, such as fibrates. In patients on concomitant fibrates, the dose of simvastatin should generally not exceed 10 mg/day). Products include:
Lofibra Tablets 1219
Lofibra Capsules 1216
Tricor Tablets 527
Triglide Tablets 3123

Fluconazole (The risk of myopathy appears to be increased by high levels of HMG-CoA reductase inhibitory activity and the drugs that share the same metabolic pathways as simvastatin, such as antifungal azoles, can raise the plasma levels of simvastatin and may increase the risk of myopathy).
No products indexed under this heading.

Fluoxetine (Description: Potent inhibators of CYP3A4 can raise the plasma levels of HMG-CoA reductase inhibitory activity and increase the risk of myopathy and rhabdomyolysis, particulary with higher doses of simvastin).
No products indexed under this heading.

Fluoxetine Hydrochloride (Description: Potent inhibators of CYP3A4 can raise the plasma levels of HMG-CoA reductase inhibitory activity and increase the risk of myopathy and rhabdomyolysis, particulary with higher doses of simvastin). Products include:
Prozac Pulvules and Liquid 1801
Symbyax Capsules 1819

Fluvoxamine Maleate (Description: Potent inhibators of CYP3A4 can raise the plasma levels of HMG-CoA reductase inhibitory activity and increase the risk of myopathy and rhabdomyolysis, particulary with higher doses of simvastin).
No products indexed under this heading.

Gemfibrozil (The incidence and severity of myopathy are increased by co-administration of HMG-CoA reductase inhibitors with drugs that cause myopathy when given alone, such as fibrates. In patients on concomitant fibrates, the dose of simvastatin should generally not exceed 10 mg/day).
No products indexed under this heading.

Indinavir Sulfate (Description: Potent inhibators of CYP3A4 can raise the plasma levels of HMG-CoA reductase inhibitory activity and increase the risk of myopathy and rhabdomyolysis, particulary with higher doses of simvastin). Products include:
Crixivan Capsules 1940

Isoniazid (Description: Potent inhibators of CYP3A4 can raise the plasma levels of HMG-CoA reductase inhibitory activity and increase the risk of myopathy and rhabdomyolysis, particulary with higher doses of simvastin).
No products indexed under this heading.

Itraconazole (Simvastatin is metabolized by CYP3A4; co-administration with potent inhibitors of CYP3A4, such as itraconazole, increases the risk of myopathy by reducing the elimination of simvastatin; concurrent use should be avoided).

No products indexed under this heading.

Ketoconazole (Simvastatin is metabolized by CYP3A4; co-administration with potent inhibitors of CYP3A4, such as ketoconazole, increases the risk of myopathy by reducing the elimination of simvastatin; concurrent use should be avoided). Products include:

Nizoral A-D Shampoo, 1% 1868

Lopinavir (Description: Potent inhibators of CYP3A4 can raise the plasma levels of HMG-CoA reductase inhibitory activity and increase the risk of myopathy and rhabdomyolysis, particulary with higher doses of simvastin). Products include:

Kaletra ... 476

Metronidazole (Description: Potent inhibators of CYP3A4 can raise the plasma levels of HMG-CoA reductase inhibitory activity and increase the risk of myopathy and rhabdomyolysis, particulary with higher doses of simvastin). Products include:

Metrogel 1% 1211
MetroGel-Vaginal Gel 1855
Vandazole Vaginal Gel 3338

Metronidazole Benzoate (Description: Potent inhibators of CYP3A4 can raise the plasma levels of HMG-CoA reductase inhibitory activity and increase the risk of myopathy and rhabdomyolysis, particulary with higher doses of simvastin).

No products indexed under this heading.

Metronidazole Hydrochloride (Description: Potent inhibitors of CYP3A4 can raise the plasma levels of HMG-CoA reductase inhibitory activity and increase the risk of myopathy and rhabdomyolysis, particulary with higher doses of simvastin).

No products indexed under this heading.

Miconazole (The risk of myopathy appears to be increased by high levels of HMG-CoA reductase inhibitory activity and the drugs that share the same metabolic pathways as simvastatin, such as antifungal azoles, can raise the plasma levels of simvastatin and may increase the risk of myopathy).

No products indexed under this heading.

Nefazodone Hydrochloride (Simvastatin is metabolized by CYP3A4; co-administration with potent inhibitors of CYP3A4, such as nefazodone, increases the risk of myopathy by reducing the elimination of simvastatin; concurrent use should be avoided).

No products indexed under this heading.

Nelfinavir Mesylate (Description: Potent inhibitors of CYP3A4 can raise the plasma levels of HMG-CoA reductase inhibitory activity and increase the risk of myopathy and rhabdomyolysis, particulary with higher doses of simvastin). Products include:

Viracept ... 2577

Niacin (The incidence and severity of myopathy are increased by co-administration of HMG-CoA reductase inhibitors with drugs that cause myopathy when given alone, such as lipid-lowering doses of niacin (greater than or equal to 1g/day); in patients on concomitant niacin, the dose of simvastatin should generally not exceed 10 mg). Products include:

Advicor Tablets 1722
Niaspan Extended-Release
Tablets ... 1730

Nifedipine (Description: Potent inhibators of CYP3A4 can raise the plasma levels of HMG-CoA reductase inhibitory activity and increase the risk of myopathy and rhabdomyolysis, particulary with higher doses of simvastin). Products include:

Adalat CC Tablets 2964

Norfloxacin (Description: Potent inhibitors of CYP3A4 can raise the plasma levels of HMG-CoA reductase inhibitory activity and increase the risk of myopathy and rhabdomyolysis, particulary with higher doses of simvastin). Products include:

Noroxin Tablets 2032

Oxiconazole Nitrate (The risk of myopathy appears to be increased by high levels of HMG-CoA reductase inhibitory activity and the drugs that share the same metabolic pathways as simvastatin, such as antifungal azoles, can raise the plasma levels of simvastatin and may increase the risk of myopathy). Products include:

Oxistat ... 2667

Paroxetine Hydrochloride (Description: Potent inhibitors of CYP3A4 can raise the plasma levels of HMG-CoA reductase inhibitory activity and increase the risk of myopathy and rhabdomyolysis, particulary with higher doses of simvastin). Products include:

Paxil CR Controlled-Release
Tablets ... 1538
Paxil ... 1530

Propranolol Hydrochloride (Significant decreases in mean Cmax, but no change in AUC). Products include:

Inderal LA Long-Acting Capsules 3429
InnoPran XL Capsules 2723

Quinine (Description: Potent inhibitors of CYP3A4 can raise the plasma levels of HMG-CoA reductase inhibitory activity and increase the risk of myopathy and rhabdomyolysis, particulary with higher doses of simvastin).

No products indexed under this heading.

Quinine Sulfate (Description: Potent inhibitors of CYP3A4 can raise the plasma levels of HMG-CoA reductase inhibitory activity and increase the risk of myopathy and rhabdomyolysis, particulary with higher doses of simvastin). Products include:

No products indexed under this heading.

Ritonavir (Description: Potent inhibators of CYP3A4 can raise the plasma levels of HMG-CoA reductase inhibitory activity and increase the risk of myopathy and rhabdomyolysis, particulary with higher doses of simvastin). Products include:

Kaletra ... 476
Norvir ... 503

Saquinavir (Description: Potent inhibitors of CYP3A4 can raise the plasma levels of HMG-CoA reductase inhibitory activity and increase the risk of myopathy and rhabdomyolysis, particulary with higher doses of simvastin).

No products indexed under this heading.

Saquinavir Mesylate (Description: Potent inhibitors of CYP3A4 can raise the plasma levels of HMG-CoA reductase inhibitory activity and increase the risk of myopathy and rhabdomyolysis, particulary with higher doses of simvastin). Products include:

Invirase ... 2772

Sertraline Hydrochloride (Description: Potent inhibitors of CYP3A4 can raise the plasma levels of HMG-CoA reductase inhibitory activity and increase the risk of myopathy and rhabdomyolysis, particulary with higher doses of simvastin). Products include:

Zoloft ... 2586

Telithromycin (Simvastatin is metabolized by CYP3A4; co-administration with potent inhibitors of CYP3A4, such as telithromycin, increases the risk of myopathy by reducing the elimination of simvastatin; concurrent use should be avoided). Products include:

Ketek Tablets 2903

Terconazole (The risk of myopathy appears to be increased by high levels of HMG-CoA reductase inhibitory activity and the drugs that share the same metabolic pathways as simvastatin, such as antifungal azoles, can raise the plasma levels of simvastatin and may increase the risk of myopathy).

No products indexed under this heading.

Troleandomycin (Description: Potent inhibitors of CYP3A4 can raise the plasma levels of HMG-CoA reductase inhibitory activity and increase the risk of myopathy and rhabdomyolysis, particulary with higher doses of simvastin).

No products indexed under this heading.

Venlafaxine Hydrochloride (Description: Potent inhibitors of CYP3A4 can raise the plasma levels of HMG-CoA reductase inhibitory activity and increase the risk of myopathy and rhabdomyolysis, particulary with higher doses of simvastin). Products include:

Effexor Tablets 3411
Effexor XR Capsules 3417

Verapamil Hydrochloride (Co-administration has resulted in myopathy, especially in patients on a higher dose of simvastatin; the dose of simvastatin should not exceed 20 mg daily in patients on concomitant verapamil). Products include:

Covera-HS Tablets 3139
Tarka Tablets 524
Verelan PM Extended-Release
Capsules, Controlled-Onset.......... 3106

Voriconazole (Description: Potent inhibitors of CYP3A4 can raise the plasma levels of HMG-CoA reductase inhibitory activity and increase the risk of myopathy and rhabdomyolysis, particulary with higher doses of simvastin). Products include:

VFEND I.V. 2564
VFEND Oral Suspension 2564
VFEND Tablets 2564

Warfarin Sodium (Simvastatin modestly potentiates the effect of coumarin anticoagulants; the prothrombin time is increased from baseline). Products include:

Coumadin for Injection 898
Coumadin Tablets 898

Zafirlukast (Description: Potent inhibitors of CYP3A4 can raise the plasma levels of HMG-CoA reductase inhibitory activity and increase the risk of myopathy and rhabdomyolysis, particulary with higher doses of simvastin). Products include:

Accolate Tablets 671

Zileuton (Description: Potent inhibitors of CYP3A4 can raise the plasma levels of HMG-CoA reductase inhibitory activity and increase the risk of myopathy and rhabdomyolysis, particulary with higher doses of simvastin). Products include:

Zyflo Tablets 1023

Food Interactions

Alcohol (Simvastatin causes persistent increases in serum transaminase in 1% of patients; therefore, it should be used with caution in patients who consume substantial quantities of alcohol).

Grapefruit (Description: Potent inhibators of CYP3A4 can raise the plasma levels of HMG-CoA reductase inhibitory activity and increase the risk of myopathy and rhabdomyolysis, particularly with higher doses of simvastin).

Grapefruit Juice (Simvastatin is a substrate for CYP4503A4 and grapefruit juice contains one or more components that inhibit CYP3A4; co-administration with grapefruit juice can increase the plasma concentrations of simvastatin and its B-hydroxyacid metabolite; large quantities of grapefruit juice (>1 quart daily) significantly increase the serum concentrations and should be avoided).

ZOFRAN INJECTION
(Ondansetron Hydrochloride) 1634
See Zofran Tablets

ZOFRAN INJECTION PREMIXED
(Ondansetron Hydrochloride) 1634
See Zofran Tablets

ZOFRAN ORAL SOLUTION
(Ondansetron Hydrochloride) 1639
See Zofran Tablets

ZOFRAN TABLETS
(Ondansetron Hydrochloride) 1639
May interact with phenytoin and certain other agents. Compounds in these categories include:

Carbamazepine (Co-administration with potent inducers of CYP3A4, such as carbamazepine, may increase the clearance and decrease ondansetron blood concentrations; based on available data, no dosage adjustment is recommended). Products include:

Carbatrol Capsules 3171
Equetro Extended-Release
Capsules....................................... 3180
Tegretol/Tegretol-XR 2295

Fosphenytoin Sodium (Co-administration with potent inducers of CYP3A4, such as phenytoin, may increase the clearance and decrease ondansetron blood concentrations; based on the available data, no dosage adjustment is recommended).

No products indexed under this heading.

Phenytoin (Co-administration with potent inducers of CYP3A4, such as phenytoin, may increase the clearance and decrease ondansetron blood concentrations; based on the available data, no dosage adjustment is recommended).
No products indexed under this heading.

Phenytoin Sodium (Co-administration with potent inducers of CYP3A4, such as phenytoin, may increase the clearance and decrease ondansetron blood concentrations; based on the available data, no dosage adjustment is recommended). Products include:
Phenytek Capsules 2160

Rifampin (Co-administration with potent inducers of CYP3A4, such as rifampin, may increase the clearance and decrease ondansetron blood concentrations; based on available data, no dosage adjustment is recommended).
No products indexed under this heading.

Tramadol Hydrochloride (Ondansetron may be associated with an increase in patient-controlled administration of tramadol). Products include:
Ultram ER Tablets 2392

Food Interactions

Food, unspecified (Bioavailability slightly enhanced by food).

ZOFRAN ODT ORALLY DISINTEGRATING TABLETS

(Ondansetron) 1639
See Zofran Tablets

ZOLOFT ORAL CONCENTRATE

(Sertraline Hydrochloride) 2586

May interact with anticoagulants, cytochrome p450 2d6 substrates (selected), antidepressant drugs, lithium preparations, monoamine oxidase inhibitors, non-steroidal anti-inflammatory agents, phenytoin, highly protein bound drugs (selected), tricyclic antidepressants, and certain other agents. Compounds in these categories include:

Amiodarone Hydrochloride (Co-administration with drugs that are highly protein bound may cause a shift in plasma concentrations, potentially resulting in an adverse effect).
No products indexed under this heading.

Amitriptyline Hydrochloride (Concurrent use of drugs that inhibit the biochemical activity of P450IID6, such as tricyclic antidepressants, may increase plasma concentrations of co-administered drugs that are metabolized by P450IID6; changes in the dosage may be required; the duration of an appropriate washout period which should intervene before switching has not been established).
No products indexed under this heading.

Amoxapine (Concurrent use of drugs that inhibit the biochemical activity of P450IID6, such as tricyclic antidepressants, may increase plasma concentrations of co-administered drugs that are metabolized by P450IID6; changes in the dosage may be required; the duration of an appropriate washout period which should intervene before switching has not been established).
No products indexed under this heading.

Amphetamine Aspartate (Many drugs effective in the treatment of major depressive disorder, eg, the SSRIs, including sertraline, and most tricyclic antidepressant drugs effective in the treatment of major depressive disorder inhibit the biochemical activity of the drug metabolizing isoenzyme cytochrome P450 2D6, and, thus, may increase the plasma concentrations of co-administered drugs that are metabolized by CYP2D6. The drugs for which this potential interaction is of greatest concern are those metabolized by CYP2D6 and which have a narrow therapeutic index). Products include:
Adderall Tablets 3164
Adderall XR Capsules 3166

Amphetamine Aspartate Monohydrate (Many drugs effective in the treatment of major depressive disorder, eg, the SSRIs, including sertraline, and most tricyclic antidepressant drugs effective in the treatment of major depressive disorder inhibit the biochemical activity of the drug metabolizing isoenzyme cytochrome P450 2D6, and, thus, may increase the plasma concentrations of co-administered drugs that are metabolized by CYP2D6. The drugs for which this potential interaction is of greatest concern are those metabolized by CYP2D6 and which have a narrow therapeutic index).
No products indexed under this heading.

Amphetamine Sulfate (Many drugs effective in the treatment of major depressive disorder, eg, the SSRIs, including sertraline, and most tricyclic antidepressant drugs effective in the treatment of major depressive disorder inhibit the biochemical activity of the drug metabolizing isoenzyme cytochrome P450 2D6, and, thus, may increase the plasma concentrations of co-administered drugs that are metabolized by CYP2D6. The drugs for which this potential interaction is of greatest concern are those metabolized by CYP2D6 and which have a narrow therapeutic index). Products include:
Adderall Tablets 3164
Adderall XR Capsules 3166

Anisindione (Patients should be cautioned about the concomitant use of sertraline hydrochloride and drugs that affect coagulation since the combined use of psychotropic drugs that interfere with serotonin reuptake and these agents has been associated with an increased risk of bleeding). Products include:
Miradon Tablets 3042

Ardeparin Sodium (Patients should be cautioned about the concomitant use of sertraline hydrochloride and drugs that affect coagulation since the combined use of psychotropic drugs that interfere with serotonin reuptake and these agents has been associated with an increased risk of bleeding).
No products indexed under this heading.

Aspirin (Patients should be cautioned about the concomitant use of sertraline hydrochloride and aspirin since the combined use of psychotropic drugs that interfere with serotonin reuptake and these agents has been associated with an increased risk of bleeding). Products include:
Aggrenox Capsules 822
Bayer Aspirin 744
BC Allergy Sinus Cold Powder 677
BC Headache Powder 677
Arthritis Strength BC Powder 677
BC Sinus Cold Powder 677
Excedrin Extra Strength Caplets/Tablets/Geltabs 684
Excedrin Migraine Caplets/Tablets/Geltabs 609
Goody's Body Pain Formula Powder 684
Goody's Extra Strength Headache Powders 611
Goody's Extra Strength Pain Relief Tablets 685
Percodan Tablets 1132
St. Joseph 81 mg Aspirin Chewable and Enteric Coated Tablets 1869

Aspirin, Enteric Coated (Patients should be cautioned about the concomitant use of sertraline hydrochloride and aspirin since the combined use of psychotropic drugs that interfere with serotonin reuptake and these agents has been associated with an increased risk of bleeding).
No products indexed under this heading.

Aspirin Buffered (Patients should be cautioned about the concomitant use of sertraline hydrochloride and aspirin since the combined use of psychotropic drugs that interfere with serotonin reuptake and these agents has been associated with an increased risk of bleeding). Products include:
Bufferin Extra Strength Tablets 678
Bufferin Regular Strength Tablets 678

Astemizole (Sertraline has been shown to have some inhibition of P4503A4 *in vitro*, astemizole is metabolized by P4503A4 isoenzyme and inhibition of this enzyme system may result in increased serum levels of astemizole; co-administration requires caution).
No products indexed under this heading.

Atomoxetine Hydrochloride (Many drugs effective in the treatment of major depressive disorder, eg, the SSRIs, including sertraline, and most tricyclic antidepressant drugs effective in the treatment of major depressive disorder inhibit the biochemical activity of the drug metabolizing isoenzyme cytochrome P450 2D6, and, thus, may increase the plasma concentrations of co-administered drugs that are metabolized by CYP2D6. The drugs for which this potential interaction is of greatest concern are those metabolized by CYP2D6 and which have a narrow therapeutic index). Products include:
Strattera Capsules 1814

Atovaquone (Co-administration with drugs that are highly protein bound may cause a shift in plasma concentrations, potentially resulting in an adverse effect). Products include:
Malarone Pediatric Tablets 1517
Malarone Tablets 1517
Mepron Suspension 1521

Bisoprolol Fumarate (Many drugs effective in the treatment of major depressive disorder, eg, the SSRIs, including sertraline, and most tricyclic antidepressant drugs effective in the treatment of major depressive disorder inhibit the biochemical activity of the drug metabolizing isoenzyme cytochrome P450 2D6, and, thus, may increase the plasma concentrations of co-administered drugs that are metabolized by CYP2D6. The drugs for which this potential interaction is of greatest concern are those metabolized by CYP2D6 and which have a narrow therapeutic index).
No products indexed under this heading.

Bupropion Hydrochloride (Concurrent use of drugs that inhibit the biochemical activity of P450IID6, such as tricyclic antidepressants, may increase plasma concentrations of co-administered drugs that are metabolized by P450IID6; changes in the dosage may be required; the duration of an appropriate washout period which should intervene before switching has not been established). Products include:
Wellbutrin Tablets 1603
Wellbutrin SR Sustained-Release Tablets 1607
Wellbutrin XL Extended-Release Tablets 1613
Zyban Sustained-Release Tablets 1644

Captopril (Many drugs effective in the treatment of major depressive disorder, eg, the SSRIs, including sertraline, and most tricyclic antidepressant drugs effective in the treatment of major depressive disorder inhibit the biochemical activity of the drug metabolizing isoenzyme cytochrome P450 2D6, and, thus, may increase the plasma concentrations of co-administered drugs that are metabolized by CYP2D6. The drugs for which this potential interaction is of greatest concern are those metabolized by CYP2D6 and which have a narrow therapeutic index). Products include:
Captopril Tablets 2149

Carvedilol (Many drugs effective in the treatment of major depressive disorder, eg, the SSRIs, including sertraline, and most tricyclic antidepressant drugs effective in the treatment of major depressive disorder inhibit the biochemical activity of the drug metabolizing isoenzyme cytochrome P450 2D6, and, thus, may increase the plasma concentrations of co-administered drugs that are metabolized by CYP2D6. The drugs for which this potential interaction is of greatest concern are those metabolized by CYP2D6 and which have a narrow therapeutic index). Products include:
Coreg Tablets 1414

Cefonicid Sodium (Co-administration with drugs that are highly protein bound may cause a shift in plasma concentrations, potentially resulting in an adverse effect).
No products indexed under this heading.

Celecoxib (Co-administration with drugs that are highly protein bound may cause a shift in plasma concentrations, potentially resulting in an adverse effect). Products include:

Cevimeline Hydrochloride (Many drugs effective in the treatment of major depressive disorder, eg, the SSRIs, including sertraline, and most tricyclic antidepressant drugs effective in the treatment of major depressive disorder inhibit the biochemical activity of the drug metabolizing isoenzyme cytochrome P450 2D6, and, thus, may increase the plasma concentrations of co-administered drugs that are metabolized by CYP2D6. The drugs for which this potential interaction is of greatest concern are those metabolized by CYP2D6 and which have a narrow therapeutic index). Products include:

Chlordiazepoxide (Co-administration with drugs that are highly protein bound may cause a shift in plasma concentrations, potentially resulting in an adverse effect).

No products indexed under this heading.

Chlordiazepoxide Hydrochloride (Co-administration with drugs that are highly protein bound may cause a shift in plasma concentrations, potentially resulting in an adverse effect). Products include:

Chlorpromazine (Co-administration with drugs that are highly protein bound may cause a shift in plasma concentrations, potentially resulting in an adverse effect).

No products indexed under this heading.

Chlorpromazine Hydrochloride (Co-administration with drugs that are highly protein bound may cause a shift in plasma concentrations, potentially resulting in an adverse effect).

No products indexed under this heading.

Chlorpropamide (Many drugs effective in the treatment of major depressive disorder, eg, the SSRIs, including sertraline, and most tricyclic antidepressant drugs effective in the treatment of major depressive disorder inhibit the biochemical activity of the drug metabolizing isoenzyme cytochrome P450 2D6, and, thus, may increase the plasma concentrations of co-administered drugs that are metabolized by CYP2D6. The drugs for which this potential interaction is of greatest concern are those metabolized by CYP2D6 and which have a narrow therapeutic index).

No products indexed under this heading.

Cimetidine (Potential for increase in Zoloft mean AUC (50%), Cmax (24%) and half-life (26%); clinical significance is unknown). Products include:

Cimetidine Hydrochloride (Potential for increase in Zoloft mean AUC (50%), Cmax (24%) and half-life (26%); clinical significance is unknown).

No products indexed under this heading.

Cisapride (Sertraline induces the metabolism of cisapride (cisapride AUC and Cmax were reduced by about 35%)).

No products indexed under this heading.

Citalopram Hydrobromide (Concurrent use of drugs that inhibit the biochemical activity of P450IID6, such as tricyclic antidepressants, may increase plasma concentrations of co-administered drugs that are metabolized by P450IID6; changes in the dosage may be required; the duration of an appropriate washout period which should intervene before switching has not been established). Products include:

Clomipramine Hydrochloride (Concurrent use of drugs that inhibit the biochemical activity of P450IID6, such as tricyclic antidepressants, may increase plasma concentrations of co-administered drugs that are metabolized by P450IID6; changes in the dosage may be required; the duration of an appropriate washout period which should intervene before switching has not been established).

No products indexed under this heading.

Clozapine (Co-administration with drugs that are highly protein bound may cause a shift in plasma concentrations, potentially resulting in an adverse effect). Products include:

CNS-Active Drugs, unspecified (Caution is advised if Zoloft is co-administered with other CNS-active drugs).

No products indexed under this heading.

Codeine Phosphate (Many drugs effective in the treatment of major depressive disorder, eg, the SSRIs, including sertraline, and most tricyclic antidepressant drugs effective in the treatment of major depressive disorder inhibit the biochemical activity of the drug metabolizing isoenzyme cytochrome P450 2D6, and, thus, may increase the plasma concentrations of co-administered drugs that are metabolized by CYP2D6. The drugs for which this potential interaction is of greatest concern are those metabolized by CYP2D6 and which have a narrow therapeutic index). Products include:

Codeine Sulfate (Many drugs effective in the treatment of major depressive disorder, eg, the SSRIs, including sertraline, and most tricyclic antidepressant drugs effective in the treatment of major depressive disorder inhibit the biochemical activity of the drug metabolizing isoenzyme cytochrome P450 2D6, and, thus, may increase the plasma concentrations of co-administered drugs that are metabolized by CYP2D6. The drugs for which this potential interaction is of greatest concern are those metabolized by CYP2D6 and which have a narrow therapeutic index).

No products indexed under this heading.

Cyclobenzaprine Hydrochloride (Many drugs effective in the treatment of major depressive disorder, eg, the SSRIs, including sertraline, and most tricyclic antidepressant

drugs effective in the treatment of major depressive disorder inhibit the biochemical activity of the drug metabolizing isoenzyme cytochrome P450 2D6, and, thus, may increase the plasma concentrations of co-administered drugs that are metabolized by CYP2D6. The drugs for which this potential interaction is of greatest concern are those metabolized by CYP2D6 and which have a narrow therapeutic index).

No products indexed under this heading.

Cyclosporine (Co-administration with drugs that are highly protein bound may cause a shift in plasma concentrations, potentially resulting in an adverse effect). Products include:

Dalteparin Sodium (Patients should be cautioned about the concomitant use of sertraline hydrochloride and drugs that affect coagulation since the combined use of psychotropic drugs that interfere with serotonin reuptake and these agents has been associated with an increased risk of bleeding). Products include:

Danaparoid Sodium (Patients should be cautioned about the concomitant use of sertraline hydrochloride and drugs that affect coagulation since the combined use of psychotropic drugs that interfere with serotonin reuptake and these agents has been associated with an increased risk of bleeding).

No products indexed under this heading.

Desipramine Hydrochloride (Concurrent use of drugs that inhibit the biochemical activity of P450IID6, such as tricyclic antidepressants, may increase plasma concentrations of co-administered drugs that are metabolized by P450IID6; changes in the dosage may be required; the duration of an appropriate washout period which should intervene before switching has not been established).

No products indexed under this heading.

Dexfenfluramine Hydrochloride (Many drugs effective in the treatment of major depressive disorder, eg, the SSRIs, including sertraline, and most tricyclic antidepressant drugs effective in the treatment of major depressive disorder inhibit the biochemical activity of the drug metabolizing isoenzyme cytochrome P450 2D6, and, thus, may increase the plasma concentrations of co-administered drugs that are metabolized by CYP2D6. The drugs for which this potential interaction is of greatest concern are those metabolized by CYP2D6 and which have a narrow therapeutic index).

No products indexed under this heading.

Dextromethorphan Hydrobromide (Many drugs effective in the treatment of major depressive disorder, eg, the SSRIs, including sertraline, and most tricyclic antidepressant drugs effective in the treatment of major depressive disorder inhibit the biochemical activity of the drug metabolizing isoenzyme cytochrome

P450 2D6, and, thus, may increase the plasma concentrations of co-administered drugs that are metabolized by CYP2D6. The drugs for which this potential interaction is of greatest concern are those metabolized by CYP2D6 and which have a narrow therapeutic index). Products include:

Tylenol Cold Head Congestion Nighttime Caplets with Cool Burst ... 1873
Tylenol Cold Head Congestion Severe Caplets with Cool Burst ... 1873
Tylenol Cold Multi-Symptom Daytime Caplets with Cool Burst and Gelcaps ... 1874
Tylenol Cold Multi-Symptom Daytime Liquid with Citrus Burst ... 1874
Tylenol Cold Multi-Symptom Nighttime Caplets with Cool Burst ... 1874
Tylenol Cold Multi-Symptom Nighttime Liquid with Cool Burst ... 1874
Tylenol Cold Multi-Symptom Severe Caplets with Cool Burst ... 1874
Tylenol Cold Multi-Symptom Severe Daytime Liquid with Citrus Burst ... 1874
Tylenol Cough & Sore Throat Daytime Liquid with Cool Burst ... 1877
Tylenol Cough & Sore Throat Nighttime Liquid with Cool Burst ... 1877
Concentrated Tylenol Infants' Drops Plus Cold and Cough ... 1879
Vicks 44 Cough Relief Liquid ... 2679
Vicks 44D Cough & Head Congestion Relief Liquid ... 2679
Vicks 44E Cough & Chest Congestion Relief Liquid ... 2679
Pediatric Vicks 44e Cough & Chest Congestion Relief Liquid ... 2676
Vicks 44M Cough, Cold & Flu Relief Liquid ... 2680
Pediatric Vicks 44m Cough & Cold Relief Liquid ... 2676
Vicks DayQuil LiquiCaps/Liquid Multi-Symptom Cold/Flu Relief ... 761
Vicks DayQuil Multi-Symptom Cold/Flu Relief LiquiCaps ... 2678
Vicks DayQuil Multi-Symptom Cold/Flu Relief Liquid ... 2678
Vicks NyQuil Multi-Symptom Cold/Flu Relief Liquid ... 2681
Children's Vicks NyQuil Cold/Cough Relief ... 756
Vicks NyQuil Multi-Symptom Cold/Flu Relief LiquiCaps ... 2681
Vicks NyQuil LiquiCaps/Liquid Multi-Symptom Cold/Flu Relief ... 763
Vicks NyQuil Cough Liquid ... 2680
Children's Vicks NyQuil Cold/Cough Relief Liquid ... 2680
Zicam Cough Max Nighttime Cough Spray ... 767
Zicam Cough Max Cough Spray ... 767
Zicam Cough Max Cough Melts ... 767
Zicam Cough Plus D Cough Spray ... 767
Zicam Cough Relief Cough Spray ... 767
Zicam Maximum Strength Flu Daytime ... 768
Zicam Maximum Strength Flu Nighttime ... 768

Dextromethorphan Polistirex (Many drugs effective in the treatment of major depressive disorder, eg, the SSRIs, including sertraline, and most tricyclic antidepressant drugs effective in the treatment of major depressive disorder inhibit the biochemical activity of the drug metabolizing isoenzyme cytochrome P450 2D6, and, thus, may increase the plasma concentrations of co-administered drugs that are metabolized by CYP2D6. The drugs for which this potential interaction is of greatest concern are those metabolized by CYP2D6 and which have a narrow therapeutic index). Products include:
Delsym Extended-Release Suspension 12 Hour Cough Suppressant ... 611

Diazepam (Co-administration with intravenous diazepam has resulted in decrease in relative to baseline diazepam clearance and increase in Tmax for desmethyldiazepam; the clinical significance is unknown). Products include:
Diastat Rectal Delivery System ... 3343
Valium Tablets ... 2819

Diclofenac Potassium (Co-administration with drugs that are highly protein bound may cause a shift in plasma concentrations, potentially resulting in an adverse effect).
No products indexed under this heading.

Diclofenac Sodium (Co-administration with drugs that are highly protein bound may cause a shift in plasma concentrations, potentially resulting in an adverse effect). Products include:
Arthrotec Tablets ... 3129
Voltaren Ophthalmic Solution ... 2309
Voltaren Tablets ... 2307
Voltaren-XR Tablets ... 2310

Dicumarol (Patients should be cautioned about the concomitant use of sertraline hydrochloride and drugs that affect coagulation since the combined use of psychotropic drugs that interfere with serotonin reuptake and these agents has been associated with an increased risk of bleeding).
No products indexed under this heading.

Digitoxin (Co-administration with drugs that are highly protein bound, such as digitoxin, may cause a shift in plasma concentrations, potentially resulting in an adverse effect).
No products indexed under this heading.

Dipyridamole (Co-administration with drugs that are highly protein bound may cause a shift in plasma concentrations, potentially resulting in an adverse effect). Products include:
Aggrenox Capsules ... 822
Persantine Tablets ... 868

Disulfiram (Zoloft Oral Concentrate contains 12% alcohol; concurrent use with disulfiram may result in Antabuse-Alcohol reaction; co-administration of Zoloft Oral Concentrate and disulfiram is contraindicated).
No products indexed under this heading.

Dolasetron Mesylate (Many drugs effective in the treatment of major depressive disorder, eg, the SSRIs, including sertraline, and most tricyclic antidepressant drugs effective in the treatment of major depressive disorder inhibit the biochemical activity of the drug metabolizing isoenzyme cytochrome P450 2D6, and, thus, may increase the plasma concentrations of co-administered drugs that are metabolized by CYP2D6. The drugs for which this potential interaction is of greatest concern are those metabolized by CYP2D6 and which have a narrow therapeutic index). Products include:
Anzemet Injection ... 2859
Anzemet Tablets ... 2862

Donepezil Hydrochloride (Many drugs effective in the treatment of major depressive disorder, eg, the SSRIs, including sertraline, and most tricyclic antidepressant drugs effective in the treatment of major depressive disorder inhibit the biochemical activity of the drug metabolizing isoenzyme cytochrome P450 2D6, and, thus, may increase the plasma concentrations of co-administered drugs that are metabolized by CYP2D6. The drugs for which this potential interaction is of greatest concern are those metabolized by CYP2D6 and which have a narrow therapeutic index). Products include:
Aricept Tablets ... 1094
Aricept ODT Tablets ... 1094

Doxepin Hydrochloride (Concurrent use of drugs that inhibit the biochemical activity of P450IID6, such as tricyclic antidepressants, may increase plasma concentrations of co-administered drugs that are metabolized by P450IID6; changes in the dosage may be required; the duration of an appropriate washout period which should intervene before switching has not been established).
No products indexed under this heading.

Encainide Hydrochloride (Many drugs effective in the treatment of major depressive disorder, eg, the SSRIs, including sertraline, and most tricyclic antidepressant drugs effective in the treatment of major depressive disorder inhibit the biochemical activity of the drug metabolizing isoenzyme cytochrome P450 2D6, and, thus, may increase the plasma concentrations of co-administered drugs that are metabolized by CYP2D6. The drugs for which this potential interaction is of greatest concern are those metabolized by CYP2D6 and which have a narrow therapeutic index).
No products indexed under this heading.

Enoxaparin Sodium (Patients should be cautioned about the concomitant use of sertraline hydrochloride and drugs that affect coagulation since the combined use of psychotropic drugs that interfere with serotonin reuptake and these agents has been associated with an increased risk of bleeding). Products include:
Lovenox Injection ... 2915

Escitalopram Oxalate (Concurrent use of drugs that inhibit the biochemical activity of P450IID6, such as tricyclic antidepressants, may increase plasma concentrations of co-administered drugs that are metabolized by P450IID6; changes in the dosage may be required; the duration of an appropriate washout period which should intervene before switching has not been established). Products include:
Lexapro Oral Solution ... 1190
Lexapro Tablets ... 1190

Ethanol (Patients should be told that although sertraline hydrochloride has not been shown in experiments with normal subjects to increase the mental and motor skill impairments caused by alcohol, the concomitant use of sertraline hydrochloride and alcohol is not advised).
No products indexed under this heading.

Etodolac (Patients should be cautioned about the concomitant use of sertraline hydrochloride and non-selective NSAIDs (eg, NSAIDs that inhibit both cyclooxygenase isoenzymes, COX 1 and 2), since the combined use of psychotropic drugs that interfere with serotonin reuptake and these agents has been associated with an increased risk of bleeding).
No products indexed under this heading.

Fenoprofen Calcium (Co-administration with drugs that are highly protein bound may cause a shift in plasma concentrations, potentially resulting in an adverse effect). Products include:
Nalfon Capsules ... 2502

Fentanyl (Many drugs effective in the treatment of major depressive disorder, eg, the SSRIs, including sertraline, and most tricyclic antidepressant drugs effective in the treatment of major depressive disorder inhibit the biochemical activity of the drug metabolizing isoenzyme cytochrome P450 2D6, and, thus, may increase the plasma concentrations of co-administered drugs that are metabolized by CYP2D6. The drugs for which this potential interaction is of greatest concern are those metabolized by CYP2D6 and which have a narrow therapeutic index). Products include:
Duragesic Transdermal System ... 2373
Ionsys Transdermal System ... 2379

Fentanyl Citrate (Many drugs effective in the treatment of major depressive disorder, eg, the SSRIs, including sertraline, and most tricyclic antidepressant drugs effective in the treatment of major depressive disorder inhibit the biochemical activity of the drug metabolizing isoenzyme cytochrome P450 2D6, and, thus, may increase the plasma concentrations of co-administered drugs that are metabolized by CYP2D6. The drugs for which this potential interaction is of greatest concern are those metabolized by CYP2D6 and which have a narrow therapeutic index). Products include:
Actiq ... 979

Flecainide Acetate (Concurrent use of drugs that inhibit the biochemical activity of P450IID6, such as flecainide, may increase plasma concentrations of co-administered drugs that are metabolized by P450IID6; changes in the dosage may be required). Products include:
Tambocor Tablets ... 1856

Fluoxetine (Many drugs effective in the treatment of major depressive disorder, eg, the SSRIs, including sertraline, and most tricyclic antidepressant drugs effective in the treatment of major depressive disorder inhibit the biochemical activity of the drug metabolizing isoenzyme cytochrome P450 2D6, and, thus, may increase the plasma concentrations of co-administered drugs that are metabolized by CYP2D6. The drugs for which this potential interaction is of greatest concern are those metabolized by CYP2D6 and which have a narrow therapeutic index).
No products indexed under this heading.

Fluoxetine Hydrochloride (Concurrent use of drugs that inhibit the biochemical activity of P450IID6, such as SSRIs, may increase plasma concentrations of co-administered drugs that are metabolized by P450IID6; changes in the dosage may be required; the duration of an appropriate washout period, which should intervene before switching, has not been established). Products include:
Prozac Pulvules and Liquid ... 1801
Symbyax Capsules ... 1819

Fluphenazine Decanoate (Many drugs effective in the treatment of major depressive disorder, eg, the SSRIs, including sertraline, and most tricyclic antidepressant drugs effective in the treatment of major depres-

sive disorder inhibit the biochemical activity of the drug metabolizing isoenzyme cytochrome P450 2D6, and, thus, may increase the plasma concentrations of co-administered drugs that are metabolized by CYP2D6. The drugs for which this potential interaction is of greatest concern are those metabolized by CYP2D6 and which have a narrow therapeutic index).
No products indexed under this heading.

Fluphenazine Enanthate (Many drugs effective in the treatment of major depressive disorder, eg, the SSRIs, including sertraline, and most tricyclic antidepressant drugs effective in the treatment of major depressive disorder inhibit the biochemical activity of the drug metabolizing isoenzyme cytochrome P450 2D6, and, thus, may increase the plasma concentrations of co-administered drugs that are metabolized by CYP2D6. The drugs for which this potential interaction is of greatest concern are those metabolized by CYP2D6 and which have a narrow therapeutic index).
No products indexed under this heading.

Fluphenazine Hydrochloride (Many drugs effective in the treatment of major depressive disorder, eg, the SSRIs, including sertraline, and most tricyclic antidepressant drugs effective in the treatment of major depressive disorder inhibit the biochemical activity of the drug metabolizing isoenzyme cytochrome P450 2D6, and, thus, may increase the plasma concentrations of co-administered drugs that are metabolized by CYP2D6. The drugs for which this potential interaction is of greatest concern are those metabolized by CYP2D6 and which have a narrow therapeutic index).
No products indexed under this heading.

Flurazepam Hydrochloride (Co-administration with drugs that are highly protein bound may cause a shift in plasma concentrations, potentially resulting in an adverse effect). Products include:
Dalmane Capsules 3342

Flurbiprofen (Co-administration with drugs that are highly protein bound may cause a shift in plasma concentrations, potentially resulting in an adverse effect).
No products indexed under this heading.

Fluvoxamine Maleate (Concurrent use of drugs that inhibit the biochemical activity of P450IID6, such as SSRIs, may increase plasma concentrations of co-administered drugs that are metabolized by P450IID6; changes in the dosage may be required; the duration of an appropriate washout period, which should intervene before switching, has not been established).
No products indexed under this heading.

Fondaparinux Sodium (Patients should be cautioned about the concomitant use of sertraline hydrochloride and drugs that affect coagulation since the combined use of psychotropic drugs that interfere with serotonin reuptake and these agents has been associated with an increased risk of bleeding). Products include:
Arixtra Injection 1351

Formoterol Fumarate (Many drugs effective in the treatment of major depressive disorder, eg, the SSRIs, including sertraline, and most tricyclic antidepressant drugs effective in the treatment of major depressive disorder inhibit the biochemical activity of the drug metabolizing isoenzyme cytochrome P450 2D6, and, thus, may increase the plasma concentrations of co-administered drugs that are metabolized by CYP2D6. The drugs for which this potential interaction is of greatest concern are those metabolized by CYP2D6 and which have a narrow therapeutic index). Products include:
Foradil Aerolizer 3010

Fosphenytoin Sodium (It is recommended that plasma phenytoin concentrations be monitored following initiation of sertraline hydrochloride therapy with appropriate adjustments to the phenytoin dose).
No products indexed under this heading.

Galantamine Hydrobromide (Many drugs effective in the treatment of major depressive disorder, eg, the SSRIs, including sertraline, and most tricyclic antidepressant drugs effective in the treatment of major depressive disorder inhibit the biochemical activity of the drug metabolizing isoenzyme cytochrome P450 2D6, and, thus, may increase the plasma concentrations of co-administered drugs that are metabolized by CYP2D6. The drugs for which this potential interaction is of greatest concern are those metabolized by CYP2D6 and which have a narrow therapeutic index). Products include:
Razadyne 2399
Razadyne ER Extended-Release Capsules 2399

Glipizide (Co-administration with drugs that are highly protein bound may cause a shift in plasma concentrations, potentially resulting in an adverse effect).
No products indexed under this heading.

Haloperidol (Many drugs effective in the treatment of major depressive disorder, eg, the SSRIs, including sertraline, and most tricyclic antidepressant drugs effective in the treatment of major depressive disorder inhibit the biochemical activity of the drug metabolizing isoenzyme cytochrome P450 2D6, and, thus, may increase the plasma concentrations of co-administered drugs that are metabolized by CYP2D6. The drugs for which this potential interaction is of greatest concern are those metabolized by CYP2D6 and which have a narrow therapeutic index).
No products indexed under this heading.

Haloperidol Decanoate (Many drugs effective in the treatment of major depressive disorder, eg, the SSRIs, including sertraline, and most tricyclic antidepressant drugs effective in the treatment of major depressive disorder inhibit the biochemical activity of the drug metabolizing isoenzyme cytochrome P450 2D6, and, thus, may increase the plasma concentrations of co-administered drugs that are metabolized by CYP2D6. The drugs for which this potential interaction is of greatest concern are those metabolized by CYP2D6 and which have a narrow therapeutic index).
No products indexed under this heading.

Heparin Calcium (Patients should be cautioned about the concomitant use of sertraline hydrochloride and drugs that affect coagulation since the combined use of psychotropic drugs that interfere with serotonin reuptake and these agents has been associated with an increased risk of bleeding).
No products indexed under this heading.

Heparin Sodium (Patients should be cautioned about the concomitant use of sertraline hydrochloride and drugs that affect coagulation since the combined use of psychotropic drugs that interfere with serotonin reuptake and these agents has been associated with an increased risk of bleeding).
No products indexed under this heading.

Hydrocodone Bitartrate (Many drugs effective in the treatment of major depressive disorder, eg, the SSRIs, including sertraline, and most tricyclic antidepressant drugs effective in the treatment of major depressive disorder inhibit the biochemical activity of the drug metabolizing isoenzyme cytochrome P450 2D6, and, thus, may increase the plasma concentrations of co-administered drugs that are metabolized by CYP2D6. The drugs for which this potential interaction is of greatest concern are those metabolized by CYP2D6 and which have a narrow therapeutic index). Products include:
Hycodan 1116
Hycotuss Expectorant Syrup 1117
Vicodin Tablets 535
Vicodin ES Tablets 536
Vicodin HP Tablets 538
Vicoprofen Tablets 539
Zydone Tablets 1139

Ibuprofen (Co-administration with drugs that are highly protein bound may cause a shift in plasma concentrations, potentially resulting in an adverse effect). Products include:
Advil Allergy Sinus Caplets .... ▣ 770
Advil .... ▣ 674
Children's Advil Oral Suspension .... ▣ 603
Children's Advil Chewable Tablets .. ▣ 603
Advil Cold & Sinus .... ▣ 723
Infants' Advil Concentrated Drops .. ▣ 604
Infants' Advil Concentrated Drops - White Grape (Dye-Free) .... ▣ 604
Junior Strength Advil Swallow Tablets .... ▣ 605
Advil Migraine Liquigels .... ▣ 608
Advil Multi-Symptom Cold Caplets .... ▣ 770
Advil PM Caplets .... ▣ 615
Motrin IB Tablets and Caplets 1866
Children's Motrin Oral Suspension ... 1867
Children's Motrin Non-Staining Dye-Free Oral Suspension 1867
Children's Motrin Cold Oral Suspension 1867
Infants' Motrin Concentrated Drops 1867
Infants' Motrin Non-Staining Dye-Free Concentrated Drops 1867
Junior Strength Motrin Caplets and Chewable Tablets 1867
Vicoprofen Tablets 539

Imipramine Hydrochloride (Concurrent use of drugs that inhibit the biochemical activity of P450IID6, such as tricyclic antidepressants, may increase plasma concentrations of co-administered drugs that are metabolized by P450IID6; changes in the dosage may be required; the duration of an appropriate washout period which should intervene before switching has not been established).
No products indexed under this heading.

Imipramine Pamoate (Concurrent use of drugs that inhibit the biochemical activity of P450IID6, such as tricyclic antidepressants, may increase plasma concentrations of co-administered drugs that are metabolized by P450IID6; changes in the dosage may be required; the duration of an appropriate washout period which should intervene before switching has not been established).
No products indexed under this heading.

Indomethacin (Co-administration with drugs that are highly protein bound may cause a shift in plasma concentrations, potentially resulting in an adverse effect). Products include:
Indocin 1995

Indomethacin Sodium Trihydrate (Co-administration with drugs that are highly protein bound may cause a shift in plasma concentrations, potentially resulting in an adverse effect). Products include:
Indocin I.V. 2465

Indoramin Hydrochloride (Many drugs effective in the treatment of major depressive disorder, eg, the SSRIs, including sertraline, and most tricyclic antidepressant drugs effective in the treatment of major depressive disorder inhibit the biochemical activity of the drug metabolizing isoenzyme cytochrome P450 2D6, and, thus, may increase the plasma concentrations of co-administered drugs that are metabolized by CYP2D6. The drugs for which this potential interaction is of greatest concern are those metabolized by CYP2D6 and which have a narrow therapeutic index).
No products indexed under this heading.

Isocarboxazid (Co-administration has resulted in serious, sometimes fatal, reactions including hyperthermia, rigidity, myoclonus, autonomic instability, extreme agitation progressing to delirium and coma; concurrent and/or sequential use is contraindicated).
No products indexed under this heading.

Ketoprofen (Co-administration with drugs that are highly protein bound may cause a shift in plasma concentrations, potentially resulting in an adverse effect).
No products indexed under this heading.

Ketorolac Tromethamine (Co-administration with drugs that are highly protein bound may cause a shift in plasma concentrations, potentially resulting in an adverse effect). Products include:
Acular Ophthalmic Solution .... ⊙ 565
Acular LS Ophthalmic Solution .... ⊙ 566

Labetalol Hydrochloride (Many drugs effective in the treatment of major depressive disorder, eg, the SSRIs, including sertraline, and most tricyclic antidepressant drugs effective in the treatment of major depressive disorder inhibit the biochemical activity of the drug metabolizing isoenzyme cytochrome P450 2D6, and, thus, may increase the plasma concentrations of co-administered drugs that are metabolized by CYP2D6. The drugs for which this potential interaction is of greatest concern are those metabolized by CYP2D6 and which have a narrow therapeutic index).

No products indexed under this heading.

Lidocaine (Many drugs effective in the treatment of major depressive disorder, eg, the SSRIs, including sertraline, and most tricyclic antidepressant drugs effective in the treatment of major depressive disorder inhibit the biochemical activity of the drug metabolizing isoenzyme cytochrome P450 2D6, and, thus, may increase the plasma concentrations of co-administered drugs that are metabolized by CYP2D6. The drugs for which this potential interaction is of greatest concern are those metabolized by CYP2D6 and which have a narrow therapeutic index). Products include:

Lidoderm Patch **1118**
Synera Topical Patch **1137**

Lidocaine Hydrochloride (Many drugs effective in the treatment of major depressive disorder, eg, the SSRIs, including sertraline, and most tricyclic antidepressant drugs effective in the treatment of major depressive disorder inhibit the biochemical activity of the drug metabolizing isoenzyme cytochrome P450 2D6, and, thus, may increase the plasma concentrations of co-administered drugs that are metabolized by CYP2D6. The drugs for which this potential interaction is of greatest concern are those metabolized by CYP2D6 and which have a narrow therapeutic index).

No products indexed under this heading.

Lithium (No significant alteration in plasma lithium levels or renal clearance; nonetheless, plasma lithium levels should be monitored).

No products indexed under this heading.

Lithium Carbonate (No significant alteration in plasma lithium levels or renal clearance; nonetheless, plasma lithium levels should be monitored). Products include:

Lithobid Tablets **1692**

Lithium Citrate (No significant alteration in plasma lithium levels or renal clearance; nonetheless, plasma lithium levels should be monitored).

No products indexed under this heading.

Low Molecular Weight Heparins (Patients should be cautioned about the concomitant use of sertraline hydrochloride and drugs that affect coagulation since the combined use of psychotropic drugs that interfere with serotonin reuptake and these agents has been associated with an increased risk of bleeding).

No products indexed under this heading.

Maprotiline Hydrochloride (Concurrent use of drugs that inhibit the biochemical activity of P450IID6; such as tricyclic antidepressants, may increase plasma concentrations of co-administered drugs that are metabolized by P450IID6; changes in the dosage may be required; the duration of an appropriate washout period which should intervene before switching has not been established).

No products indexed under this heading.

Meclofenamate Sodium (Co-administration with drugs that are highly protein bound may cause a shift in plasma concentrations, potentially resulting in an adverse effect).

No products indexed under this heading.

Mefenamic Acid (Co-administration with drugs that are highly protein bound may cause a shift in plasma concentrations, potentially resulting in an adverse effect).

No products indexed under this heading.

Meloxicam (Patients should be cautioned about the concomitant use of sertraline hydrochloride and non-selective NSAIDs (eg, NSAIDs that inhibit both cyclooxygenase isoenzymes, COX 1 and 2), since the combined use of psychotropic drugs that interfere with serotonin reuptake and these agents has been associated with an increased risk of bleeding). Products include:

Mobic Oral Suspension **863**
Mobic Tablets **863**

Meperidine Hydrochloride (Many drugs effective in the treatment of major depressive disorder, eg, the SSRIs, including sertraline, and most tricyclic antidepressant drugs effective in the treatment of major depressive disorder inhibit the biochemical activity of the drug metabolizing isoenzyme cytochrome P450 2D6, and, thus, may increase the plasma concentrations of co-administered drugs that are metabolized by CYP2D6. The drugs for which this potential interaction is of greatest concern are those metabolized by CYP2D6 and which have a narrow therapeutic index).

No products indexed under this heading.

Methadone Hydrochloride (Many drugs effective in the treatment of major depressive disorder, eg, the SSRIs, including sertraline, and most tricyclic antidepressant drugs effective in the treatment of major depressive disorder inhibit the biochemical activity of the drug metabolizing isoenzyme cytochrome P450 2D6, and, thus, may increase the plasma concentrations of co-administered drugs that are metabolized by CYP2D6. The drugs for which this potential interaction is of greatest concern are those metabolized by CYP2D6 and which have a narrow therapeutic index).

No products indexed under this heading.

Methamphetamine Hydrochloride (Many drugs effective in the treatment of major depressive disorder, eg, the SSRIs, including sertraline, and most tricyclic antidepressant drugs effective in the treatment of major depressive disorder inhibit the biochemical activity of the drug metabolizing isoenzyme cytochrome P450 2D6, and, thus, may increase the plasma concentrations of co-administered drugs that are metabolized by CYP2D6. The drugs for which this potential interaction is of greatest concern are those metabolized by CYP2D6 and which have a narrow therapeutic index). Products include:

Desoxyn Tablets, USP **2462**

Metoprolol Succinate (Many drugs effective in the treatment of major depressive disorder, eg, the SSRIs, including sertraline, and most tricyclic antidepressant drugs effective in the treatment of major depressive disorder inhibit the biochemical activity of the drug metabolizing isoenzyme cytochrome P450 2D6, and, thus, may increase the plasma concentrations of co-administered drugs that are metabolized by CYP2D6. The drugs for which this potential interaction is of greatest concern are those metabolized by CYP2D6 and which have a narrow therapeutic index). Products include:

Toprol-XL Tablets **668**

Metoprolol Tartrate (Many drugs effective in the treatment of major depressive disorder, eg, the SSRIs, including sertraline, and most tricyclic antidepressant drugs effective in the treatment of major depressive disorder inhibit the biochemical activity of the drug metabolizing isoenzyme cytochrome P450 2D6, and, thus, may increase the plasma concentrations of co-administered drugs that are metabolized by CYP2D6. The drugs for which this potential interaction is of greatest concern are those metabolized by CYP2D6 and which have a narrow therapeutic index). Products include:

Lopressor Injection **2238**
Lopressor Tablets **2238**
Lopressor HCT 50/25 Tablets **2241**
Lopressor HCT 100/25 Tablets **2241**
Lopressor HCT 100/50 Tablets **2241**

Mexiletine Hydrochloride (Many drugs effective in the treatment of major depressive disorder, eg, the SSRIs, including sertraline, and most tricyclic antidepressant drugs effective in the treatment of major depressive disorder inhibit the biochemical activity of the drug metabolizing isoenzyme cytochrome P450 2D6, and, thus, may increase the plasma concentrations of co-administered drugs that are metabolized by CYP2D6. The drugs for which this potential interaction is of greatest concern are those metabolized by CYP2D6 and which have a narrow therapeutic index).

No products indexed under this heading.

Midazolam Hydrochloride (Co-administration with drugs that are highly protein bound may cause a shift in plasma concentrations, potentially resulting in an adverse effect).

No products indexed under this heading.

Mirtazapine (Concurrent use of drugs that inhibit the biochemical activity of P450IID6, such as tricyclic antidepressants, may increase plasma concentrations of co-administered drugs that are metabolized by P450IID6; changes in the dosage may be required; the duration of an appropriate washout period which should intervene before switching has not been established).

No products indexed under this heading.

Moclobemide (Concomitant use in patients taking MAO inhibitors and SSRIs, such as sertraline, has resulted in cases of serious fatal reactions including hyperthermia, rigidity, myoclonus, autonomic instability, delirium and coma; concurrent and/or sequential use is contraindicated).

No products indexed under this heading.

Morphine Sulfate (Many drugs effective in the treatment of major depressive disorder, eg, the SSRIs, including sertraline, and most tricyclic antidepressant drugs effective in the treatment of major depressive disorder inhibit the biochemical activity of the drug metabolizing isoenzyme cytochrome P450 2D6, and, thus, may increase the plasma concentrations of co-administered drugs that are metabolized by CYP2D6. The drugs for which this potential interaction is of greatest concern are those metabolized by CYP2D6 and which have a narrow therapeutic index). Products include:

Avinza Capsules **1741**
Kadian Capsules **577**
MS Contin Tablets **2701**

Nabumetone (Patients should be cautioned about the concomitant use of sertraline hydrochloride and non-selective NSAIDs (eg, NSAIDs that inhibit both cyclooxygenase isoenzymes, COX 1 and 2), since the combined use of psychotropic drugs that interfere with serotonin reuptake and these agents has been associated with an increased risk of bleeding).

No products indexed under this heading.

Naproxen (Co-administration with drugs that are highly protein bound may cause a shift in plasma concentrations, potentially resulting in an adverse effect). Products include:

EC-Naprosyn Delayed-Release Tablets **2761**
Naprosyn Suspension **2761**
Naprosyn Tablets **2761**
Prevacid NapraPAC **3280**

Naproxen Sodium (Co-administration with drugs that are highly protein bound may cause a shift in plasma concentrations, potentially resulting in an adverse effect). Products include:

Aleve Caplets **742**
Aleve Gelcaps **743**
Aleve Tablets **743**
Aleve Cold & Sinus Caplets **744**
Anaprox Tablets **2761**
Anaprox DS Tablets **2761**

Nefazodone Hydrochloride (Care and prudent medical judgment should be exercised regarding the optimal timing of switching from another antidepressant to Zoloft; the duration of an appropriate washout period, which should intervene before switching, has not been established).

No products indexed under this heading.

Nelfinavir Mesylate (Many drugs effective in the treatment of major depressive disorder, eg, the SSRIs, including sertraline, and most tricyclic antidepressant drugs effective in the treatment of major depressive disorder inhibit the biochemical activity of the drug metabolizing isoenzyme cytochrome P450 2D6, and, thus, may increase the plasma concentrations of co-administered drugs that are metabolized by CYP2D6. The drugs for which this potential interaction is of greatest concern are those metabolized by CYP2D6 and which have a narrow therapeutic index). Products include:

Nortriptyline Hydrochloride (Concurrent use of drugs that inhibit the biochemical activity of P450IID6, such as tricyclic antidepressants, may increase plasma concentrations of co-administered drugs that are metabolized by P450IID6; changes in the dosage may be required; the duration of an appropriate washout period which should intervene before switching has not been established).

No products indexed under this heading.

Olanzapine (Many drugs effective in the treatment of major depressive disorder, eg, the SSRIs, including sertraline, and most tricyclic antidepressant drugs effective in the treatment of major depressive disorder inhibit the biochemical activity of the drug metabolizing isoenzyme cytochrome P450 2D6, and, thus, may increase the plasma concentrations of co-administered drugs that are metabolized by CYP2D6. The drugs for which this potential interaction is of greatest concern are those metabolized by CYP2D6 and which have a narrow therapeutic index). Products include:

Omeprazole (Many drugs effective in the treatment of major depressive disorder, eg, the SSRIs, including sertraline, and most tricyclic antidepressant drugs effective in the treatment of major depressive disorder inhibit the biochemical activity of the drug metabolizing isoenzyme cytochrome P450 2D6, and, thus, may increase the plasma concentrations of co-administered drugs that are metabolized by CYP2D6. The drugs for which this potential interaction is of greatest concern are those metabolized by CYP2D6 and which have a narrow therapeutic index). Products include:

Ondansetron (Many drugs effective in the treatment of major depressive disorder, eg, the SSRIs, including sertraline, and most tricyclic antidepressant drugs effective in the treat-

ment of major depressive disorder inhibit the biochemical activity of the drug metabolizing isoenzyme cytochrome P450 2D6, and, thus, may increase the plasma concentrations of co-administered drugs that are metabolized by CYP2D6. The drugs for which this potential interaction is of greatest concern are those metabolized by CYP2D6 and which have a narrow therapeutic index). Products include:

Ondansetron Hydrochloride (Many drugs effective in the treatment of major depressive disorder, eg, the SSRIs, including sertraline, and most tricyclic antidepressant drugs effective in the treatment of major depressive disorder inhibit the biochemical activity of the drug metabolizing isoenzyme cytochrome P450 2D6, and, thus, may increase the plasma concentrations of co-administered drugs that are metabolized by CYP2D6. The drugs for which this potential interaction is of greatest concern are those metabolized by CYP2D6 and which have a narrow therapeutic index). Products include:

Oxaprozin (Co-administration with drugs that are highly protein bound may cause a shift in plasma concentrations, potentially resulting in an adverse effect).

No products indexed under this heading.

Oxazepam (Co-administration with drugs that are highly protein bound may cause a shift in plasma concentrations, potentially resulting in an adverse effect).

No products indexed under this heading.

Oxycodone Hydrochloride (Many drugs effective in the treatment of major depressive disorder, eg, the SSRIs, including sertraline, and most tricyclic antidepressant drugs effective in the treatment of major depressive disorder inhibit the biochemical activity of the drug metabolizing isoenzyme cytochrome P450 2D6, and, thus, may increase the plasma concentrations of co-administered drugs that are metabolized by CYP2D6. The drugs for which this potential interaction is of greatest concern are those metabolized by CYP2D6 and which have a narrow therapeutic index). Products include:

Paclitaxel (Many drugs effective in the treatment of major depressive disorder, eg, the SSRIs, including sertraline, and most tricyclic antidepressant drugs effective in the treatment of major depressive disorder inhibit the biochemical activity of the drug metabolizing isoenzyme cytochrome P450 2D6, and, thus, may increase the plasma concentrations of co-administered drugs that are metabolized by CYP2D6. The drugs for which this potential interaction is of greatest concern are those metabolized by CYP2D6 and which

have a narrow therapeutic index).
No products indexed under this heading.

Pargyline Hydrochloride (Concomitant use in patients taking MAO inhibitors and SSRIs, such as sertraline, has resulted in cases of serious fatal reactions including hyperthermia, rigidity, myoclonus, autonomic instability, delirium and coma; concurrent and/or sequential use is contraindicated).

No products indexed under this heading.

Paroxetine Hydrochloride (Concurrent use of drugs that inhibit the biochemical activity of P450II6, such as SSRIs, may increase plasma concentrations of co-administered drugs that are metabolized by P450IID6; changes in the dosage may be required; the duration of an appropriate washout period, which should intervene before switching, has not been established). Products include:

Phenelzine Sulfate (Co-administration has resulted in serious, sometimes fatal, reactions including hyperthermia, rigidity, myoclonus, autonomic instability, extreme agitation progressing to delirium and coma; concurrent and/or sequential use is contraindicated).

No products indexed under this heading.

Phenylbutazone (Co-administration with drugs that are highly protein bound may cause a shift in plasma concentrations, potentially resulting in an adverse effect).

No products indexed under this heading.

Phenytoin (It is recommended that plasma phenytoin concentrations be monitored following initiation of sertraline hydrochloride therapy with appropriate adjustments to the phenytoin dose).

No products indexed under this heading.

Phenytoin Sodium (It is recommended that plasma phenytoin concentrations be monitored following initiation of sertraline hydrochloride therapy with appropriate adjustments to the phenytoin dose). Products include:

Pimozide (Co-administration of 2 mg pimozide and 200 mg sertraline (q.d.) was associated with an increase in pimozide AUC and Cmax, but was not associated with any changes in EKG. Due to the narrow therapeutic index of pimozide and the interaction noted at a low dose of pimozide, concomitant use should be contraindicated).

No products indexed under this heading.

Pindolol (Many drugs effective in the treatment of major depressive disorder, eg, the SSRIs, including sertraline, and most tricyclic antidepressant drugs effective in the treatment of major depressive disorder inhibit the biochemical activity of the drug metabolizing isoenzyme cytochrome P450 2D6, and, thus, may increase the plasma concentrations of co-administered drugs that are metabolized by CYP2D6. The drugs for which this potential interaction is of greatest concern are those

metabolized by CYP2D6 and which have a narrow therapeutic index).
No products indexed under this heading.

Piroxicam (Co-administration with drugs that are highly protein bound may cause a shift in plasma concentrations, potentially resulting in an adverse effect).

No products indexed under this heading.

Procarbazine Hydrochloride (Concomitant use in patients taking MAO inhibitors and SSRIs, such as sertraline, has resulted in cases of serious fatal reactions including hyperthermia, rigidity, myoclonus, autonomic instability, delirium and coma; concurrent and/or sequential use is contraindicated). Products include:

Propafenone Hydrochloride (Concurrent use of drugs that inhibit the biochemical activity of P450IID6, such as propafenone, may increase plasma concentrations of co-administered drugs that are metabolized by P450IID6; changes in the dosage may be required). Products include:

Propoxyphene Hydrochloride (Many drugs effective in the treatment of major depressive disorder, eg, the SSRIs, including sertraline, and most tricyclic antidepressant drugs effective in the treatment of major depressive disorder inhibit the biochemical activity of the drug metabolizing isoenzyme cytochrome P450 2D6, and, thus, may increase the plasma concentrations of co-administered drugs that are metabolized by CYP2D6. The drugs for which this potential interaction is of greatest concern are those metabolized by CYP2D6 and which have a narrow therapeutic index).

No products indexed under this heading.

Propoxyphene Napsylate (Many drugs effective in the treatment of major depressive disorder, eg, the SSRIs, including sertraline, and most tricyclic antidepressant drugs effective in the treatment of major depressive disorder inhibit the biochemical activity of the drug metabolizing isoenzyme cytochrome P450 2D6, and, thus, may increase the plasma concentrations of co-administered drugs that are metabolized by CYP2D6. The drugs for which this potential interaction is of greatest concern are those metabolized by CYP2D6 and which have a narrow therapeutic index).

No products indexed under this heading.

Propranolol Hydrochloride (Co-administration with drugs that are highly protein bound may cause a shift in plasma concentrations, potentially resulting in an adverse effect). Products include:

Protriptyline Hydrochloride (Concurrent use of drugs that inhibit the biochemical activity of P450IID6, such as tricyclic antidepressants, may increase plasma concentrations of co-administered drugs that are metabolized by P450IID6; changes in the dosage may be required; the duration of an appropriate washout period which should intervene before switching has not been established).

No products indexed under this heading.

Quetiapine Fumarate (Many drugs effective in the treatment of major depressive disorder, eg, the SSRIs, including sertraline, and most tricyclic antidepressant drugs effective in the treatment of major depressive disorder inhibit the biochemical activity of the drug metabolizing isoenzyme cytochrome P450 2D6, and, thus, may increase the plasma concentrations of co-administered drugs that are metabolized by CYP2D6. The drugs for which this potential interaction is of greatest concern are those metabolized by CYP2D6 and which have a narrow therapeutic index). Products include:

Seroquel Tablets 690

Quinidine Gluconate (Many drugs effective in the treatment of major depressive disorder, eg, the SSRIs, including sertraline, and most tricyclic antidepressant drugs effective in the treatment of major depressive disorder inhibit the biochemical activity of the drug metabolizing isoenzyme cytochrome P450 2D6, and, thus, may increase the plasma concentrations of co-administered drugs that are metabolized by CYP2D6. The drugs for which this potential interaction is of greatest concern are those metabolized by CYP2D6 and which have a narrow therapeutic index).

No products indexed under this heading.

Quinidine Hydrochloride (Many drugs effective in the treatment of major depressive disorder, eg, the SSRIs, including sertraline, and most tricyclic antidepressant drugs effective in the treatment of major depressive disorder inhibit the biochemical activity of the drug metabolizing isoenzyme cytochrome P450 2D6, and, thus, may increase the plasma concentrations of co-administered drugs that are metabolized by CYP2D6. The drugs for which this potential interaction is of greatest concern are those metabolized by CYP2D6 and which have a narrow therapeutic index).

No products indexed under this heading.

Quinidine Polygalacturonate (Many drugs effective in the treatment of major depressive disorder, eg, the SSRIs, including sertraline, and most tricyclic antidepressant drugs effective in the treatment of major depressive disorder inhibit the biochemical activity of the drug metabolizing isoenzyme cytochrome P450 2D6, and, thus, may increase the plasma concentrations of co-administered drugs that are metabolized by CYP2D6. The drugs for which this potential interaction is of greatest concern are those metabolized by CYP2D6 and which have a narrow therapeutic index).

No products indexed under this heading.

Quinidine Sulfate (Many drugs effective in the treatment of major depressive disorder, eg, the SSRIs, including sertraline, and most tricyclic antidepressant drugs effective in the treatment of major depressive disorder inhibit the biochemical activity of the drug metabolizing isoenzyme cytochrome P450 2D6, and, thus, may increase the plasma concentrations of co-administered drugs that are metabolized by CYP2D6. The drugs for which this potential interaction is of greatest concern are those metabolized by CYP2D6 and which have a narrow therapeutic index).

No products indexed under this heading.

Risperidone (Many drugs effective in the treatment of major depressive disorder, eg, the SSRIs, including sertraline, and most tricyclic antidepressant drugs effective in the treatment of major depressive disorder inhibit the biochemical activity of the drug metabolizing isoenzyme cytochrome P450 2D6, and, thus, may increase the plasma concentrations of co-administered drugs that are metabolized by CYP2D6. The drugs for which this potential interaction is of greatest concern are those metabolized by CYP2D6 and which have a narrow therapeutic index). Products include:

Risperdal ... 1676
Risperdal Consta Long-Acting
 Injection .. 1682
Risperdal M-Tab Orally
 Disintegrating Tablets.................. 1676

Ritonavir (Many drugs effective in the treatment of major depressive disorder, eg, the SSRIs, including sertraline, and most tricyclic antidepressant drugs effective in the treatment of major depressive disorder inhibit the biochemical activity of the drug metabolizing isoenzyme cytochrome P450 2D6, and, thus, may increase the plasma concentrations of co-administered drugs that are metabolized by CYP2D6. The drugs for which this potential interaction is of greatest concern are those metabolized by CYP2D6 and which have a narrow therapeutic index). Products include:

Kaletra ... 476
Norvir ... 503

Rofecoxib (Patients should be cautioned about the concomitant use of sertraline hydrochloride and non-selective NSAIDs (eg, NSAIDs that inhibit both cyclooxygenase isoenzymes, COX 1 and 2), since the combined use of psychotropic drugs that interfere with serotonin reuptake and these agents has been associated with an increased risk of bleeding).

No products indexed under this heading.

Selegiline Hydrochloride (Concomitant use in patients taking MAO inhibitors and SSRIs, such as sertraline, has resulted in cases of serious fatal reactions including hyperthermia, rigidity, myoclonus, autonomic instability, delirium and coma; concurrent and/or sequential use is contraindicated). Products include:

Eldepryl Capsules 3208
Zelapar Tablets 3372

Sulindac (Co-administration with drugs that are highly protein bound

may cause a shift in plasma concentrations, potentially resulting in an adverse effect). Products include:

Clinoril Tablets 1924

Sumatriptan (Co-administration of SSRIs and sumatriptan has resulted in rare reports of weakness, hyperreflexia, and incoordination). Products include:

Imitrex Nasal Spray 1467

Sumatriptan Succinate (Co-administration of SSRIs and sumatriptan has resulted in rare reports of weakness, hyperreflexia, and incoordination). Products include:

Imitrex Injection 1463
Imitrex Tablets 1471

Tamoxifen Citrate (Many drugs effective in the treatment of major depressive disorder, eg, the SSRIs, including sertraline, and most tricyclic antidepressant drugs effective in the treatment of major depressive disorder inhibit the biochemical activity of the drug metabolizing isoenzyme cytochrome P450 2D6, and, thus, may increase the plasma concentrations of co-administered drugs that are metabolized by CYP2D6. The drugs for which this potential interaction is of greatest concern are those metabolized by CYP2D6 and which have a narrow therapeutic index). Products include:

Soltamox Oral Solution 3527

Temazepam (Co-administration with drugs that are highly protein bound may cause a shift in plasma concentrations, potentially resulting in an adverse effect). Products include:

Restoril Capsules 1860

Teniposide (Many drugs effective in the treatment of major depressive disorder, eg, the SSRIs, including sertraline, and most tricyclic antidepressant drugs effective in the treatment of major depressive disorder inhibit the biochemical activity of the drug metabolizing isoenzyme cytochrome P450 2D6, and, thus, may increase the plasma concentrations of co-administered drugs that are metabolized by CYP2D6. The drugs for which this potential interaction is of greatest concern are those metabolized by CYP2D6 and which have a narrow therapeutic index).

No products indexed under this heading.

Testosterone (Many drugs effective in the treatment of major depressive disorder, eg, the SSRIs, including sertraline, and most tricyclic antidepressant drugs effective in the treatment of major depressive disorder inhibit the biochemical activity of the drug metabolizing isoenzyme cytochrome P450 2D6, and, thus, may increase the plasma concentrations of co-administered drugs that are metabolized by CYP2D6. The drugs for which this potential interaction is of greatest concern are those metabolized by CYP2D6 and which have a narrow therapeutic index). Products include:

AndroGel\.................. 3329
Striant Mucoadhesive 1007
Testim 1% Gel 695

Testosterone Cypionate (Many drugs effective in the treatment of major depressive disorder, eg, the SSRIs, including sertraline, and most tricyclic antidepressant drugs effective in the treatment of major depressive disorder inhibit the biochemical

activity of the drug metabolizing isoenzyme cytochrome P450 2D6, and, thus, may increase the plasma concentrations of co-administered drugs that are metabolized by CYP2D6. The drugs for which this potential interaction is of greatest concern are those metabolized by CYP2D6 and which have a narrow therapeutic index).

No products indexed under this heading.

Testosterone Enanthate (Many drugs effective in the treatment of major depressive disorder, eg, the SSRIs, including sertraline, and most tricyclic antidepressant drugs effective in the treatment of major depressive disorder inhibit the biochemical activity of the drug metabolizing isoenzyme cytochrome P450 2D6, and, thus, may increase the plasma concentrations of co-administered drugs that are metabolized by CYP2D6. The drugs for which this potential interaction is of greatest concern are those metabolized by CYP2D6 and which have a narrow therapeutic index).

No products indexed under this heading.

Testosterone Propionate (Many drugs effective in the treatment of major depressive disorder, eg, the SSRIs, including sertraline, and most tricyclic antidepressant drugs effective in the treatment of major depressive disorder inhibit the biochemical activity of the drug metabolizing isoenzyme cytochrome P450 2D6, and, thus, may increase the plasma concentrations of co-administered drugs that are metabolized by CYP2D6. The drugs for which this potential interaction is of greatest concern are those metabolized by CYP2D6 and which have a narrow therapeutic index).

No products indexed under this heading.

Thioridazine (Many drugs effective in the treatment of major depressive disorder, eg, the SSRIs, including sertraline, and most tricyclic antidepressant drugs effective in the treatment of major depressive disorder inhibit the biochemical activity of the drug metabolizing isoenzyme cytochrome P450 2D6, and, thus, may increase the plasma concentrations of co-administered drugs that are metabolized by CYP2D6. The drugs for which this potential interaction is of greatest concern are those metabolized by CYP2D6 and which have a narrow therapeutic index).

No products indexed under this heading.

Thioridazine Hydrochloride (Many drugs effective in the treatment of major depressive disorder, eg, the SSRIs, including sertraline, and most tricyclic antidepressant drugs effective in the treatment of major depressive disorder inhibit the biochemical activity of the drug metabolizing isoenzyme cytochrome P450 2D6, and, thus, may increase the plasma concentrations of co-administered drugs that are metabolized by CYP2D6. The drugs for which this potential interaction is of greatest concern are those metabolized by CYP2D6 and which have a narrow therapeutic index). Products include:

Thioridazine Hydrochloride
 Tablets...................................... 2163

IMPORTANT NOTE: Always consult each drug listing in the patient's regimen for possible interactions.

Timolol Maleate (Many drugs effective in the treatment of major depressive disorder, eg, the SSRIs, including sertraline, and most tricyclic antidepressant drugs effective in the treatment of major depressive disorder inhibit the biochemical activity of the drug metabolizing isoenzyme cytochrome P450 2D6, and, thus, may increase the plasma concentrations of co-administered drugs that are metabolized by CYP2D6. The drugs for which this potential interaction is of greatest concern are those metabolized by CYP2D6 and which have a narrow therapeutic index). Products include:
- Blocadren Tablets ... 1916
- Cosopt Sterile Ophthalmic Solution ... 1931
- Timolide Tablets ... 2086
- Timoptic Sterile Ophthalmic Solution ... 2088
- Timoptic in Ocudose ... 2091
- Timoptic-XE Sterile Ophthalmic Gel Forming Solution ... 2092

Tinzaparin Sodium (Patients should be cautioned about the concomitant use of sertraline hydrochloride and drugs that affect coagulation since the combined use of psychotropic drugs that interfere with serotonin reuptake and these agents has been associated with an increased risk of bleeding).
No products indexed under this heading.

Tolbutamide (Co-administration has caused a statistically significant 16% decrease from baseline in the clearance of tolbutamide; the clinical significance of this finding is unknown).
No products indexed under this heading.

Tolmetin Sodium (Co-administration with drugs that are highly protein bound may cause a shift in plasma concentrations, potentially resulting in an adverse effect).
No products indexed under this heading.

Tolterodine Tartrate (Many drugs effective in the treatment of major depressive disorder, eg, the SSRIs, including sertraline, and most tricyclic antidepressant drugs effective in the treatment of major depressive disorder inhibit the biochemical activity of the drug metabolizing isoenzyme cytochrome P450 2D6, and, thus, may increase the plasma concentrations of co-administered drugs that are metabolized by CYP2D6. The drugs for which this potential interaction is of greatest concern are those metabolized by CYP2D6 and which have a narrow therapeutic index). Products include:
- Detrol Tablets ... 2628
- Detrol LA Capsules ... 2631

Tramadol Hydrochloride (Many drugs effective in the treatment of major depressive disorder, eg, the SSRIs, including sertraline, and most tricyclic antidepressant drugs effective in the treatment of major depressive disorder inhibit the biochemical activity of the drug metabolizing isoenzyme cytochrome P450 2D6, and, thus, may increase the plasma concentrations of co-administered drugs that are metabolized by CYP2D6. The drugs for which this potential interaction is of greatest concern are those metabolized by CYP2D6 and which have a narrow therapeutic index). Products include:
- Ultram ER Tablets ... 2392

Tranylcypromine Sulfate (Concomitant use in patients taking MAO inhibitors and SSRIs, such as sertraline, has resulted in cases of serious fatal reactions including hyperthermia, rigidity, myoclonus, autonomic instability, delirium and coma; concurrent and/or sequential use is contraindicated). Products include:
- Parnate Tablets ... 1527

Trazodone Hydrochloride (Concurrent use of drugs that inhibit the biochemical activity of P450IID6, such as tricyclic antidepressants, may increase plasma concentrations of co-administered drugs that are metabolized by P450IID6; changes in the dosage may be required; the duration of an appropriate washout period which should intervene before switching has not been established).
No products indexed under this heading.

Triazolam (Many drugs effective in the treatment of major depressive disorder, eg, the SSRIs, including sertraline, and most tricyclic antidepressant drugs effective in the treatment of major depressive disorder inhibit the biochemical activity of the drug metabolizing isoenzyme cytochrome P450 2D6, and, thus, may increase the plasma concentrations of co-administered drugs that are metabolized by CYP2D6. The drugs for which this potential interaction is of greatest concern are those metabolized by CYP2D6 and which have a narrow therapeutic index).
No products indexed under this heading.

Trimipramine Maleate (Concurrent use of drugs that inhibit the biochemical activity of P450IID6, such as tricyclic antidepressants, may increase plasma concentrations of co-administered drugs that are metabolized by P450IID6; changes in the dosage may be required; the duration of an appropriate washout period which should intervene before switching has not been established).
No products indexed under this heading.

Valdecoxib (Patients should be cautioned about the concomitant use of sertraline hydrochloride and nonselective NSAIDs (eg, NSAIDs that inhibit both cyclooxygenase isoenzymes, COX 1 and 2), since the combined use of psychotropic drugs that interfere with serotonin reuptake and these agents has been associated with an increased risk of bleeding).
No products indexed under this heading.

Valproate Sodium (It is recommended that plasma valproate concentrations be monitored following initiation of sertraline hydrochloride therapy with appropriate adjustments to the valproate dose). Products include:
- Depacon Injection ... 412

Venlafaxine Hydrochloride (Concurrent use of drugs that inhibit the biochemical activity of P450IID6, such as SSRIs, may increase plasma concentrations of co-administered drugs that are metabolized by P450IID6; changes in the dosage may be required; the duration of an appropriate washout period, which should intervene before switching, has not been established). Products include:
- Effexor Tablets ... 3411
- Effexor XR Capsules ... 3417

Vinblastine Sulfate (Many drugs effective in the treatment of major depressive disorder, eg, the SSRIs, including sertraline, and most tricyclic antidepressant drugs effective in the treatment of major depressive disorder inhibit the biochemical activity of the drug metabolizing isoenzyme cytochrome P450 2D6, and, thus, may increase the plasma concentrations of co-administered drugs that are metabolized by CYP2D6. The drugs for which this potential interaction is of greatest concern are those metabolized by CYP2D6 and which have a narrow therapeutic index).
No products indexed under this heading.

Warfarin Sodium (Co-administration has resulted in a mean increase in prothrombin time of 8% relative to baseline for sertraline; the clinical significance of this change is not known). Products include:
- Coumadin for Injection ... 898
- Coumadin Tablets ... 898

Zonisamide (Many drugs effective in the treatment of major depressive disorder, eg, the SSRIs, including sertraline, and most tricyclic antidepressant drugs effective in the treatment of major depressive disorder inhibit the biochemical activity of the drug metabolizing isoenzyme cytochrome P450 2D6, and, thus, may increase the plasma concentrations of co-administered drugs that are metabolized by CYP2D6. The drugs for which this potential interaction is of greatest concern are those metabolized by CYP2D6 and which have a narrow therapeutic index). Products include:
- Zonegran Capsules ... 1101

Food Interactions

Alcohol (Patients should be told that although sertraline hydrochloride has not been shown in experiments with normal subjects to increase the mental and motor skill impairments caused by alcohol, the concomitant use of sertraline hydrochloride and alcohol is not advised).

Food, unspecified (Co-administration of Zoloft Tablets with food slightly increased AUC but the Cmax was 25% greater, while time to reach peak plasma concentration (Tmax) decreased from 8 hours to 5.5 hours; for oral concentrate, Tmax was slightly prolonged from 5.9 hours to 7 hours with food).

ZOLOFT TABLETS

(Sertraline Hydrochloride) ... 2586

See Zoloft Oral Concentrate

ZOMETA FOR INTRAVENOUS INFUSION

(Zoledronic acid) ... 2315

May interact with aminoglycosides and loop diuretics. Compounds in these categories include:

Amikacin Sulfate (Co-administration with aminoglycosides may have an additive effect to lower serum calcium for prolonged period).
No products indexed under this heading.

Bumetanide (Increased risk of hypocalcemia). Products include:
- Bumex Tablets ... 2746

Ethacrynic Acid (Increased risk of hypocalcemia). Products include:
- Edecrin Tablets ... 1959

Furosemide (Increased risk of hypocalcemia). Products include:
- Furosemide Tablets ... 2154

Gentamicin Sulfate (Co-administration with aminoglycosides may have an additive effect to lower serum calcium for prolonged period). Products include:
- Garamycin Injectable ... 3014
- Pred-G Ophthalmic Ointment ... ⊙237
- Pred-G Ophthalmic Suspension ... ⊙236

Kanamycin Sulfate (Co-administration with aminoglycosides may have an additive effect to lower serum calcium for prolonged period).
No products indexed under this heading.

Streptomycin Sulfate (Co-administration with aminoglycosides may have an additive effect to lower serum calcium for prolonged period).
No products indexed under this heading.

Tobramycin (Co-administration with aminoglycosides may have an additive effect to lower serum calcium for prolonged period). Products include:
- TOBI Solution for Inhalation ... 2298
- TobraDex Ophthalmic Ointment ... 562
- TobraDex Ophthalmic Suspension ... 563
- Zylet Ophthalmic Suspension ... ⊙259

Tobramycin Sulfate (Co-administration with aminoglycosides may have an additive effect to lower serum calcium for prolonged period).
No products indexed under this heading.

Torsemide (Increased risk of hypocalcemia). Products include:
- Demadex Injection ... 2759
- Demadex Tablets ... 2759

ZOMIG TABLETS

(Zolmitriptan) ... 3519

May interact with 5HT1-receptor agonists, ergot-containing drugs, monoamine oxidase inhibitors, and selective serotonin reuptake inhibitors. Compounds in these categories include:

Citalopram Hydrobromide (Cases of life-threatening serotonin syndrome, including mental status changes, autonomic instability, neuromuscular aberrations, and/or GI symptoms, have been reported during combination use of selective serotonin reuptake inhibitors and triptans. If concomitant treatment with zolmitriptan and an SSRI is clinically warranted, careful observation of the patient is advised, particularly during treatment initiation and dose increases). Products include:
- Celexa ... 1176

Dihydroergotamine Mesylate (Ergot-containing drugs have been reported to cause prolonged vasospastic reactions; use of ergot-type medications and zolmitriptan within 24 hours of each other should be avoided). Products include:
- Migranal Nasal Spray ... 3348

3-Diphenylacrylate (Concomitant use with other 5-HT1 agonists within 24 hours of each other is containdicated because the vasospastic effects may be additive).
No products indexed under this heading.

Ergonovine Maleate (Ergot-containing drugs have been reported to cause prolonged vasospastic reactions; use of ergot-type medications and zolmitriptan within 24 hours of each other should be avoided).
No products indexed under this heading.

Ergotamine Tartrate (Ergot-containing drugs have been reported to cause prolonged vasospastic reactions; use of ergot-type medications and zolmitriptan within 24 hours of each other should be avoided).
No products indexed under this heading.

Escitalopram Oxalate (Cases of life-threatening serotonin syndrome, including mental status changes, autonomic instability, neuromuscular aberrations, and/or GI symptoms, have been reported during combination use of selective serotonin reuptake inhibitors and triptans. If concomitant treatment with zolmitriptan and an SSRI is clinically warranted, careful observation of the patient is advised, particularly during treatment initiation and dose increases). Products include:
Lexapro Oral Solution 1190
Lexapro Tablets 1190

Fluoxetine Hydrochloride (Cases of life-threatening serotonin syndrome, including mental status changes, autonomic instability, neuromuscular aberrations, and/or GI symptoms, have been reported during combination use of selective serotonin reuptake inhibitors and triptans. If concomitant treatment with zolmitriptan and an SSRI is clinically warranted, careful observation of the patient is advised, particularly during treatment initiation and dose increases). Products include:
Prozac Pulvules and Liquid 1801
Symbyax Capsules 1819

Fluvoxamine Maleate (Cases of life-threatening serotonin syndrome, including mental status changes, autonomic instability, neuromuscular aberrations, and/or GI symptoms, have been reported during combination use of selective serotonin reuptake inhibitors and triptans. If concomitant treatment with zolmitriptan and an SSRI is clinically warranted, careful observation of the patient is advised, particularly during treatment initiation and dose increases).
No products indexed under this heading.

Isocarboxazid (MAO-A inhibitors increase systemic exposure of zolmitriptan).
No products indexed under this heading.

Methylergonovine Maleate (Ergot-containing drugs have been reported to cause prolonged vasospastic reactions; use of ergot-type medications and zolmitriptan within 24 hours of each other should be avoided).
No products indexed under this heading.

Methysergide Maleate (Ergot-containing drugs have been reported to cause prolonged vasospastic reactions; use of ergot-type medications and zolmitriptan within 24 hours of each other should be avoided).
No products indexed under this heading.

Moclobemide (MAO-A inhibitors increase systemic exposure of zolmitriptan).
No products indexed under this heading.

Naratriptan Hydrochloride (Concomitant use with other 5-HT1 agonists within 24 hours of each other is containdicated because the vasospastic effects may be additive). Products include:
Amerge Tablets 1339

Pargyline Hydrochloride (MAO-A inhibitors increase systemic exposure of zolmitriptan).
No products indexed under this heading.

Paroxetine Hydrochloride (Cases of life-threatening serotonin syndrome, including mental status changes, autonomic instability, neuromuscular aberrations, and/or GI symptoms, have been reported during combination use of selective serotonin reuptake inhibitors and triptans. If concomitant treatment with zolmitriptan and an SSRI is clinically warranted, careful observation of the patient is advised, particularly during treatment initiation and dose increases). Products include:
Paxil CR Controlled-Release Tablets 1538
Paxil 1530

Phenelzine Sulfate (MAO-A inhibitors increase systemic exposure of zolmitriptan).
No products indexed under this heading.

Procarbazine Hydrochloride (MAO-A inhibitors increase systemic exposure of zolmitriptan). Products include:
Matulane Capsules 3191

Rizatriptan Benzoate (Concomitant use with other 5-HT1 agonists within 24 hours of each other is containdicated because the vasospastic effects may be additive). Products include:
Maxalt Tablets 2008
Maxalt-MLT Orally Disintegrating Tablets 2008

Selegiline Hydrochloride (MAO-A inhibitors increase systemic exposure of zolmitriptan). Products include:
Eldepryl Capsules 3208
Zelapar Tablets 3372

Sertraline Hydrochloride (Cases of life-threatening serotonin syndrome, including mental status changes, autonomic instability, neuromuscular aberrations, and/or GI symptoms, have been reported during combination use of selective serotonin reuptake inhibitors and triptans. If concomitant treatment with zolmitriptan and an SSRI is clinically warranted, careful observation of the patient is advised, particularly during treatment initiation and dose increases). Products include:
Zoloft 2586

Sumatriptan (Concomitant use with other 5-HT1 agonists within 24 hours of each other is containdicated because the vasospastic effects may be additive). Products include:
Imitrex Nasal Spray 1467

Sumatriptan Succinate (Concomitant use with other 5-HT1 agonists within 24 hours of each other is containdicated because the vasospastic effects may be additive). Products include:
Imitrex Injection 1463
Imitrex Tablets 1471

Tranylcypromine Sulfate (MAO-A inhibitors increase systemic exposure of zolmitriptan). Products include:
Parnate Tablets 1527

ZOMIG NASAL SPRAY

(Zolmitriptan) 3523
May interact with 5HT1-receptor agonists, ergot-containing drugs, monoamine oxidase inhibitors, oral contraceptives, selective serotonin reuptake inhibitors, and certain other agents. Compounds in these categories include:

Acetaminophen (Zolmitriptan delayed the Tmax of acetaminophen by one hour in a single dose study). Products include:
Comtrex Maximum Strength Cold & Cough Day/Night Caplets - Day Formulation .... ■ 726
Comtrex Maximum Strength Cold & Cough Day/Night Caplets - Night Formulation .... ■ 726
Comtrex Maximum Strength Non-Drowsy Cold & Cough Caplets .... ■ 725
Comtrex Maximum Strength Day/Night Severe Cold & Sinus Caplets - Day Formulation .... ■ 725
Comtrex Maximum Strength Day/Night Severe Cold & Sinus Caplets - Night Formulation .... ■ 725
Contac Cold and Flu Maximum Strength Caplets .... ■ 728
Contac Cold and Flu Day and Night Caplets (Day Formulation Only) .... ■ 727
Contac Cold and Flu Day and Night Caplets (Night Formulation Only) .... ■ 727
Contac Cold and Flu Non-Drowsy Caplets .... ■ 728
Excedrin Extra Strength Caplets/Tablets/Geltabs .... ■ 684
Excedrin Migraine Caplets/Tablets/Geltabs .... ■ 609
Excedrin PM Caplets/Tablets/Geltabs .... ■ 610
Excedrin Sinus Headache Caplets/Tablets .... ■ 610
Excedrin Tension Headache Caplets/Tablets/Geltabs .... ■ 611
Goody's Body Pain Formula Powder .... ■ 684
Goody's Extra Strength Headache Powders .... ■ 611
Goody's Extra Strength Pain Relief Tablets .... ■ 685
Goody's PM Powder for Pain with Sleeplessness .... ■ 612
Percocet Tablets 1131
Robitussin Cough, Cold & Flu Nighttime Liquid .... ■ 738
TheraFlu Cold & Sore Throat Hot Liquid .... ■ 741
TheraFlu Flu & Chest Congestion Hot Liquid .... ■ 741
TheraFlu Flu & Sore Throat Hot Liquid .... ■ 742
TheraFlu Daytime Severe Cold Hot Liquid .... ■ 742
TheraFlu Nighttime Severe Cold Hot Liquid .... ■ 740
TheraFlu Warming Relief Daytime Severe Cold .... ■ 743
TheraFlu Warming Relief Nighttime Severe Cold .... ■ 743
Triaminic Cough & Sore Throat Liquid .... ■ 747
Regular Strength Tylenol Tablets 1870
Children's Tylenol with Flavor Creator .... ■ 679
Children's Tylenol Plus Flu Oral Suspension .... ■ 749
Tylenol Cold Head Congestion Daytime Caplets with Cool Burst and Gelcaps .... ■ 750
Tylenol Cold Multi-Symptom Daytime Liquid .... ■ 752
Tylenol Cold Multi-Symptom Severe Daytime Liquid .... ■ 752
Tylenol 8 Hour Extended Release Caplets 1870
Tylenol 1870
Extra Strength Tylenol PM Caplets, Vanilla Caplets, Geltabs, Gelcaps and Liquid 1875
Extra Strength Tylenol Rapid Release Gels 1870
Concentrated Tylenol Infants' Drops Plus Cold & Cough .... ■ 754
Tylenol with Codeine Tablets 2391
Tylenol Allergy Multi-Symptom Caplets with Cool Burst and Gelcaps 1872
Tylenol Allergy Multi-Symptom Nighttime Caplets with Cool Burst 1872
Tylenol Severe Allergy Caplets 1872
Tylenol Arthritis Pain Extended Release Caplets and Geltabs 1870
Tylenol Chest Congestion Caplets with Cool Burst 1872
Tylenol Chest Congestion Liquid with Cool Burst 1872
Children's Tylenol Suspension Liquid and Meltaways 1878
Children's Tylenol Plus Cold Suspension Liquid 1879
Children's Tylenol Plus Cold & Allergy Suspension Liquid 1878
Children's Tylenol Plus Cough & Runny Nose Suspension Liquid 1879
Children's Tylenol Plus Cough & Sore Throat Suspension Liquid 1879
Children's Tylenol Suspension with Flavor Creator 1878
Children's Tylenol Plus Flu Suspension Liquid 1881
Children's Tylenol Plus Multi-Symptom Cold Suspension Liquid 1879
Tylenol Cold Severe Congestion Non-Drowsy Caplets with Cool Burst 1874
Tylenol Cold Head Congestion Daytime Caplets with Cool Burst 1873
Tylenol Cold Head Congestion Nighttime Caplets with Cool Burst 1873
Tylenol Cold Head Congestion Severe Caplets with Cool Burst 1873
Tylenol Cold Multi-Symptom Daytime Caplets with Cool Burst and Gelcaps 1874
Tylenol Cold Multi-Symptom Daytime Liquid with Citrus Burst 1874
Tylenol Cold Multi-Symptom Nighttime Caplets with Cool Burst 1874
Tylenol Cold Multi-Symptom Nighttime Liquid with Cool Burst 1874
Tylenol Cold Multi-Symptom Severe Caplets with Cool Burst 1874
Tylenol Cold Multi-Symptom Severe Daytime Liquid with Citrus Burst 1874
Tylenol Cough & Sore Throat Daytime Liquid with Cool Burst 1877
Tylenol Cough & Sore Throat Nighttime Liquid with Cool Burst 1877
Concentrated Tylenol Infants' Drops 1878
Concentrated Tylenol Infants' Drops Plus Cold 1879
Concentrated Tylenol Infants' Drops Plus Cold and Cough 1879
Jr. Tylenol Meltaways 1878
Tylenol Sinus Severe Congestion Caplets with Cool Burst 1876
Tylenol Sinus Congestion & Pain Daytime Caplets with Cool Burst and Gelcaps 1876
Tylenol Sinus Congestion & Pain Nighttime Caplets with Cool Burst 1876
Tylenol Sinus Congestion & Pain Severe Caplets with Cool Burst 1876
Tylenol Sore Throat Daytime Liquid with Cool Burst 1877
Tylenol Sore Throat Nighttime Liquid with Cool Burst 1877
Women's Tylenol Menstrual Relief Caplets 1877
Vicks 44M Cough, Cold & Flu Relief Liquid 2680
Vicks DayQuil LiquiCaps/Liquid Multi-Symptom Cold/Flu Relief .... ■ 761

Cimetidine (Following administration of cimetidine, the half-life and AUC of zolmitriptan and its active metabolites were approximately doubled). Products include:

Cimetidine Hydrochloride (Following administration of cimetidine, the half-life and AUC of zolmitriptan and its active metabolites were approximately doubled).

No products indexed under this heading.

Citalopram Hydrobromide (Cases of life-threatening serotonin syndrome, including mental status changes, autonomic instability, neuromuscular aberrations, and/or GI symptoms, have been reported during combination use of selective serotonin reuptake inhibitors and triptans. If concomitant treatment with zolmitriptan and an SSRI is clinically warranted, careful observation of the patient is advised, particularly during treatment initiation and dose increases). Products include:

Desogestrel (Retrospective analysis of pharmacokinetic data indicates the mean plasma concentrations, Cmax and AUC, of zolmitriptan were generally higher in females taking oral contraceptives, Tmax was delayed by one-half hour in these females). Products include:

Dihydroergotamine Mesylate (Ergot-containing drugs have been reported to cause prolonged vasospastic reactions; because there is a theoretical basis that these effects may be additive, use of ergot-type agents and zolmitriptan within 24 hours is contraindicated). Products include:

3-Diphenylacrylate (Co-administration with other 5-HT1 agonists within 24 hours of each other is contraindicated).

No products indexed under this heading.

Duloxetine Hydrochloride (Cases of life-threatening serotonin syndrome, including mental status changes, autonomic instability, neuromuscular aberrations, and/or GI symptoms, have been reported during combination use of serotonin and norepinephrine reuptake inhibitors and triptans. If concomitant treatment with zolmitriptan and an SNRI is clinically warranted, careful observation of the patient is advised, particularly during treatment initiation and dose increases). Products include:

Ergonovine Maleate (Ergot-containing drugs have been reported to cause prolonged vasospastic reactions; because there is a theoretical basis that these effects may be additive, use of ergot-type agents and zolmitriptan within 24 hours is contraindicated).

No products indexed under this heading.

Ergotamine Tartrate (Ergot-containing drugs have been reported to cause prolonged vasospastic reactions; because there is a theoretical basis that these effects may be additive, use of ergot-type agents and zolmitriptan within 24 hours is contraindicated).

No products indexed under this heading.

Escitalopram Oxalate (Cases of life-threatening serotonin syndrome, including mental status changes, autonomic instability, neuromuscular aberrations, and/or GI symptoms, have been reported during combination use of selective serotonin reuptake inhibitors and triptans. If concomitant treatment with zolmitriptan and an SSRI is clinically warranted, careful observation of the patient is advised, particularly during treatment initiation and dose increases). Products include:

Ethinyl Estradiol (Retrospective analysis of pharmacokinetic data indicates the mean plasma concentrations, Cmax and AUC, of zolmitriptan were generally higher in females taking oral contraceptives, Tmax was delayed by one-half hour in these females). Products include:

Ethynodiol Diacetate (Retrospective analysis of pharmacokinetic data indicates the mean plasma concentrations, Cmax and AUC, of zolmitriptan were generally higher in females taking oral contraceptives, Tmax was delayed by one-half hour in these females).

No products indexed under this heading.

Fluoxetine Hydrochloride (Cases of life-threatening serotonin syndrome, including mental status changes, autonomic instability, neuromuscular aberrations, and/or GI symptoms, have been reported during combination use of selective serotonin reuptake inhibitors and triptans. If concomitant treatment with zolmitriptan and an SSRI is clinically warranted, careful observation of the patient is advised, particularly during treatment initiation and dose increases). Products include:

Fluvoxamine Maleate (Cases of life-threatening serotonin syndrome, including mental status changes, autonomic instability, neuromuscular aberrations, and/or GI symptoms, have been reported during combination use of selective serotonin reuptake inhibitors and triptans. If concomitant treatment with zolmitriptan and an SSRI is clinically war-

ranted, careful observation of the patient is advised, particularly during treatment initiation and dose increases).

No products indexed under this heading.

Isocarboxazid (MAO-A inhibitors increase the systemic exposure of zolmitriptan; concurrent and/or sequential use is contraindicated).

No products indexed under this heading.

Levonorgestrel (Retrospective analysis of pharmacokinetic data indicates the mean plasma concentrations, Cmax and AUC, of zolmitriptan were generally higher in females taking oral contraceptives, Tmax was delayed by one-half hour in these females). Products include:

Mestranol (Retrospective analysis of pharmacokinetic data indicates the mean plasma concentrations, Cmax and AUC, of zolmitriptan were generally higher in females taking oral contraceptives, Tmax was delayed by one-half hour in these females).

No products indexed under this heading.

Methylergonovine Maleate (Ergot-containing drugs have been reported to cause prolonged vasospastic reactions; because there is a theoretical basis that these effects may be additive, use of ergot-type agents and zolmitriptan within 24 hours is contraindicated).

No products indexed under this heading.

Methysergide Maleate (Ergot-containing drugs have been reported to cause prolonged vasospastic reactions; because there is a theoretical basis that these effects may be additive, use of ergot-type agents and zolmitriptan within 24 hours is contraindicated).

No products indexed under this heading.

Moclobemide (MAO-A inhibitors increase the systemic exposure of zolmitriptan; concurrent and/or sequential use is contraindicated).

No products indexed under this heading.

Naratriptan Hydrochloride (Co-administration with other 5-HT1 agonists within 24 hours of each other is contraindicated). Products include:

Nefazodone Hydrochloride (Cases of life-threatening serotonin syndrome, including mental status changes, autonomic instability, neuromuscular aberrations, and/or GI symptoms, have been reported during combination use of serotonin and norepinephrine reuptake inhibitors and triptans. If concomitant treatment with zolmitriptan and an SNRI is clinically warranted, careful observation of the patient is advised, particularly during treatment initiation and dose increases).

No products indexed under this heading.

Norethindrone (Retrospective analysis of pharmacokinetic data indicates the mean plasma concentrations, Cmax and AUC, of zolmitriptan were generally higher in females

taking oral contraceptives, Tmax was delayed by one-half hour in these females). Products include:

Norethynodrel (Retrospective analysis of pharmacokinetic data indicates the mean plasma concentrations, Cmax and AUC, of zolmitriptan were generally higher in females taking oral contraceptives, Tmax was delayed by one-half hour in these females).

No products indexed under this heading.

Norgestimate (Retrospective analysis of pharmacokinetic data indicates the mean plasma concentrations, Cmax and AUC, of zolmitriptan were generally higher in females taking oral contraceptives, Tmax was delayed by one-half hour in these females). Products include:

Norgestrel (Retrospective analysis of pharmacokinetic data indicates the mean plasma concentrations, Cmax and AUC, of zolmitriptan were generally higher in females taking oral contraceptives, Tmax was delayed by one-half hour in these females).

No products indexed under this heading.

Pargyline Hydrochloride (MAO-A inhibitors increase the systemic exposure of zolmitriptan; concurrent and/or sequential use is contraindicated).

No products indexed under this heading.

Paroxetine Hydrochloride (Cases of life-threatening serotonin syndrome, including mental status changes, autonomic instability, neuromuscular aberrations, and/or GI symptoms, have been reported during combination use of selective serotonin reuptake inhibitors and triptans. If concomitant treatment with zolmitriptan and an SSRI is clinically warranted, careful observation of the patient is advised, particularly during treatment initiation and dose increases). Products include:

Phenelzine Sulfate (MAO-A inhibitors increase the systemic exposure of zolmitriptan; concurrent and/or sequential use is contraindicated).

No products indexed under this heading.

Procarbazine Hydrochloride (MAO-A inhibitors increase the systemic exposure of zolmitriptan; concurrent and/or sequential use is contraindicated). Products include:

Propanolol (Cmax and AUC of zolmitriptan increased after one week of dosing with propanolol; Cmax and AUC of N-desmethyl metabolite was reduced).

No products indexed under this heading.

Rizatriptan Benzoate (Co-administration with other 5-HT1 agonists within 24 hours of each other is contraindicated). Products include:

Selegiline Hydrochloride (MAO-A inhibitors increase the systemic exposure of zolmitriptan; concurrent and/or sequential use is contraindicated). Products include:

Eldepryl Capsules 3208
Zelapar Tablets 3372

Sertraline Hydrochloride (Cases of life-threatening serotonin syndrome, including mental status changes, autonomic instability, neuromuscular aberrations, and/or GI symptoms, have been reported during combination use of selective serotonin reuptake inhibitors and triptans. If concomitant treatment with zolmitriptan and an SSRI is clinically warranted, careful observation of the patient is advised, particularly during treatment initiation and dose increases). Products include:

Zoloft 2586

Sumatriptan (Co-administration with other 5-HT1 agonists within 24 hours of each other is contraindicated). Products include:

Imitrex Nasal Spray 1467

Sumatriptan Succinate (Co-administration with other 5-HT1 agonists within 24 hours of each other is contraindicated). Products include:

Imitrex Injection 1463
Imitrex Tablets 1471

Tranylcypromine Sulfate (MAO-A inhibitors increase the systemic exposure of zolmitriptan; concurrent and/or sequential use is contraindicated). Products include:

Parnate Tablets 1527

Venlafaxine Hydrochloride (Cases of life-threatening serotonin syndrome, including mental status changes, autonomic instability, neuromuscular aberrations, and/or GI symptoms, have been reported during combination use of serotonin and norepinephrine reuptake inhibitors and triptans. If concomitant treatment with zolmitriptan and an SNRI is clinically warranted, careful observation of the patient is advised, particularly during treatment initiation and dose increases). Products include:

Effexor Tablets 3411
Effexor XR Capsules 3417

ZOMIG-ZMT TABLETS

(Zolmitriptan) 3519

See Zomig Tablets

ZONEGRAN CAPSULES

(Zonisamide) 1101

May interact with phenytoin, valproate, and certain other agents. Compounds in these categories include:

Carbamazepine (Co-administration with drugs that induce liver enzymes increases the metabolism and clearance of zonisamide and decreases the half-life to 38 hours). Products include:

Carbatrol Capsules 3171
Equetro Extended-Release Capsules 3180
Tegretol/Tegretol-XR 2295

Divalproex Sodium (The half-life of zonisamide in patients concurrently on the non-enzyme inducing AED, valproate, was 46 hours). Products include:

Depakote Sprinkle Capsules 422
Depakote Tablets 427
Depakote ER Tablets 434

Fosphenytoin Sodium (Co-administration with drugs that induce liver enzymes increases the metabolism and clearance of zonisamide and decreases the half-life to 27 hours).

No products indexed under this heading.

Phenobarbital (Co-administration with drugs that induce liver enzymes increases the metabolism and clearance of zonisamide and decreases the half-life to 38 hours). Products include:

Donnatal Extentabs 2493

Phenytoin (Co-administration with drugs that induce liver enzymes increases the metabolism and clearance of zonisamide and decreases the half-life to 27 hours).

No products indexed under this heading.

Phenytoin Sodium (Co-administration with drugs that induce liver enzymes increases the metabolism and clearance of zonisamide and decreases the half-life to 27 hours). Products include:

Phenytek Capsules 2160

Valproate Sodium (The half-life of zonisamide in patients concurrently on the non-enzyme inducing AED, valproate, was 46 hours). Products include:

Depacon Injection 412

Valproic Acid (The half-life of zonisamide in patients concurrently on the non-enzyme inducing AED, valproate, was 46 hours). Products include:

Depakene 417

ZOSTAVAX INJECTION

(Zoster Vaccine Live) 2111

None cited in PDR database.

ZOSYN

(Piperacillin Sodium, Tazobactam Sodium) 3492

May interact with aminoglycosides, anticoagulants, nondepolarizing neuromuscular blocking agents, and certain other agents. Compounds in these categories include:

Amikacin Sulfate (The mixing of beta-lactam antibiotics with aminoglycosides in-vitro can result in substantial inactivation of the aminoglycoside. However, amikacin and gentamicin have been shown to be compatible in vitro with reformulated Zosyn containing EDTA supplied in vials or bulk pharmacy containers in certain diluents at specific concentrations for a simultaneous Y-site infusion. Reformulated Zosyn containing EDTA is not compatible with tobramycin for simultaneous administration via Y-site infusion).

No products indexed under this heading.

Anisindione (Coagulation parameters should be tested more frequently and monitored regularly during simultaneous administration; effect of concurrent use is not specified). Products include:

Miradon Tablets 3042

Ardeparin Sodium (Coagulation parameters should be tested more frequently and monitored regularly during simultaneous administration; effect of concurrent use is not specified).

No products indexed under this heading.

Atracurium Besylate (Due to similar mechanism of action as vecuronium, it is expected that the neuromuscular blockade produced by other non-depolarizing muscle relaxants could be prolonged in the presence of piperacillin).

No products indexed under this heading.

Cisatracurium Besylate (Due to similar mechanism of action as vecuronium, it is expected that the neuromuscular blockade produced by other non-depolarizing muscle relaxants could be prolonged in the presence of piperacillin). Products include:

Nimbex Injection 498

Dalteparin Sodium (Coagulation parameters should be tested more frequently and monitored regularly during simultaneous administration; effect of concurrent use is not specified). Products include:

Fragmin Injection 1097

Danaparoid Sodium (Coagulation parameters should be tested more frequently and monitored regularly during simultaneous administration; effect of concurrent use is not specified).

No products indexed under this heading.

Dicumarol (Coagulation parameters should be tested more frequently and monitored regularly during simultaneous administration; effect of concurrent use is not specified).

No products indexed under this heading.

Enoxaparin Sodium (Coagulation parameters should be tested more frequently and monitored regularly during simultaneous administration; effect of concurrent use is not specified). Products include:

Lovenox Injection 2915

Fondaparinux Sodium (Coagulation parameters should be tested more frequently and monitored regularly during simultaneous administration; effect of concurrent use is not specified). Products include:

Arixtra Injection 1351

Gentamicin Sulfate (The mixing of beta-lactam antibiotics with aminoglycosides in-vitro can result in substantial inactivation of the aminoglycoside. However, amikacin and gentamicin have been shown to be compatible in vitro with reformulated Zosyn containing EDTA supplied in vials or bulk pharmacy containers in certain diluents at specific concentrations for a simultaneous Y-site infusion. Reformulated Zosyn containing EDTA is not compatible with tobramycin for simultaneous administration via Y-site infusion). Products include:

Garamycin Injectable 3014
Pred-G Ophthalmic Ointment .... ⊙237
Pred-G Ophthalmic Suspension .... ⊙236

Heparin Calcium (Coagulation parameters should be tested more frequently and monitored regularly during simultaneous administration; effect of concurrent use is not specified).

No products indexed under this heading.

Heparin Sodium (Coagulation parameters should be tested more frequently and monitored regularly during simultaneous administration; effect of concurrent use is not specified).

No products indexed under this heading.

Kanamycin Sulfate (The mixing of beta-lactam antibiotics with aminoglycosides in-vitro can result in substantial inactivation of the aminoglycoside. However, amikacin and gentamicin have been shown to be compatible in vitro with reformulated Zosyn containing EDTA supplied in vials or bulk pharmacy containers in certain diluents at specific concentrations for a simultaneous Y-site infusion. Reformulated Zosyn containing EDTA is not compatible with tobramycin for simultaneous administration via Y-site infusion).

No products indexed under this heading.

Low Molecular Weight Heparins (Coagulation parameters should be tested more frequently and monitored regularly during simultaneous administration; effect of concurrent use is not specified).

No products indexed under this heading.

Methotrexate (Limited data suggests that co-administration of methotrexate and piperacillin may reduce the clearance of methotrexate due to competition for renal excretion).

No products indexed under this heading.

Metocurine Iodide (Due to similar mechanism of action as vecuronium, it is expected that the neuromuscular blockade produced by other non-depolarizing muscle relaxants could be prolonged in the presence of piperacillin).

No products indexed under this heading.

Mivacurium Chloride (Due to similar mechanism of action as vecuronium, it is expected that the neuromuscular blockade produced by other non-depolarizing muscle relaxants could be prolonged in the presence of piperacillin). Products include:

Mivacron Injection 493

Pancuronium Bromide (Due to similar mechanism of action as vecuronium, it is expected that the neuromuscular blockade produced by other non-depolarizing muscle relaxants could be prolonged in the presence of piperacillin).

No products indexed under this heading.

Probenecid (Concomitant administration prolongs half-life of piperacillin by 21% and of tazobactam by 71%).

No products indexed under this heading.

Rapacuronium Bromide (Due to similar mechanism of action as vecuronium, it is expected that the neuromuscular blockade produced by other non-depolarizing muscle relaxants could be prolonged in the presence of piperacillin).

No products indexed under this heading.

Rocuronium Bromide (Due to similar mechanism of action as vecuronium, it is expected that the neuromuscular blockade produced by other non-depolarizing muscle relaxants could be prolonged in the presence of piperacillin). Products include:

Zemuron Injection 2346

Streptomycin Sulfate (The mixing of beta-lactam antibiotics with aminoglycosides in-vitro can result in substantial inactivation of the aminoglycoside. However, amikacin and gentamicin have been shown to be compatible in vitro with reformulated Zosyn containing EDTA supplied in vials or bulk pharmacy containers in certain diluents at specific concentrations for a simultaneous Y-site infusion. Reformulated Zosyn containing EDTA is not compatible with tobramycin for simultaneous administration via Y-site infusion).

No products indexed under this heading.

Tinzaparin Sodium (Coagulation parameters should be tested more frequently and monitored regularly during simultaneous administration; effect of concurrent use is not specified).

No products indexed under this heading.

Tobramycin (The mixing of beta-lactam antibiotics with aminoglycosides in-vitro can result in substantial inactivation of the aminoglycoside. However, amikacin and gentamicin have been shown to be compatible in vitro with reformulated Zosyn containing EDTA supplied in vials or bulk pharmacy containers in certain diluents at specific concentrations for a simultaneous Y-site infusion. Reformulated Zosyn containing EDTA is not compatible with tobramycin for simultaneous administration via Y-site infusion). Products include:

TOBI Solution for Inhalation 2298
TobraDex Ophthalmic Ointment 562
TobraDex Ophthalmic Suspension ... 563
Zylet Ophthalmic Suspension .... ⊙259

Tobramycin Sulfate (Co-administration has resulted in the alteration of tobramycin pharmacokinetics which may be due to *in vitro* and *in vivo* inactivation of tobramycin).

No products indexed under this heading.

Vecuronium Bromide (Co-administration of piperacillin and vecuronium has been implicated in the prolongation of the neuromuscular blockade).

No products indexed under this heading.

Warfarin Sodium (Coagulation parameters should be tested more frequently and monitored regularly during simultaneous administration; effect of concurrent use is not specified). Products include:

Coumadin for Injection 898
Coumadin Tablets 898

ZOVIRAX CAPSULES

(Acyclovir) 1643

May interact with nephrotoxic agents and certain other agents. Compounds in these categories include:

Abacavir Sulfate (Caution should be exercised when administering acyclovir to patients receiving potentially nephrotoxic agents since this may increase the risk of renal dysfunction and/or the risk of reversible CNS symptoms such as those that have been reported in patients treated with intravenous acyclovir. Adequate hydration should be maintained). Products include:

Epzicom Tablets 1436
Trizivir Tablets 1589
Ziagen 1626

Acyclovir Sodium (Caution should be exercised when administering acyclovir to patients receiving potentially nephrotoxic agents since this may increase the risk of renal dysfunction and/or the risk of reversible CNS symptoms such as those that have been reported in patients treated with intravenous acyclovir. Adequate hydration should be maintained).

No products indexed under this heading.

Alatrofloxacin Mesylate (Caution should be exercised when administering acyclovir to patients receiving potentially nephrotoxic agents since this may increase the risk of renal dysfunction and/or the risk of reversible CNS symptoms such as those that have been reported in patients treated with intravenous acyclovir. Adequate hydration should be maintained).

No products indexed under this heading.

Aldesleukin (Caution should be exercised when administering acyclovir to patients receiving potentially nephrotoxic agents since this may increase the risk of renal dysfunction and/or the risk of reversible CNS symptoms such as those that have been reported in patients treated with intravenous acyclovir. Adequate hydration should be maintained). Products include:

Proleukin for Injection 2266

Amikacin Sulfate (Caution should be exercised when administering acyclovir to patients receiving potentially nephrotoxic agents since this may increase the risk of renal dysfunction and/or the risk of reversible CNS symptoms such as those that have been reported in patients treated with intravenous acyclovir. Adequate hydration should be maintained).

No products indexed under this heading.

Amoxicillin (Caution should be exercised when administering acyclovir to patients receiving potentially nephrotoxic agents since this may increase the risk of renal dysfunction and/or the risk of reversible CNS symptoms such as those that have been reported in patients treated with intravenous acyclovir. Adequate hydration should be maintained). Products include:

Amoxil Capsules 1343
Amoxil Chewable Tablets 1343
Amoxil Pediatric Drops for Oral Suspension 1343
Amoxil Powder for Oral Suspension 1343
Amoxil Tablets 1343
Augmentin 1360
Augmentin Tablets 1363
Augmentin XR Extended-Release Tablets 1369
Augmentin ES-600 Powder for Oral Suspension 1366
PREVPAC 3284

Amoxicillin Trihydrate (Caution should be exercised when administering acyclovir to patients receiving potentially nephrotoxic agents since this may increase the risk of renal dysfunction and/or the risk of reversible CNS symptoms such as those that have been reported in patients treated with intravenous acyclovir. Adequate hydration should be maintained).

No products indexed under this heading.

Amphotericin B (Caution should be exercised when administering acyclovir to patients receiving potentially nephrotoxic agents since this may increase the risk of renal dysfunction and/or the risk of reversible CNS symptoms such as those that have been reported in patients treated with intravenous acyclovir. Adequate hydration should be maintained).

No products indexed under this heading.

Amphotericin B, liposomal (Caution should be exercised when administering acyclovir to patients receiving potentially nephrotoxic agents since this may increase the risk of renal dysfunction and/or the risk of reversible CNS symptoms such as those that have been reported in patients treated with intravenous acyclovir. Adequate hydration should be maintained). Products include:

AmBisome for Injection 620

Amphotericin B Cholesteryl Sulfate (Caution should be exercised when administering acyclovir to patients receiving potentially nephrotoxic agents since this may increase the risk of renal dysfunction and/or the risk of reversible CNS symptoms such as those that have been reported in patients treated with intravenous acyclovir. Adequate hydration should be maintained).

No products indexed under this heading.

Amphotericin B Lipid Complex (Caution should be exercised when administering acyclovir to patients receiving potentially nephrotoxic agents since this may increase the risk of renal dysfunction and/or the risk of reversible CNS symptoms such as those that have been reported in patients treated with intravenous acyclovir. Adequate hydration should be maintained). Products include:

Abelcet Injection 1141

Ampicillin (Caution should be exercised when administering acyclovir to patients receiving potentially nephrotoxic agents since this may increase the risk of renal dysfunction and/or the risk of reversible CNS symptoms such as those that have been reported in patients treated with intravenous acyclovir. Adequate hydration should be maintained).

No products indexed under this heading.

Ampicillin Sodium (Caution should be exercised when administering acyclovir to patients receiving potentially nephrotoxic agents since this may increase the risk of renal dysfunction and/or the risk of reversible CNS symptoms such as those that have been reported in patients treated with intravenous acyclovir. Adequate hydration should be maintained).

No products indexed under this heading.

Ampicillin Trihydrate (Caution should be exercised when administering acyclovir to patients receiving potentially nephrotoxic agents since this may increase the risk of renal dysfunction and/or the risk of reversible CNS symptoms such as those that have been reported in patients treated with intravenous acyclovir. Adequate hydration should be maintained).

No products indexed under this heading.

Amprenavir (Caution should be exercised when administering acyclovir to patients receiving potentially nephrotoxic agents since this may increase the risk of renal dysfunction and/or the risk of reversible CNS symptoms such as those that have been reported in patients treated with intravenous acyclovir. Adequate hydration should be maintained). Products include:

Agenerase Capsules 1327
Agenerase Oral Solution 1332

Aspirin (Caution should be exercised when administering acyclovir to patients receiving potentially nephrotoxic agents since this may increase the risk of renal dysfunction and/or the risk of reversible CNS symptoms such as those that have been reported in patients treated with intravenous acyclovir. Adequate hydration should be maintained). Products include:

Aggrenox Capsules 822
Bayer Aspirin 744
BC Allergy Sinus Cold Powder .... ▣677
BC Headache Powder .... ▣677
Arthritis Strength BC Powder .... ▣677
BC Sinus Cold Powder .... ▣677
Excedrin Extra Strength Caplets/Tablets/Geltabs .... ▣684
Excedrin Migraine Caplets/Tablets/Geltabs .... ▣609
Goody's Body Pain Formula Powder .... ▣684
Goody's Extra Strength Headache Powders .... ▣611
Goody's Extra Strength Pain Relief Tablets .... ▣685
Percodan Tablets 1132
St. Joseph 81 mg Aspirin Chewable and Enteric Coated Tablets 1869

Atazanavir (Caution should be exercised when administering acyclovir to patients receiving potentially nephrotoxic agents since this may increase the risk of renal dysfunction and/or the risk of reversible CNS symptoms such as those that have been reported in patients treated with intravenous acyclovir. Adequate hydration should be maintained).

No products indexed under this heading.

Atorvastatin Calcium (Caution should be exercised when administering acyclovir to patients receiving potentially nephrotoxic agents since this may increase the risk of renal dysfunction and/or the risk of reversible CNS symptoms such as those that have been reported in patients treated with intravenous acyclovir. Adequate hydration should be maintained). Products include:

Caduet Tablets 2508
Lipitor Tablets 2483

Azithromycin Dihydrate (Caution should be exercised when administering acyclovir to patients receiving potentially nephrotoxic agents since this may increase the risk of renal dysfunction and/or the risk of reversible CNS symptoms such as those that have been reported in patients treated with intravenous acyclovir. Adequate hydration should be maintained).
No products indexed under this heading.

Azlocillin Sodium (Caution should be exercised when administering acyclovir to patients receiving potentially nephrotoxic agents since this may increase the risk of renal dysfunction and/or the risk of reversible CNS symptoms such as those that have been reported in patients treated with intravenous acyclovir. Adequate hydration should be maintained).
No products indexed under this heading.

Aztreonam (Caution should be exercised when administering acyclovir to patients receiving potentially nephrotoxic agents since this may increase the risk of renal dysfunction and/or the risk of reversible CNS symptoms such as those that have been reported in patients treated with intravenous acyclovir. Adequate hydration should be maintained).
No products indexed under this heading.

Bacampicillin Hydrochloride (Caution should be exercised when administering acyclovir to patients receiving potentially nephrotoxic agents since this may increase the risk of renal dysfunction and/or the risk of reversible CNS symptoms such as those that have been reported in patients treated with intravenous acyclovir. Adequate hydration should be maintained).
No products indexed under this heading.

Balsalazide Disodium (Caution should be exercised when administering acyclovir to patients receiving potentially nephrotoxic agents since this may increase the risk of renal dysfunction and/or the risk of reversible CNS symptoms such as those that have been reported in patients treated with intravenous acyclovir. Adequate hydration should be maintained). Products include:
Colazal Capsules **2838**

Benazepril Hydrochloride (Caution should be exercised when administering acyclovir to patients receiving potentially nephrotoxic agents since this may increase the risk of renal dysfunction and/or the risk of reversible CNS symptoms such as those that have been reported in patients treated with intravenous acyclovir. Adequate hydration should be maintained). Products include:
Lotensin Tablets **2243**
Lotensin HCT Tablets **2246**
Lotrel Capsules **2249**

Bendroflumethiazide (Caution should be exercised when administering acyclovir to patients receiving potentially nephrotoxic agents since this may increase the risk of renal dysfunction and/or the risk of reversible CNS symptoms such as those that have been reported in patients treated with intravenous acyclovir. Adequate hydration should be maintained).
No products indexed under this heading.

Caffeine (Caution should be exercised when administering acyclovir to patients receiving potentially nephrotoxic agents since this may increase the risk of renal dysfunction and/or the risk of reversible CNS symptoms such as those that have been reported in patients treated with intravenous acyclovir. Adequate hydration should be maintained). Products include:
BC Headache Powder **677**
Arthritis Strength BC Powder **677**
Excedrin Extra Strength Caplets/Tablets/Geltabs **684**
Excedrin Migraine Caplets/Tablets/Geltabs **609**
Excedrin Tension Headache Caplets/Tablets/Geltabs **611**
Goody's Extra Strength Headache Powders **611**
Goody's Extra Strength Pain Relief Tablets **685**
Vivarin **602**
Winrgy Dietary Supplement **823**

Captopril (Caution should be exercised when administering acyclovir to patients receiving potentially nephrotoxic agents since this may increase the risk of renal dysfunction and/or the risk of reversible CNS symptoms such as those that have been reported in patients treated with intravenous acyclovir. Adequate hydration should be maintained). Products include:
Captopril Tablets **2149**

Carbenicillin Disodium (Caution should be exercised when administering acyclovir to patients receiving potentially nephrotoxic agents since this may increase the risk of renal dysfunction and/or the risk of reversible CNS symptoms such as those that have been reported in patients treated with intravenous acyclovir. Adequate hydration should be maintained).
No products indexed under this heading.

Carbenicillin Indanyl Sodium (Caution should be exercised when administering acyclovir to patients receiving potentially nephrotoxic agents since this may increase the risk of renal dysfunction and/or the risk of reversible CNS symptoms such as those that have been reported in patients treated with intravenous acyclovir. Adequate hydration should be maintained).
No products indexed under this heading.

Carboplatin (Caution should be exercised when administering acyclovir to patients receiving potentially nephrotoxic agents since this may increase the risk of renal dysfunction and/or the risk of reversible CNS symptoms such as those that have been reported in patients treated with intravenous acyclovir. Adequate hydration should be maintained).
No products indexed under this heading.

Carmustine (BCNU) (Caution should be exercised when administering acyclovir to patients receiving potentially nephrotoxic agents since this may increase the risk of renal dysfunction and/or the risk of reversible CNS symptoms such as those that have been reported in patients treated with intravenous acyclovir. Adequate hydration should be maintained).
No products indexed under this heading.

Cefaclor (Caution should be exercised when administering acyclovir to patients receiving potentially nephrotoxic agents since this may increase the risk of renal dysfunction and/or the risk of reversible CNS symptoms such as those that have been reported in patients treated with intravenous acyclovir. Adequate hydration should be maintained).
No products indexed under this heading.

Cefadroxil (Caution should be exercised when administering acyclovir to patients receiving potentially nephrotoxic agents since this may increase the risk of renal dysfunction and/or the risk of reversible CNS symptoms such as those that have been reported in patients treated with intravenous acyclovir. Adequate hydration should be maintained).
No products indexed under this heading.

Cefamandole Nafate (Caution should be exercised when administering acyclovir to patients receiving potentially nephrotoxic agents since this may increase the risk of renal dysfunction and/or the risk of reversible CNS symptoms such as those that have been reported in patients treated with intravenous acyclovir. Adequate hydration should be maintained).
No products indexed under this heading.

Cefazolin Sodium (Caution should be exercised when administering acyclovir to patients receiving potentially nephrotoxic agents since this may increase the risk of renal dysfunction and/or the risk of reversible CNS symptoms such as those that have been reported in patients treated with intravenous acyclovir. Adequate hydration should be maintained).
No products indexed under this heading.

Cefdinir (Caution should be exercised when administering acyclovir to patients receiving potentially nephrotoxic agents since this may increase the risk of renal dysfunction and/or the risk of reversible CNS symptoms such as those that have been reported in patients treated with intravenous acyclovir. Adequate hydration should be maintained). Products include:
Omnicef Capsules **511**
Omnicef for Oral Suspension **511**

Cefepime Hydrochloride (Caution should be exercised when administering acyclovir to patients receiving potentially nephrotoxic agents since this may increase the risk of renal dysfunction and/or the risk of reversible CNS symptoms such as those that have been reported in patients treated with intravenous acyclovir. Adequate hydration should be maintained). Products include:
Maxipime for Injection **1105**

Cefixime (Caution should be exercised when administering acyclovir to patients receiving potentially nephrotoxic agents since this may increase the risk of renal dysfunction and/or the risk of reversible CNS symptoms such as those that have been reported in patients treated with intravenous acyclovir. Adequate hydration should be maintained). Products include:
Suprax **1843**

Cefmetazole Sodium (Caution should be exercised when administering acyclovir to patients receiving potentially nephrotoxic agents since this may increase the risk of renal dysfunction and/or the risk of reversible CNS symptoms such as those that have been reported in patients treated with intravenous acyclovir. Adequate hydration should be maintained).
No products indexed under this heading.

Cefonicid Sodium (Caution should be exercised when administering acyclovir to patients receiving potentially nephrotoxic agents since this may increase the risk of renal dysfunction and/or the risk of reversible CNS symptoms such as those that have been reported in patients treated with intravenous acyclovir. Adequate hydration should be maintained).
No products indexed under this heading.

Cefoperazone Sodium (Caution should be exercised when administering acyclovir to patients receiving potentially nephrotoxic agents since this may increase the risk of renal dysfunction and/or the risk of reversible CNS symptoms such as those that have been reported in patients treated with intravenous acyclovir. Adequate hydration should be maintained).
No products indexed under this heading.

Ceforanide (Caution should be exercised when administering acyclovir to patients receiving potentially nephrotoxic agents since this may increase the risk of renal dysfunction and/or the risk of reversible CNS symptoms such as those that have been reported in patients treated with intravenous acyclovir. Adequate hydration should be maintained).
No products indexed under this heading.

Cefotaxime Sodium (Caution should be exercised when administering acyclovir to patients receiving potentially nephrotoxic agents since this may increase the risk of renal dysfunction and/or the risk of reversible CNS symptoms such as those that have been reported in patients treated with intravenous acyclovir. Adequate hydration should be maintained).
No products indexed under this heading.

Cefotetan (Caution should be exercised when administering acyclovir to patients receiving potentially nephrotoxic agents since this may increase the risk of renal dysfunction and/or the risk of reversible CNS symptoms such as those that have been reported in patients treated with intravenous acyclovir. Adequate hydration should be maintained).
No products indexed under this heading.

Cefoxitin Sodium (Caution should be exercised when administering acyclovir to patients receiving potentially nephrotoxic agents since this may increase the risk of renal dysfunction and/or the risk of reversible CNS symptoms such as those that have been reported in patients treated with intravenous acyclovir. Adequate hydration should be maintained). Products include:

Mefoxin for Injection 2012
Mefoxin Premixed Intravenous Solution.. 2016

Cefpodoxime Proxetil (Caution should be exercised when administering acyclovir to patients receiving potentially nephrotoxic agents since this may increase the risk of renal dysfunction and/or the risk of reversible CNS symptoms such as those that have been reported in patients treated with intravenous acyclovir. Adequate hydration should be maintained). Products include:

Vantin Tablets and Oral Suspension 2645

Cefprozil (Caution should be exercised when administering acyclovir to patients receiving potentially nephrotoxic agents since this may increase the risk of renal dysfunction and/or the risk of reversible CNS symptoms such as those that have been reported in patients treated with intravenous acyclovir. Adequate hydration should be maintained).

No products indexed under this heading.

Ceftazidime (Caution should be exercised when administering acyclovir to patients receiving potentially nephrotoxic agents since this may increase the risk of renal dysfunction and/or the risk of reversible CNS symptoms such as those that have been reported in patients treated with intravenous acyclovir. Adequate hydration should be maintained). Products include:

Fortaz 1453

Ceftizoxime Sodium (Caution should be exercised when administering acyclovir to patients receiving potentially nephrotoxic agents since this may increase the risk of renal dysfunction and/or the risk of reversible CNS symptoms such as those that have been reported in patients treated with intravenous acyclovir. Adequate hydration should be maintained).

No products indexed under this heading.

Ceftriaxone Sodium (Caution should be exercised when administering acyclovir to patients receiving potentially nephrotoxic agents since this may increase the risk of renal dysfunction and/or the risk of reversible CNS symptoms such as those that have been reported in patients treated with intravenous acyclovir. Adequate hydration should be maintained). Products include:

Rocephin Injectable Vials, ADD-Vantage, Galaxy, Bulk........... 2800

Cefuroxime Axetil (Caution should be exercised when administering acyclovir to patients receiving potentially nephrotoxic agents since this may increase the risk of renal dysfunction and/or the risk of reversible CNS symptoms such as those that have been reported in patients treated with intravenous acyclovir. Adequate hydration should be maintained). Products include:

Ceftin 1407

Cefuroxime Sodium (Caution should be exercised when administering acyclovir to patients receiving potentially nephrotoxic agents since this may increase the risk of renal dysfunction and/or the risk of reversible CNS symptoms such as those that have been reported in patients treated with intravenous acyclovir. Adequate hydration should be maintained).

No products indexed under this heading.

Celecoxib (Caution should be exercised when administering acyclovir to patients receiving potentially nephrotoxic agents since this may increase the risk of renal dysfunction and/or the risk of reversible CNS symptoms such as those that have been reported in patients treated with intravenous acyclovir. Adequate hydration should be maintained). Products include:

Celebrex Capsules 3134

Cephalexin (Caution should be exercised when administering acyclovir to patients receiving potentially nephrotoxic agents since this may increase the risk of renal dysfunction and/or the risk of reversible CNS symptoms such as those that have been reported in patients treated with intravenous acyclovir. Adequate hydration should be maintained). Products include:

Keflex Capsules 549

Cephalothin Sodium (Caution should be exercised when administering acyclovir to patients receiving potentially nephrotoxic agents since this may increase the risk of renal dysfunction and/or the risk of reversible CNS symptoms such as those that have been reported in patients treated with intravenous acyclovir. Adequate hydration should be maintained).

No products indexed under this heading.

Cephapirin Sodium (Caution should be exercised when administering acyclovir to patients receiving potentially nephrotoxic agents since this may increase the risk of renal dysfunction and/or the risk of reversible CNS symptoms such as those that have been reported in patients treated with intravenous acyclovir. Adequate hydration should be maintained).

No products indexed under this heading.

Cephradine (Caution should be exercised when administering acyclovir to patients receiving potentially nephrotoxic agents since this may increase the risk of renal dysfunction and/or the risk of reversible CNS symptoms such as those that have been reported in patients treated with intravenous acyclovir. Adequate hydration should be maintained).

No products indexed under this heading.

Cerivastatin Sodium (Caution should be exercised when administering acyclovir to patients receiving potentially nephrotoxic agents since this may increase the risk of renal dysfunction and/or the risk of reversible CNS symptoms such as those that have been reported in patients treated with intravenous acyclovir. Adequate hydration should be maintained).

No products indexed under this heading.

Chlorothiazide (Caution should be exercised when administering acyclovir to patients receiving potentially nephrotoxic agents since this may increase the risk of renal dysfunction and/or the risk of reversible CNS symptoms such as those that have been reported in patients treated with intravenous acyclovir. Adequate hydration should be maintained). Products include:

Diuril Oral Suspension 1954

Chlorothiazide Sodium (Caution should be exercised when administering acyclovir to patients receiving potentially nephrotoxic agents since this may increase the risk of renal dysfunction and/or the risk of reversible CNS symptoms such as those that have been reported in patients treated with intravenous acyclovir. Adequate hydration should be maintained). Products include:

Diuril Sodium Intravenous 2467

Chlorpropamide (Caution should be exercised when administering acyclovir to patients receiving potentially nephrotoxic agents since this may increase the risk of renal dysfunction and/or the risk of reversible CNS symptoms such as those that have been reported in patients treated with intravenous acyclovir. Adequate hydration should be maintained).

No products indexed under this heading.

Cidofovir (Caution should be exercised when administering acyclovir to patients receiving potentially nephrotoxic agents since this may increase the risk of renal dysfunction and/or the risk of reversible CNS symptoms such as those that have been reported in patients treated with intravenous acyclovir. Adequate hydration should be maintained).

No products indexed under this heading.

Cilastatin Sodium (Caution should be exercised when administering acyclovir to patients receiving potentially nephrotoxic agents since this may increase the risk of renal dysfunction and/or the risk of reversible CNS symptoms such as those that have been reported in patients treated with intravenous acyclovir. Adequate hydration should be maintained). Products include:

Primaxin I.M. 2045
Primaxin I.V. 2048

Cimetidine (Caution should be exercised when administering acyclovir to patients receiving potentially nephrotoxic agents since this may increase the risk of renal dysfunction and/or the risk of reversible CNS symptoms such as those that have been reported in patients treated with intravenous acyclovir. Adequate hydration should be maintained). Products include:

Tagamet HB 200 Tablets .... ■□664

Cimetidine Hydrochloride (Caution should be exercised when administering acyclovir to patients receiving potentially nephrotoxic agents since this may increase the risk of renal dysfunction and/or the risk of reversible CNS symptoms such as those that have been reported in patients treated with intravenous acyclovir. Adequate hydration should be maintained).

No products indexed under this heading.

Cisplatin (Caution should be exercised when administering acyclovir to patients receiving potentially nephrotoxic agents since this may increase the risk of renal dysfunction and/or the risk of reversible CNS symptoms such as those that have been reported in patients treated with intravenous acyclovir. Adequate hydration should be maintained).

No products indexed under this heading.

Cladribine (Caution should be exercised when administering acyclovir to patients receiving potentially nephrotoxic agents since this may increase the risk of renal dysfunction and/or the risk of reversible CNS symptoms such as those that have been reported in patients treated with intravenous acyclovir. Adequate hydration should be maintained). Products include:

Leustatin Injection 2357

Clozapine (Caution should be exercised when administering acyclovir to patients receiving potentially nephrotoxic agents since this may increase the risk of renal dysfunction and/or the risk of reversible CNS symptoms such as those that have been reported in patients treated with intravenous acyclovir. Adequate hydration should be maintained). Products include:

Clozaril Tablets 2184
FazaClo Orally Disintegrating Tablets 551

Colistimethate Sodium (Caution should be exercised when administering acyclovir to patients receiving potentially nephrotoxic agents since this may increase the risk of renal dysfunction and/or the risk of reversible CNS symptoms such as those that have been reported in patients treated with intravenous acyclovir. Adequate hydration should be maintained).

No products indexed under this heading.

Colistin Sulfate (Caution should be exercised when administering acyclovir to patients receiving potentially nephrotoxic agents since this may increase the risk of renal dysfunction and/or the risk of reversible CNS symptoms such as those that have been reported in patients treated with intravenous acyclovir. Adequate hydration should be maintained).

No products indexed under this heading.

Cyclophosphamide (Caution should be exercised when administering acyclovir to patients receiving potentially nephrotoxic agents since this may increase the risk of renal dysfunction and/or the risk of reversible CNS symptoms such as those that have been reported in patients treated with intravenous acyclovir. Adequate hydration should be maintained).

No products indexed under this heading.

Cyclosporine (Caution should be exercised when administering acyclovir to patients receiving potentially nephrotoxic agents since this may increase the risk of renal dysfunction and/or the risk of reversible CNS symptoms such as those that have been reported in patients treated with intravenous acyclovir. Adequate hydration should be maintained). Products include:

Gengraf Capsules **459**
Neoral Oral Solution **2259**
Neoral Soft Gelatin Capsules **2259**
Restasis Ophthalmic Emulsion **575**
Sandimmune **2275**

Cytarabine (Caution should be exercised when administering acyclovir to patients receiving potentially nephrotoxic agents since this may increase the risk of renal dysfunction and/or the risk of reversible CNS symptoms such as those that have been reported in patients treated with intravenous acyclovir. Adequate hydration should be maintained).
No products indexed under this heading.

Cytarabine Liposome (Caution should be exercised when administering acyclovir to patients receiving potentially nephrotoxic agents since this may increase the risk of renal dysfunction and/or the risk of reversible CNS symptoms such as those that have been reported in patients treated with intravenous acyclovir. Adequate hydration should be maintained). Products include:
DepoCyt Injection **1143**

Delavirdine Mesylate (Caution should be exercised when administering acyclovir to patients receiving potentially nephrotoxic agents since this may increase the risk of renal dysfunction and/or the risk of reversible CNS symptoms such as those that have been reported in patients treated with intravenous acyclovir. Adequate hydration should be maintained). Products include:
Rescriptor Tablets **2551**

Diatrizoate Meglumine (Caution should be exercised when administering acyclovir to patients receiving potentially nephrotoxic agents since this may increase the risk of renal dysfunction and/or the risk of reversible CNS symptoms such as those that have been reported in patients treated with intravenous acyclovir. Adequate hydration should be maintained).
No products indexed under this heading.

Diatrizoate Sodium (Caution should be exercised when administering acyclovir to patients receiving potentially nephrotoxic agents since this may increase the risk of renal dysfunction and/or the risk of reversible CNS symptoms such as those that have been reported in patients treated with intravenous acyclovir. Adequate hydration should be maintained).
No products indexed under this heading.

Diclofenac Potassium (Caution should be exercised when administering acyclovir to patients receiving potentially nephrotoxic agents since this may increase the risk of renal dysfunction and/or the risk of reversible CNS symptoms such as those that have been reported in patients treated with intravenous acyclovir. Adequate hydration should be maintained).
No products indexed under this heading.

Diclofenac Sodium (Caution should be exercised when administering acyclovir to patients receiving potentially nephrotoxic agents since this may increase the risk of renal dysfunction and/or the risk of reversible CNS symptoms such as those that have been reported in patients treated with intravenous acyclovir. Adequate hydration should be maintained). Products include:
Arthrotec Tablets **3129**
Voltaren Ophthalmic Solution **2309**
Voltaren Tablets **2307**
Voltaren-XR Tablets **2310**

Dicloxacillin Sodium (Caution should be exercised when administering acyclovir to patients receiving potentially nephrotoxic agents since this may increase the risk of renal dysfunction and/or the risk of reversible CNS symptoms such as those that have been reported in patients treated with intravenous acyclovir. Adequate hydration should be maintained).
No products indexed under this heading.

Didanosine (Caution should be exercised when administering acyclovir to patients receiving potentially nephrotoxic agents since this may increase the risk of renal dysfunction and/or the risk of reversible CNS symptoms such as those that have been reported in patients treated with intravenous acyclovir. Adequate hydration should be maintained).
No products indexed under this heading.

Efavirenz (Caution should be exercised when administering acyclovir to patients receiving potentially nephrotoxic agents since this may increase the risk of renal dysfunction and/or the risk of reversible CNS symptoms such as those that have been reported in patients treated with intravenous acyclovir. Adequate hydration should be maintained). Products include:
Atripla Tablets **945**
Sustiva Capsules **930**
Sustiva Tablets **930**

Emtricitabine (Caution should be exercised when administering acyclovir to patients receiving potentially nephrotoxic agents since this may increase the risk of renal dysfunction and/or the risk of reversible CNS symptoms such as those that have been reported in patients treated with intravenous acyclovir. Adequate hydration should be maintained). Products include:
Atripla Tablets **945**
Emtriva Capsules **1287**
Emtriva Oral Solution **1287**
Truvada Tablets **1296**

Enalapril Maleate (Caution should be exercised when administering acyclovir to patients receiving potentially nephrotoxic agents since this may increase the risk of renal dysfunction and/or the risk of reversible CNS symptoms such as those that have been reported in patients treated with intravenous acyclovir. Adequate hydration should be maintained). Products include:
Vasotec I.V. Injection **2103**

Enalaprilat (Caution should be exercised when administering acyclovir to patients receiving potentially nephrotoxic agents since this may increase the risk of renal dysfunction and/or the risk of reversible CNS symptoms such as those that have been reported in patients treated with intravenous acyclovir. Adequate hydration should be maintained).
No products indexed under this heading.

Enfuvirtide (Caution should be exercised when administering acyclovir to patients receiving potentially nephrotoxic agents since this may increase the risk of renal dysfunction and/or the risk of reversible CNS symptoms such as those that have been reported in patients treated with intravenous acyclovir. Adequate hydration should be maintained). Products include:
Fuzeon Injection **2767**

Ethiodized Oil (Caution should be exercised when administering acyclovir to patients receiving potentially nephrotoxic agents since this may increase the risk of renal dysfunction and/or the risk of reversible CNS symptoms such as those that have been reported in patients treated with intravenous acyclovir. Adequate hydration should be maintained).
No products indexed under this heading.

Etodolac (Caution should be exercised when administering acyclovir to patients receiving potentially nephrotoxic agents since this may increase the risk of renal dysfunction and/or the risk of reversible CNS symptoms such as those that have been reported in patients treated with intravenous acyclovir. Adequate hydration should be maintained).
No products indexed under this heading.

Fenoprofen Calcium (Caution should be exercised when administering acyclovir to patients receiving potentially nephrotoxic agents since this may increase the risk of renal dysfunction and/or the risk of reversible CNS symptoms such as those that have been reported in patients treated with intravenous acyclovir. Adequate hydration should be maintained). Products include:
Nalfon Capsules **2502**

Filgrastim (Caution should be exercised when administering acyclovir to patients receiving potentially nephrotoxic agents since this may increase the risk of renal dysfunction and/or the risk of reversible CNS symptoms such as those that have been reported in patients treated with intravenous acyclovir. Adequate hydration should be maintained). Products include:
Neupogen for Injection **603**

Fluorouracil (Caution should be exercised when administering acyclovir to patients receiving potentially nephrotoxic agents since this may increase the risk of renal dysfunction and/or the risk of reversible CNS symptoms such as those that have been reported in patients treated with intravenous acyclovir. Adequate hydration should be maintained). Products include:
Carac Cream, 0.5% **2879**
Efudex **3363**

Flurbiprofen (Caution should be exercised when administering acyclovir to patients receiving potentially nephrotoxic agents since this may increase the risk of renal dysfunction and/or the risk of reversible CNS symptoms such as those that have been reported in patients treated with intravenous acyclovir. Adequate hydration should be maintained).
No products indexed under this heading.

Fluvastatin Sodium (Caution should be exercised when administering acyclovir to patients receiving potentially nephrotoxic agents since this may increase the risk of renal dysfunction and/or the risk of reversible CNS symptoms such as those that have been reported in patients treated with intravenous acyclovir. Adequate hydration should be maintained). Products include:
Lescol Capsules **2233**
Lescol XL Tablets **2233**

Foscarnet Sodium (Caution should be exercised when administering acyclovir to patients receiving potentially nephrotoxic agents since this may increase the risk of renal dysfunction and/or the risk of reversible CNS symptoms such as those that have been reported in patients treated with intravenous acyclovir. Adequate hydration should be maintained).
No products indexed under this heading.

Fosinopril Sodium (Caution should be exercised when administering acyclovir to patients receiving potentially nephrotoxic agents since this may increase the risk of renal dysfunction and/or the risk of reversible CNS symptoms such as those that have been reported in patients treated with intravenous acyclovir. Adequate hydration should be maintained).
No products indexed under this heading.

Furosemide (Caution should be exercised when administering acyclovir to patients receiving potentially nephrotoxic agents since this may increase the risk of renal dysfunction and/or the risk of reversible CNS symptoms such as those that have been reported in patients treated with intravenous acyclovir. Adequate hydration should be maintained). Products include:
Furosemide Tablets **2154**

Gadopentetate Dimeglumine (Caution should be exercised when administering acyclovir to patients receiving potentially nephrotoxic agents since this may increase the risk of renal dysfunction and/or the risk of reversible CNS symptoms such as those that have been reported in patients treated with intravenous acyclovir. Adequate hydration should be maintained).
No products indexed under this heading.

Gentamicin (Caution should be exercised when administering acyclovir to patients receiving potentially nephrotoxic agents since this may increase the risk of renal dysfunction and/or the risk of reversible CNS symptoms such as those that have been reported in patients treated with intravenous acyclovir. Adequate hydration should be maintained).
No products indexed under this heading.

Gentamicin Sulfate (Caution should be exercised when administering acyclovir to patients receiving potentially nephrotoxic agents since this may increase the risk of renal dysfunction and/or the risk of reversible CNS symptoms such as those that have been reported in patients treated with intravenous acyclovir. Adequate hydration should be maintained). Products include:
Garamycin Injectable **3014**
Pred-G Ophthalmic Ointment .... ⊙**237**
Pred-G Ophthalmic Suspension ...... ⊙**236**

Glipizide (Caution should be exercised when administering acyclovir to patients receiving potentially nephrotoxic agents since this may increase the risk of renal dysfunction and/or the risk of reversible CNS symptoms such as those that have been reported in patients treated with intravenous acyclovir. Adequate hydration should be maintained).
No products indexed under this heading.

Globulin, Immune (Human) (Caution should be exercised when administering acyclovir to patients receiving potentially nephrotoxic agents since this may increase the risk of renal dysfunction and/or the risk of reversible CNS symptoms such as those that have been reported in patients treated with intravenous acyclovir. Adequate hydration should be maintained). Products include:
Flebogamma 5%, Immune Globulin Intravenous (Human)........ 1658
GamaSTAN 3234

Glyburide (Caution should be exercised when administering acyclovir to patients receiving potentially nephrotoxic agents since this may increase the risk of renal dysfunction and/or the risk of reversible CNS symptoms such as those that have been reported in patients treated with intravenous acyclovir. Adequate hydration should be maintained).
No products indexed under this heading.

Gold Therapy (Caution should be exercised when administering acyclovir to patients receiving potentially nephrotoxic agents since this may increase the risk of renal dysfunction and/or the risk of reversible CNS symptoms such as those that have been reported in patients treated with intravenous acyclovir. Adequate hydration should be maintained).
No products indexed under this heading.

HMG-CoA Reductase Inhibitors (Caution should be exercised when administering acyclovir to patients receiving potentially nephrotoxic agents since this may increase the risk of renal dysfunction and/or the risk of reversible CNS symptoms such as those that have been reported in patients treated with intravenous acyclovir. Adequate hydration should be maintained).
No products indexed under this heading.

Hydrochlorothiazide (Caution should be exercised when administering acyclovir to patients receiving potentially nephrotoxic agents since this may increase the risk of renal dysfunction and/or the risk of reversible CNS symptoms such as those that have been reported in patients treated with intravenous acyclovir. Adequate hydration should be maintained). Products include:
Aldoril Tablets 1910
Atacand HCT 651
Avalide Tablets 888
Avalide Tablets 2874
Benicar HCT Tablets 1044
Diovan HCT Tablets 2196
Dyazide Capsules 1423
Hyzaar 50-12.5 Tablets 1990
Hyzaar 100-12.5 Tablets 1990
Hyzaar 100-25 Tablets 1990
Lopressor HCT 50/25 Tablets 2241
Lopressor HCT 100/25 Tablets 2241
Lopressor HCT 100/50 Tablets 2241
Lotensin HCT Tablets 2246
Micardis HCT Tablets 856
Moduretic Tablets 2028
Prinzide Tablets 2056
Teveten HCT Tablets 1737
Timolide Tablets 2086
Uniretic Tablets 3100

Hydroflumethiazide (Caution should be exercised when administering acyclovir to patients receiving potentially nephrotoxic agents since this may increase the risk of renal dysfunction and/or the risk of reversible CNS symptoms such as those that have been reported in patients treated with intravenous acyclovir. Adequate hydration should be maintained).
No products indexed under this heading.

Ibuprofen (Caution should be exercised when administering acyclovir to patients receiving potentially nephrotoxic agents since this may increase the risk of renal dysfunction and/or the risk of reversible CNS symptoms such as those that have been reported in patients treated with intravenous acyclovir. Adequate hydration should be maintained). Products include:
Advil Allergy Sinus Caplets .... ■ 770
Advil .... ■ 674
Children's Advil Oral Suspension .... ■ 603
Children's Advil Chewable Tablets .... ■ 603
Advil Cold & Sinus .... ■ 723
Infants' Advil Concentrated Drops .... ■ 604
Infants' Advil Concentrated Drops - White Grape (Dye-Free)........ ■ 604
Junior Strength Advil Swallow Tablets........ ■ 605
Advil Migraine Liquigels .... ■ 608
Advil Multi-Symptom Cold Caplets........ ■ 770
Advil PM Caplets .... ■ 615
Motrin IB Tablets and Caplets 1866
Children's Motrin Oral Suspension 1867
Children's Motrin Non-Staining Dye-Free Oral Suspension........ 1867
Children's Motrin Cold Oral Suspension 1867
Infants' Motrin Concentrated Drops 1867
Infants' Motrin Non-Staining Dye-Free Concentrated Drops........ 1867
Junior Strength Motrin Caplets and Chewable Tablets........ 1867
Vicoprofen Tablets 539

Idarubicin Hydrochloride (Caution should be exercised when administering acyclovir to patients receiving potentially nephrotoxic agents since this may increase the risk of renal dysfunction and/or the risk of reversible CNS symptoms such as those that have been reported in patients treated with intravenous acyclovir. Adequate hydration should be maintained).
No products indexed under this heading.

Ifosfamide (Caution should be exercised when administering acyclovir to patients receiving potentially nephrotoxic agents since this may increase the risk of renal dysfunction and/or the risk of reversible CNS symptoms such as those that have been reported in patients treated with intravenous acyclovir. Adequate hydration should be maintained).
No products indexed under this heading.

Imipenem (Caution should be exercised when administering acyclovir to patients receiving potentially nephrotoxic agents since this may increase the risk of renal dysfunction and/or the risk of reversible CNS symptoms such as those that have been reported in patients treated with intravenous acyclovir. Adequate hydration should be maintained). Products include:
Primaxin I.M. 2045
Primaxin I.V. 2048

Immune Globulin Intravenous (Human) (Caution should be exercised when administering acyclovir to patients receiving potentially nephrotoxic agents since this may increase the risk of renal dysfunction and/or the risk of reversible CNS symptoms such as those that have been reported in patients treated with intravenous acyclovir. Adequate hydration should be maintained). Products include:
Carimune NF 3499
Gammagard Liquid 721
Gammagard S/D 724
Gamunex Immune Globulin I.V., 10%........ 3235

Indinavir Sulfate (Caution should be exercised when administering acyclovir to patients receiving potentially nephrotoxic agents since this may increase the risk of renal dysfunction and/or the risk of reversible CNS symptoms such as those that have been reported in patients treated with intravenous acyclovir. Adequate hydration should be maintained). Products include:
Crixivan Capsules 1940

Indomethacin (Caution should be exercised when administering acyclovir to patients receiving potentially nephrotoxic agents since this may increase the risk of renal dysfunction and/or the risk of reversible CNS symptoms such as those that have been reported in patients treated with intravenous acyclovir. Adequate hydration should be maintained). Products include:
Indocin 1995

Indomethacin Sodium Trihydrate (Caution should be exercised when administering acyclovir to patients receiving potentially nephrotoxic agents since this may increase the risk of renal dysfunction and/or the risk of reversible CNS symptoms such as those that have been reported in patients treated with intravenous acyclovir. Adequate hydration should be maintained). Products include:
Indocin I.V. 2465

Interferon Beta-1b (Caution should be exercised when administering acyclovir to patients receiving potentially nephrotoxic agents since this may increase the risk of renal dysfunction and/or the risk of reversible CNS symptoms such as those that have been reported in patients treated with intravenous acyclovir. Adequate hydration should be maintained). Products include:
Betaseron for SC Injection 767

Interleukin-2 (Caution should be exercised when administering acyclovir to patients receiving potentially nephrotoxic agents since this may increase the risk of renal dysfunction and/or the risk of reversible CNS symptoms such as those that have been reported in patients treated with intravenous acyclovir. Adequate hydration should be maintained).
No products indexed under this heading.

Iodamide Meglumine (Caution should be exercised when administering acyclovir to patients receiving potentially nephrotoxic agents since this may increase the risk of renal dysfunction and/or the risk of reversible CNS symptoms such as those that have been reported in patients treated with intravenous acyclovir. Adequate hydration should be maintained).
No products indexed under this heading.

Iohexol (Caution should be exercised when administering acyclovir to patients receiving potentially nephrotoxic agents since this may increase the risk of renal dysfunction and/or the risk of reversible CNS symptoms such as those that have been reported in patients treated with intravenous acyclovir. Adequate hydration should be maintained).
No products indexed under this heading.

Iopamidol (Caution should be exercised when administering acyclovir to patients receiving potentially nephrotoxic agents since this may increase the risk of renal dysfunction and/or the risk of reversible CNS symptoms such as those that have been reported in patients treated with intravenous acyclovir. Adequate hydration should be maintained).
No products indexed under this heading.

Iopanoic Acid (Caution should be exercised when administering acyclovir to patients receiving potentially nephrotoxic agents since this may increase the risk of renal dysfunction and/or the risk of reversible CNS symptoms such as those that have been reported in patients treated with intravenous acyclovir. Adequate hydration should be maintained).
No products indexed under this heading.

Iothalamate Meglumine (Caution should be exercised when administering acyclovir to patients receiving potentially nephrotoxic agents since this may increase the risk of renal dysfunction and/or the risk of reversible CNS symptoms such as those that have been reported in patients treated with intravenous acyclovir. Adequate hydration should be maintained).
No products indexed under this heading.

Ioxaglate Meglumine (Caution should be exercised when administering acyclovir to patients receiving potentially nephrotoxic agents since this may increase the risk of renal dysfunction and/or the risk of reversible CNS symptoms such as those that have been reported in patients treated with intravenous acyclovir. Adequate hydration should be maintained).
No products indexed under this heading.

Ioxaglate Sodium (Caution should be exercised when administering acyclovir to patients receiving potentially nephrotoxic agents since this may increase the risk of renal dysfunction and/or the risk of reversible CNS symptoms such as those that have been reported in patients treated with intravenous acyclovir. Adequate hydration should be maintained).
No products indexed under this heading.

Kanamycin Sulfate (Caution should be exercised when administering acyclovir to patients receiving potentially nephrotoxic agents since this may increase the risk of renal dysfunction and/or the risk of reversible CNS symptoms such as those that have been reported in patients treated with intravenous acyclovir. Adequate hydration should be maintained).

No products indexed under this heading.

Ketoprofen (Caution should be exercised when administering acyclovir to patients receiving potentially nephrotoxic agents since this may increase the risk of renal dysfunction and/or the risk of reversible CNS symptoms such as those that have been reported in patients treated with intravenous acyclovir. Adequate hydration should be maintained).

No products indexed under this heading.

Ketorolac Tromethamine (Caution should be exercised when administering acyclovir to patients receiving potentially nephrotoxic agents since this may increase the risk of renal dysfunction and/or the risk of reversible CNS symptoms such as those that have been reported in patients treated with intravenous acyclovir. Adequate hydration should be maintained). Products include:

Lamium album (Caution should be exercised when administering acyclovir to patients receiving potentially nephrotoxic agents since this may increase the risk of renal dysfunction and/or the risk of reversible CNS symptoms such as those that have been reported in patients treated with intravenous acyclovir. Adequate hydration should be maintained).

No products indexed under this heading.

Lisinopril (Caution should be exercised when administering acyclovir to patients receiving potentially nephrotoxic agents since this may increase the risk of renal dysfunction and/or the risk of reversible CNS symptoms such as those that have been reported in patients treated with intravenous acyclovir. Adequate hydration should be maintained). Products include:

Lithium (Caution should be exercised when administering acyclovir to patients receiving potentially nephrotoxic agents since this may increase the risk of renal dysfunction and/or the risk of reversible CNS symptoms such as those that have been reported in patients treated with intravenous acyclovir. Adequate hydration should be maintained).

No products indexed under this heading.

Lithium Carbonate (Caution should be exercised when administering acyclovir to patients receiving potentially nephrotoxic agents since this may increase the risk of renal dysfunction and/or the risk of reversible CNS symptoms such as those

that have been reported in patients treated with intravenous acyclovir. Adequate hydration should be maintained). Products include:

Lithium Citrate (Caution should be exercised when administering acyclovir to patients receiving potentially nephrotoxic agents since this may increase the risk of renal dysfunction and/or the risk of reversible CNS symptoms such as those that have been reported in patients treated with intravenous acyclovir. Adequate hydration should be maintained).

No products indexed under this heading.

Lopinavir (Caution should be exercised when administering acyclovir to patients receiving potentially nephrotoxic agents since this may increase the risk of renal dysfunction and/or the risk of reversible CNS symptoms such as those that have been reported in patients treated with intravenous acyclovir. Adequate hydration should be maintained). Products include:

Loracarbef (Caution should be exercised when administering acyclovir to patients receiving potentially nephrotoxic agents since this may increase the risk of renal dysfunction and/or the risk of reversible CNS symptoms such as those that have been reported in patients treated with intravenous acyclovir. Adequate hydration should be maintained).

No products indexed under this heading.

Lovastatin (Caution should be exercised when administering acyclovir to patients receiving potentially nephrotoxic agents since this may increase the risk of renal dysfunction and/or the risk of reversible CNS symptoms such as those that have been reported in patients treated with intravenous acyclovir. Adequate hydration should be maintained). Products include:

Meclofenamate Sodium (Caution should be exercised when administering acyclovir to patients receiving potentially nephrotoxic agents since this may increase the risk of renal dysfunction and/or the risk of reversible CNS symptoms such as those that have been reported in patients treated with intravenous acyclovir. Adequate hydration should be maintained).

No products indexed under this heading.

Mefenamic Acid (Caution should be exercised when administering acyclovir to patients receiving potentially nephrotoxic agents since this may increase the risk of renal dysfunction and/or the risk of reversible CNS symptoms such as those that have been reported in patients treated with intravenous acyclovir. Adequate hydration should be maintained).

No products indexed under this heading.

Meloxicam (Caution should be exercised when administering acyclovir to patients receiving potentially nephrotoxic agents since this may increase the risk of renal dysfunction and/or the risk of reversible CNS symptoms such as those that have been reported in patients treated with intravenous acyclovir. Adequate hydration should be maintained). Products include:

Melphalan Hydrochloride (Caution should be exercised when administering acyclovir to patients receiving potentially nephrotoxic agents since this may increase the risk of renal dysfunction and/or the risk of reversible CNS symptoms such as those that have been reported in patients treated with intravenous acyclovir. Adequate hydration should be maintained). Products include:

Mesalamine (Caution should be exercised when administering acyclovir to patients receiving potentially nephrotoxic agents since this may increase the risk of renal dysfunction and/or the risk of reversible CNS symptoms such as those that have been reported in patients treated with intravenous acyclovir. Adequate hydration should be maintained). Products include:

Methimazole (Caution should be exercised when administering acyclovir to patients receiving potentially nephrotoxic agents since this may increase the risk of renal dysfunction and/or the risk of reversible CNS symptoms such as those that have been reported in patients treated with intravenous acyclovir. Adequate hydration should be maintained).

No products indexed under this heading.

Methotrexate (Caution should be exercised when administering acyclovir to patients receiving potentially nephrotoxic agents since this may increase the risk of renal dysfunction and/or the risk of reversible CNS symptoms such as those that have been reported in patients treated with intravenous acyclovir. Adequate hydration should be maintained).

No products indexed under this heading.

Methotrexate Sodium (Caution should be exercised when administering acyclovir to patients receiving potentially nephrotoxic agents since this may increase the risk of renal dysfunction and/or the risk of reversible CNS symptoms such as those that have been reported in patients treated with intravenous acyclovir. Adequate hydration should be maintained).

No products indexed under this heading.

Methyclothiazide (Caution should be exercised when administering acyclovir to patients receiving potentially nephrotoxic agents since this may increase the risk of renal dysfunction and/or the risk of reversible CNS symptoms such as those that have been reported in patients treated with intravenous acyclovir. Adequate hydration should be maintained).

No products indexed under this heading.

Mezlocillin Sodium (Caution should be exercised when administering acyclovir to patients receiving potentially nephrotoxic agents since this may increase the risk of renal dysfunction and/or the risk of reversible CNS symptoms such as those that have been reported in patients treated with intravenous acyclovir. Adequate hydration should be maintained).

No products indexed under this heading.

Minocycline Hydrochloride (Caution should be exercised when administering acyclovir to patients receiving potentially nephrotoxic agents since this may increase the risk of renal dysfunction and/or the risk of reversible CNS symptoms such as those that have been reported in patients treated with intravenous acyclovir. Adequate hydration should be maintained). Products include:

Mitomycin (Mitomycin-C) (Caution should be exercised when administering acyclovir to patients receiving potentially nephrotoxic agents since this may increase the risk of renal dysfunction and/or the risk of reversible CNS symptoms such as those that have been reported in patients treated with intravenous acyclovir. Adequate hydration should be maintained).

No products indexed under this heading.

Moexipril Hydrochloride (Caution should be exercised when administering acyclovir to patients receiving potentially nephrotoxic agents since this may increase the risk of renal dysfunction and/or the risk of reversible CNS symptoms such as those that have been reported in patients treated with intravenous acyclovir. Adequate hydration should be maintained). Products include:

Muromonab-CD3 (Caution should be exercised when administering acyclovir to patients receiving potentially nephrotoxic agents since this may increase the risk of renal dysfunction and/or the risk of reversible CNS symptoms such as those that have been reported in patients treated with intravenous acyclovir. Adequate hydration should be maintained). Products include:

IMPORTANT NOTE: Always consult each drug listing in the patient's regimen for possible interactions.

Nabumetone (Caution should be exercised when administering acyclovir to patients receiving potentially nephrotoxic agents since this may increase the risk of renal dysfunction and/or the risk of reversible CNS symptoms such as those that have been reported in patients treated with intravenous acyclovir. Adequate hydration should be maintained).

No products indexed under this heading.

Nafcillin Sodium (Caution should be exercised when administering acyclovir to patients receiving potentially nephrotoxic agents since this may increase the risk of renal dysfunction and/or the risk of reversible CNS symptoms such as those that have been reported in patients treated with intravenous acyclovir. Adequate hydration should be maintained).

No products indexed under this heading.

Naproxen (Caution should be exercised when administering acyclovir to patients receiving potentially nephrotoxic agents since this may increase the risk of renal dysfunction and/or the risk of reversible CNS symptoms such as those that have been reported in patients treated with intravenous acyclovir. Adequate hydration should be maintained). Products include:

EC-Naprosyn Delayed-Release Tablets 2761
Naprosyn Suspension 2761
Naprosyn Tablets 2761
Prevacid NapraPAC 3280

Naproxen Sodium (Caution should be exercised when administering acyclovir to patients receiving potentially nephrotoxic agents since this may increase the risk of renal dysfunction and/or the risk of reversible CNS symptoms such as those that have been reported in patients treated with intravenous acyclovir. Adequate hydration should be maintained). Products include:

Aleve Caplets 742
Aleve Gelcaps 743
Aleve Tablets 743
Aleve Cold & Sinus Caplets 744
Anaprox Tablets 2761
Anaprox DS Tablets 2761

Nelfinavir Mesylate (Caution should be exercised when administering acyclovir to patients receiving potentially nephrotoxic agents since this may increase the risk of renal dysfunction and/or the risk of reversible CNS symptoms such as those that have been reported in patients treated with intravenous acyclovir. Adequate hydration should be maintained). Products include:

Viracept 2577

Neomycin (Caution should be exercised when administering acyclovir to patients receiving potentially nephrotoxic agents since this may increase the risk of renal dysfunction and/or the risk of reversible CNS symptoms such as those that have been reported in patients treated with intravenous acyclovir. Adequate hydration should be maintained). Products include:

Neosporin Antibiotic Ointment .... ▣643
Neosporin + Pain Relief Antibiotic Cream and Ointment (Maximum Strength) .... ▣643

Neomycin, oral (Caution should be exercised when administering acyclovir to patients receiving potentially nephrotoxic agents since this may increase the risk of renal dysfunction and/or the risk of reversible CNS symptoms such as those that have been reported in patients treated with intravenous acyclovir. Adequate hydration should be maintained).

No products indexed under this heading.

Neomycin Sulfate (Caution should be exercised when administering acyclovir to patients receiving potentially nephrotoxic agents since this may increase the risk of renal dysfunction and/or the risk of reversible CNS symptoms such as those that have been reported in patients treated with intravenous acyclovir. Adequate hydration should be maintained). Products include:

Neosporin Ophthalmic Solution Sterile .... ⊙265
Poly-Pred Ophthalmic Suspension .... ⊙233

Nephrotoxic Drugs (Caution should be exercised when administering acyclovir to patients receiving potentially nephrotoxic agents since this may increase the risk of renal dysfunction and/or the risk of reversible CNS symptoms such as those that have been reported in patients treated with intravenous acyclovir. Adequate hydration should be maintained).

No products indexed under this heading.

Nevirapine (Caution should be exercised when administering acyclovir to patients receiving potentially nephrotoxic agents since this may increase the risk of renal dysfunction and/or the risk of reversible CNS symptoms such as those that have been reported in patients treated with intravenous acyclovir. Adequate hydration should be maintained). Products include:

Viramune Oral Suspension 873
Viramune Tablets 873

Norfloxacin (Caution should be exercised when administering acyclovir to patients receiving potentially nephrotoxic agents since this may increase the risk of renal dysfunction and/or the risk of reversible CNS symptoms such as those that have been reported in patients treated with intravenous acyclovir. Adequate hydration should be maintained). Products include:

Noroxin Tablets 2032

Olsalazine Sodium (Caution should be exercised when administering acyclovir to patients receiving potentially nephrotoxic agents since this may increase the risk of renal dysfunction and/or the risk of reversible CNS symptoms such as those that have been reported in patients treated with intravenous acyclovir. Adequate hydration should be maintained).

No products indexed under this heading.

Omeprazole (Caution should be exercised when administering acyclovir to patients receiving potentially nephrotoxic agents since this may increase the risk of renal dysfunction and/or the risk of reversible CNS symptoms such as those that have been reported in patients treated with intravenous acyclovir. Adequate hydration should be maintained). Products include:

Zegerid Capsules 2958
Zegerid Powder for Oral Solution 2958

Oxaprozin (Caution should be exercised when administering acyclovir to patients receiving potentially nephrotoxic agents since this may increase the risk of renal dysfunction and/or the risk of reversible CNS symptoms such as those that have been reported in patients treated with intravenous acyclovir. Adequate hydration should be maintained).

No products indexed under this heading.

Pamidronate Disodium (Caution should be exercised when administering acyclovir to patients receiving potentially nephrotoxic agents since this may increase the risk of renal dysfunction and/or the risk of reversible CNS symptoms such as those that have been reported in patients treated with intravenous acyclovir. Adequate hydration should be maintained). Products include:

Aredia for Injection 2179

Paroxetine Hydrochloride (Caution should be exercised when administering acyclovir to patients receiving potentially nephrotoxic agents since this may increase the risk of renal dysfunction and/or the risk of reversible CNS symptoms such as those that have been reported in patients treated with intravenous acyclovir. Adequate hydration should be maintained). Products include:

Paxil CR Controlled-Release Tablets 1538
Paxil 1530

Penicillamine (Caution should be exercised when administering acyclovir to patients receiving potentially nephrotoxic agents since this may increase the risk of renal dysfunction and/or the risk of reversible CNS symptoms such as those that have been reported in patients treated with intravenous acyclovir. Adequate hydration should be maintained). Products include:

Cuprimine Capsules 1947

Penicillin G Benzathine (Caution should be exercised when administering acyclovir to patients receiving potentially nephrotoxic agents since this may increase the risk of renal dysfunction and/or the risk of reversible CNS symptoms such as those that have been reported in patients treated with intravenous acyclovir. Adequate hydration should be maintained). Products include:

Bicillin C-R Injectable Suspension 1706

Penicillin G Potassium (Caution should be exercised when administering acyclovir to patients receiving potentially nephrotoxic agents since this may increase the risk of renal dysfunction and/or the risk of reversible CNS symptoms such as those that have been reported in patients treated with intravenous acyclovir. Adequate hydration should be maintained).

No products indexed under this heading.

Penicillin G Procaine (Caution should be exercised when administering acyclovir to patients receiving potentially nephrotoxic agents since this may increase the risk of renal dysfunction and/or the risk of reversible CNS symptoms such as those that have been reported in patients treated with intravenous acyclovir. Adequate hydration should be maintained). Products include:

Bicillin C-R Injectable Suspension 1706

Penicillin G Sodium (Caution should be exercised when administering acyclovir to patients receiving potentially nephrotoxic agents since this may increase the risk of renal dysfunction and/or the risk of reversible CNS symptoms such as those that have been reported in patients treated with intravenous acyclovir. Adequate hydration should be maintained).

No products indexed under this heading.

Penicillin V Potassium (Caution should be exercised when administering acyclovir to patients receiving potentially nephrotoxic agents since this may increase the risk of renal dysfunction and/or the risk of reversible CNS symptoms such as those that have been reported in patients treated with intravenous acyclovir. Adequate hydration should be maintained).

No products indexed under this heading.

Pentamidine Isethionate (Caution should be exercised when administering acyclovir to patients receiving potentially nephrotoxic agents since this may increase the risk of renal dysfunction and/or the risk of reversible CNS symptoms such as those that have been reported in patients treated with intravenous acyclovir. Adequate hydration should be maintained).

No products indexed under this heading.

Perindopril Erbumine (Caution should be exercised when administering acyclovir to patients receiving potentially nephrotoxic agents since this may increase the risk of renal dysfunction and/or the risk of reversible CNS symptoms such as those that have been reported in patients treated with intravenous acyclovir. Adequate hydration should be maintained). Products include:

Aceon Tablets (2 mg, 4 mg, 8 mg) 3194

Phenylbutazone (Caution should be exercised when administering acyclovir to patients receiving potentially nephrotoxic agents since this may increase the risk of renal dysfunction and/or the risk of reversible CNS symptoms such as those that have been reported in patients treated with intravenous acyclovir. Adequate hydration should be maintained).

No products indexed under this heading.

Piroxicam (Caution should be exercised when administering acyclovir to patients receiving potentially nephrotoxic agents since this may increase the risk of renal dysfunction and/or the risk of reversible CNS symptoms such as those that have been reported in patients treated with intravenous acyclovir. Adequate hydration should be maintained).

No products indexed under this heading.

Plicamycin (Caution should be exercised when administering acyclovir to patients receiving potentially nephrotoxic agents since this may increase the risk of renal dysfunction and/or the risk of reversible CNS symptoms such as those that have been reported in patients treated with intravenous acyclovir. Adequate hydration should be maintained).

No products indexed under this heading.

Polymyxin (Caution should be exercised when administering acyclovir to patients receiving potentially nephrotoxic agents since this may increase the risk of renal dysfunction and/or the risk of reversible CNS symptoms such as those that have been reported in patients treated with intravenous acyclovir. Adequate hydration should be maintained).

No products indexed under this heading.

Polymyxin B Sulfate (Caution should be exercised when administering acyclovir to patients receiving potentially nephrotoxic agents since this may increase the risk of renal dysfunction and/or the risk of reversible CNS symptoms such as those that have been reported in patients treated with intravenous acyclovir. Adequate hydration should be maintained). Products include:

Neosporin Antibiotic Ointment ◫**643**
Neosporin Ophthalmic Solution
　Sterile.. ⊙ **265**
Neosporin + Pain Relief Antibiotic
　Cream and Ointment
　(Maximum Strength).................... ◫**643**
Poly-Pred Ophthalmic
　Suspension ⊙ **233**
Polysporin First Aid Antibiotic
　Ointment.. ◫**643**
Polytrim Ophthalmic Solution **574**

Polythiazide (Caution should be exercised when administering acyclovir to patients receiving potentially nephrotoxic agents since this may increase the risk of renal dysfunction and/or the risk of reversible CNS symptoms such as those that have been reported in patients treated with intravenous acyclovir. Adequate hydration should be maintained).

No products indexed under this heading.

Pravastatin Sodium (Caution should be exercised when administering acyclovir to patients receiving potentially nephrotoxic agents since this may increase the risk of renal dysfunction and/or the risk of reversible CNS symptoms such as those that have been reported in patients treated with intravenous acyclovir. Adequate hydration should be maintained).

No products indexed under this heading.

Probenecid (Co-administration of probenecid with intravenous acyclovir has been shown to increase acyclovir half-life and systemic exposure; urinary excretion and renal clearance were correspondingly reduced).

No products indexed under this heading.

Quinapril Hydrochloride (Caution should be exercised when administering acyclovir to patients receiving potentially nephrotoxic agents since this may increase the risk of renal dysfunction and/or the risk of reversible CNS symptoms such as those that have been reported in patients treated with intravenous acyclovir. Adequate hydration should be maintained).

No products indexed under this heading.

Rabeprazole Sodium (Caution should be exercised when administering acyclovir to patients receiving potentially nephrotoxic agents since this may increase the risk of renal dysfunction and/or the risk of reversible CNS symptoms such as those that have been reported in patients treated with intravenous acyclovir. Adequate hydration should be maintained). Products include:

Aciphex Tablets **1090**

Ramipril (Caution should be exercised when administering acyclovir to patients receiving potentially nephrotoxic agents since this may increase the risk of renal dysfunction and/or the risk of reversible CNS symptoms such as those that have been reported in patients treated with intravenous acyclovir. Adequate hydration should be maintained). Products include:

Altace Capsules **1702**

Rifampin (Caution should be exercised when administering acyclovir to patients receiving potentially nephrotoxic agents since this may increase the risk of renal dysfunction and/or the risk of reversible CNS symptoms such as those that have been reported in patients treated with intravenous acyclovir. Adequate hydration should be maintained).

No products indexed under this heading.

Riluzole (Caution should be exercised when administering acyclovir to patients receiving potentially nephrotoxic agents since this may increase the risk of renal dysfunction and/or the risk of reversible CNS symptoms such as those that have been reported in patients treated with intravenous acyclovir. Adequate hydration should be maintained). Products include:

Rilutek Tablets **2930**

Ritonavir (Caution should be exercised when administering acyclovir to patients receiving potentially nephrotoxic agents since this may increase the risk of renal dysfunction and/or the risk of reversible CNS symptoms such as those that have been reported in patients treated with intravenous acyclovir. Adequate hydration should be maintained). Products include:

Kaletra ... **476**
Norvir ... **503**

Rofecoxib (Caution should be exercised when administering acyclovir to patients receiving potentially nephrotoxic agents since this may increase the risk of renal dysfunction and/or the risk of reversible CNS symptoms such as those that have been reported in patients treated with intravenous acyclovir. Adequate hydration should be maintained).

No products indexed under this heading.

Saquinavir (Caution should be exercised when administering acyclovir to patients receiving potentially nephrotoxic agents since this may increase the risk of renal dysfunction and/or the risk of reversible CNS symptoms such as those that have been reported in patients treated with intravenous acyclovir. Adequate hydration should be maintained).

No products indexed under this heading.

Sibutramine Hydrochloride Monohydrate (Caution should be exercised when administering acyclovir to patients receiving potentially nephrotoxic agents since this may increase the risk of renal dysfunction and/or the risk of reversible CNS symptoms such as those that have been reported in patients treated with intravenous acyclovir. Adequate hydration should be maintained). Products include:

Meridia Capsules **489**

Simvastatin (Caution should be exercised when administering acyclovir to patients receiving potentially nephrotoxic agents since this may increase the risk of renal dysfunction and/or the risk of reversible CNS symptoms such as those that have been reported in patients treated with intravenous acyclovir. Adequate hydration should be maintained). Products include:

Vytorin 10/10 Tablets **2114**
Vytorin 10/10 Tablets **3077**
Vytorin 10/20 Tablets **2114**
Vytorin 10/20 Tablets **3077**
Vytorin 10/40 Tablets **2114**
Vytorin 10/40 Tablets **3077**
Vytorin 10/80 Tablets **2114**
Vytorin 10/80 Tablets **3077**
Zocor Tablets **2105**

Spirapril Hydrochloride (Caution should be exercised when administering acyclovir to patients receiving potentially nephrotoxic agents since this may increase the risk of renal dysfunction and/or the risk of reversible CNS symptoms such as those that have been reported in patients treated with intravenous acyclovir. Adequate hydration should be maintained).

No products indexed under this heading.

Stavudine (Caution should be exercised when administering acyclovir to patients receiving potentially nephrotoxic agents since this may increase the risk of renal dysfunction and/or the risk of reversible CNS symptoms such as those that have been reported in patients treated with intravenous acyclovir. Adequate hydration should be maintained).

No products indexed under this heading.

Streptomycin Sulfate (Caution should be exercised when administering acyclovir to patients receiving potentially nephrotoxic agents since this may increase the risk of renal dysfunction and/or the risk of reversible CNS symptoms such as those that have been reported in patients treated with intravenous acyclovir. Adequate hydration should be maintained).

No products indexed under this heading.

Streptozocin (Caution should be exercised when administering acyclovir to patients receiving potentially nephrotoxic agents since this may increase the risk of renal dysfunction and/or the risk of reversible CNS symptoms such as those that have been reported in patients treated with intravenous acyclovir. Adequate hydration should be maintained).

No products indexed under this heading.

Sulfacytine (Caution should be exercised when administering acyclovir to patients receiving potentially nephrotoxic agents since this may increase the risk of renal dysfunction and/or the risk of reversible CNS symptoms such as those that have been reported in patients treated with intravenous acyclovir. Adequate hydration should be maintained).

No products indexed under this heading.

Sulfamethizole (Caution should be exercised when administering acyclovir to patients receiving potentially nephrotoxic agents since this may increase the risk of renal dysfunction and/or the risk of reversible CNS symptoms such as those that have been reported in patients treated with intravenous acyclovir. Adequate hydration should be maintained).

No products indexed under this heading.

Sulfamethoxazole (Caution should be exercised when administering acyclovir to patients receiving potentially nephrotoxic agents since this may increase the risk of renal dysfunction and/or the risk of reversible CNS symptoms such as those that have been reported in patients treated with intravenous acyclovir. Adequate hydration should be maintained).

No products indexed under this heading.

Sulfasalazine (Caution should be exercised when administering acyclovir to patients receiving potentially nephrotoxic agents since this may increase the risk of renal dysfunction and/or the risk of reversible CNS symptoms such as those that have been reported in patients treated with intravenous acyclovir. Adequate hydration should be maintained).

No products indexed under this heading.

Sulfinpyrazone (Caution should be exercised when administering acyclovir to patients receiving potentially nephrotoxic agents since this may increase the risk of renal dysfunction and/or the risk of reversible CNS symptoms such as those that have been reported in patients treated with intravenous acyclovir. Adequate hydration should be maintained).

No products indexed under this heading.

IMPORTANT NOTE: Always consult each drug listing in the patient's regimen for possible interactions.

Sulfisoxazole Acetyl (Caution should be exercised when administering acyclovir to patients receiving potentially nephrotoxic agents since this may increase the risk of renal dysfunction and/or the risk of reversible CNS symptoms such as those that have been reported in patients treated with intravenous acyclovir. Adequate hydration should be maintained).

No products indexed under this heading.

Sulfisoxazole Diolamine (Caution should be exercised when administering acyclovir to patients receiving potentially nephrotoxic agents since this may increase the risk of renal dysfunction and/or the risk of reversible CNS symptoms such as those that have been reported in patients treated with intravenous acyclovir. Adequate hydration should be maintained).

No products indexed under this heading.

Sulindac (Caution should be exercised when administering acyclovir to patients receiving potentially nephrotoxic agents since this may increase the risk of renal dysfunction and/or the risk of reversible CNS symptoms such as those that have been reported in patients treated with intravenous acyclovir. Adequate hydration should be maintained). Products include:

Clinoril Tablets 1924

Tacrolimus (Caution should be exercised when administering acyclovir to patients receiving potentially nephrotoxic agents since this may increase the risk of renal dysfunction and/or the risk of reversible CNS symptoms such as those that have been reported in patients treated with intravenous acyclovir. Adequate hydration should be maintained). Products include:

Prograf Capsules and Injection 632
Protopic Ointment 638

Tenofovir Disoproxil Fumarate (Caution should be exercised when administering acyclovir to patients receiving potentially nephrotoxic agents since this may increase the risk of renal dysfunction and/or the risk of reversible CNS symptoms such as those that have been reported in patients treated with intravenous acyclovir. Adequate hydration should be maintained). Products include:

Atripla Tablets 945
Truvada Tablets 1296
Viread Tablets 1301

Thioguanine (Caution should be exercised when administering acyclovir to patients receiving potentially nephrotoxic agents since this may increase the risk of renal dysfunction and/or the risk of reversible CNS symptoms such as those that have been reported in patients treated with intravenous acyclovir. Adequate hydration should be maintained). Products include:

Tabloid Tablets 1575

Ticarcillin Disodium (Caution should be exercised when administering acyclovir to patients receiving potentially nephrotoxic agents since this may increase the risk of renal dysfunction and/or the risk of reversible CNS symptoms such as those that have been reported in patients

treated with intravenous acyclovir. Adequate hydration should be maintained). Products include:

Timentin ADD-Vantage 1580
Timentin Injection Galaxy Container 1583
Timentin IV Infusion 1577
Timentin Pharmacy Bulk Package 1586

Tobramycin (Caution should be exercised when administering acyclovir to patients receiving potentially nephrotoxic agents since this may increase the risk of renal dysfunction and/or the risk of reversible CNS symptoms such as those that have been reported in patients treated with intravenous acyclovie. Adequate hydration should be maintained). Products include:

TOBI Solution for Inhalation 2298
TobraDex Ophthalmic Ointment 562
TobraDex Ophthalmic Suspension ... 563
Zylet Ophthalmic Suspension ⊙ 259

Tobramycin Sulfate (Caution should be exercised when administering acyclovir to patients receiving potentially nephrotoxic agents since this may increase the risk of renal dysfunction and/or the risk of reversible CNS symptoms such as those that have been reported in patients treated with intravenous acyclovir. Adequate hydration should be maintained).

No products indexed under this heading.

Tolazamide (Caution should be exercised when administering acyclovir to patients receiving potentially nephrotoxic agents since this may increase the risk of renal dysfunction and/or the risk of reversible CNS symptoms such as those that have been reported in patients treated with intravenous acyclovir. Adequate hydration should be maintained).

No products indexed under this heading.

Tolbutamide (Caution should be exercised when administering acyclovir to patients receiving potentially nephrotoxic agents since this may increase the risk of renal dysfunction and/or the risk of reversible CNS symptoms such as those that have been reported in patients treated with intravenous acyclovir. Adequate hydration should be maintained).

No products indexed under this heading.

Tolmetin Sodium (Caution should be exercised when administering acyclovir to patients receiving potentially nephrotoxic agents since this may increase the risk of renal dysfunction and/or the risk of reversible CNS symptoms such as those that have been reported in patients treated with intravenous acyclovir. Adequate hydration should be maintained).

No products indexed under this heading.

Trandolapril (Caution should be exercised when administering acyclovir to patients receiving potentially nephrotoxic agents since this may increase the risk of renal dysfunction and/or the risk of reversible CNS symptoms such as those that have been reported in patients treated with intravenous acyclovir. Adequate hydration should be maintained). Products include:

Mavik Tablets 486
Tarka Tablets 524

Triamterene (Caution should be exercised when administering acy-

clovir to patients receiving potentially nephrotoxic agents since this may increase the risk of renal dysfunction and/or the risk of reversible CNS symptoms such as those that have been reported in patients treated with intravenous acyclovir. Adequate hydration should be maintained). Products include:

Dyazide Capsules 1423
Dyrenium Capsules 3400

Trimethadione (Caution should be exercised when administering acyclovir to patients receiving potentially nephrotoxic agents since this may increase the risk of renal dysfunction and/or the risk of reversible CNS symptoms such as those that have been reported in patients treated with intravenous acyclovir. Adequate hydration should be maintained).

No products indexed under this heading.

Trovafloxacin Mesylate (Caution should be exercised when administering acyclovir to patients receiving potentially nephrotoxic agents since this may increase the risk of renal dysfunction and/or the risk of reversible CNS symptoms such as those that have been reported in patients treated with intravenous acyclovir. Adequate hydration should be maintained).

No products indexed under this heading.

Tyropanoate Sodium (Caution should be exercised when administering acyclovir to patients receiving potentially nephrotoxic agents since this may increase the risk of renal dysfunction and/or the risk of reversible CNS symptoms such as those that have been reported in patients treated with intravenous acyclovir. Adequate hydration should be maintained).

No products indexed under this heading.

Valacyclovir Hydrochloride (Caution should be exercised when administering acyclovir to patients receiving potentially nephrotoxic agents since this may increase the risk of renal dysfunction and/or the risk of reversible CNS symptoms such as those that have been reported in patients treated with intravenous acyclovir. Adequate hydration should be maintained). Products include:

Valtrex Caplets 1597

Valdecoxib (Caution should be exercised when administering acyclovir to patients receiving potentially nephrotoxic agents since this may increase the risk of renal dysfunction and/or the risk of reversible CNS symptoms such as those that have been reported in patients treated with intravenous acyclovir. Adequate hydration should be maintained).

No products indexed under this heading.

Vancomycin Hydrochloride (Caution should be exercised when administering acyclovir to patients receiving potentially nephrotoxic agents since this may increase the risk of renal dysfunction and/or the risk of reversible CNS symptoms such as those that have been reported in patients treated with intravenous acyclovir. Adequate hydration should be maintained). Products include:

Vancocin HCl Capsules, USP 3380

Voriconazole (Caution should be exercised when administering acyclovir to patients receiving potentially nephrotoxic agents since this may increase the risk of renal dysfunction and/or the risk of reversible CNS symptoms such as those that have been reported in patients treated with intravenous acyclovir. Adequate hydration should be maintained). Products include:

VFEND I.V. 2564
VFEND Oral Suspension 2564
VFEND Tablets 2564

Zalcitabine (Caution should be exercised when administering acyclovir to patients receiving potentially nephrotoxic agents since this may increase the risk of renal dysfunction and/or the risk of reversible CNS symptoms such as those that have been reported in patients treated with intravenous acyclovir. Adequate hydration should be maintained).

No products indexed under this heading.

Zidovudine (Caution should be exercised when administering acyclovir to patients receiving potentially nephrotoxic agents since this may increase the risk of renal dysfunction and/or the risk of reversible CNS symptoms such as those that have been reported in patients treated with intravenous acyclovir. Adequate hydration should be maintained). Products include:

Combivir Tablets 1411
Retrovir 1560
Retrovir IV Infusion 1564
Trizivir Tablets 1589

Zoledronic acid (Caution should be exercised when administering acyclovir to patients receiving potentially nephrotoxic agents since this may increase the risk of renal dysfunction and/or the risk of reversible CNS symptoms such as those that have been reported in patients treated with intravenous acyclovir. Adequate hydration should be maintained). Products include:

Zometa for Intravenous Infusion 2315

ZOVIRAX CREAM

(Acyclovir) 820
None cited in PDR database.

ZOVIRAX OINTMENT

(Acyclovir) 821
None cited in PDR database.

ZOVIRAX SUSPENSION

(Acyclovir) 1643
See Zovirax Capsules

ZOVIRAX TABLETS

(Acyclovir) 1643
See Zovirax Capsules

ZYBAN SUSTAINED-RELEASE TABLETS

(Bupropion Hydrochloride) 1644
May interact with benzodiazepines, corticosteroids, antidepressant drugs, hypnotics and sedatives, monoamine oxidase inhibitors, antipsychotic agents, phenytoin, drugs which lower seizure threshold, xanthines, and certain other agents. Compounds in these categories include:

Alprazolam (Bupropion is associated with a dose-related risk of seizures; excessive use of benzodiazepine sedatives is associated with increased risk of seizures; bupropion

is contraindicated in patients undergoing abrupt discontinuation of benzodiazepine sedatives). Products include:
Niravam Orally Disintegrating Tablets 3092

Amantadine Hydrochloride (Limited clinical data suggests higher incidence of adverse experiences with co-administration; use small initial dose and gradually increase doses). Products include:
Symmetrel Tablets 1135

Aminophylline (Bupropion is associated with a dose-related risk of seizures; co-administration with drugs that lower seizure threshold may increase the risk of seizures with bupropion; concurrent use should be undertaken with extreme caution).
No products indexed under this heading.

Amitriptyline Hydrochloride (Bupropion is associated with dose-dependent risk of seizures; co-administration with drugs that lower seizure threshold may increase the risk of seizure with bupropion).
No products indexed under this heading.

Amoxapine (Bupropion is associated with dose-dependent risk of seizures; co-administration with drugs that lower seizure threshold may increase the risk of seizure with bupropion).
No products indexed under this heading.

Aripiprazole (Bupropion is associated with dose-dependent risk of seizures; co-administration with drugs that lower seizure threshold, such as antipsychotics, may increase the risk of seizure with bupropion). Products include:
Abilify Oral Solution 882
Abilify Oral Solution 2450
Abilify Discmelt Orally Disintegrating Tablets 882
Abilify Discmelt Orally Disintegrating Tablets 2450
Abilify Tablets 882
Abilify Tablets 2450

Atazanavir (Co-administration with fosamprenavir/ritonavir combination may lead to decreased levels of atazanavir).
No products indexed under this heading.

Atazanavir sulfate (Co-administration with fosamprenavir/ritonavir combination may lead to decreased levels of atazanavir). Products include:
Reyataz Capsules 921

Betamethasone Acetate (Concurrent administration of bupropion hydrochloride and agents that lower seizure threshold, such as systemic steroids, should be undertaken only with extreme caution).
No products indexed under this heading.

Betamethasone Sodium Phosphate (Concurrent administration of bupropion hydrochloride and agents that lower seizure threshold, such as systemic steroids, should be undertaken only with extreme caution).
No products indexed under this heading.

Bupropion (Zyban should not be used in combination with any other medications containing bupropion, such as Wellbutrin or Wellbutrin SR).
No products indexed under this heading.

Carbamazepine (May induce the metabolism of bupropion). Products include:
Carbatrol Capsules 3171
Equetro Extended-Release Capsules 3180
Tegretol/Tegretol-XR 2295

Chlordiazepoxide (Bupropion is associated with a dose-related risk of seizures; excessive use of benzodiazepine sedatives is associated with increased risk of seizures; bupropion is contraindicated in patients undergoing abrupt discontinuation of benzodiazepine sedatives).
No products indexed under this heading.

Chlordiazepoxide Hydrochloride (Bupropion is associated with a dose-related risk of seizures; excessive use of benzodiazepine sedatives is associated with increased risk of seizures; bupropion is contraindicated in patients undergoing abrupt discontinuation of benzodiazepine sedatives). Products include:
Librium Capsules 3347

Chlorpromazine (Bupropion is associated with dose-dependent risk of seizures; co-administration with drugs that lower seizure threshold, such as antipsychotics, may increase the risk of seizure with bupropion).
No products indexed under this heading.

Chlorpromazine Hydrochloride (Bupropion is associated with dose-dependent risk of seizures; co-administration with drugs that lower seizure threshold, such as antipsychotics, may increase the risk of seizure with bupropion).
No products indexed under this heading.

Chlorprothixene (Bupropion is associated with dose-dependent risk of seizures; co-administration with drugs that lower seizure threshold, such as antipsychotics, may increase the risk of seizure with bupropion).
No products indexed under this heading.

Chlorprothixene Hydrochloride (Bupropion is associated with dose-dependent risk of seizures; co-administration with drugs that lower seizure threshold, such as antipsychotics, may increase the risk of seizure with bupropion).
No products indexed under this heading.

Cimetidine (May inhibit the metabolism of bupropion). Products include:
Tagamet HB 200 Tablets 664

Cimetidine Hydrochloride (May inhibit the metabolism of bupropion).
No products indexed under this heading.

Citalopram Hydrobromide (Bupropion is associated with dose-dependent risk of seizures; co-administration with drugs that lower seizure threshold, such as antidepressants, may increase the risk of seizure with bupropion). Products include:
Celexa 1176

Clorazepate Dipotassium (Bupropion is associated with a dose-related risk of seizures; excessive use of benzodiazepine sedatives is associated with increased risk of seizures; bupropion is contraindicated in patients undergoing abrupt discontinuation of benzodiazepine sedatives). Products include:
Tranxene 2474

Clozapine (Bupropion is associated with dose-dependent risk of seizures; co-administration with drugs that lower seizure threshold, such as antipsychotics, may increase the risk of seizure with bupropion). Products include:
Clozaril Tablets 2184
FazaClo Orally Disintegrating Tablets 551

Cortisone Acetate (Concurrent administration of bupropion hydrochloride and agents that lower seizure threshold, such as systemic steroids, should be undertaken only with extreme caution).
No products indexed under this heading.

Cyclophosphamide (Bupropion is primarily metabolized, based on in vitro studies, to hydroxybupropion by the CYP2B6 isoenzyme, therefore the potential exists for a drug interaction with agents that affect the CYP2B6 isoenzyme metabolism, such as cyclophosphamide).
No products indexed under this heading.

Desipramine Hydrochloride (Co-administration in male subjects who were extensive metabolizers of the CYP2D6 isoenzyme with daily doses of bupropion followed by a single dose of desipramine increased the Cmax, AUC and t1/2 of desipramine by an average of approximately two-, five-, and two-fold respectively; co-administration should be initiated at the lower end of the dose range of desipramine; potential for increased risk of seizures).
No products indexed under this heading.

Dexamethasone (Concurrent administration of bupropion hydrochloride and agents that lower seizure threshold, such as systemic steroids, should be undertaken only with extreme caution). Products include:
Ciprodex Otic Suspension 559
Decadron Tablets 1951
TobraDex Ophthalmic Ointment 562
TobraDex Ophthalmic Suspension ... 563

Dexamethasone Acetate (Concurrent administration of bupropion hydrochloride and agents that lower seizure threshold, such as systemic steroids, should be undertaken only with extreme caution).
No products indexed under this heading.

Dexamethasone Sodium Phosphate (Concurrent administration of bupropion hydrochloride and agents that lower seizure threshold, such as systemic steroids, should be undertaken only with extreme caution).
No products indexed under this heading.

Diazepam (Bupropion is associated with a dose-related risk of seizures; excessive use of benzodiazepine sedatives is associated with increased risk of seizures; bupropion is contraindicated in patients undergoing abrupt discontinuation of benzodiazepine sedatives). Products include:
Diastat Rectal Delivery System 3343
Valium Tablets 2819

Doxepin Hydrochloride (Bupropion is associated with dose-dependent risk of seizures; co-administration with drugs that lower seizure threshold may increase the risk of seizure with bupropion).
No products indexed under this heading.

Dyphylline (Bupropion is associated with a dose-related risk of seizures; co-administration with drugs that lower seizure threshold may increase the risk of seizures with bupropion; concurrent use should be undertaken with extreme caution).
No products indexed under this heading.

Escitalopram Oxalate (Bupropion is associated with dose-dependent risk of seizures; co-administration with drugs that lower seizure threshold, such as antidepressants, may increase the risk of seizure with bupropion). Products include:
Lexapro Oral Solution 1190
Lexapro Tablets 1190

Estazolam (Bupropion is associated with a dose-related risk of seizures; excessive use of benzodiazepine sedatives is associated with increased risk of seizures; bupropion is contraindicated in patients undergoing abrupt discontinuation of benzodiazepine sedatives). Products include:
ProSom Tablets 517

Ethchlorvynol (Bupropion hydrochloride is contraindicated in patients undergoing abrupt discontinuation of sedatives).
No products indexed under this heading.

Ethinamate (Bupropion hydrochloride is contraindicated in patients undergoing abrupt discontinuation of sedatives).
No products indexed under this heading.

Flecainide Acetate (Co-administration of bupropion with drugs that are metabolized by CYP2D6 isoenzyme, such as flecainide, may result in, based on data with desipramine, increased Cmax, AUC and t1/2; co-administration should be initiated at the lower end of the dose range of flecainide). Products include:
Tambocor Tablets 1856

Fludrocortisone Acetate (Concurrent administration of bupropion hydrochloride and agents that lower seizure threshold, such as systemic steroids, should be undertaken only with extreme caution).
No products indexed under this heading.

Fluoxetine Hydrochloride (Co-administration of bupropion with drugs that are metabolized by CYP2D6 isoenzyme, such as fluoxetine, may result in, based on data with desipramine, increased Cmax, AUC and t1/2; co-administration should be initiated at the lower end of the dose range of fluoxetine). Products include:
Prozac Pulvules and Liquid 1801
Symbyax Capsules 1819

IMPORTANT NOTE: Always consult each drug listing in the patient's regimen for possible interactions.

Fluphenazine Decanoate (Bupropion is associated with dose-dependent risk of seizures; co-administration with drugs that lower seizure threshold, such as antipsychotics, may increase the risk of seizure with bupropion).
No products indexed under this heading.

Fluphenazine Enanthate (Bupropion is associated with dose-dependent risk of seizures; co-administration with drugs that lower seizure threshold, such as antipsychotics, may increase the risk of seizure with bupropion).
No products indexed under this heading.

Fluphenazine Hydrochloride (Bupropion is associated with dose-dependent risk of seizures; co-administration with drugs that lower seizure threshold, such as antipsychotics, may increase the risk of seizure with bupropion).
No products indexed under this heading.

Flurazepam Hydrochloride (Bupropion is associated with a dose-related risk of seizures; excessive use of benzodiazepine sedatives is associated with increased risk of seizures; bupropion is contraindicated in patients undergoing abrupt discontinuation of benzodiazepine sedatives). Products include:
Dalmane Capsules 3342

Fosphenytoin Sodium (May induce the metabolism of bupropion).
No products indexed under this heading.

Glutethimide (Bupropion hydrochloride is contraindicated in patients undergoing abrupt discontinuation of sedatives).
No products indexed under this heading.

Halazepam (Bupropion is associated with a dose-related risk of seizures; excessive use of benzodiazepine sedatives is associated with increased risk of seizures; bupropion is contraindicated in patients undergoing abrupt discontinuation of benzodiazepine sedatives).
No products indexed under this heading.

Haloperidol (Co-administration of bupropion with drugs that are metabolized by CYP2D6 isoenzyme, such as haloperidol, may result in, based on data with desipramine, increased Cmax, AUC and t1/2; co-administration should be initiated at the lower end of the dose range of haloperidol; potential for increased risk of seizures).
No products indexed under this heading.

Haloperidol Decanoate (Co-administration of bupropion with drugs that are metabolized by CYP2D6 isoenzyme, such as haloperidol, may result in, based on data with desipramine, increased Cmax, AUC and t1/2; co-administration should be initiated at the lower end of the dose range of haloperidol; potential for increased risk of seizures).
No products indexed under this heading.

Hydrocortisone (Concurrent administration of bupropion hydrochloride and agents that lower seizure threshold, such as systemic steroids, should be undertaken only with extreme caution). Products include:
Colocort Rectal Suspension, USP (Retention) 100 mg/60 mL 2476
Hydrocortone Tablets 1989
Preparation H Hydrocortisone Cream .... ■ 646

Hydrocortisone Acetate (Concurrent administration of bupropion hydrochloride and agents that lower seizure threshold, such as systemic steroids, should be undertaken only with extreme caution). Products include:
Analpram-HC 1159
Pramosone 1161
ProctoFoam-HC 3099

Hydrocortisone Sodium Phosphate (Concurrent administration of bupropion hydrochloride and agents that lower seizure threshold, such as systemic steroids, should be undertaken only with extreme caution).
No products indexed under this heading.

Hydrocortisone Sodium Succinate (Concurrent administration of bupropion hydrochloride and agents that lower seizure threshold, such as systemic steroids, should be undertaken only with extreme caution).
No products indexed under this heading.

Imipramine Hydrochloride (Co-administration of bupropion with drugs that are metabolized by CYP2D6 isoenzyme, such as imipramine, may result in, based on data with desipramine, increased Cmax, AUC and t1/2; co-administration should be initiated at the lower end of the dose range of imipramine; potential for increased risk of seizures).
No products indexed under this heading.

Imipramine Pamoate (Co-administration of bupropion with drugs that are metabolized by CYP2D6 isoenzyme, such as imipramine, may result in, based on data with desipramine, increased Cmax, AUC and t1/2; co-administration should be initiated at the lower end of the dose range of imipramine; potential for increased risk of seizures).
No products indexed under this heading.

Isocarboxazid (Concurrent and/or sequential use with MAO inhibitors is contraindicated).
No products indexed under this heading.

Levodopa (Limited clinical data suggests higher incidence of adverse experiences with co-administration; use small initial dose and gradually increase doses). Products include:
Parcopa Orally Disintegrating Tablets 3097
Stalevo Tablets 2287

Lithium Carbonate (Bupropion is associated with dose-dependent risk of seizures; co-administration with drugs that lower seizure threshold, such as antipsychotics, may increase the risk of seizure with bupropion). Products include:
Lithobid Tablets 1692

Lithium Citrate (Bupropion is associated with dose-dependent risk of seizures; co-administration with drugs that lower seizure threshold, such as antipsychotics, may increase the risk of seizure with bupropion).
No products indexed under this heading.

Lorazepam (Bupropion is associated with a dose-related risk of seizures; excessive use of benzodiazepine sedatives is associated with increased risk of seizures; bupropion is contraindicated in patients undergoing abrupt discontinuation of benzodiazepine sedatives).
No products indexed under this heading.

Loxapine Hydrochloride (Bupropion is associated with dose-dependent risk of seizures; co-administration with drugs that lower seizure threshold, such as antipsychotics, may increase the risk of seizure with bupropion).
No products indexed under this heading.

Loxapine Succinate (Bupropion is associated with dose-dependent risk of seizures; co-administration with drugs that lower seizure threshold, such as antipsychotics, may increase the risk of seizure with bupropion).
No products indexed under this heading.

Maprotiline Hydrochloride (Bupropion is associated with dose-dependent risk of seizures; co-administration with drugs that lower seizure threshold may increase the risk of seizure with bupropion).
No products indexed under this heading.

Mesoridazine Besylate (Bupropion is associated with dose-dependent risk of seizures; co-administration with drugs that lower seizure threshold, such as antipsychotics, may increase the risk of seizure with bupropion).
No products indexed under this heading.

Methotrimeprazine (Bupropion is associated with dose-dependent risk of seizures; co-administration with drugs that lower seizure threshold, such as antipsychotics, may increase the risk of seizure with bupropion).
No products indexed under this heading.

Methylprednisolone Acetate (Concurrent administration of bupropion hydrochloride and agents that lower seizure threshold, such as systemic steroids, should be undertaken only with extreme caution). Products include:
Depo-Medrol Injectable Suspension 2617
Depo-Medrol Single-Dose Vial 2619

Methylprednisolone Sodium Succinate (Concurrent administration of bupropion hydrochloride and agents that lower seizure threshold, such as systemic steroids, should be undertaken only with extreme caution).
No products indexed under this heading.

Metoprolol Succinate (Co-administration of bupropion with drugs that are metabolized by CYP2D6 isoenzyme, such as metoprolol, may result in, based on data with desipramine, increased Cmax, AUC and t1/2; co-administration should be initiated at the lower end of the dose range of metoprolol). Products include:
Toprol-XL Tablets 668

Metoprolol Tartrate (Co-administration of bupropion with drugs that are metabolized by CYP2D6 isoenzyme, such as metoprolol, may result in, based on data with desipramine, increased Cmax, AUC and t1/2; co-administration should be initiated at the lower end of the dose range of metoprolol). Products include:
Lopressor Injection 2238
Lopressor Tablets 2238
Lopressor HCT 50/25 Tablets 2241
Lopressor HCT 100/25 Tablets 2241
Lopressor HCT 100/50 Tablets 2241

Midazolam Hydrochloride (Bupropion is associated with a dose-related risk of seizures; excessive use of benzodiazepine sedatives is associated with increased risk of seizures; bupropion is contraindicated in patients undergoing abrupt discontinuation of benzodiazepine sedatives).
No products indexed under this heading.

Mirtazapine (Bupropion is associated with dose-dependent risk of seizures; co-administration with drugs that lower seizure threshold, such as antidepressants, may increase the risk of seizure with bupropion).
No products indexed under this heading.

Moclobemide (Concurrent and/or sequential use with MAO inhibitors is contraindicated).
No products indexed under this heading.

Molindone Hydrochloride (Bupropion is associated with dose-dependent risk of seizures; co-administration with drugs that lower seizure threshold, such as antipsychotics, may increase the risk of seizure with bupropion). Products include:
Moban Tablets 1119

Nefazodone Hydrochloride (Bupropion is associated with dose-dependent risk of seizures; co-administration with drugs that lower seizure threshold, such as antidepressants, may increase the risk of seizure with bupropion).
No products indexed under this heading.

Nicotine (Co-administration of bupropion and nicotine transdermal system has resulted in a higher incidence of treatment-emergent hypertension). Products include:
NicoDerm CQ Clear Patch .... ■ 622

Nortriptyline Hydrochloride (Co-administration of bupropion with drugs that are metabolized by CYP2D6 isoenzyme, such as nortriptyline, may result in, based on data with desipramine, increased Cmax, AUC and t1/2; co-administration should be initiated at the lower end of the dose range of nortriptyline; potential for increased risk of seizures).
No products indexed under this heading.

Olanzapine (Bupropion is associated with dose-dependent risk of seizures; co-administration with drugs that lower seizure threshold, such as antipsychotics, may increase the risk of seizure with bupropion). Products include:

Orphenadrine Citrate (Bupropion is primarily metabolized, based on in vitro studies, to hydroxybupropion by the CYP2B6 isoenzyme; therefore the potential exists for a drug inter-action with agents that affect the CYP2B6 isoenzyme metabolism, such as orphenadrine). Products include:

Oxazepam (Bupropion is associat-ed with a dose-related risk of sei-zures; excessive use of benzodiaz-epine sedatives is associated with increased risk of seizures; bupropion is contraindicated in patients under-going abrupt discontinuation of ben-zodiazepine sedatives).

 No products indexed under this heading.

Pargyline Hydrochloride (Concur-rent and/or sequential use with MAO inhibitors is contraindicated).

 No products indexed under this heading.

Paroxetine Hydrochloride (Co-administration of bupropion with drugs that are metabolized by CYP2D6 isoenzyme, such as parox-etine, may result in, based on data with desipramine, increased Cmax, AUC and t1/2; co-administration should be initiated at the lower end of the dose range of paroxetine). Products include:

Perphenazine (Bupropion is asso-ciated with dose-dependent risk of seizures; co-administration with drugs that lower seizure threshold, such as antipsychotics, may increase the risk of seizure with bupropion).

 No products indexed under this heading.

Phenelzine Sulfate (Concurrent and/or sequential use with MAO inhibitors is contraindicated; acute toxicity of bupropion is enhanced by phenelzine in animal models).

 No products indexed under this heading.

Phenobarbital (May induce the metabolism of bupropion). Products include:

Phenytoin (May induce the metabo-lism of bupropion).

 No products indexed under this heading.

Phenytoin Sodium (May induce the metabolism of bupropion). Products include:

Pimozide (Bupropion is associated with dose-dependent risk of sei-zures; co-administration with drugs that lower seizure threshold, such as antipsychotics, may increase the risk of seizure with bupropion).

 No products indexed under this heading.

Prazepam (Bupropion is associated with a dose-related risk of seizures; excessive use of benzodiazepine sedatives is associated with increased risk of seizures; bupropion is contraindicated in patients under-going abrupt discontinuation of ben-zodiazepine sedatives).

 No products indexed under this heading.

Prednisolone Acetate (Concurrent administration of bupropion hydro-chloride and agents that lower sei-zure threshold, such as systemic steroids, should be undertaken only with extreme caution). Products include:

Prednisolone Sodium Phosphate (Concurrent administration of bupro-pion hydrochloride and agents that lower seizure threshold, such as sys-temic steroids, should be undertak-en only with extreme caution).

 No products indexed under this heading.

Prednisolone Tebutate (Concur-rent administration of bupropion hydrochloride and agents that lower seizure threshold, such as systemic steroids, should be undertaken only with extreme caution).

 No products indexed under this heading.

Prednisone (Concurrent administra-tion of bupropion hydrochloride and agents that lower seizure threshold, such as systemic steroids, should be undertaken only with extreme caution).

 No products indexed under this heading.

Procarbazine Hydrochloride (Concurrent and/or sequential use with MAO inhibitors is contraindi-cated). Products include:

Prochlorperazine (Bupropion is associated with dose-dependent risk of seizures; co-administration with drugs that lower seizure threshold, such as antipsychotics, may increase the risk of seizure with bupropion).

 No products indexed under this heading.

Promethazine Hydrochloride (Bupropion is associated with dose-dependent risk of seizures; co-administration with drugs that lower seizure threshold, such as antipsy-chotics, may increase the risk of seizure with bupropion). Products include:

Propafenone Hydrochloride (Co-administration of bupropion with drugs that are metabolized by CYP2D6 isoenzyme, such as pro-pafenone, may result in, based on data with desipramine, increased Cmax, AUC and t1/2; co-administration should be initiated at the lower end of the dose range of propafenone). Products include:

Propofol (Bupropion hydrochloride is contraindicated in patients under-going abrupt discontinuation of sedatives).

 No products indexed under this heading.

Protriptyline Hydrochloride (Bupropion is associated with dose-dependent risk of seizures; co-administration with drugs that lower seizure threshold may increase the risk of seizure with bupropion).

 No products indexed under this heading.

Quazepam (Bupropion is associat-ed with a dose-related risk of sei-zures; excessive use of benzodiaz-epine sedatives is associated with increased risk of seizures; bupropion is contraindicated in patients under-going abrupt discontinuation of ben-zodiazepine sedatives).

 No products indexed under this heading.

Quetiapine Fumarate (Bupropion is associated with dose-dependent risk of seizures; co-administration with drugs that lower seizure thresh-old, such as antipsychotics, may increase the risk of seizure with bupropion). Products include:

Ramelteon (Bupropion hydrochlo-ride is contraindicated in patients undergoing abrupt discontinuation of sedatives). Products include:

Risperidone (Co-administration of bupropion with drugs that are metab-olized by CYP2D6 isoenzyme, such as risperidone, may result in, based on data with desipramine, increased Cmax, AUC and t1/2; co-administration should be initiated at the lower end of the dose range of risperidone; potential for increased risk of seizures). Products include:

Secobarbital Sodium (Bupropion hydrochloride is contraindicated in patients undergoing abrupt discon-tinuation of sedatives).

 No products indexed under this heading.

Selegiline Hydrochloride (Concur-rent and/or sequential use with MAO inhibitors is contraindicated). Products include:

Sertraline Hydrochloride (Co-administration of bupropion with drugs that are metabolized by CYP2D6 isoenzyme, such as sertra-line, may result in, based on data with desipramine, increased Cmax, AUC and t1/2; co-administration should be initiated at the lower end of the dose range of sertraline). Products include:

Temazepam (Bupropion is associ-ated with a dose-related risk of sei-zures; excessive use of benzodiaz-epine sedatives is associated with increased risk of seizures; bupropion is contraindicated in patients under-going abrupt discontinuation of ben-zodiazepine sedatives). Products include:

Theophylline (Bupropion is associ-ated with a dose-related risk of sei-zures; co-administration with drugs that lower seizure threshold may increase the risk of seizures with bupropion; concurrent use should be undertaken with extreme caution).

 No products indexed under this heading.

Theophylline Anhydrous (Bupro-pion is associated with a dose-related risk of seizures; co-administration with drugs that lower seizure threshold may increase the risk of seizures with bupropion; con-current use should be undertaken with extreme caution). Products include:

Theophylline Calcium Salicylate (Bupropion is associated with a dose-related risk of seizures; co-administration with drugs that lower seizure threshold may increase the risk of seizures with bupropion; con-current use should be undertaken with extreme caution).

 No products indexed under this heading.

Theophylline Dihydroxypropyl (Glyceryl) (Bupropion is associated with a dose-related risk of seizures; co-administration with drugs that lower seizure threshold may increase the risk of seizures with bupropion; concurrent use should be undertaken with extreme caution).

 No products indexed under this heading.

Theophylline Ethylenediamine (Bupropion is associated with a dose-related risk of seizures; co-administration with drugs that lower seizure threshold may increase the risk of seizures with bupropion; con-current use should be undertaken with extreme caution).

 No products indexed under this heading.

Theophylline Sodium Glycinate (Bupropion is associated with a dose-related risk of seizures; co-administration with drugs that lower seizure threshold may increase the risk of seizures with bupropion; con-current use should be undertaken with extreme caution).

 No products indexed under this heading.

Thioridazine Hydrochloride (Co-administration of bupropion with drugs that are metabolized by CYP2D6 isoenzyme, such as thiorid-azine, may result in, based on data with desipramine, increased Cmax, AUC and t1/2; co-administration should be initiated at the lower end of the dose range of thioridazine; potential for increased risk of sei-zures). Products include:

Thiotepa (Bupropion is primarily metabolized, based on in vitro stud-ies, to hydroxybupropion by the CYP2B6 isoenzyme; therefore the potential exists for a drug interaction with agents that affect the CYP2B6 isoenzyme metabolism, such as thiotepa).

 No products indexed under this heading.

Thiothixene (Bupropion is associat-ed with dose-dependent risk of seizures; co-administration with drugs that lower seizure threshold, such as

antipsychotics, may increase the risk of seizure with bupropion). Products include:
Thiothixene Capsules 2165

Tranylcypromine Sulfate (Concurrent and/or sequential use with MAO inhibitors is contraindicated). Products include:
Parnate Tablets 1527

Trazodone Hydrochloride (Bupropion is associated with dose-dependent risk of seizures; co-administration with drugs that lower seizure threshold may increase the risk of seizure with bupropion).
No products indexed under this heading.

Triamcinolone (Concurrent administration of bupropion hydrochloride and agents that lower seizure threshold, such as systemic steroids, should be undertaken only with extreme caution).
No products indexed under this heading.

Triamcinolone Acetonide (Concurrent administration of bupropion hydrochloride and agents that lower seizure threshold, such as systemic steroids, should be undertaken only with extreme caution). Products include:
Azmacort Inhalation Aerosol 1726
Nasacort AQ Nasal Spray 2922

Triamcinolone Diacetate (Concurrent administration of bupropion hydrochloride and agents that lower seizure threshold, such as systemic steroids, should be undertaken only with extreme caution).
No products indexed under this heading.

Triamcinolone Hexacetonide (Concurrent administration of bupropion hydrochloride and agents that lower seizure threshold, such as systemic steroids, should be undertaken only with extreme caution).
No products indexed under this heading.

Triazolam (Bupropion is associated with a dose-related risk of seizures; excessive use of benzodiazepine sedatives is associated with increased risk of seizures; bupropion is contraindicated in patients undergoing abrupt discontinuation of benzodiazepine sedatives).
No products indexed under this heading.

Trifluoperazine Hydrochloride (Bupropion is associated with dose-dependent risk of seizures; co-administration with drugs that lower seizure threshold, such as antipsychotics, may increase the risk of seizure with bupropion).
No products indexed under this heading.

Trimipramine Maleate (Bupropion is associated with dose-dependent risk of seizures; co-administration with drugs that lower seizure threshold may increase the risk of seizure with bupropion).
No products indexed under this heading.

Venlafaxine Hydrochloride (Bupropion is associated with dose-dependent risk of seizures; co-administration with drugs that lower seizure threshold, such as antidepressants, may increase the risk of seizure with bupropion). Products include:
Effexor Tablets 3411
Effexor XR Capsules 3417

Warfarin Sodium (Altered PT and/or INR infrequently associated with hemorrhagic or thrombotic complications were observed when bupropion was co-administered with warfarin). Products include:
Coumadin for Injection 898
Coumadin Tablets 898

Zaleplon (Bupropion hydrochloride is contraindicated in patients undergoing abrupt discontinuation of sedatives). Products include:
Sonata Capsules 1717

Ziprasidone Hydrochloride (Bupropion is associated with dose-dependent risk of seizures; co-administration with drugs that lower seizure threshold, such as antipsychotics, may increase the risk of seizure with bupropion). Products include:
Geodon Capsules 2529

Zolpidem Tartrate (Bupropion hydrochloride is contraindicated in patients undergoing abrupt discontinuation of sedatives). Products include:
Ambien Tablets 2851
Ambien CR Tablets 2855

Food Interactions

Alcohol (Bupropion hydrochloride is contraindicated in patients undergoing abrupt discontinuation of alcohol. The consumption of alcohol during treatment with bupropion hydrochloride should be minimized or avoided).

Food, unspecified (Food increases Cmax and AUC of bupropion by 11% and 17% respectively. The mean time to peak concentration Tmax was prolonged by 1 hour; this effect was of no clinical significance).

ZYDONE TABLETS

(Acetaminophen, Hydrocodone Bitartrate)... 1139
May interact with anticholinergics, central nervous system depressants, monoamine oxidase inhibitors, narcotic analgesics, tricyclic antidepressants, and certain other agents. Compounds in these categories include:

Alfentanil Hydrochloride (Co-administration may exhibit additive CNS depression).
No products indexed under this heading.

Alprazolam (Co-administration may exhibit additive CNS depression). Products include:
Niravam Orally Disintegrating Tablets 3092

Amitriptyline Hydrochloride (Co-administration of tricyclic antidepressants with hydrocodone may increase the effect of either hydrocodone or antidepressant).
No products indexed under this heading.

Amoxapine (Co-administration of tricyclic antidepressants with hydrocodone may increase the effect of either hydrocodone or antidepressant).
No products indexed under this heading.

Aprobarbital (Co-administration may exhibit additive CNS depression).
No products indexed under this heading.

Atropine Sulfate (Co-administration may produce paralytic ileus). Products include:
Donnatal Extentabs 2493

Belladonna Alkaloids (Co-administration may produce paralytic ileus). Products include:
Hyland's Teething Tablets .... ▣830

Benztropine Mesylate (Co-administration may produce paralytic ileus).
No products indexed under this heading.

Biperiden Hydrochloride (Co-administration may produce paralytic ileus).
No products indexed under this heading.

Buprenorphine Hydrochloride (Co-administration may exhibit additive CNS depression). Products include:
Buprenex Injectable 2716
Suboxone Tablets 2717
Subutex Tablets 2717

Buspirone Hydrochloride (Co-administration may exhibit additive CNS depression).
No products indexed under this heading.

Butabarbital (Co-administration may exhibit additive CNS depression).
No products indexed under this heading.

Butalbital (Co-administration may exhibit additive CNS depression).
No products indexed under this heading.

Chlordiazepoxide (Co-administration may exhibit additive CNS depression).
No products indexed under this heading.

Chlordiazepoxide Hydrochloride (Co-administration may exhibit additive CNS depression). Products include:
Librium Capsules 3347

Chlorpromazine (Co-administration may exhibit additive CNS depression).
No products indexed under this heading.

Chlorpromazine Hydrochloride (Co-administration may exhibit additive CNS depression).
No products indexed under this heading.

Chlorprothixene (Co-administration may exhibit additive CNS depression).
No products indexed under this heading.

Chlorprothixene Hydrochloride (Co-administration may exhibit additive CNS depression).
No products indexed under this heading.

Chlorprothixene Lactate (Co-administration may exhibit additive CNS depression).
No products indexed under this heading.

Clidinium Bromide (Co-administration may produce paralytic ileus).
No products indexed under this heading.

Clomipramine Hydrochloride (Co-administration of tricyclic antidepressants with hydrocodone may increase the effect of either hydrocodone or antidepressant).
No products indexed under this heading.

Clorazepate Dipotassium (Co-administration may exhibit additive CNS depression). Products include:
Tranxene 2474

Clozapine (Co-administration may exhibit additive CNS depression). Products include:
Clozaril Tablets 2184
FazaClo Orally Disintegrating Tablets 551

Codeine Phosphate (Co-administration may exhibit additive CNS depression). Products include:
Tylenol with Codeine Tablets 2391

Desflurane (Co-administration may exhibit additive CNS depression).
No products indexed under this heading.

Desipramine Hydrochloride (Co-administration of tricyclic antidepressants with hydrocodone may increase the effect of either hydrocodone or antidepressant).
No products indexed under this heading.

Dezocine (Co-administration may exhibit additive CNS depression).
No products indexed under this heading.

Diazepam (Co-administration may exhibit additive CNS depression). Products include:
Diastat Rectal Delivery System 3343
Valium Tablets 2819

Dicyclomine Hydrochloride (Co-administration may produce paralytic ileus). Products include:
Bentyl Capsules 697
Bentyl Injection 697
Bentyl Syrup 697
Bentyl Tablets 697

Doxepin Hydrochloride (Co-administration of tricyclic antidepressants with hydrocodone may increase the effect of either hydrocodone or antidepressant).
No products indexed under this heading.

Droperidol (Co-administration may exhibit additive CNS depression).
No products indexed under this heading.

Enflurane (Co-administration may exhibit additive CNS depression).
No products indexed under this heading.

Estazolam (Co-administration may exhibit additive CNS depression). Products include:
ProSom Tablets 517

Ethanol (Co-administration may exhibit additive CNS depression).
No products indexed under this heading.

Ethchlorvynol (Co-administration may exhibit additive CNS depression).
No products indexed under this heading.

Ethinamate (Co-administration may exhibit additive CNS depression).
No products indexed under this heading.

Ethyl Alcohol (Co-administration may exhibit additive CNS depression).
No products indexed under this heading.

Fentanyl (Co-administration may exhibit additive CNS depression). Products include:
Duragesic Transdermal System 2373
Ionsys Transdermal System 2379

Fentanyl Citrate (Co-administration may exhibit additive CNS depression). Products include:
Actiq 979

Fluphenazine Decanoate (Co-administration may exhibit additive CNS depression).
No products indexed under this heading.

Fluphenazine Enanthate (Co-administration may exhibit additive CNS depression).
No products indexed under this heading.

Fluphenazine Hydrochloride (Co-administration may exhibit additive CNS depression).
No products indexed under this heading.

Flurazepam Hydrochloride (Co-administration may exhibit additive CNS depression). Products include:
Dalmane Capsules 3342

Glutethimide (Co-administration may exhibit additive CNS depression).
No products indexed under this heading.

Glycopyrrolate (Co-administration may produce paralytic ileus).
No products indexed under this heading.

Haloperidol (Co-administration may exhibit additive CNS depression).
No products indexed under this heading.

Haloperidol Decanoate (Co-administration may exhibit additive CNS depression).
No products indexed under this heading.

Hydrocodone Polistirex (Co-administration may exhibit additive CNS depression). Products include:
Tussionex Pennkinetic Extended-Release Suspension 3327

Hydromorphone Hydrochloride (Co-administration may exhibit additive CNS depression). Products include:
Dilaudid ... 440
Dilaudid Non-Sterile Powder 440
Dilaudid Oral Liquid 445
Dilaudid Rectal Suppositories 440
Dilaudid Tablets 440
Dilaudid Tablets - 8 mg 445
Dilaudid-HP 442

Hydroxyzine Hydrochloride (Co-administration may exhibit additive CNS depression).
No products indexed under this heading.

Hyoscyamine (Co-administration may produce paralytic ileus).
No products indexed under this heading.

Hyoscyamine Sulfate (Co-administration may produce paralytic ileus). Products include:
Donnatal Extentabs 2493
Prosed/DS Tablets 1157

Imipramine Hydrochloride (Co-administration of tricyclic antidepressants with hydrocodone may increase the effect of either hydrocodone or antidepressant).
No products indexed under this heading.

Imipramine Pamoate (Co-administration of tricyclic antidepressants with hydrocodone may increase the effect of either hydrocodone or antidepressant).
No products indexed under this heading.

Ipratropium Bromide (Co-administration may produce paralytic ileus). Products include:
Atrovent Inhalation Solution 835
Atrovent HFA Inhalation Aerosol 841

Atrovent Nasal Spray 0.03% 837
Atrovent Nasal Spray 0.06% 839
Combivent Inhalation Aerosol 847
DuoNeb Inhalation Solution 1058

Isocarboxazid (Co-administration of MAO inhibitors with hydrocodone may increase the effect of either hydrocodone or MAO inhibitor).
No products indexed under this heading.

Isoflurane (Co-administration may exhibit additive CNS depression).
No products indexed under this heading.

Ketamine Hydrochloride (Co-administration may exhibit additive CNS depression).
No products indexed under this heading.

Levomethadyl Acetate Hydrochloride (Co-administration may exhibit additive CNS depression).
No products indexed under this heading.

Levorphanol Tartrate (Co-administration may exhibit additive CNS depression).
No products indexed under this heading.

Lorazepam (Co-administration may exhibit additive CNS depression).
No products indexed under this heading.

Loxapine Hydrochloride (Co-administration may exhibit additive CNS depression).
No products indexed under this heading.

Loxapine Succinate (Co-administration may exhibit additive CNS depression).
No products indexed under this heading.

Maprotiline Hydrochloride (Co-administration of tricyclic antidepressants with hydrocodone may increase the effect of either hydrocodone or antidepressant).
No products indexed under this heading.

Mepenzolate Bromide (Co-administration may produce paralytic ileus).
No products indexed under this heading.

Meperidine Hydrochloride (Co-administration may exhibit additive CNS depression).
No products indexed under this heading.

Mephobarbital (Co-administration may exhibit additive CNS depression).
No products indexed under this heading.

Meprobamate (Co-administration may exhibit additive CNS depression).
No products indexed under this heading.

Mesoridazine Besylate (Co-administration may exhibit additive CNS depression).
No products indexed under this heading.

Methadone Hydrochloride (Co-administration may exhibit additive CNS depression).
No products indexed under this heading.

Methohexital Sodium (Co-administration may exhibit additive CNS depression).
No products indexed under this heading.

Methotrimeprazine (Co-administration may exhibit additive CNS depression).
No products indexed under this heading.

Methoxyflurane (Co-administration may exhibit additive CNS depression).
No products indexed under this heading.

Midazolam Hydrochloride (Co-administration may exhibit additive CNS depression).
No products indexed under this heading.

Moclobemide (Co-administration of MAO inhibitors with hydrocodone may increase the effect of either hydrocodone or MAO inhibitor).
No products indexed under this heading.

Molindone Hydrochloride (Co-administration may exhibit additive CNS depression). Products include:
Moban Tablets 1119

Morphine Sulfate (Co-administration may exhibit additive CNS depression). Products include:
Avinza Capsules 1741
Kadian Capsules 577
MS Contin Tablets 2701

Nortriptyline Hydrochloride (Co-administration of tricyclic antidepressants with hydrocodone may increase the effect of either hydrocodone or antidepressant).
No products indexed under this heading.

Olanzapine (Co-administration may exhibit additive CNS depression). Products include:
Symbyax Capsules 1819
Zyprexa Tablets 1830
Zyprexa IntraMuscular 1830
Zyprexa ZYDIS Orally Disintegrating Tablets 1830

Oxazepam (Co-administration may exhibit additive CNS depression).
No products indexed under this heading.

Oxybutynin Chloride (Co-administration may produce paralytic ileus). Products include:
Ditropan XL Extended-Release Tablets 2413

Oxycodone Hydrochloride (Co-administration may exhibit additive CNS depression). Products include:
OxyContin Tablets 2703
OxyFast Oral Concentrate Solution 2708
OxyIR Capsules 2708
Percocet Tablets 1131
Percodan Tablets 1132

Pargyline Hydrochloride (Co-administration of MAO inhibitors with hydrocodone may increase the effect of either hydrocodone or MAO inhibitor).
No products indexed under this heading.

Pentobarbital Sodium (Co-administration may exhibit additive CNS depression). Products include:
Nembutal Sodium Solution, USP 2470

Perphenazine (Co-administration may exhibit additive CNS depression).
No products indexed under this heading.

Phenelzine Sulfate (Co-administration of MAO inhibitors with hydrocodone may increase the effect of either hydrocodone or MAO inhibitor).
No products indexed under this heading.

Phenobarbital (Co-administration may exhibit additive CNS depression). Products include:
Donnatal Extentabs 2493

Prazepam (Co-administration may exhibit additive CNS depression).
No products indexed under this heading.

Procarbazine Hydrochloride (Co-administration of MAO inhibitors with hydrocodone may increase the effect of either hydrocodone or MAO inhibitor). Products include:
Matulane Capsules 3191

Prochlorperazine (Co-administration may exhibit additive CNS depression).
No products indexed under this heading.

Procyclidine Hydrochloride (Co-administration may produce paralytic ileus).
No products indexed under this heading.

Promethazine Hydrochloride (Co-administration may exhibit additive CNS depression). Products include:
Phenergan Tablets and Suppositories 3440

Propantheline Bromide (Co-administration may produce paralytic ileus).
No products indexed under this heading.

Propofol (Co-administration may exhibit additive CNS depression).
No products indexed under this heading.

Propoxyphene Hydrochloride (Co-administration may exhibit additive CNS depression).
No products indexed under this heading.

Propoxyphene Napsylate (Co-administration may exhibit additive CNS depression).
No products indexed under this heading.

Protriptyline Hydrochloride (Co-administration of tricyclic antidepressants with hydrocodone may increase the effect of either hydrocodone or antidepressant).
No products indexed under this heading.

Quazepam (Co-administration may exhibit additive CNS depression).
No products indexed under this heading.

Quetiapine Fumarate (Co-administration may exhibit additive CNS depression). Products include:
Seroquel Tablets 690

Remifentanil Hydrochloride (Co-administration may exhibit additive CNS depression).
No products indexed under this heading.

Risperidone (Co-administration may exhibit additive CNS depression). Products include:
Risperdal 1676
Risperdal Consta Long-Acting Injection 1682
Risperdal M-Tab Orally Disintegrating Tablets 1676

Scopolamine (Co-administration may produce paralytic ileus). Products include:
Transderm Scōp Transdermal Therapeutic System 2177

Scopolamine Hydrobromide (Co-administration may produce paralytic ileus). Products include:
Donnatal Extentabs 2493

IMPORTANT NOTE: Always consult each drug listing in the patient's regimen for possible interactions.

Secobarbital Sodium (Co-administration may exhibit additive CNS depression).
No products indexed under this heading.

Selegiline Hydrochloride (Co-administration of MAO inhibitors with hydrocodone may increase the effect of either hydrocodone or MAO inhibitor). Products include:
Eldepryl Capsules 3208
Zelapar Tablets 3372

Sevoflurane (Co-administration may exhibit additive CNS depression). Products include:
Ultane Liquid for Inhalation 531

Sodium Oxybate (Co-administration may exhibit additive CNS depression). Products include:
Xyrem Oral Solution 1688

Sufentanil Citrate (Co-administration may exhibit additive CNS depression).
No products indexed under this heading.

Temazepam (Co-administration may exhibit additive CNS depression). Products include:
Restoril Capsules 1860

Thiamylal Sodium (Co-administration may exhibit additive CNS depression).
No products indexed under this heading.

Thioridazine Hydrochloride (Co-administration may exhibit additive CNS depression). Products include:
Thioridazine Hydrochloride Tablets 2163

Thiothixene (Co-administration may exhibit additive CNS depression). Products include:
Thiothixene Capsules 2165

Tolterodine Tartrate (Co-administration may produce paralytic ileus). Products include:
Detrol Tablets 2628
Detrol LA Capsules 2631

Tranylcypromine Sulfate (Co-administration of MAO inhibitors with hydrocodone may increase the effect of either hydrocodone or MAO inhibitor). Products include:
Parnate Tablets 1527

Triazolam (Co-administration may exhibit additive CNS depression).
No products indexed under this heading.

Tridihexethyl Chloride (Co-administration may produce paralytic ileus).
No products indexed under this heading.

Trifluoperazine Hydrochloride (Co-administration may exhibit additive CNS depression).
No products indexed under this heading.

Trihexyphenidyl Hydrochloride (Co-administration may produce paralytic ileus).
No products indexed under this heading.

Trimipramine Maleate (Co-administration of tricyclic antidepressants with hydrocodone may increase the effect of either hydrocodone or antidepressant).
No products indexed under this heading.

Zaleplon (Co-administration may exhibit additive CNS depression). Products include:
Sonata Capsules 1717

Ziprasidone Hydrochloride (Co-administration may exhibit additive CNS depression). Products include:
Geodon Capsules 2529

Zolpidem Tartrate (Co-administration may exhibit additive CNS depression). Products include:
Ambien Tablets 2851
Ambien CR Tablets 2855

Food Interactions

Alcohol (Co-administration may exhibit additive CNS depression).

ZYFLO TABLETS

(Zileuton) 1023

May interact with xanthines and certain other agents. Compounds in these categories include:

Aminophylline (Co-administration with theophylline results in, on average, an approximate doubling of serum theophylline concentrations; theophylline dosage in these patients should be reduced and serum theophylline concentrations monitored closely).
No products indexed under this heading.

Dyphylline (Co-administration with theophylline results in, on average, an approximate doubling of serum theophylline concentrations; theophylline dosage in these patients should be reduced and serum theophylline concentrations monitored closely).
No products indexed under this heading.

Propranolol Hydrochloride (Co-administration results in a significant increase in propranolol concentrations and consequent increase in beta-blocker activity). Products include:
Inderal LA Long-Acting Capsules 3429
InnoPran XL Capsules 2723

Terfenadine (Co-administration of multiple doses for 7 days has resulted in a decrease in clearance of terfenadine by 22% leading to a statistically significant increase in mean AUC and Cmax of terfenadine).
No products indexed under this heading.

Theophylline (Co-administration with theophylline results in, on average, an approximate doubling of serum theophylline concentrations; theophylline dosage in these patients should be reduced and serum theophylline concentrations monitored closely).
No products indexed under this heading.

Theophylline Anhydrous (Co-administration with theophylline results in, on average, an approximate doubling of serum theophylline concentrations; theophylline dosage in these patients should be reduced and serum theophylline concentrations monitored closely). Products include:
Uniphyl Tablets 2710

Theophylline Calcium Salicylate (Co-administration with theophylline results in, on average, an approximate doubling of serum theophylline concentrations; theophylline dosage in these patients should be reduced and serum theophylline concentrations monitored closely).
No products indexed under this heading.

Theophylline Dihydroxypropyl (Glyceryl) (Co-administration with theophylline results in, on average, an approximate doubling of serum theophylline concentrations; theophylline dosage in these patients should be reduced and serum theophylline concentrations monitored closely).
No products indexed under this heading.

Theophylline Ethylenediamine (Co-administration with theophylline results in, on average, an approximate doubling of serum theophylline concentrations; theophylline dosage in these patients should be reduced and serum theophylline concentrations monitored closely).
No products indexed under this heading.

Theophylline Sodium Glycinate (Co-administration with theophylline results in, on average, an approximate doubling of serum theophylline concentrations; theophylline dosage in these patients should be reduced and serum theophylline concentrations monitored closely).
No products indexed under this heading.

Warfarin Sodium (Co-administration results in a clinically significant increase in prothrombin time). Products include:
Coumadin for Injection 898
Coumadin Tablets 898

Food Interactions

Food, unspecified (Co-administration has resulted in a small but statistically significant increase (27%) in zileuton Cmax without significant changes in the extent of absorption (AUC) or Tmax; zileuton can be administered with or without food).

ZYLET OPHTHALMIC SUSPENSION

(Loteprednol Etabonate, Tobramycin) .... ⊙259

ZYMAR OPHTHALMIC SOLUTION

(Gatifloxacin) 575
None cited in PDR database.

ZYPREXA TABLETS

(Olanzapine) 1830

May interact with antihypertensives, central nervous system depressants, cytochrome p450 1a2 inducers (selected), cytochrome p450 1a2 inhibitors (selected), dopamine agonists, drugs that elevate levels of glucuronosyl transferase, and certain other agents. Compounds in these categories include:

Acebutolol Hydrochloride (Olanzapine, because of its potential for inducing hypotension, may enhance the effects of certain antihypertensive agents).
No products indexed under this heading.

Alatrofloxacin Mesylate (Can potentially inhibit olanzapine clearance; therefore, a dosage decrease might be considered).
No products indexed under this heading.

Alfentanil Hydrochloride (Given the primary CNS effects of olanzapine, caution should be used when olanzapine is taken in combination with other centrally-acting drugs).
No products indexed under this heading.

Alprazolam (Given the primary CNS effects of olanzapine, caution should be used when olanzapine is taken in combination with other centrally-acting drugs). Products include:
Niravam Orally Disintegrating Tablets 3092

Amiodarone Hydrochloride (Can potentially inhibit olanzapine clearance; therefore, a dosage decrease might be considered).
No products indexed under this heading.

Amlodipine Besylate (Olanzapine, because of its potential for inducing hypotension, may enhance the effects of certain antihypertensive agents). Products include:
Caduet Tablets 2508
Lotrel Capsules 2249
Norvasc Tablets 2545

Anastrozole (Can potentially inhibit olanzapine clearance; therefore, a dosage decrease might be considered). Products include:
Arimidex Tablets 673

Aprobarbital (Given the primary CNS effects of olanzapine, caution should be used when olanzapine is taken in combination with other centrally-acting drugs).
No products indexed under this heading.

Atenolol (Olanzapine, because of its potential for inducing hypotension, may enhance the effects of certain antihypertensive agents).
No products indexed under this heading.

Benazepril Hydrochloride (Olanzapine, because of its potential for inducing hypotension, may enhance the effects of certain antihypertensive agents). Products include:
Lotensin Tablets 2243
Lotensin HCT Tablets 2246
Lotrel Capsules 2249

Bendroflumethiazide (Olanzapine, because of its potential for inducing hypotension, may enhance the effects of certain antihypertensive agents).
No products indexed under this heading.

Betaxolol Hydrochloride (Olanzapine, because of its potential for inducing hypotension, may enhance the effects of certain antihypertensive agents). Products include:
Betoptic S Ophthalmic Suspension 558

Bisoprolol Fumarate (Olanzapine, because of its potential for inducing hypotension, may enhance the effects of certain antihypertensive agents).
No products indexed under this heading.

Bromocriptine Mesylate (Olanzapine may antagonize the effects of dopamine agonists).
No products indexed under this heading.

Buprenorphine Hydrochloride (Given the primary CNS effects of olanzapine, caution should be used when olanzapine is taken in combination with other centrally-acting drugs). Products include:
Buprenex Injectable 2716
Suboxone Tablets 2717
Subutex Tablets 2717

Buspirone Hydrochloride (Given the primary CNS effects of olanzapine, caution should be used when olanzapine is taken in combination with other centrally-acting drugs).
No products indexed under this heading.

Butabarbital (Given the primary CNS effects of olanzapine, caution should be used when olanzapine is taken in combination with other centrally-acting drugs).
No products indexed under this heading.

Butalbital (Given the primary CNS effects of olanzapine, caution should be used when olanzapine is taken in combination with other centrally-acting drugs).
No products indexed under this heading.

Candesartan Cilexetil (Olanzapine, because of its potential for inducing hypotension, may enhance the effects of certain antihypertensive agents). Products include:
Atacand Tablets 649
Atacand HCT 651

Captopril (Olanzapine, because of its potential for inducing hypotension, may enhance the effects of certain antihypertensive agents). Products include:
Captopril Tablets 2149

Carbamazepine (Causes an approximately 50% increase in the clearance of olanzapine at 400 mg daily; higher daily doses of carbamazepine may cause an even greater increase in olanzapine clearance). Products include:
Carbatrol Capsules 3171
Equetro Extended-Release Capsules 3180
Tegretol/Tegretol-XR 2295

Carteolol Hydrochloride (Olanzapine, because of its potential for inducing hypotension, may enhance the effects of certain antihypertensive agents). Products include:
Carteolol Hydrochloride Ophthalmic Solution USP, 1%....... ⊙ 249

Charcoal, Activated (Co-administration with activated charcoal reduces the Cmax and AUC of olanzapine by about 60%).
No products indexed under this heading.

Chlordiazepoxide (Given the primary CNS effects of olanzapine, caution should be used when olanzapine is taken in combination with other centrally-acting drugs).
No products indexed under this heading.

Chlordiazepoxide Hydrochloride (Given the primary CNS effects of olanzapine, caution should be used when olanzapine is taken in combination with other centrally-acting drugs). Products include:
Librium Capsules 3347

Chlorothiazide (Olanzapine, because of its potential for inducing hypotension, may enhance the effects of certain antihypertensive agents). Products include:
Diuril Oral Suspension 1954

Chlorothiazide Sodium (Olanzapine, because of its potential for inducing hypotension, may enhance the effects of certain antihypertensive agents). Products include:
Diuril Sodium Intravenous 2467

Chlorpromazine (Given the primary CNS effects of olanzapine, caution should be used when olanzapine is taken in combination with other centrally-acting drugs).
No products indexed under this heading.

Chlorpromazine Hydrochloride (Given the primary CNS effects of olanzapine, caution should be used when olanzapine is taken in combination with other centrally-acting drugs).
No products indexed under this heading.

Chlorprothixene (Given the primary CNS effects of olanzapine, caution should be used when olanzapine is taken in combination with other centrally-acting drugs).
No products indexed under this heading.

Chlorprothixene Hydrochloride (Given the primary CNS effects of olanzapine, caution should be used when olanzapine is taken in combination with other centrally-acting drugs).
No products indexed under this heading.

Chlorprothixene Lactate (Given the primary CNS effects of olanzapine, caution should be used when olanzapine is taken in combination with other centrally-acting drugs).
No products indexed under this heading.

Chlorthalidone (Olanzapine, because of its potential for inducing hypotension, may enhance the effects of certain antihypertensive agents). Products include:
Clorpres Tablets 2153

Cimetidine (Can potentially inhibit olanzapine clearance; therefore, a dosage decrease might be considered). Products include:
Tagamet HB 200 Tablets 664

Cimetidine Hydrochloride (Can potentially inhibit olanzapine clearance; therefore, a dosage decrease might be considered).
No products indexed under this heading.

Ciprofloxacin (Can potentially inhibit olanzapine clearance; therefore, a dosage decrease might be considered). Products include:
Cipro Oral Suspension 2977
Cipro I.V. 2984
Cipro XR Tablets 2990
Ciprodex Otic Suspension 559

Ciprofloxacin Hydrochloride (Can potentially inhibit olanzapine clearance; therefore, a dosage decrease might be considered). Products include:
Ciloxan Ophthalmic Ointment 559
Ciloxan Ophthalmic Solution .... ⊙ 206
Cipro Tablets 2977
Proquin XR Tablets 1153

Citalopram Hydrobromide (May cause an increase in olanzapine clearance; therefore, a dosage increase might be considered). Products include:
Celexa 1176

Clarithromycin (Can potentially inhibit olanzapine clearance; therefore, a dosage decrease might be considered). Products include:
Biaxin/Biaxin XL 402
PREVPAC 3284

Clonidine (Olanzapine, because of its potential for inducing hypotension, may enhance the effects of certain antihypertensive agents). Products include:
Catapres-TTS 844

Clonidine Hydrochloride (Olanzapine, because of its potential for inducing hypotension, may enhance the effects of certain antihypertensive agents). Products include:
Catapres Tablets 843
Clorpres Tablets 2153

Clorazepate Dipotassium (Given the primary CNS effects of olanzapine, caution should be used when olanzapine is taken in combination with other centrally-acting drugs). Products include:
Tranxene 2474

Clozapine (Given the primary CNS effects of olanzapine, caution should be used when olanzapine is taken in combination with other centrally-acting drugs). Products include:
Clozaril Tablets 2184
FazaClo Orally Disintegrating Tablets 551

Codeine Phosphate (Given the primary CNS effects of olanzapine, caution should be used when olanzapine is taken in combination with other centrally-acting drugs). Products include:
Tylenol with Codeine Tablets 2391

Deserpidine (Olanzapine, because of its potential for inducing hypotension, may enhance the effects of certain antihypertensive agents).
No products indexed under this heading.

Desflurane (Given the primary CNS effects of olanzapine, caution should be used when olanzapine is taken in combination with other centrally-acting drugs).
No products indexed under this heading.

Desogestrel (Can potentially inhibit olanzapine clearance; therefore, a dosage decrease might be considered). Products include:
Mircette Tablets 1066

Dezocine (Given the primary CNS effects of olanzapine, caution should be used when olanzapine is taken in combination with other centrally-acting drugs).
No products indexed under this heading.

Diazepam (Co-administration of diazepam with olanzapine may potentiate orthostatic hypotension). Products include:
Diastat Rectal Delivery System 3343
Valium Tablets 2819

Diazoxide (Olanzapine, because of its potential for inducing hypotension, may enhance the effects of certain antihypertensive agents). Products include:
Hyperstat I.V. 3017

Diltiazem Hydrochloride (Olanzapine, because of its potential for inducing hypotension, may enhance the effects of certain antihypertensive agents). Products include:
Cardizem LA Extended Release Tablets 1728
Tiazac Capsules 1201

Diltiazem Maleate (May cause an increase in olanzapine clearance; therefore, a dosage increase might be considered).
No products indexed under this heading.

Dopamine Hydrochloride (Olanzapine may antagonize the effects of dopamine agonists).
No products indexed under this heading.

Doxazosin Mesylate (Olanzapine, because of its potential for inducing hypotension, may enhance the effects of certain antihypertensive agents). Products include:
Cardura XL Tablets 2515

Droperidol (Given the primary CNS effects of olanzapine, caution should be used when olanzapine is taken in combination with other centrally-acting drugs).
No products indexed under this heading.

Enalapril Maleate (Olanzapine, because of its potential for inducing hypotension, may enhance the effects of certain antihypertensive agents). Products include:
Vasotec I.V. Injection 2103

Enalaprilat (Olanzapine, because of its potential for inducing hypotension, may enhance the effects of certain antihypertensive agents).
No products indexed under this heading.

Enflurane (Given the primary CNS effects of olanzapine, caution should be used when olanzapine is taken in combination with other centrally-acting drugs).
No products indexed under this heading.

Enoxacin (Can potentially inhibit olanzapine clearance; therefore, a dosage decrease might be considered).
No products indexed under this heading.

Eprosartan Mesylate (Olanzapine, because of its potential for inducing hypotension, may enhance the effects of certain antihypertensive agents). Products include:
Teveten Tablets 1735
Teveten HCT Tablets 1737

Erythromycin (May cause an increase in olanzapine clearance; therefore, a dosage increase might be considered). Products include:
Ery-Tab Tablets 449
Erythromycin Base Filmtab Tablets 455
Erythromycin Delayed-Release Capsules, USP 457
PCE Dispertab Tablets 515

Erythromycin Estolate (May cause an increase in olanzapine clearance; therefore, a dosage increase might be considered).
No products indexed under this heading.

Erythromycin Ethylsuccinate (May cause an increase in olanzapine clearance; therefore, a dosage increase might be considered). Products include:
E.E.S. 451
EryPed 447

Erythromycin Gluceptate (May cause an increase in olanzapine clearance; therefore, a dosage increase might be considered).
No products indexed under this heading.

Erythromycin Lactobionate (May cause an increase in olanzapine clearance; therefore, a dosage increase might be considered).
No products indexed under this heading.

Erythromycin Stearate (May cause an increase in olanzapine clearance; therefore, a dosage increase might be considered). Products include:
Erythrocin Stearate Filmtab Tablets 453

Esmolol Hydrochloride (Olanzapine, because of its potential for inducing hypotension, may enhance the effects of certain antihypertensive agents).
No products indexed under this heading.

Estazolam (Given the primary CNS effects of olanzapine, caution should be used when olanzapine is taken in combination with other centrally-acting drugs). Products include:
ProSom Tablets 517

Ethanol (Given the primary CNS effects of olanzapine, caution should be used when olanzapine is taken in combination with other centrally-acting drugs).
No products indexed under this heading.

Ethchlorvynol (Given the primary CNS effects of olanzapine, caution should be used when olanzapine is taken in combination with other centrally-acting drugs).
No products indexed under this heading.

Ethinamate (Given the primary CNS effects of olanzapine, caution should be used when olanzapine is taken in combination with other centrally-acting drugs).
No products indexed under this heading.

Ethinyl Estradiol (Can potentially inhibit olanzapine clearance; therefore, a dosage decrease might be considered). Products include:
Mircette Tablets 1066
NuvaRing 2340
Ortho-Cyclen/Ortho Tri-Cyclen 2429
Ortho Evra Transdermal System 2417
Ortho Tri-Cyclen Lo Tablets 2436
Seasonique Tablets 1077
Yasmin 28 Tablets 796
Yaz Tablets 803

Ethyl Alcohol (Given the primary CNS effects of olanzapine, caution should be used when olanzapine is taken in combination with other centrally-acting drugs).
No products indexed under this heading.

Felodipine (Olanzapine, because of its potential for inducing hypotension, may enhance the effects of certain antihypertensive agents).
No products indexed under this heading.

Fentanyl (Given the primary CNS effects of olanzapine, caution should be used when olanzapine is taken in combination with other centrally-acting drugs). Products include:
Duragesic Transdermal System 2373
Ionsys Transdermal System 2379

Fentanyl Citrate (Given the primary CNS effects of olanzapine, caution should be used when olanzapine is taken in combination with other centrally-acting drugs). Products include:
Actiq 979

Fluoxetine Hydrochloride (Co-administration causes a small increase in the maximum concentration of olanzapine and a small decrease in olanzapine clearance; the magnitude of the impact of this factor is small in comparison to the overall variability between individuals and, therefore, dose modification is not routinely recommended). Products include:
Prozac Pulvules and Liquid 1801
Symbyax Capsules 1819

Fluphenazine Decanoate (Given the primary CNS effects of olanzapine, caution should be used when olanzapine is taken in combination with other centrally-acting drugs).
No products indexed under this heading.

Fluphenazine Enanthate (Given the primary CNS effects of olanzapine, caution should be used when olanzapine is taken in combination with other centrally-acting drugs).
No products indexed under this heading.

Fluphenazine Hydrochloride (Given the primary CNS effects of olanzapine, caution should be used when olanzapine is taken in combination with other centrally-acting drugs).
No products indexed under this heading.

Flurazepam Hydrochloride (Given the primary CNS effects of olanzapine, caution should be used when olanzapine is taken in combination with other centrally-acting drugs). Products include:
Dalmane Capsules 3342

Fluvoxamine (Can potentially inhibit olanzapine clearance; therefore, a dosage decrease might be considered).
No products indexed under this heading.

Fluvoxamine Maleate (Decreases the clearance of olanzapine leading to a mean increase in olanzapine Cmax and AUC; lower doses of olanzapine should be considered or co-administered).
No products indexed under this heading.

Fosinopril Sodium (Olanzapine, because of its potential for inducing hypotension, may enhance the effects of certain antihypertensive agents).
No products indexed under this heading.

Furosemide (Olanzapine, because of its potential for inducing hypotension, may enhance the effects of certain antihypertensive agents). Products include:
Furosemide Tablets 2154

Gatifloxacin (Can potentially inhibit olanzapine clearance; therefore, a dosage decrease might be considered). Products include:
Tequin Injection 938
Tequin Injection in 5% Dextrose 938
Tequin Tablets 938
Zymar Ophthalmic Solution 575

Gemifloxacin Mesylate (Can potentially inhibit olanzapine clearance; therefore, a dosage decrease might be considered).
No products indexed under this heading.

Glutethimide (Given the primary CNS effects of olanzapine, caution should be used when olanzapine is taken in combination with other centrally-acting drugs).
No products indexed under this heading.

Grepafloxacin Hydrochloride (Can potentially inhibit olanzapine clearance; therefore, a dosage decrease might be considered).
No products indexed under this heading.

Guanabenz Acetate (Olanzapine, because of its potential for inducing hypotension, may enhance the effects of certain antihypertensive agents).
No products indexed under this heading.

Guanethidine Monosulfate (Olanzapine, because of its potential for inducing hypotension, may enhance the effects of certain antihypertensive agents).
No products indexed under this heading.

Haloperidol (Given the primary CNS effects of olanzapine, caution should be used when olanzapine is taken in combination with other centrally-acting drugs).
No products indexed under this heading.

Haloperidol Decanoate (Given the primary CNS effects of olanzapine, caution should be used when olanzapine is taken in combination with other centrally-acting drugs).
No products indexed under this heading.

Hydralazine Hydrochloride (Olanzapine, because of its potential for inducing hypotension, may enhance the effects of certain antihypertensive agents). Products include:
BiDil Tablets 2171

Hydrochlorothiazide (Olanzapine, because of its potential for inducing hypotension, may enhance the effects of certain antihypertensive agents). Products include:
Aldoril Tablets 1910
Atacand HCT 651
Avalide Tablets 888
Avalide Tablets 2874
Benicar HCT Tablets 1044
Diovan HCT Tablets 2196
Dyazide Capsules 1423
Hyzaar 50-12.5 Tablets 1990
Hyzaar 100-12.5 Tablets 1990
Hyzaar 100-25 Tablets 1990
Lopressor HCT 50/25 Tablets 2241
Lopressor HCT 100/25 Tablets 2241
Lopressor HCT 100/50 Tablets 2241
Lotensin HCT Tablets 2246
Micardis HCT Tablets 856
Moduretic Tablets 2028
Prinzide Tablets 2056
Teveten HCT Tablets 1737
Timolide Tablets 2086
Uniretic Tablets 3100

Hydrocodone Bitartrate (Given the primary CNS effects of olanzapine, caution should be used when olanzapine is taken in combination with other centrally-acting drugs). Products include:
Hycodan 1116
Hycotuss Expectorant Syrup 1117
Vicodin Tablets 535
Vicodin ES Tablets 536
Vicodin HP Tablets 538
Vicoprofen Tablets 539
Zydone Tablets 1139

Hydrocodone Polistirex (Given the primary CNS effects of olanzapine, caution should be used when olanzapine is taken in combination with other centrally-acting drugs). Products include:
Tussionex Pennkinetic Extended-Release Suspension 3327

Hydroflumethiazide (Olanzapine, because of its potential for inducing hypotension, may enhance the effects of certain antihypertensive agents).
No products indexed under this heading.

Hydromorphone Hydrochloride (Given the primary CNS effects of olanzapine, caution should be used when olanzapine is taken in combination with other centrally-acting drugs). Products include:
Dilaudid 440
Dilaudid Non-Sterile Powder 440
Dilaudid Oral Liquid 445
Dilaudid Rectal Suppositories 440
Dilaudid Tablets 440
Dilaudid Tablets - 8 mg 445
Dilaudid-HP 442

Hydroxyzine Hydrochloride (Given the primary CNS effects of olanzapine, caution should be used when olanzapine is taken in combination with other centrally-acting drugs).
No products indexed under this heading.

Hypericum (May cause an increase in olanzapine clearance; therefore, a dosage increase might be considered). Products include:
Satiete Tablets .... ■ 832

Indapamide (Olanzapine, because of its potential for inducing hypotension, may enhance the effects of certain antihypertensive agents). Products include:
Indapamide Tablets 2156

Insulin (May cause an increase in olanzapine clearance; therefore, a dosage increase might be considered).
No products indexed under this heading.

Irbesartan (Olanzapine, because of its potential for inducing hypotension, may enhance the effects of certain antihypertensive agents). Products include:
Avalide Tablets 888
Avalide Tablets 2874
Avapro Tablets 891
Avapro Tablets 2871

Isoflurane (Given the primary CNS effects of olanzapine, caution should be used when olanzapine is taken in combination with other centrally-acting drugs).
No products indexed under this heading.

Isoniazid (Can potentially inhibit olanzapine clearance; therefore, a dosage decrease might be considered).
No products indexed under this heading.

Isradipine (Olanzapine, because of its potential for inducing hypotension, may enhance the effects of certain antihypertensive agents). Products include:
DynaCirc CR Tablets 2721

Ketamine Hydrochloride (Given the primary CNS effects of olanzapine, caution should be used when olanzapine is taken in combination with other centrally-acting drugs).
No products indexed under this heading.

Ketoconazole (Can potentially inhibit olanzapine clearance; therefore, a dosage decrease might be considered). Products include:
Nizoral A-D Shampoo, 1% 1868

Labetalol Hydrochloride (Olanzapine, because of its potential for inducing hypotension, may enhance the effects of certain antihypertensive agents).
No products indexed under this heading.

Lansoprazole (May cause an increase in olanzapine clearance; therefore, a dosage increase might be considered). Products include:
Prevacid Delayed-Release Capsules 3271
Prevacid for Delayed-Release Oral Suspension 3271

Levodopa (Olanzapine may antagonize the effects of levodopa). Products include:

Levofloxacin (Can potentially inhibit olanzapine clearance; therefore, a dosage decrease might be considered). Products include:

Levomethadyl Acetate Hydrochloride (Given the primary CNS effects of olanzapine, caution should be used when olanzapine is taken in combination with other centrally-acting drugs).

No products indexed under this heading.

Levonorgestrel (Can potentially inhibit olanzapine clearance; therefore, a dosage decrease might be considered). Products include:

Levorphanol Tartrate (Given the primary CNS effects of olanzapine, caution should be used when olanzapine is taken in combination with other centrally-acting drugs).

No products indexed under this heading.

Lisinopril (Olanzapine, because of its potential for inducing hypotension, may enhance the effects of certain antihypertensive agents). Products include:

Lomefloxacin Hydrochloride (Can potentially inhibit olanzapine clearance; therefore, a dosage decrease might be considered).

No products indexed under this heading.

Lorazepam (Given the primary CNS effects of olanzapine, caution should be used when olanzapine is taken in combination with other centrally-acting drugs).

No products indexed under this heading.

Losartan Potassium (Olanzapine, because of its potential for inducing hypotension, may enhance the effects of certain antihypertensive agents). Products include:

Loxapine Hydrochloride (Given the primary CNS effects of olanzapine, caution should be used when olanzapine is taken in combination with other centrally-acting drugs).

No products indexed under this heading.

Loxapine Succinate (Given the primary CNS effects of olanzapine, caution should be used when olanzapine is taken in combination with other centrally-acting drugs).

No products indexed under this heading.

Mecamylamine Hydrochloride (Olanzapine, because of its potential for inducing hypotension, may enhance the effects of certain antihypertensive agents).

No products indexed under this heading.

Meperidine Hydrochloride (Given the primary CNS effects of olanzapine, caution should be used when olanzapine is taken in combination with other centrally-acting drugs).

No products indexed under this heading.

Mephobarbital (Given the primary CNS effects of olanzapine, caution should be used when olanzapine is taken in combination with other centrally-acting drugs).

No products indexed under this heading.

Meprobamate (Given the primary CNS effects of olanzapine, caution should be used when olanzapine is taken in combination with other centrally-acting drugs).

No products indexed under this heading.

Mesoridazine Besylate (Given the primary CNS effects of olanzapine, caution should be used when olanzapine is taken in combination with other centrally-acting drugs).

No products indexed under this heading.

Mestranol (Can potentially inhibit olanzapine clearance; therefore, a dosage decrease might be considered).

No products indexed under this heading.

Methadone Hydrochloride (Given the primary CNS effects of olanzapine, caution should be used when olanzapine is taken in combination with other centrally-acting drugs).

No products indexed under this heading.

Methohexital Sodium (Given the primary CNS effects of olanzapine, caution should be used when olanzapine is taken in combination with other centrally-acting drugs).

No products indexed under this heading.

Methotrimeprazine (Given the primary CNS effects of olanzapine, caution should be used when olanzapine is taken in combination with other centrally-acting drugs).

No products indexed under this heading.

Methoxsalen (Can potentially inhibit olanzapine clearance; therefore, a dosage decrease might be considered). Products include:

Methoxyflurane (Given the primary CNS effects of olanzapine, caution should be used when olanzapine is taken in combination with other centrally-acting drugs).

No products indexed under this heading.

Methyclothiazide (Olanzapine, because of its potential for inducing hypotension, may enhance the effects of certain antihypertensive agents).

No products indexed under this heading.

Methyldopa (Olanzapine, because of its potential for inducing hypotension, may enhance the effects of certain antihypertensive agents). Products include:

Methyldopate Hydrochloride (Olanzapine, because of its potential for inducing hypotension, may enhance the effects of certain antihypertensive agents).

No products indexed under this heading.

Metolazone (Olanzapine, because of its potential for inducing hypotension, may enhance the effects of certain antihypertensive agents).

No products indexed under this heading.

Metoprolol Succinate (Olanzapine, because of its potential for inducing hypotension, may enhance the effects of certain antihypertensive agents). Products include:

Metoprolol Tartrate (Olanzapine, because of its potential for inducing hypotension, may enhance the effects of certain antihypertensive agents). Products include:

Metyrosine (Olanzapine, because of its potential for inducing hypotension, may enhance the effects of certain antihypertensive agents). Products include:

Mexiletine Hydrochloride (Can potentially inhibit olanzapine clearance; therefore, a dosage decrease might be considered).

No products indexed under this heading.

Mibefradil Dihydrochloride (Olanzapine, because of its potential for inducing hypotension, may enhance the effects of certain antihypertensive agents).

No products indexed under this heading.

Midazolam Hydrochloride (Given the primary CNS effects of olanzapine, caution should be used when olanzapine is taken in combination with other centrally-acting drugs).

No products indexed under this heading.

Minoxidil (Olanzapine, because of its potential for inducing hypotension, may enhance the effects of certain antihypertensive agents). Products include:

Moexipril Hydrochloride (Olanzapine, because of its potential for inducing hypotension, may enhance the effects of certain antihypertensive agents). Products include:

Molindone Hydrochloride (Given the primary CNS effects of olanzapine, caution should be used when olanzapine is taken in combination with other centrally-acting drugs). Products include:

Morphine Sulfate (Given the primary CNS effects of olanzapine, caution should be used when olanzapine is taken in combination with other centrally-acting drugs). Products include:

Moxifloxacin Hydrochloride (Can potentially inhibit olanzapine clearance; therefore, a dosage decrease might be considered). Products include:

Nadolol (Olanzapine, because of its potential for inducing hypotension, may enhance the effects of certain antihypertensive agents). Products include:

Nafcillin Sodium (May cause an increase in olanzapine clearance; therefore, a dosage increase might be considered).

No products indexed under this heading.

Nalidixic Acid (Can potentially inhibit olanzapine clearance; therefore, a dosage decrease might be considered).

No products indexed under this heading.

Nicardipine Hydrochloride (Olanzapine, because of its potential for inducing hypotension, may enhance the effects of certain antihypertensive agents). Products include:

Nicotine (May cause an increase in olanzapine clearance; therefore, a dosage increase might be considered). Products include:

Nicotine Polacrilex (May cause an increase in olanzapine clearance; therefore, a dosage increase might be considered).

No products indexed under this heading.

Nicotine Salicylate (May cause an increase in olanzapine clearance; therefore, a dosage increase might be considered).

No products indexed under this heading.

Nicotine Sulfate (May cause an increase in olanzapine clearance; therefore, a dosage increase might be considered).

No products indexed under this heading.

Nifedipine (Olanzapine, because of its potential for inducing hypotension, may enhance the effects of certain antihypertensive agents). Products include:

Nisoldipine (Olanzapine, because of its potential for inducing hypotension, may enhance the effects of certain antihypertensive agents). Products include:

Nitroglycerin (Olanzapine, because of its potential for inducing hypotension, may enhance the effects of certain antihypertensive agents). Products include:

Norethindrone (Can potentially inhibit olanzapine clearance; therefore, a dosage decrease might be considered). Products include:

Norfloxacin (Can potentially inhibit olanzapine clearance; therefore, a dosage decrease might be considered). Products include:

IMPORTANT NOTE: Always consult each drug listing in the patient's regimen for possible interactions.

Tacrine Hydrochloride (Can potentially inhibit olanzapine clearance; therefore, a dosage decrease might be considered).

No products indexed under this heading.

Telmisartan (Olanzapine, because of its potential for inducing hypotension, may enhance the effects of certain antihypertensive agents).
Products include:

Temazepam (Given the primary CNS effects of olanzapine, caution should be used when olanzapine is taken in combination with other centrally-acting drugs). Products include:

Terazosin Hydrochloride (Olanzapine, because of its potential for inducing hypotension, may enhance the effects of certain antihypertensive agents). Products include:

Thiamylal Sodium (Given the primary CNS effects of olanzapine, caution should be used when olanzapine is taken in combination with other centrally-acting drugs).

No products indexed under this heading.

Thioridazine Hydrochloride (Given the primary CNS effects of olanzapine, caution should be used when olanzapine is taken in combination with other centrally-acting drugs). Products include:

Thiothixene (Given the primary CNS effects of olanzapine, caution should be used when olanzapine is taken in combination with other centrally-acting drugs). Products include:

Ticlopidine Hydrochloride (Can potentially inhibit olanzapine clearance; therefore, a dosage decrease might be considered). Products include:

Timolol Maleate (Olanzapine, because of its potential for inducing hypotension, may enhance the effects of certain antihypertensive agents). Products include:

Tobacco (May cause an increase in olanzapine clearance; therefore, a dosage increase might be considered).

No products indexed under this heading.

Torsemide (Olanzapine, because of its potential for inducing hypotension, may enhance the effects of certain antihypertensive agents). Products include:

Trandolapril (Olanzapine, because of its potential for inducing hypotension, may enhance the effects of certain antihypertensive agents). Products include:

Triazolam (Given the primary CNS effects of olanzapine, caution should be used when olanzapine is taken in combination with other centrally-acting drugs).

No products indexed under this heading.

Trifluoperazine Hydrochloride (Given the primary CNS effects of olanzapine, caution should be used when olanzapine is taken in combination with other centrally-acting drugs).

No products indexed under this heading.

Trimethaphan Camsylate (Olanzapine, because of its potential for inducing hypotension, may enhance the effects of certain antihypertensive agents).

No products indexed under this heading.

Troleandomycin (Can potentially inhibit olanzapine clearance; therefore, a dosage decrease might be considered).

No products indexed under this heading.

Trovafloxacin Mesylate (Can potentially inhibit olanzapine clearance; therefore, a dosage decrease might be considered).

No products indexed under this heading.

Valsartan (Olanzapine, because of its potential for inducing hypotension, may enhance the effects of certain antihypertensive agents). Products include:

Verapamil Hydrochloride (Olanzapine, because of its potential for inducing hypotension, may enhance the effects of certain antihypertensive agents). Products include:

Zaleplon (Given the primary CNS effects of olanzapine, caution should be used when olanzapine is taken in combination with other centrally-acting drugs). Products include:

Zileuton (Can potentially inhibit olanzapine clearance; therefore, a dosage decrease might be considered). Products include:

Ziprasidone Hydrochloride (Given the primary CNS effects of olanzapine, caution should be used when olanzapine is taken in combination with other centrally-acting drugs). Products include:

Zolpidem Tartrate (Given the primary CNS effects of olanzapine, caution should be used when olanzapine is taken in combination with other centrally-acting drugs). Products include:

Food Interactions

Alcohol (Co-administration of alcohol with olanzapine potentiates orthostatic hypotension; concurrent use should be avoided).

Broccoli (May cause an increase in olanzapine clearance; therefore, a dosage increase might be considered).

Brussel Sprouts (May cause an increase in olanzapine clearance; therefore, a dosage increase might be considered).

Charbroiled Food (May cause an increase in olanzapine clearance; therefore, a dosage increase might be considered).

Grapefruit Juice (Can potentially inhibit olanzapine clearance; therefore, a dosage decrease might be considered).

ZYPREXA INTRAMUSCULAR

May interact with antihypertensives, benzodiazepines, central nervous system depressants, cytochrome p450 1a2 inducers (selected), cytochrome p450 1a2 inhibitors (selected), dopamine agonists, drugs that elevate levels of glucuronosyl transferase, and certain other agents. Compounds in these categories include:

Acebutolol Hydrochloride (Olanzapine, because of its potential for inducing hypotension, may enhance the effects of certain antihypertensive agents).

No products indexed under this heading.

Alatrofloxacin Mesylate (Can potentially inhibit olanzapine clearance; therefore, a dosage decrease might be considered).

No products indexed under this heading.

Alfentanil Hydrochloride (Given the primary CNS effects of olanzapine, caution should be used when olanzapine is taken in combination with other centrally-acting drugs).

No products indexed under this heading.

Alprazolam (Given the primary CNS effects of olanzapine, caution should be used when olanzapine is taken in combination with other centrally-acting drugs). Products include:

Amiodarone Hydrochloride (Can potentially inhibit olanzapine clearance; therefore, a dosage decrease might be considered).

No products indexed under this heading.

Amlodipine Besylate (Olanzapine, because of its potential for inducing hypotension, may enhance the effects of certain antihypertensive agents). Products include:

Anastrozole (Can potentially inhibit olanzapine clearance; therefore, a dosage decrease might be considered). Products include:

Aprobarbital (Given the primary CNS effects of olanzapine, caution should be used when olanzapine is taken in combination with other centrally-acting drugs).

No products indexed under this heading.

Atenolol (Olanzapine, because of its potential for inducing hypotension, may enhance the effects of certain antihypertensive agents).

No products indexed under this heading.

Benazepril Hydrochloride (Olanzapine, because of its potential for inducing hypotension, may enhance the effects of certain antihypertensive agents). Products include:

Bendroflumethiazide (Olanzapine, because of its potential for inducing hypotension, may enhance the effects of certain antihypertensive agents).

No products indexed under this heading.

Betaxolol Hydrochloride (Olanzapine, because of its potential for inducing hypotension, may enhance the effects of certain antihypertensive agents). Products include:

Bisoprolol Fumarate (Olanzapine, because of its potential for inducing hypotension, may enhance the effects of certain antihypertensive agents).

No products indexed under this heading.

Bromocriptine Mesylate (Olanzapine may antagonize the effects of dopamine agonists).

No products indexed under this heading.

Buprenorphine Hydrochloride (Given the primary CNS effects of olanzapine, caution should be used when olanzapine is taken in combination with other centrally-acting drugs). Products include:

Buspirone Hydrochloride (Given the primary CNS effects of olanzapine, caution should be used when olanzapine is taken in combination with other centrally-acting drugs).

No products indexed under this heading.

Butabarbital (Given the primary CNS effects of olanzapine, caution should be used when olanzapine is taken in combination with other centrally-acting drugs).

No products indexed under this heading.

Butalbital (Given the primary CNS effects of olanzapine, caution should be used when olanzapine is taken in combination with other centrally-acting drugs).

No products indexed under this heading.

Candesartan Cilexetil (Olanzapine, because of its potential for inducing hypotension, may enhance the effects of certain antihypertensive agents). Products include:

Captopril (Olanzapine, because of its potential for inducing hypotension, may enhance the effects of certain antihypertensive agents). Products include:

Carbamazepine (Causes an approximately 50% increase in the clearance of olanzapine at 400 mg daily; higher daily doses of carbamazepine may cause an even greater increase in olanzapine clearance). Products include:

Carteolol Hydrochloride (Olanzapine, because of its potential for inducing hypotension, may enhance the effects of certain antihypertensive agents). Products include:

IMPORTANT NOTE: Always consult each drug listing in the patient's regimen for possible interactions.

Chlordiazepoxide (Given the primary CNS effects of olanzapine, caution should be used when olanzapine is taken in combination with other centrally-acting drugs).
No products indexed under this heading.

Chlordiazepoxide Hydrochloride (Given the primary CNS effects of olanzapine, caution should be used when olanzapine is taken in combination with other centrally-acting drugs). Products include:
Librium Capsules 3347

Chlorothiazide (Olanzapine, because of its potential for inducing hypotension, may enhance the effects of certain antihypertensive agents). Products include:
Diuril Oral Suspension 1954

Chlorothiazide Sodium (Olanzapine, because of its potential for inducing hypotension, may enhance the effects of certain antihypertensive agents). Products include:
Diuril Sodium Intravenous 2467

Chlorpromazine (Given the primary CNS effects of olanzapine, caution should be used when olanzapine is taken in combination with other centrally-acting drugs).
No products indexed under this heading.

Chlorpromazine Hydrochloride (Given the primary CNS effects of olanzapine, caution should be used when olanzapine is taken in combination with other centrally-acting drugs).
No products indexed under this heading.

Chlorprothixene (Given the primary CNS effects of olanzapine, caution should be used when olanzapine is taken in combination with other centrally-acting drugs).
No products indexed under this heading.

Chlorprothixene Hydrochloride (Given the primary CNS effects of olanzapine, caution should be used when olanzapine is taken in combination with other centrally-acting drugs).
No products indexed under this heading.

Chlorprothixene Lactate (Given the primary CNS effects of olanzapine, caution should be used when olanzapine is taken in combination with other centrally-acting drugs).
No products indexed under this heading.

Chlorthalidone (Olanzapine, because of its potential for inducing hypotension, may enhance the effects of certain antihypertensive agents). Products include:
Clorpres Tablets 2153

Cimetidine (Can potentially inhibit olanzapine clearance; therefore, a dosage decrease might be considered). Products include:
Tagamet HB 200 Tablets .... ◘664

Cimetidine Hydrochloride (Can potentially inhibit olanzapine clearance; therefore, a dosage decrease might be considered).
No products indexed under this heading.

Ciprofloxacin (Can potentially inhibit olanzapine clearance; therefore, a dosage decrease might be considered). Products include:
Cipro Oral Suspension 2977
Cipro I.V. 2984
Cipro XR Tablets 2990
Ciprodex Otic Suspension 559

Ciprofloxacin Hydrochloride (Can potentially inhibit olanzapine clearance; therefore, a dosage decrease might be considered). Products include:
Ciloxan Ophthalmic Ointment 559
Ciloxan Ophthalmic Solution .... ⊙206
Cipro Tablets 2977
Proquin XR Tablets 1153

Citalopram Hydrobromide (May cause an increase in olanzapine clearance; therefore, a dosage increase might be considered). Products include:
Celexa 1176

Clarithromycin (Can potentially inhibit olanzapine clearance; therefore, a dosage decrease might be considered). Products include:
Biaxin/Biaxin XL 402
PREVPAC 3284

Clonidine (Olanzapine, because of its potential for inducing hypotension, may enhance the effects of certain antihypertensive agents). Products include:
Catapres-TTS 844

Clonidine Hydrochloride (Olanzapine, because of its potential for inducing hypotension, may enhance the effects of certain antihypertensive agents). Products include:
Catapres Tablets 843
Clorpres Tablets 2153

Clorazepate Dipotassium (Given the primary CNS effects of olanzapine, caution should be used when olanzapine is taken in combination with other centrally-acting drugs). Products include:
Tranxene 2474

Clozapine (Given the primary CNS effects of olanzapine, caution should be used when olanzapine is taken in combination with other centrally-acting drugs). Products include:
Clozaril Tablets 2184
FazaClo Orally Disintegrating Tablets 551

Codeine Phosphate (Given the primary CNS effects of olanzapine, caution should be used when olanzapine is taken in combination with other centrally-acting drugs). Products include:
Tylenol with Codeine Tablets 2391

Deserpidine (Olanzapine, because of its potential for inducing hypotension, may enhance the effects of certain antihypertensive agents).
No products indexed under this heading.

Desflurane (Given the primary CNS effects of olanzapine, caution should be used when olanzapine is taken in combination with other centrally-acting drugs).
No products indexed under this heading.

Desogestrel (Can potentially inhibit olanzapine clearance; therefore, a dosage decrease might be considered). Products include:
Mircette Tablets 1066

Dezocine (Given the primary CNS effects of olanzapine, caution should be used when olanzapine is taken in combination with other centrally-acting drugs).
No products indexed under this heading.

Diazepam (Co-administration of diazepam with olanzapine may potentiate orthostatic hypotension. Concomitant administration of intramuscular olanzapine and parenteral benzodiazepine has not been studied and is therefore not recommended. If use of intramuscular olanzapine in combination with parenteral benzodiazepines is considered, careful evaluation of clinical status for excessive sedation and cardiorespiratory depression is recommended). Products include:
Diastat Rectal Delivery System 3343
Valium Tablets 2819

Diazoxide (Olanzapine, because of its potential for inducing hypotension, may enhance the effects of certain antihypertensive agents). Products include:
Hyperstat I.V. 3017

Diltiazem Hydrochloride (Olanzapine, because of its potential for inducing hypotension, may enhance the effects of certain antihypertensive agents). Products include:
Cardizem LA Extended Release Tablets 1728
Tiazac Capsules 1201

Diltiazem Maleate (May cause an increase in olanzapine clearance; therefore, a dosage increase might be considered).
No products indexed under this heading.

Dopamine Hydrochloride (Olanzapine may antagonize the effects of dopamine agonists).
No products indexed under this heading.

Doxazosin Mesylate (Olanzapine, because of its potential for inducing hypotension, may enhance the effects of certain antihypertensive agents). Products include:
Cardura XL Tablets 2515

Droperidol (Given the primary CNS effects of olanzapine, caution should be used when olanzapine is taken in combination with other centrally-acting drugs).
No products indexed under this heading.

Enalapril Maleate (Olanzapine, because of its potential for inducing hypotension, may enhance the effects of certain antihypertensive agents). Products include:
Vasotec I.V. Injection 2103

Enalaprilat (Olanzapine, because of its potential for inducing hypotension, may enhance the effects of certain antihypertensive agents).
No products indexed under this heading.

Enflurane (Given the primary CNS effects of olanzapine, caution should be used when olanzapine is taken in combination with other centrally-acting drugs).
No products indexed under this heading.

Enoxacin (Can potentially inhibit olanzapine clearance; therefore, a dosage decrease might be considered).
No products indexed under this heading.

Eprosartan Mesylate (Olanzapine, because of its potential for inducing hypotension, may enhance the effects of certain antihypertensive agents). Products include:
Teveten Tablets 1735
Teveten HCT Tablets 1737

Erythromycin (May cause an increase in olanzapine clearance; therefore, a dosage increase might be considered). Products include:
Ery-Tab Tablets 449
Erythromycin Base Filmtab Tablets 455
Erythromycin Delayed-Release Capsules, USP 457
PCE Dispertab Tablets 515

Erythromycin Estolate (May cause an increase in olanzapine clearance; therefore, a dosage increase might be considered).
No products indexed under this heading.

Erythromycin Ethylsuccinate (May cause an increase in olanzapine clearance; therefore, a dosage increase might be considered). Products include:
E.E.S. 451
EryPed 447

Erythromycin Gluceptate (May cause an increase in olanzapine clearance; therefore, a dosage increase might be considered).
No products indexed under this heading.

Erythromycin Lactobionate (May cause an increase in olanzapine clearance; therefore, a dosage increase might be considered).
No products indexed under this heading.

Erythromycin Stearate (May cause an increase in olanzapine clearance; therefore, a dosage increase might be considered). Products include:
Erythrocin Stearate Filmtab Tablets 453

Esmolol Hydrochloride (Olanzapine, because of its potential for inducing hypotension, may enhance the effects of certain antihypertensive agents).
No products indexed under this heading.

Estazolam (Given the primary CNS effects of olanzapine, caution should be used when olanzapine is taken in combination with other centrally-acting drugs). Products include:
ProSom Tablets 517

Ethanol (Given the primary CNS effects of olanzapine, caution should be used when olanzapine is taken in combination with other centrally-acting drugs).
No products indexed under this heading.

Ethchlorvynol (Given the primary CNS effects of olanzapine, caution should be used when olanzapine is taken in combination with other centrally-acting drugs).
No products indexed under this heading.

Ethinamate (Given the primary CNS effects of olanzapine, caution should be used when olanzapine is taken in combination with other centrally-acting drugs).
No products indexed under this heading.

Ethinyl Estradiol (Can potentially inhibit olanzapine clearance; therefore, a dosage decrease might be considered). Products include:
Mircette Tablets 1066
NuvaRing 2340
Ortho-Cyclen/Ortho Tri-Cyclen 2429
Ortho Evra Transdermal System 2417
Ortho Tri-Cyclen Lo Tablets 2436
Seasonique Tablets 1077
Yasmin 28 Tablets 796
Yaz Tablets 803

Ethyl Alcohol (Given the primary CNS effects of olanzapine, caution should be used when olanzapine is taken in combination with other centrally-acting drugs).
No products indexed under this heading.

Felodipine (Olanzapine, because of its potential for inducing hypotension, may enhance the effects of certain antihypertensive agents).
No products indexed under this heading.

Fentanyl (Given the primary CNS effects of olanzapine, caution should be used when olanzapine is taken in combination with other centrally-acting drugs). Products include:
Duragesic Transdermal System 2373
Ionsys Transdermal System 2379

Fentanyl Citrate (Given the primary CNS effects of olanzapine, caution should be used when olanzapine is taken in combination with other centrally-acting drugs). Products include:
Actiq ... 979

Fluoxetine Hydrochloride (Co-administration causes a small increase in the maximum concentration of olanzapine and a small decrease in olanzapine clearance; the magnitude of the impact of this factor is small in comparison to the overall variability between individuals and, therefore, dose modification is not routinely recommended). Products include:
Prozac Pulvules and Liquid 1801
Symbyax Capsules 1819

Fluphenazine Decanoate (Given the primary CNS effects of olanzapine, caution should be used when olanzapine is taken in combination with other centrally-acting drugs).
No products indexed under this heading.

Fluphenazine Enanthate (Given the primary CNS effects of olanzapine, caution should be used when olanzapine is taken in combination with other centrally-acting drugs).
No products indexed under this heading.

Fluphenazine Hydrochloride (Given the primary CNS effects of olanzapine, caution should be used when olanzapine is taken in combination with other centrally-acting drugs).
No products indexed under this heading.

Flurazepam Hydrochloride (Given the primary CNS effects of olanzapine, caution should be used when olanzapine is taken in combination with other centrally-acting drugs). Products include:
Dalmane Capsules 3342

Fluvoxamine (Can potentially inhibit olanzapine clearance; therefore, a dosage decrease might be considered).
No products indexed under this heading.

Fluvoxamine Maleate (Decreases the clearance of olanzapine leading to a mean increase in olanzapine Cmax and AUC; lower doses of olanzapine should be considered or co-administered).
No products indexed under this heading.

Fosinopril Sodium (Olanzapine, because of its potential for inducing hypotension, may enhance the effects of certain antihypertensive agents).
No products indexed under this heading.

Furosemide (Olanzapine, because of its potential for inducing hypotension, may enhance the effects of certain antihypertensive agents). Products include:
Furosemide Tablets 2154

Gatifloxacin (Can potentially inhibit olanzapine clearance; therefore, a dosage decrease might be considered). Products include:
Tequin Injection 938
Tequin Injection in 5% Dextrose 938
Tequin Tablets 938
Zymar Ophthalmic Solution 575

Gemifloxacin Mesylate (Can potentially inhibit olanzapine clearance; therefore, a dosage decrease might be considered).
No products indexed under this heading.

Glutethimide (Given the primary CNS effects of olanzapine, caution should be used when olanzapine is taken in combination with other centrally-acting drugs).
No products indexed under this heading.

Grepafloxacin Hydrochloride (Can potentially inhibit olanzapine clearance; therefore, a dosage decrease might be considered).
No products indexed under this heading.

Guanabenz Acetate (Olanzapine, because of its potential for inducing hypotension, may enhance the effects of certain antihypertensive agents).
No products indexed under this heading.

Guanethidine Monosulfate (Olanzapine, because of its potential for inducing hypotension, may enhance the effects of certain antihypertensive agents).
No products indexed under this heading.

Halazepam (Concomitant administration of intramuscular olanzapine and parenteral benzodiazepine has not been studied and is therefore not recommended. If use of intramuscular olanzapine in combination with parenteral benzodiazepines is considered, careful evaluation of clinical status for excessive sedation and cardiorespiratory depression is recommended).
No products indexed under this heading.

Haloperidol (Given the primary CNS effects of olanzapine, caution should be used when olanzapine is taken in combination with other centrally-acting drugs).
No products indexed under this heading.

Haloperidol Decanoate (Given the primary CNS effects of olanzapine, caution should be used when olanzapine is taken in combination with other centrally-acting drugs).
No products indexed under this heading.

Hydralazine Hydrochloride (Olanzapine, because of its potential for inducing hypotension, may enhance the effects of certain antihypertensive agents). Products include:
BiDil Tablets 2171

Hydrochlorothiazide (Olanzapine, because of its potential for inducing hypotension, may enhance the effects of certain antihypertensive agents). Products include:
Aldoril Tablets 1910
Atacand HCT 651
Avalide Tablets 888
Avalide Tablets 2874
Benicar HCT Tablets 1044
Diovan HCT Tablets 2196
Dyazide Capsules 1423
Hyzaar 50-12.5 Tablets 1990
Hyzaar 100-12.5 Tablets 1990
Hyzaar 100-25 Tablets 1990

Lopressor HCT 50/25 Tablets 2241
Lopressor HCT 100/25 Tablets 2241
Lopressor HCT 100/50 Tablets 2241
Lotensin HCT Tablets 2246
Micardis HCT Tablets 856
Moduretic Tablets 2028
Prinzide Tablets 2056
Teveten HCT Tablets 1737
Timolide Tablets 2086
Uniretic Tablets 3100

Hydrocodone Bitartrate (Given the primary CNS effects of olanzapine, caution should be used when olanzapine is taken in combination with other centrally-acting drugs). Products include:
Hycodan 1116
Hycotuss Expectorant Syrup 1117
Vicodin Tablets 535
Vicodin ES Tablets 536
Vicodin HP Tablets 538
Vicoprofen Tablets 539
Zydone Tablets 1139

Hydrocodone Polistirex (Given the primary CNS effects of olanzapine, caution should be used when olanzapine is taken in combination with other centrally-acting drugs). Products include:
Tussionex Pennkinetic
Extended-Release Suspension 3327

Hydroflumethiazide (Olanzapine, because of its potential for inducing hypotension, may enhance the effects of certain antihypertensive agents).
No products indexed under this heading.

Hydromorphone Hydrochloride (Given the primary CNS effects of olanzapine, caution should be used when olanzapine is taken in combination with other centrally-acting drugs). Products include:
Dilaudid 440
Dilaudid Non-Sterile Powder 440
Dilaudid Oral Liquid 445
Dilaudid Rectal Suppositories 440
Dilaudid Tablets 440
Dilaudid Tablets - 8 mg 445
Dilaudid-HP 442

Hydroxyzine Hydrochloride (Given the primary CNS effects of olanzapine, caution should be used when olanzapine is taken in combination with other centrally-acting drugs).
No products indexed under this heading.

Hypericum (May cause an increase in olanzapine clearance; therefore, a dosage increase might be considered). Products include:
Satiete Tablets ◧832

Indapamide (Olanzapine, because of its potential for inducing hypotension, may enhance the effects of certain antihypertensive agents). Products include:
Indapamide Tablets 2156

Insulin (May cause an increase in olanzapine clearance; therefore, a dosage increase might be considered).
No products indexed under this heading.

Irbesartan (Olanzapine, because of its potential for inducing hypotension, may enhance the effects of certain antihypertensive agents). Products include:
Avalide Tablets 888
Avalide Tablets 2874
Avapro Tablets 891
Avapro Tablets 2871

Isoflurane (Given the primary CNS effects of olanzapine, caution should be used when olanzapine is taken in combination with other centrally-acting drugs).
No products indexed under this heading.

Isoniazid (Can potentially inhibit olanzapine clearance; therefore, a dosage decrease might be considered).
No products indexed under this heading.

Isradipine (Olanzapine, because of its potential for inducing hypotension, may enhance the effects of certain antihypertensive agents). Products include:
DynaCirc CR Tablets 2721

Ketamine Hydrochloride (Given the primary CNS effects of olanzapine, caution should be used when olanzapine is taken in combination with other centrally-acting drugs).
No products indexed under this heading.

Ketoconazole (Can potentially inhibit olanzapine clearance; therefore, a dosage decrease might be considered). Products include:
Nizoral A-D Shampoo, 1% 1868

Labetalol Hydrochloride (Olanzapine, because of its potential for inducing hypotension, may enhance the effects of certain antihypertensive agents).
No products indexed under this heading.

Lansoprazole (May cause an increase in olanzapine clearance; therefore, a dosage increase might be considered). Products include:
Prevacid Delayed-Release
Capsules 3271
Prevacid for Delayed-Release Oral
Suspension 3271
Prevacid SoluTab
Delayed-Release Orally
Disintegrating Tablets 3271
Prevacid I.V. for Injection 3277
Prevacid NapraPAC 3280
PREVPAC 3284

Levodopa (Olanzapine may antagonize the effects of levodopa). Products include:
Parcopa Orally Disintegrating
Tablets 3097
Stalevo Tablets 2287

Levofloxacin (Can potentially inhibit olanzapine clearance; therefore, a dosage decrease might be considered). Products include:
Levaquin 2384
Levaquin in 5% Dextrose Injection 2384
Quixin Ophthalmic Solution 3383

Levomethadyl Acetate Hydrochloride (Given the primary CNS effects of olanzapine, caution should be used when olanzapine is taken in combination with other centrally-acting drugs).
No products indexed under this heading.

Levonorgestrel (Can potentially inhibit olanzapine clearance; therefore, a dosage decrease might be considered). Products include:
Climara Pro Transdermal System 776
Mirena Intrauterine System 787
Plan B Tablets 1076
Seasonique Tablets 1077

Levorphanol Tartrate (Given the primary CNS effects of olanzapine, caution should be used when olanzapine is taken in combination with other centrally-acting drugs).
No products indexed under this heading.

IMPORTANT NOTE: Always consult each drug listing in the patient's regimen for possible interactions.

Lisinopril (Olanzapine, because of its potential for inducing hypotension, may enhance the effects of certain antihypertensive agents). Products include:
- Prinivil Tablets 2052
- Prinzide Tablets 2056

Lomefloxacin Hydrochloride (Can potentially inhibit olanzapine clearance; therefore, a dosage decrease might be considered).
No products indexed under this heading.

Lorazepam (Co-administration added to the somnolence observed with either intramuscular drug alone).
No products indexed under this heading.

Losartan Potassium (Olanzapine, because of its potential for inducing hypotension, may enhance the effects of certain antihypertensive agents). Products include:
- Cozaar Tablets 1935
- Hyzaar 50-12.5 Tablets 1990
- Hyzaar 100-12.5 Tablets 1990
- Hyzaar 100-25 Tablets 1990

Loxapine Hydrochloride (Given the primary CNS effects of olanzapine, caution should be used when olanzapine is taken in combination with other centrally-acting drugs).
No products indexed under this heading.

Loxapine Succinate (Given the primary CNS effects of olanzapine, caution should be used when olanzapine is taken in combination with other centrally-acting drugs).
No products indexed under this heading.

Mecamylamine Hydrochloride (Olanzapine, because of its potential for inducing hypotension, may enhance the effects of certain antihypertensive agents).
No products indexed under this heading.

Meperidine Hydrochloride (Given the primary CNS effects of olanzapine, caution should be used when olanzapine is taken in combination with other centrally-acting drugs).
No products indexed under this heading.

Mephobarbital (Given the primary CNS effects of olanzapine, caution should be used when olanzapine is taken in combination with other centrally-acting drugs).
No products indexed under this heading.

Meprobamate (Given the primary CNS effects of olanzapine, caution should be used when olanzapine is taken in combination with other centrally-acting drugs).
No products indexed under this heading.

Mesoridazine Besylate (Given the primary CNS effects of olanzapine, caution should be used when olanzapine is taken in combination with other centrally-acting drugs).
No products indexed under this heading.

Mestranol (Can potentially inhibit olanzapine clearance; therefore, a dosage decrease might be considered).
No products indexed under this heading.

Methadone Hydrochloride (Given the primary CNS effects of olanzapine, caution should be used when olanzapine is taken in combination with other centrally-acting drugs).
No products indexed under this heading.

Methohexital Sodium (Given the primary CNS effects of olanzapine, caution should be used when olanzapine is taken in combination with other centrally-acting drugs).
No products indexed under this heading.

Methotrimeprazine (Given the primary CNS effects of olanzapine, caution should be used when olanzapine is taken in combination with other centrally-acting drugs).
No products indexed under this heading.

Methoxsalen (Can potentially inhibit olanzapine clearance; therefore, a dosage decrease might be considered). Products include:
- Oxsoralen Lotion 1% 3352
- Oxsoralen-Ultra Capsules 3353

Methoxyflurane (Given the primary CNS effects of olanzapine, caution should be used when olanzapine is taken in combination with other centrally-acting drugs).
No products indexed under this heading.

Methyclothiazide (Olanzapine, because of its potential for inducing hypotension, may enhance the effects of certain antihypertensive agents).
No products indexed under this heading.

Methyldopa (Olanzapine, because of its potential for inducing hypotension, may enhance the effects of certain antihypertensive agents). Products include:
- Aldoril Tablets 1910

Methyldopate Hydrochloride (Olanzapine, because of its potential for inducing hypotension, may enhance the effects of certain antihypertensive agents).
No products indexed under this heading.

Metolazone (Olanzapine, because of its potential for inducing hypotension, may enhance the effects of certain antihypertensive agents).
No products indexed under this heading.

Metoprolol Succinate (Olanzapine, because of its potential for inducing hypotension, may enhance the effects of certain antihypertensive agents). Products include:
- Toprol-XL Tablets 668

Metoprolol Tartrate (Olanzapine, because of its potential for inducing hypotension, may enhance the effects of certain antihypertensive agents). Products include:
- Lopressor Injection 2238
- Lopressor Tablets 2238
- Lopressor HCT 50/25 Tablets 2241
- Lopressor HCT 100/25 Tablets 2241
- Lopressor HCT 100/50 Tablets 2241

Metyrosine (Olanzapine, because of its potential for inducing hypotension, may enhance the effects of certain antihypertensive agents). Products include:
- Demser Capsules 1953

Mexiletine Hydrochloride (Can potentially inhibit olanzapine clearance; therefore, a dosage decrease might be considered).
No products indexed under this heading.

Mibefradil Dihydrochloride (Olanzapine, because of its potential for inducing hypotension, may enhance the effects of certain antihypertensive agents).
No products indexed under this heading.

Midazolam Hydrochloride (Given the primary CNS effects of olanzapine, caution should be used when olanzapine is taken in combination with other centrally-acting drugs).
No products indexed under this heading.

Minoxidil (Olanzapine, because of its potential for inducing hypotension, may enhance the effects of certain antihypertensive agents). Products include:
- Men's Rogaine Extra Strength Hair Regrowth Treatment Topical Solution, Ocean Rush Scent and Original Unscented .... ▣ 633
- Men's Rogaine Foam Hair Regrowth Treatment .... ▣ 633
- Women's Rogaine Hair Regrowth Treatment Topical Solution, Spring Bloom Scent and Original Unscented .... ▣ 634

Moexipril Hydrochloride (Olanzapine, because of its potential for inducing hypotension, may enhance the effects of certain antihypertensive agents). Products include:
- Uniretic Tablets 3100
- Univasc Tablets 3104

Molindone Hydrochloride (Given the primary CNS effects of olanzapine, caution should be used when olanzapine is taken in combination with other centrally-acting drugs). Products include:
- Moban Tablets 1119

Morphine Sulfate (Given the primary CNS effects of olanzapine, caution should be used when olanzapine is taken in combination with other centrally-acting drugs). Products include:
- Avinza Capsules 1741
- Kadian Capsules 577
- MS Contin Tablets 2701

Moxifloxacin Hydrochloride (Can potentially inhibit olanzapine clearance; therefore, a dosage decrease might be considered). Products include:
- Avelox 2970
- Vigamox Ophthalmic Solution 564

Nadolol (Olanzapine, because of its potential for inducing hypotension, may enhance the effects of certain antihypertensive agents). Products include:
- Nadolol Tablets 2159

Nafcillin Sodium (May cause an increase in olanzapine clearance; therefore, a dosage increase might be considered).
No products indexed under this heading.

Nalidixic Acid (Can potentially inhibit olanzapine clearance; therefore, a dosage decrease might be considered).
No products indexed under this heading.

Nicardipine Hydrochloride (Olanzapine, because of its potential for inducing hypotension, may enhance the effects of certain antihypertensive agents). Products include:
- Cardene I.V. 2497

Nicotine (May cause an increase in olanzapine clearance; therefore, a dosage increase might be considered). Products include:
- NicoDerm CQ Clear Patch .... ▣ 622

Nicotine Polacrilex (May cause an increase in olanzapine clearance; therefore, a dosage increase might be considered).
No products indexed under this heading.

Nicotine Salicylate (May cause an increase in olanzapine clearance; therefore, a dosage increase might be considered).
No products indexed under this heading.

Nicotine Sulfate (May cause an increase in olanzapine clearance; therefore, a dosage increase might be considered).
No products indexed under this heading.

Nifedipine (Olanzapine, because of its potential for inducing hypotension, may enhance the effects of certain antihypertensive agents). Products include:
- Adalat CC Tablets 2964

Nisoldipine (Olanzapine, because of its potential for inducing hypotension, may enhance the effects of certain antihypertensive agents). Products include:
- Sular Tablets 3122

Nitroglycerin (Olanzapine, because of its potential for inducing hypotension, may enhance the effects of certain antihypertensive agents). Products include:
- Nitro-Dur Transdermal Infusion System 3046
- Nitrolingual Pumpspray 3120

Norethindrone (Can potentially inhibit olanzapine clearance; therefore, a dosage decrease might be considered). Products include:
- Ortho Micronor Tablets 2426

Norfloxacin (Can potentially inhibit olanzapine clearance; therefore, a dosage decrease might be considered). Products include:
- Noroxin Tablets 2032

Norgestrel (Can potentially inhibit olanzapine clearance; therefore, a dosage decrease might be considered).
No products indexed under this heading.

Ofloxacin (Can potentially inhibit olanzapine clearance; therefore, a dosage decrease might be considered). Products include:
- Floxin Otic Solution 1049

Omeprazole (May cause an increase in olanzapine clearance by inducing CYP1A2 or glucuronyl transferase clearance). Products include:
- Zegerid Capsules 2958
- Zegerid Powder for Oral Solution 2958

Oxazepam (Given the primary CNS effects of olanzapine, caution should be used when olanzapine is taken in combination with other centrally-acting drugs).
No products indexed under this heading.

Oxycodone Hydrochloride (Given the primary CNS effects of olanzapine, caution should be used when olanzapine is taken in combination with other centrally-acting drugs). Products include:
- OxyContin Tablets 2703
- OxyFast Oral Concentrate Solution 2708
- OxyIR Capsules 2708
- Percocet Tablets 1131
- Percodan Tablets 1132

Paroxetine Hydrochloride (Can potentially inhibit olanzapine clearance; therefore, a dosage decrease might be considered). Products include:

Paxil CR Controlled-Release
 Tablets .. 1538
Paxil ... 1530

Penbutolol Sulfate (Olanzapine, because of its potential for inducing hypotension, may enhance the effects of certain antihypertensive agents).

No products indexed under this heading.

Pentobarbital Sodium (Given the primary CNS effects of olanzapine, caution should be used when olanzapine is taken in combination with other centrally-acting drugs). Products include:

Nembutal Sodium Solution, USP 2470

Pergolide Mesylate (Olanzapine may antagonize the effects of dopamine agonists). Products include:

Permax Tablets 3356

Perindopril Erbumine (Olanzapine, because of its potential for inducing hypotension, may enhance the effects of certain antihypertensive agents). Products include:

Aceon Tablets (2 mg, 4 mg,
 8 mg).. 3194

Perphenazine (Given the primary CNS effects of olanzapine, caution should be used when olanzapine is taken in combination with other centrally-acting drugs).

No products indexed under this heading.

Phenobarbital (Given the primary CNS effects of olanzapine, caution should be used when olanzapine is taken in combination with other centrally-acting drugs). Products include:

Donnatal Extentabs 2493

Phenoxybenzamine Hydrochloride (Olanzapine, because of its potential for inducing hypotension, may enhance the effects of certain antihypertensive agents). Products include:

Dibenzyline Capsules 3399

Phentolamine Mesylate (Olanzapine, because of its potential for inducing hypotension, may enhance the effects of certain antihypertensive agents).

No products indexed under this heading.

Phenytoin (May cause an increase in olanzapine clearance; therefore, a dosage increase might be considered).

No products indexed under this heading.

Phenytoin Sodium (May cause an increase in olanzapine clearance; therefore, a dosage increase might be considered). Products include:

Phenytek Capsules 2160

Pindolol (Olanzapine, because of its potential for inducing hypotension, may enhance the effects of certain antihypertensive agents).

No products indexed under this heading.

Polythiazide (Olanzapine, because of its potential for inducing hypotension, may enhance the effects of certain antihypertensive agents).

No products indexed under this heading.

Pramipexole Dihydrochloride (Olanzapine may antagonize the effects of dopamine agonists). Products include:

Mirapex Tablets 859

Prazepam (Given the primary CNS effects of olanzapine, caution should be used when olanzapine is taken in combination with other centrally-acting drugs).

No products indexed under this heading.

Prazosin Hydrochloride (Olanzapine, because of its potential for inducing hypotension, may enhance the effects of certain antihypertensive agents).

No products indexed under this heading.

Primidone (May cause an increase in olanzapine clearance; therefore, a dosage increase might be considered).

No products indexed under this heading.

Prochlorperazine (Given the primary CNS effects of olanzapine, caution should be used when olanzapine is taken in combination with other centrally-acting drugs).

No products indexed under this heading.

Promethazine Hydrochloride (Given the primary CNS effects of olanzapine, caution should be used when olanzapine is taken in combination with other centrally-acting drugs). Products include:

Phenergan Tablets and
 Suppositories............................... 3440

Propofol (Given the primary CNS effects of olanzapine, caution should be used when olanzapine is taken in combination with other centrally-acting drugs).

No products indexed under this heading.

Propoxyphene Hydrochloride (Given the primary CNS effects of olanzapine, caution should be used when olanzapine is taken in combination with other centrally-acting drugs).

No products indexed under this heading.

Propoxyphene Napsylate (Given the primary CNS effects of olanzapine, caution should be used when olanzapine is taken in combination with other centrally-acting drugs).

No products indexed under this heading.

Propranolol Hydrochloride (Olanzapine, because of its potential for inducing hypotension, may enhance the effects of certain antihypertensive agents). Products include:

Inderal LA Long-Acting Capsules 3429
InnoPran XL Capsules 2723

Quazepam (Given the primary CNS effects of olanzapine, caution should be used when olanzapine is taken in combination with other centrally-acting drugs).

No products indexed under this heading.

Quetiapine Fumarate (Given the primary CNS effects of olanzapine, caution should be used when olanzapine is taken in combination with other centrally-acting drugs). Products include:

Seroquel Tablets 690

Quinapril Hydrochloride (Olanzapine, because of its potential for inducing hypotension, may enhance the effects of certain antihypertensive agents).

No products indexed under this heading.

Ramipril (Olanzapine, because of its potential for inducing hypoten-

sion, may enhance the effects of certain antihypertensive agents). Products include:

Altace Capsules 1702

Ranitidine Hydrochloride (Can potentially inhibit olanzapine clearance; therefore, a dosage decrease might be considered). Products include:

Zantac .. 1624
Zantac Injection 1619
Zantac Injection Pharmacy Bulk
 Package...................................... 1622

Rauwolfia Serpentina (Olanzapine, because of its potential for inducing hypotension, may enhance the effects of certain antihypertensive agents).

No products indexed under this heading.

Remifentanil Hydrochloride (Given the primary CNS effects of olanzapine, caution should be used when olanzapine is taken in combination with other centrally-acting drugs).

No products indexed under this heading.

Rescinnamine (Olanzapine, because of its potential for inducing hypotension, may enhance the effects of certain antihypertensive agents).

No products indexed under this heading.

Reserpine (Olanzapine, because of its potential for inducing hypotension, may enhance the effects of certain antihypertensive agents).

No products indexed under this heading.

Rifampicin (May cause an increase in olanzapine clearance; therefore, a dosage increase might be considered).

No products indexed under this heading.

Rifampin (May cause an increase in olanzapine clearance by inducing CYP1A2 or glucuronyl tranferase clearance).

No products indexed under this heading.

Risperidone (Given the primary CNS effects of olanzapine, caution should be used when olanzapine is taken in combination with other centrally-acting drugs). Products include:

Risperdal 1676
Risperdal Consta Long-Acting
 Injection 1682
Risperdal M-Tab Orally
 Disintegrating Tablets................... 1676

Ritonavir (May cause an increase in olanzapine clearance; therefore, a dosage increase might be considered). Products include:

Kaletra .. 476
Norvir ... 503

Ropinirole Hydrochloride (Olanzapine may antagonize the effects of dopamine agonists). Products include:

Requip Tablets 1555

Secobarbital Sodium (Given the primary CNS effects of olanzapine, caution should be used when olanzapine is taken in combination with other centrally-acting drugs).

No products indexed under this heading.

Sevoflurane (Given the primary CNS effects of olanzapine, caution should be used when olanzapine is taken in combination with other centrally-acting drugs). Products include:

Ultane Liquid for Inhalation 531

Sodium Nitroprusside (Olanzapine, because of its potential for inducing hypotension, may enhance the effects of certain antihypertensive agents).

No products indexed under this heading.

Sodium Oxybate (Given the primary CNS effects of olanzapine, caution should be used when olanzapine is taken in combination with other centrally-acting drugs). Products include:

Xyrem Oral Solution 1688

Sotalol Hydrochloride (Olanzapine, because of its potential for inducing hypotension, may enhance the effects of certain antihypertensive agents).

No products indexed under this heading.

Sparfloxacin (Can potentially inhibit olanzapine clearance; therefore, a dosage decrease might be considered).

No products indexed under this heading.

Spirapril Hydrochloride (Olanzapine, because of its potential for inducing hypotension, may enhance the effects of certain antihypertensive agents).

No products indexed under this heading.

Sufentanil Citrate (Given the primary CNS effects of olanzapine, caution should be used when olanzapine is taken in combination with other centrally-acting drugs).

No products indexed under this heading.

Tacrine Hydrochloride (Can potentially inhibit olanzapine clearance; therefore, a dosage decrease might be considered).

No products indexed under this heading.

Telmisartan (Olanzapine, because of its potential for inducing hypotension, may enhance the effects of certain antihypertensive agents). Products include:

Micardis Tablets 854
Micardis HCT Tablets 856

Temazepam (Given the primary CNS effects of olanzapine, caution should be used when olanzapine is taken in combination with other centrally-acting drugs). Products include:

Restoril Capsules 1860

Terazosin Hydrochloride (Olanzapine, because of its potential for inducing hypotension, may enhance the effects of certain antihypertensive agents). Products include:

Hytrin Capsules 471

Thiamylal Sodium (Given the primary CNS effects of olanzapine, caution should be used when olanzapine is taken in combination with other centrally-acting drugs).

No products indexed under this heading.

Thioridazine Hydrochloride (Given the primary CNS effects of olanzapine, caution should be used when olanzapine is taken in combination with other centrally-acting drugs). Products include:

Thioridazine Hydrochloride
 Tablets.. 2163

Thiothixene (Given the primary CNS effects of olanzapine, caution should be used when olanzapine is taken in combination with other centrally-acting drugs). Products include:

IMPORTANT NOTE: Always consult each drug listing in the patient's regimen for possible interactions.

Thiothixene Capsules 2165

Ticlopidine Hydrochloride (Can potentially inhibit olanzapine clearance; therefore, a dosage decrease might be considered). Products include:

Ticlid Tablets 2810

Timolol Maleate (Olanzapine, because of its potential for inducing hypotension, may enhance the effects of certain antihypertensive agents). Products include:

Blocadren Tablets 1916
Cosopt Sterile Ophthalmic Solution 1931
Timolide Tablets 2086
Timoptic Sterile Ophthalmic Solution 2088
Timoptic in Ocudose 2091
Timoptic-XE Sterile Ophthalmic Gel Forming Solution 2092

Tobacco (May cause an increase in olanzapine clearance; therefore, a dosage increase might be considered).

No products indexed under this heading.

Torsemide (Olanzapine, because of its potential for inducing hypotension, may enhance the effects of certain antihypertensive agents). Products include:

Demadex Injection 2759
Demadex Tablets 2759

Trandolapril (Olanzapine, because of its potential for inducing hypotension, may enhance the effects of certain antihypertensive agents). Products include:

Mavik Tablets 486
Tarka Tablets 524

Triazolam (Given the primary CNS effects of olanzapine, caution should be used when olanzapine is taken in combination with other centrally-acting drugs).

No products indexed under this heading.

Trifluoperazine Hydrochloride (Given the primary CNS effects of olanzapine, caution should be used when olanzapine is taken in combination with other centrally-acting drugs).

No products indexed under this heading.

Trimethaphan Camsylate (Olanzapine, because of its potential for inducing hypotension, may enhance the effects of certain antihypertensive agents).

No products indexed under this heading.

Troleandomycin (Can potentially inhibit olanzapine clearance; therefore, a dosage decrease might be considered).

No products indexed under this heading.

Trovafloxacin Mesylate (Can potentially inhibit olanzapine clearance; therefore, a dosage decrease might be considered).

No products indexed under this heading.

Valsartan (Olanzapine, because of its potential for inducing hypotension, may enhance the effects of certain antihypertensive agents). Products include:

Diovan Tablets 2193
Diovan HCT Tablets 2196

Verapamil Hydrochloride (Olanzapine, because of its potential for inducing hypotension, may enhance the effects of certain antihypertensive agents). Products include:

Covera-HS Tablets 3139
Tarka Tablets 524
Verelan PM Extended-Release Capsules, Controlled-Onset 3106

Zaleplon (Given the primary CNS effects of olanzapine, caution should be used when olanzapine is taken in combination with other centrally-acting drugs). Products include:

Sonata Capsules 1717

Zileuton (Can potentially inhibit olanzapine clearance; therefore, a dosage decrease might be considered). Products include:

Zyflo Tablets 1023

Ziprasidone Hydrochloride (Given the primary CNS effects of olanzapine, caution should be used when olanzapine is taken in combination with other centrally-acting drugs). Products include:

Geodon Capsules 2529

Zolpidem Tartrate (Given the primary CNS effects of olanzapine, caution should be used when olanzapine is taken in combination with other centrally-acting drugs). Products include:

Ambien Tablets 2851
Ambien CR Tablets 2855

Food Interactions

Alcohol (Co-administration of alcohol with olanzapine potentiates orthostatic hypotension; concurrent use should be avoided).

Broccoli (May cause an increase in olanzapine clearance; therefore, a dosage increase might be considered).

Brussel Sprouts (May cause an increase in olanzapine clearance; therefore, a dosage increase might be considered).

Charbroiled Food (May cause an increase in olanzapine clearance; therefore, a dosage increase might be considered).

Grapefruit Juice (Can potentially inhibit olanzapine clearance; therefore, a dosage decrease might be considered).

ZYPREXA ZYDIS ORALLY DISINTEGRATING TABLETS

(Olanzapine) 1830

See Zyprexa Tablets

ZYRTEC CHEWABLE TABLETS

(Cetirizine Hydrochloride) 2594

See Zyrtec Tablets

ZYRTEC SYRUP

(Cetirizine Hydrochloride) 2594

See Zyrtec Tablets

ZYRTEC TABLETS

(Cetirizine Hydrochloride) 2594

May interact with central nervous system depressants, xanthines, and certain other agents. Compounds in these categories include:

Alfentanil Hydrochloride (Concurrent use may result in additional impairment of CNS performance and reduction in mental alertness).

No products indexed under this heading.

Alprazolam (Concurrent use may result in additional impairment of CNS performance and reduction in mental alertness). Products include:

Niravam Orally Disintegrating Tablets 3092

Aminophylline (Small decrease in the clearance of cetirizine caused by a larger dose, e.g., 400 mg dose of theophylline).

No products indexed under this heading.

Aprobarbital (Concurrent use may result in additional impairment of CNS performance and reduction in mental alertness).

No products indexed under this heading.

Buprenorphine Hydrochloride (Concurrent use may result in additional impairment of CNS performance and reduction in mental alertness). Products include:

Buprenex Injectable 2716
Suboxone Tablets 2717
Subutex Tablets 2717

Buspirone Hydrochloride (Concurrent use may result in additional impairment of CNS performance and reduction in mental alertness).

No products indexed under this heading.

Butabarbital (Concurrent use may result in additional impairment of CNS performance and reduction in mental alertness).

No products indexed under this heading.

Butalbital (Concurrent use may result in additional impairment of CNS performance and reduction in mental alertness).

No products indexed under this heading.

Chlordiazepoxide (Concurrent use may result in additional impairment of CNS performance and reduction in mental alertness).

No products indexed under this heading.

Chlordiazepoxide Hydrochloride (Concurrent use may result in additional impairment of CNS performance and reduction in mental alertness). Products include:

Librium Capsules 3347

Chlorpromazine (Concurrent use may result in additional impairment of CNS performance and reduction in mental alertness).

No products indexed under this heading.

Chlorpromazine Hydrochloride (Concurrent use may result in additional impairment of CNS performance and reduction in mental alertness).

No products indexed under this heading.

Chlorprothixene (Concurrent use may result in additional impairment of CNS performance and reduction in mental alertness).

No products indexed under this heading.

Chlorprothixene Hydrochloride (Concurrent use may result in additional impairment of CNS performance and reduction in mental alertness).

No products indexed under this heading.

Chlorprothixene Lactate (Concurrent use may result in additional impairment of CNS performance and reduction in mental alertness).

No products indexed under this heading.

Clorazepate Dipotassium (Concurrent use may result in additional impairment of CNS performance and reduction in mental alertness). Products include:

Tranxene 2474

Clozapine (Concurrent use may result in additional impairment of CNS performance and reduction in mental alertness). Products include:

Clozaril Tablets 2184
FazaClo Orally Disintegrating Tablets 551

Codeine Phosphate (Concurrent use may result in additional impairment of CNS performance and reduction in mental alertness). Products include:

Tylenol with Codeine Tablets 2391

Desflurane (Concurrent use may result in additional impairment of CNS performance and reduction in mental alertness).

No products indexed under this heading.

Dezocine (Concurrent use may result in additional impairment of CNS performance and reduction in mental alertness).

No products indexed under this heading.

Diazepam (Concurrent use may result in additional impairment of CNS performance and reduction in mental alertness). Products include:

Diastat Rectal Delivery System 3343
Valium Tablets 2819

Droperidol (Concurrent use may result in additional impairment of CNS performance and reduction in mental alertness).

No products indexed under this heading.

Dyphylline (Small decrease in the clearance of cetirizine caused by a larger dose, e.g., 400 mg dose of theophylline).

No products indexed under this heading.

Enflurane (Concurrent use may result in additional impairment of CNS performance and reduction in mental alertness).

No products indexed under this heading.

Estazolam (Concurrent use may result in additional impairment of CNS performance and reduction in mental alertness). Products include:

ProSom Tablets 517

Ethanol (Concurrent use may result in additional impairment of CNS performance and reduction in mental alertness).

No products indexed under this heading.

Ethchlorvynol (Concurrent use may result in additional impairment of CNS performance and reduction in mental alertness).

No products indexed under this heading.

Ethinamate (Concurrent use may result in additional impairment of CNS performance and reduction in mental alertness).

No products indexed under this heading.

Ethyl Alcohol (Concurrent use may result in additional impairment of CNS performance and reduction in mental alertness).

No products indexed under this heading.

Fentanyl (Concurrent use may result in additional impairment of CNS performance and reduction in mental alertness). Products include:

Duragesic Transdermal System 2373
Ionsys Transdermal System 2379

Fentanyl Citrate (Concurrent use may result in additional impairment

of CNS performance and reduction in mental alertness). Products include:
Actiq ... 979

Fluphenazine Decanoate (Concurrent use may result in additional impairment of CNS performance and reduction in mental alertness).
No products indexed under this heading.

Fluphenazine Enanthate (Concurrent use may result in additional impairment of CNS performance and reduction in mental alertness).
No products indexed under this heading.

Fluphenazine Hydrochloride (Concurrent use may result in additional impairment of CNS performance and reduction in mental alertness).
No products indexed under this heading.

Flurazepam Hydrochloride (Concurrent use may result in additional impairment of CNS performance and reduction in mental alertness). Products include:
Dalmane Capsules ... 3342

Glutethimide (Concurrent use may result in additional impairment of CNS performance and reduction in mental alertness).
No products indexed under this heading.

Haloperidol (Concurrent use may result in additional impairment of CNS performance and reduction in mental alertness).
No products indexed under this heading.

Haloperidol Decanoate (Concurrent use may result in additional impairment of CNS performance and reduction in mental alertness).
No products indexed under this heading.

Hydrocodone Bitartrate (Concurrent use may result in additional impairment of CNS performance and reduction in mental alertness). Products include:
Hycodan ... 1116
Hycotuss Expectorant Syrup ... 1117
Vicodin Tablets ... 535
Vicodin ES Tablets ... 536
Vicodin HP Tablets ... 538
Vicoprofen Tablets ... 539
Zydone Tablets ... 1139

Hydrocodone Polistirex (Concurrent use may result in additional impairment of CNS performance and reduction in mental alertness). Products include:
Tussionex Pennkinetic Extended-Release Suspension ... 3327

Hydromorphone Hydrochloride (Concurrent use may result in additional impairment of CNS performance and reduction in mental alertness). Products include:
Dilaudid ... 440
Dilaudid Non-Sterile Powder ... 440
Dilaudid Oral Liquid ... 445
Dilaudid Rectal Suppositories ... 440
Dilaudid Tablets ... 440
Dilaudid Tablets - 8 mg ... 445
Dilaudid-HP ... 442

Hydroxyzine Hydrochloride (Concurrent use may result in additional impairment of CNS performance and reduction in mental alertness).
No products indexed under this heading.

Isoflurane (Concurrent use may result in additional impairment of CNS performance and reduction in mental alertness).
No products indexed under this heading.

Ketamine Hydrochloride (Concurrent use may result in additional impairment of CNS performance and reduction in mental alertness).
No products indexed under this heading.

Levomethadyl Acetate Hydrochloride (Concurrent use may result in additional impairment of CNS performance and reduction in mental alertness).
No products indexed under this heading.

Levorphanol Tartrate (Concurrent use may result in additional impairment of CNS performance and reduction in mental alertness).
No products indexed under this heading.

Lorazepam (Concurrent use may result in additional impairment of CNS performance and reduction in mental alertness).
No products indexed under this heading.

Loxapine Hydrochloride (Concurrent use may result in additional impairment of CNS performance and reduction in mental alertness).
No products indexed under this heading.

Loxapine Succinate (Concurrent use may result in additional impairment of CNS performance and reduction in mental alertness).
No products indexed under this heading.

Meperidine Hydrochloride (Concurrent use may result in additional impairment of CNS performance and reduction in mental alertness).
No products indexed under this heading.

Mephobarbital (Concurrent use may result in additional impairment of CNS performance and reduction in mental alertness).
No products indexed under this heading.

Meprobamate (Concurrent use may result in additional impairment of CNS performance and reduction in mental alertness).
No products indexed under this heading.

Mesoridazine Besylate (Concurrent use may result in additional impairment of CNS performance and reduction in mental alertness).
No products indexed under this heading.

Methadone Hydrochloride (Concurrent use may result in additional impairment of CNS performance and reduction in mental alertness).
No products indexed under this heading.

Methohexital Sodium (Concurrent use may result in additional impairment of CNS performance and reduction in mental alertness).
No products indexed under this heading.

Methotrimeprazine (Concurrent use may result in additional impairment of CNS performance and reduction in mental alertness).
No products indexed under this heading.

Methoxyflurane (Concurrent use may result in additional impairment of CNS performance and reduction in mental alertness).
No products indexed under this heading.

Midazolam Hydrochloride (Concurrent use may result in additional impairment of CNS performance and reduction in mental alertness).
No products indexed under this heading.

Molindone Hydrochloride (Concurrent use may result in additional impairment of CNS performance and reduction in mental alertness). Products include:
Moban Tablets ... 1119

Morphine Sulfate (Concurrent use may result in additional impairment of CNS performance and reduction in mental alertness). Products include:
Avinza Capsules ... 1741
Kadian Capsules ... 577
MS Contin Tablets ... 2701

Olanzapine (Concurrent use may result in additional impairment of CNS performance and reduction in mental alertness). Products include:
Symbyax Capsules ... 1819
Zyprexa Tablets ... 1830
Zyprexa IntraMuscular ... 1830
Zyprexa ZYDIS Orally Disintegrating Tablets ... 1830

Oxazepam (Concurrent use may result in additional impairment of CNS performance and reduction in mental alertness).
No products indexed under this heading.

Oxycodone Hydrochloride (Concurrent use may result in additional impairment of CNS performance and reduction in mental alertness). Products include:
OxyContin Tablets ... 2703
OxyFast Oral Concentrate Solution ... 2708
OxyIR Capsules ... 2708
Percocet Tablets ... 1131
Percodan Tablets ... 1132

Pentobarbital Sodium (Concurrent use may result in additional impairment of CNS performance and reduction in mental alertness). Products include:
Nembutal Sodium Solution, USP ... 2470

Perphenazine (Concurrent use may result in additional impairment of CNS performance and reduction in mental alertness).
No products indexed under this heading.

Phenobarbital (Concurrent use may result in additional impairment of CNS performance and reduction in mental alertness). Products include:
Donnatal Extentabs ... 2493

Prazepam (Concurrent use may result in additional impairment of CNS performance and reduction in mental alertness).
No products indexed under this heading.

Prochlorperazine (Concurrent use may result in additional impairment of CNS performance and reduction in mental alertness).
No products indexed under this heading.

Promethazine Hydrochloride (Concurrent use may result in additional impairment of CNS performance and reduction in mental alertness). Products include:
Phenergan Tablets and Suppositories ... 3440

Propofol (Concurrent use may result in additional impairment of CNS performance and reduction in mental alertness).
No products indexed under this heading.

Propoxyphene Hydrochloride (Concurrent use may result in additional impairment of CNS performance and reduction in mental alertness).
No products indexed under this heading.

Propoxyphene Napsylate (Concurrent use may result in additional impairment of CNS performance and reduction in mental alertness).
No products indexed under this heading.

Quazepam (Concurrent use may result in additional impairment of CNS performance and reduction in mental alertness).
No products indexed under this heading.

Quetiapine Fumarate (Concurrent use may result in additional impairment of CNS performance and reduction in mental alertness). Products include:
Seroquel Tablets ... 690

Remifentanil Hydrochloride (Concurrent use may result in additional impairment of CNS performance and reduction in mental alertness).
No products indexed under this heading.

Risperidone (Concurrent use may result in additional impairment of CNS performance and reduction in mental alertness). Products include:
Risperdal ... 1676
Risperdal Consta Long-Acting Injection ... 1682
Risperdal M-Tab Orally Disintegrating Tablets ... 1676

Secobarbital Sodium (Concurrent use may result in additional impairment of CNS performance and reduction in mental alertness).
No products indexed under this heading.

Sevoflurane (Concurrent use may result in additional impairment of CNS performance and reduction in mental alertness). Products include:
Ultane Liquid for Inhalation ... 531

Sodium Oxybate (Concurrent use may result in additional impairment of CNS performance and reduction in mental alertness). Products include:
Xyrem Oral Solution ... 1688

Sufentanil Citrate (Concurrent use may result in additional impairment of CNS performance and reduction in mental alertness).
No products indexed under this heading.

Temazepam (Concurrent use may result in additional impairment of CNS performance and reduction in mental alertness). Products include:
Restoril Capsules ... 1860

Theophylline (Small decrease in the clearance of cetirizine caused by a larger dose, e.g., 400 mg dose of theophylline).
No products indexed under this heading.

Theophylline Anhydrous (Small decrease in the clearance of cetirizine caused by a larger dose, e.g., 400 mg dose of theophylline). Products include:
Uniphyl Tablets ... 2710

Theophylline Calcium Salicylate
(Small decrease in the clearance of cetirizine caused by a larger dose, e.g., 400 mg dose of theophylline).
No products indexed under this heading.

Theophylline Dihydroxypropyl (Glyceryl) (Small decrease in the clearance of cetirizine caused by a larger dose, e.g., 400 mg dose of theophylline).
No products indexed under this heading.

Theophylline Ethylenediamine
(Small decrease in the clearance of cetirizine caused by a larger dose, e.g., 400 mg dose of theophylline).
No products indexed under this heading.

Theophylline Sodium Glycinate
(Small decrease in the clearance of cetirizine caused by a larger dose, e.g., 400 mg dose of theophylline).
No products indexed under this heading.

Thiamylal Sodium (Concurrent use may result in additional impairment of CNS performance and reduction in mental alertness).
No products indexed under this heading.

Thioridazine Hydrochloride (Concurrent use may result in additional impairment of CNS performance and reduction in mental alertness). Products include:
Thioridazine Hydrochloride Tablets .. **2163**

Thiothixene (Concurrent use may result in additional impairment of CNS performance and reduction in mental alertness). Products include:
Thiothixene Capsules **2165**

Triazolam (Concurrent use may result in additional reduction of CNS performance and reduction in mental alertness).
No products indexed under this heading.

Trifluoperazine Hydrochloride
(Concurrent use may result in additional impairment of CNS performance and reduction in mental alertness).
No products indexed under this heading.

Zaleplon (Concurrent use may result in additional reduction of CNS performance and reduction in mental alertness). Products include:
Sonata Capsules **1717**

Ziprasidone Hydrochloride (Concurrent use may result in additional impairment of CNS performance and reduction in mental alertness). Products include:
Geodon Capsules **2529**

Zolpidem Tartrate (Concurrent use may result in additional impairment of CNS performance and reduction in mental alertness). Products include:
Ambien Tablets **2851**
Ambien CR Tablets **2855**

Food Interactions

Alcohol (Concurrent use may result in additional impairment of CNS performance and reduction in mental alertness).

Food, unspecified (Food has no effect on the extent of cetirizine absorption, but Tmax may be delayed and Cmax may be decreased in the presence of food).

ZYRTEC-D 12 HOUR EXTENDED RELEASE TABLETS

(Cetirizine Hydrochloride, Pseudoephedrine Hydrochloride)........ **2597**
May interact with central nervous system depressants, cardiac glycosides, histamine H2-receptor antagonists, monoamine oxidase inhibitors, proton pump inhibitor, sympathomimetics, xanthines, and certain other agents. Compounds in these categories include:

Albuterol (Co-administration with other sympathomimetic agents may result in harmful cardiovascular effects). Products include:
Proventil Inhalation Aerosol **3053**

Albuterol Sulfate (Co-administration with other sympathomimetic agents may result in harmful cardiovascular effects). Products include:
AccuNeb Inhalation Solution **1055**
Combivent Inhalation Aerosol **847**
DuoNeb Inhalation Solution **1058**
ProAir HFA Inhalation Aerosol **3300**
Proventil Inhalation Solution 0.083% **3055**
Proventil HFA Inhalation Aerosol **3056**
Ventolin HFA Inhalation Aerosol **1600**
VoSpire ER Tablets **1052**

Alfentanil Hydrochloride (Concurrent use may result in additional reduction in alertness impairment of CNS performance).
No products indexed under this heading.

Alprazolam (Concurrent use may result in additional reduction in alertness impairment of CNS performance). Products include:
Niravam Orally Disintegrating Tablets ... **3092**

Aminophylline (Small decrease in the clearance of cetirizine caused by a 400 mg dose of theophylline; it is possible that larger theophylline doses could have a greater effect).
No products indexed under this heading.

Aprobarbital (Concurrent use may result in additional reduction in alertness impairment of CNS performance).
No products indexed under this heading.

Buprenorphine Hydrochloride
(Concurrent use may result in additional reduction in alertness impairment of CNS performance). Products include:
Buprenex Injectable **2716**
Suboxone Tablets **2717**
Subutex Tablets **2717**

Buspirone Hydrochloride (Concurrent use may result in additional reduction in alertness impairment of CNS performance).
No products indexed under this heading.

Butabarbital (Concurrent use may result in additional reduction in alertness impairment of CNS performance).
No products indexed under this heading.

Butalbital (Concurrent use may result in additional reduction in alertness impairment of CNS performance).
No products indexed under this heading.

Chlordiazepoxide (Concurrent use may result in additional reduction in alertness impairment of CNS performance).
No products indexed under this heading.

Chlordiazepoxide Hydrochloride
(Concurrent use may result in additional reduction in alertness impairment of CNS performance). Products include:
Librium Capsules **3347**

Chlorpromazine (Concurrent use may result in additional reduction in alertness impairment of CNS performance).
No products indexed under this heading.

Chlorpromazine Hydrochloride
(Concurrent use may result in additional reduction in alertness impairment of CNS performance).
No products indexed under this heading.

Chlorprothixene (Concurrent use may result in additional reduction in alertness impairment of CNS performance).
No products indexed under this heading.

Chlorprothixene Hydrochloride
(Concurrent use may result in additional reduction in alertness impairment of CNS performance).
No products indexed under this heading.

Chlorprothixene Lactate (Concurrent use may result in additional reduction in alertness impairment of CNS performance).
No products indexed under this heading.

Cimetidine (H2 antagonists increase gastric pH and may reduce the absorption of delavirdine; chronic use of these drugs with delavirdine is not recommended). Products include:
Tagamet HB 200 Tablets ▣▣**664**

Cimetidine Hydrochloride (H2 antagonists increase gastric pH and may reduce the absorption of delavirdine; chronic use of these drugs with delavirdine is not recommended).
No products indexed under this heading.

Clorazepate Dipotassium (Concurrent use may result in additional reduction in alertness impairment of CNS performance). Products include:
Tranxene .. **2474**

Clozapine (Concurrent use may result in additional reduction in alertness impairment of CNS performance). Products include:
Clozaril Tablets **2184**
FazaClo Orally Disintegrating Tablets **551**

Codeine Phosphate (Concurrent use may result in additional reduction in alertness impairment of CNS performance). Products include:
Tylenol with Codeine Tablets **2391**

Desflurane (Concurrent use may result in additional reduction in alertness impairment of CNS performance).
No products indexed under this heading.

Deslanoside (Co-administration of pseudoephedrine may increase ectopic pacemaker activity).
No products indexed under this heading.

Dezocine (Concurrent use may result in additional reduction in alertness impairment of CNS performance).
No products indexed under this heading.

Diazepam (Concurrent use may result in additional reduction in alertness impairment of CNS performance). Products include:
Diastat Rectal Delivery System **3343**
Valium Tablets **2819**

Digitalis Glycoside Preparations
(Co-administration of pseudoephedrine may increase ectopic pacemaker activity).
No products indexed under this heading.

Digitoxin (Co-administration of pseudoephedrine may increase ectopic pacemaker activity).
No products indexed under this heading.

Digoxin (Co-administration of pseudoephedrine may increase ectopic pacemaker activity). Products include:
Lanoxicaps Capsules **1490**
Lanoxin Injection **1494**
Lanoxin Injection Pediatric **1497**
Lanoxin Tablets **1500**

Dobutamine Hydrochloride (Co-administration with other sympathomimetic agents may result in harmful cardiovascular effects).
No products indexed under this heading.

Dopamine Hydrochloride (Co-administration with other sympathomimetic agents may result in harmful cardiovascular effects).
No products indexed under this heading.

Droperidol (Concurrent use may result in additional reduction in alertness impairment of CNS performance).
No products indexed under this heading.

Dyphylline (Small decrease in the clearance of cetirizine caused by a 400 mg dose of theophylline; it is possible that larger theophylline doses could have a greater effect).
No products indexed under this heading.

Enflurane (Concurrent use may result in additional reduction in alertness impairment of CNS performance).
No products indexed under this heading.

Ephedrine Hydrochloride (Co-administration with other sympathomimetic agents may result in harmful cardiovascular effects).
No products indexed under this heading.

Ephedrine Sulfate (Co-administration with other sympathomimetic agents may result in harmful cardiovascular effects).
No products indexed under this heading.

Ephedrine Tannate (Co-administration with other sympathomimetic agents may result in harmful cardiovascular effects).
No products indexed under this heading.

Epinephrine (Co-administration with other sympathomimetic agents may result in harmful cardiovascular effects). Products include:
EpiPen ... **1061**
Primatene Mist ▣▣**719**
Twinject 0.15 **3379**
Twinject 0.3 **3378**

Epinephrine Bitartrate (Co-administration with other sympathomimetic agents may result in harmful cardiovascular effects).
No products indexed under this heading.

Epinephrine Hydrochloride (Co-administration with other sympathomimetic agents may result in harmful cardiovascular effects).
No products indexed under this heading.

Esomeprazole Magnesium (Proton pump inhibitors increase gastric pH and may reduce the absorption of delavirdine chronic use of these drugs with delavirdine is not recommended). Products include:
Nexium Delayed-Release Capsules 655

Estazolam (Concurrent use may result in additional reduction in alertness impairment of CNS performance). Products include:
ProSom Tablets 517

Ethanol (Concurrent use may result in additional reduction in alertness impairment of CNS performance).
No products indexed under this heading.

Ethchlorvynol (Concurrent use may result in additional reduction in alertness impairment of CNS performance).
No products indexed under this heading.

Ethinamate (Concurrent use may result in additional reduction in alertness impairment of CNS performance).
No products indexed under this heading.

Ethyl Alcohol (Concurrent use may result in additional reduction in alertness impairment of CNS performance).
No products indexed under this heading.

Famotidine (H2 antagonists increase gastric pH and may reduce the absorption of delavirdine; chronic use of these drugs with delavirdine is not recommended). Products include:
Pepcid Injection 2040
Pepcid 2038
Pepcid AC Gelcaps 1701
Pepcid AC Tablets 1701
Maximum Strength Pepcid AC Tablets 1701
Pepcid Complete Chewable Tablets 1701

Fentanyl (Concurrent use may result in additional reduction in alertness impairment of CNS performance). Products include:
Duragesic Transdermal System 2373
Ionsys Transdermal System 2379

Fentanyl Citrate (Concurrent use may result in additional reduction in alertness impairment of CNS performance). Products include:
Actiq 979

Fluphenazine Decanoate (Concurrent use may result in additional reduction in alertness impairment of CNS performance).
No products indexed under this heading.

Fluphenazine Enanthate (Concurrent use may result in additional reduction in alertness impairment of CNS performance).
No products indexed under this heading.

Fluphenazine Hydrochloride (Concurrent use may result in additional reduction in alertness impairment of CNS performance).
No products indexed under this heading.

Flurazepam Hydrochloride (Concurrent use may result in additional reduction in alertness impairment of CNS performance). Products include:
Dalmane Capsules 3342

Glutethimide (Concurrent use may result in additional reduction in alertness impairment of CNS performance).
No products indexed under this heading.

Haloperidol (Concurrent use may result in additional reduction in alertness impairment of CNS performance).
No products indexed under this heading.

Haloperidol Decanoate (Concurrent use may result in additional reduction in alertness impairment of CNS performance).
No products indexed under this heading.

Hydrocodone Bitartrate (Concurrent use may result in additional reduction in alertness impairment of CNS performance). Products include:
Hycodan 1116
Hycotuss Expectorant Syrup 1117
Vicodin Tablets 535
Vicodin ES Tablets 536
Vicodin HP Tablets 538
Vicoprofen Tablets 539
Zydone Tablets 1139

Hydrocodone Polistirex (Concurrent use may result in additional reduction in alertness impairment of CNS performance). Products include:
Tussionex Pennkinetic Extended-Release Suspension 3327

Hydromorphone Hydrochloride (Concurrent use may result in additional reduction in alertness impairment of CNS performance). Products include:
Dilaudid 440
Dilaudid Non-Sterile Powder 440
Dilaudid Oral Liquid 445
Dilaudid Rectal Suppositories 440
Dilaudid Tablets 440
Dilaudid Tablets - 8 mg 445
Dilaudid-HP 442

Hydroxyzine Hydrochloride (Concurrent use may result in additional reduction in alertness impairment of CNS performance).
No products indexed under this heading.

Isocarboxazid (Concurrent and/or sequential use with MAO inhibitors is contraindicated).
No products indexed under this heading.

Isoflurane (Concurrent use may result in additional reduction in alertness impairment of CNS performance).
No products indexed under this heading.

Isoproterenol Hydrochloride (Co-administration with other sympathomimetic agents may result in harmful cardiovascular effects).
No products indexed under this heading.

Isoproterenol Sulfate (Co-administration with other sympathomimetic agents may result in harmful cardiovascular effects).
No products indexed under this heading.

Ketamine Hydrochloride (Concurrent use may result in additional reduction in alertness impairment of CNS performance).
No products indexed under this heading.

Lansoprazole (Proton pump inhibitors increase gastric pH and may reduce the absorption of delavirdine chronic use of these drugs with delavirdine is not recommended). Products include:
Prevacid Delayed-Release Capsules 3271
Prevacid for Delayed-Release Oral Suspension 3271
Prevacid SoluTab Delayed-Release Orally Disintegrating Tablets 3271
Prevacid I.V. for Injection 3277
Prevacid NapraPAC 3280
PREVPAC 3284

Levalbuterol Hydrochloride (Co-administration with other sympathomimetic agents may result in harmful cardiovascular effects). Products include:
Xopenex Inhalation Solution 3146
Xopenex Inhalation Solution Concentrate 3150

Levomethadyl Acetate Hydrochloride (Concurrent use may result in additional reduction in alertness impairment of CNS performance).
No products indexed under this heading.

Levorphanol Tartrate (Concurrent use may result in additional reduction in alertness impairment of CNS performance).
No products indexed under this heading.

Lorazepam (Concurrent use may result in additional reduction in alertness impairment of CNS performance).
No products indexed under this heading.

Loxapine Hydrochloride (Concurrent use may result in additional reduction in alertness impairment of CNS performance).
No products indexed under this heading.

Loxapine Succinate (Concurrent use may result in additional reduction in alertness impairment of CNS performance).
No products indexed under this heading.

Mecamylamine Hydrochloride (Pseudoephedrine may reduce the antihypertensive effect).
No products indexed under this heading.

Meperidine Hydrochloride (Concurrent use may result in additional reduction in alertness impairment of CNS performance).
No products indexed under this heading.

Mephobarbital (Concurrent use may result in additional reduction in alertness impairment of CNS performance).
No products indexed under this heading.

Meprobamate (Concurrent use may result in additional reduction in alertness impairment of CNS performance).
No products indexed under this heading.

Mesoridazine Besylate (Concurrent use may result in additional reduction in alertness impairment of CNS performance).
No products indexed under this heading.

Metaproterenol Sulfate (Co-administration with other sympathomimetic agents may result in harmful cardiovascular effects). Products include:
Alupent Inhalation Aerosol 826

Metaraminol Bitartrate (Co-administration with other sympathomimetic agents may result in harmful cardiovascular effects).
No products indexed under this heading.

Methadone Hydrochloride (Concurrent use may result in additional reduction in alertness impairment of CNS performance).
No products indexed under this heading.

Methohexital Sodium (Concurrent use may result in additional reduction in alertness impairment of CNS performance).
No products indexed under this heading.

Methotrimeprazine (Concurrent use may result in additional reduction in alertness impairment of CNS performance).
No products indexed under this heading.

Methoxamine Hydrochloride (Co-administration with other sympathomimetic agents may result in harmful cardiovascular effects).
No products indexed under this heading.

Methoxyflurane (Concurrent use may result in additional reduction in alertness impairment of CNS performance).
No products indexed under this heading.

Methyldopa (Pseudoephedrine may reduce the antihypertensive effect). Products include:
Aldoril Tablets 1910

Methyldopate Hydrochloride (Pseudoephedrine may reduce the antihypertensive effect).
No products indexed under this heading.

Midazolam Hydrochloride (Concurrent use may result in additional reduction in alertness impairment of CNS performance).
No products indexed under this heading.

Moclobemide (Concurrent and/or sequential use with MAO inhibitors is contraindicated).
No products indexed under this heading.

Molindone Hydrochloride (Concurrent use may result in additional reduction in alertness impairment of CNS performance). Products include:
Moban Tablets 1119

Morphine Sulfate (Concurrent use may result in additional reduction in alertness impairment of CNS performance). Products include:
Avinza Capsules 1741
Kadian Capsules 577
MS Contin Tablets 2701

Nizatidine (H2 antagonists increase gastric pH and may reduce the absorption of delavirdine; chronic use of these drugs with delavirdine is not recommended). Products include:
Axid Oral Solution 879

Norepinephrine Bitartrate (Co-administration with other sympathomimetic agents may result in harmful cardiovascular effects).
No products indexed under this heading.

Olanzapine (Concurrent use may result in additional reduction in alertness impairment of CNS performance). Products include:
Symbyax Capsules 1819
Zyprexa Tablets 1830

Zyprexa IntraMuscular 1830
Zyprexa ZYDIS Orally Disintegrating Tablets 1830

Omeprazole (Proton pump inhibitors increase gastric pH and may reduce the absorption of delavirdine chronic use of these drugs with delavirdine is not recommended). Products include:
Zegerid Capsules 2958
Zegerid Powder for Oral Solution 2958

Oxazepam (Concurrent use may result in additional reduction in alertness impairment of CNS performance).
No products indexed under this heading.

Oxycodone Hydrochloride (Concurrent use may result in additional reduction in alertness impairment of CNS performance). Products include:
OxyContin Tablets 2703
OxyFast Oral Concentrate Solution 2708
OxyIR Capsules 2708
Percocet Tablets 1131
Percodan Tablets 1132

Pantoprazole Sodium (Proton pump inhibitors increase gastric pH and may reduce the absorption of delavirdine chronic use of these drugs with delavirdine is not recommended). Products include:
Protonix I.V. 3472
Protonix Tablets 3469

Pargyline Hydrochloride (Concurrent and/or sequential use with MAO inhibitors is contraindicated).
No products indexed under this heading.

Pentobarbital Sodium (Concurrent use may result in additional reduction in alertness impairment of CNS performance). Products include:
Nembutal Sodium Solution, USP 2470

Perphenazine (Concurrent use may result in additional reduction in alertness impairment of CNS performance).
No products indexed under this heading.

Phenelzine Sulfate (Concurrent and/or sequential use with MAO inhibitors is contraindicated).
No products indexed under this heading.

Phenobarbital (Concurrent use may result in additional reduction in alertness impairment of CNS performance). Products include:
Donnatal Extentabs 2493

Phenylephrine Bitartrate (Co-administration with other sympathomimetic agents may result in harmful cardiovascular effects).
No products indexed under this heading.

Phenylephrine Hydrochloride (Co-administration with other sympathomimetic agents may result in harmful cardiovascular effects). Products include:
Comtrex Maximum Strength Non-Drowsy Cold & Cough Caplets .... ▣725
Comtrex Maximum Strength Day/Night Severe Cold & Sinus Caplets - Day Formulation .... ▣725
Comtrex Maximum Strength Day/Night Severe Cold & Sinus Caplets - Night Formulation .... ▣725
Contac Cold and Flu Maximum Strength Caplets .... ▣728
Contac Cold and Flu Day and Night Caplets (Day Formulation Only) .... ▣727
Contac Cold and Flu Day and Night Caplets (Night Formulation Only) .... ▣727
Contac Cold and Flu Non-Drowsy Caplets .... ▣728
Contac-D Cold Non-Drowsy Tablets .... ▣729
Children's Dimetapp Cold & Allergy Elixir .... ▣730
Children's Dimetapp Cold & Allergy Chewable Tablets .... ▣730
Children's Dimetapp DM Cold & Cough Elixir .... ▣731
Toddler's Dimetapp Cold and Cough Drops .... ▣732
Excedrin Sinus Headache Caplets/Tablets .... ▣610
4-Way Fast Acting Nasal Spray ...... ▣775
4-Way Menthol Nasal Spray .... ▣775
Preparation H Maximum Strength Cream .... ▣666
Preparation H Cooling Gel .... ▣666
Preparation H .... ▣666
Refenesen PE Caplets .... ▣721
Robitussin Cough & Allergy Syrup .. ▣736
Robitussin Cough & Cold Nighttime Liquid .... ▣736
Robitussin Cough, Cold & Flu Nighttime Liquid .... ▣738
Robitussin Head & Chest Congestion PE Syrup .... ▣739
Robitussin Pediatric Cough & Cold Nighttime Liquid .... ▣736
TheraFlu Cold & Cough Hot Liquid .... ▣740
TheraFlu Cold & Sore Throat Hot Liquid .... ▣741
TheraFlu Flu & Sore Throat Hot Liquid .... ▣742
TheraFlu Daytime Severe Cold Hot Liquid .... ▣742
TheraFlu Nighttime Severe Cold Hot Liquid .... ▣740
TheraFlu Warming Relief Daytime Severe Cold .... ▣743
TheraFlu Warming Relief Nighttime Severe Cold .... ▣743
Triaminic Chest & Nasal Congestion Liquid .... ▣746
Triaminic Cold & Allergy Liquid .... ▣746
Triaminic Daytime Cold & Cough Liquid .... ▣745
Triaminic Nighttime Cold & Cough Liquid .... ▣746
Triaminic Thin Strips Cold .... ▣748
Triaminic Thin Strips Cold & Cough .... ▣778
Triaminic Infant Thin Strips Decongestant .... ▣747
Triaminic Infant Thin Strips Decongestant Plus Cough .... ▣747
Children's Tylenol Plus Flu Oral Suspension .... ▣749
Tylenol Cold Head Congestion Daytime Caplets with Cool Burst and Gelcaps .... ▣750
Tylenol Cold Multi-Symptom Daytime Liquid .... ▣752
Tylenol Cold Multi-Symptom Severe Daytime Liquid .... ▣752
Concentrated Tylenol Infants' Drops Plus Cold & Cough .... ▣754
Tylenol Allergy Multi-Symptom Caplets with Cool Burst and Gelcaps 1872
Tylenol Allergy Multi-Symptom Nighttime Caplets with Cool Burst 1872
Children's Tylenol Plus Cold Suspension Liquid 1879
Children's Tylenol Plus Cold & Allergy Suspension Liquid 1878
Children's Tylenol Plus Flu Suspension Liquid 1881
Children's Tylenol Plus Multi-Symptom Cold Suspension Liquid 1879
Tylenol Cold Head Congestion Daytime Caplets with Cool Burst 1873
Tylenol Cold Head Congestion Nighttime Caplets with Cool Burst 1873
Tylenol Cold Head Congestion Severe Caplets with Cool Burst..... 1873
Tylenol Cold Multi-Symptom Daytime Caplets with Cool Burst and Gelcaps 1874
Tylenol Cold Multi-Symptom Daytime Liquid with Citrus Burst ... 1874
Tylenol Cold Multi-Symptom Nighttime Caplets with Cool Burst 1874
Tylenol Cold Multi-Symptom Nighttime Liquid with Cool Burst ... 1874
Tylenol Cold Multi-Symptom Severe Caplets with Cool Burst..... 1874
Tylenol Cold Multi-Symptom Severe Daytime Liquid with Citrus Burst 1874
Tylenol Sinus Congestion & Pain Daytime Caplets with Cool Burst and Gelcaps 1876
Tylenol Sinus Congestion & Pain Nighttime Caplets with Cool Burst 1876
Tylenol Sinus Congestion & Pain Severe Caplets with Cool Burst..... 1876
Vicks 44D Cough & Head Congestion Relief Liquid .... ▣760
Vicks DayQuil LiquiCaps/Liquid Multi-Symptom Cold/Flu Relief..... ▣761
Zicam Cough Plus D Cough Spray .... ▣767

Phenylephrine Tannate (Co-administration with other sympathomimetic agents may result in harmful cardiovascular effects).
No products indexed under this heading.

Phenylpropanolamine Hydrochloride (Co-administration with other sympathomimetic agents may result in harmful cardiovascular effects).
No products indexed under this heading.

Pirbuterol Acetate (Co-administration with other sympathomimetic agents may result in harmful cardiovascular effects). Products include:
Maxair Autohaler 1852

Prazepam (Concurrent use may result in additional reduction in alertness impairment of CNS performance).
No products indexed under this heading.

Procarbazine Hydrochloride (Concurrent and/or sequential use with MAO inhibitors is contraindicated). Products include:
Matulane Capsules 3191

Prochlorperazine (Concurrent use may result in additional reduction in alertness impairment of CNS performance).
No products indexed under this heading.

Promethazine Hydrochloride (Concurrent use may result in additional reduction in alertness impairment of CNS performance). Products include:
Phenergan Tablets and Suppositories 3440

Propofol (Concurrent use may result in additional reduction in alertness impairment of CNS performance).
No products indexed under this heading.

Propoxyphene Hydrochloride (Concurrent use may result in additional reduction in alertness impairment of CNS performance).
No products indexed under this heading.

Propoxyphene Napsylate (Concurrent use may result in additional reduction in alertness impairment of CNS performance).
No products indexed under this heading.

Pseudoephedrine Sulfate (Co-administration with other sympathomimetic agents may result in harmful cardiovascular effects). Products include:
Alavert Allergy & Sinus D-12 Hour Tablets .... ▣771
Clarinex-D 24-Hour Extended-Release Tablets 2998
Claritin-D Non-Drowsy 12 Hour Tablets .... ▣772
Claritin-D Non-Drowsy 24 Hour Tablets .... ▣772

Quazepam (Concurrent use may result in additional reduction in alertness impairment of CNS performance).
No products indexed under this heading.

Quetiapine Fumarate (Concurrent use may result in additional reduction in alertness impairment of CNS performance). Products include:
Seroquel Tablets 690

Rabeprazole Sodium (Proton pump inhibitors increase gastric pH and may reduce the absorption of delavirdine chronic use of these drugs with delavirdine is not recommended). Products include:
Aciphex Tablets 1090

Ranitidine Bismuth Citrate (H2 antagonists increase gastric pH and may reduce the absorption of delavirdine; chronic use of these drugs with delavirdine is not recommended).
No products indexed under this heading.

Ranitidine Hydrochloride (H2 antagonists increase gastric pH and may reduce the absorption of delavirdine; chronic use of these drugs with delavirdine is not recommended). Products include:
Zantac 1624
Zantac Injection 1619
Zantac Injection Pharmacy Bulk Package 1622

Remifentanil Hydrochloride (Concurrent use may result in additional reduction in alertness impairment of CNS performance).
No products indexed under this heading.

Reserpine (Pseudoephedrine may reduce the antihypertensive effect).
No products indexed under this heading.

Risperidone (Concurrent use may result in additional reduction in alertness impairment of CNS performance). Products include:
Risperdal 1676
Risperdal Consta Long-Acting Injection 1682
Risperdal M-Tab Orally Disintegrating Tablets 1676

Salmeterol Xinafoate (Co-administration with other sympathomimetic agents may result in harmful cardiovascular effects). Products include:
Advair Diskus 100/50 1308
Advair Diskus 250/50 1308
Advair Diskus 500/50 1308
Advair HFA Inhalation Aerosol 1318
Serevent Diskus 1568

Secobarbital Sodium (Concurrent use may result in additional reduction in alertness impairment of CNS performance).
No products indexed under this heading.

Selegiline Hydrochloride (Concurrent and/or sequential use with MAO inhibitors is contraindicated). Products include:
Eldepryl Capsules 3208
Zelapar Tablets 3372

Sevoflurane (Concurrent use may result in additional reduction in alertness impairment of CNS performance). Products include:
Ultane Liquid for Inhalation 531

Sufentanil Citrate (Concurrent use may result in additional reduction in alertness impairment of CNS performance).
No products indexed under this heading.

Temazepam (Concurrent use may result in additional reduction in alertness impairment of CNS performance). Products include:
Restoril Capsules 1860

Terbutaline Sulfate (Co-administration with other sympathomimetic agents may result in harmful cardiovascular effects).
No products indexed under this heading.

Theophylline (Small decrease in the clearance of cetirizine caused by a 400 mg dose of theophylline; it is possible that larger theophylline doses could have a greater effect).
No products indexed under this heading.

Theophylline Anhydrous (Small decrease in the clearance of cetirizine caused by a 400 mg dose of theophylline; it is possible that larger theophylline doses could have a greater effect). Products include:
Uniphyl Tablets 2710

Theophylline Calcium Salicylate (Small decrease in the clearance of cetirizine caused by a 400 mg dose of theophylline; it is possible that larger theophylline doses could have a greater effect).
No products indexed under this heading.

Theophylline Dihydroxypropyl (Glyceryl) (Small decrease in the clearance of cetirizine caused by a 400 mg dose of theophylline; it is possible that larger theophylline doses could have a greater effect).
No products indexed under this heading.

Theophylline Ethylenediamine (Small decrease in the clearance of cetirizine caused by a 400 mg dose of theophylline; it is possible that larger theophylline doses could have a greater effect).
No products indexed under this heading.

Theophylline Sodium Glycinate (Small decrease in the clearance of cetirizine caused by a 400 mg dose of theophylline; it is possible that larger theophylline doses could have a greater effect).
No products indexed under this heading.

Thiamylal Sodium (Concurrent use may result in additional reduction in alertness impairment of CNS performance).
No products indexed under this heading.

Thioridazine Hydrochloride (Concurrent use may result in additional reduction in alertness impairment of CNS performance). Products include:
Thioridazine Hydrochloride Tablets 2163

Thiothixene (Concurrent use may result in additional reduction in alertness impairment of CNS performance). Products include:
Thiothixene Capsules 2165

Tranylcypromine Sulfate (Concurrent and/or sequential use with MAO inhibitors is contraindicated). Products include:
Parnate Tablets 1527

Triazolam (Concurrent use may result in additional reduction in alertness impairment of CNS performance).
No products indexed under this heading.

Trifluoperazine Hydrochloride (Concurrent use may result in additional reduction in alertness impairment of CNS performance).
No products indexed under this heading.

Zaleplon (Concurrent use may result in additional reduction in alertness impairment of CNS performance). Products include:
Sonata Capsules 1717

Ziprasidone Hydrochloride (Concurrent use may result in additional reduction in alertness impairment of CNS performance). Products include:
Geodon Capsules 2529

Zolpidem Tartrate (Concurrent use may result in additional reduction in alertness impairment of CNS performance). Products include:
Ambien Tablets 2851
Ambien CR Tablets 2855

Food Interactions

Alcohol (Concurrent use may result in additional reduction in alertness impairment of CNS performance).

ZYVOX FOR ORAL SUSPENSION

(Linezolid) 2652
See Zyvox Tablets

ZYVOX INJECTION

(Linezolid) 2652
See Zyvox Tablets

ZYVOX TABLETS

(Linezolid) 2652
May interact with serotoninergic agents, sympathomimetics, and certain other agents. Compounds in these categories include:

Albuterol (Linezolid is a reversible nonselective inhibitor of MAO; therefore, linezolid has the potential for interaction with adrenergic agents). Products include:
Proventil Inhalation Aerosol 3053

Albuterol Sulfate (Linezolid is a reversible nonselective inhibitor of MAO; therefore, linezolid has the potential for interaction with adrenergic agents). Products include:
AccuNeb Inhalation Solution 1055
Combivent Inhalation Aerosol 847
DuoNeb Inhalation Solution 1058
ProAir HFA Inhalation Aerosol 3300
Proventil Inhalation Solution 0.083% 3055
Proventil HFA Inhalation Aerosol 3056
Ventolin HFA Inhalation Aerosol 1600
VoSpire ER Tablets 1052

Citalopram Hydrobromide (Linezolid is a reversible nonselective inhibitor of monoamine oxidase. Therefore, linezolid has the potential for interaction with serotonergic agents. Spontaneous reports of serotonin syndrome associated with co-administration of linezolid and serotinergic agents, including antidepressants such as selective serotonin reuptake inhibitors (SSRIs), have been reported. Patients who are treated with linezolid and concomitant serotinergic agents should be closely observed for signs and symptoms of serotonin syndrome (e.g., cognitive dysfunction, hyperpyrexia, hyperreflexia, incoordination). If any signs or symptoms occur, physicians should consider discontinuation of either one or both agents (linezolid or concomitant serotinergic agents)). Products include:
Celexa 1176

Dobutamine Hydrochloride (Linezolid is a reversible nonselective inhibitor of MAO; therefore, linezolid has the potential for interaction with adrenergic agents).
No products indexed under this heading.

Dopamine Hydrochloride (Some patients receiving Zyvox with dopaminergic agents may experience a reversible enhancement of pressor response; initial dose of dopamine should be reduced and titrated to achieve the desired response).
No products indexed under this heading.

Ephedrine Hydrochloride (Linezolid is a reversible nonselective inhibitor of MAO; therefore, linezolid has the potential for interaction with adrenergic agents).
No products indexed under this heading.

Ephedrine Sulfate (Linezolid is a reversible nonselective inhibitor of MAO; therefore, linezolid has the potential for interaction with adrenergic agents).
No products indexed under this heading.

Ephedrine Tannate (Linezolid is a reversible nonselective inhibitor of MAO; therefore, linezolid has the potential for interaction with adrenergic agents).
No products indexed under this heading.

Epinephrine (Linezolid is a reversible nonselective inhibitor of MAO; therefore, linezolid has the potential for interaction with adrenergic agents). Products include:
EpiPen 1061
Primatene Mist 719
Twinject 0.15 3379
Twinject 0.3 3378

Epinephrine Bitartrate (Linezolid is a reversible nonselective inhibitor of MAO; therefore, linezolid has the potential for interaction with adrenergic agents).
No products indexed under this heading.

Epinephrine Hydrochloride (Some patients receiving Zyvox with vasopressors may experience a reversible enhancement of pressor response; initial dose of epinephrine should be reduced and titrated to achieve the desired response).
No products indexed under this heading.

Escitalopram Oxalate (Linezolid is a reversible nonselective inhibitor of monoamine oxidase. Therefore, linezolid has the potential for interaction with serotonergic agents. Spontaneous reports of serotonin syndrome associated with co-administration of linezolid and serotinergic agents, including antidepressants such as selective serotonin reuptake inhibitors (SSRIs), have been reported. Patients who are treated with linezolid and concomitant serotinergic agents should be closely observed for signs and symptoms of serotonin syndrome (e.g., cognitive dysfunction, hyperpyrexia, hyperreflexia, incoordination). If any signs or symptoms occur, physicians should consider discontinuation of either one or both agents (linezolid or concomitant serotinergic agents)). Products include:
Lexapro Oral Solution 1190
Lexapro Tablets 1190

Fluoxetine Hydrochloride (Linezolid is a reversible nonselective inhibitor of monoamine oxidase. Therefore, linezolid has the potential for interaction with serotonergic agents. Spontaneous reports of serotonin syndrome associated with co-administration of linezolid and serotinergic agents, including antidepressants such as selective serotonin reuptake inhibitors (SSRIs), have been reported. Patients who are treated with linezolid and concomitant serotinergic agents should be closely observed for signs and symptoms of serotonin syndrome (e.g., cognitive dysfunction, hyperpyrexia, hyperreflexia, incoordination). If any signs or symptoms occur, physicians should consider discontinuation of either one or both agents (linezolid or concomitant serotinergic agents)). Products include:
Prozac Pulvules and Liquid 1801
Symbyax Capsules 1819

Fluvoxamine Maleate (Linezolid is a reversible nonselective inhibitor of monoamine oxidase. Therefore, linezolid has the potential for interaction with serotonergic agents. Spontaneous reports of serotonin syndrome associated with co-administration of linezolid and serotinergic agents, including antidepressants such as selective serotonin reuptake inhibitors (SSRIs), have been reported. Patients who are treated with linezolid and concomitant serotinergic agents should be closely observed for signs and symptoms of serotonin syndrome (e.g., cognitive dysfunction, hyperpyrexia, hyperreflexia, incoordination). If any signs or symptoms occur, physicians should consider discontinuation of either one or both agents (linezolid or concomitant serotinergic agents)).
No products indexed under this heading.

Isoproterenol Hydrochloride (Linezolid is a reversible nonselective inhibitor of MAO; therefore, linezolid has the potential for interaction with adrenergic agents).
No products indexed under this heading.

Isoproterenol Sulfate (Linezolid is a reversible nonselective inhibitor of MAO; therefore, linezolid has the potential for interaction with adrenergic agents).
No products indexed under this heading.

Levalbuterol Hydrochloride (Linezolid is a reversible nonselective inhibitor of MAO; therefore, linezolid has the potential for interaction with adrenergic agents). Products include:
Xopenex Inhalation Solution 3146
Xopenex Inhalation Solution Concentrate 3150

Metaproterenol Sulfate (Linezolid is a reversible nonselective inhibitor of MAO; therefore, linezolid has the potential for interaction with adrenergic agents). Products include:
Alupent Inhalation Aerosol 826

Metaraminol Bitartrate (Linezolid is a reversible nonselective inhibitor of MAO; therefore, linezolid has the potential for interaction with adrenergic agents).
No products indexed under this heading.

Methoxamine Hydrochloride (Linezolid is a reversible nonselective inhibitor of MAO; therefore, linezolid has the potential for interaction with adrenergic agents).
No products indexed under this heading.

Norepinephrine Bitartrate (Linezolid is a reversible nonselective inhibitor of MAO; therefore, linezolid has the potential for interaction with adrenergic agents).
No products indexed under this heading.

Paroxetine Hydrochloride (Linezolid is a reversible nonselective inhibitor of monoamine oxidase. Therefore, linezolid has the potential for interaction with serotonergic agents. Spontaneous reports of serotonin syndrome associated with co-administration of linezolid and serotinergic agents, including antidepressants such as selective serotonin reuptake inhibitors (SSRIs), have been reported. Patients who are treated with linezolid and concomitant serotinergic agents should be closely observed for signs and symptoms of serotonin syndrome (e.g., cognitive dysfunction, hyperpyrexia, hyperreflexia, incoordination). If any signs or symptoms occur, physicians should consider discontinuation of either one or both agents (linezolid or concomitant serotinergic agents)). Products include:
- Paxil CR Controlled-Release Tablets ... 1538
- Paxil ... 1530

Phenylephrine Bitartrate (Linezolid is a reversible nonselective inhibitor of MAO; therefore, linezolid has the potential for interaction with adrenergic agents).
No products indexed under this heading.

Phenylephrine Hydrochloride (Linezolid is a reversible nonselective inhibitor of MAO; therefore, linezolid has the potential for interaction with adrenergic agents). Products include:
- Comtrex Maximum Strength Non-Drowsy Cold & Cough Caplets ... ▣725
- Comtrex Maximum Strength Day/Night Severe Cold & Sinus Caplets - Day Formulation ... ▣725
- Comtrex Maximum Strength Day/Night Severe Cold & Sinus Caplets - Night Formulation ... ▣725
- Contac Cold and Flu Maximum Strength Caplets ... ▣728
- Contac Cold and Flu Day and Night Caplets (Day Formulation Only) ... ▣727
- Contac Cold and Flu Day and Night Caplets (Night Formulation Only) ... ▣727
- Contac Cold and Flu Non-Drowsy Caplets ... ▣728
- Contac-D Cold Non-Drowsy Tablets ... ▣729
- Children's Dimetapp Cold & Allergy Elixir ... ▣730
- Children's Dimetapp Cold & Allergy Chewable Tablets ... ▣730
- Children's Dimetapp DM Cold & Cough Elixir ... ▣731
- Toddler's Dimetapp Cold and Cough Drops ... ▣732
- Excedrin Sinus Headache Caplets/Tablets ... ▣610
- 4-Way Fast Acting Nasal Spray ... ▣775
- 4-Way Menthol Nasal Spray ... ▣775
- Preparation H Maximum Strength Cream ... ▣666
- Preparation H Cooling Gel ... ▣666
- Preparation H ... ▣666
- Refenesen PE Caplets ... ▣721
- Robitussin Cough & Allergy Syrup ... ▣736
- Robitussin Cough & Cold Nighttime Liquid ... ▣736
- Robitussin Cough, Cold & Flu Nighttime Liquid ... ▣738
- Robitussin Head & Chest Congestion PE Syrup ... ▣739
- Robitussin Pediatric Cough & Cold Nighttime Liquid ... ▣736
- TheraFlu Cold & Cough Hot Liquid ... ▣740
- TheraFlu Cold & Sore Throat Hot Liquid ... ▣741
- TheraFlu Flu & Sore Throat Hot Liquid ... ▣742
- TheraFlu Daytime Severe Cold Hot Liquid ... ▣742
- TheraFlu Nighttime Severe Cold Hot Liquid ... ▣740
- TheraFlu Warming Relief Daytime Severe Cold ... ▣743
- TheraFlu Warming Relief Nighttime Severe Cold ... ▣743
- Triaminic Chest & Nasal Congestion Liquid ... ▣746
- Triaminic Cold & Allergy Liquid ... ▣746
- Triaminic Daytime Cold & Cough Liquid ... ▣745
- Triaminic Nighttime Cold & Cough Liquid ... ▣746
- Triaminic Thin Strips Cold ... ▣748
- Triaminic Thin Strips Cold & Cough ... ▣778
- Triaminic Infant Thin Strips Decongestant ... ▣747
- Triaminic Infant Thin Strips Decongestant Plus Cough ... ▣747
- Children's Tylenol Plus Flu Oral Suspension ... ▣749
- Tylenol Cold Head Congestion Daytime Caplets with Cool Burst and Gelcaps ... ▣750
- Tylenol Cold Multi-Symptom Daytime Liquid ... ▣752
- Tylenol Cold Multi-Symptom Severe Daytime Liquid ... ▣752
- Concentrated Tylenol Infants' Drops Plus Cold & Cough ... ▣754
- Tylenol Allergy Multi-Symptom Caplets with Cool Burst and Gelcaps ... 1872
- Tylenol Allergy Multi-Symptom Nighttime Caplets with Cool Burst ... 1872
- Children's Tylenol Plus Cold Suspension Liquid ... 1879
- Children's Tylenol Plus Cold & Allergy Suspension Liquid ... 1878
- Children's Tylenol Plus Flu Suspension Liquid ... 1881
- Children's Tylenol Plus Multi-Symptom Cold Suspension Liquid ... 1879
- Tylenol Cold Head Congestion Daytime Caplets with Cool Burst ... 1873
- Tylenol Cold Head Congestion Nighttime Caplets with Cool Burst ... 1873
- Tylenol Cold Head Congestion Severe Caplets with Cool Burst ... 1873
- Tylenol Cold Multi-Symptom Daytime Caplets with Cool Burst and Gelcaps ... 1874
- Tylenol Cold Multi-Symptom Daytime Liquid with Citrus Burst ... 1874
- Tylenol Cold Multi-Symptom Nighttime Caplets with Cool Burst ... 1874
- Tylenol Cold Multi-Symptom Nighttime Liquid with Cool Burst ... 1874
- Tylenol Cold Multi-Symptom Severe Caplets with Cool Burst ... 1874
- Tylenol Cold Multi-Symptom Severe Daytime Liquid with Citrus Burst ... 1874
- Tylenol Sinus Congestion & Pain Daytime Caplets with Cool Burst and Gelcaps ... 1876
- Tylenol Sinus Congestion & Pain Nighttime Caplets with Cool Burst ... 1876
- Tylenol Sinus Congestion & Pain Severe Caplets with Cool Burst ... 1876
- Vicks 44D Cough & Head Congestion Relief Liquid ... ▣760
- Vicks DayQuil LiquiCaps/Liquid Multi-Symptom Cold/Flu Relief ... ▣761
- Zicam Cough Plus D Cough Spray ... ▣767

Phenylephrine Tannate (Linezolid is a reversible nonselective inhibitor of MAO; therefore, linezolid has the potential for interaction with adrenergic agents).
No products indexed under this heading.

Phenylpropanolamine Hydrochloride (Co-administration has resulted in a reversible enhancement of pressor response of phenylpropanolamine).
No products indexed under this heading.

Pirbuterol Acetate (Linezolid is a reversible nonselective inhibitor of MAO; therefore, linezolid has the potential for interaction with adrenergic agents). Products include:
- Maxair Autohaler ... 1852

Pseudoephedrine Hydrochloride (Co-administration has resulted in a reversible enhancement of pressor response of pseudoephedrine). Products include:
- Advil Allergy Sinus Caplets ... ▣770
- Advil Cold & Sinus ... ▣723
- Advil Multi-Symptom Cold Caplets ... ▣770
- Aleve Cold & Sinus Caplets ... 744
- Allegra-D 12 Hour Extended-Release Tablets ... 2846
- Allegra-D 24 Hour Extended-Release Tablets ... 2849
- BC Cold Powder ... ▣677
- Comtrex Maximum Strength Cold & Cough Day/Night Caplets - Day Formulation ... ▣726
- Comtrex Maximum Strength Cold & Cough Day/Night Caplets - Night Formulation ... ▣726
- Children's Motrin Cold Oral Suspension ... 1867
- Mucinex D Extended-Release Bi-Layer Tablets ... ▣776
- Robitussin Cough & Cold CF Liquid ... ▣735
- Robitussin Cough & Cold Pediatric Drops ... ▣735
- Tylenol Sinus Congestion & Pain Nighttime Caplets with Cool Burst ... ▣778
- Tylenol Cold Severe Congestion Non-Drowsy Caplets with Cool Burst ... 1874
- Tylenol Sinus Severe Congestion Caplets with Cool Burst ... 1876
- Vicks 44D Cough & Head Congestion Relief Liquid ... 2679
- Vicks 44M Cough, Cold & Flu Relief Liquid ... 2680
- Vicks DayQuil Multi-Symptom Cold/Flu Relief LiquiCaps ... 2678
- Vicks DayQuil Multi-Symptom Cold/Flu Relief Liquid ... 2678
- Vicks NyQuil Multi-Symptom Cold/Flu Relief Liquid ... 2681
- Vicks NyQuil Multi-Symptom Cold/Flu Relief LiquiCaps ... 2681
- Children's Vicks NyQuil Cold/Cough Relief Liquid ... 2680
- Zyrtec-D 12 Hour Extended Release Tablets ... 2597

Pseudoephedrine Sulfate (Linezolid is a reversible nonselective inhibitor of MAO; therefore, linezolid has the potential for interaction with adrenergic agents). Products include:
- Alavert Allergy & Sinus D-12 Hour Tablets ... ▣771
- Clarinex-D 24-Hour Extended-Release Tablets ... 2998
- Claritin-D Non-Drowsy 12 Hour Tablets ... ▣772
- Claritin-D Non-Drowsy 24 Hour Tablets ... ▣772

Salmeterol Xinafoate (Linezolid is a reversible nonselective inhibitor of MAO; therefore, linezolid has the potential for interaction with adrenergic agents). Products include:
- Advair Diskus 100/50 ... 1308
- Advair Diskus 250/50 ... 1308
- Advair Diskus 500/50 ... 1308
- Advair HFA Inhalation Aerosol ... 1318
- Serevent Diskus ... 1568

Sertraline Hydrochloride (Linezolid is a reversible nonselective inhibitor of monoamine oxidase. Therefore, linezolid has the potential for interaction with serotonergic agents. Spontaneous reports of serotonin syndrome associated with co-administration of linezolid and serotinergic agents, including antidepressants such as selective serotonin reuptake inhibitors (SSRIs), have been reported. Patients who are treated with linezolid and concomitant serotinergic agents should be closely observed for signs and symptoms of serotonin syndrome (e.g., cognitive dysfunction, hyperpyrexia, hyperreflexia, incoordination). If any signs or symptoms occur, physicians should consider discontinuation of either one or both agents (linezolid or concomitant serotinergic agents)). Products include:
- Zoloft ... 2586

Terbutaline Sulfate (Linezolid is a reversible nonselective inhibitor of MAO; therefore, linezolid has the potential for interaction with adrenergic agents).
No products indexed under this heading.

Tyramine (Co-administration has resulted in a significant pressor response).
No products indexed under this heading.

Venlafaxine Hydrochloride (Linezolid is a reversible nonselective inhibitor of monoamine oxidase. Therefore, linezolid has the potential for interaction with serotonergic agents. Spontaneous reports of serotonin syndrome associated with co-administration of linezolid and serotinergic agents, including antidepressants such as selective serotonin reuptake inhibitors (SSRIs), have been reported. Patients who are treated with linezolid and concomitant serotinergic agents should be closely observed for signs and symptoms of serotonin syndrome (e.g., cognitive dysfunction, hyperpyrexia, hyperreflexia, incoordination). If any signs or symptoms occur, physicians should consider discontinuation of either one or both agents (linezolid or concomitant serotinergic agents)). Products include:
- Effexor Tablets ... 3411
- Effexor XR Capsules ... 3417

Food Interactions

Beverages with high tyramine (Co-administration has resulted in a significant pressor response; patients receiving linezolid should avoid consuming large amounts of beverages containing tyramine).

Food, unspecified (The time to reach maximum concentration is delayed from 1.5 hours to 2.2 hours and Cmax is decreased by about 17% when linezolid is co-administered with high fat food; linezolid may be administered without regard to the timing of meals).

Food high in tyramine (Co-administration has resulted in a significant pressor response; patients receiving linezolid should avoid consuming large amounts of food containing tyramine).

SECTION 2

FOOD INTERACTIONS CROSS-REFERENCE

In this section, drug/food and drug/alcohol interactions listed in the preceding index are cross-referenced by dietary item. Under each entry is an alphabetical list, by brand name, of drugs said to interact with the item. A brief description of the interaction follows each brand, along with the page number of the underlying text. Page numbers refer to the 2007 editions of *PDR®*, *PDR for Ophthalmic Medicines™* and the *PDR for Nonprescription Drugs, Dietary Supplements and Herbs™*, which is published later each year. A key to the symbols denoting the companion volumes appears in the bottom margin.

Entries in this section are limited to drug/food and drug/alcohol interactions listed in official prescribing information as published by *PDR®*.

Alcohol

Abilify Tablets (Given the primary CNS effects of aripiprazole, caution should be use when co-administered with alcohol; patients should be advised to avoid alcohol while taking aripiprazole)........ 882

Abilify Tablets (Given the primary CNS effects of aripiprazole, caution should be use when co-administered with alcohol; patients should be advised to avoid alcohol while taking aripiprazole)........ 2450

Actiq (Concurrent use with alcoholic beverages may result in increased depressant effects; hypoventilation, hypotension, and profound sedation may occur)........ 979

ActoPlus Met Tablets (Alcohol is known to potentiate the effect of metformin on lactate metabolism. Patients, therefore, should be warned against excessive alcohol intake, acute or chronic, while receiving Actoplus Met)........ 3214

Adipex-P Tablets (May result in adverse drug interaction)........ 1215

Advicor Tablets (Concomitant alcohol may increase the flushing and its use should be avoided around the time of Advicor administration)........ 1722

Advil Allergy Sinus Caplets (Consuming 3 or more alcoholic beverages while using this product may increase the risk of stomach bleeding)........ ▣ 770

Advil Caplets (Consuming 3 or more alcoholic beverages while using this product may increase the risk of stomach bleeding)........ ▣ 674

Advil Migraine Liquigels (Consumption of 3 or more alcoholic beverage the risk of stomach bleeding)........ ▣ 608

Advil PM Caplets (Having 3 or more alcoholic beverages will increase the chances of stomach bleeding)........ ▣ 615

Agenerase Oral Solution (Concurrent use of Agenerase Oral Solution with alcoholic beverages is not recommended)........ 1332

Aggrenox Capsules (Patients who consume three or more alcoholic drinks every day should be counseled about the bleeding risks involved with chronic, heavy alcohol use while taking aspirin)........ 822

Aldoril Tablets (Aggravates orthostatic hypotension)........ 1910

Aleve Caplets (Taking with alcohol may increase chances of stomach bleeding)........ ▣ 675

Aleve Caplets (Taking with alcohol may increase chances of stomach bleeding)........ 742

Aleve Gelcaps (Taking with alcohol may increase chances of stomach bleeding)........ ▣ 675

Aleve Gelcaps (Taking with alcohol may increase chances of stomach bleeding)........ 743

Aleve Cold & Sinus Caplets (Taking with alcohol may increase chances of stomach bleeding)........ 744

Aleve Tablets (Taking with alcohol may increase chances of stomach bleeding)........ ▣ 676

Aleve Tablets (Taking with alcohol may increase chances of stomach bleeding)........ 743

Aleve Cold & Sinus Caplets (Taking with alcohol may increase chances of stomach bleeding)........ ▣ 724

Alphagan P Ophthalmic Solution (Possible additive or potentiating effect with CNS depressants)........ 567

Ambien Tablets (Co-administration produces additive effects on psychomotor performance)........ 2851

Ambien CR Tablets (An additive effect on psychomotor performance between alcohol and zolpidem tartrate was demonstrated)........ 2855

Apidra Injection (Alcohol may either potentiate or weaken the blood glucose-lowering effect of insulin)........ 2864

Astelin Nasal Spray (Concurrent use may result in additional reduction in alertness and impairment of CNS performance; alcohol intake should be avoided)........ 1904

Atacand HCT 16-12.5 Tablets (May aggravate orthostatic hypotension produced by hydrochlorothiazide)........ 651

Avalide Tablets (Potentiation of orthostatic hypotension)........ 888

Avalide Tablets (Potentiation of orthostatic hypotension)........ 2874

Avandamet Tablets (Alcohol potentiates the effect of metformin on lactate metabolism; patients should be warned against excessive alcohol intake, acute or chronic)........ 1373

Avinza Capsules (Patients must not consume alcoholic beverages, prescription or non-prescription medications containing alcohol while on morphine sulfate therapy. Consumption of alcohol while taking morphine sulfate may result in the rapid release and absoption of a potentially fatal dose of morphine)........ 1741

Bayer Aspirin Comprehensive Prescribing Information (Chronic heavy alcohol users, 3 or more drinks per day, should consult their physicians for advice on when and how they should take pain relievers/fever reducers including aspirin)........ ▣ 796

BC Allergy Sinus Cold Powder (Individuals consuming 3 or more alcohol-containing drinks per day should consult their physician for advice on when and how they should take this product; increases drowsiness; avoid concurrent use)........ ▣ 677

Benicar HCT Tablets (Concurrent administration could cause potentiation of orthostatic hypotension)........ 1044

BiDil Tablets (The effects of BiDil on vasodilators, including alcohol, may be additive)........ 2171

Bufferin Extra Strength Tablets (Concomitant consumption of alcohol may cause liver damage)........ ▣ 678

Buprenex Injectable (Increased CNS depression)....2716

Captopril Tablets (Drugs having vasodilator activity should, if possible, be discontinued before starting captopril)....2149

Catapres Tablets (Clonidine may potentiate the CNS-depressive effects)....843

Catapres-TTS (Clonidine may potentiate the CNS-depressive effects)....844

Celexa Tablets (Although citalopram did not potentiate cognitive and motor effects of alcohol, concurrent use is not recommended)....1176

Cesamet Capsules (Co-administration is cautioned in individuals receiving concomitant therapy with alcohol because of the potential for additive or synergistic CNS effects; also reported to increase the positive subjective mood effects of smoked marijuana)....3340

Cialis Tablets (Both tadalafil and alcohol act as mild vasodilators. When mild vasodilators are taken in combination, blood-pressure lowering effects of each individual compound may be increased. Substantial consumption of alcohol in combination with tadalafil may increase the potential for orthostatic signs and symptoms, including increase in heart rate, decrease in standing blood pressure, dizziness, and headache)....1838

Clorpres Tablets (Clonidine may enhance the CNS-depressive effects of alcohol; orthostatic hypotension may be aggravated by alcohol)....2153

Clozaril Tablets (Given the primary CNS effect of clozapine, caution is advised in using it concomitantly with alcohol)....2184

Comtan Tablets (Possible additive sedative effects)....2189

Comtrex Maximum Strength Cold & Cough Day/Night Caplets - Day Formulation (Concurrent use may increase drowsiness)....■□ 726

Comtrex Maximum Strength Cold & Cough Day/Night Caplets - Night Formulation (Concurrent use may increase drowsiness)....■□ 726

Comtrex Maximum Strength Non-Drowsy Cold & Cough Caplets (Chronic heavy alcohol users, 3 or more alcoholic drinks per day, should consult their physicians for advice on when and how to use pain relievers including acetaminophen)....■□ 725

Comtrex Maximum Strength Day/Night Severe Cold & Sinus Caplets - Day Formulation (Chronic heavy alcohol users, 3 or more alcoholic drinks per day, should consult their physicians for advice on when and how to use pain relievers including acetaminophen)....■□ 725

Comtrex Maximum Strength Day/Night Severe Cold & Sinus Caplets - Night Formulation (Chronic heavy alcohol users, 3 or more alcoholic drinks per day, should consult their physicians for advice on when and how to use pain relievers including acetaminophen; concurrent use may increase drowsiness effect)....■□ 725

Contac Cold and Flu Maximum Strength Caplets (Concomitant consumption of alcohol may cause liver damage; may increase drowsiness effect)....■□ 728

Contac Cold and Flu Day and Night Caplets (Day Formulation Only) (Concomitant consumption of alcohol may cause liver damage; may increase drowsiness effect)....■□ 727

Contac Cold and Flu Day and Night Caplets (Night Formulation Only) (Concomitant consumption of alcohol may cause liver damage; may increase drowsiness effect)....■□ 727

Contac Cold and Flu Non-Drowsy Caplets (Concomitant consumption of alcohol may cause liver damage; may increase drowsiness effect)....■□ 728

Coumadin Tablets (Decreased or increased prothrombin time response)....898

Covera-HS Tablets (Verapamil may increase blood alcohol concentrations and prolong its effect)....3139

Cymbalta Delayed-Release Capsules (Use of duloxetine concomitantly with heavy alcohol intake may be associated with severe liver injury; therefore, duloxetine should ordinarily not be prescribed for patients with substantial alcohol use)....1757

Dantrium Capsules (Co-administration may result in increased drowsiness; caution should be exercised)....2694

Demser Capsules (Additive sedative effects)....1953

Depacon Injection (Co-administration may result in additive CNS depression)....412

Depakene Capsules (Valproate produces CNS depression, especially when combined with another CNS depressant, such as alcohol)....417

Depakote Tablets (Valproate produces CNS depression, especially when combined with another CNS depressant, such as alcohol)....427

Depakote ER Tablets (Valproate produces CNS depression, especially when combined with another CNS depressant, such as alcohol)....434

DepoDur Extended-Release Injection (The concurrent use of other central nervous system (CNS) depressants, including alcohol, increases the risk of respiratory depression, hypotension, profound sedation or coma. Use with caution and with vigilant monitoring in patients taking these agents)....1110

Diastat Rectal Delivery System (Potential for synergistic CNS-depressant effect)....3343

Dilaudid Ampules (Additive CNS depression)....440

Dilaudid Oral Liquid (May exhibit an additive CNS depression)....445

Children's Dimetapp Cold & Allergy Elixir (May increase drowsiness effect)....■□ 730

Children's Dimetapp DM Cold & Cough Elixir (Increases drowsiness effect; avoid concurrent use)....■□ 731

Diovan HCT Tablets (Co-administration of thiazide diuretics and alcohol may result in potentiation of orthostatic hypotension)....2196

Ditropan XL Extended-Release Tablets (Enhances the drowsiness effect caused by anticholinergic agents such as oxybutynin)....2413

Diuril Oral Suspension (Potentiation of orthostatic hypotension may occur)....1954

Diuril Sodium Intravenous (Potentiation of orthostatic hypotension may occur)....2467

Duragesic Transdermal System (The concomitant use of fentanyl with other CNS depressants, including alcohol, may cause respiratory depression, hypotension, and profound sedation or potentially result in coma. When such combined therapy is contemplated, the dose of one or both agents should be significantly reduced)....2373

Effexor XR Capsules (Co-administration of venlafaxine as a stable regimen did not exaggerate the psychomotor and psychometric effects of alcohol; however, patients should be advised to avoid alcohol while taking venlafaxine)....3417

Emsam Transdermal System (The use of alcohol is not recommended while using selegiline transdermal system.)....903

Equetro Extended-Release Capsules (Because of its primary CNS effect, caution should be used when carbamazepine is taken with alcohol)....3180

Excedrin Extra Strength Caplets/Tablets/Geltabs (Concomitant consumption of alcohol may cause liver damage)....■□ 684

Excedrin Migraine Caplets/Tablets/Geltabs (Concomitant consumption of alcohol may cause liver damage)....■□ 609

Excedrin PM Caplets/Tablets/Geltabs (Concomitant consumption of alcohol may cause liver damage)....■□ 610

Excedrin Sinus Headache Caplets/Tablets (Having 3 or more alcoholic beverages may cause liver damage)....■□ 610

Excedrin Tension Headache Caplets/Tablets/Geltabs (Concomitant consumption of alcohol may cause liver damage)....■□ 611

Exubera Inhalation Powder (Alcohol may either increase or reduce the blood glucose-lowering effect of insulin. Co-administration may require insulin dose adjustment and particularly close monitoring)....2524

FazaClo Orally Disintegrating Tablets (Given the primary CNS effect of clozapine, caution is advised in using it concomitantly with alcohol)....551

Fortamet Extended-Release Tablets (Alcohol is known to potentiate the effect of metformin on lactate metabolism; therefore, patients should be warned against excessive acute or chronic intake)....3115

Furosemide Tablets (Aggravates orthostatic hypotension)....2154

Gabitril Tablets (Possible additive depressive effects)....984

Geodon Capsules (Somnolence was a commonly reported adverse event in patients treated with ziprasidone; concurrent use with alcohol or other CNS active drugs, such as depressants, should be undertaken with caution)....2529

Goody's Extra Strength Pain Relief Tablets (Individuals consuming 3 or more alcohol-containing drinks per day should consult their physicians for advice on when and how they should take this product)....■□ 685

Goody's PM Powder for Pain with Sleeplessness (Individuals consuming 3 or more alcohol-containing drinks per day should consult their physicians for advice on when and how they should take this product; avoid alcoholic beverages since diphenhydramine causes drowsiness)....■□ 612

Gris-PEG Tablets (The effects of alcohol may be potentiated by griseofulvin, producing such effects as tachycardia and flushing)....2502

Humalog-Pen (Co-administration with drugs with hypoglycemic activity may result in decreased insulin requirements)....1781

Humalog Mix 50/50-Pen (Insulin requirements may be decreased in the presence of drugs with hypoglycemic activity, such as alcohol)....1783

Hycodan Tablets (Exhibits an additive CNS depression)....1116

Hycotuss Expectorant Syrup (Exhibits an additive CNS depression)....1117

Hyzaar 50-12.5 Tablets (Potentiation of orthostatic hypotension)....1990

Imdur Tablets (Additive vasodilating effects)....3018

Indapamide Tablets (Aggravates orthostatic hypotension)....2156

Inderal LA Long-Acting Capsules (Slows the rate of absorption of propranolol)....3429

Ionsys Transdermal System (The concomitant use of other central nervous system depressants, such as alcoholic beverages, may produce additive depressant effects. Hypoventilation, hypotension, profound sedation, and coma may occur. Therefore, use of concomitant CNS depressants requires individual adjustment of dosage of the concomitant medication and observation of a given patient)....2379

Kadian Capsules (Co-administration may increase the risk of respiratory depression, hypotension and profound sedation and coma)....577

Klonopin Tablets (Potentiates CNS-depressant action)....2778

Lantus Injection (May either potentiate or weaken the blood-glucose-lowering effect of insulin)....2909

Levemir Injection (Co-administration may either potentiate or weaken the blood-glucose lowering effect of insulin)....2320

Lexapro Tablets (Given the primary CNS effects of escitalopram, concurrent use is not recommended)....1190

Lithostat Tablets (Acetohydroxamic acid taken in association with alcoholic beverages has resulted in rash)....2140

Lotensin HCT Tablets (Orthostatic hypotension produced by thiazides may be potentiated by alcohol)....2246

Lunesta Tablets (An additive effect on psychomotor performance was seen with co-administration of eszopiclone and alcohol 0.70 g/kg for up to 4 hours after alcohol consumption)....3142

Lyrica Capsules (Alcohol consumption should be avoided while taking pregabalin, as pregabalin may potentiate the impairment of motor skills and sedation of alcohol)....2539

Marinol Capsules (Co-administration results in additive drowsiness and CNS depression)....3333

Matulane Capsules (Concurrent use may produce an Antabuse-like reaction; concomitant use should be avoided) 3191

Meridia Capsules (Concurrent use has not resulted in psychomotor reactions of clinical significance, however, concomitant use with excessive alcohol is not recommended) 489

MetroGel-Vaginal Gel (Possibility of a disulfiram-like reaction) 1855

Mevacor Tablets (Lovastatin should be used with caution in patients who have consumed substantial quantity of alcohol and have a past history of liver disease; active liver disease and unexplained elevation in transaminase are contraindications to the use of lovastatin) 2021

Micardis HCT Tablets (Potentiation of orthostatic hypotension) 856

Miradon Tablets (Has been reported to diminish and/or increase oral anticoagulant response, i.e., decreased prothrombin time response significantly) 3042

Moduretic Tablets (Potentiation of orthostatic hypotension) 2028

MS Contin Tablets (Respiratory depression, hypotension and profound sedation or coma may result) 2701

Nembutal Sodium Solution, USP (Concomitant use of other CNS depressants may produce additive depressant effects) 2470

Niaspan Extended-Release Tablets (Concomitant alcohol may increase the side effects of flushing and pruritus and should be avoided around the time of Niaspan ingestion) 1730

Nitro-Dur Transdermal Infusion System (Enhances sensitivity to the hypotensive effects) 3046

Nitrolingual Pumpspray (Enhanced sensitivity to hypotensive effects) 3120

NovoLog Injection (May either potentiate or weaken the blood-glucose-lowering effect of insulin) 2326

Numorphan Injection (Concomitant use may produce additive CNS depressant effects) 1120

Nytol QuickGels Softgels Maximum Strength (Concurrent use will heighten the depressant effect of Nytol; avoid alcoholic beverages while taking this product) .... ▣ 616

Opana Tablets (The concomitant use of other CNS depressants including sedatives, hypnotics, tranquilizers, general anesthetics, phenothiazines, other opioids, and alcohol may produce additive CNS depressant effects. Additive effects resulting in respiratory depression, hypotension, profound sedation or coma may result if these drugs are taken in combination with the usual doses of oxymorphone hydrochloride) 1122

OxyContin Tablets (Concurrent use with the usual dose of OxyContin may result in respiratory depression, profound sedation or coma) 2703

OxyIR Capsules (Concomitant use may exhibit an additive CNS depression) 2708

Oxytrol Transdermal System (May enhance drowsiness caused by anticholinergic agents such as oxybutynin) 3392

Parnate Tablets (Concurrent use is contraindicated; a marked potentiating effect on alcohol has been reported) 1527

Paxil Tablets (Concurrent use should be avoided) 1530

Percocet Tablets (Additive CNS depression) 1131

Percodan Tablets (Additive CNS depression) 1132

Permax Tablets (Pergolide may cause somnolence; concurrent use with alcohol may result in additive sedative effects) 3356

Pexeva Tablets (Avoid the use of alcohol while taking Pexeva) 1694

Phenergan Tablets and Suppositories (Promethazine may increase, prolong, or intensify the sedative action of other CNS depressants, such as alcohol) 3440

Phenytek Capsules (Acute alcohol intake may increase phenytoin serum levels; chronic alcohol abuse may decrease phenytoin serum levels) 2160

Photofrin for Injection (Compounds that quench active oxygen species or scavenge radicals, such as ethanol, would be expected to decrease photodynamic therapy; no human data available to support or rebut this possibility) 702

Prinzide Tablets (Co-administration of thiazide and alcohol may potentiate orthostatic hypotension) 2056

ProSom Tablets (Co-administration may result in increased CNS depression) 517

Provigil Tablets (The use of modafinil in combination with alcohol has not been studied. It is advisable to avoid alcohol while taking modafinil) 988

Prozac Pulvules and Liquid (Concurrent use with CNS active agents, such as alcohol, requires caution) 1801

Requip Tablets (Possible additive sedative effects) 1555

Rilutek Tablets (Alcohol may increase the risk of hepatotoxicity; patients on riluzole should be discouraged from drinking excessive amounts of alcohol) 2930

Risperdal Tablets (Caution should be used when risperidone is taken in combination with alcohol) 1676

Robitussin Cough & Cold Long-Acting Liquid (Avoid alcoholic beverages. Consumption of alcohol may increase the drowsiness effect) .... ▣ 735

Robitussin Cough & Allergy Syrup (Avoid alcoholic beverages when using this product) .... ▣ 736

Robitussin Cough & Cold Nighttime Liquid (Avoid alcoholic beverages when using this product) .... ▣ 736

Robitussin Cough, Cold & Flu Nighttime Liquid (Chronic heavy alcohol users, 3 or more drinks per day, should consult their physicians for advice on when and how they should take pain relievers/fever reducers including acetaminophen; increases drowsiness effect) .... ▣ 738

Robitussin Pediatric Cough & Cold Nighttime Liquid (Avoid alcoholic beverages when using this product) .... ▣ 736

Rozerem Tablets (With single-dose, daytime co-administration of ramelteon 32 mg and alcohol (0.6 g/kg), there were no clinically meaningful or statistically significant effects on peak or total exposure to ramelteon. However, an additive effect was seen on some measures of psychomotor performance (ie. the Digit Symbol Substitution Test, the Psychomotor Vigilance Task Test, and a Visual Analog Scale of sedation) at some post-dose time points. No additive effect was seen on the Delayed Word Recognition Test. Because alcohol by itself impairs performance, and the intended effect of ramelteon is to promote sleep, patients should be cautioned not to consume alcohol when using ramelteon) 3231

Seromycin Capsules (Concurrent use increases the possibility and risk of epileptic episodes) 1813

Seroquel Tablets (The cognitive and motor effect of alcohol is potentiated; alcohol use should be avoided) 690

Simply Sleep Caplets (Diphenhydramine is an antihistamine with sedative properties; concurrent use with alcoholic beverages should be avoided) 1868

Skelaxin Tablets (Skelaxin may enhance the effects of alcohol, barbiturates and other CNS depressants) 1716

Sleep-Tite Caplets (Concurrent use is not recommended) .... ▣ 832

Sominex Original Formula Tablets (Concurrent use of alcoholic beverages is not recommended) .... ▣ 616

Sonata Capsules (Concurrent use may produce additive CNS depressant effects) 1717

Soriatane Capsules (Clinical evidence has shown that etretinate can be formed with concurrent ingestion of acitretin and ethanol) 1013

St. Joseph 81 mg Aspirin Chewable and Enteric Coated Tablets (Chronic heavy alcohol users, 3 or more drinks per day, in combination with analgesic/antipyretic drug products containing aspirin increases the risk of adverse GI events, including stomach bleeding) 1869

St. Joseph 81 mg Aspirin (Consuming 3 or more alcoholic beverages can increase the risk of stomach bleeding) .... ▣ 688

Sustiva Capsules (Potential for additive central nervous system effects when Sustiva is used concomitantly with alcohol) 930

Symbyax Capsules (Alcohol may potentiate the orthostatic effect of olanzapine, increasing the risk of orthostatic hypotension. Therefore, patients should be advised to avoid alcohol while taking Symbyax) 1819

Symmetrel Tablets (May increase the potential for CNS effects such as dizziness, confusion, light-headedness and orthostatic hypotension; avoid excessive alcohol usage) 1135

Tasmar Tablets (Possible additive sedative effects when used in combination with CNS depressants, such as alcohol) 3358

Teveten HCT Tablets (May potentiate orthostatic hypotension) 1737

Thalomid Capsules (Thalidomide has been reported to enhance the sedative activity of alcohol) 965

TheraFlu Cold & Cough Hot Liquid (Concurrent use may increase drowsiness; avoid alcoholic drinks) .... ▣ 740

TheraFlu Cold & Sore Throat Hot Liquid (Concurrent use may increase drowsiness; avoid alcoholic drinks) .... ▣ 741

TheraFlu Flu & Chest Congestion Hot Liquid (Avoid alcoholic drinks) .... ▣ 741

TheraFlu Flu & Sore Throat Hot Liquid (Concurrent use may increase drowsiness; avoid alcoholic drinks) .... ▣ 742

TheraFlu Daytime Severe Cold Hot Liquid (Chronic heavy alcohol users, 3 or more drinks per day, should consult their physicians for advice on when and how they should take pain relievers/fever reducers, including acetaminophen; may increase the drowsiness effect) .... ▣ 742

TheraFlu Nighttime Severe Cold Hot Liquid (Concurrent use may increase drowsiness; avoid alcoholic drinks) .... ▣ 740

TheraFlu Warming Relief Daytime Severe Cold (Consuming 3 or more alcoholic beverages with this product may cause hepatotoxicity) .... ▣ 743

TheraFlu Warming Relief Nighttime Severe Cold (Consuming 3 or more alcoholic beverages with this product may cause hepatotoxicity) .... ▣ 743

TheraFlu Thin Strips Multi Symptom (Co-administration with alcohol may increase drowsiness) .... ▣ 744

Thioridazine Hydrochloride Tablets (Thioridazine is capable of potentiating CNS depressants) 2163

Thiothixene Capsules (Possible additive effects which may include hypotension) 2165

Tindamax Tablets (Alcoholic beverages should be avoided during tinidazole therapy and for three days afterward because abdominal cramps, nausea, vomiting, headaches and flushing may occur) 2142

Topamax Tablets (Potential for increased CNS depression) 2404

Transderm Scōp Transdermal Therapeutic System (Scopolamine is an anticholinergic agent and causes certain CNS effects, such as drowsiness and dizziness, and hence it should be used with care in patients on concomitant therapy) 2177

Tranxene T-TAB Tablets (Actions of benzodiazepines may be potentiated; prolonged sleeping time) 2474

Trecator Tablets (Excessive ethanol ingestion should be avoided because a psychotic reaction has been reported) 3487

Triaminic Nighttime Cold & Cough Liquid (Concomitant consumption of alcohol may cause liver damage) .... ▣ 746

Triaminic Cough & Runny Nose Softchews (May increase drowsiness effect) .... ▣ 748

Trileptal Tablets (Oxcarbazepine causes dizziness and somnolence, concurrent use with alcohol could result in possible additive sedative effect) 2300

Tri-Luma Cream (Patients should avoid topical products containing high alcohol concentrations) 1213

Trizivir Tablets (Concurrent use decreases the elimination of abacavir causing an increase in overall exposure) **1589**

Tussionex Pennkinetic Extended-Release Suspension (Combined use may result in additive CNS depression) **3327**

Regular Strength Tylenol Tablets (Chronic heavy alcohol users, 3 or more drinks per day, should consult their physicians for advice on when and how they should take pain relievers including acetaminophen) **1870**

Tylenol 8 Hour Extended Release Caplets (Chronic heavy alcohol users, 3 or more drinks per day, should consult their physicians for advice on when and how they should take pain relievers including acetaminophen) .... ▣ **695**

Tylenol Chest Congestion Caplets with Cool Burst (Consuming 3 or more alcoholic beverages with this product may cause hepatotoxicity) .... ▣ **722**

Tylenol Cold Head Congestion Daytime Caplets with Cool Burst and Gelcaps (Concomitant consumption of alcohol may cause liver damage) .... ▣ **750**

Tylenol Cold Head Congestion Nighttime Caplets with Cool Burst (Concomitant consumption of alcohol may cause liver damage) .... ▣ **750**

Tylenol Cold Head Congestion Severe Caplets with Cool Burst (Concomitant consumption of alcohol with acetaminophen may cause liver damage; alcohol may increase drowsiness effect) .... ▣ **750**

Tylenol Cold Multi-Symptom Daytime Caplets with Cool Burst and Gelcaps (Concomitant consumption of alcohol may cause liver damage) .... ▣ **752**

Tylenol Cold Multi-Symptom Daytime Liquid (Chronic heavy alcohol users, 3 or more drinks per day, should consult their physicians for advice on when and how they should take pain relievers including acetaminophen) .... ▣ **752**

Tylenol Cold Multi-Symptom NightTime Caplets with Cool Burst (Concomitant consumption of alcohol may cause liver damage) .... ▣ **752**

Tylenol Cold Multi-Symptom NightTime Liquid with Cool Burst (Concomitant consumption of alcohol may cause liver damage) .... ▣ **752**

Tylenol Cold Multi-Symptom Severe Caplets with Cool Burst (Chronic heavy alcohol users, 3 or more drinks per day, should consult their physicians for advice on when and how they should take pain relievers including acetaminophen) .... ▣ **752**

Tylenol Cold Multi-Symptom Severe Daytime Liquid (Concomitant consumption of alcohol may cause liver damage) .... ▣ **752**

Tylenol Cough & Sore Throat Daytime Liquid with Cool Burst (Concomitant consumption of alcohol may cause liver damage) .... ▣ **790**

Tylenol Cough & Sore Throat Nighttime Liquid with Cool Burst (Concomitant consumption of alcohol may cause liver damage) .... ▣ **790**

Extra Strength Tylenol PM Caplets, Vanilla Caplets, Geltabs, Gelcaps and Liquid (Concurrent use may increase drowsiness effect; chronic heavy alcohol abusers, 3 or more drinks per day, may be at increased risk of liver toxicity from excessive acetaminophen use) **1875**

Tylenol Sinus Severe Congestion Caplets with Cool Burst (Chronic heavy alcohol users, 3 or more drinks per day, should consult their physicians for advice on when and how they should take pain relievers including acetaminophen) .... ▣ **778**

Tylenol Sore Throat Daytime Liquid with Cool Burst (Concomitant consumption of alcohol may cause liver damage) .... ▣ **790**

Tylenol Sore Throat Nighttime Liquid with Cool Burst (Concomitant consumption of alcohol with acetaminophen may cause liver damage; alcohol may increase drowsiness effect) .... ▣ **790**

Tylenol with Codeine Tablets (Concurrent use with other CNS depressants may exhibit an additive CNS depression) **2391**

Tylenol Severe Allergy Caplets (Concurrent use may increase drowsiness effect; chronic heavy alcohol abusers, 3 or more drinks per day, may be at increased risk of liver toxicity from excessive acetaminophen use) **1872**

Tylenol Chest Congestion Caplets with Cool Burst (Concurrent use may increase drowsiness effect; chronic heavy alcohol abusers, 3 or more drinks per day, may be at increased risk of liver toxicity from excessive acetaminophen use) **1872**

Tylenol Cold Severe Congestion Non-Drowsy Caplets with Cool Burst (Chronic heavy alcohol abusers, 3 or more drinks per day, may be at increased risk of liver toxicity from acetaminophen use) **1874**

Tylenol Cold Head Congestion Daytime Caplets with Cool Burst (Concurrent use may increase drowsiness effect; chronic heavy alcohol abusers, 3 or more drinks per day, may be at increased risk of liver toxicity from excessive acetaminophen use) **1873**

Tylenol Cold Head Congestion Nighttime Caplets with Cool Burst (Concurrent use may increase drowsiness effect; chronic heavy alcohol abusers, 3 or more drinks per day, may be at increased risk of liver toxicity from excessive acetaminophen use) **1873**

Tylenol Cold Multi-Symptom Daytime Caplets with Cool Burst and Gelcaps (Consumption of 3 or more alcoholic drinks every day, need to ask your doctor whether you should take acetaminophen; may be at increased risk of liver toxicity from acetaminophen use) **1874**

Tylenol Cough & Sore Throat Daytime Liquid with Cool Burst (Consumption of 3 or more alcoholic drinks everyday, need to ask your doctor whether you should take acetaminophen; may be at increased risk of liver toxicity from acetaminophen use) **1877**

Tylenol Sinus Severe Congestion Caplets with Cool Burst (Concurrent use may increase drowsiness effect; chronic heavy alcohol abusers, 3 or more drinks per day, may be at increased risk of liver toxicity from excessive acetaminophen use) **1876**

Tylenol Sinus Congestion & Pain Daytime Caplets with Cool Burst and Gelcaps (Concurrent use may increase drowsiness effect; chronic heavy alcohol abusers, 3 or more drinks per day, may be at increased risk of liver toxicity from excessive acetaminophen use) **1876**

Tylenol Sinus Congestion & Pain Nighttime Caplets with Cool Burst (May increase drowsiness effect) **1876**

Tylenol Sinus Congestion & Pain Severe Caplets with Cool Burst (Avoid concurrent use; chronic heavy alcohol abusers, 3 or more drinks per day, may be at increased risk of liver toxicity from acetaminophen use) **1876**

Tylenol Sore Throat Nighttime Liquid with Cool Burst (Concurrent use may increase drowsiness effect; chronic heavy alcohol abusers, 3 or more drinks perday, may be at increased risk of liver toxicity from excessive acetaminophen use) **1877**

Women's Tylenol Menstrual Relief Caplets (Chronic heavy alcohol users, 3 or more drinks per day, should consult their physicians for advice on when and how they should take pain relievers, including acetaminophen) **1877**

Ultram ER Tablets (Tramadol hydrochloride is contraindicated in acute intoxication with alcohol. Tramadol hydrochloride should be used with caution and in reduced dosages when administered to patients receiving CNS depressants, such as alcohol. Tramadol may be expected to have additive effects when used in conjunction with alcohol) **2392**

Uniphyl Tablets (Concurrent use with a single dose of alcohol (3mL/kg of whiskey) decreases theophylline clearance for up to 24 hours) **2710**

Uniretic Tablets (Co-administration of alcohol with thiazide diuretics may result in potentiation of orthostatic hypotension) **3100**

Valium Tablets (May potentiate the actions of diazepam) **2819**

Vandazole Vaginal Gel (The patient should be cautioned about drinking alcohol while being treated with metronidazole vaginal gel) **3338**

Ventavis Inhalation Solution (Iloprost has the potential to increase the hypotensive effect of vasodilators and antihypertensive agents) **1020**

Verelan PM Extended-Release Capsules, Controlled-Onset (Verapamil has been found to significantly inhibit ethanol elimination resulting in elevated blood ethanol concentration that may prolong the intoxicating effects of alcohol) **3106**

Vicks 44M Cough, Cold & Flu Relief Liquid (May increase drowsiness effect; patients consuming 3 or more alcoholic drinks per day should consult their physician for advice on when and how they should take this medication) **2680**

Pediatric Vicks 44m Cough & Cold Relief Liquid (May increase drowsiness effect) **2676**

Pediatric Vicks 44m Cough & Cold Relief Liquid (Concomitant consumption of alcohol may cause liver damage) .... ▣ **759**

Vicks DayQuil LiquiCaps/Liquid Multi-Symptom Cold/Flu Relief (Concomitant consumption of alcohol may cause liver damage) .... ▣ **761**

Vicks DayQuil Multi-Symptom Cold/Flu Relief LiquiCaps (Patients consuming 3 or more alcoholic drinks per day should consult their physician for advice on when and how they should take this medication) **2678**

Vicks NyQuil Multi-Symptom Cold/Flu Relief LiquiCaps (May increase drowsiness effect; patients consuming 3 or more alcoholic drinks per day should consult their physician for advice on when and how they should take this medication) **2681**

Vicks NyQuil LiquiCaps/Liquid Multi-Symptom Cold/Flu Relief (Chronic heavy alcohol users, 3 or more drinks per day, are at increased risk of liver toxicity from excessive acetaminophen use; alcohol increases drowsiness effect and concurrent use of alcoholic beverages should be avoided) .... ▣ **763**

Children's Vicks NyQuil Cold/Cough Relief Liquid (May increase drowsiness effect) **2680**

Vicodin Tablets (May exhibit an additive CNS depression) **535**

Vicodin ES Tablets (Additive CNS depression) **536**

Vicodin HP Tablets (Concurrent use results in an additive CNS depression) **538**

Vicoprofen Tablets (May exhibit additive CNS depression) **539**

Visudyne for Injection (Co-administration with compounds that quench active oxygen species or scavenge radicals, such as ethanol, would be expected to decrease verteporfin activity) **2305**

Wellbutrin SR Sustained-Release Tablets (Bupropion hydrochloride is contraindicated in patients undergoing abrupt discontinuation of alcohol. The consumption of alcohol during treatment with bupropion hydrochloride should be minimized or avoided) **1607**

Xyrem Oral Solution (The combined use of alcohol with sodium oxybate may result in potentiation of the central nervous system-depressant effects of sodium oxybate and alcohol) **1688**

Ziagen Tablets (Decreases the elimination of abacavir causing an increase in overall exposure) **1626**

Zicam Maximum Strength Flu Daytime (Concurrent use may increase drowsiness; avoid alcoholic beverages) .... ▣ **768**

Zicam Maximum Strength Flu Nighttime (Concurrent use may increase drowsiness; avoid alcoholic beverages) .... ▣ **768**

Zocor Tablets (Simvastatin causes persistent increases in serum transaminase in 1% of patients; therefore, it should be used with caution in patients who consume substantial quantities of alcohol) **2105**

Zoloft Oral Concentrate (Patients should be told that although sertraline hydrochloride has not been shown in experiments with normal subjects to increase the mental and motor skill impairments caused by alcohol, the concomitant use of sertraline hydrochloride and alcohol is not advised) **2586**

Zyban Sustained-Release Tablets (Bupropion hydrochloride is contraindicated in patients undergoing abrupt discontinuation of alcohol. The consumption of alcohol during treatment with bupropion hydrochloride should be minimized or avoided) 1644
Zydone Tablets (Co-administration may exhibit additive CNS depression) 1139
Zyprexa Tablets (Co-administration of alcohol with olanzapine potentiates orthostatic hypotension; concurrent use should be avoided) 1830
Zyprexa IntraMuscular (Co-administration of alcohol with olanzapine potentiates orthostatic hypotension; concurrent use should be avoided) 1830
Zyrtec Tablets (Concurrent use may result in additional impairment of CNS performance and reduction in mental alertness) 2594
Zyrtec-D 12 Hour Extended Release Tablets (Concurrent use may result in additional reduction in alertness impairment of CNS performance) 2597

Anchovies

Parnate Tablets (Potential for hypertensive crisis; concurrent use is contraindicated) 1527

Avocados

Parnate Tablets (Potential for hypertensive crisis; concurrent use is contraindicated) 1527

Bananas

Matulane Capsules (Procarbazine exhibits some MAO inhibitory activity: concurrent use should be avoided) 3191
Parnate Tablets (Potential for hypertensive crisis; concurrent use is contraindicated) 1527

Beans, broad

Parnate Tablets (Potential for hypertensive crisis; concurrent use is contraindicated) 1527

Beans, Fava

Parnate Tablets (Potential for hypertensive crisis; concurrent use is contraindicated) 1527

Beer, alcohol-free

Parnate Tablets (Potential for hypertensive crisis; concurrent use is contraindicated) 1527

Beer, unspecified

Parnate Tablets (Potential for hypertensive crisis; concurrent use is contraindicated) 1527

Beverages, caffeine-containing

Fosamax Tablets (Concomitant administration of alendronate with coffee reduces bioavailability by approximately 60%) 1969
Fosamax Plus D Tablets (Concomitant administration of alendronate with coffee reduces bioavailability by approximately 60%) 1977
Parnate Tablets (Potential for hypertensive crisis; concurrent use is contraindicated) 1527

Beverages with high tyramine

Azilect Tablets (Severe hypertensive reactions have followed the administration of tyramine rich beverages and non-selective MAO inhibitors) 3293
Emsam Transdermal System (As a class, MAO inhibitors have been associated with hypertensive crises caused by the ingestion of foods with a high concentration of tyramine) 903
Zyvox Tablets (Co-administration has resulted in a significant pressor response; patients receiving linezolid should avoid consuming large amounts of beverages containing tyramine) 2652

Broccoli

Biltricide Tablets (Concomitant administration of drugs that increase the activity of drug metabolizing liver enzymes (Cytochrome P450) may reduce plasma levels of praziquantel) 2976
Cafcit Injection (Caffeine has the potential to interact with drugs that induce CYP1A2) 1886
Rozerem Tablets (Efficacy may be reduced when ramelteon is used in combination with strong CYP enzyme inducers such as rifampin) 3231
Symbyax Capsules (Agents that induce CYP1A2 or glucuronyl transferase enzymes may cause an increase in olanzapine concentration) 1819
Zyprexa Tablets (May cause an increase in olanzapine clearance; therefore, a dosage increase might be considered) 1830
Zyprexa IntraMuscular (May cause an increase in olanzapine clearance; therefore, a dosage increase might be considered) 1830

Brussel Sprouts

Biltricide Tablets (Concomitant administration of drugs that increase the activity of drug metabolizing liver enzymes (Cytochrome P450) may reduce plasma levels of praziquantel) 2976
Cafcit Injection (Caffeine has the potential to interact with drugs that induce CYP1A2) 1886
Rozerem Tablets (Efficacy may be reduced when ramelteon is used in combination with strong CYP enzyme inducers such as rifampin) 3231
Symbyax Capsules (Agents that induce CYP1A2 or glucuronyl transferase enzymes may cause an increase in olanzapine concentration) 1819
Zyprexa Tablets (May cause an increase in olanzapine clearance; therefore, a dosage increase might be considered) 1830
Zyprexa IntraMuscular (May cause an increase in olanzapine clearance; therefore, a dosage increase might be considered) 1830

Caviar

Parnate Tablets (Potential for hypertensive crisis; concurrent use is contraindicated) 1527

Charbroiled Food

Biltricide Tablets (Concomitant administration of drugs that increase the activity of drug metabolizing liver enzymes (Cytochrome P450) may reduce plasma levels of praziquantel) 2976
Cafcit Injection (Caffeine has the potential to interact with drugs that induce CYP1A2) 1886
Rozerem Tablets (Efficacy may be reduced when ramelteon is used in combination with strong CYP enzyme inducers such as rifampin) 3231
Symbyax Capsules (Agents that induce CYP1A2 or glucuronyl transferase enzymes may cause an increase in olanzapine concentration) 1819
Zyprexa Tablets (May cause an increase in olanzapine clearance; therefore, a dosage increase might be considered) 1830
Zyprexa IntraMuscular (May cause an increase in olanzapine clearance; therefore, a dosage increase might be considered) 1830

Cheese, aged

Matulane Capsules (Procarbazine exhibits some MAO inhibitory activity: concurrent use should be avoided) 3191
Parnate Tablets (Potential for hypertensive crisis; concurrent use is contraindicated) 1527

Cheese, strong, unpasteurized

Parnate Tablets (Potential for hypertensive crisis; concurrent use is contraindicated) 1527

Cheese, unspecified

Parnate Tablets (Potential for hypertensive crisis; concurrent use is contraindicated) 1527

Chocolate

Parnate Tablets (Potential for hypertensive crisis; concurrent use is contraindicated) 1527

Cotton seed meal

Levoxyl Tablets (Concurrent use of cotton seed meal may bind and decrease the absorption of levothyroxine sodium from GI tract) 1712

Cream, sour

Parnate Tablets (Potential for hypertensive crisis; concurrent use is contraindicated) 1527

Dairy products

Cipro Tablets (Oral ciprofloxacin should not be taken concurrently with milk or yogurt alone, since absorption of ciprofloxacin may be significantly reduced; dietary calcium as part of a meal, however, does not significantly affect ciprofloxacin absorption) 2977
Cipro I.V. (Oral ciprofloxacin should not be taken concurrently with milk or yogurt alone, since absorption of ciprofloxacin may be significantly reduced; dietary calcium as part of a meal; however, does not significantly affect ciprofloxacin absorption) 2984
Cipro XR Tablets (Concurrent administration of ciprofloxacin with dairy products should be avoided since decreased absorption of ciprofloxacin is possible) 2990
Cuprimine Capsules (In all patients receiving penicillamine, it is important that penicillamine be given at least one hour apart from milk. This permits maximim absorption and reduces the likelihood of inactivation by metal binding in the gastrointestinal tract) 1947
Dulcolax Tablets (Dulcolax should not be taken within one hour of taking milk) .... ▣ 649
Emcyt Capsules (Calcium-rich foods may impair the absorption of estramustine) 2634
Fleet Phospho-soda ACCU-PREP (Concurrent use within one hour should be avoided) 1168
Fleet Prep Kits (Concurrent use within one hour should be avoided) 1170
Noroxin Tablets (Avoid simultaneous ingestion; administer norfloxacin at least one hour before or two hours after ingestion of milk and/or other dairy products) 2032
Tambocor Tablets (Milk may inhibit absorption in infants; a reduction in Tambocor dosage should be considered when milk is removed from the diet of infants) 1856

Diet, high-lipid

Adalat CC Tablets (High-fat meal increases peak plasma nifedipine concentrations by 60%, a prolongation in the time to peak concentration, but no significant change in the AUC; administer on an empty stomach) 2964
Albenza Tablets (Oral bioavailability appears to be enhanced when albendazole is co-administered with a fatty meal) 1338
Allegra-D 12 Hour Extended-Release Tablets (Co-administration with a high-fat meal decreased fexofenadine plasma concentrations Cmax and AUC, and Tmax was delayed by 50%; the rate of extent of pseudoephedrine absorption was not affected by food; administration of Allegra-D with food should be avoided) 2846
Gengraf Capsules (A high fat meal within one-half hour before cyclosporine administration decreases the AUC by 13% and Cmax by 33%) 459
Neoral Soft Gelatin Capsules (A high-fat meal consumed within one-half hour before Neoral administration decreased the AUC by 13% and Cmax by 33%) 2259
Rilutek Tablets (Co-administration with high-fat meal decreases absorption, reduces AUC by about 20% and peak blood levels by about 45%) 2930
Sular Tablets (Food with a high fat content has a pronounced effect on the release of nisoldipine resulting in a significant increase in peak concentration (Cmax) by up to 300%; concomitant intake of high-fat meal should be avoided) 3122
Uniphyl Tablets (Co-administration with a standardized high-fat meal results in increased peak plasma concentration and bioavailability; however, a precipitous increase in the rate and extent of absorption was not evident; the dosing should be ideally administered consistently either with or without food) 2710

Diet, potassium-rich

Midamor Tablets (Potential for rapid increases in serum potassium levels) 2026
Moduretic Tablets (Potential for rapid increases in serum potassium levels) 2028

Diet high in vitamin K

Coumadin Tablets (Decreased prothrombin time) 898
Miradon Tablets (Has been reported to diminish oral anticoagulant response, i.e., decreased prothrombin time response significantly) 3042

Dietary Fiber

Levoxyl Tablets (Concurrent use of dietary fiber may bind and decrease the absorption of levothyroxine sodium from GI tract) 1712

Drinks, hot, unspecified

Advicor Tablets (Concomitant hot drinks may increase the flushing and its use should be avoided around the time of Advicor administration) 1722
Niaspan Extended-Release Tablets (Concomitant hot drinks may increase the side effects of flushing and pruritus and should be avoided around the time of Niaspan ingestion) 1730

Figs, canned

Parnate Tablets (Potential for hypertensive crisis; concurrent use is contraindicated)....1527

Food, calcium-rich

Cipro XR Tablets (Concurrent administration of ciprofloxacin with calcium-fortified juices should be avoided since decreased absorption of ciprofloxacin is possible)....2990

Emcyt Capsules (Calcium-rich foods may impair the absorption of estramustine)....2634

Food, charcoal-broiled

Rilutek Tablets (Potential inducers of CYP1A2, such as charcoal-broiled food, could increase the rate of riluzole elimination)....2930

Food, unspecified

Accolate Tablets (Co-administration with food reduces mean bioavailability by approximately 40%; patients should be instructed to take Accolate at least 1 hour before or 2 hours after meals).... 671

Aceon Tablets (2 mg, 4 mg, 8 mg) (The presence of food in the GI tract does not affect the rate or extent of absorption of perindopril but reduces bioavailability of perindoprilat by about 35%; in clinical trials, perindopril was generally administered in a non-fasting state)....3194

Actonel Tablets (Mean oral bioavailability is decreased when risedronate is administered with food; risedronate sodium is effective when administered at least 30 minutes before breakfast)....2683

Actonel with Calcium Tablets (Mean oral bioavailability is decreased when risedronate is administered with food; risedronate sodium is effective when administered at least 30 minutes before breakfast)....2688

Adderall XR Capsules (Concurrent use with food prolongs T_{max} by 2.5 hours, however, food does not affect the extent of absorption)....3166

Agenerase Oral Solution (High-fat meals may decrease the absorption of Agenerase and should be avoided; Agenerase may be taken with meals of normal fat content)....1332

Altace Capsules (The rate of absorption is reduced, not the extent of absorption)....1702

Altoprev Extended-Release Tablets (Decreases the bioavailability of Altoprev)....3109

Aromasin Tablets (Exemestane plasma levels increased approximately 40% after high-fat breakfast)....2600

Avandamet Tablets (Food decreases the extent and slightly delays the absorption of metformin)....1373

Biaxin Filmtab Tablets (Food slightly delays both the onset of absorption and the formation of the active metabolite, but does not affect the extent of bioavailability; Biaxin may be administered without regard to food).... 402

Captopril Tablets (Reduces absorption by about 30% to 40%; should be given one hour before meals)....2149

Carbatrol Capsules (A high fat meal increased the rat of absorption of a single 400 mg dose but not the AUC; elimination half-life remains unchanged between fasting and fed states)....3171

Ceftin Tablets (Absorption is greater when taken after food)....1407

Celebrex Capsules (Co-administration with a high-fat meal delayed peak plasma levels for about 1 to 2 hours with an increase in total absorption (AUC) of 10% to 20%; Celebrex can be administered without regard to the timing of meals)....3134

CellCept Capsules (Food has no effect on MPA AUC, but has been shown to decrease MPA Cmax by 40%; it is recommended that CellCept be administered on an empty stomach)....2747

Cipro Tablets (Delays the oral absorption of the drug resulting in peak concentrations that are closer to two hours after dosing)....2977

Cipro I.V. (Delays the oral absorption of the drug resulting in peak concentrations that are closer to two hours after dosing)....2984

Clinoril Tablets (The peak plasma concentrations of biologically active sulfide metabolite is delayed slightly in the presence of food)....1924

Coreg Tablets (When carvedilol is administered with food, the rate of absorption is slowed, as evidenced by a delay in the time to reach peak plasma levels, with no significant difference in extent of bioavailability; patients should be instructed to take Coreg with food in order to minimize the risk of hypotension)....1414

Crixivan Capsules (Co-administration with a meal high in calories, fat, and protein has resulted in a 77% ± 8% reduction in AUC and an 84% +/- 7% reduction in Cmax; administer without food 1 hour before or 2 hours after a meal)....1940

Cuprimine Capsules (Food reduces the absorption of penicillamine. In all patients receiving penicillamine, it is important that penicillamine be given on an empty stomach, at least one hour before meals or two hours after meals. This permits maximum absorption and reduces the likelihood of inactivation by metal binding in the gastrointestinal tract)....1947

Demadex Tablets (Simultaneous food intake delays the time to Cmax by about 30 minutes, but overall bioavailability (AUC) and diuretic activity are unchanged)....2759

Diovan Tablets (Decreases the exposure (as measured by AUC) to valsartan about 40% and peak plasma concentration by about 50%)....2193

EC-Naprosyn Delayed-Release Tablets (The presence of food prolonged the time the EC-Naprosyn remained in the stomach, time to first detectable serum naproxen levels, and time to maximal naproxen levels (Tmax), but did not affect peak naproxen levels (Cmax))....2761

Eldepryl Capsules (The bioavailability of selegiline is increased 3 to 4 fold when it is taken with food)....3208

Epivir Tablets (Absorption of lamivudine was slower in the fed state compared with fasted state; there was no significant difference in systemic exposure in the fed state and fasted states; Epivir may be given with or without food)....1427

Erythromycin Delayed-Release Capsules, USP (Lowers the blood levels of systemically available erythromycin).... 457

Evista Tablets (Administration of raloxifene with a standardized, high fat meal increases the absorption of raloxifene, but does not lead to clinically meaningful changes in systemic exposure; Evista can be administered without regard to meals)....1763

Evoxac Capsules (Co-administration with food decreases the rate of absorption, with a fasting Tmax of 1.53 hours and a Tmax of 2.86 hours after a meal; the peak concentration is reduced by 17.3%)....1047

Exelon Capsules (Co-administration with food delays absorption (Tmax) by 90 minutes, lowers Cmax by approximately 30% and increases AUC by approximately 30%)....2206

Flomax Capsules (Tmax is reached by 4 to 5 hours under fasting conditions and by 6 to 7 hours when tamsulosin is administered with food; taking tamsulosin under fasted conditions results in a 30% increase in AUC and 40% to 70% increase in Cmax compared to fed conditions; Flomax should be taken approximately 30 minutes following the meal).... 850

Gabitril Tablets (A high fat meal decreases the rate (mean Tmax was prolonged to 2.5 hours, and Cmax was reduced by about 40%) but not the extent (AUC) of tiagabine).... 984

Gengraf Capsules (The administration of food with Gengraf decreases the cyclosporine AUC and Cmax).... 459

Hytrin Capsules (Delays the time to peak concentration by about 40 minutes; minimal effect on the extent of absorption).... 471

Imdur Tablets (May decrease the rate (increase in Tmax) but not the extent (AUC) of absorption)....3018

Imitrex Tablets (Delays the Tmax slightly by about 0.5 hour with no significant effect on the bioavailability)....1471

Invirase Capsules (Saquinavir 24-hour AUC and Cmax following the administration of a high calorie meal were an average two times higher than after a lower calorie, lower fat meal; the effect of food has been shown to persist for up to 2 hours)....2772

Kadian Capsules (Slows the rate of absorption of Kadian, the extent of absorption is not affected and Kadian can be administered without regard to meals; the pellets in Kadian should not be dissolved).... 577

Kaletra Tablets (Co-administration with moderate fat meal was associated with a mean increase in AUC and Cmax; to enhance bioavailability Kaletra should be taken with food).... 476

Keppra Tablets (Decreases Cmax by 20% and delays Tmax by 1.5 hours; does not affect the extent of absorption)....3314

Kytril Tablets (When oral granisetron was administered with food, AUC was decreased by 5% and Cmax increased by 30% in non-fasted individuals)....2784

Lamisil Tablets (Co-administration has resulted in an increase in the AUC of terbinafine of less than 20%)....2232

Lescol Capsules (Administration of regular formulation of fluvastatin with food reduces the rate but not the extent of absorption; administration with evening meal results in a two-fold decrease in Cmax and more than a two-fold increase in tmax as compared to administration 4 hours after the evening meal; administration of Lescol XL with a high fat meal delayed the absorption and increased the bioavailability by 50%)....2233

Levaquin Injection (Co-administration slightly prolongs the time to peak concentration by approximately 1 hour and slightly decreases the peak concentration by approximately 14%; levofloxacin can be administered without regard to food)....2384

Levaquin Tablets (Co-administration slightly prolongs the time to peak concentration by approximately 1 hour and slightly decreases the peak concentration by approximately 14%; levofloxacin can be administered without regard to food)....2384

Lofibra Tablets (The absorption of fenofibrate is increased when administered with food; Lofibra should be given with meals)....1219

Lotronex Tablets (Alosetron absorption is decreased by approximately 25% by co-administration with food with a mean delay in time to peak concentration of 15 minutes; Lotronex can be taken with or without food)....1512

Malarone Tablets (Dietary fat intake with atovaquone increases the rate and extent of absorption; Malarone should be taken with food or milky drink)....1517

Mavik Tablets (Slows absorption of trandolapril but does not affect AUC or Cmax).... 486

Maxalt Tablets (Delays the time to reach peak concentration by an hour; no significant effect on the bioavailability)....2008

Mepron Suspension (Food enhances absorption by approximately two-fold)....1521

Meridia Capsules (Co-administration with a standard breakfast has resulted in reduced peak M1 and M2 amine concentrations and delayed the time to peak by approximately three hours; the AUCs of M1 and M2 were not significantly altered).... 489

Micardis Tablets (Slightly reduces the bioavailability of telmisartan; Micardis tablets may be administered with or without food).... 854

Micardis HCT Tablets (Slightly reduces the bioavailability of telmisartan with reduction in AUC of about 6%).... 856

Mirapex Tablets (Food does not affect the extent of pramipexole absorption, although the time of maximum plasma concentration is increased by about 1 hour when the drug is taken with a meal).... 859

Mobic Tablets (Co-administration with a high-fat breakfast did not affect extent of absorption of meloxicam capsules but led to 22% higher Cmax values; mean Cmax values were achieved between 5 to 6 hours; Mobic tablets can be administered without regard to timing of meals).... 863

Neoral Soft Gelatin Capsules (Administration of food with Neoral decreases the AUC and Cmax)....2259

Noroxin Tablets (Co-administration may decrease the absorption of norfloxacin; administer at least one hour before or two hours after a meal) 2032

Omnicef Capsules (Although Cmax and AUC of cefdinir absorption from capsules are reduced by 44% and 33%, respectively, when given with a high-fat meal, the magnitude of these reductions is not likely to be clinically significant; therefore, cefdinir may be taken without regard to food) 511

Paxil Tablets (Co-administration with food resulted in a slight increase (6%) in AUC, but Cmax was 29% greater; time to reach peak plasma concentration decreased from 6.4 hours post-dosing to 4.9 hours) 1530

Pepcid for Oral Suspension (Bioavailability may be slightly increased by antacids) 2038

Pletal Tablets (Co-administration with a high-fat meal increases absorption, with an approximately 90% increase in Cmax and a 25% increase in AUC; patients should be advised to take Pletal at least one hour before or two hours after breakfast and dinner) 2455

Premphase Tablets (Administration with a high fat breakfast decreased total estrone Cmax and increased total equilin Cmax compared to fasting state, no other effect on rate or extent of absorption; administration with food doubles MPA Cmax and increases MPA AUC) 3456

Prempro Tablets (Administration with food decreased Cmax of total estrone compared to fasting state, no other effect on rate or extent of absorption; administration with food doubles MPA Cmax and increases MPA AUC) 3456

Prevacid Delayed-Release Capsules (Cmax and AUC are diminished by about 50% if the drug is given 30 minutes after food as opposed to the fasting condition; Prevacid should be taken before eating) 3271

PREVPAC (Both Cmax and AUC are diminished by about 50% if the lansoprazole is given 30 minutes after food as opposed to the fasting condition) 3284

Prilosec OTC Delayed-Release Tablets (Absorption begins only after the granules leave the stomach; Prilosec should be taken before eating) 2677

Prograf Capsules and Injection (The presence and composition of food has decreased both the rate and extent of tacrolimus absorption; this effect was most pronounced with a high-fat meal; the rate and extent of tacrolimus absorption were greatest under fasted conditions) 632

Prometrium Capsules (100 mg, 200 mg) (Concomitant food ingestion increases the bioavailability of Prometrium Capsules relative to the fasting state) 3203

Provigil Tablets (Delays the absorption (tmax) by approximately one hour; no effect on overall bioavailability) 988

Prozac Pulvules and Liquid (May delay absorption of fluoxetine inconsequentially; Prozac may be administered with or without food) 1801

Rapamune Oral Solution and Tablets (A high-fat meal altered the bioavailability characteristics of sirolimus compared to fasting; 34% decrease in the peak blood sirolimus concentration, a 3.5-fold increase in the time-to-peak concentration and 35% increase in total exposure; to minimize variability, Rapamune should be taken consistently with or without food) 3475

Rebetron Combination Therapy (Both AUC and Cmax increased by 70% when Rebetron was administered with a high-fat meal in a single-dose pharmacokinetic study; there are insufficient data to address the clinical relevance of these results) 3063

Requip Tablets (Food does not affect the extent of absorption of ropinirole, although Tmax is increased by 2.5 hours and Cmax is decreased by 25% when taken with a high fat meal) 1555

Ritalin LA Capsules (When Ritalin LA was administered with a high fat breakfast to adults, Ritalin LA had a longer lag time until absorption began and variable delays in the time until the peak concentration, the time until the interpeak minimum, and the time until the second peak; administration times relative to meals and meal composition may need to be individually titrated) 2271

Romazicon Injection (Ingestion of food during an IV infusion results in a 50% increase in clearance) 2804

Rythmol SR Capsules (Increased peak blood level and bioavailability in a single dose study) 2727

Seroquel Tablets (The bioavailability of quetiapine is marginally affected by administration with food, with Cmax and AUC values increased by 25% and 15%, respectively) 690

Sonata Capsules (A high-fat/heavy meal prolongs the absorption of zaleplon compared to fasting state, delays tmax by approximately 2 hours and reduces Cmax approximately 35%; the effect of Sonata on sleep onset may be reduced if it is taken with or immediately after a high-fat/heavy meal) 1717

Starlix Tablets (Administration of nateglinide with liquid meal significantly reduces peak plasma levels) 2292

Suprax (Increases time to maximal absorption approximately 0.8 hour) 1843

Sustiva Capsules (High fat meal may increase the absorption of Sustiva and should be avoided; it can be taken with or without meals of normal composition) 930

Targretin Capsules (Co-administration with a fat-containing meal has resulted in higher plasma bexarotene AUC and Cmax values; because safety and efficacy data are based upon administration with food, it is recommended that Targretin capsules be administered with or immediately following a meal) 1747

Tarka Tablets (Co-administration with food decreases verapamil bioavailability and the time to peak plasma concentration is delayed; bioavailability of trandolapril is not altered; Tarka should be administered with food) 524

Tasmar Tablets (Food given within 1 hour before and 2 hours after dosing of tolcapone decreases the relative bioavailability by 10% to 20%; Tasmar may be taken with or without food) 3358

Temodar Capsules (Co-administration with a modified high-fat breakfast has resulted in decrease in mean plasma concentration and AUC by 32% and 9%, respectively, and 2-fold increase in Tmax) 3073

Teveten Tablets (Co-administration with food delays absorption and causes variable changes in Cmax and AUC values which do not appear clinically important) 1735

Thalomid Capsules (Co-administration of Thalomid with a high fat meal causes minor changes in the observed AUC and Cmax values; however, it causes an increase in Tmax to approximately 6 hours) 965

Tricor Tablets (The absorption of fenofibrate is increased when administered with food; Tricor should be given with meals) 527

Uniretic Tablets (Bioavailability varies with formulation and food intake which reduces Cmax and AUC of moexiprilat by about 70% and 40% respectively after ingestion of low-fat breakfast or by 80% and 50% respectively after the ingestion of a high-fat breakfast; patients should be advised to take Uniretic one hour before a meal) 3100

Univasc Tablets (Food reduces Cmax and AUC by about 70% and 40% respectively after ingestion of a low-fat breakfast or by 80% and 50% respectively after the ingestion of high-fat breakfast) 3104

Valcyte Tablets (Co-administration with high fat meals has resulted in increased steady-state ganciclovir AUC and Cmax without any prolongation in time to peak plasma concentrations; Valcyte should be administered with food) 2813

Vantin Tablets and Oral Suspension (The extent of absorption and the mean peak plasma concentration increased when film-coated tablets were administered with food) 2645

Vesanoid Capsules (The absorption of retinoids as a class has been shown to be enhanced when taken with food) 2820

VFEND Tablets (When multiple doses of voriconazole are administered with high fat meals, the mean Cmax and AUC are reduced; VFEND tablets should be taken at least one hour before or one hour following a meal) 2564

Viagra Tablets (When Viagra is taken with a high fat meal, the rate of absorption is reduced with a mean delay in Tmax of 60 minutes and a mean reduction in Cmax of 29%) 2573

Viracept Tablets (Maximum plasma concentrations and AUC were 2- to 3-fold higher under fed conditions compared to fasting; Viracept should be taken with a meal or light snack) 2577

Viread Tablets (Increases the bioavailability and delays the time to tenofovir Cmax; Viread should be taken with a meal) 1301

Wellbutrin SR Sustained-Release Tablets (Food increases Cmax and AUC of bupropion by 11% and 17%, respectively; no clinically significant food effect) 1607

Xeloda Tablets (Reduces both rate and extent of absorption of capecitabine and delays Tmax of both parent and 5-FU) 2822

Xenical Capsules (Gastrointestinal events may increase when orlistat is taken with a diet high in fat) 2831

Zelnorm Tablets (Reduces the bioavailability of tegaserod; Zelnorm should be taken before meals) 2312

Zofran Tablets (Bioavailability slightly enhanced by food) 1639

Zoloft Oral Concentrate (Co-administration of Zoloft Tablets with food slightly increased AUC but the Cmax was 25% greater, while time to reach peak plasma concentration (Tmax) decreased from 8 hours to 5.5 hours; for oral concentrate, Tmax was slightly prolonged from 5.9 hours to 7 hours with food) 2586

Zyban Sustained-Release Tablets (Food increases Cmax and AUC of bupropion by 11% and 17% respectively. The mean time to peak concentration Tmax was prolonged by 1 hour; this effect was of no clinical significance) 1644

Zyflo Tablets (Co-administration has resulted in a small but statistically significant increase (27%) in zileuton Cmax without significant changes in the extent of absorption (AUC) or Tmax; zileuton can be administered with or without food) 1023

Zyrtec Tablets (Food has no effect on the extent of cetirizine absorption, but Tmax may be delayed and Cmax may be decreased in the presence of food) 2594

Zyvox Tablets (The time to reach maximum concentration is delayed from 1.5 hours to 2.2 hours and Cmax is decreased by about 17% when linezolid is co-administered with high fat food; linezolid may be administered without regard to the timing of meals) 2652

Food having a pH greater than 5.5

Creon 5 Capsules (Can dissolve the protective coating resulting in early release of enzymes, irritation of oral mucosa, and/or loss of enzyme activity) 3198

Ultrase Capsules (Can dissolve the protective coating resulting in early release of enzymes, irritation of oral mucosa, and/or loss of enzyme activity) 708

Ultrase MT Capsules (Can dissolve the protective enteric shell) 709

Food high in tyramine

Azilect Tablets (Severe hypertensive reactions have followed the administration of tyramine rich foods and non-selective MAO inhibitors) 3293

Emsam Transdermal System (As a class, MAO inhibitors have been associated with hypertensive crises caused by the ingestion of foods with a high concentration of tyramine) 903

Zyvox Tablets (Co-administration has resulted in a significant pressor response; patients receiving linezolid should avoid consuming large amounts of food containing tyramine) 2652

Food with high concentration of tyramine

Emsam Transdermal System (As a class, MAO inhibitors have been associated with hypertensive crises caused by the ingestion of foods with a high concentration of tyramine) 903

Matulane Capsules (Procarbazine exhibits some MAO inhibitory activity: concurrent use should be avoided).....................**3191**

Parnate Tablets (Potential for hypertensive crisis; concurrent use is contraindicated)...................**1527**

Fruit juices, unspecified

Allegra Capsules (Grapefruit, orange and apple may reduce the bioavailability and exposure of fexofenadine; it is recommended that fexofenadine should be taken with water)......................**2844**

Dexedrine Spansule Capsules (Lowers absorption of amphetamines)**1420**

DextroStat Tablets (Lowers absorption of amphetamines by acting as gastrointestinal acidifying agent)............................**3179**

Fruits, dried

Parnate Tablets (Potential for hypertensive crisis; concurrent use is contraindicated)...................**1527**

Fruits, overripe

Parnate Tablets (Potential for hypertensive crisis; concurrent use is contraindicated)...................**1527**

Grapefruit

Abilify Tablets (Inhibitors of CYP3A4 or CYP2D6 can inhibit aripiprazole elimination and cause increased blood levels) **882**

Abilify Tablets (Inhibitors of CYP3A4 can inhibit aripiprazole elimination and cause increased blood levels)**2450**

Adalat CC Tablets (Nifedipine is mainly eliminated by metabolism and is a substrate of CYP3A4. Inhibitors of CYP3A4 can impact the exposure to nifedipine and consequently its desirable and undesirable effects)......................**2964**

Angeliq Tablets (Inhibitors of CYP3A4 such as erythromycin, clarithromycin, ketoconazole, itraconazole, ritonavir and grapefruit juice may increase plasma concentrations of estrogens and may result in side effects) **762**

Avodart Soft Gelatin Capsules (Blood concentrations of dutasteride may increase in the presence of CYP3A4 inhibitors)**1390**

Biltricide Tablets (Grapefruit juice was reported to produce a 1.6-fold increase in the Cmax and a 1.9-fold increase in the AUC of praziquantel)......................**2976**

Buprenex Injectable (Buprenorphine is metabolized by the CYP3A4 isoenzyme; co-administration with inhibitors of CYP3A4 may cause decrease in clearance of buprenorphine)**2716**

Carbatrol Capsules (Carbamazepine is metabolized mainly by cytochrome P450 (CYP) 3A4 to the active carbamazepine 10,11 -epoxide, which is further metabolized to the trans-diol by epoxide hydrolase. Therefore, the potential exists for interaction between carbamazepine and any agent that inhibits CYP3A4 and/or epoxide hydrolase)**3171**

Cardizem LA Extended Release Tablets (Diltiazem is both a substrate and an inhibitor of the CYP3A4 enzyme system. Other drugs that are specific substrates, inhibitors, or inducers of this enzyme system may have a significant impact on the efficacy and side effect profile of diltiazem)**1728**

Cialis Tablets (Tadalafil is metabolized predominantly by CYP3A4 in the liver. The dose of tadalafil should be limited to 10 mg no more than once every 72 hours in patients taking potent inhibitors of CYP3A4)**1838**

Climara Transdermal System (Inhibitors of CYP3A4 such as erythromycin, clarithromycin, ketoconazole, itraconazole, ritonavir and grapefruit juice may increase plasma concentrations of estrogens and may result in side effects) **771**

Climara Pro Transdermal System (Inhibitors of CYP3A4 such as erythromycin, clarithromycin, ketoconazole, itraconazole, ritonavir and grapefruit juice may increase plasma concentrations of estrogens and may result in side effects) **776**

Covera-HS Tablets (Clinically significant interactions have been reported with inhibitors of CYP3A4 causing elevation of plasma levels of verapamil while inducers of CYP3A4 have caused a lowering of plasma levels of verapamil)**3139**

Crixivan Capsules (Co-administration of indinavir and other drugs that inhibit CYP3A4 may decrease the clearance of indinavir and may result in increased plasma concentrations of indinavir)**1940**

Decadron Tablets (Drugs which inhibit cytochrome P450 3A4 enzyme activity have the potential to result in increased plasma concentrations of corticosteroids)**1951**

Diastat Rectal Delivery System (Studies suggest that CYP2C19 and CYP3A4 are the principal enzymes involved in the initial oxidative metabolism of diazepam. Therefore, potential interactions may occur when diazepam is given concurrently with agents that affect CYP2C19 and CYP3A4 activity. Potential inhibitors of CYP3A4 could decrease the rate of diazepam elimination)...................**3343**

Duragesic Transdermal System (The concurrent use of CYP3A4 inhibitors with transdermal fentanyl may result in an increase in fentanyl plasma concentrations, which could increase or prolong adverse drug effects and may cause serious respiratory depression. In this situation, special patient care and observation are appropriate)..................................**2373**

Emend Capsules (Co-administration of EMEND with drugs that inhibit CYP3A4 activity may result in increased plasma concentrations of aprepitant and should be approached with caution)**1963**

Enjuvia Tablets (Inhibitors of CYP3A4 such as erythromycin, clarithromycin, ketoconazole, itraconazole, ritonavir and grapefruit juice may increase plasma concentrations of estrogens and may result in side effects)......................**1062**

Entocort EC Capsules (Concurrent use with extensive intake of grapefruit juice has caused rise in systemic exposure of budesonide by two-fold; ingestion of grapefruit should be avoided)................................**2698**

Equetro Extended-Release Capsules (Carbamazepine is metabolized mainly by CYP3A4 the active carbamazepine 10,11-epoxide, which is futher metabolized to the trans-diol by epoxide hydrolase. Therefore, the potential exists for interaction between carbamazepine and any agent that inhibits CYP3A4 and/or epoxide hydrolase. Agents that are CYP3A4 inhibitors may increase the plasma levels of carbamazepine. Thus, if a patient has been titrated to a stable dosage of carbamazepine, and then begins a course of treatment with a CYP3A4 or epoxide hydrolase inhibitor, it is reasonable to expect that a dose reduction for carbamazepine may be necessary)............................**3180**

Estrasorb Topical Emulsion (Inhibitors of CYP3A4 may increase plasma concentrations of estrogens and may result in side effects)**1147**

Estratest H.S. Tablets (Co-administration with inhibitors of CYP3A4 may increase plasma concentrations of estrogens and may result in side effects)**3199**

Evoxac Capsules (Drugs which inhibit CYP3A3/4 also inhibit the metabolism of cevimeline)........**1047**

Flonase Nasal Spray (Caution should be exercised when potent cytochrome P450 3A4 inhibitors are co-administered with fluticasone propionate)**1440**

Gengraf Capsules (Affects the metabolism of cyclosporine by increasing blood concentration of cyclosporine; concurrent use should be avoided)....................... **459**

Gleevec Tablets (Caution is recommended when administering Gleevec with inhibitors of the CYP3A4 family. Substances that inhibit CYP3A4 activity may decrease metabolism and increase imatinib concentrations. There is a significant increase in exposure to imatinib when Gleevec is co-administered with ketoconazole)**2227**

Hectorol Capsules (Cytochrome P450 inhibitors may inhibit the 25-hydroxylation of doxercalciferol. Hence, formation of the active doxercalciferol moiety may be hindered)**1275**

Inspra Tablets (Eplerenone should not be used with strong inhibitors of CYP450 3A4. Potent inhibitors of CYP3A4 caused increased exposure of about 5-fold, while less potent CYP3A4 inhibitors (e.g., erythromycin, saquinavir, verapamil, fluconazole) gave approximately 2-fold increases in exposure. Grapefruit juice caused only a small increase (about 25%) in exposure)**2536**

Ionsys Transdermal System (The concomitant use of fentanyl with CYP3A4 inhibitors may result in a decreases in fentanyl clearance, which could increase or prolong adverse drug effects including serious respiratory depression. In this situation, special patient care and observation is appropriate)**2379**

Iressa Tablets (Substances that are potent inhibitors of CYP3A4 (e.g., ketoconazole and itraconazole) decrease gefitinib metabolism and increase gefitinib plasma concentrations)..... **684**

Levitra Tablets (Concomitant use with moderate/strong CYP 3A4 inhibitors results in significant increases in plasma levels of vardenafil)**3034**

Lexiva Tablets (Amprenavir, the active metabolite of fosamprenavir, is metabolized in the liver by the cytochrome P450 enzyme system. Amprenavir may inhibit or induce CYP3A4. Caution should be used when co-administering medications that are substrates, inhibitors, or inducers of CYP3A4, or potentially toxic medications that are metabolized by CYP3A4)**1505**

Lotronex Tablets (Co-administration of alosetron and strong CYP3A4 inhibitors has not been evaluated but should be undertaken with caution because of similar potential drug interactions)**1512**

Menostar Transdermal System (Inhibitors of CYP3A4 may increase plasma concentrations of estrogens and may result in side effects) **782**

Mevacor Tablets (The risk of myopathy/rhabdomyolysis is increased by concomitant use of lovastatin with potent inhibitors of CYP3A4, particularly with higher doses of lovastatin; concomitant use should be avoided unless the benefits of combined therapy outweigh the increased risk)..........**2021**

Migranal Nasal Spray (Co-administration of dihydroergotamin with potent CYP3A4 inhibitors results in vasospasm that can lead to cerebral ischemia and/or ischemia of the extremities, therefore it is contraindicated).......**3348**

Neoral Soft Gelatin Capsules (Affects the metabolism of cyclosporine and should be avoided) ..**2259**

Niravam Orally Disintegrating Tablets (Available data from clinical studies of benzodiazepines, other than alprazolam, suggest a possible drug interaction with alprazolam and grapefruit juice; caution is recommended during co-administration)**3092**

NuvaRing (CYP3A4 inhibitors may increase plasma hormone levels) ...**2340**

Pletal Tablets (A reduced dose of cilostazol should be considered when taken concomitantly with CYP3A4 inhibitors)**2455**

Premarin Tablets (Co-administration of inhibitors of CYP3A4 with estrogens may affect estrogen drug metabolism. Inhibitors of CYP3A4 may increase plasma concentrations of estrogens and may result in side effects)**3446**

Premphase Tablets (Co-administration of estrogens with inhibitors of CYP3A4 may increase plasma concentrations of estrogens and may result in side effects)**3456**

Prempro Tablets (Co-administration of estrogens with inhibitors of CYP3A4 may increase plasma concentrations of estrogens and may result in side effects)**3456**

Prograf Capsules and Injection (Since tacrolimus is metabolized mainly by the CYP3A enzyme systems, substances known to inhibit these enzymes may decrease the metabolism or increase bioavailability of tacrolimus as indicated by increased whole blood or plasma concentrations. Monitoring of blood concentrations and appropriate dosage adjustments are essential when such drugs are used concomitantly) ... 632

Provigil Tablets (Co-administration of potent inhibitors of CYP3A4 could alter the plasma levels of modafinil) ... 988

Pulmicort Respules (Concomitant administration of budesonide with known inhibitors of CYP3A4 may inhibit the metabolism of, and increase the systemic exposure to, budesonide; care should be exercised) ... 661

Ranexa Tablets (Ranolazine is primarily metabolized by CYP3A. Use of ranolazine with potent or moderately potent inhibitors of CYP3A, such as grapefruit juice or grapefruit containing products, is contraindicated because concomitant administration will increase ranolazine plasma levels and QTc prolongation) ... 1035

Rapamune Oral Solution and Tablets (Sirolimus is extensively metabolized by the CYP3A4 isoenzyme in the gut wall and liver. Co-administration with inhibitors of CYP3A4 may decrease the metabolism of sirolimus and increase sirolimus levels. Co-administration with strong inducers of CYP3A4 is not recommended) ... 3475

Relpax Tablets (Eletriptan should not be used within 72 hours of drugs that have demonstrated potent CYP3A4 inhibition) ... 2548

Rescriptor Tablets (Co-administration with drugs that inhibit CYP3A may increase delavirdine plasma concentrations) ... 2551

Revatio Tablets (Sildenafil metabolism is principally mediated by the CYP3A4 (major route) and CYP2C9 (minor route) cytochrome P450 isoforms. Therefore, inhibitors of these isoenzymes may reduce sildenafil clearance) ... 2557

Reyataz Capsules (Co-administration of atazanavir sulfate and other drugs that inhibit CYP3A may increase atazanavir sulfate plasma concentrations) ... 921

Rhinocort Aqua Nasal Spray (Co-administration with inhibitors of CYP4503A4 may inhibit the metabolism of, and increase the systemic exposure to budesonide) ... 665

Rozerem Tablets (Ramelteon should be administered with caution in subjects taking strong CYP2C9 inhibitors such as fluconazole) ... 3231

Rythmol SR Capsules (Drugs that inhibit CYP3A4 might lead to increased plasma levels of propafenone; patients should be closely monitored and the propafenone dose adjusted accordingly) ... 2727

Sandimmune I.V. Ampuls for Infusion (Co-administration results in increased blood concentrations of cyclosporine; concurrent use should be avoided) ... 2275

Seasonique Tablets (CYP3A4 inhibitors may increase plasma ethinyl estradiol levels) ... 1077

Sensipar Tablets (Since cinacalcet hydrochloride is metabolized in part by CYP3A4, dose adjustment of cinacalcet hydrochloride may be required and PTH and serum calcium concentrations closely monitored if a patient initiates or discontinues therapy with a strong CYP3A4 inhibitor) ... 608

Seroquel Tablets (Co-administration with an inhibitor of CYP4503A may reduce oral clearance of quetiapine, resulting in an increase in maximum plasma concentration of quetiapine; dose adjustment of quetiapine will be necessary) ... 690

Sonata Capsules (CYP3A4 inhibitors may decrease zaleplon's clearance, possibly increasing its concentration) ... 1717

Suboxone Tablets (Buprenorphine is metabolized to norbuprenorphine by cytochrome CYP3A4. Because CYP3A4 inhibitors may increase plasma concentrations of buprenorphine, patients already on CYP3A4 inhibitors should have their dose of Subutex or Subuxone adjusted.) ... 2717

Subutex Tablets (Buprenorphine is metabolized to norbuprenorphine by cytochrome CYP3A4. Because CYP3A4 inhibitors may increase plasma concentrations of buprenorphine, patients already on CYP3A4 inhibitors should have their dose of Subutex or Subuxone adjusted.) ... 2717

Sutent Capsules (Grapefruit may increase plasma concentrations of sunitinib maleate) ... 2560

Symbicort 80/4.5 Inhalation Aerosol (Concomitant administration of CYP3A4 inhibitors (e.g., itraconazole, clarithromycin, erythromycin, etc.) may inhibit the metabolism of, and increase the systemic exposure to, budesonide. Caution should be exercised with co-administration of Symbicort with potent CYP3A4 inhibitors) ... 3511

Tarceva Tablets (Caution when administering or taking erlotinib with strong CYP3A4 inhibitors such as atazanavir, clarithromycin, indinavir, itraconazole, nefazodone, nelfinavir, ritonavir, saquinavir, telithromycin, troleandomycin, and voriconazole) ... 1259

Tarceva Tablets (Caution when administering or taking erlotinib with strong CYP3A4 inhibitors such as atazanavir, clarithromycin, indinavir, itraconazole, nefazodone, nelfinavir, ritonavir, saquinavir, telithromycin, troleandomycin, and voriconazole) ... 2444

Taxotere Injection Concentrate (Metabolism of docetaxel may be inhibited by co-administration with CYP3A4 inhibitors, thereby leading to substantial increases in docetaxel blood concentrations) ... 2932

Tracleer Tablets (Co-administration of both a CYP2C9 inhibitor and a CYP3A4 inhibitor with bosentan will likely lead to large increases in plasma concentrations of bosentan and is not recommended) ... 545

Ultram ER Tablets (Administration of CYP3A4 inhibitors, such as ketoconazole and erythromycin, with tramadol hydrochloride may effect the meatbolism of tramadol leading to altered tramadol exposure) ... 2392

Uroxatral Tablets (Uroxatral should not be co-administered with potent CYP3A4 inhibitors such as ketoconazole, itraconazole, and ritonavir, since alfuzosin blood levels are increased) ... 2943

Vaprisol (Conivaptan is a substrate of CYP3A4. Co-administration of conivaptan with CYP3A4 inhibitors could lead to an increase in conivaptan concentrations. Concomitant use of conivaptan with potent CYP3A4 inhibitors is contraindicated) ... 643

Velcade for Injection (Patients who are concomitantly receiving Velcade and drugs that are inhibitors or inducers of cytochrome P450 3A4 should be closely monitored for either toxicities or reduced efficacy) ... 2133

Verelan PM Extended-Release Capsules, Controlled-Onset (Grapefruit juice may significantly increase concentrations of verapamil) ... 3106

Vesanoid Capsules (Tretinoin is metaboized by the hepatic P450 system; therefore, there is a potential for alteration of pharmacokinetic parameters in patients administered concomitant medications that are also inducers of this system. To date, there is no data to suggest that co-use with these medications increases or decreases either efficacy or toxicity of tretinoin) ... 2820

VFEND Tablets (CYP3A4 inhibitors may increase voriconazole systemic exposure (plasma concentrations)) ... 2564

Viracept Tablets (Nelfinavir is metabolized by CYP3A and CYP2C19; co-administration of Viracept and drugs that inhibit CYP3A or CYP2C19 may increase nelfinavir plasma concentrations) ... 2577

Vytorin 10/10 Tablets (Concomitant use of Vytorin and large quantities of grapefruit juice should be avoided) ... 2114

Zocor Tablets (Description: Potent inhibators of CYP3A4 can raise the plasma levels of HMG-CoA reductase inhibitory activity and increase the risk of myopathy and rhabdomyolysis, particulary with higher doses of simvastin) ... 2105

Grapefruit Juice

Abilify Tablets (Inhibitors of CYP3A4 or CYP2D6 can inhibit aripiprazole elimination and cause increased blood levels) ... 882

Abilify Tablets (Inhibitors of CYP3A4 can inhibit aripiprazole elimination and cause increased blood levels) ... 2450

Adalat CC Tablets (Co-administration of nifedipine with grapefruit juice results in up to a 2-fold increase in AUC and Cmax, due to inhibition of CYP3A4-related first-pass metabolism. This effect of grapefruit juice may last for at least 3 days; co-administration should beavoided) ... 2964

Advicor Tablets (Inhibits CYP3A4 and can increase the plasma concentration of lovastatin; concurrent use should be avoided) ... 1722

Agrylin Capsules (Anagrelide is metabolized at least in part by CYP1A2. Therefore, CYP1A2 inhibitors could theoretically adversely influence the clearance of anagrelide) ... 3169

Allegra-D 12 Hour Extended-Release Tablets (Co-administration with grapefruit, orange or apple juice will reduce the bioavailability and exposure or fexofenadine) ... 2846

Altoprev Extended-Release Tablets (Co-administration with potent CYP3A4 inhibitors, such as large quantities of grapefruit juice (greater than 1 quart daily), increases the risk of myopathy/rhabdomyolysis; concurrent use should be avoided) ... 3109

Angeliq Tablets (Inhibitors of CYP3A4 such as erythromycin, clarithromycin, ketoconazole, itraconazole, ritonavir and grapefruit juice may increase plasma concentrations of estrogens and may result in side effects) ... 762

Avodart Soft Gelatin Capsules (Blood concentrations of dutasteride may increase in the presence of CYP3A4 inhibitors) ... 1390

Azilect Tablets (Rasagiline plasma concentrations may increase up to 2 fold in patients using concomitant CYP1A2 inhibitors) ... 3293

Biltricide Tablets (Grapefruit juice was reported to produce a 1.6-fold increase in the Cmax and a 1.9-fold increase in the AUC of praziquantel) ... 2976

Buprenex Injectable (Buprenorphine is metabolized by the CYP3A4 isoenzyme; co-administration with inhibitors of CYP3A4 may cause decrease in clearance of buprenorphine) ... 2716

Cafcit Injection (Caffeine has the potential to interact with drugs that inhibit CYP1A2) ... 1886

Carbatrol Capsules (Carbamazepine is metabolized mainly by cytochrome P450 (CYP) 3A4 to the active carbamazepine 10,11 -epoxide, which is further metabolized to the trans-diol by epoxide hydrolase. Therefore, the potential exists for interaction between carbamazepine and any agent that inhibits CYP3A4 and/or epoxide hydrolase) ... 3171

Cardizem LA Extended Release Tablets (Diltiazem is both a substrate and an inhibitor of the CYP3A4 enzyme system. Other drugs that are specific substrates, inhibitors, or inducers of this enzyme system may have a significant impact on the efficacy and side effect profile of diltiazem) ... 1728

Cialis Tablets (YP3A4 inhibitors such as grapefruit juice may likely increase tadalafil exposure) ... 1838

Climara Transdermal System (Inducers of CYP3A4, such as grapefruit juice, may increase plasma concentrations of estrogens and may result in side effects) ... 771

Climara Pro Transdermal System (Inhibitors of CYP3A4 such as erythromycin, clarithromycin, ketoconazole, itraconazole, ritonavir and grapefruit juice may increase plasma concentrations of estrogens and may result in side effects) ... 776

Covera-HS Tablets (Grapefruit juice may significantly increase concentrations of verapamil) ... 3139

Crixivan Capsules (Potential for decrease in indinavir AUC) ... 1940

Cymbalta Delayed-Release Capsules (Concomitant use of duloxetine with fluvoxamine, an inhibitor of CYP1A2, results in a 6-fold increase in AUC, about 2.5-fold increase in Cmax, and an approximately 3-fold increase in t1/2 of duloxetine. Since duloxetine is metabolized in part by CYP1A2, concomitant use of duloxetine with other inhibitors of CYP1A2, would be expected to have the same effects; these combinations should be avoided) ... 1757

Decadron Tablets (Drugs which inhibit cytochrome P450 3A4 enzyme activity have the potential to result in increased plasma concentrations of corticosteroids) **1951**

Diastat Rectal Delivery System (Studies suggest that CYP2C19 and CYP3A4 are the principal enzymes involved in the initial oxidative metabolism of diazepam. Therefore, potential interactions may occur when diazepam is given concurrently with agents that affect CYP2C19 and CYP3A4 activity. Potential inhibitors of CYP3A4 could decrease the rate of diazepam elimination) **3343**

Duragesic Transdermal System (The concurrent use of CYP3A4 inhibitors with transdermal fentanyl may result in an increase in fentanyl plasma concentrations, which could increase or prolong adverse drug effects and may cause serious respiratory depression. In this situation, special patient care and observation are appropriate) **2373**

Emend Capsules (Co-administration of EMEND with drugs that inhibit CYP3A4 activity may result in increased plasma concentrations of aprepitant and should be approached with caution) **1963**

Enjuvia Tablets (Inhibitors of CYP3A4 such as erythromycin, clarithromycin, ketoconazole, itraconazole, ritonavir and grapefruit juice may increase plasma concentrations of estrogens and may result in side effects) **1062**

Entocort EC Capsules (Concurrent use with extensive intake of grapefruit juice has caused rise in systemic exposure of budesonide by two-fold; ingestion of grapefruit juice should be avoided) **2698**

Equetro Extended-Release Capsules (Carbamazepine is metabolized mainly by CYP3A4 the active carbamazepine 10,11-epoxide, which is futher metabolized to the trans-diol by epoxide hydrolase. Therefore, the potential exists for interaction between carbamazepine and any agent that inhibits CYP3A4 and/or epoxide hydrolase. Agents that are CYP3A4 inhibitors may increase the plasma levels of carbamazepine. Thus, if a patient has been titrated to a stable dosage of carbamazepine, and then begins a course of treatment with a CYP3A4 or epoxide hydrolase inhibitor, it is reasonable to expect that a dose reduction for carbamazepine may be necessary) **3180**

Estrasorb Topical Emulsion (Inhibitors of CYP3A4 may increase plasma concentrations of estrogens and may result in side effects) **1147**

Estratest H.S. Tablets (Co-administration with inhibitors of CYP3A4 may increase plasma concentrations of estrogens and may result in side effects) **3199**

Evoxac Capsules (Co-administration with drugs which inhibit CYP3A3/4, such as grapefruit juice, may inhibit the metabolism of cevimeline resulting in a higher risk of adverse events) **1047**

Flonase Nasal Spray (Caution should be exercised when potent cytochrome P450 3A4 inhibitors are co-administered with fluticasone propionate) **1440**

Gengraf Capsules (Affects the metabolism of cyclosporine by increasing blood concentration of cyclosporine; concurrent use should be avoided) **459**

Gleevec Tablets (Caution is recommended when administering Gleevec with inhibitors of the CYP3A4 family. Substances that inhibit CYP3A4 activity may decrease metabolism and increase imatinib concentrations. There is a significant increase in exposure to imatinib when Gleevec is co-administered with ketoconazole) **2227**

Hectorol Capsules (Cytochrome P450 inhibitors may inhibit the 25-hydroxylation of doxercalciferol. Hence, formation of the active doxercalciferol moiety may be hindered) **1275**

InnoPran XL Capsules (Blood levels and/or toxicity of propranolol may be increased by administration of propranolol hydrochloride extended-release capsules with inhibitors of CYP1A2) **2723**

Inspra Tablets (Eplerenone should not be used with strong inhibitors of CYP450 3A4. Potent inhibitors of CYP3A4 caused increased exposure of about 5-fold, while less potent CYP3A4 inhibitors (e.g., erythromycin, saquinavir, verapamil, fluconazole) gave approximately 2-fold increases in exposure. Grapefruit juice caused only a small increase (about 25%) in exposure) **2536**

Ionsys Transdermal System (The concomitant use of fentanyl with CYP3A4 inhibitors may result in a decreases in fentanyl clearance, which could increase or prolong adverse drug effects including serious respiratory depression. In this situation, special patient care and observation is appropriate) **2379**

Iressa Tablets (Substances that are potent inhibitors of CYP3A4 (e.g., ketoconazole and itraconazole) decrease gefitinib metabolism and increase gefitinib plasma concentrations) **684**

Levitra Tablets (Concomitant use with moderate/strong CYP 3A4 inhibitors results in significant increases in plasma levels of vardenafil) **3034**

Lexiva Tablets (Amprenavir, the active metabolite of fosamprenavir, is metabolized in the liver by the cytochrome P450 enzyme system. Amprenavir may inhibit or induce CYP3A4. Caution should be used when co-administering medications that are substrates, inhibitors, or inducers of CYP3A4, or potentially toxic medications that are metabolized by CYP3A4) **1505**

Lotronex Tablets (Co-administration of alosetron and strong CYP3A4 inhibitors has not been evaluated but should be undertaken with caution because of similar potential drug interactions) **1512**

Menostar Transdermal System (Inhibitors of CYP3A4 may increase plasma concentrations of estrogens and may result in side effects) **782**

Mevacor Tablets (The risk of myopathy/rhabdomyolysis is increased by concomitant use of lovastatin with potent inhibitors of CYP3A4, particularly with higher doses of lovastatin; concomitant use should be avoided unless the benefits of combined therapy outweigh the increased risk) **2021**

Migranal Nasal Spray (Co-administration of dihydroergotamin with potent CYP3A4 inhibitors results in vasospasm that can lead to cerebral ischemia and/or ischemia of the extremities, therefore it is contraindicated) **3348**

Neoral Soft Gelatin Capsules (Affects the metabolism of cyclosporine and should be avoided) **2259**

Niravam Orally Disintegrating Tablets (Available data from clinical studies of benzodiazepines, other than alprazolam, suggest a possible drug interaction with alprazolam and grapefruit juice; caution is recommended during co-administration) **3092**

NuvaRing (CYP3A4 inhibitors may increase plasma hormone levels) **2340**

Pletal Tablets (Co-administration of cilostazol with inhibitors of CYP3A4, such as grapefruit juice, increase cilostazol plasma concentration by 50%; concurrent consumption of grapefruit juice should be avoided) **2455**

Premarin Tablets (Co-administration of grapefruit juice with estrogens may increase plasma concentrations of estrogens and may result in side effects) **3446**

Premphase Tablets (Co-administration of estrogens with inhibitors of CYP3A4, such as grapefruit juice, may increase plasma concentrations of estrogens and may result in side effects) **3456**

Prempro Tablets (Co-administration of estrogens with inhibitors of CYP3A4, such as grapefruit juice, may increase plasma concentrations of estrogens and may result in side effects) **3456**

Prograf Capsules and Injection (Co-administered grapefruit juice has been reported to increase tacrolimus blood trough concentrations in liver transplant patients; grapefruit juice should be avoided) **632**

Provigil Tablets (Co-administration of potent inhibitors of CYP3A4 could alter the plasma levels of modafinil) **988**

Pulmicort Respules (Concomitant administration of budesonide with known inhibitors of CYP3A4 may inhibit the metabolism of, and increase the systemic exposure to, budesonide; care should be exercised) **661**

Ranexa Tablets (Ranolazine is primarily metabolized by CYP3A. Use of ranolazine with potent or moderately potent inhibitors of CYP3A, such as grapefruit juice or grapefruit containing products, is contraindicated because concomitant administration will increase ranolazine plasma levels and QTc prolongation) **1035**

Rapamune Oral Solution and Tablets (Induces CYP3A4-mediated metabolism of sirolimus; Rapamune must not be administered or diluted with grapefruit juice) **3475**

Relpax Tablets (Eletriptan should not be used within 72 hours of drugs that have demonstrated potent CYP3A4 inhibition) **2548**

Requip Tablets (If therapy with a drug known to be a potent inhibitor of CYP1A2 is stopped or started during treatment with ropinirole hydrochloride, adjustment of the dose of ropinirole hydrocholoride may be required) **1555**

Revatio Tablets (Sildenafil metabolism is principally mediated by the CYP3A4 (major route) and CYP2C9 (minor route) cytochrome P450 isoforms. Therefore, inhibitors of these isoenzymes may reduce sildenafil clearance) **2557**

Rhinocort Aqua Nasal Spray (Co-administration with inhibitors of CYP4503A4 may inhibit the metabolism of, and increase the systemic exposure to budesonide) **665**

Rozerem Tablets (Ramelteon should be administered with caution in subjects taking strong CYP2C9 inhibitors such as fluconazole) **3231**

Rythmol SR Capsules (Drugs that inhibit CYP1A2 might lead to increased plasma levels of propafenone; patients should be closely monitored and the propafenone dose adjusted accordingly) **2727**

Sandimmune I.V. Ampuls for Infusion (Co-administration results in increased blood concentrations of cyclosporine; concurrent use should be avoided) **2275**

Seasonique Tablets (CYP3A4 inhibitors may increase plasma ethinyl estradiol levels) **1077**

Seroquel Tablets (Co-administration with an inhibitor of CYP4503A may reduce oral clearance of quetiapine, resulting in an increase in maximum plasma concentration of quetiapine; dose adjustment of quetiapine will be necessary) **690**

Sonata Capsules (CYP3A4 inhibitors may decrease zaleplon's clearance, possibly increasing its concentration) **1717**

Suboxone Tablets (Buprenorphine is metabolized to norbuprenorphine by cytochrome CYP3A4. Because CYP3A4 inhibitors may increase plasma concentrations of buprenorphine, patients already on CYP3A4 inhibitors should have their dose of Subutex or Subuxone adjusted.) **2717**

Subutex Tablets (Buprenorphine is metabolized to norbuprenorphine by cytochrome CYP3A4. Because CYP3A4 inhibitors may increase plasma concentrations of buprenorphine, patients already on CYP3A4 inhibitors should have their dose of Subutex or Subuxone adjusted.) **2717**

Sutent Capsules (Grapefruit may increase plasma concentrations of sunitinib maleate) **2560**

Symbicort 80/4.5 Inhalation Aerosol (Concomitant administration of CYP3A4 inhibitors (e.g., itraconazole, clarithromycin, erythromycin, etc.) may inhibit the metabolism of, and increase the systemic exposure to, budesonide. Caution should be exercised with co-administration of Symbicort with potent CYP3A4 inhibitors) **3511**

Tarceva Tablets (Caution when administering or taking erlotinib with strong CYP3A4 inhibitors such as atazanavir, clarithromycin, indinavir, itraconazole, nefazodone, nelfinavir, ritonavir, saquinavir, telithromycin, troleandomycin, and voriconazole) **1259**

Tarceva Tablets (Caution when administering or taking erlotinib with strong CYP3A4 inhibitors such as atazanavir, clarithromycin, indinavir, itraconazole, nefazodone, nelfinavir, ritonavir, saquinavir, telithromycin, troleandomycin, and voriconazole) **2444**

Targretin Capsules (Bexarotene is metabolized by CYP403A4; co-administration with inhibitors of CYP4503A4, such as grapefruit juice, would be expected to lead to an increase in plasma bexarotene concentrations) **1747**

Taxotere Injection Concentrate (Metabolism of docetaxel may be inhibited by co-administration with CYP3A4 inhibitors, thereby leading to substantial increases in docetaxel blood concentrations) **2932**

Tracleer Tablets (Co-administration of both a CYP2C9 inhibitor and a CYP3A4 inhibitor with bosentan will likely lead to large increases in plasma concentrations of bosentan and is not recommended) **545**

Ultram ER Tablets (Administration of CYP3A4 inhibitors, such as ketoconazole and erythromycin, with tramadol hydrochloride may effect the meatbolism of tramadol leading to altered tramadol exposure) **2392**

Uroxatral Tablets (Uroxatral should not be co-administered with potent CYP3A4 inhibitors such as ketoconazole, itraconazole, and ritonavir, since alfuzosin blood levels are increased) **2943**

Vaprisol (Conivaptan is a substrate of CYP3A4. Co-administration of conivaptan with CYP3A4 inhibitors could lead to an increase in conivaptan concentrations. Concomitant use of conivaptan with potent CYP3A4 inhibitors is contraindicated) **643**

Velcade for Injection (Patients who are concomitantly receiving Velcade and drugs that are inhibitors or inducers of cytochrome P450 3A4 should be closely monitored for either toxicities or reduced efficacy) **2133**

Verelan PM Extended-Release Capsules, Controlled-Onset (Grapefruit juice may significantly increase concentrations of verapamil) **3106**

Vesanoid Capsules (Tretinoin is metaboized by the hepatic P450 system; therefore, there is a potential for alteration of pharmacokinetic parameters in patients administered concomitant medications that are also inducers of this system. To date, there is no data to suggest that co-use with these medications increases or decreases either efficacy or toxicity of tretinoin) **2820**

VFEND Tablets (CYP3A4 inhibitors may increase voriconazole systemic exposure (plasma concentrations)) **2564**

Vytorin 10/10 Tablets (Concomitant use of Vytorin and large quantities of grapefruit juice should be avoided) **2114**

Vytorin 10/10 Tablets (Co-administration with potent CYP3A4 inhibitors, such as large quantities of grapefruit juice (greater than 1 quart daily), increases the risk of myopathy/rhabdomyolysis; concurrent use should be avoided) **3077**

Zocor Tablets (Simvastatin is a substrate for CYP4503A4 and grapefruit juice contains one or more components that inhibit CYP3A4; co-administration with grapefruit juice can increase the plasma concentrations of simvastatin and its B-hydroxyacid metabolite; large quantities of grapefruit juice (>1 quart daily) significantly increase the serum concentrations and should be avoided) **2105**

Zyprexa Tablets (Can potentially inhibit olanzapine clearance; therefore, a dosage decrease might be considered) **1830**

Zyprexa IntraMuscular (Can potentially inhibit olanzapine clearance; therefore, a dosage decrease might be considered) **1830**

Herring, pickled

Parnate Tablets (Potential for hypertensive crisis; concurrent use is contraindicated) **1527**

Liqueurs

Parnate Tablets (Potential for hypertensive crisis; concurrent use is contraindicated) **1527**

Liver

Parnate Tablets (Potential for hypertensive crisis; concurrent use is contraindicated) **1527**

Meal, high in bran fiber

Lanoxin Tablets (The amount of digoxin from an oral dose may be reduced) **1500**

Meal, unspecified

Ambien Tablets (Mean AUC and Cmax decreased by 15% and 25% respectively, while Tmax was prolonged by 60%; for faster sleep onset, Ambien should not be administered with or immediately after meal) **2851**

Avandaryl Tablets (When glimepiride is given with meals the mean Tmax is slightly increased (12%) and mean Cmax and AUC are slightly decreased) **1379**

Cozaar Tablets (A meal slows absorption and decreases Cmax, but has minor effects on losartan AUC or on the AUC of the metabolite) **1935**

Famvir Tablets (Penciclovir Cmax decreased approximately 50% and Tmax was delayed by 1.5 hours when a capsule formulation of famciclovir was administered with food; there is no effect on the extent of availability (AUC) of penciclovir) **2211**

Fosamax Tablets (Standardized breakfast decreases bioavailability by approximately 40% when alendronate is administered either one-half or 1 hour before breakfast) **1969**

Fosamax Plus D Tablets (Bioavailability was decreased (by approximately 40%) when 10 mg alendronate was administered either 0.5 or 1 hour before a standardized breakfast, when compared to dosing 2 hours before eating) **1977**

Hyzaar 50-12.5 Tablets (Meal slows absorption and decreases Cmax but has minor effects on losartan AUC or on the AUC of the metabolite) **1990**

Lanoxin Tablets (Slows the rate of absorption) **1500**

Mevacor Tablets (When lovastatin was given under fasting conditions, plasma concentrations of total inhibitors were on average about two-thirds those found when lovastatin was administered immediately after a standard meal) **2021**

Nimotop Capsules (Administration of nimodipine capsules following a standard breakfast resulted in 68% lower peak plasma concentration and 38% lower bioavailability) **749**

Norvir Soft Gelatin Capsules (Relative to fasting conditions, the extent of absorption of ritonavir from capsule formulation was 15% higher when administered with a meal; decreased peak ritonavir concentrations when oral solution was given under non-fasting condition) **503**

PCE Dispertab Tablets (Presence of food results in lower blood levels; optimal blood levels are obtained when PCE is given in the fasting state (at least ½ hour and preferably 2 hours before meals)) **515**

Ticlid Tablets (Administration after meals results in a 20% increase in the AUC of ticlopidine) **2810**

Meat extracts

Parnate Tablets (Potential for hypertensive crisis; concurrent use is contraindicated) **1527**

Meat prepared with tenderizers

Parnate Tablets (Potential for hypertensive crisis; concurrent use is contraindicated) **1527**

Milk, low fat

Dyazide Capsules (Concurrent use of low-salt milk with triamterene may result in hyperkalemia, especially in patients with renal insufficiency) **1423**

Milk, low salt

Dyrenium Capsules (Co-administration may promote serum potassium accumulation and possibly result in hyperkalemia) **3400**

Orange Juice

Allegra-D 12 Hour Extended-Release Tablets (Co-administration with grapefruit, orange or apple juice will reduce the bioavailability and exposure or fexofenadine) **2846**

Fosamax Tablets (Concomitant administration of alendronate with orange juice reduces bioavailability by approximately 60%) **1969**

Fosamax Plus D Tablets (Concomitant administration of alendronate with orange juice reduces bioavailability by approximately 60%) **1977**

Prunes

Parnate Tablets (Potential for hypertensive crisis; concurrent use is contraindicated) **1527**

Raisins

Parnate Tablets (Potential for hypertensive crisis; concurrent use is contraindicated) **1527**

Raspberries

Parnate Tablets (Potential for hypertensive crisis; concurrent use is contraindicated) **1527**

Salt Substitutes, Potassium-Containing

Altace Capsules (Increases risk of hyperkalemia) **1702**

Inspra Tablets (Eplerenone is contraindicated in patients treated concomitantly with salt substitutes containing potassium) **2536**

Prinivil Tablets (Use of lisinopril with potassium-sparing diuretics (such as spironolactone, triamterene or amiloride), potassium supplements or potassium-containing salt substitutes may lead to significant increases in serum potassium. Therefore, if concomitant use of these agents is indicated because of demonstrated hypokalemia, they should be used with caution and with frequent monitoring of serum potassium. Potassium-sparing agents should generally not be used in patients with heart failure who are receiving lisinopril) **2052**

Prinzide Tablets (Risk factors for the development of hyperkalemia include the concomitant use of potassium-sparing diuretics, potassium supplements and/or potassium-containing salt substitutes. Hyperkalemia can cause serious, sometimes, fatal, arrhythmias. Prinzide should be used cautiously, if at all, with these agents and with frequent monitoring of serum potassium) **2056**

Sauerkraut

Parnate Tablets (Potential for hypertensive crisis; concurrent use is contraindicated) **1527**

Sherry

Parnate Tablets (Potential for hypertensive crisis; concurrent use is contraindicated) **1527**

Soy Sauce

Parnate Tablets (Potential for hypertensive crisis; concurrent use is contraindicated) **1527**

Soybean Formula, Children's

Levoxyl Tablets (Concurrent use of soybean flour may bind and decrease the absorption of levothyroxine sodium from GI tract) **1712**

Synthroid Tablets (Binds and decreases absorption of levothyroxine sodium from the gastrointestinal tract) **520**

Vegetables, green leafy

Coumadin Tablets (Large amounts of green leafy vegetables may affect warfarin therapy) **898**

Walnuts

Levoxyl Tablets (Concurrent use of walnuts may bind and decrease the absorption of levothyroxine sodium from GI tract) **1712**

Wine, Chianti

Parnate Tablets (Potential for hypertensive crisis; concurrent use is contraindicated) **1527**

Wine, unspecified

Matulane Capsules (Procarbazine exhibits some MAO inhibitory activity: concurrent use should be avoided) **3191**

Yeast Extract

Parnate Tablets (Potential for hypertensive crisis; concurrent use is contraindicated) **1527**

Yogurt

Matulane Capsules (Procarbazine exhibits some MAO inhibitory activity: concurrent use should be avoided) **3191**

Parnate Tablets (Potential for hypertensive crisis; concurrent use is contraindicated) **1527**

SECTION 3

SIDE EFFECTS INDEX

Presented in this section is an alphabetical list of every side effect reported in the "Adverse Reactions" section of the product descriptions in *PDR®* and its companion volumes. Under each side effect is an alphabetical list of brands associated with the reaction.

If noted in the underlying text, incidence is shown in parentheses immediately after the brand name. Products reporting an incidence rate of 3% or more are marked with a ▲ symbol at their left. Because incidence data are sometimes drawn from controlled clinical trials, the rates seen in actual clinical practice may vary from those found in the published reports.

This index lists only side effects noted in official prescribing information as published by *PDR®*. To alert you to the full range of possibilities, the entries include adverse effects shared by an entire class of drugs, but not necessarily reported for the specific drug in question. The index is restricted to reactions that may be expected to occur at recommended dosages in the general patient population. Precautions to be taken under special circumstances are not listed, nor are the effects of overdosage.

The page numbers shown for the products refer to the 2007 editions of *PDR®*, *PDR for Ophthalmic Medicines™*, and the *PDR for Nonprescription Drugs, Dietary Supplements and Herbs™*, which is published later in the year. A key to the symbols denoting the companion volumes appears in the bottom margin.

A

Abdomen, enlarged

Abilify Oral Solution (Infrequent)........ 882
Abilify Oral Solution (Infrequent)....... 2450
Abilify Discmelt Orally Disintegrating Tablets (Infrequent)................................. 882
Abilify Discmelt Orally Disintegrating Tablets (Infrequent)................................. 2450
Abilify Tablets (Infrequent)................ 882
Abilify Tablets (Infrequent)................ 2450
▲ Angeliq Tablets (7%) 762
Campral Tablets (Rare)..................... 1174
▲ Camptosar Injection (0% to 10%) 2604
Estring Vaginal Ring........................ 2635
▲ Follistim AQ Cartridge (8%) 2338
Ionsys Transdermal System (.1% to less than 1%)........................... 2379
▲ I.V. Busulfex (23%) 2493
Omacor Capsules............................ 2725
Prevacid NapraPAC (Less than 1%).. 3280
Relpax Tablets (Rare)....................... 2548
Reyataz Capsules (Less than 3%)..... 921

Abdomen, redistribution/accumulation of body fat

Kaletra.. 476
Retrovir.. 1560

Abdominal bloating

Abilify Oral Solution (Infrequent)........ 882
Abilify Oral Solution (Infrequent)....... 2450
Abilify Discmelt Orally Disintegrating Tablets (Infrequent)................................. 882
Abilify Discmelt Orally Disintegrating Tablets (Infrequent)................................. 2450
Abilify Tablets (Infrequent)................ 882
Abilify Tablets (Infrequent)................ 2450
Aciphex Tablets (Rare)..................... 1090
Actonel with Calcium Tablets............ 2688
Aerobid/Aerobid-M (Less than 1%)... 1171
Angeliq Tablets................................ 762
Aralast (Greater than or equal to 0.2%).. 717
Aricept Tablets (Frequent)................ 1094
Aricept ODT Tablets (Frequent)........ 1094
Asacol Delayed-Release Tablets (2% or greater)........................... 2692
Bentyl Capsules............................... 697
Bentyl Injection................................ 697
Bentyl Syrup.................................... 697
Bentyl Tablets.................................. 697
Climara Transdermal System........... 771
Climara Pro Transdermal System..... 776
Colazal Capsules............................ 2838
▲ Colyte with Flavor Packs for Oral Solution (Up to 50%)..................... 3088
Coumadin for Injection (Infrequent)... 898
Coumadin Tablets (Infrequent).......... 898
▲ Creon 5 Capsules (Among most frequent)..................................... 3198
▲ Creon 10 Capsules (Among most frequent)..................................... 3198
▲ Creon 20 Capsules (Among most frequent)..................................... 3199
▲ Depo-Provera Contraceptive Injection (1% to 5%)..................... 2622
Donnatal Extentabs.......................... 2493
Enjuvia Tablets................................ 1062
Estrasorb Topical Emulsion............. 1147
Estratest Tablets............................. 3199
Estratest H.S. Tablets...................... 3199
Fansidar Tablets.............................. 2765
▲ HalfLytely and Bisacodyl Tablets Bowel Prep Kit with Flavors Packs (22.3% to 50%)................. 881
Imitrex Nasal Spray......................... 1467
Indocin Capsules (Less than 1%)...... 1995
Indocin I.V. (Less than 1%).............. 2465
Indocin (Less than 1%).................... 1995
Lexapro Oral Solution (Infrequent).... 1190
Lexapro Tablets (Infrequent)............ 1190
Limbrel Capsules (0.006%).............. 2672
Menostar Transdermal System........ 782
MetroGel-Vaginal Gel (Less than 1%).. 1855
Midamor Tablets (Less than or equal to 1%)............................... 2026
Mircette Tablets.............................. 1066
Moduretic Tablets (Less than or equal to 1%)............................... 2028
Nadolol Tablets (1 to 5 of 1000 patients)..................................... 2159
Noroxin Tablets (Less frequent)........ 2032
Norvir (Less than 2%)...................... 503
Ortho-Cyclen Tablets....................... 2429
Ortho Evra Transdermal System...... 2417
Ortho Tri-Cyclen Tablets.................. 2429
Ortho Tri-Cyclen Lo Tablets............. 2436
▲ OsmoPrep Tablets (31% to 39%) 2840
Premarin Intravenous...................... 3442
Premarin Tablets............................ 3446
Premarin Vaginal Cream................. 3452
Premphase Tablets......................... 3456
Prempro Tablets............................. 3456
Prilosec OTC Delayed-Release Tablets (Less than 1%)................. 2677
▲ Prochieve 4% Gel (7%) 1003
▲ Prochieve 8% Gel (7%) 1003
▲ Prometrium Capsules (100 mg, 200 mg) (12%)............................ 3203
ProNutra Protein Supplement.......... 1668
Seasonique Tablets........................ 1077
▲ Thiola Tablets (16.7%) 2141
▲ Thrombate III (1 of 17) 3257
Ticlid Tablets (0.5% to 1.0%)........... 2810
▲ TriLyte with Flavor Packs for Oral Solution (Up to 50%)................... 3100
Yasmin 28 Tablets......................... 796
Yaz Tablets................................... 803
Zegerid Capsules (Less than 1%)..... 2958
Zegerid Powder for Oral Solution (Less than 1%)............................ 2958

Abdominal discomfort
(see also under Distress, abdominal; Distress, gastrointestinal)

Ambien CR Tablets (1%).................. 2855
▲ Amitiza Capsules (1.5% to 3.4%) 3224
Biaxin/Biaxin XL (2%)..................... 402
Carafate Tablets (Less than 0.5%).... 701
▲ Chantix Tablets (5% to 7%) 2517
Cipro (Less than 1%)....................... 2977
Cipro I.V. (1.7%)............................. 2984
Cipro XR Tablets (Less than 1%)....... 2990
▲ Clozaril Tablets (4%) 2184
▲ Depo-Provera Contraceptive Injection (Greater than 5%)........... 2622
Dulcolax Stool Softener................. ▣648
Dulcolax Suppositories.................. ▣648
Dulcolax Tablets........................... ▣649
▲ DynaCirc CR Tablets (1.3% to 5.1%).. 2721
▲ Epivir-HBV (16%) 1432
▲ FazaClo Orally Disintegrating Tablets (4%).................................. 551
Fleet Bisacodyl Laxatives................ 1165
Fleet Prep Kits.............................. 1170
▲ Flovent Diskus (3%) 1443
▲ Gengraf Capsules (Up to 7%) 459
Hyperstat I.V. 3017
Imitrex Nasal Spray (Infrequent)....... 1467
Imitrex Tablets............................... 1471
K-Dur Extended-Relase Tablets......... 3033
Klonopin (Infrequent)...................... 2778
Lexapro Oral Solution (Infrequent).... 1190
Lexapro Tablets (Infrequent)............ 1190
Lithobid Tablets............................. 1692
▲ Lotronex Tablets (7%) 1512
Children's Motrin Oral Suspension.. ▣685
Children's Motrin Non-Staining Dye-Free Oral Suspension.......... ▣685
Children's Motrin Oral Suspension.... 1867
Children's Motrin Non-Staining Dye-Free Oral Suspension............ 1867
Infants' Motrin Concentrated Drops... 1867
Infants' Motrin Non-Staining Dye-Free Concentrated Drops....... 1867
Junior Strength Motrin Caplets and Chewable Tablets........................ 1867
Nadolol Tablets (1 to 5 of 1000 patients)..................................... 2159
▲ Neoral Oral Solution (Up to 7%) 2259
▲ Neoral Soft Gelatin Capsules (Up to 7%)... 2259

- ▲ Niravam Orally Disintegrating Tablets (18.3%) 3092
- Oracea Capsules (1.1%) 1000
- Pepcid Injection (Infrequent) 2040
- Pepcid (Infrequent) 2038
- Relpax Tablets (1% to 2%) 2548
- Restoril Capsules (1.5%) 1860
- ▲ Sandimmune (Less than 1% to 7%) 2275
- ▲ Sandostatin Injection (34% to 61%) 2278
- Symbicort 80/4.5 Inhalation Aerosol (1.1%) 3511
- ▲ Symbicort 160/4.5 Inhalation Aerosol (6.5%) 3511
- ▲ Trisenox Injection (8%) 993
- Urocit-K Tablets (Some patients) 2144
- Vantas (Less than 2%) 3375
- ▲ Xenical Capsules (25.5%) 2831
- Zelnorm Tablets 2312

Abdominal distention

- Actiq (1% or greater) 979
- Aldoril Tablets 1910
- Aloprim for Injection (Less than 1%) 2167
- AmBisome for Injection (Less common) 620
- ▲ Amitiza Capsules (0% to 7.1%) 3224
- Aptivus Capsules (Less than 2%) 826
- ▲ Arranon Injection (0% to 6%) 1357
- Avalide Tablets 888
- Avalide Tablets 2874
- Avapro Tablets (Less than 1%) 891
- Avapro Tablets (Less than 1%) 2871
- Byetta Injection 611
- ▲ CellCept Capsules (3% to less than 20%) 2747
- ▲ CellCept Intravenous (3% to less than 20%) 2747
- ▲ CellCept Oral Suspension (3% to less than 20%) 2747
- ▲ CellCept Tablets (3% to less than 20%) 2747
- ▲ Chantix Tablets (5% to 7%) 2517
- Clozaril Tablets (Less than 1%) 2184
- Colocort Rectal Suspension, USP (Retention) 100 mg/60 mL 2476
- Crixivan Capsules 1940
- Cubicin for Injection (Less than 1%) 1026
- ▲ Dacogen Injection (5%) 2129
- Decadron Tablets 1951
- ▲ DepoDur Extended-Release Injection (2% to 5%) 1110
- Depo-Medrol Injectable Suspension 2617
- Depo-Medrol Single-Dose Vial 2619
- ▲ depo-subQ provera 104 Injectable Suspension (1% to less than 5%) 2624
- ▲ Doxil Injection (1% to 10%) 2351
- Duragesic Transdermal System (Less than 1%) 2373
- DynaCirc CR Tablets (1.2%) 2721
- Effexor Tablets (Infrequent) 3411
- ▲ Eloxatin for Injection (2% to 5%) 2892
- Evoxac Capsules 1047
- FazaClo Orally Disintegrating Tablets (Less than 1%) 551
- Follistim AQ Cartridge 2338
- Fosamax (Up to 1.4%) 1969
- Fosamax Plus D Tablets (0% to 1.4%) 1977
- Gengraf Capsules (1% to less than 3%) 459
- Gleevec Tablets (Less common) 2227
- Hydrocortone Tablets 1989
- Imitrex Nasal Spray 1467
- ▲ Indocin I.V. (1% to 3%) 2465
- ▲ Intron A for Injection (Less than 5%) 3024
- Invanz for Injection (Greater than 0.1%) 1999
- Kaletra (Less than 2%) 476
- Ketek Tablets (Greater than or equal to 0.2% to less than 2%) 2903
- Lamictal (Rare) 1481
- ▲ Leukine (4%) 814
- Lotronex Tablets (2%) 1512
- Mavik Tablets (0.3% to 1.0%) 486
- Merrem I.V. (Greater than 0.1% to 1%) 686
- Mirapex Tablets (Less than 1%) 859
- ▲ MoviPrep Oral Solution (59.8%) 2839
- ▲ Myfortic Tablets (3% to less than 20%) 2255
- NeoProfen Injection 2472
- Neoral Oral Solution (1% to less than 3%) 2259
- Neoral Soft Gelatin Capsules (1% to less than 3%) 2259
- Nexium Delayed-Release Capsules (Less than 1%) 655
- Nexium I.V. (Less than 1%) 659
- ▲ Opana Tablets (1% to less than 10%) 1122
- ▲ Opana ER Tablets (1% to less than 10%) 1126
- Oracea Capsules (1.1%) 1000
- Pentasa Capsules (Less than 1%) 3185
- Permax Tablets (Infrequent) 3356
- Prevacid Delayed-Release Capsules (Less than 1%) 3271
- Prevacid for Delayed-Release Oral Suspension (Less than 1%) 3271
- Prevacid SoluTab Delayed-Release Orally Disintegrating Tablets (Less than 1%) 3271
- PREVPAC (Less than 1%) 3284
- Prezista Tablets (Less than 2%) 3306
- ▲ Prograf Capsules and Injection (3% to 15%) 632
- ▲ Proleukin for Injection (10%) 2266
- ▲ Prometrium Capsules (100 mg, 200 mg) (6% to 8%) 3203
- ▲ Rapamune Oral Solution and Tablets (3% to 20%) 3475
- ReoPro Vials (0.1%) 1809
- Requip Tablets (Infrequent) 1555
- Rescriptor Tablets 2551
- Rilutek Tablets (Infrequent) 2930
- Risperdal (Rare) 1676
- Risperdal M-Tab Orally Disintegrating Tablets (Rare) 1676
- ▲ Rituxan I.V. (1% to 5%) 1254
- Rythmol SR Capsules 2727
- Sanctura Tablets (Greater than or equal to 0.5%) 1151
- ▲ Sandostatin Injection (Less than 10% to 35%) 2278
- Sandostatin LAR Depot (Rare) 2280
- Seroquel Tablets (Rare) 690
- ▲ Simulect for Injection (3% to 10%) 2284
- ▲ Taxotere Injection Concentrate (6%) 2932
- Thalomid Capsules 965
- Tiazac Capsules (2%) 1201
- Topamax Sprinkle Capsules (Infrequent) 2404
- Topamax Tablets (Infrequent) 2404
- ▲ Trisenox Injection (8%) 993
- ▲ Valcyte Tablets (Less than 5%) 2813
- Vantin Tablets and Oral Suspension (Less than 1%) 2645
- ▲ Vesanoid Capsules (11%) 2820
- VFEND I.V. (Less than 2%) 2564
- VFEND Oral Suspension (Less than 2%) 2564
- VFEND Tablets (Less than 2%) 2564
- ▲ Xeloda Tablets (Less than 5%) 2822
- Xifaxan Tablets (Less than 2%) 2842
- Xyrem Oral Solution (Infrequent) 1688
- ▲ Zelnorm Tablets (3% to 4%) 2312
- Zyprexa Tablets (Infrequent) 1830
- Zyprexa ZYDIS Orally Disintegrating Tablets (Infrequent) 1830
- Zyrtec Chewable Tablets (Less than 2%) 2594
- Zyrtec (Less than 2%) 2594
- Zyrtec-D 12 Hour Extended Release Tablets (Less than 2%) 2597

Abdominal guarding

- Sandostatin Injection (Rare) 2278
- Sandostatin LAR Depot (Rare) 2280

Abdominal mass

- Estratest Tablets 3199
- Estratest H.S. Tablets 3199

Abdominal pain, gynecological

- ▲ Follistim AQ Cartridge (25%) 2338

Abdominal pain, upper

- ▲ Dacogen Injection (5%) 2129
- ▲ MoviPrep Oral Solution (5.8%) 2839
- ▲ Vivitrol (11% to 16%) 995

Abdominal pain/cramps

- ▲ Abelcet Injection (4%) 1141
- Abilify Oral Solution 882
- Abilify Oral Solution 2450
- Abilify Discmelt Orally Disintegrating Tablets 882
- Abilify Discmelt Orally Disintegrating Tablets 2450
- Abilify Tablets 882
- Abilify Tablets 2450
- Accolate Tablets (1.8% to 2.8%) 671
- Aceon Tablets (2 mg, 4 mg, 8 mg) (2.7%) 3194
- Aciphex Tablets 1090
- ▲ Actimmune (8%) 1671
- Actiq (1% or greater) 979
- ▲ Actonel Tablets (7.3% to 11.6%) 2683
- ▲ Actonel with Calcium Tablets (7.3% to 11.6%) 2688
- Adalat CC Tablets (Less than 1%) 2964
- ▲ Adderall XR Capsules (11% to 14%) 3166
- Advair Diskus 100/50 1308
- Advair Diskus 250/50 1308
- Advair Diskus 500/50 1308
- ▲ Advair HFA Inhalation Aerosol (1% to 3%) 1318
- Advate Injection (0.6%) 712
- ▲ Advicor Tablets (4%) 1722
- ▲ Aerobid/Aerobid-M (3% to 9%) 1171
- ▲ Agenerase Capsules (14%) 1327
- Agenerase Oral Solution 1332
- ▲ Aggrenox Capsules (17.5%) 822
- ▲ Agrylin Capsules (16.4%) 3169
- ▲ Albenza Tablets (Up to 6.0%) 1338
- Aldoril Tablets 1910
- ▲ Alinia for Oral Suspension (7.8%) 2835
- ▲ Alinia Tablets (7.8%) 2835
- Allegra-D 12 Hour Extended-Release Tablets (1.4%) 2846
- Allegra-D 24 Hour Extended-Release Tablets (1.4%) 2849
- Aloxi Injection (Less than 1%) 2127
- Altace Capsules (Less than 1%) 1702
- Altoprev Extended-Release Tablets (2% to 2.5%) 3109
- Ambien Tablets (2%) 2851
- Ambien CR Tablets (Frequent) 2855
- ▲ AmBisome for Injection (9.9% to 19.8%) 620
- Amerge Tablets (Infrequent) 1339
- Aminohippurate Sodium PAH Injection 1913
- ▲ Amitiza Capsules (0% to 6.8%) 3224
- ▲ Anaprox Tablets (3% to 9%) 2761
- ▲ Anaprox DS Tablets (3% to 9%) 2761
- ▲ Angeliq Tablets (11%) 762
- ▲ Anzemet Injection (3.2%) 2859
- Anzemet Tablets (Rare) 2862
- Aptivus Capsules (2.8%) 826
- ▲ Aranesp for Injection (12%) 581
- ▲ Aredia for Injection (22.6%) 2179
- ▲ Argatroban Injection (2.6% to 3.6%) 1346
- Aricept Tablets 1094
- Aricept ODT Tablets 1094
- ▲ Arimidex Tablets (6% to 9%) 673
- Arixtra Injection (1.4%) 1351
- ▲ Aromasin Tablets (6% to 11%) 2600
- ▲ Arranon Injection (0% to 9%) 1357
- ▲ Arthrotec Tablets (21%) 3129
- ▲ Asacol Delayed-Release Tablets (18%) 2692
- ▲ Asmanex Twisthaler (2% to 3%) 2966
- Astelin Nasal Spray (Infrequent) 1904
- Atacand Tablets (More than 1%) 649
- Atacand HCT (0.5% or greater) 651
- Atripla Tablets (Greater than or equal to 2%) 945
- Augmentin XR Extended-Release Tablets (1.6%) 1369
- Avalide Tablets (2%) 888
- Avalide Tablets (2%) 2874
- ▲ Avandamet Tablets (5%) 1373
- Avandaryl Tablets (Less than 1%) 1379
- ▲ Avandia Tablets (3%) 1384
- Avapro Tablets (1% or greater) 891
- Avapro Tablets (1% or greater) 2871
- ▲ Avastin IV (8% to 61%) 1227
- Avelox (0.1% to less than 2%) 2970
- ▲ Avinza Capsules (5% to 10%) 1741
- Axert Tablets (Infrequent) 2396
- ▲ Axid Oral Solution (7.5%) 879
- ▲ Azilect Tablets (5%) 3293
- ▲ Azmacort Inhalation Aerosol (1% to 3%) 1726
- Bactroban Cream (Less than 1%) 1394
- Benicar Tablets (Greater than 0.5%) 1043
- Benicar HCT Tablets (Greater than 1%) 1044
- Bentyl Capsules 697
- Bentyl Injection 697
- Bentyl Syrup 697
- Bentyl Tablets 697
- ▲ Betaseron for SC Injection (19%) 767
- ▲ Bexxar (3% to 15%) 1398
- ▲ Biaxin/Biaxin XL (2% to 3%) 402
- Biltricide Tablets 2976
- Blocadren Tablets 1916
- ▲ Boniva Injection (5.3% to 7.8%) 2738
- ▲ Boniva Tablets (5.3% to 7.8%) 2741
- ▲ Boostrix (3% to 26%) 1404
- Bumex Tablets (0.2% to 2.9%) 2746
- Byetta Injection 611
- ▲ Caduet Tablets (1.6% to 3.8%) 2508
- ▲ Campath Ampules (2% to 11%) 811
- Campral Tablets (Frequent) 1174
- ▲ Camptosar Injection (9% to 67.7%) 2604
- ▲ Canasa Rectal Suppositories (5.2%) 699
- ▲ Cancidas for Injection (0% to 3.6%) 1918
- Captopril Tablets (About 0.5% to 2%) 2149
- Carbatrol Capsules 3171
- Cardene I.V. (0.7%) 2497
- Cardura XL Tablets (1.8%) 2515
- Carimune NF 3499
- ▲ Carnitor Injection (5% to 21%) 3188
- Carnitor Tablets and Oral Solution 3190
- Catapres Tablets (Rare) 843
- Ceftin (0.1% to 1%) 1407
- ▲ Celebrex Capsules (4.1%) 3134
- ▲ Celexa (3%) 1176
- ▲ CellCept Capsules (24.7% to 62.5%) 2747
- ▲ CellCept Intravenous (24.7% to 62.5%) 2747
- ▲ CellCept Oral Suspension (24.7% to 62.5%) 2747
- ▲ CellCept Tablets (24.7% to 62.5%) 2747
- ▲ Cerezyme for Injection (Approximately 6.5%) 1270
- Cervidil Vaginal Insert (Less than 1%) 1181
- Cesamet Capsules 3340
- ▲ Chantix Tablets (5% to 7%) 2517
- ▲ Chemet Capsules (5.2% to 15.7%) 2458
- Cialis Tablets (Less than 2%) 1838
- ▲ Cipro (Less than 1% to 3.3%) 2977
- ▲ Cipro I.V. (1% or less to 3.3%) 2984
- Cipro XR Tablets (Less than 1%) 2990
- Cleocin Vaginal Ovules (Less than 1%) 2616
- ▲ Climara Transdermal System (11% to 16%) 771
- ▲ Climara Pro Transdermal System (4.2%) 776
- Clindagel 1203
- ▲ Clinoril Tablets (10%) 1924
- ▲ Clolar for Intravenous Infusion (36%) 1271
- ▲ Colazal Capsules (6%) 2838
- Colyte with Flavor Packs for Oral Solution (Less frequent) 3088
- ▲ Combivir Tablets (6% to 9%) 1411
- ▲ Comtan Tablets (8%) 2189
- ▲ Concerta Extended-Release Tablets (0.7% to 7%) 1881
- Copaxone for Injection (At least 2%) 3297
- ▲ Copegus Tablets (8%) 2754
- Cosmegen for Injection 2459
- ▲ Cosopt Sterile Ophthalmic Solution (1% to 5%) 1931
- Coumadin for Injection (Infrequent) 898
- Coumadin Tablets (Infrequent) 898
- Cozaar Tablets (1% or greater) 1935
- ▲ Creon 5 Capsules (Among most frequent) 3198
- ▲ Creon 10 Capsules (Among most frequent) 3198
- ▲ Creon 20 Capsules (Among most frequent) 3199
- Crestor Tablets (Greater than or equal to 2%) 678
- ▲ Crixivan Capsules (16.6%) 1940
- ▲ Cubicin for Injection (1% to 5.8%) 1026
- Cymbalta Delayed-Release Capsules (Infrequent) 1757
- ▲ Dacogen Injection (14%) 2129
- Dalmane Capsules 3342
- Dantrium Capsules (Less frequent) 2694
- Dapsone Tablets USP 1673
- Daytrana Transdermal Patch 3174
- Demser Capsules (Infrequent) 1953
- ▲ Depacon Injection (1.1% to 23%) 412
- ▲ Depakene (12% to 23%) 417
- ▲ Depakote Sprinkle Capsules (9% to 23%) 422
- ▲ Depakote Tablets (9% to 23%) 427
- ▲ Depakote ER Tablets (7% to 23%) 434
- ▲ Depo-Provera Contraceptive Injection (Greater than 5%) 2622
- ▲ depo-subQ provera 104 Injectable Suspension (1% to less than 5%) 2624
- ▲ Detrol Tablets (5%) 2628
- ▲ Detrol LA Capsules (4%) 2631
- Diastat Rectal Delivery System (1% or more) 3343
- Dilaudid-HP (Less frequent) 442
- Diovan Tablets (2%) 2193
- Diovan HCT Tablets (Greater than 0.2%) 2196
- ▲ Ditropan XL Extended-Release Tablets (2% to less than 5%) 2413
- Diuril Sodium Intravenous 2467
- ▲ Doxil Injection (1% to 33.5%) 2351
- Duac Topical Gel 3212
- ▲ Duragesic Transdermal System (3% to 10%) 2373
- Dyazide Capsules 1423
- ▲ EC-Naprosyn Delayed-Release Tablets (3% to 9%) 2761
- Edecrin 1959

▲ E.E.S. (Among most frequent) 451
▲ Effexor Tablets (2.2% to 8.0%) 3411
▲ Effexor XR Capsules (4%) 3417
▲ Eldepryl Capsules (4 of 49 patients).. 3208
▲ Elitek (20%) 2890
Elmiron Capsules (2%)........................ 2415
▲ Eloxatin for Injection (1% to 33%) 2892
Elspar for Injection............................ 2463
Elspar for Injection............................ 1960
▲ Emend Capsules (4.6%) 1963
Emsam Transdermal System........... 903
▲ Emtriva Capsules (8% to 14%) 1287
▲ Emtriva Oral Solution (8% to 14%) ... 1287
▲ Enablex Extended-Release Tablets (2.4% to 3.9%)................. 2203
▲ Enbrel for Injection (5% to 19%) 584
Engerix-B Vaccine (Less than 1%)..... 1425
▲ Enjuvia Tablets (4% to 15%) 1062
▲ Entocort EC Capsules (6%) 2698
▲ Epivir (6% to 9%) 1427
▲ Epivir-HBV (16%) 1432
Epogen for Injection........................ 591
▲ Epzicom Tablets (4% to 5%) 1436
Equetro Extended-Release Capsules.. 3180
Eraxis for Injection (Less than 1% to less than 2%).............................. 2521
▲ Erbitux (8% to 45%) 910
▲ EryPed (Among most frequent) 447
▲ Ery-Tab Tablets (Among most frequent).. 449
▲ Erythrocin Stearate Filmtab Tablets (Among most frequent)..... 453
▲ Erythromycin Base Filmtab Tablets (Among most frequent)...... 455
▲ Erythromycin Delayed-Release Capsules, USP (Among most frequent).. 457
Estrasorb Topical Emulsion............. 1147
Estratest Tablets 3199
Estratest H.S. Tablets...................... 3199
▲ Estring Vaginal Ring (4%) 2635
▲ Evista Tablets (6.6%) 1763
Evoclin Foam (1%)............................ 1009
▲ Evoxac Capsules (7.6%) 1047
▲ Exelon Capsules (4% to 13%) 2206
▲ Exelon Oral Solution (4% to 13%) ... 2206
▲ Famvir Tablets (1.1% to 7.9%) 2211
Fansidar Tablets 2765
▲ Faslodex Injection (11.8%) 681
▲ Femara Tablets (4% to 6%) 2214
▲ Ferrlecit Injection (3% to 15%) 3388
Flebogamma 5%, Immune Globulin Intravenous (Human).................... 1658
Fleet Bisacodyl Laxatives................. 1165
Fleet Prep Kits................................... 1170
▲ Flonase Nasal Spray (1% to 3%) 1440
▲ Flovent Diskus (3%) 1443
Floxin Otic Solution (Single report)... 1049
Fluarix... 1451
Flumadine (1.4%).............................. 1183
▲ Flumist Vaccine (3.7%) 1901
▲ Focalin Tablets (15%) 2220
Focalin XR Capsules 2223
▲ Follistim AQ Cartridge (5% to 28%)... 2338
▲ Fortamet Extended-Release Tablets (3.3%)............................. 3115
Fortaz (1 in 416)............................... 1453
▲ Fortical Nasal Spray (1% to 3%) 3337
▲ Fosamax (0.9% to 6.6%) 1969
▲ Fosamax Plus D Tablets (0.9% to 6.6%).. 1977
▲ Fosrenol Chewable Tablets (5% to 17%)... 3183
Frova Tablets (Frequent).................. 1113
Furosemide Tablets.......................... 2154
▲ Fuzeon Injection (3.9%) 2767
▲ Gabitril Tablets (5% to 7%) 984
Gammagard Liquid........................... 721
Gammagard S/D................................ 724
▲ Gamunex Immune Globulin I.V., 10% (4%)... 3235
Gantrisin Pediatric Suspension......... 2770
▲ Gengraf Capsules (2.7% to 15%) 459
Geodon (Frequent)............................ 2529
▲ Gleevec Tablets (1% to 40%) 2227
Guanidine Hydrochloride Tablets...... 3016
▲ HalfLytely and Bisacodyl Tablets Bowel Prep Kit with Flavors Packs (9.1% to 50%).................. 881
Havrix Vaccine (Less than 1%).......... 1456
▲ Hepsera Tablets (2% to 9%) 1292
▲ Herceptin I.V. (22%) 1233
▲ Humira Injection (7%) 466
▲ Hycamtin for Injection (Less than 1% to 33%)...................................... 1458
Hytrin Capsules (At least 1%)........... 471
Hyzaar 50-12.5 Tablets (1.2%)......... 1990
Hyzaar 100-12.5 Tablets (1.2%)....... 1990
Hyzaar 100-25 Tablets (1.2%).......... 1990
▲ Imdur Tablets (Less than or equal to 5%)... 3018
Imitrex Injection................................. 1463
Imitrex Nasal Spray........................... 1467
Imitrex Tablets.................................. 1471
Indapamide Tablets (Less than 5%).. 2156
Inderal LA Long-Acting Capsules...... 3429
Indocin (Greater than 1%)................. 1995
Infed Injection................................... 3390
▲ Infergen (24% to 41%) 3364
InnoPran XL Capsules...................... 2723
Inspra Tablets (1%)........................... 2536
▲ Intron A for Injection (1% to 21%) 3024
▲ Invanz for Injection (1% to 4.7%) 1999
▲ Invirase (0.3% to 6.1%) 2772
▲ Ionsys Transdermal System (1% to less than 10%)........................... 2379
▲ I.V. Busulfex (3% to 72%) 2493
Kadian Capsules (Less than 3%)....... 577
▲ Kaletra (4% to 10%) 476
K-Dur Extended-Relase Tablets......... 3033
Keflex Capsules................................ 549
Keppra Injection................................ 3320
Keppra Oral Solution (1% to 2%)...... 3314
Keppra Tablets (1% to 2%).............. 3314
Ketek Tablets (Greater than or equal to 0.2% to less than 2%) 2903
▲ Kineret Injection (5%) 599
Klonopin (1%) 2778
▲ K-Lor Oral Solution (Among most common) 474
Kristalose for Oral Solution 1034
▲ Kytril Injection (6%) 2781
▲ Kytril (4% to 6%) 2784
▲ Lamictal (5% to 10%) 1481
Lamisil Tablets (2.4%) 2232
Lanoxicaps Capsules (Rare) 1490
Lanoxin Injection (Rare) 1494
Lanoxin Injection Pediatric (Rare) 1497
Lanoxin Tablets (Rare) 1500
▲ Lariam Tablets (Among most frequent) 2786
▲ Lescol Capsules (4.9%) 2233
▲ Lescol XL Tablets (3.7%) 2233
▲ Leukine (38%) 814
▲ Leustatin Injection (6%) 2357
Levaquin (0.4% to 2.5%) 2384
Levaquin in 5% Dextrose Injection (0.4% to 2.5%)............................. 2384
Levitra Tablets (Less than 2%) 3034
Levothroid Tablets 1186
Levoxyl Tablets 1712
Lexapro Oral Solution (2%) 1190
Lexapro Tablets (2%) 1190
▲ Lexiva Tablets (Less than 1% to 11%)... 1505
▲ Lipitor Tablets (Up to 3.8%) 2483
Lithobid Tablets 1692
▲ Lofibra Tablets (4.6%) 1219
▲ Lofibra Capsules (4.6%) 1216
Lopressor Injection (Less than 1%) .. 2238
Lopressor Tablets (Less than 1%) 2238
Lotensin HCT Tablets (0.3% to 1%) .. 2246
Lotrel Capsules 2249
▲ Lotronex Tablets (7%) 1512
Lunesta Tablets 3142
Lyrica Capsules (Greather than or equal to 1%) 2539
▲ Malarone Pediatric Tablets (2% to 31%) 1517
▲ Malarone Tablets (2% to 31%) 1517
▲ Marinol Capsules (3% to 10%) 3333
Matulane Capsules 3191
Mavik Tablets (0.3% to 1.0%) 486
Maxair Autohaler 1852
Mefoxin for Injection 2012
Mefoxin Premixed Intravenous Solution 2016
▲ Megace ES Oral Suspension (1% to 3%) 2481
▲ Menostar Transdermal System (8%) 782
▲ Mepron Suspension (4% to 21%) 1521
▲ Meridia Capsules (4.5%) 489
Merrem I.V. (Greater than 0.1% to 1%) 686
▲ Metadate CD Capsules (7%) 3323
▲ Mevacor Tablets (2.0% to 5.7%) 2021
Miacalcin Injection 2252
▲ Miacalcin Nasal Spray (1% to 3%) ... 2253
Micardis Tablets (1%) 854
Micardis HCT Tablets (Less than 2%) 856
▲ Midamor Tablets (Between 1% and 3%) 2026
Migranal Nasal Spray (Rare) 3348
Mintezol 2027
Miradon Tablets 3042
Mirapex Tablets (1% or more) 859
Mircette Tablets 1066
▲ Mirena Intrauterine System (5% or more) 787
▲ Mobic Oral Suspension (1.9% to 4.7%) 863
▲ Mobic Tablets (1.9% to 4.7%) 863
Moduretic Tablets (Greater than 1%, less than 3%) 2028
▲ MoviPrep Oral Solution (13.3%) 2839
MS Contin Tablets (Less frequent) 2701
Mycamine for Injection (0.5% to 1.9%)... 628
▲ Myfortic Tablets (3% to less than 20%) 2255
▲ Mylotarg for Injection (26% to 39%) 3431
Myozyme for Intravenous Infusion.... 1279
Nabi-HB 2169
Nalfon Capsules (2%)....................... 2502
▲ Naprosyn Suspension (3% to 9%) 2761
▲ Naprosyn Tablets (3% to 9%) 2761
▲ Natrecor for Injection (1% to 3%) 3127
▲ Neoral Oral Solution (2.7% to 15%)... 2259
▲ Neoral Soft Gelatin Capsules (2.7% to 15%)................................ 2259
▲ Neulasta Injection (15% to 72%) 601
▲ Neumega for Injection (Greater than or equal to 10%).................... 3435
Neupogen for Injection (Infrequent).. 603
Neurontin Capsules (2.7%).............. 2487
Neurontin Oral Solution (2.7%) 2487
Neurontin Tablets (2.7%) 2487
▲ Nexavar Tablets (0% to 11%) 746
▲ Nexium Delayed-Release Capsules (Greater than or equal to 1% to 3.8%) 655
▲ Nexium I.V. (Greater than or equal to 1% to 3.8%) 659
▲ Niaspan Extended-Release Tablets (2% to 5%) 1730
▲ Nipent for Injection (4% to 16%) 1863
Noroxin Tablets (0.3% to 1.6%) 2032
Norvasc Tablets (1.6%) 2545
▲ Norvir (6% to 8.3%) 503
Numorphan Injection 1120
NuvaRing 2340
Omnicef Capsules (1%) 511
Omnicef for Oral Suspension (0.8%) 511
▲ Oncaspar (Greater than 1% but less than 5%) 1145
Opana Tablets (Less than 1%) 1122
Opana ER Tablets (2.5%) 1126
Oracea Capsules (1.1% to 1.9%) 1000
Ortho-Cyclen Tablets 2429
▲ Ortho Evra Transdermal System (9% to 22%) 2417
Ortho Tri-Cyclen Tablets 2429
Ortho Tri-Cyclen Lo Tablets 2436
Orthoclone OKT3 Sterile Solution 2360
▲ OsmoPrep Tablets (23% to 24%) 2840
▲ OxyContin Tablets (Between 1% and 5%) 2703
▲ Oxytrol Transdermal System (Greater than 1%) 3392
▲ Pancrease MT Capsules (Among most frequent) 1885
Parcopa Orally Disintegrating Tablets 3097
Parnate Tablets 1527
▲ Paser Granules (Among most common) 1674
▲ Paxil CR Controlled-Release Tablets (4%) 1538
▲ Paxil (4%) 1530
▲ PCE Dispertab Tablets (Among most frequent) 515
Pediarix Vaccine 1548
▲ Pegasys (15%) 2789
▲ PEG-Intron Powder for Injection (15%) 3048
Pentasa Capsules (1.1% to 1.7%) 3185
Percodan Tablets 1132
▲ Permax Tablets (5.8%) 3356
▲ Pexeva Tablets (4%) 1694
▲ Photofrin for Injection (12% to 20%) 702
▲ Plan B Tablets (17.6%) 1076
▲ Plavix Tablets (5.6%) 917
▲ Plavix Tablets (5.6%) 2926
▲ Pletal Tablets (4% to 5%) 2455
▲ Precose Tablets (19%) 751
Premarin Intravenous 3442
▲ Premarin Tablets (15% to 17%) 3446
Premarin Vaginal Cream 3452
▲ Premphase Tablets (13% to 23%) 3456
▲ Prempro Tablets (13% to 23%) 3456
▲ Prevacid Delayed-Release Capsules (2.1% to 5%) 3271
▲ Prevacid for Delayed-Release Oral Suspension (2.1% to 5%) 3271
▲ Prevacid SoluTab Delayed-Release Orally Disintegrating Tablets (2.1% to 5%) 3271
Prevacid I.V. for Injection (Less than 1%) 3277
▲ Prevacid NapraPAC (2.1% to 9%) 3280
▲ PREVPAC (1.8% to 3%) 3284
Prezista Tablets (1.2% to 2.3%) 3306
▲ Prilosec OTC Delayed-Release Tablets (2.4% to 5.2%) 2677
Primaxin I.M. 2045
Primaxin I.V. (Less than 0.2%) 2048
▲ Prinivil Tablets (0.3% to 4.0%) 2052
Prinzide Tablets (0.3% to 1%)........... 2056
▲ Prochieve 4% Gel (12% to 15%) 1003
▲ Prochieve 8% Gel (12% to 15%) 1003
▲ Prograf Capsules and Injection (29% to 59%)................................ 632
▲ Proleukin for Injection (11%) 2266
▲ Prometrium Capsules (100 mg, 200 mg) (10% to 20%)................... 3203
ProNutra Protein Supplement 1668
ProQuad... 2064
Proquin XR Tablets (Less than 1%)... 1153
ProSom Tablets (1%)........................ 517
▲ Protonix I.V. (12%) 3472
▲ Protonix Tablets (1% to 4%) 3469
▲ Protopic Ointment (1% to 5%) 638
Provigil Tablets (At least 1%)............ 988
Prozac Pulvules and Liquid............... 1801
▲ Pulmicort Respules (2% to 3%) 661
Pulmozyme Inhalation Solution......... 1248
▲ Quadramet Injection (6%) 1040
Ranexa Tablets (Greater than 0.5% to less than 2%)............................. 1035
Raniclor Tablets, Chewable.............. 2505
▲ Rapamune Oral Solution and Tablets (28% to 36%)................... 3475
▲ Razadyne (5%) 2399
▲ Razadyne ER Extended-Release Capsules (5%)............................... 2399
▲ Rebetol (13%) 3058
▲ Rebif Prefilled Syringe for Injection (20% to 22%)................. 3159
Recombivax HB (Less than 1%)........ 2071
ReFacto Vials.................................... 3484
Relenza Rotadisk (Less than 1.5%).. 1552
Relpax Tablets (1% to 2%)............... 2548
▲ Remicade for IV Injection (12%) 971
Renagel Tablets................................. 1282
▲ Requip Tablets (3% to 9%) 1555
▲ Rescriptor Tablets (2.4% to 5%) 2551
▲ Retrovir Capsules (3.2%) 1560
▲ Retrovir IV Infusion (4%) 1564
▲ Retrovir (3.2%) 1560
▲ Revlimid Capsules (8.1% to 12.2%)... 958
▲ Reyataz Capsules (5% to 10%) 921
▲ Ribavirin, USP Capsules (13%) 3068
▲ Rilutek Tablets (6.8% to 7.8%) 2930
▲ Risperdal (1% to 4%) 1676
Risperdal Consta Long-Acting Injection (Frequent)....................... 1682
▲ Risperdal M-Tab Orally Disintegrating Tablets (1% to 4%).. 1676
Ritalin Hydrochloride Tablets............ 2269
Ritalin LA Capsules........................... 2271
Ritalin-SR Tablets.............................. 2269
▲ Rituxan I.V. (1% to 14%) 1254
Rocaltrol Capsules............................ 2798
Rocaltrol Oral Solution..................... 2798
Rocephin Injectable Vials, ADD-Vantage, Galaxy, Bulk (Rare).. 2800
Rythmol SR Capsules........................ 2727
Sanctura Tablets (1.5%)................... 1151
▲ Sandostatin LAR Depot (29.1%) 2280
Seasonique Tablets........................... 1077
▲ Seroquel Tablets (4%) 690
▲ Simulect for Injection (Greater than or equal to 10%).................... 2284
Singulair (Greater than or equal to 2% to 2.9%)................................... 2077
Soltamox Oral Solution (1%)............ 3527
▲ Sonata Capsules (6%) 1717
▲ Soriatane Capsules (1% to 10%) 1013
▲ Spiriva HandiHaler (5% to 6%) 869
▲ Stalevo Tablets (5% to 8%) 2287
▲ Strattera Capsules (2% to 20%) 1814
Striant Mucoadhesive....................... 1007
Stromectol Tablets (0.9%)................ 2083
▲ Suboxone Tablets (11.20%) 2717
▲ Subutex Tablets (11.7%) 2717
▲ Suprax (3%) 1843
▲ Sustiva Capsules (1% to 3%) 930
▲ Sustiva Tablets (1% to 3%) 930
▲ Sutent Capsules (3% to 33%) 2560
▲ Symlin Injection (2% to 8%) 613
▲ Tambocor Tablets (3.3%) 1856
▲ Tamiflu Capsules (2% to 5%) 2807
▲ Tamiflu Oral Suspension (2% to 5%).. 2807
▲ Tarceva Tablets (Less than 1% to 46%)... 1259
▲ Tarceva Tablets (Less than 1% to 46%)... 2444
▲ Targretin Capsules (3.8% to 10.7%)... 1747
▲ Tasmar Tablets (5% to 6%) 3358
▲ Taxotere Injection Concentrate (1.8% to 10.9%)............................ 2932
Tegretol/Tegretol-XR......................... 2295
▲ Temodar Capsules (5% to 9%) 3073
▲ Tequin Injection (0.1% to 3%) 938
▲ Tequin Injection in 5% Dextrose (0.1% to 3%).................................. 938
▲ Tequin Tablets (0.1% to 3%) 938
Teveten Tablets (2%)........................ 1735

Teveten HCT Tablets (Less than 1%) 1737
▲ Thalomid Capsules (4.2%) 965
▲ Thiola Tablets (16.7%) 2141
▲ Thymoglobulin for Intravenous Infusion (37.8%) 1284
Tindamax Tablets 2142
▲ TOBI Solution for Inhalation (12.8%) 2298
▲ Topamax Sprinkle Capsules (5% to 7%) 2404
▲ Topamax Tablets (5% to 7%) 2404
Toprol-XL Tablets (Greater than 1%) 668
Tracleer Tablets 545
Trecator Tablets 3487
Trelstar LA Suspension (1.1%) 3397
▲ Tricor Tablets (4.6%) 527
▲ Triglide Tablets (4.6%) 3123
▲ Trileptal Tablets (3% to 13%) 2300
▲ Trileptal Oral Suspension (3% to 13%) 2300
TriLyte with Flavor Packs for Oral Solution 3100
▲ Trisenox Injection (58%) 993
▲ Trizivir Tablets (6% to 9%) 1589
▲ Truvada Tablets (Greater than 5%) 1296
Twinrix Vaccine (Less than 1%) 1595
▲ Tygacil for Injection (6.8%) 3488
Tylenol with Codeine Tablets 2391
▲ Ultram ER Tablets (1% to greater than 5%) 2392
Ultrase Capsules 708
▲ Ultrase MT Capsules (5.7%) 709
Uniretic Tablets (More than 1%) 3100
Univasc Tablets (Less than 1%) 3104
Uroxatral Tablets (1% to 2%) 2943
▲ Vagifem Tablets (7%) 2334
▲ Valcyte Tablets (15%) 2813
▲ Valtrex Caplets (1% to 11%) 1597
▲ Vandazole Vaginal Gel (5%) 3338
Vantin Tablets and Oral Suspension (Less than 1% to 1.6%) 2645
Vaqta (1.1% to 1.6%) 2097
Varivax (Greater than or equal to 1%) 2100
Vasotec I.V. Injection (1.6%) 2103
▲ Velcade for Injection (16%) 2133
▲ Vesanoid Capsules (31%) 2820
VESIcare Tablets (1.2% to 1.9%) 646
VFEND I.V. (Less than 2%) 2564
VFEND Oral Suspension (Less than 2%) 2564
VFEND Tablets (Less than 2%) 2564
Viadur Implant (Less than 2%) 757
Viagra Tablets (Less than 2%) 2573
▲ Vicoprofen Tablets (3% to 9%) 539
Viracept (Less than 2%) 2577
Viramune Oral Suspension (1%) 873
Viramune Tablets (1%) 873
▲ Viread Tablets (4% to 7%) 1301
▲ Vivitrol (11% to 16%) 995
Vivotif 819
▲ Voltaren Ophthalmic Solution (Less than or equal to 3%) 2309
▲ Voltaren Tablets (1% to 10%) 2307
▲ Voltaren-XR Tablets (1% to 10%) 2310
Vytorin 10/10 Tablets 2114
Vytorin 10/10 Tablets 3077
Vytorin 10/20 Tablets 2114
Vytorin 10/20 Tablets 3077
Vytorin 10/40 Tablets 2114
Vytorin 10/40 Tablets 3077
Vytorin 10/80 Tablets 2114
Vytorin 10/80 Tablets 3077
▲ WelChol Tablets (5%) 1050
▲ Wellbutrin SR Sustained-Release Tablets (3% to 9%) 1607
▲ Wellbutrin XL Extended-Release Tablets (3% to 9%) 1613
WinRho SDF 732
▲ Xeloda Tablets (9% to 35%) 2822
▲ Xenical Capsules (25.5%) 2831
▲ Xifaxan Tablets (7.2%) 2842
Xopenex Inhalation Solution (1.5%) 3146
Xopenex Inhalation Solution Concentrate (1.5%) 3150
Xopenex HFA Inhalation Aerosol (1.5%) 3154
▲ Xyrem Oral Solution (3% to 11.4%) 1688
Yasmin 28 Tablets (Greater than 1%) 796
Yaz Tablets (Greater than 1%) 803
Zantac 1624
Zantac Injection 1619
Zantac Injection Pharmacy Bulk Package (Frequent) 1622
Zantac Injection Premixed 1619
Zantac 1624
▲ Zegerid Capsules (2.4% to 5.2%) 2958
▲ Zegerid Powder for Oral Solution (2.4% to 5.2%) 2958
▲ Zelnorm Tablets (2% to 12%) 2312
Zemaira (0.2% to 0.4%) 3509
▲ Zetia Tablets (2.7% to 3.5%) 2120
▲ Zetia Tablets (2.7% to 3%) 3083
▲ Ziagen (6%) 1626
Zinacef for Injection 1631
Zinacef Injection 1631
Zmax for Oral Suspension (2.7%) 2583
▲ Zocor Tablets (3.2%) 2105
Zofran Injection (2%) 1634
▲ Zofran (1% to 3%) 1639
▲ Zofran ODT Orally Disintegrating Tablets (1% to 3%) 1639
▲ Zoloft (2% to 7%) 2586
▲ Zometa for Intravenous Infusion (14% to 16.3%) 2315
Zomig Tablets (Rare) 3519
Zomig Nasal Spray (Very rare to less than 2%) 3523
Zomig-ZMT Tablets (Rare) 3519
▲ Zonegran Capsules (6%) 1101
Zosyn (1.3%) 3492
▲ Zyban Sustained-Release Tablets (3%) 1644
▲ Zyflo Tablets (4.6%) 1023
▲ Zyprexa Tablets (4%) 1830
Zyprexa IntraMuscular (Infrequent) 1830
▲ Zyprexa ZYDIS Orally Disintegrating Tablets (4%) 1830
▲ Zyrtec Chewable Tablets (4.4% to 5.6%) 2594
▲ Zyrtec (4.4% to 5.6%) 2594
▲ Zyrtec-D 12 Hour Extended Release Tablets (4.4% to 5.6%) 2597
Zyvox (0% to 2.4%) 2652

Abdominal surgeries, increased risk of
Zelnorm Tablets (0.3%) 2312

Abdominal symptom complex, acute
Permax Tablets (Rare) 3356
Prozac Pulvules and Liquid (Rare) 1801

Abdominal symptoms, unspecified
▲ Agenerase Oral Solution (14%) 1332

Abdominal tenderness
Ambien CR Tablets (1%) 2855
▲ Chantix Tablets (5% to 7%) 2517
Sandostatin Injection (Rare) 2278

Abortion
Copaxone for Injection (Infrequent) 3297
Effexor Tablets (Rare) 3411
Effexor XR Capsules (Rare) 3417
Gabitril Tablets (Infrequent) 984
Imitrex Injection 1463
Imitrex Nasal Spray 1467
Imitrex Tablets (Rare) 1471
Paxil CR Controlled-Release Tablets (Infrequent) 1538
Paxil (Infrequent) 1530
Permax Tablets (Infrequent) 3356
Pexeva Tablets (rare) 1694
Prozac Pulvules and Liquid (Infrequent) 1801

Abortion, septic
ParaGard T 380A Intrauterine Copper Contraceptive 1073

Abortion, spontaneous
Celexa 1176
Lexapro Oral Solution 1190
Lexapro Tablets 1190
Limbrel Capsules (0.003%) 2672
Lupron Depot-PED 7.5 mg, 11.25 mg and 15 mg (Possible) 3269
Rebif Prefilled Syringe for Injection 3159

Abrasion
▲ Dacogen Injection (5%) 2129
Neurontin Oral Solution (1.3%) 2487

Abscess
Actiq (Less than 1%) 979
Aldurazyme for Intravenous Infusion (2%) 1268
Ambien Tablets (Rare) 2851
Ambien CR Tablets (Rare) 2855
▲ Aranesp for Injection (27%) 581
Aricept Tablets (Infrequent) 1094
Aricept ODT Tablets (Infrequent) 1094
Campath Ampules 811
Campral Tablets (Infrequent) 1174
Capastat Sulfate for Injection 1755
▲ CellCept Capsules (3% to less than 20%) 2747
▲ CellCept Intravenous (3% to less than 20%) 2747
▲ CellCept Oral Suspension (3% to less than 20%) 2747
▲ CellCept Tablets (3% to less than 20%) 2747
Colazal Capsules 2838
Depo-Medrol Single-Dose Vial 2619
Doxil Injection (Less than 1%) 2351
Enbrel for Injection 584
▲ Evoxac Capsules (1% to 3%) 1047
Ferrlecit Injection 3388
Gabitril Tablets (Infrequent) 984
▲ Gengraf Capsules (4.4%) 459
▲ Hectorol Capsules (3.3%) 1275
▲ Hectorol Injection (3.3%) 1278
Infed Injection 3390
▲ Intron A for Injection (Less than 5%) 3024
Invirase (Less than 2%) 2772
Ionsys Transdermal System (.1% to less than 1%) 2379
Lamictal (Rare) 1481
Levaquin (0.1% to 0.9%) 2384
Levaquin in 5% Dextrose Injection (0.1% to 0.9%) 2384
▲ Lupron Depot-PED 7.5 mg, 11.25 mg and 15 mg (5%) 3269
Lyrica Capsules (0.1% to 1%) 2539
Micardis Tablets (More than 0.3%) 854
Micardis HCT Tablets 856
Myobloc Injection (Greater than 2%) 3192
▲ Neoral Soft Gelatin Capsules (1% to 4.4%) 2259
Neurontin Capsules (Infrequent) 2487
Neurontin Oral Solution (Infrequent) 2487
Neurontin Tablets (Infrequent) 2487
Nipent for Injection (2%) 1863
Paxil CR Controlled-Release Tablets (Rare) 1538
Paxil (Rare) 1530
PEG-Intron Powder for Injection (Less than or equal to 1%) 3048
Permax Tablets (Infrequent) 3356
▲ Prograf Capsules and Injection (3% to 15%) 632
▲ Prometrium Capsules (100 mg, 200 mg) (Less than 5%) 3203
Protonix I.V. (Less than 1%) 3472
Protonix Tablets (Less than 1%) 3469
Protopic Ointment (0.2% to less than 1%) 638
▲ Rapamune Oral Solution and Tablets (3% to 20%) 3475
Raptiva for Injection 1250
Relpax Tablets (Rare) 2548
▲ Remicade for IV Injection (15%) 971
ReoPro Vials (0.2%) 1809
Requip Tablets (Infrequent) 1555
Rescriptor Tablets 2551
Rilutek Tablets (Infrequent) 2930
Risperdal Consta Long-Acting Injection (Infrequent) 1682
▲ Sandimmune (4.4% to 5.3%) 2275
Suboxone Tablets (2%) 2717
Subutex Tablets (2%) 2717
Tasmar Tablets (Infrequent) 3358
▲ Tygacil for Injection (3.2%) 3488
Uniretic Tablets (Less than 1%) 3100
Vantin Tablets and Oral Suspension (Less than 1%) 2645

Abscess, abdominal
Enbrel for Injection 584
Invanz for Injection (1%) 1999

Abscess, dental
Vivitrol 995
Xyrem Oral Solution (Infrequent) 1688

Abscess, foot
Enbrel for Injection 584

Abscess, peridiverticular
Dacogen Injection 2129

Abscess, periodontal
Abilify Oral Solution (Infrequent) 882
Abilify Oral Solution (Infrequent) 2450
Abilify Discmelt Orally Disintegrating Tablets (Infrequent) 882
Abilify Discmelt Orally Disintegrating Tablets (Infrequent) 2450
Abilify Tablets (Infrequent) 882
Abilify Tablets (Infrequent) 2450
Actiq (1% or greater) 979
Aricept Tablets (Infrequent) 1094
Aricept ODT Tablets (Infrequent) 1094
Copaxone for Injection (At least 2%) 3297
Crestor Tablets (Greater than or equal to 1%) 678
▲ Depacon Injection (1% to 5%) 412
▲ Depakene (1% to 5%) 417
▲ Depakote Sprinkle Capsules (1% to 5%) 422
▲ Depakote Tablets (1% to 5%) 427
Depakote ER Tablets (Greater than 1%) 434
Doxil Injection (Less than 1%) 2351
Gabitril Tablets (Infrequent) 984
Neurontin Capsules (Infrequent) 2487
Neurontin Oral Solution (Infrequent) 2487
Neurontin Tablets (Infrequent) 2487
Norvir (Less than 2%) 503
Permax Tablets (Infrequent) 3356
Pletal Tablets (Less than 2%) 2455
Protonix I.V. (Less than 1%) 3472
Protonix Tablets (Less than 1%) 3469
▲ Protopic Ointment (Up to 3%) 638
Provigil Tablets (Greater than or equal to 1%) 988
Rescriptor Tablets 2551
Symbyax Capsules (Infrequent) 1819
Uniretic Tablets (Less than 1%) 3100
Zyprexa Tablets (Infrequent) 1830
Zyprexa ZYDIS Orally Disintegrating Tablets (Infrequent) 1830

Abscess, perirectal
Revlimid Capsules 958

Abscess, peritonsillar
Amevive 626
Tamiflu Capsules (Less than 1%) 2807
Tamiflu Oral Suspension (Less than 1%) 2807

Abscess, renal
Gengraf Capsules (1% to less than 3%) 459
Neoral Oral Solution (1% to less than 3%) 2259
▲ Sandostatin LAR Depot (1% to 4%) 2280

Abscess at injection site
ADACEL Vaccine (Very rare) 2945
Bicillin C-R Injectable Suspension 1706
Cerezyme for Injection (Less than 1%) 1270
Copaxone for Injection (Frequent) 3297
Fluarix 1451
Lupron Depot 3.75 mg 3260
Lupron Depot 7.5 mg 3264
Lupron Depot–3 Month 11.25 mg 3265
▲ Lupron Injection Pediatric (5%) 3259
Liquid PedvaxHIB 2035

Abuse
Ambien Tablets (Rare) 2851
Prozac Pulvules and Liquid 1801
Sonata Capsules 1717

Acanthosis nigricans
Advicor Tablets 1722
Niaspan Extended-Release Tablets 1730

Accident, road traffic
Xyrem Oral Solution (Infrequent) 1688

Accommodation, changes in
Ambien CR Tablets (Rare) 2855
Avandaryl Tablets 1379

Accommodation, impaired
Ambien Tablets (Rare) 2851
Blephamide Ophthalmic Ointment (Occasional) 568
Blephamide Ophthalmic Suspension 569
Caduet Tablets (Less than or equal to 0.1%) 2508
Celexa (Frequent) 1176
Concerta Extended-Release Tablets 1881
Detrol Tablets (2%) 2628
▲ Effexor Tablets (5.6% to 9.1%) 3411
Effexor XR Capsules (Frequent) 3417
FML Ophthalmic Ointment (Occasional) ⊙228
FML Ophthalmic Suspension (Occasional) ⊙227
FML Forte Ophthalmic Suspension (Occasional) ⊙226
Focalin Tablets 2220
Imitrex Nasal Spray 1467
Lamictal (Infrequent) 1481
Lyrica Capsules (0.1% to 1%) 2539
Metadate CD Capsules 3323
▲ Mirapex Tablets (Greater than 1% to 4%) 859
Neurontin Capsules (Rare) 2487
Neurontin Oral Solution (Rare) 2487
Neurontin Tablets (Rare) 2487
Norvasc Tablets (Less than 0.1%) 2545
Paxil CR Controlled-Release Tablets (Infrequent) 1538
Paxil (Infrequent) 1530

Pred Mild Ophthalmic Suspension (Occasional) ⊙238
Pred Forte Ophthalmic Suspension (Occasional) ⊙235
Relpax Tablets (Rare) 2548
Requip Tablets (Infrequent) 1555
Risperdal (Infrequent) 1676
Risperdal Consta Long-Acting Injection (Infrequent) 1682
Risperdal M-Tab Orally Disintegrating Tablets (Infrequent) 1676
Ritalin Hydrochloride Tablets 2269
Ritalin LA Capsules 2271
Ritalin-SR Tablets 2269
Seroquel Tablets (Rare) 690
Sonata Capsules (Rare) 1717
Symbyax Capsules (Infrequent) 1819
Topamax Sprinkle Capsules (Greater than 1%) 2404
Topamax Tablets (Greater than 1%) 2404
Transderm Scōp Transdermal Therapeutic System 2177
Trileptal Tablets (Up to 2%) 2300
Trileptal Oral Suspension (Up to 2%) 2300
VFEND I.V. (Less than 2%) 2564
VFEND Oral Suspension (Less than 2%) 2564
VFEND Tablets (Less than 2%) 2564
Wellbutrin SR Sustained-Release Tablets (Infrequent) 1607
Wellbutrin XL Extended-Release Tablets (Infrequent) 1613
Zantac (Rare) 1624
Zantac Injection (Rare) 1619
Zantac (Rare) 1624
Zofran Injection 1634
Zoloft (Infrequent) 2586
Zyban Sustained-Release Tablets (Infrequent) 1644
Zyprexa Tablets (Rare) 1830
Zyprexa ZYDIS Orally Disintegrating Tablets (Rare) 1830
Zyrtec Chewable Tablets (Less than 2%) 2594
Zyrtec (Less than 2%) 2594
Zyrtec-D 12 Hour Extended Release Tablets (Less than 2%) 2597

Accommodation paresis
DAPTACEL Vaccine 2950
Miradon Tablets 3042

Aches
▲ ADACEL Vaccine (1.2% to 30.4%) 2945
Asacol Delayed-Release Tablets 2692
Cipro (Less than 1%) 2977
Cipro I.V. (1% or less) 2984
Cipro XR Tablets 2990
Cosopt Sterile Ophthalmic Solution 1931
Eldepryl Capsules (1 of 49 patients) 3208
▲ Flonase Nasal Spray (1% to 3%) 1440
Inderal LA Long-Acting Capsules 3429
Midamor Tablets (Less than or equal to 1%) 2026
▲ Nabi-HB (3%) 2169
Nadolol Tablets 2159
Orthoclone OKT3 Sterile Solution 2360
Proquin XR Tablets 1153
Recombivax HB (Less than 1%) 2071
▲ Serevent Diskus (1% to 3%) 1568
Tamiflu Capsules 2807
Timoptic Sterile Ophthalmic Solution 2088
Timoptic in Ocudose 2091
Timoptic-XE Sterile Ophthalmic Gel Forming Solution 2092
Toprol-XL Tablets 668

Aches, joints
(*see under* Arthralgia)

Acholia
Reyataz Capsules (Less than 3%) 921

Acid-base disturbances
Demadex Injection 2759
Demadex Tablets 2759

Acidosis
▲ Abelcet Injection (3%) 1141
Actiq (Less than 1%) 979
AmBisome for Injection (Less common) 620
Cafcit (2.2%) 1886
Campath Ampules 811
▲ CellCept Capsules (3% to less than 20%) 2747
▲ CellCept Intravenous (3% to less than 20%) 2747
▲ CellCept Oral Suspension (3% to less than 20%) 2747
▲ CellCept Tablets (3% to less than 20%) 2747
Cipro (Less than 1%) 2977
Cipro I.V. (1% or less) 2984
Cipro XR Tablets 2990
Dyazide Capsules 1423
Fleet Enema 1165
Fleet Phospho-soda 1166
Fleet Phospho-soda ACCU-PREP 1168
Fleet Phospho-soda EZ-PREP 1169
Fleet Prep Kits 1170
Indocin I.V. (Less than 3%) 2465
Mycamine for Injection 628
Percodan Tablets 1132
Permax Tablets (Rare) 3356
▲ Prograf Capsules and Injection (3% to 15%) 632
▲ Proleukin for Injection (12%) 2266
▲ Rapamune Oral Solution and Tablets (3% to 20%) 3475
Requip Tablets (Infrequent) 1555
▲ Simulect for Injection (3% to 10%) 2284
Symbyax Capsules (Rare) 1819
Topamax Sprinkle Capsules (Infrequent) 2404
Topamax Tablets (Infrequent) 2404
Trasylol Injection (1% to 2%) 754
▲ Trisenox Injection (5%) 993
Tygacil for Injection 3488
Ultane Liquid for Inhalation (Less than 1%) 531
▲ Vesanoid Capsules (3%) 2820
Zyprexa Tablets (Frequent) 1830
Zyprexa ZYDIS Orally Disintegrating Tablets (Frequent) 1830

Acidosis, hypochloremic metabolic
Gengraf Capsules 459
Sandimmune (Occasional) 2275
▲ Topamax Sprinkle Capsules (2% to 67%) 2404
▲ Topamax Tablets (2% to 67%) 2404

Acidosis, metabolic
Aggrenox Capsules 822
Aloprim for Injection (Less than 1%) 2167
Aloxi Injection (Less than 1%) 2127
Bayer Aspirin 744
Bayer Aspirin Comprehensive Prescribing Information ▣796
Daranide Tablets 1950
Eloxatin for Injection 2892
Foradil Aerolizer 3010
Oncaspar 1145
Percodan Tablets 1132
St. Joseph 81 mg Aspirin Chewable and Enteric Coated Tablets 1869
St. Joseph 81 mg Aspirin ▣688
Sulfamylon Cream 2162
Sulfamylon for 5% Topical Solution 2162
Topamax Sprinkle Capsules 2404
Topamax Tablets 2404
Viracept 2577

Acidosis, renal tubular
Abelcet Injection 1141
Topamax Sprinkle Capsules 2404
Topamax Tablets 2404

Acidosis, respiratory
▲ CellCept Capsules (3% to less than 20%) 2747
▲ CellCept Intravenous (3% to less than 20%) 2747
▲ CellCept Oral Suspension (3% to less than 20%) 2747
▲ CellCept Tablets (3% to less than 20%) 2747
Rilutek Tablets (Infrequent) 2930

Acne
(*see under* Acneiform eruptions)

Acne, cystic, flare-up
Parnate Tablets 1527

Acne, flare-up of
Differin Cream (Less than 1%) 1210

Acne, transient exacerbation of
Oxandrin Tablets 2962

Acne fulminaris
Accutane Capsules 2731

Acneiform eruptions
Abilify Oral Solution (Infrequent) 882
Abilify Oral Solution (Infrequent) 2450
Abilify Discmelt Orally Disintegrating Tablets (Infrequent) 882
Abilify Discmelt Orally Disintegrating Tablets (Infrequent) 2450
Abilify Tablets (Infrequent) 882
Abilify Tablets (Infrequent) 2450
Aclovate Cream (Infrequent) 2660
▲ Aerobid/Aerobid-M (1% to 3%) 1171
Ambien Tablets (Rare) 2851
Ambien CR Tablets (Rare) 2855
Amerge Tablets (Rare) 1339
Analpram-HC 1159
▲ AndroGel (1% to 8%) 3329
Androxy Tablets 3335
Apexicon E Cream 2661
Arthrotec Tablets (Rare) 3129
Asacol Delayed-Release Tablets (1% to 2%) 2692
Caduet Tablets (Less than 2%) 2508
Campral Tablets (Infrequent) 1174
Canasa Rectal Suppositories (1.2%) 699
Celexa (Infrequent) 1176
▲ CellCept Capsules (3% to less than 20%) 2747
▲ CellCept Intravenous (3% to less than 20%) 2747
▲ CellCept Oral Suspension (3% to less than 20%) 2747
▲ CellCept Tablets (3% to less than 20%) 2747
Chantix Tablets (Infrequent) 2517
Clobevate Gel 3211
Clobex Lotion 1204
Clobex Shampoo 1206
Clobex Spray (Less than 1%) 1208
Copaxone for Injection (At least 2%) 3297
Cosmegen for Injection 2459
Cutivate Cream (Infrequent) 2662
Cutivate Ointment (Infrequent to more frequent) 2665
Cymbalta Delayed-Release Capsules (Infrequent) 1757
Dantrium Capsules (Less frequent) 2694
Decadron Tablets 1951
▲ Depo-Provera Contraceptive Injection (1% to 5%) 2622
▲ depo-subQ provera 104 Injectable Suspension (1% to less than 5%) 2624
Diprolene Gel 0.05% 3001
Diprolene Lotion 0.05% (1%) 3002
Diprolene Ointment 0.05% (Infrequent) 3003
Diprolene AF Cream 0.05% (Infrequent) 3000
Diprosone Cream, USP 0.05% 3004
▲ Doxil Injection (1% to 10%) 2351
Effexor Tablets (Infrequent) 3411
Effexor XR Capsules (Infrequent) 3417
Elidel Cream 1% (0.9% to 1.8%) 2200
Elocon Cream 0.1% (Infrequent) 3005
Elocon Lotion 0.1% (Infrequent) 3006
Elocon Ointment 0.1% (Infrequent) 3007
Emend Capsules (Greater than 0.5%) 1963
▲ Entocort EC Capsules (15%) 2698
Estratest Tablets 3199
Estratest H.S. Tablets 3199
Evoxac Capsules (Less than 1%) 1047
Finacea Gel (1% or less) 1669
▲ Flovent Diskus (1% to 3%) 1443
Gabitril Tablets (1% or more) 984
▲ Gengraf Capsules (1% to 6%) 459
Herceptin I.V. (2%) 1233
▲ Humatrope Vials and Cartridges (Up to 5.8%) 1787
▲ Imdur Tablets (Less than or equal to 5%) 3018
▲ Intron A for Injection (Less than 5%) 3024
Invirase (Less than 2%) 2772
▲ Iressa Tablets (25% to 37%) 684
Kaletra (Less than 2%) 476
Lamictal (1.3%) 1481
Lexapro Oral Solution (Infrequent) 1190
Lexapro Tablets (Infrequent) 1190
Lipitor Tablets (Less than 2%) 2483
Lithobid Tablets 1692
Locoid Lipocream Cream (Infrequent) 1160
Lofibra Tablets 1219
Lofibra Capsules 1216
Lotrisone 3040
Lotronex Tablets (Rare) 1512
Lunesta Tablets (Infrequent) 3142
▲ Lupron Depot–3 Month 11.25 mg (Up to 10%) 3265
Lupron Depot-PED 7.5 mg, 11.25 mg and 15 mg (2%) 3269
Lupron Injection Pediatric (2%) 3259
Luxíq Foam (One patient) 1010
Maxalt Tablets (Rare) 2008
Maxalt-MLT Orally Disintegrating Tablets (Rare) 2008
Meridia Capsules (1%) 489
Mircette Tablets 1066
▲ Mirena Intrauterine System (5% or more) 787
▲ Myfortic Tablets (3% to less than 20%) 2255
Namenda (More than one patient) 1195
▲ Neoral Oral Solution (1% to 6%) 2259
▲ Neoral Soft Gelatin Capsules (1% to 6%) 2259
Neurontin Capsules 2487
Neurontin Oral Solution 2487
Neurontin Tablets 2487
▲ Nexavar Tablets (Common) 746
Nexium Delayed-Release Capsules (Less than 1%) 655
Nexium I.V. (Less than 1%) 659
Nimotop Capsules (Up to 1.4%) 749
Nipent for Injection (Less than 3%) 1863
Norvir (Less than 2%) 503
NuvaRing 2340
Olux Foam 1012
Ortho-Cyclen Tablets 2429
Ortho Evra Transdermal System 2417
Ortho Micronor Tablets (Rare) 2426
Ortho Tri-Cyclen Tablets 2429
Ortho Tri-Cyclen Lo Tablets 2436
Oxandrin Tablets 2962
Paxil CR Controlled-Release Tablets (Infrequent) 1538
Paxil (Infrequent) 1530
Pentasa Capsules (0.2%) 3185
Pepcid Injection (Infrequent) 2040
Pepcid (Infrequent) 2038
Permax Tablets (Infrequent) 3356
Pexeva Tablets (infrequent) 1694
Pramosone 1161
Premphase Tablets 3456
Prempro Tablets 3456
Prevacid Delayed-Release Capsules (Less than 1%) 3271
Prevacid for Delayed-Release Oral Suspension (Less than 1%) 3271
Prevacid SoluTab Delayed-Release Orally Disintegrating Tablets (Less than 1%) 3271
Prevacid NapraPAC (Less than 1%) 3280
PREVPAC (Less than 1%) 3284
Prochieve 4% Gel 1003
Prochieve 8% Gel 1003
ProctoFoam-HC 3099
▲ Prograf Capsules and Injection (3% to 15%) 632
▲ Prometrium Capsules (100 mg, 200 mg) (Less than 5%) 3203
ProSom Tablets (Rare) 517
Protonix I.V. (Less than 1%) 3472
Protonix Tablets (Less than 1%) 3469
▲ Protopic Ointment (2% to 7%) 638
Prozac Pulvules and Liquid (Infrequent) 1801
▲ Rapamune Oral Solution and Tablets (20% to 31%) 3475
▲ Raptiva for Injection (4%) 1250
ReFacto Vials 3484
Retrovir Capsules 1560
Retrovir IV Infusion 1564
Retrovir 1560
Risperdal (Infrequent to 2%) 1676
Risperdal Consta Long-Acting Injection (2%) 1682
Risperdal M-Tab Orally Disintegrating Tablets (Infrequent to 2%) 1676
▲ Sandimmune (1% to 6%) 2275
Sandostatin LAR Depot (1% to 4%) 2280
Seasonique Tablets 1077
Seroquel Tablets (Infrequent) 690
▲ Simulect for Injection (Greater than or equal to 10%) 2284
Sonata Capsules (Infrequent) 1717
Soriatane Capsules (Less than 1%) 1013
Striant Mucoadhesive 1007
Sular Tablets (Less than or equal to 1%) 3122
Symbyax Capsules (Infrequent) 1819
Targretin Capsules 1747
Temovate Cream 2668
Temovate Gel (Infrequent) 2669
Temovate Ointment 2668
Temovate Scalp Application (Infrequent) 2670
Temovate E Emollient (Infrequent) 2671
Testim 1% Gel (Less than 1%) 695
▲ Thalomid Capsules (3.1% to 11.1%) 965
▲ Topamax Sprinkle Capsules (2% to 3%) 2404

▲ Topamax Tablets (2% to 3%) 2404
Trecator Tablets 3487
Tricor Tablets 527
Trileptal Tablets (1% to 2%) 2300
Trileptal Oral Suspension (1% to 2%) 2300
▲ Tri-Luma Cream (5%) 1213
Uniretic Tablets (Less than 1%) 3100
▲ Valcyte Tablets (Less than 5%) 2813
Vandazole Vaginal Gel (Less than 1%) 3338
Vanos Cream 1893
Vantin Tablets and Oral Suspension (Less than 1%) 2645
Wellbutrin Tablets (Rare) 1603
Wellbutrin SR Sustained-Release Tablets (At least 1%) 1607
Wellbutrin XL Extended-Release Tablets (At least 1%) 1613
Xyrem Oral Solution (Infrequent) 1688
Yasmin 28 Tablets (Greater than 1%) 796
Yaz Tablets (Greater than 1%) 803
Zoloft (Infrequent) 2586
Zonegran Capsules (Infrequent) 1101
Zyban Sustained-Release Tablets (Infrequent) 1644
Zyprexa Tablets (2%) 1830
Zyprexa ZYDIS Orally Disintegrating Tablets (2%) 1830
Zyrtec Chewable Tablets (Less than 2%) 2594
Zyrtec (Less than 2%) 2594
Zyrtec-D 12 Hour Extended Release Tablets (Less than 2%) 2597

Acneiform reactions
Cutivate Lotion 0.05% (Rare) 2664
Elocon Lotion 0.1% (2 in 209 patients) 3006
▲ Erbitux (8% to 90%) 910
▲ I.V. Busulfex (7%) 2493

Acrocyanosis, exacerbation
R-Gene 10 for Intravenous Use (One patient) 2641

Adams-Stokes syndrome
Exelon Capsules (Infrequent) 2206
Exelon Oral Solution (Infrequent) 2206

Addiction
Lyrica Capsules (Rare) 2539

Adenitis
Clinoril Tablets 1924
Dolobid Tablets (Less than 1 in 100) 1955
Pneumovax 23 (Rare) 2043

Adenoma, prostatic
Exelon Capsules (Infrequent) 2206
Exelon Oral Solution (Infrequent) 2206

Adenoma, unspecified
▲ Humira Injection (Less than 5%) 466

Adenomas, benign pituitary
Lupron Depot 3.75 mg 3260
Risperdal 1676
Risperdal Consta Long-Acting Injection 1682
Risperdal M-Tab Orally Disintegrating Tablets 1676

Adenomas, endocrine system
Permax Tablets (Infrequent) 3356

Adenopathy
Carbatrol Capsules 3171
Enbrel for Injection 584
Equetro Extended-Release Capsules 3180
Kogenate FS 738
Kogenate FS with Bio-Set 740
Rescriptor Tablets 2551
Tegretol/Tegretol-XR 2295
▲ Thiola Tablets (4%) 2141

ADH syndrome, inappropriate
Avandaryl Tablets 1379
Carbatrol Capsules 3171
Celexa (Several cases) 1176
Depacon Injection 412
Depakene 417
Depakote Sprinkle Capsules 422
Depakote Tablets 427
Depakote ER Tablets 434
Duetact Tablets 3226
Effexor Tablets 3411
Effexor XR Capsules 3417
Equetro Extended-Release Capsules 3180
Kadian Capsules (Less than 3%) 577
Lexapro Oral Solution 1190
Lexapro Tablets 1190
OxyContin Tablets (Less than 1%) 2703
Parnate Tablets 1527
Paxil CR Controlled-Release Tablets 1538
Paxil 1530
Permax Tablets (Infrequent) 3356
Pexeva Tablets (infrequent) 1694
Requip Tablets (Rare) 1555
Seroquel Tablets 690
Tegretol/Tegretol-XR 2295
Thalomid Capsules 965
Wellbutrin Tablets 1603
Wellbutrin SR Sustained-Release Tablets 1607
Wellbutrin XL Extended-Release Tablets 1613
Zyban Sustained-Release Tablets 1644

Adnexal torsion, ovarian
Follistim AQ Cartridge 2338

Adrenal crisis
Advair Diskus 100/50 1308
Advair Diskus 250/50 1308
Advair Diskus 500/50 1308

Adrenal insufficiency
Azmacort Inhalation Aerosol 1726
Beconase AQ Nasal Spray 1396
Cutivate Ointment 2665
▲ NeoProfen Injection (7%) 2472
Pulmicort Respules (Less than 1%) 661
Revlimid Capsules 958
VFEND I.V. (Less than 2%) 2564
VFEND Oral Suspension (Less than 2%) 2564
VFEND Tablets (Less than 2%) 2564

Adrenal suppression
(*see also under* HPA axis suppression)

Adrenergic syndrome, unspecified
Paxil CR Controlled-Release Tablets (Rare) 1538
Paxil (Rare) 1530

Adrenocortical unresponsiveness, secondary
Colocort Rectal Suspension, USP (Retention) 100 mg/60 mL 2476
Decadron Tablets 1951
Depo-Medrol Injectable Suspension 2617
Depo-Medrol Single-Dose Vial 2619
Hydrocortone Tablets 1989

Affect, blunted
Abilify Oral Solution (Rare) 882
Abilify Oral Solution (Rare) 2450
Abilify Discmelt Orally Disintegrating Tablets (Rare) 882
Abilify Discmelt Orally Disintegrating Tablets (Rare) 2450
Abilify Tablets (Rare) 882
Abilify Tablets (Rare) 2450

Affect lability
▲ Daytrana Transdermal Patch (6%) 3174
Xyrem Oral Solution (Infrequent) 1688

Afibrinogenemia
Depacon Injection (One infant) 412
Depakene (One infant) 417
Depakote Tablets (One infant) 427
Depakote ER Tablets (One infant) 434

Ageusia
▲ Aerobid/Aerobid-M (3% to 9%) 1171
Aggrenox Capsules (Less than 1%) 822
Arthrotec Tablets (Rare) 3129
Astelin Nasal Spray (Infrequent) 1904
Beconase AQ Nasal Spray (Rare) 1396
Bentyl Capsules 697
Bentyl Injection 697
Bentyl Syrup 697
Bentyl Tablets 697
Caduet Tablets (Less than 2%) 2508
Campath Ampules 811
Captopril Tablets (Approximately 2 to 4 of 100 patients) 2149
Celexa (Rare) 1176
Cipro 2977
Cipro I.V. 2984
Cipro XR Tablets 2990
Clinoril Tablets (Less than 1 in 100) 1924
Copaxone for Injection (Infrequent) 3297
Donnatal Extentabs 2493
Doxil Injection (Less than 1%) 2351
Effexor Tablets (Infrequent) 3411
Effexor XR Capsules (Infrequent) 3417
Exelon Capsules (Infrequent) 2206
Exelon Oral Solution (Infrequent) 2206
Flonase Nasal Spray 1440
Flumadine (Less than 0.3%) 1183
Gabitril Tablets (Infrequent) 984
▲ Intron A for Injection (Less than 5%) 3024
Kaletra (Less than 2%) 476
Klonopin (Infrequent) 2778
Lamictal (Rare) 1481
Lamisil Tablets (Uncommon) 2232
Lipitor Tablets (Less than 2%) 2483
Lyrica Capsules (0.1% to 1%) 2539
Neurontin Capsules (Infrequent) 2487
Neurontin Oral Solution (Infrequent) 2487
Neurontin Tablets (Infrequent) 2487
Nexium Delayed-Release Capsules (Less than 1%) 655
Nexium I.V. (Less than 1%) 659
Norvir (Less than 2%) 503
Paxil CR Controlled-Release Tablets (Infrequent) 1538
Paxil (Infrequent) 1530
Pexeva Tablets (rare) 1694
Prevacid Delayed-Release Capsules (Less than 1%) 3271
Prevacid for Delayed-Release Oral Suspension (Less than 1%) 3271
Prevacid SoluTab Delayed-Release Orally Disintegrating Tablets (Less than 1%) 3271
Prevacid NapraPAC (Less than 1%) 3280
PREVPAC (Less than 1%) 3284
Proquin XR Tablets 1153
Prozac Pulvules and Liquid (Rare) 1801
Rilutek Tablets (Rare) 2930
Soltamox Oral Solution (Infrequently) 3527
Sonata Capsules (Rare) 1717
Soriatane Capsules (Less than 1%) 1013
Tequin Injection (Less than 0.1%) 938
Tequin Injection in 5% Dextrose (Less than 0.1%) 938
Tequin Tablets (Less than 0.1%) 938
Topamax Sprinkle Capsules (1% to 2%) 2404
Topamax Tablets (1% to 2%) 2404
Vantin Tablets and Oral Suspension (Less than 1%) 2645
VFEND I.V. (Less than 2%) 2564
VFEND Oral Suspension (Less than 2%) 2564
VFEND Tablets (Less than 2%) 2564
▲ Xeloda Tablets (Less than 5%) 2822
Xifaxan Tablets (Less than 2%) 2842
Zelapar Tablets 3372
Zyrtec Chewable Tablets (Less than 2%) 2594
Zyrtec (Less than 2%) 2594
Zyrtec-D 12 Hour Extended Release Tablets (Less than 2%) 2597

Aggression
Accutane Capsules 2731
Adderall XR Capsules 3166
Advair Diskus 100/50 1308
Advair Diskus 250/50 1308
Advair Diskus 500/50 1308
Advair HFA Inhalation Aerosol 1318
Ambien Tablets (Rare) 2851
Amerge Tablets (Rare) 1339
Aricept Tablets (Frequent) 1094
Aricept ODT Tablets (Frequent) 1094
Celexa (Infrequent) 1176
Chantix Tablets (Infrequent) 2517
Concerta Extended-Release Tablets 1881
Copegus Tablets (Less than 1%) 2754
Depacon Injection 412
Depakene 417
Depakote Sprinkle Capsules 422
Depakote Tablets 427
Depakote ER Tablets 434
DextroStat Tablets 3179
Effexor Tablets 3411
Effexor XR Capsules 3417
Evoxac Capsules 1047
▲ Exelon Capsules (3%) 2206
▲ Exelon Oral Solution (3%) 2206
Flovent Diskus 1443
Flovent HFA 1447
Genotropin Lyophilized Powder 2638
Imitrex Injection 1463
Imitrex Tablets (Rare) 1471
▲ Intron A for Injection (Less than 5%) 3024
Klonopin (Infrequent) 2778
Levaquin (0.1% to 0.9%) 2384
Levaquin in 5% Dextrose Injection (0.1% to 0.9%) 2384
Lexapro Oral Solution (Infrequent) 1190
Lexapro Tablets (Infrequent) 1190
Neurontin Capsules 2487
Neurontin Oral Solution 2487
Neurontin Tablets 2487
Niravam Orally Disintegrating Tablets (Rare) 3092
Paxil CR Controlled-Release Tablets 1538
Paxil 1530
Pegasys (Less than 1%) 2789
PEG-Intron Powder for Injection (Less than or equal to 1%) 3048
Prilosec OTC Delayed-Release Tablets (Less than 1%) 2677
Prochieve 4% Gel 1003
Prochieve 8% Gel 1003
Prozac Pulvules and Liquid 1801
Pulmicort Respules (Less than 1%) 661
Razadyne 2399
Razadyne ER Extended-Release Capsules 2399
Requip Tablets (Infrequent) 1555
▲ Risperdal (1% to 3%) 1676
▲ Risperdal M-Tab Orally Disintegrating Tablets (1% to 3%) 1676
Ritalin Hydrochloride Tablets 2269
Ritalin LA Capsules 2271
Ritalin-SR Tablets 2269
Seromycin Capsules 1813
Singulair 2077
Soriatane Capsules 1013
Strattera Capsules (0.50%) 1814
Sustiva Capsules (0.4%) 930
Sustiva Tablets (0.4%) 930
Symbyax Capsules 1819
Symmetrel Tablets 1135
▲ Topamax Sprinkle Capsules (2% to 9%) 2404
▲ Topamax Tablets (2% to 9%) 2404
Trileptal Tablets 2300
Trileptal Oral Suspension 2300
Wellbutrin Tablets 1603
Wellbutrin SR Sustained-Release Tablets 1607
Wellbutrin XL Extended-Release Tablets 1613
Zegerid Capsules (Less than 1%) 2958
Zegerid Powder for Oral Solution (Less than 1%) 2958
Zoloft (Infrequent to 2%) 2586
Zyban Sustained-Release Tablets 1644

Aggressive reaction
Ambien CR Tablets (Rare) 2855
Atripla Tablets 945
Namenda (Frequent) 1195
Zmax for Oral Suspension 2583
Zyrtec Chewable Tablets (Rare) 2594
Zyrtec (Rare) 2594
Zyrtec-D 12 Hour Extended Release Tablets (Rare) 2597

Agitation
▲ Abilify Oral Solution (25%) 882
▲ Abilify Oral Solution (25%) 2450
▲ Abilify Discmelt Orally Disintegrating Tablets (25%) 882
▲ Abilify Discmelt Orally Disintegrating Tablets (25%) 2450
▲ Abilify Tablets (25%) 882
▲ Abilify Tablets (25%) 2450
Aciphex Tablets (Rare) 1090
Actiq (Less than 1%) 979
▲ Adderall XR Capsules (8%) 3166
Advair Diskus 100/50 1308
Advair Diskus 250/50 1308
Advair Diskus 500/50 1308
Advair HFA Inhalation Aerosol 1318
Aggrenox Capsules (Less than 1%) 822
Aldara Cream, 5% 1846
Allegra-D 12 Hour Extended-Release Tablets (1.9%) 2846
Allegra-D 24 Hour Extended-Release Tablets (1.9%) 2849
Aloprim for Injection (Less than 1%) 2167
Ambien Tablets (Infrequent) 2851
Ambien CR Tablets (Infrequent) 2855
AmBisome for Injection (Less common) 620
Amerge Tablets (Rare) 1339
Amoxil Capsules (Rare) 1343
Amoxil Chewable Tablets (Rare) 1343
Amoxil Pediatric Drops for Oral Suspension (Rare) 1343
Amoxil Powder for Oral Suspension (Rare) 1343
Amoxil Tablets (Rare) 1343
Anzemet Injection (Infrequently) 2859

Anzemet Tablets (Infrequently) 2862
Aricept Tablets 1094
Aricept ODT Tablets 1094
Atripla Tablets 945
Augmentin (Rare) 1360
Augmentin Tablets (Rare) 1363
Augmentin XR Extended-Release Tablets (Rare) 1369
Augmentin ES-600 Powder for Oral Suspension (Rare) 1366
Avelox (Less than 0.1%) 2970
▲ Avinza Capsules (Less than 5%) 1741
Azilect Tablets (Infrequent) 3293
Bayer Aspirin 744
Bayer Aspirin Comprehensive Prescribing Information ◙ 796
Bicillin C-R Injectable Suspension 1706
Buprenex Injectable (Rare) 2716
Caduet Tablets (Less than or equal to 0.1%) 2508
Campral Tablets (Infrequent) 1174
Carbatrol Capsules 3171
Cardura XL Tablets 2515
Catapres Tablets (About 3 in 100 patients) 843
Catapres-TTS (0.5% or less) 844
▲ Celexa (3%) 1176
▲ CellCept Capsules (3% to less than 20%) 2747
▲ CellCept Intravenous (3% to less than 20%) 2747
▲ CellCept Oral Suspension (3% to less than 20%) 2747
▲ CellCept Tablets (3% to less than 20%) 2747
Chantix Tablets (Infrequent) 2517
Cipro 2977
Cipro I.V. 2984
Cipro XR Tablets 2990
▲ Clorpres Tablets (About 3%) 2153
▲ Clozaril Tablets (4%) 2184
Comtan Tablets (1%) 2189
Comvax 1928
▲ Copaxone for Injection (4%) 3297
Cuprimine Capsules 1947
Depacon Injection (1% or more) 412
Depakene (1% or more) 417
Depakote Sprinkle Capsules 422
▲ Depakote Tablets (1% to 5%) 427
Depakote ER Tablets (Greater than 1%) 434
Dexedrine 1420
Diastat Rectal Delivery System (Greater than or equal to 1%) 3343
Dilaudid 440
Dilaudid Non-Sterile Powder 440
Dilaudid Oral Liquid (Less frequent) 445
Dilaudid Rectal Suppositories 440
Dilaudid Tablets 440
Dilaudid Tablets - 8 mg (Less frequent) 445
Dilaudid-HP (Less frequent) 442
Donnatal Extentabs 2493
▲ Doxil Injection (1% to 10%) 2351
Duragesic Transdermal System (1% or greater) 2373
▲ Effexor Tablets (2% to 4.5%) 3411
▲ Effexor XR Capsules (4%) 3417
Eldepryl Capsules 3208
Elspar for Injection 2463
Elspar for Injection 1960
Engerix-B Vaccine (Less than 1%) 1425
▲ Entocort EC Capsules (Less than 5%) 2698
Equetro Extended-Release Capsules 3180
Evoxac Capsules (Less than 1%) 1047
Exelon Capsules (2% or more) 2206
Exelon Oral Solution (2% or more) 2206
▲ FazaClo Orally Disintegrating Tablets (4%) 551
Ferrlecit Injection 3388
Flovent Diskus 1443
Flovent HFA 1447
Flumadine (0.3% to 1%) 1183
Fortical Nasal Spray (Less than 1%) 3337
Frova Tablets (Infrequent) 1113
Gabitril Tablets (1%) 984
Geodon Capsules (Frequent) 2529
Imitrex Injection (Infrequent) 1463
Imitrex Nasal Spray (Infrequent) 1467
Imitrex Tablets (Up to 2%) 1471
▲ Indapamide Tablets (Greater than or equal to 5%) 2156
▲ Infergen (4% to 6%) 3364
▲ Intron A for Injection (Less than 5%) 3024
▲ Invanz for Injection (3.3% to 5.1%) 1999
Invirase (Less than 2%) 2772
Ionsys Transdermal System (.1% to less than 1%) 2379
I.V. Busulfex (2%) 2493
Kadian Capsules (Less than 3%) 577
Kaletra (Less than 2%) 476
Keflex Capsules 549
▲ Keppra Oral Solution (6%) 3314
▲ Keppra Tablets (6%) 3314
Klonopin 2778
Kytril Injection (Less than 2%) 2781
Lamictal (Infrequent) 1481
Lariam Tablets (Occasional) 2786
Leukeran Tablets (Rare) 1504
Levaquin (0.1% to 0.9%) 2384
Levaquin in 5% Dextrose Injection (0.1% to 0.9%) 2384
Lexapro Oral Solution (Infrequent) 1190
Lexapro Tablets (Infrequent) 1190
Lunesta Tablets (Infrequent) 3142
▲ Lupron Depot 7.5 mg (Less than 5%) 3264
Lupron Depot–3 Month 11.25 mg 3265
Lyrica Capsules (0.1% to 1%) 2539
Maxalt Tablets (Infrequent) 2008
Maxalt-MLT Orally Disintegrating Tablets (Infrequent) 2008
Meridia Capsules (Greater than or equal to 1%) 489
Merrem I.V. (Greater than 0.1% to 1%) 686
Miacalcin Nasal Spray (Less than 1%) 2253
Mirapex Tablets (Less than 1%) 859
MS Contin Tablets (Less frequent) 2701
Myozyme for Intravenous Infusion 1279
Namenda (Greater than or equal to 2%) 1195
Nembutal Sodium Solution, USP (Less than 1%) 2470
Neurontin Capsules (Infrequent) 2487
Neurontin Oral Solution (Infrequent) 2487
Neurontin Tablets (Infrequent) 2487
Niravam Orally Disintegrating Tablets (2.9%) 3092
Norflex Injection 1856
Norvasc Tablets (Less than 0.1%) 2545
Norvir (Less than 2%) 503
Opana Tablets (Less than 1%) 1122
Opana ER Tablets (Less than 1%) 1126
Orthoclone OKT3 Sterile Solution 2360
OxyContin Tablets (Less than 1%) 2703
Parcopa Orally Disintegrating Tablets 3097
Parnate Tablets 1527
▲ Paxil CR Controlled-Release Tablets (1.1% to 5%) 1538
▲ Paxil (1.1% to 5%) 1530
PEG-Intron Powder for Injection (2%) 3048
Pepcid Injection (Infrequent) 2040
Pepcid (Infrequent) 2038
Percodan Tablets 1132
Permax Tablets (Infrequent) 3356
▲ Pexeva Tablets (1.1% to 5%) 1694
Phenergan Tablets and Suppositories 3440
Prevacid Delayed-Release Capsules (Less than 1%) 3271
Prevacid for Delayed-Release Oral Suspension (Less than 1%) 3271
Prevacid SoluTab Delayed-Release Orally Disintegrating Tablets (Less than 1%) 3271
Prevacid NapraPAC (Less than 1%) 3280
PREVPAC (Less than 1%) 3284
▲ Prograf Capsules and Injection (3% to 15%) 632
Proleukin for Injection 2266
ProQuad 2064
Proquin XR Tablets 1153
ProSom Tablets (Infrequent) 517
Provigil Tablets (1%) 988
Prozac Pulvules and Liquid (At least 2%) 1801
Raniclor Tablets, Chewable (Rare) 2505
Razadyne (Greater than or equal to 2%) 2399
Razadyne ER Extended-Release Capsules (Greater than or equal to 2%) 2399
▲ Rebetol (5% to 8%) 3058
Recombivax HB 2071
Relpax Tablets (Infrequent) 2548
ReoPro Vials (0.7%) 1809
Requip Tablets (Infrequent) 1555
Rescriptor Tablets 2551
Restoril Capsules (Less than 0.5%) 1860
Reyataz Capsules (Less than 3%) 921
▲ Ribavirin, USP Capsules (5% to 8%) 3068
Rilutek Tablets (Frequent) 2930
▲ Risperdal (8% to 26%) 1676
Risperdal Consta Long-Acting Injection (Frequent) 1682
▲ Risperdal M-Tab Orally Disintegrating Tablets (8% to 26%) 1676
▲ Romazicon Injection (3% to 9%) 2804
▲ Seroquel Tablets (4%) 690
▲ Simulect for Injection (3% to 10%) 2284
Singulair 2077
Sonata Capsules (Infrequent) 1717
St. Joseph 81 mg Aspirin Chewable and Enteric Coated Tablets 1869
St. Joseph 81 mg Aspirin ◙ 688
Stalevo Tablets (1%) 2287
Sustiva Capsules (Less than 2%) 930
Sustiva Tablets (Less than 2%) 930
Symbyax Capsules 1819
▲ Symmetrel Tablets (1% to 5%) 1135
Targretin Capsules 1747
Tasmar Tablets (1%) 3358
Tegretol/Tegretol-XR 2295
Tequin Injection (Less than 0.1%) 938
Tequin Injection in 5% Dextrose (Less than 0.1%) 938
Tequin Tablets (Less than 0.1%) 938
Thalomid Capsules 965
Thioridazine Hydrochloride Tablets 2163
Thiothixene Capsules 2165
▲ Topamax Sprinkle Capsules (1% to 3%) 2404
▲ Topamax Tablets (1% to 3%) 2404
Trasylol Injection (1% to 2%) 754
Trileptal Tablets (1% to 2%) 2300
Trileptal Oral Suspension (1% to 2%) 2300
▲ Trisenox Injection (5%) 993
Twinrix Vaccine (Less than 1%) 1595
▲ Ultane Liquid for Inhalation (7% to 15%) 531
▲ Ultram ER Tablets (1% to greater than 5%) 2392
▲ Valcyte Tablets (Less than 5%) 2813
Valtrex Caplets 1597
▲ Vesanoid Capsules (9%) 2820
VFEND I.V. (Less than 2%) 2564
VFEND Oral Suspension (Less than 2%) 2564
VFEND Tablets (Less than 2%) 2564
Vicoprofen Tablets (Less than 1%) 539
▲ Vivitrol (8% to 12%) 995
▲ Wellbutrin Tablets (31.9%) 1603
▲ Wellbutrin SR Sustained-Release Tablets (3% to 9%) 1607
▲ Wellbutrin XL Extended-Release Tablets (2% to 9%) 1613
Zantac (Rare) 1624
Zantac Injection 1619
Zantac Injection Pharmacy Bulk Package (Rare) 1622
Zantac Injection Premixed 1619
Zantac (Rare) 1624
Zelapar Tablets 3372
Zmax for Oral Suspension 2583
▲ Zofran Injection (2% to 6%) 1634
▲ Zofran (6%) 1639
▲ Zofran ODT Orally Disintegrating Tablets (6%) 1639
▲ Zoloft (1% to 6%) 2586
▲ Zometa for Intravenous Infusion (12.8%) 2315
Zomig Tablets (Infrequent) 3519
Zomig Nasal Spray (Infrequent to less than 2%) 3523
Zomig-ZMT Tablets (Infrequent) 3519
▲ Zonegran Capsules (9%) 1101
▲ Zosyn (2.1% to 7.1%) 3492
Zovirax 1643
Zyban Sustained-Release Tablets (Frequent) 1644
▲ Zyprexa Tablets (23%) 1830
▲ Zyprexa ZYDIS Orally Disintegrating Tablets (23%) 1830
Zyrtec Chewable Tablets (Less than 2%) 2594
Zyrtec (Less than 2%) 2594
Zyrtec-D 12 Hour Extended Release Tablets (Less than 2%) 2597

Agnosia

▲ Vesanoid Capsules (3%) 2820

Agranulocytosis

Accolate Tablets 671
Accutane Capsules 2731
Aceon Tablets (2 mg, 4 mg, 8 mg) 3194
Aciphex Tablets 1090
Albenza Tablets (Rare) 1338
Aldoril Tablets 1910
Altace Capsules (Rare) 1702
AmBisome for Injection (Infrequent) 620
Amoxil Capsules 1343
Amoxil Chewable Tablets 1343
Amoxil Pediatric Drops for Oral Suspension 1343
Amoxil Powder for Oral Suspension 1343
Amoxil Tablets 1343
Anaprox Tablets (Less than 1%) 2761
Anaprox DS Tablets (Less than 1%) 2761
Arthrotec Tablets (Rare) 3129
Asacol Delayed-Release Tablets (Rare) 2692
Atacand Tablets (Very rare) 649
Atacand HCT 651
Augmentin 1360
Augmentin Tablets 1363
Augmentin XR Extended-Release Tablets 1369
Augmentin ES-600 Powder for Oral Suspension 1366
Avalide Tablets 888
Avalide Tablets 2874
Avandaryl Tablets 1379
BiDil Tablets 2171
▲ Blephamide Ophthalmic Ointment (Among most often) 568
Blephamide Ophthalmic Suspension 569
Blocadren Tablets 1916
Campath Ampules 811
Captopril Tablets 2149
Carbatrol Capsules 3171
Ceftin 1407
Cipro 2977
Cipro I.V. (1% or less) 2984
Cipro XR Tablets 2990
Cleocin Vaginal Ovules 2616
Clinoril Tablets (Less than 1%) 1924
Clorpres Tablets 2153
Clozaril Tablets (1% to 1.3%) 2184
Cosmegen for Injection 2459
Cosopt Sterile Ophthalmic Solution 1931
Cuprimine Capsules 1947
Dapsone Tablets USP 1673
Daranide Tablets 1950
Didronel Tablets (Rare) 2697
Diovan HCT Tablets 2196
Diuril Oral Suspension 1954
Diuril Sodium Intravenous 2467
Dolobid Tablets (Less than 1 in 100) 1955
Duetact Tablets 3226
Dyazide Capsules 1423
EC-Naprosyn Delayed-Release Tablets (Less than 1%) 2761
Edecrin 1959
Effexor Tablets 3411
Effexor XR Capsules 3417
Equetro Extended-Release Capsules 3180
Fansidar Tablets 2765
FazaClo Orally Disintegrating Tablets (1%) 551
FML-S Ophthalmic Suspension ⊙ 229
Fortaz (Very rare) 1453
Furosemide Tablets 2154
Gantrisin Pediatric Suspension 2770
Garamycin Injectable 3014
▲ Humira Injection (Less than 5%) 466
Hyzaar 50-12.5 Tablets 1990
Hyzaar 100-12.5 Tablets 1990
Hyzaar 100-25 Tablets 1990
Indapamide Tablets 2156
Inderal LA Long-Acting Capsules 3429
Indocin Capsules (Less than 1%) 1995
Indocin I.V. (Less than 1%) 2465
Indocin (Less than 1%) 1995
InnoPran XL Capsules 2723
Keflex Capsules 549
Lamictal 1481
Lamisil Tablets (Rare) 2232
▲ Leukine (6%) 814
Levaquin (0.1% to 0.9%) 2384
Levaquin in 5% Dextrose Injection (0.1% to 0.9%) 2384
Lofibra Tablets (Rare) 1219
Lofibra Capsules (Rare) 1216
Lopressor Injection (Rare) 2238
Lopressor Tablets (Rare) 2238
Lopressor HCT 50/25 Tablets 2241
Lopressor HCT 100/25 Tablets 2241
Lopressor HCT 100/50 Tablets 2241
Lotensin HCT Tablets 2246
Lotrel Capsules 2249
Mavik Tablets (Rare) 486
Maxipime for Injection 1105
Mefoxin for Injection 2012
Mefoxin Premixed Intravenous Solution 2016
Micardis HCT Tablets 856
Miradon Tablets 3042
Mobic Oral Suspension (Less than 0.1%) 863

Mobic Tablets (Less than 0.1%) 863
Moduretic Tablets 2028
Mustargen for Injection (Relatively infrequent) 2468
Nadolol Tablets 2159
Nalfon Capsules (Less than 1%) 2502
Naprosyn Suspension (Less than 1%) 2761
Naprosyn Tablets (Less than 1%) 2761
Nexium I.V. (Rare) 659
▲ Nipent for Injection (3% to 10%) 1863
Noroxin Tablets 2032
Omnicef Capsules 511
Omnicef for Oral Suspension 511
Oncaspar 1145
Parcopa Orally Disintegrating Tablets 3097
Parnate Tablets 1527
Paser Granules 1674
Paxil CR Controlled-Release Tablets 1538
Paxil 1530
Pentasa Capsules 3185
Pepcid Injection (Rare) 2040
Pepcid (Rare) 2038
Pexeva Tablets 1694
Phenergan Tablets and Suppositories 3440
Phenytek Capsules (Occasional) 2160
Plavix Tablets (Less than 1%) 917
Plavix Tablets (Less than 1%) 2926
Pletal Tablets (Very rare) 2455
Prevacid Delayed-Release Capsules (Less than 1%) 3271
Prevacid for Delayed-Release Oral Suspension (Less than 1%) 3271
Prevacid SoluTab Delayed-Release Orally Disintegrating Tablets (Less than 1%) 3271
Prevacid NapraPAC (Less than 1%) 3280
PREVPAC 3284
Prilosec OTC Delayed-Release Tablets (Rare) 2677
Primaxin I.M. 2045
Primaxin I.V. 2048
Prinivil Tablets (Rare to frequent) 2052
Prinzide Tablets (Rare) 2056
Proquin XR Tablets 1153
ProSom Tablets (Rare) 517
Provigil Tablets 988
Raniclor Tablets, Chewable 2505
Rocephin Injectable Vials, ADD-Vantage, Galaxy, Bulk 2800
Seroquel Tablets 690
Stalevo Tablets 2287
Suprax 1843
Tegretol/Tegretol-XR (Very low incidence) 2295
Teveten HCT Tablets 1737
Thioridazine Hydrochloride Tablets (Infrequent) 2163
Thiothixene Capsules 2165
Ticlid Tablets (Rare) 2810
Timolide Tablets 2086
Timoptic Sterile Ophthalmic Solution 2088
Timoptic in Ocudose 2091
Timoptic-XE Sterile Ophthalmic Gel Forming Solution 2092
Toprol-XL Tablets (Rare) 668
Tricor Tablets (Rare) 527
Trusopt Sterile Ophthalmic Solution (Rare) 2095
Uniretic Tablets (More than 1%) 3100
Vantin Tablets and Oral Suspension 2645
Vasotec I.V. Injection (Several cases) 2103
VFEND I.V. (Less than 2%) 2564
VFEND Oral Suspension (Less than 2%) 2564
VFEND Tablets (Less than 2%) 2564
Vicodin Tablets 535
Vicodin ES Tablets 536
Vicodin HP Tablets 538
Voltaren Tablets (Rarely) 2307
Voltaren-XR Tablets (Rarely) 2310
▲ Xeloda Tablets (Less than 5%) 2822
Zantac (Rare) 1624
Zantac Injection (Rare) 1619
Zantac Injection Pharmacy Bulk Package (Rare) 1622
Zantac Injection Premixed (Rare) 1619
Zantac (Rare) 1624
Zegerid Capsules (Rare) 2958
Zegerid Powder for Oral Solution (Rare) 2958
Zinacef for Injection 1631
Zinacef Injection 1631
Zoloft 2586
Zonegran Capsules (Rare) 1101
Zosyn (1% or less) 3492

Airway constriction
Amerge Tablets (Rare) 1339

Airway obstruction
Altace Capsules 1702
Amerge Tablets (Rare) 1339
Captopril Tablets 2149
Erbitux 910
▲ Infasurf Intratracheal Suspension (39%) 1184
Levaquin (0.1% to 0.9%) 2384
Levaquin in 5% Dextrose Injection (0.1% to 0.9%) 2384
Orthoclone OKT3 Sterile Solution 2360
Prinivil Tablets 2052
Prinzide Tablets 2056
Revlimid Capsules 958
▲ Ultane Liquid for Inhalation (8%) 531
Vasotec I.V. Injection 2103

Akathisia
▲ Abilify Oral Solution (12% to 17%) 882
▲ Abilify Oral Solution (12% to 17%) 2450
▲ Abilify Discmelt Orally Disintegrating Tablets (12% to 17%) 882
▲ Abilify Discmelt Orally Disintegrating Tablets (12% to 17%) 2450
▲ Abilify Tablets (12% to 17%) 882
▲ Abilify Tablets (12% to 17%) 2450
Celexa 1176
Cesamet Capsules 3340
▲ Clozaril Tablets (3%) 2184
Effexor Tablets (Infrequent) 3411
Effexor XR Capsules (Infrequent) 3417
▲ FazaClo Orally Disintegrating Tablets (3%) 551
▲ Geodon (8% to 10%) 2529
Lamictal (Infrequent) 1481
Lexapro Oral Solution 1190
Lexapro Tablets 1190
▲ Mirapex Tablets (2% to 3%) 859
Moban Tablets 1119
▲ Niravam Orally Disintegrating Tablets (1.6% to 3%) 3092
Paxil CR Controlled-Release Tablets 1538
Paxil 1530
Permax Tablets (1.6%) 3356
Pexeva Tablets 1694
Prozac Pulvules and Liquid (Infrequent) 1801
▲ Risperdal (16% to 34%) 1676
▲ Risperdal Consta Long-Acting Injection (2% to 9%) 1682
▲ Risperdal M-Tab Orally Disintegrating Tablets (16% to 34%) 1676
Symbyax Capsules 1819
Thioridazine Hydrochloride Tablets 2163
Thiothixene Capsules 2165
VFEND I.V. (Less than 2%) 2564
VFEND Oral Suspension (Less than 2%) 2564
VFEND Tablets (Less than 2%) 2564
Wellbutrin Tablets (1.5%) 1603
Wellbutrin XL Extended-Release Tablets (2%) 1613
Zoloft 2586
Zomig Tablets (Rare) 3519
Zomig-ZMT Tablets (Rare) 3519
▲ Zyprexa Tablets (3% to 27%) 1830
▲ Zyprexa IntraMuscular (2% to 5%) 1830
▲ Zyprexa ZYDIS Orally Disintegrating Tablets (3% to 27%) 1830

Akinesia
Abilify Oral Solution (Infrequent) 882
Abilify Oral Solution (Infrequent) 2450
Abilify Discmelt Orally Disintegrating Tablets (Infrequent) 882
Abilify Discmelt Orally Disintegrating Tablets (Infrequent) 2450
Abilify Tablets (Infrequent) 882
Abilify Tablets (Infrequent) 2450
▲ Clozaril Tablets (4%) 2184
Effexor Tablets (Rare) 3411
Effexor XR Capsules (Rare) 3417
▲ FazaClo Orally Disintegrating Tablets (4%) 551
Geodon Capsules (Frequent) 2529
Maxalt Tablets (Rare) 2008
Maxalt-MLT Orally Disintegrating Tablets (Rare) 2008
Moban Tablets 1119
Parnate Tablets 1527
Paxil CR Controlled-Release Tablets (Infrequent) 1538
Paxil (Infrequent) 1530
Permax Tablets (1.1%) 3356
Pexeva Tablets (rare) 1694
Thioridazine Hydrochloride Tablets 2163
▲ Wellbutrin Tablets (8.0%) 1603
Wellbutrin SR Sustained-Release Tablets 1607
Wellbutrin XL Extended-Release Tablets 1613
Zelapar Tablets 3372
Zyban Sustained-Release Tablets 1644
▲ Zyprexa Tablets (8% to 20%) 1830
▲ Zyprexa IntraMuscular (2% to 4%) 1830
▲ Zyprexa ZYDIS Orally Disintegrating Tablets (8% to 20%) 1830

Alanine aminotransferase levels, changes in
Bumex Tablets (0.5%) 2746
Parcopa Orally Disintegrating Tablets 3097
Prozac Pulvules and Liquid (Infrequent) 1801
▲ Sutent Capsules (2% to 39%) 2560
▲ Zyvox (0% to 10.1%) 2652

Alanine aminotransferase levels, elevation of
Abelcet Injection 1141
Abilify Oral Solution (Infrequent) 882
Abilify Oral Solution (Infrequent) 2450
Abilify Discmelt Orally Disintegrating Tablets (Infrequent) 882
Abilify Discmelt Orally Disintegrating Tablets (Infrequent) 2450
Abilify Tablets (Infrequent) 882
Abilify Tablets (Infrequent) 2450
Accolate Tablets (1.5%) 671
Accutane Capsules 2731
Aceon Tablets (2 mg, 4 mg, 8 mg) (1.6% to 1.7%) 3194
Aciphex Tablets (0.2%) 1090
Actos Tablets (0.3%) 3219
Adalat CC Tablets (Rare) 2964
▲ Alimta for Injection (1% to 10%) 1750
Alinia for Oral Suspension (Less than 1.1%) 2835
Alinia Tablets (Less than 1.1%) 2835
Aloxi Injection (Less than 1%) 2127
Altoprev Extended-Release Tablets 3109
Ambien Tablets (Infrequent) 2851
Ambien CR Tablets (Infrequent) 2855
▲ AmBisome for Injection (14.6%) 620
Amevive (1.7%) 626
Amoxil Capsules 1343
Amoxil Chewable Tablets 1343
Amoxil Pediatric Drops for Oral Suspension 1343
Amoxil Powder for Oral Suspension 1343
Amoxil Tablets 1343
Anaprox Tablets (Less than 1%) 2761
Anaprox DS Tablets (Less than 1%) 2761
Anzemet Injection 2859
Anzemet Tablets 2862
▲ Aptivus Capsules (2.7% to 17.5%) 826
▲ Aralast (11.1%) 717
▲ Arimidex Tablets (2% to 5%) 673
Arixtra Injection (0.3% to 2.6%) 1351
Arthrotec Tablets (1.6%) 3129
Asacol Delayed-Release Tablets 2692
Astelin Nasal Spray (Infrequently) 1904
Atripla Tablets (2%) 945
Augmentin (Infrequent) 1360
Augmentin Tablets (Infrequent) 1363
Augmentin XR Extended-Release Tablets (Infrequent) 1369
Augmentin ES-600 Powder for Oral Suspension 1366
Avandamet Tablets (0.2%) 1373
Avandia Tablets (0.2%) 1384
Axid Oral Solution (Less common) 879
▲ Baraclude (2% to 12%) 894
BeneFix Vials (1.6%) 3408
Benicar HCT Tablets (Greater than 1%) 1044
▲ Betaseron for SC Injection (10%) 767
Biaxin/Biaxin XL 402
Calcijex Injection 411
Calcium Disodium Versenate Injection 1851
Campral Tablets (Infrequent) 1174
▲ Cancidas for Injection (3.7% to 10.8%) 1918
Cardizem LA Extended Release Tablets (Less than 2%) 1728
Ceftin (0.1% to 1%) 1407
Celebrex Capsules (0.1% to 1.9%) 3134
▲ CellCept Capsules (3% to less than 20%) 2747
▲ CellCept Intravenous (3% to less than 20%) 2747
▲ CellCept Oral Suspension (3% to less than 20%) 2747
▲ CellCept Tablets (3% to less than 20%) 2747
▲ Chemet Capsules (4.2% to 10.4%) 2458
Cipro (1.9%) 2977
▲ Cipro I.V. (Among most frequent) 2984
▲ Clolar for Intravenous Infusion (44%) 1271
Colazal Capsules 2838
Combivir Tablets 1411
▲ Coreg Tablets (Greater than 1% to 3%) 1414
Covera-HS Tablets (1.4%) 3139
▲ Crixivan Capsules (4.9%) 1940
Cubicin for Injection (Less than 1%) 1026
Cutivate Lotion 0.05% (Rare) 2664
Cymbalta Delayed-Release Capsules 1757
Dalmane Capsules (Rare) 3342
▲ Depacon Injection (1% to 5%) 412
Depakene (Frequent) 417
▲ Depakote Sprinkle Capsules (1% to 5%) 422
▲ Depakote Tablets (Frequent) 427
Depakote ER Tablets (Greater than 1%) 434
Depo-Medrol Single-Dose Vial 2619
Dolobid Tablets 1955
▲ Doxil Injection (1% to 5%) 2351
EC-Naprosyn Delayed-Release Tablets (Less than 1%) 2761
Effexor Tablets (Infrequent) 3411
Effexor XR Capsules (Rare) 3417
▲ Eloxatin for Injection (0% to 36%) 2892
Elspar for Injection 2463
Elspar for Injection 1960
▲ Emend Capsules (6%) 1963
▲ Emtriva Capsules (2% to 5%) 1287
▲ Emtriva Oral Solution (2% to 5%) 1287
▲ Epivir (3.7% to 4%) 1427
▲ Epivir-HBV (11%) 1432
Eraxis for Injection (2.3%) 2521
Eulexin Capsules 3009
Evoxac Capsules (Less than 1%) 1047
▲ Famvir Tablets (3.2%) 2211
Femara Tablets 2214
▲ Fortaz (1 in 15) 1453
Fuzeon Injection 2767
▲ Gamunex Immune Globulin I.V., 10% (7% to 18%) 3235
Garamycin Injectable 3014
▲ Gemzar for Injection (38% to 72%) 1771
▲ Gleevec Tablets (0% to 7%) 2227
Hectorol Capsules 1275
▲ Hepsera Tablets (2% to 20%) 1292
▲ Humatrope Vials and Cartridges (6.25% to 6.67%) 1787
▲ Hycamtin for Injection (Less than 1% to 5%) 1458
▲ Imdur Tablets (Less than or equal to 5%) 3018
Increlex Injection 3291
Inspra Tablets (15 patients) 2536
▲ Intron A for Injection (Up to 15% of patients) 3024
▲ Invanz for Injection (3.8% to 8.8%) 1999
▲ Invirase (Less than 1% to 4%) 2772
▲ I.V. Busulfex (7% to 31%) 2493
▲ Kaletra (4% to 10%) 476
Keflex Capsules 549
▲ Kytril Injection (3.3%) 2781
▲ Kytril (9%) 2784
▲ Leukine (13%) 814
▲ Lexiva Tablets (6%) 1505
▲ Lofibra Tablets (Up to 3.4%) 1219
▲ Lofibra Capsules (3.4%) 1216
Lotronex Tablets (1%) 1512
▲ Lovenox Injection (Up to 5.5%) 2915
Malarone Pediatric Tablets 1517
Malarone Tablets 1517
Marinol Capsules (Less than 1%) 3333
Mavik Tablets (0.3% to 1.0%) 486
Maxipime for Injection (2.8%) 1105
Mefoxin for Injection 2012
Mefoxin Premixed Intravenous Solution 2016
▲ Mepron Suspension (6%) 1521
Meridia Capsules (1.6%) 489
Merrem I.V. (Greater than 0.2%) 686
Mevacor Tablets 2021
Mobic Oral Suspension (Less than 2%) 863
Mobic Tablets (Less than 2%) 863
Mycamine for Injection (0.4% to 2.6%) 628
▲ Mylotarg for Injection (9%) 3431
Naprosyn Suspension (Less than 1%) 2761

Naprosyn Tablets (Less than 1%) 2761
Nexium Delayed-Release Capsules (Less than 1%) 655
Nexium I.V. (Less than 1%) 659
Niaspan Extended-Release Tablets 1730
Nimotop Capsules (0.2%; rare) 749
Noroxin Tablets (1.4%) 2032
▲ Norvir (7.8% to 8.5%) 503
Omacor Capsules 2725
Omnicef Capsules (0.7%) 511
Omnicef for Oral Suspension (0.4%) 511
▲ Oncaspar (Greater than 5%) 1145
Orthoclone OKT3 Sterile Solution 2360
Oxandrin Tablets 2962
Paxil CR Controlled-Release Tablets (Infrequent) 1538
Paxil (Infrequent) 1530
Pegasys (Less than 1%) 2789
▲ PEG-Intron Powder for Injection (10%) 3048
Pentasa Capsules (Less than 1%) 3185
Pexeva Tablets (infrequent) 1694
Precose Tablets 751
Prevacid Delayed-Release Capsules 3271
Prevacid for Delayed-Release Oral Suspension 3271
Prevacid SoluTab Delayed-Release Orally Disintegrating Tablets 3271
Prevacid NapraPAC 3280
PREVPAC (Less than 1%) 3284
▲ Prezista Tablets (5.6% to 6.9%) 3306
Prilosec OTC Delayed-Release Tablets (Rare) 2677
Primaxin I.M. 2045
Primaxin I.V. 2048
▲ Prograf Capsules and Injection (3% to 15%) 632
Proquin XR Tablets (Less than 1%) 1153
Protonix I.V. (Greater than or equal to 1%) 3472
Protonix Tablets (Greater than or equal to 1%) 3469
Protopic Ointment (Greater than or equal to 1%) 638
Prozac Pulvules and Liquid (Rare) 1801
Raniclor Tablets, Chewable 2505
▲ Rapamune Oral Solution and Tablets (3% to 20%) 3475
▲ Rebif Prefilled Syringe for Injection (20% to 27%) 3159
▲ Remicade for IV Injection (Less than 1% to 42%) 971
▲ Rescriptor Tablets (4.1% to 5.1%) 2551
▲ Revlimid Capsules (8.1%) 958
Risperdal (Infrequent) 1676
Risperdal Consta Long-Acting Injection (Infrequent) 1682
Risperdal M-Tab Orally Disintegrating Tablets (Infrequent) 1676
Rocaltrol Capsules 2798
Rocaltrol Oral Solution 2798
▲ Rocephin Injectable Vials, ADD-Vantage, Galaxy, Bulk (3.3%) 2800
Rythmol SR Capsules 2727
▲ Seroquel Tablets (5%) 690
Singulair (1% to 2.1%) 2077
Somavert Injection (0.8% to 1.2%) 2642
Sonata Capsules (Rare) 1717
▲ Soriatane Capsules (Approximately 1 in 3 patients) 1013
Stromectol Tablets (2%) 2083
Suprax (Less than 2%) 1843
Sustiva Capsules (2%) 930
Sustiva Tablets (2%) 930
▲ Symbyax Capsules (6.3%) 1819
Symmetrel Tablets 1135
Synagis (More than 1%) 1897
Tarceva Tablets 1259
Tarceva Tablets 2444
Targretin Capsules 1747
Tarka Tablets 524
▲ Tasmar Tablets (1% to 5%) 3358
▲ Taxotere Injection Concentrate (4.3%) 2932
Tequin Injection (Less than 0.1%) 938
Tequin Injection in 5% Dextrose (Less than 0.1%) 938
Tequin Tablets (Less than 0.1%) 938
Teveten Tablets (Less than 1%) 1735
Teveten HCT Tablets (Less than 1%) 1737
Thalomid Capsules 965
Tiazac Capsules (Less than 2%) 1201
Ticlid Tablets (Rare) 2810
Timentin ADD-Vantage 1580
Timentin Injection Galaxy Container 1583
Timentin IV Infusion 1577
Timentin Pharmacy Bulk Package 1586
Topamax Sprinkle Capsules (Infrequent) 2404
Topamax Tablets (Infrequent) 2404
▲ Tracleer Tablets (11%) 545
Trasylol Injection 754
Trecator Tablets 3487
▲ Tricor Tablets (3.0%) 527
▲ Triglide Tablets (3%) 3123
▲ Trisenox Injection (20%) 993
▲ Trizivir Tablets (3.7%) 1589
Truvada Tablets (2%) 1296
▲ Tygacil for Injection (5.6%) 3488
Ultane Liquid for Inhalation (Less than 1%) 531
▲ Ultram ER Tablets (1% to greater than 5%) 2392
Uniretic Tablets (More than 1%) 3100
▲ Valtrex Caplets (14%) 1597
Vantin Tablets and Oral Suspension 2645
Verelan PM Extended-Release Capsules, Controlled-Onset 3106
▲ VFEND I.V. (1.8% to 18.9%) 2564
▲ VFEND Oral Suspension (1.8% to 18.9%) 2564
▲ VFEND Tablets (1.8% to 18.9%) 2564
Viracept (Less than 2%) 2577
▲ Viramune Oral Suspension (3.4%) 873
▲ Viramune Tablets (3.4%) 873
▲ Viread Tablets (2% to 4%) 1301
Vivitrol 995
Xeloda Tablets (1.6%) 2822
Xyrem Oral Solution (Infrequent) 1688
Zantac 1624
Zantac Injection 1619
Zantac 1624
Zegerid Capsules (Rare) 2958
Zegerid Powder for Oral Solution (Rare) 2958
Zelapar Tablets 3372
▲ Ziagen (6%) 1626
▲ Zinacef for Injection (1 in 25 patients) 1631
▲ Zinacef Injection (1 in 25 patients) 1631
Zmax for Oral Suspension (Less then 1%) 2583
Zocor Tablets (1%) 2105
▲ Zofran Injection (Approximately 5% of patients) 1634
Zofran (Approximately 1% to 2%) 1639
Zofran ODT Orally Disintegrating Tablets (Approximately 1% to 2%) 1639
Zoloft (Infrequent) 2586
Zonegran Capsules (Rare) 1101
Zosyn 3492
Zyflo Tablets (1.9%) 1023
Zyprexa Tablets (2%) 1830
Zyprexa IntraMuscular 1830
Zyprexa ZYDIS Orally Disintegrating Tablets (2%) 1830

Albuminuria
Abilify Oral Solution (Infrequent) 882
Abilify Oral Solution (Infrequent) 2450
Abilify Discmelt Orally Disintegrating Tablets (Infrequent) 882
Abilify Discmelt Orally Disintegrating Tablets (Infrequent) 2450
Abilify Tablets (Infrequent) 882
Abilify Tablets (Infrequent) 2450
Aciphex Tablets 1090
Astelin Nasal Spray (Infrequent) 1904
Atacand Tablets (More than 1%) 649
Atacand HCT 651
Azilect Tablets (Greater than 1%) 3293
Caduet Tablets (Greater than or equal to 2%) 2508
Calcijex Injection 411
Carbatrol Capsules 3171
Cardizem LA Extended Release Tablets (Less than 2%) 1728
▲ CellCept Capsules (3% to less than 20%) 2747
▲ CellCept Intravenous (3% to less than 20%) 2747
▲ CellCept Oral Suspension (3% to less than 20%) 2747
▲ CellCept Tablets (3% to less than 20%) 2747
Cipro 2977
Cipro I.V. 2984
▲ Coreg Tablets (Greater than 1% to 3%) 1414
▲ Dacogen Injection (7%) 2129
Dapsone Tablets USP 1673
▲ Doxil Injection (1% to 5%) 2351
Effexor Tablets (Infrequent) 3411
Effexor XR Capsules (Infrequent) 3417
Equetro Extended-Release Capsules 3180
Evoxac Capsules (Less than 1%) 1047
Exelon Capsules (Infrequent) 2206
Exelon Oral Solution (Infrequent) 2206
Geodon Capsules (Infrequent) 2529
Hectorol Capsules 1275
Hectorol Injection 1278
Inspra Tablets (1%) 2536
▲ Intron A for Injection (Less than 5%) 3024
▲ Keppra Oral Solution (4%) 3314
▲ Keppra Tablets (4%) 3314
Lipitor Tablets (Less than 2%) 2483
Lithobid Tablets 1692
Lyrica Capsules (0.1% to 1%) 2539
▲ Megace ES Oral Suspension (1% to 3%) 2481
Miradon Tablets 3042
Mobic Oral Suspension (Less than 2%) 863
Mobic Tablets (Less than 2%) 863
Nexium Delayed-Release Capsules (Less than 1%) 655
Nexium I.V. (Less than 1%) 659
Noroxin Tablets 2032
▲ Ontak Vials (10%) 1745
Pentasa Capsules (Less than 1%) 3185
Pletal Tablets (Less than 2%) 2455
Prevacid Delayed-Release Capsules (Less than 1%) 3271
Prevacid for Delayed-Release Oral Suspension 3271
Prevacid SoluTab Delayed-Release Orally Disintegrating Tablets (Less than 1%) 3271
Prevacid NapraPAC 3280
PREVPAC (Less than 1%) 3284
▲ Prograf Capsules and Injection (3% to 15%) 632
Protonix I.V. (Less than 1%) 3472
Protonix Tablets (Less than 1%) 3469
Provigil Tablets (1%) 988
Prozac Pulvules and Liquid (Infrequent) 1801
▲ Rapamune Oral Solution and Tablets (3% to 20%) 3475
Requip Tablets (Infrequent) 1555
Rocaltrol Capsules 2798
Rocaltrol Oral Solution 2798
▲ Sandostatin LAR Depot (1% to 4%) 2280
▲ Simulect for Injection (3% to 10%) 2284
Sonata Capsules (Rare) 1717
Targretin Capsules 1747
Tegretol/Tegretol-XR 2295
Teveten Tablets (Less than 1%) 1735
Teveten HCT Tablets (Less than 1%) 1737
▲ Thalomid Capsules (3.1% to 8.3%) 965
Topamax Sprinkle Capsules (Infrequent) 2404
Topamax Tablets (Infrequent) 2404
Ultane Liquid for Inhalation (Less than 1%) 531
Uniretic Tablets (Less than 1%) 3100
Uroqid-Acid No. 2 Tablets 760
VFEND I.V. (Less than 2%) 2564
VFEND Oral Suspension (Less than 2%) 2564
VFEND Tablets (Less than 2%) 2564
▲ Visudyne for Injection (1% to 10%) 2305
Zelapar Tablets 3372
Zonegran Capsules (Rare) 1101
Zyprexa Tablets (Rare) 1830
Zyprexa ZYDIS Orally Disintegrating Tablets (Rare) 1830

Alcohol, increased sensitivity to
Catapres Tablets 843
Celexa (Infrequent) 1176
Clorpres Tablets 2153
Copaxone for Injection (Infrequent) 3297
Effexor Tablets (Rare) 3411
Effexor XR Capsules (Rare) 3417
Lamictal (Rare) 1481
Neurontin Capsules (Rare) 2487
Neurontin Oral Solution (Rare) 2487
Neurontin Tablets (Rare) 2487
▲ Protopic Ointment (Up to 7%) 638
Prozac Pulvules and Liquid (Rare) 1801
Rescriptor Tablets 2551
Seroquel Tablets (Infrequent) 690
Soriatane Capsules (Less than 1%) 1013
Symbyax Capsules (Infrequent) 1819
Tequin Injection (Less than 0.1%) 938
Tequin Injection in 5% Dextrose (Less than 0.1%) 938
Tequin Tablets (Less than 0.1%) 938
Teveten Tablets (Less than 1%) 1735
Teveten HCT Tablets (Less than 1%) 1737
Topamax Sprinkle Capsules (Rare) 2404
Topamax Tablets (Rare) 2404

Alcohol abuse
Effexor Tablets (Rare) 3411
Effexor XR Capsules (Rare) 3417
Paxil CR Controlled-Release Tablets (Infrequent) 1538
Paxil (Infrequent) 1530
Pexeva Tablets (infrequent) 1694
Zyprexa Tablets (Infrequent) 1830
Zyprexa ZYDIS Orally Disintegrating Tablets (Infrequent) 1830

Alcohol craving
Campral Tablets (Rare) 1174

Alkalosis
▲ CellCept Capsules (3% to less than 20%) 2747
▲ CellCept Intravenous (3% to less than 20%) 2747
▲ CellCept Oral Suspension (3% to less than 20%) 2747
▲ CellCept Tablets (3% to less than 20%) 2747
Percodan Tablets 1132
▲ Prograf Capsules and Injection (3% to 15%) 632
▲ Proleukin for Injection (4%) 2266

Alkalosis, metabolic
Indocin I.V. (Less than 3%) 2465

Alkalosis, respiratory
Adenocard Injection 617
Bayer Aspirin 744
Bayer Aspirin Comprehensive Prescribing Information ..... ▣ 796
Percodan Tablets 1132
St. Joseph 81 mg Aspirin ..... ▣ 688

Allergic reactions
Hurricaine Topical Anesthetic Spray, 2 oz. Wild Cherry (Rare) ..... ▣ 712
Abelcet Injection 1141
Abilify Oral Solution (Rare) 882
Abilify Oral Solution (Rare) 2450
Abilify Discmelt Orally Disintegrating Tablets (Rare) 882
Abilify Discmelt Orally Disintegrating Tablets (Rare) 2450
Abilify Tablets (Rare) 882
Abilify Tablets (Rare) 2450
AccuNeb Inhalation Solution (0.9% to 3.4%) 1055
Accutane Capsules 2731
Aceon Tablets (2 mg, 4 mg, 8 mg) (2.0%) 3194
Aciphex Tablets 1090
Actiq (Less than 1%) 979
Activase I.V. (Very rare) 1223
Actonel Tablets (1.9% to 2.5%) 2683
Actonel with Calcium Tablets (1.9% to 2.5%) 2688
▲ Acular Ophthalmic Solution (Approximately 1% to 10%) 565
▲ Acular LS Ophthalmic Solution (1% to 10%) 566
ADACEL Vaccine 2945
Adalat CC Tablets (Less than 1%) 2964
Adipex-P 1215
▲ Advair Diskus 100/50 (1% to 3%) 1308
▲ Advair Diskus 250/50 (1% to 3%) 1308
▲ Advair Diskus 500/50 (1% to 3%) 1308
▲ Advair HFA Inhalation Aerosol (1% to 3%) 1318
Advil Caplets ..... ▣ 674
Children's Advil Oral Suspension ..... ▣ 603
Children's Advil Chewable Tablets ..... ▣ 603
Advil Cold & Sinus ..... ▣ 723
Advil Gel Caplets ..... ▣ 674
Infants' Advil Concentrated Drops ..... ▣ 604
Infants' Advil Concentrated Drops - White Grape (Dye-Free) ..... ▣ 604
Junior Strength Advil Swallow Tablets ..... ▣ 605
Advil Liqui-Gels ..... ▣ 674
Advil Migraine Liquigels ..... ▣ 608
Advil Tablets ..... ▣ 674
Aggrastat 1907
Aggrenox Capsules (Less than 1%) 822
▲ Alamast Ophthalmic Solution (Less than 5%) 3381
Albenza Tablets (Rare) 1338
Albutein 5%, Albumin (Human) 1652
Albutein 25%, Albumin (Human) 1653
▲ Alimta for Injection (Up to 8%) 1750
Alinia for Oral Suspension (Less than 1%) 2835
Alinia Tablets (Less than 1%) 2835
Alkeran for Injection 955
Alkeran Tablets 956
▲ Alphagan P Ophthalmic Solution (1% to 4%) 567

Alphanate, Antihemophilic Factor (Human) 1654
AlphaNine SD, Coagulation Factor IX (Human) 1656
Ambien Tablets (Rare) 2851
Ambien CR Tablets (Rare) 2855
AmBisome for Injection (Less common) 620
Amerge Tablets (Rare) 1339
Amoxil Capsules 1343
Amoxil Chewable Tablets 1343
Amoxil Pediatric Drops for Oral Suspension 1343
Amoxil Powder for Oral Suspension 1343
Amoxil Tablets 1343
Antivenin (Micrurus fulvius) 3407
Antivenin Polyvalent 3405
Apidra Injection 2864
Aranesp for Injection (Rare) 581
Aredia for Injection (Rare) 2179
Argatroban Injection 1346
Arimidex Tablets (Very rare) 673
Arthrotec Tablets (Less than 0.1%) 3129
Astelin Nasal Spray (Infrequent) 1904
▲ Atripla Tablets (Greater than or equal to 5%) 945
Atrovent HFA Inhalation Aerosol 841
Attenuvax (Rare) 1914
Augmentin 1360
Augmentin Tablets 1363
Avelox (0.1% to less than 2%) 2970
Azilect Tablets (Greater than 1%) 3293
Azopt Ophthalmic Suspension (Less than 1%) 557
BeneFix Vials (1.5%) 3408
Bentyl Capsules 697
Bentyl Injection 697
Bentyl Syrup 697
Bentyl Tablets 697
▲ Betimol Ophthalmic Solution (1% to 5%) 3382
▲ Betimol Ophthalmic Solution (1% to 5%) ⊙295
Betoptic S Ophthalmic Suspension 558
Bexxar 1398
Biaxin/Biaxin XL 402
Bicillin C-R Injectable Suspension 1706
BiDil Tablets (1% to less than 2%) 2171
Biltricide Tablets 2976
Boniva Injection (2.5%) 2738
Boniva Tablets (2.5%) 2741
▲ Brimonidine Tartrate Ophthalmic Solution 0.2% (10% to 30%) ⊙248
Caduet Tablets (Greater than 0.1% to 2.8%) 2508
Campath Ampules 811
Campral Tablets (Infrequent) 1174
Carac Cream, 0.5% (1.2%) 2879
Cardizem LA Extended Release Tablets (Less than 2%) 1728
▲ Carnitor Injection (2% to 6%) 3188
Catapres Tablets 843
Ceftin 1407
Celebrex Capsules (0.1% to 1.9%) 3134
Celexa 1176
Cesamet Capsules 3340
Cetacaine Topical Anesthetic 999
Ciloxan Ophthalmic Ointment (Less than 1%) 559
Ciloxan Ophthalmic Solution (Less than 1%) ⊙206
Cipro (Less than 1%) 2977
Cipro I.V. (1% or less) 2984
Cipro XR Tablets 2990
Colyte with Flavor Packs for Oral Solution (Isolated cases) 3088
Copaxone for Injection (Rare) 3297
▲ Coreg Tablets (Greater than 1% to 3%) 1414
Cosopt Sterile Ophthalmic Solution 1931
Coumadin for Injection (Infrequent) 898
Coumadin Tablets (Infrequent) 898
Creon 5 Capsules (Less frequent) 3198
Creon 10 Capsules (Less frequent) 3198
Creon 20 Capsules (Less frequent) 3199
Cutivate Lotion 0.05% (Less than 1%) 2664
CytoGam Intravenous (Rare) 1895
Cytomel Tablets (Rare) 1710
Depacon Injection 412
Depakene 417
Depakote Sprinkle Capsules 422
▲ Depakote Tablets (1% to 5%) 427
Depakote ER Tablets 434
Depo-Medrol Single-Dose Vial 2619
Depo-Provera Contraceptive Injection (Less than 1%) 2622
depo-subQ provera 104 Injectable Suspension 2624
Digibind for Injection (Rare) 1421
Dilaudid Oral Liquid 445
Dilaudid Tablets - 8 mg 445
Diovan Tablets 2193
Diovan HCT Tablets (Greater than 0.2%) 2196
▲ Doxil Injection (1% to 5%) 2351
Duragesic Transdermal System (1% or greater) 2373
E.E.S. 451
Effexor Tablets (Infrequent) 3411
Effexor XR Capsules (Infrequent) 3417
Elitek 2890
Elmiron Capsules (Less than or equal to 1%) 2415
▲ Eloxatin for Injection (3% to 10%) 2892
Elspar for Injection 2463
Elspar for Injection 1960
Emcyt Capsules 2634
▲ Emtriva Capsules (17% to 30%) 1287
▲ Emtriva Oral Solution (17% to 30%) 1287
Enbrel for Injection (Less than 0.5%) 584
Epogen for Injection (Rare) 591
▲ Equetro Extended-Release Capsules (Less than 5%) 3180
EryPed 447
Ery-Tab Tablets 449
Erythrocin Stearate Filmtab Tablets 453
Erythromycin Delayed-Release Capsules, USP 457
Estring Vaginal Ring (1%) 2635
Ethyol for Injection 1898
▲ Evoxac Capsules (1% to 3%) 1047
Exelon Capsules (Frequent) 2206
Exelon Oral Solution (Frequent) 2206
Feiba VH 718
Ferrlecit Injection (0.5%) 3388
Fleet Phospho-soda ACCU-PREP 1168
Fleet Phospho-soda EZ-PREP 1169
Flomax Capsules 850
FML Ophthalmic Suspension ⊙227
Focalin Tablets 2220
▲ Fortaz (Among most common) 1453
Fortical Nasal Spray 3337
Fragmin Injection (Rare) 1097
Gabitril Tablets (Frequent) 984
Gantrisin Pediatric Suspension 2770
Gengraf Capsules (1% to less than 3%) 459
Geodon 2529
GlucaGen 761
Glucagon for Injection Vials and Emergency Kit 1778
Hemofil M (Extremely rare) 728
▲ Herceptin I.V. (3%) 1233
Humalog-Pen (Less common) 1781
Humalog Mix 50/50-Pen 1783
Humalog Mix 75/25-Pen 1785
Humate-P (Rare) 3502
Humulin 50/50, 100 Units (Less common to occasional) 1791
Humulin 70/30 Pen 1793
Humulin L, 100 Units 1794
Humulin N Pen 1797
Hurricaine Topical Anesthetic Gel, 1 oz. Wild Cherry, Pina Colada, Watermelon, and Fresh Mint, 5.25 g. Wild Cherry (Rare) ▣712
Hurricaine Topical Anesthetic Liquid, 1 oz. Wild Cherry, Pina Colada, 0.005 fl. oz. Snap-n-Go Swabs Wild Cherry (Rare) ▣712
Hurricaine Topical Anesthetic Spray Extension Tubes (200) (Rare) ▣712
Hurricaine Topical Anesthetic Spray Kit, 2 oz. Wild Cherry with disposable Extension Tubes (200) (Rare) ▣712
Hyalgan Solution (Three cases) 2901
▲ Hycamtin for Injection (Infrequent to 6%) 1458
Hytrin Capsules (Rare) 471
Increlex Injection 3291
Infanrix Vaccine 1476
▲ Infergen (3% to 7%) 3364
Integrilin Injection 3020
Invirase (Less than 2%) 2772
Iressa Tablets (Very rare) 684
▲ I.V. Busulfex (2% to 26%) 2493
Kaletra (Less than 2%) 476
Keppra Oral Solution (2%) 3314
Keppra Tablets (2%) 3314
Ketek Tablets (Rare) 2903
Klonopin (2%) 2778
Koāte-DVI 3250
Kogenate FS 738
Kytril Injection (Rare) 2781
Lamictal (Infrequent) 1481
Lamisil Tablets (Rare) 2232
Lantus Injection 2909
Lescol Capsules (2.3%) 2233
Lescol XL Tablets (1%) 2233
Leukeran Tablets 1504
▲ Leukine (12%) 814
Levaquin (0.1% to 0.9%) 2384
Levaquin in 5% Dextrose Injection (0.1% to 0.9%) 2384
Levemir Injection 2320
Lexapro Oral Solution (Frequent) 1190
Lexapro Tablets (Frequent) 1190
Lipitor Tablets (Up to 2.8%) 2483
Lofibra Tablets 1219
Lofibra Capsules 1216
Lotronex Tablets (Rare) 1512
Lovenox Injection 2915
Lunesta Tablets (Infrequent) 3142
Lyrica Capsules (Greater than or equal to 1%) 2539
Matulane Capsules 3191
Mefoxin for Injection 2012
Mefoxin Premixed Intravenous Solution 2016
Mepron Suspension (0.8% to 1.1%) 1521
Meridia Capsules (1.5%) 489
Merrem I.V. 686
Metamucil 2675
Miacalcin Injection (A few cases) 2252
Miacalcin Nasal Spray (Less than 1%) 2253
Micardis Tablets (More than 0.3%) 854
Micardis HCT Tablets 856
Mirapex Tablets (1% or more) 859
Mivacron Injection 493
Mobic Oral Suspension (Less than 2%) 863
Mobic Tablets (Less than 2%) 863
Motrin IB Tablets and Caplets 1866
Children's Motrin Oral Suspension ▣685
Children's Motrin Non-Staining Dye-Free Oral Suspension ▣685
Children's Motrin Oral Suspension 1867
Children's Motrin Non-Staining Dye-Free Oral Suspension 1867
Children's Motrin Cold Oral Suspension 1867
Infants' Motrin Concentrated Drops 1867
Infants' Motrin Non-Staining Dye-Free Concentrated Drops 1867
Junior Strength Motrin Caplets and Chewable Tablets 1867
Mumpsvax (Extremely rare) 2031
Myobloc Injection (2% or greater) 3192
Namenda (Infrequent) 1195
Natacyn Antifungal Ophthalmic Suspension (One case) ⊙208
Neoral Oral Solution (1% to less than 3%) 2259
Neoral Soft Gelatin Capsules (1% to less than 3%) 2259
Neulasta Injection 601
Neumega for Injection 3435
Neupogen for Injection (Less than 1 in 4000) 603
Neurontin Capsules (Infrequent) 2487
Neurontin Oral Solution 2487
Neurontin Tablets (Infrequent) 2487
Nexium Delayed-Release Capsules (Less than 1%) 655
Nexium I.V. (Less than 1%) 659
▲ Nipent for Injection (2% to 11%) 1863
Nitro-Dur Transdermal Infusion System (Uncommon) 3046
Noroxin Tablets (Less frequent) 2032
Norvasc Tablets (More than 0.1% to 1%) 2545
Norvir (Less than 2%) 503
NovoLog Injection 2326
NovoLog Mix 70/30 2328
NovoSeven (1%) 2331
Numorphan Injection 1120
Nutropin for Injection 1239
Nutropin AQ Injection 1243
Nutropin AQ Pen 1243
Nutropin AQ Pen Cartridge 1243
Omnicef Capsules 511
Omnicef for Oral Suspension 511
▲ Oncaspar (Greater than 5%) 1145
Opana Tablets (Less than 1%) 1122
Opana ER Tablets (Less than 1%) 1126
OptiPranolol Metipranolol Ophthalmic Solution 0.3% (A small number of patients) ⊙256
Paxil CR Controlled-Release Tablets (Infrequent) 1538
Paxil (Infrequent) 1530
PCE Dispertab Tablets 515
Pentasa Capsules 3185
Pexeva Tablets (Infrequent) 1694
PhosLo GelCaps 2169
Plasbumin-5 (Rare) 3251
Plasbumin-20 (Rare) 3252
Plasbumin-25 (Rare) 3253
Plavix Tablets (Less than 1%) 917
Plavix Tablets (Less than 1%) 2926
Pred Mild Ophthalmic Suspension ⊙238
Pred Forte Ophthalmic Suspension ⊙235
Prevacid Delayed-Release Capsules (Less than 1%) 3271
Prevacid for Delayed-Release Oral Suspension (Less than 1%) 3271
Prevacid SoluTab Delayed-Release Orally Disintegrating Tablets (Less than 1%) 3271
Prevacid NapraPAC (Less than 1%) 3280
PREVPAC 3284
Prilosec OTC Delayed-Release Tablets 2677
Primaxin I.M. 2045
Prochieve 4% Gel 1003
Prochieve 8% Gel 1003
Procrit for Injection (Rare) 2364
▲ Prograf Capsules and Injection (3% to 15%) 632
Prolastin (Occasional) 3255
Proleukin for Injection (1%) 2266
Propine Ophthalmic Solution ⊙239
Proquin XR Tablets 1153
ProSom Tablets (Infrequent) 517
Protonix I.V. (Less than 1%) 3472
Protonix Tablets (Less than 1%) 3469
▲ Protopic Ointment (6% to 22%) 638
▲ Proventil HFA Inhalation Aerosol (6%) 3056
Provigil Tablets (At least 1%) 988
Psoriatec Cream (Very few instances) 1089
▲ Pulmicort Respules (1% to 3%) 661
Quixin Ophthalmic Solution (Less than 1%) 3383
Recombinate (Extremely rare) 729
ReFacto Vials 3484
▲ Refludan for Injection (3.5%) 792
Relpax Tablets (Rare) 2548
Remicade for IV Injection (Greater than or equal to 0.2%) 971
ReoPro Vials 1809
Rescriptor Tablets 2551
Retavase (3 patients) 2499
Reyataz Capsules (Less than 3%) 921
R-Gene 10 for Intravenous Use (One patient) 2641
Rhophylac (Rare) 3505
Risperdal (Rare) 1676
Risperdal M-Tab Orally Disintegrating Tablets (Rare) 1676
Rocaltrol Capsules (One case) 2798
Rocaltrol Oral Solution (One case) 2798
Sandimmune (2% or less) 2275
Sandostatin Injection (Less than 1%) 2278
▲ Sandostatin LAR Depot (5% to 15%) 2280
Seromycin Capsules 1813
Soltamox Oral Solution (2.5%) 3527
Sonata Capsules 1717
▲ Spiriva HandiHaler (1% to 3%) 869
Suprax 1843
Sustiva Capsules 930
Sustiva Tablets 930
▲ Symlin Injection (Less than 1% to 6%) 613
Symmetrel Tablets 1135
Synera Topical Patch (Less than or equal to 1%) 1137
Tasmar Tablets (Infrequent) 3358
▲ Taxotere Injection Concentrate (1.8% to 10.4%) 2932
▲ Temodar Capsules (3%) 3073
▲ Tequin Injection (0.1% to 3%) 938
▲ Tequin Injection in 5% Dextrose (0.1% to 3%) 938
▲ Tequin Tablets (0.1% to 3%) 938
Thalomid Capsules 965
Thiothixene Capsules 2165
Tiazac Capsules (1%) 1201
Ticlid Tablets 2810
Timoptic Sterile Ophthalmic Solution 2088
Timoptic in Ocudose 2091
Timoptic-XE Sterile Ophthalmic Gel Forming Solution 2092
TNKase I.V. (Rare) 1264
▲ Topamax Sprinkle Capsules (Less than 1% to 3%) 2404
▲ Topamax Tablets (Less than 1% to 3%) 2404
Trasylol Injection (0.3%) 754
Traumeel Injection Solution (Rare) 1664
Tricor Tablets 527
Trileptal Tablets (Up to 2%) 2300

(▣ Described in PDR For Nonprescription Drugs) Incidence data in parenthesis; ▲ 3% or more (⊙ Described in PDR For Ophthalmic Medicines™)

Trileptal Oral Suspension (Up to 2%) 2300
Trusopt Sterile Ophthalmic Solution 2095
▲ Truvada Tablets (Greater than 5%) 1296
Twinrix Vaccine 1595
Tygacil for Injection (0.2% to less than 2%) 3488
Tylenol with Codeine Tablets 2391
Ultane Liquid for Inhalation (Less than 1%) 531
Ultrase Capsules (Less frequent) 708
Ultrase MT Capsules (Less frequent) 709
Uniretic Tablets (Less than 1%) 3100
▲ Vagifem Tablets (3% to 5%) 2334
Vandazole Vaginal Gel (Less than 1%) 3338
Vantin Tablets and Oral Suspension 2645
Varivax (Greater than or equal to 1%) 2100
VFEND I.V. (Less than 2%) 2564
VFEND Oral Suspension (Less than 2%) 2564
VFEND Tablets (Less than 2%) 2564
Viagra Tablets (Less than 2%) 2573
Vicodin Tablets 535
Vicodin ES Tablets 536
Vicodin HP Tablets 538
Vicoprofen Tablets (Less than 1%) 539
Viracept (Less than 2%) 2577
Viramune Oral Suspension 873
Viramune Tablets 873
▲ Vivaglobin (11%) 3506
Vivitrol 995
Wellbutrin Tablets 1603
Wellbutrin SR Sustained-Release Tablets 1607
Wellbutrin XL Extended-Release Tablets 1613
Yasmin 28 Tablets 796
Yaz Tablets (Greater than 1%) 803
Zeel Solution 1665
Zegerid Capsules 2958
Zegerid Powder for Oral Solution 2958
Zelapar Tablets 3372
Zelnorm Tablets 2312
Zemplar Capsules (Rare) 541
Zemplar Injection (Rare) 543
Zemuron Injection (Rare) 2346
Zinacef for Injection 1631
Zinacef Injection 1631
Zoloft (Rare) 2586
Zomig Tablets (Infrequent) 3519
Zomig Nasal Spray (Infrequent) 3523
Zomig-ZMT Tablets (Infrequent) 3519
Zonegran Capsules (Infrequent) 1101
Zosyn 3492
Zyban Sustained-Release Tablets (1%) 1644

Allergic sensitization

▲ Alferon N Injection (1% to 18%) 1665
Animi-3 Capsules 2492
▲ Blephamide Ophthalmic Ointment (Among most often) 568
▲ Blephamide Ophthalmic Suspension (Most often) 569
▲ Catapres-TTS (5 of 101 patients) 844
Citracal Prenatal Rx Tablets 2139
▲ FML-S Ophthalmic Suspension (Among most often) ⊙ 229
Metamucil Capsules 2675
▲ Poly-Pred Ophthalmic Suspension (Most often) ⊙ 233
Pred-G Ophthalmic Ointment ⊙ 237
▲ Pred-G Ophthalmic Suspension (Most often) ⊙ 236
Prenate Elite Tablets 3121

Allergy

(*see under* Allergic reactions)

Alopecia

Abilify Oral Solution (Infrequent) 882
Abilify Oral Solution (Infrequent) 2450
Abilify Discmelt Orally Disintegrating Tablets (Infrequent) 882
Abilify Discmelt Orally Disintegrating Tablets (Infrequent) 2450
Abilify Tablets (Infrequent) 882
Abilify Tablets (Infrequent) 2450
Accutane Capsules 2731
Aciphex Tablets 1090
Actiq (Less than 1%) 979
Adalat CC Tablets (Rare) 2964
Advicor Tablets 1722
Aggrenox Capsules 822
▲ Agrylin Capsules (1% to 5%) 3169
Albenza Tablets (Less than 1.0% to 1.6%) 1338
Aldara Cream, 5% (1.4%) 1846
Aldoril Tablets 1910
▲ Alimta for Injection (11%) 1750
Alkeran for Injection 955
Alkeran Tablets 956
Aloprim for Injection (Less than 1%) 2167
Altoprev Extended-Release Tablets 3109
AmBisome for Injection (Less common) 620
Amerge Tablets (Rare) 1339
Anaprox Tablets (Less than 1%) 2761
Anaprox DS Tablets (Less than 1%) 2761
AndroGel (1%) 3329
Aricept Tablets (Infrequent) 1094
Aricept ODT Tablets (Infrequent) 1094
▲ Aromasin Tablets (2% to 15%) 2600
Arthrotec Tablets (Rare) 3129
Asacol Delayed-Release Tablets 2692
Atacand HCT 651
▲ Avastin IV (6% to 32%) 1227
Azilect Tablets (Greater than 1%) 3293
Azopt Ophthalmic Suspension (Less than 1%) 557
Benicar Tablets 1043
Benicar HCT Tablets (Rare) 1044
Betagan Ophthalmic Solution, USP ⊙ 220
▲ Betaseron for SC Injection (4%) 767
▲ Betimol Ophthalmic Solution (More than 5%) 3382
▲ Betimol Ophthalmic Solution (More than 5%) ⊙ 295
Betoptic S Ophthalmic Suspension (Rare) 558
BiDil Tablets (1% to less than 2%) 2171
Blocadren Tablets (Less than 1%) 1916
Caduet Tablets (Less than 2%) 2508
Campral Tablets (Infrequent) 1174
▲ Camptosar Injection (60%) 2604
Canasa Rectal Suppositories 699
Captopril Tablets (About 0.5% to 2%) 2149
Carbatrol Capsules 3171
Cardizem LA Extended Release Tablets (Infrequent) 1728
Cardura XL Tablets 2515
Catapres Tablets 843
Catapres-TTS 844
Celebrex Capsules (0.1% to 1.9%) 3134
Celexa (Infrequent) 1176
▲ CellCept Capsules (3% to less than 20%) 2747
▲ CellCept Intravenous (3% to less than 20%) 2747
▲ CellCept Oral Suspension (3% to less than 20%) 2747
▲ CellCept Tablets (3% to less than 20%) 2747
Climara Transdermal System 771
Climara Pro Transdermal System 776
Clinoril Tablets (Less than 1%) 1924
Clobex Shampoo 1206
Clorpres Tablets (About 2 in 1,000) 2153
Colazal Capsules 2838
Combivent Inhalation Aerosol 847
Combivir Tablets 1411
Comvax 1928
Concerta Extended-Release Tablets 1881
Copaxone for Injection (At least 2%) 3297
▲ Copegus Tablets (28%) 2754
Coreg Tablets (Less than or equal to 0.1%) 1414
Cosmegen for Injection 2459
Cosopt Sterile Ophthalmic Solution 1931
Coumadin for Injection (Infrequent) 898
Coumadin Tablets (Infrequent) 898
Covera-HS Tablets (Less than 2%) 3139
Cozaar Tablets (Less than 1%) 1935
Crixivan Capsules 1940
Cuprimine Capsules (Rare) 1947
Cymbalta Delayed-Release Capsules (Infrequent) 1757
▲ Dacogen Injection (8%) 2129
Daytrana Transdermal Patch 3174
▲ Depacon Injection (6% to 24%) 412
▲ Depakene (6% to 24%) 417
▲ Depakote Sprinkle Capsules (6% to 24%) 422
▲ Depakote Tablets (1% to 24%) 427
▲ Depakote ER Tablets (6% to 24%) 434
▲ Depo-Provera Contraceptive Injection (1% to 5%) 2622
Didronel Tablets 2697
Diovan Tablets 2193
Diovan HCT Tablets 2196
Diuril Oral Suspension 1954
Diuril Sodium Intravenous 2467
▲ Doxil Injection (8.9% to 19.2%) 2351
EC-Naprosyn Delayed-Release Tablets (Less than 1%) 2761
Effexor Tablets (Infrequent) 3411
Effexor XR Capsules (Infrequent) 3417
Efudex 3363
Eldepryl Capsules 3208
Eligard 7.5 mg (Less than 2%) 2880
Eligard 30 mg (2.2%) 2885
▲ Elmiron Capsules (4%) 2415
▲ Eloxatin for Injection (3% to 30%) 2892
Emcyt Capsules (1%) 2634
▲ Emend Capsules (24%) 1963
▲ Enbrel for Injection (1% to 6%) 584
Engerix-B Vaccine 1425
Enjuvia Tablets 1062
▲ Entocort EC Capsules (Less than 5%) 2698
Epivir 1427
Epivir-HBV 1432
Epzicom Tablets 1436
▲ Equetro Extended-Release Capsules (Less than 5%) 3180
▲ Erbitux (4% to 21%) 910
Estrasorb Topical Emulsion 1147
Estratest Tablets 3199
Estratest H.S. Tablets 3199
Evoxac Capsules (Less than 1%) 1047
Exelon Capsules (Infrequent) 2206
Exelon Oral Solution (Infrequent) 2206
▲ Femara Tablets (5%) 2214
Focalin Tablets 2220
Focalin XR Capsules 2223
Follistim AQ Cartridge 2338
Fortical Nasal Spray (Less than 1%) 3337
Gabitril Tablets (Frequent) 984
Garamycin Injectable 3014
▲ Gemzar for Injection (15% to 49%) 1771
▲ Gengraf Capsules (4%) 459
Genotropin Lyophilized Powder 2638
Geodon Capsules (Infrequent) 2529
Gleevec Tablets (Less common) 2227
▲ Hycamtin for Injection (31% to 62%) 1458
Hyzaar 50-12.5 Tablets 1990
Hyzaar 100-12.5 Tablets 1990
Hyzaar 100-25 Tablets 1990
Inderal LA Long-Acting Capsules (Rare) 3429
Indocin Capsules (Less than 1%) 1995
Indocin I.V. (Less than 1%) 2465
Indocin (Less than 1%) 1995
▲ Infergen (10% to 14%) 3364
InnoPran XL Capsules (Rare) 2723
▲ Intron A for Injection (Up to 38%) 3024
Invirase (Less than 2%) 2772
▲ I.V. Busulfex (2% to 15%) 2493
Kaletra (Less than 2%) 476
Keppra Injection 3320
Keppra Oral Solution (1% to 2%) 3314
Keppra Tablets (1% to 2%) 3314
Klonopin (Infrequent) 2778
▲ Kytril (3%) 2784
Lamictal (1.3%) 1481
Lamisil Tablets 2232
Lariam Tablets (Less than 1%) 2786
Lescol Capsules 2233
Lescol XL Tablets 2233
▲ Leukine (37% to 73%) 814
Levaquin (0.1% to 0.9%) 2384
Levaquin in 5% Dextrose Injection (0.1% to 0.9%) 2384
Levothroid Tablets 1186
Levoxyl Tablets 1712
Lexapro Oral Solution (Infrequent) 1190
Lexapro Tablets (Infrequent) 1190
Lipitor Tablets (Less than 2%) 2483
Lithobid Tablets 1692
Lithostat Tablets 2140
Lofibra Tablets (Less than 1%) 1219
Lofibra Capsules (Less than 1%) 1216
Lopressor Injection (Rare) 2238
Lopressor Tablets (Rare) 2238
Lopressor HCT 50/25 Tablets 2241
Lopressor HCT 100/25 Tablets 2241
Lopressor HCT 100/50 Tablets 2241
Lotensin Tablets (Less than 1%) 2243
Lotensin HCT Tablets (0.3% or more) 2246
Lotrel Capsules (Infrequent) 2249
Lotronex Tablets (Rare) 1512
Lunesta Tablets (Infrequent) 3142
▲ Lupron Depot 3.75 mg (Among most frequent) 3260
▲ Lupron Depot–3 Month 11.25 mg (Less than 5%) 3265
Lupron Depot-PED 7.5 mg, 11.25 mg and 15 mg (Less than 2%) 3269
Lupron Injection Pediatric (Less than 2%) 3259
Luxíq Foam (One patient) 1010
Lyrica Capsules (0.1% to 1%) 2539
Matulane Capsules 3191
Maxair Autohaler 1852
▲ Megace ES Oral Suspension (1% to 3%) 2481
Menostar Transdermal System 782
Meridia Capsules 489
Metadate CD Capsules 3323
Mevacor Tablets (0.5% to 1.0%) 2021
Miacalcin Nasal Spray (Less than 1%) 2253
Midamor Tablets (Less than or equal to 1%) 2026
Miradon Tablets 3042
Mobic Oral Suspension (Less than 2%) 863
Mobic Tablets (Less than 2%) 863
Moduretic Tablets 2028
Mustargen for Injection (Infrequent) 2468
Myleran Tablets (Rare) 1525
Nadolol Tablets (Infrequent) 2159
Nalfon Capsules (Less than 1%) 2502
Namenda (Infrequent) 1195
Naprosyn Suspension (Less than 1%) 2761
Naprosyn Tablets (Less than 1%) 2761
▲ Neoral Oral Solution (4%) 2259
▲ Neoral Soft Gelatin Capsules (4%) 2259
▲ Neulasta Injection (15% to 72%) 601
▲ Neumega for Injection (Greater than or equal to 10%) 3435
▲ Neupogen for Injection (18%) 603
Neurontin Capsules (Infrequent) 2487
Neurontin Oral Solution (Infrequent) 2487
Neurontin Tablets (Infrequent) 2487
▲ Nexavar Tablets (0% to 27%) 746
Nexium I.V. (Rare) 659
Nipent for Injection (Less than 3%) 1863
Norvasc Tablets (Less than 0.1%) 2545
Omacor Capsules 2725
Oncaspar 1145
Ortho-Cyclen Tablets 2429
Ortho Evra Transdermal System 2417
Ortho Tri-Cyclen Tablets 2429
Ortho Tri-Cyclen Lo Tablets 2436
Parcopa Orally Disintegrating Tablets 3097
Parnate Tablets 1527
Paxil CR Controlled-Release Tablets (Infrequent) 1538
Paxil (Infrequent) 1530
Pediarix Vaccine 1548
▲ Pegasys (23%) 2789
▲ PEG-Intron Powder for Injection (22%) 3048
Pentasa Capsules (Less than 1%) 3185
Pepcid Injection (Infrequent) 2040
Pepcid (Infrequent) 2038
Permax Tablets (Infrequent) 3356
Persantine Tablets (Rare) 868
Pexeva Tablets (infrequent) 1694
Premarin Intravenous 3442
Premarin Tablets 3446
Premarin Vaginal Cream 3452
Premphase Tablets 3456
Prempro Tablets 3456
Prevacid Delayed-Release Capsules (Less than 1%) 3271
Prevacid for Delayed-Release Oral Suspension (Less than 1%) 3271
Prevacid SoluTab Delayed-Release Orally Disintegrating Tablets (Less than 1%) 3271
Prevacid NapraPAC (Less than 1%) 3280
PREVPAC (Less than 1%) 3284
Prezista Tablets (Less than 2%) 3306
Prilosec OTC Delayed-Release Tablets (Less than 1%) 2677
Prinivil Tablets (0.3% to 1.0%) 2052
Prinzide Tablets 2056
▲ Prograf Capsules and Injection (3% to 15%) 632
Proleukin for Injection (1%) 2266
Protonix I.V. (Less than 1%) 3472
Protonix Tablets (Less than 1%) 3469
Protopic Ointment (1%) 638
Prozac Pulvules and Liquid (Infrequent) 1801
▲ Rebetol (23% to 36%) 3058
▲ Rebetron Combination Therapy (27% to 32%) 3063
Relpax Tablets (Rare) 2548
Requip Tablets (Infrequent) 1555
Rescriptor Tablets 2551
Reyataz Capsules (Less than 3%) 921
▲ Ribavirin, USP Capsules (23% to 36%) 3068
Rilutek Tablets (Up to 1.2%) 2930
Risperdal (Infrequent) 1676
Risperdal Consta Long-Acting Injection (Infrequent) 1682

Risperdal M-Tab Orally Disintegrating Tablets (Infrequent) 1676
Ritalin Hydrochloride Tablets (A few instances) 2269
Ritalin LA Capsules 2271
Ritalin-SR Tablets (A few instances) 2269
Rythmol SR Capsules 2727
▲ Sandostatin Injection (1% to 4%) 2278
▲ Sandostatin LAR Depot (1% to 4%) 2280
▲ Soltamox Oral Solution (Infrequent to 5.2%) 3527
Sonata Capsules (Infrequent) 1717
▲ Soriatane Capsules (50% to 75%) 1013
Stalevo Tablets 2287
Sular Tablets (Less than or equal to 1%) 3122
Sustiva Capsules (Less than 2%) 930
Sustiva Tablets (Less than 2%) 930
▲ Sutent Capsules (0% to 12%) 2560
Symbyax Capsules (Infrequent) 1819
Synthroid Tablets 520
Tambocor Tablets (Less than 1%) 1856
▲ Tarceva Tablets (0% to 14%) 1259
▲ Tarceva Tablets (0% to 14%) 2444
▲ Targretin Capsules (3.6% to 11.3%) 1747
Tarka Tablets 524
Tasmar Tablets (1%) 3358
▲ Taxotere Injection Concentrate (Less than 1% to 75.8%) 2932
Tegretol/Tegretol-XR 2295
▲ Temodar Capsules (55%) 3073
Temovate Scalp Application (1 of 294 patients) 2670
Teveten HCT Tablets 1737
Thalomid Capsules 965
Thyrolar Tablets 1199
Tiazac Capsules (Infrequent) 1201
Timolide Tablets 2086
Timoptic Sterile Ophthalmic Solution (Less frequent) 2088
Timoptic in Ocudose (Less frequent) 2091
Timoptic-XE Sterile Ophthalmic Gel Forming Solution 2092
▲ Topamax Sprinkle Capsules (Greater than 1% to 5%) 2404
▲ Topamax Tablets (Greater than 1% to 5%) 2404
Toprol-XL Tablets (Rare) 668
Tricor Tablets 527
Trileptal Tablets 2300
Trileptal Oral Suspension 2300
Trizivir Tablets 1589
Twinrix Vaccine 1595
Uniretic Tablets (Less than 1%) 3100
Univasc Tablets (Less than 1%) 3104
Valtrex Caplets 1597
Vantin Tablets and Oral Suspension (Less than 1%) 2645
Vasotec I.V. Injection (0.5% to 1.0%) 2103
Verelan PM Extended-Release Capsules, Controlled-Onset (2% or less) 3106
▲ Vesanoid Capsules (14%) 2820
VFEND I.V. (Less than 2%) 2564
VFEND Oral Suspension (Less than 2%) 2564
VFEND Tablets (Less than 2%) 2564
Viadur Implant (2.3%) 757
Voltaren Tablets (Occasionally) 2307
Voltaren-XR Tablets (Occasionally) 2310
Vytorin 10/10 Tablets 2114
Vytorin 10/10 Tablets 3077
Vytorin 10/20 Tablets 2114
Vytorin 10/20 Tablets 3077
Vytorin 10/40 Tablets 2114
Vytorin 10/40 Tablets 3077
Vytorin 10/80 Tablets 2114
Vytorin 10/80 Tablets 3077
Wellbutrin Tablets (Infrequent) 1603
Wellbutrin SR Sustained-Release Tablets 1607
Wellbutrin XL Extended-Release Tablets 1613
Xyrem Oral Solution (Infrequent) 1688
Yasmin 28 Tablets 796
Zantac (Rare) 1624
Zantac Injection (Rare) 1619
Zantac Injection Pharmacy Bulk Package (Rare) 1622
Zantac Injection Premixed (Rare) 1619
Zantac (Rare) 1624
Zegerid Capsules (Less than 1%) 2958
Zegerid Powder for Oral Solution (Less than 1%) 2958
▲ Zinecard for Injection (94% to 100%) 2650
Zocor Tablets 2105
Zoloft (Infrequent) 2586
▲ Zometa for Intravenous Infusion (12%) 2315
Zonegran Capsules (Infrequent) 1101
Zovirax 1643
Zyprexa Tablets (Infrequent) 1830
Zyprexa ZYDIS Orally Disintegrating Tablets (Infrequent) 1830
Zyrtec Chewable Tablets (Less than 2%) 2594
Zyrtec (Less than 2%) 2594
Zyrtec-D 12 Hour Extended Release Tablets (Less than 2%) 2597

Alopecia hereditaria
Androxy Tablets 3335
Estratest Tablets 3199
Estratest H.S. Tablets 3199
Oxandrin Tablets 2962

Alpha-glutamyl transferase, elevation
Eulexin Capsules 3009

ALT elevation
(*see under* Alanine aminotransferase levels, elevation of)

Altered saliva
Ambien CR Tablets (Rare) 2855

Alveolitis
Cuprimine Capsules 1947

Alveolitis, allergic
Fansidar Tablets 2765
Paxil CR Controlled-Release Tablets 1538
Paxil 1530
Pexeva Tablets 1694
Tricor Tablets 527

Alveolitis, fibrosing
Canasa Rectal Suppositories 699

Amaurosis
Zofran Injection (One patient) 1634

Amblyopia
Abilify Oral Solution (Rare) 882
Abilify Oral Solution (Rare) 2450
Abilify Discmelt Orally Disintegrating Tablets (Rare) 882
Abilify Discmelt Orally Disintegrating Tablets (Rare) 2450
Abilify Tablets (Rare) 882
Abilify Tablets (Rare) 2450
Aciphex Tablets 1090
▲ Actonel Tablets (3.3%) 2683
Adalat CC Tablets (Less than 1%) 2964
Advicor Tablets 1722
▲ Agrylin Capsules (1% to 5%) 3169
Aloxi Injection (Less than 1%) 2127
Arthrotec Tablets (Rare) 3129
Avelox (Less then 0.1%) 2970
▲ Avinza Capsules (Less than 5%) 1741
Axid Oral Solution (1.0%) 879
▲ BiDil Tablets (3%) 2171
Buprenex Injectable (Infrequent) 2716
Caduet Tablets (Less than 2%) 2508
Campral Tablets (Infrequent) 1174
Cardizem LA Extended Release Tablets (Less than 2%) 1728
▲ Carnitor Injection (3% to 6%) 3188
▲ CellCept Capsules (3% to less than 20%) 2747
▲ CellCept Intravenous (3% to less than 20%) 2747
▲ CellCept Oral Suspension (3% to less than 20%) 2747
▲ CellCept Tablets (3% to less than 20%) 2747
Cesamet Capsules 3340
Copaxone for Injection (At least 2%) 3297
▲ Depacon Injection (4% to 12%) 412
▲ Depakene (8% to 12%) 417
▲ Depakote Sprinkle Capsules (4% to 12%) 422
▲ Depakote Tablets (1% to 12%) 427
▲ Depakote ER Tablets (4% to 12%) 434
Doxil Injection (Less than 1%) 2351
Duragesic Transdermal System (Less than 1%) 2373
Elmiron Capsules (Less than or equal to 1%) 2415
▲ Equetro Extended-Release Capsules (6%) 3180
Flomax Capsules (0.2% to 2.0%) 850
▲ Gabitril Tablets (1% to 9%) 984
Herceptin I.V. (At least one of the 958 patients) 1233
Hytrin Capsules (0.6% to 1.3%) 471
Iressa Tablets (2%) 684
Kadian Capsules (Less than 3%) 577
Keppra Injection 3320
Keppra Oral Solution (1% or 2%) 3314
Keppra Tablets (1% or 2%) 3314
Lipitor Tablets (Less than 2%) 2483
Lofibra Tablets 1219
Lofibra Capsules 1216
▲ Megace ES Oral Suspension (1% to 3%) 2481
Meridia Capsules (Greater than or equal to 1%) 489
Myobloc Injection (Greater than 2%) 3192
Natrecor for Injection (Greater than or equal to 1%) 3127
Neumega for Injection 3435
▲ Neurontin Capsules (2.7% to 4.2%) 2487
▲ Neurontin Oral Solution (2.7% to 4.2%) 2487
▲ Neurontin Tablets (2.7% to 4.2%) 2487
Niaspan Extended-Release Tablets 1730
Nipent for Injection (Less than 3%) 1863
Norvir (Less than 2%) 503
Paxil CR Controlled-Release Tablets (Rare) 1538
Paxil (Rare) 1530
Pexeva Tablets (rare) 1694
Pletal Tablets (Less than 2%) 2455
Prevacid Delayed-Release Capsules (Less than 1%) 3271
Prevacid for Delayed-Release Oral Suspension (Less than 1%) 3271
Prevacid SoluTab Delayed-Release Orally Disintegrating Tablets (Less than 1%) 3271
PREVPAC (Less than 1%) 3284
▲ Prograf Capsules and Injection (3% to 15%) 632
Protonix I.V. (Less than 1%) 3472
Protonix Tablets (Less than 1%) 3469
Provigil Tablets (1%) 988
Retrovir Capsules 1560
Retrovir IV Infusion 1564
Retrovir 1560
Rilutek Tablets (Infrequent) 2930
Seroquel Tablets (2%) 690
Sular Tablets (Less than or equal to 1%) 3122
▲ Symbyax Capsules (4% to 5%) 1819
Thalomid Capsules 965
Tiazac Capsules (Less than 2%) 1201
Tricor Tablets 527
Ultane Liquid for Inhalation (Less than 1%) 531
▲ Wellbutrin SR Sustained-Release Tablets (2% to 3%) 1607
▲ Wellbutrin XL Extended-Release Tablets (2% to 3%) 1613
Zelapar Tablets 3372
Zomig Nasal Spray (Infrequent) 3523
Zonegran Capsules (Frequent) 1101
Zyban Sustained-Release Tablets (Frequent) 1644
▲ Zyprexa Tablets (3% to 9%) 1830
▲ Zyprexa ZYDIS Orally Disintegrating Tablets (3% to 9%) 1830

Amelia
Thalomid Capsules 965

Amenorrhea
Abilify Oral Solution (Infrequent) 882
Abilify Oral Solution (Infrequent) 2450
Abilify Discmelt Orally Disintegrating Tablets (Infrequent) 882
Abilify Discmelt Orally Disintegrating Tablets (Infrequent) 2450
Abilify Tablets (Infrequent) 882
Abilify Tablets (Infrequent) 2450
Aldoril Tablets 1910
Alinia for Oral Suspension (Less than 1%) 2835
Alinia Tablets (Less than 1%) 2835
Alkeran for Injection 955
Alkeran Tablets (A significant number of patients) 956
▲ Androxy Tablets (Most Common) 3335
Astelin Nasal Spray (Infrequent) 1904
Celexa (Frequent) 1176
▲ Depacon Injection (1% to 5%) 412
▲ Depakene (1% to 5%) 417
▲ Depakote Sprinkle Capsules (1% to 5%) 422
▲ Depakote Tablets (1% to 5%) 427
▲ Depakote ER Tablets (1% to 5%) 434
▲ depo-subQ provera 104 Injectable Suspension (6%) 2624
Effexor Tablets (Infrequent) 3411
Effexor XR Capsules (Infrequent) 3417
▲ Estratest Tablets (Among most common) 3199
▲ Estratest H.S. Tablets (Among most common) 3199
Evoxac Capsules (Less than 1%) 1047
Gabitril Tablets (Infrequent) 984
Geodon Capsules (Infrequent) 2529
▲ Intron A for Injection (Less than 5%) 3024
I.V. Busulfex 2493
Kadian Capsules (Less than 3%) 577
Kaletra (0% to 2%) 476
Lamictal (1.9%) 1481
Leukeran Tablets 1504
Lunesta Tablets (Infrequent) 3142
Lyrica Capsules (0.1% to 1%) 2539
Mircette Tablets 1066
▲ Mirena Intrauterine System (20%) 787
Moban Tablets (Infrequent) 1119
Mustargen for Injection 2468
Neurontin Capsules (Infrequent) 2487
Neurontin Oral Solution (Infrequent) 2487
Neurontin Tablets (Infrequent) 2487
Nipent for Injection (Less than 3%) 1863
NuvaRing 2340
Ortho-Cyclen Tablets 2429
Ortho Evra Transdermal System 2417
Ortho Micronor Tablets 2426
Ortho Tri-Cyclen Tablets 2429
Ortho Tri-Cyclen Lo Tablets 2436
OxyContin Tablets 2703
Paxil CR Controlled-Release Tablets (Infrequent) 1538
Paxil (Infrequent) 1530
Pentasa Capsules (Less than 1%) 3185
Permax Tablets (Rare) 3356
Pexeva Tablets (infrequent) 1694
Premarin Intravenous 3442
Premarin Vaginal Cream 3452
Premphase Tablets 3456
Prempro Tablets 3456
Prometrium Capsules (100 mg, 200 mg) 3203
Prozac Pulvules and Liquid (Infrequent) 1801
Requip Tablets (Infrequent) 1555
Rescriptor Tablets 2551
Reyataz Capsules (Less than 3%) 921
Rilutek Tablets (Rare) 2930
Risperdal (Infrequent) 1676
Risperdal Consta Long-Acting Injection (Frequent) 1682
Risperdal M-Tab Orally Disintegrating Tablets (Infrequent) 1676
Sandostatin Injection (Less than 1%) 2278
Seasonique Tablets 1077
Seroquel Tablets (Infrequent) 690
▲ Soltamox Oral Solution (16%) 3527
Symbyax Capsules (Infrequent) 1819
▲ Taxotere Injection Concentrate (61.7%) 2932
Thalomid Capsules 965
Thioridazine Hydrochloride Tablets 2163
Thiothixene Capsules 2165
Topamax Sprinkle Capsules (2%) 2404
Topamax Tablets (2%) 2404
Yasmin 28 Tablets 796
Yaz Tablets 803
Zoloft (Infrequent) 2586
Zonegran Capsules (Infrequent) 1101
Zyprexa Tablets (Infrequent) 1830
Zyprexa ZYDIS Orally Disintegrating Tablets (Infrequent) 1830

Amentia
Clozaril Tablets (Less than 1%) 2184
FazaClo Orally Disintegrating Tablets (Less than 1%) 551

Amnesia
Abilify Oral Solution (Infrequent) 882
Abilify Oral Solution (Infrequent) 2450
Abilify Discmelt Orally Disintegrating Tablets (Infrequent) 882
Abilify Discmelt Orally Disintegrating Tablets (Infrequent) 2450
Abilify Tablets (Infrequent) 882
Abilify Tablets (Infrequent) 2450
Aceon Tablets (2 mg, 4 mg, 8 mg) (0.3% to 1%) 3194
Aciphex Tablets (Rare) 1090
Actiq (Less than 1%) 979
Aggrenox Capsules (2.4%) 822
▲ Agrylin Capsules (1% to 5%) 3169
Altace Capsules (Less than 1%) 1702

Ambien Tablets (1%) 2851
Ambien CR Tablets (Infrequent) 2855
AndroGel (Fewer than 1%) 3329
▲ Arranon Injection (0% to 3%) 1357
Avelox (Less than 0.1%) 2970
▲ Avinza Capsules (Less than 5%) 1741
Caduet Tablets (Less than 2%) 2508
Campral Tablets (Frequent) 1174
Cardizem LA Extended Release Tablets (Less than 2%) 1728
Celexa (Frequent) 1176
Chantix Tablets (Infrequent) 2517
Clozaril Tablets (Less than 1%) 2184
Copaxone for Injection (At least 2%) 3297
Coreg Tablets (Less than or equal to 0.1%) 1414
▲ Depacon Injection (4% to 7%) 412
▲ Depakene (5% to 7%) 417
▲ Depakote Sprinkle Capsules (4% to 7%) 422
▲ Depakote Tablets (1% to 7%) 427
▲ Depakote ER Tablets (4% to 7%) 434
Didronel Tablets 2697
Duragesic Transdermal System (1% or greater) 2373
Effexor Tablets 3411
Effexor XR Capsules (Frequent) 3417
▲ Equetro Extended-Release Capsules (8%) 3180
Evoxac Capsules 1047
Exelon Capsules (Infrequent) 2206
Exelon Oral Solution (Infrequent) 2206
FazaClo Orally Disintegrating Tablets (Less than 1%) 551
Frova Tablets (Infrequent) 1113
Geodon Capsules (Frequent) 2529
▲ Infergen (2% to 10%) 3364
▲ Intron A for Injection (Up to 14%) 3024
Invirase (Less than 2%) 2772
Kadian Capsules (Less than 3%) 577
Kaletra (Less than 2%) 476
Keppra Injection (2%) 3320
Keppra Oral Solution (2%) 3314
Keppra Tablets (2%) 3314
Klonopin 2778
Lamictal (Frequent) 1481
Lexapro Oral Solution (Infrequent) 1190
Lexapro Tablets (Infrequent) 1190
Lipitor Tablets (Less than 2%) 2483
▲ Lyrica Capsules (1% to 6%) 2539
Marinol Capsules (Greater than 1%) 3333
Meridia Capsules 489
▲ Mirapex Tablets (4% to 6%) 859
Namenda (Infrequent) 1195
Neurontin Capsules (1.2% to 2.2%) 2487
Neurontin Oral Solution (1.2% to 2.2%) 2487
Neurontin Tablets (1.2% to 2.2%) 2487
Niravam Orally Disintegrating Tablets 3092
Norvasc Tablets (Less than 0.1%) 2545
Norvir (Less than 2%) 503
OxyContin Tablets (Less than 1%) 2703
Paxil CR Controlled-Release Tablets (2%) 1538
Paxil (2%) 1530
Permax Tablets (Frequent) 3356
Pexeva Tablets (2%) 1694
Prevacid Delayed-Release Capsules (Less than 1%) 3271
Prevacid for Delayed-Release Oral Suspension (Less than 1%) 3271
Prevacid SoluTab Delayed-Release Orally Disintegrating Tablets (Less than 1%) 3271
Prevacid NapraPAC (Less than 1%) 3280
PREVPAC (Less than 1%) 3284
▲ Prograf Capsules and Injection (3% to 15%) 632
ProSom Tablets (Infrequent) 517
Provigil Tablets (1%) 988
Prozac Pulvules and Liquid (Frequent) 1801
Relpax Tablets (Rare) 2548
▲ Requip Tablets (3%) 1555
Rescriptor Tablets 2551
Restoril Capsules (Less than 0.5%) 1860
Reyataz Capsules (Less than 3%) 921
Rilutek Tablets (Infrequent) 2930
Risperdal (Infrequent) 1676
Risperdal Consta Long-Acting Injection (Infrequent) 1682
Risperdal M-Tab Orally Disintegrating Tablets (Infrequent) 1676
Sandostatin Injection (Less than 1%) 2278
Seroquel Tablets (Infrequent) 690
▲ Sonata Capsules (2% to 4%) 1717
Sular Tablets (Less than or equal to 1%) 3122
Sustiva Capsules (Less than 2%) 930
Sustiva Tablets (Less than 2%) 930
▲ Symbyax Capsules (1% to 3%) 1819
Symmetrel Tablets (0.1% to 1%) 1135
Tambocor Tablets (Less than 1%) 1856
Tasmar Tablets (Infrequent) 3358
▲ Temodar Capsules (10%) 3073
Thalomid Capsules 965
Tiazac Capsules (Less than 2%) 1201
▲ Trileptal Tablets (1% to 5%) 2300
▲ Trileptal Oral Suspension (1% to 5%) 2300
Uniretic Tablets (Less than 1%) 3100
VFEND I.V. (Less than 2%) 2564
VFEND Oral Suspension (Less than 2%) 2564
VFEND Tablets (Less than 2%) 2564
Viadur Implant (Less than 2%) 757
Vytorin 10/10 Tablets 2114
Vytorin 10/10 Tablets 3077
Vytorin 10/20 Tablets 2114
Vytorin 10/20 Tablets 3077
Vytorin 10/40 Tablets 2114
Vytorin 10/40 Tablets 3077
Vytorin 10/80 Tablets 2114
Vytorin 10/80 Tablets 3077
Wellbutrin SR Sustained-Release Tablets (Rare) 1607
Wellbutrin XL Extended-Release Tablets (Rare) 1613
Zoloft (Infrequent) 2586
Zomig Tablets (Rare) 3519
Zomig Nasal Spray (Infrequent) 3523
Zomig-ZMT Tablets (Rare) 3519
Zyban Sustained-Release Tablets (Rare) 1644
▲ Zyprexa Tablets (5%) 1830
▲ Zyprexa ZYDIS Orally Disintegrating Tablets (5%) 1830
Zyrtec Chewable Tablets (Less than 2%) 2594
Zyrtec (Less than 2%) 2594
Zyrtec-D 12 Hour Extended Release Tablets (Less than 2%) 2597

Amyloidosis

Thalomid Capsules 965

ANA, positive

Aceon Tablets (2 mg, 4 mg, 8 mg) 3194
Adalat CC Tablets (Rare) 2964
Advicor Tablets 1722
Aldoril Tablets 1910
Altace Capsules (Less than 1%) 1702
Altoprev Extended-Release Tablets (Rare) 3109
Captopril Tablets 2149
▲ Enbrel for Injection (11%) 584
▲ Humira Injection (12%) 466
Lescol Capsules (Rare) 2233
Lescol XL Tablets 2233
Mevacor Tablets (Rare) 2021
Prinivil Tablets (0.3% to 1.0%) 2052
Prinzide Tablets 2056
Ticlid Tablets (Rare) 2810
Vasotec I.V. Injection (0.5% to 1.0%) 2103
Vytorin 10/10 Tablets 2114
Vytorin 10/10 Tablets 3077
Vytorin 10/20 Tablets 2114
Vytorin 10/20 Tablets 3077
Vytorin 10/40 Tablets 2114
Vytorin 10/40 Tablets 3077
Vytorin 10/80 Tablets 2114
Vytorin 10/80 Tablets 3077
Zocor Tablets (Rare) 2105

Anaphylactic reactions

Abilify Oral Solution (Rare) 882
Abilify Oral Solution (Rare) 2450
Abilify Discmelt Orally Disintegrating Tablets (Rare) 882
Abilify Discmelt Orally Disintegrating Tablets (Rare) 2450
Abilify Tablets (Rare) 882
Abilify Tablets (Rare) 2450
Aceon Tablets (2 mg, 4 mg, 8 mg) (0.3% to 1%) 3194
▲ Acetadote Injection (14% to 19%) 1031
ADACEL Vaccine 2945
Adalat CC Tablets (Rare) 2964
Advair Diskus 100/50 (Very rare) 1308
Advair Diskus 250/50 (Very rare) 1308
Advair Diskus 500/50 (Very rare) 1308
Aggrastat 1907
Aldoril Tablets 1910
Amoxil Capsules 1343
Amoxil Chewable Tablets 1343
Amoxil Pediatric Drops for Oral Suspension 1343
Amoxil Powder for Oral Suspension 1343
Amoxil Tablets 1343
Antivenin (Black Widow Spider Antivenin) 1913
Anzemet Injection (Rare) 2859
Anzemet Tablets (Rare) 2862
Atacand HCT 651
Atrovent HFA Inhalation Aerosol 841
Atrovent Nasal Spray 0.06% 839
Augmentin 1360
Augmentin Tablets 1363
Augmentin ES-600 Powder for Oral Suspension 1366
Avalide Tablets 888
Avalide Tablets 2874
Avelox 2970
Beconase AQ Nasal Spray 1396
Bexxar 1398
Boostrix (Rarely) 1404
Byetta Injection 611
Camptosar Injection 2604
Celebrex Capsules (Less than 0.1%) 3134
Cipro 2977
Cipro I.V. (1% or less) 2984
Cipro XR Tablets (Rare) 2990
Climara Transdermal System 771
Climara Pro Transdermal System 776
Combivent Inhalation Aerosol (Less than 2%) 847
Cozaar Tablets 1935
Dacogen Injection 2129
depo-subQ provera 104 Injectable Suspension (Infrequent) 2624
Digibind for Injection 1421
Dilaudid Oral Liquid 445
Dilaudid Tablets - 8 mg 445
Diuril Oral Suspension 1954
Diuril Sodium Intravenous 2467
Dolobid Tablets (Less than 1 in 100) 1955
Elidel Cream 1% 2200
Eligard 22.5 mg 2883
Eligard 30 mg 2885
Elspar for Injection 2463
Elspar for Injection 1960
Enjuvia Tablets 1062
Flovent HFA (Very rare) 1447
Fluarix 1451
Foradil Aerolizer (Rare) 3010
Fortaz 1453
GamaSTAN 3234
Gammagard Liquid 721
Gammagard S/D (A remote possibility) 724
Gamunex Immune Globulin I.V., 10% 3235
HalfLytely and Bisacodyl Tablets Bowel Prep Kit with Flavors Packs (Rare) 881
HibTITER 3426
Humalog-Pen (Less common) 1781
Humalog Mix 50/50-Pen 1783
Humalog Mix 75/25-Pen 1785
Humate-P (Rare) 3502
HyperHep B S/D (Rare) 3240
Hyzaar 50-12.5 Tablets 1990
Hyzaar 100-12.5 Tablets 1990
Hyzaar 100-25 Tablets 1990
Indapamide Tablets 2156
Inderal LA Long-Acting Capsules 3429
Infanrix Vaccine 1476
Infed Injection 3390
Kogenate FS 738
Levitra Tablets (Less than 2%) 3034
Lotensin HCT Tablets 2246
Mefoxin Premixed Intravenous Solution 2016
Menostar Transdermal System 782
Meruvax II 2019
Micardis HCT Tablets 856
Mintezol 2027
Mivacron Injection 493
Moduretic Tablets 2028
Nabi-HB (Rare) 2169
Nexium Delayed-Release Capsules (Rare) 655
Nexium I.V. (Rare) 659
Nimbex Injection 498
Norflex Injection (Rare) 1856
Noroxin Tablets (Occasional) 2032
NovoSeven 2331
▲ Oncaspar (Greater than 1% but less than 5%) 1145
Orthoclone OKT3 Sterile Solution 2360
OxyContin Tablets (Less than 1%) 2703
Pediarix Vaccine (Rare) 1548
Pegasys 2789
Pred Mild Ophthalmic Suspension ⊙238
Premarin Vaginal Cream 3452
Prevnar for Injection 3463
PREVPAC 3284
Primaxin I.M. 2045
Primaxin I.V. 2048
Prinzide Tablets 2056
Prograf Capsules and Injection (A few patients) 632
Proquin XR Tablets 1153
Rapamune Oral Solution and Tablets 3475
Refludan for Injection 792
Rhophylac (Rare) 3505
Risperdal 1676
Risperdal Consta Long-Acting Injection 1682
Risperdal M-Tab Orally Disintegrating Tablets 1676
Rituxan I.V. 1254
Sanctura Tablets 1151
Sandimmune I.V. Ampuls for Infusion (Rare) 2275
Seasonique Tablets 1077
Sonata Capsules 1717
Symmetrel Tablets 1135
Tequin Injection 938
Tequin Injection in 5% Dextrose 938
Tequin Tablets 938
Teveten HCT Tablets 1737
Timentin ADD-Vantage 1580
Timentin Injection Galaxy Container 1583
Timentin IV Infusion 1577
Timentin Pharmacy Bulk Package 1586
Timolide Tablets 2086
Trasylol Injection (Less than 0.5%) 754
Traumeel Injection Solution (Rare) 1664
Voltaren Tablets (Rarely) 2307
Voltaren-XR Tablets (Rarely) 2310
Zeel Solution 1665
Zemuron Injection (Rare) 2346
Zosyn (Occasional) 3492

Anaphylactic shock

Ambien Tablets (Rare) 2851
Ambien CR Tablets (Rare) 2855
Aredia for Injection (Very rare) 2179
Avelox 2970
CytoGam Intravenous (A possibility) 1895
Eloxatin for Injection 2892
Fortical Nasal Spray (1 patient) 3337
GlucaGen (Rare) 761
HyperRAB (Rare) 3242
HyperTET (Few isolated cases) 3248
Levaquin 2384
Levaquin in 5% Dextrose Injection 2384
Maxipime for Injection 1105
Meridia Capsules 489
Miacalcin Injection (A few cases) 2252
Orthoclone OKT3 Sterile Solution 2360
Protonix I.V. 3472
Protonix Tablets 3469
Sandostatin Injection 2278
Sandostatin LAR Depot (Rare) 2280
Taxotere Injection Concentrate (Rare) 2932
Trasylol Injection 754
Vantin Tablets and Oral Suspension (Less than 1%) 2645
Wellbutrin Tablets (Rare) 1603
Wellbutrin SR Sustained-Release Tablets (Rare) 1607
Wellbutrin XL Extended-Release Tablets (Rare) 1613
Zosyn (1% or less) 3492
Zyban Sustained-Release Tablets (Rare) 1644

Anaphylactoid reactions

Abelcet Injection 1141
Activase I.V. (Very rare) 1223
Altace Capsules (Less than 1%) 1702
Amerge Tablets 1339
Amoxil Capsules (Occasional) 1343
Amoxil Chewable Tablets (Occasional) 1343
Amoxil Pediatric Drops for Oral Suspension (Occasional) 1343
Amoxil Powder for Oral Suspension (Occasional) 1343
Amoxil Tablets (Occasional) 1343
Anaprox Tablets (Less than 1%) 2761
Anaprox DS Tablets (Less than 1%) 2761
Androxy Tablets (Rare) 3335
Angeliq Tablets 762
Arthrotec Tablets 3129
Astelin Nasal Spray 1904
Attenuvax 1914
Beconase AQ Nasal Spray 1396
Campath Ampules 811
Camptosar Injection 2604
Captopril Tablets 2149
Carimune NF 3499
Cerezyme for Injection 1270

Cleocin Vaginal Ovules (A few cases) 2616
Climara Transdermal System 771
Climara Pro Transdermal System 776
Copaxone for Injection (Rare) 3297
Crixivan Capsules 1940
Decadron Tablets 1951
Depo-Provera Contraceptive Injection 2622
Detrol Tablets 2628
Detrol LA Capsules 2631
Digibind for Injection 1421
Dolobid Tablets 1955
Doxil Injection (Less than 1%) 2351
EC-Naprosyn Delayed-Release Tablets (Less than 1%) 2761
Engerix-B Vaccine 1425
Enjuvia Tablets 1062
Epogen for Injection 591
Estrasorb Topical Emulsion 1147
Estratest Tablets (Rare) 3199
Estratest H.S. Tablets (Rare) 3199
Ethyol for Injection (Rare) 1898
Fansidar Tablets 2765
Feiba VH 718
Flonase Nasal Spray 1440
Fluarix 1451
Fortaz 1453
Fragmin Injection (Few cases) 1097
Garamycin Injectable 3014
Gemzar for Injection (Rare) 1771
Havrix Vaccine (Rare) 1456
Herceptin I.V. (At least one of the 958 patients) 1233
HibTITER 3426
Hyalgan Solution 2901
Hycamtin for Injection (Rare) 1458
Imitrex Injection (Rare) 1463
Imitrex Nasal Spray 1467
Imitrex Tablets (Rare) 1471
Inderal LA Long-Acting Capsules 3429
Invanz for Injection (Very rare) 1999
Kytril Injection (Rare) 2781
Levaquin 2384
Levaquin in 5% Dextrose Injection 2384
Lotrel Capsules 2249
Lovenox Injection 2915
Lupron Depot 3.75 mg (Rare) 3260
Lupron Depot–3 Month 11.25 mg 3265
Lupron Depot-PED 7.5 mg, 11.25 mg and 15 mg (Rare) 3269
Lyrica Capsules (Rare) 2539
Mavik Tablets 486
Menostar Transdermal System 782
Mephyton Tablets 2018
Meridia Capsules 489
Meruvax II 2019
Mivacron Injection 493
M-M-R II 2006
Mobic Oral Suspension (Less than 0.1%) 863
Mobic Tablets (Less than 0.1%) 863
Mumpsvax 2031
Naprosyn Suspension (Less than 1%) 2761
Naprosyn Tablets (Less than 1%) 2761
Nimbex Injection 498
Nitro-Dur Transdermal Infusion System (A few reports) 3046
Noroxin Tablets (Occasional) 2032
Orencia Powder for Intravenous Infusion (2 cases) 914
Orthoclone OKT3 Sterile Solution 2360
OxyContin Tablets (Less than 1%) 2703
Plavix Tablets (Very rare) 917
Plavix Tablets (Very rare) 2926
Pneumovax 23 (Rare) 2043
Premarin Vaginal Cream 3452
Premphase Tablets 3456
Prempro Tablets 3456
Prevacid Delayed-Release Capsules 3271
Prevacid for Delayed-Release Oral Suspension 3271
Prevacid SoluTab Delayed-Release Orally Disintegrating Tablets 3271
Prevacid NapraPAC (Less than 1%) 3280
Prevnar for Injection 3463
PREVPAC 3284
Prinivil Tablets (0.3% to 1.0%) 2052
Prinzide Tablets 2056
Procrit for Injection 2364
Prometrium Capsules (100 mg, 200 mg) 3203
ProQuad 2064
Protopic Ointment (Greater than or equal to 1%) 638
Rapamune Oral Solution and Tablets 3475
Retavase (2 patients) 2499
Rituxan I.V. 1254
Sandostatin Injection 2278
Sandostatin LAR Depot (Rare) 2280
Seasonique Tablets 1077
Skelaxin Tablets (Rare) 1716
Suprax 1843
Trasylol Injection 754
TriLyte with Flavor Packs for Oral Solution (Rare) 3100
Twinrix Vaccine 1595
Ultane Liquid for Inhalation (Less than 1%) 531
Uniretic Tablets (More than 1%) 3100
Vasotec I.V. Injection (0.5% to 1.0%) 2103
VFEND I.V. (Less than 2%) 2564
VFEND Oral Suspension (Less than 2%) 2564
VFEND Tablets (Less than 2%) 2564
Vivaglobin 3506
Wellbutrin Tablets 1603
Wellbutrin SR Sustained-Release Tablets 1607
Wellbutrin XL Extended-Release Tablets 1613
Zemuron Injection (Rare) 2346
Zofran Injection 1634
Zofran 1639
Zofran ODT Orally Disintegrating Tablets 1639
Zoloft 2586
Zomig Tablets (Very rare) 3519
Zomig Nasal Spray (Very rare) 3523
Zomig-ZMT Tablets (Very rare) 3519
Zosyn 3492
Zyban Sustained-Release Tablets 1644
Zyprexa Tablets 1830
Zyprexa ZYDIS Orally Disintegrating Tablets 1830

Anaphylaxis

Abelcet Injection (Less than 0.1%) 1141
Aciphex Tablets 1090
Adderall Tablets (Rare) 3164
Adderall XR Capsules 3166
Advicor Tablets (Rare) 1722
Aggrastat 1907
Aldurazyme for Intravenous Infusion 1268
Alferon N Injection 1665
Alkeran for Injection (2.4%) 955
Alkeran Tablets (Rare) 956
Allegra (Rare) 2844
Allegra-D 12 Hour Extended-Release Tablets (Rare) 2846
Allegra-D 24 Hour Extended-Release Tablets (Rare) 2849
Altoprev Extended-Release Tablets (Rare) 3109
Amerge Tablets 1339
Aminohippurate Sodium PAH Injection 1913
Amoxil Capsules 1343
Amoxil Chewable Tablets 1343
Amoxil Pediatric Drops for Oral Suspension 1343
Amoxil Powder for Oral Suspension 1343
Amoxil Tablets 1343
Antivenin (Black Widow Spider Antivenin) 1913
Antivenin (Micrurus fulvius) 3407
Antivenin Polyvalent 3405
Arimidex Tablets (Very rare) 673
Atrovent Inhalation Solution (A single case) 835
Atrovent HFA Inhalation Aerosol 841
Attenuvax 1914
Axid Oral Solution (Rare) 879
Azmacort Inhalation Aerosol 1726
Bayer Aspirin 744
BeneFix Vials 3408
Bentyl Capsules 697
Bentyl Injection 697
Bentyl Syrup 697
Bentyl Tablets 697
Betaseron for SC Injection 767
Bexxar 1398
Biaxin/Biaxin XL (Rare) 402
Bicillin C-R Injectable Suspension 1706
Blocadren Tablets 1916
Caduet Tablets 2508
Cancidas for Injection (0%) 1918
Ceftin 1407
Celexa 1176
Clarinex Syrup (Rare) 2995
Clarinex Tablets (Rare) 2995
Clarinex Reditabs Tablets (Rare) 2995
Clarinex-D 24-Hour Extended-Release Tablets 2998
Clinoril Tablets 1924
Colyte with Flavor Packs for Oral Solution (Rare) 3088
Combivent Inhalation Aerosol (Rare) 847
Combivir Tablets 1411
Comvax 1928
Coreg Tablets (Less than or equal to 0.1%) 1414
Cosopt Sterile Ophthalmic Solution 1931
Cubicin for Injection 1026
CytoGam Intravenous 1895
Dantrium Capsules (Less frequent) 2694
Dantrium Intravenous (One case) 2695
Daraprim Tablets 1419
Decadron Tablets 1951
Depakene 417
Depakote Sprinkle Capsules 422
Depakote Tablets 427
Depakote ER Tablets 434
Depo-Medrol Single-Dose Vial 2619
Depo-Provera Contraceptive Injection 2622
depo-subQ provera 104 Injectable Suspension (Infrequent) 2624
Digibind for Injection 1421
Diovan HCT Tablets (Less frequent) 2196
Donnatal Extentabs 2493
Dyazide Capsules 1423
Dyrenium Capsules 3400
E.E.S. 451
Effexor Tablets 3411
Effexor XR Capsules 3417
Elitek (Less than 1%) 2890
Elspar for Injection 2463
Elspar for Injection 1960
Engerix-B Vaccine 1425
Epivir 1427
Epivir-HBV 1432
Epzicom Tablets 1436
EryPed 447
Ery-Tab Tablets 449
Erythrocin Stearate Filmtab Tablets 453
Erythromycin Base Filmtab Tablets 455
Erythromycin Delayed-Release Capsules, USP 457
Flonase Nasal Spray 1440
Fluarix 1451
Flumist Vaccine 1901
Fluorescite Injection ⊙ 207
Fortaz (Very rare) 1453
GamaSTAN (Rare) 3234
Gammagard S/D 724
Gantrisin Pediatric Suspension 2770
Havrix Vaccine (Rare) 1456
Herceptin I.V. 1233
Humira Injection 466
Hytrin Capsules (Rare) 471
Imitrex Injection (Rare) 1463
Imitrex Nasal Spray 1467
Imitrex Tablets (Rare) 1471
Indocin Capsules (Less than 1%) 1995
Indocin I.V. (Less than 1%) 2465
Indocin (Less than 1%) 1995
Infed Injection 3390
Integrilin Injection (One patient) 3020
Intron A for Injection (Rare) 3024
Invanz for Injection (Very rare) 1999
Ketek Tablets (Rare) 2903
Kytril Injection (Rare) 2781
Kytril (Rare) 2784
Lamisil Tablets (Rare) 2232
Lescol Capsules (Rare) 2233
Lescol XL Tablets 2233
Lexapro Oral Solution (Infrequent) 1190
Lexapro Tablets (Infrequent) 1190
Lipitor Tablets 2483
Malarone Pediatric Tablets (One case) 1517
Malarone Tablets (One case) 1517
Maxipime for Injection 1105
Mefoxin for Injection 2012
Mefoxin Premixed Intravenous Solution 2016
Meruvax II 2019
Mevacor Tablets (Rare) 2021
Miacalcin Injection (One case) 2252
Miacalcin Nasal Spray (One case) 2253
Mintezol 2027
M-M-R II 2006
MS Contin Tablets (Extremely rare) 2701
Mumpsvax 2031
Mustargen for Injection 2468
Mylotarg for Injection 3431
Nalfon Capsules (Less than 1%) 2502
Nasonex Nasal Spray 3043
Neosporin Ophthalmic Solution Sterile (Rare) ⊙ 265
Neulasta Injection 601
Neumega for Injection 3435
Norvir (Rare) 503
Omnicef Capsules 511
Omnicef for Oral Suspension 511
Oncaspar 1145
Oracea Capsules 1000
Orencia Powder for Intravenous Infusion (2 cases) 914
Orthoclone OKT3 Sterile Solution 2360
Paxil CR Controlled-Release Tablets 1538
Paxil 1530
PCE Dispertab Tablets 515
Pepcid Injection (Infrequent) 2040
Pepcid (Infrequent) 2038
Pexeva Tablets 1694
Poly-Pred Ophthalmic Suspension ⊙ 233
Premarin Tablets 3446
Premphase Tablets 3456
Prempro Tablets 3456
PREVPAC (Rare) 3284
Prilosec OTC Delayed-Release Tablets (Rare) 2677
Prograf Capsules and Injection (A small percentage of patients) 632
Proleukin for Injection 2266
Prometrium Capsules (100 mg, 200 mg) 3203
ProQuad 2064
Protonix I.V. 3472
Protonix Tablets 3469
Raniclor Tablets, Chewable (Rare) 2505
Rebetron Combination Therapy 3063
Recombivax HB (Less than 1%) 2071
ReFacto Vials 3484
Remicade for IV Injection (Less than 1%) 971
ReoPro Vials 1809
Retrovir Capsules (One patient) 1560
Retrovir IV Infusion (One patient) 1564
Retrovir (One patient) 1560
Rocephin Injectable Vials, ADD-Vantage, Galaxy, Bulk (Rare) 2800
Serevent Diskus 1568
Seroquel Tablets 690
Simulect for Injection 2284
Singulair 2077
Solodyn Extended Release Tablets 1890
St. Joseph 81 mg Aspirin Chewable and Enteric Coated Tablets 1869
St. Joseph 81 mg Aspirin ■ 688
Suprax 1843
Synagis (Less than 1 case per 100,000 patients) 1897
Tamiflu Capsules (Rare) 2807
Tamiflu Oral Suspension (Rare) 2807
Temodar Capsules (Rare) 3073
Thiothixene Capsules (Rare) 2165
Ticlid Tablets 2810
Timoptic Sterile Ophthalmic Solution 2088
Timoptic in Ocudose 2091
Timoptic-XE Sterile Ophthalmic Gel Forming Solution 2092
TNKase I.V. (Rare) 1264
Trasylol Injection 754
Trizivir Tablets 1589
Twinrix Vaccine 1595
Valtrex Caplets 1597
Vancocin HCl Capsules, USP 3380
Varivax 2100
Viramune Oral Suspension 873
Viramune Tablets 873
Vytorin 10/10 Tablets 2114
Vytorin 10/10 Tablets 3077
Vytorin 10/20 Tablets 2114
Vytorin 10/20 Tablets 3077
Vytorin 10/40 Tablets 2114
Vytorin 10/40 Tablets 3077
Vytorin 10/80 Tablets 2114
Vytorin 10/80 Tablets 3077
Xenical Capsules 2831
Xolair 1266
Xopenex Inhalation Solution 3146
Xopenex Inhalation Solution Concentrate 3150
Xopenex HFA Inhalation Aerosol 3154
Zantac (Rare) 1624
Zantac Injection (Rare) 1619
Zantac Injection Pharmacy Bulk Package (Rare) 1622
Zantac Injection Premixed (Rare) 1619
Zantac (Rare) 1624
Zegerid Capsules (Rare) 2958
Zegerid Powder for Oral Solution (Rare) 2958
Zetia Tablets 2120
Ziagen 1626
Zinacef for Injection (Rare) 1631
Zinacef Injection (Rare) 1631
Zmax for Oral Suspension 2583

Zocor Tablets (Rare) 2105
Zofran Injection (Rare) 1634
Zofran (Rare) 1639
Zofran ODT Orally Disintegrating Tablets (Rare) 1639
Zomig Tablets (Very rare) 3519
Zomig Nasal Spray (Very rare) 3523
Zomig-ZMT Tablets (Very rare) 3519
Zosyn (1.0% or less) 3492
Zovirax Capsules (Rare) 1643
Zovirax Cream 820
Zovirax (Rare) 1643
Zyrtec Chewable Tablets (Rare) 2594
Zyrtec (Rare) 2594
Zyrtec-D 12 Hour Extended Release Tablets (Rare) 2597

Anasarca
▲ Gleevec Tablets (2% to 16%) 2227

Anastomotic disruption
Avastin IV (Rare) 1227
Rapamune Oral Solution and Tablets 3475

Anastomotic leak
Invanz for Injection (1.5%) 1999

Androgen excess, signs or symptoms of
▲ Lupron Depot 3.75 mg (Less than 5%) 3260
▲ Lupron Depot–3 Month 11.25 mg (Less than 5%) 3265

Anemia
▲ Abelcet Injection (4%) 1141
Abilify Oral Solution (Frequent) 882
Abilify Oral Solution (Frequent) 2450
Abilify Discmelt Orally Disintegrating Tablets (Frequent) 882
Abilify Discmelt Orally Disintegrating Tablets (Frequent) 2450
Abilify Tablets (Frequent) 882
Abilify Tablets (Frequent) 2450
Accutane Capsules 2731
Aceon Tablets (2 mg, 4 mg, 8 mg) 3194
Aciphex Tablets 1090
Actiq (Less than 1%) 979
Actonel Tablets (2.4%) 2683
Actonel with Calcium Tablets (2.4%) 2688
Actos Tablets (Less than or equal to 2%) 3219
Adalat CC Tablets (Rare) 2964
Aggrenox Capsules (1.6%) 822
▲ Agrylin Capsules (1% to 5%) 3169
▲ Alimta for Injection (1% to 33%) 1750
Alinia for Oral Suspension (Less than 1%) 2835
Alinia Tablets (Less than 1%) 2835
Alkeran for Injection 955
Alkeran Tablets 956
Aloprim for Injection (Less than 1%) 2167
Ambien Tablets (Rare) 2851
Ambien CR Tablets (Rare) 2855
AmBisome for Injection (Less common) 620
Amerge Tablets (Rare) 1339
Amoxil Capsules 1343
Amoxil Chewable Tablets 1343
Amoxil Pediatric Drops for Oral Suspension 1343
Amoxil Powder for Oral Suspension 1343
Amoxil Tablets 1343
Anaprox Tablets (Less than 1%) 2761
Anaprox DS Tablets (Less than 1%) 2761
Anzemet Injection (Infrequently) 2859
Anzemet Tablets (Infrequently) 2862
Aptivus Capsules (Less than 2%) 826
▲ Aredia for Injection (42.5%) 2179
Aricept Tablets (Infrequent) 1094
Aricept ODT Tablets (Infrequent) 1094
▲ Arimidex Tablets (2% to 5%) 673
▲ Arixtra Injection (1.5% to 19.6%) 1351
▲ Arranon Injection (10% to 99%) 1357
Arthrotec Tablets (Rare) 3129
Asacol Delayed-Release Tablets 2692
Atacand Tablets 649
Augmentin 1360
Augmentin Tablets 1363
Augmentin XR Extended-Release Tablets 1369
Augmentin ES-600 Powder for Oral Suspension 1366
▲ Avandamet Tablets (7.1%) 1373
Avandaryl Tablets (0.6% to 2.3%) 1379
Avandia Tablets (1.9%) 1384
Avelox (0.1% to less than 2%) 2970
▲ Avinza Capsules (Less than 5%) 1741
Axid Oral Solution (More frequent) 879
Betaseron for SC Injection 767
Bexxar 1398
Caduet Tablets (Less than 2%) 2508
Calcium Disodium Versenate Injection 1851
▲ Campath Ampules (38% to 80%) 811
Campral Tablets (Infrequent) 1174
▲ Camptosar Injection (4.5% to 96.9%) 2604
▲ Cancidas for Injection (0% to 3.8%) 1918
Captopril Tablets 2149
▲ Carnitor Injection (3% to 12%) 3188
Celebrex Capsules (0.1% to 1.9%) 3134
▲ Celexa (Infrequent) 1176
▲ CellCept Capsules (25.6% to 43%) 2747
▲ CellCept Intravenous (25.6% to 43%) 2747
▲ CellCept Oral Suspension (25.6% to 43%) 2747
▲ CellCept Tablets (25.6% to 43%) 2747
Cesamet Capsules 3340
Chantix Tablets (Infrequent) 2517
Cipro (Less than 0.1%) 2977
Cipro XR Tablets 2990
Clinoril Tablets (Less than 1%) 1924
Clolar for Intravenous Infusion 1271
Clozaril Tablets (Less than 1%) 2184
Colazal Capsules 2838
Combivir Tablets (2.9%) 1411
Concerta Extended-Release Tablets 1881
▲ Copegus Tablets (11% to 22%) 2754
▲ Coreg Tablets (Greater than 0.1% to greater than 3%) 1414
Cosmegen for Injection 2459
▲ Cozaar Tablets (Less than 1% to 14%) 1935
Crestor Tablets (Greater than or equal to 1%) 678
Crixivan Capsules (0.6%) 1940
▲ Cubicin for Injection (2.1% to 12.5%) 1026
▲ Dacogen Injection (82%) 2129
Daytrana Transdermal Patch 3174
Demser Capsules (Rare) 1953
Depacon Injection 412
Depakene 417
Depakote Sprinkle Capsules 422
Depakote Tablets 427
Depakote ER Tablets (Greater than 1%) 434
DepoCyt Injection (1%) 1143
▲ DepoDur Extended-Release Injection (Greater than 10%) 1110
Depo-Provera Contraceptive Injection (Less than 1%) 2622
depo-subQ provera 104 Injectable Suspension 2624
Diastat Rectal Delivery System (Less than 1%) 3343
Dolobid Tablets 1955
▲ Doxil Injection (5.8% to 52.6%) 2351
Duetact Tablets (Less than 2%) 3226
EC-Naprosyn Delayed-Release Tablets (Less than 1%) 2761
Effexor Tablets (Infrequent) 3411
Effexor XR Capsules (Infrequent) 3417
Eldepryl Capsules 3208
Elmiron Capsules (Less than or equal to 1%) 2415
▲ Eloxatin for Injection (1% to 81%) 2892
▲ Emend Capsules (Greater than 0.5%) 1963
Enbrel for Injection 584
Epivir 1427
Epivir-HBV 1432
Epogen for Injection 591
Epzicom Tablets 1436
▲ Erbitux (3% to 16%) 910
▲ Eulexin Capsules (6%) 3009
▲ Evoxac Capsules (1% to 3%) 1047
Exelon Capsules (Frequent) 2206
Exelon Oral Solution (Frequent) 2206
Famvir Tablets (0.1%) 2211
▲ Faslodex Injection (4.5%) 681
FazaClo Orally Disintegrating Tablets (Less than 1%) 551
Ferrlecit Injection 3388
Focalin Tablets 2220
Focalin XR Capsules 2223
Fortical Nasal Spray (Less than 1%) 3337
Furosemide Tablets 2154
Gabitril Tablets (Infrequent) 984
Gantrisin Pediatric Suspension 2770
Garamycin Injectable 3014
▲ Gemzar for Injection (45% to 86%) 1771
Gengraf Capsules (1% to less than 3%) 459
Geodon Capsules (Infrequent) 2529
▲ Gleevec Tablets (0% to 42%) 2227
Guanidine Hydrochloride Tablets 3016
▲ Hectorol Capsules (Greater than or equal to 5%) 1275
▲ Herceptin I.V. (4%) 1233
▲ Hycamtin for Injection (40% to 95%) 1458
Hyzaar 50-12.5 Tablets 1990
Hyzaar 100-12.5 Tablets 1990
Hyzaar 100-25 Tablets 1990
Imitrex Injection 1463
Imitrex Nasal Spray 1467
Imitrex Tablets (Rare) 1471
Indocin Capsules (Less than 1%) 1995
Indocin I.V. (Less than 1%) 2465
Indocin (Less than 1%) 1995
▲ Intron A for Injection (Less than 5% to 22%) 3024
▲ Invanz for Injection (5.7%) 1999
Invirase (Less than or equal to 2%) 2772
▲ Ionsys Transdermal System (3%) 2379
I.V. Busulfex (100%) 2493
Kadian Capsules (Less than 3%) 577
Kaletra (Less than 2%) 476
Klonopin 2778
Kogenate FS 738
Kogenate FS with Bio-Set 740
▲ Kytril Injection (9.4%) 2781
▲ Kytril (4%) 2784
Lamictal (Infrequent) 1481
▲ Leustatin Injection (37%) 2357
Levaquin (0.1% to 0.9%) 2384
Levaquin in 5% Dextrose Injection (0.1% to 0.9%) 2384
Lexapro Oral Solution (Infrequent) 1190
Lexapro Tablets (Infrequent) 1190
Lipitor Tablets (Less than 2%) 2483
Lofibra Tablets 1219
Lofibra Capsules 1216
▲ Lovenox Injection (2% to 16%) 2915
▲ Lucentis Injection (3% to 8%) 1237
Lunesta Tablets (Infrequent) 3142
Lyrica Capsules (0.1% to 1%) 2539
Malarone Pediatric Tablets 1517
Malarone Tablets 1517
Matulane Capsules (Frequent) 3191
Mefoxin for Injection 2012
Mefoxin Premixed Intravenous Solution 2016
▲ Megace ES Oral Suspension (0% to 5%) 2481
▲ Mepron Suspension (4% to 6%) 1521
Meridia Capsules 489
▲ Merrem I.V. (Greater than 1% to 5.5%) 686
Metadate CD Capsules 3323
Miacalcin Nasal Spray (Less than 1%) 2253
Miradon Tablets 3042
▲ Mobic Oral Suspension (0% to 4.1%) 863
▲ Mobic Tablets (0% to 4.1%) 863
Mycamine for Injection (0.8% to 1.2%) 628
▲ Myfortic Tablets (3% to 21.6%) 2255
Myleran Tablets 1525
▲ Mylotarg for Injection (22%) 3431
▲ Myozyme for Intravenous Infusion (31%) 1279
Namenda (Frequent) 1195
Naprosyn Suspension (Less than 1%) 2761
Naprosyn Tablets (Less than 1%) 2761
Natrecor for Injection (Greater than or equal to 1%) 3127
▲ NeoProfen Injection (32%) 2472
Neoral Oral Solution (1% to less than 3%) 2259
Neoral Soft Gelatin Capsules (1% to less than 3%) 2259
▲ Neupogen for Injection (Approximately 10%) 603
Neurontin Capsules (Infrequent) 2487
Neurontin Oral Solution (Infrequent) 2487
Neurontin Tablets (Infrequent) 2487
▲ Nexavar Tablets (Common) 746
Nexium Delayed-Release Capsules (Less than 1%) 655
Nexium I.V. (Less than 1%) 659
Nimotop Capsules (Less than 1%) 749
▲ Nipent for Injection (8% to 35%) 1863
Norvir (Less than 2%) 503
Oncaspar 1145
▲ Ontak Vials (18%) 1745
ParaGard T 380A Intrauterine Copper Contraceptive 1073
Parnate Tablets 1527
Paxil CR Controlled-Release Tablets (Infrequent) 1538
Paxil (Infrequent) 1530
Pegasys (2%) 2789
PEG-Intron Powder for Injection 3048
Pentasa Capsules 3185
Permax Tablets (1.1%) 3356
Pexeva Tablets (infrequent) 1694
▲ Photofrin for Injection (32%) 702
Plavix Tablets (1% to 2.5%) 917
Plavix Tablets (1% to 2.5%) 2926
Pletal Tablets (Less than 2%) 2455
Prevacid Delayed-Release Capsules (Less than 1%) 3271
Prevacid for Delayed-Release Oral Suspension (Less than 1%) 3271
Prevacid SoluTab Delayed-Release Orally Disintegrating Tablets (Less than 1%) 3271
Prevacid NapraPAC (Less than 1%) 3280
PREVPAC (Less than 1%) 3284
Prilosec OTC Delayed-Release Tablets (Rare) 2677
Prinivil Tablets 2052
Prochieve 4% Gel 1003
Prochieve 8% Gel 1003
▲ Prograf Capsules and Injection (5% to 47%) 632
▲ Proleukin for Injection (29%) 2266
Proquin XR Tablets 1153
Protonix I.V. (Less than 1%) 3472
Protonix Tablets (Less than 1%) 3469
Protopic Ointment (0.2% to less than 1%) 638
Provigil Tablets (At least 1%) 988
Prozac Pulvules and Liquid (Infrequent) 1801
▲ Rapamune Oral Solution and Tablets (23% to 37%) 3475
Raptiva for Injection 1250
▲ Razadyne (3%) 2399
▲ Razadyne ER Extended-Release Capsules (3%) 2399
▲ Rebetol (12% to 17%) 3058
▲ Rebetron Combination Therapy (10%) 3063
▲ Rebif Prefilled Syringe for Injection (3% to 5%) 3159
▲ Refludan for Injection (12.4%) 792
Relpax Tablets (Rare) 2548
▲ Remicade for IV Injection (Greater than or equal to 0.2% to 11%) 971
ReoPro Vials (1.2%) 1809
Requip Tablets (1% or more) 1555
Rescriptor Tablets (0.7% to 1.0%) 2551
Retavase (0.9% to 2.6%) 2499
▲ Retrovir Capsules (1.1% to 29%) 1560
▲ Retrovir IV Infusion (1.1% to 29%) 1564
▲ Retrovir (1.1% to 29%) 1560
▲ Revlimid Capsules (6.1% to 24.3%) 958
▲ Ribavirin, USP Capsules (12% to 17%) 3068
Rilutek Tablets (Infrequent) 2930
Risperdal (Infrequent) 1676
Risperdal Consta Long-Acting Injection (Frequent) 1682
Risperdal M-Tab Orally Disintegrating Tablets (Infrequent) 1676
Ritalin Hydrochloride Tablets 2269
Ritalin LA Capsules 2271
Ritalin-SR Tablets 2269
▲ Rituxan I.V. (3% to 8%) 1254
Rocephin Injectable Vials, ADD-Vantage, Galaxy, Bulk (Less than 1%) 2800
Rythmol SR Capsules 2727
Sandimmune (2% or less) 2275
Sandostatin Injection (Less than 1%) 2278
▲ Sandostatin LAR Depot (5% to 15%) 2280
Seroquel Tablets (Infrequent) 690
▲ Simulect for Injection (Greater than or equal to 10%) 2284
Sonata Capsules (Infrequent) 1717
Stromectol Tablets (One patient) 2083
Sular Tablets (Less than or equal to 1%) 3122
▲ Sutent Capsules (2% to 26%) 2560
Symbyax Capsules (Infrequent) 1819
Synagis (More than 1%) 1897
Tabloid Tablets 1575
Tamiflu Capsules (Less than 1%) 2807
Tamiflu Oral Suspension (Less than 1%) 2807
▲ Targretin Capsules (6% to 24.5%) 1747
Tasmar Tablets (Infrequent) 3358
▲ Taxotere Injection Concentrate (7.7% to 97.8%) 2932
Temodar Capsules 3073
Teveten Tablets (Less than 1%) 1735
Teveten HCT Tablets (Less than 1%) 1737
▲ Thalomid Capsules (5.6% to 12.5%) 965
▲ Thiola Tablets (4%) 2141
Thioridazine Hydrochloride Tablets 2163
Ticlid Tablets 2810
Topamax Sprinkle Capsules (1% to 2%) 2404

Topamax Tablets (1% to 2%) 2404
▲ Tracleer Tablets (3%) 545
Trasylol Injection (2%) 754
Trelstar Depot (1.4%) 3394
Tricor Tablets 527
Triglide Tablets 3123
▲ Trisenox Injection (20%) 993
Trizivir Tablets (2.9%) 1589
▲ Tygacil for Injection (4.2%) 3488
Uniretic Tablets (Less than 1%) 3100
▲ Valcyte Tablets (8% to 26%) 2813
Valtrex Caplets (Up to 0.8%) 1597
Vantas (Less than 2%) 3375
Vantin Tablets and Oral Suspension (Less than 1%) 2645
▲ Vaprisol (3.8%) 643
Vasotec I.V. Injection 2103
▲ Velcade for Injection (26%) 2133
VFEND I.V. (0.1%) 2564
VFEND Oral Suspension (0.1%) 2564
VFEND Tablets (0.1%) 2564
Viadur Implant (2.3%) 757
Viagra Tablets (Less than 2%) 2573
Viracept (Less than 2%) 2577
Viramune Oral Suspension 873
Viramune Tablets 873
Virazole for Inhalation Solution 3370
▲ Visudyne for Injection (1% to 10%) 2305
▲ Voltaren Tablets (1% to 10%) 2307
▲ Voltaren-XR Tablets (1% to 10%) 2310
Wellbutrin Tablets (Rare) 1603
Wellbutrin SR Sustained-Release Tablets 1607
Wellbutrin XL Extended-Release Tablets 1613
▲ Xeloda Tablets (1% to 80%) 2822
▲ Zegerid Capsules (7.9%) 2958
▲ Zegerid Powder for Oral Solution (7.9%) 2958
Zelapar Tablets 3372
Ziagen (0% to less than 1%) 1626
Zoloft (Rare) 2586
▲ Zometa for Intravenous Infusion (22.1% to 33%) 2315
Zonegran Capsules (Infrequent) 1101
Zosyn (1% or less) 3492
Zovirax 1643
Zyban Sustained-Release Tablets 1644
Zyprexa Tablets (Infrequent) 1830
Zyprexa ZYDIS Orally Disintegrating Tablets (Infrequent) 1830
▲ Zyvox (0% to 5.6%) 2652

Anemia, aplastic

Aceon Tablets (2 mg, 4 mg, 8 mg) 3194
Aggrenox Capsules 822
Aldoril Tablets 1910
Anaprox Tablets (Less than 1%) 2761
Anaprox DS Tablets (Less than 1%) 2761
Arthrotec Tablets (Rare) 3129
Asacol Delayed-Release Tablets (Rare) 2692
Atacand HCT 651
Avalide Tablets 888
Avalide Tablets 2874
Avandaryl Tablets 1379
▲ Blephamide Ophthalmic Ointment (Among most often) 568
Blephamide Ophthalmic Suspension 569
Carbatrol Capsules 3171
Ceftin 1407
Clinoril Tablets (Less than 1 in 100) 1924
Clorpres Tablets 2153
Copegus Tablets (Less than 1%) 2754
Coreg Tablets (Rare) 1414
Cosmegen for Injection 2459
Cuprimine Capsules 1947
Dantrium Capsules (Less frequent) 2694
Dantrium Intravenous 2695
Dapsone Tablets USP 1673
Depacon Injection 412
Depakene 417
Depakote Sprinkle Capsules 422
Depakote Tablets 427
Depakote ER Tablets 434
Diovan HCT Tablets 2196
Diuril Oral Suspension 1954
Diuril Sodium Intravenous 2467
Duetact Tablets 3226
Dyazide Capsules 1423
EC-Naprosyn Delayed-Release Tablets (Less than 1%) 2761
Effexor Tablets 3411
Effexor XR Capsules 3417
Enbrel for Injection 584
Epzicom Tablets 1436
Equetro Extended-Release Capsules 3180
Fansidar Tablets 2765
FML-S Ophthalmic Suspension ⊙229
Fortaz 1453
Furosemide Tablets 2154
Gantrisin Pediatric Suspension 2770
Gleevec Tablets (Rare) 2227
Humira Injection 466
Hyzaar 50-12.5 Tablets 1990
Hyzaar 100-12.5 Tablets 1990
Hyzaar 100-25 Tablets 1990
Indapamide Tablets 2156
Indocin Capsules (Less than 1%) 1995
Indocin I.V. (Less than 1%) 2465
Indocin (Less than 1%) 1995
Intron A for Injection (Very rare) 3024
Keflex Capsules 549
Lamictal (Rare) 1481
Leustatin Injection (Some reports) 2357
Levaquin (Rare) 2384
Levaquin in 5% Dextrose Injection (Rare) 2384
Lopressor HCT 50/25 Tablets 2241
Lopressor HCT 100/25 Tablets 2241
Lopressor HCT 100/50 Tablets 2241
Lotensin HCT Tablets 2246
Maxipime for Injection 1105
Mefoxin for Injection 2012
Mefoxin Premixed Intravenous Solution 2016
Micardis HCT Tablets 856
Midamor Tablets (Rare) 2026
Moduretic Tablets 2028
Myleran Tablets 1525
Nalfon Capsules (Less than 1%) 2502
Naprosyn Suspension (Less than 1%) 2761
Naprosyn Tablets (Less than 1%) 2761
Nipent for Injection (Less than 3%) 1863
Norflex Injection (Very rare) 1856
Omnicef Capsules 511
Omnicef for Oral Suspension 511
Orthoclone OKT3 Sterile Solution 2360
Paxil CR Controlled-Release Tablets 1538
Paxil 1530
Pentasa Capsules 3185
Pexeva Tablets 1694
Plavix Tablets (Less than 1%) 917
Plavix Tablets (Less than 1%) 2926
Prevacid Delayed-Release Capsules (Less than 1%) 3271
Prevacid for Delayed-Release Oral Suspension (Less than 1%) 3271
Prevacid SoluTab Delayed-Release Orally Disintegrating Tablets (Less than 1%) 3271
Prevacid NapraPAC (Less than 1%) 3280
PREVPAC 3284
Prinzide Tablets 2056
Prozac Pulvules and Liquid 1801
Raniclor Tablets, Chewable (Rare) 2505
Rebetron Combination Therapy (Very rare) 3063
Retrovir Capsules 1560
Retrovir IV Infusion 1564
Retrovir 1560
Rilutek Tablets (Rare) 2930
Rituxan I.V. (One case) 1254
Suprax 1843
Tegretol/Tegretol-XR (Very low incidence) 2295
Teveten HCT Tablets 1737
Thalomid Capsules 965
Thioridazine Hydrochloride Tablets 2163
Ticlid Tablets (Rare) 2810
Timolide Tablets 2086
Trizivir Tablets 1589
Trusopt Sterile Ophthalmic Solution (Rare) 2095
▲ Valcyte Tablets (Less than 5%) 2813
Valtrex Caplets 1597
Vantin Tablets and Oral Suspension 2645
VFEND I.V. (Less than 2%) 2564
VFEND Oral Suspension (Less than 2%) 2564
VFEND Tablets (Less than 2%) 2564
Voltaren Tablets (Rarely) 2307
Voltaren-XR Tablets (Rarely) 2310
Zantac (Rare) 1624
Zantac Injection (Rare) 1619
Zantac Injection Pharmacy Bulk Package (Rare) 1622
Zantac Injection Premixed (Rare) 1619
Zantac (Rare) 1624
Zinacef for Injection 1631
Zinacef Injection 1631
Zoloft 2586
Zonegran Capsules (Rare) 1101

Anemia, dilutional

Neumega for Injection 3435
Prolastin 3255

Anemia, hemolytic

Aceon Tablets (2 mg, 4 mg, 8 mg) 3194
Aciphex Tablets 1090
Advicor Tablets 1722
Agenerase Capsules 1327
Agenerase Oral Solution 1332
Aldoril Tablets 1910
Alkeran for Injection 955
Alkeran Tablets 956
Alphanate, Antihemophilic Factor (Human) (Rare) 1654
Altace Capsules (Less than 1%) 1702
Altoprev Extended-Release Tablets (Rare) 3109
Amoxil Capsules 1343
Amoxil Chewable Tablets 1343
Amoxil Pediatric Drops for Oral Suspension 1343
Amoxil Powder for Oral Suspension 1343
Amoxil Tablets 1343
Anaprox Tablets (Less than 1%) 2761
Anaprox DS Tablets (Less than 1%) 2761
Aricept Tablets (Rare) 1094
Aricept ODT Tablets (Rare) 1094
Arthrotec Tablets (Rare) 3129
Atacand HCT 651
Augmentin 1360
Augmentin Tablets 1363
Augmentin XR Extended-Release Tablets 1369
Augmentin ES-600 Powder for Oral Suspension 1366
Avalide Tablets 888
Avalide Tablets 2874
Avandaryl Tablets 1379
Bicillin C-R Injectable Suspension 1706
Campath Ampules 811
Captopril Tablets 2149
Cardizem LA Extended Release Tablets (Infrequent) 1728
Ceftin 1407
Celexa 1176
Cipro 2977
Cipro I.V. (Rare) 2984
Cipro XR Tablets 2990
Clinoril Tablets (Less than 1 in 100) 1924
Crixivan Capsules 1940
Cuprimine Capsules 1947
Diovan HCT Tablets 2196
Diuril Oral Suspension 1954
Diuril Sodium Intravenous 2467
Dolobid Tablets (Less than 1 in 100) 1955
Duetact Tablets 3226
Dyazide Capsules 1423
EC-Naprosyn Delayed-Release Tablets (Less than 1%) 2761
Eloxatin for Injection 2892
Eulexin Capsules 3009
Fansidar Tablets 2765
Fortaz (Rare) 1453
Furosemide Tablets 2154
Gamunex Immune Globulin I.V., 10% (Very rare) 3235
Gantrisin Pediatric Suspension 2770
Gengraf Capsules 459
Hyzaar 50-12.5 Tablets 1990
Hyzaar 100-12.5 Tablets 1990
Hyzaar 100-25 Tablets 1990
Imitrex Injection 1463
Imitrex Tablets 1471
Indocin Capsules (Less than 1%) 1995
Indocin I.V. (Less than 1%) 2465
Indocin (Less than 1%) 1995
▲ Intron A for Injection (Less than 5%) 3024
Invirase (Rare) 2772
Keflex Capsules 549
Lamictal 1481
Lescol Capsules (Rare) 2233
Lescol XL Tablets 2233
Leustatin Injection (Some reports) 2357
Levaquin (Rare) 2384
Levaquin in 5% Dextrose Injection (Rare) 2384
Lexapro Oral Solution 1190
Lexapro Tablets 1190
▲ Lithostat Tablets (3% to 15%) 2140
Lotensin Tablets (Less than 1%) 2243
Lotensin HCT Tablets (Rare) 2246
Lotrel Capsules (Rare) 2249
Matulane Capsules 3191
Maxipime for Injection 1105
Mefoxin for Injection 2012
Mefoxin Premixed Intravenous Solution 2016
Mevacor Tablets (Rare) 2021
Micardis HCT Tablets 856
Moduretic Tablets 2028
Mustargen for Injection (Rare) 2468
Mycamine for Injection 628
Nalfon Capsules (Less than 1 %) 2502
Naprosyn Suspension (Less than 1%) 2761
Naprosyn Tablets (Less than 1%) 2761
Neoral Oral Solution 2259
Neoral Soft Gelatin Capsules 2259
Nipent for Injection (Less than 3%) 1863
Noroxin Tablets (Rare) 2032
Omnicef Capsules 511
Omnicef for Oral Suspension 511
▲ Oncaspar (Greater than 1% but less than 5%) 1145
Oracea Capsules 1000
Orthoclone OKT3 Sterile Solution 2360
Parcopa Orally Disintegrating Tablets 3097
Paser Granules 1674
Paxil CR Controlled-Release Tablets 1538
Paxil 1530
PEG-Intron Powder for Injection 3048
Pexeva Tablets 1694
Pneumovax 23 (Rare) 2043
Prevacid Delayed-Release Capsules (Less than 1%) 3271
Prevacid for Delayed-Release Oral Suspension (Less than 1%) 3271
Prevacid SoluTab Delayed-Release Orally Disintegrating Tablets (Less than 1%) 3271
Prevacid NapraPAC (Less than 1%) 3280
PREVPAC 3284
Prilosec OTC Delayed-Release Tablets (Rare) 2677
Primaxin I.M. 2045
Primaxin I.V. 2048
Prinivil Tablets (Rare) 2052
Prinzide Tablets 2056
Prograf Capsules and Injection 632
Proquin XR Tablets 1153
Raniclor Tablets, Chewable (Rare) 2505
Raptiva for Injection 1250
▲ Rebetol (10%) 3058
▲ Rebetron Combination Therapy (10%) 3063
Remicade for IV Injection (Greater than or equal to 0.2%) 971
ReoPro Vials (0.3%) 1809
Rescriptor Tablets 2551
Retrovir Capsules 1560
Retrovir IV Infusion 1564
Retrovir 1560
Revlimid Capsules 958
Rituxan I.V. (Two cases) 1254
Rocephin Injectable Vials, ADD-Vantage, Galaxy, Bulk (Less than 1%) 2800
Skelaxin Tablets 1716
Solodyn Extended Release Tablets 1890
Stalevo Tablets 2287
Sulfamylon Cream 2162
Sulfamylon for 5% Topical Solution 2162
Suprax 1843
Teveten HCT Tablets 1737
Thiothixene Capsules 2165
Tiazac Capsules (Infrequent) 1201
Ticlid Tablets (Rare) 2810
Timolide Tablets 2086
Uniretic Tablets (Less than 1%) 3100
Univasc Tablets (Less than 1%) 3104
Vantin Tablets and Oral Suspension 2645
Vasotec I.V. Injection 2103
VFEND I.V. (Less than 2%) 2564
VFEND Oral Suspension (Less than 2%) 2564
VFEND Tablets (Less than 2%) 2564
Virazole for Inhalation Solution 3370
Voltaren Tablets (Rarely) 2307
Voltaren-XR Tablets (Rarely) 2310
Vytorin 10/10 Tablets 2114
Vytorin 10/10 Tablets 3077
Vytorin 10/20 Tablets 2114
Vytorin 10/20 Tablets 3077
Vytorin 10/40 Tablets 2114
Vytorin 10/40 Tablets 3077
Vytorin 10/80 Tablets 2114
Vytorin 10/80 Tablets 3077
Zegerid Capsules (Rare) 2958
Zegerid Powder for Oral Solution (Rare) 2958
Zinacef for Injection 1631
Zinacef Injection 1631
Zocor Tablets (Rare) 2105
Zosyn 3492
Zyrtec Chewable Tablets (Rare) 2594
Zyrtec (Rare) 2594
Zyrtec-D 12 Hour Extended Release Tablets (Rare) 2597

Anemia, hemolytic, autoimmune
Fluarix 1451

Anemia, hemolytic, immune
Campath Ampules 811
Prozac Pulvules and Liquid 1801
Zantac (Exceedingly rare) 1624
Zantac Injection (Exceedingly rare) 1619
Zantac Injection Pharmacy Bulk Package (Rare) 1622
Zantac Injection Premixed (Exceedingly rare) 1619
Zantac (Exceedingly rare) 1624

Anemia, hypochromic
Abilify Oral Solution (Infrequent) 882
Abilify Oral Solution (Infrequent) 2450
Abilify Discmelt Orally Disintegrating Tablets (Infrequent) 882
Abilify Discmelt Orally Disintegrating Tablets (Infrequent) 2450
Abilify Tablets (Infrequent) 882
Abilify Tablets (Infrequent) 2450
Aciphex Tablets 1090
Celexa (Rare) 1176
▲ CellCept Capsules (24.6%) 2747
▲ CellCept Intravenous (24.6%) 2747
▲ CellCept Oral Suspension (24.6%) 2747
▲ CellCept Tablets (24.6%) 2747
▲ Doxil Injection (5.2% to 9.8%) 2351
Evoxac Capsules (Less than 1%) 1047
Exelon Capsules (Infrequent) 2206
Exelon Oral Solution (Infrequent) 2206
Geodon Capsules (Rare) 2529
▲ Imdur Tablets (Less than or equal to 5%) 3018
Lovenox Injection (2%) 2915
Lyrica Capsules (0.1% to 1%) 2539
Merrem I.V. (Greater than 0.1% to 1%) 686
Nexium Delayed-Release Capsules (Less than 1%) 655
Nexium I.V. (Less than 1%) 659
Paxil CR Controlled-Release Tablets (Rare) 1538
Paxil (Rare) 1530
Pexeva Tablets (rare) 1694
Plavix Tablets (Less than 1%) 917
Plavix Tablets (Less than 1%) 2926
▲ Prograf Capsules and Injection (3% to 15%) 632
Protonix I.V. (Less than 1%) 3472
Protonix Tablets (Less than 1%) 3469
Prozac Pulvules and Liquid (Rare) 1801
Requip Tablets (Infrequent) 1555
Rilutek Tablets (Rare) 2930
Risperdal (Infrequent) 1676
Risperdal M-Tab Orally Disintegrating Tablets (Infrequent) 1676
Seroquel Tablets (Infrequent) 690
▲ Targretin Capsules (3.6% to 13.2%) 1747
Thalomid Capsules 965
Uniretic Tablets (Less than 1%) 3100

Anemia, iron deficiency
Abilify Oral Solution (Infrequent) 882
Abilify Oral Solution (Infrequent) 2450
Abilify Discmelt Orally Disintegrating Tablets (Infrequent) 882
Abilify Discmelt Orally Disintegrating Tablets (Infrequent) 2450
Abilify Tablets (Infrequent) 882
Abilify Tablets (Infrequent) 2450
Lamictal (Rare) 1481
Paxil CR Controlled-Release Tablets (Rare) 1538
Paxil (Rare) 1530
Percodan Tablets 1132
Permax Tablets (Infrequent) 3356
Pexeva Tablets (rare) 1694
Pletal Tablets (Less than 2%) 2455
Protonix I.V. (Less than 1%) 3472
Protonix Tablets (Less than 1%) 3469
Rilutek Tablets (Rare) 2930
Viadur Implant (Less than 2%) 757
Zyprexa IntraMuscular 1830

Anemia, macrocytic
Abilify Oral Solution (Infrequent) 882
Abilify Oral Solution (Infrequent) 2450
Abilify Discmelt Orally Disintegrating Tablets (Infrequent) 882
Abilify Discmelt Orally Disintegrating Tablets (Infrequent) 2450
Abilify Tablets (Infrequent) 882
Abilify Tablets (Infrequent) 2450
Ambien Tablets (Rare) 2851
Ambien CR Tablets (Rare) 2855
Azilect Tablets (Infrequent) 3293
Depacon Injection 412
Depakene 417
Depakote Tablets 427
Depakote ER Tablets 434
Eulexin Capsules 3009
Lamictal (Rare) 1481
Thalomid Capsules 965
VFEND I.V. (Less than 2%) 2564
VFEND Oral Suspension (Less than 2%) 2564
VFEND Tablets (Less than 2%) 2564

Anemia, megaloblastic
Daraprim Tablets 1419
Dyazide Capsules 1423
Dyrenium Capsules (Rare) 3400
Fansidar Tablets 2765
Nembutal Sodium Solution, USP 2470
Permax Tablets (Infrequent) 3356
Phenytek Capsules 2160
Thalomid Capsules 965
VFEND I.V. (Less than 2%) 2564
VFEND Oral Suspension (Less than 2%) 2564
VFEND Tablets (Less than 2%) 2564

Anemia, microangiopathic hemolytic
Gengraf Capsules 459
Plavix Tablets 917
Plavix Tablets 2926
Sandimmune (Occasional) 2275

Anemia, microcytic
Paxil CR Controlled-Release Tablets (Rare) 1538
Paxil (Rare) 1530
Pexeva Tablets (rare) 1694
Thalomid Capsules 965
VFEND I.V. (Less than 2%) 2564
VFEND Oral Suspension (Less than 2%) 2564
VFEND Tablets (Less than 2%) 2564
Zonegran Capsules (Rare) 1101

Anemia, nonhemolytic
Parcopa Orally Disintegrating Tablets 3097
Stalevo Tablets 2287

Anemia, normocytic
Paxil CR Controlled-Release Tablets (Rare) 1538
Paxil (Rare) 1530
Pexeva Tablets (rare) 1694
Risperdal (Rare) 1676
Risperdal M-Tab Orally Disintegrating Tablets (Rare) 1676
VFEND I.V. (Less than 2%) 2564
VFEND Oral Suspension (Less than 2%) 2564
VFEND Tablets (Less than 2%) 2564
Zyprexa Tablets (Infrequent) 1830
Zyprexa ZYDIS Orally Disintegrating Tablets (Infrequent) 1830

Anemia, refractory
Revlimid Capsules 958

Anemia, sideroblastic
Cuprimine Capsules 1947

Anemia with thrombocytopenia, hemolytic, microangiopathic
Tarceva Tablets (0.8%) 1259
Tarceva Tablets (0.8%) 2444

Anesthesia, local
Denavir Cream (0.9%) 2174
Migranal Nasal Spray (Infrequent) 3348

Anesthetic effect
Lithobid Tablets 1692

Anetoderma
Cuprimine Capsules (Rare) 1947

Aneurysm
Requip Tablets (Infrequent) 1555
Sandostatin LAR Depot (Rare) 2280
Vivitrol 995

Aneurysm, aortic
Effexor Tablets (Rare) 3411
Effexor XR Capsules (Rare) 3417
Imitrex Nasal Spray (Rare) 1467

Anger
Meridia Capsules 489

Angiectases, cutaneous
Adalat CC Tablets (Less than 1%) 2964

Angiitis
Indocin Capsules (Less than 1%) 1995
Indocin I.V. (Less than 1%) 2465
Indocin (Less than 1%) 1995
Timolide Tablets 2086

Angina
Amerge Tablets 1339
Aromasin Tablets (1.6%) 2600
Caduet Tablets 2508
Cardizem LA Extended Release Tablets (Less than 2%) 1728
Clozaril Tablets (1%) 2184
Combivent Inhalation Aerosol (Less than 2%) 847
Concerta Extended-Release Tablets 1881
Copegus Tablets (Less than 1%) 2754
Daytrana Transdermal Patch 3174
FazaClo Orally Disintegrating Tablets (1%) 551
Femara Tablets (Less than or equal to 2%) 2214
Focalin Tablets 2220
Focalin XR Capsules 2223
Foradil Aerolizer 3010
Hyperstat I.V. 3017
Imitrex Nasal Spray 1467
Imitrex Tablets (Rare) 1471
▲ Intron A for Injection (Less than 5%) 3024
Levothroid Tablets 1186
Levoxyl Tablets 1712
Lofibra Tablets 1219
Lofibra Capsules 1216
▲ Lupron Depot 7.5 mg (Less than 5%) 3264
Metadate CD Capsules 3323
Migranal Nasal Spray (Rare) 3348
OptiPranolol Metipranolol Ophthalmic Solution 0.3% (A small number of patients) ⊙256
Orthoclone OKT3 Sterile Solution (Less than 1%) 2360
PEG-Intron Powder for Injection (Less than or equal to 1%) 3048
Prevacid Delayed-Release Capsules (Less than 1%) 3271
Prevacid for Delayed-Release Oral Suspension (Less than 1%) 3271
Prevacid SoluTab Delayed-Release Orally Disintegrating Tablets (Less than 1%) 3271
Prevacid NapraPAC (Less than 1%) 3280
PREVPAC (Less than 1%) 3284
Prilosec OTC Delayed-Release Tablets (Less than 1%) 2677
Proleukin for Injection 2266
Proventil Inhalation Aerosol 3053
Proventil HFA Inhalation Aerosol 3056
Ritalin Hydrochloride Tablets 2269
Ritalin LA Capsules 2271
Ritalin-SR Tablets 2269
Rituxan I.V. (One patient) 1254
Tamiflu Capsules (Less than 1%) 2807
Tamiflu Oral Suspension (Less than 1%) 2807
Tarka Tablets (0.3% or more) 524
Taxotere Injection Concentrate (Rare) 2932
Tiazac Capsules (Less than 2%) 1201
Tricor Tablets 527
Triglide Tablets 3123
Univasc Tablets (Less than 1%) 3104
Ventolin HFA Inhalation Aerosol 1600
VoSpire ER Tablets 1052
Zegerid Capsules (Less than 1%) 2958
Zegerid Powder for Oral Solution (Less than 1%) 2958
Zofran Injection (Rare) 1634
Zofran (Rare) 1639
Zofran ODT Orally Disintegrating Tablets (Rare) 1639

Angina, crescendo
BiDil Tablets 2171
Nitro-Dur Transdermal Infusion System (Uncommon) 3046

Angina, increased
Lotrel Capsules (Rare) 2249
Nitro-Dur Transdermal Infusion System (2%) 3046
Norvasc Tablets (Rare) 2545

Angina, Prinzmetal's, episodes of
Imitrex Injection 1463
Imitrex Nasal Spray 1467

Angina pectoris
Abilify Oral Solution (Infrequent) 882
Abilify Oral Solution (Infrequent) 2450
Abilify Discmelt Orally Disintegrating Tablets (Infrequent) 882
Abilify Discmelt Orally Disintegrating Tablets (Infrequent) 2450
Abilify Tablets (Infrequent) 882
Abilify Tablets (Infrequent) 2450
Aciphex Tablets 1090
Actiq (Less than 1%) 979
Actonel Tablets (2.5%) 2683
Actonel with Calcium Tablets (2.5%) 2688
Aggrenox Capsules 822
Agrylin Capsules (1% to 5%) 3169
▲ Altace Capsules (3%) 1702
Ambien Tablets (Rare) 2851
Ambien CR Tablets (Rare) 2855
▲ Aranesp for Injection (8%) 581
Argatroban Injection (1.8%) 1346
Aricept Tablets (Infrequent) 1094
Aricept ODT Tablets (Infrequent) 1094
Arimidex Tablets (1.7%) 673
Atacand Tablets (Less frequently) 649
Atacand HCT (Less than 0.5%) 651
Avalide Tablets 888
Avalide Tablets 2874
Avapro Tablets (Less than 1%) 891
Avapro Tablets (Less than 1%) 2871
Azilect Tablets (Greater than 1%) 3293
Caduet Tablets (Less than 2%) 2508
Campath Ampules 811
Campral Tablets (Infrequent) 1174
Camptosar Injection 2604
Captopril Tablets (2 to 3 of 1000 patients) 2149
Cardene I.V. (Rare) 2497
Cardura XL Tablets (Less than 1%) 2515
Celebrex Capsules (0.1% to 1.9%) 3134
Celexa (Infrequent) 1176
▲ CellCept Capsules (3% to less than 20%) 2747
▲ CellCept Intravenous (3% to less than 20%) 2747
▲ CellCept Oral Suspension (3% to less than 20%) 2747
▲ CellCept Tablets (3% to less than 20%) 2747
Chantix Tablets (Infrequent) 2517
Cialis Tablets (Less than 2%) 1838
Cipro (Less than 1%) 2977
Cipro I.V. (1% or less) 2984
Cipro XR Tablets 2990
▲ Coreg Tablets (2% to 6%) 1414
Cosopt Sterile Ophthalmic Solution 1931
Covera-HS Tablets (2% or less) 3139
Cozaar Tablets (Less than 1%) 1935
Crestor Tablets (Greater than or equal to 1%) 678
Crixivan Capsules 1940
Doxil Injection (Less than 1%) 2351
Effexor Tablets (Infrequent) 3411
Effexor XR Capsules (Infrequent) 3417
Eldepryl Capsules 3208
Evoxac Capsules (Less than 1%) 1047
Exelon Capsules (Frequent) 2206
Exelon Oral Solution (Frequent) 2206
Exubera Inhalation Powder (0.7%) 2524
Ferrlecit Injection 3388
Forteo for Injection (2.5%) 1767
▲ Fortical Nasal Spray (1% to 3%) 3337
Fuzeon Injection 2767
Gabitril Tablets (Infrequent) 984
Geodon Capsules (Infrequent) 2529
Hyzaar 50-12.5 Tablets 1990
Hyzaar 100-12.5 Tablets 1990
Hyzaar 100-25 Tablets 1990
Imitrex Injection 1463
Imitrex Tablets 1471
Inspra Tablets 2536
Kytril (Rare) 2784
Lamictal (Rare) 1481
Levaquin (0.1% to 0.9%) 2384
Levaquin in 5% Dextrose Injection (0.1% to 0.9%) 2384
Levitra Tablets (Less than 2%) 3034
Lipitor Tablets (Less than 2%) 2483
Lofibra Tablets 1219
Lofibra Capsules 1216
Maxalt Tablets (Rare) 2008
Maxalt-MLT Orally Disintegrating Tablets (Rare) 2008
Meridia Capsules 489

▲ Miacalcin Nasal Spray (1% to 3%) ... 2253
Micardis Tablets (More than 0.3%).... 854
Micardis HCT Tablets 856
Midamor Tablets (Less than or equal to 1%) 2026
Mirapex Tablets (Less than 1%)........ 859
Mobic Oral Suspension (Less than 2%).................................. 863
Mobic Tablets (Less than 2%)........... 863
Moduretic Tablets (Less than or equal to 1%) 2028
Namenda (Infrequent) 1195
▲ Natrecor for Injection (2% to 6%) 3127
Neurontin Capsules (Infrequent)....... 2487
Neurontin Oral Solution (Infrequent)................................ 2487
Neurontin Tablets (Infrequent).......... 2487
Nipent for Injection (Less than 3%)... 1863
Omacor Capsules (1.3%)................ 2725
Ortho-Cyclen/Ortho Tri-Cyclen 2429
Ortho Tri-Cyclen Lo Tablets 2436
Paxil CR Controlled-Release Tablets (Rare) 1538
Paxil (Rare).................................. 1530
Permax Tablets (Infrequent)............ 3356
Persantine Tablets (Rare)................ 868
Pexeva Tablets (rare)..................... 1694
Photofrin for Injection.................... 702
Pletal Tablets (2% or greater).......... 2455
Prinivil Tablets (Greater than 1%)...... 2052
Prinzide Tablets 2056
▲ Prograf Capsules and Injection (3% to 15%)............................. 632
▲ Prometrium Capsules (100 mg, 200 mg) (less than 5%)............... 3203
Proquin XR Tablets........................ 1153
Protonix I.V. (Less than 1%)............. 3472
Protonix Tablets (Less than 1%)........ 3469
Protopic Ointment (Greater than or equal to 1%)............................ 638
Prozac Pulvules and Liquid (Infrequent)............................. 1801
ReFacto Vials............................... 3484
Relpax Tablets (Rare)...................... 2548
Requip Tablets (Infrequent).............. 1555
Revlimid Capsules 958
Rilutek Tablets (Infrequent).............. 2930
Risperdal (Rare)............................ 1676
Risperdal Consta Long-Acting Injection (Infrequent) 1682
Risperdal M-Tab Orally Disintegrating Tablets (Rare)......... 1676
Rythmol SR Capsules (2%)............... 2727
Seroquel Tablets (Infrequent)........... 690
▲ Simulect for Injection (3% to 10%) ... 2284
Sonata Capsules (Infrequent)............ 1717
▲ Spiriva HandiHaler (1% to 3%) 869
Symbyax Capsules (Rare)................. 1819
Tambocor Tablets (Less than 1%)..... 1856
Targretin Capsules......................... 1747
Tasmar Tablets (Infrequent).............. 3358
Teveten Tablets (Less than 1%)........ 1735
Teveten HCT Tablets (Less than 1%)..................................... 1737
Thalomid Capsules......................... 965
Timolide Tablets 2086
Topamax Sprinkle Capsules (Infrequent) 2404
Topamax Tablets (Infrequent)........... 2404
▲ Travatan Ophthalmic Solution (1% to 5%).................................. 563
Tricor Tablets 527
Triglide Tablets 3123
Uroxatral Tablets 2943
Vasotec I.V. Injection (1.5%)............ 2103
Verelan PM Extended-Release Capsules, Controlled-Onset (2% or less)................................... 3106
Viagra Tablets (Less than 2%).......... 2573
Vivitrol 995
Xalatan Sterile Ophthalmic Solution (1% to 2%)................... 2649
Zelapar Tablets 3372
Zelnorm Tablets 2312
Zomig Tablets (Rare)...................... 3519
Zomig Nasal Spray (Rare)................ 3523
Zomig-ZMT Tablets (Rare)............... 3519
Zostavax Injection (0.3% to 0.9%)..... 2111

Angina pectoris, aggravation

Aldoril Tablets.............................. 1910
Blocadren Tablets (Less than 1%)..... 1916
▲ Coreg Tablets (Greater than 1% to 3%).................................... 1414
Eldepryl Capsules.......................... 3208
▲ Imdur Tablets (Less than or equal to 5%).................................. 3018
Sandostatin LAR Depot (Rare).......... 2280
▲ Spiriva HandiHaler (1% to 3%) 869
Timoptic Sterile Ophthalmic Solution (Less frequent)............... 2088
Timoptic in Ocudose (Less frequent).................................. 2091
Timoptic-XE Sterile Ophthalmic Gel Forming Solution 2092

Angina pectoris, exacerbation of, post-abrupt discontinuation

Inderal LA Long-Acting Capsules...... 3429
Toprol-XL Tablets 668

Angina tonsillaris

Invirase (Less than 2%)................... 2772

Angina, unstable

Rythmol SR Capsules...................... 2727
Tamiflu Capsules (Less than 1%)...... 2807
Vivitrol 995

Angioedema

(*see also under* Edema, angioneurotic)

Abilify Oral Solution (Rare)............... 882
Abilify Oral Solution (Rare)............... 2450
Abilify Discmelt Orally Disintegrating Tablets (Rare)......... 882
Abilify Discmelt Orally Disintegrating Tablets (Rare) 2450
Abilify Tablets (Rare) 882
Abilify Tablets (Rare) 2450
Aceon Tablets (2 mg, 4 mg, 8 mg) (0.1%) 3194
▲ Acetadote Injection (1.62% to 7.73%) 1031
Aciphex Tablets 1090
Actonel Tablets (Very rare) 2683
Actonel with Calcium Tablets (Very rare) 2688
Adderall Tablets (Rare) 3164
Adderall XR Capsules 3166
Advair HFA Inhalation Aerosol (Rare) 1318
Advicor Tablets (Rare) 1722
Aldara Cream, 5% 1846
Aldurazyme for Intravenous Infusion 1268
Allegra (Rare) 2844
Allegra-D 12 Hour Extended-Release Tablets (Rare) ... 2846
Allegra-D 24 Hour Extended-Release Tablets (Rare) ... 2849
AmBisome for Injection (Infrequent) 620
Amevive 626
Aminohippurate Sodium PAH Injection 1913
Angeliq Tablets 762
Aredia for Injection (Rare) 2179
Arimidex Tablets (Very rare) 673
Arthrotec Tablets (Rare) 3129
Atacand Tablets (Less frequently) 649
Atacand HCT (Less than 0.5%) 651
Atrovent HFA Inhalation Aerosol 841
Avalide Tablets (Rare) 888
Avalide Tablets (Rare) 2874
Avandaryl Tablets (Rare) 1379
Avapro Tablets (Rare) 891
Avapro Tablets (Rare) 2871
Avelox 2970
Bayer Aspirin 744
Beconase AQ Nasal Spray (Rare) 1396
BeneFix Vials 3408
Benicar Tablets 1043
Benicar HCT Tablets (Rare) 1044
BiDil Tablets (1% to less than 2%) 2171
Caduet Tablets (Greater than 0.1% to less than or equal to 1%) 2508
Campath Ampules 811
Captopril Tablets (Approximately 1 in 1000 patients) 2149
Cardizem LA Extended Release Tablets (Infrequent) 1728
Catapres Tablets 843
Ceftin 1407
Celebrex Capsules (Less than 0.1%) 3134
Celexa 1176
▲ Cerezyme for Injection (Approximately 6.6%) 1270
Cipro (Less than 1%) 2977
Cipro I.V. (1% or less) 2984
Colazal Capsules 2838
Comvax 1928
Copaxone for Injection (Infrequent) .. 3297
Cosopt Sterile Ophthalmic Solution 1931
Cozaar Tablets (Rare) 1935
Crestor Tablets (Less than 1%) 678
Decadron Tablets 1951
Demadex Injection 2759
Demadex Tablets 2759
depo-subQ provera 104 Injectable Suspension 2624
Detrol LA Capsules 2631
Didronel Tablets 2697
Diovan Tablets (Rare) 2193
Diovan HCT Tablets (Rare)................ 2196
DynaCirc CR Tablets....................... 2721
Eloxatin for Injection 2892
Emcyt Capsules............................. 2634
Emend Capsules (One patient)......... 1963
Enbrel for Injection......................... 584
Enjuvia Tablets.............................. 1062
Estrasorb Topical Emulsion.............. 1147
Estratest Tablets 3199
Estratest H.S. Tablets..................... 3199
Faslodex Injection (Less than 1%)..... 681
Flovent Diskus (Rare)...................... 1443
Flovent HFA 1447
Fluarix 1451
Foradil Aerolizer (Rare).................... 3010
Fortaz (Very rare)........................... 1453
Fosamax (Rare).............................. 1969
Fosamax Plus D Tablets (Rarely)....... 1977
GamaSTAN................................... 3234
Gantrisin Pediatric Suspension......... 2770
Gleevec Tablets (Rare) 2227
Herceptin I.V. 1233
Hycamtin for Injection (Rare) 1458
Hyzaar 50-12.5 Tablets (Rare) 1990
Hyzaar 100-12.5 Tablets (Rare) 1990
Hyzaar 100-25 Tablets (Rare) 1990
Indocin (Less than 1%) 1995
Keflex Capsules 549
Ketek Tablets (Rare) 2903
Lamisil Tablets (Rare) 2232
Levaquin 2384
Levaquin in 5% Dextrose Injection 2384
Levothroid Tablets 1186
Levoxyl Tablets 1712
Lexapro Oral Solution 1190
Lexapro Tablets 1190
Lithobid Tablets 1692
Lotensin Tablets (Less than 1%) 2243
Lotensin HCT Tablets (0.3%) 2246
Lotrel Capsules (About 0.5%) 2249
Lyrica Capsules (Rare) 2539
Maxalt Tablets 2008
Maxalt-MLT Orally Disintegrating Tablets 2008
Menostar Transdermal System 782
Merrem I.V. 686
Micardis Tablets (Single case) 854
Micardis HCT Tablets 856
Mintezol 2027
Mobic Oral Suspension (Less than 2%) 863
Mobic Tablets (Less than 2%) 863
Nalfon Capsules (Less than 1%) 2502
Nasonex Nasal Spray 3043
Nembutal Sodium Solution, USP 2470
Neurontin Capsules 2487
Neurontin Oral Solution 2487
Neurontin Tablets 2487
Nexium Delayed-Release Capsules (Less than 1%) 655
Nexium I.V. (Less than 1%) 659
Noroxin Tablets 2032
Norvasc Tablets (More than 0.1% to 1%) 2545
Parcopa Orally Disintegrating Tablets 3097
Pediarix Vaccine 1548
Persantine Tablets (Rare) 868
Pexeva Tablets (rare) 1694
Plavix Tablets 917
Plavix Tablets 2926
Premarin Intravenous 3442
Premarin Tablets 3446
Premarin Vaginal Cream 3452
Premphase Tablets 3456
Prempro Tablets 3456
Prinivil Tablets (0.1% to 1.0%) 2052
Proquin XR Tablets 1153
Protonix I.V. 3472
Protonix Tablets 3469
Protopic Ointment (Greater than or equal to 1%) 638
Proventil Inhalation Aerosol 3053
Qvar Inhalation Aerosol (Rare) 3303
Raniclor Tablets, Chewable (Rare) 2505
Rebetron Combination Therapy 3063
Recombivax HB (Less than 1%) 2071
Reyataz Capsules (Less than 3%) 921
Rhinocort Aqua Nasal Spray (Rare) .. 665
Risperdal 1676
Risperdal Consta Long-Acting Injection 1682
Risperdal M-Tab Orally Disintegrating Tablets 1676
▲ Rituxan I.V. (1% to 11%) 1254
Seasonique Tablets 1077
Singulair 2077
Spiriva HandiHaler (Less than 1%) 869
St. Joseph 81 mg Aspirin Chewable and Enteric Coated Tablets 1869
St. Joseph 81 mg Aspirin.................. ▣ 688
Stalevo Tablets.............................. 2287
Suprax 1843
Synera Topical Patch...................... 1137
Thalomid Capsules......................... 965
Timoptic Sterile Ophthalmic Solution 2088
Timoptic in Ocudose....................... 2091
Timoptic-XE Sterile Ophthalmic Gel Forming Solution 2092
Tindamax Tablets........................... 2142
TNKase I.V. (Rare).......................... 1264
Trusopt Sterile Ophthalmic Solution 2095
Twinrix Vaccine............................. 1595
Uniretic Tablets (Less than 0.5% to more than 1%)........................... 3100
Univasc Tablets (Less than 1%)......... 3104
Uroxatral Tablets........................... 2943
Valtrex Caplets 1597
Vasotec I.V. Injection...................... 2103
Ventolin HFA Inhalation Aerosol 1600
VFEND I.V. (Less than 2%) 2564
VFEND Oral Suspension (Less than 2%) 2564
VFEND Tablets (Less than 2%) 2564
Viramune Oral Suspension 873
Viramune Tablets 873
Voltaren Tablets (Rarely) 2307
Voltaren-XR Tablets (Rarely) 2310
VoSpire ER Tablets (Rare) 1052
Vytorin 10/40 Tablets 2114
Xenical Capsules 2831
Xopenex Inhalation Solution 3146
Xopenex Inhalation Solution Concentrate 3150
Xopenex HFA Inhalation Aerosol 3154
Zetia Tablets 2120
Zetia Tablets 3083
Zinacef for Injection 1631
Zinacef Injection 1631
Zmax for Oral Suspension 2583
Zofran Injection 1634
Zofran 1639
Zofran ODT Orally Disintegrating Tablets 1639
Zoloft 2586
Zyprexa Tablets 1830
Zyprexa ZYDIS Orally Disintegrating Tablets 1830

Angioedema, extremities

Aceon Tablets (2 mg, 4 mg, 8 mg) (0.1%) 3194
Altace Capsules 1702
Captopril Tablets (Approximately 1 in 1000 patients) 2149
Lotensin Tablets 2243
Lotrel Capsules 2249
Mavik Tablets 486
Pegasys 2789
Prinivil Tablets (0.1%) 2052
Prinzide Tablets (Rare) 2056
Uniretic Tablets 3100
Vasotec I.V. Injection 2103

Angioedema, eyes

▲ Advair HFA Inhalation Aerosol (1% to 3%) 1318
Altace Capsules 1702
Captopril Tablets 2149
Uniretic Tablets 3100

Angioedema, face

Aceon Tablets (2 mg, 4 mg, 8 mg) (0.3% to 1%) 3194
Altace Capsules 1702
Atrovent HFA Inhalation Aerosol 841
Atrovent Nasal Spray 0.06% 839
Avalide Tablets (Rare) 888
Avalide Tablets (Rare) 2874
Avapro Tablets (Rare) 891
Avapro Tablets (Rare) 2871
Captopril Tablets (Approximately 1 in 1000 patients) 2149
Catapres-TTS (2 of 3,539 patients) 844
Cozaar Tablets (Rare) 1935
Crestor Tablets (Less than 1%) 678
Flomax Capsules 850
Hyzaar 50-12.5 Tablets (Rare) 1990
Hyzaar 100-12.5 Tablets (Rare) 1990
Hyzaar 100-25 Tablets (Rare) 1990
Lotensin Tablets 2243
Lotrel Capsules (About 0.5%) 2249
Mavik Tablets (0.13%) 486
Prinivil Tablets 2052
Prinzide Tablets (Rare) 2056
Uniretic Tablets (Less than 0.5%) 3100
Vasotec I.V. Injection 2103

Angioedema, glottis
Aceon Tablets (2 mg, 4 mg, 8 mg) (0.1%) 3194
Altace Capsules 1702
Captopril Tablets (Approximately 1 in 1000 patients) 2149
Cozaar Tablets (Rare) 1935
Hyzaar 50-12.5 Tablets (Rare) 1990
Hyzaar 100-12.5 Tablets (Rare) 1990
Hyzaar 100-25 Tablets (Rare) 1990
Lotensin Tablets 2243
Lotrel Capsules (About 0.5%) 2249
Mavik Tablets (0.3% to 1.0%) 486
Prinivil Tablets 2052
Prinzide Tablets (Rare) 2056
Tarka Tablets 524
Uniretic Tablets 3100
Vasotec I.V. Injection 2103

Angioedema, intestinal
Aceon Tablets (2 mg, 4 mg, 8 mg) 3194
Altace Capsules 1702
Captopril Tablets 2149
Lotensin Tablets 2243
Mavik Tablets 486
Prinivil Tablets (Rare) 2052
Prinzide Tablets (Rare) 2056

Angioedema, larynx
Aceon Tablets (2 mg, 4 mg, 8 mg) (0.1%) 3194
Activase I.V. 1223
Altace Capsules 1702
Captopril Tablets (Approximately 1 in 1000 patients) 2149
Levaquin 2384
Levaquin in 5% Dextrose Injection 2384
Lotensin Tablets 2243
Mavik Tablets 486
Prinivil Tablets 2052
Prinzide Tablets (Rare) 2056
Uniretic Tablets 3100
Vasotec I.V. Injection 2103

Angioedema, lips
Aceon Tablets (2 mg, 4 mg, 8 mg) (0.1%) 3194
Altace Capsules 1702
Atrovent HFA Inhalation Aerosol 841
Atrovent Nasal Spray 0.06% 839
Avalide Tablets (Rare) 888
Avalide Tablets (Rare) 2874
Avapro Tablets (Rare) 891
Avapro Tablets (Rare) 2871
Captopril Tablets (Approximately 1 in 1000 patients) 2149
Cozaar Tablets (Rare) 1935
Flomax Capsules 850
Hyzaar 50-12.5 Tablets (Rare) 1990
Hyzaar 100-12.5 Tablets (Rare) 1990
Hyzaar 100-25 Tablets (Rare) 1990
Lotensin Tablets 2243
Lotrel Capsules 2249
Mavik Tablets 486
Prinivil Tablets 2052
Prinzide Tablets (Rare) 2056
Uniretic Tablets 3100
Vasotec I.V. Injection 2103

Angioedema, mucous membranes of the mouth
Activase I.V. 1223
Captopril Tablets 2149

Angioedema, oropharyngeal
Avalide Tablets (Rare) 888
Avalide Tablets (Rare) 2874
Avapro Tablets (Rare) 891
Avapro Tablets (Rare) 2871
Cozaar Tablets (Rare) 1935
Hyzaar 50-12.5 Tablets (Rare) 1990
Hyzaar 100-12.5 Tablets (Rare) 1990
Hyzaar 100-25 Tablets (Rare) 1990

Angioedema, throat
Levaquin 2384
Levaquin in 5% Dextrose Injection 2384

Angioedema of tongue
Aceon Tablets (2 mg, 4 mg, 8 mg) (0.1%) 3194
Altace Capsules 1702
Atrovent HFA Inhalation Aerosol 841
Atrovent Nasal Spray 0.06% 839
Avalide Tablets (Rare) 888
Avalide Tablets (Rare) 2874
Avapro Tablets (Rare) 891
Avapro Tablets (Rare) 2871
Captopril Tablets (Approximately 1 in 1000 patients) 2149
Catapres-TTS (One case) 844
Cozaar Tablets (Rare) 1935
Flomax Capsules 850
Hyzaar 50-12.5 Tablets (Rare) 1990
Hyzaar 100-12.5 Tablets (Rare) 1990
Hyzaar 100-25 Tablets (Rare) 1990
Levaquin 2384
Levaquin in 5% Dextrose Injection 2384
Lotensin Tablets 2243
Lotrel Capsules (About 0.5%) 2249
Mavik Tablets 486
Prinivil Tablets 2052
Prinzide Tablets (Rare) 2056
Uniretic Tablets 3100
Vasotec I.V. Injection 2103

Angitis, necrotizing
Lopressor HCT 50/25 Tablets 2241
Lopressor HCT 100/25 Tablets 2241
Lopressor HCT 100/50 Tablets 2241

Anhidrosis
Cesamet Capsules 3340

Anisocoria
Betoptic S Ophthalmic Suspension 558
Lyrica Capsules (Rare) 2539
Paxil CR Controlled-Release Tablets (Rare) 1538
Paxil (Rare) 1530
Pexeva Tablets (Rare) 1694

Anophthalmos
Thalomid Capsules 965

Anorexia
Abelcet Injection 1141
Abilify Oral Solution 882
Abilify Oral Solution 2450
Abilify Discmelt Orally Disintegrating Tablets 882
Abilify Discmelt Orally Disintegrating Tablets 2450
Abilify Tablets 882
Abilify Tablets 2450
Aciphex Tablets 1090
▲ Actimmune (3%) 1671
Actiq (Less than 1%) 979
Adderall Tablets 3164
▲ Adderall XR Capsules (2.9% to 33%) 3166
Advicor Tablets 1722
Aggrenox Capsules (1.2%) 822
▲ Agrylin Capsules (7.7%) 3169
Aldoril Tablets 1910
▲ Alferon N Injection (1% to 68%) 1665
▲ Alimta for Injection (1% to 62%) 1750
Alinia for Oral Suspension (Less than 1%) 2835
Alinia Tablets (Less than 1%) 2835
Aloxi Injection (Less than 1%) 2127
Altace Capsules (Less than 1%) 1702
Altoprev Extended-Release Tablets (Rare) 3109
Ambien Tablets (1%) 2851
Ambien CR Tablets (Infrequent) 2855
AmBisome for Injection (Less common) 620
Anzemet Injection (Rare) 2859
Anzemet Tablets (Rare) 2862
Aptivus Capsules (Less than 2%) 826
▲ Aredia for Injection (1% to 20.8%) 2179
▲ Aricept Tablets (3% to 7%) 1094
▲ Aricept ODT Tablets (3% to 7%) 1094
▲ Arimidex Tablets (5% to 8%) 673
▲ Aromasin Tablets (6%) 2600
▲ Arranon Injection (0% to 9%) 1357
Arthrotec Tablets (Rare) 3129
Asacol Delayed-Release Tablets 2692
Asmanex Twisthaler (1% to less than 3%) 2966
Atacand HCT 651
Atripla Tablets (Greater than or equal to 2%) 945
Avalide Tablets 888
Avalide Tablets 2874
▲ Avastin IV (35% to 43%) 1227
Avelox (0.1% to less than 2%) 2970
▲ Avinza Capsules (5% to 10%) 1741
Axid Oral Solution (1.2%) 879
▲ Azilect Tablets (5%) 3293
Bentyl Capsules 697
Bentyl Injection 697
Bentyl Syrup 697
Bentyl Tablets 697
▲ Bexxar (0% to 14%) 1398
Biaxin/Biaxin XL 402
Biltricide Tablets 2976
Buprenex Injectable (Rare) 2716
Caduet Tablets (Greater than 0.1% to less than 2%) 2508
Calcijex Injection 411
Calcium Disodium Versenate Injection 1851
▲ Campath Ampules (20%) 811
▲ Campral Tablets (2% to 5%) 1174
▲ Camptosar Injection (5% to 55%%) 2604
Cancidas for Injection (0% to 1.3%) 1918
Captopril Tablets (About 0.5% to 2%) 2149
Carbatrol Capsules 3171
Cardizem LA Extended Release Tablets (Less than 2%) 1728
Cardura XL Tablets 2515
▲ Carnitor Injection (3% to 6%) 3188
Catapres Tablets (About 1 in 100 patients) 843
Catapres-TTS (0.5% or less) 844
Ceftin Tablets (0.1% to 1%) 1407
Celebrex Capsules (0.1% to 1.9%) 3134
▲ Celexa (4%) 1176
▲ CellCept Capsules (3% to 25.3%) 2747
▲ CellCept Intravenous (3% to 25.3%) 2747
▲ CellCept Oral Suspension (3% to 25.3%) 2747
▲ CellCept Tablets (3% to 25.3%) 2747
▲ Cesamet Capsules (8%) 3340
Chantix Tablets (1% to 2%) 2517
Cipro (Less than 1%) 2977
Cipro I.V. (1% or less) 2984
Cipro XR Tablets (Less than 1%) 2990
▲ Clarinex Syrup (4.5%) 2995
Clarinex-D 24-Hour Extended-Release Tablets (2%) 2998
Clinoril Tablets (Greater than 1%) 1924
▲ Clolar for Intravenous Infusion (31%) 1271
Clorpres Tablets (About 1%) 2153
Clozaril Tablets (1%) 2184
Colazal Capsules (2%) 2838
▲ Combivir Tablets (10%) 1411
▲ Comvax (0.8% to 3.9%) 1928
▲ Concerta Extended-Release Tablets (0.7% to 4%) 1881
▲ Copaxone for Injection (8%) 3297
▲ Copegus Tablets (24%) 2754
Cosmegen for Injection 2459
Cosopt Sterile Ophthalmic Solution 1931
Cozaar Tablets (Less than 1%) 1935
Crixivan Capsules (2.7%) 1940
Cuprimine Capsules 1947
▲ Cymbalta Delayed-Release Capsules (3% to 5%) 1757
▲ Dacogen Injection (16%) 2129
Dalmane Capsules (Rare) 3342
Dantrium Capsules (Rare) 2694
▲ DAPTACEL Vaccine (9% to 17.6%) 2950
▲ Daranide Tablets (Among the most common effects) 1950
Daraprim Tablets 1419
▲ Daytrana Transdermal Patch (4% to 46%) 3174
▲ Depacon Injection (4% to 12%) 412
▲ Depakene (11% to 12%) 417
▲ Depakote Sprinkle Capsules (4% to 12%) 422
▲ Depakote Tablets (1% to 12%) 427
▲ Depakote ER Tablets (11% to 12%) 434
Dexedrine 1420
DextroStat Tablets 3179
Diastat Rectal Delivery System (Less than 1%) 3343
Dilaudid 440
Dilaudid Non-Sterile Powder 440
Dilaudid Oral Liquid 445
Dilaudid Rectal Suppositories 440
Dilaudid Tablets 440
Dilaudid Tablets - 8 mg 445
Dilaudid-HP (Less frequent) 442
Diovan Tablets (Less frequent) 2193
Diovan HCT Tablets (Less frequent) 2196
Diuril Oral Suspension 1954
Diuril Sodium Intravenous 2467
Dolobid Tablets (Less than 1 in 100) 1955
▲ Doxil Injection (1% to 20.1%) 2351
▲ Duragesic Transdermal System (3% to 10%) 2373
Edecrin 1959
▲ E.E.S. (Among most frequent) 451
▲ Effexor Tablets (11% to 17.0%) 3411
▲ Effexor XR Capsules (5% to 20%) 3417
Eldepryl Capsules 3208
Elmiron Capsules (Less than or equal to 1%) 2415
▲ Eloxatin for Injection (1% to 29%) 2892
Elspar for Injection 2463
Elspar for Injection 1960
▲ Emcyt Capsules (4%) 2634
▲ Emend Capsules (4.3% to 10.1%) 1963
Enbrel for Injection 584
Engerix-B Vaccine (Less than 1%) 1425
▲ Epivir (10%) 1427
Equetro Extended-Release Capsules 3180
▲ Erbitux (2% to 36%) 910
▲ EryPed (Among most frequent) 447
▲ Ery-Tab Tablets (Among most frequent) 449
▲ Erythrocin Stearate Filmtab Tablets (Among most frequent) 453
▲ Erythromycin Base Filmtab Tablets (Among most frequent) 455
▲ Erythromycin Delayed-Release Capsules, USP (Among most frequent) 457
▲ Eulexin Capsules (4%) 3009
▲ Evoxac Capsules (1% to 3%) 1047
▲ Exelon Capsules (6% to 17%) 2206
▲ Exelon Oral Solution (6% to 17%) 2206
Famvir Tablets (1.1% to 2.6%) 2211
▲ Faslodex Injection (9%) 681
FazaClo Orally Disintegrating Tablets (1%) 551
▲ Femara Tablets (3% to 5%) 2214
Ferrlecit Injection 3388
Flumadine (1.6%) 1183
▲ Focalin Tablets (6%) 2220
Focalin XR Capsules 2223
Fortical Nasal Spray (Less than 1%) 3337
Frova Tablets (Infrequent) 1113
Furosemide Tablets 2154
Fuzeon Injection (2.3%) 2767
Gabitril Tablets (1% or more) 984
Gantrisin Pediatric Suspension 2770
▲ Gemzar for Injection (16%) 1771
▲ Gengraf Capsules (Less than 2% to 3%) 459
Geodon (2% to frequent) 2529
▲ Gleevec Tablets (0% to 17%) 2227
Guanidine Hydrochloride Tablets 3016
▲ Havrix Vaccine (1% to 19%) 1456
▲ Hectorol Capsules (4.9%) 1275
▲ Hectorol Injection (4.9%) 1278
▲ Herceptin I.V. (14%) 1233
HibTITER 3426
▲ Hycamtin for Injection (Up to 19%) 1458
Hyperstat I.V. 3017
Hyzaar 50-12.5 Tablets 1990
Hyzaar 100-12.5 Tablets 1990
Hyzaar 100-25 Tablets 1990
▲ Indapamide Tablets (Less than 5%) 2156
Indocin (Less than 1%) 1995
▲ Infergen (21% to 24%) 3364
▲ Intron A for Injection (1% to 69%) 3024
Invanz for Injection (Greater than 0.1%) 1999
Invirase (Less than 2%) 2772
▲ Iressa Tablets (7% to 11%) 684
▲ I.V. Busulfex (21% to 85%) 2493
Kadian Capsules (Less than 3%) 577
Kaletra (Up to 2%) 476
▲ Keppra Injection (3%) 3320
▲ Keppra Oral Solution (3% to 13%) 3314
▲ Keppra Tablets (3% to 13%) 3314
Ketek Tablets (Greater than or equal to 0.2% to less than 2%) 2903
Kionex Powder 2477
Klonopin 2778
Lamictal (2%) 1481
Lamisil Tablets 2232
Lanoxicaps Capsules (Common) 1490
Lanoxin Injection (Common) 1494
Lanoxin Injection Pediatric 1497
Lanoxin Tablets 1500
▲ Lariam Tablets (Among most frequent) 2786
Lescol Capsules 2233
Lescol XL Tablets 2233
▲ Leukine (13% to 54%) 814
Levaquin (0.1% to 0.9%) 2384
Levaquin in 5% Dextrose Injection (0.1% to 0.9%) 2384
Lexapro Oral Solution 1190
Lexapro Tablets 1190
Lipitor Tablets (Less than 2%) 2483
Lithobid Tablets 1692
▲ Lithostat Tablets (20% to 25%) 2140
Lofibra Tablets 1219
Lofibra Capsules 1216
Lopressor HCT 50/25 Tablets 2241
Lopressor HCT 100/25 Tablets 2241
Lopressor HCT 100/50 Tablets 2241
Lotensin HCT Tablets (0.3% to 1%) 2246
Lunesta Tablets (Infrequent) 3142
Lupron Depot 7.5 mg (Less than 5%) 3264
▲ Malarone Pediatric Tablets (5%) 1517
▲ Malarone Tablets (5%) 1517
Marinol Capsules (Less than 1%) 3333
Matulane Capsules 3191
Maxair Autohaler 1852
Maxalt Tablets (Rare) 2008
Maxalt-MLT Orally Disintegrating Tablets (Rare) 2008
▲ Menactra Vaccine (0.3% to 11.8%) 2954
▲ Mepron Suspension (7%) 1521
▲ Meridia Capsules (13%) 489

Merrem I.V. (Greater than 0.1% to 1%) 686
▲ Metadate CD Capsules (9%) 3323
Mevacor Tablets (Rare) 2021
Miacalcin Nasal Spray (Less than 1%) 2253
▲ Midamor Tablets (3% to 8%) 2026
Migranal Nasal Spray (Rare) 3348
Mintezol 2027
Miradon Tablets 3042
▲ Mirapex Tablets (Greater than or equal to 1% to 4%) 859
▲ Moduretic Tablets (3% to 8%) 2028
MS Contin Tablets (Less frequent) 2701
Mustargen for Injection 2468
Mycamine for Injection 628
Myleran Tablets 1525
▲ Mylotarg for Injection (22% to 27%) 3431
Nadolol Tablets (1 to 5 of 1000 patients) 2159
Nalfon Capsules (Less than 1%) 2502
Namenda (Greater than or equal to 2%) 1195
Neoral Oral Solution (2% or less to 3%) 2259
Neoral Soft Gelatin Capsules (2% or less to 3%) 2259
▲ Neulasta Injection (15% to 72%) 601
▲ Neumega for Injection (Greater than or equal to 10%) 3435
▲ Neupogen for Injection (9%) 603
Neurontin Capsules (Frequent) 2487
Neurontin Oral Solution (More than 2%) 2487
Neurontin Tablets (Frequent) 2487
▲ Nexavar Tablets (0% to 16%) 746
Nexium Delayed-Release Capsules (Less than 1%) 655
Nexium I.V. (Less than 1%) 659
▲ Nipent for Injection (13% to 16%) 1863
Niravam Orally Disintegrating Tablets 3092
Noroxin Tablets (Less frequent) 2032
Norvasc Tablets (More than 0.1% to 1%) 2545
▲ Norvir (1.7% to 7.8%) 503
Omacor Capsules 2725
Omnicef Capsules (0.3%) 511
Omnicef for Oral Suspension (0.3%) 511
▲ Oncaspar (Greater than 1% but less than 5%) 1145
▲ Ontak Vials (36%) 1745
Oracea Capsules 1000
Ortho-Cyclen/Ortho Tri-Cyclen 2429
Ortho Tri-Cyclen Lo Tablets 2436
Orthoclone OKT3 Sterile Solution (Less than 1%) 2360
▲ OxyContin Tablets (Between 1% and 5%) 2703
Parcopa Orally Disintegrating Tablets 3097
Parnate Tablets 1527
Paser Granules (Less frequent) 1674
▲ PCE Dispertab Tablets (Among most frequent) 515
Pediarix Vaccine 1548
▲ Pegasys (17%) 2789
▲ PEG-Intron Powder for Injection (20%) 3048
Pentasa Capsules (Less than 1% to 1.1%) 3185
Pepcid Injection (Infrequent) 2040
Pepcid (Infrequent) 2038
Percodan Tablets 1132
▲ Permax Tablets (4.8%) 3356
PhosLo GelCaps 2169
▲ Photofrin for Injection (4% to 8%) 702
Pletal Tablets (Less than 2%) 2455
Potaba (Infrequent) 1650
Prevacid Delayed-Release Capsules (Less than 1%) 3271
Prevacid for Delayed-Release Oral Suspension (Less than 1%) 3271
Prevacid SoluTab Delayed-Release Orally Disintegrating Tablets (Less than 1%) 3271
Prevacid NapraPAC (Less than 1%) 3280
PREVPAC (Less than 1%) 3284
Prezista Tablets (Less than 2%) 3306
Prilosec OTC Delayed-Release Tablets (Less than 1%) 2677
Prinivil Tablets (Greater than 1%) 2052
Prinzide Tablets 2056
▲ Prograf Capsules and Injection (3% to 34%) 632
▲ Proleukin for Injection (20%) 2266
Prometrium Capsules (100 mg, 200 mg) 3203
ProQuad (Greater than or equal to 0.2% to less than 1%) 2064
Protonix I.V. (Less than 1%) 3472
Protonix Tablets (Less than 1%) 3469
Protopic Ointment (Greater than or equal to 1%) 638
▲ Provigil Tablets (4%) 988
▲ Prozac Pulvules and Liquid (8% to 17%) 1801
▲ Pulmicort Respules (1% to 3%) 661
▲ Rapamune Oral Solution and Tablets (3% to 20%) 3475
▲ Razadyne (7% to 9%) 2399
▲ Razadyne ER Extended-Release Capsules (7% to 9%) 2399
▲ Rebetol (21% to 51%) 3058
▲ Rebetron Combination Therapy (21% to 27%) 3063
ReFacto Vials 3484
Relpax Tablets (Infrequent) 2548
▲ Requip Tablets (4%) 1555
Rescriptor Tablets 2551
Restoril Capsules (0.5% to 0.9%) 1860
▲ Retrovir Capsules (11% to 20.1%) 1560
▲ Retrovir IV Infusion (11% to 20.1%) 1564
▲ Retrovir (11% to 20.1%) 1560
▲ Revlimid Capsules (10.1% to 13.6%) 958
Reyataz Capsules (Less than 3%) 921
▲ Ribavirin, USP Capsules (21% to 51%) 3068
▲ Rilutek Tablets (3.8% to 8.6%) 2930
Risperdal (Frequent) 1676
Risperdal Consta Long-Acting Injection (Infrequent) 1682
Risperdal M-Tab Orally Disintegrating Tablets (Frequent) 1676
Ritalin Hydrochloride Tablets 2269
▲ Ritalin LA Capsules (3.1%) 2271
Ritalin-SR Tablets 2269
Rocaltrol Capsules 2798
Rocaltrol Oral Solution 2798
Rythmol SR Capsules 2727
Sandimmune (2% or less) 2275
▲ Sandostatin LAR Depot (5% to 15%) 2280
▲ Sensipar Tablets (6%) 608
Seroquel Tablets (Frequent) 690
Soltamox Oral Solution (1%) 3527
Sonata Capsules (Less than 1% to 2%) 1717
▲ Soriatane Capsules (1% to 10%) 1013
Stalevo Tablets 2287
Strattera Capsules 1814
Stromectol Tablets (0.9%) 2083
Sular Tablets (Less than or equal to 1%) 3122
Sustiva Capsules (Less than 1% to 2%) 930
Sustiva Tablets (Less than 1% to 2%) 930
▲ Sutent Capsules (1% to 33%) 2560
▲ Symlin Injection (0% to 17%) 613
▲ Symmetrel Tablets (1% to 5%) 1135
Tabloid Tablets (Less frequent) 1575
Tambocor Tablets (1% to 3%) 1856
▲ Tarceva Tablets (Less than 1% to 52%) 1259
▲ Tarceva Tablets (Less than 1% to 52%) 2444
▲ Targretin Capsules (2.4% to 22.6%) 1747
▲ Tasmar Tablets (19% to 23%) 3358
▲ Taxotere Injection Concentrate (5% to 50.7%) 2932
Tegretol/Tegretol-XR 2295
▲ Temodar Capsules (9% to 27%) 3073
Tequin Injection (Less than 0.1%) 938
Tequin Injection in 5% Dextrose (Less than 0.1%) 938
Tequin Tablets (Less than 0.1%) 938
Teveten Tablets (Less than 1%) 1735
Teveten HCT Tablets (Less than 1%) 1737
▲ Thalomid Capsules (2.8% to 9.4%) 965
▲ Thiola Tablets (16.7%) 2141
Thioridazine Hydrochloride Tablets 2163
Thiothixene Capsules 2165
Tiazac Capsules (Less than 2%) 1201
Ticlid Tablets (1.0%) 2810
Timolide Tablets 2086
Timoptic Sterile Ophthalmic Solution (Less frequent) 2088
Timoptic in Ocudose (Less frequent) 2091
Timoptic-XE Sterile Ophthalmic Gel Forming Solution 2092
Tindamax Tablets (1.5% to 2.5%) 2142
▲ TOBI Solution for Inhalation (18.6%) 2298
▲ Topamax Sprinkle Capsules (4% to 24%) 2404
▲ Topamax Tablets (4% to 24%) 2404
Trecator Tablets 3487
Trelstar LA Suspension (1.7%) 3397
Tricor Tablets 527
Triglide Tablets 3123
▲ Trileptal Tablets (3% to 5%) 2300
▲ Trileptal Oral Suspension (3% to 5%) 2300
▲ Trisenox Injection (23%) 993
▲ Trizivir Tablets (15%) 1589
Truvada Tablets 1296
Twinrix Vaccine (Less than 1%) 1595
Tygacil for Injection (0.2% to less than 2%) 3488
▲ Ultram ER Tablets (0.7% to 5.9%) 2392
Uniretic Tablets (Less than 1%) 3100
Valtrex Caplets (Less than 1% to 2%) 1597
Vandazole Vaginal Gel (Less than 1%) 3338
Vantin Tablets and Oral Suspension (Less than 1%) 2645
Vaqta (1.2%) 2097
Vasotec I.V. Injection (0.5% to 1.0%) 2103
▲ Velcade for Injection (34%) 2133
▲ Vesanoid Capsules (17%) 2820
VFEND I.V. (Less than 2%) 2564
VFEND Oral Suspension (Less than 2%) 2564
VFEND Tablets (Less than 2%) 2564
Vicoprofen Tablets (Less than 3%) 539
Viracept (Less than 2%) 2577
▲ Viread Tablets (3% to 4%) 1301
▲ Vivitrol (6% to 20%) 995
Vytorin 10/10 Tablets 2114
Vytorin 10/10 Tablets 3077
Vytorin 10/20 Tablets 2114
Vytorin 10/20 Tablets 3077
Vytorin 10/40 Tablets 2114
Vytorin 10/40 Tablets 3077
Vytorin 10/80 Tablets 2114
Vytorin 10/80 Tablets 3077
▲ Wellbutrin Tablets (18.3%) 1603
▲ Wellbutrin SR Sustained-Release Tablets (3% to greater than or equal to 5%) 1607
▲ Wellbutrin XL Extended-Release Tablets (3% to greater than or equal to 5%) 1613
▲ Xeloda Tablets (1% to 13%) 2822
Xifaxan Tablets (Less than 2%) 2842
Xyrem Oral Solution (Frequent) 1688
Zegerid Capsules (Less than 1%) 2958
Zegerid Powder for Oral Solution (Less than 1%) 2958
Zelapar Tablets 3372
▲ Zinecard for Injection (27% to 42%) 2650
Zmax for Oral Suspension 2583
Zocor Tablets 2105
▲ Zoloft (3% to 11%) 2586
▲ Zometa for Intravenous Infusion (9.3% to 22%) 2315
Zomig Tablets (Rare) 3519
Zomig-ZMT Tablets (Rare) 3519
▲ Zonegran Capsules (13%) 1101
▲ Zyban Sustained-Release Tablets (1% to 3%) 1644
Zyprexa Tablets 1830
Zyprexa ZYDIS Orally Disintegrating Tablets 1830
Zyrtec Chewable Tablets (Less than 2%) 2594
Zyrtec (Less than 2%) 2594
Zyrtec-D 12 Hour Extended Release Tablets (Less than 2%) 2597

Anorgasmia

Abilify Oral Solution (Rare) 882
Abilify Oral Solution (Rare) 2450
Abilify Discmelt Orally Disintegrating Tablets (Rare) 882
Abilify Discmelt Orally Disintegrating Tablets (Rare) 2450
Abilify Tablets (Rare) 882
Abilify Tablets (Rare) 2450
▲ Depo-Provera Contraceptive Injection (1% to 5%) 2622
▲ Duragesic Transdermal System (4%) 2373
Effexor Tablets 3411
▲ Effexor XR Capsules (3% to 17%) 3417
Eldepryl Capsules 3208
Emsam Transdermal System (0.2%) 903
Geodon Capsules (Infrequent) 2529
Lamictal (Rare) 1481
▲ Lexapro Oral Solution (2% to 6%) 1190
▲ Lexapro Tablets (2% to 6%) 1190
Lyrica Capsules (Greater than or equal to 1%) 2539
Neurontin Capsules (Infrequent) 2487
Neurontin Oral Solution (Infrequent) 2487
Neurontin Tablets (Infrequent) 2487
▲ Paxil CR Controlled-Release Tablets (2% to 10.0%) 1538
▲ Paxil (2% to 10.0%) 1530
Prozac Pulvules and Liquid (Infrequent) 1801
Risperdal (Frequent) 1676
Risperdal M-Tab Orally Disintegrating Tablets (Frequent) 1676
▲ Symbyax Capsules (1% to 3%) 1819
Viagra Tablets (Less than 2%) 2573

Anosmia

▲ Aerobid/Aerobid-M (3% to 9%) 1171
Astelin Nasal Spray (Infrequently) 1904
Beconase AQ Nasal Spray (Rare) 1396
Cipro 2977
Cipro I.V. (1% or less) 2984
Cipro XR Tablets 2990
Flonase Nasal Spray 1440
Proquin XR Tablets 1153
Rhinocort Aqua Nasal Spray (Rare) 665
Vasotec I.V. Injection (0.5% to 1.0%) 2103

Anotia

Thalomid Capsules 965

Anotia, fetal

Accutane Capsules 2731

Anovulation, prolonged

depo-subQ provera 104 Injectable Suspension 2624

Antibodies, development of

Elspar for Injection 2463
Elspar for Injection 1960
NovoLog Injection 2326

Anticholinergic syndrome

Clozaril Tablets 2184

Antidiuretic effect

Dilaudid 440
Dilaudid Non-Sterile Powder 440
Dilaudid Rectal Suppositories 440
Dilaudid Tablets 440
Dilaudid-HP (Less frequent) 442
MS Contin Tablets (Less frequent) 2701
Risperdal (Rare) 1676
Risperdal M-Tab Orally Disintegrating Tablets (Rare) 1676

Antisocial reaction

Pexeva Tablets (Rare) 1694
Prozac Pulvules and Liquid (Rare) 1801
Zyprexa Tablets (Infrequent) 1830
Zyprexa ZYDIS Orally Disintegrating Tablets (Infrequent) 1830

Antithrombin, decrease

Estratest Tablets 3199
Estratest H.S. Tablets 3199
Oncaspar 1145
Ortho-Cyclen/Ortho Tri-Cyclen 2429
Premarin Tablets 3446

Anuria

Abelcet Injection 1141
Campath Ampules 811
Carimune NF 3499
CytoGam Intravenous 1895
Effexor Tablets (Rare) 3411
Effexor XR Capsules (Rare) 3417
Fansidar Tablets 2765
Flebogamma 5%, Immune Globulin Intravenous (Human) 1658
Gammagard S/D (Some patients) 724
Gantrisin Pediatric Suspension 2770
Invanz for Injection (Greater than 0.1%) 1999
Miradon Tablets 3042
Mycamine for Injection 628
Nalfon Capsules (Less than 1%) 2502
Neurontin Capsules (Rare) 2487
Neurontin Oral Solution (Rare) 2487
Neurontin Tablets (Rare) 2487
Orthoclone OKT3 Sterile Solution (Less than 1%) 2360
Primaxin I.M. 2045
Primaxin I.V. (2.2%) 2048
Prinivil Tablets (0.3% to 1.0%) 2052
Prinzide Tablets 2056
▲ Proleukin for Injection (5%) 2266
VFEND I.V. (Less than 2%) 2564
VFEND Oral Suspension (Less than 2%) 2564
VFEND Tablets (Less than 2%) 2564

Anuria, neonatal

Aceon Tablets (2 mg, 4 mg, 8 mg) 3194
Altace Capsules 1702
Avapro Tablets 891
Avapro Tablets 2871

Captopril Tablets 2149
Cozaar Tablets 1935
Hyzaar 50-12.5 Tablets 1990
Hyzaar 100-12.5 Tablets 1990
Hyzaar 100-25 Tablets 1990
Lotrel Capsules 2249
Prinivil Tablets 2052
Prinzide Tablets 2056
Vasotec I.V. Injection 2103

Anxiety

▲ Abilify Oral Solution (20%) 882
▲ Abilify Oral Solution (20%) 2450
▲ Abilify Discmelt Orally Disintegrating Tablets (20%) 882
▲ Abilify Discmelt Orally Disintegrating Tablets (20%) 2450
▲ Abilify Tablets (20%) 882
▲ Abilify Tablets (20%) 2450
Aceon Tablets (2 mg, 4 mg, 8 mg) (0.3% to 1%) 3194
Aciphex Tablets 1090
▲ Actonel Tablets (0.6% to 4.3%) 2683
▲ Actonel with Calcium Tablets (0.6% to 4.7%) 2688
Adalat CC Tablets (Less than 1%) 2964
▲ Adderall XR Capsules (8%) 3166
Advair HFA Inhalation Aerosol 1318
Advicor Tablets 1722
▲ Aerobid/Aerobid-M (1% to 3%) 1171
Allegra-D 12 Hour Extended-Release Tablets (1.4%) 2846
Allegra-D 24 Hour Extended-Release Tablets (1.4%) 2849
Aloxi Injection (1%) 2127
Altace Capsules (Less than 1%) 1702
Altoprev Extended-Release Tablets 3109
Ambien Tablets (1%) 2851
▲ Ambien CR Tablets (2% to 3%) 2855
▲ AmBisome for Injection (7.4% to 13.7%) 620
Amerge Tablets (Infrequent) 1339
Amitiza Capsules (0% to 1.4%) 3224
Amoxil Capsules (Rare) 1343
Amoxil Chewable Tablets (Rare) 1343
Amoxil Pediatric Drops for Oral Suspension (Rare) 1343
Amoxil Powder for Oral Suspension (Rare) 1343
Amoxil Tablets (Rare) 1343
Anaprox Tablets (Less than 1%) 2761
Anaprox DS Tablets (Less than 1%) 2761
AndroGel (Fewer than 1%) 3329
Androxy Tablets 3335
Anzemet Injection (Infrequently) 2859
Anzemet Tablets (Infrequently) 2862
▲ Aredia for Injection (14.3%) 2179
▲ Arimidex Tablets (2% to 6%) 673
Arixtra Injection (0.8%) 1351
▲ Aromasin Tablets (4.1% to 10%) 2600
Arthrotec Tablets (Rare) 3129
Asacol Delayed-Release Tablets (2% or greater) 2692
Astelin Nasal Spray (Infrequent) 1904
Atacand Tablets (0.5% or greater) 649
Atacand HCT (0.5% or greater) 651
Atripla Tablets (Greater than or equal to 2%) 945
Augmentin (Rare) 1360
Augmentin Tablets (Rare) 1363
Augmentin XR Extended-Release Tablets (Rare) 1369
Augmentin ES-600 Powder for Oral Suspension (Rare) 1366
Avalide Tablets (1% or greater) 888
Avalide Tablets (1% or greater) 2874
Avapro Tablets (Less than 1%) 891
Avapro Tablets (Less than 1%) 2871
Avelox (0.1% to less than 2%) 2970
▲ Avinza Capsules (Less than 5%) 1741
Axert Tablets (Infrequent) 2396
Axid Oral Solution (1.8%) 879
Azilect Tablets (Frequent) 3293
▲ Betaseron for SC Injection (10%) 767
Biaxin/Biaxin XL 402
Bicillin C-R Injectable Suspension 1706
▲ BOTOX Purified Neurotoxin Complex (3% to 10%) 570
Brimonidine Tartrate Ophthalmic Solution 0.2% (Less than 3%) .... ⊙ 248
Caduet Tablets (Greater than 0.1% to less than or equal to 1%) 2508
▲ Campral Tablets (5% to 8%) 1174
Carnitor Injection (1% to 2%) 3188
Catapres Tablets 843
Catapres-TTS (0.5% or less) 844
Celebrex Capsules (0.1% to 1.9%) 3134
▲ Celexa (4%) 1176
▲ CellCept Capsules (3% to 28.4%) 2747
▲ CellCept Intravenous (3% to 28.4%) 2747
▲ CellCept Oral Suspension (3% to 28.4%) 2747
▲ CellCept Tablets (3% to 28.4%) 2747
Cesamet Capsules 3340
Chantix Tablets (Frequent) 2517
Cipro 2977
Cipro I.V. (1% or less) 2984
Cipro XR Tablets 2990
▲ Clolar for Intravenous Infusion (22%) 1271
Clorpres Tablets 2153
Clozaril Tablets (1%) 2184
Colazal Capsules 2838
Comtan Tablets (2%) 2189
▲ Copaxone for Injection (23%) 3297
▲ Copegus Tablets (33%) 2754
Cosopt Sterile Ophthalmic Solution 1931
Cozaar Tablets (Less than 1%) 1935
Crestor Tablets (Greater than or equal to 1%) 678
Crixivan Capsules (Less than 2%) 1940
▲ Cubicin for Injection (1% to 5%) 1026
Cuprimine Capsules 1947
▲ Cymbalta Delayed-Release Capsules (3%) 1757
▲ Dacogen Injection (11%) 2129
▲ DAPTACEL Vaccine (23.6% to 39.6%) 2950
Demser Capsules 1953
▲ Depacon Injection (1% to 5%) 412
▲ Depakene (1% to 5%) 417
▲ Depakote Sprinkle Capsules (1% to 5%) 422
▲ Depakote Tablets (1% to 5%) 427
▲ Depakote ER Tablets (1% to 5%) 434
▲ DepoDur Extended-Release Injection (2% to 5%) 1110
▲ depo-subQ provera 104 Injectable Suspension (1% to less than 5%) 2624
Detrol LA Capsules (1%) 2631
Dilaudid 440
Dilaudid Non-Sterile Powder 440
Dilaudid Rectal Suppositories 440
Dilaudid Tablets 440
Diovan Tablets 2193
Diovan HCT Tablets (Greater than 0.2%) 2196
▲ Doxil Injection (Less than 1% to 10%) 2351
▲ Duragesic Transdermal System (3% to 10%) 2373
EC-Naprosyn Delayed-Release Tablets (Less than 1%) 2761
▲ Effexor Tablets (2% to 11.2%) 3411
Effexor XR Capsules (1%) 3417
Eldepryl Capsules (1 of 49 patients) 3208
▲ Eloxatin for Injection (2% to 5%) 2892
Emcyt Capsules (1%) 2634
Emend Capsules (Greater than 0.5%) 1963
Emsam Transdermal System 903
EpiPen 1061
▲ Epogen for Injection (2% to 7%) 591
▲ Epzicom Tablets (3% to 5%) 1436
▲ Equetro Extended-Release Capsules (7%) 3180
Estratest Tablets 3199
Estratest H.S. Tablets 3199
▲ Estring Vaginal Ring (1% to 3%) 2635
Eulexin Capsules (1%) 3009
Evoxac Capsules (1.3%) 1047
▲ Exelon Capsules (4% to 5%) 2206
▲ Exelon Oral Solution (4% to 5%) 2206
▲ Fabrazyme for Intravenous Infusion (8%) 1274
▲ Faslodex Injection (5%) 681
FazaClo Orally Disintegrating Tablets (1%) 551
Femara Tablets (Less frequent) 2214
Flebogamma 5%, Immune Globulin Intravenous (Human) 1658
▲ Focalin XR Capsules (5% to 11%) 2223
Foradil Aerolizer (1.5%) 3010
Fortical Nasal Spray (Less than 1%) 3337
Frova Tablets (Frequent) 1113
Fuzeon Injection 2767
Gabitril Tablets (1% or more) 984
Gantrisin Pediatric Suspension 2770
Gengraf Capsules (1% to less than 3%) 459
▲ Geodon (5%) 2529
▲ Gleevec Tablets (0% to 12%) 2227
Hycodan 1116
Hycotuss Expectorant Syrup 1117
Hyperstat I.V. 3017
Hytrin Capsules (At least 1%) 471
Hyzaar 50-12.5 Tablets 1990
Hyzaar 100-12.5 Tablets 1990
Hyzaar 100-25 Tablets 1990
▲ Imdur Tablets (Less than or equal to 5%) 3018
Imitrex Injection (Frequent) 1463
Imitrex Nasal Spray (Infrequent) 1467
Imitrex Tablets 1471
▲ Indapamide Tablets (Greater than or equal to 5%) 2156
Indocin (Less than 1%) 1995
▲ Infanrix Vaccine (3.3% to 9.2%) 1476
▲ Infergen (10% to 19%) 3364
▲ Intron A for Injection (Up to 5%) 3024
Invanz for Injection (0.8% to 1.1%) 1999
Invirase (Greater than or equal to 2%) 2772
▲ Ionsys Transdermal System (1% to less than 10%) 2379
▲ I.V. Busulfex (72% to 75%) 2493
▲ Kadian Capsules (Less than 3% to 6%) 577
Kaletra (Less than 2%) 476
Keppra Injection (2%) 3320
Keppra Oral Solution (2%) 3314
Keppra Tablets (2%) 3314
Ketek Tablets (Less than 0.2%) 2903
Klonopin (Infrequent) 2778
▲ Kytril Injection (Less than 2% to 3.4%) 2781
Kytril (2%) 2784
▲ Lamictal (3.8%) 1481
Lanoxicaps Capsules 1490
Lanoxin Injection 1494
Lanoxin Injection Pediatric 1497
Lanoxin Tablets 1500
Lariam Tablets (Occasional) 2786
Lescol Capsules 2233
Lescol XL Tablets 2233
▲ Leukine (11%) 814
Levaquin (1.2%) 2384
Levaquin in 5% Dextrose Injection (1.2%) 2384
Levothroid Tablets 1186
Levoxyl Tablets 1712
Lexapro Oral Solution (At least 2%) 1190
Lexapro Tablets (At least 2%) 1190
▲ Lithostat Tablets (20%) 2140
Lofibra Tablets 1219
Lofibra Capsules 1216
Lotensin Tablets (Less than 1%) 2243
Lotrel Capsules 2249
Lotronex Tablets (Infrequent) 1512
Lunesta Tablets (Infrequent) 3142
▲ Lupron Depot 3.75 mg (3%) 3260
▲ Lupron Depot–3 Month 11.25 mg (Less than 5%) 3265
Lyrica Capsules (Greater than or equal to 1%) 2539
Malarone Pediatric Tablets (Less than 1%) 1517
Malarone Tablets (Less than 1%) 1517
Marinol Capsules (Greater than 1%) 3333
Mavik Tablets (0.3% to 1.0%) 486
Maxair Autohaler 1852
Maxalt Tablets (Infrequent) 2008
Maxalt-MLT Orally Disintegrating Tablets (Infrequent) 2008
▲ Mepron Suspension (7%) 1521
▲ Meridia Capsules (4.5%) 489
Merrem I.V. (Greater than 0.1% to 1%) 686
Mevacor Tablets (0.5% to 1.0%) 2021
Miacalcin Nasal Spray (Less than 1%) 2253
Micardis Tablets (More than 0.3%) 854
Micardis HCT Tablets 856
Migranal Nasal Spray (Rare) 3348
Mirapex Tablets (1% or more) 859
Mobic Oral Suspension (Less than 2%) 863
Mobic Tablets (Less than 2%) 863
▲ Myfortic Tablets (3% to less than 20%) 2255
▲ Mylotarg for Injection (7% to 10%) 3431
Myobloc Injection (Greater than 2%) 3192
Namenda (Greater than or equal to 2%) 1195
Naprosyn Suspension (Less than 1%) 2761
Naprosyn Tablets (Less than 1%) 2761
▲ Natrecor for Injection (2% to 3%) 3127
Nembutal Sodium Solution, USP (Less than 1%) 2470
Neoral Oral Solution (1% to less than 3%) 2259
Neoral Soft Gelatin Capsules (1% to less than 3%) 2259
Neurontin Capsules (Frequent) 2487
Neurontin Oral Solution (Frequent) 2487
Neurontin Tablets (Frequent) 2487
▲ Nipent for Injection (3% to 10%) 1863
▲ Niravam Orally Disintegrating Tablets (16.6% to 19.2%) 3092
Noroxin Tablets (Less frequent) 2032
Norvasc Tablets (More than 0.1% to 1%) 2545
Norvir (0 to 1.7%) 503
▲ Opana Tablets (1% to less than 10%) 1122
▲ Opana ER Tablets (1% to less than 10%) 1126
OptiPranolol Metipranolol Ophthalmic Solution 0.3% (A small number of patients) .... ⊙ 256
Oracea Capsules (1.5%) 1000
▲ OxyContin Tablets (Between 1% and 5%) 2703
Parcopa Orally Disintegrating Tablets 3097
Parnate Tablets 1527
▲ Paxil CR Controlled-Release Tablets (1% to 5.9%) 1538
▲ Paxil (1% to 5.9%) 1530
▲ Pegasys (19%) 2789
▲ PEG-Intron Powder for Injection (28%) 3048
Pepcid Injection (Infrequent) 2040
Pepcid (Infrequent) 2038
Percodan Tablets 1132
▲ Permax Tablets (6.4%) 3356
▲ Pexeva Tablets (2% to 5.9%) 1694
▲ Photofrin for Injection (3% to 7%) 702
Plavix Tablets (1% to 2.5%) 917
Plavix Tablets (1% to 2.5%) 2926
Pletal Tablets (Less than 2%) 2455
▲ Premphase Tablets (2% to 5%) 3456
▲ Prempro Tablets (2% to 5%) 3456
Prevacid Delayed-Release Capsules (Less than 1%) 3271
Prevacid for Delayed-Release Oral Suspension (Less than 1%) 3271
Prevacid SoluTab Delayed-Release Orally Disintegrating Tablets (Less than 1%) 3271
Prevacid NapraPAC (Less than 1%) 3280
PREVPAC (Less than 1%) 3284
Prezista Tablets (Less than 2%) 3306
Prilosec OTC Delayed-Release Tablets (Less than 1%) 2677
ProAir HFA Inhalation Aerosol (Less than 3%) 3300
ProAmatine Tablets (Less frequent) 3186
▲ Procrit for Injection (2% to 11%) 2364
▲ Prograf Capsules and Injection (3% to 15%) 632
▲ Proleukin for Injection (12%) 2266
Prometrium Capsules (100 mg, 200 mg) (Less than 5%) 3203
Proquin XR Tablets 1153
ProSom Tablets (Frequent) 517
Protonix I.V. (Greater than or equal to 1%) 3472
Protonix Tablets (Greater than or equal to 1%) 3469
Proventil HFA Inhalation Aerosol (Less than 3%) 3056
▲ Provigil Tablets (5%) 988
▲ Prozac Pulvules and Liquid (4% to 17%) 1801
Pulmicort Respules (Less than 1%) 661
▲ Rapamune Oral Solution and Tablets (3% to 20%) 3475
Razadyne (Greater than or equal to 2%) 2399
Razadyne ER Extended-Release Capsules (Greater than or equal to 2%) 2399
▲ Rebetol (47%) 3058
Relpax Tablets (Infrequent) 2548
ReoPro Vials (1.7%) 1809
Requip Tablets (1% or more) 1555
▲ Rescriptor Tablets (2.4% to 6.7%) 2551
Restoril Capsules (2%) 1860
Retrovir Capsules 1560
Retrovir IV Infusion 1564
Retrovir 1560
Reyataz Capsules (Less than 3%) 921
▲ Ribavirin, USP Capsules (47%) 3068
▲ Risperdal (4% to 20%) 1676
Risperdal Consta Long-Acting Injection (Frequent) 1682
▲ Risperdal M-Tab Orally Disintegrating Tablets (4% to 20%) 1676
▲ Rituxan I.V. (1% to 5%) 1254
▲ Romazicon Injection (3% to 9%) 2804
▲ Rythmol SR Capsules (10% to 13%) 2727
Sandimmune (Rare) 2275
Sandostatin Injection (Less than 1%) 2278
▲ Sandostatin LAR Depot (5% to 15%) 2280
Serevent Diskus (1% to less than 3%) 1568
▲ Seroquel Tablets (4%) 690
▲ Simulect for Injection (3% to 10%) 2284
Sonata Capsules (Frequent) 1717
Soriatane Capsules (Less than 1%) 1013
Stalevo Tablets (2%) 2287

Striant Mucoadhesive ... 1007
▲ Suboxone Tablets (12%) ... 2717
▲ Subutex Tablets (12%) ... 2717
Sular Tablets (Less than or equal to 1%) ... 3122
▲ Sustiva Capsules (2% to 13%) ... 930
▲ Sustiva Tablets (2% to 13%) ... 930
Symbyax Capsules ... 1819
▲ Symmetrel Tablets (1% to 5%) ... 1135
Tambocor Tablets (1% to 3%) ... 1856
▲ Tarceva Tablets (0% to 13%) ... 1259
▲ Tarceva Tablets (0% to 13%) ... 2444
Tarka Tablets (0.3% or more) ... 524
Tasmar Tablets (1% or more) ... 3358
▲ Temodar Capsules (7%) ... 3073
Tequin Injection (Less than 0.1%) ... 938
Tequin Injection in 5% Dextrose (Less than 0.1%) ... 938
Tequin Tablets (Less than 0.1%) ... 938
Teveten Tablets (Less than 1%) ... 1735
Teveten HCT Tablets (Less than 1%) ... 1737
Thalomid Capsules ... 965
Thyrolar Tablets ... 1199
Timoptic Sterile Ophthalmic Solution (Less frequent) ... 2088
Timoptic in Ocudose (Less frequent) ... 2091
Timoptic-XE Sterile Ophthalmic Gel Forming Solution ... 2092
▲ Topamax Sprinkle Capsules (4% to 24%) ... 2404
▲ Topamax Tablets (4% to 24%) ... 2404
Toprol-XL Tablets ... 668
Trasylol Injection (1% to 2%) ... 754
▲ Travatan Ophthalmic Solution (1% to 5%) ... 563
Tricor Tablets ... 527
▲ Trileptal Tablets (5% to 7%) ... 2300
▲ Trileptal Oral Suspension (5% to 7%) ... 2300
▲ Trisenox Injection (30%) ... 993
Truvada Tablets ... 1296
Tussionex Pennkinetic Extended-Release Suspension ... 3327
Twinject 0.3 ... 3378
Twinject 0.15 ... 3379
▲ Ultram ER Tablets (1% to greater than 5%) ... 2392
Uniretic Tablets (Less than 1%) ... 3100
Univasc Tablets (Less than 1%) ... 3104
Vantin Tablets and Oral Suspension (Less than 1%) ... 2645
▲ Velcade for Injection (14%) ... 2133
▲ Vesanoid Capsules (17%) ... 2820
VFEND I.V. (Less than 2%) ... 2564
VFEND Oral Suspension (Less than 2%) ... 2564
VFEND Tablets (Less than 2%) ... 2564
Viadur Implant (Less than 2%) ... 757
Viagra Tablets ... 2573
Vicodin Tablets ... 535
Vicodin ES Tablets ... 536
Vicodin HP Tablets ... 538
▲ Vicoprofen Tablets (3% to 9%) ... 539
Viracept (Less than 2%) ... 2577
▲ Viread Tablets (6%) ... 1301
▲ Vivitrol (8% to 12%) ... 995
Voltaren Tablets (Occasionally) ... 2307
Voltaren-XR Tablets (Occasionally) ... 2310
Vytorin 10/10 Tablets ... 2114
Vytorin 10/10 Tablets ... 3077
Vytorin 10/20 Tablets ... 2114
Vytorin 10/20 Tablets ... 3077
Vytorin 10/40 Tablets ... 2114
Vytorin 10/40 Tablets ... 3077
Vytorin 10/80 Tablets ... 2114
Vytorin 10/80 Tablets ... 3077
▲ Wellbutrin Tablets (3.1%) ... 1603
▲ Wellbutrin SR Sustained-Release Tablets (5% to 6%) ... 1607
▲ Wellbutrin XL Extended-Release Tablets (5% to 7%) ... 1613
▲ Xenical Capsules (2.8% to 4.4%) ... 2831
Xopenex Inhalation Solution (2.7%) ... 3146
Xopenex Inhalation Solution Concentrate (2.7%) ... 3150
Xopenex HFA Inhalation Aerosol (2.7%) ... 3154
Zegerid Capsules (Less than 1%) ... 2958
Zegerid Powder for Oral Solution (Less than 1%) ... 2958
▲ Ziagen (5%) ... 1626
Zmax for Oral Suspension ... 2583
Zocor Tablets ... 2105
▲ Zofran Injection (2% to 6%) ... 1634
▲ Zofran (6%) ... 1639
▲ Zofran ODT Orally Disintegrating Tablets (6%) ... 1639
▲ Zoloft (4%) ... 2586
▲ Zometa for Intravenous Infusion (11% to 14%) ... 2315
Zomig Tablets (Infrequent) ... 3519
Zomig Nasal Spray (Infrequent) ... 3523
Zomig-ZMT Tablets (Infrequent) ... 3519
▲ Zonegran Capsules (3%) ... 1101
▲ Zosyn (1.2% to 3.2%) ... 3492
▲ Zyban Sustained-Release Tablets (8%) ... 1644
Zydone Tablets ... 1139
▲ Zyprexa Tablets (9%) ... 1830
▲ Zyprexa ZYDIS Orally Disintegrating Tablets (9%) ... 1830
Zyrtec Chewable Tablets (Less than 2%) ... 2594
Zyrtec (Less than 2%) ... 2594
Zyrtec-D 12 Hour Extended Release Tablets (Less than 2%) ... 2597

Anxiety, paradoxical
Diastat Rectal Delivery System ... 3343
Valium Tablets ... 2819

Aortic valve disease
Revlimid Capsules ... 958

Apathy
Abilify Oral Solution (Infrequent) ... 882
Abilify Oral Solution (Infrequent) ... 2450
Abilify Discmelt Orally Disintegrating Tablets (Infrequent) ... 882
Abilify Discmelt Orally Disintegrating Tablets (Infrequent) ... 2450
Abilify Tablets (Infrequent) ... 882
Abilify Tablets (Infrequent) ... 2450
Ambien Tablets (Rare) ... 2851
Ambien CR Tablets (Rare) ... 2855
Azilect Tablets (Rare) ... 3293
Caduet Tablets (Less than or equal to 0.1%) ... 2508
Campath Ampules ... 811
Campral Tablets (Infrequent) ... 1174
Celexa (Infrequent) ... 1176
Cesamet Capsules ... 3340
Effexor Tablets (Infrequent) ... 3411
Effexor XR Capsules (Infrequent) ... 3417
Eldepryl Capsules ... 3208
Evoxac Capsules ... 1047
Exelon Capsules (Infrequent) ... 2206
Exelon Oral Solution (Infrequent) ... 2206
Fansidar Tablets ... 2765
Gabitril Tablets (Infrequent) ... 984
Gantrisin Pediatric Suspension ... 2770
Hectorol Capsules ... 1275
Hectorol Injection ... 1278
Imitrex Injection ... 1463
Imitrex Nasal Spray (Rare) ... 1467
Imitrex Tablets (Rare) ... 1471
▲ Intron A for Injection (Less than 5%) ... 3024
Kadian Capsules (Less than 3%) ... 577
Keppra Oral Solution ... 3314
Keppra Tablets ... 3314
Klonopin (Infrequent) ... 2778
Lamictal (Infrequent) ... 1481
Lanoxicaps Capsules ... 1490
Lanoxin Injection ... 1494
Lanoxin Injection Pediatric ... 1497
Lanoxin Tablets ... 1500
Lexapro Oral Solution (Infrequent) ... 1190
Lexapro Tablets (Infrequent) ... 1190
Lunesta Tablets ... 3142
Lyrica Capsules (0.1% to 1%) ... 2539
Mirapex Tablets (1% or more) ... 859
Namenda (Infrequent) ... 1195
Neurontin Capsules (Infrequent) ... 2487
Neurontin Oral Solution (Infrequent) ... 2487
Neurontin Tablets (Infrequent) ... 2487
Nexium Delayed-Release Capsules (Less than 1%) ... 655
Nexium I.V. (Less than 1%) ... 659
Norvasc Tablets (Less than 0.1%) ... 2545
Permax Tablets (Infrequent) ... 3356
Prevacid Delayed-Release Capsules (Less than 1%) ... 3271
Prevacid for Delayed-Release Oral Suspension (Less than 1%) ... 3271
Prevacid SoluTab Delayed-Release Orally Disintegrating Tablets (Less than 1%) ... 3271
Prevacid NapraPAC (Less than 1%) ... 3280
PREVPAC (Less than 1%) ... 3284
Prilosec OTC Delayed-Release Tablets (Less than 1%) ... 2677
ProQuad ... 2064
ProSom Tablets (Infrequent) ... 517
Prozac Pulvules and Liquid (Infrequent) ... 1801
Razadyne (Infrequent) ... 2399
Razadyne ER Extended-Release Capsules (Infrequent) ... 2399
Relpax Tablets (Infrequent) ... 2548
Requip Tablets (Infrequent) ... 1555
Rilutek Tablets (Infrequent) ... 2930
Risperdal (Infrequent) ... 1676
Risperdal Consta Long-Acting Injection (Frequent) ... 1682
Risperdal M-Tab Orally Disintegrating Tablets (Infrequent) ... 1676
Rocaltrol Capsules ... 2798
Rocaltrol Oral Solution ... 2798
Seroquel Tablets (Infrequent) ... 690
Sonata Capsules (Frequent) ... 1717
Sustiva Capsules (Less than 2%) ... 930
Sustiva Tablets (Less than 2%) ... 930
Tambocor Tablets (Less than 1%) ... 1856
Tasmar Tablets (Infrequent) ... 3358
▲ Topamax Sprinkle Capsules (1% to 3%) ... 2404
▲ Topamax Tablets (1% to 3%) ... 2404
Trileptal Tablets ... 2300
Trileptal Oral Suspension ... 2300
Zegerid Capsules (Less than 1%) ... 2958
Zegerid Powder for Oral Solution (Less than 1%) ... 2958
Zoloft (Infrequent) ... 2586
Zomig Tablets (Rare) ... 3519
Zomig Nasal Spray (Rare) ... 3523
Zomig-ZMT Tablets (Rare) ... 3519
▲ Zyprexa Tablets (4%) ... 1830
▲ Zyprexa ZYDIS Orally Disintegrating Tablets (4%) ... 1830

Aphasia
Amerge Tablets (Rare) ... 1339
Aricept Tablets (Frequent) ... 1094
Aricept ODT Tablets (Frequent) ... 1094
Arranon Injection (1%) ... 1357
Avelox (Less than 0.1%) ... 2970
Azilect Tablets (Infrequent) ... 3293
Campath Ampules ... 811
Colazal Capsules ... 2838
Duragesic Transdermal System (Less than 1%) ... 2373
Effexor Tablets (Rare) ... 3411
Effexor XR Capsules (Rare) ... 3417
Evoxac Capsules ... 1047
Exelon Capsules (Infrequent) ... 2206
Exelon Oral Solution (Infrequent) ... 2206
▲ Intron A for Injection (Less than 5%) ... 3024
Lamictal (Infrequent) ... 1481
Lyrica Capsules (0.1% to 1%) ... 2539
Namenda (Infrequent) ... 1195
Neurontin Capsules (Infrequent) ... 2487
Neurontin Oral Solution (Infrequent) ... 2487
Neurontin Tablets (Infrequent) ... 2487
Norvir (Less than 2%) ... 503
Orthoclone OKT3 Sterile Solution (Less than 1%) ... 2360
Paxil CR Controlled-Release Tablets (Rare) ... 1538
Paxil (Rare) ... 1530
Pexeva Tablets (rare) ... 1694
Razadyne (Infrequent) ... 2399
Razadyne ER Extended-Release Capsules (Infrequent) ... 2399
Relpax Tablets (Rare) ... 2548
Requip Tablets (Infrequent) ... 1555
Revlimid Capsules ... 958
Risperdal (Rare) ... 1676
Risperdal M-Tab Orally Disintegrating Tablets (Rare) ... 1676
Sandostatin LAR Depot (Rare) ... 2280
Seroquel Tablets (Rare) ... 690
Symbyax Capsules (Rare) ... 1819
Trileptal Tablets ... 2300
Trileptal Oral Suspension ... 2300
▲ Vesanoid Capsules (3%) ... 2820
Wellbutrin Tablets (Rare) ... 1603
Wellbutrin SR Sustained-Release Tablets ... 1607
Wellbutrin XL Extended-Release Tablets ... 1613
Zelapar Tablets ... 3372
Zyban Sustained-Release Tablets ... 1644

Aphonia
Advair Diskus 100/50 ... 1308
Advair Diskus 250/50 ... 1308
Advair Diskus 500/50 ... 1308
Advair HFA Inhalation Aerosol ... 1318
Flovent Diskus ... 1443
Flovent HFA ... 1447
Klonopin ... 2778
Migranal Nasal Spray (Rare) ... 3348

Aphthous stomatitis
(*see under* Stomatitis, ulcerative)

Aplasia, bone marrow
Paxil CR Controlled-Release Tablets ... 1538
Paxil ... 1530
Pexeva Tablets ... 1694

Aplasia, red cell
Combivir Tablets ... 1411
Cuprimine Capsules ... 1947
Epivir ... 1427
Epivir-HBV ... 1432
▲ Epogen for Injection (4 to 11%) ... 591
Lamictal (Rare) ... 1481
Miradon Tablets ... 3042
Retrovir Capsules ... 1560
Retrovir IV Infusion ... 1564
Retrovir ... 1560
Trizivir Tablets ... 1589

Aplasia, unspecified
Campath Ampules ... 811

Aplastic anemia
(*see under* Anemia, aplastic)

Apnea
Abilify Oral Solution (Rare) ... 882
Abilify Oral Solution (Rare) ... 2450
Abilify Discmelt Orally Disintegrating Tablets (Rare) ... 882
Abilify Discmelt Orally Disintegrating Tablets (Rare) ... 2450
Abilify Tablets (Rare) ... 882
Abilify Tablets (Rare) ... 2450
Aciphex Tablets (Rare) ... 1090
Actiq ... 979
Aloprim for Injection (Less than 1%) ... 2167
Alphagan P Ophthalmic Solution ... 567
Aricept Tablets (Infrequent) ... 1094
Aricept ODT Tablets (Infrequent) ... 1094
Bentyl Capsules ... 697
Bentyl Injection ... 697
Bentyl Syrup ... 697
Bentyl Tablets ... 697
Bicillin C-R Injectable Suspension ... 1706
Brimonidine Tartrate Ophthalmic Solution 0.2% ... ⊙ 248
Buprenex Injectable (Infrequent) ... 2716
Carimune NF ... 3499
▲ CellCept Capsules (3% to less than 20%) ... 2747
▲ CellCept Intravenous (3% to less than 20%) ... 2747
▲ CellCept Oral Suspension (3% to less than 20%) ... 2747
▲ CellCept Tablets (3% to less than 20%) ... 2747
Dilaudid Oral Liquid ... 445
Dilaudid Tablets - 8 mg ... 445
Dilaudid-HP ... 442
▲ Doxil Injection (1% to 10%) ... 2351
▲ Duragesic Transdermal System (3% to 10%) ... 2373
Effexor XR Capsules (Rare) ... 3417
Ethyol for Injection ... 1898
Evoxac Capsules ... 1047
Exelon Capsules (Infrequent) ... 2206
Exelon Oral Solution (Infrequent) ... 2206
Flebogamma 5%, Immune Globulin Intravenous (Human) ... 1658
Gabitril Tablets (Infrequent) ... 984
Gammagard Liquid ... 721
Gammagard S/D (Rare) ... 724
Gamunex Immune Globulin I.V., 10% (Rare) ... 3235
Herceptin I.V. (At least one of the 958 patients) ... 1233
HibTITER ... 3426
Indocin I.V. (Less than 3%) ... 2465
▲ Infasurf Intratracheal Suspension (61% to 76%) ... 1184
Ionsys Transdermal System (.1% to less than 1%) ... 2379
Lamictal ... 1481
Lyrica Capsules (Rare) ... 2539
Merrem I.V. (1.3%) ... 686
MS Contin Tablets ... 2701
Mycamine for Injection ... 628
Namenda (Infrequent) ... 1195
Natrecor for Injection (Greater than or equal to 1%) ... 3127
Nembutal Sodium Solution, USP (Less than 1%) ... 2470
▲ NeoProfen Injection (28%) ... 2472
Neurontin Capsules (Infrequent) ... 2487
Neurontin Oral Solution (Infrequent) ... 2487
Neurontin Tablets (Infrequent) ... 2487
Orthoclone OKT3 Sterile Solution (Less than 1%) ... 2360
OxyContin Tablets ... 2703
Permax Tablets (Infrequent) ... 3356
Phenergan Tablets and Suppositories ... 3440
Proleukin for Injection (1%) ... 2266
Prozac Pulvules and Liquid (Rare) ... 1801
Pulmozyme Inhalation Solution ... 1248

Rilutek Tablets (More than 2%) 2930
Risperdal 1676
Risperdal Consta Long-Acting Injection 1682
Risperdal M-Tab Orally Disintegrating Tablets 1676
Sonata Capsules (Rare) 1717
Striant Mucoadhesive 1007
Symbyax Capsules (Infrequent) 1819
Synagis (More than 1%) 1897
Tasmar Tablets (Rare) 3358
Thalomid Capsules 965
▲ Trasylol Injection (3%) 754
Ultane Liquid for Inhalation (Less than 1% to 2%) 531
Virazole for Inhalation Solution 3370
Xyrem Oral Solution (Infrequent) 1688
Zomig Tablets (Rare) 3519
Zomig-ZMT Tablets (Rare) 3519
Zonegran Capsules (Rare) 1101
Zyprexa Tablets (Infrequent) 1830
Zyprexa ZYDIS Orally Disintegrating Tablets (Infrequent) 1830
Zyvox (0% to 2.3%) 2652

Appendicitis

▲ Advair Diskus 100/50 (1% to 3%) 1308
▲ Advair Diskus 250/50 (1% to 3%) 1308
▲ Advair Diskus 500/50 (1% to 3%) 1308
Amevive 626
Effexor Tablets (Rare) 3411
Effexor XR Capsules (Rare) 3417
Enbrel for Injection 584
Evoxac Capsules (Less than 1%) 1047
Gardasil Injection (0.02%) 1984
Sandostatin Injection (Less than 1%) 2278
Sandostatin LAR Depot (Rare) 2280
▲ Ultram ER Tablets (1% to greater than 5%) 2392

Appetite, changes

Anaprox Tablets (Less than 1%) 2761
Anaprox DS Tablets (Less than 1%) 2761
Arthrotec Tablets (Rare) 3129
Decadron Tablets 1951
Depo-Provera Contraceptive Injection (Less than 1%) 2622
EC-Naprosyn Delayed-Release Tablets (Less than 1%) 2761
▲ Effexor Tablets (1% to 6%) 3411
▲ Effexor XR Capsules (1% to 6%) 3417
Eldepryl Capsules 3208
Gleevec Tablets (Infrequent) 2227
Hydrocortone Tablets 1989
Invirase (Greater than or equal to 2%) 2772
Lupron Depot 3.75 mg (2%) 3260
Lupron Depot–3 Month 11.25 mg (Less than 5%) 3265
▲ Midamor Tablets (Between 1% and 3%) 2026
Mircette Tablets 1066
Moduretic Tablets (Less than or equal to 1%) 2028
Naprosyn Suspension (Less than 1%) 2761
Naprosyn Tablets (Less than 1%) 2761
NuvaRing 2340
Ortho-Cyclen Tablets 2429
Ortho Evra Transdermal System 2417
Ortho Tri-Cyclen Tablets 2429
Ortho Tri-Cyclen Lo Tablets 2436
Premphase Tablets 3456
Prempro Tablets 3456
Seasonique Tablets 1077
▲ Sutent Capsules (9%) 2560
Univasc Tablets (Less than 1%) 3104
Voltaren Tablets (Rarely) 2307
Voltaren-XR Tablets (Rarely) 2310
▲ Wellbutrin Tablets (3.7%) 1603
Yasmin 28 Tablets 796
Yaz Tablets 803

Appetite, decreased

Adderall Tablets 3164
▲ Adderall XR Capsules (22% to 36%) 3166
▲ Aerobid/Aerobid-M (3% to 9%) 1171
Aloxi Injection (Less than 1%) 2127
Ambien CR Tablets (Rare) 2855
Amitiza Capsules (Less than 0.2%) 3224
Aptivus Capsules (Less than 2%) 826
▲ Byetta Injection (Greater than or equal to 1% to less than 5%) 611
Chantix Tablets (1% to 2%) 2517
▲ Clolar for Intravenous Infusion (11%) 1271
▲ Combivir Tablets (10%) 1411
Cubicin for Injection (Less than 1% to 2%) 1026
▲ Cymbalta Delayed-Release Capsules (3% to 11%) 1757
▲ Dacogen Injection (16%) 2129
▲ Daytrana Transdermal Patch (26%) 3174
DynaCirc CR Tablets (0.5% to 1%) 2721
Emend Capsules (Greater than 0.5%) 1963
▲ Epivir (10%) 1427
▲ Femara Tablets (4%) 2214
▲ Focalin XR Capsules (30%) 2223
▲ Fuzeon Injection (3.2%) 2767
Garamycin Injectable 3014
Imitrex Injection (Rare) 1463
Imitrex Nasal Spray (Rare) 1467
Imitrex Tablets (Rare) 1471
Invirase (Greater than or equal to 2%) 2772
Klonopin (1%) 2778
▲ Kytril (5%) 2784
▲ Leustatin Injection (17%) 2357
▲ Lexapro Oral Solution (3%) 1190
▲ Lexapro Tablets (3%) 1190
MetroGel-Vaginal Gel (1%) 1855
Mycamine for Injection (0.7%) 628
▲ Nexavar Tablets (Common) 746
▲ Niravam Orally Disintegrating Tablets (12.8% to 27.8%) 3092
Oncaspar 1145
Opana Tablets (Less than 1%) 1122
Opana ER Tablets (2.9%) 1126
▲ Paxil CR Controlled-Release Tablets (2.0% to 9%) 1538
▲ Paxil (2.0% to 9%) 1530
▲ Pexeva Tablets (2% to 9%) 1694
▲ Prevnar for Injection (0% to 30%) 3463
Prezista Tablets (Less than 2%) 3306
Prochieve 4% Gel 1003
Prochieve 8% Gel 1003
ProSom Tablets (Infrequent) 517
Recombivax HB (Greater than 1%) 2071
Rescriptor Tablets 2551
Ritalin LA Capsules 2271
▲ Strattera Capsules (5% to 23%) 1814
▲ Trisenox Injection (15%) 993
▲ Ultram ER Tablets (1% to greater than 5%) 2392
▲ Valcyte Tablets (Less than 5%) 2813
Vandazole Vaginal Gel 3338
Vantin Tablets and Oral Suspension (Less than 1%) 2645
▲ Velcade for Injection (43%) 2133
▲ Vivitrol (6% to 20%) 995
▲ Wellbutrin XL Extended-Release Tablets (4%) 1613
Xyrem Oral Solution (Infrequent) 1688
▲ Zometa for Intravenous Infusion (13%) 2315

Appetite, increased

Abilify Oral Solution (Infrequent) 882
Abilify Oral Solution (Infrequent) 2450
Abilify Discmelt Orally Disintegrating Tablets (Infrequent) 882
Abilify Discmelt Orally Disintegrating Tablets (Infrequent) 2450
Abilify Tablets (Infrequent) 882
Abilify Tablets (Infrequent) 2450
Aceon Tablets (2 mg, 4 mg, 8 mg) (0.3% to 1%) 3194
Aciphex Tablets 1090
Aerobid/Aerobid-M (1% to 3%) 1171
Alinia for Oral Suspension (Less than 1%) 2835
Alinia Tablets (Less than 1%) 2835
Ambien Tablets (Rare) 2851
Aricept Tablets (Infrequent) 1094
Aricept ODT Tablets (Infrequent) 1094
▲ Aromasin Tablets (3%) 2600
Asacol Delayed-Release Tablets 2692
Astelin Nasal Spray (Infrequent) 1904
Caduet Tablets (Less than 2%) 2508
Campral Tablets (Frequent) 1174
Celebrex Capsules (0.1% to 1.9%) 3134
Celexa (Frequent) 1176
Cesamet Capsules (2%) 3340
▲ Chantix Tablets (3% to 4%) 2517
▲ Clarinex Syrup (3.1%) 2995
Clozaril Tablets (Less than 1%) 2184
Copaxone for Injection (Infrequent) 3297
Crixivan Capsules (2.1%) 1940
Cymbalta Delayed-Release Capsules (Frequent) 1757
Decadron Tablets 1951
▲ Depacon Injection (1% to 5%) 412
▲ Depakene (1% to 5%) 417
▲ Depakote Sprinkle Capsules (1% to 5%) 422
▲ Depakote Tablets (1% to 6%) 427
▲ Depakote ER Tablets (Greater than 1% to 6%) 434
Diovan HCT Tablets (Less than frequent) 2196
Doxil Injection (Less than 1%) 2351
DynaCirc CR Tablets (0.5% to 1%) 2721
▲ Entocort EC Capsules (Less than 5%) 2698
Evoxac Capsules (Less than 1%) 1047
FazaClo Orally Disintegrating Tablets (Less than 1%) 551
Fortical Nasal Spray (Less than 1%) 3337
Gabitril Tablets (2%) 984
Gengraf Capsules (1% to less than 3%) 459
▲ Intron A for Injection (Less than 5%) 3024
Kaletra (Less than 2%) 476
Klonopin (Infrequent) 2778
Lamictal (Infrequent) 1481
Levothroid Tablets 1186
Levoxyl Tablets 1712
Lexapro Oral Solution (Frequent) 1190
Lexapro Tablets (Frequent) 1190
Lipitor Tablets (Less than 2%) 2483
Lofibra Tablets 1219
Lofibra Capsules 1216
Lunesta Tablets (Infrequent) 3142
▲ Lyrica Capsules (1% to 6%) 2539
Maxalt Tablets (Rare) 2008
Maxalt-MLT Orally Disintegrating Tablets (Rare) 2008
▲ Meridia Capsules (8.7%) 489
Miacalcin Nasal Spray (Less than 1%) 2253
Namenda (Infrequent) 1195
Neoral Oral Solution (1% to less than 3%) 2259
Neoral Soft Gelatin Capsules (1% to less than 3%) 2259
Neurontin Capsules (1.1%) 2487
Neurontin Oral Solution (1.1%) 2487
Neurontin Tablets (1.1%) 2487
Nexium Delayed-Release Capsules (Less than 1%) 655
Nexium I.V. (Less than 1%) 659
▲ Niravam Orally Disintegrating Tablets (32.7%) 3092
Norvasc Tablets (Less than 0.1%) 2545
Omacor Capsules 2725
Oncaspar (Less than 1%) 1145
OxyContin Tablets (Less than 1%) 2703
▲ Paxil CR Controlled-Release Tablets (4%) 1538
▲ Paxil (4%) 1530
Permax Tablets (Infrequent) 3356
▲ Pexeva Tablets (2% to 4%) 1694
Prevacid Delayed-Release Capsules (Less than 1%) 3271
Prevacid for Delayed-Release Oral Suspension (Less than 1%) 3271
Prevacid SoluTab Delayed-Release Orally Disintegrating Tablets (Less than 1%) 3271
Prevacid NapraPAC (Less than 1%) 3280
PREVPAC (Less than 1%) 3284
Prochieve 4% Gel 1003
Prochieve 8% Gel 1003
▲ Prograf Capsules and Injection (3% to 15%) 632
Prometrium Capsules (100 mg, 200 mg) 3203
ProSom Tablets (Infrequent) 517
Protonix I.V. (Less than 1%) 3472
Protonix Tablets (Less than 1%) 3469
Provigil Tablets (At least 1%) 988
Prozac Pulvules and Liquid (Frequent) 1801
Relpax Tablets (Rare) 2548
Rescriptor Tablets 2551
Reyataz Capsules (Less than 3%) 921
Rilutek Tablets (Infrequent) 2930
Risperdal (Infrequent) 1676
Risperdal Consta Long-Acting Injection (Infrequent) 1682
Risperdal M-Tab Orally Disintegrating Tablets (Infrequent) 1676
Seroquel Tablets (Infrequent) 690
Sonata Capsules (Infrequent) 1717
▲ Soriatane Capsules (1% to 10%) 1013
Sular Tablets (Less than or equal to 1%) 3122
▲ Symbyax Capsules (Greater than or equal to 5% to 16%) 1819
Testim 1% Gel (Less than 1%) 695
Thalomid Capsules 965
Thiothixene Capsules 2165
Topamax Sprinkle Capsules (1%) 2404
Topamax Tablets (1%) 2404
Tricor Tablets 527
Triglide Tablets 3123
Trileptal Tablets 2300
Trileptal Oral Suspension 2300
Uniretic Tablets (Less than 1%) 3100
Vantas (Less than 2%) 3375
Vivitrol 995
Wellbutrin SR Sustained-Release Tablets (At least 1%) 1607
▲ Wellbutrin XL Extended-Release Tablets (4%) 1613
Xyrem Oral Solution (Infrequent) 1688
Zelnorm Tablets 2312
Zoloft (Frequent) 2586
Zomig Tablets (Infrequent) 3519
Zomig Nasal Spray (Rare) 3523
Zomig-ZMT Tablets (Infrequent) 3519
Zyban Sustained-Release Tablets (2%) 1644
▲ Zyprexa Tablets (2% to 24%) 1830
▲ Zyprexa ZYDIS Orally Disintegrating Tablets (2% to 24%) 1830
Zyrtec Chewable Tablets (Less than 2%) 2594
Zyrtec (Less than 2%) 2594
Zyrtec-D 12 Hour Extended Release Tablets (Less than 2%) 2597

Appetite, loss of

(*see also under* Anorexia)

▲ Chemet Capsules (12.0% to 20.9%) 2458
▲ Concerta Extended-Release Tablets (4%) 1881
▲ Focalin Tablets (Among more frequent) 2220
Focalin XR Capsules 2223
HibTITER (23 of 1,118 vaccinations) 3426
▲ Infanrix Vaccine (6.0% to 27.8%) 1476
Metadate CD Capsules 3323
Miacalcin Injection 2252
Numorphan Injection 1120
▲ Pediarix Vaccine (21.6% or less) 1548
Tasmar Tablets 3358
Varivax (Greater than or equal to 1%) 2100
Ziagen 1626

Appetite disorder, unspecified

Ambien CR Tablets (1%) 2855
▲ Vivitrol (6% to 20%) 995

Application site macules

Oxytrol Transdermal System (2.5%) 3392

Application site rash

▲ Aldara Cream, 5% (20.5%) 1846
Authia Cream (Occasional) 3404
▲ Oxytrol Transdermal System (3.3%) 3392
ThermaCare Heat Wraps 2677

Application site reaction, unspecified

▲ Aldara Cream, 5% (33%) 1846
▲ Climara Pro Transdermal System (40.6%) 776
▲ Daytrana Transdermal Patch (6%) 3174
▲ Duragesic Transdermal System (3% to 10%) 2373
▲ Emsam Transdermal System (24%) 903
▲ Erbitux (18%) 910
Evoclin Foam, 1% (1%) 1009
Loprox Shampoo 1888
▲ Menostar Transdermal System (9%) 782
Synera Topical Patch (Less than or equal to 1%) 1137
▲ Tri-Luma Cream (5.45%) 1213
Vanos Cream (0.4% to 1.4%) 1893

Apprehension

Adenocard Injection (Less than 1%) 617
Dalmane Capsules 3342
Dilaudid Oral Liquid (Less frequent) 445
Dilaudid Tablets - 8 mg (Less frequent) 445
Dilaudid-HP (Less frequent) 442
Edecrin 1959
EpiPen 1061
Hyperstat I.V. 3017
Lidoderm Patch 1118
Matulane Capsules 3191
Maxalt Tablets (Rare) 2008
Maxalt-MLT Orally Disintegrating Tablets (Rare) 2008
MS Contin Tablets (Less frequent) 2701
Synera Topical Patch 1137
Twinject 0.3 3378
Twinject 0.15 3379

Apraxia

Eldepryl Capsules 3208
Exelon Capsules (Infrequent) 2206

Exelon Oral Solution (Infrequent) 2206
Neurontin Capsules (Rare) 2487
Neurontin Oral Solution (Rare) 2487
Neurontin Tablets (Rare) 2487
Razadyne (Infrequent) 2399
Razadyne ER Extended-Release Capsules (Infrequent) 2399
Risperdal Consta Long-Acting Injection (Infrequent) 1682
Topamax Sprinkle Capsules (Infrequent) 2404
Topamax Tablets (Infrequent) 2404

Arachnoiditis
Depo-Medrol Single-Dose Vial 2619

Areflexia
Neurontin Capsules (Frequent) 2487
Neurontin Oral Solution 2487
Neurontin Tablets (Frequent) 2487

Arm, stiffness of
Engerix-B Vaccine (Less than 1%) 1425

Arrhythmia, exacerbation of
Toprol-XL Tablets (Greater than 1%) 668

Arrhythmia, nodal
Pexeva Tablets (Rare) 1694
Pletal Tablets (Less than 2%) 2455
ReoPro Vials (0.2%) 1809
Rythmol SR Capsules 2727
VFEND I.V. (Less than 2%) 2564
VFEND Oral Suspension (Less than 2%) 2564
VFEND Tablets (Less than 2%) 2564

Arrhythmias
Abelcet Injection (Rare) 1141
Activase I.V. 1223
Actonel Tablets (2%) 2683
Adenocard Injection 617
Adenoscan (1%) 619
Advair Diskus 100/50 1308
Advair Diskus 250/50 1308
Advair Diskus 500/50 1308
▲ Advair HFA Inhalation Aerosol (1% to 3%) 1318
Advicor Tablets 1722
Aggrenox Capsules (Less than 1%) 822
▲ Agrylin Capsules (1% to 5%) 3169
Aldara Cream, 5% 1846
Allegra-D 12 Hour Extended-Release Tablets 2846
Allegra-D 24 Hour Extended-Release Tablets 2849
Ambien Tablets (Rare) 2851
Ambien CR Tablets (Rare) 2855
AmBisome for Injection (Less common) 620
Anaprox Tablets (Less than 1%) 2761
Anaprox DS Tablets (Less than 1%) 2761
▲ Aranesp for Injection (10%) 581
Arthrotec Tablets (Rare) 3129
Avalide Tablets 888
Avalide Tablets 2874
Avapro Tablets (Less than 1%) 891
Avapro Tablets (Less than 1%) 2871
Bayer Aspirin 744
Betagan Ophthalmic Solution, USP ⊙220
Betimol Ophthalmic Solution 3382
Betimol Ophthalmic Solution ⊙295
Biltricide Tablets 2976
Blocadren Tablets (Greater than 1.1%) 1916
Brimonidine Tartrate Ophthalmic Solution 0.2% (Less than 3%) ⊙248
Caduet Tablets (Greater than 0.1% to less than 2%) 2508
Calcijex Injection 411
Campath Ampules 811
Carbatrol Capsules 3171
Cardizem LA Extended Release Tablets (Less than 2%) 1728
Cardura XL Tablets 2515
▲ Carnitor Injection (2% to 3%) 3188
Carteolol Hydrochloride Ophthalmic Solution USP, 1% (Occasional) ⊙249
Catapres Tablets (Rare) 843
Catapres-TTS (0.5% or less) 844
▲ CellCept Capsules (3% to less than 20%) 2747
▲ CellCept Intravenous (3% to less than 20%) 2747
▲ CellCept Oral Suspension (3% to less than 20%) 2747
▲ CellCept Tablets (3% to less than 20%) 2747
Cesamet Capsules 3340
Chantix Tablets (Infrequent) 2517
Chemet Capsules (Up to 1.8%) 2458
Cipro I.V. (1% or less) 2984
Cipro XR Tablets 2990
Clinoril Tablets (Rare) 1924
Clorpres Tablets (Rare) 2153
Clozaril Tablets (Several patients) 2184
Combivent Inhalation Aerosol (Less than 2%) 847
Concerta Extended-Release Tablets 1881
Copaxone for Injection 3297
Copegus Tablets (Less than 1%) 2754
Cosopt Sterile Ophthalmic Solution 1931
Cozaar Tablets (Less than 1%) 1935
Crestor Tablets (Less than 1%) 678
Daytrana Transdermal Patch 3174
Decadron Tablets 1951
Depakote ER Tablets (Greater than 1%) 434
Ditropan XL Extended-Release Tablets (Rare) 2413
Doxil Injection (Less than 1%) 2351
Duragesic Transdermal System (1% or greater) 2373
Dyazide Capsules 1423
EC-Naprosyn Delayed-Release Tablets (Less than 1%) 2761
Effexor Tablets 3411
Effexor XR Capsules (Infrequent) 3417
Eldepryl Capsules 3208
Elitek (Less than or equal to 1%) 2890
EpiPen 1061
Equetro Extended-Release Capsules 3180
Ery-Tab Tablets (Occasional reports) 449
Erythrocin Stearate Filmtab Tablets (Occasional reports) 453
Erythromycin Base Filmtab Tablets (Occasional reports) 455
Erythromycin Delayed-Release Capsules, USP (Occasional reports) 457
Ethyol for Injection (Rare) 1898
Evoxac Capsules (Less than 1%) 1047
Fabrazyme for Intravenous Infusion 1274
Focalin Tablets 2220
Focalin XR Capsules 2223
Foradil Aerolizer 3010
Furosemide Tablets 2154
Gemzar for Injection (2%) 1771
Gengraf Capsules (2%) 459
Hectorol Capsules 1275
Hectorol Injection 1278
Herceptin I.V. (At least one of the 958 patients) 1233
▲ Humira Injection (Less than 5%) 466
Hytrin Capsules (At least 1%) 471
Hyzaar 50-12.5 Tablets 1990
Hyzaar 100-12.5 Tablets 1990
Hyzaar 100-25 Tablets 1990
▲ Imdur Tablets (Less than or equal to 5%) 3018
Imitrex Injection (Rare) 1463
Imitrex Nasal Spray (Infrequent) 1467
Imitrex Tablets (Rare to infrequent) 1471
Indocin Capsules (Less than 1%) 1995
Indocin I.V. (Less than 1%) 2465
Indocin (Less than 1%) 1995
Infed Injection 3390
▲ Intron A for Injection (Less than 5%) 3024
Invanz for Injection (Greater than 0.1%) 1999
Ionsys Transdermal System (.1% to less than 1%) 2379
▲ I.V. Busulfex (5%) 2493
Kytril Injection (Rare) 2781
Lanoxicaps Capsules 1490
Lanoxin Injection 1494
Lanoxin Injection Pediatric 1497
Leukine 814
Levaquin (0.1% to 0.9%) 2384
Levaquin in 5% Dextrose Injection (0.1% to 0.9%) 2384
Levothroid Tablets 1186
Levoxyl Tablets 1712
Lipitor Tablets (Less than 2%) 2483
Lithobid Tablets 1692
Lofibra Tablets 1219
Lofibra Capsules 1216
Lotronex Tablets (Rare) 1512
Maxalt Tablets (Infrequent) 2008
Maxalt-MLT Orally Disintegrating Tablets (Infrequent) 2008
Metadate CD Capsules 3323
Midamor Tablets (Less than or equal to 1%) 2026
Mirapex Tablets (Less than 1%) 859
Mivacron Injection (Less than 1%) 493
Moban Tablets 1119
Mobic Oral Suspension (Less than 2%) 863
Mobic Tablets (Less than 2%) 863
Moduretic Tablets (Greater than 1%, less than 3%) 2028
Mycamine for Injection 628
Naprosyn Suspension (Less than 1%) 2761
Naprosyn Tablets (Less than 1%) 2761
Neoral Oral Solution (2%) 2259
Neoral Soft Gelatin Capsules (2%) 2259
▲ Neupogen for Injection (11 of 375 cancer patients) 603
Nexavar Tablets (Infrequent) 746
Niaspan Extended-Release Tablets 1730
Nipent for Injection (Less than 3%) 1863
Norvasc Tablets (More than 0.1% to 1%) 2545
Omacor Capsules 2725
▲ Ontak Vials (6%) 1745
Orthoclone OKT3 Sterile Solution (Less than 1%) 2360
Paxil CR Controlled-Release Tablets (Rare) 1538
Paxil (Rare) 1530
Pepcid Injection (Infrequent) 2040
Pepcid (Infrequent) 2038
Permax Tablets (1.1%) 3356
Phenergan Tablets and Suppositories 3440
Prevacid Delayed-Release Capsules (Less than 1%) 3271
Prevacid for Delayed-Release Oral Suspension (Less than 1%) 3271
Prevacid SoluTab Delayed-Release Orally Disintegrating Tablets (Less than 1%) 3271
Prevacid NapraPAC (Less than 1%) 3280
PREVPAC (Less than 1%) 3284
Prinivil Tablets (0.3% to 1.0%) 2052
Prinzide Tablets 2056
Prograf Capsules and Injection 632
▲ Proleukin for Injection (10%) 2266
Propine Ophthalmic Solution ⊙239
Proquin XR Tablets 1153
ProSom Tablets (Rare) 517
Protonix I.V. (Less than 1%) 3472
Protonix Tablets (Less than 1%) 3469
Protopic Ointment (Greater than or equal to 1%) 638
Proventil Inhalation Aerosol 3053
Provigil Tablets (1%) 988
Prozac Pulvules and Liquid (Infrequent) 1801
▲ Quadramet Injection (5%) 1040
Relpax Tablets (Rare) 2548
Remicade for IV Injection (Greater than or equal to 0.2%) 971
Rescriptor Tablets 2551
Retavase 2499
Risperdal 1676
Risperdal M-Tab Orally Disintegrating Tablets 1676
Ritalin Hydrochloride Tablets 2269
Ritalin LA Capsules 2271
Ritalin-SR Tablets 2269
Rituxan I.V. (Four patients) 1254
Rocaltrol Capsules 2798
Rocaltrol Oral Solution 2798
Romazicon Injection (Less than 1%) 2804
Rythmol SR Capsules 2727
▲ Sandostatin Injection (9%) 2278
Serevent Diskus 1568
Seroquel Tablets 690
Symbyax Capsules (Infrequent) 1819
Symmetrel Tablets 1135
Tamiflu Capsules 2807
Tamiflu Oral Suspension 2807
Tasmar Tablets (Infrequent) 3358
▲ Taxotere Injection Concentrate (4.5%) 2932
Tegretol/Tegretol-XR 2295
Thalomid Capsules 965
Timolide Tablets (Less than 1%) 2086
Timoptic Sterile Ophthalmic Solution (Less frequent) 2088
Timoptic in Ocudose (Less frequent) 2091
Timoptic-XE Sterile Ophthalmic Gel Forming Solution 2092
TNKase I.V. 1264
▲ Trasylol Injection (4%) 754
Tricor Tablets 527
Triglide Tablets 3123
Ultane Liquid for Inhalation (Less than 1%) 531
Uniphyl Tablets 2710
Uniretic Tablets (Less than 1%) 3100
Vasotec I.V. Injection (0.5% to 1.0%) 2103
Ventolin HFA Inhalation Aerosol 1600
▲ Vesanoid Capsules (23%) 2820
Vicoprofen Tablets (Less than 1%) 539
Voltaren Tablets (Rarely) 2307
Voltaren-XR Tablets (Rarely) 2310
▲ Wellbutrin Tablets (5.3%) 1603
▲ Wellbutrin XL Extended-Release Tablets (5%) 1613
Xopenex Inhalation Solution 3146
Xopenex Inhalation Solution Concentrate 3150
Xopenex HFA Inhalation Aerosol 3154
Zantac (Rare) 1624
Zantac Injection (Rare) 1619
Zantac Injection Pharmacy Bulk Package (Rare) 1622
Zantac Injection Premixed (Rare) 1619
Zantac (Rare) 1624
Zemuron Injection (Less than 1%) 2346
Zofran Injection 1634
Zomig Tablets (Infrequent) 3519
Zomig Nasal Spray (Infrequent) 3523
Zomig-ZMT Tablets (Infrequent) 3519
Zosyn (1.0% or less) 3492
Zyrtec-D 12 Hour Extended Release Tablets 2597

Arrhythmias, junctional
Proleukin for Injection (1%) 2266

Arrhythmias, malignant
Symmetrel Tablets 1135

Arrhythmias, sinus
Aloxi Injection (Less than 1%) 2127
Anzemet Injection 2859
Anzemet Tablets 2862
Eraxis for Injection (Less than 1% to less than 2%) 2521
Imitrex Injection (Infrequent) 1463
Imitrex Nasal Spray 1467
Imitrex Tablets 1471
Rythmol SR Capsules 2727

Arrhythmias, supraventricular
Cubicin for Injection (Less than 1%) 1026
Cymbalta Delayed-Release Capsules (Very rare) 1757
Intron A for Injection (Rare) 3024
Leukine (Occasional) 814
Pegasys (Less than 1%) 2789
PEG-Intron Powder for Injection (Less than or equal to 1%) 3048
▲ Proleukin for Injection (5%) 2266
Revlimid Capsules 958
Rituxan I.V. (Four patients) 1254
Sanctura Tablets 1151

Arrhythmias, ventricular
Adenoscan (Less than 1%) 619
Biaxin/Biaxin XL 402
Campath Ampules 811
Celexa 1176
Doxil Injection (Less than 1%) 2351
E.E.S. (Rare) 451
EryPed (Rare) 447
Erythrocin Stearate Filmtab Tablets (Rare) 453
Erythromycin Base Filmtab Tablets (Rare) 455
Erythromycin Delayed-Release Capsules, USP 457
Hyperstat I.V. 3017
Lanoxicaps Capsules (Less common) 1490
Lanoxin Injection 1494
Lanoxin Injection Pediatric (Less common) 1497
Lanoxin Tablets (Less common) 1500
Lexapro Oral Solution 1190
Lexapro Tablets 1190
Neumega for Injection 3435
Noroxin Tablets (Rare) 2032
PCE Dispertab Tablets 515
PREVPAC (Rare) 3284
▲ Proleukin for Injection (3%) 2266
Prozac Pulvules and Liquid (Rare) 1801
Relpax Tablets (Rare) 2548
ReoPro Vials (0.3%) 1809
Revatio Tablets 2557
Rituxan I.V. (Four patients) 1254
Rythmol SR Capsules 2727
▲ Tambocor Tablets (7% to 13%) 1856
Tequin Injection 938
Tequin Injection in 5% Dextrose 938
Tequin Tablets 938
Trasylol Injection (1% to 2%) 754
VFEND I.V. (Less than 2%) 2564
VFEND Oral Suspension (Less than 2%) 2564
VFEND Tablets (Less than 2%) 2564

Viagra Tablets 2573
Zofran Injection 1634
Zofran 1639
Zofran ODT Orally Disintegrating Tablets 1639

Arterial carbon dioxide, decrease

Sulfamylon Cream 2162

Arterial insufficiency

Blocadren Tablets 1916
Cosopt Sterile Ophthalmic Solution 1931
Inderal LA Long-Acting Capsules 3429
InnoPran XL Capsules 2723
Lopressor Injection (1%) 2238
Lopressor Tablets (1%) 2238
Lopressor HCT 50/25 Tablets 2241
Lopressor HCT 100/25 Tablets 2241
Lopressor HCT 100/50 Tablets 2241
Timolide Tablets 2086
Timoptic Sterile Ophthalmic Solution 2088
Timoptic in Ocudose 2091
Timoptic-XE Sterile Ophthalmic Gel Forming Solution 2092
Toprol-XL Tablets (About 1 of 100 patients) 668

Arteriosclerosis

Tasmar Tablets (Rare) 3358

Arteriospasm

Fortaz 1453
Tasmar Tablets (Infrequent) 3358

Arteritis

Ambien Tablets (Rare) 2851
Ambien CR Tablets (Rare) 2855
Aricept Tablets (Infrequent) 1094
Aricept ODT Tablets (Infrequent) 1094
Effexor Tablets (Rare) 3411
Effexor XR Capsules (Rare) 3417
Gantrisin Pediatric Suspension 2770
Zyprexa Tablets (Rare) 1830
Zyprexa ZYDIS Orally Disintegrating Tablets (Rare) 1830

Arteritis, temporal

Imitrex Nasal Spray 1467
Imitrex Tablets 1471
Orthoclone OKT3 Sterile Solution (Less than 1%) 2360

Arthralgia

Abelcet Injection 1141
Abilify Oral Solution (Infrequent) 882
Abilify Oral Solution (Infrequent) 2450
Abilify Discmelt Orally Disintegrating Tablets (Infrequent) 882
Abilify Discmelt Orally Disintegrating Tablets (Infrequent) 2450
Abilify Tablets (Infrequent) 882
Abilify Tablets (Infrequent) 2450
Accutane Capsules 2731
Aceon Tablets (2 mg, 4 mg, 8 mg) (0.3% to 1.1%) 3194
Actimmune (2%) 1671
Actiq (1% or greater) 979
▲ Actonel Tablets (11.5% to 32.8%) 2683
▲ Actonel with Calcium Tablets (11.5% to 23.7%) 2688
▲ ADACEL Vaccine (0.3% to 14%) 2945
Adalat CC Tablets (Less than 1%) 2964
▲ Advair Diskus 100/50 (1% to 3%) 1308
▲ Advair Diskus 250/50 (1% to 3%) 1308
▲ Advair Diskus 500/50 (1% to 3%) 1308
▲ Advair HFA Inhalation Aerosol (1% to 3%) 1318
▲ Advate Injection (23.3%) 712
Advicor Tablets 1722
▲ Aggrenox Capsules (5.5%) 822
Agrylin Capsules (1% to 5%) 3169
Aldara Cream, 5% (0.9%) 1846
Aldoril Tablets 1910
▲ Alferon N Injection (3% to 10%) 1665
▲ Alimta for Injection (Up to 8%) 1750
Aloprim for Injection (Less than 1%) 2167
Aloxi Injection (Less than 1%) 2127
Altace Capsules (Less than 1%) 1702
▲ Altoprev Extended-Release Tablets (5%) 3109
▲ Ambien Tablets (4%) 2851
Ambien CR Tablets (2% to frequent) 2855
AmBisome for Injection (Less common) 620
Amerge Tablets (Infrequent) 1339
▲ Amitiza Capsules (0% to 3.1%) 3224
Angeliq Tablets 762
Anzemet Injection (Rare) 2859
Anzemet Tablets (Rare) 2862
▲ Aranesp for Injection (11% to 13%) 581
▲ Aredia for Injection (11.5% to 26%) 2179
▲ Arimidex Tablets (2% to 15%) 673
▲ Aromasin Tablets (2% to 28.8%) 2600
▲ Arranon Injection (0% to 9%) 1357
Arthrotec Tablets (Rare) 3129
▲ Asacol Delayed-Release Tablets (5%) 2692
▲ Asmanex Twisthaler (13%) 2966
Atacand Tablets (More than 1%) 649
Atacand HCT (0.5% or greater) 651
▲ Atripla Tablets (Greater than or equal to 5%) 945
Augmentin 1360
Augmentin Tablets 1363
Augmentin XR Extended-Release Tablets 1369
Augmentin ES-600 Powder for Oral Suspension 1366
Avalide Tablets 888
Avalide Tablets 2874
▲ Avandamet Tablets (5%) 1373
Avapro Tablets (Less than 1%) 891
Avapro Tablets (Less than 1%) 2871
Avelox (0.1% to less than 2%) 2970
Axert Tablets (Rare) 2396
▲ Azilect Tablets (7% to 8%) 3293
Azmacort Inhalation Aerosol 1726
Beconase AQ Nasal Spray 1396
Benicar Tablets (Greater than 0.5%) 1043
Benicar HCT Tablets (Greater than 1%) 1044
▲ Betaseron for SC Injection (31%) 767
▲ Bexxar (1% to 10%) 1398
Bicillin C-R Injectable Suspension 1706
BiDil Tablets (1% to less than 2%) 2171
Blocadren Tablets (Less than 1%) 1916
▲ Boniva Injection (3.5% to 5.6%) 2738
▲ Boniva Tablets (3.5% to 5.6%) 2741
Boostrix 1404
Bumex Tablets (0.2% to 2.9%) 2746
▲ Caduet Tablets (Greater than 0.1% to 5.1%) 2508
Calcium Disodium Versenate Injection 1851
Campral Tablets (Frequent) 1174
▲ Captopril Tablets (About 4 to 7 of 100 patients) 2149
Carbatrol Capsules 3171
Cardura XL Tablets (Less than 1%) 2515
Catapres Tablets (About 6 in 1,000 patients) 843
Catapres-TTS (0.5% or less) 844
Ceftin for Oral Suspension (0.1% to 1%) 1407
Celebrex Capsules (0.1% to 1.9%) 3134
Celexa (2%) 1176
▲ CellCept Capsules (3% to less than 20%) 2747
▲ CellCept Intravenous (3% to less than 20%) 2747
▲ CellCept Oral Suspension (3% to less than 20%) 2747
▲ CellCept Tablets (3% to less than 20%) 2747
Cesamet Capsules 3340
Chantix Tablets (Frequent) 2517
Cialis Tablets (Less than 2%) 1838
Cipro (Less than 1%) 2977
Cipro I.V. (1% or less) 2984
Cipro XR Tablets 2990
Climara Transdermal System (1% to 5%) 771
▲ Climara Pro Transdermal System (4.2%) 776
Clinoril Tablets (Less than 1 in 100) 1924
▲ Clolar for Intravenous Infusion (11%) 1271
Clorpres Tablets (About 6 in 1,000) 2153
Clozaril Tablets (Less than 1%) 2184
▲ Colazal Capsules (4%) 2838
Combivent Inhalation Aerosol (Less than 2%) 847
▲ Combivir Tablets (5%) 1411
Comvax 1928
Concerta Extended-Release Tablets 1881
▲ Copaxone for Injection (24%) 3297
▲ Copegus Tablets (22%) 2754
▲ Coreg Tablets (1% to 6%) 1414
Cosopt Sterile Ophthalmic Solution 1931
Coumadin for Injection 898
Coumadin Tablets 898
Covera-HS Tablets (Less than 2%) 3139
Cozaar Tablets (Less than 1%) 1935
Crestor Tablets (Greater than or equal to 2%) 678
Crixivan Capsules 1940
▲ Cubicin for Injection (0.9% to 3.3%) 1026
Cuprimine Capsules 1947
CytoGam Intravenous (Less than 5.0%) 1895
▲ Dacogen Injection (20%) 2129
Dalmane Capsules 3342
Daytrana Transdermal Patch 3174
Demadex Injection (1.8%) 2759
Demadex Tablets (1.8%) 2759
▲ Depacon Injection (1% to 5%) 412
▲ Depakene (1% to 5%) 417
▲ Depakote Sprinkle Capsules (1% to 5%) 422
▲ Depakote Tablets (1% to 5%) 427
Depakote ER Tablets (Greater than 1%) 434
▲ Depo-Provera Contraceptive Injection (1% to 5%) 2622
▲ depo-subQ provera 104 Injectable Suspension (1% to less than 5%) 2624
Detrol Tablets (2%) 2628
Didronel Tablets (Infrequent) 2697
▲ Diovan Tablets (1% to 3%) 2193
Diovan HCT Tablets (Greater than 0.2%) 2196
Dolobid Tablets (Less than 1 in 100) 1955
▲ Doxil Injection (1% to 10%) 2351
DynaCirc CR Tablets (0.5% to 1%) 2721
Effexor Tablets 3411
Effexor XR Capsules (Frequent) 3417
Elidel Cream 1% (Up to 1.5%) 2200
Eligard 7.5 mg (Less than 2%) 2880
▲ Eligard 22.5 mg (3.4%) 2883
▲ Eloxatin for Injection (7% to 10%) 2892
Elspar for Injection 2463
Elspar for Injection 1960
Emend Capsules (Greater than 0.5%) 1963
▲ Emtriva Capsules (3% to 5%) 1287
▲ Emtriva Oral Solution (3% to 5%) 1287
Enablex Extended-Release Tablets (Greater than or equal to 1%) 2203
Enbrel for Injection 584
Engerix-B Vaccine (Less than 1%) 1425
Enjuvia Tablets 1062
▲ Epivir (5%) 1427
▲ Epivir-HBV (7%) 1432
Epogen for Injection (Rare) 591
Equetro Extended-Release Capsules 3180
Estrasorb Topical Emulsion 1147
Estratest Tablets 3199
Estratest H.S. Tablets 3199
▲ Estring Vaginal Ring (3%) 2635
▲ Euflexxa (6.9% to 8.75%) 1162
▲ Evista Tablets (10.7% to 15.5%) 1763
▲ Evoxac Capsules (3.7%) 1047
Exelon Capsules (2% or more) 2206
Exelon Oral Solution (2% or more) 2206
Famvir Tablets (1.3% to 1.5%) 2211
Fansidar Tablets 2765
FazaClo Orally Disintegrating Tablets (Less than 1%) 551
▲ Femara Tablets (1% to 22%) 2214
Ferrlecit Injection 3388
Flebogamma 5%, Immune Globulin Intravenous (Human) 1658
▲ Flovent Diskus (1% to 17%) 1443
▲ Fluarix (6.4% to 11%) 1451
Focalin XR Capsules 2223
Follistim AQ Cartridge 2338
▲ Forteo for Injection (10.1%) 1767
▲ Fortical Nasal Spray (3.8%) 3337
▲ Fosamax (0.4% to approximately 6%) 1969
▲ Fosamax Plus D Tablets (0.4% to 4.1%) 1977
Frova Tablets (Infrequent) 1113
▲ Gamunex Immune Globulin I.V., 10% (4%) 3235
Gantrisin Pediatric Suspension 2770
Garamycin Injectable 3014
Gardasil Injection (1.2%) 1984
▲ Gengraf Capsules (1% to 6%) 459
Genotropin Lyophilized Powder 2638
Geodon Capsules 2529
▲ Gleevec Tablets (0% to 40%) 2227
Havrix Vaccine (Less than 1%) 1456
▲ Hectorol Capsules (4.9%) 1275
▲ Hectorol Injection (4.9%) 1278
▲ Herceptin I.V. (6%) 1233
▲ Humatrope Vials and Cartridges (10.8% to 17.3%) 1787
Hycamtin for Injection (0.2% to 0.9%) 1458
Hytrin Capsules (At least 1%) 471
Hyzaar 50-12.5 Tablets 1990
Hyzaar 100-12.5 Tablets 1990
Hyzaar 100-25 Tablets 1990
▲ Imdur Tablets (Less than or equal to 5%) 3018
Imitrex Injection (Infrequent) 1463
▲ Increlex Injection (Greater than or equal to 5%) 3291
Infed Injection 3390
▲ Infergen (43% to 51%) 3364
▲ Intron A for Injection (Up to 19%) 3024
Invanz for Injection (Greater than 0.5%) 1999
Invirase (Less than 2%) 2772
▲ I.V. Busulfex (13%) 2493
Kadian Capsules (Less than 3%) 577
Kaletra (Less than 2%) 476
Keflex Capsules 549
▲ Kepivance (10%) 597
Keppra Injection 3320
Keppra Oral Solution (1% or more) 3314
Keppra Tablets (1% or more) 3314
▲ Kineret Injection (6%) 599
Klonopin (Infrequent) 2778
K-Phos Original (Sodium Free) Tablets (Less frequent) 760
K-Phos Neutral Tablets 760
Lamictal (2.0%) 1481
Lamisil Tablets 2232
Lariam Tablets (Infrequent) 2786
▲ Lescol Capsules (4.0%) 2233
Lescol XL Tablets (1.3%) 2233
▲ Leukine (11% to 21%) 814
▲ Leustatin Injection (5%) 2357
Levaquin (0.1% to 0.9%) 2384
Levaquin in 5% Dextrose Injection (0.1% to 0.9%) 2384
Levitra Tablets (Less than 2%) 3034
Levothroid Tablets 1186
Levoxyl Tablets 1712
Lexapro Oral Solution (Frequent) 1190
Lexapro Tablets (Frequent) 1190
Limbrel Capsules (0.009%) 2672
▲ Lipitor Tablets (Up to 5.1%) 2483
Lithobid Tablets 1692
Lofibra Tablets 1219
Lofibra Capsules 1216
Lopressor Injection 2238
Lopressor Tablets 2238
Lopressor HCT 50/25 Tablets 2241
Lopressor HCT 100/25 Tablets 2241
Lopressor HCT 100/50 Tablets 2241
Lotensin Tablets (Less than 1%) 2243
Lotensin HCT Tablets (0.3% to 1%) 2246
▲ Lucentis Injection (3% to 11%) 1237
Lunesta Tablets (Infrequent) 3142
Lupron Depot 7.5 mg 3264
Lupron Depot–3 Month 11.25 mg 3265
Lupron Injection Pediatric 3259
Lyrica Capsules (Greather than or equal to 1%) 2539
Matulane Capsules 3191
Maxalt Tablets (Infrequent) 2008
Maxalt-MLT Orally Disintegrating Tablets (Infrequent) 2008
▲ Menactra Vaccine (0.3% to 19.8%) 2954
▲ Menostar Transdermal System (12%) 782
▲ Meridia Capsules (5.9%) 489
Meruvax II 2019
Metadate CD Capsules 3323
Mevacor Tablets (0.5% to 1.0%) 2021
▲ Miacalcin Nasal Spray (3.8%) 2253
Micardis Tablets (More than 0.3%) 854
Micardis HCT Tablets 856
Midamor Tablets (Less than or equal to 1%) 2026
Migranal Nasal Spray (Rare) 3348
Mirapex Tablets (Greater than or equal to 1%) 859
M-M-R II 2006
▲ Mobic Oral Suspension (0% to 5.3%) 863
▲ Mobic Tablets (0% to 5.3%) 863
Moduretic Tablets (Less than or equal to 1%) 2028
Mycamine for Injection 628
▲ Myfortic Tablets (3% to less than 20%) 2255
▲ Myobloc Injection (4% to 10%) 3192
Namenda (Greater than or equal to 2%) 1195
Nasonex Nasal Spray (Greater than or equal to 2%) 3043
▲ Neoral Oral Solution (1% to 6%) 2259
▲ Neoral Soft Gelatin Capsules (1% to 6%) 2259
▲ Neulasta Injection (15% to 72%) 601
Neupogen for Injection (Infrequent) 603
Neurontin Capsules (Frequent) 2487
Neurontin Oral Solution (Frequent) 2487
Neurontin Tablets (Frequent) 2487
▲ Nexavar Tablets (Common to 10%) 746
Nexium Delayed-Release Capsules (Less than 1%) 655

Nexium I.V. (Less than 1%) 659
▲ Nipent for Injection (3% to 10%) 1863
▲ Norditropin Cartridges (19%) 2323
Noroxin Tablets 2032
Norvasc Tablets (More than 0.1% to 1%) 2545
Norvir (0 to1.7%) 503
NovoSeven 2331
▲ Nutropin for Injection (0.1% to 27%) 1239
▲ Nutropin AQ Injection (0.1% to 27%) 1243
▲ Nutropin AQ Pen (0.1% to 27%) 1243
▲ Nutropin AQ Pen Cartridge (0.1% to 27%) 1243
Omacor Capsules 2725
▲ Oncaspar (Greater than 1% but less than 5%) 1145
▲ Ontak Vials (8%) 1745
Orthoclone OKT3 Sterile Solution (Less than 1%) 2360
Paxil CR Controlled-Release Tablets (Frequent) 1538
Paxil (Frequent) 1530
Pediarix Vaccine 1548
▲ Pegasys (28%) 2789
▲ PEG-Intron Powder for Injection (23%) 3048
Pentasa Capsules (Less than 1%) 3185
Pepcid Injection (Infrequent) 2040
Pepcid (Infrequent) 2038
Permax Tablets (1.6%) 3356
Pexeva Tablets (frequent) 1694
Phenytek Capsules 2160
▲ Photofrin for Injection (31%) 702
▲ Plavix Tablets (6.3%) 917
▲ Plavix Tablets (6.3%) 2926
Pletal Tablets (Less than 2%) 2455
Pneumovax 23 (Rare) 2043
▲ Premarin Tablets (7% to 14%) 3446
Premarin Vaginal Cream 3452
▲ Premphase Tablets (7% to 13%) 3456
▲ Prempro Tablets (7% to 13%) 3456
Prevacid Delayed-Release Capsules (Less than 1%) 3271
Prevacid for Delayed-Release Oral Suspension (Less than 1%) 3271
Prevacid SoluTab Delayed-Release Orally Disintegrating Tablets (Less than 1%) 3271
Prevacid NapraPAC (Less than 1%) 3280
PREVPAC (Less than 1%) 3284
Prezista Tablets (Less than 2%) 3306
Prilosec OTC Delayed-Release Tablets (Less than 1%) 2677
Prinivil Tablets (0.3% to 1.0%) 2052
Prinzide Tablets 2056
▲ Prochieve 4% Gel (8%) 1003
▲ Prochieve 8% Gel (8%) 1003
▲ Procrit for Injection (Rare to 11%) 2364
▲ Prograf Capsules and Injection (3% to 25%) 632
▲ Proleukin for Injection (6%) 2266
▲ Prometrium Capsules (100 mg, 200 mg) (20%) 3203
ProQuad 2064
Proquin XR Tablets 1153
ProSom Tablets (Rare) 517
Protonix I.V. (Greater than or equal to 1%) 3472
Protonix Tablets (Greater than or equal to 1%) 3469
▲ Protopic Ointment (Greater than or equal to 1% to 3%) 638
Provigil Tablets (At least 1%) 988
Prozac Pulvules and Liquid 1801
Raniclor Tablets, Chewable 2505
▲ Rapamune Oral Solution and Tablets (25% to 31%) 3475
Raptiva for Injection 1250
▲ Rebetol (15% to 34%) 3058
▲ Rebetron Combination Therapy (29% to 33%) 3063
Recombivax HB (Less than 1%) 2071
Relenza Rotadisk (Less than 1.5%) 1552
Relpax Tablets (Infrequent) 2548
▲ Remicade for IV Injection (8%) 971
▲ Renagel Tablets (12.1%) 1282
▲ Requip Tablets (4% to 7%) 1555
Rescriptor Tablets 2551
▲ Retisert Implant (5% to 15%) ☉258
Retrovir Capsules 1560
Retrovir IV Infusion 1564
Retrovir 1560
▲ Revlimid Capsules (1.4% to 21.6%) 958
▲ Reyataz Capsules (Less than 1% to 4%) 921
▲ Ribavirin, USP Capsules (15% to 33%) 3068
▲ Rilutek Tablets (1.6% to 5.1%) 2930
▲ Risperdal (2% to 3%) 1676
Risperdal Consta Long-Acting Injection (Frequent) 1682
▲ Risperdal M-Tab Orally Disintegrating Tablets (2% to 3%) 1676
Ritalin Hydrochloride Tablets 2269
Ritalin LA Capsules 2271
Ritalin-SR Tablets 2269
▲ Rituxan I.V. (1% to 10%) 1254
Rozerem Tablets (2%) 3231
Sandimmune (Rare) 2275
▲ Sandostatin Injection (1% to 4%) 2278
▲ Sandostatin LAR Depot (5% to 15%) 2280
Serevent Diskus (1% to 2%) 1568
Seroquel Tablets (Infrequent) 690
▲ Simulect for Injection (3% to 10%) 2284
Singulair 2077
Solodyn Extended Release Tablets (1%) 1890
Sonata Capsules (Frequent) 1717
▲ Soriatane Capsules (10% to 25%) 1013
▲ Strattera Capsules (2% or greater) 1814
▲ Stromectol Tablets (9.3%) 2083
Sular Tablets (Less than or equal to 1%) 3122
Sustiva Capsules (Less than 2%) 930
Sustiva Tablets (Less than 2%) 930
▲ Sutent Capsules (1% to 28%) 2560
▲ Symbyax Capsules (3% to 5%) 1819
▲ Symlin Injection (2% to 7%) 613
Tambocor Tablets (Less than 1%) 1856
Targretin Capsules 1747
Tarka Tablets (0.3% to 1.7%) 524
Tasmar Tablets (1% or more) 3358
▲ Taxotere Injection Concentrate (3.4% to 19.4%) 2932
Tegretol/Tegretol-XR 2295
▲ Temodar Capsules (6%) 3073
Tequin Injection (Less than 0.1%) 938
Tequin Injection in 5% Dextrose (Less than 0.1%) 938
Tequin Tablets (Less than 0.1%) 938
Teveten Tablets (2%) 1735
Teveten HCT Tablets (Less than 1%) 1737
Thalomid Capsules 965
▲ Thiola Tablets (4%) 2141
Thyrolar Tablets 1199
Timentin ADD-Vantage 1580
Timentin Injection Galaxy Container 1583
Timentin IV Infusion 1577
Timentin Pharmacy Bulk Package 1586
Timolide Tablets 2086
Timoptic Sterile Ophthalmic Solution 2088
Timoptic in Ocudose 2091
Timoptic-XE Sterile Ophthalmic Gel Forming Solution 2092
Tindamax Tablets 2142
▲ Topamax Sprinkle Capsules (1% to 7%) 2404
▲ Topamax Tablets (1% to 7%) 2404
Toprol-XL Tablets 668
Trasylol Injection (1% to 2%) 754
Trelstar LA Suspension (2.3%) 3397
Tricor Tablets 527
Trileptal Tablets 2300
Trileptal Oral Suspension 2300
▲ Trisenox Injection (33%) 993
▲ Trizivir Tablets (5%) 1589
Truvada Tablets 1296
Twinrix Vaccine (Less than 1%) 1595
▲ Ultram ER Tablets (1% to greater than 5%) 2392
Uniretic Tablets (Less than 1%) 3100
Univasc Tablets (Less than 1%) 3104
Uroqid-Acid No. 2 Tablets 760
▲ Valcyte Tablets (Less than 5%) 2813
▲ Valtrex Caplets (Less than 1% to 6%) 1597
Vantas (Less than 2%) 3375
Varivax (Greater than or equal to 1%) 2100
Vasotec I.V. Injection (0.5% to 1.0%) 2103
▲ Velcade for Injection (14%) 2133
Verelan PM Extended-Release Capsules, Controlled-Onset (2% or less) 3106
VFEND I.V. (Less than 2%) 2564
VFEND Oral Suspension (Less than 2%) 2564
VFEND Tablets (Less than 2%) 2564
Viagra Tablets (Greater than 2%) 2573
Vicoprofen Tablets (Less than 1%) 539
Viracept (Less than 2%) 2577
▲ Viramune Oral Suspension (2% to 6%) 873
▲ Viramune Tablets (2% to 6%) 873
▲ Viread Tablets (5%) 1301
▲ Visudyne for Injection (1% to 10%) 2305
▲ Vivitrol (4% to 12%) 995
Vytorin 10/10 Tablets 2114
Vytorin 10/10 Tablets 3077
Vytorin 10/20 Tablets 2114
Vytorin 10/20 Tablets 3077
Vytorin 10/40 Tablets 2114
Vytorin 10/40 Tablets 3077
Vytorin 10/80 Tablets 2114
Vytorin 10/80 Tablets 3077
Wellbutrin Tablets 1603
▲ Wellbutrin SR Sustained-Release Tablets (1% to 4%) 1607
▲ Wellbutrin XL Extended-Release Tablets (1% to 4%) 1613
WinRho SDF 732
Xalatan Sterile Ophthalmic Solution (1% to 2%) 2649
Xifaxan Tablets (Less than 2%) 2842
▲ Xolair (8%) 1266
Xyrem Oral Solution (Frequent) 1688
Zantac (Rare) 1624
Zantac Injection (Rare) 1619
Zantac Injection Pharmacy Bulk Package (Rare) 1622
Zantac Injection Premixed (Rare) 1619
Zantac (Rare) 1624
Zegerid Capsules (Less than 1%) 2958
Zegerid Powder for Oral Solution (Less than 1%) 2958
Zelapar Tablets 3372
▲ Zetia Tablets (3.4% to 3.8%) 2120
▲ Zetia Tablets (3.8%) 3083
Ziagen 1626
Zmax for Oral Suspension 2583
Zocor Tablets 2105
Zofran Injection (2%) 1634
Zoloft (Infrequent) 2586
▲ Zometa for Intravenous Infusion (5% to 21%) 2315
Zomig Nasal Spray (Infrequent) 3523
Zonegran Capsules (Infrequent) 1101
Zosyn (1.0% or less) 3492
▲ Zyban Sustained-Release Tablets (4% to 5%) 1644
Zyflo Tablets (Greater than 1%) 1023
▲ Zyprexa Tablets (5%) 1830
▲ Zyprexa ZYDIS Orally Disintegrating Tablets (5%) 1830
Zyrtec Chewable Tablets (Less than 2%) 2594
Zyrtec (Less than 2%) 2594
Zyrtec-D 12 Hour Extended Release Tablets (Less than 2%) 2597

Arthralgia, monoarticular

Recombivax HB (Less than 1%) 2071

Arthritis

Abilify Oral Solution (Infrequent) 882
Abilify Oral Solution (Infrequent) 2450
Abilify Discmelt Orally Disintegrating Tablets (Infrequent) 882
Abilify Discmelt Orally Disintegrating Tablets (Infrequent) 2450
Abilify Tablets (Infrequent) 882
Abilify Tablets (Infrequent) 2450
Accutane Capsules 2731
Aceon Tablets (2 mg, 4 mg, 8 mg) (1.0%) 3194
Aciphex Tablets 1090
Actiq (Less than 1%) 979
▲ Actonel Tablets (4.1% to 4.8%) 2683
▲ Actonel with Calcium Tablets (4.1% to 4.8%) 2688
Adalat CC Tablets (Less than 1%) 2964
Advicor Tablets 1722
Aggrenox Capsules (2.1%) 822
Aldara Cream, 5% (0.9%) 1846
Altace Capsules (Less than 1%) 1702
Altoprev Extended-Release Tablets (Rare) 3109
Ambien Tablets (Infrequent) 2851
Ambien CR Tablets (Infrequent) 2855
Aricept Tablets (2%) 1094
Aricept ODT Tablets (2%) 1094
▲ Arimidex Tablets (12% to 17%) 673
Asacol Delayed-Release Tablets (1% to 2%) 2692
Atacand HCT (0.5% or greater) 651
Atrovent Inhalation Solution (0.9%) 835
Augmentin 1360
Augmentin Tablets 1363
Augmentin XR Extended-Release Tablets 1369
Augmentin ES-600 Powder for Oral Suspension 1366
Avalide Tablets 888
Avalide Tablets 2874
Avapro Tablets (Less than 1%) 891
Avapro Tablets (Less than 1%) 2871
Avelox (Less than 0.1%) 2970
Axert Tablets (Rare) 2396
Azilect Tablets (2%) 3293
Benicar Tablets (Greater than 0.5%) 1043
Benicar HCT Tablets (Greater than 1%) 1044
▲ Boniva Injection (3.2%) 2738
▲ Boniva Tablets (3.2%) 2741
Caduet Tablets (Greater than or equal to 2%) 2508
Campath Ampules 811
Celexa (Infrequent) 1176
Chantix Tablets (Infrequent) 2517
Clinoril Tablets (Less than 1 in 100) 1924
Colazal Capsules 2838
Comvax 1928
Copaxone for Injection (Infrequent) 3297
▲ Coreg Tablets (Greater than 1% to 3%) 1414
Cozaar Tablets (Less than 1%) 1935
Crestor Tablets (Greater than or equal to 2%) 678
Demadex Injection 2759
Demadex Tablets 2759
Didronel Tablets 2697
▲ Ditropan XL Extended-Release Tablets (2% to less than 5%) 2413
Dolobid Tablets (Less than 1 in 100) 1955
Effexor Tablets (Infrequent) 3411
Effexor XR Capsules (Infrequent) 3417
Engerix-B Vaccine (Less than 1%) 1425
▲ Estring Vaginal Ring (4%) 2635
Evoxac Capsules (Less than 1%) 1047
Exelon Capsules (Frequent) 2206
Exelon Oral Solution (Frequent) 2206
Faslodex Injection (2.8%) 681
▲ Femara Tablets (0.4% to 6.7%) 2214
Fortical Nasal Spray (Less than 1%) 3337
Gabitril Tablets (Infrequent) 984
▲ Humira Injection (Less than 5%) 466
Hytrin Capsules (At least 1%) 471
Hyzaar 50-12.5 Tablets 1990
Hyzaar 100-12.5 Tablets 1990
Hyzaar 100-25 Tablets 1990
Imitrex Nasal Spray (Infrequent) 1467
Imitrex Tablets 1471
Infed Injection 3390
▲ Intron A for Injection (Less than 5%) 3024
Invirase (Less than 2%) 2772
Keflex Capsules 549
Lamictal (Rare) 1481
Lescol Capsules (2.1%) 2233
Lescol XL Tablets (1.3%) 2233
Levaquin (0.1% to 0.9%) 2384
Levaquin in 5% Dextrose Injection (0.1% to 0.9%) 2384
Lexapro Oral Solution (Infrequent) 1190
Lexapro Tablets (Infrequent) 1190
Lipitor Tablets (Greater than or equal to 2%) 2483
Lofibra Tablets 1219
Lofibra Capsules 1216
Lopressor Injection 2238
Lopressor Tablets 2238
Lopressor HCT 50/25 Tablets (Very rare) 2241
Lopressor HCT 100/25 Tablets (Very rare) 2241
Lopressor HCT 100/50 Tablets (Very rare) 2241
Lotensin Tablets (Less than 1%) 2243
Lotensin HCT Tablets (0.3% or more) 2246
▲ Lucentis Injection (0% to 8%) 1237
Lunesta Tablets (Infrequent) 3142
▲ Macugen Injection (1% to 5%) ☉261
▲ Menostar Transdermal System (5%) 782
Meridia Capsules (Greater than or equal to 1%) 489
Meruvax II (Rare) 2019
Mevacor Tablets (Rare) 2021
Miacalcin Nasal Spray (Less than 1%) 2253
Micardis Tablets (More than 0.3%) 854
Micardis HCT Tablets 856
▲ Mirapex Tablets (3%) 859
M-M-R II 2006
Myobloc Injection (Greater than 2%) 3192
Neurontin Capsules (Infrequent) 2487
Neurontin Oral Solution (Infrequent) 2487
Neurontin Tablets (Infrequent) 2487
Nipent for Injection (Less than 3%) 1863
Noroxin Tablets 2032
Nutropin for Injection (0.1%) 1239
Nutropin AQ Injection (0.1%) 1243
Nutropin AQ Pen (0.1%) 1243
Nutropin AQ Pen Cartridge (0.1%) 1243

Omacor Capsules 2725
OptiPranolol Metipranolol Ophthalmic Solution 0.3% (A small number of patients) ⊙256
Orthoclone OKT3 Sterile Solution (Less than 1%) 2360
Paxil CR Controlled-Release Tablets (Infrequent) 1538
Paxil (Infrequent) 1530
Permax Tablets (Infrequent) 3356
Persantine Tablets (Rare) 868
Pexeva Tablets (infrequent) 1694
Plavix Tablets (1% to 2.5%) 917
Plavix Tablets (1% to 2.5%) 2926
Pletal Tablets (2% or greater) 2455
Pneumovax 23 2043
Prevacid Delayed-Release Capsules (Less than 1%) 3271
Prevacid for Delayed-Release Oral Suspension (Less than 1%) 3271
Prevacid SoluTab Delayed-Release Orally Disintegrating Tablets (Less than 1%) 3271
Prevacid NapraPAC (Less than 1%) 3280
PREVPAC (Less than 1%) 3284
Prinivil Tablets (0.3% to 1.0%) 2052
Prinzide Tablets 2056
Proleukin for Injection (1%) 2266
Prometrium Capsules (100 mg, 200 mg) (Less than 5%) 3203
ProQuad 2064
ProSom Tablets (Infrequent) 517
Protonix I.V. (Less than 1%) 3472
Protonix Tablets (Less than 1%) 3469
Protopic Ointment (Greater than or equal to 1%) 638
Provigil Tablets (At least 1%) 988
Prozac Pulvules and Liquid (Infrequent) 1801
Raniclor Tablets, Chewable 2505
Raptiva for Injection 1250
Recombivax HB (Greater than 1%) 2071
Relpax Tablets (Infrequent) 2548
Requip Tablets (1% or more) 1555
Rescriptor Tablets 2551
Revlimid Capsules 958
Risperdal (Rare) 1676
Risperdal Consta Long-Acting Injection (Infrequent) 1682
Risperdal M-Tab Orally Disintegrating Tablets (Rare) 1676
Rythmol SR Capsules 2727
Sandostatin Injection (Less than 1%) 2278
Sandostatin LAR Depot (Rare) 2280
Seroquel Tablets (Infrequent) 690
Sonata Capsules (Frequent) 1717
▲ Soriatane Capsules (1% to 10%) 1013
▲ Spiriva HandiHaler (Greater than or equal to 3%) 869
Sular Tablets (Less than or equal to 1%) 3122
Symbyax Capsules (Infrequent) 1819
Tasmar Tablets (1% to 2%) 3358
Teveten Tablets (Less than 1%) 1735
Teveten HCT Tablets (Less than 1%) 1737
Thalomid Capsules 965
Tindamax Tablets 2142
▲ Travatan Ophthalmic Solution (1% to 5%) 563
Tricor Tablets 527
Twinrix Vaccine 1595
Uniretic Tablets (Less than 1%) 3100
Vasotec I.V. Injection (0.5% to 1.0%) 2103
VFEND I.V. (Less than 2%) 2564
VFEND Oral Suspension (Less than 2%) 2564
VFEND Tablets (Less than 2%) 2564
Viadur Implant (Less than 2%) 757
Viagra Tablets (Less than 2%) 2573
Viracept (Less than 2%) 2577
▲ Vivitrol (4% to 12%) 995
Vytorin 10/10 Tablets 2114
Vytorin 10/10 Tablets 3077
Vytorin 10/20 Tablets 2114
Vytorin 10/20 Tablets 3077
Vytorin 10/40 Tablets 2114
Vytorin 10/40 Tablets 3077
Vytorin 10/80 Tablets 2114
Vytorin 10/80 Tablets 3077
▲ Wellbutrin Tablets (3.1%) 1603
Wellbutrin SR Sustained-Release Tablets (Up to 2%) 1607
Wellbutrin XL Extended-Release Tablets (0% to 2%) 1613
▲ Xeloda Tablets (Less than 5%) 2822
▲ Xenical Capsules (5.4%) 2831
Xyrem Oral Solution (Infrequent) 1688
Zelapar Tablets 3372
Zocor Tablets (Rare) 2105
Zomig Tablets (Rare) 3519
Zomig-ZMT Tablets (Rare) 3519
Zonegran Capsules (Infrequent) 1101
Zyban Sustained-Release Tablets 1644
Zyprexa Tablets (Infrequent) 1830
Zyprexa ZYDIS Orally Disintegrating Tablets (Infrequent) 1830
Zyrtec Chewable Tablets (Less than 2%) 2594
Zyrtec (Less than 2%) 2594
Zyrtec-D 12 Hour Extended Release Tablets (Less than 2%) 2597

Arthritis, acute gouty, precipitation of

Revlimid Capsules 958

Arthritis, exacerbation of

Bicillin C-R Injectable Suspension 1706
Campath Ampules 811
▲ Entocort EC Capsules (Less than 5%) 2698
Evoxac Capsules (Less than 1%) 1047
Nexium Delayed-Release Capsules (Less than 1%) 655
Nexium I.V. (Less than 1%) 659
Revlimid Capsules 958
Teveten Tablets (Less than 1%) 1735
Teveten HCT Tablets (Less than 1%) 1737

Arthritis, inflammatory

Raptiva for Injection (0.4%) 1250

Arthritis, polyarticular

Rituxan I.V. 1254

Arthritis, psoriatic

Raptiva for Injection 1250

Arthritis, pyogenic

▲ Humira Injection (Less than 5%) 466

Arthritis, tuberculous

Enbrel for Injection 584

Arthritis, septic

Elidel Cream 1% 2200
Enbrel for Injection 584
▲ Humira Injection (Less than 5%) 466
Raptiva for Injection 1250

Arthropathy, Charcot-like

Depo-Medrol Single-Dose Vial 2619

Arthropathy, unspecified

Campath Ampules 811
Colazal Capsules 2838
Didronel Tablets 2697
Evoxac Capsules (Less than 1%) 1047
▲ Gengraf Capsules (4%) 459
▲ Lescol XL Tablets (3.2%) 2233
Lexapro Oral Solution (Infrequent) 1190
Lexapro Tablets (Infrequent) 1190
▲ Neoral Oral Solution (4%) 2259
▲ Neoral Soft Gelatin Capsules (4%) 2259
Nexium Delayed-Release Capsules (Less than 1%) 655
Nexium I.V. (Less than 1%) 659
Risperdal Consta Long-Acting Injection (Infrequent) 1682
▲ Simulect for Injection (3% to 10%) 2284
▲ Starlix Tablets (3.3%) 2292
Ticlid Tablets (Rare) 2810
Zelnorm Tablets 2312

Arthrosis

Abilify Oral Solution (Infrequent) 882
Abilify Oral Solution (Infrequent) 2450
Abilify Discmelt Orally Disintegrating Tablets (Infrequent) 882
Abilify Discmelt Orally Disintegrating Tablets (Infrequent) 2450
Abilify Tablets (Infrequent) 882
Abilify Tablets (Infrequent) 2450
Aciphex Tablets 1090
Aggrenox Capsules (1.1%) 822
Ambien Tablets (Rare) 2851
Ambien CR Tablets (Rare) 2855
▲ Aredia for Injection (At least 10%) 2179
▲ Arimidex Tablets (4% to 7%) 673
Atacand HCT (0.5% or greater) 651
Azilect Tablets (Rare) 3293
Caduet Tablets (Greater than 0.1% to less than or equal to 1%) 2508
Celebrex Capsules (0.1% to 1.9%) 3134
Depacon Injection (1% or more) 412
Depakene (1% or more) 417
Depakote Sprinkle Capsules 422
▲ Depakote Tablets (1% to 5%) 427
Depakote ER Tablets (Greater than 1%) 434
Effexor Tablets (Infrequent) 3411
Effexor XR Capsules (Infrequent) 3417
Euflexxa (1.25%) 1162
▲ Fabrazyme for Intravenous Infusion (3%) 1274
▲ Fortical Nasal Spray (1% to 3%) 3337
Frova Tablets (Infrequent) 1113
Gabitril Tablets (Infrequent) 984
▲ Humatrope Vials and Cartridges (10.8%) 1787
▲ Intron A for Injection (Less than 5%) 3024
Kaletra (Less than 2%) 476
Levaquin (0.1% to 0.9%) 2384
Levaquin in 5% Dextrose Injection (0.1% to 0.9%) 2384
Lofibra Tablets 1219
Lofibra Capsules 1216
Lunesta Tablets (Rare) 3142
Lyrica Capsules (0.1% to 1%) 2539
Meridia Capsules 489
▲ Miacalcin Nasal Spray (1% to 3%) 2253
Neurontin Capsules (Infrequent) 2487
Neurontin Oral Solution (Infrequent) 2487
Neurontin Tablets (Infrequent) 2487
Norvasc Tablets (More than 0.1% to 1%) 2545
Norvir (Less than 2%) 503
NovoSeven (1%) 2331
Paxil CR Controlled-Release Tablets (Rare) 1538
Paxil (Rare) 1530
Pexeva Tablets (infrequent) 1694
Plavix Tablets (1% to 2.5%) 917
Plavix Tablets (1% to 2.5%) 2926
Protonix I.V. (Less than 1%) 3472
Protonix Tablets (Less than 1%) 3469
Protopic Ointment (0.2% to less than 1%) 638
Prozac Pulvules and Liquid (Rare) 1801
▲ Rapamune Oral Solution and Tablets (3% to 20%) 3475
Relpax Tablets (Infrequent) 2548
Requip Tablets (1% or more) 1555
Rilutek Tablets (Infrequent) 2930
Risperdal (Rare) 1676
Risperdal Consta Long-Acting Injection (Infrequent) 1682
Risperdal M-Tab Orally Disintegrating Tablets (Rare) 1676
Sonata Capsules (Infrequent) 1717
▲ Soriatane Capsules (1% to 10%) 1013
Symbyax Capsules (Rare) 1819
Targretin Capsules 1747
Tasmar Tablets (Infrequent) 3358
Teveten Tablets (Less than 1%) 1735
Teveten HCT Tablets (Less than 1%) 1737
Topamax Sprinkle Capsules (Infrequent) 2404
Topamax Tablets (Infrequent) 2404
Tricor Tablets 527
Uniretic Tablets (Less than 1%) 3100
Viagra Tablets (Less than 2%) 2573
▲ Visudyne for Injection (1% to 10%) 2305
Zelapar Tablets 3372
Zoloft (Infrequent) 2586
Zyprexa Tablets (Infrequent) 1830
Zyprexa ZYDIS Orally Disintegrating Tablets (Infrequent) 1830
Zyrtec Chewable Tablets (Less than 2%) 2594
Zyrtec (Less than 2%) 2594
Zyrtec-D 12 Hour Extended Release Tablets (Less than 2%) 2597

Ascaris, appearance in mouth and nose

Mintezol 2027

Ascites

Actiq (1% or greater) 979
Campath Ampules 811
Campral Tablets (Rare) 1174
▲ Camptosar Injection (9%) 2604
▲ CellCept Capsules (24.2%) 2747
▲ CellCept Intravenous (24.2%) 2747
▲ CellCept Oral Suspension (24.2%) 2747
▲ CellCept Tablets (24.2%) 2747
Cosmegen for Injection 2459
▲ Dacogen Injection (10%) 2129
▲ Doxil Injection (1% to 10%) 2351
▲ Eloxatin for Injection (2% to 5%) 2892
Follistim AQ Cartridge 2338
▲ Gleevec Tablets (3% to 15%) 2227
Herceptin I.V. (At least one of the 958 patients) 1233
▲ Intron A for Injection (Less than 5%) 3024
Invirase (Rare) 2772
Levaquin (0.1% to 0.9%) 2384
Levaquin in 5% Dextrose Injection (0.1% to 0.9%) 2384
Lyrica Capsules (Rare) 2539
Mylotarg for Injection (Observed in 8 out of 274 patients) 3431
Oncaspar 1145
▲ Prograf Capsules and Injection (7% to 27%) 632
▲ Proleukin for Injection (4%) 2266
▲ Rapamune Oral Solution and Tablets (3% to 20%) 3475
Requip Tablets (Rare) 1555
Risperdal (Rare) 1676
Risperdal M-Tab Orally Disintegrating Tablets (Rare) 1676
▲ Sandostatin LAR Depot (1% to 4%) 2280
Tabloid Tablets 1575
Taxotere Injection Concentrate (Less frequent) 2932
Thalomid Capsules 965
▲ Valcyte Tablets (Less than 5%) 2813
▲ Vesanoid Capsules (3%) 2820
VFEND I.V. (Less than 2%) 2564
VFEND Oral Suspension (Less than 2%) 2564
VFEND Tablets (Less than 2%) 2564
▲ Xeloda Tablets (Less than 5%) 2822

Aseptic meningitis syndrome

Carimune NF 3499
Clinoril Tablets (Less than 1 in 100) 1924
CytoGam Intravenous (Infrequent) 1895
Gammagard Liquid (Infrequent) 721
Orthoclone OKT3 Sterile Solution (Less than 1%) 2360

Aseptic necrosis of femoral/humeral heads

Colocort Rectal Suspension, USP (Retention) 100 mg/60 mL 2476
Decadron Tablets 1951
Depo-Medrol Injectable Suspension 2617
Depo-Medrol Single-Dose Vial 2619
Hydrocortone Tablets 1989

Aspartate aminotransferase levels, changes in

Abilify Oral Solution (Infrequent) 882
Abilify Oral Solution (Infrequent) 2450
Abilify Discmelt Orally Disintegrating Tablets (Infrequent) 882
Abilify Discmelt Orally Disintegrating Tablets (Infrequent) 2450
Abilify Tablets (Infrequent) 882
Abilify Tablets (Infrequent) 2450
Bumex Tablets (0.6%) 2746
▲ Emcyt Capsules (2% to 34%) 2634
Parcopa Orally Disintegrating Tablets 3097
Prozac Pulvules and Liquid (Infrequent) 1801
▲ Sutent Capsules (2% to 39%) 2560
▲ Zyvox (1.7% to 5%) 2652

Aspartate aminotransferase levels, elevation of

Abelcet Injection 1141
Accutane Capsules 2731
Aceon Tablets (2 mg, 4 mg, 8 mg) (0.3% to 1%) 3194
Aciphex Tablets (0.2%) 1090
Adalat CC Tablets (Rare) 2964
▲ Alimta for Injection (Less than 1% to 8%) 1750
Aloxi Injection (Less than 1%) 2127
Altoprev Extended-Release Tablets 3109
Ambien Tablets (Rare) 2851
Ambien CR Tablets (Rare) 2855
▲ AmBisome for Injection (12.8%) 620
Amevive (1.7%) 626
Amoxil Capsules 1343
Amoxil Chewable Tablets 1343
Amoxil Pediatric Drops for Oral Suspension 1343
Amoxil Powder for Oral Suspension 1343
Amoxil Tablets 1343
Anaprox Tablets (Less than 1%) 2761
Anaprox DS Tablets (Less than 1%) 2761
Anzemet Injection 2859
Anzemet Tablets 2862
▲ Aptivus Capsules (0.7% to 17.5%) 826
▲ Aralast (11.1%) 717
▲ Arimidex Tablets (2% to 5%) 673
Arixtra Injection (0.2% to 2.6%) 1351
▲ Arranon Injection (1% to 6%) 1357
Arthrotec Tablets 3129
Asacol Delayed-Release Tablets 2692
▲ Atripla Tablets (3%) 945
Augmentin (Infrequent) 1360

Augmentin Tablets (Infrequent) 1363
Augmentin XR Extended-Release Tablets (Infrequent) 1369
Augmentin ES-600 Powder for Oral Suspension 1366
Axid Oral Solution (Less common) 879
▲ Baraclude (5%) 894
BeneFix Vials (1.6%) 3408
Benicar HCT Tablets (Greater than 1%) 1044
▲ Betaseron for SC Injection (3%) 767
Biaxin/Biaxin XL (Less than 1%) 402
Bicillin C-R Injectable Suspension 1706
Calcijex Injection 411
Calcium Disodium Versenate Injection 1851
Campral Tablets (Infrequent) 1174
▲ Camptosar Injection (1% to 10%) 2604
▲ Cancidas for Injection (1.9% to 13%) 1918
Cardizem LA Extended Release Tablets (Less than 2%) 1728
Ceftin (0.1% to 1%) 1407
Celebrex Capsules (0.1% to 1.9%) 3134
▲ CellCept Capsules (3% to less than 20%) 2747
▲ CellCept Intravenous (3% to less than 20%) 2747
▲ CellCept Oral Suspension (3% to less than 20%) 2747
▲ CellCept Tablets (3% to less than 20%) 2747
▲ Chemet Capsules (4.2% to 10.4%) 2458
Cipro (1.7%) 2977
▲ Cipro I.V. (Among most frequent) 2984
▲ Clolar for Intravenous Infusion (38%) 1271
Colazal Capsules 2838
Combivir Tablets 1411
▲ Coreg Tablets (Greater than 1% to 3%) 1414
Covera-HS Tablets (1.4%) 3139
▲ Crixivan Capsules (3.7%) 1940
Cubicin for Injection (Less than 1%) 1026
Cutivate Lotion 0.05% (Rare) 2664
Cymbalta Delayed-Release Capsules 1757
▲ Dacogen Injection (10%) 2129
Dalmane Capsules (Rare) 3342
Demser Capsules (Rare) 1953
▲ Depacon Injection (1% to 5%) 412
Depakene (Frequent) 417
▲ Depakote Sprinkle Capsules (1% to 5%) 422
Depakote Tablets (Frequent) 427
Depakote ER Tablets (Greater than 1%) 434
Depo-Medrol Single-Dose Vial 2619
Dolobid Tablets 1955
EC-Naprosyn Delayed-Release Tablets (Less than 1%) 2761
Effexor Tablets (Infrequent) 3411
Effexor XR Capsules (Infrequent) 3417
▲ Eloxatin for Injection (0% to 54%) 2892
Elspar for Injection 2463
Elspar for Injection 1960
▲ Emend Capsules (3%) 1963
▲ Emtriva Capsules (3% to 6%) 1287
▲ Emtriva Oral Solution (3% to 6%) 1287
Epivir (Up to 1.7%) 1427
Eraxis for Injection (0.3% to 0.8%) 2521
Eulexin Capsules 3009
Evoxac Capsules (Less than 1%) 1047
Famvir Tablets (2.3%) 2211
Femara Tablets 2214
▲ Fortaz (1 in 16) 1453
Fuzeon Injection 2767
Gamunex Immune Globulin I.V., 10% 3235
Garamycin Injectable 3014
▲ Gemzar for Injection (52% to 78%) 1771
▲ Gleevec Tablets (0% to 4.8%) 2227
Hectorol Capsules 1275
Hectorol Injection 1278
▲ Hepsera Tablets (2% to 8%) 1292
▲ Humatrope Vials and Cartridges (6.67% to 12.50%) 1787
▲ Hycamtin for Injection (Less than 1% to 5%) 1458
▲ Imdur Tablets (Less than or equal to 5%) 3018
Increlex Injection 3291
▲ Intron A for Injection (Up to 63% of patients) 3024
▲ Invanz for Injection (3.8% to 8.4%) 1999
▲ Invirase (Less than 1% to 4%) 2772
▲ Kaletra (2% to 10%) 476
Keflex Capsules 549
Kytril Injection (2.8%) 2781
Kytril (2%) 2784
▲ Lexiva Tablets (6%) 1505
▲ Lofibra Tablets (Up to 3%) 1219
▲ Lofibra Capsules (3%) 1216
Lotronex Tablets 1512
▲ Lovenox Injection (Up to 3.9%) 2915
Lupron Depot 3.75 mg (One patient) 3260
▲ Lupron Depot 7.5 mg (Greater than or equal to 5%) 3264
Malarone Pediatric Tablets 1517
Malarone Tablets 1517
Marinol Capsules (Less than 1%) 3333
Maxipime for Injection (2.4%) 1105
Mefoxin for Injection 2012
Mefoxin Premixed Intravenous Solution 2016
▲ Mepron Suspension (4%) 1521
Meridia Capsules (1.6%) 489
Merrem I.V. (Greater than 0.2%) 686
Mevacor Tablets 2021
Mobic Oral Suspension (Less than 2%) 863
Mobic Tablets (Less than 2%) 863
Mycamine for Injection (0.8% to 2.7%) 628
▲ Mylotarg for Injection (18%) 3431
Nabi-HB (2%) 2169
Nalfon Capsules (Less than 1%) 2502
Naprosyn Suspension (Less than 1%) 2761
Naprosyn Tablets (Less than 1%) 2761
Nexium Delayed-Release Capsules (Less than 1%) 655
Nexium I.V. (Less than 1%) 659
Niaspan Extended-Release Tablets 1730
Noroxin Tablets (1.4% to 1.6%) 2032
▲ Norvir (6.4% to 9.5%) 503
Omacor Capsules 2725
Omnicef Capsules (0.4%) 511
Omnicef for Oral Suspension (0.2%) 511
▲ Oncaspar (Greater than 1% but less than 5%) 1145
Oracea Capsules (2.2%) 1000
Orthoclone OKT3 Sterile Solution (Less than 1%) 2360
Oxandrin Tablets 2962
Paxil CR Controlled-Release Tablets (Infrequent) 1538
Paxil (Infrequent) 1530
Pentasa Capsules (Less than 1%) 3185
Pexeva Tablets (infrequent) 1694
Precose Tablets 751
Prevacid Delayed-Release Capsules 3271
Prevacid for Delayed-Release Oral Suspension 3271
Prevacid SoluTab Delayed-Release Orally Disintegrating Tablets 3271
Prevacid NapraPAC 3280
PREVPAC (Less than 1%) 3284
▲ Prezista Tablets (5.3% to 10%) 3306
Prilosec OTC Delayed-Release Tablets (Rare) 2677
Primaxin I.M. 2045
Primaxin I.V. 2048
▲ Prograf Capsules and Injection (3% to 15%) 632
▲ Proleukin for Injection (23%) 2266
Proquin XR Tablets (Less than 1%) 1153
ProSom Tablets (Rare) 517
Protonix I.V. (Greater than or equal to 1%) 3472
Protonix Tablets (Less than 1%) 3469
Protopic Ointment (Greater than or equal to 1%) 638
Provigil Tablets (At least 1%) 988
Raniclor Tablets, Chewable 2505
▲ Rapamune Oral Solution and Tablets (3% to 20%) 3475
▲ Rebif Prefilled Syringe for Injection (10% to 17%) 3159
Remicade for IV Injection 971
▲ Rescriptor Tablets (2.3% to 3.4%) 2551
Risperdal (Infrequent) 1676
Risperdal Consta Long-Acting Injection (Rare) 1682
Risperdal M-Tab Orally Disintegrating Tablets (Infrequent) 1676
Rocaltrol Capsules 2798
Rocaltrol Oral Solution 2798
▲ Rocephin Injectable Vials, ADD-Vantage, Galaxy, Bulk (3.1%) 2800
Rythmol SR Capsules 2727
▲ Seroquel Tablets (3%) 690
Singulair (1.6%) 2077
▲ Soltamox Oral Solution (5%) 3527
Somavert Injection (0.8%) 2642
Sonata Capsules (Rare) 1717
▲ Soriatane Capsules (Approximately 1 in 3 patients) 1013
Stromectol Tablets (2%) 2083
Suprax (Less than 2%) 1843
Sustiva Capsules (2%) 930
Sustiva Tablets (2%) 930
Symbyax Capsules (2%) 1819
Symmetrel Tablets 1135
▲ Synagis (3.0%) 1897
Tarceva Tablets 1259
Tarceva Tablets 2444
Targretin Capsules 1747
Tarka Tablets 524
Tasmar Tablets (1% to 5%) 3358
▲ Taxotere Injection Concentrate (4.3%) 2932
Tequin Injection (Less than 0.1%) 938
Tequin Injection in 5% Dextrose (Less than 0.1%) 938
Tequin Tablets (Less than 0.1%) 938
Teveten Tablets (Less than 1%) 1735
Teveten HCT Tablets (Less than 1%) 1737
▲ Thalomid Capsules (2.8% to 12.5%) 965
Tiazac Capsules (Less than 2%) 1201
Ticlid Tablets (Rare) 2810
Timentin ADD-Vantage 1580
Timentin Injection Galaxy Container 1583
Timentin IV Infusion 1577
Timentin Pharmacy Bulk Package 1586
Topamax Sprinkle Capsules (Infrequent) 2404
Topamax Tablets (Infrequent) 2404
▲ Tracleer Tablets (11%) 545
Trecator Tablets 3487
▲ Tricor Tablets (3.4%) 527
▲ Triglide Tablets (3.4%) 3123
▲ Trisenox Injection (13%) 993
Trizivir Tablets (1.7%) 1589
▲ Truvada Tablets (3%) 1296
▲ Tygacil for Injection (4.3%) 3488
Ultane Liquid for Inhalation (Less than 1%) 531
▲ Ultram ER Tablets (1% to greater than 5%) 2392
Uniretic Tablets (Less than 1%) 3100
▲ Valtrex Caplets (1% to 16%) 1597
Vantas (Less than 2%) 3375
Vantin Tablets and Oral Suspension 2645
Verelan PM Extended-Release Capsules, Controlled-Onset 3106
▲ VFEND I.V. (1.9% to 20.3%) 2564
▲ VFEND Oral Suspension (1.9% to 20.3%) 2564
▲ VFEND Tablets (1.9% to 20.3%) 2564
Viracept (Less than 2%) 2577
Viramune Oral Suspension (2.0%) 873
Viramune Tablets (2.0%) 873
▲ Viread Tablets (3% to 5%) 1301
Vivitrol (1.5%) 995
Xifaxan Tablets (Less than 2%) 2842
Zegerid Capsules (Rare) 2958
Zegerid Powder for Oral Solution (Rare) 2958
▲ Ziagen (6%) 1626
▲ Zinacef for Injection (1 in 25 patients) 1631
▲ Zinacef Injection (1 in 25 patients) 1631
Zmax for Oral Suspension (Less then 1%) 2583
Zocor Tablets (1%) 2105
▲ Zofran Injection (Approximately 5% of patients) 1634
Zofran (Approximately 1% to 2%) 1639
Zofran ODT Orally Disintegrating Tablets (Approximately 1% to 2%) 1639
Zoloft (Infrequent) 2586
Zonegran Capsules (Rare) 1101
Zosyn 3492
Zyprexa Tablets 1830
Zyprexa IntraMuscular 1830
Zyprexa ZYDIS Orally Disintegrating Tablets 1830

Aspergillosis, bronchopulmonary

Dacogen Injection 2129

Asphyxia

Bentyl Capsules 697
Bentyl Injection 697
Bentyl Syrup 697
Bentyl Tablets 697

Aspiration

Clozaril Tablets 2184
FazaClo Orally Disintegrating Tablets 551
Levaquin (0.1% to 0.9%) 2384
Levaquin in 5% Dextrose Injection (0.1% to 0.9%) 2384
Percodan Tablets 1132
Risperdal (Rare) 1676
Risperdal M-Tab Orally Disintegrating Tablets (Rare) 1676
Seroquel Tablets 690

AST elevation

(*see under* Aspartate aminotransferase levels, elevation of)

Asterixis

Bumex Tablets (0.1%) 2746
Depacon Injection 412
Depakene 417
Depakote Sprinkle Capsules 422
Depakote Tablets 427
Depakote ER Tablets 434
Fortaz 1453
Orthoclone OKT3 Sterile Solution (Less than 1%) 2360
Phenytek Capsules (Rare) 2160
▲ Vesanoid Capsules (3%) 2820

Asthenia

▲ Abilify Oral Solution (Infrequent to 8%) 882
▲ Abilify Oral Solution (Infrequent to 8%) 2450
▲ Abilify Discmelt Orally Disintegrating Tablets (Infrequent to 8%) 882
▲ Abilify Discmelt Orally Disintegrating Tablets (Infrequent to 8%) 2450
▲ Abilify Tablets (Infrequent to 8%) 882
▲ Abilify Tablets (Infrequent to 8%) 2450
Accolate Tablets (1.8%) 671
Accutane Capsules 2731
▲ Aceon Tablets (2 mg, 4 mg, 8 mg) (7.9%) 3194
Aciphex Tablets 1090
▲ Actiq (4% to 38%) 979
▲ Actonel Tablets (3.5% to 5.1%) 2683
▲ Actonel with Calcium Tablets (3.5% to 5.4%) 2688
▲ ADACEL Vaccine (1.2% to 30.4%) 2945
Adalat CC Tablets (Less than 1%) 2964
▲ Adderall XR Capsules (2% to 6%) 3166
Adenoscan (Less than 1%) 619
▲ Advicor Tablets (5%) 1722
▲ Aerobid/Aerobid-M (1% to 3%) 1171
Aggrenox Capsules (1.8%) 822
▲ Agrylin Capsules (23.1%) 3169
Albalon Ophthalmic Solution ⊙ 218
Aldoril Tablets 1910
Alinia for Oral Suspension (Less than 1%) 2835
Alinia Tablets (Less than 1%) 2835
Allegra-D 12 Hour Extended-Release Tablets 2846
Allegra-D 24 Hour Extended-Release Tablets 2849
Aloxi Injection (1%) 2127
▲ Alphagan P Ophthalmic Solution (1% to 4%) 567
Altace Capsules (0.3% to 2.0%) 1702
▲ Altoprev Extended-Release Tablets (3%) 3109
Ambien Tablets (Frequent) 2851
Ambien CR Tablets (1% to frequent) 2855
▲ AmBisome for Injection (6.2% to 13.1%) 620
Amitiza Capsules (Less than 0.2%) 3224
AndroGel (0% to 3%) 3329
Aptivus Capsules (1.5%) 826
▲ Aranesp for Injection (5%) 581
▲ Aredia for Injection (22.2%) 2179
▲ Arimidex Tablets (13% to 19%) 673
Aromasin Tablets (Less frequent) 2600
▲ Arranon Injection (0% to 17%) 1357
Arthrotec Tablets (Rare) 3129
▲ Asacol Delayed-Release Tablets (7%) 2692
Atacand Tablets (0.5% or greater) 649
Atacand HCT (0.5% or greater) 651
Atripla Tablets 945
Avalide Tablets 888
Avalide Tablets 2874
Avandaryl Tablets (1.6%) 1379
Avapro Tablets (1% or greater) 891
Avapro Tablets (1% or greater) 2871
▲ Avastin IV (10% to 74%) 1227
Avelox (0.1% to less than 2%) 2970
▲ Avinza Capsules (5% to 10%) 1741
Axert Tablets (Infrequent) 2396
▲ Axid Oral Solution (3.1%) 879
Azilect Tablets (Frequent) 3293
Benicar Tablets 1043
Benicar HCT Tablets (Rare) 1044
▲ Bentyl Capsules (7%) 697
▲ Bentyl Injection (7%) 697
▲ Bentyl Syrup (7%) 697
▲ Bentyl Tablets (7%) 697
Betagan Ophthalmic Solution, USP ⊙ 220

▲ Betaseron for SC Injection (61%) 767
▲ Betimol Ophthalmic Solution (1% to 5%) 3382
▲ Betimol Ophthalmic Solution (1% to 5%) ⊙ 295
▲ Bexxar (2% to 46%) 1398
Bicillin C-R Injectable Suspension 1706
▲ BiDil Tablets (14%) 2171
Biltricide Tablets 2976
Blocadren Tablets (0.6%) 1916
▲ Boniva Injection (3.5%) 2738
▲ Boniva Tablets (3.5%) 2741
▲ BOTOX Purified Neurotoxin Complex (2% to 10%) 570
▲ Brimonidine Tartrate Ophthalmic Solution 0.2% (3% to 9%) ⊙ 248
Bumex Tablets (0.2% to 2.9%) 2746
▲ Byetta Injection (Greater than or equal to 1% to less than 5%) 611
▲ Caduet Tablets (Less than 1% to 3.8%) 2508
Calcijex Injection 411
▲ Campath Ampules (4% to 13%) 811
▲ Campral Tablets (5% to 7%) 1174
▲ Camptosar Injection (12% to 76%) 2604
Cancidas for Injection (0%) 1918
Captopril Tablets 2149
Cardene I.V. (0.7%) 2497
Cardizem LA Extended Release Tablets (2.6%) 1728
▲ Cardura XL Tablets (3.9%) 2515
▲ Carnitor Injection (8% to 12%) 3188
Carteolol Hydrochloride Ophthalmic Solution USP, 1% (Occasional) ⊙ 249
▲ Catapres Tablets (About 10 in 100 patients) 843
Catapres-TTS (0.5% or less) 844
Cathflo Activase (2%) 1231
Caverject Impulse Injection (Less than 1%) 2612
Celebrex Capsules (0.1% to 1.9%) 3134
Celexa (At least 2%) 1176
▲ CellCept Capsules (35.4% to 43.3%) 2747
▲ CellCept Intravenous (35.4% to 43.3%) 2747
▲ CellCept Oral Suspension (35.4% to 43.3%) 2747
▲ CellCept Tablets (35.4% to 43.3%) 2747
▲ Cesamet Capsules (8%) 3340
▲ Chantix Tablets (4% to 7%) 2517
Cialis Tablets (Less than 2%) 1838
Cipro (Less than 1%) 2977
Cipro I.V. (1% or less) 2984
Cipro XR Tablets (Less than 1%) 2990
Clinoril Tablets (Less than 1 in 100) 1924
▲ Clorpres Tablets (About 10%) 2153
Clozaril Tablets (1%) 2184
Colazal Capsules 2838
Combivent Inhalation Aerosol 847
Combivir Tablets 1411
Comtan Tablets (2%) 2189
▲ Copaxone for Injection (41%) 3297
▲ Copegus Tablets (65%) 2754
▲ Coreg Tablets (7% to 11%) 1414
Cosopt Sterile Ophthalmic Solution 1931
Coumadin for Injection (Infrequent) 898
Coumadin Tablets (Infrequent) 898
Cozaar Tablets (1% or greater) 1935
Crestor Tablets (2.7%) 678
Crixivan Capsules (2.1%) 1940
▲ Cubicin for Injection (Less than 1% to 5%) 1026
▲ Cymbalta Delayed-Release Capsules (2% to 8%) 1757
Dacogen Injection 2129
Dalmane Capsules 3342
▲ Dantrium Capsules (Among most frequent) 2694
Dapsone Tablets USP 1673
Daranide Tablets 1950
Decadron Tablets 1951
Demadex Injection (2%) 2759
Demadex Tablets (2%) 2759
▲ Depacon Injection (10% to 27%) 412
▲ Depakene (21% to 27%) 417
▲ Depakote Sprinkle Capsules (10% to 27%) 422
▲ Depakote Tablets (10% to 27%) 427
▲ Depakote ER Tablets (6% to 27%) 434
▲ DepoCyt Injection (5% to 19%) 1143
▲ Depo-Provera Contraceptive Injection (Greater than 5%) 2622
depo-subQ provera 104 Injectable Suspension 2624
Diastat Rectal Delivery System (At least 1%) 3343
Dilaudid 440
Dilaudid Non-Sterile Powder 440
Dilaudid Oral Liquid (Less frequent) 445
Dilaudid Rectal Suppositories 440
Dilaudid Tablets 440
Dilaudid Tablets - 8 mg (Less frequent) 445
Dilaudid-HP (Less frequent) 442
Diovan Tablets 2193
Diovan HCT Tablets (Greater than 0.2%) 2196
▲ Ditropan XL Extended-Release Tablets (3% to 7%) 2413
Diuril Oral Suspension 1954
Diuril Sodium Intravenous 2467
Dolobid Tablets (Less than 1 in 100) 1955
Donnatal Extentabs 2493
▲ Doxil Injection (6.5% to 40.2%) 2351
Duetact Tablets (1.6%) 3226
▲ Duragesic Transdermal System (10% or more) 2373
Dyazide Capsules 1423
DynaCirc CR Tablets 2721
Dyrenium Capsules (Rare) 3400
▲ Effexor Tablets (2% to 16.9%) 3411
▲ Effexor XR Capsules (1% to 17%) 3417
Eldepryl Capsules 3208
Eligard 22.5 mg (Less than 2%) 2883
▲ Eligard 45 mg (3.6%) 2888
▲ Emend Capsules (3.4% to 17.8%) 1963
Emsam Transdermal System 903
▲ Emtriva Capsules (12% to 16%) 1287
▲ Emtriva Oral Solution (12% to 16%) 1287
Enablex Extended-Release Tablets (1.5% to 2.7%) 2203
▲ Enbrel for Injection (5% to 11%) 584
Engerix-B Vaccine (Less than 1%) 1425
▲ Entocort EC Capsules (Less than 5%) 2698
EpiPen 1061
Epivir 1427
Epivir-HBV 1432
▲ Epogen for Injection (7% to 13%) 591
Epzicom Tablets 1436
▲ Equetro Extended-Release Capsules (8%) 3180
▲ Erbitux (4% to 56%) 910
▲ Euflexxa (3%) 1162
Evoxac Capsules (0.5%) 1047
▲ Exelon Capsules (2% to 6%) 2206
▲ Exelon Oral Solution (2% to 6%) 2206
Fansidar Tablets 2765
▲ Faslodex Injection (22.7%) 681
FazaClo Orally Disintegrating Tablets (1%) 551
▲ Femara Tablets (0.6% to 33.6%) 2214
▲ Ferrlecit Injection (7%) 3388
▲ Flomax Capsules (7.8% to 8.5%) 850
Fluarix 1451
Flumadine (1.4%) 1183
▲ Flumist Vaccine (25.7%) 1901
▲ Forteo for Injection (8.7%) 1767
Fosamax 1969
Fosamax Plus D Tablets 1977
Frova Tablets (Infrequent) 1113
Furosemide Tablets 2154
Fuzeon Injection 2767
▲ Gabitril Tablets (18% to 23%) 984
▲ Gamunex Immune Globulin I.V., 10% (4% to 10%) 3235
Gantrisin Pediatric Suspension 2770
Gemzar for Injection (Common) 1771
Gengraf Capsules (Rare) 459
▲ Geodon (5% to 6%) 2529
▲ Gleevec Tablets (0.2% to 21%) 2227
Hectorol Capsules 1275
Hectorol Injection 1278
▲ Hepsera Tablets (2% to 13%) 1292
▲ Herceptin I.V. (42%) 1233
▲ Humatrope Vials and Cartridges (3.33% to 6.25%) 1787
▲ Hycamtin for Injection (Less than 1% to 25%) 1458
Hyperstat I.V. (2%) 3017
▲ Hytrin Capsules (1.6% to 11.3%) 471
Hyzaar 50-12.5 Tablets (1% or greater) 1990
Hyzaar 100-12.5 Tablets (1% or greater) 1990
Hyzaar 100-25 Tablets (1% or greater) 1990
▲ Imdur Tablets (Less than or equal to 5%) 3018
▲ Imitrex Injection (5%) 1463
Imitrex Nasal Spray (Infrequent) 1467
Imitrex Tablets (Less than 1% to 2%) 1471
▲ Indapamide Tablets (Less than 5%) 2156
Inderal LA Long-Acting Capsules 3429
Infed Injection 3390
▲ Infergen (9% to 10%) 3364
InnoPran XL Capsules 2723
▲ Intron A for Injection (Up to 40%) 3024
Invanz for Injection (1.2%) 1999
▲ Invirase (0.3% to 9.2%) 2772
Ionsys Transdermal System (.1% to less than 1%) 2379
▲ Iressa Tablets (5% to 6%) 684
▲ I.V. Busulfex (2% to 51%) 2493
Kadian Capsules (Less than 3%) 577
▲ Kaletra (3% to 9%) 476
▲ Keppra Injection (15%) 3320
▲ Keppra Oral Solution (8.9% to 15%) 3314
▲ Keppra Tablets (8.9% to 15%) 3314
K-Phos Neutral Tablets 760
▲ Kytril Injection (5%) 2781
▲ Kytril (14% to 18%) 2784
▲ Lamictal (2% to 8%) 1481
Lanoxicaps Capsules 1490
Lanoxin Injection 1494
Lanoxin Injection Pediatric 1497
Lanoxin Tablets 1500
Lariam Tablets (Less than 1%) 2786
Lescol Capsules (Rare) 2233
Lescol XL Tablets 2233
▲ Leukine (17% to 66%) 814
▲ Leustatin Injection (9%) 2357
Levaquin (0.1% to 0.9%) 2384
Levaquin in 5% Dextrose Injection (0.1% to 0.9%) 2384
Levitra Tablets (Less than 2%) 3034
Levothroid Tablets 1186
Lexapro Oral Solution (Infrequent) 1190
Lexapro Tablets (Infrequent) 1190
Lidoderm Patch 1118
▲ Lipitor Tablets (Up to 3.8%) 2483
Lofibra Tablets (2.1%) 1219
Lofibra Capsules (2.1%) 1216
Lopressor HCT 50/25 Tablets 2241
Lopressor HCT 100/25 Tablets 2241
Lopressor HCT 100/50 Tablets 2241
Lotensin Tablets (Less than 1%) 2243
Lotensin HCT Tablets (0.3% to1%) 2246
Lotrel Capsules 2249
▲ Lumigan Ophthalmic Solution (1% to 5%) 573
Lunesta Tablets 3142
▲ Lupron Depot 3.75 mg (9%) 3260
Lupron Depot 7.5 mg (Less than 5%) 3264
▲ Lupron Depot–3 Month 11.25 mg (9%) 3265
▲ Lyrica Capsules (2% to 7%) 2539
▲ Malarone Pediatric Tablets (3% to 8%) 1517
▲ Malarone Tablets (3% to 8%) 1517
Marinol Capsules (Greater than 1%) 3333
Matulane Capsules 3191
▲ Mavik Tablets (3.3%) 486
Maxair Autohaler 1852
▲ Maxalt Tablets (4% to 7%) 2008
▲ Maxalt-MLT Orally Disintegrating Tablets (4% to 7%) 2008
▲ Megace ES Oral Suspension (2% to 6%) 2481
▲ Mepron Suspension (8% to 31%) 1521
▲ Meridia Capsules (5.9%) 489
Mevacor Tablets (1.2% to 1.7%) 2021
Micardis Tablets 854
Micardis HCT Tablets 856
▲ Midamor Tablets (Between 1% and 3%) 2026
Migranal Nasal Spray (1%) 3348
Mintezol 2027
▲ Mirapex Tablets (10% to 14%) 859
▲ Moduretic Tablets (3% to 8%) 2028
MS Contin Tablets (Less frequent) 2701
Mustargen for Injection 2468
Myleran Tablets 1525
▲ Mylotarg for Injection (37%) 3431
▲ Myobloc Injection (0% to 6%) 3192
▲ Nalfon Capsules (5.4%) 2502
Neoral Oral Solution (Rare) 2259
Neoral Soft Gelatin Capsules (Rare) 2259
▲ Neulasta Injection (15% to 72%) 601
▲ Neumega for Injection (14%) 3435
▲ Neupogen for Injection (4%) 603
▲ Neurontin Capsules (5.7%) 2487
▲ Neurontin Oral Solution (5.7%) 2487
▲ Neurontin Tablets (5.7%) 2487
▲ Nexavar Tablets (Very Common) 746
Nexium Delayed-Release Capsules (Less than 1%) 655
Nexium I.V. (Less than 1%) 659
Niaspan Extended-Release Tablets 1730
▲ Nipent for Injection (10% to 13%) 1863
▲ Niravam Orally Disintegrating Tablets (5.8% to 7.1%) 3092
Nitrolingual Pumpspray 3120
Norditropin Cartridges 2323
Norflex Injection 1856
Noroxin Tablets (Less frequent) 2032
Norvasc Tablets (Less than 1% to 2%) 2545
▲ Norvir (10.3% to 15.3%) 503
Numorphan Injection 1120
Omacor Capsules 2725
Omnicef Capsules (0.2%) 511
Omnicef for Oral Suspension (0.2%) 511
▲ Ontak Vials (66%) 1745
Opana Tablets (Less than 1%) 1122
Opana ER Tablets (Less than 1%) 1126
OptiPranolol Metipranolol Ophthalmic Solution 0.3% (A small number of patients) ⊙ 256
Ortho-Cyclen Tablets 2429
Ortho Evra Transdermal System 2417
Ortho Tri-Cyclen Tablets 2429
Ortho Tri-Cyclen Lo Tablets 2436
Orthoclone OKT3 Sterile Solution (Less than 1%) 2360
▲ OxyContin Tablets (6%) 2703
Parcopa Orally Disintegrating Tablets 3097
Parnate Tablets 1527
▲ Patanol Ophthalmic Solution (Less than 5%) 561
▲ Paxil CR Controlled-Release Tablets (1.6% to 22%) 1538
▲ Paxil (1.6% to 22%) 1530
Pediarix Vaccine 1548
▲ Pegasys (56%) 2789
▲ PEG-Intron Powder for Injection (52%) 3048
Pentasa Capsules (Less than 1%) 3185
Pepcid Injection (Infrequent) 2040
Pepcid (Infrequent) 2038
Percodan Tablets 1132
▲ Permax Tablets (4.2%) 3356
▲ Pexeva Tablets (1.6% to 22%) 1694
▲ Photofrin for Injection (6%) 702
Plavix Tablets (1% to 2.5%) 917
Plavix Tablets (1% to 2.5%) 2926
Pletal Tablets (2% or greater) 2455
Pneumovax 23 2043
▲ Premarin Tablets (7% to 8%) 3446
▲ Premphase Tablets (6% to 10%) 3456
▲ Prempro Tablets (6% to 10%) 3456
Prevacid Delayed-Release Capsules (Less than 1%) 3271
Prevacid for Delayed-Release Oral Suspension (Less than 1%) 3271
Prevacid SoluTab Delayed-Release Orally Disintegrating Tablets (Less than 1%) 3271
Prevacid NapraPAC (Less than 1%) 3280
PREVPAC (Less than 1%) 3284
Prezista Tablets (Less than 2%) 3306
Prilosec OTC Delayed-Release Tablets (1.1% to 1.3%) 2677
Primaxin I.M. 2045
Primaxin I.V. (Less than 0.2%) 2048
Prinivil Tablets (Greater than 1%) 2052
Prinzide Tablets (1.8%) 2056
ProAmatine Tablets (Rare) 3186
Prochieve 4% Gel 1003
Prochieve 8% Gel 1003
▲ Procrit for Injection (7% to 13%) 2364
▲ Prograf Capsules and Injection (11% to 52%) 632
▲ Proleukin for Injection (23%) 2266
Prometrium Capsules (100 mg, 200 mg) 3203
Proquin XR Tablets 1153
▲ ProSom Tablets (11%) 517
ProstaScint Kit 1037
Protonix I.V. (Greater than or equal to 1%) 3472
Protonix Tablets (Greater than or equal to 1%) 3469
▲ Protopic Ointment (1% to 3%) 638
Provigil Tablets (At least 1%) 988
▲ Prozac Pulvules and Liquid (7% to 21%) 1801
Pulmozyme Inhalation Solution 1248
Ranexa Tablets 1035
Raniclor Tablets, Chewable (Rare) 2505
▲ Rapamune Oral Solution and Tablets (22% to 40%) 3475
Raptiva for Injection 1250
Razadyne (Frequent) 2399
Razadyne ER Extended-Release Capsules (Greater than or equal to 2%) 2399
▲ Rebetol (5% to 66%) 3058
▲ Rebetron Combination Therapy (4% to 9%) 3063
Recombivax HB (Equal to or greater than 1%) 2071
ReFacto Vials 3484
▲ Relpax Tablets (4% to 10%) 2548
ReoPro Vials (0.7%) 1809
Requip Tablets (Infrequent) 1555
▲ Rescriptor Tablets (5.3% to 16%) 2551
Restoril Capsules (1.4%) 1860
▲ Retrovir Capsules (8.6% to 69%) 1560
▲ Retrovir IV Infusion (8.6% to 69%) 1564

▲ Retrovir (8.6% to 69%) 1560
▲ Revlimid Capsules (1.4% to 23.4%) 958
Reyataz Capsules (Less than 3%)..... 921
▲ Ribavirin, USP Capsules (5% to 10%) 3068
▲ Rilutek Tablets (14.8% to 20.1%) 2930
Risperdal 1676
Risperdal Consta Long-Acting Injection (Frequent) 1682
Risperdal M-Tab Orally Disintegrating Tablets 1676
▲ Rituxan I.V. (1% to 26%) 1254
Rocaltrol Capsules 2798
Rocaltrol Oral Solution 2798
▲ Romazicon Injection (1% to 3%) 2804
▲ Rythmol SR Capsules (3% to 4%) 2727
Sandimmune (Rare) 2275
▲ Sandostatin Injection (1% to 4%) 2278
▲ Sandostatin LAR Depot (5% to 15%) 2280
▲ Sensipar Tablets (7%) 608
▲ Seroquel Tablets (5%) 690
▲ Simulect for Injection (3% to 10%) ... 2284
Singulair (1.8%) 2077
▲ Sonata Capsules (5% to 7%) 1717
Stalevo Tablets (2%) 2287
Stromectol Tablets (0.9%) 2083
▲ Suboxone Tablets (6.5% to 14%) 2717
▲ Subutex Tablets (4.9% to 14%) 2717
Sustiva Capsules (Less than 2%) 930
Sustiva Tablets (Less than 2%) 930
▲ Sutent Capsules (5% to 22%) 2560
▲ Symbyax Capsules (Up to 15%) 1819
Symmetrel Tablets (0.1% to 1%) 1135
▲ Tambocor Tablets (Less than 1% to 4.9%) 1856
▲ Targretin Capsules (20.2% to 45.3%) 1747
Tarka Tablets (0.3% or more) 524
Tasmar Tablets (1% or more) 3358
▲ Taxotere Injection Concentrate (12.8% to 80.8%) 2932
▲ Temodar Capsules (7% to 13%) 3073
Tequin Injection (Less than 0.1%) 938
Tequin Injection in 5% Dextrose (Less than 0.1%) 938
Tequin Tablets (Less than 0.1%) 938
Teveten Tablets (Less than 1%) 1735
Teveten HCT Tablets (Less than 1%) 1737
▲ Thalomid Capsules (8.3%) 965
▲ Thiola Tablets (4%) 2141
Thiothixene Capsules 2165
▲ Thymoglobulin for Intravenous Infusion (26.8%) 1284
▲ Thyrogen for Injection (3.4%) 1286
Thyrolar Tablets 1199
Tiazac Capsules (1% to 4%) 1201
Ticlid Tablets (0.5% to 1.0%) 2810
Timolide Tablets (1.9%) 2086
Timoptic Sterile Ophthalmic Solution (Less frequent) 2088
Timoptic in Ocudose (Less frequent) 2091
Timoptic-XE Sterile Ophthalmic Gel Forming Solution 2092
Tindamax Tablets (1.1% to 2.1%) 2142
▲ TOBI Solution for Inhalation (35.7%) 2298
▲ Topamax Sprinkle Capsules (Less than 1% to 6%) 2404
▲ Topamax Tablets (Less than 1% to 6%) 2404
Trasylol Injection (2%) 754
Trelstar LA Suspension (1.1%) 3397
Tricor Tablets (2.1%) 527
Triglide Tablets (2.1%) 3123
▲ Trileptal Tablets (3% to 6%) 2300
▲ Trileptal Oral Suspension (3% to 6%) 2300
▲ Trisenox Injection (10%) 993
▲ Trizivir Tablets (Greater than or equal to 5%) 1589
Trusopt Sterile Ophthalmic Solution (Infrequent) 2095
▲ Truvada Tablets (Greater than 5%) ... 1296
Twinject 0.3 3378
Twinject 0.15 3379
Twinrix Vaccine (Less than 1%) 1595
Tygacil for Injection (2.5%) 3488
Ultane Liquid for Inhalation (Less than 1%) 531
▲ Ultram ER Tablets (0.7% to 6.5%) ... 2392
Uniretic Tablets (Less than 1%) 3100
Uroqid-Acid No. 2 Tablets 760
▲ Urso 250 Tablets (11.7%) 710
▲ Urso Forte Tablets (11.7%) 710
▲ Valcyte Tablets (Less than 5%) 2813
▲ Valtrex Caplets (1% to 4%) 1597
Vantas (Less than 2%) 3375
Vantin Tablets and Oral Suspension (Less than 1%) 2645
▲ Vaqta (3.9%) 2097
Vasotec I.V. Injection (1.1% to 1.6%) 2103
Verelan PM Extended-Release Capsules, Controlled-Onset (2%) ... 3106
Vesanoid Capsules 2820
VFEND I.V. (Less than 2%) 2564
VFEND Oral Suspension (Less than 2%) 2564
VFEND Tablets (Less than 2%) 2564
▲ Viadur Implant (7.6%) 757
Viagra Tablets (Less than 2%) 2573
▲ Vicoprofen Tablets (3% to 9%) 539
Viracept (Less than 2%) 2577
Virazole for Inhalation Solution 3370
▲ Viread Tablets (6% to 11%) 1301
▲ Visudyne for Injection (1% to 10%) .. 2305
▲ Vivaglobin (0.1% to 5%) 3506
▲ Vivitrol (12% to 23%) 995
▲ Voltaren Ophthalmic Solution (Less than or equal to 3%) 2309
Voltaren Tablets (Occasionally) 2307
Voltaren-XR Tablets (Occasionally) 2310
VoSpire ER Tablets (Less frequent) .. 1052
Vytorin 10/10 Tablets 2114
Vytorin 10/10 Tablets 3077
Vytorin 10/20 Tablets 2114
Vytorin 10/20 Tablets 3077
Vytorin 10/40 Tablets 2114
Vytorin 10/40 Tablets 3077
Vytorin 10/80 Tablets 2114
Vytorin 10/80 Tablets 3077
▲ WelChol Tablets (4%) 1050
▲ Wellbutrin SR Sustained-Release Tablets (2% to 4%) 1607
▲ Wellbutrin XL Extended-Release Tablets (2% to 4%) 1613
WinRho SDF 732
▲ Xeloda Tablets (Less than 1% to 26%) 2822
Xifaxan Tablets (Less than 2%) 2842
▲ Xopenex Inhalation Solution (3%) 3146
▲ Xopenex Inhalation Solution Concentrate (3%) 3150
▲ Xopenex HFA Inhalation Aerosol (3%) 3154
▲ Xyrem Oral Solution (3% to 5.9%) ... 1688
Yasmin 28 Tablets (Greater than 1%) 796
Yaz Tablets (Greater than 1%) 803
Zegerid Capsules (1.1% to 1.3%) 2958
Zegerid Powder for Oral Solution (1.1% to 1.3%) 2958
Zemaira (0.6%) 3509
▲ Zemplar Capsules (3%) 541
▲ Zemplar Injection (3%) 543
Zmax for Oral Suspension (Less then 1%) 2583
Zocor Tablets (1.6%) 2105
Zofran (Up to 2%) 1639
Zofran ODT Orally Disintegrating Tablets (Up to 2%) 1639
Zoloft (Frequent) 2586
▲ Zometa for Intravenous Infusion (5% to 24%) 2315
▲ Zomig Tablets (Common) 3519
▲ Zomig Nasal Spray (0% to 3%) 3523
▲ Zomig-ZMT Tablets (Common) 3519
Zonegran Capsules (Frequent) 1101
Zostavax Injection (1%) 2111
Zyban Sustained-Release Tablets (Frequent) 1644
▲ Zyflo Tablets (3.8%) 1023
▲ Zyprexa Tablets (8% to 20%) 1830
Zyprexa IntraMuscular (2%) 1830
▲ Zyprexa ZYDIS Orally Disintegrating Tablets (8% to 20%) 1830
Zyrtec Chewable Tablets (Less than 2%) 2594
Zyrtec (Less than 2%) 2594
Zyrtec-D 12 Hour Extended Release Tablets (Less than 2%) 2597

Asthenopia

Ambien CR Tablets (1%) 2855
▲ Lumigan Ophthalmic Solution (1% to 3%) 573

Asthma, allergic

Abelcet Injection 1141
Bicillin C-R Injectable Suspension 1706
Fluarix 1451

Asthma, bronchial

Advair HFA Inhalation Aerosol 1318
Agrylin Capsules (1% to 5%) 3169
Aralast (Greater than or equal to 0.2%) 717
BeneFix Vials (1.6%) 3408
Caduet Tablets (Less than 2%) 2508
Chantix Tablets (Infrequent) 2517
Cipro I.V. (1.8%) 2984
Coreg Tablets (Greater than 0.1% to 1%) 1414
Cuprimine Capsules 1947
Doxil Injection (Less than 1%) 2351
▲ Gamunex Immune Globulin I.V., 10% (3% to 29%) 3235
▲ I.V. Busulfex (8%) 2493
Kadian Capsules (Less than 3%) 577
Kaletra (Less than 2%) 476
Levaquin (0.1% to 0.9%) 2384
Levaquin in 5% Dextrose Injection (0.1% to 0.9%) 2384
Lipitor Tablets (Less than 2%) 2483
Norvir (Less than 2%) 503
Omacor Capsules 2725
Permax Tablets (Infrequent) 3356
Prevacid Delayed-Release Capsules (Less than 1%) 3271
Prevacid for Delayed-Release Oral Suspension (Less than 1%) 3271
Prevacid SoluTab Delayed-Release Orally Disintegrating Tablets (Less than 1%) 3271
Prevacid NapraPAC (Less than 1%) .. 3280
PREVPAC (Less than 1%) 3284
Prinivil Tablets (0.3% to 1.0%) 2052
Prochieve 4% Gel 1003
Prochieve 8% Gel 1003
Prozac Pulvules and Liquid (Infrequent) 1801
St. Joseph 81 mg Aspirin .... ▣ 688
Tasmar Tablets (Infrequent) 3358
Uniretic Tablets (Less than 1%) 3100
Vandazole Vaginal Gel (Less than 1%) 3338
Vaqta (Less than 1%) 2097
Vasotec I.V. Injection (0.5% to 1.0%) 2103
▲ Vesanoid Capsules (3%) 2820
Vicoprofen Tablets (Less than 1%) 539
Voltaren Tablets (Occasionally) 2307
Voltaren-XR Tablets (Occasionally) 2310
Xyrem Oral Solution (Infrequent) 1688

Asthma, worsening of

▲ AccuNeb Inhalation Solution (1.3% to 11.1%) 1055
Advair HFA Inhalation Aerosol 1318
Angeliq Tablets 762
▲ Asacol Delayed-Release Tablets (5% or greater) 2692
Climara Transdermal System 771
Climara Pro Transdermal System 776
▲ Elidel Cream 1% (Up to 3.9%) 2200
Enjuvia Tablets 1062
Estrasorb Topical Emulsion 1147
Estratest Tablets 3199
Estratest H.S. Tablets 3199
Finacea Gel (Rare) 1669
▲ Flebogamma 5%, Immune Globulin Intravenous (Human) (18%) 1658
Flovent Diskus 1443
Flovent HFA 1447
Foradil Aerolizer 3010
Menostar Transdermal System 782
Nexium Delayed-Release Capsules (Less than 1%) 655
Nexium I.V. (Less than 1%) 659
Premarin Intravenous 3442
Premarin Tablets 3446
Premarin Vaginal Cream 3452
Premphase Tablets 3456
Prempro Tablets 3456
Qvar Inhalation Aerosol (Up to 4%) ... 3303
Striant Mucoadhesive 1007
Stromectol Tablets 2083
▲ Tamiflu Capsules (3.5%) 2807
▲ Tamiflu Oral Suspension (1% to 3%) 2807
Vaqta 2097
Xalatan Sterile Ophthalmic Solution 2649
▲ Xopenex Inhalation Solution (9%) 3146
▲ Xopenex Inhalation Solution Concentrate (9%) 3150
▲ Xopenex HFA Inhalation Aerosol (9%) 3154

Asthmatic episodes

Abilify Oral Solution (Frequent) 882
Abilify Oral Solution (Frequent) 2450
Abilify Discmelt Orally Disintegrating Tablets (Frequent) ... 882
Abilify Discmelt Orally Disintegrating Tablets (Frequent) ... 2450
Abilify Tablets (Frequent) 882
Abilify Tablets (Frequent) 2450
Aciphex Tablets 1090
Actiq (Less than 1%) 979
Aggrenox Capsules (Less than 1%) .. 822
▲ Alupent Inhalation Aerosol (1% to 4%) 826
AmBisome for Injection (Less common) 620
Amerge Tablets (Rare) 1339
Amitiza Capsules (Less than 0.2%) .. 3224
Anaprox Tablets 2761
Anaprox DS Tablets 2761
Arthrotec Tablets (Rare) 3129
Avelox (Less than 1%) 2970
Azilect Tablets (Greater than 1%) 3293
Bayer Aspirin 744
Betoptic S Ophthalmic Suspension (Rare) 558
Campath Ampules 811
Campral Tablets (Infrequent) 1174
Celexa (Rare) 1176
▲ CellCept Capsules (3% to less than 20%) 2747
▲ CellCept Intravenous (3% to less than 20%) 2747
▲ CellCept Oral Suspension (3% to less than 20%) 2747
▲ CellCept Tablets (3% to less than 20%) 2747
Cipro (1.8%) 2977
Copaxone for Injection (Infrequent) .. 3297
Crestor Tablets (Greater than or equal to 1%) 678
depo-subQ provera 104 Injectable Suspension 2624
Diastat Rectal Delivery System (2%) 3343
Dilaudid Oral Liquid 445
Dilaudid Tablets - 8 mg 445
Doxil Injection (Less than 1%) 2351
Duragesic Transdermal System (Less than 1%) 2373
EC-Naprosyn Delayed-Release Tablets 2761
Effexor Tablets (Infrequent) 3411
Effexor XR Capsules (Infrequent) 3417
Eldepryl Capsules 3208
▲ Elidel Cream 1% (0.7% to 3.3%) 2200
Engerix-B Vaccine 1425
Evoxac Capsules (Less than 1%) 1047
Exubera Inhalation Powder (1.3% to 2%) 2524
▲ Flonase Nasal Spray (3.3% to 7.2%) 1440
Fluarix 1451
Flumist Vaccine 1901
Gabitril Tablets (Infrequent) 984
Gardasil Injection (2 cases) 1984
Gengraf Capsules (1% to less than 3%) 459
Herceptin I.V. (At least one of the 958 patients) 1233
▲ Humira Injection (Less than 5%) 466
Imitrex Injection 1463
Imitrex Nasal Spray (Rare) 1467
Imitrex Tablets (Infrequent) 1471
Indocin Capsules (Less than 1%) 1995
Indocin I.V. (Less than 1%) 2465
Indocin (Less than 1%) 1995
Invanz for Injection (Greater than 0.1%) 1999
Ionsys Transdermal System (.1% to less than 1%) 2379
Keppra Oral Solution (2%) 3314
Keppra Tablets (2%) 3314
Klonopin (Infrequent) 2778
Levaquin (0.1% to 0.9%) 2384
Levaquin in 5% Dextrose Injection (0.1% to 0.9%) 2384
Lexapro Oral Solution (Infrequent) 1190
Lexapro Tablets (Infrequent) 1190
Lofibra Tablets 1219
Lofibra Capsules 1216
Lotensin Tablets (Less than 1%) 2243
Lunesta Tablets (Infrequent) 3142
Lupron Depot 3.75 mg (Rare) 3260
Lupron Depot–3 Month 11.25 mg 3265
Lupron Depot-PED 7.5 mg, 11.25 mg and 15 mg (Rare) 3269
Merrem I.V. (Greater than 0.1% to 1%) 686
Micardis Tablets (More than 0.3%) ... 854
Micardis HCT Tablets 856
Mobic Oral Suspension (Less than 2%) 863
Mobic Tablets (Less than 2%) 863
Motrin IB Tablets and Caplets 1866
Children's Motrin Oral Suspension .. ▣ 685
Children's Motrin Non-Staining Dye-Free Oral Suspension .... ▣ 685
Children's Motrin Oral Suspension 1867
Children's Motrin Non-Staining Dye-Free Oral Suspension 1867
Children's Motrin Cold Oral Suspension 1867
Infants' Motrin Concentrated Drops 1867
Infants' Motrin Non-Staining Dye-Free Concentrated Drops 1867
Junior Strength Motrin Caplets and Chewable Tablets 1867
Namenda (Infrequent) 1195

Naprosyn Suspension 2761
Naprosyn Tablets 2761
Nasacort AQ Nasal Spray 2922
Nasonex Nasal Spray (Greater than or equal to 2%) 3043
Neurontin Capsules (Infrequent) 2487
Neurontin Oral Solution (Infrequent) 2487
Neurontin Tablets (Infrequent) 2487
▲ Nipent for Injection (3% to 10%) 1863
Omnicef Capsules 511
Omnicef for Oral Suspension 511
Paxil CR Controlled-Release Tablets (Infrequent) 1538
Paxil (Infrequent) 1530
Pexeva Tablets (infrequent) 1694
Phenergan Tablets and Suppositories 3440
Pletal Tablets (Less than 2%) 2455
Pred Mild Ophthalmic Suspension ⊙238
Prevnar for Injection 3463
Prinzide Tablets 2056
▲ Prograf Capsules and Injection (3% to 15%) 632
Proleukin for Injection 2266
ProSom Tablets (Infrequent) 517
Protonix I.V. (Less than 1%) 3472
Protonix Tablets (Less than 1%) 3469
▲ Protopic Ointment (4% to 16%) 638
Provigil Tablets (1%) 988
▲ Rapamune Oral Solution and Tablets (3% to 20%) 3475
Raptiva for Injection 1250
Relenza Rotadisk (Less than 1%) 1552
Relpax Tablets (Infrequent) 2548
Requip Tablets (Infrequent) 1555
Rilutek Tablets (Infrequent) 2930
Risperdal (Rare) 1676
Risperdal M-Tab Orally Disintegrating Tablets (Rare) 1676
Rituxan I.V. (0.3%) 1254
▲ Serevent Diskus (3% to 4%) 1568
Seroquel Tablets (Rare) 690
Sonata Capsules (Infrequent) 1717
St. Joseph 81 mg Aspirin Chewable and Enteric Coated Tablets 1869
Sular Tablets (Less than or equal to 1%) 3122
Sustiva Capsules (Less than 2%) 930
Sustiva Tablets (Less than 2%) 930
Symbyax Capsules (Infrequent) 1819
Synagis (More than 1%) 1897
▲ Tamiflu Capsules (3.5%) 2807
▲ Tamiflu Oral Suspension (3.5%) 2807
Tequin Injection (Less than 0.1%) 938
Tequin Injection in 5% Dextrose (Less than 0.1%) 938
Tequin Tablets (Less than 0.1%) 938
Teveten Tablets (Less than 1%) 1735
Teveten HCT Tablets (Less than 1%) 1737
Thioridazine Hydrochloride Tablets 2163
▲ TOBI Solution for Inhalation (15.9%) 2298
Topamax Sprinkle Capsules (Greater than 1%) 2404
Topamax Tablets (Greater than 1%) 2404
Trasylol Injection (2%) 754
Tricor Tablets 527
Trileptal Tablets 2300
Trileptal Oral Suspension 2300
Twinrix Vaccine 1595
Vantin Tablets and Oral Suspension (Less than 1%) 2645
Vaqta 2097
Viagra Tablets (Less than 2%) 2573
Viokase 711
Xalatan Sterile Ophthalmic Solution 2649
▲ Xeloda Tablets (Less than 5%) 2822
Zelapar Tablets 3372
Zemuron Injection (Less than 1%) 2346
Zyprexa Tablets (Infrequent) 1830
Zyprexa ZYDIS Orally Disintegrating Tablets (Infrequent) 1830

Asystole

Adenocard Injection 617
Cardizem LA Extended Release Tablets (Infrequent) 1728
Invanz for Injection (Greater than 0.1%) 1999
Lanoxicaps Capsules 1490
Lanoxin Injection 1494
Lanoxin Injection Pediatric 1497
Lanoxin Tablets 1500
TriLyte with Flavor Packs for Oral Solution 3100
Zantac Injection (Rare) 1619
Zantac Injection Pharmacy Bulk Package (Rare) 1622
Zantac Injection Premixed (Rare) 1619

Ataxia

Abilify Oral Solution (Rare to Infrequent) 882
Abilify Oral Solution (Rare to Infrequent) 2450
Abilify Discmelt Orally Disintegrating Tablets (Rare to Infrequent) 882
Abilify Discmelt Orally Disintegrating Tablets (Rare to Infrequent) 2450
Abilify Tablets (Rare to Infrequent) 882
Abilify Tablets (Rare to Infrequent) 2450
Actiq (Less than 1%) 979
Ambien Tablets (Frequent) 2851
Ambien CR Tablets (1% to frequent) 2855
Anzemet Injection (Rare) 2859
Anzemet Tablets (Rare) 2862
Aricept Tablets (Frequent) 1094
Aricept ODT Tablets (Frequent) 1094
▲ Arranon Injection (0% to 9%) 1357
Atripla Tablets 945
Attenuvax (Rare) 1914
▲ Avinza Capsules (Less than 5%) 1741
Axert Tablets (Rare) 2396
▲ Azilect Tablets (3%) 3293
Betagan Ophthalmic Solution, USP (Rare) ⊙220
▲ Betaseron for SC Injection (21%) 767
Buprenex Injectable (Rare) 2716
Caduet Tablets (Less than 2%) 2508
Captopril Tablets 2149
Celebrex Capsules (Less than 0.1%) 3134
Celexa (Infrequent) 1176
▲ Cesamet Capsules (13% to 14%) 3340
Cipro (Less than 1%) 2977
Cipro I.V. (1% or less) 2984
Cipro XR Tablets (Less than 1%) 2990
Clozaril Tablets (1%) 2184
Copaxone for Injection (At least 2%) 3297
Cozaar Tablets (Less than 1%) 1935
Cymbalta Delayed-Release Capsules (Infrequent) 1757
Dalmane Capsules 3342
Daranide Tablets 1950
▲ Depacon Injection (8%) 412
▲ Depakene (8%) 417
▲ Depakote Sprinkle Capsules (1% to 8%) 422
▲ Depakote Tablets (1% to 8%) 427
▲ Depakote ER Tablets (8%) 434
▲ Diastat Rectal Delivery System (3%) 3343
Doxil Injection (Less than 1%) 2351
Effexor Tablets (Infrequent) 3411
Effexor XR Capsules (Infrequent) 3417
▲ Eloxatin for Injection (2% to 5%) 2892
▲ Equetro Extended-Release Capsules (5% to 15%) 3180
Exelon Capsules (Frequent) 2206
Exelon Oral Solution (Frequent) 2206
Fabrazyme for Intravenous Infusion 1274
Fansidar Tablets 2765
FazaClo Orally Disintegrating Tablets (1%) 551
Flumadine (0.3% to 1%) 1183
Frova Tablets (Infrequent) 1113
▲ Gabitril Tablets (5%) 984
Gantrisin Pediatric Suspension 2770
Garamycin Injectable 3014
Geodon Capsules (Frequent) 2529
Guanidine Hydrochloride Tablets 3016
Herceptin I.V. (At least one of the 958 patients) 1233
Hyzaar 50-12.5 Tablets 1990
Hyzaar 100-12.5 Tablets 1990
Hyzaar 100-25 Tablets 1990
Imitrex Tablets (Infrequent) 1471
▲ Intron A for Injection (Less than 5%) 3024
Invirase (Less than 2%) 2772
Kadian Capsules (Less than 3%) 577
Kaletra (Less than 2%) 476
▲ Keppra Injection (3%) 3320
▲ Keppra Oral Solution (2% to 3%) 3314
▲ Keppra Tablets (2% to 3%) 3314
▲ Klonopin (30%) 2778
▲ Lamictal (5% to 28%) 1481
Lariam Tablets (Occasional) 2786
Leukeran Tablets (Rare) 1504
Levaquin (0.1% to 0.9%) 2384
Levaquin in 5% Dextrose Injection (0.1% to 0.9%) 2384
Librium Capsules 3347
Lithobid Tablets 1692
Lunesta Tablets (Infrequent) 3142
▲ Lyrica Capsules (1% to 20%) 2539
Marinol Capsules (Greater than 1%) 3333
Matulane Capsules 3191
Maxalt Tablets (Infrequent) 2008
Maxalt-MLT Orally Disintegrating Tablets (Infrequent) 2008
Mintezol 2027
Mirapex Tablets (1% or more) 859
M-M-R II (Rare) 2006
Namenda (Frequent) 1195
Nembutal Sodium Solution, USP (Less than 1%) 2470
▲ Neurontin Capsules (3.3% to 12.5%) 2487
▲ Neurontin Oral Solution (3.3% to 12.5%) 2487
▲ Neurontin Tablets (3.3% to 12.5%) 2487
Nipent for Injection (Less than 3%) 1863
Niravam Orally Disintegrating Tablets 3092
Noroxin Tablets 2032
Norvasc Tablets (Less than 0.1%) 2545
Norvir (Less than 2%) 503
Parcopa Orally Disintegrating Tablets 3097
Parnate Tablets 1527
Paxil CR Controlled-Release Tablets (Rare to infrequent) 1538
Paxil (Rare to infrequent) 1530
Permax Tablets (1.6%) 3356
Pexeva Tablets (infrequent) 1694
Phenergan Tablets and Suppositories 3440
▲ Phenytek Capsules (Among most common) 2160
Prinivil Tablets (0.3% to 1.0%) 2052
Prinzide Tablets 2056
▲ Prograf Capsules and Injection (3% to 15%) 632
Proquin XR Tablets 1153
ProSom Tablets (Rare) 517
Proventil HFA Inhalation Aerosol (Less than 3%) 3056
Provigil Tablets (1%) 988
Prozac Pulvules and Liquid (Infrequent) 1801
Razadyne (Infrequent) 2399
Razadyne ER Extended-Release Capsules (Infrequent) 2399
Relpax Tablets (Infrequent) 2548
Restoril Capsules (0.5% to 0.9%) 1860
Rilutek Tablets (Infrequent) 2930
▲ Risperdal (17% to 34%) 1676
Risperdal Consta Long-Acting Injection (Infrequent) 1682
▲ Risperdal M-Tab Orally Disintegrating Tablets (17% to 34%) 1676
▲ Romazicon Injection (10%) 2804
Rythmol SR Capsules 2727
Seroquel Tablets (Infrequent) 690
Sonata Capsules (Infrequent) 1717
Stalevo Tablets 2287
Sular Tablets (Less than or equal to 1%) 3122
Sustiva Capsules 930
Sustiva Tablets 930
Symbyax Capsules (Infrequent) 1819
▲ Symmetrel Tablets (1% to 5%) 1135
▲ Tambocor Tablets (1% to 3%) 1856
Targretin Capsules 1747
▲ Temodar Capsules (8%) 3073
▲ Tequin Injection (Less than 0.1%) 938
▲ Tequin Injection in 5% Dextrose (Less than 0.1%) 938
▲ Tequin Tablets (Less than 0.1%) 938
Teveten Tablets (Less than 1%) 1735
Teveten HCT Tablets (Less than 1%) 1737
Thalomid Capsules 965
Tindamax Tablets 2142
▲ Topamax Sprinkle Capsules (1% to 16%) 2404
▲ Topamax Tablets (1% to 16%) 2404
Tranxene 2474
▲ Trileptal Tablets (5% to 31%) 2300
▲ Trileptal Oral Suspension (5% to 31%) 2300
Uniretic Tablets (Less than 1%) 3100
Valcyte Tablets 2813
▲ Valium Tablets (Among most common) 2819
Valtrex Caplets 1597
Varivax 2100
Vasotec I.V. Injection (0.5% to 1.0%) 2103
VFEND I.V. (Less than 2%) 2564
VFEND Oral Suspension (Less than 2%) 2564
VFEND Tablets (Less than 2%) 2564
Viagra Tablets (Less than 2%) 2573
Wellbutrin Tablets (Frequent) 1603
Wellbutrin SR Sustained-Release Tablets (Rare) 1607
Wellbutrin XL Extended-Release Tablets (Rare) 1613
▲ Xeloda Tablets (Less than 5%) 2822
▲ Zelapar Tablets (3%) 3372
Zoloft (Infrequent) 2586
Zomig Tablets (Rare) 3519
Zomig Nasal Spray (Infrequent) 3523
Zomig-ZMT Tablets (Rare) 3519
▲ Zonegran Capsules (6%) 1101
Zovirax 1643
Zyban Sustained-Release Tablets (Rare) 1644
Zyprexa Tablets (2%) 1830
Zyprexa ZYDIS Orally Disintegrating Tablets (2%) 1830
Zyrtec Chewable Tablets (Less than 2%) 2594
Zyrtec (Less than 2%) 2594
Zyrtec-D 12 Hour Extended Release Tablets (Less than 2%) 2597
Zyvox 2652

Ataxia, cerebellar

Vaqta (Very rare) 2097

Atelectasis

AmBisome for Injection (Less common) 620
▲ CellCept Capsules (3% to less than 20%) 2747
▲ CellCept Intravenous (3% to less than 20%) 2747
▲ CellCept Oral Suspension (3% to less than 20%) 2747
▲ CellCept Tablets (3% to less than 20%) 2747
Effexor Tablets (Rare) 3411
Effexor XR Capsules (Rare) 3417
Evoxac Capsules 1047
▲ Invanz for Injection (3.4%) 1999
Ionsys Transdermal System (.1% to less than 1%) 2379
I.V. Busulfex (2%) 2493
Kadian Capsules (Less than 3%) 577
Lyrica Capsules (Rare) 2539
▲ NeoProfen Injection (4%) 2472
Numorphan Injection 1120
▲ Prograf Capsules and Injection (5% to 28%) 632
Prozac Pulvules and Liquid (Rare) 1801
▲ Rapamune Oral Solution and Tablets (3% to 20%) 3475
Rythmol SR Capsules 2727
▲ Trasylol Injection (5%) 754
Virazole for Inhalation Solution (Infrequent) 3370
Zyprexa Tablets (Rare) 1830
Zyprexa ZYDIS Orally Disintegrating Tablets (Rare) 1830

Atherosclerosis

Imitrex Injection 1463
Imitrex Nasal Spray 1467

Atrial arrhythmias

Hyperstat I.V. 3017
▲ Imdur Tablets (Less than or equal to 5%) 3018
Ketek Tablets 2903
Mirapex Tablets (Less than 1%) 859
▲ Neumega for Injection (15%) 3435
Proleukin for Injection (Less than 1%) 2266
Razadyne (Infrequent) 2399
Romazicon Injection (Less than 1%) 2804
Symbyax Capsules (Rare) 1819
▲ Trasylol Injection (3%) 754
Ultane Liquid for Inhalation (Less than 1%) 531
VFEND I.V. (Less than 2%) 2564
VFEND Oral Suspension (Less than 2%) 2564
VFEND Tablets (Less than 2%) 2564
Zoloft 2586

Atrial contractions, premature

Adenocard Injection 617
Neurontin Capsules (Rare) 2487
Neurontin Oral Solution (Rare) 2487
Neurontin Tablets (Rare) 2487
▲ Proleukin for Injection (4%) 2266
Risperdal (Rare) 1676
Risperdal M-Tab Orally Disintegrating Tablets (Rare) 1676

Atrial fibrillations

Abilify Oral Solution (Infrequent) 882
Abilify Oral Solution (Infrequent) 2450

Abilify Discmelt Orally Disintegrating Tablets (Infrequent) 882
Abilify Discmelt Orally Disintegrating Tablets (Infrequent) 2450
Abilify Tablets (Infrequent) 882
Abilify Tablets (Infrequent) 2450
Adalat CC Tablets (Less than 1%) 2964
Adenocard Injection 617
Advair Diskus 100/50 1308
Advair Diskus 250/50 1308
Advair Diskus 500/50 1308
Advair HFA Inhalation Aerosol 1318
Advicor Tablets 1722
Agrylin Capsules 3169
Aldara Cream, 5% (1.4%) 1846
AmBisome for Injection (Less common) 620
Amerge Tablets (Infrequent) 1339
Anzemet Injection 2859
Anzemet Tablets 2862
Aredia for Injection (Up to 6%) 2179
▲ Argatroban Injection (3%) 1346
Aricept Tablets (Frequent) 1094
Aricept ODT Tablets (Frequent) 1094
Arthrotec Tablets (Rare) 3129
Atrovent HFA Inhalation Aerosol 841
Avelox (Less than 0.1%) 2970
Caduet Tablets (Greater than 0.1% to less than or equal to 1%) 2508
Campath Ampules 811
▲ Carnitor Injection (2% to 6%) 3188
Celexa (Rare) 1176
▲ CellCept Capsules (3% to less than 20%) 2747
▲ CellCept Intravenous (3% to less than 20%) 2747
▲ CellCept Oral Suspension (3% to less than 20%) 2747
▲ CellCept Tablets (3% to less than 20%) 2747
Chantix Tablets (Rare) 2517
Clozaril Tablets 2184
Copaxone for Injection (Infrequent) 3297
Cozaar Tablets (Less than 1%) 1935
Cubicin for Injection (Less than 1%) 1026
Cymbalta Delayed-Release Capsules (Infrequent) 1757
Dacogen Injection (Greater than or equal to 1%) 2129
Demadex Injection 2759
Demadex Tablets 2759
DynaCirc CR Tablets (0.5% to 1%) 2721
Effexor Tablets 3411
Effexor XR Capsules 3417
Eraxis for Injection (Less than 1% to less than 2%) 2521
Ethyol for Injection (Rare) 1898
Exelon Capsules (Frequent) 2206
Exelon Oral Solution (Frequent) 2206
FazaClo Orally Disintegrating Tablets 551
Geodon Capsules (Infrequent) 2529
Guanidine Hydrochloride Tablets 3016
▲ Humira Injection (Less than 5%) 466
Hyzaar 50-12.5 Tablets 1990
Hyzaar 100-12.5 Tablets 1990
Hyzaar 100-25 Tablets 1990
▲ Imdur Tablets (Less than or equal to 5%) 3018
Imitrex Injection (Extremely rare) 1463
Imitrex Nasal Spray 1467
Imitrex Tablets (Rare) 1471
▲ Intron A for Injection (Less than 5%) 3024
Invanz for Injection (Greater than 0.1%) 1999
Ionsys Transdermal System (.1% to less than 1%) 2379
I.V. Busulfex (2%) 2493
Kadian Capsules (Less than 3%) 577
Kaletra (Less than 2%) 476
Kytril Injection (Rare) 2781
Kytril (Rare) 2784
Lamictal (Rare) 1481
Levaquin (0.1% to 0.9%) 2384
Levaquin in 5% Dextrose Injection (0.1% to 0.9%) 2384
Lexapro Oral Solution 1190
Lexapro Tablets 1190
Lofibra Tablets 1219
Lofibra Capsules 1216
Lovenox Injection (0.7%) 2915
Meridia Capsules 489
Micardis Tablets 854
Micardis HCT Tablets 856
Mirapex Tablets (Less than 1%) 859
Nalfon Capsules (Less than 1%) 2502
Namenda (Infrequent) 1195
Natrecor for Injection (Greater than or equal to 1%) 3127
▲ Neumega for Injection (12%) 3435
Neurontin Capsules (Rare) 2487
Neurontin Oral Solution (Rare) 2487
Neurontin Tablets (Rare) 2487
Niaspan Extended-Release Tablets 1730
Norvasc Tablets (More than 0.1% to 1%) 2545
OptiPranolol Metipranolol Ophthalmic Solution 0.3% (A small number of patients) ⊙256
Paxil CR Controlled-Release Tablets (Rare) 1538
Paxil (Rare) 1530
Permax Tablets (Infrequent) 3356
Pexeva Tablets (rare) 1694
▲ Photofrin for Injection (10%) 702
Plavix Tablets (1% to 2.5%) 917
Plavix Tablets (1% to 2.5%) 2926
Pletal Tablets (Less than 2%) 2455
Prinivil Tablets (0.3% to 1.0%) 2052
Prinzide Tablets 2056
Prograf Capsules and Injection 632
Protonix I.V. (Less than 1%) 3472
Protonix Tablets (Less than 1%) 3469
Proventil Inhalation Aerosol 3053
Prozac Pulvules and Liquid (Rare) 1801
▲ Rapamune Oral Solution and Tablets (3% to 20%) 3475
Razadyne (Infrequent) 2399
Razadyne ER Extended-Release Capsules (Infrequent) 2399
Relpax Tablets (Rare) 2548
▲ ReoPro Vials (3.5%) 1809
Requip Tablets (2%) 1555
Revlimid Capsules (0.3% to 2.6%) 958
Rilutek Tablets (Infrequent) 2930
Risperdal 1676
Risperdal Consta Long-Acting Injection 1682
Risperdal M-Tab Orally Disintegrating Tablets 1676
Sandostatin LAR Depot (Rare) 2280
Serevent Diskus 1568
Seroquel Tablets (Rare) 690
▲ Simulect for Injection (3% to 10%) 2284
Spiriva HandiHaler (Less than 1%) 869
Sular Tablets (Less than or equal to 1%) 3122
Symbyax Capsules (Rare) 1819
Tasmar Tablets (Infrequent) 3358
Taxotere Injection Concentrate 2932
Teveten Tablets (Less than 1%) 1735
Teveten HCT Tablets (Less than 1%) 1737
Thalomid Capsules 965
▲ Trasylol Injection (21%) 754
Tricor Tablets 527
Triglide Tablets 3123
Ultane Liquid for Inhalation (Less than 1%) 531
Uniretic Tablets (Less than 1%) 3100
Vaprisol (2.7%) 643
Vasotec I.V. Injection (0.5% to 1.0%) 2103
Ventolin HFA Inhalation Aerosol 1600
VFEND I.V. (Less than 2%) 2564
VFEND Oral Suspension (Less than 2%) 2564
VFEND Tablets (Less than 2%) 2564
▲ Visudyne for Injection (1% to 10%) 2305
Vivitrol 995
▲ Xeloda Tablets (Less than 5%) 2822
Xopenex Inhalation Solution 3146
Xopenex Inhalation Solution Concentrate 3150
Xopenex HFA Inhalation Aerosol 3154
▲ Zegerid Capsules (6.2%) 2958
▲ Zegerid Powder for Oral Solution (6.2%) 2958
Zelapar Tablets 3372
Zofran Injection 1634
Zomig Nasal Spray (Rare) 3523
Zonegran Capsules (Rare) 1101
Zosyn (1.0% or less) 3492
Zyprexa Tablets (Infrequent) 1830
Zyprexa ZYDIS Orally Disintegrating Tablets (Infrequent) 1830

Atrial flutter

Abilify Oral Solution (Rare) 882
Abilify Oral Solution (Rare) 2450
Abilify Discmelt Orally Disintegrating Tablets (Rare) 882
Abilify Discmelt Orally Disintegrating Tablets (Rare) 2450
Abilify Tablets (Rare) 882
Abilify Tablets (Rare) 2450
Amerge Tablets (Infrequent) 1339
Anzemet Injection 2859
Anzemet Tablets 2862
Aredia for Injection (Up to 1%) 2179
▲ CellCept Capsules (3% to less than 20%) 2747
▲ CellCept Intravenous (3% to less than 20%) 2747
▲ CellCept Oral Suspension (3% to less than 20%) 2747
▲ CellCept Tablets (3% to less than 20%) 2747
Cipro (Less than 1%) 2977
Cipro I.V. (1% or less) 2984
Cipro XR Tablets 2990
Cubicin for Injection (Less than 1%) 1026
Ethyol for Injection (Rare) 1898
▲ Neumega for Injection (12%) 3435
Pletal Tablets (Less than 2%) 2455
Prograf Capsules and Injection 632
Proquin XR Tablets 1153
Protonix I.V. (Less than 1%) 3472
Protonix Tablets (Less than 1%) 3469
▲ ReoPro Vials (3.5%) 1809
Revlimid Capsules 958
Rythmol SR Capsules 2727
Taxotere Injection Concentrate (Rare) 2932
▲ Trasylol Injection (6%) 754
Uniphyl Tablets 2710
Zelapar Tablets 3372

Atrial hypertrophy

Rythmol SR Capsules 2727

Atrial tachycardia

Lanoxicaps Capsules 1490
Lanoxin Injection 1494
Lanoxin Injection Pediatric 1497
Lanoxin Tablets 1500
Prinivil Tablets (0.3% to 1.0%) 2052
Prinzide Tablets 2056
Uniphyl Tablets 2710
Vasotec I.V. Injection (0.5% to 1.0%) 2103

Atrioventricular dissociation

Covera-HS Tablets (Less than 2%) 3139
Lanoxicaps Capsules (Common) 1490
Lanoxin Injection (Common) 1494
Lanoxin Tablets (Common) 1500
Tarka Tablets 524
Verelan PM Extended-Release Capsules, Controlled-Onset (2% or less) 3106

Atrophy

Cuprimine Capsules 1947

Atrophy, cutaneous

Depo-Medrol Single-Dose Vial 2619

Atrophy, subcutaneous

Depo-Medrol Single-Dose Vial 2619
Garamycin Injectable (Rare) 3014

Atrophy, testicular

▲ Eligard 45 mg (7.2%) 2888
▲ Vantas (5.3%) 3375

Atrophy at application site

Clobex Spray (0% to 1%) 1208

Atrophy at injection site

Bicillin C-R Injectable Suspension 1706

Attention, disturbance in

Ambien CR Tablets (2%) 2855
Arranon Injection (1%) 1357
Chantix Tablets (Frequent) 2517
Proquin XR Tablets (Less than 1%) 1153
▲ Topamax Sprinkle Capsules (3% to 14%) 2404
▲ Topamax Tablets (3% to 14%) 2404
▲ Ultram ER Tablets (1% to greater than 5%) 2392
Vivitrol 995
▲ Xyrem Oral Solution (2.9% to 8.6%) 1688

Atypical measles

Attenuvax 1914
ProQuad 2064

Auditory acuity, decrease

▲ Capastat Sulfate for Injection (Approximately 11%) 1755

Auditory canals, small or absent, fetal

Accutane Capsules 2731

Auditory disturbances

▲ Wellbutrin Tablets (5.3%) 1603

Aura disappeared

Neurontin Capsules 2487
Neurontin Oral Solution 2487
Neurontin Tablets 2487

Autoimmune disorders

Ionsys Transdermal System (.1% to less than 1%) 2379
Remicade for IV Injection 971

Autoimmune disorders, life-threatening, aggravation of

Copegus Tablets (Less than 1%) 2754

Autonomic deficit, persistent

Symmetrel Tablets (Uncommon) 1135

A-V block

Abilify Oral Solution (Infrequent) 882
Abilify Oral Solution (Infrequent) 2450
Abilify Discmelt Orally Disintegrating Tablets (Infrequent) 882
Abilify Discmelt Orally Disintegrating Tablets (Infrequent) 2450
Abilify Tablets (Infrequent) 882
Abilify Tablets (Infrequent) 2450
Activase I.V. 1223
Adenocard Injection 617
Anzemet Injection 2859
Anzemet Tablets 2862
Biltricide Tablets 2976
Blocadren Tablets (Less than 1%) 1916
Carbatrol Capsules 3171
Cardene I.V. (Rare) 2497
Catapres Tablets (Rare) 843
Catapres-TTS (0.5% or less) 844
Clorpres Tablets (Rare) 2153
▲ Coreg Tablets (Greater than 1% to 3%) 1414
Covera-HS Tablets (0.8% to 2%) 3139
Equetro Extended-Release Capsules 3180
Exelon Capsules (Infrequent) 2206
Exelon Oral Solution (Infrequent) 2206
Kytril Injection (Rare) 2781
Lanoxicaps Capsules 1490
Lanoxin Injection 1494
Lanoxin Injection Pediatric (Common) 1497
Lanoxin Tablets 1500
Lariam Tablets (Infrequent) 2786
Namenda 1195
Nipent for Injection (Less than 3%) 1863
Pepcid Injection (Infrequent) 2040
Pepcid (Infrequent) 2038
Permax Tablets (Infrequent) 3356
Razadyne (Infrequent) 2399
Razadyne ER Extended-Release Capsules (Infrequent) 2399
ReoPro Vials (1.3%) 1809
Retavase 2499
Risperdal (Infrequent) 1676
Risperdal Consta Long-Acting Injection (Infrequent) 1682
Risperdal M-Tab Orally Disintegrating Tablets (Infrequent) 1676
Rythmol SR Capsules 2727
Tambocor Tablets 1856
Tegretol/Tegretol-XR 2295
▲ Tiazac Capsules (4%) 1201
Timolide Tablets 2086
TNKase I.V. 1264
Topamax Sprinkle Capsules (Infrequent) 2404
Topamax Tablets (Infrequent) 2404
Ultane Liquid for Inhalation (Less than 1%) 531
Verelan PM Extended-Release Capsules, Controlled-Onset (0.8% to 1.2%) 3106
VFEND I.V. (Less than 2%) 2564
VFEND Oral Suspension (Less than 2%) 2564
VFEND Tablets (Less than 2%) 2564
Viagra Tablets (Less than 2%) 2573
Wellbutrin SR Sustained-Release Tablets 1607
Wellbutrin XL Extended-Release Tablets 1613
Zantac (Rare) 1624
Zantac Injection (Rare) 1619
Zantac Injection Pharmacy Bulk Package (Rare) 1622
Zantac Injection Premixed (Rare) 1619
Zantac (Rare) 1624
Zoloft 2586
Zyban Sustained-Release Tablets 1644
Zyprexa IntraMuscular (Infrequent) 1830

A-V block, complete

Azilect Tablets (Rare) 3293

A-V block, first-degree

Adenocard Injection 617
▲ Adenoscan (2.9% to 3%) 619

Aricept Tablets (Infrequent) 1094
Aricept ODT Tablets (Infrequent) 1094
▲ Cardizem LA Extended Release Tablets (2.4% to 3.2%) 1728
Cathflo Activase (1.2%) 1231
Covera-HS Tablets (1.2% to 1.7%) 3139
Effexor Tablets (Rare) 3411
Effexor XR Capsules (Rare) 3417
Geodon Capsules (Rare) 2529
Lanoxicaps Capsules 1490
Lanoxin Injection 1494
Lanoxin Injection Pediatric 1497
Lanoxin Tablets 1500
Mavik Tablets (0.3% to 1.0%) 486
▲ Rythmol SR Capsules (2% to 3%) 2727
Seroquel Tablets (Infrequent) 690
Sular Tablets (Less than or equal to 1%) 3122
▲ Tarka Tablets (3.9%) 524
Uniretic Tablets (Less than 1%) 3100
Verelan PM Extended-Release Capsules, Controlled-Onset (1.2%) 3106
Zelapar Tablets 3372

A-V block, intensification of
Blocadren Tablets 1916
Inderal LA Long-Acting Capsules 3429
InnoPran XL Capsules 2723
Lopressor Injection 2238
Lopressor Tablets 2238
Lopressor HCT 50/25 Tablets 2241
Lopressor HCT 100/25 Tablets 2241
Lopressor HCT 100/50 Tablets 2241
Nadolol Tablets (Single instance) 2159
Toprol-XL Tablets 668

A-V block, second-degree
Adenocard Injection 617
Adenoscan (2.6% to 3%) 619
Azilect Tablets (Rare) 3293
Blocadren Tablets (Less than 1%) 1916
Cardizem LA Extended Release Tablets (Less than 2%) 1728
Covera-HS Tablets (0.8% to 2%) 3139
Cozaar Tablets (Less than 1%) 1935
Hyzaar 50-12.5 Tablets 1990
Hyzaar 100-12.5 Tablets 1990
Hyzaar 100-25 Tablets 1990
Lanoxicaps Capsules 1490
Lanoxin Injection 1494
Lanoxin Injection Pediatric 1497
Lanoxin Tablets 1500
Proleukin for Injection (Less than 1%) 2266
Reyataz Capsules (Rare) 921
Tambocor Tablets (Less than 1%) 1856
Tarka Tablets (Less frequent) 524
Ultane Liquid for Inhalation (Less than 1%) 531
Verelan PM Extended-Release Capsules, Controlled-Onset (0.8% to 1.2%) 3106

A-V block, third-degree
Adenocard Injection 617
Adenoscan (0.8%; less than 1%) 619
Blocadren Tablets (Less than 1%) 1916
Cardizem LA Extended Release Tablets (Less than 2%) 1728
Coreg Tablets (Less than or equal to 0.1%) 1414
Covera-HS Tablets (0.8% to 2%) 3139
Lanoxicaps Capsules 1490
Lanoxin Injection 1494
Lanoxin Injection Pediatric 1497
Lanoxin Tablets 1500
Tambocor Tablets (Less than 1%) 1856
Tarka Tablets 524
Verelan PM Extended-Release Capsules, Controlled-Onset (0.8% to 1.2%) 3106
Wellbutrin Tablets 1603

A-V conduction, prolongation
Timolide Tablets 2086

A-V conduction changes, unspecified
Natrecor for Injection (Greater than or equal to 1%) 3127
Nimotop Capsules 749

A-V shunt, thrombosis of
(*see under* Thrombosis of vascular access)

Avitaminosis
Campral Tablets (Infrequent) 1174
Kaletra (Less than 2%) 476
Norvir (Less than 2%) 503
Thalomid Capsules 965
Zelapar Tablets 3372

Awareness, heightened
Demser Capsules 1953
Imitrex Tablets (Rare) 1471
▲ Marinol Capsules (8% to 24%) 3333

Azoospermia
Mustargen for Injection 2468

Azotemia
Altace Capsules 1702
Aredia for Injection (Up to 4%) 2179
Avalide Tablets 888
Avalide Tablets 2874
▲ Bumex Tablets (10.6%) 2746
Carbatrol Capsules 3171
Cleocin Vaginal Ovules (Rare) 2616
Demadex Injection 2759
Demadex Tablets 2759
Diuril Sodium Intravenous 2467
Dyrenium Capsules (Rare) 3400
Effexor Tablets (Rare) 3411
Effexor XR Capsules (Rare) 3417
Elspar for Injection (Frequent) 2463
Elspar for Injection (Frequent) 1960
Equetro Extended-Release Capsules 3180
Furosemide Tablets 2154
Guanidine Hydrochloride Tablets 3016
Hyzaar 50-12.5 Tablets 1990
Hyzaar 100-12.5 Tablets 1990
Hyzaar 100-25 Tablets 1990
▲ Indocin I.V. (41% of infants) 2465
Lotrel Capsules 2249
Nalfon Capsules (Less than 1%) 2502
Prinivil Tablets (0.3% to 1.0%) 2052
Prinzide Tablets 2056
Requip Tablets (Rare) 1555
Revlimid Capsules 958
Tegretol/Tegretol-XR 2295
Teveten HCT Tablets 1737
Tygacil for Injection 3488
Vancocin HCl Capsules, USP 3380
Vasotec I.V. Injection 2103
VFEND I.V. (Less than 2%) 2564
VFEND Oral Suspension (Less than 2%) 2564
VFEND Tablets (Less than 2%) 2564

B

Babinski's phenomenon, bilateral
Neurontin Capsules (Infrequent) 2487
Neurontin Oral Solution (Infrequent) 2487
Neurontin Tablets (Infrequent) 2487

Back strain
Prinzide Tablets (0.3% to 1%) 2056

Backache
Abilify Oral Solution 882
Abilify Oral Solution 2450
Abilify Discmelt Orally Disintegrating Tablets 882
Abilify Discmelt Orally Disintegrating Tablets 2450
Abilify Tablets 882
Abilify Tablets 2450
Accolate Tablets (1.5%) 671
▲ Aceon Tablets (2 mg, 4 mg, 8 mg) (Up to 5.8%) 3194
Actimmune (2%) 1671
Actiq (1% or greater) 979
▲ Actonel Tablets (8.7% to 26.1%) 2683
▲ Actonel with Calcium Tablets (8.7% to 26.1%) 2688
Adenocard Injection (Less than 1%) 617
Adenoscan (Less than 1%) 619
Advair Diskus 100/50 1308
Advair Diskus 250/50 1308
Advair Diskus 500/50 1308
Advair HFA Inhalation Aerosol 1318
▲ Advicor Tablets (5%) 1722
▲ Aggrenox Capsules (4.6%) 822
▲ Agrylin Capsules (5.9%) 3169
Alamast Ophthalmic Solution (Less than 5%) 3381
Aldara Cream, 5% (1.4%) 1846
Alferon N Injection (Up to 4%) 1665
Allegra (2.2% to 2.8%) 2844
Allegra-D 12 Hour Extended-Release Tablets (1.9%) 2846
Allegra-D 24 Hour Extended-Release Tablets (1.9%) 2849
▲ Altoprev Extended-Release Tablets (5%) 3109
▲ Ambien Tablets (3%) 2851
▲ Ambien CR Tablets (4% to frequent) 2855
▲ AmBisome for Injection (12%) 620
▲ Amitiza Capsules (2.3% to 3.4%) 3224
▲ Angeliq Tablets (7%) 762
Aralast (Greater than or equal to 0.2%) 717
▲ Aranesp for Injection (8%) 581
▲ Aredia for Injection (At least 5%) 2179
▲ Argatroban Injection (8%) 1346
▲ Arimidex Tablets (8% to 12%) 673
Arixtra Injection (1.3%) 1351
▲ Aromasin Tablets (2% to 8.6%) 2600
▲ Arranon Injection (0% to 8%) 1357
▲ Asacol Delayed-Release Tablets (7%) 2692
▲ Asmanex Twisthaler (3% to 6%) 2966
Astelin Nasal Spray (Infrequent) 1904
▲ Atacand Tablets (3%) 649
▲ Atacand HCT (3.3%) 651
▲ Atripla Tablets (Greater than or equal to 5%) 945
▲ Atrovent Inhalation Solution (3.2%) 835
▲ Atrovent HFA Inhalation Aerosol (2% to 7%) 841
▲ Avandamet Tablets (5%) 1373
▲ Avandia Tablets (4% to 5.1%) 1384
Avelox (Less than 0.1%) 2970
▲ Avinza Capsules (5% to 10%) 1741
Axert Tablets (Infrequent) 2396
Axid Oral Solution (2.4%) 879
▲ Azmacort Inhalation Aerosol (2% to 4%) 1726
Benicar HCT Tablets (Greater than 1%) 1044
▲ Bexxar (1% to 8%) 1398
▲ Boniva Injection (4.3% to 13.5%) 2738
▲ Boniva Tablets (4.3% to 13.5%) 2741
Boostrix 1404
▲ BOTOX Purified Neurotoxin Complex (2% to 10%) 570
▲ Caduet Tablets (Greater than 0.1% to 3.8%) 2508
▲ Campath Ampules (3% to 10%) 811
Campral Tablets (Frequent) 1174
▲ Camptosar Injection (2% to 14%) 2604
Cancidas for Injection (0% to 0.7%) 1918
Carafate Suspension (Less than 0.5%) 701
Carafate Tablets (Less than 0.5%) 701
Cardura XL Tablets (2.9%) 2515
Carimune NF 3499
▲ Carnitor Injection (6% to 9%) 3188
Caverject Impulse Injection (1%) 2612
Celebrex Capsules (2.8%) 3134
Celexa (At least 2%) 1176
▲ CellCept Capsules (34.6% to 46.6%) 2747
▲ CellCept Intravenous (34.6% to 46.6%) 2747
▲ CellCept Oral Suspension (34.6% to 46.6%) 2747
▲ CellCept Tablets (34.6% to 46.6%) 2747
▲ Cerezyme for Injection (Approximately 6.5%) 1270
Cesamet Capsules 3340
Chantix Tablets (Frequent) 2517
▲ Chemet Capsules (5.2% to 15.7%) 2458
▲ Cialis Tablets (3% to 6%) 1838
Cipro (Less than 1%) 2977
Cipro I.V. (1% or less) 2984
Cipro XR Tablets 2990
▲ Climara Transdermal System (4% to 9%) 771
▲ Climara Pro Transdermal System (6.1%) 776
▲ Clolar for Intravenous Infusion (13%) 1271
Clozaril Tablets (1%) 2184
Colazal Capsules (2%) 2838
Comtan Tablets (2%) 2189
▲ Copaxone for Injection (16%) 3297
▲ Copegus Tablets (5%) 2754
Cosopt Sterile Ophthalmic Solution (1% to 5%) 1931
▲ Cozaar Tablets (2% to 12%) 1935
Crestor Tablets (2.6%) 678
▲ Crixivan Capsules (8.4%) 1940
▲ Cubicin for Injection (1% to 6.7%) 1026
CytoGam Intravenous (Less than 5.0%) 1895
▲ Dacogen Injection (17%) 2129
Dantrium Capsules (Less frequent) 2694
▲ Depacon Injection (1% to 5%) 412
▲ Depakene (1% to 5%) 417
▲ Depakote Sprinkle Capsules (1% to 5%) 422
▲ Depakote Tablets (1% to 8%) 427
▲ Depakote ER Tablets (Greater than 1% to 8%) 434
▲ DepoCyt Injection (7%) 1143
▲ DepoDur Extended-Release Injection (2% to 5%) 1110
▲ Depo-Provera Contraceptive Injection (1% to 5%) 2622
▲ depo-subQ provera 104 Injectable Suspension (1% to less than 5%) 2624
Detrol Tablets (2.7%) 2628
▲ Diovan Tablets (3%) 2193
Diovan HCT Tablets (More than 2%) 2196
▲ Ditropan XL Extended-Release Tablets (2% to less than 5%) 2413
▲ Doxil Injection (6.8% to 11.7%) 2351
DuoNeb Inhalation Solution 1058
Duragesic Transdermal System (Greater than or equal to 1%) 2373
DynaCirc CR Tablets (0.5% to 1%) 2721
Edex Injection (2%) 3089
Effexor Tablets 3411
Effexor XR Capsules 3417
Eldepryl Capsules (1 of 49 patients) 3208
Elidel Cream 1% (0.3% to 1.8%) 2200
Eligard 7.5 mg (Less than 2%) 2880
▲ Eloxatin for Injection (11% to 19%) 2892
Emend Capsules (Greater than 0.5%) 1963
Emsam Transdermal System 903
Enablex Extended-Release Tablets (Greater than or equal to 1%) 2203
Engerix-B Vaccine (Less than 1%) 1425
▲ Entocort EC Capsules (7%) 2698
▲ Equetro Extended-Release Capsules (5%) 3180
Eraxis for Injection (Less than 1% to less than 2%) 2521
▲ Erbitux (3% to 16%) 910
▲ Estring Vaginal Ring (6%) 2635
▲ Euflexxa (0.63% to 6%) 1162
▲ Evoxac Capsules (4.5%) 1047
Exelon Capsules (2% or more) 2206
Exelon Oral Solution (2% or more) 2206
Famvir Tablets (1.5% to 1.9%) 2211
▲ Faslodex Injection (14.4%) 681
FazaClo Orally Disintegrating Tablets (1%) 551
▲ Femara Tablets (0.3% to 22%) 2214
Ferrlecit Injection (0.4%) 3388
Flebogamma 5%, Immune Globulin Intravenous (Human) 1658
▲ Flomax Capsules (7.0% to 8.3%) 850
▲ Follistim AQ Cartridge (7%) 2338
▲ Foradil Aerolizer (4.2%) 3010
▲ Fortical Nasal Spray (5%) 3337
Frova Tablets (Infrequent) 1113
Gabitril Tablets (1% or more) 984
Gammagard Liquid 721
Gammagard S/D (Occasional) 724
▲ Gamunex Immune Globulin I.V., 10% (6%) 3235
Geodon for Injection (Up to 1%) 2529
▲ Gleevec Tablets (0% to 26%) 2227
▲ Herceptin I.V. (22%) 1233
▲ Humatrope Vials and Cartridges (9.1% to 9.6%) 1787
▲ Humira Injection (6%) 466
▲ Hycamtin for Injection (2% to 23%) 1458
Hyperstat I.V. 3017
Hytrin Capsules (2.4%) 471
Hyzaar 50-12.5 Tablets (2.1%) 1990
Hyzaar 100-12.5 Tablets (2.1%) 1990
Hyzaar 100-25 Tablets (2.1%) 1990
▲ Imdur Tablets (Less than or equal to 5%) 3018
Imitrex Injection (Rare) 1463
Imitrex Nasal Spray (Infrequent) 1467
Imitrex Tablets 1471
▲ Indapamide Tablets (Greater than or equal to 5%) 2156
Infed Injection 3390
▲ Infergen (29% to 42%) 3364
▲ Intron A for Injection (Up to 19%) 3024
Invirase (Less than or equal to 2%) 2772
Ionsys Transdermal System (2%) 2379
▲ I.V. Busulfex (23%) 2493
Kadian Capsules (Less than 3%) 577
Kaletra (Less than 2%) 476
Keppra Injection 3320
Keppra Oral Solution (1% or more) 3314
Keppra Tablets (1% or more) 3314
Klonopin (Infrequent) 2778
▲ Lamictal (8%) 1481
▲ Lescol Capsules (5.7%) 2233
▲ Lescol XL Tablets (4.7%) 2233
▲ Leukine (9%) 814
Levaquin (1.2%) 2384
Levaquin in 5% Dextrose Injection (1.2%) 2384
Levitra Tablets (Less than or equal to 2%) 3034
Lexapro Oral Solution (At least 2%) 1190
Lexapro Tablets (At least 2%) 1190
▲ Lipitor Tablets (Up to 3.8%) 2483
▲ Lofibra Tablets (3.4%) 1219
▲ Lofibra Capsules (3.4%) 1216

Lotensin HCT Tablets (More than 1%)........ 2246
Lotrel Capsules........ 2249
▲ Lucentis Injection (1% to 10%)........ 1237
Lunesta Tablets........ 3142
Lyrica Capsules (1% to 2%)........ 2539
▲ Meridia Capsules (8.2%)........ 489
Merrem I.V. (Greater than 0.1% to 1%)........ 686
Metrogel 1% (0.5%)........ 1211
▲ Miacalcin Nasal Spray (5.0%)........ 2253
▲ Micardis Tablets (3%)........ 854
Micardis HCT Tablets (Less than 2%)........ 856
Midamor Tablets (Less than or equal to 1%)........ 2026
Mirapex Tablets (Greater than or equal to 1%)........ 859
▲ Mirena Intrauterine System (5% or more)........ 787
▲ Mobic Oral Suspension (0.4% to 3%)........ 863
▲ Mobic Tablets (0.4% to 3%)........ 863
Moduretic Tablets (Less than or equal to 1%)........ 2028
▲ Myfortic Tablets (3% to less than 20%)........ 2255
▲ Mylotarg for Injection (12% to 16%)........ 3431
▲ Myobloc Injection (3% to 7%)........ 3192
▲ Namenda (3%)........ 1195
▲ Natrecor for Injection (1% to 4%)........ 3127
Neurontin Capsules (1% to 1.8%)........ 2487
Neurontin Oral Solution (1% to 1.8%)........ 2487
Neurontin Tablets (1% to 1.8%)........ 2487
Nexium Delayed-Release Capsules (Less than 1%)........ 655
Nexium I.V. (Less than 1%)........ 659
Noroxin Tablets (0.3% to 1.0%)........ 2032
Norvasc Tablets (More than 0.1% to 1%)........ 2545
Norvir (Less than 2%)........ 503
Omacor Capsules (2.2%)........ 2725
Oracea Capsules (1.1%)........ 1000
▲ Orencia Powder for Intravenous Infusion (7%)........ 914
▲ Oxytrol Transdermal System (Greater than 1%)........ 3392
ParaGard T 380A Intrauterine Copper Contraceptive........ 1073
Parcopa Orally Disintegrating Tablets........ 3097
▲ Paxil CR Controlled-Release Tablets (3%)........ 1538
▲ Paxil (3%)........ 1530
▲ Pegasys (9%)........ 2789
Permax Tablets (1.6%)........ 3356
▲ Pexeva Tablets (3%)........ 1694
▲ Photofrin for Injection (5% to 11%)........ 702
Plasmanate (Occasional)........ 3255
▲ Plavix Tablets (5.8%)........ 917
▲ Plavix Tablets (5.8%)........ 2926
▲ Pletal Tablets (6% to 7%)........ 2455
▲ Premarin Tablets (13% to 14%)........ 3446
▲ Premphase Tablets (13% to 16%)........ 3456
▲ Prempro Tablets (13% to 16%)........ 3456
Prevacid Delayed-Release Capsules (Less than 1%)........ 3271
Prevacid for Delayed-Release Oral Suspension (Less than 1%)........ 3271
Prevacid SoluTab Delayed-Release Orally Disintegrating Tablets (Less than 1%)........ 3271
Prevacid NapraPAC (Less than 1%)........ 3280
PREVPAC (Less than 1%)........ 3284
Prilosec OTC Delayed-Release Tablets (1.1%)........ 2677
Prinivil Tablets (0.3% to greater than 1.0%)........ 2052
Prinzide Tablets (0.3% to 1%)........ 2056
ProAmatine Tablets (Rare)........ 3186
Prochieve 4% Gel........ 1003
Prochieve 8% Gel........ 1003
▲ Prograf Capsules and Injection (17% to 30%)........ 632
▲ Proleukin for Injection (9%)........ 2266
▲ Prometrium Capsules (100 mg, 200 mg) (8%)........ 3203
Proquin XR Tablets........ 1153
ProSom Tablets (2%)........ 517
Protonix I.V. (Greater than or equal to 1%)........ 3472
Protonix Tablets (Greater than or equal to 1%)........ 3469
▲ Protopic Ointment (1% to 3%)........ 638
▲ Proventil HFA Inhalation Aerosol (4%)........ 3056
▲ Provigil Tablets (6%)........ 988
Prozac Pulvules and Liquid........ 1801
▲ Qvar Inhalation Aerosol (Less than 1% to 4%)........ 3303
▲ Rapamune Oral Solution and Tablets (16% to 26%)........ 3475
▲ Raptiva for Injection (4%)........ 1250
Razadyne (Greater than or equal to 2%)........ 2399
Razadyne ER Extended-Release Capsules (Greater than or equal to 2%)........ 2399
▲ Rebif Prefilled Syringe for Injection (23% to 25%)........ 3159
Recombivax HB (Less than 1%)........ 2071
Relpax Tablets (Frequent)........ 2548
▲ Remicade for IV Injection (8%)........ 971
▲ Renagel Tablets (4%)........ 1282
Requip Tablets (1% or more)........ 1555
Restoril Capsules (0.5% to 0.9%)........ 1860
▲ Retisert Implant (5% to 15%)........ ⊙258
Retrovir Capsules........ 1560
Retrovir IV Infusion........ 1564
Retrovir........ 1560
▲ Revlimid Capsules (4.7% to 20.9%)........ 958
▲ Reyataz Capsules (2% to 6%)........ 921
▲ Rilutek Tablets (1.7% to 4.1%)........ 2930
Risperdal (Up to 2%)........ 1676
Risperdal Consta Long-Acting Injection (Frequent)........ 1682
Risperdal M-Tab Orally Disintegrating Tablets (Up to 2%)........ 1676
▲ Rituxan I.V. (1% to 10%)........ 1254
▲ Sandostatin Injection (1% to 4%)........ 2278
▲ Seroquel Tablets (3%)........ 690
▲ Simulect for Injection (3% to 10%)........ 2284
▲ Somavert Injection (4% to 8%)........ 2642
Sonata Capsules (Frequent)........ 1717
▲ Soriatane Capsules (1% to 10%)........ 1013
▲ Stalevo Tablets (2% to 4%)........ 2287
▲ Starlix Tablets (4%)........ 2292
▲ Strattera Capsules (2% or greater)........ 1814
Stromectol Tablets........ 2083
▲ Suboxone Tablets (3.7% to 14%)........ 2717
▲ Subutex Tablets (7.8% to 14%)........ 2717
▲ Sutent Capsules (1% to 17%)........ 2560
▲ Symbicort 80/4.5 Inhalation Aerosol (3.2%)........ 3511
Symbicort 160/4.5 Inhalation Aerosol (1.6%)........ 3511
▲ Targretin Capsules (2.4% to 11.3%)........ 1747
Tarka Tablets (2.2%)........ 524
Taxotere Injection Concentrate........ 2932
▲ Temodar Capsules (8%)........ 3073
▲ Tequin Injection (0.1% to 3%)........ 938
▲ Tequin Injection in 5% Dextrose (0.1% to 3%)........ 938
▲ Tequin Tablets (0.1% to 3%)........ 938
Teveten Tablets (Less than 1%)........ 1735
Teveten HCT Tablets (2.6%)........ 1737
Thalomid Capsules (4.2%)........ 965
▲ TOBI Solution for Inhalation (7%)........ 2298
▲ Topamax Sprinkle Capsules (1% to 5%)........ 2404
▲ Topamax Tablets (1% to 5%)........ 2404
Travatan Ophthalmic Solution (1% to 5%)........ 563
Trelstar LA Suspension (2.9%)........ 3397
▲ Tricor Tablets (3.4%)........ 527
▲ Triglide Tablets (3.4%)........ 3123
▲ Trileptal Tablets (2% to 4%)........ 2300
▲ Trileptal Oral Suspension (2% to 4%)........ 2300
▲ Trisenox Injection (18%)........ 993
Truvada Tablets........ 1296
Twinrix Vaccine (Less than 1%)........ 1595
Tygacil for Injection (1.2%)........ 3488
▲ Ultram ER Tablets (1% to greater than 5%)........ 2392
Uniretic Tablets (More than 1%)........ 3100
▲ Vagifem Tablets (7%)........ 2334
▲ Valcyte Tablets (Less than 5%)........ 2813
Vancocin HCl Capsules, USP........ 3380
Vandazole Vaginal Gel (Less than 1%)........ 3338
Vantas (Less than 2%)........ 3375
Vantin Tablets and Oral Suspension (Less than 1%)........ 2645
Vaqta (1.1%)........ 2097
▲ Velcade for Injection (14%)........ 2133
▲ Ventavis Inhalation Solution (7%)........ 1020
VFEND I.V. (Less than 2%)........ 2564
VFEND Oral Suspension (Less than 2%)........ 2564
VFEND Tablets (Less than 2%)........ 2564
Viagra Tablets (Greater than 2%)........ 2573
Viracept (Less than 2%)........ 2577
▲ Viread Tablets (3% to 9%)........ 1301
▲ Visudyne for Injection (1% to 10%)........ 2305
▲ Vivitrol (4% to 7%)........ 995
Vytorin 10/10 Tablets........ 2114
Vytorin 10/10 Tablets........ 3077
Vytorin 10/20 Tablets........ 2114
Vytorin 10/20 Tablets........ 3077
Vytorin 10/40 Tablets........ 2114
Vytorin 10/40 Tablets........ 3077
Vytorin 10/80 Tablets........ 2114
Vytorin 10/80 Tablets........ 3077
▲ WelChol Tablets (3%)........ 1050
Wellbutrin SR Sustained-Release Tablets (At least 1%)........ 1607
Wellbutrin XL Extended-Release Tablets (At least 1%)........ 1613
WinRho SDF........ 732
Xalatan Sterile Ophthalmic Solution (1% to 2%)........ 2649
▲ Xeloda Tablets (Less than 1% to 12%)........ 2822
▲ Xenical Capsules (13.90%)........ 2831
▲ Xyrem Oral Solution (5.7% to 6.1%)........ 1688
Yasmin 28 Tablets (Greater than 1%)........ 796
Yaz Tablets (Greater than 1%)........ 803
Zegerid Capsules (1.1%)........ 2958
Zegerid Powder for Oral Solution (1.1%)........ 2958
▲ Zelapar Tablets (5%)........ 3372
▲ Zelnorm Tablets (2% to 5%)........ 2312
Zemaira (0.2% to 0.4%)........ 3509
▲ Zetia Tablets (3.4% to 4.3%)........ 2120
▲ Zetia Tablets (3.4% to 4.1%)........ 3083
Zoloft (Frequent)........ 2586
▲ Zometa for Intravenous Infusion (15%)........ 2315
Zomig Tablets (Infrequent)........ 3519
Zomig Nasal Spray (Infrequent)........ 3523
Zomig-ZMT Tablets (Infrequent)........ 3519
Zosyn (1.0% or less)........ 3492
Zyban Sustained-Release Tablets (Infrequent)........ 1644
▲ Zyprexa Tablets (4% to 8%)........ 1830
▲ Zyprexa ZYDIS Orally Disintegrating Tablets (4% to 8%)........ 1830
Zyrtec Chewable Tablets (Less than 2%)........ 2594
Zyrtec (Less than 2%)........ 2594
Zyrtec-D 12 Hour Extended Release Tablets (Less than 2%)........ 2597

Bacteremia
▲ Aranesp for Injection (27%)........ 581
Bexxar........ 1398
▲ Clolar for Intravenous Infusion (10%)........ 1271
Crixivan Capsules........ 1940
▲ Cubicin for Injection (5%)........ 1026
▲ Dacogen Injection (5%)........ 2129
Effexor Tablets (Rare)........ 3411
Enbrel for Injection........ 584
Retrovir Capsules (1.6%)........ 1560
Retrovir IV Infusion (2%)........ 1564
Retrovir (1.6%)........ 1560
Revlimid Capsules........ 958

Bacteriuria
Primaxin I.M........ 2045

Bad breath
(*see under* Halitosis)

Balance, loss of
(*see also under* Equilibrium dysfunction)
Dalmane Capsules........ 3342
Eldepryl Capsules........ 3208
Rythmol SR Capsules........ 2727
Tarka Tablets (Less frequent)........ 524
Tasmar Tablets (2% to 3%)........ 3358

Balance disorder
Ambien CR Tablets (2%)........ 2855
Arranon Injection (0% to 2%)........ 1357
Chantix Tablets (Rare)........ 2517
Xyrem Oral Solution (Frequent)........ 1688

Balanitis
Doxil Injection (Less than 1%)........ 2351
Effexor XR Capsules (Rare)........ 3417
▲ Lupron Depot 7.5 mg (Less than 5%)........ 3264
Lyrica Capsules (Rare)........ 2539
Protonix I.V. (Less than 1%)........ 3472
Protonix Tablets (Less than 1%)........ 3469
Solodyn Extended Release Tablets........ 1890

Balanoposthitis
Requip Tablets (Infrequent)........ 1555
Zoloft (Rare)........ 2586

Baldness, male pattern
(*see under* Alopecia hereditaria)

Barrett's esophagus
Nexium Delayed-Release Capsules (Less than 1%)........ 655
Nexium I.V. (Less than 1%)........ 659

Bartter's syndrome
Capastat Sulfate for Injection (1 patient)........ 1755

Basedow's disease
Revlimid Capsules........ 958

Basophils, increase
Effexor Tablets (Rare)........ 3411
Effexor XR Capsules (Rare)........ 3417
Geodon Capsules (Rare)........ 2529
Paxil CR Controlled-Release Tablets (Rare)........ 1538
Paxil (Rare)........ 1530
Pexeva Tablets (rare)........ 1694
Primaxin I.M........ 2045
Primaxin I.V........ 2048
Rocephin Injectable Vials, ADD-Vantage, Galaxy, Bulk (Rare)........ 2800
Vantin Tablets and Oral Suspension........ 2645
Vesanoid Capsules (Isolated cases)........ 2820

Behavior, abnormal
Mirapex Tablets........ 859

Behavior, hostile
Focalin Tablets........ 2220
Focalin XR Capsules........ 2223
Niravam Orally Disintegrating Tablets (Rare)........ 3092

Behavior, inappropriate
Phenergan Tablets and Suppositories........ 3440
ProSom Tablets........ 517
Ritalin Hydrochloride Tablets........ 2269
Ritalin LA Capsules........ 2271
Ritalin-SR Tablets........ 2269
Symmetrel Tablets........ 1135
Tessalon Capsules (Isolated instances)........ 1199
Tessalon Perles (Isolated instances)........ 1199

Behavior, schizophrenic
Zonegran Capsules (2%)........ 1101

Behavior, violent
Accutane Capsules........ 2731
Invanz for Injection (Greater than 0.1%)........ 1999
Prozac Pulvules and Liquid........ 1801
Zovirax........ 1643

Behavioral changes
Advair HFA Inhalation Aerosol (Very Rare)........ 1318
Ambien Tablets........ 2851
Amoxil Capsules (Rare)........ 1343
Amoxil Chewable Tablets (Rare)........ 1343
Amoxil Pediatric Drops for Oral Suspension (Rare)........ 1343
Amoxil Powder for Oral Suspension (Rare)........ 1343
Amoxil Tablets (Rare)........ 1343
Augmentin (Rare)........ 1360
Augmentin Tablets (Rare)........ 1363
Augmentin XR Extended-Release Tablets (Rare)........ 1369
Augmentin ES-600 Powder for Oral Suspension (Rare)........ 1366
Biaxin/Biaxin XL........ 402
Catapres Tablets........ 843
Catapres-TTS (0.5% or less)........ 844
Clorpres Tablets........ 2153
Cosopt Sterile Ophthalmic Solution........ 1931
Effexor Tablets........ 3411
Effexor XR Capsules........ 3417
Eldepryl Capsules........ 3208
▲ Keppra Oral Solution (38%)........ 3314
▲ Keppra Tablets (38%)........ 3314
▲ Klonopin (5% to 25%)........ 2778
Nadolol Tablets (6 of 1000 patients)........ 2159
Neurontin Capsules........ 2487
Neurontin Oral Solution........ 2487
Neurontin Tablets........ 2487
Paxil CR Controlled-Release Tablets........ 1538
Paxil........ 1530
PREVPAC........ 3284
Thioridazine Hydrochloride Tablets........ 2163
Timoptic Sterile Ophthalmic Solution (Less frequent)........ 2088
Timoptic in Ocudose (Less frequent)........ 2091
Timoptic-XE Sterile Ophthalmic Gel Forming Solution........ 2092
Uniphyl Tablets........ 2710
Valtrex Caplets........ 1597

Zoloft 2586
Zyprexa Tablets 1830
Zyprexa ZYDIS Orally Disintegrating Tablets 1830

Behavioral deterioration
Depacon Injection 412
Depakene 417
Depakote Sprinkle Capsules 422
Depakote Tablets 427
Depakote ER Tablets 434

Behavioral disturbances, exacerbation of
Focalin XR Capsules 2223
Ritalin LA Capsules 2271

Belching
▲ Actonel Tablets (3.3%) 2683
Lexapro Oral Solution (Infrequent) 1190
Lexapro Tablets (Infrequent) 1190

Bell's palsy
Aldoril Tablets 1910
▲ Altoprev Extended-Release Tablets (0.5% to 1%) 3109
Comvax 1928
Depo-Provera Contraceptive Injection (Less than 1%) 2622
Engerix-B Vaccine 1425
Flumist Vaccine 1901
▲ Intron A for Injection (Less than 5%) 3024
Mevacor Tablets (0.5% to 1.0%) 2021
Permax Tablets (Rare) 3356
ProQuad 2064
Recombivax HB 2071
Sandostatin Injection (Less than 1%) 2278
Sandostatin LAR Depot (Rare) 2280
▲ Soriatane Capsules (Less than 5%) 1013
Thalomid Capsules 965
Twinrix Vaccine 1595
Varivax 2100
Zocor Tablets 2105

Benign prostatic hyperplasia
▲ Actonel Tablets (5%) 2683

Benzyl alcohol, sensitivity to
Depo-Medrol Injectable Suspension 2617
Epogen for Injection 591
Herceptin I.V. 1233
Leukine 814
Leustatin Injection 2357
Mivacron Injection 493
Nimbex Injection 498
Norditropin Cartridges 2323
Nutropin for Injection 1239
Procrit for Injection 2364

Bezoar
Carafate Suspension 701
Carafate Tablets 701
Prevacid Delayed-Release Capsules (Less than 1%) 3271
Prevacid for Delayed-Release Oral Suspension (Less than 1%) 3271
Prevacid SoluTab Delayed-Release Orally Disintegrating Tablets (Less than 1%) 3271
Prevacid NapraPAC (Less than 1%) 3280
PREVPAC (Less than 1%) 3284
St. Joseph 81 mg Aspirin Chewable and Enteric Coated Tablets 1869

Bigeminy
Azilect Tablets (Rare) 3293
Effexor Tablets (Rare) 3411
Effexor XR Capsules (Rare) 3417
Ionsys Transdermal System (.1% to less than 1%) 2379
Lanoxicaps Capsules 1490
Lanoxin Injection 1494
Lanoxin Injection Pediatric 1497
Lanoxin Tablets 1500
Sonata Capsules (Rare) 1717
Ultane Liquid for Inhalation (Less than 1%) 531
Uniretic Tablets (Less than 1%) 3100
VFEND I.V. (Less than 2%) 2564
VFEND Oral Suspension (Less than 2%) 2564
VFEND Tablets (Less than 2%) 2564
Virazole for Inhalation Solution (Infrequent) 3370
Zelapar Tablets 3372

Bile duct obstruction
Thalomid Capsules 965
Zelnorm Tablets 2312

Bile duct sludge, presence of metabolites
Clinoril Tablets (Rare) 1924

Biliary lithiasis
Rocephin 2800

Biliary sludge
Sandostatin Injection (Frequent) 2278

Biliary stasis
Thioridazine Hydrochloride Tablets 2163

Bilirubin, indirect, changes
▲ Sutent Capsules (0% to 15%) 2560

Bilirubin, total, decrease
▲ Avastin IV (1% to 6%) 1227
▲ Dacogen Injection (5%) 2129

Bilirubin, total, increase
Aloxi Injection (Less than 1%) 2127
▲ Arranon Injection (2% to 10%) 1357
▲ Atripla Tablets (Up to 3%) 945
▲ Baraclude (2% to 3%) 894
Epzicom Tablets 1436
Maxipime for Injection (Greater than 0.1% to less than 1%) 1105
Soltamox Oral Solution (2%) 3527
▲ Truvada Tablets (1% to 12%) 1296

Bilirubinemia
▲ Abelcet Injection (4%) 1141
Abilify Oral Solution (Infrequent) 882
Abilify Oral Solution (Infrequent) 2450
Abilify Discmelt Orally Disintegrating Tablets (Infrequent) 882
Abilify Discmelt Orally Disintegrating Tablets (Infrequent) 2450
Abilify Tablets (Infrequent) 882
Abilify Tablets (Infrequent) 2450
Aldurazyme for Intravenous Infusion (2%) 1268
Ambien Tablets (Rare) 2851
Ambien CR Tablets (Rare) 2855
▲ AmBisome for Injection (11.1% to 18.1%) 620
Arthrotec Tablets (Rare) 3129
Asacol Delayed-Release Tablets 2692
Campral Tablets (Infrequent) 1174
▲ Cancidas for Injection (0% to 3.8%) 1918
Celexa (Rare) 1176
▲ CellCept Capsules (3% to less than 20%) 2747
▲ CellCept Intravenous (3% to less than 20%) 2747
▲ CellCept Oral Suspension (3% to less than 20%) 2747
▲ CellCept Tablets (3% to less than 20%) 2747
Coreg Tablets (Greater than 0.1% to 1%) 1414
Doxil Injection (Less than 1%) 2351
Effexor Tablets (Rare) 3411
Effexor XR Capsules (Rare) 3417
▲ Eloxatin for Injection (1% to 20%) 2892
Eraxis for Injection (Less than 1% to less than 2%) 2521
Gengraf Capsules (1% to less than 3%) 459
▲ Intron A for Injection (Less than 5%) 3024
Lamictal (Rare) 1481
Lexapro Oral Solution 1190
Lexapro Tablets 1190
Lotronex Tablets (Rare) 1512
Mefoxin for Injection 2012
Mefoxin Premixed Intravenous Solution 2016
Mobic Oral Suspension (Less than 2%) 863
Mobic Tablets (Less than 2%) 863
▲ Mylotarg for Injection (11% to 13%) 3431
Neoral Oral Solution (1% to less than 3%) 2259
Neoral Soft Gelatin Capsules (1% to less than 3%) 2259
Nexium Delayed-Release Capsules (Less than 1%) 655
Nexium I.V. (Less than 1%) 659
Niaspan Extended-Release Tablets 1730
▲ Oncaspar (Greater than 1% but less than 5%) 1145
Paxil CR Controlled-Release Tablets (Rare) 1538
Paxil (Rare) 1530
Pexeva Tablets (rare) 1694
Plavix Tablets (Less than 1%) 917
Plavix Tablets (Less than 1%) 2926
Prevacid Delayed-Release Capsules 3271
Prevacid for Delayed-Release Oral Suspension 3271
Prevacid SoluTab Delayed-Release Orally Disintegrating Tablets 3271
Prevacid NapraPAC 3280
PREVPAC 3284
▲ Prograf Capsules and Injection (3% to 15%) 632
▲ Proleukin for Injection (40%) 2266
Protonix I.V. (Less than 1%) 3472
Protonix Tablets (Less than 1%) 3469
Protopic Ointment (Greater than or equal to 1%) 638
▲ Rebif Prefilled Syringe for Injection (2% to 3%) 3159
ReFacto Vials 3484
Relpax Tablets (Rare) 2548
Requip Tablets (Infrequent) 1555
Rescriptor Tablets 2551
Risperdal Consta Long-Acting Injection (Rare) 1682
Sonata Capsules (Rare) 1717
Symbyax Capsules (Rare) 1819
Thalomid Capsules 965
Tygacil for Injection (2.3%) 3488
Ultane Liquid for Inhalation (Less than 1%) 531
Uniretic Tablets (Less than 1%) 3100
VFEND I.V. (0.5% to 1.1%) 2564
VFEND Oral Suspension (0.5% to 1.1%) 2564
VFEND Tablets (0.5% to 1.1%) 2564
Viracept 2577
Zyprexa Tablets (Infrequent) 1830
Zyprexa ZYDIS Orally Disintegrating Tablets (Infrequent) 1830

Bilirubinuria
Primaxin I.M. 2045
Primaxin I.V. 2048

Binge eating, unspecified
Ambien CR Tablets (1%) 2855

Bipolar illness
DextroStat Tablets 3179
Ritalin Hydrochloride Tablets 2269
Ritalin-SR Tablets 2269

Birth, premature
Accutane Capsules 2731
Paxil CR Controlled-Release Tablets 1538
Sandimmune 2275

Birth defects, increased risk of
Coumadin for Injection 898
Coumadin Tablets 898
Cuprimine Capsules 1947
Depacon Injection (Multiple reports) 412
Depakene (Multiple reports) 417
Depakote Tablets (Multiple reports) 427
Depakote ER Tablets (Multiple reports) 434
Efudex 3363
Klonopin 2778
Phenytek Capsules 2160
Podocon-25 Liquid 2478
Premarin Intravenous 3442
Premarin Vaginal Cream 3452
Premphase Tablets 3456
Prempro Tablets 3456
Rebetol 3058
Rebetron Combination Therapy 3063
Soriatane Capsules 1013
Thalomid Capsules 965
Tracleer Tablets 545

Birth weight, low
Adderall Tablets 3164
Adderall XR Capsules 3166
Aggrenox Capsules 822
Bayer Aspirin 744
Dexedrine 1420
Percodan Tablets 1132
Sandimmune 2275
St. Joseph 81 mg Aspirin Chewable and Enteric Coated Tablets 1869
St. Joseph 81 mg Aspirin ▣ 688

Blackout spells
Lithobid Tablets 1692

Bladder, irritability
Oxandrin Tablets 2962

Bladder, neurogenic
Bicillin C-R Injectable Suspension 1706
Exelon Capsules (Infrequent) 2206
Exelon Oral Solution (Infrequent) 2206

Bladder, spasms
▲ DepoDur Extended-Release Injection (2% to 5%) 1110
Furosemide Tablets 2154
Midamor Tablets (Less than or equal to 1%) 2026
Moduretic Tablets 2028
▲ Myfortic Tablets (3% to less than 20%) 2255

Bladder dysfunction
Aricept Tablets (Infrequent) 1094
Aricept ODT Tablets (Infrequent) 1094
DepoCyt Injection 1143
Depo-Medrol Single-Dose Vial 2619
Invanz for Injection (Greater than 0.1%) 1999

Blanching
Catapres-TTS (1 of 101 patients) 844
▲ Synera Topical Patch (12%) 1137

Blebs, filtering (ocular)
Blephamide Ophthalmic Ointment (Increased incidence) 568
FML Ophthalmic Ointment ⊙228
FML Ophthalmic Suspension ⊙227
FML Forte Ophthalmic Suspension ⊙226
Pred Mild Ophthalmic Suspension ⊙238
Pred Forte Ophthalmic Suspension ⊙235

Bleeding
Abilify Oral Solution (Infrequent) 882
Abilify Oral Solution (Infrequent) 2450
Abilify Discmelt Orally Disintegrating Tablets (Infrequent) 882
Abilify Discmelt Orally Disintegrating Tablets (Infrequent) 2450
Abilify Tablets (Infrequent) 882
Abilify Tablets (Infrequent) 2450
Accolate Tablets 671
▲ Activase I.V. (Most common complication) 1223
▲ Aggrastat (Among most common) 1907
▲ Aggrenox Capsules (3.2%) 822
Agrylin Capsules (1% to 5%) 3169
Aldara Cream, 5% (More than 1%) 1846
Alkeran for Injection 955
Alkeran Tablets 956
Aloprim for Injection (Less than 1%) 2167
AmBisome for Injection (Less common) 620
▲ Arixtra Injection (0% to 3.4%) 1351
Azilect Tablets (2%) 3293
Bexxar 1398
Cafcit (2.2%) 1886
▲ Camptosar Injection (1% to 5%) 2604
▲ Carnitor Injection (2% to 9%) 3188
▲ Cathflo Activase (Among most frequent) 1231
Ceftin 1407
▲ CellCept Capsules (3% to less than 20%) 2747
▲ CellCept Intravenous (3% to less than 20%) 2747
▲ CellCept Oral Suspension (3% to less than 20%) 2747
▲ CellCept Tablets (3% to less than 20%) 2747
Colazal Capsules 2838
Coumadin for Injection 898
Coumadin Tablets 898
Crixivan Capsules 1940
Depacon Injection 412
Depakene 417
Depakote Sprinkle Capsules 422
Depakote Tablets 427
Depakote ER Tablets 434
▲ Doxil Injection (1% to 5%) 2351
Effexor Tablets 3411
Effexor XR Capsules 3417
Elitek (Less than or equal to 1%) 2890
Elspar for Injection 2463
Elspar for Injection 1960
Emend Capsules (Greater than 0.5%) 1963
Ferrlecit Injection (Two or more patients) 3388
Fortaz 1453
▲ Fragmin Injection (0.43% to 3.6%) 1097
Gabitril Tablets (Infrequent) 984
▲ Gamunex Immune Globulin I.V., 10% (29%) 3235

- ▲ Gemzar for Injection (Up to 17%) 1771
- ▲ Gleevec Tablets (0% to 53%) 2227
- Herceptin I.V. (At least one of the 958 patients) 1233
- ▲ Hycamtin for Injection (Rare to 15%) 1458
- ▲ Integrilin Injection (10.5% to 14.2%) 3020
- ▲ Intron A for Injection (8%) 3024
- Invanz for Injection (Greater than 0.1%) 1999
- Ionsys Transdermal System (.1% to less than 1%) 2379
- Iressa Tablets 684
- I.V. Busulfex 2493
- Keflex Capsules 549
- Lamictal (2%) 1481
- Leukeran Tablets 1504
- ▲ Leukine (23% to 29%) 814
- ▲ Levulan Kerastick for Topical Solution, 20% (2% to 4%) 1085
- Lotronex Tablets (Rare) 1512
- ▲ Lovenox Injection (1% to 13%) 2915
- Maxipime for Injection 1105
- Mefoxin for Injection 2012
- Mefoxin Premixed Intravenous Solution 2016
- Meridia Capsules 489
- Miradon Tablets 3042
- Mustargen for Injection 2468
- ▲ Mylotarg for Injection (9% to 13%) 3431
- Nalfon Capsules (Less than 1%) 2502
- ▲ NeoProfen Injection (6% to 32%) 2472
- ▲ Nipent for Injection (3% to 10%) 1863
- Norvir (Less than 2%) 503
- NovoSeven (Greater than or equal to 2%) 2331
- Omnicef Capsules 511
- Omnicef for Oral Suspension 511
- Oncaspar 1145
- Percodan Tablets 1132
- Pexeva Tablets 1694
- Pletal Tablets (Less than 2%) 2455
- ▲ Prograf Capsules and Injection (3% to 15%) 632
- Proleukin for Injection (Less than 1%) 2266
- Protonix I.V. (Less than 1%) 3472
- Protonix Tablets (Less than 1%) 3469
- Prozac Pulvules and Liquid (Frequent) 1801
- Raniclor Tablets, Chewable 2505
- ▲ Rapamune Oral Solution and Tablets (3% to 20%) 3475
- ReFacto Vials 3484
- ▲ ReoPro Vials (10.6% to 16.8%) 1809
- ▲ Retavase (21.1%) 2499
- Rilutek Tablets (Rare) 2930
- Risperdal (Rare) 1676
- Risperdal M-Tab Orally Disintegrating Tablets (Rare) 1676
- Rythmol SR Capsules 2727
- ▲ Simulect for Injection (3% to 10%) 2284
- Soriatane Capsules (Less than 1%) 1013
- Suprax 1843
- ▲ Sutent Capsules (1% to 26%) 2560
- Targretin Capsules 1747
- Tasmar Tablets (1%) 3358
- Taxotere Injection Concentrate 2932
- Ticlid Tablets 2810
- ▲ TNKase I.V. (4.7% to 21.8%) 1264
- Trasylol Injection (1% to 2%) 754
- ▲ Trisenox Injection (8%) 993
- Ultane Liquid for Inhalation (Less than 1%) 531
- Uniretic Tablets (Less than 1%) 3100
- ▲ Valcyte Tablets (Less than 5%) 2813
- Vantin Tablets and Oral Suspension 2645
- ▲ Vesanoid Capsules (60%) 2820
- ▲ Xeloda Tablets (Less than 5%) 2822
- ▲ Xigris Powder for Intravenous Infusion (Most common) 1828
- Zemaira (0.2% to 0.4%) 3509
- Zinacef for Injection 1631
- Zinacef Injection 1631
- ▲ Zinecard for Injection (2% to 3%) 2650
- Zoloft 2586
- Zosyn (1.0% or less) 3492
- Zyprexa Tablets (Infrequent) 1830
- Zyprexa ZYDIS Orally Disintegrating Tablets (Infrequent) 1830

Bleeding, antepartum

- Aggrenox Capsules 822
- Bayer Aspirin 744
- Bayer Aspirin Comprehensive Prescribing Information ▣796
- Percodan Tablets 1132
- St. Joseph 81 mg Aspirin Chewable and Enteric Coated Tablets 1869
- St. Joseph 81 mg Aspirin ▣688

Bleeding, at invaded sites

- Fragmin Injection (3 cases) 1097

Bleeding, at site of administration

- ▲ Aldara Cream, 5% (3.3%) 1846
- ▲ Aranesp for Injection (6%) 581
- ▲ Copaxone for Injection (5%) 3297
- Dacogen Injection 2129
- Doxil Injection (Less than 1%) 2351
- Enbrel for Injection 584
- Genotropin Lyophilized Powder (Infrequent) 2638
- ▲ Intron A for Injection (Less than 5%) 3024
- Kogenate FS with Bio-Set 740
- ReoPro Vials (1 to 50 events) 1809

Bleeding, breakthrough

- Angeliq Tablets 762
- Climara Transdermal System 771
- Climara Pro Transdermal System 776
- Enjuvia Tablets 1062
- Estrasorb Topical Emulsion 1147
- Estratest Tablets 3199
- Estratest H.S. Tablets 3199
- Menostar Transdermal System 782
- Mircette Tablets 1066
- NuvaRing 2340
- Ortho-Cyclen Tablets 2429
- Ortho Evra Transdermal System 2417
- Ortho Tri-Cyclen Tablets 2429
- Ortho Tri-Cyclen Lo Tablets 2436
- Premarin Intravenous 3442
- Premarin Tablets 3446
- Premarin Vaginal Cream 3452
- Premphase Tablets 3456
- Prempro Tablets 3456
- Prometrium Capsules (100 mg, 200 mg) 3203
- Seasonique Tablets 1077
- Yasmin 28 Tablets 796
- Yaz Tablets 803

Bleeding, dental

- Abilify Oral Solution (Rare) 882
- Abilify Oral Solution (Rare) 2450
- Abilify Discmelt Orally Disintegrating Tablets (Rare) 882
- Abilify Discmelt Orally Disintegrating Tablets (Rare) 2450
- Abilify Tablets (Rare) 882
- Abilify Tablets (Rare) 2450
- Accutane Capsules 2731
- Actiq (Less than 1%) 979
- Activase I.V. (Less than 1%) 1223
- Aggrenox Capsules (Less than 1%) 822
- AmBisome for Injection (Less common) 620
- ▲ Avastin IV (6%) 1227
- Celexa (Rare) 1176
- ▲ Clolar for Intravenous Infusion (15%) 1271
- Copaxone for Injection (Infrequent) 3297
- Coumadin for Injection 898
- Coumadin Tablets 898
- Crixivan Capsules (Less than 2%) 1940
- ▲ Dacogen Injection (8%) 2129
- Depakote ER Tablets (Greater than 1%) 434
- Doxil Injection (Less than 1%) 2351
- Effexor Tablets (Rare) 3411
- Effexor XR Capsules (Rare) 3417
- Elmiron Capsules (Less than or equal to 1%) 2415
- Gengraf Capsules (1% to less than 3%) 459
- Geodon Capsules (Rare) 2529
- ▲ Intron A for Injection (Less than 5%) 3024
- Lamictal (Rare) 1481
- Lipitor Tablets (Less than 2%) 2483
- Mustargen for Injection 2468
- Neoral Oral Solution (1% to less than 3%) 2259
- Neoral Soft Gelatin Capsules (1% to less than 3%) 2259
- Neurontin Capsules (Infrequent) 2487
- Neurontin Oral Solution (Infrequent) 2487
- Neurontin Tablets (Infrequent) 2487
- Pletal Tablets (Less than 2%) 2455
- Prevacid Delayed-Release Capsules (Less than 1%) 3271
- Prevacid for Delayed-Release Oral Suspension (Less than 1%) 3271
- Prevacid SoluTab Delayed-Release Orally Disintegrating Tablets (Less than 1%) 3271
- PREVPAC (Less than 1%) 3284
- Prozac Pulvules and Liquid (Infrequent) 1801
- Rescriptor Tablets 2551
- Retrovir Capsules 1560
- Retrovir IV Infusion 1564
- Retrovir 1560
- Rilutek Tablets (Infrequent) 2930
- Rythmol SR Capsules 2727
- Seroquel Tablets (Infrequent) 690
- Sonata Capsules (Rare) 1717
- ▲ Soriatane Capsules (1% to 10%) 1013
- Sutent Capsules 2560
- Topamax Sprinkle Capsules (Infrequent) 2404
- Topamax Tablets (Infrequent) 2404
- Trileptal Tablets 2300
- Trileptal Oral Suspension 2300
- VFEND I.V. (Less than 2%) 2564
- VFEND Oral Suspension (Less than 2%) 2564
- VFEND Tablets (Less than 2%) 2564
- Wellbutrin SR Sustained-Release Tablets 1607
- Wellbutrin XL Extended-Release Tablets 1613
- Zonegran Capsules (Infrequent) 1101
- Zyban Sustained-Release Tablets 1644

Bleeding, duodenal ulcer

- Emend Capsules (Isolated cases) 1963

Bleeding, gastrointestinal

- ▲ Abelcet Injection (4%) 1141
- Abilify Oral Solution (Infrequent) 882
- Abilify Oral Solution (Infrequent) 2450
- Abilify Discmelt Orally Disintegrating Tablets (Infrequent) 882
- Abilify Discmelt Orally Disintegrating Tablets (Infrequent) 2450
- Abilify Tablets (Infrequent) 882
- Abilify Tablets (Infrequent) 2450
- Aciphex Tablets (Rare) 1090
- Actimmune (Rare) 1671
- Actiq (1% or greater) 979
- ▲ Activase I.V. (5%) 1223
- Adalat CC Tablets (Less than 1%) 2964
- Advil Allergy Sinus Caplets ▣770
- Advil Caplets ▣674
- Children's Advil Oral Suspension ▣603
- Children's Advil Chewable Tablets ▣603
- Advil Cold & Sinus ▣723
- Advil Gel Caplets ▣674
- Infants' Advil Concentrated Drops ▣604
- Infants' Advil Concentrated Drops - White Grape (Dye-Free) ▣604
- Junior Strength Advil Swallow Tablets ▣605
- Advil Liqui-Gels ▣674
- Advil Migraine Liquigels ▣608
- Advil Multi-Symptom Cold Caplets ▣770
- Advil PM Caplets ▣615
- Advil Tablets ▣674
- Aggrastat (0.1%) 1907
- ▲ Aggrenox Capsules (1.2% to 4.1%) 822
- ▲ Agrylin Capsules (1% to 5%) 3169
- Aleve Caplets 742
- Aleve Gelcaps 743
- Aleve Cold & Sinus Caplets 744
- Aleve Tablets 743
- Aleve Cold & Sinus Caplets ▣724
- Aloprim for Injection (Less than 1%) 2167
- ▲ AmBisome for Injection (9.9%) 620
- Anaprox Tablets (Less than 1%) 2761
- Anaprox DS Tablets (Less than 1%) 2761
- ▲ Aredia for Injection (Up to 6%) 2179
- ▲ Argatroban Injection (2.3% to 14.4%) 1346
- Aricept Tablets (Frequent) 1094
- Aricept ODT Tablets (Frequent) 1094
- Arthrotec Tablets (Rare) 3129
- ▲ Asacol Delayed-Release Tablets (2% to 5%) 2692
- ▲ Avastin IV (19% to 24%) 1227
- Azilect Tablets (Frequent) 3293
- Bayer Aspirin 744
- Bayer Aspirin Comprehensive Prescribing Information ▣796
- BC Headache Powder ▣677
- BC Allergy Sinus Cold Powder ▣677
- Arthritis Strength BC Powder ▣677
- BC Sinus Cold Powder ▣677
- Cafcit (2.2%) 1886
- Campath Ampules 811
- Campral Tablets (Infrequent) 1174
- Cathflo Activase 1231
- Celebrex Capsules (Less than 0.1%) 3134
- Celexa 1176
- ▲ CellCept Capsules (1.7% to less than 20%) 2747
- ▲ CellCept Intravenous (1.7% to less than 20%) 2747
- ▲ CellCept Oral Suspension (1.7% to less than 20%) 2747
- ▲ CellCept Tablets (1.7% to less than 20%) 2747
- Chantix Tablets (Infrequent) 2517
- Cipro (Less than 1%) 2977
- Cipro I.V. (Less than 1%) 2984
- Cipro XR Tablets 2990
- Clinoril Tablets (Less than 1%) 1924
- Copegus Tablets (Less than 1%) 2754
- Coreg Tablets (Less than or equal to 0.1%) 1414
- Cubicin for Injection (1.7%) 1026
- Dacogen Injection 2129
- Dantrium Capsules (Rare) 2694
- Demadex Injection 2759
- Demadex Tablets 2759
- Dolobid Tablets (Less than 1 in 100) 1955
- Doxil Injection (Less than 1%) 2351
- EC-Naprosyn Delayed-Release Tablets (Less than 1%) 2761
- Edecrin 1959
- Effexor Tablets (Rare) 3411
- Effexor XR Capsules (Rare) 3417
- Eldepryl Capsules 3208
- Emcyt Capsules (1%) 2634
- Enbrel for Injection (Infrequent) 584
- Evoxac Capsules (Less than 1%) 1047
- Exelon Capsules (Infrequent) 2206
- Exelon Oral Solution (Infrequent) 2206
- Fosamax (Occasional) 1969
- Fragmin Injection (1 case) 1097
- Gabitril Tablets (Infrequent) 984
- Gantrisin Pediatric Suspension 2770
- Gengraf Capsules (1% to less than 3%) 459
- ▲ Gleevec Tablets (0.4% to 8%) 2227
- Goody's Body Pain Formula Powder ▣684
- Goody's Extra Strength Headache Powders ▣611
- Goody's Extra Strength Pain Relief Tablets ▣685
- ▲ Humira Injection (Less than 5%) 466
- Imitrex Injection 1463
- Imitrex Nasal Spray (Rare) 1467
- Imitrex Tablets (Rare) 1471
- Indocin Capsules (Less than 1%) 1995
- ▲ Indocin I.V. (3% to 9%) 2465
- Indocin (Less than 1%) 1995
- Integrilin Injection 3020
- ▲ Intron A for Injection (Less than 5%) 3024
- Invanz for Injection (Greater than 0.1%) 1999
- Ionsys Transdermal System (.1% to less than 1%) 2379
- K-Dur Extended-Relase Tablets 3033
- K-Tab Tablets 475
- Lamictal (Rare) 1481
- ▲ Leukine (11% to 27%) 814
- Levaquin (0.1% to 0.9%) 2384
- Levaquin in 5% Dextrose Injection (0.1% to 0.9%) 2384
- Lexapro Oral Solution 1190
- Lexapro Tablets 1190
- Lyrica Capsules (0.1% to 1%) 2539
- Meridia Capsules 489
- Merrem I.V. (0.5%) 686
- Midamor Tablets (Less than or equal to 1%) 2026
- Mobic Oral Suspension (Less than 2%) 863
- Mobic Tablets (Less than 2%) 863
- Moduretic Tablets (Less than or equal to 1%) 2028
- Motrin IB Tablets and Caplets 1866
- Children's Motrin Oral Suspension 1867
- Children's Motrin Non-Staining Dye-Free Oral Suspension 1867
- Children's Motrin Cold Oral Suspension 1867
- Infants' Motrin Concentrated Drops 1867
- Infants' Motrin Non-Staining Dye-Free Concentrated Drops 1867
- Junior Strength Motrin Caplets and Chewable Tablets 1867
- Mustargen for Injection 2468
- Myfortic Tablets 2255
- Mylotarg for Injection 3431
- Nalfon Capsules (Less than 1%) 2502
- Namenda (Infrequent) 1195
- Naprosyn Suspension (Less than 1%) 2761
- Naprosyn Tablets (Less than 1%) 2761
- Neoral Oral Solution (1% to less than 3%) 2259
- Neoral Soft Gelatin Capsules (1% to less than 3%) 2259

Nexium Delayed-Release Capsules (Less than 1%) ... 655
Nexium I.V. (Less than 1%) ... 659
Nimotop Capsules (Less than 1%) ... 749
Norvir (Less than 2%) ... 503
NovoSeven ... 2331
Omnicef Capsules ... 511
Omnicef for Oral Suspension ... 511
Orthoclone OKT3 Sterile Solution (Less than 1%) ... 2360
Parcopa Orally Disintegrating Tablets ... 3097
Pegasys (Less than 1%) ... 2789
Pentasa Capsules (Less than 1%) ... 3185
Percodan Tablets ... 1132
Plavix Tablets (1% to 2.5%) ... 917
Plavix Tablets (1% to 2.5%) ... 2926
Pletal Tablets (Very rare) ... 2455
Prevacid Delayed-Release Capsules (Less than 1%) ... 3271
Prevacid for Delayed-Release Oral Suspension (Less than 1%) ... 3271
Prevacid SoluTab Delayed-Release Orally Disintegrating Tablets (Less than 1%) ... 3271
Prevacid NapraPAC (Less than 1%) ... 3280
PREVPAC (Less than 1%) ... 3284
▲ Prograf Capsules and Injection (3% to 15%) ... 632
▲ Proleukin for Injection (13%) ... 2266
Proquin XR Tablets ... 1153
Protonix I.V. (Less than 1%) ... 3472
Protonix Tablets (Less than 1%) ... 3469
Prozac Pulvules and Liquid (Rare) ... 1801
Razadyne ... 2399
Razadyne ER Extended-Release Capsules ... 2399
▲ Refludan for Injection (5.3%) ... 792
Remicade for IV Injection (Greater than or equal to 0.2%) ... 971
ReoPro Vials (11 events) ... 1809
Requip Tablets (Infrequent) ... 1555
Rescriptor Tablets ... 2551
▲ Retavase (1.8% to 9%) ... 2499
Revlimid Capsules ... 958
Rilutek Tablets (Infrequent) ... 2930
Risperdal (Rare) ... 1676
Risperdal M-Tab Orally Disintegrating Tablets (Rare) ... 1676
Sandimmune (Rare) ... 2275
Sandostatin Injection (Less than 1%) ... 2278
Sandostatin LAR Depot (Rare) ... 2280
▲ Simulect for Injection (3% to 10%) ... 2284
St. Joseph 81 mg Aspirin Chewable and Enteric Coated Tablets ... 1869
St. Joseph 81 mg Aspirin ... ▣ 688
Stalevo Tablets ... 2287
Sular Tablets (Less than or equal to 1%) ... 3122
Sutent Capsules ... 2560
Symbyax Capsules (Rare) ... 1819
Tarceva Tablets (Infrequent) ... 1259
Tarceva Tablets (Infrequent) ... 2444
Tasmar Tablets (Infrequent) ... 3358
Taxotere Injection Concentrate (One patient) ... 2932
Tequin Injection (Less than 0.1%) ... 938
Tequin Injection in 5% Dextrose (Less than 0.1%) ... 938
Tequin Tablets (Less than 0.1%) ... 938
Thalomid Capsules ... 965
Ticlid Tablets ... 2810
TNKase I.V. (1%) ... 1264
Trasylol Injection (1% to 2%) ... 754
TriLyte with Flavor Packs for Oral Solution ... 3100
▲ Trisenox Injection (8%) ... 993
Uniretic Tablets (Less than 1%) ... 3100
▲ Vesanoid Capsules (34%) ... 2820
VFEND I.V. (Less than 2%) ... 2564
VFEND Oral Suspension (Less than 2%) ... 2564
VFEND Tablets (Less than 2%) ... 2564
Viracept (Less than 2%) ... 2577
Vivitrol ... 995
Voltaren Tablets (Occasionally) ... 2307
Voltaren-XR Tablets (Occasionally) ... 2310
Wellbutrin Tablets (Rare) ... 1603
Wellbutrin SR Sustained-Release Tablets ... 1607
Wellbutrin XL Extended-Release Tablets ... 1613
▲ Xeloda Tablets (1% to 6%) ... 2822
▲ Xigris Powder for Intravenous Infusion (5%) ... 1828
▲ Zemplar Capsules (5%) ... 541
▲ Zemplar Injection (5%) ... 543
Zyban Sustained-Release Tablets ... 1644
Zyprexa IntraMuscular ... 1830
Zyvox (0% to 2.3%) ... 2652

Bleeding, genital
Sutent Capsules ... 2560

Bleeding, genitourinary tract
▲ Activase I.V. (4%) ... 1223
Aggrastat (0.1%) ... 1907
Argatroban Injection (1.8%) ... 1346
Premphase Tablets ... 3456
Prempro Tablets ... 3456
ReoPro Vials (5 to 8 events) ... 1809
▲ Retavase (0.9% to 9.5%) ... 2499
Xigris Powder for Intravenous Infusion (2%) ... 1828

Bleeding, gingival
(*see under* Bleeding, dental)

Bleeding, gums
Adalat CC Tablets (Less than 1%) ... 2964
Caduet Tablets (Less than 2%) ... 2508
▲ Mylotarg for Injection (5% to 14%) ... 3431
Pexeva Tablets (rare) ... 1694
Prevacid NapraPAC (Less than 1%) ... 3280
Raptiva for Injection ... 1250
Symbyax Capsules (Rare) ... 1819

Bleeding, intermenstrual
Arthrotec Tablets (Rare) ... 3129
▲ depo-subQ provera 104 Injectable Suspension (7%) ... 2624
▲ Entocort EC Capsules (Less than 5%) ... 2698
Estring Vaginal Ring ... 2635
Evoxac Capsules (Less than 1%) ... 1047
Imitrex Injection ... 1463
Imitrex Nasal Spray ... 1467
Imitrex Tablets (Infrequent) ... 1471
Risperdal (Infrequent) ... 1676
Risperdal M-Tab Orally Disintegrating Tablets (Infrequent) ... 1676
Topamax Sprinkle Capsules (Greater than 1%) ... 2404
Topamax Tablets (Greater than 1%) ... 2404
Trileptal Tablets ... 2300
Trileptal Oral Suspension ... 2300
▲ Trisenox Injection (8%) ... 993
Yasmin 28 Tablets (Greater than 1%) ... 796
Yaz Tablets (Greater than 1%) ... 803
Zoloft (Infrequent) ... 2586
Zyrtec Chewable Tablets (Less than 2%) ... 2594
Zyrtec (Less than 2%) ... 2594
Zyrtec-D 12 Hour Extended Release Tablets (Less than 2%) ... 2597

Bleeding, internal
Activase I.V. ... 1223

Bleeding, intra-abdominal
Xigris Powder for Intravenous Infusion (2%) ... 1828

Bleeding, intracerebral
Gleevec Tablets (0% to 1%) ... 2227
Revatio Tablets ... 2557
Ticlid Tablets (Rare) ... 2810
Viagra Tablets ... 2573

Bleeding, intracranial
Abilify Oral Solution (Rare) ... 882
Abilify Oral Solution (Rare) ... 2450
Abilify Discmelt Orally Disintegrating Tablets (Rare) ... 882
Abilify Discmelt Orally Disintegrating Tablets (Rare) ... 2450
Abilify Tablets (Rare) ... 882
Abilify Tablets (Rare) ... 2450
Activase I.V. (0.4% to 1.3%) ... 1223
Aggrastat (0.1%) ... 1907
Aggrenox Capsules (0.6% to less than 1%) ... 822
▲ Argatroban Injection (1% to 4.3%) ... 1346
Aricept Tablets (Infrequent) ... 1094
Aricept ODT Tablets (Infrequent) ... 1094
Arranon Injection (1%) ... 1357
Bayer Aspirin ... 744
Bayer Aspirin Comprehensive Prescribing Information ... ▣ 796
Campath Ampules ... 811
Cardene I.V. (0.7%) ... 2497
Elspar for Injection ... 2463
Elspar for Injection ... 1960
Exelon Capsules (Infrequent) ... 2206
Exelon Oral Solution (Infrequent) ... 2206
▲ Indocin I.V. (3% to 9%) ... 2465
▲ Infasurf Intratracheal Suspension (29% to 36%) ... 1184
Integrilin Injection (Rare) ... 3020
Invirase (Rare) ... 2772
Lovenox Injection ... 2915
Mylotarg for Injection (1%) ... 3431
Namenda ... 1195
Neurontin Capsules (Infrequent) ... 2487
Neurontin Oral Solution (Infrequent) ... 2487
Neurontin Tablets (Infrequent) ... 2487
Percodan Tablets ... 1132
Plavix Tablets (Less than 1%) ... 917
Plavix Tablets (Less than 1%) ... 2926
Pletal Tablets (Very rare) ... 2455
Refludan for Injection ... 792
ReoPro Vials (1 to 3 events) ... 1809
Retavase (0.8%) ... 2499
Sandostatin LAR Depot (Rare) ... 2280
St. Joseph 81 mg Aspirin Chewable and Enteric Coated Tablets ... 1869
Xigris (2%) ... 1828

Bleeding, lip
Neurontin Capsules (Rare) ... 2487
Neurontin Oral Solution (Rare) ... 2487
Neurontin Tablets (Rare) ... 2487

Bleeding, menstrual, heavy
depo-subQ provera 104 ... 2624

Bleeding, menstrual, prolonged
ParaGard T 380A Intrauterine Copper Contraceptive ... 1073

Bleeding, mouth
Evoxac Capsules (Less than 1%) ... 1047
▲ Intron A for Injection (Less than 5%) ... 3024
ReoPro Vials (4 events) ... 1809

Bleeding, mucosal
Effexor Tablets (Rare) ... 3411

Bleeding, nasal
(*see also under* Epistaxis)
Cesamet Capsules ... 3340

Bleeding, oropharyngeal
Integrilin Injection ... 3020

Bleeding, otic
Relenza Rotadisk (Less than 1%) ... 1552
ReoPro Vials (9 to 11 events) ... 1809

Bleeding, pericardial
Activase I.V. ... 1223

Bleeding, perioperative
Ticlid Tablets ... 2810

Bleeding, pharyngeal
▲ TNKase I.V. (3.1%) ... 1264

Bleeding, postoperative
▲ Advair HFA Inhalation Aerosol (1% to 3%) ... 1318
▲ Arixtra Injection (4.3%) ... 1351
Dacogen Injection ... 2129
Ionsys Transdermal System (.1% to less than 1%) ... 2379
Persantine Tablets (Rare) ... 868
Revlimid Capsules ... 958

Bleeding, postpartum
Percodan Tablets ... 1132
St. Joseph 81 mg Aspirin ... ▣ 688

Bleeding, puncture site
Capastat Sulfate for Injection ... 1755
TNKase I.V. (Less than 1%) ... 1264

Bleeding, renal-pelvic
Cipro I.V. (1% or less) ... 2984

Bleeding, respiratory tract
TNKase I.V. (Less than 1%) ... 1264

Bleeding, retroperitoneal
Activase I.V. (Less than 1%) ... 1223
Aggrastat (0.6%) ... 1907
Argatroban Injection (0.9%) ... 1346
Integrilin Injection ... 3020
Lovenox Injection ... 2915
Plavix Tablets (Less than 1%) ... 917
Plavix Tablets (Less than 1%) ... 2926
Pletal Tablets (Less than 2%) ... 2455
Proleukin for Injection ... 2266
ReoPro Vials (2 to 12 events) ... 1809
TNKase I.V. (Less than 1%) ... 1264
▲ Xigris (3%) ... 1828

Bleeding, subarachnoid
Revlimid Capsules ... 958

Bleeding, subcutaneous
Imitrex Injection ... 1463

Bleeding, subdural
Bayer Aspirin ... 744
Bayer Aspirin Comprehensive Prescribing Information ... ▣ 796

Bleeding, superficial
Activase I.V. ... 1223

Bleeding, upper GI
(*see under* Bleeding, gastrointestinal)

Bleeding, urethral
Ceftin Tablets (0.1% to 1%) ... 1407
Cipro (Less than 1%) ... 2977
Cipro XR Tablets ... 2990
Dacogen Injection ... 2129
Klonopin (Infrequent) ... 2778
Proquin XR Tablets ... 1153

Bleeding, urinary tract
Amerge Tablets (Rare) ... 1339
Eligard 22.5 mg (Less than 2%) ... 2883
Lotronex Tablets ... 1512
▲ TNKase I.V. (Less than 1% to 3.7%) ... 1264

Bleeding, uterine
Abilify Oral Solution (Rare) ... 882
Abilify Oral Solution (Rare) ... 2450
Abilify Discmelt Orally Disintegrating Tablets (Rare) ... 882
Abilify Discmelt Orally Disintegrating Tablets (Rare) ... 2450
Abilify Tablets (Rare) ... 882
Abilify Tablets (Rare) ... 2450
Aggrenox Capsules (Less than 1%) ... 822
Caduet Tablets (Less than 2%) ... 2508
Climara Transdermal System ... 771
▲ depo-subQ provera 104 Injectable Suspension (1% to less than 5%) ... 2624
Effexor Tablets (Rare) ... 3411
Effexor XR Capsules (Infrequent) ... 3417
Estratest Tablets ... 3199
Estratest H.S. Tablets ... 3199
Evoxac Capsules (Less than 1%) ... 1047
Gengraf Capsules (1% to less than 3%) ... 459
Geodon Capsules (Rare) ... 2529
▲ Intron A for Injection (Less than 5%) ... 3024
Lipitor Tablets (Less than 2%) ... 2483
Lunesta Tablets ... 3142
Neoral Oral Solution (1% to less than 3%) ... 2259
Neoral Soft Gelatin Capsules (1% to less than 3%) ... 2259
Permax Tablets (Infrequent) ... 3356
Premarin Intravenous ... 3442
Premarin Vaginal Cream ... 3452
Premphase Tablets ... 3456
Prempro Tablets ... 3456
Prozac Pulvules and Liquid (Rare) ... 1801
Requip Tablets (Rare) ... 1555
Rilutek Tablets (Rare) ... 2930
Tasmar Tablets (Rare) ... 3358
VFEND I.V. (Less than 2%) ... 2564
VFEND Oral Suspension (Less than 2%) ... 2564
VFEND Tablets (Less than 2%) ... 2564

Bleeding, uterine, irregularities
depo-subQ provera 104 Injectable Suspension ... 2624
Estrasorb Topical Emulsion ... 1147

Bleeding, vaginal
Abilify Oral Solution (Infrequent) ... 882
Abilify Oral Solution (Infrequent) ... 2450
Abilify Discmelt Orally Disintegrating Tablets (Infrequent) ... 882
Abilify Discmelt Orally Disintegrating Tablets (Infrequent) ... 2450
Abilify Tablets (Infrequent) ... 882
Abilify Tablets (Infrequent) ... 2450
Actiq (Less than 1%) ... 979
AmBisome for Injection (Less common) ... 620
▲ Angeliq Tablets (9.3%) ... 762
▲ Arimidex Tablets (1% to 5%) ... 673
Arthrotec Tablets (Rare) ... 3129
▲ Avastin IV (6%) ... 1227
Caduet Tablets (Less than 2%) ... 2508
Celebrex Capsules (0.1% to 1.9%) ... 3134
Celexa (Infrequent) ... 1176
Climara Transdermal System ... 771
▲ Climara Pro Transdermal System (36.8%) ... 776
Clinoril Tablets (Less than 1%) ... 1924
Coumadin for Injection ... 898
Coumadin Tablets ... 898
Depacon Injection (1% or more) ... 412
Depakene (1% or more) ... 417

Depakote Sprinkle Capsules............ 422
▲ Depakote Tablets (1% to 5%) 427
Depakote ER Tablets (1% or more)... 434
▲ depo-subQ provera 104 Injectable Suspension (1% to less than 5%)............................ 2624
▲ Doxil Injection (1% to 10%) 2351
Effexor Tablets (Infrequent).............. 3411
Effexor XR Capsules (Infrequent)...... 3417
▲ Eloxatin for Injection (2% to 5%) 2892
Enjuvia Tablets.................................. 1062
Estratest Tablets 3199
Estratest H.S. Tablets........................ 3199
▲ Estring Vaginal Ring (4%) 2635
▲ Evista Tablets (2.5% to 6.2%) 1763
Evoxac Capsules (Less than 1%)...... 1047
Faslodex Injection (Less than 1%)..... 681
Gabitril Tablets (Infrequent) 984
Geodon Capsules (Rare)................... 2529
Indocin Capsules (Less than 1%)...... 1995
Indocin I.V. (Less than 1%)................ 2465
Indocin (Less than 1%)...................... 1995
Inspra Tablets (0.4%)........................ 2536
Lipitor Tablets (Less than 2%).......... 2483
Lunesta Tablets (Infrequent)............. 3142
Lupron Depot-PED 7.5 mg, 11.25 mg and 15 mg (2%)........... 3269
Lupron Injection Pediatric (2%)......... 3259
Menostar Transdermal System......... 782
▲ Mylotarg for Injection (4% to 13%) ... 3431
Neurontin Capsules (Infrequent)....... 2487
Neurontin Oral Solution (Infrequent)..................................... 2487
Neurontin Tablets (Infrequent).......... 2487
Ortho-Cyclen/Ortho Tri-Cyclen 2429
Ortho Tri-Cyclen Lo Tablets.............. 2436
Paxil CR Controlled-Release Tablets (Rare)................................ 1538
Paxil (Rare).. 1530
Permax Tablets (Infrequent)............. 3356
Pexeva Tablets (Rare)...................... 1694
Pletal Tablets (Less than 2%)........... 2455
▲ Premarin Tablets (2% to 14%) 3446
▲ Premphase Tablets (1% to 6%) 3456
▲ Prempro Tablets (1% to 6%) 3456
Prozac Pulvules and Liquid (Infrequent)..................................... 1801
Refludan for Injection (1.8%)........... 792
Requip Tablets (Infrequent).............. 1555
Risperdal (Infrequent)....................... 1676
Risperdal M-Tab Orally Disintegrating Tablets (Infrequent)..................................... 1676
Seroquel Tablets (Infrequent)........... 690
▲ Soltamox Oral Solution (2% to 23%)... 3527
Sonata Capsules (Rare)................... 1717
Sular Tablets (Less than or equal to 1%).. 3122
Symbyax Capsules (Infrequent)........ 1819
▲ Topamax Sprinkle Capsules (0% to 3%)... 2404
▲ Topamax Tablets (0% to 3%) 2404
▲ Trisenox Injection (13%) 993
Uniretic Tablets (Less than 1%)........ 3100
VFEND I.V. (Less than 2%)............... 2564
VFEND Oral Suspension (Less than 2%).. 2564
VFEND Tablets (Less than 2%).......... 2564
Wellbutrin SR Sustained-Release Tablets (Up to 2%)....................... 1607
Wellbutrin XL Extended-Release Tablets (0% to 2%)....................... 1613
Xyrem Oral Solution (Infrequent)....... 1688
Zoloft (Infrequent)............................. 2586

Bleeding, wound

▲ Fragmin Injection (0.1% to 3.4%) 1097
▲ Ionsys Transdermal System (1% to less than 10%)......................... 2379
Sutent Capsules............................. 2560

Bleeding at injection site

▲ Amevive (4%) 626
Bicillin C-R Injectable Suspension..... 1706
▲ BOTOX Purified Neurotoxin Complex (3% to 10%).................. 570
▲ Edex Injection (6% to 15%) 3089
▲ Humira Injection (20%) 466
▲ Lovenox Injection (3% to 5%) 2915
ProQuad... 2064
▲ Retavase (4.6% to 48.6%) 2499
▲ Visudyne for Injection (10% to 30%)... 2305
Zemaira (0.9%)................................ 3509

Bleeding diathesis

Cipro (Less than 0.1%).................... 2977
Cipro I.V. (Rare)............................... 2984
Cipro XR Tablets.............................. 2990
Proquin XR Tablets........................... 1153

Bleeding irregularities

Climara Transdermal System........... 771
Climara Pro Transdermal System..... 776
Menostar Transdermal System........ 782
Mirena Intrauterine System.............. 787
Ortho Micronor Tablets..................... 2426
Plavix Tablets (1% to 2.5%)............. 917
Plavix Tablets (1% to 2.5%)............. 2926
Premphase Tablets.......................... 3456
Prempro Tablets.............................. 3456

Bleeding secondary to eczema

Bactroban Cream (One report)......... 1394

Bleeding tendency, increased

Alphanate, Antihemophilic Factor (Human) (Rare)............................ 1654
Pletal Tablets (Very rare)................. 2455
Singulair.. 2077
▲ Thiola Tablets (4%) 2141

Bleeding time, prolongation

Actiq (Less than 1%)........................ 979
Acular LS Ophthalmic Solution......... 566
Advate Injection (0.6%)................... 712
▲ Anaprox Tablets (1% to 10%) 2761
▲ Anaprox DS Tablets (1% to 10%) 2761
Arthrotec Tablets............................. 3129
Bayer Aspirin Comprehensive Prescribing Information............... ■ 796
Cardizem LA Extended Release Tablets (Infrequent)...................... 1728
Depakote ER Tablets (Greater than 1%)... 434
Dolobid Tablets................................ 1955
▲ EC-Naprosyn Delayed-Release Tablets (1% to 10%)..................... 2761
Elmiron Capsules............................. 2415
▲ Naprosyn Suspension (1% to 10%)... 2761
▲ Naprosyn Tablets (1% to 10%) 2761
Neurontin Capsules (Rare)............... 2487
Neurontin Oral Solution (Rare).......... 2487
Neurontin Tablets (Rare).................. 2487
Paxil CR Controlled-Release Tablets (Rare)............................... 1538
Paxil (Rare)...................................... 1530
Pexeva Tablets (rare)....................... 1694
Soriatane Capsules (Less than 1%).. 1013
Tiazac Capsules (Infrequent)............ 1201
Timentin ADD-Vantage 1580
Timentin Injection Galaxy Container...................................... 1583
Timentin IV Infusion......................... 1577
Timentin Pharmacy Bulk Package.... 1586
VFEND I.V. (Less than 2%)............... 2564
VFEND Oral Suspension (Less than 2%)... 2564
VFEND Tablets (Less than 2%).......... 2564
▲ Voltaren Tablets (1% to 10%) 2307
▲ Voltaren-XR Tablets (1% to 10%) 2310
Zosyn.. 3492

Blepharitis

Abilify Oral Solution (Infrequent)....... 882
Abilify Oral Solution (Infrequent)....... 2450
Abilify Discmelt Orally Disintegrating Tablets (Infrequent)................................... 882
Abilify Discmelt Orally Disintegrating Tablets (Infrequent)................................... 2450
Abilify Tablets (Infrequent)............... 882
Abilify Tablets (Infrequent)............... 2450
▲ Alphagan P Ophthalmic Solution (1% to 4%).................................. 567
Aricept Tablets (Infrequent)............. 1094
Aricept ODT Tablets (Infrequent)...... 1094
Azopt Ophthalmic Suspension (1% to 5%)... 557
Bactroban Nasal (Less than 1%)....... 1394
▲ Betimol Ophthalmic Solution (1% to 5%)... 3382
▲ Betimol Ophthalmic Solution (1% to 5%)... ⊙ 295
▲ Brimonidine Tartrate Ophthalmic Solution 0.2% (3% to 9%)............ ⊙ 248
▲ Cosopt Sterile Ophthalmic Solution (1% to 5%)..................... 1931
Doxil Injection (Less than 1%).......... 2351
Effexor Tablets (Rare)..................... 3411
Effexor XR Capsules (Rare).............. 3417
Evoxac Capsules (Less than 1%)...... 1047
Exelon Capsules (Infrequent)............ 2206
Exelon Oral Solution (Infrequent)...... 2206
Gabitril Tablets (Infrequent)............. 984
Geodon Capsules (Infrequent).......... 2529
Invirase (Less than 2%).................... 2772
▲ Lucentis Injection (3% to 36%) 1237
▲ Lumigan Ophthalmic Solution (3% to 10%).. 573
Lyrica Capsules (0.1% to 1%).......... 2539
▲ Macugen Injection (6% to 10%) ...... ⊙ 261
Namenda (Infrequent)...................... 1195
Norvir (Less than 2%)...................... 503
OptiPranolol Metipranolol Ophthalmic Solution 0.3% (A small number of patients)........... ⊙ 256
Paxil CR Controlled-Release Tablets (Rare)............................... 1538
Paxil (Rare)..................................... 1530
Pexeva Tablets (rare)....................... 1694
Protopic Ointment (0.2% to less than 1%).. 638
Prozac Pulvules and Liquid (Rare)..... 1801
Requip Tablets (Infrequent).............. 1555
Rescriptor Tablets............................ 2551
▲ Retisert Implant (5% to 9%) .... ⊙ 258
Rilutek Tablets (Rare)...................... 2930
Risperdal (Rare)............................... 1676
Risperdal M-Tab Orally Disintegrating Tablets (Rare)........ 1676
Seroquel Tablets (Infrequent)........... 690
Sonata Capsules (Rare).................. 1717
▲ Soriatane Capsules (Less than 5%)... 1013
Sular Tablets (Less than or equal to 1%)... 3122
Targretin Capsules.......................... 1747
Timoptic Sterile Ophthalmic Solution (Less frequent)............... 2088
Timoptic in Ocudose (Less frequent)...................................... 2091
Timoptic-XE Sterile Ophthalmic Gel Forming Solution......................... 2092
Travatan Ophthalmic Solution (1% to 4%)... 563
VFEND I.V. (Less than 2%)............... 2564
VFEND Oral Suspension (Less than 2%)... 2564
VFEND Tablets (Less than 2%)......... 2564
▲ Visudyne for Injection (1% to 10%) .. 2305
Zyprexa Tablets (Infrequent)............ 1830
Zyprexa ZYDIS Orally Disintegrating Tablets (Infrequent)................................. 1830

Blepharoconjunctivitis

▲ Alphagan P Ophthalmic Solution (1% to 4%).................................. 567
▲ Betagan Ophthalmic Solution, USP (About 1 in 20 patients)........ ⊙ 220
Carteolol Hydrochloride Ophthalmic Solution USP, 1% (Occasional)................................ ⊙ 249
▲ Flovent Diskus (1% to 3%) 1443

Blepharoptosis
(see also under Ptosis, eyelids)

Betagan Ophthalmic Solution, USP.. ⊙ 220
Betimol Ophthalmic Solution............ 3382
Betimol Ophthalmic Solution............ ⊙ 295

Blepharospasm

Eldepryl Capsules............................ 3208
Exelon Capsules (Infrequent)........... 2206
Exelon Oral Solution (Infrequent)...... 2206
Parcopa Orally Disintegrating Tablets.. 3097
Requip Tablets (Infrequent).............. 1555
Stalevo Tablets................................ 2287

Blindness

Bicillin C-R Injectable Suspension..... 1706
DepoCyt Injection............................ 1143
Doxil Injection (Less than 1%).......... 2351
Gabitril Tablets (Infrequent)............. 984
Imitrex Nasal Spray......................... 1467
Imitrex Tablets................................ 1471
Lithobid Tablets.............................. 1692
Lyrica Capsules (Rare)..................... 2539
Neoral Oral Solution........................ 2259
Neoral Soft Gelatin Capsules........... 2259
Neurontin Capsules (Rare)................ 2487
Neurontin Oral Solution (Rare).......... 2487
Neurontin Tablets (Rare).................. 2487
Ortho-Cyclen/Ortho Tri-Cyclen (Rare)... 2429
Orthoclone OKT3 Sterile Solution (Less than 1%)............................ 2360
PEG-Intron Powder for Injection (Less than or equal to 1%)........... 3048
Permax Tablets (Rare)...................... 3356
Pletal Tablets (Less than 2%)........... 2455
Prograf Capsules and Injection......... 632
Proleukin for Injection (Less than 1%)... 2266
Revlimid Capsules........................... 958
Sandimmune.................................... 2275
Zelapar Tablets................................ 3372
Zofran (Rare)................................... 1639
Zofran ODT Orally Disintegrating Tablets (Rare)............................... 1639
Zoloft.. 2586
Zyrtec Chewable Tablets (Less than 2%).. 2594
Zyrtec (Less than 2%)...................... 2594
Zyrtec-D 12 Hour Extended Release Tablets (Less than 2%)..... 2597

Blindness, color

VFEND I.V. (Less than 2%)............... 2564
VFEND Oral Suspension (Less than 2%)... 2564
VFEND Tablets (Less than 2%).......... 2564

Blindness, cortical

Prograf Capsules and Injection......... 632
Sutent Capsules.............................. 2560

Blindness, night
(see under Nyctalopia)

Blindness, transient

Adalat CC Tablets (Rare).................. 2964
Chantix Tablets (Rare)..................... 2517
Imitrex Tablets................................ 1471
Proleukin for Injection (Less than 1%)... 2266
Zofran Injection............................... 1634
Zofran.. 1639
Zofran ODT Orally Disintegrating Tablets 1639

Blistering

Accolate Tablets 671
Cutivate Cream (0.8%) 2662
Efudex (Infrequent) 3363
Lotrimin 3039
Lotrisone 3040
Motrin IB Tablets and Caplets 1866
Children's Motrin Oral Suspension 1867
Children's Motrin Non-Staining Dye-Free Oral Suspension 1867
Children's Motrin Cold Oral Suspension 1867
Infants' Motrin Concentrated Drops 1867
Infants' Motrin Non-Staining Dye-Free Concentrated Drops 1867
Junior Strength Motrin Caplets and Chewable Tablets 1867
Somavert Injection 2642
Striant Mucoadhesive 1007
Sulfamylon Cream 2162
Sulfamylon for 5% Topical Solution .. 2162
▲ Sutent Capsules (7%) 2560
Viramune Oral Suspension 873
Viramune Tablets 873

Blisters at application site

Lidoderm Patch 1118
Synera Topical Patch (Less than or equal to 1%) 1137

Bloating
(see under Abdominal bloating)

Blood carbon dioxide, changes

▲ Bumex Tablets (4.3%) 2746

Blood clotting, mechanisms, disorders of

Plavix Tablets (Less than 1%) 917
Plavix Tablets (Less than 1%) 2926

Blood dyscrasias

Abelcet Injection 1141
Asacol Delayed-Release Tablets 2692
BiDil Tablets 2171
▲ Blephamide Ophthalmic Ointment (Among most often) 568
Blephamide Ophthalmic Suspension 569
Campath Ampules 811
Dapsone Tablets USP 1673
Depo-Provera Contraceptive Injection (Less than 1%) 2622
depo-subQ provera 104 Injectable Suspension 2624
Furosemide Tablets 2154
▲ Leukine (25%) 814
Librium Capsules 3347
Prozac Pulvules and Liquid (Rare) 1801
Tambocor Tablets (Extremely rare) .. 1856
Trusopt Sterile Ophthalmic Solution (Rare) 2095
Zonegran Capsules (Rare) 1101

Blood glucose, elevation
(see under Hyperglycinemia)

Blood glucose, reduction
(see under Hypoglycemia)

Blood loss, increase
(see under Bleeding)

Blood pressure, changes

Clozaril Tablets 2184

Covera-HS Tablets (1.4%) ... 3139
Curosurf Intratracheal Suspension ... 1057
Decadron Tablets ... 1951
Depacon Injection ... 412
Depakene ... 417
Depakote Sprinkle Capsules ... 422
Depakote Tablets ... 427
Depakote ER Tablets ... 434
▲ DepoDur Extended-Release Injection (2% to 5%) ... 1110
Diastat Rectal Delivery System (Infrequent) ... 3343
Dilaudid ... 440
Dilaudid Non-Sterile Powder ... 440
Dilaudid Oral Liquid ... 445
Dilaudid Rectal Suppositories ... 440
Dilaudid Tablets ... 440
Dilaudid Tablets - 8 mg ... 445
Dilaudid-HP (Less frequent) ... 442
Doxil Injection (Less than 1%) ... 2351
Duragesic Transdermal System (Less than 1%) ... 2373
Effexor Tablets (Rare) ... 3411
Effexor XR Capsules (Rare) ... 3417
Emend Capsules (Isolated cases) ... 1963
Ethyol for Injection ... 1898
Exelon Capsules (Frequent) ... 2206
Exelon Oral Solution (Frequent) ... 2206
Fabrazyme for Intravenous Infusion ... 1274
FazaClo Orally Disintegrating Tablets (Less than 1%) ... 551
Ferrlecit Injection ... 3388
Frova Tablets (Rare) ... 1113
Geodon Capsules (Infrequent) ... 2529
▲ Hectorol Capsules (6.6%) ... 1275
▲ Hectorol Injection (6.6%) ... 1278
Hyperstat I.V. ... 3017
▲ Imdur Tablets (Less than or equal to 5%) ... 3018
Imitrex Injection (Infrequent) ... 1463
Imitrex Nasal Spray (Rare) ... 1467
Imitrex Tablets (Rare) ... 1471
Inderal LA Long-Acting Capsules ... 3429
Indocin I.V. (Less than 3%) ... 2465
▲ Infasurf Intratracheal Suspension (34%) ... 1184
Infed Injection ... 3390
InnoPran XL Capsules ... 2723
▲ Intron A for Injection (Less than 5%) ... 3024
Invanz for Injection (Greater than 0.1%) ... 1999
Ionsys Transdermal System (.1% to less than 1%) ... 2379
Kadian Capsules (Less than 3%) ... 577
Kaletra ... 476
Ketek Tablets (Less than 0.2%) ... 2903
▲ Kytril Injection (4.5%) ... 2781
Lariam Tablets (Less than 1%) ... 2786
Levaquin (0.1% to 0.9%) ... 2384
Levaquin in 5% Dextrose Injection (0.1% to 0.9%) ... 2384
Lexapro Oral Solution (Infrequent) ... 1190
Lexapro Tablets (Infrequent) ... 1190
Lidoderm Patch ... 1118
Lithobid Tablets ... 1692
▲ Lopressor Injection (3% to 15.9%) ... 2238
▲ Lopressor Tablets (3% to 15.9%) ... 2238
▲ Lopressor HCT 50/25 Tablets (3% to 6%) ... 2241
▲ Lopressor HCT 100/25 Tablets (3% to 6%) ... 2241
▲ Lopressor HCT 100/50 Tablets (3% to 6%) ... 2241
▲ Mavik Tablets (0.3% to 4.7%) ... 486
Maxalt Tablets (Infrequent) ... 2008
Maxalt-MLT Orally Disintegrating Tablets (Infrequent) ... 2008
Merrem I.V. (Greater than 0.1% to 1%) ... 686
Midamor Tablets ... 2026
Mirena Intrauterine System ... 787
Mivacron Injection (Less than 1%) ... 493
MS Contin Tablets (Less frequent) ... 2701
Mylotarg for Injection ... 3431
▲ Myozyme for Intravenous Infusion (21%) ... 1279
Nadolol Tablets (Common) ... 2159
Namenda (Infrequent) ... 1195
▲ Natrecor for Injection (1% to 5%) ... 3127
Nembutal Sodium Solution, USP (Less than 1%) ... 2470
Neurontin Capsules (Rare) ... 2487
Neurontin Oral Solution (Rare) ... 2487
Neurontin Tablets (Rare) ... 2487
Nimbex Injection (0.4%) ... 498
Nimotop Capsules (Up to 1.0%) ... 749
Nipent for Injection (Less than 3%) ... 1863
Norvasc Tablets (More than 0.1% to 1%) ... 2545
NovoSeven (1%) ... 2331
Numorphan Injection ... 1120
Opana Tablets (Less than 1%) ... 1122
Opana ER Tablets (Less than 1%) ... 1126
OptiPranolol Metipranolol Ophthalmic Solution 0.3% (A small number of patients) ... ⊙256
Orthoclone OKT3 Sterile Solution (Less than 1%) ... 2360
Paxil CR Controlled-Release Tablets (Infrequent) ... 1538
Paxil (Infrequent) ... 1530
Percodan Tablets ... 1132
Permax Tablets (Infrequent) ... 3356
Pexeva Tablets (infrequent) ... 1694
Phenergan Tablets and Suppositories ... 3440
Photofrin for Injection ... 702
Prevacid Delayed-Release Capsules (Less than 1%) ... 3271
Prevacid for Delayed-Release Oral Suspension (Less than 1%) ... 3271
Prevacid SoluTab Delayed-Release Orally Disintegrating Tablets (Less than 1%) ... 3271
Prevacid NapraPAC (Less than 1%) ... 3280
PREVPAC (Less than 1%) ... 3284
Prilosec OTC Delayed-Release Tablets (Less than 1%) ... 2677
Prinivil Tablets (0.3% to 1.0%) ... 2052
Prinzide Tablets ... 2056
▲ Proleukin for Injection (7%) ... 2266
Provigil Tablets (At least 1%) ... 988
Prozac Pulvules and Liquid (Rare) ... 1801
Ranexa Tablets (Less than or equal 0.5%) ... 1035
Razadyne (2%) ... 2399
Razadyne ER Extended-Release Capsules (2%) ... 2399
Relpax Tablets (Rare) ... 2548
Remicade for IV Injection (Greater than or equal to 0.2%) ... 971
▲ ReoPro Vials (5.2%) ... 1809
Requip Tablets (Infrequent) ... 1555
Revlimid Capsules ... 958
Rilutek Tablets (Rare) ... 2930
Risperdal ... 1676
Risperdal Consta Long-Acting Injection (Infrequent) ... 1682
Risperdal M-Tab Orally Disintegrating Tablets ... 1676
▲ Rituxan I.V. (1% to 5%) ... 1254
Romazicon Injection (Less than 1%) ... 2804
▲ Rythmol SR Capsules (3% to 4%) ... 2727
Seroquel Tablets (Infrequent) ... 690
Symbyax Capsules (Infrequent) ... 1819
Synera Topical Patch ... 1137
Tambocor Tablets (Less than 1%) ... 1856
Tarka Tablets (1.8%) ... 524
Tasmar Tablets (Infrequent) ... 3358
Tequin Injection (Less than 0.1%) ... 938
Tequin Injection in 5% Dextrose (Less than 0.1%) ... 938
Tequin Tablets (Less than 0.1%) ... 938
Teveten Tablets (Less than 1%) ... 1735
Teveten HCT Tablets (Less than 1%) ... 1737
Thalomid Capsules ... 965
Timolide Tablets (1.2%) ... 2086
Timoptic Sterile Ophthalmic Solution (Less frequent) ... 2088
Timoptic in Ocudose (Less frequent) ... 2091
Timoptic-XE Sterile Ophthalmic Gel Forming Solution ... 2092
Topamax Sprinkle Capsules (1%) ... 2404
Topamax Tablets (1%) ... 2404
Toprol-XL Tablets (1.5% to approximately 3 of 100 patients) ... 668
Trasylol Injection (1% to 2%) ... 754
Travatan Ophthalmic Solution (1% to 5%) ... 563
Trileptal Tablets ... 2300
Trileptal Oral Suspension ... 2300
Tygacil for Injection (0.2% to less than 2%) ... 3488
▲ Ultane Liquid for Inhalation (5%) ... 531
Uniretic Tablets (Less than 1%) ... 3100
Vasotec I.V. Injection (0.5% to 1.0%) ... 2103
Verelan PM Extended-Release Capsules, Controlled-Onset (1.4%) ... 3106
VFEND I.V. (Less than 2%) ... 2564
VFEND Oral Suspension (Less than 2%) ... 2564
VFEND Tablets (Less than 2%) ... 2564
Virazole for Inhalation Solution (Infrequent) ... 3370
▲ Xeloda Tablets (Less than 5%) ... 2822
Zantac (Rare) ... 1624
Zantac Injection (Rare) ... 1619
Zantac Injection Pharmacy Bulk Package (Rare) ... 1622
Zantac Injection Premixed (Rare) ... 1619
Zantac (Rare) ... 1624
▲ Zegerid Capsules (3.9%) ... 2958
▲ Zegerid Powder for Oral Solution (3.9%) ... 2958
Zofran Injection (Rare) ... 1634
▲ Zofran (6%) ... 1639
▲ Zofran ODT Orally Disintegrating Tablets (6%) ... 1639
Zoloft ... 2586
Zometa for Intravenous Infusion ... 2315
Zomig Tablets (Rare) ... 3519
Zomig Nasal Spray (Rare) ... 3523
Zomig-ZMT Tablets (Rare) ... 3519
Zonegran Capsules (Infrequent) ... 1101
Zosyn (1.0% or less) ... 3492
Zyprexa Tablets (Infrequent) ... 1830
Zyprexa IntraMuscular ... 1830
Zyprexa ZYDIS Orally Disintegrating Tablets (Infrequent) ... 1830

Bradycardia, symptomatic

Nadolol Tablets (2 of 100 patients) .. 2159

Bradycardia, transient

Covera-HS Tablets (1.4%) ... 3139

Bradykinesia

Abilify Oral Solution (Infrequent) ... 882
Abilify Oral Solution (Infrequent) ... 2450
Abilify Discmelt Orally Disintegrating Tablets (Infrequent) ... 882
Abilify Discmelt Orally Disintegrating Tablets (Infrequent) ... 2450
Abilify Tablets (Infrequent) ... 882
Abilify Tablets (Infrequent) ... 2450
Effexor Tablets (Rare) ... 3411
Effexor XR Capsules (Rare) ... 3417
Eldepryl Capsules ... 3208
▲ Exelon Capsules (Frequent) ... 2206
▲ Exelon Oral Solution (Frequent) ... 2206
Maxalt Tablets (Rare) ... 2008
Maxalt-MLT Orally Disintegrating Tablets (Rare) ... 2008
Paxil CR Controlled-Release Tablets ... 1538
Paxil ... 1530
Pexeva Tablets ... 1694
Risperdal Consta Long-Acting Injection (Infrequent) ... 1682
▲ Wellbutrin Tablets (8.0%) ... 1603

Bradykinetic episodes

Parcopa Orally Disintegrating Tablets ... 3097
Stalevo Tablets ... 2287

Bradylogia

Imitrex Tablets (Rare) ... 1471

Bradypnea

Zoloft (Rare) ... 2586

Brain damage

Rythmol SR Capsules ... 2727

Brain syndrome, acute

Actiq (Less than 1%) ... 979
Doxil Injection (Less than 1%) ... 2351
Permax Tablets (Infrequent) ... 3356
Prozac Pulvules and Liquid (Infrequent) ... 1801
Rilutek Tablets (Rare) ... 2930
Symbyax Capsules (Rare) ... 1819
VFEND I.V. (Less than 2%) ... 2564
VFEND Oral Suspension (Less than 2%) ... 2564
VFEND Tablets (Less than 2%) ... 2564
Virazole for Inhalation Solution ... 3370

Brain syndrome, organic, acute

Garamycin Injectable ... 3014

Breast, redistribution/accumulation of body fat

Retrovir ... 1560

Breast abscess

Lamictal (Rare) ... 1481
Rilutek Tablets (Rare) ... 2930

Breast atrophy

Paxil CR Controlled-Release Tablets (Rare) ... 1538
Paxil (Rare) ... 1530
Pexeva Tablets ... 1694

Breast changes, unspecified

▲ Emcyt Capsules (Up to 66%) ... 2634
▲ Lupron Depot 3.75 mg (3%) ... 3260
▲ Lupron Depot-3 Month 11.25 mg (3%) ... 3265
Lupron Depot-PED 7.5 mg, 11.25 mg and 15 mg (Less than 2%) ... 3269
Lupron Injection Pediatric (Less than 2%) ... 3259
Ortho-Cyclen Tablets ... 2429
▲ Ortho Evra Transdermal System (9% to 22%) ... 2417
Ortho Tri-Cyclen Tablets ... 2429
Ortho Tri-Cyclen Lo Tablets ... 2436
Premphase Tablets ... 3456
Prempro Tablets ... 3456

Breast discharge

Climara Transdermal System ... 771
Climara Pro Transdermal System ... 776
Effexor Tablets (Rare) ... 3411
Effexor XR Capsules (Rare) ... 3417
Estrasorb Topical Emulsion ... 1147
Menostar Transdermal System ... 782
Premarin Tablets ... 3446
Premphase Tablets ... 3456
Prempro Tablets ... 3456

Breast engorgement

Adalat CC Tablets (Less than 1%) ... 2964
Copaxone for Injection (Infrequent) .. 3297
Effexor Tablets (Rare) ... 3411
Effexor XR Capsules (Rare) ... 3417
Estring Vaginal Ring ... 2635
Permax Tablets (Rare) ... 3356
Prozac Pulvules and Liquid (Rare) ... 1801
Symbyax Capsules (Rare) ... 1819
Thioridazine Hydrochloride Tablets .. 2163

Breast enlargement

Aciphex Tablets (Rare) ... 1090
Aldoril Tablets ... 1910
Angeliq Tablets ... 762
Aptivus Capsules ... 826
Caduet Tablets (Less than 2%) ... 2508
Catapres-TTS (0.5% or less) ... 844
Celexa (Infrequent) ... 1176
Climara Transdermal System ... 771
Climara Pro Transdermal System ... 776
Combivir Tablets ... 1411
Copaxone for Injection (Infrequent) .. 3297
Crixivan Capsules ... 1940
Demser Capsules (Infrequent) ... 1953
Depacon Injection ... 412
Depakene ... 417
Depakote Sprinkle Capsules ... 422
Depakote Tablets ... 427
Depakote ER Tablets ... 434
Effexor Tablets (Rare) ... 3411
Effexor XR Capsules (Rare) ... 3417
Eligard 30 mg (1.1%) ... 2885
▲ Emcyt Capsules (60%) ... 2634
Enjuvia Tablets ... 1062
Estrasorb Topical Emulsion ... 1147
Estratest Tablets ... 3199
Estratest H.S. Tablets ... 3199
Estring Vaginal Ring ... 2635
Gabitril Tablets (Infrequent) ... 984
Gleevec Tablets (Infrequent) ... 2227
Imitrex Nasal Spray ... 1467
Indocin Capsules (Less than 1%) ... 1995
Indocin I.V. (Less than 1%) ... 2465
Indocin (Less than 1%) ... 1995
Invirase ... 2772
Lipitor Tablets (Less than 2%) ... 2483
Lunesta Tablets (Infrequent) ... 3142
Lupron Depot 7.5 mg (Less than 5%) ... 3264
Menostar Transdermal System ... 782
Mircette Tablets ... 1066
Norvir ... 503
Ortho-Cyclen Tablets ... 2429
Ortho Evra Transdermal System ... 2417
Ortho Tri-Cyclen Tablets ... 2429
Ortho Tri-Cyclen Lo Tablets ... 2436
Paxil CR Controlled-Release Tablets (Rare) ... 1538
Paxil (Rare) ... 1530
Pexeva Tablets (rare) ... 1694
Premarin Intravenous ... 3442
Premarin Tablets ... 3446
Premarin Vaginal Cream ... 3452
▲ Premphase Tablets (2% to 5%) ... 3456
▲ Prempro Tablets (2% to 5%) ... 3456
Prevacid Delayed-Release Capsules (Less than 1%) ... 3271

Prevacid for Delayed-Release Oral Suspension (Less than 1%) 3271
Prevacid SoluTab Delayed-Release Orally Disintegrating Tablets (Less than 1%) 3271
Prevacid NapraPAC (Less than 1%) 3280
PREVPAC (Less than 1%) 3284
▲ Prochieve 4% Gel (40%) 1003
▲ Prochieve 8% Gel (40%) 1003
Prometrium Capsules (100 mg, 200 mg) 3203
Propecia Tablets (0.5% to 1.8%) 2060
Proscar Tablets (0.5% to 1.8%) 2067
ProSom Tablets (Rare) 517
Prozac Pulvules and Liquid (Infrequent) 1801
Requip Tablets (Rare) 1555
Rescriptor Tablets 2551
Seasonique Tablets 1077
Striant Mucoadhesive 1007
Symbyax Capsules (Infrequent) 1819
Thiothixene Capsules 2165
Trizivir Tablets 1589
Truvada Tablets 1296
Uniretic Tablets (Less than 1%) 3100
Vandazole Vaginal Gel (Less than 1%) 3338
▲ Viadur Implant (6.9%) 757
Viagra Tablets (Less than 2%) 2573
Viracept 2577
Viramune Oral Suspension 873
Viramune Tablets 873
Viread Tablets 1301
Yasmin 28 Tablets 796
Yaz Tablets 803
Ziagen 1626
Zoloft (Rare) 2586
Zyprexa Tablets (Rare) 1830
Zyprexa ZYDIS Orally Disintegrating Tablets (Rare) 1830

Breast fibroadenosis

Ambien Tablets (Rare) 2851
Ambien CR Tablets (Rare) 2855
Aricept Tablets (Infrequent) 1094
Aricept ODT Tablets (Infrequent) 1094
Celebrex Capsules (0.1% to 1.9%) 3134
Gengraf Capsules (1% to less than 3%) 459
Neoral Oral Solution (1% to less than 3%) 2259
Neoral Soft Gelatin Capsules (1% to less than 3%) 2259

Breast fibrocystic

Angeliq Tablets 762
Aricept Tablets (Infrequent) 1094
Aricept ODT Tablets (Infrequent) 1094
Caduet Tablets (Less than 2%) 2508
Climara Transdermal System 771
Climara Pro Transdermal System 776
Copaxone for Injection (Infrequent) 3297
Effexor Tablets (Rare) 3411
Effexor XR Capsules (Rare) 3417
Enjuvia Tablets 1062
Estrasorb Topical Emulsion 1147
Estratest Tablets 3199
Estratest H.S. Tablets 3199
Gabitril Tablets (Infrequent) 984
Lipitor Tablets (Less than 2%) 2483
Menostar Transdermal System 782
Ortho-Cyclen/Ortho Tri-Cyclen 2429
Ortho Tri-Cyclen Lo Tablets 2436
Paxil CR Controlled-Release Tablets (Rare) 1538
Paxil (Rare) 1530
Permax Tablets (Infrequent) 3356
Pexeva Tablets (rare) 1694
Premarin Tablets 3446
Premarin Vaginal Cream 3452
Premphase Tablets 3456
Prempro Tablets 3456
Prozac Pulvules and Liquid (Infrequent) 1801
Symbyax Capsules (Infrequent) 1819
Zomig Nasal Spray (Rare) 3523

Breast lumps

Amerge Tablets (Rare) 1339
Depo-Provera Contraceptive Injection (Less than 1%) 2622
depo-subQ provera 104 Injectable Suspension 2624
Imitrex Nasal Spray 1467
Nipent for Injection (Less than 3%) 1863
Ortho-Cyclen Tablets 2429
Ortho Evra Transdermal System 2417
Ortho Tri-Cyclen Tablets 2429
Ortho Tri-Cyclen Lo Tablets 2436

Breast milk, maternal, excreted in

Accolate Tablets 671
Adalat CC Tablets 2964
Adderall Tablets 3164
Adderall XR Capsules 3166
Advicor Tablets 1722
Aggrenox Capsules 822
Aldoril Tablets 1910
Aloprim for Injection 2167
Altace Capsules 1702
Ambien Tablets 2851
Anaprox Tablets 2761
Anaprox DS Tablets 2761
Arthrotec Tablets 3129
Asacol Delayed-Release Tablets 2692
Augmentin 1360
Augmentin Tablets 1363
Augmentin XR Extended-Release Tablets 1369
Augmentin ES-600 Powder for Oral Suspension 1366
Avalide Tablets 888
Avalide Tablets 2874
Avinza Capsules 1741
Axid Oral Solution 879
Biltricide Tablets 2976
Blocadren Tablets 1916
Captopril Tablets 2149
Carbatrol Capsules 3171
Catapres Tablets 843
Catapres-TTS 844
Ceftin Tablets 1407
Celexa 1176
Cipro 2977
Cipro I.V. 2984
Cipro XR Tablets 2990
Clarinex Tablets 2995
Clarinex Reditabs Tablets 2995
Cleocin Vaginal Ovules 2616
Clorpres Tablets 2153
Clozaril Tablets 2184
Cosopt Sterile Ophthalmic Solution 1931
Coumadin for Injection 898
Covera-HS Tablets 3139
Dapsone Tablets USP 1673
Daraprim Tablets 1419
Decadron Tablets 1951
Depacon Injection 412
Depakene 417
Depakote Sprinkle Capsules 422
Depakote Tablets 427
Depakote ER Tablets 434
Desoxyn Tablets, USP 2462
Dexedrine 1420
DextroStat Tablets 3179
Diastat Rectal Delivery System 3343
Dilaudid Oral Liquid 445
Dilaudid Tablets - 8 mg 445
Dilaudid-HP 442
Diovan HCT Tablets 2196
Diuril Oral Suspension 1954
Diuril Sodium Intravenous 2467
Dolobid Tablets 1955
Duragesic Transdermal System 2373
Dyazide Capsules 1423
Dyrenium Capsules 3400
EC-Naprosyn Delayed-Release Tablets 2761
E.E.S. 451
Effexor Tablets 3411
Effexor XR Capsules 3417
EryPed 447
Ery-Tab Tablets 449
Erythrocin Stearate Filmtab Tablets 453
Fluorescite Injection ⊙ 207
Fortaz 1453
Furosemide Tablets 2154
Gengraf Capsules 459
Hydrocortone Tablets 1989
Imitrex Injection 1463
Imitrex Nasal Spray 1467
Imitrex Tablets 1471
Inderal LA Long-Acting Capsules 3429
Indocin 1995
Infed Injection 3390
Invanz for Injection 1999
Kadian Capsules 577
Lamictal 1481
Lamisil Tablets 2232
Lanoxicaps Capsules 1490
Lanoxin Injection 1494
Lanoxin Injection Pediatric 1497
Lanoxin Tablets 1500
Lariam Tablets 2786
Lescol Capsules 2233
Lescol XL Tablets 2233
Levoxyl Tablets 1712
Lexapro Oral Solution 1190
Lexapro Tablets 1190
Lotensin Tablets 2243
Lotensin HCT Tablets 2246
Lotrel Capsules 2249
Marinol Capsules 3333
Mefoxin for Injection 2012
Mefoxin Premixed Intravenous Solution 2016
Meruvax II 2019
Midamor Tablets 2026
Migranal Nasal Spray 3348
Moduretic Tablets 2028
MS Contin Tablets 2701
Naprosyn Suspension 2761
Naprosyn Tablets 2761
Nembutal Sodium Solution, USP 2470
Neoral Oral Solution 2259
Neoral Soft Gelatin Capsules 2259
Neurontin Capsules 2487
Neurontin Oral Solution 2487
Neurontin Tablets 2487
Niaspan Extended-Release Tablets 1730
Ortho-Cyclen Tablets 2429
Ortho Evra Transdermal System 2417
Ortho Micronor Tablets 2426
Ortho Tri-Cyclen Tablets 2429
Ortho Tri-Cyclen Lo Tablets 2436
Oxistat 2667
OxyContin Tablets 2703
OxyFast Oral Concentrate Solution 2708
OxyIR Capsules 2708
Paxil CR Controlled-Release Tablets 1538
Paxil 1530
PCE Dispertab Tablets 515
Pentasa Capsules 3185
Pepcid Injection 2040
Pepcid 2038
Persantine Tablets 868
Phenytek Capsules 2160
Premphase Tablets 3456
Prempro Tablets 3456
Prevacid Delayed-Release Capsules 3271
Prevacid for Delayed-Release Oral Suspension 3271
Prevacid SoluTab Delayed-Release Orally Disintegrating Tablets 3271
PREVPAC 3284
Prinzide Tablets 2056
Prograf Capsules and Injection 632
Protopic Ointment 638
Pulmicort Respules 661
Qvar Inhalation Aerosol 3303
Retrovir Capsules 1560
Retrovir IV Infusion 1564
Retrovir 1560
Rocaltrol Capsules 2798
Rocaltrol Oral Solution 2798
Rocephin Injectable Vials, ADD-Vantage, Galaxy, Bulk 2800
Sandimmune 2275
Sonata Capsules 1717
St. Joseph 81 mg Aspirin Chewable and Enteric Coated Tablets 1869
Stromectol Tablets 2083
Symmetrel Tablets 1135
Synthroid Tablets 520
Tambocor Tablets 1856
Tarka Tablets 524
Tegretol/Tegretol-XR 2295
Tiazac Capsules 1201
Timolide Tablets 2086
Timoptic Sterile Ophthalmic Solution 2088
Timoptic in Ocudose 2091
Timoptic-XE Sterile Ophthalmic Gel Forming Solution 2092
Toprol-XL Tablets 668
Tranxene 2474
Trileptal Tablets 2300
Trileptal Oral Suspension 2300
Trisenox Injection 993
Trizivir Tablets 1589
Tylenol with Codeine Tablets 2391
Uniphyl Tablets 2710
Uniretic Tablets 3100
Uroqid-Acid No. 2 Tablets 760
Vancocin HCl Capsules, USP 3380
Vantin Tablets and Oral Suspension 2645
Vasotec I.V. Injection 2103
Verelan PM Extended-Release Capsules, Controlled-Onset 3106
Vicodin Tablets 535
Vicodin ES Tablets 536
Vicodin HP Tablets 538
Viramune Oral Suspension 873
Viramune Tablets 873
Wellbutrin SR Sustained-Release Tablets 1607
Wellbutrin XL Extended-Release Tablets 1613
Yasmin 28 Tablets 796
Zantac 1624
Zantac Injection 1619
Zantac 1624
Zinacef for Injection 1631
Zinacef Injection 1631
Zosyn 3492
Zovirax 1643
Zyban Sustained-Release Tablets 1644
Zyrtec Chewable Tablets 2594
Zyrtec 2594
Zyrtec-D 12 Hour Extended Release Tablets 2597

Breast nipple bleeding

Depo-Provera Contraceptive Injection (Less than 1%) 2622
depo-subQ provera 104 Injectable Suspension 2624

Breast pain

Abilify Oral Solution (Infrequent) 882
Abilify Oral Solution (Infrequent) 2450
Abilify Discmelt Orally Disintegrating Tablets (Infrequent) 882
Abilify Discmelt Orally Disintegrating Tablets (Infrequent) 2450
Abilify Tablets (Infrequent) 882
Abilify Tablets (Infrequent) 2450
Actiq (1% or greater) 979
Ambien Tablets (Rare) 2851
Ambien CR Tablets (Rare) 2855
▲ AndroGel (1% to 3%) 3329
▲ Angeliq Tablets (18.9%) 762
▲ Arimidex Tablets (8%) 673
Arthrotec Tablets (Rare) 3129
Astelin Nasal Spray (Infrequent) 1904
Celebrex Capsules (0.1% to 1.9%) 3134
Celexa (Infrequent) 1176
Cipro (0.3% to 1%) 2977
Cipro I.V. (1% or less) 2984
Cipro XR Tablets 2990
▲ Climara Transdermal System (5% to 29%) 771
▲ Climara Pro Transdermal System (18.9%) 776
Clozaril Tablets (Less than 1%) 2184
Copaxone for Injection (At least 2%) 3297
▲ Depo-Provera Contraceptive Injection (1% to 5%) 2622
▲ depo-subQ provera 104 Injectable Suspension (1% to less than 5%) 2624
Doxil Injection (Less than 1%) 2351
Effexor Tablets (Infrequent) 3411
Effexor XR Capsules (Infrequent) 3417
▲ Enjuvia Tablets (0% to 14%) 1062
▲ Estrasorb Topical Emulsion (10%) 1147
Estratest Tablets 3199
Estratest H.S. Tablets 3199
Estring Vaginal Ring (1%) 2635
▲ Evista Tablets (4.4%) 1763
Evoxac Capsules (Less than 1%) 1047
Exelon Capsules (Infrequent) 2206
Exelon Oral Solution (Infrequent) 2206
FazaClo Orally Disintegrating Tablets (Less than 1%) 551
▲ Femara Tablets (7%) 2214
▲ Follistim AQ Cartridge (15%) 2338
Gabitril Tablets (Infrequent) 984
Gengraf Capsules (1% to less than 3%) 459
▲ Imdur Tablets (Less than or equal to 5%) 3018
Infergen (2%) 3364
Klonopin (Infrequent) 2778
Lamictal (Infrequent) 1481
Lunesta Tablets (Infrequent) 3142
▲ Lupron Depot 3.75 mg (3%) 3260
▲ Lupron Depot–3 Month 11.25 mg (3%) 3265
▲ Menostar Transdermal System (5%) 782
▲ Mirena Intrauterine System (5% or more) 787
Neoral Oral Solution (1% to less than 3%) 2259
Neoral Soft Gelatin Capsules (1% to less than 3%) 2259
Neurontin Capsules (Rare) 2487
Neurontin Oral Solution (Rare) 2487
Neurontin Tablets (Rare) 2487
Paxil CR Controlled-Release Tablets (Infrequent) 1538
Paxil (Infrequent) 1530
Pentasa Capsules (Less than 1%) 3185
Permax Tablets (Infrequent) 3356
Pexeva Tablets (infrequent) 1694
▲ Premarin Tablets (7% to 12%) 3446
▲ Premphase Tablets (13% to 38%) 3456
▲ Prempro Tablets (13% to 38%) 3456

Prevacid Delayed-Release Capsules (Less than 1%).............. 3271
Prevacid for Delayed-Release Oral Suspension (Less than 1%)........... 3271
Prevacid SoluTab Delayed-Release Orally Disintegrating Tablets (Less than 1%)............................. 3271
Prevacid NapraPAC (Less than 1%).. 3280
PREVPAC (Less than 1%)................ 3284
Prinivil Tablets (0.3% to 1.0%)......... 2052
Prinzide Tablets.............................. 2056
▲ Prochieve 4% Gel (13%) 1003
▲ Prochieve 8% Gel (13%) 1003
▲ Prometrium Capsules (100 mg, 200 mg) (6% to 16%).................... 3203
Proquin XR Tablets......................... 1153
Protonix I.V. (Less than 1%)............ 3472
Protonix Tablets (Less than 1%)....... 3469
Protopic Ointment (Greater than or equal to 1%)............................. 638
Prozac Pulvules and Liquid (Infrequent)................................ 1801
Relpax Tablets (Rare)...................... 2548
Rilutek Tablets (Rare)...................... 2930
Risperdal (Rare to infrequent)........... 1676
Risperdal Consta Long-Acting Injection (Infrequent).................. 1682
Risperdal M-Tab Orally Disintegrating Tablets (Rare to infrequent)................................. 1676
Rythmol SR Capsules...................... 2727
▲ Sandostatin LAR Depot (1% to 4%).. 2280
Sonata Capsules (Infrequent)........... 1717
Soriatane Capsules (Less than 1%).. 1013
Striant Mucoadhesive..................... 1007
Symbyax Capsules (Frequent).......... 1819
Targretin Capsules.......................... 1747
▲ Temodar Capsules (6%) 3073
▲ Topamax Sprinkle Capsules (4%) 2404
▲ Topamax Tablets (4%) 2404
Trelstar LA Suspension (2.3%).......... 3397
Uniretic Tablets (Less than 1%)........ 3100
Vandazole Vaginal Gel (1%)............. 3338
Vantas (Less than 2%)..................... 3375
▲ Viadur Implant (3.1%) 757
Yasmin 28 Tablets (Greater than 1%).. 796
Yaz Tablets (Greater than 1%).......... 803
Zoloft (Rare)................................... 2586
Zyprexa Tablets (Infrequent)............ 1830
Zyprexa ZYDIS Orally Disintegrating Tablets (Infrequent)................................. 1830
Zyrtec Chewable Tablets (Less than 2%)................................... 2594
Zyrtec (Less than 2%)..................... 2594
Zyrtec-D 12 Hour Extended Release Tablets (Less than 2%)..... 2597

Breast secretion
Amerge Tablets (Rare)...................... 1339
Estratest Tablets............................ 3199
Estratest H.S. Tablets...................... 3199
Imitrex Nasal Spray........................ 1467
Imitrex Tablets (Rare)...................... 1471
Mircette Tablets.............................. 1066
Ortho-Cyclen Tablets....................... 2429
Ortho Evra Transdermal System...... 2417
Ortho Tri-Cyclen Tablets.................. 2429
Ortho Tri-Cyclen Lo Tablets............. 2436
Premarin Intravenous...................... 3442
Premarin Vaginal Cream.................. 3452
Seasonique Tablets......................... 1077
Topamax Sprinkle Capsules (Infrequent)................................. 2404
Topamax Tablets (Infrequent).......... 2404
Yasmin 28 Tablets........................... 796
Yaz Tablets...................................... 803

Breast size, changes
Depo-Provera Contraceptive Injection (Less than 1%)................ 2622

Breast tenderness
Angeliq Tablets................................ 762
Climara Transdermal System........... 771
Climara Pro Transdermal System..... 776
▲ depo-subQ provera 104 Injectable Suspension (1% to less than 5%)............................. 2624
Eligard 22.5 mg (Less than 2%)...... 2883
▲ Emcyt Capsules (66%) 2634
Enjuvia Tablets................................ 1062
Estrasorb Topical Emulsion............. 1147
Estratest Tablets............................. 3199
Estratest H.S. Tablets..................... 3199
Follistim AQ Cartridge..................... 2338
Imitrex Nasal Spray......................... 1467
Imitrex Tablets (Infrequent)............. 1471
Indocin Capsules (Less than 1%)..... 1995
Indocin I.V. (Less than 1%).............. 2465
Indocin (Less than 1%).................... 1995
▲ Lupron Depot 3.75 mg (3%) 3260
▲ Lupron Depot–3 Month 11.25 mg (3%).. 3265
Menostar Transdermal System........ 782
Mircette Tablets.............................. 1066
NuvaRing.. 2340
Ortho-Cyclen Tablets....................... 2429
Ortho Evra Transdermal System...... 2417
Ortho Micronor Tablets................... 2426
Ortho Tri-Cyclen Tablets.................. 2429
Ortho Tri-Cyclen Lo Tablets............. 2436
▲ Plan B Tablets (10.7%) 1076
Premarin Intravenous...................... 3442
Premarin Tablets............................. 3446
Premarin Vaginal Cream.................. 3452
Premphase Tablets.......................... 3456
Prempro Tablets............................. 3456
Prevacid Delayed-Release Capsules (Less than 1%).............. 3271
Prevacid for Delayed-Release Oral Suspension (Less than 1%)........... 3271
Prevacid SoluTab Delayed-Release Orally Disintegrating Tablets (Less than 1%)............................. 3271
Prevacid NapraPAC (Less than 1%).. 3280
PREVPAC (Less than 1%)................ 3284
▲ Prometrium Capsules (100 mg, 200 mg) (27%).............................. 3203
Propecia Tablets (0.4% to 0.7%)...... 2060
Proscar Tablets (0.4% to 0.7%)........ 2067
Seasonique Tablets......................... 1077
Vantas (Less than 2%)..................... 3375
Yasmin 28 Tablets........................... 796
Yaz Tablets...................................... 803

Breath sounds, abnormal
▲ Dacogen Injection (10%) 2129
Epivir... 1427
Epivir-HBV...................................... 1432
▲ Trisenox Injection (10%) 993
Trizivir Tablets................................ 1589

Breathholding
▲ Ultane Liquid for Inhalation (2% to 5%).. 531

Breathing, difficult
(*see under* Dyspnea)

Breathing, irregular
Dilaudid.. 440
Dilaudid Non-Sterile Powder............ 440
Dilaudid Rectal Suppositories........... 440
Dilaudid Tablets.............................. 440
Dilaudid-HP..................................... 442
Imitrex Nasal Spray......................... 1467
Lotronex Tablets (Infrequent)........... 1512
Parcopa Orally Disintegrating Tablets.. 3097
Stalevo Tablets............................... 2287
Vicodin Tablets............................... 535
Vicodin ES Tablets.......................... 536
Vicoprofen Tablets.......................... 539
Zydone Tablets............................... 1139

Breathing, labored
(*see under* Dyspnea)

Breathing, shallow
(*see under* Hypopnea)

Breathing, stertorous
Duragesic Transdermal System (Less than 1%)............................. 2373
Neurontin Capsules (Rare)............... 2487
▲ Neurontin Oral Solution (3.4%) 2487
Neurontin Tablets (Rare).................. 2487

Breathing sound, abnormal
Combivir Tablets............................. 1411
Epzicom Tablets............................. 1436

Bromsulphalein retention, increase
(*see under* BSP retention, increase)

Bronchial anastomotic dehiscence
Rapamune Oral Solution and Tablets.. 3475

Bronchial constriction
Vaqta (Less than 1%)...................... 2097

Bronchial obstruction
Blocadren Tablets............................ 1916
Cosopt Sterile Ophthalmic Solution.. 1931
Timoptic Sterile Ophthalmic Solution.. 2088
Timoptic in Ocudose........................ 2091
Timoptic-XE Sterile Ophthalmic Gel Forming Solution......................... 2092

Bronchial secretions, thickening
Betoptic S Ophthalmic Suspension (Rare)... 558

Bronchiectasis
Pulmozyme Inhalation Solution......... 1248

Bronchiolitis
Comvax (Two vaccinees)................. 1928
Cuprimine Capsules........................ 1947
Flumist Vaccine.............................. 1901
Lyrica Capsules (Rare)..................... 2539
▲ Myozyme for Intravenous Infusion (23%).. 1279
Prevnar for Injection........................ 3463
RotaTeq (0.6% to 1.4%).................. 2074
Synagis (More than 1%)................... 1897
Thiola Tablets (2%)......................... 2141
Vaqta... 2097

Bronchiolitis, obliterative
PEG-Intron Powder for Injection........ 3048
Pentasa Capsules (One case)........... 3185
Rituxan I.V. (0.3%).......................... 1254
Tarceva Tablets............................... 1259
Tarceva Tablets............................... 2444

Bronchiolitis obliterans
Pegasys.. 2789
Raptiva for Injection (1 case)............ 1250

Bronchiolitis obliterans organizing pneumonia
Rapamune Oral Solution and Tablets (Infrequent)...................... 3475

Bronchitis
AccuNeb Inhalation Solution (0.9% to 1.7%)..................................... 1055
Aceon Tablets (2 mg, 4 mg, 8 mg) (0.3% to 1%)............................. 3194
Actiq (1% or greater)....................... 979
▲ Actonel Tablets (2.3% to 4.9%) 2683
▲ Actonel with Calcium Tablets (2.3% to 4.9%)............................. 2688
Advair Diskus 100/50 (2%)............. 1308
▲ Advair Diskus 250/50 (8%) 1308
▲ Advair Diskus 500/50 (2% to 8%) ... 1308
Aerobid/Aerobid-M (1% to 3%)......... 1171
Agrylin Capsules (1% to 5%)............ 3169
▲ Alamast Ophthalmic Solution (Less than 5%)............................ 3381
Aldara Cream, 5% (0.9%)................ 1846
Alphagan P Ophthalmic Solution (1% to 4%)................................. 567
Ambien Tablets (Infrequent)............. 2851
Ambien CR Tablets (Infrequent)........ 2855
Amerge Tablets (Infrequent)............. 1339
▲ Amitiza Capsules (1.6% to 3.4%) 3224
Aptivus Capsules (2.9%).................. 826
Aralast (Greater than or equal to 0.2%).. 717
▲ Aranesp for Injection (6%) 581
Aricept Tablets (Frequent)............... 1094
Aricept ODT Tablets (Frequent)........ 1094
▲ Arimidex Tablets (2% to 5%) 673
Aromasin Tablets (Less frequent)..... 2600
Asacol Delayed-Release Tablets (2% or greater)............................. 2692
Astelin Nasal Spray (Infrequently)..... 1904
Atacand Tablets (More than 1%)....... 649
Atacand HCT (0.5% or greater)......... 651
▲ Atrovent Inhalation Solution (14.6%)... 835
▲ Atrovent HFA Inhalation Aerosol (10% to 23%)................................ 841
Axert Tablets (Infrequent)................. 2396
Bexxar.. 1398
▲ BiDil Tablets (8%) 2171
▲ Boniva Injection (2.5% to 10%) 2738
▲ Boniva Tablets (2.5% to 10%) 2741
Caduet Tablets (Greater than or equal to 2%)................................ 2508
▲ Campath Ampules (13% to 21%) 811
Campral Tablets (Frequent)............. 1174
▲ Carnitor Injection (3% to 5%) 3188
Celebrex Capsules (0.1% to 1.9%)... 3134
Celexa (Infrequent)......................... 1176
▲ CellCept Capsules (3% to less than 20%)...................................... 2747
▲ CellCept Intravenous (3% to less than 20%)...................................... 2747
▲ CellCept Oral Suspension (3% to less than 20%).............................. 2747
▲ CellCept Tablets (3% to less than 20%).. 2747
▲ Clarinex Syrup (6.1%) 2995
▲ Climara Pro Transdermal System (4.2%).. 776
Clozaril Tablets (Less than 1%)........ 2184
▲ Combivent Inhalation Aerosol (12.3%).. 847
▲ Copaxone for Injection (9%) 3297
▲ Coreg Tablets (5%) 1414
▲ Cosopt Sterile Ophthalmic Solution (1% to 5%)...................... 1931
▲ Cozaar Tablets (Less than 1% to 10%)....................................... 1935
Crestor Tablets (Greater than or equal to 2%)................................ 678
▲ Depacon Injection (5%) 412
▲ Depakene (5%) 417
▲ Depakote Sprinkle Capsules (5%) 422
▲ Depakote Tablets (5%) 427
▲ Depakote ER Tablets (5%) 434
▲ depo-subQ provera 104 Injectable Suspension (1% to less than 5%)............................. 2624
Detrol Tablets (2.1%)...................... 2628
Diovan HCT Tablets (Greater than 0.2%).. 2196
▲ Ditropan XL Extended-Release Tablets (2% to less than 5%)......... 2413
Doxil Injection (Less than 1%).......... 2351
DuoNeb Inhalation Solution (1.7%)... 1058
Duragesic Transdermal System (Greater than or equal to 1%)........ 2373
Effexor Tablets (Frequent)............... 3411
▲ Elidel Cream 1% (0.4% to 10.7%) 2200
Enablex Extended-Release Tablets (Greater than or equal to 1%)........ 2203
Enbrel for Injection.......................... 584
▲ Enjuvia Tablets (0% to 7%) 1062
▲ Entocort EC Capsules (Less than 5%)... 2698
▲ Epivir-HBV (Among most common).. 1432
▲ Equetro Extended-Release Capsules (Less than 5%).............. 3180
▲ Estring Vaginal Ring (1% to 3%) 2635
Euflexxa (0.63%)............................ 1162
▲ Evoxac Capsules (4.1%) 1047
Exelon Capsules (2% or more)........ 2206
Exelon Oral Solution (2% or more).... 2206
▲ Exubera Inhalation Powder (3.2% to 5.4%)..................................... 2524
▲ Fabrazyme for Intravenous Infusion (3%)................................ 1274
FazaClo Orally Disintegrating Tablets (Less than 1%)................. 551
▲ Flebogamma 5%, Immune Globulin Intravenous (Human) (20%).. 1658
▲ Flonase Nasal Spray (1% to 3%) 1440
▲ Flovent Diskus (3%) 1443
Flovent HFA (2%)........................... 1447
Flumist Vaccine.............................. 1901
▲ Foradil Aerolizer (4.6%) 3010
Fortical Nasal Spray (Less than 1%)... 3337
▲ Fosrenol Chewable Tablets (5%) 3183
Gabitril Tablets (Frequent)................ 984
Gengraf Capsules (1%).................... 459
▲ Humira Injection (Less than 5%) 466
Hytrin Capsules (At least 1%)........... 471
Hyzaar 50-12.5 Tablets (1% or greater).. 1990
Hyzaar 100-12.5 Tablets (1% or greater).. 1990
Hyzaar 100-25 Tablets (1% or greater).. 1990
▲ Imdur Tablets (Less than or equal to 5%).. 3018
Imitrex Nasal Spray......................... 1467
▲ Infergen (2% to 6%) 3364
Intron A for Injection (Less than or equal to 5%)................................ 3024
Invirase (Less than 2% to 2.7%)....... 2772
Kaletra (Up to 2%)........................... 476
Keppra Injection............................. 3320
Keppra Oral Solution (1% or more)... 3314
Keppra Tablets (1% or more)............ 3314
Kionex Powder (Rare)...................... 2477
Klonopin (1%)................................. 2778
▲ Lamictal (2% to 7%) 1481
Lescol Capsules (1.8%)................... 2233
Lescol XL Tablets (2.6%)................. 2233
Levaquin (0.1% to 0.9%).................. 2384
Levaquin in 5% Dextrose Injection (0.1% to 0.9%)............................. 2384
Lexapro Oral Solution (Frequent)...... 1190
Lexapro Tablets (Frequent).............. 1190
Lipitor Tablets (Greater than or equal to 2%)................................ 2483
Lofibra Tablets................................ 1219
Lofibra Capsules............................. 1216
Lotensin Tablets (Less than 1%)....... 2243
Lotensin HCT Tablets (0.3% or more)... 2246
▲ Lucentis Injection (3% to 10%) 1237
Lunesta Tablets (Infrequent)............ 3142
▲ Lyrica Capsules (1% to 3%) 2539
▲ Macugen Injection (6% to 10%) ...... ⊙261
▲ Menostar Transdermal System (6%).. 782
Meridia Capsules (Greater than or equal to 1%)................................ 489
Metrogel 1% (1.1%)........................ 1211

Miacalcin Nasal Spray (Less than 1%)........ 2253
Micardis Tablets (More than 0.3%).... 854
Micardis HCT Tablets (Less than 2%)........ 856
Migranal Nasal Spray (Rare)........ 3348
Namenda (Greater than or equal to 2%)........ 1195
Nasonex Nasal Spray (Greater than or equal to 2%)........ 3043
Neoral Oral Solution (1%)........ 2259
Neoral Soft Gelatin Capsules (1%).... 2259
▲ Neurontin Capsules (3.4%) 2487
▲ Neurontin Oral Solution (3.4%) 2487
▲ Neurontin Tablets (3.4%) 2487
▲ Nipent for Injection (3%) 1863
▲ Norditropin Cartridges (9%) 2323
Omacor Capsules........ 2725
OptiPranolol Metipranolol Ophthalmic Solution 0.3% (A small number of patients)........ ⊙256
▲ Orencia Powder for Intravenous Infusion (0.2% to 13%)........ 914
Paxil CR Controlled-Release Tablets (Infrequent)........ 1538
Paxil (Infrequent)........ 1530
Permax Tablets (Infrequent)........ 3356
Pexeva Tablets (infrequent)........ 1694
▲ Photofrin for Injection (4%) 702
▲ Plavix Tablets (3.7%) 917
▲ Plavix Tablets (3.7%) 2926
Pletal Tablets (2% or greater)........ 2455
Prevacid Delayed-Release Capsules (Less than 1%)........ 3271
Prevacid for Delayed-Release Oral Suspension (Less than 1%)........ 3271
Prevacid SoluTab Delayed-Release Orally Disintegrating Tablets (Less than 1%)........ 3271
Prevacid NapraPAC (Less than 1%).. 3280
PREVPAC (Less than 1%)........ 3284
Prinivil Tablets (0.3% to 1.0%)........ 2052
Prinzide Tablets (0.3% to 1%)........ 2056
▲ Prograf Capsules and Injection (3% to 17%)........ 632
▲ Prometrium Capsules (100 mg, 200 mg) (Less than 5%)........ 3203
ProQuad........ 2064
Protonix I.V. (Greater than or equal to 1%)........ 3472
Protonix Tablets (Greater than or equal to 1%)........ 3469
▲ Protopic Ointment (2% to 6%) 638
▲ Proventil Inhalation Solution 0.083% (1.5% to 4%)........ 3055
Provigil Tablets (At least 1%)........ 988
Pulmozyme Inhalation Solution........ 1248
▲ Quadramet Injection (4%) 1040
▲ Rapamune Oral Solution and Tablets (3% to 20%)........ 3475
Raptiva for Injection........ 1250
Razadyne (Greater than or equal to 2%)........ 2399
Razadyne ER Extended-Release Capsules (Greater than or equal to 2%)........ 2399
Relenza Rotadisk (2%)........ 1552
Relpax Tablets (Rare)........ 2548
▲ Remicade for IV Injection (10%) 971
▲ Renagel Tablets (11.1%) 1282
ReoPro Vials (0.3%)........ 1809
▲ Requip Tablets (3%) 1555
▲ Rescriptor Tablets (3.5% to 6.7%) ... 2551
▲ Revlimid Capsules (6.1%) 958
Rilutek Tablets (More than 2%)........ 2930
▲ Rituxan I.V. (1% to 5%) 1254
▲ Sandostatin LAR Depot (1% to 4%)........ 2280
▲ Serevent Diskus (4% to 7%) 1568
▲ Simulect for Injection (3% to 10%) ... 2284
Singulair (Greater than or equal to 2%)........ 2077
Sonata Capsules (Frequent)........ 1717
Starlix Tablets (2.7%)........ 2292
Symbyax Capsules (Frequent)........ 1819
Synagis (More than 1%)........ 1897
Tamiflu Capsules (1% to 2%)........ 2807
Tamiflu Oral Suspension (1% to 2%)........ 2807
Targretin Capsules........ 1747
Tarka Tablets (1.5%)........ 524
Tasmar Tablets (Frequent)........ 3358
Teveten Tablets (1% or greater)........ 1735
Teveten HCT Tablets (Less than 1%)........ 1737
▲ Tiazac Capsules (1% to 4%) 1201
▲ Topamax Sprinkle Capsules (2% to 7%)........ 2404
▲ Topamax Tablets (2% to 7%) 2404
▲ Travatan Ophthalmic Solution (1% to 5%)........ 563
Tricor Tablets........ 527
▲ Trileptal Tablets (Up to 3%) 2300
▲ Trileptal Oral Suspension (Up to 3%)........ 2300
▲ Ultram ER Tablets (1% to greater than 5%)........ 2392
Uniretic Tablets (More than 1%)........ 3100
Uroxatral Tablets (1% to 2%)........ 2943
▲ Vagifem Tablets (3% to 5%) 2334
Vantin Tablets and Oral Suspension (Less than 1%)........ 2645
Vasotec I.V. Injection (0.5% to 1.0%)........ 2103
Viagra Tablets (Less than 2%)........ 2573
Vicoprofen Tablets (Less than 1%).... 539
Vivitrol........ 995
Wellbutrin Tablets (Infrequent)........ 1603
Wellbutrin SR Sustained-Release Tablets (At least 1%)........ 1607
Wellbutrin XL Extended-Release Tablets (At least 1%)........ 1613
▲ Xeloda Tablets (Less than 5%) 2822
Xyrem Oral Solution (Frequent)........ 1688
Yasmin 28 Tablets (Greater than 1%)........ 796
Yaz Tablets (Greater than 1%)........ 803
Zelapar Tablets........ 3372
Zemaira (0.8%)........ 3509
▲ Ziagen (4%) 1626
Zoloft (Rare)........ 2586
Zomig Tablets (Infrequent)........ 3519
Zomig Nasal Spray (Infrequent)........ 3523
Zomig-ZMT Tablets (Infrequent)........ 3519
Zyban Sustained-Release Tablets (2%)........ 1644
Zyrtec Chewable Tablets (Less than 2%)........ 2594
Zyrtec (Less than 2%)........ 2594
Zyrtec-D 12 Hour Extended Release Tablets (Less than 2%)..... 2597

Bronchoconstriction

Intron A for Injection (Rare)........ 3024
Invanz for Injection (Greater than 0.1%)........ 1999
Pegasys........ 2789
Rebetron Combination Therapy........ 3063

Bronchopneumonia

Kionex Powder (Rare)........ 2477
Revlimid Capsules........ 958
▲ Xeloda Tablets (Less than 5%) 2822

Bronchopulmonary dysplasia

I.V. Busulfex (Rare)........ 2493
Myleran Tablets........ 1525

Bronchospasm

Abelcet Injection (Rare)........ 1141
Accutane Capsules........ 2731
▲ Acetadote Injection (1.23% to 5.85%)........ 1031
Actimmune (Rare)........ 1671
Adenocard Injection........ 617
Advair Diskus 100/50........ 1308
Advair Diskus 250/50........ 1308
Advair Diskus 500/50........ 1308
Advair HFA Inhalation Aerosol (Rare)........ 1318
Aggrenox Capsules (Less than 1%).. 822
Aldurazyme for Intravenous Infusion........ 1268
Alkeran for Injection (In some patients)........ 955
Ambien Tablets (Rare)........ 2851
Ambien CR Tablets (Rare)........ 2855
Anzemet Injection (Rare)........ 2859
Anzemet Tablets (Rare)........ 2862
Astelin Nasal Spray (Infrequent)........ 1904
Atrovent Inhalation Solution (2.3%)... 835
Atrovent HFA Inhalation Aerosol........ 841
Atrovent Nasal Spray 0.06% (Rare).. 839
Attenuvax........ 1914
Axid Oral Solution (Rare)........ 879
Bayer Aspirin........ 744
Beconase AQ Nasal Spray (Rare)..... 1396
Betagan Ophthalmic Solution, USP........ ⊙220
Betaseron for SC Injection........ 767
▲ Betimol Ophthalmic Solution (More than 5%)........ 3382
▲ Betimol Ophthalmic Solution (More than 5%)........ ⊙295
Betoptic S Ophthalmic Suspension (Rare)........ 558
Bexxar........ 1398
Blocadren Tablets (0.6%)........ 1916
▲ Campath Ampules (2% to 9%) 811
Captopril Tablets........ 2149
Carimune NF........ 3499
Carteolol Hydrochloride Ophthalmic Solution USP, 1%....... ⊙249
Celebrex Capsules (0.1% to 1.9%)... 3134
Celexa (Rare)........ 1176
Cipro (Less than 1%)........ 2977
Cipro I.V. (1% or less)........ 2984
Cipro XR Tablets........ 2990
Clinoril Tablets (Less than 1 in 100)........ 1924
Colazal Capsules........ 2838
Combivent Inhalation Aerosol (0.3%; rare)........ 847
Coreg Tablets (Less than or equal to 0.1%)........ 1414
Cosopt Sterile Ophthalmic Solution........ 1931
Dilaudid........ 440
Dilaudid Non-Sterile Powder........ 440
Dilaudid Oral Liquid........ 445
Dilaudid Rectal Suppositories........ 440
Dilaudid Tablets........ 440
Dilaudid Tablets - 8 mg........ 445
Dilaudid-HP (Less frequent)........ 442
Diovan HCT Tablets (Less frequent)........ 2196
Dolobid Tablets (Less than 1 in 100)........ 1955
Elitek........ 2890
Eloxatin for Injection (Rare)........ 2892
Engerix-B Vaccine........ 1425
Evoxac Capsules (Less than 1%)...... 1047
Exelon Capsules (Infrequent)........ 2206
Exelon Oral Solution (Infrequent)...... 2206
Fabrazyme for Intravenous Infusion (2%)........ 1274
Flebogamma 5%, Immune Globulin Intravenous (Human)........ 1658
Flonase Nasal Spray........ 1440
Flovent HFA........ 1447
Fluarix........ 1451
Flumadine (Less than 0.3%)........ 1183
Fluorescite Injection........ ⊙207
Fortaz (Very rare)........ 1453
▲ Fortical Nasal Spray (1% to 3%) 3337
Gammagard Liquid........ 721
Gammagard S/D........ 724
Gamunex Immune Globulin I.V., 10%........ 3235
Gardasil Injection (1 case)........ 1984
Gemzar for Injection (Less than 2%)........ 1771
▲ Gengraf Capsules (1% to 5%) 459
Herceptin I.V........ 1233
▲ Humira Injection (Less than 5%) 466
▲ Imdur Tablets (Less than or equal to 5%)........ 3018
Imitrex Injection........ 1463
Imitrex Nasal Spray........ 1467
Inderal LA Long-Acting Capsules...... 3429
Infed Injection........ 3390
InnoPran XL Capsules........ 2723
▲ Intron A for Injection (Less than or equal to 5%)........ 3024
Lamictal (2%)........ 1481
Levaquin (0.1% to 0.9%)........ 2384
Levaquin in 5% Dextrose Injection (0.1% to 0.9%)........ 2384
Lopressor Injection (1%)........ 2238
Lopressor Tablets (1%)........ 2238
Lopressor HCT 50/25 Tablets (Less than 1%)........ 2241
Lopressor HCT 100/25 Tablets (Less than 1%)........ 2241
Lopressor HCT 100/50 Tablets (Less than 1%)........ 2241
Meruvax II........ 2019
Miacalcin Injection (A few cases)...... 2252
▲ Miacalcin Nasal Spray (1% to 3%) ... 2253
Migranal Nasal Spray (Rare)........ 3348
Mivacron Injection (Less than 1%) 493
M-M-R II........ 2006
Mobic Oral Suspension (Less than 2%)........ 863
Mobic Tablets (Less than 2%)........ 863
Mumpsvax........ 2031
Myozyme for Intravenous Infusion 1279
Nadolol Tablets (1 of 1000 patients)........ 2159
▲ Neoral Oral Solution (1% to 5%) 2259
▲ Neoral Soft Gelatin Capsules (1% to 5%)........ 2259
Neurontin Capsules (Rare)........ 2487
Neurontin Oral Solution (Rare)........ 2487
Neurontin Tablets (Rare)........ 2487
Nimbex Injection (0.2%)........ 498
Nipent for Injection (Less than 3%)... 1863
Norvir........ 503
Numorphan Injection........ 1120
▲ Oncaspar (Less than 1% to greater than 5%)........ 1145
Orthoclone OKT3 Sterile Solution (Less than 1%)........ 2360
Pepcid Injection (Infrequent)........ 2040
Pepcid (Infrequent)........ 2038
Percodan Tablets........ 1132
Persantine Tablets (Rare)........ 868
Photofrin for Injection........ 702
Plavix Tablets (Very rare)........ 917
Plavix Tablets (Very rare)........ 2926
Prevnar for Injection........ 3463
Prinivil Tablets (0.3% to 1.0%)........ 2052
Prinzide Tablets........ 2056
ProQuad........ 2064
Proquin XR Tablets........ 1153
Proventil Inhalation Aerosol........ 3053
▲ Proventil Inhalation Solution 0.083% (8% to 15.4%)........ 3055
Proventil HFA Inhalation Aerosol (Rare)........ 3056
Pulmicort Respules (Less than 1%).. 661
Qvar Inhalation Aerosol (Rare)........ 3303
Recombivax HB (Less than 1%)........ 2071
Refludan for Injection (Common)...... 792
Relenza Rotadisk (Less than 1%)...... 1552
Remicade for IV Injection........ 971
ReoPro Vials (0.3%)........ 1809
Rhinocort Aqua Nasal Spray (2%)..... 665
Risperdal (Infrequent)........ 1676
Risperdal M-Tab Orally Disintegrating Tablets (Infrequent)........ 1676
▲ Rituxan I.V. (1% to 8%) 1254
Rocephin Injectable Vials, ADD-Vantage, Galaxy, Bulk (Rare)........ 2800
RotaTeq (1.1%)........ 2074
▲ Simulect for Injection (3% to 10%) ... 2284
St. Joseph 81 mg Aspirin Chewable and Enteric Coated Tablets........ 1869
St. Joseph 81 mg Aspirin........ ▣688
Synera Topical Patch........ 1137
Tambocor Tablets (Less than 1%)..... 1856
Taxotere Injection Concentrate (0.9%)........ 2932
Tequin Injection (Less than 0.1%)..... 938
Tequin Injection in 5% Dextrose (Less than 0.1%)........ 938
Tequin Tablets (Less than 0.1%)....... 938
Tessalon Capsules........ 1199
Tessalon Perles........ 1199
Timolide Tablets (1.6%)........ 2086
Timoptic Sterile Ophthalmic Solution (Less frequent)........ 2088
Timoptic in Ocudose (Less frequent)........ 2091
Timoptic-XE Sterile Ophthalmic Gel Forming Solution........ 2092
Tindamax Tablets (Rare)........ 2142
TOBI Solution for Inhalation........ 2298
Toprol-XL Tablets (About 1 of 100 patients)........ 668
Trusopt Sterile Ophthalmic Solution........ 2095
Twinrix Vaccine........ 1595
Ultane Liquid for Inhalation (Less than 1%)........ 531
Univasc Tablets (Less than 1%)........ 3104
Vasotec I.V. Injection (0.5% to 1.0%)........ 2103
Ventolin HFA Inhalation Aerosol........ 1600
Viracept........ 2577
Virazole for Inhalation Solution (Infrequent)........ 3370
VoSpire ER Tablets (Rare)........ 1052
Wellbutrin SR Sustained-Release Tablets (Rare)........ 1607
Wellbutrin XL Extended-Release Tablets (Rare)........ 1613
Zantac (Rare)........ 1624
Zantac Injection........ 1619
Zantac Injection Pharmacy Bulk Package (Rare)........ 1622
Zantac Injection Premixed........ 1619
Zantac (Rare)........ 1624
Zemaira (0.5%)........ 3509
Zemuron Injection (Less than 1%)..... 2346
Zofran Injection (Rare to less than 1%)........ 1634
Zofran (Rare)........ 1639
Zofran ODT Orally Disintegrating Tablets (Rare)........ 1639
Zoloft (Infrequent)........ 2586
Zomig Tablets (Infrequent)........ 3519
Zomig-ZMT Tablets (Infrequent)........ 3519
Zosyn (1.0% or less)........ 3492
Zyban Sustained-Release Tablets (Rare)........ 1644
▲ Zyrtec Chewable Tablets (1.9% to 3.1%)........ 2594
▲ Zyrtec (1.9% to 3.1%) 2594
▲ Zyrtec-D 12 Hour Extended Release Tablets (1.9% to 3.1%)..... 2597

Bronchospasm, exacerbation of

AccuNeb Inhalation Solution........ 1055
Cardura XL Tablets........ 2515

Celebrex Capsules (0.1% to 1.9%)... 3134
Didronel Tablets (Rare) 2697
Serevent Diskus 1568

Bronchospasm, paradoxical
AccuNeb Inhalation Solution 1055
Advair Diskus 100/50 1308
Advair Diskus 250/50 1308
Advair Diskus 500/50 1308
Advair HFA Inhalation Aerosol 1318
Alupent Inhalation Aerosol 826
Combivent Inhalation Aerosol (Less than 2%) 847
DuoNeb Inhalation Solution 1058
Flovent Diskus 1443
Flovent HFA 1447
Proventil HFA Inhalation Aerosol 3056
Serevent Diskus 1568
Ventolin HFA Inhalation Aerosol 1600
Xopenex Inhalation Solution 3146
Xopenex Inhalation Solution Concentrate 3150
Xopenex HFA Inhalation Aerosol 3154

Browache
OptiPranolol Metipranolol Ophthalmic Solution 0.3% (A small number of patients) ⊙256

Bruising
Accolate Tablets 671
Accutane Capsules 2731
Arixtra Injection (1%) 1351
Arthrotec Tablets (Rare) 3129
Azmacort Inhalation Aerosol 1726
Carbatrol Capsules 3171
Clozaril Tablets (Less than 1%) 2184
Coumadin for Injection 898
Coumadin Tablets 898
Covera-HS Tablets (Less than 2%) 3139
Cymbalta Delayed-Release Capsules (Infrequent) 1757
Depacon Injection 412
Depakene 417
Depakote Sprinkle Capsules 422
Depakote Tablets 427
Depakote ER Tablets 434
▲ Eligard 22.5 mg (3.4%) 2883
Elocon Cream 0.1% (1 in 97 patients) 3005
▲ Emcyt Capsules (3%) 2634
Enbrel for Injection 584
▲ Entocort EC Capsules (15%) 2698
FazaClo Orally Disintegrating Tablets (Less than 1%) 551
Hycamtin for Injection 1458
Imitrex Injection 1463
▲ Increlex Injection (Greater than or equal to 5%) 3291
Lexapro Oral Solution (Infrequent) 1190
Lexapro Tablets (Infrequent) 1190
Maxair Autohaler (0.6%) 1852
Nalfon Capsules (Less than 1%) 2502
Neurontin Capsules (Frequent) 2487
Neurontin Oral Solution (Frequent) 2487
Neurontin Tablets (Frequent) 2487
Oncaspar 1145
Raptiva for Injection 1250
ReFacto Vials 3484
Rescriptor Tablets 2551
▲ Sandostatin Injection (1% to 4%) 2278
Singulair 2077
Tarka Tablets 524
Tegretol/Tegretol-XR 2295
Trileptal Tablets 2300
Trileptal Oral Suspension 2300
Verelan PM Extended-Release Capsules, Controlled-Onset (2% or less) 3106

Bruising at application site
Lidoderm Patch 1118

Bruising at injection site
ADACEL Vaccine (Very rare) 2945
Eligard 45 mg (Less than 1% to 2.3%) 2888
▲ Vantas (7.2%) 3375
Xolair 1266

Bruising at insertion site
▲ Vantas (7.2%) 3375

Bruit, abdominal aortic
Proquin XR Tablets (Less than 1%) 1153

Bruxism
Effexor Tablets (Infrequent) 3411
Effexor XR Capsules (Infrequent) 3417
Eldepryl Capsules 3208
Lexapro Oral Solution (Infrequent) 1190
Lexapro Tablets (Infrequent) 1190
Parcopa Orally Disintegrating Tablets 3097
Paxil CR Controlled-Release Tablets (Infrequent) 1538
Paxil (Infrequent) 1530
Pexeva Tablets (Infrequent) 1694
Seroquel Tablets (Infrequent) 690
Sonata Capsules (Rare) 1717
Stalevo Tablets 2287
Wellbutrin Tablets (Infrequent) 1603
Wellbutrin SR Sustained-Release Tablets (Infrequent) 1607
Wellbutrin XL Extended-Release Tablets (Infrequent) 1613
Zyban Sustained-Release Tablets (Infrequent) 1644

BSP retention
Capastat Sulfate for Injection 1755

BSP retention, increase
Estratest Tablets 3199
Estratest H.S. Tablets 3199
Oxandrin Tablets 2962

Buccoglossal syndrome
Abilify Oral Solution (Rare) 882
Abilify Oral Solution (Rare) 2450
Abilify Discmelt Orally Disintegrating Tablets (Rare) 882
Abilify Discmelt Orally Disintegrating Tablets (Rare) 2450
Abilify Tablets (Rare) 882
Abilify Tablets (Rare) 2450
Effexor Tablets (Rare) 3411
Effexor XR Capsules (Rare) 3417
Geodon Capsules (Frequent) 2529
Prozac Pulvules and Liquid (Infrequent) 1801
Seroquel Tablets (Rare) 690
Symbyax Capsules (Infrequent) 1819
Zyprexa Tablets (1% to 2%) 1830
Zyprexa ZYDIS Orally Disintegrating Tablets (1% to 2%) 1830

Budd-Chiari syndrome
Mircette Tablets 1066
NuvaRing 2340
Ortho-Cyclen Tablets 2429
Ortho Evra Transdermal System 2417
Ortho Tri-Cyclen Tablets 2429
Ortho Tri-Cyclen Lo Tablets 2436
Seasonique Tablets 1077
Yasmin 28 Tablets 796
Yaz Tablets 803

Buffalo hump
(*see under* Dorsocervical fat enlargement)

Bulbus oculi, perforation
Alrex Ophthalmic Suspension 0.2% ⊙246
Blephamide Ophthalmic Ointment 568
Blephamide Ophthalmic Suspension 569
FML Ophthalmic Ointment ⊙228
FML Ophthalmic Suspension ⊙227
FML Forte Ophthalmic Suspension ⊙226
FML-S Ophthalmic Suspension ⊙229
Lotemax Ophthalmic Suspension 0.5% ⊙251
Poly-Pred Ophthalmic Suspension ⊙233
Pred Mild Ophthalmic Suspension ⊙238
Pred Forte Ophthalmic Suspension ⊙235
Retisert Implant ⊙258
TobraDex Ophthalmic Ointment 562
TobraDex Ophthalmic Suspension 563

Bulimia
Paxil CR Controlled-Release Tablets (Rare) 1538
Paxil (Rare) 1530
Pexeva Tablets (Rare) 1694

BUN, increased
Demadex Injection 2759
Demadex Tablets 2759

BUN levels, abnormal
Zyvox (0.2% to 2.1%) 2652

BUN levels, changes
Colocort Rectal Suspension, USP (Retention) 100 mg/60 mL 2476
Decadron Tablets 1951
Depo-Medrol Injectable Suspension 2617
Depo-Medrol Single-Dose Vial 2619
▲ Intron A for Injection (Up to 12%) 3024
Moban Tablets 1119
Neurontin Capsules (Rare) 2487
Neurontin Oral Solution (Rare) 2487
Neurontin Tablets (Rare) 2487
Parcopa Orally Disintegrating Tablets 3097
▲ Vasotec I.V. Injection (About 0.2% to 20%) 2103

BUN levels, decrease
Cipro I.V. (Infrequent) 2984

BUN levels, elevation
Abilify Oral Solution (Infrequent) 882
Abilify Oral Solution (Infrequent) 2450
Abilify Discmelt Orally Disintegrating Tablets (Infrequent) 882
Abilify Discmelt Orally Disintegrating Tablets (Infrequent) 2450
Abilify Tablets (Infrequent) 882
Abilify Tablets (Infrequent) 2450
Aceon Tablets (2 mg, 4 mg, 8 mg) 3194
Aggrenox Capsules 822
Aldoril Tablets 1910
▲ Altace Capsules (0.5% to 3%) 1702
Ambien Tablets (Rare) 2851
Ambien CR Tablets (Rare) 2855
▲ AmBisome for Injection (21%) 620
Aredia for Injection 2179
Arthrotec Tablets (Rare) 3129
Asacol Delayed-Release Tablets 2692
Atacand Tablets (Infrequent) 649
Atacand HCT (0.5% or greater) 651
Avalide Tablets 888
Avalide Tablets 2874
Avapro Tablets (Less than 0.7%) 891
Avapro Tablets (Less than 0.7%) 2871
Bayer Aspirin 744
Bayer Aspirin Comprehensive Prescribing Information ▣796
Benicar HCT Tablets (1.3%) 1044
▲ Biaxin/Biaxin XL (4%) 402
Bicillin C-R Injectable Suspension 1706
Blocadren Tablets 1916
Calcijex Injection 411
▲ Capastat Sulfate for Injection (36%) 1755
Captopril Tablets 2149
Carbatrol Capsules 3171
Carimune NF 3499
Ceftin 1407
Celebrex Capsules (0.1% to 1.9%) 3134
▲ CellCept Capsules (34.6%) 2747
▲ CellCept Intravenous (34.6%) 2747
▲ CellCept Oral Suspension (34.6%) 2747
▲ CellCept Tablets (34.6%) 2747
Cipro (0.9%) 2977
Cipro I.V. 2984
▲ Coreg Tablets (Less than or equal to 1% to 6%) 1414
Cozaar Tablets (Less than 0.1%) 1935
CytoGam Intravenous 1895
▲ Diovan Tablets (16.6%) 2193
▲ Diovan HCT Tablets (15%) 2196
Doxil Injection (Less than 1%) 2351
Dyazide Capsules 1423
Dyrenium Capsules (Rare) 3400
Effexor Tablets (Rare) 3411
Effexor XR Capsules (Rare) 3417
▲ Emend Capsules (4.4% to 4.7%) 1963
Equetro Extended-Release Capsules 3180
Eulexin Capsules 3009
Evoxac Capsules (Less than 1%) 1047
Fansidar Tablets 2765
Flebogamma 5%, Immune Globulin Intravenous (Human) 1658
Fortaz (Occasional) 1453
Gammagard S/D 724
Gantrisin Pediatric Suspension 2770
Garamycin Injectable 3014
▲ Gemzar for Injection (8% to 16%) 1771
Gengraf Capsules (1% to less than 3%) 459
Geodon Capsules (Rare) 2529
Hectorol Capsules 1275
Hectorol Injection 1278
Hyzaar 50-12.5 Tablets (0.6%) 1990
Hyzaar 100-12.5 Tablets (0.6%) 1990
Hyzaar 100-25 Tablets (0.6%) 1990
Indapamide Tablets (Less than 5%) 2156
Indocin Capsules (Less than 1%) 1995
▲ Indocin I.V. (41% of infants) 2465
Indocin (Less than 1%) 1995
Inspra Tablets (0.5%) 2536
▲ Intron A for Injection (Less than 5%) 3024
Invanz for Injection (0.1% to 1%) 1999
▲ I.V. Busulfex (2% to 3%) 2493
Keflex Capsules 549
▲ Leukine (23%) 814
Lotensin HCT Tablets 2246
Lotrel Capsules 2249
▲ Lupron Depot 7.5 mg (Greater than or equal to 5%) 3264
▲ Mavik Tablets (0.6% to 9%) 486
Maxipime for Injection (Greater than 0.1% to less than 1%) 1105
Mefoxin for Injection 2012
Mefoxin Premixed Intravenous Solution 2016
Mepron Suspension (1%) 1521
Merrem I.V. (Greater than 0.2%) 686
Micardis HCT Tablets 856
Mobic Oral Suspension (Less than 2%) 863
Mobic Tablets (Less than 2%) 863
Mycamine for Injection (0.5%) 628
▲ NeoProfen Injection (1% to 7%) 2472
Neoral Oral Solution (1% to less than 3%) 2259
Neoral Soft Gelatin Capsules (1% to less than 3%) 2259
Noroxin Tablets (Less frequent) 2032
Omnicef Capsules (0.3%) 511
Omnicef for Oral Suspension (0.2%) 511
Oracea Capsules 1000
Paxil CR Controlled-Release Tablets (Rare) 1538
Paxil (Rare) 1530
Pexeva Tablets (Rare) 1694
Pletal Tablets (Very rare) 2455
▲ PREVPAC (4%) 3284
Primaxin I.M. 2045
Primaxin I.V. 2048
▲ Prinivil Tablets (2.0% to 11.6%) 2052
Prinzide Tablets 2056
▲ Prograf Capsules and Injection (3% to 15%) 632
▲ Proleukin for Injection (63%) 2266
Prozac Pulvules and Liquid (Rare) 1801
Ranexa Tablets 1035
Raniclor Tablets, Chewable 2505
▲ Rapamune Oral Solution and Tablets (3% to 20%) 3475
Requip Tablets (Frequent) 1555
Rocaltrol Capsules 2798
Rocaltrol Oral Solution 2798
Rocephin Injectable Vials, ADD-Vantage, Galaxy, Bulk (1.2%) 2800
Sandimmune 2275
St. Joseph 81 mg Aspirin Chewable and Enteric Coated Tablets 1869
Sular Tablets (Less than or equal to 1%) 3122
Suprax (Less than 2%) 1843
Symmetrel Tablets 1135
Tegretol/Tegretol-XR 2295
Teveten Tablets (0.6%) 1735
Teveten HCT Tablets (1.3%) 1737
Thalomid Capsules 965
Timentin ADD-Vantage 1580
Timentin Injection Galaxy Container 1583
Timentin IV Infusion 1577
Timentin Pharmacy Bulk Package 1586
Tygacil for Injection (2.1%) 3488
Ultane Liquid for Inhalation (Less than 1%) 531
Uniretic Tablets (Less than 1%) 3100
Univasc Tablets (1%) 3104
Vancocin HCl Capsules, USP (Rare) 3380
Vantin Tablets and Oral Suspension 2645
VFEND I.V. (Less than 2%) 2564
VFEND Oral Suspension (Less than 2%) 2564
VFEND Tablets (Less than 2%) 2564
Zinacef for Injection 1631
Zinacef Injection 1631
Zmax for Oral Suspension (Less then 1%) 2583
Zonegran Capsules 1101
Zosyn 3492
Zovirax 1643

Bundle branch block
Abilify Oral Solution (Rare) 882
Abilify Oral Solution (Rare) 2450
Abilify Discmelt Orally Disintegrating Tablets (Rare) 882
Abilify Discmelt Orally Disintegrating Tablets (Rare) 2450
Abilify Tablets (Rare) 882
Abilify Tablets (Rare) 2450
Aciphex Tablets 1090
Anzemet Injection 2859
Anzemet Tablets 2862
Azilect Tablets (Frequent) 3293
Cardizem LA Extended Release Tablets (Less than 2%) 1728

Celexa (Rare) 1176
Coreg Tablets (Less than or equal to 0.1%) 1414
Cymbalta Delayed-Release Capsules (Infrequent) 1757
Doxil Injection (Less than 1%) 2351
Effexor Tablets (Rare) 3411
Effexor XR Capsules (Infrequent) 3417
Eraxis for Injection (Less than 1% to less than 2%) 2521
Evoxac Capsules 1047
Exelon Capsules (Infrequent) 2206
Exelon Oral Solution (Infrequent) 2206
Fortical Nasal Spray (Less than 1%) 3337
Geodon Capsules (Rare) 2529
▲ Imdur Tablets (Less than or equal to 5%) 3018
Lexapro Oral Solution 1190
Lexapro Tablets 1190
Miacalcin Nasal Spray (Less than 1%) 2253
Paxil CR Controlled-Release Tablets (Rare) 1538
Paxil (Rare) 1530
Pexeva Tablets (rare) 1694
Razadyne (Infrequent) 2399
Razadyne ER Extended-Release Capsules (Infrequent) 2399
Rilutek Tablets (Infrequent) 2930
Risperdal Consta Long-Acting Injection (Infrequent) 1682
Rythmol SR Capsules (Greater than or equal to 2%) 2727
Seroquel Tablets (Infrequent) 690
Sonata Capsules (Infrequent) 1717
Symbyax Capsules (Rare) 1819
Tarka Tablets (Less frequent) 524
Tiazac Capsules (Less than 2%) 1201
Trasylol Injection (1% to 2%) 754
Uniretic Tablets (Less than 1%) 3100
VFEND I.V. (Less than 2%) 2564
VFEND Oral Suspension (Less than 2%) 2564
VFEND Tablets (Less than 2%) 2564

Burn wound infection
Amevive 626

Burning
Aclovate Cream (Approximately 2%) 2660
▲ Acular Ophthalmic Solution (Up to 40%) 565
▲ Acular LS Ophthalmic Solution (20% to 40%) 566
Analpram-HC 1159
Apexicon E Cream 2661
Bactroban Nasal (2%) 1394
Bactroban Ointment (1.5%) 1395
▲ Brimonidine Tartrate Ophthalmic Solution 0.2% (10% to 30%) ⊙ 248
Catapres-TTS (3 of 101 patients) 844
Clobevate Gel (Less than 2%) 3211
Clobex Shampoo 1206
Cutivate Cream (0.6% to 1.6%) 2662
Cutivate Lotion 0.05% (2%) 2664
Cutivate Ointment (Less than 1%) 2665
Elocon Cream 0.1% (1.6%) 3005
Elocon Lotion 0.1% (4 in 209 patients) 3006
▲ Elocon Ointment 0.1% (4.8%) 3007
Evoxac Capsules (Less than 1%) 1047
▲ Finacea Gel (4% to 20%) 1669
Fleet Bisacodyl Laxatives 1165
Fleet Prep Kits 1170
Garamycin Injectable 3014
Lotrimin 3039
▲ Metrogel 1% (1.3% to 7.2%) 1211
▲ Naftin Gel (5.0%) 2126
Olux Foam (Less than 2%) 1012
Ophthetic Ophthalmic Solution (Occasional) ⊙ 232
Panafil Ointment (Occasional) 1663
Panafil SE Spray Emulsion 1663
▲ Panretin Gel (0% to 34%) 1747
Pramosone 1161
Pred-G Ophthalmic Suspension ⊙ 236
Tasmar Tablets (1% to 2%) 3358
Temovate Cream (1%) 2668
▲ Temovate Gel (Among most frequent) 2669
Temovate Scalp Application (Infrequent) 2670
▲ Temovate E Emollient (5%) 2671
Tindamax Tablets 2142
Vanos Cream 1893
Zantac Injection 1619
Zantac Injection Pharmacy Bulk Package (Frequent) 1622
Zantac Injection Premixed 1619
▲ Zovirax Ointment (28.3%) 821

Burning, local
▲ Aldara Cream, 5% (More than 1% to 26%) 1846
▲ Alphagan P Ophthalmic Solution (Approximately 5% to 9%) 567
Bactroban Cream (Less than 1% to 3.6%) 1394
Colocort Rectal Suspension, USP (Retention) 100 mg/60 mL (Rare) 2476
▲ Efudex (Among most frequent) 3363
▲ Elidel Cream 1% (1.5% to 25.9%) 2200
Klaron Lotion 10% 2909
Locoid Lipocream Cream (Infrequent) 1160
Mentax Cream (Approximately 1%) 2158
Mumpsvax 2031
▲ Naftin Cream (6%) 2126
Sulfamylon for 5% Topical Solution 2162

Burning, vaginal
(*see under* Vaginal burning)

Burning, vulvovaginal
(*see under* Vaginal burning)

Burning at application site
▲ Aldara Cream, 5% (5.6%) 1846
▲ Clobex Spray (40% to 47%) 1208
▲ Cutivate Lotion 0.05% (5%) 2664
▲ Evoclin Foam, 1% (6%) 1009
Ionsys Transdermal System (.1% to less than 1%) 2379
Levulan Kerastick for Topical Solution, 20% 1085
Lidoderm Patch 1118
▲ Oxytrol Transdermal System (Greater than 1%) 3392
Premarin Vaginal Cream 3452
ThermaCare Heat Wraps ▣ 692
▲ Vanos Cream (1.8% to 6.6%) 1893

Burning at injection site
Aloxi Injection (Very rare) 2127
Anzemet Injection 2859
Attenuvax 1914
Cerezyme for Injection (Less than 1%) 1270
Cipro I.V. (1% or less) 2984
▲ Eligard 22.5 mg (21.7%) 2883
▲ Eligard 30 mg (20%) 2885
▲ Eligard 45 mg (16%) 2888
Genotropin Lyophilized Powder (Infrequent) 2638
▲ Intron A for Injection (Less than 5%) 3024
Invanz for Injection (1.3%) 1999
Meruvax II 2019
M-M-R II 2006
Mumpsvax 2031
ProQuad 2064
ThermaCare Heat Wraps 2677
Timentin ADD-Vantage 1580
Timentin Injection Galaxy Container 1583
Timentin IV Infusion 1577
Timentin Pharmacy Bulk Package 1586
Xolair 1266
▲ Zofran Injection (4%) 1634

Burning sensation
Accuzyme Debriding Ointment (A small percentage) 1662
Accuzyme SE Spray Emulsion (Small Percentage) 1662
Adenocard Injection (Less than 1%) 617
Ambien CR Tablets (1%) 2855
Amerge Tablets (Infrequent) 1339
Arranon Injection (1%) 1357
BeneFIX Vials (1.5%) 3408
Clobevate Gel (1.8%) 3211
Copaxone for Injection (Infrequent) 3297
Doxil Injection 2351
Fleet Glycerin Laxatives 1165
Fleet Glycerin Suppositories 1165
▲ Imitrex Injection (7%) 1463
Imitrex Nasal Spray (0.4% to 1.4%) 1467
Imitrex Tablets (Frequent) 1471
▲ Olux Foam (10%) 1012
ProstaScint Kit 1037
Reyataz Capsules (Less than 3%) 921
▲ Sulfamylon Cream (One of two most frequent) 2162
Temovate Cream (1%) 2668
Temovate Gel (1.8%) 2669
Temovate Ointment (0.5%) 2668
▲ Temovate Scalp Application (29 of 294 patients) 2670

Bursitis
Abilify Oral Solution (Infrequent) 882
Abilify Oral Solution (Infrequent) 2450
Abilify Discmelt Orally Disintegrating Tablets (Infrequent) 882
Abilify Discmelt Orally Disintegrating Tablets (Infrequent) 2450
Abilify Tablets (Infrequent) 882
Abilify Tablets (Infrequent) 2450
Aciphex Tablets 1090
▲ Actonel Tablets (1.3% to 3%) 2683
▲ Actonel with Calcium Tablets (1.3% to 3%) 2688
Avalide Tablets 888
Avalide Tablets 2874
Avapro Tablets (Less than 1%) 891
Avapro Tablets (Less than 1%) 2871
▲ Azmacort Inhalation Aerosol (1% to 3%) 1726
Caduet Tablets (Less than 2%) 2508
Celexa (Rare) 1176
Copaxone for Injection (Infrequent) 3297
Effexor Tablets (Infrequent) 3411
Effexor XR Capsules (Infrequent) 3417
Enbrel for Injection (Infrequent) 584
Evoxac Capsules (Less than 1%) 1047
Gabitril Tablets (Infrequent) 984
Gengraf Capsules (1% to less than 3%) 459
Lamictal (Rare) 1481
Lipitor Tablets (Less than 2%) 2483
Lofibra Tablets 1219
Lofibra Capsules 1216
Lunesta Tablets (Infrequent) 3142
Meridia Capsules 489
Mirapex Tablets (2%) 859
Neoral Oral Solution (1% to less than 3%) 2259
Neoral Soft Gelatin Capsules (1% to less than 3%) 2259
Neurontin Capsules (Rare) 2487
Neurontin Oral Solution (Rare) 2487
Neurontin Tablets (Rare) 2487
Noroxin Tablets (Less frequent) 2032
Paxil CR Controlled-Release Tablets (Rare) 1538
Paxil (Rare) 1530
Permax Tablets (1.6%) 3356
Pexeva Tablets (Rare) 1694
Pletal Tablets (Less than 2%) 2455
Protonix I.V. (Less than 1%) 3472
Protonix Tablets (Less than 1%) 3469
Protopic Ointment (0.2% to less than 1%) 638
Prozac Pulvules and Liquid (Infrequent) 1801
Requip Tablets (Infrequent) 1555
Revlimid Capsules 958
Risperdal (Rare) 1676
Risperdal M-Tab Orally Disintegrating Tablets (Rare) 1676
Rythmol SR Capsules 2727
Sonata Capsules (Infrequent) 1717
Symbyax Capsules (Rare) 1819
Tricor Tablets 527
Uniretic Tablets (Less than 1%) 3100
Zelapar Tablets 3372
Zyprexa Tablets (Rare) 1830
Zyprexa ZYDIS Orally Disintegrating Tablets (Rare) 1830

C

Cachexia
Actiq (1% or greater) 979
▲ Doxil Injection (1% to 10%) 2351
Exelon Capsules (Infrequent) 2206
Exelon Oral Solution (Infrequent) 2206
▲ Intron A for Injection (Less than or equal to 5%) 3024
Norvir (Less than 2%) 503
Permax Tablets (Rare) 3356
Risperdal (Rare) 1676
Risperdal M-Tab Orally Disintegrating Tablets (Rare) 1676
▲ Sandostatin LAR Depot (1% to 4%) 2280
▲ Xeloda Tablets (Less than 5%) 2822

Calcification, ectopic
Calcijex Injection 411
Hectorol Capsules 1275
Hectorol Injection 1278
Rocaltrol Capsules 2798
Rocaltrol Oral Solution 2798

Calcification, soft tissue
Rocaltrol Capsules 2798
Rocaltrol Oral Solution 2798

Calcium, metabolism, disorders of
Lotronex Tablets (Rare) 1512

Calcium retention
Androxy Tablets 3335
Estratest Tablets 3199
Estratest H.S. Tablets 3199
Oxandrin Tablets 2962

Calf muscles, need to flex
Imitrex Injection (Rare) 1463

Callus formation, post bone fracture
Miradon Tablets 3042

Cancer, breast
Climara Pro Transdermal System 776
Depo-Provera Contraceptive Injection (Less than 1%) 2622
depo-subQ provera 104 Injectable Suspension 2624
Estrasorb Topical Emulsion 1147
Menostar Transdermal System 782
Neurontin Capsules (Infrequent) 2487
Neurontin Oral Solution (Infrequent) 2487
Neurontin Tablets (Infrequent) 2487
Premarin Tablets 3446
Premarin Vaginal Cream 3452
Propecia Tablets (Four cases) 2060
Proscar Tablets (Four cases) 2067

Cancer, cervical
Depo-Provera Contraceptive Injection (Less than 1%) 2622
depo-subQ provera 104 Injectable Suspension 2624
Estratest Tablets 3199
Estratest H.S. Tablets 3199
Ortho-Cyclen/Ortho Tri-Cyclen 2429
Ortho Tri-Cyclen Lo Tablets 2436
Permax Tablets (Infrequent) 3356
Premarin Intravenous 3442
Premarin Vaginal Cream 3452

Cancer, skin, non-melanoma
Myfortic Tablets (0.9% to 1.8%) 2255
Raptiva for Injection 1250

Cancer, vaginal
Estratest Tablets 3199
Estratest H.S. Tablets 3199
Premarin Intravenous 3442
Premarin Vaginal Cream 3452

Candidiasis
Abilify Oral Solution (Rare) 882
Abilify Oral Solution (Rare) 2450
Abilify Discmelt Orally Disintegrating Tablets (Rare) 882
Abilify Discmelt Orally Disintegrating Tablets (Rare) 2450
Abilify Tablets (Rare) 882
Abilify Tablets (Rare) 2450
▲ Advair Diskus 100/50 (3%) 1308
▲ Advair Diskus 250/50 (1% to 3%) 1308
Advair Diskus 500/50 (Up to 3%) 1308
▲ Advair HFA Inhalation Aerosol (1% to 3%) 1318
▲ Aerobid/Aerobid-M (3% to 9%) 1171
▲ Aredia for Injection (Up to 6%) 2179
Augmentin 1360
Augmentin Tablets 1363
Augmentin XR Extended-Release Tablets 1369
Augmentin ES-600 Powder for Oral Suspension (1.4%) 1366
Avelox (0.1% to less than 2%) 2970
Biaxin/Biaxin XL 402
▲ Campath Ampules (1% to 8%) 811
Ceftin for Oral Suspension (0.1% to 1%) 1407
Celebrex Capsules (0.1% to 1.9%) 3134
▲ CellCept Capsules (17% to 22.4%) 2747
▲ CellCept Intravenous (17% to 22.4%) 2747
▲ CellCept Oral Suspension (17% to 22.4%) 2747
▲ CellCept Tablets (17% to 22.4%) 2747
▲ Chemet Capsules (5.2% to 15.7%) 2458
Cipro (Less than 1%) 2977
Cipro I.V. (1% or less) 2984
Cipro XR Tablets 2990
Cleocin Vaginal Ovules (Less than 1%) 2616
Colazal Capsules 2838
▲ Doxil Injection (23.5%) 2351
Effexor Tablets (Infrequent) 3411
Elocon Cream 0.1% (1 in 182 patients) 3005
Emend Capsules (Greater than 0.5%) 1963
Eraxis for Injection (Less than 1% to less than 2%) 2521
▲ Evoxac Capsules (1% to 3%) 1047
Fortaz (Less than 1%) 1453

▲ Imdur Tablets (Less than or equal to 5%) 3018
▲ Intron A for Injection (Up to 17%) 3024
Invanz for Injection (Greater than 0.1%) 1999
Invirase (Less than 2%) 2772
Klonopin (Infrequent) 2778
Levaquin (0.1% to 0.9%) 2384
Levaquin in 5% Dextrose Injection (0.1% to 0.9%) 2384
▲ Megace ES Oral Suspension (1% to 3%) 2481
Merrem I.V. (0.1% to 2.0%) 686
▲ Myfortic Tablets (Less than or equal to 5.6%) 2255
Nipent for Injection (2%) 1863
Norvir (Less than 2%) 503
Omnicef Capsules (0.2%) 511
Omnicef for Oral Suspension (1%) 511
Paxil CR Controlled-Release Tablets (Infrequent) 1538
Paxil (Infrequent) 1530
Pentasa Capsules (Less than 1%) 3185
Permax Tablets (Infrequent) 3356
Pexeva Tablets (Rare) 1694
▲ Photofrin for Injection (9%) 702
Prevacid Delayed-Release Capsules (Less than 1%) 3271
Prevacid for Delayed-Release Oral Suspension (Less than 1%) 3271
Prevacid SoluTab Delayed-Release Orally Disintegrating Tablets (Less than 1%) 3271
Prevacid NapraPAC (Less than 1%) 3280
PREVPAC (Less than 1%) 3284
Primaxin I.M. 2045
Primaxin I.V. (Less than 0.2%) 2048
ProQuad 2064
Protonix I.V. (Less than 1%) 3472
Protonix Tablets (Less than 1%) 3469
Protopic Ointment (0.2% to less than 1%) 638
▲ Pulmicort Respules (3% to 4%) 661
Relpax Tablets (Rare) 2548
▲ Remicade for IV Injection (5%) 971
Rilutek Tablets (0.4% to 1.2%) 2930
▲ Sandostatin LAR Depot (1% to 4%) 2280
Seasonique Tablets 1077
Seroquel Tablets (Infrequent) 690
▲ Simulect for Injection (3% to 10%) 2284
Soriatane Capsules (Less than 1%) 1013
▲ Spiriva HandiHaler (3% to 4%) 869
Suprax (Less than 2%) 1843
Symbyax Capsules (Infrequent) 1819
Targretin Capsules 1747
Thalomid Capsules 965
Uniretic Tablets (Less than 1%) 3100
Vantin Tablets and Oral Suspension (Less than 1%) 2645
▲ Xeloda Tablets (Less than 5%) 2822
Yaz Tablets (Greater than 1%) 803
▲ Zometa for Intravenous Infusion (11.6%) 2315
Zosyn (1.6%) 3492
Zyprexa Tablets (Infrequent) 1830
Zyprexa ZYDIS Orally Disintegrating Tablets (Infrequent) 1830

Candidiasis, cutaneous
Cipro XR Tablets 2990
Omnicef for Oral Suspension (0.9%) 511
Proquin XR Tablets 1153
Protopic Ointment (0.2% to less than 1%) 638

Candidiasis, esophageal
Prilosec OTC Delayed-Release Tablets (Less than 1%) 2677
▲ Zegerid Capsules (3.9%) 2958
▲ Zegerid Powder for Oral Solution (3.9%) 2958

Candidiasis, gastrointestinal
▲ CellCept Capsules (3% to less than 20%) 2747
▲ CellCept Intravenous (3% to less than 20%) 2747
▲ CellCept Oral Suspension (3% to less than 20%) 2747
▲ CellCept Tablets (3% to less than 20%) 2747
Cipro 2977
Protonix I.V. (Less than 1%) 3472
Protonix Tablets (Less than 1%) 3469
▲ Thymoglobulin for Intravenous Infusion (4.9%) 1284
Zyrtec-D 12 Hour Extended Release Tablets 2597

Candidiasis, genital
(see also under Vaginal candidiasis)
▲ Azmacort Inhalation Aerosol (1% to 3%) 1726
Celebrex Capsules (0.1% to 1.9%) 3134
Effexor Tablets (Infrequent) 3411
Effexor XR Capsules 3417
Evoxac Capsules (Less than 1%) 1047
Infergen (2%) 3364
Lamictal (Infrequent) 1481
Levaquin (0.2%) 2384
Levaquin in 5% Dextrose Injection (0.2%) 2384
Mefoxin for Injection 2012
Mefoxin Premixed Intravenous Solution 2016
Nexium Delayed-Release Capsules (Less than 1%) 655
Nexium I.V. (Less than 1%) 659
Paxil CR Controlled-Release Tablets (Rare) 1538
Paxil (Rare) 1530
PREVPAC (Less than 3%) 3284
▲ Prochieve 4% Gel (5%) 1003
▲ Prochieve 8% Gel (5%) 1003
Requip Tablets (Infrequent) 1555
Rilutek Tablets (Rare) 2930
Rocephin Injectable Vials, ADD-Vantage, Galaxy, Bulk (Occasional) 2800
▲ Vagifem Tablets (5%) 2334

Candidiasis, mouth
(see under Candidiasis, oral)

Candidiasis, nasal
Nasonex Nasal Spray (Rare) 3043

Candidiasis, oral
Abilify Oral Solution (Infrequent) 882
Abilify Oral Solution (Infrequent) 2450
Abilify Discmelt Orally Disintegrating Tablets (Infrequent) 882
Abilify Discmelt Orally Disintegrating Tablets (Infrequent) 2450
Abilify Tablets (Infrequent) 882
Abilify Tablets (Infrequent) 2450
Actiq (Less than 1%) 979
▲ Advair Diskus 100/50 (1% to 4%) 1308
▲ Advair Diskus 250/50 (1% to 4%) 1308
▲ Advair Diskus 500/50 (1% to 4%) 1308
▲ Advair HFA Inhalation Aerosol (1% to 3%) 1318
▲ Asmanex Twisthaler (4% to 22%) 2966
Augmentin ES-600 Powder for Oral Suspension 1366
Avelox (0.1% to less than 2%) 2970
Azmacort Inhalation Aerosol (A few cases) 1726
▲ CellCept Capsules (3% to less than 20%) 2747
▲ CellCept Intravenous (3% to less than 20%) 2747
▲ CellCept Oral Suspension (3% to less than 20%) 2747
▲ CellCept Tablets (3% to less than 20%) 2747
Cipro (Less than 1%) 2977
Cipro I.V. (1% or less) 2984
Cipro XR Tablets 2990
▲ Clolar for Intravenous Infusion (13%) 1271
Comvax (0.2% to 0.8%) 1928
Copaxone for Injection (Frequent) 3297
Cubicin for Injection (Less than 1%) 1026
▲ Dacogen Injection (6%) 2129
▲ Doxil Injection (1% to 10%) 2351
Effexor Tablets (Infrequent) 3411
Effexor XR Capsules (Infrequent) 3417
Eraxis for Injection (Less than 1% to less than 2%) 2521
▲ Flovent Diskus (9% to 31%) 1443
▲ Flovent HFA (4%) 1447
Fortaz (Less than 1%) 1453
Gris-PEG Tablets (Occasional) 2502
Invanz for Injection (0.1% to 1%) 1999
Ketek Tablets (Greater than or equal to 0.2% to less than 2%) 2903
Maxipime for Injection (Greater than 0.1% to less than 1%) 1105
▲ Megace ES Oral Suspension (1% to 3%) 2481
▲ Mepron Suspension (5% to 10%) 1521
Merrem I.V. (Greater than 0.1% to 1%) 686
▲ Myfortic Tablets (3% to less than 20%) 2255
▲ Myozyme for Intravenous Infusion (31%) 1279
Nasonex Nasal Spray (Rare) 3043
▲ Neumega for Injection (14%) 3435
Neurontin Capsules (Infrequent) 2487
Neurontin Oral Solution (Infrequent) 2487
Neurontin Tablets (Infrequent) 2487
Prevacid Delayed-Release Capsules (Less than 1%) 3271
Prevacid for Delayed-Release Oral Suspension (Less than 1%) 3271
Prevacid SoluTab Delayed-Release Orally Disintegrating Tablets (Less than 1%) 3271
Prevacid NapraPAC (Less than 1%) 3280
Prevnar for Injection 3463
PREVPAC (Less than 1%) 3284
▲ Prograf Capsules and Injection (3% to 15%) 632
Proquin XR Tablets 1153
Protonix I.V. (Less than 1%) 3472
Protonix Tablets (Less than 1%) 3469
Protopic Ointment (0.2% to less than 1%) 638
Quadramet Injection (2%) 1040
▲ Rapamune Oral Solution and Tablets (3% to 20%) 3475
Rescriptor Tablets 2551
Serevent Diskus (1% to less than 3%) 1568
Symbicort 80/4.5 Inhalation Aerosol (1.4%) 3511
▲ Symbicort 160/4.5 Inhalation Aerosol (3.2%) 3511
Synagis (More than 1%) 1897
▲ Tequin Injection (0.1% to 3%) 938
▲ Tequin Injection in 5% Dextrose (0.1% to 3%) 938
▲ Tequin Tablets (0.1% to 3%) 938
▲ Thalomid Capsules (4.2%) 965
▲ Thymoglobulin for Intravenous Infusion (3.7%) 1284
Tindamax Tablets 2142
▲ Trisenox Injection (5%) 993
Vantin Tablets and Oral Suspension (Less than 1%) 2645
Vaprisol (2.2%) 643
▲ Xeloda Tablets (Less than 1% to 7%) 2822
Zmax for Oral Suspension (Less then 1%) 2583
▲ Zosyn (3.9%) 3492
Zyprexa Tablets (Infrequent) 1830
Zyprexa ZYDIS Orally Disintegrating Tablets (Infrequent) 1830
Zyvox (0% to 1.1%) 2652

Candidiasis, pharynx
▲ Advair HFA Inhalation Aerosol (1% to 3%) 1318
Azmacort Inhalation Aerosol 1726
Serevent Diskus (1% to less than 3%) 1568

Candidiasis, urinary tract
Nexium Delayed-Release Capsules (Less than 1%) 655
Nexium I.V. (Less than 1%) 659

Candidiasis, vaginal
Avelox (0.1% to less than 2%) 2970
▲ Doxil Injection (1% to 10%) 2351
Enjuvia Tablets 1062
Invanz for Injection (Greater than 0.1%) 1999
Proquin XR Tablets (Less than 1%) 1153

Candiduria
Cipro 2977
Cipro I.V. 2984
Cipro XR Tablets 2990
Noroxin Tablets 2032
Proquin XR Tablets 1153
Zosyn (1.0% or less) 3492

Cannula site reaction
▲ Vaprisol (5.5%) 643

Capillary fragility
▲ Aerobid/Aerobid-M (1% to 3%) 1171
Campath Ampules 811
Neurontin Capsules (Rare) 2487
Neurontin Oral Solution (Rare) 2487
Neurontin Tablets (Rare) 2487

Capillary leak syndrome
Aldara Cream, 5% 1846
Betaseron for SC Injection 767
Clolar for Intravenous Infusion 1271
I.V. Busulfex 2493
Leukine 814
Neumega for Injection 3435
Neupogen for Injection (One event) 603
Orthoclone OKT3 Sterile Solution (Less than 1%) 2360
Proleukin for Injection 2266
Simulect for Injection 2284

Carbohydrate craving
Lexapro Oral Solution (Infrequent) 1190
Lexapro Tablets (Infrequent) 1190

Carbohydrate tolerance, decrease
Angeliq Tablets 762
Climara Transdermal System 771
Climara Pro Transdermal System 776
Decadron Tablets 1951
Depo-Medrol Injectable Suspension 2617
Depo-Medrol Single-Dose Vial 2619
Estrasorb Topical Emulsion 1147
Estratest Tablets 3199
Estratest H.S. Tablets 3199
Hydrocortone Tablets 1989
Menostar Transdermal System 782
Mircette Tablets 1066
NuvaRing 2340
Ortho-Cyclen Tablets 2429
Ortho Evra Transdermal System 2417
Ortho Tri-Cyclen Tablets 2429
Ortho Tri-Cyclen Lo Tablets 2436
Premarin Intravenous 3442
Premarin Vaginal Cream 3452
Premphase Tablets 3456
Prempro Tablets 3456
Yasmin 28 Tablets 796
Yaz Tablets 803

Carbohydrate tolerance, reduced
Enjuvia Tablets 1062

Carcinoma
Nutropin for Injection 1239
Nutropin AQ Injection 1243
Nutropin AQ Pen 1243
Nutropin AQ Pen Cartridge 1243

Carcinoma, basal cell
Aldara Cream, 5% (2.3%) 1846
Amevive (Less than 0.1%) 626
Elidel Cream 1% 2200
Evoxac Capsules (Less than 1%) 1047
Metrogel 1% (0.2%) 1211
Neoral Oral Solution (0.4%) 2259
Neoral Soft Gelatin Capsules (0.4%) 2259
Protopic Ointment 638
▲ Rapamune Oral Solution and Tablets (0.7% to 4.7%) 3475
Remicade for IV Injection (Greater than or equal to 0.2%) 971
Requip Tablets (1% or more) 1555
Sandostatin Injection (Less than 1%) 2278
Sandostatin LAR Depot (Rare) 2280

Carcinoma, bile duct
▲ Humira Injection (Less than 5%) 466

Carcinoma, bladder
Bexxar 1398
Requip Tablets (Infrequent) 1555

Carcinoma, breast
Actiq (1% or greater) 979
Ambien Tablets (Rare) 2851
Angeliq Tablets 762
Bexxar 1398
Celebrex Capsules (0.1% to 1.9%) 3134
Climara Transdermal System 771
Enbrel for Injection 584
Enjuvia Tablets 1062
Estratest Tablets 3199
Estratest H.S. Tablets 3199
Eulexin Capsules (Two reports) 3009
▲ Humira Injection (Less than 5%) 466
Imitrex Nasal Spray 1467
Lamictal (Rare) 1481
Ortho-Cyclen/Ortho Tri-Cyclen 2429
Ortho Tri-Cyclen Lo Tablets 2436
Paxil CR Controlled-Release Tablets (Rare) 1538
Paxil (Rare) 1530
Permax Tablets (Infrequent) 3356
Premarin Intravenous 3442
Premphase Tablets 3456
Prempro Tablets 3456
Prometrium Capsules (100 mg, 200 mg) (2%) 3203
Remicade for IV Injection (Greater than or equal to 0.2%) 971
Requip Tablets (Infrequent) 1555
Sandostatin LAR Depot (Rare) 2280
Symbyax Capsules (Rare) 1819
Tasmar Tablets (Infrequent) 3358
Uniretic Tablets (Less than 1%) 3100

Zelapar Tablets ... 3372
Zelnorm Tablets ... 2312
Zomig Nasal Spray (Rare) ... 3523

Carcinoma, bronchoalveolar
Revlimid Capsules ... 958

Carcinoma, cervix
Copaxone for Injection (Infrequent)... 3297
▲ Humira Injection (Less than 5%) ... 466

Carcinoma, CNS
Zelapar Tablets ... 3372

Carcinoma, colon
Enbrel for Injection ... 584
▲ Humira Injection (Less than 5%) ... 466

Carcinoma, colorectal
Bexxar ... 1398

Carcinoma, endometrial
Angeliq Tablets ... 762
Arimidex Tablets (0.1% to 0.2%) ... 673
Climara Transdermal System ... 771
Climara Pro Transdermal System ... 776
Enjuvia Tablets ... 1062
Estrasorb Topical Emulsion ... 1147
Estratest Tablets ... 3199
Estratest H.S. Tablets ... 3199
Menostar Transdermal System ... 782
Omacor Capsules ... 2725
Premarin Intravenous ... 3442
Premarin Tablets ... 3446
Premarin Vaginal Cream ... 3452
Premphase Tablets ... 3456
Prempro Tablets ... 3456
Soltamox Oral Solution ... 3527

Carcinoma, esophageal
Requip Tablets (Infrequent) ... 1555

Carcinoma, gallbladder
▲ Humira Injection (Less than 5%) ... 466

Carcinoma, gastric
Bexxar ... 1398

Carcinoma, gastrointestinal
Copaxone for Injection (Infrequent) .. 3297
▲ Humira Injection (Less than 5%) ... 466
Protonix I.V. (Less than 1%) ... 3472
Protonix Tablets (Less than 1%) ... 3469
Tasmar Tablets (Rare) ... 3358
▲ Visudyne for Injection (1% to 10%) ... 2305
Zomig Nasal Spray (Rare) ... 3523

Carcinoma, head and neck
Bexxar ... 1398

Carcinoma, hepatocellular
Ortho-Cyclen/Ortho Tri-Cyclen (Rare) ... 2429
Ortho Tri-Cyclen Lo Tablets ... 2436
Testim 1% Gel ... 695

Carcinoma, laryngeal
Prevacid Delayed-Release Capsules (Less than 1%) ... 3271
Prevacid for Delayed-Release Oral Suspension (Less than 1%) ... 3271
Prevacid SoluTab Delayed-Release Orally Disintegrating Tablets (Less than 1%) ... 3271
Prevacid NapraPAC (Less than 1%) .. 3280
PREVPAC (Less than 1%) ... 3284

Carcinoma, liver
Campral Tablets (Rare) ... 1174

Carcinoma, lung
Bexxar ... 1398
Enbrel for Injection ... 584
Matulane Capsules ... 3191
Orencia Powder for Intravenous Infusion (8 cases) ... 914
Permax Tablets (Rare) ... 3356
Prinivil Tablets (0.3% to 1.0%) ... 2052
Revlimid Capsules ... 958
Rilutek Tablets (Infrequent) ... 2930
Uniretic Tablets (Less than 1%) ... 3100
Zelapar Tablets ... 3372
Zostavax Injection (1 case) ... 2111

Carcinoma, lung, non-small cell
Emend Capsules (Greater than 0.5%) ... 1963

Carcinoma, ovarian
Angeliq Tablets ... 762
Climara Transdermal System ... 771
Climara Pro Transdermal System ... 776
Enjuvia Tablets ... 1062
Estrasorb Topical Emulsion ... 1147
Estratest Tablets ... 3199
Estratest H.S. Tablets ... 3199
Menostar Transdermal System ... 782
Premarin Intravenous ... 3442
Premarin Tablets ... 3446
Premarin Vaginal Cream ... 3452
Premphase Tablets ... 3456
Prempro Tablets ... 3456
Tasmar Tablets (Rare) ... 3358

Carcinoma, prostate
Campath Ampules ... 811
Enbrel for Injection ... 584
▲ Humira Injection (Less than 5%) ... 466
Mirapex Tablets (Less than 1%) ... 859
Paxil CR Controlled-Release Tablets (Rare) ... 1538
Paxil (Rare) ... 1530
▲ Propecia Tablets (6.4%) ... 2060
▲ Proscar Tablets (6.4%) ... 2067
Revlimid Capsules ... 958
Rilutek Tablets (Infrequent) ... 2930
Striant Mucoadhesive ... 1007
Tasmar Tablets (Infrequent) ... 3358
Testim 1% Gel ... 695
Zelapar Tablets ... 3372

Carcinoma, rectal
▲ Humira Injection (Less than 5%) ... 466
Requip Tablets (Infrequent) ... 1555

Carcinoma, skin
Actonel Tablets (2%) ... 2683
Actonel with Calcium Tablets (2%) ... 2688
Azilect Tablets (Greater than 1%) ... 3293
Bexxar ... 1398
▲ CellCept Capsules (1.6% to less than 20%) ... 2747
▲ CellCept Intravenous (1.6% to less than 20%) ... 2747
▲ CellCept Oral Suspension (1.6% to less than 20%) ... 2747
▲ CellCept Tablets (1.6% to less than 20%) ... 2747
Copaxone for Injection (Infrequent)... 3297
Gabitril Tablets (Infrequent) ... 984
▲ Humira Injection (Less than 5%) ... 466
Neurontin Capsules (Rare) ... 2487
Neurontin Oral Solution (Rare) ... 2487
Neurontin Tablets (Rare) ... 2487
Orthoclone OKT3 Sterile Solution ... 2360
Permax Tablets (Infrequent) ... 3356
Prevacid Delayed-Release Capsules (Less than 1%) ... 3271
Prevacid for Delayed-Release Oral Suspension (Less than 1%) ... 3271
Prevacid SoluTab Delayed-Release Orally Disintegrating Tablets (Less than 1%) ... 3271
Prevacid NapraPAC (Less than 1%) .. 3280
PREVPAC (Less than 1%) ... 3284
▲ Prograf Capsules and Injection (One of the two most common forms) ... 632
▲ Rapamune Oral Solution and Tablets (1.1% to 6.5%) ... 3475
Sandimmune ... 2275
Uniretic Tablets (Less than 1%) ... 3100
Zelapar Tablets ... 3372

Carcinoma, skin, benign
▲ CellCept Capsules (3% to less than 20%) ... 2747
▲ CellCept Intravenous (3% to less than 20%) ... 2747
▲ CellCept Oral Suspension (3% to less than 20%) ... 2747
▲ CellCept Tablets (3% to less than 20%) ... 2747
Copaxone for Injection (Infrequent)... 3297
Gabitril Tablets (Infrequent) ... 984
Kaletra (Less than 2%) ... 476
Permax Tablets (Rare) ... 3356
▲ Protopic Ointment (1% to 3%) ... 638
Thalomid Capsules ... 965
Virazole for Inhalation Solution ... 3370
Zelapar Tablets ... 3372

Carcinoma, squamous
▲ Aldara Cream, 5% (3.7%) ... 1846
Amevive (Less than 0.1%) ... 626
Campath Ampules ... 811
Elidel Cream 1% ... 2200
Evoxac Capsules (Less than 1%) ... 1047
Protopic Ointment ... 638
Rapamune Oral Solution and Tablets (0.4% to 2.7%) ... 3475

Carcinoma, testicular
Campath Ampules ... 811

Carcinoma, thyroid
Solodyn Extended Release Tablets... 1890

Carcinoma, unspecified
▲ Actonel Tablets (0.8% to 3.3%) ... 2683
▲ Actonel with Calcium Tablets (0.8% to 3.3%) ... 2688
Aggrenox Capsules (1.7%) ... 822
▲ Arimidex Tablets (5%) ... 673
▲ CellCept Capsules (3% to less than 20%) ... 2747
▲ CellCept Intravenous (3% to less than 20%) ... 2747
▲ CellCept Oral Suspension (3% to less than 20%) ... 2747
▲ CellCept Tablets (3% to less than 20%) ... 2747
Colazal Capsules ... 2838
Effexor Tablets (Rare) ... 3411
Effexor XR Capsules (Rare) ... 3417
Ferrlecit Injection ... 3388
Gabitril Tablets (Infrequent) ... 984
Gengraf Capsules ... 459
▲ Humira Injection (Less than 5%) ... 466
Levaquin (0.1% to 0.9%) ... 2384
Levaquin in 5% Dextrose Injection (0.1% to 0.9%) ... 2384
Lupron Depot 7.5 mg (Less than 5%) ... 3264
Myobloc Injection (Greater than 2%) ... 3192
Neoral Oral Solution (1% to less than 3%) ... 2259
Neoral Soft Gelatin Capsules (1% to less than 3%) ... 2259
Nipent for Injection (Less than 3%) ... 1863
Omacor Capsules ... 2725
Paxil CR Controlled-Release Tablets (Infrequent) ... 1538
Paxil (Infrequent) ... 1530
Permax Tablets (Infrequent) ... 3356
Prevacid Delayed-Release Capsules (Less than 1%) ... 3271
Prevacid for Delayed-Release Oral Suspension (Less than 1%) ... 3271
Prevacid SoluTab Delayed-Release Orally Disintegrating Tablets (Less than 1%) ... 3271
Prevacid NapraPAC (Less than 1%) .. 3280
PREVPAC (Less than 1%) ... 3284
Protonix I.V. (Less than 1%) ... 3472
Protonix Tablets (Less than 1%) ... 3469
Rilutek Tablets (Infrequent) ... 2930
Tasmar Tablets (Infrequent) ... 3358
Zelapar Tablets ... 3372
Zomig Nasal Spray (Rare to infrequent) ... 3523

Carcinoma, uterine
▲ Humira Injection (Less than 5%) ... 466
Requip Tablets (Rare) ... 1555

Cardiac abnormalities
Accolate Tablets (Rare) ... 671
Albalon Ophthalmic Solution ... ⊙ 218
Clozaril Tablets (1%) ... 2184
FazaClo Orally Disintegrating Tablets (1%) ... 551
Flovent Diskus ... 1443
▲ Leukine (23%) ... 814
Parcopa Orally Disintegrating Tablets ... 3097
Rythmol SR Capsules ... 2727

Cardiac anomalies
Stalevo Tablets ... 2287

Cardiac arrest
▲ Abelcet Injection (6%) ... 1141
Abilify Oral Solution (Infrequent) ... 882
Abilify Oral Solution (Infrequent) ... 2450
Abilify Discmelt Orally Disintegrating Tablets (Infrequent) ... 882
Abilify Discmelt Orally Disintegrating Tablets (Infrequent) ... 2450
Abilify Tablets (Infrequent) ... 882
Abilify Tablets (Infrequent) ... 2450
Aceon Tablets (2 mg, 4 mg, 8 mg) ... 3194
Activase I.V. ... 1223
Adalat CC Tablets (Less than 1%) ... 2964
Adenoscan ... 619
AmBisome for Injection (Less common) ... 620
Antivenin Polyvalent (Isolated cases) ... 3405
▲ Aranesp for Injection (10%) ... 581
▲ Argatroban Injection (5.8%) ... 1346
Avelox (Very rare) ... 2970
Betagan Ophthalmic Solution, USP ... ⊙ 220
Betimol Ophthalmic Solution ... 3382
Betimol Ophthalmic Solution ... ⊙ 295
Bicillin C-R Injectable Suspension ... 1706
Blocadren Tablets (Less than 1%) ... 1916
Campath Ampules ... 811
Camptosar Injection ... 2604
Captopril Tablets ... 2149
Carimune NF ... 3499
Celexa (Rare) ... 1176
▲ CellCept Capsules (3% to less than 20%) ... 2747
▲ CellCept Intravenous (3% to less than 20%) ... 2747
▲ CellCept Oral Suspension (3% to less than 20%) ... 2747
▲ CellCept Tablets (3% to less than 20%) ... 2747
Clozaril Tablets (Rare) ... 2184
Cosopt Sterile Ophthalmic Solution ... 1931
Cubicin for Injection (Less than 1%) ... 1026
Decadron Tablets ... 1951
Dilaudid ... 440
Dilaudid Oral Liquid ... 445
Dilaudid Tablets - 8 mg ... 445
Dilaudid-HP ... 442
▲ Doxil Injection (1% to 10%) ... 2351
Effexor Tablets (Rare) ... 3411
Effexor XR Capsules (Rare) ... 3417
Elitek (Less than or equal to 1%) ... 2890
Ethyol for Injection (Rare) ... 1898
Exelon Capsules (Infrequent) ... 2206
Exelon Oral Solution (Infrequent) ... 2206
Fabrazyme for Intravenous Infusion ... 1274
Flebogamma 5%, Immune Globulin Intravenous (Human) ... 1658
Fluorescite Injection ... ⊙ 207
Gammagard Liquid ... 721
Gammagard S/D (Rare) ... 724
Gamunex Immune Globulin I.V., 10% (Rare) ... 3235
Herceptin I.V. (At least one of the 958 patients) ... 1233
▲ Humira Injection (Less than 5%) ... 466
Imitrex Injection ... 1463
Imitrex Tablets ... 1471
Infed Injection ... 3390
Invanz for Injection (Greater than 0.1%) ... 1999
Kadian Capsules ... 577
K-Lor Oral Solution ... 474
K-Tab Tablets ... 475
Lanoxicaps Capsules ... 1490
Lanoxin Injection ... 1494
Lanoxin Injection Pediatric ... 1497
Lanoxin Tablets ... 1500
Levaquin (0.1% to 0.9%) ... 2384
Levaquin in 5% Dextrose Injection (0.1% to 0.9%) ... 2384
Levothroid Tablets ... 1186
Levoxyl Tablets ... 1712
Lexapro Oral Solution ... 1190
Lexapro Tablets ... 1190
Lidoderm Patch ... 1118
Meridia Capsules ... 489
Merrem I.V. (Greater than 0.1% to 1%) ... 686
MS Contin Tablets ... 2701
Mycamine for Injection ... 628
Namenda (Infrequent) ... 1195
Neumega for Injection ... 3435
Nipent for Injection (Less than 3%) ... 1863
Omacor Capsules ... 2725
Orthoclone OKT3 Sterile Solution (Less than 1%) ... 2360
Permax Tablets (Infrequent) ... 3356
Pletal Tablets (Less than 2%) ... 2455
Prinivil Tablets (0.3% to 1.0%) ... 2052
Prinzide Tablets ... 2056
Prograf Capsules and Injection ... 632
Proleukin for Injection (Less than 1% to 2%) ... 2266
Proventil Inhalation Aerosol ... 3053
Prozac Pulvules and Liquid (Rare) ... 1801
Pulmozyme Inhalation Solution ... 1248
Remicade for IV Injection (Greater than or equal to 0.2%) ... 971
Requip Tablets (Infrequent) ... 1555
Retavase ... 2499
Revlimid Capsules ... 958
Reyataz Capsules (Less than 3%) ... 921
Rilutek Tablets (More than 2%) ... 2930
Rythmol SR Capsules ... 2727
Sandostatin LAR Depot (Rare) ... 2280
Symmetrel Tablets ... 1135
▲ Tambocor Tablets (5.1%) ... 1856
Tasmar Tablets (Infrequent) ... 3358
Thalomid Capsules ... 965
Thioridazine Hydrochloride Tablets .. 2163
Timolide Tablets ... 2086
Timoptic Sterile Ophthalmic Solution (Less frequent) ... 2088
Timoptic in Ocudose (Less frequent) ... 2091

Timoptic-XE Sterile Ophthalmic Gel Forming Solution 2092
TNKase I.V. 1264
Trasylol Injection (1% to 2%) 754
Uniretic Tablets (Less than 1%) 3100
Vasotec I.V. Injection (0.5% to 1.0%) 2103
▲ Vesanoid Capsules (3%) 2820
VFEND I.V. (Less than 2%) 2564
VFEND Oral Suspension (Less than 2%) 2564
VFEND Tablets (Less than 2%) 2564
Viagra Tablets (Less than 2%) 2573
Virazole for Inhalation Solution 3370
Zosyn (1.0% or less) 3492
Zyprexa Tablets (Rare) 1830
Zyprexa ZYDIS Orally Disintegrating Tablets (Rare) 1830

Cardiac arrhythmias
(*see under* Arrhythmias)

Cardiac asystole
(*see under* Asystole)

Cardiac collapse
BOTOX Purified Neurotoxin Complex (2 patients) 570

Cardiac death
Cialis Tablets 1838
Exelon Capsules (Infrequent) 2206
Exelon Oral Solution (Infrequent) 2206
Revatio Tablets 2557
Viagra Tablets 2573

Cardiac disorders, unspecified
▲ Rituxan I.V. (29%) 1254

Cardiac dysrhythmias
(*see under* Arrhythmias)

Cardiac enlargement
Decadron Tablets 1951

Cardiac failure
(*see under* Heart failure)

Cardiac insufficiency
Rescriptor Tablets 2551

Cardiac murmur
Aceon Tablets (2 mg, 4 mg, 8 mg) (0.3% to 1%) 3194
Amerge Tablets (Rare) 1339
Avalide Tablets 888
Avalide Tablets 2874
Avapro Tablets (Less than 1%) 891
Avapro Tablets (Less than 1%) 2871
Cipro I.V. (1% or less) 2984
Cipro XR Tablets 2990
Copaxone for Injection (Infrequent) 3297
▲ Dacogen Injection (16%) 2129
Evoxac Capsules (Less than 1%) 1047
▲ Imdur Tablets (Less than or equal to 5%) 3018
▲ Increlex Injection (Greater than or equal to 5%) 3291
Invanz for Injection (Greater than 0.1%) 1999
Invirase (Less than 2%) 2772
Neurontin Capsules (Infrequent) 2487
Neurontin Oral Solution (Infrequent) 2487
Neurontin Tablets (Infrequent) 2487
Proquin XR Tablets 1153
▲ Rythmol SR Capsules (2% to 4%) 2727
Thalomid Capsules 965
▲ Vesanoid Capsules (3%) 2820

Cardiac output, decrease
Digibind for Injection (Few instances) 1421
Fabrazyme for Intravenous Infusion 1274
Paxil CR Controlled-Release Tablets (Rare) 1538
Paxil (Rare) 1530
Pexeva Tablets (rare) 1694

Cardiac rhythms, disturbances
Calcium Disodium Versenate Injection 1851
Captopril Tablets 2149
Daraprim Tablets 1419
Lanoxicaps Capsules 1490
Lanoxin Injection 1494
Lanoxin Injection Pediatric 1497
Lanoxin Tablets 1500
Nadolol Tablets (1 of 100 patients) 2159
Prinzide Tablets 2056
Rescriptor Tablets 2551
Univasc Tablets (Less than 1%) 3104
Vasotec I.V. Injection (0.5% to 1.0%) 2103

Cardiac rhythms, ectopic
Biltricide Tablets 2976

Cardiac tamponade
Activase I.V. 1223
I.V. Busulfex 2493
Myleran Tablets (A small number of patients) 1525
Retavase 2499
▲ Taxotere Injection Concentrate (6%) 2932
TNKase I.V. 1264

Cardiac toxicity, unspecified
Doxil Injection 2351
Lanoxicaps Capsules 1490
Lanoxin Injection 1494
Lanoxin Injection Pediatric 1497
Lanoxin Tablets 1500

Cardiac valve disorder, unspecified
Adipex-P 1215
Permax Tablets 3356
Protopic Ointment (0.2% to less than 1%) 638

Cardialgia
(*see under* Heartburn)

Cardiodynia
(*see under* Heartburn)

Cardiomegaly
Abilify Oral Solution (Rare) 882
Abilify Oral Solution (Rare) 2450
Abilify Discmelt Orally Disintegrating Tablets (Rare) 882
Abilify Discmelt Orally Disintegrating Tablets (Rare) 2450
Abilify Tablets (Rare) 882
Abilify Tablets (Rare) 2450
Agrylin Capsules 3169
AmBisome for Injection (Less common) 620
Doxil Injection (Less than 1%) 2351
Evoxac Capsules 1047
▲ Fabrazyme for Intravenous Infusion (3%) 1274
Geodon Capsules (Rare) 2529
▲ I.V. Busulfex (5%) 2493
▲ Neumega for Injection (21%) 3435
Requip Tablets (Infrequent) 1555
VFEND I.V. (Less than 2%) 2564
VFEND Oral Suspension (Less than 2%) 2564
VFEND Tablets (Less than 2%) 2564
Zelapar Tablets 3372

Cardiomyopathy
Abelcet Injection 1141
Adderall Tablets (Isolated reports) 3164
Adderall XR Capsules (Isolated cases) 3166
Agrylin Capsules 3169
Aldara Cream, 5% 1846
Betaseron for SC Injection 767
Campral Tablets (Rare) 1174
Clozaril Tablets 2184
Combivir Tablets 1411
Dacogen Injection 2129
Dexedrine (Isolated reports) 1420
DextroStat Tablets (Isolated reports) 3179
▲ Doxil Injection (1% to 5%) 2351
FazaClo Orally Disintegrating Tablets 551
Herceptin I.V. 1233
Imitrex Injection 1463
Imitrex Nasal Spray 1467
Imitrex Tablets 1471
▲ Intron A for Injection (Less than 5%) 3024
▲ Megace ES Oral Suspension (1% to 3%) 2481
PEG-Intron Powder for Injection (Less than or equal to 1%) 3048
Proleukin for Injection 2266
Rescriptor Tablets 2551
Retrovir Capsules (0.8%) 1560
Retrovir IV Infusion (1%) 1564
Retrovir (0.8%) 1560
Revlimid Capsules 958
Trizivir Tablets 1589
VFEND I.V. (Less than 2%) 2564
VFEND Oral Suspension (Less than 2%) 2564
VFEND Tablets (Less than 2%) 2564
Viagra Tablets (Less than 2%) 2573
Zelapar Tablets 3372

Cardiomyopathy, hypertrophic, premature infants
Decadron Tablets 1951

Cardiopulmonary arrest
Abilify Oral Solution (Infrequent to Rare) 882
Abilify Oral Solution (Infrequent to Rare) 2450
Abilify Discmelt Orally Disintegrating Tablets (Infrequent to Rare) 882
Abilify Discmelt Orally Disintegrating Tablets (Infrequent to Rare) 2450
Abilify Tablets (Infrequent to Rare) 882
Abilify Tablets (Infrequent to Rare) 2450
Cipro (Less than 1%) 2977
Cipro I.V. (1% or less) 2984
Cipro XR Tablets 2990
Erbitux (2%) 910
Fortaz 1453
Lariam Tablets (One patient) 2786
Proquin XR Tablets 1153
Pulmozyme Inhalation Solution 1248
Risperdal 1676
Risperdal Consta Long-Acting Injection 1682
Risperdal M-Tab Orally Disintegrating Tablets 1676
Zofran Injection 1634
Zofran 1639
Zofran ODT Orally Disintegrating Tablets 1639

Cardiorespiratory arrest
Aloprim for Injection (Less than 1%) 2167
Avalide Tablets 888
Avalide Tablets 2874
Avapro Tablets (Less than 1%) 891
Avapro Tablets (Less than 1%) 2871
Dacogen Injection (Greater than or equal to 1%) 2129
Orthoclone OKT3 Sterile Solution 2360
Revlimid Capsules 958

Cardiospasm
Paxil CR Controlled-Release Tablets (Rare) 1538
Paxil (Rare) 1530
Pexeva Tablets (Rare) 1694
Prevacid Delayed-Release Capsules (Less than 1%) 3271
Prevacid for Delayed-Release Oral Suspension (Less than 1%) 3271
Prevacid SoluTab Delayed-Release Orally Disintegrating Tablets (Less than 1%) 3271
Prevacid NapraPAC (Less than 1%) 3280
PREVPAC (Less than 1%) 3284
Protonix I.V. (Less than 1%) 3472
Protonix Tablets (Less than 1%) 3469
Sonata Capsules (Rare) 1717

Cardiovascular abnormalities, fetal
Accutane Capsules 2731
Clinoril Tablets 1924
Dolobid Tablets 1955

Cardiovascular collapse
Allegra-D 12 Hour Extended-Release Tablets 2846
Allegra-D 24 Hour Extended-Release Tablets 2849
Carbatrol Capsules 3171
Cipro 2977
Cipro I.V. (1% or less) 2984
Cipro XR Tablets 2990
Clarinex-D 24-Hour Extended-Release Tablets 2998
Diastat Rectal Delivery System (Infrequent) 3343
Equetro Extended-Release Capsules 3180
Infed Injection 3390
Levaquin 2384
Levaquin in 5% Dextrose Injection 2384
Lidoderm Patch 1118
Lupron Injection Pediatric 3259
Noroxin Tablets 2032
Orthoclone OKT3 Sterile Solution 2360
Proquin XR Tablets 1153
Synera Topical Patch 1137
Tegretol/Tegretol-XR 2295
Tessalon Capsules 1199
Tessalon Perles 1199
Zyrtec-D 12 Hour Extended Release Tablets 2597

Cardiovascular disorders
Actonel Tablets (2.5%) 2683
Actonel with Calcium Tablets (2.5%) 2688
Agrylin Capsules (1% to 5%) 3169
Allegra-D 12 Hour Extended-Release Tablets (Rare) 2846
Allegra-D 24 Hour Extended-Release Tablets (Rare) 2849
Aloprim for Injection (Less than 1%) 2167
Argatroban Injection (2.3%) 1346
▲ Carnitor Injection (3% to 6%) 3188
▲ CellCept Capsules (3% to 25.6%) 2747
▲ CellCept Intravenous (3% to 25.6%) 2747
▲ CellCept Oral Suspension (3% to 25.6%) 2747
▲ CellCept Tablets (3% to 25.6%) 2747
▲ Clozaril Tablets (Greater than 5%) 2184
Crixivan Capsules 1940
Evoxac Capsules (Less than 1%) 1047
▲ Humira Injection (Less than 5%) 466
▲ Hycamtin for Injection (25%) 1458
Lofibra Tablets 1219
Lofibra Capsules 1216
Menostar Transdermal System (10%) 782
▲ Neoral Oral Solution (28.0%) 2259
▲ Neoral Soft Gelatin Capsules (28.0%) 2259
Neumega for Injection 3435
Protonix I.V. (Less than 1%) 3472
Protonix Tablets (Less than 1%) 3469
Risperdal 1676
Risperdal Consta Long-Acting Injection 1682
Risperdal M-Tab Orally Disintegrating Tablets 1676
Singulair 2077
Tasmar Tablets (Rare) 3358
Tricor Tablets 527
Zelapar Tablets 3372
Zostavax Injection (0.3%) 2111
Zyban Sustained-Release Tablets 1644

Cardiovascular events
DextroStat Tablets 3179
Rituxan I.V. (1.7%) 1254

Cardiovascular toxicity, unspecified
Sutent Capsules (1 patient) 2560

Carnitine concentrations, decreased
Depacon Injection 412
Depakene 417
Depakote Sprinkle Capsules 422
Depakote Tablets 427
Depakote ER Tablets 434

Carotid artery occlusion
▲ Macugen Injection (1% to 5%) ⊙261

Carotid bruit
Rythmol SR Capsules 2727

Carotid sinus hypersensitivity
Aldoril Tablets 1910

Carpal tunnel syndrome
Aromasin Tablets (2.4%) 2600
Evoxac Capsules (Less than 1%) 1047
Humatrope Vials and Cartridges (Rare) 1787
▲ Intron A for Injection (Less than 5%) 3024
Lexapro Oral Solution (Infrequent) 1190
Lexapro Tablets (Infrequent) 1190
Namenda (More than one patient) 1195
▲ Nutropin for Injection (27%) 1239
▲ Nutropin AQ Injection (27%) 1243
▲ Nutropin AQ Pen (27%) 1243
▲ Nutropin AQ Pen Cartridge (27%) 1243
Prograf Capsules and Injection 632
Prozac Pulvules and Liquid 1801
Thalomid Capsules 965

Cataplexy
Clozaril Tablets 2184
FazaClo Orally Disintegrating Tablets 551
Provigil Tablets (Greater than or equal to 1%) 988
▲ Xyrem Oral Solution (8.6%) 1688

Cataracts
Abilify Oral Solution (Infrequent) 882
Abilify Oral Solution (Infrequent) 2450

Abilify Discmelt Orally Disintegrating Tablets (Infrequent) 882
Abilify Discmelt Orally Disintegrating Tablets (Infrequent) 2450
Abilify Tablets (Infrequent) 882
Abilify Tablets (Infrequent) 2450
Accutane Capsules 2731
Aciphex Tablets 1090
▲ Actonel Tablets (1.9% to 5.9%) 2683
▲ Actonel with Calcium Tablets (1.9% to 5.9%) 2688
Advair Diskus 100/50 1308
Advair Diskus 250/50 1308
Advair Diskus 500/50 1308
Advair HFA Inhalation Aerosol 1318
▲ Alphagan P Ophthalmic Solution (1% to 4%) 567
Altoprev Extended-Release Tablets 3109
Aricept Tablets (Frequent) 1094
Aricept ODT Tablets (Frequent) 1094
▲ Arimidex Tablets (4% to 6%) 673
Azmacort Inhalation Aerosol (Rare) 1726
Beconase AQ Nasal Spray (Rare) 1396
▲ Betimol Ophthalmic Solution (1% to 5%) 3382
▲ Betimol Ophthalmic Solution (1% to 5%) ⊙295
Celebrex Capsules (0.1% to 1.9%) 3134
Celexa (Rare) 1176
▲ CellCept Capsules (3% to less than 20%) 2747
▲ CellCept Intravenous (3% to less than 20%) 2747
▲ CellCept Oral Suspension (3% to less than 20%) 2747
▲ CellCept Tablets (3% to less than 20%) 2747
Chantix Tablets (Rare) 2517
Copaxone for Injection (Infrequent) 3297
▲ Cozaar Tablets (7%) 1935
Effexor Tablets (Infrequent) 3411
Effexor XR Capsules (Infrequent) 3417
Evoxac Capsules (Less than 1%) 1047
Exelon Capsules (Frequent) 2206
Exelon Oral Solution (Frequent) 2206
Flonase Nasal Spray 1440
Flovent Diskus 1443
Flovent HFA 1447
Gengraf Capsules (1% to less than 3%) 459
Geodon Capsules (Infrequent) 2529
▲ Humira Injection (Less than 5%) 466
Hyperstat I.V. 3017
Lescol Capsules 2233
Lescol XL Tablets 2233
Levaquin 2384
Levaquin in 5% Dextrose Injection 2384
Lofibra Tablets 1219
Lofibra Capsules 1216
▲ Lucentis Injection (5% to 16%) 1237
▲ Lumigan Ophthalmic Solution (3% to 10%) 573
▲ Macugen Injection (10% to 40%) ⊙261
Mirapex Tablets (Less than 1%) 859
Mircette Tablets 1066
Myleran Tablets (Rare) 1525
Namenda (Frequent) 1195
Neoral Oral Solution (1% to less than 3%) 2259
Neoral Soft Gelatin Capsules (1% to less than 3%) 2259
Neurontin Capsules (Infrequent) 2487
Neurontin Oral Solution (Infrequent) 2487
Neurontin Tablets (Infrequent) 2487
NuvaRing 2340
Omacor Capsules 2725
Ortho-Cyclen Tablets 2429
Ortho Evra Transdermal System 2417
Ortho Tri-Cyclen Tablets 2429
Ortho Tri-Cyclen Lo Tablets 2436
Paxil CR Controlled-Release Tablets (Rare) 1538
Paxil (Rare) 1530
Permax Tablets (Rare) 3356
Pexeva Tablets (rare) 1694
Photofrin for Injection 702
Plavix Tablets (1% to 2.5%) 917
Plavix Tablets (1% to 2.5%) 2926
Protonix I.V. (Less than 1%) 3472
Protonix Tablets (Less than 1%) 3469
Protopic Ointment (0.2% to less than 1%) 638
Prozac Pulvules and Liquid 1801
Pulmicort Respules (Rare) 661
▲ Rapamune Oral Solution and Tablets (3% to 20%) 3475
▲ Retisert Implant (50% to 90%) ⊙258
Rilutek Tablets (Rare) 2930
Seasonique Tablets 1077
Soltamox Oral Solution 3527
Sonata Capsules (Rare) 1717
▲ Spiriva HandiHaler (1% to 3%) 869
Tasmar Tablets (Rare) 3358
Travatan Ophthalmic Solution (1% to 4%) 563
Tricor Tablets 527
Trileptal Tablets 2300
Trileptal Oral Suspension 2300
Uniretic Tablets (Less than 1%) 3100
Viagra Tablets (Less than 2%) 2573
▲ Visudyne for Injection (1% to 10%) 2305
Vytorin 10/10 Tablets 2114
Vytorin 10/10 Tablets 3077
Vytorin 10/20 Tablets 2114
Vytorin 10/20 Tablets 3077
Vytorin 10/40 Tablets 2114
Vytorin 10/40 Tablets 3077
Vytorin 10/80 Tablets 2114
Vytorin 10/80 Tablets 3077
Yasmin 28 Tablets 796
Yaz Tablets 803
Zelapar Tablets 3372
Zoloft 2586
Zyprexa Tablets (Infrequent) 1830
Zyprexa ZYDIS Orally Disintegrating Tablets (Infrequent) 1830

Cataracts, posterior subcapsular
Alrex Ophthalmic Suspension 0.2% ⊙246
Blephamide Ophthalmic Ointment (Infrequent) 568
Blephamide Ophthalmic Suspension 569
Colocort Rectal Suspension, USP (Retention) 100 mg/60 mL 2476
▲ Cosopt Sterile Ophthalmic Solution (1% to 5%) 1931
Decadron Tablets 1951
Depo-Medrol Injectable Suspension 2617
Depo-Medrol Single-Dose Vial 2619
FML Ophthalmic Ointment (Infrequent) ⊙228
FML Ophthalmic Suspension ⊙227
FML Forte Ophthalmic Suspension (Infrequent) ⊙226
FML-S Ophthalmic Suspension ⊙229
Hydrocortone Tablets 1989
Lotemax Ophthalmic Suspension 0.5% ⊙251
Poly-Pred Ophthalmic Suspension ⊙233
Pred Mild Ophthalmic Suspension (Infrequent) ⊙238
Pred Forte Ophthalmic Suspension ⊙235
Pred-G Ophthalmic Ointment ⊙237
Pred-G Ophthalmic Suspension ⊙236
Retisert Implant ⊙258
▲ Soriatane Capsules (1% to 5%) 1013
TobraDex Ophthalmic Ointment 562
TobraDex Ophthalmic Suspension 563

Cataracts, traumatic, iatrogenic
Lucentis Injection (Less than 0.1%) 1237

Catatonia
Blocadren Tablets 1916
Celexa (Rare) 1176
Cosopt Sterile Ophthalmic Solution 1931
Depacon Injection (1% or more) 412
Depakene (1% or more) 417
Depakote Sprinkle Capsules 422
▲ Depakote Tablets (1% to 5%) 427
Depakote ER Tablets (Greater than 1%) 434
Effexor Tablets 3411
Effexor XR Capsules 3417
Inderal LA Long-Acting Capsules 3429
InnoPran XL Capsules 2723
Lopressor Injection 2238
Lopressor Tablets 2238
Lopressor HCT 50/25 Tablets 2241
Lopressor HCT 100/25 Tablets 2241
Lopressor HCT 100/50 Tablets 2241
Nadolol Tablets 2159
Phenergan Tablets and Suppositories 3440
Relpax Tablets (Rare) 2548
Risperdal (Infrequent) 1676
Risperdal M-Tab Orally Disintegrating Tablets (Infrequent) 1676
Seroquel Tablets (Infrequent) 690
Timolide Tablets 2086
Timoptic Sterile Ophthalmic Solution 2088
Timoptic in Ocudose 2091
Timoptic-XE Sterile Ophthalmic Gel Forming Solution 2092
Toprol-XL Tablets 668

Causalgia
Thalomid 965

Cellulitis
Actiq (1% or greater) 979
Adalat CC Tablets (Less than 1%) 2964
Aloprim for Injection (Less than 1%) 2167
AmBisome for Injection (Less common) 620
Aricept Tablets (Infrequent) 1094
Aricept ODT Tablets (Infrequent) 1094
Bactroban Cream (Less than 1%) 1394
BeneFix Vials (1.5%) 3408
Campath Ampules 811
Celebrex Capsules (0.1% to 1.9%) 3134
Celexa (Rare) 1176
▲ CellCept Capsules (3% to less than 20%) 2747
▲ CellCept Intravenous (3% to less than 20%) 2747
▲ CellCept Oral Suspension (3% to less than 20%) 2747
▲ CellCept Tablets (3% to less than 20%) 2747
▲ Clolar for Intravenous Infusion (11%) 1271
Copaxone for Injection (Infrequent) 3297
▲ Cozaar Tablets (7%) 1935
Cubicin for Injection (1% to 2%) 1026
▲ Dacogen Injection (12%) 2129
Doxil Injection (Less than 1%) 2351
Effexor Tablets (Rare) 3411
Effexor XR Capsules (Rare) 3417
Elitek (Less than or equal to 1%) 2890
Enbrel for Injection 584
Evoxac Capsules (Less than 1%) 1047
Exelon Capsules (Infrequent) 2206
Exelon Oral Solution (Infrequent) 2206
Gabitril Tablets (Infrequent) 984
Gemzar for Injection (Rare) 1771
Gengraf Capsules (1% to less than 3%) 459
Herceptin I.V. (At least one of the 958 patients) 1233
▲ Humira Injection (Less than 5%) 466
Hyperstat I.V. 3017
Infanrix Vaccine 1476
▲ Intron A for Injection (Less than 5%) 3024
Invanz for Injection (1.5%) 1999
Invirase (Less than 2%) 2772
Kineret Injection 599
Klonopin (Infrequent) 2778
Lunesta Tablets (Infrequent) 3142
▲ Lupron Depot 7.5 mg (Less than 5%) 3264
Lyrica Capsules (0.1% to 1%) 2539
Namenda (Infrequent) 1195
Neoral Oral Solution (1% to less than 3%) 2259
Neoral Soft Gelatin Capsules (1% to less than 3%) 2259
Neurontin Capsules (Infrequent) 2487
Neurontin Oral Solution (Infrequent) 2487
Neurontin Tablets (Infrequent) 2487
▲ Nipent for Injection (6%) 1863
Orencia Powder for Intravenous Infusion (0.2% to 0.5%) 914
Paxil CR Controlled-Release Tablets (Rare) 1538
Paxil (Rare) 1530
Pediarix Vaccine 1548
PEG-Intron Powder for Injection (Less than or equal to 1%) 3048
Permax Tablets (Infrequent) 3356
Pexeva Tablets (Rare) 1694
▲ Prograf Capsules and Injection (3% to 15%) 632
Proleukin for Injection 2266
ProQuad 2064
Protopic Ointment (Greater than or equal to 1%) 638
▲ Rapamune Oral Solution and Tablets (3% to 20%) 3475
Raptiva for Injection 1250
Remicade for IV Injection (Greater than or equal to 0.2%) 971
ReoPro Vials (0.3%) 1809
Requip Tablets (Infrequent) 1555
▲ Revlimid Capsules (5.4%) 958
Reyataz Capsules (Less than 3%) 921
Rilutek Tablets (Infrequent) 2930
Sandostatin Injection (Less than 1%) 2278
▲ Sandostatin LAR Depot (1% to 4%) 2280
Sular Tablets (Less than or equal to 1%) 3122
Symbyax Capsules (Infrequent) 1819
Targretin Capsules 1747
Tasmar Tablets (Infrequent) 3358
Thalomid Capsules 965
▲ Ultram ER Tablets (1% to greater than 5%) 2392
Uniretic Tablets (Less than 1%) 3100
Varivax 2100
▲ Vesanoid Capsules (8%) 2820
VFEND I.V. (Less than 2%) 2564
VFEND Oral Suspension (Less than 2%) 2564
VFEND Tablets (Less than 2%) 2564
Vivitrol 995
Xyrem Oral Solution (Infrequent) 1688
Zelapar Tablets 3372
Zomig Nasal Spray (Rare) 3523

Cellulitis, injection site
Bicillin C-R Injectable Suspension 1706
Fluarix 1451
Infed Injection 3390

Cellulitis, pre-septal
Amevive 626

Cellulitis-like reactions
Pneumovax 23 (Rare) 2043

Central nervous system demyelinating disorders
ADACEL Vaccine 2945

Centrilobular sinusoidal fibrosis
Myleran Tablets 1525

Cephalin flocculation test, positive
Cuprimine Capsules 1947

Cerebellar dysfunction
Neurontin Capsules (Infrequent) 2487
Neurontin Oral Solution (Infrequent) 2487
Neurontin Tablets (Infrequent) 2487

Cerebellar infarction
Revlimid Capsules 958

Cerebellar malformation, fetal
Accutane Capsules 2731

Cerebellar syndrome, acute
Lamictal (Rare) 1481
Lyrica Capsules (Rare) 2539
Topamax Sprinkle Capsules (Rare) 2404
Topamax Tablets (Rare) 2404

Cerebral abnormalities, fetal
Accutane Capsules 2731

Cerebral arterial insufficiency, symptoms
Carbatrol Capsules 3171
Equetro Extended-Release Capsules 3180
Tegretol/Tegretol-XR 2295

Cerebral arteritis
Concerta Extended-Release Tablets (Isolated cases) 1881
Daytrana Transdermal Patch 3174
Focalin Tablets 2220
Focalin XR Capsules 2223
Metadate CD Capsules (Isolated cases) 3323
Ritalin Hydrochloride Tablets (Isolated cases) 2269
Ritalin LA Capsules 2271
Ritalin-SR Tablets (Isolated cases) 2269

Cerebral atrophy
Depacon Injection (Several cases) 412
Depakene (Several reports) 417
Depakote Sprinkle Capsules (Several reports) 422
Depakote Tablets (Several reports) 427
Depakote ER Tablets (Several reports) 434

Cerebral bleeding
(*see under* Cerebral hemorrhage)

Cerebral embolism
Prozac Pulvules and Liquid (Rare) 1801
Rilutek Tablets (Rare) 2930
Trasylol Injection (1% to 2%) 754

Cerebral hemorrhage
Arranon Injection (1%) 1357

Azilect Tablets (Rare) 3293
Cafcit (2.2%) 1886
Campath Ampules 811
Copegus Tablets (Less than 1%) 2754
Imitrex Injection 1463
Imitrex Tablets 1471
I.V. Busulfex (One patient) 2493
Kaletra (Less than 2%) 476
Mircette Tablets 1066
Mylotarg for Injection (2%) 3431
Namenda (Infrequent) 1195
Nexavar Tablets (Infrequent) 746
NuvaRing 2340
Ortho-Cyclen Tablets 2429
Ortho Evra Transdermal System 2417
Ortho Tri-Cyclen Tablets 2429
Ortho Tri-Cyclen Lo Tablets 2436
Pegasys (Less than 1%) 2789
Permax Tablets (Rare) 3356
Pletal Tablets (Very rare) 2455
Proleukin for Injection 2266
Rilutek Tablets (Infrequent) 2930
Seasonique Tablets 1077
Tasmar Tablets (Infrequent) 3358
Trileptal Tablets 2300
Trileptal Oral Suspension 2300
▲ Vesanoid Capsules (9%) 2820
VFEND I.V. (Less than 2%) 2564
VFEND Oral Suspension (Less than 2%) 2564
VFEND Tablets (Less than 2%) 2564
Yasmin 28 Tablets 796
Yaz Tablets 803

Cerebral herniation
Activase I.V. 1223

Cerebral infarction
Activase I.V. 1223
Aloprim for Injection (Less than 1%) 2167
Amerge Tablets 1339
Camptosar Injection 2604
Geodon Capsules (Rare) 2529
Hyperstat I.V. 3017
Namenda 1195
NovoSeven 2331
Pletal Tablets (Less than 2%) 2455
Prevacid Delayed-Release Capsules (Less than 1%) 3271
Prevacid for Delayed-Release Oral Suspension (Less than 1%) 3271
Prevacid SoluTab Delayed-Release Orally Disintegrating Tablets (Less than 1%) 3271
Prevacid NapraPAC (Less than 1%) 3280
PREVPAC (Less than 1%) 3284
Prograf Capsules and Injection 632
Remicade for IV Injection (Greater than or equal to 0.2%) 971
Revlimid Capsules 958
Uniretic Tablets (Less than 1%) 3100

Cerebral ischemia
(*see under* Ischemia, cerebral)

Cerebral lesions
Proleukin for Injection 2266

Cerebral occlusion
Concerta Extended-Release Tablets (Isolated cases) 1881
Daytrana Transdermal Patch 3174
Focalin Tablets 2220
Focalin XR Capsules 2223
Metadate CD Capsules (Isolated cases) 3323
Ritalin Hydrochloride Tablets (Isolated cases) 2269
Ritalin LA Capsules 2271
Ritalin-SR Tablets (Isolated cases) 2269

Cerebral thrombosis
Cipro (Less than 1%) 2977
Cipro I.V. (1% or less) 2984
Cipro XR Tablets 2990
Lamictal (Rare) 1481
Mircette Tablets 1066
NuvaRing 2340
Ortho-Cyclen Tablets 2429
Ortho Evra Transdermal System 2417
Ortho Tri-Cyclen Tablets 2429
Ortho Tri-Cyclen Lo Tablets 2436
Proquin XR Tablets 1153
Seasonique Tablets 1077
Trasylol Injection (0.5%) 754
Viagra Tablets (Less than 2%) 2573
Yasmin 28 Tablets 796
Yaz Tablets 803

Cerebrospinal fluid proteins, changes
Thiothixene Capsules 2165

Cerebrovascular accident
Abelcet Injection 1141
Abilify Oral Solution (Infrequent) 882
Abilify Oral Solution (Infrequent) 2450
Abilify Discmelt Orally Disintegrating Tablets (Infrequent) 882
Abilify Discmelt Orally Disintegrating Tablets (Infrequent) 2450
Abilify Tablets (Infrequent) 882
Abilify Tablets (Infrequent) 2450
Aceon Tablets (2 mg, 4 mg, 8 mg) (0.2%) 3194
▲ Agrylin Capsules (1% to 5%) 3169
Aldara Cream, 5% 1846
Amerge Tablets 1339
Aricept Tablets (Infrequent) 1094
Aricept ODT Tablets (Infrequent) 1094
Arimidex Tablets (1%) 673
Avalide Tablets 888
Avalide Tablets 2874
Avapro Tablets (Less than 1%) 891
Avapro Tablets (Less than 1%) 2871
Betagan Ophthalmic Solution, USP ⊙220
Betimol Ophthalmic Solution 3382
Betimol Ophthalmic Solution ⊙295
Bicillin C-R Injectable Suspension 1706
Blocadren Tablets (Less than 1%) 1916
Camptosar Injection 2604
Captopril Tablets 2149
Cardura XL Tablets 2515
Carteolol Hydrochloride Ophthalmic Solution USP, 1% ⊙249
Catapres-TTS (0.5% or less) 844
Celebrex Capsules (Less than 0.1%) 3134
Celexa (Infrequent) 1176
Cesamet Capsules 3340
Chantix Tablets (Rare) 2517
▲ Coreg Tablets (Greater than 1% to 3%) 1414
Cosopt Sterile Ophthalmic Solution (Less than 1%) 1931
Covera-HS Tablets (Less than 2%) 3139
Cozaar Tablets (Less than 1%) 1935
Effexor Tablets (Rare) 3411
Effexor XR Capsules (Rare) 3417
Emcyt Capsules (2%) 2634
Epogen for Injection (0.4%) 591
Fortical Nasal Spray (Less than 1%) 3337
Gammagard S/D 724
Gemzar for Injection (2%) 1771
Geodon Capsules (Rare) 2529
Hyzaar 50-12.5 Tablets 1990
Hyzaar 100-12.5 Tablets 1990
Hyzaar 100-25 Tablets 1990
Imitrex Injection 1463
Imitrex Nasal Spray 1467
Imitrex Tablets 1471
Lamictal (Rare) 1481
▲ Macugen Injection (1% to 5%) ⊙261
Maxalt Tablets (Very rare) 2008
Maxalt-MLT Orally Disintegrating Tablets (Very rare) 2008
Meridia Capsules 489
Miacalcin Nasal Spray (Less than 1%) 2253
Namenda (Frequent) 1195
Neurontin Capsules (Rare) 2487
Neurontin Oral Solution (Rare) 2487
Neurontin Tablets (Rare) 2487
Orthoclone OKT3 Sterile Solution 2360
Paxil CR Controlled-Release Tablets (Rare) 1538
Paxil (Rare) 1530
Permax Tablets (Infrequent) 3356
Pexeva Tablets (Rare) 1694
Pletal Tablets (Very rare) 2455
Prevacid Delayed-Release Capsules (Less than 1%) 3271
Prevacid for Delayed-Release Oral Suspension (Less than 1%) 3271
Prevacid SoluTab Delayed-Release Orally Disintegrating Tablets (Less than 1%) 3271
Prevacid NapraPAC (Less than 1%) 3280
PREVPAC (Less than 1%) 3284
Prinivil Tablets (0.3% to 1.0%) 2052
Prinzide Tablets 2056
▲ Procrit for Injection (0.4% to 3.2%) 2364
ProQuad 2064
Protopic Ointment (Greater than or equal to 1%) 638
Prozac Pulvules and Liquid (Rare) 1801
Quadramet Injection (1%) 1040
Razadyne (Infrequent) 2399
Revlimid Capsules 958
Risperdal 1676
Risperdal Consta Long-Acting Injection 1682
Risperdal M-Tab Orally Disintegrating Tablets 1676
Rythmol SR Capsules 2727
Seroquel Tablets (Infrequent) 690
Sular Tablets (Less than or equal to 1%) 3122
Tarceva Tablets (2.3%) 1259
Tarceva Tablets (2.3%) 2444
Targretin Capsules 1747
Tarka Tablets 524
Tasmar Tablets (Infrequent) 3358
Thalomid Capsules 965
Timolide Tablets 2086
Timoptic Sterile Ophthalmic Solution (Less frequent) 2088
Timoptic in Ocudose (Less frequent) 2091
Timoptic-XE Sterile Ophthalmic Gel Forming Solution 2092
Trasylol Injection (1% to 2%) 754
Univasc Tablets (Less than 1%) 3104
Varivax 2100
Vasotec I.V. Injection (0.5% to 1.0%) 2103
Verelan PM Extended-Release Capsules, Controlled-Onset (2% or less) 3106
Vesanoid Capsules 2820
VFEND I.V. (Less than 2%) 2564
VFEND Oral Suspension (Less than 2%) 2564
VFEND Tablets (Less than 2%) 2564
Zonegran Capsules (Infrequent) 1101
Zosyn (1.0% or less) 3492
Zyprexa Tablets (Infrequent) 1830
Zyprexa ZYDIS Orally Disintegrating Tablets (Infrequent) 1830

Cerebrovascular disorders
Abilify Oral Solution 882
Abilify Oral Solution 2450
Abilify Discmelt Orally Disintegrating Tablets 882
Abilify Discmelt Orally Disintegrating Tablets 2450
Abilify Tablets 882
Abilify Tablets 2450
Aldoril Tablets 1910
Ambien Tablets (Infrequent) 2851
Ambien CR Tablets (Infrequent) 2855
Campath Ampules 811
Coreg Tablets (Less than or equal to 0.1%) 1414
Crixivan Capsules 1940
Elitek (Less than or equal to 1%) 2890
Flumadine (Less than 0.3%) 1183
Levaquin (0.1% to 0.9%) 2384
Levaquin in 5% Dextrose Injection (0.1% to 0.9%) 2384
Micardis Tablets (More than 0.3%) 854
Micardis HCT Tablets (More than 0.3%) 856
Ortho-Cyclen/Ortho Tri-Cyclen 2429
Ortho Tri-Cyclen Lo Tablets 2436
Relpax Tablets (Rare) 2548
Risperdal 1676
Risperdal Consta Long-Acting Injection 1682
Risperdal M-Tab Orally Disintegrating Tablets 1676
Toprol-XL Tablets (Greater than 1%) 668
Zoloft (Rare) 2586

Cerebrovascular events
Symbyax Capsules 1819

Cerebrovascular insufficiency
Captopril Tablets 2149

Cerumen, increased
Norvir (Less than 2%) 503

Cervical disorders
(*see under* Cervical irregularities)

Cervical dysplasia
Campath Ampules 811

Cervical ectropion, changes
(*see also under* Cervical erosion, changes)
Angeliq Tablets 762
Climara Transdermal System 771
Climara Pro Transdermal System 776
Enjuvia Tablets 1062
Estrasorb Topical Emulsion 1147
Menostar Transdermal System 782
Premarin Tablets 3446
Seasonique Tablets 1077

Cervical erosion, changes
(*see also under* Cervical ectropion, changes)
Estratest Tablets 3199
Estratest H.S. Tablets 3199
Mircette Tablets 1066
NuvaRing 2340
Ortho-Cyclen/Ortho Tri-Cyclen 2429
Ortho Tri-Cyclen Lo Tablets 2436
Premarin Intravenous 3442
Premarin Vaginal Cream 3452
Premphase Tablets 3456
Prempro Tablets 3456
Yasmin 28 Tablets 796
Yaz Tablets 803

Cervical eversion, changes in
(*see under* Cervical ectropion, changes; Cervical erosion, changes)

Cervical irregularities
Lupron Depot-PED 7.5 mg, 11.25 mg and 15 mg (Less than 2%) 3269
Lupron Injection Pediatric (Less than 2%) 3259
▲ Premphase Tablets (4% to 5%) 3456
▲ Prempro Tablets (4% to 5%) 3456

Cervical secretion, changes
Angeliq Tablets 762
Climara Transdermal System 771
Climara Pro Transdermal System 776
Enjuvia Tablets 1062
Estrasorb Topical Emulsion 1147
Estratest Tablets 3199
Estratest H.S. Tablets 3199
Menostar Transdermal System 782
Mircette Tablets 1066
Ortho-Cyclen/Ortho Tri-Cyclen 2429
Ortho Tri-Cyclen Lo Tablets 2436
Premarin Intravenous 3442
Premarin Tablets 3446
Premarin Vaginal Cream 3452
Premphase Tablets 3456
Prempro Tablets 3456
Prometrium Capsules (100 mg, 200 mg) 3203
Seasonique Tablets 1077
Yasmin 28 Tablets 796
Yaz 803

Cervical smear test, abnormal
Zomig Nasal Spray (Rare) 3523

Cervical smear test, positive
Evoxac Capsules (Less than 1%) 1047

Cervicitis
Abilify Oral Solution (Rare) 882
Abilify Oral Solution (Rare) 2450
Abilify Discmelt Orally Disintegrating Tablets (Rare) 882
Abilify Discmelt Orally Disintegrating Tablets (Rare) 2450
Abilify Tablets (Rare) 882
Abilify Tablets (Rare) 2450
Effexor Tablets (Rare) 3411
Effexor XR Capsules (Rare) 3417
Lyrica Capsules (Rare) 2539

Chalazion
Invirase (Less than 2%) 2772
Soriatane Capsules (Less than 1%) 1013

Changes in blood glucose levels
Neurontin Capsules 2487
Neurontin Oral Solution 2487
Neurontin Tablets 2487
Ortho-Cyclen/Ortho Tri-Cyclen 2429

Character changes
Seromycin Capsules 1813

Charcot's syndrome
▲ Imdur Tablets (Less than or equal to 5%) 3018
▲ Mavik Tablets (3.8%) 486
ReoPro Vials (0.4%) 1809
Risperdal Consta Long-Acting Injection (Rare) 1682
Soriatane Capsules (Less than 1%) 1013
Timolide Tablets 2086

Cheek puffing
Moban Tablets 1119
Thiothixene Capsules 2165

Cheilitis
Accutane Capsules 2731

Actiq (Less than 1%) 979
Caduet Tablets (Less than 2%) 2508
Cosmegen for Injection 2459
Effexor Tablets (Rare) 3411
Effexor XR Capsules (Rare) 3417
Frova Tablets (Rare) 1113
Invirase (Less than 2%) 2772
Lipitor Tablets (Less than 2%) 2483
Norvir (Less than 2%) 503
Protopic Ointment (Greater than or equal to 1%) 638
Rilutek Tablets (Rare) 2930
Sonata Capsules (Rare) 1717
▲ Soriatane Capsules (More than 75%) 1013
Targretin Capsules 1747
Tequin Injection (Less than 0.1%) 938
Tequin Injection in 5% Dextrose (Less than 0.1%) 938
Tequin Tablets (Less than 0.1%) 938
Uniretic Tablets (Less than 1%) 3100
VFEND I.V. (Less than 2%) 2564
VFEND Oral Suspension (Less than 2%) 2564
VFEND Tablets (Less than 2%) 2564

Cheilosis
Calcium Disodium Versenate Injection 1851
Cuprimine Capsules (Rare) 1947

Chemosis
▲ Alrex Ophthalmic Suspension 0.2% (5% to 15%) ⊙246
▲ Lotemax Ophthalmic Suspension 0.5% (5% to 15%) ⊙251
▲ Zymar Ophthalmic Solution (1% to 4%) 575

Chest, pressure
Imitrex Injection (2%) 1463
▲ Imitrex Nasal Spray (2% to 3%) 1467
▲ Imitrex Tablets (2% to 3%) 1471

Chest congestion
Advair Diskus 100/50 1308
Advair Diskus 250/50 1308
Advair Diskus 500/50 1308
Advair HFA Inhalation Aerosol 1318
Aerobid/Aerobid-M (3% to 9%) 1171
▲ Azmacort Inhalation Aerosol (1% to 3%) 1726
Effexor Tablets (Infrequent) 3411
Effexor XR Capsules (Infrequent) 3417
Klonopin 2778
Rescriptor Tablets 2551

Chest numbness
Tessalon Capsules 1199
Tessalon Perles 1199

Chest pain, musculoskeletal
▲ Trelstar LA Suspension (13.2%) 3397
Wellbutrin SR Sustained-Release Tablets (Infrequent) 1607
▲ Wellbutrin XL Extended-Release Tablets (3% to 4%) 1613

Chest pain, substernal
Aciphex Tablets 1090
Adalat CC Tablets (Less than 1%) 2964
Effexor Tablets (Frequent) 3411
Effexor XR Capsules (Frequent) 3417
▲ Intron A for Injection (Less than 5%) 3024
Kaletra (Less than 2%) 476
Nexium Delayed-Release Capsules (Less than 1%) 655
Nexium I.V. (Less than 1%) 659
Norvir (Less than 2%) 503
▲ Photofrin for Injection (5%) 702
Protonix I.V. (Less than 1%) 3472
Protonix Tablets (Less than 1%) 3469
Reyataz Capsules (Less than 3%) 921
Tequin Injection (Less than 0.1%) 938
Tequin Injection in 5% Dextrose (Less than 0.1%) 938
Tequin Tablets (Less than 0.1%) 938
VFEND I.V. (Less than 2%) 2564
VFEND Oral Suspension (Less than 2%) 2564
VFEND Tablets (Less than 2%) 2564
Zoloft (Rare) 2586

Chest sound, abnormalities
Gengraf Capsules (1% to less than 3%) 459
▲ Imdur Tablets (Less than or equal to 5%) 3018
▲ Leustatin Injection (9%) 2357
Neoral Oral Solution (1% to less than 3%) 2259
Neoral Soft Gelatin Capsules (1% to less than 3%) 2259
Orthoclone OKT3 Sterile Solution 2360
Prinivil Tablets (Greater than 1%) 2052
Prinzide Tablets 2056
▲ Simulect for Injection (3% to 10%) 2284

Chest tightness
Abilify Oral Solution (Infrequent) 882
Abilify Oral Solution (Infrequent) 2450
Abilify Discmelt Orally Disintegrating Tablets (Infrequent) 882
Abilify Discmelt Orally Disintegrating Tablets (Infrequent) 2450
Abilify Tablets (Infrequent) 882
Abilify Tablets (Infrequent) 2450
Acetadote Injection (1%) 1031
▲ Adenocard Injection (7%) 617
Advair Diskus 100/50 1308
Advair Diskus 250/50 1308
Advair Diskus 500/50 1308
Advair HFA Inhalation Aerosol 1318
▲ Aerobid/Aerobid-M (1% to 3%) 1171
Alferon N Injection 1665
Allegra (Rare) 2844
Allegra-D 12 Hour Extended-Release Tablets (Rare) 2846
Allegra-D 24 Hour Extended-Release Tablets (Rare) 2849
BeneFix Vials (1.5%) 3408
Carimune NF 3499
Ceftin Tablets (0.1% to 1%) 1407
▲ Doxil Injection (Approximately 6.8%) 2351
Elitek 2890
Ethyol for Injection (Rare) 1898
Flebogamma 5%, Immune Globulin Intravenous (Human) 1658
Flovent Diskus 1443
Flovent HFA 1447
Gammagard Liquid 721
▲ Humate-P (6%) 3502
Hyperstat I.V. 3017
▲ Imitrex Injection (3%) 1463
Imitrex Nasal Spray (Infrequent) 1467
Imitrex Tablets (Frequent) 1471
Infed Injection 3390
Lexapro Oral Solution (Infrequent) 1190
Lexapro Tablets (Infrequent) 1190
Lithobid Tablets 1692
Maxair Autohaler (1.3%) 1852
▲ Maxalt Tablets (Less than 2% to 3%) 2008
▲ Maxalt-MLT Orally Disintegrating Tablets (Less than 2% to 3%) 2008
Meridia Capsules 489
Ortho-Cyclen/Ortho Tri-Cyclen 2429
Ortho Tri-Cyclen Lo Tablets 2436
Orthoclone OKT3 Sterile Solution 2360
▲ Relpax Tablets (1% to 4%) 2548
Sular Tablets (Very rare) 3122
Taxotere Injection Concentrate 2932
▲ Thrombate III (3 of 17) 3257
Tussionex Pennkinetic Extended-Release Suspension (Occasional) 3327
Ventavis Inhalation Solution 1020
Vivitrol 995
▲ Zomig Tablets (Common) 3519
Zomig Nasal Spray (1% to less than 2%) 3523
▲ Zomig-ZMT Tablets (Common) 3519

Chewing movements
Moban Tablets 1119
Thioridazine Hydrochloride Tablets 2163
Thiothixene Capsules 2165

CHF
(*see under* Congestive heart failure)

Chills
▲ Abelcet Injection (18%) 1141
Abilify Oral Solution (Infrequent) 882
Abilify Oral Solution (Infrequent) 2450
Abilify Discmelt Orally Disintegrating Tablets (Infrequent) 882
Abilify Discmelt Orally Disintegrating Tablets (Infrequent) 2450
Abilify Tablets (Infrequent) 882
Abilify Tablets (Infrequent) 2450
Aceon Tablets (2 mg, 4 mg, 8 mg) (0.3% to 1%) 3194
Aciphex Tablets 1090
▲ Actimmune (14%) 1671
Actiq (1% or greater) 979
▲ ADACEL Vaccine (0.5% to 15.1%) 2945
Adalat CC Tablets (Less than 1%) 2964
Advicor Tablets 1722
▲ Aerobid/Aerobid-M (1% to 3%) 1171
Aggrastat 1907
▲ Agrylin Capsules (1% to 5%) 3169
Albutein 5%, Albumin (Human) 1652
Albutein 25% , Albumin (Human) 1653
▲ Alferon N Injection (14% to 87%) 1665
Alinia for Oral Suspension (Less than 1%) 2835
Alinia Tablets (Less than 1%) 2835
Aloprim for Injection (Less than 1%) 2167
Alphanate, Antihemophilic Factor (Human) 1654
AlphaNine SD, Coagulation Factor IX (Human) 1656
Altoprev Extended-Release Tablets (Rare) 3109
▲ AmBisome for Injection (40% to 48.1%) 620
Amerge Tablets (Infrequent) 1339
▲ Amevive (6%) 626
Anaprox Tablets (Less than 1%) 2761
Anaprox DS Tablets (Less than 1%) 2761
Anzemet Injection (2%) 2859
Anzemet Tablets (1.3%) 2862
Aralast (0.1%) 717
Aricept Tablets (Infrequent) 1094
Aricept ODT Tablets (Infrequent) 1094
▲ Asacol Delayed-Release Tablets (3%) 2692
Avalide Tablets (2%) 888
Avalide Tablets (2%) 2874
Avapro Tablets (Less than 1%) 891
Avapro Tablets (Less than 1%) 2871
Axert Tablets (Infrequent) 2396
Azilect Tablets (Infrequent) 3293
BeneFix Vials (1.6%) 3408
▲ Betaseron for SC Injection (25%) 767
▲ Bexxar (1% to 18%) 1398
Bicillin C-R Injectable Suspension 1706
Buprenex Injectable (Less than 1%) 2716
Calcium Disodium Versenate Injection 1851
Campral Tablets (Frequent) 1174
▲ Camptosar Injection (0% to 14%) 2604
▲ Cancidas for Injection (0% to 13.8%) 1918
Carbatrol Capsules 3171
Carimune NF 3499
Ceftin Tablets (0.1% to 1%) 1407
▲ CellCept Capsules (3% to less than 20%) 2747
▲ CellCept Intravenous (3% to less than 20%) 2747
▲ CellCept Oral Suspension (3% to less than 20%) 2747
▲ CellCept Tablets (3% to less than 20%) 2747
▲ Cerezyme for Injection (Approximately 6.5%) 1270
Cesamet Capsules 3340
Chantix Tablets (Infrequent) 2517
▲ Chemet Capsules (5.2% to 15.7%) 2458
Cipro (Less than 1%) 2977
Cipro I.V. (1% or less) 2984
Cipro XR Tablets 2990
Clinoril Tablets (Less than 1 in 100) 1924
Clozaril Tablets (Less than 1%) 2184
Colazal Capsules 2838
▲ Combivir Tablets (10%) 1411
▲ Copaxone for Injection (4%) 3297
Coumadin for Injection (Infrequent) 898
Coumadin Tablets (Infrequent) 898
▲ CytoGam Intravenous (Less than 5%) 1895
Dantrium Capsules (Less frequent) 2694
Depacon Injection (1% or more) 412
Depakene (1% or more) 417
Depakote Sprinkle Capsules 422
▲ Depakote Tablets (1% to 5%) 427
Depakote ER Tablets (Greater than 1%) 434
Depo-Provera Contraceptive Injection (Less than 1%) 2622
Dilaudid 440
Dilaudid Non-Sterile Powder 440
Dilaudid Oral Liquid 445
Dilaudid Rectal Suppositories 440
Dilaudid Tablets 440
Dilaudid Tablets - 8 mg 445
Dilaudid-HP (Less frequent) 442
Dolobid Tablets (Less than 1 in 100) 1955
▲ Doxil Injection (1% to 5%) 2351
EC-Naprosyn Delayed-Release Tablets (Less than 1%) 2761
Edecrin 1959
▲ Effexor Tablets (2.2% to 6.8%) 3411
Effexor XR Capsules (Frequent) 3417
Eldepryl Capsules 3208
Elspar for Injection 2463
Elspar for Injection 1960
Engerix-B Vaccine (Less than 1%) 1425
▲ Epivir (10%) 1427
▲ Epivir-HBV (7%) 1432
Equetro Extended-Release Capsules 3180
▲ Erbitux (16%) 910
Ethyol for Injection 1898
Fansidar Tablets 2765
FazaClo Orally Disintegrating Tablets (Less than 1%) 551
Ferrlecit Injection 3388
Flebogamma 5%, Immune Globulin Intravenous (Human) 1658
Flexbumin I.V. (Occasional) 720
Fluarix 1451
▲ Flumist Vaccine (2.5% to 8.6%) 1901
Follistim AQ Cartridge 2338
Gabitril Tablets (Frequent) 984
▲ Gammagard Liquid (1.69% to 13.1%) 721
Gammagard S/D (Occasional) 724
Gantrisin Pediatric Suspension 2770
Gemzar for Injection (Common) 1771
Geodon Capsules (Frequent) 2529
Hemofil M (Extremely rare) 728
▲ Herceptin I.V. (32%) 1233
Human Albumin Grifols 20%, Albumin (Human) 1651
Human Albumin Grifols 25%, Albumin (Human) 1652
Humate-P (2%) 3502
▲ Hycamtin for Injection (69%) 1458
Imitrex Injection (Infrequent) 1463
Imitrex Nasal Spray (Infrequent) 1467
▲ Imitrex Tablets (2% to 3%) 1471
Infed Injection 3390
▲ Intron A for Injection (Up to 54%) 3024
Invanz for Injection (Greater than 0.1%) 1999
Ionsys Transdermal System (.1% to less than 1%) 2379
▲ I.V. Busulfex (46%) 2493
Kadian Capsules (Less than 3%) 577
Kaletra (Up to 2%) 476
Lamictal (1.3%) 1481
▲ Lariam Tablets (Among most frequent) 2786
Lescol Capsules (Rare) 2233
Lescol XL Tablets 2233
▲ Leukine (19% to 25%) 814
▲ Leustatin Injection (9%) 2357
Lexapro Oral Solution (Infrequent) 1190
Lexapro Tablets (Infrequent) 1190
Lotensin HCT Tablets (0.3% or more) 2246
Lyrica Capsules (0.1% to 1%) 2539
Marinol Capsules (Less than 1%) 3333
Matulane Capsules 3191
Maxalt Tablets (Infrequent) 2008
Maxalt-MLT Orally Disintegrating Tablets (Infrequent) 2008
▲ Menactra Vaccine (0.2% to 9.7%) 2954
Merrem I.V. (Greater than 0.1% to 1%) 686
Mevacor Tablets (Rare) 2021
Mintezol 2027
MS Contin Tablets (Less frequent) 2701
▲ Mylotarg for Injection (64% to 68%) 3431
Myobloc Injection (Greater than 2%) 3192
Nabi-HB 2169
Naprosyn Suspension (Less than 1%) 2761
Naprosyn Tablets (Less than 1%) 2761
▲ Neumega for Injection (Greater than or equal to 10%) 3435
Neurontin Capsules (Infrequent) 2487
Neurontin Oral Solution (Infrequent) 2487
Neurontin Tablets (Infrequent) 2487
Niaspan Extended-Release Tablets 1730
▲ Nipent for Injection (11% to 19%) 1863
Noroxin Tablets (Less frequent) 2032
Norvir (Less than 2%) 503
Omacor Capsules 2725
▲ Oncaspar (Greater than 5%) 1145
▲ Ontak Vials (81%) 1745
▲ Orthoclone OKT3 Sterile Solution (59%) 2360
▲ OxyContin Tablets (Between 1% and 5%) 2703
Parnate Tablets 1527
Paxil CR Controlled-Release Tablets (2%) 1538
Paxil (2%) 1530
Permax Tablets (1.1%) 3356
Pexeva Tablets (Infrequent to 2%) 1694
Plasbumin-5 (Rare) 3251
Plasbumin-20 (Rare) 3252
Plasbumin-25 (Rare) 3253
Pletal Tablets (Less than 2%) 2455
Pneumovax 23 (Common) 2043

Prevacid Delayed-Release Capsules (Less than 1%)............ 3271
Prevacid for Delayed-Release Oral Suspension (Less than 1%)........ 3271
Prevacid NapraPAC (Less than 1%).. 3280
Prevacid SoluTab Delayed-Release Orally Disintegrating Tablets (Less than 1%)............ 3271
PREVPAC (Less than 1%)............ 3284
Prinivil Tablets (0.3% to 1.0%)........ 2052
Prinzide Tablets............ 2056
▲ ProAmatine Tablets (4.9%)............ 3186
Profilnine SD, Factor IX Complex (Human)............ 1660
▲ Prograf Capsules and Injection (3% to 15%)............ 632
Prolastin (Occasional)............ 3255
▲ Proleukin for Injection (52%)............ 2266
Proquin XR Tablets............ 1153
ProSom Tablets (Infrequent)............ 517
Protonix I.V. (Less than 1%)............ 3472
Protonix Tablets (Less than 1%)............ 3469
Protopic Ointment (Greater than or equal to 1%)............ 638
Provigil Tablets (1%)............ 988
Prozac Pulvules and Liquid (Frequent)............ 1801
▲ Quadramet Injection (8.5%)............ 1040
▲ Rapamune Oral Solution and Tablets (3% to 20%)............ 3475
▲ Raptiva for Injection (13%)............ 1250
Recombinate (Extremely rare)............ 729
Recombivax HB (Less than 1%)............ 2071
ReFacto Vials............ 3484
Refludan for Injection (Uncommon)... 792
Relpax Tablets (Frequent)............ 2548
Rescriptor Tablets............ 2551
Retrovir Capsules............ 1560
Retrovir IV Infusion............ 1564
Retrovir............ 1560
Rhophylac (Occasionally)............ 3505
Rilutek Tablets (Infrequent)............ 2930
▲ Rituxan I.V. (3% to 33%)............ 1254
Rocephin Injectable Vials, ADD-Vantage, Galaxy, Bulk (Less than 1%)............ 2800
Seroquel Tablets (Infrequent)............ 690
Sonata Capsules (Infrequent)............ 1717
▲ Suboxone Tablets (6% to 7.5%)............ 2717
▲ Subutex Tablets (6% to 7.8%)............ 2717
Sular Tablets (Less than or equal to 1%)............ 3122
Symbyax Capsules (Frequent)............ 1819
▲ Targretin Capsules (9.5% to 13.2%)............ 1747
Tasmar Tablets (Infrequent)............ 3358
Taxotere Injection Concentrate............ 2932
Tegretol/Tegretol-XR............ 2295
▲ Tequin Injection (0.1% to 3%)............ 938
▲ Tequin Injection in 5% Dextrose (0.1% to 3%)............ 938
▲ Tequin Tablets (0.1% to 3%)............ 938
Tessalon Capsules............ 1199
Tessalon Perles............ 1199
▲ Thalomid Capsules (4.2%)............ 965
▲ Thiola Tablets (4%)............ 2141
▲ Thrombate III (2 of 17)............ 3257
▲ Thymoglobulin for Intravenous Infusion (57.3%)............ 1284
Thyrogen for Injection (1%)............ 1286
Ticlid Tablets............ 2810
Timentin ADD-Vantage............ 1580
Timentin Injection Galaxy Container............ 1583
Timentin IV Infusion............ 1577
Timentin Pharmacy Bulk Package.... 1586
▲ Trizivir Tablets (20%)............ 1589
Tygacil for Injection (0.2% to less than 2%)............ 3488
Uniretic Tablets (Less than 1%)............ 3100
Vancocin HCl Capsules, USP (Infrequent)............ 3380
Vantin Tablets and Oral Suspension (Less than 1%)............ 2645
Varivax (Greater than or equal to 1%)............ 2100
▲ VFEND I.V. (0.2% to 3.7%)............ 2564
▲ VFEND Oral Suspension (0.2% to 3.7%)............ 2564
▲ VFEND Tablets (0.2% to 3.7%)............ 2564
Viadur Implant (Less than 2%)............ 757
Viagra Tablets (Less than 2%)............ 2573
Vytorin 10/10 Tablets............ 2114
Vytorin 10/10 Tablets............ 3077
Vytorin 10/20 Tablets............ 2114
Vytorin 10/20 Tablets............ 3077
Vytorin 10/40 Tablets............ 2114
Vytorin 10/40 Tablets............ 3077
Vytorin 10/80 Tablets............ 2114
Vytorin 10/80 Tablets............ 3077
Wellbutrin Tablets (1.2%)............ 1603
Wellbutrin SR Sustained-Release Tablets (Infrequent)............ 1607
Wellbutrin XL Extended-Release Tablets (Infrequent)............ 1613
WinRho SDF (Less than 2%)............ 732
Xopenex Inhalation Solution (Less than 2%)............ 3146
Xopenex Inhalation Solution Concentrate (Less than 2%)............ 3150
Xopenex HFA Inhalation Aerosol (Less than 2%)............ 3154
▲ Zemplar Capsules (5%)............ 541
▲ Zemplar Injection (5%)............ 543
▲ Ziagen (6% to 9 %)............ 1626
Zocor Tablets (Rare)............ 2105
Zometa for Intravenous Infusion............ 2315
Zomig Tablets (Infrequent)............ 3519
Zomig Nasal Spray (Infrequent)............ 3523
Zomig-ZMT Tablets (Infrequent)............ 3519
Zyban Sustained-Release Tablets (Infrequent)............ 1644
Zyprexa Tablets (Infrequent)............ 1830
Zyprexa ZYDIS Orally Disintegrating Tablets (Infrequent)............ 1830

Chloasma

Angeliq Tablets............ 762
Climara Transdermal System............ 771
Climara Pro Transdermal System............ 776
Depo-Provera Contraceptive Injection (Less than 1%)............ 2622
depo-subQ provera 104 Injectable Suspension............ 2624
Enjuvia Tablets............ 1062
Estratest Tablets............ 3199
Estratest H.S. Tablets............ 3199
Menostar Transdermal System............ 782
Mircette Tablets............ 1066
NuvaRing............ 2340
Ortho-Cyclen Tablets............ 2429
Ortho Evra Transdermal System............ 2417
Ortho Tri-Cyclen Tablets............ 2429
Ortho Tri-Cyclen Lo Tablets............ 2436
Premarin Intravenous............ 3442
Premarin Vaginal Cream............ 3452
Premphase Tablets............ 3456
Prempro Tablets............ 3456
Prometrium Capsules (100 mg, 200 mg)............ 3203
Topamax Sprinkle Capsules (Rare)... 2404
Topamax Tablets (Rare)............ 2404

Chloasma, possibly persistent

Estrasorb Topical Emulsion............ 1147
Seasonique Tablets............ 1077

Chloride retention

Androxy Tablets............ 3335
Estratest Tablets............ 3199
Estratest H.S. Tablets............ 3199
Oxandrin Tablets............ 2962

Choking sensation

Advair Diskus 100/50............ 1308
Advair Diskus 250/50............ 1308
Advair Diskus 500/50............ 1308
Advair HFA Inhalation Aerosol............ 1318
Dantrium Intravenous............ 2695
Evoxac Capsules (Less than 1%)............ 1047
Hyperstat I.V.............. 3017
Relpax Tablets (Rare)............ 2548
Risperdal Consta Long-Acting Injection (Infrequent)............ 1682
Serevent Diskus (Rare)............ 1568

Cholangitis

Abelcet Injection............ 1141
Aciphex Tablets (Rare)............ 1090
▲ CellCept Capsules (3% to less than 20%)............ 2747
▲ CellCept Intravenous (3% to less than 20%)............ 2747
▲ CellCept Oral Suspension (3% to less than 20%)............ 2747
▲ CellCept Tablets (3% to less than 20%)............ 2747
Copegus Tablets (Less than 1%)............ 2754
Kaletra (Less than 2%)............ 476
Norvir (Less than 2%)............ 503
Pegasys (Less than 1%)............ 2789
▲ Prograf Capsules and Injection (3% to 15%)............ 632
Thalomid Capsules............ 965
Zonegran Capsules (Rare)............ 1101

Cholangitis, sclerosing

Doxil Injection (Less than 1%)............ 2351

Cholecystectomy

Prometrium Capsules (100 mg, 200 mg) (2%)............ 3203

Cholecystitis

Abelcet Injection............ 1141
Abilify Oral Solution (Infrequent)............ 882
Abilify Oral Solution (Infrequent)............ 2450
Abilify Discmelt Orally Disintegrating Tablets (Infrequent)............ 882
Abilify Discmelt Orally Disintegrating Tablets (Infrequent)............ 2450
Abilify Tablets (Infrequent)............ 882
Abilify Tablets (Infrequent)............ 2450
Aciphex Tablets............ 1090
Amevive............ 626
Aricept Tablets............ 1094
Aricept ODT Tablets............ 1094
Asacol Delayed-Release Tablets............ 2692
BiDil Tablets (1% to less than 2%)............ 2171
Campral Tablets (Rare)............ 1174
Celexa (Rare)............ 1176
Copaxone for Injection (Infrequent)... 3297
Dacogen Injection............ 2129
Effexor Tablets (Rare)............ 3411
Effexor XR Capsules (Rare)............ 3417
Enbrel for Injection (Infrequent)............ 584
Evoxac Capsules............ 1047
Exelon Capsules (Infrequent)............ 2206
Exelon Oral Solution (Infrequent)............ 2206
▲ Flovent Diskus (1% to 3%)............ 1443
Gabitril Tablets (Infrequent)............ 984
▲ Humira Injection (Less than 5%)............ 466
Kaletra (Less than 2%)............ 476
Lofibra Tablets............ 1219
Lofibra Capsules............ 1216
Lotronex Tablets (Rare)............ 1512
Lyrica Capsules (0.1% to 1%)............ 2539
Meridia Capsules............ 489
Neurontin Capsules (Rare)............ 2487
Neurontin Oral Solution (Rare)............ 2487
Neurontin Tablets (Rare)............ 2487
Permax Tablets (Rare)............ 3356
Proleukin for Injection............ 2266
Protonix I.V. (Less than 1%)............ 3472
Protonix Tablets (Less than 1%)............ 3469
Prozac Pulvules and Liquid (Rare)............ 1801
Remicade for IV Injection (Greater than or equal to 0.2%)............ 971
Requip Tablets (Infrequent)............ 1555
Revlimid Capsules............ 958
Rilutek Tablets (Rare)............ 2930
Risperdal (Rare)............ 1676
Risperdal M-Tab Orally Disintegrating Tablets (Rare)............ 1676
Tasmar Tablets (Rare)............ 3358
Tricor Tablets............ 527
Triglide Tablets............ 3123
▲ Ultram ER Tablets (1% to greater than 5%)............ 2392
VFEND I.V. (Less than 2%)............ 2564
VFEND Oral Suspension (Less than 2%)............ 2564
VFEND Tablets (Less than 2%)............ 2564
Vivitrol............ 995
Vytorin 10/10 Tablets............ 2114
Vytorin 10/10 Tablets............ 3077
Vytorin 10/20 Tablets............ 2114
Vytorin 10/20 Tablets............ 3077
Vytorin 10/40 Tablets............ 2114
Vytorin 10/40 Tablets............ 3077
Vytorin 10/80 Tablets............ 2114
Vytorin 10/80 Tablets............ 3077
Zelapar Tablets............ 3372
Zelnorm Tablets............ 2312
Zetia Tablets............ 2120
Zetia Tablets............ 3083
Zonegran Capsules (Rare)............ 1101

Cholelithiasis

Abilify Oral Solution (Infrequent)............ 882
Abilify Oral Solution (Infrequent)............ 2450
Abilify Discmelt Orally Disintegrating Tablets (Infrequent)............ 882
Abilify Discmelt Orally Disintegrating Tablets (Infrequent)............ 2450
Abilify Tablets (Infrequent)............ 882
Abilify Tablets (Infrequent)............ 2450
Aciphex Tablets............ 1090
Aggrenox Capsules (Less than 1%)............ 822
Aricept Tablets (Infrequent)............ 1094
Aricept ODT Tablets (Infrequent)............ 1094
Celebrex Capsules (Less than 0.1%)............ 3134
Celexa (Rare)............ 1176
Effexor Tablets (Rare)............ 3411
Effexor XR Capsules (Rare)............ 3417
Evoxac Capsules (Less than 1%)............ 1047
Fortical Nasal Spray (Less than 1%)............ 3337
Gabitril Tablets (Infrequent)............ 984
▲ Humira Injection (Less than 5%)............ 466
Invanz for Injection (Greater than 0.1%)............ 1999
Levaquin (0.1% to 0.9%)............ 2384
Levaquin in 5% Dextrose Injection (0.1% to 0.9%)............ 2384
Lofibra Tablets............ 1219
Lofibra Capsules............ 1216
Lunesta Tablets (Infrequent)............ 3142
Lyrica Capsules (0.1% to 1%)............ 2539
Meridia Capsules............ 489
Miacalcin Nasal Spray (Less than 1%)............ 2253
Neurontin Capsules (Rare)............ 2487
Neurontin Oral Solution (Rare)............ 2487
Neurontin Tablets (Rare)............ 2487
Paxil CR Controlled-Release Tablets (Rare)............ 1538
Paxil (Rare)............ 1530
Permax Tablets (Infrequent)............ 3356
Persantine Tablets (Rare)............ 868
Pexeva Tablets (rare)............ 1694
Pletal Tablets (Less than 2%)............ 2455
Prevacid Delayed-Release Capsules (Less than 1%)............ 3271
Prevacid for Delayed-Release Oral Suspension (Less than 1%)............ 3271
Prevacid NapraPAC (Less than 1%).. 3280
Prevacid SoluTab Delayed-Release Orally Disintegrating Tablets (Less than 1%)............ 3271
PREVPAC (Less than 1%)............ 3284
Protonix I.V. (Less than 1%)............ 3472
Protonix Tablets (Less than 1%)............ 3469
Prozac Pulvules and Liquid (Infrequent)............ 1801
Remicade for IV Injection (Greater than or equal to 0.2%)............ 971
Requip Tablets (Infrequent)............ 1555
Risperdal (Rare)............ 1676
Risperdal M-Tab Orally Disintegrating Tablets (Rare)............ 1676
Sonata Capsules (Rare)............ 1717
Symbyax Capsules (Infrequent)............ 1819
Tasmar Tablets (Infrequent)............ 3358
Tricor Tablets............ 527
Triglide Tablets............ 3123
Trileptal Tablets............ 2300
Trileptal Oral Suspension............ 2300
▲ Ultram ER Tablets (1% to greater than 5%)............ 2392
Uniretic Tablets (Less than 1%)............ 3100
VFEND I.V. (Less than 2%)............ 2564
VFEND Oral Suspension (Less than 2%)............ 2564
VFEND Tablets (Less than 2%)............ 2564
Vivitrol............ 995
Vytorin 10/10 Tablets............ 2114
Vytorin 10/10 Tablets............ 3077
Vytorin 10/20 Tablets............ 2114
Vytorin 10/20 Tablets............ 3077
Vytorin 10/40 Tablets............ 2114
Vytorin 10/40 Tablets............ 3077
Vytorin 10/80 Tablets............ 2114
Vytorin 10/80 Tablets............ 3077
Zelapar Tablets............ 3372
Zelnorm Tablets............ 2312
Zetia Tablets............ 2120
Zetia Tablets............ 3083
Zonegran Capsules (Infrequent)............ 1101

Cholestasis

Avandaryl Tablets............ 1379
Captopril Tablets (Rare)............ 2149
Ceftin............ 1407
Clinoril Tablets (Less than 1%)............ 1924
Clozaril Tablets............ 2184
Dolobid Tablets (Less than 1 in 100)............ 1955
Eraxis for Injection (Less than 1% to less than 2%)............ 2521
FazaClo Orally Disintegrating Tablets............ 551
Fortaz............ 1453
Maxipime for Injection............ 1105
Mefoxin for Injection............ 2012
Mefoxin Premixed Intravenous Solution............ 2016
Mintezol............ 2027
NeoProfen Injection............ 2472
Norvasc Tablets............ 2545
Omnicef Capsules............ 511
Omnicef for Oral Suspension............ 511
Suprax............ 1843
Tambocor Tablets (Rare)............ 1856
Ticlid Tablets............ 2810
Vantin Tablets and Oral Suspension............ 2645
Zinacef for Injection............ 1631
Zinacef Injection............ 1631
Zyrtec Chewable Tablets (Rare)............ 2594
Zyrtec (Rare)............ 2594
Zyrtec-D 12 Hour Extended Release Tablets (Rare)............ 2597

Cholestasis, intrahepatic
Amoxil Capsules 1343
Amoxil Chewable Tablets 1343
Amoxil Pediatric Drops for Oral Suspension 1343
Amoxil Powder for Oral Suspension 1343
Amoxil Tablets 1343
Cuprimine Capsules (Rare) 1947

Cholestatic hepatic injury
Axid Oral Solution (Rare) 879
Coumadin for Injection (Infrequent) 898
Coumadin Tablets (Infrequent) 898

Cholesterol, systemic, microembolism
Coumadin for Injection (Infrequent) 898
Coumadin Tablets (Infrequent) 898

Cholinergic reactions
Camptosar Injection 2604
Evoxac Capsules 1047
Risperdal (Rare) 1676
Risperdal M-Tab Orally Disintegrating Tablets (Rare) 1676

Choluria
Xifaxan Tablets (Less than 2%) 2842

Chondrocalcinosis pyrophosphate
Revlimid Capsules 958

Chondrodystrophy
Prozac Pulvules and Liquid (Rare) 1801

Chorea
Angeliq Tablets 762
Climara Transdermal System 771
Climara Pro Transdermal System 776
Dilaudid-HP 442
Eldepryl Capsules 3208
Enjuvia Tablets 1062
Estrasorb Topical Emulsion 1147
Estratest Tablets 3199
Estratest H.S. Tablets 3199
Klonopin 2778
Menostar Transdermal System 782
Phenytek Capsules (Rare) 2160
Premarin Intravenous 3442
Premarin Tablets 3446
Premarin Vaginal Cream 3452
Premphase Tablets 3456
Prempro Tablets 3456

Chorea, exacerbation of
Seasonique Tablets 1077

Choreiform
Parcopa Orally Disintegrating Tablets (Common) 3097

Choreoathetosis
Celexa 1176
Gabitril Tablets (Infrequent) 984
Geodon Capsules (Frequent) 2529
Lexapro Oral Solution 1190
Lexapro Tablets 1190
Neurontin Capsules (Rare) 2487
Neurontin Oral Solution (Rare) 2487
Neurontin Tablets (Rare) 2487
Pexeva Tablets (Rare) 1694
Requip Tablets (Infrequent) 1555
Seroquel Tablets (Rare) 690

Choreoathetotic movements
Aldoril Tablets 1910
Lamictal (Rare) 1481
Lithobid Tablets 1692
Neurontin Capsules (Rare) 2487
Neurontin Oral Solution (Rare) 2487
Neurontin Tablets (Rare) 2487
Paxil CR Controlled-Release Tablets (Rare) 1538
Paxil (Rare) 1530
Permax Tablets (Frequent) 3356
Risperdal (Rare) 1676
Risperdal M-Tab Orally Disintegrating Tablets (Rare) 1676
Tasmar Tablets (Infrequent) 3358
Thioridazine Hydrochloride Tablets 2163
Zoloft (Rare) 2586
Zyprexa Tablets (1% to 2%) 1830
Zyprexa ZYDIS Orally Disintegrating Tablets (1% to 2%) 1830

Chorioretinitis
Neurontin Capsules (Rare) 2487
Neurontin Oral Solution (Rare) 2487
Neurontin Tablets (Rare) 2487
Stromectol Tablets 2083

Choroidal detachment
▲ Retisert Implant (5% to 9%) ⊙258

Choroidal detachment, post-filtration procedures
Cosopt Sterile Ophthalmic Solution 1931
Timoptic Sterile Ophthalmic Solution 2088
Timoptic in Ocudose 2091
Timoptic-XE Sterile Ophthalmic Gel Forming Solution 2092
Trusopt Sterile Ophthalmic Solution 2095

Choroiditis
Stromectol Tablets 2083

Chromatopsia
Cipro (Less than 1%) 2977
Cipro I.V. (1% or less) 2984
Cipro XR Tablets 2990
Effexor Tablets (Rare) 3411
Effexor XR Capsules (Rare) 3417
Levitra Tablets (Less than 2%) 3034
Proquin XR Tablets 1153
VFEND I.V. (0.4% to 1.2%) 2564
VFEND Oral Suspension (0.4% to 1.2%) 2564
VFEND Tablets (0.4% to 1.2%) 2564

Chromaturia
Rescriptor Tablets 2551
Xyrem Oral Solution (Infrequent) 1688

Chromosomal abnormalities
Mustargen for Injection 2468

Churg-Strauss syndrome
Accolate Tablets (Rare) 671
Advair Diskus 100/50 (Rare) 1308
Advair Diskus 250/50 (Rare) 1308
Advair Diskus 500/50 (Rare) 1308
Flovent Diskus (Rare) 1443
Flovent HFA (Rare) 1447
Singulair 2077

Circulatory collapse
Amerge Tablets 1339
Decadron Tablets 1951
Furosemide Tablets 2154

Circulatory collapse, peripheral
▲ Intron A for Injection (Less than or equal to 5%) 3024
Lithobid Tablets 1692

Circulatory depression
Actiq 979
Dilaudid 440
Dilaudid Oral Liquid 445
Dilaudid Tablets - 8 mg 445
Dilaudid-HP 442
MS Contin Tablets 2701
OxyContin Tablets 2703

Circulatory failure
Ambien Tablets (Rare) 2851
Ambien CR Tablets (Rare) 2855
Dilaudid 440
Levaquin (0.1% to 0.9%) 2384
Levaquin in 5% Dextrose Injection (0.1% to 0.9%) 2384
Prevacid Delayed-Release Capsules (Less than 1%) 3271
Prevacid for Delayed-Release Oral Suspension (Less than 1%) 3271
Prevacid NapraPAC (Less than 1%) 3280
Prevacid SoluTab Delayed-Release Orally Disintegrating Tablets (Less than 1%) 3271
PREVPAC (Less than 1%) 3284
Remicade for IV Injection (Greater than or equal to 0.2%) 971
Trasylol Injection 754
Zosyn (1.0% or less) 3492

Circulatory overload
Albutein 5%, Albumin (Human) 1652
Albutein 25% , Albumin (Human) 1653

Cirrhosis, hepatic
(*see under* Cirrhosis of liver)

Cirrhosis of liver
Advicor Tablets (Rare) 1722
Altoprev Extended-Release Tablets 3109
Campral Tablets (Infrequent) 1174
Colazal Capsules 2838
Lescol Capsules (Rare) 2233
Lescol XL Tablets (Rare) 2233
Mevacor Tablets (Rare) 2021
Pentasa Capsules 3185
Tracleer Tablets (Rare) 545
Vytorin 10/10 Tablets (Rare) 2114
Vytorin 10/10 Tablets (Rare) 3077
Vytorin 10/20 Tablets (Rare) 2114
Vytorin 10/20 Tablets (Rare) 3077
Vytorin 10/40 Tablets (Rare) 2114
Vytorin 10/40 Tablets (Rare) 3077
Vytorin 10/80 Tablets (Rare) 2114
Vytorin 10/80 Tablets (Rare) 3077
Zocor Tablets (Rare) 2105

Clamminess
Eligard 22.5 mg (Less than 2%) 2883
▲ Eligard 30 mg (4.4%) 2885
Evoxac Capsules (Less than 1%) 1047
Exelon Capsules (Infrequent) 2206
Exelon Oral Solution (Infrequent) 2206
▲ Intron A for Injection (Less than 5%) 3024
Migranal Nasal Spray (Infrequent) 3348
Norvasc Tablets (Less than 0.1%) 2545
Opana Tablets (Less than 1%) 1122
Opana ER Tablets (Less than 1%) 1126
▲ Ultram ER Tablets (1% to greater than 5%) 2392
Xifaxan Tablets (Less than 2%) 2842
Zoloft (Infrequent) 2586

Claudication
Blocadren Tablets 1916
Cosopt Sterile Ophthalmic Solution 1931
Covera-HS Tablets (Less than 2%) 3139
Lopressor Injection 2238
Lopressor Tablets 2238
Namenda (More than one patient) 1195
Tarka Tablets 524
Timolide Tablets 2086
Timoptic Sterile Ophthalmic Solution 2088
Timoptic in Ocudose 2091
Timoptic-XE Sterile Ophthalmic Gel Forming Solution 2092
Verelan PM Extended-Release Capsules, Controlled-Onset (2% or less) 3106

Claudication, intermittent
(*see under* Charcot's syndrome)

Cleft palate, neonatal
Accutane Capsules 2731
Proventil Inhalation Aerosol 3053
Proventil Inhalation Solution 0.083% 3055

Clitoris, enlargement
(*see under* Clitoromegaly)

Clitoromegaly
▲ Androxy Tablets (Most Common) 3335
Estratest Tablets 3199
Estratest H.S. Tablets 3199
Oxandrin Tablets 2962

Clotting disorder, intravascular
Cosmegen for Injection 2459

Clotting factors, suppression of
Androxy Tablets 3335

Clotting time, prolongation
Oncaspar (Less than 1%) 1145
Testim 1% Gel (Less than 1%) 695
Zosyn 3492

CNS, unresponsiveness, unspecified
Cipro I.V. 2984
Cipro XR Tablets 2990

CNS abnormalities, fetal
Accutane Capsules 2731

CNS depression
Anaprox Tablets (Less than 1%) 2761
Anaprox DS Tablets (Less than 1%) 2761
Cesamet Capsules 3340
Depacon Injection 412
Depakene 417
Depakote Tablets 427
Depakote ER Tablets 434
Diastat Rectal Delivery System 3343
EC-Naprosyn Delayed-Release Tablets (Less than 1%) 2761
▲ Klonopin (Most frequent) 2778
Lamictal (Infrequent) 1481
Lidoderm Patch 1118
Naprosyn Suspension (Less than 1%) 2761
Naprosyn Tablets (Less than 1%) 2761
Nembutal Sodium Solution, USP (Less than 1%) 2470
Neurontin Capsules 2487
Neurontin Oral Solution 2487
Neurontin Tablets 2487
Opana Tablets (Less than 1%) 1122
Opana ER Tablets (Less than 1%) 1126
Prozac Pulvules and Liquid (Infrequent) 1801
Rilutek Tablets (Rare) 2930
Synera Topical Patch 1137
▲ Vesanoid Capsules (3%) 2820

CNS reactions
Attenuvax 1914
Clozaril Tablets 2184
▲ Intron A for Injection (Less than 5%) 3024
Lanoxicaps Capsules (Rare) 1490
Lanoxin Injection 1494
Lanoxin Injection Pediatric 1497
Lanoxin Tablets 1500
Lariam Tablets 2786
▲ Leukine (11%) 814
▲ Nipent for Injection (1% to 11%) 1863
Noroxin Tablets 2032
Orthoclone OKT3 Sterile Solution 2360
Stalevo Tablets 2287

CNS stimulation
Adipex-P 1215
Avelox 2970
Axert Tablets (Infrequent) 2396
Cafcit 1886
Cesamet Capsules 3340
Cipro 2977
Cipro I.V. 2984
Cipro XR Tablets 2990
Clarinex-D 24-Hour Extended-Release Tablets 2998
Combivent Inhalation Aerosol 847
Effexor Tablets (Infrequent) 3411
Effexor XR Capsules (Infrequent) 3417
Kytril Injection (Less than 2%) 2781
Lamictal (Rare) 1481
Lidoderm Patch 1118
Meridia Capsules (1.5%) 489
Mirapex Tablets (Less than 1%) 859
Noroxin Tablets 2032
Paxil CR Controlled-Release Tablets (Frequent) 1538
Paxil (Frequent) 1530
Proventil Inhalation Aerosol 3053
Proventil HFA Inhalation Aerosol 3056
Prozac Pulvules and Liquid (Infrequent) 1801
Synera Topical Patch 1137
Tequin Injection 938
Tequin Injection in 5% Dextrose 938
Tequin Tablets 938
Ventolin HFA Inhalation Aerosol 1600
VoSpire ER Tablets 1052
Wellbutrin SR Sustained-Release Tablets (1% to 2%) 1607
Wellbutrin XL Extended-Release Tablets (1% to 2%) 1613
Zyban Sustained-Release Tablets (Infrequent) 1644
Zyprexa Tablets (Infrequent) 1830
Zyprexa ZYDIS Orally Disintegrating Tablets (Infrequent) 1830
Zyrtec-D 12 Hour Extended Release Tablets 2597

CNS stimulation, paradoxical
Diastat Rectal Delivery System 3343
Niravam Orally Disintegrating Tablets (Rare) 3092
Numorphan Injection 1120

CNS toxicity
DepoCyt Injection 1143
▲ Nipent for Injection (1% to 11%) 1863

Coagulation defects, neonatal
Phenytek Capsules 2160

Coagulation dysfunction
Abelcet Injection 1141
AmBisome for Injection (Less common) 620
Campath Ampules 811
Celexa (Rare) 1176
▲ CellCept Capsules (3% to less than 20%) 2747
▲ CellCept Intravenous (3% to less than 20%) 2747

▲ CellCept Oral Suspension (3% to less than 20%) 2747
▲ CellCept Tablets (3% to less than 20%) 2747
Depacon Injection 412
Depakene 417
Depakote Tablets 427
Depakote ER Tablets 434
Elspar for Injection 2463
Elspar for Injection 1960
Estratest Tablets 3199
Estratest H.S. Tablets 3199
Herceptin I.V. (At least one of the 958 patients) 1233
▲ Leukine (19%) 814
Neurontin Capsules 2487
Neurontin Oral Solution 2487
Neurontin Tablets 2487
Nimotop Capsules (Less than 1%) 749
NovoSeven (1%) 2331
Omnicef Capsules 511
Omnicef for Oral Suspension 511
Oncaspar (Less than 1%) 1145
Orthoclone OKT3 Sterile Solution 2360
Plavix Tablets (1% to 2.5%) 917
Plavix Tablets (1% to 2.5%) 2926
Premarin Intravenous 3442
Premarin Vaginal Cream 3452
▲ Prograf Capsules and Injection (3% to 15%) 632
▲ Proleukin for Injection (10%) 2266
Quadramet Injection (1.5%) 1040
Rituxan I.V. (0.3%) 1254
Symbyax Capsules (Rare) 1819
▲ Xeloda Tablets (Less than 5%) 2822

Coagulation tests, altered results
Zosyn 3492

Coagulation time, increase in
Arthrotec Tablets (Rare) 3129
Zoloft 2586

Coagulopathy
Aggrenox Capsules 822
Bayer Aspirin 744
Bayer Aspirin Comprehensive Prescribing Information ▣796
Enbrel for Injection 584
Eraxis for Injection (Less than 1% to less than 2%) 2521
Mycamine for Injection 628
NovoSeven 2331
Oncaspar 1145
Revlimid Capsules 958
St. Joseph 81 mg Aspirin Chewable and Enteric Coated Tablets 1869
St. Joseph 81 mg Aspirin ▣688

Coccidioidomycosis, disseminated
Remicade for IV Injection 971

Cochlear lesion
DAPTACEL Vaccine 2950

Cognition, decreased
Ambien CR Tablets (Infrequent) 2855

Cognitive dysfunction
Ambien Tablets (Infrequent) 2851
Amerge Tablets (Infrequent) 1339
Anaprox Tablets (Rare) 2761
Anaprox DS Tablets (Rare) 2761
EC-Naprosyn Delayed-Release Tablets (Rare) 2761
Naprosyn Suspension (Rare) 2761
Naprosyn Tablets (Rare) 2761
▲ Niravam Orally Disintegrating Tablets (10.3% to 28.8%) 3092
Orthoclone OKT3 Sterile Solution 2360
Prevacid NapraPAC (Less than 1%) 3280
Rescriptor Tablets 2551
Risperdal 1676
Risperdal M-Tab Orally Disintegrating Tablets 1676
▲ Topamax Sprinkle Capsules (0% to 7%) 2404
▲ Topamax Tablets (0% to 7%) 2404
Zyvox 2652

Cogwheel rigidity
Abilify Oral Solution (Infrequent) 882
Abilify Oral Solution (Infrequent) 2450
Abilify Discmelt Orally Disintegrating Tablets (Infrequent) 882
Abilify Discmelt Orally Disintegrating Tablets (Infrequent) 2450
Abilify Tablets (Infrequent) 882
Abilify Tablets (Infrequent) 2450
Geodon (Frequent) 2529
Lithobid Tablets 1692
Lyrica Capsules (Rare) 2539
Paxil CR Controlled-Release Tablets 1538
Paxil 1530
Pexeva Tablets 1694
Symbyax Capsules (Infrequent) 1819
Thioridazine Hydrochloride Tablets 2163
Thiothixene Capsules 2165
▲ Zyprexa Tablets (8% to 20%) 1830
▲ Zyprexa IntraMuscular (2% to 4%) 1830
▲ Zyprexa ZYDIS Orally Disintegrating Tablets (8% to 20%) 1830

Cold, reduced tolerance
Coumadin for Injection (Infrequent) 898
Coumadin Tablets (Infrequent) 898

Cold sensations
Aceon Tablets (2 mg, 4 mg, 8 mg) (0.3% to 1%) 3194
Aricept Tablets (Infrequent) 1094
Aricept ODT Tablets (Infrequent) 1094
Buprenex Injectable (Less than 1%) 2716
Coumadin for Injection (Infrequent) 898
Coumadin Tablets (Infrequent) 898
Ethyol for Injection 1898
▲ Frova Tablets (3%) 1113
Guanidine Hydrochloride Tablets 3016
Imitrex Injection (Rare) 1463
▲ Imitrex Nasal Spray (2% to 3%) 1467
▲ Imitrex Tablets (2% to 3%) 1471
Migranal Nasal Spray (Infrequent) 3348
Prograf Capsules and Injection 632
Synera Topical Patch 1137
Xyrem Oral Solution (Infrequent) 1688
Zofran Injection (2%) 1634

Cold sore, non-herpetic
▲ Intron A for Injection (Less than 5%) 3024
Varivax (Greater than or equal to 1%) 2100

Cold symptoms, unspecified
▲ AccuNeb Inhalation Solution (Up to 3.4%) 1055
▲ Aerobid/Aerobid-M (15%) 1171
▲ Alamast Ophthalmic Solution (10% to 25%) 3381
Carac Cream, 0.5% (2.3%) 2879
▲ Cutivate Lotion 0.05% (4%) 2664
▲ Elestat Ophthalmic Solution (Approximately 10%) 1669
▲ Geodon Capsules (8%) 2529
Patanol Ophthalmic Solution (Less than 5%) 561
Paxil CR Controlled-Release Tablets 1538
Paxil 1530
Prinivil Tablets (1.1%) 2052
▲ ProSom Tablets (3%) 517
▲ Sandostatin Injection (1% to 4%) 2278
Somavert Injection 2642
▲ Trizivir Tablets (Greater than or equal to 5%) 1589
▲ Xalatan Sterile Ophthalmic Solution (Approximately 4%) 2649

Coldness of extremities
▲ Blocadren Tablets (8%) 1916
Cosopt Sterile Ophthalmic Solution 1931
Effexor Tablets (Infrequent) 3411
Effexor XR Capsules (Infrequent) 3417
Gleevec Tablets (Infrequent) 2227
Lithobid Tablets 1692
Lopressor Injection (1%) 2238
Lopressor Tablets (1%) 2238
Lopressor HCT 50/25 Tablets 2241
Lopressor HCT 100/25 Tablets 2241
Lopressor HCT 100/50 Tablets 2241
Maxalt Tablets (Infrequent) 2008
Maxalt-MLT Orally Disintegrating Tablets (Infrequent) 2008
ReoPro Vials (0.2%) 1809
Rythmol SR Capsules 2727
Strattera Capsules 1814
Timolide Tablets 2086
Timoptic Sterile Ophthalmic Solution 2088
Timoptic in Ocudose 2091
Timoptic-XE Sterile Ophthalmic Gel Forming Solution 2092
Toprol-XL Tablets (About 1 of 100 patients) 668
Xyrem Oral Solution (Infrequent) 1688

Colds, susceptibility
Betimol Ophthalmic Solution (1% to 5%) 3382
Betimol Ophthalmic Solution (1% to 5%) ⊙295
Hytrin Capsules (At least 1%) 471
Prinzide Tablets (0.3% to 1%) 2056

Colic
Invirase (Less than 2%) 2772
Prevnar for Injection 3463

Colic, biliary
Kadian Capsules (Less than 3%) 577

Colitis
Abilify Oral Solution (Frequent) 882
Abilify Oral Solution (Frequent) 2450
Abilify Discmelt Orally Disintegrating Tablets (Frequent) 882
Abilify Discmelt Orally Disintegrating Tablets (Frequent) 2450
Abilify Tablets (Frequent) 882
Abilify Tablets (Frequent) 2450
Accutane Capsules 2731
Aciphex Tablets 1090
▲ Actonel Tablets (0.8% to 3.3%) 2683
Actonel with Calcium Tablets (0.8% to 2.5%) 2688
Aldoril Tablets 1910
Alimta for Injection (Rare) 1750
Anaprox Tablets (Less than 1%) 2761
Anaprox DS Tablets (Less than 1%) 2761
▲ Avastin IV (1% to 6%) 1227
Azilect Tablets (Infrequent) 3293
Benzaclin Topical Gel 2877
Caduet Tablets (Less than 2%) 2508
Campath Ampules 811
Campral Tablets (Rare) 1174
Camptosar Injection (Rare) 2604
Canasa Rectal Suppositories (1.2%) 699
Celebrex Capsules (Less than 0.1%) 3134
Celexa (Rare) 1176
CellCept Capsules 2747
CellCept Intravenous 2747
CellCept Oral Suspension 2747
CellCept Tablets 2747
Cleocin Vaginal Ovules 2616
Clindagel 1203
Clinoril Tablets (Less than 1%) 1924
Copaxone for Injection (Infrequent) 3297
Copegus Tablets (Less than 1%) 2754
Doxil Injection (Less than 1%) 2351
Duac Topical Gel 3212
EC-Naprosyn Delayed-Release Tablets (Less than 1%) 2761
Effexor Tablets (Infrequent) 3411
Effexor XR Capsules (Infrequent) 3417
Eligard 7.5 mg (2.5%) 2880
Elmiron Capsules (Less than or equal to 1%) 2415
Eloxatin for Injection 2892
Evoclin Foam, 1% (Rarely) 1009
Exelon Capsules (Infrequent) 2206
Exelon Oral Solution (Infrequent) 2206
Fleet Prep Kits 1170
Fortaz 1453
Gleevec Tablets (Rare) 2227
Herceptin I.V. (At least one of the 958 patients) 1233
▲ Imitrex Nasal Spray (2% to 3%) 1467
Imitrex Tablets 1471
Invanz for Injection (1.7%) 1999
Keflex Capsules 549
Lipitor Tablets (Less than 2%) 2483
Lofibra Tablets 1219
Lofibra Capsules 1216
Lotronex Tablets (Rare) 1512
Lunesta Tablets (Rare) 3142
Lyrica Capsules (0.1% to 1%) 2539
Maxipime for Injection (Greater than 0.1% to less than 1%) 1105
Mefoxin for Injection 2012
Mefoxin Premixed Intravenous Solution 2016
Mircette Tablets 1066
Mobic Oral Suspension (Less than 2%) 863
Mobic Tablets (Less than 2%) 863
Myfortic Tablets 2255
Namenda 1195
Naprosyn Suspension (Less than 1%) 2761
Naprosyn Tablets (Less than 1%) 2761
Neurontin Capsules (Rare) 2487
Neurontin Oral Solution (Rare) 2487
Neurontin Tablets (Rare) 2487
Norvir (Less than 2%) 503
NuvaRing 2340
Omacor Capsules 2725
Oncaspar 1145
Ortho-Cyclen Tablets 2429
Ortho Evra Transdermal System 2417
Ortho Tri-Cyclen Tablets 2429
Ortho Tri-Cyclen Lo Tablets 2436
Paxil CR Controlled-Release Tablets (Rare) 1538
Paxil (Rare) 1530
Permax Tablets (Rare) 3356
Pexeva Tablets (Infrequent) 1694
Plavix Tablets 917
Plavix Tablets 2926
Pletal Tablets (Less than 2%) 2455
Prevacid Delayed-Release Capsules (Less than 1%) 3271
Prevacid for Delayed-Release Oral Suspension (Less than 1%) 3271
Prevacid NapraPAC (Less than 1%) 3280
Prevacid SoluTab Delayed-Release Orally Disintegrating Tablets (Less than 1%) 3271
Prevnar for Injection 3463
PREVPAC (Less than 1%) 3284
Prograf Capsules and Injection 632
Proleukin for Injection 2266
Protonix I.V. (Less than 1%) 3472
Protonix Tablets (Less than 1%) 3469
Protopic Ointment (0.2% to less than 1%) 638
Prozac Pulvules and Liquid (Infrequent) 1801
Requip Tablets (Infrequent) 1555
Rescriptor Tablets 2551
Reyataz Capsules (Less than 3%) 921
Risperdal Consta Long-Acting Injection (Infrequent) 1682
Rocephin Injectable Vials, ADD-Vantage, Galaxy, Bulk (Rare) 2800
▲ Sandostatin LAR Depot (1% to 4%) 2280
Seasonique Tablets 1077
Sonata Capsules (Less than 1%) 1717
Sular Tablets (Less than or equal to 1%) 3122
Suprax 1843
Symbyax Capsules (Infrequent) 1819
Targretin Capsules 1747
Tasmar Tablets (Infrequent) 3358
Tequin Injection (Less than 0.1%) 938
Tequin Injection in 5% Dextrose (Less than 0.1%) 938
Tequin Tablets (Less than 0.1%) 938
Thalomid Capsules 965
Ticlid Tablets 2810
Tricor Tablets 527
Triglide Tablets 3123
Trileptal Tablets 2300
Trileptal Oral Suspension 2300
Uniretic Tablets (Less than 1%) 3100
Vivitrol 995
Voltaren Tablets (Rarely) 2307
Voltaren-XR Tablets (Rarely) 2310
Wellbutrin Tablets (Rare) 1603
Wellbutrin SR Sustained-Release Tablets 1607
Wellbutrin XL Extended-Release Tablets 1613
Yasmin 28 Tablets 796
Yaz Tablets 803
Zelapar Tablets 3372
Zinacef for Injection 1631
Zinacef Injection 1631
Zoloft (Rare) 2586
Zomig Nasal Spray (Rare) 3523
Zonegran Capsules (Rare) 1101
Zyban Sustained-Release Tablets 1644

Colitis, hemorrhagic
Augmentin ES-600 Powder for Oral Suspension 1366
Pegasys (Less than 1%) 2789
PEG-Intron Powder for Injection 3048

Colitis, ischemic
Blocadren Tablets 1916
Cosopt Sterile Ophthalmic Solution 1931
Imitrex Injection 1463
Imitrex Nasal Spray 1467
Imitrex Tablets 1471
InnoPran XL Capsules 2723
Lotronex Tablets (Infrequent) 1512
Nadolol Tablets 2159
Pegasys (Less than 1%) 2789
PEG-Intron Powder for Injection 3048
Revlimid Capsules 958
Timoptic-XE Sterile Ophthalmic Gel Forming Solution 2092
Zelnorm Tablets 2312
Zomig Nasal Spray (Very rare) 3523

Colitis, lymphocytic
Plavix Tablets 917
Plavix Tablets 2926

Colitis, pseudomembranous
Amoxil Capsules 1343
Amoxil Chewable Tablets 1343
Amoxil Pediatric Drops for Oral Suspension 1343
Amoxil Powder for Oral Suspension 1343
Amoxil Tablets 1343
Augmentin 1360
Augmentin Tablets 1363
Augmentin XR Extended-Release Tablets 1369
Augmentin ES-600 Powder for Oral Suspension 1366
Avelox (Less than 0.1%) 2970
Benzaclin Topical Gel 2877
Biaxin/Biaxin XL 402
Bicillin C-R Injectable Suspension 1706
Campath Ampules 811
Ceftin 1407
Cipro 2977
Cipro I.V. (1% or less) 2984
Cipro XR Tablets 2990
Cleocin Vaginal Ovules 2616
Clindagel 1203
Duac Topical Gel 3212
E.E.S. 451
EryPed 447
Ery-Tab Tablets (Rare) 449
Erythrocin Stearate Filmtab Tablets (Rare) 453
Erythromycin Base Filmtab Tablets (Rare) 455
Erythromycin Delayed-Release Capsules, USP (Rare) 457
Evoclin Foam, 1% (Rarely) 1009
Fortaz (Less frequent) 1453
Gantrisin Pediatric Suspension 2770
Invanz for Injection 1999
Keflex Capsules 549
Levaquin (0.1% to 0.9%) 2384
Levaquin in 5% Dextrose Injection (0.1% to 0.9%) 2384
Maxipime for Injection (Greater than 0.1% to less than 1%) 1105
Mefoxin for Injection 2012
Mefoxin Premixed Intravenous Solution 2016
Merrem I.V. 686
Noroxin Tablets 2032
Omnicef Capsules 511
Omnicef for Oral Suspension 511
PCE Dispertab Tablets 515
PREVPAC 3284
Primaxin I.M. 2045
Primaxin I.V. (Less than 0.2%) 2048
Proquin XR Tablets 1153
Raniclor Tablets, Chewable (Rare) 2505
Revlimid Capsules 958
Rocephin Injectable Vials, ADD-Vantage, Galaxy, Bulk 2800
Suprax (Several patients) 1843
Tamiflu Capsules (Less than 1%) 2807
Tamiflu Oral Suspension (Less than 1%) 2807
Tequin Injection (Less than 0.1%) 938
Tequin Injection in 5% Dextrose (Less than 0.1%) 938
Tequin Tablets (Less than 0.1%) 938
Timentin ADD-Vantage 1580
Timentin Injection Galaxy Container 1583
Timentin IV Infusion 1577
Timentin Pharmacy Bulk Package 1586
Tygacil for Injection 3488
Vantin Tablets and Oral Suspension (Less than 1%) 2645
VFEND I.V. (Less than 2%) 2564
VFEND Oral Suspension (Less than 2%) 2564
VFEND Tablets (Less than 2%) 2564
Zinacef for Injection 1631
Zinacef Injection 1631
Zmax for Oral Suspension 2583
Zosyn (One patient) 3492
Zyvox 2652

Colitis, ulcerative
Camptosar Injection 2604
Evoxac Capsules (Less than 1%) 1047
Indocin (Less than 1%) 1995
Lotronex Tablets (Rare) 1512
Pegasys (Less than 1%) 2789
Plavix Tablets 917
Plavix Tablets 2926
Prevacid Delayed-Release Capsules (Less than 1%) 3271
Prevacid for Delayed-Release Oral Suspension (Less than 1%) 3271
Prevacid NapraPAC (Less than 1%) 3280
Prevacid SoluTab Delayed-Release Orally Disintegrating Tablets (Less than 1%) 3271
PREVPAC (Less than 1%) 3284
Protonix I.V. (Less than 1%) 3472
Protonix Tablets (Less than 1%) 3469
Vantin Tablets and Oral Suspension 2645

Colitis, ulcerative, worsening of
▲ Asacol Delayed-Release Tablets (3%) 2692
Colazal Capsules 2838
Pentasa Capsules (0.4%) 3185

Collagen disease, unspecified
Rythmol SR Capsules 2727

Collapse
Carbatrol Capsules 3171
Clozaril Tablets (Rare) 2184
Mintezol 2027
Nitrolingual Pumpspray 3120
Tegretol/Tegretol-XR 2295
▲ Xeloda Tablets (Less than 5%) 2822

Colon, irritable
Aricept Tablets (Infrequent) 1094
Aricept ODT Tablets (Infrequent) 1094
Prilosec OTC Delayed-Release Tablets (Less than 1%) 2677
Zegerid Capsules (Less than 1%) 2958
Zegerid Powder for Oral Solution (Less than 1%) 2958

Colon obstruction
VESIcare Tablets 646

Colonic strictures
Creon 5 Capsules 3198
Creon 10 Capsules 3198
Creon 20 Capsules 3199
Revlimid Capsules 958
Ultrase Capsules 708
Ultrase MT Capsules 709

Color perception, disturbed
Cesamet Capsules 3340
Cialis Tablets (Less than 2%) 1838
Cipro (Less than 1%) 2977
Cipro XR Tablets 2990
Proquin XR Tablets 1153

Color vision, changes
Levitra Tablets (Less than 2%) 3034
▲ VFEND I.V. (Approximately 21%) 2564
▲ VFEND Oral Suspension (Approximately 21%) 2564
▲ VFEND Tablets (Approximately 21%) 2564

Coma
Aciphex Tablets 1090
Aggrenox Capsules (Less than 1%) 822
Aloprim for Injection (Less than 1%) 2167
AmBisome for Injection (Less common) 620
Anaprox Tablets (Less than 1%) 2761
Anaprox DS Tablets (Less than 1%) 2761
Arranon Injection (1%) 1357
Arthrotec Tablets (Rare) 3129
Avinza Capsules (Less than 5%) 1741
Bayer Aspirin 744
Bayer Aspirin Comprehensive Prescribing Information ▣796
Bicillin C-R Injectable Suspension 1706
Buprenex Injectable (Infrequent) 2716
Campath Ampules 811
Carimune NF 3499
Copaxone for Injection (Infrequent) 3297
Copegus Tablets (Less than 1%) 2754
Dalmane Capsules 3342
Depacon Injection (Rare) 412
▲ Depakene (Rare) 417
Depakote Sprinkle Capsules (Rare) 422
Depakote Tablets (Rare) 427
Depakote ER Tablets (Rare) 434
EC-Naprosyn Delayed-Release Tablets (Less than 1%) 2761
Elspar for Injection 2463
Elspar for Injection 1960
Evoxac Capsules (Less than 1%) 1047
Flebogamma 5%, Immune Globulin Intravenous (Human) 1658
Fortaz 1453
Gabitril Tablets (Infrequent) 984
Gammagard Liquid 721
Gammagard S/D (Rare) 724
Gamunex Immune Globulin I.V., 10% (Rare) 3235
Indocin Capsules (Less than 1%) 1995
Indocin I.V. (Less than 1%) 2465
Indocin (Less than 1%) 1995
▲ Intron A for Injection (Less than 5%) 3024
I.V. Busulfex (One patient) 2493
Klonopin 2778
Levaquin (0.1% to 0.9%) 2384
Levaquin in 5% Dextrose Injection (0.1% to 0.9%) 2384
Lithobid Tablets 1692
Lyrica Capsules (Rare) 2539
Matulane Capsules 3191
Maxipime for Injection 1105
Naprosyn Suspension (Less than 1%) 2761
Naprosyn Tablets (Less than 1%) 2761
Oncaspar 1145
Orthoclone OKT3 Sterile Solution 2360
Pegasys (Less than 1%) 2789
Percodan Tablets 1132
Permax Tablets (Infrequent) 3356
PhosLo GelCaps 2169
Podocon-25 Liquid 2478
Prograf Capsules and Injection 632
Proleukin for Injection (1%) 2266
Prozac Pulvules and Liquid (Rare) 1801
ReoPro Vials (0.4%) 1809
Requip Tablets (Infrequent) 1555
Rilutek Tablets (Infrequent) 2930
Risperdal (Rare) 1676
Risperdal M-Tab Orally Disintegrating Tablets (Rare) 1676
Seromycin Capsules 1813
St. Joseph 81 mg Aspirin Chewable and Enteric Coated Tablets 1869
St. Joseph 81 mg Aspirin ▣688
Stromectol Tablets 2083
Symbyax Capsules (Infrequent) 1819
Symmetrel Tablets 1135
Tindamax Tablets (Rare) 2142
▲ Trisenox Injection (5%) 993
Valtrex Caplets 1597
▲ Vesanoid Capsules (3%) 2820
VFEND I.V. (Less than 2%) 2564
VFEND Oral Suspension (Less than 2%) 2564
VFEND Tablets (Less than 2%) 2564
Voltaren Tablets (Rarely) 2307
Voltaren-XR Tablets (Rarely) 2310
Wellbutrin Tablets 1603
Wellbutrin SR Sustained-Release Tablets 1607
Wellbutrin XL Extended-Release Tablets 1613
Zoloft (Rare) 2586
Zovirax 1643
Zyban Sustained-Release Tablets 1644
Zyprexa Tablets (Rare) 1830
Zyprexa ZYDIS Orally Disintegrating Tablets (Rare) 1830

Coma, hyperosmolar
FazaClo Orally Disintegrating Tablets 551

Coma, hepatic
Concerta Extended-Release Tablets 1881
Daytrana Transdermal Patch 3174
Focalin Tablets 2220
Focalin XR Capsules 2223
Levaquin (0.1% to 0.9%) 2384
Levaquin in 5% Dextrose Injection (0.1% to 0.9%) 2384
Metadate CD Capsules 3323
Prinzide Tablets 2056
Ritalin Hydrochloride Tablets (Some instances) 2269
Ritalin LA Capsules 2271
Ritalin-SR Tablets (Some instances) 2269
VFEND I.V. (Less than 2%) 2564
VFEND Oral Suspension (Less than 2%) 2564
VFEND Tablets (Less than 2%) 2564
▲ Xeloda Tablets (Less than 5%) 2822

Coma, hyperosmolar non-ketonic
Hyperstat I.V. 3017

Combativeness
Orthoclone OKT3 Sterile Solution 2360
Zosyn (1.0% or less) 3492

Complement activation
Visudyne for Injection (Less than 1%) 2305

Concentration, impaired
Abilify Oral Solution (Infrequent) 882
Abilify Oral Solution (Infrequent) 2450
Abilify Discmelt Orally Disintegrating Tablets (Infrequent) 882
Abilify Discmelt Orally Disintegrating Tablets (Infrequent) 2450
Abilify Tablets (Infrequent) 882
Abilify Tablets (Infrequent) 2450
Ambien CR Tablets (Infrequent) 2855
Atripla Tablets (Greater than or equal to 2%) 945
▲ Cesamet Capsules (12%) 3340
▲ Copegus Tablets (10%) 2754
Coreg Tablets (Greater than 0.1% to 1%) 1414
▲ Imdur Tablets (Less than or equal to 5%) 3018
Imitrex Injection (Rare) 1463
Levaquin (0.1% to 0.9%) 2384
Levaquin in 5% Dextrose Injection (0.1% to 0.9%) 2384
Lunesta Tablets (Infrequent) 3142
Niravam Orally Disintegrating Tablets 3092
▲ Pegasys (8%) 2789
▲ PEG-Intron Powder for Injection (10%) 3048
▲ Pexeva Tablets (3%) 1694
Prevacid NapraPAC (Less than 1%) 3280
▲ Rebetol (5% to 21%) 3058
Rescriptor Tablets 2551
▲ Ribavirin, USP Capsules (5% to 21%) 3068
Risperdal (2%) 1676
Risperdal Consta Long-Acting Injection (Infrequent) 1682
Risperdal M-Tab Orally Disintegrating Tablets (2%) 1676
▲ Topamax Sprinkle Capsules (3% to 14%) 2404
▲ Topamax Tablets (3% to 14%) 2404
Wellbutrin Tablets 1603
Wellbutrin SR Sustained-Release Tablets 1607
Wellbutrin XL Extended-Release Tablets 1613

Concussion
Xyrem Oral Solution (Infrequent) 1688

Condition aggravated
Denavir Cream 2174
Levaquin (0.1% to 0.9%) 2384
Levaquin in 5% Dextrose Injection (0.1% to 0.9%) 2384

Conduction disturbances
Aceon Tablets (2 mg, 4 mg, 8 mg) (0.3% to 1%) 3194
Avalide Tablets 888
Avalide Tablets 2874
Avapro Tablets (Less than 1%) 891
Avapro Tablets (Less than 1%) 2871
Blocadren Tablets 1916
Catapres-TTS 844
Clorpres Tablets (Rare) 2153
▲ Lanoxicaps Capsules (Among most common) 1490
▲ Lanoxin Injection (Among most common) 1494
▲ Lanoxin Injection Pediatric (Among most common) 1497
▲ Lanoxin Tablets (Among most common) 1500
Lariam Tablets (Infrequent) 2786
Nadolol Tablets (1 of 100 patients) 2159
Paxil CR Controlled-Release Tablets (Infrequent) 1538
Paxil (Infrequent) 1530
Reyataz Capsules (Rare) 921
Rythmol SR Capsules (Greater than or equal to 2%) 2727

Confusion
Abilify Oral Solution (Frequent) 882
Abilify Oral Solution (Frequent) 2450
Abilify Discmelt Orally Disintegrating Tablets (Frequent) 882
Abilify Discmelt Orally Disintegrating Tablets (Frequent) 2450
Abilify Tablets (Frequent) 882
Abilify Tablets (Frequent) 2450
Aciphex Tablets (Rare) 1090
Actimmune (Rare) 1671
▲ Actiq (1% to 6%) 979
Adalat CC Tablets (Less than 1%) 2964
Aggrenox Capsules (1.1%) 822
Agrylin Capsules (1% to 5%) 3169
Aldoril Tablets 1910
▲ Alferon N Injection (One patient to 3%) 1665
Ambien Tablets (Frequent) 2851
Ambien CR Tablets (Frequent) 2855
▲ AmBisome for Injection (8.6% to 12.9%) 620
Amerge Tablets (Rare) 1339
Amoxil Capsules (Rare) 1343
Amoxil Chewable Tablets (Rare) 1343

Amoxil Pediatric Drops for Oral Suspension (Rare)........ 1343
Amoxil Powder for Oral Suspension (Rare)........ 1343
Amoxil Tablets (Rare)........ 1343
Anaprox Tablets (Less than 1%)........ 2761
Anaprox DS Tablets (Less than 1%)........ 2761
Anzemet Injection (Infrequently)........ 2859
Anzemet Tablets (Infrequently)........ 2862
Aricept Tablets........ 1094
Aricept ODT Tablets........ 1094
▲ Arimidex Tablets (2% to 5%)........ 673
▲ Arixtra Injection (1.2% to 3.1%)........ 1351
▲ Aromasin Tablets (2% to 5%)........ 2600
▲ Arranon Injection (0% to 8%)........ 1357
Arthrotec Tablets (Rare)........ 3129
Asacol Delayed-Release Tablets........ 2692
Astelin Nasal Spray........ 1904
Augmentin (Rare)........ 1360
Augmentin Tablets (Rare)........ 1363
Augmentin XR Extended-Release Tablets (Rare)........ 1369
Augmentin ES-600 Powder for Oral Suspension (Rare)........ 1366
Avalide Tablets........ 888
Avalide Tablets........ 2874
▲ Avastin IV (1% to 6%)........ 1227
Avelox (Less than 0.1%)........ 2970
▲ Avinza Capsules (Less than 5%)........ 1741
Axid Oral Solution (Rare)........ 879
Bayer Aspirin........ 744
Bayer Aspirin Comprehensive Prescribing Information........ ▣ 796
Bentyl Capsules........ 697
Bentyl Injection........ 697
Bentyl Syrup........ 697
Bentyl Tablets........ 697
Betagan Ophthalmic Solution, USP........ ⊙ 220
Betaseron for SC Injection........ 767
Biaxin/Biaxin XL........ 402
Bicillin C-R Injectable Suspension........ 1706
Campath Ampules........ 811
Campral Tablets (Infrequent)........ 1174
Camptosar Injection (0% to 2.7%)........ 2604
Captopril Tablets........ 2149
Carbatrol Capsules........ 3171
Cardene I.V. (Rare)........ 2497
Celexa (Frequent)........ 1176
▲ CellCept Capsules (3% to less than 20%)........ 2747
▲ CellCept Intravenous (3% to less than 20%)........ 2747
▲ CellCept Oral Suspension (3% to less than 20%)........ 2747
▲ CellCept Tablets (3% to less than 20%)........ 2747
Cesamet Capsules........ 3340
Cipro........ 2977
Cipro I.V. (1% or less)........ 2984
Cipro XR Tablets........ 2990
▲ Clozaril Tablets (3%)........ 2184
Copaxone for Injection (2%)........ 3297
Cosopt Sterile Ophthalmic Solution........ 1931
Covera-HS Tablets (Less than 2%)........ 3139
Cozaar Tablets (Less than 1%)........ 1935
Cubicin for Injection (1% to 2%)........ 1026
▲ Dacogen Injection (12%)........ 2129
Dalmane Capsules (Rare)........ 3342
Dantrium Capsules (Less frequent)........ 2694
Daranide Tablets........ 1950
Daytrana Transdermal Patch........ 3174
Demser Capsules........ 1953
▲ Depacon Injection (1% to 5%)........ 412
▲ Depakene (1% to 5%)........ 417
▲ Depakote Sprinkle Capsules (1% to 5%)........ 422
▲ Depakote Tablets (1% to 5%)........ 427
▲ Depakote ER Tablets (1% to 5%)........ 434
▲ DepoCyt Injection (4% to 14%)........ 1143
Diastat Rectal Delivery System (Greater than or equal to 1%)........ 3343
Didronel Tablets........ 2697
Diovan HCT Tablets........ 2196
▲ Ditropan XL Extended-Release Tablets (2% to less than 5%)........ 2413
Diuril Oral Suspension........ 1954
Diuril Sodium Intravenous........ 2467
Dolobid Tablets (Less than 1 in 100)........ 1955
▲ Doxil Injection (1% to 10%)........ 2351
▲ Duragesic Transdermal System (10% or more)........ 2373
Dyazide Capsules........ 1423
EC-Naprosyn Delayed-Release Tablets (Less than 1%)........ 2761
Edecrin........ 1959
Effexor Tablets (2%)........ 3411
Effexor XR Capsules (Frequent)........ 3417
▲ Eldepryl Capsules (3 of 49 patients)........ 3208
Elspar for Injection........ 2463
Elspar for Injection........ 1960
Emend Capsules (Greater than 0.5%)........ 1963
▲ Entocort EC Capsules (Less than 5%)........ 2698
Equetro Extended-Release Capsules........ 3180
Erbitux (2%)........ 910
Ery-Tab Tablets (Isolated reports)........ 449
Erythrocin Stearate Filmtab Tablets (Isolated reports)........ 453
Erythromycin Base Filmtab Tablets (Isolated reports)........ 455
Erythromycin Delayed-Release Capsules, USP (Isolated reports)........ 457
Eulexin Capsules (1%)........ 3009
Evoxac Capsules (Less than 1%)........ 1047
▲ Exelon Capsules (8%)........ 2206
▲ Exelon Oral Solution (8%)........ 2206
Famvir Tablets (Infrequent)........ 2211
▲ FazaClo Orally Disintegrating Tablets (3%)........ 551
Flovent HFA........ 1447
Flumadine (Less than 0.3%)........ 1183
Frova Tablets (Infrequent)........ 1113
▲ Gabitril Tablets (5%)........ 984
Garamycin Injectable........ 3014
Gengraf Capsules (1% to less than 3%)........ 459
Geodon Capsules (Frequent)........ 2529
Gleevec Tablets (Rare)........ 2227
Gris-PEG Tablets (Occasional)........ 2502
Guanidine Hydrochloride Tablets........ 3016
Herceptin I.V. (At least one of the 958 patients)........ 1233
▲ Humira Injection (Less than 5%)........ 466
Hyperstat I.V........ 3017
Hyzaar 50-12.5 Tablets........ 1990
Hyzaar 100-12.5 Tablets........ 1990
Hyzaar 100-25 Tablets........ 1990
▲ Imdur Tablets (Less than or equal to 5%)........ 3018
Imitrex Injection (Infrequent)........ 1463
Imitrex Nasal Spray (Infrequent)........ 1467
Imitrex Tablets (Infrequent)........ 1471
Indocin (Less than 1%)........ 1995
▲ Infergen (4%)........ 3364
▲ Intron A for Injection (Up to 12%)........ 3024
▲ Invanz for Injection (3.3% to 5.1%)........ 1999
Invirase (Less than 2%)........ 2772
Ionsys Transdermal System (.1% to less than 1%)........ 2379
▲ I.V. Busulfex (11%)........ 2493
Kadian Capsules (Less than 3%)........ 577
Kaletra (Less than 2%)........ 476
Keflex Capsules........ 549
Keppra Injection........ 3320
Keppra Oral Solution (1% to 2%)........ 3314
Keppra Tablets (1% to 2%)........ 3314
Klonopin (1%)........ 2778
K-Phos Original (Sodium Free) Tablets (Less frequent)........ 760
K-Phos Neutral Tablets........ 760
Lamictal (1.8%)........ 1481
Lanoxicaps Capsules........ 1490
Lanoxin Injection........ 1494
Lanoxin Injection Pediatric........ 1497
Lanoxin Tablets........ 1500
Lariam Tablets (Occasional)........ 2786
Leukeran Tablets (Rare)........ 1504
Levaquin (0.1% to 0.9%)........ 2384
Levaquin in 5% Dextrose Injection (0.1% to 0.9%)........ 2384
Lexapro Oral Solution (Infrequent)........ 1190
Lexapro Tablets (Infrequent)........ 1190
Librium Capsules........ 3347
Lidoderm Patch........ 1118
Lithobid Tablets........ 1692
Lopressor Injection........ 2238
Lopressor Tablets........ 2238
Lopressor HCT 50/25 Tablets........ 2241
Lopressor HCT 100/25 Tablets........ 2241
Lopressor HCT 100/50 Tablets........ 2241
Lotronex Tablets (Rare)........ 1512
Lovenox Injection (2.2%)........ 2915
▲ Lunesta Tablets (0% to 3%)........ 3142
Lupron Depot 3.75 mg........ 3260
▲ Lyrica Capsules (1% to 7%)........ 2539
Marinol Capsules (Greater than 1%)........ 3333
Matulane Capsules........ 3191
Maxair Autohaler........ 1852
Maxalt Tablets (Infrequent)........ 2008
Maxalt-MLT Orally Disintegrating Tablets (Infrequent)........ 2008
Maxipime for Injection........ 1105
▲ Megace ES Oral Suspension (1% to 3%)........ 2481
Meridia Capsules........ 489
Merrem I.V. (Greater than 0.1% to 1%)........ 686
Midamor Tablets (Less than or equal to 1%)........ 2026
Migranal Nasal Spray (Infrequent)........ 3348
Mintezol........ 2027
▲ Mirapex Tablets (4% to 10%)........ 859
Mobic Oral Suspension (Less than 2%)........ 863
Mobic Tablets (Less than 2%)........ 863
Moduretic Tablets (Less than or equal to 1%)........ 2028
Myobloc Injection (Greater than 2%)........ 3192
Nalfon Capsules (1.4%)........ 2502
▲ Namenda (6%)........ 1195
Naprosyn Suspension (Less than 1%)........ 2761
Naprosyn Tablets (Less than 1%)........ 2761
Natrecor for Injection (Greater than or equal to 1%)........ 3127
Nembutal Sodium Solution, USP (Less than 1%)........ 2470
Neoral Oral Solution (1% to less than 3%)........ 2259
Neoral Soft Gelatin Capsules (1% to less than 3%)........ 2259
Neumega for Injection........ 3435
Neurontin Capsules........ 2487
Neurontin Oral Solution........ 2487
Neurontin Tablets........ 2487
Nexium Delayed-Release Capsules (Less than 1%)........ 655
Nexium I.V. (Less than 1%)........ 659
▲ Niravam Orally Disintegrating Tablets (5% to 10.4%)........ 3092
Norflex Injection (Infrequent)........ 1856
Noroxin Tablets........ 2032
Norvir (0.6% to 0.9%)........ 503
Numorphan Injection........ 1120
Oncaspar (Less than 1%)........ 1145
▲ Ontak Vials (8%)........ 1745
Opana Tablets (2.7%)........ 1122
Orthoclone OKT3 Sterile Solution........ 2360
▲ OxyContin Tablets (Between 1% and 5%)........ 2703
Parcopa Orally Disintegrating Tablets........ 3097
Parnate Tablets........ 1527
Paxil CR Controlled-Release Tablets (1%)........ 1538
Paxil (1%)........ 1530
Pepcid Injection (Infrequent)........ 2040
Pepcid (Infrequent)........ 2038
Percodan Tablets........ 1132
▲ Permax Tablets (11.1%)........ 3356
Pexeva Tablets (1%)........ 1694
Phenergan Tablets and Suppositories........ 3440
▲ Phenytek Capsules (Among most common)........ 2160
PhosLo GelCaps........ 2169
▲ Photofrin for Injection (8%)........ 702
Plavix Tablets........ 917
Plavix Tablets........ 2926
Prevacid Delayed-Release Capsules (Less than 1%)........ 3271
Prevacid for Delayed-Release Oral Suspension (Less than 1%)........ 3271
Prevacid NapraPAC (Less than 1%)........ 3280
Prevacid SoluTab Delayed-Release Orally Disintegrating Tablets (Less than 1%)........ 3271
▲ PREVPAC (Less than 1% to 3%)........ 3284
Prezista Tablets (Less than 2%)........ 3306
Prilosec OTC Delayed-Release Tablets (Less than 1%)........ 2677
Primaxin I.M........ 2045
Primaxin I.V. (Less than 0.2%)........ 2048
Prinivil Tablets (0.3% to 1.0%)........ 2052
Prinzide Tablets........ 2056
ProAmatine Tablets (Less frequent)........ 3186
▲ Prograf Capsules and Injection (3% to 15%)........ 632
▲ Proleukin for Injection (34%)........ 2266
Prometrium Capsules (100 mg, 200 mg) (Less than 5%)........ 3203
Proquin XR Tablets........ 1153
ProSom Tablets (2%)........ 517
Protonix I.V. (Less than 1%)........ 3472
Protonix Tablets (Less than 1%)........ 3469
Provigil Tablets (1%)........ 988
Prozac Pulvules and Liquid (Frequent)........ 1801
Raniclor Tablets, Chewable (Rare)........ 2505
▲ Rapamune Oral Solution and Tablets (3% to 20%)........ 3475
Razadyne (Greater than or equal to 2%)........ 2399
Razadyne ER Extended-Release Capsules (Greater than or equal to 2%)........ 2399
Relpax Tablets (Infrequent)........ 2548
Remicade for IV Injection (Greater than or equal to 0.2%)........ 971
ReoPro Vials (0.6%)........ 1809
▲ Requip Tablets (5%)........ 1555
Rescriptor Tablets........ 2551
Restoril Capsules (1.3%)........ 1860
Retrovir Capsules........ 1560
Retrovir IV Infusion........ 1564
Retrovir........ 1560
Revlimid Capsules (1.7% to 2.3%)........ 958
Reyataz Capsules (Less than 3%)........ 921
Rilutek Tablets (Infrequent)........ 2930
Risperdal (Infrequent)........ 1676
Risperdal Consta Long-Acting Injection (Infrequent)........ 1682
Risperdal M-Tab Orally Disintegrating Tablets (Infrequent)........ 1676
Romazicon Injection (Less than 1%)........ 2804
Sandimmune (2% or less)........ 2275
▲ Sandostatin LAR Depot (5% to 15%)........ 2280
Seromycin Capsules........ 1813
Seroquel Tablets (Infrequent)........ 690
Sonata Capsules (1% or less)........ 1717
St. Joseph 81 mg Aspirin Chewable and Enteric Coated Tablets........ 1869
St. Joseph 81 mg Aspirin........ ▣ 688
Stalevo Tablets........ 2287
Stromectol Tablets........ 2083
Sular Tablets (Less than or equal to 1%)........ 3122
Sustiva Capsules (Less than 2%)........ 930
Sustiva Tablets (Less than 2%)........ 930
Symbyax Capsules (Infrequent)........ 1819
▲ Symmetrel Tablets (0.1% to 5%)........ 1135
Synera Topical Patch........ 1137
Tambocor Tablets (Less than 1%)........ 1856
Tamiflu Capsules........ 2807
Tamiflu Oral Suspension........ 2807
Targretin Capsules........ 1747
Tarka Tablets........ 524
▲ Tasmar Tablets (10% to 11%)........ 3358
Taxotere Injection Concentrate........ 2932
Tegretol/Tegretol-XR........ 2295
▲ Temodar Capsules (5%)........ 3073
Tequin Injection (Less than 0.1%)........ 938
Tequin Injection in 5% Dextrose (Less than 0.1%)........ 938
Tequin Tablets (Less than 0.1%)........ 938
Tessalon Capsules........ 1199
Tessalon Perles........ 1199
Thalomid Capsules........ 965
Timolide Tablets (Less than 1%)........ 2086
Timoptic Sterile Ophthalmic Solution (Less frequent)........ 2088
Timoptic in Ocudose (Less frequent)........ 2091
Timoptic-XE Sterile Ophthalmic Gel Forming Solution........ 2092
Tindamax Tablets (Rare)........ 2142
▲ Topamax Sprinkle Capsules (2% to 14%)........ 2404
▲ Topamax Tablets (2% to 14%)........ 2404
Toprol-XL Tablets........ 668
Transderm Scōp Transdermal Therapeutic System (Infrequent)........ 2177
Tranxene (Less common)........ 2474
▲ Trasylol Injection (4%)........ 754
Tricor Tablets........ 527
Trileptal Tablets (1% to 2%)........ 2300
Trileptal Oral Suspension (1% to 2%)........ 2300
▲ Trisenox Injection (5%)........ 993
Ultane Liquid for Inhalation (Less than 1%)........ 531
▲ Ultram ER Tablets (1% to greater than 5%)........ 2392
Uroqid-Acid No. 2 Tablets........ 760
▲ Valcyte Tablets (Less than 5%)........ 2813
Valium Tablets (Infrequent)........ 2819
Valtrex Caplets........ 1597
Vantin Tablets and Oral Suspension (Less than 1%)........ 2645
▲ Vaprisol (3.8%)........ 643
Vasotec I.V. Injection (0.5% to 1%)........ 2103
Verelan PM Extended-Release Capsules, Controlled-Onset (2% or less)........ 3106
▲ Vesanoid Capsules (14%)........ 2820
VFEND I.V. (Less than 2%)........ 2564
VFEND Oral Suspension (Less than 2%)........ 2564
VFEND Tablets (Less than 2%)........ 2564
Vicoprofen Tablets (Less than 3%)........ 539
Voltaren Tablets (Occasionally)........ 2307
Voltaren-XR Tablets (Occasionally)........ 2310
▲ Wellbutrin Tablets (8.4%)........ 1603
Wellbutrin SR Sustained-Release Tablets........ 1607

▲ Wellbutrin XL Extended-Release Tablets (8%)..... 1613
▲ Xeloda Tablets (Less than 5%)..... 2822
▲ Xyrem Oral Solution (Less than 1% to 5.9%)..... 1688
Zantac (Rare)..... 1624
Zantac Injection (Rare)..... 1619
Zantac Injection Pharmacy Bulk Package (Rare)..... 1622
Zantac Injection Premixed (Rare)..... 1619
Zantac (Rare)..... 1624
Zegerid Capsules (Less than 1%)..... 2958
Zegerid Powder for Oral Solution (Less than 1%)..... 2958
Zoloft (Infrequent)..... 2586
▲ Zometa for Intravenous Infusion (7% to 12.8%)..... 2315
Zomig Nasal Spray (Infrequent)..... 3523
▲ Zonegran Capsules (6%)..... 1101
Zosyn (1.0% or less)..... 3492
Zovirax..... 1643
Zyban Sustained-Release Tablets (Infrequent)..... 1644
▲ Zyprexa Tablets (4%)..... 1830
Zyprexa IntraMuscular (Infrequent)..... 1830
▲ Zyprexa ZYDIS Orally Disintegrating Tablets (4%)..... 1830
Zyrtec Chewable Tablets (Less than 2%)..... 2594
Zyrtec (Less than 2%)..... 2594
Zyrtec-D 12 Hour Extended Release Tablets (Less than 2%)..... 2597

Confusion, mental
(*see under* Confusion)

Confusion, nocturnal

Thioridazine Hydrochloride Tablets (Extremely rare)..... 2163

Confusional state
(*see under* Confusion)

Congelation

Eldepryl Capsules..... 3208

Congenital anomalies

Altoprev Extended-Release Tablets (Rare)..... 3109
Arthrotec Tablets..... 3129
Depacon Injection..... 412
Depakene..... 417
Depakote Tablets..... 427
Depakote ER Tablets..... 434
Effexor Tablets..... 3411
Effexor XR Capsules..... 3417
Havrix Vaccine (Rare)..... 1456
Lescol Capsules (Rare)..... 2233
Lescol XL Tablets..... 2233
Mevacor Tablets (Rare)..... 2021
Permax Tablets..... 3356
Premarin Intravenous..... 3442
Proventil Inhalation Aerosol..... 3053
Proventil Inhalation Solution 0.083%..... 3055
Retrovir Capsules..... 1560
Retrovir IV Infusion..... 1564
Retrovir..... 1560
Twinrix Vaccine..... 1595
Zocor Tablets..... 2105

Congenital malformation

Carbatrol Capsules..... 3171
Diastat Rectal Delivery System..... 3343
Follistim AQ Cartridge..... 2338
Phenytek Capsules..... 2160
Singulair (Rare)..... 2077
Tegretol/Tegretol-XR..... 2295
Tranxene..... 2474
Valium Tablets..... 2819

Congestion

▲ Advair Diskus 100/50 (1% to 3%)..... 1308
▲ Advair Diskus 250/50 (1% to 3%)..... 1308
▲ Advair Diskus 500/50 (1% to 3%)..... 1308
▲ Advair HFA Inhalation Aerosol (1% to 3%)..... 1318
Avalide Tablets..... 888
Avalide Tablets..... 2874
Avapro Tablets (Less than 1%)..... 891
Avapro Tablets (Less than 1%)..... 2871
▲ Infergen (5% to 12%)..... 3364
Tricor Tablets..... 527

Congestion, nasal
(*see under* Nasal congestion)

Congestion, upper respiratory tract

Xyrem Oral Solution (Infrequent)..... 1688

Congestive heart failure

Actos Tablets (1.1%)..... 3219
Agrylin Capsules..... 3169
Aldoril Tablets..... 1910
Aminohippurate Sodium PAH Injection..... 1913
Anaprox Tablets (Less than 1%)..... 2761
Anaprox DS Tablets (Less than 1%)..... 2761
▲ Aranesp for Injection (6%)..... 581
Aricept Tablets (Infrequent)..... 1094
Aricept ODT Tablets (Infrequent)..... 1094
Arthrotec Tablets (Rare)..... 3129
Avandia Tablets..... 1384
Avastin IV..... 1227
Betagan Ophthalmic Solution, USP..... ⊙ 220
Betoptic S Ophthalmic Suspension (Rare)..... 558
Captopril Tablets (2 to 3 of 1000 patients)..... 2149
Carbatrol Capsules..... 3171
Cardizem LA Extended Release Tablets (Less than 2%)..... 1728
Carteolol Hydrochloride Ophthalmic Solution USP, 1%..... ⊙ 249
Catapres Tablets (Rare)..... 843
Catapres-TTS (0.5% or less)..... 844
Celebrex Capsules (Less than 0.1%)..... 3134
▲ CellCept Capsules (3% to less than 20%)..... 2747
▲ CellCept Intravenous (3% to less than 20%)..... 2747
▲ CellCept Oral Suspension (3% to less than 20%)..... 2747
▲ CellCept Tablets (3% to less than 20%)..... 2747
Clinoril Tablets (Less than 1%)..... 1924
Clorpres Tablets (Rare)..... 2153
Clozaril Tablets..... 2184
Colocort Rectal Suspension, USP (Retention) 100 mg/60 mL..... 2476
Covera-HS Tablets (1.8% to 2%)..... 3139
Cymbalta Delayed-Release Capsules (Infrequent)..... 1757
Dacogen Injection..... 2129
Decadron Tablets..... 1951
Depo-Medrol Injectable Suspension..... 2617
Depo-Medrol Single-Dose Vial..... 2619
Digibind for Injection (Few instances)..... 1421
Dolobid Tablets..... 1955
▲ Doxil Injection (1% to 5%)..... 2351
EC-Naprosyn Delayed-Release Tablets (Less than 1%)..... 2761
Effexor Tablets (Rare)..... 3411
Effexor XR Capsules (Infrequent)..... 3417
▲ Emcyt Capsules (3%)..... 2634
Enbrel for Injection..... 584
Equetro Extended-Release Capsules..... 3180
Gemzar for Injection (Very rare)..... 1771
▲ Herceptin I.V. (7%)..... 1233
▲ Humira Injection (Less than 5%)..... 466
Hydrocortone Tablets..... 1989
Inderal LA Long-Acting Capsules..... 3429
Indocin Capsules (Less than 1%)..... 1995
Indocin I.V. (Less than 1%)..... 2465
Indocin (Less than 1%)..... 1995
InnoPran XL Capsules..... 2723
Lopressor Injection (1%)..... 2238
Lopressor Tablets (1%)..... 2238
Lopressor HCT 50/25 Tablets..... 2241
Lopressor HCT 100/25 Tablets..... 2241
Lopressor HCT 100/50 Tablets..... 2241
Lupron Depot 7.5 mg (Less than 5%)..... 3264
Meridia Capsules..... 489
Micardis Tablets..... 854
Micardis HCT Tablets..... 856
Naprosyn Suspension (Less than 1%)..... 2761
Naprosyn Tablets (Less than 1%)..... 2761
Neumega for Injection..... 3435
Neurontin Capsules (Infrequent)..... 2487
Neurontin Oral Solution (Infrequent)..... 2487
Neurontin Tablets (Infrequent)..... 2487
Nimotop Capsules (Less than 1%)..... 749
Paxil CR Controlled-Release Tablets (Rare)..... 1538
Paxil (Rare)..... 1530
Permax Tablets (Frequent)..... 3356
Pexeva Tablets (rare)..... 1694
Pletal Tablets (Less than 2%)..... 2455
Prevacid NapraPAC (Less than 1%)..... 3280
Prevnar for Injection..... 3463
Proleukin for Injection (1%)..... 2266
Protonix I.V. (Less than 1%)..... 3472
Protonix Tablets (Less than 1%)..... 3469
Prozac Pulvules and Liquid (Infrequent)..... 1801
▲ Rapamune Oral Solution and Tablets (3% to 20%)..... 3475
Remicade for IV Injection..... 971
Retrovir Capsules (0.8%)..... 1560
Retrovir IV Infusion (1%)..... 1564
Retrovir (0.8%)..... 1560
Revlimid Capsules..... 958
Rilutek Tablets (Infrequent)..... 2930
Rythmol SR Capsules (1% to 2%)..... 2727
Sandostatin Injection (Less than 1%)..... 2278
Seromycin Capsules..... 1813
Seroquel Tablets (Infrequent)..... 690
Sular Tablets (Less than or equal to 1%)..... 3122
Symbyax Capsules (Rare)..... 1819
Symmetrel Tablets (0.1% to 1%)..... 1135
Tambocor Tablets..... 1856
Tarka Tablets..... 524
Tegretol/Tegretol-XR..... 2295
Thalomid Capsules..... 965
Tiazac Capsules (Less than 2%)..... 1201
Toprol-XL Tablets (About 1 of 100 patients)..... 668
Trasylol Injection (1% to 2%)..... 754
Vantin Tablets and Oral Suspension (Less than 1%)..... 2645
▲ Velcade for Injection (5%)..... 2133
Ventavis Inhalation Solution..... 1020
Verelan PM Extended-Release Capsules, Controlled-Onset (1.8%)..... 3106
VFEND I.V. (Less than 2%)..... 2564
VFEND Oral Suspension (Less than 2%)..... 2564
VFEND Tablets (Less than 2%)..... 2564
Vivitrol..... 995
Voltaren Tablets (Occasionally)..... 2307
Voltaren-XR Tablets (Occasionally)..... 2310
Zelapar Tablets..... 3372
Zostavax Injection (0.3% to 1.5%)..... 2111
Zyprexa Tablets (Infrequent)..... 1830
Zyprexa ZYDIS Orally Disintegrating Tablets (Infrequent)..... 1830

Conjunctiva, suffusion

Brimonidine Tartrate Ophthalmic Solution 0.2% (Less than 3%)..... ⊙ 248

Conjunctival blanching

▲ Brimonidine Tartrate Ophthalmic Solution 0.2% (3% to 9%)..... ⊙ 248

Conjunctival chemosis

Natacyn Antifungal Ophthalmic Suspension (One case)..... ⊙ 208
▲ Retisert Implant (5% to 9%)..... ⊙ 258

Conjunctival deposits

Propine Ophthalmic Solution..... ⊙ 239

Conjunctival erythema

Poly-Pred Ophthalmic Suspension..... ⊙ 233

Conjunctival follicles

▲ Brimonidine Tartrate Ophthalmic Solution 0.2% (10% to 30%)..... ⊙ 248
▲ Cosopt Sterile Ophthalmic Solution (1% to 5%)..... 1931

Conjunctival hyperemia

▲ Lumigan Ophthalmic Solution (15% to 45%)..... 573
Poly-Pred Ophthalmic Suspension..... ⊙ 233
▲ Retisert Implant (10% to 35%)..... ⊙ 258

Conjunctival injection

▲ Betimol Ophthalmic Solution (More than 5%)..... 3382
▲ Betimol Ophthalmic Solution (More than 5%)..... ⊙ 295
▲ Cosopt Sterile Ophthalmic Solution (1% to 5%)..... 1931
Fansidar Tablets..... 2765
Gantrisin Pediatric Suspension..... 2770
Mintezol..... 2027
▲ Neumega for Injection (19% to 58%)..... 3435
Pepcid Injection (Infrequent)..... 2040
Pepcid (Infrequent)..... 2038
▲ Visudyne for Injection (1% to 10%)..... 2305

Conjunctival irritation

▲ Brimonidine Tartrate Ophthalmic Solution 0.2% (3% to 9%)..... ⊙ 248
Efudex (Infrequent)..... 3363
▲ Zymar Ophthalmic Solution (5% to 10%)..... 575

Conjunctival microhemorrhage

Brimonidine Tartrate Ophthalmic Solution 0.2% (Less than 3%)..... ⊙ 248
▲ Lucentis Injection (43% to 77%)..... 1237

Conjunctivitis

Abilify Oral Solution (Frequent)..... 882
Abilify Oral Solution (Frequent)..... 2450
Abilify Discmelt Orally Disintegrating Tablets (Frequent)..... 882
Abilify Discmelt Orally Disintegrating Tablets (Frequent)..... 2450
Abilify Tablets (Frequent)..... 882
Abilify Tablets (Frequent)..... 2450
Accutane Capsules..... 2731
Aceon Tablets (2 mg, 4 mg, 8 mg) (0.3% to 1%)..... 3194
Actiq (1% or greater)..... 979
▲ Actonel Tablets (3.1%)..... 2683
▲ Actonel with Calcium Tablets (3.1%)..... 2688
Adalat CC Tablets (Less than 1%)..... 2964
▲ Advair Diskus 100/50 (1% to 3%)..... 1308
▲ Advair Diskus 250/50 (1% to 3%)..... 1308
▲ Advair Diskus 500/50 (1% to 3%)..... 1308
▲ Advair HFA Inhalation Aerosol (1% to 3%)..... 1318
Aldara Cream, 5% (0.5%)..... 1846
▲ Alphagan P Ophthalmic Solution (1% to 4%)..... 567
▲ Alrex Ophthalmic Suspension 0.2% (Less than 5%)..... ⊙ 246
Ambien Tablets (Rare)..... 2851
Ambien CR Tablets (Rare)..... 2855
AmBisome for Injection (Less common)..... 620
Anaprox Tablets (Less than 1%)..... 2761
Anaprox DS Tablets (Less than 1%)..... 2761
Arthrotec Tablets (Rare)..... 3129
Asacol Delayed-Release Tablets (1% to 2%)..... 2692
Astelin Nasal Spray (Infrequent)..... 1904
Atacand HCT (0.5% or greater)..... 651
Atrovent Nasal Spray 0.03% (Less than 2%)..... 837
Atrovent Nasal Spray 0.06% (Less than 1%)..... 839
Attenuvax..... 1914
Avalide Tablets..... 888
Avalide Tablets..... 2874
Avapro Tablets (Less than 1%)..... 891
Avapro Tablets (Less than 1%)..... 2871
Axert Tablets (Rare)..... 2396
▲ Azilect Tablets (3%)..... 3293
Azopt Ophthalmic Suspension (Less than 1%)..... 557
Betimol Ophthalmic Solution..... 3382
Betimol Ophthalmic Solution..... ⊙ 295
BiDil Tablets..... 2171
Buprenex Injectable (Less than 1%)..... 2716
Caduet Tablets (Greater than 0.1% to less than or equal to 1%)..... 2508
Carbatrol Capsules..... 3171
Cardene I.V. (Rare)..... 2497
Celebrex Capsules (0.1% to 1.9%)..... 3134
Celexa (Infrequent)..... 1176
▲ CellCept Capsules (3% to less than 20%)..... 2747
▲ CellCept Intravenous (3% to less than 20%)..... 2747
▲ CellCept Oral Suspension (3% to less than 20%)..... 2747
▲ CellCept Tablets (3% to less than 20%)..... 2747
Chantix Tablets (Infrequent)..... 2517
Cialis Tablets (Less than 2%)..... 1838
Clinoril Tablets (Less than 1 in 100)..... 1924
Colazal Capsules..... 2838
Comvax..... 1928
Copaxone for Injection (At least 2%)..... 3297
▲ Cosopt Sterile Ophthalmic Solution (1% to 5%)..... 1931
Cozaar Tablets (Less than 1%)..... 1935
Depacon Injection (1% or more)..... 412
Depakene (1% or more)..... 417
Depakote Sprinkle Capsules..... 422
▲ Depakote Tablets (1% to 5%)..... 427
▲ Depakote ER Tablets (Greater than 1% to 5%)..... 434
Differin Cream (Less than 1%)..... 1210
▲ Doxil Injection (1% to 10%)..... 2351
EC-Naprosyn Delayed-Release Tablets (Less than 1%)..... 2761
Effexor Tablets (Infrequent)..... 3411
Effexor XR Capsules (Infrequent)..... 3417
Elmiron Capsules (Less than or equal to 1%)..... 2415
▲ Eloxatin for Injection (2% to 9%)..... 2892
Emend Capsules (Greater than 0.5%)..... 1963
Engerix-B Vaccine..... 1425
Equetro Extended-Release Capsules..... 3180
▲ Erbitux (Less than 1% to 14%)..... 910
▲ Evoxac Capsules (4.3%)..... 1047
Exelon Capsules (Infrequent)..... 2206
Exelon Oral Solution (Infrequent)..... 2206

Ferrlecit Injection 3388
Flonase Nasal Spray 1440
▲ Flovent Diskus (1% to 3%) 1443
Fluarix 1451
Flumist Vaccine 1901
FML Ophthalmic Ointment (Occasional) ⊙228
FML Ophthalmic Suspension (Occasional) ⊙227
FML Forte Ophthalmic Suspension (Occasional) ⊙226
FML-S Ophthalmic Suspension ⊙229
▲ Fortical Nasal Spray (1% to 3%) 3337
Frova Tablets (Infrequent) 1113
Fuzeon Injection (2%) 2767
Gabitril Tablets (1% or more) 984
Gengraf Capsules (1% to less than 3%) 459
Geodon Capsules (Infrequent) 2529
Gleevec Tablets (Less common) 2227
Hectorol Capsules 1275
Hectorol Injection 1278
Hytrin Capsules (At least 1%) 471
Hyzaar 50-12.5 Tablets 1990
Hyzaar 100-12.5 Tablets 1990
Hyzaar 100-25 Tablets 1990
▲ Imdur Tablets (Less than or equal to 5%) 3018
Imitrex Injection 1463
Imitrex Nasal Spray 1467
▲ Indapamide Tablets (Less than 5%) 2156
▲ Infergen (4% to 8%) 3364
▲ Intron A for Injection (Less than 5%) 3024
Iressa Tablets (2%) 684
Kadian Capsules (Less than 3%) 577
Lamictal (Infrequent) 1481
Levaquin (0.1% to 0.9%) 2384
Levaquin in 5% Dextrose Injection (0.1% to 0.9%) 2384
Levitra Tablets (Less than 2%) 3034
Lexapro Oral Solution (Infrequent) 1190
Lexapro Tablets (Infrequent) 1190
Lofibra Tablets 1219
Lofibra Capsules 1216
▲ Lotemax Ophthalmic Suspension 0.5% (Less than 5%) ⊙251
Lotensin HCT Tablets (0.3% or more) 2246
Lunesta Tablets (Infrequent) 3142
▲ Lupron Depot 3.75 mg (Less than 5%) 3260
▲ Lupron Depot–3 Month 11.25 mg (Less than 5%) 3265
Luxiq Foam (One patient) 1010
Lyrica Capsules (Greater than or equal to 1%) 2539
▲ Macugen Injection (6% to 10%) ⊙261
Marinol Capsules (0.3% to 1%) 3333
Meruvax II 2019
▲ Miacalcin Nasal Spray (1% to 3%) 2253
Micardis Tablets (More than 0.3%) 854
Micardis HCT Tablets 856
Migranal Nasal Spray (Infrequent) 3348
Mirapex Tablets (1% or more) 859
M-M-R II 2006
Mobic Oral Suspension (Less than 2%) 863
Mobic Tablets (Less than 2%) 863
Mumpsvax 2031
Namenda (Frequent) 1195
Naprosyn Suspension (Less than 1%) 2761
Naprosyn Tablets (Less than 1%) 2761
Nasonex Nasal Spray (Greater than or equal to 2%) 3043
Neoral Oral Solution (1% to less than 3%) 2259
Neoral Soft Gelatin Capsules (1% to less than 3%) 2259
Neurontin Capsules (1.2%) 2487
Neurontin Oral Solution (1.2%) 2487
Neurontin Tablets (1.2%) 2487
Nexium Delayed-Release Capsules (Less than 1%) 655
Nexium I.V. (Less than 1%) 659
▲ Nipent for Injection (4%) 1863
Norvasc Tablets (More than 0.1% to 1%) 2545
Omnicef Capsules 511
Omnicef for Oral Suspension 511
OptiPranolol Metipranolol Ophthalmic Solution 0.3% (A small number of patients) ⊙256
Orthoclone OKT3 Sterile Solution 2360
Ovide .5% Lotion 3290
Paxil CR Controlled-Release Tablets (Infrequent) 1538
Paxil (Infrequent) 1530
▲ PEG-Intron Powder for Injection (4%) 3048
Pentasa Capsules (Less than 1%) 3185
Permax Tablets (Infrequent) 3356
Pexeva Tablets (Infrequent) 1694
Plavix Tablets (1% to 2.5%) 917
Plavix Tablets (1% to 2.5%) 2926
Pletal Tablets (Less than 2%) 2455
Poly-Pred Ophthalmic Suspension ⊙233
Pred Mild Ophthalmic Suspension (Occasional) ⊙238
Pred Forte Ophthalmic Suspension (Occasional) ⊙235
Prevacid Delayed-Release Capsules (Less than 1%) 3271
Prevacid for Delayed-Release Oral Suspension (Less than 1%) 3271
Prevacid NapraPAC (Less than 1%) 3280
Prevacid SoluTab Delayed-Release Orally Disintegrating Tablets (Less than 1%) 3271
Prevnar for Injection 3463
PREVPAC (Less than 1%) 3284
Prochieve 4% Gel 1003
Prochieve 8% Gel 1003
▲ Proleukin for Injection (4%) 2266
▲ Protopic Ointment (2% to 4%) 638
Provigil Tablets (Greater than or equal to 1%) 988
Prozac Pulvules and Liquid (Infrequent) 1801
▲ Pulmicort Respules (Less than 1% to 4%) 661
▲ Pulmozyme Inhalation Solution (1% to 5%) 1248
▲ Rapamune Oral Solution and Tablets (3% to 20%) 3475
▲ Rebetol (4% to 5%) 3058
Recombivax HB 2071
Relpax Tablets (Infrequent) 2548
Requip Tablets (Infrequent) 1555
Rescriptor Tablets 2551
▲ Ribavirin, USP Capsules (4% to 5%) 3068
Risperdal Consta Long-Acting Injection (Infrequent) 1682
Rocaltrol Capsules 2798
Rocaltrol Oral Solution 2798
Sandimmune (2% or less) 2275
Serevent Diskus (1% to less than 3%) 1568
Seroquel Tablets (Infrequent) 690
▲ Simulect for Injection (3% to 10%) 2284
Singulair (Greater than or equal to 2%) 2077
Sonata Capsules (Frequent) 1717
▲ Soriatane Capsules (1% to 10%) 1013
Stromectol Tablets 2083
Sular Tablets (Less than or equal to 1%) 3122
Symbyax Capsules (Infrequent) 1819
Synagis (More than 1%) 1897
Tamiflu Capsules (1%) 2807
Tamiflu Oral Suspension (1%) 2807
▲ Tarceva Tablets (0% to 12%) 1259
▲ Tarceva Tablets (0% to 12%) 2444
Targretin Capsules 1747
Taxotere Injection Concentrate 2932
Tegretol/Tegretol-XR 2295
Teveten Tablets (Less than 1%) 1735
Teveten HCT Tablets (Less than 1%) 1737
Tiazac Capsules (2%) 1201
Timoptic Sterile Ophthalmic Solution (Less frequent) 2088
Timoptic in Ocudose (Less frequent) 2091
▲ Timoptic-XE Sterile Ophthalmic Gel Forming Solution (1% to 5%) 2092
Topamax Sprinkle Capsules (1% to 2%) 2404
Topamax Tablets (1% to 2%) 2404
▲ Travatan Ophthalmic Solution (1% to 4%) 563
Trelstar LA Suspension (1.1%) 3397
Tricor Tablets 527
Trizivir Tablets 1589
▲ Trusopt Sterile Ophthalmic Solution (Approximately 1% to 5%) 2095
Twinrix Vaccine 1595
Ultane Liquid for Inhalation (Less than 1%) 531
Uniretic Tablets (Less than 1%) 3100
Vaqta (1.3%) 2097
Vasotec I.V. Injection (0.5% to 1.0%) 2103
VFEND I.V. (Less than 2%) 2564
VFEND Oral Suspension (Less than 2%) 2564
VFEND Tablets (Less than 2%) 2564
Viagra Tablets (Less than 2%) 2573
▲ Vigamox Ophthalmic Solution (1% to 6%) 564
Viramune Oral Suspension 873
Viramune Tablets 873
Virazole for Inhalation Solution 3370
▲ Visudyne for Injection (1% to 10%) 2305
Vivitrol 995
▲ Voltaren Ophthalmic Solution (Less than or equal to 5%) 2309
Voltaren Tablets (Rarely) 2307
Voltaren-XR Tablets (Rarely) 2310
Xalatan Sterile Ophthalmic Solution (Less than 1%) 2649
▲ Xeloda Tablets (Less than 5%) 2822
Xyrem Oral Solution (Infrequent) 1688
Zelapar Tablets 3372
Ziagen 1626
Zoloft (Infrequent) 2586
Zomig Nasal Spray (Rare) 3523
Zonegran Capsules (Infrequent) 1101
Zyflo Tablets (Greater than 1%) 1023
▲ Zymar Ophthalmic Solution (5% to 10%) 575
Zyprexa Tablets 1830
Zyprexa ZYDIS Orally Disintegrating Tablets 1830
Zyrtec Chewable Tablets (Less than 2%) 2594
Zyrtec (Less than 2%) 2594
Zyrtec-D 12 Hour Extended Release Tablets (Less than 2%) 2597

Conjunctivitis, allergic
▲ Alphagan P Ophthalmic Solution (Approximately 10% to 20%) 567
▲ Lumigan Ophthalmic Solution (1% to 3%) 573
▲ Macugen Injection (1% to 5%) ⊙261

Conjunctivitis, calcific
Calcijex Injection 411

Conjunctivitis, follicular
▲ Alphagan P Ophthalmic Solution (Approximately 5% to 9%) 567
Propine Ophthalmic Solution ⊙239

Conjunctivitis, hemorrhagic
▲ Alphagan P Ophthalmic Solution (1% to 4%) 567

Conjunctivitis, nonspecific
▲ Keppra Oral Solution (3%) 3314
▲ Keppra Tablets (3%) 3314

Conjunctivitis sicca
Cymbalta Delayed-Release Capsules (Infrequent) 1757
Thyrolar Tablets 1199

Consciousness, decreased
Abilify Oral Solution (Infrequent) 882
Abilify Oral Solution (Infrequent) 2450
Abilify Discmelt Orally Disintegrating Tablets (Infrequent) 882
Abilify Discmelt Orally Disintegrating Tablets (Infrequent) 2450
Abilify Tablets (Infrequent) 882
Abilify Tablets (Infrequent) 2450
▲ Arranon Injection (0% to 6%) 1357
Opana Tablets (Less than 1%) 1122
Opana ER Tablets (Less than 1%) 1126
Revlimid Capsules 958
Xyrem Oral Solution (Infrequent) 1688

Consciousness, disorders of
Amerge Tablets (Rare) 1339
Comtan Tablets 2189
▲ Intron A for Injection (Less than 5%) 3024
Neoral Oral Solution 2259
Neoral Soft Gelatin Capsules 2259
Permax Tablets 3356
Sandimmune 2275
Symmetrel Tablets (Uncommon) 1135
Tasmar Tablets (Four cases) 3358
Valtrex Caplets 1597
Zovirax 1643

Consciousness, loss of
Adenocard Injection 617
Arranon Injection (1%) 1357
Carimune NF 3499
Cesamet Capsules 3340
Cipro 2977
Cipro I.V. (1% or less) 2984
Cipro XR Tablets 2990
Effexor Tablets (Rare) 3411
Effexor XR Capsules (Rare) 3417
Ferrlecit Injection 3388
Flebogamma 5%, Immune Globulin Intravenous (Human) 1658
Gammagard Liquid 721
Gammagard S/D (Rare) 724
Gamunex Immune Globulin I.V., 10% (Rare) 3235
Hyperstat I.V. 3017
Infed Injection 3390
Invirase (Less than 2%) 2772
Levaquin 2384
Levaquin in 5% Dextrose Injection 2384
Lidoderm Patch 1118
Neumega for Injection 3435
Noroxin Tablets 2032
Omnicef Capsules 511
Omnicef for Oral Suspension 511
Orthoclone OKT3 Sterile Solution 2360
PEG-Intron Powder for Injection (Less than or equal to 1%) 3048
Synera Topical Patch 1137
Taxotere Injection Concentrate 2932
▲ Vesanoid Capsules (3%) 2820
▲ Xeloda Tablets (Less than 5%) 2822

Constipation
▲ Abilify Oral Solution (11% to 13%) 882
▲ Abilify Oral Solution (11% to 13%) 2450
▲ Abilify Discmelt Orally Disintegrating Tablets (11% to 13%) 882
▲ Abilify Discmelt Orally Disintegrating Tablets (11% to 13%) 2450
▲ Abilify Tablets (11% to 13%) 882
▲ Abilify Tablets (11% to 13%) 2450
Aceon Tablets (2 mg, 4 mg, 8 mg) (0.3% to 1%) 3194
Aciphex Tablets 1090
Actiq (1% to 4%) 979
▲ Actonel Tablets (6.6% to 12.2%) 2683
▲ Actonel with Calcium Tablets (12.2% to 12.5%) 2688
▲ Adalat CC Tablets (1% to 3%) 2964
Adderall Tablets 3164
▲ Adderall XR Capsules (2% to 4%) 3166
Adipex-P 1215
▲ Advair Diskus 100/50 (1% to 3%) 1308
▲ Advair Diskus 250/50 (1% to 3%) 1308
▲ Advair Diskus 500/50 (1% to 3%) 1308
▲ Advair HFA Inhalation Aerosol (1% to 3%) 1318
Advicor Tablets 1722
▲ Aerobid/Aerobid-M (1% to 3%) 1171
▲ Agrylin Capsules (1% to 5%) 3169
Aldoril Tablets 1910
Alferon N Injection (One patient) 1665
▲ Alimta for Injection (Up to 44%) 1750
Alinia for Oral Suspension (Less than 1%) 2835
Alinia Tablets (Less than 1%) 2835
Aloprim for Injection (Less than 1%) 2167
▲ Aloxi Injection (5%) 2127
Altace Capsules (Less than 1%) 1702
▲ Altoprev Extended-Release Tablets (2% to 3.5%) 3109
Ambien Tablets (Infrequent) 2851
Ambien CR Tablets (Infrequent to 2%) 2855
AmBisome for Injection (Less common) 620
Amerge Tablets (Infrequent) 1339
Amitiza Capsules (0% to 1.1%) 3224
▲ Anaprox Tablets (3% to 9%) 2761
▲ Anaprox DS Tablets (3% to 9%) 2761
Anzemet Injection (Rare) 2859
Anzemet Tablets (Rare) 2862
▲ Aranesp for Injection (5% to 18%) 581
▲ Aredia for Injection (33.2%) 2179
▲ Arimidex Tablets (7% to 9%) 673
▲ Arixtra Injection (1.8% to 8.5%) 1351
▲ Aromasin Tablets (5%) 2600
▲ Arranon Injection (0% to 21%) 1357
Arthrotec Tablets (Rare) 3129
▲ Asacol Delayed-Release Tablets (5%) 2692
Astelin Nasal Spray (Infrequent) 1904
Atacand HCT 651
Atripla Tablets 945
Atrovent Inhalation Solution (0.9%) 835
Atrovent HFA Inhalation Aerosol 841
Atrovent Nasal Spray 0.03% 837
Atrovent Nasal Spray 0.06% 839
Avalide Tablets 888
Avalide Tablets 2874
▲ Avandamet Tablets (5%) 1373
Avapro Tablets (Less than 1%) 891
Avapro Tablets (Less than 1%) 2871
▲ Avastin IV (4%) 1227
Avelox (Less than 0.1%) 2970
▲ Avinza Capsules (Greater than 10%) 1741
Axid Oral Solution (2.5%) 879
▲ Azilect Tablets (9%) 3293
Bentyl Capsules 697
Bentyl Injection 697
Bentyl Syrup 697
Bentyl Tablets 697
▲ Betaseron for SC Injection (20%) 767
▲ Bexxar (1% to 6%) 1398
▲ Boniva Injection (2.5% to 4%) 2738

▲ Boniva Tablets (2.5% to 4%) 2741
Buprenex Injectable (Less than 1%) 2716
Byetta Injection 611
Caduet Tablets (Greater than 0.1% to 2.5%) 2508
Calcijex Injection 411
▲ Campath Ampules (1% to 9%) 811
Campral Tablets (Frequent) 1174
▲ Camptosar Injection (0.4% to 32.3%) 2604
Captopril Tablets (About 0.5% to 2%) 2149
Carafate Suspension (2%) 701
Carafate Tablets (2%) 701
Carbatrol Capsules 3171
Cardizem LA Extended Release Tablets (Less than 2%) 1728
▲ Carnitor Injection (3%) 3188
▲ Catapres Tablets (About 10 in 100 patients) 843
Catapres-TTS (1 of 101 patients) 844
Celebrex Capsules (0.1% to 1.9%) 3134
Celexa (At least 2%) 1176
▲ CellCept Capsules (18.5% to 41.2%) 2747
▲ CellCept Intravenous (18.5% to 41.2%) 2747
▲ CellCept Oral Suspension (18.5% to 41.2%) 2747
▲ CellCept Tablets (18.5% to 41.2%) 2747
Cesamet Capsules 3340
▲ Chantix Tablets (Greater than 5% to 8%) 2517
Cipro 2977
Cipro I.V. (1% or less) 2984
Cipro XR Tablets (Less than 1%) 2990
▲ Clinoril Tablets (3% to 9%) 1924
▲ Clolar for Intravenous Infusion (21%) 1271
▲ Clorpres Tablets (About 10%) 2153
▲ Clozaril Tablets (More than 5% to 25%) 2184
Colazal Capsules (1%) 2838
Combivent Inhalation Aerosol 847
▲ Comtan Tablets (6%) 2189
Copaxone for Injection (At least 2%) 3297
▲ Covera-HS Tablets (7.2% to 11.7%) 3139
Cozaar Tablets (Less than 1%) 1935
▲ Creon 5 Capsules (Among most frequent) 3198
▲ Creon 10 Capsules (Among most frequent) 3198
▲ Creon 20 Capsules (Among most frequent) 3199
Crestor Tablets (Greater than or equal to 2%) 678
▲ Cubicin for Injection (6.2% to 10.8%) 1026
▲ Cymbalta Delayed-Release Capsules (11%) 1757
▲ Dacogen Injection (35%) 2129
Dalmane Capsules 3342
Dantrium Capsules (Less frequent) 2694
Daranide Tablets 1950
Demadex Injection (1.8%) 2759
Demadex Tablets (1.8%) 2759
▲ Depacon Injection (Up to 5%) 412
▲ Depakene (5%) 417
▲ Depakote Sprinkle Capsules (5%) 422
▲ Depakote Tablets (1% to 5%) 427
▲ Depakote ER Tablets (Greater than 1% to 5%) 434
▲ DepoCyt Injection (7%) 1143
▲ DepoDur Extended-Release Injection (Greater than 10%) 1110
Desoxyn Tablets, USP 2462
▲ Detrol Tablets (7%) 2628
▲ Detrol LA Capsules (6%) 2631
Dexedrine 1420
DextroStat Tablets 3179
Diastat Rectal Delivery System (Infrequent) 3343
Dilaudid 440
Dilaudid Non-Sterile Powder 440
Dilaudid Oral Liquid 445
Dilaudid Rectal Suppositories 440
Dilaudid Tablets 440
Dilaudid Tablets - 8 mg 445
Dilaudid-HP (Less frequent) 442
Diovan Tablets 2193
Diovan HCT Tablets (Less frequent) 2196
▲ Ditropan XL Extended-Release Tablets (7% to 13%) 2413
Diuril Oral Suspension 1954
Diuril Sodium Intravenous 2467
Dolobid Tablets (Greater than 1 in 100) 1955
Donnatal Extentabs 2493
▲ Doxil Injection (1% to 30.1%) 2351
DuoNeb Inhalation Solution (More than 1%) 1058
▲ Duragesic Transdermal System (10% or more) 2373
Dyazide Capsules 1423
▲ DynaCirc CR Tablets (1.2% to 3.8%) 2721
▲ EC-Naprosyn Delayed-Release Tablets (3% to 9%) 2761
▲ Effexor Tablets (15%) 3411
▲ Effexor XR Capsules (5% to 10%) 3417
Eldepryl Capsules 3208
▲ Elidel Cream 1% (0.4% to 3.4%) 2200
Eligard 7.5 mg (Less than 2%) 2880
▲ Elitek (20%) 2890
Elmiron Capsules (Less than or equal to 1%) 2415
▲ Eloxatin for Injection (22% to 32%) 2892
▲ Emend Capsules (10.3% to 12.3%) 1963
▲ Enablex Extended-Release Tablets (14.8% to 21.3%) 2203
Engerix-B Vaccine (Less than 1%) 1425
▲ Epogen for Injection (42% to 43%) 591
▲ Equetro Extended-Release Capsules (5%) 3180
Eraxis for Injection (Less than 1% to less than 2%) 2521
▲ Erbitux (2% to 35%) 910
▲ Evoxac Capsules (1% to 3%) 1047
▲ Exelon Capsules (5%) 2206
▲ Exelon Oral Solution (5%) 2206
▲ Famvir Tablets (1.4% to 4.4%) 2211
▲ Faslodex Injection (12%) 681
▲ FazaClo Orally Disintegrating Tablets (Greater than 5% to 25%) 551
▲ Femara Tablets (0.2% to 11.3%) 2214
Flomax Capsules (Infrequent) 850
Flumadine 1183
▲ Follistim AQ Cartridge (5%) 2338
▲ Forteo for Injection (5.4%) 1767
▲ Fortical Nasal Spray (1% to 3%) 3337
▲ Fosamax (Up to 3.1%) 1969
▲ Fosamax Plus D Tablets (0% to 3.1%) 1977
▲ Fosrenol Chewable Tablets (6% to 14%) 3183
Frova Tablets (Infrequent) 1113
Furosemide Tablets 2154
▲ Fuzeon Injection (3.9%) 2767
Gabitril Tablets (1% or more) 984
▲ Gemzar for Injection (10% to 42%) 1771
Gengraf Capsules (1% to less than 3%) 459
▲ Geodon (9%) 2529
▲ Gleevec Tablets (0% to 16%) 2227
▲ Hectorol Capsules (3.3% to greater than or equal to 5%) 1275
▲ Hectorol Injection (3.3%) 1278
▲ Hycamtin for Injection (Less than 1% to 39%) 1458
Hycodan 1116
Hyperstat I.V. 3017
Hytrin Capsules (At least 1%) 471
Hyzaar 50-12.5 Tablets 1990
Hyzaar 100-12.5 Tablets 1990
Hyzaar 100-25 Tablets 1990
▲ Imdur Tablets (Less than or equal to 5%) 3018
Imitrex Nasal Spray (Infrequent) 1467
Imitrex Tablets (Infrequent) 1471
▲ Indapamide Tablets (Less than 5%) 2156
Inderal LA Long-Acting Capsules 3429
Indocin Capsules (Greater than 1%) 1995
▲ Indocin I.V. (1% to 3%) 2465
Indocin (Greater than 1%) 1995
▲ Infergen (5% to 9%) 3364
▲ InnoPran XL Capsules (1% to 3%) 2723
▲ Intron A for Injection (Up to 10%) 3024
▲ Invanz for Injection (2.3% to 4%) 1999
Invirase (Greater than or equal to 2%) 2772
▲ Ionsys Transdermal System (1% to less than 10%) 2379
▲ I.V. Busulfex (35% to 38%) 2493
▲ Kadian Capsules (Virtually all patients) 577
Kaletra (Less than 2%) 476
Keppra Injection 3320
▲ Keppra Oral Solution (1% to 3%) 3314
▲ Keppra Tablets (1% to 3%) 3314
Ketek Tablets (Greater than or equal to 0.2% to less than 2%) 2903
Kionex Powder 2477
Klonopin (2%) 2778
Kogenate FS 738
Kogenate FS with Bio-Set 740
▲ Kytril Injection (3% to 9.4%) 2781
▲ Kytril (3% to 18%) 2784
▲ Lamictal (4%) 1481
▲ Lescol Capsules (3.1%) 2233
Lescol XL Tablets (2.3%) 2233
▲ Leukine (8%) 814
▲ Leustatin Injection (9%) 2357
▲ Levaquin (0.1% to 3.1%) 2384
▲ Levaquin in 5% Dextrose Injection (0.1% to 3.1%) 2384
▲ Lexapro Oral Solution (3% to 6%) 1190
▲ Lexapro Tablets (3% to 6%) 1190
Librium Capsules 3347
Lipitor Tablets (Up to 2.5%) 2483
Lofibra Tablets (2.1%) 1219
Lofibra Capsules (2.1%) 1216
Lopressor Injection (1%) 2238
Lopressor Tablets (1%) 2238
Lopressor HCT 50/25 Tablets (1%) 2241
Lopressor HCT 100/25 Tablets (1%) 2241
Lopressor HCT 100/50 Tablets (1%) 2241
Lotensin Tablets (Less than 1%) 2243
Lotensin HCT Tablets (0.3% to 1%) 2246
Lotrel Capsules 2249
▲ Lotronex Tablets (29%) 1512
▲ Lucentis Injection (3% to 7%) 1237
▲ Lyrica Capsules (1% to 7%) 2539
Matulane Capsules 3191
Mavik Tablets (0.3% to 1.0%) 486
Maxalt Tablets (Infrequent) 2008
Maxalt-MLT Orally Disintegrating Tablets (Infrequent) 2008
▲ Megace ES Oral Suspension (1% to 3%) 2481
▲ Menostar Transdermal System (5%) 782
▲ Mepron Suspension (3%) 1521
▲ Meridia Capsules (11.5%) 489
▲ Merrem I.V. (1.4% to 7%) 686
▲ Mevacor Tablets (2.0% to 4.9%) 2021
▲ Miacalcin Nasal Spray (1% to 3%) 2253
Micardis Tablets (More than 0.3%) 854
Micardis HCT Tablets 856
▲ Midamor Tablets (Between 1% and 3%) 2026
▲ Mirapex Tablets (10% to 14%) 859
Moban Tablets 1119
Mobic Oral Suspension (0.8% to 1.8%) 863
Mobic Tablets (0.8% to 1.8%) 863
Moduretic Tablets (Less than or equal to 1%) 2028
▲ MS Contin Tablets (Less frequent to among most frequent) 2701
Mycamine for Injection (0.2%) 628
▲ Myfortic Tablets (3% to 38%) 2255
▲ Mylotarg for Injection (23%) 3431
▲ Myozyme for Intravenous Infusion (23%) 1279
Nadolol Tablets (1 to 5 of 1000 patients) 2159
▲ Nalfon Capsules (7%) 2502
▲ Namenda (5%) 1195
▲ Naprosyn Suspension (3% to 9%) 2761
▲ Naprosyn Tablets (3% to 9%) 2761
Nembutal Sodium Solution, USP (Less than 1%) 2470
Neoral Oral Solution (1% to less than 3%) 2259
Neoral Soft Gelatin Capsules (1% to less than 3%) 2259
▲ Neulasta Injection (15% to 72%) 601
▲ Neumega for Injection (Greater than or equal to 10%) 3435
▲ Neupogen for Injection (5%) 603
▲ Neurontin Capsules (1.5% to 3.9%) 2487
▲ Neurontin Oral Solution (1.5% to 3.9%) 2487
▲ Neurontin Tablets (1.5% to 3.9%) 2487
▲ Nexavar Tablets (0% to 15%) 746
Nexium Delayed-Release Capsules (Greater than or equal to 1%) 655
Nexium I.V. (Greater than or equal to 1%) 659
Nipent for Injection (Less than 3%) 1863
▲ Niravam Orally Disintegrating Tablets (10.4% to 26.2%) 3092
Norflex Injection 1856
Noroxin Tablets (0.3% to 1.0%) 2032
Norvasc Tablets (More than 0.1% to 1%) 2545
Norvir (0% to 0.7%) 503
Numorphan Injection 1120
Omacor Capsules 2725
Omnicef Capsules (0.3%) 511
Omnicef for Oral Suspension (0.3%) 511
Oncaspar (Less than 1%) 1145
▲ Ontak Vials (9%) 1745
▲ Opana Tablets (4.1%) 1122
▲ Opana ER Tablets (5.7% to 27.6%) 1126
▲ OxyContin Tablets (23%) 2703
OxyFast Oral Concentrate Solution 2708
OxyIR Capsules 2708
▲ Oxytrol Transdermal System (3.3%) 3392
▲ Pancrease MT Capsules (Among most frequent) 1885
Parcopa Orally Disintegrating Tablets 3097
Parnate Tablets 1527
▲ Paxil CR Controlled-Release Tablets (1.1% to 16%) 1538
▲ Paxil (1.1% to 16%) 1530
PEG-Intron Powder for Injection (1%) 3048
Pentasa Capsules (Less than 1%) 3185
Pepcid Injection (1.2%) 2040
Pepcid (1.2%) 2038
Percocet Tablets 1131
Percodan Tablets 1132
▲ Permax Tablets (10.6%; frequent) 3356
▲ Pexeva Tablets (1.1% to 16%) 1694
Phenytek Capsules 2160
PhosLo GelCaps 2169
▲ Photofrin for Injection (17% to 24%) 702
Plavix Tablets (1% to 2.5%) 917
Plavix Tablets (1% to 2.5%) 2926
Prevacid Delayed-Release Capsules (1%) 3271
Prevacid for Delayed-Release Oral Suspension (1%) 3271
▲ Prevacid NapraPAC (1% to 9%) 3280
Prevacid SoluTab Delayed-Release Orally Disintegrating Tablets (1%) 3271
PREVPAC (1%) 3284
Prezista Tablets (0.6% to 2.3%) 3306
Prilosec OTC Delayed-Release Tablets (1.1% to 1.5%) 2677
Prinivil Tablets (0.3% to 1.0%) 2052
Prinzide Tablets (0.3% to 1%) 2056
▲ Prochieve 4% Gel (27%) 1003
▲ Prochieve 8% Gel (27%) 1003
▲ Procrit for Injection (42% to 53%) 2364
▲ Prograf Capsules and Injection (23% to 35%) 632
▲ Proleukin for Injection (5%) 2266
Prometrium Capsules (100 mg, 200 mg) (Less than 5%) 3203
ProSom Tablets (Frequent) 517
Protonix I.V. (Greater than or equal to 1%) 3472
Protonix Tablets (Greater than or equal to 1%) 3469
Protopic Ointment (Greater than or equal to 1%) 638
Provigil Tablets (2%) 988
▲ Prozac Pulvules and Liquid (5%) 1801
▲ Ranexa Tablets (4.5% to 8%) 1035
▲ Rapamune Oral Solution and Tablets (28% to 38%) 3475
Razadyne (Greater than or equal to 2%) 2399
Razadyne ER Extended-Release Capsules (Greater than or equal to 2%) 2399
▲ Rebetol (5%) 3058
Recombivax HB 2071
ReFacto Vials 3484
Relpax Tablets (Infrequent) 2548
Remicade for IV Injection (Greater than or equal to 0.2%) 971
▲ Renagel Tablets (2% to 8.1%) 1282
ReoPro Vials (0.3%) 1809
▲ Requip Tablets (6%) 1555
Rescriptor Tablets 2551
▲ Retrovir Capsules (6.4%) 1560
▲ Retrovir IV Infusion (6.4%) 1564
▲ Retrovir (6.4%) 1560
▲ Revlimid Capsules (23.6% to 38.7%) 958
Reyataz Capsules (Less than 3%) 921
▲ Ribavirin, USP Capsules (5%) 3068
Rilutek Tablets (More than 2%) 2930
▲ Risperdal (7% to 13%) 1676
▲ Risperdal Consta Long-Acting Injection (5% to 7%) 1682
▲ Risperdal M-Tab Orally Disintegrating Tablets (7% to 13%) 1676
Rocaltrol Capsules 2798
Rocaltrol Oral Solution 2798
▲ Rythmol SR Capsules (8% to 14%) 2727
▲ Sanctura Tablets (9.6%) 1151
Sandimmune (Rare) 2275
▲ Sandostatin Injection (Less than 10%) 2278
▲ Sandostatin LAR Depot (18.8%) 2280
▲ Seroquel Tablets (8%) 690
▲ Simulect for Injection (Greater than or equal to 10%) 2284
Slow Fe Iron Tablets ▣ 818
▲ Soltamox Oral Solution (4.4%) 3527
Sonata Capsules (Frequent) 1717
Soriatane Capsules (Less than 1%) 1013
▲ Spiriva HandiHaler (1% to 4%) 869
▲ Stalevo Tables (6%) 2287

▲ Strattera Capsules (Less than 1% to 10%) ... 1814
Stromectol Tablets (0.9%) ... 2083
▲ Suboxone Tablets (11% to 12.1%) .. 2717
▲ Subutex Tablets (7.8% to 11%) ... 2717
Sustiva Capsules ... 930
Sustiva Tablets ... 930
▲ Sutent Capsules (0% to 34%) ... 2560
▲ Symmetrel Tablets (1% to 5%) ... 1135
▲ Tambocor Tablets (4.4%) ... 1856
▲ Tarceva Tablets (1% to 31%) ... 1259
▲ Tarceva Tablets (1% to 31%) ... 2444
Targretin Capsules ... 1747
▲ Tarka Tablets (3.3%) ... 524
▲ Tasmar Tablets (6% to 8%) ... 3358
▲ Taxotere Injection Concentrate (1.8% to 25.3%) ... 2932
Tegretol/Tegretol-XR ... 2295
▲ Temodar Capsules (22% to 33%) ... 3073
▲ Tequin Injection (0.1% to 3%) ... 938
▲ Tequin Injection in 5% Dextrose (0.1% to 3%) ... 938
▲ Tequin Tablets (0.1% to 3%) ... 938
Tessalon Capsules ... 1199
Tessalon Perles ... 1199
Teveten Tablets (Less than 1%) ... 1735
Teveten HCT Tablets (Less than 1%) ... 1737
▲ Thalomid Capsules (4.2%) ... 965
Thioridazine Hydrochloride Tablets .. 2163
Thiothixene Capsules (Infrequently) .. 2165
Tiazac Capsules (Less than 2%) ... 1201
Timolide Tablets (Less than 1%) ... 2086
Tindamax Tablets (0.4% to 1.4%) ... 2142
▲ Topamax Sprinkle Capsules (Greater than 1% to 5%) ... 2404
▲ Topamax Tablets (Greater than 1% to 5%) ... 2404
Toprol-XL Tablets (About 1 of 100 patients) ... 668
▲ Trasylol Injection (4%) ... 754
Trelstar LA Suspension (1.7%) ... 3397
Tricor Tablets (2.1%) ... 527
Triglide Tablets (2.1%) ... 3123
▲ Trileptal Tablets (2% to 6%) ... 2300
▲ Trileptal Oral Suspension (2% to 6%) ... 2300
▲ Trisenox Injection (28%) ... 993
Tussionex Pennkinetic Extended-Release Suspension ... 3327
Twinrix Vaccine (Less than 1%) ... 1595
Tygacil for Injection (2.8%) ... 3488
Tylenol with Codeine Tablets ... 2391
▲ Ultram ER Tablets (12.2% to 29.7%) ... 2392
Uniretic Tablets (Less than 1%) ... 3100
Univasc Tablets (Less than 1%) ... 3104
Uroxatral Tablets (1% to 2%) ... 2943
▲ Valcyte Tablets (Less than 5%) ... 2813
Valium Tablets (Infrequent) ... 2819
▲ Valtrex Caplets (Less than 1% to 4%) ... 1597
Vandazole Vaginal Gel (Less than 1%) ... 3338
▲ Vantas (3.5%) ... 3375
▲ Vaprisol (4.9%) ... 643
Varivax (Greater than or equal to 1%) ... 2100
Vasotec I.V. Injection (0.5% to 1.0%) ... 2103
▲ Velcade for Injection (42%) ... 2133
▲ Verelan PM Extended-Release Capsules, Controlled-Onset (7.3% to 8.8%) ... 3106
▲ Vesanoid Capsules (17%) ... 2820
▲ VESIcare Tablets (5.4% to 13.4%) ... 646
VFEND I.V. (Less than 2%) ... 2564
VFEND Oral Suspension (Less than 2%) ... 2564
VFEND Tablets (Less than 2%) ... 2564
Viadur Implant (Less than 2%) ... 757
Vicodin Tablets ... 535
Vicodin ES Tablets ... 536
Vicodin HP Tablets ... 538
▲ Vicoprofen Tablets (22%) ... 539
▲ Visudyne for Injection (1% to 10%) .. 2305
Vivitrol ... 995
▲ Voltaren Tablets (1% to 10%) ... 2307
▲ Voltaren-XR Tablets (1% to 10%) ... 2310
Vytorin 10/10 Tablets ... 2114
Vytorin 10/10 Tablets ... 3077
Vytorin 10/20 Tablets ... 2114
Vytorin 10/20 Tablets ... 3077
Vytorin 10/40 Tablets ... 2114
Vytorin 10/40 Tablets ... 3077
Vytorin 10/80 Tablets ... 2114
Vytorin 10/80 Tablets ... 3077
▲ WelChol Tablets (11%) ... 1050
▲ Wellbutrin Tablets (26.0%) ... 1603
▲ Wellbutrin SR Sustained-Release Tablets (5% to 10%) ... 1607
▲ Wellbutrin XL Extended-Release Tablets (5% to 10%) ... 1613
▲ Xeloda Tablets (1% to 14%) ... 2822
▲ Xifaxan Tablets (3.8%) ... 2842
Xyrem Oral Solution (Frequent) ... 1688
Zantac ... 1624
Zantac Injection ... 1619
Zantac Injection Pharmacy Bulk Package (Frequency) ... 1622
Zantac Injection Premixed ... 1619
Zantac ... 1624
▲ Zegerid Capsules (1.1% to 4.5%) ... 2958
▲ Zegerid Powder for Oral Solution (1.1% to 4.5%) ... 2958
▲ Zelapar Tablets (4%) ... 3372
Zemplar Injection ... 543
Zmax for Oral Suspension (Less then 1%) ... 2583
Zocor Tablets (2.3%) ... 2105
▲ Zofran Injection (11%) ... 1634
▲ Zofran (6% to 9%) ... 1639
▲ Zofran ODT Orally Disintegrating Tablets (6% to 9%) ... 1639
▲ Zoloft (1% to 8%) ... 2586
▲ Zometa for Intravenous Infusion (26.7% to 31%) ... 2315
Zomig Tablets (Rare) ... 3519
Zomig Nasal Spray (Rare) ... 3523
Zomig-ZMT Tablets (Rare) ... 3519
Zonegran Capsules (2%) ... 1101
▲ Zosyn (7.7% to 8.4%) ... 3492
▲ Zyban Sustained-Release Tablets (8%) ... 1644
Zydone Tablets ... 1139
Zyflo Tablets (Greater than 1%) ... 1023
▲ Zyprexa Tablets (6% to 11%) ... 1830
▲ Zyprexa ZYDIS Orally Disintegrating Tablets (6% to 11%) ... 1830
Zyrtec Chewable Tablets (Less than 2%) ... 2594
Zyrtec (Less than 2%) ... 2594
Zyrtec-D 12 Hour Extended Release Tablets (Less than 2%) ... 2597
Zyvox (2.2%) ... 2652

Constipation, aggravation of

Nexium Delayed-Release Capsules (Less than 1%) ... 655
Nexium I.V. (Less than 1%) ... 659
Sanctura Tablets (1.4%) ... 1151
▲ Ultram ER Tablets (1% to greater than 5%) ... 2392

Constitutional symptoms, unspecified

▲ Alimta for Injection (1% to 11%) ... 1750

Constriction, pupillary

(*see under* Miosis)

Constriction, pupils

(*see under* Miosis)

Contact lenses, intolerance

Accutane Capsules ... 2731
Angeliq Tablets ... 762
Climara Transdermal System ... 771
Climara Pro Transdermal System ... 776
Enjuvia Tablets ... 1062
Estrasorb Topical Emulsion ... 1147
Estratest Tablets ... 3199
Estratest H.S. Tablets ... 3199
Menostar Transdermal System ... 782
Mircette Tablets ... 1066
NuvaRing ... 2340
Ortho-Cyclen Tablets ... 2429
Ortho Evra Transdermal System ... 2417
Ortho Tri-Cyclen Tablets ... 2429
Ortho Tri-Cyclen Lo Tablets ... 2436
Premarin Intravenous ... 3442
Premarin Tablets ... 3446
Premarin Vaginal Cream ... 3452
Premphase Tablets ... 3456
Prempro Tablets ... 3456
Seasonique Tablets ... 1077
Yasmin 28 Tablets ... 796
Yaz Tablets ... 803

Contusions

▲ Advair Diskus 100/50 (1% to 3%) ... 1308
▲ Advair Diskus 250/50 (1% to 3%) ... 1308
▲ Advair Diskus 500/50 (1% to 3%) ... 1308
Advair HFA Inhalation Aerosol ... 1318
Ambien CR Tablets (1%) ... 2855
▲ Clolar for Intravenous Infusion (11%) ... 1271
▲ Flovent Diskus (1% to 3%) ... 1443
Lotronex Tablets (Rare) ... 1512
▲ Macugen Injection (1% to 5%) ... ⊙ 261
▲ Myfortic Tablets (3% to less than 20%) ... 2255
▲ Revlimid Capsules (8.1%) ... 958
Vantas (Less than 2%) ... 3375
Xyrem Oral Solution (Frequent) ... 1688

Convulsions

Abelcet Injection ... 1141
Aciphex Tablets ... 1090
Adderall Tablets ... 3164
Aggrenox Capsules (1.7%) ... 822
Aldara Cream, 5% ... 1846
Aldoril Tablets ... 1910
Altace Capsules (Less than 1%) ... 1702
Ambien Tablets ... 2851
AmBisome for Injection (Less common) ... 620
Amerge Tablets (Rare) ... 1339
Anaprox Tablets (Less than 1%) ... 2761
Anaprox DS Tablets (Less than 1%) .. 2761
Aranesp for Injection (0.6%) ... 581
Aricept Tablets ... 1094
Aricept ODT Tablets ... 1094
▲ Arranon Injection (0% to 4%) ... 1357
Arthrotec Tablets (Rare) ... 3129
Atripla Tablets ... 945
Attenuvax (Rare) ... 1914
Augmentin (Rare) ... 1360
Augmentin Tablets (Rare) ... 1363
Augmentin XR Extended-Release Tablets (Rare) ... 1369
Augmentin ES-600 Powder for Oral Suspension (Rare) ... 1366
Avelox ... 2970
Avinza Capsules (Less than 5%) ... 1741
Azilect Tablets (Infrequent) ... 3293
Betaseron for SC Injection ... 767
Biaxin/Biaxin XL ... 402
Biltricide Tablets ... 2976
Boostrix ... 1404
Buprenex Injectable (Rare) ... 2716
Campral Tablets (Infrequent) ... 1174
Ceftin for Oral Suspension ... 1407
▲ CellCept Capsules (3% to less than 20%) ... 2747
▲ CellCept Intravenous (3% to less than 20%) ... 2747
▲ CellCept Oral Suspension (3% to less than 20%) ... 2747
▲ CellCept Tablets (3% to less than 20%) ... 2747
Cesamet Capsules ... 3340
Chantix Tablets (Rare) ... 2517
Cipro ... 2977
Cipro I.V. ... 2984
Cipro XR Tablets ... 2990
Clarinex-D 24-Hour Extended-Release Tablets ... 2998
Clinoril Tablets (Less than 1%) ... 1924
▲ Clozaril Tablets (3%) ... 2184
Colocort Rectal Suspension, USP (Retention) 100 mg/60 mL ... 2476
Coreg Tablets (Less than or equal to 0.1%) ... 1414
Decadron Tablets ... 1951
Depo-Medrol Injectable Suspension ... 2617
Depo-Medrol Single-Dose Vial ... 2619
Depo-Provera Contraceptive Injection (Less than 1%) ... 2622
depo-subQ provera 104 Injectable Suspension ... 2624
Diastat Rectal Delivery System (Greater than or equal to 1%) ... 3343
Ditropan XL Extended-Release Tablets (Rare) ... 2413
Diuril Oral Suspension ... 1954
Diuril Sodium Intravenous ... 2467
Doxil Injection (Less than 1%) ... 2351
Duragesic Transdermal System (1% or greater) ... 2373
EC-Naprosyn Delayed-Release Tablets (Less than 1%) ... 2761
E.E.S. ... 451
Effexor Tablets (Infrequent) ... 3411
Effexor XR Capsules (Infrequent) ... 3417
Elitek (Less than or equal to 1%) ... 2890
Epzicom Tablets ... 1436
Erythrocin Stearate Filmtab Tablets (Rare) ... 453
Erythromycin Delayed-Release Capsules, USP (Rare) ... 457
Ethyol for Injection ... 1898
Evoxac Capsules ... 1047
Exelon Capsules (Frequent) ... 2206
Exelon Oral Solution (Frequent) ... 2206
Fansidar Tablets ... 2765
▲ FazaClo Orally Disintegrating Tablets (3%) ... 551
Ferrlecit Injection ... 3388
Fluarix ... 1451
Flumadine (Less than 0.3%) ... 1183
Fluorescite Injection ... ⊙ 207
Gabitril Tablets ... 984
Gantrisin Pediatric Suspension ... 2770
Garamycin Injectable ... 3014
▲ Gengraf Capsules (1% to 5%) ... 459
Gleevec Tablets (Rare) ... 2227
Havrix Vaccine (Rare) ... 1456
Herceptin I.V. (At least one of the 958 patients) ... 1233
HibTITER ... 3426
Hydrocortone Tablets ... 1989
Hyperstat I.V. ... 3017
Imitrex Injection (Rare) ... 1463
Imitrex Tablets (Rare) ... 1471
▲ Increlex Injection (Greater than or equal to 5%) ... 3291
Indocin Capsules (Less than 1%) ... 1995
Indocin I.V. (Less than 1%) ... 2465
Indocin (Less than 1%) ... 1995
Infanrix Vaccine ... 1476
Infed Injection ... 3390
▲ Intron A for Injection (Less than 5%) ... 3024
Invirase (Less than 2%) ... 2772
Kaletra (Less than 2%) ... 476
Keppra Injection ... 3320
Keppra Oral Solution (1% to 2%) ... 3314
Keppra Tablets (1% to 2%) ... 3314
▲ Lamictal (2% to 3%) ... 1481
Lariam Tablets (Occasional) ... 2786
Levaquin (0.1% to 0.9%) ... 2384
Levaquin in 5% Dextrose Injection (0.1% to 0.9%) ... 2384
Lexapro Oral Solution ... 1190
Lexapro Tablets ... 1190
Lidoderm Patch ... 1118
Matulane Capsules ... 3191
▲ Megace ES Oral Suspension (1% to 3%) ... 2481
Meridia Capsules (0.1%) ... 489
Mintezol ... 2027
Mirapex Tablets (Less than 1%) ... 859
Mobic Oral Suspension (Less than 2%) ... 863
Mobic Tablets (Less than 2%) ... 863
Mycamine for Injection ... 628
Namenda (Infrequent) ... 1195
Naprosyn Suspension (Less than 1%) ... 2761
Naprosyn Tablets (Less than 1%) ... 2761
NeoProfen Injection ... 2472
▲ Neoral Oral Solution (1% to 5%) ... 2259
▲ Neoral Soft Gelatin Capsules (1% to 5%) ... 2259
Neurontin Capsules (More than 1%) ... 2487
Neurontin Oral Solution ... 2487
Neurontin Tablets (More than 1%) ... 2487
Nipent for Injection (Less than 3%) ... 1863
Noroxin Tablets ... 2032
Norvir (Less than 2%) ... 503
▲ Oncaspar (Greater than 1% but less than 5%) ... 1145
Parcopa Orally Disintegrating Tablets ... 3097
Paxil CR Controlled-Release Tablets (0.1%) ... 1538
Paxil (0.1%) ... 1530
PCE Dispertab Tablets (Rare) ... 515
Pediarix Vaccine ... 1548
Permax Tablets (Infrequent) ... 3356
Pexeva Tablets (rare) ... 1694
Prevacid Delayed-Release Capsules (Less than 1%) ... 3271
Prevacid for Delayed-Release Oral Suspension (Less than 1%) ... 3271
Prevacid NapraPAC (Less than 1%) .. 3280
Prevacid SoluTab Delayed-Release Orally Disintegrating Tablets (Less than 1%) ... 3271
PREVPAC (Less than 1%) ... 3284
Primatene Mist ... ▣ 719
▲ Primaxin I.V. (5.9%) ... 2048
▲ Prograf Capsules and Injection (3% to 15%) ... 632
ProQuad ... 2064
Proquin XR Tablets ... 1153
Protonix I.V. (Less than 1%) ... 3472
Protonix Tablets (Less than 1%) ... 3469
Prozac Pulvules and Liquid (0.1% to 0.2%) ... 1801
Razadyne (Infrequent) ... 2399
Razadyne ER Extended-Release Capsules (Infrequent) ... 2399
▲ Rebif Prefilled Syringe for Injection (4% to 5%) ... 3159
Remicade for IV Injection (Less than 1%) ... 971
Requip Tablets (Infrequent) ... 1555
Reyataz Capsules (Less than 3%) ... 921
Rilutek Tablets (Infrequent) ... 2930
Risperdal Consta Long-Acting Injection (Infrequent) ... 1682
Romazicon Injection ... 2804
▲ Sandimmune (1% to 5%) ... 2275
Sandostatin LAR Depot (Rare) ... 2280
Seromycin Capsules ... 1813
St. Joseph 81 mg Aspirin ... ▣ 688
Stalevo Tablets ... 2287
Sustiva Capsules (Less than 2%) ... 930
Sustiva Tablets (Less than 2%) ... 930
Symbyax Capsules ... 1819

Symmetrel Tablets (Less than 0.1%) 1135
Synera Topical Patch 1137
Tambocor Tablets (Less than 1%) 1856
▲ Temodar Capsules (6% to 23%) 3073
Tequin Injection (Less than 0.1%) 938
Tequin Injection in 5% Dextrose (Less than 0.1%) 938
Tequin Tablets (Less than 0.1%) 938
Thalomid Capsules 965
Timolide Tablets 2086
Tindamax Tablets 2142
Trasylol Injection (1% to 2%) 754
▲ Trisenox Injection (8%) 993
Twinrix Vaccine 1595
▲ Valcyte Tablets (Less than 5%) 2813
Valtrex Caplets 1597
Vantin Tablets and Oral Suspension 2645
▲ Vesanoid Capsules (3%) 2820
VFEND I.V. (Less than 2%) 2564
VFEND Oral Suspension (Less than 2%) 2564
VFEND Tablets (Less than 2%) 2564
Virazole for Inhalation Solution 3370
Vivitrol 995
Voltaren Tablets (Rarely) 2307
Voltaren-XR Tablets (Rarely) 2310
Zmax for Oral Suspension 2583
Zoloft 2586
Zomig Nasal Spray (Rare) 3523
Zonegran Capsules (Frequent) 1101
Zosyn (1.0% or less) 3492
Zyrtec Chewable Tablets (Rare) 2594
Zyrtec (Rare) 2594
Zyrtec-D 12 Hour Extended Release Tablets (Rare) 2597
Zyvox (0% to 2.8%) 2652

Convulsions, aggravated
Topamax Sprinkle Capsules (More than 1%) 2404
Topamax Tablets (More than 1%) 2404
Trileptal Tablets (1% to 2%) 2300
Trileptal Oral Suspension (1% to 2%) 2300

Convulsions, clonic
Seromycin Capsules 1813
Uniphyl Tablets (A few isolated reports) 2710

Convulsions, grand mal
Aranesp for Injection (0.6%) 581
Arranon Injection (0% to 1%) 1357
Campath Ampules 811
Celexa 1176
Cipro (Less than 1%) 2977
Diastat Rectal Delivery System (Fewer than 1%) 3343
Keppra Injection 3320
Keppra Oral Solution (1% or more) 3314
Keppra Tablets (1% or more) 3314
Lamictal (Rare) 1481
Lexapro Oral Solution 1190
Lexapro Tablets 1190
Namenda 1195
Norvir (Less than 2%) 503
Paxil CR Controlled-Release Tablets (Rare) 1538
Paxil (Rare) 1530
Pexeva Tablets (Rare) 1694
Proquin XR Tablets 1153
Requip Tablets (Rare) 1555
Topamax Sprinkle Capsules (1%) 2404
Topamax Tablets (1%) 2404
VFEND I.V. (Less than 2%) 2564
VFEND Oral Suspension (Less than 2%) 2564
VFEND Tablets (Less than 2%) 2564

Convulsions, local
Aranesp for Injection (0.6%) 581
▲ Temodar Capsules (6%) 3073

Convulsions, major
Seromycin Capsules 1813

Convulsions, tonic generalized
Uniphyl Tablets (A few isolated reports) 2710

Convulsive threshold, lowering
Adderall XR Capsules 3166

Coombs' test, positive
Adalat CC Tablets 2964
Aldoril Tablets 1910
Carimune NF 3499
Catapres Tablets 843
Ceftin (0.1% to 1%) 1407
Clorpres Tablets 2153
Flebogamma 5%, Immune Globulin Intravenous (Human) 1658
▲ Fortaz (1 in 23) 1453
Gammagard Liquid 721
Gammagard S/D 724
Gamunex Immune Globulin I.V., 10% 3235
▲ Maxipime for Injection (16.2%) 1105
Mefoxin for Injection 2012
Mefoxin Premixed Intravenous Solution 2016
Merrem I.V. (Greater than 0.2%) 686
Paser Granules 1674
Primaxin I.M. 2045
Primaxin I.V. 2048
Raniclor Tablets, Chewable (0.5%) 2505
Rilutek Tablets (Infrequent) 2930
Suprax 1843
Vantin Tablets and Oral Suspension (Occasional) 2645
Zinacef for Injection (Fewer than 1 in 250 patients) 1631
Zinacef Injection (Fewer than 1 in 250 patients) 1631
Zosyn 3492

Coordination, disturbed
(*see under* Coordination, impaired)

Coordination, impaired
Amerge Tablets (Rare) 1339
Arranon Injection (1%) 1357
Arthrotec Tablets (Rare) 3129
Atripla Tablets 945
Avelox (Less than 0.1%) 2970
Carbatrol Capsules 3171
Celexa (Rare) 1176
Cesamet Capsules 3340
Cipro XR Tablets (Less than 1%) 2990
Clozaril Tablets (Less than 1%) 2184
Combivent Inhalation Aerosol 847
▲ Depacon Injection (1% to 5%) 412
▲ Diastat Rectal Delivery System (3%) 3343
Duragesic Transdermal System (1% or greater) 2373
Equetro Extended-Release Capsules 3180
Evoxac Capsules (Less than 1%) 1047
FazaClo Orally Disintegrating Tablets (Less than 1%) 551
▲ Intron A for Injection (Less than 5%) 3024
▲ Klonopin (6%) 2778
▲ Lamictal (6.0%) 1481
Levaquin (0.1% to 0.9%) 2384
Levaquin in 5% Dextrose Injection (0.1% to 0.9%) 2384
Lexapro Oral Solution (Infrequent) 1190
Lexapro Tablets (Infrequent) 1190
Marinol Capsules 3333
Namenda (Infrequent) 1195
Neurontin Capsules (1.1%) 2487
Neurontin Oral Solution (1.1%) 2487
Neurontin Tablets (1.1%) 2487
▲ Niravam Orally Disintegrating Tablets (6.6% to 40.1%) 3092
▲ Phenytek Capsules (Among most common) 2160
▲ ProSom Tablets (4%) 517
▲ Rebif Prefilled Syringe for Injection (4% to 5%) 3159
Requip Tablets (Infrequent) 1555
Rescriptor Tablets 2551
Rilutek Tablets (Infrequent) 2930
Tegretol/Tegretol-XR 2295
▲ Temodar Capsules (11%) 3073
▲ Topamax Sprinkle Capsules (4%) 2404
▲ Topamax Tablets (4%) 2404
▲ Trileptal Tablets (1% to 3%) 2300
▲ Trileptal Oral Suspension (1% to 3%) 2300
Wellbutrin SR Sustained-Release Tablets (Infrequent) 1607
Wellbutrin XL Extended-Release Tablets (Infrequent) 1613
Xyrem Oral Solution (Infrequent) 1688
Zoloft (Infrequent) 2586
Zomig Nasal Spray (Infrequent) 3523
Zyban Sustained-Release Tablets (Infrequent) 1644
Zyrtec Chewable Tablets (Less than 2%) 2594
Zyrtec (Less than 2%) 2594
Zyrtec-D 12 Hour Extended Release Tablets (Less than 2%) 2597

Coordination, lack of
(*see under* Ataxia)

Coordination difficulty
(*see under* Coordination, impaired)

Cor pulmonale
Chantix Tablets (Rare) 2517
Pulmozyme Inhalation Solution 1248

Cornea, discoloration
Xalatan Sterile Ophthalmic Solution 2649

Cornea, gray, ground-glass appearance
Ophthetic Ophthalmic Solution ⊙232

Cornea, opacities
Accutane Capsules 2731
Imitrex Injection 1463
Imitrex Tablets 1471
Symmetrel Tablets (0.1% to 1%) 1135

Cornea, white crystalline precipitates, presence of
▲ Ciloxan Ophthalmic Ointment (Approximately 17%) 559
▲ Ciloxan Ophthalmic Solution (Approximately 17%) ⊙206

Corneal abrasion
▲ Macugen Injection (1% to 5%) ⊙261

Corneal changes
Efudex (Infrequent) 3363
Neurontin Capsules (Rare) 2487
Neurontin Oral Solution (Rare) 2487
Neurontin Tablets (Rare) 2487

Corneal clouding
▲ Chemet Capsules (1.0% to 3.7%) 2458

Corneal curvature, steepening
Climara Transdermal System 771
Climara Pro Transdermal System 776
Estratest Tablets 3199
Estratest H.S. Tablets 3199
Mircette Tablets 1066
NuvaRing 2340
Ortho-Cyclen Tablets 2429
Ortho Evra Transdermal System 2417
Ortho Tri-Cyclen Tablets 2429
Ortho Tri-Cyclen Lo Tablets 2436
Premarin Vaginal Cream 3452
Premphase Tablets 3456
Prempro Tablets 3456
Seasonique Tablets 1077
Yasmin 28 Tablets 796
Yaz Tablets 803

Corneal deposits
Indocin (Less than 1%) 1995
▲ Macugen Injection (1% to 5%) ⊙261
Propine Ophthalmic Solution ⊙239
Thioridazine Hydrochloride Tablets 2163
▲ Voltaren Ophthalmic Solution (Less than or equal to 5%) 2309

Corneal epithelial breakdown
Acular Ophthalmic Solution 565
Acular LS Ophthalmic Solution 566
Iressa Tablets (Very rare) 684
Voltaren Ophthalmic Solution 2309

Corneal epithelium disorder
▲ Macugen Injection (1% to 5%) ⊙261

Corneal erosion
Acular Ophthalmic Solution 565
Acular LS Ophthalmic Solution 566
Alphagan P Ophthalmic Solution (Less than 1%) 567
▲ Brimonidine Tartrate Ophthalmic Solution 0.2% (3% to 9%) ⊙248
Iressa Tablets 684
Sonata Capsules (Rare) 1717
Voltaren Ophthalmic Solution 2309
Xalatan Sterile Ophthalmic Solution 2649

Corneal infiltrate
Acular Ophthalmic Solution (Rare) 565
▲ Acular LS Ophthalmic Solution (1% to 5%) 566
Ciloxan Ophthalmic Ointment (Less than 1%) 559
Ciloxan Ophthalmic Solution (Less than 1%) ⊙206
Voltaren Ophthalmic Solution 2309

Corneal opacity
Aciphex Tablets 1090
Aldurazyme for Intravenous Infusion (2%) 1268
Anaprox Tablets 2761
Anaprox DS Tablets 2761
EC-Naprosyn Delayed-Release Tablets 2761
Evoxac Capsules (Less than 1%) 1047
Namenda (Infrequent) 1195
Naprosyn Suspension 2761
Naprosyn Tablets 2761
VFEND I.V. (Less than 2%) 2564
VFEND Oral Suspension (Less than 2%) 2564
VFEND Tablets (Less than 2%) 2564
▲ Voltaren Ophthalmic Solution (Less than or equal to 5%) 2309

Corneal perforation
Acular Ophthalmic Solution 565
Acular LS Ophthalmic Solution 566
Voltaren Ophthalmic Solution 2309

Corneal punctate, defects
Symmetrel Tablets (0.1% to 1%) 1135

Corneal punctate keratitis
Betoptic S Ophthalmic Suspension (Small number of patients) 558
Voltaren Ophthalmic Solution 2309

Corneal sensitivity, decrease
Betagan Ophthalmic Solution, USP (A small number of patients) ⊙220
Betimol Ophthalmic Solution 3382
Betimol Ophthalmic Solution ⊙295
Betoptic S Ophthalmic Suspension 558
Cosopt Sterile Ophthalmic Solution 1931
Timoptic Sterile Ophthalmic Solution (Less frequent) 2088
Timoptic in Ocudose (Less frequent) 2091
Timoptic-XE Sterile Ophthalmic Gel Forming Solution 2092

Corneal sensitivity, unspecified
Carteolol Hydrochloride Ophthalmic Solution USP, 1% (Occasional) ⊙249

Corneal staining
Betimol Ophthalmic Solution (1% to 5%) 3382
Betimol Ophthalmic Solution (1% to 5%) ⊙295
▲ Brimonidine Tartrate Ophthalmic Solution 0.2% (3% to 9%) ⊙248
Carteolol Hydrochloride Ophthalmic Solution USP, 1% (Occasional) ⊙249
Ciloxan Ophthalmic Ointment (Less than 1%) 559
Ciloxan Ophthalmic Solution (Less than 1%) ⊙206

Corneal thinning
Acular Ophthalmic Solution 565
Acular LS Ophthalmic Solution 566
Myleran Tablets 1525
Pred-G Ophthalmic Ointment ⊙237
Voltaren Ophthalmic Solution 2309

Corneal ulceration
Acular Ophthalmic Solution (Rare) 565
Ambien Tablets (Rare) 2851
Ambien CR Tablets (Rare) 2855
BOTOX Purified Neurotoxin Complex 570
Copegus Tablets (Less than 1%) 2754
Evoxac Capsules (Less than 1%) 1047
Paxil CR Controlled-Release Tablets (Rare) 1538
Paxil (Rare) 1530
Pegasys (Less than 1%) 2789
Pred Mild Ophthalmic Suspension (Occasional) ⊙238
Pred Forte Ophthalmic Suspension (Occasional) ⊙235
Soriatane Capsules (Less than 1%) 1013
Tarceva Tablets 1259
Tarceva Tablets 2444
Voltaren Ophthalmic Solution 2309

Coronary artery disease, aggravation
Carbatrol Capsules 3171
Equetro Extended-Release Capsules 3180
Tegretol/Tegretol-XR 2295

Coronary artery disease, unspecified
Amevive (Less than 1%) 626

Campath Ampules 811
Celebrex Capsules (0.1% to 1.9%) ... 3134
Chantix Tablets (Rare) 2517
Cymbalta Delayed-Release Capsules (Infrequent) 1757
Effexor Tablets (Rare) 3411
Effexor XR Capsules (Rare) 3417
▲ Humira Injection (Less than 5%) 466
▲ Intron A for Injection (Less than 5%) 3024
Lofibra Tablets 1219
Lofibra Capsules 1216
Proleukin for Injection (Less than 1%) 2266
Rythmol SR Capsules 2727
Tasmar Tablets (Infrequent) 3358
Testim 1% Gel 695
Toprol-XL Tablets (Greater than 1%) 668
Tricor Tablets 527
Triglide Tablets 3123
Zostavax Injection (0.3% to 0.9%) 2111

Coronary heart disease

Premarin Tablets 3446

Coronary occlusion

Omacor Capsules 2725
Trasylol Injection (1% to 2%) 754
Zostavax Injection (0.3%) 2111

Coronary thrombosis

Levaquin (0.1% to 0.9%) 2384
Levaquin in 5% Dextrose Injection (0.1% to 0.9%) 2384

Corpuscular volume, mean, elevation

Thalomid Capsules 965

Cortical lens opacities, scattered punctate

Carbatrol Capsules 3171
Equetro Extended-Release Capsules 3180
Tegretol/Tegretol-XR 2295

Corticosteroid binding globulin, elevated

Adderall Tablets 3164
Menostar Transdermal System 782
Premphase Tablets 3456
Prempro Tablets 3456

Costochondritis

Evoxac Capsules (Less than 1%) 1047
Neurontin Capsules (Rare) 2487
Neurontin Oral Solution (Rare) 2487
Neurontin Tablets (Rare) 2487
Rythmol SR Capsules 2727

Cough

▲ Abilify Oral Solution (3%) 882
▲ Abilify Oral Solution (3%) 2450
▲ Abilify Discmelt Orally Disintegrating Tablets (3%) 882
▲ Abilify Discmelt Orally Disintegrating Tablets (3%) 2450
▲ Abilify Tablets (3%) 882
▲ Abilify Tablets (3%) 2450
▲ Aceon Tablets (2 mg, 4 mg, 8 mg) (6.0% to 12.0%) 3194
▲ Acetadote Injection (.88% to 4.22%) 1031
Actiq (1% or greater) 979
▲ Actonel Tablets (2.5% to 3.1%) 2683
▲ Actonel with Calcium Tablets (2.5% to 3.1%) 2688
Adalat CC Tablets (Less than 1%) 2964
Adenoscan (Less than 1%) 619
▲ Advair Diskus 100/50 (3%) 1308
▲ Advair Diskus 250/50 (6%) 1308
▲ Advair Diskus 500/50 (3% to 6%) ... 1308
Advair HFA Inhalation Aerosol 1318
▲ Advate Injection (15.3%) 712
▲ Aerobid/Aerobid-M (3% to 9%) 1171
Aggrenox Capsules (1.5%) 822
▲ Agrylin Capsules (6.3%) 3169
▲ Alamast Ophthalmic Solution (Less than 5%) 3381
Aldara Cream, 5% (2.8%) 1846
Aldurazyme for Intravenous Infusion 1268
Alferon N Injection (One patient to 1%) 1665
Alkeran for Injection 955
Alkeran Tablets 956
▲ Allegra (3.8%) 2844
Alphagan P Ophthalmic Solution (1% to 4%) 567
▲ Altace Capsules (7.6% to 12%) 1702
▲ Alupent Inhalation Aerosol (3.3%) 826
Ambien Tablets (Infrequent) 2851
Ambien CR Tablets (Infrequent) 2855
▲ AmBisome for Injection (17.8%) 620
Amerge Tablets (Infrequent) 1339
Amevive (Common) 626
Amitiza Capsules (0% to 1.6%) 3224
Aptivus Capsules (0.8%) 826
▲ Aranesp for Injection (10%) 581
▲ Aredia for Injection (25.7%) 2179
Argatroban Injection (2.8%) 1346
▲ Arimidex Tablets (7% to 11%) 673
Arixtra Injection (2.1%) 1351
▲ Aromasin Tablets (6%) 2600
▲ Arranon Injection (0% to 25%) 1357
Arthrotec Tablets (Rare) 3129
Asacol Delayed-Release Tablets (1% to 2%) 2692
Astelin Nasal Spray (Infrequent) 1904
Atacand Tablets (More than 1%) 649
Atacand HCT (0.5% or greater) 651
▲ Atrovent Inhalation Solution (4.6%) 835
▲ Atrovent HFA Inhalation Aerosol (3% to 5%) 841
Atrovent Nasal Spray 0.03% (Less than 2%) 837
Atrovent Nasal Spray 0.06% (Less than 1%) 839
Attenuvax 1914
Avalide Tablets (1% or greater) 888
Avalide Tablets (1% or greater) 2874
▲ Avandia Tablets (6.1%) 1384
Avapro Tablets (2.8%) 891
Avapro Tablets (2.8%) 2871
Axid Oral Solution (2.0%) 879
Azmacort Inhalation Aerosol 1726
Bactroban Nasal (2%) 1394
BeneFix Vials (1.5%) 3408
Benicar HCT Tablets (Greater than 1%) 1044
Blocadren Tablets 1916
▲ BOTOX Purified Neurotoxin Complex (2% to 10%) 570
Caduet Tablets (Less than or equal to 0.1%) 2508
▲ Campath Ampules (2% to 25%) 811
▲ Camptosar Injection (0% to 20.2%) 2604
Captopril Tablets (0.5% to 2%) 2149
Cardizem LA Extended Release Tablets (2%) 1728
▲ Carnitor Injection (9% to 18%) 3188
Caverject Impulse Injection (1%) 2612
Ceftin for Oral Suspension (0.1% to 1%) 1407
Celebrex Capsules (0.1% to 1.9%) 3134
Celexa (Frequent) 1176
▲ Cerezyme for Injection (Approximately 6.6%) 1270
▲ Chemet Capsules (0.7% to 3.7%) 2458
▲ Clarinex Syrup (10.6% to 10.8%) 2995
▲ Clolar for Intravenous Infusion (19%) 1271
Clozaril Tablets (Less than 1%) 2184
Colazal Capsules (2%) 2838
▲ Combivent Inhalation Aerosol (4.2%) 847
▲ Combivir Tablets (18%) 1411
Comvax (0.2% to 0.9%) 1928
▲ Concerta Extended-Release Tablets (4%) 1881
Copaxone for Injection (At least 2%) 3297
▲ Copegus Tablets (10%) 2754
▲ Coreg Tablets (5% to 8%) 1414
▲ Cosopt Sterile Ophthalmic Solution (1% to 5%) 1931
Cozaar Tablets (1% or greater) 1935
Crixivan Capsules (1.5%) 1940
▲ Cubicin for Injection (1% to 3.3%) 1026
▲ Cutivate Lotion 0.05% (3%) 2664
▲ Cymbalta Delayed-Release Capsules (3% to 6%) 1757
▲ Dacogen Injection (40%) 2129
Demadex Injection (2%) 2759
Demadex Tablets (2%) 2759
▲ Depacon Injection (1% to 5%) 412
▲ Depakene (1% to 5%) 417
▲ Depakote Sprinkle Capsules (1% to 5%) 422
▲ Depakote Tablets (1% to 5%) 427
▲ Depakote ER Tablets (1% to 5%) 434
Detrol Tablets (2.1%) 2628
Diastat Rectal Delivery System (Less than 1%) 3343
Diovan Tablets (0.6% to 2.6%) 2193
Diovan HCT Tablets (Greater than 0.2%) 2196
▲ Ditropan XL Extended-Release Tablets (2% to less than 5%) 2413
▲ Doxil Injection (Less than 1% to 9.6%) 2351
Duragesic Transdermal System (1% or greater) 2373
DynaCirc CR Tablets (0.5% to 1%) 2721
Effexor Tablets 3411
▲ Effexor XR Capsules (3%) 3417
▲ Elidel Cream 1% (2.4% to 15.8%) 2200
▲ Eloxatin for Injection (11% to 19%) 2892
Emend Capsules (Greater than 0.5%) 1963
▲ Enbrel for Injection (5% to 6%) 584
▲ Epivir (18%) 1427
▲ Epivir-HBV (Among most common) 1432
▲ Epogen for Injection (18%) 591
Eraxis for Injection (Less than 1% to less than 2%) 2521
▲ Erbitux (Less than 1% to 20%) 910
▲ Evista Tablets (6% to 9.3%) 1763
▲ Evoxac Capsules (6.1%) 1047
Exelon Capsules (2% or more) 2206
Exelon Oral Solution (2% or more) 2206
▲ Faslodex Injection (10.4%) 681
FazaClo Orally Disintegrating Tablets (Less than 1%) 551
▲ Femara Tablets (5% to 13%) 2214
▲ Ferrlecit Injection (6%) 3388
▲ Flebogamma 5%, Immune Globulin Intravenous (Human) (25%) 1658
▲ Flomax Capsules (3.4% to 4.5%) 850
▲ Flonase Nasal Spray (3.6% to 3.8%) 1440
▲ Flovent Diskus (5% to 9%) 1443
▲ Flovent HFA (4%) 1447
Floxin Otic Solution (Single report) ... 1049
Fluarix 1451
Flumadine (Less than 0.3%) 1183
▲ Flumist Vaccine (13.9% to 38.5%) ... 1901
▲ Forteo for Injection (6.4%) 1767
Fortical Nasal Spray (Less than 1%) 3337
▲ Fuzeon Injection (3.9%) 2767
▲ Gabitril Tablets (4%) 984
▲ Gammagard Liquid (0.61% to 8.2%) 721
Gantrisin Pediatric Suspension 2770
Gardasil Injection (2%) 1984
Gemzar for Injection (Common) 1771
▲ Gengraf Capsules (4% to 5%) 459
▲ Gleevec Tablets (0% to 27%) 2227
Hepsera Tablets (2% or greater) 1292
▲ Herceptin I.V. (26%) 1233
▲ Humatrope Vials and Cartridges (Up to 6.25%) 1787
▲ Hycamtin for Injection (1% to 15%) 1458
Hyperstat I.V. 3017
Hytrin Capsules (At least 1%) 471
Hyzaar 50-12.5 Tablets (2.6%) 1990
Hyzaar 100-12.5 Tablets (2.6%) 1990
Hyzaar 100-25 Tablets (2.6%) 1990
▲ Imdur Tablets (Less than or equal to 5%) 3018
Imitrex Nasal Spray (Infrequent) 1467
Imitrex Tablets (Infrequent) 1471
▲ Indapamide Tablets (Less than 5%) 2156
Inspra Tablets (2%) 2536
▲ Intron A for Injection (Up to 31%) 3024
▲ Invanz for Injection (1.3% to 4.4%) 1999
Invirase (Less than 2%) 2772
▲ I.V. Busulfex (28%) 2493
▲ Keppra Oral Solution (2% to 11%) ... 3314
▲ Keppra Tablets (2% to 11%) 3314
Klonopin (2%) 2778
Kytril Injection (2.2%) 2781
▲ Lamictal (7% to 8%) 1481
Lescol Capsules (2.4%) 2233
Lescol XL Tablets (1.9%) 2233
Leukeran Tablets 1504
▲ Leustatin Injection (7% to 10%) 2357
Levaquin (0.1% to 0.9%) 2384
Levaquin in 5% Dextrose Injection (0.1% to 0.9%) 2384
Lexapro Oral Solution (Frequent) 1190
Lexapro Tablets (Frequent) 1190
Lofibra Tablets 1219
Lofibra Capsules 1216
Lotensin Tablets (1.2%) 2243
Lotensin HCT Tablets (2.1%) 2246
▲ Lotrel Capsules (3.3%) 2249
Lotronex Tablets (Rare) 1512
▲ Lucentis Injection (3% to 10%) 1237
▲ Malarone Pediatric Tablets (Less than 1% to 10%) 1517
▲ Malarone Tablets (Less than 1% to 10%) 1517
Marinol Capsules (Less than 1%) 3333
Matulane Capsules 3191
▲ Mavik Tablets (0.3% to 35%) 486
Maxair Autohaler (1.2%) 1852
Maxalt Tablets (Rare) 2008
Maxalt-MLT Orally Disintegrating Tablets (Rare) 2008
▲ Megace ES Oral Suspension (1% to 3%) 2481
▲ Mepron Suspension (25%) 1521
▲ Meridia Capsules (3.8%) 489
Meruvax II 2019
Miacalcin Nasal Spray (Less than 1%) 2253
Micardis Tablets (1% to 1.6%) 854
Micardis HCT Tablets (2% or greater) 856
▲ Midamor Tablets (Between 1% and 3%) 2026
Mirapex Tablets (1% or more) 859
M-M-R II 2006
Mobic Oral Suspension (0.2% to 2.4%) 863
Mobic Tablets (0.2% to 2.4%) 863
Moduretic Tablets 2028
Mumpsvax 2031
▲ Myfortic Tablets (3% to less than 20%) 2255
▲ Mylotarg for Injection (16% to 18%) 3431
▲ Myozyme for Intravenous Infusion (46%) 1279
Nadolol Tablets (1 to 5 of 1000 patients) 2159
▲ Namenda (4%) 1195
Nasacort AQ Nasal Spray (2.1%) 2922
▲ Nasonex Nasal Spray (7% to 13%) 3043
▲ Neoral Oral Solution (4% to 5%) 2259
▲ Neoral Soft Gelatin Capsules (4% to 5%) 2259
▲ Neumega for Injection (29%) 3435
▲ Neupogen for Injection (6%) 603
Neurontin Capsules (1.8%) 2487
Neurontin Oral Solution (1.8%) 2487
Neurontin Tablets (1.8%) 2487
▲ Nexavar Tablets (0% to 13%) 746
Nexium Delayed-Release Capsules (Less than 1%) 655
Nexium I.V. (Less than 1%) 659
▲ Nipent for Injection (17% to 20%) 1863
Norvasc Tablets (Less than 0.1%) 2545
Norvir (Less than 2%) 503
Omacor Capsules 2725
Oncaspar (Less than 1%) 1145
▲ Ontak Vials (26%) 1745
OptiPranolol Metipranolol Ophthalmic Solution 0.3% (A small number of patients) .... ⊙256
▲ Orencia Powder for Intravenous Infusion (0.1% to 8%) 914
OxyContin Tablets (Less than 1%) 2703
Parcopa Orally Disintegrating Tablets 3097
Paxil CR Controlled-Release Tablets (Frequent) 1538
Paxil (Frequent) 1530
▲ Pegasys (4%) 2789
▲ PEG-Intron Powder for Injection (8%) 3048
▲ Photofrin for Injection (7% to 9%) 702
▲ Plavix Tablets (3.1%) 917
▲ Plavix Tablets (3.1%) 2926
▲ Pletal Tablets (3% to 4%) 2455
Prevacid Delayed-Release Capsules (Less than 1%) 3271
Prevacid for Delayed-Release Oral Suspension (Less than 1%) 3271
Prevacid SoluTab Delayed-Release Orally Disintegrating Tablets (Less than 1%) 3271
PREVPAC (Less than 1%) 3284
Prezista Tablets (Less than 2%) 3306
Prilosec OTC Delayed-Release Tablets (1.1%) 2677
▲ Prinivil Tablets (1% to 3.5%) 2052
▲ Prinzide Tablets (3.9%) 2056
▲ Procrit for Injection (18%) 2364
▲ Prograf Capsules and Injection (3% to 18%) 632
▲ Proleukin for Injection (11%) 2266
▲ Prometrium Capsules (100 mg, 200 mg) (8%) 3203
ProQuad (Greater than or equal to 0.2% to less than 1%) 2064
ProSom Tablets (Infrequent) 517
Protonix I.V. (Greater than or equal to 1%) 3472
Protonix Tablets (Greater than or equal to 1%) 3469
▲ Protopic Ointment (1% to 15%) 638
▲ Proventil Inhalation Solution 0.083% (3.1% to 4%) 3055
Provigil Tablets (At least 1%) 988
Prozac Pulvules and Liquid 1801
▲ Pulmicort Respules (5% to 9%) 661
Pulmozyme Inhalation Solution 1248
▲ Rapamune Oral Solution and Tablets (3% to 20%) 3475
Razadyne (Greater than or equal to 2%) 2399
Razadyne ER Extended-Release Capsules (Greater than or equal to 2%) 2399
▲ Rebetol (16% to 23%) 3058
Recombivax HB (Less than 1%) 2071

ReFacto Vials 3484
Refludan for Injection (Common) 792
▲ Relenza Rotadisk (1% to 17%) 1552
Relpax Tablets (Rare) 2548
▲ Remicade for IV Injection (12%) 971
▲ Renagel Tablets (7.1%) 1282
▲ Requip Tablets (1% to 3%) 1555
▲ Rescriptor Tablets (3.5% to 5%) 2551
▲ Retisert Implant (5% to 15%) ⊙258
Retrovir Capsules 1560
Retrovir IV Infusion 1564
Retrovir 1560
▲ Revlimid Capsules (14.5% to 19.6%) 958
Rhinocort Aqua Nasal Spray (2%) 665
▲ Ribavirin, USP Capsules (16% to 23%) 3068
▲ Rilutek Tablets (2.1% to 3.7%) 2930
▲ Risperdal (2% to 3%) 1676
▲ Risperdal Consta Long-Acting Injection (2% to 5%) 1682
▲ Risperdal M-Tab Orally Disintegrating Tablets (2% to 3%) 1676
▲ Rituxan I.V. (1% to 13%) 1254
Rythmol SR Capsules 2727
▲ Serevent Diskus (Greater than 3%) 1568
Seroquel Tablets (Infrequent) 690
▲ Simulect for Injection (Greater than or equal to 10%) 2284
Singulair (1% to 2.7%) 2077
▲ Soltamox Oral Solution (4%) 3527
Soriatane Capsules (Less than 1%) 1013
▲ Spiriva HandiHaler (Greater than or equal to 3%) 869
Stalevo Tablets 2287
Starlix Tablets (2.4%) 2292
▲ Strattera Capsules (2% to 11%) 1814
▲ Suboxone Tablets (4%) 2717
▲ Subutex Tablets (4%) 2717
Sular Tablets (Less than or equal to 1%) 3122
▲ Sustiva Capsules (25%) 930
▲ Sustiva Tablets (25%) 930
▲ Sutent Capsules (0% to 17%) 2560
▲ Symlin Injection (2% to 6%) 613
Synagis (More than 1%) 1897
▲ Tamiflu Capsules (1.2% to 5.6%) 2807
▲ Tamiflu Oral Suspension (1.2% to 5.6%) 2807
▲ Tarceva Tablets (0% to 33%) 1259
▲ Tarceva Tablets (0% to 33%) 2444
Targretin Capsules 1747
▲ Tarka Tablets (4.6%) 524
Tasmar Tablets (Infrequent) 3358
▲ Temodar Capsules (5% to 8%) 3073
▲ Teveten Tablets (4%) 1735
Teveten HCT Tablets (Less than 1%) 1737
Thalomid Capsules 965
Tiazac Capsules (1% to 2%) 1201
Timolide Tablets 2086
Timoptic Sterile Ophthalmic Solution (Less frequent) 2088
Timoptic in Ocudose (Less frequent) 2091
Timoptic-XE Sterile Ophthalmic Gel Forming Solution 2092
▲ TOBI Solution for Inhalation (46.1%) 2298
▲ Topamax Sprinkle Capsules (2% to 4%) 2404
▲ Topamax Tablets (2% to 4%) 2404
Trelstar LA Suspension (1.7%) 3397
▲ Trileptal Tablets (Up to 5%) 2300
▲ Trileptal Oral Suspension (Up to 5%) 2300
▲ Trisenox Injection (65%) 993
▲ Trizivir Tablets (18%) 1589
Truvada Tablets 1296
▲ Ultram ER Tablets (1% to greater than 5%) 2392
▲ Uniretic Tablets (Less than 1% to 3%) 3100
▲ Valcyte Tablets (Less than 5%) 2813
Vantin Tablets and Oral Suspension (Less than 1%) 2645
▲ Vaqta (1% to 5.1%) 2097
Varivax (Greater than or equal to 1%) 2100
Vasotec I.V. Injection (1.3% to 2.2%) 2103
▲ Velcade for Injection (21%) 2133
▲ Ventolin HFA Inhalation Aerosol (5%) 1600
VESIcare Tablets (0.2% to 1.1%) 646
VFEND I.V. (Less than 2%) 2564
VFEND Oral Suspension (Less than 2%) 2564
VFEND Tablets (Less than 2%) 2564
Viagra Tablets (Less than 2%) 2573
Vicoprofen Tablets (Less than 1%) 539
▲ Vigamox Ophthalmic Solution (1% to 4%) ⊙215
▲ Visudyne for Injection (1% to 10%) 2305
Vytorin 10/10 Tablets 2114
Vytorin 10/10 Tablets 3077
Vytorin 10/20 Tablets 2114
Vytorin 10/20 Tablets 3077
Vytorin 10/40 Tablets 2114
Vytorin 10/40 Tablets 3077
Vytorin 10/80 Tablets 2114
Vytorin 10/80 Tablets 3077
WelChol Tablets (2%) 1050
Wellbutrin SR Sustained-Release Tablets (1% to 2%) 1607
Wellbutrin XL Extended-Release Tablets (1% to 2%) 1613
▲ Xeloda Tablets (Less than 5%) 2822
▲ Xopenex Inhalation Solution (1.4% to 4.1%) 3146
▲ Xopenex Inhalation Solution Concentrate (1.4% to 4.1%) 3150
▲ Xopenex HFA Inhalation Aerosol (1.4% to 4.1%) 3154
Xyrem Oral Solution (Frequent) 1688
Yaz Tablets (Greater than 1%) 803
Zegerid Capsules (1.1%) 2958
Zegerid Powder for Oral Solution (1.1%) 2958
Zetia Tablets (2.3%) 2120
Zetia Tablets (2.3%) 3083
Ziagen 1626
Zoloft (Infrequent) 2586
▲ Zometa for Intravenous Infusion (11.6% to 22%) 2315
Zosyn (1.0% or less) 3492
▲ Zyban Sustained-Release Tablets (3%) 1644
▲ Zyprexa Tablets (5%) 1830
▲ Zyprexa ZYDIS Orally Disintegrating Tablets (5%) 1830
▲ Zyrtec Chewable Tablets (2.8% to 4.4%) 2594
▲ Zyrtec (2.8% to 4.4%) 2594
Zyrtec-D 12 Hour Extended Release Tablets (2.8% to 4.4%) 2597
Zyvox 2652

Cough, increased
Aralast (0.1% to 0.6%) 717
▲ Atripla Tablets (Greater than or equal to 5%) 945
▲ Bexxar (1% to 21%) 1398
Campral Tablets (Frequent) 1174
▲ CellCept Capsules (31.1%) 2747
▲ CellCept Intravenous (31.1%) 2747
▲ CellCept Oral Suspension (31.1%) 2747
▲ CellCept Tablets (31.1%) 2747
Crestor Tablets (Greater than or equal to 2%) 678
▲ Elestat Ophthalmic Solution (1% to 3%) 1669
▲ Emtriva Capsules (14%) 1287
▲ Emtriva Oral Solution (14%) 1287
▲ Exubera Inhalation Powder (21.9% to 29.5%) 2524
▲ Gamunex Immune Globulin I.V., 10% (1.7% to 54%) 3235
▲ Geodon Capsules (3%) 2529
▲ Hectorol Capsules (Greater than or equal to 5%) 1275
Ionsys Transdermal System (.1% to less than 1%) 2379
Keppra Injection (2%) 3320
Merrem I.V. (Greater than 0.1% to 1%) 686
▲ Myobloc Injection (3% to 7%) 3192
Natrecor for Injection (Greater than or equal to 1%) 3127
▲ Premarin Tablets (4% to 7%) 3446
▲ Premphase Tablets (5% to 8%) 3456
▲ Prempro Tablets (5% to 8%) 3456
Prevacid NapraPAC (Less than 1%) 3280
▲ Quadramet Injection (4%) 1040
▲ Reyataz Capsules (1% to 5%) 921
Tricor Tablets 527
▲ Tygacil for Injection (3.7%) 3488
▲ Ultane Liquid for Inhalation (5% to 11%) 531
▲ Univasc Tablets (6.1%) 3104
▲ Ventavis Inhalation Solution (39%) 1020
▲ Vigamox Ophthalmic Solution (1% to 4%) 564
▲ Vivaglobin (10%) 3506
Zemaira (0.4%) 3509
Zomig Nasal Spray (Infrequent) 3523

Cough, productive
▲ Flebogamma 5%, Immune Globulin Intravenous (Human) (25%) 1658
Permax Tablets (Frequent) 3356

Cough reflex, depression
Kadian Capsules (Less than 3%) 577
Prozac Pulvules and Liquid (Rare) 1801

CPK, elevation
(*see under* Creatine kinase, increase)

Cramping
Advair Diskus 100/50 1308
Advair Diskus 250/50 1308
Advair Diskus 500/50 1308
Aldoril Tablets 1910
Alferon N Injection (One patient) 1665
Aminohippurate Sodium PAH Injection 1913
▲ Aromasin Tablets (3.1%) 2600
Asacol Delayed-Release Tablets 2692
Atacand HCT 651
Avalide Tablets 888
Avalide Tablets 2874
Clinoril Tablets (Greater than 1%) 1924
Clorpres Tablets 2153
Colazal Capsules (1%) 2838
Coumadin for Injection (Infrequent) 898
Coumadin Tablets (Infrequent) 898
Dilaudid 440
Dilaudid Non-Sterile Powder 440
Dilaudid Oral Liquid 445
Dilaudid Rectal Suppositories 440
Dilaudid Tablets 440
Dilaudid Tablets - 8 mg 445
Diovan HCT Tablets 2196
Diuril Oral Suspension 1954
Diuril Sodium Intravenous 2467
Exelon Capsules (Infrequent) 2206
Exelon Oral Solution (Infrequent) 2206
▲ Ferrlecit Injection (25%) 3388
▲ Gengraf Capsules (1% to 4%) 459
Hyzaar 50-12.5 Tablets 1990
Hyzaar 100-12.5 Tablets 1990
Hyzaar 100-25 Tablets 1990
Lopressor HCT 50/25 Tablets 2241
Lopressor HCT 100/25 Tablets 2241
Lopressor HCT 100/50 Tablets 2241
Lotensin HCT Tablets 2246
MetroGel-Vaginal Gel (1%) 1855
Moduretic Tablets 2028
▲ Neoral Oral Solution (1% to 4%) 2259
▲ Neoral Soft Gelatin Capsules (1% to 4%) 2259
Nexium Delayed-Release Capsules (Less than 1%) 655
Nexium I.V. (Less than 1%) 659
ParaGard T 380A Intrauterine Copper Contraceptive 1073
Prinzide Tablets 2056
Protopic Ointment (0.2% to less than 1%) 638
▲ Sandimmune (Up to 4%) 2275
Teveten HCT Tablets 1737
▲ Thrombate III (2 of 17) 3257
Timolide Tablets 2086
Tindamax Tablets (1.4% to 1.8%) 2142
Uniretic Tablets 3100

Cramping, abdominal
(*see under* Abdominal pain/cramps)

Cramping, legs
Angeliq Tablets 762
Ionsys Transdermal System (.1% to less than 1%) 2379
▲ Zelapar Tablets (3%) 3372
Zomig Tablets (Infrequent) 3519
Zomig-ZMT Tablets (Infrequent) 3519

Cramping, muscular
Abilify Oral Solution (Frequent) 882
Abilify Oral Solution (Frequent) 2450
Abilify Discmelt Orally Disintegrating Tablets (Frequent) 882
Abilify Discmelt Orally Disintegrating Tablets (Frequent) 2450
Abilify Tablets (Frequent) 882
Abilify Tablets (Frequent) 2450
Adalat CC Tablets (Rare) 2964
▲ Advair Diskus 250/50 (3%) 1308
▲ Advair HFA Inhalation Aerosol (1% to 3%) 1318
Advicor Tablets 1722
Alferon N Injection (1%) 1665
Altoprev Extended-Release Tablets (0.6% to 1.1%) 3109
Ambien CR Tablets (2%) 2855
Amerge Tablets (Infrequent) 1339
Amitiza Capsules (0% to 1%) 3224
Antivenin (Black Widow Spider Antivenin) 1913
Aptivus Capsules (Less than 2%) 826
▲ Aricept Tablets (3% to 8%) 1094
▲ Aricept ODT Tablets (3% to 8%) 1094
Asacol Delayed-Release Tablets 2692
Avalide Tablets (1% or greater) 888
Avalide Tablets (1% or greater) 2874
Avapro Tablets (Less than 1%) 891
Avapro Tablets (Less than 1%) 2871
BiDil Tablets 2171
Boniva Injection (1.8% to 2%) 2738
Boniva Tablets (1.8% to 2%) 2741
▲ Bumex Tablets (1.1% to 4.1%) 2746
Caduet Tablets (Less than 1% to 2%) 2508
Cardizem LA Extended Release Tablets (Less than 2%) 1728
Cardura XL Tablets 2515
Ceftin Tablets (0.1% to 1%) 1407
Chantix Tablets (Frequent) 2517
Climara Transdermal System 771
▲ Coreg Tablets (Greater than 1% to 3%) 1414
Covera-HS Tablets (Less than 2%) 3139
Cozaar Tablets (1%) 1935
Cubicin for Injection (Less than 1%) 1026
▲ Cymbalta Delayed-Release Capsules (4% to 5%) 1757
CytoGam Intravenous (Less than 5.0%) 1895
Diovan Tablets 2193
Diovan HCT Tablets (Greater than 0.2%) 2196
Diuril Sodium Intravenous 2467
Dolobid Tablets (Rare) 1955
Dyazide Capsules 1423
Eldepryl Capsules 3208
▲ Entocort EC Capsules (Less than 5%) 2698
Flebogamma 5%, Immune Globulin Intravenous (Human) 1658
Foradil Aerolizer 3010
▲ Fosamax (Up to approximately 6%) 1969
Fosamax Plus D Tablets (0% to 1.1%) 1977
Furosemide Tablets 2154
Gammagard Liquid 721
▲ Gleevec Tablets (28% to 62%) 2227
▲ Humira Injection (Less than 5%) 466
Hyzaar 50-12.5 Tablets 1990
Hyzaar 100-12.5 Tablets 1990
Hyzaar 100-25 Tablets 1990
Imitrex Injection (Frequent) 1463
Imitrex Nasal Spray (Rare) 1467
Imitrex Tablets (Infrequent) 1471
▲ Indapamide Tablets (Greater than or equal to 5%) 2156
Invirase (Less than 2%) 2772
Ketek Tablets 2903
Klonopin (Infrequent) 2778
K-Phos Original (Sodium Free) Tablets (Less frequent) 760
K-Phos Neutral Tablets 760
Lariam Tablets (Infrequent) 2786
Lescol Capsules 2233
Lescol XL Tablets 2233
Lexapro Oral Solution (Infrequent) 1190
Lexapro Tablets (Infrequent) 1190
Lotrel Capsules 2249
Mavik Tablets (0.3% to 1.0%) 486
Maxalt Tablets (Infrequent) 2008
Maxalt-MLT Orally Disintegrating Tablets (Infrequent) 2008
Mevacor Tablets (0.6% to 1.1%) 2021
Micardis Tablets 854
Micardis HCT Tablets 856
▲ Midamor Tablets (Between 1% and 3%) 2026
Migranal Nasal Spray (Infrequent) 3348
Moduretic Tablets (Less than or equal to 1%) 2028
▲ Myfortic Tablets (3% to less than 20%) 2255
Nimotop Capsules (Up to 1.4%) 749
Niravam Orally Disintegrating Tablets (2.4%) 3092
Norvasc Tablets (Less than 1% to 2%) 2545
Norvir (Less than 2%) 503
Oncaspar 1145
Parcopa Orally Disintegrating Tablets 3097
Pepcid Injection (Infrequent) 2040
Pepcid (Infrequent) 2038
Prilosec OTC Delayed-Release Tablets (Less than 1%) 2677
Prinivil Tablets (Greater than 1%) 2052
Prinzide Tablets (2%) 2056
▲ Prograf Capsules and Injection (3% to 15%) 632
Prozac Pulvules and Liquid (Infrequent) 1801
▲ Requip Tablets (3%) 1555
Rescriptor Tablets 2551
▲ Revlimid Capsules (2% to 30.1%) 958
Rythmol SR Capsules 2727
▲ Serevent Diskus (3%) 1568
▲ Simulect for Injection (3% to 10%) 2284
Singulair 2077

Stalevo Tablets 2287
▲ Tasmar Tablets (17% to 18%) 3358
Teveten Tablets (Less than 1%) 1735
Tiazac Capsules (Less than 2%) 1201
Timolide Tablets 2086
▲ Ultram ER Tablets (1% to greater than 5%) 2392
Uroqid-Acid No. 2 Tablets 760
▲ Valcyte Tablets (Less than 5%) 2813
Vasotec I.V. Injection (0.5% to 1.0%) 2103
▲ Velcade for Injection (12%) 2133
▲ Ventavis Inhalation Solution (6%) 1020
Verelan PM Extended-Release Capsules, Controlled-Onset (2% or less) 3106
Viracept (Less than 2%) 2577
▲ Vivitrol (2% to 8%) 995
VoSpire ER Tablets (2.7%) 1052
Vytorin 10/10 Tablets 2114
Vytorin 10/10 Tablets 3077
Vytorin 10/20 Tablets 2114
Vytorin 10/20 Tablets 3077
Vytorin 10/40 Tablets 2114
Vytorin 10/40 Tablets 3077
Vytorin 10/80 Tablets 2114
Vytorin 10/80 Tablets 3077
Zegerid Capsules (Less than 1%) 2958
Zegerid Powder for Oral Solution (Less than 1%) 2958
Zocor Tablets 2105
Zoloft (Infrequent) 2586
Zometa for Intravenous Infusion 2315

Cramps, abdominal
(*see under* Abdominal pain/cramps)

Cramps, lower limbs
Aciphex Tablets 1090
Actiq (1% or greater) 979
▲ Actonel Tablets (3.3% to 3.5%) 2683
▲ Adalat CC Tablets (3% or less) 2964
Agrylin Capsules (1% to 5%) 3169
Alinia for Oral Suspension (Less than 1%) 2835
Alinia Tablets (Less than 1%) 2835
Ambien Tablets (Infrequent) 2851
Ambien CR Tablets (Infrequent) 2855
Atacand HCT (0.5% or greater) 651
▲ Betaseron for SC Injection (4%) 767
Caduet Tablets (Less than 2%) 2508
Campral Tablets (Frequent) 1174
Carbatrol Capsules 3171
▲ Carnitor Injection (4% to 8%) 3188
Catapres Tablets (About 3 in 1,000) 843
Catapres-TTS (0.5% or less) 844
Caverject Impulse Injection (Less than 1%) 2612
Celebrex Capsules (0.1% to 1.9%) 3134
Celexa (Infrequent) 1176
▲ CellCept Capsules (3% to less than 20%) 2747
▲ CellCept Intravenous (3% to less than 20%) 2747
▲ CellCept Oral Suspension (3% to less than 20%) 2747
▲ CellCept Tablets (3% to less than 20%) 2747
Climara Transdermal System 771
Climara Pro Transdermal System 776
Clorpres Tablets (About 3 in 1,000) 2153
▲ Depacon Injection (1% to 5%) 412
▲ Depakene (1% to 5%) 417
▲ Depakote Sprinkle Capsules (1% to 5%) 422
▲ Depakote Tablets (1% to 5%) 427
▲ Depakote ER Tablets (1% to 5%) 434
▲ Depo-Provera Contraceptive Injection (1% to 5%) 2622
Didronel Tablets 2697
DuoNeb Inhalation Solution (1.4%) 1058
DynaCirc CR Tablets (0.5% to 1%) 2721
Effexor Tablets (Infrequent) 3411
Effexor XR Capsules (Infrequent) 3417
▲ Emcyt Capsules (8%) 2634
Enjuvia Tablets 1062
Equetro Extended-Release Capsules 3180
Estrasorb Topical Emulsion 1147
Estratest H.S. Tablets 3199
▲ Evista Tablets (5.9% to 7%) 1763
▲ Evoxac Capsules (1% to 3%) 1047
Exelon Capsules (Frequent) 2206
Exelon Oral Solution (Frequent) 2206
▲ Ferrlecit Injection (10%) 3388
Foradil Aerolizer (1.7%) 3010
Forteo for Injection (2.6%) 1767
Frova Tablets (Infrequent) 1113
Gabitril Tablets (Infrequent) 984
Gammagard S/D (Occasional) 724
▲ Gengraf Capsules (12%) 459
▲ Intron A for Injection (Less than 5%) 3024
Invirase (Less than 2%) 2772
Klonopin (Infrequent) 2778
Lamictal (Rare) 1481
Levaquin (0.1% to 0.9%) 2384
Levaquin in 5% Dextrose Injection (0.1% to 0.9%) 2384
Lipitor Tablets (Less than 2%) 2483
Lofibra Tablets 1219
Lofibra Capsules 1216
Lunesta Tablets (Infrequent) 3142
Lyrica Capsules (Grather than or equal to 1%) 2539
Menostar Transdermal System 782
Meridia Capsules (Greater than or equal to 1%) 489
Micardis Tablets (More than 0.3%) 854
Micardis HCT Tablets 856
Mirapex Tablets (1% or more) 859
Natrecor for Injection (Greater than or equal to 1%) 3127
▲ Neoral Oral Solution (12%) 2259
▲ Neoral Soft Gelatin Capsules (12%) 2259
Neurontin Capsules (Infrequent) 2487
Neurontin Oral Solution (Infrequent) 2487
Neurontin Tablets (Infrequent) 2487
Oxsoralen-Ultra Capsules 3353
Pentasa Capsules (Less than 1%) 3185
Plavix Tablets (1% to 2.5%) 917
Plavix Tablets (1% to 2.5%) 2926
Pletal Tablets (2% or greater) 2455
▲ Premarin Tablets (3% to 7%) 3446
Premarin Vaginal Cream 3452
▲ Premphase Tablets (3% to 7%) 3456
▲ Prempro Tablets (3% to 7%) 3456
Prevacid Delayed-Release Capsules (Less than 1%) 3271
Prevacid for Delayed-Release Oral Suspension (Less than 1%) 3271
Prevacid NapraPAC (Less than 1%) 3280
Prevacid SoluTab Delayed-Release Orally Disintegrating Tablets (Less than 1%) 3271
PREVPAC (Less than 1%) 3284
ProAmatine Tablets (Rare) 3186
Prochieve 4% Gel 1003
Prochieve 8% Gel 1003
▲ Prograf Capsules and Injection (3% to 15%) 632
Prometrium Capsules (100 mg, 200 mg) (Less than 5%) 3203
Protonix I.V. (Less than 1%) 3472
Protonix Tablets (Less than 1%) 3469
Proventil HFA Inhalation Aerosol (Less than 3%) 3056
Provigil Tablets (At least 1%) 988
Prozac Pulvules and Liquid (Infrequent) 1801
▲ Rapamune Oral Solution and Tablets (3% to 20%) 3475
Razadyne (Infrequent) 2399
Requip Tablets (1% or more) 1555
Rilutek Tablets (Infrequent) 2930
Risperdal (Rare) 1676
Risperdal Consta Long-Acting Injection (Infrequent) 1682
Risperdal M-Tab Orally Disintegrating Tablets (Rare) 1676
▲ Sandostatin LAR Depot (5% to 15%) 2280
Seroquel Tablets (Infrequent) 690
Sular Tablets (Less than or equal to 1%) 3122
Symbyax Capsules (Infrequent) 1819
Tegretol/Tegretol-XR 2295
Tequin Injection (Less than 0.1%) 938
Tequin Injection in 5% Dextrose (Less than 0.1%) 938
Tequin Tablets (Less than 0.1%) 938
Teveten HCT Tablets (Less than 1%) 1737
Thalomid Capsules 965
Topamax Sprinkle Capsules (2%) 2404
Topamax Tablets (2%) 2404
Tricor Tablets 527
VFEND I.V. (Less than 2%) 2564
VFEND Oral Suspension (Less than 2%) 2564
VFEND Tablets (Less than 2%) 2564
Wellbutrin SR Sustained-Release Tablets (Infrequent) 1607
Wellbutrin XL Extended-Release Tablets (Infrequent) 1613
Xopenex Inhalation Solution (2.7%) 3146
Xopenex Inhalation Solution Concentrate (2.7%) 3150
Xopenex HFA Inhalation Aerosol (2.7%) 3154
Zoloft (Infrequent) 2586
Zonegran Capsules (Infrequent) 1101
Zyban Sustained-Release Tablets (Infrequent) 1644
Zyprexa Tablets (Infrequent) 1830
Zyprexa ZYDIS Orally Disintegrating Tablets (Infrequent) 1830
Zyrtec Chewable Tablets (Less than 2%) 2594
Zyrtec (Less than 2%) 2594
Zyrtec-D 12 Hour Extended Release Tablets (Less than 2%) 2597

Cramps, night
Proquin XR Tablets (Less than 1%) 1153

Cranial nerve, dysfunction
Advicor Tablets 1722
Garamycin Injectable 3014
Lescol Capsules 2233
Lescol XL Tablets 2233
Zocor Tablets 2105

Cranial nerve, paralysis of
Amerge Tablets (Rare) 1339
Eloxatin for Injection 2892

Cranial nerve deficit, fetal
Accutane Capsules 2731

Craniofacial deformities
Altace Capsules 1702
Captopril Tablets 2149
Cozaar Tablets 1935
Hyzaar 50-12.5 Tablets 1990
Hyzaar 100-12.5 Tablets 1990
Hyzaar 100-25 Tablets 1990
Lotrel Capsules 2249
Prinivil Tablets 2052
Prinzide Tablets 2056
Vasotec I.V. Injection 2103

Craniosynostosis
Synthroid Tablets 520

Creatine kinase, increase
Accutane Capsules 2731
Aciphex Tablets 1090
Actos Tablets 3219
Adalat CC Tablets (Rare) 2964
Advicor Tablets 1722
▲ Altoprev Extended-Release Tablets (11%) 3109
Atacand Tablets (0.5% or greater) 649
Atacand HCT (0.5% or greater) 651
Axert Tablets (Infrequent) 2396
Cardizem LA Extended Release Tablets (Less than 2%) 1728
Clozaril Tablets 2184
Colazal Capsules 2838
Combivir Tablets 1411
Comtan Tablets 2189
▲ Cubicin for Injection (2.8% to 6.7%) 1026
Effexor Tablets 3411
Effexor XR Capsules 3417
▲ Emtriva Capsules (11% to 12%) 1287
▲ Emtriva Oral Solution (11% to 12%) 1287
Epivir 1427
▲ Epivir-HBV (9%) 1432
Evoxac Capsules 1047
Gleevec Tablets (up to 1.5%) 2227
▲ Hepsera Tablets (7%) 1292
Levitra Tablets (2%) 3034
▲ Lofibra Tablets (3%) 1219
▲ Lofibra Capsules (3%) 1216
▲ Mevacor Tablets (11%) 2021
Noroxin Tablets (Rare) 2032
Oxandrin Tablets 2962
Paxil CR Controlled-Release Tablets (Rare) 1538
Paxil (Rare) 1530
▲ Rapamune Oral Solution and Tablets (3% to 20%) 3475
ReFacto Vials 3484
Retrovir IV Infusion 1564
Sandostatin Injection (Less than 1%) 2278
Sandostatin LAR Depot (Rare) 2280
Seroquel Tablets 690
Symmetrel Tablets 1135
Tasmar Tablets (Three cases) 3358
Teveten Tablets (Less than 1%) 1735
Teveten HCT Tablets (Less than 1%) 1737
Tiazac Capsules (Less than 2%) 1201
▲ Tricor Tablets (3%) 527
Trizivir Tablets 1589
▲ Truvada Tablets (7%) 1296
Twinrix Vaccine 1595
Uniretic Tablets (Less than 1%) 3100
▲ Viread Tablets (7% to 12%) 1301
Ziagen 1626
Zmax for Oral Suspension (Less then 1%) 2583
▲ Zocor Tablets (5%) 2105

Creatine phosphokinase, increase
Effexor Tablets 3411
Eraxis for Injection (Less than 1% to less than 2%) 2521
▲ Vivitrol (11% to 16%) 995
Vytorin 10/40 Tablets 2114
Zetia Tablets 2120
Zetia Tablets 3083

Creatinine, increase
(*see under* Serum creatinine, elevation)

Creatinine clearance, changes
Bumex Tablets (0.3%) 2746

Creatinine clearance, decrease
▲ Alimta for Injection (Up to 5%) 1750
Lithobid Tablets 1692
▲ NeoProfen Injection (3%) 2472
▲ Valcyte Tablets (Less than 5%) 2813
Vantas (Less than 2%) 3375
VFEND I.V. (Less than 2%) 2564
VFEND Oral Suspension (Less than 2%) 2564
VFEND Tablets (Less than 2%) 2564
Zinacef for Injection 1631
Zinacef Injection 1631

Crepitations
▲ Dacogen Injection (5%) 2129
▲ Trisenox Injection (10%) 993

Crohn's disease, exacerbation
▲ Entocort EC Capsules (Less than 5%) 2698
Proleukin for Injection (Two patients) 2266

Croup
(*see under* Laryngotracheobronchitis)

Crusting
▲ Levulan Kerastick for Topical Solution, 20% (1% to 71%) 1085
▲ Panretin Gel (1% to 8%) 1747

Crying
Ambien Tablets 2851
Aricept Tablets (Frequent) 1094
Aricept ODT Tablets (Frequent) 1094
▲ Comvax (0.2% to 10.6%) 1928
DAPTACEL Vaccine (1% to 2.5%) 2950
Daytrana Transdermal Patch 3174
HibTITER (38 of 1,118 vaccinations) 3426
▲ Infanrix Vaccine (2.2% to 3.9%) 1476
Lexapro Oral Solution (Infrequent) 1190
Lexapro Tablets (Infrequent) 1190
Namenda (Infrequent) 1195
Paxil CR Controlled-Release Tablets 1538
Paxil 1530
▲ Pediarix Vaccine (1.4% to 24.9%) 1548
Prochieve 4% Gel 1003
Prochieve 8% Gel 1003
ProQuad (Greater than or equal to 0.2% to less than 1%) 2064
Recombivax HB (Greater than 1%) 2071
▲ Romazicon Injection (1% to 3%) 2804
Strattera Capsules (2%) 1814
Ultane Liquid for Inhalation (Less than 1%) 531
Vaqta (1.8%) 2097
Xyrem Oral Solution (Infrequent) 1688

Cryptococcosis
▲ CellCept Capsules (Less than 4%) 2747
▲ CellCept Intravenous (Less than 4%) 2747
▲ CellCept Oral Suspension (Less than 4%) 2747
▲ CellCept Tablets (Less than 4%) 2747
Doxil Injection (Less than 1%) 2351

Crystalluria
Amoxil Capsules 1343
Amoxil Chewable Tablets 1343
Amoxil Pediatric Drops for Oral Suspension 1343
Amoxil Powder for Oral Suspension 1343
Amoxil Tablets 1343
Augmentin 1360
Augmentin Tablets 1363
Augmentin XR Extended-Release Tablets 1369

Cardizem LA Extended Release Tablets (Less than 2%) 1728
Cipro (Rare) 2977
Cipro I.V. (1% or less) 2984
Cipro XR Tablets 2990
Clinoril Tablets (Less than 1 in 100) 1924
Crixivan Capsules 1940
Dantrium Capsules (Less frequent) 2694
Demser Capsules (A few patients) 1953
Effexor Tablets (Rare) 3411
Effexor XR Capsules (Rare) 3417
Fansidar Tablets 2765
Gantrisin Pediatric Suspension 2770
Levaquin 2384
Levaquin in 5% Dextrose Injection 2384
Lyrica Capsules (Rare) 2539
Mintezol 2027
Noroxin Tablets 2032
Paser Granules 1674
Reyataz Capsules (Less than 3%) 921
Uniretic Tablets (Less than 1%) 3100

Culture negative, unspecified
Revlimid Capsules 958

Cushingoid appearance
Advair Diskus 100/50 1308
Advair Diskus 250/50 1308
Advair Diskus 500/50 1308
Advair HFA Inhalation Aerosol 1318
Aptivus Capsules 826
Crixivan Capsules 1940
Retrovir 1560
Truvada Tablets 1296

Cushingoid state
(*see under* Cushing's syndrome)

Cushing's syndrome
Aclovate Cream 2660
Advair Diskus 100/50 1308
Advair Diskus 250/50 1308
Advair Diskus 500/50 1308
Advair HFA Inhalation Aerosol 1318
▲ CellCept Capsules (3% to less than 20%) 2747
▲ CellCept Intravenous (3% to less than 20%) 2747
▲ CellCept Oral Suspension (3% to less than 20%) 2747
▲ CellCept Tablets (3% to less than 20%) 2747
Clobevate Gel 3211
Clobex Shampoo 1206
Colocort Rectal Suspension, USP (Retention) 100 mg/60 mL 2476
Copaxone for Injection (Infrequent) 3297
Cutivate Cream 2662
Cutivate Lotion 0.05% (Rare) 2664
Cutivate Ointment 2665
Decadron Tablets 1951
Depo-Medrol Injectable Suspension 2617
Depo-Medrol Single-Dose Vial 2619
Diprolene Gel 0.05% 3001
Diprolene Lotion 0.05% 3002
Diprolene Ointment 0.05% (Some patients) 3003
Diprolene AF Cream 0.05% (Some patients) 3000
Diprosone Cream, USP 0.05% 3004
Elocon Cream 0.1% 3005
Elocon Lotion 0.1% 3006
Elocon Ointment 0.1% 3007
Flovent Diskus 1443
Flovent HFA 1447
Hydrocortone Tablets 1989
Kaletra (Less than 2%) 476
Lotrisone 3040
▲ Myfortic Tablets (3% to less than 20%) 2255
Neurontin Capsules (Rare) 2487
Neurontin Oral Solution (Rare) 2487
Neurontin Tablets (Rare) 2487
Olux Foam 1012
▲ Prograf Capsules and Injection (3% to 15%) 632
▲ Rapamune Oral Solution and Tablets (3% to 20%) 3475
Temovate Cream 2668
Temovate Gel 2669
Temovate Ointment 2668
Temovate Scalp Application 2670
Temovate E Emollient 2671
Vanos Cream 1893

Cushing's syndrome, manifestations of
Clobex Spray 1208

Cutaneous reactions, severe
Celexa (Rare) 1176

Cutaneous reactions, unspecified
Flebogamma 5%, Immune Globulin Intravenous (Human) 1658
Lotrisone Cream 3040
Malarone Pediatric Tablets 1517
Malarone Tablets 1517

Cutaneous tenderness
Oxsoralen-Ultra Capsules 3353

Cyanosis
Abilify Oral Solution (Infrequent) 882
Abilify Oral Solution (Infrequent) 2450
Abilify Discmelt Orally Disintegrating Tablets (Infrequent) 882
Abilify Discmelt Orally Disintegrating Tablets (Infrequent) 2450
Abilify Tablets (Infrequent) 882
Abilify Tablets (Infrequent) 2450
AmBisome for Injection (Infrequent) 620
BeneFix Vials 3408
Bicillin C-R Injectable Suspension 1706
Buprenex Injectable (Less than 1%) 2716
Campath Ampules 811
Carimune NF 3499
▲ Cerezyme for Injection (Approximately 6.6%) 1270
Clozaril Tablets (Less than 1%) 2184
Copaxone for Injection (Infrequent) 3297
Effexor Tablets (Rare) 3411
Effexor XR Capsules (Rare) 3417
Elitek (Less than or equal to 1%) 2890
FazaClo Orally Disintegrating Tablets (Less than 1%) 551
Flebogamma 5%, Immune Globulin Intravenous (Human) 1658
Gammagard Liquid 721
Gammagard S/D 724
Gamunex Immune Globulin I.V., 10% 3235
Gantrisin Pediatric Suspension 2770
Imitrex Injection 1463
Imitrex Nasal Spray 1467
Imitrex Tablets 1471
Infanrix Vaccine 1476
▲ Infasurf Intratracheal Suspension (65%) 1184
Infed Injection 3390
▲ Intron A for Injection (Less than or equal to 5%) 3024
Invirase (Less than 2%) 2772
Mephyton Tablets (Rare) 2018
Mycamine for Injection 628
Myozyme for Intravenous Infusion 1279
Pediarix Vaccine 1548
Permax Tablets (Infrequent) 3356
Primaxin I.M. 2045
Primaxin I.V. (Less than 0.2%) 2048
Relpax Tablets (Rare) 2548
Rilutek Tablets (Rare) 2930
Seroquel Tablets (Rare) 690
Sonata Capsules (Rare) 1717
Soriatane Capsules (Less than 1%) 1013
Tequin Injection (Less than 0.1%) 938
Tequin Injection in 5% Dextrose (Less than 0.1%) 938
Tequin Tablets (Less than 0.1%) 938
Thalomid Capsules 965
VFEND I.V. (Less than 2%) 2564
VFEND Oral Suspension (Less than 2%) 2564
VFEND Tablets (Less than 2%) 2564
Virazole for Inhalation Solution (Infrequent) 3370
Zelapar Tablets 3372
Zomig Tablets (Rare) 3519
Zomig Nasal Spray (Infrequent) 3523
Zomig-ZMT Tablets (Rare) 3519
Zyprexa Tablets (Infrequent) 1830
Zyprexa ZYDIS Orally Disintegrating Tablets (Infrequent) 1830

Cyanosis, hand
▲ Intron A for Injection (Less than 5%) 3024

Cycloplegia
Bentyl Capsules 697
Bentyl Injection 697
Bentyl Syrup 697
Bentyl Tablets 697
Ditropan XL Extended-Release Tablets 2413
Donnatal Extentabs 2493

Cylindruria
Cipro 2977
Cipro I.V. (1% or less) 2984
Levaquin 2384
Levaquin in 5% Dextrose Injection 2384
Noroxin Tablets 2032

Cyst, sebaceous
Rescriptor Tablets 2551

Cyst, synovial
Gengraf Capsules (1% to less than 3%) 459
Neoral Oral Solution (1% to less than 3%) 2259
Neoral Soft Gelatin Capsules (1% to less than 3%) 2259

Cyst, unspecified
Actiq (Less than 1%) 979
▲ Arimidex Tablets (5%) 673
▲ CellCept Capsules (3% to less than 20%) 2747
▲ CellCept Intravenous (3% to less than 20%) 2747
▲ CellCept Oral Suspension (3% to less than 20%) 2747
▲ CellCept Tablets (3% to less than 20%) 2747
Copaxone for Injection (2%) 3297
Gabitril Tablets (Frequent) 984
Imitrex Injection 1463
Lofibra Tablets 1219
Lofibra Capsules 1216
Myobloc Injection (Greater than 2%) 3192
Neurontin Capsules (Rare) 2487
Neurontin Oral Solution (Rare) 2487
Neurontin Tablets (Rare) 2487
Prochieve 4% Gel 1003
Prochieve 8% Gel 1003
Protonix I.V. (Less than 1%) 3472
Protonix Tablets (Less than 1%) 3469
Protopic Ointment (Up to 3%) 638
▲ Simulect for Injection (3% to 10%) 2284
Soriatane Capsules (Less than 1%) 1013
Symbyax Capsules (Infrequent) 1819
Thalomid Capsules 965
Tricor Tablets 527
Uniretic Tablets (Less than 1%) 3100
Xyrem Oral Solution (Infrequent) 1688
Zelapar Tablets 3372
Zomig Nasal Spray (Infrequent) 3523

Cystitis
Abilify Oral Solution (Infrequent) 882
Abilify Oral Solution (Infrequent) 2450
Abilify Discmelt Orally Disintegrating Tablets (Infrequent) 882
Abilify Discmelt Orally Disintegrating Tablets (Infrequent) 2450
Abilify Tablets (Infrequent) 882
Abilify Tablets (Infrequent) 2450
Aciphex Tablets 1090
▲ Actonel Tablets (4.1%) 2683
▲ Actonel with Calcium Tablets (4.1%) 2688
Ambien Tablets (Infrequent) 2851
Ambien CR Tablets (Infrequent) 2855
Anaprox Tablets (Less than 1%) 2761
Anaprox DS Tablets (Less than 1%) 2761
Aricept Tablets (Infrequent) 1094
Aricept ODT Tablets (Infrequent) 1094
Atacand HCT (0.5% or greater) 651
▲ Azmacort Inhalation Aerosol (1% to 3%) 1726
Caduet Tablets (Less than 2%) 2508
Copaxone for Injection (At least 2%) 3297
Depacon Injection (1% or more) 412
Depakene (1% or more) 417
Depakote Sprinkle Capsules 422
▲ Depakote Tablets (1% to 5%) 427
Depakote ER Tablets (Greater than 1%) 434
▲ Ditropan XL Extended-Release Tablets (2% to less than 5%) 2413
▲ Doxil Injection (Less than 1% to 10%) 2351
EC-Naprosyn Delayed-Release Tablets (Less than 1%) 2761
Effexor Tablets (Infrequent) 3411
Effexor XR Capsules (Infrequent) 3417
Estratest Tablets 3199
Estratest H.S. Tablets 3199
▲ Estring Vaginal Ring (1% to 3%) 2635
▲ Eulexin Capsules (16%) 3009
▲ Evista Tablets (3.3% to 4.6%) 1763
▲ Evoxac Capsules (1% to 3%) 1047
Exelon Capsules (Infrequent) 2206
Exelon Oral Solution (Infrequent) 2206
▲ Fortical Nasal Spray (1% to 3%) 3337
Gabitril Tablets (Infrequent) 984
▲ Humira Injection (Less than 5%) 466
▲ Intron A for Injection (Less than 5%) 3024
Klonopin (Infrequent) 2778
Lamictal (Rare) 1481
Leukeran Tablets 1504
Lipitor Tablets (Less than 2%) 2483
Lofibra Tablets 1219
Lofibra Capsules 1216
Lunesta Tablets (Infrequent) 3142
▲ Miacalcin Nasal Spray (1% to 3%) 2253
Micardis Tablets (More than 0.3%) 854
Micardis HCT Tablets 856
Migranal Nasal Spray (Infrequent) 3348
Myobloc Injection (Greater than 2%) 3192
Nalfon Capsules (Less than 1%) 2502
Naprosyn Suspension (Less than 1%) 2761
Naprosyn Tablets (Less than 1%) 2761
Neurontin Capsules (Infrequent) 2487
Neurontin Oral Solution (Infrequent) 2487
Neurontin Tablets (Infrequent) 2487
Nexium Delayed-Release Capsules (Less than 1%) 655
Nexium I.V. (Less than 1%) 659
Ortho-Cyclen Tablets 2429
Ortho Evra Transdermal System 2417
Ortho Tri-Cyclen Tablets 2429
Ortho Tri-Cyclen Lo Tablets 2436
Paxil CR Controlled-Release Tablets (Infrequent) 1538
Paxil (Infrequent) 1530
Permax Tablets (Infrequent) 3356
Pexeva Tablets (infrequent) 1694
Plavix Tablets (1% to 2.5%) 917
Plavix Tablets (1% to 2.5%) 2926
Pletal Tablets (Less than 2%) 2455
Premarin Intravenous 3442
Premarin Vaginal Cream 3452
Premphase Tablets 3456
Prempro Tablets 3456
Prochieve 4% Gel 1003
Prochieve 8% Gel 1003
▲ Prograf Capsules and Injection (3% to 15%) 632
Protonix I.V. (Less than 1%) 3472
Protonix Tablets (Less than 1%) 3469
Protopic Ointment (0.2% to less than 1%) 638
Provigil Tablets (At least 1%) 988
Prozac Pulvules and Liquid (Infrequent) 1801
Razadyne (Infrequent) 2399
Razadyne ER Extended-Release Capsules (Infrequent) 2399
Risperdal (Rare) 1676
Risperdal M-Tab Orally Disintegrating Tablets (Rare) 1676
Seroquel Tablets (Infrequent) 690
Sonata Capsules (Infrequent) 1717
Symbyax Capsules (Infrequent) 1819
Teveten Tablets (Less than 1%) 1735
Teveten HCT Tablets (Less than 1%) 1737
▲ Topamax Sprinkle Capsules (1% to 3%) 2404
▲ Topamax Tablets (1% to 3%) 2404
Tricor Tablets 527
Triglide Tablets 3123
Uniretic Tablets (Less than 1%) 3100
Viagra Tablets (Less than 2%) 2573
Vicoprofen Tablets (Less than 1%) 539
Voltaren Tablets (Occasionally) 2307
Voltaren-XR Tablets (Occasionally) 2310
Wellbutrin Tablets (Rare) 1603
Wellbutrin SR Sustained-Release Tablets 1607
Wellbutrin XL Extended-Release Tablets 1613
Yasmin 28 Tablets (Greater than 1%) 796
Yaz Tablets (Greater than 1%) 803
Zelapar Tablets 3372
Zoloft (Rare) 2586
Zomig Tablets (Infrequent) 3519
Zomig-ZMT Tablets (Infrequent) 3519
Zyban Sustained-Release Tablets 1644
Zyprexa Tablets (Infrequent) 1830
Zyprexa ZYDIS Orally Disintegrating Tablets (Infrequent) 1830
Zyrtec Chewable Tablets (Less than 2%) 2594
Zyrtec (Less than 2%) 2594
Zyrtec-D 12 Hour Extended Release Tablets (Less than 2%) 2597

Cystitis, hemorrhagic
AmBisome for Injection (Infrequent) 620

Cipro I.V. (1% or less) 2984
Cipro XR Tablets 2990
Herceptin I.V. (At least one of the 958 patients) 1233
▲ I.V. Busulfex (7%) 2493
Oncaspar 1145
Prograf Capsules and Injection 632
Proquin XR Tablets 1153
VFEND I.V. (Less than 2%) 2564
VFEND Oral Suspension (Less than 2%) 2564
VFEND Tablets (Less than 2%) 2564

Cystitis, viral
Retrovir Capsules (0.8%) 1560
Retrovir IV Infusion (1%) 1564
Retrovir (0.8%) 1560

Cystitis-like syndrome
Mircette Tablets 1066
NuvaRing 2340
Seasonique Tablets 1077
Yaz Tablets 803

Cysts, epidermal
Rescriptor Tablets 2551

Cysts, vaginal
Depo-Provera Contraceptive Injection (Less than 1%) 2622
depo-subQ provera 104 Injectable Suspension 2624

Cysts at injection site
▲ Fuzeon Injection (80%) 2767

Cytokine Released Syndrome
Orthoclone OKT3 Sterile Solution (Occasional) 2360
Simulect for Injection 2284

Cytopenia, unspecified
Bexxar 1398
Humira Injection (Infrequent) 466
Pegasys 2789

D

Deafness
Abelcet Injection 1141
Abilify Oral Solution (Infrequent) 882
Abilify Oral Solution (Infrequent) 2450
Abilify Discmelt Orally Disintegrating Tablets (Infrequent) 882
Abilify Discmelt Orally Disintegrating Tablets (Infrequent) 2450
Abilify Tablets (Infrequent) 882
Abilify Tablets (Infrequent) 2450
Aciphex Tablets 1090
Actiq (Less than 1%) 979
Aggrenox Capsules (Less than 1%) 822
Caduet Tablets (Less than 2%) 2508
Campral Tablets (Infrequent) 1174
Celebrex Capsules (0.1% to 1.9%) 3134
▲ CellCept Capsules (3% to less than 20%) 2747
▲ CellCept Intravenous (3% to less than 20%) 2747
▲ CellCept Oral Suspension (3% to less than 20%) 2747
▲ CellCept Tablets (3% to less than 20%) 2747
Chantix Tablets (Rare) 2517
Copaxone for Injection (At least 2%) 3297
▲ Depacon Injection (1% to 5%) 412
▲ Depakene (1% to 5%) 417
▲ Depakote Sprinkle Capsules (1% to 5%) 422
▲ Depakote Tablets (1% to 5%) 427
Depakote ER Tablets (Greater than 1%) 434
DepoCyt Injection 1143
Edecrin 1959
Effexor Tablets (Rare) 3411
Effexor XR Capsules (Rare) 3417
Eloxatin for Injection 2892
Evoxac Capsules (Less than 1%) 1047
Gabitril Tablets (Infrequent) 984
Gengraf Capsules (1% to less than 3%) 459
Herceptin I.V. (At least one of the 958 patients) 1233
Imitrex Injection 1463
Imitrex Nasal Spray 1467
Imitrex Tablets 1471
Indocin Capsules (Less than 1%) 1995
Indocin I.V. (Less than 1%) 2465
Indocin (Less than 1%) 1995
Lamictal (Rare) 1481
Lipitor Tablets (Less than 2%) 2483
Neoral Oral Solution (1% to less than 3%) 2259
Neoral Soft Gelatin Capsules (1% to less than 3%) 2259
Neurontin Capsules (Infrequent) 2487
Neurontin Oral Solution (Infrequent) 2487
Neurontin Tablets (Infrequent) 2487
Nipent for Injection (Less than 3%) 1863
Paxil CR Controlled-Release Tablets (Rare) 1538
Paxil (Rare) 1530
Permax Tablets (Infrequent) 3356
Pexeva Tablets (rare) 1694
Prevacid Delayed-Release Capsules (Less than 1%) 3271
Prevacid for Delayed-Release Oral Suspension (Less than 1%) 3271
Prevacid SoluTab Delayed-Release Orally Disintegrating Tablets (Less than 1%) 3271
Prevacid NapraPAC (Less than 1%) 3280
PREVPAC (Less than 1%) 3284
Prograf Capsules and Injection 632
ProQuad 2064
Protonix I.V. (Less than 1%) 3472
Protonix Tablets (Less than 1%) 3469
▲ Rapamune Oral Solution and Tablets (3% to 20%) 3475
Rilutek Tablets (Rare) 2930
Risperdal Consta Long-Acting Injection (Infrequent) 1682
Sandostatin LAR Depot (Rare) 2280
Seroquel Tablets (Infrequent) 690
Sonata Capsules (Rare) 1717
Soriatane Capsules (Less than 1%) 1013
Symbyax Capsules (Infrequent) 1819
Uniretic Tablets (Less than 1%) 3100
VFEND I.V. (Less than 2%) 2564
VFEND Oral Suspension (Less than 2%) 2564
VFEND Tablets (Less than 2%) 2564
Viagra Tablets (Less than 2%) 2573
Wellbutrin SR Sustained-Release Tablets 1607
Wellbutrin XL Extended-Release Tablets 1613
Zelapar Tablets 3372
Zmax for Oral Suspension 2583
Zonegran Capsules (Infrequent) 1101
Zyban Sustained-Release Tablets 1644
Zyprexa Tablets (Infrequent) 1830
Zyprexa ZYDIS Orally Disintegrating Tablets (Infrequent) 1830
Zyrtec Chewable Tablets (Less than 2%) 2594
Zyrtec (Less than 2%) 2594
Zyrtec-D 12 Hour Extended Release Tablets (Less than 2%) 2597

Deafness, transient
Actiq (Less than 1%) 979

Death
Abilify Oral Solution 882
Abilify Oral Solution 2450
Abilify Discmelt Orally Disintegrating Tablets 882
Abilify Discmelt Orally Disintegrating Tablets 2450
Abilify Tablets 882
Abilify Tablets 2450
Anaprox Tablets (Less than 1%) 2761
Anaprox DS Tablets (Less than 1%) 2761
▲ Aranesp for Injection (7%) 581
EC-Naprosyn Delayed-Release Tablets (Less than 1%) 2761
Gemzar for Injection (Rare) 1771
Mephyton Tablets 2018
Naprosyn Suspension (Less than 1%) 2761
Naprosyn Tablets (Less than 1%) 2761
Podocon-25 Liquid 2478
Rapamune Oral Solution and Tablets (0.8% to 1.7%) 3475
Razadyne 2399
Razadyne ER Extended-Release Capsules 2399
Symbyax Capsules (Rare) 1819
Voltaren Tablets (Rarely) 2307
Voltaren-XR Tablets (Rarely) 2310

Death, fetal
Aceon Tablets (2 mg, 4 mg, 8 mg) 3194
Altace Capsules 1702
Arthrotec Tablets 3129
Atacand Tablets 649
Atacand HCT 651
Avalide Tablets 888
Avalide Tablets 2874
Avapro Tablets 891
Avapro Tablets 2871
Captopril Tablets 2149
Cozaar Tablets 1935
Hyzaar 50-12.5 Tablets 1990
Hyzaar 100-12.5 Tablets 1990
Hyzaar 100-25 Tablets 1990
Lotrel Capsules 2249
Podocon-25 Liquid 2478
Prinivil Tablets 2052
Prinzide Tablets 2056
Prometrium Capsules (100 mg, 200 mg) (Rare) 3203
Thalomid Capsules 965
Uniretic Tablets (More than 1%) 3100
Vasotec I.V. Injection 2103
Zyrtec Chewable Tablets (Rare) 2594
Zyrtec (Rare) 2594

Death, infants
Virazole for Inhalation Solution (20 cases) 3370

Death, sudden
Aciphex Tablets 1090
Adderall Tablets 3164
Adderall XR Capsules 3166
Campral Tablets (Rare) 1174
Camptosar Injection 2604
Celebrex Capsules (Less than 0.1%) 3134
Clozaril Tablets (Rare) 2184
DextroStat Tablets 3179
Gabitril Tablets (Infrequent) 984
Imitrex Tablets 1471
Meridia Capsules 489
Namenda 1195
Phenergan Tablets and Suppositories 3440
Prozac Pulvules and Liquid 1801
Risperdal (Rare) 1676
Risperdal M-Tab Orally Disintegrating Tablets (Rare) 1676
Ritalin LA Capsules 2271
Thioridazine Hydrochloride Tablets 2163
Topamax Sprinkle Capsules (Rare) 2404
Topamax Tablets (Rare) 2404
Zyprexa Tablets (Rare) 1830
Zyprexa ZYDIS Orally Disintegrating Tablets (Rare) 1830

Deep tendon reflexes, loss
Eloxatin for Injection 2892

Defecate, desire to
Aminohippurate Sodium PAH Injection 1913

Defecation, increased
▲ Xenical Capsules (2.8% to 10.8%) 2831

Defecation, painful
Invirase (Less than 2%) 2772

Deglutition disorder
Emend Capsules (Greater than 0.5%) 1963

Dehydration
Abilify Oral Solution (Frequent) 882
Abilify Oral Solution (Frequent) 2450
Abilify Discmelt Orally Disintegrating Tablets (Frequent) 882
Abilify Discmelt Orally Disintegrating Tablets (Frequent) 2450
Abilify Tablets (Frequent) 882
Abilify Tablets (Frequent) 2450
Aciphex Tablets 1090
Actiq (1% or greater) 979
Aggrenox Capsules 822
▲ Agrylin Capsules (1% to 5%) 3169
▲ Alimta for Injection (Up to 9%) 1750
Amerge Tablets (Infrequent) 1339
Aptivus Capsules (Less than 2%) 826
▲ Aranesp for Injection (5%) 581
Aricept Tablets (Frequent) 1094
Aricept ODT Tablets (Frequent) 1094
▲ Arranon Injection (1% to 7%) 1357
Arthrotec Tablets (Rare) 3129
Bayer Aspirin 744
Bayer Aspirin Comprehensive Prescribing Information 796
Bexxar 1398
Bumex Tablets (0.1%) 2746
Byetta Injection 611
Campath Ampules 811
▲ Camptosar Injection (4% to 15%) 2604
Captopril Tablets 2149
Celexa (Rare) 1176
▲ CellCept Capsules (3% to less than 20%) 2747
▲ CellCept Intravenous (3% to less than 20%) 2747
▲ CellCept Oral Suspension (3% to less than 20%) 2747
▲ CellCept Tablets (3% to less than 20%) 2747
Cymbalta Delayed-Release Capsules (Infrequent) 1757
▲ Dacogen Injection (6%) 2129
Demadex Injection 2759
Demadex Tablets 2759
Diovan HCT Tablets (Less frequent) 2196
▲ Doxil Injection (1% to 10%) 2351
Effexor Tablets (Rare) 3411
Effexor XR Capsules (Rare) 3417
Elitek (Less than or equal to 1%) 2890
▲ Eloxatin for Injection (5% to 8%) 2892
▲ Emend Capsules (5.9%) 1963
Epivir 1427
▲ Erbitux (2% to 25%) 910
Evoxac Capsules (Less than 1%) 1047
Exelon Capsules (2% to Frequent) 2206
Exelon Oral Solution (2% to Frequent) 2206
Fleet Enema 1165
Fleet Prep Kits 1170
Frova Tablets (Infrequent) 1113
Furosemide Tablets 2154
Gabitril Tablets (Infrequent) 984
Garamycin Injectable 3014
Geodon Capsules (Infrequent) 2529
Gleevec Tablets (Infrequent) 2227
▲ Hectorol Capsules (Greater than or equal to 5%) 1275
Hectorol Injection 1278
▲ Humira Injection (Less than 5%) 466
Imitrex Injection (Rare) 1463
Imitrex Nasal Spray 1467
Imitrex Tablets 1471
▲ Intron A for Injection (Less than or equal to 5%) 3024
Invanz for Injection (Greater than 0.1%) 1999
Invirase (Less than 2%) 2772
Ionsys Transdermal System (.1% to less than 1%) 2379
Kaletra (Less than 2%) 476
Keppra Oral Solution (2%) 3314
Keppra Tablets (2%) 3314
Klonopin 2778
Levaquin (0.1% to 0.9%) 2384
Levaquin in 5% Dextrose Injection (0.1% to 0.9%) 2384
Lithobid Tablets 1692
Lunesta Tablets (Rare) 3142
Maxalt Tablets (Infrequent) 2008
Maxalt-MLT Orally Disintegrating Tablets (Infrequent) 2008
Mobic Oral Suspension (Less than 2%) 863
Mobic Tablets (Less than 2%) 863
Moduretic Tablets (Less than or equal to 1%) 2028
▲ Myfortic Tablets (3% to less than 20%) 2255
Namenda (Infrequent) 1195
Neumega for Injection 3435
Neurontin Capsules 2487
Neurontin Oral Solution 2487
Neurontin Tablets 2487
Nexavar Tablets (Uncommon) 746
Norvir (Less than 2%) 503
▲ Ontak Vials (9%) 1745
Opana Tablets (Less than 1%) 1122
Opana ER Tablets (Less than 1%) 1126
OxyContin Tablets (Less than 1%) 2703
Paxil CR Controlled-Release Tablets (Rare) 1538
Paxil (Rare) 1530
Percodan Tablets 1132
Permax Tablets (Infrequent) 3356
Pexeva Tablets (Rare) 1694
▲ Photofrin for Injection (7% to 10%) 702
Prevacid Delayed-Release Capsules (Less than 1%) 3271
Prevacid for Delayed-Release Oral Suspension (Less than 1%) 3271
Prevacid SoluTab Delayed-Release Orally Disintegrating Tablets (Less than 1%) 3271
Prevacid NapraPAC (Less than 1%) 3280
PREVPAC (Less than 1%) 3284
Prinivil Tablets (0.3% to 1.0%) 2052
Prinzide Tablets 2056
▲ Prograf Capsules and Injection (3% to 15%) 632
Protonix I.V. 3472
Protonix Tablets 3469
Protopic Ointment (Greater than or equal to 1%) 638
Prozac Pulvules and Liquid (Infrequent) 1801
▲ Rapamune Oral Solution and Tablets (3% to 20%) 3475
Razadyne 2399
Razadyne ER Extended-Release Capsules 2399
Remicade for IV Injection (Greater than or equal to 0.2%) 971

Requip Tablets (Infrequent)............... 1555
Revlimid Capsules........................... 958
Reyataz Capsules (Less than 3%)..... 921
Risperdal (Rare)............................. 1676
Risperdal Consta Long-Acting
Injection (Infrequent).................... 1682
Risperdal M-Tab Orally
Disintegrating Tablets (Rare)......... 1676
Rocaltrol Capsules.......................... 2798
Rocaltrol Oral Solution.................... 2798
Rythmol SR Capsules....................... 2727
▲ Sandostatin LAR Depot (5% to
15%).. 2280
Seroquel Tablets (Infrequent)........... 690
▲ Simulect for Injection (3% to 10%) ... 2284
St. Joseph 81 mg Aspirin
Chewable and Enteric Coated
Tablets.. 1869
St. Joseph 81 mg Aspirin............... ▣688
▲ Sutent Capsules (3% to 11%) 2560
Symbyax Capsules (Infrequent)........ 1819
Tasmar Tablets (Infrequent)............. 3358
▲ Taxotere Injection Concentrate
(25.3%).. 2932
Thalomid Capsules........................... 965
Topamax Sprinkle Capsules
(Infrequent).................................... 2404
Topamax Tablets (Infrequent)........... 2404
Uniretic Tablets (Less than 1%)........ 3100
▲ Valcyte Tablets (Less than 5%) 2813
Vantin Tablets and Oral
Suspension (Less than 1%)........... 2645
Vaprisol (2.2%)................................ 643
Vaqta.. 2097
Vasotec I.V. Injection....................... 2103
▲ Velcade for Injection (18%) 2133
Viracept (Less than 2%).................. 2577
Vivitrol... 995
▲ Xeloda Tablets (2% to 10%) 2822
Xifaxan Tablets (Less than 2%)........ 2842
Zelapar Tablets................................ 3372
Zmax for Oral Suspension................ 2583
Zoloft (Rare).................................... 2586
▲ Zometa for Intravenous Infusion
(5% to 14%)................................... 2315
Zomig Nasal Spray (Rare)................ 3523
Zonegran Capsules (Infrequent)....... 1101
Zyprexa Tablets (Infrequent)............ 1830
Zyprexa IntraMuscular (Infrequent)... 1830
Zyprexa ZYDIS Orally
Disintegrating Tablets
(Infrequent).................................... 1830
Zyrtec Chewable Tablets (Less
than 2%).. 2594
Zyrtec (Less than 2%)...................... 2594
Zyrtec-D 12 Hour Extended
Release Tablets (Less than 2%)..... 2597

Delirium
Abilify Oral Solution (Infrequent)........ 882
Abilify Oral Solution (Infrequent)....... 2450
Abilify Discmelt Orally
Disintegrating Tablets
(Infrequent).................................... 882
Abilify Discmelt Orally
Disintegrating Tablets
(Infrequent).................................... 2450
Abilify Tablets (Infrequent)............... 882
Abilify Tablets (Infrequent)............... 2450
Aciphex Tablets............................... 1090
▲ Avinza Capsules (Less than 5%) 1741
Azilect Tablets (Rare)....................... 3293
Catapres Tablets.............................. 843
Catapres-TTS (0.5% or less)........... 844
Celexa... 1176
▲ CellCept Capsules (3% to less
than 20%)....................................... 2747
▲ CellCept Intravenous (3% to less
than 20%)....................................... 2747
▲ CellCept Oral Suspension (3% to
less than 20%)............................... 2747
▲ CellCept Tablets (3% to less than
20%).. 2747
Cipro... 2977
Cipro I.V. 2984
Cipro XR Tablets............................. 2990
Clorpres Tablets.............................. 2153
Clozaril Tablets............................... 2184
Effexor Tablets................................ 3411
Effexor XR Capsules....................... 3417
Evoxac Capsules............................. 1047
Exelon Capsules (Infrequent)........... 2206
Exelon Oral Solution (Infrequent)...... 2206
Famvir Tablets (Infrequent).............. 2211
FazaClo Orally Disintegrating
Tablets... 551
Geodon Capsules (Frequent)............ 2529
I.V. Busulfex (2%)........................... 2493
Lamictal (Rare)................................ 1481
Lanoxicaps Capsules....................... 1490
Lanoxin Injection............................. 1494
Lanoxin Injection Pediatric............... 1497
Lanoxin Tablets............................... 1500
Levaquin (0.1% to 0.9%)................. 2384
Levaquin in 5% Dextrose Injection
(0.1% to 0.9%)............................... 2384
Lexapro Oral Solution...................... 1190
Lexapro Tablets............................... 1190
Lyrica Capsules (Rare).................... 2539
Merrem I.V. (Greater than 0.1% to
1%).. 686
Mycamine for Injection (0.8%).......... 628
Namenda (Infrequent)...................... 1195
Orthoclone OKT3 Sterile Solution
(Less than 1%)............................... 2360
Paxil CR Controlled-Release
Tablets (Rare)................................ 1538
Paxil (Rare)..................................... 1530
Pexeva Tablets (Rare)...................... 1694
Phenergan Tablets and
Suppositories................................. 3440
PhosLo GelCaps............................. 2169
Prograf Capsules and Injection......... 632
Proquin XR Tablets.......................... 1153
Razadyne (Infrequent)..................... 2399
Razadyne ER Extended-Release
Capsules (Infrequent)..................... 2399
Requip Tablets (Infrequent).............. 1555
Revlimid Capsules........................... 958
Rilutek Tablets (Infrequent).............. 2930
Risperdal (Rare).............................. 1676
Risperdal Consta Long-Acting
Injection (Infrequent)...................... 1682
Risperdal M-Tab Orally
Disintegrating Tablets (Rare)......... 1676
Romazicon Injection (Less than
1%).. 2804
Sanctura Tablets............................. 1151
Seroquel Tablets (Rare)................... 690
Symmetrel Tablets........................... 1135
Tasmar Tablets (Rare)...................... 3358
Topamax Sprinkle Capsules
(Infrequent).................................... 2404
Topamax Tablets (Infrequent)........... 2404
Trileptal Tablets............................... 2300
Trileptal Oral Suspension................. 2300
VFEND I.V. (Less than 2%).............. 2564
VFEND Oral Suspension (Less than
2%).. 2564
VFEND Tablets (Less than 2%)........ 2564
Vivitrol... 995
Wellbutrin Tablets............................ 1603
Wellbutrin SR Sustained-Release
Tablets... 1607
Wellbutrin XL Extended-Release
Tablets... 1613
Zovirax.. 1643
Zyban Sustained-Release Tablets..... 1644
Zyprexa Tablets (Infrequent)............ 1830
Zyprexa ZYDIS Orally
Disintegrating Tablets
(Infrequent).................................... 1830

Delivery complications, unspecified
Advil Caplets................................ ▣674
Advil Cold & Sinus........................ ▣723
Advil... ▣674
Advil Migraine Liquigels................ ▣608
Advil Tablets................................. ▣674
Bayer Aspirin.................................. 744
Bayer Aspirin Comprehensive
Prescribing Information................ ▣796
BC Headache Powder.................... ▣677
BC Allergy Sinus Cold Powder........ ▣677
Arthritis Strength BC Powder.......... ▣677
BC Sinus Cold Powder.................. ▣677
Epivir.. 1427
Goody's Body Pain Formula
Powder.. ▣684
Goody's Extra Strength Headache
Powders...................................... ▣611
Goody's Extra Strength Pain
Relief Tablets.............................. ▣685
Motrin IB Tablets and Caplets.......... 1866
St. Joseph 81 mg Aspirin
Chewable and Enteric Coated
Tablets... 1869

Delusional thinking
Ritalin Hydrochloride Tablets........... 2269
Ritalin LA Capsules........................ 2271
Ritalin-SR Tablets........................... 2269

Delusions
Abilify Oral Solution (Frequent)......... 882
Abilify Oral Solution (Frequent)......... 2450
Abilify Discmelt Orally
Disintegrating Tablets (Frequent)... 882
Abilify Discmelt Orally
Disintegrating Tablets (Frequent)... 2450
Abilify Tablets (Frequent).................. 882
Abilify Tablets (Frequent).................. 2450
Adderall Tablets.............................. 3164
Ambien Tablets (Rare)..................... 2851
Ambien CR Tablets (Rare)............... 2855
Aricept Tablets (Frequent)................ 1094
Aricept ODT Tablets (Frequent)........ 1094
Atripla Tablets................................. 945
Azilect Tablets (Infrequent)............... 3293
Celexa (Rare).................................. 1176
Clozaril Tablets (Less than 1%)........ 2184
Effexor Tablets (Rare)...................... 3411
Effexor XR Capsules (Rare)............. 3417
Eldepryl Capsules........................... 3208
Evoxac Capsules............................. 1047
Exelon Capsules (2% or more)......... 2206
Exelon Oral Solution (2% or more).... 2206
FazaClo Orally Disintegrating
Tablets (Less than 1%)................... 551
Gabitril Tablets (Infrequent).............. 984
Lamictal (Rare)................................ 1481
▲ Lupron Depot 3.75 mg (Among
most frequent)................................ 3260
▲ Lupron Depot–3 Month 11.25 mg
(Less than 5%)............................... 3265
Lyrica Capsules (Rare)..................... 2539
Mirapex Tablets (1%)....................... 859
Namenda (Infrequent)...................... 1195
Parcopa Orally Disintegrating
Tablets... 3097
Paxil CR Controlled-Release
Tablets (Rare)................................ 1538
Paxil (Rare)..................................... 1530
Permax Tablets (Infrequent)............. 3356
Pexeva Tablets (Rare)...................... 1694
Prozac Pulvules and Liquid (Rare)..... 1801
Requip Tablets (Infrequent).............. 1555
Revlimid Capsules........................... 958
Rilutek Tablets (Infrequent).............. 2930
Risperdal Consta Long-Acting
Injection (Frequent)........................ 1682
Seroquel Tablets (Infrequent)........... 690
Sonata Capsules (Rare)................... 1717
Stalevo Tablets............................... 2287
Sustiva Capsules............................. 930
Sustiva Tablets................................ 930
Symmetrel Tablets........................... 1135
Tasmar Tablets (Infrequent)............. 3358
Topamax Sprinkle Capsules
(Infrequent).................................... 2404
Topamax Tablets (Infrequent)........... 2404
Trileptal Tablets............................... 2300
Trileptal Oral Suspension................. 2300
Wellbutrin Tablets (1.2%)................. 1603
Wellbutrin SR Sustained-Release
Tablets... 1607
Wellbutrin XL Extended-Release
Tablets... 1613
Zoloft (Infrequent)........................... 2586
Zyban Sustained-Release Tablets..... 1644
Zyprexa Tablets (Frequent).............. 1830

Dementia
Ambien Tablets (Rare)..................... 2851
Ambien CR Tablets (Rare)............... 2855
Angeliq Tablets............................... 762
Azilect Tablets (Infrequent)............... 3293
Depacon Injection (Several
reports)... 412
Depakene (Several reports).............. 417
Depakote Sprinkle Capsules
(Several reports)............................ 422
Depakote Tablets (Several
reports)... 427
Depakote ER Tablets (Several
reports)... 434
Effexor Tablets (Rare)...................... 3411
Effexor XR Capsules (Rare)............. 3417
Enjuvia Tablets................................ 1062
Estrasorb Topical Emulsion.............. 1147
Estratest Tablets (1.8%).................. 3199
Estratest H.S. Tablets (1.8%)........... 3199
Evoxac Capsules............................. 1047
Exelon Capsules (Infrequent)........... 2206
Exelon Oral Solution (Infrequent)...... 2206
Menostar Transdermal System........ 782
Parcopa Orally Disintegrating
Tablets... 3097
Premarin Intravenous...................... 3442
Premarin Tablets............................. 3446
Premarin Vaginal Cream.................. 3452
Premphase Tablets......................... 3456
Prempro Tablets.............................. 3456
Relpax Tablets (Rare)...................... 2548
Requip Tablets (Infrequent).............. 1555
Rilutek Tablets (Rare)...................... 2930
Risperdal Consta Long-Acting
Injection (Infrequent)...................... 1682
Rythmol SR Capsules...................... 2727
Stalevo Tablets............................... 2287
▲ Vesanoid Capsules (3%) 2820
VFEND I.V. (Less than 2%).............. 2564
VFEND Oral Suspension (Less than
2%).. 2564
VFEND Tablets (Less than 2%)........ 2564
Zelapar Tablets................................ 3372
Zyprexa Tablets (Infrequent)............ 1830
Zyprexa ZYDIS Orally
Disintegrating Tablets
(Infrequent).................................... 1830

Demyelination
Infanrix Vaccine.............................. 1476
Proleukin for Injection...................... 2266
Remicade for IV Injection................ 971

Dental caries
Abilify Oral Solution (Infrequent)........ 882
Abilify Oral Solution (Infrequent)....... 2450
Abilify Discmelt Orally
Disintegrating Tablets
(Infrequent).................................... 882
Abilify Discmelt Orally
Disintegrating Tablets
(Infrequent).................................... 2450
Abilify Tablets (Infrequent)............... 882
Abilify Tablets (Infrequent)............... 2450
Actiq (Less than 1%)........................ 979
Ambien Tablets (Rare)..................... 2851
Ambien CR Tablets (Rare)............... 2855
Copaxone for Injection (Frequent)..... 3297
Gabitril Tablets (Infrequent).............. 984
Lithobid Tablets.............................. 1692
Paxil CR Controlled-Release
Tablets (Rare)................................ 1538
Paxil (Rare)..................................... 1530
Permax Tablets (Infrequent)............. 3356
Pexeva Tablets (rare)....................... 1694
Protopic Ointment (0.2% to less
than 1%).. 638
Seroquel Tablets (Infrequent)........... 690
Symbyax Capsules (Infrequent)........ 1819
Uniretic Tablets (Less than 1%)........ 3100
Xyrem Oral Solution (Infrequent)....... 1688
Zoloft (Infrequent)........................... 2586

Dependence, drug
Actiq.. 979
Adderall Tablets.............................. 3164
Adderall XR Capsules..................... 3166
Adipex-P... 1215
Ambien Tablets (Rare)..................... 2851
Avinza Capsules............................. 1741
▲ Carnitor Injection (2% to 6%) 3188
Celexa (Infrequent).......................... 1176
Daytrana Transdermal Patch............ 3174
Dexedrine....................................... 1420
DextroStat Tablets........................... 3179
Dilaudid.. 440
Dilaudid Non-Sterile Powder............ 440
Dilaudid Oral Liquid......................... 445
Dilaudid Rectal Suppositories.......... 440
Dilaudid Tablets.............................. 440
Dilaudid Tablets - 8 mg.................... 445
Donnatal Extentabs......................... 2493
Duragesic Transdermal System....... 2373
MS Contin Tablets........................... 2701
Nembutal Sodium Solution, USP...... 2470
OxyFast Oral Concentrate Solution.. 2708
OxyIR Capsules.............................. 2708
Paxil CR Controlled-Release
Tablets (Rare)................................ 1538
Paxil (Rare)..................................... 1530
Percocet Tablets.............................. 1131
Percodan Tablets............................ 1132
Pexeva Tablets (Rare)...................... 1694
Ritalin Hydrochloride Tablets........... 2269
Ritalin LA Capsules........................ 2271
Ritalin-SR Tablets........................... 2269
Sonata Capsules............................. 1717
Tranxene.. 2474
Tylenol with Codeine Tablets........... 2391
Valium Tablets................................ 2819
Vicoprofen Tablets.......................... 539

Dependence, physical
Cesamet Capsules.......................... 3340
Dexedrine....................................... 1420
Dilaudid Ampules............................ 440
Dilaudid Non-Sterile Powder............ 440
Dilaudid Oral Liquid......................... 445
Dilaudid Rectal Suppositories.......... 440
Dilaudid Tablets.............................. 440
Dilaudid Tablets - 8 mg.................... 445
Donnatal Extentabs......................... 2493
Duragesic Transdermal System....... 2373
Hycodan... 1116
Hycotuss Expectorant Syrup........... 1117
Klonopin... 2778
Marinol Capsules (Uncommon)......... 3333
MS Contin Tablets........................... 2701
OxyContin Tablets........................... 2703
Percocet Tablets.............................. 1131
Percodan Tablets............................ 1132
ProSom Tablets.............................. 517
Tranxene.. 2474
Tylenol with Codeine Tablets........... 2391
Vicodin HP Tablets.......................... 538
Vicoprofen Tablets.......................... 539
Xyrem Oral Solution........................ 1688

Dependence, psychic
(*see under* Dependence, psychological)

Dependence, psychological

Adderall Tablets 3164
Adderall XR Capsules 3166
Avinza Capsules 1741
Cesamet Capsules 3340
Concerta Extended-Release Tablets 1881
Desoxyn Tablets, USP 2462
Dexedrine 1420
DextroStat Tablets 3179
Dilaudid 440
Dilaudid Non-Sterile Powder 440
Dilaudid Oral Liquid 445
Dilaudid Rectal Suppositories 440
Dilaudid Tablets 440
Dilaudid Tablets - 8 mg 445
Donnatal Extentabs 2493
Duragesic Transdermal System 2373
Hycodan 1116
Hycotuss Expectorant Syrup 1117
Kadian Capsules (Very rare) 577
Klonopin 2778
Marinol Capsules (Uncommon) 3333
MS Contin Tablets (Very rare) 2701
Nembutal Sodium Solution, USP 2470
Numorphan Injection 1120
OxyContin Tablets 2703
OxyFast Oral Concentrate Solution 2708
OxyIR Capsules 2708
Percocet Tablets 1131
Percodan Tablets 1132
ProSom Tablets 517
Ritalin Hydrochloride Tablets 2269
Ritalin LA Capsules 2271
Ritalin-SR Tablets 2269
Tranxene 2474
Tussionex Pennkinetic Extended-Release Suspension 3327
Tylenol with Codeine Tablets 2391
Vicodin Tablets 535
Vicodin ES Tablets 536
Vicodin HP Tablets 538
Vicoprofen Tablets 539
Xyrem Oral Solution 1688
Zydone Tablets 1139

Depersonalization

Abilify Oral Solution (Infrequent) 882
Abilify Oral Solution (Infrequent) 2450
Abilify Discmelt Orally Disintegrating Tablets (Infrequent) 882
Abilify Discmelt Orally Disintegrating Tablets (Infrequent) 2450
Abilify Tablets (Infrequent) 882
Abilify Tablets (Infrequent) 2450
Ambien Tablets (Rare) 2851
Ambien CR Tablets (Rare to 1%) 2855
Anzemet Injection (Infrequently) 2859
Anzemet Tablets (Infrequently) 2862
Astelin Nasal Spray (Infrequent) 1904
Avelox (Less than 0.1%) 2970
Betaseron for SC Injection 767
Biaxin/Biaxin XL 402
Buprenex Injectable (Infrequent) 2716
Caduet Tablets (Greater than 0.1% to less than or equal to 1%) 2508
Campral Tablets (Rare) 1174
Celexa (Infrequent) 1176
Cesamet Capsules (2%) 3340
Cipro (Less than 1%) 2977
Cipro I.V. (1% or less) 2984
Cipro XR Tablets (Less than 1%) 2990
Copaxone for Injection (Infrequent) 3297
Duragesic Transdermal System (Less than 1%) 2373
Effexor Tablets (1%) 3411
Effexor XR Capsules (Frequent) 3417
▲ Equetro Extended-Release Capsules (Less than 5%) 3180
Evoxac Capsules (Less than 1%) 1047
Exelon Capsules (Infrequent) 2206
Exelon Oral Solution (Infrequent) 2206
Frova Tablets (Infrequent) 1113
Gabitril Tablets (Frequent) 984
Indocin (Less than 1%) 1995
Keppra Oral Solution 3314
Keppra Tablets 3314
Klonopin (Infrequent) 2778
Kogenate FS 738
Kogenate FS with Bio-Set (1 case) 740
Lamictal (Infrequent) 1481
Lexapro Oral Solution (Infrequent) 1190
Lexapro Tablets (Infrequent) 1190
Lyrica Capsules (Greather than or equal to 1%) 2539
Marinol Capsules (Greater than 1%) 3333
Maxalt Tablets (Rare) 2008
Maxalt-MLT Orally Disintegrating Tablets (Rare) 2008
Namenda (Infrequent) 1195
Neurontin Capsules (Infrequent) 2487
Neurontin Oral Solution (Infrequent) 2487
Neurontin Tablets (Infrequent) 2487
Niravam Orally Disintegrating Tablets 3092
Norvasc Tablets (More than 0.1% to 1%) 2545
OxyContin Tablets (Less than 1%) 2703
Paxil CR Controlled-Release Tablets (Infrequent) 1538
Paxil (Infrequent) 1530
▲ Pexeva Tablets (3%) 1694
Prevacid Delayed-Release Capsules (Less than 1%) 3271
Prevacid for Delayed-Release Oral Suspension (Less than 1%) 3271
Prevacid SoluTab Delayed-Release Orally Disintegrating Tablets (Less than 1%) 3271
Prevacid NapraPAC (Less than 1%) 3280
PREVPAC 3284
Prozac Pulvules and Liquid (Infrequent) 1801
Relpax Tablets (Infrequent) 2548
Requip Tablets (Infrequent) 1555
Rilutek Tablets (Infrequent) 2930
Risperdal Consta Long-Acting Injection (Infrequent) 1682
▲ Romazicon Injection (1% to 3%) 2804
Seroquel Tablets (Infrequent) 690
Sonata Capsules (Less than 1% to 2%) 1717
Symbyax Capsules (Infrequent) 1819
Tambocor Tablets (Less than 1%) 1856
Tequin Injection (Less than 0.1%) 938
Tequin Injection in 5% Dextrose (Less than 0.1%) 938
Tequin Tablets (Less than 0.1%) 938
Topamax Sprinkle Capsules (1% to 2%) 2404
Topamax Tablets (1% to 2%) 2404
VFEND I.V. (Less than 2%) 2564
VFEND Oral Suspension (Less than 2%) 2564
VFEND Tablets (Less than 2%) 2564
Wellbutrin Tablets (Infrequent) 1603
Wellbutrin SR Sustained-Release Tablets (Infrequent) 1607
Wellbutrin XL Extended-Release Tablets (Infrequent) 1613
Zoloft (Infrequent) 2586
Zomig Nasal Spray (Infrequent) 3523
Zyban Sustained-Release Tablets (Infrequent) 1644
Zyprexa Tablets (Infrequent) 1830
Zyprexa ZYDIS Orally Disintegrating Tablets (Infrequent) 1830
Zyrtec Chewable Tablets (Less than 2%) 2594
Zyrtec (Less than 2%) 2594
Zyrtec-D 12 Hour Extended Release Tablets (Less than 2%) 2597

Depigmentation

Finacea Gel (Rare) 1669
▲ Intron A for Injection (Less than 5%) 3024

Depigmentation at application site

Lidoderm Patch 1118

Depression

Abilify Oral Solution (Frequent) 882
Abilify Oral Solution (Frequent) 2450
Abilify Discmelt Orally Disintegrating Tablets (Frequent) 882
Abilify Discmelt Orally Disintegrating Tablets (Frequent) 2450
Abilify Tablets (Frequent) 882
Abilify Tablets (Frequent) 2450
Accutane Capsules 2731
Aceon Tablets (2 mg, 4 mg, 8 mg) (2.0%) 3194
Aciphex Tablets 1090
▲ Actimmune (3%) 1671
▲ Actonel Tablets (2.3% to 6.8%) 2683
▲ Actonel with Calcium Tablets (2.3% to 6.8%) 2688
Adalat CC Tablets (Less than 1%) 2964
Adderall Tablets 3164
Adderall XR Capsules (0.7%) 3166
Advair Diskus 100/50 1308
Advair Diskus 250/50 1308
Advair Diskus 500/50 1308
Advair HFA Inhalation Aerosol 1318
▲ Aerobid/Aerobid-M (1% to 3%) 1171
▲ Agenerase Capsules (4% to 16%) 1327
▲ Agenerase Oral Solution (4% to 16%) 1332
▲ Agrylin Capsules (1% to 5%) 3169
Aldara Cream, 5% 1846
Aldoril Tablets 1910
▲ Alferon N Injection (One patient to 3%) 1665
▲ Alimta for Injection (Up to 14%) 1750
Alphagan P Ophthalmic Solution 567
Altace Capsules (Less than 1%) 1702
Altoprev Extended-Release Tablets 3109
Ambien Tablets (2%) 2851
Ambien CR Tablets (1%) 2855
AmBisome for Injection (Less common) 620
Amerge Tablets (Infrequent) 1339
Amitiza Capsules (0% to 1.4%) 3224
AndroGel (Up to 1%) 3329
Androxy Tablets 3335
Angeliq Tablets 762
Aptivus Capsules (2%) 826
▲ Aricept Tablets (3%) 1094
▲ Aricept ODT Tablets (3%) 1094
▲ Arimidex Tablets (2% to 13%) 673
▲ Aromasin Tablets (6.2% to 13%) 2600
▲ Arranon Injection (0% to 6%) 1357
Arthrotec Tablets (Rare) 3129
Asacol Delayed-Release Tablets 2692
▲ Asmanex Twisthaler (11%) 2966
Astelin Nasal Spray (Infrequent) 1904
Atacand Tablets (0.5% or greater) 649
Atacand HCT (0.5% or greater) 651
▲ Atripla Tablets (4%) 945
Avalide Tablets 888
Avalide Tablets 2874
Avapro Tablets (Less than 1%) 891
Avapro Tablets (Less than 1%) 2871
Avelox 2970
Axert Tablets (Rare) 2396
▲ Azilect Tablets (5%) 3293
Azmacort Inhalation Aerosol 1726
Beconase AQ Nasal Spray 1396
Betagan Ophthalmic Solution, USP ⊙220
▲ Betaseron for SC Injection (34%) 767
Betimol Ophthalmic Solution 3382
Betimol Ophthalmic Solution ⊙295
Betoptic S Ophthalmic Suspension (Rare) 558
Blocadren Tablets 1916
Brimonidine Tartrate Ophthalmic Solution 0.2% (Less than 3%) ⊙248
Caduet Tablets (Greater than 0.1% to less than 2%) 2508
▲ Campath Ampules (1% to 7%) 811
▲ Campral Tablets (4% to 8%) 1174
Captopril Tablets 2149
Carbatrol Capsules 3171
Cardizem LA Extended Release Tablets (Less than 2%) 1728
▲ Carnitor Injection (5% to 6%) 3188
Carteolol Hydrochloride Ophthalmic Solution USP, 1% ⊙249
Catapres Tablets (About 1 in 100 patients) 843
Catapres-TTS (0.5% or less) 844
Celebrex Capsules (0.1% to 1.9%) 3134
Celexa (Frequent) 1176
▲ CellCept Capsules (3% to less than 20%) 2747
▲ CellCept Intravenous (3% to less than 20%) 2747
▲ CellCept Oral Suspension (3% to less than 20%) 2747
▲ CellCept Tablets (3% to less than 20%) 2747
▲ Cesamet Capsules (14%) 3340
Chantix Tablets (Frequent) 2517
Cipro (Less than 1%) 2977
Cipro I.V. (1% or less) 2984
Cipro XR Tablets (Less than 1%) 2990
▲ Climara Transdermal System (1% to 8%) 771
▲ Climara Pro Transdermal System (5.7%) 776
Clinoril Tablets (Less than 1%) 1924
▲ Clolar for Intravenous Infusion (11%) 1271
Clorpres Tablets (About 1%) 2153
Clozaril Tablets (1%) 2184
Colazal Capsules 2838
Concerta Extended-Release Tablets 1881
Copaxone for Injection (At least 2%) 3297
▲ Copegus Tablets (20%) 2754
▲ Coreg Tablets (Greater than 1% to 3%) 1414
Cosopt Sterile Ophthalmic Solution (Less than 1%) 1931
Cozaar Tablets (Less than 1%) 1935
Crestor Tablets (Greater than or equal to 2%) 678
Crixivan Capsules 1940
Dacogen Injection (Greater than or equal to 1%) 2129
Dalmane Capsules (Rare) 3342
Dantrium Capsules (Less frequent) 2694
Daranide Tablets 1950
Daytrana Transdermal Patch 3174
Decadron Tablets 1951
Demser Capsules 1953
▲ Depacon Injection (4% to 5%) 412
▲ Depakene (5%) 417
▲ Depakote Sprinkle Capsules (4% to 5%) 422
▲ Depakote Tablets (1% to 5%) 427
▲ Depakote ER Tablets (4% to 5%) 434
▲ Depo-Provera Contraceptive Injection (1% to 5%) 2622
▲ depo-subQ provera 104 Injectable Suspension (1% to less than 5%) 2624
Diastat Rectal Delivery System (Infrequent) 3343
Didronel Tablets 2697
Dilaudid Oral Liquid (Less frequent) 445
Dilaudid Tablets - 8 mg (Less frequent) 445
Dilaudid-HP (Less frequent) 442
Diovan HCT Tablets (Less frequent) 2196
Dolobid Tablets (Less than 1 in 100) 1955
▲ Doxil Injection (Less than 1% to 10%) 2351
▲ Duragesic Transdermal System (3% to 10%) 2373
DynaCirc CR Tablets (0.5% to 1%) 2721
Effexor Tablets (1%) 3411
▲ Effexor XR Capsules (3%) 3417
Eldepryl Capsules 3208
Eligard 7.5 mg (Less than 2%) 2880
Eligard 30 mg (1.1%) 2885
Elmiron Capsules 2415
▲ Eloxatin for Injection (2% to 5%) 2892
Elspar for Injection 2463
Elspar for Injection 1960
Emend Capsules (Greater than 0.5%) 1963
▲ Emtriva Capsules (6% to 9%) 1287
▲ Emtriva Oral Solution (6% to 9%) 1287
Enbrel for Injection (Infrequent) 584
Enjuvia Tablets 1062
▲ Epzicom Tablets (7%) 1436
▲ Equetro Extended-Release Capsules (7%) 3180
▲ Erbitux (7% to 10%) 910
Estrasorb Topical Emulsion 1147
Estratest Tablets 3199
Estratest H.S. Tablets 3199
Estring Vaginal Ring 2635
Eulexin Capsules (1%) 3009
▲ Evista Tablets (6.4%) 1763
▲ Evoxac Capsules (1% to 3%) 1047
▲ Exelon Capsules (6%) 2206
▲ Exelon Oral Solution (6%) 2206
▲ Fabrazyme for Intravenous Infusion (3%) 1274
Fansidar Tablets 2765
▲ Faslodex Injection (5.7%) 681
FazaClo Orally Disintegrating Tablets (1%) 551
Femara Tablets (Less frequent) 2214
Flovent Diskus 1443
Flovent HFA 1447
Flumadine (0.3% to 1%) 1183
Focalin Tablets 2220
Focalin XR Capsules 2223
▲ Forteo for Injection (4.1%) 1767
▲ Fortical Nasal Spray (1% to 3%) 3337
Frova Tablets (Infrequent) 1113
Fuzeon Injection 2767
▲ Gabitril Tablets (3%) 984
Gantrisin Pediatric Suspension 2770
Garamycin Injectable 3014
Gengraf Capsules (Rare) 459
Geodon Capsules 2529
▲ Gleevec Tablets (0.5% to 12.7%) 2227
▲ Hectorol Capsules (Greater than or equal to 5%) 1275
▲ Herceptin I.V. (6%) 1233
Hydrocortone Tablets 1989
Hytrin Capsules (0.3%) 471
Hyzaar 50-12.5 Tablets 1990
Hyzaar 100-12.5 Tablets 1990
Hyzaar 100-25 Tablets 1990
▲ Imdur Tablets (Less than or equal to 5%) 3018
Imitrex Injection (Rare) 1463
Imitrex Nasal Spray (Infrequent) 1467
Imitrex Tablets (Infrequent) 1471
▲ Indapamide Tablets (Less than 5%) 2156
Inderal LA Long-Acting Capsules 3429

Indocin (Greater than 1%)................ 1995
▲ Infergen (18% to 26%) 3364
InnoPran XL Capsules...................... 2723
▲ Intron A for Injection (2% to 40%) 3024
Invanz for Injection (Greater than 0.1%).. 1999
Invirase (Greater than or equal to 2%).. 2772
▲ I.V. Busulfex (23%) 2493
Kadian Capsules (Less than 3%)....... 577
Kaletra (Up to 2%).......................... 476
▲ Keppra Injection (4%) 3320
▲ Keppra Oral Solution (3% to 5%) 3314
▲ Keppra Tablets (3% to 5%) 3314
▲ Klonopin (4% to 7%) 2778
▲ Lamictal (4.2%) 1481
Lanoxicaps Capsules........................ 1490
Lanoxin Injection............................. 1494
Lanoxin Injection Pediatric 1497
Lanoxin Tablets............................... 1500
Lariam Tablets (Occasional).............. 2786
Lescol Capsules 2233
Lescol XL Tablets 2233
Levaquin (0.1% to 0.9%) 2384
Levaquin in 5% Dextrose Injection (0.1% to 0.9%) 2384
Lexapro Oral Solution (Infrequent) 1190
Lexapro Tablets (Infrequent) 1190
▲ Lexiva Tablets (Less than 1% to 11%) 1505
Lipitor Tablets (Less than 2%) 2483
▲ Lithostat Tablets (20%) 2140
Lofibra Tablets 1219
Lofibra Capsules 1216
▲ Lopressor Injection (5%) 2238
▲ Lopressor Tablets (5%) 2238
▲ Lopressor HCT 50/25 Tablets (5%) 2241
▲ Lopressor HCT 100/25 Tablets (5%) 2241
▲ Lopressor HCT 100/50 Tablets (5%) 2241
Lotronex Tablets (2%) 1512
▲ Lunesta Tablets (1% to 4%) 3142
▲ Lupron Depot 3.75 mg (16%) 3260
▲ Lupron Depot–3 Month 11.25 mg (16%) 3265
Malarone Pediatric Tablets (Less than 1%) 1517
Malarone Tablets (Less than 1%) 1517
Marinol Capsules (Less than 1%) 3333
Matulane Capsules 3191
Maxair Autohaler 1852
Maxalt Tablets (Infrequent) 2008
Maxalt-MLT Orally Disintegrating Tablets (Infrequent) 2008
▲ Megace ES Oral Suspension (1% to 3%) 2481
Menostar Transdermal System 782
▲ Meridia Capsules (4.3%) 489
Merrem I.V. (Greater than 0.1% to 1%) 686
Metadate CD Capsules 3323
MetroGel-Vaginal Gel (Less than 1%) 1855
Mevacor Tablets (0.5% to 1.0%) 2021
▲ Miacalcin Nasal Spray (1% to 3%) 2253
Micardis Tablets (More than 0.3%) ... 854
Micardis HCT Tablets 856
Midamor Tablets (Less than or equal to 1%) 2026
Migranal Nasal Spray (Rare) 3348
Mintezol 2027
Mirapex Tablets (1% or more) 859
Mircette Tablets 1066
▲ Mirena Intrauterine System (5% or more) 787
Moban Tablets (Less frequent) 1119
Mobic Oral Suspension (Less than 2%) 863
Mobic Tablets (Less than 2%) 863
Moduretic Tablets (Less than or equal to 1%) 2028
MS Contin Tablets (Less frequent) 2701
▲ Myfortic Tablets (3% to less than 20%) 2255
▲ Mylotarg for Injection (8% to 10%) ... 3431
Nadolol Tablets 2159
Nalfon Capsules (Less than 1%) 2502
Namenda (Greater than or equal to 2%) 1195
Neoral Oral Solution (1%) 2259
Neoral Soft Gelatin Capsules (1%) 2259
Neurontin Capsules (1.8%) 2487
Neurontin Oral Solution (1.8%) 2487
Neurontin Tablets (1.8%) 2487
▲ Nexavar Tablets (Common) 746
Nexium I.V. (Rare) 659
Nimotop Capsules (Up to 1.4%) 749
▲ Nipent for Injection (3% to 10%) 1863
▲ Niravam Orally Disintegrating Tablets (5.1% to 13.9%) 3092
Noroxin Tablets (Less frequent) 2032
Norvasc Tablets (More than 0.1% to 1%).. 2545
Norvir (1.7%)................................... 503
Numorphan Injection........................ 1120
NuvaRing.. 2340
Omacor Capsules 2725
Opana Tablets (Less than 1%).......... 1122
Opana ER Tablets (Less than 1%)..... 1126
OptiPranolol Metipranolol Ophthalmic Solution 0.3% (A small number of patients)........... ⊙256
Ortho-Cyclen Tablets........................ 2429
Ortho Evra Transdermal System 2417
Ortho Tri-Cyclen Tablets 2429
Ortho Tri-Cyclen Lo Tablets 2436
Oxandrin Tablets............................. 2962
Oxsoralen-Ultra Capsules................. 3353
OxyContin Tablets (Less than 1%) 2703
Parcopa Orally Disintegrating Tablets 3097
Paxil CR Controlled-Release Tablets (Frequent)........................ 1538
Paxil (Frequent) 1530
▲ Pegasys (18%) 2789
▲ PEG-Intron Powder for Injection (29%) 3048
Pentasa Capsules (Less than 1%) 3185
Pepcid Injection (Infrequent) 2040
Pepcid (Infrequent) 2038
Percodan Tablets 1132
▲ Permax Tablets (3.2%) 3356
▲ Plavix Tablets (3.6%) 917
▲ Plavix Tablets (3.6%) 2926
Premarin Intravenous 3442
▲ Premarin Tablets (5% to 8%) 3446
Premarin Vaginal Cream 3452
▲ Premphase Tablets (6% to 11%) 3456
▲ Prempro Tablets (6% to 11%) 3456
Prevacid Delayed-Release Capsules (Less than 1%) 3271
Prevacid for Delayed-Release Oral Suspension (Less than 1%) 3271
Prevacid SoluTab Delayed-Release Orally Disintegrating Tablets (Less than 1%) 3271
Prevacid NapraPAC (Less than 1%) .. 3280
PREVPAC (Less than 1%) 3284
Prilosec OTC Delayed-Release Tablets (Less than 1%) 2677
Prinivil Tablets (Greater than 1%) 2052
Prinzide Tablets (0.3% to 1%) 2056
▲ Prochieve 4% Gel (8% to 11%) 1003
▲ Prochieve 8% Gel (8% to 11%) 1003
▲ Prograf Capsules and Injection (3% to 15%) 632
Proleukin for Injection (Less than 1%) 2266
▲ Prometrium Capsules (100 mg, 200 mg) (5% to 19%) 3203
Proquin XR Tablets 1153
ProSom Tablets (2%) 517
Protonix I.V. (Less than 1%) 3472
Protonix Tablets (Less than 1%) 3469
Protopic Ointment (Greater than or equal to 1% to 2%) 638
Proventil HFA Inhalation Aerosol (Less than 3%) 3056
Provigil Tablets (2%) 988
Prozac Pulvules and Liquid 1801
Pulmicort Respules (Less than 1%) .. 661
▲ Rapamune Oral Solution and Tablets (3% to 20%) 3475
▲ Razadyne (7%) 2399
▲ Razadyne ER Extended-Release Capsules (7%) 2399
▲ Rebetol (13% to 36%) 3058
▲ Rebetron Combination Therapy (23% to 36%) 3063
▲ Rebif Prefilled Syringe for Injection (25%) 3159
Relpax Tablets (Infrequent) 2548
Requip Tablets (1% or more) 1555
Restoril Capsules (1.7%) 1860
Retrovir Capsules 1560
Retrovir IV Infusion 1564
Retrovir 1560
▲ Revlimid Capsules (0.3% to 5.4%) 958
▲ Reyataz Capsules (3% to 8%) 921
▲ Ribavirin, USP Capsules (13% to 36%) 3068
▲ Rilutek Tablets (4.2% to 6.1%) 2930
Risperdal (Infrequent) 1676
Risperdal Consta Long-Acting Injection (Frequent) 1682
Risperdal M-Tab Orally Disintegrating Tablets (Infrequent) 1676
Ritalin Hydrochloride Tablets 2269
Ritalin LA Capsules 2271
Ritalin-SR Tablets 2269
▲ Romazicon Injection (1% to 3%) 2804
Rozerem Tablets (2%) 3231
▲ Rythmol SR Capsules (1% to 3%) 2727
Sandimmune (Rare) 2275
▲ Sandostatin Injection (1% to 4%) 2278
▲ Sandostatin LAR Depot (5% to 15%) 2280
Seasonique Tablets 1077
▲ Simulect for Injection (3% to 10%) ... 2284
Soltamox Oral Solution (2%)............ 3527
Sonata Capsules (Frequent)............ 1717
▲ Soriatane Capsules (1% to 10%) 1013
▲ Spiriva HandiHaler (1% to 3%) 869
Stalevo Tablets 2287
▲ Strattera Capsules (2% to 6%) 1814
Striant Mucoadhesive 1007
▲ Suboxone Tablets (11%) 2717
▲ Subutex Tablets (11%) 2717
Sular Tablets (Less than or equal to 1%).. 3122
▲ Sustiva Capsules (2% to 19%) 930
▲ Sustiva Tablets (2% to 19%) 930
▲ Symmetrel Tablets (1% to 5%) 1135
Tambocor Tablets (1% to 3%)........... 1856
▲ Tarceva Tablets (0% to 19%) 1259
▲ Tarceva Tablets (0% to 19%) 2444
Targretin Capsules......................... 1747
Tasmar Tablets (Frequent)............... 3358
Tegretol/Tegretol-XR 2295
▲ Temodar Capsules (6%) 3073
Tequin Injection (Less than 0.1%)..... 938
Tequin Injection in 5% Dextrose (Less than 0.1%)......................... 938
Tequin Tablets (Less than 0.1%)....... 938
Testim 1% Gel................................ 695
Teveten Tablets (1%)...................... 1735
Teveten HCT Tablets (Less than 1%)... 1737
Thalomid Capsules 965
Thyrolar Tablets.............................. 1199
Tiazac Capsules (Less than 2%)....... 1201
Timolide Tablets 2086
Timoptic Sterile Ophthalmic Solution (Less frequent)............... 2088
Timoptic in Ocudose (Less frequent)....................................... 2091
Timoptic-XE Sterile Ophthalmic Gel Forming Solution 2092
Tindamax Tablets (Rare).................. 2142
▲ Topamax Sprinkle Capsules (1% to 13%)....................................... 2404
▲ Topamax Tablets (1% to 13%) 2404
▲ Toprol-XL Tablets (About 5 of 100 patients)...................................... 668
Tranxene 2474
▲ Travatan Ophthalmic Solution (1% to 5%)... 563
Trecator Tablets 3487
Tricor Tablets................................. 527
▲ Trisenox Injection (20%) 993
▲ Trizivir Tablets (9%) 1589
▲ Truvada Tablets (4%) 1296
▲ Ultram ER Tablets (1% to greater than 5%).. 2392
Uniretic Tablets (Less than 1%)........ 3100
▲ Valcyte Tablets (Less than 5%) 2813
Valium Tablets (Infrequent).............. 2819
▲ Valtrex Caplets (Less than 1% to 7%)... 1597
Vandazole Vaginal Gel (Less than 1%)... 3338
Vantas (Less than 2%)..................... 3375
Vasotec I.V. Injection (0.5% to 1%)... 2103
▲ Vesanoid Capsules (14%) 2820
VESIcare Tablets (0.8% to 1.2%)...... 646
VFEND I.V. (Less than 2%)............... 2564
VFEND Oral Suspension (Less than 2%)... 2564
VFEND Tablets (Less than 2%)......... 2564
▲ Viadur Implant (5.3%) 757
Viagra Tablets (Less than 2%).......... 2573
Vicoprofen Tablets (Less than 1%).... 539
Viracept (Less than 2%)................... 2577
▲ Viread Tablets (4% to 11%) 1301
▲ Vivitrol (3% to 8%) 995
Voltaren Tablets (Occasionally)........ 2307
Voltaren-XR Tablets (Occasionally).... 2310
Vytorin 10/10 Tablets...................... 2114
Vytorin 10/10 Tablets...................... 3077
Vytorin 10/20 Tablets...................... 2114
Vytorin 10/20 Tablets...................... 3077
Vytorin 10/40 Tablets...................... 2114
Vytorin 10/40 Tablets...................... 3077
Vytorin 10/80 Tablets...................... 2114
Vytorin 10/80 Tablets...................... 3077
Wellbutrin Tablets (Frequent)........... 1603
▲ Xeloda Tablets (Less than 5%) 2822
▲ Xenical Capsules (3.4%) 2831
▲ Xyrem Oral Solution (5.9%) 1688
Yasmin 28 Tablets (Greater than 1%)... 796
Yaz Tablets (Greater than 1%).......... 803
Zantac (Rare).................................. 1624
Zantac Injection (Rare).................... 1619
Zantac Injection Pharmacy Bulk Package (Rare)........................... 1622
Zantac Injection Premixed (Rare)...... 1619
Zantac (Rare).................................. 1624
Zegerid Capsules (Less than 1%)..... 2958
Zegerid Powder for Oral Solution (Less than 1%)............................ 2958
Zelapar Tablets (2%)....................... 3372
Zelnorm Tablets.............................. 2312
Zocor Tablets 2105
Zoloft (Infrequent)........................... 2586
▲ Zometa for Intravenous Infusion (14%)... 2315
Zomig Tablets (Infrequent)............... 3519
Zomig Nasal Spray (Infrequent)........ 3523
Zomig-ZMT Tablets (Infrequent)........ 3519
▲ Zonegran Capsules (6%) 1101
Zostavax Injection (0.9%)................ 2111
Zosyn (1.0% or less)....................... 3492
Zyban Sustained-Release Tablets (Frequent)..................................... 1644
▲ Zyprexa Tablets (18%) 1830
▲ Zyprexa ZYDIS Orally Disintegrating Tablets (18%)........ 1830
Zyrtec Chewable Tablets (Less than 2%) 2594
Zyrtec (Less than 2%) 2594
Zyrtec-D 12 Hour Extended Release Tablets (Less than 2%) 2597

Depression, aggravation of

Celexa (Frequent) 1176
Coreg Tablets (Greater than 0.1% to 1%) 1414
Evoxac Capsules (Less than 1%) 1047
Frova Tablets (Rare) 1113
▲ Intron A for Injection (Less than 5%) 3024
Lexapro Oral Solution (Infrequent) 1190
Lexapro Tablets (Infrequent) 1190
Lupron Depot 3.75 mg 3260
Lupron Depot–3 Month 11.25 mg (Possible) 3265
Meridia Capsules 489
Nexium Delayed-Release Capsules (Less than 1%) 655
Nexium I.V. (Less than 1%) 659
Sustiva Capsules (Less than 2%) 930
Sustiva Tablets (Less than 2%) 930
Tegretol-XR Tablets 2295
Ziagen (5 patients) 1626
Zoloft (Infrequent) 2586

Depression, circulatory

Kadian Capsules 577

Depression, manic

Azilect Tablets (Rare) 3293

Depression, mood

(*see under* Depression)

Depression, psychotic

Azilect Tablets (Rare) 3293
Celexa (Infrequent) 1176
Copaxone for Injection (Infrequent) .. 3297
Effexor Tablets (Rare) 3411
Effexor XR Capsules (Infrequent) 3417
Lyrica Capsules (Rare) 2539
Paxil CR Controlled-Release Tablets (Rare) 1538
Paxil (Rare) 1530
Pexeva Tablets (rare) 1694
Relpax Tablets (Rare) 2548
Rilutek Tablets (Rare) 2930
Risperdal Consta Long-Acting Injection (Infrequent) 1682

Depression, respiratory, neonatal

Dilaudid 440
Dilaudid Non-Sterile Powder 440
Dilaudid Rectal Suppositories 440
Dilaudid Tablets 440
Kadian Capsules 577
MS Contin Tablets 2701
Percocet Tablets 1131
Tussionex Pennkinetic Extended-Release Suspension 3327
Tylenol with Codeine Tablets 2391
Vicodin Tablets 535
Vicodin ES Tablets 536

Depression, worsening

Paxil CR Controlled-Release Tablets 1538
Paxil 1530
Symbyax Capsules 1819

Depressive reactions

▲ Combivir Tablets (9%) 1411
▲ Epivir (9%) 1427
▲ Rescriptor Tablets (4.9% to 12.6%) 2551
Truvada Tablets 1296
▲ Ziagen (6%) 1626

Derealization

Abilify Oral Solution (Rare) 882

Abilify Oral Solution (Rare)................ 2450
Abilify Discmelt Orally Disintegrating Tablets (Rare).......... 882
Abilify Discmelt Orally Disintegrating Tablets (Rare).......... 2450
Abilify Tablets (Rare)......................... 882
Abilify Tablets (Rare)......................... 2450
Niravam Orally Disintegrating Tablets (1.9%)............................ 3092
Wellbutrin SR Sustained-Release Tablets (Rare)................................ 1607
Wellbutrin XL Extended-Release Tablets (Rare)................................ 1613
Zyban Sustained-Release Tablets (Rare)... 1644

Dermatitis

▲ Advair HFA Inhalation Aerosol (1% to 3%)... 1318
Aldara Cream, 5% (1.4%)................... 1846
Ambien Tablets (Rare)........................ 2851
Ambien CR Tablets (Rare) 2855
Amerge Tablets (Rare) 1339
Aricept Tablets (Infrequent) 1094
Aricept ODT Tablets (Infrequent) 1094
▲ Aromasin Tablets (8.2%) 2600
Atacand HCT (0.5% or greater) 651
Avalide Tablets 888
Avalide Tablets 2874
Avapro Tablets (Less than 1%) 891
Avapro Tablets (Less than 1%) 2871
Axert Tablets (Rare) 2396
Azopt Ophthalmic Suspension (1% to 5%) 557
Bactroban Cream (Less than 1%) 1394
Caduet Tablets (Less than or equal to 0.1%) 2508
Celebrex Capsules (0.1% to 1.9%) ... 3134
Celexa (Infrequent) 1176
Chantix Tablets (Infrequent) 2517
Ciloxan Ophthalmic Ointment (Less than 1%) 559
Clindagel 1203
▲ Clolar for Intravenous Infusion (41%) 1271
Clozaril Tablets (Less than 1%) 2184
Colazal Capsules 2838
Colyte with Flavor Packs for Oral Solution (Isolated cases) 3088
Copaxone for Injection (Infrequent) .. 3297
▲ Copegus Tablets (16%) 2754
Cosopt Sterile Ophthalmic Solution 1931
Coumadin for Injection (Infrequent) ... 898
Coumadin Tablets (Infrequent) 898
Cozaar Tablets (Less than 1%) 1935
Differin Cream (Less than 1%) 1210
▲ Entocort EC Capsules (Less than 5%) 2698
▲ Estring Vaginal Ring (1% to 3%) 2635
Evoxac Capsules (Less than 1%) 1047
FazaClo Orally Disintegrating Tablets (Less than 1%) 551
▲ Flovent Diskus (1% to 3%) 1443
Floxin Otic Solution (Single report) ... 1049
Gengraf Capsules (1% to less than 3%) 459
HalfLytely and Bisacodyl Tablets Bowel Prep Kit with Flavors Packs 881
▲ Hycamtin for Injection (Rare to 16%) 1458
Hyzaar 50-12.5 Tablets 1990
Hyzaar 100-12.5 Tablets 1990
Hyzaar 100-25 Tablets 1990
▲ Intron A for Injection (Up to 8%) 3024
Invanz for Injection (1%) 1999
Invirase (Less than 2%) 2772
Lexapro Oral Solution (Infrequent) 1190
Lexapro Tablets (Infrequent) 1190
Lotensin Tablets (Less than 1%) 2243
Lotrel Capsules 2249
Lotronex Tablets (Rare) 1512
Lupron Depot 7.5 mg (Less than 5%) 3264
Maxair Autohaler 1852
Meridia Capsules 489
Micardis Tablets (More than 0.3%) ... 854
Micardis HCT Tablets 856
Miradon Tablets 3042
Namenda (Infrequent) 1195
Neoral Oral Solution (1% to less than 3%) 2259
Neoral Soft Gelatin Capsules (1% to less than 3%) 2259
Nexium Delayed-Release Capsules (Less than 1%) 655
Nexium I.V. (Less than 1%) 659
Norvasc Tablets (Less than 0.1%) 2545
Opana Tablets (Less than 1%) 1122
Opana ER Tablets (Less than 1%) 1126
Pancrease MT Capsules (Frequent) .. 1885
▲ Panretin Gel (25% to 77%) 1747
▲ Pegasys (8%) 2789
Phenergan Tablets and Suppositories.................................. 3440
Phenytek Capsules (Rare)................. 2160
Prevnar for Injection.......................... 3463
Prezista Tablets (Less than 2%)........ 3306
Prilosec OTC Delayed-Release Tablets 2677
Prinzide Tablets (0.3% to 1%).......... 2056
Requip Tablets (Infrequent)............... 1555
Rescriptor Tablets 2551
Risperdal Consta Long-Acting Injection (Infrequent)...................... 1682
Rythmol SR Capsules........................ 2727
Singulair (Greater than or equal to 2%)... 2077
▲ Soriatane Capsules (1% to 10%) 1013
▲ Strattera Capsules (2% to 4%) 1814
▲ Tamiflu Capsules (1% to 5%) 2807
Tamiflu Oral Suspension (1%).......... 2807
Temovate Scalp Application (1 of 294 patients) 2670
Thioridazine Hydrochloride Tablets (Infrequent)...................................... 2163
Topamax Sprinkle Capsules (2%) 2404
Topamax Tablets (2%) 2404
TriLyte with Flavor Packs for Oral Solution 3100
▲ Trisenox Injection (43%) 993
▲ Ultram ER Tablets (1% to greater than 5%) 2392
▲ Valcyte Tablets (Less than 5%) 2813
Vaqta (Less than 1%) 2097
Varivax (Greater than or equal to 1%) 2100
VFEND I.V. (Less than 2%)................ 2564
VFEND Oral Suspension (Less than 2%) 2564
VFEND Tablets (Less than 2%) 2564
Viracept (Less than 2%) 2577
▲ Xeloda Tablets (1% to 37%) 2822
Xolair (2%) 1266
Zegerid Capsules 2958
Zegerid Powder for Oral Solution 2958
Zoloft (Rare) 2586
▲ Zometa for Intravenous Infusion (11%) 2315
Zyrtec Chewable Tablets (Less than 2%) 2594
Zyrtec (Less than 2%) 2594
Zyrtec-D 12 Hour Extended Release Tablets (Less than 2%) 2597

Dermatitis, allergic

Aloxi Injection (Less than 1%) 2127
Decadron Tablets 1951
Hydrocortone Tablets 1989
▲ Niravam Orally Disintegrating Tablets (3.8%) 3092
Prezista Tablets (Less than 2%) 3306
ProctoFoam-HC 3099
Xifaxan Tablets 2842

Dermatitis, allergic contact

Aclovate Cream (Infrequent) 2660
Analpram-HC 1159
Apexicon E Cream 2661
▲ Catapres-TTS (About 19 in 100) 844
Clobevate Gel 3211
Clobex Lotion 1204
Clobex Shampoo (Infrequent) 1206
Clobex Spray (Less than 1%) 1208
Cutivate Cream (Infrequent) 2662
Cutivate Ointment (Infrequent to more frequent) 2665
Diprolene Gel 0.05% 3001
Diprolene Lotion 0.05% (Infrequent) 3002
Diprolene Ointment 0.05% (Infrequent) 3003
Diprolene AF Cream 0.05% (Infrequent) 3000
Diprosone Cream, USP 0.05% 3004
▲ Efudex (Among most frequent) 3363
Elocon Cream 0.1% (Infrequent) 3005
Elocon Lotion 0.1% (Infrequent) 3006
Elocon Ointment 0.1% (Infrequent) ... 3007
Locoid Lipocream Cream (Infrequent) 1160
Lotrisone 3040
Luxiq Foam 1010
Olux Foam 1012
Ophthetic Ophthalmic Solution .... ⊙ 232
Oxistat Cream 2667
Pramosone 1161
Temovate Cream 2668
Temovate Gel (Infrequent) 2669
Temovate Ointment 2668
Temovate Scalp Application (Infrequent) 2670
Temovate E Emollient (Infrequent) 2671
Triaz 1892
Triaz Pads 1892
Tri-Luma Cream 1213
Vanos Cream 1893

Dermatitis, application site

Lidoderm Patch 1118

Dermatitis, atopic

Cutivate Cream (0.8%)....................... 2662
Cutivate Lotion 0.05% (Less than 1%)... 2664
Invanz for Injection (Greater than 0.5%).. 1999

Dermatitis, bullous

Carimune NF 3499
Flebogamma 5%, Immune Globulin Intravenous (Human)...................... 1658
Gammagard Liquid 721
Gammagard S/D (Rare) 724
Gamunex Immune Globulin I.V., 10% (Rare) 3235
Phenytek Capsules 2160
Rituxan I.V. 1254

Dermatitis, contact

Advair Diskus 100/50 1308
Advair Diskus 250/50 1308
Advair Diskus 500/50 1308
Advair HFA Inhalation Aerosol........... 1318
Astelin Nasal Spray (Infrequent) 1904
▲ Augmentin ES-600 Powder for Oral Suspension (3.5%)................... 1366
Bactroban Ointment (Less than 1%)... 1395
Caduet Tablets (Less than 2%).......... 2508
▲ Catapres-TTS (About 8 to 34 in 100 patients).................................. 844
Celebrex Capsules (0.1% to 1.9%)... 3134
Claripel Cream................................... 3211
Clindagel 1203
Copaxone for Injection (Infrequent)... 3297
Cosopt Sterile Ophthalmic Solution 1931
Cutivate Lotion 0.05% (Less than 1%) 2664
Doxil Injection (Less than 1%)........... 2351
Effexor Tablets (Infrequent)............... 3411
Effexor XR Capsules (Infrequent)...... 3417
Evoxac Capsules (Less than 1%)...... 1047
Exelon Capsules (Infrequent)............ 2206
Exelon Oral Solution (Infrequent) 2206
Finacea Gel (1% or less).................. 1669
Gabitril Tablets (Infrequent) 984
Geodon Capsules (Infrequent).......... 2529
Klonopin (Infrequent)......................... 2778
▲ Lamictal (2% to 5%) 1481
Lipitor Tablets (Less than 2%)........... 2483
Lofibra Tablets................................... 1219
Lofibra Capsules 1216
Lunesta Tablets (Infrequent)............. 3142
Lustra Cream 3289
Lustra-AF Cream................................ 3289
Lustra-Ultra Cream 3289
▲ Macugen Injection (1% to 5%) .... ⊙ 261
Mentax Cream (Less than 2%).......... 2158
Metrogel 1% (1.3%).......................... 1211
Nitro-Dur Transdermal Infusion System (Uncommon)..................... 3046
Norvir (Less than 2%)........................ 503
Paxil CR Controlled-Release Tablets (Rare)................................... 1538
Paxil (Rare).. 1530
Pexeva Tablets (infrequent).............. 1694
Prevacid Delayed-Release Capsules (Less than 1%)............... 3271
Prevacid for Delayed-Release Oral Suspension (Less than 1%)........... 3271
Prevacid SoluTab Delayed-Release Orally Disintegrating Tablets (Less than 1%)............................... 3271
Prevacid NapraPAC (Less than 1%).. 3280
PREVPAC (Less than 1%)................. 3284
Protonix I.V. (Less than 1%).............. 3472
Protonix Tablets (Less than 1%)....... 3469
Protopic Ointment (1% to 3%) 638
Prozac Pulvules and Liquid (Infrequent)...................................... 1801
▲ Pulmicort Respules (1% to 3%) 661
Rilutek Tablets (Rare)........................ 2930
▲ Serevent Diskus (1% to 3%) 1568
Seroquel Tablets (Infrequent)........... 690
Sonata Capsules (Infrequent)............ 1717
Symbyax Capsules (Infrequent)........ 1819
▲ Synera Topical Patch (Less than 4%)... 1137
Thioridazine Hydrochloride Tablets... 2163
Thiothixene Capsules........................ 2165
Tricor Tablets..................................... 527
Trileptal Tablets................................. 2300
Trileptal Oral Suspension.................. 2300
Trusopt Sterile Ophthalmic Solution... 2095
Uniretic Tablets (Less than 1%)........ 3100
Varivax (Greater than or equal to 1%).. 2100
VFEND I.V. (Less than 2%)............... 2564
VFEND Oral Suspension (Less than 2%)... 2564
VFEND Tablets (Less than 2%)......... 2564
Viagra Tablets (Less than 2%).......... 2573
Xyrem Oral Solution (Infrequent)....... 1688
Zelapar Tablets.................................. 3372
Zoloft (Rare)....................................... 2586
Zovirax Cream.................................... 820
Zyprexa Tablets (Infrequent).............. 1830
Zyprexa ZYDIS Orally Disintegrating Tablets (Infrequent)..................................... 1830

Dermatitis, eczematoid

Symmetrel Tablets (Less than 0.1%)... 1135

Dermatitis, exfoliative

Abelcet Injection................................ 1141
Abilify Oral Solution (Infrequent)........ 882
Abilify Oral Solution (Infrequent) 2450
Abilify Discmelt Orally Disintegrating Tablets (Infrequent)..................................... 882
Abilify Discmelt Orally Disintegrating Tablets (Infrequent)..................................... 2450
Abilify Tablets (Infrequent) 882
Abilify Tablets (Infrequent) 2450
Aceon Tablets (2 mg, 4 mg, 8 mg) ... 3194
Actiq (Less than 1%) 979
Adalat CC Tablets (Rare) 2964
Aldara Cream, 5% 1846
Aldoril Tablets 1910
Amoxil Capsules 1343
Amoxil Chewable Tablets 1343
Amoxil Pediatric Drops for Oral Suspension 1343
Amoxil Powder for Oral Suspension 1343
Amoxil Tablets 1343
Anaprox Tablets (Less than 1%) 2761
Anaprox DS Tablets (Less than 1%) .. 2761
Arthrotec Tablets (Rare) 3129
Atacand HCT 651
Augmentin (Occasional case) 1360
Augmentin Tablets (Occasional) 1363
Augmentin XR Extended-Release Tablets (Occasional) 1369
Augmentin ES-600 Powder for Oral Suspension (Occasional) 1366
Avalide Tablets 888
Avalide Tablets 2874
▲ Avastin IV (3% to 19%) 1227
Axid Oral Solution 879
Bicillin C-R Injectable Suspension 1706
Campral Tablets (Infrequent) 1174
Camptosar Injection (Up to 0.9%) 2604
Captopril Tablets 2149
Carbatrol Capsules 3171
Cardizem LA Extended Release Tablets (Infrequent) 1728
Celebrex Capsules (Less than 0.1%) 3134
Cialis Tablets 1838
Cipro 2977
Cipro I.V. (1% or less) 2984
Cipro XR Tablets 2990
Clinoril Tablets 1924
Concerta Extended-Release Tablets 1881
Coreg Tablets (Less than or equal to 0.1%) 1414
Cuprimine Capsules 1947
Cymbalta Delayed-Release Capsules (Infrequent) 1757
Daytrana Transdermal Patch 3174
Diovan HCT Tablets 2196
Diuril Oral Suspension 1954
Diuril Sodium Intravenous 2467
Dolobid Tablets (Less than 1 in 100) 1955
▲ Doxil Injection (Less than 1% to 10%) 2351
Duragesic Transdermal System (Less than 1%) 2373
EC-Naprosyn Delayed-Release Tablets (Less than 1%) 2761
Effexor Tablets (Rare) 3411
Effexor XR Capsules (Rare) 3417
Equetro Extended-Release Capsules 3180
Ethyol for Injection 1898
Fansidar Tablets 2765
Focalin Tablets 2220
Focalin XR Capsules 2223
Furosemide Tablets 2154
Gabitril Tablets (Infrequent) 984
Gantrisin Pediatric Suspension 2770

Geodon Capsules (Infrequent) 2529
Gleevec Tablets (Infrequent) 2227
Hyzaar 50-12.5 Tablets 1990
Hyzaar 100-12.5 Tablets 1990
Hyzaar 100-25 Tablets 1990
Imitrex Tablets (Rare) 1471
Inderal LA Long-Acting Capsules 3429
Indocin Capsules (Less than 1%) 1995
Indocin I.V. (Less than 1%) 2465
Indocin (Less than 1%) 1995
▲ I.V. Busulfex (5%) 2493
Kaletra (Less than 2%) 476
Lamictal (Rare) 1481
Lyrica Capsules (Rare) 2539
Mefoxin for Injection 2012
Mefoxin Premixed Intravenous Solution 2016
Metadate CD Capsules 3323
Micardis HCT Tablets 856
Miradon Tablets 3042
Mobic Oral Suspension 863
Mobic Tablets 863
Moduretic Tablets 2028
Nalfon Capsules (Less than 1%) 2502
Naprosyn Suspension (Less than 1%) 2761
Naprosyn Tablets (Less than 1%) 2761
Nembutal Sodium Solution, USP 2470
Neumega for Injection 3435
▲ Nexavar Tablets (Common) 746
Nitrolingual Pumpspray 3120
Noroxin Tablets 2032
Omnicef Capsules 511
Omnicef for Oral Suspension 511
Oracea Capsules 1000
OxyContin Tablets (Less than 1%) 2703
▲ Panretin Gel (3% to 9%) 1747
Paser Granules 1674
Paxil CR Controlled-Release Tablets (Rare) 1538
Paxil (Rare) 1530
Pexeva Tablets (Rare) 1694
Phenytek Capsules 2160
Prinzide Tablets 2056
▲ Prograf Capsules and Injection (3% to 15%) 632
▲ Proleukin for Injection (18%) 2266
Proquin XR Tablets 1153
▲ Protopic Ointment (Up to 3%) 638
Prozac Pulvules and Liquid 1801
Relpax Tablets (Rare) 2548
Rilutek Tablets (Up to 1.2%) 2930
Risperdal (Infrequent) 1676
Risperdal M-Tab Orally Disintegrating Tablets (Infrequent) 1676
Ritalin Hydrochloride Tablets 2269
Ritalin LA Capsules 2271
Ritalin-SR Tablets 2269
Seroquel Tablets (Rare) 690
Sular Tablets (Less than or equal to 1%) 3122
▲ Sustiva Capsules (Up to 3.5%) 930
▲ Sustiva Tablets (Up to 3.5%) 930
Symbyax Capsules (Rare) 1819
Tambocor Tablets (Less than 1%) 1856
▲ Targretin Capsules (9.5% to 28.3%) 1747
Tegretol/Tegretol-XR 2295
Teveten HCT Tablets 1737
Thalomid Capsules 965
Thioridazine Hydrochloride Tablets 2163
Thiothixene Capsules 2165
Tiazac Capsules (Infrequent) 1201
Ticlid Tablets (Rare) 2810
Timolide Tablets 2086
Vancocin HCl Capsules, USP (Infrequent) 3380
Vantin Tablets and Oral Suspension (Less than 1%) 2645
Vasotec I.V. Injection (0.5% to 1.0%) 2103
VFEND I.V. (Less than 2%) 2564
VFEND Oral Suspension (Less than 2%) 2564
VFEND Tablets (Less than 2%) 2564
Viagra Tablets (Less than 2%) 2573
Voltaren Tablets (Rarely) 2307
Voltaren-XR Tablets (Rarely) 2310
Wellbutrin Tablets 1603
Wellbutrin SR Sustained-Release Tablets 1607
Wellbutrin XL Extended-Release Tablets 1613
Zyban Sustained-Release Tablets 1644

Dermatitis, eyelid
OptiPranolol Metipranolol Ophthalmic Solution 0.3% (A small number of patients) ⊙256
Vantin Tablets and Oral Suspension 2645

Dermatitis, fungal
Aricept Tablets (Infrequent) 1094
Aricept ODT Tablets (Infrequent) 1094
▲ CellCept Capsules (3% to less than 20%) 2747
▲ CellCept Intravenous (3% to less than 20%) 2747
▲ CellCept Oral Suspension (3% to less than 20%) 2747
▲ CellCept Tablets (3% to less than 20%) 2747
Clindagel 1203
Copaxone for Injection (Infrequent) 3297
▲ Doxil Injection (1% to 10%) 2351
Effexor Tablets (Rare) 3411
Geodon Capsules (2%) 2529
Lamictal (Rare) 1481
Lofibra Tablets 1219
Lofibra Capsules 1216
Neurontin Capsules (Infrequent) 2487
Neurontin Oral Solution (Infrequent) 2487
Neurontin Tablets (Infrequent) 2487
Paxil CR Controlled-Release Tablets (Rare) 1538
Paxil (Rare) 1530
Permax Tablets (Infrequent) 3356
Pexeva Tablets (rare) 1694
▲ Prograf Capsules and Injection (3% to 15%) 632
Protonix I.V. (Less than 1%) 3472
Protonix Tablets (Less than 1%) 3469
▲ Protopic Ointment (1% to 6%) 638
▲ Rapamune Oral Solution and Tablets (3% to 20%) 3475
Requip Tablets (Infrequent) 1555
Rescriptor Tablets 2551
Rilutek Tablets (Infrequent) 2930
Sular Tablets (Less than or equal to 1%) 3122
Synagis (More than 1%) 1897
▲ Thalomid Capsules (4.2%) 965
Tricor Tablets 527
Uniretic Tablets (Less than 1%) 3100
Vantin Tablets and Oral Suspension (Less than 1%) 2645
Viracept (Less than 2%) 2577
Zelapar Tablets 3372

Dermatitis, herpes simplex
Elidel Cream 1% (0.3% to 1.5%) 2200
▲ Mylotarg for Injection (21%) 3431

Dermatitis, irritant
Clobex Shampoo 1206

Dermatitis, lichenoides
Effexor Tablets (Rare) 3411
Effexor XR Capsules (Rare) 3417
Evoxac Capsules (Less than 1%) 1047
▲ Intron A for Injection (Less than 5%) 3024
Lyrica Capsules (Rare) 2539
Permax Tablets (Rare) 3356
Protonix I.V. (Less than 1%) 3472
Protonix Tablets (Less than 1%) 3469
Risperdal (Rare) 1676
Risperdal M-Tab Orally Disintegrating Tablets (Rare) 1676
Rituxan I.V. 1254

Dermatitis, maculopapular
Bicillin C-R Injectable Suspension 1706

Dermatitis, medicamentosa
Prezista Tablets (Less than 2%) 3306

Dermatitis, perioral
Aclovate Cream (Infrequent) 2660
Analpram-HC 1159
Apexicon E Cream 2661
Clobevate Gel 3211
Clobex Lotion 1204
Clobex Shampoo (Infrequent) 1206
Clobex Spray (Less than 1%) 1208
Cutivate Cream (Infrequent) 2662
Cutivate Lotion 0.05% (Rare) 2664
Cutivate Ointment (Infrequent to more frequent) 2665
Diprolene Gel 0.05% 3001
Diprolene Lotion 0.05% (Infrequent) 3002
Diprolene Ointment 0.05% (Infrequent) 3003
Diprolene AF Cream 0.05% (Infrequent) 3000
Diprosone Cream, USP 0.05% 3004
Elocon Cream 0.1% (Infrequent) 3005
Elocon Lotion 0.1% (Infrequent) 3006
Elocon Ointment 0.1% (Infrequent) 3007
Locoid Lipocream Cream (Infrequent) 1160
Lotrisone 3040
Luxíq Foam 1010
Olux Foam 1012
Pramosone 1161
ProctoFoam-HC 3099
Temovate Cream 2668
Temovate Gel (Infrequent) 2669
Temovate Ointment 2668
Temovate Scalp Application (Infrequent) 2670
Temovate E Emollient (Infrequent) 2671
Tri-Luma Cream 1213
Vanos Cream 1893

Dermatitis, photosensitive
Advair Diskus 100/50 1308
Advair Diskus 250/50 1308
Advair Diskus 500/50 1308
Amerge Tablets (Rare) 1339
Anaprox Tablets (Less than 1%) 2761
Anaprox DS Tablets (Less than 1%) 2761
EC-Naprosyn Delayed-Release Tablets (Less than 1%) 2761
▲ Flovent Diskus (1% to 3%) 1443
Naprosyn Suspension (Less than 1%) 2761
Naprosyn Tablets (Less than 1%) 2761
Prevacid NapraPAC (Less than 1%) 3280

Dermatitis, purpuric
Phenytek Capsules 2160

Dermatitis, radiation recall
▲ Erbitux (3% to 86%) 910

Dermatitis, vesicular bullous
(*see under* Dermatitis, bullous)

Dermatitis seborrhic
Imitrex Injection 1463
Imitrex Nasal Spray 1467

Dermatologic reactions, unspecified
Aceon Tablets (2 mg, 4 mg, 8 mg) 3194
Altace Capsules (Less than 1%) 1702
Captopril Tablets 2149
Clinoril Tablets (Less than 1 in 100) 1924
▲ Erbitux (1% to 90%) 910
Follistim AQ Cartridge 2338
▲ Hycamtin for Injection (48%) 1458
Nexium Delayed-Release Capsules (Rare) 655
Nexium I.V. (Rare) 659
Norflex Injection (Rare) 1856
Prinivil Tablets (0.3% to 1.0%) 2052
Prinzide Tablets 2056
Protonix I.V. 3472
Protonix Tablets 3469
Tasmar Tablets (Infrequent) 3358
Vasotec I.V. Injection (0.5% to 1.0%) 2103

Dermatomyositis
Altoprev Extended-Release Tablets 3109
Cuprimine Capsules (Rare) 1947
Mevacor Tablets 2021
Vytorin 10/10 Tablets 2114
Vytorin 10/10 Tablets 3077
Vytorin 10/20 Tablets 2114
Vytorin 10/20 Tablets 3077
Vytorin 10/40 Tablets 2114
Vytorin 10/40 Tablets 3077
Vytorin 10/80 Tablets 2114
Vytorin 10/80 Tablets 3077
Zocor Tablets 2105

Dermatomyositis, exacerbation of
Actimmune (Rare) 1671

Dermatosis
▲ Advair HFA Inhalation Aerosol (1% to 3%) 1318
Amerge Tablets (Rare) 1339
▲ Flovent Diskus (1% to 3%) 1443
Gleevec Tablets (Rare) 2227
Lotronex Tablets (Rare) 1512
Revlimid Capsules 958

Descemetitis
Ophthetic Ophthalmic Solution ⊙232

Desquamation
▲ Alimta for Injection (Up to 22%) 1750
Doxil Injection (Some patients) 2351
Invanz for Injection (Greater than 0.1%) 1999
Neurontin Capsules (Rare) 2487
Neurontin Oral Solution (Rare) 2487
Neurontin Tablets (Rare) 2487
▲ Nexavar Tablets (0% to 40%) 746
Oxistat Lotion (0.4%) 2667
Rescriptor Tablets 2551
▲ Sustiva Capsules (16.7% to 24.5%) 930
▲ Sustiva Tablets (16.7% to 24.5%) 930
▲ Taxotere Injection Concentrate (0% to 5.6%) 2932
▲ Tri-Luma Cream (25.48% to 38%) 1213
Vantin Tablets and Oral Suspension (Less than 1%) 2645
Xeloda Tablets 2822
Zovirax Cream (Less than 1%) 820

Detumescence
Edex Injection 3089

Diabetes
(*see under* Diabetes mellitus)

Diabetes, aggravation of
▲ ActoPlus Met Tablets (5.1%) 3214
Campath Ampules 811
▲ Duetact Tablets (At least 5%) 3226
Geodon 2529
Namenda (Infrequent) 1195
Premphase Tablets 3456
Prempro Tablets 3456
Tamiflu Capsules 2807
Tamiflu Oral Suspension 2807

Diabetes, unstable
Lopressor Injection 2238
Lopressor Tablets 2238
Viagra Tablets (Less than 2%) 2573

Diabetes insipidus
Sandostatin LAR Depot (Rare) 2280
VFEND I.V. (Less than 2%) 2564
VFEND Oral Suspension (Less than 2%) 2564
VFEND Tablets (Less than 2%) 2564

Diabetes insipidus, nephrogenic
Atripla Tablets 945
Truvada Tablets 1296
Viread Tablets 1301

Diabetes mellitus
Abilify Oral Solution (Infrequent) 882
Abilify Oral Solution (Infrequent) 2450
Abilify Discmelt Orally Disintegrating Tablets (Infrequent) 882
Abilify Discmelt Orally Disintegrating Tablets (Infrequent) 2450
Abilify Tablets (Infrequent) 882
Abilify Tablets (Infrequent) 2450
Accutane Capsules 2731
Aptivus Capsules (Less than 2%) 826
Aricept Tablets (Infrequent) 1094
Aricept ODT Tablets (Infrequent) 1094
Boostrix 1404
Campral Tablets (Infrequent) 1174
Celebrex Capsules (0.1% to 1.9%) 3134
▲ CellCept Capsules (3% to less than 20%) 2747
▲ CellCept Intravenous (3% to less than 20%) 2747
▲ CellCept Oral Suspension (3% to less than 20%) 2747
▲ CellCept Tablets (3% to less than 20%) 2747
Chantix Tablets (Infrequent) 2517
Copegus Tablets (Less than 1%) 2754
▲ Coreg Tablets (Greater than 1% to 3%) 1414
Crestor Tablets (Greater than or equal to 1%) 678
Crixivan Capsules 1940
Doxil Injection (Less than 1%) 2351
Dyazide Capsules 1423
Effexor Tablets (Rare) 3411
Effexor XR Capsules (Infrequent) 3417
Emend Capsules (Greater than 0.5%) 1963
Evoxac Capsules (Less than 1%) 1047
Exelon Capsules (Infrequent) 2206
Exelon Oral Solution (Infrequent) 2206
Gengraf Capsules (1% to less than 3%) 459
Geodon 2529
Havrix Vaccine (1 Case) 1456
Invirase (2.7%) 2772
Kaletra (Less than 2%) 476
Lofibra Tablets 1219
Lofibra Capsules 1216
▲ Macugen Injection (1% to 5%) ⊙261
Micardis Tablets (More than 0.3%) 854
Micardis HCT Tablets 856
M-M-R II 2006
Mumpsvax 2031
▲ Myfortic Tablets (3% to less than 20%) 2255
Neoral Oral Solution (1% to less than 3%) 2259

Neoral Soft Gelatin Capsules (1% to less than 3%) 2259
Neurontin Capsules (Infrequent) 2487
Neurontin Oral Solution (Infrequent) 2487
Neurontin Tablets (Infrequent) 2487
▲ Norditropin Cartridges (5%) 2323
Norvir (Less than 2%) 503
Nutropin for Injection (0.1%) 1239
Nutropin AQ Injection (0.1%) 1243
Nutropin AQ Pen (0.1%) 1243
Nutropin AQ Pen Cartridge (0.1%) 1243
Paxil CR Controlled-Release Tablets (Rare) 1538
Paxil (Rare) 1530
Pegasys (Less than 1%) 2789
Permax Tablets (Infrequent) 3356
Pexeva Tablets (Rare) 1694
Pletal Tablets (Less than 2%) 2455
Prevacid Delayed-Release Capsules (Less than 1%) 3271
Prevacid for Delayed-Release Oral Suspension (Less than 1%) 3271
Prevacid SoluTab Delayed-Release Orally Disintegrating Tablets (Less than 1%) 3271
Prevacid NapraPAC (Less than 1%) 3280
PREVPAC (Less than 1%) 3284
Prezista Tablets (Less than 2%) 3306
Prinivil Tablets (0.3% to 1.0%) 2052
Prinzide Tablets 2056
▲ Prograf Capsules and Injection (3% to 24%) 632
Protonix I.V. (Less than 1%) 3472
Protonix Tablets (Less than 1%) 3469
Proventil HFA Inhalation Aerosol (Less than 3%) 3056
Prozac Pulvules and Liquid (Rare) 1801
Pulmozyme Inhalation Solution 1248
▲ Rapamune Oral Solution and Tablets (3% to 20%) 3475
Rebetron Combination Therapy 3063
ReoPro Vials (0.1%) 1809
Requip Tablets (Infrequent) 1555
Revlimid Capsules 958
Reyataz Capsules (Less than 3%) 921
Rilutek Tablets (Infrequent) 2930
Risperdal (Infrequent) 1676
Risperdal Consta Long-Acting Injection (Infrequent) 1682
Risperdal M-Tab Orally Disintegrating Tablets (Infrequent) 1676
Rythmol SR Capsules 2727
Sandostatin Injection (Less than 1%) 2278
Sandostatin LAR Depot (Rare) 2280
Seroquel Tablets (Infrequent) 690
▲ Simulect for Injection (3% to 10%) 2284
Sonata Capsules (Rare) 1717
Sular Tablets (Less than or equal to 1%) 3122
Tasmar Tablets (Infrequent) 3358
Tequin Injection (Less than 0.1%) 938
Tequin Injection in 5% Dextrose (Less than 0.1%) 938
Tequin Tablets (Less than 0.1%) 938
Teveten Tablets (Less than 1%) 1735
Teveten HCT Tablets (Less than 1%) 1737
Thalomid Capsules 965
Topamax Sprinkle Capsules (Infrequent) 2404
Topamax Tablets (Infrequent) 2404
Toprol-XL Tablets (Greater than 1%) 668
Tricor Tablets 527
Triglide Tablets 3123
Uniretic Tablets (Less than 1%) 3100
Viracept 2577
Zelapar Tablets 3372
Zyprexa Tablets (Infrequent) 1830
Zyprexa ZYDIS Orally Disintegrating Tablets (Infrequent) 1830
Zyrtec Chewable Tablets (Less than 2%) 2594
Zyrtec (Less than 2%) 2594
Zyrtec-D 12 Hour Extended Release Tablets (Less than 2%) 2597

Diabetes mellitus, increase

▲ Actos Tablets (5.1%) 3219
Agenerase Capsules 1327
Agenerase Oral Solution 1332
Levaquin (0.1% to 0.9%) 2384
Levaquin in 5% Dextrose Injection (0.1% to 0.9%) 2384
Toprol-XL Tablets (Greater than 1%) 668

Diabetes mellitus, insulin-dependent, post-transplant

▲ Prograf Capsules and Injection (20%) 632

Diabetes mellitus, precipitation of latent

Colocort Rectal Suspension, USP (Retention) 100 mg/60 mL 2476
Decadron Tablets 1951
Depo-Medrol Injectable Suspension 2617
Depo-Medrol Single-Dose Vial 2619
Furosemide Tablets 2154
Hydrocortone Tablets 1989
▲ Intron A for Injection (Less than 5%) 3024
Levaquin (0.1% to 0.9%) 2384
Levaquin in 5% Dextrose Injection (0.1% to 0.9%) 2384
Prinzide Tablets 2056
Risperdal 1676
Risperdal Consta Long-Acting Injection 1682
Risperdal M-Tab Orally Disintegrating Tablets 1676
Viracept 2577

Diabetes mellitus, type I

Enbrel for Injection 584

Diabetes mellitus de novo

Agenerase Capsules (2 patients) 1327
Agenerase Oral Solution (Two patients) 1332

Diabetic acidosis

Prozac Pulvules and Liquid (Rare) 1801
Zyprexa Tablets (Rare) 1830
Zyprexa ZYDIS Orally Disintegrating Tablets (Rare) 1830

Diabetic ketoacidosis

Agenerase Capsules 1327
Agenerase Oral Solution 1332
Aptivus Capsules 826
Neurontin Capsules (Rare) 2487
Neurontin Oral Solution (Rare) 2487
Neurontin Tablets (Rare) 2487
Revlimid Capsules 958
Risperdal 1676
Risperdal Consta Long-Acting Injection 1682
Risperdal M-Tab Orally Disintegrating Tablets 1676
Viracept (Some cases) 2577

Diabetic retinopathy

Neurontin Capsules (Rare) 2487
Neurontin Oral Solution (Rare) 2487
Neurontin Tablets (Rare) 2487

Dialysis encephalopathy

Maalox Regular Strength Antacid/Anti-Gas Liquid ▣ 660
Maalox Regular Strength Antacid/Antigas Liquid 2175
Maalox Max Maximum Strength Antacid/Anti-Gas Liquid 2176

Dialysis graft complication

▲ Fosrenol (3% to 26%) 3183

Dialysis osteomalacia, results in, or worsening of

Maalox Regular Strength Antacid/Anti-Gas Liquid ▣ 660
Maalox Regular Strength Antacid/Antigas Liquid 2175
Maalox Max Maximum Strength Antacid/Anti-Gas Liquid 2176

Diaphoresis

Abilify Oral Solution (Frequent) 882
Abilify Oral Solution (Frequent) 2450
Abilify Discmelt Orally Disintegrating Tablets (Frequent) 882
Abilify Discmelt Orally Disintegrating Tablets (Frequent) 2450
Abilify Tablets (Frequent) 882
Abilify Tablets (Frequent) 2450
Accutane Capsules 2731
Aceon Tablets (2 mg, 4 mg, 8 mg) (0.3% to 1%) 3194
Acetadote Injection (.29% to 1.41%) 1031
Aciphex Tablets 1090
Actiq (1% to 2%) 979
Adalat CC Tablets (Less than 1%) 2964
▲ Adderall XR Capsules (2% to 4%) 3166
Adenocard Injection (Less than 1%) 617
Adenoscan (Less than 1%) 619
▲ Advair Diskus 100/50 (1% to 3%) 1308
▲ Advair Diskus 250/50 (1% to 3%) 1308
▲ Advair Diskus 500/50 (1% to 3%) 1308
Advicor Tablets 1722
▲ Aerobid/Aerobid-M (1% to 3%) 1171
Aggrastat (2%) 1907
Albalon Ophthalmic Solution ⊙ 218
▲ Alferon N Injection (One patient to 3%) 1665
Alinia for Oral Suspension (Less than 1%) 2835
Alinia Tablets (Less than 1%) 2835
Aloprim for Injection (Less than 1%) 2167
Altace Capsules (Less than 1%) 1702
Ambien Tablets (Infrequent) 2851
▲ AmBisome for Injection (7%) 620
Amerge Tablets (Infrequent) 1339
Anaprox Tablets (Less than 3%) 2761
Anaprox DS Tablets (Less than 3%) 2761
AndroGel (Fewer than 1%) 3329
Anzemet Injection (Rare) 2859
Anzemet Tablets (Rare) 2862
Aredia for Injection 2179
Aricept Tablets (Frequent) 1094
Aricept ODT Tablets (Frequent) 1094
▲ Arimidex Tablets (1% to 5%) 673
▲ Aromasin Tablets (4% to 17.8%) 2600
Arthrotec Tablets (Rare) 3129
▲ Asacol Delayed-Release Tablets (3%) 2692
Atacand Tablets (0.5% or greater) 649
Atacand HCT (0.5% or greater) 651
Avelox (0.1% to less than 2%) 2970
▲ Avinza Capsules (5% to 10%) 1741
Axert Tablets (Rare) 2396
Axid Oral Solution (More frequent) 879
▲ Azilect Tablets (3%) 3293
▲ Betaseron for SC Injection (8%) 767
▲ Bexxar (Less than 1% to 8%) 1398
Bicillin C-R Injectable Suspension 1706
BiDil Tablets (1% to less than 2%) 2171
Blocadren Tablets (Less than 1%) 1916
Bumex Tablets (0.1%) 2746
▲ Buprenex Injectable (1% to 5%) 2716
Caduet Tablets (Less than 2%) 2508
▲ Campath Ampules (1% to 19%) 811
▲ Campral Tablets (2% to 3%) 1174
▲ Camptosar Injection (0% to 16%) 2604
Cancidas for Injection (0% to 2.8%) 1918
Captopril Tablets 2149
Carbatrol Capsules 3171
Cardene I.V. (1.4%) 2497
Carimune NF 3499
Caverject Impulse Injection (Less than 1%) 2612
Celebrex Capsules (0.1% to 1.9%) 3134
▲ Celexa (11%) 1176
▲ CellCept Capsules (3% to less than 20%) 2747
▲ CellCept Intravenous (3% to less than 20%) 2747
▲ CellCept Oral Suspension (3% to less than 20%) 2747
▲ CellCept Tablets (3% to less than 20%) 2747
Cesamet Capsules 3340
Cialis Tablets (Less than 2%) 1838
Cipro (Less than 1%) 2977
Cipro I.V. (1% or less) 2984
Cipro XR Tablets 2990
Clinoril Tablets (Less than 1 in 100) 1924
▲ Clozaril Tablets (More than 5% to 6%) 2184
Comtan Tablets (2%) 2189
▲ Copaxone for Injection (15%) 3297
▲ Copegus Tablets (6%) 2754
Coreg Tablets (Greater than 0.1% to 1%) 1414
Cosopt Sterile Ophthalmic Solution 1931
Covera-HS Tablets (Less than 2%) 3139
Cozaar Tablets (Less than 1%) 1935
▲ Cubicin for Injection (5%) 1026
Dalmane Capsules (Rare) 3342
Dantrium Capsules (Less frequent) 2694
Decadron Tablets 1951
Depacon Injection (0.9%) 412
Depakote ER Tablets (Greater than 1%) 434
Depo-Medrol Injectable Suspension 2617
Depo-Medrol Single-Dose Vial 2619
Diastat Rectal Delivery System (Less than 1%) 3343
Dilaudid 440
Dilaudid Non-Sterile Powder 440
Dilaudid Oral Liquid 445
Dilaudid Rectal Suppositories 440
Dilaudid Tablets 440
Dilaudid Tablets - 8 mg 445
▲ Dilaudid-HP (Among most frequent) 442
Diovan HCT Tablets (Greater than 0.2%) 2196
Dolobid Tablets (Less than 1 in 100) 1955
▲ Doxil Injection (1% to 10%) 2351
▲ Duragesic Transdermal System (10% or more) 2373
Dyazide Capsules 1423
EC-Naprosyn Delayed-Release Tablets (Less than 3%) 2761
▲ Effexor Tablets (2% to 19.3%) 3411
▲ Effexor XR Capsules (1% to 14%) 3417
Eldepryl Capsules 3208
▲ Eligard 7.5 mg (25% to 56.7%) 2880
▲ Eligard 22.5 mg (56.4%) 2883
▲ Eloxatin for Injection (2% to 5%) 2892
Emend Capsules (Greater than 0.5%) 1963
Engerix-B Vaccine (Less than 1%) 1425
▲ Entocort EC Capsules (Less than 5%) 2698
Equetro Extended-Release Capsules 3180
▲ Evista Tablets (2.5% to 3.1%) 1763
▲ Evoxac Capsules (18.7%) 1047
▲ Exelon Capsules (4%) 2206
▲ Exelon Oral Solution (4%) 2206
▲ Faslodex Injection (5%) 681
▲ FazaClo Orally Disintegrating Tablets (Greater than 5% to 6%) 551
▲ Femara Tablets (Less than 0.1% to 24.2%) 2214
Ferrlecit Injection 3388
▲ Fluarix (1% to 10%) 1451
Flumadine 1183
▲ Forteo for Injection (4.2%) 1767
Fortical Nasal Spray (Less than 1%) 3337
Frova Tablets (Frequent) 1113
Gabitril Tablets (Frequent) 984
Gemzar for Injection (Infrequent) 1771
Gengraf Capsules (1% to less than 3%) 459
Geodon for Injection (Up to 2%) 2529
Guanidine Hydrochloride Tablets 3016
Humalog-Pen (Less common) 1781
Humalog Mix 50/50-Pen 1783
Humalog Mix 75/25-Pen (Less common) 1785
Humulin 50/50, 100 Units 1791
Humulin 70/30 Pen 1793
Humulin L, 100 Units (Less common) 1794
Humulin N Pen 1797
▲ Hycamtin for Injection (69%) 1458
Hydrocortone Tablets 1989
Hyperstat I.V. 3017
Hytrin Capsules (At least 1%) 471
Hyzaar 50-12.5 Tablets 1990
Hyzaar 100-12.5 Tablets 1990
Hyzaar 100-25 Tablets 1990
▲ Imdur Tablets (Less than or equal to 5%) 3018
Imitrex Injection (2%) 1463
Imitrex Nasal Spray (Infrequent) 1467
Imitrex Tablets (Infrequent) 1471
Indocin (Less than 1%) 1995
Infed Injection 3390
▲ Infergen (12% to 13%) 3364
▲ Intron A for Injection (1% to 21%) 3024
Invanz for Injection (Greater than 0.1%) 1999
Invirase (Less than 2%) 2772
▲ Ionsys Transdermal System (1% to less than 10%) 2379
Kadian Capsules (Less than 3%) 577
Kaletra (Less than 2%) 476
▲ Lamictal (2% to 5%) 1481
Lariam Tablets 2786
▲ Leukine (6%) 814
▲ Leustatin Injection (9%) 2357
Levaquin (0.1% to 0.9%) 2384
Levaquin in 5% Dextrose Injection (0.1% to 0.9%) 2384
Levitra Tablets (Less than 2%) 3034
Levoxyl Tablets 1712
▲ Lexapro Oral Solution (3% to 8%) 1190
▲ Lexapro Tablets (3% to 8%) 1190
Lipitor Tablets (Less than 2%) 2483
Lofibra Tablets 1219
Lofibra Capsules 1216
Lopressor HCT 50/25 Tablets (1%) 2241
Lopressor HCT 100/25 Tablets (1%) 2241
Lopressor HCT 100/50 Tablets (1%) 2241
Lotensin Tablets (Less than 1%) 2243
Lotensin HCT Tablets (0.3% to 1%) 2246
Lotronex Tablets (Infrequent) 1512
Lunesta Tablets 3142

▲ Lupron Depot 3.75 mg (50%) ... 3260
▲ Lupron Depot 7.5 mg (57.1%) ... 3264
▲ Lupron Depot–3 Month 11.25 mg (50%) ... 3265
Marinol Capsules (Less than 1%) ... 3333
Matulane Capsules ... 3191
Maxalt Tablets (Infrequent) ... 2008
Maxalt-MLT Orally Disintegrating Tablets (Infrequent) ... 2008
▲ Megace ES Oral Suspension (1% to 3%) ... 2481
Mephyton Tablets (Rare) ... 2018
▲ Mepron Suspension (10%) ... 1521
Meridia Capsules (2.5%) ... 489
Merrem I.V. (Greater than 0.1% to 1%) ... 686
Micardis Tablets (More than 0.3%) ... 854
Micardis HCT Tablets ... 856
Migranal Nasal Spray (Infrequent) ... 3348
Mirapex Tablets (1% or more) ... 859
Moban Tablets ... 1119
Mobic Oral Suspension (Less than 2%) ... 863
Mobic Tablets (Less than 2%) ... 863
Moduretic Tablets (Less than or equal to 1%) ... 2028
▲ MS Contin Tablets (Less frequent to among most frequent) ... 2701
Nadolol Tablets (1 to 5 of 1000 patients) ... 2159
Naprosyn Suspension (Less than 3%) ... 2761
Naprosyn Tablets (Less than 3%) ... 2761
Natrecor for Injection (Greater than or equal to 1%) ... 3127
Neoral Oral Solution (1% to less than 3%) ... 2259
Neoral Soft Gelatin Capsules (1% to less than 3%) ... 2259
Neurontin Capsules (Infrequent) ... 2487
Neurontin Oral Solution (Infrequent) ... 2487
Neurontin Tablets (Infrequent) ... 2487
Nexium Delayed-Release Capsules (Less than 1%) ... 655
Nexium I.V. (Less than 1%) ... 659
Niaspan Extended-Release Tablets ... 1730
Nimotop Capsules (Less than 1%) ... 749
▲ Nipent for Injection (8% to 10%) ... 1863
▲ Niravam Orally Disintegrating Tablets (14.4% to 15.1%) ... 3092
Nitrolingual Pumpspray ... 3120
Norvasc Tablets (More than 0.1% to 1%) ... 2545
Norvir (1.7% to 2.6%) ... 503
Numorphan Injection ... 1120
Omacor Capsules ... 2725
▲ Ontak Vials (10%) ... 1745
Orthoclone OKT3 Sterile Solution (Less than 1%) ... 2360
▲ OxyContin Tablets (5%) ... 2703
▲ Paxil CR Controlled-Release Tablets (1.1% to 19.2%) ... 1538
▲ Paxil (1.1% to 19.2%) ... 1530
▲ Pegasys (6%) ... 2789
▲ PEG-Intron Powder for Injection (6%) ... 3048
Pentasa Capsules (Less than 1%) ... 3185
Permax Tablets (2.1%) ... 3356
▲ Pexeva Tablets (1% to 14%) ... 1694
Phenergan Tablets and Suppositories ... 3440
Prevacid Delayed-Release Capsules (Less than 1%) ... 3271
Prevacid for Delayed-Release Oral Suspension (Less than 1%) ... 3271
Prevacid SoluTab Delayed-Release Orally Disintegrating Tablets (Less than 1%) ... 3271
Prevacid NapraPAC (Less than 3%) ... 3280
PREVPAC (Less than 1%) ... 3284
Prinivil Tablets (0.3% to 1.0%) ... 2052
Prinzide Tablets (0.3% to 1%) ... 2056
▲ Prograf Capsules and Injection (3% to 15%) ... 632
Prometrium Capsules (100 mg, 200 mg) ... 3203
Proquin XR Tablets ... 1153
ProSom Tablets (Infrequent) ... 517
Protonix I.V. (Less than 1%) ... 3472
Protonix Tablets (Less than 1%) ... 3469
Protopic Ointment (Greater than or equal to 1%) ... 638
Proventil HFA Inhalation Aerosol (Less than 3%) ... 3056
Provigil Tablets (1%) ... 988
▲ Prozac Pulvules and Liquid (2% to 8%) ... 1801
▲ Rapamune Oral Solution and Tablets (3% to 20%) ... 3475
▲ Rebetol (7% to 11%) ... 3058
Recombivax HB (Less than 1%) ... 2071
ReFacto Vials ... 3484
Relpax Tablets (Frequent) ... 2548
Remicade for IV Injection (Greater than or equal to 0.2%) ... 971
ReoPro Vials (1%) ... 1809
▲ Requip Tablets (6% to 7%) ... 1555
Rescriptor Tablets ... 2551
▲ Retrovir Capsules (5%) ... 1560
▲ Retrovir IV Infusion (5%) ... 1564
▲ Retrovir (5%) ... 1560
Reyataz Capsules (Less than 3%) ... 921
▲ Ribavirin, USP Capsules (7%) ... 3068
Risperdal (Infrequent) ... 1676
Risperdal M-Tab Orally Disintegrating Tablets (Infrequent) ... 1676
Rocephin Injectable Vials, ADD-Vantage, Galaxy, Bulk (Occasional) ... 2800
▲ Romazicon Injection (1% to 9%) ... 2804
▲ Sandostatin LAR Depot (5% to 15%) ... 2280
Seroquel Tablets (Frequent) ... 690
Sonata Capsules (Infrequent) ... 1717
▲ Soriatane Capsules (1% to 10%) ... 1013
▲ Suboxone Tablets (12% to 14%) ... 2717
▲ Subutex Tablets (12% to 12.6%) ... 2717
Sular Tablets (Less than or equal to 1%) ... 3122
Sustiva Capsules (1% to 2%) ... 930
Sustiva Tablets (1% to 2%) ... 930
Symmetrel Tablets ... 1135
▲ Tambocor Tablets (1% to 3%) ... 1856
Tarka Tablets ... 524
▲ Tasmar Tablets (4% to 7%) ... 3358
Tegretol/Tegretol-XR ... 2295
▲ Tequin Injection (0.1% to 3%) ... 938
▲ Tequin Injection in 5% Dextrose (0.1% to 3%) ... 938
▲ Tequin Tablets (0.1% to 3%) ... 938
Teveten Tablets (Less than 1%) ... 1735
Teveten HCT Tablets (Less than 1%) ... 1737
Thalomid Capsules ... 965
Thiothixene Capsules (Infrequently) ... 2165
Timolide Tablets ... 2086
Timoptic Sterile Ophthalmic Solution ... 2088
Timoptic in Ocudose ... 2091
Timoptic-XE Sterile Ophthalmic Gel Forming Solution ... 2092
Tindamax Tablets ... 2142
Topamax Sprinkle Capsules (2%) ... 2404
Topamax Tablets (2%) ... 2404
Tricor Tablets ... 527
▲ Trileptal Tablets (Up to 3%) ... 2300
▲ Trileptal Oral Suspension (Up to 3%) ... 2300
Truvada Tablets ... 1296
Twinject 0.3 ... 3378
Twinject 0.15 ... 3379
Twinrix Vaccine (Less than 1%) ... 1595
Tygacil for Injection (2.3%) ... 3488
Uniretic Tablets (Less than 1%) ... 3100
Univasc Tablets (Less than 1%) ... 3104
Vandazole Vaginal Gel (Less than 1%) ... 3338
Vasotec I.V. Injection (0.5% to 1.0%) ... 2103
Verelan PM Extended-Release Capsules, Controlled-Onset (2% or less) ... 3106
▲ Vesanoid Capsules (20%) ... 2820
VFEND I.V. (Less than 2%) ... 2564
VFEND Oral Suspension (Less than 2%) ... 2564
VFEND Tablets (Less than 2%) ... 2564
▲ Viadur Implant (5.3%) ... 757
Viagra Tablets (Less than 2%) ... 2573
▲ Vicoprofen Tablets (3% to 9%) ... 539
Viracept (Less than 2%) ... 2577
▲ Viread Tablets (3%) ... 1301
Vivitrol ... 995
▲ Wellbutrin Tablets (22.3%) ... 1603
▲ Wellbutrin SR Sustained-Release Tablets (5% to 6%) ... 1607
▲ Wellbutrin XL Extended-Release Tablets (5% to 6%) ... 1613
WinRho SDF ... 732
▲ Xeloda Tablets (Less than 5%) ... 2822
Xopenex Inhalation Solution ... 3146
Xopenex Inhalation Solution Concentrate ... 3150
Xopenex HFA Inhalation Aerosol ... 3154
Zelapar Tablets ... 3372
▲ Zoloft (5% to 8%) ... 2586
Zomig Nasal Spray (Infrequent) ... 3523
Zonegran Capsules (Infrequent) ... 1101
Zosyn (1.0% or less) ... 3492
Zyban Sustained-Release Tablets (Frequent) ... 1644
▲ Zyprexa Tablets (3%) ... 1830
Zyprexa IntraMuscular (Infrequent) ... 1830
▲ Zyprexa ZYDIS Orally Disintegrating Tablets (3%) ... 1830
Zyrtec Chewable Tablets (Less than 2%) ... 2594
Zyrtec (Less than 2%) ... 2594
Zyrtec-D 12 Hour Extended Release Tablets (Less than 2%) ... 2597

Diaphoresis, nocturnal

Sandimmune (Rare) ... 2275

Diaphragmatic hernia

(*see under* Hernia, hiatal)

Diarrhea

▲ Abelcet Injection (6%) ... 1141
Abilify Oral Solution ... 882
Abilify Oral Solution ... 2450
Abilify Discmelt Orally Disintegrating Tablets ... 882
Abilify Discmelt Orally Disintegrating Tablets ... 2450
Abilify Tablets ... 882
Abilify Tablets ... 2450
Accolate Tablets (2.8%) ... 671
Accutane Capsules ... 2731
▲ Aceon Tablets (2 mg, 4 mg, 8 mg) (4.3%) ... 3194
Aciphex Tablets ... 1090
▲ Actimmune (14%) ... 1671
Actiq (1% or greater) ... 979
▲ Actonel Tablets (4.9% to 19.7%) ... 2683
▲ Actonel with Calcium Tablets (4.9% to 10.6%) ... 2688
▲ ActoPlus Met Tablets (4.6% to 5.8%) ... 3214
▲ ADACEL Vaccine (0.3% to 10.3%) ... 2945
Adalat CC Tablets (Less than 1%) ... 2964
Adderall Tablets ... 3164
▲ Adderall XR Capsules (2% to 6%) ... 3166
Adipex-P ... 1215
▲ Advair Diskus 100/50 (4%) ... 1308
Advair Diskus 250/50 (2%) ... 1308
▲ Advair Diskus 500/50 (2% to 4%) ... 1308
Advate Injection (0.6%) ... 712
▲ Advicor Tablets (6%) ... 1722
▲ Aerobid/Aerobid-M (10%) ... 1171
▲ Agenerase Capsules (28% to 60%) ... 1327
▲ Agenerase Oral Solution (28% to 60%) ... 1332
▲ Aggrenox Capsules (12.7%) ... 822
▲ Agrylin Capsules (25.7%) ... 3169
Aldara Cream, 5% (More than 1%) ... 1846
Aldoril Tablets ... 1910
▲ Alferon N Injection (2% to 6%) ... 1665
▲ Alimta for Injection (Up to 26%) ... 1750
Alinia for Oral Suspension (2.1%) ... 2835
Alinia Tablets (2.1%) ... 2835
Alkeran for Injection (Infrequent) ... 955
Alkeran Tablets (Infrequent) ... 956
Aloprim for Injection (Less than 1%) ... 2167
Aloxi Injection (1%) ... 2127
Altace Capsules (Less than 1% to 1.1%) ... 1702
▲ Altoprev Extended-Release Tablets (3%) ... 3109
Ambien Tablets (1% to 3%) ... 2851
Ambien CR Tablets (Frequent) ... 2855
▲ AmBisome for Injection (15.3% to 30.3%) ... 620
Amerge Tablets (Infrequent) ... 1339
▲ Amitiza Capsules (10.3% to 13.2%) ... 3224
▲ Amoxil Capsules (8%) ... 1343
▲ Amoxil Chewable Tablets (8%) ... 1343
▲ Amoxil Pediatric Drops for Oral Suspension (8%) ... 1343
▲ Amoxil Powder for Oral Suspension (8%) ... 1343
▲ Amoxil Tablets (8%) ... 1343
Anaprox Tablets (Less than 3%) ... 2761
Anaprox DS Tablets (Less than 3%) ... 2761
▲ Anzemet Injection (12.4%) ... 2859
Anzemet Tablets (2.1%) ... 2862
▲ Aptivus Capsules (10.9%) ... 826
▲ Aranesp for Injection (16% to 22%) ... 581
▲ Aredia for Injection (28.5%) ... 2179
▲ Argatroban Injection (6.2%) ... 1346
▲ Aricept Tablets (8% to 15%) ... 1094
▲ Aricept ODT Tablets (8% to 15%) ... 1094
▲ Arimidex Tablets (6% to 8%) ... 673
Arixtra Injection (1.9% to 2.5%) ... 1351
▲ Aromasin Tablets (4% to 9.6%) ... 2600
▲ Arranon Injection (0% to 22%) ... 1357
▲ Arthrotec Tablets (19%) ... 3129
▲ Asacol Delayed-Release Tablets (7%) ... 2692
Astelin Nasal Spray (Infrequently) ... 1904
Atacand Tablets (More than 1%) ... 649
Atacand HCT (0.5% or greater) ... 651
▲ Atripla Tablets (7%) ... 945
Attenuvax (Rare) ... 1914
▲ Augmentin (9%) ... 1360
▲ Augmentin Tablets (9%) ... 1363
▲ Augmentin XR Extended-Release Tablets (14.4% to 15.6%) ... 1369
Augmentin ES-600 Powder for Oral Suspension (2.9%) ... 1366
Avalide Tablets (1% or greater) ... 888
Avalide Tablets (1% or greater) ... 2874
▲ Avandamet Tablets (12.7% to 14%) ... 1373
Avandaryl Tablets (Less than 1%) ... 1379
Avandia Tablets (1% to 2.3%) ... 1384
▲ Avapro Tablets (3%) ... 891
▲ Avapro Tablets (3%) ... 2871
▲ Avastin IV (34%) ... 1227
▲ Avelox (5%) ... 2970
▲ Avinza Capsules (5% to 10%) ... 1741
Axert Tablets (Infrequent) ... 2396
▲ Axid Oral Solution (7.2%) ... 879
▲ Azilect Tablets (5%) ... 3293
▲ Azmacort Inhalation Aerosol (1% to 3%) ... 1726
Azopt Ophthalmic Suspension (Less than 1%) ... 557
Bactroban Nasal (Less than 1%) ... 1394
Baraclude (Less than or equal to 1%) ... 894
BeneFix Vials (1.5% to 1.6%) ... 3408
Benicar HCT Tablets (Greater than 1%) ... 1044
Benzaclin Topical Gel ... 2877
Betagan Ophthalmic Solution, USP ... ⊙ 220
▲ Betaseron for SC Injection (19%) ... 767
Betimol Ophthalmic Solution ... 3382
Betimol Ophthalmic Solution ... ⊙ 295
▲ Bexxar (1% to 12%) ... 1398
▲ Biaxin/Biaxin XL (3% to 6%) ... 402
Blocadren Tablets (Less than 1%) ... 1916
▲ Boniva Injection (4.1% to 6.8%) ... 2738
▲ Boniva Tablets (4.1% to 6.8%) ... 2741
▲ Boostrix (3% to 26%) ... 1404
Bumex Tablets (0.1%) ... 2746
Buprenex Injectable (Rare) ... 2716
▲ Byetta Injection (13%) ... 611
▲ Caduet Tablets (Greater than 0.1% to 5.3%) ... 2508
▲ Campath Ampules (1% to 22%) ... 811
▲ Campral Tablets (10% to 17%) ... 1174
▲ Camptosar Injection (6.7% to 88%) ... 2604
▲ Canasa Rectal Suppositories (3.1%) ... 699
▲ Cancidas for Injection (1.3% to 3.6%) ... 1918
Captopril Tablets (About 0.5% to 2%) ... 2149
Carafate Suspension (Less than 0.5%) ... 701
Carafate Tablets (Less than 0.5%) ... 701
Carbatrol Capsules ... 3171
Cardizem LA Extended Release Tablets (Less than 2%) ... 1728
Cardura XL Tablets (Less than 1%) ... 2515
▲ Carnitor Injection (9% to 35%) ... 3188
Carnitor Tablets and Oral Solution ... 3190
▲ Ceftin (8.6%) ... 1407
▲ Celebrex Capsules (5.6%) ... 3134
▲ Celexa (8%) ... 1176
▲ CellCept Capsules (31% to 51.3%) ... 2747
▲ CellCept Intravenous (31% to 51.3%) ... 2747
▲ CellCept Oral Suspension (31% to 51.3%) ... 2747
▲ CellCept Tablets (31% to 51.3%) ... 2747
▲ Cerezyme for Injection (Approximately 6.5%) ... 1270
Cervidil Vaginal Insert (Less than 1%) ... 1181
Cesamet Capsules ... 3340
Chantix Tablets (Frequent) ... 2517
▲ Chemet Capsules (12.0% to 20.9%) ... 2458
Cialis Tablets (Less than 2%) ... 1838
▲ Cipro (1.6% to 4.8%) ... 2977
▲ Cipro I.V. (Greater than 1% to 4.8%) ... 2984
Cipro XR Tablets (2%) ... 2990
▲ Clarinex Syrup (15.4% to 19.7%) ... 2995
Cleocin Vaginal Ovules (Less than 1%) ... 2616
Clindagel ... 1203
▲ Clinoril Tablets (3% to 9%) ... 1924
▲ Clolar for Intravenous Infusion (53%) ... 1271
Clorpres Tablets ... 2153
Clozaril Tablets (2%) ... 2184
▲ Colazal Capsules (5%) ... 2838
Combivent Inhalation Aerosol (Less than 2%) ... 847
▲ Combivir Tablets (18%) ... 1411
▲ Comtan Tablets (10%) ... 2189
Comvax (0.8% to 2.2%) ... 1928
Concerta Extended-Release Tablets (2%) ... 1881
▲ Copaxone for Injection (12%) ... 3297

▲ Copegus Tablets (11%) 2754
▲ Coreg Tablets (2% to 12%) 1414
Cosmegen for Injection 2459
Cosopt Sterile Ophthalmic Solution (Less than 1%) 1931
Coumadin for Injection (Infrequent) 898
Coumadin Tablets (Infrequent) 898
Covera-HS Tablets (Less than 2%) 3139
Cozaar Tablets (1% or greater) 1935
▲ Creon 5 Capsules (Among most frequent) 3198
▲ Creon 10 Capsules (Among most frequent) 3198
▲ Creon 20 Capsules (Among most frequent) 3199
▲ Crestor Tablets (3.4%) 678
▲ Crixivan Capsules (3.3%) 1940
▲ Cubicin for Injection (5.2% to 11.7%) 1026
Cuprimine Capsules 1947
Cutivate Lotion 0.05% (1%) 2664
▲ Cymbalta Delayed-Release Capsules (7% to 13%) 1757
▲ Dacogen Injection (34%) 2129
Dalmane Capsules 3342
▲ Dantrium Capsules (Among most frequent) 2694
Demadex Injection (2%) 2759
Demadex Tablets (2%) 2759
▲ Demser Capsules (10%) 1953
▲ Depacon Injection (0.9% to 23%) 412
▲ Depakene (13% to 23%) 417
▲ Depakote Sprinkle Capsules (13% to 23%) 422
▲ Depakote Tablets (12% to 23%) 427
▲ Depakote ER Tablets (7% to 23%) 434
▲ depo-subQ provera 104 Injectable Suspension (1% to less than 5%) 2624
Desoxyn Tablets, USP 2462
▲ Detrol Tablets (4%) 2628
Dexedrine 1420
DextroStat Tablets 3179
▲ Diastat Rectal Delivery System (4%) 3343
▲ Didronel Tablets (About 1 patient in 15; possibly 2 or 3 in 10) 2697
Dilaudid 440
Dilaudid Non-Sterile Powder 440
Dilaudid Oral Liquid 445
Dilaudid Rectal Suppositories 440
Dilaudid Tablets 440
Dilaudid Tablets - 8 mg 445
Dilaudid-HP (Less frequent) 442
▲ Diovan Tablets (1% to 5%) 2193
▲ Diovan HCT Tablets (3%) 2196
▲ Ditropan XL Extended-Release Tablets (7% to 9%) 2413
Diuril Oral Suspension 1954
Diuril Sodium Intravenous 2467
▲ Dolobid Tablets (3% to 9%) 1955
▲ Doxil Injection (5.2% to 20.9%) 2351
Duac Topical Gel 3212
Duetact Tablets 3226
DuoNeb Inhalation Solution (1.8%) 1058
▲ Duragesic Transdermal System (3% to 10%) 2373
Dyazide Capsules 1423
DynaCirc CR Tablets (0.5% to 1%) 2721
Dyrenium Capsules (Rare) 3400
EC-Naprosyn Delayed-Release Tablets (Less than 3%) 2761
Edecrin 1959
▲ E.E.S. (Among most frequent) 451
▲ Effexor Tablets (8%) 3411
▲ Effexor XR Capsules (6%) 3417
Eldepryl Capsules (1 of 49 patients) 3208
▲ Elidel Cream 1% (0.6% to 7.7%) 2200
▲ Elitek (20%) 2890
▲ Elmiron Capsules (4%) 2415
▲ Eloxatin for Injection (11% to 67%) 2892
▲ Emcyt Capsules (12%) 2634
▲ Emend Capsules (5.5% to 10.3%) 1963
▲ Emsam Transdermal System (9%) 903
▲ Emtriva Capsules (23%) 1287
▲ Emtriva Oral Solution (23%) 1287
Enablex Extended-Release Tablets (0.9% to 2.1%) 2203
Enbrel for Injection 584
Engerix-B Vaccine (Less than 1%) 1425
▲ Epivir (18%) 1427
▲ Epivir-HBV (14%) 1432
▲ Epogen for Injection (0.11% to 21%) 591
▲ Epzicom Tablets (5% to 6%) 1436
▲ Equetro Extended-Release Capsules (10%) 3180
▲ Eraxis for Injection (3.1%) 2521
▲ Erbitux (2% to 72%) 910
▲ EryPed (Among most frequent) 447
▲ Ery-Tab Tablets (Among most frequent) 449
▲ Erythrocin Stearate Filmtab Tablets (Among most frequent) 453
▲ Erythromycin Base Filmtab Tablets (Among most frequent) 455
▲ Erythromycin Delayed-Release Capsules, USP (Among most frequent) 457
▲ Estring Vaginal Ring (1% to 3%) 2635
▲ Eulexin Capsules (12% to 40%) 3009
Evoclin Foam, 1% (Rarely) 1009
▲ Evoxac Capsules (10.3%) 1047
▲ Exelon Capsules (7% to 19%) 2206
▲ Exelon Oral Solution (7% to 19%) 2206
▲ Famvir Tablets (4.5% to 9%) 2211
Fansidar Tablets 2765
▲ Faslodex Injection (12.3%) 681
FazaClo Orally Disintegrating Tablets (2%) 551
▲ Femara Tablets (0.5% to 8%) 2214
▲ Ferrlecit Injection (2% to 35%) 3388
▲ Flebogamma 5%, Immune Globulin Intravenous (Human) (20%) 1658
▲ Flomax Capsules (4.3% to 6.2%) 850
▲ Flonase Nasal Spray (1% to 3%) 1440
▲ Flovent Diskus (1% to 3%) 1443
▲ Flovent HFA (1% to 3%) 1447
Floxin Otic Solution (0.6%) 1049
Fluarix (1.6%) 1451
Flumadine (0.3% to 1%) 1183
▲ Flumist Vaccine (3.7%) 1901
Follistim AQ Cartridge 2338
▲ Fortamet Extended-Release Tablets (16.7%) 3115
Fortaz (1 in 78 patients) 1453
▲ Forteo for Injection (5.1%) 1767
▲ Fortical Nasal Spray (1% to 3%) 3337
▲ Fosamax (0.6% to 3.1%) 1969
▲ Fosamax Plus D Tablets (0% to 3.1%) 1977
▲ Fosrenol Chewable Tablets (13% to 23%) 3183
Frova Tablets (Frequent) 1113
Furosemide Tablets 2154
▲ Fuzeon Injection (31.7%) 2767
▲ Gabitril Tablets (2% to 10%) 984
▲ Gammagard Liquid (0.85% to 8.2%) 721
▲ Gamunex Immune Globulin I.V., 10% (28%) 3235
Gantrisin Pediatric Suspension 2770
▲ Gardasil Injection (3.6%) 1984
▲ Gemzar for Injection (19% to 31%) 1771
▲ Gengraf Capsules (3% to 13%) 459
▲ Geodon (5%) 2529
▲ Gleevec Tablets (2% to 70%) 2227
Gris-PEG Tablets (Occasional) 2502
Guanidine Hydrochloride Tablets 3016
Havrix Vaccine (Less than 1%) 1456
▲ Hepsera Tablets (2% to 3%) 1292
▲ Herceptin I.V. (25%) 1233
HibTITER (2 of 1,118 vaccinations) 3426
▲ Hycamtin for Injection (Less than 1% to 42%) 1458
Hyperstat I.V. 3017
Hytrin Capsules (At least 1%) 471
Hyzaar 50-12.5 Tablets (1% or greater) 1990
Hyzaar 100-12.5 Tablets (1% or greater) 1990
Hyzaar 100-25 Tablets (1% or greater) 1990
▲ Imdur Tablets (Less than or equal to 5%) 3018
Imitrex Injection (Infrequent) 1463
Imitrex Nasal Spray (Infrequent) 1467
Imitrex Tablets (Frequent) 1471
▲ Indapamide Tablets (Less than 5%) 2156
Inderal LA Long-Acting Capsules 3429
Indocin Capsules (Greater than 1%) 1995
▲ Indocin I.V. (1% to 3%) 2465
Indocin (Greater than 1%) 1995
▲ Infanrix Vaccine (3.8% to 4.3%) 1476
Infed Injection 3390
▲ Infergen (24% to 29%) 3364
InnoPran XL Capsules 2723
Inspra Tablets (2%) 2536
▲ Intron A for Injection (2% to 45%) 3024
▲ Invanz for Injection (9.2% to 11.7%) 1999
▲ Invirase (1% to 8.1%) 2772
Ionsys Transdermal System (.1% to less than 1%) 2379
▲ Iressa Tablets (49% to 76%) 684
▲ I.V. Busulfex (5% to 84%) 2493
Kadian Capsules (Less than 3%) 577
▲ Kaletra (7% to 27%) 476
K-Dur Extended-Relase Tablets 3033
Keflex Capsules (Most frequent) 549
Keppra Injection 3320
▲ Keppra Oral Solution (1% to 8%) 3314
▲ Keppra Tablets (1% to 8%) 3314
▲ Ketek Tablets (10% to 10.8%) 2903
Kionex Powder (Occasional) 2477
▲ Kineret Injection (7%) 599
Klonopin 2778
▲ K-Lor Oral Solution (Among most common) 474
K-Phos Original (Sodium Free) Tablets 760
K-Phos Neutral Tablets 760
Kristalose for Oral Solution 1034
▲ K-Tab Tablets (Most common) 475
▲ Kytril Injection (3.4% to 4%) 2781
▲ Kytril (4% to 9%) 2784
▲ Lamictal (5% to 11%) 1481
▲ Lamisil Tablets (5.6%) 2232
Lanoxicaps Capsules (Less common) 1490
Lanoxin Injection (Less common) 1494
Lanoxin Injection Pediatric 1497
Lanoxin Tablets (Less common) 1500
▲ Lariam Tablets (Among most frequent) 2786
▲ Lescol Capsules (4.9%) 2233
▲ Lescol XL Tablets (3.3%) 2233
Leukeran Tablets (Infrequent) 1504
▲ Leukine (52% to 89%) 814
▲ Leustatin Injection (10%) 2357
▲ Levaquin (1.2% to 5.4%) 2384
▲ Levaquin in 5% Dextrose Injection (1.2% to 5.4%) 2384
Levitra Tablets (Less than 2%) 3034
Levothroid Tablets 1186
Levoxyl Tablets 1712
▲ Lexapro Oral Solution (6% to 14%) 1190
▲ Lexapro Tablets (6% to 14%) 1190
▲ Lexiva Tablets (5% to 52%) 1505
Limbrel Capsules (0.006%) 2672
▲ Lipitor Tablets (Up to 5.3%) 2483
Lithobid Tablets 1692
Lofibra Tablets (2.3%) 1219
Lofibra Capsules (2.3%) 1216
▲ Lopressor Injection (5%) 2238
▲ Lopressor Tablets (5%) 2238
▲ Lopressor HCT 50/25 Tablets (1% to 5%) 2241
▲ Lopressor HCT 100/25 Tablets (1% to 5%) 2241
▲ Lopressor HCT 100/50 Tablets (1% to 5%) 2241
Lotensin HCT Tablets (0.3% to 1%) 2246
Lotrel Capsules 2249
Lovenox Injection (2.2%) 2915
▲ Lunesta Tablets (2% to 4%) 3142
▲ Macugen Injection (6% to 10%) ⊙261
▲ Malarone Pediatric Tablets (1% to 8%) 1517
▲ Malarone Tablets (1% to 8%) 1517
Marinol Capsules (0.3% to 1%) 3333
Matulane Capsules 3191
Mavik Tablets (0.3% to 1.0%) 486
Maxair Autohaler (1.3%) 1852
Maxalt Tablets (Frequent) 2008
Maxalt-MLT Orally Disintegrating Tablets (Frequent) 2008
▲ Maxipime for Injection (Greater than 0.1% to 3%) 1105
Mefoxin for Injection 2012
Mefoxin Premixed Intravenous Solution 2016
▲ Megace ES Oral Suspension (6% to 13%) 2481
▲ Menactra Vaccine (0.3% to 16%) 2954
▲ Mepron Suspension (2.1% to 42%) 1521
Meridia Capsules (Greater than or equal to 1%) 489
▲ Merrem I.V. (3.5% to 7%) 686
Meruvax II 2019
MetroGel-Vaginal Gel (1%) 1855
▲ Mevacor Tablets (2.2% to 5.5%) 2021
▲ Miacalcin Nasal Spray (1% to 3%) 2253
▲ Micardis Tablets (3%) 854
▲ Micardis HCT Tablets (3%) 856
▲ Midamor Tablets (3% to 8%) 2026
Migranal Nasal Spray (2%) 3348
Mintezol 2027
Miradon Tablets 3042
Mirapex Tablets (Greater than or equal to 1%) 859
M-M-R II 2006
▲ Mobic Oral Suspension (1.9% to 7.8%) 863
▲ Mobic Tablets (1.9% to 7.8%) 863
Moduretic Tablets (Greater than 1%, less than 3%) 2028
MS Contin Tablets (Less frequent) 2701
Mumpsvax 2031
Mustargen for Injection 2468
Mycamine for Injection (1.6% to 2.1%) 628
▲ Myfortic Tablets (21.4% to 23.5%) 2255
▲ Mylotarg for Injection (30% to 36%) 3431
▲ Myozyme for Intravenous Infusion (62%) 1279
▲ Nabi-HB (3%) 2169
Nadolol Tablets (1 to 5 of 1000 patients) 2159
Nalfon Capsules (1.8%) 2502
Namenda (Greater than or equal to 2%) 1195
Naprosyn Suspension (Less than 3%) 2761
Naprosyn Tablets (Less than 3%) 2761
Nasonex Nasal Spray (Greater than or equal to 2%) 3043
▲ Neoral Oral Solution (3% to 13%) 2259
▲ Neoral Soft Gelatin Capsules (3% to 13%) 2259
▲ Neulasta Injection (15% to 72%) 601
▲ Neumega for Injection (43%) 3435
▲ Neupogen for Injection (14%) 603
▲ Neurontin Capsules (5.7%) 2487
▲ Neurontin Oral Solution (5.7%) 2487
▲ Neurontin Tablets (5.7%) 2487
▲ Nexavar Tablets (0% to 43%) 746
▲ Nexium Delayed-Release Capsules (Greater than or equal to 1% to 9.2%) 655
▲ Nexium I.V. (Greater than or equal to 1% to 9.2%) 659
▲ Niaspan Extended-Release Tablets (6% to 8%) 1730
Nicomide Tablets 1088
▲ Nimotop Capsules (Up to 4.2%) 749
▲ Nipent for Injection (15% to 17%) 1863
▲ Niravam Orally Disintegrating Tablets (10.1% to 20.6%) 3092
Noroxin Tablets (0.3% to 1.0%) 2032
Norvasc Tablets (More than 0.1% to 1%) 2545
▲ Norvir (15.4% to 23.3%) 503
▲ Omnicef Capsules (15%) 511
▲ Omnicef for Oral Suspension (8%) 511
▲ Oncaspar (Greater than 1% but less than 5%) 1145
▲ Ontak Vials (29%) 1745
Opana Tablets (Less than 1%) 1122
▲ Opana ER Tablets (4.3%) 1126
▲ Oracea Capsules (4.5%) 1000
▲ Orthoclone OKT3 Sterile Solution (14%) 2360
▲ OxyContin Tablets (Between 1% and 5%) 2703
▲ Oxytrol Transdermal System (3.2%) 3392
Paddock Nystatin USP for Oral Suspension 2478
▲ Pancrease MT Capsules (Among most frequent) 1885
Parcopa Orally Disintegrating Tablets 3097
Parnate Tablets 1527
▲ Paser Granules (Among most common) 1674
▲ Paxil CR Controlled-Release Tablets (1.0% to 12%) 1538
▲ Paxil (1.0% to 12%) 1530
▲ PCE Dispertab Tablets (Among most frequent) 515
Pediarix Vaccine 1548
Liquid PedvaxHIB (One case) 2035
▲ Pegasys (16%) 2789
▲ PEG-Intron Powder for Injection (18%) 3048
▲ Pentasa Capsules (3.4% to 3.5%) 3185
Pepcid Injection (1.7%) 2040
Pepcid (1.7%) 2038
Percodan Tablets 1132
▲ Permax Tablets (6.4%) 3356
Persantine Tablets 868
▲ Pexeva Tablets (1% to 19.2%) 1694
▲ Photofrin for Injection (5% to 9%) 702
▲ Plan B Tablets (5%) 1076
▲ Plavix Tablets (4.5%) 917
▲ Plavix Tablets (4.5%) 2926
▲ Pletal Tablets (12% to 19%) 2455
▲ Precose Tablets (31%) 751
▲ Premarin Tablets (6% to 7%) 3446
▲ Premphase Tablets (5% to 7%) 3456
▲ Prempro Tablets (5% to 7%) 3456
▲ Prevacid Delayed-Release Capsules (1.4% to 7.4%) 3271
▲ Prevacid for Delayed-Release Oral Suspension (1.4% to 7.4%) 3271
▲ Prevacid SoluTab Delayed-Release Orally Disintegrating Tablets (1.4% to 7.4%) 3271
Prevacid I.V. for Injection (Less than 1%) 3277
▲ Prevacid NapraPAC (Less than 1% to 5%) 3280
▲ Prevnar for Injection (8.3% to 13.7%) 3463
▲ PREVPAC (3% to 7.4%) 3284
Prezista Tablets (2.3% to 2.8%) 3306
▲ Prilosec OTC Delayed-Release Tablets (3.0% to 14%) 2677
Primaxin I.M. (0.6%) 2045
▲ Primaxin I.V. (1.8% to 3.9%) 2048
▲ Prinivil Tablets (3.7%) 2052
Prinzide Tablets (2.5%) 2056
ProAir HFA Inhalation Aerosol (Less than 3%) 3300

▲ Prochieve 4% Gel (8%) 1003
▲ Prochieve 8% Gel (8%) 1003
▲ Procrit for Injection (0.11% to 21%) 2364
▲ Prograf Capsules and Injection (37% to 72%) 632
▲ Proleukin for Injection (67%) 2266
▲ Prometrium Capsules (100 mg, 200 mg) (7%) 3203
ProQuad (1.2%) 2064
Proquin XR Tablets (Less than 1%) 1153
Protonix I.V. (Greater than 1%) 3472
▲ Protonix Tablets (4% to 6%) 3469
▲ Protopic Ointment (3% to 6%) 638
▲ Provigil Tablets (6%) 988
▲ Prozac Pulvules and Liquid (8% to 18%) 1801
▲ Pulmicort Respules (2% to 4%) 661
▲ Quadramet Injection (6%) 1040
Raniclor Tablets, Chewable (2.5%) 2505
▲ Rapamune Oral Solution and Tablets (25% to 42%) 3475
▲ Razadyne (6% to 12%) 2399
▲ Razadyne ER Extended-Release Capsules (6% to 12%) 2399
▲ Rebetol (17% to 22%) 3058
Recombivax HB (Greater than 1%) 2071
ReFacto Vials 3484
▲ Relenza Rotadisk (2% to 3%) 1552
Relpax Tablets (Infrequent) 2548
▲ Remicade for IV Injection (12%) 971
▲ Renagel Tablets (4% to 19.2%) 1282
ReoPro Vials (1.1%) 1809
▲ Requip Tablets (1% to 5%) 1555
▲ Rescriptor Tablets (2.4% to 5.9%) 2551
Restoril Capsules (1.7%) 1860
▲ Retrovir Capsules (0.8% to 12%) 1560
▲ Retrovir IV Infusion (1% to 12%) 1564
▲ Retrovir (0.8% to 12%) 1560
▲ Revatio Tablets (9%) 2557
▲ Revlimid Capsules (3.4% to 48.6%) 958
▲ Reyataz Capsules (6% to 25%) 921
▲ Ribavirin, USP Capsules (17% to 22%) 3068
▲ Rilutek Tablets (5.5% to 9.0%) 2930
Risperdal (Infrequent) 1676
▲ Risperdal Consta Long-Acting Injection (1% to 5%) 1682
Risperdal M-Tab Orally Disintegrating Tablets (Infrequent) 1676
▲ Rituxan I.V. (1% to 10%) 1254
Rocephin Injectable Vials, ADD-Vantage, Galaxy, Bulk (2.7%) 2800
▲ RotaTeq (3.7% to 24.1%) 2074
Rozerem Tablets (2%) 3231
▲ Rythmol SR Capsules (2% to 4%) 2727
▲ Sandimmune (3% to 8%) 2275
▲ Sandostatin Injection (22% to 61%) 2278
▲ Sandostatin LAR Depot (36%) 2280
▲ Sensipar Tablets (21%) 608
▲ Simulect for Injection (Greater than or equal to 10%) 2284
Singulair (Greater than or equal to 2%) 2077
▲ Somavert Injection (4% to 14%) 2642
▲ Soriatane Capsules (1% to 10%) 1013
▲ Stalevo Tablets (5% to 10%) 2287
▲ Starlix Tablets (3.2%) 2292
▲ Strattera Capsules (2% to 4%) 1814
Stromectol Tablets (1.8%) 2083
▲ Suboxone Tablets (3.7% to 5%) 2717
▲ Subutex Tablets (4.9% to 5%) 2717
Sular Tablets (Less than or equal to 1%) 3122
▲ Suprax (16%) 1843
▲ Sustiva Capsules (2% to 39%) 930
▲ Sustiva Tablets (2% to 39%) 930
▲ Sutent Capsules (4% to 55%) 2560
▲ Symbyax Capsules (8% to 19%) 1819
▲ Symmetrel Tablets (1% to 5%) 1135
Synagis (More than 1%) 1897
Tambocor Tablets (1% to 3%) 1856
▲ Tamiflu Capsules (1% to 10%) 2807
▲ Tamiflu Oral Suspension (1% to 10%) 2807
▲ Tarceva Tablets (Less than 1% to 54%) 1259
▲ Tarceva Tablets (Less than 1% to 54%) 2444
▲ Targretin Capsules (7.1% to 41.5%) 1747
Tarka Tablets (1.5%) 524
▲ Tasmar Tablets (16% to 18%) 3358
▲ Taxotere Injection Concentrate (2.8% to 77.8%) 2932
Tegretol/Tegretol-XR 2295
▲ Temodar Capsules (10% to 16%) 3073
▲ Tequin Injection (4%) 938
▲ Tequin Injection in 5% Dextrose (4%) 938
▲ Tequin Tablets (4%) 938
Teveten Tablets (1% or greater) 1735
Teveten HCT Tablets (Less than 1%) 1737
▲ Thalomid Capsules (4.2%) 965
▲ Thiola Tablets (16.7%) 2141
Thioridazine Hydrochloride Tablets 2163
Thiothixene Capsules 2165
▲ Thymoglobulin for Intravenous Infusion (36.6%) 1284
Tiazac Capsules (Less than 2%) 1201
▲ Ticlid Tablets (12.5%) 2810
Timentin ADD-Vantage 1580
Timentin Injection Galaxy Container 1583
Timentin IV Infusion 1577
Timentin Pharmacy Bulk Package 1586
Timolide Tablets (Less than 1%) 2086
Timoptic Sterile Ophthalmic Solution (Less frequent) 2088
Timoptic in Ocudose (Less frequent) 2091
Timoptic-XE Sterile Ophthalmic Gel Forming Solution 2092
Tindamax Tablets 2142
▲ TOBI Solution for Inhalation (6.2%) 2298
▲ Topamax Sprinkle Capsules (2% to 11%) 2404
▲ Topamax Tablets (2% to 11%) 2404
▲ Toprol-XL Tablets (About 5 of 100 patients) 668
▲ Trasylol Injection (3%) 754
Trecator Tablets 3487
Trelstar Depot (1.4%) 3394
Trelstar LA Suspension (1.1%) 3397
Tricor Tablets (2.3%) 527
Triglide Tablets (2.3%) 3123
▲ Trileptal Tablets (5% to 7%) 2300
▲ Trileptal Oral Suspension (5% to 7%) 2300
▲ Trisenox Injection (53%) 993
▲ Trizivir Tablets (12% to 26%) 1589
▲ Truvada Tablets (7%) 1296
▲ Twinrix Vaccine (4% to 6%) 1595
▲ Tygacil for Injection (12.7%) 3488
Ultrase Capsules 708
▲ Ultrase MT Capsules (0.2% to 3.6%) 709
Uniphyl Tablets 2710
Uniretic Tablets (More than 1%) 3100
▲ Univasc Tablets (3.1%) 3104
Urocit-K Tablets (Some patients) 2144
Uroqid-Acid No. 2 Tablets 760
Uroxatral Tablets 2943
Urso 250 Tablets (1%) 710
Urso Forte Tablets (1%) 710
▲ Valcyte Tablets (16% to 41%) 2813
Valtrex Caplets 1597
Vandazole Vaginal Gel (1%) 3338
▲ Vantin Tablets and Oral Suspension (1.2% to 7.2%) 2645
▲ Vaprisol (5.5%) 643
▲ Vaqta (1% to 5.9%) 2097
Varivax (Greater than or equal to 1%) 2100
Vasotec I.V. Injection (1.4% to 2.1%) 2103
▲ Velcade for Injection (57%) 2133
Ventolin HFA Inhalation Aerosol (Less than 3%) 1600
Verelan PM Extended-Release Capsules, Controlled-Onset (2.4%) 3106
▲ Vesanoid Capsules (23%) 2820
VFEND I.V. (Less than 2%) 2564
VFEND Oral Suspension (Less than 2%) 2564
VFEND Tablets (Less than 2%) 2564
Viadur Implant (2.3%) 757
▲ Viagra Tablets (3%) 2573
▲ Vicoprofen Tablets (3% to 9%) 539
Viokase 711
▲ Viracept (14% to 20%) 2577
Viramune Oral Suspension (2%) 873
Viramune Tablets (2%) 873
▲ Viread Tablets (11% to 16%) 1301
▲ Vivaglobin (10%) 3506
▲ Vivitrol (12% to 13%) 995
Vivotif 819
▲ Voltaren Tablets (1% to 10%) 2307
▲ Voltaren-XR Tablets (1% to 10%) 2310
Vytorin 10/10 Tablets 2114
Vytorin 10/10 Tablets 3077
Vytorin 10/20 Tablets 2114
Vytorin 10/20 Tablets 3077
Vytorin 10/40 Tablets 2114
Vytorin 10/40 Tablets 3077
Vytorin 10/80 Tablets 2114
Vytorin 10/80 Tablets 3077
▲ WelChol Tablets (5%) 1050
▲ Wellbutrin Tablets (6.8%) 1603
▲ Wellbutrin SR Sustained-Release Tablets (5% to 7%) 1607
▲ Wellbutrin XL Extended-Release Tablets (5% to 7%) 1613
WinRho SDF 732
▲ Xeloda Tablets (2% to 55%) 2822
Xifaxan Tablets (Less than 2%) 2842
▲ Xopenex Inhalation Solution (6%) 3146
▲ Xopenex Inhalation Solution Concentrate (1.5% to 6%) 3150
▲ Xopenex HFA Inhalation Aerosol (6%) 3154
▲ Xyrem Oral Solution (6.1% to 8.6%) 1688
Yaz Tablets (Greater than 1%) 803
Zantac 1624
Zantac Injection 1619
Zantac Injection Pharmacy Bulk Package (Frequent) 1622
Zantac Injection Premixed 1619
Zantac 1624
▲ Zegerid Capsules (3% to 7%) 2958
▲ Zegerid Powder for Oral Solution (3% to 7%) 2958
Zelapar Tablets (2%) 3372
▲ Zelnorm Tablets (4% to 9%) 2312
Zemaira (0.2% to 0.4%) 3509
▲ Zetia Tablets (2.8% to 3.7%) 2120
▲ Zetia Tablets (3.4% to 3.7%) 3083
▲ Ziagen (0% to 7%) 1626
Zinacef for Injection (1 in 220 patients) 1631
Zinacef Injection (1 in 220 patients) 1631
▲ Zinecard for Injection (14% to 21%) 2650
Zmax for Oral Suspension (11.6%) 2583
Zocor Tablets (1.9%) 2105
▲ Zofran Injection (2% to 16%) 1634
▲ Zofran (4% to 6%) 1639
▲ Zofran ODT Orally Disintegrating Tablets (4% to 6%) 1639
▲ Zoloft (13% to 24%) 2586
▲ Zometa for Intravenous Infusion (17.4% to 24%) 2315
Zomig Nasal Spray (Infrequent) 3523
▲ Zonegran Capsules (5%) 1101
Zostavax Injection (1.5%) 2111
▲ Zosyn (11.3% to 20%) 3492
Zovirax (2.4% to 3.2%) 1643
▲ Zyban Sustained-Release Tablets (4%) 1644
Zyprexa Tablets 1830
Zyprexa IntraMuscular (Infrequent) 1830
Zyprexa ZYDIS Orally Disintegrating Tablets 1830
▲ Zyrtec Chewable Tablets (1.9% to 3.1%) 2594
▲ Zyrtec (1.9% to 3.1%) 2594
▲ Zyrtec-D 12 Hour Extended Release Tablets (1.9% to 3.1%) 2597
▲ Zyvox (3.8% to 10.8%) 2652

Diarrhea, bloody

Aciphex Tablets (Rare) 1090
Asacol Delayed-Release Tablets 2692
Benzaclin Topical Gel 2877
Biltricide Tablets 2976
Canasa Rectal Suppositories 699
Cleocin Vaginal Ovules 2616
Clindagel 1203
Colazal Capsules 2838
Duac Topical Gel 3212
Evoclin Foam, 1% (Rarely) 1009
Imitrex Tablets 1471
Norvir (Less than 2%) 503
Omnicef Capsules 511
Omnicef for Oral Suspension 511
Paxil CR Controlled-Release Tablets (Rare) 1538
Paxil (Rare) 1530
Pentasa Capsules (0.9%) 3185
Pexeva Tablets (rare) 1694
Proleukin for Injection (Less than 1%) 2266
Prozac Pulvules and Liquid (Rare) 1801
Ticlid Tablets 2810
▲ Trisenox Injection (8%) 993
Vantin Tablets and Oral Suspension 2645
Zomig Tablets (Rare) 3519
Zomig Nasal Spray (Very rare) 3523
Zomig-ZMT Tablets (Rare) 3519

Diarrhea, C. difficile-associated

Cipro XR Tablets 2990
Invanz for Injection (Greater than 0.1%) 1999
Proquin XR Tablets 1153

Diarrhea, infectious

▲ Xenical Capsules (5.3%) 2831

Diastolic blood pressure, decreased

Agrylin Capsules 3169
Testim 1% Gel (1% or less) 695

Diastolic blood pressure changes

Focalin XR Capsules 2223

Digestive disorders, unspecified

Lopressor HCT 50/25 Tablets (1%) 2241
Lopressor HCT 100/25 Tablets (1%) 2241
Lopressor HCT 100/50 Tablets (1%) 2241

Digitalis toxicity

Lanoxicaps Capsules 1490
Virazole for Inhalation Solution 3370

Dim vision

Levitra Tablets (Less than 2%) 3034

Diplegia

Imitrex Injection (Rare) 1463
Imitrex Nasal Spray (Rare) 1467
Imitrex Tablets 1471

Diplopia

Abelcet Injection 1141
Abilify Oral Solution (Rare) 882
Abilify Oral Solution (Rare) 2450
Abilify Discmelt Orally Disintegrating Tablets (Rare) 882
Abilify Discmelt Orally Disintegrating Tablets (Rare) 2450
Abilify Tablets (Rare) 882
Abilify Tablets (Rare) 2450
Aciphex Tablets 1090
Adalat CC Tablets (Less than 1%) 2964
Agrylin Capsules (1% to 5%) 3169
Ambien Tablets (Frequent) 2851
Ambien CR Tablets (Frequent) 2855
Arthrotec Tablets (Rare) 3129
Axert Tablets (Rare) 2396
Azopt Ophthalmic Suspension (Less than 1%) 557
Bentyl Capsules 697
Bentyl Injection 697
Bentyl Syrup 697
Bentyl Tablets 697
Betagan Ophthalmic Solution, USP .... ⊙ 220
Betimol Ophthalmic Solution 3382
Betimol Ophthalmic Solution .... ⊙ 295
Blocadren Tablets 1916
BOTOX Purified Neurotoxin Complex (Rare) 570
Buprenex Injectable (Less than 1%) 2716
Caduet Tablets (Greater than 0.1% to less than or equal to 1%) 2508
Campral Tablets (Rare) 1174
Carbatrol Capsules 3171
Carteolol Hydrochloride Ophthalmic Solution USP, 1% .... ⊙ 249
Celexa (Rare) 1176
Cipro (Less than 1%) 2977
Cipro I.V. (1% or less) 2984
Cipro XR Tablets (Less than 1%) 2990
Copaxone for Injection (At least 2%) 3297
Cosopt Sterile Ophthalmic Solution 1931
Cymbalta Delayed-Release Capsules (Infrequent) 1757
Dantrium Capsules (Less frequent) 2694
▲ Depacon Injection (16%) 412
▲ Depakene (16%) 417
▲ Depakote Sprinkle Capsules (16%) 422
▲ Depakote Tablets (1% to 16%) 427
▲ Depakote ER Tablets (16%) 434
Dilaudid 440
Dilaudid Non-Sterile Powder 440
Dilaudid Oral Liquid (Less frequent) 445
Dilaudid Rectal Suppositories 440
Dilaudid Tablets 440
Dilaudid Tablets - 8 mg (Less frequent) 445
Dilaudid-HP (Less frequent) 442
Effexor Tablets (Infrequent) 3411
Effexor XR Capsules (Infrequent) 3417
Eldepryl Capsules 3208
▲ Equetro Extended-Release Capsules (Less than 5%) 3180
Evoxac Capsules (Less than 1%) 1047
Exelon Capsules (Infrequent) 2206
Exelon Oral Solution (Infrequent) 2206
Gabitril Tablets (1% or more) 984
Geodon Capsules (Frequent) 2529
Indocin (Less than 1%) 1995
▲ Intron A for Injection (Less than 5%) 3024
Kadian Capsules (Less than 3%) 577

Keppra Injection (2%)........................ 3320
Keppra Oral Solution (2%)................ 3314
Keppra Tablets (2%)......................... 3314
Ketek Tablets (Greater than or equal to 0.2% to less than 2%)...... 2903
Klonopin (Infrequent)........................ 2778
▲ Lamictal (5% to 49%) 1481
Levaquin (0.1% to 0.9%)................... 2384
Levaquin in 5% Dextrose Injection (0.1% to 0.9%)........................... 2384
Lexapro Oral Solution........................ 1190
Lexapro Tablets................................. 1190
Lidoderm Patch.................................. 1118
▲ Lyrica Capsules (2% to 12%) 2539
Matulane Capsules............................ 3191
Mirapex Tablets (1% or more)........... 859
MS Contin Tablets (Less frequent).... 2701
Nalfon Capsules (Less than 1%)....... 2502
Namenda (Infrequent)....................... 1195
▲ Neurontin Capsules (1.2% to 5.9%).. 2487
▲ Neurontin Oral Solution (1.2 to 5.9%).. 2487
▲ Neurontin Tablets (1.2% to 5.9%) 2487
Niravam Orally Disintegrating Tablets.. 3092
Noroxin Tablets.................................. 2032
Norvasc Tablets (More than 0.1% to 1%).. 2545
Norvir (Less than 2%)....................... 503
Numorphan Injection........................ 1120
Ortho-Cyclen/Ortho Tri-Cyclen (Rare).. 2429
Ortho Tri-Cyclen Lo Tablets............. 2436
Orthoclone OKT3 Sterile Solution..... 2360
Parcopa Orally Disintegrating Tablets.. 3097
Paxil CR Controlled-Release Tablets (Rare)............................. 1538
Paxil (Rare)... 1530
Permax Tablets (2.1%)..................... 3356
Pexeva Tablets (rare)....................... 1694
Phenergan Tablets and Suppositories............................. 3440
Photofrin for Injection....................... 702
Pletal Tablets (Less than 2%)........... 2455
Premphase Tablets........................... 3456
Prempro Tablets............................... 3456
Prevacid Delayed-Release Capsules (Less than 1%).............. 3271
Prevacid for Delayed-Release Oral Suspension (Less than 1%)........... 3271
Prevacid SoluTab Delayed-Release Orally Disintegrating Tablets (Less than 1%)............................... 3271
Prevacid NapraPAC (Less than 1%).. 3280
PREVPAC (Less than 1%)................ 3284
Prilosec OTC Delayed-Release Tablets (Less than 1%).................. 2677
Prinivil Tablets (0.3% to 1.0%).......... 2052
Prinzide Tablets................................ 2056
Proquin XR Tablets........................... 1153
ProSom Tablets (Rare)..................... 517
Protonix I.V. (Less than 1%).............. 3472
Protonix Tablets (Less than 1%)....... 3469
Prozac Pulvules and Liquid (Rare)..... 1801
Relpax Tablets (Rare)....................... 2548
ReoPro Vials (0.1%).......................... 1809
Requip Tablets (2%).......................... 1555
Rescriptor Tablets............................ 2551
Rilutek Tablets (Rare)....................... 2930
Risperdal (Rare)................................ 1676
Risperdal M-Tab Orally Disintegrating Tablets (Rare)......... 1676
▲ Romazicon Injection (1% to 3%) 2804
Sonata Capsules (Infrequent)........... 1717
▲ Soriatane Capsules (1% to 5%) 1013
Stalevo Tablets................................. 2287
Sustiva Capsules (Less than 2%)....... 930
Sustiva Tablets (Less than 2%)......... 930
Symbyax Capsules (Infrequent)......... 1819
Synera Topical Patch........................ 1137
▲ Tambocor Tablets (1% to 3%) 1856
Tasmar Tablets (Infrequent)............. 3358
Tegretol/Tegretol-XR........................ 2295
▲ Temodar Capsules (5%) 3073
Thalomid Capsules........................... 965
Timolide Tablets............................... 2086
Timoptic Sterile Ophthalmic Solution (Less frequent)................ 2088
Timoptic in Ocudose (Less frequent).. 2091
Timoptic-XE Sterile Ophthalmic Gel Forming Solution.......................... 2092
▲ Topamax Sprinkle Capsules (1% to 10%).. 2404
▲ Topamax Tablets (1% to 10%) 2404
Tranxene.. 2474
Trecator Tablets............................... 3487
▲ Trileptal Tablets (5% to 40%) 2300
▲ Trileptal Oral Suspension (5% to 40%).. 2300
Valium Tablets (Infrequent)............... 2819
VFEND I.V. (Less than 2%)................ 2564
VFEND Oral Suspension (Less than 2%).. 2564
VFEND Tablets (Less than 2%)......... 2564
Viagra Tablets.................................. 2573
▲ Visudyne for Injection (1% to 10%) .. 2305
Wellbutrin Tablets (Rare)................. 1603
Wellbutrin SR Sustained-Release Tablets.. 1607
▲ Wellbutrin XL Extended-Release Tablets (2% to 3%)...................... 1613
Xalatan Sterile Ophthalmic Solution (Less than 1%)................ 2649
Zegerid Capsules (Less than 1%)..... 2958
Zegerid Powder for Oral Solution (Less than 1%)............................ 2958
Zelapar Tablets................................. 3372
Zoloft (Rare)..................................... 2586
Zomig Tablets (Rare)........................ 3519
Zomig-ZMT Tablets (Rare)................ 3519
▲ Zonegran Capsules (6%) 1101
Zyban Sustained-Release Tablets..... 1644
Zyprexa Tablets (Infrequent)............ 1830
Zyprexa ZYDIS Orally Disintegrating Tablets (Infrequent).................................. 1830

Dipsesis

Abilify Oral Solution (Infrequent)........ 882
Abilify Oral Solution (Infrequent)....... 2450
Abilify Discmelt Orally Disintegrating Tablets (Infrequent)................................... 882
Abilify Discmelt Orally Disintegrating Tablets (Infrequent)................................... 2450
Abilify Tablets (Infrequent)............... 882
Abilify Tablets (Infrequent)............... 2450
Aciphex Tablets (Rare).................... 1090
Actiq (Less than 1%)........................ 979
Aggrenox Capsules (Less than 1%).. 822
Alferon N Injection (1%).................. 1665
Alinia for Oral Suspension (Less than 1%).. 2835
Alinia Tablets (Less than 1%)........... 2835
Ambien Tablets (Infrequent)............. 2851
Ambien CR Tablets (Infrequent)........ 2855
Amerge Tablets (Infrequent)............ 1339
Anaprox Tablets (Less than 3%)....... 2761
Anaprox DS Tablets (Less than 3%).. 2761
Aricept Tablets (Infrequent)............. 1094
Aricept ODT Tablets (Infrequent)....... 1094
Atrovent Nasal Spray 0.06% (Less than 1%).. 839
▲ Avinza Capsules (Less than 5%) 1741
Axert Tablets (Rare)........................ 2396
Bayer Aspirin.................................. 744
Bayer Aspirin Comprehensive Prescribing Information.............. ▣796
Caduet Tablets (Greater than 0.1% to less than or equal to 1%).......... 2508
Calcium Disodium Versenate Injection....................................... 1851
Campral Tablets (Infrequent)........... 1174
Cardizem LA Extended Release Tablets (Less than 2%)................. 1728
Ceftin Tablets (0.1% to 1%).............. 1407
Celexa (Infrequent).......................... 1176
▲ CellCept Capsules (3% to less than 20%)...................................... 2747
▲ CellCept Intravenous (3% to less than 20%)...................................... 2747
▲ CellCept Oral Suspension (3% to less than 20%)............................ 2747
▲ CellCept Tablets (3% to less than 20%).. 2747
Cesamet Capsules........................... 3340
Chantix Tablets (Frequent)............... 2517
Cipro XR Tablets (Less than 1%)....... 2990
Cymbalta Delayed-Release Capsules (Infrequent).................. 1757
Demadex Injection.......................... 2759
Demadex Tablets............................ 2759
Depo-Provera Contraceptive Injection (Less than 1%).............. 2622
depo-subQ provera 104 Injectable Suspension................................. 2624
Dyazide Capsules........................... 1423
EC-Naprosyn Delayed-Release Tablets (Less than 3%)............... 2761
Effexor Tablets (Infrequent)............. 3411
Effexor XR Capsules (Infrequent)...... 3417
Emcyt Capsules (1%)....................... 2634
Evoxac Capsules (Less than 1%)...... 1047
Exelon Capsules (Infrequent)............ 2206
Exelon Oral Solution (Infrequent)...... 2206
Fortical Nasal Spray (Less than 1%).. 3337
Frova Tablets (Infrequent)................ 1113
Furosemide Tablets......................... 2154
Gabitril Tablets (Infrequent).............. 984
Geodon Capsules (Infrequent).......... 2529
Imitrex Injection (Infrequent)............ 1463
Imitrex Nasal Spray (Infrequent)....... 1467
Imitrex Tablets (Infrequent).............. 1471
▲ Intron A for Injection (Less than or equal to 5%)............................... 3024
Klonopin (Infrequent)....................... 2778
K-Phos Neutral Tablets.................... 760
Lamictal (Infrequent)....................... 1481
Levaquin (0.1% to 0.9%).................. 2384
Levaquin in 5% Dextrose Injection (0.1% to 0.9%)........................... 2384
Lexapro Oral Solution (Infrequent).... 1190
Lexapro Tablets (Infrequent)............ 1190
Lithobid Tablets.............................. 1692
Lunesta Tablets (Infrequent)............ 3142
▲ Lupron Depot 3.75 mg (Among most frequent)............................. 3260
Lupron Depot–3 Month 11.25 mg (Less than 5%)............................ 3265
Maxalt Tablets (Infrequent).............. 2008
Maxalt-MLT Orally Disintegrating Tablets (Infrequent) 2008
Meridia Capsules (1.7%) 489
MetroGel-Vaginal Gel (Less than 1%) 1855
Miacalcin Nasal Spray (Less than 1%) 2253
Midamor Tablets (Less than or equal to 1%) 2026
Mirapex Tablets (Less than 1%) 859
Moduretic Tablets (Less than or equal to 1%) 2028
▲ MoviPrep Oral Solution (47.3%) 2839
Naprosyn Suspension (Less than 3%) 2761
Naprosyn Tablets (Less than 3%) 2761
Neurontin Capsules (Infrequent) 2487
Neurontin Oral Solution (Infrequent) 2487
Neurontin Tablets (Infrequent) 2487
Nexium Delayed-Release Capsules (Less than 1%) 655
Nexium I.V. (Less than 1%) 659
Norvasc Tablets (More than 0.1% to 1%) 2545
Norvir (Less than 2%) 503
Oncaspar (Less than 1%) 1145
OxyContin Tablets (Less than 1%) 2703
Paxil CR Controlled-Release Tablets (Infrequent) 1538
Paxil (Infrequent) 1530
Pentasa Capsules (Less than 1%) 3185
Percodan Tablets 1132
Permax Tablets (Infrequent) 3356
Pexeva Tablets (infrequent) 1694
Prevacid Delayed-Release Capsules (Less than 1%) 3271
Prevacid for Delayed-Release Oral Suspension (Less than 1%) 3271
Prevacid SoluTab Delayed-Release Orally Disintegrating Tablets (Less than 1%) 3271
Prevacid NapraPAC (Less than 3%) .. 3280
▲ PREVPAC (Less than 1% to 3%) 3284
Prinzide Tablets 2056
Prochieve 4% Gel 1003
Prochieve 8% Gel 1003
ProSom Tablets (Infrequent) 517
Protonix I.V. (Less than 1%) 3472
Protonix Tablets (Less than 1%) 3469
Provigil Tablets (1%) 988
Prozac Pulvules and Liquid (Infrequent to greater than or equal to 2%) 1801
Relpax Tablets (Infrequent) 2548
Requip Tablets (Infrequent) 1555
Rescriptor Tablets 2551
Rilutek Tablets (Infrequent) 2930
Risperdal (Infrequent) 1676
Risperdal M-Tab Orally Disintegrating Tablets (Infrequent) 1676
Seroquel Tablets (Infrequent) 690
Singulair 2077
Sonata Capsules (Infrequent) 1717
▲ Soriatane Capsules (1% to 10%) 1013
St. Joseph 81 mg Aspirin Chewable and Enteric Coated Tablets 1869
Symbyax Capsules (Frequent) 1819
Tasmar Tablets (Infrequent) 3358
Tequin Injection (Less than 0.1%) 938
Tequin Injection in 5% Dextrose (Less than 0.1%) 938
Tequin Tablets (Less than 0.1%) 938
Tiazac Capsules (Less than 2%) 1201
Tindamax Tablets 2142
Topamax Sprinkle Capsules (1% to 2%) 2404
Topamax Tablets (1% to 2%) 2404
Trileptal Tablets (Up to 2%) 2300
Trileptal Oral Suspension (Up to 2%).. 2300
Uniretic Tablets (Less than 1%)........ 3100
Uroqid-Acid No. 2 Tablets................ 760
Vantin Tablets and Oral Suspension (Less than 1%)........... 2645
▲ Vaprisol (9.8%) 643
Viagra Tablets (Less than 2%).......... 2573
Vicoprofen Tablets (Less than 3%).... 539
Wellbutrin SR Sustained-Release Tablets (Infrequent).................... 1607
Wellbutrin XL Extended-Release Tablets (Infrequent).................... 1613
▲ Xeloda Tablets (Less than 5%) 2822
Zoloft (Infrequent)........................... 2586
Zomig Tablets (Infrequent)............... 3519
Zomig Nasal Spray (Infrequent)........ 3523
Zomig-ZMT Tablets (Infrequent)........ 3519
Zonegran Capsules (Infrequent)....... 1101
Zosyn (1.0% or less)....................... 3492
Zyban Sustained-Release Tablets (Less than 1%).......................... 1644
▲ Zyprexa Tablets (8%) 1830
▲ Zyprexa ZYDIS Orally Disintegrating Tablets (8%) 1830
Zyrtec Chewable Tablets (Less than 2%) 2594
Zyrtec (Less than 2%) 2594
Zyrtec-D 12 Hour Extended Release Tablets (Less than 2%) 2597

Discharge, nipple

Angeliq Tablets 762
depo-subQ provera 104 Injectable Suspension 2624
Enjuvia Tablets 1062

Discoloration, application site

Lidoderm Patch 1118

Discoloration, injection site

HibTITER 3426
Neumega for Injection 3435
ProQuad 2064
▲ Visudyne for Injection (10% to 30%) 2305

Discomfort, anal

▲ MoviPrep Oral Solution (51.5%) 2839

Discomfort, arm

▲ Adenoscan (4%) 619
Imitrex Injection 1463

Discomfort, chest

▲ Adenoscan (40%) 619
Ambien CR Tablets (1%) 2855
Amerge Tablets (Frequent) 1339
▲ Amitiza Capsules (1.6% to 3.4%) 3224
▲ Cerezyme for Injection (Approximately 6.6%) 1270
Chantix Tablets (Infrequent) 2517
▲ Dacogen Injection (7%) 2129
▲ Imitrex Injection (5%) 1463
Imitrex Nasal Spray (Infrequent) 1467
Imitrex Tablets (Frequent) 1471
▲ Photofrin for Injection (11%) 702
Primaxin I.M. 2045
Primaxin I.V. (Less than 0.2%) 2048
Prinivil Tablets (0.3% to 1.0%) 2052
Prinzide Tablets (0.3% to 1%) 2056
Recombivax HB (Less than 1%) 2071
Tasmar Tablets (1% to 2%) 3358
Timentin ADD-Vantage 1580
Timentin Injection Galaxy Container 1583
Timentin IV Infusion 1577
Timentin Pharmacy Bulk Package 1586
Ventavis Inhalation Solution 1020
▲ Vesanoid Capsules (32%) 2820
VoSpire ER Tablets (Less frequent) .. 1052
Xyrem Oral Solution (Infrequent) 1688
Zomig Nasal Spray (Infrequent) 3523

Discomfort, general

Coumadin for Injection 898
Coumadin Tablets 898
Cubicin for Injection (Less than 1%) 1026
▲ HalfLytely and Bisacodyl Tablets Bowel Prep Kit with Flavors Packs (19.1%) 881
Xyrem Oral Solution (Infrequent) 1688
Zovirax Ointment 821

Discomfort, head

Xyrem Oral Solution (Infrequent) 1688

Discomfort, jaw

▲ Adenoscan (15%) 619
Imitrex Injection (2%) 1463
Zomig Nasal Spray (Rare) 3523

Discomfort, local

Albalon Ophthalmic Solution .... ⊙218

▲ Betimol Ophthalmic Solution (More than 5%) 3382
▲ Betimol Ophthalmic Solution (More than 5%) ⊙ 295
▲ Ciloxan Ophthalmic Ointment (Among most frequent) 559
▲ Ciloxan Ophthalmic Solution (Among most frequent) ⊙ 206
Efudex (Infrequent) 3363
OptiPranolol Metipranolol Ophthalmic Solution 0.3% (A small number of patients) ⊙ 256
ThermaCare Heat Wraps 2677

Discomfort, lower extremities
Adenoscan (Less than 1%) 619

Discomfort, musculoskeletal
▲ Dacogen Injection (6%) 2129
Xyrem Oral Solution (Infrequent) 1688

Discomfort, nasal
Amerge Tablets (Frequent) 1339
Imitrex Injection (2%) 1463
▲ Imitrex Nasal Spray (2.8% to 3.8%) 1467
▲ Imitrex Tablets (5% to 7%) 1471
▲ Zomig Nasal Spray (1% to 3%) 3523

Discomfort, neck
▲ Adenoscan (15%) 619

Discomfort, sinus
Imitrex Injection (2%) 1463
▲ Imitrex Nasal Spray (2.8% to 3.8%) 1467

Discomfort, throat
▲ Adenoscan (15%) 619
▲ Imitrex Injection (3%) 1463
Imitrex Nasal Spray (0.8% to 2.4%) 1467
▲ Relenza Rotadisk (8% to 19%) 1552

Discomfort, upper extremities
▲ Adenoscan (4%) 619

Discomfort, vulvovaginal
▲ Estring Vaginal Ring (5%) 2635

Discomfort at injection site
Aloxi Injection (Very rare) 2127
▲ Fuzeon Injection (96%) 2767
MICRhoGAM Ultra-Filtered 2371
Nutropin AQ Injection 1243
Nutropin AQ Pen 1243
Nutropin AQ Pen Cartridge 1243
RhoGAM Ultra-Filtered 2371

Discontinuation syndrome
Catapres-TTS 844
Clorpres Tablets (About 1%) 2153

Disease flare
Soltamox Oral Solution 3527

Disease progression, unspecified
Revlimid Capsules 958

Disinhibition
Ambien CR Tablets (1%) 2855
Niravam Orally Disintegrating Tablets (2.7%) 3092

Disorder, soft tissue, oral
▲ Dacogen Injection (6%) 2129

Disorientation
Aciphex Tablets 1090
Actimmune (Rare) 1671
Alferon N Injection (1%) 1665
▲ Ambien CR Tablets (3%) 2855
Arthrotec Tablets (Rare) 3129
Asacol Delayed-Release Tablets 2692
Biaxin/Biaxin XL 402
BiDil Tablets 2171
BOTOX Purified Neurotoxin Complex 570
Cesamet Capsules (2%) 3340
Chantix Tablets (Infrequent) 2517
Cosopt Sterile Ophthalmic Solution 1931
Dalmane Capsules 3342
Daranide Tablets 1950
Demser Capsules 1953
Dilaudid 440
Dilaudid Non-Sterile Powder 440
Dilaudid Oral Liquid (Less frequent) 445
Dilaudid Rectal Suppositories 440
Dilaudid Tablets 440
Dilaudid Tablets - 8 mg (Less frequent) 445
Dilaudid-HP (Less frequent) 442
Dolobid Tablets (Less than 1 in 100) 1955
Eldepryl Capsules 3208
Emend Capsules (Isolated cases) 1963
Famvir Tablets (Infrequent) 2211
Gantrisin Pediatric Suspension 2770
Infed Injection 3390
▲ Invanz for Injection (3.3% to 5.1%) 1999
Lexapro Oral Solution (Infrequent) 1190
Lexapro Tablets (Infrequent) 1190
Lidoderm Patch 1118
Lopressor Injection 2238
Lopressor Tablets 2238
Lopressor HCT 50/25 Tablets 2241
Lopressor HCT 100/25 Tablets 2241
Lopressor HCT 100/50 Tablets 2241
Maxalt Tablets (Infrequent) 2008
Maxalt-MLT Orally Disintegrating Tablets (Infrequent) 2008
MS Contin Tablets (Less frequent) 2701
Nalfon Capsules (Less than 1%) 2502
Oncaspar 1145
Opana Tablets (Less than 1%) 1122
Opana ER Tablets (Less than 1%) 1126
Orthoclone OKT3 Sterile Solution 2360
Parcopa Orally Disintegrating Tablets 3097
Parnate Tablets 1527
Phenergan Tablets and Suppositories 3440
PREVPAC 3284
Prezista Tablets (Less than 2%) 3306
Rescriptor Tablets 2551
Seromycin Capsules 1813
Stalevo Tablets 2287
Timoptic Sterile Ophthalmic Solution (Less frequent) 2088
Timoptic in Ocudose (Less frequent) 2091
Timoptic-XE Sterile Ophthalmic Gel Forming Solution 2092
Transderm Scōp Transdermal Therapeutic System (Infrequent) 2177
▲ Ultram ER Tablets (1% to greater than 5%) 2392
▲ Xyrem Oral Solution (2.9% to 8.6%) 1688

Disorientation, place
Blocadren Tablets 1916
Cosopt Sterile Ophthalmic Solution 1931
Inderal LA Long-Acting Capsules 3429
InnoPran XL Capsules 2723
Nadolol Tablets 2159
Timolide Tablets 2086
Timoptic Sterile Ophthalmic Solution 2088
Timoptic in Ocudose 2091
Timoptic-XE Sterile Ophthalmic Gel Forming Solution 2092
Toprol-XL Tablets 668

Disorientation, time
Blocadren Tablets 1916
Cosopt Sterile Ophthalmic Solution 1931
Inderal LA Long-Acting Capsules 3429
InnoPran XL Capsules 2723
Nadolol Tablets 2159
Timolide Tablets 2086
Timoptic Sterile Ophthalmic Solution 2088
Timoptic in Ocudose 2091
Timoptic-XE Sterile Ophthalmic Gel Forming Solution 2092
Toprol-XL Tablets 668

Distention, abdominal
(*see under* Abdominal distention)

Distress, abdominal
▲ Advair HFA Inhalation Aerosol (1% to 3%) 1318
Ambien Tablets (Rare) 2851
Augmentin (Less frequent) 1360
Augmentin Tablets (Less frequent) 1363
Ery-Tab Tablets 449
Erythrocin Stearate Filmtab Tablets 453
Imitrex Injection (Frequent) 1463
Imitrex Tablets 1471
Indocin (Greater than 1%) 1995
Invirase (0.9% to greater than or equal to 2%) 2772
▲ K-Lor Oral Solution (Among most common) 474
▲ K-Tab Tablets (Most common) 475
▲ Persantine Tablets (6.1%) 868
Stalevo Tablets 2287
▲ Ultrase MT Capsules (0.2%) 709
Zantac Injection 1619

Distress, epigastric
Abelcet Injection 1141
Aricept Tablets (Frequent) 1094
Aricept ODT Tablets (Frequent) 1094
Cipro I.V. (1% or less) 2984
Clorpres Tablets 2153
Colazal Capsules 2838
Cubicin for Injection (Less than 1%) 1026
Cuprimine Capsules 1947
▲ Emend Capsules (4%) 1963
▲ Entocort EC Capsules (Less than 5%) 2698
Ferrlecit Injection 3388
Gris-PEG Tablets (Occasional) 2502
Inderal LA Long-Acting Capsules 3429
▲ Indocin (3% to 9%) 1995
InnoPran XL Capsules 2723
▲ MetroGel-Vaginal Gel (7%) 1855
Mintezol 2027
Nexium Delayed-Release Capsules (Less than 1%) 655
Nexium I.V. (Less than 1%) 659
Oncaspar (Less than 1%) 1145
Proquin XR Tablets 1153
Sandostatin Injection (Rare) 2278
Sandostatin LAR Depot (Rare) 2280
▲ Ticlid Tablets (3.7%) 2810
Timentin ADD-Vantage 1580
Timentin Injection Galaxy Container 1583
Timentin IV Infusion 1577
Timentin Pharmacy Bulk Package 1586
Tindamax Tablets (1.4% to 1.8%) 2142
Toprol-XL Tablets (About 1 of 100 patients) 668
Viracept (Less than 2%) 2577

Distress, gastric
(*see under* Distress, gastrointestinal)

Distress, gastrointestinal
▲ Adenoscan (13%) 619
▲ Agrylin Capsules (1% to 5%) 3169
Alferon N Injection (One patient) 1665
Alupent Inhalation Aerosol (1 to 4%) 826
Amitiza Capsules (0% to 1.1%) 3224
Appearex Tablets 2125
Biltricide Tablets 2976
Bios Life Drink Mix 3328
Bumex Tablets (0.1%) 2746
Carafate Suspension (Less than 0.5%) 701
Carafate Tablets (Less than 0.5%) 701
Carbatrol Capsules 3171
Cardio Essentials Capsules 3328
▲ Chantix Tablets (5% to 7%) 2517
▲ Clinoril Tablets (10%) 1924
CM Plex Softgels 3329
Combivent Inhalation Aerosol 847
Covera-HS Tablets (Less than 2%) 3139
Cuprimine Capsules 1947
Depo-Provera Contraceptive Injection (Less than 1%) 2622
depo-subQ provera 104 Injectable Suspension 2624
▲ Dolobid Tablets (3% to 9%) 1955
▲ Emcyt Capsules (11%) 2634
Emend Capsules (Less than or equal to 0.5%) 1963
Equetro Extended-Release Capsules 3180
Evoclin Foam, 1% 1009
▲ Flovent HFA (1% to 3%) 1447
Fluorescite Injection ⊙ 207
Imitrex Tablets (Frequent) 1471
Kadian Capsules (Less than 3%) 577
K-Dur Extended-Relase Tablets 3033
▲ Lotronex Tablets (5%) 1512
▲ Lupron Depot–3 Month 11.25 mg (3% to 7%) 3265
Lupron Injection Pediatric 3259
▲ Midamor Tablets (Between 1% and 3%) 2026
Moduretic Tablets (Greater than 1%, less than 3%) 2028
Paddock Nystatin USP for Oral Suspension 2478
ProAmatine Tablets (Rare) 3186
▲ Sandostatin LAR Depot (29.1%) 2280
Tegretol/Tegretol-XR 2295
Timolide Tablets (Less than 1%) 2086
Timoptic Sterile Ophthalmic Solution 2088
Timoptic in Ocudose 2091
Verelan PM Extended-Release Capsules, Controlled-Onset (2% or less) 3106
Visutein Capsules 3329
▲ Vivitrol (11% to 16%) 995
Xifaxan Tablets (Less than 2%) 2842
Zovirax 1643

Distress, precordial
(*see under* Distress, epigastric)

Distress, stomach
(*see under* Distress, gastrointestinal)

Distress, upper GI
(*see under* Distress, epigastric)

Disturbances, emotional
(*see under* Emotional disturbances)

Disturbances, gastrointestinal
(*see under* Distress, gastrointestinal)

Disulfiram-like reactions
Avandaryl Tablets 1379

Diuresis
Amerge Tablets (Infrequent) 1339
Gantrisin Pediatric Suspension 2770
Lotronex Tablets (Rare) 1512

Diuresis, potentiation of
Uniphyl Tablets 2710

Diverticulitis
Aricept Tablets (Infrequent) 1094
Aricept ODT Tablets (Infrequent) 1094
Celebrex Capsules (0.1% to 1.9%) 3134
Celexa (Rare) 1176
Colazal Capsules 2838
Cymbalta Delayed-Release Capsules (Infrequent) 1757
Evoxac Capsules (Less than 1%) 1047
Exelon Capsules (Infrequent) 2206
Exelon Oral Solution (Infrequent) 2206
Gleevec Tablets (Rare) 2227
▲ Humira Injection (Less than 5%) 466
Lotronex Tablets (Rare) 1512
Namenda (Infrequent) 1195
Orencia Powder for Intravenous Infusion (0.2% to 0.5%) 914
Razadyne (Infrequent) 2399
Razadyne ER Extended-Release Capsules (Infrequent) 2399
Requip Tablets (Infrequent) 1555
Rescriptor Tablets 2551
Revlimid Capsules 958
Risperdal (Rare) 1676
Risperdal M-Tab Orally Disintegrating Tablets (Rare) 1676
▲ Sandostatin LAR Depot (1% to 4%) 2280
Zoloft (Rare) 2586

Dizziness
Accolate Tablets (1.6%) 671
Accutane Capsules 2731
Aciphex Tablets 1090
▲ Actiq (6% to 17%) 979
▲ Actonel Tablets (4.9% to 6.6%) 2683
▲ Actonel with Calcium Tablets (4.9% to 6.4%) 2688
▲ ActoPlus Met Tablets (4.8% to 5.4%) 3214
▲ Adalat CC Tablets (4%) 2964
Adderall Tablets 3164
▲ Adderall XR Capsules (2% to 7%) 3166
Adenocard Injection (1%) 617
▲ Adenoscan (12%) 619
Adipex-P 1215
▲ Advair Diskus 250/50 (4%) 1308
▲ Advair HFA Inhalation Aerosol (1% to 4%) 1318
Advate Injection (2%) 712
Advicor Tablets 1722
Advil Allergy Sinus Caplets ▣ 770
Advil Multi-Symptom Cold Caplets ▣ 770
▲ Aerobid/Aerobid-M (3% to 9%) 1171
▲ Aggrastat (3%) 1907
Aggrenox Capsules (Less than 1%) 822
▲ Agrylin Capsules (15.4%) 3169
Alavert Allergy & Sinus D-12 Hour Tablets ▣ 771
Albalon Ophthalmic Solution ⊙ 218
Albenza Tablets (Less than 1.0% to 1.2%) 1338
Aldara Cream, 5% (1.4%) 1846
Aldoril Tablets 1910
▲ Alferon N Injection (9%) 1665
Alinia for Oral Suspension (Less than 1%) 2835
Alinia Tablets (Less than 1%) 2835
Allegra (2.2%) 2844
Allegra-D 12 Hour Extended-Release Tablets (1.9%) 2846
Allegra-D 24 Hour Extended-Release Tablets (1.9%) 2849
Aloxi Injection (1%) 2127

▲ Alphagan P Ophthalmic Solution (1% to 4%) 567
▲ Altace Capsules (2.2% to 4.1%) 1702
Altoprev Extended-Release Tablets (2%) 3109
▲ Alupent Inhalation Aerosol (3.3%) 826
▲ Ambien Tablets (1% to 5%) 2851
▲ Ambien CR Tablets (8% to 12%) 2855
AmBisome for Injection (Less common) 620
Amerge Tablets (1% to 2%) 1339
Amevive (Common) 626
▲ Amitiza Capsules (3.4% to 4.1%) 3224
Amoxil Capsules (Rare) 1343
Amoxil Chewable Tablets (Rare) 1343
Amoxil Pediatric Drops for Oral Suspension (Rare) 1343
Amoxil Powder for Oral Suspension (Rare) 1343
Amoxil Tablets (Rare) 1343
▲ Anaprox Tablets (3% to 9%) 2761
▲ Anaprox DS Tablets (3% to 9%) 2761
AndroGel (Fewer than 1%) 3329
Angeliq Tablets 762
▲ Anzemet Injection (2.2% to 5.5%) 2859
▲ Anzemet Tablets (1.3% to 4.4%) 2862
Aptivus Capsules (Less than 2%) 826
Aralast (Greater than or equal to 0.02% to 0.1%) 717
▲ Aranesp for Injection (8% to 14%) 581
Aredia for Injection 2179
▲ Aricept Tablets (8%) 1094
▲ Aricept ODT Tablets (8%) 1094
▲ Arimidex Tablets (5% to 8%) 673
▲ Arixtra Injection (0.6% to 3.6%) 1351
▲ Aromasin Tablets (8% to 9.7%) 2600
▲ Arranon Injection (0% to 21%) 1357
Arthrotec Tablets (Rare) 3129
▲ Asacol Delayed-Release Tablets (8%) 2692
Astelin Nasal Spray (2.0%) 1904
▲ Atacand Tablets (4%) 649
Atacand HCT (2.9%) 651
▲ Atripla Tablets (8%) 945
Atrovent Inhalation Solution (2.3%) 835
▲ Atrovent HFA Inhalation Aerosol (3%) 841
Atrovent Nasal Spray 0.03% (Less than 2%) 837
Atrovent Nasal Spray 0.06% (Less than 1%) 839
Attenuvax 1914
Augmentin (Rare) 1360
Augmentin Tablets (Rare) 1363
Augmentin XR Extended-Release Tablets (Rare) 1369
Augmentin ES-600 Powder for Oral Suspension 1366
▲ Avalide Tablets (8%) 888
▲ Avalide Tablets (8%) 2874
▲ Avandamet Tablets (8%) 1373
Avandaryl Tablets (1.7%) 1379
▲ Avandia Tablets (5.1%) 1384
▲ Avapro Tablets (5.4% to 6%) 891
▲ Avapro Tablets (5.4% to 10.2%) 2871
▲ Avastin IV (19% to 26%) 1227
▲ Avelox (2%) 2970
Axert Tablets (Frequent) 2396
▲ Axid Oral Solution (4.6%) 879
Azilect Tablets (Greater than 1%) 3293
Azopt Ophthalmic Suspension (Less than 1%) 557
Bactroban Cream (Less than 1%) 1394
Baraclude (Less than 1%) 894
Bayer Aspirin 744
Bayer Aspirin Comprehensive Prescribing Information ■796
▲ BeneFix Vials (7.7%) 3408
▲ Benicar Tablets (3%) 1043
▲ Benicar HCT Tablets (9%) 1044
▲ Bentyl Capsules (29%) 697
▲ Bentyl Injection (29%) 697
▲ Bentyl Syrup (29%) 697
▲ Bentyl Tablets (29%) 697
Betagan Ophthalmic Solution, USP (Rare) ⊙220
▲ Betaseron for SC Injection (24%) 767
▲ Betimol Ophthalmic Solution (1% to 5%) 3382
▲ Betimol Ophthalmic Solution (1% to 5%) ⊙295
Betoptic S Ophthalmic Suspension (Rare) 558
▲ Bexxar (0% to 5%) 1398
Biaxin/Biaxin XL 402
Bicillin C-R Injectable Suspension 1706
▲ BiDil Tablets (32%) 2171
Biltricide Tablets 2976
BioLean II Tablets ■808
Blocadren Tablets (2.3%) 1916
▲ Boniva Injection (1% to 3.7%) 2738
▲ Boniva Tablets (1% to 3.7%) 2741
▲ BOTOX Purified Neurotoxin Complex (2% to 10%) 570
▲ Brimonidine Tartrate Ophthalmic Solution 0.2% (3% to 9%) ⊙248
▲ Bumex Tablets (1.1% to 4.1%) 2746
▲ Buprenex Injectable (5% to 10%) 2716
▲ Byetta Injection (9%) 611
▲ Caduet Tablets (1.1% to 3.4%) 2508
▲ Campath Ampules (1% to 12%) 811
▲ Campral Tablets (3% to 4%) 1174
▲ Camptosar Injection (0% to 15%) 2604
▲ Canasa Rectal Suppositories (3%) 699
Cancidas for Injection (0% to 1.5%) 1918
Captopril Tablets (About 0.5% to 2%) 2149
Carafate Suspension (Less than 0.5%) 701
Carafate Tablets (Less than 0.5%) 701
▲ Carbatrol Capsules (Among most frequent) 3171
Cardene I.V. (1.4%) 2497
▲ Cardizem LA Extended Release Tablets (3.5% to 6.4%) 1728
▲ Cardura XL Tablets (5.3%) 2515
Carimune NF 3499
▲ Carnitor Injection (5% to 6%) 3188
Carteolol Hydrochloride Ophthalmic Solution USP, 1% (Occasional) ⊙249
▲ Catapres Tablets (About 16 in 100 patients) 843
Catapres-TTS (2 of 101 patients) 844
Caverject Impulse Injection (1%) 2612
Ceftin Tablets (0.1% to 1%) 1407
Celebrex Capsules (2%) 3134
▲ Celexa (At least 2%) 1176
▲ CellCept Capsules (28.7%) 2747
▲ CellCept Intravenous (28.7%) 2747
▲ CellCept Oral Suspension (28.7%) 2747
▲ CellCept Tablets (28.7%) 2747
▲ Cerezyme for Injection (Approximately 6.5%) 1270
▲ Cesamet Capsules (59%) 3340
Chantix Tablets (Frequent) 2517
▲ Chemet Capsules (1.0% to 12.7%) 2458
Cialis Tablets (Less than 2%) 1838
Cipro (0.3% to 1%) 2977
Cipro I.V. (1% or less) 2984
Cipro XR Tablets (1% to 2%) 2990
▲ Clarinex Tablets (4%) 2995
▲ Clarinex Reditabs Tablets (4%) 2995
Clarinex-D 24-Hour Extended-Release Tablets (2%) 2998
Climara Transdermal System 771
Climara Pro Transdermal System 776
▲ Clinoril Tablets (3% to 9%) 1924
▲ Clolar for Intravenous Infusion (16%) 1271
▲ Clorpres Tablets (About 16%) 2153
▲ Clozaril Tablets (More than 5% to 27%) 2184
Colazal Capsules (1%) 2838
Combivent Inhalation Aerosol (Less than 2%) 847
▲ Combivir Tablets (10%) 1411
▲ Comtan Tablets (8%) 2189
Concerta Extended-Release Tablets (2%) 1881
Copaxone for Injection (At least 2%) 3297
▲ Copegus Tablets (14%) 2754
▲ Coreg Tablets (6% to 32%) 1414
▲ Cosopt Sterile Ophthalmic Solution (1% to 5%) 1931
Coumadin for Injection (Infrequent) 898
Coumadin Tablets (Infrequent) 898
▲ Covera-HS Tablets (3.3% to 4.7%) 3139
▲ Cozaar Tablets (3%) 1935
Crestor Tablets (Greater than or equal to 2%) 678
▲ Crixivan Capsules (3%) 1940
▲ Cubicin for Injection (2.2% to 5.8%) 1026
▲ Cymbalta Delayed-Release Capsules (6% to 17%) 1757
▲ Dacogen Injection (18%) 2129
Dalmane Capsules 3342
▲ Dantrium Capsules (Among most frequent) 2694
Daranide Tablets 1950
Daytrana Transdermal Patch 3174
▲ Demadex Injection (3.2%) 2759
▲ Demadex Tablets (3.2%) 2759
▲ Depacon Injection (5.2% to 25%) 412
▲ Depakene (18% to 25%) 417
▲ Depakote Sprinkle Capsules (13% to 25%) 422
▲ Depakote Tablets (12% to 25%) 427
▲ Depakote ER Tablets (Greater than 1% to 25%) 434
▲ DepoDur Extended-Release Injection (Greater than 10%) 1110
▲ Depo-Provera Contraceptive Injection (Greater than 5%) 2622
▲ depo-subQ provera 104 Injectable Suspension (1% to less than 5%) 2624
Desoxyn Tablets, USP (Rare) 2462
▲ Detrol Tablets (5%) 2628
Detrol LA Capsules (2%) 2631
Dexedrine 1420
DextroStat Tablets 3179
▲ Diastat Rectal Delivery System (3%) 3343
Dilaudid 440
Dilaudid Non-Sterile Powder 440
Dilaudid Oral Liquid 445
Dilaudid Rectal Suppositories 440
Dilaudid Tablets 440
Dilaudid Tablets - 8 mg 445
▲ Dilaudid-HP (Among most frequent) 442
▲ Diovan Tablets (1% to 17%) 2193
▲ Diovan HCT Tablets (9%) 2196
▲ Ditropan XL Extended-Release Tablets (4% to 6%) 2413
Diuril Oral Suspension 1954
Diuril Sodium Intravenous 2467
Dolobid Tablets (Greater than 1 in 100) 1955
Donnatal Extentabs 2493
▲ Doxil Injection (1% to 10%) 2351
Duetact Tablets (1.7%) 3226
▲ Duragesic Transdermal System (3% to 10%) 2373
Dyazide Capsules 1423
▲ DynaCirc CR Tablets (3.7% to 6.4%) 2721
Dyrenium Capsules (Rare) 3400
▲ EC-Naprosyn Delayed-Release Tablets (3% to 9%) 2761
Edex Injection (Less than 1%) 3089
▲ Effexor Tablets (3% to 23.9%) 3411
▲ Effexor XR Capsules (2% to 20%) 3417
▲ Eldepryl Capsules (7 of 49 patients) 3208
▲ Eligard 7.5 mg (3.3%) 2880
▲ Eligard 30 mg (4.4%) 2885
Elmiron Capsules (1%) 2415
▲ Eloxatin for Injection (7% to 13%) 2892
▲ Emend Capsules (3.4% to 6.6%) 1963
Emsam Transdermal System 903
▲ Emtriva Capsules (4% to 25%) 1287
▲ Emtriva Oral Solution (4% to 25%) 1287
Enablex Extended-Release Tablets (0.9% to 2.1%) 2203
▲ Enbrel for Injection (7% to 8%) 584
▲ Engerix-B Vaccine (1% to 10%) 1425
▲ Enjuvia Tablets (1% to 7%) 1062
▲ Entocort EC Capsules (7%) 2698
EpiPen 1061
▲ Epivir (10%) 1427
▲ Epogen for Injection (5% to 21%) 591
▲ Epzicom Tablets (6%) 1436
▲ Equetro Extended-Release Capsules (16% to 44%) 3180
Ery-Tab Tablets (Isolated reports) 449
Erythrocin Stearate Filmtab Tablets (Isolated reports) 453
Erythromycin Base Filmtab Tablets (Isolated reports) 455
Erythromycin Delayed-Release Capsules, USP (Isolated reports) 457
Estrasorb Topical Emulsion 1147
Estratest Tablets 3199
Estratest H.S. Tablets 3199
Estring Vaginal Ring 2635
Ethyol for Injection 1898
▲ Evoxac Capsules (4.1%) 1047
▲ Exelon Capsules (6% to 21%) 2206
▲ Exelon Oral Solution (6% to 21%) 2206
▲ Fabrazyme for Intravenous Infusion (4%) 1274
▲ Famvir Tablets (3.3% to 5.5%) 2211
▲ Faslodex Injection (6.9%) 681
▲ FazaClo Orally Disintegrating Tablets (More than 5% to 27%) 551
▲ Femara Tablets (0.4% to 14.2%) 2214
▲ Ferrlecit Injection (13%) 3388
▲ Flomax Capsules (14.9% to 17.1%) 850
▲ Flonase Nasal Spray (1% to 3%) 1440
▲ Flovent Diskus (1% to 3%) 1443
▲ Flovent HFA (1% to 3%) 1447
Floxin Otic Solution (0.6% to 1%) 1049
Fluarix 1451
Flumadine (0.7% to 1.9%) 1183
Focalin Tablets 2220
▲ Focalin XR Capsules (6%) 2223
Follistim AQ Cartridge 2338
Foradil Aerolizer (1.6%) 3010
Fortaz (Less than 1%) 1453
▲ Forteo for Injection (8%) 1767
▲ Fortical Nasal Spray (1% to 3%) 3337
Fosamax 1969
Fosamax Plus D Tablets 1977
▲ Frova Tablets (8%) 1113
Furosemide Tablets 2154
▲ Gabitril Tablets (27% to 31%) 984
▲ Gammagard Liquid (0.85% to 9.8%) 721
Gamunex Immune Globulin I.V., 10% (2%) 3235
Gantrisin Pediatric Suspension 2770
Garamycin Injectable 3014
▲ Gardasil Injection (4%) 1984
▲ Gengraf Capsules (1% to 8%) 459
▲ Geodon (8% to 16%) 2529
▲ Gleevec Tablets (0% to 16%) 2227
Gris-PEG Tablets (Occasional) 2502
Havrix Vaccine (Rare) 1456
▲ Hectorol Capsules (11.5%) 1275
▲ Hectorol Injection (11.5%) 1278
▲ Herceptin I.V. (13%) 1233
Hycodan 1116
Hycotuss Expectorant Syrup 1117
Hyperstat I.V. (2%) 3017
▲ Hytrin Capsules (2.0% to 28%) 471
▲ Hyzaar 50-12.5 Tablets (5.7%) 1990
▲ Hyzaar 100-12.5 Tablets (5.7%) 1990
▲ Hyzaar 100-25 Tablets (5.7%) 1990
▲ Imdur Tablets (8% to 11%) 3018
▲ Imitrex Injection (12%) 1463
Imitrex Nasal Spray (1% to 1.7%) 1467
Imitrex Tablets (Greater than 1%) 1471
Imodium A-D Liquid and Caplets 1865
Imodium Advanced Caplets and Chewable Tablets ■655
▲ Increlex Injection (Greater than or equal to 5%) 3291
▲ Indapamide Tablets (Greater than or equal to 5%) 2156
▲ Indocin (3% to 9%) 1995
Infed Injection 3390
▲ Infergen (18% to 22%) 3364
▲ InnoPran XL Capsules (4% to 7%) 2723
▲ Inspra Tablets (3%) 2536
▲ Intron A for Injection (7% to 24%) 3024
Invanz for Injection (1.5% to 2.1%) 1999
Invirase (0.3% to greater than or equal to 2%) 2772
Ionsys Transdermal System (3%) 2379
▲ I.V. Busulfex (30%) 2493
▲ Kadian Capsules (Among most frequent) 577
Kaletra (Less than 2%) 476
Keflex Capsules 549
▲ Keppra Injection (9%) 3320
▲ Keppra Oral Solution (7% to 9%) 3314
▲ Keppra Tablets (7% to 9%) 3314
▲ Ketek Tablets (2.8% to 3.7%) 2903
▲ Klonopin (1% to 8%) 2778
Kogenate FS 738
Kogenate FS with Bio-Set (2 cases) 740
K-Phos Original (Sodium Free) Tablets (Less frequent) 760
K-Phos Neutral Tablets 760
▲ Kytril Injection (4.1%) 2781
▲ Kytril (3% to 5%) 2784
▲ Lamictal (5% to 54%) 1481
Lanoxicaps Capsules 1490
Lanoxin Injection 1494
Lanoxin Injection Pediatric 1497
Lanoxin Tablets 1500
▲ Lariam Tablets (Among most frequent) 2786
Lescol Capsules (2.2%) 2233
Lescol XL Tablets (1.9%) 2233
▲ Leustatin Injection (9%) 2357
Levaquin (0.3% to 2.4%) 2384
Levaquin in 5% Dextrose Injection (0.3% to 2.4%) 2384
Levitra Tablets (2%) 3034
▲ Lexapro Oral Solution (4% to 7%) 1190
▲ Lexapro Tablets (4% to 7%) 1190
Lidoderm Patch 1118
Lipitor Tablets (Greater than or equal to 2%) 2483
Lithobid Tablets 1692
Lofibra Tablets 1219
Lofibra Capsules 1216
▲ Lopressor Injection (10%) 2238
▲ Lopressor Tablets (10%) 2238
▲ Lopressor HCT 50/25 Tablets (10%) 2241
▲ Lopressor HCT 100/25 Tablets (10%) 2241
▲ Lopressor HCT 100/50 Tablets (10%) 2241
▲ Lotensin Tablets (3.6%) 2243
▲ Lotensin HCT Tablets (6.3%) 2246
Lotrel Capsules (1.3%) 2249
▲ Lucentis Injection (2% to 8%) 1237
▲ Lunesta Tablets (1% to 7%) 3142
▲ Lupron Depot 3.75 mg (8%) 3260
▲ Lupron Depot–3 Month 11.25 mg (8%) 3265
▲ Lyrica Capsules (8% to 38%) 2539
▲ Macugen Injection (6% to 10%) ⊙261
▲ Malarone Pediatric Tablets (2% to 5%) 1517
▲ Malarone Tablets (2% to 5%) 1517
▲ Marinol Capsules (3% to 10%) 3333
Matulane Capsules 3191

▲ Mavik Tablets (1.3% to 23%) 486
Maxair Autohaler (0.6% to 1.2%)...... 1852
▲ Maxalt Tablets (4% to 9%) 2008
▲ Maxalt-MLT Orally Disintegrating Tablets (4% to 9%)..................... 2008
▲ Menostar Transdermal System (5%).. 782
Mephyton Tablets (Rare).................. 2018
▲ Mepron Suspension (3% to 8%) 1521
▲ Meridia Capsules (7%) 489
Merrem I.V. (Greater than 0.1% to 1%)... 686
Meruvax II.. 2019
Metadate CD Capsules.................... 3323
MetroGel-Vaginal Gel (2%)................ 1855
Mevacor Tablets (0.5% to 2.0%)....... 2021
▲ Miacalcin Nasal Spray (1% to 3%) ... 2253
Micardis Tablets (1%)........................ 854
▲ Micardis HCT Tablets (4% to 7%) 856
▲ Midamor Tablets (Between 1% and 3%).. 2026
▲ Migranal Nasal Spray (4%) 3348
Mintezol 2027
▲ Mirapex Tablets (25% to 26%) 859
Mircette Tablets.............................. 1066
Mivacron Injection (Less than 1%).... 493
M-M-R II... 2006
▲ Mobic Oral Suspension (0.4% to 3.8%)... 863
▲ Mobic Tablets (0.4% to 3.8%) 863
▲ Moduretic Tablets (3% to 8%) 2028
▲ MoviPrep Oral Solution (6.5%) 2839
▲ MS Contin Tablets (Among most frequent).. 2701
Mycamine for Injection (0% to 0.7%).. 628
▲ Myfortic Tablets (3% to less than 20%).. 2255
▲ Mylotarg for Injection (10% to 15%).. 3431
▲ Myobloc Injection (3% to 6%) 3192
Nadolol Tablets (2 of 100 patients).. 2159
▲ Nalfon Capsules (6.5%) 2502
▲ Namenda (7%) 1195
▲ Naprosyn Suspension (3% to 9%) 2761
▲ Naprosyn Tablets (3% to 9%) 2761
▲ Natrecor for Injection (3% to 6%) 3127
Nembutal Sodium Solution, USP (Less than 1%)............................ 2470
▲ Neoral Oral Solution (1% to 8%) 2259
▲ Neoral Soft Gelatin Capsules (1% to 8%).. 2259
▲ Neulasta Injection (15% to 72%) 601
▲ Neumega for Injection (38%) 3435
▲ Neurontin Capsules (2.5% to 28%).. 2487
▲ Neurontin Oral Solution (2.5% to 28%).. 2487
▲ Neurontin Tablets (2.5% to 28%) 2487
Nexium Delayed-Release Capsules (Less than 1%)............................. 655
Nexium I.V. (Less than 1%)................ 659
Niaspan Extended-Release Tablets... 1730
Nicomide Tablets............................ 1088
Nimotop Capsules (Less than 1%)..... 749
▲ Nipent for Injection (3% to 10%) 1863
▲ Niravam Orally Disintegrating Tablets (1.8% to 29.8%)............... 3092
Nitrolingual Pumpspray (Occasional)................................ 3120
Norflex Injection............................ 1856
Noroxin Tablets (1.7% to 2.6%)........ 2032
▲ Norvasc Tablets (0.1% to 3.4%) 2545
▲ Norvir (2.6% to 3.9%) 503
NuvaRing... 2340
Omacor Capsules............................ 2725
Omnicef Capsules (0.3%)................. 511
Omnicef for Oral Suspension (0.2%).. 511
Oncaspar (Less than 1%)................ 1145
▲ Ontak Vials (22%) 1745
▲ Opana Tablets (6.5%) 1122
▲ Opana ER Tablets (0% to 17.8%) 1126
OptiPranolol Metipranolol Ophthalmic Solution 0.3% (A small number of patients) .... ⊙256
▲ Orencia Powder for Intravenous Infusion (9%)................................ 914
Ortho-Cyclen Tablets...................... 2429
Ortho Evra Transdermal System...... 2417
Ortho Micronor Tablets................... 2426
Ortho Tri-Cyclen Tablets.................. 2429
Ortho Tri-Cyclen Lo Tablets............. 2436
Orthoclone OKT3 Sterile Solution..... 2360
OsmoPrep Tablets (Less frequent)... 2840
Oxsoralen-Ultra Capsules................ 3353
▲ OxyContin Tablets (13%) 2703
▲ OxyFast Oral Concentrate Solution (Among most frequent).... 2708
▲ OxyIR Capsules (Among most frequent).. 2708
Parcopa Orally Disintegrating Tablets.. 3097
Parnate Tablets.............................. 1527
▲ Paxil CR Controlled-Release Tablets (1% to 14%)...................... 1538
▲ Paxil (1% to 14%) 1530
▲ Pegasys (16%) 2789
▲ PEG-Intron Powder for Injection (12%).. 3048
Pentasa Capsules (Less than 1%).... 3185
Pepcid Injection (1.3%).................. 2040
Pepcid (1.3%)................................. 2038
▲ Percocet Tablets (Among most frequent).. 1131
▲ Percodan Tablets (Among most frequent).. 1132
▲ Permax Tablets (19.1%) 3356
▲ Persantine Tablets (13.6%) 868
▲ Pexeva Tablets (1.5% to 14%) 1694
Phenergan Tablets and Suppositories................................ 3440
Phenytek Capsules......................... 2160
▲ Plan B Tablets (11.2%) 1076
▲ Plavix Tablets (6.2%) 917
▲ Plavix Tablets (6.2%) 2926
▲ Pletal Tablets (9% to 10%) 2455
Premarin Intravenous 3442
▲ Premarin Tablets (4% to 6%) 3446
Premarin Vaginal Cream 3452
▲ Premphase Tablets (3% to 5%) 3456
▲ Prempro Tablets (3% to 5%) 3456
Prevacid Delayed-Release Capsules (Less than 1%) 3271
Prevacid for Delayed-Release Oral Suspension (Less than 1%) 3271
Prevacid SoluTab Delayed-Release Orally Disintegrating Tablets (Less than 1%) 3271
Prevacid I.V. for Injection (Less than 1%) 3277
▲ Prevacid NapraPAC (Less than 1% to 9%) 3280
▲ PREVPAC (Less than 1% to 3%) 3284
Prilosec OTC Delayed-Release Tablets (1.5%) 2677
Primaxin I.M. 2045
Primaxin I.V. (0.3%) 2048
▲ Prinivil Tablets (5.4% to 11.8%) 2052
▲ Prinzide Tablets (7.5%) 2056
▲ ProAir HFA Inhalation Aerosol (3%) .. 3300
ProAmatine Tablets (Rare) 3186
▲ Prochieve 4% Gel (5%) 1003
▲ Prochieve 8% Gel (5%) 1003
▲ Procrit for Injection (5% to 21%) 2364
▲ Prograf Capsules and Injection (3% to 19%) 632
Prolastin (0.19%) 3255
▲ Proleukin for Injection (11%) 2266
▲ Prometrium Capsules (100 mg, 200 mg) (15% to 24%) 3203
ProQuad 2064
Proquin XR Tablets (Less than 1%) ... 1153
Prosed/DS Tablets 1157
▲ ProSom Tablets (7%) 517
Protonix I.V. (Greater than 1%) 3472
Protonix Tablets (Greater than or equal to 1%) 3469
Protopic Ointment (Greater than or equal to 1%) 638
▲ Proventil Inhalation Aerosol (Less than 5%) 3053
▲ Proventil Inhalation Solution 0.083% (7%) 3055
Proventil HFA Inhalation Aerosol (Less than 3%) 3056
▲ Provigil Tablets (5%) 988
▲ Prozac Pulvules and Liquid (9%) 1801
▲ Quadramet Injection (4%) 1040
▲ Ranexa Tablets (4% to 6.2%) 1035
Raniclor Tablets, Chewable (Rare) 2505
▲ Rapamune Oral Solution and Tablets (3% to 20%) 3475
▲ Razadyne (9%) 2399
▲ Razadyne ER Extended-Release Capsules (9%) 2399
▲ Rebetol (7% to 26%) 3058
▲ Rebetron Combination Therapy (6% to 17%) 3063
ReFacto Vials 3484
Relenza Rotadisk (1% to 2%) 1552
▲ Relpax Tablets (3% to 7%) 2548
Remicade for IV Injection (Greater than or equal to 0.2%) 971
ReoPro Vials (2.9%) 1809
▲ Requip Tablets (11% to 40%) 1555
Rescriptor Tablets 2551
▲ Restoril Capsules (4.5%) 1860
▲ Retisert Implant (5% to 15%) ....⊙258
▲ Retrovir Capsules (6% to 17.9%) 1560
▲ Retrovir IV Infusion (6% to 17.9%) ...1564
▲ Retrovir (6% to 17.9%) 1560
▲ Revlimid Capsules (2.7% to 20.8%)... 958
▲ Reyataz Capsules (1% to 8%) 921
▲ Ribavirin, USP Capsules (17% to 26%) 3068
▲ Rilutek Tablets (5.1% to 12.7%) 2930
▲ Risperdal (4% to 11%) 1676
▲ Risperdal Consta Long-Acting Injection (8% to 11%).................... 1682
▲ Risperdal M-Tab Orally Disintegrating Tablets (4% to 11%).. 1676
Ritalin Hydrochloride Tablets........... 2269
Ritalin LA Capsules......................... 2271
Ritalin-SR Tablets........................... 2269
▲ Rituxan I.V. (1% to 10%) 1254
Robitussin Cough & Cold Long-Acting Liquid........................ ▣735
Robitussin Head & Chest Congestion PE Syrup................... ▣739
Robitussin Pediatric Cough & Cold Long-Acting Liquid............... ▣735
Rocephin Injectable Vials, ADD-Vantage, Galaxy, Bulk (Occasional)................................. 2800
Women's Rogaine Hair Regrowth Treatment Topical Solution, Spring Bloom Scent and Original Unscented....................... ▣634
▲ Romazicon Injection (1% to 9%) 2804
▲ Rozerem Tablets (5%) 3231
▲ Rythmol SR Capsules (21% to 23%).. 2727
▲ Sandostatin Injection (5%) 2278
Seasonique Tablets........................ 1077
▲ Sensipar Tablets (10%) 608
▲ Serevent Diskus (4%) 1568
▲ Seroquel Tablets (11%) 690
▲ Simulect for Injection (Greater than or equal to 10%)................. 2284
Singulair (1.9%).............................. 2077
▲ Skelaxin Tablets (Most frequent) 1716
▲ Solodyn Extended Release Tablets (9%)................................. 1890
Soltamox Oral Solution (Infrequently).............................. 3527
▲ Somavert Injection (4% to 8%) 2642
▲ Sonata Capsules (7% to 9%) 1717
Soriatane Capsules (Less than 1%).. 1013
St. Joseph 81 mg Aspirin Chewable and Enteric Coated Tablets 1869
St. Joseph 81 mg Aspirin.............. ▣688
▲ Stalevo Tablets (8%) 2287
Starlix Tablets (2.2%)...................... 2292
▲ Strattera Capsules (5% or greater).. 1814
Stromectol Tablets (2.8%)................ 2083
▲ Suboxone Tablets (4%) 2717
▲ Subutex Tablets (4%) 2717
▲ Sular Tablets (5%) 3122
Suprax (Less than 2%)..................... 1843
▲ Sustiva Capsules (2% to 10%) 930
▲ Sustiva Tablets (2% to 10%) 930
▲ Sutent Capsules (2% to 16%) 2560
▲ Symlin Injection (2% to 6%) 613
▲ Symmetrel Tablets (5% to 10%) 1135
Synera Topical Patch (Less than or equal to 1%)................................ 1137
▲ Tambocor Tablets (18.9%) 1856
Tamiflu Capsules (1% to 2%)............ 2807
Tamiflu Oral Suspension (1.6% to 2.1%)... 2807
▲ Tarceva Tablets (0% to 15%) 1259
▲ Tarceva Tablets (0% to 15%) 2444
Targretin Capsules.......................... 1747
▲ Tarka Tablets (3.1%) 524
▲ Tasmar Tablets (6% to 13%) 3358
▲ Taxotere Injection Concentrate (4.5% to 15.8%)............................ 2932
▲ Tegretol/Tegretol-XR (Among most frequent).............................. 2295
▲ Temodar Capsules (5% to 12%) 3073
▲ Tequin Injection (3%) 938
▲ Tequin Injection in 5% Dextrose (3%).. 938
▲ Tequin Tablets (3%) 938
Tessalon Capsules.......................... 1199
Tessalon Perles.............................. 1199
Teveten Tablets (1% or greater)........ 1735
▲ Teveten HCT Tablets (4.1%) 1737
▲ Thalomid Capsules (4.2%) 965
TheraFlu Daytime Severe Cold Hot Liquid.................................. ▣742
▲ Thrombate III (7 of 17) 3257
▲ Thymoglobulin for Intravenous Infusion (8.5%)............................ 1284
Thyrogen for Injection (1.6%)........... 1286
▲ Tiazac Capsules (5%) 1201
Ticlid Tablets (1.1%)........................ 2810
Timentin ADD-Vantage..................... 1580
Timentin Injection Galaxy Container.................................... 1583
Timentin IV Infusion........................ 1577
Timentin Pharmacy Bulk Package.... 1586
Timolide Tablets (1.2%)................... 2086
Timoptic Sterile Ophthalmic Solution (Less frequent)................ 2088
Timoptic in Ocudose (Less frequent)....................................... 2091
▲ Timoptic-XE Sterile Ophthalmic Gel Forming Solution (1% to 5%)... 2092
Tindamax Tablets (0.5% to 1.1%)..... 2142
▲ TOBI Solution for Inhalation (5.8%) .. 2298
▲ Topamax Sprinkle Capsules (4% to 32%).. 2404
▲ Topamax Tablets (4% to 32%) 2404
▲ Toprol-XL Tablets (1.8% to about 10 of 100 patients)...................... 668
▲ Transderm Scōp Transdermal Therapeutic System (12%)............ 2177
Tranxene (Less common)................. 2474
Trasylol Injection (1% to 2%)............ 754
Trecator Tablets 3487
Trelstar Depot (1.4%)...................... 3394
Trelstar LA Suspension (2.9%).......... 3397
Triaminic Chest & Nasal Congestion Liquid........................ ▣746
Tricor Tablets.................................. 527
▲ Trileptal Tablets (8% to 49%) 2300
▲ Trileptal Oral Suspension (8% to 49%)... 2300
▲ Trisenox Injection (23%) 993
▲ Trizivir Tablets (10%) 1589
Trusopt Sterile Ophthalmic Solution 2095
▲ Truvada Tablets (8%) 1296
Tussionex Pennkinetic Extended-Release Suspension 3327
Twinject 0.3 3378
Twinject 0.15 3379
Twinrix Vaccine (Less than 1%) 1595
▲ Tygacil for Injection (3.5%) 3488
Children's Tylenol Plus Cold & Allergy Oral Suspension ....▣716
Concentrated Tylenol Infants' Drops Plus Cold & Cough ....▣754
▲ Tylenol with Codeine Tablets (Among most frequent) 2391
Tylenol Allergy Multi-Symptom Caplets with Cool Burst and Gelcaps 1872
Tylenol Allergy Multi-Symptom Nighttime Caplets with Cool Burst 1872
Children's Tylenol Plus Cold Suspension Liquid 1879
Children's Tylenol Plus Flu Suspension Liquid 1881
Children's Tylenol Plus Multi-Symptom Cold Suspension Liquid 1879
Tylenol Cold Severe Congestion Non-Drowsy Caplets with Cool Burst 1874
Tylenol Cold Head Congestion Daytime Caplets with Cool Burst ...1873
Tylenol Cold Head Congestion Nighttime Caplets with Cool Burst 1873
Tylenol Cold Head Congestion Severe Caplets with Cool Burst 1873
Tylenol Cold Multi-Symptom Daytime Caplets with Cool Burst and Gelcaps 1874
Tylenol Cold Multi-Symptom Daytime Liquid with Citrus Burst ... 1874
Tylenol Cold Multi-Symptom Nighttime Caplets with Cool Burst 1874
Tylenol Cold Multi-Symptom Nighttime Liquid with Cool Burst ... 1874
Tylenol Cold Multi-Symptom Severe Caplets with Cool Burst 1874
Tylenol Cold Multi-Symptom Severe Daytime Liquid with Citrus Burst 1874
Concentrated Tylenol Infants' Drops Plus Cold 1879
Concentrated Tylenol Infants' Drops Plus Cold and Cough 1879
Tylenol Sinus Severe Congestion Caplets with Cool Burst 1876
Tylenol Sinus Congestion & Pain Daytime Caplets with Cool Burst and Gelcaps 1876
Tylenol Sinus Congestion & Pain Nighttime Caplets with Cool Burst 1876
Tylenol Sinus Congestion & Pain Severe Caplets with Cool Burst 1876
▲ Ultane Liquid for Inhalation (4%) 531
▲ Ultram ER Tablets (15.9% to 28.2%) 2392
Uniretic Tablets (Less than 1% to 1.4%) 3100
▲ Univasc Tablets (4.3%) 3104
Uroqid-Acid No. 2 Tablets 760
▲ Uroxatral Tablets (5.7%) 2943
Valcyte Tablets 2813
▲ Valtrex Caplets (2% to 4%) 1597
Vancocin HCl Capsules, USP (Rare) 3380
Vandazole Vaginal Gel (Less than 1%) 3338

Vantas (Less than 2%) 3375
Vantin Tablets and Oral Suspension (Less than 1%) 2645
Varivax 2100
▲ Vasotec I.V. Injection (4.3% to 7.9%) 2103
▲ Velcade for Injection (14%) 2133
Ventavis Inhalation Solution 1020
Ventolin HFA Inhalation Aerosol (Less than 3%) 1600
▲ Verelan PM Extended-Release Capsules, Controlled-Onset (3% to 3.3%) 3106
▲ Vesanoid Capsules (20%) 2820
VESIcare Tablets (1.8% to 1.9%) 646
VFEND I.V. (1.3% to 2.6%) 2564
VFEND Oral Suspension (1.3% to 2.6%) 2564
VFEND Tablets (1.3% to 2.6%) 2564
Viadur Implant (Less than 2%) 757
Viagra Tablets (2%) 2573
Vicks 44D Cough & Head Congestion Relief Liquid 2679
Vicks 44M Cough, Cold & Flu Relief Liquid 2680
Vicks DayQuil Multi-Symptom Cold/Flu Relief Liquid 2678
Vicks DayQuil Multi-Symptom Cold/Flu Relief LiquiCaps 2678
Vicks NyQuil Multi-Symptom Cold/Flu Relief Liquid 2681
Vicks NyQuil Multi-Symptom Cold/Flu Relief LiquiCaps 2681
Children's Vicks NyQuil Cold/Cough Relief Liquid 2680
Vicodin Tablets 535
▲ Vicodin ES Tablets (Among most frequent) 536
▲ Vicodin HP Tablets (Among most frequent) 538
▲ Vicoprofen Tablets (14%) 539
Viracept (Less than 2%) 2577
▲ Viread Tablets (1% to 3%) 1301
Visudyne for Injection 2305
▲ Vivitrol (13% to 16%) 995
▲ Voltaren Tablets (1% to 10%) 2307
▲ Voltaren-XR Tablets (1% to 10%) 2310
VoSpire ER Tablets (1.5%) 1052
Vytorin 10/10 Tablets 2114
Vytorin 10/10 Tablets 3077
Vytorin 10/20 Tablets 2114
Vytorin 10/20 Tablets 3077
Vytorin 10/40 Tablets 2114
Vytorin 10/40 Tablets 3077
Vytorin 10/80 Tablets 2114
Vytorin 10/80 Tablets 3077
▲ Wellbutrin Tablets (22.3%) 1603
▲ Wellbutrin SR Sustained-Release Tablets (5% to 11%) 1607
▲ Wellbutrin XL Extended-Release Tablets (6% to 11%) 1613
WinRho SDF 732
▲ Xeloda Tablets (1% to 12%) 2822
▲ Xenical Capsules (5.2%) 2831
Xifaxan Tablets (Less than 2%) 2842
▲ Xolair (3%) 1266
Xopenex Inhalation Solution (1.4% to 2.7%) 3146
Xopenex Inhalation Solution Concentrate (1.4% to 2.7%) 3150
Xopenex HFA Inhalation Aerosol (1.4% to 2.7%) 3154
▲ Xyrem Oral Solution (2% to 37.1%) 1688
Yasmin 28 Tablets (Greater than 1%) 796
Yaz Tablets (Greater than 1%) 803
Zantac (Rare) 1624
Zantac Injection (Rare) 1619
Zantac Injection Pharmacy Bulk Package (Rare) 1622
Zantac Injection Premixed (Rare) 1619
Zantac (Rare) 1624
Zegerid Capsules (1.5%) 2958
Zegerid Powder for Oral Solution (1.5%) 2958
▲ Zelapar Tablets (11%) 3372
▲ Zelnorm Tablets (4%) 2312
Zemaira (0.2% to 0.4%) 3509
Zetia Tablets (1.8% to 2.7%) 2120
Zetia Tablets (2.7%) 3083
▲ Ziagen (6%) 1626
Zmax for Oral Suspension (Less then 1%) 2583
Zocor Tablets 2105
▲ Zofran Injection (12%) 1634
▲ Zofran (4% to 7%) 1639
▲ Zofran ODT Orally Disintegrating Tablets (4% to 7%) 1639
▲ Zoloft (6% to 17%) 2586
▲ Zometa for Intravenous Infusion (18%) 2315
▲ Zomig Tablets (Common) 3519
▲ Zomig Nasal Spray (2% to 6%) 3523
▲ Zomig-ZMT Tablets (Common) 3519
▲ Zonegran Capsules (13%) 1101
Zosyn (1.4%) 3492
Zovirax 1643
▲ Zyban Sustained-Release Tablets (8% to 10%) 1644
▲ Zydone Tablets (Among most frequent) 1139
Zyflo Tablets (Greater than 1%) 1023
▲ Zyprexa Tablets (11% to 18%) 1830
▲ Zyprexa IntraMuscular (4%) 1830
▲ Zyprexa ZYDIS Orally Disintegrating Tablets (11% to 18%) 1830
Zyrtec Chewable Tablets (2%) 2594
Zyrtec (2%) 2594
Zyrtec-D 12 Hour Extended Release Tablets (2%) 2597
Zyvox (2%) 2652

Dizziness, aggravated

▲ Ultram ER Tablets (1% to greater than 5%) 2392

Dizziness, postural

Ambien CR Tablets (1%) 2855
Cardura XL Tablets 2515
Cesamet Capsules 3340
Diovan HCT Tablets (Greater than 0.2%) 2196
Xyrem Oral Solution (Infrequent) 1688

Dorsocervical fat enlargement

Agenerase Capsules (1 patient) 1327
Agenerase Oral Solution (1 patient) 1332
Aptivus Capsules 826
Combivir Tablets 1411
Crixivan Capsules 1940
Epivir 1427
Invirase 2772
Norvir 503
Retrovir 1560
Reyataz Capsules (Less than 3%) 921
Sustiva Capsules 930
Sustiva Tablets 930
Trizivir Tablets 1589
Truvada Tablets 1296
Viracept 2577
Viramune Oral Suspension 873
Viramune Tablets 873
Viread Tablets 1301
Ziagen 1626

Dreaming

Amerge Tablets (Rare) 1339
Dilaudid Oral Liquid (Less frequent) 445
Dilaudid Tablets - 8 mg (Less frequent) 445
▲ Malarone Pediatric Tablets (2% to 7%) 1517
▲ Malarone Tablets (2% to 7%) 1517
MS Contin Tablets (Less frequent) 2701

Dreaming, increased

Restoril Capsules (0.5% to 0.9%) 1860

Dreaming abnormalities

Abilify Oral Solution (Frequent) 882
Abilify Oral Solution (Frequent) 2450
Abilify Discmelt Orally Disintegrating Tablets (Frequent) 882
Abilify Discmelt Orally Disintegrating Tablets (Frequent) 2450
Abilify Tablets (Frequent) 882
Abilify Tablets (Frequent) 2450
Aciphex Tablets 1090
Actiq (Less than 1%) 979
Ambien Tablets (1%) 2851
Ambien CR Tablets (Infrequent) 2855
Anaprox Tablets (Less than 1%) 2761
Anaprox DS Tablets (Less than 1%) 2761
Anzemet Injection (Infrequently) 2859
Anzemet Tablets (Infrequently) 2862
▲ Aricept Tablets (3%) 1094
▲ Aricept ODT Tablets (3%) 1094
Arthrotec Tablets (Rare) 3129
▲ Atripla Tablets (4%) 945
Avelox (Less than 0.1%) 2970
▲ Avinza Capsules (Less than 5%) 1741
Axert Tablets (Rare) 2396
Axid Oral Solution (1.9%) 879
▲ Azilect Tablets (4%) 3293
Blocadren Tablets (Less than 1%) 1916
Buprenex Injectable (Less than 1%) 2716
Caduet Tablets (Greater than 0.1% to less than 2%) 2508
Campral Tablets (Infrequent) 1174
Cardizem LA Extended Release Tablets (Less than 2%) 1728
Catapres Tablets 843
Catapres-TTS (0.5% or less) 844
Cesamet Capsules 3340
▲ Chantix Tablets (9% to 13%) 2517
Cipro XR Tablets (Less than 1%) 2990
Clorpres Tablets 2153
Copaxone for Injection (Frequent) 3297
Cozaar Tablets (Less than 1%) 1935
▲ Depacon Injection (1% to 5%) 412
▲ Depakene (1% to 5%) 417
▲ Depakote Sprinkle Capsules (1% to 5%) 422
▲ Depakote Tablets (1% to 5%) 427
▲ Depakote ER Tablets (1% to 5%) 434
Dilaudid-HP (Less frequent) 442
Duragesic Transdermal System (1% or greater) 2373
EC-Naprosyn Delayed-Release Tablets (Less than 1%) 2761
▲ Effexor Tablets (4%) 3411
▲ Effexor XR Capsules (3% to 7%) 3417
▲ Eldepryl Capsules (2 of 49 patients) 3208
▲ Emtriva Capsules (2% to 11%) 1287
▲ Emtriva Oral Solution (2% to 11%) 1287
▲ Epzicom Tablets (4% to 5%) 1436
Evoxac Capsules (Less than 1%) 1047
Exelon Capsules (Infrequent) 2206
Exelon Oral Solution (Infrequent) 2206
Frova Tablets (Rare) 1113
Gabitril Tablets (Infrequent) 984
Hyzaar 50-12.5 Tablets 1990
Hyzaar 100-12.5 Tablets 1990
Hyzaar 100-25 Tablets 1990
Inderal LA Long-Acting Capsules 3429
▲ Intron A for Injection (Less than 5%) 3024
Invirase (Less than 2%) 2772
Ionsys Transdermal System (.1% to less than 1%) 2379
Kadian Capsules (Less than 3%) 577
Kaletra (Less than 2%) 476
Klonopin (Infrequent) 2778
Lamictal (Infrequent) 1481
▲ Lariam Tablets (Among most frequent) 2786
Levaquin (0.1% to 0.9%) 2384
Levaquin in 5% Dextrose Injection (0.1% to 0.9%) 2384
▲ Lexapro Oral Solution (3%) 1190
▲ Lexapro Tablets (3%) 1190
Lipitor Tablets (Less than 2%) 2483
Lotensin HCT Tablets (0.3% or more) 2246
Lotronex Tablets (Rare) 1512
▲ Lunesta Tablets (1% to 3%) 3142
Lyrica Capsules (0.1% to 1%) 2539
Maxalt Tablets (Infrequent) 2008
Maxalt-MLT Orally Disintegrating Tablets (Infrequent) 2008
Meridia Capsules 489
▲ Mirapex Tablets (Greater than or equal to 1% to 11%) 859
Naprosyn Suspension (Less than 1%) 2761
Naprosyn Tablets (Less than 1%) 2761
Neurontin Capsules (Infrequent) 2487
Neurontin Oral Solution (Infrequent) 2487
Neurontin Tablets (Infrequent) 2487
Nipent for Injection (Less than 3%) 1863
Niravam Orally Disintegrating Tablets (1.8%) 3092
Norvasc Tablets (More than 0.1% to 1%) 2545
Norvir (Less than 2%) 503
▲ OxyContin Tablets (Between 1% and 5%) 2703
Parcopa Orally Disintegrating Tablets 3097
▲ Paxil CR Controlled-Release Tablets (3% to 4%) 1538
▲ Paxil (3% to 4%) 1530
Permax Tablets (2.7%) 3356
▲ Pexeva Tablets (4%) 1694
Prevacid Delayed-Release Capsules (Less than 1%) 3271
Prevacid for Delayed-Release Oral Suspension (Less than 1%) 3271
Prevacid SoluTab Delayed-Release Orally Disintegrating Tablets (Less than 1%) 3271
Prevacid NapraPAC (Less than 1%) 3280
PREVPAC (Less than 1%) 3284
Prilosec OTC Delayed-Release Tablets (Less than 1%) 2677
▲ Prograf Capsules and Injection (3% to 15%) 632
ProQuad 2064
ProSom Tablets (2%) 517
Protonix I.V. (Less than 1%) 3472
Protonix Tablets (Less than 1%) 3469
▲ Prozac Pulvules and Liquid (1% to 5%) 1801
Relpax Tablets (Infrequent) 2548
▲ Requip Tablets (11%) 1555
Rescriptor Tablets 2551
Reyataz Capsules (Less than 3%) 921
Rilutek Tablets (Rare) 2930
Risperdal (Frequent) 1676
Risperdal Consta Long-Acting Injection (Up to 2%) 1682
Risperdal M-Tab Orally Disintegrating Tablets (Frequent) 1676
Seroquel Tablets (Infrequent) 690
Singulair (Very rare) 2077
Stalevo Tablets 2287
▲ Strattera Capsules (4%) 1814
Sular Tablets (Less than or equal to 1%) 3122
Sustiva Capsules (1% to 4%) 930
Sustiva Tablets (1% to 4%) 930
▲ Symmetrel Tablets (1% to 5%) 1135
Tambocor Tablets (Less than 1%) 1856
▲ Tasmar Tablets (16% to 21%) 3358
▲ Tequin Injection (0.1% to 3%) 938
▲ Tequin Injection in 5% Dextrose (0.1% to 3%) 938
▲ Tequin Tablets (0.1% to 3%) 938
Thioridazine Hydrochloride Tablets 2163
Tiazac Capsules (Less than 2%) 1201
Topamax Sprinkle Capsules (Infrequent) 2404
Topamax Tablets (Infrequent) 2404
▲ Truvada Tablets (4%) 1296
▲ Ultram ER Tablets (1% to greater than 5%) 2392
Vantin Tablets and Oral Suspension (Less than 1%) 2645
Vasotec I.V. Injection (0.5% to 1.0%) 2103
VFEND I.V. (Less than 2%) 2564
VFEND Oral Suspension (Less than 2%) 2564
VFEND Tablets (Less than 2%) 2564
Viagra Tablets (Less than 2%) 2573
Vicoprofen Tablets (Less than 1%) 539
Vivitrol 995
Voltaren Tablets (Occasionally) 2307
Voltaren-XR Tablets (Occasionally) 2310
Wellbutrin Tablets 1603
Wellbutrin SR Sustained-Release Tablets (At least 1%) 1607
▲ Wellbutrin XL Extended-Release Tablets (At least 1% to 3%) 1613
Xifaxan Tablets (Less than 2%) 2842
Xyrem Oral Solution (Frequent) 1688
Zegerid Capsules (Less than 1%) 2958
Zegerid Powder for Oral Solution (Less than 1%) 2958
Zoloft (Infrequent) 2586
Zomig Nasal Spray (Rare) 3523
Zonegran Capsules (Infrequent) 1101
▲ Zyban Sustained-Release Tablets (5%) 1644
Zyprexa Tablets 1830
Zyprexa ZYDIS Orally Disintegrating Tablets 1830

Drooling

Aricept Tablets 1094
Aricept ODT Tablets 1094
Dantrium Capsules (Less frequent) 2694
Demser Capsules 1953
Thioridazine Hydrochloride Tablets 2163
Thiothixene Capsules 2165

Drowsiness

▲ Abilify Oral Solution (7% to 15%) 882
▲ Abilify Oral Solution (7% to 15%) 2450
▲ Abilify Discmelt Orally Disintegrating Tablets (7% to 15%) 882
▲ Abilify Discmelt Orally Disintegrating Tablets (7% to 15%) 2450
▲ Abilify Tablets (7% to 15%) 882
▲ Abilify Tablets (7% to 15%) 2450
Accutane Capsules 2731
Aceon Tablets (2 mg, 4 mg, 8 mg) (1.3%) 3194
Aciphex Tablets 1090
▲ Actiq (9% to 20%) 979
Adalat CC Tablets (Less than 1%) 2964
▲ Adderall XR Capsules (2% to 4%) 3166
Adenoscan (Less than 1%) 619
Advil Allergy Sinus Caplets ■ 770
Advil Multi-Symptom Cold Caplets ■ 770
Advil PM Caplets ■ 615
Aggrenox Capsules (1.2%) 822
▲ Agrylin Capsules (1% to 5%) 3169
Alavert Allergy & Sinus D-12 Hour Tablets ■ 771
Albalon Ophthalmic Solution ⊙ 218
▲ Alferon N Injection (3% to 10%) 1665
Alinia for Oral Suspension (Less than 1%) 2835
Alinia Tablets (Less than 1%) 2835
Allegra (1.3% to 2.2%) 2844
Allegra-D 12 Hour Extended-Release Tablets 2846

Allegra-D 24 Hour Extended-Release Tablets ... 2849
Aloxi Injection (Less than 1%) ... 2127
▲ Alphagan P Ophthalmic Solution (1% to 4%) ... 567
Alphanate, Antihemophilic Factor (Human) ... 1654
Altace Capsules (Less than 1%) ... 1702
▲ Ambien Tablets (2% to 8%) ... 2851
▲ Ambien CR Tablets (6% to 15%) ... 2855
AmBisome for Injection (Less common) ... 620
Amerge Tablets (1% to 2%) ... 1339
▲ Anaprox Tablets (3% to 9%) ... 2761
▲ Anaprox DS Tablets (3% to 9%) ... 2761
Anzemet Injection (2.4%) ... 2859
Aptivus Capsules (Less than 2%) ... 826
Aralast (Greater than or equal to 0.2% to 0.3%) ... 717
▲ Aredia for Injection (Up to 6%) ... 2179
Aricept Tablets (2%) ... 1094
Aricept ODT Tablets (2%) ... 1094
▲ Arimidex Tablets (2% to 5%) ... 673
▲ Arranon Injection (0% to 23%) ... 1357
Arthrotec Tablets (Rare) ... 3129
Asacol Delayed-Release Tablets ... 2692
▲ Astelin Nasal Spray (0.4% to 11.5%) ... 1904
Atacand Tablets (0.5% or greater) ... 649
Atacand HCT ... 651
▲ Atripla Tablets (3%) ... 945
Avalide Tablets ... 888
Avalide Tablets ... 2874
Avapro Tablets (Less than 1%) ... 891
Avapro Tablets (Less than 1%) ... 2871
Avelox (0.1% to less than 2%) ... 2970
▲ Avinza Capsules (Greater than 10%) ... 1741
Axert Tablets (Frequent) ... 2396
Axid Oral Solution (1.9%) ... 879
▲ Azilect Tablets (6%) ... 3293
Baraclude (Less than 1%) ... 894
BC Allergy Sinus Cold Powder ... ▣677
BeneFix Vials (1.5%) ... 3408
▲ Bentyl Capsules (9%) ... 697
▲ Bentyl Injection (9%) ... 697
▲ Bentyl Syrup (9%) ... 697
▲ Bentyl Tablets (9%) ... 697
▲ Bexxar (0% to 5%) ... 1398
Bicillin C-R Injectable Suspension ... 1706
BiDil Tablets (1% to less than 2%) ... 2171
Biltricide Tablets ... 2976
Blocadren Tablets (Less than 1%) ... 1916
▲ BOTOX Purified Neurotoxin Complex (2% to 10%) ... 570
▲ Brimonidine Tartrate Ophthalmic Solution 0.2% (10% to 30%) ... ⊙248
Byetta Injection ... 611
Caduet Tablets (1.3% to less than 2%) ... 2508
Calcijex Injection ... 411
▲ Campath Ampules (1% to 5%) ... 811
Campral Tablets (Frequent) ... 1174
▲ Camptosar Injection (1.3% to 9.4%) ... 2604
Captopril Tablets ... 2149
Carafate Suspension (Less than 0.5%) ... 701
Carafate Tablets (Less than 0.5%) ... 701
▲ Carbatrol Capsules (Among most frequent) ... 3171
Cardizem LA Extended Release Tablets (Less than 2%) ... 1728
Cardura XL Tablets (1.5%) ... 2515
▲ Catapres Tablets (About 33 in 100 patients) ... 843
▲ Catapres-TTS (12 of 101 patients) ... 844
Ceftin Tablets (0.1% to 1%) ... 1407
Celebrex Capsules (0.1% to 1.9%) ... 3134
▲ Celexa (18%) ... 1176
▲ CellCept Capsules (3% to less than 20%) ... 2747
▲ CellCept Intravenous (3% to less than 20%) ... 2747
▲ CellCept Oral Suspension (3% to less than 20%) ... 2747
▲ CellCept Tablets (3% to less than 20%) ... 2747
▲ Cesamet Capsules (52% to 66%) ... 3340
▲ Chantix Tablets (3%) ... 2517
▲ Chemet Capsules (1.0% to 12.7%) ... 2458
Cialis Tablets (Less than 2%) ... 1838
Cipro (Less than 1%) ... 2977
Cipro I.V. (1% or less) ... 2984
Cipro XR Tablets (Less than 1%) ... 2990
▲ Clarinex Syrup (9.1%) ... 2995
Clarinex Tablets (2.1%) ... 2995
Clarinex Reditabs Tablets (2.1%) ... 2995
▲ Clarinex-D 24-Hour Extended-Release Tablets (3%) ... 2998
Clinoril Tablets (Less than 1%) ... 1924
▲ Clolar for Intravenous Infusion (10%) ... 1271
▲ Clorpres Tablets (About 33%) ... 2153
▲ Clozaril Tablets (More than 5% to 46%) ... 2184
Colazal Capsules ... 2838
Combivent Inhalation Aerosol ... 847
Comtan Tablets (2%) ... 2189
Comtrex Maximum Strength Cold & Cough Day/Night Caplets - Day Formulation ... ▣726
Comtrex Maximum Strength Cold & Cough Day/Night Caplets - Night Formulation ... ▣726
Comtrex Maximum Strength Day/Night Severe Cold & Sinus Caplets - Night Formulation ... ▣725
▲ Comvax (21.1% to 49.5%) ... 1928
Concerta Extended-Release Tablets ... 1881
Contac Cold and Flu Maximum Strength Caplets ... ▣728
Contac Cold and Flu Day and Night Caplets (Night Formulation Only) ... ▣727
Copaxone for Injection (At least 2%) ... 3297
▲ Coreg Tablets (Greater than 1% to 3%) ... 1414
Covera-HS Tablets (Less than 2%) ... 3139
Cozaar Tablets (Less than 1%) ... 1935
Crixivan Capsules (2.4%) ... 1940
▲ Cymbalta Delayed-Release Capsules (7% to 21%) ... 1757
CytoGam Intravenous (Infrequent) ... 1895
Dalmane Capsules ... 3342
▲ Dantrium Capsules (Among most frequent) ... 2694
▲ DAPTACEL Vaccine (13.3% to 43.2%) ... 2950
▲ Daranide Tablets (Among the most common effects) ... 1950
Daytrana Transdermal Patch ... 3174
Demadex Injection ... 2759
Demadex Tablets ... 2759
▲ Depacon Injection (1.7% to 30%) ... 412
▲ Depakene (27% to 30%) ... 417
▲ Depakote Sprinkle Capsules (18% to 30%) ... 422
▲ Depakote Tablets (17% to 30%) ... 427
▲ Depakote ER Tablets (7% to 30%) ... 434
▲ DepoCyt Injection (4% to 12%) ... 1143
▲ DepoDur Extended-Release Injection (2% to 5%) ... 1110
Depo-Provera Contraceptive Injection (Less than 1%) ... 2622
depo-subQ provera 104 Injectable Suspension ... 2624
▲ Detrol Tablets (3%) ... 2628
▲ Detrol LA Capsules (3%) ... 2631
▲ Diastat Rectal Delivery System (23%) ... 3343
Dibenzyline Capsules ... 3399
Dilaudid ... 440
Dilaudid Non-Sterile Powder ... 440
Dilaudid Rectal Suppositories ... 440
Dilaudid Tablets ... 440
Children's Dimetapp Cold & Allergy Elixir ... ▣730
Children's Dimetapp Cold & Allergy Chewable Tablets ... ▣730
Children's Dimetapp Long Acting Cough Plus Cold Syrup ... ▣731
Diovan Tablets ... 2193
Diovan HCT Tablets (Greater than 0.2%) ... 2196
▲ Ditropan XL Extended-Release Tablets (2% to 12%) ... 2413
Diuril Sodium Intravenous ... 2467
Dolobid Tablets (Greater than 1 in 100) ... 1955
Donnatal Extentabs ... 2493
▲ Doxil Injection (1% to 10%) ... 2351
DuoNeb Inhalation Solution ... 1058
▲ Duragesic Transdermal System (10% or more) ... 2373
Dyazide Capsules ... 1423
DynaCirc CR Tablets (0.5% to 1%) ... 2721
▲ EC-Naprosyn Delayed-Release Tablets (3% to 9%) ... 2761
▲ Effexor Tablets (3% to 26.1%) ... 3411
▲ Effexor XR Capsules (2% to 17%) ... 3417
Eldepryl Capsules ... 3208
▲ Eloxatin for Injection (2% to 5%) ... 2892
Elspar for Injection ... 2463
Elspar for Injection ... 1960
Emsam Transdermal System ... 903
Engerix-B Vaccine (Less than 1%) ... 1425
▲ Entocort EC Capsules (Less than 5%) ... 2698
▲ Equetro Extended-Release Capsules (12% to 32%) ... 3180
Ethyol for Injection ... 1898
Eulexin Capsules (1%) ... 3009
Evoxac Capsules (Less than 1%) ... 1047
Excedrin PM Caplets/Tablets/Geltabs ... ▣610
▲ Exelon Capsules (4% to 5%) ... 2206
▲ Exelon Oral Solution (4% to 5%) ... 2206
Famvir Tablets (1.6% to 2.6%) ... 2211
▲ FazaClo Orally Disintegrating Tablets (More than 5% to 46%) ... 551
▲ Femara Tablets (2% to 4%) ... 2214
Ferrlecit Injection ... 3388
▲ Flomax Capsules (3.0% to 4.3%) ... 850
Flumadine (0.3% to 1%) ... 1183
Focalin Tablets ... 2220
Focalin XR Capsules ... 2223
Frova Tablets (Greater than or equal to 2%) ... 1113
Furosemide Tablets ... 2154
▲ Gabitril Tablets (18%) ... 984
Gantrisin Pediatric Suspension ... 2770
▲ Gemzar for Injection (5% to 11%) ... 1771
Gengraf Capsules (1% to less than 3%) ... 459
▲ Geodon (14% to 31%) ... 2529
Gleevec Tablets (Infrequent) ... 2227
Goody's PM Powder for Pain with Sleeplessness ... ▣612
▲ Havrix Vaccine (15% to 17%) ... 1456
Hectorol Capsules ... 1275
Hectorol Injection ... 1278
HibTITER (91 of 1,118 vaccinations) ... 3426
Hycodan ... 1116
Hycotuss Expectorant Syrup ... 1117
Hyperstat I.V. ... 3017
▲ Hytrin Capsules (0.6% to 5.4%) ... 471
Hyzaar 50-12.5 Tablets ... 1990
Hyzaar 100-12.5 Tablets ... 1990
Hyzaar 100-25 Tablets ... 1990
▲ Imdur Tablets (Less than or equal to 5%) ... 3018
▲ Imitrex Injection (3%) ... 1463
Imitrex Nasal Spray (Infrequent) ... 1467
Imitrex Tablets (Greater than 1%) ... 1471
Imodium A-D Liquid and Caplets ... 1865
Imodium Advanced Caplets and Chewable Tablets ... ▣655
▲ Indapamide Tablets (Less than 5%) ... 2156
Indocin (Less than 1%) ... 1995
▲ Infanrix Vaccine (6.6% to 54%) ... 1476
▲ Infergen (4% to 5%) ... 3364
▲ Intron A for Injection (Up to 14%) ... 3024
▲ Invanz for Injection (Greater than 0.5% to 5.1%) ... 1999
Invirase (Less than 2%) ... 2772
Ionsys Transdermal System (1% to less than 10%) ... 2379
▲ Kadian Capsules (Among most frequent) ... 577
Kaletra (Less than 2%) ... 476
▲ Keppra Injection (15%) ... 3320
▲ Keppra Oral Solution (3% to 23%) ... 3314
▲ Keppra Tablets (3% to 23%) ... 3314
Ketek Tablets (Greater than or equal to 0.2% to less than 2%) ... 2903
▲ Klonopin (7% to 50%) ... 2778
▲ Kytril Injection (4%) ... 2781
Kytril (1% to 4%) ... 2784
▲ Lamictal (5% to 17%) ... 1481
▲ Lariam Tablets (Among most frequent) ... 2786
Levaquin (0.1% to 0.9%) ... 2384
Levaquin in 5% Dextrose Injection (0.1% to 0.9%) ... 2384
Levitra Tablets (Less than 2%) ... 3034
▲ Lexapro Oral Solution (4% to 13%) ... 1190
▲ Lexapro Tablets (4% to 13%) ... 1190
Librium Capsules ... 3347
Lidoderm Patch ... 1118
Lipitor Tablets (Less than 2%) ... 2483
Lithobid Tablets ... 1692
Lofibra Tablets ... 1219
Lofibra Capsules ... 1216
▲ Lopressor HCT 50/25 Tablets (10%) ... 2241
▲ Lopressor HCT 100/25 Tablets (10%) ... 2241
▲ Lopressor HCT 100/50 Tablets (10%) ... 2241
Lotensin Tablets (1.6%) ... 2243
Lotensin HCT Tablets (1.2%) ... 2246
Lotrel Capsules (Up to 0.3%) ... 2249
▲ Lunesta Tablets (8% to 10%) ... 3142
Lupron Depot-PED 7.5 mg, 11.25 mg and 15 mg (Less than 2%) ... 3269
Lupron Injection Pediatric (Less than 2%) ... 3259
▲ Lyrica Capsules (4% to 28%) ... 2539
▲ Marinol Capsules (3% to 10%) ... 3333
Matulane Capsules ... 3191
Mavik Tablets (0.3% to 1.0%) ... 486
▲ Maxalt Tablets (4% to 8%) ... 2008
▲ Maxalt-MLT Orally Disintegrating Tablets (4% to 8%) ... 2008
Meridia Capsules (1.7%) ... 489
Merrem I.V. (Greater than 0.1% to 1%) ... 686
Metadate CD Capsules ... 3323
Micardis Tablets (More than 0.3%) ... 854
Micardis HCT Tablets ... 856
Midamor Tablets (Less than or equal to 1%) ... 2026
▲ Migranal Nasal Spray (3%) ... 3348
Mintezol ... 2027
▲ Mirapex Tablets (9% to 22%) ... 859
▲ Moban Tablets (Most frequent) ... 1119
Mobic Oral Suspension (Less than 2%) ... 863
Mobic Tablets (Less than 2%) ... 863
Moduretic Tablets (Less than or equal to 1%) ... 2028
Mycamine for Injection (0.4% to 0.5%) ... 628
Myobloc Injection (Greater than 2%) ... 3192
▲ Nalfon Capsules (8.5%) ... 2502
▲ Namenda (3%) ... 1195
▲ Naprosyn Suspension (3% to 9%) ... 2761
▲ Naprosyn Tablets (3% to 9%) ... 2761
Natrecor for Injection (Greater than or equal to 1%) ... 3127
▲ Nembutal Sodium Solution, USP (1% to 3%) ... 2470
Neoral Oral Solution (1% to less than 3%) ... 2259
Neoral Soft Gelatin Capsules (1% to less than 3%) ... 2259
Neumega for Injection ... 3435
▲ Neurontin Capsules (8.4% to 21.4%) ... 2487
▲ Neurontin Oral Solution (8.4% to 21.4%) ... 2487
▲ Neurontin Tablets (8.4% to 21.4%) ... 2487
Nexium Delayed-Release Capsules (Less than 1%) ... 655
Nexium I.V. (Less than 1%) ... 659
▲ Nipent for Injection (3% to 10%) ... 1863
▲ Niravam Orally Disintegrating Tablets (41% to 76.8%) ... 3092
Norflex Injection ... 1856
Noroxin Tablets (0.3% to 1.0%) ... 2032
Norvasc Tablets (1.3% to 1.6%) ... 2545
Norvir (2.4% to 2.6%) ... 503
Numorphan Injection ... 1120
Nytol QuickGels Softgels Maximum Strength ... ▣616
Omnicef Capsules (0.2%) ... 511
Omnicef for Oral Suspension (0.2%) ... 511
Oncaspar (Less than 1%) ... 1145
▲ Opana Tablets (9.3%) ... 1122
▲ Opana ER Tablets (1.9% to 17.2%) ... 1126
OptiPranolol Metipranolol Ophthalmic Solution 0.3% (A small number of patients) ... ⊙256
▲ OxyContin Tablets (23%) ... 2703
▲ Oxytrol Transdermal System (Greater than 1%) ... 3392
Parcopa Orally Disintegrating Tablets ... 3097
Parnate Tablets ... 1527
▲ Paxil CR Controlled-Release Tablets (1.9% to 24%) ... 1538
▲ Paxil (1.9% to 24%) ... 1530
Pediarix Vaccine ... 1548
▲ Liquid PedvaxHIB (Among most frequent) ... 2035
Pentasa Capsules (Less than 1%) ... 3185
Pepcid Injection (Infrequent) ... 2040
Pepcid (Infrequent) ... 2038
Percodan Tablets ... 1132
▲ Permax Tablets (10.1%) ... 3356
▲ Pexeva Tablets (1.9% to 24%) ... 1694
Phenergan Tablets and Suppositories ... 3440
Premphase Tablets ... 3456
Prempro Tablets ... 3456
Prevacid Delayed-Release Capsules (Less than 1%) ... 3271
Prevacid for Delayed-Release Oral Suspension (Less than 1%) ... 3271
Prevacid SoluTab Delayed-Release Orally Disintegrating Tablets (Less than 1%) ... 3271
▲ Prevacid NapraPAC (Less than 1% to 9%) ... 3280
▲ Prevnar for Injection (11% to 40.7%) ... 3463
PREVPAC (Less than 1%) ... 3284
Prezista Tablets (Less than 2%) ... 3306
Prilosec OTC Delayed-Release Tablets (Less than 1%) ... 2677
Primaxin I.M. ... 2045
Primaxin I.V. (0.2%) ... 2048
Prinivil Tablets (0.3% to 1.0%) ... 2052
Prinzide Tablets (0.3% to 1%) ... 2056

(▣ Described in PDR For Nonprescription Drugs) Incidence data in parenthesis; ▲ 3% or more (⊙ Described in PDR For Ophthalmic Medicines™)

ProAmatine Tablets (Rare) ... 3186
▲ Prochieve 4% Gel (27%) ... 1003
▲ Prochieve 8% Gel (27%) ... 1003
Profilnine SD, Factor IX Complex (Human) ... 1660
▲ Prograf Capsules and Injection (3% to 15%) ... 632
▲ Proleukin for Injection (22%) ... 2266
Prometrium Capsules (100 mg, 200 mg) (Less than 5%) ... 3203
ProQuad (Greater than or equal to 0.2% to less than 1%) ... 2064
Proquin XR Tablets ... 1153
▲ ProSom Tablets (42%) ... 517
Protonix I.V. (Less than 1%) ... 3472
Protonix Tablets (Less than 1%) ... 3469
Proventil HFA Inhalation Aerosol (Less than 3%) ... 3056
Provigil Tablets (2%) ... 988
▲ Prozac Pulvules and Liquid (5% to 17%) ... 1801
Raniclor Tablets, Chewable (Rare) ... 2505
▲ Rapamune Oral Solution and Tablets (3% to 20%) ... 3475
▲ Razadyne (4%) ... 2399
▲ Razadyne ER Extended-Release Capsules (4%) ... 2399
▲ Rebif Prefilled Syringe for Injection (4% to 5%) ... 3159
Recombivax HB ... 2071
ReFacto Vials ... 3484
▲ Relpax Tablets (3% to 7%) ... 2548
▲ Requip Tablets (12% to 40%) ... 1555
Rescriptor Tablets ... 2551
▲ Restoril Capsules (9.1%) ... 1860
▲ Retrovir Capsules (8%) ... 1560
▲ Retrovir IV Infusion (8%) ... 1564
▲ Retrovir (8%) ... 1560
Reyataz Capsules (Less than 3%) ... 921
▲ Rilutek Tablets (0.8% to 4.1%) ... 2930
▲ Risperdal (3% to 41%) ... 1676
▲ Risperdal Consta Long-Acting Injection (5% to 6%) ... 1682
▲ Risperdal M-Tab Orally Disintegrating Tablets (3% to 41%) ... 1676
Ritalin Hydrochloride Tablets ... 2269
Ritalin LA Capsules ... 2271
Ritalin-SR Tablets ... 2269
Robitussin Cough & Allergy Syrup ... ▣ 736
Robitussin Cough & Cold Nighttime Liquid ... ▣ 736
Robitussin Cough, Cold & Flu Nighttime Liquid ... ▣ 738
Robitussin Pediatric Cough & Cold Nighttime Liquid ... ▣ 736
Rocaltrol Capsules ... 2798
Rocaltrol Oral Solution ... 2798
Romazicon Injection (Less than 1%) ... 2804
▲ Rozerem Tablets (5%) ... 3231
▲ Rythmol SR Capsules (1% to 3%) ... 2727
▲ Sandostatin LAR Depot (1% to 4%) ... 2280
Seromycin Capsules ... 1813
▲ Seroquel Tablets (18%) ... 690
Singulair ... 2077
▲ Skelaxin Tablets (Most frequent) ... 1716
Sleep-Tite Caplets ... ▣ 832
Solodyn Extended Release Tablets (2%) ... 1890
▲ Sonata Capsules (5%) ... 1717
▲ Soriatane Capsules (1% to 10%) ... 1013
Stalevo Tablets (2%) ... 2287
▲ Strattera Capsules (0.5% to 7%) ... 1814
Stromectol Tablets (0.9%) ... 2083
▲ Suboxone Tablets (5%) ... 2717
▲ Subutex Tablets (5%) ... 2717
Sular Tablets (Less than or equal to 1%) ... 3122
Sustiva Capsules (2% to 3%) ... 930
Sustiva Tablets (2% to 3%) ... 930
▲ Symbyax Capsules (Up to 22%) ... 1819
▲ Symmetrel Tablets (1% to 5%) ... 1135
Synera Topical Patch (Less than or equal to 1%) ... 1137
▲ Tambocor Tablets (1% to 3%) ... 1856
Tarka Tablets (0.3% or more) ... 524
▲ Tasmar Tablets (14% to 18%) ... 3358
▲ Tegretol/Tegretol-XR (Among most frequent) ... 2295
▲ Temodar Capsules (9%) ... 3073
Tequin Injection (Less than 0.1%) ... 938
Tequin Injection in 5% Dextrose (Less than 0.1%) ... 938
Tequin Tablets (Less than 0.1%) ... 938
Teveten Tablets (Less than 1%) ... 1735
Teveten HCT Tablets (Less than 1%) ... 1737
▲ Thalomid Capsules (37.5%) ... 965
TheraFlu Cold & Cough Hot Liquid ... ▣ 740
TheraFlu Cold & Sore Throat Hot Liquid ... ▣ 741
TheraFlu Flu & Sore Throat Hot Liquid ... ▣ 742
TheraFlu Nighttime Severe Cold Hot Liquid ... ▣ 740
TheraFlu Warming Relief Nighttime Severe Cold ... ▣ 743
TheraFlu Thin Strips Multi Symptom ... ▣ 744
Thioridazine Hydrochloride Tablets (Occasional) ... 2163
Thiothixene Capsules ... 2165
Tiazac Capsules (Less than 2%) ... 1201
Timolide Tablets (Less than 1%) ... 2086
Timoptic Sterile Ophthalmic Solution (Less frequent) ... 2088
Timoptic in Ocudose (Less frequent) ... 2091
Timoptic-XE Sterile Ophthalmic Gel Forming Solution ... 2092
Tindamax Tablets ... 2142
▲ Topamax Sprinkle Capsules (7% to 29%) ... 2404
▲ Topamax Tablets (7% to 29%) ... 2404
Toprol-XL Tablets ... 668
Transderm Scōp Transdermal Therapeutic System (Less than one-sixth) ... 2177
▲ Tranxene (Most frequent) ... 2474
Trecator Tablets ... 3487
Triaminic Cold & Allergy Liquid ... ▣ 746
Triaminic Nighttime Cold & Cough Liquid ... ▣ 746
Triaminic Cough & Runny Nose Softchews ... ▣ 748
Triaminic Thin Strips Cough & Runny Nose ... ▣ 749
Tricor Tablets ... 527
▲ Trileptal Tablets (5% to 36%) ... 2300
▲ Trileptal Oral Suspension (5% to 36%) ... 2300
▲ Trisenox Injection (8%) ... 993
▲ Truvada Tablets (3%) ... 1296
Tussionex Pennkinetic Extended-Release Suspension ... 3327
Twinrix Vaccine (Less than 1%) ... 1595
Tygacil for Injection (0.2% to less than 2%) ... 3488
Children's Tylenol Plus Cough & Runny Nose Suspension Liquid ... ▣ 754
Children's Tylenol Plus Cold Suspension Liquid ... ▣ 754
Children's Tylenol Plus Multi-Symptom Cold Suspension Liquid ... ▣ 754
Children's Tylenol Plus Flu Oral Suspension ... ▣ 749
Tylenol Cold Head Congestion Nighttime Caplets with Cool Burst ... ▣ 750
Tylenol Cold Head Congestion Severe Caplets with Cool Burst ... ▣ 750
Tylenol Cold Multi-Symptom NightTime ... ▣ 752
Tylenol Cough & Sore Throat Nighttime Liquid with Cool Burst ... ▣ 790
Extra Strength Tylenol PM Caplets, Vanilla Caplets, Geltabs, Gelcaps and Liquid ... 1875
Tylenol Sore Throat Nighttime Liquid with Cool Burst ... ▣ 790
Tylenol Allergy Multi-Symptom Caplets with Cool Burst and Gelcaps ... 1872
Tylenol Allergy Multi-Symptom Nighttime Caplets with Cool Burst ... 1872
Tylenol Severe Allergy Caplets ... 1872
Children's Tylenol Plus Cold Suspension Liquid ... 1879
Children's Tylenol Plus Cold & Allergy Suspension Liquid ... 1878
Children's Tylenol Plus Cough & Runny Nose Suspension Liquid ... 1879
Children's Tylenol Plus Flu Suspension Liquid ... 1881
Children's Tylenol Plus Multi-Symptom Cold Suspension Liquid ... 1879
Tylenol Cold Head Congestion Nighttime Caplets with Cool Burst ... 1873
Tylenol Cold Multi-Symptom Nighttime Caplets with Cool Burst ... 1874
Tylenol Cold Multi-Symptom Nighttime Liquid with Cool Burst ... 1874
Tylenol Cough & Sore Throat Nighttime Liquid with Cool Burst ... 1877
Tylenol Sinus Congestion & Pain Nighttime Caplets with Cool Burst ... 1876
Tylenol Sore Throat Nighttime Liquid with Cool Burst ... 1877
▲ Ultane Liquid for Inhalation (9%) ... 531
▲ Ultram ER Tablets (7.3% to 20.3%) ... 2392
Uniretic Tablets (Less than 1%) ... 3100
Univasc Tablets (Less than 1%) ... 3104
▲ Valium Tablets (Among most common) ... 2819
Vantin Tablets and Oral Suspension (Less than 1%) ... 2645
Vasotec I.V. Injection (0.5% to 1.0%) ... 2103
Verelan PM Extended-Release Capsules, Controlled-Onset (2% or less) ... 3106
▲ Vesanoid Capsules (3%) ... 2820
VFEND I.V. (Less than 2%) ... 2564
VFEND Oral Suspension (Less than 2%) ... 2564
VFEND Tablets (Less than 2%) ... 2564
Viagra Tablets (Less than 2%) ... 2573
Vicks 44M Cough, Cold & Flu Relief Liquid ... 2680
Pediatric Vicks 44m Cough & Cold Relief Liquid ... 2676
Vicks NyQuil Multi-Symptom Cold/Flu Relief Liquid ... 2681
Vicks NyQuil Multi-Symptom Cold/Flu Relief LiquiCaps ... 2681
Vicks NyQuil LiquiCaps/Liquid Multi-Symptom Cold/Flu Relief ... ▣ 763
Vicks NyQuil Cough Liquid ... 2680
Children's Vicks NyQuil Cold/Cough Relief Liquid ... 2680
Vicodin Tablets ... 535
Vicodin ES Tablets ... 536
Vicodin HP Tablets ... 538
▲ Vicoprofen Tablets (22%) ... 539
Viracept (Less than 2%) ... 2577
▲ Viramune Oral Suspension (3% to 8%) ... 873
▲ Viramune Tablets (3% to 8%) ... 873
▲ Vivitrol (4% to 12%) ... 995
Voltaren Tablets (Occasionally) ... 2307
Voltaren-XR Tablets (Occasionally) ... 2310
VoSpire ER Tablets (0.3%) ... 1052
▲ Wellbutrin SR Sustained-Release Tablets (2% to 3%) ... 1607
▲ Wellbutrin XL Extended-Release Tablets (2% to 3%) ... 1613
WinRho SDF ... 732
▲ Xyrem Oral Solution (Less than 1% to 14.3%) ... 1688
Zantac (Rare) ... 1624
Zantac Injection ... 1619
Zantac Injection Pharmacy Bulk Package (Rare) ... 1622
Zantac Injection Premixed ... 1619
Zantac (Rare) ... 1624
Zegerid Capsules (Less than 1%) ... 2958
Zegerid Powder for Oral Solution (Less than 1%) ... 2958
▲ Zelapar Tablets (3%) ... 3372
Zemplar Injection ... 543
Zicam Maximum Strength Flu Daytime ... ▣ 768
Zicam Maximum Strength Flu Nighttime ... ▣ 768
Zmax for Oral Suspension ... 2583
▲ Zofran Injection (5% to 8%) ... 1634
▲ Zofran (20%) ... 1639
▲ Zofran ODT Orally Disintegrating Tablets (20%) ... 1639
▲ Zoloft (2% to 15%) ... 2586
▲ Zometa for Intravenous Infusion (5% to 10%) ... 2315
▲ Zomig Tablets (Common) ... 3519
▲ Zomig Nasal Spray (0% to 4%) ... 3523
▲ Zomig-ZMT Tablets (Common) ... 3519
▲ Zonegran Capsules (17%) ... 1101
Zovirax ... 1643
Zyban Sustained-Release Tablets (2%) ... 1644
Zydone Tablets ... 1139
Zyflo Tablets (Greater than 1%) ... 1023
▲ Zyprexa Tablets (6% to 52%) ... 1830
▲ Zyprexa IntraMuscular (6%) ... 1830
▲ Zyprexa ZYDIS Orally Disintegrating Tablets (6% to 52%) ... 1830
▲ Zyrtec Chewable Tablets (1.9% to 13.7%) ... 2594
▲ Zyrtec (1.9% to 13.7%) ... 2594
▲ Zyrtec-D 12 Hour Extended Release Tablets (1.9% to 13.7%) ... 2597

Drug abuse

Copegus Tablets (Less than 1%) ... 2754

Drug administration site reactions, unspecified

Abelcet Injection ... 1141
Aloprim for Injection (Less than 1%) ... 2167
▲ AndroGel (3% to 5%) ... 3329
Cardene I.V. (1.4%) ... 2497
Denavir Cream (1.3%) ... 2174
Depacon Injection (2.4%) ... 412
Doxil Injection ... 2351
Duragesic Transdermal System (1% or greater) ... 2373
Engerix-B Vaccine ... 1425
▲ Epogen for Injection (7% to 25%) ... 591
▲ Floxin Otic Solution (0.6% to 16.8%) ... 1049
▲ Fortaz (Among most common) ... 1453
▲ Imitrex Injection (58.7%) ... 1463
▲ Intron A for Injection (Less than 5%) ... 3024
Leukine ... 814
▲ Leustatin Injection (9% to 19%) ... 2357
Lupron Depot 3.75 mg (1%) ... 3260
Lupron Depot–3 Month 11.25 mg (1%) ... 3265
▲ Lupron Depot-PED 7.5 mg, 11.25 mg and 15 mg (5%) ... 3269
Merrem I.V. (1.1%) ... 686
▲ Migranal Nasal Spray (6%) ... 3348
Neupogen for Injection (Infrequent) ... 603
▲ Oncaspar (Greater than 1% but less than 5%) ... 1145
▲ Ontak Vials (8%) ... 1745
▲ Ortho Evra Transdermal System (1% to 22%) ... 2417
▲ Procrit for Injection (7% to 29%) ... 2364
▲ Proleukin for Injection (3%) ... 2266
Retrovir IV Infusion (Infrequent) ... 1564
Rilutek Tablets (Infrequent) ... 2930
▲ Rocephin Injectable Vials, ADD-Vantage, Galaxy, Bulk (5% to 17%) ... 2800
Taxotere Injection Concentrate ... 2932
▲ Testim 1% Gel (2% to 4%) ... 695
▲ Vesanoid Capsules (17%) ... 2820
Zosyn (0.5%) ... 3492
▲ Zyban Sustained-Release Tablets (11%) ... 1644

Drug effect, unspecified, diminished

Mivacron ... 493

Drug fever

Aldoril Tablets ... 1910
Clozaril Tablets ... 2184
DynaCirc CR Tablets (0.5% to 1%) ... 2721
Fansidar Tablets ... 2765
Invirase (Rare) ... 2772
Leukeran Tablets ... 1504
Primaxin I.M. ... 2045
Primaxin I.V. (Less than 0.2%) ... 2048
Suprax (Less than 2%) ... 1843
Taxotere Injection Concentrate ... 2932
Timentin ADD-Vantage ... 1580
Timentin Injection Galaxy Container ... 1583
Timentin IV Infusion ... 1577
Timentin Pharmacy Bulk Package ... 1586
Vancocin HCl Capsules, USP (Infrequent) ... 3380
Zinacef for Injection (Rare) ... 1631
Zinacef Injection (Rare) ... 1631

Drug idiosyncrasies

(*see under* Allergic reactions)

Drug overdose

Campral Tablets (Infrequent) ... 1174
Copegus Tablets (Less than 1%) ... 2754
Keppra Injection ... 3320
Lyrica Capsules (0.1% to 1%) ... 2539
Pegasys (Less than 1%) ... 2789
Prozac Pulvules and Liquid (Infrequent) ... 1801
Reyataz Capsules (Less than 3%) ... 921
Symbyax Capsules (Infrequent) ... 1819

Dry mouth

(*see under* Xerostomia)

Dry skin

(*see under* Xerosis cutis)

Dry sockets

Celebrex Capsules ... 3134

Dryness

Aclovate (Approximately 2%) ... 2660
Analpram-HC ... 1159
Apexicon E Cream ... 2661
Cutivate Cream (1.2%) ... 2662
Cutivate Ointment (Infrequent to more frequent) ... 2665
Elocon Lotion 0.1% (Infrequent) ... 3006
Locoid Lipocream Cream (Infrequent) ... 1160
▲ Naftin Cream (3%) ... 2126
Olux Foam (Less than 1%) ... 1012
Ophthetic Ophthalmic Solution ... ⊙ 232
Pramosone ... 1161
ProQuad ... 2064

Temovate Cream 2668
Temovate Gel (Infrequent) 2669
Temovate Ointment 2668
Temovate Scalp Application (Infrequent) 2670
Temovate E Emollient (Infrequent) 2671
Vanos Cream 1893

Dryness, mucous membrane
Advicor Tablets 1722
Dolobid Tablets (Less than 1 in 100) 1955
Mintezol Chewable Tablets 2027
Myleran Tablets (Rare) 1525
Timolide Tablets (Less than 1%) 2086
▲ Vesanoid Capsules (77%) 2820
Vytorin 10/10 Tablets 2114
Vytorin 10/10 Tablets 3077
Vytorin 10/20 Tablets 2114
Vytorin 10/20 Tablets 3077
Vytorin 10/40 Tablets 2114
Vytorin 10/40 Tablets 3077
Vytorin 10/80 Tablets 2114
Vytorin 10/80 Tablets 3077
Zocor Tablets 2105

Dryness, nose
(*see under* Xeromycteria)

Dryness, vaginal
Effexor Tablets (Rare) 3411
Effexor XR Capsules (Rare) 3417
▲ Femara Tablets (5.3%) 2214
Soltamox Oral Solution (Infrequently) 3527

Dryness, vulvovaginal
Ambien CR Tablets (1%) 2855

Dryness at application site
Clobex Spray (0% to 2%) 1208
Evoclin Foam, 1% (1%) 1009
Ionsys Transdermal System (.1% to less than 1%) 2379

Duodenitis
Aciphex Tablets (Rare) 1090
Actonel with Calcium Tablets (0.1% to 1%) 2688
Effexor Tablets (Rare) 3411
Effexor XR Capsules (Rare) 3417
Evoxac Capsules (Less than 1%) 1047
Invanz for Injection (Greater than 0.1%) 1999
Nexium Delayed-Release Capsules (Less than 1%) 655
Nexium I.V. (Less than 1%) 659
Paxil CR Controlled-Release Tablets (Rare) 1538
Paxil (Rare) 1530
Permax Tablets (Rare) 3356
Pexeva Tablets (rare) 1694
Pletal Tablets (Less than 2%) 2455
Protonix I.V. (Less than 1%) 3472
Protonix Tablets (Less than 1%) 3469
Requip Tablets (Infrequent) 1555
Rythmol SR Capsules 2727
VFEND I.V. (Less than 2%) 2564
VFEND Oral Suspension (Less than 2%) 2564
VFEND Tablets (Less than 2%) 2564
Zonegran Capsules (Rare) 1101

Dupuytren's contracture
Requip Tablets (Rare) 1555

Dypnea
▲ Clolar for Intravenous Infusion (13%) 1271
Ionsys Transdermal System (.1% to less than 1%) 2379
▲ Ribavirin, USP Capsules (24%) 3068
Ultane Liquid for Inhalation (Less than 1%) 531

Dysarthria
Abilify Oral Solution (Infrequent) 882
Abilify Oral Solution (Infrequent) 2450
Abilify Discmelt Orally Disintegrating Tablets (Infrequent) 882
Abilify Discmelt Orally Disintegrating Tablets (Infrequent) 2450
Abilify Tablets (Infrequent) 882
Abilify Tablets (Infrequent) 2450
Ambien Tablets (Infrequent) 2851
Ambien CR Tablets (Infrequent) 2855
Aricept Tablets (Infrequent) 1094
Aricept ODT Tablets (Infrequent) 1094
Arranon Injection (1%) 1357
Azilect Tablets (Infrequent) 3293
Chantix Tablets (Rare) 2517
Clozaril Tablets (Less than 1%) 2184
Cymbalta Delayed-Release Capsules (Infrequent) 1757
Depacon Injection 412
Depakene 417
Depakote Sprinkle Capsules 422
▲ Depakote Tablets (1% to 5%) 427
Depakote ER Tablets (Greater than 1%) 434
Diastat Rectal Delivery System (Greater than or equal to 1%) 3343
Eloxatin for Injection 2892
Emend Capsules (Less than or equal to 0.5%) 1963
FazaClo Orally Disintegrating Tablets (Less than 1%) 551
Gabitril Tablets (Frequent) 984
Geodon Capsules (Frequent) 2529
Imitrex Injection (Rare) 1463
Imitrex Nasal Spray (Infrequent) 1467
Imitrex Tablets (Infrequent) 1471
Indocin Capsules (Less than 1%) 1995
Indocin I.V. (Less than 1%) 2465
Indocin (Less than 1%) 1995
Invirase (Less than 2%) 2772
Klonopin (2%) 2778
Lamictal (1.0%) 1481
Lyrica Capsules (0.1% to 1%) 2539
Maxalt Tablets (Infrequent) 2008
Maxalt-MLT Orally Disintegrating Tablets (Infrequent) 2008
Neumega for Injection 3435
Neurontin Capsules (2.4%) 2487
Neurontin Oral Solution (2.4%) 2487
Neurontin Tablets (2.4%) 2487
Nipent for Injection (Less than 3%) 1863
▲ Niravam Orally Disintegrating Tablets (23.3%) 3092
Paxil CR Controlled-Release Tablets (Rare) 1538
Paxil (Rare) 1530
Pexeva Tablets (Rare) 1694
Protonix I.V. (Less than 1%) 3472
Protonix Tablets (Less than 1%) 3469
Prozac Pulvules and Liquid (Rare) 1801
Revlimid Capsules 958
Rilutek Tablets (Infrequent) 2930
Risperdal (Infrequent) 1676
Risperdal M-Tab Orally Disintegrating Tablets (Infrequent) 1676
Seromycin Capsules 1813
Seroquel Tablets (Frequent) 690
Sonata Capsules (Rare) 1717
Symbyax Capsules (Infrequent) 1819
Valium Tablets (Infrequent) 2819
Valtrex Caplets 1597
▲ Vesanoid Capsules (3%) 2820
Wellbutrin Tablets (Infrequent) 1603
Wellbutrin SR Sustained-Release Tablets 1607
Wellbutrin XL Extended-Release Tablets 1613
▲ Xeloda Tablets (Less than 5%) 2822
Xyrem Oral Solution (Infrequent) 1688
Zonegran Capsules (Infrequent) 1101
Zovirax 1643
Zyban Sustained-Release Tablets 1644
Zyprexa Tablets (Infrequent) 1830
Zyprexa ZYDIS Orally Disintegrating Tablets (Infrequent) 1830

Dysautonomia
Azilect Tablets (Infrequent) 3293
Lyrica Capsules (Rare) 2539

Dyscrasias, blood
(*see under* Blood dyscrasias)

Dysdiadochokinesia
Klonopin 2778

Dysentery
Xifaxan Tablets (Less than 2%) 2842

Dysesthesia
AmBisome for Injection (Less common) 620
▲ Astelin Nasal Spray (7.9%) 1904
Avelox 2970
Azilect Tablets (Infrequent) 3293
Copaxone for Injection (At least 2%) 3297
Evoxac Capsules (Less than 1%) 1047
Floxin Otic Solution (Single report) 1049
Frova Tablets (Frequent) 1113
Imitrex Injection (Rare) 1463
Imitrex Nasal Spray (Rare) 1467
Imitrex Tablets (Rare) 1471
Invirase (Less than 2%) 2772
▲ Kepivance (12%) 597
Levulan Kerastick for Topical Solution, 20% (2%) 1085
Maxalt Tablets (Rare) 2008
Maxalt-MLT Orally Disintegrating Tablets (Rare) 2008
Neurontin Capsules (Infrequent) 2487
Neurontin Oral Solution (Infrequent) 2487
Neurontin Tablets (Infrequent) 2487
Prinivil Tablets (0.3% to 1.0%) 2052
Prinzide Tablets 2056
Proquin XR Tablets 1153
▲ Taxotere Injection Concentrate (7 of 134 patients) 2932
Tequin Injection 938
Tequin Injection in 5% Dextrose 938
Tequin Tablets 938
Thalomid Capsules 965
Vasotec I.V. Injection (0.5% to 1.0%) 2103
▲ Velcade for Injection (23%) 2133

Dysesthesia, hemifacial
Prilosec OTC Delayed-Release Tablets (Less than 1%) 2677
Zegerid Capsules (Less than 1%) 2958
Zegerid Powder for Oral Solution (Less than 1%) 2958

Dysgeusia
Advate Injection (2.6%) 712
Altoprev Extended-Release Tablets 3109
Amitiza Capsules (Less than 0.2%) 3224
▲ Arranon Injection (0% to 3%) 1357
Byetta Injection 611
Captopril Tablets (Approximately 2 to 4 of 100 patients) 2149
Cardizem LA Extended Release Tablets (Less than 2%) 1728
▲ Chantix Tablets (5% to 8%) 2517
Cozaar Tablets 1935
Emend Capsules (Greater than 0.5%) 1963
Ferrlecit Injection 3388
Havrix Vaccine (Less than 1%) 1456
Ketek Tablets (1.5% to 1.6%) 2903
Lithobid Tablets 1692
Maxalt Tablets 2008
Maxalt-MLT Orally Disintegrating Tablets 2008
Mevacor Tablets (0.8%) 2021
Mycamine for Injection (0.7%) 628
Noroxin Tablets 2032
▲ Revlimid Capsules (6.1% to 13.3%) 958
Rocephin Injectable Vials, ADD-Vantage, Galaxy, Bulk (Less than 1%) 2800
Rozerem Tablets (2%) 3231
Sanctura Tablets (Greater than or equal to 0.5%) 1151
Tiazac Capsules (Less than 1%) 1201
Twinrix Vaccine (Less than 1%) 1595
▲ Velcade for Injection (13%) 2133
Vivitrol 995
Xyrem Oral Solution (Infrequent) 1688

Dyskinesia
Abilify Oral Solution (Infrequent) 882
Abilify Oral Solution (Infrequent) 2450
Abilify Discmelt Orally Disintegrating Tablets (Infrequent) 882
Abilify Discmelt Orally Disintegrating Tablets (Infrequent) 2450
Abilify Tablets (Infrequent) 882
Abilify Tablets (Infrequent) 2450
Adderall Tablets 3164
Adderall XR Capsules 3166
▲ Azilect Tablets (18%) 3293
Bentyl Capsules 697
Bentyl Injection 697
Bentyl Syrup 697
Bentyl Tablets 697
Celexa 1176
▲ Comtan Tablets (25%) 2189
Concerta Extended-Release Tablets 1881
Cubicin for Injection (Less than 1%) 1026
Daytrana Transdermal Patch 3174
Dexedrine 1420
DextroStat Tablets 3179
Effexor Tablets (Rare) 3411
▲ Eldepryl Capsules (2 of 49 patients) 3208
Evoxac Capsules (Less than 1%) 1047
▲ Exelon Capsules (Frequent) 2206
▲ Exelon Oral Solution (Frequent) 2206
Focalin Tablets 2220
Focalin XR Capsules 2223
▲ Geodon Capsules (14%) 2529
Kaletra (Less than 2%) 476
Lamictal (Infrequent) 1481
Lexapro Oral Solution 1190
Lexapro Tablets 1190
Lyrica Capsules (Rare) 2539
Metadate CD Capsules 3323
▲ Mirapex Tablets (47%) 859
Namenda 1195
Neurontin Capsules 2487
Neurontin Oral Solution 2487
Neurontin Tablets 2487
Parcopa Orally Disintegrating Tablets (Common) 3097
Paxil CR Controlled-Release Tablets (Rare) 1538
Paxil (Rare) 1530
▲ Permax Tablets (62.4%) 3356
Pexeva Tablets (infrequent) 1694
Phenytek Capsules (Rare) 2160
Provigil Tablets (1%) 988
Prozac Pulvules and Liquid 1801
Requip Tablets (1% or more) 1555
Risperdal Consta Long-Acting Injection (Infrequent) 1682
Ritalin Hydrochloride Tablets 2269
Ritalin LA Capsules 2271
Ritalin-SR Tablets 2269
Seroquel Tablets (Infrequent) 690
▲ Stalevo Tablets (5% to 25%) 2287
▲ Tasmar Tablets (42% to 51%) 3358
Thalomid Capsules 965
Topamax Sprinkle Capsules (Infrequent) 2404
Topamax Tablets (Infrequent) 2404
Wellbutrin Tablets (Frequent) 1603
Wellbutrin SR Sustained-Release Tablets 1607
Wellbutrin XL Extended-Release Tablets 1613
Xyrem Oral Solution (Infrequent) 1688
▲ Zelapar Tablets (6%) 3372
Zoloft (Rare) 2586
Zonegran Capsules 1101
Zyban Sustained-Release Tablets 1644
Zyprexa Tablets (1% to 2%) 1830
Zyprexa ZYDIS Orally Disintegrating Tablets (1% to 2%) 1830

Dyskinesia, orofacial
Neurontin Capsules (Rare) 2487
Neurontin Oral Solution (Rare) 2487
Neurontin Tablets (Rare) 2487
Provigil Tablets (At least 1%) 988
Zyrtec Chewable Tablets (Rare) 2594
Zyrtec (Rare) 2594
Zyrtec-D 12 Hour Extended Release Tablets (Rare) 2597

Dyskinesia, tardive
(*see under* Tardive dyskinesia)

Dyslipidemia
Cymbalta Delayed-Release Capsules (Infrequent) 1757

Dysmenorrhea
Abilify Oral Solution 882
Abilify Oral Solution 2450
Abilify Discmelt Orally Disintegrating Tablets 882
Abilify Discmelt Orally Disintegrating Tablets 2450
Abilify Tablets 882
Abilify Tablets 2450
Aciphex Tablets 1090
▲ Adderall XR Capsules (2% to 4%) 3166
Advair Diskus 100/50 1308
Advair Diskus 250/50 1308
Advair Diskus 500/50 1308
Advair HFA Inhalation Aerosol 1318
Alamast Ophthalmic Solution (Less than 5%) 3381
Allegra (1.5%) 2844
Angeliq Tablets 762
Arthrotec Tablets (Rare) 3129
▲ Asacol Delayed-Release Tablets (3%) 2692
▲ Asmanex Twisthaler (4% to 9%) 2966
Axert Tablets (Infrequent) 2396
▲ Betaseron for SC Injection (7%) 767
Celebrex Capsules (0.1% to 1.9%) 3134
▲ Celexa (3%) 1176
Cipro XR Tablets (Less than 1%) 2990
Clarinex Tablets (2.1%) 2995
Clarinex Reditabs Tablets (2.1%) 2995
Clozaril Tablets (Less than 1%) 2184
Concerta Extended-Release Tablets (2%) 1881
▲ Copaxone for Injection (6%) 3297
▲ Depacon Injection (1% to 5%) 412
▲ Depakene (1% to 5%) 417
▲ Depakote Sprinkle Capsules (1% to 5%) 422
▲ Depakote Tablets (1% to 5%) 427
Depakote ER Tablets (Greater than 1%) 434

Depo-Provera Contraceptive Injection (Less than 1%) 2622
Effexor Tablets 3411
▲ Effexor XR Capsules (6%) 3417
Elidel Cream 1% (1.1% to 1.5%) 2200
▲ Enjuvia Tablets (1% to 8%) 1062
Estrasorb Topical Emulsion 1147
Estratest Tablets 3199
Estratest H.S. Tablets 3199
Evoxac Capsules (Less than 1%) 1047
▲ Famvir Tablets (2.2% to 7.6%) 2211
FazaClo Orally Disintegrating Tablets (Less than 1%) 551
Fluarix (1.3%) 1451
Gabitril Tablets (Frequent) 984
Geodon for Injection (Up to 2%) 2529
▲ Hycamtin for Injection (59%) 1458
Imitrex Injection (Rare) 1463
Imitrex Nasal Spray (Infrequent) 1467
Imitrex Tablets (Infrequent) 1471
▲ Infergen (2% to 9%) 3364
▲ Intron A for Injection (Less than 5%) 3024
▲ Klonopin (3%) 2778
▲ Lamictal (6.6%) 1481
Levaquin (0.1% to 0.9%) 2384
Levaquin in 5% Dextrose Injection (0.1% to 0.9%) 2384
▲ Lunesta Tablets (0% to 3%) 3142
Lyrica Capsules (0.1% to 1%) 2539
Menostar Transdermal System 782
▲ Meridia Capsules (3.5%) 489
▲ Mirena Intrauterine System (5% or more) 787
▲ Nasonex Nasal Spray (1% to 5%) 3043
Neurontin Capsules (Infrequent) 2487
Neurontin Oral Solution (Infrequent) 2487
Neurontin Tablets (Infrequent) 2487
Nexium Delayed-Release Capsules (Less than 1%) 655
Nexium I.V. (Less than 1%) 659
Noroxin Tablets (Less frequent) 2032
ParaGard T 380A Intrauterine Copper Contraceptive 1073
Paxil CR Controlled-Release Tablets (Infrequent) 1538
Paxil (Infrequent) 1530
Permax Tablets (Frequent) 3356
Premarin Intravenous 3442
Premarin Tablets 3446
Premarin Vaginal Cream 3452
▲ Premphase Tablets (3% to 13%) 3456
▲ Prempro Tablets (3% to 13%) 3456
Prevacid Delayed-Release Capsules (Less than 1%) 3271
Prevacid for Delayed-Release Oral Suspension (Less than 1%) 3271
Prevacid SoluTab Delayed-Release Orally Disintegrating Tablets (Less than 1%) 3271
Prevacid NapraPAC (Less than 1%) 3280
PREVPAC (Less than 1%) 3284
Prochieve 4% Gel 1003
Prochieve 8% Gel 1003
Protonix I.V. (Less than 1%) 3472
Protonix Tablets (Less than 1%) 3469
▲ Protopic Ointment (Up to 4%) 638
Provigil Tablets (At least 1%) 988
Prozac Pulvules and Liquid 1801
Qvar Inhalation Aerosol (1% to 3%) 3303
Risperdal (Infrequent) 1676
Risperdal Consta Long-Acting Injection (Infrequent) 1682
Risperdal M-Tab Orally Disintegrating Tablets (Infrequent) 1676
Seasonique Tablets 1077
Seroquel Tablets (Infrequent) 690
▲ Sonata Capsules (3% to 4%) 1717
▲ Strattera Capsules (5% or greater) 1814
Topamax Sprinkle Capsules (More than 1%) 2404
Topamax Tablets (More than 1%) 2404
Uniretic Tablets (Less than 1%) 3100
▲ Valtrex Caplets (Less than 1% to 8%) 1597
▲ Vandazole Vaginal Gel (3%) 3338
VFEND I.V. (Less than 2%) 2564
VFEND Oral Suspension (Less than 2%) 2564
VFEND Tablets (Less than 2%) 2564
Wellbutrin SR Sustained-Release Tablets (At least 1%) 1607
Wellbutrin XL Extended-Release Tablets (At least 1% to 2%) 1613
Yasmin 28 Tablets (Greater than 1%) 796
Yaz Tablets (Greater than 1%) 803
Zelnorm Tablets (1% to 2%) 2312
Zoloft (Infrequent) 2586
Zomig Tablets (Rare) 3519
Zomig Nasal Spray (Rare) 3523
Zomig-ZMT Tablets (Rare) 3519
Zyprexa Tablets (2%) 1830
Zyprexa ZYDIS Orally Disintegrating Tablets (2%) 1830
Zyrtec Chewable Tablets (Less than 2%) 2594
Zyrtec (Less than 2%) 2594
Zyrtec-D 12 Hour Extended Release Tablets (Less than 2%) 2597

Dysmetria

Trileptal Tablets 2300
Trileptal Oral Suspension 2300

Dyspareunia

Depo-Provera Contraceptive Injection (Less than 1%) 2622
▲ Hycamtin for Injection (59%) 1458
Lyrica Capsules (Rare) 2539
ParaGard T 380A Intrauterine Copper Contraceptive 1073
▲ Prochieve 4% Gel (6%) 1003
▲ Prochieve 8% Gel (6%) 1003
Wellbutrin Tablets (Rare) 1603
Wellbutrin SR Sustained-Release Tablets 1607
Wellbutrin XL Extended-Release Tablets 1613
Zyban Sustained-Release Tablets 1644

Dyspepsia

Abelcet Injection 1141
▲ Abilify Oral Solution (15%) 882
▲ Abilify Oral Solution (15%) 2450
▲ Abilify Discmelt Orally Disintegrating Tablets (15%) 882
▲ Abilify Discmelt Orally Disintegrating Tablets (15%) 2450
▲ Abilify Tablets (15%) 882
▲ Abilify Tablets (15%) 2450
Accolate Tablets (1.5%) 671
Aceon Tablets (2 mg, 4 mg, 8 mg) (0.3% to 1.9%) 3194
Acetadote Injection (.24% to 1.17%) 1031
Aciphex Tablets 1090
Actiq (1% or greater) 979
▲ Actonel Tablets (6.9% to 7.6%) 2683
▲ Actonel with Calcium Tablets (6.9% to 7.6%) 2688
Adalat CC Tablets (Less than 1%) 2964
Adderall XR Capsules (2%) 3166
Advair Diskus 100/50 1308
Advair Diskus 250/50 1308
Advair Diskus 500/50 1308
Advair HFA Inhalation Aerosol 1318
▲ Advicor Tablets (3%) 1722
▲ Aerobid/Aerobid-M (1% to 3%) 1171
▲ Aggrenox Capsules (18.4%) 822
▲ Agrylin Capsules (5.2%) 3169
Aldara Cream, 5% (2.8%) 1846
▲ Alferon N Injection (3%) 1665
Alinia for Oral Suspension (Less than 1%) 2835
Alinia Tablets (Less than 1%) 2835
Allegra (1.3%) 2844
Allegra-D 12 Hour Extended-Release Tablets (2.8%) 2846
Allegra-D 24 Hour Extended-Release Tablets (2.8%) 2849
Aloxi Injection (Less than 1%) 2127
▲ Alphagan P Ophthalmic Solution (1% to 4%) 567
Altace Capsules (Less than 1%) 1702
Altoprev Extended-Release Tablets (1% to 1.6%) 3109
▲ Ambien Tablets (5%) 2851
Ambien CR Tablets (Frequent) 2855
AmBisome for Injection (Less common) 620
Amerge Tablets (Infrequent) 1339
Amitiza Capsules (0% to 2.9%) 3224
Anaprox Tablets (Less than 3%) 2761
Anaprox DS Tablets (Less than 3%) 2761
▲ Anzemet Injection (3%) 2859
▲ Anzemet Tablets (3%) 2862
Aptivus Capsules (Less than 2%) 826
▲ Aredia for Injection (22.6%) 2179
▲ Arimidex Tablets (5% to 7%) 673
Arixtra Injection (0.3% to 2.4%) 1351
▲ Aromasin Tablets (2% to 5%) 2600
▲ Arthrotec Tablets (14%) 3129
▲ Asacol Delayed-Release Tablets (6%) 2692
▲ Asmanex Twisthaler (3% to 5%) 2966
Atacand Tablets (0.5% or greater) 649
Atacand HCT (0.5% or greater) 651
Atripla Tablets (Greater than or equal to 2%) 945
▲ Atrovent HFA Inhalation Aerosol (1% to 5%) 841
Avalide Tablets (2%) 888
Avalide Tablets (2%) 2874
▲ Avandamet Tablets (10%) 1373
Avapro Tablets (2%) 891
Avapro Tablets (2%) 2871
▲ Avastin IV (17% to 24%) 1227
Avelox (0.1% to less than 2%) 2970
▲ Avinza Capsules (Less than 5%) 1741
Axert Tablets (Infrequent) 2396
▲ Axid Oral Solution (3.6%) 879
▲ Azilect Tablets (5% to 7%) 3293
Azopt Ophthalmic Suspension (Less than 1%) 557
Baraclude (Less than or equal to 1%) 894
Bayer Aspirin 744
Bayer Aspirin Comprehensive Prescribing Information ▣796
Benicar Tablets (Greater than 0.5%) 1043
Benicar HCT Tablets (Greater than 1%) 1044
▲ Betaseron for SC Injection (14%) 767
▲ Bexxar (Less than 1% to 6%) 1398
Biaxin/Biaxin XL (2%) 402
Blocadren Tablets (0.6%) 1916
▲ Boniva Injection (5.6% to 11.9%) 2738
▲ Boniva Tablets (5.6% to 11.9%) 2741
Buprenex Injectable (Infrequent) 2716
▲ Byetta Injection (6%) 611
Caduet Tablets (Less than 1% to 2.8%) 2508
▲ Campath Ampules (10%) 811
Campral Tablets (Frequent) 1174
▲ Camptosar Injection (0% to 10%) 2604
Captopril Tablets 2149
Cardene I.V. (Rare) 2497
Cardura XL Tablets (1.4%) 2515
▲ Carnitor Injection (5% to 9%) 3188
Ceftin Tablets (0.1% to 1%) 1407
▲ Celebrex Capsules (8.8%) 3134
▲ Celexa (5%) 1176
▲ CellCept Capsules (22.4%) 2747
▲ CellCept Intravenous (22.4%) 2747
▲ CellCept Oral Suspension (22.4%) 2747
▲ CellCept Tablets (22.4%) 2747
Cesamet Capsules 3340
▲ Chantix Tablets (5%) 2517
▲ Cialis Tablets (4% to 10%) 1838
Cipro (2.7%) 2977
Cipro I.V. (2.7%) 2984
Cipro XR Tablets (1%) 2990
▲ Clarinex Tablets (3%) 2995
▲ Clarinex Reditabs Tablets (3%) 2995
▲ Clinoril Tablets (3% to 9%) 1924
▲ Clozaril Tablets (14%) 2184
Colazal Capsules (2%) 2838
Combivent Inhalation Aerosol (Less than 2%) 847
▲ Combivir Tablets (5%) 1411
Comtan Tablets (2%) 2189
Copaxone for Injection (At least 2%) 3297
▲ Copegus Tablets (6%) 2754
▲ Cosopt Sterile Ophthalmic Solution (1% to 5%) 1931
Cozaar Tablets (1% or greater) 1935
▲ Crestor Tablets (3.4%) 678
Crixivan Capsules (1.5%) 1940
▲ Cubicin for Injection (0.9% to 4.2%) 1026
▲ Cymbalta Delayed-Release Capsules (4%) 1757
▲ Dacogen Injection (12%) 2129
Dalmane Capsules 3342
Demadex Injection (1.6%) 2759
Demadex Tablets (1.6%) 2759
▲ Depacon Injection (8% to 11%) 412
▲ Depakene (8% to 11%) 417
▲ Depakote Sprinkle Capsules (8% to 11%) 422
▲ Depakote Tablets (8% to 13%) 427
▲ Depakote ER Tablets (7% to 23%) 434
▲ DepoDur Extended-Release Injection (2% to 5%) 1110
▲ Detrol Tablets (4%) 2628
▲ Detrol LA Capsules (3%) 2631
Diovan Tablets 2193
Diovan HCT Tablets (Greater than 0.2%) 2196
▲ Ditropan XL Extended-Release Tablets (5% to 7%) 2413
▲ Dolobid Tablets (3% to 9%) 1955
▲ Doxil Injection (Less than 1% to 12.1%) 2351
DuoNeb Inhalation Solution (1.3%) 1058
▲ Duragesic Transdermal System (3% to 10%) 2373
EC-Naprosyn Delayed-Release Tablets (Less than 3%) 2761
▲ Effexor Tablets (4.5% to 5%) 3411
Effexor XR Capsules (At least 2%) 3417
Eligard 22.5 mg (Less than 2%) 2883
Elmiron Capsules (2%) 2415
▲ Eloxatin for Injection (7% to 14%) 2892
▲ Emend Capsules (8.4%) 1963
▲ Emsam Transdermal System (4%) 903
▲ Emtriva Capsules (4% to 8%) 1287
▲ Emtriva Oral Solution (4% to 8%) 1287
▲ Enablex Extended-Release Tablets (2.7% to 8.4%) 2203
▲ Enbrel for Injection (4% to 11%) 584
Engerix-B Vaccine 1425
▲ Entocort EC Capsules (6%) 2698
▲ Epivir (5%) 1427
▲ Epogen for Injection (9% to 11%) 591
▲ Equetro Extended-Release Capsules (10%) 3180
Eraxis for Injection (0.3%) 2521
▲ Erbitux (6% to 14%) 910
▲ Estring Vaginal Ring (1% to 3%) 2635
▲ Evista Tablets (5.9%) 1763
▲ Evoxac Capsules (7.8%) 1047
▲ Exelon Capsules (9%) 2206
▲ Exelon Oral Solution (9%) 2206
▲ Fabrazyme for Intravenous Infusion (3%) 1274
▲ Famvir Tablets (1.1% to 3.4%) 2211
▲ FazaClo Orally Disintegrating Tablets (14%) 551
▲ Femara Tablets (3% to 4%) 2214
Ferrlecit Injection 3388
Floxin Otic Solution (Single report) 1049
Flumadine (0.3% to 1%) 1183
▲ Focalin XR Capsules (5% to 9%) 2223
▲ Fortamet Extended-Release Tablets (4.2%) 3115
▲ Forteo for Injection (5.2%) 1767
▲ Fortical Nasal Spray (1% to 3%) 3337
▲ Fosamax (1.1% to 3.6%) 1969
▲ Fosamax Plus D Tablets (1.1% to 3.6%) 1977
Frova Tablets (2%) 1113
Gabitril Tablets (1% or more) 984
▲ Gengraf Capsules (2.2% to 8%) 459
▲ Geodon (8%) 2529
▲ Gleevec Tablets (0% to 27%) 2227
▲ Hectorol Capsules (4.9% to greater than or equal to 5%) 1275
▲ Hectorol Injection (4.9%) 1278
▲ Hepsera Tablets (3%) 1292
Hytrin Capsules (At least 1%) 471
Hyzaar 50-12.5 Tablets 1990
Hyzaar 100-12.5 Tablets 1990
Hyzaar 100-25 Tablets 1990
▲ Imdur Tablets (Less than or equal to 5%) 3018
Imitrex Nasal Spray 1467
▲ Indapamide Tablets (Less than 5%) 2156
▲ Indocin (3% to 9%) 1995
▲ Infergen (12% to 21%) 3364
▲ Intron A for Injection (Up to 8%) 3024
Invanz for Injection (1% to 1.1%) 1999
Invirase (0.9% to greater than or equal to 2%) 2772
▲ Ionsys Transdermal System (1% to less than 10%) 2379
▲ I.V. Busulfex (44%) 2493
Kadian Capsules (Less than 3%) 577
▲ Kaletra (1% to 5%) 476
Keflex Capsules 549
Keppra Injection 3320
Keppra Oral Solution (1% or more) 3314
Keppra Tablets (1% or more) 3314
Ketek Tablets (Greater than or equal to 0.2% to less than 2%) 2903
Klonopin (Infrequent) 2778
▲ Kytril Injection (3%) 2781
▲ Kytril (4% to 6%) 2784
▲ Lamictal (2% to 7%) 1481
▲ Lamisil Tablets (4.3%) 2232
Lariam Tablets 2786
▲ Lescol Capsules (7.9%) 2233
▲ Lescol XL Tablets (3.5%) 2233
▲ Leukine (17%) 814
Levaquin (0.2% to 2.3%) 2384
Levaquin in 5% Dextrose Injection (0.2% to 2.3%) 2384
▲ Levitra Tablets (4%) 3034
Lexapro Oral Solution (Infrequent) 1190
Lexapro Tablets (Infrequent) 1190
Limbrel Capsules 2672
Lipitor Tablets (1.3% to 2.8%) 2483
Lofibra Tablets 1219
Lofibra Capsules 1216
Lotensin HCT Tablets (0.3% to 1%) 2246
Lotrel Capsules 2249
Lotronex Tablets (Infrequent) 1512
▲ Lunesta Tablets (2% to 6%) 3142
▲ Macugen Injection (1% to 5%) ⊙261
▲ Malarone Pediatric Tablets (1% to 3%) 1517
▲ Malarone Tablets (1% to 3%) 1517
▲ Mavik Tablets (0.3% to 6.4%) 486
Maxalt Tablets (Infrequent) 2008
Maxalt-MLT Orally Disintegrating Tablets (Infrequent) 2008
▲ Megace ES Oral Suspension (0% to 4%) 2481
▲ Menostar Transdermal System (5%) 782
▲ Mepron Suspension (5%) 1521
▲ Meridia Capsules (5%) 489

Merrem I.V. (Greater than 0.1% to 1%) ... 686
▲ Mevacor Tablets (1.0% to 3.9%) ... 2021
▲ Miacalcin Nasal Spray (1% to 3%) ... 2253
Micardis Tablets (1%) ... 854
Micardis HCT Tablets (Less than 2%) ... 856
▲ Midamor Tablets (Less than or equal to 1%) ... 2026
Migranal Nasal Spray (Infrequent) ... 3348
Mirapex Tablets (Greater than or equal to 1%) ... 859
▲ Mobic Oral Suspension (3.8% to 8.9%) ... 863
▲ Mobic Tablets (3.8% to 8.9%) ... 863
Moduretic Tablets ... 2028
MoviPrep Oral Solution (2.8%) ... 2839
▲ Myfortic Tablets (3% to 22.5%) ... 2255
▲ Mylotarg for Injection (8% to 27%) ... 3431
▲ Myobloc Injection (0% to 10%) ... 3192
▲ Nalfon Capsules (10.3%) ... 2502
Naprosyn Suspension (Less than 3%) ... 2761
Naprosyn Tablets (Less than 3%) ... 2761
Nasonex Nasal Spray (Greater than or equal to 2%) ... 3043
▲ Neoral Oral Solution (2.2% to 8%) ... 2259
▲ Neoral Soft Gelatin Capsules (2.2% to 8%) ... 2259
▲ Neulasta Injection (15% to 72%) ... 601
▲ Neumega for Injection (Greater than or equal to 10%) ... 3435
Neurontin Capsules (1% to 2.2%) ... 2487
Neurontin Oral Solution (1% to 2.2%) ... 2487
Neurontin Tablets (1% to 2.2%) ... 2487
▲ Nexavar Tablets (Common) ... 746
Nexium Delayed-Release Capsules (Less than 1%) ... 655
Nexium I.V. (Less than 1%) ... 659
▲ Nipent for Injection (3% to 10%) ... 1863
Noroxin Tablets (0.3% to 1.0%) ... 2032
Norvasc Tablets (Less than 1% to 2%) ... 2545
▲ Norvir (0% to 5.9%) ... 503
▲ Omacor Capsules (3.1%) ... 2725
Omnicef Capsules (0.7%) ... 511
Omnicef for Oral Suspension (0.2%) ... 511
▲ Ontak Vials (7%) ... 1745
Opana Tablets (Less than 1%) ... 1122
Opana ER Tablets (Less than 1%) ... 1126
▲ Orencia Powder for Intravenous Infusion (6%) ... 914
▲ OxyContin Tablets (Between 1% and 5%) ... 2703
Parcopa Orally Disintegrating Tablets ... 3097
▲ Paxil CR Controlled-Release Tablets (2% to 5%) ... 1538
▲ Paxil (2% to 5%) ... 1530
Pegasys (Less than 1%) ... 2789
▲ PEG-Intron Powder for Injection (6%) ... 3048
Pentasa Capsules (1.6%) ... 3185
Percodan Tablets ... 1132
▲ Permax Tablets (6.4%) ... 3356
Persantine Tablets (Rare) ... 868
Pexeva Tablets (2%) ... 1694
▲ Photofrin for Injection (6%) ... 702
▲ Plavix Tablets (5.2%) ... 917
▲ Plavix Tablets (5.2%) ... 2926
▲ Pletal Tablets (6%) ... 2455
▲ Premarin Tablets (9% to 11%) ... 3446
▲ Premphase Tablets (5% to 8%) ... 3456
▲ Prempro Tablets (5% to 8%) ... 3456
Prevacid Delayed-Release Capsules (Less than 1%) ... 3271
Prevacid for Delayed-Release Oral Suspension (Less than 1%) ... 3271
Prevacid SoluTab Delayed-Release Orally Disintegrating Tablets (Less than 1%) ... 3271
Prevacid I.V. for Injection (Less than 1%) ... 3277
Prevacid NapraPAC (Less than 3%) ... 3280
▲ PREVPAC (Less than 1% to 3%) ... 3284
Prezista Tablets (Less than 2%) ... 3306
Prinivil Tablets (0.3% to 1.0%) ... 2052
Prinzide Tablets (1.3%) ... 2056
Prochieve 4% Gel ... 1003
Prochieve 8% Gel ... 1003
▲ Procrit for Injection (7% to 11%) ... 2364
▲ Prograf Capsules and Injection (3% to 28%) ... 632
▲ Proleukin for Injection (7%) ... 2266
▲ Prometrium Capsules (100 mg, 200 mg) (Less than 5%) ... 3203
Proquin XR Tablets (Less than 1%) ... 1153
ProSom Tablets (2%) ... 517
Protonix I.V. (Greater than 1%) ... 3472
Protonix Tablets (Greater than or equal to 1%) ... 3469
▲ Protopic Ointment (1% to 4%) ... 638
Proventil Inhalation Solution 0.083% (1% to 1.5%) ... 3055
▲ Provigil Tablets (5%) ... 988
▲ Prozac Pulvules and Liquid (6% to 10%) ... 1801
▲ Pulmozyme Inhalation Solution (3%) ... 1248
▲ Rapamune Oral Solution and Tablets (17% to 25%) ... 3475
▲ Razadyne (5%) ... 2399
▲ Razadyne ER Extended-Release Capsules (5%) ... 2399
▲ Rebetol (Less than 1% to 16%) ... 3058
▲ Rebetron Combination Therapy (14% to 16%) ... 3063
Recombivax HB (Less than 1%) ... 2071
ReFacto Vials ... 3484
▲ Relpax Tablets (1% to 2%) ... 2548
▲ Remicade for IV Injection (10%) ... 971
▲ Renagel Tablets (5% to 16.2%) ... 1282
ReoPro Vials (2.1%) ... 1809
▲ Requip Tablets (4% to 10%) ... 1555
Rescriptor Tablets ... 2551
▲ Retrovir Capsules (5% to 6%) ... 1560
▲ Retrovir IV Infusion (5% to 6%) ... 1564
▲ Retrovir (5% to 6%) ... 1560
▲ Revatio Tablets (13%) ... 2557
▲ Revlimid Capsules (13.9%) ... 958
Reyataz Capsules (Less than 3%) ... 921
▲ Ribavirin, USP Capsules (Less than 1% to 16%) ... 3068
▲ Rilutek Tablets (2.5% to 6.1%) ... 2930
▲ Risperdal (5% to 11%) ... 1676
▲ Risperdal Consta Long-Acting Injection (7%) ... 1682
▲ Risperdal M-Tab Orally Disintegrating Tablets (5% to 11%) ... 1676
▲ Rituxan I.V. (3%) ... 1254
Rocephin Injectable Vials, ADD-Vantage, Galaxy, Bulk (Rare) ... 2800
Rythmol SR Capsules ... 2727
Sanctura Tablets (1.2%) ... 1151
▲ Sandostatin LAR Depot (5% to 15%) ... 2280
Serevent Diskus (1% to less than 3%) ... 1568
▲ Seroquel Tablets (5%) ... 690
▲ Simulect for Injection (Greater than or equal to 10%) ... 2284
Singulair (2.1%) ... 2077
Sonata Capsules (Frequent) ... 1717
Soriatane Capsules (Less than 1%) ... 1013
▲ Spiriva HandiHaler (1% to 6%) ... 869
St. Joseph 81 mg Aspirin Chewable and Enteric Coated Tablets ... 1869
St. Joseph 81 mg Aspirin ... ▣ 688
Stalevo Tablets (2%) ... 2287
▲ Strattera Capsules (4% to 8%) ... 1814
▲ Suboxone Tablets (3%) ... 2717
▲ Subutex Tablets (3%) ... 2717
Sular Tablets (Less than or equal to 1%) ... 3122
▲ Suprax (3%) ... 1843
Sustiva Capsules (1% to 4%) ... 930
Sustiva Tablets (1% to 4%) ... 930
▲ Sutent Capsules (1% to 46%) ... 2560
Tambocor Tablets (1% to 3%) ... 1856
Tamiflu Capsules ... 2807
▲ Tarceva Tablets (0% to 17%) ... 1259
▲ Tarceva Tablets (0% to 17%) ... 2444
Targretin Capsules ... 1747
Tarka Tablets (0.3% or more) ... 524
▲ Tasmar Tablets (3% to 4%) ... 3358
▲ Tequin Injection (0.1% to 3%) ... 938
▲ Tequin Injection in 5% Dextrose (0.1% to 3%) ... 938
▲ Tequin Tablets (0.1% to 3%) ... 938
Teveten Tablets (1% or greater) ... 1735
Teveten HCT Tablets (Less than 1%) ... 1737
Thalomid Capsules ... 965
▲ Tiazac Capsules (4%) ... 1201
▲ Ticlid Tablets (7.0%) ... 2810
Timolide Tablets (Less than 1%) ... 2086
Timoptic Sterile Ophthalmic Solution ... 2088
Timoptic in Ocudose (Less frequent) ... 2091
Timoptic-XE Sterile Ophthalmic Gel Forming Solution ... 2092
Tindamax Tablets (1.4% to 1.8%) ... 2142
▲ Topamax Sprinkle Capsules (2% to 7%) ... 2404
▲ Topamax Tablets (2% to 7%) ... 2404
▲ Tracleer Tablets (4%) ... 545
Trasylol Injection (1% to 2%) ... 754
▲ Travatan Ophthalmic Solution (1% to 5%) ... 563
Trelstar LA Suspension (1.7%) ... 3397
Tricor Tablets ... 527
Triglide Tablets ... 3123
▲ Trileptal Tablets (2% to 6%) ... 2300
▲ Trileptal Oral Suspension (2% to 6%) ... 2300
▲ Trisenox Injection (10%) ... 993
▲ Trizivir Tablets (5%) ... 1589
Truvada Tablets ... 1296
Twinrix Vaccine ... 1595
Tygacil for Injection (2.9%) ... 3488
▲ Ultram ER Tablets (1% to greater than 5%) ... 2392
Uniretic Tablets (More than 1%) ... 3100
Univasc Tablets (Greater than 1%) ... 3104
Uroxatral Tablets (1% to 2%) ... 2943
▲ Urso 250 Tablets (10%) ... 710
▲ Urso Forte Tablets (10%) ... 710
▲ Vagifem Tablets (3% to 5%) ... 2334
▲ Valcyte Tablets (Less than 5%) ... 2813
Vandazole Vaginal Gel (Less than 1%) ... 3338
Vantin Tablets and Oral Suspension (Less than 1%) ... 2645
Vasotec I.V. Injection (0.5% to 1.0%) ... 2103
▲ Velcade for Injection (13%) ... 2133
Verelan PM Extended-Release Capsules, Controlled-Onset (2.7%) ... 3106
▲ Vesanoid Capsules (14%) ... 2820
▲ VESIcare Tablets (1.4% to 3.9%) ... 646
VFEND I.V. (Less than 2%) ... 2564
VFEND Oral Suspension (Less than 2%) ... 2564
VFEND Tablets (Less than 2%) ... 2564
▲ Viagra Tablets (7%) ... 2573
▲ Vicoprofen Tablets (12%) ... 539
Viracept (Less than 2%) ... 2577
▲ Viread Tablets (3% to 4%) ... 1301
▲ Voltaren Tablets (1% to 10%) ... 2307
▲ Voltaren-XR Tablets (1% to 10%) ... 2310
Vytorin 10/10 Tablets ... 2114
Vytorin 10/10 Tablets ... 3077
Vytorin 10/20 Tablets ... 2114
Vytorin 10/20 Tablets ... 3077
Vytorin 10/40 Tablets ... 2114
Vytorin 10/40 Tablets ... 3077
Vytorin 10/80 Tablets ... 2114
Vytorin 10/80 Tablets ... 3077
▲ WelChol Tablets (8%) ... 1050
▲ Wellbutrin Tablets (3.1%) ... 1603
Wellbutrin SR Sustained-Release Tablets (At least 1%) ... 1607
▲ Wellbutrin XL Extended-Release Tablets (3%) ... 1613
Xopenex Inhalation Solution (1.4% to 2.7%) ... 3146
Xopenex Inhalation Solution Concentrate (1.4% to 2.7%) ... 3150
Xopenex HFA Inhalation Aerosol (1.4% to 2.7%) ... 3154
▲ Xyrem Oral Solution (2.9% to 9.1%) ... 1688
Yaz Tablets (Greater than 1%) ... 803
▲ Zelapar Tablets (5%) ... 3372
Zelnorm Tablets ... 2312
Zemaira (0.2% to 0.4%) ... 3509
Zmax for Oral Suspension (Less then 1%) ... 2583
Zocor Tablets (1.1%) ... 2105
▲ Zoloft (6% to 13%) ... 2586
▲ Zometa for Intravenous Infusion (10%) ... 2315
Zomig Nasal Spray (Infrequent) ... 3523
▲ Zonegran Capsules (3%) ... 1101
▲ Zosyn (1.9% to 3.3%) ... 3492
Zyban Sustained-Release Tablets (Frequent) ... 1644
▲ Zyflo Tablets (8.2%) ... 1023
▲ Zyprexa Tablets (7% to 11%) ... 1830
▲ Zyprexa ZYDIS Orally Disintegrating Tablets (7% to 11%) ... 1830
Zyrtec Chewable Tablets (Less than 2%) ... 2594
Zyrtec (Less than 2%) ... 2594
Zyrtec-D 12 Hour Extended Release Tablets (Less than 2%) ... 2597
Zyvox ... 2652

Dysphagia

Abilify Oral Solution (Infrequent) ... 882
Abilify Oral Solution (Infrequent) ... 2450
Abilify Discmelt Orally Disintegrating Tablets (Infrequent) ... 882
Abilify Discmelt Orally Disintegrating Tablets (Infrequent) ... 2450
Abilify Tablets (Infrequent) ... 882
Abilify Tablets (Infrequent) ... 2450
Aciphex Tablets ... 1090
Actiq (1% or greater) ... 979
Actonel Tablets ... 2683
Actonel with Calcium Tablets ... 2688
Adalat CC Tablets (Less than 1%) ... 2964
▲ Alimta for Injection (Up to 6%) ... 1750
Altace Capsules (Less than 1%) ... 1702
Ambien Tablets (Infrequent) ... 2851
AmBisome for Injection (Less common) ... 620
Arthrotec Tablets (Rare) ... 3129
Avelox (Less than 0.1%) ... 2970
Avinza Capsules (Less than 5%) ... 1741
▲ BOTOX Purified Neurotoxin Complex (19%) ... 570
Caduet Tablets (Greater than 0.1% to less than 2%) ... 2508
Campral Tablets (Infrequent) ... 1174
Celebrex Capsules (0.1% to 1.9%) ... 3134
Celexa (Infrequent) ... 1176
▲ CellCept Capsules (3% to less than 20%) ... 2747
▲ CellCept Intravenous (3% to less than 20%) ... 2747
▲ CellCept Oral Suspension (3% to less than 20%) ... 2747
▲ CellCept Tablets (3% to less than 20%) ... 2747
Chantix Tablets (Infrequent) ... 2517
Cialis Tablets (Less than 2%) ... 1838
Cipro (Less than 1%) ... 2977
Cipro I.V. (1% or less) ... 2984
Cipro XR Tablets ... 2990
Clozaril Tablets ... 2184
Copaxone for Injection (At least 2%) ... 3297
Cosmegen for Injection ... 2459
Cymbalta Delayed-Release Capsules (Infrequent) ... 1757
▲ Dacogen Injection (6%) ... 2129
Depakote ER Tablets (Greater than 1%) ... 434
▲ Doxil Injection (1% to 10%) ... 2351
Edecrin ... 1959
Effexor Tablets (Infrequent) ... 3411
Effexor XR Capsules (Infrequent) ... 3417
Eldepryl Capsules ... 3208
Emend Capsules (Greater than 0.5%) ... 1963
▲ Erbitux (26% to 65%) ... 910
Evoxac Capsules (Less than 1%) ... 1047
Exelon Capsules (Infrequent) ... 2206
Exelon Oral Solution (Infrequent) ... 2206
FazaClo Orally Disintegrating Tablets ... 551
Flumadine ... 1183
Fosamax (0.1% to 1%) ... 1969
Fosamax Plus D Tablets (0.1% to 1%) ... 1977
Frova Tablets (Infrequent) ... 1113
Gabitril Tablets (Infrequent) ... 984
Gengraf Capsules (1% to less than 3%) ... 459
Geodon Capsules (2%) ... 2529
Imitrex Injection (Frequent) ... 1463
Imitrex Nasal Spray (Infrequent) ... 1467
Imitrex Tablets (Infrequent) ... 1471
▲ Intron A for Injection (Less than 5%) ... 3024
Invanz for Injection (Greater than 0.1%) ... 1999
Invirase (Less than 2%) ... 2772
Kadian Capsules (Less than 3%) ... 577
Kaletra (Up to 2%) ... 476
Lamictal (Infrequent) ... 1481
▲ Leukine (11%) ... 814
Levaquin (0.1% to 0.9%) ... 2384
Levaquin in 5% Dextrose Injection (0.1% to 0.9%) ... 2384
Levitra Tablets (Less than 2%) ... 3034
Lipitor Tablets (Less than 2%) ... 2483
Lunesta Tablets (Rare) ... 3142
▲ Lupron Depot 7.5 mg (Less than 5%) ... 3264
Lupron Depot-PED 7.5 mg, 11.25 mg and 15 mg (Less than 2%) ... 3269
Lupron Injection Pediatric (Less than 2%) ... 3259
Lyrica Capsules (0.1% to 1%) ... 2539
Matulane Capsules ... 3191
Maxalt Tablets (Infrequent) ... 2008
Maxalt-MLT Orally Disintegrating Tablets (Infrequent) ... 2008
Migranal Nasal Spray (Infrequent) ... 3348
Mirapex Tablets (2%) ... 859
▲ Myobloc Injection (10% to 25%) ... 3192
Namenda ... 1195
Neoral Oral Solution (1% to less than 3%) ... 2259
Neoral Soft Gelatin Capsules (1% to less than 3%) ... 2259
Neurontin Capsules (Rare) ... 2487
Neurontin Oral Solution (Rare) ... 2487
Neurontin Tablets (Rare) ... 2487
▲ Nexavar Tablets (Common) ... 746
Nexium Delayed-Release Capsules (Less than 1%) ... 655
Nexium I.V. (Less than 1%) ... 659

Nipent for Injection (Less than 3%) 1863
Noroxin Tablets 2032
Norvasc Tablets (More than 0.1% to 1%) 2545
Norvir (Less than 2%) 503
Omacor Capsules 2725
▲ Ontak Vials (6%) 1745
Oracea Capsules 1000
OxyContin Tablets (Less than 1%) 2703
Parcopa Orally Disintegrating Tablets 3097
Paxil CR Controlled-Release Tablets (Infrequent) 1538
Paxil (Infrequent) 1530
Pentasa Capsules (Less than 1%) 3185
Permax Tablets (Frequent) 3356
Pexeva Tablets (Infrequent) 1694
▲ Photofrin for Injection (10% to 24%) 702
Prevacid Delayed-Release Capsules (Less than 1%) 3271
Prevacid for Delayed-Release Oral Suspension (Less than 1%) 3271
Prevacid SoluTab Delayed-Release Orally Disintegrating Tablets (Less than 1%) 3271
Prevacid NapraPAC (Less than 1%) 3280
PREVPAC (Less than 1%) 3284
▲ Prograf Capsules and Injection (3% to 15%) 632
Proquin XR Tablets 1153
Protonix I.V. (Less than 1%) 3472
Protonix Tablets (Less than 1%) 3469
Prozac Pulvules and Liquid (Infrequent) 1801
▲ Rapamune Oral Solution and Tablets (3% to 20%) 3475
Razadyne (Infrequent) 2399
Razadyne ER Extended-Release Capsules (Infrequent) 2399
Relpax Tablets (1% to 2%) 2548
Remicade for IV Injection 971
Requip Tablets (Infrequent) 1555
Rescriptor Tablets 2551
Retrovir Capsules 1560
Retrovir IV Infusion 1564
Retrovir 1560
Revlimid Capsules 958
Rilutek Tablets (More than 2%) 2930
Risperdal (Infrequent) 1676
Risperdal Consta Long-Acting Injection (Infrequent) 1682
Risperdal M-Tab Orally Disintegrating Tablets (Infrequent) 1676
Rythmol SR Capsules 2727
▲ Sandostatin LAR Depot (1% to 4%) 2280
Seroquel Tablets (Infrequent) 690
Solodyn Extended Release Tablets 1890
Sonata Capsules (Rare) 1717
Stalevo Tablets 2287
Sular Tablets (Less than or equal to 1%) 3122
Symbyax Capsules 1819
Symmetrel Tablets 1135
Tasmar Tablets (Infrequent) 3358
▲ Taxotere Injection Concentrate (1.8% to 16.3%) 2932
Tequin Injection (Less than 0.1%) 938
Tequin Injection in 5% Dextrose (Less than 0.1%) 938
Tequin Tablets (Less than 0.1%) 938
Thalomid Capsules 965
Topamax Sprinkle Capsules (1%) 2404
Topamax Tablets (1%) 2404
Trileptal Tablets 2300
Trileptal Oral Suspension 2300
Uniretic Tablets (Less than 1%) 3100
VFEND I.V. (Less than 2%) 2564
VFEND Oral Suspension (Less than 2%) 2564
VFEND Tablets (Less than 2%) 2564
Viagra Tablets (Less than 2%) 2573
Vicoprofen Tablets (Less than 1%) 539
Wellbutrin Tablets (Infrequent) 1603
Wellbutrin SR Sustained-Release Tablets (Up to 2%) 1607
Wellbutrin XL Extended-Release Tablets (0% to 2%) 1613
▲ Xeloda Tablets (Less than 5%) 2822
Xyrem Oral Solution (Infrequent) 1688
▲ Zinecard for Injection (Up to 8%) 2650
Zoloft (Infrequent) 2586
▲ Zometa for Intravenous Infusion (5% to 10%) 2315
Zomig Nasal Spray (1% to less than 2%) 3523
Zonegran Capsules (Infrequent) 1101
Zyban Sustained-Release Tablets (Infrequent) 1644
Zyprexa Tablets (Infrequent) 1830
Zyprexa ZYDIS Orally Disintegrating Tablets (Infrequent) 1830

Dysphasia

Ambien Tablets (Rare) 2851
Ambien CR Tablets (Rare to infrequent) 2855
Aricept Tablets (Infrequent) 1094
Aricept ODT Tablets (Infrequent) 1094
Cipro 2977
Cipro I.V. (1% or less) 2984
Cipro XR Tablets 2990
Imitrex Injection 1463
Imitrex Nasal Spray 1467
▲ Temodar Capsules (7%) 3073
▲ Xeloda Tablets (Less than 5%) 2822

Dysphonia

▲ Advair Diskus 100/50 (5%) 1308
▲ Advair Diskus 250/50 (2% to 5%) 1308
▲ Advair Diskus 500/50 (2% to 5%) 1308
▲ Advair HFA Inhalation Aerosol (1% to 3%) 1318
Colazal Capsules 2838
Combivent Inhalation Aerosol (Less than 2%) 847
Evoxac Capsules (Less than 1%) 1047
Exelon Capsules (Infrequent) 2206
Exelon Oral Solution (Infrequent) 2206
▲ Flovent Diskus (1% to 9%) 1443
Flovent HFA (2%) 1447
Foradil Aerolizer (1%) 3010
▲ Intron A for Injection (Less than 5%) 3024
Proventil HFA Inhalation Aerosol (Less than 3%) 3056
▲ Pulmicort Respules (1% to 3%) 661
▲ Qvar Inhalation Aerosol (Up to 4%) 3303
ReoPro Vials (0.3%) 1809
Requip Tablets (Infrequent) 1555
Romazicon Injection (Less than 1%) 2804
▲ Sandostatin LAR Depot (1% to 4%) 2280
Soriatane Capsules (Less than 1%) 1013
▲ Spiriva HandiHaler (1% to 3%) 869
Topamax Sprinkle Capsules (Infrequent) 2404
Topamax Tablets (Infrequent) 2404
Trileptal Tablets 2300
Trileptal Oral Suspension 2300
Zoloft (Rare) 2586
Zyrtec Chewable Tablets (Less than 2%) 2594
Zyrtec (Less than 2%) 2594
Zyrtec-D 12 Hour Extended Release Tablets (Less than 2%) 2597

Dysphoria

Abilify Oral Solution (Infrequent) 882
Abilify Oral Solution (Infrequent) 2450
Abilify Discmelt Orally Disintegrating Tablets (Infrequent) 882
Abilify Discmelt Orally Disintegrating Tablets (Infrequent) 2450
Abilify Tablets (Infrequent) 882
Abilify Tablets (Infrequent) 2450
Acetadote Injection (.39% to 1.87%) 1031
Actiq 979
Adderall Tablets 3164
Adderall XR Capsules 3166
Adipex-P 1215
Advair Diskus 100/50 1308
Advair Diskus 250/50 1308
Advair Diskus 500/50 1308
Advair HFA Inhalation Aerosol 1318
Aldoril Tablets 1910
Allegra-D 12 Hour Extended-Release Tablets 2846
Allegra-D 24 Hour Extended-Release Tablets 2849
Ambien Tablets 2851
Amerge Tablets (Rare) 1339
Aricept Tablets (Infrequent) 1094
Aricept ODT Tablets (Infrequent) 1094
Atacand HCT 651
Avalide Tablets 888
Avalide Tablets 2874
Axert Tablets (Infrequent) 2396
Buprenex Injectable (Rare) 2716
Cafcit 1886
Catapres Tablets 843
Catapres-TTS (0.5% or less) 844
▲ Cesamet Capsules (9%) 3340
Chantix Tablets (Frequent) 2517
Cipro (Less than 1.1%) 2977
Cipro I.V. (Greater than 1%) 2984
Cipro XR Tablets 2990
Clorpres Tablets 2153
▲ Clozaril Tablets (4%) 2184
Cymbalta Delayed-Release Capsules (Frequent) 1757
Dalmane Capsules (Rare) 3342
Demadex Tablets 2759
Desoxyn Tablets, USP (Rare) 2462
Dexedrine 1420
DextroStat Tablets 3179
Dilaudid 440
Dilaudid Non-Sterile Powder 440
Dilaudid Oral Liquid 445
Dilaudid Rectal Suppositories 440
Dilaudid Tablets 440
Dilaudid Tablets - 8 mg 445
Dilaudid-HP (Less frequent) 442
Diovan HCT Tablets 2196
Diuril Oral Suspension 1954
Diuril Sodium Intravenous 2467
Eldepryl Capsules 3208
▲ Exelon Capsules (Frequent) 2206
▲ Exelon Oral Solution (Frequent) 2206
▲ FazaClo Orally Disintegrating Tablets (4%) 551
Flovent Diskus 1443
Flovent HFA 1447
Furosemide Tablets 2154
Hycodan 1116
Hycotuss Expectorant Syrup 1117
Hyzaar 50-12.5 Tablets 1990
Hyzaar 100-12.5 Tablets 1990
Hyzaar 100-25 Tablets 1990
▲ Infanrix Vaccine (8.6% to 15.9%) 1476
Lamictal (Infrequent) 1481
Lariam Tablets 2786
Levaquin 2384
Levaquin in 5% Dextrose Injection 2384
Lexapro Oral Solution (Infrequent) 1190
Lexapro Tablets (Infrequent) 1190
Lithobid Tablets 1692
Lopressor HCT 50/25 Tablets 2241
Lopressor HCT 100/25 Tablets 2241
Lopressor HCT 100/50 Tablets 2241
Lotensin HCT Tablets 2246
Micardis HCT Tablets 856
Moduretic Tablets 2028
▲ MS Contin Tablets (Among most frequent) 2701
Myozyme for Intravenous Infusion 1279
Namenda 1195
Nitrolingual Pumpspray 3120
Noroxin Tablets 2032
Numorphan Injection 1120
Opana Tablets (Less than 1%) 1122
Opana ER Tablets (Less than 1%) 1126
Oxsoralen-Ultra Capsules 3353
OxyFast Oral Concentrate Solution 2708
OxyIR Capsules 2708
Parnate Tablets 1527
Percocet Tablets 1131
Percodan Tablets 1132
Prinzide Tablets 2056
Proquin XR Tablets 1153
Rescriptor Tablets 2551
Restoril Capsules (Less than 0.5%) 1860
▲ Romazicon Injection (1% to 3%) 2804
Singulair (Very rare) 2077
Tequin Injection 938
Tequin Injection in 5% Dextrose 938
Tequin Tablets 938
Teveten HCT Tablets 1737
Thioridazine Hydrochloride Tablets (Extremely rare) 2163
Thiothixene Capsules 2165
Timolide Tablets 2086
Transderm Scōp Transdermal Therapeutic System (Infrequent) 2177
Trecator Tablets 3487
Tussionex Pennkinetic Extended-Release Suspension 3327
Twinject 0.3 3378
Twinject 0.15 3379
Tylenol with Codeine Tablets 2391
▲ Ultram ER Tablets (1% to greater than 5%) 2392
Uniphyl Tablets 2710
Uniretic Tablets 3100
Vicodin Tablets 535
Vicodin ES Tablets 536
Vicodin HP Tablets 538
VoSpire ER Tablets (Less frequent) 1052
Wellbutrin Tablets (Infrequent) 1603
Wellbutrin SR Sustained-Release Tablets (Infrequent) 1607
Wellbutrin XL Extended-Release Tablets (Infrequent) 1613
Xyrem Oral Solution (Infrequent) 1688
Zelnorm Tablets 2312
Zyban Sustained-Release Tablets (Less than 1%) 1644
Zydone Tablets 1139

Dysplasia, gastrointestinal

Nexium Delayed-Release Capsules (Less than 1%) 655
Nexium I.V. (Less than 1%) 659

Dysplasia, unspecified

Reyataz Capsules (Less than 3%) 921

Dyspnea

▲ Abelcet Injection (7%) 1141
Abilify Oral Solution (Frequent) 882
Abilify Oral Solution (Frequent) 2450
Abilify Discmelt Orally Disintegrating Tablets (Frequent) 882
Abilify Discmelt Orally Disintegrating Tablets (Frequent) 2450
Abilify Tablets (Frequent) 882
Abilify Tablets (Frequent) 2450
Aceon Tablets (2 mg, 4 mg, 8 mg) (0.3% to 1%) 3194
Acetadote Injection (.54% to 2.58%) 1031
Aciphex Tablets 1090
▲ Actiq (2% to 6%) 979
▲ Actonel Tablets (3.8%) 2683
▲ Actonel with Calcium Tablets (3.8%) 2688
Actos Tablets 3219
ADACEL Vaccine 2945
Adalat CC Tablets (Less than 1%) 2964
▲ Adderall XR Capsules (2% to 4%) 3166
▲ Adenocard Injection (12%) 617
▲ Adenoscan (Approximately 28%) 619
Advair Diskus 100/50 1308
Advair Diskus 250/50 1308
Advair Diskus 500/50 1308
Advair HFA Inhalation Aerosol 1318
Advate Injection (0.6%) 712
Advicor Tablets 1722
▲ Aerobid/Aerobid-M (1% to 3%) 1171
Aggrenox Capsules 822
▲ Agrylin Capsules (11.9%) 3169
Aldara Cream, 5% 1846
Aldurazyme for Intravenous Infusion 1268
▲ Alimta for Injection (1% to 72%) 1750
Alkeran for Injection (In some patients) 955
Allegra (Rare) 2844
Allegra-D 12 Hour Extended-Release Tablets (Rare) 2846
Allegra-D 24 Hour Extended-Release Tablets (Rare) 2849
Alphagan P Ophthalmic Solution (1% to 4%) 567
Altace Capsules (Less than 1%) 1702
Altoprev Extended-Release Tablets (Rare) 3109
Ambien Tablets (Infrequent) 2851
Ambien CR Tablets (Infrequent) 2855
▲ AmBisome for Injection (17.6% to 23%) 620
Amerge Tablets 1339
▲ Amitiza Capsules (2.4% to 3.4) 3224
▲ Anaprox Tablets (3% to 9%) 2761
▲ Anaprox DS Tablets (3% to 9%) 2761
Anzemet Injection (Rare) 2859
Anzemet Tablets (Rare) 2862
Aptivus Capsules (Less than 2%) 826
Aralast (0.1%) 717
▲ Aranesp for Injection (12%) 581
▲ Aredia for Injection (Up to 23.3%) 2179
▲ Argatroban Injection (8.1%) 1346
Aricept Tablets (Frequent) 1094
Aricept ODT Tablets (Frequent) 1094
▲ Arimidex Tablets (6% to 11%) 673
▲ Aromasin Tablets (10%) 2600
▲ Arranon Injection (2% to 20%) 1357
Arthrotec Tablets (Rare) 3129
Astelin Nasal Spray (Infrequently) 1904
Atacand Tablets (0.5% or greater) 649
Atacand HCT (0.5% or greater) 651
Atripla Tablets 945
▲ Atrovent Inhalation Solution (9.6%) 835
▲ Atrovent HFA Inhalation Aerosol (7% to 8%) 841
Avalide Tablets 888
Avalide Tablets 2874
Avapro Tablets (Less than 1%) 891
Avapro Tablets (Less than 1%) 2871
▲ Avastin IV (25% to 26%) 1227
Avelox (0.1% to less than 2%) 2970
▲ Avinza Capsules (5% to 10%) 1741
Axert Tablets (Infrequent) 2396
▲ Azilect Tablets (3%) 3293
Azopt Ophthalmic Suspension (Less than 1%) 557
▲ BeneFix Vials (3.2%) 3408
Bentyl Capsules 697
Bentyl Injection 697
Bentyl Syrup 697
Bentyl Tablets 697

Betagan Ophthalmic Solution, USP ⊙220
▲ Betaseron for SC Injection (7%) 767
Betimol Ophthalmic Solution 3382
Betimol Ophthalmic Solution ⊙295
Betoptic S Ophthalmic Suspension (Rare) 558
▲ Bexxar (3% to 11%) 1398
Bicillin C-R Injectable Suspension 1706
Blocadren Tablets (1.7%) 1916
Boostrix (Rarely) 1404
BOTOX Purified Neurotoxin Complex (Rare) 570
Buprenex Injectable (Less than 1%) 2716
Caduet Tablets (Less than 1% to 2%) 2508
Cafcit (2.2%) 1886
▲ Campath Ampules (9% to 26%) 811
Campral Tablets (Frequent) 1174
▲ Camptosar Injection (2.2% to 22%) 2604
Cancidas for Injection (2%) 1918
Captopril Tablets (About 0.5% to 2%) 2149
Carbatrol Capsules 3171
Cardene I.V. (0.7%) 2497
Cardizem LA Extended Release Tablets (Less than 2%) 1728
Cardura XL Tablets (1.2%) 2515
Carimune NF 3499
▲ Carnitor Injection (3% to 11%) 3188
Carteolol Hydrochloride Ophthalmic Solution USP, 1% (Occasional) ⊙249
Celebrex Capsules (0.1% to 1.9%) 3134
Celexa (Infrequent) 1176
▲ CellCept Capsules (31% to 36.7%) 2747
▲ CellCept Intravenous (31% to 36.7%) 2747
▲ CellCept Oral Suspension (31% to 36.7%) 2747
▲ CellCept Tablets (31% to 36.7%) 2747
▲ Cerezyme for Injection (Approximately 6.6%) 1270
Cesamet Capsules 3340
Chantix Tablets (1% to 2%) 2517
Cialis Tablets (Less than 2%) 1838
Cipro (Less than 1%) 2977
Cipro I.V. (1% or less) 2984
Clarinex Syrup (Rare) 2995
Clarinex Tablets (Rare) 2995
Clarinex Reditabs Tablets (Rare) 2995
Clarinex-D 24-Hour Extended-Release Tablets 2998
Clinoril Tablets (Less than 1%) 1924
Clozaril Tablets (1%) 2184
Colazal Capsules 2838
▲ Combivent Inhalation Aerosol (4.5%) 847
▲ Comtan Tablets (3%) 2189
Comvax 1928
▲ Copaxone for Injection (19%) 3297
▲ Copegus Tablets (13%) 2754
▲ Coreg Tablets (Greater than 3%) 1414
Cosopt Sterile Ophthalmic Solution (Less than 1%) 1931
Coumadin for Injection 898
Coumadin Tablets 898
Covera-HS Tablets (1.4% to 2%) 3139
Cozaar Tablets (Less than 1%) 1935
Crestor Tablets (Greater than or equal to 1%) 678
Crixivan Capsules 1940
▲ Cubicin for Injection (2.1% to 3.3%) 1026
Dacogen Injection 2129
▲ Depacon Injection (1% to 5%) 412
▲ Depakene (5%) 417
▲ Depakote Sprinkle Capsules (1% to 5%) 422
▲ Depakote Tablets (1% to 5%) 427
▲ Depakote ER Tablets (1% to 5%) 434
▲ DepoDur Extended-Release Injection (2% to 5%) 1110
Depo-Provera Contraceptive Injection (Less than 1%) 2622
depo-subQ provera 104 Injectable Suspension 2624
Diovan Tablets 2193
Diovan HCT Tablets (Greater than 0.2%) 2196
Dolobid Tablets (Rare) 1955
▲ Doxil Injection (1% to 15.1%) 2351
▲ Duragesic Transdermal System (3% to 10%) 2373
DynaCirc CR Tablets (0.5% to 1%) 2721
▲ EC-Naprosyn Delayed-Release Tablets (3% to 9%) 2761
Effexor Tablets (Frequent) 3411
Effexor XR Capsules (Frequent) 3417
Elitek 2890
Elmiron Capsules (Less than or equal to 1%) 2415
▲ Eloxatin for Injection (5% to 20%) 2892
▲ Emcyt Capsules (11%) 2634
Emend Capsules (Greater than 0.5%) 1963
Enbrel for Injection (Infrequent) 584
▲ Entocort EC Capsules (Less than 5%) 2698
Equetro Extended-Release Capsules 3180
Eraxis for Injection 2521
▲ Erbitux (2% to 23%) 910
Ethyol for Injection 1898
Evoxac Capsules (Less than 1%) 1047
▲ Exelon Capsules (Frequent) 2206
▲ Exelon Oral Solution (Frequent) 2206
▲ Exubera Inhalation Powder (3.6% to 4.4%) 2524
Fabrazyme for Intravenous Infusion 1274
▲ Faslodex Injection (14.9%) 681
FazaClo Orally Disintegrating Tablets (1%) 551
▲ Femara Tablets (0.8% to 18%) 2214
▲ Ferrlecit Injection (11%) 3388
Flebogamma 5%, Immune Globulin Intravenous (Human) 1658
▲ Flonase Nasal Spray (1% to 3%) 1440
Flovent Diskus 1443
Flovent HFA 1447
Fluarix 1451
Flumadine (0.3% to 1%) 1183
Follistim AQ Cartridge 2338
Foradil Aerolizer (2.1%) 3010
▲ Forteo for Injection (3.6%) 1767
Fortical Nasal Spray (Less than 1%) 3337
Frova Tablets (Infrequent) 1113
Gabitril Tablets (Frequent) 984
Gammagard Liquid 721
Gammagard S/D 724
Gamunex Immune Globulin I.V., 10% 3235
▲ Gemzar for Injection (3% to 23%) 1771
▲ Gengraf Capsules (1% to 5%) 459
Geodon Capsules (2%) 2529
▲ Gleevec Tablets (0.9% to 21%) 2227
GlucaGen (Rare) 761
Havrix Vaccine (Rare) 1456
▲ Hectorol Capsules (Greater than or equal to 5% to 11.5%) 1275
▲ Hectorol Injection (11.5%) 1278
▲ Herceptin I.V. (22%) 1233
▲ Humira Injection (Less than 5%) 466
▲ Hycamtin for Injection (1.8% to 22%) 1458
Hyperstat I.V. 3017
▲ Hytrin Capsules (0.5% to 3.1%) 471
Hyzaar 50-12.5 Tablets 1990
Hyzaar 100-12.5 Tablets 1990
Hyzaar 100-25 Tablets 1990
▲ Imdur Tablets (Less than or equal to 5%) 3018
Imitrex Injection (Infrequent) 1463
Imitrex Nasal Spray (Infrequent) 1467
Imitrex Tablets (Frequent) 1471
Indocin Capsules (Less than 1%) 1995
Indocin I.V. (Less than 1%) 2465
Indocin (Less than 1%) 1995
Infanrix Vaccine 1476
Infed Injection 3390
▲ Infergen (7% to 8%) 3364
▲ Intron A for Injection (Up to 34%) 3024
Invanz for Injection (1% to 2.6%) 1999
Invirase (Less than 2%) 2772
Iressa Tablets (2%) 684
▲ I.V. Busulfex (2% to 25%) 2493
Kadian Capsules (Less than 3%) 577
Kaletra (Less than 2%) 476
Klonopin (Infrequent) 2778
K-Phos Original (Sodium Free) Tablets (Less frequent) 760
K-Phos Neutral Tablets 760
Lamictal (1.1%) 1481
Lariam Tablets 2786
Lescol Capsules (Rare) 2233
Lescol XL Tablets 2233
▲ Leukine (15% to 28%) 814
▲ Leustatin Injection (11%) 2357
Levaquin (0.1% to 1.3%) 2384
Levaquin in 5% Dextrose Injection (0.1% to 1.3%) 2384
Levitra Tablets (Less than 2%) 3034
Levothroid Tablets 1186
Levoxyl Tablets 1712
Lipitor Tablets (Less than 2%) 2483
Lofibra Tablets 1219
Lofibra Capsules 1216
Lopressor Injection (Less than 1%) 2238
Lopressor Tablets (Less than 1%) 2238
Lopressor HCT 50/25 Tablets (1%) 2241
Lopressor HCT 100/25 Tablets (1%) 2241
Lopressor HCT 100/50 Tablets (1%) 2241
Lotensin Tablets (Less than 1%) 2243
▲ Lovenox Injection (3.3%) 2915
Lunesta Tablets (Infrequent) 3142
▲ Lyrica Capsules (2% to 3%) 2539
Mavik Tablets (0.3% to 1.0%) 486
Maxalt Tablets (Frequent) 2008
Maxalt-MLT Orally Disintegrating Tablets (Frequent) 2008
Mefoxin for Injection 2012
Mefoxin Premixed Intravenous Solution 2016
▲ Megace ES Oral Suspension (1% to 3%) 2481
Mephyton Tablets (Rare) 2018
▲ Mepron Suspension (15% to 21%) 1521
Meridia Capsules (Greater than or equal to 1%) 489
Merrem I.V. (Greater than 0.1% to 1%) 686
Mevacor Tablets (Rare) 2021
Miacalcin Nasal Spray (Less than 1%) 2253
Micardis Tablets (More than 0.3%) 854
Micardis HCT Tablets 856
▲ Midamor Tablets (Between 1% and 3%) 2026
Migranal Nasal Spray (Infrequent) 3348
▲ Mirapex Tablets (Greater than or equal to 1% to 4%) 859
Mobic Oral Suspension (Less than 2%) 863
Mobic Tablets (Less than 2%) 863
Moduretic Tablets (Greater than 1%, less than 3%) 2028
Mycamine for Injection 628
▲ Myfortic Tablets (3% to less than 20%) 2255
▲ Mylotarg for Injection (26%) 3431
Myobloc Injection (Greater than 2%) 3192
Nalfon Capsules (2.8%) 2502
Namenda (2%) 1195
▲ Naprosyn Suspension (3% to 9%) 2761
▲ Naprosyn Tablets (3% to 9%) 2761
▲ Neoral Oral Solution (1% to 5.0%) 2259
▲ Neoral Soft Gelatin Capsules (1% to 5%) 2259
▲ Neumega for Injection (48%) 3435
▲ Neupogen for Injection (9%) 603
Neurontin Capsules (Infrequent) 2487
Neurontin Oral Solution (Infrequent) 2487
Neurontin Tablets (Infrequent) 2487
▲ Nexavar Tablets (Less than 1% to 14%) 746
Nexium Delayed-Release Capsules (Less than 1%) 655
Nexium I.V. (Less than 1%) 659
Niaspan Extended-Release Tablets 1730
Nimotop Capsules (Up to 1.2%) 749
▲ Nipent for Injection (8% to 11%) 1863
Noroxin Tablets 2032
Norvasc Tablets (Less than 1% to 2%) 2545
Norvir (Less than 2%) 503
Omacor Capsules 2725
▲ Oncaspar (Greater than 5%) 1145
▲ Ontak Vials (29%) 1745
Opana Tablets (Less than 1%) 1122
Opana ER Tablets (Less than 1%) 1126
OptiPranolol Metipranolol Ophthalmic Solution 0.3% (A small number of patients) ⊙256
Orencia Powder for Intravenous Infusion (Less than 0.1% to 1%) 914
▲ Orthoclone OKT3 Sterile Solution (21%) 2360
▲ OxyContin Tablets (Between 1% and 5%) 2703
Parcopa Orally Disintegrating Tablets 3097
Paxil CR Controlled-Release Tablets (Infrequent) 1538
Paxil (Infrequent) 1530
Pediarix Vaccine (Rare) 1548
▲ Pegasys (Less than 1% to 4%) 2789
▲ PEG-Intron Powder for Injection (4%) 3048
Pentasa Capsules (One case) 3185
Percodan Tablets 1132
▲ Permax Tablets (4.8%) 3356
Pexeva Tablets (infrequent) 1694
▲ Photofrin for Injection (6% to 20%) 702
▲ Plavix Tablets (4.5%) 917
▲ Plavix Tablets (4.5%) 2926
Pletal Tablets (2% or greater) 2455
Prevacid Delayed-Release Capsules (Less than 1%) 3271
Prevacid for Delayed-Release Oral Suspension (Less than 1%) 3271
Prevacid SoluTab Delayed-Release Orally Disintegrating Tablets (Less than 1%) 3271
▲ Prevacid NapraPAC (Less than 1% to 9%) 3280
PREVPAC (Less than 1%) 3284
Prezista Tablets (Less than 2%) 3306
Primaxin I.M. 2045
Primaxin I.V. (Less than 0.2%) 2048
Prinivil Tablets (Greater than 1%) 2052
Prinzide Tablets (0.3% to 1%) 2056
ProAir HFA Inhalation Aerosol (Less than 3%) 3300
Prochieve 4% Gel 1003
Prochieve 8% Gel 1003
▲ Prograf Capsules and Injection (5% to 29%) 632
Prolastin (Occasional) 3255
▲ Proleukin for Injection (43%) 2266
Proquin XR Tablets (Less than 1%) 1153
Prosed/DS Tablets 1157
ProSom Tablets (Infrequent) 517
Protonix I.V. (Greater than or equal to 1%) 3472
Protonix Tablets (Greater than or equal to 1%) 3469
Protopic Ointment (Greater than or equal to 1%) 638
Proventil Inhalation Solution 0.083% (1.5%) 3055
Provigil Tablets (Greater than or equal to 1%) 988
▲ Pulmozyme Inhalation Solution (17%) 1248
Ranexa Tablets (Greater than 0.5% to less than 2%) 1035
Raniclor Tablets, Chewable (Rare) 2505
▲ Rapamune Oral Solution and Tablets (22% to 30%) 3475
Raptiva for Injection 1250
▲ Rebetol (5% to 26%) 3058
▲ Rebetron Combination Therapy (17% to 19%) 3063
Recombivax HB (Less than 1%) 2071
ReFacto Vials 3484
Refludan for Injection (Common) 792
Relenza Rotadisk (Less than 1%) 1552
Relpax Tablets (Infrequent) 2548
Remicade for IV Injection (1%) 971
▲ Renagel Tablets (10.1%) 1282
▲ Requip Tablets (3%) 1555
Rescriptor Tablets 2551
Restoril Capsules (0.5% to 0.9%) 1860
▲ Retrovir Capsules (5%) 1560
▲ Retrovir IV Infusion (5%) 1564
▲ Retrovir (5%) 1560
▲ Revlimid Capsules (4.7% to 20.2%) 958
Reyataz Capsules (Less than 3%) 921
Rhophylac (Rare) 3505
▲ Ribavirin, USP Capsules (5% to 26%) 3068
Rilutek Tablets (More than 2%) 2930
Risperdal (Up to 1%) 1676
Risperdal Consta Long-Acting Injection (Frequent) 1682
Risperdal M-Tab Orally Disintegrating Tablets (Up to 1%) 1676
▲ Rituxan I.V. (1% to 7%) 1254
▲ Romazicon Injection (3% to 9%) 2804
▲ Rythmol SR Capsules (13% to 17%) 2727
Sandimmune 2275
Seroquel Tablets (Infrequent) 690
▲ Simulect for Injection (Greater than or equal to 10%) 2284
Sonata Capsules (Infrequent) 1717
▲ Stalevo Tablets (3%) 2287
Striant Mucoadhesive 1007
Stromectol Tablets 2083
Sular Tablets (Less than or equal to 1%) 3122
Sustiva Capsules 930
Sustiva Tablets 930
▲ Sutent Capsules (0% to 28%) 2560
Symbyax Capsules (1% to 2%) 1819
Symmetrel Tablets (0.1% to 1%) 1135
Synagis (More than 1%) 1897
▲ Tambocor Tablets (10.3%) 1856
▲ Tarceva Tablets (Less than 1% to 41%) 1259
▲ Tarceva Tablets (Less than 1% to 41%) 2444
Targretin Capsules 1747
Tarka Tablets (1.3%) 524
▲ Tasmar Tablets (3%) 3358
▲ Taxotere Injection Concentrate (6%) 2932
Tegretol/Tegretol-XR 2295
▲ Temodar Capsules (5%) 3073
▲ Tequin Injection (0.1% to 3%) 938

▲ Tequin Injection in 5% Dextrose (0.1% to 3%) 938
▲ Tequin Tablets (0.1% to 3%) 938
Thalomid Capsules 965
▲ Thiola Tablets (4%) 2141
▲ Thymoglobulin for Intravenous Infusion (28%) 1284
Tiazac Capsules (Less than 2%) 1201
Timolide Tablets (1.2%) 2086
Timoptic Sterile Ophthalmic Solution (Less frequent) 2088
Timoptic in Ocudose (Less frequent) 2091
Timoptic-XE Sterile Ophthalmic Gel Forming Solution 2092
Tindamax Tablets (Rare) 2142
▲ TOBI Solution for Inhalation (33.7%) 2298
▲ Topamax Sprinkle Capsules (1% to 3%) 2404
▲ Topamax Tablets (1% to 3%) 2404
Toprol-XL Tablets (Greater than 1%) 668
▲ Trasylol Injection (4%) 754
Trelstar LA Suspension (1.1%) 3397
Tricor Tablets 527
TriLyte with Flavor Packs for Oral Solution 3100
▲ Trisenox Injection (53%) 993
Trizivir Tablets 1589
Trusopt Sterile Ophthalmic Solution 2095
Truvada Tablets 1296
Twinrix Vaccine 1595
Tygacil for Injection (2.9%) 3488
▲ Ultram ER Tablets (1% to greater than 5%) 2392
Uniretic Tablets (Less than 1%) 3100
Univasc Tablets (Less than 1%) 3104
Uroqid-Acid No. 2 Tablets 760
▲ Valcyte Tablets (Less than 5%) 2813
Valtrex Caplets 1597
Vancocin HCl Capsules, USP 3380
Vantin Tablets and Oral Suspension (Less than 1%) 2645
Vasotec I.V. Injection (0.5% to 1.3%) 2103
▲ Velcade for Injection (20%) 2133
Ventavis Inhalation Solution 1020
Verelan PM Extended-Release Capsules, Controlled-Onset (2% or less) 3106
▲ Vesanoid Capsules (60%) 2820
VFEND I.V. (Less than 2%) 2564
VFEND Oral Suspension (Less than 2%) 2564
VFEND Tablets (Less than 2%) 2564
Viadur Implant (2.3%) 757
Viagra Tablets (Less than 2%) 2573
Vicoprofen Tablets (Less than 3%) 539
Viracept (Less than 2%) 2577
Virazole for Inhalation Solution 3370
Viread Tablets 1301
Visudyne for Injection 2305
Vivaglobin (0.1%) 3506
Vivitrol 995
Voltaren Tablets (Occasionally) 2307
Voltaren-XR Tablets (Occasionally) 2310
Vytorin 10/10 Tablets 2114
Vytorin 10/10 Tablets 3077
Vytorin 10/20 Tablets 2114
Vytorin 10/20 Tablets 3077
Vytorin 10/40 Tablets 2114
Vytorin 10/40 Tablets 3077
Vytorin 10/80 Tablets 2114
Vytorin 10/80 Tablets 3077
Wellbutrin Tablets (Infrequent) 1603
Wellbutrin SR Sustained-Release Tablets 1607
Wellbutrin XL Extended-Release Tablets 1613
Xalatan Sterile Ophthalmic Solution 2649
▲ Xeloda Tablets (Less than 5%) 2822
Xifaxan Tablets (Less than 2%) 2842
Xopenex Inhalation Solution 3146
Xopenex Inhalation Solution Concentrate 3150
Xopenex HFA Inhalation Aerosol 3154
Xyrem Oral Solution (Less than 1%) 1688
▲ Zelapar Tablets (3%) 3372
Zelnorm Tablets 2312
Zemaira (0.2% to 0.4%) 3509
Ziagen 1626
Zocor Tablets (Rare) 2105
Zoloft (Infrequent) 2586
▲ Zometa for Intravenous Infusion (22.1% to 27%) 2315
Zomig Nasal Spray (Infrequent) 3523
Zonegran Capsules (Infrequent) 1101
Zyban Sustained-Release Tablets (1%) 1644
▲ Zyprexa Tablets (3%) 1830
▲ Zyprexa ZYDIS Orally Disintegrating Tablets (3%) 1830
Zyrtec Chewable Tablets (Less than 2%) 2594
Zyrtec (Less than 2%) 2594
Zyrtec-D 12 Hour Extended Release Tablets (Less than 2%) 2597
Zyvox 2652

Dyspnea, aggravation of
▲ Revatio Tablets (7%) 2557
Toprol-XL Tablets (Greater than 1%) 668

Dyspnea, exertional
▲ Arranon Injection (0% to 7%) 1357
Clozaril Tablets 2184
▲ Copegus Tablets (4%) 2754
▲ Myfortic Tablets (3% to less than 20%) 2255
Neumega for Injection 3435
Pegasys (Less than 1%) 2789
▲ Revlimid Capsules (6.8%) 958
Vantas (Less than 2%) 3375

Dyspnea, nocturnal
Astelin Nasal Spray (Infrequently) 1904
Prinivil Tablets (0.3% to 1.0%) 2052
Prinzide Tablets 2056
Xyrem Oral Solution (Infrequent) 1688

Dyspnea, nocturnal, paroxysmal
Clozaril Tablets 2184
Herceptin I.V. 1233

Dysrhythmia
Bayer Aspirin Comprehensive Prescribing Information 796
Camptosar Injection 2604
Percodan Tablets 1132
St. Joseph 81 mg Aspirin Chewable and Enteric Coated Tablets 1869
▲ Taxotere Injection Concentrate (2.3% to 4.5%) 2932

Dysstasia
Xyrem Oral Solution (Infrequent) 1688

Dysthesias
▲ Campath Ampules (15%) 811

Dystonia
Abilify Oral Solution (Infrequent) 882
Abilify Oral Solution (Infrequent) 2450
Abilify Discmelt Orally Disintegrating Tablets (Infrequent) 882
Abilify Discmelt Orally Disintegrating Tablets (Infrequent) 2450
Abilify Tablets (Infrequent) 882
Abilify Tablets (Infrequent) 2450
Aloprim for Injection (Less than 1%) 2167
AmBisome for Injection (Less common) 620
▲ Azilect Tablets (3%) 3293
Celexa (Infrequent) 1176
Cesamet Capsules 3340
Clozaril Tablets 2184
Cuprimine Capsules 1947
Effexor Tablets (Rare) 3411
Effexor XR Capsules (Rare) 3417
Eldepryl Capsules 3208
Exelon Capsules (Infrequent) 2206
Exelon Oral Solution (Infrequent) 2206
Gabitril Tablets (Infrequent) 984
▲ Geodon Capsules (4% to 14%) 2529
Imitrex Injection (Rare) 1463
Imitrex Tablets (Rare) 1471
Lamictal (Rare) 1481
Lexapro Oral Solution 1190
Lexapro Tablets 1190
Lyrica Capsules (Rare) 2539
Migranal Nasal Spray (Infrequent) 3348
▲ Mirapex Tablets (2% to 8%) 859
Moban Tablets (Infrequent) 1119
Neurontin Capsules (Infrequent) 2487
Neurontin Oral Solution (Infrequent) 2487
Neurontin Tablets (Infrequent) 2487
Niravam Orally Disintegrating Tablets 3092
Parcopa Orally Disintegrating Tablets (Common) 3097
Paxil CR Controlled-Release Tablets (Infrequent) 1538
Paxil (Infrequent) 1530
▲ Permax Tablets (11.6%) 3356
Pexeva Tablets (infrequent) 1694
Phenytek Capsules (Rare) 2160
Prozac Pulvules and Liquid (Rare) 1801
Relpax Tablets (Rare) 2548
Requip Tablets (1% or more) 1555
▲ Risperdal (17% to 34%) 1676
Risperdal Consta Long-Acting Injection (Frequent) 1682
▲ Risperdal M-Tab Orally Disintegrating Tablets (17% to 34%) 1676
Symbyax Capsules (Rare) 1819
Syprine Capsules 2085
▲ Tasmar Tablets (19% to 22%) 3358
Thioridazine Hydrochloride Tablets 2163
Thiothixene Capsules 2165
Topamax Sprinkle Capsules (Infrequent) 2404
Topamax Tablets (Infrequent) 2404
Trileptal Tablets 2300
Trileptal Oral Suspension 2300
Wellbutrin Tablets (Frequent) 1603
Wellbutrin SR Sustained-Release Tablets 1607
Wellbutrin XL Extended-Release Tablets 1613
Zelapar Tablets 3372
Zofran Injection 1634
Zofran 1639
Zofran ODT Orally Disintegrating Tablets 1639
Zoloft (Infrequent) 2586
Zomig Tablets (Rare) 3519
Zomig-ZMT Tablets (Rare) 3519
Zonegran Capsules (Rare) 1101
Zyban Sustained-Release Tablets 1644
▲ Zyprexa Tablets (2% to 3%) 1830
▲ Zyprexa ZYDIS Orally Disintegrating Tablets (2% to 3%) 1830

Dystonia, tardive
Thioridazine Hydrochloride Tablets 2163
Thiothixene Capsules 2165

Dystonic reactions
(*see under* Dystonia)

Dystrophy
Rocaltrol Capsules 2798
Rocaltrol Oral Solution 2798

Dysuria
Abelcet Injection 1141
Abilify Oral Solution (Infrequent) 882
Abilify Oral Solution (Infrequent) 2450
Abilify Discmelt Orally Disintegrating Tablets (Infrequent) 882
Abilify Discmelt Orally Disintegrating Tablets (Infrequent) 2450
Abilify Tablets (Infrequent) 882
Abilify Tablets (Infrequent) 2450
Aciphex Tablets 1090
Actiq (Less than 1%) 979
Adalat CC Tablets (Less than 1%) 2964
Agrylin Capsules (1% to 5%) 3169
Alferon N Injection (1%) 1665
Alinia for Oral Suspension (Less than 1%) 2835
Alinia Tablets (Less than 1%) 2835
Allegra-D 12 Hour Extended-Release Tablets 2846
Allegra-D 24 Hour Extended-Release Tablets 2849
Ambien Tablets (Rare) 2851
Ambien CR Tablets (Rare to 1%) 2855
AmBisome for Injection (Less common) 620
Anaprox Tablets (Less than 1%) 2761
Anaprox DS Tablets (Less than 1%) 2761
Anzemet Injection (Rare) 2859
Anzemet Tablets (Rare) 2862
Aricept Tablets (Infrequent) 1094
Aricept ODT Tablets (Infrequent) 1094
Arthrotec Tablets (Rare) 3129
Asacol Delayed-Release Tablets 2692
▲ Avinza Capsules (Less than 5%) 1741
Caduet Tablets (Less than 2%) 2508
Cardura XL Tablets (Less than 1%) 2515
Ceftin Tablets (0.1% to 1%) 1407
Celexa (Infrequent) 1176
▲ CellCept Capsules (3% to less than 20%) 2747
▲ CellCept Intravenous (3% to less than 20%) 2747
▲ CellCept Oral Suspension (3% to less than 20%) 2747
▲ CellCept Tablets (3% to less than 20%) 2747
Cleocin Vaginal Ovules (Less than 1%) 2616
Clinoril Tablets 1924
Clorpres Tablets (Rare) 2153
Combivent Inhalation Aerosol (Less than 2%) 847
Copaxone for Injection (At least 2%) 3297
Crixivan Capsules (1.5%) 1940
Cymbalta Delayed-Release Capsules (Frequent) 1757
▲ Dacogen Injection (6%) 2129
Demser Capsules (A few patients) 1953
Depacon Injection (1% or more) 412
Depakene (1% or more) 417
Depakote Sprinkle Capsules 422
▲ Depakote Tablets (1% to 5%) 427
Depakote ER Tablets (1% or more) 434
Detrol Tablets (2%) 2628
Detrol LA Capsules (1%) 2631
Diovan HCT Tablets (Less Frequent) 2196
Dolobid Tablets (Less than 1 in 100) 1955
▲ Doxil Injection (1% to 10%) 2351
DynaCirc CR Tablets (0.5% to 1%) 2721
EC-Naprosyn Delayed-Release Tablets (Less than 1%) 2761
Effexor Tablets (Infrequent) 3411
▲ Eloxatin for Injection (1% to 6%) 2892
Emend Capsules (Greater than 0.5%) 1963
▲ Entocort EC Capsules (Less than 5%) 2698
▲ Estring Vaginal Ring (1% to 3%) 2635
Evoxac Capsules (Less than 1%) 1047
Exelon Capsules (Infrequent) 2206
Exelon Oral Solution (Infrequent) 2206
Gabitril Tablets (Frequent) 984
Gengraf Capsules (1%) 459
Imitrex Injection (Rare) 1463
Imitrex Nasal Spray (Infrequent) 1467
Imitrex Tablets (Up to 2%) 1471
▲ Intron A for Injection (Less than 5%) 3024
Invanz for Injection (1.1%) 1999
Ionsys Transdermal System (.1% to less than 1%) 2379
▲ I.V. Busulfex (7%) 2493
Klonopin (Infrequent) 2778
Lamictal (Rare) 1481
Lexapro Oral Solution (Infrequent) 1190
Lexapro Tablets (Infrequent) 1190
Lipitor Tablets (Less than 2%) 2483
Lunesta Tablets (Infrequent) 3142
▲ Lupron Depot 3.75 mg (Among most frequent) 3260
Lupron Depot–3 Month 11.25 mg (Less than 5%) 3265
Lyrica Capsules (0.1% to 1%) 2539
Maxalt Tablets (Rare) 2008
Maxalt-MLT Orally Disintegrating Tablets (Rare) 2008
Merrem I.V. (Greater than 0.1% to 1%) 686
Midamor Tablets (Less than or equal to 1%) 2026
Mirapex Tablets (Less than 1%) 859
Moduretic Tablets (Less than or equal to 1%) 2028
▲ Myfortic Tablets (3% to less than 20%) 2255
Nalfon Capsules (Less than 1%) 2502
Namenda (Infrequent) 1195
Naprosyn Suspension (Less than 1%) 2761
Naprosyn Tablets (Less than 1%) 2761
Neoral Oral Solution (1%) 2259
Neoral Soft Gelatin Capsules (1%) 2259
Neurontin Capsules (Infrequent) 2487
Neurontin Oral Solution (Infrequent) 2487
Neurontin Tablets (Infrequent) 2487
Nexium Delayed-Release Capsules (Less than 1%) 655
Nexium I.V. (Less than 1%) 659
Norvasc Tablets (Less than 0.1%) 2545
Norvir (Less than 2%) 503
OxyContin Tablets (Less than 1%) 2703
Oxytrol Transdermal System (2.4%) 3392
Paxil CR Controlled-Release Tablets (Infrequent) 1538
Paxil (Infrequent) 1530
Permax Tablets (Infrequent) 3356
Pexeva Tablets (infrequent) 1694
Prevacid Delayed-Release Capsules (Less than 1%) 3271
Prevacid for Delayed-Release Oral Suspension (Less than 1%) 3271
Prevacid SoluTab Delayed-Release Orally Disintegrating Tablets (Less than 1%) 3271
Prevacid NapraPAC (Less than 1%) 3280
PREVPAC (Less than 1%) 3284
Prinivil Tablets (0.3% to 1.0%) 2052
Prinzide Tablets 2056
▲ ProAmatine Tablets (13.4%) 3186

Prochieve 4% Gel 1003
Prochieve 8% Gel 1003
▲ Prograf Capsules and Injection (3% to 15%) 632
▲ Proleukin for Injection (3%) 2266
Proquin XR Tablets (Less than 1%) 1153
Protonix I.V. (Less than 1%) 3472
Protonix Tablets (Less than 1%) 3469
Prozac Pulvules and Liquid (Infrequent) 1801
▲ Rapamune Oral Solution and Tablets (3% to 20%) 3475
Recombivax HB (Less than 1%) 2071
ReoPro Vials (0.4%) 1809
Requip Tablets (Infrequent) 1555
Retrovir Capsules 1560
Retrovir IV Infusion 1564
Retrovir 1560
▲ Revlimid Capsules (6.8%) 958
Rilutek Tablets (Up to 1.2%) 2930
Risperdal (Infrequent) 1676
Risperdal M-Tab Orally Disintegrating Tablets (Infrequent) 1676
Rythmol SR Capsules 2727
Seroquel Tablets (Infrequent) 690
▲ Simulect for Injection (3% to 10%) 2284
Sonata Capsules (Infrequent) 1717
Soriatane Capsules (Less than 1%) 1013
Sular Tablets (Less than or equal to 1%) 3122
Symbyax Capsules (Infrequent) 1819
Tasmar Tablets (Infrequent) 3358
▲ Tequin Injection (0.1% to 3%) 938
▲ Tequin Injection in 5% Dextrose (0.1% to 3%) 938
▲ Tequin Tablets (0.1% to 3%) 938
Topamax Sprinkle Capsules (0% to 2%) 2404
Topamax Tablets (0% to 2%) 2404
▲ Trelstar LA Suspension (4.6%) 3397
Trileptal Tablets 2300
Trileptal Oral Suspension 2300
▲ Ultram ER Tablets (1% to greater than 5%) 2392
Uniretic Tablets (Less than 1%) 3100
Uroqid-Acid No. 2 Tablets (Occasional) 760
▲ Valcyte Tablets (Less than 5%) 2813
Vandazole Vaginal Gel (Less than 1%) 3338
Vantas (Less than 2%) 3375
Vantin Tablets and Oral Suspension (Less than 1%) 2645
▲ Vesanoid Capsules (9%) 2820
VFEND I.V. (Less than 2%) 2564
VFEND Oral Suspension (Less than 2%) 2564
VFEND Tablets (Less than 2%) 2564
Viadur Implant (Less than 2%) 757
Voltaren Tablets (Occasionally) 2307
Voltaren-XR Tablets (Occasionally) 2310
Wellbutrin Tablets (Rare) 1603
Wellbutrin SR Sustained-Release Tablets 1607
Wellbutrin XL Extended-Release Tablets 1613
Xifaxan Tablets (Less than 2%) 2842
Zofran Injection (2%) 1634
Zoloft (Infrequent) 2586
Zonegran Capsules (Infrequent) 1101
Zosyn (1.0% or less) 3492
Zyban Sustained-Release Tablets 1644
Zyprexa Tablets (Infrequent) 1830
Zyprexa ZYDIS Orally Disintegrating Tablets (Infrequent) 1830
Zyrtec Chewable Tablets (Less than 2%) 2594
Zyrtec (Less than 2%) 2594
Zyrtec-D 12 Hour Extended Release Tablets (Less than 2%) 2597

Dyuria
Lofibra Tablets 1219
Lofibra Capsules 1216
Targretin Capsules 1747
Tricor Tablets 527

E

Ear, discomfort
Adenoscan (Less than 1%) 619
▲ Aerobid/Aerobid-M (1% to 3%) 1171
Bumex Tablets (0.1%) 2746
▲ Ciprodex Otic Suspension (3%) 559
Invirase (Less than 2%) 2772
Levaquin (0.1% to 0.9%) 2384
Levaquin in 5% Dextrose Injection (0.1% to 0.9%) 2384
Xyrem Oral Solution (Infrequent) 1688

Ear, disorders of
▲ Advair HFA Inhalation Aerosol (1% to 3%) 1318
Ciprodex Otic Suspension (1 patient) 559
FazaClo Orally Disintegrating Tablets (Less than 1%) 551
▲ Imitrex Nasal Spray (2.5% to 3.8%) 1467
▲ I.V. Busulfex (3%) 2493
Levaquin (0.1% to 0.9%) 2384
Levaquin in 5% Dextrose Injection (0.1% to 0.9%) 2384
Prevacid NapraPAC (Less than 1%) 3280
ProAir HFA Inhalation Aerosol (Less than 3%) 3300
Relpax Tablets (Rare) 2548
▲ Risperdal Consta Long-Acting Injection (Up to 3%) 1682

Ear, external abnormalities, fetal
Accutane Capsules 2731

Ear congestion
Ciprodex (0.4%) 559

Ear disease, unspecified
Actiq (1% or greater) 979
▲ Advair Diskus 100/50 (3%) 1308
Advair Diskus 250/50 1308
▲ Advair Diskus 500/50 (3%) 1308
Asacol Delayed-Release Tablets (2% or greater) 2692
Avapro Tablets (Less than 1%) 891
Avapro Tablets (Less than 1%) 2871
Cardene I.V. (Rare) 2497
Celebrex Capsules (0.1% to 1.9%) 3134
▲ CellCept Capsules (3% to less than 20%) 2747
▲ CellCept Intravenous (3% to less than 20%) 2747
▲ CellCept Oral Suspension (3% to less than 20%) 2747
▲ CellCept Tablets (3% to less than 20%) 2747
Clozaril Tablets (Less than 1%) 2184
▲ Depakote Tablets (1% to 5%) 427
Exubera Inhalation Powder (1.3%) 2524
Ferrlecit Injection 3388
Gengraf Capsules (1%) 459
▲ Humatrope Vials and Cartridges (11.8%) 1787
Lamictal (2%) 1481
Lotronex Tablets (Rare) 1512
Neoral Oral Solution (1%) 2259
Neoral Soft Gelatin Capsules (1%) 2259
Prevacid Delayed-Release Capsules (Less than 1%) 3271
Prevacid for Delayed-Release Oral Suspension (Less than 1%) 3271
Prevacid SoluTab Delayed-Release Orally Disintegrating Tablets (Less than 1%) 3271
PREVPAC (Less than 1%) 3284
Protopic Ointment (0.2% to less than 1%) 638
Provigil Tablets (At least 1%) 988
Tamiflu Capsules (1.7%) 2807
Tamiflu Oral Suspension (2%) 2807
▲ Vesanoid Capsules (6%) 2820

Ear drum, perforated
Neurontin Capsules (Rare) 2487
Neurontin Oral Solution (Rare) 2487
Neurontin Tablets (Rare) 2487

Ear precipitate
Ciprodex Otic Suspension (0.5%) 559

Earache
Advair HFA Inhalation Aerosol 1318
Fortical Nasal Spray (Less than 1%) 3337
▲ Hycamtin for Injection (59%) 1458
Lopressor HCT 50/25 Tablets (1%) 2241
Lopressor HCT 100/25 Tablets (1%) 2241
Lopressor HCT 100/50 Tablets (1%) 2241

Ears, blocked
Asacol Delayed-Release Tablets 2692
▲ Chemet Capsules (1.0% to 3.7%) 2458
Neurontin Capsules (Infrequent) 2487
Neurontin Oral Solution (Infrequent) 2487
Neurontin Tablets (Infrequent) 2487
Orthoclone OKT3 Sterile Solution 2360

Ears, ringing
(*see under* Tinnitus)

Ears, roaring in
Garamycin Injectable 3014

Ebriety, feeling of
▲ Intron A for Injection (Less than 5%) 3024

Ecchymoses
Abilify Oral Solution (Frequent) 882
Abilify Oral Solution (Frequent) 2450
Abilify Discmelt Orally Disintegrating Tablets (Frequent) 882
Abilify Discmelt Orally Disintegrating Tablets (Frequent) 2450
Abilify Tablets (Frequent) 882
Abilify Tablets (Frequent) 2450
Aceon Tablets (2 mg, 4 mg, 8 mg) (0.3% to 1%) 3194
Aciphex Tablets 1090
Actiq (1% or greater) 979
Activase I.V. (1%) 1223
▲ Actonel Tablets (4.3%) 2683
▲ Actonel with Calcium Tablets (4.3%) 2688
Advair Diskus 100/50 1308
Advair Diskus 250/50 1308
Advair Diskus 500/50 1308
Advair HFA Inhalation Aerosol 1318
Agrylin Capsules (1% to 5%) 3169
Aloprim for Injection (Less than 1%) 2167
▲ Anaprox Tablets (3% to 9%) 2761
▲ Anaprox DS Tablets (3% to 9%) 2761
▲ Aricept Tablets (4%) 1094
▲ Aricept ODT Tablets (4%) 1094
Arthrotec Tablets (Rare) 3129
Avalide Tablets 888
Avalide Tablets 2874
Avapro Tablets (Less than 1%) 891
Avapro Tablets (Less than 1%) 2871
▲ Azilect Tablets (2% to 5%) 3293
Campral Tablets (Infrequent) 1174
Cardizem LA Extended Release Tablets (Less than 2%) 1728
Caverject Impulse Injection (2%) 2612
Celebrex Capsules (0.1% to 1.9%) 3134
Celexa 1176
▲ CellCept Capsules (3% to less than 20%) 2747
▲ CellCept Intravenous (3% to less than 20%) 2747
▲ CellCept Oral Suspension (3% to less than 20%) 2747
▲ CellCept Tablets (3% to less than 20%) 2747
Clinoril Tablets (Less than 1%) 1924
Colocort Rectal Suspension, USP (Retention) 100 mg/60 mL 2476
Comvax 1928
▲ Copaxone for Injection (8%) 3297
Covera-HS Tablets (Less than 2%) 3139
Cozaar Tablets (Less than 1%) 1935
Crestor Tablets (Greater than or equal to 1%) 678
Cymbalta Delayed-Release Capsules (Infrequent) 1757
▲ Dacogen Injection (22%) 2129
Decadron Tablets 1951
▲ Depacon Injection (4% to 5%) 412
▲ Depakene (5%) 417
▲ Depakote Sprinkle Capsules (4% to 5%) 422
▲ Depakote Tablets (1% to 5%) 427
▲ Depakote ER Tablets (Greater than 1% to 5%) 434
Depo-Medrol Injectable Suspension 2617
Depo-Medrol Single-Dose Vial 2619
▲ Doxil Injection (1% to 10%) 2351
▲ EC-Naprosyn Delayed-Release Tablets (3% to 9%) 2761
Effexor Tablets (Frequent) 3411
Effexor XR Capsules (Frequent) 3417
Elmiron Capsules (Less than or equal to 1%) 2415
Engerix-B Vaccine (Less than 1%) 1425
Flovent Diskus 1443
Flovent HFA 1447
▲ Gabitril Tablets (1% to 6%) 984
▲ Gamunex Immune Globulin I.V., 10% (40%) 3235
Geodon Capsules (Infrequent) 2529
▲ Gleevec Tablets (0.4% to 11%) 2227
Guanidine Hydrochloride Tablets 3016
▲ Hyalgan Solution (14%) 2901
Hydrocortone Tablets 1989
Hyzaar 50-12.5 Tablets 1990
Hyzaar 100-12.5 Tablets 1990
Hyzaar 100-25 Tablets 1990
Indocin Capsules (Less than 1%) 1995
Indocin I.V. (Less than 1%) 2465
Indocin (Less than 1%) 1995
▲ Infergen (4% to 6%) 3364
Keppra Injection 3320
▲ Keppra Oral Solution (1% to 4%) 3314
▲ Keppra Tablets (1% to 4%) 3314
Lamictal (Infrequent) 1481
Lexapro Oral Solution 1190
Lexapro Tablets 1190
Lipitor Tablets (Less than 2%) 2483
Lofibra Tablets 1219
Lofibra Capsules 1216
▲ Lovenox Injection (Up to 3%) 2915
▲ Lupron Depot 3.75 mg (Among most frequent) 3260
Lupron Depot 7.5 mg (Less than 5%) 3264
Lupron Depot–3 Month 11.25 mg (Less than 5%) 3265
Meridia Capsules (0.7%) 489
▲ Mylotarg for Injection (9% to 11%) 3431
Myobloc Injection (Greater than 2%) 3192
Nabi-HB (2%) 2169
▲ Naprosyn Suspension (3% to 9%) 2761
▲ Naprosyn Tablets (3% to 9%) 2761
▲ Neumega for Injection (Greater than or equal to 10%) 3435
Neurontin Capsules (Infrequent) 2487
Neurontin Oral Solution (Infrequent) 2487
Neurontin Tablets (Infrequent) 2487
Norvir (Less than 2%) 503
Oncaspar 1145
Paxil CR Controlled-Release Tablets (Infrequent) 1538
Paxil (Infrequent) 1530
Pentasa Capsules (Less than 1%) 3185
Pexeva Tablets (infrequent) 1694
Pletal Tablets (Less than 2%) 2455
▲ Prevacid NapraPAC (3% to 9%) 3280
▲ Prograf Capsules and Injection (3% to 15%) 632
Protonix I.V. (Less than 1%) 3472
Protonix Tablets (Less than 1%) 3469
Protopic Ointment (Greater than or equal to 1%) 638
Provigil Tablets (At least 1%) 988
Prozac Pulvules and Liquid (Infrequent) 1801
▲ Quadramet Injection (3%) 1040
▲ Rapamune Oral Solution and Tablets (3% to 20%) 3475
▲ Revlimid Capsules (5.4%) 958
Reyataz Capsules (Less than 3%) 921
Rilutek Tablets (Infrequent) 2930
▲ Rythmol SR Capsules (2% to 4%) 2727
Seroquel Tablets (Infrequent) 690
Sonata Capsules (Infrequent) 1717
Sular Tablets (Less than or equal to 1%) 3122
Tarka Tablets 524
Tequin Injection (Less than 0.1%) 938
Tequin Injection in 5% Dextrose (Less than 0.1%) 938
Tequin Tablets (Less than 0.1%) 938
Ticlid Tablets 2810
Tricor Tablets 527
Triglide Tablets 3123
▲ Trisenox Injection (20%) 993
Twinrix Vaccine (Less than 1%) 1595
Uniretic Tablets (Less than 1%) 3100
Vaqta (1%) 2097
Verelan PM Extended-Release Capsules, Controlled-Onset (2% or less) 3106
VFEND I.V. (Less than 2%) 2564
VFEND Oral Suspension (Less than 2%) 2564
VFEND Tablets (Less than 2%) 2564
▲ Viadur Implant (4.6%) 757
Voltaren Tablets (Occasionally) 2307
Voltaren-XR Tablets (Occasionally) 2310
Wellbutrin Tablets 1603
Wellbutrin SR Sustained-Release Tablets (Infrequent) 1607
Wellbutrin XL Extended-Release Tablets (Infrequent) 1613
Zelapar Tablets (2%) 3372
Zemaira (0.2% to 0.4%) 3509
Zomig Nasal Spray (Rare) 3523
Zonegran Capsules (2%) 1101
Zyban Sustained-Release Tablets (Infrequent) 1644
▲ Zyprexa Tablets (5%) 1830
▲ Zyprexa ZYDIS Orally Disintegrating Tablets (5%) 1830

Ecchymosis, injection site
Bicillin C-R Injectable Suspension 1706
▲ Edex Injection (4%) 3089
▲ Fluarix (1% to 10%) 1451
▲ Fuzeon Injection (52%) 2767
ProQuad (1.5%) 2064
▲ Vivitrol (4% to 7%) 995

Ecchymosis, soft eyelid tissue
BOTOX Purified Neurotoxin Complex 570

Ecchymosis, unspecified
Caduet Tablets (Less than 2%) 2508
Lyrica Capsules (Greater than or equal to 1%) 2539
Percodan Tablets 1132
Symbyax Capsules (Frequent) 1819
▲ Thiola Tablets (16.7%) 2141
Zomig Tablets (Infrequent) 3519
Zomig-ZMT Tablets (Infrequent) 3519

ECG changes
(*see under* EKG changes)

Eclampsia
Paxil CR Controlled-Release Tablets 1538
Paxil 1530
Pexeva Tablets 1694

Ectopy, ventricular
Proquin XR Tablets 1153

Ectropion
BOTOX Purified Neurotoxin Complex (Less than 1%) 570
Soriatane Capsules (Less than 1%) .. 1013

Eczema
Abilify Oral Solution (Infrequent) 882
Abilify Oral Solution (Infrequent) 2450
Abilify Discmelt Orally Disintegrating Tablets (Infrequent) 882
Abilify Discmelt Orally Disintegrating Tablets (Infrequent) 2450
Abilify Tablets (Infrequent) 882
Abilify Tablets (Infrequent) 2450
Accutane Capsules 2731
▲ Advair HFA Inhalation Aerosol (1% to 3%) 1318
▲ Aerobid/Aerobid-M (3% to 9%) 1171
Aldara Cream, 5% (1.9%) 1846
Arthrotec Tablets (Rare) 3129
Astelin Nasal Spray (Infrequent) 1904
Atacand HCT (0.5% or greater) 651
Caduet Tablets (Less than 2%) 2508
Celexa (Infrequent) 1176
Chantix Tablets (Infrequent) 2517
Clozaril Tablets (Less than 1%) 2184
Copaxone for Injection (Frequent) 3297
▲ Copegus Tablets (5%) 2754
Cubicin for Injection (Less than 1%) 1026
Cutivate Cream (0.8%) 2662
Cymbalta Delayed-Release Capsules (Infrequent) 1757
Dantrium Capsules (Less frequent) .. 2694
Differin Cream (Less than 1%) 1210
Effexor Tablets (Infrequent) 3411
Effexor XR Capsules (Infrequent) 3417
Engerix-B Vaccine 1425
▲ Entocort EC Capsules (Less than 5%) 2698
Evoxac Capsules (Less than 1%) 1047
Exelon Capsules (Frequent) 2206
Exelon Oral Solution (Frequent) 2206
FazaClo Orally Disintegrating Tablets (Less than 1%) 551
▲ Flovent Diskus (1% to 3%) 1443
Floxin Otic Solution (Single report) ... 1049
Fortical Nasal Spray (Less than 1%) 3337
Gabitril Tablets (Infrequent) 984
Gengraf Capsules (1% to less than 3%) 459
Geodon Capsules (Infrequent) 2529
Imitrex Injection 1463
Imitrex Nasal Spray 1467
▲ Intron A for Injection (Less than 5%) 3024
Invirase (Greater than or equal to 2%) 2772
Kaletra (Less than 2%) 476
Ketek Tablets (Less than 0.2%) 2903
Lamictal (2%) 1481
Levaquin (0.1% to 0.9%) 2384
Levaquin in 5% Dextrose Injection (0.1% to 0.9%) 2384
Lexapro Oral Solution (Infrequent) 1190
Lexapro Tablets (Infrequent) 1190
Lipitor Tablets (Less than 2%) 2483
Lofibra Tablets 1219
Lofibra Capsules 1216
Lotronex Tablets (Rare) 1512
Lunesta Tablets (Infrequent) 3142
Lyrica Capsules (0.1% to 1%) 2539
Miacalcin Nasal Spray (Less than 1%) 2253
Micardis Tablets (More than 0.3%) ... 854
Micardis HCT Tablets 856
Namenda (Infrequent) 1195
Neoral Oral Solution (1% to less than 3%) 2259
Neoral Soft Gelatin Capsules (1% to less than 3%) 2259
Neurontin Capsules (Infrequent) 2487
Neurontin Oral Solution (Infrequent) 2487
Neurontin Tablets (Infrequent) 2487
Nexavar Tablets (Uncommon) 746
Nipent for Injection (Less than 3%) ... 1863
Norvir (Less than 2%) 503
Olux Foam (One case) 1012
Omacor Capsules 2725
Paxil CR Controlled-Release Tablets (Infrequent) 1538
Paxil (Infrequent) 1530
Pegasys (1%) 2789
Pentasa Capsules (Less than 1%) 3185
Permax Tablets (Infrequent) 3356
Pexeva Tablets (infrequent) 1694
Plavix Tablets (1% to 2.5%) 917
Plavix Tablets (1% to 2.5%) 2926
Prezista Tablets (Less than 2%) 3306
Protonix I.V. (Less than 1%) 3472
Protonix Tablets (Less than 1%) 3469
Protopic Ointment (Up to 3%) 638
Prozac Pulvules and Liquid (Infrequent) 1801
▲ Pulmicort Respules (1% to 3%) 661
Recombivax HB 2071
Relpax Tablets (Rare) 2548
Requip Tablets (Infrequent) 1555
Reyataz Capsules (Less than 3%) 921
Rilutek Tablets (0.8% to 1.6%) 2930
Risperdal Consta Long-Acting Injection (Infrequent) 1682
Serevent Diskus (1% to 3%) 1568
Seroquel Tablets (Infrequent) 690
Singulair (Greater than or equal to 2%) 2077
Sonata Capsules (Infrequent) 1717
Soriatane Capsules (Less than 1%) .. 1013
Sustiva Capsules (Less than 2%) 930
Sustiva Tablets (Less than 2%) 930
Symbyax Capsules (Infrequent) 1819
Synagis (More than 1%) 1897
Tasmar Tablets (Infrequent) 3358
Teveten Tablets (Less than 1%) 1735
Teveten HCT Tablets (Less than 1%) 1737
Thalomid Capsules 965
Topamax Sprinkle Capsules (1%) 2404
Topamax Tablets (1%) 2404
Tricor Tablets 527
Uniretic Tablets (Less than 1%) 3100
Varivax (Greater than or equal to 1%) 2100
VFEND I.V. (Less than 2%) 2564
VFEND Oral Suspension (Less than 2%) 2564
VFEND Tablets (Less than 2%) 2564
▲ Visudyne for Injection (1% to 10%) .. 2305
Vytorin 10/10 Tablets 2114
Vytorin 10/10 Tablets 3077
Vytorin 10/20 Tablets 2114
Vytorin 10/20 Tablets 3077
Vytorin 10/40 Tablets 2114
Vytorin 10/40 Tablets 3077
Vytorin 10/80 Tablets 2114
Vytorin 10/80 Tablets 3077
Xopenex Inhalation Solution 3146
Xopenex Inhalation Solution Concentrate 3150
Xopenex HFA Inhalation Aerosol 3154
Zelapar Tablets 3372
Zoloft (Rare) 2586
Zomig Nasal Spray (Rare) 3523
Zonegran Capsules (Infrequent) 1101
▲ Zosyn (4.2%) 3492
Zovirax Cream 820
Zyprexa Tablets (Infrequent) 1830
Zyprexa ZYDIS Orally Disintegrating Tablets (Infrequent) 1830
Zyrtec Chewable Tablets (Less than 2%) 2594
Zyrtec (Less than 2%) 2594
Zyrtec-D 12 Hour Extended Release Tablets (Less than 2%) 2597

Eczema, asteatotic
Clobex Spray (0% to 2%) 1208

Eczema, dyshidrotic
Oxistat Lotion (0.4%) 2667

Eczema, exacerbation of
Cutivate (0.8% to 3.0%) 2662

Eczema at injection site
ProQuad 2064

Eczema herpeticum
Cutivate Lotion 0.05% (Rare) 2664
Protopic Ointment (Up to 2%) 638

Eczematous reactions
(*see under* Eczema)

Edema
Abilify Oral Solution (Infrequent) 882
Abilify Oral Solution (Infrequent) 2450
Abilify Discmelt Orally Disintegrating Tablets (Infrequent) 882
Abilify Discmelt Orally Disintegrating Tablets (Infrequent) 2450
Abilify Tablets (Infrequent) 882
Abilify Tablets (Infrequent) 2450
Accolate Tablets 671
Accutane Capsules 2731
▲ Aceon Tablets (2 mg, 4 mg, 8 mg) (0.3% to 3.9%) 3194
Aciphex Tablets 1090
Actiq (Less than 1%) 979
▲ ActoPlus Met Tablets (4.8% to 6%) 3214
▲ Actos Tablets (4.8% to 7.2%) 3219
▲ Advair Diskus 100/50 (1% to 3%) ... 1308
▲ Advair Diskus 250/50 (1% to 3%) ... 1308
▲ Advair Diskus 500/50 (1% to 3%) ... 1308
Advicor Tablets 1722
▲ Aerobid/Aerobid-M (3% to 9%) 1171
Aggrastat (2%) 1907
▲ Agrylin Capsules (20.6%) 3169
▲ Aldara Cream, 5% (Up to 18%) 1846
Aldoril Tablets 1910
Alferon N Injection (One patient) 1665
▲ Alimta for Injection (Up to 19%) 1750
Alkeran for Injection 955
Aloprim for Injection (Less than 1%) 2167
Altace Capsules (Less than 1%) 1702
Ambien Tablets (Infrequent) 2851
Ambien CR Tablets (Infrequent) 2855
▲ AmBisome for Injection (12.3% to 14.3%) 620
Amerge Tablets (Infrequent) 1339
Amevive (2%) 626
Amitiza Capsules (Less than 0.2%) .. 3224
▲ Anaprox Tablets (3% to 9%) 2761
▲ Anaprox DS Tablets (3% to 9%) 2761
Angeliq Tablets 762
Anzemet Injection (Rare) 2859
Anzemet Tablets (Rare) 2862
▲ Aranesp for Injection (6% to 21%) ... 581
Aredia for Injection (Up to 1%) 2179
▲ Arimidex Tablets (7% to 11%) 673
▲ Arixtra Injection (0.9% to 8.7%) 1351
▲ Aromasin Tablets (5.5% to 7%) 2600
▲ Arranon Injection (0% to 11%) 1357
Arthrotec Tablets (Rare) 3129
Asacol Delayed-Release Tablets 2692
▲ Avalide Tablets (3%) 888
▲ Avalide Tablets (3%) 2874
▲ Avandamet Tablets (2% to 14.7%) ... 1373
▲ Avandaryl Tablets (1% to 4.8%) 1379
▲ Avandia Tablets (4.8%) 1384
Avapro Tablets (1% or greater) 891
Avapro Tablets (1% or greater) 2871
▲ Avinza Capsules (Less than 5%) 1741
Bicillin C-R Injectable Suspension 1706
Blocadren Tablets (0.6%) 1916
▲ Caduet Tablets (1.8% to 14.6%) 2508
▲ Campath Ampules (1% to 13%) 811
▲ Camptosar Injection (1% to 10%) 2604
Cancidas for Injection (0%) 1918
Captopril Tablets 2149
Carbatrol Capsules 3171
▲ Cardizem LA Extended Release Tablets (Up to 4.6%) 1728
Catapres-TTS (3 of 101 patients) 844
Celebrex Capsules (0.1% to 1.9%) ... 3134
▲ CellCept Capsules (3% to 28.2%) 2747
▲ CellCept Intravenous (3% to 28.2%) 2747
▲ CellCept Oral Suspension (3% to 28.2%) 2747
▲ CellCept Tablets (3% to 28.2%) 2747
Chantix Tablets (Frequent) 2517
Clarinex Syrup (Rare) 2995
Clarinex Tablets (Rare) 2995
Clarinex Reditabs Tablets (Rare) 2995
Clarinex-D 24-Hour Extended-Release Tablets 2998
▲ Climara Transdermal System (0.5% to 13%) 771
▲ Climara Pro Transdermal System (3.8%) 776
Clinoril Tablets (Greater than 1%) 1924
Clobex Shampoo 1206
▲ Clolar for Intravenous Infusion (20%) 1271
Clozaril Tablets (Less than 1%) 2184
Colazal Capsules 2838
Colocort Rectal Suspension, USP (Retention) 100 mg/60 mL 2476
Combivent Inhalation Aerosol (Less than 2%) 847
Comvax 1928
▲ Copaxone for Injection (3%) 3297
▲ Coreg Tablets (5% to 6%) 1414
Coumadin for Injection (Infrequent) ... 898
Coumadin Tablets (Infrequent) 898
▲ Covera-HS Tablets (1.9% to 3.0%) ... 3139
Cozaar Tablets (1% or greater) 1935
▲ Cubicin for Injection (1% to 6.7%) 1026
Cutivate Lotion 0.05% (Rare) 2664
Cymbalta Delayed-Release Capsules (Infrequent) 1757
▲ Dacogen Injection (18%) 2129
Decadron Tablets 1951
Demadex Injection (1.1%) 2759
Demadex Tablets (1.1%) 2759
▲ Depakote Tablets (1% to 5%) 427
▲ Depakote ER Tablets (Greater than 1% to 5%) 434
Depo-Medrol Injectable Suspension 2617
Depo-Medrol Single-Dose Vial 2619
▲ Depo-Provera Contraceptive Injection (1% to 5%) 2622
depo-subQ provera 104 Injectable Suspension 2624
Diovan Tablets (More than 1%) 2193
Dolobid Tablets (Less than 1 in 100) 1955
▲ Doxil Injection (1% to 10%) 2351
▲ Duetact Tablets (Greater than 5%) ... 3226
Duragesic Transdermal System (1% or greater) 2373
▲ DynaCirc CR Tablets (8.9% to 35.9%) 2721
▲ EC-Naprosyn Delayed-Release Tablets (3% to 9%) 2761
Effexor Tablets (Infrequent) 3411
Effexor XR Capsules (Frequent) 3417
▲ Eloxatin for Injection (10% to 15%) 2892
▲ Emcyt Capsules (19%) 2634
Emend Capsules (Greater than 0.5%) 1963
Enjuvia Tablets 1062
▲ Epogen for Injection (6% to 17%) 591
▲ Equetro Extended-Release Capsules (Less than 5%) 3180
Estrasorb Topical Emulsion 1147
Estratest Tablets 3199
Estratest H.S. Tablets 3199
▲ Eulexin Capsules (4%) 3009
▲ Evoxac Capsules (1% to 3%) 1047
Exelon Capsules (Frequent) 2206
Exelon Oral Solution (Frequent) 2206
FazaClo Orally Disintegrating Tablets (Less than 1%) 551
▲ Femara Tablets (0.2% to 18.4%) 2214
▲ Ferrlecit Injection (5%) 3388
Finacea Gel (1% or less) 1669
Flebogamma 5%, Immune Globulin Intravenous (Human) 1658
▲ Flovent Diskus (1% to 3%) 1443
Gabitril Tablets (Frequent) 984
Gantrisin Pediatric Suspension 2770
▲ Gemzar for Injection (Less than 1% to 13%) 1771
▲ Gengraf Capsules (10%) 459
Genotropin Lyophilized Powder 2638
▲ Gleevec Tablets (0.7% to 81%) 2227
▲ Hectorol Capsules (34.4%) 1275
▲ Hectorol Injection (34.4%) 1278
▲ Herceptin I.V. (8%) 1233
▲ Humate-P (6%) 3502
▲ Humatrope Vials and Cartridges (2.5% to 21.2%) 1787
Hydrocortone Tablets 1989
Hytrin Capsules (0.9%) 471
Hyzaar 50-12.5 Tablets (1.3%) 1990
Hyzaar 100-12.5 Tablets (1.3%) 1990
Hyzaar 100-25 Tablets (1.3%) 1990
▲ Imdur Tablets (Less than or equal to 5%) 3018
Imitrex Nasal Spray (Infrequent) 1467
Imitrex Tablets (Rare to infrequent) ... 1471
Indocin Capsules (Less than 1%) 1995
Indocin I.V. (Less than 1%) 2465
Indocin (Less than 1%) 1995
▲ Intron A for Injection (Less than or equal to 5%) 3024
▲ Invanz for Injection (2.9% to 3.4%) 1999
Invirase (Less than 2%) 2772
Ionsys Transdermal System (.1% to less than 1%) 2379
▲ I.V. Busulfex (28% to 79%) 2493
Kadian Capsules (Less than 3%) 577
Kaletra (Less than 2%) 476
▲ Kepivance (28%) 597
Klaron Lotion 10% (One of 105 patients) 2909
Klonopin (Infrequent) 2778
Lamictal (2%) 1481

Lariam Tablets 2786
▲ Leukine (13% to 34%) 814
▲ Leustatin Injection (6%) 2357
Levaquin (0.1% to 0.9%) 2384
Levaquin in 5% Dextrose Injection (0.1% to 0.9%) 2384
Librium Capsules 3347
Limbrel Capsules (0.003%) 2672
Lipitor Tablets (Less than 2%) 2483
Lithobid Tablets 1692
Lofibra Tablets 1219
Lofibra Capsules 1216
Lopressor HCT 50/25 Tablets (1%) 2241
Lopressor HCT 100/25 Tablets (1%) 2241
Lopressor HCT 100/50 Tablets (1%) 2241
▲ Lotrel Capsules (0.6% to 3.2%) 2249
Lotrimin 3039
Lotrisone (Less than 1%) 3040
Lovenox Injection (2%) 2915
▲ Lupron Depot 3.75 mg (5.4%) 3260
▲ Lupron Depot 7.5 mg (14.3%) 3264
▲ Lupron Depot–3 Month 11.25 mg (5.4% to 7%) 3265
▲ Lyrica Capsules (2% to 4%) 2539
Matulane Capsules 3191
Mavik Tablets (0.3% to 1.0%) 486
Maxair Autohaler 1852
Maxalt Tablets (Rare) 2008
Maxalt-MLT Orally Disintegrating Tablets (Rare) 2008
▲ Megace ES Oral Suspension (1% to 3%) 2481
Menostar Transdermal System 782
Meridia Capsules (1.2%) 489
Micardis Tablets 854
Micardis HCT Tablets 856
Migranal Nasal Spray (Infrequent) 3348
▲ Mirapex Tablets (4% to 5%) 859
Mircette Tablets 1066
▲ Mobic Oral Suspension (0.6% to 4.5%) 863
▲ Mobic Tablets (0.6% to 4.5%) 863
MS Contin Tablets (Less frequent) 2701
▲ Myfortic Tablets (3% to less than 20%) 2255
Myobloc Injection (Greater than 2%) 3192
▲ Naprosyn Suspension (3% to 9%) 2761
▲ Naprosyn Tablets (3% to 9%) 2761
▲ NeoProfen Injection (4%) 2472
▲ Neoral Oral Solution (2% to 10%) 2259
▲ Neoral Soft Gelatin Capsules (2% to 10%) 2259
▲ Neumega for Injection (59%) 3435
Neurontin Capsules (Infrequent) 2487
Neurontin Oral Solution (Infrequent) 2487
Neurontin Tablets (Infrequent) 2487
Nexium Delayed-Release Capsules (Less than 1%) 655
Nexium I.V. (Less than 1%) 659
Niaspan Extended-Release Tablets 1730
Nimotop Capsules (Up to 1.2%) 749
▲ Niravam Orally Disintegrating Tablets (4.9%) 3092
▲ Norditropin Cartridges (25%) 2323
Noroxin Tablets (Less frequent) 2032
▲ Norvasc Tablets (1.8% to 14.6%) 2545
Norvir (Less than 2%) 503
NovoSeven (1%) 2331
▲ Nutropin for Injection (41%) 1239
▲ Nutropin AQ Injection (41%) 1243
▲ Nutropin AQ Pen (41%) 1243
▲ Nutropin AQ Pen Cartridge (41%) 1243
NuvaRing 2340
Omacor Capsules 2725
▲ Oncaspar (Greater than 5%) 1145
▲ Ontak Vials (47%) 1745
Opana Tablets (Less than 1%) 1122
Opana ER Tablets (Less than 1%) 1126
OptiPranolol Metipranolol Ophthalmic Solution 0.3% (A small number of patients) ⊙ 256
Ortho-Cyclen Tablets 2429
Ortho Evra Transdermal System 2417
Ortho Tri-Cyclen Tablets 2429
Ortho Tri-Cyclen Lo Tablets 2436
Oxandrin Tablets 2962
Oxsoralen-Ultra Capsules 3353
OxyContin Tablets (Less than 1%) 2703
▲ Panretin Gel (3% to 8%) 1747
Parcopa Orally Disintegrating Tablets 3097
Parnate Tablets 1527
Paxil CR Controlled-Release Tablets (Frequent) 1538
Paxil (Frequent) 1530
Pediarix Vaccine 1548
Pentasa Capsules (Less than 1%) 3185
Permax Tablets (1.6%) 3356
Pexeva Tablets (infrequent) 1694
▲ Photofrin for Injection (5% to 18%) 702
▲ Plavix Tablets (4.1%) 917
▲ Plavix Tablets (4.1%) 2926
Pletal Tablets (Less than 2%) 2455
Precose Tablets (Rare) 751
Premarin Intravenous 3442
Premarin Tablets 3446
Premarin Vaginal Cream 3452
Premphase Tablets 3456
Prempro Tablets 3456
Prevacid Delayed-Release Capsules (Less than 1%) 3271
Prevacid for Delayed-Release Oral Suspension (Less than 1%) 3271
Prevacid SoluTab Delayed-Release Orally Disintegrating Tablets (Less than 1%) 3271
▲ Prevacid NapraPAC (Less than 1% to 9%) 3280
PREVPAC (Less than 1%) 3284
Prinivil Tablets (0.3% to 1.0%) 2052
Prinzide Tablets 2056
Prochieve 4% Gel 1003
Prochieve 8% Gel 1003
▲ Procrit for Injection (6% to 17%) 2364
▲ Prograf Capsules and Injection (3% to 18%) 632
▲ Proleukin for Injection (15%) 2266
Prometrium Capsules (100 mg, 200 mg) (Less than 5%) 3203
ProSom Tablets (Rare) 517
Protonix I.V. (Less than 1%) 3472
Protonix Tablets (Less than 1%) 3469
Protopic Ointment (Greater than or equal to 1%) 638
Proventil HFA Inhalation Aerosol (Less than 3%) 3056
Provigil Tablets (1%) 988
Prozac Pulvules and Liquid (Infrequent) 1801
▲ Rapamune Oral Solution and Tablets (16% to 24%) 3475
Recombivax HB (Less than 1%) 2071
Relpax Tablets (Infrequent) 2548
Remicade for IV Injection (Greater than or equal to 0.2%) 971
ReoPro Vials (0.3%) 1809
▲ Requip Tablets (Infrequent) 1555
Rescriptor Tablets 2551
Retrovir Capsules (0.8%) 1560
Retrovir IV Infusion (1%) 1564
Retrovir (0.8%) 1560
▲ Revlimid Capsules (10.1%) 958
Reyataz Capsules (Less than 3%) 921
Rilutek Tablets (Rare to frequent) 2930
Risperdal (Infrequent) 1676
Risperdal M-Tab Orally Disintegrating Tablets (Infrequent) 1676
▲ Rythmol SR Capsules (5% to 13%) 2727
Sandimmune (2% or less) 2275
▲ Sandostatin Injection (1% to 4%) 2278
Sandostatin LAR Depot (Rare) 2280
Seasonique Tablets 1077
▲ Serevent Diskus (1% to 3%) 1568
▲ Simulect for Injection (Greater than or equal to 10%) 2284
Singulair 2077
▲ Soltamox Oral Solution (4% to 32%) 3527
Sonata Capsules (Infrequent) 1717
▲ Soriatane Capsules (1% to 10%) 1013
Stalevo Tablets 2287
Striant Mucoadhesive 1007
▲ Symbyax Capsules (Greater than or equal to 5%) 1819
Symmetrel Tablets 1135
▲ Synera Topical Patch (12%) 1137
▲ Tambocor Tablets (3.5%) 1856
▲ Tarceva Tablets (Less than 1% to 37%) 1259
▲ Tarceva Tablets (Less than 1% to 37%) 2444
Tarka Tablets (0.3% to 1.3%) 524
Tasmar Tablets (Infrequent) 3358
▲ Taxotere Injection Concentrate (0% to 66.7%) 2932
Tegretol/Tegretol-XR 2295
Tequin Injection (Less than 0.1%) 938
Tequin Injection in 5% Dextrose (Less than 0.1%) 938
Tequin Tablets (Less than 0.1%) 938
Thalomid Capsules 965
Thioridazine Hydrochloride Tablets 2163
Thyrogen for Injection (4 patients out of 55) 1286
Tiazac Capsules (2%) 1201
Timolide Tablets 2086
Timoptic Sterile Ophthalmic Solution 2088
Timoptic in Ocudose 2091
Timoptic-XE Sterile Ophthalmic Gel Forming Solution 2092
Topamax Sprinkle Capsules (1% to 2%) 2404
Topamax Tablets (1% to 2%) 2404
▲ Tracleer Tablets (4%) 545
Trelstar LA Suspension (2.3%) 3397
Tricor Tablets 527
Triglide Tablets 3123
Trileptal Tablets (1% to 2%) 2300
Trileptal Oral Suspension (1% to 2%) 2300
▲ Trisenox Injection (40%) 993
Trizivir Tablets 1589
Uniretic Tablets (Less than 1%) 3100
Uroxatral Tablets 2943
▲ Valcyte Tablets (Less than 5%) 2813
Vantas (Less than 2%) 3375
Vaqta (Less than 1%) 2097
▲ Velcade for Injection (11%) 2133
Verelan PM Extended-Release Capsules, Controlled-Onset (1.7% to 1.9%) 3106
▲ Vesanoid Capsules (29% to 32%) 2820
VFEND I.V. (Less than 2%) 2564
VFEND Oral Suspension (Less than 2%) 2564
VFEND Tablets (Less than 2%) 2564
Viadur Implant (Less than 2%) 757
Viagra Tablets (Less than 2%) 2573
▲ Vicoprofen Tablets (3% to 9%) 539
Viracept 2577
▲ Voltaren Tablets (1% to 10%) 2307
▲ Voltaren-XR Tablets (1% to 10%) 2310
Wellbutrin Tablets (Frequent) 1603
Wellbutrin SR Sustained-Release Tablets (Infrequent) 1607
Wellbutrin XL Extended-Release Tablets (Infrequent) 1613
▲ Xeloda Tablets (1% to 9%) 2822
Xyrem Oral Solution (Infrequent) 1688
Yasmin 28 Tablets 796
Yaz Tablets 803
Zelapar Tablets 3372
▲ Zemplar Capsules (7%) 541
▲ Zemplar Injection (7%) 543
Ziagen 1626
Zmax for Oral Suspension 2583
Zoloft (Infrequent) 2586
Zomig Tablets (Infrequent) 3519
Zomig-ZMT Tablets (Infrequent) 3519
Zonegran Capsules (Infrequent) 1101
Zosyn (0.1% to 1.9%) 3492
Zyban Sustained-Release Tablets (Infrequent) 1644
Zyprexa Tablets (2%) 1830
Zyprexa ZYDIS Orally Disintegrating Tablets (2%) 1830
Zyrtec Chewable Tablets (Less than 2%) 2594
Zyrtec (Less than 2%) 2594
Zyrtec-D 12 Hour Extended Release Tablets (Less than 2%) 2597
Zyvox (0% to 2.3%) 2652

Edema, aggravated

▲ Gleevec Tablets (2% to 16%) 2227

Edema, angioneurotic

Accolate Tablets 671
Adalat CC Tablets (Less than 1%) 2964
Altace Capsules (0.3%) 1702
Altoprev Extended-Release Tablets (Rare) 3109
Anaprox Tablets (Less than 1%) 2761
Anaprox DS Tablets (Less than 1%) 2761
Atrovent Nasal Spray 0.06% (Rare) 839
Augmentin 1360
Augmentin Tablets 1363
Augmentin XR Extended-Release Tablets 1369
Bexxar 1398
Byetta Injection 611
Caduet Tablets 2508
Carafate Suspension 701
Carafate Tablets 701
Catapres Tablets (About 5 in 1,000 patients) 843
Catapres-TTS (0.5% or less) 844
Ceftin 1407
Cipro XR Tablets 2990
Climara Transdermal System 771
Climara Pro Transdermal System 776
Clinoril Tablets (Less than 1 in 100) 1924
Clorpres Tablets (About 5 in 1,000) 2153
Colyte with Flavor Packs for Oral Solution (Rare) 3088
Combivent Inhalation Aerosol (Rare) 847
Comvax (Rare) 1928
Cozaar Tablets (Rare) 1935
CytoGam Intravenous (A possibility) 1895
Decadron Tablets 1951
Diovan Tablets (Less frequent) 2193
Diovan HCT Tablets (Less frequent) 2196
Dolobid Tablets (Less than 1 in 100) 1955
EC-Naprosyn Delayed-Release Tablets (Less than 1%) 2761
Elidel Cream 1% 2200
Engerix-B Vaccine 1425
Eraxis for Injection (Less than 1% to less than 2%) 2521
Flonase Nasal Spray 1440
Fluarix 1451
Gengraf Capsules (1% to less than 3%) 459
Gris-PEG Tablets (Rare) 2502
Havrix Vaccine (Rare) 1456
HibTITER 3426
Hydrocortone Tablets 1989
HyperHep B S/D 3240
HyperRAB (Rare) 3242
HyperTET (Few isolated cases) 3248
Imitrex Injection 1463
Imitrex Nasal Spray 1467
Imitrex Tablets 1471
Intron A for Injection (Rare) 3024
Lamictal (Rare) 1481
Lescol Capsules (Rare) 2233
Lescol XL Tablets 2233
Leukeran Tablets 1504
Lipitor Tablets 2483
Malarone Pediatric Tablets 1517
Malarone Tablets 1517
Mavik Tablets (0.13%) 486
Mefoxin for Injection 2012
Mefoxin Premixed Intravenous Solution 2016
Meridia Capsules 489
Mevacor Tablets (Rare) 2021
Micardis Tablets 854
Micardis HCT Tablets 856
M-M-R II 2006
Naprosyn Suspension (Less than 1%) 2761
Naprosyn Tablets (Less than 1%) 2761
Neoral Oral Solution (1% to less than 3%) 2259
Neoral Soft Gelatin Capsules (1% to less than 3%) 2259
Niaspan Extended-Release Tablets 1730
Noroxin Tablets 2032
Norvir 503
Oracea Capsules 1000
Orthoclone OKT3 Sterile Solution 2360
Paxil CR Controlled-Release Tablets (Rare) 1538
Paxil (Rare) 1530
Liquid PedvaxHIB (Rare) 2035
Pepcid Injection (Infrequent) 2040
Pepcid (Infrequent) 2038
Premarin Vaginal Cream 3452
Prevacid NapraPAC (Less than 1%) 3280
Prevnar for Injection 3463
Prilosec OTC Delayed-Release Tablets (Less than 1%) 2677
Primaxin I.M. 2045
Primaxin I.V. (Less than 0.2%) 2048
Prinzide Tablets (Rare) 2056
ProQuad 2064
Proventil Inhalation Solution 0.083% (Rare) 3055
Proventil HFA Inhalation Aerosol (Rare) 3056
Pulmicort Respules (Less than 1%) 661
Raptiva for Injection 1250
Rescriptor Tablets 2551
Rilutek Tablets (Rare) 2930
Risperdal 1676
Risperdal M-Tab Orally Disintegrating Tablets 1676
Sanctura Tablets (One event) 1151
Solodyn Extended Release Tablets 1890
▲ Stromectol Tablets (22.7%) 2083
Sular Tablets (Very rare) 3122
Tarka Tablets (0.15%) 524
Tequin Injection 938
Tequin Injection in 5% Dextrose 938
Tequin Tablets 938
Thioridazine Hydrochloride Tablets 2163
Trusopt Sterile Ophthalmic Solution 2095
VESIcare Tablets 646
Vivitrol 995
Vytorin 10/10 Tablets 2114
Vytorin 10/10 Tablets 3077
Vytorin 10/20 Tablets 2114
Vytorin 10/20 Tablets 3077
Vytorin 10/40 Tablets 2114

Vytorin 10/40 Tablets........ 3077
Vytorin 10/80 Tablets........ 2114
Vytorin 10/80 Tablets........ 3077
Wellbutrin Tablets........ 1603
Wellbutrin SR Sustained-Release Tablets........ 1607
Wellbutrin XL Extended-Release Tablets........ 1613
Xifaxan Tablets........ 2842
Zantac (Rare)........ 1624
Zantac Injection (Rare)........ 1619
Zantac Injection Pharmacy Bulk Package (Rare)........ 1622
Zantac Injection Premixed (Rare)........ 1619
Zantac (Rare)........ 1624
Zegerid Capsules (Less than 1%)........ 2958
Zegerid Powder for Oral Solution (Less than 1%)........ 2958
Zetia Tablets........ 2120
Zocor Tablets (Rare)........ 2105
Zofran Injection (Rare)........ 1634
Zometa for Intravenous Infusion........ 2315
Zomig Nasal Spray (Rare)........ 3523
Zovirax Cream........ 820
Zyban Sustained-Release Tablets........ 1644
Zyrtec Chewable Tablets (Less than 2%)........ 2594
Zyrtec (Less than 2%)........ 2594
Zyrtec-D 12 Hour Extended Release Tablets (Less than 2%)........ 2597

Edema, aphakic cystoid macular

Cosopt Sterile Ophthalmic Solution........ 1931
Timoptic Sterile Ophthalmic Solution (Less frequent)........ 2088
Timoptic in Ocudose (Less frequent)........ 2091
Timoptic-XE Sterile Ophthalmic Gel Forming Solution........ 2092

Edema, cerebral

Activase I.V........ 1223
Aggrenox Capsules........ 822
Bayer Aspirin........ 744
Bayer Aspirin Comprehensive Prescribing Information........ ▣796
Gleevec Tablets (Rare)........ 2227
Orthoclone OKT3 Sterile Solution........ 2360
Percodan Tablets........ 1132
Permax Tablets (Rare)........ 3356
Proleukin for Injection (Less than 1%)........ 2266
St. Joseph 81 mg Aspirin Chewable and Enteric Coated Tablets........ 1869
St. Joseph 81 mg Aspirin........ ▣688
Thiothixene Capsules........ 2165
▲ Vesanoid Capsules (3%)........ 2820
VFEND I.V. (Less than 2%)........ 2564
VFEND Oral Suspension (Less than 2%)........ 2564
VFEND Tablets (Less than 2%)........ 2564

Edema, conjunctival

▲ Alphagan P Ophthalmic Solution (1% to 4%)........ 567
▲ Brimonidine Tartrate Ophthalmic Solution 0.2% (3% to 9%)........ ⊙248
Cipro........ 2977
Cipro XR Tablets........ 2990
Cosopt Sterile Ophthalmic Solution (1% to 5%)........ 1931
Differin Cream (Less than 1%)........ 1210
Effexor Tablets (Rare)........ 3411
Effexor XR Capsules (Rare)........ 3417
▲ Lumigan Ophthalmic Solution (1% to 3%)........ 573
▲ Macugen Injection (1% to 5%)........ ⊙261
▲ Nevanac Ophthalmic Suspension 0.1% (1% to 5%)........ ⊙209
Patanol Ophthalmic Solution (Less than 5%)........ 561
Paxil CR Controlled-Release Tablets (Rare)........ 1538
Paxil (Rare)........ 1530
Pexeva Tablets (rare)........ 1694
Proquin XR Tablets........ 1153
Protopic Ointment (0.2% to less than 1%)........ 638
▲ Retisert Implant (5% to 9%)........ ⊙258
Trileptal Tablets........ 2300
Trileptal Oral Suspension........ 2300

Edema, corneal

▲ Acular Ophthalmic Solution (1% to 10%)........ 565
▲ Acular LS Ophthalmic Solution (1% to 10%)........ 566
▲ Macugen Injection (10% to 40%)........ ⊙261
▲ Nevanac Ophthalmic Suspension 0.1% (1% to 5%)........ ⊙209
▲ Retisert Implant (5% to 9%)........ ⊙258
Symmetrel Tablets (0.1% to 1%)........ 1135
▲ Voltaren Ophthalmic Solution (Less than or equal to 5%)........ 2309
Xalatan Sterile Ophthalmic Solution........ 2649

Edema, cystoid macular

Advicor Tablets........ 1722
Lumigan Ophthalmic Solution........ 573
Niaspan Extended-Release Tablets........ 1730
Travatan Ophthalmic Solution........ 563
Xalatan Sterile Ophthalmic Solution........ 2649

Edema, dependent

Aldurazyme for Intravenous Infusion (2%)........ 1268
▲ Coreg Tablets (4%)........ 1414
Diovan HCT Tablets (Greater than 0.2%)........ 2196
▲ Entocort EC Capsules (Less than 5%)........ 2698
▲ Fabrazyme for Intravenous Infusion (6%)........ 1274
Micardis Tablets (More than 0.3%)........ 854
Micardis HCT Tablets........ 856
▲ Mobic Oral Suspension (0.6% to 4.5%)........ 863
▲ Mobic Tablets (0.6% to 4.5%)........ 863
Razadyne (Infrequent)........ 2399
Razadyne ER Extended-Release Capsules (Infrequent)........ 2399
▲ Requip Tablets (6%)........ 1555
▲ Simulect for Injection (3% to 10%)........ 2284
▲ Spiriva HandiHaler (3% to 5%)........ 869
Teveten Tablets (1% or greater)........ 1735
Teveten HCT Tablets (Less than 1%)........ 1737
Zoloft (Infrequent)........ 2586

Edema, ear

Fabrazyme for Intravenous Infusion........ 1274

Edema, esophageal

▲ Photofrin for Injection (8%)........ 702

Edema, extremities

Celexa (Infrequent)........ 1176
Cipro (Less than 1%)........ 2977
Cipro I.V. (1% or less)........ 2984
Cipro XR Tablets........ 2990
Depacon Injection........ 412
Depakene........ 417
Depakote Sprinkle Capsules........ 422
Depakote Tablets........ 427
Depakote ER Tablets........ 434
Imitrex Injection (Rare)........ 1463
Lexapro Oral Solution (Infrequent)........ 1190
Lexapro Tablets (Infrequent)........ 1190
Raniclor Tablets, Chewable (Rare)........ 2505
Tarka Tablets........ 524
Taxotere Injection Concentrate........ 2932

Edema, eyelid

ProQuad........ 2064
▲ Retisert Implant (10% to 35%)........ ⊙258

Edema, facial

Abilify Oral Solution (Infrequent)........ 882
Abilify Oral Solution (Infrequent)........ 2450
Abilify Discmelt Orally Disintegrating Tablets (Infrequent)........ 882
Abilify Discmelt Orally Disintegrating Tablets (Infrequent)........ 2450
Abilify Tablets (Infrequent)........ 882
Abilify Tablets (Infrequent)........ 2450
Aciphex Tablets (Rare)........ 1090
Actiq (Less than 1%)........ 979
Adalat CC Tablets (Less than 1%)........ 2964
Advair Diskus 100/50........ 1308
Advair Diskus 250/50........ 1308
Advair Diskus 500/50........ 1308
Advair HFA Inhalation Aerosol........ 1318
▲ Aldurazyme for Intravenous Infusion (9%)........ 1268
Ambien Tablets (Rare)........ 2851
Ambien CR Tablets (Rare)........ 2855
AmBisome for Injection (Less common)........ 620
Anzemet Injection (Rare)........ 2859
Anzemet Tablets (Rare)........ 2862
Aricept Tablets (Infrequent)........ 1094
Aricept ODT Tablets (Infrequent)........ 1094
Asacol Delayed-Release Tablets........ 2692
Astelin Nasal Spray........ 1904
Attenuvax........ 1914
Avalide Tablets........ 888
Avalide Tablets........ 2874
Avapro Tablets (Less than 1%)........ 891
Avapro Tablets (Less than 1%)........ 2871
Avelox (Less than 0.1%)........ 2970
Azilect Tablets (Infrequent)........ 3293
▲ Azmacort Inhalation Aerosol (1% to 3%)........ 1726
Benicar Tablets (Five patients)........ 1043
Benicar HCT Tablets (2 out of 1,243 patients)........ 1044
Bexxar........ 1398
Caduet Tablets (Less than 2%)........ 2508
Campath Ampules........ 811
Campral Tablets (Rare)........ 1174
▲ Cancidas for Injection (0% to 3.1%)........ 1918
▲ Carac Cream, 0.5% (35.4%)........ 2879
Celebrex Capsules (0.1% to 1.9%)........ 3134
Celexa (Rare)........ 1176
▲ CellCept Capsules (3% to less than 20%)........ 2747
▲ CellCept Intravenous (3% to less than 20%)........ 2747
▲ CellCept Oral Suspension (3% to less than 20%)........ 2747
▲ CellCept Tablets (3% to less than 20%)........ 2747
Cesamet Capsules........ 3340
Cialis Tablets (Less than 2%)........ 1838
Cipro (Less than 1%)........ 2977
Cipro I.V. (1% or less)........ 2984
Cipro XR Tablets........ 2990
Colyte with Flavor Packs for Oral Solution (Rare)........ 3088
Combivent Inhalation Aerosol (Less than 2%)........ 847
▲ Copaxone for Injection (6%)........ 3297
Cozaar Tablets (Rare)........ 1935
Cymbalta Delayed-Release Capsules (Infrequent)........ 1757
Depacon Injection (1% or more)........ 412
Depakene (1% or more)........ 417
Depakote Sprinkle Capsules........ 422
▲ Depakote Tablets (1% to 5%)........ 427
Depakote ER Tablets (1% or more)........ 434
Doxil Injection (Less than 1%)........ 2351
Effexor Tablets (Infrequent)........ 3411
Effexor XR Capsules (Infrequent)........ 3417
Elidel Cream 1%........ 2200
▲ Entocort EC Capsules (Less than 5%)........ 2698
Evoxac Capsules (Less than 1%)........ 1047
Exelon Capsules (Infrequent)........ 2206
Exelon Oral Solution (Infrequent)........ 2206
Flonase Nasal Spray........ 1440
Flovent HFA........ 1447
Flumist Vaccine........ 1901
Gabitril Tablets (Infrequent)........ 984
Geodon Capsules (Frequent)........ 2529
HibTITER........ 3426
Hytrin Capsules (At least 1%)........ 471
Imitrex Nasal Spray........ 1467
Imitrex Tablets........ 1471
▲ Intron A for Injection (Up to 10%)........ 3024
Invanz for Injection (Greater than 0.1%)........ 1999
Kaletra (Less than 2%)........ 476
Keppra Oral Solution (2%)........ 3314
Keppra Tablets (2%)........ 3314
Ketek Tablets........ 2903
Klonopin........ 2778
Lamictal (2%)........ 1481
Levaquin (0.1% to 0.9%)........ 2384
Levaquin in 5% Dextrose Injection (0.1% to 0.9%)........ 2384
Levitra Tablets (Less than 2%)........ 3034
Levulan Kerastick for Topical Solution, 20% (1%)........ 1085
Lipitor Tablets (Less than 2%)........ 2483
Lofibra Tablets (Less than 1%)........ 1219
Lofibra Capsules (Less than 1%)........ 1216
Lunesta Tablets (Infrequent)........ 3142
Lupron Depot–3 Month 11.25 mg........ 3265
▲ Lyrica Capsules (1% to 3%)........ 2539
Maxalt Tablets (Infrequent)........ 2008
Maxalt-MLT Orally Disintegrating Tablets (Infrequent)........ 2008
Meridia Capsules........ 489
Meruvax II........ 2019
Micardis Tablets........ 854
Micardis HCT Tablets........ 856
M-M-R II........ 2006
Mobic Oral Suspension (Less than 2%)........ 863
Mobic Tablets (Less than 2%)........ 863
Mumpsvax........ 2031
Myozyme for Intravenous Infusion........ 1279
Neumega for Injection........ 3435
Neupogen for Injection........ 603
Neurontin Capsules (Frequent)........ 2487
Neurontin Oral Solution (Frequent)........ 2487
Neurontin Tablets (Frequent)........ 2487
Nexium Delayed-Release Capsules (Less than 1%)........ 655
Nexium I.V. (Less than 1%)........ 659
▲ Nipent for Injection (3% to 10%)........ 1863
Noroxin Tablets........ 2032
Norvir (Less than 2%)........ 503
Numorphan Injection........ 1120
Omnicef Capsules........ 511
Omnicef for Oral Suspension........ 511
Oncaspar (Less than 1%)........ 1145
OxyContin Tablets (Less than 1%)........ 2703
Paxil CR Controlled-Release Tablets (Infrequent)........ 1538
Paxil (Infrequent)........ 1530
Pepcid Injection (Infrequent)........ 2040
Pepcid (Infrequent)........ 2038
Permax Tablets (1.1%)........ 3356
Pexeva Tablets (infrequent)........ 1694
Pletal Tablets (Less than 2%)........ 2455
Prevnar for Injection........ 3463
Primaxin I.V. (Less than 0.2%)........ 2048
Prinivil Tablets (0.3% to 1.0%)........ 2052
Prinzide Tablets........ 2056
Prochieve 4% Gel........ 1003
Prochieve 8% Gel........ 1003
Propecia Tablets........ 2060
ProQuad........ 2064
Proquin XR Tablets........ 1153
Protonix I.V. (Less than 1%)........ 3472
Protonix Tablets (Less than 1%)........ 3469
Protopic Ointment (1% to 3%)........ 638
Prozac Pulvules and Liquid (Infrequent)........ 1801
Raniclor Tablets, Chewable (Rare)........ 2505
▲ Rapamune Oral Solution and Tablets (3% to 20%)........ 3475
Relenza Rotadisk........ 1552
Relpax Tablets (Infrequent)........ 2548
Remicade for IV Injection........ 971
Rilutek Tablets (Infrequent)........ 2930
Sandostatin LAR Depot (Rare)........ 2280
Seroquel Tablets (Infrequent)........ 690
▲ Simulect for Injection (3% to 10%)........ 2284
Sonata Capsules (Infrequent)........ 1717
Stromectol Tablets (1.2%)........ 2083
Sular Tablets (Less than or equal to 1%)........ 3122
Sulfamylon Cream........ 2162
Sulfamylon for 5% Topical Solution........ 2162
Suprax........ 1843
Tarka Tablets........ 524
Tasmar Tablets (Infrequent)........ 3358
Tequin Injection (Less than 0.1%)........ 938
Tequin Injection in 5% Dextrose (Less than 0.1%)........ 938
Tequin Tablets (Less than 0.1%)........ 938
Teveten HCT Tablets (Less than 1%)........ 1737
▲ Thalomid Capsules (4.2%)........ 965
Topamax Sprinkle Capsules (Infrequent)........ 2404
Topamax Tablets (Infrequent)........ 2404
Tricor Tablets........ 527
▲ Trisenox Injection (8%)........ 993
Valtrex Caplets........ 1597
Vantin Tablets and Oral Suspension (Less than 1%)........ 2645
▲ Vesanoid Capsules (6%)........ 2820
VFEND I.V (Less than 2%)........ 2564
VFEND Oral Suspension (Less than 2%)........ 2564
VFEND Tablets (Less than 2%)........ 2564
Viagra Tablets (Less than 2%)........ 2573
Viramune Oral Suspension........ 873
Viramune Tablets........ 873
▲ Voltaren Ophthalmic Solution (Less than or equal to 3%)........ 2309
Wellbutrin SR Sustained-Release Tablets (Infrequent)........ 1607
Wellbutrin XL Extended-Release Tablets (Infrequent)........ 1613
Zelapar Tablets........ 3372
Zemplar Injection........ 543
Zoloft (Infrequent)........ 2586
Zomig Tablets (Infrequent)........ 3519
Zomig Nasal Spray (Infrequent)........ 3523
Zomig-ZMT Tablets (Infrequent)........ 3519
Zonegran Capsules (Infrequent)........ 1101
Zyban Sustained-Release Tablets (Less than 1%)........ 1644
Zyprexa Tablets (Infrequent)........ 1830
Zyprexa ZYDIS Orally Disintegrating Tablets (Infrequent)........ 1830
Zyrtec Chewable Tablets (Less than 2%)........ 2594
Zyrtec (Less than 2%)........ 2594
Zyrtec-D 12 Hour Extended Release Tablets (Less than 2%)........ 2597

Edema, generalized

Caduet Tablets (Less than 2%)........ 2508
Symbyax Capsules (Frequent)........ 1819

Edema, genital

Doxil Injection (Less than 1%)........ 2351
Estring Vaginal Ring........ 2635
▲ Simulect for Injection (3% to 10%)........ 2284
Viagra Tablets (Less than 2%)........ 2573

Edema, hand
Cipro XR Tablets ... 2990
Proquin XR Tablets ... 1153
Remicade for IV Injection ... 971
Seroquel Tablets (Rare) ... 690

Edema, heart failure
(*see under* Congestive heart failure)

Edema, injection site
▲ Betaseron for SC Injection (3%) ... 767
Bicillin C-R Injectable Suspension ... 1706
Ionsys Transdermal System (.1% to less than 1%) ... 2379
Merrem I.V. (0.2%) ... 686
Premarin Intravenous ... 3442
▲ Trisenox Injection (10%) ... 993
Tygacil for Injection (0% to less than 2%) ... 3488
▲ Visudyne for Injection (10% to 30%) ... 2305

Edema, labia
Alinia for Oral Suspension (Less than 1%) ... 2835
Alinia Tablets (Less than 1%) ... 2835
Vandazole Vaginal Gel (Less than 1%) ... 3338

Edema, laryngeal
Activase I.V. (Very rare) ... 1223
Arthrotec Tablets (Rare) ... 3129
Avelox ... 2970
Axid Oral Solution (Rare) ... 879
Bayer Aspirin ... 744
BeneFix Vials ... 3408
Bicillin C-R Injectable Suspension ... 1706
Cipro (Less than 1%) ... 2977
Cipro I.V. (1% or less) ... 2984
Cipro XR Tablets ... 2990
Effexor XR Capsules (Rare) ... 3417
Ethyol for Injection (Rare) ... 1898
Fortaz ... 1453
Garamycin Injectable ... 3014
Levitra Tablets (Less than 2%) ... 3034
Lotrel Capsules (About 0.5%) ... 2249
Neumega for Injection ... 3435
Nexium Delayed-Release Capsules (Less than 1%) ... 655
Nexium I.V. (Less than 1%) ... 659
Nipent for Injection (Less than 3%) ... 1863
Numorphan Injection ... 1120
Omnicef Capsules ... 511
Omnicef for Oral Suspension ... 511
Orthoclone OKT3 Sterile Solution ... 2360
Percodan Tablets ... 1132
Permax Tablets (Rare) ... 3356
Persantine Tablets (Rare) ... 868
Prinivil Tablets (0.3% to 1.0%) ... 2052
Prinzide Tablets (Rare) ... 2056
Proquin XR Tablets ... 1153
Prozac Pulvules and Liquid (Rare) ... 1801
Remicade for IV Injection ... 971
St. Joseph 81 mg Aspirin Chewable and Enteric Coated Tablets ... 1869
St. Joseph 81 mg Aspirin ... ◘◙ 688
Tarka Tablets ... 524
▲ Thiola Tablets (4%) ... 2141
Thioridazine Hydrochloride Tablets ... 2163
Thyrogen for Injection (1 patient out of 55) ... 1286
TNKase I.V. (Rare) ... 1264
Vasotec I.V. Injection ... 2103
▲ Vesanoid Capsules (3%) ... 2820
Zofran Injection ... 1634
Zofran ... 1639
Zofran ODT Orally Disintegrating Tablets ... 1639
Zomig Nasal Spray (Infrequent) ... 3523

Edema, laryngotracheal
Photofrin for Injection ... 702

Edema, legs
▲ Estring Vaginal Ring (1% to 3%) ... 2635
▲ Trelstar LA Suspension (6.3%) ... 3397

Edema, lesional
Oncaspar (Less than 1%) ... 1145

Edema, lips
Cipro (Less than 1%) ... 2977
Cipro I.V. (1% or less) ... 2984
Cipro XR Tablets ... 2990
Combivent Inhalation Aerosol (Less than 2%) ... 847
Cozaar Tablets (Rare) ... 1935
Fabrazyme for Intravenous Infusion ... 1274
Imitrex Tablets ... 1471
▲ Oncaspar (Greater than 1% but less than 5%) ... 1145
Orthoclone OKT3 Sterile Solution ... 2360
Propecia Tablets ... 2060
Proquin XR Tablets ... 1153
Remicade for IV Injection ... 971
Rescriptor Tablets ... 2551
Retrovir Capsules ... 1560
Retrovir IV Infusion ... 1564
Retrovir ... 1560
Tarka Tablets ... 524

Edema, local
Avodart Soft Gelatin Capsules ... 1390
Cleocin Vaginal Ovules (Less than 1%) ... 2616
Denavir Cream ... 2174
Havrix Vaccine (Rare) ... 1456
Lidoderm Patch ... 1118
Oncaspar ... 1145
Rescriptor Tablets ... 2551
Striant Mucoadhesive (2.0%) ... 1007
Vantin Tablets and Oral Suspension (Less than 1%) ... 2645
Zovirax Ointment ... 821

Edema, lower extremities
▲ ActoPlus Met Tablets (2.9% to 11.3%) ... 3214
Advate Injection (0.6%) ... 712
▲ Aromasin Tablets (7%) ... 2600
▲ Cardizem LA Extended Release Tablets (5% to 8%) ... 1728
▲ Coreg Tablets (Greater than 1% to 3%) ... 1414
Eldepryl Capsules ... 3208
▲ Femara Tablets (5%) ... 2214
Ferrlecit Injection ... 3388
Miacalcin Injection ... 2252
Micardis Tablets (More than 0.3%) ... 854
Micardis HCT Tablets ... 856
▲ Mobic Oral Suspension (0.6% to 4.5%) ... 863
▲ Mobic Tablets (0.6% to 4.5%) ... 863
▲ Myfortic Tablets (3% to less than 20%) ... 2255
Nexium Delayed-Release Capsules (Less than 1%) ... 655
Nexium I.V. (Less than 1%) ... 659
▲ Norditropin Cartridges (15%) ... 2323
Proquin XR Tablets ... 1153
▲ Requip Tablets (6%) ... 1555
▲ Simulect for Injection (Greater than or equal to 10%) ... 2284
Taxotere Injection Concentrate ... 2932
▲ Tracleer Tablets (8%) ... 545
Trileptal Tablets (1% to 2%) ... 2300
Trileptal Oral Suspension (1% to 2%) ... 2300
▲ Ultram ER Tablets (1% to greater than 5%) ... 2392
VESIcare Tablets (0.3% to 1.1%) ... 646
Xenical Capsules (2.8%) ... 2831
▲ Zometa for Intravenous Infusion (5% to 21%) ... 2315
Zyprexa Tablets (1%) ... 1830
Zyprexa ZYDIS Orally Disintegrating Tablets (1%) ... 1830
Zyrtec Chewable Tablets (Less than 2%) ... 2594
Zyrtec (Less than 2%) ... 2594
Zyrtec-D 12 Hour Extended Release Tablets (Less than 2%) ... 2597

Edema, lung
Zelapar Tablets ... 3372

Edema, macular
Avandamet Tablets ... 1373
Avandaryl Tablets (Very rare) ... 1379
Avandia Tablets ... 1384
Gleevec Tablets (Rare) ... 2227
Intron A for Injection ... 3024
Lumigan Ophthalmic Solution ... 573
Pegasys ... 2789
PEG-Intron Powder for Injection ... 3048
▲ Retisert Implant (5% to 9%) ... ⊙ 258
Retrovir Capsules (A single case) ... 1560
Retrovir IV Infusion (A single case) ... 1564
Retrovir (A single case) ... 1560
Travatan Ophthalmic Solution ... 563
Xalatan Sterile Ophthalmic Solution ... 2649

Edema, mouth
Campath Ampules ... 811
Evoxac Capsules (Less than 1%) ... 1047
Frova Tablets (Rare) ... 1113
Tequin Injection (Less than 0.1%) ... 938
Tequin Injection in 5% Dextrose (Less than 0.1%) ... 938
Tequin Tablets (Less than 0.1%) ... 938
Zemplar Injection ... 543

Edema, nasal
▲ Atrovent Nasal Spray 0.03% (3.1%) ... 837
Striant Mucoadhesive ... 1007

Edema, neck
Proquin XR Tablets ... 1153

Edema, non-specific
(*see under* Edema)

Edema, oropharyngeal
Advair Diskus 100/50 ... 1308
Advair Diskus 250/50 ... 1308
Advair Diskus 500/50 ... 1308
Advair HFA Inhalation Aerosol ... 1318
Arthrotec Tablets (Rare) ... 3129
Atrovent HFA Inhalation Aerosol ... 841
Atrovent Nasal Spray 0.06% (Rare) ... 839
Cipro (Less than 1%) ... 2977
Cipro I.V. (1% or less) ... 2984
Cipro XR Tablets ... 2990
Combivent Inhalation Aerosol (Rare) ... 847
Denavir Cream ... 2174
Flovent HFA ... 1447
Proventil Inhalation Aerosol ... 3053
Proventil Inhalation Solution 0.083% (Rare) ... 3055
Proventil HFA Inhalation Aerosol (Rare) ... 3056
Relenza Rotadisk (Less than 1%) ... 1552
Ventolin HFA Inhalation Aerosol (Less than 3%) ... 1600
VoSpire ER Tablets (Rare) ... 1052

Edema, palpebral
Aredia for Injection (One patient) ... 2179
Betoptic S Ophthalmic Suspension ... 558
▲ Carteolol Hydrochloride Ophthalmic Solution USP, 1% (About 1 of 4 patients) ... ⊙ 249
Cipro I.V. (1% or less) ... 2984
Imitrex Nasal Spray ... 1467
Imitrex Tablets ... 1471
Maxalt Tablets (Infrequent) ... 2008
Maxalt-MLT Orally Disintegrating Tablets (Infrequent) ... 2008
Orthoclone OKT3 Sterile Solution ... 2360
Prinzide Tablets ... 2056
ProSom Tablets (Infrequent) ... 517
Vasotec I.V. Injection ... 2103
Viagra Tablets ... 2573
Viroptic Ophthalmic Solution (2.8%) ... ⊙ 266
▲ Zymar Ophthalmic Solution (1% to 4%) ... 575

Edema, paramacular
Viagra Tablets ... 2573

Edema, penile
Caverject Impulse Injection (1%) ... 2612

Edema, periorbital
(*see under* Edema, peripheral)

Edema, peripheral
Abilify Oral Solution (2%) ... 882
Abilify Oral Solution (2%) ... 2450
Abilify Discmelt Orally Disintegrating Tablets (2%) ... 882
Abilify Discmelt Orally Disintegrating Tablets (2%) ... 2450
Abilify Tablets (2%) ... 882
Abilify Tablets (2%) ... 2450
Aciphex Tablets ... 1090
Actiq (1% or greater) ... 979
▲ Actonel Tablets (1.6% to 8.2%) ... 2683
▲ Actonel with Calcium Tablets (1.6% to 4.2%) ... 2688
▲ ActoPlus Met Tablets (6%) ... 3214
▲ Adalat CC Tablets (18% to 29%) ... 2964
▲ Aerobid/Aerobid-M (1% to 3%) ... 1171
▲ Agrylin Capsules (8.9%) ... 3169
Ambien Tablets (Rare) ... 2851
Ambien CR Tablets (Rare) ... 2855
▲ AmBisome for Injection (14.6%) ... 620
▲ Amitiza Capsules (0% to 3.8%) ... 3224
Anaprox Tablets (Some patients) ... 2761
Anaprox DS Tablets (Some patients) ... 2761
AndroGel (Fewer than 1%) ... 3329
Angeliq Tablets (1.8%) ... 762
Anzemet Injection (Rare) ... 2859
Anzemet Tablets (Rare) ... 2862
Aralast (Greater than or equal to 0.2%) ... 717
▲ Aranesp for Injection (11%) ... 581
Aricept Tablets (Infrequent) ... 1094
Aricept ODT Tablets (Infrequent) ... 1094
▲ Arimidex Tablets (5% to 10%) ... 673
▲ Aromasin Tablets (7%) ... 2600
▲ Arranon Injection (0% to 15%) ... 1357
Arthrotec Tablets (Rare) ... 3129
▲ Asacol Delayed-Release Tablets (3%) ... 2692
Atacand HCT (0.5% or greater) ... 651
Attenuvax ... 1914
Avandamet Tablets ... 1373
Avelox (0.1%) ... 2970
▲ Avinza Capsules (5% to 10%) ... 1741
Benicar Tablets (Greater than 0.5%) ... 1043
Benicar HCT Tablets (Greater than 1%) ... 1044
▲ Betaseron for SC Injection (15%) ... 767
▲ Betimol Ophthalmic Solution (1% to 5%) ... 3382
▲ Betimol Ophthalmic Solution (1% to 5%) ... ⊙ 295
▲ Bexxar (0% to 9%) ... 1398
Caduet Tablets (Greater than or equal to 2%) ... 2508
▲ Campath Ampules (1% to 13%) ... 811
Campral Tablets (Frequent) ... 1174
Cardene I.V. (Rare) ... 2497
▲ Carnitor Injection (3% to 6%) ... 3188
Celebrex Capsules (2.1%) ... 3134
▲ CellCept Capsules (27.0% to 64%) ... 2747
▲ CellCept Intravenous (27.0% to 64%) ... 2747
▲ CellCept Oral Suspension (27.0% to 64%) ... 2747
▲ CellCept Tablets (27.0% to 64%) ... 2747
Cerezyme for Injection ... 1270
Clozaril Tablets ... 2184
▲ Copaxone for Injection (7%) ... 3297
▲ Coreg Tablets (2% to 7%) ... 1414
Crestor Tablets (Greater than or equal to 2%) ... 678
▲ Cubicin for Injection (6.7%) ... 1026
Cymbalta Delayed-Release Capsules (Infrequent) ... 1757
▲ Dacogen Injection (25%) ... 2129
Demser Capsules (Rare) ... 1953
▲ Depacon Injection (3% to 8%) ... 412
▲ Depakene (8%) ... 417
▲ Depakote Sprinkle Capsules (3% to 8%) ... 422
▲ Depakote Tablets (1% to 8%) ... 427
▲ Depakote ER Tablets (Greater than 1% to 8%) ... 434
▲ DepoCyt Injection (7%) ... 1143
Detrol Tablets ... 2628
Detrol LA Capsules ... 2631
Diovan HCT Tablets (Greater than 0.2%) ... 2196
Ditropan XL Extended-Release Tablets (Rare) ... 2413
▲ Doxil Injection (1% to 11.3%) ... 2351
▲ Duetact Tablets (Greater than 5%) ... 3226
EC-Naprosyn Delayed-Release Tablets (Some patients) ... 2761
Effexor Tablets (Frequent) ... 3411
Eldepryl Capsules ... 3208
▲ Eloxatin for Injection (5% to 10%) ... 2892
Emcyt Capsules ... 2634
Enablex Extended-Release Tablets (Greater than or equal to 1%) ... 2203
▲ Enbrel for Injection (2% to 8%) ... 584
▲ Equetro Extended-Release Capsules (Less than 5%) ... 3180
Eraxis for Injection (Less than 1% to less than 2%) ... 2521
▲ Erbitux (1% to 16%) ... 910
▲ Evista Tablets (3.3% to 5.2%) ... 1763
▲ Evoxac Capsules (Less than 1% to 3%) ... 1047
Exelon Capsules (2% or more) ... 2206
Exelon Oral Solution (2% or more) ... 2206
Fansidar Tablets ... 2765
▲ Faslodex Injection (9%) ... 681
FazaClo Orally Disintegrating Tablets ... 551
▲ Femara Tablets (5%) ... 2214
Ferrlecit Injection ... 3388
Fortical Nasal Spray (Less than 1%) ... 3337
Gabitril Tablets (Frequent) ... 984
Gantrisin Pediatric Suspension ... 2770
▲ Gemzar for Injection (20%) ... 1771
Geodon Capsules (Infrequent) ... 2529
▲ Herceptin I.V. (10%) ... 1233
▲ Humatrope Vials and Cartridges (11.5% to 18.2%) ... 1787
▲ Humira Injection (Less than 5%) ... 466
▲ Hytrin Capsules (0.6% to 5.5%) ... 471
Imitrex Nasal Spray ... 1467
Imitrex Tablets ... 1471
Indapamide Tablets (Less than 5%) ... 2156
▲ Infergen (4% to 9%) ... 3364
▲ Intron A for Injection (Less than or equal to 5%) ... 3024
Ionsys Transdermal System (.1% to less than 1%) ... 2379
Iressa Tablets (2%) ... 684
Kadian Capsules (Less than 3%) ... 577
Kaletra (Less than 2%) ... 476
Klonopin (Infrequent) ... 2778
Lamictal (Infrequent) ... 1481
▲ Leukine (11% to 15%) ... 814

Levaquin (0.1% to 0.9%) 2384
Levaquin in 5% Dextrose Injection (0.1% to 0.9%) 2384
Lipitor Tablets (Greater than or equal to 2%) 2483
Lofibra Tablets 1219
Lofibra Capsules 1216
Lopressor Injection (1%) 2238
Lopressor Tablets (1%) 2238
▲ Lovenox Injection (3% to 6%) 2915
Lunesta Tablets (Frequent) 3142
Lupron Depot-PED 7.5 mg, 11.25 mg and 15 mg (Less than 2%) 3269
Lupron Injection Pediatric (Less than 2%) 3259
▲ Lyrica Capsules (3% to 12%) 2539
▲ Megace ES Oral Suspension (1% to 3%) 2481
Meridia Capsules (Greater than or equal to 1%) 489
Merrem I.V. (Greater than 0.1% to 1%) 686
Meruvax II 2019
Miacalcin Nasal Spray (Less than 1%) 2253
Micardis Tablets (1%) 854
Micardis HCT Tablets (1%) 856
Migranal Nasal Spray (Rare) 3348
▲ Mirapex Tablets (2% to 5%) 859
M-M-R II 2006
▲ Mobic Oral Suspension (0.6% to 4.5%) 863
▲ Mobic Tablets (0.6% to 4.5%) 863
Mumpsvax 2031
▲ Myfortic Tablets (3% to less than 20%) 2255
▲ Mylotarg for Injection (8% to 19%) 3431
Myobloc Injection (Greater than 2%) 3192
Myozyme for Intravenous Infusion 1279
▲ Nalfon Capsules (5%) 2502
Namenda (Greater than or equal to 2%) 1195
Naprosyn Suspension (Some patients) 2761
Naprosyn Tablets (Some patients) 2761
▲ Neulasta Injection (15% to 72%) 601
Neumega for Injection 3435
▲ Neurontin Capsules (1.7% to 8.3%) 2487
▲ Neurontin Oral Solution (1.7% to 8.3%) 2487
▲ Neurontin Tablets (1.7% to 8.3%) 2487
Nexium Delayed-Release Capsules (Less than 1%) 655
Nexium I.V. (Less than 1%) 659
Niaspan Extended-Release Tablets 1730
▲ Nipent for Injection (3% to 10%) 1863
▲ Norditropin Cartridges (42%) 2323
Norvir (Less than 2%) 503
▲ Nutropin for Injection (41%) 1239
▲ Nutropin AQ Injection (41%) 1243
▲ Nutropin AQ Pen (41%) 1243
▲ Nutropin AQ Pen Cartridge (41%) 1243
▲ Oncaspar (Greater than 1% but less than 5%) 1145
OxyContin Tablets (Less than 1%) 2703
Paxil CR Controlled-Release Tablets (Infrequent) 1538
Paxil (Infrequent) 1530
Pepcid Injection (Infrequent) 2040
Pepcid (Infrequent) 2038
▲ Permax Tablets (7.4%) 3356
Pexeva Tablets (infrequent) 1694
▲ Photofrin for Injection (7%) 702
▲ Pletal Tablets (7% to 9%) 2455
▲ Premphase Tablets (3% to 4%) 3456
▲ Prempro Tablets (3% to 4%) 3456
Prevacid Delayed-Release Capsules (Less than 1%) 3271
Prevacid for Delayed-Release Oral Suspension (Less than 1%) 3271
Prevacid SoluTab Delayed-Release Orally Disintegrating Tablets (Less than 1%) 3271
Prevacid NapraPAC (Less than 1%) 3280
PREVPAC (Less than 1%) 3284
Prezista Tablets (Less than 2%) 3306
Prilosec OTC Delayed-Release Tablets (Less than 1%) 2677
Prinivil Tablets (0.3% to 1.0%) 2052
Prinzide Tablets 2056
▲ Prograf Capsules and Injection (12% to 36%) 632
▲ Proleukin for Injection (28%) 2266
▲ Prometrium Capsules (100 mg, 200 mg) (Less than 5%) 3203
ProQuad 2064
Protonix I.V. (Less than 1%) 3472
Protonix Tablets (Less than 1%) 3469
▲ Protopic Ointment (1% to 4%) 638
Provigil Tablets (At least 1%) 988
Prozac Pulvules and Liquid (Infrequent) 1801
Ranexa Tablets (Greater than 0.5% to less than 2%) 1035
▲ Rapamune Oral Solution and Tablets (54% to 64%) 3475
Raptiva for Injection 1250
Razadyne (Greater than or equal to 2%) 2399
Razadyne ER Extended-Release Capsules (Greater than or equal to 2%) 2399
Relpax Tablets (Infrequent) 2548
ReoPro Vials (1.6%) 1809
Requip Tablets (Infrequent) 1555
▲ Revlimid Capsules (20.3% to 21.1%) 958
Reyataz Capsules (Less than 3%) 921
▲ Rilutek Tablets (3.3% to 4.2%) 2930
▲ Risperdal Consta Long-Acting Injection (2% to 3%) 1682
▲ Rituxan I.V. (0% to 8%) 1254
▲ Sandostatin LAR Depot (5% to 15%) 2280
Seroquel Tablets (Infrequent) 690
▲ Simulect for Injection (Greater than or equal to 10%) 2284
Soltamox Oral Solution (Infrequently) 3527
▲ Somavert Injection (4% to 8%) 2642
Sonata Capsules (Less than 1%) 1717
▲ Stromectol Tablets (3.2%) 2083
▲ Sular Tablets (22%) 3122
Sustiva Capsules (Less than 2%) 930
Sustiva Tablets (Less than 2%) 930
▲ Sutent Capsules (1% to 17%) 2560
▲ Symbyax Capsules (5% to 8%) 1819
▲ Symmetrel Tablets (1% to 5%) 1135
▲ Targretin Capsules (4.8% to 11.3%) 1747
Tasmar Tablets (1% or more) 3358
▲ Taxotere Injection Concentrate (6% to 39%) 2932
▲ Temodar Capsules (11%) 3073
▲ Tequin Injection (0.1% to 3%) 938
▲ Tequin Injection in 5% Dextrose (0.1% to 3%) 938
▲ Tequin Tablets (0.1% to 3%) 938
Teveten Tablets (Less than 1%) 1735
Teveten HCT Tablets (Less than 1%) 1737
▲ Thalomid Capsules (4.2%) 965
Thioridazine Hydrochloride Tablets 2163
Thiothixene Capsules 2165
▲ Thymoglobulin for Intravenous Infusion (34.1%) 1284
▲ Tiazac Capsules (3% to 5%) 1201
Toprol-XL Tablets (About 1 of 100 patients) 668
▲ Trasylol Injection (5%) 754
Trelstar LA Suspension (1.1%) 3397
Tricor Tablets 527
Triglide Tablets 3123
▲ Tygacil for Injection (3.3%) 3488
Uniretic Tablets (More than 1%) 3100
Univasc Tablets (Greater than 1%) 3104
▲ Urso 250 Tablets (8.3%) 710
▲ Urso Forte Tablets (8.3%) 710
▲ Valcyte Tablets (Less than 5%) 2813
Vantas (Less than 2%) 3375
Vantin Tablets and Oral Suspension (Less than 1%) 2645
▲ Vaprisol (5.5%) 643
Ventavis Inhalation Solution 1020
▲ Verelan PM Extended-Release Capsules, Controlled-Onset (3.7%) 3106
▲ Vesanoid Capsules (52%) 2820
▲ VFEND I.V. (Less than 2%) 2564
▲ VFEND Oral Suspension (Less than 2%) 2564
▲ VFEND Tablets (Less than 2%) 2564
▲ Viadur Implant (3.1%) 757
Viagra Tablets (Less than 2%) 2573
Wellbutrin SR Sustained-Release Tablets (Infrequent) 1607
Wellbutrin XL Extended-Release Tablets (Infrequent) 1613
Zegerid Capsules (Less than 1%) 2958
Zegerid Powder for Oral Solution (Less than 1%) 2958
Zelnorm Tablets 2312
Zoloft (Infrequent) 2586
Zomig Nasal Spray (Rare) 3523
Zonegran Capsules (Infrequent) 1101
Zovirax 1643
Zyban Sustained-Release Tablets (Infrequent) 1644
▲ Zyprexa Tablets (2% to 6%) 1830
▲ Zyprexa ZYDIS Orally Disintegrating Tablets (2% to 6%) 1830
Zyrtec Chewable Tablets (Less than 2%) 2594
Zyrtec (Less than 2%) 2594
Zyrtec-D 12 Hour Extended Release Tablets (Less than 2%) 2597

Edema, pharyngeal

Atacand Tablets (More than 1%) 649
Avelox (Less than 0.1%) 2970
Cipro 2977
Cipro XR Tablets 2990
Cozaar Tablets (Rare) 1935
Maxalt Tablets (Rare) 2008
Maxalt-MLT Orally Disintegrating Tablets (Rare) 2008
Noroxin Tablets 2032
Remicade for IV Injection 971
Xolair 1266

Edema, pulmonary

Abelcet Injection 1141
Abilify Oral Solution (Rare) 882
Abilify Oral Solution (Rare) 2450
Abilify Discmelt Orally Disintegrating Tablets (Rare) 882
Abilify Discmelt Orally Disintegrating Tablets (Rare) 2450
Abilify Tablets (Rare) 882
Abilify Tablets (Rare) 2450
Activase I.V. 1223
Aggrenox Capsules (Less than 1%) 822
Albutein 5%, Albumin (Human) 1652
Albutein 25%, Albumin (Human) 1653
Aldara Cream, 5% 1846
Aldoril Tablets 1910
Ambien Tablets (Rare) 2851
Ambien CR Tablets (Rare) 2855
AmBisome for Injection (Less common) 620
Anaprox Tablets 2761
Anaprox DS Tablets 2761
Argatroban Injection (0.9%) 1346
Atacand HCT 651
Avalide Tablets 888
Avalide Tablets 2874
Avandaryl Tablets 1379
Avandia Tablets 1384
Bayer Aspirin 744
Bayer Aspirin Comprehensive Prescribing Information 796
Blocadren Tablets 1916
Cafcit (2.2%) 1886
Campath Ampules 811
Carimune NF 3499
▲ CellCept Capsules (3% to less than 20%) 2747
▲ CellCept Intravenous (3% to less than 20%) 2747
▲ CellCept Oral Suspension (3% to less than 20%) 2747
▲ CellCept Tablets (3% to less than 20%) 2747
Cipro (Less than 1%) 2977
Cipro I.V. (1% or less) 2984
Cipro XR Tablets 2990
Clolar for Intravenous Infusion 1271
▲ Coreg Tablets (Less than or equal to 0.1% to greater than 3%) 1414
Cosopt Sterile Ophthalmic Solution 1931
Covera-HS Tablets (1.8% to 2%) 3139
▲ Dacogen Injection (6%) 2129
Dantrium Intravenous (Rare) 2695
Decadron Tablets 1951
Diovan HCT Tablets 2196
Diuril Oral Suspension 1954
Diuril Sodium Intravenous 2467
Dyazide Capsules 1423
EC-Naprosyn Delayed-Release Tablets 2761
Elitek (Less than or equal to 1%) 2890
Ferrlecit Injection 3388
Flebogamma 5%, Immune Globulin Intravenous (Human) 1658
Gammagard Liquid 721
Gammagard S/D 724
Gamunex Immune Globulin I.V., 10% 3235
▲ Gleevec Tablets (2% to 16%) 2227
Herceptin I.V. 1233
Human Albumin Grifols 20%, Albumin (Human) 1651
Human Albumin Grifols 25%, Albumin (Human) 1652
Hyzaar 50-12.5 Tablets 1990
Hyzaar 100-12.5 Tablets 1990
Hyzaar 100-25 Tablets 1990
Indocin Capsules (Less than 1%) 1995
Indocin I.V. (Less than 1%) 2465
Indocin (Less than 1%) 1995
Kaletra (Less than 2%) 476
Levaquin (0.1% to 0.9%) 2384
Levaquin in 5% Dextrose Injection (0.1% to 0.9%) 2384
Lopressor HCT 50/25 Tablets 2241
Lopressor HCT 100/25 Tablets 2241
Lopressor HCT 100/50 Tablets 2241
Lotensin HCT Tablets 2246
Lovenox Injection (0.7%) 2915
Lupron Depot 7.5 mg (Less than 5%) 3264
Lyrica Capsules (Rare) 2539
Micardis HCT Tablets 856
Moduretic Tablets 2028
Nalfon Capsules (Less than 1%) 2502
Namenda (Infrequent) 1195
Naprosyn Suspension 2761
Naprosyn Tablets 2761
Neumega for Injection 3435
Neurontin Capsules (Rare) 2487
Neurontin Oral Solution (Rare) 2487
Neurontin Tablets (Rare) 2487
Orthoclone OKT3 Sterile Solution (Less than 2%) 2360
Paxil CR Controlled-Release Tablets (Rare) 1538
Paxil (Rare) 1530
Percodan Tablets 1132
Permax Tablets (Infrequent) 3356
Pexeva Tablets (Rare) 1694
Photofrin for Injection 702
Prinivil Tablets (Greater than 1%) 2052
Prinzide Tablets 2056
▲ Prograf Capsules and Injection (3% to 15%) 632
▲ Proleukin for Injection (Less than 1% to 10%) 2266
Proquin XR Tablets 1153
Prozac Pulvules and Liquid (Rare) 1801
▲ Rapamune Oral Solution and Tablets (3% to 20%) 3475
Remicade for IV Injection (Greater than or equal to 0.2%) 971
ReoPro Vials (1.5%) 1809
Requip Tablets (Infrequent) 1555
Retavase 2499
Revlimid Capsules 958
Rilutek Tablets (Infrequent) 2930
Risperdal Consta Long-Acting Injection (Rare) 1682
▲ Simulect for Injection (3% to 10%) 2284
Symmetrel Tablets 1135
Targretin Capsules 1747
Tarka Tablets 524
Tasmar Tablets (Rare) 3358
Taxotere Injection Concentrate (Rare) 2932
Teveten HCT Tablets 1737
Thalomid Capsules 965
Timolide Tablets 2086
Timoptic Sterile Ophthalmic Solution (Less frequent) 2088
Timoptic in Ocudose (Less frequent) 2091
Timoptic-XE Sterile Ophthalmic Gel Forming Solution 2092
TNKase I.V. 1264
Trasylol Injection (1.2%) 754
TriLyte with Flavor Packs for Oral Solution 3100
Uniretic Tablets 3100
Vasotec I.V. Injection (0.5% to 1.0%) 2103
Verelan PM Extended-Release Capsules, Controlled-Onset (1.8%) 3106
▲ Vesanoid Capsules (3%) 2820
VFEND I.V. (Less than 2%) 2564
VFEND Oral Suspension (Less than 2%) 2564
VFEND Tablets (Less than 2%) 2564
Virazole for Inhalation Solution (Infrequent) 3370
Zostavax Injection (0.2% to 1.2%) 2111
Zosyn (1.0% or less) 3492

Edema, pulmonary, non-cardiogenic

Kadian Capsules (Less than 3%) 577

Edema, retinal

Lyrica Capsules (0.1% to 1%) 2539
▲ Macugen Injection (1% to 5%) ⊙261

Edema, scrotal

Actiq (1% or greater) 979
Caverject Impulse Injection (Less than 1%) 2612
▲ CellCept Capsules (3% to less than 20%) 2747
▲ CellCept Intravenous (3% to less than 20%) 2747
▲ CellCept Oral Suspension (3% to less than 20%) 2747
▲ CellCept Tablets (3% to less than 20%) 2747
▲ Intron A for Injection (Less than or equal to 5%) 3024

Protonix I.V. (Less than 1%)............. 3472
Protonix Tablets (Less than 1%)....... 3469
▲ Rapamune Oral Solution and Tablets (3% to 20%)................... 3475
Uniretic Tablets (Less than 1%)........ 3100
VFEND I.V. (Less than 2%)................ 2564
VFEND Oral Suspension (Less than 2%)... 2564
VFEND Tablets (Less than 2%).......... 2564

Edema, skin
(*see under* Edema, angioneurotic)

Edema, stromal
Viroptic Ophthalmic Solution........... ⊙266

Edema, superficial
▲ Gleevec Tablets (1.1% to 81%) 2227

Edema, tongue
Abilify Oral Solution (Infrequent)........ 882
Abilify Oral Solution (Infrequent)....... 2450
Abilify Discmelt Orally Disintegrating Tablets (Infrequent) 882
Abilify Discmelt Orally Disintegrating Tablets (Infrequent) 2450
Abilify Tablets (Infrequent) 882
Abilify Tablets (Infrequent) 2450
Aricept Tablets (Infrequent) 1094
Aricept ODT Tablets (Infrequent) 1094
Azilect Tablets (Infrequent) 3293
Betaseron for SC Injection 767
Colyte with Flavor Packs for Oral Solution (Rare) 3088
Combivent Inhalation Aerosol (Less than 2%) 847
Cozaar Tablets (Rare) 1935
Effexor Tablets (Infrequent) 3411
Effexor XR Capsules (Infrequent) 3417
▲ Entocort EC Capsules (Less than 5%) 2698
Fleet Phospho-soda (Rare) 1166
Fleet Phospho-soda ACCU-PREP (Rare) 1168
Fleet Phospho-soda EZ-PREP (Rare) 1169
Flonase Nasal Spray 1440
▲ Geodon Capsules (3%) 2529
Lamictal (Rare) 1481
Levaquin (0.1% to 0.9%) 2384
Levaquin in 5% Dextrose Injection (0.1% to 0.9%) 2384
Lunesta Tablets (Rare) 3142
Lyrica Capsules (0.1% to 1%) 2539
Maxalt Tablets (Infrequent) 2008
Maxalt-MLT Orally Disintegrating Tablets (Infrequent) 2008
Meridia Capsules 489
Neumega for Injection 3435
Nexium Delayed-Release Capsules (Less than 1%) 655
Nexium I.V. (Less than 1%) 659
OsmoPrep Tablets (Rare) 2840
Paxil CR Controlled-Release Tablets (Rare) 1538
Paxil (Rare) 1530
Pexeva Tablets (rare) 1694
Pletal Tablets (Less than 2%) 2455
Prozac Pulvules and Liquid (Rare) 1801
Relpax Tablets (Rare) 2548
Requip Tablets (Infrequent) 1555
Retrovir Capsules 1560
Retrovir IV Infusion 1564
Retrovir 1560
Risperdal (Rare) 1676
Risperdal M-Tab Orally Disintegrating Tablets (Rare) 1676
Seroquel Tablets (Infrequent) 690
Sonata Capsules (Rare) 1717
Tarka Tablets 524
Tequin Injection (Less than 0.1%) 938
Tequin Injection in 5% Dextrose (Less than 0.1%) 938
Tequin Tablets (Less than 0.1%) 938
Topamax Sprinkle Capsules (Rare) ...2404
Topamax Tablets (Rare) 2404
Uniretic Tablets (Less than 1%) 3100
VFEND I.V. (Less than 2%) 2564
VFEND Oral Suspension (Less than 2%) 2564
VFEND Tablets (Less than 2%) 2564
Wellbutrin SR Sustained-Release Tablets (Rare) 1607
Wellbutrin XL Extended-Release Tablets (Rare) 1613
Xolair 1266
Zelapar Tablets 3372
Zoloft (Rare) 2586
Zomig Tablets (Infrequent) 3519
Zomig Nasal Spray (Infrequent) 3523
Zomig-ZMT Tablets (Infrequent)........ 3519
Zyban Sustained-Release Tablets (Rare)... 1644
Zyprexa Tablets (Infrequent)............ 1830
Zyprexa ZYDIS Orally Disintegrating Tablets (Infrequent)................................ 1830
Zyrtec Chewable Tablets (Less than 2%)................................... 2594
Zyrtec (Less than 2%)..................... 2594
Zyrtec-D 12 Hour Extended Release Tablets (Less than 2%)..... 2597

Edema, turbinate
Xopenex Inhalation Solution (1.4% to 2.8%)................................. 3146
Xopenex Inhalation Solution Concentrate (1.4% to 2.8%).......... 3150
Xopenex HFA Inhalation Aerosol (1.4% to 2.8%).............................. 3154

Edema, upper extremities
Avalide Tablets................................. 888
Avalide Tablets................................ 2874
Avapro Tablets (Less than 1%)......... 891
Avapro Tablets (Less than 1%)......... 2871
Zyprexa Tablets (Infrequent)............ 1830
Zyprexa ZYDIS Orally Disintegrating Tablets (Infrequent)................................ 1830

EEG changes
ADACEL Vaccine............................. 2945
Clozaril Tablets............................... 2184
DAPTACEL Vaccine......................... 2950
FazaClo Orally Disintegrating Tablets 551
Gabitril Tablets................................ 984
Levaquin.. 2384
Levaquin in 5% Dextrose Injection.... 2384
Librium Capsules............................. 3347
Paxil CR Controlled-Release Tablets (Rare)............................ 1538
Paxil (Rare)...................................... 1530
ProSom Tablets............................... 517
Prozac Pulvules and Liquid (Rare)..... 1801
Topamax Sprinkle Capsules (Infrequent)................................ 2404
Topamax Tablets (Infrequent)........... 2404
Trileptal Tablets (Up to 2%).............. 2300
Trileptal Oral Suspension (Up to 2%).. 2300
Valium Tablets (Infrequent).............. 2819
Wellbutrin Tablets (Rare)................. 1603
Wellbutrin SR Sustained-Release Tablets 1607
Wellbutrin XL Extended-Release Tablets (Rare)............................ 1613
Zyban Sustained-Release Tablets..... 1644

Efficacy, lack of
Cesamet Capsules.......................... 3340
Neoral Oral Solution (1.4%)............. 2259
Neoral Soft Gelatin Capsules (1.4%)... 2259

Ejaculate volume, decreased
▲ Proscar Tablets (1.5% to 3.7%) 2067

Ejaculation, delayed
▲ Cymbalta Delayed-Release Capsules (3%)................................ 1757
▲ Effexor XR Capsules (17%) 3417
▲ Lexapro Oral Solution (9%) 1190
▲ Lexapro Tablets (9%) 1190
▲ Zoloft (14%) 2586

Ejaculation, inhibition
Demser Capsules (Infrequent).......... 1953
Dibenzyline Capsules....................... 3399
Parnate Tablets 1527
▲ Paxil CR Controlled-Release Tablets (3.7% to 10.0%).............. 1538
▲ Paxil (3.7% to 10.0%) 1530
Wellbutrin Tablets (Infrequent).......... 1603

Ejaculation, premature
Bumex Tablets (0.1%)...................... 2746

Ejaculation, retrograde
Flomax 850

Ejaculation disturbances
Abilify Oral Solution (Infrequent)........ 882
Abilify Oral Solution (Infrequent)....... 2450
Abilify Discmelt Orally Disintegrating Tablets (Infrequent)................................. 882
Abilify Discmelt Orally Disintegrating Tablets (Infrequent)................................ 2450
Abilify Tablets (Infrequent)................ 882
Abilify Tablets (Infrequent)............... 2450
▲ Avinza Capsules (Less than 5%) 1741
Avodart Soft Gelatin Capsules (0.1% to 1.4%)............................ 1390
Caduet Tablets (Less than 2%)......... 2508
Campral Tablets (Rare).................... 1174
▲ Celexa (6%) 1176
Clozaril Tablets (1%)....................... 2184
▲ Cymbalta Delayed-Release Capsules (3%)................................ 1757
▲ Duragesic Transdermal System (4%).. 2373
▲ Effexor Tablets (3% to 12.5%) 3411
▲ Effexor XR Capsules (5% to 16%) 3417
Emsam Transdermal System (1%).... 903
FazaClo Orally Disintegrating Tablets (1%)................................. 551
▲ Flomax Capsules (8.4% to 18.1%) ... 850
Geodon Capsules (Infrequent).......... 2529
Kaletra (Less than 2%).................... 476
Klonopin (1%) 2778
Lamictal (Rare)................................ 1481
Levitra Tablets (Less than 2%)......... 3034
▲ Lexapro Oral Solution (5% to 14%) 1190
▲ Lexapro Tablets (5% to 14%) 1190
Lipitor Tablets (Less than 2%) 2483
Lyrica Capsules (0.1% to 1%) 2539
Meridia Capsules 489
Mirapex Tablets (Less than 1%) 859
Neurontin Capsules (Infrequent) 2487
Neurontin Oral Solution (Infrequent) 2487
Neurontin Tablets (Infrequent) 2487
▲ Paxil CR Controlled-Release Tablets (1.6% to 25%) 1538
▲ Paxil (1.6% to 25%) 1530
▲ Pexeva Tablets (1.6% to 28%) 1694
▲ Propecia Tablets (0.2% to 3.7%) 2060
Proscar Tablets (0.2% to 0.8%) 2067
Provigil Tablets (1%) 988
Prozac Pulvules and Liquid (Less than 1%) 1801
Requip Tablets (Rare) 1555
Risperdal (Infrequent) 1676
Risperdal M-Tab Orally Disintegrating Tablets (Infrequent) 1676
Seroquel Tablets (Infrequent) 690
▲ Strattera Capsules (5% or greater) 1814
▲ Symbyax Capsules (2% to 7%) 1819
Thioridazine Hydrochloride Tablets .. 2163
▲ Topamax Sprinkle Capsules (Up to 3%) 2404
▲ Topamax Tablets (Up to 3%) 2404
Viagra Tablets (Less than 2%) 2573
Wellbutrin Tablets (Rare) 1603
Wellbutrin SR Sustained-Release Tablets 1607
Wellbutrin XL Extended-Release Tablets 1613
▲ Zoloft (7% to 19%) 2586
Zyban Sustained-Release Tablets 1644
Zyprexa Tablets (Infrequent) 1830
Zyprexa ZYDIS Orally Disintegrating Tablets (Infrequent) 1830

Ejaculation failure
Flomax Capsules 850
Levaquin (0.1% to 0.9%) 2384
Levaquin in 5% Dextrose Injection (0.1% to 0.9%) 2384
Risperdal Consta Long-Acting Injection (Infrequent) 1682
▲ Strattera Capsules (5%) 1814

Ejection fraction reduction
Herceptin I.V. 1233

EKG, abnormal
Chantix Tablets (Infrequent) 2517
Xyrem Oral Solution (Infrequent) 1688

EKG changes
Aceon Tablets (2 mg, 4 mg, 8 mg) (1.8%) 3194
Aciphex Tablets 1090
Aloprim for Injection (Less than 1%) 2167
Amerge Tablets (Infrequent) 1339
Anzemet Injection (Rare) 2859
Anzemet Tablets (Rare) 2862
Atacand HCT (0.5% or greater) 651
Avelox (Less than 0.1%) 2970
Bumex Tablets (0.4% to 2.9%) 2746
Carbatrol Capsules 3171
Cardene I.V. (1.4%) 2497
Cardizem LA Extended Release Tablets (Less than 2%) 1728
▲ Carnitor Injection (2% to 6%) 3188
Catapres Tablets (Rare) 843
Catapres-TTS (0.5% or less) 844
Clorpres Tablets (Rare) 2153
Clozaril Tablets (1%) 2184
Demadex Injection (2%) 2759
Demadex Tablets (2%)..................... 2759
Effexor Tablets................................ 3411
Effexor XR Capsules....................... 3417
Eraxis for Injection (Less than 1% to less than 2%)........................... 2521
Evoxac Capsules (Less than 1%)...... 1047
FazaClo Orally Disintegrating Tablets (1%)................................. 551
Frova Tablets (Infrequent)................ 1113
Gabitril Tablets (Infrequent).............. 984
Hyperstat I.V.................................. 3017
Imitrex Nasal Spray (Infrequent)....... 1467
Imitrex Tablets (Infreqent)................ 1471
I.V. Busulfex (2%)........................... 2493
Kytril Injection (Rare)....................... 2781
Lamictal.. 1481
Lanoxicaps Capsules....................... 1490
Lanoxin Injection............................. 1494
Lanoxin Injection Pediatric 1497
Lanoxin Tablets............................... 1500
Lexapro Oral Solution (Infrequent) 1190
Lexapro Tablets (Infrequent) 1190
Lofibra Tablets 1219
Lofibra Capsules 1216
Lotensin HCT Tablets 2246
Micardis Tablets (More than 0.3%) ... 854
Micardis HCT Tablets 856
Midamor Tablets 2026
Nalfon Capsules (Less than 1%) 2502
Nimotop Capsules (Up to 1.4%) 749
Paxil CR Controlled-Release Tablets (Infrequent) 1538
Paxil (Infrequent) 1530
Permax Tablets (Infrequent) 3356
▲ Prograf Capsules and Injection (3% to 15%) 632
Protonix I.V. (Less than 1%) 3472
Protonix Tablets (Less than 1%) 3469
Retrovir Capsules (2.4%) 1560
▲ Retrovir IV Infusion (3%) 1564
Retrovir (2.4%) 1560
Seroquel Tablets (Rare) 690
Taxotere Injection Concentrate 2932
Teveten Tablets (Less than 1%) 1735
Teveten HCT Tablets (Less than 1%) 1737
Thioridazine Hydrochloride Tablets .. 2163
Tiazac Capsules (Less than 2%) 1201
Tricor Tablets 527
Triglide Tablets 3123
Uniretic Tablets (More than 1%) 3100
Verelan PM Extended-Release Capsules, Controlled-Onset (2%) ... 3106
Viagra Tablets (Less than 2%) 2573
Wellbutrin Tablets (Infrequent) 1603
Xopenex Inhalation Solution 3146
Xopenex Inhalation Solution Concentrate 3150
Xopenex HFA Inhalation Aerosol 3154
Zemuron Injection (Less than 1%) 2346
Zofran Injection 1634
Zofran 1639
Zofran ODT Orally Disintegrating Tablets 1639

EKG changes, PR prolongation
Amerge Tablets (Infrequent) 1339
Imitrex Injection (Infrequent) 1463
Imitrex Tablets 1471
Lanoxicaps Capsules 1490
Lanoxin Injection 1494
Lanoxin Injection Pediatric 1497
Lanoxin Tablets 1500
▲ Trisenox Injection (8%) 993

EKG changes, Q wave disturbances
▲ Imdur Tablets (Less than or equal to 5%) 3018

EKG changes, QRS interval prolonged
Seroquel Tablets (Infrequent) 690
▲ Trisenox Injection (8%) 993

EKG changes, QT interval prolonged
Abilify Oral Solution (Infrequent) 882
Abilify Oral Solution (Infrequent) 2450
Abilify Discmelt Orally Disintegrating Tablets (Infrequent) 882
Abilify Discmelt Orally Disintegrating Tablets (Infrequent) 2450
Abilify Tablets (Infrequent) 882
Abilify Tablets (Infrequent) 2450
Aciphex Tablets (Rare) 1090
Aloxi Injection (Less than 1%) 2127
Amerge Tablets (Infrequent) 1339
Avelox (0.1% to less than 2%) 2970
Celexa 1176
Detrol LA Capsules 2631

E.E.S. 451
Effexor Tablets (Rare) 3411
Effexor XR Capsules (Rare) 3417
Eraxis for Injection (Less than 1% to less than 2%) 2521
Erythrocin Stearate Filmtab Tablets (Rare) 453
Erythromycin Base Filmtab Tablets (Rare) 455
Erythromycin Delayed-Release Capsules, USP 457
Geodon Capsules 2529
Imitrex Injection (Infrequent) 1463
Levaquin 2384
Levaquin in 5% Dextrose Injection 2384
Lexapro Oral Solution 1190
Lexapro Tablets 1190
Namenda 1195
Noroxin Tablets (Rare) 2032
PCE Dispertab Tablets 515
Pletal Tablets (Very rare) 2455
Prograf Capsules and Injection 632
Prozac Pulvules and Liquid 1801
Razadyne (Infrequent) 2399
Razadyne ER Extended-Release Capsules (Infrequent) 2399
Rythmol SR Capsules 2727
Seroquel Tablets (Infrequent) 690
Strattera Capsules (Very Rare) 1814
▲ Sutent Capsules (11%) 2560
Symbyax Capsules (Infrequent) 1819
Tequin Injection 938
Tequin Injection in 5% Dextrose 938
Tequin Tablets 938
Thioridazine Hydrochloride Tablets 2163
▲ Trisenox Injection (40%) 993
Uniretic Tablets (Less than 1%) 3100
VFEND I.V. (Less than 2%) 2564
VFEND Oral Suspension (Less than 2%) 2564
VFEND Tablets (Less than 2%) 2564
Viracept 2577
Zofran Injection (Rare) 1634
Zofran (Rare) 1639
Zofran ODT Orally Disintegrating Tablets (Rare) 1639
Zoloft 2586
Zomig Tablets (Rare) 3519
Zomig-ZMT Tablets (Rare) 3519

EKG changes, sinus pause
Tambocor Tablets (1% to 3%) 1856

EKG changes, ST section
AccuNeb Inhalation Solution (One case) 1055
▲ Adenoscan (3%) 619
Amerge Tablets (Infrequent) 1339
Anzemet Injection 2859
Anzemet Tablets 2862
Cardene I.V. (Rare) 2497
Clozaril Tablets 2184
Imitrex Injection (Infrequent) 1463
Imitrex Tablets 1471
Lanoxicaps Capsules 1490
Lanoxin Injection 1494
Lanoxin Injection Pediatric 1497
Lanoxin Tablets 1500
OxyContin Tablets (Less than 1%) 2703
Risperdal (Rare) 1676
Risperdal M-Tab Orally Disintegrating Tablets (Rare) 1676
Seroquel Tablets (Rare) 690
Tarka Tablets (0.3% or more) 524

EKG changes, ST segment depression
Zofran Injection 1634
Zofran 1639
Zofran ODT Orally Disintegrating Tablets 1639

EKG changes, T-wave
Adenoscan (Less than 1%) 619
Amerge Tablets (Infrequent) 1339
Anzemet Injection 2859
Anzemet Tablets 2862
Cardene I.V. (Rare) 2497
Clozaril Tablets 2184
Evoxac Capsules (Less than 1%) 1047
Imitrex Injection (Infrequent) 1463
Imitrex Tablets 1471
Lithobid Tablets (Rare) 1692
Moban Tablets (Rare) 1119
Pentasa Capsules (Infrequent) 3185
Prograf Capsules and Injection 632
Razadyne (Infrequent) 2399
Razadyne ER Extended-Release Capsules (Infrequent) 2399
Risperdal (Rare) 1676
Risperdal Consta Long-Acting Injection (Rare) 1682
Risperdal M-Tab Orally Disintegrating Tablets (Rare) 1676
Sular Tablets (Less than or equal to 1%) 3122
Symbyax Capsules (Rare) 1819
Tarka Tablets (0.3% or more) 524
Uniretic Tablets (less than 1%) 3100

Elastosis perforans, serpiginosa
Cuprimine Capsules (Rare) 1947
▲ Thiola Tablets (16.7%) 2141

Elation
▲ Marinol Capsules (8% to 24%) 3333

Electrocardiogram, abnormal
Edex Injection (1%) 3089
Provigil Tablets (Greater than or equal to 1%) 988
Rythmol SR Capsules 2727
Symbyax Capsules (Infrequent) 1819

Electrocardiographic changes
(*see under* EKG changes)

Electroencephalographic changes
(*see under* EEG changes)

Electrolyte disturbances
(*see under* Electrolyte imbalance)

Electrolyte imbalance
Aldoril Tablets 1910
Aloprim for Injection (Less than 1%) 2167
Aloxi Injection (Less than 1%) 2127
Avalide Tablets 888
Avalide Tablets 2874
Benicar HCT Tablets 1044
Camptosar Injection 2604
Capastat Sulfate for Injection (1 patient) 1755
Cubicin for Injection (Less than 1%) 1026
Daranide Tablets 1950
Diovan HCT Tablets 2196
Diuril Oral Suspension 1954
Diuril Sodium Intravenous 2467
Dyazide Capsules 1423
Epivir 1427
Fleet Phospho-soda ACCU-PREP 1168
Fleet Phospho-soda EZ-PREP 1169
Fleet Prep Kits 1170
Follistim AQ Cartridge 2338
Indapamide Tablets 2156
Kionex Powder 2477
Levaquin (0.1% to 0.9%) 2384
Levaquin in 5% Dextrose Injection (0.1% to 0.9%) 2384
Moduretic Tablets 2028
Permax Tablets (Rare) 3356
Prevacid Delayed-Release Capsules 3271
Prevacid for Delayed-Release Oral Suspension 3271
Prevacid SoluTab Delayed-Release Orally Disintegrating Tablets 3271
Prevacid NapraPAC 3280
PREVPAC 3284
Prinzide Tablets 2056
Risperdal 1676
Risperdal M-Tab Orally Disintegrating Tablets 1676
Tequin Injection (Less than 0.1%) 938
Tequin Injection in 5% Dextrose (Less than 0.1%) 938
Tequin Tablets (Less than 0.1%) 938
Teveten HCT Tablets 1737
Thalomid Capsules 965
Timolide Tablets 2086
Uniretic Tablets (More than 1%) 3100
Zelnorm Tablets 2312
Zosyn 3492

Electromechanical dissociation
Retavase 2499

Electro-oculogram, abnormal
Norvir (Less than 2%) 503

Elevated bilirubin levels
(*see under* Hyperbilirubinemia)

Embolism
Activase I.V. 1223
▲ Alimta for Injection (1% to 7%) 1750
Decadron Tablets 1951
Furosemide Tablets 2154
Gleevec Tablets (Rare) 2227
Levaquin (0.1% to 0.9%) 2384
Levaquin in 5% Dextrose Injection (0.1% to 0.9%) 2384
Lithostat Tablets (3 cases) 2140
Ortho-Cyclen/Ortho Tri-Cyclen 2429
Ortho Tri-Cyclen Lo Tablets 2436
TNKase I.V. 1264
Trasylol Injection (1% to 2%) 754
Zosyn (1.0% or less) 3492

Embolism, arterial
Rythmol SR Capsules 2727

Embolism, cholesterol
Activase I.V. (Rare) 1223
TNKase I.V. 1264

Embolism, limb
ReoPro Vials (0.3%) 1809
Requip Tablets (Rare) 1555

Embolism, lower extremities
Camptosar Injection 2604
Rilutek Tablets (Infrequent) 2930

Embolism, pulmonary
Abelcet Injection 1141
Abilify Oral Solution (Rare) 882
Abilify Oral Solution (Rare) 2450
Abilify Discmelt Orally Disintegrating Tablets (Rare) 882
Abilify Discmelt Orally Disintegrating Tablets (Rare) 2450
Abilify Tablets (Rare) 882
Abilify Tablets (Rare) 2450
Aciphex Tablets (Rare) 1090
Actimmune (Rare) 1671
Aloprim for Injection (Less than 1%) 2167
Ambien Tablets (Rare) 2851
Ambien CR Tablets (Rare) 2855
Angeliq Tablets 762
Aranesp for Injection (1.3%) 581
Arthrotec Tablets (Rare) 3129
▲ Avastin IV (16%) 1227
Betaseron for SC Injection 767
Bicillin C-R Injectable Suspension 1706
Campath Ampules 811
Campral Tablets (Rare) 1174
Camptosar Injection 2604
Cathflo Activase 1231
Celebrex Capsules (Less than 0.1%) 3134
Celexa (Rare) 1176
Chantix Tablets (Rare) 2517
Cipro (Less than 1%) 2977
Cipro I.V. (1% or less) 2984
Cipro XR Tablets 2990
Climara Transdermal System 771
Climara Pro Transdermal System 776
Clozaril Tablets 2184
Copegus Tablets (Less than 1%) 2754
Dacogen Injection 2129
Depo-Provera Contraceptive Injection (Less than 1%) 2622
depo-subQ provera 104 Injectable Suspension 2624
Effexor Tablets (Rare) 3411
Effexor XR Capsules (Rare) 3417
Emcyt Capsules (2%) 2634
Emend Capsules (Greater than 0.5%) 1963
Enbrel for Injection (Infrequent) 584
Enjuvia Tablets 1062
Epogen for Injection (Rare) 591
Erbitux (1%) 910
Estrasorb Topical Emulsion 1147
Estratest Tablets 3199
Estratest H.S. Tablets 3199
Evoxac Capsules (Less than 1%) 1047
Exelon Capsules (Infrequent) 2206
Exelon Oral Solution (Infrequent) 2206
FazaClo Orally Disintegrating Tablets 551
Femara Tablets (Less than or equal to 2%) 2214
Gammagard S/D 724
Geodon Capsules (Rare) 2529
Imitrex Nasal Spray 1467
Imitrex Tablets 1471
Ionsys Transdermal System (.1% to less than 1%) 2379
Levaquin (0.1% to 0.9%) 2384
Levaquin in 5% Dextrose Injection (0.1% to 0.9%) 2384
Lexapro Oral Solution 1190
Lexapro Tablets 1190
Lithostat Tablets (3 cases) 2140
Lupron Depot 7.5 mg 3264
Lupron Depot–3 Month 11.25 mg 3265
Lupron Injection Pediatric 3259
Megace ES Oral Suspension 2481
Menostar Transdermal System 782
Merrem I.V. (Greater than 0.1% to 1%) 686
Mirapex Tablets (Less than 1%) 859
Mircette Tablets 1066
Mycamine for Injection 628
Namenda (Infrequent) 1195
Neurontin Capsules (Rare) 2487
Neurontin Oral Solution (Rare) 2487
Neurontin Tablets (Rare) 2487
Nipent for Injection (Less than 3%) 1863
NovoSeven 2331
NuvaRing 2340
Ortho-Cyclen Tablets 2429
Ortho Evra Transdermal System 2417
Ortho Tri-Cyclen Tablets 2429
Ortho Tri-Cyclen Lo Tablets 2436
Paxil CR Controlled-Release Tablets (Rare) 1538
Paxil (Rare) 1530
Pegasys (Less than 1%) 2789
Permax Tablets (Infrequent) 3356
Pexeva Tablets (rare) 1694
Premarin Intravenous 3442
Premarin Tablets 3446
Premarin Vaginal Cream 3452
Premphase Tablets (1.3%) 3456
Prempro Tablets (1.3%) 3456
Prinivil Tablets (0.3% to 1.0%) 2052
Prinzide Tablets 2056
▲ Procrit for Injection (3.2%) 2364
Proleukin for Injection (Less than 1%) 2266
Proquin XR Tablets 1153
Prozac Pulvules and Liquid 1801
Remicade for IV Injection (Greater than or equal to 0.2%) 971
ReoPro Vials (0.3%) 1809
Requip Tablets (Rare) 1555
▲ Revlimid Capsules (2% to 3.2%) 958
Risperdal 1676
Risperdal Consta Long-Acting Injection (Rare) 1682
Risperdal M-Tab Orally Disintegrating Tablets 1676
▲ Sandostatin LAR Depot (1% to 4%) 2280
Seasonique Tablets 1077
Soltamox Oral Solution (0.5%) 3527
Sonata Capsules (Rare) 1717
Sutent Capsules (2 patients) 2560
Tasmar Tablets (Infrequent) 3358
Taxotere Injection Concentrate 2932
Thalomid Capsules 965
Topamax Sprinkle Capsules (Infrequent) 2404
Topamax Tablets (Infrequent) 2404
Trasylol Injection (1% to 2%) 754
Vasotec I.V. Injection (0.5% to 1.0%) 2103
VFEND I.V. (Less than 2%) 2564
VFEND Oral Suspension (Less than 2%) 2564
VFEND Tablets (Less than 2%) 2564
Vivitrol 995
Wellbutrin Tablets (Rare) 1603
Wellbutrin SR Sustained-Release Tablets 1607
Wellbutrin XL Extended-Release Tablets 1613
▲ Xeloda Tablets (Less than 5%) 2822
Yasmin 28 Tablets 796
Yaz Tablets 803
Zonegran Capsules (Rare) 1101
Zosyn (1.0% or less) 3492
Zyban Sustained-Release Tablets 1644
Zyprexa Tablets 1830
Zyprexa ZYDIS Orally Disintegrating Tablets 1830

Embolism, retinal artery
Xalatan Sterile Ophthalmic Solution (Extremely rare) 2649

Embolism, venous
Retavase 2499

Emesis
(*see under* Vomiting)

Emotional disturbances
Accutane Capsules 2731
Avalide Tablets 888
Avalide Tablets 2874
Avapro Tablets (Less than 1%) 891
Avapro Tablets (Less than 1%) 2871
Cesamet Capsules 3340
Chantix Tablets (Frequent) 2517
Decadron Tablets 1951
Depacon Injection 412
Depakene 417

Depakote Sprinkle Capsules........... 422
Depakote Tablets........................... 427
Depakote ER Tablets....................... 434
Efudex (Infrequent)......................... 3363
Imitrex Nasal Spray (Rare).............. 1467
Lariam Tablets (Less than 1%)........ 2786
Paxil CR Controlled-Release Tablets (Infrequent).................... 1538
Paxil (Infrequent)............................ 1530
Pexeva Tablets (infrequent)............ 1694
Rythmol SR Capsules...................... 2727
Xyrem Oral Solution (Infrequent)....... 1688

Emotional lability
Abilify Oral Solution (Infrequent)........ 882
Abilify Oral Solution (Infrequent)....... 2450
Abilify Discmelt Orally Disintegrating Tablets (Infrequent)................................ 882
Abilify Discmelt Orally Disintegrating Tablets (Infrequent)............................... 2450
Abilify Tablets (Infrequent)............... 882
Abilify Tablets (Infrequent)............... 2450
Accutane Capsules......................... 2731
Actiq (Less than 1%)....................... 979
▲ Adderall XR Capsules (1% to 9%) 3166
Adenoscan (Less than 1%).............. 619
Ambien Tablets (Infrequent)............. 2851
Ambien CR Tablets (Infrequent)........ 2855
▲ AndroGel (Up to 3%) 3329
Aricept Tablets (Infrequent)............. 1094
Aricept ODT Tablets (Infrequent)........ 1094
Asacol Delayed-Release Tablets....... 2692
Atripla Tablets................................ 945
Avelox (Less than 0.1%).................. 2970
Azilect Tablets (Infrequent).............. 3293
Betaseron for SC Injection.............. 767
Blocadren Tablets........................... 1916
Caduet Tablets (Less than 2%)......... 2508
Celexa (Infrequent)......................... 1176
▲ CellCept Capsules (3% to less than 20%)....................................... 2747
▲ CellCept Intravenous (3% to less than 20%)....................................... 2747
▲ CellCept Oral Suspension (3% to less than 20%)............................. 2747
▲ CellCept Tablets (3% to less than 20%).. 2747
Cesamet Capsules.......................... 3340
▲ Clarinex Syrup (3.1%) 2995
Concerta Extended-Release Tablets (0.7%).............................. 1881
Copaxone for Injection (At least 2%).. 3297
Coreg Tablets (Greater than 0.1% to 1%).. 1414
Cosopt Sterile Ophthalmic Solution.. 1931
▲ Depacon Injection (6%) 412
▲ Depakene (6%) 417
▲ Depakote Sprinkle Capsules (6%) 422
▲ Depakote Tablets (1% to 6%) 427
▲ Depakote ER Tablets (6%) 434
Diastat Rectal Delivery System (Greater than or equal to 1%)........ 3343
▲ Doxil Injection (1% to 5%) 2351
Effexor Tablets (Infrequent).............. 3411
Effexor XR Capsules (Infrequent)...... 3417
Elmiron Capsules............................ 2415
Emcyt Capsules (2%)...................... 2634
Evoxac Capsules (Less than 1%)...... 1047
Exelon Capsules (Infrequent)............ 2206
Exelon Oral Solution (Infrequent)...... 2206
Frova Tablets (Infrequent)................ 1113
▲ Gabitril Tablets (3%) 984
Gengraf Capsules (1% to less than 3%)... 459
Guanidine Hydrochloride Tablets...... 3016
Inderal LA Long-Acting Capsules...... 3429
▲ Infergen (6% to 12%) 3364
InnoPran XL Capsules..................... 2723
▲ Intron A for Injection (Less than 5%)... 3024
Kaletra (Less than 2%)..................... 476
Keppra Injection (2%)...................... 3320
▲ Keppra Oral Solution (2% to 6%) 3314
▲ Keppra Tablets (2% to 6%) 3314
Klonopin (1%)................................. 2778
▲ Lamictal (4%) 1481
Levaquin (0.1% to 0.9%).................. 2384
Levaquin in 5% Dextrose Injection (0.1% to 0.9%)............................ 2384
Levothroid Tablets.......................... 1186
Levoxyl Tablets............................... 1712
Lexapro Oral Solution (Infrequent).... 1190
Lexapro Tablets (Infrequent)............ 1190
Lipitor Tablets (Less than 2%).......... 2483
Lopressor Injection.......................... 2238
Lopressor Tablets............................ 2238
Lopressor HCT 50/25 Tablets.......... 2241
Lopressor HCT 100/25 Tablets....... 2241
Lopressor HCT 100/50 Tablets....... 2241
Lunesta Tablets (Infrequent)............ 3142
▲ Lupron Depot 3.75 mg (16%) 3260
▲ Lupron Depot–3 Month 11.25 mg (16%)... 3265
Lupron Depot-PED 7.5 mg, 11.25 mg and 15 mg (Less than 2%)... 3269
Lupron Injection Pediatric (Less than 2%).. 3259
Meridia Capsules (1.3%)................. 489
Nadolol Tablets.............................. 2159
Namenda (Infrequent)..................... 1195
Neoral Oral Solution (1% to less than 3%).. 2259
Neoral Soft Gelatin Capsules (1% to less than 3%).......................... 2259
▲ Neurontin Capsules (4.2% to 6%) 2487
▲ Neurontin Oral Solution (4.2% to 6%)... 2487
▲ Neurontin Tablets (4.2% to 6%) 2487
Nipent for Injection (Less than 3%)... 1863
Norvir (Less than 2%) 503
Omacor Capsules 2725
Oncaspar (Less than 1%) 1145
Ortho Evra Transdermal System (1% to 2.4%) 2417
OxyContin Tablets (Less than 1%) 2703
Paxil CR Controlled-Release Tablets (Frequent) 1538
Paxil (Frequent) 1530
▲ PEG-Intron Powder for Injection (28%) 3048
Permax Tablets (Infrequent) 3356
Pexeva Tablets (frequent) 1694
Prevacid Delayed-Release Capsules (Less than 1%) 3271
Prevacid for Delayed-Release Oral Suspension (Less than 1%) 3271
Prevacid SoluTab Delayed-Release Orally Disintegrating Tablets (Less than 1%) 3271
Prevacid NapraPAC (Less than 1%) .. 3280
PREVPAC (Less than 1%) 3284
Prochieve 4% Gel 1003
Prochieve 8% Gel 1003
▲ Prograf Capsules and Injection (3% to 15%) 632
▲ Prometrium Capsules (100 mg, 200 mg) (6%) 3203
ProSom Tablets (Infrequent) 517
Protonix I.V. (Less than 1%) 3472
Protonix Tablets (Less than 1%) 3469
Provigil Tablets (1%) 988
Prozac Pulvules and Liquid (Frequent) 1801
▲ Pulmicort Respules (1% to 3%) 661
▲ Rapamune Oral Solution and Tablets (3% to 20%) 3475
▲ Rebetol (7% to 47%) 3058
▲ Rebetron Combination Therapy (7% to 12%) 3063
Relpax Tablets (Infrequent) 2548
Requip Tablets (Infrequent) 1555
Rescriptor Tablets 2551
Retrovir Capsules 1560
Retrovir IV Infusion 1564
Retrovir 1560
Reyataz Capsules (Less than 3%) 921
▲ Ribavirin, USP Capsules (7% to 47%) 3068
Rilutek Tablets (Infrequent) 2930
Risperdal (Rare) 1676
Risperdal Consta Long-Acting Injection (Infrequent) 1682
Risperdal M-Tab Orally Disintegrating Tablets (Rare) 1676
Romazicon Injection (1% to 3%) 2804
Seroquel Tablets (Rare) 690
Sonata Capsules (Frequent) 1717
Striant Mucoadhesive 1007
Sustiva Capsules (Less than 2%) 930
Sustiva Tablets (Less than 2%) 930
Symbyax Capsules (Infrequent) 1819
Tasmar Tablets (Frequent) 3358
Thalomid Capsules 965
Timolide Tablets 2086
Timoptic Sterile Ophthalmic Solution 2088
Timoptic in Ocudose 2091
Timoptic-XE Sterile Ophthalmic Gel Forming Solution 2092
▲ Topamax Sprinkle Capsules (3%) 2404
▲ Topamax Tablets (3%) 2404
Toprol-XL Tablets 668
Trelstar Depot (1.4%) 3394
▲ Trileptal Tablets (2% to 3%) 2300
▲ Trileptal Oral Suspension (2% to 3%) 2300
Uniretic Tablets (Less than 1%) 3100
Viracept (Less than 2%) 2577
Wellbutrin SR Sustained-Release Tablets (Infrequent) 1607
Wellbutrin XL Extended-Release Tablets (Infrequent)...................... 1613
Yasmin 28 Tablets 796
Yaz Tablets (Greater than 1%)......... 803
Zelapar Tablets.............................. 3372
Zoloft (Infrequent).......................... 2586
Zomig Tablets (Infrequent)............... 3519
Zomig-ZMT Tablets (Infrequent)........ 3519
Zyban Sustained-Release Tablets (Infrequent)................................ 1644
Zyprexa Tablets............................. 1830
Zyprexa IntraMuscular (Infrequent)... 1830
Zyprexa ZYDIS Orally Disintegrating Tablets................... 1830
Zyrtec Chewable Tablets (Less than 2%)....................................... 2594
Zyrtec (Less than 2%)..................... 2594
Zyrtec-D 12 Hour Extended Release Tablets (Less than 2%)..... 2597

Emphysema
Levaquin (0.1% to 0.9%)................. 2384
Levaquin in 5% Dextrose Injection (0.1% to 0.9%)............................ 2384
▲ Lupron Depot 7.5 mg (Less than 5%)... 3264
Paxil CR Controlled-Release Tablets (Rare)............................ 1538
Paxil (Rare)................................... 1530
Permax Tablets (Infrequent)............ 3356
Pexeva Tablets (rare)..................... 1694
Prozac Pulvules and Liquid (Rare)..... 1801
Symbyax Capsules (Rare)............... 1819
Thalomid Capsules......................... 965

Enanthema
Gengraf Capsules (1% to less than 3%)... 459
Neoral Oral Solution (1% to less than 3%)...................................... 2259
Neoral Soft Gelatin Capsules (1% to less than 3%)......................... 2259

Encephalitis
Attenuvax...................................... 1914
Boostrix.. 1404
M-M-R II (Very rare)........................ 2006
Mumpsvax (Very rare)..................... 2031
Nipent for Injection (Less than 3%)... 1863
Orthoclone OKT3 Sterile Solution (Less than 1%)........................... 2360
ProQuad.. 2064
Recombivax HB.............................. 2071
Vaqta (Very rare)............................ 2097
Varivax... 2100
VFEND I.V. (Less than 2%)............... 2564
VFEND Oral Suspension (Less than 2%)... 2564
VFEND Tablets (Less than 2%)......... 2564

Encephalitis, measles inclusion body
Attenuvax...................................... 1914
M-M-R II.. 2006

Encephalomyelitis
Fluarix.. 1451

Encephalopathy
Abelcet Injection............................ 1141
ADACEL Vaccine............................. 2945
Arranon Injection (1%)..................... 1357
Attenuvax...................................... 1914
▲ Bumex Tablets (0.6% to 4.1%) 2746
Campral Tablets (Rare).................... 1174
DAPTACEL Vaccine......................... 2950
Depacon Injection (Rare).................. 412
Depakene (Rare instances).............. 417
Depakote Sprinkle Capsules (Rare).. 422
Depakote Tablets (Rare instances).... 427
Depakote ER Tablets (Rare instances)...................................... 434
Fluarix.. 1451
Fortaz... 1453
Gabitril Tablets (Infrequent)............. 984
Garamycin Injectable...................... 3014
Gengraf Capsules........................... 459
Havrix Vaccine (Rare)...................... 1456
Infanrix Vaccine............................. 1476
I.V. Busulfex (2%)........................... 2493
Kaletra (Less than 2%).................... 476
Lariam Tablets............................... 2786
Levaquin (0.1% to 0.9%)................. 2384
Levaquin in 5% Dextrose Injection (0.1% to 0.9%)............................ 2384
Lyrica Capsules (Rare).................... 2539
Maxipime for Injection..................... 1105
▲ Midamor Tablets (Between 1% and 3%)...................................... 2026
M-M-R II (Very rare)........................ 2006
Moduretic Tablets........................... 2028
Mycamine for Injection.................... 628
Neoral Oral Solution....................... 2259
Neoral Soft Gelatin Capsules........... 2259
Neurontin Capsules (Rare)............... 2487
Neurontin Oral Solution (Rare).......... 2487
Neurontin Tablets (Rare).................. 2487
Orthoclone OKT3 Sterile Solution (Less than 1%)........................... 2360
Paser Granules.............................. 1674
Pediarix Vaccine............................ 1548
Primaxin I.M................................... 2045
Primaxin I.V. (Less than 0.2%).......... 2048
▲ Prograf Capsules and Injection (3% to 15%)................................ 632
Proleukin for Injection..................... 2266
ProQuad....................................... 2064
Sandimmune................................. 2275
Stromectol Tablets......................... 2083
Tasmar Tablets (Rare)..................... 3358
Topamax Sprinkle Capsules (Infrequent)................................ 2404
Topamax Tablets (Infrequent).......... 2404
Twinrix Vaccine.............................. 1595
Valtrex Caplets.............................. 1597
▲ Vesanoid Capsules (3%) 2820
VFEND I.V. (Less than 2%)............... 2564
VFEND Oral Suspension (Less than 2%)... 2564
VFEND Tablets (Less than 2%)......... 2564
▲ Xeloda Tablets (Less than 5%) 2822
Zelapar Tablets.............................. 3372
Zonegran Capsules (Rare)............... 1101
Zovirax... 1643
Zyprexa Tablets (Rare).................... 1830
Zyprexa ZYDIS Orally Disintegrating Tablets (Rare)......... 1830

Encephalopathy, hepatic
Aciphex Tablets (Rare).................... 1090
Eulexin Capsules........................... 3009
Intron A for Injection (Very rare)....... 3024
Prilosec OTC Delayed-Release Tablets (Rare)............................ 2677
Zegerid Capsules (Rare).................. 2958
Zegerid Powder for Oral Solution (Rare).. 2958

Encephalopathy, hypertensive
Catapres-TTS (Rare)....................... 844
Clorpres Tablets............................. 2153
Epogen for Injection (On occasion)... 591
▲ Humira Injection (Less than 5%) 466
Procrit for Injection (Occasional)...... 2364

Endocardial fibrosis
Myleran Tablets (One case)............. 1525

Endocarditis
▲ Copegus Tablets (3%) 2754
Oncaspar (Less than 1%)................. 1145
▲ Pegasys (3% to 5%) 2789
Proleukin for Injection (1%).............. 2266
Revlimid Capsules......................... 958
VFEND I.V. (Less than 2%)............... 2564
VFEND Oral Suspension (Less than 2%)... 2564
VFEND Tablets (Less than 2%)......... 2564

Endocarditis, infectious
CellCept Capsules (Occasional)....... 2747
CellCept Intravenous (Occasional).... 2747
CellCept Oral Suspension (Occasional)................................ 2747
CellCept Tablets (Occasional).......... 2747
Myfortic Tablets (Occasionally)........ 2255

Endocrine disturbances
Elocon Lotion 0.1% (1 in 65 patients)..................................... 3006
▲ Hycamtin for Injection (6%) 1458
Imitrex Nasal Spray........................ 1467
Permax Tablets (Rare)..................... 3356

Endodontic procedure
Xyrem Oral Solution (Infrequent)...... 1688

Endometrial carcinoma
(*see under* Carcinoma, endometrial)

Endometrial disorder, unspecified
Angeliq Tablets (1.8%).................... 762
▲ Estrasorb Topical Emulsion (15%) ... 1147
Evista Tablets................................ 1763
Evoxac Capsules (Less than 1%)...... 1047
Symbyax Capsules (Rare)................ 1819

Endometrial hyperplasia
Angeliq Tablets.............................. 762
Aromasin Tablets (1.7%)................. 2600
Climara Transdermal System........... 771
Climara Pro Transdermal System..... 776
Estrasorb Topical Emulsion............. 1147
Estratest Tablets............................ 3199
Estratest H.S. Tablets..................... 3199

Menostar Transdermal System 782
Premarin Intravenous 3442
Premarin Tablets 3446
Premarin Vaginal Cream 3452
Premphase Tablets 3456
Prempro Tablets 3456

Endometriosis
Effexor XR Capsules (Rare) 3417
Imitrex Injection 1463
Imitrex Nasal Spray (Rare) 1467
Imitrex Tablets 1471
Tarka Tablets (Less frequent) 524

Endometriosis, exacerbation of
Enjuvia Tablets 1062

Endometrium disorders, unspecified
Amerge Tablets (Rare) 1339
Pexeva Tablets (rare) 1694

Endophthalmitis
Campath Ampules 811
Lucentis Injection (Less than 0.1%) 1237
▲ Macugen Injection (Less than 1% to 5%) ⊙ 261

Endotracheal tube, reflux into
▲ Infasurf Intratracheal Suspension (21%) 1184

Endotracheal tube occlusion
Curosurf Intratracheal Suspension 1057

Energy, high
Eldepryl Capsules 3208

Energy, loss of
▲ Gabitril Tablets (20%) 984
Ortho-Cyclen/Ortho Tri-Cyclen 2429
Ortho Tri-Cyclen Lo Tablets 2436

Enteritis
Ambien Tablets (Rare) 2851
Ambien CR Tablets (Rare) 2855
Arthrotec Tablets (Rare) 3129
Caduet Tablets (Less than 2%) 2508
▲ Entocort EC Capsules (Less than 5%) 2698
Kaletra (Less than 2%) 476
Lipitor Tablets (Less than 2%) 2483
Micardis HCT Tablets 856
Paxil CR Controlled-Release Tablets (Rare) 1538
Paxil (Rare) 1530
Pexeva Tablets (rare) 1694
Prevacid Delayed-Release Capsules (Less than 1%) 3271
Prevacid for Delayed-Release Oral Suspension (Less than 1%) 3271
Prevacid SoluTab Delayed-Release Orally Disintegrating Tablets (Less than 1%) 3271
Prevacid NapraPAC (Less than 1%) 3280
PREVPAC (Less than 1%) 3284
Protonix I.V. (Less than 1%) 3472
Protonix Tablets (Less than 1%) 3469
Prozac Pulvules and Liquid (Rare) 1801
Rescriptor Tablets 2551
Sonata Capsules (Rare) 1717
Trileptal Tablets 2300
Trileptal Oral Suspension 2300
Uniretic Tablets (Less than 1%) 3100
Zostavax Injection (0.9%) 2111
Zyprexa Tablets (Rare) 1830
Zyprexa ZYDIS Orally Disintegrating Tablets (Rare) 1830

Enterocolitis
Augmentin 1360
Augmentin Tablets 1363
Augmentin XR Extended-Release Tablets 1369
Augmentin ES-600 Powder for Oral Suspension 1366
Chantix Tablets (Infrequent) 2517
Evoxac Capsules (Less than 1%) 1047
Indocin I.V. (Less than 3%) 2465
Kaletra (Less than 2%) 476
Omnicef Capsules 511
Omnicef for Oral Suspension 511
Oracea Capsules 1000
Prograf Capsules and Injection 632
ProSom Tablets (Rare) 517
Solodyn Extended Release Tablets 1890

Enterocolitis, necrotizing
▲ Cafcit (4.3%) 1886
Indocin I.V. 2465
▲ Infasurf Intratracheal Suspension (5% to 17%) 1184
▲ Xeloda Tablets (Less than 5%) 2822

Enterocolitis, neutropenic
Taxotere Injection Concentrate 2932

Enterocolitis, non-necrotizing
▲ NeoProfen Injection (22%) 2472

Entropion
BOTOX Purified Neurotoxin Complex (Less than 1%) 570

Enuresis
Aricept Tablets 1094
Aricept ODT Tablets 1094
Depacon Injection 412
Depakene 417
Depakote Sprinkle Capsules 422
Depakote Tablets 427
Depakote ER Tablets 434
Klonopin (Infrequent) 2778
Mintezol 2027
Thalomid Capsules 965
Wellbutrin Tablets (Rare) 1603
▲ Xyrem Oral Solution (3% to 17.1%) 1688
Zonegran Capsules (Rare) 1101

Eosinophilia
Abelcet Injection 1141
Abilify Oral Solution (Rare to infrequent) 882
Abilify Oral Solution (Rare to infrequent) 2450
Abilify Discmelt Orally Disintegrating Tablets (Rare to infrequent) 882
Abilify Discmelt Orally Disintegrating Tablets (Rare to infrequent) 2450
Abilify Tablets (Rare to infrequent) 882
Abilify Tablets (Rare to infrequent) 2450
Accolate Tablets (Rare) 671
Aceon Tablets (2 mg, 4 mg, 8 mg) 3194
Adalat CC Tablets (Less than 1%) 2964
Advair Diskus 100/50 (Rare) 1308
Advair Diskus 250/50 (Rare) 1308
Advair Diskus 500/50 (Rare) 1308
Advicor Tablets 1722
Aldoril Tablets 1910
Aloprim for Injection (Less than 1%) 2167
Altace Capsules (Less than 1%) 1702
Altoprev Extended-Release Tablets 3109
Amoxil Capsules 1343
Amoxil Chewable Tablets 1343
Amoxil Pediatric Drops for Oral Suspension 1343
Amoxil Powder for Oral Suspension 1343
Amoxil Tablets 1343
Anaprox Tablets (Less than 1%) 2761
Anaprox DS Tablets (Less than 1%) 2761
Aricept Tablets (Infrequent) 1094
Aricept ODT Tablets (Infrequent) 1094
Arthrotec Tablets (Rare) 3129
Asacol Delayed-Release Tablets 2692
Augmentin 1360
Augmentin Tablets 1363
Augmentin XR Extended-Release Tablets 1369
Augmentin ES-600 Powder for Oral Suspension 1366
Avelox (0.1% to less than 2%) 2970
Axid Oral Solution (Rare) 879
Bicillin C-R Injectable Suspension 1706
BiDil Tablets 2171
Campral Tablets (Infrequent) 1174
▲ Cancidas for Injection (3.1% to 3.2%) 1918
Capastat Sulfate for Injection (Majority of patients) 1755
▲ Captopril Tablets (About 4 to 7 of 100 patients) 2149
Carbatrol Capsules 3171
Ceftin (0.1% to 1%) 1407
Chemet Capsules (0.5% to 1.5%) 2458
Cipro (0.6%) 2977
Cipro I.V. (Greater than 1%) 2984
Cipro XR Tablets (Rare) 2990
Cleocin Vaginal Ovules 2616
Clinoril Tablets (Less than 1 in 100) 1924
Clozaril Tablets (1%) 2184
Colazal Capsules 2838
Copaxone for Injection (Infrequent) 3297
Cubicin for Injection (Less than 1% to 1.7%) 1026
Cuprimine Capsules 1947
Demser Capsules (Rare) 1953
Depacon Injection 412
Depakene 417
Depakote Sprinkle Capsules 422
Depakote Tablets 427
Depakote ER Tablets 434
Dolobid Tablets (Less than 1 in 100) 1955
Doxil Injection (Less than 1%) 2351
EC-Naprosyn Delayed-Release Tablets (Less than 1%) 2761
Effexor Tablets (Rare) 3411
Effexor XR Capsules (Rare) 3417
Efudex 3363
Equetro Extended-Release Capsules 3180
Evoxac Capsules (Less than 1%) 1047
Fansidar Tablets 2765
FazaClo Orally Disintegrating Tablets (1%) 551
Flovent Diskus 1443
▲ Fortaz (1 in 13) 1453
▲ Fuzeon Injection (1.8% to 8.3%) 2767
Gantrisin Pediatric Suspension 2770
Garamycin Injectable 3014
Geodon Capsules (Infrequent) 2529
Invanz for Injection (1.1% to 2.1%) 1999
Keflex Capsules 549
Kineret Injection 599
Klonopin 2778
Lamictal (Infrequent) 1481
Lescol Capsules (Rare) 2233
Lescol XL Tablets 2233
Leukine 814
Levaquin 2384
Levaquin in 5% Dextrose Injection 2384
Lofibra Tablets 1219
Lofibra Capsules 1216
Lotensin HCT Tablets 2246
Lyrica Capsules (0.1% to 1%) 2539
Matulane Capsules 3191
Mefoxin for Injection 2012
Mefoxin Premixed Intravenous Solution 2016
Merrem I.V. (Greater than 0.2%) 686
Mevacor Tablets 2021
Miradon Tablets 3042
Naprosyn Suspension (Less than 1%) 2761
Naprosyn Tablets (Less than 1%) 2761
Noroxin Tablets (0.6% to 1.5%) 2032
Omnicef Capsules (0.7%) 511
Omnicef for Oral Suspension (1%) 511
Oracea Capsules 1000
Orthoclone OKT3 Sterile Solution (Less than 1%) 2360
▲ Paser Granules (55% of 38 patients with drug-induced hepatitis) 1674
Paxil CR Controlled-Release Tablets (Rare) 1538
Paxil (Rare) 1530
Pentasa Capsules 3185
Permax Tablets (Rare) 3356
Pexeva Tablets (rare) 1694
Phenytek Capsules 2160
Prevacid Delayed-Release Capsules (Less than 1%) 3271
Prevacid for Delayed-Release Oral Suspension (Less than 1%) 3271
Prevacid SoluTab Delayed-Release Orally Disintegrating Tablets (Less than 1%) 3271
Prevacid NapraPAC (Less than 1%) 3280
PREVPAC (Less than 1%) 3284
Primaxin I.M. 2045
Primaxin I.V. 2048
Prinivil Tablets (0.3% to 1.0%) 2052
Prinzide Tablets 2056
▲ Proleukin for Injection (6%) 2266
Protonix I.V. (Less than 1%) 3472
Protonix Tablets (Less than 1%) 3469
Provigil Tablets (1%) 988
Raniclor Tablets, Chewable (2%) 2505
Requip Tablets (Infrequent) 1555
Rescriptor Tablets 2551
▲ Rocephin Injectable Vials, ADD-Vantage, Galaxy, Bulk (6%) 2800
Rythmol SR Capsules 2727
Seroquel Tablets (Infrequent) 690
Singulair (Rare) 2077
Solodyn Extended Release Tablets 1890
Sonata Capsules (Rare) 1717
▲ Stromectol Tablets (3%) 2083
Sulfamylon Cream 2162
Sulfamylon for 5% Topical Solution 2162
Suprax (Less than 2%) 1843
Targretin Capsules 1747
Tegretol/Tegretol-XR 2295
Thalomid Capsules 965
▲ Thiola Tablets (4%) 2141
Thioridazine Hydrochloride Tablets 2163
Thiothixene Capsules 2165
Ticlid Tablets 2810
Timentin ADD-Vantage 1580
Timentin Injection Galaxy Container 1583
Timentin IV Infusion 1577
Timentin Pharmacy Bulk Package 1586
Topamax Sprinkle Capsules (Infrequent) 2404
Topamax Tablets (Infrequent) 2404
Tricor Tablets 527
Triglide Tablets 3123
Trileptal Tablets 2300
Trileptal Oral Suspension 2300
Tygacil for Injection (0% to less than 2%) 3488
Uniretic Tablets (Less than 1%) 3100
Vancocin HCl Capsules, USP (Infrequent) 3380
Vantin Tablets and Oral Suspension 2645
Vaqta (Isolated reports) 2097
Vasotec I.V. Injection (0.5% to 1.0%) 2103
VFEND I.V. (Less than 2%) 2564
VFEND Oral Suspension (Less than 2%) 2564
VFEND Tablets (Less than 2%) 2564
Viramune Oral Suspension 873
Viramune Tablets 873
Voltaren Tablets (Occasionally) 2307
Voltaren-XR Tablets (Occasionally) 2310
Vytorin 10/10 Tablets 2114
Vytorin 10/10 Tablets 3077
Vytorin 10/20 Tablets 2114
Vytorin 10/20 Tablets 3077
Vytorin 10/40 Tablets 2114
Vytorin 10/40 Tablets 3077
Vytorin 10/80 Tablets 2114
Vytorin 10/80 Tablets 3077
Zantac (Rare) 1624
Zantac Injection 1619
Zantac Injection Pharmacy Bulk Package (Rare) 1622
Zantac Injection Premixed 1619
Zantac (Rare) 1624
Zelapar Tablets 3372
▲ Zinacef for Injection (1 in 14 patients) 1631
▲ Zinacef Injection (1 in 14 patients) 1631
Zocor Tablets 2105
Zomig Tablets (Rare) 3519
Zomig-ZMT Tablets (Rare) 3519
Zosyn 3492
Zyvox (0.4% to 1.4%) 2652

Eosinophilia, myoclonus
Carbatrol Capsules (One case) 3171
Tegretol/Tegretol-XR (One case) 2295

Eosinophilia, peripheral
Carbatrol Capsules (One case) 3171
Tegretol/Tegretol-XR (One case) 2295

Eosinophilia, pulmonary
Dapsone Tablets USP 1673
Daraprim Tablets (Rare) 1419
Effexor Tablets 3411
Effexor XR Capsules 3417

Eosinophilic pneumonitis
(*see under* Pneumonitis, eosinophilic)

Epidermal necrolysis
(*see under* Necrolysis, epidermal, toxic)

Epidermal shedding
Plavix Tablets 2926

Epidermolysis
Carimune NF 3499
Flebogamma 5%, Immune Globulin Intravenous (Human) 1658
Gammagard Liquid 721
Gamunex Immune Globulin I.V., 10% (Rare) 3235

Epidermolysis bullosa
Anaprox Tablets (Less than 1%) 2761
Anaprox DS Tablets (Less than 1%) 2761
EC-Naprosyn Delayed-Release Tablets (Less than 1%) 2761
Gammagard S/D (Rare) 724
Naprosyn Suspension (Less than 1%) 2761
Naprosyn Tablets (Less than 1%) 2761
Prevacid NapraPAC (Less than 1%) 3280

Epididymitis
Asacol Delayed-Release Tablets 2692
Caduet Tablets (Less than 2%) 2508
Evoxac Capsules (Less than 1%) 1047
Lamictal (Rare) 1481
Lipitor Tablets (Less than 2%) 2483
Lyrica Capsules (Rare) 2539
Neurontin Capsules (Rare) 2487
Neurontin Oral Solution (Rare) 2487

Neurontin Tablets (Rare) 2487
Omacor Capsules 2725
Oxandrin Tablets 2962
Paxil CR Controlled-Release Tablets (Rare) 1538
Paxil (Rare) 1530
Permax Tablets (Rare) 3356
Pexeva Tablets (rare) 1694
Protonix I.V. (Less than 1%) 3472
Protonix Tablets (Less than 1%) 3469
Requip Tablets (Infrequent) 1555
Rescriptor Tablets 2551
VFEND I.V. (Less than 2%) 2564
VFEND Oral Suspension (Less than 2%) 2564
VFEND Tablets (Less than 2%) 2564
Zelapar Tablets 3372

Epigastric pain
(*see under* Distress, epigastric)

Epilepsy, aggravation
Angeliq Tablets 762
Climara Transdermal System 771
Climara Pro Transdermal System 776
Enjuvia Tablets 1062
Estrasorb Topical Emulsion 1147
Estratest Tablets 3199
Estratest H.S. Tablets 3199
Exelon Capsules (Infrequent) 2206
Exelon Oral Solution (Infrequent) 2206
Indocin Capsules (Less than 1%) 1995
Indocin I.V. (Less than 1%) 2465
Indocin (Less than 1%) 1995
Menostar Transdermal System 782
Premarin Intravenous 3442
Premarin Tablets 3446
Premarin Vaginal Cream 3452
Premphase Tablets 3456
Prempro Tablets 3456

Epileptic ictal phenomenon
Trileptal Tablets 2300
Trileptal Oral Suspension 2300

Epileptiform movements, unspecified
Clozaril Tablets (1%) 2184
FazaClo Orally Disintegrating Tablets (1%) 551

Epiphora
▲ Alphagan P Ophthalmic Solution (1% to 4%) 567
▲ Alrex Ophthalmic Suspension 0.2% (5% to 15%) ⊙246
▲ Betimol Ophthalmic Solution (1% to 5%) 3382
▲ Betimol Ophthalmic Solution (1% to 5%) ⊙295
▲ Lotemax Ophthalmic Suspension 0.5% (5% to 15%) ⊙251
▲ Restasis Ophthalmic Emulsion (1% to 5%) 575

Epiphyseal closure, premature
Accutane Capsules 2731
Estratest Tablets 3199
Estratest H.S. Tablets 3199
Oxandrin Tablets 2962

Episcleritis
Aredia for Injection (Rare) 2179
Fosamax 1969
Fosamax Plus D Tablets (Rarely) 1977

Epistaxis
Abilify Oral Solution (Infrequent) 882
Abilify Oral Solution (Infrequent) 2450
Abilify Discmelt Orally Disintegrating Tablets (Infrequent) 882
Abilify Discmelt Orally Disintegrating Tablets (Infrequent) 2450
Abilify Tablets (Infrequent) 882
Abilify Tablets (Infrequent) 2450
Accutane Capsules 2731
Aceon Tablets (2 mg, 4 mg, 8 mg) (0.3% to 1%) 3194
Aciphex Tablets 1090
Actiq (1% or greater) 979
Activase I.V. (Less than 1%) 1223
▲ Adalat CC Tablets (3% or less) 2964
▲ Advair Diskus 100/50 (1% to 4%) 1308
▲ Advair Diskus 250/50 (1% to 4%) 1308
▲ Advair Diskus 500/50 (1% to 4%) 1308
▲ Advair HFA Inhalation Aerosol (1% to 3%) 1318
▲ Aerobid/Aerobid-M (1% to 3%) 1171
Aggrenox Capsules (2.4%) 822
▲ Agrylin Capsules (1% to 5%) 3169
Alferon N Injection (1%) 1665
Alinia for Oral Suspension (Less than 1%) 2835
Alinia Tablets (Less than 1%) 2835
Altace Capsules (Less than 1%) 1702
Ambien Tablets (Rare) 2851
Ambien CR Tablets (Rare) 2855
▲ AmBisome for Injection (8.6% to 14.9%) 620
Amerge Tablets (Rare) 1339
Anzemet Injection (Rare) 2859
Anzemet Tablets (Rare) 2862
Aricept Tablets (Infrequent) 1094
Aricept ODT Tablets (Infrequent) 1094
Arixtra Injection (1.3%) 1351
▲ Arranon Injection (0% to 8%) 1357
Arthrotec Tablets (Rare) 3129
Asmanex Twisthaler (1% to less than 3%) 2966
▲ Astelin Nasal Spray (2.0% to 3.2%) 1904
Atacand Tablets (0.5% or greater) 649
Atacand HCT (0.5% or greater) 651
▲ Atrovent Nasal Spray 0.03% (7.0% to 9.0%) 837
▲ Atrovent Nasal Spray 0.06% (8.2%) 839
Avalide Tablets 888
Avalide Tablets 2874
Avapro Tablets (Less than 1%) 891
Avapro Tablets (Less than 1%) 2871
▲ Avastin IV (32% to 35%) 1227
Axert Tablets (Infrequent) 2396
Bactroban Nasal (Less than 1%) 1394
Beconase AQ Nasal Spray (Fewer than 3 per 100 patients) 1396
Caduet Tablets (Greater than 0.1% to less than 2%) 2508
▲ Campath Ampules (1% to 7%) 811
Campral Tablets (Infrequent) 1174
Cardizem LA Extended Release Tablets (Less than 2%) 1728
Celebrex Capsules (0.1% to 1.9%) 3134
Celexa (Infrequent) 1176
▲ CellCept Capsules (3% to less than 20%) 2747
▲ CellCept Intravenous (3% to less than 20%) 2747
▲ CellCept Oral Suspension (3% to less than 20%) 2747
▲ CellCept Tablets (3% to less than 20%) 2747
Cesamet Capsules 3340
Chantix Tablets (Frequent) 2517
Cialis Tablets (Less than 2%) 1838
Cipro (Less than 1%) 2977
Cipro I.V. (1% or less) 2984
Cipro XR Tablets 2990
▲ Clarinex Syrup (3.1%) 2995
Clinoril Tablets (Less than 1%) 1924
▲ Clolar for Intravenous Infusion (31%) 1271
Clozaril Tablets (Less than 1%) 2184
Colazal Capsules 2838
Copaxone for Injection (Infrequent) 3297
Cosopt Sterile Ophthalmic Solution 1931
Coumadin for Injection 898
Coumadin Tablets 898
Cozaar Tablets (Less than 1%) 1935
▲ Depacon Injection (1% to 5%) 412
▲ Depakene (1% to 5%) 417
▲ Depakote Sprinkle Capsules (1% to 5%) 422
▲ Depakote Tablets (1% to 5%) 427
▲ Depakote ER Tablets (1% to 5%) 434
Diovan HCT Tablets (Less frequent) 2196
▲ Doxil Injection (1% to 10%) 2351
DynaCirc CR Tablets (0.5% to 1%) 2721
Effexor Tablets (Infrequent) 3411
Effexor XR Capsules (Infrequent) 3417
▲ Elidel Cream 1% (Up to 3.3%) 2200
Elmiron Capsules (Less than or equal to 1%) 2415
▲ Eloxatin for Injection (2% to 16%) 2892
▲ Evoxac Capsules (1% to 3%) 1047
Exelon Capsules (Frequent) 2206
Exelon Oral Solution (Frequent) 2206
Exubera Inhalation Powder (1.2% to 1.3%) 2524
FazaClo Orally Disintegrating Tablets (Less than 1%) 551
▲ Flonase Nasal Spray (6% to 6.9%) 1440
▲ Flovent Diskus (1% to 3%) 1443
Flumist Vaccine 1901
▲ Fortical Nasal Spray (3.5% to 10.6%) 3337
Frova Tablets (Infrequent) 1113
Gabitril Tablets (Frequent) 984
▲ Gamunex Immune Globulin I.V., 10% (23%) 3235
Gengraf Capsules (1% to less than 3%) 459
Geodon Capsules (Infrequent) 2529
▲ Gleevec Tablets (3% to 12%) 2227
Hytrin Capsules (At least 1%) 471
Hyzaar 50-12.5 Tablets 1990
Hyzaar 100-12.5 Tablets 1990
Hyzaar 100-25 Tablets 1990
Imitrex Nasal Spray 1467
Indocin Capsules (Less than 1%) 1995
Indocin I.V. (Less than 1%) 2465
Indocin (Less than 1%) 1995
▲ Infergen (6% to 8%) 3364
▲ Intron A for Injection (Less than or equal to 5%) 3024
Invanz for Injection (Greater than 0.1%) 1999
Invirase (Less than 2%) 2772
Iressa Tablets 684
▲ I.V. Busulfex (25%) 2493
Keppra Oral Solution (2%) 3314
Keppra Tablets (2%) 3314
Klonopin (Infrequent) 2778
Lamictal (Infrequent) 1481
▲ Leukine (17%) 814
▲ Leustatin Injection (5%) 2357
Levaquin (0.1% to 0.9%) 2384
Levaquin in 5% Dextrose Injection (0.1% to 0.9%) 2384
Levitra Tablets (Less than 2%) 3034
Lexapro Oral Solution (Infrequent) 1190
Lexapro Tablets (Infrequent) 1190
Lipitor Tablets (Less than 2%) 2483
Lofibra Tablets (Less than 1%) 1219
Lofibra Capsules (Less than 1%) 1216
Lotensin HCT Tablets (0.3% or more) 2246
Lunesta Tablets (Infrequent) 3142
Lupron Depot-PED 7.5 mg, 11.25 mg and 15 mg (Less than 2%) 3269
Lupron Injection Pediatric (Less than 2%) 3259
Matulane Capsules 3191
Mavik Tablets (0.3% to 1.0%) 486
Maxalt Tablets (Infrequent) 2008
Maxalt-MLT Orally Disintegrating Tablets (Infrequent) 2008
Meridia Capsules 489
Merrem I.V. (0.2%) 686
▲ Miacalcin Nasal Spray (3.5%) 2253
Micardis Tablets (More than 0.3%) 854
Micardis HCT Tablets 856
Migranal Nasal Spray (Rare) 3348
▲ Mylotarg for Injection (3% to 34%) 3431
Nasacort AQ Nasal Spray (2.7%) 2922
▲ Nasonex Nasal Spray (8% to 11%) 3043
Neoral Oral Solution (1% to less than 3%) 2259
Neoral Soft Gelatin Capsules (1% to less than 3%) 2259
▲ Neupogen for Injection (9% to 15%) 603
Neurontin Capsules (Infrequent) 2487
Neurontin Oral Solution (Infrequent) 2487
Neurontin Tablets (Infrequent) 2487
Nexium Delayed-Release Capsules (Less than 1%) 655
Nexium I.V. (Less than 1%) 659
Norvasc Tablets (More than 0.1% to 1%) 2545
Norvir (Less than 2%) 503
Omacor Capsules 2725
Oncaspar (Less than 1%) 1145
OptiPranolol Metipranolol Ophthalmic Solution 0.3% (A small number of patients) ⊙256
Paxil CR Controlled-Release Tablets (Infrequent) 1538
Paxil (Infrequent) 1530
Permax Tablets (1.6%) 3356
Pexeva Tablets (Infrequent) 1694
Plavix Tablets (2.9%) 917
Plavix Tablets (2.9%) 2926
Pletal Tablets (Less than 2%) 2455
Prevacid Delayed-Release Capsules (Less than 1%) 3271
Prevacid for Delayed-Release Oral Suspension (Less than 1%) 3271
Prevacid SoluTab Delayed-Release Orally Disintegrating Tablets (Less than 1%) 3271
Prevacid NapraPAC (Less than 1%) 3280
PREVPAC (Less than 1%) 3284
Prilosec OTC Delayed-Release Tablets (Less than 1%) 2677
Prinivil Tablets (0.3% to 1.0%) 2052
Prinzide Tablets 2056
ProQuad 2064
Proquin XR Tablets 1153
ProSom Tablets (Rare) 517
Protonix I.V. (Less than 1%) 3472
Protonix Tablets (Less than 1%) 3469
Protopic Ointment (Greater than or equal to 1%) 638
Provigil Tablets (1%) 988
Prozac Pulvules and Liquid (Infrequent to greater than or equal to 2%) 1801
▲ Pulmicort Respules (2% to 4%) 661
Quadramet Injection (2%) 1040
▲ Rapamune Oral Solution and Tablets (3% to 20%) 3475
Razadyne (Infrequent) 2399
Razadyne ER Extended-Release Capsules (Infrequent) 2399
Recombinate 729
▲ Refludan for Injection (4.4%) 792
Relenza Rotadisk (Less than 1%) 1552
Relpax Tablets (Rare) 2548
ReoPro Vials (9 to 11 events) 1809
Requip Tablets (Infrequent) 1555
Rescriptor Tablets 2551
Retrovir Capsules 1560
Retrovir IV Infusion 1564
Retrovir 1560
▲ Revatio Tablets (9%) 2557
▲ Revlimid Capsules (1.4% to 14.9%) 958
▲ Rhinocort Aqua Nasal Spray (8%) 665
Rilutek Tablets (Infrequent) 2930
Risperdal (Infrequent) 1676
Risperdal Consta Long-Acting Injection (Infrequent) 1682
Risperdal M-Tab Orally Disintegrating Tablets (Infrequent) 1676
Rocephin Injectable Vials, ADD-Vantage, Galaxy, Bulk (Rare) 2800
Rythmol SR Capsules 2727
Sandostatin Injection (Less than 1%) 2278
▲ Sandostatin LAR Depot (1% to 4%) 2280
Seroquel Tablets (Infrequent) 690
Singulair (Greater than or equal to 1%) 2077
Sonata Capsules (Less than 1%) 1717
▲ Spiriva HandiHaler (1% to 4%) 869
Sular Tablets (Less than or equal to 1%) 3122
Sutent Capsules 2560
Symbyax Capsules (Infrequent) 1819
▲ Tamiflu Capsules (3.1%) 2807
▲ Tamiflu Oral Suspension (1% to 3%) 2807
Tarka Tablets (Less frequent) 524
Tasmar Tablets (Infrequent) 3358
Tequin Injection (Less than 0.1%) 938
Tequin Injection in 5% Dextrose (Less than 0.1%) 938
Tequin Tablets (Less than 0.1%) 938
Teveten Tablets (Less than 1%) 1735
Teveten HCT Tablets (Less than 1%) 1737
Thalomid Capsules 965
Tiazac Capsules (Less than 2%) 1201
Ticlid Tablets (0.5% to 1.0%) 2810
TNKase I.V. (1.5%) 1264
▲ TOBI Solution for Inhalation (7%) 2298
▲ Topamax Sprinkle Capsules (1% to 4%) 2404
▲ Topamax Tablets (1% to 4%) 2404
Tricor Tablets 527
▲ Trileptal Tablets (2% to 4%) 2300
▲ Trileptal Oral Suspension (2% to 4%) 2300
▲ Trisenox Injection (25%) 993
Trusopt Sterile Ophthalmic Solution 2095
Uniretic Tablets (Less than 1%) 3100
Vantin Tablets and Oral Suspension (Less than 1%) 2645
VFEND I.V. (Less than 2%) 2564
VFEND Oral Suspension (Less than 2%) 2564
VFEND Tablets (Less than 2%) 2564
Viagra Tablets 2573
Wellbutrin Tablets (Rare) 1603
▲ Xeloda Tablets (Less than 5%) 2822
Zegerid Capsules (Less than 1%) 2958
Zegerid Powder for Oral Solution (Less than 1%) 2958
Zelapar Tablets 3372
Zoloft (Infrequent to 2%) 2586
Zomig Tablets (Infrequent) 3519
Zomig Nasal Spray (Infrequent) 3523
Zomig-ZMT Tablets (Infrequent) 3519
Zosyn (1.0% or less) 3492
Zyban Sustained-Release Tablets (2%) 1644
Zyprexa Tablets (Infrequent) 1830
Zyprexa ZYDIS Orally Disintegrating Tablets (Infrequent) 1830

▲ Zyrtec Chewable Tablets (1.9% to 3.7%) 2594
▲ Zyrtec (1.9% to 3.7%) 2594
▲ Zyrtec-D 12 Hour Extended Release Tablets (1.9% to 3.7%) 2597

Epitheliopathy
Ciloxan Ophthalmic Ointment (Less than 1%) 559

Equilibrium dysfunction
Amerge Tablets (Infrequent) 1339
Cesamet Capsules 3340
Covera-HS Tablets (Less than 2%) 3139
Lariam Tablets 2786
Lexapro Oral Solution (Infrequent) 1190
Lexapro Tablets (Infrequent) 1190
Restoril Capsules (0.5% to 0.9%) 1860
Transderm Scōp Transdermal Therapeutic System (Few patients) 2177
Verelan PM Extended-Release Capsules, Controlled-Onset (2% or less) 3106
▲ Xeloda Tablets (Less than 5%) 2822

Erectile disturbances, unspeficied
▲ Strattera Capsules (7%) 1814

Erection disturbances, unspecified
(*see also under* Impotence)
Advicor Tablets 1722
Altoprev Extended-Release Tablets 3109
▲ Cymbalta Delayed-Release Capsules (Up to 4%) 1757
Dantrium Capsules (Less frequent) 2694
Diovan HCT Tablets (Greater than 0.2%) 2196
Effexor Tablets (Rare) 3411
Effexor XR Capsules (Rare) 3417
Eligard 30 mg (1.1%) 2885
Lescol Capsules 2233
Lescol XL Tablets 2233
Mevacor Tablets (0.5% to 1.0%) 2021
Micardis Tablets 854
▲ Paxil CR Controlled-Release Tablets (3.7% to 10.0%) 1538
▲ Paxil (3.7% to 10.0%) 1530
Propecia Tablets (1.3%) 2060
Risperdal (Frequent) 1676
Risperdal M-Tab Orally Disintegrating Tablets (Frequent) 1676
▲ Vantas (3.5%) 3375
Wellbutrin Tablets (Infrequent) 1603
Wellbutrin SR Sustained-Release Tablets 1607
Wellbutrin XL Extended-Release Tablets 1613
Zocor Tablets 2105
Zyban Sustained-Release Tablets 1644

Erosion, genital
▲ Aldara (1% to 31%) 1846

Erosion, skin
▲ Levulan Kerastick for Topical Solution, 20% (1% to 14%) 1085

Eructation
Abilify Oral Solution (Infrequent) 882
Abilify Oral Solution (Infrequent) 2450
Abilify Discmelt Orally Disintegrating Tablets (Infrequent) 882
Abilify Discmelt Orally Disintegrating Tablets (Infrequent) 2450
Abilify Tablets (Infrequent) 882
Abilify Tablets (Infrequent) 2450
Aciphex Tablets 1090
Actiq (Less than 1%) 979
Adalat CC Tablets (Less than 1%) 2964
Agrylin Capsules (1% to 5%) 3169
Ambien Tablets (Rare) 2851
Ambien CR Tablets (Rare) 2855
AmBisome for Injection (Less common) 620
Anaprox Tablets (Less than 1%) 2761
Anaprox DS Tablets (Less than 1%) 2761
Aricept Tablets (Infrequent) 1094
Aricept ODT Tablets (Infrequent) 1094
Arthrotec Tablets (Rare) 3129
▲ Asacol Delayed-Release Tablets (16%) 2692
Byetta Injection 611
Caduet Tablets (Less than 2%) 2508
Campral Tablets (Infrequent) 1174
Celebrex Capsules (0.1% to 1.9%) 3134
Celexa (Infrequent) 1176
Chantix Tablets (Infrequent) 2517
Clozaril Tablets (Less than 1%) 2184
Colazal Capsules 2838
▲ Depacon Injection (1% to 5%) 412
▲ Depakene (1% to 5%) 417
▲ Depakote Sprinkle Capsules (1% to 5%) 422
▲ Depakote Tablets (1% to 5%) 427
Depakote ER Tablets (Greater than 1%) 434
Dolobid Tablets (Less than 1 in 100) 1955
Doxil Injection (Less than 1%) 2351
EC-Naprosyn Delayed-Release Tablets (Less than 1%) 2761
Effexor Tablets (Frequent) 3411
Effexor XR Capsules (2%) 3417
Emend Capsules (Greater than 0.5%) 1963
▲ Evoxac Capsules (1% to 3%) 1047
Exelon Capsules (2%) 2206
Exelon Oral Solution (2%) 2206
FazaClo Orally Disintegrating Tablets (Less than 1%) 551
Ferrlecit Injection 3388
Frova Tablets (Rare) 1113
Gabitril Tablets (Infrequent) 984
Gengraf Capsules (1% to less than 3%) 459
Imitrex Injection (Rare) 1463
Imitrex Nasal Spray (Rare) 1467
Imitrex Tablets 1471
▲ Intron A for Injection (Less than 5%) 3024
Invirase (Less than 2%) 2772
Kaletra (Less than 2%) 476
Lamictal (Rare) 1481
Lipitor Tablets (Less than 2%) 2483
Lofibra Tablets 1219
Lofibra Capsules 1216
▲ Lupron Depot 7.5 mg (Less than 5%) 3264
Maxalt Tablets (Rare) 2008
Maxalt-MLT Orally Disintegrating Tablets (Rare) 2008
Meridia Capsules 489
Mobic Oral Suspension (Less than 2%) 863
Mobic Tablets (Less than 2%) 863
Naprosyn Suspension (Less than 1%) 2761
Naprosyn Tablets (Less than 1%) 2761
Neoral Oral Solution (1% to less than 3%) 2259
Neoral Soft Gelatin Capsules (1% to less than 3%) 2259
Neurontin Capsules (Rare) 2487
Neurontin Oral Solution (Rare) 2487
Neurontin Tablets (Rare) 2487
Nexium Delayed-Release Capsules (Less than 1%) 655
Nexium I.V. (Less than 1%) 659
Niaspan Extended-Release Tablets 1730
Norvir (Less than 2%) 503
▲ Omacor Capsules (4.9%) 2725
OxyContin Tablets (Less than 1%) 2703
Paxil CR Controlled-Release Tablets (Infrequent) 1538
Paxil (Infrequent) 1530
Pentasa Capsules (Less than 1%) 3185
Percodan Tablets 1132
Permax Tablets (Infrequent) 3356
Pexeva Tablets (infrequent) 1694
▲ Photofrin for Injection (5%) 702
Prevacid Delayed-Release Capsules (Less than 1%) 3271
Prevacid for Delayed-Release Oral Suspension (Less than 1%) 3271
Prevacid SoluTab Delayed-Release Orally Disintegrating Tablets (Less than 1%) 3271
Prevacid NapraPAC (Less than 1%) 3280
PREVPAC (Less than 1%) 3284
Prochieve 4% Gel 1003
Prochieve 8% Gel 1003
Protonix I.V. (Greater than or equal to 1%) 3472
Protonix Tablets (1%) 3469
Proventil HFA Inhalation Aerosol (Less than 3%) 3056
Prozac Pulvules and Liquid (Infrequent) 1801
▲ Rapamune Oral Solution and Tablets (3% to 20%) 3475
Relpax Tablets (Infrequent) 2548
Requip Tablets (Infrequent) 1555
Rescriptor Tablets 2551
Retrovir Capsules 1560
Retrovir IV Infusion 1564
Retrovir 1560
Risperdal (Rare) 1676
Risperdal M-Tab Orally Disintegrating Tablets (Rare) 1676
Rythmol SR Capsules 2727
Sonata Capsules (Infrequent) 1717
Symbyax Capsules (Infrequent) 1819
Thalomid Capsules 965
Tricor Tablets 527
Triglide Tablets 3123
Trileptal Tablets 2300
Trileptal Oral Suspension 2300
Uniretic Tablets (Less than 1%) 3100
Vantin Tablets and Oral Suspension (Less than 1%) 2645
Voltaren Tablets (Rarely) 2307
Voltaren-XR Tablets (Rarely) 2310
Xyrem Oral Solution (Infrequent) 1688
Zoloft (Infrequent) 2586
Zomig Nasal Spray (Rare) 3523
Zyprexa Tablets (Rare) 1830
Zyprexa ZYDIS Orally Disintegrating Tablets (Rare) 1830
Zyrtec Chewable Tablets (Less than 2%) 2594
Zyrtec (Less than 2%) 2594
Zyrtec-D 12 Hour Extended Release Tablets (Less than 2%) 2597

Eruptions
Cuprimine Capsules 1947
Meridia Capsules 489
Raptiva for Injection 1250
Solodyn Extended Release Tablets 1890

Eruptions, acneiform
(*see under* Acneiform eruptions)

Eruptions, bullous
Aciphex Tablets 1090
Ambien Tablets (Rare) 2851
Ambien CR Tablets (Rare) 2855
▲ Argatroban Injection (1% to 10%) 1346
▲ Arixtra Injection (0% to 3.1%) 1351
Campath Ampules 811
Coumadin for Injection (Infrequent) 898
Coumadin Tablets (Infrequent) 898
Eulexin Capsules 3009
Evoxac Capsules (Less than 1%) 1047
Fragmin Injection (Rare) 1097
Frova Tablets (Infrequent) 1113
Gemzar for Injection (Very rare) 1771
Gengraf Capsules (1%) 459
Gleevec Tablets (Infrequent) 2227
▲ Hycamtin for Injection (Less than 1% to 16%) 1458
Indapamide Tablets 2156
Invirase (Rare) 2772
Levaquin (0.1% to 0.9%) 2384
Levaquin in 5% Dextrose Injection (0.1% to 0.9%) 2384
Mobic Oral Suspension (Less than 2%) 863
Mobic Tablets (Less than 2%) 863
Neoral Oral Solution (1%) 2259
Neoral Soft Gelatin Capsules (1%) 2259
Plavix Tablets (Less than 1%) 917
Plavix Tablets (Less than 1%) 2926
ReoPro Vials (0.1%) 1809
Risperdal (Rare) 1676
Risperdal M-Tab Orally Disintegrating Tablets (Rare) 1676
▲ Soriatane Capsules (1% to 10%) 1013
Taxotere Injection Concentrate (Rare) 2932
Viramune Oral Suspension 873
Viramune Tablets 873
Zoloft (Rare) 2586
Zyrtec Chewable Tablets (Less than 2%) 2594
Zyrtec (Less than 2%) 2594
Zyrtec-D 12 Hour Extended Release Tablets (Less than 2%) 2597

Eruptions, cutaneous
Ethyol for Injection 1898
Rhophylac (Occasionally) 3505
Taxotere Injection Concentrate 2932

Eruptions, eczematoid
(*see under* Eczema)

Eruptions, fixed
Proquin XR Tablets 1153

Eruptions, fixed drug
Anaprox Tablets 2761
Anaprox DS Tablets 2761
Cipro 2977
Cipro I.V. 2984
Cipro XR Tablets 2990
EC-Naprosyn Delayed-Release Tablets 2761
Naprosyn Suspension 2761
Naprosyn Tablets 2761
Nitro-Dur Transdermal Infusion System (Uncommon) 3046
Prevacid Delayed-Release Capsules (Less than 1%) 3271
Prevacid for Delayed-Release Oral Suspension (Less than 1%) 3271
Prevacid SoluTab Delayed-Release Orally Disintegrating Tablets (Less than 1%) 3271
Prevacid NapraPAC (Less than 1%) 3280
PREVPAC (Less than 1%) 3284
VFEND I.V. (Less than 2%) 2564
VFEND Oral Suspension (Less than 2%) 2564
VFEND Tablets (Less than 2%) 2564

Eruptions, hemorrhagic
Angeliq Tablets 762
Climara Transdermal System 771
Climara Pro Transdermal System 776
Enjuvia Tablets 1062
Estrasorb Topical Emulsion 1147
Estratest Tablets 3199
Estratest H.S. Tablets 3199
Menostar Transdermal System 782
Mircette Tablets 1066
NuvaRing 2340
Ortho-Cyclen Tablets 2429
Ortho Evra Transdermal System 2417
Ortho Tri-Cyclen Tablets 2429
Ortho Tri-Cyclen Lo Tablets 2436
Premarin Intravenous 3442
Premarin Tablets 3446
Premarin Vaginal Cream 3452
Premphase Tablets 3456
Prempro Tablets 3456
Seasonique Tablets 1077
Yasmin 28 Tablets 796
Yaz Tablets 803

Eruptions, herpetic
▲ Chemet Capsules (2.6% to 11.2%) 2458
Zostavax Injection (17 cases) 2111

Eruptions, maculopapular
Avandaryl Tablets (Less than 1%) 1379
Duetact Tablets (Less than 1%) 3226
Mustargen for Injection (Occasional) 2468
▲ Reyataz Capsules (21%) 921

Eruptions, morbilliform
Avandaryl Tablets (Less than 1%) 1379
Duetact Tablets (Less than 1%) 3226
Raniclor Tablets, Chewable (1.5%) 2505

Eruptions, mucocutaneous
▲ Chemet Capsules (2.6% to 11.2%) 2458

Erysipelas
▲ Humira Injection (Less than 5%) 466

Erythema
Accutane Capsules 2731
Aceon Tablets (2 mg, 4 mg, 8 mg) (0.3% to 1%) 3194
Aclovate Cream (Approximately 2%) 2660
▲ Aldara Cream, 5% (1% to 65%) 1846
Alphagan P Ophthalmic Solution 567
AmBisome for Injection (Infrequent) 620
Amerge Tablets (Infrequent) 1339
Aricept Tablets (Infrequent) 1094
Aricept ODT Tablets (Infrequent) 1094
Avandaryl Tablets (Less than 1%) 1379
Axert Tablets (Rare) 2396
Bactroban Ointment (Less than 1%) 1395
Benzaclin Topical Gel (2%) 2877
Betoptic S Ophthalmic Suspension (Small number of patients) 558
Brevoxyl-4 Creamy Wash 3210
Brevoxyl-4 Gel 3210
Brevoxyl-8 Creamy Wash 3210
Brevoxyl-8 Gel 3210
Brimonidine Tartrate Ophthalmic Solution 0.2% ⊙248
Cancidas for Injection (1.2% to 1.5%) 1918
▲ Carac Cream, 0.5% (93.4%) 2879
▲ Catapres-TTS (26 of 101 patients) 844
Ceftin Tablets (0.1% to 1%) 1407
Chantix Tablets (Infrequent) 2517
Ciprodex Otic Suspension (0.4%) 559
Cipro I.V. (1% or less) 2984
▲ Clarinex Syrup (3%) 2995
Climara Transdermal System 771
Clobevate Gel (Less than 2%) 3211
Clobex Lotion 1204
▲ Clolar for Intravenous Infusion (18%) 1271
Clozaril Tablets (Less than 1%) 2184

▲ Copaxone for Injection (4%) 3297
Cosmegen for Injection.................... 2459
Cozaar Tablets (Less than 1%)......... 1935
▲ Cubicin for Injection (5%) 1026
Cutivate Cream (1.6%).................... 2662
Cutivate Ointment (Less than 1%)..... 2665
Cymbalta Delayed-Release Capsules (Infrequent)................... 1757
▲ Dacogen Injection (14%) 2129
Dantrium Intravenous (Rare)............ 2695
Decadron Tablets 1951
Detrol Tablets (1.9%)...................... 2628
▲ Differin Cream (Less than 1% to 38%)... 1210
▲ Differin Gel (10% to 40%) 1211
Digibind for Injection (One patient).... 1421
Diprolene Gel 0.05%........................ 3001
Diprolene Ointment 0.05% (3 per 767 patients)................................ 3003
▲ Doxil Injection (3.4%) 2351
Duac Topical Gel (2%)...................... 3212
Duetact Tablets (Less than 1%) 3226
Duragesic Transdermal System (1% or greater) 2373
▲ Efudex (Among most frequent) 3363
Elidel Cream 1% (Up to 2.2%) 2200
Eligard 22.5 mg (1.7%) 2883
Eligard 30 mg (2.2%) 2885
Eloxatin for Injection (Less than 1%) 2892
Emsam Transdermal System 903
Engerix-B Vaccine (Less than 1%) 1425
Eraxis for Injection (Less than 1% to less than 2%) 2521
Eulexin Capsules 3009
FazaClo Orally Disintegrating Tablets (Less than 1%) 551
Finacea Gel (2% or less) 1669
Fluarix 1451
Follistim AQ Cartridge 2338
Fosamax (Rare) 1969
Hycamtin for Injection 1458
Hydrocortone Tablets 1989
Hyzaar 50-12.5 Tablets 1990
Hyzaar 100-12.5 Tablets 1990
Hyzaar 100-25 Tablets 1990
Imitrex Injection (Infrequent) 1463
Imitrex Nasal Spray 1467
Imitrex Tablets (Infrequent) 1471
Infanrix Vaccine 1476
▲ Infergen (6%) 3364
▲ Intron A for Injection (Less than 5%) 3024
Invanz for Injection (1.2% to 1.6%) ... 1999
Invirase (Less than 2%) 2772
▲ Kepivance (32%) 597
Klaron Lotion 10% (One of 105 patients) 2909
Lamictal (Infrequent) 1481
▲ Leustatin Injection (6%) 2357
Lotrimin 3039
Lotrisone 3040
Lovenox Injection 2915
Maxalt Tablets (Infrequent) 2008
Maxalt-MLT Orally Disintegrating Tablets (Infrequent) 2008
Mentax Cream (Less than 2%) 2158
Meruvax II 2019
▲ Miacalcin Nasal Spray (10.6%) 2253
Micardis Tablets 854
Miradon Tablets 3042
Mivacron Injection (less than1%) 493
M-M-R II 2006
Myozyme for Intravenous Infusion 1279
▲ Nabi-HB (12%) 2169
Naftin Cream (2%) 2126
Naftin Gel (0.5%) 2126
▲ Nexavar Tablets (Very Common) 746
Noroxin Tablets (Less frequent) 2032
Olux Foam (Less than 2%) 1012
▲ Oncaspar (Greater than 5%) 1145
Orthoclone OKT3 Sterile Solution (Less than 1%) 2360
Oxistat Cream (0.2%) 2667
Oxsoralen-Ultra Capsules 3353
▲ Panretin Gel (25% to 77%) 1747
▲ Pediarix Vaccine (0.6% to 41.9%) ... 1548
▲ Photofrin for Injection (Approximately 20%) 702
▲ Prevnar for Injection (0% to 48.3%) 3463
Prinivil Tablets (0.3% to 1.0%) 2052
Prinzide Tablets 2056
▲ Proleukin for Injection (41%) 2266
▲ Protopic Ointment (9% to 28%) 638
Prozac Pulvules and Liquid 1801
Recombivax HB (Equal to or greater than 1%) 2071
Rescriptor Tablets 2551
▲ Revatio Tablets (6%) 2557
▲ Revlimid Capsules (5.4%) 958
Rythmol SR Capsules 2727
Sulfamylon Cream 2162
Sulfamylon for 5% Topical Solution... 2162
▲ Sustiva Capsules (8.8% to 9.9%) 930
▲ Sustiva Tablets (8.8% to 9.9%) 930
▲ Synera Topical Patch (71%) 1137
Taxotere Injection Concentrate (0.9%) 2932
Temodar Capsules (1%).................. 3073
▲ Temovate Gel (Among most frequent) 2669
Temovate Ointment (Less frequent) 2668
Temovate E Emollient (Less than 2%) 2671
Thioridazine Hydrochloride Tablets... 2163
Transderm Scōp Transdermal Therapeutic System (Infrequent) ... 2177
▲ Tri-Luma Cream (29.17% to 41%) ... 1213
▲ Trisenox Injection (13%) 993
Twinrix Vaccine (Less than 1%)......... 1595
Vaprisol (2.7%) 643
Vaqta (Less than 1%) 2097
Xeloda Tablets 2822
▲ Zinecard for Injection (4% to 5%) 2650
Zomig Nasal Spray (Rare) 3523

Erythema, application site

▲ Dacogen Injection (5%) 2129
▲ Humira Injection (20%) 466
▲ Ionsys Transdermal System (14%) .. 2379
Levulan Kerastick for Topical Solution, 20% 1085
Lidoderm Patch 1118
Metrogel 1% 1211
▲ Oxytrol Transdermal System (5.6% to 8.3%) 3392

Erythema, conjunctival

Neosporin Ophthalmic Solution Sterile .... ⊙ 265
TobraDex Ophthalmic Ointment (Less than 4%) 562
TobraDex Ophthalmic Suspension (Less than 4%) 563

Erythema, facial

Acetadote Injection (.24% to 1.17%) 1031
Avalide Tablets 888
Avalide Tablets 2874
Avapro Tablets (Less than 1%) 891
Avapro Tablets (Less than 1%) 2871
▲ Carac Cream, 0.5% (89.4% to 96.5%) 2879
Colocort Rectal Suspension, USP (Retention) 100 mg/60 mL 2476
Depo-Medrol Injectable Suspension 2617
Depo-Medrol Single-Dose Vial 2619

Erythema, hemorrhagic exudative

(*see under* Henoch-Schönlein purpura)

Erythema, insertion site

Vantas (2.8%) 3375

Erythema, nasal

▲ Fortical Nasal Spray (10.6%) 3337

Erythema, oral

▲ Advair Diskus 100/50 (1% to 3%) ... 1308
▲ Advair Diskus 250/50 (1% to 3%) ... 1308
▲ Advair Diskus 500/50 (1% to 3%) ... 1308

Erythema, palmar

Acetadote Injection (.29% to 1.41%) 1031

Erythema, penile

▲ Caverject Impulse Injection (3%) 2612

Erythema, periungual

▲ Penlac (5%) 2924

Erythema at injection site

▲ Actimmune (14%) 1671
▲ ADACEL Vaccine (2.7% to 24.7%) ... 2945
Attenuvax 1914
▲ Comvax (22.4% to 27.2%) 1928
Cubicin for Injection (2.5%) 1026
▲ DAPTACEL Vaccine (12.1% to 19.7%) 2950
Daytrana Transdermal Patch 3174
Edex Injection (2%) 3089
▲ Enbrel for Injection (37%) 584
▲ Engerix-B Vaccine (1% to 10%) 1425
▲ Fuzeon Injection (91%) 2767
▲ Gardasil Injection (0.2% to 24.6%) .. 1984
HibTITER (Less than 1% to 2.0%) 3426
Humalog-Pen 1781
▲ Infergen (17% to 23%) 3364
▲ Invanz for Injection (3.9%) 1999
▲ Leustatin Injection (9%) 2357
Pediarix Vaccine 1548
Liquid PedvaxHIB (0.4% to 2.2%) 2035
Pneumovax 23 (Common)............... 2043
Primaxin I.V. (0.4%)......................... 2048
▲ ProQuad (14.4%) 2064
Risperdal Consta Long-Acting Injection (1%) 1682
Taxotere Injection Concentrate 2932
▲ Trisenox Injection (13%) 993
▲ Vaprisol (4.9%) 643
▲ Vaqta (0.8% to 13.1%) 2097
▲ Varivax (19.3% to 32.5%) 2100
▲ Zostavax Injection (33.7%) 2111

Erythema multiforme

Abelcet Injection 1141
Aciphex Tablets 1090
Advicor Tablets 1722
Aldoril Tablets 1910
Altace Capsules (Less than 1%) 1702
Altoprev Extended-Release Tablets (Rare) 3109
Amoxil Capsules 1343
Amoxil Chewable Tablets 1343
Amoxil Pediatric Drops for Oral Suspension 1343
Amoxil Powder for Oral Suspension 1343
Amoxil Tablets 1343
Anaprox Tablets (Less than 1%) 2761
Anaprox DS Tablets (Less than 1%) .. 2761
Angeliq Tablets 762
Arimidex Tablets (Very rare) 673
Arthrotec Tablets (Rare) 3129
Atacand HCT 651
Atripla Tablets 945
Attenuvax (Rare) 1914
Augmentin 1360
Augmentin Tablets 1363
Augmentin XR Extended-Release Tablets 1369
Augmentin ES-600 Powder for Oral Suspension 1366
Avalide Tablets 888
Avalide Tablets 2874
Caduet Tablets (Greater than 0.1% to less than or equal to 1%) 2508
Captopril Tablets 2149
Carbatrol Capsules 3171
Cardizem LA Extended Release Tablets (Infrequent) 1728
Carimune NF 3499
Ceftin 1407
Celebrex Capsules (Less than 0.1%) 3134
Celexa (At least 3 patients) 1176
Cipro 2977
Cipro I.V. (1% or less) 2984
Cipro XR Tablets 2990
Cleocin Vaginal Ovules (Rare) 2616
Climara Transdermal System 771
Climara Pro Transdermal System 776
Clinoril Tablets (Less than 1%) 1924
Clozaril Tablets 2184
Combivir Tablets 1411
Comvax 1928
Concerta Extended-Release Tablets 1881
Covera-HS Tablets (Less than 2%) 3139
Crixivan Capsules 1940
Daraprim Tablets 1419
Daytrana Transdermal Patch 3174
Depacon Injection 412
Depakene 417
Depakote Sprinkle Capsules 422
Depakote Tablets 427
Depakote ER Tablets 434
Diovan HCT Tablets 2196
Diuril Oral Suspension 1954
Diuril Sodium Intravenous 2467
Dolobid Tablets (Less than 1 in 100) 1955
Doxil Injection (Less than 1%) 2351
EC-Naprosyn Delayed-Release Tablets (Less than 1%) 2761
E.E.S. (Rare) 451
Effexor Tablets 3411
Effexor XR Capsules 3417
Engerix-B Vaccine (Less than 1%) 1425
Enjuvia Tablets 1062
Epzicom Tablets 1436
Equetro Extended-Release Capsules 3180
EryPed (Rare) 447
Erythromycin Delayed-Release Capsules, USP (Rare) 457
Estrasorb Topical Emulsion 1147
Estratest Tablets 3199
Estratest H.S. Tablets 3199
Ethyol for Injection 1898
Fansidar Tablets 2765
FazaClo Orally Disintegrating Tablets 551
Flebogamma 5%, Immune Globulin Intravenous (Human).................. 1658
Fluarix 1451
Focalin Tablets 2220
Focalin XR Capsules 2223
Fortaz 1453
Furosemide Tablets 2154
Gammagard Liquid 721
Gammagard S/D (Rare) 724
Gamunex Immune Globulin I.V., 10% (Rare) 3235
Gleevec Tablets 2227
Gris-PEG Tablets (Occasional) 2502
Havrix Vaccine (Rare) 1456
HibTITER 3426
Hyzaar 50-12.5 Tablets 1990
Hyzaar 100-12.5 Tablets 1990
Hyzaar 100-25 Tablets 1990
Inderal LA Long-Acting Capsules 3429
Indocin Capsules (Less than 1%) 1995
Indocin I.V. (Less than 1%) 2465
Indocin (Less than 1%) 1995
Iressa Tablets (Very rare) 684
Keflex Capsules (Rare) 549
Ketek Tablets (Less than 0.2%) 2903
Lamictal 1481
Lariam Tablets 2786
Lescol Capsules (Rare) 2233
Lescol XL Tablets 2233
Leukeran Tablets (Rare) 1504
Levaquin 2384
Levaquin in 5% Dextrose Injection 2384
Lexapro Oral Solution 1190
Lexapro Tablets 1190
Lipitor Tablets 2483
Lunesta Tablets (Rare) 3142
Lupron Depot-PED 7.5 mg, 11.25 mg and 15 mg (2%) 3269
Lupron Injection Pediatric (2%) 3259
Malarone Pediatric Tablets (Rare) 1517
Malarone Tablets (Rare) 1517
Maxipime for Injection 1105
Mefoxin for Injection 2012
Mefoxin Premixed Intravenous Solution 2016
Menostar Transdermal System 782
Mepron Suspension 1521
Merrem I.V. 686
Meruvax II (Rare) 2019
Metadate CD Capsules 3323
Mevacor Tablets (Rare) 2021
Micardis HCT Tablets 856
Mintezol 2027
Mircette Tablets 1066
M-M-R II (Rare) 2006
Mobic Oral Suspension (Less than 0.1%) 863
Mobic Tablets (Less than 0.1%) 863
Moduretic Tablets 2028
Mumpsvax (Rare) 2031
Mustargen for Injection 2468
Mycamine for Injection 628
Myleran Tablets (Rare) 1525
Naprosyn Suspension (Less than 1%) 2761
Naprosyn Tablets (Less than 1%) 2761
Neurontin Capsules 2487
Neurontin Oral Solution 2487
Neurontin Tablets 2487
Nexavar Tablets (Uncommon) 746
Nexium Delayed-Release Capsules .. 655
Nexium I.V. 659
Noroxin Tablets 2032
Norvasc Tablets (More than 0.1% to 1%) 2545
NuvaRing 2340
Omnicef Capsules 511
Omnicef for Oral Suspension 511
Ortho-Cyclen Tablets 2429
Ortho Evra Transdermal System 2417
Ortho Tri-Cyclen Tablets 2429
Ortho Tri-Cyclen Lo Tablets 2436
Paxil CR Controlled-Release Tablets (Rare) 1538
Paxil (Rare) 1530
PCE Dispertab Tablets (Rare) 515
Pediarix Vaccine 1548
PEG-Intron Powder for Injection 3048
Pexeva Tablets (rare) 1694
Plavix Tablets 917
Plavix Tablets 2926
Premarin Intravenous 3442
Premarin Tablets 3446
Premarin Vaginal Cream 3452
Premphase Tablets 3456
Prempro Tablets 3456
Prevacid NapraPAC (Less than 1%) .. 3280
Prevnar for Injection 3463
PREVPAC 3284
Prezista Tablets (Less than 2%) 3306

Prilosec OTC Delayed-Release Tablets (Very rare) 2677
Primaxin I.M. 2045
Primaxin I.V. (Less than 0.2%) 2048
Prinzide Tablets 2056
ProAmatine Tablets (Rare) 3186
ProQuad 2064
Proquin XR Tablets 1153
Protonix I.V. 3472
Protonix Tablets 3469
Provigil Tablets (Rare) 988
Raniclor Tablets, Chewable 2505
Raptiva for Injection 1250
Rescriptor Tablets 2551
Reyataz Capsules 921
Rilutek Tablets (Rare) 2930
Ritalin Hydrochloride Tablets 2269
Ritalin LA Capsules 2271
Ritalin-SR Tablets 2269
Rocaltrol Capsules (One case) 2798
Rocaltrol Oral Solution (One case) 2798
Seasonique Tablets 1077
Solodyn Extended Release Tablets 1890
Soltamox Oral Solution (Very rare) 3527
Suprax (Less than 2%) 1843
Sustiva Capsules (Up to 3.3%) 930
Sustiva Tablets (Up to 3.3%) 930
Tamiflu Capsules (Rare) 2807
Tamiflu Oral Suspension (Rare) 2807
Tarka Tablets 524
Tasmar Tablets (Infrequent) 3358
Taxotere Injection Concentrate (Rare) 2932
Tegretol/Tegretol-XR 2295
Temodar Capsules (Rare) 3073
Teveten HCT Tablets 1737
Tiazac Capsules (Infrequent) 1201
Ticlid Tablets (Rare) 2810
Timentin ADD-Vantage 1580
Timentin Injection Galaxy Container 1583
Timentin IV Infusion 1577
Timentin Pharmacy Bulk Package 1586
Timolide Tablets 2086
Topamax Sprinkle Capsules 2404
Topamax Tablets 2404
Trileptal Tablets 2300
Trileptal Oral Suspension 2300
Trizivir Tablets 1589
Twinrix Vaccine 1595
Valtrex Caplets 1597
Vantin Tablets and Oral Suspension 2645
Varivax 2100
Vasotec I.V. Injection (0.5% to 1.0%) 2103
Verelan PM Extended-Release Capsules, Controlled-Onset (2% or less) 3106
VFEND I.V. (Rare) 2564
VFEND Oral Suspension (Rare) 2564
VFEND Tablets (Rare) 2564
Voltaren Tablets (Rarely) 2307
Voltaren-XR Tablets (Rarely) 2310
Vytorin 10/10 Tablets 2114
Vytorin 10/10 Tablets 3077
Vytorin 10/20 Tablets 2114
Vytorin 10/20 Tablets 3077
Vytorin 10/40 Tablets 2114
Vytorin 10/40 Tablets 3077
Vytorin 10/80 Tablets 2114
Vytorin 10/80 Tablets 3077
Wellbutrin Tablets (Rare) 1603
Wellbutrin SR Sustained-Release Tablets (Rare) 1607
Wellbutrin XL Extended-Release Tablets (Rare) 1613
Yasmin 28 Tablets 796
Yaz Tablets 803
Zantac (Rare) 1624
Zantac Injection (Rare) 1619
Zantac (Rare) 1624
Zegerid Capsules (Very rare) 2958
Zegerid Powder for Oral Solution (Very rare) 2958
Ziagen 1626
Zinacef for Injection (Rare) 1631
Zinacef Injection (Rare) 1631
Zmax for Oral Suspension (Rare) 2583
Zocor Tablets (Rare) 2105
Zomig Nasal Spray (Rare) 3523
Zosyn (Rare) 3492
Zovirax 1643
Zyban Sustained-Release Tablets (Rare) 1644

Erythema nodosum
Accutane Capsules 2731
Anaprox Tablets 2761
Anaprox DS Tablets 2761
Angeliq Tablets 762
Asacol Delayed-Release Tablets 2692
Carbatrol Capsules 3171
Cipro (Less than 1%) 2977
Cipro I.V. (1% or less) 2984
Cipro XR Tablets 2990
Climara Transdermal System 771
Climara Pro Transdermal System 776
Colazal Capsules 2838
Copaxone for Injection (Infrequent) 3297
Depakote ER Tablets (Greater than 1%) 434
Doxil Injection (Less than 1%) 2351
EC-Naprosyn Delayed-Release Tablets 2761
Effexor Tablets (Rare) 3411
Effexor XR Capsules (Rare) 3417
Engerix-B Vaccine (Less than 1%) 1425
Enjuvia Tablets 1062
Estrasorb Topical Emulsion 1147
Estratest Tablets 3199
Estratest H.S. Tablets 3199
Indocin Capsules (Less than 1%) 1995
Indocin I.V. (Less than 1%) 2465
Indocin (Less than 1%) 1995
▲ Intron A for Injection (Less than 5%) 3024
I.V. Busulfex (2%) 2493
Menostar Transdermal System 782
Mircette Tablets 1066
Myleran Tablets (Rare) 1525
Naprosyn Suspension 2761
Naprosyn Tablets 2761
Neupogen for Injection (One event) 603
NuvaRing 2340
Omnicef Capsules 511
Omnicef for Oral Suspension 511
Ortho-Cyclen/Ortho Tri-Cyclen 2429
Ortho Tri-Cyclen Lo Tablets 2436
Paxil CR Controlled-Release Tablets (Rare) 1538
Paxil (Rare) 1530
Pentasa Capsules (Less than 1%) 3185
Pexeva Tablets (rare) 1694
Premarin Intravenous 3442
Premarin Tablets 3446
Premarin Vaginal Cream 3452
Premphase Tablets 3456
Prempro Tablets 3456
Proquin XR Tablets 1153
Recombivax HB (Less than 1%) 2071
Seasonique Tablets 1077
Tegretol/Tegretol-XR 2295
Thalomid Capsules 965
Twinrix Vaccine 1595
Uniretic Tablets (Less than 1%) 3100
Vesanoid Capsules (Isolated cases) 2820
Yasmin 28 Tablets 796
Yaz Tablets 803

Erythema simplex
Oncaspar (Less than 1%) 1145

Erythematous streaking
▲ Zinecard for Injection (4% to 5%) 2650

Erythrocytes, abnormal
▲ Ferrlecit Injection (11%) 3388
Gabitril Tablets (Infrequent) 984
Paxil CR Controlled-Release Tablets (Rare) 1538
Paxil (Rare) 1530
Pexeva Tablets (rare) 1694
Uniretic Tablets (Less than 1%) 3100

Erythrocytosis
Moban Tablets 1119

Erythrocyturia
Emend Capsules (Greater than 0.5%) 1963

Erythroderma
Cozaar Tablets 1935
Hyzaar 50-12.5 Tablets 1990
Hyzaar 100-12.5 Tablets 1990
Hyzaar 100-25 Tablets 1990

Erythroleukemia
Thalomid Capsules 965

Erythromelalgia
Adalat CC Tablets (Rare) 2964
Gammagard S/D 724

Erythropenia
Accutane Capsules 2731
Aricept Tablets (Infrequent) 1094
Aricept ODT Tablets (Infrequent) 1094
Moban Tablets 1119
Mustargen for Injection 2468
Primaxin I.M. 2045

Escharotic effect
Cetacaine Topical Anesthetic 999
▲ Panretin Gel (1% to 8%) 1747

Esophageal disease, unspecified
Myleran Tablets 1525
Nexium Delayed-Release Capsules (Less than 1%) 655
Nexium I.V. (Less than 1%) 659

Esophageal erosions
Fosamax 1969
Fosamax Plus D Tablets 1977

Esophageal perforation
Celebrex Capsules (Less than 0.1%) 3134
Fosamax (Rare) 1969
Fosamax Plus D Tablets (Rarely) 1977
Razadyne (Rare) 2399
Razadyne ER Extended-Release Capsules (Rare) 2399
TriLyte with Flavor Packs for Oral Solution 3100

Esophageal rupture
Exelon Capsules (One case) 2206
Exelon Oral Solution (One case) 2206

Esophageal stenosis
Actiq (Less than 1%) 979
Cymbalta Delayed-Release Capsules (Infrequent) 1757
Prevacid NapraPAC (Less than 1%) 3280
Rilutek Tablets (Infrequent) 2930

Esophageal stricture
Evoxac Capsules (Less than 1%) 1047
Fosamax (Rare) 1969
Fosamax Plus D Tablets (Rarely) 1977
Nexium Delayed-Release Capsules (Less than 1%) 655
Nexium I.V. (Less than 1%) 659
▲ Photofrin for Injection (6% to 38%) 702
Prevacid Delayed-Release Capsules (Less than 1%) 3271
Prevacid for Delayed-Release Oral Suspension (Less than 1%) 3271
Prevacid SoluTab Delayed-Release Orally Disintegrating Tablets (Less than 1%) 3271
PREVPAC (Less than 1%) 3284

Esophageal ulceration
Accutane Capsules 2731
Actonel with Calcium Tablets 2688
Arthrotec Tablets (Rare) 3129
Azilect Tablets (Infrequent) 3293
Fosamax Plus D Tablets (0.1% to 1.5%) 1977
Oracea Capsules (Rare) 1000
Prevacid Delayed-Release Capsules (Less than 1%) 3271
Prevacid for Delayed-Release Oral Suspension (Less than 1%) 3271
Prevacid SoluTab Delayed-Release Orally Disintegrating Tablets (Less than 1%) 3271
PREVPAC (Less than 1%) 3284
Zelapar Tablets 3372

Esophagitis
Abilify Oral Solution (Rare) 882
Abilify Oral Solution (Rare) 2450
Abilify Discmelt Orally Disintegrating Tablets (Rare) 882
Abilify Discmelt Orally Disintegrating Tablets (Rare) 2450
Abilify Tablets (Rare) 882
Abilify Tablets (Rare) 2450
Accutane Capsules 2731
Aciphex Tablets 1090
Actiq (Less than 1%) 979
Actonel with Calcium Tablets 2688
Adalat CC Tablets (Less than 1%) 2964
▲ Alimta for Injection (Up to 6%) 1750
Amerge Tablets (Rare) 1339
Anaprox Tablets (Less than 1%) 2761
Anaprox DS Tablets (Less than 1%) 2761
Arthrotec Tablets (Rare) 3129
Azilect Tablets (Infrequent) 3293
Caduet Tablets (Less than 2%) 2508
Campath Ampules 811
Campral Tablets (Infrequent) 1174
Celebrex Capsules (0.1% to 1.9%) 3134
Celexa (Infrequent) 1176
▲ CellCept Capsules (3% to less than 20%) 2747
▲ CellCept Intravenous (3% to less than 20%) 2747
▲ CellCept Oral Suspension (3% to less than 20%) 2747
▲ CellCept Tablets (3% to less than 20%) 2747
Chantix Tablets (Infrequent) 2517
Cialis Tablets (Less than 2%) 1838
Copaxone for Injection (Infrequent) 3297
Cosmegen for Injection 2459
Didronel Tablets 2697
▲ Doxil Injection (1% to 10%) 2351
EC-Naprosyn Delayed-Release Tablets (Less than 1%) 2761
Effexor Tablets (Infrequent) 3411
Effexor XR Capsules (Infrequent) 3417
Elmiron Capsules (Less than or equal to 1%) 2415
Enbrel for Injection 584
Evoxac Capsules (Less than 1%) 1047
Exelon Capsules (Infrequent) 2206
Exelon Oral Solution (Infrequent) 2206
Fosamax 1969
Fosamax Plus D Tablets 1977
Gabitril Tablets (Infrequent) 984
Gengraf Capsules (1% to less than 3%) 459
▲ Humira Injection (Less than 5%) 466
▲ Intron A for Injection (Less than 5%) 3024
Invanz for Injection (Greater than 0.1%) 1999
Invirase (Less than 2%) 2772
I.V. Busulfex (2%) 2493
Kaletra (Less than 2%) 476
Lamictal 1481
Levaquin (0.1% to 0.9%) 2384
Levaquin in 5% Dextrose Injection (0.1% to 0.9%) 2384
Levitra Tablets (Less than 2%) 3034
Lipitor Tablets (Less than 2%) 2483
Lofibra Tablets 1219
Lofibra Capsules 1216
Lotrel Capsules 2249
Lyrica Capsules (0.1% to 1%) 2539
Mobic Oral Suspension (Less than 2%) 863
Mobic Tablets (Less than 2%) 863
Myfortic Tablets 2255
Naprosyn Suspension (Less than 1%) 2761
Naprosyn Tablets (Less than 1%) 2761
Neoral Oral Solution (1% to less than 3%) 2259
Neoral Soft Gelatin Capsules (1% to less than 3%) 2259
Neurontin Capsules (Rare) 2487
Neurontin Oral Solution (Rare) 2487
Neurontin Tablets (Rare) 2487
Nexium Delayed-Release Capsules (Less than 1%) 655
Nexium I.V. (Less than 1%) 659
Norvir (Less than 2%) 503
Oracea Capsules (Rare) 1000
Paxil CR Controlled-Release Tablets (Rare) 1538
Paxil (Rare) 1530
Permax Tablets (Infrequent) 3356
Pexeva Tablets (rare) 1694
▲ Photofrin for Injection (5%) 702
Pletal Tablets (Less than 2%) 2455
Prevacid Delayed-Release Capsules (Less than 1%) 3271
Prevacid for Delayed-Release Oral Suspension (Less than 1%) 3271
Prevacid SoluTab Delayed-Release Orally Disintegrating Tablets (Less than 1%) 3271
Prevacid NapraPAC (Less than 1%) 3280
PREVPAC (Less than 1%) 3284
▲ Prograf Capsules and Injection (3% to 15%) 632
Protonix I.V. (Less than 1%) 3472
Protonix Tablets (Less than 1%) 3469
Prozac Pulvules and Liquid (Infrequent) 1801
▲ Rapamune Oral Solution and Tablets (3% to 20%) 3475
Relpax Tablets (Infrequent) 2548
Requip Tablets (Infrequent) 1555
Reyataz Capsules (Less than 3%) 921
Risperdal (Rare) 1676
Risperdal M-Tab Orally Disintegrating Tablets (Rare) 1676
▲ Simulect for Injection (3% to 10%) 2284
Sonata Capsules (Infrequent) 1717
Soriatane Capsules (Less than 1%) 1013
Symbyax Capsules (Infrequent) 1819
Tasmar Tablets (Infrequent) 3358
▲ Taxotere Injection Concentrate (1.8% to 16.3%) 2932
Teveten Tablets (Less than 1%) 1735
Teveten HCT Tablets (Less than 1%) 1737
Thalomid Capsules 965
Topamax Sprinkle Capsules (Infrequent) 2404
Topamax Tablets (Infrequent) 2404

Tricor Tablets 527
Triglide Tablets 3123
Trileptal Tablets 2300
Trileptal Oral Suspension 2300
Uniretic Tablets (Less than 1%) 3100
VFEND I.V. (Less than 2%) 2564
VFEND Oral Suspension (Less than 2%) 2564
VFEND Tablets (Less than 2%) 2564
Viagra Tablets (Less than 2%) 2573
Vicoprofen Tablets (Less than 1%) 539
Voltaren Tablets (Occasionally) 2307
Voltaren-XR Tablets (Occasionally) 2310
Wellbutrin Tablets 1603
Wellbutrin SR Sustained-Release Tablets 1607
Wellbutrin XL Extended-Release Tablets 1613
Xeloda Tablets 2822
Zelapar Tablets 3372
▲ Zinecard for Injection (3% to 6%) 2650
Zoloft (Infrequent) 2586
Zomig Tablets (Infrequent) 3519
Zomig-ZMT Tablets (Infrequent) 3519
Zonegran Capsules (Rare) 1101
Zyban Sustained-Release Tablets 1644
Zyprexa Tablets (Infrequent) 1830
Zyprexa ZYDIS Orally Disintegrating Tablets (Infrequent) 1830

Esophagitis, ulcerative
Colocort Rectal Suspension, USP (Retention) 100 mg/60 mL 2476
Decadron Tablets 1951
Depo-Medrol Injectable Suspension 2617
Depo-Medrol Single-Dose Vial 2619
Hydrocortone Tablets 1989
Indocin I.V. (Less than 1%) 2465

Esophagospasm
Ambien Tablets (Rare) 2851
Ambien CR Tablets (Rare) 2855
Effexor XR Capsules (Rare) 3417
Frova Tablets (Infrequent) 1113
Migranal Nasal Spray (Rare) 3348
Neurontin Capsules (Rare) 2487
Neurontin Oral Solution (Rare) 2487
Neurontin Tablets (Rare) 2487

Esosinophilia
Zelnorm Tablets 2312

ESR, elevation
Accutane Capsules 2731
Aceon Tablets (2 mg, 4 mg, 8 mg) 3194
Advicor Tablets 1722
Altace Capsules (Less than 1%) 1702
Altoprev Extended-Release Tablets (Rare) 3109
Ambien Tablets (Rare) 2851
Ambien CR Tablets (Rare) 2855
Captopril Tablets 2149
Cipro I.V. (Rare) 2984
Clozaril Tablets 2184
Comvax 1928
FazaClo Orally Disintegrating Tablets 551
Lescol Capsules (Rare) 2233
Lescol XL Tablets 2233
Mevacor Tablets (Rare) 2021
Prinivil Tablets (0.3% to 1.0%) 2052
Prinzide Tablets 2056
Recombivax HB 2071
Vasotec I.V. Injection (0.5% to 1.0%) 2103
Vytorin 10/10 Tablets 2114
Vytorin 10/10 Tablets 3077
Vytorin 10/20 Tablets 2114
Vytorin 10/20 Tablets 3077
Vytorin 10/40 Tablets 2114
Vytorin 10/40 Tablets 3077
Vytorin 10/80 Tablets 2114
Vytorin 10/80 Tablets 3077
Zocor Tablets (Rare) 2105

ESR decrease
Thalomid Capsules 965

Euphoria
Abilify Oral Solution (Rare) 882
Abilify Oral Solution (Rare) 2450
Abilify Discmelt Orally Disintegrating Tablets (Rare) 882
Abilify Discmelt Orally Disintegrating Tablets (Rare) 2450
Abilify Tablets (Rare) 882
Abilify Tablets (Rare) 2450
Actiq (Less than 1%) 979
Adderall Tablets 3164
Adderall XR Capsules 3166
Adipex-P 1215
Ambien Tablets (Frequent) 2851
Ambien CR Tablets (1% to frequent) 2855
Avinza Capsules (Less than 5%) 1741
Axert Tablets (Rare) 2396
Bicillin C-R Injectable Suspension 1706
Celexa (Infrequent) 1176
▲ Cesamet Capsules (11% to 38%) 3340
Chantix Tablets (Rare) 2517
Copaxone for Injection (At least 2%) 3297
Dalmane Capsules (Rare) 3342
Decadron Tablets 1951
Depacon Injection (0.9%) 412
Desoxyn Tablets, USP 2462
Dexedrine 1420
DextroStat Tablets 3179
▲ Diastat Rectal Delivery System (3%) 3343
Dilaudid 440
Dilaudid Non-Sterile Powder 440
Dilaudid Oral Liquid 445
Dilaudid Rectal Suppositories 440
Dilaudid Tablets 440
Dilaudid Tablets - 8 mg 445
Dilaudid-HP (Less frequent) 442
▲ Duragesic Transdermal System (3% to 10%) 2373
Effexor Tablets (Infrequent) 3411
Effexor XR Capsules (Infrequent) 3417
Eldepryl Capsules 3208
Flumadine (Less than 0.3%) 1183
Frova Tablets (Infrequent) 1113
Gabitril Tablets (Frequent) 984
Hydrocortone Tablets 1989
Hyperstat I.V. 3017
Imitrex Injection (Infrequent) 1463
Imitrex Nasal Spray (Infrequent) 1467
Imitrex Tablets (Infrequent) 1471
Invirase (Less than 2%) 2772
Kadian Capsules (Less than 3%) 577
Lamictal (Infrequent) 1481
Lidoderm Patch 1118
Lunesta Tablets (Rare) 3142
▲ Lyrica Capsules (2% to 3%) 2539
▲ Marinol Capsules (3% to 10%) 3333
Maxalt Tablets (Frequent) 2008
Maxalt-MLT Orally Disintegrating Tablets (Frequent) 2008
Migranal Nasal Spray (Infrequent) 3348
Moban Tablets (Less frequent) 1119
▲ MS Contin Tablets (Among most frequent) 2701
Neurontin Capsules (Infrequent) 2487
Neurontin Oral Solution (Infrequent) 2487
Neurontin Tablets (Infrequent) 2487
Norvir (Less than 2%) 503
Numorphan Injection 1120
Opana Tablets (Less than 1%) 1122
Opana ER Tablets (Less than 1%) 1126
▲ OxyContin Tablets (Between 1% and 5%) 2703
OxyFast Oral Concentrate Solution 2708
OxyIR Capsules 2708
Parcopa Orally Disintegrating Tablets 3097
Paxil CR Controlled-Release Tablets (Rare) 1538
Paxil (Rare) 1530
Percocet Tablets 1131
Percodan Tablets 1132
Permax Tablets (Infrequent) 3356
Pexeva Tablets (infrequent) 1694
Phenergan Tablets and Suppositories 3440
ProSom Tablets (Infrequent) 517
Prozac Pulvules and Liquid (Infrequent) 1801
Relpax Tablets (Infrequent) 2548
Requip Tablets (Infrequent) 1555
Rescriptor Tablets 2551
Restoril Capsules (1.5%) 1860
Rilutek Tablets (Rare) 2930
Risperdal (Infrequent) 1676
Risperdal Consta Long-Acting Injection (Infrequent) 1682
Risperdal M-Tab Orally Disintegrating Tablets (Infrequent) 1676
▲ Romazicon Injection (1% to 3%) 2804
Seroquel Tablets (Rare) 690
Sonata Capsules (Frequent) 1717
Stalevo Tablets 2287
Sustiva Capsules (Less than 2%) 930
Sustiva Tablets (Less than 2%) 930
Symbyax Capsules (Infrequent) 1819
Symmetrel Tablets (0.1% to 1%) 1135
Synera Topical Patch 1137
Tambocor Tablets (Less than 1%) 1856
Tasmar Tablets (1%) 3358
Tequin Injection (Less than 0.1%) 938
Tequin Injection in 5% Dextrose (Less than 0.1%) 938
Tequin Tablets (Less than 0.1%) 938
Thalomid Capsules 965
Topamax Sprinkle Capsules (Infrequent) 2404
Topamax Tablets (Infrequent) 2404
Trileptal Tablets 2300
Trileptal Oral Suspension 2300
Tussionex Pennkinetic Extended-Release Suspension 3327
Tylenol with Codeine Tablets 2391
▲ Ultram ER Tablets (1% to greater than 5%) 2392
VFEND I.V. (Less than 2%) 2564
VFEND Oral Suspension (Less than 2%) 2564
VFEND Tablets (Less than 2%) 2564
Vicoprofen Tablets (Less than 1%) 539
Vivitrol 995
Wellbutrin Tablets (1.2%) 1603
Wellbutrin SR Sustained-Release Tablets 1607
Wellbutrin XL Extended-Release Tablets 1613
Xyrem Oral Solution (Infrequent) 1688
Zoloft (Infrequent) 2586
Zomig Tablets (Rare) 3519
Zomig Nasal Spray (Rare) 3523
Zomig-ZMT Tablets (Rare) 3519
Zonegran Capsules (Infrequent) 1101
Zyban Sustained-Release Tablets 1644
▲ Zyprexa Tablets (2% to 3%) 1830
▲ Zyprexa ZYDIS Orally Disintegrating Tablets (2% to 3%) 1830
Zyrtec Chewable Tablets (Less than 2%) 2594
Zyrtec (Less than 2%) 2594
Zyrtec-D 12 Hour Extended Release Tablets (Less than 2%) 2597

Eustachian tube dysfunction
Neurontin Capsules (Rare) 2487
Neurontin Oral Solution (Rare) 2487
Neurontin Tablets (Rare) 2487

Exanthema
Aptivus Capsules (Less than 2%) 826
Boostrix 1404
Copaxone for Injection (Infrequent) 3297
Covera-HS Tablets (Less than 2%) 3139
Lariam Tablets (Infrequent) 2786
Tarka Tablets 524
Verelan PM Extended-Release Capsules, Controlled-Onset (2% or less) 3106

Exanthema, viral
ProQuad (1.2%) 2064
Vaqta (1%) 2097

Excitability
BC Allergy Sinus Cold Powder ▣ 677
Bentyl Capsules 697
Bentyl Injection 697
Bentyl Syrup 697
Bentyl Tablets 697
Comtrex Maximum Strength Cold & Cough Day/Night Caplets - Day Formulation ▣ 726
Comtrex Maximum Strength Cold & Cough Day/Night Caplets - Night Formulation ▣ 726
Comtrex Maximum Strength Day/Night Severe Cold & Sinus Caplets - Night Formulation ▣ 725
Contac Cold and Flu Maximum Strength Caplets ▣ 728
Contac Cold and Flu Day and Night Caplets (Night Formulation Only) ▣ 727
Children's Dimetapp Cold & Allergy Elixir ▣ 730
Children's Dimetapp Cold & Allergy Chewable Tablets ▣ 730
Children's Dimetapp Long Acting Cough Plus Cold Syrup ▣ 731
Donnatal Extentabs 2493
Klonopin (Infrequent) 2778
Lexapro Oral Solution (Infrequent) 1190
Lexapro Tablets (Infrequent) 1190
Oxandrin Tablets 2962
Phenergan Tablets and Suppositories 3440
Robitussin Cough & Allergy Syrup ▣ 736
Robitussin Cough & Cold Nighttime Liquid ▣ 736
Robitussin Cough, Cold & Flu Nighttime Liquid ▣ 738
Robitussin Pediatric Cough & Cold Long-Acting Liquid ▣ 735
Robitussin Pediatric Cough & Cold Nighttime Liquid ▣ 736
TheraFlu Cold & Cough Hot Liquid ▣ 740
TheraFlu Cold & Sore Throat Hot Liquid ▣ 741
TheraFlu Flu & Sore Throat Hot Liquid ▣ 742
TheraFlu Nighttime Severe Cold Hot Liquid ▣ 740
TheraFlu Warming Relief Nighttime Severe Cold ▣ 743
TheraFlu Thin Strips Multi Symptom ▣ 744
Triaminic Cold & Allergy Liquid ▣ 746
Triaminic Nighttime Cold & Cough Liquid ▣ 746
Triaminic Cough & Runny Nose Softchews ▣ 748
Triaminic Thin Strips Cough & Runny Nose ▣ 749
Children's Tylenol Plus Cough & Runny Nose Suspension Liquid ▣ 754
Children's Tylenol Plus Cold Suspension Liquid ▣ 754
Children's Tylenol Plus Multi-Symptom Cold Suspension Liquid ▣ 754
Children's Tylenol Plus Flu Oral Suspension ▣ 749
Tylenol Cold Head Congestion Nighttime Caplets with Cool Burst ▣ 750
Tylenol Cold Head Congestion Severe Caplets with Cool Burst ▣ 750
Tylenol Cold Multi-Symptom NightTime ▣ 752
Tylenol Cough & Sore Throat Nighttime Liquid with Cool Burst ▣ 790
Tylenol Sore Throat Nighttime Liquid with Cool Burst ▣ 790
Tylenol Allergy Multi-Symptom Caplets with Cool Burst and Gelcaps 1872
Tylenol Allergy Multi-Symptom Nighttime Caplets with Cool Burst 1872
Tylenol Severe Allergy Caplets 1872
Children's Tylenol Plus Cold Suspension Liquid 1879
Children's Tylenol Plus Cold & Allergy Suspension Liquid 1878
Children's Tylenol Plus Cough & Runny Nose Suspension Liquid 1879
Children's Tylenol Plus Flu Suspension Liquid 1881
Children's Tylenol Plus Multi-Symptom Cold Suspension Liquid 1879
Tylenol Cold Head Congestion Nighttime Caplets with Cool Burst 1873
Tylenol Cold Multi-Symptom Nighttime Caplets with Cool Burst 1874
Tylenol Cold Multi-Symptom Nighttime Liquid with Cool Burst 1874
Tylenol Cough & Sore Throat Nighttime Liquid with Cool Burst 1877
Tylenol Sinus Congestion & Pain Nighttime Caplets with Cool Burst 1876
Tylenol Sore Throat Nighttime Liquid with Cool Burst 1877
Pediatric Vicks 44m Cough & Cold Relief Liquid 2676
Vicks NyQuil Multi-Symptom Cold/Flu Relief Liquid 2681
Vicks NyQuil Multi-Symptom Cold/Flu Relief LiquiCaps 2681
Vicks NyQuil LiquiCaps/Liquid Multi-Symptom Cold/Flu Relief ▣ 763
Children's Vicks NyQuil Cold/Cough Relief Liquid 2680
Zicam Maximum Strength Flu Daytime ▣ 768
Zicam Maximum Strength Flu Nighttime ▣ 768
Zyrtec-D 12 Hour Extended Release Tablets 2597

Excitement, paradoxical
ProSom Tablets 517
Valium Tablets 2819

Excoriation
▲ Aldara Cream, 5% (Up to 25%) 1846
Catapres-TTS (3 of 101 patients) 844
Cutivate Lotion 0.05% (2%) 2664
Levulan Kerastick for Topical Solution, 20% (1%) 1085
▲ Panretin Gel (1% to 8%) 1747
Sulfamylon Cream (Rare) 2162

Exercise tolerance, decreased
Blocadren Tablets 1916
Cosopt Sterile Ophthalmic Solution 1931
Lopressor HCT 50/25 Tablets (1%) 2241
Lopressor HCT 100/25 Tablets (1%) 2241
Lopressor HCT 100/50 Tablets (1%) 2241
Timoptic Sterile Ophthalmic Solution (Less frequent) 2088
Timoptic in Ocudose (Less frequent) 2091
Timoptic-XE Sterile Ophthalmic Gel Forming Solution 2092

Exophthalmos
Colocort Rectal Suspension, USP (Retention) 100 mg/60 mL 2476
Decadron Tablets 1951
Depo-Medrol Injectable Suspension 2617
Depo-Medrol Single-Dose Vial 2619
Effexor Tablets (Rare) 3411
Effexor XR Capsules (Rare) 3417
Hydrocortone Tablets 1989
Lyrica Capsules (Rare) 2539
Paxil CR Controlled-Release Tablets (Rare) 1538
Paxil (Rare) 1530
Pexeva Tablets (rare) 1694
Prozac Pulvules and Liquid (Rare) 1801
Zoloft (Rare) 2586

Extraocular movement, impairment of
Lescol Capsules 2233
Lescol XL Tablets 2233
Vytorin 10/10 Tablets 2114
Vytorin 10/10 Tablets 3077
Vytorin 10/20 Tablets 2114
Vytorin 10/20 Tablets 3077
Vytorin 10/40 Tablets 2114
Vytorin 10/40 Tablets 3077
Vytorin 10/80 Tablets 2114
Vytorin 10/80 Tablets 3077
Zocor Tablets 2105

Extrapyramidal disorder
Lexapro Oral Solution 1190
Lexapro Tablets 1190
Namenda (Infrequent) 1195
Parcopa Orally Disintegrating Tablets 3097
Symbyax Capsules (Infrequent) 1819

Extrapyramidal symptoms
Abelcet Injection 1141
▲ Abilify Oral Solution (6% to 17%) 882
▲ Abilify Oral Solution (6% to 17%) 2450
▲ Abilify Discmelt Orally Disintegrating Tablets (6% to 17%) 882
▲ Abilify Discmelt Orally Disintegrating Tablets (6% to 17%) 2450
▲ Abilify Tablets (6% to 17%) 882
▲ Abilify Tablets (6% to 17%) 2450
Aciphex Tablets (Rare) 1090
Cardizem LA Extended Release Tablets (Infrequent) 1728
Celexa (Infrequent) 1176
Clozaril Tablets 2184
▲ Demser Capsules (10%) 1953
Effexor Tablets 3411
Effexor XR Capsules 3417
▲ Equetro Extended-Release Capsules (Less than 5%) 3180
▲ Geodon (14% to 31%) 2529
▲ Intron A for Injection (Less than 5%) 3024
Kytril Injection (Rare) 2781
Kytril (One case) 2784
Lamictal (Rare) 1481
Librium Capsules 3347
▲ Mirapex Tablets (Greater than or equal to 1% to 28%) 859
Moban Tablets 1119
Paxil CR Controlled-Release Tablets (Rare) 1538
Paxil (Rare) 1530
Permax Tablets (1.6%) 3356
Pexeva Tablets (rare) 1694
Phenergan Tablets and Suppositories 3440
Proleukin for Injection 2266
Prozac Pulvules and Liquid (Rare) 1801
Requip Tablets (Infrequent) 1555
Rilutek Tablets (Infrequent) 2930
▲ Risperdal (17% to 34%) 1676
Risperdal Consta Long-Acting Injection 1682
▲ Risperdal M-Tab Orally Disintegrating Tablets (17% to 34%) 1676
Seroquel Tablets 690
Stalevo Tablets 2287
Tasmar Tablets (Infrequent) 3358
Thioridazine Hydrochloride Tablets (Infrequent) 2163
Thiothixene Capsules 2165
Tiazac Capsules (Infrequent) 1201
Trileptal Tablets 2300
Trileptal Oral Suspension 2300
VFEND I.V. (Less than 2%) 2564
VFEND Oral Suspension (Less than 2%) 2564
VFEND Tablets (Less than 2%) 2564
Wellbutrin SR Sustained-Release Tablets 1607
Wellbutrin XL Extended-Release Tablets 1613
Zofran Injection (Rare) 1634
Zofran (Rare) 1639
Zofran ODT Orally Disintegrating Tablets (Rare) 1639
Zoloft 2586
Zyban Sustained-Release Tablets 1644
▲ Zyprexa Tablets (8% to 32%) 1830
▲ Zyprexa IntraMuscular (2% to 4%) 1830
▲ Zyprexa ZYDIS Orally Disintegrating Tablets (8% to 32%) 1830

Extrapyramidal syndrome
Lyrica Capsules (Rare) 2539

Extrasystoles
Abilify Oral Solution (Infrequent) 882
Abilify Oral Solution (Infrequent) 2450
Abilify Discmelt Orally Disintegrating Tablets (Infrequent) 882
Abilify Discmelt Orally Disintegrating Tablets (Infrequent) 2450
Abilify Tablets (Infrequent) 882
Abilify Tablets (Infrequent) 2450
Adalat CC Tablets (Less than 1%) 2964
Advair Diskus 100/50 1308
Advair Diskus 250/50 1308
Advair Diskus 500/50 1308
Advair HFA Inhalation Aerosol 1318
Aloxi Injection (Less than 1%) 2127
Ambien Tablets (Rare) 2851
Ambien CR Tablets (Rare) 2855
Anzemet Injection 2859
Anzemet Tablets 2862
Atacand HCT (0.5% or greater) 651
Caduet Tablets (Less than or equal to 0.1%) 2508
Cardene I.V. (0.7%) 2497
Celexa (Infrequent) 1176
▲ CellCept Capsules (3% to less than 20%) 2747
▲ CellCept Intravenous (3% to less than 20%) 2747
▲ CellCept Oral Suspension (3% to less than 20%) 2747
▲ CellCept Tablets (3% to less than 20%) 2747
Effexor Tablets (Infrequent) 3411
Effexor XR Capsules (Infrequent) 3417
Ethyol for Injection 1898
Evoxac Capsules (Less than 1%) 1047
Exelon Capsules (Infrequent) 2206
Exelon Oral Solution (Infrequent) 2206
▲ Imdur Tablets (Less than or equal to 5%) 3018
▲ Intron A for Injection (Less than 5%) 3024
Lariam Tablets (Occasional) 2786
Lofibra Tablets 1219
Lofibra Capsules 1216
Lotronex Tablets (Rare) 1512
Meridia Capsules 489
Norvasc Tablets (Less than 0.1%) 2545
Proventil Inhalation Aerosol 3053
Prozac Pulvules and Liquid (Rare) 1801
Requip Tablets (2%) 1555
Rythmol SR Capsules 2727
Serevent Diskus 1568
Teveten Tablets (Less than 1%) 1735
Teveten HCT Tablets (Less than 1%) 1737
Tiazac Capsules (2%) 1201
Tricor Tablets 527
Ventolin HFA Inhalation Aerosol (Less than 3%) 1600
VFEND I.V. (Less than 2%) 2564
VFEND Oral Suspension (Less than 2%) 2564
VFEND Tablets (Less than 2%) 2564
Wellbutrin SR Sustained-Release Tablets 1607
Wellbutrin XL Extended-Release Tablets 1613
▲ Xeloda Tablets (Less than 5%) 2822
Xopenex Inhalation Solution 3146
Xopenex Inhalation Solution Concentrate 3150
Xopenex HFA Inhalation Aerosol 3154
Zomig Tablets (Rare) 3519
Zomig-ZMT Tablets (Rare) 3519
Zyban Sustained-Release Tablets 1644

Extrasystoles, supraventricular
Aloxi Injection (Less than 1%) 2127
Caverject Impulse Injection (Less than 1%) 2612
▲ CellCept Capsules (3% to less than 20%) 2747
▲ CellCept Intravenous (3% to less than 20%) 2747
▲ CellCept Oral Suspension (3% to less than 20%) 2747
▲ CellCept Tablets (3% to less than 20%) 2747
Pexeva Tablets (rare) 1694
Rythmol SR Capsules 2727
Ultane Liquid for Inhalation (Less than 1%) 531

Extravasation
Cosmegen for Injection 2459
Doxil Injection 2351
Fluorescite Injection ⊙ 207
Gemzar for Injection (Infrequent) 1771
Hyperstat I.V. 3017
ProQuad 2064
Romazicon Injection 2804
Taxotere Injection Concentrate 2932
▲ Visudyne for Injection (10% to 30%) 2305
Zinecard for Injection (1% to 3%) 2650

Extremities, rigidity of
Abilify Oral Solution (Frequent) 882
Abilify Oral Solution (Frequent) 2450
Abilify Discmelt Orally Disintegrating Tablets (Frequent) 882
Abilify Discmelt Orally Disintegrating Tablets (Frequent) 2450
Abilify Tablets (Frequent) 882
Abilify Tablets (Frequent) 2450

Extroversion
Ambien Tablets 2851

Exudate, increased
Bactroban Ointment (Less than 1%) 1395
▲ Thrombate III (1 of 17) 3257
Xalatan Sterile Ophthalmic Solution (Less than 1%) 2649

Eye abnormalities, fetal
Accutane Capsules 2731

Eye abnormality, unspecified
Topamax Sprinkle Capsules (2%) 2404
Topamax Tablets (2%) 2404

Eye discharge
▲ Macugen Injection (10% to 40%) ⊙ 261
Retisert Implant (5% to 9%) ⊙ 258

Eye disorder, unspecified
Cesamet Capsules 3340
Lyrica Capsules (1% to 2%) 2539

Eye globe, perforation
(*see under* Bulbus oculi, perforation)

Eye movements, abnormal
Klonopin 2778
Mevacor Tablets (0.5% to 1.0%) 2021
Zocor Tablets 2105

Eye swelling
▲ Advair HFA Inhalation Aerosol (1% to 3%) 1318
Cesamet Capsules 3340
Fluarix 1451
Poly-Pred Ophthalmic Suspension ⊙ 233
▲ Retisert Implant (5% to 9%) ⊙ 258
Xyrem Oral Solution (Infrequent) 1688

Eyeball, perforation
(*see under* Bulbus oculi, perforation)

Eyelash changes
Xalatan Sterile Ophthalmic Solution 2649

Eyelash darkening
▲ Lumigan Ophthalmic Solution (3% to 10%) 573
▲ Travatan Ophthalmic Solution (Among most frequent) 563
Xalatan Sterile Ophthalmic Solution 2649

Eyelashes, increase in growth
Iressa Tablets 684
▲ Lumigan Ophthalmic Solution (15% to 45%) 573
▲ Travatan Ophthalmic Solution (Among most frequent) 563

Eyelashes, matting of
Betoptic S Ophthalmic Suspension (Small number of patients) 558
Lacrisert Sterile Ophthalmic Insert 2005

Eyelid, discomfort
▲ Xalatan (1% to 4%) 2649

Eyelid crusting
Brimonidine Tartrate Ophthalmic Solution 0.2% (Less than 3%) ⊙ 248
Cosopt Sterile Ophthalmic Solution 1931
Travatan Ophthalmic Solution (1% to 4%) 563
Trusopt Sterile Ophthalmic Solution 2095
▲ Xalatan Sterile Ophthalmic Solution (1% to 4%) 2649

Eyelid disorder, unspecified
Cesamet Capsules 3340

Eyelid skin darkening
▲ Lumigan Ophthalmic Solution (3% to 10%) 573
▲ Travatan Ophthalmic Solution (Among most frequent) 563
Xalatan Sterile Ophthalmic Solution 2649

Eyelid swelling
▲ Acular LS Ophthalmic Solution (1% to 5%) 566
Cialis Tablets (Less than 2%) 1838
▲ Euflexxa (3%) 1162
Fluarix 1451
▲ Voltaren Ophthalmic Solution (Less than or equal to 5%) 2309

Eyelids, deposits in
Soriatane Capsules (Less than 5%) 1013
Xalatan Sterile Ophthalmic Solution (1% to 4%) 2649

Eyelids, edema of
▲ Alphagan P Ophthalmic Solution (1% to 4%) 567
BOTOX Purified Neurotoxin Complex (2 cases) 570
▲ Brimonidine Tartrate Ophthalmic Solution 0.2% (3% to 9%) ⊙ 248
Ciloxan Ophthalmic Ointment (Less than 1%) 559
Ciloxan Ophthalmic Solution (Less than 1%) ⊙ 206
Hyzaar 50-12.5 Tablets 1990
Hyzaar 100-12.5 Tablets 1990
Hyzaar 100-25 Tablets 1990
Lacrisert Sterile Ophthalmic Insert 2005
Polytrim Ophthalmic Solution (Multiple reports) 574
Quixin Ophthalmic Solution (Less than 1%) 3383
Stromectol Tablets 2083
▲ Trisenox Injection (5%) 993
▲ Xalatan Sterile Ophthalmic Solution (1% to 4%) 2649

Eyelids, erythema
▲ Alphagan P Ophthalmic Solution (1% to 4%) 567
▲ Alrex Ophthalmic Suspension 0.2% (Less than 5%) ⊙ 246
▲ Betimol Ophthalmic Solution (More than 5%) 3382
▲ Betimol Ophthalmic Solution (More than 5%) ⊙ 295
▲ Brimonidine Tartrate Ophthalmic Solution 0.2% (3% to 9%) ⊙ 248
▲ Lotemax Ophthalmic Suspension 0.5% (Less than 5%) ⊙ 251
▲ Lumigan Ophthalmic Solution (3% to 10%) 573
Xalatan Sterile Ophthalmic Solution (1% to 4%) 2649

Eyelids, pruritis
Alphagan P Ophthalmic Solution 567

Brimonidine Tartrate Ophthalmic Solution 0.2% ⊙ 248

Eyes, burning of
▲ Alamast Ophthalmic Solution (Less than 5%) 3381
▲ Alrex Ophthalmic Suspension 0.2% (5% to 15%) ⊙ 246
▲ Betagan Ophthalmic Solution, USP (About 1 in 3 patients) ⊙ 220
▲ Betimol Ophthalmic Solution (1 in 8 patients) 3382
▲ Betimol Ophthalmic Solution (1 in 8 patients) ⊙ 295
Bleph-10 Ophthalmic Solution 10% ⊙ 222
▲ Carac Cream, 0.5% (5.4%) 2879
▲ Carteolol Hydrochloride Ophthalmic Solution USP, 1% (About 1 of 4 patients) ⊙ 249
Catapres Tablets 843
Catapres-TTS (0.5% or less) 844
▲ Ciloxan Ophthalmic Ointment (Among most frequent) 559
▲ Ciloxan Ophthalmic Solution (Among most frequent) ⊙ 206
Clorpres Tablets 2153
▲ Cosopt Sterile Ophthalmic Solution (Up to 30%) 1931
Cozaar Tablets (Less than 1%) 1935
Dalmane Capsules (Rare) 3342
▲ Elestat Ophthalmic Solution (1% to 10%) 1669
FML Ophthalmic Suspension ⊙ 227
FML Forte Ophthalmic Suspension ⊙ 226
Hyzaar 50-12.5 Tablets 1990
Hyzaar 100-12.5 Tablets 1990
Hyzaar 100-25 Tablets 1990
▲ Lotemax Ophthalmic Suspension 0.5% (5% to 15%) ⊙ 251
▲ Lumigan Ophthalmic Solution (3% to 10%) 573
Maxalt Tablets (Infrequent) 2008
Maxalt-MLT Orally Disintegrating Tablets (Infrequent) 2008
Muro 128 Ophthalmic Ointment ⊙ 253
Muro 128 Ophthalmic Solution 2% and 5% ⊙ 252
Ocufen Ophthalmic Solution ⊙ 232
Ophthetic Ophthalmic Solution ⊙ 232
▲ Patanol Ophthalmic Solution (Less than 5%) 561
▲ Polytrim Ophthalmic Solution (Among most frequent) 574
Pred Mild Ophthalmic Suspension ⊙ 238
Pred Forte Ophthalmic Suspension ⊙ 235
▲ Propine Ophthalmic Solution (6%) ⊙ 239
▲ Quixin Ophthalmic Solution (1% to 3%) 3383
▲ Restasis Ophthalmic Emulsion (17%) 575
Restoril Capsules (0.5% to 0.9%) 1860
Tessalon Capsules 1199
Tessalon Perles 1199
▲ Timoptic Sterile Ophthalmic Solution (Approximately 1 in 8 patients) 2088
▲ Timoptic in Ocudose (Approximately 1 in 8 patients) 2091
▲ Timoptic-XE Sterile Ophthalmic Gel Forming Solution (1 in 8 patients) 2092
▲ Trusopt Sterile Ophthalmic Solution (Approximately one-third of patients) 2095
Viagra Tablets 2573
▲ Viroptic Ophthalmic Solution (4.6%) ⊙ 266
Visine For Contacts Rewetting Drops ⊙ 289
▲ Xalatan Sterile Ophthalmic Solution (5% to 15%) 2649

Eyes, cotton wool spots
Intron A for Injection 3024
PEG-Intron Powder for Injection 3048

Eyes, dilatation of pupil
(*see under* Mydriasis)

Eyes, discoloration
Alinia for Oral Suspension (Less than 1%) 2835
Alinia Tablets (Less than 1%) 2835
FazaClo Orally Disintegrating Tablets (Less than 1%) 551

Eyes, disorders of
Adalat CC Tablets (Less than 1%) 2964
▲ Aerobid/Aerobid-M (1% to 3%) 1171
▲ Alphagan P Ophthalmic Solution (1% to 4%) 567
Astelin Nasal Spray (Infrequent) 1904
Avapro Tablets (Less than 1%) 891
Avapro Tablets (Less than 1%) 2871
Carbatrol Capsules 3171
▲ Carnitor Injection (3% to 6%) 3188
Clinoril Tablets (Less than 1%) 1924
▲ Copaxone for Injection (4%) 3297
Depakote ER Tablets (Greater than 1%) 434
Kaletra (Less than 2%) 476
Lofibra Tablets 1219
Lofibra Capsules 1216
▲ Lupron Depot 3.75 mg (Among most frequent) 3260
Mintezol 2027
Mirapex Tablets (Less than 1%) 859
Neurontin Capsules (Rare) 2487
Neurontin Oral Solution (Rare) 2487
Neurontin Tablets (Rare) 2487
Permax Tablets (1.1%) 3356
Protopic Ointment (Greater than or equal to 1%) 638
▲ Requip Tablets (3%) 1555
▲ Soriatane Capsules (1% to 10%) 1013
Stromectol Tablets 2083
Tambocor Tablets 1856
Tegretol/Tegretol-XR 2295
▲ Thrombate III (1 of 17) 3257
Travatan Ophthalmic Solution (1% to 4%) 563
Tricor Tablets 527
Varivax (Greater than or equal to 1%) 2100
▲ Vesanoid Capsules (17%) 2820
Viracept (Less than 2%) 2577

Eyes, dry
(*see under* Xerophthalmia)

Eyes, irritation of
▲ Acular Ophthalmic Solution (Approximately 1% to 10%) 565
▲ Acular LS Ophthalmic Solution (1% to 10%) 566
Advicor Tablets 1722
Albalon Ophthalmic Solution ⊙ 218
Aloxi Injection (Less than 1%) 2127
▲ Alphagan P Ophthalmic Solution (1% to 4%) 567
▲ Alrex Ophthalmic Suspension 0.2% (Less than 5%) ⊙ 246
Altoprev Extended-Release Tablets (0.5% to 1%) 3109
Ambien Tablets (Infrequent) 2851
Ambien CR Tablets (Infrequent) 2855
Aricept Tablets (Frequent) 1094
Aricept ODT Tablets (Frequent) 1094
Atrovent Nasal Spray 0.03% (Less than 2%) 837
Bleph-10 Ophthalmic Solution 10% ⊙ 222
Blocadren Tablets (1.1%) 1916
▲ BOTOX Purified Neurotoxin Complex (10.0%) 570
▲ Brimonidine Tartrate Ophthalmic Solution 0.2% (3% to 9%) ⊙ 248
▲ Carac Cream, 0.5% (5.4%) 2879
Cardizem LA Extended Release Tablets (Less than 2%) 1728
▲ Carteolol Hydrochloride Ophthalmic Solution USP, 1% (About 1 of 4 patients) ⊙ 249
Cesamet Capsules 3340
Chantix Tablets (Infrequent) 2517
Cubicin for Injection (Less than 1%) 1026
Flonase Nasal Spray 1440
Fluarix 1451
FML Ophthalmic Suspension ⊙ 227
FML Forte Ophthalmic Suspension ⊙ 226
Imitrex Injection (Infrequent) 1463
Imitrex Nasal Spray (Infrequent) 1467
Imitrex Tablets (Up to 2%) 1471
Invirase (Less than 2%) 2772
Klonopin (Infrequent) 2778
Lacrisert Sterile Ophthalmic Insert 2005
Lexapro Oral Solution (Infrequent) 1190
Lexapro Tablets (Infrequent) 1190
▲ Lotemax Ophthalmic Suspension 0.5% (Less than 5%) ⊙ 251
▲ Lucentis Injection (4% to 19%) 1237
▲ Lumigan Ophthalmic Solution (3% to 10%) 573
▲ Macugen Injection (10% to 40%) ⊙ 261
Maxalt Tablets (Infrequent) 2008
Maxalt-MLT Orally Disintegrating Tablets (Infrequent) 2008
Mevacor Tablets (0.5% to 1.0%) 2021
Muro 128 Ophthalmic Ointment ⊙ 253
Muro 128 Ophthalmic Solution 2% and 5% ⊙ 252
Neosporin Ophthalmic Solution Sterile ⊙ 265
Ocufen Ophthalmic Solution ⊙ 232
▲ Polytrim Ophthalmic Solution (Among most frequent) 574
Pred Mild Ophthalmic Suspension ⊙ 238
Pred Forte Ophthalmic Suspension ⊙ 235
Prilosec OTC Delayed-Release Tablets (Less than 1%) 2677
ProQuad 2064
ProSom Tablets (Infrequent) 517
▲ Retisert Implant (10% to 35%) ⊙ 258
▲ Soriatane Capsules (1% to 10%) 1013
Tambocor Tablets (Less than 1%) 1856
Temovate Scalp Application (1 of 294 patients) 2670
Tiazac Capsules (Less than 2%) 1201
Timolide Tablets 2086
Timoptic Sterile Ophthalmic Solution (Less frequent) 2088
Timoptic in Ocudose (Less frequent) 2091
Timoptic-XE Sterile Ophthalmic Gel Forming Solution 2092
▲ Trisenox Injection (10%) 993
Vaqta (Less than 1%) 2097
▲ Voltaren Ophthalmic Solution (Less than or equal to 5%) 2309
▲ Xeloda Tablets (13%) 2822
Xyrem Oral Solution (Infrequent) 1688
Zegerid Capsules (Less than 1%) 2958
Zegerid Powder for Oral Solution (Less than 1%) 2958
▲ Zymar Ophthalmic Solution (1% to 4%) 575

Eyes, nonreactive
Nipent for Injection (Less than 3%) 1863

Eyes, redness of
▲ Advair Diskus 100/50 (1% to 3%) 1308
▲ Advair Diskus 250/50 (1% to 3%) 1308
▲ Advair Diskus 500/50 (1% to 3%) 1308
Albalon Ophthalmic Solution ⊙ 218
Ambien CR Tablets (2%) 2855
Clozaril Tablets (Less than 1%) 2184
Fluarix 1451
Percodan Tablets 1132
▲ Polytrim Ophthalmic Solution (Among most frequent) 574
Transderm Scōp Transdermal Therapeutic System (Infrequent) 2177
▲ Travatan Ophthalmic Solution (35% to 50%) 563
Trusopt Sterile Ophthalmic Solution 2095
Viagra Tablets 2573
Visine For Contacts Rewetting Drops ⊙ 289
Xyrem Oral Solution (Infrequent) 1688
▲ Zymar Ophthalmic Solution (1% to 4%) 575

Eyes, "Spots" before the
Aricept Tablets (Infrequent) 1094
Aricept ODT Tablets (Infrequent) 1094
Depacon Injection 412
Depakene 417
Depakote Sprinkle Capsules 422
Depakote Tablets 427
Depakote ER Tablets 434
Tambocor Tablets 1856

Eyes, stinging
▲ Restasis Ophthalmic Emulsion (1% to 5%) 575
▲ Viroptic Ophthalmic Solution (4.6%) ⊙ 266
▲ Voltaren Ophthalmic Solution (15%) 2309
▲ Xalatan Sterile Ophthalmic Solution (5% to 15%) 2649

Eyes, swollen
▲ Macugen Injection (1% to 5%) ⊙ 261

Eyes, tearing
▲ Alphagan P Ophthalmic Solution (1% to 4%) 567
Astelin Nasal Spray (Infrequent) 1904
Beconase AQ Nasal Spray (Fewer than 3 per 100 patients) 1396
Betoptic S Ophthalmic Suspension (Small number of patients) 558
▲ Brimonidine Tartrate Ophthalmic Solution 0.2% (3% to 9%) ⊙ 248
▲ Carac Cream, 0.5% (5.4%) 2879
▲ Carteolol Hydrochloride Ophthalmic Solution USP, 1% (About 1 of 4 patients) ⊙ 249
▲ Chemet Capsules (1.0% to 3.7%) 2458
Ciloxan Ophthalmic Ointment (Less than 1%) 559
Ciloxan Ophthalmic Solution (Less than 1%) ⊙ 206
Cosopt Sterile Ophthalmic Solution 1931
Dantrium Capsules (Less frequent) 2694
Emcyt Capsules (1%) 2634
Levitra Tablets (Less than 2%) 3034
▲ Lumigan Ophthalmic Solution (1% to 3%) 573
Nipent for Injection (Less than 3%) 1863
Polytrim Ophthalmic Solution (Multiple reports) 574
▲ Retisert Implant (10% to 35%) ⊙ 258
Sonata Capsules (Infrequent) 1717
Strattera Capsules 1814
▲ Suboxone Tablets (5%) 2717
▲ Subutex Tablets (5%) 2717
Taxotere Injection Concentrate 2932
Timoptic Sterile Ophthalmic Solution (Less frequent) 2088
Timoptic in Ocudose (Less frequent) 2091
▲ Timoptic-XE Sterile Ophthalmic Gel Forming Solution (1% to 5%) 2092
Travatan Ophthalmic Solution (1% to 4%) 563
Visine For Contacts Rewetting Drops ⊙ 289
▲ Xalatan Sterile Ophthalmic Solution (1% to 4%) 2649
▲ Zymar Ophthalmic Solution (1% to 4%) 575

Eyes, watering
Astelin Nasal Spray (Infrequently) 1904

F

Face, rhythmical involuntary movements
Moban Tablets 1119
Thiothixene Capsules 2165

Facial dehiscence
Rapamune Oral Solution and Tablets 3475

Facial dysmorphia, fetal
Accutane Capsules 2731

Facial features, coarsening
Phenytek Capsules 2160

Facial wasting
Aptivus Capsules (Less than 2%) 826
Combivir Tablets 1411
Crixivan Capsules 1940
Invirase 2772
Norvir 503
Retrovir 1560
Reyataz Capsules (Less than 3%) 921
Truvada Tablets 1296
Viracept 2577
Viramune Oral Suspension 873
Viramune Tablets 873
Viread Tablets 1301

Facies, mask-like
Thiothixene Capsules 2165
▲ Zyprexa Tablets (8% to 20%) 1830
▲ Zyprexa IntraMuscular (2% to 4%) 1830
▲ Zyprexa ZYDIS Orally Disintegrating Tablets (8% to 20%) 1830

Factor VIII decrease
Advate Injection (0.6%) 712

Factors II, V, VII, X, decrease
Estratest Tablets 3199
Estratest H.S. Tablets 3199
Oxandrin Tablets 2962

Factors VII, VIII, IX, X, increase
Estratest Tablets 3199
Estratest H.S. Tablets 3199
Ortho-Cyclen/Ortho Tri-Cyclen 2429

Fainting
(*see under* Syncope)

Faintness
Fleet Prep Kits 1170
Parcopa Orally Disintegrating Tablets 3097

Falling
▲ Advate Injection (12.7%) 712
Ambien Tablets (Infrequent) 2851
Ambien CR Tablets (Infrequent) 2855
▲ Azilect Tablets (5% to 11%) 3293
▲ Dacogen Injection (8%) 2129
Dalmane Capsules 3342
Detrol Tablets (1.5%) 2628
Eldepryl Capsules 3208
Evoxac Capsules (Less than 1%) 1047
Geodon Capsules (Frequent) 2529
Klonopin (Infrequent) 2778

Lexapro Oral Solution (Infrequent).... 1190
Lexapro Tablets (Infrequent)............ 1190
Matulane Capsules.......................... 3191
Mobic Oral Suspension (0% to 2.6%)... 863
Mobic Tablets (0% to 2.6%)............. 863
Namenda (Greater than or equal to 2%).. 1195
Parcopa Orally Disintegrating Tablets 3097
Razadyne (Greater than or equal to 2%)... 2399
Razadyne ER Extended-Release Capsules (Greater than or equal to 2%)... 2399
Requip Tablets (1% or more)........... 1555
Revlimid Capsules 958
▲ Tasmar Tablets (4% to 6%) 3358
▲ Trileptal Tablets (Up to 4%) 2300
▲ Trileptal Oral Suspension (Up to 4%) 2300
Viagra Tablets (Less than 2%) 2573
Xyrem Oral Solution (Frequent) 1688

Family stress
Estring Vaginal Ring (2%) 2635

Fanconi syndrome
Atripla Tablets 945
Depacon Injection (Rare) 412
Depakene (Rare) 417
Depakote Sprinkle Capsules (Rare) .. 422
Depakote Tablets (Rare) 427
Depakote ER Tablets (Rare) 434
Garamycin Injectable 3014
Revlimid Capsules 958
Truvada Tablets 1296
Viread Tablets 1301

Fasciculations
Amerge Tablets (Rare) 1339
Aricept Tablets (Infrequent) 1094
Aricept ODT Tablets (Infrequent) 1094
Clozaril Tablets (Less than 1%) 2184
▲ Depakote Sprinkle Capsules (1% to 5%) 422
Dilaudid Oral Liquid (Less frequent) 445
Dilaudid Tablets - 8 mg (Less frequent) 445
Dilaudid-HP 442
Eldepryl Capsules 3208
Eloxatin for Injection 2892
Garamycin Injectable 3014
Leukeran Tablets (Rare) 1504
Migranal Nasal Spray (Rare) 3348
MS Contin Tablets (Less frequent) 2701
▲ Niravam Orally Disintegrating Tablets (6.9% to 7.9%) 3092
Parcopa Orally Disintegrating Tablets 3097
Parnate Tablets 1527
Paxil CR Controlled-Release Tablets (Rare) 1538
Paxil (Rare) 1530
Pexeva Tablets (rare) 1694
ReoPro Vials (0.4%) 1809
Retrovir 1560
Stalevo Tablets 2287
▲ Ultram ER Tablets (1% to greater than 5%) 2392
Uniphyl Tablets 2710
▲ Vivitrol (2% to 8%) 995
Xyrem Oral Solution (Infrequent) 1688

Fasciitis, necrotizing
Raptiva for Injection 1250

Fasciitis, necrotizing fulminant
Clinoril Tablets (Rare) 1924
Dolobid Tablets 1955
Indocin (Rare) 1995

Fat deposits, abnormal
Decadron Tablets 1951

Fat redistribution, unspecified
Agenerase Capsules (Nine patients) 1327
Agenerase Oral Solution (Nine patients) 1332
Aptivus Capsules 826
Atripla Tablets 945
Crixivan Capsules (2.1%) 1940
Epzicom Tablets 1436
Prezista Tablets (Less than 2%) 3306
Rescriptor Tablets 2551
Truvada Tablets 1296
Viracept (Less than 2%) 2577

Fatality, hepatic related
Eulexin Capsules 3009

Fatigue
Accutane Capsules 2731
▲ Actimmune (14%) 1671
▲ ADACEL Vaccine (1.2% to 30.2%) ... 2945
▲ Adalat CC Tablets (4%) 2964
▲ Advair Diskus 250/50 (3%) 1308
▲ Aerobid/Aerobid-M (1% to 3%) 1171
▲ Agenerase Capsules (7% to 14%) ... 1327
▲ Agenerase Oral Solution (7% to 14%) 1332
▲ Aggrenox Capsules (5.8%) 822
Agrylin Capsules 3169
Aldara Cream, 5% (More than 1%).... 1846
▲ Alferon N Injection (6% to 14%) 1665
▲ Alimta for Injection (Up to 87%) 1750
Allegra (1.3%) 2844
Aloxi Injection (Less than 1%) 2127
▲ Alphagan P Ophthalmic Solution (1% to 4%) 567
Altace Capsules (2%) 1702
Ambien Tablets (1%) 2851
▲ Ambien CR Tablets (3%) 2855
Amerge Tablets (2%) 1339
▲ Amitiza Capsules (2.3% to 6.9%) 3224
▲ Anzemet Injection (3.6%) 2859
Anzemet Tablets (2.6%) 2862
▲ Aptivus Capsules (4%) 826
▲ Aranesp for Injection (9% to 33%) ... 581
▲ Aredia for Injection (37.2%) 2179
▲ Aricept Tablets (3% to 8%) 1094
▲ Aricept ODT Tablets (3% to 8%) 1094
▲ Aromasin Tablets (8% to 22%) 2600
▲ Arranon Injection (2% to 50%) 1357
Arthrotec Tablets (Rare) 3129
▲ Asmanex Twisthaler (1% to 13%) 2966
Astelin Nasal Spray (2.3%) 1904
Atacand Tablets (More than 1%) 649
Atacand HCT (0.5% or greater) 651
▲ Atripla Tablets (7%) 945
▲ Avalide Tablets (7%) 888
▲ Avalide Tablets (7%) 2874
▲ Avandamet Tablets (6.2%) 1373
▲ Avandia Tablets (3.6%) 1384
▲ Avapro Tablets (4%) 891
▲ Avapro Tablets (4%) 2871
Axert Tablets (Infrequent) 2396
Azmacort Inhalation Aerosol 1726
Azopt Ophthalmic Suspension (Less than 1%) 557
▲ Baraclude (1% to 3%) 894
Benicar Tablets (Greater than 0.5%) 1043
Bicillin C-R Injectable Suspension 1706
▲ Blocadren Tablets (3.4% to 5%) 1916
▲ Boostrix (3.7% to 37%) 1404
▲ Brimonidine Tartrate Ophthalmic Solution 0.2% (10% to 30%)........ ⊙248
Bumex Tablets (0.1%) 2746
▲ Caduet Tablets (4.5%) 2508
Calcium Disodium Versenate Injection 1851
▲ Campath Ampules (5% to 34%) 811
Cancidas for Injection (0%) 1918
Captopril Tablets (About 0.5% to 2%) 2149
Carbatrol Capsules 3171
▲ Cardizem LA Extended Release Tablets (4.8%) 1728
Cardura XL Tablets 2515
▲ Catapres Tablets (About 4 in 100 patients) 843
▲ Catapres-TTS (6 of 101 patients) 844
Celebrex Capsules (0.1% to 1.9%)... 3134
▲ Celexa (5%) 1176
▲ Cerezyme for Injection (Approximately 6.5%) 1270
Cesamet Capsules 3340
▲ Chantix Tablets (4% to 7%) 2517
▲ Chemet Capsules (5.2% to 15.7%) 2458
Cialis Tablets (Less than 2%) 1838
▲ Clarinex Tablets (2.1% to 5%) 2995
▲ Clarinex Reditabs Tablets (2.1% to 5%) 2995
▲ Clarinex-D 24-Hour Extended-Release Tablets (3%)...... 2998
Clinoril Tablets (Less than 1 in 100) 1924
▲ Clolar for Intravenous Infusion (36%) 1271
▲ Clorpres Tablets (About 4%) 2153
Clozaril Tablets (2%) 2184
Colazal Capsules (2%) 2838
Combivent Inhalation Aerosol (Less than 2%) 847
▲ Combivir Tablets (10%) 1411
▲ Comtan Tablets (6%) 2189
▲ Copegus Tablets (65%) 2754
▲ Coreg Tablets (24%) 1414
Cosmegen for Injection 2459
Cosopt Sterile Ophthalmic Solution 1931
Coumadin for Injection (Infrequent)... 898
Coumadin Tablets (Infrequent) 898
▲ Covera-HS Tablets (1.7% to 4.5%) ... 3139
Cozaar Tablets (1% or greater) 1935
Crixivan Capsules (2.7%) 1940
Cubicin for Injection (Less than 1%) 1026
▲ Cymbalta Delayed-Release Capsules (2% to 12%) 1757
▲ Dantrium Capsules (Among most frequent) 2694
▲ depo-subQ provera 104 Injectable Suspension (1% to less than 5%) 2624
▲ Detrol Tablets (4%) 2628
Detrol LA Capsules (2%) 2631
Dibenzyline Capsules 3399
▲ Diovan Tablets (2% to 3%) 2193
▲ Diovan HCT Tablets (5%) 2196
Dolobid Tablets (Greater than 1 in 100) 1955
Doxil Injection 2351
▲ Duragesic Transdermal System (3% to 10%) 2373
Dyazide Capsules 1423
▲ DynaCirc CR Tablets (2.5% to 7.6%) 2721
Dyrenium Capsules (Rare) 3400
Edecrin 1959
Effexor XR Capsules 3417
Eldepryl Capsules 3208
▲ Eligard 7.5 mg (17.5%) 2880
▲ Eligard 22.5 mg (6%) 2883
▲ Eligard 30 mg (13.3%) 2885
▲ Eligard 45 mg (11.7%) 2888
▲ Eloxatin for Injection (4% to 68%) 2892
Elspar for Injection 2463
Elspar for Injection 1960
▲ Emend Capsules (17.8% to 21.9%) 1963
Enbrel for Injection 584
▲ Engerix-B Vaccine (14%) 1425
▲ Entocort EC Capsules (5%) 2698
▲ Epivir (27%) 1427
▲ Epivir-HBV (24%) 1432
▲ Epogen for Injection (9% to 25%) 591
▲ Epzicom Tablets (6% to 8%) 1436
Equetro Extended-Release Capsules 3180
Euflexxa (1.25% to 1.88%) 1162
Eulexin Capsules 3009
▲ Evoxac Capsules (3.3%) 1047
▲ Exelon Capsules (4% to 9%) 2206
▲ Exelon Oral Solution (4% to 9%) 2206
▲ Famvir Tablets (4% to 6.3%) 2211
Fansidar Tablets 2765
FazaClo Orally Disintegrating Tablets (2%) 551
▲ Femara Tablets (6% to 13%) 2214
▲ Ferrlecit Injection (6%) 3388
Flebogamma 5%, Immune Globulin Intravenous (Human) 1658
▲ Flovent Diskus (1% to 16%) 1443
▲ Fluarix (12.2% to 19.7%) 1451
Flumadine (1.0%) 1183
▲ Flumist Vaccine (25.7%) 1901
Foradil Aerolizer 3010
▲ Fortical Nasal Spray (1% to 3%) 3337
▲ Frova Tablets (5%) 1113
▲ Fuzeon Injection (20.2%) 2767
Gabitril Tablets 984
▲ Gammagard Liquid (2.18% to 16.4%) 721
Gammagard S/D (Occasional) 724
Gantrisin Pediatric Suspension 2770
▲ Gemzar for Injection (40%) 1771
▲ Gengraf Capsules (3%) 459
▲ Gleevec Tablets (1% to 53%) 2227
Gris-PEG Tablets 2502
▲ Havrix Vaccine (1% to 10%) 1456
▲ Hycamtin for Injection (Up to 37%) .. 1458
▲ Hytrin Capsules (7.4% to 11.3%) ... 471
Hyzaar 50-12.5 Tablets (1% or greater) 1990
Hyzaar 100-12.5 Tablets (1% or greater) 1990
Hyzaar 100-25 Tablets (1% or greater) 1990
▲ Imdur Tablets (Less than or equal to 5%) 3018
Imitrex Injection (1.1%) 1463
▲ Imitrex Tablets (2% to 3%) 1471
Imodium A-D Liquid and Caplets 1865
Imodium Advanced Caplets and Chewable Tablets .... ▣655
▲ Indapamide Tablets (Greater than or equal to 5%) 2156
Inderal LA Long-Acting Capsules 3429
Indocin (Greater than 1%) 1995
▲ Infergen (65% to 69%) 3364
▲ InnoPran XL Capsules (5% to 7%) 2723
Inspra Tablets (2%) 2536
▲ Intron A for Injection (4% to 96%) 3024
Invanz for Injection (1.2%) 1999
▲ Invirase (Less than 2% to 6.1%) 2772
I.V. Busulfex (2%) 2493
Keflex Capsules 549
Keppra Oral Solution 3314
▲ Keppra Tablets (5%) 3314
Ketek Tablets (Greater than or equal to 0.2% to less than 2%)...... 2903
▲ Klonopin (7%) 2778
K-Phos Original (Sodium Free) Tablets (Less frequent) 760
K-Phos Neutral Tablets 760
▲ Lamictal (8%) 1481
Lamisil Tablets 2232
▲ Lariam Tablets (Among most frequent) 2786
Lescol Capsules (2.7%) 2233
Lescol XL Tablets (1.6%) 2233
▲ Leustatin Injection (11% to 45%) 2357
Levaquin (1.2%) 2384
Levaquin in 5% Dextrose Injection (1.2%) 2384
Levothroid Tablets 1186
Levoxyl Tablets 1712
▲ Lexapro Oral Solution (2% to 8%) 1190
▲ Lexapro Tablets (2% to 8%) 1190
▲ Lexiva Tablets (Less than 1% to 18%) 1505
Lithobid Tablets 1692
Lithostat Tablets 2140
▲ Lopressor Injection (1% to 10%) 2238
▲ Lopressor Tablets (1% to 10%) 2238
▲ Lopressor HCT 50/25 Tablets (10%) 2241
▲ Lopressor HCT 100/25 Tablets (10%) 2241
▲ Lopressor HCT 100/50 Tablets (10%) 2241
Lotensin Tablets (2.4%) 2243
▲ Lotensin HCT Tablets (5.2%) 2246
Lotrel Capsules 2249
Lotronex Tablets (Rare) 1512
Mavik Tablets (More than 1%) 486
Maxair Autohaler 1852
▲ Maxalt Tablets (4% to 7%) 2008
▲ Maxalt-MLT Orally Disintegrating Tablets (4% to 7%) 2008
▲ Menactra Vaccine (0.9% to 34.7%) 2954
MetroGel-Vaginal Gel (Less than 1%) 1855
▲ Miacalcin Nasal Spray (1% to 3%) ... 2253
Micardis Tablets (1%) 854
▲ Micardis HCT Tablets (3%) 856
▲ Midamor Tablets (Between 1% and 3%) 2026
Migranal Nasal Spray (1%) 3348
Mintezol 2027
Mobic Oral Suspension (Less than 2%) 863
Mobic Tablets (Less than 2%) 863
Moduretic Tablets (Greater than 1%, less than 3%) 2028
▲ Myfortic Tablets (3% to less than 20%) 2255
Myleran Tablets 1525
Nabi-HB 2169
Nadolol Tablets (2 of 100 patients) .. 2159
Nalfon Capsules (1.7%) 2502
Namenda (2%) 1195
▲ Neoral Oral Solution (3%) 2259
▲ Neoral Soft Gelatin Capsules (3%) ... 2259
▲ Neulasta Injection (15% to 72%) 601
▲ Neupogen for Injection (11%) 603
▲ Neurontin Capsules (3.4% to 11%) 2487
▲ Neurontin Oral Solution (3.4% to 11%) 2487
▲ Neurontin Tablets (3.4% to 11%) 2487
▲ Nexavar Tablets (Less than 1% to 37%) 746
Nexium Delayed-Release Capsules (Less than 1%) 655
Nexium I.V. (Less than 1%) 659
▲ Nipent for Injection (29% to 42%) 1863
▲ Niravam Orally Disintegrating Tablets (18.4% to 48.6%) 3092
▲ Norvasc Tablets (4.5%) 2545
Numorphan Injection 1120
Oncaspar 1145
Opana Tablets (Less than 1%) 1122
▲ Opana ER Tablets (3.9%) 1126
Ortho-Cyclen Tablets 2429
Ortho Evra Transdermal System 2417
Ortho Tri-Cyclen Tablets 2429
Ortho Tri-Cyclen Lo Tablets 2436
Orthoclone OKT3 Sterile Solution 2360
▲ Oxytrol Transdermal System (Greater than 1%) 3392
Parcopa Orally Disintegrating Tablets 3097
▲ Pegasys (56%) 2789
▲ PEG-Intron Powder for Injection (52%) 3048
Pepcid Injection (Infrequent) 2040
Pepcid (Infrequent) 2038
Persantine Tablets (Rare) 868
Phenergan Tablets and Suppositories 3440
▲ Photofrin for Injection (4%) 702
▲ Plan B Tablets (16.9%) 1076

▲ Plavix Tablets (3.3%) ... 917
▲ Plavix Tablets (3.3%) ... 2926
Premphase Tablets ... 3456
Prempro Tablets ... 3456
Prezista Tablets (Less than 2%) ... 3306
Prilosec OTC Delayed-Release Tablets (Less than 1%) ... 2677
Prinivil Tablets (2.5%) ... 2052
▲ Prinzide Tablets (3.7%) ... 2056
Prochieve 4% Gel ... 1003
Prochieve 8% Gel ... 1003
▲ Procrit for Injection (9% to 25%) ... 2364
▲ Proleukin for Injection (53%) ... 2266
▲ Prometrium Capsules (100 mg, 200 mg) (8% to 9%) ... 3203
Proquin XR Tablets (Less than 1%) ... 1153
▲ Pulmicort Respules (1% to 3%) ... 661
▲ Razadyne (5%) ... 2399
▲ Razadyne ER Extended-Release Capsules (5%) ... 2399
▲ Rebetol (58% to 70%) ... 3058
▲ Rebetron Combination Therapy (62% to 70%) ... 3063
▲ Rebif Prefilled Syringe for Injection (33% to 41%) ... 3159
Recombinate ... 729
Recombivax HB (Greater than 1%) ... 2071
Relenza Rotadisk (Less than 1.5%) ... 1552
▲ Remicade for IV Injection (9%) ... 971
▲ Requip Tablets (8% to 11%) ... 1555
▲ Rescriptor Tablets (5.3% to 16%) ... 2551
▲ Restoril Capsules (4.8%) ... 1860
▲ Revlimid Capsules (4.7% to 38.4%) ... 958
▲ Reyataz Capsules (2% to 3%) ... 921
RhoGAM Ultra-Filtered ... 2371
▲ Ribavirin, USP Capsules (60% to 70%) ... 3068
▲ Risperdal (Frequent to 4%) ... 1676
▲ Risperdal Consta Long-Acting Injection (3% to 7%) ... 1682
▲ Risperdal M-Tab Orally Disintegrating Tablets (Frequent to 4%) ... 1676
Romazicon Injection (1% to 3%) ... 2804
▲ Rozerem Tablets (4%) ... 3231
▲ Rythmol SR Capsules (11% to 13%) ... 2727
Sanctura Tablets (1.9%) ... 1151
▲ Sandostatin Injection (1% to 4%) ... 2278
▲ Simulect for Injection (3% to 10%) ... 2284
Singulair (1.8%) ... 2077
▲ Solodyn Extended Release Tablets (9%) ... 1890
▲ Soltamox Oral Solution (4%) ... 3527
▲ Soriatane Capsules (1% to 10%) ... 1013
▲ Stalevo Tablets (6%) ... 2287
▲ Strattera Capsules (Greater than 5%) ... 1814
Striant Mucoadhesive ... 1007
Stromectol Tablets (0.9%) ... 2083
▲ Sustiva Capsules (2% to 8%) ... 930
▲ Sustiva Tablets (2% to 8%) ... 930
▲ Sutent Capsules (8% to 74%) ... 2560
▲ Symlin Injection (3% to 7%) ... 613
▲ Symmetrel Tablets (0.1% to 5%) ... 1135
▲ Tambocor Tablets (7.7%) ... 1856
▲ Tamiflu Capsules (1% to 8%) ... 2807
▲ Tamiflu Oral Suspension (1% to 7.9%) ... 2807
▲ Tarceva Tablets (2% to 73%) ... 1259
▲ Tarceva Tablets (2% to 73%) ... 2444
Tarka Tablets (2.8%) ... 524
▲ Tasmar Tablets (3% to 8%) ... 3358
Tegretol/Tegretol-XR ... 2295
▲ Temodar Capsules (13% to 61%) ... 3073
Teveten Tablets (2%) ... 1735
Teveten HCT Tablets (1.9%) ... 1737
▲ Thiola Tablets (4%) ... 2141
Thiothixene Capsules ... 2165
Thyrolar Tablets ... 1199
Timolide Tablets (1.9%) ... 2086
Timoptic Sterile Ophthalmic Solution (Less frequent) ... 2088
Timoptic in Ocudose (Less frequent) ... 2091
Timoptic-XE Sterile Ophthalmic Gel Forming Solution ... 2092
Tindamax Tablets (1.1% to 2.1%) ... 2142
▲ Topamax Sprinkle Capsules (9% to 30%) ... 2404
▲ Topamax Tablets (9% to 30%) ... 2404
▲ Toprol-XL Tablets (About 10 of 100 patients) ... 668
▲ Tracleer Tablets (4%) ... 545
Tranxene ... 2474
Trelstar Depot (2.1%) ... 3394
Trelstar LA Suspension (2.3%) ... 3397
▲ Tricor Tablets (5%) ... 527
▲ Trileptal Tablets (7% to 21%) ... 2300
▲ Trileptal Oral Suspension (7% to 21%) ... 2300
▲ Trisenox Injection (63%) ... 993
▲ Trizivir Tablets (44%) ... 1589
Trusopt Sterile Ophthalmic Solution (Infrequent) ... 2095
▲ Truvada Tablets (7%) ... 1296
▲ Twinrix Vaccine (11% to 14%) ... 1595
Uniretic Tablets (1%) ... 3100
Univasc Tablets (2.4%) ... 3104
Uroqid-Acid No. 2 Tablets ... 760
Uroxatral Tablets (2.7%) ... 2943
▲ Valcyte Tablets (Less than 5%) ... 2813
▲ Valium Tablets (Among most common) ... 2819
▲ Valtrex Caplets (8%) ... 1597
▲ Vantas (9.9%) ... 3375
Vantin Tablets and Oral Suspension (Less than 1%) ... 2645
▲ Vaqta (3.9%) ... 2097
Varivax (Greater than or equal to 1%) ... 2100
▲ Vasotec I.V. Injection (1.8% to 3.0%) ... 2103
▲ Velcade for Injection (65%) ... 2133
Verelan PM Extended-Release Capsules, Controlled-Onset (1.7%) ... 3106
Vesanoid Capsules ... 2820
VESIcare Tablets (1% to 2.1%) ... 646
Viadur Implant (Rare) ... 757
▲ Viramune Oral Suspension (7% to 19%) ... 873
▲ Viramune Tablets (7% to 19%) ... 873
▲ Vivitrol (12% to 23%) ... 995
Vytorin 10/10 Tablets ... 2114
Vytorin 10/10 Tablets ... 3077
Vytorin 10/20 Tablets ... 2114
Vytorin 10/20 Tablets ... 3077
Vytorin 10/40 Tablets ... 2114
Vytorin 10/40 Tablets ... 3077
Vytorin 10/80 Tablets ... 2114
Vytorin 10/80 Tablets ... 3077
▲ Wellbutrin Tablets (5.0%) ... 1603
▲ Xeloda Tablets (4% to 42%) ... 2822
▲ Xenical Capsules (3.1% to 7.2%) ... 2831
Xifaxan Tablets (Less than 2%) ... 2842
▲ Xolair (3%) ... 1266
Xyrem Oral Solution (Frequent) ... 1688
Zegerid Capsules (Less than 1%) ... 2958
Zegerid Powder for Oral Solution (Less than 1%) ... 2958
Zelnorm Tablets (1%) ... 2312
Zetia Tablets (1.9% to 2.8%) ... 2120
Zetia Tablets (1.9% to 2.2%) ... 3083
▲ Ziagen (12%) ... 1626
▲ Zinecard for Injection (48% to 61%) ... 2650
Zmax for Oral Suspension ... 2583
▲ Zofran Injection (5%) ... 1634
▲ Zofran (9% to 13%) ... 1639
▲ Zofran ODT Orally Disintegrating Tablets (9% to 13%) ... 1639
▲ Zoloft (10% to 16%) ... 2586
▲ Zometa for Intravenous Infusion (39%) ... 2315
▲ Zonegran Capsules (8%) ... 1101
▲ Zyrtec Chewable Tablets (3.6% to 5.9%) ... 2594
▲ Zyrtec (3.6% to 5.9%) ... 2594
▲ Zyrtec-D 12 Hour Extended Release Tablets (3.6% to 5.9%) ... 2597

Fatigue, muscular
Dyazide Capsules ... 1423
Furosemide Tablets ... 2154
Imitrex Injection (Rare) ... 1463
Prinzide Tablets ... 2056

Fear
Dilaudid ... 440
Dilaudid Non-Sterile Powder ... 440
Dilaudid Rectal Suppositories ... 440
Dilaudid Tablets ... 440
Hycodan ... 1116
Hycotuss Expectorant Syrup ... 1117
Niravam Orally Disintegrating Tablets (1.4%) ... 3092
Romazicon Injection ... 2804
Tussionex Pennkinetic Extended-Release Suspension ... 3327
Vicodin Tablets ... 535
Vicodin ES Tablets ... 536
Vicodin HP Tablets ... 538
Xyrem Oral Solution (Infrequent) ... 1688
Zydone Tablets ... 1139
Zyrtec-D 12 Hour Extended Release Tablets ... 2597

Febrile reactions
Capastat Sulfate for Injection ... 1755
Digibind for Injection ... 1421
Follistim AQ Cartridge ... 2338
Infed Injection ... 3390
▲ Leustatin Injection (11%) ... 2357
Liquid PedvaxHIB ... 2035
Varivax (Less than 0.1%) ... 2100

Fecal fat, increase
(*see under* Steatorrhea)

Fecal impaction
Abilify Oral Solution (Infrequent) ... 882
Abilify Oral Solution (Infrequent) ... 2450
Abilify Discmelt Orally Disintegrating Tablets (Infrequent) ... 882
Abilify Discmelt Orally Disintegrating Tablets (Infrequent) ... 2450
Abilify Tablets (Infrequent) ... 882
Abilify Tablets (Infrequent) ... 2450
Actiq (Less than 1%) ... 979
Clozaril Tablets ... 2184
Doxil Injection (Less than 1%) ... 2351
FazaClo Orally Disintegrating Tablets ... 551
Geodon Capsules (Rare) ... 2529
Kionex Powder ... 2477
Paxil CR Controlled-Release Tablets (Rare) ... 1538
Paxil (Rare) ... 1530
Pexeva Tablets (rare) ... 1694
Rilutek Tablets (Infrequent) ... 2930
VESIcare Tablets ... 646
Zyprexa Tablets (Infrequent) ... 1830
Zyprexa ZYDIS Orally Disintegrating Tablets (Infrequent) ... 1830

Fecal urgency
▲ Xenical Capsules (2.8% to 22.1%) ... 2831
▲ Xifaxan Tablets (5.9%) ... 2842

Fecaloma
Exelon Capsules (Infrequent) ... 2206
Exelon Oral Solution (Infrequent) ... 2206

Feces, color change
Prilosec OTC Delayed-Release Tablets (Less than 1%) ... 2677
Zegerid Capsules (Less than 1%) ... 2958
Zegerid Powder for Oral Solution (Less than 1%) ... 2958

Feces, discoloration
Invirase (Less than 2%) ... 2772
Ortho Evra Transdermal System ... 2417
Prevacid Delayed-Release Capsules (Less than 1%) ... 3271
Prevacid for Delayed-Release Oral Suspension (Less than 1%) ... 3271
Prevacid SoluTab Delayed-Release Orally Disintegrating Tablets (Less than 1%) ... 3271
PREVPAC (Less than 1%) ... 3284
Risperdal (Rare) ... 1676
Risperdal M-Tab Orally Disintegrating Tablets (Rare) ... 1676

Feces abnormal
Colazal Capsules ... 2838
Xifaxan Tablets (Less than 2%) ... 2842

Feeding Problems
NeoProfen Injection ... 2472

Feeling, drugged
▲ Ambien Tablets (3%) ... 2851
Ambien CR Tablets (Frequent) ... 2855
Neurontin Capsules (Infrequent) ... 2487
Neurontin Oral Solution (Infrequent) ... 2487
Neurontin Tablets (Infrequent) ... 2487
Paxil CR Controlled-Release Tablets (2%) ... 1538
Paxil (2%) ... 1530
Pexeva Tablets (2%) ... 1694

Feeling, high
Neurontin Capsules (Rare) ... 2487
Neurontin Oral Solution (Rare) ... 2487
Neurontin Tablets (Rare) ... 2487

Feeling, intoxicated
(*see also under* Inebriated feeling)
Ambien Tablets (Rare) ... 2851
Ambien CR Tablets (Rare) ... 2855
Effexor XR Capsules (Rare) ... 3417
Imitrex Injection (Rare) ... 1463
Trileptal Tablets ... 2300
Trileptal Oral Suspension ... 2300

Feeling, shaky
Koāte-DVI (0.7%) ... 3250

Feeling, strange
Ambien Tablets (Rare) ... 2851
Ambien CR Tablets (Rare) ... 2855
Amerge Tablets (Infrequent) ... 1339
Imitrex Injection (2%) ... 1463
Imitrex Nasal Spray (Infrequent) ... 1467
Imitrex Tablets ... 1471
Lexapro Oral Solution (Infrequent) ... 1190
Lexapro Tablets (Infrequent) ... 1190
MS Contin Tablets (Less frequent) ... 2701
Neurontin Capsules (Rare) ... 2487
Neurontin Oral Solution (Rare) ... 2487
Neurontin Tablets (Rare) ... 2487
Trileptal Tablets (1% to 2%) ... 2300
Trileptal Oral Suspension (1% to 2%) ... 2300

Feeling of sickness of injection
Euflexxa (1.88%) ... 1162

Fertility, impairment of
Intron A for Injection ... 3024
Levothroid Tablets ... 1186

Fertility, male, decrease
Lofibra Tablets (Less than 1%) ... 1219
Lofibra Capsules (Less than 1%) ... 1216
Reyataz Capsules (Less than 3%) ... 921
Tricor Tablets ... 527

Festination
Eldepryl Capsules ... 3208

Fetal death
(*see under* Death, fetal)

Fetal defects
Accutane Capsules ... 2731
Climara Transdermal System ... 771
Lotrel Capsules ... 2249
Nembutal Sodium Solution, USP ... 2470

Fetal harm
Accutane Capsules ... 2731
Advicor Tablets ... 1722
Advil Caplets ... ▣674
Advil Cold & Sinus ... ▣723
Advil ... ▣674
Advil Migraine Liquigels ... ▣608
Advil Tablets ... ▣674
Albenza Tablets ... 1338
Alkeran for Injection ... 955
Alkeran Tablets ... 956
Altoprev Extended-Release Tablets ... 3109
Aredia for Injection ... 2179
Arimidex Tablets ... 673
Aromasin Tablets ... 2600
Arthrotec Tablets ... 3129
Atacand Tablets ... 649
Atacand HCT ... 651
Avalide Tablets ... 888
Avalide Tablets ... 2874
Avapro Tablets ... 891
Avapro Tablets ... 2871
Bayer Aspirin Comprehensive Prescribing Information ... ▣796
BC Headache Powder ... ▣677
BC Allergy Sinus Cold Powder ... ▣677
Arthritis Strength BC Powder ... ▣677
BC Sinus Cold Powder ... ▣677
Benicar Tablets ... 1043
Camptosar Injection ... 2604
Captopril Tablets ... 2149
Carac Cream, 0.5% ... 2879
Carbatrol Capsules ... 3171
Cosmegen for Injection ... 2459
Cozaar Tablets ... 1935
Efudex ... 3363
Eligard 7.5 mg ... 2880
Eligard 22.5 mg ... 2883
Eligard 30 mg ... 2885
Estratest Tablets ... 3199
Estratest H.S. Tablets ... 3199
Eulexin Capsules ... 3009
Evista Tablets ... 1763
Faslodex Injection ... 681
Femara Tablets ... 2214
Garamycin Injectable ... 3014
Gemzar for Injection ... 1771
Goody's Body Pain Formula Powder ... ▣684
Goody's Extra Strength Headache Powders ... ▣611
Goody's Extra Strength Pain Relief Tablets ... ▣685
Hycamtin for Injection ... 1458
Hyzaar 50-12.5 Tablets ... 1990
Hyzaar 100-12.5 Tablets ... 1990
Hyzaar 100-25 Tablets ... 1990
Lescol Capsules ... 2233
Lescol XL Tablets ... 2233
Leukeran Tablets ... 1504
Lotensin Tablets ... 2243
Lotrel Capsules ... 2249
Mavik Tablets ... 486
Mevacor Tablets ... 2021
Micardis Tablets ... 854
Micardis HCT Tablets ... 856

Migranal Nasal Spray 3348
Mustargen for Injection 2468
Myleran Tablets 1525
Mylotarg for Injection 3431
Nembutal Sodium Solution, USP 2470
Niravam Orally Disintegrating Tablets 3092
Premarin Intravenous 3442
Prinivil Tablets 2052
Prinzide Tablets 2056
ProSom Tablets 517
Pulmicort Respules (Remote) 661
Rebetol 3058
ReoPro Vials 1809
Tabloid Tablets 1575
Targretin Capsules 1747
Taxotere Injection Concentrate 2932
Tegretol/Tegretol-XR 2295
Temodar Capsules 3073
Teveten HCT Tablets 1737
Thalomid Capsules 965
TOBI Solution for Inhalation 2298
Tracleer Tablets 545
Tygacil for Injection 3488
Vasotec I.V. Injection 2103
Vesanoid Capsules 2820
Viadur Implant 757
Virazole for Inhalation Solution 3370
Xeloda Tablets 2822
Zocor Tablets 2105

Fetal hemorrhage

Coumadin for Injection 898
Coumadin Tablets 898

Fetal hydantoin syndrome

Phenytek Capsules 2160

Fetal problems, unspecified

Bayer Aspirin 744
BC Headache Powder ▣677
Cipro I.V. 2984
Polytrim Ophthalmic Solution 574
Vasotec I.V. Injection 2103

Fever

▲ Abelcet Injection (14%) 1141
Abilify Oral Solution (Frequent) 882
Abilify Oral Solution (Frequent) 2450
Abilify Discmelt Orally Disintegrating Tablets (Frequent) 882
Abilify Discmelt Orally Disintegrating Tablets (Frequent) 2450
Abilify Tablets (Frequent) 882
Abilify Tablets (Frequent) 2450
Accolate Tablets (1.6%) 671
Aceon Tablets (2 mg, 4 mg, 8 mg) (0.3% to 1.5%) 3194
Aciphex Tablets 1090
▲ Actimmune (52%) 1671
Actiq (1% or greater) 979
Activase I.V. 1223
▲ ADACEL Vaccine (0% to 5%) 2945
Adalat CC Tablets (Rare) 2964
▲ Adderall XR Capsules (5%) 3166
▲ Advair Diskus 100/50 (5%) 1308
▲ Advair Diskus 250/50 (5%) 1308
▲ Advair Diskus 500/50 (5%) 1308
Advair HFA Inhalation Aerosol 1318
▲ Advate Injection (16.7%) 712
Advicor Tablets 1722
▲ Aerobid/Aerobid-M (3% to 9%) 1171
Aggrastat (Less than 1%) 1907
Aggrenox Capsules (Less than 1%) 822
▲ Agrylin Capsules (8.9%) 3169
Alamast Ophthalmic Solution (Less than 5%) 3381
Albenza Tablets (Up to 1.0%) 1338
Albutein 5%, Albumin (Human) 1652
Albutein 25%, Albumin (Human) 1653
Aldara Cream, 5% (More than 1%) 1846
Aldoril Tablets 1910
Aldurazyme for Intravenous Infusion 1268
▲ Alferon N Injection (18% to 81%) 1665
▲ Alimta for Injection (Up to 26%) 1750
Alinia for Oral Suspension (Less than 1%) 2835
Alinia Tablets (Less than 1%) 2835
Alkeran for Injection 955
Alkeran Tablets 956
Allegra (2.4%) 2844
Aloprim for Injection (Less than 1%) 2167
Aloxi Injection (Less than 1%) 2127
Alphanate, Antihemophilic Factor (Human) 1654
Altace Capsules (Less than 1%) 1702
Altoprev Extended-Release Tablets (Rare) 3109
Ambien Tablets (Infrequent) 2851
Ambien CR Tablets (Rare to 1%) 2855
Amerge Tablets (Infrequent) 1339
Amitiza Capsules (0% to 1.1%) 3224
Anaprox Tablets (Less than 1%) 2761
Anaprox DS Tablets (Less than 1%) 2761
▲ Anzemet Injection (4.3%) 2859
▲ Anzemet Tablets (3.5%) 2862
▲ Aptivus Capsules (Less than 2% to 4.6%) 826
Aralast (0.1%) 717
▲ Aranesp for Injection (7% to 19%) 581
▲ Aredia for Injection (38.5%) 2179
▲ Argatroban Injection (3.6% to 6.9%) 1346
Aricept Tablets (Infrequent) 1094
Aricept ODT Tablets (Infrequent) 1094
▲ Arimidex Tablets (2% to 5%) 673
▲ Arixtra Injection (0.3% to 13.6%) 1351
Aromasin Tablets (Less frequent) 2600
▲ Arranon Injection (0% to 23%) 1357
Arthrotec Tablets (Rare) 3129
▲ Asacol Delayed-Release Tablets (6%) 2692
Asmanex Twisthaler (1% to less than 3%) 2966
Astelin Nasal Spray (Infrequently) 1904
Atacand Tablets (0.5% or greater) 649
▲ Atripla Tablets (Greater than or equal to 5%) 945
Attenuvax (Occasional) 1914
Augmentin (Frequent) 1360
Augmentin Tablets (Frequent) 1363
Augmentin XR Extended-Release Tablets (Frequent) 1369
Augmentin ES-600 Powder for Oral Suspension 1366
Avalide Tablets 888
Avalide Tablets 2874
Avapro Tablets (Less than 1%) 891
Avapro Tablets (Less than 1%) 2871
▲ Avinza Capsules (5% to 10%) 1741
Axert Tablets (Rare) 2396
Axid Oral Solution (1.6%) 879
▲ Azilect Tablets (3%) 3293
Bayer Aspirin 744
Bayer Aspirin Comprehensive Prescribing Information ▣796
▲ BeneFix Vials (3.1%) 3408
▲ Betaseron for SC Injection (36%) 767
▲ Bexxar (2% to 37%) 1398
Bicillin C-R Injectable Suspension 1706
Blocadren Tablets 1916
▲ Boostrix (1% to 13.5%) 1404
▲ BOTOX Purified Neurotoxin Complex (2% to 10%) 570
Caduet Tablets (Less than 2%) 2508
Calcium Disodium Versenate Injection 1851
▲ Campath Ampules (19% to 86%) 811
Campral Tablets (Infrequent) 1174
▲ Camptosar Injection (0.4% to 45%) 2604
Canasa Rectal Suppositories (1.2%) 699
▲ Cancidas for Injection (2.9% to 26.2%) 1918
▲ Captopril Tablets (About 4 to 7 of 100) 2149
Carbatrol Capsules 3171
Cardene I.V. (Rare) 2497
Carimune NF 3499
▲ Carnitor Injection (5% to 12%) 3188
Catapres Tablets 843
Catapres-TTS (0.5% or less) 844
Cathflo Activase 1231
Ceftin for Oral Suspension (0.1% to 1%) 1407
Celebrex Capsules (0.1% to 1.9%) 3134
Celexa (2%) 1176
▲ CellCept Capsules (3% to 52.3%) 2747
▲ CellCept Intravenous (3% to 52.3%) 2747
▲ CellCept Oral Suspension (3% to 52.3%) 2747
▲ CellCept Tablets (3% to 52.3%) 2747
▲ Cerezyme for Injection (Approximately 6.5%) 1270
Cervidil Vaginal Insert (Less than 1%) 1181
Cesamet Capsules 3340
Chantix Tablets (Infrequent) 2517
▲ Chemet Capsules (5.2% to 15.7%) 2458
Cipro (Less than 1% to 2.1%) 2977
Cipro I.V. (1% or less to 2.1%) 2984
Cipro XR Tablets 2990
▲ Clarinex Syrup (5.5% to 16.9%) 2995
Cleocin Vaginal Ovules (Less than 1%) 2616
Clinoril Tablets (Less than 1%) 1924
▲ Clolar for Intravenous Infusion (41%) 1271
Clorpres Tablets 2153
▲ Clozaril Tablets (1% to 5% or more) 2184
Colazal Capsules (2%) 2838
▲ Combivir Tablets (10%) 1411
Comtan Tablets 2189
▲ Comvax (0.8% to 14.2%) 1928
▲ Concerta Extended-Release Tablets (3%) 1881
▲ Copaxone for Injection (8%) 3297
▲ Copegus Tablets (41%) 2754
▲ Coreg Tablets (Greater than 1% to 3%) 1414
Cosmegen for Injection 2459
Cosopt Sterile Ophthalmic Solution 1931
Coumadin for Injection (Infrequent) 898
Coumadin Tablets (Infrequent) 898
Cozaar Tablets (Less than 1%) 1935
Crixivan Capsules (1.5%) 1940
▲ Cubicin for Injection (1.9% to 6.7%) 1026
Cuprimine Capsules (Rare) 1947
▲ Cutivate Lotion 0.05% (4%) 2664
▲ Cymbalta Delayed-Release Capsules (1% to 3%) 1757
CytoGam Intravenous (Less than 5.0%) 1895
▲ Dacogen Injection (53%) 2129
Dantrium Capsules (Less frequent) 2694
Dapsone Tablets USP 1673
▲ DAPTACEL Vaccine (9.9% to 11.9%) 2950
Daranide Tablets 1950
Daytrana Transdermal Patch 3174
▲ Depacon Injection (Rare to 6%) 412
▲ Depakene (6%) 417
▲ Depakote Sprinkle Capsules (6%) 422
▲ Depakote Tablets (1% to 6%) 427
▲ Depakote ER Tablets (6%) 434
▲ DepoCyt Injection (4% to 11%) 1143
▲ DepoDur Extended-Release Injection (Greater than 10%) 1110
Depo-Provera Contraceptive Injection (Less than 1%) 2622
depo-subQ provera 104 Injectable Suspension 2624
Diovan HCT Tablets (Greater than 0.2%) 2196
Diuril Oral Suspension 1954
Diuril Sodium Intravenous 2467
Dolobid Tablets (Less than 1 in 100) 1955
Donnatal Extentabs 2493
▲ Doxil Injection (6.9% to 21.3%) 2351
▲ Duragesic Transdermal System (35%) 2373
EC-Naprosyn Delayed-Release Tablets (Less than 1%) 2761
Edecrin 1959
Effexor Tablets 3411
Effexor XR Capsules (Frequent) 3417
▲ Elidel Cream 1% (1.2% to 12.5%) 2200
▲ Elitek (46%) 2890
▲ Eloxatin for Injection (1% to 29%) 2892
Elspar for Injection 2463
Elspar for Injection 1960
Emend Capsules (2.9%) 1963
Enbrel for Injection 584
▲ Engerix-B Vaccine (1% to 10%) 1425
▲ Epivir (10%) 1427
▲ Epivir-HBV (7%) 1432
▲ Epogen for Injection (29% to 51%) 591
▲ Epzicom Tablets (3% to 5%) 1436
Equetro Extended-Release Capsules 3180
Eraxis for Injection (0.7%) 2521
▲ Erbitux (1% to 34%) 910
Ethyol for Injection 1898
▲ Evista Tablets (3.1% to 3.9%) 1763
▲ Evoxac Capsules (1% to 3%) 1047
Exelon Capsules (Frequent) 2206
Exelon Oral Solution (Frequent) 2206
▲ Fabrazyme for Intravenous Infusion (14%) 1274
▲ Famvir Tablets (0.8% to 3.3%) 2211
▲ Faslodex Injection (6.4%) 681
▲ FazaClo Orally Disintegrating Tablets (Greater than 5%) 551
▲ Ferrlecit Injection (3% to 15%) 3388
▲ Flebogamma 5%, Immune Globulin Intravenous (Human) (27%) 1658
Flexbumin I.V. (Occasional) 720
▲ Flonase Nasal Spray (1% to 3%) 1440
▲ Flovent Diskus (7%) 1443
▲ Flovent HFA (1% to 3%) 1447
Floxin Otic Solution (0.3%) 1049
Fluarix (0.4% to 1.7%) 1451
Flumadine 1183
▲ Flumist Vaccine (0% to 10.3%) 1901
▲ Focalin Tablets (5%) 2220
Focalin XR Capsules 2223
Follistim AQ Cartridge 2338
Foradil Aerolizer (2.2%) 3010
Fortaz (2%) 1453
Fortical Nasal Spray (Less than 1%) 3337
Fosamax (Rare) 1969
Fosamax Plus D Tablets (Rarely) 1977
Fragmin Injection (Rare) 1097
Frova Tablets (Infrequent) 1113
Furosemide Tablets 2154
Fuzeon Injection 2767
Gabitril Tablets (1% or more) 984
▲ Gammagard Liquid (2.3% to 21.3%) 721
Gammagard S/D (Occasional) 724
▲ Gamunex Immune Globulin I.V., 10% (0.1% to 28%) 3235
Gantrisin Pediatric Suspension 2770
Garamycin Injectable 3014
▲ Gardasil Injection (10.3% to 13%) 1984
▲ Gemzar for Injection (16% to 41%) 1771
▲ Gengraf Capsules (3%) 459
Geodon Capsules (Frequent) 2529
▲ Gleevec Tablets (0% to 41%) 2227
Guanidine Hydrochloride Tablets 3016
▲ Havrix Vaccine (1% to 10%) 1456
Hemofil M (Extremely rare) 728
Hepsera Tablets (2% or greater) 1292
▲ Herceptin I.V. (36%) 1233
HibTITER (0.6% to 1.4%) 3426
Human Albumin Grifols 20%, Albumin (Human) 1651
Human Albumin Grifols 25%, Albumin (Human) 1652
▲ Humira Injection (Less than 5%) 466
Hyalgan Solution (Seven cases) 2901
▲ Hycamtin for Injection (Less than 1% to 34%) 1458
Hyperstat I.V. 3017
Hytrin Capsules (0.5% to at least 1%) 471
Hyzaar 50-12.5 Tablets 1990
Hyzaar 100-12.5 Tablets 1990
Hyzaar 100-25 Tablets 1990
▲ Imdur Tablets (Less than or equal to 5%) 3018
Imitrex Injection (Rare) 1463
Imitrex Nasal Spray (Infrequent) 1467
Imitrex Tablets (Infrequent) 1471
Indapamide Tablets 2156
Inderal LA Long-Acting Capsules 3429
▲ Infanrix Vaccine (Up to 19.8%) 1476
Infed Injection 3390
▲ Infergen (58% to 61%) 3364
InnoPran XL Capsules 2723
▲ Intron A for Injection (3% to 86%) 3024
▲ Invanz for Injection (2.3% to 5%) 1999
▲ Invirase (Less than 2% to 3.4%) 2772
▲ Ionsys Transdermal System (9%) 2379
▲ I.V. Busulfex (3% to 80%) 2493
Kadian Capsules (Less than 3%) 577
Kaletra (Less than 2%) 476
Keflex Capsules 549
▲ Kepivance (39%) 597
Keppra Injection 3320
Keppra Oral Solution (1% to 2%) 3314
Keppra Tablets (1% to 2%) 3314
Klonopin (Infrequent) 2778
▲ Kytril Injection (3% to 7.9%) 2781
▲ Kytril (5%) 2784
▲ Lamictal (2% to 15%) 1481
▲ Lariam Tablets (Among most frequent) 2786
Lescol Capsules (Rare) 2233
Lescol XL Tablets 2233
Leukeran Tablets 1504
▲ Leukine (77% to 95%) 814
▲ Leustatin Injection (11% to 69%) 2357
Levaquin (0.1% to 0.9%) 2384
Levaquin in 5% Dextrose Injection (0.1% to 0.9%) 2384
Levothroid Tablets 1186
Levoxyl Tablets 1712
Lexapro Oral Solution (Frequent) 1190
Lexapro Tablets (Frequent) 1190
Limbrel Capsules (0.006%) 2672
Lipitor Tablets (Less than 2%) 2483
Lithobid Tablets 1692
Lofibra Tablets 1219
Lofibra Capsules 1216
Lopressor Injection 2238
Lopressor Tablets 2238
Lopressor HCT 50/25 Tablets 2241
Lopressor HCT 100/25 Tablets 2241
Lopressor HCT 100/50 Tablets 2241
Lotensin HCT Tablets (0.3% or more) 2246
▲ Lovenox Injection (8%) 2915
Lunesta Tablets (Infrequent) 3142
Lupron Depot 7.5 mg (Less than 5%) 3264
Lupron Depot-PED 7.5 mg, 11.25 mg and 15 mg (Less than 2%) 3269
Lupron Injection Pediatric (Less than 2%) 3259
Lyrica Capsules (Greater than or equal to 1%) 2539
▲ Malarone Pediatric Tablets (Less than 1% to 6%) 1517

▲ Malarone Tablets (Less than 1% to 6%) 1517
Matulane Capsules 3191
Maxalt Tablets (Rare) 2008
Maxalt-MLT Orally Disintegrating Tablets (Rare) 2008
Maxipime for Injection (Greater than 0.1% to 1%) 1105
Mefoxin for Injection 2012
Mefoxin Premixed Intravenous Solution 2016
▲ Megace ES Oral Suspension (1% to 6%) 2481
▲ Menactra Vaccine (0% to 5.1%) 2954
▲ Mepron Suspension (0.6% to 40%) 1521
Meridia Capsules (Greater than or equal to 1%) 489
Merrem I.V. (Greater than 0.1% to 1%) 686
Meruvax II 2019
Metadate CD Capsules 3323
Mevacor Tablets (Rare) 2021
Miacalcin Nasal Spray (Less than 1%) 2253
Micardis Tablets (More than 0.3%) 854
Micardis HCT Tablets 856
Migranal Nasal Spray (Infrequent) 3348
Mintezol 2027
Miradon Tablets 3042
Mirapex Tablets (1% or more) 859
M-M-R II 2006
Moban Tablets 1119
Mobic Oral Suspension (Less than 2%) 863
Mobic Tablets (Less than 2%) 863
Moduretic Tablets 2028
Mumpsvax (Uncommon) 2031
Mycamine for Injection (0.9% to 1.9%) 628
▲ Myfortic Tablets (3% to less than 20%) 2255
▲ Mylotarg for Injection (78% to 88%) 3431
Myobloc Injection (Greater than 2%) 3192
▲ Myozyme for Intravenous Infusion (92%) 1279
Nadolol Tablets 2159
Nalfon Capsules (Less than 1%) 2502
Naprosyn Suspension (Less than 1%) 2761
Naprosyn Tablets (Less than 1%) 2761
Natrecor for Injection (Greater than or equal to 1%) 3127
Nembutal Sodium Solution, USP 2470
Neoral Oral Solution (1% to less than 3%) 2259
Neoral Soft Gelatin Capsules (1% to less than 3%) 2259
▲ Neulasta Injection (15% to 72%) 601
▲ Neumega for Injection (36%) 3435
▲ Neupogen for Injection (12%) 603
▲ Neurontin Capsules (Greater than 1% to 10%) 2487
▲ Neurontin Oral Solution (10.1%) 2487
▲ Neurontin Tablets (Greater than 1% to 10%) 2487
▲ Nexavar Tablets (Common) 746
Nexium Delayed-Release Capsules (Less than 1%) 655
Nexium I.V. (Less than 1%) 659
▲ Nipent for Injection (42% to 46%) 1863
Noroxin Tablets (0.3% to 1.0%) 2032
▲ Norvir (0.9% to 5%) 503
NovoSeven (Greater than or equal to 2%) 2331
Omacor Capsules 2725
Omnicef Capsules 511
Omnicef for Oral Suspension 511
▲ Oncaspar (Greater than 5%) 1145
▲ Ontak Vials (81%) 1745
▲ Opana Tablets (14.2%) 1122
Ortho-Cyclen Tablets 2429
Ortho Evra Transdermal System 2417
Ortho Tri-Cyclen Tablets 2429
Ortho Tri-Cyclen Lo Tablets 2436
▲ Orthoclone OKT3 Sterile Solution (89% to 90%) 2360
▲ OxyContin Tablets (Between 1% and 5%) 2703
Panhematin for Injection 2473
Paser Granules 1674
Paxil CR Controlled-Release Tablets (2%) 1538
Paxil (2%) 1530
▲ Pediarix Vaccine (31.3% or less) 1548
▲ Liquid PedvaxHIB (0.5% to 18.1%) 2035
▲ Pegasys (37%) 2789
▲ PEG-Intron Powder for Injection (22%) 3048
Pentasa Capsules (0.9%) 3185
Pepcid Injection (Infrequent) 2040
Pepcid (Infrequent) 2038
Percodan Tablets 1132
Permax Tablets (Frequent) 3356
Phenergan Tablets and Suppositories 3440
Phenytek Capsules 2160
▲ Photofrin for Injection (19% to 31%) 702
Plasbumin-5 (Rare) 3251
Plasbumin-20 (Rare) 3252
Plasbumin-25 (Rare) 3253
Plavix Tablets (1% to 2.5%) 917
Plavix Tablets (1% to 2.5%) 2926
Pletal Tablets (Less than 2%) 2455
Podocon-25 Liquid 2478
Pneumovax 23 (Common) 2043
Potaba (Infrequent) 1650
Premphase Tablets 3456
Prempro Tablets 3456
Prevacid Delayed-Release Capsules (Less than 1%) 3271
Prevacid for Delayed-Release Oral Suspension (Less than 1%) 3271
Prevacid SoluTab Delayed-Release Orally Disintegrating Tablets (Less than 1%) 3271
Prevacid NapraPAC (Less than 1%) 3280
▲ Prevnar for Injection (0% to 36.7%) 3463
PREVPAC (Less than 1%) 3284
Prezista Tablets (Less than 2%) 3306
Prilosec OTC Delayed-Release Tablets (Less than 1%) 2677
Primaxin I.M. 2045
Primaxin I.V. (0.5%) 2048
Prinivil Tablets (0.3% to 1.1%) 2052
Prinzide Tablets (0.3% to 1%) 2056
Prochieve 4% Gel 1003
Prochieve 8% Gel 1003
▲ Procrit for Injection (29% to 51%) 2364
Profilnine SD, Factor IX Complex (Human) 1660
▲ Prograf Capsules and Injection (19% to 48%) 632
Prolastin (0.77%) 3255
▲ Proleukin for Injection (29%) 2266
Prometrium Capsules (100 mg, 200 mg) (Less than 5%) 3203
▲ ProQuad (21.5%) 2064
Proquin XR Tablets 1153
ProSom Tablets (Infrequent) 517
ProstaScint Kit 1037
Protonix I.V. (Less than 1%) 3472
Protonix Tablets (Less than 1%) 3469
▲ Protopic Ointment (1% to 18%) 638
▲ Proventil HFA Inhalation Aerosol (6%) 3056
Provigil Tablets (At least 1%) 988
Prozac Pulvules and Liquid (2%) 1801
▲ Pulmozyme Inhalation Solution (32%) 1248
▲ Quadramet Injection (8.5%) 1040
Quixin Ophthalmic Solution (1% to 3%) 3383
Raniclor Tablets, Chewable 2505
▲ Rapamune Oral Solution and Tablets (27% to 34%) 3475
▲ Raptiva for Injection (7%) 1250
Razadyne (Frequent) 2399
▲ Rebetol (32% to 61%) 3058
▲ Rebetron Combination Therapy (35% to 41%) 3063
▲ Rebif Prefilled Syringe for Injection (25% to 28%) 3159
Recombinate (Extremely rare) 729
Recombivax HB (Greater than 1%) 2071
ReFacto Vials 3484
▲ Refludan for Injection (4.4%) 792
Relenza Rotadisk (Less than 1.5%) 1552
Relpax Tablets (Rare) 2548
▲ Remicade for IV Injection (3% to 7%) 971
▲ Renagel Tablets (5.1%) 1282
Requip Tablets (Infrequent) 1555
▲ Rescriptor Tablets (1.6% to 7.1%) 2551
Retavase 2499
▲ Retisert Implant (5% to 15%) ⊙ 258
▲ Retrovir Capsules (3.2% to 16%) 1560
▲ Retrovir IV Infusion (4% to 16%) 1564
▲ Retrovir (3.2% to 16%) 1560
▲ Revatio Tablets (6%) 2557
▲ Revlimid Capsules (3.4% to 23.1%) 958
▲ Reyataz Capsules (4% to 6%) 921
RhoGAM Ultra-Filtered 2371
Rhophylac (Occasionally) 3505
▲ Ribavirin, USP Capsules (32% to 61%) 3068
▲ Risperdal (2% to 3%) 1676
Risperdal Consta Long-Acting Injection (1% to 2%) 1682
▲ Risperdal M-Tab Orally Disintegrating Tablets (2% to 3%) 1676
Ritalin Hydrochloride Tablets 2269
Ritalin LA Capsules 2271
Ritalin-SR Tablets 2269
▲ Rituxan I.V. (1% to 56%) 1254
Rocephin Injectable Vials, ADD-Vantage, Galaxy, Bulk (Less than 1%) 2800
RotaTeq (0.1%) 2074
Rythmol SR Capsules 2727
Sandimmune (2% or less) 2275
▲ Serevent Diskus (1% to 3%) 1568
Seroquel Tablets (2%) 690
Singulair (1.5% to greater than or equal to 2%) 2077
Sonata Capsules (Frequent) 1717
Soriatane Capsules (Less than 1%) 1013
St. Joseph 81 mg Aspirin Chewable and Enteric Coated Tablets 1869
St. Joseph 81 mg Aspirin ▣ 688
▲ Strattera Capsules (3%) 1814
▲ Stromectol Tablets (22.6%) 2083
▲ Suboxone Tablets (3%) 2717
▲ Subutex Tablets (3%) 2717
Sular Tablets (Less than or equal to 1%) 3122
▲ Sustiva Capsules (21%) 930
▲ Sustiva Tablets (21%) 930
▲ Sutent Capsules (1% to 18%) 2560
▲ Symbyax Capsules (3% to 4%) 1819
Symmetrel Tablets 1135
▲ Synagis (27.1%) 1897
Tambocor Tablets (1% to 3%) 1856
Tamiflu Capsules (Less than 1%) 2807
Tamiflu Oral Suspension (Less than 1%) 2807
▲ Tarceva Tablets (0% to 36%) 1259
▲ Tarceva Tablets (0% to 36%) 2444
▲ Targretin Capsules (4.8% to 17%) 1747
Tarka Tablets (Several cases) 524
Tasmar Tablets (1%) 3358
▲ Taxotere Injection Concentrate (1.8% to 46.5%) 2932
Tegretol/Tegretol-XR 2295
▲ Temodar Capsules (13%) 3073
▲ Tequin Injection (0.1% to 3%) 938
▲ Tequin Injection in 5% Dextrose (0.1% to 3%) 938
▲ Tequin Tablets (0.1% to 3%) 938
Teveten Tablets (Less than 1%) 1735
Teveten HCT Tablets (Less than 1%) 1737
▲ Thalomid Capsules (19.4% to 21.9%) 965
▲ Thiola Tablets (4%) 2141
Thioridazine Hydrochloride Tablets 2163
Thiothixene Capsules 2165
▲ Thrombate III (1 of 17) 3257
▲ Thymoglobulin for Intravenous Infusion (63.4%) 1284
Thyrogen for Injection (1%) 1286
Ticlid Tablets 2810
Timolide Tablets 2086
Timoptic Sterile Ophthalmic Solution 2088
Timoptic in Ocudose 2091
Timoptic-XE Sterile Ophthalmic Gel Forming Solution 2092
Tindamax Tablets 2142
TNKase I.V. 1264
▲ TOBI Solution for Inhalation (32.9%) 2298
▲ Topamax Sprinkle Capsules (0% to 9%) 2404
▲ Topamax Tablets (0% to 9%) 2404
Toprol-XL Tablets 668
Tracleer Tablets 545
▲ Trasylol Injection (15%) 754
Tricor Tablets 527
Triglide Tablets 3123
▲ Trileptal Tablets (Up to 3%) 2300
▲ Trileptal Oral Suspension (Up to 3%) 2300
▲ Trisenox Injection (63%) 993
▲ Trizivir Tablets (20%) 1589
Truvada Tablets 1296
Twinrix Vaccine (2% to 4%) 1595
▲ Tygacil for Injection (7.1%) 3488
Ultane Liquid for Inhalation (1%) 531
▲ Ultram ER Tablets (1% to greater than 5%) 2392
Uniretic Tablets (More than 1%) 3100
Urso 250 Tablets 710
Urso Forte Tablets 710
▲ Valcyte Tablets (13% to 31%) 2813
Vantin Tablets and Oral Suspension (Less than 1%) 2645
▲ Vaprisol (3.8%) 643
▲ Vaqta (2.7% to 11.3%) 2097
▲ Varivax (10.2% to 14.7%) 2100
Vasotec I.V. Injection (0.5% to 1.0%) 2103
▲ Velcade for Injection (35%) 2133
Verelan PM Extended-Release Capsules, Controlled-Onset 3106
▲ Vesanoid Capsules (83%) 2820
▲ VFEND I.V. (0% to 5.7%) 2564
▲ VFEND Oral Suspension (0% to 5.7%) 2564
▲ VFEND Tablets (0% to 5.7%) 2564
Vicoprofen Tablets (Rare; less than 3%) 539
▲ Vigamox Ophthalmic Solution (1% to 4%) 564
Viracept (Less than 2%) 2577
▲ Viramune Oral Suspension (3%) 873
▲ Viramune Tablets (3%) 873
▲ Viread Tablets (2% to 8%) 1301
▲ Visudyne for Injection (1% to 10%) 2305
▲ Vivaglobin (0.1% to 25%) 3506
Vivitrol 995
Vivotif 819
▲ Voltaren Ophthalmic Solution (Less than or equal to 3%) 2309
Voltaren Tablets (Occasionally) 2307
Voltaren-XR Tablets (Occasionally) 2310
Vytorin 10/10 Tablets 2114
Vytorin 10/10 Tablets 3077
Vytorin 10/20 Tablets 2114
Vytorin 10/20 Tablets 3077
Vytorin 10/40 Tablets 2114
Vytorin 10/40 Tablets 3077
Vytorin 10/80 Tablets 2114
Vytorin 10/80 Tablets 3077
Wellbutrin Tablets (1.2%) 1603
Wellbutrin SR Sustained-Release Tablets (1% to 2%) 1607
Wellbutrin XL Extended-Release Tablets (1% to 2%) 1613
WinRho SDF (1%) 732
▲ Xeloda Tablets (1% to 12%) 2822
▲ Xifaxan Tablets (3.1%) 2842
▲ Xopenex Inhalation Solution (3%) 3146
▲ Xopenex Inhalation Solution Concentrate (3% to 9.1%) 3150
▲ Xopenex HFA Inhalation Aerosol (3%) 3154
Xyrem Oral Solution (Frequent) 1688
Yaz Tablets (Greater than 1%) 803
Zantac (Rare) 1624
Zantac Injection 1619
Zantac Injection Pharmacy Bulk Package (Rare) 1622
Zantac Injection Premixed 1619
Zantac (Rare) 1624
Zegerid Capsules (Less than 1%) 2958
Zegerid Powder for Oral Solution (Less than 1%) 2958
Zelapar Tablets 3372
Zemaira (0.6%) 3509
▲ Zemplar Capsules (5%) 541
▲ Zemplar Injection (5%) 543
▲ Ziagen (6% to 9%) 1626
▲ Zinecard for Injection (22% to 34%) 2650
Zocor Tablets (Rare) 2105
▲ Zofran Injection (2% to 8%) 1634
▲ Zofran (8%) 1639
▲ Zofran ODT Orally Disintegrating Tablets (8%) 1639
Zoloft (Infrequent to 2%) 2586
▲ Zometa for Intravenous Infusion (32% to 44.2%) 2315
Zomig Tablets (Infrequent) 3519
Zomig Nasal Spray (Rare) 3523
Zomig-ZMT Tablets (Infrequent) 3519
Zostavax Injection (1.8%) 2111
▲ Zosyn (2.4% to 3.2%) 3492
Zovirax 1643
Zyban Sustained-Release Tablets (Frequent) 1644
Zyflo Tablets (Greater than 1%) 1023
▲ Zyprexa Tablets (6%) 1830
Zyprexa IntraMuscular (Infrequent) 1830
▲ Zyprexa ZYDIS Orally Disintegrating Tablets (6%) 1830
Zyrtec Chewable Tablets (Less than 2%) 2594
Zyrtec (Less than 2%) 2594
Zyrtec-D 12 Hour Extended Release Tablets (Less than 2%) 2597
▲ Zyvox (0% to 14.1%) 2652

Fever, intermittent

▲ Dacogen Injection (6%) 2129

Fever, neutropenic

Campath Ampules 811
▲ Camptosar Injection (2% to 5.8%) 2604
▲ Mylotarg for Injection (15% to 19%) 3431
▲ Neulasta Injection (15% to 72%) 601
▲ Neumega for Injection (48%) 3435
▲ Neupogen for Injection (13%) 603
▲ Xeloda Tablets (3% to 16%) 2822

Fibrillations

Tambocor Tablets 1856

Fibrillations, ventricular

Abelcet Injection 1141
Adenocard Injection (Rare) 617

Aloprim for Injection (Less than 1%) 2167
Azilect Tablets (Rare) 3293
Biltricide Tablets 2976
Celebrex Capsules (Less than 0.1%) 3134
Clozaril Tablets 2184
Covera-HS Tablets 3139
DynaCirc CR Tablets (0.5% to 1%) 2721
Effexor Tablets (Rare) 3411
Effexor XR Capsules (Rare) 3417
FazaClo Orally Disintegrating Tablets 551
Frova Tablets 1113
Hyzaar 50-12.5 Tablets 1990
Hyzaar 100-12.5 Tablets 1990
Hyzaar 100-25 Tablets 1990
Imitrex Injection (Rare) 1463
Imitrex Tablets (Rare) 1471
Lanoxicaps Capsules 1490
Lanoxin Injection 1494
Lanoxin Injection Pediatric 1497
Lanoxin Tablets 1500
Levaquin (0.1% to 0.9%) 2384
Levaquin in 5% Dextrose Injection (0.1% to 0.9%) 2384
Lyrica Capsules (Rare) 2539
Meridia Capsules 489
Paxil CR Controlled-Release Tablets 1538
Paxil 1530
Prograf Capsules and Injection 632
Prozac Pulvules and Liquid (Rare) 1801
Refludan for Injection 792
Relpax Tablets (Rare) 2548
Retavase 2499
Rilutek Tablets (Rare) 2930
Rituxan I.V. 1254
Trasylol Injection (2%) 754
Uniretic Tablets (Less than 1%) 3100
VFEND I.V. (Less than 2%) 2564
VFEND Oral Suspension (Less than 2%) 2564
VFEND Tablets (Less than 2%) 2564
Zomig Tablets 3519
Zomig Nasal Spray 3523
Zomig-ZMT Tablets 3519
Zosyn (1.0% or less) 3492

Fibrinolysis increased
NovoSeven (1%) 2331

Fibromyalgia
Cozaar Tablets (Less than 1%) 1935
Hyzaar 50-12.5 Tablets 1990
Hyzaar 100-12.5 Tablets 1990
Hyzaar 100-25 Tablets 1990
Lupron Depot 7.5 mg 3264
Lupron Depot–3 Month 11.25 mg 3265
Nexium Delayed-Release Capsules (Less than 1%) 655
Nexium I.V. (Less than 1%) 659
Pexeva Tablets (2%) 1694

Fibrosing colonopathy
Creon 5 Capsules 3198
Creon 10 Capsules 3198
Creon 20 Capsules 3199
Ultrase Capsules 708
Ultrase MT Capsules 709

Fibrosis
Copaxone for Injection (Infrequent) 3297
Genotropin Lyophilized Powder (Infrequent) 2638
Ocufen Ophthalmic Solution ⊙232
Permax Tablets 3356
▲ Xeloda Tablets (Less than 5%) 2822

Fibrosis, cavernous body
Edex Injection (2%) 3089

Fibrosis, hepatic
▲ Xeloda Tablets (Less than 5%) 2822

Fibrosis, interstitial pulmonary
(*see under* Pulmonary fibrosis)

Fibrosis, penile
▲ Caverject Impulse Injection (3%) 2612
▲ Edex Injection (5%) 3089

Fibrosis, perisinusoidal
Eloxatin for Injection 2892

Fibrosis, pleural
▲ Intron A for Injection (Less than or equal to 5%) 3024
Migranal Nasal Spray 3348
Permax Tablets (Rare) 3356

Fibrosis, retroperitoneal
Lopressor Injection 2238
Lopressor Tablets 2238
Lopressor HCT 50/25 Tablets (Very rare) 2241
Lopressor HCT 100/25 Tablets (Very rare) 2241
Lopressor HCT 100/50 Tablets (Very rare) 2241
Lyrica Capsules (Rare) 2539
Migranal Nasal Spray 3348
Permax Tablets (Rare) 3356
Tasmar Tablets 3358

Fibrosis, subretinal
▲ Lucentis Injection (0% to 13%) 1237

Fingernails, brittle
Gengraf Capsules (2% or less) 459
Neoral Oral Solution (2% or less) 2259
Neoral Soft Gelatin Capsules (2% or less) 2259
Sandimmune (2% or less) 2275

Fissuring, fingertips
Ophthetic Ophthalmic Solution ⊙232

Fissuring, unspecified
Clobevate Gel (Less than 2%) 3211
Olux Foam (Less than 2%) 1012
Oxistat Cream (0.1%) 2667
▲ Soriatane Capsules (1% to 10%) 1013
Temovate Cream (1 of 421 patients) 2668
▲ Temovate Gel (Among most frequent) 2669
Temovate E Emollient (Less than 2%) 2671

Fistula, arteriovenous
ReoPro Vials (0.4%) 1809

Fistula, tracheo-esophageal
▲ Photofrin for Injection (6%) 702
Proleukin for Injection (Less than 1%) 2266

Flare
Humira Injection (0.7%) 466
▲ Levulan Kerastick for Topical Solution, 20% (1% to 7%) 1085
Travatan Ophthalmic Solution (1% to 4%) 563

Flare, postinjection
Attenuvax (Rare) 1914
Depo-Medrol Single-Dose Vial 2619
Dilaudid-HP (Less frequent) 442
Meruvax II 2019
M-M-R II 2006
Mumpsvax (Rare) 2031

Flare at injection site
ProQuad 2064
▲ Quadramet Injection (7%) 1040

Flatulence
Abilify Oral Solution (Infrequent) 882
Abilify Oral Solution (Infrequent) 2450
Abilify Discmelt Orally Disintegrating Tablets (Infrequent) 882
Abilify Discmelt Orally Disintegrating Tablets (Infrequent) 2450
Abilify Tablets (Infrequent) 882
Abilify Tablets (Infrequent) 2450
Aceon Tablets (2 mg, 4 mg, 8 mg) (1.0%) 3194
Aciphex Tablets 1090
Actiq (1% or greater) 979
▲ Actonel Tablets (3.1% to 4.6%) 2683
▲ Actonel with Calcium Tablets (3.1% to 4.6%) 2688
Adalat CC Tablets (Less than 1%) 2964
▲ Advair HFA Inhalation Aerosol (1% to 3%) 1318
Advicor Tablets 1722
Aerobid/Aerobid-M (1% to 3%) 1171
▲ Agrylin Capsules (10.2%) 3169
Aldoril Tablets 1910
Alinia for Oral Suspension (Less than 1%) 2835
Alinia Tablets (Less than 1%) 2835
Aloprim for Injection (Less than 1%) 2167
Aloxi Injection (Less than 1%) 2127
▲ Altoprev Extended-Release Tablets (3.7% to 4.5%) 3109
Ambien Tablets (Infrequent) 2851
Ambien CR Tablets (Infrequent to 1%) 2855
AmBisome for Injection (Less common) 620
▲ Amitiza Capsules (3.4% to 6.1%) 3224
▲ Anaprox Tablets (1% to 10%) 2761
▲ Anaprox DS Tablets (1% to 10%) 2761
Aptivus Capsules (Less than 2%) 826
Aricept Tablets (Infrequent) 1094
Aricept ODT Tablets (Infrequent) 1094
▲ Arthrotec Tablets (9%) 3129
▲ Asacol Delayed-Release Tablets (3% to 5%) 2692
Asmanex Twisthaler (1% to less than 3%) 2966
Augmentin (Less frequent) 1360
Augmentin Tablets (Less frequent) 1363
Avalide Tablets 888
Avalide Tablets 2874
Avapro Tablets (Less than 1%) 891
Avapro Tablets (Less than 1%) 2871
▲ Avastin IV (11% to 19%) 1227
Avelox (0.1% to less than 2%) 2970
▲ Axid Oral Solution (4.9%) 879
Buprenex Injectable (Infrequent) 2716
Byetta Injection 611
Caduet Tablets (Greater than 0.1% to 2.8%) 2508
▲ Campral Tablets (1% to 4%) 1174
▲ Camptosar Injection (0% to 12%) 2604
▲ Canasa Rectal Suppositories (5.2%) 699
Carafate Suspension (Less than 0.5%) 701
Carafate Tablets (Less than 0.5%) 701
Ceftin (0.1% to 1%) 1407
Celebrex Capsules (2.2%) 3134
Celexa (Frequent) 1176
▲ CellCept Capsules (3% to less than 20%) 2747
▲ CellCept Intravenous (3% to less than 20%) 2747
▲ CellCept Oral Suspension (3% to less than 20%) 2747
▲ CellCept Tablets (3% to less than 20%) 2747
▲ Chantix Tablets (Greater than 5% to 9%) 2517
Cipro 2977
Cipro I.V. (1% or less) 2984
Cipro XR Tablets (Less than 1%) 2990
▲ Climara Transdermal System (1% to 7%) 771
▲ Climara Pro Transdermal System (3.8%) 776
▲ Clinoril Tablets (1% to 3%) 1924
Colazal Capsules (2%) 2838
Comtan Tablets (2%) 2189
Copaxone for Injection (At least 2%) 3297
Coumadin for Injection (Infrequent) 898
Coumadin Tablets (Infrequent) 898
Cozaar Tablets (Less than 1%) 1935
Crestor Tablets (Greater than or equal to 1%) 678
Cubicin for Injection (Less than 1%) 1026
▲ Depacon Injection (1% to 5%) 412
▲ Depakene (1% to 5%) 417
▲ Depakote Sprinkle Capsules (1% to 5%) 422
▲ Depakote Tablets (1% to 5%) 427
▲ Depakote ER Tablets (Greater than 1% to 5%) 434
▲ DepoDur Extended-Release Injection (5% to 10%) 1110
Detrol Tablets (1.3%) 2628
Diovan Tablets 2193
Diovan HCT Tablets (Greater than 0.2%) 2196
▲ Ditropan XL Extended-Release Tablets (2% to less than 5%) 2413
Dolobid Tablets (Greater than 1 in 100) 1955
▲ Doxil Injection (1% to 10%) 2351
Duragesic Transdermal System (1% or greater) 2373
▲ EC-Naprosyn Delayed-Release Tablets (1% to 10%) 2761
▲ Effexor Tablets (3%) 3411
▲ Effexor XR Capsules (4% to 5%) 3417
Eligard 7.5 mg (Less than 2%) 2880
Elmiron Capsules (Less than or equal to 1%) 2415
▲ Eloxatin for Injection (3% to 5%) 2892
Emcyt Capsules (2%) 2634
Emend Capsules (Greater than 0.5%) 1963
▲ Enjuvia Tablets (4% to 7%) 1062
▲ Entocort EC Capsules (6%) 2698
▲ Estring Vaginal Ring (1% to 3%) 2635
▲ Evista Tablets (3.1%) 1763
▲ Evoxac Capsules (1% to 3%) 1047
▲ Exelon Capsules (4%) 2206
▲ Exelon Oral Solution (4%) 2206
Famvir Tablets (1.5% to 1.9%) 2211
Ferrlecit Injection 3388
▲ Follistim AQ Cartridge (27%) 2338
▲ Fortamet Extended-Release Tablets (3.5%) 3115
Fortical Nasal Spray (Less than 1%) 3337
▲ Fosamax (Up to 4.1%) 1969
▲ Fosamax Plus D Tablets (0% to 4.1%) 1977
Frova Tablets (Infrequent) 1113
Gabitril Tablets (1% or more) 984
Gantrisin Pediatric Suspension 2770
▲ Gengraf Capsules (4%) 459
▲ Gleevec Tablets (0% to 34%) 2227
▲ Hepsera Tablets (2% to 4%) 1292
Hytrin Capsules (At least 1%) 471
Hyzaar 50-12.5 Tablets 1990
Hyzaar 100-12.5 Tablets 1990
Hyzaar 100-25 Tablets 1990
▲ Imdur Tablets (Less than or equal to 5%) 3018
Imitrex Injection (Rare) 1463
Imitrex Nasal Spray (Rare) 1467
Imitrex Tablets 1471
Indocin Capsules (Less than 1%) 1995
Indocin I.V. (Less than 1%) 2465
Indocin (Less than 1%) 1995
▲ Infergen (6% to 8%) 3364
▲ Intron A for Injection (Less than 5%) 3024
Invanz for Injection (Greater than 0.1%) 1999
Invirase (Less than 2%) 2772
▲ Ionsys Transdermal System (1% to less than 10%) 2379
▲ Kaletra (1% to 4%) 476
K-Dur Extended-Relase Tablets 3033
Ketek Tablets (Greater than or equal to 0.2% to less than 2%) 2903
Klonopin (Infrequent) 2778
▲ K-Lor Oral Solution (Among most common) 474
Kristalose for Oral Solution 1034
▲ K-Tab Tablets (Most common) 475
▲ Kytril Injection (3%) 2781
Lamictal (More than 1%) 1481
Lamisil Tablets (2.2%) 2232
Lescol Capsules (2.6%) 2233
Lescol XL Tablets (1.4%) 2233
Levaquin (0.2% to 1.2%) 2384
Levaquin in 5% Dextrose Injection (0.2% to 1.2%) 2384
Lexapro Oral Solution (2%) 1190
Lexapro Tablets (2%) 1190
Limbrel Capsules (0.006%) 2672
Lipitor Tablets (1.1% to 2.8%) 2483
Lithobid Tablets 1692
Lofibra Tablets 1219
Lofibra Capsules 1216
Lopressor Injection (1%) 2238
Lopressor Tablets (1%) 2238
Lopressor HCT 50/25 Tablets (Less than or equal to 1%) 2241
Lopressor HCT 100/25 Tablets (Less than or equal to 1%) 2241
Lopressor HCT 100/50 Tablets (Less than or equal to 1%) 2241
Lotensin HCT Tablets (0.3% or more) 2246
▲ Lotronex Tablets (3%) 1512
▲ Lyrica Capsules (1% to 3%) 2539
Maxalt Tablets (Infrequent) 2008
Maxalt-MLT Orally Disintegrating Tablets (Infrequent) 2008
▲ Megace ES Oral Suspension (0% to 10%) 2481
Meridia Capsules (Greater than or equal to 1%) 489
Merrem I.V. (Greater than 0.1% to 1%) 686
MetroGel-Vaginal Gel (Less than 1%) 1855
▲ Mevacor Tablets (3.7% to 6.4%) 2021
Miacalcin Nasal Spray (Less than 1%) 2253
Micardis Tablets (More than 0.3%) 854
Micardis HCT Tablets 856
Midamor Tablets (Less than or equal to 1%) 2026
Mirapex Tablets (Greater than or equal to 1%) 859
▲ Mobic Oral Suspension (0.4% to 3.2%) 863
▲ Mobic Tablets (0.4% to 3.2%) 863
Moduretic Tablets (Less than or equal to 1%) 2028
▲ Myfortic Tablets (3% to less than 20%) 2255
Nadolol Tablets (1 to 5 of 1000 patients) 2159
Nalfon Capsules (Less than 1%) 2502
▲ Naprosyn Suspension (1% to 10%) 2761
▲ Naprosyn Tablets (1% to 10%) 2761
▲ Neoral Oral Solution (4%) 2259
▲ Neoral Soft Gelatin Capsules (4%) 2259
Neurontin Capsules (2.1%) 2487
Neurontin Oral Solution (2.1%) 2487

Neurontin Tablets (2.1%) 2487
Nexium Delayed-Release Capsules (Greater than or equal to 1%) 655
Nexium I.V. (Greater than or equal to 1%) 659
Niaspan Extended-Release Tablets 1730
▲ Nipent for Injection (3% to 10%) 1863
Noroxin Tablets (0.3% to 1.0%) 2032
Norvasc Tablets (More than 0.1% to 1%) 2545
Norvir (0.9% to 1.7%) 503
Omnicef Capsules (0.7%) 511
Omnicef for Oral Suspension (0.6%) 511
Oncaspar (Less than 1%) 1145
▲ Opana Tablets (1% to less than 10%) 1122
▲ Opana ER Tablets (1% to less than 10%) 1126
OxyContin Tablets (Less than 1%) 2703
▲ Oxytrol Transdermal System (Greater than 1%) 3392
Parcopa Orally Disintegrating Tablets 3097
▲ Paxil CR Controlled-Release Tablets (4.0%) 1538
▲ Paxil (4.0%) 1530
Permax Tablets (Infrequent) 3356
▲ Pexeva Tablets (4%) 1694
▲ Pletal Tablets (2% to 3%) 2455
▲ Precose Tablets (74%) 751
▲ Premarin Tablets (6% to 7%) 3446
▲ Premphase Tablets (5% to 9%) 3456
▲ Prempro Tablets (5% to 9%) 3456
Prevacid Delayed-Release Capsules (Less than 1%) 3271
Prevacid for Delayed-Release Oral Suspension (Less than 1%) 3271
Prevacid SoluTab Delayed-Release Orally Disintegrating Tablets (Less than 1%) 3271
Prevacid NapraPAC (Less than 1%) 3280
PREVPAC (Less than 1%) 3284
Prezista Tablets (Less than 2%) 3306
Prilosec OTC Delayed-Release Tablets (Less than 1 to 2.7%) 2677
Prinivil Tablets (0.3% to 1.0%) 2052
Prinzide Tablets 2056
ProAmatine Tablets (Rare) 3186
Prochieve 4% Gel 1003
Prochieve 8% Gel 1003
▲ Prograf Capsules and Injection (3% to 15%) 632
ProQuad 2064
ProSom Tablets (Infrequent) 517
Protonix I.V. (Greater than or equal to 1%) 3472
▲ Protonix Tablets (2% to 4%) 3469
Proventil HFA Inhalation Aerosol (Less than 3%) 3056
Provigil Tablets (1%) 988
▲ Prozac Pulvules and Liquid (3%) 1801
▲ Rapamune Oral Solution and Tablets (3% to 20%) 3475
Razadyne (Frequent) 2399
Razadyne ER Extended-Release Capsules (Frequent) 2399
Relpax Tablets (Infrequent) 2548
▲ Renagel Tablets (4%) 1282
▲ Requip Tablets (2% to 3%) 1555
Rescriptor Tablets 2551
Retrovir Capsules 1560
Retrovir IV Infusion 1564
Retrovir 1560
Reyataz Capsules (Less than 3%) 921
Rilutek Tablets (2.0% to 2.5%) 2930
Risperdal (Infrequent) 1676
Risperdal Consta Long-Acting Injection (Infrequent) 1682
Risperdal M-Tab Orally Disintegrating Tablets (Infrequent) 1676
Rocephin Injectable Vials, ADD-Vantage, Galaxy, Bulk (Rare) 2800
Rythmol SR Capsules (1% to 2%) 2727
Sanctura Tablets (1.2%) 1151
▲ Sandostatin Injection (Less than 10%) 2278
▲ Sandostatin LAR Depot (25.7%) 2280
Seroquel Tablets (Infrequent) 690
▲ Simulect for Injection (3% to 10%) 2284
Sonata Capsules (Infrequent) 1717
Stalevo Tablets (2%) 2287
Strattera Capsules (2%) 1814
Sular Tablets (Less than or equal to 1%) 3122
▲ Suprax (4%) 1843
Sustiva Capsules (1% to 2%) 930
Sustiva Tablets (1% to 2%) 930
▲ Sutent Capsules (0% to 14%) 2560
Tambocor Tablets (Less than 1%) 1856
▲ Tarceva Tablets (0% to 13%) 1259
▲ Tarceva Tablets (0% to 13%) 2444
Targretin Capsules 1747
▲ Tasmar Tablets (2% to 4%) 3358
Tequin Injection (Less than 0.1%) 938
Tequin Injection in 5% Dextrose (Less than 0.1%) 938
Tequin Tablets (Less than 0.1%) 938
Teveten Tablets (Less than 1%) 1735
Teveten HCT Tablets (Less than 1%) 1737
▲ Thalomid Capsules (8.3%) 965
▲ Thiola Tablets (16.7%) 2141
Ticlid Tablets (1.5%) 2810
Timentin ADD-Vantage 1580
Timentin Injection Galaxy Container 1583
Timentin IV Infusion 1577
Timentin Pharmacy Bulk Package 1586
Topamax Sprinkle Capsules (1% to frequent) 2404
Topamax Tablets (1% to frequent) 2404
Toprol-XL Tablets (About 1 of 100 patients) 668
▲ Tricor Tablets (3%) 527
Triglide Tablets 3123
Trileptal Tablets 2300
Trileptal Oral Suspension 2300
Truvada Tablets 1296
▲ Ultram ER Tablets (1% to greater than 5%) 2392
Ultrase MT Capsules (1.5%) 709
Uniretic Tablets (Less than 1%) 3100
Vandazole Vaginal Gel (Less than 1%) 3338
Vantin Tablets and Oral Suspension (Less than 1%) 2645
VFEND I.V. (Less than 2%) 2564
VFEND Oral Suspension (Less than 2%) 2564
VFEND Tablets (Less than 2%) 2564
▲ Vicoprofen Tablets (3% to 9%) 539
▲ Viracept (1% to 5%) 2577
▲ Viread Tablets (3% to 4%) 1301
Vivitrol 995
▲ Voltaren Tablets (1% to 10%) 2307
▲ Voltaren-XR Tablets (1% to 10%) 2310
Vytorin 10/10 Tablets 2114
Vytorin 10/10 Tablets 3077
Vytorin 10/20 Tablets 2114
Vytorin 10/20 Tablets 3077
Vytorin 10/40 Tablets 2114
Vytorin 10/40 Tablets 3077
Vytorin 10/80 Tablets 2114
Vytorin 10/80 Tablets 3077
▲ WelChol Tablets (12%) 1050
Wellbutrin SR Sustained-Release Tablets (At least 1%) 1607
▲ Wellbutrin XL Extended-Release Tablets (At least 1% to 6%) 1613
▲ Xifaxan Tablets (11.3%) 2842
Xyrem Oral Solution (Infrequent) 1688
▲ Zegerid Capsules (4.5% to 20.2%) 2958
▲ Zegerid Powder for Oral Solution (4.5% to 20.2%) 2958
Zelapar Tablets (2%) 3372
▲ Zelnorm Tablets (6%) 2312
Zmax for Oral Suspension (Less then 1%) 2583
Zocor Tablets (1.9%) 2105
▲ Zoloft (3%) 2586
Zonegran Capsules (Infrequent) 1101
Zosyn (1.0% or less to 1.3%) 3492
Zyban Sustained-Release Tablets (Frequent) 1644
Zyflo Tablets (Greater than 1%) 1023
Zyprexa Tablets (Frequent) 1830
Zyprexa ZYDIS Orally Disintegrating Tablets (Frequent) 1830
Zyrtec Chewable Tablets (Less than 2%) 2594
Zyrtec (Less than 2%) 2594
Zyrtec-D 12 Hour Extended Release Tablets (Less than 2%) 2597

Flatus with discharge
▲ Xenical Capsules (2.1% to 23.9%) 2831

Floating feeling
Dilaudid Oral Liquid (Less frequent) 445
Dilaudid Tablets - 8 mg (Less frequent) 445
Dilaudid-HP (Less frequent) 442
Mintezol 2027
MS Contin Tablets (Less frequent) 2701

Flu Syndrome
Abilify Oral Solution (Frequent) 882
Abilify Oral Solution (Frequent) 2450
Abilify Discmelt Orally Disintegrating Tablets (Frequent) 882
Abilify Discmelt Orally Disintegrating Tablets (Frequent) 2450
Abilify Tablets (Frequent) 882
Abilify Tablets (Frequent) 2450
▲ Actonel with Calcium Tablets (7.1% to 8.7%) 2688
Alinia for Oral Suspension (Less than 1%) 2835
Alinia Tablets (Less than 1%) 2835
▲ Arimidex Tablets (2% to 7%) 673
▲ Caduet Tablets (2.2% to 3.2%) 2508
Campral Tablets (Frequent) 1174
▲ Climara Pro Transdermal System (4.7%) 776
Crestor Tablets (2.3%) 678
▲ Depakote ER Tablets (Greater than 1% to 5%) 434
▲ Enablex Extended-Release Tablets (1% to 3%) 2203
▲ Enjuvia Tablets (4% to 7%) 1062
▲ Humira Injection (7%) 466
Keppra Injection 3320
▲ Levitra Tablets (3%) 3034
▲ Lopressor HCT 50/25 Tablets (10%) 2241
▲ Lopressor HCT 100/25 Tablets (10%) 2241
▲ Lopressor HCT 100/50 Tablets (10%) 2241
Lunesta Tablets 3142
Mirapex Tablets (Greater than or equal to 1%) 859
▲ Omacor Capsules (3.5%) 2725
▲ Premphase Tablets (8% to 13%) 3456
▲ Prempro Tablets (8% to 13%) 3456
Prevacid NapraPAC (Less than 1%) 3280
▲ Raptiva for Injection (7%) 1250
Relpax Tablets (Rare) 2548
▲ Somavert Injection (4% to 12%) 2642
Triglide Tablets (2.1%) 3123
▲ Univasc Tablets (3.1%) 3104
Vandazole Vaginal Gel (Less than 1%) 3338
▲ Ventavis Inhalation Solution (14%) 1020
Yaz Tablets (Greater than 1%) 803
Zomig Nasal Spray (Infrequent) 3523

Fluid accumulation in the knee
▲ Limbrel Capsules (Greater than or equal to 2%) 2672

Fluid depletion
Captopril Tablets 2149
Kristalose for Oral Solution 1034

Fluid imbalance
Benicar HCT Tablets 1044
Imitrex Nasal Spray 1467
Lotronex Tablets (Rare) 1512
Photofrin for Injection 702
Prinzide Tablets 2056
▲ Vesanoid Capsules (6%) 2820

Fluid overload
AmBisome for Injection (Less common) 620
▲ Aranesp for Injection (6%) 581
▲ Aredia for Injection (Up to at least 15%) 2179
Campath Ampules 811
▲ Coreg Tablets (Greater than 1% to 3%) 1414
Levaquin (0.1% to 0.9%) 2384
Levaquin in 5% Dextrose Injection (0.1% to 0.9%) 2384
▲ Myfortic Tablets (3% to less than 20%) 2255
Orthoclone OKT3 Sterile Solution 2360
Prinivil Tablets (0.3% to 1.0%) 2052
▲ Simulect for Injection (3% to 10%) 2284
▲ Zegerid Capsules (5.1%) 2958
▲ Zegerid Powder for Oral Solution (5.1%) 2958
Zosyn (1.9%) 3492

Fluid retention
(*see under* Edema)

Flu-like symptoms
AccuNeb Inhalation Solution (2.6%) 1055
▲ Actimmune (Most common) 1671
Actiq (Less than 1%) 979
▲ Actonel Tablets (7.1% to 9.8%) 2683
Advair Diskus 100/50 1308
Advair Diskus 250/50 1308
Advair Diskus 500/50 1308
▲ Advicor Tablets (6%) 1722
▲ Aerobid/Aerobid-M (10%) 1171
Agrylin Capsules (1% to 5%) 3169
▲ Alamast Ophthalmic Solution (10% to 25%) 3381
▲ Aldara Cream, 5% (1% to 3%) 1846
▲ Alferon N Injection (30%) 1665
Allegra (2.5%) 2844
Aloxi Injection (Less than 1%) 2127
▲ Alphagan P Ophthalmic Solution (1% to 4%) 567
Altace Capsules 1702
▲ Altoprev Extended-Release Tablets (5%) 3109
Ambien Tablets (2%) 2851
Ambien CR Tablets (1% to frequent) 2855
AmBisome for Injection (Less common) 620
▲ Angeliq Tablets (7%) 762
Aptivus Capsules (Less than 2%) 826
▲ Aranesp for Injection (6%) 581
Aricept Tablets (Frequent) 1094
Aricept ODT Tablets (Frequent) 1094
▲ Aromasin Tablets (6%) 2600
Arthrotec Tablets 3129
▲ Asacol Delayed-Release Tablets (3% to 5%) 2692
Asmanex Twisthaler (1% to less than 3%) 2966
Atacand HCT (2.5%) 651
▲ Atrovent Inhalation Solution (3.7%) 835
▲ Atrovent HFA Inhalation Aerosol (4% to 8%) 841
▲ Avalide Tablets (3%) 888
▲ Avalide Tablets (3%) 2874
Avapro Tablets (1% or greater) 891
Avapro Tablets (1% or greater) 2871
▲ Avinza Capsules (5% to 10%) 1741
▲ Azilect Tablets (5%) 3293
▲ Azmacort Inhalation Aerosol (2% to 5%) 1726
▲ Betaseron for SC Injection (60%) 767
Bexxar 1398
▲ Boniva Injection (0.8% to 3.3%) 2738
▲ Boniva Tablets (0.8% to 3.3%) 2741
▲ BOTOX Purified Neurotoxin Complex (2% to 10%) 570
Campath Ampules 811
▲ Cancidas for Injection (0% to 3.1%) 1918
▲ Carnitor Injection (15% to 29%) 3188
Caverject Impulse Injection (2%) 2612
Celebrex Capsules (0.1% to 1.9%) 3134
Celexa (Infrequent) 1176
▲ CellCept Capsules (3% to less than 20%) 2747
▲ CellCept Intravenous (3% to less than 20%) 2747
▲ CellCept Oral Suspension (3% to less than 20%) 2747
▲ CellCept Tablets (3% to less than 20%) 2747
Chantix Tablets (Frequent) 2517
▲ Chemet Capsules (5.2% to 15.7%) 2458
Clozaril Tablets 2184
Colazal Capsules (1%) 2838
Combivent Inhalation Aerosol (1.4%) 847
▲ Copaxone for Injection (19%) 3297
▲ Coreg Tablets (Greater than 1% to 3%) 1414
▲ Cozaar Tablets (10%) 1935
Cymbalta Delayed-Release Capsules (Infrequent) 1757
▲ Depacon Injection (12%) 412
▲ Depakene (12%) 417
▲ Depakote Sprinkle Capsules (12%) 422
▲ Depakote Tablets (At least 5% to 12%) 427
▲ Depakote ER Tablets (12%) 434
▲ Detrol Tablets (3%) 2628
▲ Ditropan XL Extended-Release Tablets (2% to less than 5%) 2413
Doxil Injection (Less than 1%) 2351
▲ Duragesic Transdermal System (3% to 10%) 2373
▲ Edex Injection (3%) 3089
Effexor Tablets 3411
▲ Effexor XR Capsules (6%) 3417
▲ Elidel Cream 1% (6.6% to 13.2%) 2200
Emsam Transdermal System 903
Enbrel for Injection 584
Engerix-B Vaccine (Less than 1%) 1425
▲ Entocort EC Capsules (Less than 5%) 2698
Epogen for Injection (Rare) 591
▲ Estring Vaginal Ring (3%) 2635
Eulexin Capsules 3009
▲ Evista Tablets (13.5% to 14.6%) 1763
▲ Evoxac Capsules (1% to 3%) 1047
▲ Exelon Capsules (3%) 2206
▲ Exelon Oral Solution (3%) 2206
▲ Faslodex Injection (7.1%) 681
▲ Femara Tablets (6%) 2214
Ferrlecit Injection 3388
▲ Flonase Nasal Spray (1% to 3%) 1440
Fluarix (1.6%) 1451
Follistim AQ Cartridge 2338
▲ Fortical Nasal Spray (1% to 3%) 3337
Fosamax 1969
Fuzeon Injection (2.3%) 2767
▲ Gabitril Tablets (1% to 9%) 984
▲ Gemzar for Injection (19%) 1771
Gengraf Capsules (2%) 459

Geodon (Frequent) 2529
▲ Gleevec Tablets (0.2% to 11.1%) 2227
▲ Herceptin I.V. (10%) 1233
▲ Humatrope Vials and Cartridges (3.9% to 15.6%) 1787
Hytrin Capsules (At least 1% to 2.4%) 471
▲ Imdur Tablets (Less than or equal to 5%) 3018
Imitrex Injection (Rare) 1463
Imitrex Nasal Spray 1467
Imitrex Tablets 1471
▲ Indapamide Tablets (Less than 5%) 2156
▲ Infergen (8% to 15%) 3364
Inspra Tablets (2%) 2536
▲ Intron A for Injection (Up to 79%) 3024
Invirase (Less than 2%) 2772
Kadian Capsules (Less than 3%) 577
Kaletra (Less than 2%) 476
▲ Keppra Oral Solution (1% to 3%) 3314
▲ Keppra Tablets (1% to 3%) 3314
▲ Kineret Injection (6%) 599
▲ Klonopin (4%) 2778
▲ Lamictal (5% to 7.0%) 1481
▲ Lescol Capsules (5.1%) 2233
▲ Lescol XL Tablets (7.1%) 2233
Levaquin (0.1% to 0.9%) 2384
Levaquin in 5% Dextrose Injection (0.1% to 0.9%) 2384
▲ Lexapro Oral Solution (5%) 1190
▲ Lexapro Tablets (5%) 1190
Limbrel Capsules (0.006%) 2672
▲ Lipitor Tablets (Up to 3.2%) 2483
Lofibra Tablets (2.1%) 1219
Lofibra Capsules (2.1%) 1216
Lotensin HCT Tablets (More than 1%) 2246
▲ Lupron Depot 3.75 mg (Less than 5%) 3260
Lupron Depot–3 Month 11.25 mg (Less than 5%) 3265
Lyrica Capsules (1% to 2%) 2539
▲ Meridia Capsules (8.2%) 489
▲ Miacalcin Nasal Spray (1% to 3%) 2253
Micardis Tablets (1%) 854
Micardis HCT Tablets (2%) 856
Migranal Nasal Spray (Rare) 3348
▲ Mobic Oral Suspension (2.3% to 5.8%) 863
▲ Mobic Tablets (2.3% to 5.8%) 863
▲ Myobloc Injection (6% to 9%) 3192
Namenda (Greater than or equal to 2%) 1195
Nasonex Nasal Spray (Greater than or equal to 2%) 3043
▲ Neoral Oral Solution (3% to 9.9%) 2259
▲ Neoral Soft Gelatin Capsules (3% to 9.9%) 2259
Neumega for Injection 3435
Neurontin Capsules (More than 1%) 2487
Neurontin Oral Solution (More than 1%) 2487
Neurontin Tablets (More than 1%) 2487
▲ Nexavar Tablets (Common) 746
Nexium Delayed-Release Capsules (Less than 1%) 655
Nexium I.V. (Less than 1%) 659
Nipent for Injection (Less than 3%) 1863
▲ Norditropin Cartridges (8%) 2323
Norvir (Less than 2%) 503
▲ Ontak Vials (8%) 1745
Orthoclone OKT3 Sterile Solution 2360
Paxil CR Controlled-Release Tablets (Infrequent) 1538
Paxil (Infrequent) 1530
▲ PEG-Intron Powder for Injection (46%) 3048
▲ Permax Tablets (3.2%) 3356
Pexeva Tablets (infrequent) 1694
▲ Plavix Tablets (7.9%) 917
▲ Plavix Tablets (7.5%) 2926
Pletal Tablets (2% or greater) 2455
▲ Premarin Tablets (10% to 11%) 3446
Prevacid Delayed-Release Capsules (Less than 1%) 3271
Prevacid for Delayed-Release Oral Suspension (Less than 1%) 3271
Prevacid SoluTab Delayed-Release Orally Disintegrating Tablets (Less than 1%) 3271
Prevnar for Injection 3463
PREVPAC (Less than 1%) 3284
Prilosec OTC Delayed-Release Tablets (1%) 2677
Prinivil Tablets (0.3%) 2052
Prinzide Tablets (0.3% to 1%) 2056
Prochieve 4% Gel 1003
Prochieve 8% Gel 1003
Procrit for Injection (Rare) 2364
▲ Prograf Capsules and Injection (3% to 15%) 632
Prolastin (Occasional) 3255
Protonix I.V. (Greater than or equal to 1%) 3472
Protonix Tablets (Greater than or equal to 1%) 3469
▲ Protopic Ointment (22% to 35%) 638
▲ Provigil Tablets (4%) 988
▲ Prozac Pulvules and Liquid (3% to 10%) 1801
▲ Pulmicort Respules (1% to 3%) 661
Pulmozyme Inhalation Solution 1248
▲ Rapamune Oral Solution and Tablets (3% to 20%) 3475
▲ Rebetol (13% to 31%) 3058
▲ Rebetron Combination Therapy (14% to 18%) 3063
▲ Rebif Prefilled Syringe for Injection (56% to 59%) 3159
Recombivax HB (Less than 1%) 2071
Requip Tablets (Infrequent) 1555
▲ Rescriptor Tablets (2.4% to 7.3%) 2551
Retrovir Capsules 1560
Retrovir IV Infusion 1564
Retrovir 1560
▲ Ribavirin, USP Capsules (13% to 31%) 3068
Rilutek Tablets (More than 2%) 2930
Risperdal (Infrequent) 1676
Risperdal M-Tab Orally Disintegrating Tablets (Infrequent) 1676
▲ Sandostatin Injection (1% to 4%) 2278
▲ Serevent Diskus (5%) 1568
Seroquel Tablets (Frequent) 690
Soriatane Capsules (Less than 1%) 1013
▲ Spiriva HandiHaler (Greater than or equal to 3%) 869
▲ Starlix Tablets (3.6%) 2292
▲ Suboxone Tablets (6%) 2717
▲ Subutex Tablets (6%) 2717
Sular Tablets (Less than or equal to 1%) 3122
Synagis (More than 1%) 1897
▲ Targretin Capsules (3.6% to 13.2%) 1747
▲ Tasmar Tablets (3% to 4%) 3358
Teveten Tablets (Less than 1%) 1735
Teveten HCT Tablets (Less than 1%) 1737
Thalomid Capsules 965
Thyrogen for Injection (1%) 1286
Tiazac Capsules (2%) 1201
▲ Topamax Sprinkle Capsules (Less than 1% to 4%) 2404
▲ Topamax Tablets (Less than 1% to 4%) 2404
Tricor Tablets (2.1%) 527
Twinrix Vaccine (Less than 1%) 1595
Ultram ER Tablets (0.2% to 2%) 2392
Uniretic Tablets (More than 1%) 3100
▲ Verelan PM Extended-Release Capsules, Controlled-Onset (3.7%) 3106
VFEND I.V. (Less than 2%) 2564
VFEND Oral Suspension (Less than 2%) 2564
VFEND Tablets (Less than 2%) 2564
Viagra Tablets (Greater than 2%) 2573
Vicoprofen Tablets (Less than 3%) 539
▲ Visudyne for Injection (1% to 10%) 2305
▲ WelChol Tablets (3%) 1050
Wellbutrin Tablets (Frequent) 1603
Wellbutrin SR Sustained-Release Tablets (At least 1%) 1607
Wellbutrin XL Extended-Release Tablets (At least 1%) 1613
▲ Xalatan Sterile Ophthalmic Solution (Approximately 4%) 2649
▲ Xeloda Tablets (Less than 5%) 2822
▲ Xenical Capsules (39.7%) 2831
▲ Xopenex Inhalation Solution (1.4% to 4.2%) 3146
▲ Xopenex Inhalation Solution Concentrate (1.4% to 4.2%) 3150
▲ Xopenex HFA Inhalation Aerosol (1.4% to 4.2%) 3154
Xyrem Oral Solution (Frequent) 1688
Yasmin 28 Tablets (Greater than 1%) 796
Zegerid Capsules (1%) 2958
Zegerid Powder for Oral Solution (1%) 2958
▲ Zemplar Capsules (5%) 541
▲ Zemplar Injection (5%) 543
▲ Zometa for Intravenous Infusion (Less than 15%) 2315
▲ Zonegran Capsules (4%) 1101
Zostavax Injection (1.7%) 2111
Zyprexa Tablets (Frequent) 1830
Zyprexa ZYDIS Orally Disintegrating Tablets (Frequent) 1830

Fluorosis

Ultane Liquid for Inhalation (Less than 1%) 531

Flushing

Accutane Capsules 2731
▲ Acetadote Injection (2% to 4%) 1031
▲ Adalat CC Tablets (4%) 2964
▲ Adenoscan (44%) 619
▲ Advicor Tablets (71%) 1722
Aggrenox Capsules (Less than 1%) 822
▲ Aldurazyme for Intravenous Infusion (5%) 1268
Allegra (Rare) 2844
Allegra-D 12 Hour Extended-Release Tablets (Rare) 2846
Allegra-D 24 Hour Extended-Release Tablets (Rare) 2849
Aloprim for Injection (Less than 1%) 2167
Altoprev Extended-Release Tablets (Rare) 3109
Ambien Tablets (Rare) 2851
Ambien CR Tablets (Rare) 2855
AmBisome for Injection (Less common) 620
Aminohippurate Sodium PAH Injection 1913
Amitiza Capsules (Less than 0.2%) 3224
Anzemet Injection (Infrequently) 2859
Anzemet Tablets (Infrequently) 2862
Astelin Nasal Spray (Infrequent) 1904
Atripla Tablets 945
Avalide Tablets 888
Avalide Tablets 2874
Avapro Tablets (Less than 1%) 891
Avapro Tablets (Less than 1%) 2871
▲ BeneFix Vials (3.1%) 3408
BiDil Tablets 2171
Buprenex Injectable (Less than 1%) 2716
▲ Caduet Tablets (0.7% to 4.5%) 2508
Camptosar Injection 2604
Cancidas for Injection (1.8% to 2.9%) 1918
Captopril Tablets (2 to 5 of 1000 patients) 2149
Cardizem LA Extended Release Tablets (1.4%) 1728
Celexa (Infrequent) 1176
▲ Cerezyme for Injection (Approximately 6.6%) 1270
Cesamet Capsules 3340
▲ Cialis Tablets (2% to 3%) 1838
Cipro (Less than 1%) 2977
Cipro I.V. (1% or less) 2984
Cipro XR Tablets 2990
Clinoril Tablets (Less than 1 in 100) 1924
▲ Clolar for Intravenous Infusion (18%) 1271
Combivent Inhalation Aerosol 847
Covera-HS Tablets (0.6% to 0.8%) 3139
Cozaar Tablets (Less than 1%) 1935
Cubicin for Injection (Less than 1%) 1026
CytoGam Intravenous (Less than 5.0%) 1895
Dalmane Capsules (Rare) 3342
Dilaudid 440
Dilaudid Non-Sterile Powder 440
Dilaudid Oral Liquid 445
Dilaudid Rectal Suppositories 440
Dilaudid Tablets 440
Dilaudid Tablets - 8 mg 445
Diovan HCT Tablets (Less frequent) 2196
Dolobid Tablets 1955
▲ Doxil Injection (Approximately 6.8%) 2351
DuoNeb Inhalation Solution 1058
Duragesic Transdermal System (1% or greater) 2373
DynaCirc CR Tablets (1.2% to 3.8%) 2721
Effexor Tablets 3411
▲ Eloxatin for Injection (3% to 10%) 2892
Emcyt Capsules (1%) 2634
Emend Capsules (Greater than 0.5%) 1963
Enbrel for Injection 584
Engerix-B Vaccine (Less than 1%) 1425
▲ Entocort EC Capsules (Less than 5%) 2698
Eraxis for Injection 2521
Ethyol for Injection 1898
Evoxac Capsules (0.3%) 1047
Exelon Capsules (Infrequent) 2206
Exelon Oral Solution (Infrequent) 2206
▲ Femara Tablets (0.1% to 49.7%) 2214
Ferrlecit Injection (Two cases) 3388
Floxin Otic Solution (Single report) 1049
Fortical Nasal Spray (Less than 1%) 3337
▲ Frova Tablets (4%) 1113
Gammagard Liquid 721
Gammagard S/D (Occasional) 724
Gantrisin Pediatric Suspension 2770
▲ Gengraf Capsules (Less than 1% to 5%) 459
Gleevec Tablets (Infrequent) 2227
Hyperstat I.V. 3017
Hyzaar 50-12.5 Tablets 1990
Hyzaar 100-12.5 Tablets 1990
Hyzaar 100-25 Tablets 1990
▲ Imdur Tablets (Less than or equal to 5%) 3018
▲ Imitrex Injection (7%) 1463
Imitrex Nasal Spray (Infrequent) 1467
▲ Imitrex Tablets (Up to 4%) 1471
▲ Indapamide Tablets (Less than 5%) 2156
Indocin Capsules (Less than 1%) 1995
Indocin I.V. (Less than 1%) 2465
Indocin (Less than 1%) 1995
Infed Injection 3390
▲ Intron A for Injection (Less than 5%) 3024
Invanz for Injection (Greater than 0.1%) 1999
▲ I.V. Busulfex (25%) 2493
Ketek Tablets (Less than 0.2%) 2903
Klonopin (Infrequent) 2778
Lamictal (Infrequent) 1481
Lariam Tablets (Infrequent) 2786
Lescol Capsules (Rare) 2233
Lescol XL Tablets 2233
Leukine 814
Levaquin (0.1% to 0.9%) 2384
Levaquin in 5% Dextrose Injection (0.1% to 0.9%) 2384
▲ Levitra Tablets (11%) 3034
Levothroid Tablets 1186
Levoxyl Tablets 1712
Lexapro Oral Solution (Infrequent) 1190
Lexapro Tablets (Infrequent) 1190
Lidoderm Patch 1118
Lotensin Tablets (Less than 1%) 2243
Lotensin HCT Tablets (0.3% to 1%) 2246
Lotrel Capsules (Up to 0.3%) 2249
Marinol Capsules (0.3% to 1%) 3333
Matulane Capsules 3191
Mavik Tablets (0.3% to 1.0%) 486
Maxair Autohaler 1852
Maxalt Tablets (Frequent) 2008
Maxalt-MLT Orally Disintegrating Tablets (Frequent) 2008
Mefoxin for Injection 2012
Mefoxin Premixed Intravenous Solution 2016
Mephyton Tablets 2018
Mevacor Tablets (Rare) 2021
Miacalcin Nasal Spray (Less than 1%) 2253
Micardis Tablets (More than 0.3%) 854
Micardis HCT Tablets 856
▲ Mivacron Injection (16%) 493
Moduretic Tablets (Less than or equal to 1%) 2028
Mycamine for Injection (0.2% to 0.5%) 628
▲ Myozyme for Intravenous Infusion (21%) 1279
▲ Neoral Oral Solution (1% to 5%) 2259
▲ Neoral Soft Gelatin Capsules (1% to 5%) 2259
Neumega for Injection 3435
▲ Nexavar Tablets (Common) 746
Nexium Delayed-Release Capsules (Less than 1%) 655
Nexium I.V. (Less than 1%) 659
▲ Niaspan Extended-Release Tablets (Among most common) 1730
Nicomide Tablets 1088
Nimbex Injection (0.2%) 498
Nimotop Capsules (Less than 1% to 2.1%) 749
Nitrolingual Pumpspray 3120
Norvasc Tablets (0.7% to 4.5%) 2545
Numorphan Injection 1120
Opana Tablets (Less than 1%) 1122
Opana ER Tablets (Less than 1%) 1126
Orencia Powder for Intravenous Infusion (Less than 0.1% to 1%) 914
Orthoclone OKT3 Sterile Solution 2360
▲ Oxytrol Transdermal System (Greater than 1%) 3392
Parcopa Orally Disintegrating Tablets 3097
▲ PEG-Intron Powder for Injection (6%) 3048
Pepcid Injection (Infrequent) 2040
Pepcid (Infrequent) 2038
Percodan Tablets 1132
Persantine Tablets 868
Plasmanate (Occasional) 3255
Pletal Tablets (Very rare) 2455
Primaxin I.M. 2045
Primaxin I.V. (Less than 0.2%) 2048
Prinivil Tablets (0.3% to 1.0%) 2052

Prinzide Tablets (0.3% to 1%) 2056
Profilnine SD, Factor IX Complex (Human) 1660
Prograf Capsules and Injection 632
Proquin XR Tablets 1153
Prosed/DS Tablets 1157
ProSom Tablets (Infrequent) 517
▲ Rebetol (3% to 4%) 3058
Recombinate 729
Recombivax HB (Less than 1%) 2071
ReFacto Vials 3484
Refludan for Injection (Uncommon) 792
▲ Remicade for IV Injection (9%) 971
▲ Requip Tablets (3%) 1555
▲ Revatio Tablets (10%) 2557
▲ R-Gene 10 for Intravenous Use (3%) 2641
▲ Ribavirin, USP Capsules (3% to 4%) 3068
Risperdal (Rare) 1676
Risperdal Consta Long-Acting Injection (Rare) 1682
Risperdal M-Tab Orally Disintegrating Tablets (Rare) 1676
▲ Rituxan I.V. (0% to 5%) 1254
Rocephin Injectable Vials, ADD-Vantage, Galaxy, Bulk (Occasional) 2800
▲ Romazicon Injection (1% to 3%) 2804
Rythmol SR Capsules 2727
▲ Sandimmune (Less than 1% to 4%) 2275
▲ Sandostatin Injection (1% to 4%) 2278
▲ Soltamox Oral Solution (33%) 3527
▲ Soriatane Capsules (1% to 10%) 1013
Stalevo Tablets 2287
▲ Strattera Capsules (3%) 1814
Sustiva Capsules (Less than 2%) 930
Sustiva Tablets (Less than 2%) 930
▲ Tambocor Tablets (1% to 3%) 1856
Tarka Tablets (0.3% or more) 524
Taxotere Injection Concentrate 2932
Thyrogen for Injection 1286
Tindamax Tablets 2142
Topamax Sprinkle Capsules (Infrequent) 2404
Topamax Tablets (Infrequent) 2404
▲ Tracleer Tablets (9%) 545
Trileptal Tablets 2300
Trileptal Oral Suspension 2300
▲ Trisenox Injection (10%) 993
Twinrix Vaccine (Less than 1%) 1595
▲ Ultram ER Tablets (7.7% to 15.8%) 2392
Uniretic Tablets (Less than 1%) 3100
Univasc Tablets (1.6%) 3104
Uroxatral Tablets 2943
Vantas (Less than 2%) 3375
Vantin Tablets and Oral Suspension (Less than 1%) 2645
Vasotec I.V. Injection (0.5% to 1.0%) 2103
Verelan PM Extended-Release Capsules, Controlled-Onset (0.6%) 3106
▲ Vesanoid Capsules (23%) 2820
▲ Viagra Tablets (10%) 2573
Visudyne for Injection 2305
VoSpire ER Tablets (Less frequent) 1052
Vytorin 10/10 Tablets 2114
Vytorin 10/10 Tablets 3077
Vytorin 10/20 Tablets 2114
Vytorin 10/20 Tablets 3077
Vytorin 10/40 Tablets 2114
Vytorin 10/40 Tablets 3077
Vytorin 10/80 Tablets 2114
Vytorin 10/80 Tablets 3077
Wellbutrin Tablets (Rare) 1603
▲ Wellbutrin SR Sustained-Release Tablets (1% to 4%) 1607
▲ Wellbutrin XL Extended-Release Tablets (1% to 4%) 1613
▲ Xeloda Tablets (5%) 2822
Zelnorm Tablets 2312
Zocor Tablets (Rare) 2105
Zofran Injection 1634
Zofran 1639
Zofran ODT Orally Disintegrating Tablets 1639
Zoloft (Infrequent) 2586
Zosyn (1.0% or less) 3492
Zyban Sustained-Release Tablets (Infrequent) 1644
Zyrtec Chewable Tablets (Less than 2%) 2594
Zyrtec (Less than 2%) 2594
Zyrtec-D 12 Hour Extended Release Tablets (Less than 2%) 2597

Flushing, cutaneous
Elidel Cream 1% 2200
Kadian Capsules (Less than 3%) 577
▲ Mivacron Injection (About 25%) 493
Nitrolingual Pumpspray 3120

Flushing, facial
▲ Adenocard Injection (18%) 617
Alferon N Injection (One patient) 1665
Carimune NF 3499
Dilaudid-HP (Less frequent) 442
Doxil Injection 2351
Ferrlecit Injection 3388
Imitrex Nasal Spray 1467
Imitrex Tablets 1471
Kadian Capsules (Less than 3%) 577
Marinol Capsules (Greater than 1%) 3333
▲ Miacalcin Injection (About 2% to 5%) 2252
Mintezol 2027
MS Contin Tablets (Less frequent) 2701
ProAmatine Tablets (Less frequent) 3186
Relpax Tablets (2%) 2548
Sandimmune 2275

Flushing, hands
▲ Miacalcin Injection (About 2% to 5%) 2252

Flushing, upper thorax
Sandimmune 2275

Folliculitis
Aclovate Cream (Infrequent) 2660
Amerge Tablets (Rare) 1339
Analpram-HC 1159
Apexicon E Cream 2661
Clindagel 1203
Clobevate Gel (Less than 2%) 3211
Clobex Lotion 1204
Clobex Shampoo 1206
Clobex Spray (Less than 1%) 1208
Cutivate Cream (0.8%) 2662
Cutivate Lotion 0.05% (Less than 1%) 2664
Cutivate Ointment (Infrequent to more frequent) 2665
Didronel Tablets 2697
Diprolene Lotion 0.05% (2%) 3002
Diprolene Ointment 0.05% (2 per 767 patients) 3003
Diprolene AF Cream 0.05% (Infrequent) 3000
Diprosone Cream, USP 0.05% 3004
▲ Elidel Cream 1% (0.9% to 6.1%) 2200
Elocon Cream 0.1% (Infrequent) 3005
Elocon Lotion 0.1% (4 in 156 subjects) 3006
Elocon Ointment 0.1% (Infrequent) 3007
Evoclin Foam, 1% 1009
▲ Flovent Diskus (1% to 3%) 1443
Fuzeon Injection (2.4%) 2767
Gengraf Capsules (1% to less than 3%) 459
Guanidine Hydrochloride Tablets 3016
▲ Intron A for Injection (Less than 5%) 3024
Invirase (Less than 2%) 2772
Lexapro Oral Solution (Infrequent) 1190
Lexapro Tablets (Infrequent) 1190
Lithobid Tablets 1692
Locoid Lipocream Cream (Infrequent) 1160
Lotrisone 3040
Lotronex Tablets (Rare) 1512
Luxíq Foam 1010
Neoral Oral Solution (1% to less than 3%) 2259
Neoral Soft Gelatin Capsules (1% to less than 3%) 2259
Nexavar Tablets (Uncommon) 746
Norvir (Less than 2%) 503
Olux Foam (Less than 2%) 1012
Oxistat Cream (0.3%) 2667
Oxsoralen-Ultra Capsules 3353
Pramosone 1161
Prezista Tablets (Less than 2%) 3306
ProctoFoam-HC 3099
▲ Protopic Ointment (4% to 11%) 638
Rescriptor Tablets 2551
Sustiva Capsules (Less than 2%) 930
Sustiva Tablets (Less than 2%) 930
▲ Temovate Gel (Among most frequent) 2669
Temovate Ointment (Less frequent) 2668
Temovate Scalp Application (2 of 294 patients; infrequent) 2670
Temovate E Emollient (Less than 2%) 2671
Tri-Luma Cream 1213
Vanos Cream 1893
Viracept (Less than 2%) 2577

Folliculosis
▲ Elestat Ophthalmic Solution (1% to 10%) 1669

Fontanels, bulging
Solodyn Extended Release Tablets 1890

Food craving
Vantas (Less than 2%) 3375

Foot drop
Actiq (Less than 1%) 979
Azilect Tablets (Infrequent) 3293
▲ Copaxone for Injection (3%) 3297
Kadian Capsules (Less than 3%) 577
Matulane Capsules 3191
Prozac Pulvules and Liquid (Rare) 1801
Thalomid Capsules 965

Forceps delivery, increased incidence

Foreign body reaction
▲ Alamast Ophthalmic Solution (Less than 5%) 3381
▲ Alphagan P Ophthalmic Solution (1% to 4%) 567
▲ Alrex Ophthalmic Suspension 0.2% (5% to 15%) ⊙246
▲ Ciloxan Ophthalmic Ointment (Less than 10%) 559
▲ Ciloxan Ophthalmic Solution (Less than 10%) ⊙206
▲ Lotemax Ophthalmic Suspension 0.5% (5% to 15%) ⊙251
▲ Lumigan Ophthalmic Solution (3% to 10%) 573
▲ Travatan Ophthalmic Solution (5% to 10%) 563
▲ Xalatan Sterile Ophthalmic Solution (5% to 15%) 2649

Foreign body sensation
Xyrem Oral Solution (Infrequent) 1688

Forgetfulness
Lariam Tablets (Occasional) 2786
Lexapro Oral Solution (Infrequent) 1190
Lexapro Tablets (Infrequent) 1190
Prochieve 4% Gel 1003
Prochieve 8% Gel 1003

Fracture, ankle
Xyrem Oral Solution (Infrequent) 1688

Fracture, humerus
Tamiflu Capsules (Less than 1%) 2807
Tamiflu Oral Suspension (Less than 1%) 2807

Fracture, pathological
Actiq (Less than 1%) 979
▲ Arimidex Tablets (2% to 5%) 673
Aromasin Tablets (Less frequent) 2600
Depo-Medrol Injectable Suspension 2617
▲ Doxil Injection (1% to 10%) 2351
Effexor Tablets (Rare) 3411
Effexor XR Capsules (Rare) 3417
Herceptin I.V. (At least one of the 958 patients) 1233
Lamictal (Rare) 1481
Quadramet Injection (2.5%) 1040
Seroquel Tablets (Infrequent) 690

Fractures, long bones
Colocort Rectal Suspension, USP (Retention) 100 mg/60 mL 2476
Decadron Tablets 1951
Depo-Medrol Injectable Suspension 2617
Depo-Medrol Single-Dose Vial 2619
Hydrocortone Tablets 1989
Revlimid Capsules 958

Fractures, osteoporotic
depo-subQ provera 104 Injectable Suspension (Rare) 2624

Fractures, unspecified
Celebrex Capsules (0.1% to 1.9%) 3134
Crestor Tablets (Greater than or equal to 1%) 678
Exelon Capsules (2% or more) 2206
Exelon Oral Solution (2% or more) 2206
Femara Tablets 2214
Klonopin (Infrequent) 2778
Levaquin (0.1% to 0.9%) 2384
Levaquin in 5% Dextrose Injection (0.1% to 0.9%) 2384
Neurontin Capsules (1.1%) 2487
Neurontin Oral Solution (1.1%) 2487
Neurontin Tablets (1.1%) 2487
Nutropin for Injection 1239
Nutropin AQ Injection 1243
Nutropin AQ Pen 1243
Nutropin AQ Pen Cartridge 1243
Omacor Capsules 2725
▲ Pulmicort Respules (1% to 3%) 661
▲ Simulect for Injection (3% to 10%) 2284
Tasmar Tablets (1% or more) 3358
Xolair (2%) 1266

Fractures, vertebral compression
Decadron Tablets 1951
Depo-Medrol Single-Dose Vial 2619
Hydrocortone Tablets 1989

Free T3 resin uptake, decrease
(*see under* T3, decrease)

Freezing phenomenon
Exelon Capsules (Infrequent) 2206
Exelon Oral Solution (Infrequent) 2206

Frequent blinking
Abilify Oral Solution (Rare) 882
Abilify Oral Solution (Rare) 2450
Abilify Discmelt Orally Disintegrating Tablets (Rare) 882
Abilify Discmelt Orally Disintegrating Tablets (Rare) 2450
Abilify Tablets (Rare) 882
Abilify Tablets (Rare) 2450

Fretfulness
(*see under* Anxiety)

Frigidity, unspecified
Wellbutrin Tablets (Infrequent) 1603

Fullness, abdominal
(*see under* Abdominal bloating)

Fundi with microhemorrhage, ocular
Neurontin Capsules (Rare) 2487
Neurontin Oral Solution (Rare) 2487
Neurontin Tablets (Rare) 2487

Fungal invasion
Blephamide Ophthalmic Ointment 568
Blephamide Ophthalmic Suspension 569
FML Ophthalmic Ointment (Possibility) ⊙228
FML Ophthalmic Suspension (Possibility) ⊙227
FML Forte Ophthalmic Suspension (Possibility) ⊙226
FML-S Ophthalmic Suspension ⊙229
Pred Mild Ophthalmic Suspension ⊙238
Pred-G Ophthalmic Ointment ⊙237
Pred-G Ophthalmic Suspension ⊙236
TobraDex Ophthalmic Ointment 562
TobraDex Ophthalmic Suspension 563

Fungemia
Cubicin for Injection (Less than 1%) 1026
Eraxis for Injection (Less than 1% to less than 2%) 2521

Furunculosis
Ambien Tablets (Rare) 2851
Ambien CR Tablets (Rare) 2855
Astelin Nasal Spray (Infrequent) 1904
Copaxone for Injection (Infrequent) 3297
Depacon Injection (1% or more) 412
Depakene (1% or more) 417
Depakote Sprinkle Capsules 422
▲ Depakote Tablets (1% to 5%) 427
Depakote ER Tablets (Greater than 1%) 434
▲ Doxil Injection (1% to 10%) 2351
Effexor Tablets (Rare) 3411
Effexor XR Capsules (Rare) 3417
▲ Elocon Cream 0.1% (Approximately 7%) 3005
▲ Elocon Ointment 0.1% (4.8% to approximately 7%) 3007
Evoxac Capsules (Less than 1%) 1047
Gabitril Tablets (Infrequent) 984
Geodon for Injection (Up to 2%) 2529
▲ Intron A for Injection (Less than 5%) 3024
Invirase (Less than 2%) 2772
Kaletra (Less than 2%) 476
Lexapro Oral Solution (Infrequent) 1190
Lexapro Tablets (Infrequent) 1190
Lunesta Tablets (Rare) 3142
Neurontin Capsules (Infrequent) 2487
Neurontin Oral Solution (Infrequent) 2487
Neurontin Tablets (Infrequent) 2487
▲ Nipent for Injection (4%) 1863
Paxil CR Controlled-Release Tablets (Infrequent) 1538
Paxil (Infrequent) 1530
Pexeva Tablets (Rare) 1694
Pletal Tablets (Less than 2%) 2455

Protopic Ointment (Greater than or equal to 1%) 638
Prozac Pulvules and Liquid (Rare) 1801
Requip Tablets (Infrequent) 1555
Rilutek Tablets (Rare) 2930
Risperdal (Rare) 1676
Risperdal M-Tab Orally Disintegrating Tablets (Rare) 1676
Soriatane Capsules (Less than 1%) 1013
Tasmar Tablets (Infrequent) 3358
Teveten Tablets (Less than 1%) 1735
Teveten HCT Tablets (Less than 1%) 1737
Uniretic Tablets (Less than 1%) 3100
VFEND I.V. (Less than 2%) 2564
VFEND Oral Suspension (Less than 2%) 2564
VFEND Tablets (Less than 2%) 2564
Zyrtec Chewable Tablets (Less than 2%) 2594
Zyrtec (Less than 2%) 2594
Zyrtec-D 12 Hour Extended Release Tablets (Less than 2%) 2597

Fussiness
▲ Prevnar for Injection (16.7% to 54.1%) 3463

G

Gagging
Lexapro Oral Solution (Infrequent) 1190
Lexapro Tablets (Infrequent) 1190

Gait, abnormal
Abilify Oral Solution (Frequent) 882
Abilify Oral Solution (Frequent) 2450
Abilify Discmelt Orally Disintegrating Tablets (Frequent) 882
Abilify Discmelt Orally Disintegrating Tablets (Frequent) 2450
Abilify Tablets (Frequent) 882
Abilify Tablets (Frequent) 2450
Acetadote Injection (.24% to 1.17%) 1031
Actimmune (Rare) 1671
▲ Actiq (1% to 4%) 979
Ambien Tablets (Rare) 2851
Ambien CR Tablets (Rare) 2855
Aricept Tablets (Infrequent) 1094
Aricept ODT Tablets (Infrequent) 1094
▲ Arranon Injection (0% to 6%) 1357
▲ Avastin IV (1% to 5%) 1227
▲ Avinza Capsules (Less than 5%) 1741
Azilect Tablets (Frequent) 3293
Campath Ampules 811
Cardizem LA Extended Release Tablets (Less than 2%) 1728
Celexa (Infrequent) 1176
Cipro (Less than 1%) 2977
Cipro I.V. (1% or less) 2984
Cipro XR Tablets 2990
Colazal Capsules 2838
Copaxone for Injection (At least 2%) 3297
▲ Depacon Injection (1% to 5%) 412
▲ Depakene (1% to 5%) 417
▲ Depakote Sprinkle Capsules (1% to 5%) 422
▲ Depakote Tablets (1% to 5%) 427
▲ Depakote ER Tablets (Greater than 1% to 5%) 434
▲ DepoCyt Injection (1% to 4%) 1143
Duragesic Transdermal System (1% or greater) 2373
Effexor Tablets (Rare) 3411
Effexor XR Capsules (Rare) 3417
Evoxac Capsules 1047
Exelon Capsules (Frequent) 2206
Exelon Oral Solution (Frequent) 2206
Flumadine (Less than 0.3%) 1183
Frova Tablets (Infrequent) 1113
▲ Gabitril Tablets (3%) 984
Geodon Capsules (Frequent) 2529
▲ Intron A for Injection (Less than 5%) 3024
▲ Lamictal (4%) 1481
Levaquin (0.1% to 0.9%) 2384
Levaquin in 5% Dextrose Injection (0.1% to 0.9%) 2384
Lexapro Oral Solution 1190
Lexapro Tablets 1190
Lunesta Tablets (Rare) 3142
▲ Lyrica Capsules (1% to 8%) 2539
Maxalt Tablets (Infrequent) 2008
Maxalt-MLT Orally Disintegrating Tablets (Infrequent) 2008
Meridia Capsules 489
Migranal Nasal Spray (Rare) 3348
▲ Mirapex Tablets (Greater than or equal to 1% to 7%) 859
Namenda (Greater than or equal to 2%) 1195
Neurontin Capsules (1.5%) 2487
Neurontin Oral Solution (1.5%) 2487
Neurontin Tablets (1.5%) 2487
Norvir (Less than 2%) 503
OxyContin Tablets (Less than 1%) 2703
Parcopa Orally Disintegrating Tablets 3097
Paxil CR Controlled-Release Tablets (Rare) 1538
Paxil (Rare) 1530
Permax Tablets (1.6%) 3356
Pexeva Tablets (rare) 1694
Proquin XR Tablets 1153
Prozac Pulvules and Liquid (Infrequent) 1801
Relpax Tablets (Rare) 2548
Requip Tablets (Infrequent) 1555
Revlimid Capsules 958
Reyataz Capsules (Less than 3%) 921
Rilutek Tablets (Infrequent) 2930
▲ Risperdal (17% to 34%) 1676
Risperdal Consta Long-Acting Injection (Infrequent) 1682
▲ Risperdal M-Tab Orally Disintegrating Tablets (17% to 34%) 1676
Rythmol SR Capsules 2727
▲ Sandostatin LAR Depot (1% to 4%) 2280
Seroquel Tablets (Infrequent) 690
Sonata Capsules (Infrequent) 1717
Soriatane Capsules (Less than 1%) 1013
Stalevo Tablets 2287
Symbyax Capsules (Infrequent) 1819
Symmetrel Tablets 1135
Tasmar Tablets (1% or more) 3358
▲ Temodar Capsules (6%) 3073
Thalomid Capsules 965
Tiazac Capsules (Less than 2%) 1201
▲ Topamax Sprinkle Capsules (2% to 8%) 2404
▲ Topamax Tablets (2% to 8%) 2404
▲ Trileptal Tablets (5% to 17%) 2300
▲ Trileptal Oral Suspension (5% to 17%) 2300
▲ Vesanoid Capsules (3%) 2820
▲ Xeloda Tablets (Less than 5%) 2822
Xyrem Oral Solution (Infrequent) 1688
Zantac Injection 1619
Zantac 150 Tablets 1624
Zelapar Tablets 3372
Zoloft (Infrequent) 2586
Zonegran Capsules (Frequent) 1101
▲ Zyprexa Tablets (6%) 1830
Zyprexa IntraMuscular (Infrequent) 1830
▲ Zyprexa ZYDIS Orally Disintegrating Tablets (6%) 1830

Galactorrhea
Angeliq Tablets 762
Celexa (Infrequent) 1176
Climara Transdermal System 771
Climara Pro Transdermal System 776
Covera-HS Tablets (Less than 2%) 3139
Demser Capsules (Infrequent) 1953
Depacon Injection 412
Depakene 417
Depakote Sprinkle Capsules 422
Depakote Tablets 427
Depakote ER Tablets 434
Depo-Provera Contraceptive Injection (Less than 1%) 2622
depo-subQ provera 104 Injectable Suspension 2624
Enjuvia Tablets 1062
Estrasorb Topical Emulsion 1147
Estratest Tablets 3199
Estratest H.S. Tablets 3199
Geodon 2529
Imitrex Injection 1463
Imitrex Nasal Spray (Rare) 1467
Imitrex Tablets (Rare) 1471
Menostar Transdermal System 782
Moban Tablets (Infrequent) 1119
Niravam Orally Disintegrating Tablets 3092
Paxil CR Controlled-Release Tablets 1538
Paxil 1530
Pexeva Tablets 1694
Premarin Tablets 3446
Premphase Tablets 3456
Prempro Tablets 3456
Sandostatin Injection (Less than 1%) 2278
Sandostatin LAR Depot (Rare) 2280
Tarka Tablets 524
Thalomid Capsules 965
Thioridazine Hydrochloride Tablets 2163
Verelan PM Extended-Release Capsules, Controlled-Onset (2% or less) 3106
Zoloft 2586

Gallbladder, sonographic abnormalities
Rocephin Injectable Vials, ADD-Vantage, Galaxy, Bulk 2800

Gallbladder disease
Angeliq Tablets 762
Chantix Tablets (Infrequent) 2517
Climara Transdermal System 771
Climara Pro Transdermal System 776
Enjuvia Tablets 1062
Estrasorb Topical Emulsion 1147
Estratest Tablets 3199
Estratest H.S. Tablets 3199
Menostar Transdermal System 782
Mircette Tablets 1066
NuvaRing 2340
Ortho-Cyclen Tablets 2429
Ortho Evra Transdermal System 2417
Ortho Tri-Cyclen Tablets 2429
Ortho Tri-Cyclen Lo Tablets 2436
Premarin Intravenous 3442
Premarin Tablets 3446
Premarin Vaginal Cream 3452
Premphase Tablets 3456
Prempro Tablets 3456
Pulmozyme Inhalation Solution 1248
Rocephin Injectable Vials, ADD-Vantage, Galaxy, Bulk 2800
Sandostatin Injection (Frequent) 2278
Sandostatin LAR Depot (Rare) 2280
Seasonique Tablets 1077
Yasmin 28 Tablets 796
Yaz Tablets 803

Gallstones
Imitrex Injection (Rare) 1463
Imitrex Nasal Spray 1467
Imitrex Tablets 1471
▲ Intron A for Injection (Less than 5%) 3024
Sandostatin Injection (Frequent) 2278

Gambling, pathological
Requip Tablets 1555

Gamma-glutamyl transferase, abnormal
Vytorin 10/10 Tablets 2114
Vytorin 10/10 Tablets 3077
Vytorin 10/20 Tablets 2114
Vytorin 10/20 Tablets 3077
Vytorin 10/40 Tablets 2114
Vytorin 10/40 Tablets 3077
Vytorin 10/80 Tablets 2114
Vytorin 10/80 Tablets 3077

Gamma-glutamyl transferase, increase
Eraxis for Injection (1.3%) 2521
▲ Prezista Tablets (8.4% to 9.2%) 3306
Zosyn 3492

Gamma-glutamyl transpeptidase, elevation
Accutane Capsules 2731
Adalat CC Tablets (Less than 1%) 2964
Advicor Tablets 1722
Altoprev Extended-Release Tablets 3109
▲ Arimidex Tablets (2% to 5%) 673
Asacol Delayed-Release Tablets 2692
Avelox (0.1% to less than 2%) 2970
Axert Tablets (Rare) 2396
Benicar HCT Tablets (Greater than 1%) 1044
Betaseron for SC Injection 767
Biaxin/Biaxin XL (Less than 1%) 402
▲ CellCept Capsules (3% to less than 20%) 2747
▲ CellCept Intravenous (3% to less than 20%) 2747
▲ CellCept Oral Suspension (3% to less than 20%) 2747
▲ CellCept Tablets (3% to less than 20%) 2747
Cialis Tablets (Less than 2%) 1838
Cipro (Less than 0.1%) 2977
Cipro I.V. (Infrequent) 2984
▲ Coreg Tablets (Greater than 1% to 3%) 1414
Effexor Tablets 3411
Effexor XR Capsules 3417
Epzicom Tablets 1436
Evoxac Capsules (Less than 1%) 1047
Exelon Capsules (Infrequent) 2206
Exelon Oral Solution (Infrequent) 2206
▲ Fortaz (1 in 19) 1453
Fuzeon Injection 2767
Gemzar for Injection (Rare) 1771
Geodon Capsules (Rare) 2529
Inspra Tablets 2536
▲ Kaletra (6% to 29%) 476
Lescol Capsules 2233
Lescol XL Tablets 2233
Levitra Tablets (Less than 2%) 3034
Lofibra Tablets 1219
Lofibra Capsules 1216
Mevacor Tablets 2021
Mobic Oral Suspension (Less than 2%) 863
Mobic Tablets (Less than 2%) 863
Neurontin Capsules (Rare) 2487
Neurontin Oral Solution (Rare) 2487
Neurontin Tablets (Rare) 2487
Omnicef Capsules (1%) 511
Oncaspar 1145
Pentasa Capsules (Less than 1%) 3185
Prevacid Delayed-Release Capsules 3271
Prevacid for Delayed-Release Oral Suspension 3271
Prevacid SoluTab Delayed-Release Orally Disintegrating Tablets 3271
Prevacid NapraPAC 3280
PREVPAC (Less than 1%) 3284
Prilosec OTC Delayed-Release Tablets (Rare) 2677
▲ Prograf Capsules and Injection (3% to 15%) 632
Protonix I.V. (Less than 1%) 3472
Protonix Tablets (Less than 1%) 3469
Provigil Tablets (At least 1%) 988
Rescriptor Tablets (Up to 1.8%) 2551
Rilutek Tablets (Infrequent) 2930
Risperdal Consta Long-Acting Injection (Rare) 1682
Rythmol SR Capsules 2727
Seroquel Tablets (Infrequent to 1%) 690
▲ Soriatane Capsules (Approximately 1 in 3 patients) 1013
Symmetrel Tablets 1135
Ticlid Tablets (Rare) 2810
▲ Topamax Sprinkle Capsules (1% to 3%) 2404
▲ Topamax Tablets (1% to 3%) 2404
Tricor Tablets 527
Trileptal Tablets 2300
Trileptal Oral Suspension 2300
Vantin Tablets and Oral Suspension 2645
▲ Ventavis Inhalation Solution (6%) 1020
VFEND I.V. (Less than 2%) 2564
VFEND Oral Suspension (Less than 2%) 2564
VFEND Tablets (Less than 2%) 2564
Viracept (Less than 2%) 2577
Viramune Oral Suspension (2.4%) 873
Viramune Tablets (2.4%) 873
Zegerid Capsules (Rare) 2958
Zegerid Powder for Oral Solution (Rare) 2958
Zelapar Tablets 3372
Ziagen 1626
Zocor Tablets 2105
Zyprexa Tablets 1830
Zyprexa ZYDIS Orally Disintegrating Tablets 1830

Gangrene
Bicillin C-R Injectable Suspension 1706
Gemzar for Injection (Very rare) 1771
Levaquin (0.1% to 0.9%) 2384
Levaquin in 5% Dextrose Injection (0.1% to 0.9%) 2384
Lopressor Injection (Very rare) 2238
Lopressor Tablets (Very rare) 2238
Lopressor HCT 50/25 Tablets (Very rare) 2241
Lopressor HCT 100/25 Tablets (Very rare) 2241
Lopressor HCT 100/50 Tablets (Very rare) 2241
Proleukin for Injection (1%) 2266
Requip Tablets (Rare) 1555

Gangrene, cutaneous
Miradon Tablets 3042

Gangrene, peripheral
Celebrex Capsules (Less than 0.1%) 3134
Requip Tablets (Infrequent) 1555

Gastric acid, regurgitation
Crixivan Capsules (2.7%) 1940
▲ Fosamax (Up to 4.1%) 1969
▲ Fosamax Plus D Tablets (0% to 4.2%) 1977
Prilosec OTC Delayed-Release Tablets (1.9%) 2677
Zegerid Capsules (1.7%) 2958
Zegerid Powder for Oral Solution (1.7%) 2958

Gastric discomfort
(*see under* Distress, gastrointestinal)

Gastric disorder
(*see under* Distress, gastrointestinal)

Gastric emptying, impaired
- Cymbalta Delayed-Release Capsules (Infrequent) 1757
- Donnatal Extentabs 2493
- Prograf Capsules and Injection 632

Gastric nodule
- Prevacid NapraPAC (Less than 1%) 3280

Gastric regurgitation
- Wellbutrin SR Sustained-Release Tablets (Infrequent) 1607
- Wellbutrin XL Extended-Release Tablets (Infrequent) 1613

Gastric ulcer, nonsteroidal anti-inflammatory drug-induced
- Percodan Tablets 1132

Gastritis
- Abilify Oral Solution (Infrequent) 882
- Abilify Oral Solution (Infrequent) 2450
- Abilify Discmelt Orally Disintegrating Tablets (Infrequent) 882
- Abilify Discmelt Orally Disintegrating Tablets (Infrequent) 2450
- Abilify Tablets (Infrequent) 882
- Abilify Tablets (Infrequent) 2450
- Actonel Tablets (2.5%) 2683
- Actonel with Calcium Tablets (2.5%) 2688
- Aggrenox Capsules (Less than 1%) 822
- ▲ Agrylin Capsules (1% to 5%) 3169
- Ambien Tablets (Rare) 2851
- Ambien CR Tablets (Rare) 2855
- Amerge Tablets (Rare) 1339
- Anaprox Tablets (Less than 1%) 2761
- Anaprox DS Tablets (Less than 1%) 2761
- Aricept Tablets (Infrequent) 1094
- Aricept ODT Tablets (Infrequent) 1094
- Arthrotec Tablets (Rare) 3129
- Asacol Delayed-Release Tablets 2692
- Atacand HCT (0.5% or greater) 651
- Augmentin 1360
- Augmentin Tablets 1363
- Augmentin XR Extended-Release Tablets 1369
- Augmentin ES-600 Powder for Oral Suspension 1366
- Avelox (Less than 0.1%) 2970
- Axert Tablets (Rare) 2396
- Boniva Injection (2.2%) 2738
- Boniva Tablets (2.2%) 2741
- Caduet Tablets (Less than 2%) 2508
- Cafcit (2.2%) 1886
- Campral Tablets (Infrequent) 1174
- Cancidas for Injection (0%) 1918
- Carnitor Injection (Less frequent) 3188
- Celebrex Capsules (0.1% to 1.9%) 3134
- Celexa (Infrequent) 1176
- ▲ CellCept Capsules (3% to less than 20%) 2747
- ▲ CellCept Intravenous (3% to less than 20%) 2747
- ▲ CellCept Oral Suspension (3% to less than 20%) 2747
- ▲ CellCept Tablets (3% to less than 20%) 2747
- Cesamet Capsules 3340
- Chantix Tablets (Infrequent) 2517
- Cialis Tablets (Less than 2%) 1838
- Clinoril Tablets (Less than 1%) 1924
- Comtan Tablets (1%) 2189
- Copaxone for Injection (At least 2%) 3297
- ▲ Cozaar Tablets (Less than 1% to 5%) 1935
- Crestor Tablets (Greater than or equal to 1%) 678
- Cymbalta Delayed-Release Capsules (Frequent) 1757
- Didronel Tablets 2697
- Dolobid Tablets (Less than 1 in 100) 1955
- Doxil Injection (Less than 1%) 2351
- EC-Naprosyn Delayed-Release Tablets (Less than 1%) 2761
- Effexor Tablets (Infrequent) 3411
- Effexor XR Capsules (Infrequent) 3417
- Elmiron Capsules (Less than or equal to 1%) 2415
- ▲ Emend Capsules (4.2%) 1963
- Enbrel for Injection 584
- ▲ Estring Vaginal Ring (1% to 3%) 2635
- Evoxac Capsules (Less than 1%) 1047
- Exelon Capsules (Frequent) 2206
- Exelon Oral Solution (Frequent) 2206
- Fortical Nasal Spray (Less than 1%) 3337
- Fosamax (0.2% to 1.1%) 1969
- Fosamax Plus D Tablets (0.2% to 1.1%) 1977
- Gabitril Tablets (Infrequent) 984
- Gengraf Capsules (1% to less than 3%) 459
- Gleevec Tablets (Infrequent) 2227
- ▲ Humatrope Vials and Cartridges (Up to 6.67%) 1787
- Hyzaar 50-12.5 Tablets 1990
- Hyzaar 100-12.5 Tablets 1990
- Hyzaar 100-25 Tablets 1990
- ▲ Imdur Tablets (Less than or equal to 5%) 3018
- Imitrex Injection 1463
- Imitrex Nasal Spray 1467
- ▲ Intron A for Injection (Less than 5%) 3024
- Invanz for Injection (Greater than 0.1%) 1999
- Invirase (Less than 2%) 2772
- Kaletra (Less than 2%) 476
- Keflex Capsules 549
- Ketek Tablets (Greater than or equal to 0.2% to less than 2%) 2903
- Klonopin 2778
- Lamictal (Rare) 1481
- Levaquin (0.1% to 0.9%) 2384
- Levaquin in 5% Dextrose Injection (0.1% to 0.9%) 2384
- Levitra Tablets (Less than 2%) 3034
- Lexapro Oral Solution (Infrequent) 1190
- Lexapro Tablets (Infrequent) 1190
- Lipitor Tablets (Less than 2%) 2483
- Lithobid Tablets 1692
- Lofibra Tablets 1219
- Lofibra Capsules 1216
- Lotensin Tablets (Less than 1%) 2243
- Lotronex Tablets (Rare) 1512
- Lunesta Tablets (Rare) 3142
- Lyrica Capsules (0.1% to 1%) 2539
- ▲ Malarone Pediatric Tablets (2% to 3%) 1517
- ▲ Malarone Tablets (2% to 3%) 1517
- ▲ Mavik Tablets (4.2%) 486
- Maxalt Tablets (Rare) 2008
- Maxalt-MLT Orally Disintegrating Tablets (Rare) 2008
- Meridia Capsules (1.7%) 489
- Miacalcin Nasal Spray (Less than 1%) 2253
- Micardis Tablets (More than 0.3%) 854
- Micardis HCT Tablets 856
- Mobic Oral Suspension (Less than 2%) 863
- Mobic Tablets (Less than 2%) 863
- Nalfon Capsules (Less than 1%) 2502
- Namenda 1195
- Naprosyn Suspension (Less than 1%) 2761
- Naprosyn Tablets (Less than 1%) 2761
- NeoProfen Injection 2472
- Neoral Oral Solution (1% to less than 3%) 2259
- Neoral Soft Gelatin Capsules (1% to less than 3%) 2259
- Neurontin Capsules (Infrequent) 2487
- Neurontin Oral Solution (Infrequent) 2487
- Neurontin Tablets (Infrequent) 2487
- Nexavar Tablets (Uncommon) 746
- Norvasc Tablets (Less than 0.1%) 2545
- Norvir (Less than 2%) 503
- Omacor Capsules 2725
- ▲ OxyContin Tablets (Between 1% and 5%) 2703
- Permax Tablets (Infrequent) 3356
- Pexeva Tablets (Infrequent) 1694
- Pletal Tablets (Less than 2%) 2455
- Prevacid Delayed-Release Capsules (Less than 1%) 3271
- Prevacid for Delayed-Release Oral Suspension (Less than 1%) 3271
- Prevacid SoluTab Delayed-Release Orally Disintegrating Tablets (Less than 1%) 3271
- Prevacid NapraPAC (Less than 1%) 3280
- PREVPAC (Less than 1%) 3284
- Prinivil Tablets (0.3% to 1.0%) 2052
- Prinzide Tablets 2056
- Prochieve 4% Gel 1003
- Prochieve 8% Gel 1003
- ▲ Prograf Capsules and Injection (3% to 15%) 632
- Proleukin for Injection 2266
- ProSom Tablets (Infrequent) 517
- Protopic Ointment (Greater than or equal to 1%) 638
- Prozac Pulvules and Liquid (Infrequent) 1801
- ▲ Rapamune Oral Solution and Tablets (3% to 20%) 3475
- Razadyne (Infrequent) 2399
- Razadyne ER Extended-Release Capsules (Infrequent) 2399
- ReFacto Vials 3484
- Relpax Tablets (Infrequent) 2548
- Requip Tablets (Infrequent) 1555
- ▲ Revatio Tablets (3%) 2557
- Revlimid Capsules 958
- Reyataz Capsules (Less than 3%) 921
- Rilutek Tablets (Infrequent) 2930
- Risperdal (Infrequent) 1676
- Risperdal Consta Long-Acting Injection (Infrequent) 1682
- Risperdal M-Tab Orally Disintegrating Tablets (Infrequent) 1676
- Rythmol SR Capsules 2727
- Sanctura Tablets 1151
- Sandimmune (2% or less) 2275
- ▲ Sandostatin LAR Depot (1% to 4%) 2280
- Seroquel Tablets (Infrequent) 690
- Sonata Capsules (Infrequent) 1717
- Soriatane Capsules (Less than 1%) 1013
- Stalevo Tablets (1%) 2287
- Sular Tablets (Less than or equal to 1%) 3122
- Symbyax Capsules (Infrequent) 1819
- Tequin Injection (Less than 0.1%) 938
- Tequin Injection in 5% Dextrose (Less than 0.1%) 938
- Tequin Tablets (Less than 0.1%) 938
- Teveten Tablets (Less than 1%) 1735
- Teveten HCT Tablets (Less than 1%) 1737
- Thymoglobulin for Intravenous Infusion (1.2%) 1284
- ▲ Topamax Sprinkle Capsules (0% to 3%) 2404
- ▲ Topamax Tablets (0% to 3%) 2404
- Tricor Tablets 527
- Triglide Tablets 3123
- Trileptal Tablets (1% to 2%) 2300
- Trileptal Oral Suspension (1% to 2%) 2300
- Uniretic Tablets (Less than 1%) 3100
- Vantin Tablets and Oral Suspension (Less than 1%) 2645
- Viagra Tablets (Less than 2%) 2573
- Vicoprofen Tablets (Less than 3%) 539
- Voltaren Tablets (Occasionally) 2307
- Voltaren-XR Tablets (Occasionally) 2310
- Xeloda Tablets 2822
- Zelapar Tablets 3372
- Zelnorm Tablets 2312
- Zmax for Oral Suspension (Less then 1%) 2583
- Zoloft (Rare) 2586
- Zomig Tablets (Rare) 3519
- Zomig Nasal Spray (Rare) 3523
- Zomig-ZMT Tablets (Rare) 3519
- Zonegran Capsules (Infrequent) 1101
- Zosyn (1.0% or less) 3492
- Zyprexa Tablets (Infrequent) 1830
- Zyprexa ZYDIS Orally Disintegrating Tablets (Infrequent) 1830
- Zyrtec Chewable Tablets (Less than 2%) 2594
- Zyrtec (Less than 2%) 2594
- Zyrtec-D 12 Hour Extended Release Tablets (Less than 2%) 2597

Gastritis, atrophic
- Protonix Tablets 3469

Gastritis, hemorrhagic
- Azilect Tablets (Rare) 3293
- Plavix Tablets (Less than 1%) 917
- Plavix Tablets (Less than 1%) 2926
- Requip Tablets (Rare) 1555

Gastroduodenitis
- Lotronex Tablets (Rare) 1512

Gastroenteritis
- Abilify Oral Solution (Infrequent) 882
- Abilify Oral Solution (Infrequent) 2450
- Abilify Discmelt Orally Disintegrating Tablets (Infrequent) 882
- Abilify Discmelt Orally Disintegrating Tablets (Infrequent) 2450
- Abilify Tablets (Infrequent) 882
- Abilify Tablets (Infrequent) 2450
- AccuNeb Inhalation Solution (0.9% to 3.4%) 1055
- Aceon Tablets (2 mg, 4 mg, 8 mg) (0.3% to 1%) 3194
- Aciphex Tablets 1090
- Actiq (Less than 1%) 979
- ▲ Actonel Tablets (3.5% to 3.8%) 2683
- ▲ Actonel with Calcium Tablets (3.5% to 3.8%) 2688
- ▲ Advair Diskus 100/50 (1% to 3%) 1308
- ▲ Advair Diskus 250/50 (1% to 3%) 1308
- ▲ Advair Diskus 500/50 (1% to 3%) 1308
- Altace Capsules (Less than 1%) 1702
- Ambien Tablets (Infrequent) 2851
- Ambien CR Tablets (Infrequent to 1%) 2855
- Amerge Tablets (Infrequent) 1339
- Amevive 626
- Aricept Tablets (Infrequent) 1094
- Aricept ODT Tablets (Infrequent) 1094
- Asacol Delayed-Release Tablets (2% or greater) 2692
- Asmanex Twisthaler (1% to less than 3%) 2966
- Astelin Nasal Spray (Infrequent) 1904
- Atacand Tablets (0.5% or greater) 649
- Atacand HCT (0.5% or greater) 651
- Avalide Tablets 888
- Avalide Tablets 2874
- Avapro Tablets (Less than 1%) 891
- Avapro Tablets (Less than 1%) 2871
- ▲ Avinza Capsules (Less than 5%) 1741
- Axert Tablets (Rare) 2396
- ▲ Azilect Tablets (3%) 3293
- Benicar Tablets (Greater than 0.5%) 1043
- Benicar HCT Tablets (Greater than 1%) 1044
- Caduet Tablets (Less than 2%) 2508
- Campath Ampules 811
- Campral Tablets (Infrequent) 1174
- Celebrex Capsules (0.1% to 1.9%) 3134
- Celexa (Infrequent) 1176
- ▲ CellCept Capsules (3% to less than 20%) 2747
- ▲ CellCept Intravenous (3% to less than 20%) 2747
- ▲ CellCept Oral Suspension (3% to less than 20%) 2747
- ▲ CellCept Tablets (3% to less than 20%) 2747
- Clinoril Tablets (Less than 1%) 1924
- Clozaril Tablets (Less than 1%) 2184
- Colazal Capsules 2838
- ▲ Copaxone for Injection (3%) 3297
- Crestor Tablets (Greater than or equal to 2%) 678
- Depacon Injection (1% or more) 412
- Depakene (1% or more) 417
- Depakote Sprinkle Capsules 422
- ▲ Depakote Tablets (1% to 5%) 427
- Depakote ER Tablets (Greater than 1%) 434
- Diovan HCT Tablets (Greater than 0.2%) 2196
- Effexor Tablets (Infrequent) 3411
- Effexor XR Capsules (Infrequent) 3417
- ▲ Elidel Cream 1% (1.8% to 7.4%) 2200
- Eligard 7.5 mg (2.5%) 2880
- Enbrel for Injection 584
- Epivir 1427
- Evista Tablets (2.6%) 1763
- Evoxac Capsules (Less than 1%) 1047
- Exelon Capsules (Infrequent) 2206
- Exelon Oral Solution (Infrequent) 2206
- FazaClo Orally Disintegrating Tablets (Less than 1%) 551
- ▲ Flovent Diskus (1% to 3%) 1443
- Gabitril Tablets (1% or more) 984
- Gardasil Injection (0.03%) 1984
- Gengraf Capsules (1% to less than 3%) 459
- Gleevec Tablets (Infrequent) 2227
- Herceptin I.V. (At least one of the 958 patients) 1233
- ▲ Humira Injection (Less than 5%) 466
- Imitrex Injection 1463
- Imitrex Nasal Spray (Rare) 1467
- Indocin Capsules (Less than 1%) 1995
- Indocin I.V. (Less than 1%) 2465
- Indocin (Less than 1%) 1995
- ▲ Intron A for Injection (Less than 5%) 3024
- Invirase (Less than 2%) 2772
- Kaletra (Less than 2%) 476
- Keppra Injection 3320
- ▲ Keppra Oral Solution (1% to 4%) 3314
- ▲ Keppra Tablets (1% to 4%) 3314
- Ketek Tablets (Greater than or equal to 0.2% to less than 2%) 2903
- Kogenate FS 738
- Kogenate FS with Bio-Set 740
- Levaquin (0.1% to 0.9%) 2384

Levaquin in 5% Dextrose Injection (0.1% to 0.9%)........ 2384
Lexapro Oral Solution (Frequent)...... 1190
Lexapro Tablets (Frequent)........ 1190
Lipitor Tablets (Less than 2%).......... 2483
Lofibra Tablets........ 1219
Lofibra Capsules........ 1216
Lotensin HCT Tablets (0.3% or more)........ 2246
Lotronex Tablets (Rare)........ 1512
Lyrica Capsules (Greater than or equal to 1%)........ 2539
Meridia Capsules (Greater than or equal to 1%)........ 489
Micardis Tablets (More than 0.3%).... 854
Micardis HCT Tablets........ 856
▲ Myozyme for Intravenous Infusion (41%)........ 1279
Namenda (Infrequent)........ 1195
Neoral Oral Solution (1% to less than 3%)........ 2259
Neoral Soft Gelatin Capsules (1% to less than 3%)........ 2259
Neurontin Capsules (Infrequent)....... 2487
Neurontin Oral Solution (Infrequent)........ 2487
Neurontin Tablets (Infrequent).......... 2487
Nexium Delayed-Release Capsules (Less than 1%)........ 655
Nexium I.V. (Less than 1%)........ 659
▲ Norditropin Cartridges (8%) 2323
Norvir (Less than 2%)........ 503
Omacor Capsules........ 2725
Paxil CR Controlled-Release Tablets (Rare)........ 1538
Paxil (Rare)........ 1530
PEG-Intron Powder for Injection (Less than or equal to 1%)........ 3048
Permax Tablets (Infrequent)........ 3356
Pexeva Tablets (Infrequent)........ 1694
Pletal Tablets (Less than 2%)........ 2455
Prevacid Delayed-Release Capsules (Less than 1%)........ 3271
Prevacid for Delayed-Release Oral Suspension (Less than 1%)........ 3271
Prevacid SoluTab Delayed-Release Orally Disintegrating Tablets (Less than 1%)........ 3271
Prevacid NapraPAC (Less than 1%).. 3280
Prevnar for Injection........ 3463
PREVPAC (Less than 1%)........ 3284
Primaxin I.M........ 2045
Primaxin I.V. (Less than 0.2%)........ 2048
Prograf Capsules and Injection........ 632
Prometrium Capsules (100 mg, 200 mg) (Less than 5%)........ 3203
Protonix I.V. (Greater than or equal to 1%)........ 3472
Protonix Tablets (Greater than or equal to 1%)........ 3469
▲ Protopic Ointment (2% to 4%) 638
Provigil Tablets (At least 1%)........ 988
Prozac Pulvules and Liquid (Infrequent)........ 1801
▲ Pulmicort Respules (5%) 661
▲ Rapamune Oral Solution and Tablets (3% to 20%)........ 3475
Raptiva for Injection........ 1250
Razadyne (Infrequent)........ 2399
Razadyne ER Extended-Release Capsules (Infrequent)........ 2399
ReFacto Vials........ 3484
Rescriptor Tablets........ 2551
Revlimid Capsules........ 958
Reyataz Capsules (Less than 3%)..... 921
Risperdal (Rare)........ 1676
Risperdal M-Tab Orally Disintegrating Tablets (Rare)........ 1676
RotaTeq (0.2%)........ 2074
▲ Sandostatin LAR Depot (1% to 4%)........ 2280
Seroquel Tablets (Infrequent to 2%)........ 690
▲ Simulect for Injection (3% to 10%) ... 2284
Singulair (Greater than or equal to 2%)........ 2077
Sonata Capsules (Infrequent)........ 1717
Soriatane Capsules (Less than 1%).. 1013
Symbyax Capsules (Infrequent)........ 1819
Synagis (More than 1%)........ 1897
Targretin Capsules........ 1747
Tasmar Tablets (Infrequent)........ 3358
Teveten Tablets (Less than 1%)........ 1735
Teveten HCT Tablets (Less than 1%)........ 1737
Thalomid Capsules........ 965
▲ Topamax Sprinkle Capsules (1% to 3%)........ 2404
▲ Topamax Tablets (1% to 3%) 2404
Tricor Tablets........ 527
Triglide Tablets........ 3123
Trizivir Tablets........ 1589
▲ Ultram ER Tablets (1% to greater than 5%)........ 2392
Uniretic Tablets (Less than 1%)........ 3100
Vaqta........ 2097
VFEND I.V. (Less than 2%)........ 2564
VFEND Oral Suspension (Less than 2%)........ 2564
VFEND Tablets (Less than 2%)........ 2564
Viagra Tablets (Less than 2%)........ 2573
Vicoprofen Tablets (Less than 1%).... 539
Vivitrol........ 995
▲ Xeloda Tablets (Less than 5%) 2822
Xopenex Inhalation Solution........ 3146
Xopenex Inhalation Solution Concentrate........ 3150
Xopenex HFA Inhalation Aerosol........ 3154
Xyrem Oral Solution (Infrequent)....... 1688
Yasmin 28 Tablets (Greater than 1%)........ 796
Yaz Tablets (Greater than 1%)........ 803
Zelapar Tablets........ 3372
Zoloft (Infrequent)........ 2586
Zomig Tablets (Infrequent)........ 3519
Zomig-ZMT Tablets (Infrequent)........ 3519
Zonegran Capsules (Infrequent)........ 1101
Zyprexa Tablets (Infrequent)........ 1830
Zyprexa ZYDIS Orally Disintegrating Tablets (Infrequent)........ 1830

Gastroenteritis, infectious

Singulair (1.5%)........ 2077

Gastroenteritis, viral

▲ Amitiza Capsules (1% to 3.4%) 3224
▲ Flovent Diskus (3%) 1443
▲ Strattera Capsules (2% or greater)........ 1814
▲ Ultram ER Tablets (1% to greater than 5%)........ 2392
▲ Xyrem Oral Solution (6.1%) 1688

Gastroesophageal reflux

Abilify Oral Solution (Infrequent) 882
Abilify Oral Solution (Infrequent) 2450
Abilify Discmelt Orally Disintegrating Tablets (Infrequent)........ 882
Abilify Discmelt Orally Disintegrating Tablets (Infrequent)........ 2450
Abilify Tablets (Infrequent)........ 882
Abilify Tablets (Infrequent)........ 2450
Aldara Cream, 5% (1.4%)........ 1846
Ambien CR Tablets (1%)........ 2855
Amerge Tablets (Rare)........ 1339
Amitiza Capsules (0% to 1.8%) 3224
Aptivus Capsules (Less than 2%) 826
Axert Tablets (Rare)........ 2396
▲ Byetta Injection (Greater than or equal to 1% to less than 5%) 611
Celebrex Capsules (0.1% to 1.9%) ... 3134
Celexa (Rare)........ 1176
Chantix Tablets (1%)........ 2517
Cialis Tablets (Less than 2%)........ 1838
▲ Dacogen Injection (5%)........ 2129
▲ Ditropan XL Extended-Release Tablets (2% to less than 5%) 2413
▲ Eloxatin for Injection (1% to 5%) 2892
Emend Capsules (Greater than 0.5%)........ 1963
▲ Evoxac Capsules (1% to 3%)........ 1047
Exelon Capsules (Infrequent)........ 2206
Exelon Oral Solution (Infrequent) 2206
Fosamax (0.7% to 2.8%)........ 1969
Fosamax Plus D Tablets (0.7% to 2.8%)........ 1977
Frova Tablets (Rare)........ 1113
Gleevec Tablets (Less common) 2227
Imitrex Injection (Infrequent)........ 1463
Imitrex Nasal Spray (Infrequent) 1467
Imitrex Tablets (Infrequent)........ 1471
Kadian Capsules (Less than 3%) 577
Levaquin (0.1% to 0.9%)........ 2384
Levaquin in 5% Dextrose Injection (0.1% to 0.9%)........ 2384
Levitra Tablets (Less than 2%) 3034
Lexapro Oral Solution (Frequent) 1190
Lexapro Tablets (Frequent)........ 1190
Micardis Tablets (More than 0.3%) ... 854
Micardis HCT Tablets 856
Mobic Oral Suspension (Less than 2%)........ 863
Mobic Tablets (Less than 2%)........ 863
▲ Myfortic Tablets (3% to less than 20%)........ 2255
▲ Myozyme for Intravenous Infusion (26%)........ 1279
Namenda........ 1195
NeoProfen Injection........ 2472
Prograf Capsules and Injection 632
ReoPro Vials (0.1%)........ 1809
Requip Tablets (Infrequent)........ 1555
Rescriptor Tablets........ 2551
Revlimid Capsules........ 958
Risperdal (Rare)........ 1676
Risperdal Consta Long-Acting Injection (Infrequent)........ 1682
Risperdal M-Tab Orally Disintegrating Tablets (Rare)........ 1676
Rythmol SR Capsules........ 2727
Seroquel Tablets (Infrequent)........ 690
▲ Spiriva HandiHaler (1% to 3%) 869
Topamax Sprinkle Capsules (Greater than 1%)........ 2404
Topamax Tablets (Greater than 1%)........ 2404
Vivitrol........ 995
Xyrem Oral Solution (Infrequent)....... 1688
Zelnorm Tablets........ 2312

Gastrointestinal anomaly, unspecified

Prevacid Delayed-Release Capsules (Less than 1%)........ 3271
Prevacid for Delayed-Release Oral Suspension (Less than 1%)........ 3271
Prevacid SoluTab Delayed-Release Orally Disintegrating Tablets (Less than 1%)........ 3271
Prevacid NapraPAC (Less than 1%).. 3280
PREVPAC (Less than 1%)........ 3284

Gastrointestinal bleeding

(*see under* Bleeding, gastrointestinal)

Gastrointestinal concretions

Kionex Powder........ 2477

Gastrointestinal disorders

Accutane Capsules........ 2731
Actonel Tablets (1.9% to 2.3%)........ 2683
Actonel with Calcium Tablets (1.9% to 2.5%)........ 2688
Adalat CC Tablets (Less than 1%)..... 2964
Adderall Tablets........ 3164
Adderall XR Capsules........ 3166
▲ Adenoscan (13%) 619
Adipex-P........ 1215
▲ Advair Diskus 100/50 (1% to 4%) ... 1308
Advair Diskus 250/50 (1%)........ 1308
▲ Advair Diskus 500/50 (1% to 4%) ... 1308
▲ Advair HFA Inhalation Aerosol (1% to 3%)........ 1318
▲ Aerobid/Aerobid-M (1% to 10%) 1171
Alkeran for Injection (Infrequent)....... 955
Alkeran Tablets (Infrequent)........ 956
▲ Alphagan P Ophthalmic Solution (1% to 4%)........ 567
▲ Amerge Tablets (6% to 7%) 1339
Anaprox Tablets........ 2761
Anaprox DS Tablets........ 2761
Argatroban Injection (0.9%)........ 1346
▲ Arimidex Tablets (4% to 34%) 673
Arthrotec Tablets........ 3129
Avelox (Less than 0.1%)........ 2970
Axid Oral Solution (1.1%)........ 879
▲ Boostrix (3% to 26%) 1404
▲ Brimonidine Tartrate Ophthalmic Solution 0.2% (3% to 9%)........ ⊙248
Captopril Tablets........ 2149
▲ Carnitor Injection (2% to 6%) 3188
Carnitor Tablets and Oral Solution.... 3190
▲ CellCept Capsules (3% to less than 20%)........ 2747
▲ CellCept Intravenous (3% to less than 20%)........ 2747
▲ CellCept Oral Suspension (3% to less than 20%)........ 2747
▲ CellCept Tablets (3% to less than 20%)........ 2747
▲ Chemet Capsules (About 10%) 2458
Clindagel........ 1203
▲ Clinoril Tablets (3% to 9%) 1924
▲ Clozaril Tablets (Greater than 5%) ... 2184
Comtan Tablets (1%)........ 2189
▲ Copaxone for Injection (5%) 3297
Cosopt Sterile Ophthalmic Solution........ 1931
▲ Creon 5 Capsules (Among most frequent)........ 3198
▲ Cuprimine Capsules (17%) 1947
▲ Daranide Tablets (Among the most common effects)........ 1950
Depacon Injection........ 412
Depakene........ 417
▲ Depakote Tablets (1% to 5%) 427
Depakote ER Tablets........ 434
Dexedrine........ 1420
DextroStat Tablets........ 3179
Didronel Tablets........ 2697
Dyazide Capsules........ 1423
EC-Naprosyn Delayed-Release Tablets........ 2761
▲ Eulexin Capsules (6%) 3009
▲ Evista Tablets (3.3%) 1763
Ferrlecit Injection........ 3388
▲ Flovent Diskus (4%) 1443
▲ Flovent HFA (1% to 3%) 1447
▲ Fortaz (Among most common) 1453
Forteo for Injection (2.3%)........ 1767
Furosemide Tablets........ 2154
▲ Gengraf Capsules (4% to 19.8%) 459
▲ Humira Injection (Less than 5%) 466
▲ Hyalgan Solution (29%) 2901
Ionsys Transdermal System (.1% to less than 1%)........ 2379
Kaletra (Less than 2%)........ 476
K-Dur Extended-Relase Tablets........ 3033
Ketek Tablets (Greater than or equal to 0.2% to less than 2%)...... 2903
Klonopin (Infrequent)........ 2778
K-Phos Neutral Tablets........ 760
Lanoxicaps Capsules........ 1490
Leukeran Tablets (Infrequent)........ 1504
▲ Leukine (37%) 814
▲ Lithostat Tablets (20% to 25%) 2140
Lofibra Tablets........ 1219
Lofibra Capsules........ 1216
Lupron Depot 3.75 mg (2%)........ 3260
▲ Lupron Depot 7.5 mg (14.3%) 3264
Lupron Depot–3 Month 11.25 mg (2%)........ 3265
Micardis Tablets (More than 0.3%) ... 854
Micardis HCT Tablets 856
Midamor Tablets (Less than or equal to 1%)........ 2026
Mircette Tablets 1066
Moduretic Tablets (Less than or equal to 1%)........ 2028
Myobloc Injection (2% or greater) 3192
Naprosyn Suspension 2761
Naprosyn Tablets 2761
▲ Neoral Oral Solution (4% to 19.8%)........ 2259
▲ Neoral Soft Gelatin Capsules (4% to 19.8%)........ 2259
Neurontin Capsules (Infrequent) 2487
Neurontin Oral Solution (Infrequent)........ 2487
Neurontin Tablets (Infrequent) 2487
Nexium Delayed-Release Capsules (Less than 1%)........ 655
Nexium I.V. (Less than 1%) 659
Nimotop Capsules (Up to 2.4%) 749
Nipent for Injection 1863
Norvir (Less than 2%) 503
NuvaRing 2340
Omacor Capsules 2725
Omnicef Capsules 511
Omnicef for Oral Suspension 511
Ortho-Cyclen/Ortho Tri-Cyclen 2429
Ortho Tri-Cyclen Lo Tablets 2436
Oxsoralen-Ultra Capsules 3353
OxyContin Tablets (Less than 1%) 2703
▲ Pancrease MT Capsules (Among most frequent)........ 1885
▲ Plavix Tablets (About 27.1%) 917
▲ Plavix Tablets (About 27.1%) 2926
▲ Precose Tablets (Among most common)........ 751
Prevacid Delayed-Release Capsules (Less than 1%)........ 3271
Prevacid for Delayed-Release Oral Suspension (Less than 1%)........ 3271
Prevacid SoluTab Delayed-Release Orally Disintegrating Tablets (Less than 1%)........ 3271
Prevacid NapraPAC (Less than 1%) .. 3280
PREVPAC (Less than 1%) 3284
Prinzide Tablets (0.3% to 1%)........ 2056
Proleukin for Injection (Less than 1%)........ 2266
Protonix I.V. (Greater than or equal to 1%)........ 3472
Protonix Tablets (Greater than or equal to 1%)........ 3469
Protopic Ointment (0.2% to less than 1%)........ 638
Provigil Tablets (At least 1%) 988
Relpax Tablets (Infrequent)........ 2548
Rescriptor Tablets 2551
▲ Retrovir Capsules (20%) 1560
▲ Retrovir IV Infusion (20%) 1564
▲ Retrovir (20%) 1560
Reyataz Capsules (Less than 3%) 921
Seasonique Tablets 1077
▲ Simulect for Injection (3% to 10%) ... 2284
▲ Skelaxin Tablets (Most frequent) 1716
▲ Spiriva HandiHaler (1% to 3%) 869
St. Joseph 81 mg Aspirin Chewable and Enteric Coated Tablets........ 1869
Stalevo Tablets (1%) 2287
Striant Mucoadhesive 1007
▲ Suprax (30%) 1843
Taxotere Injection Concentrate 2932
Tessalon Capsules 1199
Tessalon Perles 1199
Thalomid Capsules 965
▲ Ticlid Tablets (30% to 40%) 2810
Timoptic-XE Sterile Ophthalmic Gel Forming Solution 2092
Topamax Sprinkle Capsules (1%) 2404

Topamax Tablets (1%) 2404
Toprol-XL Tablets 668
Tranxene (Less common) 2474
Travatan Ophthalmic Solution (1% to 5%) 563
Trecator Tablets 3487
Tricor Tablets 527
Triglide Tablets 3123
▲ Ultrase Capsules (Most frequent) 708
Uroqid-Acid No. 2 Tablets 760
▲ Urso 250 Tablets (5%) 710
▲ Urso Forte Tablets (5%) 710
Vantin Tablets and Oral Suspension 2645
▲ Vesanoid Capsules (26%) 2820
Viokase 711
▲ Vivitrol (12% to 13%) 995
▲ Xenical Capsules (Among most frequent) 2831
Yaz Tablets 803
Zinacef for Injection (1 in 150 patients) 1631
Zinacef Injection (1 in 150 patients) 1631
Zomig Nasal Spray (Infrequent) 3523
Zosyn 3492

Gastrointestinal disorders, unspecified
▲ Focalin XR Capsules (28% to 44%) 2223
▲ Hycamtin for Injection (63%) 1458
Merrem I.V. (Greater than 1%) 686
▲ Vivaglobin (0.1% to 37%) 3506

Gastrointestinal fistula
▲ Entocort EC Capsules (Less than 5%) 2698

Gastrointestinal impaction
Lotronex Tablets 1512

Gastrointestinal infarction
Zomig Nasal Spray (Very rare) 3523

Gastrointestinal inflammation
Arthrotec Tablets 3129
Mobic Oral Suspension 863
Mobic Tablets 863
Voltaren Tablets 2307

Gastrointestinal motility, decreased
Enablex Extended-Release Tablets 2203
Lotronex Tablets (Rare) 1512

Gastrointestinal neoplasm, benign
Arthrotec Tablets (Rare) 3129

Gastrointestinal obstruction
K-Dur Extended-Relase Tablets 3033
K-Tab Tablets 475
Lotronex Tablets (Rare) 1512
Sandostatin Injection (Rare) 2278

Gastrointestinal perforation
Aggrenox Capsules (Less than 1%) 822
▲ Anaprox Tablets (Approximately 1% to 4%) 2761
▲ Anaprox DS Tablets (Approximately 1% to 4%) 2761
Arthrotec Tablets 3129
Avastin IV 1227
Bayer Aspirin 744
CellCept Capsules (Rare) 2747
CellCept Intravenous (Rare) 2747
CellCept Oral Suspension (Rare) 2747
CellCept Tablets (Rare) 2747
Clinoril Tablets (Rare) 1924
Dolobid Tablets (Less than 1 in 100) 1955
▲ EC-Naprosyn Delayed-Release Tablets (Approximately 1% to 4%) 2761
Gleevec Tablets (Rare) 2227
Indocin Capsules (Approximately 1%) 1995
Indocin I.V. 2465
Indocin (Approximately 1%) 1995
K-Dur Extended-Relase Tablets 3033
K-Tab Tablets 475
Lotronex Tablets 1512
Mobic Oral Suspension 863
Mobic Tablets 863
▲ Naprosyn Suspension (Approximately 1% to 4%) 2761
▲ Naprosyn Tablets (Approximately 1% to 4%) 2761
Prevacid NapraPAC (Less than 1%) 3280
▲ Prograf Capsules and Injection (3%) 632
St. Joseph 81 mg Aspirin Chewable and Enteric Coated Tablets 1869
Taxotere Injection Concentrate 2932
▲ Voltaren Tablets (1% to 10%) 2307
▲ Voltaren-XR Tablets (1% to 10%) 2310

Gastrointestinal reactions
(*see under* Gastrointestinal disorders)

Gastrointestinal reflux
Arthrotec Tablets (Rare) 3129
Lotronex Tablets (Rare) 1512
Nexavar Tablets (Uncommon) 746

Gastrointestinal symptoms
(*see under* Gastrointestinal disorders)

Gastrointestinal toxicity
Alkeran for Injection 955
Alkeran Tablets 956
Anaprox Tablets 2761
Anaprox DS Tablets 2761
EC-Naprosyn Delayed-Release Tablets 2761
I.V. Busulfex (Frequent) 2493
Naprosyn Suspension 2761
Naprosyn Tablets 2761

Gastrointestinal upset
(*see under* Gastrointestinal disorders)

Genital abnormalities
▲ Pexeva Tablets (2% to 10%) 1694
Vesanoid Capsules 2820

Genital bacterial growth, asymptomatic
▲ Estring (4%) 2635

Genital malformation
Thalomid Capsules 965

Genital moniliasis
Augmentin XR Extended-Release Tablets (2.1%) 1369
▲ Estring Vaginal Ring (6%) 2635
Keflex Capsules 549
Levaquin (0.1% to 0.9%) 2384
Levaquin in 5% Dextrose Injection (0.1% to 0.9%) 2384
Topamax Sprinkle Capsules (Greater than 1%) 2404
Topamax Tablets (Greater than 1%) 2404

Genitalia, male, external, abnormalities of
Propecia Tablets 2060
Proscar Tablets 2067

Genitourinary disturbances
Adalat CC Tablets (Less than 1%) 2964
Dalmane Capsules 3342
Eulexin Capsules (2%) 3009
▲ Hycamtin for Injection (36%) 1458
▲ Leukine (50%) 814
▲ Nipent for Injection (Up to 15%) 1863
▲ Paxil CR Controlled-Release Tablets (3%) 1538
▲ Paxil (3%) 1530
Tranxene 2474

Germinal aplasia
Mustargen for Injection 2468

GGTP, elevation
(*see under* Gamma-glutamyl transpeptidase, elevation)

Giardiasis
Colazal Capsules 2838

Giddiness
(*see under* Dizziness)

Gingival disorder, unspecified
Adalat CC Tablets (Less than 1%) 2964
Cubicin for Injection (Less than 1%) 1026
Xenical Capsules (2%) 2831
Xifaxan Tablets (Less than 2%) 2842

Gingival hyperplasia
Adalat CC Tablets (Rare) 2964
Caduet Tablets (Greater than 0.1% to less than or equal to 1%) 2508
Cardizem LA Extended Release Tablets (Infrequent) 1728
▲ CellCept Capsules (3% to less than 20%) 2747
▲ CellCept Intravenous (3% to less than 20%) 2747
▲ CellCept Oral Suspension (3% to less than 20%) 2747
▲ CellCept Tablets (3% to less than 20%) 2747
Covera-HS Tablets (Less than 2%) 3139
Evoxac Capsules 1047
Gabitril Tablets (Infrequent) 984
▲ Gengraf Capsules (4% to 16%) 459
▲ Intron A for Injection (Less than 5%) 3024
Lamictal (Infrequent) 1481
▲ Myfortic Tablets (3% to less than 20%) 2255
▲ Neoral Oral Solution (3.8% to 16%) 2259
▲ Neoral Soft Gelatin Capsules (3.8% to 16%) 2259
Norvasc Tablets (More than 0.1% to 1%) 2545
Phenytek Capsules 2160
Rapamune Oral Solution and Tablets 3475
▲ Sandimmune (4% to 16%) 2275
▲ Simulect for Injection (3% to 10%) 2284
Soriatane Capsules (Less than 1%) 1013
Sular Tablets (Less than or equal to 1%) 3122
Tarka Tablets 524
Tiazac Capsules (Infrequent) 1201
Topamax Sprinkle Capsules (Infrequent to 1%) 2404
Topamax Tablets (Infrequent to 1%) 2404
Trileptal Tablets 2300
Trileptal Oral Suspension 2300
Verelan PM Extended-Release Capsules, Controlled-Onset (2% or less) 3106
VFEND I.V. (Less than 2%) 2564
VFEND Oral Suspension (Less than 2%) 2564
VFEND Tablets (Less than 2%) 2564
Zoloft (Rare) 2586
Zonegran Capsules (Infrequent) 1101

Gingivitis
Abilify Oral Solution (Infrequent) 882
Abilify Oral Solution (Infrequent) 2450
Abilify Discmelt Orally Disintegrating Tablets (Infrequent) 882
Abilify Discmelt Orally Disintegrating Tablets (Infrequent) 2450
Abilify Tablets (Infrequent) 882
Abilify Tablets (Infrequent) 2450
Accutane Capsules 2731
Aciphex Tablets 1090
Actiq (1% or greater) 979
Aricept Tablets (Infrequent) 1094
Aricept ODT Tablets (Infrequent) 1094
Azilect Tablets (2%) 3293
Campath Ampules 811
Celexa (Infrequent) 1176
▲ CellCept Capsules (3% to less than 20%) 2747
▲ CellCept Intravenous (3% to less than 20%) 2747
▲ CellCept Oral Suspension (3% to less than 20%) 2747
▲ CellCept Tablets (3% to less than 20%) 2747
Chantix Tablets (Frequent) 2517
Copaxone for Injection (At least 2%) 3297
Cymbalta Delayed-Release Capsules (Infrequent) 1757
▲ Doxil Injection (1% to 10%) 2351
Effexor Tablets (Infrequent) 3411
Effexor XR Capsules (Infrequent) 3417
▲ Eloxatin for Injection (2% to 5%) 2892
Evoxac Capsules (Less than 1%) 1047
Exelon Capsules (Infrequent) 2206
Exelon Oral Solution (Infrequent) 2206
Gabitril Tablets (Frequent) 984
Gengraf Capsules 459
▲ Intron A for Injection (Up to 14%) 3024
Invirase (Less than 2%) 2772
Keppra Injection 3320
Keppra Oral Solution (1% or more) 3314
Keppra Tablets (1% or more) 3314
Klonopin 2778
Lamictal (Infrequent) 1481
Lupron Depot-PED 7.5 mg, 11.25 mg and 15 mg (Less than 2%) 3269
Lupron Injection Pediatric (Less than 2%) 3259
Neoral Oral Solution 2259
Neoral Soft Gelatin Capsules 2259
Neurontin Capsules (Frequent) 2487
Neurontin Oral Solution (Frequent) 2487
Neurontin Tablets (Frequent) 2487
▲ Nipent for Injection (3% to 10%) 1863
Norvir (Less than 2%) 503
Paxil CR Controlled-Release Tablets (Rare) 1538
Paxil (Rare) 1530
Permax Tablets (Infrequent) 3356
Pexeva Tablets (infrequent) 1694
Protonix I.V. (Less than 1%) 3472
Protonix Tablets (Less than 1%) 3469
Provigil Tablets (1%) 988
▲ Rapamune Oral Solution and Tablets (3% to 20%) 3475
Relpax Tablets (Rare) 2548
Requip Tablets (1% or more) 1555
Rescriptor Tablets 2551
Risperdal (Rare) 1676
Risperdal Consta Long-Acting Injection (Infrequent) 1682
Risperdal M-Tab Orally Disintegrating Tablets (Rare) 1676
Sandostatin LAR Depot (1% to 4%) 2280
Seroquel Tablets (Infrequent) 690
Sonata Capsules (Infrequent) 1717
▲ Soriatane Capsules (1% to 10%) 1013
Striant Mucoadhesive 1007
Symbyax Capsules (Infrequent) 1819
Targretin Capsules 1747
Tequin Injection (Less than 0.1%) 938
Tequin Injection in 5% Dextrose (Less than 0.1%) 938
Tequin Tablets (Less than 0.1%) 938
Teveten Tablets (Less than 1%) 1735
Teveten HCT Tablets (Less than 1%) 1737
Topamax Sprinkle Capsules (1%) 2404
Topamax Tablets (1%) 2404
Uniretic Tablets (Less than 1%) 3100
Vandazole Vaginal Gel (Less than 1%) 3338
VFEND I.V. (Less than 2%) 2564
VFEND Oral Suspension (Less than 2%) 2564
VFEND Tablets (Less than 2%) 2564
Viagra Tablets (Less than 2%) 2573
Wellbutrin SR Sustained-Release Tablets (Infrequent) 1607
Wellbutrin XL Extended-Release Tablets (Infrequent) 1613
Zelapar Tablets 3372
Zomig Nasal Spray (Rare) 3523
Zonegran Capsules (Infrequent) 1101
Zyban Sustained-Release Tablets (Infrequent) 1644
Zyprexa Tablets (Infrequent) 1830
Zyprexa ZYDIS Orally Disintegrating Tablets (Infrequent) 1830

Gingivostomatitis
Cuprimine Capsules (Rare) 1947

Glassy-eyed appearance
Klonopin 2778

Glaucoma
(*see also under* IOP, elevation of)
Aciphex Tablets 1090
Advair Diskus 100/50 1308
Advair Diskus 250/50 1308
Advair Diskus 500/50 1308
Advair HFA Inhalation Aerosol 1318
Ambien Tablets (Rare) 2851
Ambien CR Tablets (Rare) 2855
Aricept Tablets (Infrequent) 1094
Aricept ODT Tablets (Infrequent) 1094
Arthrotec Tablets (Rare) 3129
Azmacort Inhalation Aerosol (Rare) 1726
Beconase AQ Nasal Spray (Rare) 1396
Blephamide Ophthalmic Ointment (A possibility) 568
Blephamide Ophthalmic Suspension 569
Celebrex Capsules (0.1% to 1.9%) 3134
Clozaril Tablets 2184
Colocort Rectal Suspension, USP (Retention) 100 mg/60 mL 2476
Cymbalta Delayed-Release Capsules (Infrequent) 1757
Decadron Tablets 1951
Depo-Medrol Injectable Suspension 2617
Depo-Medrol Single-Dose Vial 2619
Effexor XR Capsules (Rare) 3417
Evoxac Capsules (Less than 1%) 1047
Exelon Capsules (Infrequent) 2206
Exelon Oral Solution (Infrequent) 2206
Flonase Nasal Spray 1440
FML Forte Ophthalmic Suspension ⊙226
Hydrocortone Tablets 1989

Levitra Tablets (Less than 2%).......... 3034
Lipitor Tablets (Less than 2%)........... 2483
▲ Lucentis Injection (8% to 24%) 1237
▲ Macugen Injection (10% to 40%) .... ⊙ 261
Midamor Tablets (Less than or equal to 1%)................................ 2026
Mirapex Tablets (Less than 1%)........ 859
Moduretic Tablets.......................... 2028
Namenda (Infrequent)...................... 1195
Neurontin Capsules (Rare)................ 2487
Neurontin Oral Solution (Rare).......... 2487
Neurontin Tablets (Rare).................. 2487
Pexeva Tablets (rare)...................... 1694
Poly-Pred Ophthalmic Suspension... ⊙ 233
Pred-G Ophthalmic Ointment.............. ⊙ 237
Pred-G Ophthalmic Suspension....... ⊙ 236
Protonix I.V. (Less than 1%)............ 3472
Protonix Tablets (Less than 1%)....... 3469
Prozac Pulvules and Liquid (Rare)..... 1801
Pulmicort Respules (Rare)............... 661
Requip Tablets (Infrequent) 1555
▲ Retisert Implant (50% to 90%) .... ⊙ 258
Rilutek Tablets (Rare) 2930
Sandostatin LAR Depot (Rare) 2280
Seroquel Tablets (Rare) 690
Sonata Capsules (Rare) 1717
Sular Tablets (Less than or equal to 1%) 3122
Tasmar Tablets (Rare) 3358
TobraDex Ophthalmic Ointment 562
TobraDex Ophthalmic Suspension 563
Uniretic Tablets (Less than 1%) 3100
Viroptic Ophthalmic Solution .... ⊙ 266
Zelapar Tablets 3372
Zoloft (Rare) 2586
Zonegran Capsules (Infrequent) 1101
Zyprexa Tablets (Rare) 1830
Zyprexa ZYDIS Orally Disintegrating Tablets (Rare) 1830
Zyrtec Chewable Tablets (Less than 2%) 2594
Zyrtec (Less than 2%) 2594

Glaucoma, angle closure precipitation

Atrovent Nasal Spray 0.03% 837
Atrovent Nasal Spray 0.06% 839
BOTOX Purified Neurotoxin Complex (One report) 570
Combivent Inhalation Aerosol 847
DuoNeb Inhalation Solution 1058
Effexor Tablets 3411
Transderm Scōp Transdermal Therapeutic System (Infrequent) ... 2177

Glaucoma, corticosteroid-induced

Blephamide Ophthalmic Suspension 569
FML Ophthalmic Ointment .... ⊙ 228
FML Ophthalmic Suspension .... ⊙ 227
FML Forte Ophthalmic Suspension .... ⊙ 226
FML-S Ophthalmic Suspension .... ⊙ 229
Poly-Pred Ophthalmic Suspension ... ⊙ 233
Pred Mild Ophthalmic Suspension ... ⊙ 238
Pred Forte Ophthalmic Suspension .... ⊙ 235
Pred-G Ophthalmic Suspension .... ⊙ 236
TobraDex Ophthalmic Ointment 562
TobraDex Ophthalmic Suspension 563

Glaucoma, narrow-angle

Atrovent HFA Inhalation Aerosol 841
FazaClo Orally Disintegrating Tablets 551

Glaucoma, secondary

Topamax Sprinkle Capsules 2404
Topamax Tablets 2404

Glaucoma, worsening of narrow angle

Atrovent Inhalation Solution 835
Atrovent HFA Inhalation Aerosol 841
Atrovent Nasal Spray 0.03% 837
Atrovent Nasal Spray 0.06% 839
Combivent Inhalation Aerosol 847
DuoNeb Inhalation Solution 1058

Globus hystericus

Daranide Tablets 1950
Imitrex Injection (Rare) 1463

Glomerular filtration rate, decrease

Captopril Tablets 2149

Glomerulitis

Lyrica Capsules (Rare) 2539

Glomerulonephritis

Accutane Capsules 2731
Anaprox Tablets (Less than 1%)....... 2761
Anaprox DS Tablets (Less than 1%).. 2761
Cuprimine Capsules........................ 1947
EC-Naprosyn Delayed-Release Tablets (Less than 1%)................. 2761
Fuzeon Injection............................. 2767
Naprosyn Suspension (Less than 1%).. 2761
Naprosyn Tablets (Less than 1%)..... 2761
Orthoclone OKT3 Sterile Solution..... 2360
Prevacid NapraPAC (Less than 1%).. 3280
Zyrtec Chewable Tablets (Rare)........ 2594
Zyrtec (Rare) 2594
Zyrtec-D 12 Hour Extended Release Tablets (Rare)................. 2597

Glomerulonephropathy, membranous

Enbrel for Injection (Infrequent)......... 584

Glomerulopathy

Herceptin I.V. (Rare)........................ 1233
Plavix Tablets 917
Plavix Tablets 2926

Glossitis

Abilify Oral Solution (Rare) 882
Abilify Oral Solution (Rare) 2450
Abilify Discmelt Orally Disintegrating Tablets (Rare) 882
Abilify Discmelt Orally Disintegrating Tablets (Rare) 2450
Abilify Tablets (Rare) 882
Abilify Tablets (Rare) 2450
Aciphex Tablets 1090
Actiq (1% or greater) 979
Actonel with Calcium Tablets (0.1% to 1%) 2688
Aerobid/Aerobid-M (1% to 3%) 1171
Anaprox Tablets (Less than 1%) 2761
Anaprox DS Tablets (Less than 1%) .. 2761
Arthrotec Tablets (Rare) 3129
Astelin Nasal Spray (Infrequent) 1904
Augmentin 1360
Augmentin Tablets 1363
Augmentin XR Extended-Release Tablets 1369
Augmentin ES-600 Powder for Oral Suspension 1366
Avelox (0.1% to less than 2%) 2970
Betoptic S Ophthalmic Suspension (Rare) 558
Biaxin/Biaxin XL 402
Caduet Tablets (Less than 2%) 2508
Captopril Tablets 2149
Carbatrol Capsules 3171
Celexa (Rare) 1176
Clinoril Tablets (Less than 1%) 1924
Colazal Capsules 2838
Cuprimine Capsules 1947
Daraprim Tablets 1419
Depacon Injection (1% or more) 412
Depakene (1% or more) 417
Depakote Sprinkle Capsules 422
▲ Depakote Tablets (1% to 5%) 427
Depakote ER Tablets (Greater than 1%) 434
Didronel Tablets 2697
▲ Doxil Injection (1% to 5%) 2351
EC-Naprosyn Delayed-Release Tablets (Less than 1%) 2761
Effexor Tablets (Infrequent) 3411
Effexor XR Capsules (Infrequent) 3417
▲ Entocort EC Capsules (Less than 5%) 2698
Equetro Extended-Release Capsules 3180
Evoxac Capsules (Less than 1%) 1047
Exelon Capsules (Infrequent) 2206
Exelon Oral Solution (Infrequent) 2206
Fansidar Tablets 2765
Gabitril Tablets (Infrequent) 984
Gantrisin Pediatric Suspension 2770
Gengraf Capsules (1% to less than 3%) 459
▲ Imdur Tablets (Less than or equal to 5%) 3018
Invirase (Less than 2%) 2772
Ketek Tablets (Greater than or equal to 0.2% to less than 2%) 2903
Lamictal (Infrequent) 1481
Lipitor Tablets (Less than 2%) 2483
Lupron Depot 3.75 mg 3260
Lupron Depot–3 Month 11.25 mg 3265
Maxair Autohaler 1852
Merrem I.V. (1.0%) 686
Myobloc Injection (Greater than 2%) 3192
Naprosyn Suspension (Less than 1%) 2761
Naprosyn Tablets (Less than 1%) 2761
Neoral Oral Solution (1% to less than 3%) 2259
Neoral Soft Gelatin Capsules (1% to less than 3%)........................... 2259
Neurontin Capsules (Infrequent)....... 2487
Neurontin Oral Solution (Infrequent)................................... 2487
Neurontin Tablets (Infrequent).......... 2487
Nipent for Injection (Less than 3%)... 1863
Oracea Capsules............................ 1000
Paxil CR Controlled-Release Tablets (Infrequent)...................... 1538
Paxil (Infrequent)............................ 1530
Permax Tablets (Rare)..................... 3356
Pexeva Tablets (Infrequent).............. 1694
Prevacid Delayed-Release Capsules (Less than 1%).............. 3271
Prevacid for Delayed-Release Oral Suspension (Less than 1%).......... 3271
Prevacid SoluTab Delayed-Release Orally Disintegrating Tablets (Less than 1%)............................ 3271
Prevacid NapraPAC (Less than 1%).. 3280
PREVPAC (Less than 1%) 3284
Primaxin I.M................................. 2045
Primaxin I.V. (Less than 0.2%).......... 2048
ProAir HFA Inhalation Aerosol (Less than 3%)............................ 3300
Protonix I.V. (Less than 1%)............. 3472
Protonix Tablets (Less than 1%) 3469
Prozac Pulvules and Liquid (Infrequent)................................... 1801
Relpax Tablets (Infrequent).............. 2548
Requip Tablets (Infrequent).............. 1555
Rilutek Tablets (Infrequent).............. 2930
Rythmol SR Capsules...................... 2727
▲ Sandostatin LAR Depot (1% to 4%).. 2280
Seroquel Tablets (Infrequent)........... 690
Solodyn Extended Release Tablets... 1890
Sonata Capsules (Infrequent)........... 1717
Soriatane Capsules (Less than 1%).. 1013
Sular Tablets (Less than or equal to 1%)... 3122
Tegretol/Tegretol-XR....................... 2295
▲ Tequin Injection (0.1% to 3%) 938
▲ Tequin Injection in 5% Dextrose (0.1% to 3%).............................. 938
▲ Tequin Tablets (0.1% to 3%) 938
Topamax Sprinkle Capsules (1%)..... 2404
Topamax Tablets (1%)..................... 2404
Uniretic Tablets (Less than 1%)........ 3100
Vasotec I.V. Injection (0.5% to 1.0%)... 2103
VFEND I.V. (Less than 2%)............... 2564
VFEND Oral Suspension (Less than 2%)... 2564
VFEND Tablets (Less than 2%)......... 2564
Viagra Tablets (Less than 2%).......... 2573
Vicoprofen Tablets (Less than 1%).... 539
Voltaren Tablets (Occasionally)......... 2307
Voltaren-XR Tablets (Occasionally).... 2310
Wellbutrin Tablets (Rare).................. 1603
Wellbutrin SR Sustained-Release Tablets (Infrequent)...................... 1607
Wellbutrin XL Extended-Release Tablets (Infrequent)...................... 1613
Zoloft (Rare)................................... 2586
Zonegran Capsules (Infrequent)....... 1101
Zyban Sustained-Release Tablets (Infrequent)................................ 1644
Zyprexa Tablets (Infrequent)............ 1830
Zyprexa ZYDIS Orally Disintegrating Tablets (Infrequent)................................ 1830

Glossodynia

Adenoscan (Less than 1%).............. 619
Aldoril Tablets................................ 1910
Clozaril Tablets (1%)....................... 2184
▲ Dacogen Injection (5%) 2129
▲ Imitrex Injection (4.9%) 1463
Imitrex Tablets............................... 1471
Nexavar Tablets (Common)............... 746
Rythmol SR Capsules...................... 2727
▲ Sutent Capsules (0% to 15%) 2560

Glossoncus

Altace Capsules............................. 1702
Ceftin Tablets (0.1% to 1%)............. 1407
Fluarix.. 1451
Fortical Nasal Spray....................... 3337
Maxalt Tablets............................... 2008
Maxalt-MLT Orally Disintegrating Tablets 2008
Miacalcin Injection (A few cases)...... 2252
Miacalcin Nasal Spray (Few reports)... 2253
Romazicon Injection (Less than 1%)... 2804
Tambocor Tablets (Less than 1%)..... 1856
Tamiflu Capsules............................ 2807
Tamiflu Oral Suspension.................. 2807

Glossoplegia

Risperdal (Rare)............................. 1676
Risperdal M-Tab Orally Disintegrating Tablets (Rare)......... 1676

Glossotrichia

Augmentin..................................... 1360
Augmentin Tablets.......................... 1363
Augmentin XR Extended-Release Tablets 1369
Augmentin ES-600 Powder for Oral Suspension 1366
Klonopin (Infrequent)...................... 2778
PREVPAC....................................... 3284

Glucocorticoids, decreased

Elocon Cream 0.1% (2 in 182 subjects)....................................... 3005
▲ Elocon Lotion 0.1% (4 in 65 subjects)....................................... 3006
Elocon Ointment 0.1% (1 in 63 patients)....................................... 3007

Glucocorticoids, increased

Evoxac Capsules (Less than 1%)...... 1047
Prevacid NapraPAC 3280

Glucose tolerance, changes

Celexa (Infrequent) 1176
Estratest Tablets 3199
Estratest H.S. Tablets 3199
Furosemide Tablets 2154
Oncaspar 1145
Premarin Intravenous 3442

Glucose tolerance, decreased

Decadron Tablets 1951
depo-subQ provera 104 Injectable Suspension 2624
Emcyt Capsules 2634
Kaletra (Less than 2%) 476
Lyrica Capsules (Rare) 2539
Niaspan Extended-Release Tablets ... 1730
Nutropin for Injection 1239
Nutropin AQ Injection 1243
Nutropin AQ Pen 1243
Nutropin AQ Pen Cartridge 1243
Ortho-Cyclen/Ortho Tri-Cyclen 2429
Ortho Tri-Cyclen Lo Tablets 2436
Oxandrin Tablets 2962
Premarin Intravenous 3442
Premarin Vaginal Cream 3452
Uniretic Tablets (Less than 1%) 3100
VFEND I.V. (Less than 2%) 2564
VFEND Oral Suspension (Less than 2%) 2564
VFEND Tablets (Less than 2%) 2564

Glucose tolerance, impaired

Megace ES Oral Suspension 2481
Menostar Transdermal System 782
▲ Norditropin Cartridges (6%) 2323
Premarin Tablets 3446
Premphase Tablets 3456
Prempro Tablets 3456

Glucosuria

Aclovate Cream 2660
Bumex Tablets (0.7%) 2746
Clobex Lotion 1204
Clobex Shampoo 1206
Clobex Spray 1208
Clorpres Tablets (Rare) 2153
Diprolene Gel 0.05% 3001
Diprolene Lotion 0.05% 3002
Diprolene Ointment 0.05% (Some patients) 3003
Diprolene AF Cream 0.05% (Some patients) 3000
Elspar for Injection (Low) 2463
Elspar for Injection (Low) 1960
Humatrope Vials and Cartridges (Infrequent) 1787
Lotrisone 3040
Norditropin Cartridges 2323
Olux Foam 1012
Temovate Cream 2668
Temovate Gel 2669
Temovate Ointment 2668
Temovate Scalp Application 2670
Vanos Cream 1893

Glycosuria

Abilify Oral Solution (Rare) 882
Abilify Oral Solution (Rare) 2450
Abilify Discmelt Orally Disintegrating Tablets (Rare) 882
Abilify Discmelt Orally Disintegrating Tablets (Rare) 2450
Abilify Tablets (Rare) 882
Abilify Tablets (Rare) 2450
Aldoril Tablets 1910
Aloprim for Injection (Less than 1%) 2167
Aloxi Injection (Less than 1%) 2127
Amerge Tablets (Rare) 1339

Arthrotec Tablets (Rare) 3129
Avalide Tablets 888
Avalide Tablets 2874
▲ Baraclude (4%) 894
Calcium Disodium Versenate Injection 1851
Carbatrol Capsules 3171
Clorpres Tablets 2153
▲ Coreg Tablets (Greater than 1% to 3%) 1414
Cutivate Lotion 0.05% (Rare) 2664
Decadron Tablets 1951
Diovan HCT Tablets 2196
Diprosone Cream, USP 0.05% 3004
Diuril Oral Suspension 1954
Diuril Sodium Intravenous 2467
Doxil Injection (Less than 1%) 2351
Dyazide Capsules 1423
Effexor Tablets (Rare) 3411
Effexor XR Capsules (Infrequent) 3417
Elocon Cream 0.1% 3005
Elocon Lotion 0.1% 3006
Elocon Ointment 0.1% 3007
Equetro Extended-Release Capsules 3180
Evoxac Capsules 1047
Furosemide Tablets 2154
Geodon Capsules (Infrequent) 2529
Hepsera Tablets (1%) 1292
Hyzaar 50-12.5 Tablets 1990
Hyzaar 100-12.5 Tablets 1990
Hyzaar 100-25 Tablets 1990
▲ Indapamide Tablets (Less than 5%) 2156
Indocin Capsules (Less than 1%) 1995
Indocin I.V. (Less than 1%) 2465
Indocin (Less than 1%) 1995
Lithobid Tablets 1692
Lopressor HCT 50/25 Tablets 2241
Lopressor HCT 100/25 Tablets 2241
Lopressor HCT 100/50 Tablets 2241
Lotensin HCT Tablets 2246
Micardis HCT Tablets 856
Moduretic Tablets 2028
Neurontin Capsules (Rare) 2487
Neurontin Oral Solution (Rare) 2487
Neurontin Tablets (Rare) 2487
Nexium Delayed-Release Capsules (Less than 1%) 655
Nexium I.V. (Less than 1%) 659
Noroxin Tablets (Less frequent) 2032
Norvir (Less than 2%) 503
Prevacid Delayed-Release Capsules (Less than 1%) 3271
Prevacid for Delayed-Release Oral Suspension 3271
Prevacid SoluTab Delayed-Release Orally Disintegrating Tablets (Less than 1%) 3271
Prevacid NapraPAC 3280
PREVPAC (Less than 1%) 3284
Prilosec OTC Delayed-Release Tablets (Less than 1%) 2677
Prograf Capsules and Injection 632
Protonix I.V. (Less than 1%) 3472
Protonix Tablets (Less than 1%) 3469
Prozac Pulvules and Liquid (Rare) 1801
▲ Rapamune Oral Solution and Tablets (3% to 20%) 3475
Requip Tablets (Infrequent) 1555
Risperdal Consta Long-Acting Injection (Infrequent) 1682
Rocephin Injectable Vials, ADD-Vantage, Galaxy, Bulk (Rare) 2800
Rythmol SR Capsules 2727
Seroquel Tablets (Infrequent) 690
Symbyax Capsules (Infrequent) 1819
Tegretol/Tegretol-XR 2295
Teveten Tablets (Less than 1%) 1735
Teveten HCT Tablets (Less than 1%) 1737
Thiothixene Capsules 2165
Timolide Tablets 2086
Ultane Liquid for Inhalation (Less than 1%) 531
Uniretic Tablets (Less than 1%) 3100
VFEND I.V. (Less than 2%) 2564
VFEND Oral Suspension (Less than 2%) 2564
VFEND Tablets (Less than 2%) 2564
Vicoprofen Tablets (Less than 1%) 539
Wellbutrin Tablets (Rare) 1603
Wellbutrin SR Sustained-Release Tablets 1607
Wellbutrin XL Extended-Release Tablets 1613
Zegerid Capsules (Less than 1%) 2958
Zegerid Powder for Oral Solution (Less than 1%) 2958
Zyban Sustained-Release Tablets 1644

Goiter
Abilify Oral Solution (Rare) 882
Abilify Oral Solution (Rare) 2450
Abilify Discmelt Orally Disintegrating Tablets (Rare) 882
Abilify Discmelt Orally Disintegrating Tablets (Rare) 2450
Abilify Tablets (Rare) 882
Abilify Tablets (Rare) 2450
Aricept Tablets (Infrequent) 1094
Aricept ODT Tablets (Infrequent) 1094
Campral Tablets (Rare) 1174
Celexa (Rare) 1176
Copaxone for Injection (Infrequent) 3297
Effexor Tablets (Rare) 3411
Effexor XR Capsules (Rare) 3417
Evoxac Capsules (Less than 1%) 1047
Exelon Capsules (Infrequent) 2206
Exelon Oral Solution (Infrequent) 2206
Fortical Nasal Spray (Less than 1%) 3337
Gabitril Tablets (Infrequent) 984
Gantrisin Pediatric Suspension 2770
Gengraf Capsules (1% to less than 3%) 459
Lamictal (Rare) 1481
Meridia Capsules 489
Miacalcin Nasal Spray (Less than 1%) 2253
Neoral Oral Solution (1% to less than 3%) 2259
Neoral Soft Gelatin Capsules (1% to less than 3%) 2259
Neurontin Capsules (Rare) 2487
Neurontin Oral Solution (Rare) 2487
Neurontin Tablets (Rare) 2487
Nexium Delayed-Release Capsules (Less than 1%) 655
Nexium I.V. (Less than 1%) 659
Paxil CR Controlled-Release Tablets (Rare) 1538
Paxil (Rare) 1530
Pexeva Tablets (Rare) 1694
Prevacid Delayed-Release Capsules (Less than 1%) 3271
Prevacid for Delayed-Release Oral Suspension (Less than 1%) 3271
Prevacid SoluTab Delayed-Release Orally Disintegrating Tablets (Less than 1%) 3271
Prevacid NapraPAC (Less than 1%) 3280
PREVPAC (Less than 1%) 3284
Protonix I.V. (Less than 1%) 3472
Protonix Tablets (Less than 1%) 3469
Relpax Tablets (Rare) 2548
▲ Sandostatin Injection (6%) 2278
▲ Sandostatin LAR Depot (8%) 2280
Sonata Capsules (Rare) 1717
Uniretic Tablets (Less than 1%) 3100
Zyprexa Tablets (Infrequent) 1830
Zyprexa ZYDIS Orally Disintegrating Tablets (Infrequent) 1830

Goiter, euthyroid
Lithobid Tablets 1692
Zomig Nasal Spray (Rare) 3523

Goiter production
(*see under* Goiter)

Gonadotropin secretion, inhibition
▲ Androxy Tablets (Most Common) 3335
▲ Estratest Tablets (Among most common) 3199
▲ Estratest H.S. Tablets (Among most common) 3199
Oxandrin Tablets 2962

Goodpasture's syndrome
Campath Ampules 811
Cuprimine Capsules 1947

Goosebumps
(*see under* Piloerection)

Gout
Abilify Oral Solution (Rare) 882
Abilify Oral Solution (Rare) 2450
Abilify Discmelt Orally Disintegrating Tablets (Rare) 882
Abilify Discmelt Orally Disintegrating Tablets (Rare) 2450
Abilify Tablets (Rare) 882
Abilify Tablets (Rare) 2450
Aceon Tablets (2 mg, 4 mg, 8 mg) (0.3% to 1%) 3194
Aciphex Tablets 1090
Adalat CC Tablets (Less than 1%) 2964
Advicor Tablets 1722
Ambien Tablets (Rare) 2851
Ambien CR Tablets (Rare) 2855
Aricept Tablets (Infrequent) 1094
Aricept ODT Tablets (Infrequent) 1094
Arthrotec Tablets (Rare) 3129
Asacol Delayed-Release Tablets 2692
Avalide Tablets 888
Avalide Tablets 2874
Avapro Tablets (Less than 1%) 891
Avapro Tablets (Less than 1%) 2871
Caduet Tablets (Less than 2%) 2508
Campral Tablets (Infrequent) 1174
▲ CellCept Capsules (3% to less than 20%) 2747
▲ CellCept Intravenous (3% to less than 20%) 2747
▲ CellCept Oral Suspension (3% to less than 20%) 2747
▲ CellCept Tablets (3% to less than 20%) 2747
Cipro (Less than 1%) 2977
Cipro I.V. (1% or less) 2984
Clorpres Tablets 2153
Copaxone for Injection (Infrequent) 3297
▲ Coreg Tablets (Greater than 1% to 3%) 1414
Cozaar Tablets (Less than 1%) 1935
Demadex Injection 2759
Demadex Tablets 2759
Diovan HCT Tablets (Less frequent) 2196
Edecrin 1959
Effexor Tablets (Rare) 3411
Effexor XR Capsules (Rare) 3417
Evoxac Capsules 1047
Exelon Capsules (Infrequent) 2206
Exelon Oral Solution (Infrequent) 2206
Furosemide Tablets 2154
Geodon Capsules (Rare) 2529
Gleevec Tablets (Infrequent) 2227
Hytrin Capsules (At least 1%) 471
Hyzaar 50-12.5 Tablets 1990
Hyzaar 100-12.5 Tablets 1990
Hyzaar 100-25 Tablets 1990
Invanz for Injection (Greater than 0.1%) 1999
Klonopin (Infrequent) 2778
Levaquin (0.1% to 0.9%) 2384
Levaquin in 5% Dextrose Injection (0.1% to 0.9%) 2384
Lexapro Oral Solution (Infrequent) 1190
Lexapro Tablets (Infrequent) 1190
Lipitor Tablets (Less than 2%) 2483
Lofibra Tablets 1219
Lofibra Capsules 1216
Lopressor HCT 50/25 Tablets (1%) 2241
Lopressor HCT 100/25 Tablets (1%) 2241
Lopressor HCT 100/50 Tablets (1%) 2241
Lotensin HCT Tablets (0.3% to 1%) 2246
Lotrel Capsules (Infrequent) 2249
Lunesta Tablets (Rare) 3142
Mavik Tablets (0.3% to 1.0%) 486
Micardis Tablets (More than 0.3%) 854
Micardis HCT Tablets 856
Moduretic Tablets (Less than or equal to 1%) 2028
Neurontin Capsules (Infrequent) 2487
Neurontin Oral Solution (Infrequent) 2487
Neurontin Tablets (Infrequent) 2487
Niaspan Extended-Release Tablets 1730
Nipent for Injection (Less than 3%) 1863
Norvir (Less than 2%) 503
Paxil CR Controlled-Release Tablets (Rare) 1538
Paxil (Rare) 1530
PEG-Intron Powder for Injection (Less than or equal to 1%) 3048
Permax Tablets (Infrequent) 3356
Pexeva Tablets (rare) 1694
Plavix Tablets (1% to 2.5%) 917
Plavix Tablets (1% to 2.5%) 2926
Pletal Tablets (Less than 2%) 2455
Prevacid Delayed-Release Capsules (Less than 1%) 3271
Prevacid for Delayed-Release Oral Suspension (Less than 1%) 3271
Prevacid SoluTab Delayed-Release Orally Disintegrating Tablets (Less than 1%) 3271
Prevacid NapraPAC (Less than 1%) 3280
PREVPAC (Less than 1%) 3284
Prinivil Tablets (0.3% to 1.0%) 2052
Prinzide Tablets 2056
Proquin XR Tablets 1153
Protonix I.V. (Less than 1%) 3472
Protonix Tablets (Less than 1%) 3469
Prozac Pulvules and Liquid (Infrequent) 1801
Requip Tablets (1% or more) 1555
Revlimid Capsules 958
Reyataz Capsules (Less than 3%) 921
Rilutek Tablets (Infrequent) 2930
Rythmol SR Capsules 2727
Sandostatin LAR Depot (1% to 4%) 2280
Seroquel Tablets (Infrequent) 690
Sonata Capsules (Infrequent) 1717
Sular Tablets (Less than or equal to 1%) 3122
Symbyax Capsules (Rare) 1819
Tarka Tablets (Less frequent) 524
Teveten Tablets (Less than 1%) 1735
Teveten HCT Tablets (Less than 1%) 1737
Tiazac Capsules (1% to 2%) 1201
Timolide Tablets 2086
Tricor Tablets 527
Triglide Tablets 3123
Uniretic Tablets (Less than 1%) 3100
Vantin Tablets and Oral Suspension (Less than 1%) 2645
Viagra Tablets (Less than 2%) 2573
Zelapar Tablets 3372
Zyprexa Tablets (Rare) 1830
Zyprexa ZYDIS Orally Disintegrating Tablets (Rare) 1830

Gout, exacerbation of
Cipro XR Tablets 2990

Graft dysfunction, primary
Prograf Capsules and Injection 632

Graft loss
▲ Rapamune Oral Solution and Tablets (3.4% to 6.3%) 3475

Graft versus host reaction
▲ I.V. Busulfex (18%) 2493
▲ Valcyte Tablets (24%) 2813
VFEND I.V. (Less than 2%) 2564
VFEND Oral Suspension (Less than 2%) 2564
VFEND Tablets (Less than 2%) 2564

Granulocytopenia
Albenza Tablets (Rare) 1338
Aldoril Tablets 1910
Anaprox Tablets (Less than 1%) 2761
Anaprox DS Tablets (Less than 1%) 2761
▲ Aredia for Injection (19.8%) 2179
Celexa (Rare) 1176
Colazal Capsules 2838
Dalmane Capsules (Rare) 3342
EC-Naprosyn Delayed-Release Tablets (Less than 1%) 2761
Evoxac Capsules (Less than 1%) 1047
Garamycin Injectable 3014
Gris-PEG Tablets 2502
▲ Humira Injection (Less than 5%) 466
▲ Infergen (23% to 42%) 3364
▲ Intron A for Injection (Less than 5%) 3024
▲ I.V. Busulfex (100%) 2493
Levaquin (0.1% to 0.9%) 2384
Levaquin in 5% Dextrose Injection (0.1% to 0.9%) 2384
Mefoxin for Injection 2012
Mefoxin Premixed Intravenous Solution 2016
Mustargen for Injection 2468
Naprosyn Suspension (Less than 1%) 2761
Naprosyn Tablets (Less than 1%) 2761
▲ Neulasta Injection (15% to 72%) 601
Omnicef Capsules 511
Omnicef for Oral Suspension 511
Phenytek Capsules (Occasional) 2160
Plavix Tablets (Less than 1%) 917
Plavix Tablets (Less than 1%) 2926
Pletal Tablets (Very rare) 2455
Prevacid NapraPAC (Less than 1%) 3280
▲ Retrovir Capsules (1.8% to 47%) 1560
▲ Retrovir IV Infusion (1.8% to 47%) 1564
▲ Retrovir (1.8% to 47%) 1560
Revlimid Capsules (2%) 958
Risperdal Consta Long-Acting Injection (Rare) 1682
Thalomid Capsules 965
Topamax Sprinkle Capsules (Infrequent) 2404
Topamax Tablets (Infrequent) 2404
Viramune Oral Suspension 873
Viramune Tablets 873
▲ Xeloda Tablets (2% to 86%) 2822
Zantac (A few patients) 1624
Zantac Injection (Few patients) 1619
Zantac Injection Pharmacy Bulk Package (Infrequent) 1622
Zantac Injection Premixed (Few patients) 1619
Zantac (A few patients) 1624
Zinecard for Injection 2650
▲ Zometa for Intravenous Infusion (5% to 10%) 2315

Granulocytosis
Rescriptor Tablets ... 2551
Vantin Tablets and Oral Suspension ... 2645

Granuloma, subcutaneous
Fluorescite Injection ... ⊙207

Granuloma, unspecified
Actiq (Less than 1%) ... 979
Lyrica Capsules (Rare) ... 2539
VFEND I.V. (Less than 2%) ... 2564
VFEND Oral Suspension (Less than 2%) ... 2564
VFEND Tablets (Less than 2%) ... 2564

Granulomatosis, Wegener's
Accutane Capsules ... 2731

Grave's Disease
Campath Ampules ... 811

Groin pain
Ferrlecit Injection ... 3388

Growth, abnormal
Nutropin for Injection ... 1239
Nutropin AQ Injection ... 1243
Nutropin AQ Pen ... 1243
Nutropin AQ Pen Cartridge ... 1243

Growth, temporary slowing in
Adderall XR Capsules ... 3166
Concerta Extended-Release Tablets ... 1881

Growth rate, decrease
Adderall Tablets ... 3164
Advair HFA Inhalation Aerosol ... 1318
Rocaltrol Capsules ... 2798
Rocaltrol Oral Solution ... 2798
▲ Sandostatin Injection (37%) ... 2278

Growth retardation
Advair Diskus 100/50 ... 1308
Advair Diskus 250/50 ... 1308
Advair Diskus 500/50 ... 1308
Cosmegen for Injection ... 2459
Elocon Cream 0.1% ... 3005
Elocon Lotion 0.1% ... 3006
Elocon Ointment 0.1% ... 3007
Hectorol Capsules ... 1275
Hectorol Injection ... 1278
Herceptin I.V. (At least one of the 958 patients) ... 1233
Lotrisone Cream ... 3040
Phenytek Capsules ... 2160

Growth retardation, intrauterine
Altace Capsules ... 1702
Captopril Tablets ... 2149
Cozaar Tablets ... 1935
Hyzaar 50-12.5 Tablets ... 1990
Hyzaar 100-12.5 Tablets ... 1990
Hyzaar 100-25 Tablets ... 1990
Prinivil Tablets ... 2052
Prinzide Tablets ... 2056
Vasotec I.V. Injection ... 2103

Growth suppression
Azmacort Inhalation Aerosol ... 1726
Beconase AQ Nasal Spray ... 1396
Colocort Rectal Suspension, USP (Retention) 100 mg/60 mL ... 2476
Decadron Tablets ... 1951
Depo-Medrol Injectable Suspension ... 2617
Depo-Medrol Single-Dose Vial ... 2619
Desoxyn Tablets, USP ... 2462
DextroStat Tablets ... 3179
Flonase Nasal Spray ... 1440
Flovent Diskus ... 1443
Flovent HFA ... 1447
Focalin XR Capsules ... 2223
Hydrocortone Tablets ... 1989
Pulmicort Respules ... 661
Rhinocort Aqua Nasal Spray ... 665
Ritalin Hydrochloride Tablets ... 2269
Ritalin LA Capsules ... 2271
Ritalin-SR Tablets ... 2269

Guillain-Barré syndrome
ADACEL Vaccine ... 2945
Asacol Delayed-Release Tablets (Rare) ... 2692
Attenuvax (Rare) ... 1914
Boostrix ... 1404
Campath Ampules ... 811
Comvax ... 1928
Cuprimine Capsules ... 1947
DAPTACEL Vaccine ... 2950
Effexor Tablets (Rare) ... 3411
Effexor XR Capsules (Rare) ... 3417
Engerix-B Vaccine (Less than 1%) ... 1425
Fluarix ... 1451
Flumist Vaccine ... 1901
Fuzeon Injection ... 2767
Havrix Vaccine (Rare) ... 1456
HibTITER ... 3426
Infanrix Vaccine ... 1476
Lyrica Capsules (Rare) ... 2539
Menactra Vaccine ... 2954
Meruvax II (Isolated reports) ... 2019
M-M-R II (Rare) ... 2006
Mumpsvax ... 2031
Noroxin Tablets ... 2032
Paxil CR Controlled-Release Tablets ... 1538
Paxil ... 1530
Pediarix Vaccine ... 1548
Liquid PedvaxHIB ... 2035
Pexeva Tablets ... 1694
Pneumovax 23 (Rare) ... 2043
ProQuad ... 2064
Recombivax HB ... 2071
Remicade for IV Injection ... 971
Twinrix Vaccine ... 1595
Vaqta (Very rare) ... 2097
Varivax ... 2100
VFEND I.V. (Less than 2%) ... 2564
VFEND Oral Suspension (Less than 2%) ... 2564
VFEND Tablets (Less than 2%) ... 2564

Gums, sore
Rythmol SR Capsules ... 2727
▲ Striant Mucoadhesive (3.1%) ... 1007
Wellbutrin Tablets (Infrequent) ... 1603

Gustatory Disturbances
▲ Wellbutrin XL Extended-Release Tablets (3%) ... 1613

Gustatory sensation
▲ Wellbutrin Tablets (3.1%) ... 1603

Gynecological disorders, unspecified
▲ Zofran (7%) ... 1639
▲ Zofran ODT Orally Disintegrating Tablets (7%) ... 1639

Gynecomastia
Abilify Oral Solution (Infrequent) ... 882
Abilify Oral Solution (Infrequent) ... 2450
Abilify Discmelt Orally Disintegrating Tablets (Infrequent) ... 882
Abilify Discmelt Orally Disintegrating Tablets (Infrequent) ... 2450
Abilify Tablets (Infrequent) ... 882
Abilify Tablets (Infrequent) ... 2450
Adalat CC Tablets (Rare) ... 2964
Advicor Tablets ... 1722
Aldoril Tablets ... 1910
Altoprev Extended-Release Tablets ... 3109
AndroGel (Up to 3%) ... 3329
▲ Androxy Tablets (Most Common) ... 3335
Atripla Tablets ... 945
Avodart Soft Gelatin Capsules (0.5% to 1.1%) ... 1390
Axid Oral Solution (Rare) ... 879
Caduet Tablets ... 2508
Captopril Tablets ... 2149
Cardizem LA Extended Release Tablets (Less than 2%) ... 1728
Cardura XL Tablets ... 2515
Catapres Tablets (About 1 in 1,000 patients) ... 843
Catapres-TTS (0.5% or less) ... 844
Celexa (Rare) ... 1176
Cipro I.V. (1% or less) ... 2984
Cipro XR Tablets ... 2990
Clinoril Tablets (Rare) ... 1924
Clorpres Tablets (About 1 in 1,000) ... 2153
Covera-HS Tablets (Less than 2%) ... 3139
Effexor Tablets (Rare) ... 3411
Effexor XR Capsules (Rare) ... 3417
Eligard 7.5 mg (Less than 2%) ... 2880
Eligard 22.5 mg (Less than 2%) ... 2883
Eligard 30 mg (2.2%) ... 2885
▲ Eligard 45 mg (3.6%) ... 2888
▲ Eulexin Capsules (9%) ... 3009
▲ Gengraf Capsules (Less than 1% to 4%) ... 459
Geodon Capsules (Rare) ... 2529
▲ Humatrope Vials and Cartridges (Rare to 5.4%) ... 1787
Indocin Capsules (Less than 1%) ... 1995
Indocin I.V. (Less than 1%) ... 2465
Indocin (Less than 1%) ... 1995
Inspra Tablets (0.4% to 1%) ... 2536
▲ Intron A for Injection (Less than 5%) ... 3024
Kadian Capsules (Less than 3%) ... 577
Kaletra (Less than 2%) ... 476
Lanoxicaps Capsules (Occasional) ... 1490
Lanoxin Injection (Occasional) ... 1494
Lanoxin Injection Pediatric (Occasional) ... 1497
Lanoxin Tablets (Occasional) ... 1500
Lescol Capsules ... 2233
Lescol XL Tablets ... 2233
Lofibra Tablets ... 1219
Lofibra Capsules ... 1216
Lotrel Capsules ... 2249
▲ Lunesta Tablets (0% to 3%) ... 3142
Lupron Depot-PED 7.5 mg, 11.25 mg and 15 mg (Less than 2%) ... 3269
Lupron Injection Pediatric (Less than 2%) ... 3259
Matulane Capsules ... 3191
▲ Megace ES Oral Suspension (1% to 3%) ... 2481
Mevacor Tablets (0.5% to 1.0%) ... 2021
Midamor Tablets ... 2026
Moban Tablets (Infrequent) ... 1119
Moduretic Tablets ... 2028
Myleran Tablets (Rare) ... 1525
▲ Neoral Oral Solution (Less than 1% to 4%) ... 2259
▲ Neoral Soft Gelatin Capsules (Less than 1% to 4%) ... 2259
Neurontin Capsules (Rare) ... 2487
Neurontin Oral Solution (Rare) ... 2487
Neurontin Tablets (Rare) ... 2487
Nexavar Tablets (Uncommon) ... 746
Niravam Orally Disintegrating Tablets ... 3092
Norvasc Tablets (Infrequent) ... 2545
Nutropin for Injection (0.1%) ... 1239
Nutropin AQ Injection (0.1%) ... 1243
Nutropin AQ Pen (0.1%) ... 1243
Nutropin AQ Pen Cartridge (0.1%) ... 1243
Oxandrin Tablets ... 2962
Pepcid Injection (Rare) ... 2040
Pepcid (Rare) ... 2038
Prevacid Delayed-Release Capsules (Less than 1%) ... 3271
Prevacid for Delayed-Release Oral Suspension (Less than 1%) ... 3271
Prevacid SoluTab Delayed-Release Orally Disintegrating Tablets (Less than 1%) ... 3271
Prevacid NapraPAC (Less than 1%) ... 3280
PREVPAC (Less than 1%) ... 3284
Prezista Tablets (Less than 2%) ... 3306
Prilosec OTC Delayed-Release Tablets (Less than 1%) ... 2677
Proquin XR Tablets ... 1153
Prozac Pulvules and Liquid ... 1801
Requip Tablets (Infrequent) ... 1555
Retrovir Capsules ... 1560
Retrovir IV Infusion ... 1564
Retrovir ... 1560
Reyataz Capsules (Less than 3%) ... 921
Risperdal (Rare) ... 1676
Risperdal Consta Long-Acting Injection (Infrequent) ... 1682
Risperdal M-Tab Orally Disintegrating Tablets (Rare) ... 1676
▲ Sandimmune (Less than 1% to 4%) ... 2275
Sandostatin Injection (Less than 1%) ... 2278
Sandostatin LAR Depot (Rare) ... 2280
Seroquel Tablets (Rare) ... 690
Striant Mucoadhesive ... 1007
Sular Tablets ... 3122
Sustiva Capsules ... 930
Sustiva Tablets ... 930
Symbyax Capsules (Rare) ... 1819
Tarka Tablets ... 524
Testim 1% Gel (1% or less) ... 695
Thalomid Capsules ... 965
Thioridazine Hydrochloride Tablets ... 2163
Thiothixene Capsules ... 2165
Tiazac Capsules (Less than 2%) ... 1201
Trecator Tablets ... 3487
Trelstar LA Suspension (1.7%) ... 3397
Tricor Tablets ... 527
Trizivir Tablets ... 1589
▲ Vantas (4.1%) ... 3375
Vasotec I.V. Injection (0.5% to 1.0%) ... 2103
Verelan PM Extended-Release Capsules, Controlled-Onset (2% or less) ... 3106
▲ Viadur Implant (6.9%) ... 757
Vytorin 10/10 Tablets ... 2114
Vytorin 10/10 Tablets ... 3077
Vytorin 10/20 Tablets ... 2114
Vytorin 10/20 Tablets ... 3077
Vytorin 10/40 Tablets ... 2114
Vytorin 10/40 Tablets ... 3077
Vytorin 10/80 Tablets ... 2114
Vytorin 10/80 Tablets ... 3077
Wellbutrin Tablets (Infrequent) ... 1603
Wellbutrin SR Sustained-Release Tablets ... 1607
Wellbutrin XL Extended-Release Tablets ... 1613
Zantac (Occasional) ... 1624
Zantac Injection ... 1619
Zantac Injection Pharmacy Bulk Package (Infrequent) ... 1622
Zantac Injection Premixed ... 1619
Zantac (Occasional) ... 1624
Zegerid Capsules (Less than 1%) ... 2958
Zegerid Powder for Oral Solution (Less than 1%) ... 2958
Zocor Tablets ... 2105
Zoloft (Rare) ... 2586
Zonegran Capsules (Rare) ... 1101
Zyban Sustained-Release Tablets ... 1644
Zyprexa Tablets (Infrequent) ... 1830
Zyprexa ZYDIS Orally Disintegrating Tablets (Infrequent) ... 1830

Gynecomastia, aggravated
Vantas (Less than 2%) ... 3375

H

Haemophilus B disease
Liquid PedvaxHIB ... 2035

Hair, abnormal growth
(*see under* Hirsutism)

Hair, dry brittle
Gengraf Capsules (Rare) ... 459
Lithobid Tablets ... 1692
Neoral Oral Solution (Rare) ... 2259
Neoral Soft Gelatin Capsules (Rare) ... 2259
Sandimmune (Rare) ... 2275

Hair discoloration
Effexor Tablets (Rare) ... 3411
Effexor XR Capsules (Rare) ... 3417
Psoriatec Cream ... 1089
Men's Rogaine Extra Strength Hair Regrowth Treatment Topical Solution, Ocean Rush Scent and Original Unscented ... ▣633
Women's Rogaine Hair Regrowth Treatment Topical Solution, Spring Bloom Scent and Original Unscented ... ▣634
Soriatane Capsules (Less than 1%) ... 1013
▲ Sutent Capsules (0% to 17%) ... 2560
Wellbutrin Tablets (Rare) ... 1603

Hair growth, unwanted
Lupron Injection Pediatric ... 3259
Women's Rogaine Hair Regrowth Treatment Topical Solution, Spring Bloom Scent and Original Unscented ... ▣634

Hair loss
(*see under* Alopecia)

Hair problems, unspecified
Accutane Capsules ... 2731
Advicor Tablets ... 1722
Altoprev Extended-Release Tablets ... 3109
Emcyt Capsules (1%) ... 2634
Invirase (Less than 2%) ... 2772
Lescol Capsules ... 2233
Lescol XL Tablets ... 2233
▲ Lupron Depot 3.75 mg (Among most frequent) ... 3260
▲ Lupron Depot 7.5 mg (Less than 5%) ... 3264
▲ Lupron Depot–3 Month 11.25 mg (Less than 5%) ... 3265
Mevacor Tablets ... 2021
Neurontin Capsules (Rare) ... 2487
Neurontin Oral Solution (Rare) ... 2487
Neurontin Tablets (Rare) ... 2487
Prevacid Delayed-Release Capsules (Less than 1%) ... 3271
Prevacid for Delayed-Release Oral Suspension (Less than 1%) ... 3271
Prevacid SoluTab Delayed-Release Orally Disintegrating Tablets (Less than 1%) ... 3271
Prevacid NapraPAC (Less than 1%) ... 3280
PREVPAC (Less than 1%) ... 3284
Vytorin 10/10 Tablets ... 2114
Vytorin 10/10 Tablets ... 3077
Vytorin 10/20 Tablets ... 2114

Vytorin 10/20 Tablets 3077
Vytorin 10/40 Tablets 2114
Vytorin 10/40 Tablets 3077
Vytorin 10/80 Tablets 2114
Vytorin 10/80 Tablets 3077
Zocor Tablets 2105
Zomig Nasal Spray (Rare) 3523

Hair texture, abnormal

▲ Imdur Tablets (Less than or equal to 5%) 3018
▲ Intron A for Injection (Less than 5%) 3024
Men's Rogaine Extra Strength Hair Regrowth Treatment Topical Solution, Ocean Rush Scent and Original Unscented .... ▣633
Women's Rogaine Hair Regrowth Treatment Topical Solution, Spring Bloom Scent and Original Unscented .... ▣634
▲ Soriatane Capsules (1% to 10%) 1013
Topamax Sprinkle Capsules (Infrequent) 2404
Topamax Tablets (Infrequent) 2404
Zoloft (Rare) 2586

Hair thinning

Accutane Capsules 2731
▲ Arimidex Tablets (2% to 5%) 673
Clorpres Tablets 2153
Fansidar Tablets 2765
Intron A for Injection 3024
Lithobid Tablets 1692
Soltamox Oral Solution (Infrequently) 3527

Halitosis

Effexor Tablets (Rare) 3411
Exelon Capsules (Infrequent) 2206
Exelon Oral Solution (Infrequent) 2206
Floxin Otic Solution (Single report) 1049
Gabitril Tablets (Infrequent) 984
▲ Intron A for Injection (Less than 5%) 3024
Lamictal (Infrequent) 1481
Lunesta Tablets (Infrequent) 3142
Prevacid Delayed-Release Capsules (Less than 1%) 3271
Prevacid for Delayed-Release Oral Suspension (Less than 1%) 3271
Prevacid SoluTab Delayed-Release Orally Disintegrating Tablets (Less than 1%) 3271
Prevacid NapraPAC (Less than 1%) 3280
PREVPAC (Less than 1%) 3284
Protonix I.V. (Less than 1%) 3472
Protonix Tablets (Less than 1%) 3469
Relpax Tablets (Rare) 2548
Rythmol SR Capsules 2727
Tequin Injection (Less than 0.1%) 938
Tequin Injection in 5% Dextrose (Less than 0.1%) 938
Tequin Tablets (Less than 0.1%) 938

Hallucinations

Abilify Oral Solution (Infrequent to frequent) 882
Abilify Oral Solution (Infrequent to frequent) 2450
Abilify Discmelt Orally Disintegrating Tablets (Infrequent to frequent) 882
Abilify Discmelt Orally Disintegrating Tablets (Infrequent to frequent) 2450
Abilify Tablets (Infrequent to frequent) 882
Abilify Tablets (Infrequent to frequent) 2450
Actimmune (Rare) 1671
Actiq (1% to 2%) 979
Adderall Tablets 3164
Allegra-D 12 Hour Extended-Release Tablets 2846
Allegra-D 24 Hour Extended-Release Tablets 2849
Ambien Tablets (Infrequent) 2851
▲ Ambien CR Tablets (Infrequent to 4%) 2855
AmBisome for Injection (Less common) 620
Amerge Tablets (Rare) 1339
Anaprox Tablets (Less than 1%) 2761
Anaprox DS Tablets (Less than 1%) 2761
Aricept Tablets 1094
Aricept ODT Tablets 1094
Arthrotec Tablets (Rare) 3129
Avelox (Less than 0.1%) 2970
▲ Avinza Capsules (Less than 5%) 1741
▲ Azilect Tablets (4%) 3293
Biaxin/Biaxin XL 402
Blocadren Tablets (Less than 1%) 1916
Buprenex Injectable (Infrequent) 2716
Campath Ampules 811
Campral Tablets (Infrequent) 1174
Cardizem LA Extended Release Tablets (Less than 2%) 1728
Catapres Tablets 843
Celexa (Infrequent) 1176
▲ CellCept Capsules (3% to less than 20%) 2747
▲ CellCept Intravenous (3% to less than 20%) 2747
▲ CellCept Oral Suspension (3% to less than 20%) 2747
▲ CellCept Tablets (3% to less than 20%) 2747
Cesamet Capsules 3340
Chantix Tablets (Rare) 2517
Cipro (Less than 1%) 2977
Cipro I.V. (1% or less) 2984
Cipro XR Tablets 2990
Clozaril Tablets (Less than 1%) 2184
Comtan Tablets 2189
Copaxone for Injection (Infrequent) 3297
Cosopt Sterile Ophthalmic Solution 1931
Cubicin for Injection (Less than 1%) 1026
Cymbalta Delayed-Release Capsules 1757
Dalmane Capsules (Rare) 3342
Demser Capsules 1953
Depacon Injection 412
Depakene 417
Depakote Sprinkle Capsules 422
▲ Depakote Tablets (1% to 5%) 427
Depakote ER Tablets (Greater than 1%) 434
Detrol Tablets 2628
Didronel Tablets 2697
Dilaudid 440
Dilaudid Non-Sterile Powder 440
Dilaudid Oral Liquid (Less frequent) 445
Dilaudid Rectal Suppositories 440
Dilaudid Tablets 440
Dilaudid Tablets - 8 mg (Less frequent) 445
Dilaudid-HP (Less frequent) 442
Ditropan XL Extended-Release Tablets (Rare) 2413
Dolobid Tablets (Less than 1 in 100) 1955
▲ Duragesic Transdermal System (3% to 10%) 2373
EC-Naprosyn Delayed-Release Tablets (Less than 1%) 2761
Effexor Tablets (Infrequent) 3411
Effexor XR Capsules (Infrequent) 3417
▲ Eldepryl Capsules (3 of 49 patients) 3208
Elspar for Injection 2463
Elspar for Injection 1960
Equetro Extended-Release Capsules 3180
Ery-Tab Tablets (Isolated reports) 449
Erythrocin Stearate Filmtab Tablets (Isolated reports) 453
Erythromycin Base Filmtab Tablets (Isolated reports) 455
Erythromycin Delayed-Release Capsules, USP (Isolated reports) 457
Evoxac Capsules (Less than 1%) 1047
▲ Exelon Capsules (4%) 2206
▲ Exelon Oral Solution (4%) 2206
Famvir Tablets (Infrequent) 2211
Fansidar Tablets 2765
FazaClo Orally Disintegrating Tablets (Less than 1%) 551
Flumadine (Less than 0.3%) 1183
Focalin Tablets 2220
Gabitril Tablets (Frequent) 984
Gantrisin Pediatric Suspension 2770
Guanidine Hydrochloride Tablets 3016
Imitrex Injection 1463
Imitrex Tablets (Rare) 1471
Inderal LA Long-Acting Capsules 3429
InnoPran XL Capsules 2723
Invanz for Injection (Very rare) 1999
Invirase (Less than 2%) 2772
▲ I.V. Busulfex (5%) 2493
Kadian Capsules (Less than 3%) 577
Keflex Capsules 549
Klonopin 2778
Lamictal (Infrequent) 1481
Lanoxicaps Capsules 1490
Lanoxin Injection 1494
Lanoxin Injection Pediatric 1497
Lanoxin Tablets 1500
Lariam Tablets (Occasional) 2786
Leukeran Tablets (Rare) 1504
Levaquin (0.1% to 0.9%) 2384
Levaquin in 5% Dextrose Injection (0.1% to 0.9%) 2384
Lithobid Tablets 1692
Lopressor Injection 2238
Lopressor Tablets 2238
Lopressor HCT 50/25 Tablets 2241
Lopressor HCT 100/25 Tablets 2241
Lopressor HCT 100/50 Tablets 2241
▲ Lunesta Tablets (1% to 3%) 3142
Lyrica Capsules (0.1% to 1%) 2539
Marinol Capsules (Greater than 1%) 3333
Matulane Capsules 3191
Maxipime for Injection 1105
Merrem I.V. (Greater than 0.1% to 1%) 686
▲ Mirapex Tablets (9% to 17%) 859
MS Contin Tablets (Less frequent) 2701
Nadolol Tablets 2159
Naprosyn Suspension (Less than 1%) 2761
Naprosyn Tablets (Less than 1%) 2761
Nembutal Sodium Solution, USP (Less than 1%) 2470
Neurontin Capsules (Infrequent) 2487
Neurontin Oral Solution (Infrequent) 2487
Neurontin Tablets (Infrequent) 2487
Nipent for Injection (Less than 3%) 1863
Niravam Orally Disintegrating Tablets 3092
Norflex Injection 1856
Noroxin Tablets 2032
Norvir (Less than 2%) 503
Numorphan Injection 1120
Opana Tablets (Less than 1%) 1122
Opana ER Tablets (Less than 1%) 1126
OxyContin Tablets (Less than 1%) 2703
Parcopa Orally Disintegrating Tablets 3097
Paxil CR Controlled-Release Tablets (Infrequent) 1538
Paxil (Infrequent) 1530
Pepcid Injection (Infrequent) 2040
Pepcid (Infrequent) 2038
Percodan Tablets 1132
▲ Permax Tablets (13.8%) 3356
Pexeva Tablets (Infrequent) 1694
Phenergan Tablets and Suppositories 3440
Plavix Tablets 917
Plavix Tablets 2926
Prevacid Delayed-Release Capsules (Less than 1%) 3271
Prevacid for Delayed-Release Oral Suspension (Less than 1%) 3271
Prevacid SoluTab Delayed-Release Orally Disintegrating Tablets (Less than 1%) 3271
Prevacid NapraPAC (Less than 1%) 3280
PREVPAC (Less than 1%) 3284
Prilosec OTC Delayed-Release Tablets (Less than 1%) 2677
Primaxin I.M. 2045
Primaxin I.V. 2048
▲ Prograf Capsules and Injection (3% to 15%) 632
Proquin XR Tablets 1153
ProSom Tablets (Rare) 517
Protonix I.V. (Less than 1%) 3472
Protonix Tablets (Less than 1%) 3469
Provigil Tablets (At least 1%) 988
Prozac Pulvules and Liquid (Infrequent) 1801
Raniclor Tablets, Chewable (Rare) 2505
Razadyne (Greater than or equal to 2%) 2399
Razadyne ER Extended-Release Capsules (Greater than or equal to 2%) 2399
Relpax Tablets (Rare) 2548
▲ Requip Tablets (5% to 10%) 1555
Rescriptor Tablets 2551
Restoril Capsules (Less than 0.5%) 1860
Reyataz Capsules (Less than 3%) 921
Rilutek Tablets (Infrequent) 2930
▲ Risperdal Consta Long-Acting Injection (6% to 7%) 1682
Ritalin Hydrochloride Tablets 2269
Ritalin LA Capsules 2271
Ritalin-SR Tablets 2269
Sanctura Tablets 1151
▲ Sandostatin LAR Depot (1% to 4%) 2280
Seroquel Tablets (Infrequent) 690
Singulair 2077
Sonata Capsules (Less than 1%) 1717
▲ Stalevo Tablets (4%) 2287
Sustiva Capsules (Less than 2%) 930
Sustiva Tablets (Less than 2%) 930
▲ Symmetrel Tablets (1% to 5%) 1135
▲ Tasmar Tablets (8% to 10%) 3358
Tequin Injection (Less than 0.1%) 938
Tequin Injection in 5% Dextrose (Less than 0.1%) 938
Tequin Tablets (Less than 0.1%) 938
Tiazac Capsules (Less than 2%) 1201
Timolide Tablets 2086
Timoptic Sterile Ophthalmic Solution (Less frequent) 2088
Timoptic in Ocudose (Less frequent) 2091
Timoptic-XE Sterile Ophthalmic Gel Forming Solution 2092
Topamax Sprinkle Capsules (Frequent) 2404
Topamax Tablets (Frequent) 2404
Toprol-XL Tablets 668
Transderm Scōp Transdermal Therapeutic System (Infrequent) 2177
▲ Valcyte Tablets (Less than 5%) 2813
Valium Tablets 2819
Vantin Tablets and Oral Suspension (Less than 1%) 2645
▲ Vesanoid Capsules (6%) 2820
VFEND I.V. (0% to 2.8%) 2564
VFEND Oral Suspension (0% to 2.8%) 2564
VFEND Tablets (0% to 2.8%) 2564
Voltaren Tablets (Rarely) 2307
Voltaren-XR Tablets (Rarely) 2310
Wellbutrin Tablets (Frequent) 1603
Wellbutrin SR Sustained-Release Tablets 1607
Wellbutrin XL Extended-Release Tablets 1613
Zantac (Rare) 1624
Zantac Injection 1619
Zantac Injection Pharmacy Bulk Package (Rare) 1622
Zantac Injection Premixed 1619
Zantac (Rare) 1624
Zegerid Capsules (Less than 1%) 2958
Zegerid Powder for Oral Solution (Less than 1%) 2958
▲ Zelapar Tablets (4%) 3372
Zoloft (Infrequent) 2586
Zomig Tablets (Rare) 3519
Zomig-ZMT Tablets (Rare) 3519
Zosyn (1.0% or less) 3492
Zovirax 1643
Zyban Sustained-Release Tablets 1644
Zyprexa Tablets 1830
Zyprexa ZYDIS Orally Disintegrating Tablets 1830
Zyrtec Chewable Tablets (Rare) 2594
Zyrtec (Rare) 2594
Zyrtec-D 12 Hour Extended Release Tablets 2597

Hallucinations, auditory

Bicillin C-R Injectable Suspension 1706
Catapres Tablets (Rare) 843
Catapres-TTS (0.5% or less) 844
Clorpres Tablets 2153
Lexapro Oral Solution (Infrequent) 1190
Lexapro Tablets (Infrequent) 1190
Orthoclone OKT3 Sterile Solution 2360
Valtrex Caplets 1597
Xyrem (Infrequent) 1688

Hallucinations, paradoxical

Diastat Rectal Delivery System 3343
Niravam Orally Disintegrating Tablets (Rare) 3092

Hallucinations, visual

Bicillin C-R Injectable Suspension 1706
Carbatrol Capsules 3171
Catapres Tablets (Rare) 843
Catapres-TTS (0.5% or less) 844
Clorpres Tablets 2153
Lexapro Oral Solution 1190
Lexapro Tablets 1190
Orthoclone OKT3 Sterile Solution 2360
Tegretol/Tegretol-XR 2295
Tessalon Capsules 1199
Tessalon Perles 1199
Valtrex Caplets 1597

Hand-foot syndrome

(*see under* Palmar-plantar erythrodysesthesia syndrome)

Hangover

Aciphex Tablets (Rare) 1090
▲ Advair HFA Inhalation Aerosol (0% to 3%) 1318
Effexor Tablets (Infrequent) 3411
Effexor XR Capsules (Infrequent) 3417
Lyrica Capsules (Rare) 2539
Maxalt Tablets (Infrequent) 2008
Maxalt-MLT Orally Disintegrating Tablets (Infrequent) 2008
Neurontin Capsules (Rare) 2487
Neurontin Oral Solution (Rare) 2487
Neurontin Tablets (Rare) 2487
Nipent for Injection (Less than 3%) 1863

▲ ProSom Tablets (3%) 517
Restoril Capsules (2.5%) 1860
Sonata Capsules (Infrequent) 1717
Thalomid Capsules 965
Xyrem Oral Solution (Infrequent) 1688
Zyprexa Tablets (Infrequent) 1830
Zyprexa ZYDIS Orally Disintegrating Tablets (Infrequent) 1830

HDL, decrease

▲ AndroGel (3% to 6%) 3329
Coreg Tablets (Less than or equal to 0.1%) 1414
Premphase Tablets 3456
Prempro Tablets 3456
Targretin Capsules 1747

HDL, increase

Equetro Extended-Release Capsules 3180
Menostar Transdermal System 782
Premarin Tablets 3446
Premphase Tablets 3456
Prempro Tablets 3456

Head, tight feeling

Adenocard Injection (Less than 1%) 617
Aricept Tablets (Infrequent) 1094
Aricept ODT Tablets (Infrequent) 1094
Imitrex Injection (2.2%) 1463
Imitrex Tablets (Infrequent) 1471
Klonopin (Infrequent) 2778
ProAmatine Tablets (Less frequent) 3186

Headache

▲ Abelcet Injection (6%) 1141
▲ Abilify Oral Solution (31%) 882
▲ Abilify Oral Solution (31%) 2450
▲ Abilify Discmelt Orally Disintegrating Tablets (31%) 882
▲ Abilify Discmelt Orally Disintegrating Tablets (31%) 2450
▲ Abilify Tablets (31%) 882
▲ Abilify Tablets (31%) 2450
▲ Accolate Tablets (4.5% to 12.9%) 671
Accutane Capsules 2731
▲ Aceon Tablets (2 mg, 4 mg, 8 mg) (23.8%) 3194
Aciphex Tablets (2.4%) 1090
▲ Actimmune (33%) 1671
▲ Actiq (3% to 6%) 979
▲ Actonel Tablets (7.2% to 18%) 2683
▲ Actonel with Calcium Tablets (7.2% to 7.3%) 2688
▲ ActoPlus Met Tablets (4.6% to 6%) 3214
▲ Actos Tablets (9.1%) 3219
Acular Ophthalmic Solution (Rare) 565
▲ Acular LS Ophthalmic Solution (1% to 5%) 566
▲ ADACEL Vaccine (2% to 44%) 2945
▲ Adalat CC Tablets (19%) 2964
Adderall Tablets 3164
▲ Adderall XR Capsules (26%) 3166
Adenocard Injection (2%) 617
▲ Adenoscan (18%) 619
Adipex-P 1215
▲ Advair Diskus 100/50 (12% to 20%) 1308
▲ Advair Diskus 250/50 (12% to 20%) 1308
▲ Advair Diskus 500/50 (12% to 20%) 1308
▲ Advair HFA Inhalation Aerosol (15% to 21%) 1318
▲ Advate Injection (29.3%) 712
▲ Advicor Tablets (9%) 1722
▲ Aerobid/Aerobid-M (25%) 1171
▲ Agenerase Capsules (12% to 16%) 1327
▲ Agenerase Oral Solution (12% to 16%) 1332
Aggrastat (Less than 1%) 1907
▲ Aggrenox Capsules (39.2%) 822
▲ Agrylin Capsules (43.5%) 3169
▲ Alamast Ophthalmic Solution (10% to 25%) 3381
Albalon Ophthalmic Solution .... ⊙ 218
▲ Albenza Tablets (1.3% to 11.0%) 1338
▲ Aldara Cream, 5% (More than 1% to 5%) 1846
Aldoril Tablets 1910
Aldurazyme for Intravenous Infusion 1268
▲ Alferon N Injection (3% to 31%) 1665
Alinia for Oral Suspension (1.1%) 2835
Alinia Tablets (1.1%) 2835
▲ Allegra (7.2% to 10.6%) 2844
▲ Allegra-D 12 Hour Extended-Release Tablets (13.8%) 2846
▲ Allegra-D 24 Hour Extended-Release Tablets (13.8%) 2849
Aloprim for Injection (Less than 1%) 2167
▲ Aloxi Injection (9%) 2127
Alphagan P Ophthalmic Solution (1% to 4%) 567
Alphanate, Antihemophilic Factor (Human) 1654
▲ Altace Capsules (1.2% to 5.4%) 1702
▲ Altoprev Extended-Release Tablets (2.1% to 3.2%) 3109
▲ Alupent Inhalation Aerosol (3.3%) 826
▲ Ambien Tablets (7% to 19%) 2851
▲ Ambien CR Tablets (14% to 19%) 2855
▲ AmBisome for Injection (9.4% to 19.8%) 620
Amevive (0.20%) 626
▲ Amitiza Capsules (3.4% to 13.2%) 3224
▲ Amoxil Capsules (7%) 1343
▲ Amoxil Chewable Tablets (7%) 1343
▲ Amoxil Pediatric Drops for Oral Suspension (7%) 1343
▲ Amoxil Powder for Oral Suspension (7%) 1343
▲ Amoxil Tablets (7%) 1343
▲ Anaprox Tablets (3% to 9%) 2761
▲ Anaprox DS Tablets (3% to 9%) 2761
AndroGel (Up to 3%) 3329
Androxy Tablets 3335
▲ Angeliq Tablets (5.3%) 762
▲ Anzemet Injection (9.4% to 24.3%) 2859
▲ Anzemet Tablets (7% to 17.9%) 2862
▲ Aptivus Capsules (3.1%) 826
Aralast (0.3% to 0.7%) 717
▲ Aranesp for Injection (12% to 16%) 581
▲ Aredia for Injection (10% to 26.2%) 2179
▲ Argatroban Injection (5.4%) 1346
▲ Aricept Tablets (10%) 1094
▲ Aricept ODT Tablets (10%) 1094
▲ Arimidex Tablets (7% to 18%) 673
▲ Arixtra Injection (0% to 4.5%) 1351
▲ Aromasin Tablets (6.9% to 13.1%) 2600
▲ Arranon Injection (0% to 17%) 1357
Arthrotec Tablets (Rare) 3129
▲ Asacol Delayed-Release Tablets (35%) 2692
▲ Asmanex Twisthaler (17% to 22%) 2966
▲ Astelin Nasal Spray (7.9% to 14.8%) 1904
Atacand Tablets (More than 1%) 649
▲ Atripla Tablets (5%) 945
▲ Atrovent Inhalation Solution (6.4%) 835
▲ Atrovent HFA Inhalation Aerosol (6% to 7%) 841
▲ Atrovent Nasal Spray 0.03% (9.8%) 837
Attenuvax 1914
Augmentin (Less frequent) 1360
Augmentin Tablets (Less frequent) 1363
▲ Augmentin XR Extended-Release Tablets (3.5%) 1369
Avalide Tablets (1% or greater) 888
Avalide Tablets (1% or greater) 2874
▲ Avandamet Tablets (6.5% to 11%) 1373
▲ Avandaryl Tablets (1.5% to greater than or equal to 5%) 1379
▲ Avandia Tablets (5.9% to 17.2%) 1384
Avapro Tablets (1% or greater) 891
Avapro Tablets (1% or greater) 2871
▲ Avastin IV (26%) 1227
Avelox (2%) 2970
▲ Avinza Capsules (Greater than 10%) 1741
Axert Tablets (Frequent) 2396
▲ Axid Oral Solution (16.6%) 879
▲ Azilect Tablets (11% to 14%) 3293
▲ Azmacort Inhalation Aerosol (7% to 21%) 1726
▲ Azopt Ophthalmic Suspension (1% to 5%) 557
▲ Bactroban Cream (1.7% to 3.6%) 1394
▲ Bactroban Nasal (9%) 1394
▲ Baraclude (2% to 5%) 894
Bayer Aspirin 744
Bayer Aspirin Comprehensive Prescribing Information .... ▣ 796
Beconase AQ Nasal Spray (Fewer than 5 per 100 patients) 1396
▲ BeneFix Vials (10.8%) 3408
Benicar HCT Tablets (Greater than 2%) 1044
Bentyl Capsules 697
Bentyl Injection 697
Bentyl Syrup 697
Bentyl Tablets 697
Betagan Ophthalmic Solution, USP (Rare) .... ⊙ 220
▲ Betaseron for SC Injection (57%) 767
▲ Betimol Ophthalmic Solution (More than 5%) 3382
▲ Betimol Ophthalmic Solution (More than 5%) .... ⊙ 295
Betoptic S Ophthalmic Suspension (Rare) 558
▲ Bexxar (0% to 16%) 1398
Biaxin/Biaxin XL (2%) 402
Bicillin C-R Injectable Suspension 1706
▲ BiDil Tablets (50%) 2171
Biltricide Tablets 2976
BioLean II Tablets .... ▣ 808
Blocadren Tablets (Greater than 1%) 1916
▲ Boniva Injection (3.3% to 6.5%) 2738
▲ Boniva Tablets (3.3% to 6.5%) 2741
▲ Boostrix (3.7% to 43.1%) 1404
▲ BOTOX Purified Neurotoxin Complex (3% to 11%) 570
▲ Brimonidine Tartrate Ophthalmic Solution 0.2% (10% to 30%) .... ⊙ 248
▲ Bumex Tablets (0.6% to 4.1%) 2746
▲ Buprenex Injectable (1% to 5%) 2716
▲ Byetta Injection (9%) 611
▲ Caduet Tablets (2.5% to 16.7%) 2508
Calcijex Injection 411
Calcium Disodium Versenate Injection 1851
▲ Campath Ampules (1% to 24%) 811
Campral Tablets (Frequent) 1174
▲ Camptosar Injection (1% to 17%) 2604
▲ Canasa Rectal Suppositories (14.4%) 699
▲ Cancidas for Injection (4.3% to 11.3%) 1918
Captopril Tablets (About 0.5% to 2%) 2149
▲ Carac Cream, 0.5% (3.1%) 2879
Carafate Suspension (Less than 0.5%) 701
Carafate Tablets (Less than 0.5%) 701
Carbatrol Capsules 3171
▲ Cardene I.V. (14.6%) 2497
▲ Cardizem LA Extended Release Tablets (Up to 4.6%) 1728
▲ Cardura XL Tablets (6%) 2515
Carimune NF 3499
▲ Carnitor Injection (3% to 37%) 3188
Carteolol Hydrochloride Ophthalmic Solution USP, 1% (Occasional) .... ⊙ 249
Catapres Tablets (About 1 in 100 patients) 843
▲ Catapres-TTS (5 of 101 patients) 844
Caverject Impulse Injection (2%) 2612
Ceftin Tablets (0.1% to 1%) 1407
▲ Celebrex Capsules (15.8%) 3134
Celexa (At least 2%) 1176
▲ CellCept Capsules (16.1% to 54.3%) 2747
▲ CellCept Intravenous (16.1% to 54.3%) 2747
▲ CellCept Oral Suspension (16.1% to 54.3%) 2747
▲ CellCept Tablets (16.1% to 54.3%) 2747
▲ Cerezyme for Injection (Approximately 6.5%) 1270
▲ Cesamet Capsules (6% to 7%) 3340
▲ Chantix Tablets (15% to 19%) 2517
▲ Chemet Capsules (5.2% to 15.7%) 2458
▲ Cialis Tablets (11% to 15%) 1838
Cipro (Less than 1%) 2977
Cipro I.V. (Greater than 1%) 2984
▲ Cipro XR Tablets (1% to 3%) 2990
▲ Clarinex Tablets (14%) 2995
▲ Clarinex Reditabs Tablets (14%) 2995
▲ Clarinex-D 24-Hour Extended-Release Tablets (6%) 2998
Cleocin Vaginal Ovules (Less than 1%) 2616
▲ Climara Transdermal System (5% to 18%) 771
▲ Climara Pro Transdermal System (5.2%) 776
▲ Clinoril Tablets (3% to 9%) 1924
Clobex Shampoo (1.8%) 1206
▲ Clolar for Intravenous Infusion (46%) 1271
Clorpres Tablets (About 1 in 100) 2153
▲ Clozaril Tablets (More than 5% to 7%) 2184
▲ Colazal Capsules (8%) 2838
Colocort Rectal Suspension, USP (Retention) 100 mg/60 mL 2476
▲ Combivent Inhalation Aerosol (5.6%) 847
▲ Combivir Tablets (35%) 1411
▲ Concerta Extended-Release Tablets (9% to 14%) 1881
Copaxone for Injection (At least 2%) 3297
▲ Copegus Tablets (43%) 2754
▲ Coreg Tablets (5% to 8%) 1414
▲ Cosopt Sterile Ophthalmic Solution (1% to 5%) 1931
Coumadin for Injection (Infrequent) 898
Coumadin Tablets (Infrequent) 898
▲ Covera-HS Tablets (2.2% to 6.6%) 3139
Cozaar Tablets (1% or greater) 1935
▲ Crestor Tablets (5.5%) 678
▲ Crixivan Capsules (5.4%) 1940
▲ Cubicin for Injection (5.4% to 6.7%) 1026
Cutivate Lotion 0.05% (2%) 2664
▲ Cymbalta Delayed-Release Capsules (13% to 15%) 1757
CytoGam Intravenous (Infrequent) 1895
▲ Dacogen Injection (28%) 2129
Dalmane Capsules 3342
Dantrium Capsules (Less frequent) 2694
Dapsone Tablets USP 1673
Daranide Tablets 1950
▲ Daytrana Transdermal Patch (28%) 3174
Decadron Tablets 1951
▲ Demadex Injection (7.3%) 2759
▲ Demadex Tablets (7.3%) 2759
Demser Capsules (Infrequent) 1953
Denavir Cream 2174
▲ Depacon Injection (4.3% to 31%) 412
▲ Depakene (31%) 417
▲ Depakote Sprinkle Capsules (31%) 422
▲ Depakote Tablets (31%) 427
▲ Depakote ER Tablets (31%) 434
▲ DepoCyt Injection (18% to 53%) 1143
▲ DepoDur Extended-Release Injection (Greater than 10%) 1110
Depo-Medrol Injectable Suspension 2617
Depo-Medrol Single-Dose Vial 2619
▲ Depo-Provera Contraceptive Injection (Greater than 5%) 2622
▲ depo-subQ provera 104 Injectable Suspension (9%) 2624
Desoxyn Tablets, USP 2462
▲ Detrol Tablets (11%) 2628
▲ Detrol LA Capsules (6%) 2631
Dexedrine 1420
DextroStat Tablets 3179
▲ Diastat Rectal Delivery System (5%) 3343
Didronel Tablets 2697
Dilaudid 440
Dilaudid Non-Sterile Powder 440
Dilaudid Oral Liquid (Less frequent) 445
Dilaudid Rectal Suppositories 440
Dilaudid Tablets 440
Dilaudid Tablets - 8 mg (Less frequent) 445
Dilaudid-HP (Less frequent) 442
Diovan Tablets (More than 1%) 2193
Diovan HCT Tablets (More than 2%) 2196
▲ Ditropan XL Extended-Release Tablets (6% to 10%) 2413
Diuril Oral Suspension 1954
Diuril Sodium Intravenous 2467
▲ Dolobid Tablets (3% to 9%) 1955
Donnatal Extentabs 2493
▲ Doxil Injection (Approximately 5.3% to 10.5%) 2351
Duetact Tablets 3226
▲ Duragesic Transdermal System (3% to 10%) 2373
Dyazide Capsules 1423
▲ DynaCirc CR Tablets (10.3% to 18.3%) 2721
Dyrenium Capsules (Rare) 3400
▲ EC-Naprosyn Delayed-Release Tablets (3% to 9%) 2761
Edecrin 1959
Edex Injection (2%) 3089
▲ Effexor Tablets (3% to 25%) 3411
▲ Effexor XR Capsules (2% to 34%) 3417
▲ Eldepryl Capsules (2 of 49 patients) 3208
▲ Elestat Ophthalmic Solution (1% to 3%) 1669
▲ Elidel Cream 1% (7% to 16%) 2200
▲ Elitek (26%) 2890
▲ Elmiron Capsules (3%) 2415
▲ Eloxatin for Injection (7% to 17%) 2892
Elspar for Injection 2463
Elspar for Injection 1960
Emcyt Capsules (1%) 2634
▲ Emend Capsules (5% to 16.4%) 1963
▲ Emsam Transdermal System (18%) 903
▲ Emtriva Capsules (13% to 22%) 1287
▲ Emtriva Oral Solution (13% to 22%) 1287
▲ Enablex Extended-Release Tablets (6.7%) 2203
▲ Enbrel for Injection (17% to 24%) 584
▲ Engerix-B Vaccine (1% to 10%) 1425
▲ Enjuvia Tablets (15% to 25%) 1062
▲ Entocort EC Capsules (21%) 2698
EpiPen 1061
▲ Epivir (35%) 1427
▲ Epivir-HBV (21%) 1432
▲ Epogen for Injection (0.4% to 19%) 591

▲ Epzicom Tablets (6% to 7%) 1436
▲ Equetro Extended-Release Capsules (22%) 3180
Eraxis for Injection (1.3%) 2521
▲ Erbitux (Less than 1% to 25%) 910
▲ Estrasorb Topical Emulsion (9%) 1147
Estratest Tablets 3199
Estratest H.S. Tablets 3199
▲ Estring Vaginal Ring (13%) 2635
Euflexxa (0.63%) 1162
▲ Evoclin Foam, 1% (3%) 1009
▲ Evoxac Capsules (14.4%) 1047
▲ Exelon Capsules (4% to 17%) 2206
▲ Exelon Oral Solution (4% to 17%) 2206
▲ Fabrazyme for Intravenous Infusion (13%) 1274
▲ Famvir Tablets (16% to 39.3%) 2211
Fansidar Tablets 2765
▲ Faslodex Injection (15.4%) 681
▲ FazaClo Orally Disintegrating Tablets (Greater than 5% to 7%).... 551
▲ Femara Tablets (0.7% to 20%) 2214
▲ Ferrlecit Injection (7% to 29%) 3388
▲ Flebogamma 5%, Immune Globulin Intravenous (Human) (53%) 1658
▲ Flomax Capsules (19.3% to 21.1%) 850
▲ Flonase Nasal Spray (6.6% to 16.1%) 1440
▲ Flovent Diskus (12%) 1443
▲ Flovent HFA (11%) 1447
Floxin Otic Solution (0.2% to 0.3%) .. 1049
▲ Fluarix (14.3% to 19.3%) 1451
Flumadine (1.4%) 1183
▲ Flumist Vaccine (6.8% to 40.4%) 1901
Fluorescite Injection .... ⊙ 207
Focalin Tablets 2220
▲ Focalin XR Capsules (25% to 39%) 2223
▲ Follistim AQ Cartridge (5%) 2338
Foradil Aerolizer 3010
▲ Fortamet Extended-Release Tablets (4.7%) 3115
Fortaz (Less than 1%) 1453
▲ Forteo for Injection (7.5%) 1767
▲ Fortical Nasal Spray (3.2%) 3337
Fosamax (Up to 2.6%) 1969
Fosamax Plus D Tablets (0% to 2.6%) 1977
▲ Fosrenol Chewable Tablets (5% to 21%) 3183
▲ Frova Tablets (4%) 1113
Furosemide Tablets 2154
Gabitril Tablets (1% or more) 984
▲ Gammagard Liquid (6.9% to 36.1%) 721
Gammagard S/D (Occasional) 724
▲ Gamunex Immune Globulin I.V., 10% (0.8% to 58%) 3235
Gantrisin Pediatric Suspension 2770
Garamycin Injectable 3014
Gardasil Injection (0.03%) 1984
Gemzar for Injection (Common) 1771
▲ Gengraf Capsules (2% to 25%) 459
Genotropin Lyophilized Powder 2638
▲ Geodon (18%) 2529
▲ Gleevec Tablets (0% to 39%) 2227
Gris-PEG Tablets (Occasional) 2502
▲ Havrix Vaccine (9% to 14%) 1456
▲ Hectorol Capsules (27.9%) 1275
▲ Hectorol Injection (27.9%) 1278
▲ Hepsera Tablets (2% to 9%) 1292
▲ Herceptin I.V. (26%) 1233
HibTITER 3426
Human Albumin Grifols 20%, Albumin (Human) 1651
Human Albumin Grifols 25%, Albumin (Human) 1652
▲ Humatrope Vials and Cartridges (6.07% to 9.38%) 1787
▲ Humira Injection (12%) 466
▲ Hyalgan Solution (18%) 2901
▲ Hycamtin for Injection (0.2% to 21%) 1458
Hydrocortone Tablets 1989
Hyperstat I.V. 3017
▲ Hytrin Capsules (1.1% to 16.2%) 471
Hyzaar 50-12.5 Tablets (1% or greater) 1990
Hyzaar 100-12.5 Tablets (1% or greater) 1990
Hyzaar 100-25 Tablets (1% or greater) 1990
▲ Imdur Tablets (38% to 57%) 3018
Imitrex Injection (2%) 1463
Imitrex Tablets (Greater than 1%) 1471
▲ Increlex Injection (Greater than or equal to 5%) 3291
▲ Indapamide Tablets (Greater than or equal to 5%) 2156
▲ Indocin (11.7%) 1995
Infed Injection 3390
▲ Infergen (78% to 82%) 3364
Inspra Tablets 2536
▲ Intron A for Injection (4% to 62%) 3024
▲ Invanz for Injection (4.4% to 6.8%) 1999
Invirase (Greater than or equal to 2%) 2772
▲ Ionsys Transdermal System (9%) 2379
▲ I.V. Busulfex (5% to 69%) 2493
Kadian Capsules (Less than 3%) 577
▲ Kaletra (2% to 7%) 476
Keflex Capsules 549
▲ Keppra Injection (14%) 3320
▲ Keppra Oral Solution (2% to 14%) 3314
▲ Keppra Tablets (2% to 14%) 3314
▲ Ketek Tablets (2% to 5.5%) 2903
▲ Kineret Injection (12%) 599
Klonopin 2778
Koāte-DVI (0.7%) 3250
K-Phos Neutral Tablets 760
▲ Kytril Injection (8.6% to 14%) 2781
▲ Kytril (14% to 21%) 2784
▲ Lamictal (29.1%) 1481
▲ Lamisil Tablets (12.9%) 2232
Lanoxicaps Capsules 1490
Lanoxin Injection 1494
Lanoxin Injection Pediatric 1497
Lanoxin Tablets 1500
▲ Lariam Tablets (Among most frequent) 2786
▲ Lescol Capsules (8.9%) 2233
▲ Lescol XL Tablets (4.7%) 2233
▲ Leukine (26% to 36%) 814
▲ Leustatin Injection (7% to 22%) 2357
▲ Levaquin (0.1% to 5.8%) 2384
▲ Levaquin in 5% Dextrose Injection (0.1% to 5.8%) 2384
▲ Levitra Tablets (15%) 3034
Levothroid Tablets 1186
Levoxyl Tablets 1712
▲ Lexapro Oral Solution (24%) 1190
▲ Lexapro Tablets (24%) 1190
▲ Lexiva Tablets (2% to 27%) 1505
Lidoderm Patch 1118
▲ Lipitor Tablets (2.5% to 16.7%) 2483
Lithobid Tablets 1692
▲ Lithostat Tablets (30%) 2140
▲ Lofibra Tablets (3.2%) 1219
▲ Lofibra Capsules (3.2%) 1216
Lopressor Injection 2238
Lopressor Tablets 2238
▲ Lopressor HCT 50/25 Tablets (10%) 2241
▲ Lopressor HCT 100/25 Tablets (10%) 2241
▲ Lopressor HCT 100/50 Tablets (10%) 2241
Loprox Shampoo 1888
▲ Lotemax Ophthalmic Suspension 0.5% (Less than 15%) .... ⊙ 251
▲ Lotensin Tablets (6.2%) 2243
▲ Lotensin HCT Tablets (3.1%) 2246
Lotrel Capsules (2.2%) 2249
Lotronex Tablets 1512
▲ Lucentis Injection (2% to 15%) 1237
▲ Lumigan Ophthalmic Solution (1% to 5%) 573
▲ Lunesta Tablets (13% to 21%) 3142
▲ Lupron Depot 3.75 mg (33%) 3260
Lupron Depot 7.5 mg (Less than 5%) 3264
▲ Lupron Depot–3 Month 11.25 mg (33%) 3265
Lupron Depot-PED 7.5 mg, 11.25 mg and 15 mg (Less than 2%) 3269
Lupron Injection Pediatric (Less than 2%) 3259
▲ Lyrica Capsules (5% to 8%) 2539
▲ Macugen Injection (6% to 10%) .... ⊙ 261
▲ Malarone Pediatric Tablets (3% to 22%) 1517
▲ Malarone Tablets (3% to 22%) 1517
Marinol Capsules (Less than 1%) 3333
Matulane Capsules 3191
Mavik Tablets (More than 1%) 486
Maxair Autohaler (1.3% to 2.0%) 1852
Maxalt Tablets (Less than 2%) 2008
Maxalt-MLT Orally Disintegrating Tablets (Less than 2%) 2008
Maxipime for Injection (Greater than 0.1% to 1%) 1105
▲ Megace ES Oral Suspension (1% to 10%) 2481
▲ Menactra Vaccine (1.1% to 41.8%) 2954
Menostar Transdermal System 782
▲ Mepron Suspension (16% to 31%) .. 1521
▲ Meridia Capsules (30.3%) 489
▲ Merrem I.V. (2.3% to 7.8%) 686
Meruvax II 2019
▲ Metadate CD Capsules (12%) 3323
Metrogel 1% (2.2%) 1211
▲ MetroGel-Vaginal Gel (5%) 1855
▲ Mevacor Tablets (2.1% to 9.3%) 2021
▲ Miacalcin Nasal Spray (3.2%) 2253
Micardis Tablets (1%) 854
Micardis HCT Tablets (2% or greater) 856
▲ Midamor Tablets (3% to 8%) 2026
Mintezol 2027
Miradon Tablets 3042
Mirapex Tablets (1% or more) 859
Mircette Tablets 1066
▲ Mirena Intrauterine System (5% or more) 787
M-M-R II 2006
▲ Mobic Oral Suspension (2.4% to 8.3%) 863
▲ Mobic Tablets (2.4% to 8.3%) 863
▲ Moduretic Tablets (3% to 8%) 2028
MoviPrep Oral Solution (1.8%) 2839
MS Contin Tablets (Less frequent) 2701
Mycamine for Injection (0.9% to 2.7%) 628
▲ Myfortic Tablets (3% to less than 20%) 2255
▲ Mylotarg for Injection (27% to 50%) 3431
▲ Myobloc Injection (2% to 16%) 3192
Myozyme for Intravenous Infusion 1279
▲ Nabi-HB (14%) 2169
Nadolol Tablets (1 to 5 of 1000 patients) 2159
▲ Nalfon Capsules (8.7%) 2502
▲ Namenda (6%) 1195
▲ Naprosyn Suspension (3% to 9%) 2761
▲ Naprosyn Tablets (3% to 9%) 2761
Nasacort AQ Nasal Spray (2% or greater) 2922
▲ Nasonex Nasal Spray (17% to 26%) 3043
▲ Natrecor for Injection (7% to 9%) 3127
Nembutal Sodium Solution, USP 2470
▲ Neoral Oral Solution (2% to 25%) 2259
▲ Neoral Soft Gelatin Capsules (2% to 25%) 2259
▲ Neulasta Injection (15% to 72%) 601
▲ Neumega for Injection (41%) 3435
▲ Neupogen for Injection (7%) 603
▲ Neurontin Capsules (3.3%) 2487
▲ Neurontin Oral Solution (3.3%) 2487
▲ Neurontin Tablets (3.3%) 2487
▲ Nexavar Tablets (0% to 10%) 746
▲ Nexium Delayed-Release Capsules (3.8% to 5.5%) 655
▲ Nexium I.V. (3.8% to 5.5%) 659
▲ Niaspan Extended-Release Tablets (5% to 11%) 1730
Nicomide Tablets 1088
Nimotop Capsules (Up to 4.1%) 749
▲ Nipent for Injection (13% to 17%) 1863
▲ Niravam Orally Disintegrating Tablets (12.9% to 29.2%) 3092
▲ Nitro-Dur Transdermal Infusion System (63%) 3046
▲ Nitrolingual Pumpspray (50%) 3120
▲ Norditropin Cartridges (Small number of patients -9%) 2323
Norflex Injection 1856
Noroxin Tablets (2.0% to 2.8%) 2032
▲ Norvasc Tablets (7.3%) 2545
▲ Norvir (6% to 6.5%) 503
NovoSeven (1%) 2331
Numorphan Injection 1120
Nutropin for Injection (A small number of patients) 1239
Nutropin AQ Injection (A small number of patients) 1243
Nutropin AQ Pen (A small number of patients) 1243
Nutropin AQ Pen Cartridge (A small number of patients) 1243
▲ NuvaRing (5% to 14%) 2340
Omnicef Capsules (2%) 511
Omnicef for Oral Suspension (2%) 511
▲ Oncaspar (Greater than 1% but less than 5%) 1145
▲ Ontak Vials (26%) 1745
▲ Opana Tablets (7.9%) 1122
▲ Opana ER Tablets (2.9% to 12.2%) 1126
OptiPranolol Metipranolol Ophthalmic Solution 0.3% (A small number of patients) .... ⊙ 256
▲ Orencia Powder for Intravenous Infusion (18%) 914
Ortho-Cyclen Tablets 2429
▲ Ortho Evra Transdermal System (9% to 22%) 2417
Ortho Micronor Tablets 2426
Ortho Tri-Cyclen Tablets 2429
Ortho Tri-Cyclen Lo Tablets 2436
▲ Orthoclone OKT3 Sterile Solution (11% to 44%) 2360
OsmoPrep Tablets (Less frequent) 2840
Oxsoralen-Ultra Capsules 3353
▲ OxyContin Tablets (7%) 2703
▲ Oxytrol Transdermal System (Greater than 1%) 3392
Parcopa Orally Disintegrating Tablets 3097
Parnate Tablets 1527
▲ Patanol Ophthalmic Solution (7%) 561
▲ Paxil CR Controlled-Release Tablets (17% to 18%) 1538
▲ Paxil (17% to 18%) 1530
Pediarix Vaccine 1548
▲ Pegasys (54%) 2789
▲ PEG-Intron Powder for Injection (56%) 3048
Pentasa Capsules (2.0% to 2.2%) 3185
▲ Pepcid Injection (4.7%) 2040
▲ Pepcid (4.7%) 2038
Percodan Tablets 1132
▲ Permax Tablets (5.3%) 3356
Persantine Tablets (2.3%) 868
▲ Pexeva Tablets (18%) 1694
Phenytek Capsules 2160
▲ Photofrin for Injection (6%) 702
▲ Plan B Tablets (16.8%) 1076
Plasmanate (Occasional) 3255
▲ Plavix Tablets (7.6%) 917
▲ Plavix Tablets (7.6%) 2926
▲ Pletal Tablets (27% to 34%) 2455
Pneumovax 23 2043
Premarin Intravenous 3442
▲ Premarin Tablets (26% to 32%) 3446
Premarin Vaginal Cream 3452
▲ Premphase Tablets (28% to 37%) 3456
▲ Prempro Tablets (28% to 37%) 3456
▲ Prevacid Delayed-Release Capsules (Greater than 1% to 7%) 3271
▲ Prevacid for Delayed-Release Oral Suspension (Greater than 1% to 7%) 3271
▲ Prevacid SoluTab Delayed-Release Orally Disintegrating Tablets (Greater than 1% to 7%) 3271
Prevacid I.V. for Injection (1%) 3277
▲ Prevacid NapraPAC (3% to 9%) 3280
▲ PREVPAC (1% to 6%) 3284
▲ Prezista Tablets (0.9% to 3.8%) 3306
▲ Prilosec OTC Delayed-Release Tablets (2.9% to 7%) 2677
Primaxin I.M. 2045
Primaxin I.V. (Less than 0.2%) 2048
▲ Prinivil Tablets (4.4% to 5.7%) 2052
▲ Prinzide Tablets (5.2%) 2056
▲ ProAir HFA Inhalation Aerosol (7%) .. 3300
ProAmatine Tablets (Less frequent) 3186
▲ Prochieve 4% Gel (13%) 1003
▲ Prochieve 8% Gel (13%) 1003
▲ Procrit for Injection (0.40% to 19%) 2364
Profilnine SD, Factor IX Complex (Human) 1660
▲ Prograf Capsules and Injection (37% to 64%) 632
▲ Proleukin for Injection (12%) 2266
▲ Prometrium Capsules (100 mg, 200 mg) (10% to 31%) 3203
Propine Ophthalmic Solution .... ⊙ 239
ProQuad 2064
Proquin XR Tablets (Less than 1% to 2.4%) 1153
▲ ProSom Tablets (16%) 517
ProstaScint Kit 1037
Protonix I.V. (Greater than 1%) 3472
▲ Protonix Tablets (5% to 9%) 3469
▲ Protopic Ointment (10% to 20%) 638
Proventil Inhalation Aerosol 3053
▲ Proventil Inhalation Solution 0.083% (3% to 3.1%) 3055
Proventil HFA Inhalation Aerosol 3056
▲ Provigil Tablets (34%) 988
▲ Prozac Pulvules and Liquid (21%) 1801
Quixin Ophthalmic Solution (1% to 3%) 3383
▲ Qvar Inhalation Aerosol (8% to 25%) 3303
▲ Ranexa Tablets (3% to 5.5%) 1035
▲ Rapamune Oral Solution and Tablets (23% to 34%) 3475
▲ Raptiva for Injection (32%) 1250
▲ Razadyne (8%) 2399
▲ Razadyne ER Extended-Release Capsules (8%) 2399
▲ Rebetol (58% to 69%) 3058
▲ Rebetron Combination Therapy (63% to 67%) 3063
▲ Rebif Prefilled Syringe for Injection (65% to 70%) 3159
Recombivax HB (Greater than or equal to 1%) 2071
ReFacto Vials 3484
▲ Relenza Rotadisk (2% to 24%) 1552
▲ Relpax Tablets (3% to 4%) 2548
▲ Remicade for IV Injection (18%) 971
▲ Renagel Tablets (9.1%) 1282
Requip Tablets (1% or more) 1555
▲ Rescriptor Tablets (11.2% to 16.8%) 2551
▲ Restoril Capsules (8.5%) 1860
▲ Retisert Implant (31%) .... ⊙ 258
▲ Retrovir Capsules (1.6% to 62.5%) 1560
▲ Retrovir IV Infusion (2% to 62.5%) ... 1564

▲ Retrovir (1.6% to 62.5%) 1560
▲ Revatio Tablets (46%) 2557
▲ Revlimid Capsules (1.4% to 21.4%) 958
▲ Reyataz Capsules (8% to 14%) 921
▲ R-Gene 10 for Intravenous Use (3%) 2641
Rhophylac (Occasionally) 3505
▲ Ribavirin, USP Capsules (58% to 69%) 3068
▲ Rilutek Tablets (7.0% to 8.0%) 2930
▲ Risperdal (12% to 14%) 1676
▲ Risperdal Consta Long-Acting Injection (15% to 22%) 1682
▲ Risperdal M-Tab Orally Disintegrating Tablets (12% to 14%) 1676
Ritalin Hydrochloride Tablets 2269
Ritalin LA Capsules 2271
Ritalin-SR Tablets 2269
▲ Rituxan I.V. (1% to 19%) 1254
Rocaltrol Capsules 2798
Rocaltrol Oral Solution 2798
Rocephin Injectable Vials, ADD-Vantage, Galaxy, Bulk (Occasional) 2800
▲ Romazicon Injection (1% to 9%) 2804
▲ Rozerem Tablets (7%) 3231
▲ Rythmol SR Capsules (6% to 10%) 2727
▲ Sanctura Tablets (4.2%) 1151
▲ Sandimmune (2% to 15%) 2275
▲ Sandostatin Injection (6%) 2278
Seasonique Tablets 1077
▲ Serevent Diskus (13% to 17%) 1568
Seromycin Capsules 1813
▲ Seroquel Tablets (21%) 690
▲ Simulect for Injection (Greater than or equal to 10%) 2284
▲ Singulair (1% to 18.4%) 2077
▲ Skelaxin Tablets (Most frequent) 1716
▲ Solodyn Extended Release Tablets (23%) 1890
Soltamox Oral Solution (Infrequently) 3527
▲ Sonata Capsules (30% to 42%) 1717
▲ Soriatane Capsules (1% to 10%) 1013
St. Joseph 81 mg Aspirin Chewable and Enteric Coated Tablets 1869
St. Joseph 81 mg Aspirin .... ■□ 688
Stalevo Tablets 2287
▲ Strattera Capsules (17% to 27%) 1814
▲ Striant Mucoadhesive (3.1%) 1007
Stromectol Tablets (0.2%) 2083
▲ Suboxone Tablets (30% to 36.4%) 2717
▲ Subutex Tablets (29.1% to 30%) 2717
▲ Sular Tablets (22%) 3122
Suprax (Less than 2%) 1843
▲ Sustiva Capsules (5% to 11%) 930
▲ Sustiva Tablets (5% to 11%) 930
▲ Sutent Capsules (1% to 25%) 2560
▲ Symbicort 80/4.5 Inhalation Aerosol (6.5%) 3511
▲ Symbicort 160/4.5 Inhalation Aerosol (11.3%) 3511
▲ Symlin Injection (5% to 13%) 613
▲ Symmetrel Tablets (1% to 5%) 1135
Synera Topical Patch (Less than or equal to 1%) 1137
▲ Tambocor Tablets (9.6%) 1856
▲ Tamiflu Capsules (2% to 18%) 2807
▲ Tamiflu Oral Suspension (1.8% to 20.1%) 2807
▲ Tarceva Tablets (0% to 15%) 1259
▲ Tarceva Tablets (0% to 15%) 2444
▲ Targretin Capsules (29.8% to 41.5%) 1747
▲ Tarka Tablets (8.9%) 524
▲ Tasmar Tablets (10% to 11%) 3358
Tegretol/Tegretol-XR 2295
▲ Temodar Capsules (5% to 41%) 3073
Temovate Scalp Application (1 of 294 patients) 2670
▲ Tequin Injection (3%) 938
▲ Tequin Injection in 5% Dextrose (3%) 938
▲ Tequin Tablets (3%) 938
Tessalon Capsules 1199
Tessalon Perles 1199
Testim 1% Gel (1%) 695
Teveten Tablets (1% or greater) 1735
▲ Teveten HCT Tablets (3.4%) 1737
Tev-Tropin for Injection (Infrequently) 1222
▲ Thalomid Capsules (12.5%) 965
Thioridazine Hydrochloride Tablets (Extremely rare) 2163
▲ Thymoglobulin for Intravenous Infusion (40.2%) 1284
▲ Thyrogen for Injection (7.3%) 1286
Thyrolar Tablets 1199
▲ Tiazac Capsules (8%) 1201
Ticlid Tablets (0.5% to 1.0%) 2810
Timentin ADD-Vantage 1580
Timentin Injection Galaxy Container 1583
Timentin IV Infusion 1577
Timentin Pharmacy Bulk Package 1586
Timolide Tablets (Less than 1%) 2086
Timoptic Sterile Ophthalmic Solution (Less frequent) 2088
Timoptic in Ocudose (Less frequent) 2091
▲ Timoptic-XE Sterile Ophthalmic Gel Forming Solution (1% to 5%) 2092
Tindamax Tablets (0.7% to 1.3%) 2142
▲ TOBI Solution for Inhalation (26.7%) 2298
Topamax Sprinkle Capsules (More than 1%) 2404
Topamax Tablets (More than 1%) 2404
Toprol-XL Tablets 668
▲ Tracleer Tablets (22%) 545
Transderm Scōp Transdermal Therapeutic System (Few patients) 2177
Tranxene (Less common) 2474
▲ Travatan Ophthalmic Solution (1% to 5%) 563
Trecator Tablets 3487
▲ Trelstar Depot (5%) 3394
▲ Trelstar LA Suspension (6.9%) 3397
▲ Tricor Tablets (3.2%) 527
▲ Triglide Tablets (3.2%) 3123
▲ Trileptal Tablets (15% to 32%) 2300
▲ Trileptal Oral Suspension (15% to 32%) 2300
▲ Trisenox Injection (60%) 993
▲ Trizivir Tablets (28%) 1589
Trusopt Sterile Ophthalmic Solution (Infrequent) 2095
▲ Truvada Tablets (5%) 1296
▲ Twinrix Vaccine (13% to 22%) 1595
▲ Tygacil for Injection (5.9%) 3488
Ultane Liquid for Inhalation (1%) 531
Uniphyl Tablets 2710
Uniretic Tablets (More than 1%) 3100
Univasc Tablets (Greater than 1%) 3104
Uroqid-Acid No. 2 Tablets 760
▲ Uroxatral Tablets (3%) 2943
▲ Vagifem Tablets (9% to 10%) 2334
▲ Valcyte Tablets (9% to 22%) 2813
Valium Tablets (Infrequent) 2819
▲ Valtrex Caplets (13% to 38%) 1597
▲ Vandazole Vaginal Gel (7%) 3338
▲ Vanos Cream (2.8% to 4%) 1893
Vantas (2.9%) 3375
Vantin Tablets and Oral Suspension (Less than 1% to 1.1%) 2645
▲ Vaprisol (12%) 643
▲ Vaqta (0.4% to 16%) 2097
Varivax (Greater than or equal to 1%) 2100
Vasotec I.V. Injection (1.8% to 5.2%) 2103
▲ Velcade for Injection (26%) 2133
▲ Ventavis Inhalation Solution (30%) 1020
Ventolin HFA Inhalation Aerosol 1600
▲ Verelan PM Extended-Release Capsules, Controlled-Onset (2.2% to 12.1%) 3106
▲ Vesanoid Capsules (86%) 2820
▲ VFEND I.V. (0% to 3%) 2564
▲ VFEND Oral Suspension (0% to 3%) 2564
▲ VFEND Tablets (0% to 3%) 2564
▲ Viadur Implant (4.6%) 757
▲ Viagra Tablets (16%) 2573
▲ Vicoprofen Tablets (27%) 539
Viracept (Less than 2%) 2577
▲ Viramune Oral Suspension (3%) 873
▲ Viramune Tablets (3%) 873
▲ Viread Tablets (5% to 14%) 1301
Visudyne for Injection 2305
▲ Vivaglobin (0% to 48%) 3506
▲ Vivitrol (16% to 36%) 995
Vivotif 819
▲ Voltaren Ophthalmic Solution (Less than or equal to 3%) 2309
▲ Voltaren Tablets (1% to 10%) 2307
▲ Voltaren-XR Tablets (1% to 10%) 2310
▲ VoSpire ER Tablets (18.8%) 1052
▲ Vytorin 10/10 Tablets (6.8%) 2114
▲ Vytorin 10/10 Tablets (6.8%) 3077
▲ Vytorin 10/20 Tablets (6.8%) 2114
▲ Vytorin 10/20 Tablets (6.8%) 3077
▲ Vytorin 10/40 Tablets (6.8%) 2114
▲ Vytorin 10/40 Tablets (6.8%) 3077
▲ Vytorin 10/80 Tablets (6.8%) 2114
▲ Vytorin 10/80 Tablets (6.8%) 3077
▲ WelChol Tablets (6%) 1050
▲ Wellbutrin SR Sustained-Release Tablets (25% to 26%) 1607
▲ Wellbutrin XL Extended-Release Tablets (25% to 34%) 1613
WinRho SDF (2%) 732
▲ Xeloda Tablets (1% to 9%) 2822
▲ Xenical Capsules (30.6%) 2831
▲ Xifaxan Tablets (9.7%) 2842
▲ Xolair (15%) 1266
▲ Xopenex Inhalation Solution (11.9%) 3146
▲ Xopenex Inhalation Solution Concentrate (7.6% to 11.9%) 3150
▲ Xopenex HFA Inhalation Aerosol (11.9%) 3154
▲ Xyrem Oral Solution (8.8% to 37.1%) 1688
Yasmin 28 Tablets (Greater than 1%) 796
Yaz Tablets (Greater than 1%) 803
Zantac 1624
Zantac Injection 1619
Zantac Injection Pharmacy Bulk Package (Frequent) 1622
Zantac Injection Premixed 1619
Zantac 1624
▲ Zegerid Capsules (2.9% to 7%) 2958
▲ Zegerid Powder for Oral Solution (2.9% to 7%) 2958
▲ Zelapar Tablets (7%) 3372
▲ Zelnorm Tablets (1% to 15%) 2312
Zemaira (2.5%) 3509
Zemplar Injection 543
▲ Zetia Tablets (8%) 2120
▲ Zetia Tablets (8%) 3083
▲ Ziagen (1% to 13%) 1626
Zmax for Oral Suspension (1.3%) 2583
▲ Zocor Tablets (3.5%) 2105
▲ Zofran Injection (17% to 25%) 1634
▲ Zofran (9% to 27%) 1639
▲ Zofran ODT Orally Disintegrating Tablets (9% to 27%) 1639
▲ Zoloft (26%) 2586
▲ Zometa for Intravenous Infusion (5% to 19%) 2315
Zomig Tablets (Rare) 3519
Zomig Nasal Spray (Rare to less than 2%) 3523
Zomig-ZMT Tablets (Rare) 3519
▲ Zonegran Capsules (10%) 1101
Zostavax Injection (1.4%) 2111
▲ Zosyn (4.5% to 7.7%) 3492
Zovirax (2.2%) 1643
Zyban Sustained-Release Tablets (Frequent) 1644
▲ Zyflo Tablets (24.6%) 1023
▲ Zymar Ophthalmic Solution (1% to 4%) 575
▲ Zyprexa Tablets (17%) 1830
▲ Zyprexa ZYDIS Orally Disintegrating Tablets (17%) 1830
▲ Zyrtec Chewable Tablets (11.0% to 14.0%) 2594
▲ Zyrtec (11.0% to 14.0%) 2594
Zyrtec-D 12 Hour Extended Release Tablets 2597
▲ Zyvox (0% to 6.5%) 2652

Headache, migraine

(*see under* Migraine)

Headache, sinus

Arranon Injection (1%) 1357
Cesamet Capsules 3340
▲ Flebogamma 5%, Immune Globulin Intravenous (Human) (53%) 1658
Lexapro Oral Solution (Frequent) 1190
Lexapro Tablets (Frequent) 1190
Oracea Capsules (1.1%) 1000
▲ Serevent Diskus (1% to 3%) 1568
▲ Strattera Capsules (3%) 1814
▲ Vivitrol (16% to 36%) 995
Xyrem (Infrequent) 1688

Headache, throbbing

Hyperstat I.V. 3017

Headache, vascular

Meridia Capsules 489
Paxil CR Controlled-Release Tablets 1538
Paxil 1530
Pexeva Tablets (rare) 1694
Prozac Pulvules and Liquid (Infrequent) 1801

Healing, abnormal

Cafcit (2.2%) 1886
▲ CellCept Capsules (3% to less than 20%) 2747
▲ CellCept Intravenous (3% to less than 20%) 2747
▲ CellCept Oral Suspension (3% to less than 20%) 2747
▲ CellCept Tablets (3% to less than 20%) 2747
▲ Humira Injection (Less than 5%) 466
Ionsys Transdermal System (.1% to less than 1%) 2379
▲ Prograf Capsules and Injection (3% to 15%) 632
Soriatane Capsules (Less than 1%) 1013
▲ Tygacil for Injection (3.5%) 3488

Hearing, impaired

Accutane Capsules 2731
Anaprox Tablets (Less than 1%) 2761
Anaprox DS Tablets (Less than 1%) 2761
Arthrotec Tablets (Rare) 3129
Bumex Tablets (0.5% to 2.9%) 2746
EC-Naprosyn Delayed-Release Tablets (Less than 1%) 2761
Lariam Tablets 2786
Lupron Injection Pediatric 3259
Mustargen for Injection 2468
Naprosyn Suspension (Less than 1%) 2761
Naprosyn Tablets (Less than 1%) 2761
Norvir (Less than 2%) 503
Pegasys 2789
PEG-Intron Powder for Injection 3048
Prevacid NapraPAC (Less than 1%) 3280
Requip Tablets (Infrequent) 1555
Rythmol SR Capsules 2727
▲ Taxotere Injection Concentrate (0% to 6.3%) 2932
Vesanoid Capsules (Less than 1%) 2820
Vicodin Tablets (Very rare) 535
Vicodin ES Tablets (Very rare) 536
Vicodin HP Tablets (Very rare) 538
Voltaren Tablets (Rarely) 2307
Voltaren-XR Tablets (Rarely) 2310

Hearing, loss of

Abelcet Injection 1141
Aggrenox Capsules 822
Altace Capsules (Less than 1%) 1702
Bayer Aspirin 744
Bayer Aspirin Comprehensive Prescribing Information .... ■□ 796
▲ Capastat Sulfate for Injection (3%) 1755
Cipro (Less than 1%) 2977
Cipro I.V. (1% or less) 2984
Cipro XR Tablets 2990
Coreg Tablets (Less than or equal to 0.1%) 1414
Demadex Injection 2759
Demadex Tablets 2759
Depacon Injection 412
Depakene 417
Depakote Sprinkle Capsules 422
Depakote Tablets 427
Depakote ER Tablets 434
Dolobid Tablets (Rare) 1955
Fabrazyme for Intravenous Infusion 1274
Floxin Otic Solution (Single report) 1049
Fortical Nasal Spray (Less than 1%) 3337
Furosemide Tablets 2154
Gantrisin Pediatric Suspension 2770
Garamycin Injectable 3014
Gengraf Capsules (2% or less) 459
Imitrex Nasal Spray 1467
Maalox Maximum Strength Total Stomach Relief Peppermint Liquid .... ■□ 660
▲ Macugen Injection (1% to 5%) .... ⊙ 261
Matulane Capsules 3191
Miacalcin Nasal Spray (Less than 1%) 2253
Neoral Oral Solution (2% or less) 2259
Neoral Soft Gelatin Capsules (2% or less) 2259
Neurontin Capsules (Infrequent) 2487
Neurontin Oral Solution (Infrequent) 2487
Neurontin Tablets (Infrequent) 2487
Orthoclone OKT3 Sterile Solution 2360
Pegasys 2789
PEG-Intron Powder for Injection 3048
Percodan Tablets 1132
PREVPAC 3284
Primaxin I.M. 2045
Primaxin I.V. (Less than 0.2%) 2048
Prograf Capsules and Injection 632
Proquin XR Tablets 1153
Prozac Pulvules and Liquid (Rare) 1801
Raptiva for Injection (1 case) 1250
Retrovir Capsules 1560
Retrovir IV Infusion 1564
Retrovir 1560
Sandimmune (2% or less) 2275
Sandostatin Injection (Less than 1%) 2278
St. Joseph 81 mg Aspirin Chewable and Enteric Coated Tablets 1869
Taxotere Injection Concentrate (Rare) 2932
TOBI Solution for Inhalation 2298
Vancocin HCl Capsules, USP (A few dozen cases) 3380
▲ Vesanoid Capsules (6%) 2820
Zinacef for Injection (A few pediatric patients) 1631

Zinacef Injection (A few pediatric patients) 1631
Zmax for Oral Suspension 2583

Hearing decreased
Aricept Tablets (Infrequent) 1094
Aricept ODT Tablets (Infrequent) 1094
Campath Ampules 811
Ciprodex Otic Suspension (1 patient) 559
Clinoril Tablets (Less than 1%) 1924
Evoxac Capsules (Less than 1%) 1047
Invirase (Less than 2%) 2772
Nalfon Capsules (1.6%) 2502
Namenda (Infrequent) 1195
ProSom Tablets (Rare) 517
Risperdal (Rare) 1676
Risperdal Consta Long-Acting Injection (Infrequent) 1682
Risperdal M-Tab Orally Disintegrating Tablets (Rare) 1676
Solodyn Extended Release Tablets 1890
Topamax Sprinkle Capsules (1% to 2%) 2404
Topamax Tablets (1% to 2%) 2404
▲ Visudyne for Injection (1% to 10%) 2305

Hearing disturbances
Amerge Tablets (Infrequent) 1339
Anaprox Tablets (Less than 3%) 2761
Anaprox DS Tablets (Less than 3%) 2761
Avalide Tablets 888
Avalide Tablets 2874
Avapro Tablets (Less than 1%) 891
Avapro Tablets (Less than 1%) 2871
EC-Naprosyn Delayed-Release Tablets (Less than 3%) 2761
Imitrex Nasal Spray (Infrequent) 1467
Imitrex Tablets (Infrequent) 1471
Indocin Capsules (Less than 1%) 1995
Indocin I.V. (Less than 1%) 2465
Indocin (Less than 1%) 1995
▲ Intron A for Injection (Less than 5%) 3024
Naprosyn Suspension (Less than 3%) 2761
Naprosyn Tablets (Less than 3%) 2761
Prevacid NapraPAC (Less than 3%) 3280
Rebetol 3058
Ribavirin, USP Capsules 3068
Taxotere Injection Concentrate (Rare) 2932
Zmax for Oral Suspension 2583

Hearing loss, reversible
Depacon Injection 412
Depakene 417
Depakote Tablets 427
Depakote ER Tablets 434
E.E.S. (Isolated reports) 451
EryPed (Isolated reports) 447
Ery-Tab Tablets (Isolated reports) 449
Erythrocin Stearate Filmtab Tablets (Isolated reports) 453
Erythromycin Base Filmtab Tablets (Isolated reports) 455
Erythromycin Delayed-Release Capsules, USP (Isolated reports) 457
Hyperstat I.V. 3017
PCE Dispertab Tablets (Isolated reports) 515
Romazicon Injection (Less than 1%) 2804
St. Joseph 81 mg Aspirin ■ 688

Heart beat, irregular
Adenocard Injection 617
▲ Indapamide Tablets (Less than 5%) 2156
K-Phos Original (Sodium Free) Tablets (Less frequent) 760
K-Phos Neutral Tablets 760
Children's Motrin Oral Suspension ■ 685
Children's Motrin Non-Staining Dye-Free Oral Suspension ■ 685
Children's Motrin Oral Suspension 1867
Children's Motrin Non-Staining Dye-Free Oral Suspension 1867
Infants' Motrin Concentrated Drops 1867
Infants' Motrin Non-Staining Dye-Free Concentrated Drops 1867
Junior Strength Motrin Caplets and Chewable Tablets 1867
Rythmol SR Capsules 2727
Uroqid-Acid No. 2 Tablets 760

Heart beats, ectopic
Imitrex Injection (Infrequent) 1463
Imitrex Nasal Spray 1467
Imitrex Tablets 1471

Heart block
(*see also under* Sinoatrial block)
Actimmune (Rare) 1671
Adenocard Injection 617
Agrylin Capsules 3169
Aricept Tablets 1094
Aricept ODT Tablets 1094
Betagan Ophthalmic Solution, USP ⊙ 220
Betimol Ophthalmic Solution 3382
Betimol Ophthalmic Solution ⊙ 295
Betoptic S Ophthalmic Suspension (Rare) 558
Carteolol Hydrochloride Ophthalmic Solution USP, 1% ⊙ 249
Imitrex Nasal Spray 1467
Imitrex Tablets (Rare) 1471
Lanoxicaps Capsules 1490
Lanoxin Injection 1494
Lanoxin Injection Pediatric 1497
Lanoxin Tablets 1500
Levaquin (0.1% to 0.9%) 2384
Levaquin in 5% Dextrose Injection (0.1% to 0.9%) 2384
Paxil CR Controlled-Release Tablets (Rare) 1538
Paxil (Rare) 1530
Permax Tablets (Rare) 3356
Pexeva Tablets (rare) 1694
Prozac Pulvules and Liquid (Rare) 1801
Relpax Tablets (Rare) 2548
Reyataz Capsules (Less than 3%) 921
Timoptic Sterile Ophthalmic Solution (Less frequent) 2088
Timoptic in Ocudose (Less frequent) 2091
Trasylol Injection (1% to 2%) 754
Zyprexa IntraMuscular (Infrequent) 1830

Heart block, first degree
▲ Lopressor Injection (5.3%) 2238
▲ Lopressor Tablets (5.3%) 2238

Heart block, second degree
▲ Lopressor Injection (4.7%) 2238
▲ Lopressor Tablets (4.7%) 2238
Toprol-XL Tablets 668
Zofran Injection 1634

Heart block, third degree
I.V. Busulfex (2%) 2493
▲ Lopressor Injection (4.7%) 2238
▲ Lopressor Tablets (4.7%) 2238
Nadolol Tablets (Single instance) 2159
Toprol-XL Tablets 668
Wellbutrin Tablets 1603

Heart defects, congenital
Thalomid Capsules 965

Heart failure
Abelcet Injection 1141
Abilify Oral Solution (Infrequent) 882
Abilify Oral Solution (Infrequent) 2450
Abilify Discmelt Orally Disintegrating Tablets (Infrequent) 882
Abilify Discmelt Orally Disintegrating Tablets (Infrequent) 2450
Abilify Tablets (Infrequent) 882
Abilify Tablets (Infrequent) 2450
Actimmune (Rare) 1671
Activase I.V. 1223
Aggrenox Capsules (1.6%) 822
▲ Agrylin Capsules (1% to 5%) 3169
Aldara Cream, 5% 1846
Aloprim for Injection (Less than 1%) 2167
Altace Capsules (2%) 1702
Aredia for Injection (Up to 1%) 2179
Aromasin Tablets (0.4%) 2600
Avalide Tablets 888
Avalide Tablets 2874
Avapro Tablets (Less than 1%) 891
Avapro Tablets (Less than 1%) 2871
Azilect Tablets (Infrequent) 3293
Betimol Ophthalmic Solution 3382
Betimol Ophthalmic Solution ⊙ 295
Blocadren Tablets 1916
Caduet Tablets (Less than or equal to 0.1%) 2508
Campath Ampules 811
Campral Tablets (Rare) 1174
Carteolol Hydrochloride Ophthalmic Solution USP, 1% (In some cases) ⊙ 249
Celexa (Infrequent) 1176
▲ CellCept Capsules (3% to less than 20%) 2747
▲ CellCept Intravenous (3% to less than 20%) 2747
▲ CellCept Oral Suspension (3% to less than 20%) 2747
▲ CellCept Tablets (3% to less than 20%) 2747
Coreg Tablets 1414
Cosopt Sterile Ophthalmic Solution (Less than 1%) 1931
Cubicin for Injection (1% to 2%) 1026
Cymbalta Delayed-Release Capsules (Infrequent) 1757
Dantrium Capsules (Less frequent) 2694
Dantrium Intravenous 2695
Doxil Injection (Less than 1%) 2351
DynaCirc CR Tablets (0.5% to 1%) 2721
Elitek (Less than or equal to 1%) 2890
Enbrel for Injection (Infrequent) 584
Exelon Capsules (Frequent) 2206
Exelon Oral Solution (Frequent) 2206
Flumadine (Less than 0.3%) 1183
Gengraf Capsules (1% to less than 3%) 459
Gleevec Tablets (Infrequent) 2227
Herceptin I.V. 1233
▲ Imdur Tablets (Less than or equal to 5%) 3018
▲ Intron A for Injection (Less than 5%) 3024
Invanz for Injection (Greater than 0.1%) 1999
I.V. Busulfex (2%) 2493
Levothroid Tablets 1186
Levoxyl Tablets 1712
▲ Lopressor Injection (27.5%) 2238
▲ Lopressor Tablets (27.5%) 2238
Lovenox Injection (0.95%) 2915
Lyrica Capsules (0.1% to 1%) 2539
Merrem I.V. (Greater than 0.1% to 1%) 686
Mirapex Tablets (Less than 1%) 859
Mobic Oral Suspension (Less than 2%) 863
Mobic Tablets (Less than 2%) 863
Myozyme for Intravenous Infusion 1279
Nadolol Tablets (1 of 100 patients) 2159
Namenda (Frequent) 1195
NeoProfen Injection 2472
Neoral Oral Solution (1% to less than 3%) 2259
Neoral Soft Gelatin Capsules (1% to less than 3%) 2259
Neurontin Capsules (Rare) 2487
Neurontin Oral Solution (Rare) 2487
Neurontin Tablets (Rare) 2487
Nexavar Tablets (Infrequent) 746
Nipent for Injection (Less than 3%) 1863
Norvasc Tablets (Less than 0.1%) 2545
Omnicef Capsules 511
Omnicef for Oral Suspension 511
Orthoclone OKT3 Sterile Solution 2360
▲ Photofrin for Injection (7%) 702
Plavix Tablets (1% to 2.5%) 917
Plavix Tablets (1% to 2.5%) 2926
Pulmozyme Inhalation Solution 1248
Razadyne (Infrequent) 2399
Razadyne ER Extended-Release Capsules (Infrequent) 2399
▲ Refludan for Injection (3%) 792
Requip Tablets (Infrequent) 1555
Retavase 2499
Revlimid Capsules 958
Rilutek Tablets (Infrequent) 2930
Risperdal 1676
Risperdal Consta Long-Acting Injection 1682
Risperdal M-Tab Orally Disintegrating Tablets 1676
Rituxan I.V. (Rare) 1254
▲ Sandostatin LAR Depot (1% to 4%) 2280
▲ Simulect for Injection (3% to 10%) 2284
Targretin Capsules 1747
Tasmar Tablets (Infrequent) 3358
Taxotere Injection Concentrate (Rare) 2932
Thalomid Capsules 965
Timolide Tablets (Less than 1%) 2086
Timoptic Sterile Ophthalmic Solution (Less frequent) 2088
Timoptic in Ocudose (Less frequent) 2091
Timoptic-XE Sterile Ophthalmic Gel Forming Solution 2092
TNKase I.V. 1264
Toprol-XL Tablets 668
▲ Trasylol Injection (5%) 754
Trileptal Tablets 2300
Trileptal Oral Suspension 2300
Verelan PM Extended-Release Capsules, Controlled-Onset 3106
▲ Vesanoid Capsules (6%) 2820
Viagra Tablets (Less than 2%) 2573
Zelapar Tablets 3372
Zonegran Capsules (Rare) 1101
Zosyn (1.0% or less) 3492
Zyprexa Tablets 1830
Zyprexa ZYDIS Orally Disintegrating Tablets 1830
Zyrtec Chewable Tablets (Less than 2%) 2594
Zyrtec (Less than 2%) 2594
Zyrtec-D 12 Hour Extended Release Tablets (Less than 2%) 2597

Heart failure, congestive
(*see under* Congestive heart failure)

Heart failure, worsening of
Avandaryl Tablets 1379
Avandia Tablets 1384
Prinivil Tablets (Greater than 1%) 2052
Prinzide Tablets 2056
Toprol-XL Tablets 668
Velcade for Injection 2133

Heart rate, abnormal
Rescriptor Tablets 2551
Thyrolar Tablets 1199

Heart rate, changes
▲ Blocadren Tablets (5%) 1916
Invirase Capsules (Less than 2%) 2772
Invirase Tablets (Less than 2%) 2772
Transderm Scōp Transdermal Therapeutic System 2177
Visudyne for Injection 2305
Zemuron Injection 2346

Heart rate, decrease
Betagan Ophthalmic Solution, USP ⊙ 220
ProAmatine Tablets 3186

Heart rate, increased
Abilify Oral Solution 882
Abilify Oral Solution 2450
Abilify Discmelt Orally Disintegrating Tablets 882
Abilify Discmelt Orally Disintegrating Tablets 2450
Abilify Tablets 882
Abilify Tablets 2450
Effexor Tablets 3411
Levaquin (0.1% to 0.9%) 2384
Levaquin in 5% Dextrose Injection (0.1% to 0.9%) 2384
Levothroid Tablets 1186
Meridia Capsules 489
Primatene Mist ■ 719
Ritalin LA Capsules 2271
Women's Rogaine Hair Regrowth Treatment Topical Solution, Spring Bloom Scent and Original Unscented ■ 634
Thyrolar Tablets 1199
▲ Ultram ER Tablets (1% to greater than 5%) 2392
▲ Xopenex Inhalation Solution (0.8% to 6%) 3146
▲ Xopenex Inhalation Solution Concentrate (0.8% to 6%) 3150
▲ Xopenex HFA Inhalation Aerosol (0.8% to 6%) 3154
Xyrem Oral Solution (Infrequent) 1688

Heart sounds, abnormal
Gengraf Capsules (1% to less than 3%) 459
Neoral Oral Solution (1% to less than 3%) 2259
Neoral Soft Gelatin Capsules (1% to less than 3%) 2259
Rythmol SR Capsules 2727
▲ Simulect for Injection (3% to 10%) 2284

Heart spasms
(*see under* Cardiospasm)

Heartburn
▲ Aerobid/Aerobid-M (3% to 9%) 1171
▲ Alferon N Injection (3%) 1665
Altoprev Extended-Release Tablets 3109
▲ Anaprox Tablets (3% to 9%) 2761
▲ Anaprox DS Tablets (3% to 9%) 2761
Arthrotec Tablets (Rare) 3129
Avalide Tablets (2%) 888
Avalide Tablets (2%) 2874
Avapro Tablets (2%) 891
Avapro Tablets (2%) 2871
Bayer Aspirin 744
Bayer Aspirin Comprehensive Prescribing Information ■ 796
▲ Clozaril Tablets (4%) 2184
Combivent Inhalation Aerosol 847
Dalmane Capsules 3342
▲ EC-Naprosyn Delayed-Release Tablets (3% to 9%) 2761
Eldepryl Capsules 3208
▲ Emend Capsules (5.3%) 1963

▲ FazaClo Orally Disintegrating Tablets (4%) 551
▲ Indocin (3% to 9%) 1995
Klonopin (Infrequent) 2778
Lexapro Oral Solution (Frequent) 1190
Lexapro Tablets (Frequent) 1190
Limbrel Capsules 2672
Lopressor Injection (1%) 2238
Lopressor Tablets (1%) 2238
Lopressor HCT 50/25 Tablets (Less than or equal to 1%) 2241
Lopressor HCT 100/25 Tablets (Less than or equal to 1%) 2241
Lopressor HCT 100/50 Tablets (Less than or equal to 1%) 2241
Mevacor Tablets (1.6%) 2021
Midamor Tablets (Less than or equal to 1%) 2026
Moduretic Tablets 2028
▲ Naprosyn Suspension (3% to 9%) 2761
▲ Naprosyn Tablets (3% to 9%) 2761
Noroxin Tablets (0.3% to 1.0%) 2032
Parcopa Orally Disintegrating Tablets 3097
▲ Prevacid NapraPAC (3% to 9%) 3280
Primaxin I.M. 2045
Primaxin I.V. (Less than 0.2%) 2048
Prinivil Tablets (0.3% to 1.0%) 2052
Prinzide Tablets (0.3% to 1%) 2056
ProAmatine Tablets (Rare) 3186
▲ Proventil Inhalation Aerosol (Less than 5%) 3053
St. Joseph 81 mg Aspirin Chewable and Enteric Coated Tablets 1869
Stalevo Tablets 2287
Syprine Capsules 2085
Toprol-XL Tablets (About 1 of 100 patients) 668
▲ Voltaren Tablets (1% to 10%) 2307
▲ Voltaren-XR Tablets (1% to 10%) 2310

Heat intolerance
Alferon N Injection (1%) 1665
Imitrex Tablets 1471
Levothroid Tablets 1186
Levoxyl Tablets 1712
Reyataz Capsules (Less than 3%) 921

Heat sensations
Prograf Capsules and Injection 632
Synera Topical Patch 1137

Heat stroke
Abilify Oral Solution (Rare) 882
Abilify Oral Solution (Rare) 2450
Abilify Discmelt Orally Disintegrating Tablets (Rare) 882
Abilify Discmelt Orally Disintegrating Tablets (Rare) 2450
Abilify Tablets (Rare) 882
Abilify Tablets (Rare) 2450
Clozaril Tablets 2184
Donnatal Extentabs 2493
Evoxac Capsules (Less than 1%) 1047
Lunesta Tablets (Infrequent) 3142
Protonix I.V. (Less than 1%) 3472
Protonix Tablets (Less than 1%) 3469
Vivitrol 995

Heaviness
▲ Imitrex Injection (7%) 1463
Xyrem Oral Solution (Infrequent) 1688

Heaviness, head
Abilify Oral Solution (Rare) 882
Abilify Oral Solution (Rare) 2450
Abilify Discmelt Orally Disintegrating Tablets (Rare) 882
Abilify Discmelt Orally Disintegrating Tablets (Rare) 2450
Abilify Tablets (Rare) 882
Abilify Tablets (Rare) 2450

Heavy sensation, arms
Adenocard Injection (Less than 1%) 617

Heavy sensation, legs
Eldepryl Capsules 3208
K-Phos Original (Sodium Free) Tablets (Less frequent) 760
K-Phos Neutral Tablets 760

Hemarthrosis
Kaletra 476
NovoSeven (Greater than or equal to 2%) 2331

Hematemesis
Abilify Oral Solution (Rare) 882
Abilify Oral Solution (Rare) 2450
Abilify Discmelt Orally Disintegrating Tablets (Rare) 882
Abilify Discmelt Orally Disintegrating Tablets (Rare) 2450
Abilify Tablets (Rare) 882
Abilify Tablets (Rare) 2450
Aggrenox Capsules 822
AmBisome for Injection (Less common) 620
Anaprox Tablets (Less than 1%) 2761
Anaprox DS Tablets (Less than 1%) 2761
Argatroban Injection (2.6%) 1346
Arthrotec Tablets (Rare) 3129
Azilect Tablets (Rare) 3293
Campath Ampules 811
Campral Tablets (Infrequent) 1174
Clozaril Tablets (Less than 1%) 2184
Copaxone for Injection (Infrequent) 3297
▲ Depacon Injection (1% to 5%) 412
▲ Depakene (1% to 5%) 417
▲ Depakote Sprinkle Capsules (1% to 5%) 422
▲ Depakote Tablets (1% to 5%) 427
Depakote ER Tablets (Greater than 1%) 434
EC-Naprosyn Delayed-Release Tablets (Less than 1%) 2761
Effexor Tablets (Rare) 3411
Effexor XR Capsules (Rare) 3417
Exelon Capsules (Infrequent) 2206
Exelon Oral Solution (Infrequent) 2206
FazaClo Orally Disintegrating Tablets (Less than 1%) 551
Geodon Capsules (Rare) 2529
Herceptin I.V. (At least one of the 958 patients) 1233
Imitrex Injection 1463
Imitrex Nasal Spray (Rare) 1467
Imitrex Tablets (Rare) 1471
I.V. Busulfex (2%) 2493
Lamictal 1481
▲ Leukine (13%) 814
Matulane Capsules 3191
Mobic Oral Suspension (Less than 2%) 863
Mobic Tablets (Less than 2%) 863
Naprosyn Suspension (Less than 1%) 2761
Naprosyn Tablets (Less than 1%) 2761
Neurontin Capsules (Rare) 2487
Neurontin Oral Solution (Rare) 2487
Neurontin Tablets (Rare) 2487
Paxil CR Controlled-Release Tablets (Rare) 1538
Paxil (Rare) 1530
Permax Tablets (Infrequent) 3356
Pexeva Tablets (rare) 1694
▲ Photofrin for Injection (8%) 702
Pletal Tablets (Less than 2%) 2455
Prevacid Delayed-Release Capsules (Less than 1%) 3271
Prevacid for Delayed-Release Oral Suspension (Less than 1%) 3271
Prevacid SoluTab Delayed-Release Orally Disintegrating Tablets (Less than 1%) 3271
Prevacid NapraPAC (Less than 1%) 3280
PREVPAC (Less than 1%) 3284
Proleukin for Injection (Less than 1%) 2266
Protonix I.V. (Less than 1%) 3472
Protonix Tablets (Less than 1%) 3469
Prozac Pulvules and Liquid (Rare) 1801
Relpax Tablets (Rare) 2548
ReoPro Vials (5 to 11 events) 1809
Requip Tablets (Rare) 1555
Rilutek Tablets (Rare) 2930
Risperdal (Rare) 1676
Risperdal M-Tab Orally Disintegrating Tablets (Rare) 1676
Seroquel Tablets (Infrequent) 690
Tarceva Tablets 1259
Tarceva Tablets 2444
Tequin Injection (Less than 0.1%) 938
Tequin Injection in 5% Dextrose (Less than 0.1%) 938
Tequin Tablets (Less than 0.1%) 938
Tricor Tablets 527
Trileptal Tablets 2300
Trileptal Oral Suspension 2300
VFEND I.V. (Less than 2%) 2564
VFEND Oral Suspension (Less than 2%) 2564
VFEND Tablets (Less than 2%) 2564
Voltaren Tablets (Occasionally) 2307
Voltaren-XR Tablets (Occasionally) 2310
Xeloda Tablets 2822
Zomig Tablets (Rare) 3519
Zomig-ZMT Tablets (Rare) 3519
Zonegran Capsules (Rare) 1101

Hematochezia
Bicillin C-R Injectable Suspension 1706
Camptosar Injection 2604
Coumadin for Injection 898
Cymbalta Delayed-Release Capsules (Infrequent) 1757
Invirase (Less than 2%) 2772
Nalfon Capsules (Less than 1%) 2502
Neurontin Capsules (Infrequent) 2487
Neurontin Oral Solution (Infrequent) 2487
Neurontin Tablets (Infrequent) 2487
ProQuad 2064
▲ Remicade for IV Injection (10%) 971
Rescriptor Tablets 2551
Tarceva Tablets 1259
Tarceva Tablets 2444
Trileptal Tablets 2300
Trileptal Oral Suspension 2300
Xifaxan Tablets (Less than 2%) 2842

Hematocrit, decrease
Aceon Tablets (2 mg, 4 mg, 8 mg) 3194
ActoPlus Met Tablets 3214
Actos Tablets 3219
Advate Injection (0.6%) 712
Aggrastat (2.2%) 1907
Aggrenox Capsules 822
Alphanate, Antihemophilic Factor (Human) 1654
Altace Capsules (Rare) 1702
▲ Argatroban Injection (10.4%) 1346
Atacand Tablets 649
Atacand HCT 651
Avandamet Tablets 1373
Avandaryl Tablets 1379
Avandia Tablets 1384
Benicar Tablets 1043
Benicar HCT Tablets (One patient) 1044
Blocadren Tablets 1916
▲ Cancidas for Injection (0.9% to 11.1%) 1918
▲ Cipro I.V. (Among most frequent) 2984
▲ DepoDur Extended-Release Injection (2% to 5%) 1110
Diovan Tablets (0.8%) 2193
Diovan HCT Tablets (Less than 0.1%) 2196
Eligard 7.5 mg (Less than 2%) 2880
Hyzaar 50-12.5 Tablets 1990
Hyzaar 100-12.5 Tablets 1990
Hyzaar 100-25 Tablets 1990
Infergen (1% or less) 3364
▲ Invanz for Injection (3% to 3.4%) 1999
▲ Lariam Tablets (Among most frequent) 2786
Lofibra Tablets 1219
Lofibra Capsules 1216
▲ Lupron Depot 7.5 mg (Greater than or equal to 5%) 3264
Maxipime for Injection (Greater than 0.1% to less than 1%) 1105
Merrem I.V. (Greater than 0.2%) 686
Micardis HCT Tablets (0.6%) 856
Neumega for Injection 3435
Noroxin Tablets (Less frequent) 2032
Omnicef for Oral Suspension (0.2%) 511
Panhematin for Injection 2473
Parcopa Orally Disintegrating Tablets 3097
Precose Tablets 751
Primaxin I.M. 2045
Primaxin I.V. 2048
Prinivil Tablets (Frequent) 2052
Prinzide Tablets (Frequent) 2056
ReoPro Vials (7 to 11 events) 1809
Teveten HCT Tablets (0.1%) 1737
Timentin ADD-Vantage 1580
Timentin Injection Galaxy Container 1583
Timentin IV Infusion 1577
Timentin Pharmacy Bulk Package 1586
Tracleer Tablets 545
Tranxene 2474
Vantin Tablets and Oral Suspension 2645
Vasotec I.V. Injection (Frequent) 2103
▲ Zinacef for Injection (1 in 10 patients) 1631
▲ Zinacef Injection (1 in 10 patients) 1631
Zosyn 3492

Hematocrit, increase
▲ AndroGel (3% to 6%) 3329
Clozaril Tablets 2184
Epogen for Injection 591
FazaClo Orally Disintegrating Tablets 551
Procrit for Injection 2364
Striant Mucoadhesive 1007
Testim 1% Gel (1% to 2%) 695

Hematocrit content, deviation
Bumex Tablets (0.6%) 2746

Hematologic abnormalities
Depakote ER Tablets 434

Hematologic reactions
Dapsone Tablets USP 1673
Daraprim Tablets 1419
Lamictal 1481
Rebif Prefilled Syringe for Injection 3159

Hematologic toxicity
Bexxar 1398
Doxil Injection 2351
Retrovir IV Infusion 1564

Hematoma
Aceon Tablets (2 mg, 4 mg, 8 mg) (0.3% to 1%) 3194
▲ Advair Diskus 100/50 (1% to 3%) 1308
▲ Advair Diskus 250/50 (1% to 3%) 1308
▲ Advair Diskus 500/50 (1% to 3%) 1308
Advate Injection (0.6%) 712
Aggrenox Capsules (Less than 1%) 822
Anzemet Injection (Infrequently) 2859
Anzemet Tablets (Infrequently) 2862
▲ Argatroban Injection (3.6%) 1346
Arixtra Injection (2.1% to 2.8%) 1351
Campath Ampules 811
Caverject Impulse Injection 2612
Copaxone for Injection (Infrequent) 3297
▲ Dacogen Injection (5%) 2129
Depacon Injection 412
Depakene 417
Depakote Sprinkle Capsules 422
Depakote Tablets 427
Depakote ER Tablets 434
Eldepryl Capsules 3208
Emend Capsules (Greater than 0.5%) 1963
Evoxac Capsules (Less than 1%) 1047
Exelon Capsules (Infrequent) 2206
Exelon Oral Solution (Infrequent) 2206
▲ Flovent Diskus (1% to 3%) 1443
Havrix Vaccine (Less than 1%) 1456
Imitrex Injection 1463
Imitrex Tablets (Rare) 1471
Invanz for Injection (Greater than 0.1%) 1999
Levaquin (0.1% to 0.9%) 2384
Levaquin in 5% Dextrose Injection (0.1% to 0.9%) 2384
Lexapro Oral Solution (Infrequent) 1190
Lexapro Tablets (Infrequent) 1190
Lotronex Tablets (Rare) 1512
Lovenox Injection 2915
Nimotop Capsules (Less than 1%) 749
Paxil CR Controlled-Release Tablets (Infrequent) 1538
Paxil (Infrequent) 1530
Pexeva Tablets (infrequent) 1694
Plavix Tablets (1% to 2.5%) 917
Plavix Tablets (1% to 2.5%) 2926
ReFacto Vials 3484
▲ Refludan for Injection (10.6%) 792
ReoPro Vials 1809
Risperdal Consta Long-Acting Injection (Rare) 1682
Rythmol SR Capsules 2727
▲ Sandostatin Injection (1% to 4%) 2278
▲ Sandostatin LAR Depot (1% to 4%) 2280
▲ Simulect for Injection (3% to 10%) 2284
▲ Thrombate III (1 of 17) 3257
▲ TNKase I.V. (1.7% to 12.3%) 1264
Topamax Sprinkle Capsules (1%) 2404
Topamax Tablets (1%) 2404
Vantas (Less than 2%) 3375
Vantin Tablets and Oral Suspension (Less than 1%) 2645
▲ Varivax (24.4% to 32.5%) 2100

Hematoma, periorbital
▲ Macugen Injection (1% to 5%) ⊙261

Hematoma, spinal-epidural
Aggrastat 1907
Fragmin Injection (9 cases) 1097

Hematoma, splenic
NovoSeven 2331

Hematoma, subdermal
Neurontin Oral Solution (Infrequent) 2487
Seroquel Tablets (Rare) 690

Hematoma, subdural
Actiq (Less than 1%) 979
▲ Humira Injection (Less than 5%) 466
Neurontin 2487
Pletal Tablets (Very rare) 2455
Rilutek Tablets (Infrequent) 2930
Zelapar Tablets 3372

Hematoma at injection site
▲ Edex Injection (5%) 3089
▲ Fragmin Injection (0.2% to 4.7%) 1097

ProQuad 2064
Zostavax Injection (1.4%) 2111

Hematopoietic depression
Cosmegen for Injection 2459
Mustargen for Injection (Occasional) 2468

Hematuria
Abilify Oral Solution (Infrequent) 882
Abilify Oral Solution (Infrequent) 2450
Abilify Discmelt Orally Disintegrating Tablets (Infrequent) 882
Abilify Discmelt Orally Disintegrating Tablets (Infrequent) 2450
Abilify Tablets (Infrequent) 882
Abilify Tablets (Infrequent) 2450
Accutane Capsules 2731
Aceon Tablets (2 mg, 4 mg, 8 mg) (0.3% to 1%) 3194
Aciphex Tablets (Rare) 1090
Actiq (Less than 1%) 979
Aggrenox Capsules (Less than 1%) 822
▲ Agrylin Capsules (1% to 5%) 3169
Aloprim for Injection (Less than 1%) 2167
▲ AmBisome for Injection (14%) 620
Anaprox Tablets (Less than 1%) 2761
Anaprox DS Tablets (Less than 1%) 2761
Anzemet Injection (Rare) 2859
Anzemet Tablets (Rare) 2862
▲ Argatroban Injection (0.9% to 11.8%) 1346
Aricept Tablets (Infrequent) 1094
Aricept ODT Tablets (Infrequent) 1094
Arthrotec Tablets (Rare) 3129
Asacol Delayed-Release Tablets 2692
Astelin Nasal Spray (Infrequent) 1904
Atacand Tablets (0.5% or greater) 649
Atacand HCT (0.5% or greater) 651
Atripla Tablets (2%) 945
Augmentin (Rare) 1360
Augmentin Tablets (Rare) 1363
Augmentin XR Extended-Release Tablets (Rare) 1369
Augmentin ES-600 Powder for Oral Suspension (Rare) 1366
▲ Baraclude (9%) 894
Benicar HCT Tablets (Greater than 1%) 1044
Bicillin C-R Injectable Suspension 1706
Caduet Tablets (Greater than or equal to 2%) 2508
Campath Ampules 811
Campral Tablets (Rare) 1174
Cancidas for Injection (2.2%) 1918
Cardene I.V. (0.7%) 2497
Cardura XL Tablets 2515
Caverject Impulse Injection (Less than 1%) 2612
Celebrex Capsules (0.1% to 1.9%) 3134
Celexa (Rare) 1176
▲ CellCept Capsules (3% to less than 20%) 2747
▲ CellCept Intravenous (3% to less than 20%) 2747
▲ CellCept Oral Suspension (3% to less than 20%) 2747
▲ CellCept Tablets (3% to less than 20%) 2747
Cipro 2977
Cipro I.V. (1% or less) 2984
Cipro XR Tablets (Less than 1%) 2990
Clinoril Tablets (Less than 1%) 1924
▲ Clolar for Intravenous Infusion (17%) 1271
Colazal Capsules 2838
▲ Coreg Tablets (Greater than 1% to 3%) 1414
Coumadin for Injection 898
Coumadin Tablets 898
▲ Crixivan Capsules (Approximately 12.4%) 1940
Cuprimine Capsules 1947
Dantrium Capsules (Less frequent) 2694
Daraprim Tablets 1419
Demser Capsules (A few patients) 1953
Diuril Sodium Intravenous (1 case) 2467
Dolobid Tablets (Less than 1 in 100) 1955
▲ Doxil Injection (1% to 10%) 2351
EC-Naprosyn Delayed-Release Tablets (Less than 1%) 2761
Edecrin 1959
Effexor Tablets (Infrequent) 3411
Effexor XR Capsules (Infrequent) 3417
Eloxatin for Injection 2892
▲ Eulexin Capsules (7%) 3009
Evoxac Capsules (Less than 1%) 1047
Exelon Capsules (Frequent) 2206
Exelon Oral Solution (Frequent) 2206
Fortical Nasal Spray (Less than 1%) 3337
Fragmin Injection (2.9%) 1097
Gabitril Tablets (Infrequent) 984
Gantrisin Pediatric Suspension 2770
▲ Gemzar for Injection (Up to 35%) 1771
Gengraf Capsules (1% to less than 3%) 459
Genotropin Lyophilized Powder (Infrequent) 2638
Geodon Capsules (Infrequent) 2529
Gleevec Tablets (Infrequent) 2227
▲ Hepsera Tablets (11%) 1292
Herceptin I.V. (At least one of the 958 patients) 1233
▲ Humira Injection (5%) 466
Imitrex Nasal Spray 1467
Imitrex Tablets (Rare) 1471
Indocin Capsules (Less than 1%) 1995
Indocin I.V. (Less than 1%) 2465
Indocin (Less than 1%) 1995
Infed Injection 3390
▲ Intron A for Injection (Less than 5%) 3024
Invanz for Injection (Greater than 0.1%) 1999
Ionsys Transdermal System (.1% to less than 1%) 2379
Iressa Tablets 684
Lamictal (Infrequent) 1481
▲ Leukine (9%) 814
Levaquin (0.1% to 0.9%) 2384
Levaquin in 5% Dextrose Injection (0.1% to 0.9%) 2384
Lexapro Oral Solution (Infrequent) 1190
Lexapro Tablets (Infrequent) 1190
Lipitor Tablets (Less than 2%) 2483
Lovenox Injection (Less than 2%) 2915
Lunesta Tablets (Infrequent) 3142
Lyrica Capsules (0.1% to 1%) 2539
Matulane Capsules 3191
Meridia Capsules 489
Miacalcin Nasal Spray (Less than 1%) 2253
Mintezol 2027
Mirapex Tablets (Less than 1%) 859
Mobic Oral Suspension (Less than 2%) 863
Mobic Tablets (Less than 2%) 863
▲ Myfortic Tablets (3% to less than 20%) 2255
▲ Mylotarg for Injection (1% to 37%) 3431
Nalfon Capsules (Less than 1%) 2502
Namenda (Infrequent) 1195
Naprosyn Suspension (Less than 1%) 2761
Naprosyn Tablets (Less than 1%) 2761
NeoProfen Injection (1%) 2472
Neoral Oral Solution (1% to less than 3%) 2259
Neoral Soft Gelatin Capsules (1% to less than 3%) 2259
Neupogen for Injection (Infrequent) 603
Neurontin Capsules (Infrequent) 2487
Neurontin Oral Solution (Infrequent) 2487
Neurontin Tablets (Infrequent) 2487
Nexium Delayed-Release Capsules (Less than 1%) 655
Nexium I.V. (Less than 1%) 659
Noroxin Tablets 2032
Norvir (Less than 2%) 503
Oncaspar (Less than 1%) 1145
▲ Ontak Vials (10%) 1745
OxyContin Tablets (Less than 1%) 2703
Parcopa Orally Disintegrating Tablets 3097
Paxil CR Controlled-Release Tablets (Infrequent) 1538
Paxil (Infrequent) 1530
Pentasa Capsules (Less than 1%) 3185
Permax Tablets (1.1%) 3356
Pexeva Tablets (Infrequent) 1694
Plavix Tablets (Less than 1%) 917
Plavix Tablets (Less than 1%) 2926
Pletal Tablets (2% or greater) 2455
Prevacid Delayed-Release Capsules (Less than 1%) 3271
Prevacid for Delayed-Release Oral Suspension 3271
Prevacid SoluTab Delayed-Release Orally Disintegrating Tablets (Less than 1%) 3271
Prevacid NapraPAC (Less than 1%) 3280
PREVPAC (Less than 1%) 3284
Prilosec OTC Delayed-Release Tablets (Less than 1%) 2677
Primaxin I.M. 2045
Primaxin I.V. 2048
▲ Prograf Capsules and Injection (3% to 15%) 632
▲ Proleukin for Injection (9%) 2266
Proquin XR Tablets 1153
ProSom Tablets (Rare) 517
Protonix I.V. (Less than 1%) 3472
Protonix Tablets (Less than 1%) 3469
Provigil Tablets (1%) 988
Prozac Pulvules and Liquid (Infrequent) 1801
▲ Quadramet Injection (5%) 1040
Ranexa Tablets (Less than or equal to 0.5%) 1035
▲ Rapamune Oral Solution and Tablets (3% to 20%) 3475
▲ Razadyne (3%) 2399
▲ Razadyne ER Extended-Release Capsules (3%) 2399
▲ Refludan for Injection (4.4%) 792
ReoPro Vials (4 events) 1809
Requip Tablets (Infrequent) 1555
Rescriptor Tablets 2551
Retrovir Capsules (0.8%) 1560
Retrovir IV Infusion (1%) 1564
Retrovir (0.8%) 1560
Revlimid Capsules 958
Reyataz Capsules (Less than 3%) 921
Rilutek Tablets (Infrequent) 2930
Risperdal (Infrequent) 1676
Risperdal Consta Long-Acting Injection (Infrequent) 1682
Risperdal M-Tab Orally Disintegrating Tablets (Infrequent) 1676
Rocephin Injectable Vials, ADD-Vantage, Galaxy, Bulk (Rare) 2800
▲ Rythmol SR Capsules (1% to 3%) 2727
Sandimmune (Rare) 2275
Sandostatin Injection (Less than 1%) 2278
Sandostatin LAR Depot (Rare) 2280
▲ Simulect for Injection (3% to 10%) 2284
Sonata Capsules (Infrequent) 1717
Sular Tablets (Less than or equal to 1%) 3122
Sustiva Capsules (Up to 1%) 930
Sustiva Tablets (Up to 1%) 930
Symbyax Capsules (Infrequent) 1819
Targretin Capsules 1747
Tarka Tablets (Less frequent) 524
▲ Tasmar Tablets (4% to 5%) 3358
▲ Tequin Injection (0.1% to 3%) 938
▲ Tequin Injection in 5% Dextrose (0.1% to 3%) 938
▲ Tequin Tablets (0.1% to 3%) 938
Teveten Tablets (Less than 1%) 1735
Teveten HCT Tablets (Less than 1%) 1737
Thalomid Capsules 965
▲ Thiola Tablets (5%) 2141
Ticlid Tablets 2810
Topamax Sprinkle Capsules (Less than 1% to 2%) 2404
Topamax Tablets (Less than 1% to 2%) 2404
Trileptal Tablets 2300
Trileptal Oral Suspension 2300
Truvada Tablets (2%) 1296
▲ Ultram ER Tablets (1% to greater than 5%) 2392
Uniretic Tablets (Less than 1%) 3100
Uroqid-Acid No. 2 Tablets (Rare) 760
▲ Vagifem Tablets (3% to 5%) 2334
Vantin Tablets and Oral Suspension (Less than 1%) 2645
Vaprisol (2.2%) 643
VFEND I.V. (Less than 2%) 2564
VFEND Oral Suspension (Less than 2%) 2564
VFEND Tablets (Less than 2%) 2564
Viagra Tablets 2573
▲ Viread Tablets (2% to 7%) 1301
Voltaren Tablets (Occasionally) 2307
Voltaren-XR Tablets (Occasionally) 2310
Xifaxan Tablets (Less than 2%) 2842
Xyrem Oral Solution (Infrequent) 1688
Zegerid Capsules (Less than 1%) 2958
Zegerid Powder for Oral Solution (Less than 1%) 2958
Zoloft (Rare) 2586
Zometa for Intravenous Infusion 2315
Zomig Tablets (Infrequent) 3519
Zomig-ZMT Tablets (Infrequent) 3519
Zonegran Capsules (Infrequent) 1101
Zosyn (1.0% or less) 3492
Zovirax 1643
Zyprexa Tablets (Infrequent) 1830
Zyprexa ZYDIS Orally Disintegrating Tablets (Infrequent) 1830
Zyrtec Chewable Tablets (Less than 2%) 2594
Zyrtec (Less than 2%) 2594
Zyrtec-D 12 Hour Extended Release Tablets (Less than 2%) 2597

Hematuria, aggravated
Vantas (Less than 2%) 3375

Hematuria, microscopic
Calcium Disodium Versenate Injection 1851
▲ Crixivan Capsules (Approximately 12.4%) 1940
▲ Ontak Vials (Less than 5%) 1745

Hemianopsia
Trileptal Tablets 2300
Trileptal Oral Suspension 2300

Hemiparesis
Arranon Injection (1%) 1357
Exelon Capsules (Infrequent) 2206
Exelon Oral Solution (Infrequent) 2206
Femara Tablets (Less than or equal to 2%) 2214
Klonopin 2778
Orthoclone OKT3 Sterile Solution 2360
Prograf Capsules and Injection 632
Requip Tablets (Rare) 1555
Sandostatin LAR Depot (Rare) 2280
▲ Temodar Capsules (18%) 3073
Thyrogen for Injection (4 patients out of 55) 1286

Hemiplegia
Actiq (Less than 1%) 979
Azilect Tablets (Infrequent) 3293
DepoCyt Injection 1143
Doxil Injection (Less than 1%) 2351
Gabitril Tablets (Infrequent) 984
Imitrex Injection (Rare) 1463
Imitrex Tablets 1471
Lamictal (Rare) 1481
Namenda (Infrequent) 1195
Neurontin Capsules (Infrequent) 2487
Neurontin Oral Solution (Infrequent) 2487
Neurontin Tablets (Infrequent) 2487
Orthoclone OKT3 Sterile Solution 2360
Permax Tablets (Rare) 3356
Prevacid Delayed-Release Capsules (Less than 1%) 3271
Prevacid for Delayed-Release Oral Suspension (Less than 1%) 3271
Prevacid SoluTab Delayed-Release Orally Disintegrating Tablets (Less than 1%) 3271
Prevacid NapraPAC (Less than 1%) 3280
PREVPAC (Less than 1%) 3284
Relpax Tablets (Rare) 2548
Requip Tablets (Rare) 1555
Rilutek Tablets (Infrequent) 2930
Seroquel Tablets (Infrequent) 690
Tasmar Tablets (Rare) 3358
Thyrogen for Injection (4 patients out of 55) 1286
Trileptal Tablets 2300
Trileptal Oral Suspension 2300
▲ Vesanoid Capsules (3%) 2820

Hemochromatosis
Effexor Tablets (Rare) 3411
Effexor XR Capsules (Rare) 3417

Hemoconcentration
Follistim AQ Cartridge 2338

Hemoglobin, decrease
Aceon Tablets (2 mg, 4 mg, 8 mg) 3194
ActoPlus Met Tablets 3214
Actos Tablets 3219
Aggrastat (2.1%) 1907
Aggrenox Capsules 822
Altace Capsules (Rare) 1702
▲ Argatroban Injection (10.4%) 1346
Atacand Tablets 649
Atacand HCT 651
Avalide Tablets 888
Avalide Tablets 2874
Avandamet Tablets 1373
Avandaryl Tablets 1379
Avandia Tablets 1384
Avapro Tablets (Less than 0.2%) 891
Avapro Tablets (Less than 0.2%) 2871
Benicar Tablets 1043
Blocadren Tablets 1916
▲ Cancidas for Injection (0.9% to 12.3%) 1918
Cipro (Less than 0.1%) 2977
▲ Cipro I.V. (Among most frequent) 2984
▲ Copegus Tablets (13%) 2754
Crixivan Capsules (0.6%) 1940
▲ Dapsone Tablets USP (Almost all patients) 1673
▲ Diovan HCT Tablets (Greater than 20%) 2196
Eligard 7.5 mg (Less than 2%) 2880
▲ Emend Capsules (3.8%) 1963
Hyzaar 50-12.5 Tablets 1990

Hyzaar 100-12.5 Tablets 1990
Hyzaar 100-25 Tablets 1990
Infergen (1% or less) 3364
▲ Invanz for Injection (4.5% to 4.9%) 1999
Invirase (Up to 1%) 2772
Lofibra Tablets 1219
Lofibra Capsules 1216
▲ Lupron Depot 7.5 mg (Greater than or equal to 5%) 3264
Merrem I.V. (Greater than 0.2%) 686
Micardis Tablets 854
Micardis HCT Tablets (1.2%) 856
Mustargen for Injection 2468
▲ Myfortic Tablets (3% to less than 20%) 2255
Neumega for Injection 3435
Noroxin Tablets (0.6%) 2032
Omnicef Capsules (0.3%) 511
Omnicef for Oral Suspension (0.4%) 511
Parcopa Orally Disintegrating Tablets 3097
▲ Pegasys (17%) 2789
▲ PEG-Intron Powder for Injection (30%) 3048
Primaxin I.M. 2045
Primaxin I.V. 2048
Prinivil Tablets (Frequent) 2052
Prinzide Tablets (Frequent) 2056
▲ Quadramet Injection (40.7%) 1040
Rebetol 3058
Rebetron Combination Therapy 3063
Refludan for Injection 792
ReoPro Vials (7 to 11 events) 1809
Revlimid Capsules 958
Rythmol SR Capsules 2727
▲ Temodar Capsules (51%) 3073
Teveten Tablets (0.1%) 1735
Teveten HCT Tablets (0.1%) 1737
Timentin ADD-Vantage 1580
Timentin Injection Galaxy Container 1583
Timentin IV Infusion 1577
Timentin Pharmacy Bulk Package 1586
Tracleer Tablets 545
Valtrex Caplets (Up to 0.8%) 1597
Vantin Tablets and Oral Suspension 2645
Vasotec I.V. Injection (Frequent) 2103
Viramune Oral Suspension (1.2%) 873
Viramune Tablets (1.2%) 873
WinRho SDF 732
Xeloda Tablets (1%) 2822
▲ Zinacef for Injection (1 in 10 patients) 1631
▲ Zinacef Injection (1 in 10 patients) 1631
Zosyn 3492

Hemoglobin, increase
FazaClo Orally Disintegrating Tablets 551
Fuzeon Injection (0.6% to 1.5%) 2767
Testim 1% Gel (1% to 2%) 695

Hemoglobin content, deviation
Amerge Tablets (Rare) 1339
Bumex Tablets (0.8%) 2746
Diovan Tablets (0.4%) 2193
Diovan HCT Tablets (0.004%) 2196
▲ Intron A for Injection (Up to 32%) 3024
Lotronex Tablets (Rare) 1512

Hemoglobinemia
▲ AndroGel (3% to 6%) 3329
Clozaril Tablets 2184
Stromectol Tablets (1%) 2083

Hemoglobinuria
Mycamine for Injection 628
Raptiva for Injection 1250
WinRho SDF 732

Hemolysis
Alphanate, Antihemophilic Factor (Human) 1654
Campath Ampules 811
Carimune NF 3499
Cozaar Tablets 1935
▲ Dapsone Tablets USP (Most common) 1673
▲ Doxil Injection (1% to 5%) 2351
Elitek (Less than 1%) 2890
Flebogamma 5%, Immune Globulin Intravenous (Human) 1658
Gammagard Liquid 721
Gammagard S/D 724
Gamunex Immune Globulin I.V., 10% 3235
Hyzaar 50-12.5 Tablets (One subject) 1990
Hyzaar 100-12.5 Tablets (One subject) 1990
Hyzaar 100-25 Tablets (One subject) 1990
Mycamine for Injection 628
Prevacid Delayed-Release Capsules (Less than 1%) 3271
Prevacid for Delayed-Release Oral Suspension (Less than 1%) 3271
Prevacid SoluTab Delayed-Release Orally Disintegrating Tablets (Less than 1%) 3271
Prevacid NapraPAC (Less than 1%) 3280
PREVPAC (Less than 1%) 3284
Rebetron Combination Therapy 3063
Revlimid Capsules 958
Seroquel Tablets (Rare) 690
Trasylol Injection (0.3%) 754
Uniretic Tablets (Less than 1%) 3100
Vasotec I.V. Injection (A few cases) 2103

Hemolysis, neonatal
Dapsone Tablets USP 1673
Mephyton Tablets 2018

Hemolytic icterus
(*see under* Jaundice)

Hemolytic-uremic syndrome
Eloxatin for Injection 2892
Gemzar for Injection (Rare) 1771
Gengraf Capsules 459
Mircette Tablets 1066
Neoral Oral Solution 2259
Neoral Soft Gelatin Capsules 2259
NuvaRing 2340
Ortho-Cyclen Tablets 2429
Ortho Evra Transdermal System 2417
Ortho Tri-Cyclen Tablets 2429
Ortho Tri-Cyclen Lo Tablets 2436
Prograf Capsules and Injection 632
▲ Rapamune Oral Solution and Tablets (3% to 20%) 3475
Seasonique Tablets 1077
Valtrex Caplets 1597
Yasmin 28 Tablets 796
Yaz Tablets 803

Hemopericardium
Aggrastat 1907
Cardene I.V. (0.7%) 2497

Hemoperitoneum
Follistim AQ Cartridge 2338
Merrem I.V. (0.2%) 686
Trasylol Injection (1% to 2%) 754

Hemophilus
▲ Intron A for Injection (Less than 5%) 3024

Hemoptysis
Abelcet Injection 1141
Abilify Oral Solution (Rare) 882
Abilify Oral Solution (Rare) 2450
Abilify Discmelt Orally Disintegrating Tablets (Rare) 882
Abilify Discmelt Orally Disintegrating Tablets (Rare) 2450
Abilify Tablets (Rare) 882
Abilify Tablets (Rare) 2450
Actiq (Less than 1%) 979
Aggrenox Capsules (Less than 1%) 822
AmBisome for Injection (Less common) 620
Argatroban Injection (2.9%) 1346
Campath Ampules 811
▲ CellCept Capsules (3% to less than 20%) 2747
▲ CellCept Intravenous (3% to less than 20%) 2747
▲ CellCept Oral Suspension (3% to less than 20%) 2747
▲ CellCept Tablets (3% to less than 20%) 2747
Cipro (Less than 1%) 2977
Cipro I.V. (1% or less) 2984
Cipro XR Tablets 2990
Colazal Capsules 2838
Dacogen Injection 2129
Duragesic Transdermal System (1% or greater) 2373
Effexor Tablets (Rare) 3411
Effexor XR Capsules (Rare) 3417
▲ Eloxatin for Injection (2% to 5%) 2892
Evoxac Capsules (Less than 1%) 1047
Gabitril Tablets (Infrequent) 984
▲ Intron A for Injection (Less than or equal to 5%) 3024
Invanz for Injection (Greater than 0.1%) 1999
Invirase (Less than 2%) 2772
▲ I.V. Busulfex (3%) 2493
Levaquin (0.1% to 0.9%) 2384
Levaquin in 5% Dextrose Injection (0.1% to 0.9%) 2384
Lupron Depot 7.5 mg (Less than 5%) 3264
Matulane Capsules 3191
Namenda (Infrequent) 1195
Natrecor for Injection (Greater than or equal to 1%) 3127
Neurontin Capsules (Rare) 2487
Neurontin Oral Solution (Rare) 2487
Neurontin Tablets (Rare) 2487
Paxil CR Controlled-Release Tablets (Rare) 1538
Paxil (Rare) 1530
Permax Tablets (Infrequent) 3356
Pexeva Tablets (Rare) 1694
Photofrin for Injection (One patient) 702
Plavix Tablets (Less than 1%) 917
Plavix Tablets (Less than 1%) 2926
Pletal Tablets (Less than 2%) 2455
Prevacid Delayed-Release Capsules (Less than 1%) 3271
Prevacid for Delayed-Release Oral Suspension (Less than 1%) 3271
Prevacid SoluTab Delayed-Release Orally Disintegrating Tablets (Less than 1%) 3271
Prevacid NapraPAC (Less than 1%) 3280
PREVPAC (Less than 1%) 3284
Prinivil Tablets (0.3% to 1.0%) 2052
Prinzide Tablets 2056
Proleukin for Injection (1%) 2266
Proquin XR Tablets 1153
Prozac Pulvules and Liquid (Rare) 1801
Pulmozyme Inhalation Solution 1248
ReoPro Vials (9 to 11 events) 1809
Rilutek Tablets (Infrequent) 2930
Risperdal Consta Long-Acting Injection (Infrequent) 1682
Rythmol SR Capsules 2727
Symbyax Capsules (Rare) 1819
Targretin Capsules 1747
Thiola Tablets (2%) 2141
▲ TOBI Solution for Inhalation (19.4%) 2298
▲ Trisenox Injection (8%) 993
Uniretic Tablets (Less than 1%) 3100
▲ Ventavis Inhalation Solution (5%) 1020
VFEND I.V. (Less than 2%) 2564
VFEND Oral Suspension (Less than 2%) 2564
VFEND Tablets (Less than 2%) 2564
▲ Xeloda Tablets (Less than 5%) 2822
Zoloft (Rare) 2586
Zonegran Capsules (Rare) 1101
Zyprexa Tablets (Infrequent) 1830
Zyprexa ZYDIS Orally Disintegrating Tablets (Infrequent) 1830

Hemorrhage
(*see under* Bleeding)

Hemorrhage, all sites
▲ Nexavar Tablets (0% to 15%) 746

Hemorrhage, cerebral
(*see under* Cerebral hemorrhage)

Hemorrhage, cerebrovascular
Mycamine for Injection 628
Revatio Tablets 2557
Viagra Tablets 2573

Hemorrhage, CNS
▲ Gleevec Tablets (0% to 9%) 2227

Hemorrhage, colon
Actiq (Less than 1%) 979
Prozac Pulvules and Liquid (Rare) 1801

Hemorrhage, conjunctival
Exelon Capsules (Infrequent) 2206
Exelon Oral Solution (Infrequent) 2206
Gleevec Tablets (Infrequent) 2227
Macugen Injection ⊙261
Namenda (Infrequent) 1195
Plavix Tablets 917
Plavix Tablets 2926
▲ Retisert Implant (10% to 35%) ⊙258
Stromectol Tablets 2083
Trileptal Tablets 2300
Trileptal Oral Suspension 2300
▲ Zymar Ophthalmic Solution (1% to 4%) 575

Hemorrhage, ear
Imitrex Nasal Spray 1467

Hemorrhage, esophageal
Demadex Injection 2759
Demadex Tablets 2759
Pletal Tablets (Less than 2%) 2455
Protonix I.V. (Less than 1%) 3472
Protonix Tablets (Less than 1%) 3469

Hemorrhage, eye, anterior chamber
Evoxac Capsules (Less than 1%) 1047
Zoloft (Rare) 2586

Hemorrhage, eyes
Abilify Oral Solution (Infrequent) 882
Abilify Oral Solution (Infrequent) 2450
Abilify Discmelt Orally Disintegrating Tablets (Infrequent) 882
Abilify Discmelt Orally Disintegrating Tablets (Infrequent) 2450
Abilify Tablets (Infrequent) 882
Abilify Tablets (Infrequent) 2450
Actiq (Less than 1%) 979
Adalat CC Tablets (Less than 1%) 2964
AmBisome for Injection (Less common) 620
Amerge Tablets (Rare) 1339
Caduet Tablets (Less than 2%) 2508
▲ CellCept Capsules (3% to less than 20%) 2747
▲ CellCept Intravenous (3% to less than 20%) 2747
▲ CellCept Oral Suspension (3% to less than 20%) 2747
▲ CellCept Tablets (3% to less than 20%) 2747
Effexor Tablets 3411
Effexor XR Capsules 3417
Imitrex Nasal Spray 1467
Iressa Tablets (Very rare) 684
▲ Leukine (11%) 814
Lipitor Tablets (Less than 2%) 2483
Lyrica Capsules (0.1% to 1%) 2539
Neumega for Injection 3435
Neurontin Capsules (Infrequent) 2487
Neurontin Oral Solution (Infrequent) 2487
Neurontin Tablets (Infrequent) 2487
Ocufen Ophthalmic Solution ⊙232
Paxil CR Controlled-Release Tablets (Rare) 1538
Paxil (Rare) 1530
Permax Tablets (Infrequent) 3356
Pexeva Tablets (Rare) 1694
Plavix Tablets 917
Plavix Tablets 2926
Pletal Tablets (Less than 2%) 2455
Prozac Pulvules and Liquid (Rare) 1801
Relpax Tablets (Rare) 2548
ReoPro Vials (9 to 11 events) 1809
Rythmol SR Capsules 2727
Sonata Capsules (Rare) 1717
Soriatane Capsules (Less than 1%) 1013
Symbyax Capsules (Rare) 1819
Tasmar Tablets (Infrequent) 3358
Ticlid Tablets 2810
Uniretic Tablets (Less than 1%) 3100
VFEND I.V. (Less than 2%) 2564
VFEND Oral Suspension (Less than 2%) 2564
VFEND Tablets (Less than 2%) 2564
Viagra Tablets (Less than 2%) 2573
Zelapar Tablets 3372
Zyprexa Tablets (Infrequent) 1830
Zyprexa ZYDIS Orally Disintegrating Tablets (Infrequent) 1830
Zyrtec Chewable Tablets (Less than 2%) 2594
Zyrtec (Less than 2%) 2594
Zyrtec-D 12 Hour Extended Release Tablets (Less than 2%) 2597

Hemorrhage, focal
Thyrogen for Injection (4 patients out of 55) 1286

Hemorrhage, gastrointestinal
(*see under* Bleeding, gastrointestinal)

Hemorrhage, intra-alveolar
▲ I.V. Busulfex (5%) 2493

Hemorrhage, intracerebral
(*see under* Bleeding, intracerebral)

Hemorrhage, intracranial
Aptivus Capsules (Less than 2%) 826
Dacogen Injection (Greater than or equal to 1%) 2129

Hemorrhage, intraventricular
▲ NeoProfen Injection (15% to 29%) 2472

Hemorrhage, postpartum
Aggrenox Capsules 822
Bayer Aspirin 744
Bayer Aspirin Comprehensive Prescribing Information ▣796

St. Joseph 81 mg Aspirin Chewable and Enteric Coated Tablets 1869

Hemorrhage, pulmonary
Aggrastat 1907
Mylotarg for Injection 3431
Photofrin for Injection 702
Plavix Tablets (Less than 1%) 917
Plavix Tablets (Less than 1%) 2926
Pletal Tablets (Very rare) 2455
ReoPro Vials (9 to 11 events) 1809
Revatio Tablets 2557
Sutent Capsules (2 patients) 2560
Viagra Tablets 2573

Hemorrhage, purpuric
Carbatrol Capsules 3171
Tegretol/Tegretol-XR 2295

Hemorrhage, rectal
Ambien CR Tablets (Rare) 2855
Caduet Tablets (Less than 2%) 2508
Campral Tablets (Infrequent) 1174
Demadex Injection 2759
Demadex Tablets 2759
depo-subQ provera 104 Injectable Suspension 2624
Lyrica Capsules (0.1% to 1%) 2539
Prevacid NapraPAC (Less than 1%) 3280
Prozac Pulvules and Liquid (Rare) 1801
Risperdal Consta Long-Acting Injection (Infrequent) 1682
Sutent Capsules 2560
Tricor Tablets 527
Zelnorm Tablets 2312

Hemorrhage, retinal
Aricept Tablets (Infrequent) 1094
Aricept ODT Tablets (Infrequent) 1094
Effexor Tablets (Rare) 3411
Effexor XR Capsules (Rare) 3417
Elitek (Less than or equal to 1%) 2890
Elmiron Capsules (Less than or equal to 1%) 2415
Gleevec Tablets (Rare) 2227
Intron A for Injection (Rare) 3024
▲ Lucentis Injection (15% to 26%) 1237
Matulane Capsules 3191
Namenda (Infrequent) 1195
Paxil CR Controlled-Release Tablets (Rare) 1538
Paxil (Rare) 1530
Pegasys 2789
PEG-Intron Powder for Injection 3048
Pexeva Tablets (Rare) 1694
Plavix Tablets 917
Plavix Tablets 2926
Pletal Tablets (Less than 2%) 2455
▲ Retisert Implant (5% to 9%) ⊙258
Revatio Tablets (1.4% to 1.9%) 2557
VFEND I.V. (Less than 2%) 2564
VFEND Oral Suspension (Less than 2%) 2564
VFEND Tablets (Less than 2%) 2564
Viagra Tablets 2573
▲ Visudyne for Injection (1% to 10%) 2305

Hemorrhage, subarachnoid
Aggrenox Capsules (Less than 1%) 822
Amerge Tablets 1339
Campath Ampules 811
Imitrex Injection 1463
Imitrex Nasal Spray 1467
Imitrex Tablets 1471
Orthoclone OKT3 Sterile Solution 2360
Requip Tablets (Rare) 1555
Revatio Tablets 2557
Rilutek Tablets (Rare) 2930
Symbyax Capsules (Rare) 1819
Viagra Tablets 2573
Zyprexa Tablets (Rare) 1830
Zyprexa ZYDIS Orally Disintegrating Tablets (Rare) 1830

Hemorrhage, subconjunctival
Effexor Tablets (Rare) 3411
Effexor XR Capsules (Rare) 3417
Travatan Ophthalmic Solution (1% to 4%) 563
▲ Vigamox Ophthalmic Solution (1% to 6%) 564
▲ Visudyne for Injection (1% to 10%) 2305

Hemorrhage, subcutaneous
Mustargen for Injection 2468
Pletal Tablets (Very rare) 2455
Ticlid Tablets 2810

Hemorrhage, throat
Imitrex Nasal Spray 1467

Hemorrhage, tumor
▲ Gleevec Tablets (Rare to 4%) 2227

Hemorrhage, uterine
Prozac Pulvules and Liquid (Rare) 1801

Hemorrhage, vaginal
▲ Femara Tablets (Less than 0.1% to 4.8%) 2214

Hemorrhage, vitreous
Gleevec Tablets (Rare) 2227
▲ Macugen Injection (1% to 5%) ⊙261
▲ Retisert Implant (10% to 35%) ⊙258
▲ Visudyne for Injection (1% to 10%) 2305
Xalatan Sterile Ophthalmic Solution (Extremely rare) 2649

Hemorrhagic colitis
Amoxil Capsules 1343
Amoxil Chewable Tablets 1343
Amoxil Pediatric Drops for Oral Suspension 1343
Amoxil Powder for Oral Suspension 1343
Amoxil Tablets 1343
Augmentin 1360
Augmentin Tablets 1363
Augmentin XR Extended-Release Tablets 1369
Kaletra (Less than 2%) 476
Lamictal (Rare) 1481
Omnicef Capsules 511
Omnicef for Oral Suspension 511
Primaxin I.M. 2045
Primaxin I.V. (Less than 0.2%) 2048

Hemorrhagic complications
Coumadin for Injection 898
Coumadin Tablets 898
Lovenox Injection (Low incidence) 2915

Hemorrhagic eruptions
(*see under* Eruptions, hemorrhagic)

Hemorrhagic tendency
Mustargen for Injection 2468

Hemorrhoids
Abilify Oral Solution (Infrequent) 882
Abilify Oral Solution (Infrequent) 2450
Abilify Discmelt Orally Disintegrating Tablets (Infrequent) 882
Abilify Discmelt Orally Disintegrating Tablets (Infrequent) 2450
Abilify Tablets (Infrequent) 882
Abilify Tablets (Infrequent) 2450
Aggrenox Capsules (1%) 822
Ambien Tablets (Rare) 2851
Ambien CR Tablets (Rare) 2855
AmBisome for Injection (Less common) 620
Amerge Tablets (Rare) 1339
Aricept Tablets (Infrequent) 1094
Aricept ODT Tablets (Infrequent) 1094
Arthrotec Tablets (Rare) 3129
Campath Ampules 811
Celebrex Capsules (0.1% to 1.9%) 3134
Celexa (Infrequent) 1176
▲ Chemet Capsules (12.0% to 20.9%) 2458
Colazal Capsules 2838
▲ Dacogen Injection (8%) 2129
Effexor Tablets (Infrequent) 3411
Effexor XR Capsules (Infrequent) 3417
▲ Eloxatin for Injection (2% to 5%) 2892
▲ Entocort EC Capsules (Less than 5%) 2698
▲ Estring Vaginal Ring (1% to 3%) 2635
Evoxac Capsules (Less than 1%) 1047
Exelon Capsules (Infrequent) 2206
Exelon Oral Solution (Infrequent) 2206
▲ Imdur Tablets (Less than or equal to 5%) 3018
▲ Infergen (1% to 6%) 3364
Invanz for Injection (Greater than 0.1%) 1999
Invirase (Less than 2%) 2772
Klonopin (Infrequent) 2778
Lexapro Oral Solution (Infrequent) 1190
Lexapro Tablets (Infrequent) 1190
Lotronex Tablets (2%) 1512
Micardis Tablets (More than 0.3%) 854
Micardis HCT Tablets 856
Neurontin Capsules (Infrequent) 2487
Neurontin Oral Solution (Infrequent) 2487
Neurontin Tablets (Infrequent) 2487
Requip Tablets (Infrequent) 1555
Risperdal (Infrequent) 1676
Risperdal Consta Long-Acting Injection (Infrequent) 1682
Risperdal M-Tab Orally Disintegrating Tablets (Infrequent) 1676
Sandostatin Injection (Less than 1%) 2278
▲ Sandostatin LAR Depot (5% to 15%) 2280
Seroquel Tablets (Infrequent) 690
Soriatane Capsules (Less than 1%) 1013
Topamax Sprinkle Capsules (Infrequent) 2404
Topamax Tablets (Infrequent) 2404
Trileptal Tablets 2300
Trileptal Oral Suspension 2300
Vivitrol 995
Zelnorm Tablets 2312
Zyrtec Chewable Tablets (Less than 2%) 2594
Zyrtec (Less than 2%) 2594
Zyrtec-D 12 Hour Extended Release Tablets (Less than 2%) 2597

Hemospermia
Rescriptor Tablets 2551

Hemostasis, interference
Depacon Injection 412
Depakote Tablets 427

Hemothorax
Permax Tablets (Rare) 3356
Plavix Tablets (Less than 1%) 917
Plavix Tablets (Less than 1%) 2926
Refludan for Injection 792

Henoch-Schönlein purpura
Boostrix 1404
Cozaar Tablets 1935
Fluarix 1451
Hyzaar 50-12.5 Tablets 1990
Hyzaar 100-12.5 Tablets 1990
Hyzaar 100-25 Tablets 1990
Parcopa Orally Disintegrating Tablets 3097
Paxil CR Controlled-Release Tablets 1538
Paxil 1530
Pexeva Tablets 1694
ProQuad 2064
Stalevo Tablets 2287
Varivax 2100

Hepatic adenoma
Estratest Tablets (Rare) 3199
Estratest H.S. Tablets (Rare) 3199
Mircette Tablets 1066
Ortho-Cyclen Tablets 2429
Ortho Evra Transdermal System 2417
Ortho Tri-Cyclen Tablets 2429
Ortho Tri-Cyclen Lo Tablets 2436
Premarin Intravenous 3442
Premarin Vaginal Cream 3452
Seasonique Tablets 1077
Yasmin 28 Tablets 796
Yaz Tablets 803

Hepatic coma
(*see also under* Coma, hepatic)
Androxy Tablets (Rare) 3335

Hepatic dysfunction
Accolate Tablets 671
Actimmune (Rare) 1671
▲ Advair Diskus 100/50 (1% to 3%) 1308
▲ Advair Diskus 250/50 (1% to 3%) 1308
▲ Advair Diskus 500/50 (1% to 3%) 1308
Advicor Tablets 1722
Aggrenox Capsules (Less than 1%) 822
▲ Albenza Tablets (Less than 1.0% to 15.6%) 1338
Aldara Cream, 5% 1846
Aldoril Tablets 1910
Alkeran for Injection 955
Alkeran Tablets 956
Altoprev Extended-Release Tablets 3109
Ambien Tablets (Infrequent) 2851
Ambien CR Tablets (Infrequent) 2855
AmBisome for Injection (Less common) 620
Amerge Tablets (Rare) 1339
Amoxil Capsules 1343
Amoxil Chewable Tablets 1343
Amoxil Pediatric Drops for Oral Suspension 1343
Amoxil Powder for Oral Suspension 1343
Amoxil Tablets 1343
Anaprox Tablets (Less than 1%) 2761
Anaprox DS Tablets (Less than 1%) 2761
▲ Anzemet Injection (3.6%) 2859
Arixtra Injection (0.4%) 1351
Arthrotec Tablets (Rare) 3129
Atacand Tablets 649
Atacand HCT 651
Augmentin (Infrequent) 1360
Augmentin Tablets (Infrequent) 1363
Augmentin XR Extended-Release Tablets (Infrequent) 1369
Augmentin ES-600 Powder for Oral Suspension (Infrequently) 1366
Avandaryl Tablets 1379
Avelox (1%) 2970
Avinza Capsules (Less than 5%) 1741
Biaxin/Biaxin XL (Infrequent) 402
Blocadren Tablets 1916
Capastat Sulfate for Injection 1755
Captopril Tablets 2149
Carbatrol Capsules 3171
Carimune NF 3499
Catapres Tablets 843
Ceftin 1407
Celebrex Capsules (0.1% to 1.9%) 3134
▲ CellCept Capsules (3% to less than 20%) 2747
▲ CellCept Intravenous (3% to less than 20%) 2747
▲ CellCept Oral Suspension (3% to less than 20%) 2747
▲ CellCept Tablets (3% to less than 20%) 2747
▲ Cipro I.V. (Among most frequent) 2984
Cleocin Vaginal Ovules 2616
Clinoril Tablets (Less than 1 in 100) 1924
Concerta Extended-Release Tablets 1881
Copegus Tablets (Less than 1%) 2754
Cosmegen for Injection 2459
Crixivan Capsules 1940
Cuprimine Capsules 1947
Dantrium Capsules 2694
Daranide Tablets 1950
Daytrana Transdermal Patch 3174
Depacon Injection 412
Depakene 417
Depakote Sprinkle Capsules (Occasional) 422
Depakote Tablets 427
Depakote ER Tablets 434
Diovan Tablets (Occasional) 2193
Dolobid Tablets (Less than 1 in 100) 1955
Dyazide Capsules 1423
EC-Naprosyn Delayed-Release Tablets (Less than 1%) 2761
Edecrin (Rare) 1959
E.E.S. 451
Effexor Tablets 3411
Effexor XR Capsules 3417
Elmiron Capsules (1%) 2415
Emcyt Capsules 2634
Engerix-B Vaccine 1425
Epivir 1427
EryPed 447
Ery-Tab Tablets 449
Erythrocin Stearate Filmtab Tablets 453
Erythromycin Base Filmtab Tablets 455
Erythromycin Delayed-Release Capsules, USP 457
Estratest Tablets 3199
Estratest H.S. Tablets 3199
Eulexin Capsules 3009
Evoxac Capsules (Less than 1%) 1047
Exelon Capsules (Infrequent) 2206
Exelon Oral Solution (Infrequent) 2206
Flebogamma 5%, Immune Globulin Intravenous (Human) 1658
Focalin Tablets 2220
Focalin XR Capsules 2223
Fortaz 1453
Gabitril Tablets (Infrequent) 984
Gammagard Liquid 721
Gammagard S/D 724
Gamunex Immune Globulin I.V., 10% 3235
Guanidine Hydrochloride Tablets 3016
Hepsera Tablets (2% or greater) 1292
▲ Hycamtin for Injection (24%) 1458
Imitrex Injection (Infrequent) 1463
Imitrex Nasal Spray 1467
Imitrex Tablets 1471
▲ Intron A for Injection (Less than 5%) 3024
Invirase (Rare) 2772
Kaletra 476
Ketek Tablets 2903
Lamictal (Infrequent) 1481
▲ Lamisil Tablets (3.3%) 2232
Leukine 814
Levaquin (0.1% to 0.9%) 2384
Levaquin in 5% Dextrose Injection (0.1% to 0.9%) 2384
Librium Capsules 3347
Lipitor Tablets (Less than 2%) 2483
▲ Lofibra Tablets (7.5%) 1219

▲ Lofibra Capsules (7.5%) 1216
Lopressor Injection 2238
Lopressor Tablets 2238
Lopressor HCT 50/25 Tablets (Very rare) 2241
Lopressor HCT 100/25 Tablets (Very rare) 2241
Lopressor HCT 100/50 Tablets (Very rare) 2241
▲ Lumigan Ophthalmic Solution (1% to 5%) 573
Lupron Injection Pediatric 3259
Matulane Capsules 3191
Maxipime for Injection 1105
Mefoxin for Injection 2012
Mefoxin Premixed Intravenous Solution 2016
Metadate CD Capsules 3323
Mevacor Tablets 2021
Midamor Tablets (Rare) 2026
Mintezol (Rare) 2027
Moban Tablets (Rare) 1119
Moduretic Tablets 2028
Mycamine for Injection 628
Naprosyn Suspension (Less than 1%) 2761
Naprosyn Tablets (Less than 1%) 2761
Neurontin Capsules 2487
Neurontin Oral Solution 2487
Neurontin Tablets 2487
Nexium Delayed-Release Capsules (Less than 1%) 655
Nexium I.V. (Less than 1%) 659
Niaspan Extended-Release Tablets 1730
Nimotop Capsules (Up to 1.2%) 749
▲ Nipent for Injection (2% to 19%) 1863
Norvir (Less than 2%) 503
Omnicef Capsules 511
Omnicef for Oral Suspension 511
▲ Oncaspar (Greater than 1% but less than 5%) 1145
Oxandrin Tablets 2962
Paxil CR Controlled-Release Tablets 1538
Paxil 1530
PCE Dispertab Tablets 515
Pediarix Vaccine 1548
Pegasys (Less than 1%) 2789
Permax Tablets (Infrequent) 3356
Persantine Tablets (Rare) 868
Pexeva Tablets 1694
Phenytek Capsules 2160
Plavix Tablets 917
Plavix Tablets 2926
Premarin Vaginal Cream 3452
Prevacid Delayed-Release Capsules 3271
Prevacid for Delayed-Release Oral Suspension 3271
Prevacid SoluTab Delayed-Release Orally Disintegrating Tablets 3271
PREVPAC (Infrequent) 3284
▲ Prograf Capsules and Injection (5% to 36%) 632
Proleukin for Injection 2266
Protopic Ointment (Greater than or equal to 1%) 638
▲ Provigil Tablets (2% to 3%) 988
Prozac Pulvules and Liquid (Infrequent) 1801
▲ Rapamune Oral Solution and Tablets (3% to 20%) 3475
▲ Rebif Prefilled Syringe for Injection (4% to 18%) 3159
▲ Refludan for Injection (5.3%) 792
Relpax Tablets (Infrequent) 2548
Remicade for IV Injection (Rare) 971
Rilutek Tablets (Infrequent) 2930
Ritalin Hydrochloride Tablets (Some instances) 2269
Ritalin LA Capsules 2271
Ritalin-SR Tablets (Some instances) 2269
▲ Somavert Injection (4% to 12%) 2642
Sonata Capsules (Rare) 1717
Soriatane Capsules (Less than 1%) 1013
Strattera Capsules 1814
Striant Mucoadhesive 1007
Sular Tablets (Less than or equal to 1%) 3122
Suprax 1843
Synagis (More than 1%) 1897
Tabloid Tablets (Occasional) 1575
Tambocor Tablets (Rare) 1856
Tamiflu Capsules 2807
Tamiflu Oral Suspension 2807
Tasmar Tablets 3358
Tegretol/Tegretol-XR 2295
Thalomid Capsules 965
Ticlid Tablets (1.0%) 2810
Timolide Tablets 2086
▲ Tracleer Tablets (8%) 545
Tranxene 2474
▲ Trasylol Injection (3%) 754
Trelstar LA Suspension (1.1%) 3397
Trileptal Tablets 2300
Trileptal Oral Suspension 2300
Ultane Liquid for Inhalation (Less than 1%) 531
▲ Valcyte Tablets (Less than 5%) 2813
Valtrex Caplets 1597
Vantas (Less than 2%) 3375
Vantin Tablets and Oral Suspension 2645
Vaqta (Isolated reports) 2097
▲ Vesanoid Capsules (50% to 60%) 2820
VFEND I.V. (2.7%) 2564
VFEND Oral Suspension (2.7%) 2564
VFEND Tablets (2.7%) 2564
Viagra Tablets (Less than 2%) 2573
Viracept 2577
Viramune Oral Suspension 873
Viramune Tablets 873
Wellbutrin SR Sustained-Release Tablets (Infrequent) 1607
Wellbutrin XL Extended-Release Tablets (Infrequent) 1613
Zinacef for Injection 1631
Zinacef Injection 1631
Zmax for Oral Suspension 2583
Zofran Injection 1634
Zofran 1639
Zofran ODT Orally Disintegrating Tablets 1639
Zoloft (Rare) 2586
Zovirax 1643
Zyban Sustained-Release Tablets (Infrequent) 1644
Zyrtec Chewable Tablets (Less than 2%) 2594
Zyrtec (Less than 2%) 2594
Zyrtec-D 12 Hour Extended Release Tablets (Less than 2%) 2597
Zyvox (0.4% to 1.3%) 2652

Hepatic enzymes, elevation

(*see also under* Serum transaminase, elevation)
Accolate Tablets (Rare) 671
Accutane Capsules 2731
Aggrenox Capsules 822
Agrylin Capsules (2 of 551 patients) 3169
Altace Capsules (Rare) 1702
▲ Anaprox Tablets (Up to 15%) 2761
▲ Anaprox DS Tablets (Up to 15%) 2761
Arixtra Injection (0.3%) 1351
Asacol Delayed-Release Tablets 2692
Atacand Tablets (Infrequent) 649
Atacand HCT 651
Avandamet Tablets 1373
Avandia Tablets 1384
Avapro Tablets 891
Avapro Tablets (Very rare) 2871
Benicar Tablets (Infrequently) 1043
Betaseron for SC Injection 767
Biaxin/Biaxin XL (Infrequent) 402
Biltricide Tablets 2976
Caduet Tablets 2508
▲ Camptosar Injection (Fewer than 10%) 2604
Canasa Rectal Suppositories 699
Captopril Tablets 2149
Ceftin for Oral Suspension (0.1% to 1%) 1407
Celexa (Infrequent) 1176
Clarinex Syrup (Rare) 2995
Clarinex Tablets (Rare) 2995
Clarinex Reditabs Tablets (Rare) 2995
Colazal Capsules 2838
Comvax 1928
Coreg Tablets (Greater than 0.1% to 1%) 1414
Coumadin for Injection (Infrequent) 898
Coumadin Tablets (Infrequent) 898
Covera-HS Tablets (1.4%) 3139
Dantrium Capsules 2694
Depacon Injection 412
Depakene 417
Depakote Tablets 427
Depakote ER Tablets 434
Diovan Tablets 2193
Diovan HCT Tablets 2196
Dyazide Capsules 1423
DynaCirc CR Tablets (0.5% to 1%) 2721
Dyrenium Capsules (Rare) 3400
▲ EC-Naprosyn Delayed-Release Tablets (Up to 15%) 2761
EryPed 447
Evoxac Capsules (Less than 1%) 1047
▲ Hycamtin for Injection (Less than 1% to 8%) 1458
Hyzaar 50-12.5 Tablets (Occasional) 1990
Hyzaar 100-12.5 Tablets (Occasional) 1990
Hyzaar 100-25 Tablets (Occasional) 1990
Imitrex Nasal Spray 1467
Imitrex Tablets 1471
Ketek Tablets (Greater than or equal to 0.2% to less than 2%) 2903
Lescol Capsules 2233
Lescol XL Tablets 2233
Lotrel Capsules (Scattered incidents) 2249
Micardis HCT Tablets 856
MS Contin Tablets 2701
Nadolol Tablets 2159
▲ Naprosyn Suspension (Up to 15%) 2761
▲ Naprosyn Tablets (Up to 15%) 2761
Niaspan Extended-Release Tablets 1730
Niravam Orally Disintegrating Tablets 3092
Noroxin Tablets 2032
Norvasc Tablets (Infrequent) 2545
Paxil CR Controlled-Release Tablets 1538
Paxil 1530
Percodan Tablets 1132
Persantine Tablets 868
Plavix Tablets (1% to 2.5%) 917
Plavix Tablets (1% to 2.5%) 2926
PREVPAC (Infrequent) 3284
Prinivil Tablets (Rare) 2052
Prinzide Tablets (Rare) 2056
Provigil Tablets (At least 1%) 988
Rebif Prefilled Syringe for Injection 3159
Recombivax HB 2071
Risperdal Consta Long-Acting Injection (Frequent) 1682
Sandostatin Injection (Less than 1%) 2278
Sandostatin LAR Depot (Rare) 2280
St. Joseph 81 mg Aspirin Chewable and Enteric Coated Tablets 1869
St. Joseph 81 mg Aspirin ▣ 688
Sustiva Capsules 930
Sustiva Tablets 930
Tabloid Tablets (Occasional) 1575
Tarka Tablets (2.8%) 524
Tasmar Tablets 3358
Tegretol/Tegretol-XR 2295
Thalomid Capsules 965
Trileptal Tablets 2300
Trileptal Oral Suspension 2300
Trizivir Tablets 1589
Vasotec I.V. Injection 2103
Verelan PM Extended-Release Capsules, Controlled-Onset 3106
VFEND I.V. (1.5% to 2.4%) 2564
VFEND Oral Suspension (1.5% to 2.4%) 2564
VFEND Tablets (1.5% to 2.4%) 2564
▲ Vicoprofen Tablets (Up to 15%) 539
▲ Visudyne for Injection (1% to 10%) 2305
▲ Voltaren Tablets (1% to 10%) 2307
▲ Voltaren-XR Tablets (1% to 10%) 2310
Zoloft (One or more patients) 2586
Zovirax 1643

Hepatic enzymes, increased

Aptivus Capsules (Less than 2%) 826
Atripla Tablets 945
Bayer Aspirin Comprehensive Prescribing Information ▣ 796
Eraxis for Injection (1.5%) 2521
Lexapro Oral Solution (Infrequent) 1190
Lexapro Tablets (Infrequent) 1190
MS Contin Tablets (Less frequent) 2701
Nicomide Tablets 1088
Univasc Tablets 3104

Hepatic eosinophilic infiltration

Singulair (Very rare) 2077

Hepatic failure

Abelcet Injection 1141
Accolate Tablets (Rare) 671
Aceon Tablets (2 mg, 4 mg, 8 mg) 3194
Aloprim for Injection (Less than 1%) 2167
Altace Capsules 1702
Anaprox Tablets (Less than 1%) 2761
Anaprox DS Tablets (Less than 1%) 2761
Aptivus Capsules (Less than 2%) 826
Arthrotec Tablets (Rare) 3129
Asacol Delayed-Release Tablets (Rare) 2692
Atripla Tablets 945
Biaxin/Biaxin XL (Very rare) 402
Campath Ampules 811
Captopril Tablets (Rare) 2149
Celebrex Capsules (Less than 0.1%) 3134
Cipro 2977
Cipro I.V. 2984
Cipro XR Tablets 2990
Clinoril Tablets (Less than 1 in 100) 1924
Colazal Capsules 2838
Copegus Tablets (2%) 2754
Cosmegen for Injection 2459
Crixivan Capsules 1940
Depacon Injection 412
Depakene 417
Depakote Sprinkle Capsules 422
Depakote Tablets 427
Depakote ER Tablets 434
Dolobid Tablets 1955
Doxil Injection (Less than 1%) 2351
EC-Naprosyn Delayed-Release Tablets (Less than 1%) 2761
Effexor Tablets 3411
Effexor XR Capsules 3417
Elspar for Injection 2463
Elspar for Injection 1960
Eulexin Capsules (Rare) 3009
Gemzar for Injection (Rare) 1771
Gleevec Tablets (Rare) 2227
Hepsera Tablets (2% or greater) 1292
Herceptin I.V. (At least one of the 958 patients) 1233
Intron A for Injection (Very rare) 3024
Lamisil Tablets (Rare) 2232
Levaquin (0.1% to 0.9%) 2384
Levaquin in 5% Dextrose Injection (0.1% to 0.9%) 2384
Mavik Tablets (Rare) 486
Merrem I.V. (Greater than 0.1% to 1%) 686
Mintezol (Rare) 2027
Mobic Oral Suspension (Less than 0.1%) 863
Mobic Tablets (Less than 0.1%) 863
Mycamine for Injection 628
Mylotarg for Injection 3431
Namenda 1195
Naprosyn Suspension (Less than 1%) 2761
Naprosyn Tablets (Less than 1%) 2761
Niravam Orally Disintegrating Tablets 3092
Omnicef Capsules 511
Omnicef for Oral Suspension 511
Oncaspar 1145
Pentasa Capsules 3185
Persantine Tablets 868
Plavix Tablets 917
PREVPAC (Very rare) 3284
Prilosec OTC Delayed-Release Tablets (Rare) 2677
Prinivil Tablets (Rare) 2052
Prinzide Tablets (Rare) 2056
Proleukin for Injection (Less than 1%) 2266
Proquin XR Tablets 1153
Protonix I.V. 3472
Protonix Tablets 3469
Prozac Pulvules and Liquid 1801
Rebif Prefilled Syringe for Injection (Very rare) 3159
Remicade for IV Injection 971
Rescriptor Tablets 2551
Revlimid Capsules 958
Risperdal (Rare) 1676
Risperdal M-Tab Orally Disintegrating Tablets (Rare) 1676
Solodyn Extended Release Tablets 1890
Sustiva Capsules 930
Sustiva Tablets 930
Tambocor Tablets (Rare) 1856
Targretin Capsules 1747
Tasmar Tablets 3358
Tegretol/Tegretol-XR (Very rare) 2295
Topamax Sprinkle Capsules 2404
Topamax Tablets 2404
Tracleer Tablets 545
Trasylol Injection (1% to 2%) 754
Trizivir Tablets 1589
Vasotec I.V. Injection (0.5% to 1.0%) 2103
VFEND I.V. (Less than 2%) 2564
VFEND Oral Suspension (Less than 2%) 2564
VFEND Tablets (Less than 2%) 2564
Viramune Oral Suspension 873
Viramune Tablets 873
Voltaren Tablets (Rarely) 2307
Voltaren-XR Tablets (Rarely) 2310
▲ Xeloda Tablets (Less than 5%) 2822
Zantac (Rare) 1624
Zantac Injection (Rare) 1619
Zantac Injection Pharmacy Bulk Package (Rare) 1622
Zantac Injection Premixed (Rare) 1619

Zantac (Rare) 1624
Zegerid Capsules (Rare) 2958
Zegerid Powder for Oral Solution (Rare) 2958
Ziagen 1626
Zofran Injection 1634
Zofran 1639
Zofran ODT Orally Disintegrating Tablets 1639
Zoloft (One or more patients) 2586

Hepatic failure, fulminant

Elspar for Injection 2463
Elspar for Injection 1960
Tasmar Tablets (Three cases) 3358
Zofran Injection Premixed 1634

Hepatic function tests, impaired

(*see under* Hepatic dysfunction)

Hepatic hemangioma, enlargement

Angeliq Tablets 762
Enjuvia Tablets 1062
Estrasorb Topical Emulsion 1147
Menostar Transdermal System 782
Premarin Intravenous 3442
Premarin Tablets 3446
Premarin Vaginal Cream 3452
Premphase Tablets 3456
Prempro Tablets 3456

Hepatic necrosis

Aceon Tablets (2 mg, 4 mg, 8 mg) (Rare) 3194
Advicor Tablets 1722
Altace Capsules (Rare) 1702
Altoprev Extended-Release Tablets (Rare) 3109
Asacol Delayed-Release Tablets (Rare) 2692
▲ Blephamide Ophthalmic Ointment (Among most often) 568
Blephamide Ophthalmic Suspension 569
Captopril Tablets (Rare) 2149
Celebrex Capsules (Rare) 3134
Celexa 1176
Cipro (Rare) 2977
Cipro I.V. (1% or less) 2984
Cipro XR Tablets (Rare) 2990
Colazal Capsules 2838
Dolobid Tablets 1955
Effexor Tablets 3411
Effexor XR Capsules 3417
Eraxis for Injection (Less than 1% to less than 2%) 2521
Eulexin Capsules 3009
Fansidar Tablets 2765
FML-S Ophthalmic Suspension ⊙229
Gantrisin Pediatric Suspension 2770
▲ Humira Injection (Less than 5%) 466
Lescol Capsules (Rare) 2233
Lescol XL Tablets 2233
Levaquin (Rare) 2384
Levaquin in 5% Dextrose Injection (Rare) 2384
Lexapro Oral Solution 1190
Lexapro Tablets 1190
Lotrel Capsules (Rare) 2249
Mavik Tablets (Rare) 486
Mevacor Tablets (Rare) 2021
Myleran Tablets 1525
Niaspan Extended-Release Tablets 1730
Noroxin Tablets 2032
Oxandrin Tablets (Rare) 2962
Paxil CR Controlled-Release Tablets 1538
Paxil 1530
Pentasa Capsules 3185
Pexeva Tablets 1694
Prilosec OTC Delayed-Release Tablets (Rare) 2677
Prinivil Tablets (Rare) 2052
Prinzide Tablets (Rare) 2056
Prograf Capsules and Injection 632
Proquin XR Tablets 1153
Rapamune Oral Solution and Tablets 3475
Tabloid Tablets 1575
Tarka Tablets (Rare) 524
Ticlid Tablets (Rare) 2810
Trusopt Sterile Ophthalmic Solution (Rare) 2095
Uniretic Tablets (Rare) 3100
Vasotec I.V. Injection (Rare) 2103
Viramune Oral Suspension 873
Viramune Tablets 873
Vytorin 10/10 Tablets (Rare) 2114
Vytorin 10/10 Tablets (Rare) 3077
Vytorin 10/20 Tablets (Rare) 2114
Vytorin 10/20 Tablets (Rare) 3077
Vytorin 10/40 Tablets (Rare) 2114
Vytorin 10/40 Tablets (Rare) 3077
Vytorin 10/80 Tablets (Rare) 2114
Vytorin 10/80 Tablets (Rare) 3077
Zegerid Capsules (Rare) 2958
Zegerid Powder for Oral Solution (Rare) 2958
Zocor Tablets (Rare) 2105
Zonegran Capsules (Rare) 1101

Hepatic veno-occlusive disease

Abelcet Injection 1141
Alkeran for Injection 955
AmBisome for Injection (Less common) 620
Cosmegen for Injection 2459
▲ I.V. Busulfex (8%) 2493
Myleran Tablets 1525
▲ Mylotarg for Injection (5%) 3431
Tabloid Tablets 1575

Hepatitis

Abelcet Injection 1141
Abilify Oral Solution (Rare) 882
Abilify Oral Solution (Rare) 2450
Abilify Discmelt Orally Disintegrating Tablets (Rare) 882
Abilify Discmelt Orally Disintegrating Tablets (Rare) 2450
Abilify Tablets (Rare) 882
Abilify Tablets (Rare) 2450
Accutane Capsules 2731
Aciphex Tablets (Rare) 1090
Advicor Tablets 1722
Aldoril Tablets 1910
Alkeran for Injection 955
Alkeran Tablets 956
Altace Capsules (Less than 1%) 1702
Altoprev Extended-Release Tablets 3109
Amevive (1 case) 626
Anaprox Tablets (Less than 1%) 2761
Anaprox DS Tablets (Less than 1%) 2761
Aptivus Capsules (Less than 2%) 826
Aricept Tablets 1094
Aricept ODT Tablets 1094
Arthrotec Tablets (Rare) 3129
Asacol Delayed-Release Tablets (Rare) 2692
Atacand Tablets 649
Atacand HCT 651
Atripla Tablets 945
Augmentin (Rare) 1360
Augmentin Tablets (Rare) 1363
Avalide Tablets 888
Avandamet Tablets 1373
Avandaryl Tablets 1379
Avandia Tablets 1384
Avapro Tablets 891
Avapro Tablets (Very rare) 2871
Avelox 2970
Axid Oral Solution 879
Bayer Aspirin 744
Bayer Aspirin Comprehensive Prescribing Information ■□796
Betaseron for SC Injection 767
BiDil Tablets 2171
Caduet Tablets (Less than 2%) 2508
Campral Tablets (Infrequent) 1174
Captopril Tablets 2149
Carbatrol Capsules 3171
Cardura XL Tablets 2515
Catapres Tablets (Rare) 843
Ceftin 1407
Celebrex Capsules (Less than 0.1%) 3134
Celexa (Rare) 1176
▲ CellCept Capsules (3% to less than 20%) 2747
▲ CellCept Intravenous (3% to less than 20%) 2747
▲ CellCept Oral Suspension (3% to less than 20%) 2747
▲ CellCept Tablets (3% to less than 20%) 2747
Cipro (Less than 1%) 2977
Cipro I.V. (1% or less) 2984
Cipro XR Tablets 2990
Clarinex-D 24-Hour Extended-Release Tablets (Very rare) 2998
Clinoril Tablets (Less than 1%) 1924
Clorpres Tablets (Rare) 2153
Clozaril Tablets 2184
Cosmegen for Injection 2459
Coumadin for Injection (Infrequent) 898
Coumadin Tablets (Infrequent) 898
Cozaar Tablets (Rare) 1935
Crestor Tablets (Less than 1%) 678
Crixivan Capsules 1940
Dantrium Capsules (Less frequent) 2694
Depakote ER Tablets 434
Diovan Tablets (Very rare) 2193
Diovan HCT Tablets (Very rare) 2196
Dolobid Tablets (Less than 1 in 100) 1955
Doxil Injection (Less than 1%) 2351
Duetact Tablets (Rare) 3226
EC-Naprosyn Delayed-Release Tablets (Less than 1%) 2761
E.E.S. 451
Effexor Tablets (Rare) 3411
Effexor XR Capsules (Rare) 3417
Enbrel for Injection 584
Equetro Extended-Release Capsules 3180
EryPed 447
Erythromycin Delayed-Release Capsules, USP 457
Eulexin Capsules (Less than 1%) 3009
Fansidar Tablets 2765
FazaClo Orally Disintegrating Tablets 551
Fortical Nasal Spray (Less than 1%) 3337
Gantrisin Pediatric Suspension 2770
Gleevec Tablets (Uncommon) 2227
Havrix Vaccine (Rare) 1456
Herceptin I.V. (At least one of the 958 patients) 1233
Hyzaar 50-12.5 Tablets (Rare) 1990
Hyzaar 100-12.5 Tablets (Rare) 1990
Hyzaar 100-25 Tablets (Rare) 1990
Invirase (Less than 2%) 2772
Keflex Capsules (Rare) 549
Keppra Injection 3320
▲ Keppra Oral Solution (5%) 3314
Keppra Tablets 3314
Ketek Tablets (Greater than or equal to 0.2% to less than 2%) 2903
Lamictal (Rare) 1481
Lescol Capsules 2233
Lescol XL Tablets 2233
Levaquin (Rare) 2384
Levaquin in 5% Dextrose Injection (Rare) 2384
Lexapro Oral Solution 1190
Lexapro Tablets 1190
Lipitor Tablets (Less than 2%) 2483
Lofibra Tablets 1219
Lofibra Capsules 1216
Lopressor Injection 2238
Lopressor Tablets 2238
Lopressor HCT 50/25 Tablets (Very rare) 2241
Lopressor HCT 100/25 Tablets (Very rare) 2241
Lopressor HCT 100/50 Tablets (Very rare) 2241
Lotronex Tablets (A single case) 1512
Lunesta Tablets (Rare) 3142
Malarone Pediatric Tablets (Very rare) 1517
Malarone Tablets (Very rare) 1517
Mevacor Tablets 2021
Miacalcin Nasal Spray (Less than 1%) 2253
Miradon Tablets 3042
Mobic Oral Suspension (Less than 2%) 863
Mobic Tablets (Less than 2%) 863
Naprosyn Suspension (Less than 1%) 2761
Naprosyn Tablets (Less than 1%) 2761
Neurontin Capsules 2487
Neurontin Oral Solution 2487
Neurontin Tablets 2487
Nexium Delayed-Release Capsules (Very rare) 655
Nexium I.V. (Very rare) 659
Nimotop Capsules (Less than 1%) 749
Niravam Orally Disintegrating Tablets 3092
Noroxin Tablets 2032
Norvasc Tablets (Less than 0.1%) 2545
Norvir (Less than 2%) 503
Omnicef Capsules 511
Omnicef for Oral Suspension 511
Orthoclone OKT3 Sterile Solution 2360
Parnate Tablets (Rare) 1527
Paser Granules 1674
Paxil CR Controlled-Release Tablets (Rare) 1538
Paxil (Rare) 1530
PCE Dispertab Tablets 515
Pentasa Capsules (Infrequent) 3185
Percodan Tablets 1132
Permax Tablets (Infrequent) 3356
Persantine Tablets (Rare) 868
Pexeva Tablets (Rare) 1694
Plavix Tablets 917
Plavix Tablets 2926
Prilosec OTC Delayed-Release Tablets (Rare) 2677
Primaxin I.M. 2045
Primaxin I.V. (Less than 0.2%) 2048
Prinivil Tablets (0.3% to 1.0%) 2052
Prinzide Tablets 2056
▲ Prograf Capsules and Injection (3% to 15%) 632
Proleukin for Injection 2266
Prometrium Capsules (100 mg, 200 mg) 3203
Proquin XR Tablets 1153
Protonix I.V. (Less than 1%) 3472
Protonix Tablets (Less than 1%) 3469
Prozac Pulvules and Liquid (Rare) 1801
Raniclor Tablets, Chewable (Rare) 2505
Rebif Prefilled Syringe for Injection (Rare) 3159
Remicade for IV Injection (Greater than or equal to 0.2%) 971
Rescriptor Tablets 2551
Retrovir Capsules (Rare) 1560
Retrovir IV Infusion (Rare) 1564
Retrovir (Rare) 1560
Reyataz Capsules (Less than 3%) 921
Rilutek Tablets (Infrequent) 2930
Risperdal (Rare) 1676
Risperdal Consta Long-Acting Injection (Rare) 1682
Risperdal M-Tab Orally Disintegrating Tablets (Rare) 1676
Sandostatin Injection (Less than 1%) 2278
Sandostatin LAR Depot (Rare) 2280
Solodyn Extended Release Tablets 1890
Soriatane Capsules (Less than 1%) 1013
St. Joseph 81 mg Aspirin Chewable and Enteric Coated Tablets 1869
St. Joseph 81 mg Aspirin ■□688
Suprax 1843
Sustiva Capsules (Less than 2%) 930
Sustiva Tablets (Less than 2%) 930
Tamiflu Capsules 2807
Tamiflu Oral Suspension 2807
Taxotere Injection Concentrate (Rare) 2932
Tegretol/Tegretol-XR 2295
Tequin Injection 938
Tequin Injection in 5% Dextrose 938
Tequin Tablets 938
Thalomid Capsules 965
Ticlid Tablets (Rare) 2810
Timentin ADD-Vantage (Rare) 1580
Timentin Injection Galaxy Container (Rare) 1583
Timentin IV Infusion (Rare) 1577
Timentin Pharmacy Bulk Package (Rare) 1586
Topamax Sprinkle Capsules 2404
Topamax Tablets 2404
Toprol-XL Tablets 668
Trecator Tablets 3487
Tricor Tablets 527
Truvada Tablets 1296
Twinrix Vaccine 1595
Ultane Liquid for Inhalation (Less than 1%) 531
Univasc Tablets (Less than 1%) 3104
Valtrex Caplets 1597
Vasotec I.V. Injection (0.5% to 1.0%) 2103
▲ Vesanoid Capsules (3%) 2820
VFEND I.V. (Less than 2%) 2564
VFEND Oral Suspension (Less than 2%) 2564
VFEND Tablets (Less than 2%) 2564
Viracept (Less than 2%) 2577
Viramune Oral Suspension (1%) 873
Viramune Tablets (1%) 873
Voltaren Tablets (Occasionally) 2307
Voltaren-XR Tablets (Occasionally) 2310
Vytorin 10/10 Tablets 2114
Vytorin 10/10 Tablets 3077
Vytorin 10/20 Tablets 2114
Vytorin 10/20 Tablets 3077
Vytorin 10/40 Tablets 2114
Vytorin 10/40 Tablets 3077
Vytorin 10/80 Tablets 2114
Vytorin 10/80 Tablets 3077
Wellbutrin Tablets 1603
Wellbutrin SR Sustained-Release Tablets 1607
Wellbutrin XL Extended-Release Tablets 1613
▲ Xeloda Tablets (Less than 5%) 2822
Zantac (Occasional) 1624
Zantac Injection 1619
Zantac Injection Pharmacy Bulk Package (Infrequent) 1622
Zantac Injection Premixed 1619
Zantac (Occasional) 1624
Zegerid Capsules (Rare) 2958

Zegerid Powder for Oral Solution (Rare) 2958
Zelapar Tablets 3372
Zetia Tablets 2120
Zetia Tablets 3083
Zmax for Oral Suspension 2583
Zocor Tablets 2105
Zoloft (One or more patients) 2586
Zosyn 3492
Zovirax 1643
Zyban Sustained-Release Tablets 1644
Zyprexa Tablets (Infrequent) 1830
Zyprexa ZYDIS Orally Disintegrating Tablets (Infrequent) 1830
Zyrtec Chewable Tablets (Rare) 2594
Zyrtec (Rare) 2594
Zyrtec-D 12 Hour Extended Release Tablets (Rare) 2597

Hepatitis, allergic

Adalat CC Tablets (Rare) 2964

Hepatitis, autoimmune

Remicade for IV Injection 971

Hepatitis, cholestatic

Avelox 2970
Biaxin/Biaxin XL (Infrequent) 402
Cardura XL Tablets 2515
EryPed 447
Estratest Tablets 3199
Estratest H.S. Tablets 3199
Ketek Tablets 2903
Lamisil Tablets (Rare) 2232
Nalfon Capsules (Less than 1%) 2502
Oxandrin Tablets 2962
PREVPAC (Infrequent) 3284
Prilosec OTC Delayed-Release Tablets (Rare) 2677
Risperdal (Rare) 1676
Risperdal M-Tab Orally Disintegrating Tablets (Rare) 1676
Singulair (Rare) 2077
Viramune Oral Suspension 873
Viramune Tablets 873
▲ Xeloda Tablets (Less than 5%) 2822
Zantac (Occasional) 1624
Zantac Injection (Occasional) 1619
Zantac Injection Pharmacy Bulk Package (Infrequent) 1622
Zantac Injection Premixed (Occasional) 1619
Zantac (Occasional) 1624
Zegerid Capsules (Rare) 2958
Zegerid Powder for Oral Solution (Rare) 2958
Zosyn 3492

Hepatitis, cytolytic

Amoxil Capsules 1343
Amoxil Chewable Tablets 1343
Amoxil Pediatric Drops for Oral Suspension 1343
Amoxil Powder for Oral Suspension 1343
Amoxil Tablets 1343
PREVPAC 3284
Prograf Capsules and Injection 632

Hepatitis, fulminant

Celebrex Capsules (Less than 0.1%) 3134
Omnicef Capsules 511
Omnicef for Oral Suspension 511
Precose Tablets (Few cases) 751
Primaxin I.M. (0.2%) 2045
Primaxin I.V. (0.2%) 2048
Rituxan I.V. 1254
Viramune Oral Suspension 873
Viramune Tablets 873

Hepatitis, hepatocellular

Ketek Tablets 2903

Hepatitis, idiopathic

Raptiva for Injection (1 case) 1250

Hepatitis, infectious

Plavix Tablets (Less than 1%) 917
Plavix Tablets (Less than 1%) 2926

Hepatitis, overt

Prilosec OTC Delayed-Release Tablets (Rare) 2677
Zegerid Capsules (Rare) 2958
Zegerid Powder for Oral Solution (Rare) 2958

Hepatitis, post-treatment exacerbations of

Combivir Tablets 1411
Epivir 1427
Epivir-HBV 1432
Epzicom Tablets 1436
Trizivir Tablets 1589

Hepatitis, reactivation

Remicade for IV Injection 971
Rituxan I.V. 1254

Hepatitis, symptomatic

Accolate Tablets (Rare) 671

Hepatitis, toxic

Alkeran for Injection 955
Cuprimine Capsules (Rare) 1947
Dapsone Tablets USP 1673
Indocin Capsules (Less than 1%) 1995
Indocin I.V. (Less than 1%) 2465
Indocin (Less than 1%) 1995
Phenytek Capsules 2160

Hepatitis, viral

Evoxac Capsules (Less than 1%) 1047
Prolastin 3255

Hepatobiliary dysfunction

Lamisil Tablets (Rare) 2232

Hepatocellular atrophy

Myleran Tablets 1525

Hepatocellular damage

Mycamine for Injection 628

Hepatomas

Aciphex Tablets (Rare) 1090
Advicor Tablets 1722
Altoprev Extended-Release Tablets (Rare) 3109
Lescol Capsules (Rare) 2233
Lescol XL Tablets 2233
Mevacor Tablets (Rare) 2021
NuvaRing 2340
Premarin Intravenous 3442
Premarin Vaginal Cream 3452
Vytorin 10/10 Tablets (Rare) 2114
Vytorin 10/10 Tablets (Rare) 3077
Vytorin 10/20 Tablets (Rare) 2114
Vytorin 10/20 Tablets (Rare) 3077
Vytorin 10/40 Tablets (Rare) 2114
Vytorin 10/40 Tablets (Rare) 3077
Vytorin 10/80 Tablets (Rare) 2114
Vytorin 10/80 Tablets (Rare) 3077
Zocor Tablets (Rare) 2105

Hepatomas, benign

Mircette Tablets 1066
Ortho-Cyclen/Ortho Tri-Cyclen (Rare) 2429
Ortho Tri-Cyclen Lo Tablets 2436
Seasonique Tablets 1077
Yaz Tablets 803

Hepatomegaly

Abelcet Injection 1141
Abilify Oral Solution (Rare) 882
Abilify Oral Solution (Rare) 2450
Abilify Discmelt Orally Disintegrating Tablets (Rare) 882
Abilify Discmelt Orally Disintegrating Tablets (Rare) 2450
Abilify Tablets (Rare) 882
Abilify Tablets (Rare) 2450
Aloprim for Injection (Less than 1%) 2167
AmBisome for Injection (Less common) 620
Blocadren Tablets 1916
Camptosar Injection 2604
▲ Clolar for Intravenous Infusion (15%) 1271
Combivir Tablets 1411
Copaxone for Injection (Infrequent) 3297
Cosmegen for Injection 2459
Cosopt Sterile Ophthalmic Solution 1931
Decadron Tablets 1951
Epivir 1427
Epivir-HBV 1432
Epzicom Tablets 1436
Gabitril Tablets (Infrequent) 984
Garamycin Injectable 3014
Geodon Capsules (Rare) 2529
▲ Infergen (3% to 5%) 3364
Invirase (Less than 2%) 2772
▲ I.V. Busulfex (6%) 2493
Klonopin 2778
Lofibra Tablets (Less than 1%) 1219
Lofibra Capsules (Less than 1%) 1216
Lunesta Tablets (Rare) 3142
▲ Megace ES Oral Suspension (1% to 3%) 2481
Mycamine for Injection 628
Neupogen for Injection (Infrequent) 603
Neurontin Capsules (Infrequent) 2487
Neurontin Oral Solution (Infrequent) 2487
Neurontin Tablets (Infrequent) 2487
Norvir (Less than 2%) 503
Oncaspar (Less than 1%) 1145
Orthoclone OKT3 Sterile Solution 2360
Paser Granules 1674
▲ PEG-Intron Powder for Injection (6%) 3048
Permax Tablets (Infrequent) 3356
Proleukin for Injection (1%) 2266
▲ Rebetol (4%) 3058
Rescriptor Tablets 2551
Retrovir Capsules (Rare) 1560
Retrovir IV Infusion (Rare) 1564
Retrovir (Rare) 1560
Reyataz Capsules (Less than 3%) 921
▲ Ribavirin, USP Capsules (4%) 3068
Risperdal Consta Long-Acting Injection (Infrequent) 1682
Rythmol SR Capsules 2727
Sular Tablets (Less than or equal to 1%) 3122
Symbyax Capsules (Infrequent) 1819
Tabloid Tablets 1575
Thalomid Capsules 965
Timolide Tablets 2086
Timoptic Sterile Ophthalmic Solution 2088
Timoptic in Ocudose 2091
Timoptic-XE Sterile Ophthalmic Gel Forming Solution 2092
Tricor Tablets 527
Trizivir Tablets 1589
Truvada Tablets 1296
Viread Tablets 1301
Zoloft (One or more patients) 2586

Hepatorenal syndrome, unspecified

Actiq (Less than 1%) 979
Depakote ER Tablets 434

Hepatosplenomegaly

Doxil Injection (Less than 1%) 2351
Invirase (Less than 2%) 2772
Mylotarg for Injection 3431
Proleukin for Injection 2266
Reyataz Capsules (Less than 3%) 921
Tegretol/Tegretol-XR 2295
▲ Vesanoid Capsules (9%) 2820

Hepatotoxicity

Accutane Capsules 2731
Advicor Tablets 1722
Alkeran Tablets (Rare) 956
Arthrotec Tablets 3129
Asacol Delayed-Release Tablets (Rare) 2692
Avandaryl Tablets 1379
Campath Ampules 811
Carbatrol Capsules 3171
▲ CellCept Capsules (3% to less than 20%) 2747
▲ CellCept Intravenous (3% to less than 20%) 2747
▲ CellCept Oral Suspension (3% to less than 20%) 2747
▲ CellCept Tablets (3% to less than 20%) 2747
Combivir Tablets 1411
Comtrex Maximum Strength Cold & Cough Day/Night Caplets - Day Formulation .... ▣ 726
Comtrex Maximum Strength Cold & Cough Day/Night Caplets - Night Formulation .... ▣ 726
Comtrex Maximum Strength Non-Drowsy Cold & Cough Caplets .... ▣ 725
Comtrex Maximum Strength Day/Night Severe Cold & Sinus Caplets - Day Formulation .... ▣ 725
Comtrex Maximum Strength Day/Night Severe Cold & Sinus Caplets - Night Formulation .... ▣ 725
Cosmegen for Injection 2459
Dantrium Capsules 2694
Depacon Injection 412
Depakene 417
Depakote Sprinkle Capsules 422
Depakote Tablets 427
Depakote ER Tablets 434
Effexor Tablets 3411
Effexor XR Capsules 3417
Eloxatin for Injection 2892
Estratest Tablets 3199
Estratest H.S. Tablets 3199
Excedrin Sinus Headache Caplets/Tablets .... ▣ 610
Furosemide Tablets 2154
Gemzar for Injection (Rare) 1771
▲ Gengraf Capsules (Less than 1% to 7%) 459
▲ Gleevec Tablets (3% to 12%) 2227
Goody's Body Pain Formula Powder .... ▣ 684
Goody's Extra Strength Headache Powders .... ▣ 611
Goody's Extra Strength Pain Relief Tablets .... ▣ 685
Goody's PM Powder for Pain with Sleeplessness .... ▣ 612
Intron A for Injection (Rare) 3024
I.V. Busulfex 2493
Lamisil Tablets 2232
Leukeran Tablets 1504
▲ Leukine (13%) 814
Lunesta Tablets (Rare) 3142
Mintezol 2027
Miradon Tablets 3042
Mylotarg for Injection 3431
Nembutal Sodium Solution, USP 2470
▲ Neoral Oral Solution (Less than 1% to 7%) 2259
▲ Neoral Soft Gelatin Capsules (Less than 1% to 7%) 2259
Nicomide Tablets 1088
Norvir (Less than 2%) 503
Oracea Capsules (Rare) 1000
Pentasa Capsules 3185
Percodan Tablets 1132
Phenytek Capsules 2160
Prevacid Delayed-Release Capsules 3271
Prevacid for Delayed-Release Oral Suspension 3271
Prevacid SoluTab Delayed-Release Orally Disintegrating Tablets 3271
Prevacid NapraPAC 3280
PREVPAC 3284
▲ Prograf Capsules and Injection (3% to 15%) 632
Rapamune Oral Solution and Tablets 3475
Reyataz Capsules (Less than 3%) 921
Risperdal (Rare) 1676
Risperdal Consta Long-Acting Injection (Rare) 1682
Risperdal M-Tab Orally Disintegrating Tablets (Rare) 1676
Robitussin Cough, Cold & Flu Nighttime Liquid .... ▣ 738
▲ Sandimmune (Less than 1% to 7%) 2275
Soriatane Capsules 1013
Tegretol/Tegretol-XR 2295
TheraFlu Daytime Severe Cold Hot Liquid .... ▣ 742
TheraFlu Warming Relief Daytime Severe Cold .... ▣ 743
TheraFlu Warming Relief Nighttime Severe Cold .... ▣ 743
Trasylol Injection (0.5%) 754
Regular Strength Tylenol Tablets 1870
Tylenol 8 Hour Extended Release Caplets .... ▣ 695
Tylenol Chest Congestion Caplets with Cool Burst .... ▣ 722
Tylenol Chest Congestion Liquid with Cool Burst .... ▣ 722
Children's Tylenol with Flavor Creator .... ▣ 679
Tylenol Cold Multi-Symptom Daytime Liquid .... ▣ 752
Tylenol Cold Multi-Symptom Severe Caplets with Cool Burst .... ▣ 752
Tylenol Cough & Sore Throat Daytime Liquid with Cool Burst .... ▣ 790
Tylenol Cough & Sore Throat Nighttime Liquid with Cool Burst .... ▣ 790
Tylenol 8 Hour Extended Release Caplets 1870
Tylenol 1870
Extra Strength Tylenol PM Caplets, Vanilla Caplets, Geltabs, Gelcaps and Liquid 1875
Extra Strength Tylenol Rapid Release Gels 1870
Tylenol Sinus Severe Congestion Caplets with Cool Burst .... ▣ 778
Tylenol Allergy Multi-Symptom Caplets with Cool Burst and Gelcaps 1872
Tylenol Allergy Multi-Symptom Nighttime Caplets with Cool Burst 1872
Tylenol Severe Allergy Caplets 1872
Tylenol Arthritis Pain Extended Release Caplets and Geltabs 1870
Tylenol Chest Congestion Caplets with Cool Burst 1872
Tylenol Chest Congestion Liquid with Cool Burst 1872

Tylenol Cold Severe Congestion Non-Drowsy Caplets with Cool Burst 1874
Tylenol Cold Head Congestion Daytime Caplets with Cool Burst 1873
Tylenol Cold Head Congestion Nighttime Caplets with Cool Burst 1873
Tylenol Cold Head Congestion Severe Caplets with Cool Burst 1873
Tylenol Cough & Sore Throat Daytime Liquid with Cool Burst 1877
Tylenol Cough & Sore Throat Nighttime Liquid with Cool Burst 1877
Tylenol Sinus Severe Congestion Caplets with Cool Burst 1876
Tylenol Sinus Congestion & Pain Daytime Caplets with Cool Burst and Gelcaps 1876
Tylenol Sinus Congestion & Pain Nighttime Caplets with Cool Burst 1876
Tylenol Sinus Congestion & Pain Severe Caplets with Cool Burst 1876
Tylenol Sore Throat Daytime Liquid with Cool Burst 1877
Tylenol Sore Throat Nighttime Liquid with Cool Burst 1877
Women's Tylenol Menstrual Relief Caplets 1877
Vicks 44M Cough, Cold & Flu Relief Liquid 2680
Vicks DayQuil Multi-Symptom Cold/Flu Relief LiquiCaps 2678
Vicks DayQuil Multi-Symptom Cold/Flu Relief Liquid 2678
Vicks NyQuil Multi-Symptom Cold/Flu Relief Liquid 2681
Vicks NyQuil Multi-Symptom Cold/Flu Relief LiquiCaps 2681
Viramune Oral Suspension 873
Viramune Tablets 873
Wellbutrin Tablets (Infrequent) 1603
Wellbutrin SR Sustained-Release Tablets 1607
Wellbutrin XL Extended-Release Tablets 1613
▲ Xeloda Tablets (Less than 5%) 2822
Zicam Maximum Strength Flu Daytime ▣ 768
Zicam Maximum Strength Flu Nighttime ▣ 768
Zyban Sustained-Release Tablets 1644

Hernia, hiatal
Aricept Tablets (Infrequent) 1094
Aricept ODT Tablets (Infrequent) 1094
Celebrex Capsules (0.1% to 1.9%) 3134
Neurontin Capsules (Rare) 2487
Neurontin Oral Solution (Rare) 2487
Neurontin Tablets (Rare) 2487
Prometrium Capsules (100 mg, 200 mg) (Less than 5%) 3203
Remicade for IV Injection (Greater than or equal to 0.2%) 971
Triglide Tablets 3123

Hernia, inguinal
Edex Injection (1%) 3089
NeoProfen Injection 2472
Prevnar for Injection 3463
Revlimid Capsules 958
Xifaxan Tablets (Less than 2%) 2842
Zyban Sustained-Release Tablets (Infrequent) 1644

Hernia, unspecified
Actonel Tablets (2.9%) 2683
Actonel with Calcium Tablets (2.9%) 2688
Azilect Tablets (2%) 3293
Campral Tablets (Infrequent) 1174
▲ CellCept Capsules (3% to less than 20%) 2747
▲ CellCept Intravenous (3% to less than 20%) 2747
▲ CellCept Oral Suspension (3% to less than 20%) 2747
▲ CellCept Tablets (3% to less than 20%) 2747
Effexor XR Capsules 3417
Exelon Capsules (Infrequent) 2206
Exelon Oral Solution (Infrequent) 2206
Gabitril Tablets (Infrequent) 984
Lofibra Tablets 1219
Lofibra Capsules 1216
Lunesta Tablets (Infrequent) 3142
Myobloc Injection (2% or greater) 3192
Neurontin Capsules (Rare) 2487
Neurontin Oral Solution (Rare) 2487
Neurontin Tablets (Rare) 2487
Nexium Delayed-Release Capsules (Less than 1%) 655
Nexium I.V. (Less than 1%) 659
Permax Tablets (Infrequent) 3356
Plavix Tablets (1% to 2.5%) 917
Plavix Tablets (1% to 2.5%) 2926
▲ Prograf Capsules and Injection (3% to 15%) 632
Protonix I.V. (Less than 1%) 3472
Protonix Tablets (Less than 1%) 3469
Protopic Ointment (Greater than or equal to 1%) 638
▲ Rapamune Oral Solution and Tablets (3% to 20%) 3475
Relpax Tablets (Rare) 2548
Rilutek Tablets (Infrequent) 2930
▲ Simulect for Injection (3% to 10%) 2284
Symbyax Capsules (Infrequent) 1819
▲ Synagis (4.1%) 1897
Tasmar Tablets (Infrequent) 3358
Thalomid Capsules 965
Tricor Tablets 527
Uniretic Tablets (Less than 1%) 3100
Zelapar Tablets 3372

Herpes, precipitation
Oxsoralen-Ultra Capsules 3353

Herpes, unspecified
Bexxar 1398
Imitrex Nasal Spray (Rare) 1467
Matulane Capsules 3191
▲ Megace ES Oral Suspension (1% to 3%) 2481

Herpes labialis
Alferon N Injection (1%) 1665
Finacea Gel (Rare) 1669

Herpes simplex
Aceon Tablets (2 mg, 4 mg, 8 mg) (0.3% to 1%) 3194
Aldara Cream, 5% (1.9%) 1846
Alrex Ophthalmic Suspension 0.2% ⊙ 246
Ambien Tablets (Rare) 2851
Ambien CR Tablets (Rare) 2855
AmBisome for Injection (Less common) 620
Amevive 626
Aptivus Capsules (Less than 2%) 826
Aricept Tablets (Infrequent) 1094
Aricept ODT Tablets (Infrequent) 1094
Astelin Nasal Spray (Infrequent) 1904
Blephamide Ophthalmic Ointment 568
▲ Campath Ampules (1% to 11%) 811
Celebrex Capsules (0.1% to 1.9%) 3134
▲ CellCept Capsules (10.1% to 20.8%) 2747
▲ CellCept Intravenous (10.1% to 20.8%) 2747
▲ CellCept Oral Suspension (10.1% to 20.8%) 2747
▲ CellCept Tablets (10.1% to 20.8%) 2747
▲ Clolar for Intravenous Infusion (11%) 1271
▲ Copaxone for Injection (4%) 3297
Cutivate Cream (0.8%) 2662
▲ Doxil Injection (1% to 10%) 2351
Effexor XR Capsules 3417
Efudex (Infrequent) 3363
▲ Elidel Cream 1% (0.4% to 4%) 2200
Emend Capsules (Greater than 0.5%) 1963
▲ Euflexxa (3%) 1162
Evoxac Capsules (Less than 1%) 1047
Exelon Capsules (Infrequent) 2206
Exelon Oral Solution (Infrequent) 2206
FML Ophthalmic Ointment ⊙ 228
▲ Fuzeon Injection (3.5% to 4.1%) 2767
Gabitril Tablets (Infrequent) 984
Gengraf Capsules (1% to less than 3%) 459
Gleevec Tablets (Infrequent) 2227
Herceptin I.V. (2%) 1233
▲ Intron A for Injection (Up to 5%) 3024
Invanz for Injection (1%) 1999
Invirase (Less than 2%) 2772
Klonopin (Infrequent) 2778
Levaquin (0.1% to 0.9%) 2384
Levaquin in 5% Dextrose Injection (0.1% to 0.9%) 2384
Lofibra Tablets 1219
Lofibra Capsules 1216
Lotemax Ophthalmic Suspension 0.5% ⊙ 251
Meridia Capsules (1.3%) 489
Migranal Nasal Spray (Rare) 3348
▲ Myfortic Tablets (1.3% to less than 20%) 2255
▲ Mylotarg for Injection (2% to 25%) 3431
Neoral Oral Solution (1% to less than 3%) 2259
Neoral Soft Gelatin Capsules (1% to less than 3%) 2259
Neurontin Capsules (Infrequent) 2487
Neurontin Oral Solution (Infrequent) 2487
Neurontin Tablets (Infrequent) 2487
▲ Nipent for Injection (4%) 1863
Oncaspar 1145
▲ Orencia Powder for Intravenous Infusion (Less than 5%) 914
Paxil CR Controlled-Release Tablets (Rare) 1538
Paxil (Rare) 1530
Permax Tablets (Infrequent) 3356
Pexeva Tablets (Infrequent) 1694
▲ Prograf Capsules and Injection (3% to 15%) 632
▲ Prometrium Capsules (100 mg, 200 mg) (Less than 5%) 3203
ProQuad 2064
Protonix I.V. (Less than 1%) 3472
Protonix Tablets (Less than 1%) 3469
▲ Protopic Ointment (4% to 12%) 638
Provigil Tablets (1%) 988
▲ Pulmicort Respules (1% to 3%) 661
Requip Tablets (Infrequent) 1555
Rescriptor Tablets 2551
▲ Simulect for Injection (3% to 10%) 2284
Soriatane Capsules (Less than 1%) 1013
Sular Tablets (Less than or equal to 1%) 3122
Tasmar Tablets (Infrequent) 3358
Teveten Tablets (Less than 1%) 1735
Teveten HCT Tablets (Less than 1%) 1737
Thalomid Capsules 965
▲ Thymoglobulin for Intravenous Infusion (4.9%) 1284
Tricor Tablets 527
▲ Trisenox Injection (13%) 993
Uniretic Tablets (Less than 1%) 3100
VFEND I.V. (Less than 2%) 2564
VFEND Oral Suspension (Less than 2%) 2564
VFEND Tablets (Less than 2%) 2564
Viagra Tablets (Less than 2%) 2573
Xyrem Oral Solution (Infrequent) 1688
Zelapar Tablets 3372

Herpes simplex, disseminated
Accutane Capsules 2731

Herpes zoster
Aciphex Tablets (Rare) 1090
Actiq (Less than 1%) 979
Ambien Tablets (Rare) 2851
Ambien CR Tablets (Rare) 2855
Aptivus Capsules (Less than 2%) 826
Aricept Tablets (Infrequent) 1094
Aricept ODT Tablets (Infrequent) 1094
Campath Ampules 811
Celebrex Capsules (0.1% to 1.9%) 3134
▲ CellCept Capsules (4% to 10.7%) 2747
▲ CellCept Intravenous (4% to 10.7%) 2747
▲ CellCept Oral Suspension (4% to 10.7%) 2747
▲ CellCept Tablets (4% to 10.7%) 2747
Copaxone for Injection (Frequent) 3297
▲ Doxil Injection (Less than 1% to 10%) 2351
Effexor XR Capsules 3417
Engerix-B Vaccine 1425
▲ Euflexxa (3%) 1162
Evoxac Capsules (Less than 1%) 1047
Gabitril Tablets (Infrequent) 984
Gengraf Capsules (1% to less than 3%) 459
Gleevec Tablets (Infrequent) 2227
Herceptin I.V. (At least one of the 958 patients) 1233
▲ Humira Injection (Less than 5%) 466
▲ Intron A for Injection (Less than 5%) 3024
Invirase (Less than 2%) 2772
Lamictal (Rare) 1481
Leustatin Injection (8 episodes) 2357
Lofibra Tablets 1219
Lofibra Capsules 1216
Lunesta Tablets (Rare) 3142
Mustargen for Injection 2468
▲ Myfortic Tablets (1.9% to less than 20%) 2255
Neoral Oral Solution (1% to less than 3%) 2259
Neoral Soft Gelatin Capsules (1% to less than 3%) 2259
Neurontin Capsules (Rare) 2487
Neurontin Oral Solution (Rare) 2487
Neurontin Tablets (Rare) 2487
▲ Nipent for Injection (8%) 1863
Orencia Powder for Intravenous Infusion (0.7%) 914
Paxil CR Controlled-Release Tablets (Rare) 1538
Paxil (Rare) 1530
Permax Tablets (Infrequent) 3356
Pexeva Tablets (rare) 1694
Prinivil Tablets (0.3% to 1.0%) 2052
Prinzide Tablets 2056
ProQuad 2064
Protonix I.V. (Less than 1%) 3472
Protonix Tablets (Less than 1%) 3469
Protopic Ointment (Up to 3%) 638
Prozac Pulvules and Liquid (Rare) 1801
▲ Rapamune Oral Solution and Tablets (3% to 20%) 3475
Recombivax HB 2071
Remicade for IV Injection 971
Requip Tablets (Infrequent) 1555
Rescriptor Tablets 2551
▲ Simulect for Injection (3% to 10%) 2284
▲ Spiriva HandiHaler (1% to 3%) 869
Sular Tablets (Less than or equal to 1%) 3122
Tasmar Tablets (Infrequent) 3358
Tricor Tablets 527
▲ Trisenox Injection (8%) 993
Twinrix Vaccine 1595
Uniretic Tablets (Less than 1%) 3100
Varivax 2100
Vasotec I.V. Injection (0.5% to 1.0%) 2103
▲ Velcade for Injection (13%) 2133
Xyrem Oral Solution (Infrequent) 1688
Zelapar Tablets 3372

Herxheimer's reaction
▲ Ceftin Tablets (5.6%) 1407

Hiccups
Abilify Oral Solution (Infrequent) 882
Abilify Oral Solution (Infrequent) 2450
Abilify Discmelt Orally Disintegrating Tablets (Infrequent) 882
Abilify Discmelt Orally Disintegrating Tablets (Infrequent) 2450
Abilify Tablets (Infrequent) 882
Abilify Tablets (Infrequent) 2450
Aciphex Tablets 1090
Actiq (Less than 1%) 979
Aloxi Injection (Less than 1%) 2127
Ambien Tablets (Frequent) 2851
Ambien CR Tablets (Frequent) 2855
AmBisome for Injection (Less common) 620
Avinza Capsules (Less than 5%) 1741
Celexa (Rare) 1176
▲ CellCept Capsules (3% to less than 20%) 2747
▲ CellCept Intravenous (3% to less than 20%) 2747
▲ CellCept Oral Suspension (3% to less than 20%) 2747
▲ CellCept Tablets (3% to less than 20%) 2747
Cipro (Less than 1%) 2977
Cipro I.V. (1% or less) 2984
Cipro XR Tablets 2990
Decadron Tablets 1951
Depakote ER Tablets (Greater than 1%) 434
Diastat Rectal Delivery System (Greater than or equal to 1%) 3343
Doxil Injection (Less than 1%) 2351
Duragesic Transdermal System (1% or greater) 2373
▲ Eloxatin for Injection (2% to 5%) 2892
▲ Emend Capsules (10.8%) 1963
Ethyol for Injection 1898
▲ Evoxac Capsules (1% to 3%) 1047
Frova Tablets (Rare) 1113
Gabitril Tablets (Infrequent) 984
Gengraf Capsules (2% or less) 459
Imitrex Injection (Rare) 1463
Imitrex Nasal Spray 1467
Imitrex Tablets (Rare) 1471
Invanz for Injection (Greater than 0.1%) 1999
Ionsys Transdermal System (.1% to less than 1%) 2379
▲ I.V. Busulfex (18%) 2493
Kadian Capsules (Less than 3%) 577
Lamictal (Rare) 1481
Lunesta Tablets (Infrequent) 3142
Lyrica Capsules (Rare) 2539
Maxalt Tablets (Rare) 2008
Maxalt-MLT Orally Disintegrating Tablets (Rare) 2008
Migranal Nasal Spray (Infrequent) 3348
Moduretic Tablets (Less than or equal to 1%) 2028
Mycamine for Injection (0.2%) 628
Neoral Oral Solution (2% or less) 2259
Neoral Soft Gelatin Capsules (2% or less) 2259
Neurontin Capsules (Rare) 2487
Neurontin Oral Solution (Rare) 2487
Neurontin Tablets (Rare) 2487

Nexium Delayed-Release Capsules (Less than 1%) 655
Nexium I.V. (Less than 1%) 659
Norvir (Less than 2%) 503
▲ OxyContin Tablets (Between 1% and 5%) 2703
Parcopa Orally Disintegrating Tablets 3097
Paxil CR Controlled-Release Tablets (Rare) 1538
Paxil (Rare) 1530
Permax Tablets (1.1%) 3356
Pexeva Tablets (Rare) 1694
▲ Photofrin for Injection (6%) 702
Prevacid Delayed-Release Capsules (Less than 1%) 3271
Prevacid for Delayed-Release Oral Suspension (Less than 1%) 3271
Prevacid SoluTab Delayed-Release Orally Disintegrating Tablets (Less than 1%) 3271
Prevacid NapraPAC (Less than 1%) 3280
PREVPAC (Less than 1%) 3284
Prezista Tablets (Less than 2%) 3306
Proquin XR Tablets 1153
Protonix I.V. (Less than 1%) 3472
Protonix Tablets (Less than 1%) 3469
Prozac Pulvules and Liquid (Infrequent) 1801
Razadyne (Infrequent) 2399
Razadyne ER Extended-Release Capsules (Infrequent) 2399
Relpax Tablets (Rare) 2548
Requip Tablets (Infrequent) 1555
Rescriptor Tablets 2551
Reyataz Capsules (Less than 3%) 921
Rilutek Tablets (Infrequent) 2930
Romazicon Injection (Less than 1%) 2804
Sandimmune (2% or less) 2275
Seroquel Tablets (Rare) 690
Sonata Capsules (Rare) 1717
Stalevo Tablets 2287
Symbyax Capsules (Infrequent) 1819
Tasmar Tablets (Infrequent) 3358
Trileptal Tablets 2300
Trileptal Oral Suspension 2300
Ultane Liquid for Inhalation (Less than 1%) 531
Vicoprofen Tablets (Less than 3%) 539
Xyrem Oral Solution (Infrequent) 1688
Zelapar Tablets 3372
Zemuron Injection (Less than 1%) 2346
Zofran Injection 1634
Zofran 1639
Zofran ODT Orally Disintegrating Tablets 1639
Zoloft (Rare) 2586
Zomig Tablets (Infrequent) 3519
Zomig Nasal Spray (Rare) 3523
Zomig-ZMT Tablets (Infrequent) 3519
Zosyn (1.0% or less to 2.6%) 3492
Zyprexa Tablets (Rare) 1830
Zyprexa ZYDIS Orally Disintegrating Tablets (Rare) 1830

Hip fracture
Arimidex Tablets (1%) 673
Revlimid Capsules 958

Hirsutism
Accutane Capsules 2731
AndroGel (Fewer than 1%) 3329
Androxy Tablets 3335
Angeliq Tablets 762
Aricept Tablets (Infrequent) 1094
Aricept ODT Tablets (Infrequent) 1094
Carbatrol Capsules (Isolated cases) 3171
▲ CellCept Capsules (3% to less than 20%) 2747
▲ CellCept Intravenous (3% to less than 20%) 2747
▲ CellCept Oral Suspension (3% to less than 20%) 2747
▲ CellCept Tablets (3% to less than 20%) 2747
Climara Transdermal System 771
Climara Pro Transdermal System 776
Dantrium Capsules (Less frequent) 2694
Decadron Tablets 1951
Depo-Provera Contraceptive Injection (Less than 1%) 2622
Effexor Tablets (Rare) 3411
Effexor XR Capsules (Rare) 3417
Eldepryl Capsules 3208
Enjuvia Tablets 1062
▲ Entocort EC Capsules (5%) 2698
Equetro Extended-Release Capsules 3180
Estrasorb Topical Emulsion 1147
Estratest Tablets 3199
Estratest H.S. Tablets 3199
Gabitril Tablets (Infrequent) 984
▲ Gengraf Capsules (21% to 45%) 459
Hydrocortone Tablets 1989
Hyperstat I.V. 3017
▲ Intron A for Injection (Less than 5%) 3024
Klonopin 2778
Lamictal (Infrequent) 1481
▲ Lumigan Ophthalmic Solution (1% to 5%) 573
Lunesta Tablets (Rare) 3142
Lupron Depot–3 Month 11.25 mg (0.6% to 1%) 3265
Lyrica Capsules (0.1% to 1%) 2539
Menostar Transdermal System 782
Mircette Tablets 1066
▲ Myfortic Tablets (3% to less than 20%) 2255
▲ Neoral Oral Solution (21% to 45%) 2259
▲ Neoral Soft Gelatin Capsules (21% to 45%) 2259
Neurontin Capsules (Infrequent) 2487
Neurontin Oral Solution (Infrequent) 2487
Neurontin Tablets (Infrequent) 2487
NuvaRing 2340
Ortho-Cyclen Tablets 2429
Ortho Evra Transdermal System 2417
Ortho Micronor Tablets (Rare) 2426
Ortho Tri-Cyclen Tablets 2429
Ortho Tri-Cyclen Lo Tablets 2436
Oxandrin Tablets 2962
Paxil CR Controlled-Release Tablets (Rare) 1538
Paxil (Rare) 1530
Permax Tablets (Infrequent) 3356
Pexeva Tablets (Rare) 1694
Photofrin for Injection 702
Premarin Intravenous 3442
Premarin Tablets 3446
Premarin Vaginal Cream 3452
Premphase Tablets 3456
Prempro Tablets 3456
▲ Prograf Capsules and Injection (3% to 15%) 632
Prozac Pulvules and Liquid (Rare) 1801
▲ Rapamune Oral Solution and Tablets (3% to 20%) 3475
▲ Sandimmune (21% to 45%) 2275
Seasonique Tablets 1077
Tegretol/Tegretol-XR (Isolated cases) 2295
Viadur Implant (Less than 2%) 757
Wellbutrin Tablets (Rare) 1603
Wellbutrin SR Sustained-Release Tablets 1607
Wellbutrin XL Extended-Release Tablets 1613
Yasmin 28 Tablets 796
Yaz Tablets 803
Zonegran Capsules (Infrequent) 1101
Zyban Sustained-Release Tablets 1644
Zyprexa Tablets (Infrequent) 1830
Zyprexa ZYDIS Orally Disintegrating Tablets (Infrequent) 1830

Histoplasmosis
Remicade for IV Injection 971

Histrionic movements
FazaClo Orally Disintegrating Tablets (Less than 1%) 551

HIV viral load increase
Thalomid Capsules 965

Hives
(*see under* Urticaria)

Hives at injection site
Prevnar for Injection 3463
Xolair 1266

Hoarseness
Aceon Tablets (2 mg, 4 mg, 8 mg) (0.3% to 1%) 3194
▲ Advair Diskus 100/50 (5%) 1308
▲ Advair Diskus 250/50 (2% to 8%) 1308
▲ Advair Diskus 500/50 (2% to 5%) 1308
▲ Aerobid/Aerobid-M (3% to 9%) 1171
Atrovent Nasal Spray 0.03% (Less than 2%) 837
Atrovent Nasal Spray 0.06% (Less than 1%) 839
Azmacort Inhalation Aerosol 1726
Captopril Tablets 2149
Depo-Provera Contraceptive Injection (Less than 1%) 2622
depo-subQ provera 104 Injectable Suspension 2624
Emcyt Capsules (1%) 2634
Flonase Nasal Spray 1440
▲ Flovent Diskus (1% to 9%) 1443
Flovent HFA (2%) 1447
Klonopin (Infrequent) 2778
Levaquin 2384
Levaquin in 5% Dextrose Injection 2384
Matulane Capsules 3191
Maxalt Tablets (Rare) 2008
Maxalt-MLT Orally Disintegrating Tablets (Rare) 2008
Neurontin Capsules 2487
Neurontin Oral Solution 2487
Neurontin Tablets 2487
▲ Nexavar Tablets (Common) 746
Oxandrin Tablets 2962
Parcopa Orally Disintegrating Tablets 3097
Proventil Inhalation Aerosol 3053
Retrovir Capsules 1560
Retrovir IV Infusion 1564
Retrovir 1560
Spiriva HandiHaler 869
Stalevo Tablets 2287
Vasotec I.V. Injection (0.5% to 1.0%) 2103
Ventolin HFA Inhalation Aerosol 1600
Vicoprofen Tablets (Less than 1%) 539
▲ Xeloda Tablets (Less than 5%) 2822

Hodgkin's disease
Phenytek Capsules 2160

Hodgkin's disease, nodular sclerosing
Thalomid Capsules 965

Hoigne's syndrome
Bicillin C-R Injectable Suspension 1706

Hordeolum
Alphagan P Ophthalmic Solution (Less than 1%) 567

Hormonal imbalance
Norvir (Less than 2%) 503
Wellbutrin Tablets (Rare) 1603

Horner's syndrome
Parcopa Orally Disintegrating Tablets 3097
Stalevo Tablets 2287

Hostility
Abilify Oral Solution (Frequent) 882
Abilify Oral Solution (Frequent) 2450
Abilify Discmelt Orally Disintegrating Tablets (Frequent) 882
Abilify Discmelt Orally Disintegrating Tablets (Frequent) 2450
Abilify Tablets (Frequent) 882
Abilify Tablets (Frequent) 2450
Adderall XR Capsules 3166
Amerge Tablets (Rare) 1339
Aricept Tablets (Infrequent) 1094
Aricept ODT Tablets (Infrequent) 1094
Azilect Tablets (Rare) 3293
Campral Tablets (Infrequent) 1174
Copaxone for Injection (Infrequent) 3297
Depacon Injection 412
Depakene 417
Depakote Sprinkle Capsules 422
Depakote Tablets 427
Depakote ER Tablets 434
Duragesic Transdermal System (Less than 1%) 2373
Effexor Tablets (Infrequent) 3411
Effexor XR Capsules (Infrequent) 3417
Gabitril Tablets (2%) 984
Geodon Capsules (Frequent) 2529
Keppra Injection (2%) 3320
▲ Keppra Oral Solution (2% to 12%) 3314
▲ Keppra Tablets (2% to 12%) 3314
Klonopin 2778
Lamictal (Frequent) 1481
Lunesta Tablets (Infrequent) 3142
Lyrica Capsules (0.1% to 1%) 2539
▲ Neurontin Capsules (5.2% to 7.6%) 2487
▲ Neurontin Oral Solution (5.2% to 7.6%) 2487
▲ Neurontin Tablets (5.2% to 7.6%) 2487
Nipent for Injection (Less than 3%) 1863
Paxil CR Controlled-Release Tablets (Infrequent) 1538
Paxil (Infrequent) 1530
Permax Tablets (Infrequent) 3356
Pexeva Tablets (Infrequent) 1694
Prevacid Delayed-Release Capsules (Less than 1%) 3271
Prevacid for Delayed-Release Oral Suspension (Less than 1%) 3271
Prevacid SoluTab Delayed-Release Orally Disintegrating Tablets (Less than 1%) 3271
Prevacid NapraPAC (Less than 1%) 3280
PREVPAC (Less than 1%) 3284
ProSom Tablets (Infrequent) 517
Prozac Pulvules and Liquid (Infrequent) 1801
Reyataz Capsules (Less than 3%) 921
Rilutek Tablets (Frequent) 2930
Ritalin LA Capsules 2271
Sonata Capsules (Rare) 1717
Strattera Capsules 1814
Symbyax Capsules (Infrequent) 1819
Tasmar Tablets (Infrequent) 3358
Tequin Injection (Less than 0.1%) 938
Tequin Injection in 5% Dextrose (Less than 0.1%) 938
Tequin Tablets (Less than 0.1%) 938
Thalomid Capsules 965
▲ Wellbutrin Tablets (5.6%) 1603
Wellbutrin SR Sustained-Release Tablets (Infrequent) 1607
Wellbutrin XL Extended-Release Tablets (Infrequent) 1613
Zoloft 2586
Zyban Sustained-Release Tablets (Infrequent) 1644
▲ Zyprexa Tablets (15%) 1830
▲ Zyprexa ZYDIS Orally Disintegrating Tablets (15%) 1830

Hot flashes
Advate Injection (1.3%) 712
Alferon N Injection (1%) 1665
Aloxi Injection (Less than 1%) 2127
Ambien Tablets (Rare) 2851
Ambien CR Tablets (Rare) 2855
Aricept Tablets (Frequent) 1094
Aricept ODT Tablets (Frequent) 1094
▲ Arimidex Tablets (11% to 36%) 673
▲ Aromasin Tablets (13%) 2600
Caduet Tablets (Greater than 0.1% to less than or equal to 1%) 2508
Celebrex Capsules (0.1% to 1.9%) 3134
Celexa (Infrequent) 1176
Cesamet Capsules 3340
Clozaril Tablets (Less than 1%) 2184
Colazal Capsules 2838
▲ Depo-Provera Contraceptive Injection (1% to 5%) 2622
▲ Effexor XR Capsules (4%) 3417
▲ Eligard 7.5 mg (25% to 56.7%) 2880
▲ Eligard 22.5 mg (56.4%) 2883
▲ Eligard 30 mg (73.3%) 2885
▲ Eligard 45 mg (57.7%) 2888
Elitek (Less than or equal to 1%) 2890
▲ Eloxatin for Injection (2% to 5%) 2892
Eraxis for Injection (Less than 1% to less than 2%) 2521
Estring Vaginal Ring (2%) 2635
▲ Eulexin Capsules (46% to 61%) 3009
▲ Evista Tablets (9.7% to 24.6%) 1763
Evoxac Capsules (2.4%) 1047
Exelon Capsules (Frequent) 2206
Exelon Oral Solution (Frequent) 2206
FazaClo Orally Disintegrating Tablets (Less than 1%) 551
▲ Femara Tablets (5% to 19%) 2214
Floxin Otic Solution (Single report) 1049
Fluarix 1451
Frova Tablets (Infrequent) 1113
Gengraf Capsules (1% to less than 3%) 459
▲ Imdur Tablets (Less than or equal to 5%) 3018
▲ Infergen (7% to 13%) 3364
▲ Intron A for Injection (Less than 5%) 3024
Invirase (Less than 2%) 2772
▲ I.V. Busulfex (25%) 2493
Lamictal (1.3%) 1481
Levaquin (0.1% to 0.9%) 2384
Levaquin in 5% Dextrose Injection (0.1% to 0.9%) 2384
Lexapro Oral Solution (Frequent) 1190
Lexapro Tablets (Frequent) 1190
Limbrel Capsules (0.003%) 2672
Lotrel Capsules 2249
▲ Lupron Depot 3.75 mg (50%) 3260
▲ Lupron Depot 7.5 mg (57.1%) 3264
▲ Lupron Depot–3 Month 11.25 mg (58% to 98%) 3265
Maxalt Tablets (Frequent) 2008
Maxalt-MLT Orally Disintegrating Tablets (Frequent) 2008
Migranal Nasal Spray (1%) 3348
Mobic Oral Suspension (Less than 2%) 863
Mobic Tablets (Less than 2%) 863
Myozyme for Intravenous Infusion 1279
Neoral Oral Solution (1% to less than 3%) 2259
Neoral Soft Gelatin Capsules (1% to less than 3%) 2259
Nexium Delayed-Release Capsules (Less than 1%) 655
Nexium I.V. (Less than 1%) 659

Norvasc Tablets (More than 0.1% to 1%) 2545
Opana Tablets (Less than 1%) 1122
Opana ER Tablets (Less than 1%) 1126
Parcopa Orally Disintegrating Tablets 3097
Prochieve 4% Gel 1003
Prochieve 8% Gel 1003
▲ Prometrium Capsules (100 mg, 200 mg) (11%) 3203
Requip Tablets (1% or more) 1555
▲ Romazicon Injection (1% to 3%) 2804
Sandostatin LAR Depot (1% to 4%) 2280
▲ Soltamox Oral Solution (2.8% to 80%) 3527
▲ Soriatane Capsules (1% to 10%) 1013
Stalevo Tablets 2287
Sustiva Capsules (Less than 2%) 930
Sustiva Tablets (Less than 2%) 930
Testim 1% Gel (1% or less) 695
Teveten Tablets (Less than 1%) 1735
Teveten HCT Tablets (Less than 1%) 1737
Topamax Sprinkle Capsules (1% to 2%) 2404
Topamax Tablets (1% to 2%) 2404
▲ Trelstar Depot (58.6%) 3394
▲ Trelstar LA Suspension (73%) 3397
Trileptal Tablets (1% to 2%) 2300
Trileptal Oral Suspension (1% to 2%) 2300
▲ Ultram ER Tablets (1% to greater than 5%) 2392
▲ Vagifem Tablets (3% to 5%) 2334
▲ Vantas (65.5%) 3375
▲ Wellbutrin SR Sustained-Release Tablets (1% to 3%) 1607
▲ Wellbutrin XL Extended-Release Tablets (6%) 1613
▲ Xeloda Tablets (Less than 5%) 2822
Xifaxan Tablets (Less than 2%) 2842
Zoloft (2%) 2586
Zyban Sustained-Release Tablets (1%) 1644
Zyrtec Chewable Tablets (Less than 2%) 2594
Zyrtec (Less than 2%) 2594
Zyrtec-D 12 Hour Extended Release Tablets (Less than 2%) 2597

Hot flushes
▲ Arimidex Tablets (13% to 26%) 673
▲ Aromasin Tablets (21.2% to 32.9%) 2600
Cardura XL Tablets 2515
Chantix Tablets (Frequent) 2517
Cymbalta Delayed-Release Capsules (2%) 1757
▲ depo-subQ provera 104 Injectable Suspension (1% to less than 5%) 2624
▲ Emend Capsules (3%) 1963
Prograf Capsules and Injection 632
Vivitrol 995

HPA axis suppression
Aclovate Cream 2660
Advair Diskus 100/50 1308
Advair Diskus 250/50 1308
Advair Diskus 500/50 1308
Clobex Shampoo 1206
Clobex Spray 1208
Cutivate Cream 2662
Cutivate Ointment 2665
Diprolene Gel 0.05% 3001
Diprolene Lotion 0.05% 3002
Diprolene Ointment 0.05% (Some patients) 3003
Diprolene AF Cream 0.05% (Some patients) 3000
Diprosone Cream, USP 0.05% 3004
▲ Elocon Cream 0.1% (16%) 3005
Elocon Lotion 0.1% 3006
▲ Elocon Ointment 0.1% (27%) 3007
Lotrisone 3040
▲ Olux Foam (5 of 13 patients) 1012
Temovate Cream 2668
Temovate Gel 2669
Temovate Ointment 2668
Temovate Scalp Application 2670
Temovate E Emollient 2671
Vanos Cream 1893

HPA function suppression
Azmacort Inhalation Aerosol 1726

Hunger
Imitrex Injection (Rare) 1463
Imitrex Nasal Spray (Rare) 1467
Imitrex Tablets (Rare) 1471
Klonopin (Infrequent) 2778
▲ MoviPrep Oral Solution (30.2%) 2839

Hydrocephalus
Arranon Injection (1%) 1357
DepoCyt Injection 1143
Herceptin I.V. (At least one of the 958 patients) 1233

Hydrocephalus, fetal
Accutane Capsules 2731

Hydronephrosis
Actiq (1% or greater) 979
▲ CellCept Capsules (3% to less than 20%) 2747
▲ CellCept Intravenous (3% to less than 20%) 2747
▲ CellCept Oral Suspension (3% to less than 20%) 2747
▲ CellCept Tablets (3% to less than 20%) 2747
Crixivan Capsules (2.8%) 1940
Doxil Injection (Less than 1%) 2351
Herceptin I.V. (At least one of the 958 patients) 1233
▲ Myfortic Tablets (3% to less than 20%) 2255
▲ Prograf Capsules and Injection (3% to 15%) 632
▲ Rapamune Oral Solution and Tablets (3% to 20%) 3475
VFEND I.V. (Less than 2%) 2564
VFEND Oral Suspension (Less than 2%) 2564
VFEND Tablets (Less than 2%) 2564

Hydrothorax
Follistim AQ Cartridge 2338

Hypalgesia
Lyrica Capsules (Rare) 2539

Hyperacidity
Lotronex Tablets (Rare) 1512

Hyperactive deep tendon reflexes
Lithobid Tablets 1692

Hyperactivity
Abilify Oral Solution (Infrequent) 882
Abilify Oral Solution (Infrequent) 2450
Abilify Discmelt Orally Disintegrating Tablets (Infrequent) 882
Abilify Discmelt Orally Disintegrating Tablets (Infrequent) 2450
Abilify Tablets (Infrequent) 882
Abilify Tablets (Infrequent) 2450
Advair HFA Inhalation Aerosol (Very Rare) 1318
▲ Aerobid/Aerobid-M (1% to 3%) 1171
Amerge Tablets (Rare) 1339
Amoxil Capsules (Rare) 1343
Amoxil Chewable Tablets (Rare) 1343
Amoxil Pediatric Drops for Oral Suspension (Rare) 1343
Amoxil Powder for Oral Suspension (Rare) 1343
Amoxil Tablets (Rare) 1343
Augmentin (Rare) 1360
Augmentin Tablets (Rare) 1363
Augmentin XR Extended-Release Tablets (Rare) 1369
Augmentin ES-600 Powder for Oral Suspension (Rare) 1366
Ceftin for Oral Suspension (0.1% to 1%) 1407
Cesamet Capsules 3340
Clarinex-D 24-Hour Extended-Release Tablets (2%) 2998
Dalmane Capsules (Rare) 3342
Depacon Injection 412
Depakene 417
Depakote Sprinkle Capsules 422
Depakote Tablets 427
Depakote ER Tablets 434
Klonopin (Infrequent) 2778
Levothroid Tablets 1186
Levoxyl Tablets 1712
Moban Tablets (Less frequent) 1119
Neurontin Capsules 2487
Neurontin Oral Solution 2487
Neurontin Tablets 2487
PREVPAC 3284
Raniclor Tablets, Chewable (Rare) 2505
Tasmar Tablets (1%) 3358
Thioridazine Hydrochloride Tablets (Extremely rare) 2163
Zmax for Oral Suspension 2583

Hyperactivity, psychomotor
Xyrem Oral Solution (Infrequent) 1688

Hyperacusis
Axert Tablets (Infrequent) 2396
Carbatrol Capsules 3171
Effexor Tablets (Infrequent) 3411
Effexor XR Capsules (Infrequent) 3417
Equetro Extended-Release Capsules 3180
Frova Tablets (Infrequent) 1113
Gabitril Tablets (Infrequent) 984
Lunesta Tablets (Rare) 3142
Lyrica Capsules (0.1% to 1%) 2539
Maxalt Tablets (Rare) 2008
Maxalt-MLT Orally Disintegrating Tablets (Rare) 2008
Paxil CR Controlled-Release Tablets (Rare) 1538
Paxil (Rare) 1530
Pexeva Tablets (Rare) 1694
Prozac Pulvules and Liquid (Rare) 1801
Rilutek Tablets (Rare) 2930
Risperdal (Rare) 1676
Risperdal M-Tab Orally Disintegrating Tablets (Rare) 1676
Romazicon Injection (Less than 1%) 2804
Sonata Capsules (2%) 1717
Tegretol/Tegretol-XR 2295
Zoloft (Rare) 2586
Zomig Tablets (Infrequent) 3519
Zomig-ZMT Tablets (Infrequent) 3519

Hyperaesthesia
Xyrem Oral Solution (Infrequent) 1688

Hyperalgesia
Lamictal (Rare) 1481
Lyrica Capsules (0.1% to 1%) 2539
Paxil CR Controlled-Release Tablets (Rare) 1538
Paxil (Rare) 1530
Pexeva Tablets (rare) 1694
Relpax Tablets (Rare) 2548
Retrovir Capsules 1560
Retrovir IV Infusion 1564
Retrovir 1560
Thalomid Capsules 965

Hyperammonemia
Aciphex Tablets 1090
Depacon Injection 412
Depakene 417
Depakote Sprinkle Capsules 422
Depakote Tablets 427
Depakote ER Tablets 434
Oncaspar (Less than 1%) 1145

Hyperammonemic encephalopathy
Depacon Injection 412
Depakene 417
Depakote Sprinkle Capsules 422
Depakote Tablets 427
Depakote ER Tablets 434

Hyperamylasemia
Aptivus Capsules (Less than 2%) 826

Hyperbilirubinemia
Abelcet Injection 1141
Accolate Tablets (Rare) 671
Advicor Tablets 1722
Aloprim for Injection (Less than 1%) 2167
Altace Capsules 1702
Altoprev Extended-Release Tablets 3109
▲ AndroGel (3% to 6%) 3329
Anzemet Injection (Less than 1%) 2859
Anzemet Tablets (Less than 1%) 2862
▲ Aromasin Tablets (0.9% to 6.9%) 2600
Atacand Tablets (Infrequent) 649
Atacand HCT 651
Augmentin (Infrequent) 1360
Augmentin Tablets (Infrequent) 1363
Augmentin XR Extended-Release Tablets (Infrequent) 1369
Augmentin ES-600 Powder for Oral Suspension (Infrequently) 1366
Avelox (Greater than or equal to 2%) 2970
Benicar Tablets (Infrequently) 1043
Biaxin/Biaxin XL (Less than 1%) 402
Campath Ampules 811
▲ Camptosar Injection (7.2% to 83.9%) 2604
Captopril Tablets 2149
Ceftin 1407
Cipro (0.3%) 2977
▲ Cipro I.V. (Among most frequent) 2984
Clarinex Tablets (Rare) 2995
Clarinex Reditabs Tablets (Rare) 2995
Clarinex-D 24-Hour Extended-Release Tablets 2998
▲ Clolar for Intravenous Infusion (15%) 1271
Colazal Capsules 2838
Covera-HS Tablets 3139
▲ Crixivan Capsules (11.9% to 14%) 1940
▲ Dacogen Injection (14%) 2129
Dapsone Tablets USP 1673
Depacon Injection (Occasional) 412
Depakene 417
Depakote Sprinkle Capsules (Occasional) 422
Depakote Tablets (Occasional) 427
Depakote ER Tablets 434
▲ Doxil Injection (1% to 5%) 2351
▲ Eloxatin for Injection (13%) 2892
Elspar for Injection 2463
Elspar for Injection 1960
Emend Capsules (Greater than 0.5%) 1963
Emtriva Capsules (Less than 1% to 1%) 1287
Emtriva Oral Solution (Less than 1% to 1%) 1287
Epivir (0.8%) 1427
Eulexin Capsules 3009
Famvir Tablets (1.9%) 2211
Fortaz 1453
Garamycin Injectable 3014
▲ Gemzar for Injection (13% to 26%) 1771
Gengraf Capsules (1% to less than 3%) 459
▲ Gleevec Tablets (0% to 3.8%) 2227
Hycamtin for Injection (Less than 3%) 1458
HyperRho S/D Full Dose 3246
Hyperstat I.V. 3017
Hyzaar 50-12.5 Tablets (Occasional) 1990
Hyzaar 100-12.5 Tablets (Occasional) 1990
Hyzaar 100-25 Tablets (Occasional) 1990
Invanz for Injection (0.6% to 1.7%) 1999
▲ Invirase (Less than 1% to 4%) 2772
▲ I.V. Busulfex (30% to 49%) 2493
Kaletra (Up to 1%) 476
Keflex Capsules 549
Ketek Tablets (Less than 0.2%) 2903
Lescol Capsules 2233
Lescol XL Tablets 2233
▲ Leukine (30%) 814
Leustatin Injection 2357
Levaquin (0.1% to 0.9%) 2384
Levaquin in 5% Dextrose Injection (0.1% to 0.9%) 2384
Lexapro Oral Solution (Infrequent) 1190
Lexapro Tablets (Infrequent) 1190
Lotrel Capsules (Rare) 2249
Lotronex Tablets 1512
Mavik Tablets (0.2% of patients) 486
Mephyton Tablets (Rare) 2018
Meridia Capsules (1.6%) 489
Merrem I.V. (Greater than 0.2%) 686
Mevacor Tablets 2021
Micardis HCT Tablets (Occasional) 856
Mycamine for Injection (1% to 2.8%) 628
Myleran Tablets 1525
▲ Mylotarg for Injection (29%) 3431
Neoral Oral Solution (1% to less than 3%) 2259
Neoral Soft Gelatin Capsules (1% to less than 3%) 2259
Nexavar Tablets (Uncommon) 746
Niravam Orally Disintegrating Tablets 3092
Omnicef Capsules (0.2%) 511
Omnicef for Oral Suspension (0.2%) 511
Oncaspar 1145
Oxandrin Tablets 2962
Pegasys 2789
▲ PEG-Intron Powder for Injection (10% to 14%) 3048
Pentasa Capsules 3185
PREVPAC (Less than 1%) 3284
Prezista Tablets (0.9% to 2.3%) 3306
Prilosec OTC Delayed-Release Tablets (Rare) 2677
Primaxin I.M. 2045
Primaxin I.V. 2048
Prinivil Tablets (Rare) 2052
Prinzide Tablets (Rare) 2056
▲ Prograf Capsules and Injection (12% to 30%) 632
▲ Proleukin for Injection (64%) 2266
Proquin XR Tablets (Less than 1%) 1153
ProstaScint Kit (1%) 1037
Protonix Tablets (Less than 1%) 3469
Raniclor Tablets, Chewable 2505
▲ Rebetol (10% to 14%) 3058
Rebetron Combination Therapy 3063
Rescriptor Tablets (0.5% to 1.0%) 2551
Retrovir Capsules (Rare) 1560
Retrovir IV Infusion (Rare) 1564

Retrovir (Rare) 1560
Revlimid Capsules 958
RhoGAM Ultra-Filtered 2371
Rocephin Injectable Vials, ADD-Vantage, Galaxy, Bulk (Less than 1%) 2800
Rythmol SR Capsules 2727
Strattera Capsules 1814
Stromectol Tablets 2083
Suprax 1843
Symmetrel Tablets 1135
Tarceva Tablets 1259
Tarceva Tablets 2444
Tarka Tablets 524
Tequin Injection (Less than 0.1%) 938
Tequin Injection in 5% Dextrose (Less than 0.1%) 938
Tequin Tablets (Less than 0.1%) 938
Ticlid Tablets (Rare) 2810
Timentin ADD-Vantage 1580
Timentin Injection Galaxy Container 1583
Timentin IV Infusion 1577
Timentin Pharmacy Bulk Package 1586
Tracleer Tablets 545
Trecator Tablets 3487
Trizivir Tablets (0.8%) 1589
Vantin Tablets and Oral Suspension 2645
Vasotec I.V. Injection 2103
Verelan PM Extended-Release Capsules, Controlled-Onset 3106
▲ VFEND I.V. (4.3% to 19.4%) 2564
▲ VFEND Oral Suspension (4.3% to 19.4%) 2564
▲ VFEND Tablets (4.3% to 19.4%) 2564
Viramune Oral Suspension (0.4%) 873
Viramune Tablets (0.4%) 873
▲ Xeloda Tablets (2% to 22%) 2822
Zegerid Capsules (Rare) 2958
Zegerid Powder for Oral Solution (Rare) 2958
Zinacef for Injection (1 in 500 patients) 1631
Zinacef Injection (1 in 500 patients) 1631
Zmax for Oral Suspension (Less then 1%) 2583
Zocor Tablets 2105
Zoloft (One or more patients) 2586
Zosyn 3492
Zovirax 1643
Zyrtec Chewable Tablets (A single case) 2594
Zyrtec (A single case) 2594
Zyrtec-D 12 Hour Extended Release Tablets (A single case) 2597

Hypercalcemia

Abelcet Injection 1141
Actiq (Less than 1%) 979
Aloprim for Injection (Less than 1%) 2167
Avelox (Greater than or equal to 2%) 2970
Benicar HCT Tablets 1044
Calcijex Injection 411
Calcium Disodium Versenate Injection 1851
▲ Carnitor Injection (6% to 15%) 3188
▲ CellCept Capsules (3% to less than 20%) 2747
▲ CellCept Intravenous (3% to less than 20%) 2747
▲ CellCept Oral Suspension (3% to less than 20%) 2747
▲ CellCept Tablets (3% to less than 20%) 2747
Cipro I.V. (Infrequent) 2984
Climara Transdermal System 771
▲ Doxil Injection (1% to 10%) 2351
Eraxis for Injection (Less than 1% to less than 2%) 2521
Estratest Tablets 3199
Estratest H.S. Tablets 3199
Evoxac Capsules (Less than 1%) 1047
Femara Tablets (Less frequent) 2214
▲ Forteo for Injection (6% to 11.1%) 1767
▲ Fosrenol Chewable Tablets (0% to 4%) 3183
Hectorol Capsules 1275
Hectorol Injection 1278
Herceptin I.V. (At least one of the 958 patients) 1233
Hyzaar 50-12.5 Tablets 1990
Hyzaar 100-12.5 Tablets 1990
Hyzaar 100-25 Tablets 1990
▲ Intron A for Injection (Less than or equal to 5%) 3024
▲ Invirase (Less than 1% to 4%) 2772
Lithobid Tablets 1692
Maxipime for Injection (Greater than 0.1% to less than 1%) 1105
Micardis HCT Tablets 856
▲ Myfortic Tablets (3% to less than 20%) 2255
Nipent for Injection (Less than 3%) 1863
Oxandrin Tablets 2962
Paxil CR Controlled-Release Tablets (Rare) 1538
Paxil (Rare) 1530
Pexeva Tablets (Rare) 1694
PhosLo GelCaps 2169
Premarin Intravenous 3442
Premarin Vaginal Cream 3452
Premphase Tablets 3456
Prempro Tablets 3456
Prinzide Tablets 2056
▲ Prograf Capsules and Injection (3% to 15%) 632
Proleukin for Injection (1%) 2266
▲ Rapamune Oral Solution and Tablets (3% to 20%) 3475
Rilutek Tablets (Rare) 2930
▲ Rocaltrol Capsules (1 in 3) 2798
▲ Rocaltrol Oral Solution (1 in 3) 2798
▲ Simulect for Injection (3% to 10%) 2284
Soltamox Oral Solution (Infrequently) 3527
Timolide Tablets 2086
Uniretic Tablets (Less than 1%) 3100
Vantas (Less than 2%) 3375
Vesanoid Capsules (Isolated cases) 2820
VFEND I.V. (Less than 2%) 2564
VFEND Oral Suspension (Less than 2%) 2564
VFEND Tablets (Less than 2%) 2564
Xeloda Tablets (1.1%) 2822
Zemplar Capsules 541
Zemplar Injection 543
Zosyn 3492

Hypercalciuria

Calcijex Injection 411
Effexor XR Capsules (Rare) 3417
Hectorol Capsules 1275
▲ Rocaltrol Capsules (1 in 7) 2798
▲ Rocaltrol Oral Solution (1 in 7) 2798

Hypercapnia

▲ DepoDur Extended-Release Injection (2% to 5%) 1110

Hyperchloremia

Avelox (Greater than or equal to 2%) 2970
▲ Bumex Tablets (14.9%) 2746
Daranide Tablets 1950
Demadex Injection 2759
Demadex Tablets 2759
Geodon Capsules (Rare) 2529
Primaxin I.M. 2045
Primaxin I.V. 2048
Sulfamylon Cream 2162
Sulfamylon for 5% Topical Solution 2162
Topamax Sprinkle Capsules (Infrequent) 2404
Topamax Tablets (Infrequent) 2404

Hyperchlorhydria

Effexor Tablets (Rare) 3411
Effexor XR Capsules (Rare) 3417
Prozac Pulvules and Liquid (Infrequent) 1801

Hypercholesterolemia

Abilify Oral Solution (Infrequent) 882
Abilify Oral Solution (Infrequent) 2450
Abilify Discmelt Orally Disintegrating Tablets (Infrequent) 882
Abilify Discmelt Orally Disintegrating Tablets (Infrequent) 2450
Abilify Tablets (Infrequent) 882
Abilify Tablets (Infrequent) 2450
Accutane Capsules 2731
Aceon Tablets (2 mg, 4 mg, 8 mg) (0.3% to 1%) 3194
Aciphex Tablets 1090
Agenerase Capsules 1327
Aldara Cream, 5% (1.9%) 1846
▲ Alphagan P Ophthalmic Solution (1% to 4%) 567
Ambien Tablets (Rare) 2851
Ambien CR Tablets (Rare) 2855
Amerge Tablets (Rare) 1339
Androxy Tablets 3335
▲ Aptivus Capsules (0.8% to 11.3%) 826
▲ Arimidex Tablets (2% to 9%) 673
Arthrotec Tablets (Rare) 3129
▲ Atripla Tablets (25%) 945
Axert Tablets (Rare) 2396
Benicar Tablets (Greater than 0.5%) 1043
Benicar HCT Tablets 1044
BiDil Tablets (1% to less than 2%) 2171
▲ Boniva Injection (4.8%) 2738
▲ Boniva Tablets (4.8%) 2741
Bumex Tablets (0.4%) 2746
Calcijex Injection 411
Carbatrol Capsules (Occasional) 3171
Celebrex Capsules (0.1% to 1.9%) 3134
▲ CellCept Capsules (3% to 41.2%) 2747
▲ CellCept Intravenous (3% to 41.2%) 2747
▲ CellCept Oral Suspension (3% to 41.2%) 2747
▲ CellCept Tablets (3% to 41.2%) 2747
▲ Chemet Capsules (4.2% to 10.4%) 2458
Cipro 2977
Cipro I.V. (Infrequent) 2984
Clozaril Tablets (Rare) 2184
▲ Coreg Tablets (1% to 4%) 1414
Crixivan Capsules (0.9%) 1940
Cymbalta Delayed-Release Capsules (Infrequent) 1757
Edex Injection (1%) 3089
▲ Effexor Tablets (5.3%) 3411
▲ Effexor XR Capsules (5.3%) 3417
Equetro Extended-Release Capsules 3180
Estratest Tablets 3199
Estratest H.S. Tablets 3199
Evoxac Capsules (Less than 1%) 1047
Exelon Capsules (Infrequent) 2206
Exelon Oral Solution (Infrequent) 2206
FazaClo Orally Disintegrating Tablets (Very Rare) 551
▲ Femara Tablets (Less than 0.1% to 15.6%) 2214
Gabitril Tablets (Infrequent) 984
Gengraf Capsules (Less than 3%) 459
Geodon Capsules (Infrequent) 2529
Hectorol Capsules 1275
Hectorol Injection 1278
▲ Humira Injection (6%) 466
Hyzaar 50-12.5 Tablets 1990
Hyzaar 100-12.5 Tablets 1990
Hyzaar 100-25 Tablets 1990
Inspra Tablets (0.3% to 1%) 2536
▲ Kaletra (9% to 39%) 476
▲ Leukine (17%) 814
Lexapro Oral Solution (Infrequent) 1190
Lexapro Tablets (Infrequent) 1190
Lunesta Tablets (Infrequent) 3142
▲ Lupron Depot 3.75 mg (7%) 3260
▲ Lupron Depot 7.5 mg (Greater than or equal to 5%) 3264
Micardis Tablets (More than 0.3%) 854
Micardis HCT Tablets 856
▲ Myfortic Tablets (3% to less than 20%) 2255
Myobloc Injection (Greater than 2%) 3192
Neoral Oral Solution (Less than 3%) 2259
Neoral Soft Gelatin Capsules (Less than 3%) 2259
Neurontin Capsules (Rare) 2487
Neurontin Oral Solution (Rare) 2487
Neurontin Tablets (Rare) 2487
Noroxin Tablets 2032
▲ Norvir (36.5% to 44.8%) 503
Oxandrin Tablets 2962
Paxil CR Controlled-Release Tablets (Rare) 1538
Paxil (Rare) 1530
Permax Tablets (Infrequent) 3356
Pexeva Tablets (Rare) 1694
▲ Plavix Tablets (4%) 917
▲ Plavix Tablets (4%) 2926
Prevacid Delayed-Release Capsules 3271
Prevacid for Delayed-Release Oral Suspension 3271
Prevacid SoluTab Delayed-Release Orally Disintegrating Tablets 3271
Prevacid NapraPAC 3280
PREVPAC 3284
Prezista Tablets (Less than 2%) 3306
Prinzide Tablets 2056
▲ Prograf Capsules and Injection (3% to 15%) 632
Protopic Ointment (0.2% to less than 1%) 638
Prozac Pulvules and Liquid (Infrequent) 1801
▲ Rapamune Oral Solution and Tablets (38% to 46%) 3475
Requip Tablets (Infrequent) 1555
Rilutek Tablets (Rare) 2930
Risperdal Consta Long-Acting Injection (Infrequent) 1682
Rituxan I.V. 1254
Rocaltrol Capsules 2798
Rocaltrol Oral Solution 2798
Rythmol SR Capsules 2727
Sonata Capsules (Infrequent) 1717
▲ Spiriva HandiHaler (1% to 3%) 869
Sustiva Capsules 930
Sustiva Tablets 930
▲ Targretin Capsules (32.1% to 62.3%) 1747
Tasmar Tablets (Infrequent) 3358
Tegretol/Tegretol-XR (Occasional) 2295
Teveten Tablets (Less than 1%) 1735
Teveten HCT Tablets (Less than 1%) 1737
Thalomid Capsules 965
Ticlid Tablets 2810
Timolide Tablets 2086
Travatan Ophthalmic Solution (1% to 5%) 563
▲ Truvada Tablets (15%) 1296
Uniretic Tablets (Less than 1%) 3100
Vantas (Less than 2%) 3375
▲ Vesanoid Capsules (Up to 60%) 2820
VFEND I.V. (Less than 2%) 2564
VFEND Oral Suspension (Less than 2%) 2564
VFEND Tablets (Less than 2%) 2564
▲ Viread Tablets (19%) 1301
Vivitrol 995
Xyrem Oral Solution (Infrequent) 1688
Zelapar Tablets 3372
▲ Zoloft (Approximately 3%) 2586
Zyprexa Tablets (Rare) 1830
Zyprexa ZYDIS Orally Disintegrating Tablets (Rare) 1830

Hypercorticism

Advair Diskus 100/50 1308
Advair Diskus 250/50 1308
Advair Diskus 500/50 1308
Advair HFA Inhalation Aerosol 1318
Beconase AQ Nasal Spray 1396
Blephamide Ophthalmic Ointment (Rare) 568
Blephamide Ophthalmic Suspension (Rare) 569
Entocort EC Capsules 2698
FML Ophthalmic Ointment (Rare) ⊙228
FML Ophthalmic Suspension (Rare) ⊙227
Pred Mild Ophthalmic Suspension (Rare) ⊙238
Pred Forte Ophthalmic Suspension (Rare) ⊙235
Pulmicort Respules (Less than 1%) 661

Hypercorticoidism

Poly-Pred Ophthalmic Suspension ⊙233

Hyperdipsia

(*see under* Dipsesis)

Hyperemia

Azopt Ophthalmic Suspension (1% to 5%) 557
▲ Elestat Ophthalmic Solution (1% to 10%) 1669
Lacrisert Sterile Ophthalmic Insert 2005
▲ Patanol Ophthalmic Solution (Less than 5%) 561
Topamax Sprinkle Capsules 2404
Topamax Tablets 2404
Viroptic Ophthalmic Solution ⊙266

Hyperemia, conjunctival

▲ Acular LS Ophthalmic Solution (1% to 5%) 566
▲ Alphagan P Ophthalmic Solution (Approximately 10% to 20%) 567
▲ Brimonidine Tartrate Ophthalmic Solution 0.2% (10% to 30%) ⊙248
▲ Carteolol Hydrochloride Ophthalmic Solution USP, 1% (About 1 of 4 patients) ⊙249
▲ Ciloxan Ophthalmic Ointment (Less than 10%) 559
▲ Ciloxan Ophthalmic Solution (Less than 10%) ⊙206
▲ Cosopt Sterile Ophthalmic Solution (5% to 30%) 1931
FML Ophthalmic Ointment (Occasional) ⊙228
FML Ophthalmic Suspension (Occasional) ⊙227
FML Forte Ophthalmic Suspension (Occasional) ⊙226
FML-S Ophthalmic Suspension ⊙229
▲ Lucentis Injection (0% to 9%) 1237
▲ Lumigan Ophthalmic Solution (15% to 45%) 573
Natacyn Antifungal Ophthalmic Suspension (One case) ⊙208
Neurontin Capsules (Rare) 2487
Neurontin Oral Solution (Rare) 2487
Neurontin Tablets (Rare) 2487
Ophthetic Ophthalmic Solution ⊙232
Pred Mild Ophthalmic Suspension (Occasional) ⊙238

Pred Forte Ophthalmic Suspension (Occasional)............ ⊙235
▲ Restasis Ophthalmic Emulsion (1% to 5%).................... 575
▲ Travatan Ophthalmic Solution (15% to 45%).................... 563
▲ Vigamox Ophthalmic Solution (1% to 6%).................... 564
▲ Xalatan Sterile Ophthalmic Solution (5% to 15%).................... 2649

Hypereosinophilia

Ketek Tablets (Less than 0.2%).......... 2903
Leustatin Injection.......................... 2357
Maxipime for Injection (1.7%).......... 1105
Vivitrol.................................... 995
Zyprexa Tablets (0.3%).................. 1830
Zyprexa IntraMuscular (0.3%).......... 1830
Zyprexa ZYDIS Orally Disintegrating Tablets (0.3%)........ 1830

Hyperesthesia

Abilify Oral Solution (Infrequent)........ 882
Abilify Oral Solution (Infrequent) 2450
Abilify Discmelt Orally Disintegrating Tablets (Infrequent) 882
Abilify Discmelt Orally Disintegrating Tablets (Infrequent) 2450
Abilify Tablets (Infrequent) 882
Abilify Tablets (Infrequent) 2450
Amerge Tablets (Rare) 1339
Arthrotec Tablets (Rare) 3129
Asacol Delayed-Release Tablets 2692
Axert Tablets (Infrequent) 2396
Celexa (Rare) 1176
Cipro 2977
Cipro I.V. 2984
Cipro XR Tablets 2990
▲ Dacogen Injection (11%) 2129
Diprolene Lotion 0.05% (Less than 1%) 3002
Doxil Injection (Less than 1%) 2351
Effexor Tablets (Infrequent) 3411
Effexor XR Capsules (Frequent) 3417
Evoxac Capsules 1047
Frova Tablets (Frequent) 1113
Gengraf Capsules 459
Imitrex Injection (Rare) 1463
Imitrex Tablets (Rare) 1471
▲ Intron A for Injection (Less than 5%) 3024
Invirase (Less than 2%) 2772
▲ Kepivance (12%) 597
Lamictal (Rare) 1481
Lidoderm Patch 1118
Lunesta Tablets (Rare) 3142
Lyrica Capsules (0.1% to 1%) 2539
Maxalt Tablets (Infrequent) 2008
Maxalt-MLT Orally Disintegrating Tablets (Infrequent) 2008
Myobloc Injection (Greater than 2%) 3192
Neoral Oral Solution 2259
Neoral Soft Gelatin Capsules 2259
Neurontin Capsules (Rare) 2487
Neurontin Oral Solution (Rare) 2487
Neurontin Tablets (Rare) 2487
Norvir (Less than 2%) 503
Pletal Tablets (2% or greater) 2455
ProAmatine Tablets (Rare) 3186
Proquin XR Tablets 1153
▲ Protopic Ointment (Up to 7%) 638
Prozac Pulvules and Liquid (Rare) 1801
Relpax Tablets (Frequent) 2548
▲ Requip Tablets (4%) 1555
Rescriptor Tablets 2551
Sonata Capsules (Infrequent) 1717
▲ Soriatane Capsules (10% to 25%) ... 1013
Targretin Capsules 1747
Tequin Injection (Less than 0.1%) 938
Tequin Injection in 5% Dextrose (Less than 0.1%) 938
Tequin Tablets (Less than 0.1%) 938
Thalomid Capsules 965
Topamax Sprinkle Capsules (Rare) ... 2404
Topamax Tablets (Rare) 2404
Tri-Luma Cream (2%) 1213
Zoloft (Infrequent) 2586
Zometa for Intravenous Infusion 2315
Zomig Tablets (Infrequent) 3519
▲ Zomig Nasal Spray (0% to 5%) 3523
Zomig-ZMT Tablets (Infrequent) 3519
Zonegran Capsules (Rare) 1101
Zyrtec Chewable Tablets (Less than 2%) 2594
Zyrtec (Less than 2%) 2594
Zyrtec-D 12 Hour Extended Release Tablets (Less than 2%) 2597

Hyperesthesia, tongue

Alferon N Injection (1%) 1665

Hyperexcitability

Phenergan Tablets and Suppositories 3440

Hyperexcitability, paradoxical

Diastat Rectal Delivery System........ 3343

Hyperfibrinogenemia

Alphanate, Antihemophilic Factor (Human) (Rare)............................ 1654
Colazal Capsules............................ 2838
Menostar Transdermal System........ 782
Neumega for Injection 3435
Premarin Tablets............................. 3446
Premphase Tablets 3456
Prempro Tablets 3456

Hypergammaglobulinemia

Pexeva Tablets (Rare)...................... 1694
Prevacid Delayed-Release Capsules 3271
Prevacid for Delayed-Release Oral Suspension 3271
Prevacid SoluTab Delayed-Release Orally Disintegrating Tablets 3271
PREVPAC.. 3284

Hyperglycemia

Abelcet Injection.............................. 1141
Abilify Oral Solution (Infrequent)......... 882
Abilify Oral Solution (Infrequent)....... 2450
Abilify Discmelt Orally Disintegrating Tablets (Infrequent)................................ 882
Abilify Discmelt Orally Disintegrating Tablets (Infrequent)................................ 2450
Abilify Tablets (Infrequent)................ 882
Abilify Tablets (Infrequent)................ 2450
Accutane Capsules.......................... 2731
Aceon Tablets (2 mg, 4 mg, 8 mg) (0.3% to 1%).................................. 3194
Aciphex Tablets............................... 1090
Aclovate Cream............................... 2660
Actimmune (Rare)............................ 1671
Actiq (1% or greater)........................ 979
Adalat CC Tablets (Rare).................. 2964
Advair Diskus 100/50....................... 1308
Advair Diskus 250/50....................... 1308
Advair Diskus 500/50....................... 1308
Advair HFA Inhalation Aerosol.......... 1318
▲ Advicor Tablets (4%)..................... 1722
▲ Agenerase Capsules (2% to 3%) 1327
Agenerase Oral Solution (2.3%)....... 1332
Aggrenox Capsules (Less than 1%).. 822
Albalon Ophthalmic Solution .... ⊙218
Aldoril Tablets................................. 1910
Aloprim for Injection (Less than 1%).. 2167
Aloxi Injection (Less than 1%)........... 2127
Altace Capsules.............................. 1702
Ambien Tablets (Infrequent)............. 2851
Ambien CR Tablets (Infrequent)........ 2855
▲ AmBisome for Injection (8.2% to 23%).. 620
Amerge Tablets (Rare)..................... 1339
Anaprox Tablets (Less than 1%)....... 2761
Anaprox DS Tablets (Less than 1%).. 2761
▲ AndroGel (3% to 6%) 3329
Aptivus Capsules (Less than 2%)...... 826
Aricept Tablets (Infrequent).............. 1094
Aricept ODT Tablets (Infrequent)....... 1094
▲ Arranon Injection (0% to 6%) 1357
Arthrotec Tablets (Rare)................... 3129
Atacand Tablets (0.5% or greater)..... 649
Atacand HCT (0.5% or greater)........ 651
Avalide Tablets................................ 888
Avalide Tablets................................ 2874
▲ Avandamet Tablets (5.9%) 1373
▲ Avandia Tablets (8.1%) 1384
Avelox (Less than 0.1%)................... 2970
Axert Tablets (Infrequent)................. 2396
Baraclude (2%)................................ 894
Bayer Aspirin.................................. 744
Bayer Aspirin Comprehensive Prescribing Information.............. ▣796
Benicar HCT Tablets (Greater than 1%).. 1044
▲ BiDil Tablets (4%) 2171
Blocadren Tablets........................... 1916
▲ Bumex Tablets (6.6%) 2746
Caduet Tablets (Greater than 0.1% to less than 2%)......................... 2508
Cafcit... 1886
Campath Ampules........................... 811
Campral Tablets (Infrequent)............ 1174
Camptosar Injection........................ 2604
Cardizem LA Extended Release Tablets (Less than 2%)................. 1728
Catapres Tablets (Rare).................. 843
Celebrex Capsules (0.1% to 1.9%)... 3134
▲ CellCept Capsules (43.7% to 46.7%).. 2747
▲ CellCept Intravenous (43.7% to 46.7%).. 2747
▲ CellCept Oral Suspension (43.7% to 46.7%).................................... 2747
▲ CellCept Tablets (43.7% to 46.7%).. 2747
Cipro.. 2977
▲ Cipro I.V. (Among most frequent) 2984
Cipro XR Tablets (Less than 1%)....... 2990
Clinoril Tablets (Rare)...................... 1924
Clobex Lotion 1204
Clobex Shampoo............................. 1206
Clobex Spray.................................. 1208
Clorpres Tablets.............................. 2153
Clozaril Tablets............................... 2184
Combivir Tablets.............................. 1411
▲ Coreg Tablets (5% to 12%) 1414
Cosopt Sterile Ophthalmic Solution.. 1931
Crixivan Capsules............................ 1940
Cubicin for Injection (1% to 2%)........ 1026
Cutivate Lotion 0.05% (Rare) 2664
▲ Dacogen Injection (33%) 2129
Decadron Tablets 1951
Demadex Injection 2759
Demadex Tablets 2759
Diovan HCT Tablets 2196
Diprolene Gel 0.05% 3001
Diprolene Lotion 0.05% 3002
Diprolene Ointment 0.05% (Some patients) 3003
Diprolene AF Cream 0.05% (Some patients) 3000
Diprosone Cream, USP 0.05% 3004
Diuril Oral Suspension 1954
Diuril Sodium Intravenous 2467
▲ Doxil Injection (1% to 10%) 2351
Dyazide Capsules 1423
EC-Naprosyn Delayed-Release Tablets (Less than 1%) 2761
Edecrin 1959
Edex Injection (1%) 3089
Effexor Tablets (Infrequent) 3411
Effexor XR Capsules (Infrequent) 3417
Elocon Cream 0.1% 3005
Elocon Lotion 0.1% 3006
Elocon Ointment 0.1% 3007
Elspar for Injection (Low) 2463
Elspar for Injection (Low) 1960
Emend Capsules (Greater than 0.5%) 1963
Epivir 1427
Epivir-HBV 1432
Epzicom Tablets 1436
Eraxis for Injection (Less than 1% to less than 2%) 2521
Evoxac Capsules (Less than 1%) 1047
Exelon Capsules (Infrequent) 2206
Exelon Oral Solution (Infrequent) 2206
FazaClo Orally Disintegrating Tablets 551
Flovent Diskus 1443
Flovent HFA 1447
Foradil Aerolizer 3010
Furosemide Tablets 2154
Fuzeon Injection 2767
Gabitril Tablets (Infrequent) 984
Gengraf Capsules (2% or less) 459
Genotropin Lyophilized Powder (Infrequent) 2638
Geodon Capsules (Infrequent) 2529
Humatrope Vials and Cartridges (Infrequent) 1787
Hydrocortone Tablets 1989
Hyperstat I.V. 3017
Hyzaar 50-12.5 Tablets 1990
Hyzaar 100-12.5 Tablets 1990
Hyzaar 100-25 Tablets 1990
Imitrex Injection 1463
Imitrex Nasal Spray 1467
Imitrex Tablets (Rare) 1471
Indapamide Tablets (Less than 5%) .. 2156
Indocin Capsules (Less than 1%) 1995
Indocin I.V. (Less than 1%) 2465
Indocin (Less than 1%) 1995
▲ Intron A for Injection (Less than or equal to 5%) 3024
Invanz for Injection (1.2% to 1.7%) ... 1999
▲ Invirase (2.7% to less than or equal to 5%) 2772
Ionsys Transdermal System (.1% to less than 1%) 2379
▲ I.V. Busulfex (15% to 67%) 2493
▲ Kaletra (1% to 5%) 476
Lamictal (Rare) 1481
▲ Leukine (25% to 41%) 814
Levaquin (0.1% to 0.9%) 2384
Levaquin in 5% Dextrose Injection (0.1% to 0.9%) 2384
Lexapro Oral Solution (Infrequent) 1190
Lexapro Tablets (Infrequent) 1190
Lexiva Tablets (Less than 1%) 1505
Lipitor Tablets (Less than 2%).......... 2483
Lithobid Tablets.............................. 1692
Lopressor HCT 50/25 Tablets.......... 2241
Lopressor HCT 100/25 Tablets........ 2241
Lopressor HCT 100/50 Tablets........ 2241
Lotensin HCT Tablets...................... 2246
Lotrisone.. 3040
Lotronex Tablets (Rare)................... 1512
▲ Lupron Depot 7.5 mg (Greater than or equal to 5%)..................... 3264
▲ Megace ES Oral Suspension (0% to 6%).. 2481
▲ Mepron Suspension (9%) 1521
Meridia Capsules............................ 489
Micardis HCT Tablets...................... 856
Mintezol 2027
Moduretic Tablets........................... 2028
▲ Myfortic Tablets (3% to less than 20%)... 2255
▲ Mylotarg for Injection (10% to 11%)... 3431
Naprosyn Suspension (Less than 1%).. 2761
Naprosyn Tablets (Less than 1%)..... 2761
NeoProfen Injection........................ 2472
Neoral Oral Solution (2% or less)...... 2259
Neoral Soft Gelatin Capsules (2% or less)....................................... 2259
Neurontin Capsules (1.2%)............... 2487
Neurontin Oral Solution (1.2%)......... 2487
Neurontin Tablets (1.2%)................. 2487
Niaspan Extended-Release Tablets... 1730
Nicomide Tablets............................ 1088
Nimotop Capsules (0.8%; rare)......... 749
Norditropin Cartridges..................... 2323
Noroxin Tablets............................... 2032
Norvasc Tablets (More than 0.1% to 1%)... 2545
Norvir... 503
Olux Foam...................................... 1012
Omacor Capsules............................ 2725
Omnicef Capsules (0.9%)................. 511
Omnicef for Oral Suspension (0.9%)... 511
▲ Oncaspar (Greater than 1% but less than 5%)............................. 1145
Oracea Capsules (1.1%)................... 1000
Paxil CR Controlled-Release Tablets (Infrequent)...................... 1538
Paxil (Infrequent)............................ 1530
Pegasys.. 2789
PEG-Intron Powder for Injection (Less than or equal to 1%).......... 3048
Percodan Tablets............................ 1132
Permax Tablets (Infrequent)............ 3356
Pexeva Tablets (Rare)...................... 1694
Phenytek Capsules.......................... 2160
Prevacid Delayed-Release Capsules (Less than 1%).............. 3271
Prevacid for Delayed-Release Oral Suspension (Less than 1%).......... 3271
Prevacid SoluTab Delayed-Release Orally Disintegrating Tablets (Less than 1%).............................. 3271
Prevacid NapraPAC (Less than 1%).. 3280
PREVPAC (Less than 1%)................. 3284
▲ Prezista Tablets (2.3% to 5.9%) 3306
Prinzide Tablets.............................. 2056
▲ Prograf Capsules and Injection (Many patients; 13% to 47%)......... 632
Proleukin for Injection (2%).............. 2266
Protonix I.V. (Less than or equal to 1%).. 3472
Protonix Tablets (Less than or equal to 1%).................................. 3469
Protopic Ointment (Greater than or equal to 1%).................................. 638
Provigil Tablets (Greater than or equal to 1%).................................. 988
▲ Rapamune Oral Solution and Tablets (3% to 20%)..................... 3475
Razadyne (Infrequent)..................... 2399
Razadyne ER Extended-Release Capsules (Infrequent).................... 2399
Rebetron Combination Therapy........ 3063
Relpax Tablets (Rare)...................... 2548
Requip Tablets (1% or more)............ 1555
Rescriptor Tablets........................... 2551
▲ Revlimid Capsules (15%) 958
Risperdal.. 1676
Risperdal Consta Long-Acting Injection (Infrequent)...................... 1682
Risperdal M-Tab Orally Disintegrating Tablets..................... 1676
▲ Rituxan I.V. (1% to 9%) 1254
Rythmol SR Capsules...................... 2727
Sandimmune (2% or less)................. 2275
▲ Sandostatin Injection (3% to 16%) ... 2278
▲ Sandostatin LAR Depot (15% to 27%).. 2280
Serevent Diskus (1% to less than 3%).. 1568
Seroquel Tablets (Infrequent)............ 690

▲ Simulect for Injection (Greater than or equal to 10%) 2284
Sonata Capsules (Rare) 1717
▲ Spiriva HandiHaler (1% to 3%) 869
St. Joseph 81 mg Aspirin Chewable and Enteric Coated Tablets 1869
St. Joseph 81 mg Aspirin ▣688
Symbyax Capsules 1819
Targretin Capsules 1747
Temovate Cream 2668
Temovate Gel 2669
Temovate Ointment 2668
Temovate Scalp Application 2670
Tequin Injection (Less than 0.1%) 938
Tequin Injection in 5% Dextrose (Less than 0.1%) 938
Tequin Tablets (Less than 0.1%) 938
Teveten Tablets (Less than 1%) 1735
Teveten HCT Tablets (Less than 1%) 1737
Thalomid Capsules 965
Thiothixene Capsules 2165
Tiazac Capsules (Less than 2%) 1201
Timolide Tablets 2086
Timoptic Sterile Ophthalmic Solution 2088
Timoptic in Ocudose 2091
Timoptic-XE Sterile Ophthalmic Gel Forming Solution 2092
Topamax Sprinkle Capsules (Infrequent) 2404
Topamax Tablets (Infrequent) 2404
Trasylol Injection (1% to 2%) 754
Trileptal Tablets 2300
Trileptal Oral Suspension 2300
▲ Trisenox Injection (45%) 993
Trizivir Tablets 1589
Truvada Tablets (1%) 1296
Tygacil for Injection (1.8%) 3488
Ultane Liquid for Inhalation (Less than 1%) 531
▲ Ultram ER Tablets (1% to greater than 5%) 2392
Uniretic Tablets (More than 1%) 3100
Urso 250 Tablets (1%) 710
Urso Forte Tablets (1%) 710
▲ Valcyte Tablets (Less than 5%) 2813
Vanos Cream 1893
Vantas (Less than 2%) 3375
Vantin Tablets and Oral Suspension 2645
Vaprisol (2.7%) 643
VFEND I.V. (Less than 2%) 2564
VFEND Oral Suspension (Less than 2%) 2564
VFEND Tablets (Less than 2%) 2564
Viagra Tablets (Less than 2%) 2573
Viracept (Less than 2%) 2577
▲ Viread Tablets (2% to 3%) 1301
Voltaren Tablets (Rarely) 2307
Voltaren-XR Tablets (Rarely) 2310
Wellbutrin Tablets 1603
Wellbutrin SR Sustained-Release Tablets 1607
Wellbutrin XL Extended-Release Tablets 1613
▲ Xopenex Inhalation Solution (2.6% to 5.2%) 3146
▲ Xopenex Inhalation Solution Concentrate (2.6% to 5.2%) 3150
▲ Xopenex HFA Inhalation Aerosol (2.6% to 5.2%) 3154
Xyrem Oral Solution (Infrequent) 1688
Zegerid Capsules (0.7%) 2958
Zegerid Powder for Oral Solution (0.7%) 2958
Zelapar Tablets 3372
Ziagen (Less than 1%) 1626
Zoloft 2586
Zomig Tablets (Rare) 3519
Zomig-ZMT Tablets (Rare) 3519
Zosyn 3492
Zyprexa Tablets (Infrequent) 1830
Zyprexa ZYDIS Orally Disintegrating Tablets (Infrequent) 1830

Hyperglycemia, hyperosmolar nonketotic
Tequin Injection 938
Tequin Injection in 5% Dextrose 938
Tequin Tablets 938

Hyperglycemia, transient
▲ Rituxan I.V. (1% to 5%) 1254

Hyperglycinemia
Atripla Tablets (1%) 945
Depacon Injection 412
Depakene 417
Depakote Sprinkle Capsules 422
Depakote Tablets 427
Depakote ER Tablets 434
▲ Emtriva Capsules (2% to 3%) 1287
▲ Emtriva Oral Solution (2% to 3%) 1287
Moban Tablets 1119
Parcopa Orally Disintegrating Tablets 3097
Pletal Tablets (Very rare) 2455
Rythmol SR Capsules 2727

Hyperhemoglobinemia
Ambien Tablets (Rare) 2851
Ambien CR Tablets (Rare) 2855
Evoxac Capsules 1047
Prevacid NapraPAC 3280

Hyperheparinemia
Mustargen for Injection (Rare) 2468

Hyperhidrosis
Accutane Capsules 2731
Amitiza Capsules (Less than 0.2%) 3224
Byetta Injection (Greater than or equal to 1% to less than 5%) 611
Chantix Tablets (Frequent) 2517
▲ Cymbalta Delayed-Release Capsules (6% to 8%) 1757
Diovan HCT Tablets (Greater than 0.2%) 2196
DynaCirc CR Tablets (0.5% to 1%) 2721
Havrix Vaccine (Rare) 1456
Miacalcin Nasal Spray (Less than 1%) 2253
Myozyme for Intravenous Infusion 1279
Noroxin Tablets (0.3% to 1.0%) 2032
Prezista Tablets (Less than 2%) 3306
Prilosec OTC Delayed-Release Tablets (Less than 1%) 2677
Primaxin I.M. 2045
Primaxin I.V. (Less than 0.2%) 2048
Prinivil Tablets 2052
Prinzide Tablets (0.3% to 1%) 2056
▲ Requip Tablets (3%) 1555
Restoril Capsules (0.5% to 0.9%) 1860
Thyrolar Tablets 1199
Vasotec I.V. Injection 2103
▲ Xyrem Oral Solution (2.9% to 5.7%) 1688
Zegerid Capsules (Less than 1%) 2958
Zegerid Powder for Oral Solution (Less than 1%) 2958

Hyperhistaminemia
▲ Vesanoid Capsules (3%) 2820

Hyperirritability
Mintezol 2027
Seromycin Capsules 1813

Hyperirritability, muscle
Lithobid Tablets 1692

Hyperirritability, neuromuscular
Timentin ADD-Vantage 1580
Timentin Injection Galaxy Container 1583
Timentin IV Infusion 1577
Timentin Pharmacy Bulk Package 1586

Hyperkalemia
Abelcet Injection 1141
Abilify Oral Solution (Infrequent) 882
Abilify Oral Solution (Infrequent) 2450
Abilify Discmelt Orally Disintegrating Tablets (Infrequent) 882
Abilify Discmelt Orally Disintegrating Tablets (Infrequent) 2450
Abilify Tablets (Infrequent) 882
Abilify Tablets (Infrequent) 2450
Aceon Tablets (2 mg, 4 mg, 8 mg) (1.4%) 3194
Aggrenox Capsules 822
Aloprim for Injection (Less than 1%) 2167
Aloxi Injection (1%) 2127
Altace Capsules (Approximately 1%) 1702
AmBisome for Injection (Less common) 620
Anaprox Tablets (Less than 1%) 2761
Anaprox DS Tablets (Less than 1%) 2761
Androxy Tablets 3335
Atacand Tablets 649
Atacand HCT (Very rare) 651
Avalide Tablets 888
Avalide Tablets 2874
▲ Avapro Tablets (18.6%) 891
▲ Avapro Tablets (18.6%) 2871
Bayer Aspirin 744
Bayer Aspirin Comprehensive Prescribing Information ▣796
Blocadren Tablets 1916
Campath Ampules 811
Cancidas for Injection (0% to 0.9%) 1918
Captopril Tablets 2149
▲ Carnitor Injection (6%) 3188
▲ CellCept Capsules (22%) 2747
▲ CellCept Intravenous (22%) 2747
▲ CellCept Oral Suspension (22%) 2747
▲ CellCept Tablets (22%) 2747
Chantix Tablets (Rare) 2517
Cipro 2977
Cipro I.V. (Infrequent) 2984
Clinoril Tablets (Less than 1 in 100) 1924
▲ Coreg Tablets (Greater than 1% to 3%) 1414
▲ Cozaar Tablets (7%) 1935
▲ Cubicin for Injection (5%) 1026
▲ Dacogen Injection (13%) 2129
Demadex Injection 2759
Demadex Tablets 2759
▲ Diovan Tablets (2% to 4.4%) 2193
Diovan HCT Tablets 2196
Doxil Injection (Less than 1%) 2351
Dyazide Capsules 1423
Dyrenium Capsules (Rare) 3400
EC-Naprosyn Delayed-Release Tablets (Less than 1%) 2761
Effexor Tablets (Rare) 3411
Effexor XR Capsules (Rare) 3417
Epogen for Injection (Approximately 0.11%) 591
Eraxis for Injection (Less than 1% to less than 2%) 2521
Estratest Tablets 3199
Estratest H.S. Tablets 3199
Evoxac Capsules 1047
▲ Ferrlecit Injection (6%) 3388
Gengraf Capsules (1% to less than 3%) 459
Geodon Capsules (Rare) 2529
Gleevec Tablets (Rare) 2227
Hyzaar 50-12.5 Tablets (0.4%) 1990
Hyzaar 100-12.5 Tablets (0.4%) 1990
Hyzaar 100-25 Tablets (0.4%) 1990
Indocin Capsules (Less than 1%) 1995
Indocin I.V. (Less than 1%) 2465
Indocin (Less than 1%) 1995
▲ Inspra Tablets (3.4% to 15.6%) 2536
Invanz for Injection (0.5% to 1.3%) 1999
▲ Invirase (Less than 1% to 4%) 2772
K-Dur Extended-Relase Tablets 3033
▲ K-Lor Oral Solution (Among most severe) 474
▲ K-Tab Tablets (Most common) 475
Levaquin (0.1% to 0.9%) 2384
Levaquin in 5% Dextrose Injection (0.1% to 0.9%) 2384
Lotensin Tablets 2243
Lotrel Capsules (Approximately 1.5%) 2249
▲ Mavik Tablets (0.3% to 5.3%) 486
Maxipime for Injection (Greater than 0.1% to less than 1%) 1105
Micardis Tablets 854
▲ Midamor Tablets (Between 1% and 3%) 2026
Moduretic Tablets (Greater than 1%, less than 3%) 2028
▲ Myfortic Tablets (3% to less than 20%) 2255
Naprosyn Suspension (Less than 1%) 2761
Naprosyn Tablets (Less than 1%) 2761
Neoral Oral Solution (1% to less than 3%) 2259
Neoral Soft Gelatin Capsules (1% to less than 3%) 2259
Noroxin Tablets 2032
Omnicef Capsules (0.2%) 511
Omnicef for Oral Suspension (0.2%) 511
Oxandrin Tablets 2962
Paxil CR Controlled-Release Tablets (Rare) 1538
Paxil (Rare) 1530
Percodan Tablets 1132
Pexeva Tablets (Rare) 1694
Prevacid NapraPAC (Less than 1%) 3280
Primaxin I.M. 2045
Primaxin I.V. 2048
▲ Prinivil Tablets (Approximately 2.2% to 4.8%) 2052
Prinzide Tablets (Approximately 1.4%) 2056
Procrit for Injection (0.11%) 2364
▲ Prograf Capsules and Injection (13% to 45%) 632
▲ Proleukin for Injection (4%) 2266
Prozac Pulvules and Liquid (Rare) 1801
▲ Rapamune Oral Solution and Tablets (12% to 17%) 3475
ReoPro Vials (0.1%) 1809
Requip Tablets (Infrequent) 1555
Rescriptor Tablets 2551
Rituxan I.V. 1254
Sandimmune (Occasional) 2275
▲ Simulect for Injection (Greater than or equal to 10%) 2284
St. Joseph 81 mg Aspirin Chewable and Enteric Coated Tablets 1869
St. Joseph 81 mg Aspirin ▣688
▲ Sutent Capsules (6%) 2560
Symbyax Capsules (Rare) 1819
Targretin Capsules 1747
Tarka Tablets 524
Teveten Tablets (Less than 1%) 1735
Teveten HCT Tablets (Less than 1%) 1737
Thalomid Capsules 965
▲ Thymoglobulin for Intravenous Infusion (26.8%) 1284
▲ Trisenox Injection (18%) 993
Uniretic Tablets (Less than 1%) 3100
Univasc Tablets 3104
▲ Valcyte Tablets (Less than 5%) 2813
Vasotec I.V. Injection (Approximately 1%) 2103
VFEND I.V. (Less than 2%) 2564
VFEND Oral Suspension (Less than 2%) 2564
VFEND Tablets (Less than 2%) 2564
Zegerid Capsules (2.2%) 2958
Zegerid Powder for Oral Solution (2.2%) 2958
Zelapar Tablets 3372
Zmax for Oral Suspension (Less then 1%) 2583
Zometa for Intravenous Infusion 2315
Zosyn 3492
Zyprexa Tablets (Infrequent) 1830
Zyprexa IntraMuscular (Infrequent) 1830
Zyprexa ZYDIS Orally Disintegrating Tablets (Infrequent) 1830

Hyperkalemia, neonatal
Altace Capsules 1702
Prograf Capsules and Injection 632

Hyperkeratosis
▲ Aldara Cream, 5% (8.8%) 1846
Aricept Tablets (Infrequent) 1094
Aricept ODT Tablets (Infrequent) 1094
Covera-HS Tablets (Less than 2%) 3139
Cymbalta Delayed-Release Capsules (Infrequent) 1757
Evoxac Capsules (Less than 1%) 1047
Requip Tablets (Infrequent) 1555
Risperdal (Infrequent) 1676
Risperdal M-Tab Orally Disintegrating Tablets (Infrequent) 1676
Soriatane Capsules (Less than 1%) 1013
Tarka Tablets 524
Zyrtec Chewable Tablets (Less than 2%) 2594
Zyrtec (Less than 2%) 2594
Zyrtec-D 12 Hour Extended Release Tablets (Less than 2%) 2597

Hyperkinesia
Abilify Oral Solution (Infrequent) 882
Abilify Oral Solution (Infrequent) 2450
Abilify Discmelt Orally Disintegrating Tablets (Infrequent) 882
Abilify Discmelt Orally Disintegrating Tablets (Infrequent) 2450
Abilify Tablets (Infrequent) 882
Abilify Tablets (Infrequent) 2450
Aciphex Tablets (Rare) 1090
AndroGel (One patient) 3329
Astelin Nasal Spray (Infrequent) 1904
Azilect Tablets (Frequent) 3293
Caduet Tablets (Less than 2%) 2508
Campral Tablets (Rare) 1174
Celexa (Infrequent) 1176
Clozaril Tablets (1%) 2184
▲ Comtan Tablets (10%) 2189
Diastat Rectal Delivery System (Greater than or equal to 1%) 3343
Effexor Tablets (Infrequent) 3411
Effexor XR Capsules (Infrequent) 3417
▲ Entocort EC Capsules (Less than 5%) 2698
Evoxac Capsules (Less than 1%) 1047
Exelon Capsules (Infrequent) 2206
Exelon Oral Solution (Infrequent) 2206
FazaClo Orally Disintegrating Tablets (1%) 551
Floxin Otic Solution (Single report) 1049
Flumadine (Less than 0.3%) 1183
Gabitril Tablets (Frequent) 984
Geodon Capsules (Frequent) 2529

▲ Intron A for Injection (Less than 5%) 3024
Keppra Oral Solution (2%) 3314
Keppra Tablets (2%) 3314
Lamictal (Infrequent) 1481
Levaquin (0.1% to 0.9%) 2384
Levaquin in 5% Dextrose Injection (0.1% to 0.9%) 2384
Lipitor Tablets (Less than 2%) 2483
Lyrica Capsules (0.1% to 1%) 2539
Maxair Autohaler 1852
Maxalt Tablets (Rare) 2008
Maxalt-MLT Orally Disintegrating Tablets (Rare) 2008
Mirapex Tablets (Less than 1%) 859
Namenda (Infrequent) 1195
Nembutal Sodium Solution, USP (Less than 1%) 2470
▲ Neurontin Capsules (2.5% to 4.7%) 2487
▲ Neurontin Oral Solution (2.5% to 4.7%) 2487
▲ Neurontin Tablets (2.5% to 4.7%) 2487
Nipent for Injection (Less than 3%) 1863
Omnicef for Oral Suspension (0.2%) 511
OxyContin Tablets (Less than 1%) 2703
Paxil CR Controlled-Release Tablets (Infrequent) 1538
Paxil (Infrequent) 1530
Permax Tablets (Infrequent) 3356
Prevacid Delayed-Release Capsules (Less than 1%) 3271
Prevacid for Delayed-Release Oral Suspension (Less than 1%) 3271
Prevacid SoluTab Delayed-Release Orally Disintegrating Tablets (Less than 1%) 3271
Prevacid NapraPAC (Less than 1%) 3280
PREVPAC (Less than 1%) 3284
Protonix I.V. (Less than 1%) 3472
Protonix Tablets (Less than 1%) 3469
Proventil HFA Inhalation Aerosol (Less than 3%) 3056
Provigil Tablets (1%) 988
Prozac Pulvules and Liquid (At least 2%) 1801
▲ Pulmicort Respules (1% to 3%) 661
Razadyne (Infrequent) 2399
Razadyne ER Extended-Release Capsules (Infrequent) 2399
Relpax Tablets (Infrequent) 2548
Requip Tablets (2%) 1555
Reyataz Capsules (Less than 3%) 921
▲ Risperdal (17% to 34%) 1676
▲ Risperdal M-Tab Orally Disintegrating Tablets (17% to 34%) 1676
▲ Sandostatin LAR Depot (1% to 4%) 2280
Seroquel Tablets (Infrequent) 690
Sonata Capsules (Infrequent) 1717
▲ Stalevo Tablets (5% to 10%) 2287
Symbyax Capsules (1% to 2%) 1819
Symmetrel Tablets (0.1% to 1%) 1135
▲ Tasmar Tablets (2% to 3%) 3358
▲ Topamax Sprinkle Capsules (5%) 2404
▲ Topamax Tablets (5%) 2404
Trileptal Tablets 2300
Trileptal Oral Suspension 2300
Vantin Tablets and Oral Suspension (Less than 1%) 2645
Viracept (Less than 2%) 2577
Wellbutrin SR Sustained-Release Tablets (Infrequent) 1607
Wellbutrin XL Extended-Release Tablets (Infrequent) 1613
WinRho SDF 732
Zelapar Tablets 3372
Zoloft (Infrequent to 2%) 2586
Zomig Tablets (Rare) 3519
Zomig-ZMT Tablets (Rare) 3519
Zonegran Capsules (Infrequent) 1101
Zyban Sustained-Release Tablets (Infrequent) 1644
▲ Zyprexa Tablets (5% to 11%) 1830
Zyprexa IntraMuscular (2%) 1830
▲ Zyprexa ZYDIS Orally Disintegrating Tablets (5% to 11%) 1830
Zyrtec Chewable Tablets (Less than 2%) 2594
Zyrtec (Less than 2%) 2594
Zyrtec-D 12 Hour Extended Release Tablets (Less than 2%) 2597

Hyperlipemia
Abilify Oral Solution (Infrequent) 882
Abilify Oral Solution (Infrequent) 2450
Abilify Discmelt Orally Disintegrating Tablets (Infrequent) 882
Abilify Discmelt Orally Disintegrating Tablets (Infrequent) 2450
Abilify Tablets (Infrequent) 882
Abilify Tablets (Infrequent) 2450
Benicar HCT Tablets (Greater than 1%) 1044
Lunesta Tablets (Rare) 3142
Omacor Capsules 2725
Prevacid NapraPAC 3280
Prozac Pulvules and Liquid (Infrequent) 1801
Risperdal Consta Long-Acting Injection (Infrequent) 1682
Symbyax Capsules (Infrequent) 1819

Hyperlipidemia
Aciphex Tablets 1090
Ambien Tablets (Rare) 2851
Ambien CR Tablets (Rare) 2855
Amerge Tablets (Rare) 1339
▲ AndroGel (3% to 6%) 3329
Avelox (Less than 0.1%) 2970
Benicar Tablets (Greater than 0.5%) 1043
▲ BiDil Tablets (3%) 2171
▲ CellCept Capsules (3% to less than 20%) 2747
▲ CellCept Intravenous (3% to less than 20%) 2747
▲ CellCept Oral Suspension (3% to less than 20%) 2747
▲ CellCept Tablets (3% to less than 20%) 2747
Chantix Tablets (Infrequent) 2517
Cymbalta Delayed-Release Capsules (Infrequent) 1757
Doxil Injection (Less than 1%) 2351
Effexor Tablets (Infrequent) 3411
Effexor XR Capsules (Infrequent) 3417
Evoxac Capsules (Less than 1%) 1047
Exelon Capsules (Infrequent) 2206
Exelon Oral Solution (Infrequent) 2206
Gabitril Tablets (Infrequent) 984
Geodon Capsules (Rare) 2529
▲ Humatrope Vials and Cartridges (8.1%) 1787
▲ Humira Injection (7%) 466
Lovenox Injection (Rare) 2915
▲ Myfortic Tablets (3% to less than 20%) 2255
Namenda (More than one patient) 1195
Neurontin Capsules (Rare) 2487
Neurontin Oral Solution (Rare) 2487
Neurontin Tablets (Rare) 2487
▲ Norvir (1.7% to 4.1%) 503
Pletal Tablets (Less than 2%) 2455
Prevacid Delayed-Release Capsules 3271
Prevacid for Delayed-Release Oral Suspension 3271
Prevacid SoluTab Delayed-Release Orally Disintegrating Tablets 3271
PREVPAC 3284
Prezista Tablets (Less than 2%) 3306
▲ Prograf Capsules and Injection (3% to 31%) 632
Protonix I.V. (Greater than or equal to 1%) 3472
Protonix Tablets (Greater than or equal to 1%) 3469
▲ Rapamune Oral Solution and Tablets (38% to 57%) 3475
Rythmol SR Capsules 2727
Sandimmune 2275
Seroquel Tablets (Infrequent) 690
▲ Targretin Capsules (76.6% to 79.2%) 1747
▲ Thalomid Capsules (5.6% to 9.4%) 965
Topamax Sprinkle Capsules (Infrequent) 2404
Topamax Tablets (Infrequent) 2404
Uniretic Tablets (Less than 1%) 3100
Viracept (Less than 2%) 2577
Zelapar Tablets 3372
Zyprexa Tablets (Rare) 1830
Zyprexa ZYDIS Orally Disintegrating Tablets (Rare) 1830

Hypermagnesemia
Doxil Injection (Less than 1%) 2351
VFEND I.V. (Less than 2%) 2564
VFEND Oral Suspension (Less than 2%) 2564
VFEND Tablets (Less than 2%) 2564
Zometa for Intravenous Infusion (2%) 2315

Hypernatremia
Abilify Oral Solution (Rare) 882
Abilify Oral Solution (Rare) 2450
Abilify Discmelt Orally Disintegrating Tablets (Rare) 882
Abilify Discmelt Orally Disintegrating Tablets (Rare) 2450
Abilify Tablets (Rare) 882
Abilify Tablets (Rare) 2450
Aloprim for Injection (Less than 1%) 2167
▲ AmBisome for Injection (4.1%) 620
Demadex Injection 2759
Demadex Tablets 2759
Doxil Injection (Less than 1%) 2351
Eraxis for Injection (Less than 1% to less than 2%) 2521
Fleet Enema 1165
Fleet Phospho-soda 1166
Fleet Phospho-soda ACCU-PREP 1168
Fleet Phospho-soda EZ-PREP 1169
Fleet Prep Kits 1170
Invanz for Injection (0.1% to 1%) 1999
▲ Invirase (Less than 1% to 4%) 2772
▲ Kaletra (3%) 476
Kristalose for Oral Solution 1034
Levaquin (0.1% to 0.9%) 2384
Levaquin in 5% Dextrose Injection (0.1% to 0.9%) 2384
▲ NeoProfen Injection (7%) 2472
Prezista Tablets (0% to 2.3%) 3306
Proleukin for Injection (1%) 2266
Revlimid Capsules 958
▲ Sutent Capsules (0% to 10%) 2560
Timentin ADD-Vantage 1580
Timentin Injection Galaxy Container 1583
Timentin IV Infusion 1577
Timentin Pharmacy Bulk Package 1586
Topamax Sprinkle Capsules (Rare) 2404
Topamax Tablets (Rare) 2404
VFEND I.V. (Less than 2%) 2564
VFEND Oral Suspension (Less than 2%) 2564
VFEND Tablets (Less than 2%) 2564
Viagra Tablets (Less than 2%) 2573
Xyrem Oral Solution (Infrequent) 1688
Zegerid Capsules (1.7%) 2958
Zegerid Powder for Oral Solution (1.7%) 2958
Zometa for Intravenous Infusion 2315
Zosyn 3492
Zyprexa Tablets (Rare) 1830
Zyprexa ZYDIS Orally Disintegrating Tablets (Rare) 1830

Hyperosmolarity
Revlimid Capsules 958

Hyperostosis, skeletal
Accutane Capsules 2731
▲ Soriatane Capsules (Less than 1% to 25%) 1013

Hyperparathyroidism
Lithobid Tablets 1692
Nutropin for Injection 1239
Nutropin AQ Injection 1243
Nutropin AQ Pen 1243
Nutropin AQ Pen Cartridge 1243
Prinzide Tablets 2056

Hyperperistalsis, intestinal
Camptosar Injection 2604

Hyperphenylalaninemia
Daraprim Tablets (Rare) 1419

Hyperphosphatemia
Aloprim for Injection (Less than 1%) 2167
AmBisome for Injection (Less common) 620
Androxy Tablets 3335
Cancidas for Injection (0%) 1918
Didronel Tablets 2697
Effexor Tablets (Rare) 3411
Effexor XR Capsules (Rare) 3417
Estratest Tablets 3199
Estratest H.S. Tablets 3199
Fleet Enema 1165
Fleet Phospho-soda 1166
Fleet Phospho-soda ACCU-PREP 1168
Fleet Phospho-soda EZ-PREP 1169
Fleet Prep Kits 1170
Hectorol Capsules 1275
Hectorol Injection 1278
▲ Myfortic Tablets (3% to less than 20%) 2255
Oxandrin Tablets 2962
Paxil CR Controlled-Release Tablets (Rare) 1538
Paxil (Rare) 1530
Pexeva Tablets (Rare) 1694
▲ Prograf Capsules and Injection (3% to 15%) 632
Proleukin for Injection (1%) 2266
▲ Rapamune Oral Solution and Tablets (3% to 20%) 3475
Requip Tablets (Infrequent) 1555
Risperdal (Rare) 1676
Risperdal M-Tab Orally Disintegrating Tablets (Rare) 1676
Rituxan I.V. 1254
Zelapar Tablets 3372

Hyperpigmentation
Accutane Capsules 2731
Advicor Tablets 1722
Aldara Cream, 5% 1846
Blocadren Tablets 1916
▲ Catapres-TTS (5 of 101 patients) 844
Cipro (Less than 1%) 2977
Cipro I.V. (1% or less) 2984
Cipro XR Tablets 2990
Crixivan Capsules 1940
Depo-Medrol Single-Dose Vial 2619
▲ Efudex (Among most frequent) 3363
▲ Levulan Kerastick for Topical Solution, 20% (20% to 36%) 1085
Matulane Capsules 3191
▲ Myleran Tablets (5% to10%) 1525
Niaspan Extended-Release Tablets 1730
Proquin XR Tablets 1153
Taxotere Injection Concentrate 2932
Tri-Luma Cream (18 occurrences in 27 patients) 1213
▲ Trisenox Injection (8%) 993

Hyperplasia, endometrial
Enjuvia Tablets 1062
Premarin Tablets 3446

Hyperplasia, gingival
(*see under* Gingival hyperplasia)

Hyperplasia, mammary
Cuprimine Capsules (Rare) 1947

Hyperplasia, uterine
Depo-Provera Contraceptive Injection (Less than 1%) 2622
depo-subQ provera 104 Injectable Suspension 2624

Hyperpnea
Aggrenox Capsules (Less than 1%) 822
Bayer Aspirin 744
Bayer Aspirin Comprehensive Prescribing Information ▣ 796
Percodan Tablets 1132

Hyperprolactinemia
Aldoril Tablets 1910
Celexa 1176
Covera-HS Tablets (Less than 2%) 3139
Effexor Tablets 3411
Effexor XR Capsules 3417
Lexapro Oral Solution 1190
Lexapro Tablets 1190
Moban Tablets 1119
Niravam Orally Disintegrating Tablets 3092
Paxil CR Controlled-Release Tablets 1538
Paxil 1530
Prozac Pulvules and Liquid 1801
Risperdal 1676
Risperdal Consta Long-Acting Injection (Infrequent) 1682
Risperdal M-Tab Orally Disintegrating Tablets 1676
Rythmol SR Capsules 2727
Symbyax Capsules 1819
Tarka Tablets 524
Verelan PM Extended-Release Capsules, Controlled-Onset (2% or less) 3106
Zoloft 2586
Zyprexa Tablets 1830
Zyprexa IntraMuscular 1830
Zyprexa ZYDIS Orally Disintegrating Tablets 1830

Hyperproteinemia
Evoxac Capsules 1047

Hyperprothrombinemia
AmBisome for Injection (Less common) 620
Avelox (Less than 0.1%) 2970
▲ Doxil Injection (1% to 10%) 2351
Estratest Tablets 3199
Estratest H.S. Tablets 3199
Rythmol SR Capsules 2727
Topamax Sprinkle Capsules (1%) 2404
Topamax Tablets (1%) 2404

Hyperpyrexia
(*see under* Fever)

Hyperreflexia
Abilify Oral Solution (Infrequent) 882

Abilify Oral Solution (Infrequent) 2450
Abilify Discmelt Orally Disintegrating Tablets (Infrequent) 882
Abilify Discmelt Orally Disintegrating Tablets (Infrequent) 2450
Abilify Tablets (Infrequent) 882
Abilify Tablets (Infrequent) 2450
▲ Aldurazyme for Intravenous Infusion (3%) 1268
Depacon Injection (1% or more) 412
Depakene (1% or more) 417
Depakote Sprinkle Capsules 422
▲ Depakote Tablets (1% to 5%) 427
Depakote ER Tablets (Greater than 1%) 434
Effexor Tablets (Rare) 3411
Effexor XR Capsules (Rare) 3417
Exelon Capsules (Infrequent) 2206
Exelon Oral Solution (Infrequent) 2206
Gabitril Tablets (Infrequent) 984
Geodon Capsules (Rare) 2529
Invirase (Less than 2%) 2772
Keppra Oral Solution (2%) 3314
Keppra Tablets (2%) 3314
Lexapro Oral Solution (Infrequent) 1190
Lexapro Tablets (Infrequent) 1190
Neurontin Capsules (Frequent) 2487
Neurontin Oral Solution (Frequent) 2487
Neurontin Tablets (Frequent) 2487
Orthoclone OKT3 Sterile Solution 2360
Paxil CR Controlled-Release Tablets (Rare) 1538
Paxil (Rare) 1530
Pexeva Tablets (rare) 1694
Prozac Pulvules and Liquid (Rare) 1801
Rescriptor Tablets 2551
Reyataz Capsules (Less than 3%) 921
Risperdal (Rare) 1676
Risperdal M-Tab Orally Disintegrating Tablets (Rare) 1676
Seromycin Capsules 1813
Sonata Capsules (Rare) 1717
Topamax Sprinkle Capsules (Infrequent) 2404
Topamax Tablets (Infrequent) 2404
Trileptal Tablets 2300
Trileptal Oral Suspension 2300
Zonegran Capsules (Infrequent) 1101
Zyvox 2652

Hypersalivation
(*see under* Sialism)

Hypersecretion
Klonopin 2778

Hypersensitivity
▲ Alimta for Injection (Up to 8%) 1750
Alkeran for Injection 955
Aloxi Injection (Very rare) 2127
Amoxil Capsules 1343
Amoxil Chewable Tablets 1343
Amoxil Pediatric Drops for Oral Suspension 1343
Amoxil Powder for Oral Suspension 1343
Amoxil Tablets 1343
Androxy Tablets 3335
Aptivus Capsules (Less than 2%) 826
Betagan Ophthalmic Solution, USP ⊙220
Bleph-10 Ophthalmic Solution 10% ⊙222
Carteolol Hydrochloride Ophthalmic Solution USP, 1% ⊙249
Chantix Tablets (Infrequent) 2517
Clinoril Tablets (Less than 1%) 1924
Cubicin for Injection (Less than 1%) 1026
Cymbalta Delayed-Release Capsules (Very rare) 1757
Dacogen Injection 2129
Daranide Tablets 1950
Demser Capsules (Rare) 1953
Dolobid Tablets (Less than 1 in 100) 1955
▲ Elspar for Injection (32.5% to 75%) 2463
▲ Elspar for Injection (32.5% to 75%) 1960
Estratest Tablets (Rare) 3199
Estratest H.S. Tablets (Rare) 3199
Fluarix 1451
Fluorescite Injection ⊙207
FML-S Ophthalmic Suspension ⊙229
Fortaz (Immediate in 1 in 285 patients) 1453
Human Albumin Grifols 20%, Albumin (Human) 1651
Human Albumin Grifols 25%, Albumin (Human) 1652
Hydrocortone Tablets 1989
Hyperstat I.V. 3017
Imitrex Injection (Infrequent) 1463
Imitrex Nasal Spray (Rare) 1467
Imitrex Tablets (Frequent) 1471
Indocin (Less than 1%) 1995
Lacrisert Sterile Ophthalmic Insert 2005
Leukeran Tablets 1504
Micardis Tablets 854
Mustargen for Injection 2468
Nembutal Sodium Solution, USP 2470
Norflex Injection 1856
Noroxin Tablets (A few patients) 2032
Opana Tablets (Less than 1%) 1122
Opana ER Tablets (Less than 1%) 1126
Pediarix Vaccine 1548
Plavix Tablets 2926
Premarin Vaginal Cream 3452
PREVPAC 3284
Prinzide Tablets 2056
Proquin XR Tablets (Less than 1%) 1153
Raniclor Tablets, Chewable (1.5%) 2505
Recombivax HB 2071
Ritalin Hydrochloride Tablets 2269
Ritalin LA Capsules 2271
Ritalin-SR Tablets 2269
Rocephin Injectable Vials, ADD-Vantage, Galaxy, Bulk 2800
Rosac Cream with Sunscreens (Rare) 3213
Seromycin Capsules 1813
Solodyn Extended Release Tablets 1890
Thyrolar Tablets 1199
Timoptic Sterile Ophthalmic Solution (Less frequent) 2088
Timoptic in Ocudose (Less frequent) 2091
TobraDex Ophthalmic Ointment (Less than 4%) 562
TobraDex Ophthalmic Suspension (Less than 4%) 563
Viramune Oral Suspension 873
Viramune Tablets 873
Xyrem Oral Solution (Infrequent) 1688
Zantac (Rare) 1624
Zantac Injection (Rare) 1619
Zantac Injection Pharmacy Bulk Package (Rare) 1622
Zantac Injection Premixed (Rare) 1619
Zantac (Rare) 1624
Zinacef for Injection (Fewer than 1%) 1631
Zinacef Injection (Fewer than 1%) 1631
Zomig Tablets (Rare) 3519
Zomig-ZMT Tablets (Rare) 3519

Hypersensitivity at injection site
Aloxi Injection (Very rare) 2127
Amevive (Less than 1%) 626
▲ Betaseron for SC Injection (3%) 767
Bexxar 1398
Bicillin C-R Injectable Suspension 1706
HibTITER 3426

Hypersensitivity reactions, Arthus-type
ADACEL Vaccine 2945
Boostrix 1404
Pediarix Vaccine 1548

Hypersensitivity reactions, general
Accolate Tablets 671
Actonel Tablets (Very rare) 2683
Actonel with Calcium Tablets (Very rare) 2688
Adderall XR Capsules 3166
Advair Diskus 100/50 1308
Advair Diskus 250/50 1308
Advair Diskus 500/50 1308
Advair HFA Inhalation Aerosol (Rare) 1318
Alferon N Injection 1665
Alkeran Tablets 956
Altace Capsules (Less than 1%) 1702
Altoprev Extended-Release Tablets (Rare) 3109
Aminohippurate Sodium PAH Injection 1913
Antivenin (Black Widow Spider Antivenin) 1913
Asacol Delayed-Release Tablets (Some patients) 2692
Atrovent HFA Inhalation Aerosol 841
Augmentin 1360
Augmentin Tablets 1363
Augmentin XR Extended-Release Tablets 1369
Augmentin ES-600 Powder for Oral Suspension 1366
Axid Oral Solution (Rare) 879
Beconase AQ Nasal Spray (Rare) 1396
Benicar HCT Tablets 1044
▲ Betimol Ophthalmic Solution (More than 5%) 3382
▲ Betimol Ophthalmic Solution (More than 5%) ⊙295
Bexxar 1398
Carafate Suspension 701
Carafate Tablets 701
Carimune NF 3499
Ceftin 1407
Cialis Tablets 1838
Cipro 2977
Cipro XR Tablets (Rare) 2990
Clarinex Syrup (Rare) 2995
Clarinex-D 24-Hour Extended-Release Tablets 2998
Cleocin Vaginal Ovules 2616
Clozaril Tablets 2184
Comvax 1928
Coumadin for Injection (Infrequent) 898
Coumadin Tablets (Infrequent) 898
Cozaar Tablets 1935
Crestor Tablets (Less than 1%) 678
Daytrana Transdermal Patch 3174
Depakote ER Tablets 434
Didronel Tablets 2697
Digibind for Injection 1421
Faslodex Injection (Less than 1%) 681
FazaClo Orally Disintegrating Tablets 551
Ferrlecit Injection 3388
Fleet Phospho-soda (Rare) 1166
Fleet Phospho-soda ACCU-PREP (Rare) 1168
Fleet Phospho-soda EZ-PREP (Rare) 1169
Flovent HFA (Rare) 1447
Flumist Vaccine 1901
Focalin XR Capsules 2223
Fosamax 1969
Fosamax Plus D Tablets 1977
Furosemide Tablets 2154
Gammagard Liquid 721
Humira Injection 466
Hyzaar 50-12.5 Tablets 1990
Hyzaar 100-12.5 Tablets 1990
Hyzaar 100-25 Tablets 1990
Inderal LA Long-Acting Capsules 3429
Infanrix Vaccine 1476
Infed Injection 3390
Kytril Injection (Rare) 2781
Kytril (Rare) 2784
Lescol Capsules (Rare) 2233
Lescol XL Tablets (Rare) 2233
Levothroid Tablets 1186
Mephyton Tablets 2018
Mevacor Tablets (Rare) 2021
Mylotarg for Injection 3431
Neosporin Ophthalmic Solution Sterile (Rare) ⊙265
Neumega for Injection 3435
Nexavar Tablets (Uncommon) 746
Nimbex Injection 498
▲ Oncaspar (Greater than 1% but less than 5%) 1145
Orencia Powder for Intravenous Infusion (Less than 0.1% to 1%) 914
Orthoclone OKT3 Sterile Solution 2360
Polytrim Ophthalmic Solution (Multiple reports) 574
Propecia Tablets 2060
Proscar Tablets 2067
Rapamune Oral Solution and Tablets 3475
▲ Raptiva for Injection (8%) 1250
Remicade for IV Injection 971
ReoPro Vials 1809
Rituxan I.V. 1254
Rocaltrol Capsules 2798
Rocaltrol Oral Solution 2798
Singulair 2077
Skelaxin Tablets 1716
Soltamox Oral Solution (Very rare) 3527
Sular Tablets (Very rare) 3122
Synagis (Rare) 1897
▲ Taxotere Injection Concentrate (Up to 33.3%) 2932
Tessalon Capsules 1199
Tessalon Perles 1199
Timoptic-XE Sterile Ophthalmic Gel Forming Solution 2092
Trasylol Injection 754
Trecator Tablets (Rare) 3487
Trileptal Tablets 2300
Trileptal Oral Suspension 2300
▲ Trizivir Tablets (Greater than or equal to 5%) 1589
Univasc Tablets (Less than 1%) 3104
▲ Valcyte Tablets (Less than 5%) 2813
Viracept 2577
Viroptic Ophthalmic Solution ⊙266
Visudyne for Injection (Less than 1%) 2305
Vivaglobin 3506
Vivitrol 995
Vytorin 10/10 Tablets 2114
Vytorin 10/10 Tablets 3077
Vytorin 10/20 Tablets 2114
Vytorin 10/20 Tablets 3077
Vytorin 10/40 Tablets 2114
Vytorin 10/40 Tablets 3077
Vytorin 10/80 Tablets 2114
Vytorin 10/80 Tablets 3077
▲ Xeloda Tablets (Less than 5%) 2822
Xifaxan Tablets 2842
Zelnorm Tablets 2312
Zetia Tablets 2120
Zetia Tablets 3083
▲ Ziagen (2% to 9%) 1626
Zocor Tablets (Rare) 2105
Zofran Injection (Rare) 1634
Zometa for Intravenous Infusion 2315
Zomig Nasal Spray (Rare) 3523
Zosyn (1% or less) 3492

Hypersensitivity reactions, multi-organ
Depakene (Rare) 417
Depakote Sprinkle Capsules (Rare) 422
Depakote Tablets (Rare) 427
▲ Epzicom Tablets (2% to 9%) 1436
Tegretol/Tegretol-XR 2295

Hypersensitivity vasculitis
Aldoril Tablets 1910
Clinoril Tablets (Less than 1 in 100) 1924
Dolobid Tablets (Less than 1 in 100) 1955
Lovenox Injection (Rare) 2915
PREVPAC 3284

Hypersomnia
Abilify Oral Solution (Infrequent) 882
Abilify Oral Solution (Infrequent) 2450
Abilify Discmelt Orally Disintegrating Tablets (Infrequent) 882
Abilify Discmelt Orally Disintegrating Tablets (Infrequent) 2450
Abilify Tablets (Infrequent) 882
Abilify Tablets (Infrequent) 2450
Aloxi Injection (Less than 1%) 2127
Maxalt Tablets (Rare) 2008
Maxalt-MLT Orally Disintegrating Tablets (Rare) 2008
Permax Tablets 3356
Prinivil Tablets (0.3% to 1.0%) 2052
Prinzide Tablets 2056
ProQuad 2064

Hypertension
▲ Abelcet Injection (5%) 1141
Abilify Oral Solution (2%) 882
Abilify Oral Solution (2%) 2450
Abilify Discmelt Orally Disintegrating Tablets (2%) 882
Abilify Discmelt Orally Disintegrating Tablets (2%) 2450
Abilify Tablets (2%) 882
Abilify Tablets (2%) 2450
Aciphex Tablets 1090
Actiq (Less than 1%) 979
Activase I.V. 1223
▲ Actonel Tablets (4.9% to 5.8%) 2683
▲ Actonel with Calcium Tablets (4.9% to 10%) 2688
Adderall Tablets 3164
▲ Adderall XR Capsules (12% to 35%) 3166
Adenocard Injection 617
Adenoscan (Less than 1%) 619
Adipex-P 1215
Advair HFA Inhalation Aerosol 1318
▲ Aerobid/Aerobid-M (1% to 3%) 1171
▲ Agrylin Capsules (1% to 5%) 3169
Albalon Ophthalmic Solution ⊙218
Aldara Cream, 5% (1.4%) 1846
▲ Alimta for Injection (3% to 11%) 1750
Alinia for Oral Suspension (Less than 1%) 2835
Alinia Tablets (Less than 1%) 2835
Aloprim for Injection (Less than 1%) 2167
Aloxi Injection (Less than 1%) 2127
▲ Alphagan P Ophthalmic Solution (Approximately 5% to 9%) 567
Alupent Inhalation Aerosol (Less frequent) 826

Ambien Tablets (Infrequent) 2851
Ambien CR Tablets (Infrequent to 1%) 2855
▲ AmBisome for Injection (7.9% to 19.8%) 620
Amerge Tablets (Infrequent) 1339
Amitiza Capsules (0% to 1%) 3224
Anaprox Tablets (Less than 1%) 2761
Anaprox DS Tablets (Less than 1%) 2761
Angeliq Tablets 762
Anzemet Injection (2.9%) 2859
Anzemet Tablets (2.2%) 2862
▲ Aranesp for Injection (3.7% to 23%) 581
▲ Aredia for Injection (Up to at least 15%) 2179
Aricept Tablets (Frequent) 1094
Aricept ODT Tablets (Frequent) 1094
▲ Arimidex Tablets (2% to 13%) 673
Arixtra Injection (2.4%) 1351
▲ Aromasin Tablets (5% to 15.1%) 2600
Arthrotec Tablets (Rare) 3129
Astelin Nasal Spray (Infrequent) 1904
Atrovent Inhalation Solution (0.9%) 835
Avalide Tablets 888
Avalide Tablets 2874
Avapro Tablets (Less than 1%) 891
Avapro Tablets (Less than 1%) 2871
▲ Avastin IV (12% to 34%) 1227
Avelox (0.1% to less than 2%) 2970
Avinza Capsules (Less than 5%) 1741
Axert Tablets (Rare) 2396
▲ Betaseron for SC Injection (7%) 767
Betimol Ophthalmic Solution (1% to 5%) 3382
Betimol Ophthalmic Solution (1% to 5%) ⊙295
▲ Boniva Injection (6.3% to 7.3%) 2738
▲ Boniva Tablets (6.3% to 7.3%) 2741
Brimonidine Tartrate Ophthalmic Solution 0.2% (Less than 3%) ⊙248
Buprenex Injectable (Less than 1%) 2716
Caduet Tablets (Less than 2%) 2508
Calcijex Injection 411
▲ Campath Ampules (2% to 11%) 811
Campral Tablets (Frequent) 1174
Cancidas for Injection (1.1% to 1.8%) 1918
Carbatrol Capsules 3171
Cardene I.V. (0.7%) 2497
▲ Carnitor Injection (18% to 12%) 3188
Catapres-TTS (0.5% or less) 844
Caverject Impulse Injection (2%) 2612
Celexa (Infrequent) 1176
▲ CellCept Capsules (28.2% to 77.5%) 2747
▲ CellCept Intravenous (28.2% to 77.5%) 2747
▲ CellCept Oral Suspension (28.2% to 77.5%) 2747
▲ CellCept Tablets (28.2% to 77.5%) 2747
Cesamet Capsules 3340
Chantix Tablets (Frequent) 2517
Cialis Tablets (Less than 2%) 1838
Cipro (Less than 1%) 2977
Cipro I.V. (1% or less) 2984
Cipro XR Tablets 2990
Climara Transdermal System 771
▲ Climara Pro Transdermal System (3.3%) 776
Clinoril Tablets (Less than 1%) 1924
▲ Clolar for Intravenous Infusion (11%) 1271
▲ Clozaril Tablets (4%) 2184
Colazal Capsules 2838
Colocort Rectal Suspension, USP (Retention) 100 mg/60 mL 2476
Combivent Inhalation Aerosol (Less than 2%) 847
Concerta Extended-Release Tablets 1881
Copaxone for Injection (Frequent) 3297
▲ Coreg Tablets (Greater than 1% to 3%) 1414
▲ Cosopt Sterile Ophthalmic Solution (1% to 5%) 1931
Crestor Tablets (Greater than or equal to 2%) 678
▲ Cubicin for Injection (1.1% to 5.8%) 1026
Daytrana Transdermal Patch 3174
Decadron Tablets 1951
▲ Depacon Injection (1% to 5%) 412
Depakene (1% or more) 417
▲ Depakote Sprinkle Capsules (1% to 5%) 422
▲ Depakote Tablets (1% to 5%) 427
▲ Depakote ER Tablets (Greater than 1% to 5%) 434
▲ DepoDur Extended-Release Injection (2% to 5%) 1110
Depo-Medrol Injectable Suspension 2617
Depo-Medrol Single-Dose Vial 2619
Desoxyn Tablets, USP 2462
▲ Detrol Tablets (7%) 2628
Dexedrine 1420
DextroStat Tablets 3179
Dilaudid 440
Dilaudid Non-Sterile Powder 440
Dilaudid Oral Liquid 445
Dilaudid Rectal Suppositories 440
Dilaudid Tablets 440
Dilaudid Tablets - 8 mg 445
Dilaudid-HP (Less frequent) 442
▲ Ditropan XL Extended-Release Tablets (2% to less than 5%) 2413
Dolobid Tablets 1955
Doxil Injection (Less than 1%) 2351
▲ Duragesic Transdermal System (1% to 3%) 2373
EC-Naprosyn Delayed-Release Tablets (Less than 1%) 2761
Edex Injection (2%) 3089
▲ Effexor Tablets (3% to 13%) 3411
▲ Effexor XR Capsules (4% to 5%) 3417
Eldepryl Capsules 3208
Eligard 22.5 mg (Less than 2%) 2883
Emcyt Capsules 2634
Emend Capsules (Greater than 0.5%) 1963
Enablex Extended-Release Tablets (Greater than or equal to 1%) 2203
Enbrel for Injection (Infrequent) 584
Enjuvia Tablets 1062
▲ Entocort EC Capsules (Less than 5%) 2698
▲ Epogen for Injection (0.75% to 24%) 591
Equetro Extended-Release Capsules 3180
Eraxis for Injection (Less than 1% to less than 2%) 2521
Estrasorb Topical Emulsion 1147
Estratest Tablets (Common) 3199
Estratest H.S. Tablets (Common) 3199
Ethyol for Injection 1898
▲ Euflexxa (1.88% to 3.75%) 1162
Eulexin Capsules (1%) 3009
Evoxac Capsules (Less than 1%) 1047
▲ Exelon Capsules (3%) 2206
▲ Exelon Oral Solution (3%) 2206
▲ Fabrazyme for Intravenous Infusion (3%) 1274
▲ FazaClo Orally Disintegrating Tablets (4%) 551
▲ Femara Tablets (5% to 8%) 2214
▲ Ferrlecit Injection (0.6% to 23%) 3388
Floxin Otic Solution (Single report) 1049
Flumadine (Less than 0.3%) 1183
Focalin Tablets 2220
Focalin XR Capsules 2223
Foradil Aerolizer 3010
▲ Forteo for Injection (7.1%) 1767
▲ Fortical Nasal Spray (1% to 3%) 3337
Gabitril Tablets (Frequent) 984
Gammagard S/D (Occasional) 724
Garamycin Injectable 3014
Gemzar for Injection (2%) 1771
▲ Gengraf Capsules (25% to 50%) 459
▲ Geodon (3%) 2529
Gleevec Tablets (Infrequent) 2227
GlucaGen 761
Hectorol Capsules 1275
Hectorol Injection 1278
Herceptin I.V. 1233
▲ Humatrope Vials and Cartridges (2.7% to 7.7%) 1787
▲ Humira Injection (5%) 466
Hycotuss Expectorant Syrup 1117
Hydrocortone Tablets 1989
▲ Imdur Tablets (Less than or equal to 5%) 3018
Imitrex Injection (Infrequent) 1463
Imitrex Nasal Spray (Infrequent) 1467
Imitrex Tablets (Infrequent) 1471
Indocin Capsules (Less than 1%) 1995
Indocin I.V. (Less than 1%) 2465
Indocin (Less than 1%) 1995
Infed Injection 3390
▲ Infergen (2% to 5%) 3364
▲ Intron A for Injection (Less than 5% to 9%) 3024
Invanz for Injection (0.7% to 1.6%) 1999
Invirase (Less than 2%) 2772
▲ Ionsys Transdermal System (1% to less than 10%) 2379
▲ I.V. Busulfex (7% to 36%) 2493
Kadian Capsules (Less than 3%) 577
Kaletra (Less than 2%) 476
▲ Kepivance (7% to 14%) 597
Kogenate FS 738
Kogenate FS with Bio-Set (1 case) 740
Kytril Injection (2.6%) 2781
Kytril (1%) 2784
Lamictal (Rare) 1481
Lariam Tablets (Infrequent) 2786
▲ Leukine (25% to 34%) 814
Levaquin (0.1% to 0.9%) 2384
Levaquin in 5% Dextrose Injection (0.1% to 0.9%) 2384
Levitra Tablets (Less than 2%) 3034
Levothroid Tablets 1186
Levoxyl Tablets 1712
Lexapro Oral Solution (Frequent) 1190
Lexapro Tablets (Frequent) 1190
▲ Limbrel Capsules (Greater than or equal to 2%) 2672
Lipitor Tablets (Less than 2%) 2483
Lofibra Tablets 1219
Lofibra Capsules 1216
Lotronex Tablets (Rare) 1512
▲ Lucentis Injection (5% to 23%) 1237
Lunesta Tablets (Frequent) 3142
▲ Macugen Injection (10% to 40%) ⊙261
Maxalt Tablets (Infrequent) 2008
Maxalt-MLT Orally Disintegrating Tablets (Infrequent) 2008
▲ Megace ES Oral Suspension (0% to 8%) 2481
Menostar Transdermal System 782
Meridia Capsules (2.1%) 489
Merrem I.V. (Greater than 0.1% to 1%) 686
Metadate CD Capsules 3323
Metrogel 1% (1.1%) 1211
▲ Miacalcin Nasal Spray (1% to 3%) 2253
Micardis Tablets (1%) 854
Micardis HCT Tablets 856
Migranal Nasal Spray (Rare) 3348
Mirapex Tablets (1% or more) 859
Mircette Tablets 1066
▲ Mirena Intrauterine System (5% or more) 787
Mobic Oral Suspension (Less than 2%) 863
Mobic Tablets (Less than 2%) 863
MS Contin Tablets (Less frequent) 2701
Mycamine for Injection (0.6%) 628
▲ Myfortic Tablets (3% to less than 20%) 2255
▲ Mylotarg for Injection (13% to 17%) 3431
Myozyme for Intravenous Infusion 1279
▲ Namenda (4%) 1195
Naprosyn Suspension (Less than 1%) 2761
Naprosyn Tablets (Less than 1%) 2761
▲ Neoral Oral Solution (Approximately 25% to 50% most patients) 2259
▲ Neoral Soft Gelatin Capsules (25% to 50%) 2259
▲ Neupogen for Injection (4%) 603
Neurontin Capsules (Frequent) 2487
Neurontin Oral Solution (Frequent) 2487
Neurontin Tablets (Frequent) 2487
▲ Nevanac Ophthalmic Suspension 0.1% (1% to 4%) ⊙209
▲ Nexavar Tablets (Less than 1% to 17%) 746
Nexium Delayed-Release Capsules (Less than 1%) 655
Nexium I.V. (Less than 1%) 659
NicoDerm CQ Clear Patch ▣622
Nimotop Capsules (Less than 1%) 749
Nipent for Injection (Less than 3%) 1863
▲ Norditropin Cartridges (8%) 2323
NovoSeven (Greater than or equal to 2%) 2331
NuvaRing 2340
Omacor Capsules 2725
Omnicef Capsules 511
Omnicef for Oral Suspension 511
Oncaspar (Less than 1%) 1145
▲ Ontak Vials (6%) 1745
Opana Tablets (Less than 1%) 1122
Opana ER Tablets (Less than 1%) 1126
OptiPranolol Metipranolol Ophthalmic Solution 0.3% (A small number of patients) ⊙256
▲ Oracea Capsules (1.5% to 3%) 1000
▲ Orencia Powder for Intravenous Infusion (0.1% to 7%) 914
Ortho-Cyclen Tablets 2429
Ortho Evra Transdermal System 2417
Ortho Tri-Cyclen Tablets 2429
Ortho Tri-Cyclen Lo Tablets 2436
▲ Orthoclone OKT3 Sterile Solution (8%) 2360
Parcopa Orally Disintegrating Tablets 3097
Paxil CR Controlled-Release Tablets (Frequent) 1538
Paxil (Frequent) 1530
Pegasys 2789
Permax Tablets (1.6%) 3356
Pexeva Tablets (frequent) 1694
Phenergan Tablets and Suppositories 3440
▲ Photofrin for Injection (37% to 6%) 702
▲ Plavix Tablets (4.3%) 917
▲ Plavix Tablets (4.3%) 2926
Pletal Tablets (2% or greater) 2455
Premarin Intravenous 3442
Premarin Tablets 3446
Premarin Vaginal Cream 3452
Premphase Tablets 3456
Prempro Tablets 3456
Prevacid Delayed-Release Capsules (Less than 1%) 3271
Prevacid for Delayed-Release Oral Suspension (Less than 1%) 3271
Prevacid SoluTab Delayed-Release Orally Disintegrating Tablets (Less than 1%) 3271
Prevacid NapraPAC (Less than 1%) 3280
PREVPAC (Less than 1%) 3284
Prezista Tablets (Less than 2%) 3306
Prilosec OTC Delayed-Release Tablets (Less than 1%) 2677
Primatene Mist ▣719
▲ Procrit for Injection (0.75% to 24%) 2364
▲ Prograf Capsules and Injection (Common; 38% to 62%) 632
Prometrium Capsules (100 mg, 200 mg) (Less than 5%) 3203
Propine Ophthalmic Solution ⊙239
Proquin XR Tablets 1153
ProstaScint Kit (1%) 1037
Protonix I.V. (Less than 1%) 3472
Protonix Tablets (Less than 1%) 3469
Protopic Ointment (Greater than or equal to 1% to 2%) 638
▲ Proventil Inhalation Aerosol (Less than 5%) 3053
Proventil Inhalation Solution 0.083% (1% to 3.1%) 3055
Proventil HFA Inhalation Aerosol 3056
▲ Provigil Tablets (3%) 988
Prozac Pulvules and Liquid (Frequent) 1801
▲ Quadramet Injection (3%) 1040
▲ Rapamune Oral Solution and Tablets (39% to 49%) 3475
Razadyne (Greater than or equal to 2%) 2399
Razadyne ER Extended-Release Capsules (Greater than or equal to 2%) 2399
Relpax Tablets (Infrequent) 2548
▲ Remicade for IV Injection (7%) 971
▲ Renagel Tablets (10.1%) 1282
▲ Requip Tablets (5%) 1555
Rescriptor Tablets 2551
Revatio Tablets 2557
▲ Revlimid Capsules (6.1%) 958
Reyataz Capsules (Less than 3%) 921
▲ Rilutek Tablets (3.3% to 6.8%) 2930
▲ Risperdal (Infrequent to 3%) 1676
▲ Risperdal Consta Long-Acting Injection (3%) 1682
▲ Risperdal M-Tab Orally Disintegrating Tablets (Infrequent to 3%) 1676
Ritalin LA Capsules 2271
▲ Rituxan I.V. (1% to 8%) 1254
Rocaltrol Capsules 2798
Rocaltrol Oral Solution 2798
Romazicon Injection (Less than 1%) 2804
Rythmol SR Capsules 2727
▲ Sandimmune (13% to 53%) 2275
Sandostatin Injection (Less than 1%) 2278
▲ Sandostatin LAR Depot (5% to 15%) 2280
Seasonique Tablets 1077
▲ Sensipar Tablets (7%) 608
▲ Serevent Diskus (4%) 1568
▲ Simulect for Injection (Greater than or equal to 10%) 2284
▲ Somavert Injection (8%) 2642
Sonata Capsules (Infrequent) 1717
St. Joseph 81 mg Aspirin Chewable and Enteric Coated Tablets 1869
Stalevo Tablets 2287
Strattera Capsules 1814
Striant Mucoadhesive 1007
Sular Tablets (Less than or equal to 1%) 3122
▲ Sutent Capsules (4% to 28%) 2560
Symbyax Capsules (2%) 1819
Symmetrel Tablets (0.1% to 1%) 1135
Tambocor Tablets (Less than 1%) 1856
Targretin Capsules 1747
Tasmar Tablets (Infrequent) 3358
Taxotere Injection Concentrate (Rare) 2932

Tegretol/Tegretol-XR 2295
Tequin Injection (Less than 0.1%) 938
Tequin Injection in 5% Dextrose (Less than 0.1%) 938
Tequin Tablets (Less than 0.1%) 938
Testim 1% Gel (1%) 695
Thalomid Capsules 965
▲ Thymoglobulin for Intravenous Infusion (36.6%) 1284
Thyrolar Tablets 1199
Timoptic Sterile Ophthalmic Solution (Less frequent) 2088
Timoptic in Ocudose (Less frequent) 2091
Timoptic-XE Sterile Ophthalmic Gel Forming Solution 2092
Topamax Sprinkle Capsules (1% to 2%) 2404
Topamax Tablets (1% to 2%) 2404
▲ Trasylol Injection (4%) 754
Travatan Ophthalmic Solution (1% to 5%) 563
▲ Trelstar Depot (3.6%) 3394
▲ Trelstar LA Suspension (4%) 3397
Tricor Tablets 527
Triglide Tablets 3123
Trileptal Tablets 2300
Trileptal Oral Suspension 2300
▲ Trisenox Injection (10%) 993
Twinject 0.3 3378
Twinject 0.15 3379
▲ Tygacil for Injection (4.9%) 3488
Ultane Liquid for Inhalation (2%) 531
▲ Ultram ER Tablets (1% to greater than 5%) 2392
▲ Urso 250 Tablets (8.3%) 710
▲ Urso Forte Tablets (8.3%) 710
▲ Valcyte Tablets (18%) 2813
Valtrex Caplets 1597
Vantin Tablets and Oral Suspension (Less than 1%) 2645
▲ Vaprisol (5.5%) 643
Ventolin HFA Inhalation Aerosol 1600
Verelan PM Extended-Release Capsules, Controlled-Onset (1.7%) 3106
▲ Vesanoid Capsules (11%) 2820
VESIcare Tablets (0.5% to 1.4%) 646
VFEND I.V. (Less than 2%) 2564
VFEND Oral Suspension (Less than 2%) 2564
VFEND Tablets (Less than 2%) 2564
Viadur Implant (Rare) 757
Viagra Tablets 2573
▲ Visudyne for Injection (1% to 10%) 2305
Vivitrol 995
Voltaren Tablets (Occasionally) 2307
Voltaren-XR Tablets (Occasionally) 2310
VoSpire ER Tablets 1052
▲ Wellbutrin Tablets (4.3%) 1603
Wellbutrin SR Sustained-Release Tablets (At least 1%) 1607
▲ Wellbutrin XL Extended-Release Tablets (2% to 4%) 1613
WinRho SDF 732
Xeloda Tablets 2822
Xopenex Inhalation Solution 3146
Xopenex Inhalation Solution Concentrate 3150
Xopenex HFA Inhalation Aerosol 3154
▲ Xyrem Oral Solution (6.1%) 1688
Yasmin 28 Tablets 796
Yaz Tablets 803
▲ Zegerid Capsules (7.9%) 2958
▲ Zegerid Powder for Oral Solution (7.9%) 2958
▲ Zelapar Tablets (3%) 3372
Zemuron Injection (0.1%; 2%) 2346
Zoloft (Infrequent) 2586
Zometa for Intravenous Infusion 2315
Zomig Tablets (Infrequent) 3519
Zomig Nasal Spray (Infrequent) 3523
Zomig-ZMT Tablets (Infrequent) 3519
Zonegran Capsules (Infrequent) 1101
Zosyn (1.3% to 1.6%) 3492
Zyban Sustained-Release Tablets (1% to 2.5%) 1644
Zyprexa Tablets (2%) 1830
Zyprexa ZYDIS Orally Disintegrating Tablets (2%) 1830
Zyrtec Chewable Tablets (Less than 2%) 2594
Zyrtec (Less than 2%) 2594
Zyrtec-D 12 Hour Extended Release Tablets (Less than 2%) 2597
Zyvox 2652

Hypertension, aggravation

Ambien Tablets (Rare) 2851
Ambien CR Tablets (Rare) 2855
Atrovent Inhalation Solution (0.9%) 835
Brimonidine Tartrate Ophthalmic Solution 0.2% ⊙248
Carbatrol Capsules 3171
Celebrex Capsules (0.1% to 1.9%) 3134
Dolobid Tablets 1955
Equetro Extended-Release Capsules 3180
Ethyol for Injection 1898
Evoxac Capsules (Less than 1%) 1047
Micardis Tablets 854
▲ Myfortic Tablets (3% to less than 20%) 2255
▲ Sandostatin LAR Depot (1% to 4%) 2280
Tegretol/Tegretol-XR 2295
▲ Ultram ER Tablets (1% to greater than 5%) 2392
Zoloft (Rare) 2586

Hypertension, intracranial

Aclovate Cream 2660
Cutivate Cream 2662
Cutivate Ointment 2665
Diprolene Gel 0.05% 3001
Diprolene Lotion 0.05% 3002
Diprolene Ointment 0.05% (Some patients) 3003
Elocon Cream 0.1% 3005
Elocon Ointment 0.1% 3007
Entocort EC Capsules (Three cases) 2698
Gantrisin Pediatric Suspension 2770
Genotropin Lyophilized Powder (A small number of patients) 2638
Humatrope Vials and Cartridges 1787
Increlex Injection (3 subjects) 3291
Lithobid Tablets 1692
Lotrisone Cream 3040
Lyrica Capsules (Rare) 2539
Nutropin for Injection 1239
Nutropin AQ Injection 1243
Nutropin AQ Pen 1243
Nutropin AQ Pen Cartridge 1243
Permax Tablets (Rare) 3356
▲ Vesanoid Capsules (9%) 2820
VFEND I.V. (Less than 2%) 2564
VFEND Oral Suspension (Less than 2%) 2564
VFEND Tablets (Less than 2%) 2564

Hypertension, portal

Invirase (Rare) 2772
Myleran Tablets 1525
Tabloid Tablets 1575

Hypertension, rebound

Nitro-Dur Transdermal Infusion System (Uncommon) 3046

Hypertension, supine

▲ ProAmatine Tablets (7.3%) 3186

Hypertensive crises

Avalide Tablets 888
Avalide Tablets 2874
Avapro Tablets (Less than 1%) 891
Avapro Tablets (Less than 1%) 2871
Avastin IV 1227
Cymbalta Delayed-Release Capsules (Very rare) 1757
Imitrex Injection (Rare) 1463
Nexavar Tablets (Uncommon) 746
Rythmol SR Capsules 2727
Sanctura Tablets 1151

Hyperthermia

Ambien CR Tablets (1%) 2855
Biltricide Tablets 2976
Calcijex Injection 411
Effexor Tablets 3411
Elspar for Injection 2463
Elspar for Injection 1960
Hectorol Capsules 1275
Hectorol Injection 1278
Humate-P (Rare) 3502
HyperRAB 3242
HyperRho S/D Mini-Dose 3244
HyperRho S/D Full Dose 3246
HyperTET 3248
MICRhoGAM Ultra-Filtered 2371
Prezista Tablets (Less than 2%) 3306
Proquin XR Tablets (Less than 1%) 1153
Risperdal 1676
Risperdal M-Tab Orally Disintegrating Tablets 1676
Rocaltrol Capsules 2798
Rocaltrol Oral Solution 2798
▲ RotaTeq (14.8% to 42.6%) 2074

Hyperthyroidism

Abilify Oral Solution (Rare) 882
Abilify Oral Solution (Rare) 2450
Abilify Discmelt Orally Disintegrating Tablets (Rare) 882
Abilify Discmelt Orally Disintegrating Tablets (Rare) 2450
Abilify Tablets (Rare) 882
Abilify Tablets (Rare) 2450
Aciphex Tablets 1090
Betaseron for SC Injection 767
Campath Ampules 811
Copaxone for Injection (Infrequent) 3297
Copegus Tablets (Less than 1%) 2754
Cytomel Tablets 1710
Effexor Tablets (Rare) 3411
Effexor XR Capsules (Rare) 3417
Fortical Nasal Spray (Less than 1%) 3337
▲ Intron A for Injection (Less than 5%) 3024
Levoxyl Tablets 1712
Lithobid Tablets 1692
Meridia Capsules 489
Miacalcin Nasal Spray (Less than 1%) 2253
Naturethroid Tablets 3401
Neurontin Capsules (Rare) 2487
Neurontin Oral Solution (Rare) 2487
Neurontin Tablets (Rare) 2487
▲ Ontak Vials (Less than 5%) 1745
Paxil CR Controlled-Release Tablets (Rare) 1538
Paxil (Rare) 1530
Pegasys (Less than 1%) 2789
PEG-Intron Powder for Injection (Less than or equal to 1%) 3048
Pexeva Tablets (rare) 1694
Proleukin for Injection 2266
Requip Tablets (Infrequent) 1555
Seroquel Tablets (Rare) 690
▲ Sutent Capsules (4%) 2560
Synthroid Tablets (Rare) 520
VFEND I.V. (Less than 2%) 2564
VFEND Oral Suspension (Less than 2%) 2564
VFEND Tablets (Less than 2%) 2564
Westhroid Tablets 3403
Zomig Nasal Spray (Rare) 3523

Hypertonia

Abilify Oral Solution 882
Abilify Oral Solution 2450
Abilify Discmelt Orally Disintegrating Tablets 882
Abilify Discmelt Orally Disintegrating Tablets 2450
Abilify Tablets 882
Abilify Tablets 2450
Aceon Tablets (2 mg, 4 mg, 8 mg) (0.2% to 2.7%) 3194
Aciphex Tablets 1090
Actonel Tablets (2.2%) 2683
Actonel with Calcium Tablets (2.2%) 2688
Adalat CC Tablets (Less than 1%) 2964
Aricept Tablets (Infrequent) 1094
Aricept ODT Tablets (Infrequent) 1094
▲ Arimidex Tablets (3%) 673
Arranon Injection (1%) 1357
Arthrotec Tablets (Rare) 3129
▲ Asacol Delayed-Release Tablets (5%) 2692
Avelox (Less than 0.1%) 2970
Axert Tablets (Rare) 2396
Azilect Tablets (Frequent) 3293
Azopt Ophthalmic Suspension (Less than 1%) 557
▲ Betaseron for SC Injection (50%) 767
▲ BOTOX Purified Neurotoxin Complex (2% to 10%) 570
Caduet Tablets (Less than 2%) 2508
Cardene I.V. (Rare) 2497
▲ Carnitor Injection (1% to 3%) 3188
Celebrex Capsules (0.1% to 1.9%) 3134
Celexa (Infrequent) 1176
▲ CellCept Capsules (3% to less than 20%) 2747
▲ CellCept Intravenous (3% to less than 20%) 2747
▲ CellCept Oral Suspension (3% to less than 20%) 2747
▲ CellCept Tablets (3% to less than 20%) 2747
Cipro 2977
Cipro I.V. 2984
Cipro XR Tablets 2990
Colazal Capsules 2838
▲ Copaxone for Injection (22%) 3297
Crestor Tablets (Greater than or equal to 2%) 678
▲ Depacon Injection (1% to 5%) 412
▲ Depakene (1% to 5%) 417
▲ Depakote Sprinkle Capsules (1% to 5%) 422
▲ Depakote Tablets (1% to 5%) 427
▲ Depakote ER Tablets (Greater than 1% to 5%) 434
▲ Doxil Injection (1% to 10%) 2351
Duragesic Transdermal System (Less than 1%) 2373
▲ Effexor Tablets (3%; Infrequent) 3411
Effexor XR Capsules (Infrequent) 3417
▲ Evoxac Capsules (1% to 3%) 1047
Exelon Capsules (Infrequent) 2206
Exelon Oral Solution (Infrequent) 2206
Ferrlecit Injection (Two or more patients) 3388
Frova Tablets (Rare) 1113
Gabitril Tablets (Frequent) 984
▲ Geodon (3% to 14%) 2529
Havrix Vaccine (Less than 1%) 1456
▲ Hectorol Capsules (Greater than or equal to 5%) 1275
Indapamide Tablets (Less than 5%) 2156
▲ Infergen (6% to 7%) 3364
▲ Intron A for Injection (Less than 5%) 3024
▲ Ionsys Transdermal System (1% to less than 10%) 2379
Kaletra (Less than 2%) 476
Klonopin (Infrequent) 2778
Lamictal (Rare) 1481
Levaquin (0.1% to 0.9%) 2384
Levaquin in 5% Dextrose Injection (0.1% to 0.9%) 2384
Levitra Tablets (Less than 2%) 3034
Lexapro Oral Solution (Infrequent) 1190
Lexapro Tablets (Infrequent) 1190
Lipitor Tablets (Less than 2%) 2483
Lithobid Tablets 1692
Lofibra Tablets 1219
Lofibra Capsules 1216
Lotensin Tablets (Less than 1%) 2243
Lotensin HCT Tablets (1.5%) 2246
Lunesta Tablets (Infrequent) 3142
Lyrica Capsules (Greater than or equal to 1%) 2539
Meridia Capsules (Greater than or equal to 1%) 489
Mirapex Tablets (Greater than or equal to 1%) 859
Namenda (Infrequent) 1195
Neurontin Capsules (Rare) 2487
Neurontin Oral Solution (Rare) 2487
Neurontin Tablets (Rare) 2487
Nexium Delayed-Release Capsules (Less than 1%) 655
Nexium I.V. (Less than 1%) 659
Norvasc Tablets (Less than 0.1%) 2545
Paxil CR Controlled-Release Tablets (Infrequent) 1538
Paxil (Infrequent) 1530
▲ PEG-Intron Powder for Injection (5%) 3048
Permax Tablets (1.1%) 3356
Pexeva Tablets (Infrequent) 1694
▲ Premphase Tablets (3%) 3456
▲ Prempro Tablets (3% to 4%) 3456
Prevacid Delayed-Release Capsules (Less than 1%) 3271
Prevacid for Delayed-Release Oral Suspension (Less than 1%) 3271
Prevacid SoluTab Delayed-Release Orally Disintegrating Tablets (Less than 1%) 3271
Prevacid NapraPAC (Less than 1%) 3280
PREVPAC (Less than 1%) 3284
▲ Prograf Capsules and Injection (3% to 15%) 632
Prometrium Capsules (100 mg, 200 mg) (Less than 5%) 3203
Proquin XR Tablets 1153
Protonix I.V. (Greater than or equal to 1%) 3472
Protonix Tablets (Greater than or equal to 1%) 3469
Protopic Ointment (0.2% to less than 1%) 638
Provigil Tablets (1%) 988
Prozac Pulvules and Liquid (Infrequent) 1801
Raniclor Tablets, Chewable (Rare) 2505
▲ Rapamune Oral Solution and Tablets (3% to 20%) 3475
Razadyne (Infrequent) 2399
Razadyne ER Extended-Release Capsules (Infrequent) 2399
▲ Rebif Prefilled Syringe for Injection (6% to 7%) 3159
Relpax Tablets (Frequent) 2548
ReoPro Vials (0.2%) 1809
Requip Tablets (Infrequent) 1555
Rescriptor Tablets 2551
▲ Rilutek Tablets (5.3% to 5.9%) 2930
▲ Risperdal (17% to 34%) 1676
Risperdal Consta Long-Acting Injection (Frequent) 1682
▲ Risperdal M-Tab Orally Disintegrating Tablets (17% to 34%) 1676
Rythmol SR Capsules 2727

▲ Sandostatin LAR Depot (1% to 4%) 2280
Seroquel Tablets (Frequent) 690
Sonata Capsules (1%) 1717
▲ Soriatane Capsules (1% to 10%) 1013
Sular Tablets (Less than or equal to 1%) 3122
Symmetrel Tablets 1135
Tasmar Tablets (1%) 3358
Tequin Injection (Less than 0.1%) 938
Tequin Injection in 5% Dextrose (Less than 0.1%) 938
Tequin Tablets (Less than 0.1%) 938
Thalomid Capsules 965
▲ Topamax Sprinkle Capsules (0% to 3%) 2404
▲ Topamax Tablets (0% to 3%) 2404
Tricor Tablets 527
Ultane Liquid for Inhalation (Less than 1%) 531
Uniretic Tablets (More than 1%) 3100
VFEND I.V. (Less than 2%) 2564
VFEND Oral Suspension (Less than 2%) 2564
VFEND Tablets (Less than 2%) 2564
Viagra Tablets (Less than 2%) 2573
Vicoprofen Tablets (Less than 3%) 539
Wellbutrin SR Sustained-Release Tablets (Infrequent) 1607
Wellbutrin XL Extended-Release Tablets (Infrequent) 1613
Zelapar Tablets 3372
Zoloft (Frequent) 2586
Zomig Tablets (Rare) 3519
Zomig Nasal Spray (Rare to infrequent) 3523
Zomig-ZMT Tablets (Rare) 3519
Zonegran Capsules (Infrequent) 1101
Zyban Sustained-Release Tablets (Infrequent) 1644
Zyflo Tablets (Greater than 1%) 1023
▲ Zyprexa Tablets (4% to 20%) 1830
▲ Zyprexa IntraMuscular (2% to 4%) 1830
▲ Zyprexa ZYDIS Orally Disintegrating Tablets (4% to 20%) 1830
Zyrtec Chewable Tablets (Less than 2%) 2594
Zyrtec (Less than 2%) 2594
Zyrtec-D 12 Hour Extended Release Tablets (Less than 2%) 2597

Hypertrichosis
Analpram-HC 1159
Apexicon E Cream 2661
Celexa (Rare) 1176
Clobevate Gel 3211
Cutivate Ointment (Less than 1%) 2665
Decadron Tablets 1951
Diprolene Lotion 0.05% (Infrequent) 3002
Diprolene Ointment 0.05% (Infrequent) 3003
Diprolene AF Cream 0.05% (Infrequent) 3000
Diprosone Cream, USP 0.05% 3004
Elocon Cream 0.1% (Infrequent) 3005
Elocon Lotion 0.1% (Infrequent) 3006
Elocon Ointment 0.1% (Infrequent) 3007
Finacea Gel (Rare) 1669
▲ Gengraf Capsules (6.6% to 15%) 459
Locoid Lipocream Cream (Infrequent) 1160
Lotrisone 3040
▲ Neoral Oral Solution (6.6% to 15%) 2259
▲ Neoral Soft Gelatin Capsules (6.6% to 15%) 2259
Olux Foam 1012
Phenytek Capsules 2160
Pramosone 1161
ProctoFoam-HC 3099
Risperdal (Rare) 1676
Risperdal M-Tab Orally Disintegrating Tablets (Rare) 1676
▲ Simulect for Injection (3% to 10%) 2284
Soriatane Capsules (Less than 1%) 1013
Temovate Gel (Infrequent) 2669
Temovate Scalp Application (Infrequent) 2670
Temovate E Emollient (Infrequent) 2671
Topamax Sprinkle Capsules (2%) 2404
Topamax Tablets (2%) 2404
Vanos Cream 1893
Zoloft (Rare) 2586
Zyrtec Chewable Tablets (Less than 2%) 2594
Zyrtec (Less than 2%) 2594
Zyrtec-D 12 Hour Extended Release Tablets (Less than 2%) 2597

Hypertriglyceridemia
Accutane Capsules 2731
Aceon Tablets (2 mg, 4 mg, 8 mg) (1.3%) 3194
▲ Agenerase Capsules (8% to 13%) 1327
▲ Agenerase Oral Solution (8% to 13%) 1332
▲ AndroGel (3% to 6%) 3329
Angeliq Tablets 762
▲ Aptivus Capsules (6.1% to 26.2%) 826
Atacand Tablets (0.5% or greater) 649
Atacand HCT 651
▲ Atripla Tablets (4%) 945
Benicar HCT Tablets 1044
Betaseron for SC Injection 767
Blocadren Tablets 1916
Carbatrol Capsules (Occasional) 3171
Cipro 2977
▲ Cipro I.V. (Among most frequent) 2984
Climara Transdermal System 771
Climara Pro Transdermal System 776
Clozaril Tablets (Rare) 2184
Coreg Tablets (Greater than 0.1% to 1%) 1414
Crixivan Capsules 1940
Cymbalta Delayed-Release Capsules (Infrequent) 1757
Edex Injection (2%) 3089
▲ Emtriva Capsules (9% to 10%) 1287
▲ Emtriva Oral Solution (9% to 10%) 1287
Enjuvia Tablets 1062
Epzicom Tablets 1436
Equetro Extended-Release Capsules 3180
Estrasorb Topical Emulsion 1147
Estratest Tablets 3199
Estratest H.S. Tablets 3199
Evoxac Capsules (Less than 1%) 1047
FazaClo Orally Disintegrating Tablets (Very Rare) 551
Fuzeon Injection 2767
▲ Gengraf Capsules (About 15%) 459
Hyzaar 50-12.5 Tablets 1990
Hyzaar 100-12.5 Tablets 1990
Hyzaar 100-25 Tablets 1990
▲ Infergen (5% to 6%) 3364
▲ Inspra Tablets (1% to 15%) 2536
▲ Intron A for Injection (Less than 5%) 3024
▲ Kaletra (9% to 36%) 476
Lovenox Injection 2915
▲ Lupron Depot 3.75 mg (12%) 3260
▲ Lupron Depot–3 Month 11.25 mg (32%) 3265
Menostar Transdermal System 782
▲ Neoral Oral Solution (About 15%) 2259
▲ Neoral Soft Gelatin Capsules (About 15%) 2259
Noroxin Tablets 2032
▲ Norvir (1.3% to 33.6%) 503
Ortho-Cyclen/Ortho Tri-Cyclen 2429
Ortho Tri-Cyclen Lo Tablets 2436
▲ Pegasys (20%) 2789
PEG-Intron Powder for Injection 3048
Premarin Intravenous 3442
Premarin Tablets 3446
Premarin Vaginal Cream 3452
Premphase Tablets 3456
Prempro Tablets 3456
▲ Prezista Tablets (18.9% to 25.4%) 3306
Prinzide Tablets 2056
Rapamune Oral Solution and Tablets 3475
Rebetron Combination Therapy 3063
Rescriptor Tablets 2551
Risperdal (Rare) 1676
Risperdal M-Tab Orally Disintegrating Tablets (Rare) 1676
Rythmol SR Capsules 2727
▲ Simulect for Injection (3% to 10%) 2284
Soltamox Oral Solution (Very rare) 3527
Soriatane Capsules (Less common) 1013
Sustiva Capsules 930
Sustiva Tablets 930
▲ Targretin Capsules (Approximately 70%) 1747
Tegretol/Tegretol-XR (Occasional) 2295
Teveten Tablets (1%) 1735
Teveten HCT Tablets (Less than 1%) 1737
Ticlid Tablets 2810
Timolide Tablets 2086
Trizivir Tablets 1589
▲ Truvada Tablets (4%) 1296
▲ Vesanoid Capsules (Up to 60%) 2820
▲ Viread Tablets (8% to 11%) 1301
WelChol Tablets 1050
▲ Xeloda Tablets (Less than 5%) 2822
▲ Ziagen (2% to 6%) 1626
▲ Zoloft (Approximately 5%) 2586
Zyprexa Tablets (Rare) 1830
Zyprexa IntraMuscular (Rare) 1830
Zyprexa ZYDIS Orally Disintegrating Tablets (Rare) 1830

Hypertrophic papillae of the tongue
Primaxin I.M. 2045
Primaxin I.V. (Less than 0.2%) 2048

Hypertrophy, endometrial
Exelon Capsules (Infrequent) 2206
Exelon Oral Solution (Infrequent) 2206

Hypertrophy, thymus
▲ Increlex (Greater than or equal to 5%) 3291

Hypertrophy, unspecified
Kaletra (Less than 2%) 476

Hyperuricemia
Abelcet Injection 1141
Abilify Oral Solution (Infrequent) 882
Abilify Oral Solution (Infrequent) 2450
Abilify Discmelt Orally Disintegrating Tablets (Infrequent) 882
Abilify Discmelt Orally Disintegrating Tablets (Infrequent) 2450
Abilify Tablets (Infrequent) 882
Abilify Tablets (Infrequent) 2450
Accutane Capsules 2731
Aceon Tablets (2 mg, 4 mg, 8 mg) (0.3% to 1%) 3194
Advicor Tablets 1722
Aldoril Tablets 1910
Aloprim for Injection (Less than 1%) 2167
Altace Capsules 1702
Arthrotec Tablets (Rare) 3129
Atacand Tablets (0.6%) 649
Atacand HCT (0.5% or greater) 651
Avalide Tablets 888
Avalide Tablets 2874
Avelox (Less than 0.1%) 2970
Axid Oral Solution 879
Benicar Tablets (Greater than 0.5%) 1043
▲ Benicar HCT Tablets (4%) 1044
Betaseron for SC Injection 767
Blocadren Tablets 1916
▲ Bumex Tablets (18.4%) 2746
Campral Tablets (Infrequent) 1174
Cardizem LA Extended Release Tablets (Less than 2%) 1728
▲ CellCept Capsules (3% to less than 20%) 2747
▲ CellCept Intravenous (3% to less than 20%) 2747
▲ CellCept Oral Suspension (3% to less than 20%) 2747
▲ CellCept Tablets (3% to less than 20%) 2747
Cipro (Less than 0.1%) 2977
▲ Cipro I.V. (Among most frequent) 2984
Clorpres Tablets 2153
Clozaril Tablets 2184
▲ Coreg Tablets (Greater than 1% to 3%) 1414
Creon 5 Capsules 3198
Creon 10 Capsules 3198
Creon 20 Capsules 3199
Daranide Tablets 1950
Demadex Injection 2759
Demadex Tablets 2759
Diovan HCT Tablets 2196
Diuril Oral Suspension 1954
Diuril Sodium Intravenous 2467
▲ Doxil Injection (1% to 5%) 2351
Dyazide Capsules 1423
Edecrin 1959
Effexor Tablets (Infrequent) 3411
Effexor XR Capsules (Infrequent) 3417
Evoxac Capsules (Less than 1%) 1047
FazaClo Orally Disintegrating Tablets 551
Furosemide Tablets 2154
Gengraf Capsules (1% to less than 3%) 459
Geodon Capsules (Rare) 2529
Hyzaar 50-12.5 Tablets 1990
Hyzaar 100-12.5 Tablets 1990
Hyzaar 100-25 Tablets 1990
▲ Imdur Tablets (Less than or equal to 5%) 3018
▲ Indapamide Tablets (Less than 5%) 2156
Inspra Tablets (0.3%) 2536
▲ Kaletra (Up to 3%) 476
Lofibra Tablets 1219
Lofibra Capsules 1216
Lopressor HCT 50/25 Tablets 2241
Lopressor HCT 100/25 Tablets 2241
Lopressor HCT 100/50 Tablets 2241
Lotensin HCT Tablets 2246
Lotrel Capsules (Rare) 2249
▲ Lupron Depot 7.5 mg (Greater than or equal to 5%) 3264
Lupron Injection Pediatric 3259
▲ Mavik Tablets (15%) 486
Micardis HCT Tablets 856
Moduretic Tablets 2028
▲ Myfortic Tablets (3% to less than 20%) 2255
Myleran Tablets 1525
Neoral Oral Solution (1% to less than 3%) 2259
Neoral Soft Gelatin Capsules (1% to less than 3%) 2259
▲ Neulasta Injection (8%) 601
▲ Neupogen for Injection (27% to 58%) 603
Nexium Delayed-Release Capsules (Less than 1%) 655
Nexium I.V. (Less than 1%) 659
▲ Norvir (3.8%) 503
▲ Oncaspar (Greater than 1% but less than 5%) 1145
Pancrease MT Capsules 1885
▲ PEG-Intron Powder for Injection (33% to 38%) 3048
Permax Tablets (Rare) 3356
Plavix Tablets (1% to 2.5%) 917
Plavix Tablets (1% to 2.5%) 2926
Pletal Tablets (Less than 2%) 2455
▲ Prezista Tablets (2.2% to 6.9%) 3306
Prinzide Tablets 2056
▲ Prograf Capsules and Injection (3% to 15%) 632
▲ Proleukin for Injection (9%) 2266
Prozac Pulvules and Liquid (Rare) 1801
Rapamune Oral Solution and Tablets 3475
▲ Rebetol (33% to 38%) 3058
Rebetron Combination Therapy 3063
Requip Tablets (Infrequent) 1555
Rescriptor Tablets 2551
Risperdal (Rare) 1676
Risperdal Consta Long-Acting Injection (Infrequent) 1682
Risperdal M-Tab Orally Disintegrating Tablets (Rare) 1676
Rituxan I.V. 1254
Rythmol SR Capsules 2727
Sandimmune (Occasional) 2275
▲ Simulect for Injection (Greater than or equal to 10%) 2284
Sonata Capsules (Rare) 1717
St. Joseph 81 mg Aspirin Chewable and Enteric Coated Tablets 1869
Starlix Tablets 2292
▲ Sutent Capsules (10%) 2560
Tabloid Tablets (Frequent) 1575
Teveten HCT Tablets 1737
Thalomid Capsules 965
Tiazac Capsules (Less than 2%) 1201
Timolide Tablets 2086
Tricor Tablets 527
Triglide Tablets 3123
Ultrase Capsules 708
Ultrase MT Capsules 709
Uniretic Tablets (More than 1%) 3100
Univasc Tablets 3104
VFEND I.V. (Less than 2%) 2564
VFEND Oral Suspension (Less than 2%) 2564
VFEND Tablets (Less than 2%) 2564
Viagra Tablets (Less than 2%) 2573
Viokase 711
Viracept (Less than 2%) 2577
Xyrem Oral Solution (Infrequent) 1688
Zyprexa Tablets (Infrequent) 1830
Zyprexa ZYDIS Orally Disintegrating Tablets (Infrequent) 1830

Hyperuricosuria
Creon 5 Capsules 3198
Creon 10 Capsules 3198
Creon 20 Capsules 3199
Myleran Tablets 1525
Pancrease MT Capsules 1885
Ultrase Capsules 708
Ultrase MT Capsules 709

Hyperuricuria
Viokase 711

Hyperventilation
Aciphex Tablets 1090
Actiq (Less than 1%) 979
Adenocard Injection (Less than 1%) 617
AmBisome for Injection (Less common) 620
Aricept Tablets (Infrequent) 1094
Aricept ODT Tablets (Infrequent) 1094
Arthrotec Tablets (Rare) 3129
Axert Tablets (Rare) 2396
Bumex Tablets (0.1%) 2746
Clozaril Tablets (Less than 1%) 2184

Copaxone for Injection (Frequent)..... 3297
Doxil Injection (Less than 1%)........... 2351
Effexor Tablets (Infrequent)............. 3411
Effexor XR Capsules (Infrequent)...... 3417
FazaClo Orally Disintegrating Tablets (Less than 1%)................. 551
Frova Tablets (Infrequent)................ 1113
Gabitril Tablets (Infrequent).............. 984
Ionsys Transdermal System (.1% to less than 1%)........................... 2379
▲ I.V. Busulfex (2% to 3%) 2493
Lamictal (Infrequent)....................... 1481
Neurontin Capsules (Rare)............... 2487
Neurontin Oral Solution (Rare).......... 2487
Neurontin Tablets (Rare).................. 2487
▲ Niravam Orally Disintegrating Tablets (9.7%)........................... 3092
Orthoclone OKT3 Sterile Solution..... 2360
Paxil CR Controlled-Release Tablets (Infrequent)...................... 1538
Paxil (Infrequent)............................. 1530
Permax Tablets (Infrequent)............ 3356
Pexeva Tablets (infrequent)............. 1694
Primaxin I.M.................................... 2045
Primaxin I.V. (Less than 0.2%).......... 2048
Prochieve 4% Gel........................... 1003
Prochieve 8% Gel........................... 1003
ProSom Tablets (Rare).................... 517
Prozac Pulvules and Liquid (Infrequent)................................ 1801
Relpax Tablets (Rare)...................... 2548
Rilutek Tablets (Infrequent)............... 2930
Risperdal (Infrequent)...................... 1676
Risperdal M-Tab Orally Disintegrating Tablets (Infrequent)................................ 1676
▲ Romazicon Injection (3% to 9%) 2804
Seroquel Tablets (Rare).................. 690
Sonata Capsules (Rare)................... 1717
Sulfamylon Cream........................... 2162
Sulfamylon for 5% Topical Solution... 2162
Symbyax Capsules (Infrequent)......... 1819
Tasmar Tablets (Infrequent)............. 3358
Tequin Injection (Less than 0.1%)..... 938
Tequin Injection in 5% Dextrose (Less than 0.1%)........................ 938
Tequin Tablets (Less than 0.1%)....... 938
▲ TOBI Solution for Inhalation (5.4%) .. 2298
Ultane Liquid for Inhalation (Less than 1%).................................. 531
Xyrem Oral Solution (Infrequent)....... 1688
Zoloft (Rare)..................................... 2586
Zomig Nasal Spray (Rare)................ 3523
Zyprexa Tablets (Infrequent)............ 1830
Zyprexa ZYDIS Orally Disintegrating Tablets (Infrequent)............................... 1830
Zyrtec Chewable Tablets (Less than 2%)................................ 2594
Zyrtec (Less than 2%)...................... 2594
Zyrtec-D 12 Hour Extended Release Tablets (Less than 2%)..... 2597

Hyperviscosity syndrome

Rituxan I.V. 1254

Hypervolemia

Aloprim for Injection (Less than 1%)... 2167
▲ AmBisome for Injection (8.2% to 12.2%)... 620
▲ Carnitor Injection (3% to 12%) 3188
▲ CellCept Capsules (3% to less than 20%).................................... 2747
▲ CellCept Intravenous (3% to less than 20%).................................... 2747
▲ CellCept Oral Suspension (3% to less than 20%)............................ 2747
▲ CellCept Tablets (3% to less than 20%).. 2747
▲ Coreg Tablets (Greater than 1% to 3%).. 1414
Ferrlecit Injection............................. 3388
I.V. Busulfex.................................... 2493
Merrem I.V. (Greater than 0.1% to 1%).. 686
▲ Prograf Capsules and Injection (3% to 15%)................................. 632
▲ Rapamune Oral Solution and Tablets (3% to 20%).................... 3475
Trasylol Injection (1% to 2%)............ 754
VFEND I.V. (Less than 2%)............... 2564
VFEND Oral Suspension (Less than 2%)... 2564
VFEND Tablets (Less than 2%).......... 2564

Hypesthesia

(*see also under* Hypoesthesia)

Ionsys Transdermal System (.1% to less than 1%).......................... 2379

Hypnagogic effects

▲ Advair Diskus 100/50 (1% to 3%) ... 1308
▲ Advair Diskus 250/50 (1% to 3%) ... 1308
▲ Advair Diskus 500/50 (1% to 3%) ... 1308
Lotronex Tablets (Infrequent)............ 1512

Hypoactivity

▲ Aerobid/Aerobid-M (1% to 3%) 1171
▲ Flumist Vaccine (10.6 to 14%) 1901

Hypoacusis

▲ Increlex Injection (Greater than or equal to 5%)................................ 3291
VFEND I.V. (Less than 2%)................ 2564
VFEND Oral Suspension (Less than 2%)... 2564
VFEND Tablets (Less than 2%).......... 2564

Hypoadrenalism

Sandostatin Injection (Less than 1%).. 2278
Sandostatin LAR Depot (Rare).......... 2280

Hypoadrenalism, neonatal

Azmacort Inhalation Aerosol............ 1726
Decadron Tablets............................. 1951
Hydrocortone Tablets....................... 1989
Pulmicort Respules.......................... 661

Hypoalbuminemia

▲ Arranon Injection (1% to 10%) 1357
Baraclude (0% to less than 1%)......... 894
Campath Ampules............................. 811
▲ Cancidas for Injection (4.6% to 8.6%).. 1918
▲ Dacogen Injection (24%) 2129
Dapsone Tablets USP...................... 1673
Emend Capsules (Greater than 0.5%)... 1963
Evista Tablets.................................. 1763
▲ Gleevec Tablets (0% to 4%) 2227
▲ Leukine (27%) 814
▲ Lupron Depot 7.5 mg (Greater than or equal to 5%).................... 3264
Oncaspar 1145
▲ Ontak Vials (83%) 1745
▲ Prezista Tablets (3.1% to 4.3%) 3306
▲ Proleukin for Injection (8%) 2266
Vantin Tablets and Oral Suspension 2645
Zosyn.. 3492

Hypoalbuminuria

Elspar for Injection........................... 2463
Elspar for Injection........................... 1960
Invanz for Injection (0.9% to 1.7%)... 1999

Hypoasthesia

▲ Revlimid Capsules (6.8%) 958

Hypocalcemia

Abelcet Injection.............................. 1141
Actiq (Less than 1%)........................ 979
Actonel Tablets (0.8%)..................... 2683
Actonel with Calcium Tablets (0.8%)... 2688
Aloprim for Injection (Less than 1%)... 2167
▲ AmBisome for Injection (4.9% to 18.4%)... 620
Angeliq Tablets................................ 762
▲ Aredia for Injection (Up to 12%) 2179
▲ Arranon Injection (1% to 8%) 1357
Azilect Tablets (Infrequent)............... 3293
Betaseron for SC Injection............... 767
Cancidas for Injection (0% to 1.9%)... 1918
▲ CellCept Capsules (3% to 30%) 2747
▲ CellCept Intravenous (3% to 30%) ... 2747
▲ CellCept Oral Suspension (3% to 30%).. 2747
▲ CellCept Tablets (3% to 30%) 2747
Climara Transdermal System........... 771
Climara Pro Transdermal System..... 776
Colazal Capsules............................ 2838
Cosmegen for Injection.................... 2459
▲ Doxil Injection (1% to 5%) 2351
Enjuvia Tablets................................ 1062
Equetro Extended-Release Capsules.................................... 3180
Estrasorb Topical Emulsion.............. 1147
Estratest Tablets.............................. 3199
Estratest H.S. Tablets...................... 3199
Ethyol for Injection (Rare)................. 1898
Evista Tablets.................................. 1763
Fleet Enema.................................... 1165
Fleet Phospho-soda......................... 1166
Fleet Phospho-soda ACCU-PREP...... 1168
Fleet Phospho-soda EZ-PREP........... 1169
Fleet Prep Kits................................. 1170
▲ Fosamax (Approximately 18%) 1969
▲ Fosamax Plus D Tablets (18%) 1977
Frova Tablets (Rare)......................... 1113
Furosemide Tablets.......................... 2154
Garamycin Injectable........................ 3014
Geodon Capsules (Rare).................. 2529
▲ Invirase (Less than 1% to 4%) 2772
Ionsys Transdermal System (.1% to less than 1%).......................... 2379
▲ I.V. Busulfex (3% to 49%) 2493
Kionex Powder 2477
Leukine (2%).................................... 814
▲ Mavik Tablets (4.7%) 486
Maxipime for Injection (Greater than 0.1% to less than 1%)........... 1105
Menostar Transdermal System........ 782
Mycamine for Injection (1.2% to 1.9%)... 628
▲ Myfortic Tablets (3% to less than 20%).. 2255
▲ Mylotarg for Injection (10% to 12%)... 3431
▲ NeoProfen Injection (12%) 2472
Omnicef for Oral Suspension (0.5%)... 511
▲ Ontak Vials (17%) 1745
Paxil CR Controlled-Release Tablets (Rare)............................ 1538
Paxil (Rare)..................................... 1530
Pexeva Tablets (Rare)..................... 1694
Precose Tablets............................... 751
Premarin Tablets.............................. 3446
Premarin Vaginal Cream.................. 3452
Premphase Tablets.......................... 3456
Prempro Tablets.............................. 3456
▲ Prezista Tablets (0% to 4%) 3306
▲ Prograf Capsules and Injection (3% to 15%)................................ 632
▲ Proleukin for Injection (11%) 2266
Prozac Pulvules and Liquid (Rare)..... 1801
▲ Rapamune Oral Solution and Tablets (3% to 20%)..................... 3475
Rescriptor Tablets............................ 2551
Revlimid Capsules (0.3% to 2.3%).... 958
Rituxan I.V. 1254
▲ Simulect for Injection (3% to 10%) ... 2284
Targretin Capsules.......................... 1747
Tegretol-XR Tablets......................... 2295
Thalomid Capsules.......................... 965
Topamax Sprinkle Capsules (Infrequent)............................... 2404
Topamax Tablets (Infrequent).......... 2404
Trileptal Tablets............................... 2300
Trileptal Oral Suspension................. 2300
▲ Trisenox Injection (10%) 993
Tygacil for Injection (0% to less than 2%).. 3488
Uniretic Tablets (Less than 1%)........ 3100
▲ Valcyte Tablets (Less than 5%) 2813
VFEND I.V. (Less than 2%)............... 2564
VFEND Oral Suspension (Less than 2%)... 2564
VFEND Tablets (Less than 2%)......... 2564
Xeloda Tablets (2.3%)...................... 2822
Xyrem Oral Solution (Infrequent)...... 1688
▲ Zometa for Intravenous Infusion (0.6% to less than 15%)............... 2315
Zosyn.. 3492

Hypochloremia

▲ CellCept Capsules (3% to less than 20%).................................... 2747
▲ CellCept Intravenous (3% to less than 20%).................................... 2747
▲ CellCept Oral Suspension (3% to less than 20%)............................ 2747
▲ CellCept Tablets (3% to less than 20%).. 2747
Demadex Injection........................... 2759
Demadex Tablets............................. 2759
Doxil Injection (Less than 1%)........... 2351
Dyazide Capsules............................ 1423
Geodon Capsules (Rare).................. 2529
▲ Indapamide Tablets (Less than 5%)... 2156
Requip Tablets (Rare)...................... 1555
Uniretic Tablets (Less than 1%)........ 3100

Hypochloremic alkalosis

Diuril Sodium Intravenous................ 2467
Furosemide Tablets.......................... 2154
Prinzide Tablets............................... 2056
Teveten HCT Tablets........................ 1737

Hypocholesterolemia

Bumex Tablets (0.4%)....................... 2746
Evista Tablets.................................. 1763
Geodon Capsules (Rare).................. 2529
Prevacid Delayed-Release Capsules.. 3271
Prevacid for Delayed-Release Oral Suspension.................................... 3271
Prevacid SoluTab Delayed-Release Orally Disintegrating Tablets......... 3271
Prevacid NapraPAC.......................... 3280
PREVPAC... 3284
Proleukin for Injection (1%)............... 2266
▲ Simulect for Injection (Greater than or equal to 10%).................. 2284
Topamax Sprinkle Capsules (Rare)... 2404
Topamax Tablets (Rare)................... 2404

Hypoesthesia

Abilify Oral Solution (Infrequent)....... 882
Abilify Oral Solution (Infrequent)....... 2450
Abilify Discmelt Orally Disintegrating Tablets (Infrequent)....................................... 882
Abilify Discmelt Orally Disintegrating Tablets (Infrequent)....................................... 2450
Abilify Tablets (Infrequent)................ 882
Abilify Tablets (Infrequent)................ 2450
Actiq (1% or greater)......................... 979
ADACEL Vaccine.............................. 2945
Adalat CC Tablets (Less than 1%)..... 2964
Alinia for Oral Suspension (Less than 1%).. 2835
Alinia Tablets (Less than 1%)............ 2835
Ambien Tablets (Infrequent).............. 2851
Ambien CR Tablets (Infrequent to 2%)... 2855
Amerge Tablets (Rare)..................... 1339
▲ Amitiza Capsules (0.5% to 3.4%) 3224
▲ Aromasin Tablets (2% to 5%) 2600
▲ Arranon Injection (0% to 17%) 1357
Arthrotec Tablets (Rare)................... 3129
Astelin Nasal Spray (Infrequent) 1904
Atacand HCT (0.5% or greater) 651
Atripla Tablets 945
Avelox (Less than 0.1%) 2970
Azilect Tablets (Infrequent) 3293
Caduet Tablets (Greater than 0.1% to less than 2%)............................ 2508
Campral Tablets (Infrequent) 1174
Cardene I.V. (0.7%) 2497
Cardura XL Tablets 2515
Caverject Impulse Injection (Less than 1%) 2612
Celebrex Capsules (0.1% to 1.9%) ... 3134
Celexa (Infrequent) 1176
Cialis Tablets (Less than 2%) 1838
Cipro 2977
Cipro I.V. 2984
Cipro XR Tablets 2990
Colazal Capsules 2838
Copaxone for Injection (At least 2%) 3297
▲ Coreg Tablets (Greater than 1% to 3%) 1414
▲ Cozaar Tablets (Less than 1% to 5%) 1935
Cymbalta Delayed-Release Capsules (Infrequent) 1757
Denavir Cream (0.9%) 2174
Depacon Injection (0.6%) 412
Depakene 417
Depakote Sprinkle Capsules 422
Depakote Tablets 427
Depakote ER Tablets 434
▲ DepoDur Extended-Release Injection (2% to 5%) 1110
Effexor Tablets 3411
▲ Emend Capsules (Greater than 0.5%) 1963
Engerix-B Vaccine 1425
▲ Evoxac Capsules (1% to 3%) 1047
Exelon Capsules (Infrequent) 2206
Exelon Oral Solution (Infrequent) 2206
Ferrlecit Injection 3388
Floxin Otic Solution (Single report) ... 1049
Fluarix 1451
Flumadine 1183
Frova Tablets (Infrequent) 1113
Gabitril Tablets (Frequent) 984
Gengraf Capsules (1% to less than 3%) 459
Geodon Capsules (2%) 2529
▲ Humatrope Vials and Cartridges (Up to 6.25%) 1787
Hyzaar 50-12.5 Tablets 1990
Hyzaar 100-12.5 Tablets 1990
Hyzaar 100-25 Tablets 1990
▲ Imdur Tablets (Less than or equal to 5%) 3018
▲ Infergen (8% to 10%) 3364
▲ Intron A for Injection (Up to 10%) 3024
Invanz for Injection (Greater than 0.1%) 1999
Kadian Capsules (Less than 3%) 577
▲ Kepivance (12%) 597
Klonopin (Infrequent) 2778
Lamictal (Infrequent) 1481
Levaquin (0.1% to 0.9%) 2384
Levaquin in 5% Dextrose Injection (0.1% to 0.9%) 2384
Levitra Tablets (Less than 2%) 3034
Lidoderm Patch 1118
Lipitor Tablets (Less than 2%) 2483
Lotensin HCT Tablets (0.3% or more) 2246
Lotronex Tablets (Rare) 1512
Lunesta Tablets (Infrequent) 3142
Lupron Depot 3.75 mg 3260
Lupron Depot–3 Month 11.25 mg 3265
Lyrica Capsules (Greater than or equal to 1%) 2539

Maxalt Tablets (Frequent) 2008
Maxalt-MLT Orally Disintegrating Tablets (Frequent) 2008
▲ Megace ES Oral Suspension (1% to 3%) 2481
Meridia Capsules 489
Micardis Tablets (More than 0.3%) 854
Micardis HCT Tablets 856
Migranal Nasal Spray (Infrequent) 3348
▲ Mirapex Tablets (Greater than or equal to 1% to 3%) 859
Namenda (Infrequent) 1195
Neoral Oral Solution (1% to less than 3%) 2259
Neoral Soft Gelatin Capsules (1% to less than 3%) 2259
Neurontin Capsules (1.2%) 2487
Neurontin Oral Solution (1.2%) 2487
Neurontin Tablets (1.2%) 2487
Nexium Delayed-Release Capsules (Less than 1%) 655
Nexium I.V. (Less than 1%) 659
Noroxin Tablets 2032
Norvasc Tablets (More than 0.1% to 1%) 2545
OxyContin Tablets (Less than 1%) 2703
Paxil CR Controlled-Release Tablets (Infrequent) 1538
Paxil (Infrequent) 1530
Pexeva Tablets (infrequent) 1694
Plavix Tablets (1% to 2.5%) 917
Plavix Tablets (1% to 2.5%) 2926
Prevacid Delayed-Release Capsules (Less than 1%) 3271
Prevacid for Delayed-Release Oral Suspension (Less than 1%) 3271
Prevacid SoluTab Delayed-Release Orally Disintegrating Tablets (Less than 1%) 3271
Prevacid NapraPAC (Less than 1%) 3280
PREVPAC (Less than 1%) 3284
Prezista Tablets (Less than 2%) 3306
Proquin XR Tablets 1153
Protonix I.V. (Less than 1%) 3472
Protonix Tablets (Less than 1%) 3469
Prozac Pulvules and Liquid (Infrequent) 1801
Ranexa Tablets (Less than or equal to 0.5%) 1035
▲ Rapamune Oral Solution and Tablets (3% to 20%) 3475
Recombivax HB 2071
ReoPro Vials (0.3%) 1809
Requip Tablets (Infrequent) 1555
Rescriptor Tablets 2551
Reyataz Capsules (Less than 3%) 921
Rilutek Tablets (Infrequent) 2930
Risperdal (Rare to 2%) 1676
Risperdal Consta Long-Acting Injection (Up to 2%) 1682
Risperdal M-Tab Orally Disintegrating Tablets (Rare to 2%) 1676
▲ Romazicon Injection (1% to 3%) 2804
▲ Sandostatin LAR Depot (5% to 15%) 2280
▲ Simulect for Injection (3% to 10%) 2284
Singulair 2077
Sonata Capsules (Less than 1% to 2%) 1717
Soriatane Capsules (Less than 1%) 1013
Sular Tablets (Less than or equal to 1%) 3122
Sustiva Capsules (1% to 2%) 930
Sustiva Tablets (1% to 2%) 930
Symbyax Capsules (Infrequent) 1819
▲ Tambocor Tablets (1% to 3%) 1856
Targretin Capsules 1747
Tarka Tablets (Less frequent) 524
Tasmar Tablets (Frequent) 3358
Tequin Injection 938
Tequin Injection in 5% Dextrose 938
Tequin Tablets 938
▲ Topamax Sprinkle Capsules (1% to 8%) 2404
▲ Topamax Tablets (1% to 8%) 2404
▲ Trileptal Tablets (1% to 3%) 2300
▲ Trileptal Oral Suspension (1% to 3%) 2300
▲ Ultram ER Tablets (1% to greater than 5%) 2392
Uniretic Tablets (Less than 1%) 3100
VFEND I.V. (Less than 2%) 2564
VFEND Oral Suspension (Less than 2%) 2564
VFEND Tablets (Less than 2%) 2564
Viagra Tablets (Less than 2%) 2573
▲ Visudyne for Injection (1% to 10%) 2305
Wellbutrin SR Sustained-Release Tablets (Infrequent) 1607
Wellbutrin XL Extended-Release Tablets (Infrequent) 1613
▲ Xeloda Tablets (Less than 1% to 4%) 2822
Xopenex Inhalation Solution 3146
Xopenex Inhalation Solution Concentrate 3150
Xopenex HFA Inhalation Aerosol 3154
▲ Xyrem Oral Solution (Less than 1% to 5.9%) 1688
Zoloft (Frequent) 2586
▲ Zometa for Intravenous Infusion (12%) 2315
Zyban Sustained-Release Tablets (Infrequent) 1644
Zyprexa Tablets (Infrequent) 1830
Zyprexa ZYDIS Orally Disintegrating Tablets (Infrequent) 1830
Zyrtec Chewable Tablets (Less than 2%) 2594
Zyrtec (Less than 2%) 2594
Zyrtec-D 12 Hour Extended Release Tablets (Less than 2%) 2597

Hypoestrogeneism

▲ Lupron Depot 3.75 mg (Among most frequent) 3260
Lupron Depot–3 Month 11.25 mg 3265
Neurontin Capsules (Rare) 2487
Neurontin Oral Solution (Rare) 2487
Neurontin Tablets (Rare) 2487

Hypofibrinogenemia

Depacon Injection 412
Depakene 417
Depakote Sprinkle Capsules 422
Depakote Tablets 427
Depakote ER Tablets 434
Elspar for Injection 2463
Elspar for Injection 1960
Gantrisin Pediatric Suspension 2770
Lamictal (Rare) 1481
NovoSeven (Greater than or equal to 2%) 2331
Oncaspar 1145
Panhematin for Injection 2473

Hypogeusia

Cuprimine Capsules (Some patients) 1947
Thiola Tablets 2141

Hypoglycemia

Abelcet Injection 1141
Abilify Oral Solution (Infrequent) 882
Abilify Oral Solution (Infrequent) 2450
Abilify Discmelt Orally Disintegrating Tablets (Infrequent) 882
Abilify Discmelt Orally Disintegrating Tablets (Infrequent) 2450
Abilify Tablets (Infrequent) 882
Abilify Tablets (Infrequent) 2450
Actiq (Less than 1%) 979
▲ Actos Tablets (8% to 15%) 3219
Aggrenox Capsules 822
Anaprox Tablets (Less than 1%) 2761
Anaprox DS Tablets (Less than 1%) 2761
Apidra Injection 2864
▲ Arranon Injection (0% to 6%) 1357
Arthrotec Tablets (Rare) 3129
▲ Avandamet Tablets (3%) 1373
Avandaryl Tablets (0.9% to 1.7%) 1379
▲ Avandia Tablets (0.6% to 4%) 1384
Avelox (Greater than or equal to 2%) 2970
Bayer Aspirin 744
Bayer Aspirin Comprehensive Prescribing Information ■796
Biaxin/Biaxin XL (Rare) 402
Blocadren Tablets 1916
▲ Byetta Injection (3.3% to 35.7%) 611
Caduet Tablets (Less than 2%) 2508
Cafcit 1886
Campath Ampules 811
Celebrex Capsules (Less than 0.1%) 3134
Celexa (Rare) 1176
▲ CellCept Capsules (3% to less than 20%) 2747
▲ CellCept Intravenous (3% to less than 20%) 2747
▲ CellCept Oral Suspension (3% to less than 20%) 2747
▲ CellCept Tablets (3% to less than 20%) 2747
Chantix Tablets (Rare) 2517
Cipro (Less than 0.1%) 2977
Cipro I.V. (Rare) 2984
Cipro XR Tablets 2990
▲ Coreg Tablets (5% to 12%) 1414
Cosopt Sterile Ophthalmic Solution 1931
▲ Cozaar Tablets (14%) 1935
Cubicin for Injection (1% to 2%) 1026
Cuprimine Capsules 1947
Cymbalta Delayed-Release Capsules (Frequent) 1757
Doxil Injection (Less than 1%) 2351
▲ Duetact Tablets (Greater than 5%) 3226
EC-Naprosyn Delayed-Release Tablets (Less than 1%) 2761
Edecrin (In 2 uremic patients) 1959
Effexor Tablets (Infrequent) 3411
Effexor XR Capsules (Infrequent) 3417
Epivir 1427
Evoxac Capsules (Less than 1%) 1047
Exelon Capsules (Infrequent) 2206
Exelon Oral Solution (Infrequent) 2206
Exubera Inhalation Powder 2524
Ferrlecit Injection 3388
Frova Tablets (Rare) 1113
Gabitril Tablets (Infrequent) 984
Gantrisin Pediatric Suspension 2770
Gengraf Capsules (1% to less than 3%) 459
Geodon Capsules (Rare) 2529
Herceptin I.V. (At least one of the 958 patients) 1233
▲ Humalog-Pen (Most common) 1781
Humalog Mix 50/50-Pen 1783
Humalog Mix 75/25-Pen 1785
Humulin 50/50, 100 Units 1791
Humulin 70/30 Pen 1793
Humulin L, 100 Units 1794
Humulin N Pen 1797
Humulin R, 100 Units 1798
Humulin U, 100 Units 1800
Imitrex Nasal Spray 1467
Imitrex Tablets (Rare) 1471
▲ Increlex Injection (5% to 42%) 3291
▲ Indocin I.V. (1% to 3%) 2465
▲ Invirase (Less than 1% to 4%) 2772
Lantus Injection 2909
Levaquin (0.1% to 0.9%) 2384
Levaquin in 5% Dextrose Injection (0.1% to 0.9%) 2384
Levemir Injection 2320
Lipitor Tablets (Less than 2%) 2483
Lofibra Tablets 1219
Lofibra Capsules 1216
Lotronex Tablets (Rare) 1512
▲ Lyrica Capsules (1% to 3%) 2539
Mepron Suspension (1%) 1521
Meridia Capsules 489
Merrem I.V. (Greater than 1%) 686
Moban Tablets 1119
Namenda 1195
Naprosyn Suspension (Less than 1%) 2761
Naprosyn Tablets (Less than 1%) 2761
▲ NeoProfen Injection (12%) 2472
Neoral Oral Solution (1% to less than 3%) 2259
Neoral Soft Gelatin Capsules (1% to less than 3%) 2259
Neurontin Capsules (Infrequent) 2487
Neurontin Oral Solution (Infrequent) 2487
Neurontin Tablets (Infrequent) 2487
Noroxin Tablets 2032
NovoLog Injection 2326
NovoLog Mix 70/30 2328
Omnicef Capsules (0.2%) 511
Omnicef for Oral Suspension (0.2%) 511
▲ Oncaspar (Greater than 1% but less than 5%) 1145
Paser Granules 1674
Paxil CR Controlled-Release Tablets (Rare) 1538
Paxil (Rare) 1530
Pegasys (Less than 1%) 2789
Percodan Tablets 1132
Permax Tablets (Infrequent) 3356
Pexeva Tablets (Rare) 1694
Precose Tablets 751
Prevacid Delayed-Release Capsules (Less than 1%) 3271
Prevacid for Delayed-Release Oral Suspension (Less than 1%) 3271
Prevacid SoluTab Delayed-Release Orally Disintegrating Tablets (Less than 1%) 3271
Prevacid NapraPAC (Less than 1%) 3280
PREVPAC (Less than 1%) 3284
▲ Prezista Tablets (1.5% to 3.7%) 3306
Prilosec OTC Delayed-Release Tablets (Less than 1%) 2677
Prinivil Tablets 2052
▲ Prograf Capsules and Injection (3% to 15%) 632
Proleukin for Injection (2%) 2266
Protopic Ointment (Greater than or equal to 1%) 638
Prozac Pulvules and Liquid 1801
▲ Rapamune Oral Solution and Tablets (3% to 20%) 3475
Requip Tablets (Infrequent) 1555
Revlimid Capsules 958
Risperdal (Rare) 1676
Risperdal M-Tab Orally Disintegrating Tablets (Rare) 1676
▲ Sandostatin Injection (3% to 16%) 2278
▲ Sandostatin LAR Depot (2% to 4%) 2280
Seroquel Tablets (Infrequent) 690
Sonata Capsules (Rare) 1717
St. Joseph 81 mg Aspirin Chewable and Enteric Coated Tablets 1869
St. Joseph 81 mg Aspirin ■688
Starlix Tablets (2.4%) 2292
Symbyax Capsules (Infrequent) 1819
▲ Symlin Injection (0.4% to 16.8%) 613
Tequin Injection (Less than 0.1%) 938
Tequin Injection in 5% Dextrose (Less than 0.1%) 938
Tequin Tablets (Less than 0.1%) 938
Thiothixene Capsules 2165
Timolide Tablets 2086
Timoptic-XE Sterile Ophthalmic Gel Forming Solution 2092
Topamax Sprinkle Capsules (1%) 2404
Topamax Tablets (1%) 2404
Trecator Tablets 3487
Tricor Tablets 527
Triglide Tablets 3123
Trileptal Tablets 2300
Trileptal Oral Suspension 2300
▲ Trisenox Injection (8%) 993
▲ Truvada Tablets (1% to 12%) 1296
Tygacil for Injection (0% to less than 2%) 3488
Vantin Tablets and Oral Suspension 2645
▲ Vaprisol (3.3%) 643
VFEND I.V. (Less than 2%) 2564
VFEND Oral Suspension (Less than 2%) 2564
VFEND Tablets (Less than 2%) 2564
Viagra Tablets (Less than 2%) 2573
Viracept (Less than 2%) 2577
Wellbutrin Tablets 1603
Wellbutrin SR Sustained-Release Tablets 1607
Wellbutrin XL Extended-Release Tablets 1613
▲ Zegerid Capsules (3.4%) 2958
▲ Zegerid Powder for Oral Solution (3.4%) 2958
Zelapar Tablets 3372
Zoloft (Rare) 2586
Zonegran Capsules (Rare) 1101
Zosyn (1.0% or less) 3492
Zyprexa Tablets (Infrequent) 1830
Zyprexa ZYDIS Orally Disintegrating Tablets (Infrequent) 1830

Hypoglycemia, masked symptoms of

Betagan Ophthalmic Solution, USP ⊙220
Betimol Ophthalmic Solution 3382
Betimol Ophthalmic Solution ⊙295
Timoptic in Ocudose (Less frequent) 2091
Timoptic-XE Sterile Ophthalmic Gel Forming Solution 2092

Hypoglycemic reactions

Abilify Oral Solution (Rare) 882
Abilify Oral Solution (Rare) 2450
Abilify Discmelt Orally Disintegrating Tablets (Rare) 882
Abilify Discmelt Orally Disintegrating Tablets (Rare) 2450
Abilify Tablets (Rare) 882
Abilify Tablets (Rare) 2450
Symbyax Capsules (Rare) 1819

Hypogonadism

Permax Tablets (Rare) 3356
Virazole for Inhalation Solution 3370

Hypogonadism, male

Kaletra (Up to 2%) 476

Hypohidrosis

Bentyl Capsules 697
Bentyl Injection 697
Bentyl Syrup 697
Bentyl Tablets 697
Celexa (Rare) 1176
Donnatal Extentabs 2493
Paxil CR Controlled-Release Tablets (Rare) 1538
Paxil (Rare) 1530

Pexeva Tablets (Rare) ... 1694
Risperdal (Infrequent) ... 1676
Risperdal M-Tab Orally Disintegrating Tablets (Infrequent) ... 1676
Zonegran Capsules ... 1101

Hypokalemia

▲ Abelcet Injection (5%) ... 1141
Abilify Oral Solution (Infrequent) ... 882
Abilify Oral Solution (Infrequent) ... 2450
Abilify Discmelt Orally Disintegrating Tablets (Infrequent) ... 882
Abilify Discmelt Orally Disintegrating Tablets (Infrequent) ... 2450
Abilify Tablets (Infrequent) ... 882
Abilify Tablets (Infrequent) ... 2450
Aceon Tablets (2 mg, 4 mg, 8 mg) (0.3% to 1%) ... 3194
Aciphex Tablets ... 1090
Actiq (1% or greater) ... 979
Aggrenox Capsules ... 822
Aldoril Tablets ... 1910
Aloprim for Injection (Less than 1%) ... 2167
▲ AmBisome for Injection (37.6% to 43.2%) ... 620
▲ AndroGel (3% to 6%) ... 3329
▲ Aredia for Injection (4% to 18%) ... 2179
Aricept Tablets (Infrequent) ... 1094
Aricept ODT Tablets (Infrequent) ... 1094
▲ Arixtra Injection (0% to 4.2%) ... 1351
▲ Arranon Injection (2% to 11%) ... 1357
Atacand HCT (0.5% or greater) ... 651
Avalide Tablets ... 888
Avalide Tablets ... 2874
▲ Avastin IV (12% to 16%) ... 1227
Benicar HCT Tablets ... 1044
▲ Bumex Tablets (14.7%) ... 2746
Campath Ampules ... 811
▲ Cancidas for Injection (0.9% to 10.8%) ... 1918
Capastat Sulfate for Injection ... 1755
Cardene I.V. (0.7%) ... 2497
Celebrex Capsules (0.1% to 1.9%) ... 3134
Celexa (Rare) ... 1176
▲ CellCept Capsules (31.8% to 37.2%) ... 2747
▲ CellCept Intravenous (31.8% to 37.2%) ... 2747
▲ CellCept Oral Suspension (31.8% to 37.2%) ... 2747
▲ CellCept Tablets (31.8% to 37.2%) ... 2747
Chantix Tablets (Infrequent) ... 2517
Cipro I.V. (Infrequent) ... 2984
Clorpres Tablets ... 2153
Colazal Capsules ... 2838
Colocort Rectal Suspension, USP (Retention) 100 mg/60 mL ... 2476
▲ Coreg Tablets (Greater than 1% to 3%) ... 1414
▲ Cubicin for Injection (1% to 9.2%) ... 1026
▲ Dacogen Injection (22%) ... 2129
Daranide Tablets ... 1950
Decadron Tablets ... 1951
Demadex Injection ... 2759
Demadex Tablets ... 2759
▲ DepoDur Extended-Release Injection (2% to 5%) ... 1110
Depo-Medrol Injectable Suspension ... 2617
Depo-Medrol Single-Dose Vial ... 2619
Digibind for Injection ... 1421
▲ Diovan HCT Tablets (4.5%) ... 2196
Diuril Sodium Intravenous ... 2467
▲ Doxil Injection (1% to 10%) ... 2351
Dyazide Capsules (Uncommon) ... 1423
Dyrenium Capsules (Rare) ... 3400
Effexor Tablets (Infrequent) ... 3411
Effexor XR Capsules (Infrequent) ... 3417
▲ Eloxatin for Injection (3% to 9%) ... 2892
Emend Capsules (Greater than 0.5%) ... 1963
▲ Entocort EC Capsules (Less than 5%) ... 2698
▲ Eraxis for Injection (3.1%) ... 2521
Evoxac Capsules (Less than 1%) ... 1047
Exelon Capsules (Frequent) ... 2206
Exelon Oral Solution (Frequent) ... 2206
Ferrlecit Injection ... 3388
Fleet Enema for Children ... 1165
Fleet Phospho-soda ... 1166
Fleet Phospho-soda ACCU-PREP ... 1168
Fleet Phospho-soda EZ-PREP ... 1169
Fleet Prep Kits ... 1170
Foradil Aerolizer ... 3010
Furosemide Tablets ... 2154
Gabitril Tablets (Infrequent) ... 984
Garamycin Injectable ... 3014
Geodon Capsules (Infrequent) ... 2529
▲ Gleevec Tablets (0.8% to 13%) ... 2227
Humalog-Pen ... 1781
Humalog Mix 50/50-Pen ... 1783
Humalog Mix 75/25-Pen ... 1785
Hydrocortone Tablets ... 1989
▲ Hyzaar 50-12.5 Tablets (6.7%) ... 1990
▲ Hyzaar 100-12.5 Tablets (6.7%) ... 1990
▲ Hyzaar 100-25 Tablets (6.7%) ... 1990
▲ Imdur Tablets (Less than or equal to 5%) ... 3018
▲ Indapamide Tablets (3% to 7%) ... 2156
▲ Inspra Tablets (0.6% to 8.4%) ... 2536
Invanz for Injection (1.7% to 1.8%) ... 1999
▲ Invirase (Less than 1% to 4%) ... 2772
▲ Ionsys Transdermal System (1% to less than 10%) ... 2379
▲ I.V. Busulfex (2% to 64%) ... 2493
Kionex Powder ... 2477
Kristalose for Oral Solution ... 1034
Lanoxicaps Capsules ... 1490
Levaquin (0.1% to 0.9%) ... 2384
Levaquin in 5% Dextrose Injection (0.1% to 0.9%) ... 2384
▲ Lopressor HCT 50/25 Tablets (Less than 10%) ... 2241
▲ Lopressor HCT 100/25 Tablets (Less than 10%) ... 2241
▲ Lopressor HCT 100/50 Tablets (Less than 10%) ... 2241
Lotrel Capsules ... 2249
Lunesta Tablets (Rare) ... 3142
Micardis HCT Tablets (Less than 2%) ... 856
Mycamine for Injection (0.9% to 1.1%) ... 628
▲ Myfortic Tablets (3% to less than 20%) ... 2255
▲ Mylotarg for Injection (24% to 29%) ... 3431
NovoLog Injection ... 2326
NovoLog Mix 70/30 ... 2328
▲ Ontak Vials (6%) ... 1745
Parcopa Orally Disintegrating Tablets ... 3097
Paxil CR Controlled-Release Tablets (Rare) ... 1538
Paxil (Rare) ... 1530
Permax Tablets (Infrequent) ... 3356
Pexeva Tablets (Rare) ... 1694
Prinzide Tablets ... 2056
▲ Prograf Capsules and Injection (13% to 29%) ... 632
▲ Proleukin for Injection (9%) ... 2266
Proventil HFA Inhalation Aerosol (Some patients) ... 3056
Prozac Pulvules and Liquid (Infrequent) ... 1801
▲ Rapamune Oral Solution and Tablets (11% to 21%) ... 3475
Razadyne ... 2399
Razadyne ER Extended-Release Capsules ... 2399
Requip Tablets (Infrequent) ... 1555
▲ Revlimid Capsules (10.8% to 11.3%) ... 958
Rilutek Tablets (Infrequent) ... 2930
Risperdal (Rare) ... 1676
Risperdal Consta Long-Acting Injection (Infrequent) ... 1682
Risperdal M-Tab Orally Disintegrating Tablets (Rare) ... 1676
Rythmol SR Capsules ... 2727
Sandostatin LAR Depot (1% to 4%) ... 2280
Seroquel Tablets (Rare) ... 690
▲ Simulect for Injection (Greater than or equal to 10%) ... 2284
Sular Tablets (Less than or equal to 1%) ... 3122
▲ Sutent Capsules (1% to 12%) ... 2560
Symbyax Capsules (Infrequent) ... 1819
Teveten Tablets (Less than 1%) ... 1735
Teveten HCT Tablets (Less than 1%) ... 1737
Timentin ADD-Vantage (Rare) ... 1580
Timentin Injection Galaxy Container ... 1583
Timentin IV Infusion (Rare) ... 1577
Timentin Pharmacy Bulk Package (Rare) ... 1586
Timolide Tablets ... 2086
Topamax Sprinkle Capsules (Infrequent) ... 2404
Topamax Tablets (Infrequent) ... 2404
Trasylol Injection (1% to 2%) ... 754
Trileptal Tablets ... 2300
Trileptal Oral Suspension ... 2300
▲ Trisenox Injection (50%) ... 993
Tygacil for Injection (2.1%) ... 3488
Uniretic Tablets (More than 1%) ... 3100
▲ Valcyte Tablets (Less than 5%) ... 2813
▲ Vaprisol (9.8%) ... 643
▲ VFEND I.V. (0% to 16.7%) ... 2564
▲ VFEND Oral Suspension (0% to 16.7%) ... 2564
▲ VFEND Tablets (0% to 16.7%) ... 2564
▲ Xeloda Tablets (Less than 5%) ... 2822
Xopenex Inhalation Solution ... 3146
Xopenex Inhalation Solution Concentrate ... 3150
Xopenex HFA Inhalation Aerosol ... 3154
Zelapar Tablets (2%) ... 3372
Zofran Injection (Rare) ... 1634
Zofran (Rare) ... 1639
Zofran ODT Orally Disintegrating Tablets (Rare) ... 1639
▲ Zometa for Intravenous Infusion (Less than 15%) ... 2315
Zosyn ... 3492
Zyprexa Tablets (Infrequent) ... 1830
Zyprexa ZYDIS Orally Disintegrating Tablets (Infrequent) ... 1830
Zyvox (0% to 2.8%) ... 2652

Hypokalemic alkalosis

Colocort Rectal Suspension, USP (Retention) 100 mg/60 mL ... 2476
Decadron Tablets ... 1951
Depo-Medrol Injectable Suspension ... 2617
Depo-Medrol Single-Dose Vial ... 2619
Hydrocortone Tablets ... 1989

Hypokinesia

Abilify Oral Solution (Infrequent) ... 882
Abilify Oral Solution (Infrequent) ... 2450
Abilify Discmelt Orally Disintegrating Tablets (Infrequent) ... 882
Abilify Discmelt Orally Disintegrating Tablets (Infrequent) ... 2450
Abilify Tablets (Infrequent) ... 882
Abilify Tablets (Infrequent) ... 2450
Actiq (1% or greater) ... 979
Ambien Tablets (Rare) ... 2851
Ambien CR Tablets (Rare) ... 2855
Aricept Tablets (Infrequent) ... 1094
Aricept ODT Tablets (Infrequent) ... 1094
Celexa (Infrequent) ... 1176
▲ Clozaril Tablets (4%) ... 2184
▲ Comtan Tablets (9%) ... 2189
Copaxone for Injection (Infrequent) ... 3297
Coreg Tablets (Greater than 0.1% to 1%) ... 1414
Depacon Injection (1% or more) ... 412
Depakene (1% or more) ... 417
Depakote Sprinkle Capsules ... 422
▲ Depakote Tablets (1% to 5%) ... 427
Depakote ER Tablets (Greater than 1%) ... 434
Doxil Injection (Less than 1%) ... 2351
Effexor Tablets (Rare) ... 3411
Effexor XR Capsules (Rare) ... 3417
Exelon Capsules (Infrequent) ... 2206
Exelon Oral Solution (Infrequent) ... 2206
▲ FazaClo Orally Disintegrating Tablets (4%) ... 551
Gabitril Tablets (Frequent) ... 984
▲ Geodon Capsules (14%) ... 2529
▲ Intron A for Injection (Less than 5%) ... 3024
Lamictal (Rare) ... 1481
Lunesta Tablets (Rare) ... 3142
Lyrica Capsules (0.1% to 1%) ... 2539
Mirapex Tablets (1% or more) ... 859
Namenda (Frequent) ... 1195
Neurontin Capsules (Rare) ... 2487
Neurontin Oral Solution (Rare) ... 2487
Neurontin Tablets (Rare) ... 2487
Paxil CR Controlled-Release Tablets (Rare) ... 1538
Paxil (Rare) ... 1530
Permax Tablets (Infrequent) ... 3356
Pexeva Tablets (Infrequent) ... 1694
▲ ProSom Tablets (8%) ... 517
Protonix I.V. ... 3472
Razadyne (Infrequent) ... 2399
Razadyne ER Extended-Release Capsules (Infrequent) ... 2399
Relpax Tablets (Rare) ... 2548
Rilutek Tablets (Infrequent) ... 2930
▲ Risperdal (17% to 34%) ... 1676
Risperdal Consta Long-Acting Injection (Infrequent) ... 1682
▲ Risperdal M-Tab Orally Disintegrating Tablets (17% to 34%) ... 1676
Sonata Capsules (Rare) ... 1717
▲ Stalevo Tablets (9%) ... 2287
Symbyax Capsules (Infrequent) ... 1819
Symmetrel Tablets ... 1135
▲ Tasmar Tablets (1% to 3%) ... 3358
Topamax Sprinkle Capsules (Frequent) ... 2404
Topamax Tablets (Frequent) ... 2404
Trileptal Tablets ... 2300
Trileptal Oral Suspension ... 2300
Uniretic Tablets (Less than 1%) ... 3100
Wellbutrin SR Sustained-Release Tablets ... 1607
Wellbutrin XL Extended-Release Tablets ... 1613
Zelapar Tablets ... 3372
Zoloft (Infrequent) ... 2586
Zonegran Capsules (Rare) ... 1101
Zyban Sustained-Release Tablets ... 1644
▲ Zyprexa Tablets (8% to 20%) ... 1830
▲ Zyprexa IntraMuscular (2% to 4%) ... 1830
▲ Zyprexa ZYDIS Orally Disintegrating Tablets (8% to 20%) ... 1830

Hypomagnesemia

Abelcet Injection ... 1141
Actiq (1% or greater) ... 979
Aloprim for Injection (Less than 1%) ... 2167
▲ AmBisome for Injection (15.3% to 25.9%) ... 620
▲ Aredia for Injection (3.8% to at least 15%) ... 2179
▲ Arranon Injection (0% to 6%) ... 1357
Avalide Tablets ... 888
Avalide Tablets ... 2874
Benicar HCT Tablets ... 1044
Cancidas for Injection (2.3%) ... 1918
▲ CellCept Capsules (39%) ... 2747
▲ CellCept Intravenous (39%) ... 2747
▲ CellCept Oral Suspension (39%) ... 2747
▲ CellCept Tablets (39%) ... 2747
Cubicin for Injection (Less than 1%) ... 1026
▲ Dacogen Injection (24%) ... 2129
Diovan HCT Tablets ... 2196
Diuril Sodium Intravenous ... 2467
Doxil Injection (Less than 1%) ... 2351
Eraxis for Injection (Less than 1% to less than 2%) ... 2521
Furosemide Tablets ... 2154
Garamycin Injectable ... 3014
Gengraf Capsules ... 459
Geodon Capsules (Rare) ... 2529
Herceptin I.V. (At least one of the 958 patients) ... 1233
Hyzaar 50-12.5 Tablets ... 1990
Hyzaar 100-12.5 Tablets ... 1990
Hyzaar 100-25 Tablets ... 1990
Ionsys Transdermal System (.1% to less than 1%) ... 2379
▲ I.V. Busulfex (77%) ... 2493
Lanoxicaps Capsules ... 1490
▲ Leukine (15%) ... 814
Levaquin (0.1% to 0.9%) ... 2384
Levaquin in 5% Dextrose Injection (0.1% to 0.9%) ... 2384
Micardis HCT Tablets ... 856
Mycamine for Injection (0% to 1.2%) ... 628
▲ Myfortic Tablets (3% to less than 20%) ... 2255
▲ Mylotarg for Injection (3% to 10%) ... 3431
▲ Neoral Oral Solution (6%) ... 2259
▲ Neoral Soft Gelatin Capsules (6%) ... 2259
Prinzide Tablets ... 2056
▲ Prograf Capsules and Injection (16% to 48%) ... 632
▲ Proleukin for Injection (12%) ... 2266
▲ Rapamune Oral Solution and Tablets (3% to 20%) ... 3475
▲ Revlimid Capsules (6.1%) ... 958
Sandimmune (In some patients) ... 2275
▲ Simulect for Injection (3% to 10%) ... 2284
Thalomid Capsules ... 965
Timolide Tablets ... 2086
▲ Trisenox Injection (45%) ... 993
Uniretic Tablets ... 3100
▲ Valcyte Tablets (Less than 5%) ... 2813
Vaprisol (2.2%) ... 643
VFEND I.V. (Less than 2%) ... 2564
VFEND Oral Suspension (Less than 2%) ... 2564
VFEND Tablets (Less than 2%) ... 2564
▲ Xeloda Tablets (Less than 5%) ... 2822
Zegerid Capsules (0.1%) ... 2958
Zegerid Powder for Oral Solution (0.1%) ... 2958
Zometa for Intravenous Infusion (0.1% to 0.2%) ... 2315

Hypomania

Celexa ... 1176
Effexor Tablets (0.5%) ... 3411
Effexor XR Capsules (0.3%) ... 3417
Lamictal (Rare) ... 1481
Lexapro Oral Solution ... 1190
Paxil CR Controlled-Release Tablets (Approximately 1.0%) ... 1538
Paxil (Approximately 1.0%) ... 1530
Prozac Pulvules and Liquid (0.1% to 1.8%) ... 1801
Symbyax Capsules ... 1819
Wellbutrin Tablets (Frequent) ... 1603

Wellbutrin SR Sustained-Release Tablets (Rare) 1607
Wellbutrin XL Extended-Release Tablets (Rare) 1613
Zoloft (Approximately 0.4%) 2586
Zyban Sustained-Release Tablets (Rare) 1644

Hypomenorrhea
Effexor Tablets (Rare) 3411
Effexor XR Capsules (Rare) 3417
Pentasa Capsules (Less than 1%) 3185
Prozac Pulvules and Liquid (Rare) 1801
Symbyax Capsules (Infrequent) 1819

Hyponatremia
Abilify Oral Solution (Infrequent) 882
Abilify Oral Solution (Infrequent) 2450
Abilify Discmelt Orally Disintegrating Tablets (Infrequent) 882
Abilify Discmelt Orally Disintegrating Tablets (Infrequent) 2450
Abilify Tablets (Infrequent) 882
Abilify Tablets (Infrequent) 2450
Aceon Tablets (2 mg, 4 mg, 8 mg) 3194
Aciphex Tablets 1090
Actimmune (Rare) 1671
Actiq (Less than 1%) 979
Aloprim for Injection (Less than 1%) 2167
Altace Capsules 1702
AmBisome for Injection (Less common) 620
Aricept Tablets 1094
Aricept ODT Tablets 1094
Arthrotec Tablets (Rare) 3129
Atacand Tablets 649
Atacand HCT (Very rare) 651
Avandaryl Tablets 1379
Avastin IV (Rare) 1227
Benicar HCT Tablets 1044
▲ Bumex Tablets (9.2%) 2746
Campath Ampules 811
Campral Tablets (Rare) 1174
Cancidas for Injection (1.5% to 1.9%) 1918
Captopril Tablets 2149
Carbatrol Capsules 3171
Celebrex Capsules (Less than 0.1%) 3134
Celexa (Several cases) 1176
▲ CellCept Capsules (3% to less than 20%) 2747
▲ CellCept Intravenous (3% to less than 20%) 2747
▲ CellCept Oral Suspension (3% to less than 20%) 2747
▲ CellCept Tablets (3% to less than 20%) 2747
Clozaril Tablets 2184
Coreg Tablets (Greater than 1% to 3%) 1414
Cozaar Tablets 1935
▲ Dacogen Injection (19%) 2129
Demadex Injection 2759
Demadex Tablets 2759
Depacon Injection 412
Depakene 417
Depakote Sprinkle Capsules 422
Depakote Tablets 427
Depakote ER Tablets 434
Diuril Sodium Intravenous 2467
▲ Doxil Injection (1% to 10%) 2351
Duetact Tablets 3226
Dyazide Capsules 1423
Effexor Tablets (Rare) 3411
Effexor XR Capsules 3417
Emend Capsules (Greater than 0.5%) 1963
Equetro Extended-Release Capsules 3180
Evoxac Capsules (Less than 1%) 1047
Exelon Capsules (Infrequent) 2206
Exelon Oral Solution (Infrequent) 2206
FazaClo Orally Disintegrating Tablets 551
Furosemide Tablets 2154
Gabitril Tablets (Infrequent) 984
Garamycin Injectable 3014
Geodon Capsules (Rare) 2529
Gleevec Tablets (Rare) 2227
Herceptin I.V. (At least one of the 958 patients) 1233
Hyzaar 50-12.5 Tablets 1990
Hyzaar 100-12.5 Tablets 1990
Hyzaar 100-25 Tablets 1990
▲ Indapamide Tablets (Less than 5%) 2156
▲ Indocin I.V. (3% to 9%) 2465
Inspra Tablets (2.4%) 2536
▲ Invirase (Less than 1% to 4%) 2772
Ionsys Transdermal System (.1% to less than 1%) 2379
I.V. Busulfex (2%) 2493
Kadian Capsules (Less than 3%) 577
▲ Kaletra (3%) 476
Levaquin 2384
Levaquin in 5% Dextrose Injection 2384
Lexapro Oral Solution (One case) 1190
Lexapro Tablets (One case) 1190
Lotensin HCT Tablets 2246
Malarone Pediatric Tablets 1517
Malarone Tablets 1517
Mavik Tablets (0.3% to 1.0%) 486
▲ Mepron Suspension (7% to 10%) 1521
Moduretic Tablets 2028
Mycamine for Injection 628
Namenda (Infrequent) 1195
Neurontin Capsules 2487
Neurontin Oral Solution 2487
Neurontin Tablets 2487
Nexavar Tablets (Uncommon) 746
Nexium Delayed-Release Capsules (Less than 1%) 655
Nexium I.V. (Less than 1%) 659
Nimotop Capsules (Less than 1%) 749
Nipent for Injection (Less than 3%) 1863
Oncaspar (Less than 1%) 1145
OxyContin Tablets (Less than 1%) 2703
Paxil CR Controlled-Release Tablets (Rare) 1538
Paxil (Rare) 1530
Pexeva Tablets 1694
Prezista Tablets (Less than 2%) 3306
Prilosec OTC Delayed-Release Tablets (Less than 1%) 2677
Primaxin I.M. 2045
Primaxin I.V. 2048
Prinivil Tablets 2052
Prinzide Tablets 2056
▲ Prograf Capsules and Injection (3% to 15%) 632
▲ Proleukin for Injection (4%) 2266
Prozac Pulvules and Liquid 1801
▲ Rapamune Oral Solution and Tablets (3% to 20%) 3475
Requip Tablets (Infrequent) 1555
Rescriptor Tablets 2551
Rilutek Tablets (Infrequent) 2930
Risperdal (Infrequent) 1676
Risperdal Consta Long-Acting Injection (Infrequent) 1682
Risperdal M-Tab Orally Disintegrating Tablets (Infrequent) 1676
Rythmol SR Capsules 2727
Seroquel Tablets 690
▲ Sutent Capsules (6%) 2560
Symbyax Capsules 1819
Tarka Tablets 524
Tegretol/Tegretol-XR 2295
Teveten Tablets (Less than 1%) 1735
Teveten HCT Tablets (Less than 1%) 1737
Thalomid Capsules 965
Ticlid Tablets (Rare) 2810
Topamax Sprinkle Capsules (Rare) 2404
Topamax Tablets (Rare) 2404
Trileptal Tablets (2.5%) 2300
Trileptal Oral Suspension (2.5%) 2300
Tygacil for Injection (0% to less than 2%) 3488
Uniretic Tablets (Less than 1%) 3100
Univasc Tablets 3104
▲ Vaprisol (3.3%) 643
Vasotec I.V. Injection 2103
VFEND I.V. (Less than 2%) 2564
VFEND Oral Suspension (Less than 2%) 2564
VFEND Tablets (Less than 2%) 2564
▲ Zegerid Capsules (3.9%) 2958
▲ Zegerid Powder for Oral Solution (3.9%) 2958
Zelapar Tablets 3372
Zoloft (Several cases) 2586
Zonegran Capsules (Rare) 1101
Zosyn 3492
Zyprexa Tablets (Infrequent) 1830
Zyprexa ZYDIS Orally Disintegrating Tablets (Infrequent) 1830

Hyponatremia, dilutional
Diuril Sodium Intravenous 2467
Hyzaar 50-12.5 Tablets 1990
Hyzaar 100-12.5 Tablets 1990
Hyzaar 100-25 Tablets 1990
Prinzide Tablets 2056

Hypoparathyroidism
▲ Rocaltrol Capsules (1 in 3) 2798
▲ Rocaltrol Oral Solution (1 in 3) 2798

Hypophosphatemia
Abelcet Injection 1141
Actonel Tablets (2.7%) 2683
Advicor Tablets 1722
AmBisome for Injection (Less common) 620
▲ Aredia for Injection (Up to 18%) 2179
Atripla Tablets 945
Cardene I.V. (Rare) 2497
▲ CellCept Capsules (3% to less than 20%) 2747
▲ CellCept Intravenous (3% to less than 20%) 2747
▲ CellCept Oral Suspension (3% to less than 20%) 2747
▲ CellCept Tablets (3% to less than 20%) 2747
Doxil Injection (Less than 1%) 2351
Effexor Tablets (Rare) 3411
Evista Tablets 1763
▲ Fosamax (Approximately 10%) 1969
▲ Fosamax Plus D Tablets (10%) 1977
Gleevec Tablets (Infrequent) 2227
▲ Invirase (Less than 1% to 4%) 2772
Ionsys Transdermal System (.1% to less than 1%) 2379
▲ I.V. Busulfex (17%) 2493
Levaquin (0.1% to 0.9%) 2384
Levaquin in 5% Dextrose Injection (0.1% to 0.9%) 2384
Maalox Regular Strength Antacid/Anti-Gas Liquid ▣ 660
Maalox Regular Strength Antacid/Antigas Liquid 2175
Maalox Max Maximum Strength Antacid/Anti-Gas Liquid 2176
Mycamine for Injection (1.4%) 628
▲ Myfortic Tablets (3% to less than 20%) 2255
▲ Mylotarg for Injection (6% to 10%) 3431
▲ Nexavar Tablets (Very Common) 746
Niaspan Extended-Release Tablets 1730
▲ Prograf Capsules and Injection (3% to 49%) 632
▲ Proleukin for Injection (11%) 2266
▲ Rapamune Oral Solution and Tablets (15% to 23%) 3475
Rescriptor Tablets 2551
▲ Simulect for Injection (Greater than or equal to 10%) 2284
▲ Sutent Capsules (9% to 10%) 2560
Timolide Tablets 2086
Topamax Sprinkle Capsules (Rare) 2404
Topamax Tablets (Rare) 2404
Truvada Tablets 1296
Tygacil for Injection 3488
Ultane Liquid for Inhalation (Less than 1%) 531
▲ Valcyte Tablets (Less than 5%) 2813
VFEND I.V. (Less than 2%) 2564
VFEND Oral Suspension (Less than 2%) 2564
VFEND Tablets (Less than 2%) 2564
Viread Tablets 1301
▲ Zegerid Capsules (6.2%) 2958
▲ Zegerid Powder for Oral Solution (6.2%) 2958
▲ Zometa for Intravenous Infusion (0.5% to 11.8%) 2315

Hypopigmentation
Accutane Capsules 2731
Aclovate Cream (Infrequent) 2660
Aldara Cream, 5% (More than 1%) 1846
Analpram-HC 1159
Apexicon E Cream 2661
Catapres-TTS (0.5% or less) 844
Clobevate Gel 3211
Clobex Lotion 1204
Clobex Shampoo (Infrequent) 1206
Clobex Spray (Less than 1%) 1208
Cutivate Cream (Infrequent) 2662
Cutivate Lotion 0.05% (Rare) 2664
Cutivate Ointment (Infrequent to more frequent) 2665
Depo-Medrol Single-Dose Vial 2619
Diprolene Gel 0.05% 3001
Diprolene Lotion 0.05% (Infrequent) 3002
Diprolene Ointment 0.05% (Infrequent) 3003
Diprolene AF Cream 0.05% (Infrequent) 3000
Diprosone Cream, USP 0.05% 3004
Elocon Cream 0.1% (Infrequent) 3005
Elocon Lotion 0.1% (Infrequent) 3006
Elocon Ointment 0.1% (Infrequent) 3007
▲ Levulan Kerastick for Topical Solution, 20% (20% to 36%) 1085
Locoid Lipocream Cream (Infrequent) 1160
Lotrisone 3040
Luxíq Foam 1010
Olux Foam 1012
Oxsoralen-Ultra Capsules 3353
Pramosone 1161
ProctoFoam-HC 3099
Taxotere Injection Concentrate 2932
Temovate Cream 2668
Temovate Gel (Infrequent) 2669
Temovate Ointment 2668
Temovate Scalp Application (Infrequent) 2670
Temovate E Emollient (Infrequent) 2671
Tri-Luma Cream (11 occurrences in 27 patients) 1213
Vanos Cream 1893

Hypoplasia, erythroid
Captopril Tablets 2149

Hypoplasia, myeloid
(*see under* Bone marrow hypoplasia)

Hypoplastic anemia
(*see under* Anemia, hypoplastic)

Hypopnea
Vicoprofen Tablets (Less than 1%) 539

Hypoproteinemia
Actiq (Less than 1%) 979
AmBisome for Injection (Less common) 620
▲ CellCept Capsules (3% to less than 20%) 2747
▲ CellCept Intravenous (3% to less than 20%) 2747
▲ CellCept Oral Suspension (3% to less than 20%) 2747
▲ CellCept Tablets (3% to less than 20%) 2747
Cipro I.V. 2984
Colazal Capsules 2838
▲ Dacogen Injection (5%) 2129
Depakote ER Tablets (Greater than 1%) 434
Doxil Injection (Less than 1%) 2351
Effexor Tablets (Rare) 3411
Effexor XR Capsules (Rare) 3417
Evista Tablets 1763
Geodon Capsules (Rare) 2529
▲ Lupron Depot 7.5 mg (Greater than or equal to 5%) 3264
▲ Oncaspar (Greater than 1% but less than 5%) 1145
▲ Prograf Capsules and Injection (3% to 15%) 632
▲ Proleukin for Injection (7%) 2266
Risperdal (Rare) 1676
Risperdal M-Tab Orally Disintegrating Tablets (Rare) 1676
Sandostatin LAR Depot (1% to 4%) 2280
▲ Simulect for Injection (3% to 10%) 2284
Targretin Capsules 1747
Thalomid Capsules 965
▲ Tygacil for Injection (4.5%) 3488
Uniretic Tablets (Less than 1%) 3100
Vantin Tablets and Oral Suspension 2645
Zelapar Tablets 3372
Zosyn 3492
Zyprexa Tablets (Rare) 1830
Zyprexa ZYDIS Orally Disintegrating Tablets (Rare) 1830

Hypoprothrombinemia
AmBisome for Injection (Less common) 620
Arixtra Injection (1.3%) 1351
Celexa 1176
Cipro I.V. (Rare) 2984
Cipro XR Tablets (Less than 1%) 2990
Colazal Capsules 2838
▲ Coreg Tablets (Greater than 1% to 3%) 1414
Fansidar Tablets 2765
Gantrisin Pediatric Suspension 2770
Levaquin 2384
Levaquin in 5% Dextrose Injection 2384
Lexapro Oral Solution 1190
Lexapro Tablets 1190
Lyrica Capsules (Rare) 2539
Merrem I.V. (Greater than 0.2%) 686
Neurontin Capsules (Rare) 2487
Neurontin Oral Solution (Rare) 2487
Neurontin Tablets (Rare) 2487
NovoSeven (1%) 2331
Paser Granules 1674
▲ Prograf Capsules and Injection (3% to 15%) 632
Rocephin Injectable Vials, ADD-Vantage, Galaxy, Bulk (Rare) 2800
Rythmol SR Capsules 2727

Hypoptyalism
▲ Advair HFA Inhalation Aerosol (1% to 3%) 1318
Amerge Tablets (Frequent) 1339
Demser Capsules 1953
▲ Flovent HFA (1% to 3%) 1447
Imitrex Injection 1463
Imitrex Nasal Spray 1467
Imitrex Tablets (Greater than 1%) 1471
▲ Infergen (4% to 6%) 3364
Lotronex Tablets (Infrequent) 1512
▲ Niravam Orally Disintegrating Tablets (10.6% to 32.8%) 3092
Risperdal (Frequent) 1676
Risperdal M-Tab Orally Disintegrating Tablets (Frequent) 1676
Serevent Diskus (1% to less than 3%) 1568
Vantin Tablets and Oral Suspension (Less than 1%) 2645

Hyporeflexia
Abilify Oral Solution (Rare) 882
Abilify Oral Solution (Rare) 2450
Abilify Discmelt Orally Disintegrating Tablets (Rare) 882
Abilify Discmelt Orally Disintegrating Tablets (Rare) 2450
Abilify Tablets (Rare) 882
Abilify Tablets (Rare) 2450
Arranon Injection (1%) 1357
Axert Tablets (Rare) 2396
Effexor Tablets (Rare) 3411
▲ Evoxac Capsules (1% to 3%) 1047
Gabitril Tablets (Frequent) 984
Invirase (Less than 2%) 2772
Lunesta Tablets (Infrequent) 3142
Matulane Capsules 3191
Maxalt Tablets (Rare) 2008
Maxalt-MLT Orally Disintegrating Tablets (Rare) 2008
Neurontin Capsules (Frequent) 2487
Neurontin Oral Solution (Frequent) 2487
Neurontin Tablets (Frequent) 2487
Paxil CR Controlled-Release Tablets (Rare) 1538
Paxil (Rare) 1530
Pexeva Tablets (rare) 1694
ProSom Tablets (Rare) 517
Protonix I.V. (Less than 1%) 3472
Protonix Tablets (Less than 1%) 3469
Prozac Pulvules and Liquid (Rare) 1801
▲ Retrovir Capsules (5.6%) 1560
▲ Retrovir IV Infusion (7%) 1564
▲ Retrovir (5.6%) 1560
▲ Risperdal (17% to 34%) 1676
▲ Risperdal M-Tab Orally Disintegrating Tablets (17% to 34%) 1676
Sonata Capsules (Rare) 1717
Thalomid Capsules 965
Thiothixene Capsules 2165
Topamax Sprinkle Capsules (2%) 2404
Topamax Tablets (2%) 2404
Trileptal Tablets 2300
Trileptal Oral Suspension 2300
▲ Vesanoid Capsules (3%) 2820
Viagra Tablets (Less than 2%) 2573
Zelapar Tablets 3372
Zoloft (Rare) 2586

Hyporesponsive episode, unspecified
HibTITER (One case) 3426

Hyposalivation
(*see under* Hypoptyalism)

Hypospadias
Topamax Sprinkle Capsules 2404
Topamax Tablets 2404

Hypotaxia
▲ Vesanoid Capsules (3%) 2820

Hypotension
▲ Abelcet Injection (8%) 1141
Abilify Oral Solution (Frequent) 882
Abilify Oral Solution (Frequent) 2450
Abilify Discmelt Orally Disintegrating Tablets (Frequent) 882
Abilify Discmelt Orally Disintegrating Tablets (Frequent) 2450
Abilify Tablets (Frequent) 882
Abilify Tablets (Frequent) 2450
Aceon Tablets (2 mg, 4 mg, 8 mg) (0.3% to 1%) 3194
▲ Acetadote Injection (.78% to 3.75%) 1031
Actimmune (Rare) 1671
Actiq (Less than 1%) 979
Activase I.V. 1223
ADACEL Vaccine 2945
Adalat CC Tablets (Less than 1%) 2964
Adenocard Injection (Less than 1%) 617
Adenoscan (2%) 619
Advicor Tablets 1722
Aggrenox Capsules (Less than 1%) 822
Albutein 5%, Albumin (Human) 1652
Albutein 25% , Albumin (Human) 1653
Aldoril Tablets 1910
Aldurazyme for Intravenous Infusion (2%) 1268
▲ Alferon N Injection (6%) 1665
Alkeran for Injection (In some patients) 955
Allegra-D 12 Hour Extended-Release Tablets 2846
Allegra-D 24 Hour Extended-Release Tablets 2849
Aloprim for Injection (Less than 1%) 2167
Aloxi Injection (1%) 2127
Alphagan P Ophthalmic Solution 567
▲ Altace Capsules (11%) 1702
Ambien Tablets (Rare) 2851
Ambien CR Tablets (Rare) 2855
▲ AmBisome for Injection (7.4% to 14.3%) 620
Amerge Tablets (Infrequent) 1339
Anaprox Tablets (Less than 1%) 2761
Anaprox DS Tablets (Less than 1%) 2761
Anzemet Injection (Infrequently) 2859
▲ Anzemet Tablets (5.3%) 2862
▲ Aranesp for Injection (22%) 581
Aredia for Injection (Rare) 2179
▲ Argatroban Injection (7.2% to 10.7%) 1346
Aricept Tablets (Frequent) 1094
Aricept ODT Tablets (Frequent) 1094
▲ Arixtra Injection (0.3% to 3.5%) 1351
▲ Arranon Injection (1% to 8%) 1357
Arthrotec Tablets (Rare) 3129
Atacand Tablets 649
Atacand HCT (Rare) 651
Atrovent HFA Inhalation Aerosol 841
Avalide Tablets 888
Avalide Tablets 2874
Avapro Tablets (0.4%) 891
Avapro Tablets (0.4%) 2871
▲ Avastin IV (7% to 15%) 1227
Avelox (Less than 0.1%) 2970
Avinza Capsules (Less than 5%) 1741
Bayer Aspirin 744
Bayer Aspirin Comprehensive Prescribing Information ▣ 796
BeneFix Vials 3408
Benicar Tablets 1043
Betagan Ophthalmic Solution, USP ⊙ 220
Betimol Ophthalmic Solution 3382
Betimol Ophthalmic Solution ⊙ 295
▲ Bexxar (1% to 7%) 1398
Bicillin C-R Injectable Suspension 1706
▲ BiDil Tablets (8%) 2171
▲ Blocadren Tablets (3%) 1916
Boostrix (Rarely) 1404
Brimonidine Tartrate Ophthalmic Solution 0.2% ⊙ 248
▲ Bumex Tablets (0.8% to 4.1%) 2746
▲ Buprenex Injectable (1% to 5%) 2716
Caduet Tablets (Greater than 0.1% to less than or equal to 1%) 2508
Calcium Disodium Versenate Injection 1851
▲ Campath Ampules (5% to 32%) 811
Campral Tablets (Infrequent) 1174
▲ Camptosar Injection (1.7% to 5.8%) 2604
Cancidas for Injection (0.9%) 1918
Captopril Tablets (Rare) 2149
Carbatrol Capsules 3171
▲ Cardene I.V. (5.6%) 2497
Cardizem LA Extended Release Tablets (Less than 2%) 1728
Cardura XL Tablets (1.7%) 2515
Carimune NF 3499
▲ Carnitor Injection (3% to 19%) 3188
Carteolol Hydrochloride Ophthalmic Solution USP, 1% ⊙ 249
Caverject Impulse Injection (Less than 1%) 2612
Celexa (Frequent) 1176
▲ CellCept Capsules (3% to 32.5%) 2747
▲ CellCept Intravenous (3% to 32.5%) 2747
▲ CellCept Oral Suspension (3% to 32.5%) 2747
▲ CellCept Tablets (3% to 32.5%) 2747
▲ Cerezyme for Injection (Approximately 6.6%) 1270
▲ Cesamet Capsules (8%) 3340
Chantix Tablets (Infrequent) 2517
Cialis Tablets (Less than 2%) 1838
Cipro (Less than 1%) 2977
Cipro I.V. (1% or less) 2984
Cipro XR Tablets 2990
Clinoril Tablets (Less than 1 in 100) 1924
▲ Clolar for Intravenous Infusion (29%) 1271
▲ Clozaril Tablets (More than 5% to 9%) 2184
Combivent Inhalation Aerosol 847
Comtan Tablets 2189
Comvax 1928
Concerta Extended-Release Tablets 1881
Copaxone for Injection (Infrequent) 3297
▲ Coreg Tablets (9% to 14%) 1414
Cosopt Sterile Ophthalmic Solution (Less than 1%) 1931
Coumadin for Injection 898
Coumadin Tablets 898
Covera-HS Tablets (0.7% to 2.5%) 3139
▲ Cozaar Tablets (Less than 1% to 7%) 1935
▲ Cubicin for Injection (2.4% to 5%) 1026
Curosurf Intratracheal Suspension 1057
CytoGam Intravenous 1895
▲ Dacogen Injection (6%) 2129
Dalmane Capsules (Rare) 3342
Daytrana Transdermal Patch 3174
Demadex Injection 2759
Demadex Tablets 2759
Depacon Injection (1% or more) 412
Depakene (1% or more) 417
Depakote Sprinkle Capsules 422
▲ Depakote Tablets (1% to 5%) 427
Depakote ER Tablets (Greater than 1%) 434
▲ DepoDur Extended-Release Injection (Greater than 10%) 1110
Diastat Rectal Delivery System (At least 1%) 3343
Dilaudid 440
Dilaudid Non-Sterile Powder 440
Dilaudid Oral Liquid 445
Dilaudid Rectal Suppositories 440
Dilaudid Tablets 440
Dilaudid Tablets - 8 mg 445
Dilaudid-HP (Less frequent) 442
▲ Diovan Tablets (1.4% to 7%) 2193
Diovan HCT Tablets (Greater than 0.2%) 2196
Diuril Oral Suspension 1954
Diuril Sodium Intravenous 2467
▲ Doxil Injection (1% to 10%) 2351
▲ Duragesic Transdermal System (1% to 3%) 2373
Dyazide Capsules 1423
DynaCirc CR Tablets (0.5% to 1%) 2721
EC-Naprosyn Delayed-Release Tablets (Less than 1%) 2761
Edex Injection (Less than 1%) 3089
▲ Effexor Tablets (3% to 13%) 3411
Effexor XR Capsules (Infrequent) 3417
Eldepryl Capsules 3208
Eligard 22.5 mg (Less than 2%) 2883
Elitek 2890
Eloxatin for Injection (Rare) 2892
▲ Emend Capsules (Greater than 0.5%) 1963
▲ Emsam Transdermal System (3% to 6.2%) 903
Enbrel for Injection (Infrequent) 584
Engerix-B Vaccine (Less than 1%) 1425
Equetro Extended-Release Capsules 3180
Eraxis for Injection 2521
▲ Ethyol for Injection (3% to 61%) 1898
Evoxac Capsules (Less than 1%) 1047
Exelon Capsules (Frequent) 2206
Exelon Oral Solution (Frequent) 2206
▲ Fabrazyme for Intravenous Infusion (4%) 1274
▲ FazaClo Orally Disintegrating Tablets (Greater than 5% to 9%) 551
▲ Ferrlecit Injection (1.3% to 41%) 3388
Flebogamma 5%, Immune Globulin Intravenous (Human) 1658
Fluorescite Injection ⊙ 207
Focalin Tablets 2220
Focalin XR Capsules 2223
Foradil Aerolizer (Rare) 3010
Fortaz (Very rare) 1453
▲ Fosrenol Chewable Tablets (8% to 16%) 3183
Furosemide Tablets 2154
Gabitril Tablets (Infrequent) 984
Gammagard Liquid 721
Gammagard S/D 724
Gamunex Immune Globulin I.V., 10% 3235
Garamycin Injectable 3014
Gleevec Tablets (Infrequent) 2227
GlucaGen (Rare) 761
Glucagon for Injection Vials and Emergency Kit 1778
Guanidine Hydrochloride Tablets 3016
Herceptin I.V. (At least one of the 958 patients) 1233
Humalog-Pen (Less common) 1781
Humalog Mix 50/50-Pen 1783
Humalog Mix 75/25-Pen (Less common) 1785
Human Albumin Grifols 20%, Albumin (Human) 1651
Human Albumin Grifols 25%, Albumin (Human) 1652
Humulin 50/50, 100 Units 1791
Humulin 70/30 Pen (Less common) 1793
Humulin L, 100 Units (Less common) 1794
Humulin N Pen (Less common) 1797
▲ Hyperstat I.V. (7%) 3017
▲ Hytrin Capsules (0.6%; 21%) 471
Hyzaar 50-12.5 Tablets 1990
Hyzaar 100-12.5 Tablets 1990
Hyzaar 100-25 Tablets 1990
▲ Imdur Tablets (Less than or equal to 5%) 3018
Imitrex Injection (Infrequent) 1463
Imitrex Nasal Spray (Rare) 1467
Imitrex Tablets (Infrequent) 1471
Inderal LA Long-Acting Capsules 3429
Indocin Capsules (Less than 1%) 1995
Indocin I.V. (Less than 1%) 2465
Indocin (Less than 1%) 1995
Infanrix Vaccine 1476
Infed Injection 3390
InnoPran XL Capsules 2723
▲ Integrilin Injection (7%) 3020
▲ Intron A for Injection (Less than 5%) 3024
Invanz for Injection (1% to 2%) 1999
Invirase (Less than 2%) 2772
Ionsys Transdermal System (2%) 2379
▲ I.V. Busulfex (3% to 11%) 2493
Kadian Capsules (Less than 3%) 577
Ketek Tablets (Less than 0.2%) 2903
Kogenate FS (Very rare) 738
▲ Kytril Injection (3.4%) 2781
Kytril (Rare) 2784
Lariam Tablets (Infrequent) 2786
▲ Leukine (13%) 814
Levaquin (0.1% to 0.9%) 2384
Levaquin in 5% Dextrose Injection (0.1% to 0.9%) 2384
Levitra Tablets (Less than 2%) 3034
Lexapro Oral Solution 1190
Lexapro Tablets 1190
Lidoderm Patch 1118
Lithobid Tablets 1692
Lofibra Tablets 1219
Lofibra Capsules 1216
▲ Lopressor Injection (1% to 27.4%) 2238
▲ Lopressor Tablets (1% to 27.4%) 2238
Lotensin HCT Tablets (0.6%) 2246
Lotrel Capsules (Rare) 2249
Lupron Depot 3.75 mg 3260
Lupron Depot 7.5 mg 3264
Lupron Depot–3 Month 11.25 mg 3265
Lupron Depot-PED 7.5 mg, 11.25 mg and 15 mg 3269
Lupron Injection Pediatric 3259
Lyrica Capsules (0.1% to 1%) 2539
Marinol Capsules (0.3 to 1%) 3333
Matulane Capsules 3191
▲ Mavik Tablets (0.3% to 11%) 486
Maxair Autohaler 1852
Mefoxin for Injection 2012
Mefoxin Premixed Intravenous Solution 2016
Mephyton Tablets (Rare) 2018
Mepron Suspension (1%) 1521
Merrem I.V. (Greater than 0.1% to 1%) 686
Metadate CD Capsules 3323
Micardis Tablets 854
Migranal Nasal Spray (Rare) 3348
Mintezol 2027
Mirapex Tablets (Greater than or equal to 1%) 859
Mivacron Injection (Less than 1%) 493
Moban Tablets (Rare) 1119
Mobic Oral Suspension (Less than 2%) 863
Mobic Tablets (Less than 2%) 863
MS Contin Tablets (Less frequent) 2701
Mycamine for Injection (0.2%) 628
▲ Myfortic Tablets (3% to less than 20%) 2255
▲ Mylotarg for Injection (18% to 23%) 3431
Myozyme for Intravenous Infusion 1279
Nadolol Tablets (2 of 100 patients) 2159
Namenda (Infrequent) 1195

Naprosyn Suspension (Less than 1%) 2761
Naprosyn Tablets (Less than 1%) 2761
▲ Natrecor for Injection (4% to 35%) 3127
Nembutal Sodium Solution, USP (Less than 1%) 2470
NeoProfen Injection 2472
Neumega for Injection 3435
Neupogen for Injection (7 of 176 patients) 603
Neurontin Capsules (Infrequent) 2487
Neurontin Oral Solution (Infrequent) 2487
Neurontin Tablets (Infrequent) 2487
Niaspan Extended-Release Tablets 1730
Nimbex Injection (0.2%) 498
▲ Nimotop Capsules (1.2% to 50.0%) 749
▲ Nipent for Injection (3% to 10%) 1863
▲ Niravam Orally Disintegrating Tablets (4.7%) 3092
▲ Nitro-Dur Transdermal Infusion System (4%) 3046
Nitrolingual Pumpspray 3120
Norvasc Tablets (0.1% to 1%; rare) 2545
Norvir (Less than 2%) 503
NovoLog Injection 2326
NovoSeven (1%) 2331
Numorphan Injection 1120
▲ Oncaspar (Greater than 1% but less than 5%) 1145
▲ Ontak Vials (36%) 1745
▲ Opana Tablets (1% to less than 10%) 1122
▲ Opana ER Tablets (1% to less than 10%) 1126
Orencia Powder for Intravenous Infusion (Less than 0.1% to 1%) 914
Orthoclone OKT3 Sterile Solution 2360
Oxsoralen-Ultra Capsules 3353
OxyContin Tablets 2703
OxyFast Oral Concentrate Solution 2708
OxyIR Capsules 2708
Parcopa Orally Disintegrating Tablets 3097
Paxil CR Controlled-Release Tablets (Infrequent) 1538
Paxil (Infrequent) 1530
Pediarix Vaccine (Rare) 1548
Percodan Tablets 1132
Permax Tablets (2.1%) 3356
Persantine Tablets (Rare) 868
Pexeva Tablets (Infrequent) 1694
Phenergan Tablets and Suppositories 3440
▲ Photofrin for Injection (7%) 702
Plasmanate 3255
Plavix Tablets 917
Plavix Tablets 2926
Pletal Tablets (Less than 2%) 2455
Premarin Intravenous 3442
Prevacid Delayed-Release Capsules (Less than 1%) 3271
Prevacid for Delayed-Release Oral Suspension (Less than 1%) 3271
Prevacid SoluTab Delayed-Release Orally Disintegrating Tablets (Less than 1%) 3271
Prevacid NapraPAC (Less than 1%) 3280
PREVPAC (Less than 1%) 3284
Primaxin I.M. 2045
Primaxin I.V. (0.4%) 2048
▲ Prinivil Tablets (0.3% to 4.4%; rare) 2052
Prinzide Tablets (1.4%) 2056
▲ Prograf Capsules and Injection (3% to 15%) 632
Prolastin (Rare) 3255
▲ Proleukin for Injection (3% to 71%) 2266
Prometrium Capsules (100 mg, 200 mg) (Rare) 3203
Proquin XR Tablets 1153
ProstaScint Kit (1%) 1037
Protonix I.V. (Less than 1%) 3472
Protonix Tablets (Less than 1%) 3469
Provigil Tablets (Greater than or equal to 1%) 988
Prozac Pulvules and Liquid (Infrequent) 1801
Quadramet Injection (2%) 1040
Ranexa Tablets (Less than or equal to 0.5%) 1035
Raniclor Tablets, Chewable (Rare) 2505
▲ Rapamune Oral Solution and Tablets (3% to 20%) 3475
Razadyne (Infrequent) 2399
Razadyne ER Extended-Release Capsules (Infrequent) 2399
Recombivax HB (Less than 1%) 2071
ReFacto Vials 3484
Refludan for Injection 792
Relpax Tablets (Rare) 2548
Remicade for IV Injection (Greater than or equal to 0.2%) 971
▲ Renagel Tablets (11%) 1282
▲ ReoPro Vials (21.1%) 1809
Requip Tablets (2%) 1555
Retavase 2499
Revlimid Capsules 958
Rhophylac (Rare) 3505
Rilutek Tablets (Infrequent) 2930
Risperdal (Infrequent to 2%) 1676
Risperdal Consta Long-Acting Injection (Frequent) 1682
Risperdal M-Tab Orally Disintegrating Tablets (Infrequent to 2%) 1676
▲ Rituxan I.V. (1% to 10%) 1254
Rythmol SR Capsules (Greater than or equal to 2%) 2727
▲ Simulect for Injection (3% to 10%) 2284
Sonata Capsules (Infrequent) 1717
St. Joseph 81 mg Aspirin Chewable and Enteric Coated Tablets 1869
Stalevo Tablets 2287
Sular Tablets (Less than or equal to 1%; very rare) 3122
Symbyax Capsules (Infrequent) 1819
Symmetrel Tablets 1135
Synera Topical Patch 1137
Tambocor Tablets (Less than 1%) 1856
Tarka Tablets (0.3% to 0.6%) 524
Tasmar Tablets (2%) 3358
▲ Taxotere Injection Concentrate (0.9% to 3.6%) 2932
Tegretol/Tegretol-XR 2295
Tequin Injection 938
Tequin Injection in 5% Dextrose 938
Tequin Tablets 938
Teveten Tablets (Less than 1%) 1735
Teveten HCT Tablets (Less than 1%) 1737
Thalomid Capsules 965
Thioridazine Hydrochloride Tablets 2163
Thiothixene Capsules 2165
Tiazac Capsules (Less than 2%) 1201
Timolide Tablets (1.6%) 2086
Timoptic Sterile Ophthalmic Solution (Less frequent) 2088
Timoptic in Ocudose (Less frequent) 2091
Timoptic-XE Sterile Ophthalmic Gel Forming Solution 2092
TNKase I.V. 1264
Topamax Sprinkle Capsules (Infrequent) 2404
Topamax Tablets (Infrequent) 2404
Toprol-XL Tablets (About 1 of 100 patients) 668
▲ Tracleer Tablets (7%) 545
Tranxene 2474
▲ Trasylol Injection (8%) 754
Travatan Ophthalmic Solution (1% to 5%) 563
Tricor Tablets 527
Triglide Tablets 3123
Trileptal Tablets (1% to 2%) 2300
Trileptal Oral Suspension (1% to 2%) 2300
▲ Trisenox Injection (25%) 993
Trizivir Tablets 1589
Twinrix Vaccine (Less than 1%) 1595
Tygacil for Injection (2.3%) 3488
▲ Ultane Liquid for Inhalation (4% to 11%) 531
Uniretic Tablets (More than 1%) 3100
▲ Valcyte Tablets (Less than 5%) 2813
Valium Tablets (Infrequent) 2819
Vancocin HCl Capsules, USP 3380
Vantin Tablets and Oral Suspension (Less than 1%) 2645
Vaprisol (2.7%) 643
▲ Vasotec I.V. Injection (0.5% to 6.7%) 2103
▲ Velcade for Injection (11%-12%) 2133
▲ Ventavis Inhalation Solution (11%) 1020
Verelan PM Extended-Release Capsules, Controlled-Onset (2.5%) 3106
▲ Vesanoid Capsules (14%; occasional) 2820
VFEND I.V. (Less than 2%) 2564
VFEND Oral Suspension (Less than 2%) 2564
VFEND Tablets (Less than 2%) 2564
Viagra Tablets (Less than 2%) 2573
Vicoprofen Tablets (Less than 1%) 539
Virazole for Inhalation Solution 3370
Voltaren Tablets (Rarely) 2307
Voltaren-XR Tablets (Rarely) 2310
Wellbutrin Tablets (2.5%) 1603
Wellbutrin SR Sustained-Release Tablets 1607
Wellbutrin XL Extended-Release Tablets 1613
WinRho SDF 732
Xeloda Tablets 2822
Xopenex Inhalation Solution 3146
Xopenex Inhalation Solution Concentrate 3150
Xopenex HFA Inhalation Aerosol 3154
Xyrem Oral Solution (Infrequent) 1688
Zantac Injection 1619
▲ Zegerid Capsules (9.6%) 2958
▲ Zegerid Powder for Oral Solution (9.6%) 2958
Zelapar Tablets 3372
Zelnorm Tablets (0.04%) 2312
Zemuron Injection (0.1%; 2%) 2346
Ziagen 1626
Zmax for Oral Suspension 2583
Zofran Injection (Rare) 1634
▲ Zofran (5%) 1639
▲ Zofran ODT Orally Disintegrating Tablets (5%) 1639
Zoloft (Infrequent) 2586
▲ Zometa for Intravenous Infusion (10.5%) 2315
Zonegran Capsules (Infrequent) 1101
Zosyn (1.0% or less to 1.3%) 3492
Zyban Sustained-Release Tablets 1644
Zyprexa Tablets (2%) 1830
Zyprexa IntraMuscular (2%) 1830
Zyprexa ZYDIS Orally Disintegrating Tablets (2%) 1830
Zyrtec Chewable Tablets (Rare) 2594
Zyrtec (Rare) 2594
Zyrtec-D 12 Hour Extended Release Tablets (Rare) 2597

Hypotension, neonatal

Aceon Tablets (2 mg, 4 mg, 8 mg) 3194
Altace Capsules 1702
Captopril Tablets 2149
Cozaar Tablets 1935
Hyzaar 50-12.5 Tablets 1990
Hyzaar 100-12.5 Tablets 1990
Hyzaar 100-25 Tablets 1990
Lotrel Capsules 2249
Prinivil Tablets 2052
Prinzide Tablets 2056
Vasotec I.V. Injection 2103

Hypotension, orthostatic

Aceon Tablets (2 mg, 4 mg, 8 mg) (0.3% to 1%) 3194
Actiq (Less than 1%) 979
Adalat CC Tablets (Less than 1%) 2964
Advicor Tablets 1722
Agrylin Capsules (1% to 5%) 3169
Aldoril Tablets 1910
Altace Capsules (2%) 1702
Ambien Tablets (Infrequent) 2851
Ambien CR Tablets (Infrequent) 2855
AmBisome for Injection (Less common) 620
Anzemet Injection (Rare) 2859
Anzemet Tablets (Rare) 2862
Aricept Tablets (Infrequent) 1094
Aricept ODT Tablets (Infrequent) 1094
Atacand HCT 651
Avalide Tablets 888
Avalide Tablets 2874
▲ Avapro Tablets (5.4%) 891
▲ Avapro Tablets (5.4%) 2871
▲ Azilect Tablets (9%) 3293
Caduet Tablets (Greater than 0.1% to less than 2%) 2508
Campral Tablets (Infrequent) 1174
Camptosar Injection 2604
Captopril Tablets 2149
Cardene I.V. (1.4%) 2497
Cardura XL Tablets (1.2%) 2515
Catapres-TTS (0.5% or less) 844
Celexa (Frequent) 1176
▲ CellCept Capsules (3% to less than 20%) 2747
▲ CellCept Intravenous (3% to less than 20%) 2747
▲ CellCept Oral Suspension (3% to less than 20%) 2747
▲ CellCept Tablets (3% to less than 20%) 2747
Cesamet Capsules 3340
Cialis Tablets (Less than 2%) 1838
Cipro 2977
Cipro I.V. 2984
Cipro XR Tablets 2990
▲ Clorpres Tablets (About 3 in 100) 2153
Clozaril Tablets 2184
Comtan Tablets 2189
Copaxone for Injection (Infrequent) 3297
▲ Coreg Tablets (1% to 3%) 1414
Covera-HS Tablets (0.4%) 3139
▲ Cozaar Tablets (4%) 1935
Depacon Injection (1% or more) 412
Depakene (1% or more) 417
Depakote Sprinkle Capsules 422
▲ Depakote Tablets (1% to 5%) 427
Depakote ER Tablets (Greater than 1%) 434
Dibenzyline Capsules 3399
Dilaudid Multiple Dose Vials 440
Diovan Tablets (2%) 2193
Diovan HCT Tablets (Less than 0.1%) 2196
Diuril Oral Suspension 1954
Diuril Sodium Intravenous 2467
Doxil Injection (Less than 1%) 2351
Dyazide Capsules 1423
Effexor Tablets (1%) 3411
Effexor XR Capsules (Frequent) 3417
Eldepryl Capsules 3208
▲ Emsam Transdermal System (9.8%) 903
Evoxac Capsules 1047
Exelon Capsules (Frequent) 2206
Exelon Oral Solution (Frequent) 2206
FazaClo Orally Disintegrating Tablets 551
Flomax Capsules (0.2% to 0.4%) 850
Furosemide Tablets 2154
Gabitril Tablets (Infrequent) 984
Geodon (Frequent) 2529
Hycotuss Expectorant Syrup 1117
Hyperstat I.V. 3017
Hytrin Capsules 471
▲ Indapamide Tablets (Less than 5%) 2156
▲ Intron A for Injection (Less than 5%) 3024
Ionsys Transdermal System (.1% to less than 1%) 2379
Kadian Capsules 577
Kaletra (Less than 2%) 476
Klonopin (Infrequent) 2778
Lamictal (Infrequent) 1481
Levaquin (0.1% to 0.9%) 2384
Levaquin in 5% Dextrose Injection (0.1% to 0.9%) 2384
Levitra Tablets (Less than 2%) 3034
Lexapro Oral Solution 1190
Lexapro Tablets 1190
Lipitor Tablets (Less than 2%) 2483
Lopressor HCT 50/25 Tablets 2241
Lopressor HCT 100/25 Tablets 2241
Lopressor HCT 100/50 Tablets 2241
Lotensin Tablets (0.4%) 2243
Lotensin HCT Tablets (0.3%) 2246
Lyrica Capsules (0.1% to 1%) 2539
Micardis Tablets 854
Micardis HCT Tablets (Less than 2%) 856
Midamor Tablets (Less than or equal to 1%) 2026
▲ Mirapex Tablets (Greater than or equal to 1% to 53%) 859
Moduretic Tablets (Less than or equal to 1%) 2028
MS Contin Tablets 2701
Namenda (Infrequent) 1195
Niaspan Extended-Release Tablets 1730
Nitrolingual Pumpspray (Occasional) 3120
Noroxin Tablets 2032
Norvasc Tablets (More than 0.1% to 1%) 2545
Norvir (Less than 2%) 503
Numorphan Injection 1120
Opana Tablets (Less than 1%) 1122
Opana ER Tablets (Less than 1%) 1126
▲ OxyContin Tablets (Between 1% and 5%) 2703
Parcopa Orally Disintegrating Tablets 3097
Paxil CR Controlled-Release Tablets (1.2%) 1538
Paxil (1.2%) 1530
Percodan Tablets 1132
▲ Permax Tablets (9.0% to 10.0%) 3356
Pletal Tablets (Less than 2%) 2455
Prinivil Tablets (0.3% to 1.2%) 2052
Prinzide Tablets (0.5% to 1.0%) 2056
▲ Prograf Capsules and Injection (3% to 15%) 632
Prometrium Capsules (100 mg, 200 mg) (Rare) 3203
Proquin XR Tablets 1153
Prozac Pulvules and Liquid (Infrequent) 1801
Ranexa Tablets (Less than or equal to 0.5%) 1035
▲ Rapamune Oral Solution and Tablets (3% to 20%) 3475
Razadyne (Infrequent) 2399
Razadyne ER Extended-Release Capsules (Infrequent) 2399
▲ Requip Tablets (6%) 1555
Rescriptor Tablets 2551
Rilutek Tablets (0.8% to 1.6%) 2930

Risperdal ... 1676
Risperdal Consta Long-Acting Injection (Infrequent to 2%) ... 1682
Risperdal M-Tab Orally Disintegrating Tablets ... 1676
▲ Rituxan I.V. (1% to 5%) ... 1254
Sandostatin Injection (Less than 1%) ... 2278
Sandostatin LAR Depot (Rare) ... 2280
▲ Seroquel Tablets (4%) ... 690
Sonata Capsules (Rare) ... 1717
Stalevo Tablets ... 2287
Stromectol Tablets (1.1%) ... 2083
Sular Tablets (Less than or equal to 1%) ... 3122
Symbyax Capsules ... 1819
▲ Symmetrel Tablets (1% to 5%) ... 1135
▲ Tasmar Tablets (13% to 14%) ... 3358
Teveten Tablets (Less than 1%) ... 1735
Teveten HCT Tablets (Less than 1%) ... 1737
Thalomid Capsules ... 965
Timolide Tablets ... 2086
Topamax Sprinkle Capsules (Infrequent) ... 2404
Topamax Tablets (Infrequent) ... 2404
Trecator Tablets ... 3487
Trileptal Tablets ... 2300
Trileptal Oral Suspension ... 2300
▲ Ultram ER Tablets (1.7% to 5.4%) ... 2392
Uniretic Tablets ... 3100
Univasc Tablets (0.51%) ... 3104
Uroxatral Tablets (0.4%) ... 2943
▲ Vaprisol (5.5%) ... 643
Vasotec I.V. Injection (0.5% to 1.6%) ... 2103
▲ Velcade for Injection (12%) ... 2133
VFEND I.V. (Less than 2%) ... 2564
VFEND Oral Suspension (Less than 2%) ... 2564
VFEND Tablets (Less than 2%) ... 2564
Viagra Tablets (Less than 2%) ... 2573
Wellbutrin Tablets ... 1603
Wellbutrin SR Sustained-Release Tablets (Infrequent) ... 1607
Wellbutrin XL Extended-Release Tablets (Infrequent) ... 1613
▲ Xeloda Tablets (Less than 5%) ... 2822
Zoloft (Infrequent) ... 2586
Zomig Tablets (Rare) ... 3519
Zomig-ZMT Tablets (Rare) ... 3519
Zyban Sustained-Release Tablets (Infrequent) ... 1644
▲ Zyprexa Tablets (3% to 5%) ... 1830
Zyprexa IntraMuscular (1%) ... 1830
▲ Zyprexa ZYDIS Orally Disintegrating Tablets (3% to 5%) ... 1830

Hypotension, postural
(*see under* Hypotension, orthostatic)

Hypotension, symptomatic
Aceon Tablets (2 mg, 4 mg, 8 mg) ... 3194
Altace Capsules (0.5%) ... 1702
Benicar HCT Tablets ... 1044
Covera-HS Tablets ... 3139
Cozaar Tablets ... 1935
Hyzaar 50-12.5 Tablets ... 1990
Hyzaar 100-12.5 Tablets ... 1990
Hyzaar 100-25 Tablets ... 1990
Lotensin Tablets (0.3%) ... 2243
Lotrel Capsules ... 2249
Mavik Tablets (Rare; 0.6%) ... 486
Prinivil Tablets ... 2052
Tarka Tablets ... 524
Uniretic Tablets ... 3100
Univasc Tablets (0.51%) ... 3104

Hypotensive crisis
Cymbalta Delayed-Release Capsules (Infrequent) ... 1757
Hyalgan Solution (One case) ... 2901

Hypothalamic-pituitary dysfunction
Lotronex Tablets (Rare) ... 1512

Hypothermia
Aggrenox Capsules ... 822
Alphagan P Ophthalmic Solution ... 567
Bayer Aspirin ... 744
Bayer Aspirin Comprehensive Prescribing Information ... ▣ 796
Brimonidine Tartrate Ophthalmic Solution 0.2% ... ⊙ 248
Clozaril Tablets (Less than 1%) ... 2184
Depacon Injection ... 412
Depakene ... 417
Depakote Sprinkle Capsules ... 422
Depakote Tablets ... 427
Depakote ER Tablets ... 434
Doxil Injection (Less than 1%) ... 2351
Emend Capsules (Greater than 0.5%) ... 1963
Exelon Capsules (Infrequent) ... 2206
Exelon Oral Solution (Infrequent) ... 2206
FazaClo Orally Disintegrating Tablets (Less than 1%) ... 551
Geodon Capsules (Frequent) ... 2529
Invanz for Injection (1.6%) ... 1999
Ionsys Transdermal System (.1% to less than 1%) ... 2379
Namenda (Infrequent) ... 1195
Norvir (Less than 2%) ... 503
Percodan Tablets ... 1132
Permax Tablets (Infrequent) ... 3356
Proleukin for Injection (Less than 1%) ... 2266
Provigil Tablets (At least 1%) ... 988
Prozac Pulvules and Liquid (Rare) ... 1801
Relpax Tablets (Rare) ... 2548
Rilutek Tablets (Rare) ... 2930
Risperdal ... 1676
Risperdal M-Tab Orally Disintegrating Tablets ... 1676
St. Joseph 81 mg Aspirin Chewable and Enteric Coated Tablets ... 1869
St. Joseph 81 mg Aspirin ... ▣ 688
Ultane Liquid for Inhalation (1%) ... 531
▲ Vesanoid Capsules (3%) ... 2820

Hypothesia
Rythmol SR Capsules ... 2727

Hypothyroidism
Abilify Oral Solution (Infrequent) ... 882
Abilify Oral Solution (Infrequent) ... 2450
Abilify Discmelt Orally Disintegrating Tablets (Infrequent) ... 882
Abilify Discmelt Orally Disintegrating Tablets (Infrequent) ... 2450
Abilify Tablets (Infrequent) ... 882
Abilify Tablets (Infrequent) ... 2450
Aciphex Tablets ... 1090
▲ Advair Diskus 250/50 (1% to 3%) ... 1308
Amerge Tablets (Rare) ... 1339
▲ Aredia for Injection (Up to 6%) ... 2179
Betaseron for SC Injection ... 767
▲ Bexxar (0% to 7%) ... 1398
Campral Tablets (Rare) ... 1174
Celexa (Rare) ... 1176
▲ CellCept Capsules (3% to less than 20%) ... 2747
▲ CellCept Intravenous (3% to less than 20%) ... 2747
▲ CellCept Oral Suspension (3% to less than 20%) ... 2747
▲ CellCept Tablets (3% to less than 20%) ... 2747
Climara Transdermal System ... 771
Copaxone for Injection (Infrequent) ... 3297
▲ Copegus Tablets (Less than 1% to 4%) ... 2754
Effexor Tablets (Rare) ... 3411
Effexor XR Capsules (Rare) ... 3417
Evoxac Capsules (Less than 1%) ... 1047
Exelon Capsules (Infrequent) ... 2206
Exelon Oral Solution (Infrequent) ... 2206
Gabitril Tablets (Infrequent) ... 984
Genotropin Lyophilized Powder (Infrequent) ... 2638
Herceptin I.V. (At least one of the 958 patients) ... 1233
▲ Humatrope Vials and Cartridges (11%) ... 1787
Imitrex Injection ... 1463
Imitrex Nasal Spray (Rare) ... 1467
Imitrex Tablets (Rare) ... 1471
▲ Intron A for Injection (Less than 5%) ... 3024
Kaletra (Less than 2%) ... 476
Lamictal (Rare) ... 1481
Lithobid Tablets ... 1692
Meridia Capsules ... 489
Neurontin Capsules (Rare) ... 2487
Neurontin Oral Solution (Rare) ... 2487
Neurontin Tablets (Rare) ... 2487
Nexavar Tablets (Uncommon) ... 746
▲ Ontak Vials (Less than 5%) ... 1745
Paxil CR Controlled-Release Tablets (Rare) ... 1538
Paxil (Rare) ... 1530
▲ Pegasys (3% to 4%) ... 2789
▲ PEG-Intron Powder for Injection (5%) ... 3048
Permax Tablets (Infrequent) ... 3356
Pexeva Tablets (rare) ... 1694
Premarin Tablets ... 3446
Prevacid Delayed-Release Capsules (Less than 1%) ... 3271
Prevacid for Delayed-Release Oral Suspension (Less than 1%) ... 3271
Prevacid SoluTab Delayed-Release Orally Disintegrating Tablets (Less than 1%) ... 3271
Prevacid NapraPAC (Less than 1%) ... 3280
PREVPAC (Less than 1%) ... 3284
Proleukin for Injection (Less than 1%) ... 2266
Protopic Ointment (0.2% to less than 1%) ... 638
Prozac Pulvules and Liquid (Infrequent) ... 1801
▲ Rebetol (4% to 5%) ... 3058
Requip Tablets (Infrequent) ... 1555
▲ Revlimid Capsules (6.8%) ... 958
▲ Ribavirin, USP Capsules (4% to 5%) ... 3068
Risperdal Consta Long-Acting Injection (Infrequent) ... 1682
▲ Sandostatin Injection (12%) ... 2278
▲ Sandostatin LAR Depot (12%) ... 2280
Seroquel Tablets (Infrequent) ... 690
Sonata Capsules (Rare) ... 1717
▲ Sutent Capsules (4% to 7%) ... 2560
Symbyax Capsules (Infrequent) ... 1819
▲ Targretin Capsules (28.6% to 52.8%) ... 1747
Thalomid Capsules ... 965
Thyrolar Tablets ... 1199
VFEND I.V. (Less than 2%) ... 2564
VFEND Oral Suspension (Less than 2%) ... 2564
VFEND Tablets (Less than 2%) ... 2564
Zoloft ... 2586

Hypotonia
Abilify Oral Solution (Rare) ... 882
Abilify Oral Solution (Rare) ... 2450
Abilify Discmelt Orally Disintegrating Tablets (Rare) ... 882
Abilify Discmelt Orally Disintegrating Tablets (Rare) ... 2450
Abilify Tablets (Rare) ... 882
Abilify Tablets (Rare) ... 2450
Aloprim for Injection (Less than 1%) ... 2167
Alphagan P Ophthalmic Solution ... 567
Ambien Tablets (Rare) ... 2851
Ambien CR Tablets (Rare) ... 2855
Brimonidine Tartrate Ophthalmic Solution 0.2% ... ⊙ 248
Cesamet Capsules ... 3340
▲ Coreg Tablets (Greater than 1% to 3%) ... 1414
Doxil Injection (Less than 1%) ... 2351
Duragesic Transdermal System (Less than 1%) ... 2373
Effexor Tablets (Infrequent) ... 3411
Effexor XR Capsules (Infrequent) ... 3417
Frova Tablets (Rare) ... 1113
Gabitril Tablets (Frequent) ... 984
Geodon Capsules (Frequent) ... 2529
HibTITER ... 3426
Infanrix Vaccine ... 1476
Klonopin ... 2778
Lamictal (Rare) ... 1481
Lyrica Capsules (0.1% to 1%) ... 2539
Neurontin Capsules (Infrequent) ... 2487
Neurontin Oral Solution (Infrequent) ... 2487
Neurontin Tablets (Infrequent) ... 2487
Orthoclone OKT3 Sterile Solution (Less than 1%) ... 2360
OxyContin Tablets (Less than 1%) ... 2703
Pediarix Vaccine ... 1548
Permax Tablets (Infrequent) ... 3356
▲ Rapamune Oral Solution and Tablets (3% to 20%) ... 3475
Requip Tablets (Infrequent) ... 1555
Rilutek Tablets (Rare) ... 2930
Risperdal (Rare) ... 1676
Risperdal M-Tab Orally Disintegrating Tablets (Rare) ... 1676
Sonata Capsules (Infrequent) ... 1717
Trileptal Tablets ... 2300
Trileptal Oral Suspension ... 2300
Zelapar Tablets ... 3372
Zoloft (Rare) ... 2586
Zomig Tablets (Rare) ... 3519
Zomig-ZMT Tablets (Rare) ... 3519
Zonegran Capsules (Infrequent) ... 1101
Zyprexa Tablets (Infrequent) ... 1830
Zyprexa ZYDIS Orally Disintegrating Tablets (Infrequent) ... 1830

Hypotonic-hyporesponsive episode
DAPTACEL Vaccine (0.39%) ... 2950
Infanrix Vaccine ... 1476

Hypotrichosis
Vantas (Less than 2%) ... 3375

Hypouresis
▲ Chemet Capsules (Up to 3.7%) ... 2458
Cymbalta Delayed-Release Capsules (Infrequent) ... 1757
Dilaudid-HP ... 442
▲ Indocin I.V. (41% of infants) ... 2465
K-Phos Neutral Tablets ... 760
▲ NeoProfen Injection (3%) ... 2472
Prograf Capsules and Injection ... 632
Uroqid-Acid No. 2 Tablets ... 760

Hypouricemia
Cipro I.V. (Infrequent) ... 2984
Timentin ADD-Vantage ... 1580
Timentin Injection Galaxy Container ... 1583
Timentin IV Infusion ... 1577
Timentin Pharmacy Bulk Package ... 1586
Zoloft ... 2586

Hypoventilation
Aciphex Tablets (Rare) ... 1090
Avinza Capsules (Less than 5%) ... 1741
▲ Buprenex Injectable (1% to 5%) ... 2716
Copaxone for Injection (Infrequent) ... 3297
Diastat Rectal Delivery System (Two patients) ... 3343
▲ Duragesic Transdermal System (2% to 10%) ... 2373
Effexor XR Capsules (Rare) ... 3417
Ionsys Transdermal System (.1% to less than 1%) ... 2379
Nembutal Sodium Solution, USP (Less than 1%) ... 2470
Neurontin Capsules (Rare) ... 2487
Neurontin Oral Solution (Rare) ... 2487
Neurontin Tablets (Rare) ... 2487
Norvir (Less than 2%) ... 503
Percodan Tablets ... 1132
Permax Tablets (Rare) ... 3356
Prozac Pulvules and Liquid (Rare) ... 1801
Rilutek Tablets (Infrequent) ... 2930
Ultane Liquid for Inhalation (Less than 1%) ... 531
Virazole for Inhalation Solution (Infrequent) ... 3370
Zyprexa Tablets (Rare) ... 1830
Zyprexa ZYDIS Orally Disintegrating Tablets (Rare) ... 1830

Hypovolemia
Campath Ampules ... 811
▲ CellCept Capsules (3% to less than 20%) ... 2747
▲ CellCept Intravenous (3% to less than 20%) ... 2747
▲ CellCept Oral Suspension (3% to less than 20%) ... 2747
▲ CellCept Tablets (3% to less than 20%) ... 2747
▲ Coreg Tablets (Greater than 1% to 3%) ... 1414
Demadex Injection ... 2759
Demadex Tablets ... 2759
Emend Capsules (Greater than 0.5%) ... 1963
Estratest Tablets ... 3199
Estratest H.S. Tablets ... 3199
Follistim AQ Cartridge ... 2338
Zelnorm Tablets (0.04%) ... 2312

Hypoxemia
Carimune NF ... 3499
Flebogamma 5%, Immune Globulin Intravenous (Human) ... 1658
Gammagard Liquid ... 721
Gammagard S/D ... 724
Gamunex Immune Globulin I.V., 10% ... 3235
Invanz for Injection (Greater than 0.1%) ... 1999
Mivacron Injection (Less than 1%) ... 493
Orthoclone OKT3 Sterile Solution ... 2360

Hypoxia
Abilify Oral Solution (Rare) ... 882
Abilify Oral Solution (Rare) ... 2450
Abilify Discmelt Orally Disintegrating Tablets (Rare) ... 882
Abilify Discmelt Orally Disintegrating Tablets (Rare) ... 2450
Abilify Tablets (Rare) ... 882
Abilify Tablets (Rare) ... 2450
Ambien Tablets (Rare) ... 2851
Ambien CR Tablets (Rare) ... 2855
▲ AmBisome for Injection (6.2% to 7.5%) ... 620
Aricept Tablets (Infrequent) ... 1094
Aricept ODT Tablets (Infrequent) ... 1094
BeneFix Vials (1.5%) ... 3408
Bicillin C-R Injectable Suspension ... 1706

Campath Ampules 811
Carbatrol Capsules 3171
▲ CellCept Capsules (3% to less than 20%) 2747
▲ CellCept Intravenous (3% to less than 20%) 2747
▲ CellCept Oral Suspension (3% to less than 20%) 2747
▲ CellCept Tablets (3% to less than 20%) 2747
▲ Dacogen Injection (10%) 2129
▲ DepoDur Extended-Release Injection (5% to 10%) 1110
Effexor Tablets (Rare) 3411
Effexor XR Capsules (Rare) 3417
Elitek 2890
Emend Capsules (Greater than 0.5%) 1963
Ethyol for Injection (Rare) 1898
Herceptin I.V. (At least one of the 958 patients) 1233
▲ Ionsys Transdermal System (1% to less than 10%) 2379
I.V. Busulfex (2%) 2493
Kadian Capsules (Less than 3%) 577
Leukine 814
Levaquin (0.1% to 0.9%) 2384
Levaquin in 5% Dextrose Injection (0.1% to 0.9%) 2384
Merrem I.V. (Greater than 0.1% to 1%) 686
Mycamine for Injection 628
▲ Mylotarg for Injection (5%) 3431
Neulasta Injection (Single case) 601
▲ Opana Tablets (1% to less than 10%) 1122
▲ Opana ER Tablets (1% to less than 10%) 1126
Orthoclone OKT3 Sterile Solution 2360
Permax Tablets (Rare) 3356
Protopic Ointment (Greater than or equal to 1%) 638
Prozac Pulvules and Liquid (Rare) 1801
Pulmozyme Inhalation Solution 1248
▲ Rapamune Oral Solution and Tablets (3% to 20%) 3475
Revlimid Capsules (1.4%) 958
Reyataz Capsules (Less than 3%) 921
Rilutek Tablets (Infrequent) 2930
Rituxan I.V. (0.3%) 1254
Targretin Capsules 1747
Tasmar Tablets (Rare) 3358
Tegretol/Tegretol-XR 2295
Trasylol Injection (2%) 754
▲ Trisenox Injection (23%) 993
Ultane Liquid for Inhalation (Less than 1%) 531
VFEND I.V. (Less than 2%) 2564
VFEND Oral Suspension (Less than 2%) 2564
VFEND Tablets (Less than 2%) 2564
▲ Zofran (9%) 1639
▲ Zofran ODT Orally Disintegrating Tablets (9%) 1639
Zyprexa Tablets (Infrequent) 1830
Zyprexa ZYDIS Orally Disintegrating Tablets (Infrequent) 1830

Hysteria
Ambien Tablets (Rare) 2851
Imitrex Injection (Rare) 1463
Imitrex Tablets (Rare) 1471
Klonopin 2778
Neurontin Capsules (Rare) 2487
Neurontin Oral Solution (Rare) 2487
Neurontin Tablets (Rare) 2487
Paxil CR Controlled-Release Tablets (Rare) 1538
Paxil (Rare) 1530
Pexeva Tablets (Rare) 1694
Phenergan Tablets and Suppositories 3440
Relpax Tablets (Rare) 2548
Trileptal Tablets 2300
Trileptal Oral Suspension 2300

I

Ichthyosis
▲ Advair Diskus 100/50 (1% to 3%) 1308
▲ Advair Diskus 250/50 (1% to 3%) 1308
▲ Advair Diskus 500/50 (1% to 3%) 1308
Efudex (Infrequent) 3363
▲ Metrogel 1% (0.6% to 16.2%) 1211
Thalomid Capsules 965
Tricor Tablets 527

Icterus
(*see under* Jaundice)

Idiosyncrasy
Furosemide Tablets 2154

Idiosyncratic reactions
(*see under* Idiosyncrasy)

Idioventricular rhythm, accelerated
Retavase 2499

Idioventricular rhythms
Activase I.V. 1223

Ileitis, regional
Accutane Capsules 2731
Effexor XR Capsules (Rare) 3417
Indocin (Less than 1%) 1995
Norvir (Less than 2%) 503
Paxil CR Controlled-Release Tablets (Rare) 1538
Paxil (Rare) 1530
Pexeva Tablets (Rare) 1694

Ileus
Aricept Tablets (Infrequent) 1094
Aricept ODT Tablets (Infrequent) 1094
Camptosar Injection (Rare) 2604
Celebrex Capsules (Less than 0.1%) 3134
▲ CellCept Capsules (3% to less than 20%) 2747
▲ CellCept Intravenous (3% to less than 20%) 2747
▲ CellCept Oral Suspension (3% to less than 20%) 2747
▲ CellCept Tablets (3% to less than 20%) 2747
Cipro I.V. (1% or less) 2984
Cipro XR Tablets 2990
Dilaudid 440
Dilaudid Non-Sterile Powder 440
Dilaudid Oral Liquid 445
Dilaudid Rectal Suppositories 440
Dilaudid Tablets 440
Dilaudid Tablets - 8 mg 445
▲ Doxil Injection (1% to 10%) 2351
Effexor Tablets (Rare) 3411
Effexor XR Capsules 3417
Elitek (Less than or equal to 1%) 2890
Eloxatin for Injection 2892
Evoxac Capsules (Less than 1%) 1047
Fleet Prep Kits 1170
Herceptin I.V. (At least one of the 958 patients) 1233
Hyperstat I.V. 3017
Indocin I.V. (1% to 3%) 2465
Invanz for Injection (Greater than 0.1%) 1999
▲ Ionsys Transdermal System (1% to less than 10%) 2379
▲ I.V. Busulfex (2% to 8%) 2493
Lotronex Tablets (Rare) 1512
Merrem I.V. (Greater than 0.1% to 1%) 686
MS Contin Tablets (Less frequent) 2701
Myfortic Tablets 2255
Namenda 1195
NeoProfen Injection 2472
Nimotop Capsules (Rare) 749
Nipent for Injection (Less than 3%) 1863
Omnicef Capsules 511
Omnicef for Oral Suspension 511
Opana Tablets (Less than 1%) 1122
Opana ER Tablets (Less than 1%) 1126
OxyContin Tablets (Less than 1%) 2703
Paxil CR Controlled-Release Tablets (Rare) 1538
Paxil (Rare) 1530
Percodan Tablets 1132
Pexeva Tablets (Rare) 1694
▲ Photofrin for Injection (Less than 5%) 702
▲ Prograf Capsules and Injection (3% to 15%) 632
Proleukin for Injection (2%) 2266
Proquin XR Tablets 1153
▲ Rapamune Oral Solution and Tablets (3% to 20%) 3475
Remicade for IV Injection (Greater than or equal to 0.2%) 971
ReoPro Vials (0.3%) 1809
Rilutek Tablets (Rare) 2930
Taxotere Injection Concentrate 2932
Vasotec I.V. Injection (0.5% to 1.0%) 2103
▲ Xeloda Tablets (1% to 6%) 2822
Zosyn (1.0% or less) 3492
Zyprexa Tablets (Rare) 1830
Zyprexa ZYDIS Orally Disintegrating Tablets (Rare) 1830

Ileus, adynamic
Thiothixene Capsules 2165

Ileus, paralytic
BiDil Tablets 2171
Campath Ampules 811
Clozaril Tablets 2184
Covera-HS Tablets (Infrequent) 3139
▲ DepoDur Extended-Release Injection (5% to 10%) 1110
FazaClo Orally Disintegrating Tablets 551
Numorphan Injection 1120
Podocon-25 Liquid 2478
Tarka Tablets (Infrequent) 524
Thioridazine Hydrochloride Tablets 2163
Vivitrol 995

Illusion, unspecified
Ambien Tablets (Infrequent) 2851
Ambien CR Tablets (Infrequent) 2855
Evoxac Capsules 1047
Klonopin (Infrequent) 2778
Zoloft (Rare) 2586

Immobility
Moban Tablets 1119

Immune reconstitution syndrome
Epivir 1427
Epzicom Tablets 1436
Lexiva Tablets 1505
Norvir 503
Rescriptor Tablets 2551
Retrovir Capsules 1560
Retrovir IV Infusion 1564
Retrovir 1560
Viread Tablets 1301
Ziagen 1626

Immunogenicity
▲ Bexxar (1% to 7%) 1398
▲ Enbrel for Injection (6%) 584
Epogen for Injection 591
▲ Erbitux (5%) 910
Forteo for Injection (2.8%) 1767
Neumega for Injection (2%) 3435
NovoLog Injection 2326
Orencia Powder for Intravenous Infusion (1.7%) 914
PEG-Intron Powder for Injection 3048
Procrit for Injection 2364
▲ Raptiva for Injection (6.3%) 1250
Remicade for IV Injection 971
▲ Rituxan I.V. (1.1% to 5%) 1254
Synagis 1897

Immunoglobulin, abnormalities
Phenytek Capsules 2160
Rilutek Tablets (Infrequent) 2930
Xolair 1266

Immunosuppression
Cutivate Lotion 0.05% (Rare) 2664

Immunosuppression, progressive
Lamictal 1481

Impetigo
Cutivate Cream (0.8%) 2662
▲ Elidel Cream 1% (1.9% to 4%) 2200
ProQuad 2064
Varivax 2100

Impetigo, bullous
Protopic Ointment 638

Impotence
(*see also under* Sexual dysfunction)
Abelcet Injection 1141
Abilify Oral Solution (Infrequent) 882
Abilify Oral Solution (Infrequent) 2450
Abilify Discmelt Orally Disintegrating Tablets (Infrequent) 882
Abilify Discmelt Orally Disintegrating Tablets (Infrequent) 2450
Abilify Tablets (Infrequent) 882
Abilify Tablets (Infrequent) 2450
Aciphex Tablets (Rare) 1090
▲ Adalat CC Tablets (3% or less) 2964
Adderall Tablets 3164
▲ Adderall XR Capsules (2% to 4%) 3166
Adipex-P 1215
Advicor Tablets 1722
Aldoril Tablets 1910
Altace Capsules (Less than 1%) 1702
Ambien Tablets (Rare) 2851
Ambien CR Tablets (Rare) 2855
Arthrotec Tablets (Rare) 3129
Atacand HCT 651
▲ Avinza Capsules (Less than 5%) 1741
▲ Avodart Soft Gelatin Capsules (0.8% to 4.7%) 1390
Axid Oral Solution 879
Azilect Tablets (Greater than 1%) 3293
Betagan Ophthalmic Solution, USP ⊙220
▲ Betaseron for SC Injection (9%) 767
Betimol Ophthalmic Solution 3382
Betimol Ophthalmic Solution ⊙295
Bicillin C-R Injectable Suspension 1706
Blocadren Tablets (Less than 1%) 1916
Caduet Tablets (Less than 2%) 2508
Campral Tablets (Frequent) 1174
Captopril Tablets 2149
Carbatrol Capsules 3171
Cardizem LA Extended Release Tablets (Less than 2%) 1728
Cardura XL Tablets (Less than 1%) 2515
▲ Catapres Tablets (About 3 in 100 patients) 843
Catapres-TTS (2 of 101 patients) 844
▲ Celexa (3%) 1176
▲ CellCept Capsules (3% to less than 20%) 2747
▲ CellCept Intravenous (3% to less than 20%) 2747
▲ CellCept Oral Suspension (3% to less than 20%) 2747
▲ CellCept Tablets (3% to less than 20%) 2747
Chantix Tablets (Infrequent) 2517
▲ Clorpres Tablets (About 3%) 2153
Clozaril Tablets (Less than 1%) 2184
▲ Coreg Tablets (Greater than 1% to 3%) 1414
Cosopt Sterile Ophthalmic Solution 1931
Covera-HS Tablets (Less than 2%) 3139
Cozaar Tablets (Less than 1%) 1935
Demadex Injection 2759
Demadex Tablets 2759
Demser Capsules (Infrequent) 1953
Desoxyn Tablets, USP 2462
Dexedrine 1420
DextroStat Tablets 3179
Diovan Tablets 2193
Diovan HCT Tablets (Greater than 0.2%) 2196
Ditropan XL Extended-Release Tablets (Rare) 2413
Diuril Oral Suspension 1954
Diuril Sodium Intravenous 2467
Donnatal Extentabs 2493
Dyazide Capsules 1423
DynaCirc CR Tablets (0.5% to 1%) 2721
▲ Effexor Tablets (2.1% to 6%) 3411
▲ Effexor XR Capsules (3% to 10%) 3417
Eligard 7.5 mg (Less than 2%) 2880
Eligard 22.5 mg (Less than 2%) 2883
Eligard 30 mg 2885
Emsam Transdermal System (0.7%) 903
Equetro Extended-Release Capsules 3180
▲ Eulexin Capsules (33%) 3009
Evoxac Capsules 1047
Exelon Capsules (Infrequent) 2206
Exelon Oral Solution (Infrequent) 2206
FazaClo Orally Disintegrating Tablets (Less than 1%) 551
Gabitril Tablets (Infrequent) 984
Geodon Capsules (Infrequent) 2529
Hytrin Capsules (1.2% to 1.6%) 471
Hyzaar 50-12.5 Tablets 1990
Hyzaar 100-12.5 Tablets 1990
Hyzaar 100-25 Tablets 1990
▲ Imdur Tablets (Less than or equal to 5%) 3018
▲ Indapamide Tablets (Less than 5%) 2156
Inderal LA Long-Acting Capsules (Rare) 3429
InnoPran XL Capsules (Rare) 2723
▲ Intron A for Injection (Less than 5%) 3024
Invirase (Less than 2%) 2772
Klonopin (1%) 2778
▲ Lamictal (13%) 1481
Levaquin (0.1% to 0.9%) 2384
Levaquin in 5% Dextrose Injection (0.1% to 0.9%) 2384
▲ Lexapro Oral Solution (Less than 1% to 3%) 1190
▲ Lexapro Tablets (Less than 1% to 3%) 1190
Lipitor Tablets (Less than 2%) 2483
Lithobid Tablets 1692
Lopressor HCT 50/25 Tablets (1%) 2241
Lopressor HCT 100/25 Tablets (1%) 2241
Lopressor HCT 100/50 Tablets (1%) 2241
Lotensin Tablets (Less than 1%) 2243
Lotensin HCT Tablets (1.2%) 2246
Lotrel Capsules 2249
▲ Lupron Depot 7.5 mg (5.4%) 3264

Lyrica Capsules (Greater than or equal to 1%) ... 2539
Mavik Tablets (0.3% to 1.0%) ... 486
▲ Megace ES Oral Suspension (4% to 14%) ... 2481
Meridia Capsules ... 489
Micardis Tablets (More than 0.3%) ... 854
Micardis HCT Tablets ... 856
▲ Midamor Tablets (Between 1% and 3%) ... 2026
Mirapex Tablets (2%) ... 859
Moduretic Tablets (Less than or equal to 1%) ... 2028
MS Contin Tablets (Less frequent) ... 2701
Nadolol Tablets (1 to 5 of 1000 patients) ... 2159
Namenda (More than one patient) ... 1195
Neurontin Capsules (1.5%) ... 2487
Neurontin Oral Solution (1.5%) ... 2487
Neurontin Tablets (1.5%) ... 2487
Nexium Delayed-Release Capsules (Less than 1%) ... 655
Nexium I.V. (Less than 1%) ... 659
Nipent for Injection (Less than 3%) ... 1863
Norvir (Less than 2%) ... 503
Omacor Capsules ... 2725
Oxandrin Tablets ... 2962
OxyContin Tablets (Less than 1%) ... 2703
Parnate Tablets ... 1527
▲ Paxil CR Controlled-Release Tablets (4% to 10.0%) ... 1538
▲ Paxil (4% to 10.0%) ... 1530
Pepcid Injection (Rare) ... 2040
Pepcid (Rare) ... 2038
Permax Tablets (Infrequent) ... 3356
▲ Pexeva Tablets (1.5% to 8%) ... 1694
Prevacid Delayed-Release Capsules (Less than 1%) ... 3271
Prevacid for Delayed-Release Oral Suspension (Less than 1%) ... 3271
Prevacid SoluTab Delayed-Release Orally Disintegrating Tablets (Less than 1%) ... 3271
Prevacid NapraPAC (Less than 1%) ... 3280
PREVPAC (Less than 1%) ... 3284
Prinivil Tablets (1.0%) ... 2052
Prinzide Tablets (1.2%) ... 2056
▲ Propecia Tablets (5.1% to 8.1%) ... 2060
▲ Proscar Tablets (5.15 to 8.1%) ... 2067
Protonix I.V. (Less than 1%) ... 3472
Protonix Tablets (Less than 1%) ... 3469
Prozac Pulvules and Liquid (Less than 1%) ... 1801
▲ Rapamune Oral Solution and Tablets (3% to 20%) ... 3475
Relpax Tablets (Infrequent) ... 2548
▲ Requip Tablets (3%) ... 1555
Rescriptor Tablets ... 2551
Reyataz Capsules (Less than 3%) ... 921
Rilutek Tablets (Infrequent) ... 2930
Risperdal Consta Long-Acting Injection (Infrequent) ... 1682
Rythmol SR Capsules ... 2727
▲ Sandostatin LAR Depot (1% to 4%) ... 2280
Seroquel Tablets (Infrequent) ... 690
▲ Simulect for Injection (3% to 10%) ... 2284
Soltamox Oral Solution ... 3527
Sonata Capsules (Infrequent) ... 1717
▲ Strattera Capsules (3%) ... 1814
Sular Tablets (Less than or equal to 1%) ... 3122
▲ Symbyax Capsules (2% to 4%) ... 1819
Tambocor Tablets (Less than 1%) ... 1856
Tarka Tablets (0.3% or more) ... 524
Tasmar Tablets (Frequent) ... 3358
Tegretol/Tegretol-XR ... 2295
Teveten HCT Tablets ... 1737
▲ Thalomid Capsules (8.3%) ... 965
Thiothixene Capsules (Infrequently) ... 2165
Tiazac Capsules (Less than 2%) ... 1201
Timolide Tablets ... 2086
Timoptic Sterile Ophthalmic Solution (Less frequent) ... 2088
Timoptic in Ocudose (Less frequent) ... 2091
Timoptic-XE Sterile Ophthalmic Gel Forming Solution ... 2092
Topamax Sprinkle Capsules (Frequent) ... 2404
Topamax Tablets (Frequent) ... 2404
Toprol-XL Tablets ... 668
Trecator Tablets ... 3487
▲ Trelstar Depot (7.1%) ... 3394
Trelstar LA Suspension (2.3%) ... 3397
Uniretic Tablets (More than 1%) ... 3100
Uroxatral Tablets (1% to 2%) ... 2943
Vasotec I.V. Injection (0.5% to 1.0%) ... 2103
Verelan PM Extended-Release Capsules, Controlled-Onset (2% or less) ... 3106
VFEND I.V. (Less than 2%) ... 2564
VFEND Oral Suspension (Less than 2%) ... 2564
VFEND Tablets (Less than 2%) ... 2564
Viadur Implant (2.3%) ... 757
Vicoprofen Tablets (Less than 1%) ... 539
Vytorin 10/10 Tablets ... 2114
Vytorin 10/10 Tablets ... 3077
Vytorin 10/20 Tablets ... 2114
Vytorin 10/20 Tablets ... 3077
Vytorin 10/40 Tablets ... 2114
Vytorin 10/40 Tablets ... 3077
Vytorin 10/80 Tablets ... 2114
Vytorin 10/80 Tablets ... 3077
▲ Wellbutrin Tablets (3.4%) ... 1603
Wellbutrin SR Sustained-Release Tablets (Infrequent) ... 1607
Wellbutrin XL Extended-Release Tablets (Infrequent) ... 1613
Zantac (Occasional) ... 1624
Zantac Injection ... 1619
Zantac Injection Pharmacy Bulk Package (Infrequent) ... 1622
Zantac Injection Premixed ... 1619
Zantac (Occasional) ... 1624
Zoloft (Frequent) ... 2586
Zonegran Capsules (Infrequent) ... 1101
Zyban Sustained-Release Tablets (Infrequent) ... 1644
Zyprexa Tablets (Infrequent) ... 1830
Zyprexa ZYDIS Orally Disintegrating Tablets (Infrequent) ... 1830

Impulse control, impaired
Effexor Tablets (Rare) ... 3411
Paxil CR Controlled-Release Tablets ... 1538
Paxil ... 1530
Prozac Pulvules and Liquid ... 1801
Symbyax Capsules ... 1819
Zoloft ... 2586

Incontinence
Eraxis for Injection (Less than 1% to less than 2%) ... 2521
Moduretic Tablets (Less than or equal to 1%) ... 2028
Namenda (Greater than or equal to 2%) ... 1195
Niravam Orally Disintegrating Tablets (1.5%) ... 3092
Razadyne (Frequent) ... 2399
Razadyne ER Extended-Release Capsules (Frequent) ... 2399
▲ Sandostatin LAR Depot (1% to 4%) ... 2280
Valium Tablets (Infrequent) ... 2819

Incontinence, fecal
Abilify Oral Solution ... 882
Abilify Oral Solution ... 2450
Abilify Discmelt Orally Disintegrating Tablets ... 882
Abilify Discmelt Orally Disintegrating Tablets ... 2450
Abilify Tablets ... 882
Abilify Tablets ... 2450
Actiq (Less than 1%) ... 979
AmBisome for Injection (Less common) ... 620
Amitiza Capsules (Less than 0.2%) ... 3224
Aricept Tablets (Frequent) ... 1094
Aricept ODT Tablets (Frequent) ... 1094
Azilect Tablets (Infrequent) ... 3293
Colazal Capsules ... 2838
Copaxone for Injection (At least 2%) ... 3297
Depacon Injection (1% or more) ... 412
Depakene (1% or more) ... 417
Depakote Sprinkle Capsules ... 422
▲ Depakote Tablets (1% to 5%) ... 427
Depakote ER Tablets (Greater than 1%) ... 434
Exelon Capsules (Frequent) ... 2206
Exelon Oral Solution (Frequent) ... 2206
Gabitril Tablets (Infrequent) ... 984
Kaletra (Less than 2%) ... 476
Klonopin ... 2778
Lithobid Tablets ... 1692
Marinol Capsules (Less than 1%) ... 3333
Neurontin Capsules (Infrequent) ... 2487
Neurontin Oral Solution (Infrequent) ... 2487
Neurontin Tablets (Infrequent) ... 2487
Omacor Capsules ... 2725
Paxil CR Controlled-Release Tablets (Rare) ... 1538
Paxil (Rare) ... 1530
Pentasa Capsules (Less than 1%) ... 3185
Permax Tablets (Rare) ... 3356
Pexeva Tablets (rare) ... 1694
Prozac Pulvules and Liquid (Rare) ... 1801
Requip Tablets (Infrequent) ... 1555
Rilutek Tablets (Infrequent) ... 2930
Risperdal (Rare) ... 1676
Risperdal Consta Long-Acting Injection (Infrequent) ... 1682
Risperdal M-Tab Orally Disintegrating Tablets (Rare) ... 1676
Seroquel Tablets (Infrequent) ... 690
Stromectol Tablets ... 2083
Symbyax Capsules (Rare) ... 1819
Topamax Sprinkle Capsules (Infrequent to 1%) ... 2404
Topamax Tablets (Infrequent to 1%) ... 2404
▲ Trisenox Injection (8%) ... 993
▲ Xenical Capsules (1.8% to 7.7%) ... 2831
Xyrem Oral Solution (Infrequent) ... 1688
Zelnorm Tablets ... 2312
Zoloft (Rare) ... 2586
Zonegran Capsules (Rare) ... 1101
Zyprexa Tablets (Infrequent) ... 1830
Zyprexa ZYDIS Orally Disintegrating Tablets (Infrequent) ... 1830

Incoordination
(*see under* Ataxia)

Indigestion
Asacol Delayed-Release Tablets ... 2692
Augmentin ... 1360
Augmentin Tablets ... 1363
Augmentin XR Extended-Release Tablets ... 1369
Augmentin ES-600 Powder for Oral Suspension ... 1366
Carafate Suspension (Less than 0.5%) ... 701
Carafate Tablets (Less than 0.5%) ... 701
Ceftin Tablets (0.1% to 1%) ... 1407
▲ Depacon Injection (Among most common) ... 412
Depakote Sprinkle Capsules ... 422
▲ Depakote Tablets (Among most common) ... 427
Depakote ER Tablets ... 434
▲ Indocin (3% to 9%) ... 1995
▲ Lexapro Oral Solution (2% to 6%) ... 1190
▲ Lexapro Tablets (2% to 6%) ... 1190
Lithobid Tablets ... 1692
Nadolol Tablets (1 to 5 of 1000 patients) ... 2159
Oncaspar ... 1145

Induration at injection site
Aloxi Injection (Very rare) ... 2127
▲ Aredia for Injection (Up to 41%) ... 2179
Boostrix ... 1404
▲ Cancidas for Injection (0% to 3.1%) ... 1918
Capastat Sulfate for Injection ... 1755
▲ Comvax (27.2% to 27.6%) ... 1928
▲ Copaxone for Injection (13%) ... 3297
▲ Engerix-B Vaccine (1% to 10 %) ... 1425
▲ Fluarix (1% to 10%) ... 1451
▲ Fuzeon Injection (90%) ... 2767
▲ Havrix Vaccine (1% to 10%) ... 1456
HibTITER ... 3426
Imitrex Injection ... 1463
Invanz for Injection (1%) ... 1999
Lupron Depot 3.75 mg ... 3260
Lupron Depot 7.5 mg ... 3264
Lupron Depot–3 Month 11.25 mg ... 3265
Lupron Depot-PED 7.5 mg, 11.25 mg and 15 mg ... 3269
▲ Menactra Vaccine (0.3% to 17.1%) ... 2954
Meruvax II ... 2019
▲ MICRhoGAM Ultra-Filtered (Frequent) ... 2371
M-M-R II ... 2006
Oncaspar ... 1145
Liquid PedvaxHIB ... 2035
Pneumovax 23 (Common) ... 2043
▲ Prevnar for Injection (0% to 48.3%) ... 3463
Primaxin I.V. (0.2%) ... 2048
ProQuad ... 2064
▲ RhoGAM Ultra-Filtered (Frequent) ... 2371
Risperdal Consta Long-Acting Injection (1%) ... 1682
Rocephin Injectable Vials, ADD-Vantage, Galaxy, Bulk (1%) ... 2800
Timentin ADD-Vantage ... 1580
Timentin Injection Galaxy Container ... 1583
Timentin IV Infusion ... 1577
Timentin Pharmacy Bulk Package ... 1586
▲ Twinrix Vaccine (1% to 10%) ... 1595
▲ Varivax (19.35% to 32.5%) ... 2100
▲ Vivitrol (25% to 35%) ... 995
Xolair ... 1266

Inebriated feeling
Cesamet Capsules ... 3340
Klonopin (Infrequent) ... 2778
▲ Xyrem Oral Solution (8.6%) ... 1688

Infection, access site
▲ Dacogen Injection (8%) ... 2129
▲ Myozyme for Intravenous Infusion (28%) ... 1279
▲ Sensipar Tablets (5%) ... 608

Infection, acquired immunodeficiency syndrome
Thalomid Capsules ... 965

Infection, aspergillus
Myfortic Tablets (Rare) ... 2255

Infection, bacterial
Actiq (Less than 1%) ... 979
▲ Advair Diskus 100/50 (1% to 3%) ... 1308
▲ Advair Diskus 250/50 (1% to 3%) ... 1308
▲ Advair Diskus 500/50 (1% to 3%) ... 1308
▲ Advair HFA Inhalation Aerosol (1% to 3%) ... 1318
Campath Ampules ... 811
Celebrex Capsules (0.1% to 1.9%) ... 3134
Cesamet Capsules ... 3340
Comtan Tablets (1%) ... 2189
▲ Copaxone for Injection (5%) ... 3297
▲ Copegus Tablets (Less than 1% to 3%) ... 2754
Elidel Cream 1% (1.1% to 1.8%) ... 2200
Elocon Cream 0.1% (1 in 182 patients) ... 3005
Elocon Ointment 0.1% (1 in 63 patients) ... 3007
Enbrel for Injection ... 584
▲ Equetro Extended-Release Capsules (Less than 5%) ... 3180
Evoxac Capsules (Less than 1%) ... 1047
▲ Flovent Diskus (1% to 3%) ... 1443
Gengraf Capsules (1% to less than 3%) ... 459
▲ Humira Injection (Less than 5%) ... 466
▲ Imdur Tablets (Less than or equal to 5%) ... 3018
▲ Intron A for Injection (Less than 5%) ... 3024
Invirase (Less than 2%) ... 2772
Kaletra (Less than 2%) ... 476
▲ Leustatin Injection (42%) ... 2357
Levaquin (0.1% to 0.9%) ... 2384
Levaquin in 5% Dextrose Injection (0.1% to 0.9%) ... 2384
Neoral Oral Solution (1% to less than 3%) ... 2259
Neoral Soft Gelatin Capsules (1% to less than 3%) ... 2259
▲ Nipent for Injection (5%) ... 1863
Orthoclone OKT3 Sterile Solution ... 2360
Pegasys ... 2789
▲ Remicade for IV Injection (6%) ... 971
Rituxan I.V. ... 1254
▲ Sandostatin LAR Depot (1% to 4%) ... 2280
Stalevo Tablets (1%) ... 2287
▲ Targretin Capsules (1.2% to 13.2%) ... 1747
Tasmar Tablets (Infrequent) ... 3358
▲ Trisenox Injection (8%) ... 993
Vantin Tablets and Oral Suspension (Less than 1%) ... 2645
Varivax ... 2100
VFEND I.V. (Less than 2%) ... 2564
VFEND Oral Suspension (Less than 2%) ... 2564
VFEND Tablets (Less than 2%) ... 2564

Infection, bacterial, ocular, secondary
Poly-Pred Ophthalmic Suspension ... ⊙233

Infection, bladder
Advate Injection (0.6%) ... 712
Xyrem Oral Solution (Infrequent) ... 1688

Infection, C. diff
Invanz for Injection (1.7%) ... 1999

Infection, candida albicans
Aerobid/Aerobid-M ... 1171
Cubicin for Injection (1% to 2%) ... 1026
▲ Dacogen Injection (10%) ... 2129
Myfortic Tablets (0.6% to 2.3%) ... 2255
Zosyn (1% or less) ... 3492

Infection, central line
Dacogen Injection (Greater than or equal to 1%) ... 2129
Revlimid Capsules ... 958

Infection, clostridial
Eraxis for Injection (Less than 1% to less than 2%) ... 2521
Revlimid Capsules ... 958

Infection, corneal, fungal
Blephamide Ophthalmic Ointment ... 568
Pred Mild Ophthalmic Suspension ... ⊙238

Pred Forte Ophthalmic Suspension .... ⊙ 235
Pred-G Ophthalmic Suspension .... ⊙ 236
TobraDex Ophthalmic Ointment 562
TobraDex Ophthalmic Suspension 563

Infection, cryptococcus
Myfortic Tablets (Rare) 2255
Orthoclone OKT3 Sterile Solution (1.6%) 2360

Infection, cytomegalovirus
▲ CellCept Capsules (Less than 4% to 14.1%) 2747
▲ CellCept Intravenous (Less than 4% to 14.1%) 2747
▲ CellCept Oral Suspension (Less than 4% to 14.1%) 2747
▲ CellCept Tablets (Less than 4% to 14.1%) 2747
▲ Doxil Injection (20.1%) 2351
Fuzeon Injection 2767
▲ Gengraf Capsules (4.8%) 459
▲ Myfortic Tablets (1.9% to 21.6%) 2255
▲ Neoral Oral Solution (4.8%) 2259
▲ Neoral Soft Gelatin Capsules (4.8%) 2259
▲ Orthoclone OKT3 Sterile Solution (3% to 19%) 2360
Remicade for IV Injection 971
▲ Sandimmune (4.8% to 12.3%) 2275
▲ Simulect for Injection (14%) 2284
▲ Thymoglobulin for Intravenous Infusion (13.4%) 1284

Infection, decreased resistance
Decadron Tablets 1951
Orthoclone OKT3 Sterile Solution 2360
Prograf Capsules and Injection 632
Sandimmune 2275

Infection, dental
Xyrem Oral Solution (Infrequent) 1688

Infection, ears
Aceon Tablets (2 mg, 4 mg, 8 mg) (Up to 1.3%) 3194
▲ Advair Diskus 100/50 (1% to 4%) 1308
▲ Advair Diskus 250/50 (1% to 4%) 1308
▲ Advair Diskus 500/50 (1% to 4%) 1308
▲ Aerobid/Aerobid-M (3% to 9%) 1171
Amerge Tablets (Frequent) 1339
Avalide Tablets 888
Avalide Tablets 2874
Avapro Tablets (Less than 1%) 891
Avapro Tablets (Less than 1%) 2871
Ciprodex Otic Suspension (0.6%) 559
Colazal Capsules 2838
Cutivate Lotion 0.05% (1%) 2664
▲ Elidel Cream 1% (0.6% to 5.7%) 2200
▲ Entocort EC Capsules (Less than 5%) 2698
▲ Epivir-HBV (25%) 1432
Imitrex Nasal Spray (Infrequent) 1467
Invanz for Injection (Greater than 0.5%) 1999
Lotronex Tablets (Rare) 1512
▲ Myozyme for Intravenous Infusion (33%) 1279
Neurontin Capsules (Infrequent) 2487
Neurontin Oral Solution (Infrequent) 2487
Neurontin Tablets (Infrequent) 2487
▲ Liquid PedvaxHIB (Among most frequent) 2035
▲ Pulmicort Respules (2% to 5%) 661
Revlimid Capsules 958
Somavert Injection 2642
▲ Strattera Capsules (3%) 1814
▲ Trizivir Tablets (Greater than or equal to 5%) 1589
▲ Ultram ER Tablets (1% to greater than 5%) 2392
Xyrem Oral Solution (Infrequent) 1688
▲ Ziagen (5%) 1626

Infection, Epstein-Barr virus
Rapamune Oral Solution and Tablets (Less frequent) 3475

Infection, eyes
▲ Acular Ophthalmic Solution (Approximately 1% to 10%) 565
▲ Acular LS Ophthalmic Solution (1% to 10%) 566
▲ Advair Diskus 250/50 (1% to 3%) 1308
Aerobid/Aerobid-M (1% to 3%) 1171
Elidel Cream 1% (Up to 1.1%) 2200
▲ Evoxac Capsules (1% to 3%) 1047
Lexapro Oral Solution (Infrequent) 1190
Lexapro Tablets (Infrequent) 1190
▲ Pulmicort Respules (1% to 3%) 661

Infection, fungal
Actiq (1% or greater) 979
Blephamide Ophthalmic Suspension 569
Campath Ampules 811
Celebrex Capsules (0.1% to 1.9%) 3134
Cleocin Vaginal Ovules (1%) 2616
Cubicin for Injection (2.6%) 1026
Dacogen Injection 2129
▲ Depakote ER Tablets (Greater than 1% to 5%) 434
Detrol Tablets (1.1%) 2628
Enbrel for Injection 584
▲ Equetro Extended-Release Capsules (Less than 5%) 3180
▲ Evoxac Capsules (1% to 3%) 1047
Floxin Otic Solution (Single report) 1049
FML Ophthalmic Ointment .... ⊙ 228
FML Ophthalmic Suspension .... ⊙ 227
FML Forte Ophthalmic Suspension .... ⊙ 226
FML-S Ophthalmic Suspension .... ⊙ 229
Gengraf Capsules (1% to less than 3%) 459
Humira Injection 466
▲ Intron A for Injection (Less than 5%) 3024
Invirase (Less than 2%) 2772
Keppra Injection 3320
Keppra Oral Solution (1% or more) 3314
Keppra Tablets (1% or more) 3314
Klonopin (Infrequent) 2778
▲ Leustatin Injection (20%) 2357
Levaquin (0.1% to 0.9%) 2384
Levaquin in 5% Dextrose Injection (0.1% to 0.9%) 2384
Lotronex Tablets (Rare) 1512
Micardis Tablets (More than 0.3%) 854
Micardis HCT Tablets 856
▲ Myfortic Tablets (2.5% to 10.8%) 2255
Neoral Oral Solution (1% to less than 3%) 2259
Neoral Soft Gelatin Capsules (1% to less than 3%) 2259
Omacor Capsules 2725
Oracea Capsules (1.9%) 1000
▲ Orthoclone OKT3 Sterile Solution (4% to 34%) 2360
PEG-Intron Powder for Injection (Less than 1%) 3048
Proquin XR Tablets (1.6% to 2.6%) 1153
▲ Rebetol (1% to 6%) 3058
Remicade for IV Injection 971
Requip Tablets (Infrequent) 1555
Revlimid Capsules 958
Reyataz Capsules (Less than 3%) 921
▲ Ribavirin, USP Capsules (1% to 6%) 3068
Soriatane Capsules (Less than 1%) 1013
Tasmar Tablets (Infrequent) 3358
▲ Vandazole Vaginal Gel (9.1% to 12%) 3338
VFEND I.V. (Less than 2%) 2564
VFEND Oral Suspension (Less than 2%) 2564
VFEND Tablets (Less than 2%) 2564
▲ Xeloda Tablets (Less than 5%) 2822
Xyrem Oral Solution (Infrequent) 1688
Zelapar Tablets 3372
Zelnorm Tablets (Up to 1%) 2312
Zyvox (0.1% to 1.5%) 2652

Infection, fungal, corneal, secondary
Poly-Pred Ophthalmic Suspension .... ⊙ 233

Infection, fungal, local
Aceon Tablets (2 mg, 4 mg, 8 mg) (0.3% to 1%) 3194
▲ Aldara Cream, 5% (2% to 11%) 1846
Doxil Injection (Less than 1%) 2351
▲ Gengraf Capsules (7.5%) 459
▲ Neoral Oral Solution (7.5%) 2259
▲ Neoral Soft Gelatin Capsules (7.5%) 2259
▲ Sandimmune (7.5% to 9.6%) 2275
Vantin Tablets and Oral Suspension (Less than 1% to 3.1%) 2645

Infection, fungal, systemic
Gengraf Capsules (2.2%) 459
Neoral Oral Solution (2.2%) 2259
Neoral Soft Gelatin Capsules (2.2%) 2259
▲ Sandimmune (2.2% to 3.9%) 2275

Infection, gastrointestinal
▲ Advair Diskus 100/50 (1% to 3%) 1308
Advair Diskus 250/50 1308
Advair Diskus 500/50 (Up to 3%) 1308
▲ Advair HFA Inhalation Aerosol (1% to 4%) 1318
Ceftin for Oral Suspension (0.1% to 1%) 1407
▲ Flovent Diskus (1% to 3%) 1443
Revlimid Capsules 958
Serevent Diskus (1% to less than 3%) 1568

Infection, genitourinary
depo-subQ provera 104 Injectable Suspension 2624

Infection, gram-negative bacteria
▲ Orthoclone OKT3 (1.6% to 7.5%) 2360

Infection, helminthic
▲ Xolair (58%) 1266

Infection, herpes simplex
▲ Orthoclone OKT3 Sterile Solution (5% to 31%) 2360
Revlimid 958

Infection, Legionella
Orthoclone OKT3 Sterile Solution (0.7% to 1.6%) 2360
Raptiva for Injection 1250

Infection, localized
Orencia Powder for Intravenous Infusion (0.2%) 914
▲ Proleukin for Injection (23%) 2266
Revlimid Capsules 958
▲ Valcyte Tablets (Less than 5%) 2813
Vantas (2 patients) 3375
Xyrem Oral Solution (Infrequent) 1688

Infection, lower respiratory tract
▲ Advair Diskus 100/50 (1% to 3%) 1308
▲ Advair Diskus 250/50 (1% to 3%) 1308
▲ Advair Diskus 500/50 (1% to 3%) 1308
▲ Advair HFA Inhalation Aerosol (3% to 5%) 1318
Ambien CR Tablets (1%) 2855
▲ Aralast (96.3%) 717
Emend Capsules (Greater than 0.5%) 1963
▲ Flovent Diskus (1% to 3%) 1443
Foradil Aerolizer (2.1%) 3010
Imitrex Injection 1463
Imitrex Tablets 1471
Remicade for IV Injection (Greater than or equal to 0.2%) 971
▲ Velcade for Injection (15%) 2133
▲ Xenical Capsules (7.8%) 2831

Infection, masking signs of
Blephamide Ophthalmic Ointment 568
Blephamide Ophthalmic Suspension 569
FML Ophthalmic Ointment .... ⊙ 228
FML Ophthalmic Suspension .... ⊙ 227
FML Forte Ophthalmic Suspension .... ⊙ 226
FML-S Ophthalmic Suspension .... ⊙ 229
Pred Mild Ophthalmic Suspension .... ⊙ 238
Pred Forte Ophthalmic Suspension .... ⊙ 235
TobraDex Ophthalmic Ointment 562
TobraDex Ophthalmic Suspension 563

Infection, mononucleosis-like syndrome
Klonopin (Infrequent) 2778
Neurontin Capsules 2487
Neurontin Oral Solution 2487
Neurontin Tablets 2487
Paser Granules 1674

Infection, mycobacterial
CellCept Capsules 2747
CellCept Intravenous 2747
CellCept Oral Suspension 2747
CellCept Tablets 2747
Dacogen Injection (Greater than or equal to 1%) 2129
Fuzeon Injection 2767
Myfortic Tablets 2255
Rapamune Oral Solution and Tablets (Less frequent) 3475
Remicade for IV Injection 971

Infection, mycobacterium tuberculosis
Rescriptor Tablets 2551

Infection, nasal
▲ Advair Diskus 100/50 (1% to 4%) 1308
▲ Advair Diskus 250/50 (1% to 4%) 1308
▲ Advair Diskus 500/50 (1% to 4%) 1308
Amerge Tablets (Frequent) 1339
Cutivate Lotion 0.05% (Less than 1%) 2664
▲ Epivir-HBV (25%) 1432
▲ Fortical Nasal Spray (10.6%) 3337
Lotronex Tablets (Rare) 1512
▲ Miacalcin Nasal Spray (1% to 10.6%) 2253
▲ Trizivir Tablets (Greater than or equal to 5%) 1589
▲ Ziagen (5%) 1626

Infection, neutropenic
Camptosar Injection (1% to 2.2%) 2604
▲ Taxotere Injection Concentrate (15.9%) 2932

Infection, ocular, secondary
Poly-Pred Ophthalmic Suspension .... ⊙ 233

Infection, ophthalmic, bacterial
Retisert Implant .... ⊙ 258

Infection, ophthalmic, fungal
Blephamide Ophthalmic Suspension 569
Pred-G Ophthalmic Ointment .... ⊙ 237
Retisert Implant .... ⊙ 258

Infection, ophthalmic, viral
Pred-G Ophthalmic Ointment .... ⊙ 237
Retisert Implant .... ⊙ 258
Revlimid Capsules 958

Infection, opportunistic
Campath Ampules 811
CellCept Capsules 2747
CellCept Intravenous 2747
CellCept Oral Suspension 2747
CellCept Tablets 2747
▲ Doxil Injection (50.4%) 2351
Fuzeon Injection 2767
Kineret Injection (Rare) 599
Leustatin Injection 2357

Infection, oral
Revlimid Capsules 958

Infection, parasitic
▲ Clarinex Syrup (3.1%) 2995
▲ Intron A for Injection (Less than 5%) 3024
Vantin Tablets and Oral Suspension (Less than 1%) 2645

Infection, pelvis
ParaGard T 380A Intrauterine Copper Contraceptive 1073
Wellbutrin Tablets (Rare) 1603

Infection, pharyngeal
▲ Epivir-HBV (25%) 1432
Lotronex Tablets (Rare) 1512

Infection, Pneumocystis carinii
(*see under* Pneumocystis carinii, susceptibility)

Infection, post-operative
Emend Capsules (Greater than 0.5%) 1963
Invanz for Injection (2.3%) 1999

Infection, post-surgical
Amevive 626
Humira 466

Infection, prosthetic
▲ Myfortic Tablets (3% to less than 20%) 2255

Infection, protozoan
Campath Ampules 811
Enbrel for Injection 584
Orthoclone OKT3 Sterile Solution 2360
Remicade for IV Injection 971

Infection, pseudomonal, lung
Dacogen Injection 2129
Revlimid Capsules 958

Infection, respiratory
Accutane Capsules 2731
▲ Alphagan P Ophthalmic Solution (1% to 4%) 567
▲ Aromasin Tablets (2% to 5%) 2600
Betimol Ophthalmic Solution (1% to 5%) 3382
Betimol Ophthalmic Solution (1% to 5%) .... ⊙ 295
▲ Cardura XL Tablets (4.8%) 2515
▲ CellCept Capsules (22% to 37%) 2747
▲ CellCept Intravenous (22% to 37%) 2747
▲ CellCept Oral Suspension (22% to 37%) 2747
▲ CellCept Tablets (22% to 37%) 2747
▲ Depacon Injection (12% to 20%) 412
▲ Depakene (12% to 20%) 417
▲ Depakote Sprinkle Capsules (12% to 20%) 422
▲ Depakote Tablets (12% to 20%) 427
▲ Depakote ER Tablets (12% to 20%) 434
▲ Entocort EC Capsules (11%) 2698

Epivir ... 1427
▲ Epivir-HBV (Among most common) ... 1432
▲ Flovent Diskus (5%) ... 1443
▲ Geodon Capsules (8%) ... 2529
Imitrex Nasal Spray (Infrequent) ... 1467
Infanrix Vaccine ... 1476
Lotronex Tablets (Rare) ... 1512
Myozyme for Intravenous Infusion ... 1279
▲ NeoProfen Injection (19%) ... 2472
Neurontin Capsules (2.5%) ... 2487
Neurontin Oral Solution (2.5%) ... 2487
Neurontin Tablets (2.5%) ... 2487
Pediarix Vaccine ... 1548
ProQuad ... 2064
▲ Pulmicort Respules (34% to 38%) ... 661
Relpax Tablets (Infrequent) ... 2548
Remicade for IV Injection ... 971
Revlimid Capsules (1.4%) ... 958
▲ TOBI Solution for Inhalation (5.8%) .. 2298
▲ Ventolin HFA Inhalation Aerosol (7%) ... 1600
VFEND I.V. (Less than 2%) ... 2564
VFEND Oral Suspension (Less than 2%) ... 2564
VFEND Tablets (Less than 2%) ... 2564
Viagra Tablets (Greater than 2%) ... 2573
Xifaxan Tablets (Less than 2%) ... 2842

Infection, secondary

Aclovate Cream (Infrequent) ... 2660
Alrex Ophthalmic Suspension 0.2% ... ⊙ 246
Analpram-HC ... 1159
Apexicon E Cream ... 2661
Bactroban Cream (Less than 1%) ... 1394
Blephamide Ophthalmic Ointment ... 568
Blephamide Ophthalmic Suspension ... 569
Clobevate Gel ... 3211
Clobex Lotion ... 1204
Clobex Shampoo (Infrequent) ... 1206
Clobex Spray (Less than 1%) ... 1208
Cutivate Cream (Infrequent) ... 2662
Cutivate Lotion 0.05% (Rare) ... 2664
Cutivate Ointment (Infrequent to more frequent) ... 2665
Diprolene Gel 0.05% ... 3001
Diprolene Lotion 0.05% (Infrequent) ... 3002
Diprolene Ointment 0.05% (Infrequent) ... 3003
Diprolene AF Cream 0.05% (Infrequent) ... 3000
Diprosone Cream, USP 0.05% ... 3004
Elocon Cream 0.1% (Infrequent) ... 3005
Elocon Lotion 0.1% (Infrequent) ... 3006
Elocon Ointment 0.1% (Infrequent) ... 3007
EryPed 200 & EryPed 400 Oral Suspension ... 447
Ery-Tab Tablets ... 449
Erythrocin Stearate Filmtab Tablets ... 453
FML Ophthalmic Ointment ... ⊙ 228
FML Ophthalmic Suspension ... ⊙ 227
FML Forte Ophthalmic Suspension ... ⊙ 226
FML-S Ophthalmic Suspension ... ⊙ 229
Locoid Lipocream Cream (Infrequent) ... 1160
Lotemax Ophthalmic Suspension 0.5% ... ⊙ 251
Lotrisone (Less than 1%) ... 3040
Luxíq Foam ... 1010
Olux Foam ... 1012
Pramosone ... 1161
Pred Mild Ophthalmic Suspension ... ⊙ 238
Pred Forte Ophthalmic Suspension ... ⊙ 235
Pred-G Ophthalmic Ointment ... ⊙ 237
Pred-G Ophthalmic Suspension ... ⊙ 236
ProctoFoam-HC ... 3099
Temovate Cream ... 2668
Temovate Gel (Infrequent) ... 2669
Temovate Ointment ... 2668
Temovate Scalp Application (Infrequent) ... 2670
Temovate E Emollient (Infrequent) ... 2671
TobraDex Ophthalmic Ointment ... 562
TobraDex Ophthalmic Suspension ... 563
Tri-Luma Cream ... 1213
Vanos Cream ... 1893
Varivax ... 2100

Infection, serious

Raptiva for Injection (0.4%) ... 1250

Infection, Serratia

Alkeran Tablets ... 956
Orthoclone OKT3 Sterile Solution (1.6%) ... 2360

Infection, sinus

▲ Alphagan P Ophthalmic Solution (1% to 4%) ... 567
▲ Flovent Diskus (10% to 33%) ... 1443
▲ Flovent HFA (1% to 6%) ... 1447

Infection, skin

Accutane Capsules ... 2731
Aceon Tablets (2 mg, 4 mg, 8 mg) (0.3% to 1%) ... 3194
Bexxar ... 1398
Cutivate Cream (0.8%) ... 2662
Cutivate Lotion 0.05% (Less than 1%) ... 2664
▲ Flovent HFA (1% to 3%) ... 1447
▲ Gengraf Capsules (7%) ... 459
▲ Neoral Oral Solution (7%) ... 2259
▲ Neoral Soft Gelatin Capsules (7.0%) ... 2259
Prinivil Tablets (0.3% to 1.0%) ... 2052
Prinzide Tablets ... 2056
ProQuad ... 2064
▲ Sandimmune (7.0% to 10.1%) ... 2275
Singulair (Greater than or equal to 2%) ... 2077

Infection, skin and soft tissue

AccuNeb Inhalation Solution (Up to 1.7%) ... 1055
Celebrex Capsules (0.1% to 1.9%) ... 3134
▲ Elidel Cream 1% (2.2% to 6.4%) ... 2200
Enbrel for Injection ... 584
▲ Flovent Diskus (1% to 3%) ... 1443
▲ Gengraf Capsules (7%) ... 459
Lotronex Tablets (Rare) ... 1512
▲ Protopic Ointment (5% to 12%) ... 638
Varivax ... 2100

Infection, Staphylococcus epidermidis

▲ Clolar for Intravenous Infusion (13%) ... 1271
▲ Dacogen Injection (7%) ... 2129
Elidel Cream 1% (0.4% to 2.1%) ... 2200
▲ Orthoclone OKT3 Sterile Solution (4.8%) ... 2360

Infection, superimposed

Zelapar Tablets ... 3372

Infection, throat

▲ Trizivir Tablets (Greater than or equal to 5%) ... 1589
▲ Ziagen (5%) ... 1626

Infection, tooth

Singulair (Greater than or equal to 2%) ... 2077

Infection, unspecified

▲ Abelcet Injection (5%) ... 1141
▲ Accolate Tablets (3.5%) ... 671
Actiq (1% or greater) ... 979
▲ Actonel Tablets (19% to 29.9%) ... 2683
▲ Actonel with Calcium Tablets (19% to 29.9%) ... 2688
▲ Adderall XR Capsules (2% to 4%) ... 3166
▲ Advicor Tablets (20%) ... 1722
▲ Alimta for Injection (Less than 1% to 23%) ... 1750
Alinia for Oral Suspension (Less than 1%) ... 2835
Alinia Tablets (Less than 1%) ... 2835
Alkeran for Injection ... 955
Aloprim for Injection (Less than 1%) ... 2167
▲ Altoprev Extended-Release Tablets (11%) ... 3109
Ambien Tablets (1%) ... 2851
Ambien CR Tablets (Infrequent) ... 2855
▲ AmBisome for Injection (11.1%) ... 620
Amevive (0.7% to 1.5%) ... 626
Anaprox Tablets (Less than 1%) ... 2761
Anaprox DS Tablets (Less than 1%) .. 2761
▲ Aranesp for Injection (27%) ... 581
▲ Argatroban Injection (3.7%) ... 1346
▲ Arimidex Tablets (2% to 9%) ... 673
▲ Arranon Injection (1% to 9%) ... 1357
Arthrotec Tablets (Rare) ... 3129
Asacol Delayed-Release Tablets (2% or greater) ... 2692
Asmanex Twisthaler (1% to less than 3%) ... 2966
Atacand HCT (0.5% or greater) ... 651
▲ Avinza Capsules (5% to 10%) ... 1741
Axid Oral Solution (1.7%) ... 879
▲ Azilect Tablets (3%) ... 3293
▲ Bexxar (Less than 1% to 21%) ... 1398
▲ Boniva Injection (4.3%) ... 2738
▲ Boniva Tablets (4.3%) ... 2741
▲ BOTOX Purified Neurotoxin Complex (3% to 10%) ... 570
▲ Caduet Tablets (2.8% to 10.3%) ... 2508
▲ Campath Ampules (1% to 7%) ... 811
Campral Tablets (Frequent) ... 1174
▲ Camptosar Injection (0% to 14%) ... 2604
▲ Carnitor Injection (10% to 24%) ... 3188
▲ CellCept Capsules (18.2% to 27.1%) ... 2747
▲ CellCept Intravenous (18.2% to 27.1%) ... 2747
▲ CellCept Oral Suspension (18.2% to 27.1%) ... 2747
▲ CellCept Tablets (18.2% to 27.1%) ... 2747
▲ Climara Pro Transdermal System (3.3%) ... 776
▲ Clolar for Intravenous Infusion (85%) ... 1271
Clozaril Tablets ... 2184
Colazal Capsules ... 2838
▲ Copaxone for Injection (50%) ... 3297
Cosmegen for Injection ... 2459
Coumadin for Injection ... 898
Coumadin Tablets ... 898
▲ Cozaar Tablets (5%) ... 1935
Crestor Tablets (Greater than or equal to 2%) ... 678
▲ Depakote ER Tablets (Greater than 1% to 15%) ... 434
Detrol Tablets (1%) ... 2628
Diastat Rectal Delivery System (Less than 1%) ... 3343
▲ Doxil Injection (1% to 11.7%) ... 2351
EC-Naprosyn Delayed-Release Tablets (Less than 1%) ... 2761
Edex Injection (2%) ... 3089
▲ Effexor Tablets (2.2% to 6%) ... 3411
▲ Effexor XR Capsules (10%) ... 3417
▲ Elestat Ophthalmic Solution (Approximately 10%) ... 1669
Elitek (Less than or equal to 1%) ... 2890
▲ Eloxatin for Injection (4% to 25%) ... 2892
Emsam Transdermal System ... 903
▲ Enbrel for Injection (35% to 64%) ... 584
▲ Equetro Extended-Release Capsules (12%) ... 3180
▲ Erbitux (1% to 16%) ... 910
▲ Estrasorb Topical Emulsion (12%) ... 1147
Euflexxa (1.25%) ... 1162
▲ Evista Tablets (15.1%) ... 1763
▲ Evoxac Capsules (1% to 3%) ... 1047
Exelon Capsules (2% or more) ... 2206
Exelon Oral Solution (2% or more) ... 2206
Ferrlecit Injection (8%) ... 3388
▲ Flomax Capsules (9.0% to 10.8%) ... 850
▲ Fortamet Extended-Release Tablets (20.5%) ... 3115
▲ Fortical Nasal Spray (1% to 3%) ... 3337
▲ Gabitril Tablets (1% to 19%) ... 984
▲ Gemzar for Injection (3% to 16%) ... 1771
▲ Gengraf Capsules (1% to 24.7%) ... 459
▲ Hectorol Capsules (Greater than or equal to 5%) ... 1275
▲ Herceptin I.V. (20%) ... 1233
▲ Hycamtin for Injection (26% to 28%) ... 1458
▲ Indapamide Tablets (Greater than or equal to 5%) ... 2156
▲ Infergen (2% to 3%) ... 3364
▲ Intron A for Injection (Less than 5%) ... 3024
Ionsys Transdermal System (.1% to less than 1%) ... 2379
▲ I.V. Busulfex (51%) ... 2493
▲ Keppra Injection (13%) ... 3320
▲ Keppra Oral Solution (2% to 13%) ... 3314
▲ Keppra Tablets (2% to 13%) ... 3314
▲ Kineret Injection (39%) ... 599
▲ Kytril Injection (3%) ... 2781
▲ Lamictal (5% to 20%) ... 1481
Lescol Capsules ... 2233
Lescol XL Tablets ... 2233
▲ Leukine (65%) ... 814
▲ Leustatin Injection (28%) ... 2357
▲ Lipitor Tablets (2.8% to 10.3%) ... 2483
Lofibra Tablets ... 1219
Lofibra Capsules ... 1216
Lotensin Tablets (Less than 1%) ... 2243
Lotensin HCT Tablets (0.3% or more) ... 2246
▲ Lunesta Tablets (5% to 10%) ... 3142
▲ Lupron Depot 7.5 mg (5.4%) ... 3264
Lupron Depot-PED 7.5 mg, 11.25 mg and 15 mg (Less than 2%) ... 3269
Lupron Injection Pediatric (Less than 2%) ... 3259
▲ Lyrica Capsules (3% to 14%) ... 2539
▲ Megace ES Oral Suspension (1% to 3%) ... 2481
▲ Menostar Transdermal System (5%) ... 782
▲ Mepron Suspension (18% to 22%) ... 1521
▲ Miacalcin Nasal Spray (1% to 3%) ... 2253
Micardis Tablets (More than 0.3%) ... 854
Micardis HCT Tablets ... 856
Mirapex Tablets (Greater than or equal to 1%) ... 859
Mycamine for Injection ... 628
Myleran Tablets ... 1525
▲ Mylotarg for Injection (3% to 10%) ... 3431
▲ Myobloc Injection (13% to 19%) ... 3192
Naprosyn Suspension (Less than 1%) ... 2761
Naprosyn Tablets (Less than 1%) ... 2761
Nasacort AQ Nasal Spray ... 2922
NeoProfen Injection ... 2472
▲ Neoral Oral Solution (1% to 24.7%) ... 2259
▲ Neoral Soft Gelatin Capsules (1% to 24.7%) ... 2259
▲ Neumega for Injection (Greater than or equal to 10%) ... 3435
▲ Neurontin Capsules (5.1%) ... 2487
▲ Neurontin Oral Solution (5.1%) ... 2487
▲ Neurontin Tablets (5.1%) ... 2487
Nexavar Tablets (Uncommon) ... 746
▲ Nipent for Injection (7% to 36%) ... 1863
Niravam Orally Disintegrating Tablets (1.3%) ... 3092
▲ Norditropin Cartridges (13%) ... 2323
▲ Ontak Vials (48%) ... 1745
Panhematin for Injection ... 2473
▲ Paxil CR Controlled-Release Tablets (5% to 6%) ... 1538
▲ Paxil (5% to 6%) ... 1530
PEG-Intron Powder for Injection (Less than or equal to 1%) ... 3048
Permax Tablets (1.1%) ... 3356
▲ Pletal Tablets (10% to 14%) ... 2455
▲ Premarin Tablets (18% to 23%) ... 3446
▲ Premphase Tablets (16% to 18%) ... 3456
▲ Prempro Tablets (16% to 18%) ... 3456
Prevacid Delayed-Release Capsules (Less than 1%) ... 3271
Prevacid for Delayed-Release Oral Suspension (Less than 1%) ... 3271
Prevacid SoluTab Delayed-Release Orally Disintegrating Tablets (Less than 1%) ... 3271
Prevacid NapraPAC (Less than 1%) .. 3280
PREVPAC (Less than 1%) ... 3284
ProAir HFA Inhalation Aerosol (Less than 3%) ... 3300
Prochieve 4% Gel ... 1003
Prochieve 8% Gel ... 1003
▲ Prograf Capsules and Injection (45%) ... 632
▲ Proleukin for Injection (13%) ... 2266
ProQuad ... 2064
Protonix I.V. (Greater than or equal to 1%) ... 3472
Protonix Tablets (Greater than or equal to 1%) ... 3469
▲ Protopic Ointment (1% to 14%) ... 638
Provigil Tablets (At least 1%) ... 988
Prozac Pulvules and Liquid ... 1801
▲ Pulmicort Respules (1% to 3%) ... 661
▲ Quadramet Injection (7%) ... 1040
▲ Rapamune Oral Solution and Tablets (3% to 20%) ... 3475
▲ Raptiva for Injection (29%) ... 1250
Refludan for Injection (1.8%) ... 792
▲ Remicade for IV Injection (56%) ... 971
▲ Renagel Tablets (15%) ... 1282
Rescriptor Tablets ... 2551
Revlimid Capsules ... 958
Reyataz Capsules (Less than 3%) ... 921
▲ Rituxan I.V. (4% to 31%) ... 1254
▲ Simulect for Injection (3% to 10%) ... 2284
▲ Soltamox Oral Solution (6%) ... 3527
▲ Somavert Injection (23%) ... 2642
▲ Soriatane Capsules (1% to 10%) ... 1013
▲ Spiriva HandiHaler (1% to 4%) ... 869
Striant Mucoadhesive ... 1007
▲ Suboxone Tablets (5.6% to 20%) ... 2717
▲ Subutex Tablets (11.7% to 20%) ... 2717
Symbyax Capsules (Frequent) ... 1819
Synera Topical Patch (Less than or equal to 1%) ... 1137
▲ Tarceva Tablets (0% to 33%) ... 1259
▲ Tarceva Tablets (0% to 33%) ... 2444
▲ Targretin Capsules (13.1% to 22.6%) ... 1747
Tasmar Tablets (Frequent) ... 3358
▲ Taxotere Injection Concentrate (6.1% to 42%) ... 2932
▲ Thalomid Capsules (6.3% to 8.3%) ... 965
▲ Thymoglobulin for Intravenous Infusion (17.1%) ... 1284
Tiazac Capsules (2%) ... 1201
▲ Topamax Sprinkle Capsules (1% to 7%) ... 2404
▲ Topamax Tablets (1% to 7%) ... 2404
▲ Trasylol Injection (6%) ... 754
▲ Travatan Ophthalmic Solution (1% to 5%) ... 563
Tricor Tablets ... 527
Trileptal Tablets (Up to 2%) ... 2300
Trileptal Oral Suspension (Up to 2%) ... 2300
▲ Tygacil for Injection (8.3%) ... 3488
Uniretic Tablets (More than 1%) ... 3100
▲ Valcyte Tablets (Less than 5%) ... 2813
Vandazole Vaginal Gel (1%) ... 3338

▲ Verelan PM Extended-Release Capsules, Controlled-Onset (12.1%) ... 3106
▲ Vesanoid Capsules (58%) ... 2820
VFEND I.V. (Less than 2%) ... 2564
VFEND Oral Suspension (Less than 2%) ... 2564
VFEND Tablets (Less than 2%) ... 2564
▲ Vicoprofen Tablets (3% to 9%) ... 539
▲ Vigamox Ophthalmic Solution (1% to 4%) ... 564
Voltaren Tablets (Occasionally) ... 2307
Voltaren-XR Tablets (Occasionally) ... 2310
▲ WelChol Tablets (10%) ... 1050
Wellbutrin Tablets (Rare) ... 1603
▲ Wellbutrin SR Sustained-Release Tablets (8% to 9%) ... 1607
▲ Wellbutrin XL Extended-Release Tablets (8% to 9%) ... 1613
Yasmin 28 Tablets (Greater than 1%) ... 796
Yaz Tablets (Greater than 1%) ... 803
Zemaira (0.4%) ... 3509
▲ Zinecard for Injection (19% to 23%) ... 2650
▲ Zometa for Intravenous Infusion (5% to 10%) ... 2315
Zomig Nasal Spray (Infrequent) ... 3523

Infection, upper respiratory tract

Abilify Oral Solution ... 882
Abilify Oral Solution ... 2450
Abilify Discmelt Orally Disintegrating Tablets ... 882
Abilify Discmelt Orally Disintegrating Tablets ... 2450
Abilify Tablets ... 882
Abilify Tablets ... 2450
▲ Aceon Tablets (2 mg, 4 mg, 8 mg) (8.6%) ... 3194
▲ ActoPlus Met Tablets (12.4% to 15.5%) ... 3214
▲ Actos Tablets (13.2%) ... 3219
▲ Advair Diskus 100/50 (10% to 27%) ... 1308
▲ Advair Diskus 250/50 (10% To 27%) ... 1308
▲ Advair Diskus 500/50 (10% to 27%) ... 1308
▲ Advair HFA Inhalation Aerosol (16% to 24%) ... 1318
▲ Aerobid/Aerobid-M (25%) ... 1171
Aggrenox Capsules (1%) ... 822
▲ Aldara Cream, 5% (15.3%) ... 1846
▲ Aldurazyme for Intravenous Infusion (7%) ... 1268
▲ Allegra (3.2% to 4.3%) ... 2844
Allegra-D 12 Hour Extended-Release Tablets (1.4%) ... 2846
Allegra-D 24 Hour Extended-Release Tablets (1.4%) ... 2849
Altace Capsules ... 1702
▲ Ambien Tablets (5%) ... 2851
Ambien CR Tablets (1% to frequent) ... 2855
▲ Amitiza Capsules (0% to 3.7%) ... 3224
▲ Angeliq Tablets (18.9%) ... 762
▲ Aralast (96.3%) ... 717
▲ Aranesp for Injection (14%) ... 581
▲ Aredia for Injection (24.1%) ... 2179
▲ Asmanex Twisthaler (8% to 15%) ... 2966
▲ Atacand Tablets (6%) ... 649
▲ Atacand HCT (3.6%) ... 651
▲ Atripla Tablets (3%) ... 945
▲ Atrovent Inhalation Solution (13.2%) ... 835
▲ Atrovent HFA Inhalation Aerosol (9% to 34%) ... 841
▲ Atrovent Nasal Spray 0.03% (9.8%) ... 837
Avalide Tablets (1% or greater) ... 888
Avalide Tablets (1% or greater) ... 2874
▲ Avandamet Tablets (9% to 16%) ... 1373
▲ Avandaryl Tablets (Greater than or equal to 5%) ... 1379
▲ Avandia Tablets (6.1% to 9.9%) ... 1384
▲ Avapro Tablets (9%) ... 891
▲ Avapro Tablets (9%) ... 2871
▲ Avastin IV (40% to 47%) ... 1227
▲ Benicar HCT Tablets (7%) ... 1044
Bexxar ... 1398
▲ Boniva Injection (2% to 33.7%) ... 2738
▲ Boniva Tablets (2% to 33.7%) ... 2741
▲ BOTOX Purified Neurotoxin Complex (12%) ... 570
▲ Caverject Impulse Injection (4%) ... 2612
Ceftin for Oral Suspension (0.1% to 1%) ... 1407
▲ Celebrex Capsules (8.1%) ... 3134
▲ Celexa (5%) ... 1176
▲ Clarinex Syrup (10.8% to 21.2%) ... 2995
▲ Climara Transdermal System (6% to 17%) ... 771
▲ Climara Pro Transdermal System (13.2%) ... 776
▲ Clobex Spray (2% to 8%) ... 1208
▲ Combivent Inhalation Aerosol (10.9%) ... 847
Comvax (0.5% to 1.3%) ... 1928
▲ Concerta Extended-Release Tablets (8%) ... 1881
Cosopt Sterile Ophthalmic Solution (1% to 5%) ... 1931
▲ Covera-HS Tablets (5.4%) ... 3139
▲ Cozaar Tablets (8%) ... 1935
Crixivan Capsules ... 1940
▲ Cutivate Lotion 0.05% (3%) ... 2664
Dacogen Injection ... 2129
▲ depo-subQ provera 104 Injectable Suspension (1% to less than 5%) ... 2624
▲ Detrol Tablets (5.9%) ... 2628
Diovan Tablets (More than 1%) ... 2193
Diovan HCT Tablets (Greater than 0.2%) ... 2196
▲ Ditropan XL Extended-Release Tablets (2% to less than 5%) ... 2413
▲ Duetact Tablets (Greater than 5%) ... 3226
DuoNeb Inhalation Solution ... 1058
▲ Duragesic Transdermal System (3% to 10%) ... 2373
▲ Edex Injection (5%) ... 3089
▲ Elestat Ophthalmic Solution (Approximately 10%) ... 1669
▲ Elidel Cream 1% (4.3% to 19.4%) ... 2200
▲ Eloxatin for Injection (7% to 10%) ... 2892
Emend Capsules (Greater than 0.5%) ... 1963
▲ Enbrel for Injection (12% to 31%) ... 584
▲ Epogen for Injection (11%) ... 591
▲ Estring Vaginal Ring (5%) ... 2635
▲ Euflexxa (12%) ... 1162
▲ Evoxac Capsules (11.4%) ... 1047
Exelon Capsules (2% or more) ... 2206
Exelon Oral Solution (2% or more) ... 2206
▲ Exubera Inhalation Powder (29.2% to 43.3%) ... 2524
▲ Famvir Tablets (0.7% to 3.3%) ... 2211
▲ Ferrlecit Injection (6%) ... 3388
▲ Flebogamma 5%, Immune Globulin Intravenous (Human) (33%) ... 1658
▲ Flovent Diskus (18% to 31%) ... 1443
▲ Flovent HFA (18%) ... 1447
▲ Fluarix (3.9%) ... 1451
▲ Follistim AQ Cartridge (5%) ... 2338
▲ Foradil Aerolizer (7.4%) ... 3010
▲ Fortical Nasal Spray (1% to 3%) ... 3337
Gardasil Injection (1.5%) ... 1984
▲ Gengraf Capsules (7.7%) ... 459
▲ Gleevec Tablets (0% to 19%) ... 2227
Havrix Vaccine (Less than 1%) ... 1456
Herceptin I.V. ... 1233
▲ Humira Injection (17%) ... 466
▲ Hyzaar 50-12.5 Tablets (6.1%) ... 1990
▲ Hyzaar 100-12.5 Tablets (6.1%) ... 1990
▲ Hyzaar 100-25 Tablets (6.1%) ... 1990
▲ Infergen (16% to 31%) ... 3364
Invanz for Injection (2.3%) ... 1999
Invirase (Less than 2%) ... 2772
Ionsys Transdermal System (.1% to less than 1%) ... 2379
▲ Kineret Injection (14%) ... 599
▲ Klonopin (8%) ... 2778
▲ Lescol Capsules (16.2%) ... 2233
▲ Lescol XL Tablets (12.5%) ... 2233
Levaquin (0.1% to 0.9%) ... 2384
Levaquin in 5% Dextrose Injection (0.1% to 0.9%) ... 2384
Lexapro Oral Solution (At least 2%) ... 1190
Lexapro Tablets (At least 2%) ... 1190
Lotensin HCT Tablets (More than 1%) ... 2246
Lotrel Capsules ... 2249
Lotronex Tablets (1%) ... 1512
▲ Lucentis Injection (2% to 15%) ... 1237
▲ Lumigan Ophthalmic Solution (Approximately 10%) ... 573
Mavik Tablets (0.3% to 1.0%) ... 486
Maxalt Tablets (Infrequent) ... 2008
Maxalt-MLT Orally Disintegrating Tablets (Infrequent) ... 2008
▲ Menostar Transdermal System (16%) ... 782
Metrogel 1% (2.5%) ... 1211
▲ Miacalcin Nasal Spray (1% to 3%) ... 2253
▲ Micardis Tablets (7%) ... 854
▲ Micardis HCT Tablets (8%) ... 856
Migranal Nasal Spray (Infrequent) ... 3348
▲ Mirena Intrauterine System (5% or more) ... 787
▲ Mobic Oral Suspension (0% to 8.3%) ... 863
▲ Mobic Tablets (0% to 8.3%) ... 863
▲ Myfortic Tablets (3% to less than 20%) ... 2255
▲ Myozyme for Intravenous Infusion (44%) ... 1279
Nalfon Capsules (1.5%) ... 2502
Namenda (Greater than or equal to 2%) ... 1195
▲ Nasonex Nasal Spray (5% to 7%) ... 3043
▲ Neoral Oral Solution (7.7% to 13%) ... 2259
▲ Neoral Soft Gelatin Capsules (7.7% to 13%) ... 2259
Neurontin Oral Solution (More than 2%) ... 2487
▲ Nipent for Injection (13% to 16%) ... 1863
▲ Niravam Orally Disintegrating Tablets (4.3%) ... 3092
▲ NuvaRing (5% to 14%) ... 2340
Oncaspar (Less than 1%) ... 1145
▲ Orencia Powder for Intravenous Infusion (5% to 13%) ... 914
▲ Ortho Evra Transdermal System (9% to 22%) ... 2417
Parcopa Orally Disintegrating Tablets ... 3097
▲ Liquid PedvaxHIB (Among most frequent) ... 2035
▲ Plavix Tablets (8.7%) ... 917
▲ Plavix Tablets (8.7%) ... 2926
▲ Premarin Tablets (9% to 12%) ... 3446
▲ Premphase Tablets (9% to 11%) ... 3456
▲ Prempro Tablets (9% to 11%) ... 3456
Prevacid Delayed-Release Capsules (Less than 1%) ... 3271
Prevacid for Delayed-Release Oral Suspension (Less than 1%) ... 3271
Prevacid SoluTab Delayed-Release Orally Disintegrating Tablets (Less than 1%) ... 3271
Prevacid NapraPAC (Less than 1%) ... 3280
PREVPAC (Less than 1%) ... 3284
Prilosec OTC Delayed-Release Tablets (1.9%) ... 2677
Prinivil Tablets (1.2% to 1.5%) ... 2052
Prinzide Tablets (2.2%) ... 2056
Prochieve 4% Gel ... 1003
Prochieve 8% Gel ... 1003
▲ Procrit for Injection (11%) ... 2364
▲ Prometrium Capsules (100 mg, 200 mg) (5%) ... 3203
ProQuad (1.3%) ... 2064
Protonix I.V. (Greater than or equal to 1%) ... 3472
Protonix Tablets (Greater than or equal to 1%) ... 3469
▲ Proventil HFA Inhalation Aerosol (21%) ... 3056
▲ Qvar Inhalation Aerosol (5% to 11%) ... 3303
▲ Rapamune Oral Solution and Tablets (Greater than 20%) ... 3475
Razadyne (Greater than or equal to 2%) ... 2399
Razadyne ER Extended-Release Capsules (Greater than or equal to 2%) ... 2399
Recombivax HB (Equal to or greater than 1%) ... 2071
ReFacto Vials ... 3484
▲ Relenza Rotadisk (1% to 5%) ... 1552
▲ Remicade for IV Injection (32%) ... 971
▲ Renagel Tablets (5.1%) ... 1282
Requip Tablets (1% or more) ... 1555
▲ Rescriptor Tablets (4.7% to 7.6%) ... 2551
▲ Retisert Implant (5% to 15%) ... ⊙ 258
▲ Revlimid Capsules (1.4% to 14.9%) ... 958
▲ Risperdal (3%) ... 1676
Risperdal Consta Long-Acting Injection (Up to 2%) ... 1682
▲ Risperdal M-Tab Orally Disintegrating Tablets (3%) ... 1676
▲ Rituxan I.V. (7%) ... 1254
▲ Rozerem Tablets (3%) ... 3231
▲ Rythmol SR Capsules (8% to 12%) ... 2727
▲ Serevent Diskus (Greater than 3%) ... 1568
▲ Simulect for Injection (Greater than or equal to 10%) ... 2284
Singulair (1% to 1.9%) ... 2077
Somavert Injection ... 2642
▲ Spiriva HandiHaler (41% to 43%) ... 869
Stalevo Tablets ... 2287
▲ Starlix Tablets (10.5%) ... 2292
Strattera Capsules (2% or greater) ... 1814
▲ Symbicort 80/4.5 Inhalation Aerosol (7.6%) ... 3511
▲ Symbicort 160/4.5 Inhalation Aerosol (10.5%) ... 3511
▲ Synagis (50.6%) ... 1897
Tamiflu Capsules ... 2807
Tarka Tablets (0.3% to 5.4%) ... 524
▲ Tasmar Tablets (5% to 7%) ... 3358
▲ Temodar Capsules (8%) ... 3073
▲ Teveten Tablets (8%) ... 1735
Teveten HCT Tablets (0.4%) ... 1737
Thalomid Capsules ... 965
Timoptic Sterile Ophthalmic Solution (Less frequent) ... 2088
Timoptic in Ocudose (Less frequent) ... 2091
Timoptic-XE Sterile Ophthalmic Gel Forming Solution (1% to 5%) ... 2092
▲ Topamax Sprinkle Capsules (12% to 18%) ... 2404
▲ Topamax Tablets (12% to 18%) ... 2404
▲ Trileptal Tablets (5% to 10%) ... 2300
▲ Trileptal Oral Suspension (5% to 10%) ... 2300
▲ Trisenox Injection (13%) ... 993
▲ Truvada Tablets (3%) ... 1296
▲ Twinrix Vaccine (1% to 10%) ... 1595
▲ Ultram ER Tablets (1% to greater than 5%) ... 2392
Uniretic Tablets (More than 1%) ... 3100
Univasc Tablets (Greater than 1%) ... 3104
▲ Uroxatral Tablets (3%) ... 2943
▲ Vagifem Tablets (5% to 11%) ... 2334
▲ Valcyte Tablets (Less than 5%) ... 2813
Valtrex Caplets ... 1597
▲ Vaqta (1.1% to 10.1%) ... 2097
Vasotec I.V. Injection (0.5% to 1.0%) ... 2103
▲ Verelan PM Extended-Release Capsules, Controlled-Onset (12.1%) ... 3106
▲ Vivitrol (12% to 13%) ... 995
▲ Vytorin 10/10 Tablets (3.9%) ... 2114
▲ Vytorin 10/10 Tablets (3.9%) ... 3077
▲ Vytorin 10/20 Tablets (3.9%) ... 2114
▲ Vytorin 10/20 Tablets (3.9%) ... 3077
▲ Vytorin 10/40 Tablets (3.9%) ... 2114
▲ Vytorin 10/40 Tablets (3.9%) ... 3077
▲ Vytorin 10/80 Tablets (3.9%) ... 2114
▲ Vytorin 10/80 Tablets (3.9%) ... 3077
▲ Wellbutrin XL Extended-Release Tablets (9%) ... 1613
▲ Xalatan Sterile Ophthalmic Solution (Approximately 4%) ... 2649
▲ Xeloda Tablets (4%) ... 2822
▲ Xenical Capsules (26.1% to 38.1%) ... 2831
Xifaxan Tablets (Less than 2%) ... 2842
▲ Xolair (20%) ... 1266
▲ Xyrem Oral Solution (2.9% to 6.1%) ... 1688
Yasmin 28 Tablets ... 796
Yaz Tablets (Greater than 1%) ... 803
Zegerid Capsules (1.9%) ... 2958
Zegerid Powder for Oral Solution (1.9%) ... 2958
▲ Zelnorm Tablets (3% to 4%) ... 2312
Zemaira (1.6%) ... 3509
▲ Zetia Tablets (11.8% to 13%) ... 2120
▲ Zetia Tablets (13%) ... 3083
Zocor Tablets (2.1%) ... 2105
Zoloft (Infrequent) ... 2586
▲ Zometa for Intravenous Infusion (10%) ... 2315
Zostavax Injection (1.9%) ... 2111
Zyrtec Chewable Tablets (Less than 2%) ... 2594
Zyrtec (Less than 2%) ... 2594
Zyrtec-D 12 Hour Extended Release Tablets (Less than 2%) ... 2597
▲ Zyvox (3.7% to 4.2%) ... 2652

Infection, urinary tract

Aceon Tablets (2 mg, 4 mg, 8 mg) (2.8%) ... 3194
Actiq (Less than 1%) ... 979
▲ Actonel Tablets (2.9% to 10.9%) ... 2683
▲ Actonel with Calcium Tablets (2.9% to 10.9%) ... 2688
▲ ActoPlus Met Tablets (5.3% to 5.8%) ... 3214
▲ Adderall XR Capsules (5%) ... 3166
▲ Advair HFA Inhalation Aerosol (1% to 3%) ... 1318
Aldara Cream, 5% (1.4%) ... 1846
Aloprim for Injection (Less than 1%) ... 2167
Altoprev Extended-Release Tablets (2%) ... 3109
Ambien Tablets (2%) ... 2851
Ambien CR Tablets (Frequent) ... 2855
▲ Amitiza Capsules (3.4% to 4.4%) ... 3224
▲ Aredia for Injection (18.5%) ... 2179
▲ Argatroban Injection (4.6%) ... 1346
▲ Arimidex Tablets (2% to 8%) ... 673
▲ Arixtra Injection (2.3% to 4%) ... 1351
Aromasin Tablets (Less frequent) ... 2600
Arthrotec Tablets (Rare) ... 3129
Asmanex Twisthaler (1% to less than 3%) ... 2966
Atacand HCT (0.5% or greater) ... 651
Atrovent Inhalation Solution (Less than 3%) ... 835
▲ Atrovent HFA Inhalation Aerosol (2% to 10%) ... 841
Avalide Tablets (1% or greater) ... 888
Avalide Tablets (1% or greater) ... 2874
Avapro Tablets (1% or greater) ... 891
Avapro Tablets (1% or greater) ... 2871
▲ Avinza Capsules (5% to 10%) ... 1741
▲ Azmacort Inhalation Aerosol (1% to 3%) ... 1726
Benicar Tablets (Greater than 0.5%) ... 1043

Benicar HCT Tablets (Greater than 2%) ... 1044
Betaseron for SC Injection ... 767
▲ Boniva Injection (1.8% to 5.5%) ... 2738
▲ Boniva Tablets (1.8% to 5.5%) ... 2741
Caduet Tablets (Greater than or equal to 2%) ... 2508
Campath Ampules ... 811
Campral Tablets (Infrequent) ... 1174
Cardura XL Tablets (1.4%) ... 2515
▲ Carnitor Injection (2% to 3%) ... 3188
Ceftin for Oral Suspension (0.1% to 1%) ... 1407
Celebrex Capsules (0.1% to 1.9%) ... 3134
▲ CellCept Capsules (37% to 37.2%) ... 2747
▲ CellCept Intravenous (37% to 37.2%) ... 2747
▲ CellCept Oral Suspension (37% to 37.2%) ... 2747
▲ CellCept Tablets (37% to 37.2%) ... 2747
▲ Clarinex Syrup (3.6%) ... 2995
▲ Climara Pro Transdermal System (3.3%) ... 776
Combivent Inhalation Aerosol (Less than 2%) ... 847
Cosopt Sterile Ophthalmic Solution (1% to 5%) ... 1931
▲ Cozaar Tablets (Less than 1% to 16%) ... 1935
Crestor Tablets (2.3%) ... 678
▲ Cubicin for Injection (2.4% to 6.7%) ... 1026
▲ Dacogen Injection (7%) ... 2129
Depacon Injection ... 412
Depakene ... 417
Depakote Sprinkle Capsules ... 422
Depakote Tablets ... 427
▲ Depakote ER Tablets (Greater than 1% to 5%) ... 434
▲ depo-subQ provera 104 Injectable Suspension (1% to less than 5%) ... 2624
▲ Detrol Tablets (5.5%) ... 2628
Diastat Rectal Delivery System (Less than 1%) ... 3343
Diovan HCT Tablets (Greater than 0.2%) ... 2196
▲ Ditropan XL Extended-Release Tablets (5%) ... 2413
▲ Doxil Injection (1% to 10%) ... 2351
Duetact Tablets ... 3226
DuoNeb Inhalation Solution (1.6%) ... 1058
Effexor Tablets ... 3411
▲ Emend Capsules (Greater than 0.5%) ... 1963
▲ Enablex Extended-Release Tablets (3.7% to 4.7%) ... 2203
Enbrel for Injection ... 584
Epivir ... 1427
▲ Epogen for Injection (3% to 12%) ... 591
▲ Equetro Extended-Release Capsules (Less than 5%) ... 3180
Estring Vaginal Ring (2%) ... 2635
▲ Evista Tablets (4%) ... 1763
▲ Evoxac Capsules (6.1%) ... 1047
▲ Exelon Capsules (7%) ... 2206
▲ Exelon Oral Solution (7%) ... 2206
▲ Faslodex Injection (6.1%) ... 681
▲ Femara Tablets (6%) ... 2214
Ferrlecit Injection ... 3388
▲ Flovent Diskus (1% to 3%) ... 1443
▲ Flovent HFA (1% to 3%) ... 1447
Gabitril Tablets (1% or more) ... 984
▲ Gengraf Capsules (3% to 21.1%) ... 459
Hectorol Capsules ... 1275
Hectorol Injection ... 1278
▲ Herceptin I.V. (5%) ... 1233
▲ Humira Injection (8%) ... 466
Hytrin Capsules (0.5% to 1.3%) ... 471
Hyzaar 50-12.5 Tablets ... 1990
Hyzaar 100-12.5 Tablets ... 1990
Hyzaar 100-25 Tablets ... 1990
▲ Imdur Tablets (Less than or equal to 5%) ... 3018
Imitrex Injection ... 1463
Imitrex Nasal Spray ... 1467
▲ Intron A for Injection (Less than 5% to 15%) ... 3024
▲ Invanz for Injection (3.8%) ... 1999
Invirase (Less than 2%) ... 2772
Ionsys Transdermal System (.1% to less than 1%) ... 2379
Keppra Injection ... 3320
Keppra Oral Solution (1% or more) ... 3314
Keppra Tablets (1% or more) ... 3314
Klonopin (1%) ... 2778
Kytril Injection (2.6%) ... 2781
▲ Lamictal (3%) ... 1481
Lescol Capsules (1.6%) ... 2233
Lescol XL Tablets (2.7%) ... 2233
Levaquin (0.1% to 0.9%) ... 2384
Levaquin in 5% Dextrose Injection (0.1% to 0.9%) ... 2384
Lexapro Oral Solution (Frequent) ... 1190
Lexapro Tablets (Frequent) ... 1190
Lipitor Tablets (Greater than or equal to 2%) ... 2483
Lotensin Tablets (Less than 1%) ... 2243
Lotensin HCT Tablets (0.3% or more) ... 2246
Lotronex Tablets (Rare) ... 1512
▲ Lucentis Injection (4% to 9%) ... 1237
▲ Lunesta Tablets (0% to 3%) ... 3142
Lupron Depot 7.5 mg (Less than 5%) ... 3264
▲ Macugen Injection (6% to 10%) ... ⊙261
▲ Megace ES Oral Suspension (1% to 3%) ... 2481
Meridia Capsules (2.3%) ... 489
Metrogel 1% (1.1%) ... 1211
Micardis Tablets (1%) ... 854
Micardis HCT Tablets (2% or greater) ... 856
▲ Mirapex Tablets (Greater than or equal to 1% to 4%) ... 859
▲ Mobic Oral Suspension (0.3% to 4.7%) ... 863
▲ Mobic Tablets (0.3% to 4.7%) ... 863
▲ Myfortic Tablets (29.1%) ... 2255
Myobloc Injection (Greater than 2%) ... 3192
Namenda (Greater than or equal to 2%) ... 1195
▲ NeoProfen Injection (9%) ... 2472
▲ Neoral Oral Solution (3% to 21.1%) ... 2259
▲ Neoral Soft Gelatin Capsules (3% to 21.1%) ... 2259
Neurontin Capsules (Infrequent) ... 2487
Neurontin Oral Solution (Infrequent) ... 2487
Neurontin Tablets (Infrequent) ... 2487
▲ Nipent for Injection (3%) ... 1863
▲ Orencia Powder for Intravenous Infusion (0.2% to 6%) ... 914
Parcopa Orally Disintegrating Tablets ... 3097
Paxil CR Controlled-Release Tablets (2%) ... 1538
Paxil (2%) ... 1530
Permax Tablets (2.7%) ... 3356
Pexeva Tablets (2%) ... 1694
▲ Photofrin for Injection (7%) ... 702
▲ Plavix Tablets (3.1%) ... 917
▲ Plavix Tablets (3.1%) ... 2926
Pletal Tablets (2% or greater) ... 2455
Prevacid Delayed-Release Capsules (Less than 1%) ... 3271
Prevacid for Delayed-Release Oral Suspension (Less than 1%) ... 3271
Prevacid SoluTab Delayed-Release Orally Disintegrating Tablets (Less than 1%) ... 3271
Prevacid NapraPAC (Less than 1%) ... 3280
Prevnar for Injection ... 3463
PREVPAC (Less than 1%) ... 3284
Prilosec OTC Delayed-Release Tablets (Less than 1%) ... 2677
Prinivil Tablets (0.3% to 1.0%) ... 2052
Prinzide Tablets (0.3% to 1%) ... 2056
ProAir HFA Inhalation Aerosol (Less than 3%) ... 3300
Prochieve 4% Gel ... 1003
Prochieve 8% Gel ... 1003
▲ Procrit for Injection (3% to 12%) ... 2364
▲ Prograf Capsules and Injection (16% to 34%) ... 632
▲ Proleukin for Injection (23%) ... 2266
Prometrium Capsules (100 mg, 200 mg) (Less than 5%) ... 3203
Proquin XR Tablets (Less than 1%) ... 1153
Protonix I.V. (Greater than or equal to 1%) ... 3472
Protonix Tablets (Greater than or equal to 1%) ... 3469
Protopic Ointment (1% to 2%) ... 638
▲ Proventil HFA Inhalation Aerosol (3%) ... 3056
Provigil Tablets (At least 1%) ... 988
▲ Rapamune Oral Solution and Tablets (23% to 33%) ... 3475
▲ Razadyne (8%) ... 2399
▲ Razadyne ER Extended-Release Capsules (8%) ... 2399
▲ Remicade for IV Injection (8%) ... 971
ReoPro Vials (1.9%) ... 1809
▲ Requip Tablets (5%) ... 1555
Rescriptor Tablets ... 2551
▲ Revlimid Capsules (10.8%) ... 958
Reyataz Capsules (Less than 3%) ... 921
▲ Rilutek Tablets (2.5% to 4.5%) ... 2930
Rituxan I.V. ... 1254
Rocaltrol Capsules ... 2798
Rocaltrol Oral Solution ... 2798
RotaTeq (0.1%) ... 2074
▲ Sandimmune (20.2% to 21.1%) ... 2275
▲ Sandostatin Injection (1% to 4%) ... 2278
▲ Sandostatin LAR Depot (5% to 15%) ... 2280
▲ Simulect for Injection (Greater than or equal to 10%) ... 2284
▲ Spiriva HandiHaler (4% to 7%) ... 869
Stalevo Tablets ... 2287
Symbyax Capsules (Frequent) ... 1819
Targretin Capsules ... 1747
▲ Tasmar Tablets (5%) ... 3358
▲ Temodar Capsules (8%) ... 3073
Testim 1% Gel ... 695
Teveten Tablets (1%) ... 1735
Teveten HCT Tablets (Less than 1%) ... 1737
▲ Thymoglobulin for Intravenous Infusion (18.3%) ... 1284
▲ Topamax Sprinkle Capsules (1% to 4%) ... 2404
▲ Topamax Tablets (1% to 4%) ... 2404
Trasylol Injection (2%) ... 754
Travatan Ophthalmic Solution (1% to 5%) ... 563
Trelstar Depot (1.4%) ... 3394
▲ Trileptal Tablets (1% to 5%) ... 2300
▲ Trileptal Oral Suspension (1% to 5%) ... 2300
▲ Ultram ER Tablets (1% to greater than 5%) ... 2392
Uniretic Tablets (More than 1%) ... 3100
▲ Valcyte Tablets (Less than 5%) ... 2813
Vandazole Vaginal Gel (Less than 1%) ... 3338
▲ Vaprisol (3.3%) ... 643
Vasotec I.V. Injection (1.3%) ... 2103
▲ VESIcare Tablets (2.8% to 4.8%) ... 646
VFEND I.V. (Less than 2%) ... 2564
VFEND Oral Suspension (Less than 2%) ... 2564
VFEND Tablets (Less than 2%) ... 2564
Viadur Implant (Less than 2%) ... 757
▲ Viagra Tablets (3%) ... 2573
Vivitrol ... 995
Wellbutrin Tablets (Infrequent) ... 1603
Wellbutrin SR Sustained-Release Tablets (Up to 1%) ... 1607
Wellbutrin XL Extended-Release Tablets (0% to 1%) ... 1613
▲ Xeloda Tablets (Less than 1% to 6%) ... 2822
▲ Xenical Capsules (5.9% to 7.5%) ... 2831
Xyrem Oral Solution (Frequent) ... 1688
Yasmin 28 Tablets ... 796
Yaz Tablets (Greater than 1%) ... 803
Zegerid Capsules (2.2%) ... 2958
Zegerid Powder for Oral Solution (2.2%) ... 2958
Zelnorm Tablets (1% to 2%) ... 2312
▲ Zometa for Intravenous Infusion (12% to 14%) ... 2315
Zomig Nasal Spray (Rare) ... 3523
Zyflo Tablets (Greater than 1%) ... 1023
Zyprexa Tablets (2%) ... 1830
Zyprexa ZYDIS Orally Disintegrating Tablets (2%) ... 1830
Zyrtec Chewable Tablets (Less than 2%) ... 2594
Zyrtec (Less than 2%) ... 2594
Zyrtec-D 12 Hour Extended Release Tablets (Less than 2%) ... 2597

Infection, urinary tract, fungal

Cubicin for Injection (Less than 1%) ... 1026
Nexium Delayed-Release Capsules (Less than 1%) ... 655
Nexium I.V. (Less than 1%) ... 659

Infection, vagina

Cleocin Vaginal Ovules (Less than 1%) ... 2616
Clozaril Tablets (Less than 1%) ... 2184
FazaClo Orally Disintegrating Tablets (Less than 1%) ... 551
Ortho-Cyclen Tablets ... 2429
Ortho Evra Transdermal System ... 2417
Ortho Tri-Cyclen Tablets ... 2429
Ortho Tri-Cyclen Lo Tablets ... 2436
Proquin XR Tablets (Less than 1%) ... 1153
Xyrem Oral Solution (Infrequent) ... 1688

Infection, viral

▲ Aceon Tablets (2 mg, 4 mg, 8 mg) (0.3% to 3.4%) ... 3194
Actiq (1% or greater) ... 979
Adderall XR Capsules (2%) ... 3166
▲ Advair Diskus 100/50 (4%) ... 1308
▲ Advair Diskus 250/50 (1% to 6%) ... 1308
▲ Advair Diskus 500/50 (4%) ... 1308
▲ Advair HFA Inhalation Aerosol (2% to 5%) ... 1318
Aldara Cream, 5% (1.4%) ... 1846
Allegra (2.5%) ... 2844
▲ Amitiza Capsules (0.5% to 3.4%) ... 3224
Aralast (Greater than or equal to 0.2%) ... 717
Astelin Nasal Spray (Infrequent) ... 1904
Atacand HCT (0.5% or greater) ... 651
▲ Avandamet Tablets (5%) ... 1373
Bexxar ... 1398
Blephamide Ophthalmic Ointment ... 568
Blephamide Ophthalmic Suspension ... 569
Campath Ampules ... 811
Celebrex Capsules (0.1% to 1.9%) ... 3134
Colazal Capsules ... 2838
▲ Daytrana Transdermal Patch (28%) ... 3174
▲ Depakote ER Tablets (Greater than 1% to 5%) ... 434
▲ Diovan Tablets (3%) ... 2193
Diovan HCT Tablets (Less frequent) ... 2196
▲ Elidel Cream 1% (0.7% to 6.6%) ... 2200
Enbrel for Injection ... 584
▲ Epivir-HBV (Among most common) ... 1432
▲ Equetro Extended-Release Capsules (Less than 5%) ... 3180
Evoxac Capsules (Less than 1%) ... 1047
▲ Femara Tablets (5% to 6%) ... 2214
▲ Flovent Diskus (2% to 9%) ... 1443
▲ Flovent HFA (1% to 3%) ... 1447
FML Ophthalmic Ointment ... ⊙228
FML Ophthalmic Suspension ... ⊙227
FML Forte Ophthalmic Suspension ... ⊙226
▲ Foradil Aerolizer (17.2%) ... 3010
▲ Gengraf Capsules (1% to 15.9%) ... 459
▲ Imdur Tablets (Less than or equal to 5%) ... 3018
▲ Intron A for Injection (Less than 5% to 7%) ... 3024
Kaletra (Less than 2%) ... 476
Keppra Oral Solution (2%) ... 3314
Keppra Tablets (2%) ... 3314
Klonopin (Infrequent) ... 2778
▲ Leustatin Injection (20%) ... 2357
Lotronex Tablets (Rare) ... 1512
▲ Lunesta Tablets (3%) ... 3142
Myobloc Injection (Greater than 2%) ... 3192
▲ Nasonex Nasal Spray (8% to 14%) ... 3043
▲ Neoral Oral Solution (1% to 15.9%) ... 2259
▲ Neoral Soft Gelatin Capsules (1% to 15.9%) ... 2259
▲ Neurontin Capsules (Rare to 10%) ... 2487
▲ Neurontin Oral Solution (Rare to 10.9%) ... 2487
▲ Neurontin Tablets (Rare to 10.9%) ... 2487
▲ Nipent for Injection (Up to 8%) ... 1863
Omacor Capsules ... 2725
Orthoclone OKT3 Sterile Solution (1.5%) ... 2360
▲ PEG-Intron Powder for Injection (11%) ... 3048
Prinivil Tablets (0.3% to 1.0%) ... 2052
Prinzide Tablets (0.3% to 1%) ... 2056
Prolastin ... 3255
▲ Prometrium Capsules (100 mg, 200 mg) (7% to 12%) ... 3203
ProQuad (Greater than or equal to 0.2% to less than 1%) ... 2064
Provigil Tablets (Greater than or equal to 1%) ... 988
▲ Pulmicort Respules (3% to 5%) ... 661
▲ Rebetol (12%) ... 3058
▲ Relenza Rotadisk (3% to 13%) ... 1552
▲ Remicade for IV Injection (8%) ... 971
▲ Requip Tablets (11%) ... 1555
Rescriptor Tablets ... 2551
▲ Ribavirin, USP Capsules (12%) ... 3068
Rituxan I.V. ... 1254
▲ Sandimmune (15.9% to 18.4%) ... 2275
▲ Sandostatin LAR Depot (5% to 15%) ... 2280
▲ Simulect for Injection (Greater than or equal to 10%) ... 2284
Singulair (Greater than or equal to 2%) ... 2077
Synagis (More than 1%) ... 1897
Tasmar Tablets (Infrequent) ... 3358
▲ Temodar Capsules (11%) ... 3073
Teveten Tablets (2%) ... 1735
Teveten HCT Tablets (Less than 1%) ... 1737
Thalomid Capsules ... 965
▲ Topamax Sprinkle Capsules (Less than 1% to 9%) ... 2404
▲ Topamax Tablets (Less than 1% to 9%) ... 2404
▲ Trileptal Tablets (5% to 7%) ... 2300
▲ Trileptal Oral Suspension (5% to 7%) ... 2300
▲ Ultram ER Tablets (1% to greater than 5%) ... 2392
▲ Ventolin HFA Inhalation Aerosol (7%) ... 1600
▲ Voltaren Ophthalmic Solution (Less than or equal to 3%) ... 2309

Vytorin 10/10 Tablets 2114
Vytorin 10/10 Tablets 3077
Vytorin 10/20 Tablets 2114
Vytorin 10/20 Tablets 3077
Vytorin 10/40 Tablets 2114
Vytorin 10/40 Tablets 3077
Vytorin 10/80 Tablets 2114
Vytorin 10/80 Tablets 3077
▲ Xolair (23%) 1266
▲ Xopenex Inhalation Solution (6.9% to 12.3%) 3146
▲ Xopenex Inhalation Solution Concentrate (6.9% to 12.3%) 3150
▲ Xopenex HFA Inhalation Aerosol (6.9% to 12.3%) 3154
Zelapar Tablets 3372
Zetia Tablets (2.2%) 2120
Zetia Tablets (2.2%) 3083
▲ Ziagen (5%) 1626

Infection at injection site
▲ Aranesp for Injection (6%) 581
Depo-Medrol Single-Dose Vial 2619
I.V. Busulfex 2493
▲ Valcyte Tablets (3%) 2813
VFEND I.V. (Less than 2%) 2564
VFEND Oral Suspension (Less than 2%) 2564
VFEND Tablets (Less than 2%) 2564
Xolair 1266

Infection with grade 3/4 neutropenia
▲ Alimta (Up to 6%) 1750

Infectious disorders, life-threatening, aggravation of
Bicillin C-R Injectable Suspension 1706

Infectious-mononucleosis-like syndrome
Dapsone Tablets USP 1673

Infertility
Anaprox Tablets 2761
Anaprox DS Tablets 2761
EC-Naprosyn Delayed-Release Tablets 2761
Leukeran Tablets 1504
Levoxyl Tablets 1712
Naprosyn Suspension 2761
Naprosyn Tablets 2761

Infertility, male
Dapsone Tablets USP 1673

Infertility, temporary
Mircette Tablets 1066
NuvaRing 2340
Ortho-Cyclen Tablets 2429
Ortho Evra Transdermal System 2417
Ortho Tri-Cyclen Tablets 2429
Seasonique Tablets 1077
Yasmin 28 Tablets 796

Inflammation, ear
Reyataz Capsules (Less than 3%) 921

Inflammation, eye, anterior chamber
▲ Macugen Injection (10% to 40%) ⊙ 261

Inflammation, mucosal
▲ Clolar for Intravenous Infusion (18%) 1271
Dacogen Injection 2129
Emend Capsules (2.5%) 1963

Inflammation, mycosal
Mycamine for Injection (0.2%) 628

Inflammation, nasal
Imitrex Nasal Spray 1467

Inflammation, ocular
▲ Acular Ophthalmic Solution (1% to 10%) 565
▲ Acular LS Ophthalmic Solution (1% to 10%) 566
Betoptic S Ophthalmic Suspension (Small number of patients) 558
Depo-Medrol Single-Dose Vial 2619
Enbrel for Injection 584
▲ Retisert Implant (10% to 35%) ⊙ 258
Rilutek Tablets (Infrequent) 2930
Rythmol SR Capsules 2727
Tasmar Tablets (1%) 3358
Zyprexa Tablets (Infrequent) 1830
Zyprexa ZYDIS Orally Disintegrating Tablets (Infrequent) 1830

Inflammation, oral
(*see under* Stomatitis)

Inflammation, periocular
Depo-Medrol Single-Dose Vial 2619

Inflammation, unspecified
▲ Advair HFA Inhalation Aerosol (1% to 3%) 1318
Floxin Otic Solution (Single report) 1049
Klonopin (Infrequent) 2778
▲ Panretin Gel (3% to 8%) 1747
Permax Tablets 3356
Prilosec OTC Delayed-Release Tablets (Less than 1%) 2677
ProQuad 2064
ReoPro Vials (0.1%) 1809
Zegerid Capsules (Less than 1%) 2958
Zegerid Powder for Oral Solution (Less than 1%) 2958

Inflammation, upper respiratory tract
▲ Advair Diskus 100/50 (7%) 1308
▲ Advair Diskus 250/50 (6%) 1308
▲ Advair Diskus 500/50 (6% to 7%) 1308
▲ Advair HFA Inhalation Aerosol (4%) 1318
Amerge Tablets (Infrequent) 1339
▲ Flovent Diskus (5%) 1443
Flovent HFA (2%) 1447
Imitrex Nasal Spray 1467
Prevacid Delayed-Release Capsules (Less than 1%) 3271
Prevacid for Delayed-Release Oral Suspension (Less than 1%) 3271
Prevacid SoluTab Delayed-Release Orally Disintegrating Tablets (Less than 1%) 3271
Prevacid NapraPAC (Less than 1%) 3280
PREVPAC (Less than 1%) 3284
▲ Ventolin HFA Inhalation Aerosol (5%) 1600

Inflammation, wound
Ionsys Transdermal System (.1% to less than 1%) 2379

Inflammation at application site
Aldara Cream, 5% 1846
▲ Tri-Luma Cream (5.45%) 1213
Zovirax Cream 820

Inflammation at injection site
Abelcet Injection 1141
Ambien Tablets (Rare) 2851
Ambien CR Tablets (Rare) 2855
AmBisome for Injection (Less common) 620
▲ Amevive (4% to common) 626
▲ Aredia for Injection (Up to 41%) 2179
▲ Betaseron for SC Injection (53%) 767
Bicillin C-R Injectable Suspension 1706
Boostrix 1404
▲ Copaxone for Injection (49%) 3297
Depacon Injection (0.6%) 412
Doxil Injection (Less than 1%) 2351
Estratest Tablets 3199
Estratest H.S. Tablets 3199
Fortaz (1 in 69 patients) 1453
Genotropin Lyophilized Powder (Infrequent) 2638
▲ Havrix Vaccine (1% to 10%) 1456
HibTITER 3426
Humalog-Pen 1781
Humulin 50/50, 100 Units 1791
Humulin 70/30 Pen 1793
Humulin L, 100 Units 1794
Humulin N Pen 1797
Imitrex Injection 1463
▲ Infanrix Vaccine (1.0% to 39.5%) 1476
Infed Injection 3390
▲ Intron A for Injection (Up to 5%) 3024
▲ I.V. Busulfex (25%) 2493
Levaquin (0.1%) 2384
Levaquin in 5% Dextrose Injection (0.1%) 2384
Maxipime for Injection (0.6%) 1105
Merrem I.V. (2.4%) 686
▲ Miacalcin Injection (About 10%) 2252
Mycamine for Injection (1.5%) 628
▲ PEG-Intron Powder for Injection (47%) 3048
▲ Rebetron Combination Therapy (5%) 3063
▲ Ribavirin, USP Capsules (6% to 18%) 3068
Romazicon Injection 2804
▲ Sandostatin LAR Depot (1% to 4%) 2280
Taxotere Injection Concentrate 2932
Tygacil for Injection (0% to less than 2%) 3488
Varivax (Less than 0.05%) 2100
VFEND I.V. (Less than 2%) 2564
VFEND Oral Suspension (Less than 2%) 2564
VFEND Tablets (Less than 2%) 2564
▲ Visudyne for Injection (10% to 30%) 2305
Xolair 1266
▲ Zofran Injection (4%) 1634
Zosyn (0.2% to 1.3%) 3492

Inflammation at insertion site
Vantas (2 patients) 3375

Influenza
Advair Diskus 100/50 1308
Advair Diskus 250/50 1308
Advair Diskus 500/50 1308
Advair HFA Inhalation Aerosol 1318
▲ Ambien CR Tablets (3%) 2855
Amitiza Capsules (0% to 2%) 3224
Avandamet Tablets (1%) 1373
▲ Avandia Tablets (7.1%) 1384
▲ Boniva Injection (3.8% to 4%) 2738
▲ Boniva Tablets (3.8% to 4%) 2741
Clobex Spray (0% to 2%) 1208
Cutivate Lotion 0.05% (2%) 2664
▲ depo-subQ provera 104 Injectable Suspension (1% to less than 5%) 2624
Diovan HCT Tablets (Greater than 0.2%) 2196
Fuzeon Injection (2.4%) 2767
Invirase (2.7%) 2772
Lescol Capsules 2233
Lescol XL Tablets 2233
▲ Lucentis Injection (2% to 10%) 1237
Metrogel 1% (1.4%) 1211
▲ Myfortic Tablets (3% to less than 20%) 2255
Oracea Capsules (1.9%) 1000
▲ Orencia Powder for Intravenous Infusion (5% to 13%) 914
ProQuad 2064
▲ Requip Tablets (3%) 1555
▲ Retisert Implant (5% to 15%) ⊙ 258
Revlimid Capsules 958
Rozerem Tablets (1%) 3231
▲ Singulair (4.2%) 2077
▲ Strattera Capsules (2% to 3%) 1814
▲ Symbicort 80/4.5 Inhalation Aerosol (3.2%) 3511
Symbicort 160/4.5 Inhalation Aerosol (2.4%) 3511
▲ Ultram ER Tablets (1% to greater than 5%) 2392
VESIcare Tablets (0.9% to 2.2%) 646
Vivitrol 995
Vytorin 10/10 Tablets (2.6%) 2114
Vytorin 10/10 Tablets (2.6%) 3077
Vytorin 10/20 Tablets (2.6%) 2114
Vytorin 10/20 Tablets (2.6%) 3077
Vytorin 10/40 Tablets (2.6%) 2114
Vytorin 10/40 Tablets (2.6%) 3077
Vytorin 10/80 Tablets (2.6%) 2114
Vytorin 10/80 Tablets (2.6%) 3077
Xyrem Oral Solution (Frequent) 1688

Infused vein complications
▲ Cancidas for Injection (1.5% to 12%) 1918

Infusion reaction
▲ Erbitux (2% to 19%) 910
Myozyme for Intravenous Infusion 1279
Orencia Powder for Intravenous Infusion 914
▲ Remicade for IV Injection (18%) 971
▲ Rituxan I.V. (9% to 23%) 1254

Inhalation site sensation
▲ Proventil HFA Inhalation Aerosol (6%) 3056

Injury, accidental
▲ Abilify Oral Solution (5%) 882
▲ Abilify Oral Solution (5%) 2450
▲ Abilify Discmelt Orally Disintegrating Tablets (5%) 882
▲ Abilify Discmelt Orally Disintegrating Tablets (5%) 2450
▲ Abilify Tablets (5%) 882
▲ Abilify Tablets (5%) 2450
▲ Advate Injection (17.3%) 712
▲ Angeliq Tablets (5.7%) 762
▲ Arimidex Tablets (2% to 10%) 673
▲ Azilect Tablets (12%) 3293
▲ Climara Pro Transdermal System (3.3%) 776
▲ Concerta Extended-Release Tablets (6%) 1881
▲ Duetact Tablets (Greater than 5%) 3226
▲ Effexor XR Capsules (5%) 3417
Emsam Transdermal System 903
▲ Equetro Extended-Release Capsules (7%) 3180
▲ Flumist Vaccine (2.3%) 1901
▲ Humira Injection (10%) 466
Keppra Injection 3320
▲ Keppra Oral Solution (17%) 3314
▲ Keppra Tablets (17%) 3314
▲ Levitra Tablets (3%) 3034
▲ Lunesta Tablets (0% to 3%) 3142
▲ Lyrica Capsules (2% to 11%) 2539
▲ Menostar Transdermal System (14%) 782
▲ Mirapex Tablets (17%) 859
▲ Myobloc Injection (0% to 5%) 3192
▲ Premarin Tablets (6% to 12%) 3446
▲ Premphase Tablets (4% to 5%) 3456
▲ Prempro Tablets (4% to 5%) 3456
▲ Prilosec OTC Delayed-Release Tablets (3.8%) 2677
ProAir HFA Inhalation Aerosol (Less than 3%) 3300
Prozac Pulvules and Liquid 1801
Relpax Tablets (Rare) 2548
▲ Suboxone Tablets (3%) 2717
▲ Subutex Tablets (3%) 2717
▲ Symbyax Capsules (3% to 5%) 1819
Yaz Tablets (Greater than 1%) 803
▲ Zegerid Capsules (3.8%) 2958
▲ Zegerid Powder for Oral Solution (3.8%) 2958
Zelapar Tablets 3372
Zemaira (0.2% to 0.4%) 3509
▲ Zyprexa Tablets (4% to 12%) 1830
▲ Zyprexa ZYDIS Orally Disintegrating Tablets (4% to 12%) 1830

Injury, back
Xyrem (Infrequent) 1688

Injury, intentional
▲ Aldara Cream, 5% (8.8%) 1846
Campral Tablets (Infrequent) 1174
Lyrica Capsules (Rare) 2539
Symbyax Capsules (Infrequent) 1819
Zyprexa Tablets (Infrequent) 1830
Zyprexa ZYDIS Orally Disintegrating Tablets (Infrequent) 1830

Injury, limb
▲ Advate Injection (34.7%) 712
Xyrem (Infrequent) 1688

INR, abnormal
Nexavar Tablets (Uncommon) 746

INR, increase
Avelox (0.1% to less than 2%) 2970
Cubicin for Injection (1.7%) 1026
Levaquin 2384
Levaquin in 5% Dextrose Injection 2384
Tygacil for Injection (0% to less than 2%) 3488

Insomnia
▲ Abilify Oral Solution (20%) 882
▲ Abilify Oral Solution (20%) 2450
▲ Abilify Discmelt Orally Disintegrating Tablets (20%) 882
▲ Abilify Discmelt Orally Disintegrating Tablets (20%) 2450
▲ Abilify Tablets (20%) 882
▲ Abilify Tablets (20%) 2450
Accolate Tablets 671
Accutane Capsules 2731
Aciphex Tablets 1090
Actiq (1% to 2%) 979
▲ Actonel Tablets (4.7%) 2683
▲ Actonel with Calcium Tablets (4.3%) 2688
Adalat CC Tablets (Less than 1%) 2964
Adderall Tablets 3164
▲ Adderall XR Capsules (1.5% to 27%) 3166
Adipex-P 1215
Advicor Tablets 1722
Advil Allergy Sinus Caplets ▣ 770
Advil Multi-Symptom Cold Caplets ▣ 770
▲ Aerobid/Aerobid-M (1% to 3%) 1171
▲ Agrylin Capsules (1% to 5%) 3169
Alavert Allergy & Sinus D-12 Hour Tablets ▣ 771
Aldara Cream, 5% 1846
Alferon N Injection (2%) 1665
Alinia for Oral Suspension (Less than 1%) 2835
Alinia Tablets (Less than 1%) 2835
Allegra (Less than 1%) 2844
▲ Allegra-D 12 Hour Extended-Release Tablets (12.6%) 2846
▲ Allegra-D 24 Hour Extended-Release Tablets (12.6%) 2849
Aloxi Injection (Less than 1%) 2127
▲ Alphagan P Ophthalmic Solution (1% to 4%) 567
Altace Capsules (Less than 1%) 1702
Altoprev Extended-Release Tablets 3109
Ambien Tablets (Frequent) 2851
Ambien CR Tablets (Frequent) 2855
Amitiza Capsules (0% to 1.4%) 3224
Amoxil Capsules (Rare) 1343
Amoxil Chewable Tablets (Rare) 1343

Amoxil Pediatric Drops for Oral Suspension (Rare) 1343
Amoxil Powder for Oral Suspension (Rare) 1343
Amoxil Tablets (Rare) 1343
Anaprox Tablets (Less than 1%) 2761
Anaprox DS Tablets (Less than 1%) 2761
Aptivus Capsules (1.2% to less than 2%) 826
▲ Aredia for Injection (22.2%) 2179
▲ Aricept Tablets (6% to 14%) 1094
▲ Aricept ODT Tablets (6% to 14%) 1094
▲ Arimidex Tablets (2% to 10%) 673
▲ Arixtra Injection (0.9% to 5%) 1351
▲ Aromasin Tablets (11% to 13.7%) 2600
▲ Arranon Injection (0% to 7%) 1357
Arthrotec Tablets (Rare) 3129
Asacol Delayed-Release Tablets (2%) 2692
Asmanex Twisthaler (1% to less than 3%) 2966
Atacand HCT (0.5% or greater) 651
▲ Atripla Tablets (4%) 945
Atrovent Inhalation Solution (0.9%) 835
Augmentin (Rare) 1360
Augmentin Tablets (Rare) 1363
Augmentin XR Extended-Release Tablets (Rare) 1369
Augmentin ES-600 Powder for Oral Suspension (Rare) 1366
Avelox (0.1% to less than 2%) 2970
▲ Avinza Capsules (5% to 10%) 1741
Axert Tablets (Infrequent) 2396
Axid Oral Solution (2.7%) 879
Baraclude (Less than 1%) 894
Benicar Tablets (Greater than 0.5%) 1043
Bentyl Capsules 697
Bentyl Injection 697
Bentyl Syrup 697
Bentyl Tablets 697
▲ Betaseron for SC Injection (24%) 767
Betoptic S Ophthalmic Suspension (Rare) 558
Biaxin/Biaxin XL 402
BioLean II Tablets ▣808
Blocadren Tablets (Less than 1%) 1916
Boniva Injection (0.8% to 2%) 2738
Boniva Tablets (0.8% to 2%) 2741
Brimonidine Tartrate Ophthalmic Solution 0.2% (Less than 3%) ⊙248
Caduet Tablets (Greater than 0.1%) 2508
▲ Campath Ampules (10%) 811
▲ Campral Tablets (6% to 9%) 1174
▲ Camptosar Injection (0% to 19%) 2604
Cancidas for Injection (0% to 1.2%) 1918
Captopril Tablets (About 0.5 to 2%) 2149
Carafate Suspension (Less than 0.5%) 701
Carafate Tablets (Less than 0.5%) 701
Cardizem LA Extended Release Tablets (Less than 2%) 1728
▲ Carnitor Injection (1% to 3%) 3188
Carteolol Hydrochloride Ophthalmic Solution USP, 1% (Occasional) ⊙249
Catapres Tablets (About 5 in 1,000 patients) 843
Catapres-TTS (2 of 101 patients) 844
Celebrex Capsules (2.3%) 3134
▲ Celexa (15%) 1176
▲ CellCept Capsules (40.8%) 2747
▲ CellCept Intravenous (40.8%) 2747
▲ CellCept Oral Suspension (40.8%) 2747
▲ CellCept Tablets (40.8%) 2747
Cesamet Capsules 3340
▲ Chantix Tablets (18% to 19%) 2517
Cialis Tablets (Less than 2%) 1838
Cipro (Less than 1%) 2977
Cipro I.V. (1% or less) 2984
Cipro XR Tablets (Less than 1%) 2990
▲ Clarinex Syrup (4.5%) 2995
▲ Clarinex-D 24-Hour Extended-Release Tablets (5%) 2998
Clinoril Tablets (Less than 1%) 1924
Clorpres Tablets (About 5 in 1,000) 2153
▲ Clozaril Tablets (2% to 20%) 2184
Colazal Capsules (2%) 2838
Combivent Inhalation Aerosol (Less than 2%) 847
▲ Combivir Tablets (11%) 1411
▲ Concerta Extended-Release Tablets (1.5% to 5%) 1881
Copaxone for Injection (At least 2%) 3297
▲ Copegus Tablets (30%) 2754
Coreg Tablets (2%) 1414
Cosopt Sterile Ophthalmic Solution 1931
Covera-HS Tablets (Less than 2%) 3139
Cozaar Tablets (1% or greater) 1935
Crestor Tablets (Greater than or equal to 2%) 678
▲ Cubicin for Injection (4.5% to 11.2%) 1026
▲ Cymbalta Delayed-Release Capsules (8% to 13%) 1757
▲ Dacogen Injection (28%) 2129
Dantrium Capsules (Less frequent) 2694
Dapsone Tablets USP 1673
▲ Daytrana Transdermal Patch (4% to 30%) 3174
Decadron Tablets 1951
Demadex Injection (1.2%) 2759
Demadex Tablets (1.2%) 2759
Demser Capsules 1953
▲ Depacon Injection (9% to 15%) 412
▲ Depakene (15%) 417
▲ Depakote Sprinkle Capsules (9% to 15%) 422
▲ Depakote Tablets (1% to 15%) 427
▲ Depakote ER Tablets (Greater than 1% to 15%) 434
▲ DepoDur Extended-Release Injection (5% to 10%) 1110
▲ Depo-Provera Contraceptive Injection (1% to 5%) 2622
▲ depo-subQ provera 104 Injectable Suspension (1% to less than 5%) 2624
Desoxyn Tablets, USP 2462
Dexedrine 1420
DextroStat Tablets 3179
Dilaudid 440
Dilaudid Non-Sterile Powder 440
Dilaudid Oral Liquid (Less frequent) 445
Dilaudid Rectal Suppositories 440
Dilaudid Tablets 440
Dilaudid Tablets - 8 mg (Less frequent) 445
Dilaudid-HP (Less frequent) 442
Diovan Tablets 2193
Diovan HCT Tablets (Greater than 0.2%) 2196
▲ Ditropan XL Extended-Release Tablets (2% to less than 5%) 2413
Dolobid Tablets (Greater than 1 in 100) 1955
Donnatal Extentabs 2493
▲ Doxil Injection (Less than 1% to 10%) 2351
▲ Duragesic Transdermal System (3% to 10%) 2373
DynaCirc CR Tablets (0.5% to 1%) 2721
EC-Naprosyn Delayed-Release Tablets (Less than 1%) 2761
▲ Effexor Tablets (3% to 22.5%) 3411
▲ Effexor XR Capsules (3% to 23%) 3417
Efudex 3363
Eldepryl Capsules (1 of 49 patients) 3208
Eligard 7.5 mg (Less than 2%) 2880
Eligard 30 mg (1.1%) 2885
Elmiron Capsules 2415
▲ Eloxatin for Injection (9% to 11%) 2892
▲ Emcyt Capsules (3%) 2634
▲ Emend Capsules (2.1% to 4.1 %) 1963
▲ Emsam Transdermal System (12%) 903
▲ Emtriva Capsules (7% to 16%) 1287
▲ Emtriva Oral Solution (7% to 16%) 1287
Engerix-B Vaccine (Less than 1%) 1425
▲ Entocort EC Capsules (Less than 5%) 2698
▲ Epivir (11%) 1427
▲ Epogen for Injection (13% to 21%) 591
▲ Epzicom Tablets (7% to 9%) 1436
▲ Equetro Extended-Release Capsules (Less than 5%) 3180
▲ Erbitux (Less than 1% to 12%) 910
▲ Estring Vaginal Ring (4%) 2635
▲ Evista Tablets (5.5%) 1763
Evoxac Capsules (2.4%) 1047
▲ Exelon Capsules (3% to 9%) 2206
▲ Exelon Oral Solution (3% to 9%) 2206
Famvir Tablets (1.5% to 2.5%) 2211
Fansidar Tablets 2765
▲ Faslodex Injection (6.9%) 681
▲ FazaClo Orally Disintegrating Tablets (2% to 20%) 551
▲ Femara Tablets (Less than 0.1% to 7%) 2214
Flomax Capsules (1.4% to 2.4%) 850
Floxin Otic Solution (Single report) 1049
Flumadine (2.1% to 3.4%) 1183
▲ Focalin Tablets (Among most common) 2220
Focalin XR Capsules 2223
Foradil Aerolizer (1.5%) 3010
▲ Forteo for Injection (4.3%) 1767
Fortical Nasal Spray (Less than 1%) 3337
Frova Tablets (Frequent) 1113
Fuzeon Injection 2767
▲ Gabitril Tablets (6%) 984
Gantrisin Pediatric Suspension 2770
Gardasil Injection (1.2%) 1984
Gemzar for Injection (Infrequent) 1771
Gengraf Capsules (1% to less than 3%) 459
Geodon 2529
▲ Gleevec Tablets (0% to 19%) 2227
Gris-PEG Tablets (Occasional) 2502
Havrix Vaccine (Less than 1%) 1456
▲ Hectorol Capsules (Greater than or equal to 5%) 1275
▲ Herceptin I.V. (14%) 1233
Hydrocortone Tablets 1989
Hytrin Capsules (At least 1%) 471
Hyzaar 50-12.5 Tablets 1990
Hyzaar 100-12.5 Tablets 1990
Hyzaar 100-25 Tablets 1990
▲ Imdur Tablets (Less than or equal to 5%) 3018
▲ Indapamide Tablets (Less than 5%) 2156
Inderal LA Long-Acting Capsules 3429
Indocin (Less than 1%) 1995
▲ Infergen (24% to 39%) 3364
InnoPran XL Capsules 2723
▲ Intron A for Injection (Up to 12%) 3024
▲ Invanz for Injection (3% to 3.2%) 1999
Invirase (Greater than or equal to 2%) 2772
▲ Ionsys Transdermal System (3%) 2379
▲ I.V. Busulfex (84%) 2493
Kadian Capsules (Less than 3%) 577
Kaletra (Up to 2%) 476
Keppra Injection 3320
Keppra Oral Solution (1% to 2%) 3314
Keppra Tablets (1% to 2%) 3314
Ketek Tablets (Greater than or equal to 0.2% to less than 2%) 2903
Klonopin (Infrequent) 2778
▲ Kytril Injection (Less than 2% to 4.9%) 2781
▲ Kytril (3% to 5%) 2784
▲ Lamictal (5.6%) 1481
▲ Lariam Tablets (Among most frequent) 2786
Lescol Capsules (2.7%) 2233
Lescol XL Tablets (0.8%) 2233
▲ Leukine (11%) 814
▲ Leustatin Injection (7%) 2357
▲ Levaquin (0.4% to 4.6%) 2384
▲ Levaquin in 5% Dextrose Injection (0.4% to 4.6%) 2384
Levitra Tablets (Less than 2%) 3034
Levothroid Tablets 1186
Levoxyl Tablets 1712
▲ Lexapro Oral Solution (5% to 14%) 1190
▲ Lexapro Tablets (5% to 14%) 1190
Lipitor Tablets (Greater than or equal to 2%) 2483
Lofibra Tablets 1219
Lofibra Capsules 1216
Lopressor Injection 2238
Lopressor Tablets 2238
Lopressor HCT 50/25 Tablets 2241
Lopressor HCT 100/25 Tablets 2241
Lopressor HCT 100/50 Tablets 2241
Lotensin Tablets (Less than 1%) 2243
Lotensin HCT Tablets (0.3% to 1%) 2246
Lotrel Capsules 2249
Lunesta Tablets (Infrequent) 3142
▲ Lupron Depot 3.75 mg (16%) 3260
Lupron Depot 7.5 mg (Less than 5%) 3264
▲ Lupron Depot–3 Month 11.25 mg (16%) 3265
▲ Malarone Pediatric Tablets (2% to 3%) 1517
▲ Malarone Tablets (2% to 3%) 1517
Matulane Capsules 3191
Mavik Tablets (0.3% to 1.0%) 486
Maxair Autohaler 1852
Maxalt Tablets (Infrequent) 2008
Maxalt-MLT Orally Disintegrating Tablets (Infrequent) 2008
▲ Megace ES Oral Suspension (0% to 6%) 2481
▲ Mepron Suspension (10% to 19%) 1521
▲ Meridia Capsules (10.7%) 489
Merrem I.V. (Greater than 0.1% to 1%) 686
▲ Metadate CD Capsules (5%) 3323
Mevacor Tablets (0.5% to 1.0%) 2021
Miacalcin Nasal Spray (Less than 1%) 2253
Micardis Tablets (More than 0.3%) 854
Micardis HCT Tablets 856
Midamor Tablets (Less than or equal to 1%) 2026
Migranal Nasal Spray (Infrequent) 3348
▲ Mirapex Tablets (17% to 27%) 859
▲ Mobic Oral Suspension (0% to 3.6%) 863
▲ Mobic Tablets (0% to 3.6%) 863
Moduretic Tablets (Less than or equal to 1%) 2028
MS Contin Tablets (Less frequent) 2701
▲ Myfortic Tablets (23.5%) 2255
▲ Mylotarg for Injection (11% to 13%) 3431
Nalfon Capsules (Less than 1%) 2502
Namenda (Greater than or equal to 2%) 1195
Naprosyn Suspension (Less than 1%) 2761
Naprosyn Tablets (Less than 1%) 2761
▲ Natrecor for Injection (2% to 6%) 3127
Nembutal Sodium Solution, USP (Less than 1%) 2470
Neoral Oral Solution (1% to 3%) 2259
▲ Neoral Soft Gelatin Capsules (1% to 3%) 2259
▲ Neulasta Injection (15% to 72%) 601
▲ Neumega for Injection (33%) 3435
Neurontin Capsules 2487
Neurontin Oral Solution 2487
Neurontin Tablets 2487
Nexium Delayed-Release Capsules (Less than 1%) 655
Nexium I.V. (Less than 1%) 659
Niaspan Extended-Release Tablets 1730
▲ Nipent for Injection (3% to 10%) 1863
▲ Niravam Orally Disintegrating Tablets (8.9% to 29.5%) 3092
Noroxin Tablets (Less frequent) 2032
Norvasc Tablets (More than 0.1% to 1%) 2545
Norvir (2% to 2.6%) 503
Omacor Capsules 2725
Omnicef Capsules (0.2%) 511
Omnicef for Oral Suspension (0.2%) 511
▲ Ontak Vials (9%) 1745
Opana Tablets (Less than 1%) 1122
▲ Opana ER Tablets (4%) 1126
Ortho-Cyclen/Ortho Tri-Cyclen 2429
Ortho Tri-Cyclen Lo Tablets 2436
Oxandrin Tablets 2962
Oxsoralen-Ultra Capsules 3353
▲ OxyContin Tablets (Between 1% and 5%) 2703
Parcopa Orally Disintegrating Tablets 3097
Parnate Tablets 1527
▲ Paxil CR Controlled-Release Tablets (1.3% to 24%) 1538
▲ Paxil (1.3% to 24%) 1530
▲ Pegasys (19%) 2789
▲ PEG-Intron Powder for Injection (23%) 3048
Pentasa Capsules (Less than 1%) 3185
Pepcid Injection (Infrequent) 2040
Pepcid (Infrequent) 2038
▲ Permax Tablets (7.9%) 3356
▲ Pexeva Tablets (1.3% to 24%) 1694
Phenergan Tablets and Suppositories 3440
Phenytek Capsules 2160
▲ Photofrin for Injection (4% to 14%) 702
Plavix Tablets (1% to 2.5%) 917
Plavix Tablets (1% to 2.5%) 2926
Pletal Tablets (Less than 2%) 2455
▲ Premarin Tablets (6% to 7%) 3446
▲ Premphase Tablets (6% to 7%) 3456
▲ Prempro Tablets (6% to 7%) 3456
Prevacid NapraPAC (Less than 1%) 3280
PREVPAC 3284
Prilosec OTC Delayed-Release Tablets (Less than 1%) 2677
Primatene Mist ▣719
Prinivil Tablets (0.3% to 1.0%) 2052
Prinzide Tablets 2056
ProAmatine Tablets (Rare) 3186
Prochieve 4% Gel 1003
Prochieve 8% Gel 1003
▲ Procrit for Injection (13% to 21%) 2364
▲ Prograf Capsules and Injection (32% to 64%) 632
Proleukin for Injection 2266
▲ Prometrium Capsules (100 mg, 200 mg) (Less than 5%) 3203
ProQuad (Greater than or equal to 0.2% to less than 1%) 2064
Proquin XR Tablets 1153
Protonix I.V. (Greater than or equal to 1%) 3472
Protonix Tablets (Less than or equal to 1%) 3469
▲ Protopic Ointment (Up to 4%) 638
Proventil Inhalation Aerosol 3053
▲ Proventil Inhalation Solution 0.083% (1% to 3.1%) 3055
Proventil HFA Inhalation Aerosol 3056
▲ Provigil Tablets (5%) 988

▲ Prozac Pulvules and Liquid (10% to 33%) 1801
Raniclor Tablets, Chewable (Rare) 2505
▲ Rapamune Oral Solution and Tablets (13% to 22%) 3475
▲ Razadyne (5%) 2399
▲ Razadyne ER Extended-Release Capsules (5%) 2399
▲ Rebetol (14% to 41%) 3058
▲ Rebetron Combination Therapy (26% to 39%) 3063
Recombivax HB (Less to greater than 1%) 2071
ReFacto Vials 3484
Relpax Tablets (Infrequent) 2548
ReoPro Vials (0.3%) 1809
Requip Tablets (1% or more) 1555
▲ Rescriptor Tablets (1.2% to 5%) 2551
▲ Retrovir Capsules (2.4% to 5%) 1560
▲ Retrovir IV Infusion (3% to 5%) 1564
▲ Retrovir (2.4% to 5%) 1560
▲ Revatio Tablets (7%) 2557
▲ Revlimid Capsules (10.1% to 32.1%) 958
▲ Reyataz Capsules (Less than 1% to 5%) 921
▲ Ribavirin, USP Capsules (14% to 41%) 3068
Rilutek Tablets (2.1% to 2.9%) 2930
▲ Risperdal (23% to 26%) 1676
▲ Risperdal Consta Long-Acting Injection (13% to 16%) 1682
▲ Risperdal M-Tab Orally Disintegrating Tablets (23% to 26%) 1676
▲ Ritalin Hydrochloride Tablets (One of the two most common) 2269
▲ Ritalin LA Capsules (3.1%) 2271
▲ Ritalin-SR Tablets (One of the two most common) 2269
Robitussin Cough & Cold Long-Acting Liquid ▣735
Robitussin Head & Chest Congestion PE Syrup ▣739
Robitussin Pediatric Cough & Cold Long-Acting Liquid ▣735
▲ Romazicon Injection (3% to 9%) 2804
▲ Rozerem Tablets (3%) 3231
Rythmol SR Capsules 2727
▲ Sandostatin LAR Depot (5% to 15%) 2280
▲ Simulect for Injection (Greater than or equal to 10%) 2284
Singulair 2077
Sonata Capsules (Infrequent) 1717
▲ Soriatane Capsules (1% to 10%) 1013
Stalevo Tablets 2287
▲ Strattera Capsules (5% to 16%) 1814
▲ Suboxone Tablets (14% to 25%) 2717
▲ Subutex Tablets (21.4% to 25%) 2717
Sular Tablets (Less than or equal to 1%) 3122
▲ Sustiva Capsules (1% to 7%) 930
▲ Sustiva Tablets (1% to 7%) 930
Symbyax Capsules 1819
▲ Symmetrel Tablets (5% to 10%) 1135
Tambocor Tablets (1% to 3%) 1856
Tamiflu Capsules (1%) 2807
Tamiflu Oral Suspension (1.1% to 1.2%) 2807
▲ Tarceva Tablets (0% to 15%) 1259
▲ Tarceva Tablets (0% to 15%) 2444
▲ Targretin Capsules (4.8% to 11.3%) 1747
Tarka Tablets (Less frequent) 524
▲ Temodar Capsules (4% to 10%) 3073
▲ Tequin Injection (0.1% to 3%) 938
▲ Tequin Injection in 5% Dextrose (0.1% to 3%) 938
▲ Tequin Tablets (0.1% to 3%) 938
Testim 1% Gel (1% or less) 695
Teveten Tablets (Less than 1%) 1735
Teveten HCT Tablets (Less than 1%) 1737
Thalomid Capsules 965
TheraFlu Daytime Severe Cold Hot Liquid ▣742
Thiothixene Capsules 2165
Thyrolar Tablets 1199
Tiazac Capsules (Less than 2%) 1201
Timolide Tablets (Less than 1%) 2086
Timoptic Sterile Ophthalmic Solution 2088
Timoptic in Ocudose (Less frequent) 2091
Timoptic-XE Sterile Ophthalmic Gel Forming Solution 2092
Tindamax Tablets 2142
▲ Topamax Sprinkle Capsules (6% to 9%) 2404
▲ Topamax Tablets (6% to 9%) 2404
Toprol-XL Tablets 668
Tranxene 2474
▲ Trasylol Injection (3%) 754
Trelstar Depot (2.1%) 3394
Trelstar LA Suspension (1.7%) 3397
Triaminic Chest & Nasal Congestion Liquid ▣746
Tricor Tablets 527
▲ Trileptal Tablets (2% to 4%) 2300
▲ Trileptal Oral Suspension (2% to 4%) 2300
▲ Trisenox Injection (43%) 993
▲ Trizivir Tablets (7% to 13%) 1589
▲ Truvada Tablets (4%) 1296
Twinrix Vaccine (Less than 1%) 1595
Tygacil for Injection (2.3%) 3488
Children's Tylenol Plus Cold & Allergy Oral Suspension ▣716
Extra Strength Tylenol PM Caplets, Vanilla Caplets, Geltabs, Gelcaps and Liquid 1875
Concentrated Tylenol Infants' Drops Plus Cold & Cough ▣754
Tylenol Allergy Multi-Symptom Caplets with Cool Burst and Gelcaps 1872
Tylenol Allergy Multi-Symptom Nighttime Caplets with Cool Burst 1872
Children's Tylenol Plus Cold Suspension Liquid 1879
Children's Tylenol Plus Flu Suspension Liquid 1881
Children's Tylenol Plus Multi-Symptom Cold Suspension Liquid 1879
Tylenol Cold Severe Congestion Non-Drowsy Caplets with Cool Burst 1874
Tylenol Cold Head Congestion Daytime Caplets with Cool Burst 1873
Tylenol Cold Head Congestion Nighttime Caplets with Cool Burst 1873
Tylenol Cold Head Congestion Severe Caplets with Cool Burst 1873
Tylenol Cold Multi-Symptom Daytime Caplets with Cool Burst and Gelcaps 1874
Tylenol Cold Multi-Symptom Daytime Liquid with Citrus Burst 1874
Tylenol Cold Multi-Symptom Nighttime Caplets with Cool Burst 1874
Tylenol Cold Multi-Symptom Nighttime Liquid with Cool Burst 1874
Tylenol Cold Multi-Symptom Severe Caplets with Cool Burst 1874
Tylenol Cold Multi-Symptom Severe Daytime Liquid with Citrus Burst 1874
Concentrated Tylenol Infants' Drops Plus Cold 1879
Concentrated Tylenol Infants' Drops Plus Cold and Cough 1879
Tylenol Sinus Severe Congestion Caplets with Cool Burst 1876
Tylenol Sinus Congestion & Pain Daytime Caplets with Cool Burst and Gelcaps 1876
Tylenol Sinus Congestion & Pain Nighttime Caplets with Cool Burst 1876
Tylenol Sinus Congestion & Pain Severe Caplets with Cool Burst 1876
Ultane Liquid for Inhalation (Less than 1%) 531
▲ Ultram ER Tablets (6.5% to 10.9%) 2392
Uniphyl Tablets 2710
Uniretic Tablets (Less than 1%) 3100
▲ Vagifem Tablets (3% to 5%) 2334
▲ Valcyte Tablets (16%) 2813
Valium Tablets 2819
Vandazole Vaginal Gel (Less than 1%) 3338
Vantas (2.9%) 3375
Vantin Tablets and Oral Suspension (Less than 1%) 2645
▲ Vaprisol (3.3%) 643
Vasotec I.V. Injection (0.5% to 1.0%) 2103
▲ Velcade for Injection (18%) 2133
▲ Ventavis Inhalation Solution (8%) 1020
Ventolin HFA Inhalation Aerosol 1600
Verelan PM Extended-Release Capsules, Controlled-Onset (2% or less) 3106
▲ Vesanoid Capsules (14%) 2820
VFEND I.V. (Less than 2%) 2564
VFEND Oral Suspension (Less than 2%) 2564
VFEND Tablets (Less than 2%) 2564
Viagra Tablets (Less than 2%) 2573
Vicks 44D Cough & Head Congestion Relief Liquid 2679
Vicks DayQuil Multi-Symptom Cold/Flu Relief Liquid 2678
Vicks DayQuil Multi-Symptom Cold/Flu Relief LiquiCaps 2678
Children's Vicks NyQuil Cold/Cough Relief Liquid 2680
▲ Vicoprofen Tablets (3% to 9%) 539
Viracept (Less than 2%) 2577
▲ Viread Tablets (3% to 4%) 1301
▲ Vivitrol (8% to 14%) 995
▲ Voltaren Ophthalmic Solution (Less than or equal to 3%) 2309
Voltaren Tablets (Occasionally) 2307
Voltaren-XR Tablets (Occasionally) 2310
VoSpire ER Tablets (2.4%) 1052
Vytorin 10/10 Tablets 2114
Vytorin 10/10 Tablets 3077
Vytorin 10/20 Tablets 2114
Vytorin 10/20 Tablets 3077
Vytorin 10/40 Tablets 2114
Vytorin 10/40 Tablets 3077
Vytorin 10/80 Tablets 2114
Vytorin 10/80 Tablets 3077
▲ Wellbutrin Tablets (18.6%) 1603
▲ Wellbutrin SR Sustained-Release Tablets (5% to 16%) 1607
▲ Wellbutrin XL Extended-Release Tablets (11% to 20%) 1613
▲ Xeloda Tablets (Less than 5%) 2822
Xifaxan Tablets (Less than 2%) 2842
Xopenex Inhalation Solution 3146
Xopenex Inhalation Solution Concentrate 3150
Xopenex HFA Inhalation Aerosol 3154
Xyrem Oral Solution (Frequent) 1688
Zantac (Rare) 1624
Zantac Injection 1619
Zantac Injection Pharmacy Bulk Package (Rare) 1622
Zantac Injection Premixed 1619
Zantac (Rare) 1624
Zegerid Capsules (Less than 1%) 2958
Zegerid Powder for Oral Solution (Less than 1%) 2958
▲ Zelapar Tablets (7%) 3372
Zelnorm Tablets (1% to 2%) 2312
Zocor Tablets 2105
▲ Zoloft (12% to 28%) 2586
▲ Zometa for Intravenous Infusion (15.1% to 16%) 2315
Zomig Tablets (Infrequent) 3519
Zomig Nasal Spray (Infrequent to less than 2%) 3523
Zomig-ZMT Tablets (Infrequent) 3519
▲ Zonegran Capsules (6%) 1101
▲ Zosyn (4.5% to 6.6%) 3492
▲ Zyban Sustained-Release Tablets (31% to 40%) 1644
Zyflo Tablets (Greater than 1%) 1023
▲ Zyprexa Tablets (12% to 20%) 1830
▲ Zyprexa ZYDIS Orally Disintegrating Tablets (12% to 20%) 1830
▲ Zyrtec Chewable Tablets (Less than 2% to 9%) 2594
▲ Zyrtec (Less than 2% to 9%) 2594
▲ Zyrtec-D 12 Hour Extended Release Tablets (4%) 2597
Zyvox (2.5%) 2652

Insomnia, early morning

▲ Strattera Capsules (1% to 3%) 1814

Insomnia, paradoxical

Diastat Rectal Delivery System 3343

Instability, postural

Risperdal Consta Long-Acting Injection 1682

Insulin requirement, changes

Decadron Tablets 1951
Depo-Medrol Single-Dose Vial 2619
Hydrocortone Tablets 1989
Prinzide Tablets 2056

Interstitial lung disease

Effexor Tablets 3411
Effexor XR Capsules 3417
Erbitux (0.5%) 910
Iressa Tablets (1%) 684
Myfortic Tablets (Rare) 2255
Rapamune Oral Solution and Tablets 3475
Revlimid Capsules 958
Tarceva Tablets 1259
Tarceva Tablets 2444
Zemaira (1 Patient) 3509

Intervertebral disk disorder, unspecified

Imitrex Nasal Spray (Rare) 1467

Intervertebral disk herniation

Remicade for IV Injection (Greater than or equal to 0.2%) 971

Intestinal obstruction

Abilify Oral Solution (Rare) 882
Abilify Oral Solution (Rare) 2450
Abilify Discmelt Orally Disintegrating Tablets (Rare) 882
Abilify Discmelt Orally Disintegrating Tablets (Rare) 2450
Abilify Tablets (Rare) 882
Abilify Tablets (Rare) 2450
Aloprim for Injection (Less than 1%) 2167
Ambien Tablets (Rare) 2851
Ambien CR Tablets (Rare) 2855
Avastin IV (Rare) 1227
Azilect Tablets (Infrequent) 3293
Campath Ampules 811
Celebrex Capsules (Less than 0.1%) 3134
Chantix Tablets (Rare) 2517
Clozaril Tablets 2184
Dantrium Capsules (Rare) 2694
▲ Doxil Injection (11.3%) 2351
Effexor Tablets (Rare) 3411
Effexor XR Capsules (Rare) 3417
Elitek (Less than or equal to 1%) 2890
▲ Eloxatin for Injection (2% to 5%) 2892
▲ Entocort EC Capsules (Less than 5%) 2698
Evoxac Capsules 1047
Exelon Capsules (Infrequent) 2206
Exelon Oral Solution (Infrequent) 2206
FazaClo Orally Disintegrating Tablets 551
Gleevec Tablets (Rare) 2227
Herceptin I.V. (At least one of the 958 patients) 1233
▲ Hycamtin for Injection (1.1% to 4.5%) 1458
Imitrex Injection 1463
Imitrex Nasal Spray (Rare) 1467
Imitrex Tablets 1471
Invanz for Injection (2.1%) 1999
Invirase (Rare) 2772
Kionex Powder 2477
Levaquin (0.1% to 0.9%) 2384
Levaquin in 5% Dextrose Injection (0.1% to 0.9%) 2384
Meridia Capsules 489
Merrem I.V. (Greater than 0.1% to 1%) 686
MS Contin Tablets (Less frequent) 2701
Neurontin Capsules (Rare) 2487
Neurontin Oral Solution (Rare) 2487
Neurontin Tablets (Rare) 2487
Omacor Capsules 2725
▲ Pancrease MT Capsules (Among most frequent) 1885
Paxil CR Controlled-Release Tablets (Rare) 1538
Paxil (Rare) 1530
Percodan Tablets 1132
Permax Tablets (Infrequent) 3356
Pexeva Tablets (rare) 1694
Proleukin for Injection 2266
Prozac Pulvules and Liquid (Rare) 1801
Pulmozyme Inhalation Solution 1248
Remicade for IV Injection (Greater than or equal to 0.2%) 971
Revlimid Capsules 958
Rilutek Tablets (Infrequent) 2930
Risperdal 1676
Risperdal Consta Long-Acting Injection 1682
Risperdal M-Tab Orally Disintegrating Tablets 1676
Rythmol SR Capsules 2727
Sandostatin Injection (Rare) 2278
Sandostatin LAR Depot (Rare) 2280
Seroquel Tablets (Rare) 690
Sonata Capsules (Rare) 1717
Symbyax Capsules (Rare) 1819
Taxotere Injection Concentrate 2932
Thalomid Capsules 965
VESIcare Tablets 646
Xeloda Tablets 2822
Zelapar Tablets 3372
Zomig Nasal Spray (Rare) 3523
Zyprexa Tablets (Rare) 1830
Zyprexa ZYDIS Orally Disintegrating Tablets (Rare) 1830

Intestinal obstruction, pseudo

Catapres Tablets (Rare) 843
Nimotop Capsules (Rare) 749

Intestinal perforation

Arthrotec Tablets (Rare) 3129
Azilect Tablets (Rare) 3293
Campath Ampules 811

Celebrex Capsules (Less than 0.1%) 3134
Cipro (Less than 1%) 2977
Cipro I.V. (Less than 1%) 2984
Cipro XR Tablets 2990
Enbrel for Injection 584
Hydrocortone Tablets 1989
Mobic Oral Suspension (Less than 2%) 863
Mobic Tablets (Less than 2%) 863
Myfortic Tablets 2255
Percodan Tablets 1132
Proleukin for Injection (Less than 1%) 2266
Proquin XR Tablets 1153
Remicade for IV Injection (Greater than or equal to 0.2%) 971
Revlimid Capsules 958
Tabloid Tablets 1575
VFEND I.V. (Less than 2%) 2564
VFEND Oral Suspension (Less than 2%) 2564
VFEND Tablets (Less than 2%) 2564
Wellbutrin Tablets (Rare) 1603
Wellbutrin SR Sustained-Release Tablets 1607
Wellbutrin XL Extended-Release Tablets 1613
Zyban Sustained-Release Tablets 1644

Intestinal strictures
Clinoril Tablets (Rare) 1924
Indocin Capsules (Less than 1%) 1995
Indocin I.V. (Less than 1%) 2465
▲ Pancrease MT Capsules (Among most frequent) 1885

Intestinal villous atrophy
CellCept Capsules (Isolated cases) 2747
CellCept Intravenous (Isolated cases) 2747
CellCept Oral Suspension (Isolated cases) 2747
CellCept Tablets (Isolated cases) 2747

Intestines, hemorrhagic necrosis of
Lanoxicaps Capsules 1490
Lanoxin Injection 1494
Lanoxin Injection Pediatric 1497
Lanoxin Tablets 1500

Intoxication, state of
▲ Advair HFA Inhalation Aerosol (0% to 3%) 1318

Intracranial hypertension with papilledema
Colocort Rectal Suspension, USP (Retention) 100 mg/60 mL 2476
Neoral Oral Solution 2259
Neoral Soft Gelatin Capsules 2259
Norditropin Cartridges (Small number of patients) 2323
Nutropin for Injection (A small number of patients) 1239
Nutropin AQ Injection (A small number of patients) 1243
Nutropin AQ Pen (A small number of patients) 1243
Nutropin AQ Pen Cartridge (A small number of patients) 1243
Tev-Tropin for Injection (Small number of patients) 1222

Intracranial pressure, increase
Albenza Tablets (Up to 1.5%) 1338
Cipro 2977
Cipro I.V. 2984
Cipro XR Tablets 2990
Decadron Tablets 1951
Depo-Medrol Injectable Suspension 2617
Depo-Medrol Single-Dose Vial 2619
Dilaudid 440
Dilaudid Non-Sterile Powder 440
Dilaudid Oral Liquid (Less frequent) 445
Dilaudid Rectal Suppositories 440
Dilaudid Tablets 440
Dilaudid Tablets - 8 mg (Less frequent) 445
Dilaudid-HP (Less frequent) 442
Gleevec Tablets (Rare) 2227
Hydrocortone Tablets 1989
Levaquin (0.1% to 0.9%) 2384
Levaquin in 5% Dextrose Injection (0.1% to 0.9%) 2384
MS Contin Tablets (Less frequent) 2701
Noroxin Tablets 2032
Proquin XR Tablets 1153
Tequin Injection 938
Tequin Injection in 5% Dextrose 938
Tequin Tablets 938

Intraocular disorders
Amerge Tablets (Rare) 1339
Imitrex Tablets 1471

Intraocular pressure, increase
(*see under* Glaucoma)
Advair Diskus 100/50 1308
▲ Nevanac Ophthalmic Suspension 0.1% (5% to 10%) .... ⊙209

Intraocular pressure, paradoxical increase
Pulmicort Respules (Rare) 661

Intraoperative floppy iris syndrome
Cardura XL Tablets 2515
Uroxatral Tablets 2943

Intravascular coagulation, disseminated
Aggrenox Capsules 822
Aloprim for Injection (Less than 1%) 2167
AlphaNine SD, Coagulation Factor IX (Human) 1656
Bayer Aspirin 744
Bayer Aspirin Comprehensive Prescribing Information .... ▣796
Cafcit (2.2%) 1886
Campath Ampules 811
Clinoril Tablets (Less than 1 in 100) 1924
Dolobid Tablets (Less than 1 in 100) 1955
Indocin Capsules (Less than 1%) 1995
Indocin I.V. 2465
Indocin (Less than 1%) 1995
Lamictal 1481
Mylotarg for Injection (1%) 3431
NovoSeven 2331
Omnicef Capsules 511
Omnicef for Oral Suspension 511
▲ Oncaspar (Greater than 1% but less than 5%) 1145
Percodan Tablets 1132
Profilnine SD, Factor IX Complex (Human) 1660
Prograf Capsules and Injection 632
St. Joseph 81 mg Aspirin Chewable and Enteric Coated Tablets 1869
St. Joseph 81 mg Aspirin .... ▣688
Sulfamylon Cream 2162
Sulfamylon for 5% Topical Solution 2162
Trasylol Injection (1% to 2%) 754
▲ Trisenox Injection (8%) 993
Vantin Tablets and Oral Suspension 2645
▲ Vesanoid Capsules (26%) 2820
VFEND I.V. (Less than 2%) 2564
VFEND Oral Suspension (Less than 2%) 2564
VFEND Tablets (Less than 2%) 2564

Intussusception, gastrointestinal
Infanrix Vaccine 1476
Lotronex Tablets (Rare) 1512
Pediarix Vaccine 1548

Involuntary movements, abnormal
Carbatrol Capsules 3171
Clozaril Tablets (Less than 1%) 2184
Effexor Tablets 3411
Eldepryl Capsules 3208
▲ Equetro Extended-Release Capsules (Less than 5%) 3180
FazaClo Orally Disintegrating Tablets (Less than 1%) 551
Moban Tablets 1119
▲ Niravam Orally Disintegrating Tablets (14.8% to 17.3%) 3092
Omnicef Capsules 511
Omnicef for Oral Suspension 511
Seroquel Tablets (Infrequent) 690
Symmetrel Tablets (Uncommon) 1135
Tegretol/Tegretol-XR 2295

Involuntary movements, extremities
Moban Tablets 1119

IOP, elevation of
Albalon Ophthalmic Solution .... ⊙218
Alrex Ophthalmic Suspension 0.2% (2%) .... ⊙246
Beconase AQ Nasal Spray (Rare) 1396
Blephamide Ophthalmic Ointment 568
Blephamide Ophthalmic Suspension 569
Caduet Tablets (Less than 2%) 2508
Depo-Medrol Injectable Suspension 2617
Effexor Tablets (Rare) 3411
Flonase Nasal Spray 1440
FML Ophthalmic Ointment .... ⊙228
FML Ophthalmic Suspension .... ⊙227
FML Forte Ophthalmic Suspension .... ⊙226
FML-S Ophthalmic Suspension .... ⊙229
Gleevec Tablets (Rare) 2227
Lotemax Ophthalmic Suspension 0.5% .... ⊙251
Meridia Capsules 489
Paxil CR Controlled-Release Tablets (Rare) 1538
Paxil (Rare) 1530
Permax Tablets (Infrequent) 3356
Poly-Pred Ophthalmic Suspension .... ⊙233
Pred Mild Ophthalmic Suspension .... ⊙238
Pred Forte Ophthalmic Suspension .... ⊙235
Pred-G Ophthalmic Suspension .... ⊙236
Sandostatin Injection (Less than 1%) 2278
TobraDex Ophthalmic Ointment 562
TobraDex Ophthalmic Suspension 563
Viagra Tablets 2573
▲ Voltaren Ophthalmic Solution (Less than or equal to 5% to 15%) 2309

Iridocyclitis
(*see also under* Iritis)
Betagan Ophthalmic Solution, USP (Rare) .... ⊙220
Cosopt Sterile Ophthalmic Solution (Less than 1%) 1931
Trusopt Sterile Ophthalmic Solution (Rare) 2095

Iris pigmentation, increase in
▲ Lumigan Ophthalmic Solution (1% to 3%) 573
▲ Travatan Ophthalmic Solution (1% to 4%) 563
▲ Xalatan Sterile Ophthalmic Solution (5% to 15%) 2649

Iritis
(*see also under* Uveitis)
Actonel Tablets (Very rare) 2683
Actonel with Calcium Tablets (Very rare) 2688
▲ Acular Ophthalmic Solution (1% to 10%) 565
▲ Acular LS Ophthalmic Solution (1% to 10%) 566
Alphagan P Ophthalmic Solution 567
Aredia for Injection (Rare) 2179
Arthrotec Tablets (Rare) 3129
Brimonidine Tartrate Ophthalmic Solution 0.2% .... ⊙248
Colazal Capsules 2838
Lumigan Ophthalmic Solution (Less than 1%) 573
Lunesta Tablets (Rare) 3142
Lyrica Capsules (Rare) 2539
Neurontin Capsules (Rare) 2487
Neurontin Oral Solution (Rare) 2487
Neurontin Tablets (Rare) 2487
Norvir (Less than 2%) 503
Ophthetic Ophthalmic Solution (Sometimes) .... ⊙232
Prozac Pulvules and Liquid (Rare) 1801
Topamax Sprinkle Capsules (Rare) 2404
Topamax Tablets (Rare) 2404
Uniretic Tablets (Less than 1%) 3100
Viracept (Less than 2%) 2577
Xalatan Sterile Ophthalmic Solution 2649
Zonegran Capsules (Rare) 1101

Iron deficiency
Cuprimine Capsules 1947
Epogen for Injection 591
Prozac Pulvules and Liquid (Rare) 1801
Risperdal (Rare) 1676
Risperdal M-Tab Orally Disintegrating Tablets (Rare) 1676
Sandostatin Injection (Less than 1%) 2278
Syprine Capsules 2085

Irritability
Advair HFA Inhalation Aerosol (Very Rare) 1318
▲ Aerobid/Aerobid-M (3% to 9%) 1171
Angeliq Tablets 762
Aricept Tablets (Frequent) 1094
Aricept ODT Tablets (Frequent) 1094
Arthrotec Tablets (Rare) 3129
Attenuvax 1914
Cafcit 1886
Catapres-TTS (0.5% or less) 844
Ceftin for Oral Suspension (0.1% to 1%) 1407
Cesamet Capsules 3340
Chantix Tablets (Frequent) 2517
Cipro (Less than 1%) 2977
Ciprodex Otic Suspension (0.5%) 559
Cipro I.V. (1% or less) 2984
Cipro XR Tablets 2990
▲ Clarinex Syrup (12.1%) 2995
Climara Transdermal System 771
Climara Pro Transdermal System 776
▲ Clolar for Intravenous Infusion (11%) 1271
Clozaril Tablets (Less than 1%) 2184
▲ Comvax (32.2% to 57.0%) 1928
▲ Copegus Tablets (33%) 2754
Cymbalta Delayed-Release Capsules (Frequent) 1757
Dalmane Capsules 3342
▲ DAPTACEL Vaccine (36.9% to 41.4%) 2950
Daytrana Transdermal Patch 3174
▲ depo-subQ provera 104 Injectable Suspension (1% to less than 5%) 2624
Effexor Tablets 3411
Effexor XR Capsules 3417
Efudex 3363
Eldepryl Capsules 3208
Elspar for Injection 2463
Elspar for Injection 1960
Engerix-B Vaccine (Less than 1%) 1425
Enjuvia Tablets 1062
Estrasorb Topical Emulsion 1147
Estratest Tablets 3199
Estratest H.S. Tablets 3199
FazaClo Orally Disintegrating Tablets (Less than 1%) 551
▲ Flumist Vaccine (9.9% to 17.8%) 1901
▲ Gabitril Tablets (10%) 984
Guanidine Hydrochloride Tablets 3016
▲ Havrix Vaccine (24% to 36%) 1456
HibTITER (133 of 1,118 vaccinations) 3426
▲ Indapamide Tablets (Greater than or equal to 5%) 2156
▲ Infanrix Vaccine (28.8% to 61.5%) 1476
▲ Intron A for Injection (Up to 16%) 3024
Invirase (Less than 2%) 2772
▲ Lamictal (3.0%) 1481
Levothroid Tablets 1186
Levoxyl Tablets 1712
Lexapro Oral Solution (Frequent) 1190
Lexapro Tablets (Frequent) 1190
Maxalt Tablets (Infrequent) 2008
Maxalt-MLT Orally Disintegrating Tablets (Infrequent) 2008
Menostar Transdermal System 782
Meruvax II 2019
M-M-R II 2006
Mumpsvax 2031
Myozyme for Intravenous Infusion 1279
▲ Niravam Orally Disintegrating Tablets (10.5% to 33.1%) 3092
Paxil CR Controlled-Release Tablets 1538
Paxil Tablets 1530
▲ Pediarix Vaccine (1.7% to 63.8%) 1548
Liquid PedvaxHIB 2035
▲ Pegasys (19%) 2789
▲ PEG-Intron Powder for Injection (28%) 3048
Premarin Tablets 3446
Premarin Vaginal Cream 3452
Premphase Tablets 3456
Prempro Tablets 3456
▲ Prevnar for Injection (44.2% to 58.7%) 3463
Prezista Tablets (Less than 2%) 3306
Prinivil Tablets (0.3% to 1.0%) 2052
Prinzide Tablets 2056
Proleukin for Injection 2266
▲ Prometrium Capsules (100 mg, 200 mg) (5% to 8%) 3203
▲ ProQuad (6.7%) 2064
Prozac Pulvules and Liquid 1801
Pulmicort Respules (Less than 1%) 661
▲ Rebetol (10% to 47%) 3058
▲ Rebetron Combination Therapy (23% to 32%) 3063
Recombivax HB (Greater than 1%) 2071
Retrovir Capsules (1.6%) 1560
Retrovir IV Infusion (2%) 1564
Retrovir (1.6%) 1560
▲ Ribavirin, USP Capsules (10% to 47%) 3068
▲ RotaTeq (2.9% to 8.1%) 2074

Singulair (Very rare) 2077
▲ Skelaxin Tablets (Most frequent) 1716
▲ Strattera Capsules (0.5% to 8%) 1814
Symbyax Capsules 1819
▲ Symmetrel Tablets (1% to 5%) 1135
Tasmar Tablets (1%) 3358
Tranxene 2474
Twinrix Vaccine (Less than 1%) 1595
▲ Ultram ER Tablets (1% to greater than 5%) 2392
Uniphyl Tablets 2710
Vantas (Less than 2%) 3375
▲ Vaqta (10.8%) 2097
Varivax (Greater than or equal to 1%) 2100
Vivitrol 995
VoSpire ER Tablets (Less frequent) 1052
▲ Wellbutrin SR Sustained-Release Tablets (2% to 3%) 1607
▲ Wellbutrin XL Extended-Release Tablets (2% to 3%) 1613
▲ Xeloda Tablets (Less than 5%) 2822
Zoloft 2586
Zomig Tablets (Rare) 3519
Zomig Nasal Spray (Rare) 3523
Zomig-ZMT Tablets (Rare) 3519
▲ Zonegran Capsules (9%) 1101
Zyban Sustained-Release Tablets (Frequent) 1644
Zyrtec Chewable Tablets 2594
Zyrtec 2594

Irritation
Aclovate (Approximately 2%) 2660
Analpram-HC 1159
Apexicon E Cream 2661
Bleph-10 Ophthalmic Solution 10% ⊙ 222
Climara Pro Transdermal System 776
Cutivate Cream (Infrequent) 2662
Cutivate Lotion 0.05% (Rare) 2664
Cutivate Ointment (Less than 1%) 2665
Diprolene Gel 0.05% 3001
Diprolene Lotion 0.05% (Less than 1%) 3002
▲ Efudex (Among most frequent) 3363
Lotrisone 3040
Olux Foam (Less than 2%) 1012
Pramosone 1161
Pred-G Ophthalmic Suspension ⊙ 236
Temovate Cream 2668
▲ Temovate Gel (Among most frequent) 2669
Temovate Ointment (0.5%) 2668
Temovate Scalp Application (Infrequent) 2670
Temovate E Emollient (Less than 2%) 2671
Vanos Cream 1893
Viroptic Ophthalmic Solution ⊙ 266

Irritation, anal
Colyte with Flavor Packs for Oral Solution (Less frequent) 3088
Fleet Glycerin Laxatives 1165
Fleet Glycerin Suppositories 1165
TriLyte with Flavor Packs for Oral Solution 3100
Zosyn (1.0% or less) 3492

Irritation, eyelid
▲ Macugen Injection (1% to 5%) ⊙ 261

Irritation, gastric
Aldoril Tablets 1910
Atacand HCT 651
Avalide Tablets 888
Avalide Tablets 2874
Captopril Tablets (About 0.5% to 2%) 2149
Clorpres Tablets 2153
Cymbalta Delayed-Release Capsules (Infrequent) 1757
Dantrium Capsules (Rare) 2694
Diovan HCT Tablets 2196
Diuril Oral Suspension 1954
Diuril Sodium Intravenous 2467
Furosemide Tablets 2154
Guanidine Hydrochloride Tablets 3016
Hyzaar 50-12.5 Tablets 1990
Hyzaar 100-12.5 Tablets 1990
Hyzaar 100-25 Tablets 1990
Indapamide Tablets (Less than 5%) 2156
Kionex Powder 2477
Lopressor HCT 50/25 Tablets 2241
Lopressor HCT 100/25 Tablets 2241
Lopressor HCT 100/50 Tablets 2241
Lotensin HCT Tablets 2246
Micardis HCT Tablets 856
Moduretic Tablets 2028
Norflex Injection 1856
Prinzide Tablets 2056
Teveten HCT Tablets 1737
Timolide Tablets 2086
Uniretic Tablets 3100

Irritation, gastrointestinal
Dibenzyline Capsules 3399
▲ K-Lor Oral Solution (Among most common) 474
Paddock Nystatin USP for Oral Suspension 2478
Urocit-K Tablets (Some patients) 2144

Irritation, glossal
(*see under* Irritation, oral)

Irritation, local
Aldara Cream, 5% (More than 1%) 1846
Arixtra Injection 1351
Avar Cleanser (Rare) 1085
Avar Gel (Rare) 1085
Avar Green Gel 1085
Avar-e Emollient Cream (Rare) 1085
Avar-e Green Cream (Rare) 1085
Bentyl Injection 697
Bleph-10 Ophthalmic Solution 10% ⊙ 222
Blephamide Ophthalmic Ointment 568
Blephamide Ophthalmic Suspension 569
▲ Carac Cream, 0.5% (94.6%) 2879
Climara Transdermal System 771
Desenex ▣ 635
Desenex Jock Itch Spray Powder ▣ 635
Edecrin Sodium Intravenous (Occasionally) 1959
▲ Elidel Cream 1% (0.4% to 6.4%) 2200
Euflexxa (0.63%) 1162
Garamycin Injectable (Rare) 3014
HibTITER 3426
Klaron Lotion 10% 2909
Lidoderm Patch 1118
Locoid Lipocream Cream (Infrequent) 1160
Lovenox Injection 2915
Mentax Cream (Less than 2%) 2158
Metrogel 1% 1211
Naftin Cream (2%) 2126
▲ NeoProfen Injection (16%) 2472
Nitro-Dur Transdermal Infusion System 3046
Ortho Evra Transdermal System 2417
Plexion (Rare) 1889
▲ Polytrim Ophthalmic Solution (Most frequent) 574
Rosac Cream with Sunscreens (Rare) 3213
▲ Striant Mucoadhesive (9.2%) 1007
Xyrem Oral Solution (Infrequent) 1688

Irritation, nasal
▲ Advair Diskus 100/50 (1% to 3%) 1308
▲ Advair Diskus 250/50 (1% to 3%) 1308
▲ Advair Diskus 500/50 (1% to 3%) 1308
Aerobid/Aerobid-M (1% to 3%) 1171
Asmanex Twisthaler (1% to less than 3%) 2966
Atrovent Nasal Spray 0.03% (2.0%) 837
Beconase AQ Nasal Spray 1396
Efudex (Infrequent) 3363
▲ Flonase Nasal Spray (1% to 3%) 1440
▲ Fortical Nasal Spray (10.6%) 3337
Maxalt Tablets (Infrequent) 2008
Maxalt-MLT Orally Disintegrating Tablets (Infrequent) 2008
▲ Miacalcin Nasal Spray (10.6%) 2253
Nasonex Nasal Spray (Greater than or equal to 2%) 3043
Xifaxan Tablets (Less than 2%) 2842

Irritation, nasopharyngeal
▲ Beconase AQ Nasal Spray (24% of patients) 1396
Rhinocort Aqua Nasal Spray (2%) 665

Irritation, oral
Aerobid/Aerobid-M (1% to 3%) 1171
Amerge Tablets (Rare) 1339
Axert Tablets (Rare) 2396
Cesamet Capsules 3340
Furosemide Tablets 2154
Imitrex Nasal Spray 1467
Sandimmune (Rare) 2275
▲ Striant Mucoadhesive (9.2%) 1007

Irritation, oropharynx
Proventil Inhalation Aerosol 3053
Proventil HFA Inhalation Aerosol 3056
▲ Serevent Diskus (7%) 1568
Ventolin HFA Inhalation Aerosol 1600
VoSpire ER Tablets 1052

Irritation, perianal
(*see under* Irritation, anal)

Irritation, scalp
Women's Rogaine Hair Regrowth Treatment Topical Solution, Spring Bloom Scent and Original Unscented ▣ 634

Irritation, skin
(*see under* Irritation, local)

Irritation, vaginal
Ceftin for Oral Suspension (0.1% to 1%) 1407
▲ MetroGel-Vaginal Gel (9%) 1855
Vagistat-1 ▣ 804

Irritation, vulvovaginal
(*see under* Irritation, vaginal)

Irritation at application site
Clobex Spray (0% to 1%) 1208

Irritation at injection site
▲ Eligard 22.5 mg (21.7%) 2883
▲ Eligard 30 mg (20%) 2885
▲ Eulexin Capsules (3%) 3009
▲ Gammagard S/D (16%) 724
Nembutal Sodium Solution, USP 2470
▲ Pegasys (22%) 2789
Pepcid Injection Premixed (Infrequent) 2040
Retrovir IV Infusion (Infrequent) 1564
Romazicon Injection 2804
Xolair 1266

Ischemia
Aldara Cream, 5% 1846
Camptosar Injection 2604
Gammagard S/D 724
Revlimid Capsules 958
Sandostatin Injection (Less than 1%) 2278
▲ Vesanoid Capsules (3%) 2820

Ischemia, arteria basilaris
Fluorescite Injection ⊙ 207

Ischemia, cerebral
Abilify Oral Solution (Infrequent) 882
Abilify Oral Solution (Infrequent) 2450
Abilify Discmelt Orally Disintegrating Tablets (Infrequent) 882
Abilify Discmelt Orally Disintegrating Tablets (Infrequent) 2450
Abilify Tablets (Infrequent) 882
Abilify Tablets (Infrequent) 2450
Actiq (Less than 1%) 979
Arimidex Tablets (1%) 673
Betagan Ophthalmic Solution, USP ⊙ 220
Betimol Ophthalmic Solution 3382
Betimol Ophthalmic Solution ⊙ 295
Carteolol Hydrochloride Ophthalmic Solution USP, 1% ⊙ 249
Cosopt Sterile Ophthalmic Solution 1931
Effexor Tablets (Rare) 3411
Effexor XR Capsules (Rare) 3417
Enbrel for Injection (Infrequent) 584
Gabitril Tablets (Infrequent) 984
Hyperstat I.V. 3017
Imitrex Injection 1463
Imitrex Nasal Spray 1467
Imitrex Tablets (Rare) 1471
Nitrolingual Pumpspray (Occasional) 3120
NovoSeven 2331
Paxil CR Controlled-Release Tablets (Rare) 1538
Paxil (Rare) 1530
Permax Tablets (Infrequent) 3356
Pexeva Tablets (rare) 1694
Pletal Tablets (Less than 2%) 2455
Prozac Pulvules and Liquid (Rare) 1801
ReoPro Vials (0.3%) 1809
Rilutek Tablets (Rare) 2930
Seroquel Tablets (Infrequent) 690
Sonata Capsules (Rare) 1717
Sular Tablets (Less than or equal to 1%) 3122
Symbyax Capsules (Infrequent) 1819
Tasmar Tablets (Infrequent) 3358
Thalomid Capsules 965
Timolide Tablets 2086
Timoptic Sterile Ophthalmic Solution (Less frequent) 2088
Timoptic in Ocudose 2091
Timoptic-XE Sterile Ophthalmic Gel Forming Solution 2092
VFEND I.V. (Less than 2%) 2564
VFEND Oral Suspension (Less than 2%) 2564
VFEND Tablets (Less than 2%) 2564
Zelapar Tablets 3372
Zomig Tablets (Rare) 3519
Zomig-ZMT Tablets (Rare) 3519

Ischemia, colonic
Imitrex Tablets 1471

Ischemia, gastrointestinal
Zomig Tablets (Rare) 3519
Zomig Nasal Spray (Very rare) 3523
Zomig-ZMT Tablets (Rare) 3519

Ischemia, intestinal
Amerge Tablets 1339
Imitrex Nasal Spray 1467
Lanoxicaps Capsules 1490
Lanoxin Injection 1494
Lanoxin Injection Pediatric 1497
Lanoxin Tablets 1500
Zelnorm Tablets 2312

Ischemia, mesenteric
Lotronex Tablets 1512
Zelnorm Tablets 2312

Ischemia, myocardial
Abilify Oral Solution (Infrequent) 882
Abilify Oral Solution (Infrequent) 2450
Abilify Discmelt Orally Disintegrating Tablets (Infrequent) 882
Abilify Discmelt Orally Disintegrating Tablets (Infrequent) 2450
Abilify Tablets (Infrequent) 882
Abilify Tablets (Infrequent) 2450
▲ Alimta for Injection (1% to 3%) 1750
Aloxi Injection (Less than 1%) 2127
Anzemet Injection (Rare) 2859
Anzemet Tablets (Rare) 2862
Argatroban Injection (1.8%) 1346
▲ Arimidex Tablets (3%) 673
Aromasin Tablets (1.6%) 2600
BiDil Tablets 2171
Camptosar Injection 2604
Coreg Tablets (Less than or equal to 0.1%) 1414
Enbrel for Injection (Infrequent) 584
Ethyol for Injection 1898
Femara Tablets (Less than or equal to 2%) 2214
Frova Tablets 1113
Hyperstat I.V. 3017
Imitrex Injection (Extremely rare) 1463
Imitrex Nasal Spray 1467
Imitrex Tablets (Rare) 1471
Levitra Tablets (Less than 2%) 3034
Maxalt Tablets (Very rare) 2008
Maxalt-MLT Orally Disintegrating Tablets (Very rare) 2008
Nexavar Tablets (Uncommon) 746
NovoSeven 2331
Omacor Capsules 2725
Paxil CR Controlled-Release Tablets (Rare) 1538
Paxil (Rare) 1530
PEG-Intron Powder for Injection 3048
Pexeva Tablets (rare) 1694
Pletal Tablets (Less than 2%) 2455
Prograf Capsules and Injection 632
▲ Proleukin for Injection (3%) 2266
Protonix I.V. (Less than 1%) 3472
Protonix Tablets (Less than 1%) 3469
Razadyne (Infrequent) 2399
Relpax Tablets (Rare) 2548
Revlimid Capsules 958
Rilutek Tablets (Infrequent) 2930
Risperdal Consta Long-Acting Injection (Infrequent) 1682
Sutent Capsules (2 patients) 2560
Tasmar Tablets (Infrequent) 3358
Taxotere Injection Concentrate (0% to 0.9%) 2932
TNKase I.V. 1264
Trasylol Injection (1% to 2%) 754
Uniretic Tablets (Less than 1%) 3100
Viagra Tablets (Less than 2%) 2573
Zelapar Tablets 3372
Zomig Tablets 3519
Zomig Nasal Spray 3523
Zomig-ZMT Tablets 3519
Zostavax Injection (0.3%) 2111

Ischemia, peripheral
Anzemet Injection (Rare) 2859
Anzemet Tablets (Rare) 2862
Caduet Tablets (Greater than 0.1% to less than or equal to 1%) 2508
Chantix Tablets (Infrequent) 2517
Coreg Tablets (Greater than 0.1% to 1%) 1414
Evoxac Capsules (Less than 1%) 1047
Exelon Capsules (Infrequent) 2206
Exelon Oral Solution (Infrequent) 2206
Gengraf Capsules (1% to less than 3%) 459
Imitrex Tablets 1471
▲ Intron A for Injection (Less than 5%) 3024
Migranal Nasal Spray (Rare) 3348

Neoral Oral Solution (1% to less than 3%) 2259
Neoral Soft Gelatin Capsules (1% to less than 3%) 2259
Norvasc Tablets (More than 0.1% to 1%) 2545
▲ Requip Tablets (3%) 1555
Soriatane Capsules (Less than 1%) .. 1013
Teveten Tablets (Less than 1%) 1735
Teveten HCT Tablets (Less than 1%) 1737
▲ Ultram ER Tablets (1% to greater than 5%) 2392
Zoloft (Infrequent) 2586

Ischemia, recurrent
Activase I.V. 1223
Retavase 2499

Ischemia, small bowel
Lotronex Tablets 1512

Ischemia, transient
Imitrex Tablets 1471

Ischemic attacks, transient
Abilify Oral Solution 882
Abilify Oral Solution 2450
Abilify Discmelt Orally Disintegrating Tablets 882
Abilify Discmelt Orally Disintegrating Tablets 2450
Abilify Tablets 882
Abilify Tablets 2450
Actimmune (Rare) 1671
Amerge Tablets 1339
Aranesp for Injection (1%) 581
Aricept Tablets (Infrequent) 1094
Aricept ODT Tablets (Infrequent) 1094
Avalide Tablets 888
Avalide Tablets 2874
Avapro Tablets (Less than 1%) 891
Avapro Tablets (Less than 1%) 2871
Celexa (Rare) 1176
Chantix Tablets (Rare) 2517
Clozaril Tablets (Several patients) 2184
DynaCirc CR Tablets (0.5% to 1%) 2721
Epogen for Injection (0.4%) 591
▲ Exelon Capsules (Frequent) 2206
▲ Exelon Oral Solution (Frequent) 2206
▲ Femara Tablets (6.8%) 2214
Gammagard S/D 724
Imitrex Injection 1463
▲ Macugen Injection (1% to 5%) .... ⊙261
Meridia Capsules 489
Namenda (Frequent) 1195
Nexavar Tablets (Infrequent) 746
Orthoclone OKT3 Sterile Solution (Less than 1%) 2360
PEG-Intron Powder for Injection (Less than or equal to 1%) 3048
Prezista Tablets (Less than 2%) 3306
Prinivil Tablets (0.3% to 1.0%) 2052
Prinzide Tablets 2056
Procrit for Injection (0.4%) 2364
Proleukin for Injection (Less than 1%) 2266
Razadyne (Infrequent) 2399
Revatio Tablets 2557
Revlimid Capsules 958
Risperdal 1676
Risperdal Consta Long-Acting Injection 1682
Risperdal M-Tab Orally Disintegrating Tablets 1676
Viagra Tablets 2573

Ischemic colitis
Imitrex Injection 1463
Imitrex Nasal Spray 1467
Imitrex Tablets 1471
Inderal LA Long-Acting Capsules 3429
Timolide Tablets 2086
Timoptic Sterile Ophthalmic Solution 2088
Timoptic in Ocudose 2091
Zomig Tablets (Rare) 3519
Zomig-ZMT Tablets (Rare) 3519

Itching
(*see under* Pruritus)

Itching, eyes
(*see also under* Pruritus, ocular)
Transderm Scōp Transdermal Therapeutic System 2177

Itching, vulvovaginal
Ceftin Tablets (0.1% to 1%) 1407
Clozaril Tablets (Less than 1%) 2184
Vagistat-1 .... ▣804

Itching at application site
Levulan Kerastick for Topical Solution, 20% 1085

Itching at injection site
Humalog Mix 50/50-Pen 1783
▲ Humira Injection (20%) 466
Symlin Injection 613
Xolair 1266

IUD, expulsion (complete)
ParaGard T 380A 1073

J

Jarisch-Herxheimer's reaction
(*see under* Herxheimer's reaction)

Jaundice
Abelcet Injection 1141
Aceon Tablets (2 mg, 4 mg, 8 mg) .. 3194
Aciphex Tablets 1090
Actiq (1% or greater) 979
Adalat CC Tablets (Rare) 2964
Advicor Tablets 1722
Aggrenox Capsules (Less than 1%) .. 822
Aldoril Tablets 1910
Alkeran for Injection 955
Alkeran Tablets 956
Aloprim for Injection (Less than 1%) 2167
Altace Capsules 1702
Anaprox Tablets (Rare; less than 1%) 2761
Anaprox DS Tablets (Rare; less than 1%) 2761
Aricept Tablets (Infrequent) 1094
Aricept ODT Tablets (Infrequent) 1094
Arthrotec Tablets (Rare) 3129
Asacol Delayed-Release Tablets (Rare) 2692
Atacand HCT 651
Avalide Tablets 888
Avalide Tablets 2874
Avandaryl Tablets 1379
Avandia Tablets (Very rare) 1384
Avapro Tablets 891
Avapro Tablets (Very rare) 2871
Avelox (Less than 0.1%) 2970
Axid Oral Solution 879
Azilect Tablets (Rare) 3293
Biaxin/Biaxin XL (Infrequent) 402
Caduet Tablets 2508
▲ Camptosar Injection (9%) 2604
Cancidas for Injection (0.9%) 1918
Captopril Tablets 2149
Cardura XL Tablets 2515
Ceftin 1407
Celebrex Capsules 3134
Celexa (Rare) 1176
▲ CellCept Capsules (3% to less than 20%) 2747
▲ CellCept Intravenous (3% to less than 20%) 2747
▲ CellCept Oral Suspension (3% to less than 20%) 2747
▲ CellCept Tablets (3% to less than 20%) 2747
Cipro (Rare) 2977
Cipro I.V. (1% or less) 2984
Cipro XR Tablets (Rare) 2990
Cleocin Vaginal Ovules 2616
Clinoril Tablets (Less than 1%) 1924
▲ Clolar for Intravenous Infusion (15%) 1271
Clorpres Tablets 2153
Clozaril Tablets 2184
Colazal Capsules 2838
Coumadin for Injection (Infrequent) ... 898
Coumadin Tablets (Infrequent) 898
Crestor Tablets (Very rare) 678
Crixivan Capsules (1.5%) 1940
Cubicin for Injection (Less than 1%) 1026
Dantrium Capsules 2694
Dapsone Tablets USP 1673
Depo-Provera Contraceptive Injection (Less than 1%) 2622
depo-subQ provera 104 Injectable Suspension 2624
Diastat Rectal Delivery System (Infrequent) 3343
Diovan HCT Tablets 2196
Dolobid Tablets (Less than 1 in 100) 1955
Doxil Injection (Less than 1%) 2351
Duetact Tablets (Rare) 3226
Dyazide Capsules 1423
Dyrenium Capsules (Rare) 3400
EC-Naprosyn Delayed-Release Tablets (Rare; less than 1%) 2761
Edecrin (Rare) 1959
Effexor Tablets (Rare) 3411
Effexor XR Capsules (Rare) 3417
Epivir 1427
EryPed 447
Ery-Tab Tablets 449
Erythrocin Stearate Filmtab Tablets 453
Eulexin Capsules (Less than 1%) 3009
FazaClo Orally Disintegrating Tablets 551
Fortaz 1453
Furosemide Tablets 2154
Gantrisin Pediatric Suspension 2770
Geodon Capsules (Rare) 2529
Havrix Vaccine (Rare) 1456
Hyzaar 50-12.5 Tablets 1990
Hyzaar 100-12.5 Tablets 1990
Hyzaar 100-25 Tablets 1990
Indapamide Tablets 2156
Indocin Capsules (Less than 1%) 1995
Indocin I.V. (Less than 1%) 2465
Indocin (Less than 1%) 1995
▲ Intron A for Injection (Less than 5%) 3024
Invanz for Injection (Greater than 0.1%) 1999
Invirase (Rare) 2772
▲ I.V. Busulfex (12%) 2493
Kaletra (Less than 2%) 476
Lamisil Tablets 2232
Leukeran Tablets 1504
Levaquin (0.1% to 0.9%) 2384
Levaquin in 5% Dextrose Injection (0.1% to 0.9%) 2384
Librium Capsules 3347
Lopressor Injection 2238
Lopressor Tablets 2238
Lopressor HCT 50/25 Tablets (Very rare) 2241
Lopressor HCT 100/25 Tablets (Very rare) 2241
Lopressor HCT 100/50 Tablets (Very rare) 2241
Lotensin HCT Tablets 2246
Matulane Capsules 3191
Mavik Tablets (Rare) 486
Mefoxin for Injection 2012
Mefoxin Premixed Intravenous Solution 2016
Merrem I.V. (Greater than 0.1% to 1%) 686
Micardis HCT Tablets 856
Midamor Tablets (Less than or equal to 1%) 2026
Mintezol 2027
Miradon Tablets 3042
Mobic Oral Suspension (Less than 0.1%) 863
Mobic Tablets (Less than 0.1%) 863
Moduretic Tablets 2028
Mustargen for Injection (Infrequent) .. 2468
Mycamine for Injection 628
Mylotarg for Injection 3431
Nalfon Capsules (Less than 1%) 2502
Naprosyn Suspension (Rare; less than 1%) 2761
Naprosyn Tablets (Rare; less than 1%) 2761
NeoProfen Injection 2472
Neurontin Capsules 2487
Neurontin Oral Solution 2487
Neurontin Tablets 2487
Nexavar Tablets (Uncommon) 746
Nexium Delayed-Release Capsules (Very rare) 655
Nexium I.V. (Very rare) 659
Niaspan Extended-Release Tablets ... 1730
Nimotop Capsules (Less than 1%) 749
Niravam Orally Disintegrating Tablets 3092
Noroxin Tablets 2032
Norvasc Tablets (Infrequent) 2545
Norvir 503
Omnicef Capsules 511
Omnicef for Oral Suspension 511
▲ Oncaspar (Greater than 1% but less than 5%) 1145
Ortho-Cyclen Tablets 2429
Ortho Evra Transdermal System 2417
Ortho Tri-Cyclen Tablets 2429
Ortho Tri-Cyclen Lo Tablets 2436
Oxandrin Tablets 2962
Paser Granules 1674
Paxil CR Controlled-Release Tablets (Rare) 1538
Paxil (Rare) 1530
Pediarix Vaccine 1548
Pentasa Capsules 3185
Permax Tablets (Rare) 3356
Pexeva Tablets (rare) 1694
Phenergan Tablets and Suppositories 3440
▲ Photofrin for Injection (Less than 5%) 702
Pletal Tablets (Very rare) 2455
Precose Tablets 751
Prevacid NapraPAC (Less than 1%) .. 3280
PREVPAC (Infrequent) 3284
Prilosec OTC Delayed-Release Tablets (Rare) 2677
Primaxin I.M. 2045
Primaxin I.V. (Less than 0.2%) 2048
Prinivil Tablets 2052
Prinzide Tablets 2056
▲ Prograf Capsules and Injection (3% to 15%) 632
▲ Proleukin for Injection (11%) 2266
Proquin XR Tablets 1153
Protonix I.V. 3472
Protonix Tablets 3469
Raptiva for Injection 1250
Rebif Prefilled Syringe for Injection (Rare) 3159
Remicade for IV Injection (Rare) 971
Rescriptor Tablets 2551
Retrovir IV Infusion 1564
▲ Reyataz Capsules (Less than 1% to 7%) 921
Rilutek Tablets (Infrequent) 2930
Risperdal 1676
Risperdal Consta Long-Acting Injection (Rare) 1682
Risperdal M-Tab Orally Disintegrating Tablets 1676
Rocephin Injectable Vials, ADD-Vantage, Galaxy, Bulk (Rare) 2800
Sandostatin Injection (Less than 1%) 2278
▲ Sandostatin LAR Depot (1% to 4%) 2280
Skelaxin Tablets 1716
Soriatane Capsules (2 of 525 patients) 1013
Suprax 1843
Tabloid Tablets (A few cases) 1575
Tambocor Tablets 1856
Tasmar Tablets 3358
Teveten HCT Tablets 1737
Thiola Tablets 2141
Thioridazine Hydrochloride Tablets ... 2163
Tracleer Tablets 545
Trasylol Injection (1% to 2%) 754
Twinrix Vaccine 1595
Tygacil for Injection (0% to less than 2%) 3488
Ultane Liquid for Inhalation (Less than 1%) 531
Uniretic Tablets (Less than 1%) 3100
Valium Tablets (Isolated reports) 2819
Vasotec I.V. Injection 2103
VFEND I.V. (Less than 2%) 2564
VFEND Oral Suspension (Less than 2%) 2564
VFEND Tablets (Less than 2%) 2564
Viracept 2577
Viramune Oral Suspension 873
Viramune Tablets 873
Voltaren Tablets (Occasionally) 2307
Voltaren-XR Tablets (Occasionally) 2310
Wellbutrin Tablets (Infrequent) 1603
Wellbutrin SR Sustained-Release Tablets (Infrequent) 1607
Wellbutrin XL Extended-Release Tablets (Infrequent) 1613
▲ Xeloda Tablets (Less than 5%) 2822
Zantac (Occasional) 1624
Zantac Injection 1619
Zantac Injection Pharmacy Bulk Package (Infrequent) 1622
Zantac Injection Premixed 1619
Zantac (Occasional) 1624
Zegerid Capsules (Rare) 2958
Zegerid Powder for Oral Solution (Rare) 2958
Zoloft (One or more patients) 2586
Zomig Nasal Spray (Rare) 3523
Zovirax 1643
Zyban Sustained-Release Tablets (Infrequent) 1644

Jaundice, cholestatic
Aceon Tablets (2 mg, 4 mg, 8 mg) (Rare) 3194
Altace Capsules (Rare) 1702
Altoprev Extended-Release Tablets ... 3109
Amoxil Capsules 1343
Amoxil Chewable Tablets 1343
Amoxil Pediatric Drops for Oral Suspension 1343
Amoxil Powder for Oral Suspension 1343
Amoxil Tablets 1343
Androxy Tablets 3335
Angeliq Tablets 762

Asacol Delayed-Release Tablets (Rare) ... 2692
Augmentin ... 1360
Augmentin Tablets ... 1363
Augmentin XR Extended-Release Tablets ... 1369
Augmentin ES-600 Powder for Oral Suspension ... 1366
Avelox (Less than 0.1%) ... 2970
Axid Oral Solution (Rare) ... 879
Caduet Tablets (Less than 2%) ... 2508
Captopril Tablets (Rare) ... 2149
Carbatrol Capsules ... 3171
Ceftin ... 1407
▲ CellCept Capsules (3% to less than 20%) ... 2747
▲ CellCept Intravenous (3% to less than 20%) ... 2747
▲ CellCept Oral Suspension (3% to less than 20%) ... 2747
▲ CellCept Tablets (3% to less than 20%) ... 2747
Cipro ... 2977
Cipro XR Tablets ... 2990
Climara Transdermal System ... 771
Climara Pro Transdermal System ... 776
Colazal Capsules ... 2838
Dapsone Tablets USP ... 1673
Doxil Injection (Less than 1%) ... 2351
Duetact Tablets (Rare) ... 3226
Enjuvia Tablets ... 1062
Equetro Extended-Release Capsules ... 3180
Estrasorb Topical Emulsion ... 1147
Estratest Tablets ... 3199
Estratest H.S. Tablets ... 3199
Eulexin Capsules (Less than 1%) ... 3009
Geodon Capsules (Rare) ... 2529
Keflex Capsules (Rare) ... 549
Lescol Capsules ... 2233
Lescol XL Tablets ... 2233
Lipitor Tablets (Less than 2%) ... 2483
Lotrel Capsules (Rare) ... 2249
Mavik Tablets (Rare) ... 486
Menostar Transdermal System ... 782
Merrem I.V. (Greater than 0.1% to 1%) ... 686
Mevacor Tablets ... 2021
Mircette Tablets ... 1066
Myleran Tablets (Rare) ... 1525
Noroxin Tablets ... 2032
NuvaRing ... 2340
Ortho-Cyclen Tablets ... 2429
Ortho Evra Transdermal System ... 2417
Ortho Tri-Cyclen Tablets ... 2429
Ortho Tri-Cyclen Lo Tablets ... 2436
Oxandrin Tablets ... 2962
Pentasa Capsules ... 3185
Pepcid Injection (Infrequent) ... 2040
Pepcid (Infrequent) ... 2038
Phenergan Tablets and Suppositories ... 3440
Premarin Intravenous ... 3442
Premarin Tablets ... 3446
Premarin Vaginal Cream ... 3452
Premphase Tablets ... 3456
Prempro Tablets ... 3456
PREVPAC ... 3284
Prilosec OTC Delayed-Release Tablets (Rare) ... 2677
Prinivil Tablets (0.3% to 1.0%) ... 2052
Prinzide Tablets (Rare) ... 2056
▲ Prograf Capsules and Injection (3% to 15%) ... 632
Prometrium Capsules (100 mg, 200 mg) ... 3203
Proquin XR Tablets ... 1153
Protonix I.V. (Less than 1%) ... 3472
Protonix Tablets (Less than 1%) ... 3469
Prozac Pulvules and Liquid ... 1801
Raniclor Tablets, Chewable (Rare) ... 2505
Seasonique Tablets ... 1077
Tarka Tablets (Rare) ... 524
Tegretol/Tegretol-XR ... 2295
Thalomid Capsules ... 965
Ticlid Tablets (Rare) ... 2810
Timentin ADD-Vantage (Rare) ... 1580
Timentin Injection Galaxy Container (Rare) ... 1583
Timentin IV Infusion (Rare) ... 1577
Timentin Pharmacy Bulk Package (Rare) ... 1586
Uniretic Tablets (Rare) ... 3100
Vasotec I.V. Injection (0.5% to 1.0%) ... 2103
VFEND I.V. (1% to 1.7%) ... 2564
VFEND Oral Suspension (1% to 1.7%) ... 2564
VFEND Tablets (1% to 1.7%) ... 2564
Vytorin 10/10 Tablets ... 2114
Vytorin 10/10 Tablets ... 3077
Vytorin 10/20 Tablets ... 2114
Vytorin 10/20 Tablets ... 3077
Vytorin 10/40 Tablets ... 2114
Vytorin 10/40 Tablets ... 3077
Vytorin 10/80 Tablets ... 2114
Vytorin 10/80 Tablets ... 3077
Yasmin 28 Tablets ... 796
Yaz Tablets ... 803
Zegerid Capsules (Rare) ... 2958
Zegerid Powder for Oral Solution (Rare) ... 2958
Zmax for Oral Suspension ... 2583
Zocor Tablets ... 2105
Zonegran Capsules (Rare) ... 1101
Zosyn ... 3492

Jaundice, fetal
Diuril Oral Suspension ... 1954
Diuril Sodium Intravenous ... 2467

Jaundice, hepatocellular
Aceon Tablets (2 mg, 4 mg, 8 mg) ... 3194
Augmentin ... 1360
Augmentin Tablets ... 1363
Augmentin XR Extended-Release Tablets ... 1369
Augmentin ES-600 Powder for Oral Suspension ... 1366
Axid Oral Solution (Rare) ... 879
Biaxin/Biaxin XL (Infrequent) ... 402
Carbatrol Capsules ... 3171
Equetro Extended-Release Capsules ... 3180
PREVPAC (Infrequent) ... 3284
Prilosec OTC Delayed-Release Tablets (Rare) ... 2677
Prinivil Tablets (0.3% to 1.0%) ... 2052
Prinzide Tablets ... 2056
Tegretol/Tegretol-XR ... 2295
Ticlid Tablets (Rare) ... 2810
Vasotec I.V. Injection (0.5% to 1.0%) ... 2103
Zantac (Occasional) ... 1624
Zegerid Capsules (Rare) ... 2958
Zegerid Powder for Oral Solution (Rare) ... 2958

Jaundice, intrahepatic

Jaundice, intrahepatic cholestatic
Atacand HCT ... 651
Augmentin ... 1360
Augmentin Tablets ... 1363
Augmentin XR Extended-Release Tablets ... 1369
Augmentin ES-600 Powder for Oral Suspension ... 1366
Avalide Tablets ... 888
Avalide Tablets ... 2874
Clorpres Tablets ... 2153
Diovan HCT Tablets ... 2196
Diuril Oral Suspension ... 1954
Diuril Sodium Intravenous ... 2467
Furosemide Tablets ... 2154
Hyzaar 50-12.5 Tablets ... 1990
Hyzaar 100-12.5 Tablets ... 1990
Hyzaar 100-25 Tablets ... 1990
Indapamide Tablets ... 2156
Lotensin HCT Tablets ... 2246
Micardis HCT Tablets ... 856
Moduretic Tablets ... 2028
Prinzide Tablets ... 2056
Teveten HCT Tablets ... 1737
Timolide Tablets ... 2086
Uniretic Tablets ... 3100

Jaundice, neonatal
Aldoril Tablets ... 1910
Diuril Oral Suspension ... 1954
Diuril Sodium Intravenous ... 2467
Dyazide Capsules ... 1423
Mephyton Tablets ... 2018
Moduretic Tablets ... 2028
Prinzide Tablets ... 2056
Timolide Tablets ... 2086

Jaw tightness
Abilify Oral Solution (Infrequent) ... 882
Abilify Oral Solution (Infrequent) ... 2450
Abilify Discmelt Orally Disintegrating Tablets (Infrequent) ... 882
Abilify Discmelt Orally Disintegrating Tablets (Infrequent) ... 2450
Abilify Tablets (Infrequent) ... 882
Abilify Tablets (Infrequent) ... 2450
Imitrex Injection (Relatively common) ... 1463
▲ Imitrex Tablets (Less than 1% to 3%) ... 1471
Lexapro Oral Solution (Infrequent) ... 1190
Lexapro Tablets (Infrequent) ... 1190
Zomig Nasal Spray (Infrequent) ... 3523

Jerks
(*see under* Twitching)

Jitteriness
▲ Byetta Injection (9%) ... 611
Cafcit ... 1886
Cubicin for Injection (Less than 1%) ... 1026
Cymbalta Delayed-Release Capsules (Infrequent) ... 1757
▲ Focalin XR Capsules (12%) ... 2223
Guanidine Hydrochloride Tablets ... 3016
Lexapro Oral Solution (Infrequent) ... 1190
Lexapro Tablets (Infrequent) ... 1190
Opana Tablets (Less than 1%) ... 1122
Opana ER Tablets (Less than 1%) ... 1126
Prograf Capsules and Injection ... 632
▲ Ultram ER Tablets (1% to greater than 5%) ... 2392
▲ Wellbutrin XL Extended-Release Tablets (3%) ... 1613
Xyrem Oral Solution (Infrequent) ... 1688

Joint dislocation
Evoxac Capsules (Less than 1%) ... 1047

Joint disorder, unspecified
Actiq (1% or greater) ... 979
▲ Actonel Tablets (6.8%) ... 2683
▲ Actonel with Calcium Tablets (6.8%) ... 2688
Adalat CC Tablets (Less than 1%) ... 2964
▲ Arimidex Tablets (6%) ... 673
Asacol Delayed-Release Tablets (2% or greater) ... 2692
Bicillin C-R Injectable Suspension ... 1706
▲ Boniva Injection (3.6%) ... 2738
▲ Boniva Tablets (3.6%) ... 2741
▲ CellCept Capsules (3% to less than 20%) ... 2747
▲ CellCept Intravenous (3% to less than 20%) ... 2747
▲ CellCept Oral Suspension (3% to less than 20%) ... 2747
▲ CellCept Tablets (3% to less than 20%) ... 2747
Euflexxa (1.25%) ... 1162
▲ Humatrope Vials and Cartridges (2.3% to 5.8%) ... 1787
▲ Humira Injection (Less than 5%) ... 466
Hytrin Capsules (At least 1%) ... 471
Imitrex Nasal Spray (Infrequent) ... 1467
Keflex Capsules ... 549
Lamictal (1.3%) ... 1481
Lofibra Tablets ... 1219
Lofibra Capsules ... 1216
Lunesta Tablets (Infrequent) ... 3142
▲ Lupron Depot 3.75 mg (7.8%) ... 3260
▲ Lupron Depot–3 Month 11.25 mg (7.8% to 8%) ... 3265
Meridia Capsules (1.1%) ... 489
Mirapex Tablets (Less than 1%) ... 859
Mobic Oral Suspension (1.5% to 2.3%) ... 863
Mobic Tablets (1.5% to 2.3%) ... 863
Myobloc Injection (Greater than 2%) ... 3192
Neurontin Capsules (Rare) ... 2487
Neurontin Oral Solution (Rare) ... 2487
Neurontin Tablets (Rare) ... 2487
Norvir (Less than 2%) ... 503
Oncaspar (Less than 1%) ... 1145
Prevacid Delayed-Release Capsules (Less than 1%) ... 3271
Prevacid for Delayed-Release Oral Suspension (Less than 1%) ... 3271
Prevacid SoluTab Delayed-Release Orally Disintegrating Tablets (Less than 1%) ... 3271
Prevacid NapraPAC (Less than 1%) ... 3280
PREVPAC (Less than 1%) ... 3284
▲ Prograf Capsules and Injection (3% to 15%) ... 632
Protonix I.V. (Less than 1%) ... 3472
Protonix Tablets (Less than 1%) ... 3469
Protopic Ointment (0.2% to less than 1%) ... 638
Provigil Tablets (1%) ... 988
Relpax Tablets (Rare) ... 2548
Rythmol SR Capsules ... 2727
Sonata Capsules (Infrequent) ... 1717
Symbyax Capsules (1% to 2%) ... 1819
Tasmar Tablets (Infrequent) ... 3358
Thalomid Capsules ... 965
Tricor Tablets ... 527
Xenical Capsules (2.3%) ... 2831
Zomig Nasal Spray (Infrequent) ... 3523
Zyprexa IntraMuscular (Infrequent) ... 1830

Joint disturbances
Imitrex Injection (Infrequent) ... 1463

Joint effusion
Euflexxa (0.63%) ... 1162
Sandostatin Injection (Less than 1%) ... 2278
Sandostatin LAR Depot (Rare) ... 2280

Joint pain
(*see under* Arthralgia)

Joint sprain
▲ Ultram ER Tablets (1% to greater than 5%) ... 2392
Xyrem Oral Solution (Infrequent) ... 1688

Joint stiffness
Amerge Tablets (Infrequent) ... 1339
Arimidex Tablets ... 673
Avalide Tablets ... 888
Avalide Tablets ... 2874
Avapro Tablets (Less than 1%) ... 891
Avapro Tablets (Less than 1%) ... 2871
Cipro (Less than 1%) ... 2977
Cipro I.V. (1% or less) ... 2984
Cipro XR Tablets ... 2990
Gleevec Tablets (Infrequent) ... 2227
Imitrex Injection (Infrequent) ... 1463
Lexapro Oral Solution (Infrequent) ... 1190
Lexapro Tablets (Infrequent) ... 1190
Lunesta Tablets (Infrequent) ... 3142
Nabi-HB (2%) ... 2169
Neurontin Capsules (Infrequent) ... 2487
Neurontin Oral Solution (Infrequent) ... 2487
Neurontin Tablets (Infrequent) ... 2487
Oncaspar ... 1145
Proquin XR Tablets ... 1153
▲ Ultram ER Tablets (1% to greater than 5%) ... 2392
▲ Vivitrol (4% to 12%) ... 995
Xeloda Tablets ... 2822
Xyrem Oral Solution (Infrequent) ... 1688
Zyprexa Tablets ... 1830
Zyprexa ZYDIS Orally Disintegrating Tablets ... 1830

Joints, swollen
▲ ADACEL Vaccine (0.3% to 14%) ... 2945
Lithobid Tablets ... 1692
Proquin XR Tablets (Less than 1%) ... 1153

K

Kawasaki-like syndrome
Asacol Delayed-Release Tablets (One case) ... 2692
Pentasa Capsules (Less than 1%) ... 3185

Kawasaki's disease
Havrix Vaccine (1 Case) ... 1456

Keratitis
Acular Ophthalmic Solution (Less than 5%) ... 565
▲ Advair Diskus 100/50 (1% to 3%) ... 1308
▲ Advair Diskus 250/50 (1% to 3%) ... 1308
▲ Advair Diskus 500/50 (1% to 3%) ... 1308
▲ Alphagan P Ophthalmic Solution (1% to 4%) ... 567
Azopt Ophthalmic Suspension (1% to 5%) ... 557
Betagan Ophthalmic Solution, USP ... ⊙ 220
Betimol Ophthalmic Solution (1% to 5%) ... 3382
Betimol Ophthalmic Solution (1% to 5%) ... ⊙ 295
Betoptic S Ophthalmic Suspension (Rare) ... 558
BOTOX Purified Neurotoxin Complex (Less than 1%) ... 570
Carteolol Hydrochloride Ophthalmic Solution USP, 1% ... ⊙ 249
Celexa (Rare) ... 1176
Ciloxan Ophthalmic Ointment (Less than 1%) ... 559
Ciloxan Ophthalmic Solution (Less than 1%) ... ⊙ 206
Effexor Tablets (Rare) ... 3411
Effexor XR Capsules (Rare) ... 3417
Engerix-B Vaccine ... 1425
Evoxac Capsules (Less than 1%) ... 1047
▲ Flovent Diskus (1% to 3%) ... 1443
FML Ophthalmic Ointment (Occasional) ... ⊙ 228
FML Ophthalmic Suspension (Occasional) ... ⊙ 227
FML Forte Ophthalmic Suspension (Occasional) ... ⊙ 226
FML-S Ophthalmic Suspension ... ⊙ 229
Geodon Capsules (Rare) ... 2529
Imitrex Injection ... 1463
Imitrex Nasal Spray ... 1467
Lyrica Capsules (Rare) ... 2539
Patanol Ophthalmic Solution (Less than 5%) ... 561
Poly-Pred Ophthalmic Suspension ... ⊙ 233

Pred Mild Ophthalmic Suspension (Occasional) ⊙238
Pred Forte Ophthalmic Suspension (Occasional) ⊙235
Serevent Diskus (1% to less than 3%) 1568
Stromectol Tablets 2083
Symmetrel Tablets 1135
Tarceva Tablets (Infrequent) 1259
Tarceva Tablets (Infrequent) 2444
Targretin Capsules 1747
Timoptic Sterile Ophthalmic Solution (Less frequent) 2088
Timoptic-XE Sterile Ophthalmic Gel Forming Solution 2092
▲ Travatan Ophthalmic Solution (1% to 4%) 563
Twinrix Vaccine 1595
VFEND I.V. (Less than 2%) 2564
VFEND Oral Suspension (Less than 2%) 2564
VFEND Tablets (Less than 2%) 2564
▲ Vigamox Ophthalmic Solution (1% to 6%) 564
▲ Voltaren Ophthalmic Solution (28%) 2309
▲ Zymar Ophthalmic Solution (5% to 10%) 575

Keratitis, bacterial
Trusopt Sterile Ophthalmic Solution 2095
Xalatan Sterile Ophthalmic Solution 2649

Keratitis, epithelial
Ophthetic Ophthalmic Solution ⊙232

Keratitis, punctate
Albalon Ophthalmic Solution ⊙218
▲ Cosopt Sterile Ophthalmic Solution (5% to 30%) 1931
▲ Lumigan Ophthalmic Solution (3% to 10%) 573
▲ Macugen Injection (10% to 40%) ⊙261
Pred-G Ophthalmic Ointment ⊙237
Pred-G Ophthalmic Suspension (Occasional) ⊙236

Keratitis, superficial punctate
Acular Ophthalmic Solution 565
▲ Acular LS Ophthalmic Solution (1% to 10%) 566
▲ Trusopt Sterile Ophthalmic Solution (10% to 15%) 2095

Keratitis nigricans
Timoptic in Ocudose (Less frequent) 2091

Keratitis sicca
Viroptic Ophthalmic Solution ⊙266

Keratoconjunctivitis
Alrex Ophthalmic Suspension 0.2% (Less than 5%) ⊙246
Azopt Ophthalmic Suspension (Less than 1%) 557
Evoxac Capsules (Less than 1%) 1047
Gabitril Tablets (Infrequent) 984
Geodon Capsules (Rare) 2529
▲ Lotemax Ophthalmic Suspension 0.5% (Less than 5%) ⊙251
Lyrica Capsules (Rare) 2539
Paxil CR Controlled-Release Tablets (Rare) 1538
Paxil (Rare) 1530
Pexeva Tablets (infrequent) 1694
Sular Tablets (Less than or equal to 1%) 3122
VFEND I.V. (Less than 2%) 2564
VFEND Oral Suspension (Less than 2%) 2564
VFEND Tablets (Less than 2%) 2564
▲ Xeloda Tablets (Less than 5%) 2822
Xyrem Oral Solution (Infrequent) 1688
Zyprexa Tablets (Rare) 1830
Zyprexa ZYDIS Orally Disintegrating Tablets (Rare) 1830

Keratoconjunctivitis sicca
Alphagan P Ophthalmic Solution (Less than 1%) 567
▲ Tarceva Tablets (0% to 12%) 1259
▲ Tarceva Tablets (0% to 12%) 2444

Keratopathy
Alphagan P Ophthalmic Solution (1% to 4%) 567
Ciloxan Ophthalmic Ointment (Less than 1%) 559
Ciloxan Ophthalmic Solution (Less than 1%) ⊙206

Keratopathy, epithelial
Viroptic Ophthalmic Solution ⊙266
▲ Xalatan Sterile Ophthalmic Solution (5% to 15%) 2649

Keratopathy, superficial punctate
Viroptic Ophthalmic Solution ⊙266

Keratopathy, vortex
Mepron Suspension 1521

Keratosis
Gengraf Capsules (1% to less than 3%) 459
Neoral Oral Solution (1% to less than 3%) 2259
Neoral Soft Gelatin Capsules (1% to less than 3%) 2259

Keratosis pilaris
Finacea Gel (Rare) 1669

Kernicterus, neonatal
Blephamide Ophthalmic Ointment 568

Ketoacidosis
FazaClo Orally Disintegrating Tablets 551

Ketoniuria
Amerge Tablets (Rare) 1339

Ketosis
Clozaril Tablets (Sometimes) 2184
Doxil Injection (Less than 1%) 2351
Geodon Capsules (Rare) 2529
▲ Humira Injection (Less than 5%) 466
Paxil CR Controlled-Release Tablets (Rare) 1538
Paxil (Rare) 1530
Pexeva Tablets (rare) 1694
Sonata Capsules (Rare) 1717
Zyprexa Tablets (Infrequent) 1830
Zyprexa ZYDIS Orally Disintegrating Tablets (Infrequent) 1830

Kidney calculus
▲ Humira Injection (Less than 5%) 466
Lyrica Capsules (0.1% to 1%) 2539

Kidney damage
Furosemide Tablets 2154

Kidney failure, acute
Lyrica Capsules (Rare) 2539

Kidney function, abnormal
Avelox (0.1% to less than 2%) 2970
Cipro XR Tablets (Less than 1%) 2990
Tricor Tablets 527
VFEND I.V. (0.5% to 1.3%) 2564
VFEND Oral Suspension (0.5% to 1.3%) 2564
VFEND Tablets (0.5% to 1.3%) 2564

Kidney pain
(*see under* Pain, renal)

Kidney stones
(*see under* Nephrolithiasis)

Knee replacement
▲ Euflexxa (3%) 1162

L

Lab test, abnormal, unspecified
▲ Humira Injection (8%) 466
▲ Ventavis Inhalation Solution (7%) 1020

Labor, prolonged
Bayer Aspirin 744
Bayer Aspirin Comprehensive Prescribing Information ▣796
Percodan Tablets 1132
St. Joseph 81 mg Aspirin ▣688

Labor, slowing
Aggrenox Capsules 822
Kadian Capsules (Less than 3%) 577
Proventil Inhalation Solution 0.083% (Some reports) 3055

Laboratory abnormalities, unspecified
Adalat CC Tablets (Less than 1%) 2964
▲ Hycamtin for Injection (39%) 1458
Zomig Nasal Spray (Infrequent) 3523

Labyrinth disorder
▲ Intron A for Injection (Less than 5%) 3024
Zoloft (Rare) 2586

Labyrinthitis
Ambien CR Tablets (1%) 2855
Amerge Tablets (Rare) 1339
Effexor Tablets (Rare) 3411
Effexor XR Capsules (Rare) 3417
Neurontin Capsules (Rare) 2487
Neurontin Oral Solution (Rare) 2487
Neurontin Tablets (Rare) 2487
Nipent for Injection (Less than 3%) 1863
Sonata Capsules (Rare) 1717

Laceration
▲ Advair Diskus 100/50 (1% to 3%) 1308
▲ Advair Diskus 250/50 (1% to 3%) 1308
▲ Advair Diskus 500/50 (1% to 3%) 1308
▲ Advair HFA Inhalation Aerosol (1% to 3%) 1318
Asmanex Twisthaler (1% to less than 3%) 2966
Astelin Nasal Spray (Infrequently) 1904
Elidel Cream 1% (0.7% to 1.5%) 2200
▲ Flovent Diskus (1% to 3%) 1443
Xyrem Oral Solution (Infrequent) 1688

Lacrimal duct, stenosis
Taxotere Injection Concentrate (Rare) 2932
Xeloda Tablets 2822

Lacrimal gland, disorders
▲ Intron A for Injection (Less than 5%) 3024
Neurontin Capsules (Rare) 2487
Neurontin Oral Solution (Rare) 2487
Neurontin Tablets (Rare) 2487

Lacrimation
Albalon Ophthalmic Solution ⊙218
▲ Avastin IV (6% to 18%) 1227
Azopt Ophthalmic Suspension (Less than 1%) 557
BiDil Tablets 2171
▲ BOTOX Purified Neurotoxin Complex (10.0%) 570
Camptosar Injection 2604
Ciloxan Ophthalmic Ointment (Less than 1%) 559
Ciloxan Ophthalmic Solution (Less than 1%) ⊙206
Efudex 3363
▲ Eloxatin for Injection (1% to 7%) 2892
Hyperstat I.V. 3017
Imitrex Injection (Infrequent) 1463
Imitrex Nasal Spray (Infrequent) 1467
Imitrex Tablets (Infrequent) 1471
Maxalt Tablets (Infrequent) 2008
Maxalt-MLT Orally Disintegrating Tablets (Infrequent) 2008
Neurontin Capsules (Rare) 2487
Neurontin Oral Solution (Rare) 2487
Neurontin Tablets (Rare) 2487
Nipent for Injection (Less than 3%) 1863
OptiPranolol Metipranolol Ophthalmic Solution 0.3% (A small number of patients) ⊙256
Tasmar Tablets (Infrequent) 3358
Taxotere Injection Concentrate 2932
Testim 1% Gel (1% or less) 695
▲ Trusopt Sterile Ophthalmic Solution (Approximately 1% to 5%) 2095
Vasotec I.V. Injection (0.5% to 1.0%) 2103
▲ Vigamox Ophthalmic Solution (1% to 6%) 564
▲ Voltaren Ophthalmic Solution (Less than or equal to 5% to 30%) 2309
Zomig Tablets (Rare) 3519
Zomig-ZMT Tablets (Rare) 3519

Lacrimation, abnormal
Ambien Tablets (Rare) 2851
Ambien CR Tablets (Rare) 2855
Arthrotec Tablets (Rare) 3129
Celexa (Infrequent) 1176
▲ CellCept Capsules (3% to less than 20%) 2747
▲ CellCept Intravenous (3% to less than 20%) 2747
▲ CellCept Oral Suspension (3% to less than 20%) 2747
▲ CellCept Tablets (3% to less than 20%) 2747
Flumadine 1183
▲ Fortical Nasal Spray (1% to 3%) 3337
Frova Tablets (Infrequent) 1113
▲ Gleevec Tablets (0% to 18%) 2227
Lamictal (Rare) 1481
▲ Miacalcin Nasal Spray (1% to 3%) 2253
Migranal Nasal Spray (Infrequent) 3348
Mirapex Tablets (Greater than or equal to 1%) 859
Namenda (Infrequent) 1195
Relpax Tablets (Infrequent) 2548
Requip Tablets (Infrequent) 1555
Risperdal (Rare) 1676
Risperdal M-Tab Orally Disintegrating Tablets (Rare) 1676
▲ Romazicon Injection (1% to 3%) 2804
Soriatane Capsules (Less than 1%) 1013
Topamax Sprinkle Capsules (1%) 2404
Topamax Tablets (1%) 2404
▲ Visudyne for Injection (1% to 10%) 2305
Zoloft (Rare) 2586
Zomig Nasal Spray (Infrequent) 3523

Lacrimation, increased
Cialis Tablets (Less than 2%) 1838
▲ Lucentis Injection (3% to 17%) 1237
Myozyme for Intravenous Infusion 1279
▲ Sutent Capsules (6%) 2560
▲ Zymar Ophthalmic Solution (5% to 10%) 575

Lactation
Abilify Oral Solution (Rare) 882
Abilify Oral Solution (Rare) 2450
Abilify Discmelt Orally Disintegrating Tablets (Rare) 882
Abilify Discmelt Orally Disintegrating Tablets (Rare) 2450
Abilify Tablets (Rare) 882
Abilify Tablets (Rare) 2450
Aldoril Tablets 1910
Effexor Tablets (Rare) 3411
Effexor XR Capsules (Rare) 3417
Geodon Capsules (Infrequent) 2529
Lamictal (Rare) 1481
▲ Lupron Depot 3.75 mg (Among most frequent) 3260
Lupron Depot–3 Month 11.25 mg (Less than 5%) 3265
Paxil CR Controlled-Release Tablets (Rare) 1538
Paxil (Rare) 1530
Permax Tablets (Infrequent) 3356
Pexeva Tablets (rare) 1694
Prozac Pulvules and Liquid (Infrequent) 1801
Symbyax Capsules (Infrequent) 1819
Thioridazine Hydrochloride Tablets 2163
Thiothixene Capsules 2165
Vandazole Vaginal Gel (Less than 1%) 3338
Zyprexa Tablets (Infrequent) 1830
Zyprexa ZYDIS Orally Disintegrating Tablets (Infrequent) 1830

Lactation, female
Lunesta Tablets (Infrequent) 3142
Lyrica Capsules (Rare) 2539

Lactation, non-puerperal
Flumadine (Less than 0.3%) 1183
Risperdal (Infrequent) 1676
Risperdal Consta Long-Acting Injection (Infrequent) 1682
Risperdal M-Tab Orally Disintegrating Tablets (Infrequent) 1676
Sandostatin LAR Depot (Rare) 2280

Lactation, possible diminution
Mircette Tablets 1066
NuvaRing 2340
Ortho-Cyclen Tablets 2429
Ortho Evra Transdermal System 2417
Ortho Tri-Cyclen Tablets 2429
Ortho Tri-Cyclen Lo Tablets 2436
Seasonique Tablets 1077
Yaz Tablets 803

Lactation, prevention of
depo-subQ provera 104 Injectable Suspension 2624

Lactation, suppression
Bentyl Capsules 697
Bentyl Injection 697
Bentyl Syrup 697
Bentyl Tablets 697
Depo-Provera Contraceptive Injection (Less than 1%) 2622
Ditropan XL Extended-Release Tablets 2413
Donnatal Extentabs 2493

Lactation abnormalities
Seroquel Tablets (Infrequent) 690

Lactic acidosis
ActoPlus Met Tablets 3214

Aloprim for Injection (Less than 1%) 2167
Atripla Tablets 945
Combivir Tablets 1411
Epivir 1427
Epivir-HBV 1432
Epzicom Tablets 1436
Kaletra (Less than 2%) 476
Retrovir Capsules (Rare) 1560
Retrovir IV Infusion (Rare) 1564
Retrovir (Rare) 1560
Reyataz Capsules (Less than 3%) 921
Trizivir Tablets 1589
Truvada Tablets 1296
▲ Viread Tablets (5%) 1301
Ziagen 1626
Zyvox 2652

Lactic dehydrogenase increased
Abilify Oral Solution (Rare) 882
Abilify Oral Solution (Rare) 2450
Abilify Discmelt Orally Disintegrating Tablets (Rare) 882
Abilify Discmelt Orally Disintegrating Tablets (Rare) 2450
Abilify Tablets (Rare) 882
Abilify Tablets (Rare) 2450
Campral Tablets (Rare) 1174
▲ Dacogen Injection (8%) 2129
Lopressor Injection 2238
Lopressor Tablets 2238
Lopressor HCT 50/25 Tablets 2241
Lopressor HCT 100/25 Tablets 2241
Lopressor HCT 100/50 Tablets 2241
Mycamine for Injection (0.5% to 0.8%) 628
Oracea Capsules (1.5%) 1000
Pexeva Tablets (rare) 1694
▲ Tygacil for Injection (4%) 3488
Viracept (Less than 2%) 2577

Lactose, intolerance to
Sonata Capsules (Rare) 1717

Lagophthalmos
BOTOX Purified Neurotoxin Complex 570

Language problems, unspecified
▲ Topamax Sprinkle Capsules (2% to 10%) 2404
▲ Topamax Tablets (2% to 10%) 2404

Laryngeal stridor
Lotrel Capsules (About 0.5%) 2249

Laryngismus
Axert Tablets (Infrequent) 2396
Bexxar 1398
Campral Tablets (Rare) 1174
▲ Copaxone for Injection (5%) 3297
Effexor Tablets (Infrequent) 3411
Effexor XR Capsules (Infrequent) 3417
Lyrica Capsules (Rare) 2539
Paxil CR Controlled-Release Tablets 1538
Paxil 1530
Pexeva Tablets 1694
Rescriptor Tablets 2551
Symbyax Capsules (Rare) 1819
Trileptal Tablets 2300
Trileptal Oral Suspension 2300
Zoloft (Rare) 2586

Laryngitis
Abilify Oral Solution (Infrequent) 882
Abilify Oral Solution (Infrequent) 2450
Abilify Discmelt Orally Disintegrating Tablets (Infrequent) 882
Abilify Discmelt Orally Disintegrating Tablets (Infrequent) 2450
Abilify Tablets (Infrequent) 882
Abilify Tablets (Infrequent) 2450
Aciphex Tablets 1090
▲ Advair Diskus 250/50 (1% to 3%) 1308
▲ Advair HFA Inhalation Aerosol (1% to 3%) 1318
▲ Aerobid/Aerobid-M (1% to 3%) 1171
Ambien Tablets (Rare) 2851
Ambien CR Tablets (Rare) 2855
Astelin Nasal Spray (Infrequent) 1904
Axert Tablets (Rare) 2396
Celebrex Capsules (0.1% to 1.9%) 3134
Celexa (Rare) 1176
Clozaril Tablets (Less than 1%) 2184
Copaxone for Injection (At least 2%) 3297
Doxil Injection (Less than 1%) 2351
Effexor Tablets (Infrequent) 3411
Effexor XR Capsules (Infrequent) 3417
Evista Tablets (2.2%) 1763
Evoxac Capsules (Less than 1%) 1047
Exelon Capsules (Infrequent) 2206
Exelon Oral Solution (Infrequent) 2206
Exubera Inhalation Powder (0.5% to 1.1%) 2524
Fabrazyme for Intravenous Infusion (2%) 1274
FazaClo Orally Disintegrating Tablets (Less than 1%) 551
▲ Flovent Diskus (1% to 3%) 1443
▲ Flovent HFA (1% to 3%) 1447
Frova Tablets (Infrequent) 1113
Gabitril Tablets (Infrequent) 984
Herceptin I.V. (At least one of the 958 patients) 1233
Invirase (Less than 2%) 2772
Lexapro Oral Solution (Infrequent) 1190
Lexapro Tablets (Infrequent) 1190
Lofibra Tablets 1219
Lofibra Capsules 1216
Lotronex Tablets (Rare) 1512
Lunesta Tablets (Infrequent) 3142
Lupron Depot–3 Month 11.25 mg 3265
Meridia Capsules (1.3%) 489
Neurontin Capsules (Rare) 2487
Neurontin Oral Solution (Rare) 2487
Neurontin Tablets (Rare) 2487
▲ Norditropin Cartridges (6%) 2323
Omacor Capsules 2725
Permax Tablets (Infrequent) 3356
Prinivil Tablets (0.3% to 1.0%) 2052
Prinzide Tablets 2056
ProSom Tablets (Rare) 517
Protonix I.V. (Less than 1%) 3472
Protonix Tablets (Less than 1%) 3469
Protopic Ointment (Greater than or equal to 1%) 638
▲ Pulmozyme Inhalation Solution (3% to 4%) 1248
Relpax Tablets (Rare) 2548
Requip Tablets (Infrequent) 1555
Rilutek Tablets (Infrequent) 2930
Singulair (Greater than or equal to 2%) 2077
Sonata Capsules (Infrequent) 1717
Soriatane Capsules (Less than 1%) 1013
▲ Spiriva HandiHaler (1% to 3%) 869
Sular Tablets (Less than or equal to 1%) 3122
Symbyax Capsules (Infrequent) 1819
Tasmar Tablets (Infrequent) 3358
Tricor Tablets 527
Uniretic Tablets (Less than 1%) 3100
Ventolin HFA Inhalation Aerosol (Less than 3%) 1600
Viagra Tablets (Less than 2%) 2573
▲ Vivitrol (12% to 13%) 995
▲ Xeloda Tablets (Less than 5%) 2822
Xyrem Oral Solution (Infrequent) 1688
Zoloft (Rare) 2586
Zomig Tablets (Infrequent) 3519
Zomig Nasal Spray (Rare) 3523
Zomig-ZMT Tablets (Infrequent) 3519
Zyprexa Tablets (Rare) 1830
Zyprexa ZYDIS Orally Disintegrating Tablets (Rare) 1830

Laryngospasm
Abilify Oral Solution (Rare) 882
Abilify Oral Solution (Rare) 2450
Abilify Discmelt Orally Disintegrating Tablets (Rare) 882
Abilify Discmelt Orally Disintegrating Tablets (Rare) 2450
Abilify Tablets (Rare) 882
Abilify Tablets (Rare) 2450
Advair Diskus 100/50 1308
Advair Diskus 250/50 1308
Advair Diskus 500/50 1308
Atrovent HFA Inhalation Aerosol 841
Atrovent Nasal Spray 0.06% 839
Blocadren Tablets 1916
Carafate Suspension 701
Carafate Tablets 701
Combivent Inhalation Aerosol (Less than 2%) 847
Cosopt Sterile Ophthalmic Solution 1931
Dilaudid 440
Dilaudid Non-Sterile Powder 440
Dilaudid Oral Liquid 445
Dilaudid Rectal Suppositories 440
Dilaudid Tablets 440
Dilaudid Tablets - 8 mg 445
Dilaudid-HP (Less frequent) 442
Inderal LA Long-Acting Capsules 3429
InnoPran XL Capsules 2723
Lopressor Injection 2238
Lopressor Tablets 2238
Lopressor HCT 50/25 Tablets 2241
Lopressor HCT 100/25 Tablets 2241
Lopressor HCT 100/50 Tablets 2241
MS Contin Tablets (Less frequent) 2701
Nadolol Tablets 2159
Numorphan Injection 1120
Orthoclone OKT3 Sterile Solution (Less than 1%) 2360
Raptiva for Injection 1250
Serevent Diskus (Rare) 1568
Tessalon Capsules 1199
Tessalon Perles 1199
Timolide Tablets 2086
Timoptic Sterile Ophthalmic Solution 2088
Timoptic in Ocudose 2091
Timoptic-XE Sterile Ophthalmic Gel Forming Solution 2092
Toprol-XL Tablets 668
▲ Ultane Liquid for Inhalation (2% to 8%) 531
Zofran Injection 1634
Zofran 1639
Zofran ODT Orally Disintegrating Tablets 1639

Laryngotracheobronchitis
Flumist Vaccine 1901
Prevnar for Injection 3463
Synagis (More than 1%) 1897
Vaqta (1.2%) 2097

Lassitude
Azmacort Inhalation Aerosol 1726
Beconase AQ Nasal Spray 1396
Daranide Tablets 1950
Dexedrine 1420
Gantrisin Pediatric Suspension 2770
▲ Hytrin Capsules (7.4% to 11.3%) 471
Inderal LA Long-Acting Capsules 3429
InnoPran XL Capsules 2723
Neurontin Capsules (Rare) 2487
Neurontin Oral Solution (Rare) 2487
Neurontin Tablets (Rare) 2487
Phenergan Tablets and Suppositories 3440
Risperdal 1676
Risperdal M-Tab Orally Disintegrating Tablets 1676

Laughing, easy
▲ Marinol Capsules (8% to 24%) 3333

Laxative effect
Beelith Tablets 759
Robitussin Sugar Free Throat Drops ▣ 737

LDH abnormalities
Bumex Tablets (1%) 2746
Ceftin Tablets (1.0%) 1407
▲ Emcyt Capsules (2% to 31%) 2634
Nimotop Capsules (0.4%; rare) 749
Parcopa Orally Disintegrating Tablets 3097
Zyvox (0.2% to 1.8%) 2652

LDH increase
Abelcet Injection 1141
Accutane Capsules 2731
Adalat CC Tablets (Rare) 2964
Advicor Tablets 1722
AmBisome for Injection (Less common) 620
Aricept Tablets (Infrequent) 1094
Aricept ODT Tablets (Infrequent) 1094
Arthrotec Tablets (Rare) 3129
Asacol Delayed-Release Tablets 2692
Avelox (0.1% to less than 2%) 2970
Biaxin/Biaxin XL (Less than 1%) 402
Cardizem LA Extended Release Tablets (Less than 2%) 1728
▲ CellCept Capsules (3% to 23.2%) 2747
▲ CellCept Intravenous (3% to 23.2%) 2747
▲ CellCept Oral Suspension (3% to 23.2%) 2747
▲ CellCept Tablets (3% to 23.2%) 2747
Cipro (0.4%) 2977
▲ Cipro I.V. (Among most frequent) 2984
Colazal Capsules 2838
Cubicin for Injection (Less than 1%) 1026
Cuprimine Capsules (Few cases) 1947
Depacon Injection (Frequent) 412
Depakene (Frequent) 417
Depakote Sprinkle Capsules 422
▲ Depakote Tablets (Frequent) 427
Depakote ER Tablets (Frequent) 434
Doxil Injection (Less than 1%) 2351
Effexor Tablets 3411
Effexor XR Capsules 3417
Evoxac Capsules 1047
▲ Fortaz (1 in 18) 1453
Garamycin Injectable 3014
Geodon Capsules (Infrequent) 2529
Gleevec Tablets (Infrequent) 2227
Increlex Injection 3291
▲ Intron A for Injection (Less than 5%) 3024
Keflex Capsules 549
Levaquin (0.1% to 0.9%) 2384
Levaquin in 5% Dextrose Injection (0.1% to 0.9%) 2384
▲ Lupron Depot 3.75 mg (Approximately 5% to 8%) 3260
▲ Lupron Depot 7.5 mg (Greater than or equal to 5%) 3264
Mefoxin for Injection 2012
Mefoxin Premixed Intravenous Solution 2016
▲ Megace ES Oral Suspension (1% to 3%) 2481
Meridia Capsules (1.6%) 489
Merrem I.V. (Greater than 0.2%) 686
▲ Mylotarg for Injection (14% to 18%) 3431
Nalfon Capsules (Less than 1%) 2502
▲ Neulasta Injection (19%) 601
▲ Neupogen for Injection (27% to 58%) 603
Neurontin Capsules (Rare) 2487
Neurontin Oral Solution (Rare) 2487
Neurontin Tablets (Rare) 2487
Niaspan Extended-Release Tablets 1730
Noroxin Tablets (Less frequent) 2032
Omnicef Capsules (0.2%) 511
Omnicef for Oral Suspension (1%) 511
Paxil CR Controlled-Release Tablets (Rare) 1538
Paxil (Rare) 1530
Pentasa Capsules (Less than 1%) 3185
Prevacid Delayed-Release Capsules 3271
Prevacid for Delayed-Release Oral Suspension 3271
Prevacid SoluTab Delayed-Release Orally Disintegrating Tablets 3271
Prevacid NapraPAC 3280
PREVPAC (Less than 1%) 3284
Primaxin I.M. 2045
Primaxin I.V. 2048
▲ Prograf Capsules and Injection (3% to 15%) 632
Raniclor Tablets, Chewable 2505
▲ Rapamune Oral Solution and Tablets (3% to 20%) 3475
Requip Tablets (Infrequent) 1555
Retrovir IV Infusion 1564
Rilutek Tablets (Rare) 2930
▲ Rituxan I.V. (0% to 7%) 1254
Rythmol SR Capsules 2727
▲ Soriatane Capsules (Approximately 1 in 3 patients) 1013
Suprax 1843
Symmetrel Tablets 1135
▲ Targretin Capsules (7.1% to 13.2%) 1747
Tarka Tablets 524
Thalomid Capsules 965
Tiazac Capsules (Less than 2%) 1201
Timentin ADD-Vantage 1580
Timentin Injection Galaxy Container 1583
Timentin IV Infusion 1577
Timentin Pharmacy Bulk Package 1586
Toprol-XL Tablets 668
Ultane Liquid for Inhalation (Less than 1%) 531
Vantin Tablets and Oral Suspension 2645
VFEND I.V. (Less than 2%) 2564
VFEND Oral Suspension (Less than 2%) 2564
VFEND Tablets (Less than 2%) 2564
Viracept 2577
WinRho SDF 732
Zinacef for Injection (1 in 75 patients) 1631
Zinacef Injection (1 in 75 patients) 1631
Zonegran Capsules (Rare) 1101

LDL, increase
Premphase Tablets 3456
Prempro Tablets 3456

LDL, decrease
Menostar Transdermal System 782
Premarin Tablets 3446
Premphase Tablets 3456
Prempro Tablets 3456

LE cells test positive
(*see under* Lupus erythematosus)

Left ventricular dysfunction
▲ Clolar for Intravenous Infusion (27%) 1271

Orthoclone OKT3 Sterile Solution (Less than 1%) 2360

Left ventricular ejection fraction, decrease
▲ Sutent Capsules (1% to 15%) 2560

Leg cramps, nocturnal
▲ Actonel with Calcium Tablets (3.5%) 2688
Niaspan Extended-Release Tablets 1730
Trelstar LA Suspension (1.7%) 3397

Legs, heaviness
Uroqid-Acid No. 2 Tablets 760

Legs, restless
Abilify Oral Solution (Infrequent) 882
Abilify Oral Solution (Infrequent) 2450
Abilify Discmelt Orally Disintegrating Tablets (Infrequent) 882
Abilify Discmelt Orally Disintegrating Tablets (Infrequent) 2450
Abilify Tablets (Infrequent) 882
Abilify Tablets (Infrequent) 2450
Ambien Tablets (Rare) 2851
Ambien CR Tablets (Rare) 2855
Lexapro Oral Solution (Infrequent) 1190
Lexapro Tablets (Infrequent) 1190

Legs, stiffness
Colazal Capsules 2838

Leiomyoma
(*see under* Uterine fibroids)

LE-like reactions
(*see under* Lupus erythematosus)

Lens, pigmentation
Zyprexa Tablets (Rare) 1830
Zyprexa ZYDIS Orally Disintegrating Tablets (Rare) 1830

Lens changes, unspecified
Myleran Tablets 1525

Lens opacities, changes
Altoprev Extended-Release Tablets 3109
▲ Cosopt Sterile Ophthalmic Solution (1% to 5%) 1931
Lamisil Tablets 2232
Lescol Capsules 2233
Lescol XL Tablets 2233
Levaquin 2384
Levaquin in 5% Dextrose Injection 2384
Mevacor Tablets 2021
Vytorin 10/10 Tablets 2114
Vytorin 10/10 Tablets 3077
Vytorin 10/20 Tablets 2114
Vytorin 10/20 Tablets 3077
Vytorin 10/40 Tablets 2114
Vytorin 10/40 Tablets 3077
Vytorin 10/80 Tablets 2114
Vytorin 10/80 Tablets 3077
Zocor Tablets 2105

Lens opacities, irregular
Thioridazine Hydrochloride Tablets 2163

Lenticular deposits
Thioridazine Hydrochloride Tablets 2163

Lesions, anogenital
Oracea Capsules 1000

Lesions, bullous
Parcopa Orally Disintegrating Tablets 3097
Stalevo Tablets 2287

Lesions, cerebrovascular
Imitrex Nasal Spray 1467

Lesions, corneal
Effexor Tablets (Infrequent) 3411
Effexor XR Capsules (Infrequent) 3417
▲ Soriatane Capsules (1% to 5%) 1013
Targretin Capsules 1747
▲ Voltaren Ophthalmic Solution (Less than or equal to 5%) 2309
Zyprexa Tablets (Rare) 1830
Zyprexa ZYDIS Orally Disintegrating Tablets (Rare) 1830

Lesions, gastrointestinal
K-Dur Extended-Relase Tablets 3033
K-Tab Tablets 475
Lotronex Tablets (Infrequent) 1512

Lesions, nerve root
Boniva Injection (2.2%) 2738
Boniva Tablets (2.2%) 2741

Lesions, neuro-ocular
Premphase Tablets 3456
Prempro Tablets 3456

Lesions, oral
▲ Advair Diskus 250/50 (1% to 3%) 1308
Avapro Tablets (Less than 1%) 891
Avapro Tablets (Less than 1%) 2871
Striant Mucoadhesive 1007
▲ Trisenox Injection (8%) 993
Vantin Tablets and Oral Suspension (Less than 1%) 2645
Viramune Oral Suspension 873
Viramune Tablets 873

Lesions, retinal vascular
Ortho-Cyclen/Ortho Tri-Cyclen 2429
Ortho Tri-Cyclen Lo Tablets 2436
Premphase Tablets 3456
Prempro Tablets 3456

Lesions, upper motor neuron
Topamax Sprinkle Capsules (Rare) 2404
Topamax Tablets (Rare) 2404

Lethargy
Accutane Capsules 2731
Alphanate, Antihemophilic Factor (Human) 1654
▲ Ambien Tablets (3%) 2851
Ambien CR Tablets (Frequent) 2855
Arimidex Tablets (1%) 673
Arranon Injection (1%) 1357
Arthrotec Tablets 3129
Asacol Delayed-Release Tablets 2692
▲ Avinza Capsules (Less than 5%) 1741
Bayer Aspirin 744
Bayer Aspirin Comprehensive Prescribing Information ▣ 796
BeneFix Vials 3408
Bentyl Capsules 697
Bentyl Injection 697
Bentyl Syrup 697
Bentyl Tablets 697
Betagan Ophthalmic Solution, USP (Rare) ⊙ 220
Betoptic S Ophthalmic Suspension (Rare) 558
Catapres-TTS (3 of 101 patients) 844
Cathflo Activase 1231
Celebrex Capsules 3134
Chantix Tablets (1% to 2%) 2517
Cipro (Less than 1%) 2977
Cipro I.V. (1% or less) 2984
Cipro XR Tablets 2990
▲ Clolar for Intravenous Infusion (11%) 1271
Clozaril Tablets (1%) 2184
Copegus Tablets 2754
Cosmegen for Injection 2459
Coumadin for Injection (Infrequent) 898
Coumadin Tablets (Infrequent) 898
Cymbalta Delayed-Release Capsules (Frequent) 1757
▲ Dacogen Injection (12%) 2129
Dalmane Capsules 3342
Demadex Injection 2759
Demadex Tablets 2759
Depacon Injection 412
Depakote Sprinkle Capsules 422
Depakote Tablets 427
Depakote ER Tablets 434
Diastat Rectal Delivery System 3343
Dilaudid 440
Dilaudid Non-Sterile Powder 440
Dilaudid Rectal Suppositories 440
Dilaudid Tablets 440
Diovan HCT Tablets 2196
Diuril Sodium Intravenous 2467
Dyazide Capsules 1423
DynaCirc CR Tablets (0.5% to 1%) 2721
Eldepryl Capsules (1 of 49 patients) 3208
Eligard 22.5 mg (Less than 2%) 2883
Eligard 30 mg (1.1%) 2885
Eligard 45 mg (1%) 2888
▲ Emcyt Capsules (4%) 2634
FazaClo Orally Disintegrating Tablets (1%) 551
Furosemide Tablets 2154
Garamycin Injectable 3014
Gengraf Capsules (Rare) 459
HibTITER 3426
▲ Hycamtin for Injection (69%) 1458
Hycodan 1116
Hycotuss Expectorant Syrup 1117
Hyperstat I.V. 3017
Inderal LA Long-Acting Capsules 3429
Invirase (Less than 2%) 2772
▲ I.V. Busulfex (7%) 2493
Kadian Capsules (Less than 3%) 577
▲ Lexapro Oral Solution (3%) 1190
▲ Lexapro Tablets (3%) 1190
Lithobid Tablets 1692
Lithostat Tablets 2140
▲ Lopressor HCT 50/25 Tablets (10%) 2241
▲ Lopressor HCT 100/25 Tablets (10%) 2241
▲ Lopressor HCT 100/50 Tablets (10%) 2241
Matulane Capsules 3191
Neoral Oral Solution (Rare) 2259
Neoral Soft Gelatin Capsules (Rare) 2259
Opana Tablets (Less than 1%) 1122
Opana ER Tablets (Less than 1%) 1126
Orthoclone OKT3 Sterile Solution (Less than 1%) 2360
Pediarix Vaccine 1548
Percodan Tablets 1132
Prinzide Tablets 2056
Profilnine SD, Factor IX Complex (Human) 1660
Proleukin for Injection 2266
Proquin XR Tablets 1153
ReFacto Vials 3484
▲ Restoril Capsules (4.5%) 1860
RhoGAM Ultra-Filtered 2371
Sandimmune (Rare) 2275
St. Joseph 81 mg Aspirin Chewable and Enteric Coated Tablets 1869
St. Joseph 81 mg Aspirin ▣ 688
Stromectol Tablets 2083
Tasmar Tablets (1% or more) 3358
Taxotere Injection Concentrate (21.3% to 62.9%) 2932
Thioridazine Hydrochloride Tablets (Extremely rare) 2163
Tracleer Tablets 545
Trizivir Tablets 1589
Tussionex Pennkinetic Extended-Release Suspension 3327
▲ Ultram ER Tablets (1% to greater than 5%) 2392
Vantas (Less than 2%) 3375
Vicodin Tablets 535
Vicodin ES Tablets 536
Vicodin HP Tablets 538
▲ Vivitrol (12% to 23%) 995
▲ Xeloda Tablets (Up to 7%) 2822
▲ Xyrem Oral Solution (5.9%) 1688
Ziagen 1626
Zydone Tablets 1139

Leucocytosis
Lithobid Tablets 1692
Ultane Liquid for Inhalation (Less than 1%) 531

Leukemia, acute
Herceptin I.V. (At least one of the 958 patients) 1233
I.V. Busulfex (Four cases) 2493
Leukeran Tablets 1504
Nipent for Injection (Less than 3%) 1863
Revlimid Capsules 958

Leukemia, lymphoblastic
Permax Tablets (Rare) 3356

Leukemia, lymphocytic
Mustargen for Injection 2468

Leukemia, myeloblastic, acute
Invirase (Rare) 2772

Leukemia, myelocytic, acute
Matulane Capsules 3191
Revlimid Capsules 958
Zelapar Tablets 3372

Leukemia, myelogenous
Temodar Capsules 3073
Thalomid Capsules 965

Leukemia, polymorphocytic
Campath Ampules 811

Leukemia, secondary
Bexxar 1398
Campath Ampules 811

Leukemia, unspecified
Genotropin Lyophilized Powder (A small number of children) 2638
Humatrope Vials and Cartridges 1787
Indocin (Rare) 1995
Norditropin Cartridges (A small number of children) 2323
Nutropin for Injection (A small number of patients) 1239
Nutropin AQ Injection (A small number of patients) 1243
Nutropin AQ Pen (A small number of patients) 1243
Nutropin AQ Pen Cartridge (A small number of patients) 1243
Plavix Tablets (Less than 1%) 917
Plavix Tablets (Less than 1%) 2926
Tasmar Tablets (Rare) 3358
Tev-Tropin for Injection 1222
Thalomid Capsules 965
Ticlid Tablets (Rare) 2810

Leukocyte agglutinins
Miradon Tablets 3042

Leukocyte count, abnormal
Bumex Tablets (0.3%) 2746
▲ Zyvox (0.2% to 12.4%) 2652

Leukocyte count, elevated
Agrylin Capsules 3169
Vivitrol 995

Leukocytosis
Abelcet Injection 1141
Abilify Oral Solution (Infrequent) 882
Abilify Oral Solution (Infrequent) 2450
Abilify Discmelt Orally Disintegrating Tablets (Infrequent) 882
Abilify Discmelt Orally Disintegrating Tablets (Infrequent) 2450
Abilify Tablets (Infrequent) 882
Abilify Tablets (Infrequent) 2450
Aceon Tablets (2 mg, 4 mg, 8 mg) 3194
Aciphex Tablets 1090
Alinia for Oral Suspension (Less than 1%) 2835
Alinia Tablets (Less than 1%) 2835
Amerge Tablets (Infrequent) 1339
Arthrotec Tablets (Rare) 3129
Attenuvax 1914
Capastat Sulfate for Injection 1755
Carbatrol Capsules 3171
Celexa (Infrequent) 1176
▲ CellCept Capsules (22.4% to 40.5%) 2747
▲ CellCept Intravenous (22.4% to 40.5%) 2747
▲ CellCept Oral Suspension (22.4% to 40.5%) 2747
▲ CellCept Tablets (22.4% to 40.5%) 2747
Chantix Tablets (Rare) 2517
Cipro (Less than 0.1%) 2977
Cipro I.V. (Rare) 2984
Clinoril Tablets (Less than 1 in 100) 1924
Clozaril Tablets (Less than 1%) 2184
Colazal Capsules 2838
Cubicin for Injection (Less than 1%) 1026
Cuprimine Capsules 1947
Effexor Tablets (Infrequent) 3411
Effexor XR Capsules (Infrequent) 3417
▲ Efudex (Among most frequent) 3363
Emend Capsules (Greater than 0.5%) 1963
▲ Entocort EC Capsules (Less than 5%) 2698
Equetro Extended-Release Capsules 3180
Evoxac Capsules (Less than 1%) 1047
Exelon Capsules (Infrequent) 2206
Exelon Oral Solution (Infrequent) 2206
FazaClo Orally Disintegrating Tablets (Less than 1%) 551
Ferrlecit Injection 3388
Geodon Capsules (Infrequent) 2529
Infed Injection 3390
Ionsys Transdermal System (.1% to less than 1%) 2379
▲ Kytril Injection (3.7%) 2781
Lamictal (Infrequent) 1481
Lariam Tablets (Occasional) 2786
Levaquin (0.1% to 0.9%) 2384
Levaquin in 5% Dextrose Injection (0.1% to 0.9%) 2384
Lyrica Capsules (0.1% to 1%) 2539
Meruvax II 2019
MetroGel-Vaginal Gel (1.7%) 1855
Miradon Tablets 3042
M-M-R II 2006
Moban Tablets 1119
Mumpsvax 2031
Neulasta Injection (Less than 1%) 601
Neupogen for Injection (Approximately 2%) 603
Nexium Delayed-Release Capsules (Less than 1%) 655

Nexium I.V. (Less than 1%) 659
Omnicef Capsules (0.7%) 511
Omnicef for Oral Suspension (0.3%) 511
Orthoclone OKT3 Sterile Solution (Less than 1%) 2360
Panhematin for Injection 2473
▲ Paser Granules (79% of 38 patients with drug-induced hepatitis) 1674
Paxil CR Controlled-Release Tablets (Rare) 1538
Paxil (Rare) 1530
Permax Tablets (Infrequent) 3356
Pexeva Tablets (rare) 1694
Prilosec OTC Delayed-Release Tablets (Rare) 2677
Primaxin I.V. 2048
Prinivil Tablets (0.3% to 1.0%) 2052
Prinzide Tablets 2056
▲ Prograf Capsules and Injection (3% to 32%) 632
Prolastin 3255
▲ Proleukin for Injection (9%) 2266
Protonix I.V. (Less than 1%) 3472
Protonix Tablets (Less than 1%) 3469
Protopic Ointment (Greater than or equal to 1%) 638
Provigil Tablets (At least 1%) 988
Prozac Pulvules and Liquid 1801
▲ Rapamune Oral Solution and Tablets (3% to 20%) 3475
▲ Raptiva for Injection (26%) 1250
ReoPro Vials (1.0%) 1809
Requip Tablets (Infrequent) 1555
Rilutek Tablets (Infrequent) 2930
Risperdal (Rare) 1676
Risperdal Consta Long-Acting Injection (Rare) 1682
Risperdal M-Tab Orally Disintegrating Tablets (Rare) 1676
Rocephin Injectable Vials, ADD-Vantage, Galaxy, Bulk (Less than 0.1%) 2800
Seroquel Tablets (Infrequent) 690
Sonata Capsules (Rare) 1717
Symbyax Capsules (Infrequent) 1819
Symmetrel Tablets 1135
Tegretol/Tegretol-XR 2295
Thiothixene Capsules (Occasional) 2165
Trasylol Injection (1% to 2%) 754
▲ Trisenox Injection (50%) 993
▲ Tygacil for Injection (3.7%) 3488
Vantin Tablets and Oral Suspension 2645
Vasotec I.V. Injection (0.5% to 1.0%) 2103
▲ Vesanoid Capsules (About 40%) 2820
Wellbutrin Tablets 1603
Wellbutrin SR Sustained-Release Tablets 1607
Wellbutrin XL Extended-Release Tablets 1613
Zegerid Capsules (Rare) 2958
Zegerid Powder for Oral Solution (Rare) 2958
Zyban Sustained-Release Tablets 1644
Zyprexa Tablets (Infrequent) 1830
Zyprexa ZYDIS Orally Disintegrating Tablets (Infrequent) 1830

Leukocytosis, chronic

Zelapar Tablets 3372

Leukocyturia

Crixivan Capsules 1940
Emend Capsules (Greater than 0.5%) 1963
Omnicef Capsules (2%) 511
Primaxin I.M. 2045
Primaxin I.V. 2048

Leukoderma

Effexor Tablets (Rare) 3411
Effexor XR Capsules (Rare) 3417
Lamictal (Rare) 1481
Protopic Ointment (0.2% to less than 1%) 638

Leukoencephalopathy

Arranon Injection (1%) 1357
Revlimid Capsules 958

Leukoencephalopathy, multifocal progressive

Invirase (Less than 2%) 2772

Leukoencephalopathy, posterior

Sutent Capsules (Less than 1%) 2560

Leukoencephalopathy, unspecified

Prograf Capsules and Injection 632

Leukopenia

▲ Abelcet Injection (4%) 1141
Abilify Oral Solution (Infrequent) 882
Abilify Oral Solution (Infrequent) 2450
Abilify Discmelt Orally Disintegrating Tablets (Infrequent) 882
Abilify Discmelt Orally Disintegrating Tablets (Infrequent) 2450
Abilify Tablets (Infrequent) 882
Abilify Tablets (Infrequent) 2450
Accutane Capsules 2731
Aceon Tablets (2 mg, 4 mg, 8 mg) (0.1%) 3194
Aciphex Tablets 1090
Actiq (Less than 1%) 979
Adalat CC Tablets (Rare) 2964
Advicor Tablets 1722
Aldara Cream, 5% 1846
Aldoril Tablets 1910
▲ Alferon N Injection (11%) 1665
▲ Alimta for Injection (Less than 1% to 55%) 1750
Alkeran Tablets 956
Aloprim for Injection (Less than 1%) 2167
Altace Capsules 1702
Altoprev Extended-Release Tablets 3109
Ambien Tablets (Rare) 2851
Ambien CR Tablets (Rare) 2855
Amoxil Capsules 1343
Amoxil Chewable Tablets 1343
Amoxil Pediatric Drops for Oral Suspension 1343
Amoxil Powder for Oral Suspension 1343
Amoxil Tablets 1343
Anaprox Tablets (Less than 1%) 2761
Anaprox DS Tablets (Less than 1%) 2761
▲ Aptivus Capsules (3.6%) 826
▲ Aredia for Injection (Up to 4%) 2179
▲ Arimidex Tablets (2% to 5%) 673
▲ Arranon Injection (7% to 38%) 1357
Arthrotec Tablets (Rare) 3129
Asacol Delayed-Release Tablets 2692
Atacand Tablets (Very rare) 649
Atacand HCT 651
Augmentin 1360
Augmentin Tablets 1363
Augmentin XR Extended-Release Tablets 1369
Augmentin ES-600 Powder for Oral Suspension 1366
Avalide Tablets 888
Avalide Tablets 2874
Avandaryl Tablets 1379
▲ Avastin IV (37%) 1227
Avelox (0.1% to less than 2%) 2970
Azilect Tablets (Greater than 1%) 3293
▲ Betaseron for SC Injection (14%) 767
Bicillin C-R Injectable Suspension 1706
Caduet Tablets (Greater than 0.1% to less than or equal to 1%) 2508
Campral Tablets (Rare) 1174
▲ Camptosar Injection (14% to 96.4%) 2604
Canasa Rectal Suppositories (One patient) 699
▲ Cancidas for Injection (4.6% to 6.2%) 1918
Capastat Sulfate for Injection 1755
Carbatrol Capsules 3171
Cardizem LA Extended Release Tablets (Infrequent) 1728
Cardura XL Tablets 2515
Carimune NF 3499
Ceftin 1407
Celexa (Infrequent) 1176
▲ CellCept Capsules (23.2% to 45.8%) 2747
▲ CellCept Intravenous (23.2% to 45.8%) 2747
▲ CellCept Oral Suspension (23.2% to 45.8%) 2747
▲ CellCept Tablets (23.2% to 45.8%) 2747
Cesamet Capsules 3340
Cipro (0.4%) 2977
Cipro I.V. (Infrequent) 2984
Cleocin Vaginal Ovules 2616
Clinoril Tablets (Less than 1%) 1924
Clolar for Intravenous Infusion 1271
Clorpres Tablets 2153
▲ Clozaril Tablets (3%) 2184
Colazal Capsules 2838
Concerta Extended-Release Tablets 1881
Copaxone for Injection (Infrequent) 3297
Coreg Tablets (Greater than 0.1% to 1%) 1414
Cosmegen for Injection 2459
Crestor Tablets (Less than 1%) 678
Cuprimine Capsules (2%) 1947
Cutivate Lotion 0.05% (Rare) 2664
▲ Dacogen Injection (28%) 2129
Dalmane Capsules (Rare) 3342
Dantrium Capsules (Less frequent) 2694
Dantrium Intravenous 2695
Daranide Tablets 1950
Daraprim Tablets 1419
Daytrana Transdermal Patch 3174
Depacon Injection 412
Depakene 417
Depakote Sprinkle Capsules 422
Depakote Tablets 427
Depakote ER Tablets (Greater than 1%) 434
Didronel Tablets (One report) 2697
Diovan HCT Tablets 2196
Diuril Oral Suspension 1954
Diuril Sodium Intravenous 2467
Dolobid Tablets (Less than 1 in 100) 1955
▲ Doxil Injection (About 42.2% to 60%) 2351
Duetact Tablets 3226
Dyazide Capsules 1423
DynaCirc CR Tablets (0.5% to 1%) 2721
EC-Naprosyn Delayed-Release Tablets (Less than 1%) 2761
Effexor Tablets (Infrequent) 3411
Effexor XR Capsules (Infrequent) 3417
Elmiron Capsules (Less than or equal to 1%) 2415
▲ Eloxatin for Injection (0% to 85%) 2892
Elspar for Injection 2463
Elspar for Injection 1960
▲ Emcyt Capsules (4%) 2634
Enbrel for Injection 584
▲ Equetro Extended-Release Capsules (Up to 5%) 3180
Eraxis for Injection (0.7%) 2521
▲ Erbitux (Less than 1% to 25%) 910
▲ Eulexin Capsules (3%) 3009
Evoxac Capsules (Less than 1%) 1047
Famvir Tablets (1.3%) 2211
Fansidar Tablets 2765
Faslodex Injection (Less than 1%) 681
▲ FazaClo Orally Disintegrating Tablets (3%) 551
Flebogamma 5%, Immune Globulin Intravenous (Human) 1658
Focalin Tablets 2220
Focalin XR Capsules 2223
Fortaz (Very rare) 1453
Furosemide Tablets 2154
Gabitril Tablets (Infrequent) 984
Gammagard Liquid 721
Gammagard S/D (Rare) 724
Gamunex Immune Globulin I.V., 10% (Rare) 3235
Gantrisin Pediatric Suspension 2770
Garamycin Injectable 3014
▲ Gemzar for Injection (15% to 86%) 1771
▲ Gengraf Capsules (1% to 6%) 459
Geodon Capsules (Infrequent) 2529
Gris-PEG Tablets (Rare) 2502
Guanidine Hydrochloride Tablets 3016
▲ Herceptin I.V. (3%) 1233
▲ Humira Injection (Less than 5%) 466
▲ Hycamtin for Injection (32% to 98%) 1458
Hyperstat I.V. 3017
Hyzaar 50-12.5 Tablets 1990
Hyzaar 100-12.5 Tablets 1990
Hyzaar 100-25 Tablets 1990
Indapamide Tablets 2156
Indocin Capsules (Less than 1%) 1995
Indocin I.V. (Less than 1%) 2465
Indocin (Less than 1%) 1995
▲ Infergen (15% to 19%) 3364
▲ Intron A for Injection (Less than 5% to 68%) 3024
▲ Invirase (1% to 8%) 2772
Kadian Capsules (Less than 3%) 577
Kaletra (Less than 2%) 476
Keflex Capsules 549
Keppra Injection 3320
Keppra Oral Solution 3314
Keppra Tablets 3314
Klonopin 2778
▲ Kytril (11%) 2784
Lamictal (Infrequent) 1481
▲ Lariam Tablets (Among most frequent) 2786
Lescol Capsules (Rare) 2233
Lescol XL Tablets 2233
▲ Leukine (17%) 814
Levaquin (0.1% to 0.9%) 2384
Levaquin in 5% Dextrose Injection (0.1% to 0.9%) 2384
Lofibra Tablets 1219
Lofibra Capsules 1216
Lopressor HCT 50/25 Tablets 2241
Lopressor HCT 100/25 Tablets 2241
Lopressor HCT 100/50 Tablets 2241
Lotensin HCT Tablets 2246
▲ Lupron Depot 7.5 mg (Greater than or equal to 5%) 3264
Lyrica Capsules (0.1% to 1%) 2539
Matulane Capsules (Frequent) 3191
Mavik Tablets (Rare) 486
Maxipime for Injection (Greater than 0.1% to less than 1%) 1105
Mefoxin for Injection 2012
Mefoxin Premixed Intravenous Solution 2016
▲ Megace ES Oral Suspension (1% to 3%) 2481
▲ Mepron Suspension (4%) 1521
Meridia Capsules 489
Metadate CD Capsules 3323
MetroGel-Vaginal Gel (1.7%) 1855
Mevacor Tablets (Rare) 2021
Micardis HCT Tablets 856
Mintezol 2027
Miradon Tablets 3042
Moban Tablets 1119
Mobic Oral Suspension (Less than 2%) 863
Mobic Tablets (Less than 2%) 863
Moduretic Tablets 2028
Mycamine for Injection (0.9% to 2.7%) 628
▲ Myfortic Tablets (3% to less than 20%) 2255
Myleran Tablets 1525
▲ Mylotarg for Injection (43% to 52%) 3431
Namenda (Infrequent) 1195
Naprosyn Suspension (Less than 1%) 2761
Naprosyn Tablets (Less than 1%) 2761
▲ Neoral Oral Solution (1% to 6%) 2259
▲ Neoral Soft Gelatin Capsules (1% to 6%) 2259
Neurontin Capsules (1.1%) 2487
Neurontin Oral Solution (1.1%) 2487
Neurontin Tablets (1.1%) 2487
▲ Nexavar Tablets (Very Common) 746
Nexium Delayed-Release Capsules (Less than 1%) 655
Nexium I.V. (Less than 1%) 659
▲ Nipent for Injection (22% to 60%) 1863
Noroxin Tablets 2032
Norvasc Tablets (More than 0.1% to 1%) 2545
▲ Norvir (0.9% to 36.9%) 503
Omnicef Capsules (0.9%) 511
Omnicef for Oral Suspension (0.3%) 511
▲ Oncaspar (Greater than 1% but less than 5%) 1145
▲ Ontak Vials (6%) 1745
Orthoclone OKT3 Sterile Solution (Less than 1%) 2360
Parcopa Orally Disintegrating Tablets 3097
Parnate Tablets 1527
Paser Granules 1674
Paxil CR Controlled-Release Tablets (Infrequent) 1538
Paxil (Infrequent) 1530
▲ PEG-Intron Powder for Injection (4%) 3048
Pentasa Capsules 3185
Pepcid Injection (Rare) 2040
Pepcid (Rare) 2038
Percodan Tablets 1132
Permax Tablets (Infrequent) 3356
Pexeva Tablets (Infrequent) 1694
Phenergan Tablets and Suppositories 3440
Phenytek Capsules (Occasional) 2160
Plavix Tablets (Less than 1%) 917
Plavix Tablets (Less than 1%) 2926
Pletal Tablets (Very rare) 2455
Podocon-25 Liquid 2478
Prevacid Delayed-Release Capsules (Less than 1%) 3271
Prevacid for Delayed-Release Oral Suspension (Less than 1%) 3271
Prevacid SoluTab Delayed-Release Orally Disintegrating Tablets (Less than 1%) 3271
Prevacid NapraPAC (Less than 1%) 3280
PREVPAC 3284
▲ Prezista Tablets (13% to 15.4%) 3306
Primaxin I.M. 2045
Primaxin I.V. (Less than 0.2%) 2048
Prinivil Tablets (Rare) 2052
Prinzide Tablets 2056
▲ Prograf Capsules and Injection (3% to 15%) 632
▲ Proleukin for Injection (16%) 2266
ProSom Tablets (Rare) 517
Protonix I.V. (Less than 1%) 3472
Protonix Tablets (Less than 1%) 3469

Protopic Ointment (Greater than or equal to 1%) 638
Prozac Pulvules and Liquid (Rare) 1801
▲ Quadramet Injection (59.3%) 1040
Raniclor Tablets, Chewable 2505
▲ Rapamune Oral Solution and Tablets (9% to 13%) 3475
▲ Rebetol (5% to 6%) 3058
▲ Rebif Prefilled Syringe for Injection (6% to 36%) 3159
Relpax Tablets (Rare) 2548
▲ Remicade for IV Injection (Greater than or equal to 0.2% to 9%) 971
Requip Tablets (Infrequent) 1555
Rescriptor Tablets 2551
Retrovir Capsules 1560
Retrovir IV Infusion 1564
Retrovir 1560
▲ Revlimid Capsules (3.5% to 8.1%) 958
▲ Ribavirin, USP Capsules (5% to 6%) 3068
Rilutek Tablets (Infrequent) 2930
Risperdal (Rare) 1676
Risperdal Consta Long-Acting Injection (Infrequent) 1682
Risperdal M-Tab Orally Disintegrating Tablets (Rare) 1676
Ritalin Hydrochloride Tablets 2269
Ritalin LA Capsules 2271
Ritalin-SR Tablets 2269
▲ Rituxan I.V. (4% to 14%) 1254
Rocephin Injectable Vials, ADD-Vantage, Galaxy, Bulk (2.1%) 2800
▲ Sandimmune (Up to 6%) 2275
Seroquel Tablets 690
▲ Simulect for Injection (3% to 10%) 2284
Skelaxin Tablets 1716
Stalevo Tablets 2287
Stromectol Tablets (One patient) 2083
Sular Tablets (Less than or equal to 1%) 3122
Suprax (Less than 2%) 1843
▲ Sutent Capsules (0% to 7%) 2560
Symbyax Capsules (Rare) 1819
Symmetrel Tablets (Less than 0.1%) 1135
Tabloid Tablets 1575
Tambocor Tablets (Less than 1%) 1856
▲ Targretin Capsules (16.7% to 47.2%) 1747
Tarka Tablets (0.3% or more) 524
▲ Taxotere Injection Concentrate (6.1% to 98.6%) 2932
Tegretol/Tegretol-XR 2295
▲ Temodar Capsules (58%) 3073
Teveten Tablets (0.3%) 1735
Teveten HCT Tablets 1737
▲ Thalomid Capsules (16.7% to 25.5%) 965
▲ Thiola Tablets (4%) 2141
Thioridazine Hydrochloride Tablets (Infrequent) 2163
Thiothixene Capsules (Occasional) 2165
▲ Thymoglobulin for Intravenous Infusion (57.3%) 1284
Tiazac Capsules (Infrequent) 1201
Timentin ADD-Vantage 1580
Timentin Injection Galaxy Container 1583
Timentin IV Infusion 1577
Timentin Pharmacy Bulk Package 1586
Timolide Tablets 2086
Topamax Sprinkle Capsules (1% to 2%) 2404
Topamax Tablets (1% to 2%) 2404
Tricor Tablets 527
Triglide Tablets 3123
Trileptal Tablets 2300
Trileptal Oral Suspension 2300
Uniretic Tablets (Less than 1%) 3100
Urso 250 Tablets (2%) 710
Urso Forte Tablets (2%) 710
▲ Valcyte Tablets (14%) 2813
Valtrex Caplets (0.7% to 1.3%) 1597
Vantin Tablets and Oral Suspension 2645
VFEND I.V. (Less than 2%) 2564
VFEND Oral Suspension (Less than 2%) 2564
VFEND Tablets (Less than 2%) 2564
Viagra Tablets (Less than 2%) 2573
Viracept (Less than 2%) 2577
Voltaren Tablets (Occasionally) 2307
Voltaren-XR Tablets (Occasionally) 2310
Vytorin 10/10 Tablets 2114
Vytorin 10/10 Tablets 3077
Vytorin 10/20 Tablets 2114
Vytorin 10/20 Tablets 3077
Vytorin 10/40 Tablets 2114
Vytorin 10/40 Tablets 3077
Vytorin 10/80 Tablets 2114
Vytorin 10/80 Tablets 3077
Wellbutrin Tablets 1603
Wellbutrin SR Sustained-Release Tablets 1607
Wellbutrin XL Extended-Release Tablets 1613
▲ Xeloda Tablets (24% to 91%) 2822
Xyrem Oral Solution (Infrequent) 1688
Zantac (A few patients) 1624
Zantac Injection (Few patients) 1619
Zantac Injection Pharmacy Bulk Package (Infrequent) 1622
Zantac Injection Premixed (Few patients) 1619
Zantac (A few patients) 1624
Ziagen (Less than 1%) 1626
Zinacef for Injection (1 in 750 patients) 1631
Zinacef Injection (1 in 750 patients) 1631
Zinecard for Injection 2650
Zmax for Oral Suspension (Less then 1%) 2583
Zocor Tablets (Rare) 2105
Zoloft 2586
Zomig Tablets (Rare) 3519
Zomig Nasal Spray (Rare) 3523
Zomig-ZMT Tablets (Rare) 3519
Zonegran Capsules (Infrequent) 1101
Zosyn 3492
Zovirax 1643
Zyban Sustained-Release Tablets 1644
Zyprexa Tablets (Infrequent) 1830
Zyprexa ZYDIS Orally Disintegrating Tablets (Infrequent) 1830

Leukopenia, transient

Maxipime for Injection 1105
Tindamax Tablets 2142

Leukoplakia, oral

Doxil Injection (Less than 1%) 2351
Geodon Capsules (Rare) 2529
▲ Intron A for Injection (Less than 5%) 3024

Leukorrhea

Abilify Oral Solution (Infrequent) 882
Abilify Oral Solution (Infrequent) 2450
Abilify Discmelt Orally Disintegrating Tablets (Infrequent) 882
Abilify Discmelt Orally Disintegrating Tablets (Infrequent) 2450
Abilify Tablets (Infrequent) 882
Abilify Tablets (Infrequent) 2450
Aciphex Tablets (Rare) 1090
Angeliq Tablets (1.3%) 762
▲ Arimidex Tablets (2% to 9%) 673
Arthrotec Tablets (Rare) 3129
▲ Climara Transdermal System (1% to 7%) 771
▲ Depo-Provera Contraceptive Injection (1% to 5%) 2622
▲ Doxil Injection (1% to 10%) 2351
Effexor Tablets (Infrequent) 3411
Effexor XR Capsules (Infrequent) 3417
▲ Estring Vaginal Ring (7%) 2635
▲ Evista Tablets (3.3%) 1763
Evoxac Capsules (Less than 1%) 1047
Gengraf Capsules (1%) 459
▲ Intron A for Injection (Less than 5%) 3024
Levaquin (0.1% to 0.9%) 2384
Levaquin in 5% Dextrose Injection (0.1% to 0.9%) 2384
Lyrica Capsules (0.1% to 1%) 2539
▲ Menostar Transdermal System (11%) 782
▲ Mirena Intrauterine System (5% or more) 787
Neoral Oral Solution (1%) 2259
Neoral Soft Gelatin Capsules (1%) 2259
Neurontin Capsules (Rare) 2487
Neurontin Oral Solution (Rare) 2487
Neurontin Tablets (Rare) 2487
Omnicef Capsules (0.2%) 511
Omnicef for Oral Suspension (0.2%) 511
ParaGard T 380A Intrauterine Copper Contraceptive 1073
Paxil CR Controlled-Release Tablets (Rare) 1538
Paxil (Rare) 1530
Permax Tablets (Rare) 3356
Pexeva Tablets (rare) 1694
▲ Premarin Tablets (4% to 7%) 3446
▲ Premphase Tablets (3% to 9%) 3456
▲ Prempro Tablets (3% to 9%) 3456
Prevacid Delayed-Release Capsules (Less than 1%) 3271
Prevacid for Delayed-Release Oral Suspension (Less than 1%) 3271
Prevacid SoluTab Delayed-Release Orally Disintegrating Tablets (Less than 1%) 3271
Prevacid NapraPAC (Less than 1%) 3280
PREVPAC (Less than 1%) 3284
Prometrium Capsules (100 mg, 200 mg) (Less than 5%) 3203
Prozac Pulvules and Liquid (Infrequent) 1801
Relpax Tablets (Rare) 2548
Risperdal (Infrequent) 1676
Risperdal Consta Long-Acting Injection (Infrequent) 1682
Risperdal M-Tab Orally Disintegrating Tablets (Infrequent) 1676
Seroquel Tablets (Infrequent) 690
Sonata Capsules (Rare) 1717
Soriatane Capsules (Less than 1%) 1013
Symbyax Capsules (Infrequent) 1819
Topamax Sprinkle Capsules (2% to frequent) 2404
Topamax Tablets (2% to frequent) 2404
Trileptal Tablets 2300
Trileptal Oral Suspension 2300
Tygacil for Injection (0% to less than 2%) 3488
Uniretic Tablets (Less than 1%) 3100
Vandazole Vaginal Gel (Less than 1%) 3338
Yasmin 28 Tablets (Greater than 1%) 796
Yaz Tablets (Greater than 1%) 803
Zoloft (Infrequent) 2586
Zosyn (1.0% or less) 3492
Zyrtec Chewable Tablets (Less than 2%) 2594
Zyrtec (Less than 2%) 2594
Zyrtec-D 12 Hour Extended Release Tablets (Less than 2%) 2597

Lhermitte's sign

Copaxone for Injection (At least 2%) 3297
Eloxatin for Injection 2892

Libido, changes

Adderall Tablets 3164
Adderall XR Capsules 3166
Adipex-P 1215
Avalide Tablets 888
Avalide Tablets 2874
Avapro Tablets (Less than 1%) 891
Avapro Tablets (Less than 1%) 2871
Climara Transdermal System 771
Climara Pro Transdermal System 776
Desoxyn Tablets, USP 2462
Dexedrine 1420
DextroStat Tablets 3179
Diastat Rectal Delivery System (Infrequent) 3343
Enjuvia Tablets 1062
Estrasorb Topical Emulsion 1147
Estratest Tablets 3199
Estratest H.S. Tablets 3199
Invirase (Greater than or equal to 2%) 2772
▲ Lupron Depot 3.75 mg (16%) 3260
▲ Lupron Depot–3 Month 11.25 mg (16%) 3265
Menostar Transdermal System 782
Mircette Tablets 1066
Neurontin Capsules (Infrequent) 2487
Neurontin Oral Solution (Infrequent) 2487
Neurontin Tablets (Infrequent) 2487
Nipent for Injection (Less than 3%) 1863
▲ Niravam Orally Disintegrating Tablets (7.1%) 3092
Ortho-Cyclen Tablets 2429
Ortho Evra Transdermal System 2417
Ortho Tri-Cyclen Tablets 2429
Ortho Tri-Cyclen Lo Tablets 2436
Oxandrin Tablets 2962
Premarin Intravenous 3442
Premarin Tablets 3446
Premarin Vaginal Cream 3452
Premphase Tablets 3456
Prempro Tablets 3456
Seasonique Tablets 1077
Thioridazine Hydrochloride Tablets 2163
Valium Tablets (Infrequent) 2819
Yasmin 28 Tablets 796
Yaz Tablets 803

Libido, decreased

Abilify Oral Solution (Infrequent) 882
Abilify Oral Solution (Infrequent) 2450
Abilify Discmelt Orally Disintegrating Tablets (Infrequent) 882
Abilify Discmelt Orally Disintegrating Tablets (Infrequent) 2450
Abilify Tablets (Infrequent) 882
Abilify Tablets (Infrequent) 2450
Aciphex Tablets 1090
Actiq (Less than 1%) 979
Adalat CC Tablets (Less than 1%) 2964
▲ Adderall XR Capsules (2% to 4%) 3166
Aldoril Tablets 1910
Ambien Tablets (Rare) 2851
Ambien CR Tablets (Rare) 2855
Amerge Tablets (Rare) 1339
▲ AndroGel (Up to 3%) 3329
Androxy Tablets 3335
Aricept Tablets (Infrequent) 1094
Aricept ODT Tablets (Infrequent) 1094
Asacol Delayed-Release Tablets 2692
▲ Avinza Capsules (Less than 5%) 1741
▲ Avodart Soft Gelatin Capsules (0.3% to 3%) 1390
Axid Oral Solution 879
Azilect Tablets (Greater than 1%) 3293
Blocadren Tablets (0.6%) 1916
Caduet Tablets (Less than 2%) 2508
Calcijex Injection 411
Campral Tablets (Frequent) 1174
Cardura XL Tablets (Less than 1%) 2515
Celexa (2%) 1176
Chantix Tablets (Infrequent) 2517
Clozaril Tablets (Less than 1%) 2184
Copaxone for Injection (Infrequent) 3297
Coreg Tablets (Greater than 0.1% to 1%) 1414
Cosopt Sterile Ophthalmic Solution 1931
Cozaar Tablets (Less than 1%) 1935
▲ Cymbalta Delayed-Release Capsules (1% to 6%) 1757
▲ Depo-Provera Contraceptive Injection (1% to 5%) 2622
▲ depo-subQ provera 104 Injectable Suspension (1% to less than 5%) 2624
Diovan HCT Tablets (Less frequent) 2196
Duragesic Transdermal System (Less than 1%) 2373
DynaCirc CR Tablets (0.5% to 1%) 2721
▲ Effexor Tablets (2% to 5.7%) 3411
▲ Effexor XR Capsules (3% to 9%) 3417
Eligard 7.5 mg (Less than 2%) 2880
▲ Eligard 30 mg (3.3%) 2885
Eligard 45 mg (1%) 2888
Emsam Transdermal System (0.7%) 903
Estring Vaginal Ring 2635
Exelon Capsules (Infrequent) 2206
Exelon Oral Solution (Infrequent) 2206
FazaClo Orally Disintegrating Tablets (Less than 1%) 551
Flomax Capsules (1.0% to 2.0%) 850
Gabitril Tablets (Infrequent) 984
Gengraf Capsules (1% to less than 3%) 459
Hectorol Capsules 1275
Hectorol Injection 1278
Hyperstat I.V. 3017
Hytrin Capsules (0.6%) 471
Hyzaar 50-12.5 Tablets 1990
Hyzaar 100-12.5 Tablets 1990
Hyzaar 100-25 Tablets 1990
▲ Imdur Tablets (Less than or equal to 5%) 3018
Indapamide Tablets (Less than 5%) 2156
▲ Infergen (5%) 3364
▲ Intron A for Injection (Up to 5%) 3024
Kadian Capsules (Less than 3%) 577
Kaletra (Up to 2%) 476
Klonopin (1%) 2778
Lamictal (Rare) 1481
▲ Lexapro Oral Solution (3% to 7%) 1190
▲ Lexapro Tablets (3% to 7%) 1190
Librium Capsules 3347
Lipitor Tablets (Less than 2%) 2483
Lofibra Tablets 1219
Lofibra Capsules 1216
Lopressor Injection 2238
Lopressor Tablets 2238
Lotensin HCT Tablets (0.3% to 1%) 2246
Lotrel Capsules 2249
▲ Lunesta Tablets (0% to 3%) 3142
▲ Lupron Depot 3.75 mg (Less than 5%) 3260
▲ Lupron Depot 7.5 mg (5.4%) 3264
▲ Lupron Depot–3 Month 11.25 mg (1.8% to 11%) 3265
Lyrica Capsules (Greater than or equal to 1%) 2539
Mavik Tablets (0.3% to 1.0%) 486
▲ Megace ES Oral Suspension (0% to 5%) 2481
Meridia Capsules 489

Midamor Tablets (Less than or equal to 1%)... 2026
Mirapex Tablets (1%)... 859
▲ Mirena Intrauterine System (5% or more)... 787
Moduretic Tablets... 2028
MS Contin Tablets (Less frequent)... 2701
Nadolol Tablets (1 to 5 of 1000 patients)... 2159
Neoral Oral Solution (1% to less than 3%)... 2259
Neoral Soft Gelatin Capsules (1% to less than 3%)... 2259
Neurontin Capsules (Infrequent)... 2487
Neurontin Oral Solution (Infrequent)... 2487
Neurontin Tablets (Infrequent)... 2487
▲ Niravam Orally Disintegrating Tablets (14.4%)... 3092
Norvir (Less than 2%)... 503
OxyContin Tablets... 2703
▲ Paxil CR Controlled-Release Tablets (3% to 9%)... 1538
▲ Paxil (3% to 9%)... 1530
Pepcid Injection (Infrequent)... 2040
Pepcid (Infrequent)... 2038
Permax Tablets (Infrequent)... 3356
▲ Pexeva Tablets (1% to 14%)... 1694
Prevacid Delayed-Release Capsules (Less than 1%)... 3271
Prevacid for Delayed-Release Oral Suspension (Less than 1%)... 3271
Prevacid SoluTab Delayed-Release Orally Disintegrating Tablets (Less than 1%)... 3271
Prevacid NapraPAC (Less than 1%)... 3280
PREVPAC (Less than 1%)... 3284
Prinivil Tablets (0.4%)... 2052
Prinzide Tablets (0.3% to 1%)... 2056
▲ Prochieve 4% Gel (10%)... 1003
▲ Prochieve 8% Gel (10%)... 1003
▲ Propecia Tablets (1.8% - 6.4%)... 2060
▲ Proscar Tablets (2.6% to 6.4%)... 2067
ProSom Tablets (Rare)... 517
Protonix I.V. (Less than 1%)... 3472
Protonix Tablets (Less than 1%)... 3469
Provigil Tablets (At least 1%)... 988
▲ Prozac Pulvules and Liquid (1% to 11%)... 1801
Requip Tablets (Infrequent)... 1555
Rescriptor Tablets... 2551
Reyataz Capsules (Less than 3%)... 921
Rilutek Tablets (Infrequent)... 2930
Risperdal Consta Long-Acting Injection (Infrequent)... 1682
Rocaltrol Capsules... 2798
Rocaltrol Oral Solution... 2798
Rythmol SR Capsules... 2727
Sandostatin Injection (Less than 1%)... 2278
Sandostatin LAR Depot (Rare)... 2280
Seroquel Tablets (Rare)... 690
Sonata Capsules (Infrequent)... 1717
Soriatane Capsules (Less than 1%)... 1013
▲ Strattera Capsules (5% or greater)... 1814
Sular Tablets (Less than or equal to 1%)... 3122
▲ Symbyax Capsules (2% to 4%)... 1819
Symmetrel Tablets (0.1% to 1%)... 1135
Tambocor Tablets (Less than 1%)... 1856
Tarka Tablets... 524
Tasmar Tablets (Infrequent)... 3358
Thalomid Capsules... 965
Timolide Tablets (Less than 1%)... 2086
Timoptic Sterile Ophthalmic Solution... 2088
Timoptic in Ocudose... 2091
Timoptic-XE Sterile Ophthalmic Gel Forming Solution... 2092
▲ Topamax Sprinkle Capsules (0% to 3%)... 2404
▲ Topamax Tablets (0% to 3%)... 2404
Toprol-XL Tablets... 668
Trelstar LA Suspension (2.3%)... 3397
Tricor Tablets... 527
Trileptal Tablets... 2300
Trileptal Oral Suspension... 2300
▲ Ultram ER Tablets (1% to greater than 5%)... 2392
Uniretic Tablets (Less than 1%)... 3100
Vantas (2.3%)... 3375
VFEND I.V. (Less than 2%)... 2564
VFEND Oral Suspension (Less than 2%)... 2564
VFEND Tablets (Less than 2%)... 2564
Vicoprofen Tablets (Less than 1%)... 539
Vivitrol... 995
▲ Wellbutrin Tablets (3.1%)... 1603
Wellbutrin SR Sustained-Release Tablets (Infrequent)... 1607
▲ Wellbutrin XL Extended-Release Tablets (3%)... 1613
Yaz Tablets (Greater than 1%)... 803
Zantac Injection... 1619
Zantac Injection Pharmacy Bulk Package (Infrequent)... 1622
Zantac Injection Premixed... 1619
▲ Zoloft (1% to 11%)... 2586
Zonegran Capsules (Infrequent)... 1101
Zyban Sustained-Release Tablets (Infrequent)... 1644
Zyprexa Tablets (Infrequent)... 1830
Zyprexa ZYDIS Orally Disintegrating Tablets (Infrequent)... 1830
Zyrtec Chewable Tablets (Less than 2%)... 2594
Zyrtec (Less than 2%)... 2594
Zyrtec-D 12 Hour Extended Release Tablets (Less than 2%)... 2597

Libido, increased
Abilify Oral Solution (Infrequent)... 882
Abilify Oral Solution (Infrequent)... 2450
Abilify Discmelt Orally Disintegrating Tablets (Infrequent)... 882
Abilify Discmelt Orally Disintegrating Tablets (Infrequent)... 2450
Abilify Tablets (Infrequent)... 882
Abilify Tablets (Infrequent)... 2450
AndroGel (One patient)... 3329
Androxy Tablets... 3335
Aricept Tablets (Frequent)... 1094
Aricept ODT Tablets (Frequent)... 1094
Campral Tablets (Infrequent)... 1174
Celexa (Infrequent)... 1176
Clozaril Tablets (Less than 1%)... 2184
Depo-Provera Contraceptive Injection (Less than 1%)... 2622
depo-subQ provera 104 Injectable Suspension... 2624
Effexor Tablets (Infrequent)... 3411
Effexor XR Capsules (Infrequent)... 3417
Exelon Capsules (Infrequent)... 2206
Exelon Oral Solution (Infrequent)... 2206
FazaClo Orally Disintegrating Tablets (Less than 1%)... 551
Gabitril Tablets (Infrequent)... 984
Gengraf Capsules (1% to less than 3%)... 459
Klonopin (Infrequent)... 2778
Lamictal (Rare)... 1481
Librium Capsules... 3347
Lotensin Tablets (Less than 1%)... 2243
Lyrica Capsules (0.1% to 1%)... 2539
Meridia Capsules... 489
Moban Tablets... 1119
Namenda (Infrequent)... 1195
Neoral Oral Solution (1% to less than 3%)... 2259
Neoral Soft Gelatin Capsules (1% to less than 3%)... 2259
Neurontin Capsules (Rare)... 2487
Neurontin Oral Solution (Rare)... 2487
Neurontin Tablets (Rare)... 2487
▲ Niravam Orally Disintegrating Tablets (7.7%)... 3092
Parcopa Orally Disintegrating Tablets... 3097
Paxil CR Controlled-Release Tablets (Rare)... 1538
Paxil (Rare)... 1530
Permax Tablets (Infrequent)... 3356
Pexeva Tablets (Infrequent)... 1694
Prevacid Delayed-Release Capsules (Less than 1%)... 3271
Prevacid for Delayed-Release Oral Suspension (Less than 1%)... 3271
Prevacid SoluTab Delayed-Release Orally Disintegrating Tablets (Less than 1%)... 3271
Prevacid NapraPAC (Less than 1%)... 3280
PREVPAC (Less than 1%)... 3284
Prozac Pulvules and Liquid (Infrequent)... 1801
Razadyne (Infrequent)... 2399
Razadyne ER Extended-Release Capsules (Infrequent)... 2399
Requip Tablets (Infrequent)... 1555
Rilutek Tablets (Infrequent)... 2930
Risperdal (Infrequent)... 1676
Risperdal M-Tab Orally Disintegrating Tablets (Infrequent)... 1676
Seroquel Tablets (Infrequent)... 690
Stalevo Tablets... 2287
Symbyax Capsules (Rare)... 1819
Tasmar Tablets (Infrequent)... 3358
Topamax Sprinkle Capsules (Rare)... 2404
Topamax Tablets (Rare)... 2404
Trileptal Tablets... 2300
Trileptal Oral Suspension... 2300
Wellbutrin Tablets (Frequent)... 1603
Wellbutrin SR Sustained-Release Tablets... 1607
Wellbutrin XL Extended-Release Tablets... 1613
Xyrem Oral Solution (Infrequent)... 1688
Zoloft (Rare)... 2586
Zyban Sustained-Release Tablets... 1644
Zyprexa Tablets... 1830
Zyprexa ZYDIS Orally Disintegrating Tablets... 1830

Libido, loss of
Advicor Tablets... 1722
Altoprev Extended-Release Tablets... 3109
Catapres Tablets (About 3 in 100 patients)... 843
Catapres-TTS (0.5% or less)... 844
▲ Clorpres Tablets (About 3%)... 2153
▲ Eulexin Capsules (36%)... 3009
Klonopin (Infrequent)... 2778
Lescol Capsules... 2233
Lescol XL Tablets... 2233
Mevacor Tablets (0.5% to 1.0%)... 2021
Soltamox Oral Solution... 3527
Vytorin 10/10 Tablets... 2114
Vytorin 10/10 Tablets... 3077
Vytorin 10/20 Tablets... 2114
Vytorin 10/20 Tablets... 3077
Vytorin 10/40 Tablets... 2114
Vytorin 10/40 Tablets... 3077
Vytorin 10/80 Tablets... 2114
Vytorin 10/80 Tablets... 3077
Zantac (Occasional)... 1624
Zocor Tablets... 2105

Lichen planus
Anaprox Tablets... 2761
Anaprox DS Tablets... 2761
Cuprimine Capsules... 1947
EC-Naprosyn Delayed-Release Tablets... 2761
Evoxac Capsules (Less than 1%)... 1047
Naprosyn Suspension... 2761
Naprosyn Tablets... 2761
Pentasa Capsules (Less than 1%)... 3185
Plavix Tablets... 917
Plavix Tablets... 2926

Lid margin crusting
▲ Nevanac Ophthalmic Suspension 0.1% (1% to 5%)... ⊙209

Ligaments, calcification of
Accutane Capsules... 2731

Light-headedness
▲ Abilify Oral Solution (4% to 11%)... 882
▲ Abilify Oral Solution (11%)... 2450
▲ Abilify Discmelt Orally Disintegrating Tablets (4% to 11%)... 882
▲ Abilify Discmelt Orally Disintegrating Tablets (11%)... 2450
▲ Abilify Tablets (4% to 11%)... 882
▲ Abilify Tablets (11%)... 2450
Adenocard Injection (2%)... 617
▲ Adenoscan (12%)... 619
Alferon N Injection (One patient to 3%)... 1665
Altace Capsules... 1702
Ambien Tablets (2%)... 2851
Ambien CR Tablets (Frequent)... 2855
Anaprox Tablets (Less than 3%)... 2761
Anaprox DS Tablets (Less than 3%)... 2761
Beconase AQ Nasal Spray (Fewer than 5 per 100 patients)... 1396
Benicar HCT Tablets... 1044
▲ Bentyl Capsules (11%)... 697
▲ Bentyl Injection (11%)... 697
▲ Bentyl Syrup (11%)... 697
▲ Bentyl Tablets (11%)... 697
Captopril Tablets... 2149
Cesamet Capsules... 3340
Cipro (Less than 1%)... 2977
Cipro I.V. (1% or less)... 2984
Cipro XR Tablets... 2990
Cutivate Ointment (Less than 1%)... 2665
Dalmane Capsules... 3342
Dantrium Capsules (Less frequent)... 2694
Dantrium Intravenous... 2695
Dilaudid... 440
Dilaudid Non-Sterile Powder... 440
Dilaudid Oral Liquid... 445
Dilaudid Rectal Suppositories... 440
Dilaudid Tablets... 440
Dilaudid Tablets - 8 mg... 445
▲ Dilaudid-HP (Among most frequent)... 442
Diovan HCT Tablets... 2196
Dolobid Tablets (Less than 1 in 100)... 1955
EC-Naprosyn Delayed-Release Tablets (Less than 3%)... 2761
▲ Eldepryl Capsules (7 of 49 patients)... 3208
▲ Gabitril Tablets (27%)... 984
Gammagard S/D (Occasional)... 724
Guanidine Hydrochloride Tablets... 3016
Hyperstat I.V.... 3017
▲ Hytrin Capsules (28%)... 471
Hyzaar 50-12.5 Tablets... 1990
Hyzaar 100-12.5 Tablets... 1990
Hyzaar 100-25 Tablets... 1990
▲ Indapamide Tablets (Less than 5%)... 2156
Inderal LA Long-Acting Capsules... 3429
Indocin (Less than 1%)... 1995
InnoPran XL Capsules... 2723
Invirase (Less than 2%)... 2772
Levaquin... 2384
Levaquin in 5% Dextrose Injection... 2384
Lexapro Oral Solution (Frequent)... 1190
Lexapro Tablets (Frequent)... 1190
Lidoderm Patch... 1118
Limbrel Capsules (0.003%)... 2672
Lotensin HCT Tablets... 2246
Mavik Tablets... 486
Micardis HCT Tablets... 856
▲ MS Contin Tablets (Among most frequent)... 2701
Naprosyn Suspension (Less than 3%)... 2761
Naprosyn Tablets (Less than 3%)... 2761
Neumega for Injection... 3435
Nimotop Capsules (Less than 1%)... 749
▲ Niravam Orally Disintegrating Tablets (19.3% to 29.8%)... 3092
▲ Nitro-Dur Transdermal Infusion System (6%)... 3046
Norflex Injection... 1856
Noroxin Tablets... 2032
Numorphan Injection... 1120
▲ OxyFast Oral Concentrate Solution (Among most frequent)... 2708
▲ OxyIR Capsules (Among most frequent)... 2708
▲ Percocet Tablets (Among most frequent)... 1131
▲ Percodan Tablets (Among most frequent)... 1132
Prevacid NapraPAC (Less than 3%)... 3280
Prinivil Tablets... 2052
Prinzide Tablets... 2056
Prolastin (0.19%)... 3255
Proquin XR Tablets... 1153
Raptiva for Injection... 1250
Recombivax HB (Less than 1%)... 2071
Soltamox Oral Solution (Infrequently)... 3527
▲ Symmetrel Tablets (5% to 10%)... 1135
Synera Topical Patch... 1137
Tambocor Tablets... 1856
Tequin Injection... 938
Tequin Injection in 5% Dextrose... 938
Tequin Tablets... 938
Thiothixene Capsules... 2165
▲ Thrombate III (1 of 17)... 3257
▲ Tylenol with Codeine Tablets (Among most frequent)... 2391
Uniretic Tablets (Less than 1%)... 3100
Vasotec I.V. Injection... 2103
▲ Vicodin Tablets (Among most frequent)... 535
▲ Vicodin ES Tablets (Among most frequent)... 536
▲ Vicodin HP Tablets (Among most frequent)... 538
▲ Zemplar Capsules (5%)... 541
▲ Zemplar Injection (5%)... 543
▲ Zydone Tablets (Among most frequent)... 1139

Limb ischemia
Lovenox Injection... 2915

Limb reduction defects
Altace Capsules... 1702
Captopril Tablets... 2149
Cozaar Tablets... 1935
Hyzaar 50-12.5 Tablets... 1990
Hyzaar 100-12.5 Tablets... 1990
Hyzaar 100-25 Tablets... 1990
Lotrel Capsules... 2249
Prinivil Tablets... 2052
Prinzide Tablets... 2056
Proventil Inhalation Aerosol... 3053
Proventil Inhalation Solution 0.083%... 3055
Vasotec I.V. Injection... 2103

Limbitis
▲ Stromectol Tablets (3.5% to 5.5%)... 2083

Lip abnormality
ProQuad... 2064

Lipoatrophy
Aptivus Capsules (Less than 2%)...... 826
Imitrex Injection (Rare)...................... 1463
Prezista Tablets (Less than 2%)........ 3306

Lipodystrophy
Apidra Injection.............................. 2864
Aptivus Capsules (Less than 2%)...... 826
Genotropin Lyophilized Powder (Infrequent)....................................... 2638
Humalog-Pen.................................... 1781
Humalog Mix 50/50-Pen.................. 1783
Humalog Mix 75/25-Pen.................. 1785
Humulin 50/50, 100 Units (Rare)..... 1791
Humulin 70/30 Pen (Rare).............. 1793
Humulin L, 100 Units (Rare)............ 1794
Humulin N Pen (Rare)..................... 1797
Humulin R, 100 Units (Rare)............ 1798
▲ Invirase (5.4%) 2772
Lantus Injection 2909
Levemir Injection 2320
NovoLog Injection............................ 2326
NovoLog Mix 70/30 2328
▲ Reyataz Capsules (1% to 8%) 921
Viread Tablets (1%) 1301

Lipohypertrophy
Aptivus Capsules (Less than 2%) 826
Imitrex Injection (Rare) 1463
▲ Increlex Injection (Greater than or equal to 5%)...................................... 3291
Reyataz Capsules (Less than 3%) 921

Lipoma
Copaxone for Injection (Infrequent) .. 3297
▲ Intron A for Injection (Less than 5%)... 3024
Lexapro Oral Solution (Infrequent) 1190
Lexapro Tablets (Infrequent) 1190
Requip Tablets (Infrequent) 1555

Lipoprotein levels, changes
Accutane Capsules 2731
Carbatrol Capsules (Occasional) 3171
▲ Soriatane Capsules (25% to 50%) ... 1013
Tegretol/Tegretol-XR (Occasional) 2295
Timolide Tablets 2086

Lipoproteins, electrophoretic abnormalities
Sandimmune 2275

Lipotrophy
Humulin 50/50, 100 Units (Rare) 1791
Humulin 70/30 Pen (Rare) 1793
Humulin L, 100 Units (Rare) 1794
Humulin N Pen (Rare) 1797
Somavert Injection 2642

Lips, cracked
Zovirax Cream (Less than 1%) 820

Lips, dry
(*see under* Xerochilia)

Lips, enlargement
Phenytek Capsules 2160

Lips, swelling
Altace Capsules 1702
Levaquin 2384
Levaquin in 5% Dextrose Injection 2384
Lithobid Tablets 1692
Propecia Tablets 2060
Proscar Tablets 2067
Rocaltrol Capsules 2798
Rocaltrol Oral Solution 2798
Tambocor Tablets (Less than 1%) 1856

Listeriosis
Remicade for IV Injection 971

Listlessness
Aricept Tablets (Infrequent) 1094
Aricept ODT Tablets (Infrequent) 1094
Indocin (Greater than 1%) 1995

Livedo reticularis
Activase I.V. 1223
Myozyme for Intravenous Infusion 1279
▲ Symmetrel Tablets (1% to 5%) 1135

Liver, enlarged
VFEND I.V. (Less than 2%) 2564
VFEND Oral Suspension (Less than 2%) 2564
VFEND Tablets (Less than 2%) 2564

Liver, fatty
Aciphex Tablets (Rare) 1090
Advicor Tablets 1722
Copegus Tablets (Less than 1%) 2754
Effexor Tablets 3411
Effexor XR Capsules 3417
Geodon Capsules (Rare) 2529
Lescol Capsules............................... 2233
Lescol XL Tablets 2233
Lofibra Tablets................................. 1219
Lofibra Capsules.............................. 1216
Pegasys (Less than 1%)................... 2789
Plavix Tablets (Less than 1%) 917
Plavix Tablets (Less than 1%)........... 2926
Prograf Capsules and Injection.......... 632
Prozac Pulvules and Liquid (Rare)..... 1801
Reyataz Capsules (Less than 3%)..... 921
Risperdal Consta Long-Acting Injection (Rare)................................ 1682
Sandostatin LAR Depot (Rare).......... 2280
Symbyax Capsules (Rare)................ 1819
Tricor Tablets.................................... 527
Triglide Tablets 3123
Vytorin 10/10 Tablets....................... 2114
Vytorin 10/10 Tablets....................... 3077
Vytorin 10/20 Tablets....................... 2114
Vytorin 10/20 Tablets....................... 3077
Vytorin 10/40 Tablets 2114
Vytorin 10/40 Tablets 3077
Vytorin 10/80 Tablets 2114
Vytorin 10/80 Tablets 3077
Zocor Tablets 2105
Zyprexa Tablets (Rare) 1830
Zyprexa ZYDIS Orally Disintegrating Tablets (Rare) 1830

Liver abnormalities
Catapres Tablets (About 1 in 100 patients) 843
Clorpres Tablets 2153
Clozaril Tablets (1%) 2184
Effexor Tablets 3411
Oncaspar (Less than 1%) 1145
Pepcid Injection (Infrequent) 2040
Pepcid (Infrequent) 2038
▲ Tarka Tablets (3.2%) 524
Ziagen 1626
Zocor Tablets 2105
Zomig Tablets (Infrequent) 3519
Zomig-ZMT Tablets (Infrequent) 3519

Liver damage
(*see under* Hepatotoxicity)

Liver disease, venoocclusive
Prograf Capsules and Injection 632

Liver disorders
Aldoril Tablets 1910
Cosmegen for Injection 2459
Invirase (Rare) 2772
▲ Leukine (77%) 814
Mycamine for Injection 628
Pulmozyme Inhalation Solution 1248
▲ Vesanoid Capsules (3%) 2820

Liver dysfunction
(*see under* Hepatic dysfunction)

Liver enzymes, elevated
Avandaryl Tablets 1379
Bayer Aspirin 744
Clarinex-D 24-Hour Extended-Release Tablets 2998
Duetact Tablets (Rare) 3226
Fansidar Tablets 2765
Gantrisin Pediatric Suspension 2770
▲ Kytril Injection (5.6%) 2781
ProstaScint Kit (Less than 1%) 1037
Strattera Capsules 1814
Stromectol Tablets 2083
Truvada Tablets 1296
Ultane Liquid for Inhalation (Less than 1%) 531
Zetia Tablets 3083

Liver function, changes
(*see under* Hepatic dysfunction)

Liver function, impaired
(*see under* Hepatic dysfunction)

Liver function tests, abnormal
▲ Advair Diskus 100/50 (1% to 3%) 1308
Advair Diskus 250/50 (1% to 3%) 1308
▲ Advair Diskus 500/50 (1% to 3%) 1308
Advair HFA Inhalation Aerosol 1318
Anaprox Tablets (Less than 1%) 2761
Anaprox DS Tablets (Less than 1%) .. 2761
Androxy Tablets 3335
Aptivus Capsules (Less than 2%) 826
Atripla Tablets 945
Avelox (0.1% to less than 2%) 2970
Azilect Tablets (Greater than 1%) 3293
Caduet Tablets (Less than 2%) 2508
Campral Tablets (Infrequent) 1174
Carbatrol Capsules 3171
Cardura XL Tablets 2515
Chantix Tablets (Frequent) 2517
Cialis Tablets (Less than 2%) 1838
Cipro (1.3%).................................... 2977
Cipro I.V. (Greater than 1% to 1.3%).. 2984
Cipro XR Tablets (Less than 1%)...... 2990
Concerta Extended-Release Tablets 1881
Cosmegen for Injection.................... 2459
▲ Cubicin for Injection (1.7% to 3%) 1026
Dacogen Injection (Greater than or equal to 1%) 2129
Depakote ER Tablets........................ 434
EC-Naprosyn Delayed-Release Tablets (Less than 1%).................. 2761
Epzicom Tablets 1436
▲ Equetro Extended-Release Capsules (Less than 5%).............. 3180
Eraxis for Injection (Less than 1% to less than 2%)............................ 2521
Erythromycin Delayed-Release Capsules, USP (Rare).................... 457
FazaClo Orally Disintegrating Tablets (1%)................................. 551
Keppra Injection 3320
Keppra Oral Solution........................ 3314
Keppra Tablets................................. 3314
Ketek Tablets (Greater than or equal to 0.2% to less than 2%)...... 2903
Levitra Tablets (Less than 2%).......... 3034
Mycamine for Injection (0.7% to 1.5%).. 628
▲ Myfortic Tablets (3% to less than 20%).. 2255
▲ Mylotarg for Injection (20% to 29%)... 3431
Naprosyn Suspension (Less than 1%)... 2761
Naprosyn Tablets (Less than 1%)..... 2761
Oxandrin Tablets.............................. 2962
Pexeva Tablets (Infrequent).............. 1694
Plavix Tablets................................... 2926
Pletal Tablets (Very rare).................. 2455
Prevacid NapraPAC (Less than 1%).. 3280
Revlimid Capsules 958
Rythmol SR Capsules....................... 2727
Tamiflu Capsules 2807
Tamiflu Oral Suspension................... 2807
Tarceva Tablets................................ 1259
Tarceva Tablets................................ 2444
Thiola Tablets 2141
▲ Tricor Tablets (7.5%) 527
▲ Triglide Tablets (7.5%) 3123
▲ Ultram ER Tablets (1% to greater than 5%)....................................... 2392
▲ VFEND I.V. (2.7% to 3.2%) 2564
▲ VFEND Oral Suspension (2.7% to 3.2%)... 2564
▲ VFEND Tablets (2.7% to 3.2%) 2564
Viracept (Less than 2%).................... 2577
Xyrem Oral Solution (Infrequent)...... 1688
Zelapar Tablets................................ 3372
Zyvox (0.4% to 1.3%)....................... 2652

Liver function tests, elevated
▲ Anaprox Tablets (1% to 10%) 2761
▲ Anaprox DS Tablets (1% to 10%) 2761
Arthrotec Tablets............................. 3129
Decadron Tablets............................. 1951
Dolobid Tablets................................ 1955
▲ EC-Naprosyn Delayed-Release Tablets (1% to 10%)..................... 2761
▲ Elmiron Capsules (11.8%) 2415
Levothroid Tablets 1186
▲ Naprosyn Suspension (1% to 10%)... 2761
▲ Naprosyn Tablets (1% to 10%) 2761
Neurontin Capsules 2487
Neurontin Oral Solution.................... 2487
Neurontin Tablets............................. 2487
Pexeva Tablets................................. 1694
▲ Raptiva for Injection (3.1%) 1250
Sutent Capsules 2560
Trizivir Tablets 1589

Liver injury
Eulexin Capsules.............................. 3009
Ketek Tablets.................................... 2903
Remicade for IV Injection.................. 971
Singulair (Rare)................................ 2077
Strattera Capsules (Rare).................. 1814
Tasmar Tablets................................. 3358
Vantin Tablets and Oral Suspension................................. 2645

Liver pain
▲ Hycamtin for Injection (59%) 1458

Liver tenderness
Actiq (Less than 1%)......................... 979

Liver transplant, need for
Lamisil Tablets.................................. 2232

Liver tumors
(*see under* Hepatomas)

Loffler's syndrome
Paser Granules 1674

Loss of balance
(*see under* Balance, loss of)

Lower respiratory signs and symptoms
▲ Advair HFA Inhalation Aerosol (1% to 3%).. 1318
Serevent Diskus (1% to less than 3%)... 1568

Lumbago
Klonopin (Infrequent)........................ 2778
Prinivil Tablets (0.3% to 1.0%).......... 2052
Prinzide Tablets 2056

Lump at injection site
Bicillin C-R Injectable Suspension..... 1706
ProQuad... 2064

Lung crackles
▲ Dacogen Injection (14%) 2129

Lung development, hypoplastic
Altace Capsules................................ 1702
Captopril Tablets 2149
Cozaar Tablets 1935
Hyzaar 50-12.5 Tablets 1990
Hyzaar 100-12.5 Tablets 1990
Hyzaar 100-25 Tablets 1990
Lotrel Capsules 2249
Prinivil Tablets 2052
Prinzide Tablets 2056
Vasotec I.V. Injection 2103

Lung disorders, unspecified
Actiq (Less than 1%) 979
Alinia for Oral Suspension (Less than 1%) 2835
Alinia Tablets (Less than 1%) 2835
▲ AmBisome for Injection (13.6% to 17.8%) 620
BeneFix Vials (1.5%)........................ 3408
▲ CellCept Capsules (3% to less than 20%) 2747
▲ CellCept Intravenous (3% to less than 20%) 2747
▲ CellCept Oral Suspension (3% to less than 20%) 2747
▲ CellCept Tablets (3% to less than 20%) 2747
▲ DuoNeb Inhalation Solution (6.4%) .. 1058
▲ Humira Injection (Less than 5%) 466
Ionsys Transdermal System (.1% to less than 1%) 2379
▲ I.V. Busulfex (34%) 2493
▲ Leukine (20%) 814
▲ Megace ES Oral Suspension (1% to 3%) 2481
Myobloc Injection (Greater than 2%) 3192
Neurontin Capsules (Infrequent) 2487
Neurontin Oral Solution (Infrequent) 2487
Neurontin Tablets (Infrequent) 2487
▲ Nipent for Injection (Up to 12%) 1863
Norvir (Less than 2%) 503
▲ Ontak Vials (8%) 1745
▲ Prograf Capsules and Injection (3% to 15%) 632
▲ Proleukin for Injection (24%) 2266
Protonix I.V. (Less than 1%) 3472
Protonix Tablets (Less than 1%) 3469
Protopic Ointment (Greater than or equal to 1%) 638
Provigil Tablets (2%) 988
Pulmozyme Inhalation Solution 1248
▲ Rituxan I.V. (6% to 31%) 1254
Rythmol SR Capsules 2727
Symbyax Capsules (Frequent) 1819
Thalomid Capsules 965
▲ Trasylol Injection (7%) 754
Ventolin HFA Inhalation Aerosol (Less than 3%) 1600
Zemaira (0.2% to 0.4%) 3509

Lung function, decreased
▲ Humira Injection (Less than 5%) 466

Lung infiltration
Dacogen Injection 2129
Prograf Capsules and Injection 632
Revlimid Capsules 958
Solodyn Extended Release Tablets .. 1890
Tarceva Tablets 1259
Tarceva Tablets 2444

Lung injury, acute, infusion related
Gammagard Liquid 721

Lung injury, transfusion-associated
Carimune NF ... 3499
Flebogamma 5%, Immune Globulin Intravenous (Human) ... 1658
Gammagard S/D (Rare) ... 724
Gamunex Immune Globulin I.V., 10% (Rare) ... 3235

Lung neoplasms, malignant
Prinzide Tablets ... 2056

Lupus erythematosus
Advicor Tablets ... 1722
Aldoril Tablets ... 1910
Carbatrol Capsules (Isolated cases) ... 3171
Cosopt Sterile Ophthalmic Solution ... 1931
Cuprimine Capsules ... 1947
Dapsone Tablets USP ... 1673
Depacon Injection ... 412
Depakene ... 417
Depakote Sprinkle Capsules ... 422
▲ Depakote Tablets (1% to 5%) ... 427
Depakote ER Tablets (Greater than 1%) ... 434
Evoxac Capsules (Less than 1%) ... 1047
Gantrisin Pediatric Suspension ... 2770
Gris-PEG Tablets ... 2502
▲ Humira Injection (Less than 5%) ... 466
Inderal LA Long-Acting Capsules (Rare) ... 3429
Permax Tablets (Rare) ... 3356
Phenytek Capsules ... 2160
Recombivax HB ... 2071
Syprine Capsules ... 2085
Tegretol/Tegretol-XR (Isolated cases) ... 2295
Timoptic Sterile Ophthalmic Solution (Less frequent) ... 2088
Timoptic in Ocudose (Less frequent) ... 2091
Timoptic-XE Sterile Ophthalmic Gel Forming Solution ... 2092
Trileptal Tablets ... 2300
Trileptal Oral Suspension ... 2300
Zonegran Capsules (Rare) ... 1101

Lupus erythematosus, discoid
Enbrel for Injection ... 584
VFEND I.V. (Less than 2%) ... 2564
VFEND Oral Suspension (Less than 2%) ... 2564
VFEND Tablets (Less than 2%) ... 2564

Lupus erythematosus, disseminated, aggravation of
Equetro Extended-Release Capsules ... 3180

Lupus erythematosus, systemic
Anaprox Tablets ... 2761
Anaprox DS Tablets ... 2761
Benicar HCT Tablets ... 1044
Copegus Tablets (Less than 1%) ... 2754
Cosopt Sterile Ophthalmic Solution ... 1931
EC-Naprosyn Delayed-Release Tablets ... 2761
Inderal LA Long-Acting Capsules (Extremely rare) ... 3429
InnoPran XL Capsules (Rare) ... 2723
Lamisil Tablets (Infrequently) ... 2232
Naprosyn Suspension ... 2761
Naprosyn Tablets ... 2761
Pegasys (Less than 1%) ... 2789
Phenytek Capsules ... 2160
Recombivax HB ... 2071
Syprine Capsules ... 2085
Timoptic Sterile Ophthalmic Solution (Less frequent) ... 2088
Timoptic in Ocudose (Less frequent) ... 2091
Timoptic-XE Sterile Ophthalmic Gel Forming Solution ... 2092

Lupus erythematosus, systemic, exacerbation of
Seasonique Tablets ... 1077

Lupus erythematosus, systemic, exacerbation or activation of
Carbatrol Capsules ... 3171
Dyazide Capsules ... 1423
Furosemide Tablets ... 2154
Oracea Capsules ... 1000
Premphase Tablets ... 3456
Prempro Tablets ... 3456
Prinzide Tablets ... 2056
Solodyn Extended Release Tablets ... 1890
Tegretol/Tegretol-XR ... 2295

Lupus-like syndrome
Aldoril Tablets ... 1910
Altoprev Extended-Release Tablets (Rare) ... 3109
Asacol Delayed-Release Tablets ... 2692
Cuprimine Capsules ... 1947
Enbrel for Injection ... 584
Equetro Extended-Release Capsules ... 3180
Gris-PEG Tablets ... 2502
Humira Injection ... 466
InnoPran XL Capsules (Rare) ... 2723
Lamictal ... 1481
Lescol Capsules (Rare) ... 2233
Lescol XL Tablets ... 2233
Mevacor Tablets (Rare) ... 2021
PEG-Intron Powder for Injection (Less than or equal to 1%) ... 3048
Recombivax HB ... 2071
Remicade for IV Injection (Rare) ... 971
Rituxan I.V. ... 1254
Solodyn Extended Release Tablets ... 1890
Tegretol-XR Tablets (Isolated cases) ... 2295
Thiola Tablets ... 2141
Tricor Tablets ... 527
Vytorin 10/10 Tablets ... 2114
Vytorin 10/10 Tablets ... 3077
Vytorin 10/20 Tablets ... 2114
Vytorin 10/20 Tablets ... 3077
Vytorin 10/40 Tablets ... 2114
Vytorin 10/40 Tablets ... 3077
Vytorin 10/80 Tablets ... 2114
Vytorin 10/80 Tablets ... 3077
Zocor Tablets (Rare) ... 2105
Zoloft ... 2586

Lyell's syndrome
(*see under* Necrolysis, epidermal, toxic)

Lymph nodes, swelling
▲ ADACEL Vaccine (0.1% to 6.6%) ... 2945

Lymph nodes, tender
ProSom Tablets (Rare) ... 517
Stromectol Tablets (1.9%) ... 2083

Lymphadenitis
Boostrix ... 1404
▲ Intron A for Injection (Less than or equal to 5%) ... 3024
ProQuad ... 2064

Lymphadenopathy
Abilify Oral Solution (Infrequent) ... 882
Abilify Oral Solution (Infrequent) ... 2450
Abilify Discmelt Orally Disintegrating Tablets (Infrequent) ... 882
Abilify Discmelt Orally Disintegrating Tablets (Infrequent) ... 2450
Abilify Tablets (Infrequent) ... 882
Abilify Tablets (Infrequent) ... 2450
AccuNeb Inhalation Solution (0.9% to 2.6%) ... 1055
Accutane Capsules ... 2731
Aciphex Tablets ... 1090
Actiq (1% or greater) ... 979
Adalat CC Tablets (Less than 1%) ... 2964
▲ Aerobid/Aerobid-M (1% to 3%) ... 1171
Alferon N Injection (1%) ... 1665
Ambien Tablets (Rare) ... 2851
Ambien CR Tablets (Rare) ... 2855
Anaprox Tablets (Less than 1%) ... 2761
Anaprox DS Tablets (Less than 1%) ... 2761
Arthrotec Tablets (Rare) ... 3129
Asacol Delayed-Release Tablets ... 2692
Attenuvax (Less common) ... 1914
▲ Betaseron for SC Injection (8%) ... 767
Bicillin C-R Injectable Suspension ... 1706
Boostrix ... 1404
Caduet Tablets (Less than 2%) ... 2508
Campath Ampules ... 811
Campral Tablets (Rare) ... 1174
Carbatrol Capsules ... 3171
Celexa (Infrequent) ... 1176
Chantix Tablets (Infrequent) ... 2517
Cipro (0.3% to 1%) ... 2977
Cipro I.V. (1% or less) ... 2984
Cipro XR Tablets ... 2990
Colazal Capsules ... 2838
Combivir Tablets ... 1411
Comvax ... 1928
▲ Copaxone for Injection (12%) ... 3297
Cubicin for Injection (Less than 1%) ... 1026
Cuprimine Capsules ... 1947
▲ Dacogen Injection (12%) ... 2129
Depakote ER Tablets ... 434
Diastat Rectal Delivery System (Less than 1%) ... 3343
Doxil Injection (Less than 1%) ... 2351
EC-Naprosyn Delayed-Release Tablets (Less than 1%) ... 2761
Effexor Tablets (Infrequent) ... 3411
Effexor XR Capsules (Infrequent) ... 3417
Enbrel for Injection ... 584
Engerix-B Vaccine (Less than 1%) ... 1425
Epivir ... 1427
Epivir-HBV ... 1432
Epzicom Tablets ... 1436
▲ Equetro Extended-Release Capsules (Less than 5%) ... 3180
Evoxac Capsules (Less than 1%) ... 1047
Exelon Capsules (Infrequent) ... 2206
Exelon Oral Solution (Infrequent) ... 2206
Ferrlecit Injection ... 3388
Fluarix ... 1451
▲ Fortical Nasal Spray (1% to 3%) ... 3337
Fuzeon Injection ... 2767
Gabitril Tablets (Frequent) ... 984
Gengraf Capsules (1% to less than 3%) ... 459
Geodon Capsules (Infrequent) ... 2529
Havrix Vaccine (Rare) ... 1456
Imitrex Nasal Spray (Rare) ... 1467
Imitrex Tablets (Rare) ... 1471
Infanrix Vaccine ... 1476
Infed Injection ... 3390
▲ Infergen (4% to 6%) ... 3364
▲ Intron A for Injection (Less than or equal to 5%) ... 3024
Invirase (Less than 2%) ... 2772
Kaletra (Less than 2%) ... 476
Klonopin ... 2778
Lamictal (2%) ... 1481
Levaquin (0.1% to 0.9%) ... 2384
Levaquin in 5% Dextrose Injection (0.1% to 0.9%) ... 2384
Lipitor Tablets (Less than 2%) ... 2483
Lofibra Tablets ... 1219
Lofibra Capsules ... 1216
Lunesta Tablets (Infrequent) ... 3142
▲ Lupron Depot 3.75 mg (Among most frequent) ... 3260
Lupron Depot–3 Month 11.25 mg (Less than 5%) ... 3265
Lyrica Capsules (0.1% to 1%) ... 2539
Meridia Capsules ... 489
Meruvax II ... 2019
▲ Miacalcin Nasal Spray (1% to 3%) ... 2253
Mintezol ... 2027
M-M-R II ... 2006
Mumpsvax ... 2031
Nalfon Capsules (Less than 1%) ... 2502
Naprosyn Suspension (Less than 1%) ... 2761
Naprosyn Tablets (Less than 1%) ... 2761
Neoral Oral Solution (1% to less than 3%) ... 2259
Neoral Soft Gelatin Capsules (1% to less than 3%) ... 2259
Neurontin Capsules (Infrequent) ... 2487
Neurontin Oral Solution (Infrequent) ... 2487
Neurontin Tablets (Infrequent) ... 2487
Norvir (Less than 2%) ... 503
Omacor Capsules ... 2725
Orthoclone OKT3 Sterile Solution (Less than 1%) ... 2360
OxyContin Tablets (Less than 1%) ... 2703
▲ Paser Granules (46% of 38 patients with drug-induced hepatitis) ... 1674
Paxil CR Controlled-Release Tablets (Infrequent) ... 1538
Paxil (Infrequent) ... 1530
Pediarix Vaccine ... 1548
Liquid PedvaxHIB ... 2035
Permax Tablets (Infrequent) ... 3356
Pexeva Tablets (Infrequent) ... 1694
Phenytek Capsules ... 2160
Prevacid Delayed-Release Capsules (Less than 1%) ... 3271
Prevacid for Delayed-Release Oral Suspension (Less than 1%) ... 3271
Prevacid SoluTab Delayed-Release Orally Disintegrating Tablets (Less than 1%) ... 3271
Prevacid NapraPAC (Less than 1%) ... 3280
PREVPAC (Less than 1%) ... 3284
▲ Prometrium Capsules (100 mg, 200 mg) (Less than 5%) ... 3203
Proquin XR Tablets ... 1153
▲ Protopic Ointment (1% to 3%) ... 638
Prozac Pulvules and Liquid ... 1801
Quadramet Injection (2%) ... 1040
Raniclor Tablets, Chewable ... 2505
▲ Rapamune Oral Solution and Tablets (3% to 20%) ... 3475
▲ Rebif Prefilled Syringe for Injection (11% to 12%) ... 3159
Recombivax HB (Less than 1%) ... 2071
Relpax Tablets (Rare) ... 2548
Remicade for IV Injection (Greater than or equal to 0.2%) ... 971
Retrovir Capsules ... 1560
Retrovir IV Infusion ... 1564
Retrovir ... 1560
Rilutek Tablets (Rare) ... 2930
Risperdal (Rare) ... 1676
Risperdal Consta Long-Acting Injection (Infrequent) ... 1682
Risperdal M-Tab Orally Disintegrating Tablets (Rare) ... 1676
Rythmol SR Capsules ... 2727
Seroquel Tablets (Infrequent) ... 690
Sonata Capsules (Infrequent) ... 1717
Symbyax Capsules (Infrequent) ... 1819
Tamiflu Capsules (1%) ... 2807
Tamiflu Oral Suspension (1%) ... 2807
Tegretol/Tegretol-XR ... 2295
Tequin Injection (Less than 0.1%) ... 938
Tequin Injection in 5% Dextrose (Less than 0.1%) ... 938
Tequin Tablets (Less than 0.1%) ... 938
▲ Thalomid Capsules (5.6% to 12.5%) ... 965
Thiola Tablets ... 2141
Topamax Sprinkle Capsules (Infrequent) ... 2404
Topamax Tablets (Infrequent) ... 2404
Tricor Tablets ... 527
Triglide Tablets ... 3123
Trileptal Tablets (Up to 2%) ... 2300
Trileptal Oral Suspension (Up to 2%) ... 2300
▲ Trisenox Injection (8%) ... 993
Trizivir Tablets ... 1589
Twinrix Vaccine (Less than 1%) ... 1595
Uniretic Tablets (Less than 1%) ... 3100
Varivax (Greater than or equal to 1%) ... 2100
VFEND I.V. (Less than 2%) ... 2564
VFEND Oral Suspension (Less than 2%) ... 2564
VFEND Tablets (Less than 2%) ... 2564
Viramune Oral Suspension ... 873
Viramune Tablets ... 873
Vivitrol ... 995
Voltaren Tablets (Rarely) ... 2307
Voltaren-XR Tablets (Rarely) ... 2310
Wellbutrin Tablets (Rare) ... 1603
Wellbutrin SR Sustained-Release Tablets ... 1607
Wellbutrin XL Extended-Release Tablets ... 1613
Xopenex Inhalation Solution ... 3146
Xopenex Inhalation Solution Concentrate ... 3150
Xopenex HFA Inhalation Aerosol ... 3154
Xyrem Oral Solution (Infrequent) ... 1688
Ziagen ... 1626
Zomig Nasal Spray (Rare) ... 3523
Zonegran Capsules (Infrequent) ... 1101
Zovirax ... 1643
Zyban Sustained-Release Tablets ... 1644
Zyflo Tablets (Greater than 1%) ... 1023
Zyprexa Tablets (Infrequent) ... 1830
Zyprexa ZYDIS Orally Disintegrating Tablets (Infrequent) ... 1830
Zyrtec Chewable Tablets (Less than 2%) ... 2594
Zyrtec (Less than 2%) ... 2594
Zyrtec-D 12 Hour Extended Release Tablets (Less than 2%) ... 2597

Lymphadenopathy, cervical
Lexapro Oral Solution (Infrequent) ... 1190
Lexapro Tablets (Infrequent) ... 1190
Nexium Delayed-Release Capsules (Less than 1%) ... 655
Nexium I.V. (Less than 1%) ... 659
▲ Pulmicort Respules (1% to 3%) ... 661
Risperdal Consta Long-Acting Injection (Infrequent) ... 1682

Lymphadenopathy, localized
Prevnar for Injection ... 3463
ProQuad ... 2064

Lymphadenopathy, post-cervical
Evoxac Capsules (Less than 1%) ... 1047

Lymphangitis, regional
Doxil Injection (Less than 1%) ... 2351
Herceptin I.V. (At least one of the 958 patients) ... 1233

Lymphangitis, unspecified
VFEND I.V. (Less than 2%) ... 2564

VFEND Oral Suspension (Less than 2%) 2564
VFEND Tablets (Less than 2%) 2564

Lymphedema
Actiq (1% or greater) 979
▲ Arimidex Tablets (9% to 10%) 673
Aromasin Tablets (Less frequent) 2600
Copaxone for Injection (Infrequent) 3297
Doxil Injection (Less than 1%) 2351
Humatrope Vials and Cartridges 1787
Paxil CR Controlled-Release Tablets (Rare) 1538
Paxil (Rare) 1530
Pexeva Tablets (Rare) 1694
Prozac Pulvules and Liquid (Rare) 1801
Requip Tablets (Infrequent) 1555
Thalomid Capsules 965
▲ Xeloda Tablets (Less than 1% to 3%) 2822

Lymphedema, post-mastectomy
▲ Femara Tablets (7%) 2214

Lymphocele
▲ Myfortic Tablets (3% to less than 20%) 2255
▲ Rapamune Oral Solution and Tablets (3% to 20%) 3475

Lymphocytes, decrease
(*see under* Lymphocytopenia)

Lymphocytes, increase
(*see under* Lymphocytosis)

Lymphocytes, atypical
Coreg Tablets (Less than or equal to 0.1%) 1414
Pexeva Tablets (Rare) 1694

Lymphocytopenia
▲ Amevive (2% to 59%) 626
▲ Betaseron for SC Injection (88%) 767
Camptosar Injection 2604
Colazal Capsules 2838
▲ Copegus Tablets (14%) 2754
Fosamax 1969
I.V. Busulfex 2493
Leukeran Tablets 1504
Levaquin (2.3%) 2384
Levaquin in 5% Dextrose Injection (2.3%) 2384
Mavik Tablets (0.3% to 1.0%) 486
Mustargen for Injection 2468
Mycamine for Injection (0.8%) 628
Nabi-HB (2%) 2169
▲ Nexavar Tablets (Very Common) 746
Omnicef Capsules (1%) 511
Omnicef for Oral Suspension (0.8%) 511
Orthoclone OKT3 Sterile Solution (Less than 1%) 2360
Paxil CR Controlled-Release Tablets (Rare) 1538
Paxil (Rare) 1530
▲ Pegasys (3% to 86%) 2789
▲ Prezista Tablets (4.6% to 10.9%) 3306
Requip Tablets (Infrequent) 1555
Risperdal Consta Long-Acting Injection (Rare) 1682
▲ Rituxan I.V. (40% to 48%) 1254
Rocephin Injectable Vials, ADD-Vantage, Galaxy, Bulk (Less than 1%) 2800
▲ Sutent Capsules (1% to 38%) 2560
Tarka Tablets 524
▲ Temodar Capsules (55% to 60%) 3073
Topamax Sprinkle Capsules (Infrequent) 2404
Topamax Tablets (Infrequent) 2404
Trizivir Tablets 1589
Vantin Tablets and Oral Suspension 2645
▲ Xeloda Tablets (13% to 99%) 2822
Ziagen 1626
Zmax for Oral Suspension (Greater then or equal to 1%) 2583

Lymphocytosis
Campral Tablets (Infrequent) 1174
Celexa (Rare) 1176
Cipro I.V. (Infrequent) 2984
Depacon Injection 412
Depakene 417
Depakote Sprinkle Capsules 422
Depakote Tablets 427
Depakote ER Tablets 434
Effexor Tablets (Rare) 3411
Evoxac Capsules 1047
Fortaz (Very rare) 1453
Geodon Capsules (Rare) 2529
▲ Infergen (5% to 11%) 3364
▲ Intron A for Injection (Less than 5%) 3024
Neurontin Capsules (Rare) 2487
Neurontin Oral Solution (Rare) 2487
Neurontin Tablets (Rare) 2487
Norvir (Less than 2%) 503
Omnicef Capsules (0.2%) 511
Omnicef for Oral Suspension (2%) 511
Paxil CR Controlled-Release Tablets (Rare) 1538
Paxil (Rare) 1530
Permax Tablets (Rare) 3356
Pexeva Tablets (Rare) 1694
Primaxin I.M. 2045
Primaxin I.V. 2048
Prozac Pulvules and Liquid (Rare) 1801
Raniclor Tablets, Chewable 2505
▲ Raptiva for Injection (40%) 1250
Requip Tablets (Infrequent) 1555
Rocephin Injectable Vials, ADD-Vantage, Galaxy, Bulk (Less than 0.1%) 2800
Sonata Capsules (Rare) 1717
Targretin Capsules 1747
Thalomid Capsules 965
Topamax Sprinkle Capsules (Rare) 2404
Topamax Tablets (Rare) 2404
Uniretic Tablets (Less than 1%) 3100
Vantin Tablets and Oral Suspension 2645
Xifaxan Tablets (Less than 2%) 2842

Lymphoma
Amevive (Less than 0.1%) 626
Campath Ampules 811
CellCept Capsules (0.4% to 1%) 2747
CellCept Intravenous (0.4% to 1%) 2747
CellCept Oral Suspension (0.4% to 1%) 2747
CellCept Tablets (0.4% to 1%) 2747
Elidel Cream 1% 2200
▲ Enbrel for Injection (9%) 584
▲ Gengraf Capsules (Less than 1% to 6%) 459
▲ Humira Injection (Less than 5%) 466
Myfortic Tablets (0.9% to 1.3%) 2255
▲ Neoral Oral Solution (Less than 1% to 6%) 2259
▲ Neoral Soft Gelatin Capsules (Less than 1% to 6%) 2259
Orencia Powder for Intravenous Infusion (4 cases) 914
Orthoclone OKT3 Sterile Solution (Less than 1%) 2360
Phenytek Capsules 2160
Prograf Capsules and Injection 632
Protopic Ointment 638
▲ Rapamune Oral Solution and Tablets (0.6% to 3.2%) 3475
Remicade for IV Injection (Greater than or equal to 0.2%) 971
Revlimid Capsules 958
▲ Sandimmune (Less than 1% to 6%) 2275
Simulect for Injection (0.3%) 2284

Lymphoma, Hodgkin's
Raptiva for Injection 1250

Lymphoma, lymphocytic
Dantrium Capsules (Less frequent) 2694
Dantrium Intravenous 2695

Lymphoma, non-Hodgkin's
Neurontin Capsules (Rare) 2487
Neurontin Oral Solution (Rare) 2487
Neurontin Tablets (Rare) 2487
Raptiva for Injection 1250

Lymphoma-like disorder
Colazal Capsules 2838
▲ Humira Injection (Less than 5%) 466
Paser Granules 1674
Tegretol/Tegretol-XR 2295
Zelapar Tablets 3372

Lymphopenia
(*see also under* Lymphocytopenia)
Amevive 626
Revlimid Capsules (2.3%) 958

Lymphoproliferative disorder
CellCept Capsules (0.4% to 1%) 2747
CellCept Intravenous (0.4% to 1%) 2747
CellCept Oral Suspension (0.4% to 1%) 2747
CellCept Tablets (0.4% to 1%) 2747
Orthoclone OKT3 Sterile Solution 2360
▲ Rapamune Oral Solution and Tablets (0.6% to 3.2%) 3475
Simulect for Injection 2284

M

Maceration
Oxistat Cream (0.1%) 2667

Maceration, skin
Analpram-HC 1159
Apexicon E Cream 2661
Diprolene Lotion 0.05% (Infrequent) 3002
Diprolene Ointment 0.05% (Infrequent) 3003
Diprolene AF Cream 0.05% (Infrequent) 3000
Locoid Lipocream Cream (Infrequent) 1160
Neurontin Capsules (Rare) 2487
Neurontin Oral Solution (Rare) 2487
Neurontin Tablets (Rare) 2487
Olux Foam 1012
Pramosone 1161
ProctoFoam-HC 3099
Sulfamylon for 5% Topical Solution 2162
Temovate Scalp Application (Infrequent) 2670
Vanos Cream 1893

Macrocytosis
Depacon Injection 412
Depakene 417
Depakote Sprinkle Capsules 422
▲ Depakote Tablets (1% to 5%) 427
Depakote ER Tablets 434
Phenytek Capsules 2160
Retrovir Capsules 1560
Retrovir IV Infusion 1564
Retrovir 1560

Macroglobulinemia, Waldenstrom's, hyperviscosity syndrome in
Rituxan I.V. 1254

Macula lutea degeneration
Namenda (Infrequent) 1195

Maculae
Covera-HS Tablets (Less than 2%) 3139
Tarka Tablets 524
Verelan PM Extended-Release Capsules, Controlled-Onset (2% or less) 3106

Macular degeneration
Cymbalta Delayed-Release Capsules (Infrequent) 1757

Macular hypopigmentation
Zyprexa Tablets (Rare) 1830
Zyprexa ZYDIS Orally Disintegrating Tablets (Rare) 1830

Maculopathy
▲ Lucentis Injection (3% to 10%) 1237
▲ Retisert Implant (10% to 35%) ⊙ 258

Malabsorption syndrome
Atripla Tablets 945
Elspar for Injection 2463
Elspar for Injection 1960
Sustiva Capsules 930
Sustiva Tablets 930

Malaise
Abelcet Injection 1141
Abilify Oral Solution (Frequent) 882
Abilify Oral Solution (Frequent) 2450
Abilify Discmelt Orally Disintegrating Tablets (Frequent) 882
Abilify Discmelt Orally Disintegrating Tablets (Frequent) 2450
Abilify Tablets (Frequent) 882
Abilify Tablets (Frequent) 2450
Accolate Tablets 671
Accutane Capsules 2731
Aceon Tablets (2 mg, 4 mg, 8 mg) (0.3% to 1%) 3194
Aciphex Tablets 1090
Actiq (1% or greater) 979
Adalat CC Tablets (Less than 1%) 2964
▲ Advair Diskus 250/50 (3%) 1308
Advicor Tablets 1722
Aerobid/Aerobid-M (1% to 3%) 1171
Aggrenox Capsules (1.6%) 822
▲ Agrylin Capsules (6.4%) 3169
Aldara Cream, 5% 1846
▲ Alferon N Injection (9% to 65%) 1665
Alinia for Oral Suspension (Less than 1%) 2835
Alinia Tablets (Less than 1%) 2835
Altace Capsules (Less than 1%) 1702
Altoprev Extended-Release Tablets (Rare) 3109
Ambien Tablets (Infrequent) 2851
Ambien CR Tablets (Infrequent) 2855
AmBisome for Injection (Less common) 620
Amerge Tablets (2%) 1339
Amitiza Capsules (Less than 0.2%) 3224
Anaprox Tablets (Less than 1%) 2761
Anaprox DS Tablets (Less than 1%) 2761
Aptivus Capsules (Less than 2%) 826
▲ Arimidex Tablets (2% to 5%) 673
Arthrotec Tablets (Rare) 3129
Asacol Delayed-Release Tablets (1% to 2%) 2692
Astelin Nasal Spray (Infrequent) 1904
Attenuvax 1914
Avelox (0.1% to less than 2%) 2970
Avinza Capsules (Less than 5%) 1741
Azilect Tablets (2%) 3293
▲ Betaseron for SC Injection (8%) 767
BiDil Tablets (1% to less than 2%) 2171
Biltricide Tablets 2976
Buprenex Injectable (Infrequent) 2716
Caduet Tablets (Greater than 0.1% to less than 2%) 2508
Calcium Disodium Versenate Injection 1851
▲ Campath Ampules (1% to 9%) 811
Campral Tablets (Infrequent) 1174
Cancidas for Injection (0%) 1918
Captopril Tablets (0.5% to 2%) 2149
Cardura XL Tablets 2515
Catapres Tablets (About 1 in 100 patients) 843
Catapres-TTS (0.5% or less) 844
▲ CellCept Capsules (3% to less than 20%) 2747
▲ CellCept Intravenous (3% to less than 20%) 2747
▲ CellCept Oral Suspension (3% to less than 20%) 2747
▲ CellCept Tablets (3% to less than 20%) 2747
Cesamet Capsules 3340
▲ Chantix Tablets (4% to 7%) 2517
Cipro (Less than 1%) 2977
Cipro I.V. (1% or less) 2984
Cipro XR Tablets (Less than 1%) 2990
Clinoril Tablets (Less than 1 in 100) 1924
Clorpres Tablets (About 1%) 2153
Clozaril Tablets (Less than 1%) 2184
Colazal Capsules 2838
▲ Combivir Tablets (27%) 1411
Copaxone for Injection (At least 2%) 3297
▲ Coreg Tablets (Greater than 1% to 3%) 1414
Cosmegen for Injection 2459
Coumadin for Injection (Infrequent) 898
Coumadin Tablets (Infrequent) 898
Crixivan Capsules (2.1%) 1940
▲ Dacogen Injection (5%) 2129
▲ Dantrium Capsules (Among most frequent) 2694
Decadron Tablets 1951
▲ Depacon Injection (1% to 5%) 412
▲ Depakene (1% to 5%) 417
▲ Depakote Sprinkle Capsules (1% to 5%) 422
▲ Depakote Tablets (1% to 5%) 427
Depakote ER Tablets (Greater than 1%) 434
Dolobid Tablets (Less than 1 in 100) 1955
▲ Doxil Injection (1% to 5%) 2351
EC-Naprosyn Delayed-Release Tablets (Less than 1%) 2761
Edecrin 1959
Effexor Tablets (Infrequent) 3411
Effexor XR Capsules (Infrequent) 3417
Eldepryl Capsules 3208
▲ Eligard 7.5 mg (17.5%) 2880
Emend Capsules (Greater than 0.5%) 1963
Engerix-B Vaccine (Less than 1%) 1425
▲ Entocort EC Capsules (Less than 5%) 2698
▲ Epivir (27%) 1427
▲ Epivir-HBV (24%) 1432
▲ Erbitux (49%) 910
Evoxac Capsules (Less than 1%) 1047
▲ Exelon Capsules (5%) 2206
▲ Exelon Oral Solution (5%) 2206
FazaClo Orally Disintegrating Tablets (Less than 1%) 551
Ferrlecit Injection 3388
Flebogamma 5%, Immune Globulin Intravenous (Human) 1658
▲ Flovent Diskus (1% to 16%) 1443
▲ Fluarix (1% to 10%) 1451
Follistim AQ Cartridge 2338
Foradil Aerolizer 3010
Fosamax 1969
Fosamax Plus D Tablets 1977
Frova Tablets (Infrequent) 1113

Gabitril Tablets (Frequent) 984
Gardasil Injection (1.4%) 1984
Gemzar for Injection (Infrequent) 1771
Gengraf Capsules (1% to less than 3%) 459
▲ Havrix Vaccine (1% to 10%) 1456
▲ Hectorol Capsules (27.9%) 1275
▲ Hectorol Injection (27.9%) 1278
HibTITER 3426
Hycamtin for Injection (0.5% to 1.8%) 1458
Hydrocortone Tablets 1989
Hyperstat I.V. 3017
▲ Imdur Tablets (Less than or equal to 5%) 3018
Imitrex Injection (1.1%) 1463
▲ Imitrex Tablets (2% to 3%) 1471
▲ Indapamide Tablets (Greater than or equal to 5%) 2156
Indocin (Greater than 1%) 1995
Infed Injection 3390
▲ Infergen (2% to 11%) 3364
▲ Intron A for Injection (Up to 14%) 3024
Invanz for Injection (Greater than 0.1%) 1999
Kadian Capsules (Less than 3%) 577
Kaletra (Less than 2%) 476
Klonopin (Infrequent) 2778
Lamictal (2.3%) 1481
Lamisil Tablets 2232
Lariam Tablets 2786
Lescol Capsules (Rare) 2233
▲ Lescol XL Tablets (3.8%) 2233
▲ Leukine (57%) 814
▲ Leustatin Injection (5% to 7%) 2357
Levaquin (0.1% to 0.9%) 2384
Levaquin in 5% Dextrose Injection (0.1% to 0.9%) 2384
Lexapro Oral Solution (Infrequent) 1190
Lexapro Tablets (Infrequent) 1190
Lipitor Tablets (Less than 2%) 2483
▲ Lithostat Tablets (20% to 25%) 2140
Lofibra Tablets 1219
Lofibra Capsules 1216
Lotronex Tablets (Rare) 1512
Lunesta Tablets (Infrequent) 3142
Lyrica Capsules (0.1% to 1%) 2539
Marinol Capsules (Less than 1%) 3333
▲ Menactra Vaccine (1.1% to 23.6%) 2954
Meruvax II 2019
Mevacor Tablets (Rare) 2021
Micardis Tablets (More than 0.3%) 854
Micardis HCT Tablets 856
▲ Mirapex Tablets (2% to 3%) 859
M-M-R II 2006
Mobic Oral Suspension (Less than 2%) 863
Mobic Tablets (Less than 2%) 863
Moduretic Tablets (Less than or equal to 1%) 2028
▲ MoviPrep Oral Solution (19.4%) 2839
Myobloc Injection (Greater than 2%) 3192
Myozyme for Intravenous Infusion 1279
▲ Nabi-HB (6%) 2169
Nalfon Capsules (Less than 1%) 2502
Namenda 1195
Naprosyn Suspension (Less than 1%) 2761
Naprosyn Tablets (Less than 1%) 2761
Neoral Oral Solution (1% to less than 3%) 2259
Neoral Soft Gelatin Capsules (1% to less than 3%) 2259
Neurontin Capsules (Frequent) 2487
Neurontin Oral Solution (Frequent) 2487
Neurontin Tablets (Frequent) 2487
Nexium Delayed-Release Capsules (Less than 1%) 655
Nexium I.V. (Less than 1%) 659
Norvasc Tablets (More than 0.1% to 1%) 2545
Norvir (0.7% to 1.7%) 503
Omacor Capsules 2725
▲ Oncaspar (Greater than 5%) 1145
Orthoclone OKT3 Sterile Solution (Less than 1%) 2360
Oxsoralen-Ultra Capsules 3353
OxyContin Tablets (Less than 1%) 2703
Parcopa Orally Disintegrating Tablets 3097
Paxil CR Controlled-Release Tablets (Frequent) 1538
Paxil (Frequent) 1530
Pediarix Vaccine 1548
▲ PEG-Intron Powder for Injection (7%) 3048
Pentasa Capsules (Less than 1%) 3185
Percodan Tablets 1132
Permax Tablets (Infrequent) 3356
Persantine Tablets (Rare) 868
Pexeva Tablets (Infrequent) 1694
Pletal Tablets (Less than 2%) 2455
Pneumovax 23 2043
Prevacid Delayed-Release Capsules (Less than 1%) 3271
Prevacid for Delayed-Release Oral Suspension (Less than 1%) 3271
Prevacid SoluTab Delayed-Release Orally Disintegrating Tablets (Less than 1%) 3271
Prevacid NapraPAC (Less than 1%) 3280
PREVPAC (Less than 1%) 3284
Prilosec OTC Delayed-Release Tablets (Less than 1%) 2677
Prinivil Tablets (0.3% to 1.0%) 2052
Prinzide Tablets 2056
▲ Proleukin for Injection (27%) 2266
ProQuad (Greater than or equal to 0.2% to less than 1%) 2064
Proquin XR Tablets 1153
▲ ProSom Tablets (5%) 517
Protonix I.V. (Less than 1%) 3472
Protonix Tablets (Less than 1%) 3469
Protopic Ointment (Greater than or equal to 1%) 638
Proventil Inhalation Solution 0.083% (1.5%) 3055
Prozac Pulvules and Liquid (Infrequent) 1801
Pulmozyme Inhalation Solution 1248
▲ Rapamune Oral Solution and Tablets (3% to 20%) 3475
Razadyne (Frequent) 2399
▲ Rebetol (4% to 6%) 3058
▲ Rebif Prefilled Syringe for Injection (4% to 5%) 3159
Recombivax HB (Equal to or greater than 1%) 2071
Relenza Rotadisk (Less than 1.5%) 1552
Relpax Tablets (Infrequent) 2548
▲ Requip Tablets (3%) 1555
Rescriptor Tablets 2551
▲ Retrovir Capsules (8% to 53.2%) 1560
▲ Retrovir IV Infusion (8% to 53.2%) 1564
▲ Retrovir (8% to 53.2%) 1560
Reyataz Capsules (Less than 3%) 921
Rhophylac (Occasionally) 3505
▲ Ribavirin, USP Capsules (4% to 6%) 3068
Rilutek Tablets (0.4% to 1.2%) 2930
Risperdal (Infrequent) 1676
Risperdal Consta Long-Acting Injection (Infrequent) 1682
Risperdal M-Tab Orally Disintegrating Tablets (Infrequent) 1676
▲ Romazicon Injection (1% to 3%) 2804
Rythmol SR Capsules 2727
Seroquel Tablets (Infrequent) 690
▲ Simulect for Injection (3% to 10%) 2284
▲ Solodyn Extended Release Tablets (4%) 1890
Sonata Capsules (Less than 1% to 2%) 1717
Soriatane Capsules (Less than 1%) 1013
Stalevo Tablets 2287
Sular Tablets (Less than or equal to 1%) 3122
Sustiva Capsules (Less than 2%) 930
Sustiva Tablets (Less than 2%) 930
Symbyax Capsules (Infrequent) 1819
▲ Tambocor Tablets (1% to 3%) 1856
Tarka Tablets (0.3% or more) 524
Tasmar Tablets (1%) 3358
Teveten Tablets (Less than 1%) 1735
Teveten HCT Tablets (Less than 1%) 1737
▲ Thalomid Capsules (8.3%) 965
▲ Thymoglobulin for Intravenous Infusion (13.4%) 1284
Tindamax Tablets (1.1% to 2.1%) 2142
▲ TOBI Solution for Inhalation (6.2%) 2298
Tricor Tablets 527
Triglide Tablets 3123
Trileptal Tablets 2300
Trileptal Oral Suspension 2300
▲ Trizivir Tablets (44%) 1589
▲ Ultram ER Tablets (1% to greater than 5%) 2392
Univasc Tablets (Less than 1%) 3104
Vantas (Less than 2%) 3375
Vantin Tablets and Oral Suspension (Less than 1%) 2645
Varivax (Greater than or equal to 1%) 2100
▲ Velcade for Injection (65%) 2133
Verelan PM Extended-Release Capsules, Controlled-Onset 3106
▲ Vesanoid Capsules (66%) 2820
Viadur Implant (Less than 2%) 757
Viracept (Less than 2%) 2577
Viramune Oral Suspension 873
Viramune Tablets 873
Visudyne for Injection 2305
▲ Vivitrol (12% to 23%) 995
Voltaren Tablets (Occasionally) 2307
Voltaren-XR Tablets (Occasionally) 2310
Vytorin 10/10 Tablets 2114
Vytorin 10/10 Tablets 3077
Vytorin 10/20 Tablets 2114
Vytorin 10/20 Tablets 3077
Vytorin 10/40 Tablets 2114
Vytorin 10/40 Tablets 3077
Vytorin 10/80 Tablets 2114
Vytorin 10/80 Tablets 3077
Wellbutrin SR Sustained-Release Tablets (Rare) 1607
Wellbutrin XL Extended-Release Tablets (Rare) 1613
Xifaxan Tablets (Less than 2%) 2842
Xyrem Oral Solution (Frequent) 1688
Zantac (Rare) 1624
Zantac Injection (Rare) 1619
Zantac Injection Pharmacy Bulk Package (Rare) 1622
Zantac Injection Premixed (Rare) 1619
Zantac (Rare) 1624
Zegerid Capsules (Less than 1%) 2958
Zegerid Powder for Oral Solution (Less than 1%) 2958
▲ Ziagen (12%) 1626
▲ Zinecard for Injection (48% to 61%) 2650
Zmax for Oral Suspension 2583
Zocor Tablets (Rare) 2105
▲ Zofran Injection (5%) 1634
▲ Zofran (9% to 13%) 1639
▲ Zofran ODT Orally Disintegrating Tablets (9% to 13%) 1639
▲ Zoloft (1% to 10%) 2586
Zomig Tablets (Infrequent) 3519
Zomig-ZMT Tablets (Infrequent) 3519
Zonegran Capsules (Infrequent) 1101
Zosyn (1.0% or less) 3492
▲ Zovirax (11.5%) 1643
Zyban Sustained-Release Tablets (Rare) 1644
Zyflo Tablets (Greater than 1%) 1023
Zyprexa Tablets (Infrequent) 1830
Zyprexa ZYDIS Orally Disintegrating Tablets (Infrequent) 1830
▲ Zyrtec Chewable Tablets (Less than 2% to 3.6%) 2594
▲ Zyrtec (Less than 2% to 3.6%) 2594
Zyrtec-D 12 Hour Extended Release Tablets (Less than 2%) 2597

Male pattern baldness
(*see under* Alopecia hereditaria)

Malignancies, secondary
I.V. Busulfex 2493
Leukeran Tablets 1504
Temodar Capsules 3073
Xolair (0.5%) 1266

Malignancies, various types
Enbrel for Injection 584
Kineret Injection (45 patients) 599
Rapamune Oral Solution and Tablets (1.1% to 2.2%) 3475
Remicade for IV Injection (18 of 1678 patients) 971
Xolair (0.5%) 1266

Malignancy
Amevive (1.3% to 1.8%) 626
Myfortic Tablets (0.5%) 2255
Raptiva for Injection 1250
Thymoglobulin for Intravenous Infusion (Reported in 3 patients) 1284

Malignant hyperthermia
Proleukin for Injection (Less than 1%) 2266
Sandostatin LAR Depot (Rare) 2280
Ultane Liquid for Inhalation (Less than 1%) 531

Malignant melanoma
Elidel Cream 1% 2200
Parcopa Orally Disintegrating Tablets 3097
Protopic Ointment 638
Raptiva for Injection 1250
Xolair (0.5%) 1266

Malignant neoplasms
CellCept Capsules (0.7% to 2.1%) 2747
CellCept Intravenous (0.7% to 2.1%) 2747
CellCept Oral Suspension (0.7% to 2.1%) 2747
CellCept Tablets (0.7% to 2.1%) 2747
Emend Capsules (Greater than 0.5%) 1963
Orthoclone OKT3 Sterile Solution (Less than 1%) 2360
Xolair (0.5%) 1266

Malignant neoplasms, aggravated
Zometa for Intravenous Infusion 2315

Mania
Adderall Tablets 3164
Atripla Tablets 945
Cymbalta Delayed-Release Capsules (Very rare) 1757
Paxil CR Controlled-Release Tablets 1538
Paxil 1530
Prozac Pulvules and Liquid 1801
Ritalin Hydrochloride Tablets 2269
Ritalin LA Capsules 2271
Ritalin-SR Tablets 2269
Symbyax Capsules 1819
Zoloft 2586

Manic behavior
Abilify Oral Solution (Frequent) 882
Abilify Oral Solution (Frequent) 2450
Abilify Discmelt Orally Disintegrating Tablets (Frequent) 882
Abilify Discmelt Orally Disintegrating Tablets (Frequent) 2450
Abilify Tablets (Frequent) 882
Abilify Tablets (Frequent) 2450
Ambien Tablets (Rare) 2851
Campral Tablets (Rare) 1174
Celexa 1176
Cipro (Less than 1%) 2977
Cipro I.V. (1% or less) 2984
Cipro XR Tablets 2990
Concerta Extended-Release Tablets 1881
Copaxone for Injection (Infrequent) 3297
Effexor Tablets (0.5%) 3411
Effexor XR Capsules (0.5%) 3417
Evoxac Capsules (Less than 1%) 1047
Herceptin I.V. (At least one of the 958 patients) 1233
▲ Intron A for Injection (Less than 5%) 3024
Lamictal (Rare) 1481
Levaquin (0.1% to 0.9%) 2384
Levaquin in 5% Dextrose Injection (0.1% to 0.9%) 2384
Neurontin Capsules (Rare) 2487
Neurontin Oral Solution (Rare) 2487
Neurontin Tablets (Rare) 2487
Orthoclone OKT3 Sterile Solution (Less than 1%) 2360
Parnate Tablets 1527
Paxil CR Controlled-Release Tablets (Infrequent) 1538
Paxil (Infrequent) 1530
Permax Tablets (Infrequent) 3356
Provigil Tablets 988
Relpax Tablets (Rare) 2548
Requip Tablets (Infrequent) 1555
Rescriptor Tablets 2551
Retrovir IV Infusion 1564
Rilutek Tablets (Infrequent) 2930
▲ Risperdal (8%) 1676
Risperdal Consta Long-Acting Injection (Infrequent) 1682
▲ Risperdal M-Tab Orally Disintegrating Tablets (8%) 1676
Seroquel Tablets (Infrequent) 690
Sustiva Capsules (0.2%) 930
Sustiva Tablets (0.2%) 930
Symmetrel Tablets 1135
Tasmar Tablets (Infrequent) 3358
Topamax Sprinkle Capsules (Rare) 2404
Topamax Tablets (Rare) 2404
Trileptal Tablets 2300
Trileptal Oral Suspension 2300
Valtrex Caplets 1597
Wellbutrin Tablets (Frequent) 1603
Wellbutrin SR Sustained-Release Tablets 1607
Wellbutrin XL Extended-Release Tablets 1613
Zomig Nasal Spray (Rare) 3523
Zyban Sustained-Release Tablets 1644
Zyprexa Tablets (Frequent) 1830
Zyprexa ZYDIS Orally Disintegrating Tablets (Frequent) 1830

Manic reaction
Ambien CR Tablets (Rare) 2855
Azilect Tablets (Infrequent) 3293
▲ Equetro Extended-Release Capsules (Less than 5%) 3180
Lyrica Capsules (Rare) 2539
Pexeva Tablets (Infrequent) 1694

Proquin XR Tablets.......................... 1153

Manic symptoms
DextroStat Tablets.......................... 3179
Ritalin Hydrochloride Tablets............ 2269
Ritalin LA Capsules.......................... 2271
Ritalin-SR Tablets............................ 2269

Manic-depressive reaction
Abilify Oral Solution (Infrequent)......... 882
Abilify Oral Solution (Infrequent)....... 2450
Abilify Discmelt Orally Disintegrating Tablets (Infrequent)................................ 882
Abilify Discmelt Orally Disintegrating Tablets (Infrequent)................................ 2450
Abilify Tablets (Infrequent)................ 882
Abilify Tablets (Infrequent)................ 2450
Azilect Tablets (Rare)....................... 3293
▲ Equetro Extended-Release Capsules (7%)............................ 3180
Pexeva Tablets (Rare)....................... 1694

Marrow aplasia
Aloprim for Injection (Less than 1%)... 2167

Masculinization, female fetus
Oxandrin Tablets.............................. 2962

Mass, abdominal
(*see under* Abdominal mass)

Mass, pulmonary
Dacogen Injection............................ 2129

Mass at injection site
Amevive (1%)................................... 626
Betaseron for SC Injection (2%)........ 767
Boostrix.. 1404
Fluarix.. 1451
HibTITER... 3426
Xolair.. 1266

Mastalgia
(*see under* Mastodynia)

Mastitis
Amerge Tablets (Rare)....................... 1339
Aricept Tablets (Infrequent)............... 1094
Aricept ODT Tablets (Infrequent)......... 1094
Doxil Injection (Less than 1%)............ 2351
Effexor Tablets (Rare)........................ 3411
Effexor XR Capsules (Rare)................. 3417
▲ Intron A for Injection (Less than or equal to 5%)................................ 3024
Lunesta Tablets (Infrequent)............... 3142
Paxil CR Controlled-Release Tablets (Rare).............................. 1538
Paxil (Rare)..................................... 1530
Pexeva Tablets (Rare)....................... 1694
Requip Tablets (Rare)....................... 1555
Risperdal (Infrequent)....................... 1676
Risperdal M-Tab Orally Disintegrating Tablets (Infrequent)................................ 1676
Zoloft (Rare).................................... 2586
Zonegran Capsules (Rare)................. 1101

Mastodynia
Climara Transdermal System........... 771
Estratest Tablets.............................. 3199
Estratest H.S. Tablets....................... 3199
Inspra Tablets (0.1%)........................ 2536
Nalfon Capsules (Less than 1%)........ 2502
Premarin Intravenous........................ 3442
Premarin Vaginal Cream.................... 3452

Mazzotti reactions, worsening of
Stromectol Tablets............................ 2083

Measles
ProQuad... 2064

Mediastinal disorders, unspecified
▲ Focalin XR Capsules (9% to 16%) 2223

Megacolon, toxic
Camptosar Injection (Rare)............... 2604
Numorphan Injection........................ 1120

Megacolon, unspecified
Azilect Tablets (Rare)....................... 3293

Megaloblastic anemia
(*see under* Anemia, megaloblastic)

Meibomianitis
▲ Macugen Injection (1% to 5%) .... ⊙261

Melancholia
Celexa (Rare).................................. 1176

Melanoma, malignant, activation of
Stalevo Tablets................................ 2287

Melanoma, skin
Paxil CR Controlled-Release Tablets... 1538
Paxil.. 1530
Rapamune Oral Solution and Tablets (0.4% to 1.4%)................... 3475
Zelapar Tablets................................ 3372

Melanoma, unspecified
Bexxar... 1398
▲ Humira Injection (Less than 5%) 466

Melanosis
Celexa (Rare).................................. 1176
Copaxone for Injection (Infrequent)... 3297
▲ Intron A for Injection (Less than 5%)... 3024
Lyrica Capsules (Rare)..................... 2539
Neurontin Capsules (Rare)................ 2487
Neurontin Oral Solution (Rare).......... 2487
Neurontin Tablets (Rare).................. 2487
Sonata Capsules (Rare).................... 1717
VFEND I.V. (Less than 2%)................ 2564
VFEND Oral Suspension (Less than 2%)... 2564
VFEND Tablets (Less than 2%).......... 2564

Melasma
(*see under* Chloasma)

Melasma, possibly persistent
Estrasorb Topical Emulsion.............. 1147
Estratest Tablets.............................. 3199
Estratest H.S. Tablets....................... 3199
Premarin Tablets.............................. 3446
Premphase Tablets........................... 3456
Prempro Tablets............................... 3456
Seasonique Tablets.......................... 1077
Yasmin 28 Tablets............................ 796
Yaz Tablets...................................... 803

Melena
Abelcet Injection.............................. 1141
Abilify Oral Solution (Rare)............... 882
Abilify Oral Solution (Rare)............... 2450
Abilify Discmelt Orally Disintegrating Tablets (Rare)......... 882
Abilify Discmelt Orally Disintegrating Tablets (Rare)......... 2450
Abilify Tablets (Rare)........................ 882
Abilify Tablets (Rare)........................ 2450
Aciphex Tablets............................... 1090
Aggrenox Capsules (1.9%)................ 822
▲ Agrylin Capsules (1% to 5%) 3169
Anaprox Tablets (Less than 1%)....... 2761
Anaprox DS Tablets (Less than 1%).. 2761
Aricept Tablets (Infrequent).............. 1094
Aricept ODT Tablets (Infrequent)....... 1094
Arthrotec Tablets (Rare)................... 3129
Azilect Tablets (Rare)....................... 3293
Caduet Tablets (Less than 2%)......... 2508
Campath Ampules............................ 811
Campral Tablets (Rare)..................... 1174
▲ Carnitor Injection (2% to 6%) 3188
Celebrex Capsules (0.1% to 1.9%).... 3134
▲ CellCept Capsules (3% to less than 20%)....................................... 2747
▲ CellCept Intravenous (3% to less than 20%)....................................... 2747
▲ CellCept Oral Suspension (3% to less than 20%).............................. 2747
▲ CellCept Tablets (3% to less than 20%).. 2747
Colazal Capsules............................. 2838
Copaxone for Injection (Infrequent)... 3297
▲ Coreg Tablets (Greater than 1% to 3%)... 1414
Cymbalta Delayed-Release Capsules (Infrequent)................... 1757
Doxil Injection (Less than 1%)........... 2351
EC-Naprosyn Delayed-Release Tablets (Less than 1%)................ 2761
Effexor Tablets (Infrequent).............. 3411
Effexor XR Capsules (Infrequent)...... 3417
▲ Eloxatin for Injection (2% to 5%) 2892
Evoxac Capsules (Less than 1%)...... 1047
Exelon Capsules (Infrequent)............ 2206
Exelon Oral Solution (Infrequent)...... 2206
Ferrlecit Injection............................ 3388
Fosamax (Up to 1.3%)...................... 1969
Fosamax Plus D Tablets (0% to 1.3%)... 1977
Gabitril Tablets (Infrequent).............. 984
Gantrisin Pediatric Suspension......... 2770
Geodon Capsules (Rare)................... 2529
▲ Imdur Tablets (Less than or equal to 5%)... 3018
Imitrex Injection............................... 1463
Imitrex Nasal Spray (Rare)............... 1467
Imitrex Tablets (Rare)...................... 1471
▲ Intron A for Injection (Less than 5%)... 3024
Invirase (Less than 2%).................... 2772
Lamictal (Rare)................................ 1481
Levaquin (0.1% to 0.9%).................. 2384
Levaquin in 5% Dextrose Injection (0.1% to 0.9%)............................ 2384
Lipitor Tablets (Less than 2%).......... 2483
Lotensin Tablets (Less than 1%)....... 2243
Lotensin HCT Tablets....................... 2246
Lunesta Tablets (Infrequent)............. 3142
Lyrica Capsules (0.1% to 1%)........... 2539
Matulane Capsules........................... 3191
Merrem I.V. (0.3%)........................... 686
Mobic Oral Suspension (Less than 2%).. 863
Mobic Tablets (Less than 2%)........... 863
Mylotarg for Injection (1%)............... 3431
Namenda (Infrequent)...................... 1195
Naprosyn Suspension (Less than 1%).. 2761
Naprosyn Tablets (Less than 1%)..... 2761
Neurontin Capsules (Rare)............... 2487
Neurontin Oral Solution (Rare)......... 2487
Neurontin Tablets (Rare).................. 2487
Nexium Delayed-Release Capsules (Less than 1%).............................. 655
Nexium I.V. (Less than 1%).............. 659
Omacor Capsules............................. 2725
Omnicef Capsules............................ 511
Omnicef for Oral Suspension........... 511
Paxil CR Controlled-Release Tablets (Rare)............................. 1538
Paxil (Rare)..................................... 1530
Permax Tablets (Infrequent)............. 3356
Pexeva Tablets (Rare)...................... 1694
▲ Photofrin for Injection (5%) 702
Pletal Tablets (Less than 2%)........... 2455
Prevacid Delayed-Release Capsules (Less than 1%)............... 3271
Prevacid for Delayed-Release Oral Suspension (Less than 1%)........... 3271
Prevacid SoluTab Delayed-Release Orally Disintegrating Tablets (Less than 1%)............................. 3271
Prevacid NapraPAC (Less than 1%).. 3280
PREVPAC (Less than 1%)................ 3284
ProSom Tablets (Rare)..................... 517
Protonix I.V. (Less than 1%)............. 3472
Protonix Tablets (Less than 1%)....... 3469
Prozac Pulvules and Liquid (Infrequent)................................... 1801
Razadyne (Infrequent)...................... 2399
Razadyne ER Extended-Release Capsules (Infrequent).................. 2399
Requip Tablets (Infrequent).............. 1555
Revlimid Capsules........................... 958
Rilutek Tablets (Rare)...................... 2930
Risperdal (Infrequent)...................... 1676
Risperdal Consta Long-Acting Injection (Infrequent)................... 1682
Risperdal M-Tab Orally Disintegrating Tablets (Infrequent)................................ 1676
Rythmol SR Capsules...................... 2727
Sandostatin LAR Depot (1% to 4%)... 2280
Seroquel Tablets (Rare)................... 690
▲ Simulect for Injection (3% to 10%) ... 2284
Sonata Capsules (Infrequent)........... 1717
Soriatane Capsules (Less than 1%).. 1013
Sular Tablets (Less than or equal to 1%).. 3122
Tarceva Tablets............................... 1259
Tarceva Tablets............................... 2444
Targretin Capsules.......................... 1747
Topamax Sprinkle Capsules (Infrequent)................................... 2404
Topamax Tablets (Infrequent)........... 2404
Uniretic Tablets (Less than 1%)........ 3100
Vasotec I.V. Injection (0.5% to 1.0%).. 2103
VFEND I.V. (Less than 2%)............... 2564
VFEND Oral Suspension (Less than 2%).. 2564
VFEND Tablets (Less than 2%)......... 2564
Vicoprofen Tablets (Less than 3%).... 539
Voltaren Tablets (Occasionally)........ 2307
Voltaren-XR Tablets (Occasionally)... 2310
Zoloft (Rare).................................... 2586
Zomig Tablets (Rare)....................... 3519
Zomig-ZMT Tablets (Rare)................ 3519
Zonegran Capsules (Infrequent)....... 1101
Zosyn (1.0% or less)........................ 3492
Zyprexa Tablets (Infrequent)............ 1830
Zyprexa ZYDIS Orally Disintegrating Tablets (Infrequent)................................ 1830
Zyrtec Chewable Tablets (Less than 2%).. 2594
Zyrtec (Less than 2%)...................... 2594
Zyrtec-D 12 Hour Extended Release Tablets (Less than 2%)..... 2597

Memory disorders, unspecified
▲ Ambien CR Tablets (1% to 3%) 2855
Cesamet Capsules........................... 3340

Memory impairment
Abilify Oral Solution (Infrequent)........ 882
Abilify Oral Solution (Infrequent)....... 2450
Abilify Discmelt Orally Disintegrating Tablets (Infrequent)................................ 882
Abilify Discmelt Orally Disintegrating Tablets (Infrequent)................................ 2450
Abilify Tablets (Infrequent)................ 882
Abilify Tablets (Infrequent)................ 2450
Copaxone for Injection (Infrequent)... 3297
▲ Copegus Tablets (6%) 2754
Cozaar Tablets (Less than 1%)......... 1935
Eldepryl Capsules............................ 3208
Gleevec Tablets (Infrequent) 2227
Hyzaar 50-12.5 Tablets 1990
Hyzaar 100-12.5 Tablets 1990
Hyzaar 100-25 Tablets 1990
Imitrex Nasal Spray (Rare) 1467
Imitrex Tablets (Rare) 1471
▲ Klonopin (4%) 2778
Lamictal (2.4%) 1481
Lithobid Tablets 1692
Lunesta Tablets (Infrequent) 3142
▲ Lupron Depot 3.75 mg (Among most frequent) 3260
Lupron Depot–3 Month 11.25 mg (Less than 5%) 3265
Maxalt Tablets (Infrequent) 2008
Maxalt-MLT Orally Disintegrating Tablets (Infrequent) 2008
▲ Niravam Orally Disintegrating Tablets (5.5% to 33.1%) 3092
Parcopa Orally Disintegrating Tablets 3097
▲ Pegasys (5%) 2789
Prezista Tablets (Less than 2%) 3306
Prinivil Tablets (0.3% to 1.0%) 2052
Prinzide Tablets 2056
Revlimid Capsules 958
Seromycin Capsules 1813
Stalevo Tablets 2287
▲ Temodar Capsules (7%) 3073
Timolide Tablets 2086
▲ Topamax Sprinkle Capsules (2% to 14%) 2404
▲ Topamax Tablets (2% to 14%) 2404
Transderm Scōp Transdermal Therapeutic System (Infrequent) ... 2177
▲ Vesanoid Capsules (3%) 2820
Wellbutrin Tablets (Infrequent) 1603
▲ Wellbutrin SR Sustained-Release Tablets (Up to 3%) 1607
▲ Wellbutrin XL Extended-Release Tablets (3%) 1613
Xyrem Oral Solution (Frequent) 1688
▲ Zonegran Capsules (6%) 1101
Zyban Sustained-Release Tablets (Infrequent) 1644

Memory loss, short-term
Altoprev Extended-Release Tablets .. 3109
Blocadren Tablets 1916
Clozaril Tablets (Less than 1%) 2184
Cosopt Sterile Ophthalmic Solution 1931
Inderal LA Long-Acting Capsules 3429
InnoPran XL Capsules 2723
Lescol Capsules 2233
Lescol XL Tablets 2233
Lopressor Injection 2238
Lopressor Tablets 2238
Lopressor HCT 50/25 Tablets 2241
Lopressor HCT 100/25 Tablets 2241
Lopressor HCT 100/50 Tablets 2241
Meridia Capsules 489
Mevacor Tablets (0.5% to 1.0%) 2021
Nadolol Tablets 2159
Parnate Tablets 1527
Timoptic Sterile Ophthalmic Solution 2088
Timoptic in Ocudose 2091
Timoptic-XE Sterile Ophthalmic Gel Forming Solution 2092
Toprol-XL Tablets 668
Zocor Tablets 2105

Mendelson's syndrome
Abilify Oral Solution (Rare) 882
Abilify Oral Solution (Rare) 2450
Abilify Discmelt Orally Disintegrating Tablets (Rare) 882
Abilify Discmelt Orally Disintegrating Tablets (Rare) 2450
Abilify Tablets (Rare) 882

Abilify Tablets (Rare) 2450

Meniere's disease
Exelon Capsules (Infrequent) 2206
Exelon Oral Solution (Infrequent) 2206

Meniere's syndrome
Chantix Tablets (Rare) 2517
Imitrex Nasal Spray (Rare) 1467
Imitrex Tablets 1471

Meningism
Albenza Tablets (Up to 1.0%) 1338
Neurontin Capsules (Rare) 2487
Neurontin Oral Solution (Rare) 2487
Neurontin Tablets (Rare) 2487
Nipent for Injection (Less than 3%) 1863

Meningitis
Arthrotec Tablets (Rare) 3129
Campath Ampules 811
CellCept Capsules (Occasional) 2747
CellCept Intravenous (Occasional) 2747
CellCept Oral Suspension (Occasional) 2747
CellCept Tablets (Occasional) 2747
Depo-Medrol Single-Dose Vial 2619
Myfortic Tablets (Occasionally) 2255
Orthoclone OKT3 Sterile Solution (Less than 1%) 2360
Paxil CR Controlled-Release Tablets (Rare) 1538
Paxil (Rare) 1530
Permax Tablets (Infrequent) 3356
Pexeva Tablets (Rare) 1694
Proleukin for Injection (Less than 1%) 2266
Remicade for IV Injection (Greater than or equal to 0.2%) 971
Tasmar Tablets (Rare) 3358
Voltaren Tablets (Rarely) 2307
Voltaren-XR Tablets (Rarely) 2310

Meningitis, aseptic
Anaprox Tablets (Less than 1%) 2761
Anaprox DS Tablets (Less than 1%) 2761
Arthrotec Tablets (Rare) 3129
Carbatrol Capsules (One case) 3171
Celebrex Capsules (Less than 0.1%) 3134
EC-Naprosyn Delayed-Release Tablets (Less than 1%) 2761
Gammagard Liquid 721
Gamunex Immune Globulin I.V., 10% (Very rare) 3235
Mumpsvax 2031
Naprosyn Suspension (Less than 1%) 2761
Naprosyn Tablets (Less than 1%) 2761
Prevacid NapraPAC (Less than 1%) 3280
ProQuad 2064
Raptiva for Injection (1 case) 1250
Tegretol/Tegretol-XR (One case) 2295
Varivax 2100
Vicoprofen Tablets (Rare) 539

Meningitis, infectious
DepoCyt Injection 1143

Menometrorrhagia
▲ depo-subQ provera 104 Injectable Suspension (1% to less than 5%) 2624

Menopause
Effexor Tablets (Rare) 3411
Effexor XR Capsules (Rare) 3417
Permax Tablets (Infrequent) 3356
Sonata Capsules (Rare) 1717
Symbyax Capsules (Infrequent) 1819
Wellbutrin Tablets (Rare) 1603
Wellbutrin SR Sustained-Release Tablets 1607
Wellbutrin XL Extended-Release Tablets 1613
Zyban Sustained-Release Tablets 1644

Menorrhagia
Abilify Oral Solution (Rare) 882
Abilify Oral Solution (Rare) 2450
Abilify Discmelt Orally Disintegrating Tablets (Rare) 882
Abilify Discmelt Orally Disintegrating Tablets (Rare) 2450
Abilify Tablets (Rare) 882
Abilify Tablets (Rare) 2450
Aciphex Tablets (Rare) 1090
Ambien CR Tablets (1%) 2855
Arthrotec Tablets (Rare) 3129
Asacol Delayed-Release Tablets 2692
▲ Betaseron for SC Injection (8%) 767
Campral Tablets (Rare) 1174
▲ depo-subQ provera 104 Injectable Suspension (1% to less than 5%) 2624
Effexor Tablets (Infrequent) 3411
Effexor XR Capsules (Infrequent) 3417
Evoxac Capsules (Less than 1%) 1047
Gabitril Tablets (Infrequent) 984
Geodon Capsules (Infrequent) 2529
Gleevec Tablets (Infrequent) 2227
▲ Intron A for Injection (Less than 5%) 3024
Lamictal (Rare) 1481
Lunesta Tablets (Infrequent) 3142
Lyrica Capsules (0.1% to 1%) 2539
Neurontin Capsules (Infrequent) 2487
Neurontin Oral Solution (Infrequent) 2487
Neurontin Tablets (Infrequent) 2487
Paxil CR Controlled-Release Tablets (Infrequent) 1538
Paxil (Infrequent) 1530
Pentasa Capsules (Less than 1%) 3185
Permax Tablets (Infrequent) 3356
Pexeva Tablets (Rare to infrequent) 1694
Plavix Tablets (Less than 1%) 917
Plavix Tablets (Less than 1%) 2926
Prevacid Delayed-Release Capsules (Less than 1%) 3271
Prevacid for Delayed-Release Oral Suspension (Less than 1%) 3271
Prevacid SoluTab Delayed-Release Orally Disintegrating Tablets (Less than 1%) 3271
Prevacid NapraPAC (Less than 1%) 3280
PREVPAC (Less than 1%) 3284
Prozac Pulvules and Liquid (At least 2%) 1801
▲ Rapamune Oral Solution and Tablets (3% to 20%) 3475
Relpax Tablets (Rare) 2548
Risperdal (Frequent) 1676
Risperdal M-Tab Orally Disintegrating Tablets (Frequent) 1676
Seroquel Tablets (Infrequent) 690
Sonata Capsules (Infrequent) 1717
Symbyax Capsules (Frequent) 1819
Topamax Sprinkle Capsules (1% to 2%) 2404
Topamax Tablets (1% to 2%) 2404
Trileptal Tablets 2300
Trileptal Oral Suspension 2300
Vandazole Vaginal Gel (Less than 1%) 3338
Zelnorm Tablets 2312
Zoloft (Rare) 2586
Zomig Nasal Spray (Infrequent) 3523
Zonegran Capsules (Rare) 1101
Zyprexa Tablets (Infrequent) 1830
Zyprexa ZYDIS Orally Disintegrating Tablets (Infrequent) 1830
Zyrtec Chewable Tablets (Less than 2%) 2594
Zyrtec (Less than 2%) 2594
Zyrtec-D 12 Hour Extended Release Tablets (Less than 2%) 2597

Menstrual cramps
Lexapro Oral Solution (Frequent) 1190
Lexapro Tablets (Frequent) 1190
▲ Ortho Evra Transdermal System (9% to 22%) 2417

Menstrual disorders
Aceon Tablets (2 mg, 4 mg, 8 mg) (1.1%) 3194
▲ Advair HFA Inhalation Aerosol (3% to 5%) 1318
▲ Aerobid/Aerobid-M (3% to 9%) 1171
Ambien Tablets (Infrequent) 2851
Ambien CR Tablets (Infrequent) 2855
Anaprox Tablets (Less than 1%) 2761
Anaprox DS Tablets (Less than 1%) 2761
Asmanex Twisthaler (1% to less than 3%) 2966
Celebrex Capsules (0.1% to 1.9%) 3134
Chantix Tablets (Frequent) 2517
Cleocin Vaginal Ovules (Less than 1%) 2616
Colazal Capsules 2838
Depakote ER Tablets (Greater than 1%) 434
EC-Naprosyn Delayed-Release Tablets (Less than 1%) 2761
Effexor Tablets (1%) 3411
▲ Entocort EC Capsules (Less than 5%) 2698
Evoxac Capsules (Less than 1%) 1047
Gengraf Capsules (1%) 459
▲ Humira Injection (Less than 5%) 466
Lamictal (More than 1%) 1481
Lexapro Oral Solution (2% to frequent) 1190
Lexapro Tablets (2% to frequent) 1190
Lotronex Tablets (Infrequent) 1512
Lupron Depot 3.75 mg (1%) 3260
Lupron Depot–3 Month 11.25 mg (1%) 3265
Maxalt Tablets (Infrequent) 2008
Maxalt-MLT Orally Disintegrating Tablets (Infrequent) 2008
Meridia Capsules (Greater than or equal to 1%) 489
Mustargen for Injection 2468
Naprosyn Suspension (Less than 1%) 2761
Naprosyn Tablets (Less than 1%) 2761
Neoral Oral Solution (1%) 2259
Neoral Soft Gelatin Capsules (1%) 2259
Neurontin Capsules (Infrequent) 2487
Neurontin Oral Solution (Infrequent) 2487
Neurontin Tablets (Infrequent) 2487
Nexium Delayed-Release Capsules (Less than 1%) 655
Nexium I.V. (Less than 1%) 659
▲ Niravam Orally Disintegrating Tablets (10.4%) 3092
▲ PEG-Intron Powder for Injection (4%) 3048
Prevacid Delayed-Release Capsules (Less than 1%) 3271
Prevacid for Delayed-Release Oral Suspension (Less than 1%) 3271
Prevacid SoluTab Delayed-Release Orally Disintegrating Tablets (Less than 1%) 3271
Prevacid NapraPAC (Less than 1%) 3280
PREVPAC (Less than 1%) 3284
Provigil Tablets (At least 1%) 988
▲ Rebetol (6% to 7%) 3058
Relpax Tablets (Rare) 2548
Reyataz Capsules (Less than 3%) 921
▲ Ribavirin, USP Capsules (6% to 7%) 3068
▲ Soltamox Oral Solution (6%) 3527
Sonata Capsules (Rare) 1717
▲ Strattera Capsules (3%) 1814
▲ Topamax Sprinkle Capsules (1% to 3%) 2404
▲ Topamax Tablets (1% to 3%) 2404
Vaqta (1.1%) 2097
▲ Wellbutrin Tablets (4.7%) 1603
Yasmin 28 Tablets (Greater than 1%) 796
Yaz Tablets (Greater than 1%) 803
Zoloft (Infrequent) 2586

Menstrual flow, changes
Coumadin for Injection 898
Coumadin Tablets 898
Estratest Tablets 3199
Estratest H.S. Tablets 3199
Moban Tablets 1119
NuvaRing 2340
Ortho-Cyclen Tablets 2429
Ortho Evra Transdermal System 2417
Ortho Tri-Cyclen Tablets 2429
Ortho Tri-Cyclen Lo Tablets 2436
▲ Plan B Tablets (12.5% to 13.8%) 1076
Premarin Intravenous 3442
Premarin Tablets 3446
Premarin Vaginal Cream 3452
Seasonique Tablets 1077
▲ Soltamox Oral Solution (13%) 3527
Strattera Capsules (2%) 1814
Tarka Tablets 524
Yaz Tablets 803

Menstrual irregularities
Accutane Capsules 2731
Advair Diskus 100/50 1308
Advair Diskus 250/50 1308
Advair Diskus 500/50 1308
Advair HFA Inhalation Aerosol 1318
▲ Androxy Tablets (Most Common) 3335
Arthrotec Tablets (Rare) 3129
Colocort Rectal Suspension, USP (Retention) 100 mg/60 mL 2476
Covera-HS Tablets (Less than 2%) 3139
Decadron Tablets 1951
Depacon Injection 412
Depakene 417
Depakote Sprinkle Capsules 422
Depakote Tablets 427
Depakote ER Tablets 434
Depo-Medrol Injectable Suspension 2617
Depo-Medrol Single-Dose Vial 2619
▲ Depo-Provera Contraceptive Injection (Greater than 5%) 2622
▲ depo-subQ provera 104 Injectable Suspension (1% to less than 5%) 2624
▲ Estratest Tablets (Among most common) 3199
▲ Estratest H.S. Tablets (Among most common) 3199
Hydrocortone Tablets 1989
Imitrex Nasal Spray 1467
▲ Infergen (2% to 6%) 3364
▲ Intron A for Injection (Less than 5%) 3024
Klonopin (Infrequent) 2778
Levothroid Tablets 1186
Levoxyl Tablets 1712
Librium Capsules 3347
Mircette Tablets 1066
Niravam Orally Disintegrating Tablets 3092
▲ Ortho Micronor Tablets (Among most frequent) 2426
Oxandrin Tablets 2962
ParaGard T 380A Intrauterine Copper Contraceptive 1073
Premphase Tablets 3456
Prempro Tablets 3456
Prevacid Delayed-Release Capsules (Less than 1%) 3271
Prevacid for Delayed-Release Oral Suspension (Less than 1%) 3271
Prevacid SoluTab Delayed-Release Orally Disintegrating Tablets (Less than 1%) 3271
Prevacid NapraPAC (Less than 1%) 3280
PREVPAC (Less than 1%) 3284
Prometrium Capsules (100 mg, 200 mg) 3203
Remicade for IV Injection (Greater than or equal to 0.2%) 971
▲ Sandostatin LAR Depot (1% to 4%) 2280
▲ Soltamox Oral Solution (25%) 3527
Strattera Capsules (2%) 1814
Thioridazine Hydrochloride Tablets 2163
Vantin Tablets and Oral Suspension (Less than 1%) 2645
▲ Wellbutrin XL Extended-Release Tablets (5%) 1613
▲ Xenical Capsules (9.8%) 2831
Zyprexa Tablets (Infrequent) 1830
Zyprexa ZYDIS Orally Disintegrating Tablets (Infrequent) 1830

Menstruation, painful
ProSom Tablets (Infrequent) 517

Mental acuity, loss of
Parcopa Orally Disintegrating Tablets 3097
Retrovir Capsules 1560
Retrovir IV Infusion 1564
Retrovir 1560
Stalevo Tablets 2287
Tasmar Tablets (1%) 3358

Mental clouding
Dilaudid Ampules 440
Dilaudid Non-Sterile Powder 440
Dilaudid Rectal Suppositories 440
Dilaudid Tablets 440
Hycodan 1116
Hycotuss Expectorant Syrup 1117
Numorphan Injection 1120
Tussionex Pennkinetic Extended-Release Suspension 3327
Vicodin Tablets 535
Vicodin ES Tablets 536
Vicodin HP Tablets 538
Zydone Tablets 1139

Mental confusion
(*see under* Confusion)

Mental depression
(*see under* Depression)

Mental perception, altered
Cesamet Capsules 3340

Mental performance, impairment
Aldoril Tablets 1910
Alferon N Injection (1%) 1665
Ambien Tablets (Infrequent) 2851
Amerge Tablets (Infrequent) 1339
Anaprox Tablets (Less than 1%) 2761
Anaprox DS Tablets (Less than 1%) 2761
Arranon Injection (1%) 1357
Arthrotec Tablets (Rare) 3129
Celexa (Frequent) 1176
Chantix Tablets (Rare) 2517
Clozaril Tablets 2184
Copaxone for Injection (Infrequent) 3297
Cosopt Sterile Ophthalmic Solution 1931
Dilaudid 440
Dilaudid Non-Sterile Powder 440

Dilaudid Rectal Suppositories ... 440
Dilaudid Tablets ... 440
EC-Naprosyn Delayed-Release Tablets (Less than 1%) ... 2761
Exelon Capsules (Infrequent) ... 2206
Exelon Oral Solution (Infrequent) ... 2206
Flumadine (0.3% to 2.1%) ... 1183
Frova Tablets (Infrequent) ... 1113
▲ Gabitril Tablets (6%) ... 984
Gengraf Capsules (1% to less than 3%) ... 459
Hycodan ... 1116
Hycotuss Expectorant Syrup ... 1117
Imitrex Injection (Rare) ... 1463
Imitrex Nasal Spray (Rare) ... 1467
Imitrex Tablets (Infrequent) ... 1471
▲ Intron A for Injection (Up to 14%) ... 3024
Invirase (Less than 2%) ... 2772
Kadian Capsules (Less than 3%) ... 577
Klonopin (1% to 2%) ... 2778
Lamictal (1.7%) ... 1481
Levaquin (0.1% to 0.9%) ... 2384
Levaquin in 5% Dextrose Injection (0.1% to 0.9%) ... 2384
Lexapro Oral Solution (Frequent) ... 1190
Lexapro Tablets (Frequent) ... 1190
Maxalt Tablets (Frequent) ... 2008
Maxalt-MLT Orally Disintegrating Tablets (Infrequent) ... 2008
Meridia Capsules ... 489
Migranal Nasal Spray (Infrequent) ... 3348
MS Contin Tablets ... 2701
Naprosyn Suspension (Less than 1%) ... 2761
Naprosyn Tablets (Less than 1%) ... 2761
Neoral Oral Solution (1% to less than 3%) ... 2259
Neoral Soft Gelatin Capsules (1% to less than 3%) ... 2259
Opana Tablets (Less than 1%) ... 1122
Opana ER Tablets (Less than 1%) ... 1126
Paxil CR Controlled-Release Tablets (Frequent) ... 1538
Paxil (Frequent) ... 1530
Percocet Tablets ... 1131
Percodan Tablets ... 1132
Phenergan Tablets and Suppositories ... 3440
Prometrium Capsules (100 mg, 200 mg) (Less than 5%) ... 3203
ProSom Tablets ... 517
Rebetron Combination Therapy ... 3063
Requip Tablets (Infrequent) ... 1555
Risperdal (Infrequent) ... 1676
Risperdal M-Tab Orally Disintegrating Tablets (Infrequent) ... 1676
Seroquel Tablets ... 690
▲ Sustiva Capsules (1% to 9%) ... 930
▲ Sustiva Tablets (1% to 9%) ... 930
Sutent Capsules ... 2560
Tarka Tablets (Less frequent) ... 524
Timolide Tablets ... 2086
Timoptic Sterile Ophthalmic Solution ... 2088
Timoptic in Ocudose ... 2091
Timoptic-XE Sterile Ophthalmic Gel Forming Solution ... 2092
▲ Topamax Sprinkle Capsules (5% to 14%) ... 2404
▲ Topamax Tablets (5% to 14%) ... 2404
Tussionex Pennkinetic Extended-Release Suspension ... 3327
Tylenol with Codeine Tablets ... 2391
Vicodin Tablets ... 535
Vicodin ES Tablets ... 536
Vicodin HP Tablets ... 538
Vivitrol ... 995
Xyrem Oral Solution (Infrequent) ... 1688
Zelnorm Tablets ... 2312
Zoloft (1.3% to 2%) ... 2586
▲ Zonegran Capsules (6%) ... 1101
▲ Zyban Sustained-Release Tablets (9%) ... 1644
Zydone Tablets ... 1139
Zyrtec Chewable Tablets (Less than 2%) ... 2594
Zyrtec (Less than 2%) ... 2594
Zyrtec-D 12 Hour Extended Release Tablets (Less than 2%) ... 2597

Mental slowness
▲ Topamax Sprinkle Capsules (8% to 15.4%) ... 2404
▲ Topamax Tablets (8% to 15.4%) ... 2404
▲ Zonegran Capsules (4%) ... 1101

Mental status, altered
Clozaril Tablets ... 2184
Cubicin for Injection (Less than 1%) ... 1026
Cuprimine Capsules ... 1947
Dacogen Injection ... 2129
Eldepryl Capsules ... 3208
▲ Invanz for Injection (3.3% to 5.1%) ... 1999
Lanoxicaps Capsules ... 1490
Lanoxin Injection ... 1494
Lanoxin Injection Pediatric ... 1497
Lanoxin Tablets ... 1500
Moban Tablets ... 1119
Neumega for Injection ... 3435
Oncaspar ... 1145
Opana Tablets (Less than 1%) ... 1122
Opana ER Tablets (Less than 1%) ... 1126
Orthoclone OKT3 Sterile Solution (Less than 1%) ... 2360
▲ Prograf Capsules and Injection (Approximately 55%) ... 632
▲ Proleukin for Injection (73%) ... 2266
Revlimid Capsules ... 958
Risperdal ... 1676
Risperdal M-Tab Orally Disintegrating Tablets ... 1676
Seroquel Tablets ... 690
Stalevo Tablets ... 2287
Stromectol Tablets ... 2083

Mesenteric arterial thrombosis
Blocadren Tablets ... 1916
Inderal LA Long-Acting Capsules ... 3429
InnoPran XL Capsules ... 2723
Rilutek Tablets (Rare) ... 2930
Timolide Tablets ... 2086
Timoptic Sterile Ophthalmic Solution ... 2088
Timoptic in Ocudose ... 2091

Metabolic acidosis
(*see under* Acidosis, metabolic)

Metabolic changes
Clinoril Tablets (Rare) ... 1924
▲ Hycamtin for Injection (39%) ... 1458
▲ Leukine (58%) ... 814
▲ Menostar Transdermal System (12%) ... 782
▲ Neoral Oral Solution (9.3%) ... 2259
▲ Neoral Soft Gelatin Capsules (9.3%) ... 2259

Metabolism disorders, unspecified
▲ Focalin XR Capsules (34%) ... 2223

Methemoglobinemia
Hurricaine Topical Anesthetic Spray, 2 oz. Wild Cherry (Extremely rare) ... ▣712
Cipro ... 2977
Cipro I.V. ... 2984
Elitek (Less than 1%) ... 2890
Eulexin Capsules ... 3009
Fansidar Tablets ... 2765
Gantrisin Pediatric Suspension ... 2770
Hurricaine Topical Anesthetic Gel, 1 oz. Wild Cherry, Pina Colada, Watermelon, and Fresh Mint, 5.25 g. Wild Cherry (Extremely rare) ... ▣712
Hurricaine Topical Anesthetic Liquid, 1 oz. Wild Cherry, Pina Colada, 0.005 fl. oz. Snap-n-Go Swabs Wild Cherry (Extremely rare) ... ▣712
Hurricaine Topical Anesthetic Spray Extension Tubes (200) (Extremely rare) ... ▣712
Hurricaine Topical Anesthetic Spray Kit, 2 oz. Wild Cherry with disposable Extension Tubes (200) (Extremely rare) ... ▣712
Mepron Suspension ... 1521
Nitro-Dur Transdermal Infusion System (Very rare) ... 3046

Metrorrhagia
Aciphex Tablets ... 1090
Alinia for Oral Suspension (Less than 1%) ... 2835
Alinia Tablets (Less than 1%) ... 2835
Aricept Tablets (Infrequent) ... 1094
Aricept ODT Tablets (Infrequent) ... 1094
▲ Betaseron for SC Injection (11%) ... 767
Caduet Tablets (Less than 2%) ... 2508
Campral Tablets (Infrequent) ... 1174
Copaxone for Injection (At least 2%) ... 3297
Depacon Injection (1% or more) ... 412
Depakene (1% or more) ... 417
Depakote Sprinkle Capsules ... 422
▲ Depakote Tablets (1% to 5%) ... 427
▲ Depakote ER Tablets (1% to 5%) ... 434
Gabitril Tablets (Frequent) ... 984
Geodon Capsules (Infrequent) ... 2529
Lipitor Tablets (Less than 2%) ... 2483
Lunesta Tablets (Infrequent) ... 3142
Lyrica Capsules (0.1% to 1%) ... 2539
Meridia Capsules (1%) ... 489
▲ Mylotarg for Injection (2% to 10%) ... 3431
Paxil CR Controlled-Release Tablets (Rare) ... 1538
Paxil (Rare) ... 1530
Pentasa Capsules (Less than 1%) ... 3185
Permax Tablets (Infrequent) ... 3356
Prozac Pulvules and Liquid (Infrequent) ... 1801
▲ Rapamune Oral Solution and Tablets (3% to 20%) ... 3475
Rescriptor Tablets ... 2551
Rilutek Tablets (Infrequent) ... 2930
Sonata Capsules (Infrequent) ... 1717
Symbyax Capsules (Infrequent) ... 1819
Tequin Injection (Less than 0.1%) ... 938
Tequin Injection in 5% Dextrose (Less than 0.1%) ... 938
Tequin Tablets (Less than 0.1%) ... 938
Thalomid Capsules ... 965
Vandazole Vaginal Gel (1%) ... 3338
Vantin Tablets and Oral Suspension (Less than 1%) ... 2645
VFEND I.V. (Less than 2%) ... 2564
VFEND Oral Suspension (Less than 2%) ... 2564
VFEND Tablets (Less than 2%) ... 2564
Zomig Nasal Spray (Rare) ... 3523
Zyprexa Tablets (Infrequent) ... 1830
Zyprexa ZYDIS Orally Disintegrating Tablets (Infrequent) ... 1830

Metyrapone test, altered results
Estratest Tablets ... 3199
Estratest H.S. Tablets ... 3199
Menostar Transdermal System ... 782
Premarin Tablets ... 3446
Premphase Tablets ... 3456
Prempro Tablets ... 3456

Microcephaly, fetal
Accutane Capsules ... 2731
Phenytek Capsules ... 2160

Microphthalmia, fetal
Accutane Capsules ... 2731

Microphthalmos
Thalomid Capsules ... 965

Micropinna, fetal
Accutane Capsules ... 2731

Micturition, difficulty
BiDil Tablets ... 2171
Blocadren Tablets ... 1916
Catapres Tablets (About 2 in 1,000 patients) ... 843
Catapres-TTS (0.5% or less) ... 844
▲ Chemet Capsules (Up to 3.7%) ... 2458
Clorpres Tablets (About 2 in 1,000) ... 2153
Combivent Inhalation Aerosol ... 847
Cosopt Sterile Ophthalmic Solution ... 1931
Dantrium Capsules (Less frequent) ... 2694
Effexor Tablets (2%) ... 3411
Effexor XR Capsules (Frequent) ... 3417
Eligard 22.5 mg (Less than 2%) ... 2883
▲ Niravam Orally Disintegrating Tablets (12.2%) ... 3092
OxyContin Tablets (Less than 1%) ... 2703
▲ Paxil CR Controlled-Release Tablets (3%) ... 1538
▲ Paxil (3%) ... 1530
ProAmatine Tablets (Rare) ... 3186
▲ Prometrium Capsules (100 mg, 200 mg) (11%) ... 3203
Prosed/DS Tablets ... 1157
Timolide Tablets ... 2086
Timoptic Sterile Ophthalmic Solution ... 2088
Timoptic in Ocudose ... 2091
Timoptic-XE Sterile Ophthalmic Gel Forming Solution ... 2092
Transderm Scōp Transdermal Therapeutic System (Infrequent) ... 2177
Uroqid-Acid No. 2 Tablets (Occasional) ... 760
VoSpire ER Tablets (Less frequent) ... 1052
Zelapar Tablets ... 3372
Zonegran Capsules (Infrequent) ... 1101
Zyprexa Tablets (Infrequent) ... 1830
Zyprexa ZYDIS Orally Disintegrating Tablets (Infrequent) ... 1830

Micturition, frequent
Ambien CR Tablets (Rare) ... 2855
Caduet Tablets (Greater than 0.1% to less than or equal to 1%) ... 2508
Campral Tablets (Infrequent) ... 1174
Cardura XL Tablets ... 2515
▲ Doxil Injection (1% to 10%) ... 2351
Estring Vaginal Ring ... 2635
Namenda (Frequent) ... 1195
Proquin XR Tablets ... 1153

Micturition, painful
Eligard 22.5 mg (Less than 2%) ... 2883
Uroqid-Acid No. 2 Tablets (Occasional) ... 760
Zoloft (Rare) ... 2586

Micturition, urgency
Cymbalta Delayed-Release Capsules (Infrequent) ... 1757
▲ Doxil Injection (1% to 10%) ... 2351
Proquin XR Tablets (Less than 1% to 2%) ... 1153

Micturition disturbances
Abilify Oral Solution (Infrequent) ... 882
Abilify Oral Solution (Infrequent) ... 2450
Abilify Discmelt Orally Disintegrating Tablets (Infrequent) ... 882
Abilify Discmelt Orally Disintegrating Tablets (Infrequent) ... 2450
Abilify Tablets (Infrequent) ... 882
Abilify Tablets (Infrequent) ... 2450
Aceon Tablets (2 mg, 4 mg, 8 mg) (0.3% to 1%) ... 3194
Aciphex Tablets ... 1090
▲ Adalat CC Tablets (3% or less) ... 2964
Ambien Tablets (Rare) ... 2851
Aricept Tablets (2%) ... 1094
Aricept ODT Tablets (2%) ... 1094
Arthrotec Tablets (Rare) ... 3129
Astelin Nasal Spray (Infrequent) ... 1904
Avalide Tablets (2%) ... 888
Avalide Tablets (2%) ... 2874
Caduet Tablets (Greater than 0.1% to less than 2%) ... 2508
Captopril Tablets (Approximately 1 to 2 of 1000 patients) ... 2149
Carbatrol Capsules ... 3171
Cardene I.V. (Rare) ... 2497
Cardura XL Tablets ... 2515
Caverject Impulse Injection (Less than 1%) ... 2612
Celebrex Capsules (0.1% to 1.9%) ... 3134
Celexa (At least 2%) ... 1176
▲ CellCept Capsules (3% to less than 20%) ... 2747
▲ CellCept Intravenous (3% to less than 20%) ... 2747
▲ CellCept Oral Suspension (3% to less than 20%) ... 2747
▲ CellCept Tablets (3% to less than 20%) ... 2747
Cesamet Capsules ... 3340
Cipro I.V. (1% or less) ... 2984
Clozaril Tablets (1%) ... 2184
Colazal Capsules ... 2838
Copaxone for Injection (At least 2%) ... 3297
Covera-HS Tablets (Less than 2%) ... 3139
Cozaar Tablets (Less than 1%) ... 1935
▲ Dacogen Injection (5%) ... 2129
Dantrium Capsules (Less frequent) ... 2694
Daranide Tablets ... 1950
▲ Depacon Injection (1% to 5%) ... 412
▲ Depakene (1% to 5%) ... 417
▲ Depakote Sprinkle Capsules (1% to 5%) ... 422
▲ Depakote Tablets (1% to 5%) ... 427
▲ Depakote ER Tablets (1% to 5%) ... 434
Detrol Tablets (1.7%) ... 2628
Diovan HCT Tablets (Greater than 0.2%) ... 2196
Duragesic Transdermal System (Greater than 1%) ... 2373
▲ Effexor Tablets (3%) ... 3411
Effexor XR Capsules (Frequent) ... 3417
Eldepryl Capsules ... 3208
▲ Eloxatin for Injection (2% to 5%) ... 2892
▲ Entocort EC Capsules (Less than 5%) ... 2698
Equetro Extended-Release Capsules ... 3180
Evoxac Capsules (0.9%; less than 1%) ... 1047
Exelon Capsules (Infrequent) ... 2206
Exelon Oral Solution (Infrequent) ... 2206
FazaClo Orally Disintegrating Tablets (1%) ... 551
Flumadine ... 1183
Frova Tablets (Infrequent) ... 1113
Gabitril Tablets (1% or more) ... 984
Gengraf Capsules (1% to less than 3%) ... 459
Hytrin Capsules (At least 1%) ... 471
Hyzaar 50-12.5 Tablets ... 1990

Hyzaar 100-12.5 Tablets 1990
Hyzaar 100-25 Tablets 1990
Imitrex Injection (Rare) 1463
Imitrex Nasal Spray (Infrequent) 1467
Imitrex Tablets (Infrequent) 1471
▲ Indapamide Tablets (Less than 5%) 2156
Indocin (Rare) 1995
▲ Intron A for Injection (Less than 5%) 3024
Invirase (Less than 2%) 2772
Klonopin (1%) 2778
▲ Lamictal (1% to 5%) 1481
Lexapro Oral Solution (Frequent) 1190
Lexapro Tablets (Frequent) 1190
Lipitor Tablets (Less than 2%) 2483
Lofibra Tablets 1219
Lofibra Capsules 1216
Lotensin HCT Tablets (0.3% to 1%) 2246
Lotronex Tablets (Rare) 1512
Lunesta Tablets (Infrequent) 3142
Lyrica Capsules (Greater than or equal to 1%) 2539
Matulane Capsules 3191
Maxalt Tablets (Infrequent) 2008
Maxalt-MLT Orally Disintegrating Tablets (Infrequent) 2008
Megace ES Oral Suspension (0% to 2%) 2481
Meridia Capsules 489
Micardis Tablets (More than 0.3%) 854
Micardis HCT Tablets 856
Midamor Tablets (Less than or equal to 1%) 2026
Migranal Nasal Spray (Infrequent) 3348
▲ Mirapex Tablets (Greater than or equal to 1% to 6%) 859
Mobic Oral Suspension (0.1% to 2.4%) 863
Mobic Tablets (0.1% to 2.4%) 863
Moduretic Tablets 2028
Neoral Oral Solution (1% to less than 3%) 2259
Neoral Soft Gelatin Capsules (1% to less than 3%) 2259
Neurontin Capsules (Infrequent) 2487
Neurontin Oral Solution (Infrequent) 2487
Neurontin Tablets (Infrequent) 2487
Nexium Delayed-Release Capsules (Less than 1%) 655
Nexium I.V. (Less than 1%) 659
Norvasc Tablets (More than 0.1% to 1%) 2545
Norvir (Less than 2%) 503
Oncaspar (Less than 1%) 1145
Opana Tablets (Less than 1%) 1122
Opana ER Tablets (Less than 1%) 1126
Parcopa Orally Disintegrating Tablets 3097
Parnate Tablets 1527
▲ Paxil CR Controlled-Release Tablets (3%) 1538
▲ Paxil (3%) 1530
Pentasa Capsules (Less than 1%) 3185
Permax Tablets (2.7%) 3356
▲ Pexeva Tablets (2% to 3%) 1694
Pletal Tablets (Less than 2%) 2455
Prevacid Delayed-Release Capsules (Less than 1%) 3271
Prevacid for Delayed-Release Oral Suspension (Less than 1%) 3271
Prevacid SoluTab Delayed-Release Orally Disintegrating Tablets (Less than 1%) 3271
Prevacid NapraPAC (Less than 1%) 3280
PREVPAC (Less than 1%) 3284
Prilosec OTC Delayed-Release Tablets (Less than 1%) 2677
▲ ProAmatine Tablets (Among most frequent) 3186
Prochieve 4% Gel 1003
Prochieve 8% Gel 1003
▲ Prograf Capsules and Injection (3% to 15%) 632
Proleukin for Injection (1%) 2266
Proquin XR Tablets (Less than 1%) 1153
ProSom Tablets (Infrequent) 517
Protonix I.V. (Less than 1%) 3472
Protonix Tablets (Less than 1%) 3469
▲ Rapamune Oral Solution and Tablets (3% to 20%) 3475
Razadyne (Infrequent) 2399
Razadyne ER Extended-Release Capsules (Infrequent) 2399
▲ Rebif Prefilled Syringe for Injection (2% to 7%) 3159
Relpax Tablets (Infrequent) 2548
ReoPro Vials (0.1%) 1809
Requip Tablets (Infrequent) 1555
Retrovir Capsules 1560
Retrovir IV Infusion 1564
Retrovir 1560
Risperdal 1676
Risperdal Consta Long-Acting Injection (Infrequent) 1682
Risperdal M-Tab Orally Disintegrating Tablets 1676
Rythmol SR Capsules 2727
Seroquel Tablets (Infrequent) 690
▲ Simulect for Injection (3% to 10%) 2284
Sonata Capsules (Infrequent) 1717
▲ Strattera Capsules (5% or greater) 1814
Symbyax Capsules (Frequent) 1819
Tarka Tablets 524
Tasmar Tablets (1% to 2%) 3358
Tegretol/Tegretol-XR 2295
▲ Temodar Capsules (6%) 3073
Teveten Tablets (Less than 1%) 1735
Teveten HCT Tablets (Less than 1%) 1737
Topamax Sprinkle Capsules (0% to 2%) 2404
Topamax Tablets (0% to 2%) 2404
Tricor Tablets 527
Trileptal Tablets (1% to 2%) 2300
Trileptal Oral Suspension (1% to 2%) 2300
▲ Ultram ER Tablets (1% to greater than 5%) 2392
Uniretic Tablets (Less than 1%) 3100
Univasc Tablets (Greater than 1%) 3104
Vandazole Vaginal Gel (Less than 1%) 3338
Vantas (Less than 2%) 3375
Verelan PM Extended-Release Capsules, Controlled-Onset (2% or less) 3106
▲ Vesanoid Capsules (3%) 2820
▲ Viadur Implant (3.8%) 757
Viagra Tablets (Less than 2%) 2573
Vicoprofen Tablets (Less than 3%) 539
Wellbutrin Tablets (2.5%) 1603
▲ Wellbutrin SR Sustained-Release Tablets (2% to 5%) 1607
▲ Wellbutrin XL Extended-Release Tablets (2% to 5%) 1613
Xifaxan Tablets (Less than 2%) 2842
Zegerid Capsules (Less than 1%) 2958
Zegerid Powder for Oral Solution (Less than 1%) 2958
Zelapar Tablets 3372
Zoloft (Infrequent) 2586
Zomig Tablets (Infrequent) 3519
Zomig Nasal Spray (Rare) 3523
Zomig-ZMT Tablets (Infrequent) 3519
Zyban Sustained-Release Tablets (Frequent) 1644
Zyprexa Tablets (Infrequent) 1830
Zyprexa ZYDIS Orally Disintegrating Tablets (Infrequent) 1830
Zyrtec Chewable Tablets (Less than 2%) 2594
Zyrtec (Less than 2%) 2594
Zyrtec-D 12 Hour Extended Release Tablets (Less than 2%) 2597

Middle ear, fluid in

▲ Increlex Injection (Greater than or equal to 5%) 3291

Migraine

Abilify Oral Solution (Infrequent) 882
Abilify Oral Solution (Infrequent) 2450
Abilify Discmelt Orally Disintegrating Tablets (Infrequent) 882
Abilify Discmelt Orally Disintegrating Tablets (Infrequent) 2450
Abilify Tablets (Infrequent) 882
Abilify Tablets (Infrequent) 2450
AccuNeb Inhalation Solution (0.9% to 1.7%) 1055
Aciphex Tablets 1090
Actiq (1% or greater) 979
ADACEL Vaccine (1.5%) 2945
Adalat CC Tablets (Less than 1%) 2964
▲ Advair HFA Inhalation Aerosol (1% to 3%) 1318
Advicor Tablets 1722
▲ Agrylin Capsules (1% to 5%) 3169
Ambien Tablets (Infrequent) 2851
Ambien CR Tablets (Infrequent) 2855
Angeliq Tablets 762
Arthrotec Tablets (Rare) 3129
Asacol Delayed-Release Tablets (2% or greater) 2692
Azilect Tablets (Infrequent) 3293
Caduet Tablets (Less than 2%) 2508
Campral Tablets (Infrequent) 1174
Celexa (Frequent) 1176
Chantix Tablets (Infrequent) 2517
Cipro (Less than 1%) 2977
Cipro I.V. (1% or less) 2984
Cipro XR Tablets (Less than 1%) 2990
Climara Transdermal System 771
Climara Pro Transdermal System 776
▲ Copaxone for Injection (5%) 3297
Coreg Tablets (Less than or equal to 0.1%) 1414
Cozaar Tablets (Less than 1%) 1935
Doxil Injection (Less than 1%) 2351
Effexor Tablets (Frequent) 3411
Effexor XR Capsules (Frequent) 3417
Eldepryl Capsules 3208
Engerix-B Vaccine 1425
Enjuvia Tablets 1062
▲ Epzicom Tablets (6% to 7%) 1436
Estrasorb Topical Emulsion 1147
Estratest Tablets 3199
Estratest H.S. Tablets 3199
▲ Estring Vaginal Ring (1% to 3%) 2635
Evista Tablets (2.4%) 1763
▲ Evoxac Capsules (1% to 3%) 1047
Exelon Capsules (Infrequent) 2206
Exelon Oral Solution (Infrequent) 2206
▲ Famvir Tablets (0.7% to 3.1%) 2211
▲ Flovent Diskus (1% to 3%) 1443
▲ Flovent HFA (1% to 3%) 1447
Fortical Nasal Spray (Less than 1%) 3337
Gabitril Tablets (Frequent) 984
▲ Gengraf Capsules (3%) 459
Gleevec Tablets (Infrequent) 2227
Hyzaar 50-12.5 Tablets 1990
Hyzaar 100-12.5 Tablets 1990
Hyzaar 100-25 Tablets 1990
▲ Imdur Tablets (Less than or equal to 5%) 3018
Imitrex Tablets 1471
▲ Intron A for Injection (Less than 5%) 3024
Ionsys Transdermal System (.1% to less than 1%) 2379
Kaletra (Less than 2%) 476
Klonopin (Infrequent) 2778
▲ Lamictal (1% to 5%) 1481
Levaquin (0.1% to 0.9%) 2384
Levaquin in 5% Dextrose Injection (0.1% to 0.9%) 2384
Lexapro Oral Solution (Frequent) 1190
Lexapro Tablets (Frequent) 1190
Lipitor Tablets (Less than 2%) 2483
Lofibra Tablets 1219
Lofibra Capsules 1216
Lunesta Tablets (Frequent) 3142
▲ Lupron Depot 3.75 mg (33%) 3260
▲ Lupron Depot–3 Month 11.25 mg (33%) 3265
Maxair Autohaler 1852
Menostar Transdermal System 782
Meridia Capsules (2.4%) 489
Miacalcin Nasal Spray (Less than 1%) 2253
Micardis Tablets (More than 0.3%) 854
Micardis HCT Tablets 856
Mircette Tablets 1066
Myobloc Injection (Greater than 2%) 3192
▲ Neoral Oral Solution (3%) 2259
▲ Neoral Soft Gelatin Capsules (3%) 2259
Neurontin Capsules (Infrequent) 2487
Neurontin Oral Solution (Infrequent) 2487
Neurontin Tablets (Infrequent) 2487
Nexium Delayed-Release Capsules (Less than 1%) 655
Nexium I.V. (Less than 1%) 659
Niaspan Extended-Release Tablets 1730
Norvasc Tablets (Less than 0.1%) 2545
Norvir (Less than 2%) 503
NuvaRing 2340
Omacor Capsules 2725
Ortho-Cyclen Tablets 2429
Ortho Evra Transdermal System 2417
Ortho Tri-Cyclen Tablets 2429
Ortho Tri-Cyclen Lo Tablets 2436
OxyContin Tablets (Less than 1%) 2703
Paxil CR Controlled-Release Tablets (Infrequent) 1538
Paxil (Infrequent) 1530
Permax Tablets (Rare) 3356
Pexeva Tablets (Infrequent) 1694
Premarin Intravenous 3442
Premarin Tablets 3446
Premarin Vaginal Cream 3452
Premphase Tablets 3456
Prempro Tablets 3456
Prevacid Delayed-Release Capsules (Less than 1%) 3271
Prevacid for Delayed-Release Oral Suspension (Less than 1%) 3271
Prevacid SoluTab Delayed-Release Orally Disintegrating Tablets (Less than 1%) 3271
Prevacid NapraPAC (Less than 1%) 3280
PREVPAC (Less than 1%) 3284
Prochieve 4% Gel 1003
Prochieve 8% Gel 1003
Proquin XR Tablets 1153
Protonix I.V. (Greater than or equal to 1%) 3472
Protonix Tablets (Greater than or equal to 1%) 3469
Protopic Ointment (Greater than or equal to 1%) 638
Provigil Tablets (At least 1%) 988
Prozac Pulvules and Liquid (Infrequent) 1801
Recombivax HB 2071
Relpax Tablets (Infrequent) 2548
Requip Tablets (Infrequent) 1555
Rescriptor Tablets 2551
Revlimid Capsules 958
Rilutek Tablets (Infrequent) 2930
Risperdal (Rare) 1676
Risperdal Consta Long-Acting Injection (Infrequent) 1682
Risperdal M-Tab Orally Disintegrating Tablets (Rare) 1676
Rituxan I.V. (2%) 1254
Sandostatin LAR Depot (Rare) 2280
Seasonique Tablets 1077
▲ Serevent Diskus (1% to 3%) 1568
Seroquel Tablets (Infrequent) 690
Soriatane Capsules (Less than 1%) 1013
Sular Tablets (Less than or equal to 1%) 3122
Sustiva Capsules (Less than 2%) 930
Sustiva Tablets (Less than 2%) 930
Symbyax Capsules (Frequent) 1819
Tasmar Tablets (Infrequent) 3358
Tequin Injection (Less than 0.1%) 938
Tequin Injection in 5% Dextrose (Less than 0.1%) 938
Tequin Tablets (Less than 0.1%) 938
Teveten Tablets (Less than 1%) 1735
Teveten HCT Tablets (Less than 1%) 1737
Thalomid Capsules 965
Tricor Tablets 527
Triglide Tablets 3123
Trileptal Tablets 2300
Trileptal Oral Suspension 2300
▲ Ultram ER Tablets (1% to greater than 5%) 2392
Uniretic Tablets (Less than 1%) 3100
Vantin Tablets and Oral Suspension (Less than 1%) 2645
Viagra Tablets (Less than 2%) 2573
Viracept (Less than 2%) 2577
▲ Vivitrol (16% to 36%) 995
▲ Wellbutrin Tablets (25.7%) 1603
▲ Wellbutrin SR Sustained-Release Tablets (1% to 4%) 1607
▲ Wellbutrin XL Extended-Release Tablets (0% to 4%) 1613
▲ Xeloda Tablets (Less than 5%) 2822
Xifaxan Tablets (Less than 2%) 2842
Xopenex Inhalation Solution (2.7%) 3146
Xopenex Inhalation Solution Concentrate (2.7%) 3150
Xopenex HFA Inhalation Aerosol (2.7%) 3154
Xyrem Oral Solution (Infrequent) 1688
Yasmin 28 Tablets (Greater than 1%) 796
Yaz Tablets (Greater than 1%) 803
Zelapar Tablets 3372
Zelnorm Tablets (2%) 2312
Zemaira (0.2% to 0.4%) 3509
▲ Ziagen (7%) 1626
Zoloft (Infrequent) 2586
Zyban Sustained-Release Tablets (Infrequent) 1644
Zyprexa Tablets (Infrequent) 1830
Zyprexa ZYDIS Orally Disintegrating Tablets (Infrequent) 1830
Zyrtec Chewable Tablets (Less than 2%) 2594
Zyrtec (Less than 2%) 2594
Zyrtec-D 12 Hour Extended Release Tablets (Less than 2%) 2597

Migraine, aggravated

Frova Tablets (Infrequent) 1113
Migranal Nasal Spray (Rare) 3348
Nexium Delayed-Release Capsules (Less than 1%) 655
Nexium I.V. (Less than 1%) 659
Premphase Tablets 3456
Prempro Tablets 3456
Topamax Sprinkle Capsules (Greater than 1%) 2404
Topamax Tablets (Greater than 1%) 2404

Migration of implant
Viadur Implant (Rare)........................ 757

Miliaria
Aclovate Cream (Infrequent)............ 2660
Analpram-HC 1159
Apexicon E Cream............................. 2661
Clobevate Gel.................................. 3211
Clobex Lotion.................................. 1204
Clobex Shampoo (Infrequent)........... 1206
Clobex Spray (Less than 1%)........... 1208
Cutivate Cream (Infrequent)............ 2662
Cutivate Lotion 0.05% (Rare)........... 2664
Cutivate Ointment (Infrequent to more frequent)............................ 2665
Diprolene Gel 0.05%......................... 3001
Diprolene Lotion 0.05% (Infrequent).................................. 3002
Diprolene Ointment 0.05% (Infrequent).................................. 3003
Diprolene AF Cream 0.05% (Infrequent).................................. 3000
Diprosone Cream, USP 0.05% 3004
Elocon Cream 0.1% (Infrequent) 3005
Elocon Lotion 0.1% (Infrequent) 3006
Elocon Ointment 0.1% (Infrequent) ... 3007
Locoid Lipocream Cream (Infrequent) 1160
Lotrisone 3040
Luxíq Foam 1010
Olux Foam 1012
Oxsoralen-Ultra Capsules 3353
Pramosone 1161
ProctoFoam-HC 3099
Temovate Cream 2668
Temovate Gel (Infrequent) 2669
Temovate Ointment 2668
Temovate Scalp Application (Infrequent) 2670
Temovate E Emollient (Infrequent) 2671
Tri-Luma Cream 1213
Vanos Cream 1893

Miliaria ruba
ProQuad (Greater than or equal to 0.2% to less than 1%) 2064

Miosis
Actiq (Less than 1%) 979
Alphagan P Ophthalmic Solution 567
Brimonidine Tartrate Ophthalmic Solution 0.2% .... ⊙ 248
▲ Buprenex Injectable (1% to 5%) 2716
Camptosar Injection 2604
Dibenzyline Capsules 3399
Dilaudid 440
Dilaudid Non-Sterile Powder 440
Dilaudid Oral Liquid (Less frequent) 445
Dilaudid Rectal Suppositories 440
Dilaudid Tablets 440
Dilaudid Tablets - 8 mg (Less frequent) 445
Dilaudid-HP (Less frequent) 442
Effexor Tablets (Rare) 3411
Effexor XR Capsules (Rare) 3417
Emend Capsules (Less than or equal to 0.5%) 1963
Kadian Capsules (Less than 3%) 577
Lyrica Capsules (Rare) 2539
MS Contin Tablets (Less frequent) 2701
Neurontin Capsules (Rare) 2487
Neurontin Oral Solution (Rare) 2487
Neurontin Tablets (Rare) 2487
Numorphan Injection 1120
Ocufen Ophthalmic Solution .... ⊙ 232
Opana Tablets (Less than 1%) 1122
Opana ER Tablets (Less than 1%) 1126
Percodan Tablets 1132
Rythmol SR Capsules 2727
Symbyax Capsules (Infrequent) 1819
Thioridazine Hydrochloride Tablets .. 2163
Thiothixene Capsules 2165
Xyrem Oral Solution (Infrequent) 1688
Zyprexa Tablets (Rare) 1830
Zyprexa ZYDIS Orally Disintegrating Tablets (Rare) 1830

Miscarriage
Efudex 3363
Vantin Tablets and Oral Suspension 2645
Zelnorm Tablets 2312
Zomig Tablets (Rare) 3519
Zomig-ZMT Tablets (Rare) 3519

Mitral insufficiency
Requip Tablets (Infrequent) 1555

Mitral regurgitation
Activase I.V. 1223
Retavase 2499
TNKase I.V. 1264

Mitral valve disease
Effexor XR (Rare)............................ 3417

Mobility disorders, non-site specific
Amerge Tablets (Rare)..................... 1339

Molluscum contagiosum
Elidel Cream 1% (Up to 1.8%).......... 2200
Norvir (Less than 2%)...................... 503

Moniliasis
(*see under* Candidiasis)

Moniliasis, enteric
Rescriptor Tablets 2551

Moniliasis, gastrointestinal
Proquin XR Tablets.......................... 1153
▲ Thymoglobulin for Intravenous Infusion (4.9%)............................ 1284

Moniliasis, genital
(*see under* Candidiasis, genital)

Moniliasis, oral
(*see under* Candidiasis, oral)
▲ Thymoglobulin for Intravenous Infusion (3.7%)............................ 1284

Moniliasis, vaginal
Abilify Oral Solution (Infrequent)........ 882
Abilify Oral Solution (Infrequent)....... 2450
Abilify Discmelt Orally Disintegrating Tablets (Infrequent) 882
Abilify Discmelt Orally Disintegrating Tablets (Infrequent)................................ 2450
Abilify Tablets (Infrequent)................ 882
Abilify Tablets (Infrequent)............... 2450
Cipro.. 2977
Cipro XR Tablets (1% to 2%)............. 2990
Cleocin Vaginal Ovules (1.5%).......... 2616
Lamictal (Rare)................................ 1481
Merrem I.V. (Greater than 0.1% to 1%).. 686
▲ Omnicef Capsules (4%) 511
Omnicef for Oral Suspension (0.3%).. 511
Pexeva Tablets (rare)....................... 1694
▲ Premarin Tablets (5% to 6%) 3446
▲ Premphase Tablets (4% to 8%) 3456
▲ Prempro Tablets (4% to 8%) 3456
Proquin XR Tablets.......................... 1153
Rescriptor Tablets........................... 2551
Symbyax Capsules (Infrequent)........ 1819
Tricor Tablets.................................. 527
Tygacil for Injection (0% to less than 2%)....................................... 3488
Yaz Tablets (Greater than 1%).......... 803
Zyvox (1% to 1.6%).......................... 2652

Monocytosis
Campral Tablets (Rare)..................... 1174
Cipro (Less than 0.1%)..................... 2977
Cuprimine Capsules......................... 1947
Geodon Capsules (Rare)................... 2529
Paxil CR Controlled-Release Tablets (Rare)............................... 1538
Paxil (Rare)..................................... 1530
Pexeva Tablets (rare)....................... 1694
Primaxin I.M.................................... 2045
Primaxin I.V..................................... 2048
Relpax Tablets (Rare)....................... 2548
Rocephin Injectable Vials, ADD-Vantage, Galaxy, Bulk (Rare)... 2800
Rythmol SR Capsules....................... 2727
Vantin Tablets and Oral Suspension 2645
Xifaxan Tablets (Less than 2%)......... 2842

Mononeuropathy
ADACEL Vaccine.............................. 2945
Infanrix Vaccine............................... 1476

Mononuclear cells, atypical
Miradon Tablets............................... 3042

Mononucleosis, infectious
Daytrana Transdermal Patch............ 3174

Monoplegia
Imitrex Injection (Rare)..................... 1463
Imitrex Nasal Spray (Rare)................ 1467
Imitrex Tablets (Infrequent)............... 1471

Mood changes
Adalat CC Tablets (Rare).................. 2964
▲ Aerobid/Aerobid-M (1% to 3%) 1171
▲ Agenerase Oral Solution (4% to 16%).. 1332
▲ Alimta for Injection (Up to 14%) 1750
Aloxi Injection (Less than 1%)........... 2127
Ambien CR Tablets (1%).................. 2855
Angeliq Tablets 762
▲ Arimidex Tablets (17% to 19%) 673
Cesamet Capsules 3340
Chantix Tablets (Infrequent).............. 2517
Climara Transdermal System........... 771
Climara Pro Transdermal System..... 776
▲ Copegus Tablets (5% to 9%) 2754
Cymbalta Delayed-Release Capsules (Infrequent)................... 1757
Decadron Tablets 1951
Dilaudid 440
Dilaudid Non-Sterile Powder............ 440
Dilaudid Oral Liquid (Less frequent).. 445
Dilaudid Rectal Suppositories........... 440
Dilaudid Tablets 440
Dilaudid Tablets - 8 mg (Less frequent)... 445
Dilaudid-HP (Less frequent)............. 442
Eldepryl Capsules 3208
Enbrel for Injection 584
Enjuvia Tablets 1062
Estrasorb Topical Emulsion 1147
Estratest Tablets 3199
Estratest H.S. Tablets 3199
Guanidine Hydrochloride Tablets 3016
Hycodan 1116
Hycotuss Expectorant Syrup 1117
Hydrocortone Tablets 1989
Lariam Tablets (Occasional) 2786
▲ Lexiva Tablets (Less than 1% to 11%) 1505
Lupron Depot 3.75 mg 3260
Marinol Capsules 3333
Meridia Capsules 489
MS Contin Tablets (Less frequent) 2701
Oncaspar 1145
Ortho-Cyclen Tablets 2429
Ortho Evra Transdermal System 2417
Ortho Tri-Cyclen Tablets 2429
Ortho Tri-Cyclen Lo Tablets 2436
Orthoclone OKT3 Sterile Solution 2360
Paxil CR Controlled-Release Tablets 1538
Paxil 1530
▲ Pegasys (3%) 2789
Premarin Tablets 3446
Premarin Vaginal Cream 3452
Premphase Tablets 3456
Prempro Tablets 3456
Prezista Tablets (Less than 2%) 3306
Seasonique Tablets 1077
▲ Solodyn Extended Release Tablets (3%) 1890
▲ Soltamox Oral Solution (11.6%) 3527
▲ Strattera Capsules (Greater than 5%) 1814
Testim 1% Gel (1% or less) 695
▲ Topamax Sprinkle Capsules (2% to 11%) 2404
▲ Topamax Tablets (2% to 11%) 2404
Tussionex Pennkinetic Extended-Release Suspension 3327
Univasc Tablets (Less than 1%) 3104
Vicodin Tablets 535
Vicodin ES Tablets 536
Vicodin HP Tablets 538
Vicoprofen Tablets (Less than 1%) ... 539
Wellbutrin Tablets (Infrequent) 1603
▲ Xeloda Tablets (5%) 2822
Xyrem Oral Solution (Infrequent) 1688
Zydone Tablets 1139

Moon face
Copaxone for Injection (Infrequent) .. 3297
Decadron Tablets 1951

Motion sickness
Aloxi Injection (Less than 1%) 2127
Aricept Tablets 1094
Aricept ODT Tablets 1094
Evoxac Capsules (Less than 1%) 1047
Klonopin (Infrequent) 2778
Xifaxan Tablets (Less than 2%) 2842

Motor and phonic tics, exacerbations
Adderall Tablets 3164
Adderall XR Capsules 3166
Dexedrine 1420
DextroStat Tablets 3179

Motor disturbances, reversible involuntary
Zantac (Rare) 1624
Zantac Injection (Rare) 1619
Zantac Injection Pharmacy Bulk Package (Rare) 1622
Zantac Injection Premixed (Rare) 1619
Zantac (Rare) 1624

Motor dysfunction
▲ Arranon Injection (0% to 4%) 1357

Motor function, loss of
Neoral Oral Solution........................ 2259
Neoral Soft Gelatin Capsules........... 2259
Sandimmune 2275

Motor restlessness
Moban Tablets................................ 1119
Paxil CR Controlled-Release Tablets 1538
Paxil Tablets 1530
▲ Pediarix Vaccine (0.6% to 41.4%) 1548
Thioridazine Hydrochloride Tablets... 2163

Motor skills, impairment
Ambien Tablets 2851
Amerge Tablets (Rare)..................... 1339
Chantix Tablets (Rare)..................... 2517
Dapsone Tablets USP 1673
Effexor Tablets 3411
Moban Tablets................................ 1119
Neurontin Capsules (Rare)............... 2487
Neurontin Oral Solution (Rare).......... 2487
Neurontin Tablets (Rare).................. 2487
▲ Prograf Capsules and Injection (Approximately 55%)..................... 632
Proleukin for Injection (2%).............. 2266
Risperdal 1676
Risperdal M-Tab Orally Disintegrating Tablets 1676

Mottling
Bicillin C-R Injectable Suspension..... 1706

Mouth, burning
Eldepryl Capsules........................... 3208

Mouth, discoloration
▲ Kepivance (17%) 597

Mouth, dry
(*see under* Xerostomia)

Mouth, fissuring in corner of
Parnate Tablets 1527

Mouth, puckering
Moban Tablets................................ 1119

Mouth, sore
Alferon N Injection (One patient)....... 1665
▲ Flovent Diskus (1% to 3%) 1443
Gengraf Capsules (Rare).................. 459
▲ Imitrex Injection (4.9%) 1463
Miradon Tablets 3042
Neoral Oral Solution (Rare)............... 2259
Neoral Soft Gelatin Capsules (Rare)... 2259
Oncaspar 1145

Mouth, thickening of
▲ Kepivance (17%) 597

Mouth ulceration
Azilect Tablets (Infrequent)............... 3293
Chantix Tablets (Infrequent).............. 2517
▲ Doxil Injection (1% to 10%) 2351
Lyrica Capsules (0.1% to 1%)........... 2539
Prograf Capsules and Injection......... 632
ProQuad 2064
Protopic Ointment (0.2% to less than 1%).. 638

Movement, abnormal
Gabitril Tablets (Infrequent)............... 984
Lamictal (Rare)................................ 1481
Neoral Oral Solution......................... 2259
Neoral Soft Gelatin Capsules 2259
Orthoclone OKT3 Sterile Solution..... 2360
Phenergan Tablets and Suppositories 3440
Prozac Pulvules and Liquid.............. 1801
Sandimmune 2275
Zonegran Capsules (Infrequent)....... 1101
▲ Zyprexa Tablets (1% to 5%) 1830
▲ Zyprexa ZYDIS Orally Disintegrating Tablets (1% to 5%)... 1830

Movement, unspecified
Ultane Liquid for Inhalation (1%)....... 531

Movement disorder
Symbyax Capsules (Infrequent)........ 1819
▲ Zyprexa IntraMuscular (2% to 4%) ... 1830

Mucocutaneous lymph node syndrome
(*see under* Kawasaki-like syndrome)

Mucocutaneous reactions
Rituxan I.V. 1254

Mucosa damage
Invirase (Greater than or equal to 2%) 2772

Mucosal pigmentation, changes
▲ Intron A for Injection (Less than 5%) 3024

Mucositis
Alferon N Injection (One patient) 1665
Aloprim for Injection (Less than 1%) 2167
AmBisome for Injection (Less common) 620
▲ Campath Ampules (1% to 14%) 811
▲ Camptosar Injection (2% to 29.6%) 2604
▲ Elitek (2% to 15%) 2890
▲ Eloxatin for Injection (2% to 7%) 2892
▲ Erbitux (6% to 93%) 910
Evoxac Capsules (Less than 1%) 1047
▲ Intron A for Injection (Less than 5%) 3024
▲ I.V. Busulfex (97%) 2493
Myleran Tablets 1525
▲ Mylotarg for Injection (25%) 3431
▲ Neulasta Injection (15% to 72%) 601
▲ Neumega for Injection (43%) 3435
▲ Neupogen for Injection (12%) 603
Neurontin Capsules (Rare) 2487
Neurontin Oral Solution (Rare) 2487
Neurontin Tablets (Rare) 2487
▲ Nexavar Tablets (Common) 746
Oncaspar 1145
▲ Sutent Capsules (1% to 53%) 2560
▲ Vesanoid Capsules (26%) 2820
▲ Zometa for Intravenous Infusion (5% to 10%) 2315

Mucous membrane, abnormalities
Aceon Tablets (2 mg, 4 mg, 8 mg) (0.3% to 1%) 3194
Actiq (Less than 1%) 979
Altoprev Extended-Release Tablets 3109
Captopril Tablets (Approximately 1 in 1000 patients) 2149
Clinoril Tablets 1924
Emend Capsules (2.6%) 1963
Lescol Capsules 2233
Lescol XL Tablets 2233
▲ Leukine (75%) 814
Mevacor Tablets 2021
Mintezol 2027
Neurontin Capsules (Infrequent) 2487
Neurontin Oral Solution (Infrequent) 2487
Neurontin Tablets (Infrequent) 2487
Vandazole Vaginal Gel (Less than 1%) 3338
Zocor Tablets 2105

Mucus, blood-tinted
Atrovent Nasal Spray 0.03% (2.0%) 837
▲ Flonase Nasal Spray (1% to 3%) 1440

Multiorgan failure
Prograf Capsules and Injection 632
Revlimid Capsules (1.4%) 958

Multiorgan system failure
Clolar for Intravenous Infusion 1271
Cosmegen for Injection 2459
Lamictal 1481
Levaquin (0.1% to 0.9%) 2384
Levaquin in 5% Dextrose Injection (0.1% to 0.9%) 2384
Tasmar Tablets (One case) 3358
VFEND I.V. (Less than 2%) 2564
VFEND Oral Suspension (Less than 2%) 2564
VFEND Tablets (Less than 2%) 2564

Muscle atrophy
Actiq (Less than 1%) 979
Azilect Tablets (Infrequent) 3293
Campath Ampules 811
Copaxone for Injection (Infrequent) 3297
Eligard 30 mg (1.1%) 2885
Permax Tablets (Rare) 3356
Reyataz Capsules (Less than 3%) 921
Virazole for Inhalation Solution 3370

Muscle contractions, involuntary
Ambien CR Tablets (1%) 2855
Dilaudid 440
Dilaudid Non-Sterile Powder 440
Dilaudid Rectal Suppositories 440
Dilaudid Tablets 440
Levaquin (0.1% to 0.9%) 2384
Levaquin in 5% Dextrose Injection (0.1% to 0.9%) 2384
Lexapro Oral Solution (Infrequent) 1190
Lexapro Tablets (Infrequent) 1190
Namenda (Infrequent) 1195
Risperdal Consta Long-Acting Injection (Infrequent) 1682
▲ Topamax Sprinkle Capsules (2% to 4%) 2404
▲ Topamax Tablets (2% to 4%) 2404

Muscle cramp
(*see under* Cramping, muscular)

Muscle hypertonia
Lexapro Oral Solution (Infrequent) 1190
Lexapro Tablets (Infrequent) 1190
Trileptal Tablets 2300
Trileptal Oral Suspension 2300

Muscle injury
▲ Advair HFA Inhalation Aerosol (0% to 3%) 1318
▲ Ultram ER Tablets (1% to greater than 5%) 2392

Muscle mass, loss
Colocort Rectal Suspension, USP (Retention) 100 mg/60 mL 2476
Decadron Tablets 1951
Depo-Medrol Injectable Suspension 2617
Depo-Medrol Single-Dose Vial 2619
Hydrocortone Tablets 1989

Muscle movement, intraoperative
Dilaudid Oral Liquid (Less frequent) 445
Dilaudid Tablets - 8 mg (Less frequent) 445

Muscle rigidity
▲ Advair Diskus 100/50 (1% to 3%) 1308
▲ Advair Diskus 250/50 (1% to 3%) 1308
▲ Advair Diskus 500/50 (1% to 3%) 1308
Amerge Tablets (Infrequent) 1339
Ceftin Tablets (0.1% to 1%) 1407
Clozaril Tablets 2184
Comtan Tablets 2189
Cozaar Tablets (Less than 1%) 1935
Dilaudid 440
Dilaudid Non-Sterile Powder 440
Dilaudid Oral Liquid (Less frequent) 445
Dilaudid Rectal Suppositories 440
Dilaudid Tablets 440
Dilaudid Tablets - 8 mg (Less frequent) 445
Dilaudid-HP (Less frequent) 442
▲ Flovent HFA (1% to 3%) 1447
Imitrex Injection (Rare) 1463
Invirase (Less than 2%) 2772
Lexapro Oral Solution (Infrequent) 1190
Lexapro Tablets (Infrequent) 1190
Lotronex Tablets (Rare) 1512
Miacalcin Nasal Spray (Less than 1%) 2253
Migranal Nasal Spray (1%; Rare) 3348
MS Contin Tablets (Less frequent) 2701
Orthoclone OKT3 Sterile Solution 2360
Permax Tablets 3356
Phenergan Tablets and Suppositories 3440
ProSom Tablets (1%) 517
Risperdal 1676
Risperdal M-Tab Orally Disintegrating Tablets 1676
▲ Serevent Diskus (1% to 3%) 1568
Seroquel Tablets 690
Symmetrel Tablets (Uncommon) 1135
Tasmar Tablets (2%) 3358
Thioridazine Hydrochloride Tablets 2163
Thiothixene Capsules 2165
▲ Vivitrol (2% to 8%) 995
Wellbutrin Tablets 1603
Wellbutrin SR Sustained-Release Tablets 1607
Wellbutrin XL Extended-Release Tablets 1613
Zyban Sustained-Release Tablets 1644

Muscle spasms
Abilify Oral Solution (Infrequent) 882
Abilify Oral Solution (Infrequent) 2450
Abilify Discmelt Orally Disintegrating Tablets (Infrequent) 882
Abilify Discmelt Orally Disintegrating Tablets (Infrequent) 2450
Abilify Tablets (Infrequent) 882
Abilify Tablets (Infrequent) 2450
ADACEL Vaccine 2945
Advair Diskus 100/50 1308
▲ Advair Diskus 250/50 (3%) 1308
Advair Diskus 500/50 1308
▲ Advair HFA Inhalation Aerosol (1% to 3%) 1318
Aldoril Tablets 1910
Amerge Tablets (Infrequent) 1339
Aricept Tablets (Infrequent) 1094
Aricept ODT Tablets (Infrequent) 1094
Atacand HCT 651
Avalide Tablets 888
Avalide Tablets 2874
Celexa 1176
Clorpres Tablets 2153
Clozaril Tablets (1%) 2184
Diovan HCT Tablets 2196
Diuril Oral Suspension 1954
Diuril Sodium Intravenous 2467
FazaClo Orally Disintegrating Tablets (1%) 551
Furosemide Tablets 2154
Hyzaar 50-12.5 Tablets 1990
Hyzaar 100-12.5 Tablets 1990
Hyzaar 100-25 Tablets 1990
▲ Indapamide Tablets (Greater than or equal to 5%) 2156
Indocin I.V. (Less than 1%) 2465
Lamictal (1.0%) 1481
Lopressor HCT 50/25 Tablets 2241
Lopressor HCT 100/25 Tablets 2241
Lopressor HCT 100/50 Tablets 2241
Lotensin HCT Tablets 2246
Maxalt Tablets (Infrequent) 2008
Maxalt-MLT Orally Disintegrating Tablets (Infrequent) 2008
Micardis HCT Tablets 856
Migranal Nasal Spray (Rare) 3348
Mivacron Injection (Less than 1%) 493
Moduretic Tablets (Less than or equal to 1%) 2028
Parnate Tablets 1527
Prinzide Tablets 2056
Proleukin for Injection (1%) 2266
Proquin XR Tablets (Less than 1%) 1153
ProSom Tablets (Infrequent) 517
Requip Tablets (1% or more) 1555
Retrovir Capsules 1560
Retrovir IV Infusion 1564
Retrovir 1560
Rythmol SR Capsules 2727
Syprine Capsules 2085
Teveten HCT Tablets 1737
Timolide Tablets 2086
▲ Ultram ER Tablets (1% to greater than 5%) 2392
Uniretic Tablets 3100
Valium Tablets 2819
Vancocin HCl Capsules, USP 3380
▲ Vivitrol (2% to 8%) 995
Wellbutrin Tablets (1.9%) 1603
Xifaxan Tablets (Less than 2%) 2842

Muscle spasms, paradoxical
Diastat Rectal Delivery System 3343
Niravam Orally Disintegrating Tablets (Rare) 3092

Muscle stiffness
▲ Advair Diskus 100/50 (1% to 3%) 1308
▲ Advair Diskus 250/50 (1% to 3%) 1308
▲ Advair Diskus 500/50 (1% to 3%) 1308
Exelon Capsules (Infrequent) 2206
Exelon Oral Solution (Infrequent) 2206
▲ Flovent HFA (1% to 3%) 1447
Gleevec Tablets (Infrequent) 2227
Imitrex Injection (Rare) 1463
Niravam Orally Disintegrating Tablets (2.2%) 3092
▲ Vivitrol (2% to 8%) 995

Muscle tightness
Xyrem Oral Solution (Infrequent) 1688

Muscle tiredness
Imitrex Injection (Rare) 1463

Muscle tone disorders
▲ Niravam Orally Disintegrating Tablets (5.9% to 6.3%) 3092

Muscle twitching
(*see under* Fasciculations)

Muscle weakness
(*see under* Myasthenia)

Muscular disturbances
Copaxone for Injection (Infrequent) 3297
▲ Gengraf Capsules (12%) 459
Lescol Capsules 2233
Lescol XL Tablets 2233
▲ Neoral Oral Solution (12%) 2259
▲ Neoral Soft Gelatin Capsules (12%) 2259
Prometrium Capsules (100 mg, 200 mg) (Less than 5%) 3203
▲ Risperdal (17% to 34%) 1676
▲ Risperdal M-Tab Orally Disintegrating Tablets (17% to 34%) 1676
Zosyn (1.0% or less) 3492

Musculoskeletal aches
Follistim AQ Cartridge 2338

Musculoskeletal contracture
Neurontin Capsules (Rare) 2487
Neurontin Oral Solution (Rare) 2487
Neurontin Tablets (Rare) 2487

Musculoskeletal stiffness
Xyrem Oral Solution (Infrequent) 1688

Musculoskeletal symptoms, unspecified
Accutane Capsules 2731
▲ Arimidex Tablets (30% to 36%) 673
▲ Epivir (12%) 1427
Flovent Diskus 1443
▲ Gengraf Capsules (13.2%) 459
▲ Hycamtin for Injection (14%) 1458
▲ Imdur Tablets (Less than or equal to 5%) 3018
▲ Infergen (4% to 7%) 3364
Invirase (0.6% to 2.0%) 2772
Mobic Oral Suspension (1.7% to 2.9%) 863
Mobic Tablets (1.7% to 2.9%) 863
▲ Neoral Oral Solution (13.2%) 2259
▲ Neoral Soft Gelatin Capsules (13.2%) 2259
Trasylol Injection (2%) 754

Musculoskeletal trauma
Avalide Tablets 888
Avalide Tablets 2874
Avapro Tablets (2%) 891
Avapro Tablets (2%) 2871

Mutism
Prograf Capsules and Injection 632

Myalgia
Abelcet Injection 1141
▲ Abilify Oral Solution (4%) 882
▲ Abilify Oral Solution (4%) 2450
▲ Abilify Discmelt Orally Disintegrating Tablets (4%) 882
▲ Abilify Discmelt Orally Disintegrating Tablets (4%) 2450
▲ Abilify Tablets (4%) 882
▲ Abilify Tablets (4%) 2450
Accolate Tablets (1.6%) 671
Aceon Tablets (2 mg, 4 mg, 8 mg) (0.3% to 1.1%) 3194
Aciphex Tablets 1090
▲ Actimmune (6%) 1671
Actiq (Less than 1%) 979
▲ Actonel Tablets (4.6% to 6.6%) 2683
▲ Actonel with Calcium Tablets (4.6% to 6.6%) 2688
▲ ActoPlus Met Tablets (5.4%) 3214
▲ Actos Tablets (5.4%) 3219
Adalat CC Tablets (Less than 1%) 2964
▲ Advair HFA Inhalation Aerosol (1% to 4%) 1318
▲ Advicor Tablets (3%) 1722
Aggrenox Capsules (1.2%) 822
▲ Agrylin Capsules (1% to 5%) 3169
Aldara Cream, 5% (1% to 1.4%) 1846
Aldoril Tablets 1910
▲ Alferon N Injection (One patient to 45%) 1665
▲ Alimta for Injection (Up to 13%) 1750
Alinia for Oral Suspension (Less than 1%) 2835
Alinia Tablets (Less than 1%) 2835
Altace Capsules (Less than 1%) 1702
▲ Altoprev Extended-Release Tablets (3%) 3109
▲ Ambien Tablets (1% to 7%) 2851
▲ Ambien CR Tablets (4% to frequent) 2855
AmBisome for Injection (Less common) 620
Amerge Tablets (Infrequent) 1339
Amevive (Common) 626
Anaprox Tablets (Less than 1%) 2761
Anaprox DS Tablets (Less than 1%) 2761
Anzemet Injection (Rare) 2859
Anzemet Tablets (Rare) 2862
Aptivus Capsules (Less than 2%) 826
▲ Aranesp for Injection (8% to 21%) 581
▲ Aredia for Injection (26%) 2179
▲ Arimidex Tablets (2% to 6%) 673
▲ Aromasin Tablets (5.5%) 2600

▲ Arranon Injection (1% to 13%) 1357
Arthrotec Tablets (Rare)................... 3129
▲ Asacol Delayed-Release Tablets (3%)... 2692
▲ Asmanex Twisthaler (2% to 3%) 2966
Astelin Nasal Spray (1.5%)............... 1904
Atacand Tablets (0.5% or greater).... 649
Atacand HCT (0.5% or greater)........ 651
▲ Atripla Tablets (Greater than or equal to 5%)................................ 945
Augmentin.. 1360
Augmentin Tablets........................... 1363
Augmentin XR Extended-Release Tablets.. 1369
Augmentin ES-600 Powder for Oral Suspension.......................... 1366
Avalide Tablets................................ 888
Avalide Tablets................................ 2874
Avapro Tablets (1% or greater)......... 891
Avapro Tablets (1% or greater)......... 2871
▲ Avastin IV (8% to 15%) 1227
Avelox (0.1% to less than 2%) 2970
Axert Tablets (Infrequent) 2396
Axid Oral Solution (1.7%) 879
▲ Azmacort Inhalation Aerosol (1% to 3%) 1726
Beconase AQ Nasal Spray 1396
Benicar Tablets (Greater than 0.5%) 1043
Benicar HCT Tablets 1044
▲ Betaseron for SC Injection (27%) 767
▲ Bexxar (Less than 1% to 13%) 1398
BiDil Tablets (1% to less than 2%) 2171
Biltricide Tablets 2976
▲ Boniva Injection (0.8% to 5.7%) 2738
▲ Boniva Tablets (0.8% to 5.7%) 2741
Boostrix 1404
▲ Brimonidine Tartrate Ophthalmic Solution 0.2% (3% to 9%) .... ⊙ 248
▲ Caduet Tablets (Greater than 0.1% to 5.6%) 2508
Calcijex Injection 411
Calcium Disodium Versenate Injection 1851
▲ Campath Ampules (11%) 811
Campral Tablets (Frequent) 1174
▲ Cancidas for Injection (0% to 3.1%) 1918
Captopril Tablets 2149
Carbatrol Capsules 3171
Cardura XL Tablets (1.4%) 2515
Catapres Tablets (About 6 in 1,000 patients) 843
Catapres-TTS (0.5% or less) 844
Celebrex Capsules (0.1% to 1.9%) ... 3134
Celexa (2%) 1176
▲ CellCept Capsules (3% to less than 20%) 2747
▲ CellCept Intravenous (3% to less than 20%) 2747
▲ CellCept Oral Suspension (3% to less than 20%) 2747
▲ CellCept Tablets (3% to less than 20%) 2747
Cesamet Capsules 3340
Chantix Tablets (Frequent) 2517
▲ Cialis Tablets (1% to 4%) 1838
Cipro 2977
Cipro I.V. 2984
Cipro XR Tablets 2990
▲ Clarinex Tablets (2.1% to 3%) 2995
▲ Clarinex Reditabs Tablets (2.1% to 3%) 2995
Clinoril Tablets (Less than 1 in 100) 1924
▲ Clolar for Intravenous Infusion (14%) 1271
Clorpres Tablets (About 6 in 1,000) 2153
Clozaril Tablets (1%) 2184
Colazal Capsules (1%) 2838
▲ Combivir Tablets (8%) 1411
Copaxone for Injection (At least 2%) 3297
▲ Copegus Tablets (40%) 2754
Cosmegen for Injection 2459
Coumadin for Injection 898
Coumadin Tablets 898
Cozaar Tablets (1% or greater) 1935
Crestor Tablets (2.8%) 678
Cubicin for Injection (Less than 1%) 1026
▲ Cymbalta Delayed-Release Capsules (1% to 4%) 1757
▲ Dacogen Injection (5%) 2129
Dantrium Capsules (Less frequent) .. 2694
Demadex Injection (1.6%) 2759
Demadex Tablets (1.6%) 2759
▲ Depacon Injection (1% to 5%) 412
▲ Depakene (1% to 5%) 417
▲ Depakote Sprinkle Capsules (1% to 5%) 422
▲ Depakote Tablets (1% to 5%) 427
▲ Depakote ER Tablets (Greater than 1% to 5%) 434
Didronel Tablets (Infrequent)............ 2697
Diovan Tablets................................. 2193
Diovan HCT Tablets (Greater than 0.2%).. 2196
Dolobid Tablets (Less than 1 in 100).. 1955
▲ Doxil Injection (Less than 1% to 10%).. 2351
▲ Duetact Tablets (At least 5%) 3226
Dyazide Capsules............................ 1423
EC-Naprosyn Delayed-Release Tablets (Less than 1%)................. 2761
Effexor Tablets 3411
▲ Effexor XR Capsules (4%) 3417
Eligard 30 mg (2.2%)....................... 2885
▲ Eligard 45 mg (4.5%) 2888
▲ Eloxatin for Injection (2% to 5%) 2892
Emend Capsules (Greater than 0.5%).. 1963
▲ Emtriva Capsules (4% to 6%) 1287
▲ Emtriva Oral Solution (4% to 6%) 1287
Engerix-B Vaccine (Less than 1%) 1425
▲ Entocort EC Capsules (Less than 5%)... 2698
▲ Epivir (8%) 1427
▲ Epivir-HBV (14%) 1432
Epogen for Injection (Rare) 591
Equetro Extended-Release Capsules 3180
▲ Evista Tablets (7.7%) 1763
▲ Evoxac Capsules (1% to 3%) 1047
Exelon Capsules (Frequent) 2206
Exelon Oral Solution (Frequent) 2206
Faslodex Injection (Less than 1%) 681
FazaClo Orally Disintegrating Tablets (1%) 551
▲ Femara Tablets (0.3% to 6.7%) 2214
Ferrlecit Injection 3388
▲ Flovent Diskus (1% to 12%) 1443
▲ Flovent HFA (1% to 3%) 1447
▲ Fluarix (10.2% to 23%) 1451
▲ Flumist Vaccine (5% to 16.7%) 1901
▲ Fortical Nasal Spray (1% to 3%) 3337
▲ Fosamax (0.4% to approximately 6%) 1969
▲ Fosamax Plus D Tablets (0.4% to 4.1%) 1977
Frova Tablets (Infrequent) 1113
Furosemide Tablets 2154
Fuzeon Injection (2.7%) 2767
▲ Gabitril Tablets (1% to 5%) 984
Gantrisin Pediatric Suspension 2770
Gardasil Injection (2%) 1984
Gemzar for Injection (Common) 1771
Gengraf Capsules (1% to less than 3%) 459
Genotropin Lyophilized Powder 2638
Geodon Capsules (2% to frequent) .. 2529
▲ Gleevec Tablets (0% to 58%) 2227
Havrix Vaccine (Less than 1%) 1456
Hectorol Capsules 1275
Hectorol Injection 1278
Humalog Mix 50/50-Pen 1783
▲ Humatrope Vials and Cartridges (9.1% to 24.3%) 1787
▲ Hycamtin for Injection (59%) 1458
Hytrin Capsules (At least 1%) 471
Hyzaar 50-12.5 Tablets 1990
Hyzaar 100-12.5 Tablets 1990
Hyzaar 100-25 Tablets 1990
▲ Imdur Tablets (Less than or equal to 5%) 3018
Imitrex Injection (2%) 1463
Imitrex Nasal Spray (Infrequent) 1467
Imitrex Tablets (Frequent) 1471
Infed Injection 3390
▲ Infergen (51% to 58%) 3364
▲ Intron A for Injection (3% to 75%) 3024
Invirase (0.3% to greater than or equal to 2%) 2772
Ionsys Transdermal System (.1% to less than 1%) 2379
▲ I.V. Busulfex (16%) 2493
Kaletra (Up to 2%) 476
Klonopin (1%) 2778
Lamictal (More than 1%) 1481
Lamisil Tablets 2232
▲ Lariam Tablets (Among most frequent) 2786
▲ Lescol Capsules (5.0%) 2233
▲ Lescol XL Tablets (3.8%) 2233
▲ Leukine (18%) 814
▲ Leustatin Injection (7%) 2357
Levaquin (0.1% to 0.9%) 2384
Levaquin in 5% Dextrose Injection (0.1% to 0.9%) 2384
Levitra Tablets (Less than 2%) 3034
Lexapro Oral Solution (Frequent) 1190
Lexapro Tablets (Frequent) 1190
▲ Lipitor Tablets (Up to 5.6%) 2483
Lithobid Tablets 1692
Lofibra Tablets 1219
Lofibra Capsules 1216
Lopressor HCT 50/25 Tablets (1%).. 2241
Lopressor HCT 100/25 Tablets (1%).. 2241
Lopressor HCT 100/50 Tablets (1%).. 2241
Lotensin Tablets (Less than 1%)....... 2243
Lotensin HCT Tablets (0.3% to 1%).. 2246
Lotrel Capsules 2249
Lotronex Tablets (Rare).................... 1512
Lunesta Tablets 3142
▲ Lupron Depot 3.75 mg (Less than 5%).. 3260
Lupron Depot 7.5 mg (Less than 5%).. 3264
Lupron Depot–3 Month 11.25 mg (0.6% to 1%)................................. 3265
Lupron Injection Pediatric 3259
Lyrica Capsules (Greater than or equal to 1%) 2539
Marinol Capsules (Less than 1%)...... 3333
Matulane Capsules 3191
▲ Mavik Tablets (4.7%) 486
Maxalt Tablets (Infrequent) 2008
Maxalt-MLT Orally Disintegrating Tablets (Infrequent) 2008
Meridia Capsules (1.9%) 489
Meruvax II 2019
Mevacor Tablets (1.8% to 2.4%) 2021
▲ Miacalcin Nasal Spray (1% to 3%) ... 2253
Micardis Tablets (1%) 854
Micardis HCT Tablets 856
Migranal Nasal Spray (Infrequent) 3348
Mirapex Tablets (Greater than or equal to 1%) 859
M-M-R II 2006
▲ Myfortic Tablets (3% to less than 20%) 2255
▲ Mylotarg for Injection (3% to 11%) ... 3431
▲ Nabi-HB (10%) 2169
Naprosyn Suspension (Less than 1%) 2761
Naprosyn Tablets (Less than 1%) 2761
Nasonex Nasal Spray (Greater than or equal to 2%) 3043
Neoral Oral Solution (1% to less than 3%) 2259
Neoral Soft Gelatin Capsules (1% to less than 3%) 2259
▲ Neulasta Injection (15% to 72%) 601
▲ Neumega for Injection (Greater than or equal to 10%) 3435
Neupogen for Injection 603
Neurontin Capsules (2.0%) 2487
Neurontin Oral Solution (2.0%) 2487
Neurontin Tablets (2.0%) 2487
▲ Nexavar Tablets (Common to Very Common) 746
Nexium Delayed-Release Capsules (Rare) 655
Nexium I.V. (Rare) 659
Niaspan Extended-Release Tablets ... 1730
Nimotop Capsules (Up to 1.4%) 749
▲ Nipent for Injection (11% to 19%) 1863
▲ Norditropin Cartridges (15%) 2323
Noroxin Tablets 2032
Norvasc Tablets (More than 0.1% to 1%) 2545
Norvir (1.7% to 2.4.%) 503
Omacor Capsules 2725
▲ Oncaspar (Greater than 1% but less than 5%) 1145
▲ Ontak Vials (17%) 1745
OptiPranolol Metipranolol Ophthalmic Solution 0.3% (A small number of patients) .... ⊙ 256
Orthoclone OKT3 Sterile Solution (Less than 1%) 2360
Paxil CR Controlled-Release Tablets (2%) 1538
Paxil (2%) 1530
▲ Pegasys (37%) 2789
▲ PEG-Intron Powder for Injection (54%) 3048
Pentasa Capsules (Less than 1%) 3185
Pepcid Injection (Infrequent) 2040
Pepcid (Infrequent) 2038
Permax Tablets (1.1%) 3356
Persantine Tablets (Rare) 868
Pexeva Tablets (2%) 1694
Plavix Tablets 917
Plavix Tablets 2926
▲ Pletal Tablets (2% to 3%) 2455
Pneumovax 23 2043
▲ Premarin Tablets (5% to 9%) 3446
▲ Premphase Tablets (4% to 5%) 3456
▲ Prempro Tablets (4% to 5%) 3456
Prevacid Delayed-Release Capsules (Less than 1%) 3271
Prevacid for Delayed-Release Oral Suspension (Less than 1%) 3271
Prevacid SoluTab Delayed-Release Orally Disintegrating Tablets (Less than 1%)............................ 3271
Prevacid NapraPAC (Less than 1%).. 3280
▲ PREVPAC (Less than 1% to 3%) 3284
Prezista Tablets (Less than 2%)........ 3306
Prilosec OTC Delayed-Release Tablets (Less than 1%)................. 2677
Prinivil Tablets (0.3% to greater than 1%).. 2052
Prinzide Tablets (0.3% to 1%)........... 2056
Prochieve 4% Gel............................. 1003
Prochieve 8% Gel............................. 1003
Procrit for Injection (Rare)................. 2364
▲ Prograf Capsules and Injection (3% to 15%).................................. 632
▲ Proleukin for Injection (6%) 2266
Prometrium Capsules (100 mg, 200 mg) (Less than 5%)................ 3203
ProQuad... 2064
Proquin XR Tablets........................... 1153
ProSom Tablets (Infrequent)............. 517
ProstaScint Kit.................................. 1037
Protonix I.V. (Less than 1%).............. 3472
Protonix Tablets (Less than 1%)....... 3469
▲ Protopic Ointment (Up to 3%) 638
Provigil Tablets (At least 1%)............ 988
Prozac Pulvules and Liquid............... 1801
▲ Pulmicort Respules (1% to 3%) 661
▲ Rapamune Oral Solution and Tablets (3% to 20%)...................... 3475
▲ Raptiva for Injection (8%) 1250
▲ Rebetol (32% to 64%) 3058
▲ Rebetron Combination Therapy (61% to 64%).................................. 3063
▲ Rebif Prefilled Syringe for Injection (25%)............................... 3159
Recombivax HB (Less than 1%)........ 2071
ReFacto Vials................................... 3484
Relenza Rotadisk (Less than 1.5%).. 1552
Relpax Tablets (Infrequent)............... 2548
Remicade for IV Injection.................. 971
ReoPro Vials (0.3%).......................... 1809
Requip Tablets (1% or more)............ 1555
Rescriptor Tablets............................. 2551
▲ Retrovir Capsules (8%) 1560
▲ Retrovir IV Infusion (8%) 1564
▲ Retrovir (8%) 1560
▲ Revatio Tablets (7%) 2557
▲ Revlimid Capsules (8.8%) 958
Reyataz Capsules (Less than 3%)..... 921
RhoGAM Ultra-Filtered...................... 2371
▲ Ribavirin, USP Capsules (32% to 64%)... 3068
▲ Risperdal (Infrequent to 5%) 1676
▲ Risperdal Consta Long-Acting Injection (2% to 4%)...................... 1682
▲ Risperdal M-Tab Orally Disintegrating Tablets (Infrequent to 5%).......................... 1676
▲ Rituxan I.V. (1% to 10%) 1254
Rocaltrol Capsules............................ 2798
Rocaltrol Oral Solution...................... 2798
Rozerem Tablets (2%)....................... 3231
Rythmol SR Capsules........................ 2727
Sandimmune (2% or less).................. 2275
Sandostatin Injection (Less than 1%).. 2278
▲ Sandostatin LAR Depot (5% to 15%).. 2280
▲ Sensipar Tablets (15%) 608
▲ Serevent Diskus (1% to 3%) 1568
▲ Simulect for Injection (3% to 10%) ... 2284
Singulair... 2077
Solodyn Extended Release Tablets (1%).. 1890
Sonata Capsules (Frequent)............. 1717
▲ Soriatane Capsules (1% to 10%) 1013
▲ Spiriva HandiHaler (4%) 869
▲ Strattera Capsules (3%) 1814
Stromectol Tablets (0.4%)................. 2083
Sular Tablets (Less than or equal to 1%).. 3122
Sustiva Capsules (Less than 2%)...... 930
Sustiva Tablets (Less than 2%)......... 930
▲ Sutent Capsules (1% to 17%) 2560
Tambocor Tablets (Less than 1%)..... 1856
▲ Tarceva Tablets (0% to 21%) 1259
▲ Tarceva Tablets (0% to 21%) 2444
Targretin Capsules............................ 1747
Tarka Tablets (0.3% or more)........... 524
Tasmar Tablets (Frequent)................ 3358
▲ Taxotere Injection Concentrate (Less than 1% to 21.1%).............. 2932
Tegretol/Tegretol-XR......................... 2295
▲ Temodar Capsules (5%) 3073
Tequin Injection (Less than 0.1%)..... 938
Tequin Injection in 5% Dextrose (Less than 0.1%)............................ 938
Tequin Tablets (Less than 0.1%)....... 938
Teveten Tablets (1% or greater)........ 1735
Teveten HCT Tablets (0.4%).............. 1737
Thalomid Capsules........................... 965
▲ Thiola Tablets (4%) 2141

Thyrolar Tablets 1199
Tiazac Capsules (2%) 1201
Timentin ADD-Vantage 1580
Timentin Injection Galaxy Container 1583
Timentin IV Infusion 1577
Timentin Pharmacy Bulk Package 1586
Timolide Tablets (Less than 1%) 2086
Tindamax Tablets 2142
Topamax Sprinkle Capsules (Greater than 1% to 2%) 2404
Topamax Tablets (Greater than 1% to 2%) 2404
Toprol-XL Tablets 668
Trelstar LA Suspension (1.1%) 3397
Tricor Tablets 527
▲ Trisenox Injection (25%) 993
▲ Trizivir Tablets (8%) 1589
Truvada Tablets 1296
Twinrix Vaccine (Less than 1%) 1595
▲ Ultram ER Tablets (1% to greater than 5%) 2392
Uniretic Tablets (Less than 1%) 3100
Univasc Tablets (1.3%) 3104
Vantas (Less than 2%) 3375
Vantin Tablets and Oral Suspension (Less than 1%) 2645
Vaqta (1.9%) 2097
Varivax (Greater than or equal to 1%) 2100
Vasotec I.V. Injection (0.5% to 1.0%) 2103
▲ Velcade for Injection (14%) 2133
▲ Vesanoid Capsules (14%) 2820
VFEND I.V. (Less than 2%) 2564
VFEND Oral Suspension (Less than 2%) 2564
VFEND Tablets (Less than 2%) 2564
Viagra Tablets (Less than 2%) 2573
Vicoprofen Tablets (Less than 1%) 539
Viracept (Less than 2%) 2577
Viramune Oral Suspension 873
Viramune Tablets 873
▲ Viread Tablets (3% to 4%) 1301
▲ Vytorin 10/10 Tablets (3.5%) 2114
▲ Vytorin 10/10 Tablets (3.5%) 3077
▲ Vytorin 10/20 Tablets (3.5%) 2114
▲ Vytorin 10/20 Tablets (3.5%) 3077
▲ Vytorin 10/40 Tablets (3.5%) 2114
▲ Vytorin 10/40 Tablets (3.5%) 3077
▲ Vytorin 10/80 Tablets (3.5%) 2114
▲ Vytorin 10/80 Tablets (3.5%) 3077
WelChol Tablets (2%) 1050
Wellbutrin Tablets 1603
▲ Wellbutrin SR Sustained-Release Tablets (2% to 6%) 1607
▲ Wellbutrin XL Extended-Release Tablets (2% to 6%) 1613
WinRho SDF 732
Xalatan Sterile Ophthalmic Solution (1% to 2%) 2649
▲ Xeloda Tablets (Less than 5% to 9%) 2822
▲ Xenical Capsules (4.2%) 2831
Xifaxan Tablets (Less than 2%) 2842
Xopenex Inhalation Solution (1.5%) 3146
Xopenex Inhalation Solution Concentrate (1.5%) 3150
Xopenex HFA Inhalation Aerosol (1.5%) 3154
Xyrem Oral Solution (Frequent) 1688
Zantac (Rare) 1624
Zantac Injection (Rare) 1619
Zantac Injection Pharmacy Bulk Package (Rare) 1622
Zantac Injection Premixed (Rare) 1619
Zantac (Rare) 1624
Zegerid Capsules (Less than 1%) 2958
Zegerid Powder for Oral Solution (Less than 1%) 2958
▲ Zelapar Tablets (3%) 3372
Zelnorm Tablets (1%) 2312
Zemaira (0.2% to 0.4%) 3509
Zemplar Injection 543
▲ Zetia Tablets (4.5% to 5%) 2120
▲ Zetia Tablets (5%) 3083
Ziagen 1626
Zocor Tablets 2105
▲ Zofran Injection (10%) 1634
Zoloft (Frequent) 2586
▲ Zometa for Intravenous Infusion (23%) 2315
Zomig Nasal Spray (Infrequent) 3523
Zonegran Capsules (Infrequent) 1101
Zosyn (1.0% or less) 3492
Zovirax 1643
▲ Zyban Sustained-Release Tablets (2% to 4%) 1644
▲ Zyflo Tablets (3.2%) 1023
Zyprexa Tablets 1830
Zyprexa ZYDIS Orally Disintegrating Tablets 1830
Zyrtec Chewable Tablets (Less than 2%) 2594
Zyrtec (Less than 2%) 2594
Zyrtec-D 12 Hour Extended Release Tablets (Less than 2%) 2597

Myasthenia

Abilify Oral Solution (Infrequent) 882
Abilify Oral Solution (Infrequent) 2450
Abilify Discmelt Orally Disintegrating Tablets (Infrequent) 882
Abilify Discmelt Orally Disintegrating Tablets (Infrequent) 2450
Abilify Tablets (Infrequent) 882
Abilify Tablets (Infrequent) 2450
Actiq (Less than 1%) 979
▲ Actonel Tablets (3.3%) 2683
Adalat CC Tablets (Less than 1%) 2964
Altoprev Extended-Release Tablets 3109
Ambien Tablets (Rare) 2851
Ambien CR Tablets (Rare) 2855
Anaprox Tablets (Less than 1%) 2761
Anaprox DS Tablets (Less than 1%) 2761
Aricept Tablets (Infrequent) 1094
Aricept ODT Tablets (Infrequent) 1094
Avalide Tablets 888
Avalide Tablets 2874
Axert Tablets (Infrequent) 2396
Azilect Tablets (2%) 3293
Betagan Ophthalmic Solution, USP ⊙ 220
▲ Betaseron for SC Injection (46%) 767
Caduet Tablets (Less than 2%) 2508
Campath Ampules 811
Carnitor Tablets and Oral Solution 3190
Carteolol Hydrochloride Ophthalmic Solution USP, 1% ⊙ 249
Celexa (Infrequent) 1176
▲ CellCept Capsules (3% to less than 20%) 2747
▲ CellCept Intravenous (3% to less than 20%) 2747
▲ CellCept Oral Suspension (3% to less than 20%) 2747
▲ CellCept Tablets (3% to less than 20%) 2747
Cipro 2977
Cipro I.V. 2984
Cipro XR Tablets 2990
Clozaril Tablets (1%) 2184
Colocort Rectal Suspension, USP (Retention) 100 mg/60 mL 2476
Combivir Tablets 1411
Copaxone for Injection (At least 2%) 3297
Cozaar Tablets (Less than 1%) 1935
Crestor Tablets (Less than 1%) 678
Decadron Tablets 1951
▲ Depakene (1% to 5%) 417
Depakote Tablets 427
▲ Depakote ER Tablets (1% to 5%) 434
Depo-Medrol Injectable Suspension 2617
Depo-Medrol Single-Dose Vial 2619
Doxil Injection (Less than 1%) 2351
EC-Naprosyn Delayed-Release Tablets (Less than 1%) 2761
Effexor XR Capsules (Infrequent) 3417
Emend Capsules (Greater than 0.5%) 1963
Epivir 1427
Epzicom Tablets 1436
Evoxac Capsules (Less than 1%) 1047
Exelon Capsules (Infrequent) 2206
Exelon Oral Solution (Infrequent) 2206
FazaClo Orally Disintegrating Tablets (1%) 551
▲ Flumist Vaccine (25.7%) 1901
Frova Tablets (Infrequent) 1113
Gabitril Tablets (1%) 984
Garamycin Injectable 3014
▲ Humira Injection (Less than 5%) 466
Hydrocortone Tablets 1989
Hyzaar 50-12.5 Tablets 1990
Hyzaar 100-12.5 Tablets 1990
Hyzaar 100-25 Tablets 1990
▲ Imdur Tablets (Less than or equal to 5%) 3018
▲ Intron A for Injection (Less than 5%) 3024
Klonopin 2778
Lariam Tablets (Infrequent) 2786
Lescol Capsules 2233
Lescol XL Tablets 2233
Levoxyl Tablets 1712
Lexapro Oral Solution (Infrequent) 1190
Lexapro Tablets (Infrequent) 1190
Lofibra Tablets 1219
Lofibra Capsules 1216
Lotensin HCT Tablets 2246
Lunesta Tablets (Infrequent) 3142
Lyrica Capsules (Greather than or equal to 1%) 2539
Mevacor Tablets 2021
Migranal Nasal Spray (Infrequent) 3348
Mirapex Tablets (Less than or equal to 1%) 859
▲ Myobloc Injection (3% to 6%) 3192
Naprosyn Suspension (Less than 1%) 2761
Naprosyn Tablets (Less than 1%) 2761
Neurontin Capsules (Infrequent) 2487
Neurontin Oral Solution (Infrequent) 2487
Neurontin Tablets (Infrequent) 2487
Niaspan Extended-Release Tablets 1730
Nimbex Injection 498
Norvasc Tablets (Less than 0.1%) 2545
Norvir (Less than 2%) 503
Pexeva Tablets (1%) 1694
Prevacid Delayed-Release Capsules (Less than 1%) 3271
Prevacid for Delayed-Release Oral Suspension (Less than 1%) 3271
Prevacid SoluTab Delayed-Release Orally Disintegrating Tablets (Less than 1%) 3271
Prevacid NapraPAC (Less than 1%) 3280
PREVPAC (Less than 1%) 3284
Prilosec OTC Delayed-Release Tablets (Less than 1%) 2677
Proquin XR Tablets 1153
Prozac Pulvules and Liquid (Rare) 1801
▲ Quadramet Injection (6.5%) 1040
Recombivax HB 2071
ReFacto Vials 3484
Relpax Tablets (Infrequent) 2548
Requip Tablets (Infrequent) 1555
Retrovir Capsules 1560
Retrovir IV Infusion 1564
Retrovir 1560
Reyataz Capsules (Less than 3%) 921
Risperdal Consta Long-Acting Injection (Infrequent) 1682
▲ Rythmol SR Capsules (1% to 4%) 2727
Sonata Capsules (Infrequent) 1717
Soriatane Capsules (Less than 1%) 1013
Symbyax Capsules (Rare) 1819
Targretin Capsules 1747
Tequin Injection (Less than 0.1%) 938
Tequin Injection in 5% Dextrose (Less than 0.1%) 938
Tequin Tablets (Less than 0.1%) 938
Thalomid Capsules 965
Timolide Tablets 2086
Topamax Sprinkle Capsules (More than 1%) 2404
Topamax Tablets (More than 1%) 2404
Tricor Tablets 527
Trileptal Tablets (1% to 2%) 2300
Trileptal Oral Suspension (1% to 2%) 2300
Trizivir Tablets 1589
VFEND I.V. (Less than 2%) 2564
VFEND Oral Suspension (Less than 2%) 2564
VFEND Tablets (Less than 2%) 2564
Viagra Tablets (Less than 2%) 2573
Viracept (Less than 2%) 2577
▲ Visudyne for Injection (1% to 10%) 2305
Wellbutrin Tablets 1603
▲ Xeloda Tablets (Less than 5%) 2822
Zegerid Capsules (Less than 1%) 2958
Zegerid Powder for Oral Solution (Less than 1%) 2958
Zelapar Tablets 3372
Zocor Tablets 2105
Zoloft (Infrequent) 2586
Zonegran Capsules (Infrequent) 1101
Zyrtec Chewable Tablets (Less than 2%) 2594
Zyrtec (Less than 2%) 2594
Zyrtec-D 12 Hour Extended Release Tablets (Less than 2%) 2597

Myasthenia gravis

Abelcet Injection 1141
Blocadren Tablets (Less than 1%) 1916
Captopril Tablets 2149
Cuprimine Capsules 1947
▲ Depacon Injection (1% to 5%) 412
▲ Depakote Sprinkle Capsules (1% to 5%) 422
▲ Depakote Tablets (1% to 5%) 427
Effexor Tablets (Infrequent) 3411
Lamictal (1.3%) 1481
Lipitor Tablets (Less than 2%) 2483
Myleran Tablets (Rare) 1525
Paxil CR Controlled-Release Tablets (1%) 1538
Paxil (1%) 1530
▲ Prograf Capsules and Injection (3% to 15%) 632
Proquin XR Tablets 1153
Rilutek Tablets (Infrequent) 2930
Sular Tablets (Less than or equal to 1%) 3122
Syprine Capsules 2085

Myasthenia gravis, exacerbation of

Betoptic S Ophthalmic Suspension 558
Cipro 2977
Cipro I.V. 2984
Cipro XR Tablets 2990
Cosopt Sterile Ophthalmic Solution 1931
Ketek Tablets 2903
Mefoxin for Injection (A possibility) 2012
Mefoxin Premixed Intravenous Solution 2016
Noroxin Tablets 2032
Timolide Tablets 2086
Timoptic Sterile Ophthalmic Solution (Less frequent) 2088
Timoptic-XE Sterile Ophthalmic Gel Forming Solution 2092

Myasthenia gravis, increase

Betagan Ophthalmic Solution, USP ⊙ 220
Betimol Ophthalmic Solution 3382
Betimol Ophthalmic Solution ⊙ 295
Timoptic in Ocudose (Less frequent) 2091

Myasthenia gravis-like syndrome

Clozaril Tablets 2184
Garamycin Injectable 3014
Seroquel Tablets (Infrequent) 690

Myasthenic syndrome

FazaClo Orally Disintegrating Tablets 551
Thiola Tablets (2%) 2141

Mydriasis

Albalon Ophthalmic Solution ⊙ 218
Atrovent HFA Inhalation Aerosol 841
Bentyl Capsules 697
Bentyl Injection 697
Bentyl Syrup 697
Bentyl Tablets 697
Blephamide Ophthalmic Ointment (Occasional) 568
Blephamide Ophthalmic Suspension 569
Caverject Impulse Injection (Less than 1%) 2612
Celexa (Rare) 1176
Clozaril Tablets (Less than 1%) 2184
Copaxone for Injection (Infrequent) 3297
Diastat Rectal Delivery System (Less than 1%) 3343
Ditropan XL Extended-Release Tablets 2413
Donnatal Extentabs 2493
Effexor Tablets (2%) 3411
Effexor XR Capsules (Frequent) 3417
Evoxac Capsules (Less than 1%) 1047
FazaClo Orally Disintegrating Tablets (Less than 1%) 551
FML Ophthalmic Ointment (Occasional) ⊙ 228
FML Ophthalmic Suspension (Occasional) ⊙ 227
FML Forte Ophthalmic Suspension (Occasional) ⊙ 226
Imitrex Nasal Spray 1467
Imitrex Tablets (Rare) 1471
Lexapro Oral Solution (Infrequent) 1190
Lexapro Tablets (Infrequent) 1190
Lunesta Tablets (Rare) 3142
Lyrica Capsules (Rare) 2539
▲ Macugen Injection (1% to 5%) ⊙ 261
Meridia Capsules 489
Norflex Injection 1856
Ocufen Ophthalmic Solution ⊙ 232
Parcopa Orally Disintegrating Tablets 3097
Paxil CR Controlled-Release Tablets (Infrequent) 1538
Paxil (Infrequent) 1530
Pexeva Tablets (infrequent) 1694
Pred Mild Ophthalmic Suspension (Occasional) ⊙ 238
Pred Forte Ophthalmic Suspension (Occasional) ⊙ 235
Propine Ophthalmic Solution ⊙ 239
Prozac Pulvules and Liquid (Infrequent) 1801
Stalevo Tablets 2287
Strattera Capsules (1% to 2%) 1814
Symmetrel Tablets 1135
Thioridazine Hydrochloride Tablets 2163
Thiothixene Capsules 2165

Topamax Sprinkle Capsules (Rare)... 2404
Topamax Tablets (Rare)... 2404
Transderm Scōp Transdermal Therapeutic System... 2177
Trileptal Tablets... 2300
Trileptal Oral Suspension... 2300
VFEND I.V. (Less than 2%)... 2564
VFEND Oral Suspension (Less than 2%)... 2564
VFEND Tablets (Less than 2%)... 2564
Viagra Tablets (Less than 2%)... 2573
Wellbutrin Tablets (Infrequent)... 1603
Wellbutrin SR Sustained-Release Tablets... 1607
Wellbutrin XL Extended-Release Tablets... 1613
Zoloft (Infrequent)... 2586
Zyban Sustained-Release Tablets... 1644
Zyprexa Tablets (Rare)... 1830
Zyprexa ZYDIS Orally Disintegrating Tablets (Rare)... 1830

Myelitis
ADACEL Vaccine... 2945
Azilect Tablets (Rare)... 3293
Fluarix... 1451
Havrix Vaccine (Rare)... 1456
Paxil CR Controlled-Release Tablets (Rare)... 1538
Paxil (Rare)... 1530
Permax Tablets (Rare)... 3356
Pexeva Tablets... 1694
Recombivax HB... 2071
Twinrix Vaccine... 1595
Zyrtec Chewable Tablets (Less than 2%)... 2594
Zyrtec (Less than 2%)... 2594
Zyrtec-D 12 Hour Extended Release Tablets (Less than 2%)... 2597

Myelitis, transverse
Asacol Delayed-Release Tablets (Rare)... 2692
Bicillin C-R Injectable Suspension... 1706
Enbrel for Injection (Rare)... 584
Engerix-B Vaccine... 1425
Menactra Vaccine... 2954
ProQuad... 2064
Raptiva for Injection (1 case)... 1250
Recombivax HB... 2071
Remicade for IV Injection... 971
Twinrix Vaccine... 1595
Varivax... 2100

Myelodysplastic syndrome
Bexxar... 1398
Neupogen for Injection (Approximately 3%)... 603
Temodar Capsules... 3073

Myelofibrosis
Lyrica Capsules (Rare)... 2539

Myeloid immaturity
Miradon Tablets... 3042

Myeloma, multiple
Effexor XR Capsules (Rare)... 3417

Myelopolyradiculoneuritis
Invirase (Less than 2%)... 2772

Myelosclerosis, malignant
Matulane Capsules... 3191

Myelosuppression
Alkeran for Injection... 955
Camptosar Injection... 2604
Dacogen Injection... 2129
Doxil Injection... 2351
Gemzar for Injection... 1771
▲ I.V. Busulfex (100%, most frequent, occurring in all patients)... 2493
Leukeran Tablets... 1504
Leustatin Injection (Frequent)... 2357
▲ Myleran Tablets (Most frequent)... 1525
Mylotarg for Injection... 3431
Sutent Capsules... 2560
▲ Tabloid Tablets (Most frequent)... 1575
Temodar Capsules... 3073
Zinecard for Injection... 2650

Myesthenia
▲ Eloxatin for Injection (2% to 5%)... 2892

Myocardial hypertrophy
Prograf Capsules and Injection (Rare)... 632

Myocardial infarction
▲ Abelcet Injection (3%)... 1141
Abilify Oral Solution (Infrequent)... 882
Abilify Oral Solution (Infrequent)... 2450
Abilify Discmelt Orally Disintegrating Tablets (Infrequent)... 882
Abilify Discmelt Orally Disintegrating Tablets (Infrequent)... 2450
Abilify Tablets (Infrequent)... 882
Abilify Tablets (Infrequent)... 2450
Aceon Tablets (2 mg, 4 mg, 8 mg) (0.3% to 1%)... 3194
Aciphex Tablets... 1090
Actimmune (Rare)... 1671
Adderall Tablets... 3164
Adderall XR Capsules... 3166
Adenoscan (Less than 1%)... 619
▲ Advair HFA Inhalation Aerosol (1% to 3%)... 1318
Agrylin Capsules... 3169
Aldara Cream, 5%... 1846
Altace Capsules (1.7%)... 1702
Ambien Tablets (Rare)... 2851
Ambien CR Tablets (Rare)... 2855
Amerge Tablets... 1339
Amevive (Less than 1%)... 626
Anaprox Tablets (Less than 1%)... 2761
Anaprox DS Tablets (Less than 1%)... 2761
Angeliq Tablets... 762
Aranesp for Injection (2%)... 581
▲ Argatroban Injection (3.6%)... 1346
Aricept Tablets (Infrequent)... 1094
Aricept ODT Tablets (Infrequent)... 1094
Arimidex Tablets (0.8%)... 673
Aromasin Tablets (1.6%)... 2600
Arthrotec Tablets (Rare)... 3129
Atacand Tablets (Less frequently)... 649
Atacand HCT (Less than 0.5%)... 651
Avalide Tablets... 888
Avalide Tablets... 2874
Avapro Tablets (Less than 1%)... 891
Avapro Tablets (Less than 1%)... 2871
Azilect Tablets (Infrequent)... 3293
Caduet Tablets... 2508
Campath Ampules... 811
Campral Tablets (Infrequent)... 1174
Camptosar Injection (0.4% to 1.3%)... 2604
Captopril Tablets (2 to 3 of 1000 patients)... 2149
Carbatrol Capsules... 3171
Cardene I.V.... 2497
Cardizem LA Extended Release Tablets... 1728
Cardura XL Tablets... 2515
Celebrex Capsules (0.1% to 1.9%)... 3134
Celexa (Infrequent)... 1176
Chantix Tablets (Infrequent)... 2517
Cialis Tablets (Less than 2%)... 1838
Cipro (Less than 1%)... 2977
Cipro I.V. (1% or less)... 2984
Cipro XR Tablets... 2990
Climara Transdermal System... 771
Climara Pro Transdermal System... 776
Clozaril Tablets (Several patients)... 2184
Coreg Tablets (0.1% to 1%)... 1414
Cosopt Sterile Ophthalmic Solution (Less than 1%)... 1931
Covera-HS Tablets (Less than 2%)... 3139
Cozaar Tablets (Less than 1%)... 1935
Crixivan Capsules... 1940
Cymbalta Delayed-Release Capsules (Infrequent)... 1757
Dacogen Injection... 2129
Dolobid Tablets... 1955
DynaCirc CR Tablets (0.5% to 1%)... 2721
EC-Naprosyn Delayed-Release Tablets (Less than 1%)... 2761
Edex Injection (1%)... 3089
Effexor Tablets (Rare)... 3411
Effexor XR Capsules (Infrequent)... 3417
Elitek (Less than or equal to 1%)... 2890
▲ Emcyt Capsules (3%)... 2634
Emend Capsules (Greater than 0.5%)... 1963
Enbrel for Injection (Infrequent)... 584
Enjuvia Tablets... 1062
Epogen for Injection (0.4%)... 591
Estrasorb Topical Emulsion... 1147
Estratest Tablets... 3199
Estratest H.S. Tablets... 3199
Ethyol for Injection (Rare)... 1898
Evoxac Capsules (Less than 1%)... 1047
Exelon Capsules (Frequent)... 2206
Exelon Oral Solution (Frequent)... 2206
Exubera Inhalation Powder (0.7%)... 2524
Feiba VH... 718
Femara Tablets (Less than or equal to 2%)... 2214
Ferrlecit Injection... 3388
Fortical Nasal Spray (Less than 1%)... 3337
Frova Tablets... 1113
Gabitril Tablets (Infrequent)... 984
Gammagard S/D... 724
Gemzar for Injection (Very rare)... 1771
Gengraf Capsules (1% to less than 3%)... 459
▲ Humira Injection (Less than 5%)... 466
Hyperstat I.V.... 3017
Hyzaar 50-12.5 Tablets... 1990
Hyzaar 100-12.5 Tablets... 1990
Hyzaar 100-25 Tablets... 1990
▲ Imdur Tablets (Less than or equal to 5%)... 3018
Imitrex Injection (Extremely rare)... 1463
Imitrex Nasal Spray... 1467
Imitrex Tablets (Rare)... 1471
Inspra Tablets... 2536
Ionsys Transdermal System (.1% to less than 1%)... 2379
Lamictal (Rare)... 1481
Levaquin (0.1% to 0.9%)... 2384
Levaquin in 5% Dextrose Injection (0.1% to 0.9%)... 2384
Levitra Tablets (Less than 2%)... 3034
Levothroid Tablets... 1186
Levoxyl Tablets... 1712
Lexapro Oral Solution... 1190
Lexapro Tablets... 1190
Lofibra Tablets... 1219
Lofibra Capsules... 1216
Lotrel Capsules (Rare)... 2249
Maxalt Tablets (Very rare)... 2008
Maxalt-MLT Orally Disintegrating Tablets (Very rare)... 2008
Menostar Transdermal System... 782
Meridia Capsules... 489
Merrem I.V. (Greater than 0.1% to 1%)... 686
Miacalcin Nasal Spray (Less than 1%)... 2253
Micardis Tablets... 854
Micardis HCT Tablets... 856
Mirapex Tablets (Less than 1%)... 859
Mircette Tablets... 1066
Mobic Oral Suspension (Less than 2%)... 863
Mobic Tablets (Less than 2%)... 863
Mycamine for Injection... 628
Namenda (Infrequent)... 1195
Naprosyn Suspension (Less than 1%)... 2761
Naprosyn Tablets (Less than 1%)... 2761
Neoral Oral Solution (1% to less than 3%)... 2259
Neoral Soft Gelatin Capsules (1% to less than 3%)... 2259
▲ Neupogen for Injection (11 of 375 cancer patients)... 603
Neurontin Capsules (Rare)... 2487
Neurontin Oral Solution (Rare)... 2487
Neurontin Tablets (Rare)... 2487
Nexavar Tablets (Uncommon)... 746
Noroxin Tablets (Less frequent)... 2032
Norvasc Tablets (Rare)... 2545
NovoSeven... 2331
NuvaRing... 2340
Omacor Capsules... 2725
Omnicef Capsules... 511
Omnicef for Oral Suspension... 511
Ontak Vials (Two patients)... 1745
OptiPranolol Metipranolol Ophthalmic Solution 0.3% (A small number of patients)... ⊙256
Ortho-Cyclen Tablets... 2429
Ortho Evra Transdermal System... 2417
Ortho Tri-Cyclen Tablets... 2429
Ortho Tri-Cyclen Lo Tablets... 2436
Orthoclone OKT3 Sterile Solution (Less than 1%)... 2360
Parcopa Orally Disintegrating Tablets... 3097
Paxil CR Controlled-Release Tablets (Rare)... 1538
Paxil (Rare)... 1530
Pegasys... 2789
PEG-Intron Powder for Injection (Less than or equal to 1%)... 3048
Permax Tablets (1.1%)... 3356
Pexeva Tablets (Rare)... 1694
Photofrin for Injection... 702
Pletal Tablets (Less than 2%)... 2455
Premarin Intravenous... 3442
Premarin Tablets... 3446
Premarin Vaginal Cream... 3452
Premphase Tablets... 3456
Prempro Tablets... 3456
Prevacid Delayed-Release Capsules (Less than 1%)... 3271
Prevacid for Delayed-Release Oral Suspension (Less than 1%)... 3271
Prevacid SoluTab Delayed-Release Orally Disintegrating Tablets (Less than 1%)... 3271
Prevacid NapraPAC (Less than 1%)... 3280
PREVPAC (Less than 1%)... 3284
Prezista Tablets (Less than 2%)... 3306
Prinivil Tablets (0.3% to 1.0%)... 2052
Prinzide Tablets... 2056
Procrit for Injection (0.4%)... 2364
Prograf Capsules and Injection... 632
Proleukin for Injection (2%)... 2266
Proquin XR Tablets... 1153
Protonix I.V. (Less than 1%)... 3472
Protonix Tablets (Less than 1%)... 3469
Prozac Pulvules and Liquid (Infrequent)... 1801
Razadyne (Infrequent)... 2399
Rebetol... 3058
Relpax Tablets (Rare)... 2548
Remicade for IV Injection (Greater than or equal to 0.2%)... 971
Revatio Tablets... 2557
Revlimid Capsules... 958
Rilutek Tablets (Infrequent)... 2930
Risperdal (Infrequent)... 1676
Risperdal Consta Long-Acting Injection (Infrequent)... 1682
Risperdal M-Tab Orally Disintegrating Tablets (Infrequent)... 1676
Ritalin LA Capsules... 2271
Rituxan I.V.... 1254
Rythmol SR Capsules... 2727
Sandimmune (Rare)... 2275
Sandostatin LAR Depot (Rare)... 2280
Seasonique Tablets... 1077
Soriatane Capsules... 1013
Stalevo Tablets... 2287
Sular Tablets (Less than or equal to 1%)... 3122
Sutent Capsules (1 patient)... 2560
Symbyax Capsules (Rare)... 1819
Tarka Tablets (Less frequent)... 524
Tasmar Tablets (Infrequent)... 3358
Taxotere Injection Concentrate... 2932
Tegretol/Tegretol-XR... 2295
Thalomid Capsules... 965
Thyrogen for Injection (One patient)... 1286
Tiazac Capsules... 1201
Toprol-XL Tablets (Greater than 1%)... 668
▲ Trasylol Injection (6%)... 754
Tricor Tablets... 527
Triglide Tablets... 3123
▲ Ultram ER Tablets (1% to greater than 5%)... 2392
Uniretic Tablets (Less than 1%)... 3100
Univasc Tablets (Less than 1%)... 3104
Vasotec I.V. Injection (0.5% to 1.2%)... 2103
Verelan PM Extended-Release Capsules, Controlled-Onset (2% or less)... 3106
▲ Vesanoid Capsules (3%)... 2820
VFEND I.V. (Less than 2%)... 2564
VFEND Oral Suspension (Less than 2%)... 2564
VFEND Tablets (Less than 2%)... 2564
Viagra Tablets... 2573
Vivitrol... 995
Voltaren Tablets (Rarely)... 2307
Voltaren-XR Tablets (Rarely)... 2310
Wellbutrin Tablets (Rare)... 1603
Wellbutrin SR Sustained-Release Tablets... 1607
Wellbutrin XL Extended-Release Tablets... 1613
Yasmin 28 Tablets... 796
Yaz Tablets... 803
Zelapar Tablets... 3372
Zoloft (Rare)... 2586
Zomig Tablets (Rare)... 3519
Zomig Nasal Spray (Rare)... 3523
Zomig-ZMT Tablets (Rare)... 3519
Zostavax Injection (0.3%)... 2111
Zosyn (1.0% or less)... 3492
Zyban Sustained-Release Tablets... 1644

Myocardial infarction, acute
Tarceva Tablets (2.3%)... 1259
Tarceva Tablets (2.3%)... 2444

Myocardial infarction, post-abrupt discontinuation
Inderal LA Long-Acting Capsules (Some cases)... 3429

Myocardial insufficiency
Orthoclone OKT3 Sterile Solution... 2360

Myocardial reinfarction
Activase I.V.... 1223

- Retavase ... 2499
- TNKase I.V. ... 1264

Myocardial rupture
- Activase I.V. ... 1223
- Decadron Tablets ... 1951
- Hydrocortone Tablets ... 1989
- Retavase ... 2499
- TNKase I.V. ... 1264

Myocarditis
- Aldoril Tablets ... 1910
- Asacol Delayed-Release Tablets (Rare) ... 2692
- Boostrix ... 1404
- Clozaril Tablets ... 2184
- Geodon Capsules (Rare) ... 2529
- Pentasa Capsules (Infrequent) ... 3185
- Proleukin for Injection (Less than 1% to 1%) ... 2266
- Reyataz Capsules (Less than 3%) ... 921
- Risperdal (Rare) ... 1676
- Risperdal M-Tab Orally Disintegrating Tablets (Rare) ... 1676
- ▲ Vesanoid Capsules (3%) ... 2820
- ▲ Xeloda Tablets (Less than 5%) ... 2822

Myocarditis, allergic
- Fansidar Tablets ... 2765
- Gantrisin Pediatric Suspension ... 2770

Myoclonia
- Abilify Oral Solution (Infrequent) ... 882
- Abilify Oral Solution (Infrequent) ... 2450
- Abilify Discmelt Orally Disintegrating Tablets (Infrequent) ... 882
- Abilify Discmelt Orally Disintegrating Tablets (Infrequent) ... 2450
- Abilify Tablets (Infrequent) ... 882
- Abilify Tablets (Infrequent) ... 2450
- Aloprim for Injection (Less than 1%) ... 2167
- Celexa ... 1176
- Cipro ... 2977
- Cipro I.V. ... 2984
- Cipro XR Tablets ... 2990
- Clozaril Tablets (1%) ... 2184
- Copaxone for Injection (Infrequent) ... 3297
- Dilaudid ... 440
- Dilaudid Non-Sterile Powder ... 440
- Dilaudid Oral Liquid ... 445
- Dilaudid Tablets - 8 mg ... 445
- Dilaudid-HP Injection ... 442
- Effexor Tablets (Infrequent) ... 3411
- Effexor XR Capsules (Infrequent) ... 3417
- Eldepryl Capsules ... 3208
- Fortaz ... 1453
- Gabitril Tablets (Frequent) ... 984
- Geodon Capsules (Rare) ... 2529
- Imitrex Injection (Rare) ... 1463
- Kadian Capsules (Less than 3%) ... 577
- Lamictal (Infrequent) ... 1481
- Leukeran Tablets (Rare) ... 1504
- Lexapro Oral Solution ... 1190
- Lexapro Tablets ... 1190
- Mirapex Tablets (1%) ... 859
- Neurontin Capsules (Rare) ... 2487
- Neurontin Oral Solution (Rare) ... 2487
- Neurontin Tablets (Rare) ... 2487
- Noroxin Tablets ... 2032
- Orthoclone OKT3 Sterile Solution ... 2360
- ▲ Paxil CR Controlled-Release Tablets (3%) ... 1538
- ▲ Paxil (3%) ... 1530
- Permax Tablets (Infrequent) ... 3356
- Primaxin I.M. ... 2045
- Primaxin I.V. (Less than 0.2%) ... 2048
- ▲ Prograf Capsules and Injection (3% to 15%) ... 632
- Rilutek Tablets (Infrequent) ... 2930
- Seroquel Tablets (Infrequent) ... 690
- Sonata Capsules (Rare) ... 1717
- Symbyax Capsules (Infrequent) ... 1819
- Tasmar Tablets (Infrequent) ... 3358
- Wellbutrin Tablets (Frequent) ... 1603
- Zonegran Capsules (Rare) ... 1101
- ▲ Zyprexa Tablets (1% to 5%) ... 1830
- ▲ Zyprexa ZYDIS Orally Disintegrating Tablets (1% to 5%) ... 1830

Myoclonus
- Azilect Tablets (Infrequent) ... 3293
- Exelon Capsules (Infrequent) ... 2206
- Exelon Oral Solution (Infrequent) ... 2206
- FazaClo Orally Disintegrating Tablets ... 551
- ▲ Lyrica Capsules (0.1% to 4%) ... 2539
- Maxipime for Injection ... 1105
- ▲ Pexeva Tablets (3%) ... 1694
- Proquin XR Tablets ... 1153
- Xyrem Oral Solution (Infrequent) ... 1688
- Zelapar Tablets ... 3372
- ▲ Zyprexa IntraMuscular (2% to 4%) ... 1830

Myoglobinemia
- Symmetrel Tablets (Uncommon) ... 1135

Myoglobinuria
- Bicillin C-R Injectable Suspension ... 1706
- Risperdal ... 1676
- Risperdal M-Tab Orally Disintegrating Tablets ... 1676
- Seroquel Tablets ... 690
- Zocor Tablets (Rare) ... 2105

Myolysis
- Trizivir Tablets ... 1589
- Ziagen ... 1626

Myopathy
- Abilify Oral Solution (Infrequent) ... 882
- Abilify Oral Solution (Infrequent) ... 2450
- Abilify Discmelt Orally Disintegrating Tablets (Infrequent) ... 882
- Abilify Discmelt Orally Disintegrating Tablets (Infrequent) ... 2450
- Abilify Tablets (Infrequent) ... 882
- Abilify Tablets (Infrequent) ... 2450
- Actiq (Less than 1%) ... 979
- Advicor Tablets ... 1722
- Altoprev Extended-Release Tablets ... 3109
- Atripla Tablets ... 945
- Axert Tablets (Rare) ... 2396
- Campral Tablets (Frequent) ... 1174
- Copaxone for Injection (Infrequent) ... 3297
- Crestor Tablets (Less than 1%) ... 678
- Effexor Tablets (Rare) ... 3411
- Effexor XR Capsules (Rare) ... 3417
- Geodon Capsules (Rare) ... 2529
- Herceptin I.V. (At least one of the 958 patients) ... 1233
- Lescol Capsules (Occasional) ... 2233
- Lescol XL Tablets ... 2233
- Lofibra Tablets ... 1219
- Lofibra Capsules ... 1216
- Lunesta Tablets (Rare) ... 3142
- Mevacor Tablets ... 2021
- Nimbex Injection ... 498
- Paxil CR Controlled-Release Tablets (2%) ... 1538
- Paxil (2%) ... 1530
- Pexeva Tablets (2%) ... 1694
- Proleukin for Injection ... 2266
- Prozac Pulvules and Liquid (Rare) ... 1801
- Relpax Tablets (Rare) ... 2548
- ReoPro Vials (0.4%) ... 1809
- Retrovir Capsules ... 1560
- Retrovir IV Infusion ... 1564
- Retrovir ... 1560
- Revlimid Capsules ... 958
- Reyataz Capsules (Less than 3%) ... 921
- Soriatane Capsules ... 1013
- Sustiva Capsules ... 930
- Sustiva Tablets ... 930
- Symbyax Capsules (Rare) ... 1819
- Trizivir Tablets ... 1589
- VFEND I.V. (Less than 2%) ... 2564
- VFEND Oral Suspension (Less than 2%) ... 2564
- VFEND Tablets (Less than 2%) ... 2564
- Viracept (Less than 2%) ... 2577
- Vytorin 10/10 Tablets ... 2114
- Vytorin 10/10 Tablets ... 3077
- Vytorin 10/20 Tablets ... 2114
- Vytorin 10/20 Tablets ... 3077
- Vytorin 10/40 Tablets ... 2114
- Vytorin 10/40 Tablets ... 3077
- Vytorin 10/80 Tablets ... 2114
- Vytorin 10/80 Tablets ... 3077
- Zetia Tablets (Very rarely) ... 2120
- Zocor Tablets (0.02% to 0.53%) ... 2105
- Zyprexa Tablets (Rare) ... 1830
- Zyprexa ZYDIS Orally Disintegrating Tablets (Rare) ... 1830

Myopathy, steroid
- Colocort Rectal Suspension, USP (Retention) 100 mg/60 mL ... 2476
- Decadron Tablets ... 1951
- Depo-Medrol Injectable Suspension ... 2617
- Depo-Medrol Single-Dose Vial ... 2619
- Hydrocortone Tablets ... 1989

Myopia
- Evoxac Capsules (Less than 1%) ... 1047
- Namenda (Infrequent) ... 1195
- Singulair (Greater than or equal to 2%) ... 2077
- Topamax Sprinkle Capsules (1%) ... 2404
- Topamax Tablets (1%) ... 2404

Myopia, transient
- Clorpres Tablets (Occasional) ... 2153
- Cosopt Sterile Ophthalmic Solution ... 1931
- Trusopt Sterile Ophthalmic Solution ... 2095

Myosis
- Doxil Injection (Less than 1%) ... 2351

Myositis
- ADACEL Vaccine ... 2945
- Advair Diskus 100/50 ... 1308
- Advair Diskus 250/50 ... 1308
- Advair Diskus 500/50 ... 1308
- Advair HFA Inhalation Aerosol ... 1318
- Caduet Tablets (Less than 2%) ... 2508
- Campath Ampules ... 811
- Chantix Tablets (Frequent) ... 2517
- Copegus Tablets (Less than 1%) ... 2754
- Crestor Tablets (Less than 1%) ... 678
- ▲ Imdur Tablets (Less than or equal to 5%) ... 3018
- Lipitor Tablets (Less than 2%) ... 2483
- Lofibra Tablets ... 1219
- Lofibra Capsules ... 1216
- Norvir (Less than 2%) ... 503
- Paxil CR Controlled-Release Tablets (Rare) ... 1538
- Paxil (Rare) ... 1530
- Pegasys (Less than 1%) ... 2789
- Permax Tablets (Infrequent) ... 3356
- Pexeva Tablets (Rare) ... 1694
- Proleukin for Injection ... 2266
- Prozac Pulvules and Liquid (Rare) ... 1801
- Retrovir Capsules ... 1560
- Retrovir IV Infusion ... 1564
- Retrovir ... 1560
- Sonata Capsules (Rare) ... 1717
- Sular Tablets (Less than or equal to 1%) ... 3122
- Ticlid Tablets (Rare) ... 2810
- Tricor Tablets ... 527
- Vasotec I.V. Injection (0.5% to 1.0%) ... 2103
- Vesanoid Capsules (Isolated cases) ... 2820

Myxedema
- Thalomid Capsules ... 965

N

Nail discoloration
- Evoxac Capsules (Less than 1%) ... 1047
- Lithobid Tablets ... 1692
- Retrovir Capsules ... 1560
- Retrovir IV Infusion ... 1564
- Retrovir ... 1560

Nail disorders, unspecified
- Atripla Tablets ... 945
- ▲ Avastin IV (2% to 8%) ... 1227
- Celebrex Capsules (0.1% to 1.9%) ... 3134
- ▲ Erbitux (Less than 1% to 16%) ... 910
- Evoxac Capsules (Less than 1%) ... 1047
- Gleevec Tablets (Infrequent) ... 2227
- Kaletra (Less than 2%) ... 476
- Lofibra Tablets ... 1219
- Lofibra Capsules ... 1216
- Lotronex Tablets (Rare) ... 1512
- Neurontin Capsules (Rare) ... 2487
- Neurontin Oral Solution (Rare) ... 2487
- Neurontin Tablets (Rare) ... 2487
- Penlac Nail Lacquer, Topical Solution, 8% (2%) ... 2924
- Prevacid Delayed-Release Capsules (Less than 1%) ... 3271
- Prevacid for Delayed-Release Oral Suspension (Less than 1%) ... 3271
- Prevacid SoluTab Delayed-Release Orally Disintegrating Tablets (Less than 1%) ... 3271
- Prevacid NapraPAC (Less than 1%) ... 3280
- PREVPAC (Less than 1%) ... 3284
- Reyataz Capsules (Less than 3%) ... 921
- Rythmol SR Capsules ... 2727
- Soriatane Capsules ... 1013
- Sustiva Capsules ... 930
- Sustiva Tablets ... 930
- Tricor Tablets ... 527

Nails, changes of
- Accutane Capsules ... 2731
- Advicor Tablets ... 1722
- Altoprev Extended-Release Tablets ... 3109
- Copaxone for Injection (At least 2%) ... 3297
- Effexor Tablets (Infrequent) ... 3411
- Effexor XR Capsules (Infrequent) ... 3417
- Gengraf Capsules (1% to less than 3%) ... 459
- ▲ Intron A for Injection (Less than 5%) ... 3024
- Invirase (Less than 2%) ... 2772
- Lescol Capsules ... 2233
- Lescol XL Tablets ... 2233
- ▲ Lupron Depot 3.75 mg (Less than 5%) ... 3260
- ▲ Lupron Depot–3 Month 11.25 mg (Less than 5%) ... 3265
- Mevacor Tablets ... 2021
- Neoral Oral Solution (1% to less than 3%) ... 2259
- Neoral Soft Gelatin Capsules (1% to less than 3%) ... 2259
- Oncaspar ... 1145
- Pentasa Capsules (Less than 1%) ... 3185
- Protopic Ointment (0.2% to less than 1%) ... 638
- Rescriptor Tablets ... 2551
- ▲ Soriatane Capsules (25% to 50%) ... 1013
- ▲ Taxotere Injection Concentrate (0% to 8.1%) ... 2932
- ▲ Thalomid Capsules (4.2%) ... 965
- Vytorin 10/10 Tablets ... 2114
- Vytorin 10/10 Tablets ... 3077
- Vytorin 10/20 Tablets ... 2114
- Vytorin 10/20 Tablets ... 3077
- Vytorin 10/40 Tablets ... 2114
- Vytorin 10/40 Tablets ... 3077
- Vytorin 10/80 Tablets ... 2114
- Vytorin 10/80 Tablets ... 3077
- ▲ Xeloda Tablets (Less than 5%) ... 2822
- Zocor Tablets ... 2105

Nasal burning
- ▲ Astelin Nasal Spray (4.1%) ... 1904
- Atrovent Nasal Spray 0.03% (2.0%) ... 837
- Atrovent Nasal Spray 0.06% (Less than 1%) ... 839
- ▲ Flonase Nasal Spray (2.4% to 3.2%) ... 1440
- 4-Way Fast Acting Nasal Spray ... ▣775
- Nasonex Nasal Spray ... 3043
- Vicks Sinex Nasal Spray and Ultra Fine Mist for Sinus Relief ... 2681
- Vicks Vapor Inhaler (Temporary) ... 2682
- Zicam Cold Remedy Gel Swabs ... ▣766
- Zicam Cold Remedy Nasal Gel ... ▣766
- Zicam Cold Remedy Swabs Kids Size ... ▣766
- Zicam Extreme Congestion Relief ... ▣767
- Zicam Intense Sinus Relief ... ▣767

Nasal congestion
- Adenoscan (Less than 1%) ... 619
- ▲ Advair Diskus 250/50 (1% to 3%) ... 1308
- ▲ Advair HFA Inhalation Aerosol (1% to 3%) ... 1318
- ▲ Aerobid/Aerobid-M (15%) ... 1171
- Alamast Ophthalmic Solution (Less than 5%) ... 3381
- Aldoril Tablets ... 1910
- Asacol Delayed-Release Tablets ... 2692
- Astelin Nasal Spray (Infrequently) ... 1904
- ▲ Atrovent Nasal Spray 0.03% (3.1%) ... 837
- Atrovent Nasal Spray 0.06% (1.1%) ... 839
- Bentyl Capsules ... 697
- Bentyl Injection ... 697
- Bentyl Syrup ... 697
- Bentyl Tablets ... 697
- Betagan Ophthalmic Solution, USP ... ⊙220
- Betimol Ophthalmic Solution ... 3382
- Betimol Ophthalmic Solution ... ⊙295
- BiDil Tablets ... 2171
- Calcium Disodium Versenate Injection ... 1851
- Cardizem LA Extended Release Tablets (Less than 2%) ... 1728
- Caverject Impulse Injection (1%) ... 2612
- Cesamet Capsules ... 3340
- ▲ Chemet Capsules (0.7% to 3.7%) ... 2458
- ▲ Cialis Tablets (2% to 3%) ... 1838
- Clozaril Tablets (1%) ... 2184
- Combivent Inhalation Aerosol ... 847
- Cosopt Sterile Ophthalmic Solution (1% to 5%) ... 1931
- Cozaar Tablets (2%) ... 1935
- ▲ Daytrana Transdermal Patch (6%) ... 3174
- Demser Capsules (Infrequent) ... 1953
- Dibenzyline Capsules ... 3399
- Diovan HCT Tablets (Greater than 0.2%) ... 2196
- DynaCirc CR Tablets (0.5% to 1%) ... 2721
- Elidel Cream 1% (0.6% to 2.6%) ... 2200
- FazaClo Orally Disintegrating Tablets (1%) ... 551

▲ Flebogamma 5%, Immune Globulin Intravenous (Human) (21%) ... 1658
▲ Flovent Diskus (16%) ... 1443
Fluarix (2.2%) ... 1451
▲ Flumist Vaccine (9.2% to 48.1%) ... 1901
▲ Fortical Nasal Spray (10.6%) ... 3337
Gardasil Injection (1.1%) ... 1984
▲ Hytrin Capsules (0.6% to 5.9%) ... 471
Hyzaar 50-12.5 Tablets ... 1990
Hyzaar 100-12.5 Tablets ... 1990
Hyzaar 100-25 Tablets ... 1990
▲ Imdur Tablets (Less than or equal to 5%) ... 3018
▲ Intron A for Injection (Up to 10%) ... 3024
Lexapro Oral Solution (Frequent) ... 1190
Lexapro Tablets (Frequent) ... 1190
Maxalt Tablets (Infrequent) ... 2008
Maxalt-MLT Orally Disintegrating Tablets (Infrequent) ... 2008
Meridia Capsules ... 489
Metrogel 1% (1.1%) ... 1211
▲ Miacalcin Nasal Spray (10.6%) ... 2253
Midamor Tablets (Less than or equal to 1%) ... 2026
Moduretic Tablets (Less than or equal to 1%) ... 2028
▲ Niravam Orally Disintegrating Tablets (7.3% to 17.4%) ... 3092
Oracea Capsules (1.5%) ... 1000
Orthoclone OKT3 Sterile Solution ... 2360
Prinivil Tablets (0.4%) ... 2052
Prinzide Tablets (0.3% to 1%) ... 2056
Prometrium Capsules (100 mg, 200 mg) (Less than 5%) ... 3203
ProQuad (Greater than or equal to 0.2% to less than 1%) ... 2064
Proventil Inhalation Solution 0.083% (1%) ... 3055
Requip Tablets (2%) ... 1555
▲ Serevent Diskus (4% to 9%) ... 1568
Singulair (1.6%) ... 2077
▲ Strattera Capsules (2% or greater) ... 1814
Symbicort 80/4.5 Inhalation Aerosol (2.5%) ... 3511
▲ Symbicort 160/4.5 Inhalation Aerosol (3.2%) ... 3511
Tessalon Capsules ... 1199
Tessalon Perles ... 1199
Thiothixene Capsules ... 2165
Tiazac Capsules (Less than 2%) ... 1201
Timoptic Sterile Ophthalmic Solution (Less frequent) ... 2088
Timoptic in Ocudose (Less frequent) ... 2091
Timoptic-XE Sterile Ophthalmic Gel Forming Solution ... 2092
Tylenol Sinus Severe Congestion Caplets with Cool Burst ... 1876
▲ Ultram ER Tablets (1% to greater than 5%) ... 2392
Vanos Cream (0% to 1.4%) ... 1893
Vaqta (1.2%) ... 2097
▲ Viagra Tablets (4%) ... 2573
Vicks Vapor Inhaler ... 2682
Xyrem Oral Solution (Frequent) ... 1688

Nasal crusts
▲ Fortical Nasal Spray (10.6%) ... 3337

Nasal discharge, increase
Aredia for Injection (One patient) ... 2179
Emend Capsules (Greater than 0.5%) ... 1963
▲ Flovent Diskus (1% to 3%) ... 1443
▲ Flumist Vaccine (9.2% to 48.1%) ... 1901
4-Way Fast Acting Nasal Spray ... ▣ 775
▲ Miacalcin Nasal Spray (10.6%) ... 2253
Vicks Sinex Nasal Spray and Ultra Fine Mist for Sinus Relief ... 2681
Vicks Vapor Inhaler (Temporary) ... 2682
Zicam Cold Remedy Gel Swabs ... ▣ 766
Zicam Cold Remedy Nasal Gel ... ▣ 766
Zicam Cold Remedy Swabs Kids Size ... ▣ 766
Zicam Extreme Congestion Relief ... ▣ 767
Zicam Intense Sinus Relief ... ▣ 767

Nasal drainage
Alferon N Injection (2%) ... 1665

Nasal drip, posterior
Aceon Tablets (2 mg, 4 mg, 8 mg) (0.3% to 1%) ... 3194
▲ Advair Diskus 100/50 (1% to 3%) ... 1308
▲ Advair Diskus 250/50 (1% to 3%) ... 1308
▲ Advair Diskus 500/50 (1% to 3%) ... 1308
Aricept Tablets (Infrequent) ... 1094
Aricept ODT Tablets (Infrequent) ... 1094
Astelin Nasal Spray (Infrequently) ... 1904
▲ Atrovent Nasal Spray 0.03% (3.1%) ... 837
▲ Dacogen Injection (5%) ... 2129
▲ Flovent HFA (1% to 3%) ... 1447
▲ Trisenox Injection (13%) ... 993

Nasal itching
(*see under* Pruritus, rhinal)

Nasal mucosa, dryness
(*see under* Xeromycteria)

Nasal obstruction
▲ Advair Diskus 250/50 (1% to 3%) ... 1308
Neurontin Oral Solution (Rare) ... 2487

Nasal passages, dry
Abilify Oral Solution (Rare) ... 882
Abilify Oral Solution (Rare) ... 2450
Abilify Discmelt Orally Disintegrating Tablets (Rare) ... 882
Abilify Discmelt Orally Disintegrating Tablets (Rare) ... 2450
Abilify Tablets (Rare) ... 882
Abilify Tablets (Rare) ... 2450
Astelin Nasal Spray (Infrequently) ... 1904

Nasal septum, perforation
Beconase AQ Nasal Spray (Rare) ... 1396
Flonase Nasal Spray (Rare) ... 1440
Nasacort AQ Nasal Spray (One patient) ... 2922
Nasonex Nasal Spray (Rare) ... 3043
Rhinocort Aqua Nasal Spray (Rare) ... 665

Nasal sores
▲ Fortical Nasal Spray (10.6%) ... 3337

Nasal stinging
4-Way Fast Acting Nasal Spray ... ▣ 775
Vicks Sinex Nasal Spray and Ultra Fine Mist for Sinus Relief ... 2681
Vicks Vapor Inhaler (Temporary) ... 2682
Zicam Cold Remedy Gel Swabs ... ▣ 766
Zicam Cold Remedy Nasal Gel ... ▣ 766
Zicam Cold Remedy Swabs Kids Size ... ▣ 766
Zicam Extreme Congestion Relief ... ▣ 767
Zicam Intense Sinus Relief ... ▣ 767

Nasal stuffiness
Beconase AQ Nasal Spray (Fewer than 3 per 100 patients) ... 1396
Nadolol Tablets (1 to 5 of 1000 patients) ... 2159
Phenergan Tablets and Suppositories ... 3440
Thioridazine Hydrochloride Tablets ... 2163

Nasal symptoms
▲ Fortical Nasal Spray (10.6%) ... 3337

Nasal ulceration
Beconase AQ Nasal Spray (Rare) ... 1396
Fortical Nasal Spray (2.8%) ... 3337
Nasonex Nasal Spray (Rare) ... 3043

Nasopharyngitis
▲ Advate Injection (14.7%) ... 712
▲ Ambien CR Tablets (6%) ... 2855
Amitiza Capsules (0% to 2.9%) ... 3224
Astelin Nasal Spray (Infrequently) ... 1904
▲ Atripla Tablets (3%) ... 945
▲ Avandamet Tablets (6%) ... 1373
▲ Avandia Tablets (3%) ... 1384
▲ Boniva Injection (3.5% to 4.3%) ... 2738
▲ Boniva Tablets (3.5% to 4.3%) ... 2741
▲ Clobex Spray (3% to 5%) ... 1208
▲ Cymbalta Delayed-Release Capsules (7% to 9%) ... 1757
▲ Daytrana Transdermal Patch (5%) ... 3174
▲ depo-subQ provera 104 Injectable Suspension (1% to less than 5%) ... 2624
Diovan HCT Tablets (2.4%) ... 2196
▲ Elidel Cream 1% (7.6% to 26.5%) ... 2200
▲ Fluarix (2.5%) ... 1451
▲ Gardasil Injection (6.4%) ... 1984
▲ Gleevec Tablets (0% to 27%) ... 2227
Invanz for Injection (1.6%) ... 1999
▲ Lucentis Injection (5% to 16%) ... 1237
▲ Metrogel 1% (3.1%) ... 1211
▲ Myfortic Tablets (3% to less than 20%) ... 2255
▲ Myozyme for Intravenous Infusion (23%) ... 1279
Nalfon Capsules (1.2%) ... 2502
▲ Oracea Capsules (4.8%) ... 1000
▲ Orencia Powder for Intravenous Infusion (12%) ... 914
Proquin XR Tablets (2.6%) ... 1153
▲ Requip Tablets (9%) ... 1555
▲ Retisert Implant (5% to 15%) ... ⊙ 258
▲ Revlimid Capsules (23%) ... 958
Rituxan I.V. ... 1254
▲ RotaTeq (6.9%) ... 2074
Strattera Capsules (2% or greater) ... 1814
▲ Symbicort 80/4.5 Inhalation Aerosol (10.5%) ... 3511
▲ Symbicort 160/4.5 Inhalation Aerosol (9.7%) ... 3511
▲ Tracleer Tablets (11%) ... 545
▲ Trisenox Injection (5%) ... 993
▲ Truvada Tablets (3%) ... 1296
▲ Ultram ER Tablets (1% to greater than 5%) ... 2392
Valtrex Caplets ... 1597
Vanos Cream (0.9% to 1.4%) ... 1893
▲ Velcade for Injection (14%) ... 2133
▲ Vivitrol (11% to 17%) ... 995
▲ Wellbutrin XL Extended-Release Tablets (13%) ... 1613
Xifaxan Tablets (Less than 2%) ... 2842
▲ Xyrem Oral Solution (2.9% to 8%) ... 1688

Nausea
▲ Abelcet Injection (9%) ... 1141
▲ Abilify Oral Solution (Frequent to 16%) ... 882
▲ Abilify Oral Solution (Frequent to 16%) ... 2450
▲ Abilify Discmelt Orally Disintegrating Tablets (Frequent to 16%) ... 882
▲ Abilify Discmelt Orally Disintegrating Tablets (Frequent to 16%) ... 2450
▲ Abilify Tablets (Frequent to 16%) ... 882
▲ Abilify Tablets (Frequent to 16%) ... 2450
▲ Accolate Tablets (3.1%) ... 671
AccuNeb Inhalation Solution (0.9% to 1.7%) ... 1055
Accutane Capsules ... 2731
Aceon Tablets (2 mg, 4 mg, 8 mg) (2.3%) ... 3194
▲ Acetadote Injection (2% to 7%) ... 1031
Aciphex Tablets ... 1090
▲ Actimmune (10%) ... 1671
▲ Actiq (11% to 23%) ... 979
Activase I.V. ... 1223
▲ Actonel Tablets (6.2% to 10.9%) ... 2683
▲ Actonel with Calcium Tablets (6.2% to 10.9%) ... 2688
▲ ActoPlus Met Tablets (3.6% to 5.8%) ... 3214
▲ ADACEL Vaccine (0.8% to 13.3%) ... 2945
Adalat CC Tablets (2%) ... 2964
▲ Adderall XR Capsules (5%) ... 3166
▲ Adenocard Injection (3%) ... 617
▲ Advair Diskus 100/50 (4% to 5%) ... 1308
▲ Advair Diskus 250/50 (4% to 5%) ... 1308
▲ Advair Diskus 500/50 (4% to 5%) ... 1308
▲ Advair HFA Inhalation Aerosol (3% to 5%) ... 1318
Advate Injection (0.6%) ... 712
▲ Advicor Tablets (7%) ... 1722
▲ Aerobid/Aerobid-M (25%) ... 1171
▲ Agenerase Capsules (23% to 74%) ... 1327
▲ Agenerase Oral Solution (23% to 74%) ... 1332
Aggrastat (Less than 1%) ... 1907
▲ Aggrenox Capsules (16%) ... 822
▲ Agrylin Capsules (17.1%) ... 3169
Albalon Ophthalmic Solution ... ⊙ 218
▲ Albenza Tablets (3.7% to 6.2%) ... 1338
Albutein 5%, Albumin (Human) ... 1652
Albutein 25% , Albumin (Human) ... 1653
Aldara Cream, 5% (1.4%) ... 1846
Aldoril Tablets ... 1910
▲ Alferon N Injection (4% to 48%) ... 1665
▲ Alimta for Injection (Up to 84%) ... 1750
Alinia for Oral Suspension (Less than 1%) ... 2835
Alinia Tablets (Less than 1%) ... 2835
Alkeran for Injection (Infrequent) ... 955
Alkeran Tablets (Infrequent) ... 956
Allegra (1.6%) ... 2844
▲ Allegra-D 12 Hour Extended-Release Tablets (7.4%) ... 2846
▲ Allegra-D 24 Hour Extended-Release Tablets (7.4%) ... 2849
Aloprim for Injection (1.3%) ... 2167
Alphanate, Antihemophilic Factor (Human) ... 1654
AlphaNine SD, Coagulation Factor IX (Human) ... 1656
Altace Capsules (Less than 1% to 2.2%) ... 1702
Altoprev Extended-Release Tablets (1.9% to 2.2%) ... 3109
▲ Alupent Inhalation Aerosol (Up to 14%) ... 826
▲ Ambien Tablets (2% to 6%) ... 2851
▲ Ambien CR Tablets (7% to frequent) ... 2855
▲ AmBisome for Injection (25.9% to 39.7%) ... 620
▲ Amerge Tablets (4% to 5%) ... 1339
▲ Amevive (0.2% to common) ... 626
Aminohippurate Sodium PAH Injection ... 1913
▲ Amitiza Capsules (13.2% to 31.1%) ... 3224
Amoxil Capsules ... 1343
Amoxil Chewable Tablets ... 1343
Amoxil Pediatric Drops for Oral Suspension ... 1343
Amoxil Powder for Oral Suspension ... 1343
Amoxil Tablets ... 1343
▲ Anaprox Tablets (3% to 9%) ... 2761
▲ Anaprox DS Tablets (3% to 9%) ... 2761
Androxy Tablets ... 3335
Angeliq Tablets ... 762
▲ Aptivus Capsules (6.7%) ... 826
▲ Aranesp for Injection (14%) ... 581
▲ Aredia for Injection (53.5%) ... 2179
▲ Argatroban Injection (4.8% to 7.1%) ... 1346
▲ Aricept Tablets (5% to 19%) ... 1094
▲ Aricept ODT Tablets (5% to 19%) ... 1094
▲ Arimidex Tablets (10% to 20%) ... 673
▲ Arixtra Injection (0.3% to 11.3%) ... 1351
▲ Aromasin Tablets (8.5% to 18%) ... 2600
▲ Arranon Injection (0% to 41%) ... 1357
▲ Arthrotec Tablets (11%) ... 3129
▲ Asacol Delayed-Release Tablets (13%) ... 2692
▲ Asmanex Twisthaler (1% to 3%) ... 2966
Astelin Nasal Spray (2.8%) ... 1904
Atacand Tablets (More than 1%) ... 649
Atacand HCT (0.5% or greater) ... 651
▲ Atripla Tablets (8%) ... 945
▲ Atrovent Inhalation Solution (4.1%) ... 835
▲ Atrovent HFA Inhalation Aerosol (4%) ... 841
Atrovent Nasal Spray 0.03% (2.2%) ... 837
▲ Augmentin (3%) ... 1360
▲ Augmentin Tablets (3%) ... 1363
▲ Augmentin XR Extended-Release Tablets (2.1% to 3.5%) ... 1369
Augmentin ES-600 Powder for Oral Suspension ... 1366
▲ Avalide Tablets (3%) ... 888
▲ Avalide Tablets (3%) ... 2874
▲ Avandamet Tablets (16%) ... 1373
Avandaryl Tablets (1.1%) ... 1379
▲ Avandia Tablets (4%) ... 1384
Avapro Tablets (1% or greater) ... 891
Avapro Tablets (1% or greater) ... 2871
Avastin IV ... 1227
▲ Avelox (6%) ... 2970
▲ Avinza Capsules (Greater than 10%) ... 1741
Axert Tablets (1% to 2%) ... 2396
▲ Axid Oral Solution (1.2% to 5.4%) ... 879
▲ Azilect Tablets (12%) ... 3293
Azopt Ophthalmic Suspension (Less than 1%) ... 557
▲ Bactroban Cream (1.1% to 4.9%) ... 1394
Bactroban Nasal (Less than 1%) ... 1394
Bactroban Ointment (Less than 1%) ... 1395
Baraclude (Less than 1%) ... 894
▲ Bayer Aspirin (7.6%) ... 744
Bayer Aspirin Comprehensive Prescribing Information ... ▣ 796
Beconase AQ Nasal Spray (Fewer than 5 in 100 patients) ... 1396
▲ BeneFix Vials (6.2%) ... 3408
Benicar Tablets (Greater than 0.5%) ... 1043
▲ Benicar HCT Tablets (3%) ... 1044
▲ Bentyl Capsules (14%) ... 697
▲ Bentyl Injection (14%) ... 697
▲ Bentyl Syrup (14%) ... 697
▲ Bentyl Tablets (14%) ... 697
Betagan Ophthalmic Solution, USP ... ⊙ 220
▲ Betaseron for SC Injection (27%) ... 767
Betimol Ophthalmic Solution (1% to 5%) ... 3382
Betimol Ophthalmic Solution (1% to 5%) ... ⊙ 295
▲ Bexxar (3% to 36%) ... 1398
▲ Biaxin/Biaxin XL (3%) ... 402
Bicillin C-R Injectable Suspension ... 1706
▲ BiDil Tablets (10%) ... 2171
Biltricide Tablets ... 2976
Blocadren Tablets (0.6%) ... 1916
▲ Boniva Injection (4.8% to 5.1%) ... 2738
▲ Boniva Tablets (4.8% to 5.1%) ... 2741
▲ Boostrix (3% to 26%) ... 1404
▲ Bumex Tablets (0.6% to 4.1%) ... 2746
▲ Buprenex Injectable (5% to 10%) ... 2716
▲ Byetta Injection (44%) ... 611
Caduet Tablets (Greater than or equal to 2%) ... 2508
Calcijex Injection ... 411
Calcium Disodium Versenate Injection ... 1851
▲ Campath Ampules (2% to 54%) ... 811
▲ Campral Tablets (3% to 4%) ... 1174

▲ Camptosar Injection (11% to 86%) 2604
▲ Canasa Rectal Suppositories (3.1%) 699
▲ Cancidas for Injection (1.8% to 6%) 1918
Captopril Tablets (About 0.5% to 2%) 2149
Carafate Suspension (Less than 0.5%) 701
Carafate Tablets (Less than 0.5%) 701
▲ Carbatrol Capsules (Among most frequent) 3171
▲ Cardene I.V. (4.9%) 2497
Cardizem LA Extended Release Tablets (1.4%) 1728
Cardura XL Tablets (1.2%) 2515
Carimune NF 3499
▲ Carnitor Injection (5% to 12%) 3188
Carnitor Tablets and Oral Solution 3190
Carteolol Hydrochloride Ophthalmic Solution USP, 1% ⊙ 249
▲ Catapres Tablets (About 5 in 100 patients) 843
Catapres-TTS (1 of 101 patients) 844
Caverject Impulse Injection (Less than 1%) 2612
Ceftin (2.6%) 1407
▲ Celebrex Capsules (3.5%) 3134
▲ Celexa (21%) 1176
▲ CellCept Capsules (19.9% to 54.5%) 2747
▲ CellCept Intravenous (19.9% to 54.5%) 2747
▲ CellCept Oral Suspension (19.9% to 54.5%) 2747
▲ CellCept Tablets (19.9% to 54.5%) 2747
▲ Cerezyme for Injection (Approximately 6.5%) 1270
Cervidil Vaginal Insert (Less than 1%) 1181
▲ Cesamet Capsules (4%) 3340
▲ Chantix Tablets (Greater than 5% to 40%) 2517
▲ Chemet Capsules (12.0% to 20.9%) 2458
Cialis Tablets (Less than 2%) 1838
Ciloxan Ophthalmic Ointment (Less than 1%) 559
Ciloxan Ophthalmic Solution (Less than 1%) ⊙ 206
Cipro (2.5% to 2.7%) 2977
Cipro I.V. (Greater than 1% to 2.7%) 2984
▲ Cipro XR Tablets (3% to 4%) 2990
▲ Clarinex Syrup (3%) 2995
▲ Clarinex Tablets (5%) 2995
▲ Clarinex Reditabs Tablets (5%) 2995
Clarinex-D 24-Hour Extended-Release Tablets (2%) 2998
Cleocin Vaginal Ovules (Less than 1%) 2616
▲ Climara Transdermal System (1% to 6%) 771
Climara Pro Transdermal System 776
▲ Clinoril Tablets (3% to 9%) 1924
▲ Clolar for Intravenous Infusion (75%) 1271
▲ Clorpres Tablets (About 5%) 2153
▲ Clozaril Tablets (3% to 17%) 2184
▲ Colazal Capsules (5%) 2838
▲ Colyte with Flavor Packs for Oral Solution (Up to 50%) 3088
Combivent Inhalation Aerosol (2.0%) 847
▲ Combivir Tablets (13% to 33%) 1411
▲ Comtan Tablets (14%) 2189
Concerta Extended-Release Tablets 1881
▲ Copaxone for Injection (22%) 3297
▲ Copegus Tablets (25%) 2754
▲ Coreg Tablets (4% to 9%) 1414
Cosmegen for Injection (Common) 2459
▲ Cosopt Sterile Ophthalmic Solution (1% to 5%) 1931
Coumadin for Injection (Infrequent) 898
Coumadin Tablets (Infrequent) 898
Covera-HS Tablets (2.1% to 2.7%) 3139
Cozaar Tablets (1% or greater) 1935
▲ Creon 5 Capsules (Among most frequent) 3198
▲ Creon 10 Capsules (Among most frequent) 3198
▲ Creon 20 Capsules (Among most frequent) 3199
▲ Crestor Tablets (3.4%) 678
▲ Crixivan Capsules (11.7%) 1940
▲ Cubicin for Injection (5.8% to 10%) 1026
Cuprimine Capsules (Greater than 1%) 1947
▲ Cymbalta Delayed-Release Capsules (5% to 30%) 1757
▲ CytoGam Intravenous (Less than 5%) 1895
▲ Dacogen Injection (42%) 2129
Dalmane Capsules 3342
Dantrium Capsules (Rare) 2694
Dapsone Tablets USP 1673
▲ Daranide Tablets (Among the most common effects) 1950
▲ Daytrana Transdermal Patch (12%) 3174
Decadron Tablets 1951
Demadex Injection (1.8%) 2759
Demadex Tablets (1.8%) 2759
Demser Capsules (Infrequent) 1953
▲ Depacon Injection (3.2% to 48%) 412
▲ Depakene (34% to 48%) 417
▲ Depakote Sprinkle Capsules (26% to 48%) 422
▲ Depakote Tablets (22% to 48%) 427
▲ Depakote ER Tablets (15% to 48%) 434
▲ DepoCyt Injection (11%) 1143
▲ DepoDur Extended-Release Injection (Greater than 10%) 1110
▲ Depo-Provera Contraceptive Injection (1% to 5%) 2622
▲ depo-subQ provera 104 Injectable Suspension (1% to less than 5%) 2624
▲ Detrol Tablets (4.2%) 2628
▲ Didronel Tablets (About 1 patient in 15; possibly 2 or 3 in 10) 2697
Dilaudid (Infrequent) 440
Dilaudid Non-Sterile Powder (Infrequent) 440
Dilaudid Oral Liquid 445
Dilaudid Rectal Suppositories (Infrequent) 440
Dilaudid Tablets (Infrequent) 440
Dilaudid Tablets - 8 mg 445
▲ Dilaudid-HP (Among most frequent) 442
Diovan Tablets (More than 1%) 2193
Diovan HCT Tablets (Greater than 0.2%) 2196
▲ Ditropan XL Extended-Release Tablets (2% to 9%) 2413
Diuril Oral Suspension 1954
Diuril Sodium Intravenous 2467
▲ Dolobid Tablets (3% to 9%) 1955
Donnatal Extentabs 2493
▲ Doxil Injection (16.9% to 46%) 2351
Duetact Tablets 3226
DuoNeb Inhalation Solution (1.4%) 1058
▲ Duragesic Transdermal System (Greater than 10% to 24%) 2373
Dyazide Capsules 1423
DynaCirc CR Tablets 2721
Dyrenium Capsules (Rare) 3400
▲ EC-Naprosyn Delayed-Release Tablets (3% to 9%) 2761
Edecrin 1959
▲ E.E.S. (Among most frequent) 451
▲ Effexor Tablets (6% to 58.0%) 3411
▲ Effexor XR Capsules (4% to 35%) 3417
▲ Eldepryl Capsules (10 of 49 patients) 3208
▲ Elidel Cream 1% (0.4% to 6.7%) 2200
▲ Eligard 22.5 mg (3.4%) 2883
Eligard 30 mg (2.2%) 2885
▲ Elitek (27%) 2890
▲ Elmiron Capsules (4%) 2415
▲ Eloxatin for Injection (5% to 74%) 2892
Elspar for Injection 2463
Elspar for Injection 1960
▲ Emcyt Capsules (15%) 2634
▲ Emend Capsules (7.1% to12.7%) 1963
Emsam Transdermal System 903
▲ Emtriva Capsules (13% to 18%) 1287
▲ Emtriva Oral Solution (13% to 18%) 1287
▲ Enablex Extended-Release Tablets (1.5% to 4.1%) 2203
▲ Enbrel for Injection (9% to 15%) 584
Engerix-B Vaccine (Less than 1%) 1425
▲ Enjuvia Tablets (7% to 12%) 1062
▲ Entocort EC Capsules (11%) 2698
EpiPen 1061
▲ Epivir (13% to 33%) 1427
▲ Epivir-HBV (15%) 1432
▲ Epogen for Injection (0.26% to 48%) 591
▲ Epzicom Tablets (5% to 6%) 1436
▲ Equetro Extended-Release Capsules (10% to 29%) 3180
Eraxis for Injection (1%) 2521
▲ Erbitux (2% to 49%) 910
▲ EryPed (Among most frequent) 447
▲ Ery-Tab Tablets (Among most frequent) 449
▲ Erythrocin Stearate Filmtab Tablets (Among most frequent) 453
▲ Erythromycin Base Filmtab Tablets (Among most frequent) 455
▲ Erythromycin Delayed-Release Capsules, USP (Among most frequent) 457
Estrasorb Topical Emulsion 1147
Estratest Tablets 3199
Estratest H.S. Tablets 3199
▲ Estring Vaginal Ring (3%) 2635
▲ Ethyol for Injection (8% to 96%) 1898
Euflexxa (0.63% to 1.88%) 1162
▲ Eulexin Capsules (9% to 11%) 3009
▲ Evista Tablets (8.3% to 8.8%) 1763
▲ Evoxac Capsules (13.8%) 1047
▲ Exelon Capsules (29% to 47%) 2206
▲ Exelon Oral Solution (29% to 47%) 2206
▲ Fabrazyme for Intravenous Infusion (8%) 1274
▲ Famvir Tablets (7.2% to 12.5%) 2211
Fansidar Tablets 2765
▲ Faslodex Injection (26%) 681
▲ FazaClo Orally Disintegrating Tablets (5% to 17%) 551
▲ Femara Tablets (0.1% to 17%) 2214
▲ Ferrlecit Injection (2% to 35%) 3388
Flexbumin I.V. (Occasional) 720
Flomax Capsules (2.0% to 3.9%) 850
▲ Flonase Nasal Spray (2.6% to 4.8%) 1440
▲ Flovent Diskus (4% to 9%) 1443
Floxin Otic Solution (Single report to 0.3%) 1049
Fluarix 1451
Flumadine (2.8%) 1183
Flumist Vaccine 1901
Fluorescite Injection ⊙ 207
▲ Focalin Tablets (9%) 2220
Focalin XR Capsules 2223
▲ Follistim AQ Cartridge (17%) 2338
Foradil Aerolizer 3010
▲ Fortamet Extended-Release Tablets (8.5%) 3115
Fortaz (1 in 156 patients) 1453
▲ Forteo for Injection (8.5%) 1767
▲ Fortical Nasal Spray (1% to 3%) 3337
▲ Fosamax (Up to 3.6%) 1969
▲ Fosamax Plus D Tablets (0% to 3.6%) 1977
▲ Fosrenol Chewable Tablets (11% to 36%) 3183
Frova Tablets (Greater than or equal to 2%) 1113
Furosemide Tablets 2154
▲ Fuzeon Injection (22.8%) 2767
▲ Gabitril Tablets (11%) 984
▲ Gammagard Liquid (1.09% to 9.8%) 721
Gammagard S/D (Occasional) 724
▲ Gamunex Immune Globulin I.V., 10% (0.5% to 21%) 3235
Gantrisin Pediatric Suspension 2770
Garamycin Injectable 3014
▲ Gardasil Injection (6.7%) 1984
▲ Gemzar for Injection (58% to 71%) 1771
▲ Gengraf Capsules (2% to 18%) 459
Genotropin Lyophilized Powder (A small number of patients) 2638
▲ Geodon (10%) 2529
▲ Gleevec Tablets (0.9% to 74%) 2227
GlucaGen (Occassional) 761
Glucagon for Injection Vials and Emergency Kit (Occasional) 1778
Gris-PEG Tablets (Occasional) 2502
Guanidine Hydrochloride Tablets 3016
▲ HalfLytely and Bisacodyl Tablets Bowel Prep Kit with Flavors Packs (17.1% to 50%) 881
▲ Havrix Vaccine (1% to 10%) 1456
▲ Hectorol Capsules (21.3%) 1275
▲ Hectorol Injection (21.3%) 1278
Hemofil M (Extremely rare) 728
▲ Hepsera Tablets (2% to 5%) 1292
▲ Herceptin I.V. (8% to 33%) 1233
Human Albumin Grifols 20%, Albumin (Human) 1651
Human Albumin Grifols 25%, Albumin (Human) 1652
Humatrope Vials and Cartridges 1787
▲ Humira Injection (9%) 466
▲ Hycamtin for Injection (Less than 1% to 77%) 1458
Hycodan 1116
Hycotuss Expectorant Syrup 1117
Hydrocortone Tablets 1989
▲ Hyperstat I.V. (4%) 3017
▲ Hytrin Capsules (0.5% to 4.4%) 471
Hyzaar 50-12.5 Tablets (1% or greater) 1990
Hyzaar 100-12.5 Tablets (1% or greater) 1990
Hyzaar 100-25 Tablets (1% or greater) 1990
▲ Imdur Tablets (Less than or equal to 5%) 3018
▲ Imitrex Injection (4%) 1463
▲ Imitrex Nasal Spray (11% to 13.5%) 1467
Imitrex Tablets (Greater than 1%) 1471
Increlex Injection 3291
▲ Indapamide Tablets (Less than 5%) 2156
Inderal LA Long-Acting Capsules 3429
▲ Indocin (3% to 9%) 1995
Infed Injection 3390
▲ Infergen (30% to 40%) 3364
InnoPran XL Capsules 2723
▲ Intron A for Injection (1% to 66%) 3024
▲ Invanz for Injection (1.6% to 8.5%) 1999
▲ Invirase (Greater than or equal to 2% to 10.8%) 2772
▲ Ionsys Transdermal System (39%) 2379
▲ Iressa Tablets (13% to 20%) 684
▲ I.V. Busulfex (7% to 98%) 2493
▲ Kadian Capsules (Among most frequent) 577
▲ Kaletra (7% to 16%) 476
K-Dur Extended-Relase Tablets 3033
Keflex Capsules (Rare) 549
Keppra Injection 3320
Keppra Oral Solution (1% to 2%) 3314
Keppra Tablets (1% to 2%) 3314
▲ Ketek Tablets (7% to 7.9%) 2903
Kionex Powder 2477
▲ Kineret Injection (8%) 599
Klonopin 2778
▲ K-Lor Oral Solution (Among most common) 474
Koāte-DVI (0.7%) 3250
Kogenate FS 738
Kogenate FS with Bio-Set (1 case) 740
K-Phos Original (Sodium Free) Tablets 760
K-Phos Neutral Tablets 760
Kristalose for Oral Solution 1034
▲ K-Tab Tablets (Most common) 475
▲ Kytril (15% to 20%) 2784
▲ Lamictal (5% to 25%) 1481
Lamisil Tablets (2.6%) 2232
Lanoxicaps Capsules (Common) 1490
Lanoxin Injection 1494
Lanoxin Injection Pediatric 1497
Lanoxin Tablets (Common) 1500
▲ Lariam Tablets (Among most frequent) 2786
▲ Lescol Capsules (3.2%) 2233
Lescol XL Tablets (2.5%) 2233
Leukeran Tablets (Infrequent) 1504
▲ Leukine (58% to 90%) 814
▲ Leustatin Injection (28%) 2357
▲ Levaquin (1.5% to 6.8%) 2384
▲ Levaquin in 5% Dextrose Injection (1.5% to 6.8%) 2384
Levothroid Tablets 1186
▲ Lexapro Oral Solution (Greater than 5% to 18%) 1190
▲ Lexapro Tablets (Greater than 5% to 18%) 1190
▲ Lexiva Tablets (3% to 39%) 1505
Librium Capsules 3347
Lidoderm Patch 1118
Limbrel Capsules (0.011%) 2672
Lipitor Tablets (Greater than or equal to 2%) 2483
Lithobid Tablets 1692
▲ Lithostat Tablets (20% to 25%) 2140
Lofibra Tablets (2.3%) 1219
Lofibra Capsules (2.3%) 1216
Lopressor Injection (Less than or equal to 1%) 2238
Lopressor Tablets (Less than or equal to 1%) 2238
Lopressor HCT 50/25 Tablets (1%) 2241
Lopressor HCT 100/25 Tablets (1%) 2241
Lopressor HCT 100/50 Tablets (1%) 2241
Lotensin Tablets (1.5%) 2243
Lotensin HCT Tablets (1.4%) 2246
Lotrel Capsules 2249
▲ Lotronex Tablets (6%) 1512
▲ Lovenox Injection (2.5% to 3%) 2915
▲ Lucentis Injection (2% to 9%) 1237
▲ Lunesta Tablets (4% to 5%) 3142
▲ Lupron Depot 3.75 mg (13%) 3260
▲ Lupron Depot–3 Month 11.25 mg (4.8% to 13%) 3265
Lupron Depot-PED 7.5 mg, 11.25 mg and 15 mg (Less than 2%) 3269
Lupron Injection Pediatric (Less than 2%) 3259
▲ Macugen Injection (6% to 10%) ⊙ 261
▲ Malarone Pediatric Tablets (Less than 1% to 12%) 1517
▲ Malarone Tablets (Less than 1% to 12%) 1517
▲ Marinol Capsules (3% to 10%) 3333
▲ Matulane Capsules (Among most frequent) 3191
Maxair Autohaler (1.3% to 1.7%) 1852

▲ Maxalt Tablets (4% to 6%) 2008
▲ Maxalt-MLT Orally Disintegrating Tablets (4% to 6%) 2008
Maxipime for Injection (Greater than 0.1% to 2%) 1105
Mefoxin for Injection (Rare) 2012
Mefoxin Premixed Intravenous Solution (Rare) 2016
▲ Megace ES Oral Suspension (0% to 5%) 2481
Menostar Transdermal System 782
▲ Mepron Suspension (2.5% to 32%) 1521
▲ Meridia Capsules (5.9%) 489
▲ Merrem I.V. (0.8% to 7.8%) 686
Meruvax II 2019
Metadate CD Capsules 3323
Metrogel 1% 1211
▲ MetroGel-Vaginal Gel (4%) 1855
▲ Mevacor Tablets (1.9% to 4.7%) 2021
▲ Miacalcin Injection (About 10%) 2252
▲ Miacalcin Nasal Spray (1% to 3%) 2253
Micardis Tablets (1%) 854
Micardis HCT Tablets (2%) 856
▲ Midamor Tablets (3% to 8%) 2026
▲ Migranal Nasal Spray (10%) 3348
Mintezol 2027
Miradon Tablets 3042
▲ Mirapex Tablets (28%) 859
Mircette Tablets 1066
▲ Mirena Intrauterine System (5% or more) 787
M-M-R II 2006
Moban Tablets (Occasional) 1119
▲ Mobic Oral Suspension (2.4% to 4.7%) 863
▲ Mobic Tablets (2.4% to 4.7%) 863
▲ Moduretic Tablets (3% to 8%) 2028
▲ MoviPrep Oral Solution (14.4%) 2839
▲ MS Contin Tablets (Among most frequent) 2701
Mustargen for Injection 2468
Mycamine for Injection (2.3% to 2.8%) 628
▲ Myfortic Tablets (24.5% to 29.1%) 2255
Myleran Tablets 1525
▲ Mylotarg for Injection (63% to 74%) 3431
▲ Myobloc Injection (3% to 10%) 3192
Myozyme for Intravenous Infusion 1279
▲ Nabi-HB (4%) 2169
Nadolol Tablets (1 to 5 of 1000 patients) 2159
▲ Nalfon Capsules (7.7%) 2502
Namenda (Greater than or equal to 2%) 1195
▲ Naprosyn Suspension (3% to 9%) 2761
▲ Naprosyn Tablets (3% to 9%) 2761
Nasonex Nasal Spray (Greater than or equal to 2%) 3043
▲ Natrecor for Injection (4% to 13%) 3127
Nembutal Sodium Solution, USP (Less than 1%) 2470
▲ Neoral Oral Solution (2% to 18%) 2259
▲ Neoral Soft Gelatin Capsules (2% to 18%) 2259
▲ Neulasta Injection (15% to 72%) 601
▲ Neumega for Injection (77%) 3435
▲ Neupogen for Injection (10% to 57%) 603
▲ Neurontin Capsules (3.9 % to 8.4%) 2487
▲ Neurontin Oral Solution (3.9% to 8.4%) 2487
▲ Neurontin Tablets (3.9% to 8.4%) 2487
▲ Nevanac Ophthalmic Suspension 0.1% (1% to 4%) .... ⊙ 209
▲ Nexavar Tablets (0% to 23%) 746
Nexium Delayed-Release Capsules (Greater than or equal to 1%) 655
Nexium I.V. (Greater than or equal to 1%) 659
▲ Niaspan Extended-Release Tablets (2% to 8%) 1730
Nicomide Tablets 1088
Nimotop Capsules (Up to 1.4%) 749
▲ Nipent for Injection (53% to 63%) 1863
▲ Niravam Orally Disintegrating Tablets (9.6% to 22%) 3092
Nitrolingual Pumpspray (Uncommon) 3120
Norditropin Cartridges (Small number of patients) 2323
Norflex Injection 1856
▲ Noroxin Tablets (2.6% to 4.2%) 2032
Norvasc Tablets (2.9%) 2545
▲ Norvir (25.6% to 29.8%) 503
NovoSeven 2331
Numorphan Injection 1120
Nutropin for Injection (A small number of patients) 1239
Nutropin AQ Injection (A small number of patients) 1243
Nutropin AQ Pen (A small number of patients) 1243
Nutropin AQ Pen Cartridge (A small number of patients) 1243
▲ NuvaRing (5% to 14%) 2340
▲ Omnicef Capsules (3%) 511
Omnicef for Oral Suspension (0.2%) 511
▲ Oncaspar (Greater than 5%) 1145
▲ Ontak Vials (64%) 1745
▲ Opana Tablets (19%) 1122
▲ Opana ER Tablets (2.9% to 33.1%) 1126
OptiPranolol Metipranolol Ophthalmic Solution 0.3% (A small number of patients) .... ⊙ 256
Oracea Capsules 1000
▲ Orencia Powder for Intravenous Infusion (Less than or equal to 0.1% to 10%) 914
Ortho-Cyclen Tablets 2429
▲ Ortho Evra Transdermal System (9% to 22%) 2417
Ortho Micronor Tablets 2426
Ortho Tri-Cyclen Tablets 2429
Ortho Tri-Cyclen Lo Tablets 2436
▲ Orthoclone OKT3 Sterile Solution (19%) 2360
▲ OsmoPrep Tablets (26% to 37%) 2840
Oxandrin Tablets 2962
▲ Oxsoralen-Ultra Capsules (10%) 3353
▲ OxyContin Tablets (Less than 1% to 23%) 2703
▲ OxyFast Oral Concentrate Solution (Among most frequent) 2708
▲ OxyIR Capsules (Among most frequent) 2708
▲ Oxytrol Transdermal System (Greater than 1%) 3392
Paddock Nystatin USP for Oral Suspension 2478
Parcopa Orally Disintegrating Tablets (Common) 3097
Parnate Tablets 1527
▲ Paser Granules (Among most common) 1674
Patanol Ophthalmic Solution (Less than 5%) 561
▲ Paxil CR Controlled-Release Tablets (1.9% to 36.3%) 1538
▲ Paxil (1.9% to 36.3%) 1530
▲ PCE Dispertab Tablets (Among most frequent) 515
Pediarix Vaccine 1548
▲ Pegasys (24%) 2789
▲ PEG-Intron Powder for Injection (26%) 3048
▲ Pentasa Capsules (1.8% to 3.1%) 3185
Pepcid Injection (Infrequent) 2040
Pepcid (Infrequent) 2038
▲ Percocet Tablets (Among most frequent) 1131
▲ Percodan Tablets (Among most frequent) 1132
▲ Permax Tablets (24.3%) 3356
Persantine Tablets (Rare) 868
▲ Pexeva Tablets (1.9% to 36.3%) 1694
Phenergan Tablets and Suppositories 3440
Phenytek Capsules 2160
PhosLo GelCaps (Occasional) 2169
▲ Photofrin for Injection (24% to 39%) 702
▲ Plan B Tablets (23.1%) 1076
Plasmanate (Occasional) 3255
▲ Plavix Tablets (3.4%) 917
▲ Plavix Tablets (3.4%) 2926
▲ Pletal Tablets (6% to 7%) 2455
Pneumovax 23 2043
Potaba (Infrequent) 1650
Premarin Intravenous 3442
▲ Premarin Tablets (6% to 9%) 3446
Premarin Vaginal Cream 3452
▲ Premphase Tablets (7% to 11%) 3456
▲ Prempro Tablets (7% to 11%) 3456
▲ Prevacid Delayed-Release Capsules (1.3% to 3%) 3271
▲ Prevacid for Delayed-Release Oral Suspension (1.3% to 3%) 3271
▲ Prevacid SoluTab Delayed-Release Orally Disintegrating Tablets (1.3% to 3%) 3271
Prevacid I.V. for Injection (1.3%) 3277
▲ Prevacid NapraPAC (Less than 1% to 9%) 3280
▲ PREVPAC (1.4% to 3%) 3284
Prezista Tablets (Less than 2%) 3306
▲ Prilosec OTC Delayed-Release Tablets (2.2% to 4.0%) 2677
Primaxin I.M. (0.6%) 2045
Primaxin I.V. (2.0%) 2048
Prinivil Tablets (Greater than 1% to 2.0%) 2052
Prinzide Tablets (2.2%) 2056
ProAmatine Tablets (Rare) 3186
▲ Prochieve 4% Gel (7% to 22%) 1003
▲ Prochieve 8% Gel (7% to 22%) 1003
▲ Procrit for Injection (0.26% to 58%) 2364
Profilnine SD, Factor IX Complex (Human) 1660
▲ Prograf Capsules and Injection (32% to 46%) 632
▲ Proleukin for Injection (35%) 2266
▲ Prometrium Capsules (100 mg, 200 mg) (8%) 3203
Proquin XR Tablets (Less than 1%) 1153
Prosed/DS Tablets 1157
▲ ProSom Tablets (4%) 517
Protonix I.V. (Greater than 1%) 3472
Protonix Tablets (2%) 3469
▲ Protopic Ointment (1% to 3%) 638
▲ Proventil Inhalation Aerosol (Less than 15%) 3053
▲ Proventil Inhalation Solution 0.083% (3.1% to 4%) 3055
▲ Proventil HFA Inhalation Aerosol (10%) 3056
▲ Provigil Tablets (11%) 988
▲ Prozac Pulvules and Liquid (12% to 22%) 1801
▲ Quadramet Injection (32.7%) 1040
Qvar Inhalation Aerosol (Less than 1% to 2%) 3303
▲ Ranexa Tablets (4% to 4.4%) 1035
Raniclor Tablets, Chewable (Rare) 2505
▲ Rapamune Oral Solution and Tablets (25% to 36%) 3475
▲ Raptiva for Injection (11%) 1250
▲ Razadyne (13% to 24%) 2399
▲ Razadyne ER Extended-Release Capsules (13% to 24%) 2399
▲ Rebetol (33% to 47%) 3058
▲ Rebetron Combination Therapy (38% to 47%) 3063
Recombinate (Extremely rare) 729
Recombivax HB (Equal to or greater than 1%) 2071
ReFacto Vials 3484
Relenza Rotadisk (Less than 3%) 1552
▲ Relpax Tablets (4% to 8%) 2548
▲ Remicade for IV Injection (21%) 971
▲ Renagel Tablets (7% to 20.2%) 1282
▲ ReoPro Vials (18.4%) 1809
▲ Requip Tablets (30% to 60%) 1555
▲ Rescriptor Tablets (14% to 20.3%) 2551
▲ Restoril Capsules (3.1%) 1860
Retavase 2499
▲ Retisert Implant (5% to 15%) .... ⊙ 258
▲ Retrovir Capsules (0.8% to 61%) 1560
▲ Retrovir IV Infusion (1% to 61%) 1564
▲ Retrovir (0.8% to 61%) 1560
▲ Revlimid Capsules (4.1% to 23.6%) 958
▲ Reyataz Capsules (6% to 16%) 921
▲ R-Gene 10 for Intravenous Use (3%) 2641
▲ Ribavirin, USP Capsules (33% to 47%) 3068
▲ Rilutek Tablets (12.2% to 20.5%) 2930
▲ Risperdal (4% to 11%) 1676
Risperdal Consta Long-Acting Injection (Frequent) 1682
▲ Risperdal M-Tab Orally Disintegrating Tablets (4% to 11%) 1676
Ritalin Hydrochloride Tablets 2269
Ritalin LA Capsules 2271
Ritalin-SR Tablets 2269
▲ Rituxan I.V. (1% to 23%) 1254
Rocaltrol Capsules 2798
Rocaltrol Oral Solution 2798
Rocephin Injectable Vials, ADD-Vantage, Galaxy, Bulk (Less than 1%) 2800
▲ Romazicon Injection (11%) 2804
▲ Rozerem Tablets (3%) 3231
▲ Rythmol SR Capsules (9% to 17%) 2727
▲ Sandimmune (2% to 10%) 2275
▲ Sandostatin Injection (34% to 61%) 2278
▲ Sandostatin LAR Depot (10.3%) 2280
Seasonique Tablets 1077
▲ Sensipar Tablets (31%) 608
Serevent Diskus (1% to 3%) 1568
▲ Simulect for Injection (Greater than or equal to 10%) 2284
Singulair (Greater than or equal to 2%) 2077
▲ Skelaxin Tablets (Most frequent) 1716
▲ Soltamox Oral Solution (5% to 26%) 3527
▲ Somavert Injection (8% to 14%) 2642
▲ Sonata Capsules (6% to 8%) 1717
▲ Soriatane Capsules (1% to 10%) 1013
St. Joseph 81 mg Aspirin Chewable and Enteric Coated Tablets 1869
St. Joseph 81 mg Aspirin .... ■ 688
▲ Stalevo Tablets (5% to 14%) 2287
Starlix Tablets 2292
▲ Strattera Capsules (7% to 12%) 1814
Striant Mucoadhesive 1007
Stromectol Tablets (1.8%) 2083
▲ Suboxone Tablets (10% to 15%) 2717
▲ Subutex Tablets (10% to 13.6%) 2717
Sular Tablets (2%) 3122
▲ Suprax (7%) 1843
▲ Sustiva Capsules (2% to 16%) 930
▲ Sustiva Tablets (2% to 16%) 930
▲ Sutent Capsules (2% to 54%) 2560
Symbyax Capsules (Infrequent) 1819
▲ Symlin Injection (28% to 48%) 613
▲ Symmetrel Tablets (5% to 10%) 1135
Synera Topical Patch (Less than or equal to 1%) 1137
Tabloid Tablets (Less frequent) 1575
▲ Tambocor Tablets (8.9%) 1856
▲ Tamiflu Capsules (3% to 10%) 2807
▲ Tamiflu Oral Suspension (3% to 10%) 2807
▲ Tarceva Tablets (0% to 60%) 1259
▲ Tarceva Tablets (0% to 60%) 2444
▲ Targretin Capsules (7.5% to 15.5%) 1747
Tarka Tablets (0.3% to 1.5%) 524
▲ Tasmar Tablets (30% to 35%) 3358
▲ Taxotere Injection Concentrate (5.1% to 73.3%) 2932
▲ Tegretol/Tegretol-XR (Among most frequent) 2295
▲ Temodar Capsules (46% to 53%) 3073
▲ Tequin Injection (8%) 938
▲ Tequin Injection in 5% Dextrose (8%) 938
▲ Tequin Tablets (8%) 938
Tessalon Capsules 1199
Tessalon Perles 1199
Teveten Tablets (Less than 1%) 1735
Teveten HCT Tablets (Less than 1%) 1737
Tev-Tropin for Injection (Small number of patients) 1222
▲ Thalomid Capsules (4.2%) 965
▲ Thiola Tablets (16.7%) 2141
Thioridazine Hydrochloride Tablets 2163
Thiothixene Capsules 2165
▲ Thrombate III (3 of 17) 3257
▲ Thymoglobulin for Intravenous Infusion (36.6%) 1284
▲ Thyrogen for Injection (10.5%) 1286
Thyrolar Tablets 1199
Tiazac Capsules (2%) 1201
▲ Ticlid Tablets (7.0%) 2810
Timentin ADD-Vantage 1580
Timentin Injection Galaxy Container 1583
Timentin IV Infusion 1577
Timentin Pharmacy Bulk Package 1586
Timolide Tablets (Less than 1%) 2086
Timoptic Sterile Ophthalmic Solution (Less frequent) 2088
Timoptic in Ocudose (Less frequent) 2091
Timoptic-XE Sterile Ophthalmic Gel Forming Solution 2092
▲ Tindamax Tablets (3.2% to 4.5%) 2142
TNKase I.V. 1264
▲ TOBI Solution for Inhalation (11.2%) 2298
▲ Topamax Sprinkle Capsules (6% to 14%) 2404
▲ Topamax Tablets (6% to 14%) 2404
Toprol-XL Tablets (About 1 of 100 patients) 668
Tracleer Tablets 545
Transderm Scōp Transdermal Therapeutic System (Few patients) 2177
▲ Trasylol Injection (11%) 754
Trecator Tablets 3487
Trelstar LA Suspension (2.9%) 3397
Tricor Tablets (2.3%) 527
Triglide Tablets (2.3%) 3123
▲ Trileptal Tablets (10% to 29%) 2300
▲ Trileptal Oral Suspension (10% to 29%) 2300
▲ TriLyte with Flavor Packs for Oral Solution (Up to 50%) 3100
▲ Trisenox Injection (75%) 993
▲ Trizivir Tablets (12% to 60%) 1589
Trusopt Sterile Ophthalmic Solution (Infrequent) 2095
▲ Truvada Tablets (8%) 1296
Tussionex Pennkinetic Extended-Release Suspension 3327
Twinject 0.3 3378
Twinject 0.15 3379
▲ Twinrix Vaccine (2% to 4%) 1595
▲ Tygacil for Injection (25.3% to 35%) 3488
▲ Tylenol with Codeine Tablets (Among most frequent) 2391
▲ Ultane Liquid for Inhalation (25%) 531
▲ Ultram ER Tablets (15.1% to 26.2%) 2392
Uniphyl Tablets 2710

Uniretic Tablets (More than 1%)........ 3100
Univasc Tablets (Greater than 1%).... 3104
Urocit-K Tablets (Some patients)...... 2144
Uroqid-Acid No. 2 Tablets.................. 760
Uroxatral Tablets (1% to 2%)........... 2943
▲ Urso 250 Tablets (8.3%) 710
▲ Urso Forte Tablets (8.3%) 710
▲ Valcyte Tablets (8% to 30%) 2813
Valium Tablets (Infrequent)............... 2819
▲ Valtrex Caplets (5% to 15%) 1597
Vancocin HCl Capsules, USP (Infrequent).................................. 3380
▲ Vandazole Vaginal Gel (3%) 3338
Vantas (Less than 2%)..................... 3375
Vantin Tablets and Oral Suspension (1.4% to 3.8%)........... 2645
Vaqta (2.3%)...................................... 2097
Varivax (Greater than or equal to 1%).. 2100
Vasotec I.V. Injection (1.3% to 1.4%).. 2103
▲ Velcade for Injection (57%) 2133
▲ Ventavis Inhalation Solution (13%) ... 1020
Verelan PM Extended-Release Capsules, Controlled-Onset (1.7% to 2.7%) 3106
▲ Vesanoid Capsules (57%) 2820
▲ VESIcare Tablets (1.7% to 3.3%) 646
▲ VFEND I.V. (1% to 5.4%) 2564
▲ VFEND Oral Suspension (1% to 5.4%) 2564
▲ VFEND Tablets (1% to 5.4%) 2564
Viadur Implant (Less than 2%) 757
▲ Vicodin Tablets (Among most frequent) 535
▲ Vicodin ES Tablets (Among most frequent) 536
▲ Vicodin HP Tablets (Among most frequent) 538
▲ Vicoprofen Tablets (21%) 539
▲ Viracept (3% to 7%) 2577
▲ Viramune Oral Suspension (5%) 873
▲ Viramune Tablets (5%) 873
▲ Viread Tablets (1% to 11%) 1301
▲ Visudyne for Injection (1% to 10%) .. 2305
▲ Vivaglobin (0.2% to 18%) 3506
▲ Vivitrol (25% to 33%) 995
Vivotif (Infrequent) 819
▲ Voltaren Ophthalmic Solution (Less than or equal to 3%) 2309
▲ Voltaren Tablets (1% to 10%) 2307
▲ Voltaren-XR Tablets (1% to 10%) 2310
▲ VoSpire ER Tablets (4.2%) 1052
Vytorin 10/10 Tablets 2114
Vytorin 10/10 Tablets 3077
Vytorin 10/20 Tablets 2114
Vytorin 10/20 Tablets 3077
Vytorin 10/40 Tablets 2114
Vytorin 10/40 Tablets 3077
Vytorin 10/80 Tablets 2114
Vytorin 10/80 Tablets 3077
▲ WelChol Tablets (4%) 1050
▲ Wellbutrin Tablets (22.9%) 1603
▲ Wellbutrin SR Sustained-Release Tablets (5% to 18%) 1607
▲ Wellbutrin XL Extended-Release Tablets (0.8% to 18%) 1613
WinRho SDF 732
▲ Xeloda Tablets (4% to 43%) 2822
▲ Xenical Capsules (3.6% to 8.1%) 2831
▲ Xifaxan Tablets (5.3%) 2842
Xopenex Inhalation Solution 3146
Xopenex Inhalation Solution Concentrate 3150
Xopenex HFA Inhalation Aerosol 3154
▲ Xyrem Oral Solution (2% to 40%) 1688
Yasmin 28 Tablets (Greater than 1%) 796
Yaz Tablets (Greater than 1%) 803
Zantac 1624
Zantac Injection 1619
Zantac Injection Pharmacy Bulk Package (Frequent) 1622
Zantac Injection Premixed 1619
Zantac 1624
▲ Zegerid Capsules (2.2% to 4.0%) 2958
▲ Zegerid Powder for Oral Solution (2.2% to 4.0%) 2958
▲ Zelapar Tablets (11%) 3372
▲ Zelnorm Tablets (5% to 8%) 2312
Zemaira (0.2% to 0.4%) 3509
▲ Zemplar Capsules (13%) 541
▲ Zemplar Injection (13%) 543
Zemuron Injection (Less than 1%) 2346
Zetia Tablets 2120
Zetia Tablets 3083
▲ Ziagen (9% to 19%) 1626
Zinacef for Injection (1 in 440 patients) 1631
Zinacef Injection (1 in 440 patients) 1631
▲ Zinecard for Injection (51% to 77%) 2650
▲ Zmax for Oral Suspension (3.9%) 2583
Zocor Tablets (1.3%) 2105
▲ Zoloft (13% to 30%) 2586
▲ Zometa for Intravenous Infusion (29.1% to 46%)............................ 2315
▲ Zomig Tablets (Common) 3519
▲ Zomig Nasal Spray (0% to 4%) 3523
▲ Zomig-ZMT Tablets (Common) 3519
▲ Zonegran Capsules (9%) 1101
▲ Zosyn (5.8% to 6.9%) 3492
Zovirax (2.4% to 4.8%)...................... 1643
▲ Zyban Sustained-Release Tablets (9%).. 1644
▲ Zydone Tablets (Among most frequent).. 1139
▲ Zyflo Tablets (5.5%) 1023
▲ Zyprexa Tablets (2% to 9%) 1830
Zyprexa IntraMuscular (Infrequent)... 1830
▲ Zyprexa ZYDIS Orally Disintegrating Tablets (2% to 9%).. 1830
Zyrtec Chewable Tablets (1.9% to 2.8%)... 2594
Zyrtec (1.9% to 2.8%)........................ 2594
Zyrtec-D 12 Hour Extended Release Tablets (1.9% to 2.8%)..... 2597
▲ Zyvox (1.4% to 6.2%) 2652

Neck, rigidity of

Abilify Oral Solution (Frequent)......... 882
Abilify Oral Solution (Frequent)......... 2450
Abilify Discmelt Orally Disintegrating Tablets (Frequent)... 882
Abilify Discmelt Orally Disintegrating Tablets (Frequent)... 2450
Abilify Tablets (Frequent).................. 882
Abilify Tablets (Frequent).................. 2450
Aciphex Tablets 1090
Amerge Tablets 1339
Axert Tablets (Infrequent)................. 2396
Caduet Tablets (Less than 2%).......... 2508
Cardizem LA Extended Release Tablets (Less than 2%).................. 1728
Depacon Injection (1% or more)....... 412
Depakene (1% or more)..................... 417
Depakote Sprinkle Capsules 422
▲ Depakote Tablets (1% to 5%) 427
Depakote ER Tablets (Greater than 1%).. 434
Effexor Tablets (Infrequent)............. 3411
Effexor XR Capsules (Infrequent)...... 3417
Eldepryl Capsules............................. 3208
▲ Imitrex Injection (5%) 1463
Imitrex Nasal Spray 1467
Imitrex Tablets.................................. 1471
Lipitor Tablets (Less than 2%)........... 2483
Lunesta Tablets (Infrequent)............. 3142
Lyrica Capsules (0.1% to 1%)............ 2539
Maxalt Tablets (Less than 2%)........... 2008
Maxalt-MLT Orally Disintegrating Tablets (Less than 2%).................. 2008
Norvir (Less than 2%)........................ 503
Paxil CR Controlled-Release Tablets (Rare) 1538
Paxil (Rare).. 1530
Pexeva Tablets (Rare)........................ 1694
Pletal Tablets (Less than 2%)............. 2455
Prevacid Delayed-Release Capsules (Less than 1%)............... 3271
Prevacid for Delayed-Release Oral Suspension (Less than 1%)........... 3271
Prevacid SoluTab Delayed-Release Orally Disintegrating Tablets (Less than 1%).............................. 3271
Prevacid NapraPAC (Less than 1%).. 3280
PREVPAC (Less than 1%)................... 3284
Protonix I.V. (Less than 1%)............... 3472
Protonix Tablets (Less than 1%)........ 3469
Provigil Tablets (1%).......................... 988
Rescriptor Tablets 2551
Symbyax Capsules (Frequent)........... 1819
▲ Thalomid Capsules (4.2%) 965
Uniretic Tablets (Less than 1%)......... 3100
Varivax (Greater than or equal to 1%).. 2100
Zonegran Capsules (Infrequent)........ 1101
Zyflo Tablets (Greater than 1%)......... 1023
▲ Zyprexa Tablets (2% to 3%) 1830
▲ Zyprexa ZYDIS Orally Disintegrating Tablets (2% to 3%)... 1830

Neck, redistribution/accumulation of body fat

Kaletra 476
Retrovir... 1560

Neck tightness

Abilify Oral Solution (Infrequent)........ 882
Abilify Oral Solution (Infrequent) 2450
Abilify Discmelt Orally Disintegrating Tablets (Infrequent)............................... 882
Abilify Discmelt Orally Disintegrating Tablets (Infrequent)............................... 2450
Abilify Tablets (Infrequent)................ 882
Abilify Tablets (Infrequent)................ 2450
Imitrex Injection (Relatively common).. 1463
▲ Zomig Tablets (Common) 3519
Zomig Nasal Spray (Infrequent)........ 3523
▲ Zomig-ZMT Tablets (Common) 3519

Necrolysis, digitus

Sustiva Capsules (Up to 3.5%)......... 930
Sustiva Tablets (Up to 3.5%)............ 930

Necrolysis, epidermal

Celexa.. 1176
Pexeva Tablets................................... 1694
Prevacid NapraPAC (Less than 1%).. 3280
Prozac Pulvules and Liquid............... 1801

Necrolysis, epidermal, toxic

Aciphex Tablets 1090
Adderall Tablets................................. 3164
Advicor Tablets.................................. 1722
Aldoril Tablets 1910
Altoprev Extended-Release Tablets (Rare) 3109
Amoxil Capsules 1343
Amoxil Chewable Tablets 1343
Amoxil Pediatric Drops for Oral Suspension 1343
Amoxil Powder for Oral Suspension 1343
Amoxil Tablets 1343
Anaprox Tablets (Less than 1%) 2761
Anaprox DS Tablets (Less than 1%) .. 2761
Arthrotec Tablets (Rare) 3129
Atacand HCT 651
Augmentin (Occasional) 1360
Augmentin Tablets (Occasional) 1363
Augmentin ES-600 Powder for Oral Suspension 1366
Avalide Tablets 888
Avalide Tablets 2874
Betoptic S Ophthalmic Suspension (Rare) 558
Biaxin/Biaxin XL 402
▲ Blephamide Ophthalmic Ointment (Among most often) 568
Blephamide Ophthalmic Suspension 569
Caduet Tablets 2508
Carbatrol Capsules (Extremely rare) 3171
Ceftin 1407
Celebrex Capsules (Less than 0.1%) 3134
Celexa (3 cases) 1176
Cipro 2977
Cipro I.V. (1% or less) 2984
Cipro XR Tablets 2990
Clinoril Tablets (Less than 1%) 1924
Clorpres Tablets 2153
Cuprimine Capsules 1947
Daraprim Tablets 1419
Depacon Injection (Rare) 412
Depakene (Rare) 417
Depakote Sprinkle Capsules (Rare) .. 422
Depakote Tablets (Rare) 427
Depakote ER Tablets (Rare) 434
Diovan HCT Tablets 2196
Diuril Oral Suspension 1954
Diuril Sodium Intravenous 2467
Dolobid Tablets (Less than 1 in 100) 1955
▲ Duac Topical Gel (0% to 17%) 3212
EC-Naprosyn Delayed-Release Tablets (Less than 1%) 2761
E.E.S. (Rare) 451
Effexor Tablets 3411
Effexor XR Capsules 3417
Emcyt Capsules (1%) 2634
Epzicom Tablets 1436
Equetro Extended-Release Capsules 3180
EryPed (Rare) 447
Erythromycin Delayed-Release Capsules, USP (Rare) 457
Ethyol for Injection 1898
Eulexin Capsules 3009
Fansidar Tablets 2765
FML-S Ophthalmic Suspension ....⊙ 229
Fortaz 1453
Fosamax (Rare) 1969
Fosamax Plus D Tablets 1977
Gantrisin Pediatric Suspension 2770
Inderal LA Long-Acting Capsules 3429
Indocin Capsules (Less than 1%) 1995
Indocin I.V. (Less than 1%) 2465
Indocin (Less than 1%) 1995
▲ Intron A for Injection (Less than 5%) 3024
Iressa Tablets (Very rare)................. 684
Keflex Capsules (Rare)..................... 549
Lamictal (Rare).................................. 1481
Lamisil Tablets (Isolated reports)...... 2232
Lescol Capsules (Rare)..................... 2233
Lescol XL Tablets 2233
Leukeran Tablets (Rare)................... 1504
Leustatin Injection (Isolated cases)... 2357
Levaquin (Rare)................................. 2384
Levaquin in 5% Dextrose Injection (Rare) 2384
Lexapro Oral Solution 1190
Lexapro Tablets 1190
Lipitor Tablets................................... 2483
Lofibra Tablets (Rare)....................... 1219
Lofibra Capsules (Rare).................... 1216
Maxalt Tablets 2008
Maxalt-MLT Orally Disintegrating Tablets 2008
Maxipime for Injection 1105
Mefoxin for Injection 2012
Mefoxin Premixed Intravenous Solution 2016
Merrem I.V... 686
Mevacor Tablets (Rare)..................... 2021
Micardis HCT Tablets 856
Mobic Oral Suspension (Less than 0.1%) 863
Mobic Tablets (Less than 0.1%)........ 863
Moduretic Tablets 2028
Nalfon Capsules (Less than 1%)....... 2502
Naprosyn Suspension (Less than 1%) 2761
Naprosyn Tablets (Less than 1%)..... 2761
Nexium Delayed-Release Capsules (Rare) 655
Nexium I.V. (Rare)............................. 659
Noroxin Tablets................................. 2032
Omnicef Capsules............................. 511
Omnicef for Oral Suspension 511
Paxil CR Controlled-Release Tablets 1538
Paxil.. 1530
PCE Dispertab Tablets (Rare)........... 515
PEG-Intron Powder for Injection........ 3048
Pepcid Injection (Very rare).............. 2040
Pepcid (Very rare)............................. 2038
Phenytek Capsules 2160
Plavix Tablets.................................... 917
Prevacid NapraPAC 3280
PREVPAC... 3284
Prilosec OTC Delayed-Release Tablets (Very rare)........................ 2677
Primaxin I.M...................................... 2045
Primaxin I.V. (Less than 0.2%).......... 2048
Prinivil Tablets (Rare)....................... 2052
Prinzide Tablets (Rare)..................... 2056
Prograf Capsules and Injection......... 632
Proquin XR Tablets 1153
Protonix I.V....................................... 3472
Protonix Tablets................................ 3469
Raniclor Tablets, Chewable (Rare).... 2505
Raptiva for Injection 1250
Retrovir IV Infusion........................... 1564
Rituxan I.V. 1254
Stromectol Tablets............................ 2083
Suprax 1843
Sustiva Capsules (Up to 3.5%).......... 930
Sustiva Tablets (Up to 3.5%)............ 930
Tamiflu Capsules (Rare).................... 2807
Tamiflu Oral Suspension (Rare)......... 2807
Taxotere Injection Concentrate (Rare) 2932
Tegretol/Tegretol-XR (Extremely rare) 2295
Teveten HCT Tablets......................... 1737
Thalomid Capsules 965
Tiazac Capsules (Less than 2%)........ 1201
Timentin ADD-Vantage 1580
Timentin Injection Galaxy Container 1583
Timentin IV Infusion.......................... 1577
Timentin Pharmacy Bulk Package 1586
Timolide Tablets 2086
Topamax Sprinkle Capsules 2404
Topamax Tablets............................... 2404
Tricor Tablets (Rare)......................... 527
Trileptal Tablets 2300
Trileptal Oral Suspension 2300
Trizivir Tablets 1589
Trusopt Sterile Ophthalmic Solution (Rare)............................ 2095
Vancocin HCl Capsules, USP (Infrequent)..................................... 3380
Vantin Tablets and Oral Suspension (Less than 1%)........... 2645
Vasotec I.V. Injection (0.5% to 1.0%) 2103
VFEND I.V. (Rare).............................. 2564
VFEND Oral Suspension (Rare)......... 2564
VFEND Tablets (Rare)....................... 2564

Viramune Oral Suspension ... 873
Viramune Tablets ... 873
Voltaren Tablets (Rarely) ... 2307
Voltaren-XR Tablets (Rarely) ... 2310
Vytorin 10/10 Tablets ... 2114
Vytorin 10/10 Tablets ... 3077
Vytorin 10/20 Tablets ... 2114
Vytorin 10/20 Tablets ... 3077
Vytorin 10/40 Tablets ... 2114
Vytorin 10/40 Tablets ... 3077
Vytorin 10/80 Tablets ... 2114
Vytorin 10/80 Tablets ... 3077
Xalatan Sterile Ophthalmic Solution ... 2649
Zegerid Capsules (Very rare) ... 2958
Zegerid Powder for Oral Solution (Very rare) ... 2958
Ziagen ... 1626
Zinacef for Injection (Rare) ... 1631
Zinacef Injection (Rare) ... 1631
Zmax for Oral Suspension (Rare) ... 2583
Zocor Tablets (Rare) ... 2105
Zonegran Capsules (Rare) ... 1101
Zosyn ... 3492
Zovirax ... 1643

Necrosis
Arthrotec Tablets ... 3129
Captopril Tablets (Rare) ... 2149
Fortaz ... 1453
Invanz for Injection (Greater than 0.1%) ... 1999
Miradon Tablets ... 3042
Sustiva Capsules (Up to 3.5%) ... 930
Sustiva Tablets (Up to 3.5%) ... 930
Zomig Tablets (Rare) ... 3519
Zomig-ZMT Tablets (Rare) ... 3519

Necrosis, avascular
Gleevec Tablets (Rare) ... 2227

Necrosis, bone
Azilect Tablets (Infrequent) ... 3293
Herceptin I.V. (At least one of the 958 patients) ... 1233
▲ Humira Injection (Less than 5%) ... 466
▲ Rapamune Oral Solution and Tablets (3% to 20%) ... 3475
Rilutek Tablets (Rare) ... 2930
VFEND I.V. (Less than 2%) ... 2564
VFEND Oral Suspension (Less than 2%) ... 2564
VFEND Tablets (Less than 2%) ... 2564

Necrosis, bowel
Proleukin for Injection (Less than 1%) ... 2266

Necrosis, colon
Kionex Powder (Rare) ... 2477

Necrosis, cutaneous
Coumadin for Injection (Less frequent) ... 898
Coumadin Tablets (Less frequent) ... 898
Doxil Injection (Less than 1%) ... 2351
Effexor Tablets ... 3411
Lovenox Injection ... 2915
Neurontin Capsules (Rare) ... 2487
Neurontin Oral Solution (Rare) ... 2487
Neurontin Tablets (Rare) ... 2487
Thalomid Capsules ... 965

Necrosis, fat
Garamycin Injectable (Rare) ... 3014

Necrosis, femoral head avascular
Evoxac Capsules (Less than 1%) ... 1047
Nutropin for Injection ... 1239
Nutropin AQ Injection ... 1243
Nutropin AQ Pen ... 1243
Nutropin AQ Pen Cartridge ... 1243
Pulmicort Respules (Less than 1%) ... 661

Necrosis, gastrointestinal
Zomig Nasal Spray (Very rare) ... 3523

Necrosis, injection sites
▲ Betaseron for SC Injection (5%) ... 767
Bicillin C-R Injectable Suspension ... 1706
Eloxatin for Injection ... 2892
PEG-Intron Powder for Injection (Less than or equal to 1%) ... 3048
▲ Rebif Prefilled Syringe for Injection (1% to 3%) ... 3159

Necrosis, intestinal
Avastin IV (Rare) ... 1227
Lanoxicaps Capsules (Very rare) ... 1490
Tabloid Tablets ... 1575

Necrosis, ischemic
Plavix Tablets (Less than 1%) ... 917
Plavix Tablets (Less than 1%) ... 2926

Necrosis, papillary
Aggrenox Capsules ... 822
Arthrotec Tablets (Rare) ... 3129
Bayer Aspirin ... 744
Bayer Aspirin Comprehensive Prescribing Information ... ▣796
Nalfon Capsules (Less than 1%) ... 2502
Percodan Tablets ... 1132
St. Joseph 81 mg Aspirin Chewable and Enteric Coated Tablets ... 1869
St. Joseph 81 mg Aspirin ... ▣688

Necrosis, renal papillary
Anaprox Tablets (Less than 1%) ... 2761
Anaprox DS Tablets (Less than 1%) .. 2761
Dapsone Tablets USP ... 1673
Dolobid Tablets ... 1955
EC-Naprosyn Delayed-Release Tablets (Less than 1%) ... 2761
Mobic Oral Suspension ... 863
Mobic Tablets ... 863
Naprosyn Suspension (Less than 1%) ... 2761
Naprosyn Tablets (Less than 1%) ... 2761
Prevacid NapraPAC (Less than 1%) .. 3280
Vicoprofen Tablets ... 539

Necrosis, renal tubular
Atripla Tablets ... 945
Calcium Disodium Versenate Injection ... 1851
Capastat Sulfate for Injection ... 1755
Carimune NF ... 3499
▲ CellCept Capsules (3% to less than 20%) ... 2747
▲ CellCept Intravenous (3% to less than 20%) ... 2747
▲ CellCept Oral Suspension (3% to less than 20%) ... 2747
▲ CellCept Tablets (3% to less than 20%) ... 2747
Flebogamma 5%, Immune Globulin Intravenous (Human) ... 1658
Fuzeon Injection ... 2767
Gammagard S/D ... 724
Guanidine Hydrochloride Tablets ... 3016
Miradon Tablets ... 3042
Mycamine for Injection ... 628
▲ Myfortic Tablets (3% to less than 20%) ... 2255
▲ Prograf Capsules and Injection (3% to 15%) ... 632
▲ Rapamune Oral Solution and Tablets (3% to 20%) ... 3475
▲ Simulect for Injection (3% to 10%) ... 2284
Trasylol Injection (1% to 2%) ... 754
Truvada Tablets ... 1296
▲ Vesanoid Capsules (3%) ... 2820
VFEND I.V. (Less than 2%) ... 2564
VFEND Oral Suspension (Less than 2%) ... 2564
VFEND Tablets (Less than 2%) ... 2564

Necrosis, skin
Augmentin XR Extended-Release Tablets ... 1369
Depakote ER Tablets (One patient) ... 434
Fragmin Injection (Rare) ... 1097
Lyrica Capsules (Rare) ... 2539
Miradon Tablets ... 3042
Mycamine for Injection ... 628

Necrosis, tissue
Coumadin for Injection (Less frequent) ... 898
Coumadin Tablets (Less frequent) ... 898
Miradon Tablets ... 3042

Necrosis, tumor
Gleevec Tablets (Rare) ... 2227

Necrotizing angiitis
Aldoril Tablets ... 1910
Atacand HCT ... 651
Avalide Tablets ... 888
Avalide Tablets ... 2874
Clorpres Tablets ... 2153
Diovan HCT Tablets ... 2196
Diuril Sodium Intravenous ... 2467
Dyazide Capsules ... 1423
Furosemide Tablets ... 2154
Hyzaar 50-12.5 Tablets ... 1990
Hyzaar 100-12.5 Tablets ... 1990
Hyzaar 100-25 Tablets ... 1990
Indapamide Tablets ... 2156
Lotensin HCT Tablets ... 2246
Micardis HCT Tablets ... 856
Moduretic Tablets ... 2028
Prinzide Tablets ... 2056
Teveten HCT Tablets ... 1737
Uniretic Tablets ... 3100

Necrotizing cellulitis
Amevive ... 626

Neonatal morbidity
Aceon Tablets (2 mg, 4 mg, 8 mg) ... 3194
Altace Capsules ... 1702
Avalide Tablets ... 888
Avalide Tablets ... 2874
Avapro Tablets ... 891
Avapro Tablets ... 2871
Captopril Tablets ... 2149
Cozaar Tablets ... 1935
Hyzaar 50-12.5 Tablets ... 1990
Hyzaar 100-12.5 Tablets ... 1990
Hyzaar 100-25 Tablets ... 1990
Lotrel Capsules ... 2249
Mavik Tablets ... 486
Prinivil Tablets ... 2052
Prinzide Tablets ... 2056
Uniretic Tablets (Several dozen cases) ... 3100
Vasotec I.V. Injection ... 2103

Neonatal prematurity
Adderall Tablets ... 3164
Altace Capsules ... 1702
Captopril Tablets ... 2149
Cozaar Tablets ... 1935
Hyzaar 50-12.5 Tablets ... 1990
Hyzaar 100-12.5 Tablets ... 1990
Hyzaar 100-25 Tablets ... 1990
Prinivil Tablets ... 2052
Prinzide Tablets ... 2056
Vasotec I.V. Injection ... 2103

Neoplasm
(*see under* Carcinoma, unspecified)

Neoplasm, bladder
Lyrica Capsules (Rare) ... 2539

Neoplasm, bone
Relpax Tablets (Rare) ... 2548

Neoplasm, brain, benign
Requip Tablets (Infrequent) ... 1555

Neoplasm, breast
Ambien CR Tablets (Rare) ... 2855
▲ Arimidex Tablets (5%) ... 673
Lunesta Tablets (Infrequent) ... 3142
Protopic Ointment (0.2% to less than 1%) ... 638

Neoplasm, breast, male
Eulexin Capsules ... 3009

Neoplasm, breast malignant
Evoxac Capsules (Less than 1%) ... 1047
Symbyax Capsules (Infrequent) ... 1819
Xolair (0.5%) ... 1266

Neoplasm, laryngeal, malignant
Requip Tablets (Infrequent) ... 1555

Neoplasm, malignant
Estratest Tablets ... 3199
Estratest H.S. Tablets ... 3199
Orthoclone OKT3 Sterile Solution ... 2360
Xolair (0.5%) ... 1266

Neoplasm, ovarian
Follistim AQ Cartridge ... 2338

Neoplasm, prostatic malignant
Xolair (0.5%) ... 1266

Neoplasm, unspecified
Protopic Ointment (0.2% to less than 1%) ... 638
Topamax Sprinkle Capsules (Less than 1% to 2%) ... 2404
Topamax Tablets (Less than 1% to 2%) ... 2404

Neoplasm, urogenital
Zomig Nasal Spray (Rare) ... 3523

Neoplasms, hepatic
Androxy Tablets (Rare) ... 3335
Estratest Tablets (Rare) ... 3199
Estratest H.S. Tablets (Rare) ... 3199
Ortho-Cyclen/Ortho Tri-Cyclen ... 2429
Ortho Tri-Cyclen Lo Tablets ... 2436
Oxandrin Tablets ... 2962
Zomig Nasal Spray (Rare) ... 3523

Nephritis
Aceon Tablets (2 mg, 4 mg, 8 mg) ... 3194
Atripla Tablets ... 945
Caduet Tablets (Less than 2%) ... 2508
Capastat Sulfate for Injection (1 patient) ... 1755
Cipro (Less than 1%) ... 2977
Cipro I.V. (1% or less) ... 2984
Cipro XR Tablets ... 2990
Depakote ER Tablets ... 434
Gantrisin Pediatric Suspension ... 2770
Kaletra (Less than 2%) ... 476
Lipitor Tablets (Less than 2%) ... 2483
Lyrica Capsules (0.1% to 1%) ... 2539
Paxil CR Controlled-Release Tablets (Rare) ... 1538
Paxil (Rare) ... 1530
Pexeva Tablets (rare) ... 1694
Proquin XR Tablets ... 1153
Rilutek Tablets (Rare) ... 2930
Timolide Tablets ... 2086
Truvada Tablets ... 1296
VFEND I.V. (Less than 2%) ... 2564
VFEND Oral Suspension (Less than 2%) ... 2564
VFEND Tablets (Less than 2%) ... 2564

Nephritis, interstitial
Aciphex Tablets ... 1090
Aggrenox Capsules ... 822
Aldoril Tablets ... 1910
Anaprox Tablets (Less than 1%) ... 2761
Anaprox DS Tablets (Less than 1%) .. 2761
Arthrotec Tablets (Rare) ... 3129
Asacol Delayed-Release Tablets ... 2692
Atacand HCT ... 651
Augmentin (Rare) ... 1360
Augmentin Tablets (Rare) ... 1363
Augmentin XR Extended-Release Tablets (Rare) ... 1369
Augmentin ES-600 Powder for Oral Suspension (Rare) ... 1366
Avalide Tablets ... 888
Avalide Tablets ... 2874
Bayer Aspirin ... 744
Bayer Aspirin Comprehensive Prescribing Information ... ▣796
Biaxin/Biaxin XL ... 402
Captopril Tablets ... 2149
Celebrex Capsules (Less than 0.1%) ... 3134
Cipro (Less than 1%) ... 2977
Cipro I.V. (1% or less) ... 2984
Cipro XR Tablets ... 2990
Clinoril Tablets (Less than 1 in 100) ... 1924
Clozaril Tablets ... 2184
Colazal Capsules ... 2838
Crixivan Capsules ... 1940
Diovan HCT Tablets ... 2196
Diuril Oral Suspension ... 1954
Diuril Sodium Intravenous ... 2467
Dolobid Tablets (Less than 1 in 100) ... 1955
Dyazide Capsules ... 1423
Dyrenium Capsules (Rare) ... 3400
EC-Naprosyn Delayed-Release Tablets (Less than 1%) ... 2761
Fansidar Tablets ... 2765
FazaClo Orally Disintegrating Tablets ... 551
Furosemide Tablets ... 2154
Guanidine Hydrochloride Tablets ... 3016
Hyzaar 50-12.5 Tablets ... 1990
Hyzaar 100-12.5 Tablets ... 1990
Hyzaar 100-25 Tablets ... 1990
Indocin (Less than 1%) ... 1995
Keflex Capsules (Rare) ... 549
Levaquin (Rare) ... 2384
Levaquin in 5% Dextrose Injection (Rare) ... 2384
Mefoxin for Injection ... 2012
Mefoxin Premixed Intravenous Solution ... 2016
Meridia Capsules (One patient) ... 489
Micardis HCT Tablets ... 856
Mobic Oral Suspension (Less than 0.1%) ... 863
Mobic Tablets (Less than 0.1%) ... 863
Moduretic Tablets ... 2028
Nalfon Capsules (Less than 1%) ... 2502
Naprosyn Suspension (Less than 1%) ... 2761
Naprosyn Tablets (Less than 1%) ... 2761
Noroxin Tablets ... 2032
Orthoclone OKT3 Sterile Solution ... 2360
Pegasys ... 2789
PEG-Intron Powder for Injection (Less than or equal to 1%) ... 3048
Pentasa Capsules (Infrequent) ... 3185
Percodan Tablets ... 1132
Prevacid NapraPAC (Less than 1%) .. 3280
Prilosec OTC Delayed-Release Tablets (Less than 1%) ... 2677
Prinzide Tablets ... 2056
Proleukin for Injection (Less than 1%) ... 2266
Proquin XR Tablets ... 1153
Protonix I.V. ... 3472
Protonix Tablets ... 3469
Raniclor Tablets, Chewable (Rare) ... 2505

St. Joseph 81 mg Aspirin Chewable and Enteric Coated Tablets ... 1869
St. Joseph 81 mg Aspirin ... ▣ 688
Teveten HCT Tablets ... 1737
Vancocin HCl Capsules, USP (Rare) ... 3380
Voltaren Tablets (Occasionally) ... 2307
Voltaren-XR Tablets (Occasionally) ... 2310
Zegerid Capsules (Less than 1%) ... 2958
Zegerid Powder for Oral Solution (Less than 1%) ... 2958
Zinacef for Injection (Rare) ... 1631
Zinacef Injection (Rare) ... 1631
Zmax for Oral Suspension ... 2583
Zosyn (Rare) ... 3492

Nephritis, purpuric
Vantin Tablets and Oral Suspension ... 2645

Nephrocalcinosis
Fleet Phospho-soda ... 1166
Fleet Prep Kits ... 1170
Rocaltrol Capsules ... 2798
Rocaltrol Oral Solution ... 2798

Nephrolithiasis
Aceon Tablets (2 mg, 4 mg, 8 mg) (0.3% to 1%) ... 3194
Aciphex Tablets ... 1090
▲ Actonel Tablets (3%) ... 2683
Axid Oral Solution ... 879
Caduet Tablets (Less than 2%) ... 2508
Celebrex Capsules (0.1% to 1.9%) ... 3134
Celexa (Rare) ... 1176
Chantix Tablets (Infrequent) ... 2517
Cipro ... 2977
Cipro I.V. (1% or less) ... 2984
Cipro XR Tablets ... 2990
Clinoril Tablets ... 1924
Copaxone for Injection (Infrequent) ... 3297
▲ Crixivan Capsules (8.7% to 12.4%) ... 1940
Daranide Tablets ... 1950
Dyazide Capsules ... 1423
Dyrenium Capsules (Rare) ... 3400
Effexor Tablets (Infrequent) ... 3411
Effexor XR Capsules (Infrequent) ... 3417
Evoxac Capsules (Less than 1%) ... 1047
Exelon Capsules (Infrequent) ... 2206
Exelon Oral Solution (Infrequent) ... 2206
▲ Humira Injection (Less than 5%) ... 466
▲ Imdur Tablets (Less than or equal to 5%) ... 3018
Imitrex Injection (Rare) ... 1463
Imitrex Nasal Spray ... 1467
Imitrex Tablets ... 1471
Invirase (Rare) ... 2772
Kaletra (Less than 2%) ... 476
Lexapro Oral Solution (Infrequent) ... 1190
Lexapro Tablets (Infrequent) ... 1190
Lipitor Tablets (Less than 2%) ... 2483
Lunesta Tablets (Infrequent) ... 3142
Miacalcin Nasal Spray (Less than 1%) ... 2253
Neurontin Capsules (Rare) ... 2487
Neurontin Oral Solution (Rare) ... 2487
Neurontin Tablets (Rare) ... 2487
Nipent for Injection (Less than 3%) ... 1863
Norvir (Less than 2%) ... 503
Paxil CR Controlled-Release Tablets (Rare) ... 1538
Paxil (Rare) ... 1530
Permax Tablets (Infrequent) ... 3356
Pexeva Tablets (rare) ... 1694
Prevacid Delayed-Release Capsules (Less than 1%) ... 3271
Prevacid for Delayed-Release Oral Suspension (Less than 1%) ... 3271
Prevacid SoluTab Delayed-Release Orally Disintegrating Tablets (Less than 1%) ... 3271
Prevacid NapraPAC (Less than 1%) ... 3280
PREVPAC (Less than 1%) ... 3284
Prezista Tablets (Less than 2%) ... 3306
Protonix I.V. (Less than 1%) ... 3472
Protonix Tablets (Less than 1%) ... 3469
Razadyne (Infrequent) ... 2399
Razadyne ER Extended-Release Capsules (Infrequent) ... 2399
Remicade for IV Injection (Greater than or equal to 0.2%) ... 971
Requip Tablets (Infrequent) ... 1555
Rescriptor Tablets ... 2551
Revlimid Capsules ... 958
Reyataz Capsules (Less than 3%) ... 921
Rilutek Tablets (Infrequent) ... 2930
Rocephin Injectable Vials, ADD-Vantage, Galaxy, Bulk ... 2800
Sandostatin Injection (Less than 1%) ... 2278
▲ Sandostatin LAR Depot (5% to 15%) ... 2280
Sonata Capsules (Infrequent) ... 1717
Sustiva Capsules (Up to 1%) ... 930
Sustiva Tablets (Up to 1%) ... 930
Symbyax Capsules (Rare) ... 1819
Tasmar Tablets (Infrequent) ... 3358
Teveten Tablets (Less than 1%) ... 1735
Teveten HCT Tablets (Less than 1%) ... 1737
Topamax Sprinkle Capsules (Frequent) ... 2404
Topamax Tablets (Frequent) ... 2404
Tricor Tablets ... 527
Trileptal Tablets ... 2300
Trileptal Oral Suspension ... 2300
Uniretic Tablets (Less than 1%) ... 3100
Viracept (Less than 2%) ... 2577
Zonegran Capsules (Rare) ... 1101

Nephropathy
AmBisome for Injection (Less common) ... 620
Asacol Delayed-Release Tablets ... 2692
Bicillin C-R Injectable Suspension ... 1706
Campath Ampules ... 811
Ceftin ... 1407
Cymbalta Delayed-Release Capsules (Infrequent) ... 1757
Eloxatin for Injection ... 2892
Fortaz ... 1453
Keflex Capsules ... 549
Maxipime for Injection ... 1105
Mefoxin for Injection ... 2012
Mefoxin Premixed Intravenous Solution ... 2016
Nipent for Injection (Less than 3%) ... 1863
Omnicef Capsules ... 511
Omnicef for Oral Suspension ... 511
Raniclor Tablets, Chewable ... 2505
▲ Rapamune Oral Solution and Tablets (3% to 20%) ... 3475
Suprax ... 1843
Vantin Tablets and Oral Suspension ... 2645
Zinacef for Injection ... 1631
Zinacef Injection ... 1631

Nephropathy, acute uric acid
Oncaspar ... 1145

Nephropathy, proximal tubular
Carimune NF ... 3499
CytoGam Intravenous ... 1895
Flebogamma 5%, Immune Globulin Intravenous (Human) ... 1658
Gammagard S/D ... 724

Nephrosis, osmotic
Carimune NF ... 3499
CytoGam Intravenous ... 1895
Flebogamma 5%, Immune Globulin Intravenous (Human) ... 1658
Gammagard S/D ... 724

Nephrosis, toxic
Calcium Disodium Versenate Injection ... 1851
Evoxac Capsules (Less than 1%) ... 1047
Fansidar Tablets ... 2765
Gantrisin Pediatric Suspension ... 2770
Neurontin Capsules (Rare) ... 2487
Neurontin Oral Solution (Rare) ... 2487
Neurontin Tablets (Rare) ... 2487
Permax Tablets (Rare) ... 3356
VFEND I.V. (Less than 2%) ... 2564
VFEND Oral Suspension (Less than 2%) ... 2564
VFEND Tablets (Less than 2%) ... 2564

Nephrosis, unspecified
Nalfon Capsules (Less than 1%) ... 2502

Nephrotic syndrome
Anaprox Tablets (Occasional; less than 1%) ... 2761
Anaprox DS Tablets (Occasional; less than 1%) ... 2761
Arthrotec Tablets (Rare) ... 3129
Avastin IV ... 1227
Captopril Tablets (Approximately 1 to 2 of 1000 patients) ... 2149
Clinoril Tablets (Less than 1 in 100) ... 1924
Cuprimine Capsules ... 1947
Dapsone Tablets USP ... 1673
Dolobid Tablets (Rare) ... 1955
EC-Naprosyn Delayed-Release Tablets (Occasional; less than 1%) ... 2761
Fabrazyme for Intravenous Infusion ... 1274
HyperRAB (Rare) ... 3242
HyperTET (Few isolated cases) ... 3248
Indocin (Less than 1%) ... 1995
Naprosyn Suspension (Occasional; less than 1%) ... 2761
Naprosyn Tablets (Occasional; less than 1%) ... 2761
Pentasa Capsules (Infrequent) ... 3185
Prevacid NapraPAC (Less than 1%) ... 3280
▲ Thiola Tablets (5%) ... 2141
Ticlid Tablets (Rare) ... 2810

Nephrotoxicity
Anaprox Tablets ... 2761
Anaprox DS Tablets ... 2761
Aredia for Injection ... 2179
Canasa Rectal Suppositories ... 699
Capastat Sulfate for Injection ... 1755
Dolobid Tablets ... 1955
EC-Naprosyn Delayed-Release Tablets ... 2761
Garamycin Injectable ... 3014
▲ Gengraf Capsules (25% to 38%) ... 459
Leustatin Injection ... 2357
Naprosyn Suspension ... 2761
Naprosyn Tablets ... 2761
▲ Neoral Oral Solution (25% to 38%) ... 2259
▲ Neoral Soft Gelatin Capsules (25% to 38%) ... 2259
▲ Prograf Capsules and Injection (36% to 52%) ... 632
Rituxan I.V. ... 1254
▲ Sandimmune (25% to 38%) ... 2275
TOBI Solution for Inhalation ... 2298
Vancocin HCl Capsules, USP ... 3380
Vicoprofen Tablets ... 539
Zinacef for Injection ... 1631
Zinacef Injection ... 1631

Nerve compression, arm
Adacel (1.5%) ... 2945

Nerve deafness
M-M-R II ... 2006
Mumpsvax ... 2031

Nerve paralysis
Arranon Injection (1%) ... 1357

Nerve syndromes, compressed
▲ Advair Diskus 100/50 (1% to 3%) ... 1308
▲ Advair Diskus 250/50 (1% to 3%) ... 1308
▲ Advair Diskus 500/50 (1% to 3%) ... 1308
Amerge Tablets (Rare) ... 1339

Nervous system disorders, unspecified
▲ Arranon Injection (0% to 4%) ... 1357
▲ Focalin XR Capsules (30% to 50%) ... 2223
▲ Hycamtin for Injection (35%) ... 1458

Nervousness
Abilify Oral Solution (Frequent) ... 882
Abilify Oral Solution (Frequent) ... 2450
Abilify Discmelt Orally Disintegrating Tablets (Frequent) ... 882
Abilify Discmelt Orally Disintegrating Tablets (Frequent) ... 2450
Abilify Tablets (Frequent) ... 882
Abilify Tablets (Frequent) ... 2450
Accutane Capsules ... 2731
Aceon Tablets (2 mg, 4 mg, 8 mg) (1.1%) ... 3194
Aciphex Tablets ... 1090
Actiq (1% to 2%) ... 979
Adalat CC Tablets (Rare) ... 2964
▲ Adderall XR Capsules (6%) ... 3166
Adenoscan (2%) ... 619
Advil Allergy Sinus Caplets ... ▣ 770
Advil Multi-Symptom Cold Caplets ... ▣ 770
▲ Aerobid/Aerobid-M (3% to 9%) ... 1171
▲ Agrylin Capsules (1% to 5%) ... 3169
Alavert Allergy & Sinus D-12 Hour Tablets ... ▣ 771
Albalon Ophthalmic Solution ... ⊙ 218
Alferon N Injection (1%) ... 1665
Allegra (Less than 1%) ... 2844
Allegra-D 12 Hour Extended-Release Tablets (1.4%) ... 2846
Allegra-D 24 Hour Extended-Release Tablets (1.4%) ... 2849
Altace Capsules (Less than 1%) ... 1702
▲ Alupent Inhalation Aerosol (14.1%) ... 826
Ambien Tablets (1%) ... 2851
Ambien CR Tablets (Infrequent) ... 2855
AmBisome for Injection (Less common) ... 620
Amitiza Capsules (Less than 0.2%) ... 3224
Anaprox Tablets (Less than 1%) ... 2761
Anaprox DS Tablets (Less than 1%) ... 2761
AndroGel (Up to 3%) ... 3329
Angeliq Tablets ... 762
Aricept Tablets (Frequent) ... 1094
Aricept ODT Tablets (Frequent) ... 1094
▲ Arimidex Tablets (2% to 5%) ... 673
Arthrotec Tablets (Rare) ... 3129
Asacol Delayed-Release Tablets (2% or greater) ... 2692
Astelin Nasal Spray (Infrequent) ... 1904
Atripla Tablets (Greater than or equal to 2%) ... 945
Atrovent Inhalation Solution (0.5%) ... 835
Avalide Tablets (1% or greater) ... 888
Avalide Tablets (1% or greater) ... 2874
Avapro Tablets (1% or greater) ... 891
Avapro Tablets (1% or greater) ... 2871
Avelox (0.1% to less than 2%) ... 2970
▲ Avinza Capsules (Less than 5%) ... 1741
Axert Tablets (Rare) ... 2396
Axid Oral Solution (1.1%) ... 879
▲ Bentyl Capsules (6%) ... 697
▲ Bentyl Injection (6%) ... 697
▲ Bentyl Syrup (6%) ... 697
▲ Bentyl Tablets (6%) ... 697
▲ Betaseron for SC Injection (7%) ... 767
Bicillin C-R Injectable Suspension ... 1706
Blocadren Tablets (Less than 1%) ... 1916
Caduet Tablets (Greater than 0.1% to less than or equal to 1%) ... 2508
Campath Ampules ... 811
Captopril Tablets ... 2149
Cardizem LA Extended Release Tablets (Less than 2%) ... 1728
Cardura XL Tablets ... 2515
▲ Catapres Tablets (About 3 in 100 patients) ... 843
Catapres-TTS (1 of 101 patients) ... 844
Celebrex Capsules (0.1% to 1.9%) ... 3134
▲ CellCept Capsules (3% to less than 20%) ... 2747
▲ CellCept Intravenous (3% to less than 20%) ... 2747
▲ CellCept Oral Suspension (3% to less than 20%) ... 2747
▲ CellCept Tablets (3% to less than 20%) ... 2747
Cesamet Capsules ... 3340
Cipro ... 2977
Cipro I.V. ... 2984
Cipro XR Tablets ... 2990
Clarinex-D 24-Hour Extended-Release Tablets (2%) ... 2998
Climara Transdermal System ... 771
Climara Pro Transdermal System ... 776
Clinoril Tablets (Greater than 1%) ... 1924
▲ Clorpres Tablets (About 3%) ... 2153
Colazal Capsules ... 2838
Combivent Inhalation Aerosol (Less than 2%) ... 847
▲ Concerta Extended-Release Tablets (Greater than 0.7%) ... 1881
Copaxone for Injection (2%) ... 3297
▲ Copegus Tablets (33%) ... 2754
Coreg Tablets (Greater than 0.1% to 1%) ... 1414
Cosopt Sterile Ophthalmic Solution ... 1931
▲ Cozaar Tablets (Less than 1% to 4%) ... 1935
Cymbalta Delayed-Release Capsules (Frequent) ... 1757
Dalmane Capsules ... 3342
Dantrium Capsules (Less frequent) ... 2694
Daranide Tablets ... 1950
Daytrana Transdermal Patch ... 3174
Demadex Injection (1.1%) ... 2759
Demadex Tablets (1.1%) ... 2759
▲ Depacon Injection (0.9% to 11%) ... 412
▲ Depakene (11%) ... 417
▲ Depakote Sprinkle Capsules (7% to 11%) ... 422
▲ Depakote Tablets (1% to 11%) ... 427
▲ Depakote ER Tablets (Greater than 1% to 11%) ... 434
▲ Depo-Provera Contraceptive Injection (Greater than 5%) ... 2622
depo-subQ provera 104 Injectable Suspension ... 2624
Detrol Tablets (1.1%) ... 2628
Diastat Rectal Delivery System (Greater than or equal to 1%) ... 3343
Dilaudid Oral Liquid (Less frequent) ... 445
Dilaudid Tablets - 8 mg (Less frequent) ... 445
Dilaudid-HP ... 442
▲ Ditropan XL Extended-Release Tablets (2% to less than 5%) ... 2413
Dolobid Tablets (Less than 1 in 100) ... 1955
Donnatal Extentabs ... 2493
Doxil Injection (Less than 1%) ... 2351
▲ Duragesic Transdermal System (3% to 10%) ... 2373
DynaCirc CR Tablets (0.5% to 1%) ... 2721

EC-Naprosyn Delayed-Release Tablets (Less than 1%) 2761
▲ Effexor Tablets (2% to 21.3%) 3411
▲ Effexor XR Capsules (5% to 11%) 3417
Eldepryl Capsules 3208
▲ Eloxatin for Injection (2% to 5%) 2892
Emsam Transdermal System 903
Enjuvia Tablets 1062
▲ Entocort EC Capsules (Less than 5%) 2698
EpiPen Jr. Auto-Injector 1061
▲ Equetro Extended-Release Capsules (Less than 5%) 3180
Estrasorb Topical Emulsion 1147
Estratest Tablets 3199
Estratest H.S. Tablets 3199
Estring Vaginal Ring 2635
Eulexin Capsules (1%) 3009
Exelon Capsules (2% or more) 2206
Exelon Oral Solution (2% or more) 2206
Fansidar Tablets 2765
Ferrlecit Injection (Two or more patients) 3388
Flumadine (1.3% to 2.1%) 1183
▲ Focalin Tablets (Among most common) 2220
Focalin XR Capsules 2223
Foradil Aerolizer 3010
Frova Tablets (Infrequent) 1113
▲ Gabitril Tablets (10%) 984
Gengraf Capsules (1% to less than 3%) 459
Hytrin Capsules (2.3%) 471
Hyzaar 50-12.5 Tablets 1990
Hyzaar 100-12.5 Tablets 1990
Hyzaar 100-25 Tablets 1990
▲ Imdur Tablets (Less than or equal to 5%) 3018
▲ Indapamide Tablets (Less than 5%) 2156
Indocin (Less than 1%) 1995
▲ Infergen (16% to 31%) 3364
▲ Intron A for Injection (Up to 3%) 3024
Invanz for Injection (Greater than 0.1%) 1999
Ionsys Transdermal System (.1% to less than 1%) 2379
Kaletra (Less than 2%) 476
▲ Keppra Injection (4%) 3320
▲ Keppra Oral Solution (4% to 10%) 3314
▲ Keppra Tablets (4% to 10%) 3314
Klonopin (1% to 3%) 2778
Lamictal (2%) 1481
Levaquin (0.1% to 0.9%) 2384
Levaquin in 5% Dextrose Injection (0.1% to 0.9%) 2384
Levothroid Tablets 1186
Levoxyl Tablets 1712
Lexapro Oral Solution (Infrequent) 1190
Lexapro Tablets (Infrequent) 1190
Lidoderm Patch 1118
▲ Lithostat Tablets (20%) 2140
Lofibra Tablets 1219
Lofibra Capsules 1216
Lotensin Tablets (Less than 1%) 2243
Lotensin HCT Tablets (0.3% to 1%) 2246
Lotrel Capsules 2249
▲ Lunesta Tablets (0% to 5%) 3142
▲ Lupron Depot 3.75 mg (4%) 3260
▲ Lupron Depot–3 Month 11.25 mg (4%) 3265
Lupron Depot-PED 7.5 mg, 11.25 mg and 15 mg (Less than 2%) 3269
Lupron Injection Pediatric (Less than 2%) 3259
Lyrica Capsules (1% to greater than or equal to 2%) 2539
Marinol Capsules (Greater than 1%) 3333
Matulane Capsules 3191
▲ Maxair Autohaler (4.5% to 6.9%) 1852
Maxalt Tablets (Infrequent) 2008
Maxalt-MLT Orally Disintegrating Tablets (Infrequent) 2008
Menostar Transdermal System 782
▲ Meridia Capsules (5.2%) 489
Merrem I.V. (Greater than 0.1% to 1%) 686
▲ Metadate CD Capsules (Among most common) 3323
Micardis HCT Tablets 856
Midamor Tablets (Less than or equal to 1%) 2026
Migranal Nasal Spray (Infrequent) 3348
Mirapex Tablets (1% or more) 859
Mircette Tablets 1066
▲ Mirena Intrauterine System (5% or more) 787
Mobic Oral Suspension (Less than 2%) 863
Mobic Tablets (Less than 2%) 863
Moduretic Tablets (Less than or equal to 1%) 2028
MS Contin Tablets (Less frequent) 2701
▲ Nalfon Capsules (5.7%) 2502
Namenda (Infrequent) 1195
Naprosyn Suspension (Less than 1%) 2761
Naprosyn Tablets (Less than 1%) 2761
Nembutal Sodium Solution, USP (Less than 1%) 2470
Neoral Oral Solution (1% to less than 3%) 2259
Neoral Soft Gelatin Capsules (1% to less than 3%) 2259
▲ Neumega for Injection (Greater than or equal to 10%) 3435
Neurontin Capsules (2.4%) 2487
Neurontin Oral Solution (2.4%) 2487
Neurontin Tablets (2.4%) 2487
Nexium Delayed-Release Capsules (Less than 1%) 655
Nexium I.V. (Less than 1%) 659
Niaspan Extended-Release Tablets 1730
▲ Nipent for Injection (3% to 10%) 1863
▲ Niravam Orally Disintegrating Tablets (4.1%) 3092
Norvasc Tablets (More than 0.1% to 1%) 2545
Norvir (Less than 2%) 503
Numorphan Injection 1120
NuvaRing 2340
▲ Ontak Vials (11%) 1745
Opana Tablets (Less than 1%) 1122
Opana ER Tablets (Less than 1%) 1126
OptiPranolol Metipranolol Ophthalmic Solution 0.3% (A small number of patients) ⊙256
Ortho-Cyclen Tablets 2429
Ortho Evra Transdermal System 2417
Ortho Tri-Cyclen Tablets 2429
Ortho Tri-Cyclen Lo Tablets 2436
Oxsoralen-Ultra Capsules 3353
▲ OxyContin Tablets (Between 1% and 5%) 2703
Parcopa Orally Disintegrating Tablets 3097
▲ Paxil CR Controlled-Release Tablets (4% to 9%) 1538
▲ Paxil (4% to 9%) 1530
▲ Pegasys (19%) 2789
▲ PEG-Intron Powder for Injection (4%) 3048
Percodan Tablets 1132
Permax Tablets (Frequent) 3356
▲ Pexeva Tablets (2.9% to 9%) 1694
Phenergan Tablets and Suppositories 3440
Phenytek Capsules 2160
Premarin Intravenous 3442
▲ Premarin Tablets (2% to 5%) 3446
Premarin Vaginal Cream 3452
▲ Premphase Tablets (2% to 3%) 3456
▲ Prempro Tablets (2% to 3%) 3456
Prevacid Delayed-Release Capsules (Less than 1%) 3271
Prevacid for Delayed-Release Oral Suspension (Less than 1%) 3271
Prevacid SoluTab Delayed-Release Orally Disintegrating Tablets (Less than 1%) 3271
Prevacid NapraPAC (Less than 1%) 3280
PREVPAC (Less than 1%) 3284
Prilosec OTC Delayed-Release Tablets (Less than 1%) 2677
Primatene Mist ▣719
Prinivil Tablets (0.3% to 1.0%) 2052
Prinzide Tablets 2056
ProAir HFA Inhalation Aerosol (Frequent) 3300
ProAmatine Tablets (Less frequent) 3186
▲ Prochieve 4% Gel (16%) 1003
▲ Prochieve 8% Gel (16%) 1003
▲ Prograf Capsules and Injection (3%) 632
Prometrium Capsules (100 mg, 200 mg) 3203
ProQuad 2064
▲ ProSom Tablets (8%) 517
Protonix I.V. (Less than 1%) 3472
Protonix Tablets (Less than 1%) 3469
▲ Proventil Inhalation Aerosol (Less than 10%) 3053
▲ Proventil Inhalation Solution 0.083% (4%) 3055
▲ Proventil HFA Inhalation Aerosol (7%) 3056
▲ Provigil Tablets (7%) 988
▲ Prozac Pulvules and Liquid (8% to 16%) 1801
Raniclor Tablets, Chewable (Rare) 2505
▲ Rebetol (3% to 6%) 3058
▲ Rebetron Combination Therapy (4% to 5%) 3063
Relpax Tablets (Infrequent) 2548
Requip Tablets (1% or more) 1555
Rescriptor Tablets 2551
▲ Restoril Capsules (4.6%) 1860
Retrovir Capsules (1.6%) 1560
Retrovir IV Infusion (2%) 1564
Retrovir (1.6%) 1560
Reyataz Capsules (Less than 3%) 921
▲ Ribavirin, USP Capsules (3% to 6%) 3068
Risperdal (Frequent) 1676
Risperdal Consta Long-Acting Injection (Frequent) 1682
Risperdal M-Tab Orally Disintegrating Tablets (Frequent) 1676
▲ Ritalin Hydrochloride Tablets (One of the two most common) 2269
▲ Ritalin LA Capsules (Among most common) 2271
▲ Ritalin-SR Tablets (One of the two most common) 2269
Robitussin Cough & Cold Long-Acting Liquid ▣735
Robitussin Head & Chest Congestion PE Syrup ▣739
Robitussin Pediatric Cough & Cold Long-Acting Liquid ▣735
▲ Romazicon Injection (3% to 9%) 2804
Sandostatin LAR Depot (1% to 4%) 2280
Seasonique Tablets 1077
▲ Skelaxin Tablets (Most frequent) 1716
Sonata Capsules (Frequent) 1717
Stalevo Tablets 2287
▲ Suboxone Tablets (6%) 2717
▲ Subutex Tablets (6%) 2717
Sular Tablets (Less than or equal to 1%) 3122
▲ Sustiva Capsules (1% to 7%) 930
▲ Sustiva Tablets (1% to 7%) 930
▲ Symmetrel Tablets (1% to 5%) 1135
Synagis (More than 1%) 1897
Synera Topical Patch 1137
Tasmar Tablets (Infrequent) 3358
Tequin Injection (Less than 0.1%) 938
Tequin Injection in 5% Dextrose (Less than 0.1%) 938
Tequin Tablets (Less than 0.1%) 938
Teveten Tablets (Less than 1%) 1735
Teveten HCT Tablets (Less than 1%) 1737
▲ Thalomid Capsules (2.8% to 9.4%) 965
TheraFlu Daytime Severe Cold Hot Liquid ▣742
Tiazac Capsules (Less than 2%) 1201
Timolide Tablets (Less than 1%) 2086
Timoptic Sterile Ophthalmic Solution (Less frequent) 2088
Timoptic in Ocudose (Less frequent) 2091
Timoptic-XE Sterile Ophthalmic Gel Forming Solution 2092
▲ Topamax Sprinkle Capsules (4% to 19%) 2404
▲ Topamax Tablets (4% to 19%) 2404
Toprol-XL Tablets 668
Tranxene (Less common) 2474
Triaminic Chest & Nasal Congestion Liquid ▣746
Tricor Tablets 527
▲ Trileptal Tablets (2% to 4%) 2300
▲ Trileptal Oral Suspension (2% to 4%) 2300
▲ Trizivir Tablets (Greater than or equal to 5%) 1589
Children's Tylenol Plus Cold & Allergy Oral Suspension ▣716
Tylenol Allergy Multi-Symptom Caplets with Cool Burst and Gelcaps 1872
Tylenol Allergy Multi-Symptom Nighttime Caplets with Cool Burst 1872
Children's Tylenol Plus Cold Suspension Liquid 1879
Children's Tylenol Plus Flu Suspension Liquid 1881
Children's Tylenol Plus Multi-Symptom Cold Suspension Liquid 1879
Tylenol Cold Severe Congestion Non-Drowsy Caplets with Cool Burst 1874
Tylenol Cold Head Congestion Daytime Caplets with Cool Burst 1873
Tylenol Cold Head Congestion Nighttime Caplets with Cool Burst 1873
Tylenol Cold Head Congestion Severe Caplets with Cool Burst 1873
Tylenol Cold Multi-Symptom Daytime Caplets with Cool Burst and Gelcaps 1874
Tylenol Cold Multi-Symptom Daytime Liquid with Citrus Burst 1874
Tylenol Cold Multi-Symptom Nighttime Caplets with Cool Burst 1874
Tylenol Cold Multi-Symptom Nighttime Liquid with Cool Burst 1874
Tylenol Cold Multi-Symptom Severe Caplets with Cool Burst 1874
Tylenol Cold Multi-Symptom Severe Daytime Liquid with Citrus Burst 1874
Concentrated Tylenol Infants' Drops Plus Cold 1879
Concentrated Tylenol Infants' Drops Plus Cold and Cough 1879
Tylenol Sinus Severe Congestion Caplets with Cool Burst 1876
Tylenol Sinus Congestion & Pain Daytime Caplets with Cool Burst and Gelcaps 1876
Tylenol Sinus Congestion & Pain Nighttime Caplets with Cool Burst 1876
Tylenol Sinus Congestion & Pain Severe Caplets with Cool Burst 1876
Ultane Liquid for Inhalation (Less than 1%) 531
▲ Ultram ER Tablets (1% to greater than 5%) 2392
Uniretic Tablets (Less than 1%) 3100
Univasc Tablets (Less than 1%) 3104
Vantin Tablets and Oral Suspension (Less than 1%) 2645
Varivax (Greater than or equal to 1%) 2100
Vasotec I.V. Injection (0.5% to 1.0%) 2103
Vicks 44D Cough & Head Congestion Relief Liquid 2679
Vicks DayQuil Multi-Symptom Cold/Flu Relief LiquiCaps 2678
Vicks DayQuil Multi-Symptom Cold/Flu Relief Liquid 2678
Children's Vicks NyQuil Cold/Cough Relief Liquid 2680
▲ Vicoprofen Tablets (3% to 9%) 539
Vivaglobin (0.1%) 3506
▲ Vivitrol (8% to 12%) 995
Voltaren Tablets (Occasionally) 2307
Voltaren-XR Tablets (Occasionally) 2310
▲ VoSpire ER Tablets (8.5%) 1052
▲ Wellbutrin SR Sustained-Release Tablets (3% to 5%) 1607
▲ Wellbutrin XL Extended-Release Tablets (3% to 5%) 1613
▲ Xopenex Inhalation Solution (2.8% to 9.6%) 3146
▲ Xopenex Inhalation Solution Concentrate (2.8% to 9.6%) 3150
▲ Xopenex HFA Inhalation Aerosol (2.8% to 9.6%) 3154
Xyrem Oral Solution (Frequent) 1688
Yasmin 28 Tablets (Greater than 1%) 796
Yaz Tablets 803
Zegerid Capsules (Less than 1%) 2958
Zegerid Powder for Oral Solution (Less than 1%) 2958
Zelapar Tablets 3372
Zmax for Oral Suspension 2583
▲ Zoloft (6%) 2586
Zomig Nasal Spray (Infrequent) 3523
Zonegran Capsules (2%) 1101
▲ Zyban Sustained-Release Tablets (4%) 1644
Zyflo Tablets (Greater than 1%) 1023
▲ Zyprexa Tablets (16%) 1830
▲ Zyprexa ZYDIS Orally Disintegrating Tablets (16%) 1830
Zyrtec Chewable Tablets (Less than 2%) 2594
Zyrtec (Less than 2%) 2594
Zyrtec-D 12 Hour Extended Release Tablets (Less than 2%) 2597

Neuralgia

Aciphex Tablets 1090
▲ Actonel Tablets (3.8%) 2683
▲ Actonel with Calcium Tablets (3.8%) 2688
Altace Capsules (Less than 1%) 1702
Ambien Tablets (Rare) 2851
Ambien CR Tablets (Rare) 2855
Amerge Tablets (Rare) 1339
Aricept Tablets (Infrequent) 1094
Aricept ODT Tablets (Infrequent) 1094
Arthrotec Tablets (Rare) 3129
Azilect Tablets (Rare) 3293
Campral Tablets (Infrequent) 1174
Celebrex Capsules (0.1% to 1.9%) 3134
Celexa (Infrequent) 1176
Coreg Tablets (Less than or equal to 0.1%) 1414

Crestor Tablets (Greater than or equal to 1%) 678
▲ Doxil Injection (1% to 10%) 2351
Effexor Tablets (Infrequent) 3411
Effexor XR Capsules (Infrequent) 3417
Evoxac Capsules (Less than 1%) 1047
Exelon Capsules (Infrequent) 2206
Exelon Oral Solution (Infrequent) 2206
Fortical Nasal Spray (Less than 1%) 3337
Imitrex Injection 1463
Imitrex Nasal Spray (Infrequent) 1467
Imitrex Tablets (Rare) 1471
▲ Intron A for Injection (Less than 5%) 3024
Lamictal (Rare) 1481
Lofibra Tablets 1219
Lofibra Capsules 1216
▲ Lunesta Tablets (0% to 3%) 3142
Lyrica Capsules (0.1% to 1%) 2539
Miacalcin Nasal Spray (Less than 1%) 2253
Namenda (Infrequent) 1195
Nipent for Injection (Less than 3%) 1863
Norvir (Less than 2%) 503
Paxil CR Controlled-Release Tablets (Rare) 1538
Paxil (Rare) 1530
Permax Tablets (1.1%) 3356
Pexeva Tablets (Rare) 1694
Plavix Tablets (1% to 2.5%) 917
Plavix Tablets (1% to 2.5%) 2926
Pletal Tablets (Less than 2%) 2455
Proleukin for Injection 2266
Protonix I.V. (Less than 1%) 3472
Protonix Tablets (Less than 1%) 3469
Prozac Pulvules and Liquid (Infrequent) 1801
Requip Tablets (Frequent) 1555
▲ Sandostatin LAR Depot (1% to 4%) 2280
Seroquel Tablets (Rare) 690
Sonata Capsules (Infrequent) 1717
Sustiva Capsules (Less than 2%) 930
Sustiva Tablets (Less than 2%) 930
Symbyax Capsules (Infrequent) 1819
Tasmar Tablets (Infrequent) 3358
Thalomid Capsules 965
Tricor Tablets 527
Trileptal Tablets 2300
Trileptal Oral Suspension 2300
Uniretic Tablets (Less than 1%) 3100
VFEND I.V. (Less than 2%) 2564
VFEND Oral Suspension (Less than 2%) 2564
VFEND Tablets (Less than 2%) 2564
Viagra Tablets (Less than 2%) 2573
Vicoprofen Tablets (Less than 1%) 539
Wellbutrin SR Sustained-Release Tablets 1607
Wellbutrin XL Extended-Release Tablets 1613
Zelapar Tablets 3372
Zyban Sustained-Release Tablets 1644
Zyprexa Tablets (Rare) 1830
Zyprexa ZYDIS Orally Disintegrating Tablets (Rare) 1830

Neuralgia, occipital
Neurontin Capsules 2487
Neurontin Oral Solution 2487
Neurontin Tablets 2487

Neuralgia, trigeminal
Nalfon Capsules (Less than 1%) 2502

Neuritis
Ambien Tablets (Rare) 2851
Ambien CR Tablets (Rare) 2855
Amerge Tablets (Rare) 1339
Azilect Tablets (Infrequent) 3293
Clinoril Tablets (Rare) 1924
Decadron Tablets 1951
Effexor Tablets (Rare) 3411
Effexor XR Capsules (Rare) 3417
Fluarix 1451
Fluorescite Injection ⊙207
Gabitril Tablets (Infrequent) 984
▲ Imdur Tablets (Less than or equal to 5%) 3018
Infanrix Vaccine 1476
▲ Intron A for Injection (Less than 5%) 3024
Lotrel Capsules (Infrequent) 2249
Lunesta Tablets (Rare) 3142
Nipent for Injection (Less than 3%) 1863
Permax Tablets (Rare) 3356
Proleukin for Injection 2266
ProSom Tablets (Rare) 517
Protonix I.V. (Less than 1%) 3472
Protonix Tablets (Less than 1%) 3469
Protopic Ointment (Greater than or equal to 1%) 638
Prozac Pulvules and Liquid (Rare) 1801
Remicade for IV Injection (Greater than or equal to 0.2%) 971
Sandostatin Injection (Less than 1%) 2278
Soriatane Capsules (Less than 1%) 1013
Teveten Tablets (Less than 1%) 1735
Teveten HCT Tablets (Less than 1%) 1737
Thalomid Capsules 965
Uniretic Tablets (Less than 1%) 3100

Neuritis, brachial
ADACEL Vaccine 2945
Boostrix 1404
DAPTACEL Vaccine 2950
Pediarix Vaccine 1548

Neuritis, optic
Accutane Capsules 2731
Attenuvax 1914
Copaxone for Injection (Infrequent) 3297
Cuprimine Capsules 1947
▲ Doxil Injection (1% to 5%) 2351
Elmiron Capsules (Less than or equal to 1%) 2415
Eloxatin for Injection 2892
Enbrel for Injection 584
Engerix-B Vaccine 1425
Estratest Tablets 3199
Estratest H.S. Tablets 3199
Fluarix 1451
Intron A for Injection 3024
Meruvax II 2019
M-M-R II (Infrequent) 2006
Mumpsvax 2031
Nalfon Capsules (Less than 1%) 2502
Ortho Evra Transdermal System 2417
Paser Granules 1674
Paxil CR Controlled-Release Tablets 1538
Paxil 1530
Pegasys 2789
PEG-Intron Powder for Injection (Less than or equal to 1%) 3048
Pexeva Tablets 1694
Premarin Intravenous 3442
Premarin Vaginal Cream 3452
Premphase Tablets 3456
Prempro Tablets 3456
Prilosec OTC Delayed-Release Tablets (Less than 1%) 2677
Proleukin for Injection (Less than 1%) 2266
ProQuad 2064
Prozac Pulvules and Liquid 1801
Recombivax HB 2071
Remicade for IV Injection (Rare) 971
Rituxan I.V. 1254
Seasonique Tablets 1077
Trecator Tablets 3487
Twinrix Vaccine 1595
VFEND I.V. (Less than 2%) 2564
VFEND Oral Suspension (Less than 2%) 2564
VFEND Tablets (Less than 2%) 2564
Yasmin 28 Tablets 796
Zegerid Capsules (Less than 1%) 2958
Zegerid Powder for Oral Solution (Less than 1%) 2958
Zoloft 2586

Neuritis, peripheral
▲ Atripla Tablets (Greater than or equal to 5%) 945
BiDil Tablets 2171
Carbatrol Capsules 3171
▲ Doxil Injection (1% to 10%) 2351
▲ Emtriva Capsules (4%) 1287
▲ Emtriva Oral Solution (4%) 1287
Equetro Extended-Release Capsules 3180
Fansidar Tablets 2765
Gabitril Tablets (Infrequent) 984
Gantrisin Pediatric Suspension 2770
Herceptin I.V. (2%) 1233
Kaletra (Less than 2%) 476
Lamictal (Rare) 1481
Lyrica Capsules (Rare) 2539
Paxil CR Controlled-Release Tablets (Rare) 1538
Paxil (Rare) 1530
Pexeva Tablets (rare) 1694
Rilutek Tablets (Rare) 2930
Tegretol/Tegretol-XR 2295
Thalomid Capsules 965
Trecator Tablets 3487
Truvada Tablets 1296
▲ Viread Tablets (1% to 5%) 1301
Zelapar Tablets 3372
Zonegran Capsules (Infrequent) 1101

Neuritis, retrobulbar
Anaprox Tablets 2761
Anaprox DS Tablets 2761
Attenuvax 1914
EC-Naprosyn Delayed-Release Tablets 2761
Meruvax II 2019
M-M-R II 2006
Mumpsvax (Infrequent) 2031
Naprosyn Suspension 2761
Naprosyn Tablets 2761
ProQuad 2064

Neurodermatitis
Aricept Tablets (Infrequent) 1094
Aricept ODT Tablets (Infrequent) 1094

Neuroleptic malignant syndrome
Celexa 1176
Clozaril Tablets (Several cases) 2184
Comtan Tablets 2189
Concerta Extended-Release Tablets (Very rare) 1881
Daytrana Transdermal Patch 3174
Effexor Tablets 3411
Effexor XR Capsules 3417
Focalin Tablets (Very rare) 2220
Focalin XR Capsules 2223
Geodon 2529
Lexapro Oral Solution 1190
Lexapro Tablets 1190
Metadate CD Capsules (Very rare) 3323
Moban Tablets 1119
Namenda 1195
Parcopa Orally Disintegrating Tablets 3097
Paxil CR Controlled-Release Tablets 1538
Paxil 1530
Permax Tablets 3356
Pexeva Tablets 1694
Phenergan Tablets and Suppositories 3440
Prozac Pulvules and Liquid (Rare) 1801
Risperdal 1676
Risperdal Consta Long-Acting Injection (Rare) 1682
Risperdal M-Tab Orally Disintegrating Tablets 1676
Ritalin Hydrochloride Tablets 2269
Ritalin LA Capsules (Very rare) 2271
Ritalin-SR Tablets 2269
Seroquel Tablets (Rare) 690
Stalevo Tablets 2287
Symbyax Capsules 1819
Symmetrel Tablets 1135
Tegretol-XR Tablets (Isolated cases) 2295
Thioridazine Hydrochloride Tablets 2163
Thiothixene Capsules 2165
Zoloft 2586

Neurological disability, unspecified
Abelcet Injection 1141
▲ Nipent for Injection (1% to 11%) 1863

Neuromotor, unspecified
▲ Taxotere Injection Concentrate (3.2% to 8.6%) 2932

Neuromuscular block, inadequate
Nimbex 498

Neuromuscular blockade
Capastat Sulfate for Injection 1755
Mivacron Injection (3 of 2,074 patients) 493
Zemuron Injection 2346

Neuromuscular disorders, unspecified
Eulexin Capsules (2%) 3009
Lupron Depot 3.75 mg (1%) 3260
Lupron Depot 7.5 mg (Less than 5%) 3264
Lupron Depot–3 Month 11.25 mg (1%) 3265

Neuromuscular excitability
Fortaz 1453
Zosyn 3492

Neuropathy
Abilify Oral Solution (Infrequent) 882
Abilify Oral Solution (Infrequent) 2450
Abilify Discmelt Orally Disintegrating Tablets (Infrequent) 882
Abilify Discmelt Orally Disintegrating Tablets (Infrequent) 2450
Abilify Tablets (Infrequent) 882
Abilify Tablets (Infrequent) 2450
Accolate Tablets (Rare) 671
Aciphex Tablets 1090
Actiq (Less than 1%) 979
▲ Alimta for Injection (Up to 29%) 1750
Altace Capsules (Less than 1%) 1702
Ambien Tablets (Rare) 2851
Ambien CR Tablets (Rare) 2855
Aromasin Tablets (0.6%) 2600
▲ Arranon Injection (0% to 4%) 1357
▲ Atripla Tablets (Greater than or equal to 5%) 945
Axert Tablets (Rare) 2396
Azilect Tablets (Frequent) 3293
Bicillin C-R Injectable Suspension 1706
Celebrex Capsules (0.1% to 1.9%) 3134
▲ CellCept Capsules (3% to less than 20%) 2747
▲ CellCept Intravenous (3% to less than 20%) 2747
▲ CellCept Oral Suspension (3% to less than 20%) 2747
▲ CellCept Tablets (3% to less than 20%) 2747
▲ Chemet Capsules (1.0% to 12.7%) 2458
▲ Combivir Tablets (12%) 1411
Cuprimine Capsules 1947
Decadron Tablets 1951
▲ Doxil Injection (1% to 10%) 2351
Effexor Tablets (Infrequent) 3411
Effexor XR Capsules (Infrequent) 3417
▲ Eloxatin for Injection (12% to 92%) 2892
▲ Emtriva Capsules (4%) 1287
▲ Emtriva Oral Solution (4%) 1287
Engerix-B Vaccine 1425
▲ Epivir (12%) 1427
Evoxac Capsules (Less than 1%) 1047
Flovent Diskus 1443
Fluarix 1451
Gengraf Capsules (1% to less than 3%) 459
Geodon Capsules (Frequent) 2529
Havrix Vaccine (Rare) 1456
Herceptin I.V. (1%) 1233
▲ Hycamtin for Injection (3%) 1458
▲ Intron A for Injection (Less than 5%) 3024
Kaletra (Less than 2%) 476
Lariam Tablets (Occasional) 2786
Lunesta Tablets (Rare) 3142
▲ Lyrica Capsules (2% to 9%) 2539
Matulane Capsules 3191
▲ Megace ES Oral Suspension (1% to 3%) 2481
Namenda (Infrequent) 1195
Neoral Oral Solution (1% to less than 3%) 2259
Neoral Soft Gelatin Capsules (1% to less than 3%) 2259
Nimotop Capsules (Less than 1%) 749
Nipent for Injection (Less than 3%) 1863
Norvir (Less than 2%) 503
Paxil CR Controlled-Release Tablets (Rare) 1538
Paxil (Rare) 1530
Permax Tablets (Infrequent) 3356
Pexeva Tablets (rare) 1694
▲ Prograf Capsules and Injection (3%) 632
Proleukin for Injection 2266
Protonix I.V. (Less than 1%) 3472
Protonix Tablets 3469
Prozac Pulvules and Liquid (Infrequent) 1801
▲ Rapamune Oral Solution and Tablets (3% to 20%) 3475
ReFacto Vials 3484
Relpax Tablets (Rare) 2548
Rescriptor Tablets 2551
Sandostatin LAR Depot (1% to 4%) 2280
▲ Simulect for Injection (3% to 10%) 2284
Singulair 2077
Sonata Capsules (Rare) 1717
Sustiva Capsules 930
Sustiva Tablets 930
Tambocor Tablets (Less than 1%) 1856
▲ Tarceva Tablets (Less than 1% to 13%) 1259
▲ Tarceva Tablets (Less than 1% to 13%) 2444
Targretin Capsules 1747
Tasmar Tablets (Infrequent) 3358
▲ Thalomid Capsules (8.3%) 965
Topamax Sprinkle Capsules (Infrequent) 2404
Topamax Tablets (Infrequent) 2404
▲ Trizivir Tablets (12%) 1589
Truvada Tablets 1296
Twinrix Vaccine 1595
VFEND I.V. (Less than 2%) 2564
VFEND Oral Suspension (Less than 2%) 2564

VFEND Tablets (Less than 2%).......... 2564
Viagra Tablets (Less than 2%).......... 2573
Wellbutrin SR Sustained-Release Tablets 1607
Wellbutrin XL Extended-Release Tablets 1613
Zelapar Tablets 3372
Zomig Nasal Spray (Rare).......... 3523
Zonegran Capsules (Infrequent).......... 1101
Zyban Sustained-Release Tablets.......... 1644
Zyprexa Tablets (Rare).......... 1830
Zyprexa ZYDIS Orally Disintegrating Tablets (Rare).......... 1830

Neuropathy, optic

Campath Ampules 811
Fluarix 1451
Imitrex Injection 1463
Imitrex Nasal Spray 1467
Imitrex Tablets 1471
Prilosec OTC Delayed-Release Tablets (Less than 1%).......... 2677
Protonix I.V. 3472
Protonix Tablets 3469
Zegerid Capsules (Less than 1%) 2958
Zegerid Powder for Oral Solution (Less than 1%) 2958
Zyvox 2652

Neuropathy, optic, anterior ischemic, non-arteritic

Cialis Tablets 1838
Levitra Tablets 3034
Revatio Tablets 2557
Viagra Tablets 2573

Neuropathy, peripheral

Abelcet Injection 1141
Advicor Tablets 1722
Altoprev Extended-Release Tablets .. 3109
Aptivus Capsules (Less than 2%) 826
▲ Arranon Injection (0% to 13%) 1357
Asacol Delayed-Release Tablets (Rare) 2692
▲ Atripla Tablets (Greater than or equal to 5%) 945
Caduet Tablets (Greater than 0.1% to less than 2%) 2508
Cipro 2977
Cipro I.V. 2984
Cipro XR Tablets 2990
Combivir Tablets 1411
Copegus Tablets (Less than 1%) 2754
Cozaar Tablets (Less than 1%) 1935
Cuprimine Capsules 1947
Dapsone Tablets USP 1673
DepoCyt Injection 1143
Emend Capsules (Greater than 0.5%) 1963
▲ Epivir (13%) 1427
Epivir-HBV 1432
Epzicom Tablets 1436
Exelon Capsules (Infrequent) 2206
Exelon Oral Solution (Infrequent) 2206
Fuzeon Injection 2767
Garamycin Injectable 3014
Gleevec Tablets (Infrequent) 2227
Hyzaar 50-12.5 Tablets 1990
Hyzaar 100-12.5 Tablets 1990
Hyzaar 100-25 Tablets 1990
Indocin Capsules (Less than 1%) 1995
Indocin I.V. (Less than 1%) 2465
Indocin (Less than 1%) 1995
Infanrix Vaccine 1476
Invirase (1% to greater than or equal to 2%) 2772
Lescol Capsules 2233
Lescol XL Tablets 2233
Leukeran Tablets 1504
Levaquin 2384
Levaquin in 5% Dextrose Injection 2384
Lipitor Tablets (Less than 2%) 2483
Lupron Depot 3.75 mg 3260
Lupron Depot 7.5 mg 3264
Lupron Depot–3 Month 11.25 mg 3265
Lupron Depot-PED 7.5 mg, 11.25 mg and 15 mg 3269
Lupron Injection Pediatric 3259
Mevacor Tablets (0.5% to 1.0%) 2021
Noroxin Tablets 2032
Norvasc Tablets (More than 0.1% to 1%) 2545
Norvir (Less than 2%) 503
Parcopa Orally Disintegrating Tablets 3097
Pegasys (Less than 1%) 2789
PEG-Intron Powder for Injection 3048
Prezista Tablets (Less than 2%) 3306
Prinivil Tablets (0.3% to 1.0%) 2052
Prinzide Tablets 2056
Proquin XR Tablets 1153
Recombivax HB 2071
Remicade for IV Injection (Greater than or equal to 0.2%) 971
Requip Tablets (Infrequent) 1555
▲ Revlimid Capsules (5.4%) 958
Rythmol SR Capsules 2727
Soriatane Capsules 1013
Stalevo Tablets 2287
Sustiva Capsules (Less than 2%) 930
Sustiva Tablets (Less than 2%) 930
▲ Sutent Capsules (10%) 2560
Tequin Injection 938
Tequin Injection in 5% Dextrose 938
Tequin Tablets 938
Thalomid Capsules 965
Ticlid Tablets (Rare) 2810
Trizivir Tablets 1589
Truvada Tablets 1296
▲ Valcyte Tablets (9%) 2813
Vasotec I.V. Injection (0.5% to 1.0%) 2103
▲ Velcade for Injection (36%) 2133
▲ Viread Tablets (1% to 5%) 1301
Vytorin 10/10 Tablets 2114
Vytorin 10/10 Tablets 3077
Vytorin 10/20 Tablets 2114
Vytorin 10/20 Tablets 3077
Vytorin 10/40 Tablets 2114
Vytorin 10/40 Tablets 3077
Vytorin 10/80 Tablets 2114
Vytorin 10/80 Tablets 3077
▲ Xeloda Tablets (Less than 5%) 2822
Zocor Tablets 2105
Zyvox 2652

Neuropathy, peripheral sensory

Emend Capsules (Greater than 0.5%) 1963
Lariam Tablets (Occasional) 2786
Norvir (Less than 2%) 503
▲ Velcade for Injection (36%) 2133
▲ Xeloda Tablets (10%) 2822

Neuropathy, sensory

▲ Gemzar for Injection (29%) 1771
▲ Nexavar Tablets (0% to 13%) 746

Neuropsychiatric disorders

Pegasys 2789

Neuropsychiatric disorders, transient

Floxin Otic Solution (Uncommon) 1049

Neuropsychometrics performance, decrease

Blocadren Tablets 1916
Cosopt Sterile Ophthalmic Solution 1931
Inderal LA Long-Acting Capsules 3429
InnoPran XL Capsules 2723
Lopressor Injection 2238
Lopressor Tablets 2238
Lopressor HCT 50/25 Tablets 2241
Lopressor HCT 100/25 Tablets 2241
Lopressor HCT 100/50 Tablets 2241
Nadolol Tablets 2159
Timoptic Sterile Ophthalmic Solution 2088
Timoptic in Ocudose 2091
Timoptic-XE Sterile Ophthalmic Gel Forming Solution 2092
Toprol-XL Tablets 668

Neurosensory, unspecified

▲ Alimta for Injection (Up to 29%) 1750
▲ Taxotere Injection Concentrate (Up to 58.3%) 2932

Neurosis, phobic

Cesamet Capsules 3340

Neurosis, unspecified

Ambien Tablets (Rare) 2851
Ambien CR Tablets (Rare) 2855
Atripla Tablets 945
Azilect Tablets (Infrequent) 3293
Campral Tablets (Infrequent) 1174
Evoxac Capsules 1047
Exelon Capsules (Infrequent) 2206
Exelon Oral Solution (Infrequent) 2206
Gabitril Tablets (Infrequent) 984
▲ Intron A for Injection (Less than 5%) 3024
Keppra Oral Solution 3314
Keppra Tablets 3314
Lamictal (Rare) 1481
Lunesta Tablets (Infrequent) 3142
Namenda (Infrequent) 1195
Neurontin Capsules (Rare) 2487
Neurontin Oral Solution (Rare) 2487
Neurontin Tablets (Rare) 2487
Nipent for Injection (Less than 3%) ... 1863
Paxil CR Controlled-Release Tablets (Infrequent) 1538
Paxil (Infrequent) 1530
Permax Tablets (Infrequent) 3356
Pexeva Tablets (Infrequent) 1694
Prevacid Delayed-Release Capsules (Less than 1%) 3271
Prevacid for Delayed-Release Oral Suspension (Less than 1%) 3271
Prevacid SoluTab Delayed-Release Orally Disintegrating Tablets (Less than 1%) 3271
Prevacid NapraPAC (Less than 1%) .. 3280
PREVPAC (Less than 1%) 3284
Prozac Pulvules and Liquid (Infrequent) 1801
Relpax Tablets (Rare) 2548
Requip Tablets (Infrequent) 1555
Rythmol SR Capsules 2727
Sustiva Capsules 930
Sustiva Tablets 930
Symbyax Capsules (Infrequent) 1819
Topamax Sprinkle Capsules (1%) 2404
Topamax Tablets (1%) 2404
Uniretic Tablets (Less than 1%) 3100

Neurotoxicity

Garamycin Injectable 3014
Leustatin Injection (Rare) 2357
▲ Prograf Capsules and Injection (Approximately 55%) 632
▲ Zinecard for Injection (10% to 17%) 2650

Neurovascular episodes

Bicillin C-R Injectable Suspension 1706

Neutropenia

Abilify Oral Solution (Infrequent) 882
Abilify Oral Solution (Infrequent) 2450
Abilify Discmelt Orally Disintegrating Tablets (Infrequent) 882
Abilify Discmelt Orally Disintegrating Tablets (Infrequent) 2450
Abilify Tablets (Infrequent) 882
Abilify Tablets (Infrequent) 2450
Accutane Capsules 2731
Aceon Tablets (2 mg, 4 mg, 8 mg) (0.1%) 3194
▲ Alimta for Injection (2% to 58%) 1750
Aloprim for Injection (Less than 1%) 2167
Altace Capsules 1702
Aptivus Capsules (Less than 2%) 826
Aredia for Injection (Up to 1%) 2179
▲ Arranon Injection (14% to 94%) 1357
Asacol Delayed-Release Tablets 2692
Atacand Tablets (Very rare) 649
Atacand HCT 651
▲ Avastin IV (21%) 1227
▲ Betaseron for SC Injection (14%) 767
Bexxar 1398
▲ Campath Ampules (64% to 85%) 811
▲ Camptosar Injection (12% to 96.4%) 2604
▲ Cancidas for Injection (1.9% to 3.1%) 1918
Captopril Tablets 2149
Ceftin 1407
▲ CellCept Capsules (2% to 3.6%) 2747
▲ CellCept Intravenous (2% to 3.6%) .. 2747
▲ CellCept Oral Suspension (2% to 3.6%) 2747
▲ CellCept Tablets (2% to 3.6%) 2747
Chemet Capsules (0.5% to 1.5%) 2458
Cleocin Vaginal Ovules 2616
Clinoril Tablets (Less than 1 in 100) 1924
▲ Clolar for Intravenous Infusion (10%) 1271
▲ Clozaril Tablets (3%) 2184
▲ Combivir Tablets (7.2%) 1411
▲ Copegus Tablets (27% to 40%) 2754
Crixivan Capsules (1.1%) 1940
▲ Dacogen Injection (90%) 2129
Depakote ER Tablets 434
▲ DepoCyt Injection (8% to 9%) 1143
Diastat Rectal Delivery System (Infrequent) 3343
Diovan Tablets (1.9%) 2193
Diovan HCT Tablets (0.1%) 2196
▲ Doxil Injection (12.1% to 45.9%) 2351
Edecrin 1959
Effexor Tablets 3411
Effexor XR Capsules (Rare) 3417
Elitek (2%) 2890
▲ Eloxatin for Injection (0% to 81%) 2892
▲ Emend Capsules (3.1% to 8.9%) 1963
Enbrel for Injection 584
▲ Epivir (7.2% to 22%) 1427
Epivir-HBV 1432
Epzicom Tablets 1436
Eraxis for Injection (1%) 2521
▲ Famvir Tablets (3.2%) 2211
▲ FazaClo Orally Disintegrating Tablets (3%) 551
Fortaz (Very rare) 1453
Fuzeon Injection 2767
▲ Gemzar for Injection (18% to 90%) 1771
▲ Gleevec Tablets (2.2% to 48%) 2227
▲ Hycamtin for Injection (26% to 98%) 1458
▲ Intron A for Injection (Less than 5% to 92%) 3024
▲ Invanz for Injection (1% to 5.8%) 1999
Invirase (1% to 2%) 2772
▲ I.V. Busulfex (100%) 2493
▲ Kaletra (1% to 5%) 476
Keflex Capsules 549
Keppra Injection 3320
Keppra Oral Solution 3314
Keppra Tablets 3314
Kineret Injection (0.4%) 599
Lamictal 1481
Lamisil Tablets (Isolated case) 2232
Leukeran Tablets 1504
▲ Leustatin Injection (70%) 2357
▲ Lexiva Tablets (3%) 1505
Lotrel Capsules 2249
Malarone Pediatric Tablets 1517
Malarone Tablets 1517
Mavik Tablets (Rare) 486
Maxipime for Injection (Greater than 0.1% to less than 1%) 1105
Mefoxin for Injection 2012
Mefoxin Premixed Intravenous Solution 2016
▲ Mepron Suspension (5%) 1521
Midamor Tablets (Rare) 2026
Moduretic Tablets 2028
Mycamine for Injection (1.2%) 628
Mylotarg for Injection 3431
NeoProfen Injection 2472
Neumega for Injection 3435
▲ Nexavar Tablets (Common) 746
Noroxin Tablets (1.4%) 2032
▲ Norvir (6%) 503
Omnicef Capsules 511
Omnicef for Oral Suspension 511
Oracea Capsules 1000
Orthoclone OKT3 Sterile Solution (Less than 1%) 2360
Parcopa Orally Disintegrating Tablets 3097
▲ Pegasys (21% to 95%) 2789
▲ PEG-Intron Powder for Injection (6%) 3048
Plavix Tablets (Less than 1%) 917
Plavix Tablets (Less than 1%) 2926
Prevacid Delayed-Release Capsules (Less than 1%) 3271
Prevacid for Delayed-Release Oral Suspension (Less than 1%) 3271
Prevacid SoluTab Delayed-Release Orally Disintegrating Tablets (Less than 1%) 3271
Prevacid NapraPAC 3280
PREVPAC 3284
▲ Prezista Tablets (6.9% to 11.5%) 3306
Prilosec OTC Delayed-Release Tablets (Rare) 2677
Primaxin I.M. 2045
Primaxin I.V. (Less than 0.2%) 2048
Prinivil Tablets (Rare) 2052
Prinzide Tablets (Rare) 2056
Prograf Capsules and Injection 632
Proleukin for Injection 2266
Raniclor Tablets, Chewable 2505
Rapamune Oral Solution and Tablets 3475
Raptiva for Injection 1250
▲ Rebetol (14% to 26%) 3058
Rebif Prefilled Syringe for Injection ... 3159
Remicade for IV Injection 971
▲ Rescriptor Tablets (Less than 2% to 5.7%) 2551
Retrovir Capsules 1560
Retrovir IV Infusion 1564
Retrovir 1560
▲ Revlimid Capsules (5.34% to 58.8%) 958
▲ Ribavirin, USP Capsules (14% to 26%) 3068
Rilutek Tablets (Three cases) 2930
▲ Rituxan I.V. (6% to 14%) 1254
Rocephin Injectable Vials, ADD-Vantage, Galaxy, Bulk (Less than 1%) 2800
Seroquel Tablets 690
Suprax 1843
▲ Sutent Capsules (1% to 53%) 2560
Symmetrel Tablets (Less than 0.1%) 1135

Tarka Tablets (Less frequent) 524
▲ Taxotere Injection Concentrate (6.3% to 98.5%) 2932
▲ Temodar Capsules (51%) 3073
Tequin Injection (Less than 0.1%) 938
Tequin Injection in 5% Dextrose (Less than 0.1%) 938
Tequin Tablets (Less than 0.1%) 938
Teveten Tablets (1.3%) 1735
Teveten HCT Tablets 1737
Thalomid Capsules 965
Ticlid Tablets (0.8% to 2.4%) 2810
Timentin ADD-Vantage 1580
Timentin Injection Galaxy Container 1583
Timentin IV Infusion 1577
Timentin Pharmacy Bulk Package 1586
▲ Trisenox Injection (10%) 993
▲ Trizivir Tablets (7.2%) 1589
▲ Truvada Tablets (3%) 1296
Uniretic Tablets (More than 1%) 3100
▲ Valcyte Tablets (11% to 27%) 2813
Valium Tablets (Isolated reports) 2819
▲ Valtrex Caplets (18%) 1597
Vancocin HCl Capsules, USP (Several dozen cases) 3380
Vantin Tablets and Oral Suspension 2645
Vasotec I.V. Injection (Rare) 2103
▲ Velcade for Injection (19%) 2133
▲ Viramune Oral Suspension (11.1%) 873
▲ Viramune Tablets (11.1%) 873
▲ Viread Tablets (3%) 1301
▲ Xeloda Tablets (2.2% to 86%) 2822
Xifaxan Tablets (Less than 2%) 2842
Zegerid Capsules (Rare) 2958
Zegerid Powder for Oral Solution (Rare) 2958
▲ Ziagen (2% to 5%) 1626
Zinacef for Injection (Fewer than 1 in 100) 1631
Zinacef Injection (Fewer than 1 in 100) 1631
Zmax for Oral Suspension (Less then 1%) 2583
▲ Zometa for Intravenous Infusion (12%) 2315
Zosyn 3492

Neutropenia, febrile
▲ Alimta for Injection (Up to 9%) 1750
▲ Arranon Injection (1% to 12%) 1357
▲ Clolar for Intravenous Infusion (57%) 1271
▲ Dacogen Injection (29%) 2129
▲ Elitek (4%) 2890
Eloxatin for Injection 2892
Emend Capsules (Greater than 0.5%) 1963
Mycamine for Injection (0.9%) 628
▲ Revlimid Capsules (4.1% to 5.4%) 958
▲ Taxotere Injection Concentrate (11% to 33.3%) 2932
▲ Trisenox Injection (13%) 993

Neutropenia, transient
Tindamax Tablets 2142

Neutrophil count, abnormal
▲ Zyvox (0% to 5.9%) 2652

Neutrophil count, low
Rythmol SR Capsules 2727
Zelnorm Tablets 2312

Neutrophilia
▲ Atripla Tablets (3%) 945
▲ Emtriva Capsules (5%) 1287
▲ Emtriva Oral Solution (5%) 1287

Neutrophils, decrease
(*see under* Neutropenia)

Nevi, pre-existing, increased growth of
Humatrope Vials and Cartridges (Rare) 1787
Nutropin for Injection (Rare) 1239
Nutropin AQ Injection (Rare) 1243
Nutropin AQ Pen (Rare) 1243
Nutropin AQ Pen Cartridge (Rare) 1243

Night blindness
(*see under* Nyctalopia)

Night sweat
Aricept Tablets (Infrequent) 1094
Aricept ODT Tablets (Infrequent) 1094
Cymbalta Delayed-Release Capsules (Frequent) 1757
Effexor Tablets (Rare) 3411
Effexor XR Capsules (Rare) 3417
Eligard 22.5 mg (Less than 2%) 2883
▲ Eligard 30 mg (3.3%) 2885
Eligard 45 mg (2.7%) 2888
Gengraf Capsules (Rare) 459
▲ Gleevec Tablets (0.2% to 17%) 2227
Invirase (Less than 2%) 2772
Neoral Oral Solution (Rare) 2259
Neoral Soft Gelatin Capsules (Rare) 2259
▲ Oncaspar (Greater than 1% but less than 5%) 1145
Prezista Tablets (Less than 2%) 3306
▲ Prometrium Capsules (100 mg, 200 mg) (7%) 3203
▲ Revlimid Capsules (8.1%) 958
▲ Rituxan I.V. (1% to 15%) 1254
Sandimmune (Rare) 2275
▲ Trisenox Injection (8%) 993
▲ Ultram ER Tablets (1% to greater than 5%) 2392
Vantas (Less than 2%) 3375
Vivitrol 995
Xyrem Oral Solution (Infrequent) 1688

Nightmares
Aldoril Tablets 1910
Axert Tablets (Rare) 2396
Biaxin/Biaxin XL 402
Blocadren Tablets 1916
Catapres Tablets 843
Catapres-TTS (0.5% or less) 844
Chantix Tablets (1% to 2%) 2517
Cipro (Less than 1%) 2977
Cipro I.V. (1% or less) 2984
Cipro XR Tablets 2990
Clorpres Tablets 2153
▲ Clozaril Tablets (4%) 2184
Cosopt Sterile Ophthalmic Solution 1931
Cymbalta Delayed-Release Capsules (Frequent) 1757
▲ Effexor XR Capsules (4% to 7%) 3417
Eldepryl Capsules 3208
▲ FazaClo Orally Disintegrating Tablets (4%) 551
Klonopin (Infrequent) 2778
Levaquin 2384
Levaquin in 5% Dextrose Injection 2384
Lopressor Injection 2238
Lopressor Tablets 2238
▲ Lopressor HCT 50/25 Tablets (10%) 2241
▲ Lopressor HCT 100/25 Tablets (10%) 2241
▲ Lopressor HCT 100/50 Tablets (10%) 2241
Marinol Capsules (Less than 1%) 3333
Matulane Capsules 3191
Meridia Capsules 489
Nembutal Sodium Solution, USP (Less than 1%) 2470
Parcopa Orally Disintegrating Tablets 3097
Phenergan Tablets and Suppositories 3440
PREVPAC 3284
Prezista Tablets (Less than 2%) 3306
Proquin XR Tablets 1153
Restoril Capsules (1.2%) 1860
Risperdal (Rare) 1676
Risperdal M-Tab Orally Disintegrating Tablets (Rare) 1676
Rythmol SR Capsules 2727
Stalevo Tablets 2287
Tequin Injection 938
Tequin Injection in 5% Dextrose 938
Tequin Tablets 938
Timolide Tablets 2086
Timoptic Sterile Ophthalmic Solution 2088
Timoptic in Ocudose 2091
Timoptic-XE Sterile Ophthalmic Gel Forming Solution 2092
Toprol-XL Tablets 668
Vantin Tablets and Oral Suspension (Less than 1%) 2645
▲ Xyrem Oral Solution (2.9% to 6.1%) 1688

Nipple, tender
Bumex Tablets (0.1%) 2746

Nipples, sensitive
Testim 1% Gel (Less than 1%) 695

Nitrogen balance, changes
(*see under* BUN levels, changes)

NMS
(*see under* Neuroleptic malignant syndrome)

Nocardiosis
Remicade for IV Injection 971

Nocturia
Abilify Oral Solution (Rare) 882
Abilify Oral Solution (Rare) 2450
Abilify Discmelt Orally Disintegrating Tablets (Rare) 882
Abilify Discmelt Orally Disintegrating Tablets (Rare) 2450
Abilify Tablets (Rare) 882
Abilify Tablets (Rare) 2450
Actiq (Less than 1%) 979
Adalat CC Tablets (Less than 1%) 2964
Ambien Tablets (Rare) 2851
Ambien CR Tablets (Rare) 2855
Aricept Tablets (Frequent) 1094
Aricept ODT Tablets (Frequent) 1094
Arthrotec Tablets (Rare) 3129
Caduet Tablets (Greater than 0.1% to less than 2%) 2508
Calcijex Injection 411
Campral Tablets (Rare) 1174
Cardizem LA Extended Release Tablets (Less than 2%) 1728
Cardura XL Tablets 2515
Catapres Tablets (About 1 in 100 patients) 843
Chantix Tablets (Infrequent) 2517
Clorpres Tablets (About 1%) 2153
Copaxone for Injection (Infrequent) 3297
Cozaar Tablets (Less than 1%) 1935
Dantrium Capsules (Less frequent) 2694
Doxil Injection (Less than 1%) 2351
DynaCirc CR Tablets (0.5% to 1%) 2721
Effexor Tablets (Infrequent) 3411
Effexor XR Capsules (Infrequent) 3417
Eldepryl Capsules 3208
Eligard 30 mg (2.2%) 2885
Eligard 45 mg (1%) 2888
▲ Entocort EC Capsules (Less than 5%) 2698
Evoxac Capsules (Less than 1%) 1047
Exelon Capsules (Infrequent) 2206
Exelon Oral Solution (Infrequent) 2206
Frova Tablets (Rare) 1113
Gabitril Tablets (Infrequent) 984
Gengraf Capsules (1% to less than 3%) 459
Geodon Capsules (Rare) 2529
Hectorol Capsules 1275
Hectorol Injection 1278
Hyperstat I.V. 3017
Hyzaar 50-12.5 Tablets 1990
Hyzaar 100-12.5 Tablets 1990
Hyzaar 100-25 Tablets 1990
▲ Indapamide Tablets (Less than 5%) 2156
▲ Intron A for Injection (Less than 5%) 3024
Klonopin 2778
Lamictal (Rare) 1481
Lipitor Tablets (Less than 2%) 2483
Matulane Capsules 3191
Miacalcin Injection 2252
Moduretic Tablets (Less than or equal to 1%) 2028
Neoral Oral Solution (1% to less than 3%) 2259
Neoral Soft Gelatin Capsules (1% to less than 3%) 2259
Neurontin Capsules (Rare) 2487
Neurontin Oral Solution (Rare) 2487
Neurontin Tablets (Rare) 2487
Norvasc Tablets (More than 0.1% to 1%) 2545
Norvir (0% to 0.2%) 503
Paxil CR Controlled-Release Tablets (Infrequent) 1538
Paxil (Infrequent) 1530
Pexeva Tablets (infrequent) 1694
▲ Prochieve 4% Gel (13%) 1003
▲ Prochieve 8% Gel (13%) 1003
▲ Prograf Capsules and Injection (3% to 15%) 632
ProSom Tablets (Rare) 517
Protonix I.V. (Less than 1%) 3472
Protonix Tablets (Less than 1%) 3469
Prozac Pulvules and Liquid (Infrequent) 1801
▲ Rapamune Oral Solution and Tablets (3% to 20%) 3475
Razadyne (Infrequent) 2399
Razadyne ER Extended-Release Capsules (Infrequent) 2399
Requip Tablets (Infrequent) 1555
Rescriptor Tablets 2551
Rilutek Tablets (Rare) 2930
Rocaltrol Capsules 2798
Rocaltrol Oral Solution 2798
Rythmol SR Capsules 2727
Seroquel Tablets (Rare) 690
Sular Tablets (Less than or equal to 1%) 3122
Tarka Tablets (Less frequent) 524
Tasmar Tablets (Infrequent) 3358
Tiazac Capsules (Less than 2%) 1201
Topamax Sprinkle Capsules (1%) 2404
Topamax Tablets (1%) 2404
Uniretic Tablets (Less than 1%) 3100
Vantin Tablets and Oral Suspension (Less than 1%) 2645
▲ Viadur Implant (3.8%) 757
Viagra Tablets (Less than 2%) 2573
Wellbutrin Tablets (Frequent) 1603
Xeloda Tablets 2822
Zoloft (Infrequent) 2586
Zonegran Capsules (Infrequent) 1101

Nodal rhythm
Covera-HS Tablets 3139
Lanoxicaps Capsules (Common) 1490
Lanoxin Injection (Common) 1494
Lanoxin Injection Pediatric (Common) 1497
Lanoxin Tablets (Common) 1500
Romazicon Injection (Less than 1%) 2804

Nodule, subcutaneous
Enbrel for Injection 584
Gabitril Tablets (Infrequent) 984
Lyrica Capsules (Rare) 2539
Neurontin Capsules (Rare) 2487
Neurontin Oral Solution (Rare) 2487
Neurontin Tablets (Rare) 2487
Permax Tablets (Rare) 3356
Uniretic Tablets (Less than 1%) 3100

Nodule at injection site
ADACEL Vaccine 2945
Boostrix 1404
▲ Fuzeon Injection (80%) 2767
Genotropin Lyophilized Powder (Infrequent) 2638
Lovenox Injection 2915
Revlimid Capsules 958
▲ Vivitrol (8% to 32%) 995

Nodulosis
Advicor Tablets 1722

Noise intolerance
Neurontin Capsules (Rare) 2487
Neurontin Oral Solution (Rare) 2487
Neurontin Tablets (Rare) 2487

Nonprotein nitrogen increase
Levaquin 2384
Levaquin in 5% Dextrose Injection 2384

Nose, runny
▲ Fortical Nasal Spray (10.6%) 3337

NPN elevation
Celebrex Capsules (0.1% to 1.9%) 3134
▲ Coreg Tablets (6%) 1414
Garamycin Injectable 3014
▲ Gengraf Capsules (18%) 459
▲ Neoral Oral Solution (18%) 2259
▲ Neoral Soft Gelatin Capsules (18%) 2259

Nuchal rigidity
CytoGam Intravenous (Infrequent) 1895

Numbness
Adenocard Injection (1%) 617
▲ Aerobid/Aerobid-M (1% to 3%) 1171
▲ Alferon N Injection (One patient to 3%) 1665
Aricept Tablets (Infrequent) 1094
Aricept ODT Tablets (Infrequent) 1094
Avalide Tablets 888
Avalide Tablets 2874
Avapro Tablets (Less than 1%) 891
Avapro Tablets (Less than 1%) 2871
Bentyl Capsules 697
Bentyl Injection 697
Bentyl Syrup 697
Bentyl Tablets 697
BiDil Tablets 2171
BOTOX Purified Neurotoxin Complex (Rare) 570
Calcium Disodium Versenate Injection 1851
Catapres-TTS (0.5% or less) 844
Cesamet Capsules 3340
Clozaril Tablets (Less than 1%) 2184
DepoCyt Injection 1143
DynaCirc CR Tablets (0.5% to 1%) 2721
FazaClo Orally Disintegrating Tablets (Less than 1%) 551
Garamycin Injectable 3014
▲ Imitrex Injection (5%) 1463
Imitrex Nasal Spray (Infrequent) 1467
Imitrex Tablets (Frequent) 1471
Infed Injection 3390
K-Phos Original (Sodium Free) Tablets (Less frequent) 760
K-Phos Neutral Tablets 760
Metrogel 1% 1211
Mintezol 2027

Moduretic Tablets (Less than or equal to 1%) 2028
Parcopa Orally Disintegrating Tablets 3097
Parnate Tablets 1527
▲ R-Gene 10 for Intravenous Use (3%) 2641
Stalevo Tablets 2287
Synera Topical Patch 1137
Tindamax Tablets 2142
Xeloda Tablets 2822

Numbness, buccal mucosa
Clozaril Tablets (1%) 2184
FazaClo Orally Disintegrating Tablets (1%) 551
Imitrex Injection 1463
Imitrex Nasal Spray (Infrequent) 1467
Rythmol SR Capsules 2727

Numbness, extremities
Bicillin C-R Injectable Suspension 1706
▲ Indapamide Tablets (Greater than or equal to 5%) 2156
Invirase (0.6% to greater than or equal to 2%) 2772
Maxair Autohaler 1852
Ortho-Cyclen Tablets 2429
Ortho Evra Transdermal System 2417
Ortho Tri-Cyclen Tablets 2429
Ortho Tri-Cyclen Lo Tablets 2436

Numbness, face
Invirase (Less than 2%) 2772

Numbness, feet
Uroqid-Acid No. 2 Tablets 760

Numbness, fingers
Alferon N Injection (One patient) 1665
Cutivate Cream (1.0%) 2662
Olux Foam (Less than 2%) 1012
▲ Temovate Gel (Among most frequent) 2669
Temovate Ointment (Less frequent) 2668
Temovate E Emollient (Less than 2%) 2671

Numbness, hands
Alferon N Injection (One patient) 1665
Hyperstat I.V. 3017
Uroqid-Acid No. 2 Tablets 760

Numbness, lips
K-Phos Original (Sodium Free) Tablets (Less frequent) 760
K-Phos Neutral Tablets 760
Oncaspar 1145
Uroqid-Acid No. 2 Tablets 760

Numbness, mouth
(*see under* Numbness, buccal mucosa)

Numbness/tingling, fingers and toes
Eldepryl Capsules 3208

Nutrition disorders, unspecified
▲ Focalin XR Capsules (34%) 2223

Nyctalopia
Accutane Capsules 2731
Arthrotec Tablets (Rare) 3129
Chantix Tablets (Rare) 2517
Lyrica Capsules (Rare) 2539
Paxil CR Controlled-Release Tablets (Rare) 1538
Paxil (Rare) 1530
Pexeva Tablets (Infrequent) 1694
▲ Soriatane Capsules (1% to 10%) 1013
VFEND I.V. (Less than 2%) 2564
VFEND Oral Suspension (Less than 2%) 2564
VFEND Tablets (Less than 2%) 2564

Nystagmus
Aricept Tablets (Infrequent) 1094
Aricept ODT Tablets (Infrequent) 1094
Arranon Injection (1%) 1357
Axert Tablets (Rare) 2396
Carbatrol Capsules 3171
Celexa 1176
Chantix Tablets (Rare) 2517
Cipro 2977
Cipro I.V. (1% or less) 2984
Cipro XR Tablets 2990
Clozaril Tablets (Less than 1%) 2184
▲ Depacon Injection (1% to 8%) 412
▲ Depakene (7% to 8%) 417
▲ Depakote Sprinkle Capsules (1% to 8%) 422
▲ Depakote Tablets (7% to 8%) 427
▲ Depakote ER Tablets (1% to 8%) 434
Diastat Rectal Delivery System (Infrequent) 3343
Dilaudid 440
Dilaudid Non-Sterile Powder 440
Dilaudid Oral Liquid (Less frequent) 445
Dilaudid Rectal Suppositories 440
Dilaudid Tablets 440
Dilaudid Tablets - 8 mg (Less frequent) 445
Dilaudid-HP (Less frequent) 442
Effexor Tablets (Rare) 3411
Effexor XR Capsules (Rare) 3417
Equetro Extended-Release Capsules 3180
Exelon Capsules (Infrequent) 2206
Exelon Oral Solution (Infrequent) 2206
FazaClo Orally Disintegrating Tablets (Less than 1%) 551
Gabitril Tablets (2%) 984
Geodon Capsules (Rare) 2529
Kadian Capsules (Less than 3%) 577
Klonopin 2778
Lamictal (1.0%) 1481
Lexapro Oral Solution 1190
Lexapro Tablets 1190
Lithobid Tablets 1692
Lunesta Tablets (Infrequent) 3142
Lyrica Capsules (Greater than or equal to 2%) 2539
Matulane Capsules 3191
MS Contin Tablets (Less frequent) 2701
▲ Neurontin Capsules (8.3%) 2487
▲ Neurontin Oral Solution (8.3%) 2487
▲ Neurontin Tablets (8.3%) 2487
Noroxin Tablets 2032
Paxil CR Controlled-Release Tablets (Rare) 1538
Paxil (Rare) 1530
Pexeva Tablets (rare) 1694
▲ Phenytek Capsules (Among most common) 2160
Proquin XR Tablets 1153
ProSom Tablets (Rare) 517
Rescriptor Tablets 2551
Sonata Capsules (Infrequent) 1717
Tambocor Tablets (Less than 1%) 1856
Tegretol/Tegretol-XR 2295
Thalomid Capsules 965
▲ Topamax Sprinkle Capsules (10% to 11%) 2404
▲ Topamax Tablets (10% to 11%) 2404
▲ Trileptal Tablets (5% to 26%) 2300
▲ Trileptal Oral Suspension (5% to 26%) 2300
VFEND I.V. (Less than 2%) 2564
VFEND Oral Suspension (Less than 2%) 2564
VFEND Tablets (Less than 2%) 2564
Zoloft (Infrequent) 2586
▲ Zonegran Capsules (4%) 1101
Zyprexa Tablets (Rare) 1830
Zyprexa ZYDIS Orally Disintegrating Tablets (Rare) 1830

Nystagmus, horizontal
(*see also under* Nystagmus)
Restoril Capsules (Less than 0.5%) 1860

O

Obesity
Abilify Oral Solution (Infrequent) 882
Abilify Oral Solution (Infrequent) 2450
Abilify Discmelt Orally Disintegrating Tablets (Infrequent) 882
Abilify Discmelt Orally Disintegrating Tablets (Infrequent) 2450
Abilify Tablets (Infrequent) 882
Abilify Tablets (Infrequent) 2450
Aptivus Capsules 826
Celexa (Rare) 1176
Crixivan Capsules 1940
Invirase 2772
Kaletra (Less than 2%) 476
Prezista Tablets (Less than 2%) 3306
Reyataz Capsules (Less than 3%) 921
Risperdal Consta Long-Acting Injection (Infrequent) 1682
Symbyax Capsules (Infrequent) 1819
Truvada Tablets 1296

Obsessive compulsive symptoms
▲ Vivitrol (8% to 12%) 995
Zyprexa Tablets (Infrequent) 1830
Zyprexa ZYDIS Orally Disintegrating Tablets (Infrequent) 1830

Obsessive thoughts
Abilify Oral Solution (Rare) 882
Abilify Oral Solution (Rare) 2450
Abilify Discmelt Orally Disintegrating Tablets (Rare) 882
Abilify Discmelt Orally Disintegrating Tablets (Rare) 2450
Abilify Tablets (Rare) 882
Abilify Tablets (Rare) 2450

Obstipation
Emend Capsules (Greater than 0.5%) 1963
Thioridazine Hydrochloride Tablets 2163

Obtundation
Orthoclone OKT3 Sterile Solution (Less than 1%) 2360
Risperdal Consta Long-Acting Injection 1682

Ocular, foreign body sensation
▲ Azopt Ophthalmic Suspension (1% to 5%) 557
▲ Betimol Ophthalmic Solution (More than 5%) 3382
▲ Betimol Ophthalmic Solution (More than 5%) ⊙295
Betoptic S Ophthalmic Suspension (Small number of patients) 558
▲ Brimonidine Tartrate Ophthalmic Solution 0.2% (10% to 30%) ⊙248
▲ Cosopt Sterile Ophthalmic Solution (1% to 5%) 1931
▲ Lucentis Injection (6% to 19%) 1237
▲ Nevanac Ophthalmic Suspension 0.1% (5% to 10%) ⊙209
▲ Patanol Ophthalmic Solution (Less than 5%) 561
▲ Quixin Ophthalmic Solution (1% to 3%) 3383
▲ Restasis Ophthalmic Emulsion (1% to 5%) 575
Timoptic Sterile Ophthalmic Solution (Less frequent) 2088
Timoptic in Ocudose (Less frequent) 2091
▲ Timoptic-XE Sterile Ophthalmic Gel Forming Solution (1% to 5%) 2092

Ocular, hyperemia
▲ Lucentis Injection (5% to 10%) 1237
▲ Nevanac (1% to 5%) ⊙209

Ocular allergy
▲ Trusopt Sterile Ophthalmic Solution (Approximately 10%) 2095
▲ Voltaren Ophthalmic Solution (Less than or equal to 5%) 2309

Ocular discomfort
▲ Alamast Ophthalmic Solution (Less than 5%) 3381
Amerge Tablets (Rare) 1339
▲ Azopt Ophthalmic Suspension (1% to 5%) 557
▲ Betoptic S Ophthalmic Suspension (Most frequent) 558
▲ Brimonidine Tartrate Ophthalmic Solution 0.2% (3% to 9%) ⊙248
▲ Evoxac Capsules (1% to 3%) 1047
▲ Lucentis Injection (0% to 8%) 1237
▲ Macugen Injection (10% to 40%) ⊙261
▲ Nevanac Ophthalmic Suspension 0.1% (1% to 5%) ⊙209
Photofrin for Injection 702
▲ Quixin Ophthalmic Solution (1% to 3%) 3383
▲ Travatan Ophthalmic Solution (5% to 10%) 563
▲ Trusopt Sterile Ophthalmic Solution (Approximately one-third of patients) 2095
▲ Vigamox Ophthalmic Solution (1% to 6%) 564

Ocular exudate
Betoptic S Ophthalmic Suspension (Small number of patients) 558
▲ Cosopt Sterile Ophthalmic Solution (1% to 5%) 1931
▲ Lucentis Injection (1% to 9%) 1237
▲ Restasis Ophthalmic Emulsion (1% to 5%) 575
Timoptic Sterile Ophthalmic Solution (Less frequent) 2088
Timoptic in Ocudose (Less frequent) 2091
▲ Timoptic-XE Sterile Ophthalmic Gel Forming Solution (1% to 5%) 2092
Xalatan Sterile Ophthalmic Solution (Less than 1%) 2649

Ocular hypotony
▲ Retisert Implant (10% to 35%) ⊙258

Ocular irritation
Elidel Cream 1% 2200
Pred-G Ophthalmic Ointment ⊙237

Ocular palsies
Attenuvax (Rare) 1914
M-M-R II (Rare) 2006
Mumpsvax 2031
ProQuad 2064

Ocular tension, increase
Bentyl Capsules 697
Bentyl Injection 697
Bentyl Syrup 697
Bentyl Tablets 697
Donnatal Extentabs 2493
Norflex Injection 1856

Ocular toxicity
▲ TobraDex Ophthalmic Ointment (Less than 4%) 562
▲ TobraDex Ophthalmic Suspension (Less than 4%) 563

Oculogyric crisis
Abilify Oral Solution (Rare) 882
Abilify Oral Solution (Rare) 2450
Abilify Discmelt Orally Disintegrating Tablets (Rare) 882
Abilify Discmelt Orally Disintegrating Tablets (Rare) 2450
Abilify Tablets (Rare) 882
Abilify Tablets (Rare) 2450
Geodon Capsules (Frequent) 2529
Parcopa Orally Disintegrating Tablets 3097
Paxil CR Controlled-Release Tablets 1538
Paxil 1530
Pexeva Tablets 1694
Phenergan Tablets and Suppositories 3440
Relpax Tablets (Rare) 2548
▲ Risperdal (17% to 34%) 1676
Risperdal Consta Long-Acting Injection (Infrequent) 1682
▲ Risperdal M-Tab Orally Disintegrating Tablets (17% to 34%) 1676
Stalevo Tablets 2287
Symmetrel Tablets (Less than 0.1%) 1135
Thioridazine Hydrochloride Tablets 2163
Thiothixene Capsules 2165
Timolide Tablets 2086
Trileptal Tablets 2300
Trileptal Oral Suspension 2300
VFEND I.V. (Less than 2%) 2564
VFEND Oral Suspension (Less than 2%) 2564
VFEND Tablets (Less than 2%) 2564
Zofran Injection 1634
Zofran 1639
Zofran ODT Orally Disintegrating Tablets 1639
Zoloft 2586
Zonegran Capsules (Rare) 1101
▲ Zyprexa Tablets (2% to 3%) 1830
▲ Zyprexa ZYDIS Orally Disintegrating Tablets (2% to 3%) 1830

Oculomotor disturbances
Carbatrol Capsules 3171
Equetro Extended-Release Capsules 3180
Tegretol/Tegretol-XR 2295

Odynophagia
▲ Alimta for Injection (Up to 6%) 1750
▲ Photofrin for Injection (5%) 702
▲ Taxotere Injection Concentrate (1.8% to 16.3%) 2932

Oily evacuation
▲ Xenical Capsules (2.3% to 11.9%) 2831

Oligohydramnios
Aceon Tablets (2 mg, 4 mg, 8 mg) 3194
Altace Capsules 1702
Avalide Tablets 888
Avalide Tablets 2874
Avapro Tablets 891
Avapro Tablets 2871
Captopril Tablets 2149
Clinoril Tablets 1924
Cozaar Tablets 1935
Dolobid Tablets 1955
Hyzaar 50-12.5 Tablets 1990
Hyzaar 100-12.5 Tablets 1990

Hyzaar 100-25 Tablets ... 1990
Lotensin Tablets ... 2243
Lotrel Capsules ... 2249
Prinivil Tablets ... 2052
Prinzide Tablets ... 2056
Uniretic Tablets ... 3100
Vasotec I.V. Injection ... 2103

Oligomenorrhea
depo-subQ provera 104 Injectable Suspension ... 2624
Mustargen for Injection ... 2468
Ortho-Cyclen/Ortho Tri-Cyclen ... 2429
Ortho Tri-Cyclen Lo Tablets ... 2436
Sandostatin Injection (Less than 1%) ... 2278
▲ Soltamox Oral Solution (9%) ... 3527

Oligospermia
Androxy Tablets ... 3335
Avodart Soft Gelatin Capsules ... 1390
Oxandrin Tablets ... 2962

Oliguria
Abelcet Injection ... 1141
Actiq (Less than 1%) ... 979
Aloprim for Injection (Less than 1%) ... 2167
Altace Capsules ... 1702
Anaprox Tablets (Less than 1%) ... 2761
Anaprox DS Tablets (Less than 1%) .. 2761
Anzemet Injection (2.6%) ... 2859
Anzemet Tablets (2.6%) ... 2862
Arthrotec Tablets (Rare) ... 3129
▲ Avinza Capsules (Less than 5%) ... 1741
Capastat Sulfate for Injection (1 patient) ... 1755
Captopril Tablets (Approximately 1 to 2 of 1000 patients) ... 2149
Carbatrol Capsules ... 3171
Carimune NF ... 3499
Celexa (Rare) ... 1176
▲ CellCept Capsules (3% to less than 20%) ... 2747
▲ CellCept Intravenous (3% to less than 20%) ... 2747
▲ CellCept Oral Suspension (3% to less than 20%) ... 2747
▲ CellCept Tablets (3% to less than 20%) ... 2747
Cleocin Vaginal Ovules (Rare) ... 2616
CytoGam Intravenous ... 1895
Demadex Injection ... 2759
Demadex Tablets ... 2759
Depakote ER Tablets ... 434
▲ DepoDur Extended-Release Injection (2% to 5%) ... 1110
Diovan HCT Tablets ... 2196
Doxil Injection (Less than 1%) ... 2351
Duragesic Transdermal System (Less than 1%) ... 2373
Dyazide Capsules ... 1423
EC-Naprosyn Delayed-Release Tablets (Less than 1%) ... 2761
Effexor Tablets (Rare) ... 3411
Equetro Extended-Release Capsules ... 3180
Evoxac Capsules ... 1047
Exelon Capsules (Infrequent) ... 2206
Exelon Oral Solution (Infrequent) ... 2206
Fansidar Tablets ... 2765
Flebogamma 5%, Immune Globulin Intravenous (Human) ... 1658
Follistim AQ Cartridge ... 2338
Furosemide Tablets ... 2154
Gammagard S/D (Some patients) ... 724
Gantrisin Pediatric Suspension ... 2770
Garamycin Injectable ... 3014
Geodon Capsules (Rare) ... 2529
Hyzaar 50-12.5 Tablets ... 1990
Hyzaar 100-12.5 Tablets ... 1990
Hyzaar 100-25 Tablets ... 1990
Invanz for Injection (Greater than 0.1%) ... 1999
Ionsys Transdermal System (.1% to less than 1%) ... 2379
▲ I.V. Busulfex (15%) ... 2493
Kytril Injection (2.2%) ... 2781
Levaquin (0.1% to 0.9%) ... 2384
Levaquin in 5% Dextrose Injection (0.1% to 0.9%) ... 2384
Lithobid Tablets ... 1692
Lotrel Capsules ... 2249
Lunesta Tablets (Rare) ... 3142
Lyrica Capsules (0.1% to 1%) ... 2539
Mycamine for Injection ... 628
Nalfon Capsules (Less than 1%) ... 2502
Naprosyn Suspension (Less than 1%) ... 2761
Naprosyn Tablets (Less than 1%) ... 2761
Orthoclone OKT3 Sterile Solution (Less than 1%) ... 2360
Paxil CR Controlled-Release Tablets (Rare) ... 1538
Paxil (Rare) ... 1530
Pexeva Tablets (Rare) ... 1694
Primaxin I.M. ... 2045
Primaxin I.V. (2.2%) ... 2048
Prinivil Tablets (0.3% to 1.0%) ... 2052
Prinzide Tablets ... 2056
▲ Prograf Capsules and Injection (3% to 19%) ... 632
▲ Proleukin for Injection (63%) ... 2266
ProSom Tablets (Rare) ... 517
Prozac Pulvules and Liquid (Rare) ... 1801
▲ Rapamune Oral Solution and Tablets (3% to 20%) ... 3475
Reyataz Capsules (Less than 3%) ... 921
Rythmol SR Capsules ... 2727
▲ Simulect for Injection (3% to 10%) ... 2284
Symbyax Capsules (Infrequent) ... 1819
Tasmar Tablets (Infrequent) ... 3358
Tegretol/Tegretol-XR ... 2295
Thalomid Capsules ... 965
Topamax Sprinkle Capsules (Infrequent) ... 2404
Topamax Tablets (Infrequent) ... 2404
Trasylol Injection (1% to 2%) ... 754
▲ Trisenox Injection (5%) ... 993
Ultane Liquid for Inhalation (Less than 1%) ... 531
Univasc Tablets (Less than 1%) ... 3104
Vasotec I.V. Injection (0.5% to 1.0%) ... 2103
VFEND I.V. (Less than 2%) ... 2564
VFEND Oral Suspension (Less than 2%) ... 2564
VFEND Tablets (Less than 2%) ... 2564
Voltaren Tablets (Occasionally) ... 2307
Voltaren-XR Tablets (Occasionally) ... 2310
Zoloft (Rare) ... 2586
Zosyn (1.0% or less) ... 3492

Oliguria, neonatal
Altace Capsules ... 1702
Captopril Tablets ... 2149

"On-off" phenomenon
Stalevo Tablets ... 2287

Onychia
Evoxac Capsules (Less than 1%) ... 1047

Onycholysis
Taxotere Injection Concentrate (0.8%) ... 2932
▲ Xeloda Tablets (1% to 5%) ... 2822

Onychomycosis
Evoxac Capsules (Less than 1%) ... 1047

Opacification, posterior capsule
▲ Lucentis Injection (0% to 8%) ... 1237

Opacity, capsular
▲ Nevanac Ophthalmic Suspension 0.1% (5% to 10%) ... ⊙209

Opacity, punctate
Stromectol Tablets (1.4% to 1.8%) ... 2083

Ophthalmitis
Campral Tablets (Rare) ... 1174

Ophthalmoplegia
Advicor Tablets ... 1722
Altoprev Extended-Release Tablets ... 3109
Lescol Capsules ... 2233
Lescol XL Tablets ... 2233
Lupron Injection Pediatric ... 3259
Lyrica Capsules (Rare) ... 2539
Mevacor Tablets ... 2021
Vytorin 10/10 Tablets ... 2114
Vytorin 10/10 Tablets ... 3077
Vytorin 10/20 Tablets ... 2114
Vytorin 10/20 Tablets ... 3077
Vytorin 10/40 Tablets ... 2114
Vytorin 10/40 Tablets ... 3077
Vytorin 10/80 Tablets ... 2114
Vytorin 10/80 Tablets ... 3077
Zocor Tablets ... 2105

Opisthotonos
Geodon Capsules (Rare) ... 2529
Thioridazine Hydrochloride Tablets ... 2163
▲ Zyprexa Tablets (2% to 3%) ... 1830
▲ Zyprexa ZYDIS Orally Disintegrating Tablets (2% to 3%) ... 1830

Optic atrophy
Lyrica Capsules (Rare) ... 2539
Prilosec OTC Delayed-Release Tablets (Less than 1%) ... 2677
VFEND I.V. (Less than 2%) ... 2564
VFEND Oral Suspension (Less than 2%) ... 2564
VFEND Tablets (Less than 2%) ... 2564
Zegerid Capsules (Less than 1%) ... 2958
Zegerid Powder for Oral Solution (Less than 1%) ... 2958

Optic disorders
Effexor Tablets (Rare) ... 3411

Optic nerve, damage
Alrex Ophthalmic Suspension 0.2% ... ⊙246
Blephamide Ophthalmic Ointment (Infrequent) ... 568
Blephamide Ophthalmic Suspension (Infrequent) ... 569
Dapsone Tablets USP ... 1673
FML Ophthalmic Ointment (Infrequent) ... ⊙228
FML Ophthalmic Suspension (Infrequent) ... ⊙227
FML Forte Ophthalmic Suspension (Infrequent) ... ⊙226
FML-S Ophthalmic Suspension (Infrequent) ... ⊙229
Lotemax Ophthalmic Suspension 0.5% ... ⊙251
Poly-Pred Ophthalmic Suspension (Infrequent) ... ⊙233
Pred Mild Ophthalmic Suspension (Infrequent) ... ⊙238
Pred Forte Ophthalmic Suspension (Infrequent) ... ⊙235
Pred-G Ophthalmic Ointment ... ⊙237
Pred-G Ophthalmic Suspension (Infrequent) ... ⊙236
Retisert Implant ... ⊙258
TobraDex Ophthalmic Ointment (Infrequent) ... 562
TobraDex Ophthalmic Suspension (Infrequent) ... 563

Optic nerve, infarction
Hyperstat I.V. ... 3017

Orchitis
Aciphex Tablets (Rare) ... 1090
Effexor Tablets (Rare) ... 3411
Effexor XR Capsules (Rare) ... 3417
M-M-R II ... 2006
Mumpsvax (Rare) ... 2031
ProQuad ... 2064
Seroquel Tablets (Infrequent) ... 690

Organomegaly
▲ Vesanoid Capsules (3%) ... 2820

Orgasm, abnormal
▲ Cymbalta Delayed-Release Capsules (2% to 4%) ... 1757
Strattera Capsules (2%) ... 1814

Orgasmic dysfunction, female
▲ Effexor XR Capsules (2% to 8%) ... 3417
▲ Pexeva Tablets (2% to 9%) ... 1694

Oropharynx, dry
Proventil Inhalation Aerosol ... 3053
Proventil HFA Inhalation Aerosol ... 3056
Tussionex Pennkinetic Extended-Release Suspension ... 3327
Ventolin HFA Inhalation Aerosol ... 1600
VoSpire ER Tablets ... 1052

Orthopnea
Clozaril Tablets ... 2184
▲ Intron A for Injection (Less than or equal to 5%) ... 3024
Prinivil Tablets (0.3% to 1.0%) ... 2052
Prinzide Tablets ... 2056

Oscillopsia
Lamictal (Rare) ... 1481

Osteoarthritis
▲ Aromasin Tablets (4.6% to 5.9%) ... 2600

Osteoarthritis, aggravated
▲ Ultram ER Tablets (1% to greater than 5%) ... 2392

Osteoarthritis, localized
▲ Boniva Injection (1.3% to 3%) ... 2738
▲ Boniva Tablets (1.3% to 3%) ... 2741

Osteoarticular pain
Cardizem LA Extended Release Tablets (Less than 2%) ... 1728
Tiazac Capsules (Less than 2%) ... 1201

Osteochondrosis
Aromasin Tablets (0.3%) ... 2600

Osteomalacia
Didronel Tablets ... 2697
Phenytek Capsules ... 2160
VFEND I.V. (Less than 2%) ... 2564
VFEND Oral Suspension (Less than 2%) ... 2564
VFEND Tablets (Less than 2%) ... 2564

Osteomalacia, phosphate-induced
K-Phos Original (Sodium Free) Tablets ... 760
K-Phos Neutral Tablets ... 760
Uroqid-Acid No. 2 Tablets ... 760

Osteomalacia syndromes
Maalox Regular Strength Antacid/Anti-Gas Liquid ... ▣660
Maalox Regular Strength Antacid/Antigas Liquid ... 2175
Maalox Max Maximum Strength Antacid/Anti-Gas Liquid ... 2176

Osteomyelitis
Campath Ampules ... 811
Copaxone for Injection (Infrequent) .. 3297
▲ Copegus Tablets (3% to 5%) ... 2754
▲ Cubicin for Injection (Less than 1% to 5%) ... 1026
Enbrel for Injection ... 584
Evoxac Capsules (Less than 1%) ... 1047
Levaquin (0.1% to 0.9%) ... 2384
Levaquin in 5% Dextrose Injection (0.1% to 0.9%) ... 2384
Nipent for Injection (1%) ... 1863
▲ Pegasys (3% to 5%) ... 2789
Permax Tablets (Rare) ... 3356
Protopic Ointment (0.2% to less than 1%) ... 638
Prozac Pulvules and Liquid (Rare) ... 1801

Osteomyelitis, vertebral
Raptiva for Injection ... 1250

Osteonecrosis
Boniva Injection ... 2738
Boniva Tablets ... 2741
Zometa for Intravenous Infusion ... 2315

Osteonecrosis, hip
Gleevec Tablets (Rare) ... 2227

Osteonecrosis, jaw
Actonel Tablets (Very rare) ... 2683
Actonel with Calcium Tablets (Very rare) ... 2688
Didronel Tablets ... 2697
Fosamax Tablets ... 1969
Fosamax Plus D Tablets (Rarely) ... 1977
Zometa for Intravenous Infusion ... 2315

Osteopenia
Prezista Tablets (Less than 2%) ... 3306

Osteoporosis
Advair Diskus 100/50 ... 1308
Advair Diskus 250/50 ... 1308
Advair Diskus 500/50 ... 1308
Advair HFA Inhalation Aerosol ... 1318
▲ Arimidex Tablets (6% to 11%) ... 673
Celexa (Rare) ... 1176
▲ CellCept Capsules (3% to less than 20%) ... 2747
▲ CellCept Intravenous (3% to less than 20%) ... 2747
▲ CellCept Oral Suspension (3% to less than 20%) ... 2747
▲ CellCept Tablets (3% to less than 20%) ... 2747
Chantix Tablets (Infrequent) ... 2517
Colocort Rectal Suspension, USP (Retention) 100 mg/60 mL ... 2476
Decadron Tablets ... 1951
Depo-Medrol Injectable Suspension ... 2617
Depo-Medrol Single-Dose Vial ... 2619
Depo-Provera Contraceptive Injection (Less than 1%) ... 2622
depo-subQ provera 104 Injectable Suspension (Rare) ... 2624
Effexor Tablets (Rare) ... 3411
Effexor XR Capsules (Rare) ... 3417
Evoxac Capsules (Less than 1%) ... 1047
▲ Femara Tablets (6.9%) ... 2214
Flovent Diskus ... 1443
Flovent HFA ... 1447
Hydrocortone Tablets ... 1989
Neupogen for Injection (Infrequent) .. 603
Neurontin Capsules (Rare) ... 2487
Neurontin Oral Solution (Rare) ... 2487
Neurontin Tablets (Rare) ... 2487
Paxil CR Controlled-Release Tablets (Rare) ... 1538
Paxil (Rare) ... 1530

Permax Tablets (Rare) 3356
Pexeva Tablets (Rare) 1694
Prezista Tablets (Less than 2%) 3306
▲ Prograf Capsules and Injection (3% to 15%) 632
Prozac Pulvules and Liquid (Rare) 1801
Pulmicort Respules (Less than 1%) 661
▲ Rapamune Oral Solution and Tablets (3% to 20%) 3475
Requip Tablets (Infrequent) 1555
Rilutek Tablets (Rare) 2930
Sonata Capsules (Rare) 1717
Symbyax Capsules (Rare) 1819
VFEND I.V. (Less than 2%) 2564
VFEND Oral Suspension (Less than 2%) 2564
VFEND Tablets (Less than 2%) 2564
Zomig Nasal Spray (Rare) 3523
Zyprexa Tablets (Rare) 1830
Zyprexa ZYDIS Orally Disintegrating Tablets (Rare) 1830

Osteosclerosis

Effexor XR Capsules (Rare) 3417

Otitis

ProQuad (Greater than or equal to 0.2% to less than 1%) 2064
Vaqta (1.8%) 2097

Otitis externa

Abilify Oral Solution (Rare) 882
Abilify Oral Solution (Rare) 2450
Abilify Discmelt Orally Disintegrating Tablets (Rare) 882
Abilify Discmelt Orally Disintegrating Tablets (Rare) 2450
Abilify Tablets (Rare) 882
Abilify Tablets (Rare) 2450
Ambien Tablets (Rare) 2851
Ambien CR Tablets (1%) 2855
Aricept Tablets (Infrequent) 1094
Aricept ODT Tablets (Infrequent) 1094
Copaxone for Injection (Infrequent) 3297
Effexor Tablets (Rare) 3411
Effexor XR Capsules (Rare) 3417
Floxin Otic Solution (Single report) 1049
Gabitril Tablets (Infrequent) 984
Imitrex Nasal Spray 1467
Infergen (1% to 2%) 3364
Lunesta Tablets (Infrequent) 3142
Meridia Capsules 489
Neurontin Capsules (Rare) 2487
Neurontin Oral Solution (Rare) 2487
Neurontin Tablets (Rare) 2487
Paxil CR Controlled-Release Tablets (Rare) 1538
Paxil (Rare) 1530
Pexeva Tablets (Rare) 1694
Protonix I.V. (Less than 1%) 3472
Protonix Tablets (Less than 1%) 3469
Protopic Ointment (0.2% to less than 1%) 638
Singulair (Greater than or equal to 2%) 2077
Soriatane Capsules (Less than 1%) 1013
Targretin Capsules 1747
Teveten Tablets (Less than 1%) 1735
Teveten HCT Tablets (Less than 1%) 1737
Trileptal Tablets 2300
Trileptal Oral Suspension 2300
VFEND I.V. (Less than 2%) 2564
VFEND Oral Suspension (Less than 2%) 2564
VFEND Tablets (Less than 2%) 2564
Xyrem Oral Solution (Infrequent) 1688
Zelapar Tablets 3372

Otitis media

Abilify Oral Solution (Infrequent) 882
Abilify Oral Solution (Infrequent) 2450
Abilify Discmelt Orally Disintegrating Tablets (Infrequent) 882
Abilify Discmelt Orally Disintegrating Tablets (Infrequent) 2450
Abilify Tablets (Infrequent) 882
Abilify Tablets (Infrequent) 2450
AccuNeb Inhalation Solution (0.9% to 4.3%) 1055
Aciphex Tablets 1090
Actonel Tablets (2.5%) 2683
Actonel with Calcium Tablets (2.5%) 2688
▲ Advair HFA Inhalation Aerosol (1% to 3%) 1318
Allegra (2.4%) 2844
Ambien Tablets (Rare) 2851
Ambien CR Tablets (Rare) 2855
Aricept Tablets (Infrequent) 1094
Aricept ODT Tablets (Infrequent) 1094
Attenuvax 1914
Axert Tablets (Rare) 2396
Campath Ampules 811
Celebrex Capsules (0.1% to 1.9%) 3134
▲ Chemet Capsules (1.0% to 3.7%) 2458
▲ Clarinex Syrup (6.1%) 2995
Comvax (0.5% to 2.7%) 1928
▲ Depacon Injection (1% to 5%) 412
▲ Depakene (1% to 5%) 417
▲ Depakote Sprinkle Capsules (1% to 5%) 422
▲ Depakote Tablets (1% to 5%) 427
Depakote ER Tablets 434
Doxil Injection (Less than 1%) 2351
Effexor Tablets (Infrequent) 3411
Effexor XR Capsules (Infrequent) 3417
▲ Elidel Cream 1% (0.6% to 3%) 2200
▲ Estring Vaginal Ring (1% to 3%) 2635
▲ Evoxac Capsules (1% to 3%) 1047
Exelon Capsules (Infrequent) 2206
Exelon Oral Solution (Infrequent) 2206
▲ Exubera Inhalation Powder (6.5%) 2524
▲ Flovent Diskus (1% to 3%) 1443
Floxin Otic Solution (Single report) 1049
Flumist Vaccine 1901
Gabitril Tablets (Frequent) 984
▲ Humatrope Vials and Cartridges (16.2% to 35.3%) 1787
▲ Increlex Injection (Greater than or equal to 5%) 3291
Infergen (1% to 2%) 3364
Invirase (Less than 2%) 2772
Kaletra (Less than 2%) 476
Keppra Injection 3320
Keppra Oral Solution (1% to 2%) 3314
Keppra Tablets (1% to 2%) 3314
Klonopin (Infrequent) 2778
Kogenate FS with Bio-Set 740
Levaquin (0.1% to 0.9%) 2384
Levaquin in 5% Dextrose Injection (0.1% to 0.9%) 2384
Lofibra Tablets 1219
Lofibra Capsules 1216
Lunesta Tablets (Infrequent) 3142
Lyrica Capsules (Greater than or equal to 1%) 2539
Meridia Capsules 489
Meruvax II 2019
Micardis Tablets (More than 0.3%) 854
Micardis HCT Tablets 856
M-M-R II 2006
Mumpsvax 2031
Myobloc Injection (Greater than 2%) 3192
▲ Myozyme for Intravenous Infusion (44%) 1279
Namenda (More than one patient) 1195
Nasacort AQ Nasal Spray 2922
Nasonex Nasal Spray (Greater than or equal to 2%) 3043
Neurontin Capsules (1.2%) 2487
Neurontin Oral Solution (1.2%) 2487
Neurontin Tablets (1.2%) 2487
Nexium Delayed-Release Capsules (Less than 1%) 655
Nexium I.V. (Less than 1%) 659
Orthoclone OKT3 Sterile Solution (Less than 1%) 2360
Paxil CR Controlled-Release Tablets (Infrequent) 1538
Paxil (Infrequent) 1530
▲ Liquid PedvaxHIB (Among most frequent) 2035
Permax Tablets (Infrequent) 3356
Pexeva Tablets (Infrequent) 1694
Prevacid Delayed-Release Capsules (Less than 1%) 3271
Prevacid for Delayed-Release Oral Suspension (Less than 1%) 3271
Prevacid SoluTab Delayed-Release Orally Disintegrating Tablets (Less than 1%) 3271
Prevacid NapraPAC (Less than 1%) 3280
Prevnar for Injection 3463
PREVPAC (Less than 1%) 3284
▲ Prilosec OTC Delayed-Release Tablets (22.6%) 2677
▲ Prograf Capsules and Injection (3% to 15%) 632
ProQuad (Greater than or equal to 0.2% to less than 1%) 2064
▲ Protopic Ointment (Up to 7%) 638
▲ Pulmicort Respules (9% to 12%) 661
▲ Rapamune Oral Solution and Tablets (3% to 20%) 3475
Relpax Tablets (Rare) 2548
Requip Tablets (Infrequent) 1555
Rescriptor Tablets 2551
▲ RotaTeq (14.5%) 2074
Sandostatin Injection (Less than 1%) 2278
▲ Sandostatin LAR Depot (5% to 15%) 2280
Singulair (Greater than or equal to 2%) 2077
Soriatane Capsules (Less than 1%) 1013
Sular Tablets (Less than or equal to 1%) 3122
Symbyax Capsules (Up to 2%) 1819
▲ Synagis (36.4%) 1897
▲ Tamiflu Capsules (8.9%) 2807
▲ Tamiflu Oral Suspension (2% to 9%) 2807
Tasmar Tablets (Infrequent) 3358
Teveten Tablets (Less than 1%) 1735
Teveten HCT Tablets (Less than 1%) 1737
Topamax Sprinkle Capsules (1% to 2%) 2404
Topamax Tablets (1% to 2%) 2404
Tricor Tablets 527
Uniretic Tablets (Less than 1%) 3100
▲ Vaqta (7.6%) 2097
Varivax (Greater than or equal to 1%) 2100
▲ Vigamox Ophthalmic Solution (1% to 4%) 564
▲ Xenical Capsules (2.9% to 4.3%) 2831
▲ Zegerid Capsules (22.6%) 2958
▲ Zegerid Powder for Oral Solution (22.6%) 2958

Otitis media, serous

Kogenate FS 738

Otorrhea

Floxin Otic Solution (0.6%) 1049

Ototoxicity

Furosemide Tablets 2154
Garamycin Injectable 3014
Taxotere Injection Concentrate (Rare) 2932
TOBI Solution for Inhalation 2298
Vancocin HCl Capsules, USP 3380
Zyrtec Chewable Tablets (Less than 2%) 2594
Zyrtec (Less than 2%) 2594
Zyrtec-D 12 Hour Extended Release Tablets (Less than 2%) 2597

Ovarian cyst

Copaxone for Injection (Infrequent) 3297
Effexor Tablets (Rare) 3411
Effexor XR Capsules (Rare) 3417
Evoxac Capsules (Less than 1%) 1047
▲ Soltamox Oral Solution (3%) 3527
Xyrem Oral Solution (Infrequent) 1688

Ovarian disorder, unspecified

Evoxac Capsules (Less than 1%) 1047
Symbyax Capsules (Infrequent) 1819
Wellbutrin Tablets (Rare) 1603
Zelapar Tablets 3372

Ovarian enlargement

Follistim AQ Cartridge 2338

Ovarian failure

Neurontin Capsules (Rare) 2487
Neurontin Oral Solution (Rare) 2487
Neurontin Tablets (Rare) 2487

Ovarian hyperstimulation syndrome

▲ Follistim AQ Cartridge (9%) 2338

Overstimulation

Adderall Tablets 3164
Adderall XR Capsules 3166
Adipex-P 1215
Desoxyn Tablets, USP 2462
Dexedrine 1420
DextroStat Tablets 3179
Eldepryl Capsules 3208
Parnate Tablets 1527
Restoril Capsules (Less than 0.5%) 1860
Twinject 0.3 3378
Twinject 0.15 3379

Ovulation

ActoPlus Met Tablets 3214

Oxygen saturation, decreased

▲ DepoDur Extended-Release Injection (Greater than 10%) 1110
▲ Myozyme for Intravenous Infusion (41%) 1279
Opana Tablets (Less than 1%) 1122
Opana ER Tablets (Less than 1%) 1126

P

Pain

▲ Abelcet Injection (5%) 1141
Accolate Tablets (1.9%) 671
Aceon Tablets (2 mg, 4 mg, 8 mg) (0.3% to 1%) 3194
Actiq (1% or greater) 979
▲ Actonel Tablets (7.7% to 13.6%) 2683
▲ Actonel with Calcium Tablets (7.7% to 13.6%) 2688
Adalat CC Tablets (Less than 1%) 2964
▲ Advair Diskus 100/50 (1% to 3%) 1308
▲ Advair Diskus 250/50 (1% to 3%) 1308
▲ Advair Diskus 500/50 (1% to 3%) 1308
▲ Advair HFA Inhalation Aerosol (1% to 3%) 1318
▲ Advicor Tablets (8%) 1722
▲ Aggrenox Capsules (6.4%) 822
▲ Agrylin Capsules (15%) 3169
Aldara Cream, 5% (1.4%) 1846
Alinia for Oral Suspension (Less than 1%) 2835
Alinia Tablets (Less than 1%) 2835
Aloprim for Injection (Less than 1%) 2167
▲ Altoprev Extended-Release Tablets (3%) 3109
Ambien Tablets (Rare) 2851
Ambien CR Tablets (Rare) 2855
▲ AmBisome for Injection (14%) 620
Amitiza Capsules (Less than 0.2%) 3224
Anzemet Injection (2.4%) 2859
Aralast (Greater than or equal to 0.2%) 717
▲ Aredia for Injection (14.3%) 2179
▲ Argatroban Injection (4.6%) 1346
▲ Aricept Tablets (9%) 1094
▲ Aricept ODT Tablets (9%) 1094
▲ Arimidex Tablets (11% to 17%) 673
Arixtra Injection (0% to 1.7%) 1351
▲ Aromasin Tablets (13%) 2600
▲ Arranon Injection (0% to 11%) 1357
▲ Asacol Delayed-Release Tablets (14%) 2692
Asmanex Twisthaler 2966
Atacand HCT (0.5% or greater) 651
▲ Atripla Tablets (Greater than or equal to 5%) 945
▲ Atrovent Inhalation Solution (4.1%) 835
▲ Avastin IV (8% to 62%) 1227
Avelox (0.1% to less than 2%) 2970
▲ Axid Oral Solution (4.2%) 879
▲ Azmacort Inhalation Aerosol (1% to 3%) 1726
Bactroban Ointment (1.5%) 1395
Benicar Tablets (Greater than 0.5%) 1043
▲ Betaseron for SC Injection (51%) 767
▲ Bexxar (1% to 19%) 1398
Bicillin C-R Injectable Suspension 1706
Caduet Tablets (Greater than 0.1% to less than or equal to 1%) 2508
▲ Campath Ampules (2% to 24%) 811
▲ Campral Tablets (2% to 4%) 1174
▲ Camptosar Injection (2% to 24%) 2604
▲ Cancidas for Injection (1.3% to 4.6%) 1918
Cardizem LA Extended Release Tablets (Less than 2%) 1728
▲ Carnitor Injection (21% to 35%) 3188
Celebrex Capsules (0.1% to 1.9%) 3134
▲ CellCept Capsules (3% to 75.8%) 2747
▲ CellCept Intravenous (3% to 75.8%) 2747
▲ CellCept Oral Suspension (3% to 75.8%) 2747
▲ CellCept Tablets (3% to 75.8%) 2747
Cesamet Capsules 3340
Cialis Tablets (Less than 2%) 1838
Cipro (Less than 1%) 2977
Cipro I.V. (1% or less) 2984
Cleocin Vaginal Ovules (Less than 1%) 2616
▲ Climara Transdermal System (1% to 11%) 771
▲ Climara Pro Transdermal System (5.2%) 776
▲ Clolar for Intravenous Infusion (19%) 1271
Colazal Capsules (2%) 2838
Combivent Inhalation Aerosol (2.5%) 847
▲ Combivir Tablets (12%) 1411
▲ Copaxone for Injection (28%) 3297
▲ Copegus Tablets (10%) 2754
Coumadin for Injection (Infrequent) 898
Coumadin Tablets (Infrequent) 898
Crestor Tablets (Greater than or equal to 2%) 678
Crixivan Capsules 1940
▲ Dacogen Injection (13%) 2129
Denavir Cream 2174
Depacon Injection (1.3%) 412
▲ DepoCyt Injection (3% to 11%) 1143
Diastat Rectal Delivery System (1% or more) 3343
▲ Ditropan XL Extended-Release Tablets (4% to 7%) 2413
▲ Doxil Injection (3.4% to 7.2%) 2351
DuoNeb Inhalation Solution (1.3%) 1058

DynaCirc CR Tablets (0.5% to 1%) 2721
Edex Injection (2%) 3089
Effexor Tablets 3411
▲ Efudex (Among most frequent) 3363
▲ Eloxatin for Injection (5% to 15%) 2892
Emend Capsules (Greater than 0.5%) 1963
Emsam Transdermal System 903
Enablex Extended-Release Tablets (Greater than or equal to 1%) 2203
Enbrel for Injection 584
▲ Enjuvia Tablets (10% to 19%) 1062
▲ Entocort EC Capsules (5%) 2698
▲ Equetro Extended-Release Capsules (12%) 3180
▲ Erbitux (2% to 55%) 910
▲ Evoxac Capsules (3.3%) 1047
Exelon Capsules (2% or more) 2206
Exelon Oral Solution (2% or more) 2206
▲ Fabrazyme for Intravenous Infusion (6%) 1274
Famvir Tablets (2.0% to 2.6%) 2211
▲ Faslodex Injection (18.9%) 681
▲ Femara Tablets (5%) 2214
▲ Ferrlecit Injection (0.7% to 10%) 3388
▲ Flebogamma 5%, Immune Globulin Intravenous (Human) (16%) 1658
▲ Flonase Nasal Spray (1% to 3%) 1440
▲ Flovent Diskus (1% to 10%) 1443
▲ Flovent HFA (1% to 3%) 1447
Floxin Otic Solution (Single report) 1049
Fluorescite Injection ⊙ 207
▲ Forteo for Injection (21.3%) 1767
Frova Tablets (Frequent) 1113
▲ Gabitril Tablets (2% to 7%) 984
▲ Gemzar for Injection (7% to 48%) 1771
▲ Gengraf Capsules (6% to 13%) 459
Hectorol Injection 1278
▲ Herceptin I.V. (47%) 1233
▲ Humatrope Vials and Cartridges (6.25% to 13.6%) 1787
Hyalgan Solution 2901
▲ Hycamtin for Injection (1.1% to 23%) 1458
Imitrex Tablets (1% to 2%) 1471
▲ Indapamide Tablets (Greater than or equal to 5%) 2156
▲ Infergen (39% to 54%) 3364
▲ Intron A for Injection (Up to 18%) 3024
Invanz for Injection (Greater than 0.1%) 1999
▲ Ionsys Transdermal System (1% to less than 10%) 2379
▲ I.V. Busulfex (2% to 44%) 2493
Kadian Capsules (Less than 3%) 577
Kaletra (0.6%) 476
▲ Kepivance (16%) 597
▲ Keppra Injection (7%) 3320
▲ Keppra Oral Solution (6% to 7%) 3314
▲ Keppra Tablets (6% to 7%) 3314
Klonopin (Infrequent) 2778
K-Phos Original (Sodium Free) Tablets (Less frequent) 760
K-Phos Neutral Tablets 760
▲ Kytril Injection (10.1%) 2781
▲ Lamictal (More than 5%) 1481
▲ Leukine (17%) 814
Levaquin (1.3%) 2384
Levaquin in 5% Dextrose Injection (1.3%) 2384
Levitra Tablets (Less than 2%) 3034
Lofibra Tablets 1219
Lofibra Capsules 1216
Lotronex Tablets (Rare) 1512
Lovenox Injection 2915
▲ Lunesta Tablets (4% to 5%) 3142
▲ Lupron Depot 3.75 mg (12%) 3260
▲ Lupron Depot 7.5 mg (23.2%) 3264
▲ Lupron Depot–3 Month 11.25 mg (12%) 3265
Lupron Depot-PED 7.5 mg, 11.25 mg and 15 mg (2%) 3269
Lupron Injection Pediatric (2%) 3259
▲ Lyrica Capsules (2% to 5%) 2539
Matulane Capsules 3191
▲ Megace ES Oral Suspension (0% to 6%) 2481
▲ Menostar Transdermal System (13%) 782
▲ Mepron Suspension (10%) 1521
▲ Merrem I.V. (Greater than 1% to 5.1%) 686
Micardis Tablets (1%) 854
Micardis HCT Tablets (2% or greater) 856
Mirapex Tablets (1% or more) 859
▲ Mobic Oral Suspension (0.9% to 3.6%) 863
▲ Mobic Tablets (0.9% to 3.6%) 863
▲ Myfortic Tablets (3% to less than 20%) 2255
▲ Mylotarg for Injection (18%) 3431
▲ Myobloc Injection (6% to 13%) 3192
▲ Namenda (3%) 1195
▲ Neoral Oral Solution (4.4% to 13%) 2259
▲ Neoral Soft Gelatin Capsules (4.4% to 13%) 2259
▲ Neumega for Injection (Greater than or equal to 10%) 3435
Neupogen for Injection (2%) 603
Neurontin Capsules (More than 1%) 2487
Neurontin Oral Solution (More than 1%) 2487
Neurontin Tablets (More than 1%) 2487
Nexium Delayed-Release Capsules (Less than 1%) 655
Nexium I.V. (Less than 1%) 659
▲ Niaspan Extended-Release Tablets (1% to 5%) 1730
▲ Nipent for Injection (8% to 20%) 1863
Norvasc Tablets (More than 0.1% to 1%) 2545
Norvir (1.7% to 2.2%) 503
NovoSeven (1%) 2331
Omacor Capsules (1.8%) 2725
▲ Oncaspar (Greater than 5%) 1145
▲ Ontak Vials (48%) 1745
Oracea Capsules (1.5%) 1000
Orthoclone OKT3 Sterile Solution (Less than 1%) 2360
Oxistat Lotion (0.4%) 2667
OxyContin Tablets (Less than 1%) 2703
▲ Panretin Gel (0% to 34%) 1747
ParaGard T 380A Intrauterine Copper Contraceptive 1073
▲ Pediarix Vaccine (0.3% to 30.5%) 1548
▲ Pegasys (11%) 2789
▲ Permax Tablets (7.0%) 3356
▲ Photofrin for Injection (8% to 22%) 702
▲ Plavix Tablets (6.4%) 917
▲ Plavix Tablets (6.4%) 2926
Pletal Tablets (Very rare) 2455
▲ Premarin Tablets (17% to 20%) 3446
Premarin Vaginal Cream 3452
▲ Premphase Tablets (11% to 20%) 3456
▲ Prempro Tablets (11% to 20%) 3456
Prevacid Delayed-Release Capsules (Less than 1%) 3271
Prevacid for Delayed-Release Oral Suspension 3271
Prevacid SoluTab Delayed-Release Orally Disintegrating Tablets (Less than 1%) 3271
Prevacid NapraPAC (Less than 1%) 3280
PREVPAC (Less than 1%) 3284
Prilosec OTC Delayed-Release Tablets (Less than 1%) 2677
Prinivil Tablets (0.3% to 1.0%) 2052
Prinzide Tablets 2056
▲ ProAir HFA Inhalation Aerosol (3%) 3300
▲ ProAmatine Tablets (4.9%) 3186
▲ Prochieve 4% Gel (8%) 1003
▲ Prochieve 8% Gel (8%) 1003
▲ Prograf Capsules and Injection (24% to 63%) 632
▲ Proleukin for Injection (12%) 2266
Proquin XR Tablets (Less than 1%) 1153
ProSom Tablets (2%) 517
Protonix Tablets (Greater than or equal to 1%) 3469
▲ Protopic Ointment (1% to 4%) 638
Prozac Pulvules and Liquid 1801
Qvar Inhalation Aerosol (1% to 5%) 3303
▲ Rapamune Oral Solution and Tablets (24% to 33%) 3475
▲ Raptiva for Injection (10%) 1250
ReFacto Vials 3484
Relpax Tablets (Frequent) 2548
▲ Remicade for IV Injection (8%) 971
Renagel Tablets 1282
▲ ReoPro Vials (3.4% to 5.4%) 1809
▲ Requip Tablets (3% to 8%) 1555
Rescriptor Tablets 2551
▲ Retisert Implant (5% to 15%) ⊙ 258
▲ Revlimid Capsules (6.8%) 958
▲ Reyataz Capsules (1% to 3%) 921
▲ Risperdal (5%) 1676
▲ Risperdal Consta Long-Acting Injection (3% to 10%) 1682
▲ Risperdal M-Tab Orally Disintegrating Tablets (5%) 1676
▲ Rituxan I.V. (1% to 12%) 1254
Rythmol SR Capsules 2727
Serevent Diskus (1% to 3%) 1568
▲ Seroquel Tablets (7%) 690
▲ Simulect for Injection (Greater than or equal to 10%) 2284
▲ Soltamox Oral Solution (3%) 3527
▲ Somavert Injection (4% to 14%) 2642
▲ Soriatane Capsules (1% to 10%) 1013
▲ Suboxone Tablets (22.4% to 24%) 2717
▲ Subutex Tablets (18.4% to 24%) 2717
Sulfamylon for 5% Topical Solution 2162
▲ Sustiva Capsules (2% to 14%) 930
▲ Sustiva Tablets (2% to 14%) 930
▲ Synagis (8.5%) 1897
Synera Topical Patch (Less than or equal to 1%) 1137
Tamiflu Capsules 2807
Tasmar Tablets (Infrequent) 3358
▲ Taxotere Injection Concentrate (7 of 134 patients) 2932
Teveten Tablets (Less than 1%) 1735
Teveten HCT Tablets (Less than 1%) 1737
▲ Thalomid Capsules (8.3%) 965
▲ Thymoglobulin for Intravenous Infusion (46.3%) 1284
Thyrogen for Injection (4 patients out of 55) 1286
▲ Tiazac Capsules (3% to 6%) 1201
Ticlid Tablets (0.5% to 1.0%) 2810
▲ TOBI Solution for Inhalation (8.1%) 2298
Topamax Sprinkle Capsules (More than 1%) 2404
Topamax Tablets (More than 1%) 2404
Travatan Ophthalmic Solution (1% to 5%) 563
Trelstar Depot (2.1%) 3394
▲ Trelstar LA Suspension (3.4%) 3397
Tricor Tablets 527
Triglide Tablets 3123
▲ Trisenox Injection (15%) 993
Truvada Tablets 1296
▲ Tygacil for Injection (3.7%) 3488
Tylenol Sinus Severe Congestion Caplets with Cool Burst 1876
Ultane Liquid for Inhalation (Less than 1%) 531
▲ Ultram ER Tablets (1% to greater than 5%) 2392
Uniretic Tablets (More than 1%) 3100
Univasc Tablets (Greater than 1%) 3104
Uroxatral Tablets (1% to 2%) 2943
▲ Vagifem Tablets (3% to 5%) 2334
▲ Valcyte Tablets (Less than 5%) 2813
Vandazole Vaginal Gel (Less than 1%) 3338
Vantas (Less than 2%) 3375
Vantin Tablets and Oral Suspension (Less than 1%) 2645
Vaprisol (2.2%) 643
Verelan PM Extended-Release Capsules, Controlled-Onset (2.4%) 3106
▲ Vesanoid Capsules (37%) 2820
VFEND I.V. (Less than 2%) 2564
VFEND Oral Suspension (Less than 2%) 2564
VFEND Tablets (Less than 2%) 2564
Viadur Implant (Less than 2%) 757
Viagra Tablets (Less than 2%) 2573
Vicoprofen Tablets (Less than 3%) 539
Viracept (Less than 2%) 2577
▲ Viread Tablets (7% to 13%) 1301
▲ Vivaglobin (10%) 3506
▲ Voltaren Ophthalmic Solution (Less than or equal to 3%) 2309
▲ WelChol Tablets (5%) 1050
Wellbutrin Tablets (Infrequent) 1603
▲ Wellbutrin SR Sustained-Release Tablets (2% to 3%) 1607
▲ Wellbutrin XL Extended-Release Tablets (2% to 3%) 1613
▲ Xeloda Tablets (Less than 5%) 2822
Xifaxan Tablets (Less than 2%) 2842
▲ Xolair (7%) 1266
Xopenex Inhalation Solution (1.4% to 2.8%) 3146
▲ Xopenex Inhalation Solution Concentrate (1.4% to 3%) 3150
Xopenex HFA Inhalation Aerosol (1.4% to 2.8%) 3154
Xyrem Oral Solution (2.9% to 5.7%) 1688
Yaz Tablets (Greater than 1%) 803
Zegerid Capsules (Less than 1%) 2958
Zegerid Powder for Oral Solution (Less than 1%) 2958
▲ Zelapar Tablets (8%) 3372
Zemaira (0.5%) 3509
Ziagen (Less than 1%) 1626
▲ Zoloft (1% to 6%) 2586
Zomig Tablets (Common) 3519
Zomig-ZMT Tablets (Common) 3519
▲ Zosyn (1.7% to 3.2%) 3492
Zovirax Capsules 1643
Zovirax Ointment 821
Zovirax 1643
Zyban Sustained-Release Tablets (Infrequent) 1644
▲ Zyflo Tablets (7.8%) 1023
Zyrtec Chewable Tablets (Less than 2%) 2594
Zyrtec (Less than 2%) 2594
Zyrtec-D 12 Hour Extended Release Tablets (Less than 2%) 2597

Pain, abdominal

(*see under* Abdominal pain/cramps)

Pain, arm

Cipro XR Tablets 2990
Cozaar Tablets (Less than 1%) 1935
Diovan HCT Tablets (Greater than 0.2%) 2196
▲ Femara Tablets (21% to 22%) 2214
Ferrlecit Injection 3388
Hyzaar 50-12.5 Tablets 1990
Hyzaar 100-12.5 Tablets 1990
Hyzaar 100-25 Tablets 1990
Prinzide Tablets 2056
Proquin XR Tablets 1153
Vaqta (1.3%) 2097
Xolair (2%) 1266

Pain, back

(*see under* Backache)

Pain, biliary

Avinza Capsules (Less than 5%) 1741
Caduet Tablets (Less than 2%) 2508
Campath Ampules 811
Lipitor Tablets (Less than 2%) 2483
Protonix I.V. (Less than 1%) 3472
Protonix Tablets (Less than 1%) 3469
Prozac Pulvules and Liquid (Rare) 1801
Remicade for IV Injection (Greater than or equal to 0.2%) 971
Requip Tablets (Rare) 1555
Rilutek Tablets (Rare) 2930
Sonata Capsules (Rare) 1717
Trileptal Tablets 2300
Trileptal Oral Suspension 2300

Pain, bone

Abelcet Injection 1141
Abilify Oral Solution (Infrequent) 882
Abilify Oral Solution (Infrequent) 2450
Abilify Discmelt Orally Disintegrating Tablets (Infrequent) 882
Abilify Discmelt Orally Disintegrating Tablets (Infrequent) 2450
Abilify Tablets (Infrequent) 882
Abilify Tablets (Infrequent) 2450
Aciphex Tablets 1090
Actiq (Less than 1%) 979
Actonel Tablets (1.4% to 2.9%) 2683
▲ Actonel with Calcium Tablets (1.4% to 4.6%) 2688
▲ Advair HFA Inhalation Aerosol (1% to 3%) 1318
AmBisome for Injection (Less common) 620
Amerge Tablets (Rare) 1339
▲ Aranesp for Injection (10%) 581
▲ Aredia for Injection (At least 5% to 59.4%) 2179
▲ Arimidex Tablets (5% to 12%) 673
Benicar Tablets (Greater than 0.5%) 1043
Boniva Injection 2738
Boniva Tablets 2741
Calcijex Injection 411
Celexa (Infrequent) 1176
Copaxone for Injection (Infrequent) 3297
Depacon Injection 412
Depakene 417
Depakote Sprinkle Capsules 422
Depakote Tablets 427
Depakote ER Tablets 434
▲ Didronel Tablets (About 1 patient in 10 to about 2 in 10) 2697
Doxil Injection (Less than 1%) 2351
Effexor Tablets (Infrequent) 3411
Effexor XR Capsules (Infrequent) 3417
▲ Fabrazyme for Intravenous Infusion (6%) 1274
▲ Faslodex Injection (15.8%) 681
▲ Femara Tablets (22%) 2214
▲ Fosamax (0.4% to approximately 6%) 1969
▲ Fosamax Plus D Tablets (0.4% to 4.1%) 1977
▲ Frova Tablets (3%) 1113
Hectorol Capsules 1275
Hectorol Injection 1278
▲ Herceptin I.V. (7%) 1233
▲ Hycamtin for Injection (59%) 1458
▲ Infergen (13% to 26%) 3364
▲ Intron A for Injection (Less than 5%) 3024
Kadian Capsules (Less than 3%) 577
K-Phos Original (Sodium Free) Tablets (Less frequent) 760
K-Phos Neutral Tablets 760
▲ Leukine (21%) 814
Levaquin (0.1% to 0.9%) 2384

Levaquin in 5% Dextrose Injection (0.1% to 0.9%) ... 2384
Lexapro Oral Solution (Frequent) ... 1190
Lexapro Tablets (Frequent) ... 1190
Lotronex Tablets (Rare) ... 1512
Lupron Depot 7.5 mg (Less than 5%) ... 3264
▲ Neulasta Injection (15% to 72%) ... 601
▲ Neumega for Injection (Greater than or equal to 10%) ... 3435
▲ Neupogen for Injection (22% to 33%) ... 603
Neurontin Capsules (Rare) ... 2487
Neurontin Oral Solution (Rare) ... 2487
Neurontin Tablets (Rare) ... 2487
▲ Nexavar Tablets (Very Common) ... 746
Oncaspar (Less than 1%) ... 1145
Permax Tablets (Infrequent) ... 3356
Pletal Tablets (Less than 2%) ... 2455
Protonix I.V. (Less than 1%) ... 3472
Protonix Tablets (Less than 1%) ... 3469
Prozac Pulvules and Liquid (Infrequent) ... 1801
Relpax Tablets (Infrequent) ... 2548
Rescriptor Tablets ... 2551
Reyataz Capsules (Less than 3%) ... 921
Risperdal (Rare) ... 1676
Risperdal M-Tab Orally Disintegrating Tablets (Rare) ... 1676
Rocaltrol Capsules ... 2798
Rocaltrol Oral Solution ... 2798
▲ Serevent Diskus (1% to 3%) ... 1568
Seroquel Tablets (Infrequent) ... 690
▲ Soltamox Oral Solution (6%) ... 3527
▲ Soriatane Capsules (1% to 10%) ... 1013
▲ Tarceva Tablets (Less than 1% to 31%) ... 1259
▲ Tarceva Tablets (Less than 1% to 31%) ... 2444
Targretin Capsules ... 1747
Tasmar Tablets (1% or more) ... 3358
Tequin Injection (Less than 0.1%) ... 938
Tequin Injection in 5% Dextrose (Less than 0.1%) ... 938
Tequin Tablets (Less than 0.1%) ... 938
Teveten HCT Tablets (Less than 1%) ... 1737
▲ Trelstar Depot (12.1%) ... 3394
▲ Trisenox Injection (23%) ... 993
Uroqid-Acid No. 2 Tablets ... 760
Vantas (Less than 2%) ... 3375
▲ Velcade for Injection (16%) ... 2133
▲ Vesanoid Capsules (77%) ... 2820
VFEND I.V. (Less than 2%) ... 2564
VFEND Oral Suspension (Less than 2%) ... 2564
VFEND Tablets (Less than 2%) ... 2564
Viadur Implant (Less than 2%) ... 757
Viagra Tablets (Less than 2%) ... 2573
▲ Xeloda Tablets (Less than 5%) ... 2822
Zelapar Tablets ... 3372
Zemplar Injection ... 543
▲ Zometa for Intravenous Infusion (11.6% to 55%) ... 2315
Zomig Nasal Spray (Rare) ... 3523
Zyprexa Tablets (Rare) ... 1830
Zyprexa ZYDIS Orally Disintegrating Tablets (Rare) ... 1830

Pain, catheter

▲ Dacogen Injection (5%) ... 2129
Natrecor for Injection (Greater than or equal to 1%) ... 3127

Pain, cervical

▲ Myobloc Injection (4% to 10%) ... 3192

Pain, chest

▲ Abelcet Injection (3%) ... 1141
Abilify Oral Solution (Frequent) ... 882
Abilify Oral Solution (Frequent) ... 2450
Abilify Discmelt Orally Disintegrating Tablets (Frequent) ... 882
Abilify Discmelt Orally Disintegrating Tablets (Frequent) ... 2450
Abilify Tablets (Frequent) ... 882
Abilify Tablets (Frequent) ... 2450
AccuNeb Inhalation Solution (0.9% to 1.7%) ... 1055
Accutane Capsules (Less frequent) ... 2731
Aceon Tablets (2 mg, 4 mg, 8 mg) (2.4%) ... 3194
Actiq (1% or greater) ... 979
▲ Actonel Tablets (2.3% to 6.6%) ... 2683
▲ Actonel with Calcium Tablets (2.3% to 5%) ... 2688
▲ Adalat CC Tablets (3% or less) ... 2964
Adenocard Injection (Less than 1%) ... 617
Advate Injection (0.6%) ... 712
Advicor Tablets ... 1722
▲ Aerobid/Aerobid-M (3% to 9%) ... 1171
Aggrenox Capsules ... 822
▲ Agrylin Capsules (7.8%) ... 3169
Aldara Cream, 5% (0.5%) ... 1846
Aldurazyme for Intravenous Infusion (2%) ... 1268
▲ Alferon N Injection (6% to 10%) ... 1665
▲ Alimta for Injection (Less than 1% to 40%) ... 1750
Altace Capsules (1.1%) ... 1702
Altoprev Extended-Release Tablets (0.5% to 1%) ... 3109
Ambien Tablets (1%) ... 2851
Ambien CR Tablets (Infrequent) ... 2855
▲ AmBisome for Injection (8.2% to 12%) ... 620
Amitiza Capsules (0% to 1.1%) ... 3224
Anzemet Injection (Rare) ... 2859
Anzemet Tablets (Rare) ... 2862
Aralast (0.1%) ... 717
▲ Aranesp for Injection (6%) ... 581
▲ Argatroban Injection (15.2%) ... 1346
Aricept Tablets (Frequent) ... 1094
Aricept ODT Tablets (Frequent) ... 1094
▲ Arimidex Tablets (5% to 7%) ... 673
Arixtra Injection (1.4%) ... 1351
▲ Aromasin Tablets (2% to 5%) ... 2600
▲ Arranon Injection (0% to 5%) ... 1357
▲ Asacol Delayed-Release Tablets (3%) ... 2692
Astelin Nasal Spray ... 1904
Atacand Tablets (More than 1%) ... 649
Atacand HCT (0.5% or greater) ... 651
▲ Atrovent Inhalation Solution (3.2%) ... 835
Avalide Tablets (2%) ... 888
Avalide Tablets (2%) ... 2874
Avapro Tablets (1% or greater) ... 891
Avapro Tablets (1% or greater) ... 2871
Avelox (Less than 0.1%) ... 2970
Axert Tablets (Infrequent) ... 2396
Axid Oral Solution (2.3%) ... 879
Azilect Tablets (Greater than 1%) ... 3293
Azopt Ophthalmic Suspension (Less than 1%) ... 557
Benicar Tablets (Greater than 0.5%) ... 1043
Benicar HCT Tablets (Greater than 1%) ... 1044
Betagan Ophthalmic Solution, USP ... ⊙220
▲ Betaseron for SC Injection (11%) ... 767
Betimol Ophthalmic Solution ... 3382
Betimol Ophthalmic Solution ... ⊙295
▲ Bexxar (0% to 7%) ... 1398
▲ BiDil Tablets (16%) ... 2171
Blocadren Tablets (0.6%) ... 1916
Bumex Tablets (0.1%) ... 2746
Caduet Tablets (Greater than or equal to 2%) ... 2508
▲ Campath Ampules (1% to 10%) ... 811
Campral Tablets (Frequent) ... 1174
Captopril Tablets (Approximately 1 in 100 patients) ... 2149
Cardene I.V. (0.7%) ... 2497
Cardura XL Tablets (Less than 1%) ... 2515
▲ Carnitor Injection (6% to 15%) ... 3188
Catapres-TTS (0.5% or less) ... 844
Ceftin Tablets (0.1% to 1%) ... 1407
Celebrex Capsules (0.1% to 1.9%) ... 3134
Celexa ... 1176
▲ CellCept Capsules (26.3%) ... 2747
▲ CellCept Intravenous (26.3%) ... 2747
▲ CellCept Oral Suspension (26.3%) ... 2747
▲ CellCept Tablets (26.3%) ... 2747
Cesamet Capsules ... 3340
Chantix Tablets (Frequent) ... 2517
Cialis Tablets (Less than 2%) ... 1838
Cipro (Less than 1%) ... 2977
Cipro I.V. (1% or less) ... 2984
Cipro XR Tablets ... 2990
Clinoril Tablets (Less than 1 in 100) ... 1924
Clozaril Tablets (1%) ... 2184
Colazal Capsules ... 2838
Combivent Inhalation Aerosol (0.3%) ... 847
▲ Copaxone for Injection (21%) ... 3297
Coreg Tablets ... 1414
Cosopt Sterile Ophthalmic Solution (Less than 1%) ... 1931
Coumadin for Injection ... 898
Coumadin Tablets ... 898
Covera-HS Tablets (Less than 2%) ... 3139
Cozaar Tablets (1% or greater) ... 1935
Crestor Tablets (Greater than or equal to 2%) ... 678
▲ Cubicin for Injection (1% to 6.7%) ... 1026
▲ Dacogen Injection (7%) ... 2129
Dalmane Capsules ... 3342
Demadex Injection (1.2%) ... 2759
Demadex Tablets (1.2%) ... 2759
▲ Depacon Injection (1% to 5%) ... 412
▲ Depakene (1% to 5%) ... 417
▲ Depakote Sprinkle Capsules (1% to 5%) ... 422
▲ Depakote Tablets (1% to 5%) ... 427
▲ Depakote ER Tablets (1% to 5%) ... 434
Depo-Provera Contraceptive Injection (Less than 1%) ... 2622
depo-subQ provera 104 Injectable Suspension ... 2624
Detrol Tablets (2%) ... 2628
Diovan Tablets (Less frequent) ... 2193
Diovan HCT Tablets (More than 2%) ... 2196
Dolobid Tablets (Rare) ... 1955
▲ Doxil Injection (1% to 5%) ... 2351
DuoNeb Inhalation Solution (2.6%) ... 1058
Duragesic Transdermal System (1% or greater) ... 2373
DynaCirc CR Tablets (0.5% to 1%) ... 2721
Effexor Tablets (2%) ... 3411
Effexor XR Capsules (Frequent) ... 3417
Elitek (Less than or equal to 1%) ... 2890
▲ Eloxatin for Injection (5% to 8%) ... 2892
Emcyt Capsules (1%) ... 2634
Enbrel for Injection ... 584
▲ Entocort EC Capsules (Less than 5%) ... 2698
▲ Epogen for Injection (7%) ... 591
▲ Equetro Extended-Release Capsules (5%) ... 3180
Ery-Tab Tablets (Isolated reports) ... 449
Erythrocin Stearate Filmtab Tablets (Isolated reports) ... 453
Erythromycin Base Filmtab Tablets (Isolated reports) ... 455
Erythromycin Delayed-Release Capsules, USP (Isolated reports) ... 457
▲ Estring Vaginal Ring (1% to 3%) ... 2635
Ethyol for Injection ... 1898
▲ Evista Tablets (4%) ... 1763
▲ Evoxac Capsules (1% to 3%) ... 1047
Exelon Capsules (2% or more) ... 2206
Exelon Oral Solution (2% or more) ... 2206
▲ Exubera Inhalation Powder (4.7%) ... 2524
▲ Fabrazyme for Intravenous Infusion (5%) ... 1274
▲ Faslodex Injection (7.1%) ... 681
FazaClo Orally Disintegrating Tablets (1%) ... 551
▲ Femara Tablets (3% to 8%) ... 2214
▲ Ferrlecit Injection (0.5% to 10%) ... 3388
▲ Flomax Capsules (4.0% to 4.1%) ... 850
Fluarix ... 1451
▲ Foradil Aerolizer (3.2%) ... 3010
Frova Tablets (2%) ... 1113
Gabitril Tablets (1% or more) ... 984
Gammagard Liquid ... 721
▲ Gengraf Capsules (6%) ... 459
▲ Geodon Capsules (3%) ... 2529
▲ Gleevec Tablets (0.4% to 11%) ... 2227
▲ Hectorol Capsules (Greater than or equal to 5%) ... 1275
▲ Humira Injection (Less than 5%) ... 466
Hycamtin for Injection (2%) ... 1458
Hytrin Capsules (At least 1%) ... 471
Hyzaar 50-12.5 Tablets ... 1990
Hyzaar 100-12.5 Tablets ... 1990
Hyzaar 100-25 Tablets ... 1990
▲ Imdur Tablets (Less than or equal to 5%) ... 3018
Imitrex Injection ... 1463
Imitrex Nasal Spray ... 1467
▲ Imitrex Tablets (2% to 3%) ... 1471
▲ Indapamide Tablets (Less than 5%) ... 2156
Indocin (Less than 1%) ... 1995
Infed Injection ... 3390
▲ Infergen (5% to 13%) ... 3364
▲ Intron A for Injection (Up to 28%) ... 3024
Invanz for Injection (1% to 1.5%) ... 1999
Invirase (Greater than or equal to 2%) ... 2772
Ionsys Transdermal System (.1% to less than 1%) ... 2379
▲ I.V. Busulfex (26%) ... 2493
Kadian Capsules (Less than 3%) ... 577
Kaletra (Less than 2%) ... 476
Keppra Injection ... 3320
Keppra Oral Solution (1% or more) ... 3314
Keppra Tablets (1% or more) ... 3314
Klonopin (Infrequent) ... 2778
Lamictal (More than 1%) ... 1481
Lariam Tablets (Infrequent) ... 2786
▲ Leukine (15%) ... 814
Levaquin (1.2%) ... 2384
Levaquin in 5% Dextrose Injection (1.2%) ... 2384
Levitra Tablets (Less than 2%) ... 3034
Lexapro Oral Solution (Frequent) ... 1190
Lexapro Tablets (Frequent) ... 1190
Lipitor Tablets (Greater than or equal to 2%) ... 2483
Lofibra Tablets ... 1219
Lofibra Capsules ... 1216
Lotensin HCT Tablets (0.3% to 1%) ... 2246
Lotrel Capsules (Infrequent) ... 2249
Lunesta Tablets (Frequent) ... 3142
▲ Lyrica Capsules (1% to 4%) ... 2539
▲ Macugen Injection (1% to 5%) ... ⊙261
Mavik Tablets (0.3% to 1.0%) ... 486
Maxair Autohaler (1.3%) ... 1852
▲ Maxalt Tablets (Less than 2% to 3%) ... 2008
▲ Maxalt-MLT Orally Disintegrating Tablets (Less than 2% to 3%) ... 2008
▲ Megace ES Oral Suspension (1% to 3%) ... 2481
▲ Meridia Capsules (1.8%) ... 489
Merrem I.V. (Greater than 0.1% to 1%) ... 686
Mevacor Tablets (0.5% to 1.0%) ... 2021
Micardis Tablets (1%) ... 854
Micardis HCT Tablets ... 856
Midamor Tablets (Less than or equal to 1%) ... 2026
▲ Mirapex Tablets (Greater than or equal to 1% to 3%) ... 859
Moduretic Tablets (Less than or equal to 1%) ... 2028
▲ Myfortic Tablets (3% to less than 20%) ... 2255
Myobloc Injection (Greater than 2%) ... 3192
Namenda ... 1195
Nasonex Nasal Spray (Greater than or equal to 2%) ... 3043
▲ Neoral Oral Solution (6%) ... 2259
▲ Neoral Soft Gelatin Capsules (6%) ... 2259
Neumega for Injection ... 3435
▲ Neupogen for Injection (5%) ... 603
Neurontin Capsules (Infrequent) ... 2487
Neurontin Oral Solution (Infrequent) ... 2487
Neurontin Tablets (Infrequent) ... 2487
▲ Nipent for Injection (3% to 10%) ... 1863
▲ Niravam Orally Disintegrating Tablets (10.6%) ... 3092
Noroxin Tablets (Less frequent) ... 2032
Norvasc Tablets (More than 0.1% to 1%) ... 2545
Norvir (Less than 2%) ... 503
Omacor Capsules ... 2725
Omnicef Capsules ... 511
Omnicef for Oral Suspension ... 511
Oncaspar (Less than 1%) ... 1145
▲ Ontak Vials (24%) ... 1745
Ortho-Cyclen Tablets ... 2429
Ortho Evra Transdermal System ... 2417
Ortho Tri-Cyclen Tablets ... 2429
Ortho Tri-Cyclen Lo Tablets ... 2436
▲ Orthoclone OKT3 Sterile Solution (14%) ... 2360
OxyContin Tablets (Less than 1%) ... 2703
Parcopa Orally Disintegrating Tablets ... 3097
▲ Paxil CR Controlled-Release Tablets (3%) ... 1538
▲ Paxil (3%) ... 1530
Pegasys ... 2789
▲ PEG-Intron Powder for Injection (6%) ... 3048
Pentasa Capsules (Infrequent) ... 3185
▲ Permax Tablets (3.7%) ... 3356
▲ Pexeva Tablets (3%) ... 1694
▲ Photofrin for Injection (22% to 35%) ... 702
▲ Plavix Tablets (8.3%) ... 917
▲ Plavix Tablets (8.3%) ... 2926
Pletal Tablets (Very rare) ... 2455
Prevacid Delayed-Release Capsules (Less than 1%) ... 3271
Prevacid for Delayed-Release Oral Suspension (Less than 1%) ... 3271
Prevacid SoluTab Delayed-Release Orally Disintegrating Tablets (Less than 1%) ... 3271
Prevacid NapraPAC (Less than 1%) ... 3280
PREVPAC (Less than 1%) ... 3284
Prilosec OTC Delayed-Release Tablets (Less than 1%) ... 2677
▲ Prinivil Tablets (3.4%) ... 2052
Prinzide Tablets (0.3% to 1%) ... 2056
ProAir HFA Inhalation Aerosol (Less than 3%) ... 3300
▲ Procrit for Injection (7%) ... 2364
▲ Prograf Capsules and Injection (3% to 19%) ... 632
▲ Proleukin for Injection (12%) ... 2266
▲ Prometrium Capsules (100 mg, 200 mg) (5% to 7%) ... 3203
Proquin XR Tablets ... 1153
ProSom Tablets (1%) ... 517
▲ Protonix I.V. (6%) ... 3472
Protonix Tablets (Greater than or equal to 1%) ... 3469
Protopic Ointment (0.2% to less than 1%) ... 638
Proventil HFA Inhalation Aerosol (Less than 3%) ... 3056
▲ Provigil Tablets (3%) ... 988
Prozac Pulvules and Liquid (Frequent) ... 1801
▲ Pulmicort Respules (1% to 3%) ... 661

▲ Pulmozyme Inhalation Solution (18% to 25%) 1248
▲ Quadramet Injection (4%) 1040
▲ Rapamune Oral Solution and Tablets (16% to 24%) 3475
Razadyne (Frequent) 2399
Razadyne ER Extended-Release Capsules (Frequent) 2399
▲ Rebetol (5% to 9%) 3058
▲ Rebetron Combination Therapy (5% to 9%) 3063
▲ Rebif Prefilled Syringe for Injection (6% to 8%) 3159
▲ Relpax Tablets (1% to 4%) 2548
Remicade for IV Injection (1%) 971
▲ Requip Tablets (4%) 1555
Retrovir Capsules 1560
Retrovir IV Infusion 1564
Retrovir 1560
▲ Revlimid Capsules (2% to 5.4%) 958
Reyataz Capsules (Less than 3%) 921
▲ Ribavirin, USP Capsules (5% to 9%) 3068
▲ Risperdal (2% to 3%) 1676
Risperdal Consta Long-Acting Injection (Frequent) 1682
▲ Risperdal M-Tab Orally Disintegrating Tablets (2% to 3%) 1676
Women's Rogaine Hair Regrowth Treatment Topical Solution, Spring Bloom Scent and Original Unscented ▣ 634
Romazicon Injection (Less than 1%) 2804
Rythmol SR Capsules 2727
Sanctura Tablets 1151
Sandimmune (Rare) 2275
Sandostatin Injection (Less than 1%) 2278
▲ Sensipar Tablets (6%) 608
▲ Simulect for Injection (3% to 10%) 2284
▲ Somavert Injection (4% to 8%) 2642
Sonata Capsules (Frequent) 1717
Soriatane Capsules (Less than 1%) 1013
▲ Spiriva HandiHaler (5% to 7%) 869
Stalevo Tablets 2287
Strattera Capsules (0.70%) 1814
Sular Tablets (2%) 3122
Symbyax Capsules (Up to 1%) 1819
▲ Tambocor Tablets (5.4%) 1856
Targretin Capsules 1747
Tarka Tablets (0.3% to 2.2%) 524
▲ Tasmar Tablets (1% to 3%) 3358
Taxotere Injection Concentrate 2932
▲ Tequin Injection (0.1% to 3%) 938
▲ Tequin Injection in 5% Dextrose (0.1% to 3%) 938
▲ Tequin Tablets (0.1% to 3%) 938
Teveten Tablets (1% or greater) 1735
Teveten HCT Tablets (Less than 1%) 1737
Thalomid Capsules 965
▲ Thrombate III (1 of 17) 3257
Thyrolar Tablets 1199
Timolide Tablets (Less than 1%) 2086
Timoptic Sterile Ophthalmic Solution (Less frequent) 2088
Timoptic in Ocudose (Less frequent) 2091
Timoptic-XE Sterile Ophthalmic Gel Forming Solution 2092
▲ TOBI Solution for Inhalation (26%) 2298
▲ Topamax Sprinkle Capsules (Greater than 1% to 4%) 2404
▲ Topamax Tablets (Greater than 1% to 4%) 2404
Toprol-XL Tablets (Greater than 1%) 668
Trasylol Injection (2%) 754
▲ Travatan Ophthalmic Solution (1% to 5%) 563
Trelstar LA Suspension (1.7%) 3397
Tricor Tablets 527
Triglide Tablets 3123
Trileptal Tablets (Up to 2%) 2300
Trileptal Oral Suspension (Up to 2%) 2300
▲ Trisenox Injection (25%) 993
Truvada Tablets 1296
▲ Ultram ER Tablets (1% to greater than 5%) 2392
Uniretic Tablets (More than 1%) 3100
Univasc Tablets (Greater than 1%) 3104
Uroxatral Tablets 2943
▲ Urso 250 Tablets (5%) 710
▲ Urso Forte Tablets (5%) 710
Vancocin HCl Capsules, USP 3380
Vantin Tablets and Oral Suspension (Less than 1%) 2645
Vasotec I.V. Injection (0.5% to 2.1%) 2103
Ventavis Inhalation Solution 1020
Verelan PM Extended-Release Capsules, Controlled-Onset (2% or less) 3106
VFEND I.V. (Less than 2%) 2564
VFEND Oral Suspension (Less than 2%) 2564
VFEND Tablets (Less than 2%) 2564
Viagra Tablets (Less than 2%) 2573
Virazole for Inhalation Solution 3370
▲ Viread Tablets (3%) 1301
Visudyne for Injection (Less than 1%) 2305
Vivitrol 995
Wellbutrin Tablets (Infrequent) 1603
▲ Wellbutrin SR Sustained-Release Tablets (3% to 4%) 1607
▲ Wellbutrin XL Extended-Release Tablets (3% to 4%) 1613
Xalatan Sterile Ophthalmic Solution (1% to 2%) 2649
▲ Xeloda Tablets (Less than 5%) 2822
Xifaxan Tablets (Less than 2%) 2842
Xopenex Inhalation Solution 3146
Xopenex Inhalation Solution Concentrate 3150
Xopenex HFA Inhalation Aerosol 3154
Xyrem Oral Solution (Frequent) 1688
Zegerid Capsules (Less than 1%) 2958
Zegerid Powder for Oral Solution (Less than 1%) 2958
Zelapar Tablets (2%) 3372
Zelnorm Tablets 2312
Zemaira (0.5%) 3509
▲ Zetia Tablets (1.8% to 3.4%) 2120
▲ Zetia Tablets (3.4%) 3083
Zmax for Oral Suspension (Less then 1%) 2583
Zofran Injection (Rare) 1634
Zofran (Rare) 1639
Zofran ODT Orally Disintegrating Tablets (Rare) 1639
Zoloft (Frequent) 2586
▲ Zometa for Intravenous Infusion (5% to 10%) 2315
Zomig Nasal Spray (Infrequent) 3523
Zonegran Capsules (Infrequent) 1101
Zyban Sustained-Release Tablets (Less than 1%) 1644
Zyflo Tablets (Greater than 1%) 1023
▲ Zyprexa Tablets (3% to 4%) 1830
▲ Zyprexa ZYDIS Orally Disintegrating Tablets (3% to 4%) 1830
Zyrtec Chewable Tablets (Less than 2%) 2594
Zyrtec (Less than 2%) 2594
Zyrtec-D 12 Hour Extended Release Tablets (Less than 2%) 2597

Pain, chest wall
Xyrem Oral Solution (Infrequent) 1688

Pain, dental
Abilify Oral Solution 882
Abilify Oral Solution 2450
Abilify Discmelt Orally Disintegrating Tablets 882
Abilify Discmelt Orally Disintegrating Tablets 2450
Abilify Tablets 882
Abilify Tablets 2450
▲ Advair Diskus 100/50 (1% to 3%) 1308
▲ Advair Diskus 250/50 (1% to 3%) 1308
▲ Advair Diskus 500/50 (1% to 3%) 1308
▲ Advair HFA Inhalation Aerosol (1% to 3%) 1318
▲ Azmacort Inhalation Aerosol (1% to 3%) 1726
Cozaar Tablets (Less than 1%) 1935
Elidel Cream 1% (0.4% to 2.6%) 2200
▲ Estring Vaginal Ring (1% to 3%) 2635
▲ Evoxac Capsules (1% to 3%) 1047
▲ Flovent Diskus (1% to 3%) 1443
Frova Tablets (Rare) 1113
Gardasil Injection (1.5%) 1984
Hyzaar 50-12.5 Tablets 1990
Hyzaar 100-12.5 Tablets 1990
Hyzaar 100-25 Tablets 1990
Imitrex Nasal Spray 1467
▲ Infergen (3% to 7%) 3364
Klonopin (Infrequent) 2778
Lexapro Oral Solution (Frequent) 1190
Lexapro Tablets (Frequent) 1190
Micardis Tablets (More than 0.3%) 854
Micardis HCT Tablets 856
Requip Tablets (Infrequent) 1555
Reyataz Capsules (Less than 3%) 921
Risperdal (Up to 2%) 1676
Risperdal M-Tab Orally Disintegrating Tablets (Up to 2%) 1676
Serevent Diskus (1% to less than 3%) 1568
Singulair (1.7%) 2077
Teveten Tablets (Less than 1%) 1735
Teveten HCT Tablets (Less than 1%) 1737
▲ Thalomid Capsules (4.2%) 965
Trileptal Tablets (1% to 2%) 2300
Trileptal Oral Suspension (1% to 2%) 2300
Vantin Tablets and Oral Suspension (Less than 1%) 2645
Wellbutrin Tablets (Infrequent) 1603
Zyprexa Tablets (Frequent) 1830
Zyprexa ZYDIS Orally Disintegrating Tablets (Frequent) 1830

Pain, ear
Abilify Oral Solution (Infrequent) 882
Abilify Oral Solution (Infrequent) 2450
Abilify Discmelt Orally Disintegrating Tablets (Infrequent) 882
Abilify Discmelt Orally Disintegrating Tablets (Infrequent) 2450
Abilify Tablets (Infrequent) 882
Abilify Tablets (Infrequent) 2450
Aceon Tablets (2 mg, 4 mg, 8 mg) (0.3% to 1%) 3194
Acetadote Injection (1%) 1031
Actiq (Less than 1%) 979
Adenoscan (Less than 1%) 619
Advair Diskus 100/50 1308
Advair Diskus 250/50 1308
Advair Diskus 500/50 1308
Alinia for Oral Suspension (Less than 1%) 2835
Alinia Tablets (Less than 1%) 2835
Aricept Tablets (Infrequent) 1094
Aricept ODT Tablets (Infrequent) 1094
Asacol Delayed-Release Tablets (2% or greater) 2692
Asmanex Twisthaler (1% to less than 3%) 2966
Avalide Tablets 888
Avalide Tablets 2874
Avapro Tablets (Less than 1%) 891
Avapro Tablets (Less than 1%) 2871
Axert Tablets (Infrequent) 2396
Bactroban Nasal (Less than 1%) 1394
Celebrex Capsules (0.1% to 1.9%) 3134
▲ CellCept Capsules (3% to less than 20%) 2747
▲ CellCept Intravenous (3% to less than 20%) 2747
▲ CellCept Oral Suspension (3% to less than 20%) 2747
▲ CellCept Tablets (3% to less than 20%) 2747
Ciprodex Otic Suspension (0.4% to 2.3%) 559
Colazal Capsules 2838
Depacon Injection 412
Depakene 417
Depakote Sprinkle Capsules 422
▲ Depakote Tablets (1% to 5%) 427
Depakote ER Tablets 434
▲ Doxil Injection (1% to 10%) 2351
Effexor Tablets (Frequent) 3411
Elidel Cream 1% (Up to 2.9%) 2200
Engerix-B Vaccine 1425
▲ Equetro Extended-Release Capsules (Less than 5%) 3180
▲ Evoxac Capsules (1% to 3%) 1047
▲ Exubera Inhalation Powder (3.9%) 2524
▲ Flovent Diskus (1% to 3%) 1443
Floxin Otic Solution (0.6% to 1%) 1049
Frova Tablets (Infrequent) 1113
Gabitril Tablets (Frequent) 984
▲ Gamunex Immune Globulin I.V., 10% (18%) 3235
▲ Imdur Tablets (Less than or equal to 5%) 3018
Imitrex Nasal Spray (Rare) 1467
Imitrex Tablets (Infrequent) 1471
▲ Increlex Injection (Greater than or equal to 5%) 3291
Infanrix Vaccine 1476
▲ Infergen (5%) 3364
▲ Intron A for Injection (Less than or equal to 5%) 3024
Invirase (Less than 2%) 2772
Keppra Oral Solution (2%) 3314
Keppra Tablets (2%) 3314
Klonopin (Infrequent) 2778
Lamictal (1.8%) 1481
Lexapro Oral Solution (Frequent) 1190
Lexapro Tablets (Frequent) 1190
Lofibra Tablets 1219
Lofibra Capsules 1216
Lunesta Tablets (Infrequent) 3142
Lupron Depot–3 Month 11.25 mg 3265
Maxalt Tablets (Infrequent) 2008
Maxalt-MLT Orally Disintegrating Tablets (Infrequent) 2008
Meridia Capsules (1.1%) 489
Miacalcin Nasal Spray (Less than 1%) 2253
Micardis Tablets (More than 0.3%) 854
Micardis HCT Tablets 856
Migranal Nasal Spray (Infrequent) 3348
Nasonex Nasal Spray (Greater than or equal to 2%) 3043
Neurontin Capsules (Infrequent) 2487
Neurontin Oral Solution (Infrequent) 2487
Neurontin Tablets (Infrequent) 2487
Nexium Delayed-Release Capsules (Less than 1%) 655
Nexium I.V. (Less than 1%) 659
Nipent for Injection (Less than 3%) 1863
Norvir (Less than 2%) 503
Paxil CR Controlled-Release Tablets (Infrequent) 1538
Paxil (Infrequent) 1530
Pediarix Vaccine 1548
Permax Tablets (Infrequent) 3356
Pexeva Tablets (Infrequent) 1694
Pletal Tablets (Less than 2%) 2455
Prinzide Tablets (0.3% to 1%) 2056
ProAir HFA Inhalation Aerosol (Less than 3%) 3300
▲ Prograf Capsules and Injection (3% to 15%) 632
Prometrium Capsules (100 mg, 200 mg) (Less than 5%) 3203
ProQuad 2064
ProSom Tablets (Infrequent) 517
Protonix I.V. (Less than 1%) 3472
Protonix Tablets (Less than 1%) 3469
Protopic Ointment (Greater than or equal to 1%) 638
Provigil Tablets (At least 1%) 988
Prozac Pulvules and Liquid (Frequent) 1801
▲ Pulmicort Respules (1% to 3%) 661
Recombivax HB (Less than 1%) 2071
Relpax Tablets (Infrequent) 2548
Requip Tablets (Infrequent) 1555
Rescriptor Tablets 2551
Rilutek Tablets (Rare) 2930
Risperdal Consta Long-Acting Injection (Infrequent) 1682
▲ Sandostatin LAR Depot (5% to 15%) 2280
Singulair (Greater than or equal to 2%) 2077
Sonata Capsules (Less than 1%) 1717
▲ Soriatane Capsules (1% to 10%) 1013
Sular Tablets (Less than or equal to 1%) 3122
Symbyax Capsules (1% to 2%) 1819
Targretin Capsules 1747
Tasmar Tablets (Infrequent) 3358
Tequin Injection (Less than 0.1%) 938
Tequin Injection in 5% Dextrose (Less than 0.1%) 938
Tequin Tablets (Less than 0.1%) 938
Timolide Tablets 2086
▲ TOBI Solution for Inhalation (7.4%) 2298
Tricor Tablets 527
Trileptal Tablets (1% to 2%) 2300
Trileptal Oral Suspension (1% to 2%) 2300
▲ Trisenox Injection (8%) 993
Twinrix Vaccine 1595
Uniretic Tablets (Less than 1%) 3100
▲ Vesanoid Capsules (23%) 2820
VFEND I.V. (Less than 2%) 2564
VFEND Oral Suspension (Less than 2%) 2564
VFEND Tablets (Less than 2%) 2564
Viagra Tablets (Less than 2%) 2573
Xifaxan Tablets (Less than 2%) 2842
Xolair (2%) 1266
Xyrem Oral Solution (Infrequent) 1688
Zoloft (Infrequent) 2586
Zomig Tablets (Infrequent) 3519
Zomig Nasal Spray (Infrequent) 3523
Zomig-ZMT Tablets (Infrequent) 3519
Zyprexa Tablets (Infrequent) 1830
Zyprexa ZYDIS Orally Disintegrating Tablets (Infrequent) 1830
Zyrtec Chewable Tablets (Less than 2%) 2594
Zyrtec (Less than 2%) 2594
Zyrtec-D 12 Hour Extended Release Tablets (Less than 2%) 2597

Pain, epigastric
(*see under* Distress, epigastric)

Pain, esophageal
▲ Photofrin for Injection (8%) 702

Pain, exacerbation of
Lidoderm Patch 1118
Vantas (Less than 2%) 3375

Pain, extremities
▲ Amitiza Capsules (1.9% to 3.4%) 3224
▲ Angeliq Tablets (8.4%) 762
▲ Aranesp for Injection (10%) 581
▲ Arranon Injection (0% to 7%) 1357
Astelin Nasal Spray (Infrequent) 1904
▲ Betimol Ophthalmic Solution (1% to 5%) 3382
▲ Betimol Ophthalmic Solution (1% to 5%) ..... ⊙295
Blocadren Tablets 1916
▲ Boniva Injection (1.3% to 7.8%) 2738
▲ Boniva Tablets (1.3% to 7.8%) 2741
Cipro (Less than 1%) 2977
Cipro I.V. (1% or less) 2984
Cipro XR Tablets 2990
Cosopt Sterile Ophthalmic Solution 1931
▲ Cubicin for Injection (9.2%) 1026
Fluarix 1451
▲ Gammagard Liquid (0.85% to 8.2%) 721
▲ Humira Injection (Less than 5%) 466
▲ Hytrin Capsules (3.5%) 471
▲ Increlex Injection (Greater than or equal to 5%) 3291
▲ Ionsys Transdermal System (1% to less than 10%) 2379
Mavik Tablets (0.3% to 1.0%) 486
▲ Oncaspar (Greater than 1% but less than 5%) 1145
▲ Orencia Powder for Intravenous Infusion (3%) 914
Prezista Tablets (Less than 2%) 3306
Proquin XR Tablets 1153
Recombivax HB 2071
Reyataz Capsules (Less than 3%) 921
Tarka Tablets (1.1%) 524
Timoptic-XE Sterile Ophthalmic Gel Forming Solution 2092
Uroqid-Acid No. 2 Tablets 760
▲ Valcyte Tablets (Less than 5%) 2813
▲ Viadur Implant (3.1%) 757
Vivitrol 995
Vytorin 10/10 Tablets (2.3%) 2114
Vytorin 10/10 Tablets (2.3%) 3077
Vytorin 10/20 Tablets (2.3%) 2114
Vytorin 10/20 Tablets (2.3%) 3077
Vytorin 10/40 Tablets (2.3%) 2114
Vytorin 10/40 Tablets (2.3%) 3077
Vytorin 10/80 Tablets (2.3%) 2114
Vytorin 10/80 Tablets (2.3%) 3077
▲ Wellbutrin XL Extended-Release Tablets (3%) 1613
Yaz Tablets (Greater than 1%) 803
▲ Zyprexa Tablets (4% to 5%) 1830
▲ Zyprexa ZYDIS Orally Disintegrating Tablets (4% to 5%) 1830

Pain, eye
Abilify Oral Solution (Infrequent) 882
Abilify Oral Solution (Infrequent) 2450
Abilify Discmelt Orally Disintegrating Tablets (Infrequent) 882
Abilify Discmelt Orally Disintegrating Tablets (Infrequent) 2450
Abilify Tablets (Infrequent) 882
Abilify Tablets (Infrequent) 2450
Acetadote Injection (.54% to 2.58%) 1031
Aciphex Tablets 1090
▲ Acular LS Ophthalmic Solution (1% to 5%) 566
▲ Alphagan P Ophthalmic Solution (1% to 4%) 567
▲ Alrex Ophthalmic Suspension 0.2% (Less than 5%) ..... ⊙246
Ambien Tablets (Infrequent) 2851
Ambien CR Tablets (Infrequent) 2855
Amerge Tablets (Rare) 1339
Asacol Delayed-Release Tablets 2692
Astelin Nasal Spray (Infrequent) 1904
Atrovent Inhalation Solution (Less than 3%) 835
Atrovent HFA Inhalation Aerosol 841
Atrovent Nasal Spray 0.06% 839
▲ Avinza Capsules (Less than 5%) 1741
Axert Tablets (Rare) 2396
▲ Azopt Ophthalmic Suspension (1% to 5%) 557
▲ Betimol Ophthalmic Solution (1% to 5%) 3382
▲ Betimol Ophthalmic Solution (1% to 5%) ..... ⊙295
Betoptic S Ophthalmic Suspension (Small number of patients) 558
▲ Brimonidine Tartrate Ophthalmic Solution 0.2% (3% to 9%) ..... ⊙248
Caduet Tablets (Greater than 0.1% to less than or equal to 1%) 2508
Celebrex Capsules (0.1% to 1.9%) 3134
Celexa (Infrequent) 1176
Chantix Tablets (Infrequent) 2517
Cialis Tablets (Less than 2%) 1838
Ciloxan Ophthalmic Ointment (Less than 1%) 559
Ciloxan Ophthalmic Solution (Less than 1%) ..... ⊙206
Cipro (Less than 1%) 2977
Cipro I.V. (1% or less) 2984
Cipro XR Tablets 2990
Combivent Inhalation Aerosol 847
▲ Copaxone for Injection (7%) 3297
▲ Cosopt Sterile Ophthalmic Solution (1% to 5%) 1931
Depacon Injection (1% or more) 412
Depakene (1% or more) 417
Depakote Sprinkle Capsules 422
▲ Depakote Tablets (1% to 5%) 427
Depakote ER Tablets (Greater than 1%) 434
Doxil Injection (Less than 1%) 2351
DuoNeb Inhalation Solution 1058
Effexor Tablets (Infrequent) 3411
Effexor XR Capsules (Infrequent) 3417
Eldepryl Capsules 3208
Eraxis for Injection (Less than 1% to less than 2%) 2521
▲ Evoxac Capsules (1% to 3%) 1047
Exelon Capsules 2206
Exelon Oral Solution 2206
Fluarix 1451
Flumadine 1183
Frova Tablets (Infrequent) 1113
Gabitril Tablets (Infrequent) 984
Gengraf Capsules (1% to less than 3%) 459
Imitrex Nasal Spray 1467
▲ Infergen (4% to 5%) 3364
▲ Intron A for Injection (Less than 5%) 3024
Iressa Tablets 684
Levaquin (0.1% to 0.9%) 2384
Levaquin in 5% Dextrose Injection (0.1% to 0.9%) 2384
Levitra Tablets (Less than 2%) 3034
Lotemax Ophthalmic Suspension 0.5% (Less than 5%) ..... ⊙251
▲ Lucentis Injection (17% to 37%) 1237
▲ Lumigan Ophthalmic Solution (3% to 10%) 573
▲ Macugen Injection (10% to 40%) ..... ⊙261
Maxalt Tablets (Infrequent) 2008
Maxalt-MLT Orally Disintegrating Tablets (Infrequent) 2008
Meridia Capsules 489
Miacalcin Injection 2252
Migranal Nasal Spray (Rare) 3348
Namenda (Infrequent) 1195
Neoral Oral Solution (1% to less than 3%) 2259
Neoral Soft Gelatin Capsules (1% to less than 3%) 2259
Neurontin Capsules (Infrequent) 2487
Neurontin Oral Solution (Infrequent) 2487
Neurontin Tablets (Infrequent) 2487
Norvasc Tablets (More than 0.1% to 1%) 2545
Norvir (Less than 2%) 503
Paxil CR Controlled-Release Tablets (Infrequent) 1538
Paxil (Infrequent) 1530
Permax Tablets (Infrequent) 3356
Pexeva Tablets (infrequent) 1694
Photofrin for Injection 702
Prevacid Delayed-Release Capsules (Less than 1%) 3271
Prevacid for Delayed-Release Oral Suspension (Less than 1%) 3271
Prevacid SoluTab Delayed-Release Orally Disintegrating Tablets (Less than 1%) 3271
Prevacid NapraPAC (Less than 1%) 3280
PREVPAC (Less than 1%) 3284
Proquin XR Tablets 1153
ProSom Tablets (Infrequent) 517
Protopic Ointment (Greater than or equal to 1%) 638
Provigil Tablets (1%) 988
Quixin Ophthalmic Solution (1% to 3%) 3383
Relpax Tablets (Infrequent) 2548
Requip Tablets (Infrequent) 1555
▲ Restasis Ophthalmic Emulsion (1% to 5%) 575
▲ Retisert Implant (50% to 90%) ..... ⊙258
Risperdal (Rare) 1676
Risperdal Consta Long-Acting Injection (Infrequent) 1682
Risperdal M-Tab Orally Disintegrating Tablets (Rare) 1676
▲ Sonata Capsules (3% to 4%) 1717
▲ Soriatane Capsules (1% to 10%) 1013
Symbyax Capsules (Infrequent) 1819
Tambocor Tablets (Less than 1%) 1856
Tasmar Tablets (Infrequent) 3358
Tequin Injection (Less than 0.1%) 938
Tequin Injection in 5% Dextrose (Less than 0.1%) 938
Tequin Tablets (Less than 0.1%) 938
Thalomid Capsules 965
Timoptic Sterile Ophthalmic Solution (Less frequent) 2088
Timoptic in Ocudose (Less frequent) 2091
Timoptic-XE Sterile Ophthalmic Gel Forming Solution (1% to 5%) 2092
Topamax Sprinkle Capsules (More than 1%) 2404
Topamax Tablets (More than 1%) 2404
▲ Travatan Ophthalmic Solution (5% to 10%) 563
Trelstar LA Suspension (1.1%) 3397
Trusopt Sterile Ophthalmic Solution 2095
VFEND I.V. (Less than 2%) 2564
VFEND Oral Suspension (Less than 2%) 2564
VFEND Tablets (Less than 2%) 2564
Viagra Tablets (Less than 2%) 2573
▲ Vigamox Ophthalmic Solution (1% to 6%) 564
▲ Xalatan Sterile Ophthalmic Solution (1% to 4%) 2649
Xyrem Oral Solution (Infrequent) 1688
Zoloft (Infrequent) 2586
Zomig Tablets (Infrequent) 3519
Zomig-ZMT Tablets (Infrequent) 3519
▲ Zymar Ophthalmic Solution (1% to 4%) 575
Zyprexa Tablets (Infrequent) 1830
Zyprexa ZYDIS Orally Disintegrating Tablets (Infrequent) 1830
Zyrtec Chewable Tablets (Less than 2%) 2594
Zyrtec (Less than 2%) 2594
Zyrtec-D 12 Hour Extended Release Tablets (Less than 2%) 2597

Pain, facial
▲ Carac Cream, 0.5% (43.6%) 2879
Imitrex Injection (Infrequent) 1463
Imitrex Nasal Spray (Rare) 1467
Imitrex Tablets (Infrequent) 1471
Invirase (Less than 2%) 2772
Levulan Kerastick for Topical Solution, 20% (1%) 1085
Norvir (Less than 2%) 503

Pain, feet
Cipro (Less than 1%) 2977

Pain, flank
Aceon Tablets (2 mg, 4 mg, 8 mg) (0.3% to 1%) 3194
Actiq (Less than 1%) 979
Azilect Tablets (Infrequent) 3293
▲ Chemet Capsules (5.2% to 15.7%) 2458
Cleocin Vaginal Ovules (Less than 1%) 2616
Copaxone for Injection (Infrequent) 3297
Crixivan Capsules (Less than 2%) 1940
Ferrlecit Injection 3388
Geodon Capsules (Frequent) 2529
Invanz for Injection (Greater than 0.1%) 1999
Neupogen for Injection (Infrequent) 603
Prinivil Tablets (0.3% to 1.0%) 2052
Prinzide Tablets 2056
Tasmar Tablets (Frequent) 3358
Vasotec I.V. Injection (0.5% to 1.0%) 2103
▲ Vesanoid Capsules (9%) 2820
VFEND I.V. (Less than 2%) 2564
VFEND Oral Suspension (Less than 2%) 2564
VFEND Tablets (Less than 2%) 2564
Zelapar Tablets 3372
Zonegran Capsules (Infrequent) 1101

Pain, foot
Proquin XR Tablets 1153

Pain, gastric
Lopressor Injection (1%) 2238
Lopressor Tablets (1%) 2238
Lopressor HCT 50/25 Tablets (Less than or equal to 1%) 2241
Lopressor HCT 100/25 Tablets (Less than or equal to 1%) 2241
Lopressor HCT 100/50 Tablets (Less than or equal to 1%) 2241

Pain, gastrointestinal
▲ Advair Diskus 100/50 (7%) 1308
▲ Advair Diskus 250/50 (7%) 1308
▲ Advair Diskus 500/50 (7%) 1308
▲ Coreg Tablets (Greater than 1% to 3%) 1414
Duetact Tablets (Less than 1%) 3226
Parcopa Orally Disintegrating Tablets 3097
Stalevo Tablets 2287
▲ Taxotere Injection Concentrate (1.8% to 11.3%) 2932
Vivaglobin (0.1%) 3506

Pain, hip
Cozaar Tablets (Less than 1%) 1935
Humatrope Vials and Cartridges (2.7%) 1787
Hyzaar 50-12.5 Tablets 1990
Hyzaar 100-12.5 Tablets 1990
Hyzaar 100-25 Tablets 1990
Prinivil Tablets (0.3% to 1.0%) 2052
Prinzide Tablets 2056
ProQuad 2064
Zyprexa Tablets (Infrequent) 1830
Zyprexa ZYDIS Orally Disintegrating Tablets (Infrequent) 1830

Pain, infusion site
▲ Vaprisol (7.7%) 643
▲ Visudyne for Injection (10% to 30%) 2305

Pain, jaw
Abilify Oral Solution (Infrequent) 882
Abilify Oral Solution (Infrequent) 2450
Abilify Discmelt Orally Disintegrating Tablets (Infrequent) 882
Abilify Discmelt Orally Disintegrating Tablets (Infrequent) 2450
Abilify Tablets (Infrequent) 882
Abilify Tablets (Infrequent) 2450
Cipro I.V. (1% or less) 2984
Cipro XR Tablets 2990
Klonopin (Infrequent) 2778
Permax Tablets (Infrequent) 3356
Proquin XR Tablets 1153
ProSom Tablets (Rare) 517
Rythmol SR Capsules 2727
Zomig Nasal Spray (Infrequent) 3523

Pain, knee
▲ Cozaar Tablets (Less than 1% to 5%) 1935
▲ Euflexxa (53%) 1162
Hyzaar 50-12.5 Tablets 1990
Hyzaar 100-12.5 Tablets 1990
Hyzaar 100-25 Tablets 1990
Klonopin (Infrequent) 2778
Prinivil Tablets (0.3% to 1.0%) 2052

Pain, leg
Arixtra Injection (1.4%) 1351
Edex Injection (1%) 3089
FazaClo Orally Disintegrating Tablets (1%) 551
Levaquin (0.1% to 0.9%) 2384
Levaquin in 5% Dextrose Injection (0.1% to 0.9%) 2384
Parcopa Orally Disintegrating Tablets 3097
Prochieve 4% Gel 1003
Prochieve 8% Gel 1003
ProQuad 2064
▲ Risperdal Consta Long-Acting Injection (1% to 4%) 1682
Trelstar Depot (2.1%) 3394
▲ Trelstar LA Suspension (5.2%) 3397
▲ Xolair (4%) 1266

Pain, limb
▲ Aromasin Tablets (9%) 2600
▲ Cialis Tablets (1% to 3%) 1838
▲ Clolar for Intravenous Infusion (29%) 1271
Cubicin for Injection (1.5%) 1026
▲ Dacogen Injection (19%) 2129
▲ depo-subQ provera 104 Injectable Suspension (1% to less than 5%) 2624
Duetact Tablets 3226
Eligard 30 mg (1.1%) 2885
Eligard 45 mg (2.7%) 2888
Euflexxa (1.25%) 1162
▲ Femara Tablets (10%) 2214
Fuzeon Injection (2.9%) 2767
Meridia Capsules 489
▲ Renagel Tablets (13.1%) 1282
▲ Retisert Implant (5% to 15%) ..... ⊙258
▲ Revlimid Capsules (1.4% to 10.8%) 958
Stalevo Tablets 2287
▲ Sutent Capsules (1% to 18%) 2560
▲ Trisenox Injection (13%) 993

▲ Ultram ER Tablets (1% to greater than 5%) ... 2392
Vantas (Less than 2%) ... 3375
▲ Velcade for Injection (15%) ... 2133
▲ Zometa for Intravenous Infusion (14%) ... 2315

Pain, localized
Colocort Rectal Suspension, USP (Retention) 100 mg/60 mL (Rare) ... 2476
▲ Havrix Vaccine (15% to 21%) ... 1456
▲ Rescriptor Tablets (1.8% to 5.7%) ... 2551
▲ Zomig Nasal Spray (0% to 4%) ... 3523
Zyvox (0.9% to 2%) ... 2652

Pain, lower extremities
▲ Aceon Tablets (2 mg, 4 mg, 8 mg) (4.7%) ... 3194
▲ Adalat CC Tablets (3% or less) ... 2964
▲ Aggrastat (3%) ... 1907
Altoprev Extended-Release Tablets (0.5% to 1%) ... 3109
Avelox (Less than 0.1%) ... 2970
▲ Chemet Capsules (Up to 3.0%) ... 2458
Cipro (0.3% to 1%) ... 2977
Cipro XR Tablets ... 2990
Clozaril Tablets (1%) ... 2184
▲ Cozaar Tablets (1% to 5%) ... 1935
Diovan HCT Tablets (Greater than 0.2%) ... 2196
DynaCirc CR Tablets (0.5% to 1%) ... 2721
Eldepryl Capsules (1 of 49 patients) ... 3208
▲ Femara Tablets (21% to 22%) ... 2214
Frova Tablets (Rare) ... 1113
Hyzaar 50-12.5 Tablets ... 1990
Hyzaar 100-12.5 Tablets ... 1990
Hyzaar 100-25 Tablets ... 1990
Invanz for Injection (0.4% to 1.1%) ... 1999
Klonopin (Infrequent) ... 2778
Lexapro Oral Solution (Infrequent) ... 1190
Lexapro Tablets (Infrequent) ... 1190
Mevacor Tablets (0.5% to 1.0%) ... 2021
Micardis Tablets (More than 0.3%) ... 854
Micardis HCT Tablets ... 856
Midamor Tablets (Less than or equal to 1%) ... 2026
Moduretic Tablets ... 2028
▲ Myfortic Tablets (3% to less than 20%) ... 2255
Ortho Evra Transdermal System ... 2417
Prilosec OTC Delayed-Release Tablets (Less than 1%) ... 2677
Prinivil Tablets (0.3% to 1.0%) ... 2052
Prinzide Tablets (0.3% to 1%) ... 2056
▲ ProSom Tablets (3%) ... 517
Seroquel Tablets (Infrequent) ... 690
▲ Simulect for Injection (3% to 10%) ... 2284
▲ Spiriva HandiHaler (1% to 3%) ... 869
Timolide Tablets ... 2086
Timoptic Sterile Ophthalmic Solution ... 2088
Timoptic in Ocudose ... 2091
▲ Topamax Sprinkle Capsules (2% to 4%) ... 2404
▲ Topamax Tablets (2% to 4%) ... 2404
▲ Xenical Capsules (10.8%) ... 2831
Zegerid Capsules (Less than 1%) ... 2958
Zegerid Powder for Oral Solution (Less than 1%) ... 2958
Zelnorm Tablets (1%) ... 2312

Pain, medullary bone
▲ Neulasta Injection (26%) ... 601
▲ Neupogen for Injection (33%) ... 603

Pain, mouth
▲ Nexavar Tablets (Very Common) ... 746
Xyrem Oral Solution (Infrequent) ... 1688

Pain, muscle
(*see under* Myalgia)

Pain, musculoskeletal
▲ Advair Diskus 100/50 (4%) ... 1308
▲ Advair Diskus 250/50 (2% to 9%) ... 1308
▲ Advair Diskus 500/50 (2% to 4%) ... 1308
▲ Advair HFA Inhalation Aerosol (5% to 7%) ... 1318
▲ Asmanex Twisthaler (4% to 22%) ... 2966
▲ Avalide Tablets (7%) ... 888
▲ Avalide Tablets (7%) ... 2874
Bumex Tablets (0.2% to 2.9%) ... 2746
Cancidas for Injection (0% to 1.3%) ... 1918
Chantix Tablets (Frequent) ... 2517
Donnatal Extentabs ... 2493
Emend Capsules (Greater than 0.5%) ... 1963
Evoxac Capsules (2.8%) ... 1047
▲ Femara Tablets (21% to 22%) ... 2214
▲ Flovent Diskus (3%) ... 1443
▲ Flovent HFA (1% to 3%) ... 1447
▲ Fosamax (0.4% to approximately 6%) ... 1969
▲ Fosamax Plus D Tablets (0.4% to 4.1%) ... 1977
▲ Gleevec Tablets (1% to 49%) ... 2227
Invirase (Greater than or equal to 2%) ... 2772
Lopressor Injection ... 2238
Lopressor Tablets ... 2238
Maxalt Tablets (Infrequent) ... 2008
Maxalt-MLT Orally Disintegrating Tablets (Infrequent) ... 2008
▲ Nasonex Nasal Spray (1% to 5%) ... 3043
▲ PEG-Intron Powder for Injection (28%) ... 3048
Prevacid NapraPAC (Less than 1%) .. 3280
Prochieve 4% Gel ... 1003
Prochieve 8% Gel ... 1003
▲ Prometrium Capsules (100 mg, 200 mg) (12%) ... 3203
ProQuad ... 2064
▲ Rebetol (19% to 28%) ... 3058
▲ Rebetron Combination Therapy (20% to 28%) ... 3063
▲ Rebif Prefilled Syringe for Injection (10% to 15%) ... 3159
▲ Ribavirin, USP Capsules (19% to 28%) ... 3068
Risperdal (2%) ... 1676
Risperdal Consta Long-Acting Injection (Frequent) ... 1682
Risperdal M-Tab Orally Disintegrating Tablets (2%) ... 1676
▲ Serevent Diskus (12%) ... 1568
▲ Soltamox Oral Solution (3%) ... 3527
▲ Spiriva HandiHaler (1% to 3%) ... 869
▲ Trizivir Tablets (12%) ... 1589
▲ Ventolin HFA Inhalation Aerosol (5%) ... 1600
Visudyne for Injection (Less than 1%) ... 2305
▲ Ziagen (5% to 6%) ... 1626

Pain, neck
(*see under* Torticollis)

Pain, neuropathic
Arranon Injection (1%) ... 1357

Pain, ocular
▲ Nevanac Ophthalmic Suspension 0.1% (1% to 5%) ... ⊙209

Pain, oral mucosa
▲ Advair Diskus 100/50 (1% to 3%) ... 1308
▲ Advair Diskus 250/50 (1% to 3%) ... 1308
▲ Advair Diskus 500/50 (1% to 3%) ... 1308
Cipro (Less than 1%) ... 2977
Cipro I.V. (1% or less) ... 2984
Cipro XR Tablets ... 2990
▲ Flovent Diskus (1% to 3%) ... 1443
Proquin XR Tablets ... 1153
▲ Sutent Capsules (6%) ... 2560

Pain, ovarian
▲ Follistim AQ Cartridge (5%) ... 2338

Pain, paranasal sinus
Advair Diskus 100/50 ... 1308
Advair Diskus 250/50 ... 1308
Advair Diskus 500/50 ... 1308
Advair HFA Inhalation Aerosol ... 1318

Pain, pelvic
Abilify Oral Solution (Frequent) ... 882
Abilify Oral Solution (Frequent) ... 2450
Abilify Discmelt Orally Disintegrating Tablets (Frequent) ... 882
Abilify Discmelt Orally Disintegrating Tablets (Frequent) ... 2450
Abilify Tablets (Frequent) ... 882
Abilify Tablets (Frequent) ... 2450
Actiq (1% or greater) ... 979
Adalat CC Tablets (Less than 1%) ... 2964
▲ Aggrastat (6%) ... 1907
Alinia for Oral Suspension (Less than 1%) ... 2835
Alinia Tablets (Less than 1%) ... 2835
▲ Arimidex Tablets (5% to 7%) ... 673
Avelox (Less than 1%) ... 2970
Caverject Impulse Injection (Less than 1%) ... 2612
▲ CellCept Capsules (3% to less than 20%) ... 2747
▲ CellCept Intravenous (3% to less than 20%) ... 2747
▲ CellCept Oral Suspension (3% to less than 20%) ... 2747
▲ CellCept Tablets (3% to less than 20%) ... 2747
Crestor Tablets (Greater than or equal to 1%) ... 678
▲ Depo-Provera Contraceptive Injection (1% to 5%) ... 2622
▲ Doxil Injection (1% to 10%) ... 2351
Effexor Tablets (Infrequent) ... 3411
Effexor XR Capsules (Infrequent) ... 3417
Emend Capsules (Greater than 0.5%) ... 1963
▲ Faslodex Injection (9.9%) ... 681
Follistim AQ Cartridge ... 2338
Gabitril Tablets (Infrequent) ... 984
▲ Humira Injection (Less than 5%) ... 466
▲ Intron A for Injection (Less than 5%) ... 3024
Invirase (Less than 2%) ... 2772
Klonopin (Infrequent) ... 2778
Lyrica Capsules (0.1% to 1%) ... 2539
Merrem I.V. (Greater than 0.1% to 1%) ... 686
Neurontin Capsules (Rare) ... 2487
Neurontin Oral Solution (Rare) ... 2487
Neurontin Tablets (Rare) ... 2487
Paxil CR Controlled-Release Tablets (Rare) ... 1538
Paxil (Rare) ... 1530
Permax Tablets (Infrequent) ... 3356
Pexeva Tablets (Rare) ... 1694
Pletal Tablets (Less than 2%) ... 2455
▲ Premphase Tablets (4% to 5%) ... 3456
▲ Prempro Tablets (4% to 5%) ... 3456
Prevacid Delayed-Release Capsules (Less than 1%) ... 3271
Prevacid for Delayed-Release Oral Suspension (Less than 1%) ... 3271
Prevacid SoluTab Delayed-Release Orally Disintegrating Tablets (Less than 1%) ... 3271
Prevacid NapraPAC (Less than 1%) .. 3280
PREVPAC (Less than 1%) ... 3284
Prinivil Tablets (0.3% to 1.0%) ... 2052
Prinzide Tablets ... 2056
Prozac Pulvules and Liquid (Infrequent) ... 1801
▲ Rapamune Oral Solution and Tablets (3% to 20%) ... 3475
Revlimid Capsules ... 958
Reyataz Capsules (Less than 3%) ... 921
Seroquel Tablets (Infrequent) ... 690
Symbyax Capsules (Infrequent) ... 1819
VFEND I.V. (Less than 2%) ... 2564
VFEND Oral Suspension (Less than 2%) ... 2564
VFEND Tablets (Less than 2%) ... 2564
Yaz Tablets (Greater than 1%) ... 803
Zyprexa Tablets (Infrequent) ... 1830
Zyprexa ZYDIS Orally Disintegrating Tablets (Infrequent) ... 1830

Pain, penile
▲ Caverject Impulse Injection (2% to 37%) ... 2612
▲ Edex Injection (11% to 41%) ... 3089

Pain, perineal
Arthrotec Tablets (Rare) ... 3129
▲ Prochieve 4% Gel (17%) ... 1003
▲ Prochieve 8% Gel (17%) ... 1003
Requip Tablets (Infrequent) ... 1555
Risperdal (Infrequent) ... 1676
Risperdal M-Tab Orally Disintegrating Tablets (Infrequent) ... 1676

Pain, peripheral
Celebrex Capsules (0.1% to 1.9%) ... 3134

Pain, pharyngeal
▲ Gammagard Liquid (0.61% to 6.5%) ... 721
Parcopa Orally Disintegrating Tablets ... 3097

Pain, pharynx
▲ Advate Injection (11.3%) ... 712
Prilosec OTC Delayed-Release Tablets (Less than 1%) ... 2677
Primaxin I.M. ... 2045
Primaxin I.V. (Less than 0.2%) ... 2048
Prinivil Tablets (0.3% to 1.0%) ... 2052
Prinzide Tablets (0.3% to 1%) ... 2056
Stalevo Tablets ... 2287
Zegerid Capsules (Less than 1%) ... 2958
Zegerid Powder for Oral Solution (Less than 1%) ... 2958

Pain, pleural
Invanz for Injection (Greater than 0.1%) ... 1999
Migranal Nasal Spray (Rare) ... 3348

Pain, postoperative
▲ Advair HFA Inhalation Aerosol (1% to 3%) ... 1318
Aldara Cream, 5% (1.4%) ... 1846
▲ Evoxac Capsules (1% to 3%) ... 1047
▲ Myfortic Tablets (3% to 23.9%) ... 2255
▲ Myozyme for Intravenous Infusion (26%) ... 1279

Pain, post-procedure
Asmanex Twisthaler (1% to less than 3%) ... 2966
Dacogen Injection ... 2129
▲ Xyrem Oral Solution (Infrequent to 5.7%) ... 1688
Zofran Injection (1%) ... 1634

Pain, precordium
Imitrex Tablets ... 1471
Trileptal Tablets ... 2300
Trileptal Oral Suspension ... 2300
Zoloft (Rare) ... 2586

Pain, prostate
Caverject Impulse Injection (2%) ... 2612
Lupron Depot 3.75 mg ... 3260
Lupron Depot 7.5 mg ... 3264
Lupron Depot–3 Month 11.25 mg ... 3265
Lupron Depot-PED 7.5 mg, 11.25 mg and 15 mg ... 3269
Lupron Injection Pediatric ... 3259

Pain, rectum
Canasa Rectal Suppositories (1.8%) ... 699
Noroxin Tablets (0.3% to 1.0%) ... 2032
▲ Xeloda Tablets (Less than 5%) ... 2822
▲ Xenical Capsules (3.3% to 5.2%) ... 2831

Pain, renal
Actiq (Less than 1%) ... 979
Alinia for Oral Suspension (Less than 1%) ... 2835
Alinia Tablets (Less than 1%) ... 2835
Ambien Tablets (Rare) ... 2851
Ambien CR Tablets (Rare) ... 2855
Azopt Ophthalmic Suspension (Less than 1%) ... 557
Ceftin Tablets (0.1% to 1%) ... 1407
Celexa (Rare) ... 1176
Copaxone for Injection (Infrequent) ... 3297
Effexor Tablets (Infrequent) ... 3411
Effexor XR Capsules (Rare) ... 3417
Evoxac Capsules (Less than 1%) ... 1047
Frova Tablets (Rare) ... 1113
Lamictal (Rare) ... 1481
Lunesta Tablets (Infrequent) ... 3142
Neurontin Capsules (Rare) ... 2487
Neurontin Oral Solution (Rare) ... 2487
Neurontin Tablets (Rare) ... 2487
Norvir (Less than 2%) ... 503
Paxil CR Controlled-Release Tablets (Rare) ... 1538
Paxil (Rare) ... 1530
Pexeva Tablets (Rare) ... 1694
Prevacid Delayed-Release Capsules (Less than 1%) ... 3271
Prevacid for Delayed-Release Oral Suspension (Less than 1%) ... 3271
Prevacid SoluTab Delayed-Release Orally Disintegrating Tablets (Less than 1%) ... 3271
Prevacid NapraPAC (Less than 1%) .. 3280
PREVPAC (Less than 1%) ... 3284
Protonix I.V. (Less than 1%) ... 3472
Protonix Tablets (Less than 1%) ... 3469
Prozac Pulvules and Liquid (Rare) ... 1801
▲ Rapamune Oral Solution and Tablets (3% to 20%) ... 3475
Relpax Tablets (Rare) ... 2548
Rescriptor Tablets ... 2551
Reyataz Capsules (Less than 3%) ... 921
Rilutek Tablets (Infrequent) ... 2930
Risperdal Consta Long-Acting Injection (Infrequent) ... 1682
Topamax Sprinkle Capsules (Infrequent) ... 2404
Topamax Tablets (Infrequent) ... 2404
Trileptal Tablets ... 2300
Trileptal Oral Suspension ... 2300
VFEND I.V. (Less than 2%) ... 2564
VFEND Oral Suspension (Less than 2%) ... 2564
VFEND Tablets (Less than 2%) ... 2564
Zoloft (Rare) ... 2586
Zomig Nasal Spray (Rare) ... 3523

Pain, retrosternal
Invirase (Less than 2%) ... 2772
Zofran Injection (2%) ... 1634

Pain, right hypochondrium
Trileptal Tablets ... 2300
Trileptal Oral Suspension ... 2300

Pain, right upper quadrant
▲ Intron A for Injection (Less than 5% to 15%) ... 3024
Invirase (Rare) ... 2772
Lamisil Tablets ... 2232
▲ PEG-Intron Powder for Injection (8%) ... 3048
▲ Rebetol (6% to 12%) ... 3058

▲ Ribavirin, USP Capsules (6% to 12%) 3068
Tarka Tablets (Several cases) 524

Pain, salivary gland
▲ Evoxac Capsules (1% to 3%) 1047
Frova Tablets (Rare) 1113

Pain, shoulder
Altoprev Extended-Release Tablets (0.5% to 1%) 3109
Cozaar Tablets (Less than 1%) 1935
Engerix-B Vaccine (Less than 1%) 1425
Hytrin Capsules (At least 1%) 471
Hyzaar 50-12.5 Tablets 1990
Hyzaar 100-12.5 Tablets 1990
Hyzaar 100-25 Tablets 1990
Klonopin (Infrequent) 2778
▲ Lexapro Oral Solution (3%) 1190
▲ Lexapro Tablets (3%) 1190
Mevacor Tablets (0.5% to 1.0%) 2021
Moduretic Tablets 2028
Parcopa Orally Disintegrating Tablets 3097
Prinivil Tablets (0.3% to 1.0%) 2052
Prinzide Tablets (0.3% to 1%) 2056
Recombivax HB (Less than 1%) 2071
Stalevo Tablets 2287
Zofran Injection (2%) 1634

Pain, skeletal
▲ Advair HFA Inhalation Aerosol (1% to 3%) 1318
Estring Vaginal Ring (2%) 2635
▲ Euflexxa (3%) 1162
▲ Hycamtin for Injection (23%) 1458
Levaquin 2384
Levaquin in 5% Dextrose Injection 2384
▲ Neulasta Injection (15% to 72%) 601
▲ Norditropin Cartridges (11%) 2323
▲ Trelstar Depot (12.1%) 3394
▲ Trelstar LA Suspension (13.2%) 3397

Pain, stomach
(*see under* Stomachache)

Pain, substernal
Evoxac Capsules (Less than 1%) 1047
Levaquin (Less than 0.5%) 2384
Levaquin in 5% Dextrose Injection (Less than 0.5%) 2384
Sonata Capsules (Infrequent) 1717
Teveten Tablets (Less than 1%) 1735
Teveten HCT Tablets (Less than 1%) 1737

Pain, suprapubic
Proquin XR Tablets (Less than 1%) 1153

Pain, testicular
Caverject Impulse Injection (Less than 1%) 2612
Edex Injection (1%) 3089
Eligard 7.5 mg (Less than 2%) 2880
Eligard 22.5 mg (Less than 2%) 2883
Eligard 30 mg (2.2%) 2885
Fabrazyme for Intravenous Infusion (2%) 1274
Neurontin Capsules (Rare) 2487
Neurontin Oral Solution (Rare) 2487
Neurontin Tablets (Rare) 2487
Prilosec OTC Delayed-Release Tablets (Less than 1%) 2677
Propecia Tablets 2060
Proscar Tablets 2067
Rescriptor Tablets 2551
▲ Viadur Implant (3.8%) 757
Zegerid Capsules (Less than 1%) 2958
Zegerid Powder for Oral Solution (Less than 1%) 2958

Pain, thoracic spine
▲ Chemet Capsules (5.2% to 15.7%) 2458
Primaxin I.M. 2045
Primaxin I.V. (Less than 0.2%) 2048

Pain, throat
Abilify Oral Solution (Infrequent) 882
Abilify Oral Solution (Infrequent) 2450
Abilify Discmelt Orally Disintegrating Tablets (Infrequent) 882
Abilify Discmelt Orally Disintegrating Tablets (Infrequent) 2450
Abilify Tablets (Infrequent) 882
Abilify Tablets (Infrequent) 2450
Amerge Tablets (1% to 2%) 1339
▲ Imitrex Tablets (Less than 1% to 3%) 1471
Lotronex Tablets (1%) 1512
▲ Zomig Nasal Spray (1% to 4%) 3523

Pain, tongue
▲ Ventavis Inhalation Solution (4%) 1020

Pain, trauma activated
Xyrem Oral Solution (Frequent) 1688

Pain, trunk
▲ Epogen for Injection (3%) 591
▲ Leustatin Injection (6%) 2357
▲ Procrit for Injection (3%) 2364
Requip Tablets (Infrequent) 1555

Pain, tumor site
▲ Aromasin Tablets (8%) 2600
Herceptin I.V. 1233
Soltamox Oral Solution 3527

Pain, unspecified
▲ Depakote ER Tablets (11%) 434

Pain, upper extremities
Aceon Tablets (2 mg, 4 mg, 8 mg) (0.2% to 2.8%) 3194
Cipro I.V. (1% or less) 2984
Engerix-B Vaccine (Less than 1%) 1425
Midamor Tablets (Less than or equal to 1%) 2026
Moduretic Tablets 2028
Prinivil Tablets (0.3% to 1.0%) 2052
ProSom Tablets (Infrequent) 517
Thalomid Capsules 965
Timolide Tablets 2086
Timoptic Sterile Ophthalmic Solution 2088
Timoptic in Ocudose 2091

Pain, urethral
Ceftin Tablets (0.1% to 1%) 1407
Permax Tablets (Rare) 3356
Prevacid Delayed-Release Capsules (Less than 1%) 3271
Prevacid for Delayed-Release Oral Suspension (Less than 1%) 3271
Prevacid SoluTab Delayed-Release Orally Disintegrating Tablets (Less than 1%) 3271
Prevacid NapraPAC (Less than 1%) 3280
PREVPAC (Less than 1%) 3284
Protonix I.V. (Less than 1%) 3472
Protonix Tablets (Less than 1%) 3469

Pain, urinary bladder
Duragesic Transdermal System (Less than 1%) 2373
Effexor Tablets (Infrequent) 3411
Effexor XR Capsules (Infrequent) 3417
▲ Rapamune Oral Solution and Tablets (3% to 20%) 3475
ReoPro Vials (0.1%) 1809
Sonata Capsules (Infrequent) 1717
Zonegran Capsules (Rare) 1101

Pain, urinary tract
Trileptal Tablets 2300
Trileptal Oral Suspension 2300

Pain, vaginal
Cleocin Vaginal Ovules (1.9%) 2616
▲ Estring Vaginal Ring (5%) 2635
Neurontin Capsules (Rare) 2487
Neurontin Oral Solution (Rare) 2487
Neurontin Tablets (Rare) 2487
Vantin Tablets and Oral Suspension (Less than 1%) 2645

Pain at application site
▲ Aldara Cream, 5% (Up to 12%) 1846
Cleocin Vaginal Ovules (Less than 1%) 2616
Clobex Spray (1% to 2%) 1208
▲ Sulfamylon Cream (One of two most frequent) 2162
Zovirax Ointment 821

Pain at injection site
Actimmune 1671
Actiq (Less than 1%) 979
▲ ADACEL Vaccine (1.1% to 80%) 2945
Aldurazyme for Intravenous Infusion (2%) 1268
▲ Alferon N Injection (12%) 1665
Aloxi Injection (Very rare) 2127
▲ Amevive (7% to common) 626
Anzemet Injection 2859
▲ Aranesp for Injection (7%) 581
▲ Aredia for Injection (Up to 41%) 2179
Attenuvax 1914
▲ Betaseron for SC Injection (18%) 767
Bicillin C-R Injectable Suspension 1706
▲ Boostrix (4.6% to 75.3%) 1404
▲ BOTOX Purified Neurotoxin Complex (2% to 10%) 570
Calcijex Injection (Occasional) 411
Calcium Disodium Versenate Injection 1851
Capastat Sulfate for Injection 1755
Cardene I.V. (0.7%) 2497
Cipro I.V. (1% or less) 2984
▲ Clolar for Intravenous Infusion (14%) 1271
▲ Comvax (23.9% to 34.5%) 1928
▲ Copaxone for Injection (73%) 3297
Depacon Injection (2.6%) 412
Depo-Provera Contraceptive Injection (Less than 1%) 2622
▲ depo-subQ provera 104 Injectable Suspension (1% to less than 5%) 2624
Dilaudid-HP (Rare) 442
Doxil Injection (Less than 1%) 2351
Edecrin Sodium Intravenous (Occasional) 1959
▲ Eligard 22.5 mg (6%) 2883
▲ Eligard 30 mg (3.3%) 2885
Eligard 45 mg (2.7%) 2888
▲ Eloxatin for Injection (9% to 10%) 2892
▲ Enbrel for Injection (34% to 37%) 584
Engerix-B Vaccine (Less than 1%) 1425
▲ Faslodex Injection (10.9%) 681
▲ Fluarix (12.2% to 54.7%) 1451
Fluorescite Injection ⊙207
Fortaz 1453
▲ Fragmin Injection (2% to 12%) 1097
▲ Fuzeon Injection (95%) 2767
GamaSTAN 3234
▲ Gammagard S/D (16%) 724
Garamycin Injectable (Occasional) 3014
▲ Gardasil Injection (0.9% to 83.9%) 1984
Genotropin Lyophilized Powder (Infrequent) 2638
▲ Geodon for Injection (7% to 9%) 2529
Humatrope Vials and Cartridges (Infrequent) 1787
▲ Humira Injection (12% to 20%) 466
▲ Hyalgan Solution (23%) 2901
HyperHep B S/D 3240
Hyperstat I.V. 3017
Imitrex Injection 1463
▲ Infanrix Vaccine (0.9% to 10.5%) 1476
Infed Injection 3390
▲ Infergen (8% to 9%) 3364
▲ Intron A for Injection (Less than 5%) 3024
▲ Invanz for Injection (7%) 1999
Ionsys Transdermal System (.1% to less than 1%) 2379
▲ I.V. Busulfex (15%) 2493
Lantus Injection (2.7%) 2909
▲ Leustatin Injection (9% to 19%) 2357
Levaquin (0.2%) 2384
Levaquin in 5% Dextrose Injection (0.2%) 2384
Lovenox Injection (2%) 2915
Maxipime for Injection (0.6%) 1105
▲ Menactra Vaccine (0.2% to 59.2%) 2954
Merrem I.V. (0.4%) 686
Meruvax II 2019
▲ MICRhoGAM Ultra-Filtered (Frequent) 2371
Mycamine for Injection (0.9%) 628
▲ Myobloc Injection (12% to 16%) 3192
▲ Nabi-HB (4%) 2169
Neumega for Injection 3435
Nutropin for Injection (Infrequent) 1239
▲ Oncaspar (Greater than 1% but less than 5%) 1145
Pediarix Vaccine 1548
Liquid PedvaxHIB 2035
Pneumovax 23 (Common) 2043
Premarin Intravenous 3442
Prevacid I.V. for Injection (1%) 3277
Primaxin I.M. (1.2%) 2045
Primaxin I.V. (0.7%) 2048
▲ ProQuad (22%) 2064
Protonix I.V. (Greater than 1%) 3472
Recombivax HB (Equal to or greater than 1%) 2071
ReoPro Vials (0.1%) 1809
Retrovir IV Infusion (Infrequent) 1564
▲ RhoGAM Ultra-Filtered (Frequent) 2371
Rhophylac 3505
Risperdal Consta Long-Acting Injection (Frequent) 1682
▲ Rituxan I.V. (Less than 5%) 1254
Rocephin Injectable Vials, ADD-Vantage, Galaxy, Bulk (1%) 2800
▲ Romazicon Injection (3% to 9%) 2804
▲ Sandostatin Injection (7.7%) 2278
▲ Sandostatin LAR Depot (2% to 11%) 2280
Timentin ADD-Vantage 1580
Timentin Injection Galaxy Container 1583
Timentin IV Infusion 1577
Timentin Pharmacy Bulk Package 1586
▲ Trelstar Depot (3.6%) 3394
▲ Trelstar LA Suspension (4%) 3397
▲ Trisenox Injection (20%) 993
Tygacil for Injection (0% to less than 2%) 3488
▲ Vaqta (1.2% to 51.1%) 2097
▲ Varivax (19.3% to 32.5%; less than 0.05%) 2100
VFEND I.V. (Less than 2%) 2564
VFEND Oral Suspension (Less than 2%) 2564
VFEND Tablets (Less than 2%) 2564
▲ Vivitrol (10% to 17%) 995
Xolair 1266
Zantac Injection 1619
Zantac Injection Pharmacy Bulk Package (Frequent) 1622
Zantac Injection Premixed 1619
▲ Zinecard for Injection (12% to 13%) 2650
▲ Zofran Injection (4%) 1634
▲ Zostavax Injection (33.4%) 2111
Zosyn (0.2%) 3492
Zyprexa IntraMuscular (Frequent) 1830

Pain at insertion site
▲ Vantas (3.6%) 3375

Pain secondary to eczema
Bactroban Cream (One report) 1394

Pain, pharyngolaryngeal
▲ Advate Injection (11.3%) 712
Amitiza Capsules (0% to 1.7%) 3224
Astelin Nasal Spray (Infrequently) 1904
Avandia Tablets (2%) 1384
▲ Cubicin for Injection (8.3%) 1026
Diovan HCT Tablets (Greater than 0.2%) 2196
▲ Emend Capsules (3%) 1963
▲ Focalin XR Capsules (4% to 7%) 2223
▲ Myfortic Tablets (3% to less than 20%) 2255
Oracea Capsules (1.1%) 1000
Vivitrol 995
Xifaxan Tablets (Less than 2%) 2842
▲ Xyrem Oral Solution (2.9% to 9.1%) 1688
Zelnorm Tablets 2312

Pain, thorax
▲ Humira Injection (Less than 5%) 466

Pallor
Abilify Oral Solution (Infrequent) 882
Abilify Oral Solution (Infrequent) 2450
Abilify Discmelt Orally Disintegrating Tablets (Infrequent) 882
Abilify Discmelt Orally Disintegrating Tablets (Infrequent) 2450
Abilify Tablets (Infrequent) 882
Abilify Tablets (Infrequent) 2450
Advair Diskus 100/50 1308
Advair Diskus 250/50 1308
Advair Diskus 500/50 1308
Advair HFA Inhalation Aerosol 1318
Allegra-D 12 Hour Extended-Release Tablets 2846
Allegra-D 24 Hour Extended-Release Tablets 2849
Ambien Tablets (Infrequent) 2851
Ambien CR Tablets (Infrequent) 2855
Bicillin C-R Injectable Suspension 1706
Buprenex Injectable (Infrequent) 2716
Captopril Tablets (2 to 5 of 1000 patients) 2149
Catapres Tablets 843
Catapres-TTS (0.5% or less) 844
▲ CellCept Capsules (3% to less than 20%) 2747
▲ CellCept Intravenous (3% to less than 20%) 2747
▲ CellCept Oral Suspension (3% to less than 20%) 2747
▲ CellCept Tablets (3% to less than 20%) 2747
Clorpres Tablets 2153
Clozaril Tablets (Less than 1%) 2184
▲ Dacogen Injection (23%) 2129
Dapsone Tablets USP 1673
▲ Doxil Injection (1% to 10%) 2351
Effexor Tablets (Rare) 3411
Effexor XR Capsules (Rare) 3417
Enbrel for Injection 584
EpiPen 1061
Evoxac Capsules (Less than 1%) 1047
▲ Fabrazyme for Intravenous Infusion (4%) 1274
FazaClo Orally Disintegrating Tablets (Less than 1%) 551
Ferrlecit Injection 3388
Flumadine (Less than 0.3%) 1183
Gabitril Tablets (Infrequent) 984
Imitrex Injection (Rare) 1463

Imitrex Nasal Spray (Rare) 1467
Imitrex Tablets (Infrequent) 1471
Kadian Capsules (Less than 3%) 577
Kogenate FS 738
Kogenate FS with Bio-Set 740
▲ Miacalcin Nasal Spray (10.6%) 2253
Myozyme for Intravenous Infusion 1279
Nitrolingual Pumpspray 3120
Paxil CR Controlled-Release Tablets (Rare) 1538
Paxil (Rare) 1530
Pediarix Vaccine 1548
Pexeva Tablets (rare) 1694
Prozac Pulvules and Liquid (Rare) 1801
ReoPro Vials (0.1%) 1809
Rescriptor Tablets 2551
Reyataz Capsules (Less than 3%) 921
Risperdal (Rare) 1676
Risperdal M-Tab Orally Disintegrating Tablets (Rare) 1676
Rythmol SR Capsules 2727
▲ Serevent Diskus (9%) 1568
Thioridazine Hydrochloride Tablets 2163
Topamax Sprinkle Capsules (1%) 2404
Topamax Tablets (1%) 2404
▲ Trisenox Injection (10%) 993
Twinject 0.3 3378
Twinject 0.15 3379
▲ Vesanoid Capsules (6%) 2820
Wellbutrin Tablets (Rare) 1603
WinRho SDF 732
Zelapar Tablets 3372
Zoloft (Rare) 2586
Zyprexa Tablets 1830
Zyprexa ZYDIS Orally Disintegrating Tablets 1830
Zyrtec Chewable Tablets (Less than 2%) 2594
Zyrtec (Less than 2%) 2594
Zyrtec-D 12 Hour Extended Release Tablets (Less than 2%) 2597

Pallor, nasal
▲ Fortical Nasal Spray (10.6%) 3337

Palmar-plantar erythrodysesthesia syndrome
▲ Clolar for Intravenous Infusion (13%) 1271
▲ Doxil Injection (3.4% to 50.6%) 2351
▲ Eloxatin for Injection (1% to 11%) 2892
▲ Sutent Capsules (3% to 14%) 2560
▲ Xeloda Tablets (17% to 54%) 2822

Palpitations
Abilify Oral Solution (Infrequent) 882
Abilify Oral Solution (Infrequent) 2450
Abilify Discmelt Orally Disintegrating Tablets (Infrequent) 882
Abilify Discmelt Orally Disintegrating Tablets (Infrequent) 2450
Abilify Tablets (Infrequent) 882
Abilify Tablets (Infrequent) 2450
Accutane Capsules 2731
Aceon Tablets (2 mg, 4 mg, 8 mg) (0.9% to 1.1%) 3194
Aciphex Tablets 1090
Actiq (1% or greater) 979
Adalat CC Tablets (Less than 1%) 2964
Adderall Tablets 3164
▲ Adderall XR Capsules (2% to 4%) 3166
Adenocard Injection (Less than 1%) 617
Adenoscan (Less than 1%) 619
Adipex-P 1215
▲ Advair Diskus 100/50 (1% to 3%) 1308
▲ Advair Diskus 250/50 (1% to 3%) 1308
▲ Advair Diskus 500/50 (1% to 3%) 1308
Advicor Tablets 1722
▲ Aerobid/Aerobid-M (3% to 9%) 1171
Aggrenox Capsules (Less than 1%) 822
▲ Agrylin Capsules (26.1%) 3169
Aldara Cream, 5% 1846
Allegra-D 12 Hour Extended-Release Tablets (1.9%) 2846
Allegra-D 24 Hour Extended-Release Tablets (1.9%) 2849
Altace Capsules (Less than 1%) 1702
Alupent Inhalation Aerosol (Less frequent) 826
Ambien Tablets (2%) 2851
Ambien CR Tablets (2% to frequent) 2855
Amerge Tablets (Infrequent) 1339
Amitiza Capsules (Less than 0.2%) 3224
Anaprox Tablets (Less than 3%) 2761
Anaprox DS Tablets (Less than 3%) 2761
Anzemet Injection (Rare) 2859
Anzemet Tablets (Rare) 2862
Arthrotec Tablets (Rare) 3129
Atacand Tablets (0.5% or greater) 649
Atacand HCT (0.5% or greater) 651
Atripla Tablets 945
Atrovent Inhalation Solution (Less than 3%) 835
Atrovent Nasal Spray 0.06% (Less than 1%) 839
Avelox (0.1% to less than 2%) 2970
▲ Avinza Capsules (Less than 5%) 1741
Axert Tablets (Infrequent) 2396
Bentyl Capsules 697
Bentyl Injection 697
Bentyl Syrup 697
Bentyl Tablets 697
Betagan Ophthalmic Solution, USP ⊙220
▲ Betaseron for SC Injection (4%) 767
Betimol Ophthalmic Solution 3382
Betimol Ophthalmic Solution ⊙295
Bicillin C-R Injectable Suspension 1706
▲ BiDil Tablets (4%) 2171
BioLean II Tablets ▣808
Blocadren Tablets 1916
Brimonidine Tartrate Ophthalmic Solution 0.2% (Less than 3%) ⊙248
▲ Caduet Tablets (Less than 2% to 4.5%) 2508
Campral Tablets (Frequent) 1174
Captopril Tablets (Approximately 1 of 100 patients) 2149
Cardizem LA Extended Release Tablets (Less than 2%) 1728
Cardura XL Tablets (Less than 1%) 2515
▲ Carnitor Injection (3% to 8%) 3188
Carteolol Hydrochloride Ophthalmic Solution USP, 1% (Occasional) ⊙249
Catapres Tablets (About 5 in 1,000 patients) 843
Catapres-TTS (0.5% or less) 844
Celebrex Capsules (0.1% to 1.9%) 3134
Celexa (At least 2%) 1176
▲ CellCept Capsules (3% to less than 20%) 2747
▲ CellCept Intravenous (3% to less than 20%) 2747
▲ CellCept Oral Suspension (3% to less than 20%) 2747
▲ CellCept Tablets (3% to less than 20%) 2747
Cesamet Capsules 3340
Chantix Tablets (Infrequent) 2517
Cialis Tablets (Less than 2%) 1838
Cipro (Less than 1%) 2977
Cipro I.V. (1% or less) 2984
Cipro XR Tablets 2990
Clarinex Syrup 2995
Clarinex Tablets 2995
Clarinex Reditabs Tablets 2995
Clarinex-D 24-Hour Extended-Release Tablets 2998
Clinoril Tablets (Less than 1 in 100) 1924
Clorpres Tablets (About 5 in 1,000) 2153
Clozaril Tablets (Less than 1%) 2184
Colazal Capsules 2838
Combivent Inhalation Aerosol (Less than 2%) 847
Concerta Extended-Release Tablets 1881
▲ Copaxone for Injection (17%) 3297
▲ Coreg Tablets (Greater than 1% to 3%) 1414
Cosopt Sterile Ophthalmic Solution 1931
Covera-HS Tablets (Less than 2%) 3139
Cozaar Tablets (Less than 1%) 1935
Crestor Tablets (Greater than or equal to 1%) 678
Dalmane Capsules 3342
Daytrana Transdermal Patch 3174
▲ Depacon Injection (1% to 5%) 412
▲ Depakene (1% to 5%) 417
▲ Depakote Sprinkle Capsules (1% to 5%) 422
▲ Depakote Tablets (1% to 5%) 427
Depakote ER Tablets (Greater than 1%) 434
Desoxyn Tablets, USP 2462
Detrol LA Capsules 2631
Dexedrine 1420
DextroStat Tablets 3179
Dilaudid Oral Liquid 445
Dilaudid Tablets - 8 mg 445
Dilaudid-HP (Less frequent) 442
Diovan Tablets 2193
Diovan HCT Tablets (Greater than 0.2%) 2196
▲ Ditropan XL Extended-Release Tablets (2% to less than 5%) 2413
Dolobid Tablets (Rare) 1955
Donnatal Extentabs 2493
Doxil Injection (Less than 1%) 2351
DuoNeb Inhalation Solution 1058
DynaCirc CR Tablets (1.2%) 2721
EC-Naprosyn Delayed-Release Tablets (Less than 3%) 2761
Effexor Tablets 3411
Effexor XR Capsules (3%) 3417
Eldepryl Capsules (1 of 49 patients) 3208
Emend Capsules (Greater than 0.5%) 1963
Emsam Transdermal System 903
Engerix-B Vaccine 1425
▲ Entocort EC Capsules (Less than 5%) 2698
EpiPen 1061
Ery-Tab Tablets (Isolated reports) 449
Erythrocin Stearate Filmtab Tablets (Isolated reports) 453
Erythromycin Base Filmtab Tablets (Isolated reports) 455
Erythromycin Delayed-Release Capsules, USP (Isolated reports) 457
▲ Evoxac Capsules (1% to 3%) 1047
Exelon Capsules (Frequent) 2206
Exelon Oral Solution (Frequent) 2206
FazaClo Orally Disintegrating Tablets (Less than 1%) 551
Flebogamma 5%, Immune Globulin Intravenous (Human) 1658
Flomax Capsules (Infrequent) 850
▲ Flovent Diskus (1% to 3%) 1443
Flumadine (Less than 0.3%) 1183
Focalin Tablets 2220
Focalin XR Capsules 2223
Foradil Aerolizer 3010
Fortical Nasal Spray (Less than 1%) 3337
Frova Tablets (Frequent) 1113
Gabitril Tablets (Frequent) 984
Gantrisin Pediatric Suspension 2770
Guanidine Hydrochloride Tablets 3016
▲ Humira Injection (Less than 5%) 466
Hycotuss Expectorant Syrup 1117
Hyperstat I.V. 3017
▲ Hytrin Capsules (0.9% to 28%) 471
Hyzaar 50-12.5 Tablets (1.4%) 1990
Hyzaar 100-12.5 Tablets (1.4%) 1990
Hyzaar 100-25 Tablets (1.4%) 1990
▲ Imdur Tablets (Less than or equal to 5%) 3018
Imitrex Injection (Infrequent) 1463
Imitrex Nasal Spray (Infrequent) 1467
Imitrex Tablets (Up to 2%) 1471
▲ Indapamide Tablets (Less than 5%) 2156
Indocin (Less than 1%) 1995
▲ Infergen (3% to 5%) 3364
▲ Intron A for Injection (Less than 5%) 3024
Kadian Capsules (Less than 3%) 577
Kaletra (Less than 2%) 476
Ketek Tablets 2903
Klonopin (Infrequent) 2778
Lamictal (1.0%) 1481
Lanoxicaps Capsules 1490
Lanoxin Injection 1494
Lanoxin Injection Pediatric 1497
Lanoxin Tablets 1500
Lariam Tablets (Infrequent) 2786
Levaquin (0.1% to 0.9%) 2384
Levaquin in 5% Dextrose Injection (0.1% to 0.9%) 2384
Levitra Tablets (Less than 2%) 3034
Levothroid Tablets 1186
Levoxyl Tablets 1712
Lexapro Oral Solution (Frequent) 1190
Lexapro Tablets (Frequent) 1190
Limbrel Capsules (0.006%) 2672
Lipitor Tablets (Less than 2%) 2483
Lofibra Tablets 1219
Lofibra Capsules 1216
Lopressor Injection (1%) 2238
Lopressor Tablets (1%) 2238
Lopressor HCT 50/25 Tablets 2241
Lopressor HCT 100/25 Tablets 2241
Lopressor HCT 100/50 Tablets 2241
Lotensin HCT Tablets (0.3% to 1%) 2246
Lotrel Capsules (0.5% to 0.3%) 2249
▲ Lupron Depot 3.75 mg (Among most frequent) 3260
▲ Lupron Depot–3 Month 11.25 mg (Less than 5%) 3265
Marinol Capsules (Greater than 1%) 3333
Mavik Tablets (0.3% to 1.0%) 486
Maxair Autohaler (1.3% to 1.7%) 1852
Maxalt Tablets (Frequent) 2008
Maxalt-MLT Orally Disintegrating Tablets (Frequent) 2008
▲ Megace ES Oral Suspension (1% to 3%) 2481
Meridia Capsules (2%) 489
Metadate CD Capsules 3323
Miacalcin Nasal Spray (Less than 1%) 2253
Micardis Tablets (More than 0.3%) 854
Micardis HCT Tablets 856
Midamor Tablets (Less than or equal to 1%) 2026
Migranal Nasal Spray (Infrequent) 3348
Mirapex Tablets (Greater than or equal to 1%) 859
Mobic Oral Suspension (Less than 2%) 863
Mobic Tablets (Less than 2%) 863
Moduretic Tablets 2028
MS Contin Tablets (Less frequent) 2701
Nalfon Capsules (2.5%) 2502
Naprosyn Suspension (Less than 3%) 2761
Naprosyn Tablets (Less than 3%) 2761
▲ Neumega for Injection (14%) 3435
Neurontin Capsules (Infrequent) 2487
Neurontin Oral Solution (Infrequent) 2487
Neurontin Tablets (Infrequent) 2487
Niaspan Extended-Release Tablets 1730
Nimotop Capsules (Less than 1%) 749
Niravam Orally Disintegrating Tablets (7.7%) 3092
Norflex Injection 1856
Noroxin Tablets (Less frequent) 2032
▲ Norvasc Tablets (0.7% to 4.5%) 2545
Norvir (Less than 2%) 503
Numorphan Injection 1120
Opana Tablets (Less than 1%) 1122
Opana ER Tablets (Less than 1%) 1126
OptiPranolol Metipranolol Ophthalmic Solution 0.3% (A small number of patients) ⊙256
Parcopa Orally Disintegrating Tablets 3097
Parnate Tablets 1527
▲ Paxil CR Controlled-Release Tablets (2% to 3%) 1538
▲ Paxil (2% to 3%) 1530
Pentasa Capsules (Less than 1%) 3185
Pepcid Injection (Infrequent) 2040
Pepcid (Infrequent) 2038
Percodan Tablets 1132
Permax Tablets (2.1%) 3356
Persantine Tablets (Rare) 868
▲ Pexeva Tablets (2% to 3%) 1694
Plavix Tablets (1% to 2.5%) 917
Plavix Tablets (1% to 2.5%) 2926
▲ Pletal Tablets (5% to 10%) 2455
Prevacid Delayed-Release Capsules (Less than 1%) 3271
Prevacid for Delayed-Release Oral Suspension (Less than 1%) 3271
Prevacid SoluTab Delayed-Release Orally Disintegrating Tablets (Less than 1%) 3271
Prevacid NapraPAC (Less than 3%) 3280
PREVPAC (Less than 1%) 3284
Prilosec OTC Delayed-Release Tablets (Less than 1%) 2677
Primaxin I.M. 2045
Primaxin I.V. (Less than 0.2%) 2048
Prinivil Tablets (0.3% to 1.0%) 2052
Prinzide Tablets (0.3% to 1%) 2056
▲ Prometrium Capsules (100 mg, 200 mg) (Less than 5%) 3203
Proquin XR Tablets 1153
ProSom Tablets (Infrequent) 517
Protonix I.V. (Less than 1%) 3472
Protonix Tablets (Less than 1%) 3469
Protopic Ointment (Greater than or equal to 1%) 638
▲ Proventil Inhalation Aerosol (Less than 10%) 3053
Proventil HFA Inhalation Aerosol (Less than 3%) 3056
Provigil Tablets (2%) 988
Prozac Pulvules and Liquid (Frequent) 1801
Ranexa Tablets (Greater than 0.5% to less than 2%) 1035
▲ Rapamune Oral Solution and Tablets (3% to 20%) 3475
Razadyne (Infrequent) 2399
Razadyne ER Extended-Release Capsules (Infrequent) 2399
Recombivax HB (Less than 1%) 2071
ReFacto Vials 3484
Relpax Tablets (Frequent) 2548
ReoPro Vials (0.7%) 1809
▲ Requip Tablets (3%) 1555
Restoril Capsules (0.5% to 0.9%) 1860
▲ Revlimid Capsules (5.4%) 958
Reyataz Capsules (Less than 3%) 921
Rhinocort Aqua Nasal Spray (Rare) 665
Rilutek Tablets (0.4% to 1.2%) 2930
Risperdal (Infrequent) 1676

Crestor Tablets (Greater than or equal to 2%) 678
Cubicin for Injection (Less than 1%) 1026
▲ Daranide Tablets (Among the most common effects) 1950
Decadron Tablets 1951
Denavir Cream 2174
▲ Depacon Injection (0.9% to 5%) 412
▲ Depakene (1% to 5%) 417
▲ Depakote Sprinkle Capsules (1% to 5%) 422
▲ Depakote Tablets (1% to 5%) 427
▲ Depakote ER Tablets (1% to 5%) 434
DepoCyt Injection 1143
▲ DepoDur Extended-Release Injection (2% to 5%) 1110
Depo-Provera Contraceptive Injection (Less than 1%) 2622
depo-subQ provera 104 Injectable Suspension 2624
Detrol Tablets (1.1%) 2628
Didronel Tablets 2697
Dilaudid 440
Dilaudid Non-Sterile Powder 440
Dilaudid Oral Liquid (Less frequent) 445
Dilaudid Rectal Suppositories 440
Dilaudid Tablets 440
Dilaudid Tablets - 8 mg (Less frequent) 445
Dilaudid-HP (Less frequent) 442
Diovan Tablets 2193
Diovan HCT Tablets (Greater than 0.2%) 2196
Diuril Oral Suspension 1954
Diuril Sodium Intravenous 2467
Dolobid Tablets (Less than 1 in 100) 1955
▲ Doxil Injection (Less than 1% to 10%) 2351
Duragesic Transdermal System (1% or greater) 2373
Dyazide Capsules 1423
DynaCirc CR Tablets (0.5% to 1%) 2721
EC-Naprosyn Delayed-Release Tablets (Less than 1%) 2761
▲ Effexor Tablets (3%) 3411
▲ Effexor XR Capsules (2% to 3%) 3417
Elitek (Less than or equal to 1%) 2890
Elocon Cream 0.1% (2 in 182 patients) 3005
Elocon Lotion 0.1% (2 in 65 patients) 3006
▲ Emtriva Capsules (5% to 6%) 1287
▲ Emtriva Oral Solution (5% to 6%) 1287
Enbrel for Injection 584
Engerix-B Vaccine 1425
▲ Enjuvia Tablets (0% to 6%) 1062
▲ Entocort EC Capsules (Less than 5%) 2698
▲ Epivir (13%) 1427
Epivir-HBV 1432
▲ Epogen for Injection (11%) 591
Epzicom Tablets 1436
Equetro Extended-Release Capsules 3180
Estratest Tablets 3199
Estratest H.S. Tablets 3199
Euflexxa (1.25%) 1162
Evoxac Capsules (Less than 1%) 1047
Exelon Capsules (Frequent) 2206
Exelon Oral Solution (Frequent) 2206
▲ Fabrazyme for Intravenous Infusion (4%) 1274
Famvir Tablets (0.9% to 2.6%) 2211
▲ Faslodex Injection (6.4%) 681
FazaClo Orally Disintegrating Tablets 551
▲ Ferrlecit Injection (6%) 3388
Floxin Otic Solution (1%) 1049
Fluarix 1451
Fortaz (Less than 1%) 1453
▲ Fortical Nasal Spray (1% to 3%) 3337
▲ Frova Tablets (4%) 1113
Furosemide Tablets 2154
▲ Gabitril Tablets (3%) 984
Gantrisin Pediatric Suspension 2770
Gemzar for Injection (Less than 1%) 1771
▲ Gengraf Capsules (1% to 11%) 459
Geodon (Frequent) 2529
Gleevec Tablets (Less common) 2227
Havrix Vaccine (Rare) 1456
▲ Hectorol Capsules (Greater than or equal to 5%) 1275
▲ Herceptin I.V. (9%) 1233
Humate-P (2%) 3502
▲ Humatrope Vials and Cartridges (13.6% to 17.3%) 1787
▲ Humira Injection (Less than 5%) 466
▲ Hycamtin for Injection (7% to 9%) 1458
Hytrin Capsules (0.8% to 1.9%) 471
Hyzaar 50-12.5 Tablets 1990
Hyzaar 100-12.5 Tablets 1990
Hyzaar 100-25 Tablets 1990
▲ Imdur Tablets (Less than or equal to 5%) 3018
Imitrex Injection (Infrequent) 1463
Imitrex Nasal Spray (Infrequent) 1467
▲ Imitrex Tablets (3% to 5%) 1471
Indapamide Tablets 2156
Indocin (Less than 1%) 1995
Infed Injection 3390
▲ Infergen (9% to 13%) 3364
▲ Intron A for Injection (1% to 21%) 3024
Invanz for Injection (Greater than 0.1%) 1999
Invirase (0.3% to greater than or equal to 2%) 2772
Ionsys Transdermal System (.1% to less than 1%) 2379
Kadian Capsules (Less than 3%) 577
Kaletra (Up to 2%) 476
▲ Kepivance (12%) 597
Keppra Injection (2%) 3320
Keppra Oral Solution (2%) 3314
Keppra Tablets (2%) 3314
Ketek Tablets (Less than 0.2%) 2903
Klonopin (Infrequent) 2778
Lamictal (More than 1%) 1481
Lariam Tablets (Occasional) 2786
Lescol Capsules 2233
Lescol XL Tablets 2233
▲ Leukine (11%) 814
Levaquin (0.1% to 0.9%) 2384
Levaquin in 5% Dextrose Injection (0.1% to 0.9%) 2384
Levitra Tablets (Less than 2%) 3034
Lexapro Oral Solution (2%) 1190
Lexapro Tablets (2%) 1190
Lidoderm Patch 1118
Lipitor Tablets (Less than 2%) 2483
Lofibra Tablets 1219
Lofibra Capsules 1216
Lopressor HCT 50/25 Tablets 2241
Lopressor HCT 100/25 Tablets 2241
Lopressor HCT 100/50 Tablets 2241
Lotensin Tablets (Less than 1%) 2243
Lotensin HCT Tablets (0.3% to 1%) 2246
Lotrisone (1.9%) 3040
Lunesta Tablets (Infrequent) 3142
▲ Lupron Depot 3.75 mg (Less than 5%) 3260
▲ Lupron Depot–3 Month 11.25 mg (1.2% to 7%) 3265
Luxiq Foam (One patient) 1010
Lyrica Capsules (Greater than or equal to 2%) 2539
Matulane Capsules 3191
Mavik Tablets (0.3% to 1.0%) 486
▲ Maxalt Tablets (3% to 4%) 2008
▲ Maxalt-MLT Orally Disintegrating Tablets (3% to 4%) 2008
▲ Megace ES Oral Suspension (1% to 3%) 2481
Meridia Capsules (2%) 489
Merrem I.V. (Greater than 0.1% to 1%) 686
Meruvax II 2019
Mevacor Tablets (0.5% to 1.0%) 2021
▲ Miacalcin Nasal Spray (1% to 3%) 2253
Micardis Tablets (More than 0.3%) 854
Micardis HCT Tablets 856
Midamor Tablets (Less than or equal to 1%) 2026
Migranal Nasal Spray (2%) 3348
Mirapex Tablets (1% or more) 859
M-M-R II 2006
Mobic Oral Suspension (Less than 2%) 863
Mobic Tablets (Less than 2%) 863
Moduretic Tablets (Less than or equal to 1%) 2028
MS Contin Tablets (Less frequent) 2701
Nadolol Tablets (6 of 1000 patients) 2159
Namenda (Infrequent) 1195
Naprosyn Suspension (Less than 1%) 2761
Naprosyn Tablets (Less than 1%) 2761
Natrecor for Injection (Greater than or equal to 1%) 3127
▲ Neoral Oral Solution (1% to 11%) 2259
▲ Neoral Soft Gelatin Capsules (1% to 11%) 2259
Neumega for Injection 3435
Neurontin Capsules (Frequent) 2487
Neurontin Oral Solution (Infrequent) 2487
Neurontin Tablets (Frequent) 2487
Nexium Delayed-Release Capsules (Less than 1%) 655
Nexium I.V. (Less than 1%) 659
Niaspan Extended-Release Tablets 1730
▲ Nipent for Injection (3% to 10%) 1863
Niravam Orally Disintegrating Tablets (2.4%) 3092
▲ Norditropin Cartridges (11%) 2323
Noroxin Tablets 2032
Norvasc Tablets (More than 0.1% to 1%) 2545
▲ Norvir (2.6% to 3%) 503
▲ Oncaspar (Greater than 1% but less than 5%) 1145
▲ Ontak Vials (13%) 1745
OxyContin Tablets (Less than 1%) 2703
▲ Panretin Gel (3% to 22%) 1747
Parcopa Orally Disintegrating Tablets 3097
Parnate Tablets 1527
▲ Paxil CR Controlled-Release Tablets (1.0% to 5.9%) 1538
▲ Paxil (1.0% to 5.9%) 1530
Pentasa Capsules (Less than 1%) 3185
Pepcid Injection (Infrequent) 2040
Pepcid (Infrequent) 2038
Percodan Tablets 1132
Permax Tablets (1.6%) 3356
Persantine Tablets (Rare) 868
▲ Pexeva Tablets (1% to 5.9%) 1694
Plavix Tablets (1% to 2.5%) 917
Plavix Tablets (1% to 2.5%) 2926
Pletal Tablets (2% or greater) 2455
Pneumovax 23 (Rare) 2043
Podocon-25 Liquid 2478
Prevacid Delayed-Release Capsules (Less than 1%) 3271
Prevacid for Delayed-Release Oral Suspension (Less than 1%) 3271
Prevacid SoluTab Delayed-Release Orally Disintegrating Tablets (Less than 1%) 3271
Prevacid I.V. for Injection (Less than 1%) 3277
Prevacid NapraPAC (Less than 1%) 3280
PREVPAC (Less than 1%) 3284
Prezista Tablets (Less than 2%) 3306
Prilosec OTC Delayed-Release Tablets (Less than 1%) 2677
Primaxin I.M. 2045
Primaxin I.V. (Less than 0.2%) 2048
Prinivil Tablets (0.3% to 1.0%) 2052
Prinzide Tablets (1.5%) 2056
▲ ProAmatine Tablets (18.3%) 3186
▲ Procrit for Injection (11%) 2364
▲ Prograf Capsules and Injection (17% to 40%) 632
ProQuad 2064
Proquin XR Tablets (Less than 1%) 1153
ProSom Tablets (Infrequent) 517
Protonix I.V. (Less than 1%) 3472
Protonix Tablets (Less than 1%) 3469
▲ Protopic Ointment (Greater than or equal to 1% to 3%) 638
Provigil Tablets (2%) 988
Prozac Pulvules and Liquid 1801
Quadramet Injection (2%) 1040
Ranexa Tablets (Less than or equal to 0.5%) 1035
Raniclor Tablets, Chewable (Rare) 2505
▲ Rapamune Oral Solution and Tablets (3% to 20%) 3475
Razadyne (Infrequent) 2399
Razadyne ER Extended-Release Capsules (Infrequent) 2399
▲ Relpax Tablets (3% to 4%) 2548
▲ Requip Tablets (3% to 5%) 1555
▲ Retrovir Capsules (6%) 1560
▲ Retrovir IV Infusion (6%) 1564
▲ Retrovir (6%) 1560
▲ Revatio Tablets (3%) 2557
▲ Revlimid Capsules (11.6%) 958
Risperdal (Infrequent) 1676
Risperdal Consta Long-Acting Injection (Infrequent) 1682
Risperdal M-Tab Orally Disintegrating Tablets (Infrequent) 1676
Rituxan I.V. (2%) 1254
▲ Romazicon Injection (1% to 3%) 2804
Rythmol SR Capsules 2727
▲ Sandimmune (1% to 3%) 2275
▲ Sandostatin LAR Depot (5% to 15%) 2280
▲ Serevent Diskus (1% to 3%) 1568
Seromycin Capsules 1813
▲ Simulect for Injection (3% to 10%) 2284
Singulair 2077
▲ Somavert Injection (7%) 2642
▲ Sonata Capsules (3%) 1717
▲ Soriatane Capsules (10% to 25%) 1013
▲ Spiriva HandiHaler (1% to 3%) 869
Stalevo Tablets 2287
▲ Strattera Capsules (4%) 1814
Sular Tablets (Less than or equal to 1%) 3122
Sustiva Capsules (Less than 2%) 930
Sustiva Tablets (Less than 2%) 930
Symmetrel Tablets 1135
Synera Topical Patch (Less than or equal to 1%) 1137
▲ Tambocor Tablets (1% to 3%) 1856
Tarka Tablets (Less frequent) 524
▲ Tasmar Tablets (1% to 3%) 3358
▲ Taxotere Injection Concentrate (7 of 134 patients) 2932
Tegretol/Tegretol-XR 2295
▲ Temodar Capsules (9%) 3073
▲ Tequin Injection (0.1% to 3%) 938
▲ Tequin Injection in 5% Dextrose (0.1% to 3%) 938
▲ Tequin Tablets (0.1% to 3%) 938
Teveten Tablets (Less than 1%) 1735
Teveten HCT Tablets (Less than 1%) 1737
▲ Thalomid Capsules (5.6% to 15.6%) 965
Thyrogen for Injection (1.6%) 1286
Tiazac Capsules (Less than 2%) 1201
Timolide Tablets 2086
Timoptic Sterile Ophthalmic Solution (Less frequent) 2088
Timoptic in Ocudose (Less frequent) 2091
Timoptic-XE Sterile Ophthalmic Gel Forming Solution 2092
Tindamax Tablets 2142
▲ Topamax Sprinkle Capsules (1% to 51%) 2404
▲ Topamax Tablets (1% to 51%) 2404
Toprol-XL Tablets 668
Tricor Tablets 527
▲ Tri-Luma Cream (3%) 1213
▲ Trisenox Injection (33%) 993
Trizivir Tablets 1589
Trusopt Sterile Ophthalmic Solution 2095
Truvada Tablets 1296
Twinrix Vaccine (Less than 1%) 1595
▲ Ultram ER Tablets (1% to greater than 5%) 2392
Uniretic Tablets (Less than 1%) 3100
▲ Valcyte Tablets (8%) 2813
Vantin Tablets and Oral Suspension (Less than 1%) 2645
Varivax 2100
Vasotec I.V. Injection (0.5% to 1.0%) 2103
▲ Velcade for Injection (27%) 2133
Verelan PM Extended-Release Capsules, Controlled-Onset (2% or less) 3106
▲ Vesanoid Capsules (17%) 2820
VFEND I.V. (Less than 2%) 2564
VFEND Oral Suspension (Less than 2%) 2564
VFEND Tablets (Less than 2%) 2564
Viadur Implant (Less than 2%) 757
Viagra Tablets (Less than 2%) 2573
Vicoprofen Tablets (Less than 3%) 539
Viracept (Less than 2%) 2577
Viramune Oral Suspension 873
Viramune Tablets 873
Voltaren Tablets (Occasionally) 2307
Voltaren-XR Tablets (Occasionally) 2310
Vytorin 10/10 Tablets 2114
Vytorin 10/10 Tablets 3077
Vytorin 10/20 Tablets 2114
Vytorin 10/20 Tablets 3077
Vytorin 10/40 Tablets 2114
Vytorin 10/40 Tablets 3077
Vytorin 10/80 Tablets 2114
Vytorin 10/80 Tablets 3077
Wellbutrin Tablets 1603
Wellbutrin SR Sustained-Release Tablets (1% to 2%) 1607
Wellbutrin XL Extended-Release Tablets (1% to 2%) 1613
▲ Xeloda Tablets (1% to 21%) 2822
Xopenex Inhalation Solution 3146
Xopenex Inhalation Solution Concentrate 3150
Xopenex HFA Inhalation Aerosol 3154
Xyrem Oral Solution (Less than 1%) 1688
Zegerid Capsules (Less than 1%) 2958
Zegerid Powder for Oral Solution (Less than 1%) 2958
Zelapar Tablets 3372
Zemaira (0.2% to 0.4%) 3509
Ziagen 1626
Zmax for Oral Suspension 2583
Zocor Tablets 2105
Zofran Injection (2%) 1634
▲ Zoloft (3%) 2586
▲ Zometa for Intravenous Infusion (15%) 2315
▲ Zomig Tablets (Common) 3519
▲ Zomig Nasal Spray (5% to 10%) 3523
▲ Zomig-ZMT Tablets (Common) 3519
▲ Zonegran Capsules (4%) 1101
Zovirax 1643

Zyban Sustained-Release Tablets (Infrequent) ... 1644
▲ Zyprexa Tablets (5%) ... 1830
▲ Zyprexa ZYDIS Orally Disintegrating Tablets (5%) ... 1830
Zyrtec Chewable Tablets (Less than 2%) ... 2594
Zyrtec (Less than 2%) ... 2594
Zyrtec-D 12 Hour Extended Release Tablets (Less than 2%) ... 2597

Paresthesia, circumoral
▲ Agenerase Oral Solution (26% to 31%) ... 1332
Azilect Tablets (Infrequent) ... 3293
Cesamet Capsules ... 3340
Copaxone for Injection (Infrequent) ... 3297
Effexor Tablets (Infrequent) ... 3411
Effexor XR Capsules (Infrequent) ... 3417
Gabitril Tablets (Infrequent) ... 984
Geodon Capsules (Rare) ... 2529
Lyrica Capsules (0.1% to 1%) ... 2539
Neurontin Capsules (Infrequent) ... 2487
Neurontin Oral Solution (Infrequent) ... 2487
Neurontin Tablets (Infrequent) ... 2487
▲ Norvir (3.4% to 6.7%) ... 503
Paxil CR Controlled-Release Tablets (Rare) ... 1538
Paxil (Rare) ... 1530
Pexeva Tablets (rare) ... 1694
ProSom Tablets (Rare) ... 517
Prozac Pulvules and Liquid (Rare) ... 1801
▲ Rilutek Tablets (1.3% to 3.3%) ... 2930
Sonata Capsules (Infrequent) ... 1717
Thalomid Capsules ... 965
Zomig Nasal Spray (Infrequent) ... 3523
Zonegran Capsules (Rare) ... 1101
Zyprexa Tablets (Rare) ... 1830
Zyprexa ZYDIS Orally Disintegrating Tablets (Rare) ... 1830

Paresthesia, facial
Guanidine Hydrochloride Tablets ... 3016

Paresthesia, feet
Gris-PEG Tablets (Rare) ... 2502
Guanidine Hydrochloride Tablets ... 3016

Paresthesia, hands
Gris-PEG Tablets (Rare) ... 2502
Guanidine Hydrochloride Tablets ... 3016
Inderal LA Long-Acting Capsules ... 3429
InnoPran XL Capsules ... 2723
Oncaspar ... 1145

Paresthesia, lip
Fleet Phospho-soda (Rare) ... 1166
Fleet Phospho-soda ACCU-PREP (Rare) ... 1168
Fleet Phospho-soda EZ-PREP (Rare) ... 1169
Guanidine Hydrochloride Tablets ... 3016
OsmoPrep Tablets (Rare) ... 2840

Paresthesia, oral
▲ Agenerase Capsules (26% to 31%) ... 1327
▲ Agenerase Oral Solution (26% to 31%) ... 1332
Crixivan Capsules ... 1940
▲ Lexiva Tablets (Less than 1% to 10%) ... 1505

Paresthesia, peripheral
▲ Agenerase Capsules (10% to 14%) ... 1327
▲ Agenerase Oral Solution (10% to 14%) ... 1332
▲ Norvir (5% to 6%) ... 503

Parkinsonism
Aldoril Tablets ... 1910
Clozaril Tablets (Less than 1%) ... 2184
Demser Capsules ... 1953
Depakene ... 417
Depakote Tablets ... 427
Depakote ER Tablets ... 434
Exelon Capsules (2%) ... 2206
Exelon Oral Solution (2%) ... 2206
FazaClo Orally Disintegrating Tablets (Less than 1%) ... 551
Indocin (Less than 1%) ... 1995
▲ Risperdal (0.6% to 6%) ... 1676
▲ Risperdal Consta Long-Acting Injection (4% to 10%) ... 1682
▲ Risperdal M-Tab Orally Disintegrating Tablets (0.6% to 6%) ... 1676
Seroquel Tablets ... 690
▲ Zyprexa Tablets (8% to 20%) ... 1830
▲ Zyprexa IntraMuscular (2% to 4%) ... 1830
▲ Zyprexa ZYDIS Orally Disintegrating Tablets (8% to 20%) ... 1830

Parkinsonism, aggravation of
Lamictal ... 1481

Requip Tablets (1% or more) ... 1555
Risperdal ... 1676
Risperdal Consta Long-Acting Injection ... 1682
Risperdal M-Tab Orally Disintegrating Tablets ... 1676

Parkinson-like symptoms
Actimmune (Rare) ... 1671
Elspar for Injection (Rare) ... 2463
Elspar for Injection (Rare) ... 1960
Moban Tablets ... 1119
Oncaspar ... 1145

Parkinson's disease worsening
▲ Exelon Capsules (3%) ... 2206
▲ Exelon Oral Solution (3%) ... 2206

Paroniria
Allegra (Less than 1%) ... 2844
Celexa (Infrequent) ... 1176
Coreg Tablets (Greater than 0.1% to 1%) ... 1414
Evoxac Capsules (Less than 1%) ... 1047
Gengraf Capsules (1% to less than 3%) ... 459
▲ Imdur Tablets (Less than or equal to 5%) ... 3018
▲ Intron A for Injection (Less than 5%) ... 3024
Levaquin ... 2384
Levaquin in 5% Dextrose Injection ... 2384
Namenda (Infrequent) ... 1195
Neoral Oral Solution (1% to less than 3%) ... 2259
Neoral Soft Gelatin Capsules (1% to less than 3%) ... 2259
Razadyne (Infrequent) ... 2399
Razadyne ER Extended-Release Capsules (Infrequent) ... 2399
Risperdal Consta Long-Acting Injection (Infrequent) ... 1682
Zoloft (Infrequent) ... 2586
Zyrtec Chewable Tablets (Less than 2%) ... 2594
Zyrtec (Less than 2%) ... 2594
Zyrtec-D 12 Hour Extended Release Tablets (Less than 2%) ... 2597

Paronychia
Accutane Capsules ... 2731
Crixivan Capsules ... 1940
Evoxac Capsules (Less than 1%) ... 1047
▲ Soriatane Capsules (10% to 25%) ... 1013

Parosmia
Ambien Tablets (Rare) ... 2851
Ambien CR Tablets (Rare) ... 2855
Astelin Nasal Spray ... 1904
Avelox (Less than 0.1%) ... 2970
Axert Tablets (Rare) ... 2396
Caduet Tablets (Less than 2%) ... 2508
Chantix Tablets (Infrequent) ... 2517
Colazal Capsules ... 2838
Denavir Cream ... 2174
Doxil Injection (Less than 1%) ... 2351
Effexor Tablets (Infrequent) ... 3411
Effexor XR Capsules (Infrequent) ... 3417
Evoxac Capsules (Less than 1%) ... 1047
Flumadine (Less than 0.3%) ... 1183
Fortical Nasal Spray (Less than 1%) ... 3337
Gabitril Tablets (Infrequent) ... 984
▲ Intron A for Injection (Less than 5%) ... 3024
Lamictal (Rare) ... 1481
Levaquin (0.1% to 0.9%) ... 2384
Levaquin in 5% Dextrose Injection (0.1% to 0.9%) ... 2384
Lipitor Tablets (Less than 2%) ... 2483
Lyrica Capsules (Rare) ... 2539
Miacalcin Nasal Spray (Less than 1%) ... 2253
Nexium Delayed-Release Capsules (Less than 1%) ... 655
Nexium I.V. (Less than 1%) ... 659
Norvasc Tablets (Less than 0.1%) ... 2545
Norvir (Less than 2%) ... 503
Paxil CR Controlled-Release Tablets (Rare) ... 1538
Paxil (Rare) ... 1530
Pexeva Tablets (rare) ... 1694
Prevacid Delayed-Release Capsules (Less than 1%) ... 3271
Prevacid for Delayed-Release Oral Suspension (Less than 1%) ... 3271
Prevacid SoluTab Delayed-Release Orally Disintegrating Tablets (Less than 1%) ... 3271
Prevacid NapraPAC (Less than 1%) ... 3280
PREVPAC (Less than 1%) ... 3284
Prozac Pulvules and Liquid (Rare) ... 1801
Relpax Tablets (Rare) ... 2548
Rescriptor Tablets ... 2551

Sonata Capsules (Less than 1% to 2%) ... 1717
Sustiva Capsules (Less than 2%) ... 930
Sustiva Tablets (Less than 2%) ... 930
Tasmar Tablets (Infrequent) ... 3358
Tequin Injection (Less than 0.1%) ... 938
Tequin Injection in 5% Dextrose (Less than 0.1%) ... 938
Tequin Tablets (Less than 0.1%) ... 938
Topamax Sprinkle Capsules (Infrequent) ... 2404
Topamax Tablets (Infrequent) ... 2404
Zomig Tablets (Infrequent) ... 3519
Zomig Nasal Spray (Infrequent) ... 3523
Zomig-ZMT Tablets (Infrequent) ... 3519
Zonegran Capsules (Infrequent) ... 1101
Zyrtec Chewable Tablets (Less than 2%) ... 2594
Zyrtec (Less than 2%) ... 2594
Zyrtec-D 12 Hour Extended Release Tablets (Less than 2%) ... 2597

Parotid gland enlargement
Depacon Injection ... 412
Depakene ... 417
Depakote Sprinkle Capsules ... 422
Depakote Tablets ... 427
Depakote ER Tablets ... 434
Hyperstat I.V. ... 3017
Thalomid Capsules ... 965
Thioridazine Hydrochloride Tablets (Rare) ... 2163
VFEND I.V. (Less than 2%) ... 2564
VFEND Oral Suspension (Less than 2%) ... 2564
VFEND Tablets (Less than 2%) ... 2564

Parotitis
Catapres Tablets (Rare) ... 843
Clorpres Tablets (Rare) ... 2153
Effexor Tablets (Rare) ... 3411
Effexor XR Capsules (Rare) ... 3417
M-M-R II ... 2006
Mumpsvax (Very low) ... 2031
ProQuad ... 2064

Partial thromboplastin time, prolonged
Tygacil for Injection (0% to less than 2%) ... 3488

Partial thromboplastin time, accelerated
Menostar Transdermal System ... 782
Premphase Tablets ... 3456
▲ Prezista Tablets (4.3% to 7.8%) ... 3306

Partial thromboplastin time, decrease
Prempro Tablets ... 3456

Patent ductus arteriosus
Altace Capsules ... 1702
Captopril Tablets ... 2149
Cozaar Tablets ... 1935
Hyzaar 50-12.5 Tablets ... 1990
Hyzaar 100-12.5 Tablets ... 1990
Hyzaar 100-25 Tablets ... 1990
▲ Infasurf Intratracheal Suspension (45% to 47%) ... 1184
Lotrel Capsules ... 2249
Percodan Tablets ... 1132
Prinivil Tablets ... 2052
Prinzide Tablets ... 2056
Vasotec I.V. Injection ... 2103

PBI decrease
Dyazide Capsules ... 1423
Estratest Tablets ... 3199
Estratest H.S. Tablets ... 3199

Peeling, epidermal
Accutane Capsules ... 2731
Benzaclin Topical Gel (2%) ... 2877
▲ Brevoxyl-4 Creamy Wash (5 of 100 patients) ... 3210
▲ Brevoxyl-4 Gel (5 of 100 patients) ... 3210
▲ Brevoxyl-8 Creamy Wash (5 of 100 patients) ... 3210
▲ Brevoxyl-8 Gel (5 of 100 patients) ... 3210
Clindagel (0.6%) ... 1203
Cozaar Tablets (One subject) ... 1935
Hyzaar 50-12.5 Tablets (One subject) ... 1990
Hyzaar 100-12.5 Tablets (One subject) ... 1990
Hyzaar 100-25 Tablets (One subject) ... 1990
Imitrex Injection (Rare) ... 1463
Imitrex Nasal Spray (Rare) ... 1467
Lotrimin ... 3039
Lotrisone ... 3040

▲ Panretin Gel (3% to 9%) ... 1747
▲ Soriatane Capsules (50% to 75%) ... 1013

Pelger-Huet anomaly
Risperdal (Rare) ... 1676
Risperdal M-Tab Orally Disintegrating Tablets (Rare) ... 1676

Peliosis hepatis
Androxy Tablets (Rare) ... 3335
Estratest Tablets ... 3199
Estratest H.S. Tablets ... 3199
Oxandrin Tablets ... 2962

Pellagra-like syndrome
Trecator Tablets ... 3487

Pelvic inflammation
Gardasil Injection (0.02%) ... 1984
Lexapro Oral Solution (Infrequent) ... 1190
Lexapro Tablets (Infrequent) ... 1190

Pelvic inflammatory disease
Advair Diskus 100/50 ... 1308
Advair Diskus 250/50 ... 1308
Advair Diskus 500/50 ... 1308
Advair HFA Inhalation Aerosol ... 1318
Migranal Nasal Spray (Rare) ... 3348
Mirena Intrauterine System ... 787

Pelvic pressure
▲ MetroGel-Vaginal Gel (3%) ... 1855

Pemphigoid-like lesion
Captopril Tablets ... 2149
Parcopa Orally Disintegrating Tablets ... 3097
Timoptic Sterile Ophthalmic Solution ... 2088
Timoptic in Ocudose ... 2091
Timoptic-XE Sterile Ophthalmic Gel Forming Solution ... 2092

Pemphigus
Arthrotec Tablets (Rare) ... 3129
Cuprimine Capsules ... 1947
Lotensin Tablets (Less than 1%) ... 2243
Lotensin HCT Tablets (Rare) ... 2246
Lotrel Capsules (Rare) ... 2249
Mavik Tablets (0.3% to 1.0%) ... 486
Prinivil Tablets (0.3% to 1.0%) ... 2052
Prinzide Tablets ... 2056
Rituxan I.V. ... 1254
▲ Thiola Tablets (16.7%) ... 2141
Topamax Sprinkle Capsules ... 2404
Topamax Tablets ... 2404
Uniretic Tablets (Less than 1%) ... 3100
Univasc Tablets (Less than 1%) ... 3104
Vasotec I.V. Injection (0.5% to 1.0%) ... 2103

Pemphigus, bullous
Aceon Tablets (2 mg, 4 mg, 8 mg) ... 3194
Captopril Tablets ... 2149
Efudex (Infrequent) ... 3363
Soltamox Oral Solution (Very rare) ... 3527

Penile angulation
▲ Edex Injection (7%) ... 3089

Penile discharge, unspecified
Alferon N Injection (1%) ... 1665
▲ Edex Injection (3%) ... 3089
ProSom Tablets (Rare) ... 517

Penile disorder, unspecified
AndroGel (Fewer than 1%) ... 3329
▲ Caverject Impulse Injection (3%) ... 2612
▲ Edex Injection (3%) ... 3089
Eligard 30 mg (1.1%) ... 2885
Lamictal (2%) ... 1481
Norvir (Less than 2%) ... 503
Prevacid Delayed-Release Capsules (Less than 1%) ... 3271
Prevacid for Delayed-Release Oral Suspension (Less than 1%) ... 3271
Prevacid SoluTab Delayed-Release Orally Disintegrating Tablets (Less than 1%) ... 3271
Prevacid NapraPAC (Less than 1%) ... 3280
PREVPAC (Less than 1%) ... 3284
Requip Tablets (Infrequent) ... 1555
Soriatane Capsules (Less than 1%) ... 1013
Testim 1% Gel (1% or less) ... 695

Penile erection, decrease
Bumex Tablets (.1%) ... 2746

Penile erection, increase
(*see under* Priapism)

Penile erection, prolonged or inappropriate
Androxy Tablets ... 3335
Oxandrin Tablets ... 2962

Striant Mucoadhesive 1007
Viagra Tablets 2573

Penile erection, spontaneous
Cialis Tablets (Less than 2%) 1838

Penile head, discoloration of
▲ Caverject Impulse (3%) 2612

Penile shrinkage
Eligard 45 mg (1%) 2888

Penile skin tear
▲ Caverject Impulse Injection (3%) 2612

Penis, decreased sensation
Eldepryl Capsules 3208

Penis, enlargement
▲ Intron A for Injection (Less than or equal to 5%) 3024
Oxandrin Tablets 2962

Penis, fibrotic plaques
(*see under* Peyronie's disease)

Penis, strange feeling of
▲ Caverject Impulse Injection (3%) 2612

Penis, swollen
Neurontin Capsules (Rare) 2487
Neurontin Oral Solution (Rare) 2487
Neurontin Tablets (Rare) 2487

Perception of time and space, alterations in
Cesamet Capsules 3340

Perforation, cervix (total)
Omacor Capsules 2725

Perforation, gastrointestinal
Bayer Aspirin Comprehensive Prescribing Information .... ■796
Gleevec Tablets (Rare) 2227
Kionex Powder 2477
Nalfon Capsules 2502
St. Joseph 81 mg Aspirin .... ■688

Perforation, uterine wall
ParaGard T 380A 1073

Periarteritis nodosum
Fansidar Tablets 2765
Gantrisin Pediatric Suspension 2770
Phenytek Capsules 2160

Pericardial effusion
Activase I.V. 1223
Agrylin Capsules 3169
▲ CellCept Capsules (3% to less than 20%) 2747
▲ CellCept Intravenous (3% to less than 20%) 2747
▲ CellCept Oral Suspension (3% to less than 20%) 2747
▲ CellCept Tablets (3% to less than 20%) 2747
▲ Clolar for Intravenous Infusion (35%) 1271
Clozaril Tablets 2184
▲ Doxil Injection (1% to 5%) 2351
▲ Gleevec Tablets (2% to 16%) 2227
Herceptin I.V. (At least one of the 958 patients) 1233
▲ Humira Injection (Less than 5%) 466
I.V. Busulfex (2%) 2493
▲ Leukine (25%) 814
Neurontin Capsules (Rare) 2487
Neurontin Oral Solution (Rare) 2487
Neurontin Tablets (Rare) 2487
Nipent for Injection (Less than 3%) 1863
PEG-Intron Powder for Injection (Less than or equal to 1%) 3048
Permax Tablets (Rare) 3356
▲ Prograf Capsules and Injection (15%) 632
Proleukin for Injection (1%) 2266
Refludan for Injection 792
Remicade for IV Injection 971
ReoPro Vials (0.4%) 1809
Retavase 2499
Sonata Capsules (Rare) 1717
Tasmar Tablets 3358
Taxotere Injection Concentrate (Less frequent) 2932
TNKase I.V. 1264
Trasylol Injection (1% to 2%) 754
Vesanoid Capsules 2820
▲ Xeloda Tablets (Less than 5%) 2822

Pericardial rub
Neurontin Capsules (Rare) 2487
Neurontin Oral Solution (Rare) 2487
Neurontin Tablets (Rare) 2487

Pericarditis
Activase I.V. 1223
Agrylin Capsules 3169
Aldoril Tablets 1910
Asacol Delayed-Release Tablets (Rare) 2692
Campath Ampules 811
Canasa Rectal Suppositories (Rare) 699
Clozaril Tablets 2184
Colazal Capsules 2838
Evoxac Capsules (Less than 1%) 1047
▲ Humira Injection (Less than 5%) 466
Neurontin Capsules (Rare) 2487
Neurontin Oral Solution (Rare) 2487
Neurontin Tablets (Rare) 2487
Oracea Capsules 1000
Paser Granules 1674
Pentasa Capsules (Infrequent to less than 1%) 3185
Permax Tablets (Rare) 3356
Proleukin for Injection (Less than 1%) 2266
Retavase 2499
Rilutek Tablets (Infrequent) 2930
Rythmol SR Capsules 2727
Solodyn Extended Release Tablets 1890
Thalomid Capsules 965
TNKase I.V. 1264
▲ Trasylol Injection (5%) 754
▲ Vesanoid Capsules (3%) 2820

Pericarditis, allergic
Fansidar Tablets 2765

Perifollicular thickening
Thalomid Capsules 965

Periodontal destruction
Evoxac Capsules (Less than 1%) 1047

Periodontitis
▲ Coreg Tablets (Greater than 1% to 3%) 1414
Effexor Tablets (Rare) 3411
Effexor XR Capsules (Rare) 3417
Kaletra (Less than 2%) 476
Protonix I.V. (Less than 1%) 3472
Protonix Tablets (Less than 1%) 3469
Requip Tablets (Infrequent) 1555
Teveten Tablets (Less than 1%) 1735
Teveten HCT Tablets (Less than 1%) 1737
Thalomid Capsules 965
VFEND I.V. (Less than 2%) 2564
VFEND Oral Suspension (Less than 2%) 2564
VFEND Tablets (Less than 2%) 2564

Periosteal disorder, unspecified
▲ Neumega for Injection (11%) 3435
Thalomid Capsules 965

Periostitis
Bicillin C-R Injectable Suspension 1706

Peripheral nerve symptoms
▲ Reyataz Capsules (1% to 8%) 921

Peripheral vascular disease
Mirapex Tablets (Less than 1%) 859

Peripheral vascular disorder, unspecified
Actiq (Less than 1%) 979
Aricept Tablets (Infrequent) 1094
Aricept ODT Tablets (Infrequent) 1094
▲ Betaseron for SC Injection (6%) 767
Camptosar Injection 2604
Caverject Impulse Injection (Less than 1%) 2612
▲ CellCept Capsules (3% to less than 20%) 2747
▲ CellCept Intravenous (3% to less than 20%) 2747
▲ CellCept Oral Suspension (3% to less than 20%) 2747
▲ CellCept Tablets (3% to less than 20%) 2747
▲ Coreg Tablets (Greater than 1% to 3%) 1414
Effexor Tablets (Infrequent) 3411
Effexor XR Capsules (Infrequent) 3417
Gabitril Tablets (Infrequent) 984
Lofibra Tablets 1219
Lofibra Capsules 1216
Lotensin HCT Tablets (0.3% or more) 2246
Merrem I.V. (Greater than 1%) 686
Neurontin Capsules (Infrequent) 2487
Neurontin Oral Solution (Infrequent) 2487
Neurontin Tablets (Infrequent) 2487
Norvir (Less than 2%) 503
Omacor Capsules 2725
Paxil CR Controlled-Release Tablets (Infrequent) 1538
Paxil (Infrequent) 1530
▲ Prograf Capsules and Injection (3% to 15%) 632
Protopic Ointment (Greater than or equal to 1%) 638
Prozac Pulvules and Liquid (Rare) 1801
▲ Rapamune Oral Solution and Tablets (3% to 20%) 3475
Relpax Tablets (Infrequent) 2548
Rescriptor Tablets 2551
Rilutek Tablets (Infrequent) 2930
Rythmol SR Capsules 2727
Symbyax Capsules (Rare) 1819
Thalomid Capsules 965
Tricor Tablets 527
Triglide Tablets 3123
Uniretic Tablets (Less than 1%) 3100
▲ Visudyne for Injection (1% to 10%) 2305

Peripheral vascular instability
Strattera Capsules (Very Rare) 1814

Peripheral wasting
Aptivus Capsules 826
Combivir Tablets 1411
Crixivan Capsules 1940
Invirase 2772
Norvir 503
Retrovir 1560
Trizivir Tablets 1589
Truvada Tablets 1296
Viracept 2577
Viramune Oral Suspension 873
Viramune Tablets 873
Viread Tablets 1301
Ziagen 1626

Peritonitis
▲ Aranesp for Injection (27%) 581
Campath Ampules 811
▲ CellCept Capsules (3% to less than 20%) 2747
▲ CellCept Intravenous (3% to less than 20%) 2747
▲ CellCept Oral Suspension (3% to less than 20%) 2747
▲ CellCept Tablets (3% to less than 20%) 2747
Epogen for Injection 591
Exelon Capsules (Infrequent) 2206
Exelon Oral Solution (Infrequent) 2206
Neupogen for Injection (2%) 603
Paxil CR Controlled-Release Tablets (Rare) 1538
Paxil (Rare) 1530
Pexeva Tablets (Rare) 1694
▲ Photofrin for Injection (Less than 5%) 702
▲ Prograf Capsules and Injection (3% to 15%) 632
▲ Rapamune Oral Solution and Tablets (3% to 20%) 3475
Remicade for IV Injection (Greater than or equal to 0.2%) 971
Rilutek Tablets (Infrequent) 2930

Perleche
Neurontin Capsules (Rare) 2487
Neurontin Oral Solution (Rare) 2487
Neurontin Tablets (Rare) 2487

Personality changes
Ambien Tablets (Rare) 2851
Cardizem LA Extended Release Tablets (Less than 2%) 1728
Decadron Tablets 1951
▲ Depacon Injection (1% to 5%) 412
▲ Depakene (1% to 5%) 417
▲ Depakote Sprinkle Capsules (1% to 5%) 422
▲ Depakote Tablets (1% to 5%) 427
▲ Depakote ER Tablets (1% to 5%) 434
Eldepryl Capsules 3208
Enbrel for Injection 584
Evoxac Capsules 1047
Exelon Capsules (Infrequent) 2206
Exelon Oral Solution (Infrequent) 2206
Frova Tablets (Rare) 1113
Gabitril Tablets (Frequent) 984
Geodon for Injection (Up to 2%) 2529
Hydrocortone Tablets 1989
Imitrex Tablets (Rare) 1471
▲ Intron A for Injection (Less than 5%) 3024
▲ Keppra Oral Solution (8%) 3314
▲ Keppra Tablets (8%) 3314
Lamictal (Infrequent) 1481
▲ Lupron Depot 3.75 mg (Among most frequent) 3260
Lupron Depot–3 Month 11.25 mg (Less than 5%) 3265
Lupron Depot-PED 7.5 mg, 11.25 mg and 15 mg (Less than 2%) 3269
Lupron Injection Pediatric (Less than 2%) 3259
Nalfon Capsules (Less than 1%) 2502
Namenda (Infrequent) 1195
Neurontin Capsules (Rare) 2487
Neurontin Oral Solution (2.8%) 2487
Neurontin Tablets (Rare) 2487
Norvir (Less than 2%) 503
Permax Tablets (2.1%) 3356
Prometrium Capsules (100 mg, 200 mg) (Less than 5%) 3203
Prozac Pulvules and Liquid (At least 2%) 1801
Requip Tablets (Infrequent) 1555
Rilutek Tablets (Infrequent) 2930
Tiazac Capsules (Less than 2%) 1201
Topamax Sprinkle Capsules (Frequent) 2404
Topamax Tablets (Frequent) 2404
Trileptal Tablets 2300
Trileptal Oral Suspension 2300
▲ Zyprexa Tablets (8%) 1830
▲ Zyprexa ZYDIS Orally Disintegrating Tablets (8%) 1830

Personality disorder
Ambien CR Tablets (Rare) 2855
Azilect Tablets (Infrequent) 3293
Symbyax Capsules (1% to 2%) 1819
▲ Topamax Sprinkle Capsules (11%) 2404
▲ Topamax Tablets (11%) 2404
Zelapar Tablets 3372

Perspiration
(*see under* Diaphoresis)

Petechia at application site
Lidoderm Patch 1118

Petechiae
Abilify Oral Solution (Rare) 882
Abilify Oral Solution (Rare) 2450
Abilify Discmelt Orally Disintegrating Tablets (Rare) 882
Abilify Discmelt Orally Disintegrating Tablets (Rare) 2450
Abilify Tablets (Rare) 882
Abilify Tablets (Rare) 2450
AmBisome for Injection (Less common) 620
▲ Arranon Injection (0% to 12%) 1357
Caduet Tablets (Less than 2%) 2508
Cardizem LA Extended Release Tablets (Less than 2%) 1728
▲ CellCept Capsules (3% to less than 20%) 2747
▲ CellCept Intravenous (3% to less than 20%) 2747
▲ CellCept Oral Suspension (3% to less than 20%) 2747
▲ CellCept Tablets (3% to less than 20%) 2747
Cipro (Less than 1%) 2977
Cipro I.V. (1% or less) 2984
Cipro XR Tablets 2990
▲ Clolar for Intravenous Infusion (29%) 1271
Clozaril Tablets (Less than 1%) 2184
Colocort Rectal Suspension, USP (Retention) 100 mg/60 mL 2476
▲ Dacogen Injection (39%) 2129
▲ Depacon Injection (1% to 5%) 412
▲ Depakene (1% to 5%) 417
▲ Depakote Sprinkle Capsules (1% to 5%) 422
▲ Depakote Tablets (1% to 5%) 427
Depakote ER Tablets (Greater than 1%) 434
Depo-Medrol Injectable Suspension 2617
Depo-Medrol Single-Dose Vial 2619
Doxil Injection (Less than 1%) 2351
Engerix-B Vaccine (Less than 1%) 1425
FazaClo Orally Disintegrating Tablets (Less than 1%) 551
Gabitril Tablets (Infrequent) 984
▲ Gamunex Immune Globulin I.V., 10% (21%) 3235
▲ Gemzar for Injection (16%) 1771
▲ Gleevec Tablets (0.9% to 10%) 2227
Guanidine Hydrochloride Tablets 3016
Hydrocortone Tablets 1989
Indocin Capsules (Less than 1%) 1995
Indocin I.V. (Less than 1%) 2465
Indocin (Less than 1%) 1995
Lamictal (Rare to infrequent) 1481
▲ Leukine (6%) 814
▲ Leustatin Injection (8%) 2357
Lipitor Tablets (Less than 2%) 2483
Matulane Capsules 3191
Meridia Capsules 489
Migranal Nasal Spray (Infrequent) 3348
Mustargen for Injection 2468
▲ Mylotarg for Injection (1% to 20%) 3431
▲ Neupogen for Injection (17%) 603

Nipent for Injection (Less than 3%) 1863
Oncaspar (Less than 1%) 1145
Pediarix Vaccine 1548
Permax Tablets (Infrequent) 3356
Prilosec OTC Delayed-Release Tablets 2677
▲ Proleukin for Injection (4%) 2266
Proquin XR Tablets 1153
Prozac Pulvules and Liquid (Rare) 1801
Raptiva for Injection 1250
Recombivax HB 2071
ReoPro Vials (0.3%) 1809
Rescriptor Tablets 2551
Rilutek Tablets (Rare) 2930
Rythmol SR Capsules 2727
Sandostatin Injection (Less than 1%) 2278
Sandostatin LAR Depot (Rare) 2280
Sular Tablets (Less than or equal to 1%) 3122
Thalomid Capsules 965
Tiazac Capsules (Less than 2%) 1201
▲ Trisenox Injection (8%) 993
Twinrix Vaccine (Less than 1%) 1595
Uniretic Tablets (Less than 1%) 3100
VFEND I.V. (Less than 2%) 2564
VFEND Oral Suspension (Less than 2%) 2564
VFEND Tablets (Less than 2%) 2564
Zegerid Capsules 2958
Zegerid Powder for Oral Solution 2958
Zonegran Capsules (Rare) 1101

Petechiae, oral mucosal
▲ Dacogen Injection (13%) 2129

Petechiae and ecchymosis
Decadron Tablets 1951

Petechial hemorrhage
Carbatrol Capsules 3171
Tegretol/Tegretol-XR 2295

Peyronie's disease
Blocadren Tablets 1916
Cosopt Sterile Ophthalmic Solution 1931
Edex Injection (1%) 3089
Inderal LA Long-Acting Capsules (Rare) 3429
InnoPran XL Capsules (Rare) 2723
Lopressor Injection 2238
Lopressor Tablets 2238
Lopressor HCT 50/25 Tablets 2241
Lopressor HCT 100/25 Tablets 2241
Lopressor HCT 100/50 Tablets 2241
Nadolol Tablets 2159
Phenytek Capsules 2160
Requip Tablets (Rare) 1555
Timolide Tablets 2086
Timoptic Sterile Ophthalmic Solution 2088
Timoptic in Ocudose 2091
Timoptic-XE Sterile Ophthalmic Gel Forming Solution 2092
Toprol-XL Tablets (Fewer than 1 of 100,000 patients) 668

Pharyngeal discomfort
Cozaar Tablets (Less than 1%) 1935
FazaClo Orally Disintegrating Tablets (1%) 551
Hyzaar 50-12.5 Tablets 1990
Hyzaar 100-12.5 Tablets 1990
Hyzaar 100-25 Tablets 1990
Invanz for Injection (Greater than 0.1%) 1999
Nexium Delayed-Release Capsules (Less than 1%) 655
Nexium I.V. (Less than 1%) 659
Prinzide Tablets (0.3% to 1.0%) 2056

Pharyngeal secretion, increase
Xyrem Oral Solution (Infrequent) 1688

Pharyngitis
▲ Abilify Oral Solution (4%) 882
▲ Abilify Oral Solution (4%) 2450
▲ Abilify Discmelt Orally Disintegrating Tablets (4%) 882
▲ Abilify Discmelt Orally Disintegrating Tablets (4%) 2450
▲ Abilify Tablets (4%) 882
▲ Abilify Tablets (4%) 2450
▲ Aceon Tablets (2 mg, 4 mg, 8 mg) (3.3%) 3194
Acetadote Injection (1%) 1031
Actiq (1% or greater) 979
▲ Actonel Tablets (2.9% to 5.8%) 2683
▲ Actonel with Calcium Tablets (2.9% to 5.8%) 2688
▲ ActoPlus Met Tablets (5.1%) 3214
▲ Actos Tablets (5.1%) 3219
Adalat CC Tablets (Less than 1%) 2964
▲ Advair Diskus 100/50 (3% to 13%) 1308
▲ Advair Diskus 250/50 (3% to 13%) 1308
▲ Advair Diskus 500/50 (3% to 13%) 1308
Aerobid/Aerobid-M (1% to 3%) 1171
▲ Agrylin Capsules (6.8%) 3169
Aldara Cream, 5% (1.9%) 1846
Alferon N Injection (1%) 1665
▲ Alimta for Injection (Up to 28%) 1750
Alinia for Oral Suspension (Less than 1%) 2835
Alinia Tablets (Less than 1%) 2835
Aloprim for Injection (Less than 1%) 2167
Alphagan P Ophthalmic Solution (1% to 4%) 567
▲ Ambien Tablets (3%) 2851
Ambien CR Tablets (Frequent) 2855
AmBisome for Injection (Less common) 620
Amevive (Common) 626
Aralast (1.6%) 717
Aricept Tablets (Infrequent) 1094
Aricept ODT Tablets (Infrequent) 1094
▲ Arimidex Tablets (10% to 23%) 673
▲ Aromasin Tablets (2% to 5%) 2600
▲ Asacol Delayed-Release Tablets (11%) 2692
▲ Asmanex Twisthaler (8% to 13%) 2966
▲ Astelin Nasal Spray (3.8%) 1904
Atacand Tablets (2%) 649
Atacand HCT (0.5% or greater) 651
▲ Atrovent Inhalation Solution (3.7%) 835
▲ Atrovent Nasal Spray 0.03% (8.1%) 837
Atrovent Nasal Spray 0.06% (Less than 1%) 839
Avalide Tablets (1% or greater) 888
Avalide Tablets (1% or greater) 2874
Avapro Tablets (1% or greater) 891
Avapro Tablets (1% or greater) 2871
Axert Tablets (Infrequent) 2396
▲ Axid Oral Solution (3.3%) 879
▲ Azmacort Inhalation Aerosol (7% to 25%) 1726
Azopt Ophthalmic Suspension (Less than 1%) 557
Bactroban Nasal (0.5% to 4%) 1394
▲ Bexxar (0% to 12%) 1398
Boniva Injection (2.5%) 2738
Boniva Tablets (2.5%) 2741
▲ BOTOX Purified Neurotoxin Complex (3% to 10%) 570
Caduet Tablets (1.3% to 2.5%) 2508
▲ Campath Ampules (12%) 811
Campral Tablets (Frequent) 1174
▲ Carnitor Injection (15% to 27%) 3188
Celebrex Capsules (2.3%) 3134
Celexa (At least 2%) 1176
▲ CellCept Capsules (3% to less than 20%) 2747
▲ CellCept Intravenous (3% to less than 20%) 2747
▲ CellCept Oral Suspension (3% to less than 20%) 2747
▲ CellCept Tablets (3% to less than 20%) 2747
Cesamet Capsules 3340
Cialis Tablets (Less than 2%) 1838
▲ Clarinex Syrup (3.1% to 4.5%) 2995
▲ Clarinex Tablets (3% to 4.1%) 2995
▲ Clarinex Reditabs Tablets (3% to 4.1%) 2995
▲ Clarinex-D 24-Hour Extended-Release Tablets (3%) 2998
▲ Climara Transdermal System (0.5% to 7%) 771
Colazal Capsules (2%) 2838
Combivent Inhalation Aerosol (2.2%) 847
▲ Concerta Extended-Release Tablets (2% to 4%) 1881
Copaxone for Injection (At least 2%) 3297
Cosmegen for Injection 2459
▲ Cosopt Sterile Ophthalmic Solution (1% to 5%) 1931
Cozaar Tablets (1% or greater) 1935
▲ Crestor Tablets (9%) 678
Crixivan Capsules (Less than 2%) 1940
▲ Dacogen Injection (16%) 2129
▲ Depacon Injection (0.6% to 8%) 412
▲ Depakene (8%) 417
▲ Depakote Sprinkle Capsules (2% to 8%) 422
▲ Depakote Tablets (At least 5% to 8%) 427
▲ Depakote ER Tablets (2% to 8%) 434
▲ depo-subQ provera 104 Injectable Suspension (1% to less than 5%) 2624
Detrol Tablets (1.5%) 2628
Diovan Tablets (More than 1%) 2193
Diovan HCT Tablets (Less frequent) 2196
▲ Ditropan XL Extended-Release Tablets (2% to less than 5%) 2413
▲ Doxil Injection (Less than 1% to 15.9%) 2351
▲ Duetact Tablets (At least 5%) 3226
▲ DuoNeb Inhalation Solution (4.4%) 1058
Duragesic Transdermal System (1% or greater) 2373
Effexor Tablets 3411
▲ Effexor XR Capsules (7%) 3417
▲ Elestat Ophthalmic Solution (1% to 3%) 1669
▲ Elidel Cream 1% (0.9% to 8.1%) 2200
Elmiron Capsules (Less than or equal to 1%) 2415
▲ Eloxatin for Injection (2% to 9%) 2892
Emend Capsules (Greater than 0.5%) 1963
▲ Emsam Transdermal System (3%) 903
Enablex Extended-Release Tablets (Greater than or equal to 1%) 2203
▲ Enbrel for Injection (6% to 7%) 584
Epogen for Injection 591
▲ Equetro Extended-Release Capsules (Less than 5%) 3180
▲ Erbitux (3% to 26%) 910
Estring Vaginal Ring (1%) 2635
▲ Evista Tablets (5.3% to 7.6%) 1763
▲ Evoxac Capsules (5.2%) 1047
Exelon Capsules (2% or more) 2206
Exelon Oral Solution (2% or more) 2206
▲ Exubera Inhalation Powder (9.5% to 18.2%) 2524
▲ Fabrazyme for Intravenous Infusion (8%) 1274
Famvir Tablets (2.6% to 2.7%) 2211
▲ Faslodex Injection (16.1%) 681
▲ Ferrlecit Injection (6% to 12%) 3388
▲ Flomax Capsules (5.1% to 5.8%) 850
▲ Flonase Nasal Spray (6% to 7.8%) 1440
▲ Flovent HFA (1% to 3%) 1447
Floxin Otic Solution (Single report) 1049
Fluarix 1451
▲ Foradil Aerolizer (3.5%) 3010
▲ Forteo for Injection (5.5%) 1767
Fortical Nasal Spray (Less than 1%) 3337
Frova Tablets (Infrequent) 1113
▲ Gabitril Tablets (7%) 984
▲ Gamunex Immune Globulin I.V., 10% (0.8% to 41%) 3235
▲ Gemzar for Injection (22%) 1771
▲ Gengraf Capsules (4%) 459
▲ Geodon Capsules (3%) 2529
▲ Gleevec Tablets (0% to 15%) 2227
Havrix Vaccine (Less than 1%) 1456
Hepsera Tablets (2% or greater) 1292
▲ Herceptin I.V. (12%) 1233
▲ Humatrope Vials and Cartridges (3.13% to 6.67%) 1787
▲ Hycamtin for Injection (6%) 1458
Hytrin Capsules (At least 1%) 471
Hyzaar 50-12.5 Tablets (1% or greater) 1990
Hyzaar 100-12.5 Tablets (1% or greater) 1990
Hyzaar 100-25 Tablets (1% or greater) 1990
▲ Imdur Tablets (Less than or equal to 5%) 3018
▲ Indapamide Tablets (Less than 5%) 2156
Inderal LA Long-Acting Capsules 3429
▲ Infergen (17% to 34%) 3364
InnoPran XL Capsules 2723
▲ Intron A for Injection (1% to 31%) 3024
Invanz for Injection (0.7% to 1.1%) 1999
Invirase (Less than 2%) 2772
▲ Ionsys Transdermal System (1% to less than 10%) 2379
▲ I.V. Busulfex (18%) 2493
Kaletra (Less than 2%) 476
▲ Keppra Injection (6%) 3320
▲ Keppra Oral Solution (6% to 10%) 3314
▲ Keppra Tablets (6% to 10%) 3314
Klonopin (2%) 2778
▲ Lamictal (10% to 14%) 1481
▲ Lescol Capsules (3.8%) 2233
Lescol XL Tablets (2.4%) 2233
▲ Leukine (23%) 814
Levaquin (1.1%) 2384
Levaquin in 5% Dextrose Injection (1.1%) 2384
Levitra Tablets (Less than 2%) 3034
Lexapro Oral Solution (At least 2%) 1190
Lexapro Tablets (At least 2%) 1190
Lipitor Tablets (Up to 2.5%) 2483
Lofibra Tablets 1219
Lofibra Capsules 1216
▲ Lotemax Ophthalmic Suspension 0.5% (Less than 15%) ⊙ 251
Lotrel Capsules 2249
Lunesta Tablets 3142
Maxalt Tablets (Infrequent) 2008
Maxalt-MLT Orally Disintegrating Tablets (Infrequent) 2008
▲ Megace ES Oral Suspension (1% to 3%) 2481
▲ Meridia Capsules (10%) 489
Merrem I.V. (Greater than 1%) 686
Miacalcin Nasal Spray (Less than 1%) 2253
Micardis Tablets (1%) 854
Micardis HCT Tablets (Less than 2%) 856
▲ Migranal Nasal Spray (3%) 3348
Mirapex Tablets (Greater than or equal to 1%) 859
▲ Mobic Oral Suspension (0.6% to 3.2%) 863
▲ Mobic Tablets (0.6% to 3.2%) 863
▲ Mylotarg for Injection (10% to 14%) 3431
▲ Myozyme for Intravenous Infusion (36%) 1279
▲ Nasacort AQ Nasal Spray (5.1%) 2922
▲ Nasonex Nasal Spray (10 % to 12%) 3043
▲ Neoral Oral Solution (4%) 2259
▲ Neoral Soft Gelatin Capsules (4%) 2259
▲ Neumega for Injection (25%) 3435
Neurontin Capsules (1.2% to 2.8%) 2487
Neurontin Oral Solution (1.2% to 2.8%) 2487
Neurontin Tablets (1.2% To 2.8%) 2487
Nexium Delayed-Release Capsules (Less than 1%) 655
Nexium I.V. (Less than 1%) 659
▲ Nipent for Injection (8% to 10%) 1863
Norvir (0.4% to 2.6%) 503
Omacor Capsules 2725
▲ Ontak Vials (17%) 1745
OxyContin Tablets (Less than 1%) 2703
▲ Patanol Ophthalmic Solution (Less than 5%) 561
Paxil CR Controlled-Release Tablets (2.1%) 1538
Paxil (2.1%) 1530
▲ PEG-Intron Powder for Injection (10%) 3048
Permax Tablets (Frequent) 3356
▲ Photofrin for Injection (11%) 702
▲ Pletal Tablets (7% to 10%) 2455
▲ Premarin Tablets (10% to 12%) 3446
▲ Premphase Tablets (8% to 13%) 3456
▲ Prempro Tablets (8% to 13%) 3456
Prevacid Delayed-Release Capsules (Less than 1%) 3271
Prevacid for Delayed-Release Oral Suspension (Less than 1%) 3271
Prevacid SoluTab Delayed-Release Orally Disintegrating Tablets (Less than 1%) 3271
Prevacid NapraPAC (Less than 1%) 3280
Prevnar for Injection 3463
PREVPAC (Less than 1%) 3284
Prilosec OTC Delayed-Release Tablets (1%) 2677
Prinivil Tablets (0.3% to 1.0%) 2052
Prinzide Tablets 2056
▲ ProAir HFA Inhalation Aerosol (14%) 3300
Prochieve 4% Gel 1003
Prochieve 8% Gel 1003
▲ Prograf Capsules and Injection (3% to 15%) 632
Prometrium Capsules (100 mg, 200 mg) (Less than 5%) 3203
ProQuad (Greater than or equal to 0.2% to less than 1%) 2064
ProSom Tablets (1%) 517
Protonix I.V. (Greater than or equal to 1%) 3472
Protonix Tablets (Greater than or equal to 1%) 3469
▲ Protopic Ointment (3% to 12%) 638
Proventil Inhalation Solution 0.083% (Less than 1%) 3055
▲ Provigil Tablets (4%) 988
▲ Prozac Pulvules and Liquid (3% to 11%) 1801
▲ Pulmozyme Inhalation Solution (32% to 40%) 1248
Quixin Ophthalmic Solution (1% to 3%) 3383
▲ Qvar Inhalation Aerosol (8% to 27%) 3303
▲ Rapamune Oral Solution and Tablets (16% to 21%) 3475
▲ Rebetol (12% to 13%) 3058
Recombivax HB (Equal to or greater than 1%) 2071
ReFacto Vials 3484
Relpax Tablets (Frequent) 2548
▲ Remicade for IV Injection (12%) 971
▲ Requip Tablets (6%) 1555

▲ Rescriptor Tablets (1.6% to 5%) 2551
Retrovir Capsules 1560
Retrovir IV Infusion 1564
Retrovir 1560
▲ Revlimid Capsules (15.5%) 958
▲ Rhinocort Aqua Nasal Spray (4%) 665
▲ Ribavirin, USP Capsules (12% to 13%) 3068
▲ Risperdal (2% to 3%) 1676
▲ Risperdal M-Tab Orally Disintegrating Tablets (2% to 3%) 1676
▲ Sandostatin LAR Depot (5% to 15%) 2280
▲ Serevent Diskus (3% to 6%) 1568
▲ Seroquel Tablets (Frequent to 4%) ... 690
▲ Simulect for Injection (3% to 10%) ... 2284
Singulair (Greater than or equal to 2%) 2077
Soriatane Capsules (Less than 1%).. 1013
▲ Spiriva HandiHaler (7% to 9%) 869
▲ Suboxone Tablets (4%) 2717
▲ Subutex Tablets (4%) 2717
Sular Tablets (Less than 1% to 5%) .. 3122
▲ Symbyax Capsules (4% to 6%) 1819
▲ Symlin Injection (3% to 5%) 613
Synagis (2.6%) 1897
Targretin Capsules 1747
Tasmar Tablets (Frequent) 3358
▲ Temodar Capsules (8%) 3073
▲ Tequin Injection (0.1% to 3%) 938
▲ Tequin Injection in 5% Dextrose (0.1% to 3%) 938
▲ Tequin Tablets (0.1% to 3%) 938
▲ Teveten Tablets (4%) 1735
Teveten HCT Tablets (Less than 1%) 1737
▲ Thalomid Capsules (4.2%) 965
▲ Thiola Tablets (16.7%) 2141
▲ Tiazac Capsules (3%) 1201
Tindamax Tablets (Rare) 2142
▲ TOBI Solution for Inhalation (38.1%) 2298
▲ Topamax Sprinkle Capsules (2% to 6%) 2404
▲ Topamax Tablets (2% to 6%) 2404
Trelstar LA Suspension (1.1%) 3397
Tricor Tablets 527
▲ Trileptal Tablets (Up to 3%) 2300
▲ Trileptal Oral Suspension (Up to 3%) 2300
Trizivir Tablets 1589
Ultane Liquid for Inhalation (Less than 1%) 531
Uniretic Tablets (More than 1%) 3100
Univasc Tablets (1.8%) 3104
Uroxatral Tablets (1% to 2%) 2943
▲ Valcyte Tablets (Less than 5%) 2813
Vandazole Vaginal Gel (2%) 3338
Vaqta (Up to 2.7%) 2097
Varivax 2100
▲ Verelan PM Extended-Release Capsules, Controlled-Onset (3%) 3106
VESIcare Tablets (0.3% to 1.1%) 646
VFEND I.V. (Less than 2%) 2564
VFEND Oral Suspension (Less than 2%) 2564
VFEND Tablets (Less than 2%) 2564
Viagra Tablets (Less than 2%) 2573
Vicoprofen Tablets (Less than 3%) ... 539
▲ Vigamox Ophthalmic Solution (1% to 4%) 564
Viracept (Less than 2%) 2577
▲ Visudyne for Injection (1% to 10%) .. 2305
▲ Vivitrol (11% to 17%) 995
Vytorin 10/10 Tablets 2114
Vytorin 10/10 Tablets 3077
Vytorin 10/20 Tablets 2114
Vytorin 10/20 Tablets 3077
Vytorin 10/40 Tablets 2114
Vytorin 10/40 Tablets 3077
Vytorin 10/80 Tablets 2114
Vytorin 10/80 Tablets 3077
▲ WelChol Tablets (3%) 1050
▲ Wellbutrin SR Sustained-Release Tablets (3% to 11%) 1607
▲ Wellbutrin XL Extended-Release Tablets (3% to 11%) 1613
Xifaxan Tablets (Less than 2%) 2842
▲ Xolair (11%) 1266
▲ Xopenex Inhalation Solution (10.4%) 3146
▲ Xopenex Inhalation Solution Concentrate (3% to 10.4%) 3150
▲ Xopenex HFA Inhalation Aerosol (10.4%) 3154
Xyrem Oral Solution (Infrequent) 1688
Yasmin 28 Tablets (Greater than 1%) 796
Yaz Tablets (Greater than 1%) 803
Zegerid Capsules (1%) 2958
Zegerid Powder for Oral Solution (1%) 2958
▲ Zelapar Tablets (4%) 3372
Zelnorm Tablets (1%) 2312
▲ Zetia Tablets (2.3% to 3.1%) 2120
▲ Zetia Tablets (2.3% to 3.1%) 3083
Ziagen 1626
▲ Zoloft (4%) 2586
Zomig Nasal Spray (Infrequent) 3523
Zonegran Capsules (Frequent) 1101
Zosyn (1.0% or less) 3492
▲ Zyban Sustained-Release Tablets (3%) 1644
▲ Zyprexa Tablets (5%) 1830
▲ Zyprexa ZYDIS Orally Disintegrating Tablets (5%) 1830
▲ Zyrtec Chewable Tablets (2% to 6.2%) 2594
▲ Zyrtec (2% to 6.2%) 2594
▲ Zyrtec-D 12 Hour Extended Release Tablets (2% to 6.2%) 2597
Zyvox (0.5% to 2.9%) 2652

Pharyngitis, streptococcal
Clobex Spray (0% to 1%) 1208
▲ Elidel Cream 1% (Up to 3%) 2200
▲ Vivitrol (11% to 17%) 995

Pharyngolaryngeal pain
▲ Cymbalta Delayed-Release Capsules (1% to 6%) 1757
▲ Gleevec Tablets (0% to 16.9%) 2227
▲ Symbicort 80/4.5 Inhalation Aerosol (6.1%) 3511
▲ Symbicort 160/4.5 Inhalation Aerosol (8.9%) 3511

Pharyngoxerosis
Carbatrol Capsules 3171
Tegretol/Tegretol-XR 2295

Pharynix, dryness of
Equetro Extended-Release Capsules 3180

Phimosis
▲ Caverject Impulse Injection (3%) 2612

Phlebitis
Abilify Oral Solution (Infrequent) 882
Abilify Oral Solution (Infrequent) 2450
Abilify Discmelt Orally Disintegrating Tablets (Infrequent) 882
Abilify Discmelt Orally Disintegrating Tablets (Infrequent) 2450
Abilify Tablets (Infrequent) 882
Abilify Tablets (Infrequent) 2450
Adalat CC Tablets (Less than 1%) 2964
Ambien Tablets (Rare) 2851
Ambien CR Tablets (Rare) 2855
Anzemet Injection (Rare) 2859
Anzemet Tablets (Rare) 2862
Arthrotec Tablets (Rare) 3129
Azilect Tablets (Infrequent) 3293
BeneFIX Vials (1.5%) 3408
Caduet Tablets (Less than 2%) 2508
Campath Ampules 811
Campral Tablets (Infrequent) 1174
▲ Cancidas for Injection (3.5% to 15.7%) 1918
Celexa (Rare) 1176
▲ CellCept Intravenous (4%) 2747
Cipro (Less than 1%) 2977
Cipro XR Tablets 2990
Clozaril Tablets (Less than 1%) 2184
Cymbalta Delayed-Release Capsules (Infrequent) 1757
Dantrium Capsules (Less frequent) .. 2694
Doxil Injection (Less than 1%) 2351
Eraxis for Injection (0.7%) 2521
Evoxac Capsules (Less than 1%) 1047
FazaClo Orally Disintegrating Tablets (Less than 1%) 551
Ferrlecit Injection 3388
Fluorescite Injection .... ⊙207
Fortaz (1 in 69 patients) 1453
Gabitril Tablets (Infrequent) 984
Geodon Capsules (Rare) 2529
Humate-P (2%) 3502
Imitrex Injection 1463
Imitrex Nasal Spray (Rare) 1467
Imitrex Tablets 1471
Infed Injection 3390
▲ Intron A for Injection (Less than or equal to 5%) 3024
Invanz for Injection (Greater than 0.5% to 1.9%) 1999
Leustatin Injection (2%) 2357
Levaquin (0.1% to 0.9%) 2384
Levaquin in 5% Dextrose Injection (0.1% to 0.9%) 2384
Lipitor Tablets (Less than 2%) 2483
Lithostat Tablets 2140
Lofibra Tablets 1219
Lofibra Capsules 1216
Maxipime for Injection (1.3%) 1105
Merrem I.V. (0.8%) 686
Mivacron Injection (Less than 1%) 493
▲ Mycamine for Injection (1.6% to 4.2%) 628
Neurontin Capsules (Rare) 2487
Neurontin Oral Solution (Rare) 2487
Neurontin Tablets (Rare) 2487
Nipent for Injection (Less than 3%) ... 1863
NovoSeven 2331
Panhematin for Injection 2473
Parcopa Orally Disintegrating Tablets 3097
Paxil CR Controlled-Release Tablets (Rare) 1538
Paxil (Rare) 1530
Pexeva Tablets (Rare) 1694
Premarin Intravenous 3442
▲ Primaxin I.V. (3.1%) 2048
▲ Prograf Capsules and Injection (3% to 15%) 632
▲ Proleukin for Injection (23%) 2266
Proquin XR Tablets 1153
Prozac Pulvules and Liquid (Rare) 1801
Requip Tablets (Infrequent) 1555
Retrovir Capsules (1.6%) 1560
Retrovir IV Infusion (2%) 1564
Retrovir (1.6%) 1560
Rilutek Tablets (0.4% to 0.8%) 2930
Risperdal (Rare) 1676
Risperdal Consta Long-Acting Injection (Infrequent) 1682
Risperdal M-Tab Orally Disintegrating Tablets (Rare) 1676
Rocephin Injectable Vials, ADD-Vantage, Galaxy, Bulk (Less than 1%) 2800
▲ Sandostatin LAR Depot (1% to 4%) 2280
Soltamox Oral Solution (0.4%) 3527
Stalevo Tablets 2287
Taxotere Injection Concentrate 2932
Topamax Sprinkle Capsules (Infrequent) 2404
Topamax Tablets (Infrequent) 2404
Trasylol Injection (1.0%) 754
Tricor Tablets 527
Triglide Tablets 3123
Tygacil for Injection (1.8%) 3488
▲ Vaprisol (4.9%) 643
▲ Vesanoid Capsules (11%) 2820
VFEND I.V. (Less than 2%) 2564
VFEND Oral Suspension (Less than 2%) 2564
VFEND Tablets (Less than 2%) 2564
Wellbutrin Tablets (Rare) 1603
Wellbutrin SR Sustained-Release Tablets 1607
Wellbutrin XL Extended-Release Tablets 1613
▲ Xeloda Tablets (Less than 5%) 2822
▲ Zinecard for Injection (3% to 6%) 2650
Zosyn (1.3%) 3492
Zyban Sustained-Release Tablets 1644

Phlebitis, injection site
Avelox (0.1% to less than 2%) 2970
Tygacil for Injection (0% to less than 2%) 3488
▲ Vaprisol (15.80%) 643

Phobia, unspecified
Cipro XR Tablets 2990
Imitrex Injection 1463
Proquin XR Tablets 1153

Phobic disorder
Cipro (Less than 1%) 2977
Cipro I.V. (1% or less) 2984
Imitrex Tablets (Rare) 1471
Zyprexa Tablets (Infrequent) 1830
Zyprexa ZYDIS Orally Disintegrating Tablets (Infrequent) 1830

Phocomelia
Thalomid Capsules 965

Phonophobia
Imitrex Tablets (Frequent) 1471

Phosphate metabolism, disorders of
Lotronex Tablets (Rare) 1512

Phosphaturia
Daranide Tablets 1950

Phospholipid concentration, increase
Estratest Tablets 3199
Estratest H.S. Tablets 3199

Phosphorus, decrease
Actonel with Calcium Tablets (2.7%) 2688
Maxipime for Injection (2.8%) 1105
Omnicef Capsules (0.3%) 511
Omnicef for Oral Suspension (0.4%) 511
Thalomid Capsules 965

Photodermatitis
Advair HFA Inhalation Aerosol 1318
Atripla Tablets 945
Serevent Diskus (1% to 2%) 1568

Photodermatosis
Advair Diskus 100/50 1308
Advair Diskus 250/50 1308
Advair Diskus 500/50 1308

Photophobia
Abilify Oral Solution (Rare) 882
Abilify Oral Solution (Rare) 2450
Abilify Discmelt Orally Disintegrating Tablets (Rare) 882
Abilify Discmelt Orally Disintegrating Tablets (Rare) 2450
Abilify Tablets (Rare) 882
Abilify Tablets (Rare) 2450
Accutane Capsules 2731
▲ Alphagan P Ophthalmic Solution (1% to 4%) 567
▲ Alrex Ophthalmic Suspension 0.2% (5% to 15%) .... ⊙246
Amerge Tablets (Frequent) 1339
▲ Betimol Ophthalmic Solution (More than 5%) 3382
▲ Betimol Ophthalmic Solution (More than 5%) .... ⊙295
Betoptic S Ophthalmic Suspension (Small number of patients) 558
BOTOX Purified Neurotoxin Complex 570
▲ Brimonidine Tartrate Ophthalmic Solution 0.2% (3% to 9%) .... ⊙248
Calcijex Injection 411
Campral Tablets (Rare) 1174
Carteolol Hydrochloride Ophthalmic Solution USP, 1% (Occasional) .... ⊙249
Celexa (Infrequent) 1176
Cesamet Capsules 3340
Chantix Tablets (Rare) 2517
Ciloxan Ophthalmic Ointment (Less than 1%) 559
Ciloxan Ophthalmic Solution (Less than 1%) .... ⊙206
Copaxone for Injection (Infrequent) ... 3297
Cosopt Sterile Ophthalmic Solution (Less than 1%) 1931
CytoGam Intravenous (Infrequent) 1895
Depakote ER Tablets (Greater than 1%) 434
Effexor Tablets (Infrequent) 3411
Effexor XR Capsules (Infrequent) 3417
Gabitril Tablets (Infrequent) 984
Geodon Capsules (Infrequent) 2529
Havrix Vaccine (Less than 1%) 1456
Hectorol Capsules 1275
Hectorol Injection 1278
▲ Imdur Tablets (Less than or equal to 5%) 3018
Imitrex Injection (Infrequent) 1463
Imitrex Tablets (Frequent) 1471
▲ Intron A for Injection (Less than 5%) 3024
Lacrisert Sterile Ophthalmic Insert ... 2005
Lamictal (Infrequent) 1481
Levitra Tablets (Less than 2%) 3034
▲ Lotemax Ophthalmic Suspension 0.5% (5% to 15%) .... ⊙251
Lotronex Tablets (Rare) 1512
▲ Lumigan Ophthalmic Solution (1% to 3%) 573
Lunesta Tablets (Rare) 3142
Lyrica Capsules (0.1% to 1%) 2539
Matulane Capsules 3191
Maxalt Tablets (Rare) 2008
Maxalt-MLT Orally Disintegrating Tablets (Rare) 2008
Migranal Nasal Spray (Infrequent) 3348
Neurontin Capsules (Infrequent) 2487
Neurontin Oral Solution (Infrequent) 2487
Neurontin Tablets (Infrequent) 2487
▲ Nevanac Ophthalmic Suspension 0.1% (1% to 5%) .... ⊙209
Nipent for Injection (Less than 3%) ... 1863
Norvir (Less than 2%) 503
OptiPranolol Metipranolol Ophthalmic Solution 0.3% (A small number of patients) .... ⊙256
▲ Orthoclone OKT3 Sterile Solution (10%) 2360

Paxil CR Controlled-Release Tablets (Rare) 1538
Paxil (Rare) 1530
Permax Tablets (Infrequent) 3356
Pexeva Tablets (Rare) 1694
Photofrin for Injection 702
Prevacid Delayed-Release Capsules (Less than 1%) 3271
Prevacid for Delayed-Release Oral Suspension (Less than 1%) 3271
Prevacid SoluTab Delayed-Release Orally Disintegrating Tablets (Less than 1%) 3271
Prevacid NapraPAC (Less than 1%) 3280
PREVPAC (Less than 1%) 3284
Prinivil Tablets (0.3% to 1.0%) 2052
Prinzide Tablets 2056
Prograf Capsules and Injection 632
ProSom Tablets (Infrequent) 517
Prozac Pulvules and Liquid (Infrequent) 1801
▲ Quixin Ophthalmic Solution (1% to 3%) 3383
Relpax Tablets (Infrequent) 2548
Requip Tablets (Infrequent) 1555
Rescriptor Tablets 2551
▲ Retisert Implant (5% to 9%) ⊙258
Retrovir Capsules 1560
Retrovir IV Infusion 1564
Retrovir 1560
Rilutek Tablets (Rare) 2930
Risperdal (Rare) 1676
Risperdal M-Tab Orally Disintegrating Tablets (Rare) 1676
Rocaltrol Capsules 2798
Rocaltrol Oral Solution 2798
Sonata Capsules (Infrequent) 1717
▲ Soriatane Capsules (1% to 10%) 1013
Tambocor Tablets (Less than 1%) 1856
Tequin Injection (Less than 0.1%) 938
Tequin Injection in 5% Dextrose (Less than 0.1%) 938
Tequin Tablets (Less than 0.1%) 938
Topamax Sprinkle Capsules (Infrequent) 2404
Topamax Tablets (Infrequent) 2404
▲ Travatan Ophthalmic Solution (1% to 4%) 563
Trileptal Tablets 2300
Trileptal Oral Suspension 2300
▲ Trusopt Sterile Ophthalmic Solution (Approximately 1% to 5%) 2095
Twinrix Vaccine (Less than 1%) 1595
▲ VFEND I.V. (1.7% to 21%) 2564
▲ VFEND Oral Suspension (1.7% to 21%) 2564
▲ VFEND Tablets (1.7% to 21%) 2564
Viagra Tablets (Less than 2%) 2573
Visine For Contacts Rewetting Drops ⊙289
▲ Xalatan Sterile Ophthalmic Solution (1% to 4%) 2649
Zoloft (Rare) 2586
Zomig Nasal Spray (Rare) 3523
Zonegran Capsules (Rare) 1101
Zosyn (1.0% or less) 3492

Photopsia

Ambien Tablets (Rare) 2851
Ambien CR Tablets (Rare) 2855
Cymbalta Delayed-Release Capsules (Infrequent) 1757
Evoxac Capsules (Less than 1%) 1047
▲ Macugen Injection (6% to 10%) ⊙261
Maxalt Tablets (Rare) 2008
Maxalt-MLT Orally Disintegrating Tablets (Rare) 2008
▲ Retisert Implant (5% to 9%) ⊙258
Risperdal (Rare) 1676
Risperdal M-Tab Orally Disintegrating Tablets (Rare) 1676

Photosensitivity

Abilify Oral Solution (Infrequent) 882
Abilify Oral Solution (Infrequent) 2450
Abilify Discmelt Orally Disintegrating Tablets (Infrequent) 882
Abilify Discmelt Orally Disintegrating Tablets (Infrequent) 2450
Abilify Tablets (Infrequent) 882
Abilify Tablets (Infrequent) 2450
Accutane Capsules 2731
Aciphex Tablets 1090
▲ Agrylin Capsules (1% to 5%) 3169
Aldoril Tablets 1910
Alferon N Injection (1%) 1665
Altace Capsules (Less than 1%) 1702
Altoprev Extended-Release Tablets (Rare) 3109
Ambien Tablets (Rare) 2851
Amerge Tablets (Rare) 1339
Anaprox Tablets (Less than 1%) 2761
Anaprox DS Tablets (Less than 1%) 2761
Arthrotec Tablets (Rare) 3129
Atacand HCT 651
Avalide Tablets 888
Avalide Tablets 2874
Axert Tablets (Rare) 2396
▲ Azmacort Inhalation Aerosol (1% to 3%) 1726
Caduet Tablets (Less than 2%) 2508
Captopril Tablets 2149
Carbatrol Capsules 3171
Cardizem LA Extended Release Tablets (Less than 2%) 1728
Celebrex Capsules (0.1% to 1.9%) 3134
Celexa (Infrequent) 1176
Cesamet Capsules 3340
Cipro (Less than 1%) 2977
Cipro I.V. (1% or less) 2984
Cipro XR Tablets (Less than 1%) 2990
Clindagel 1203
Clinoril Tablets (Less than 1 in 100) 1924
Clorpres Tablets 2153
Clozaril Tablets 2184
Copaxone for Injection (Infrequent) 3297
Coreg Tablets (Greater than 0.1% to 1%) 1414
Cozaar Tablets (Less than 1%) 1935
Dantrium Capsules 2694
Depacon Injection 412
Depakene 417
Depakote Sprinkle Capsules 422
Depakote Tablets 427
Depakote ER Tablets 434
Diovan HCT Tablets 2196
Diuril Oral Suspension 1954
Diuril Sodium Intravenous 2467
Dolobid Tablets (Less than 1 in 100) 1955
Dyazide Capsules 1423
Dyrenium Capsules (Rare) 3400
EC-Naprosyn Delayed-Release Tablets (Less than 1%) 2761
Effexor Tablets (Infrequent) 3411
Effexor XR Capsules (Infrequent) 3417
▲ Efudex (Among most frequent) 3363
Eldepryl Capsules 3208
Elmiron Capsules (Less than or equal to 1%) 2415
Eulexin Capsules 3009
Evoxac Capsules (Less than 1%) 1047
Fansidar Tablets 2765
FazaClo Orally Disintegrating Tablets 551
Fosamax (Occasional) 1969
Furosemide Tablets 2154
Gabitril Tablets (Infrequent) 984
Gantrisin Pediatric Suspension 2770
Geodon Capsules (Frequent) 2529
Gleevec Tablets (Infrequent) 2227
Gris-PEG Tablets (Occasional) 2502
Hyzaar 50-12.5 Tablets 1990
Hyzaar 100-12.5 Tablets 1990
Hyzaar 100-25 Tablets 1990
Imitrex Injection 1463
Imitrex Nasal Spray 1467
Imitrex Tablets 1471
Indapamide Tablets 2156
▲ Intron A for Injection (Less than 5%) 3024
Invirase (Less than 2%) 2772
Lamictal (2%) 1481
Lescol Capsules (Rare) 2233
Lescol XL Tablets 2233
Lipitor Tablets (Less than 2%) 2483
Lofibra Tablets 1219
Lofibra Capsules 1216
Lopressor Injection (Very rare) 2238
Lopressor Tablets (Very rare) 2238
Lopressor HCT 50/25 Tablets (Very rare) 2241
Lopressor HCT 100/25 Tablets (Very rare) 2241
Lopressor HCT 100/50 Tablets (Very rare) 2241
Lotensin Tablets (Less than 1%) 2243
Lotensin HCT Tablets (0.3% or more) 2246
Lunesta Tablets (Infrequent) 3142
Lupron Depot 3.75 mg 3260
Lupron Depot 7.5 mg 3264
Lupron Depot–3 Month 11.25 mg 3265
Lupron Injection Pediatric 3259
Malarone Pediatric Tablets 1517
Malarone Tablets 1517
Maxalt Tablets (Infrequent) 2008
Maxalt-MLT Orally Disintegrating Tablets (Infrequent) 2008
Meridia Capsules 489
Mevacor Tablets (Rare) 2021
Micardis HCT Tablets 856
Mobic Oral Suspension (Less than 2%) 863
Mobic Tablets (Less than 2%) 863
Moduretic Tablets 2028
Naprosyn Suspension (Less than 1%) 2761
Naprosyn Tablets (Less than 1%) 2761
Neurontin Capsules (Rare) 2487
Neurontin Oral Solution (Rare) 2487
Neurontin Tablets (Rare) 2487
Nipent for Injection (Less than 3%) 1863
Noroxin Tablets 2032
Norvir (Less than 2%) 503
Paxil CR Controlled-Release Tablets (Rare) 1538
Paxil (Rare) 1530
Pentasa Capsules (Less than 1%) 3185
Pexeva Tablets (infrequent) 1694
Phenergan Tablets and Suppositories 3440
▲ Photofrin for Injection (19% to 68%) 702
Polytrim Ophthalmic Solution 574
Prinivil Tablets (0.3% to 1.0%) 2052
Prinzide Tablets 2056
▲ Prograf Capsules and Injection (3% to 15%) 632
ProSom Tablets (Rare) 517
Protopic Ointment (Greater than or equal to 1%) 638
Prozac Pulvules and Liquid (Rare) 1801
Rapamune Oral Solution and Tablets 3475
Requip Tablets (Infrequent) 1555
Reyataz Capsules (Less than 3%) 921
Rilutek Tablets (Infrequent) 2930
Risperdal (Frequent) 1676
Risperdal M-Tab Orally Disintegrating Tablets (Frequent) 1676
Seroquel Tablets (Infrequent) 690
Solodyn Extended Release Tablets 1890
Sonata Capsules (Less than 1%) 1717
Soriatane Capsules (Less than 1%) 1013
Sular Tablets (One case) 3122
Targretin Capsules 1747
Tegretol/Tegretol-XR 2295
Tequin Injection (Less than 0.1%) 938
Tequin Injection in 5% Dextrose (Less than 0.1%) 938
Tequin Tablets (Less than 0.1%) 938
Teveten HCT Tablets 1737
Thalomid Capsules 965
Thioridazine Hydrochloride Tablets (Extremely rare) 2163
Thiothixene Capsules 2165
Tiazac Capsules (Less than 2%) 1201
Timolide Tablets 2086
Topamax Sprinkle Capsules (Infrequent) 2404
Topamax Tablets (Infrequent) 2404
Toprol-XL Tablets 668
Trecator Tablets (Rare) 3487
Tricor Tablets 527
Triglide Tablets 3123
Trileptal Tablets 2300
Trileptal Oral Suspension 2300
Tygacil for Injection 3488
Uniretic Tablets (Less than 1%) 3100
Univasc Tablets (Less than 1%) 3104
Valtrex Caplets 1597
Vasotec I.V. Injection (0.5% to 1.0%) 2103
VFEND I.V. (Less than 2%) 2564
VFEND Oral Suspension (Less than 2%) 2564
VFEND Tablets (Less than 2%) 2564
Viagra Tablets (Less than 2%) 2573
▲ Visudyne for Injection (1% to 10%) 2305
Voltaren Tablets (Occasionally) 2307
Voltaren-XR Tablets (Occasionally) 2310
Vytorin 10/10 Tablets 2114
Vytorin 10/10 Tablets 3077
Vytorin 10/20 Tablets 2114
Vytorin 10/20 Tablets 3077
Vytorin 10/40 Tablets 2114
Vytorin 10/40 Tablets 3077
Vytorin 10/80 Tablets 2114
Vytorin 10/80 Tablets 3077
Wellbutrin SR Sustained-Release Tablets (Infrequent) 1607
Wellbutrin XL Extended-Release Tablets (Infrequent) 1613
▲ Xeloda Tablets (Less than 5%) 2822
Zegerid Capsules 2958
Zegerid Powder for Oral Solution 2958
Zmax for Oral Suspension 2583
Zocor Tablets (Rare) 2105
Zoloft (Infrequent) 2586
Zomig Tablets (Infrequent) 3519
Zomig-ZMT Tablets (Infrequent) 3519
Zovirax 1643
Zyban Sustained-Release Tablets (Infrequent) 1644
Zyprexa Tablets (Infrequent) 1830
Zyprexa ZYDIS Orally Disintegrating Tablets (Infrequent) 1830
Zyrtec Chewable Tablets (Less than 2%) 2594
Zyrtec (Less than 2%) 2594
Zyrtec-D 12 Hour Extended Release Tablets (Less than 2%) 2597

Photosensitivity, cutaneous

Agrylin Capsules 3169
Fosamax Plus D Tablets 1977

Photosensitivity reaction

Adalat CC Tablets (Less than 1%) 2964
▲ Adderall XR Capsules (2% to 4%) 3166
Aldara Cream, 5% (0.9%) 1846
Ambien CR Tablets (Rare) 2855
Avandaryl Tablets 1379
Azilect Tablets (Infrequent) 3293
BeneFix Vials (1.6%) 3408
Campral Tablets (Rare) 1174
Chantix Tablets (Rare) 2517
Crestor Tablets (Less than 1%) 678
Cymbalta Delayed-Release Capsules (Infrequent) 1757
Duetact Tablets (Less than 1%) 3226
▲ Equetro Extended-Release Capsules (Less than 5%) 3180
Levitra Tablets (Less than 2%) 3034
Lupron Depot-PED 7.5 mg, 11.25 mg and 15 mg 3269
Lyrica Capsules (0.1% to 1%) 2539
Protonix I.V. (Less than 1%) 3472
Raptiva for Injection 1250
Risperdal Consta Long-Acting Injection (Infrequent) 1682
Symbyax Capsules (Frequent) 1819

Phototoxicity

Avelox (Less than 0.1%) 2970
Cipro 2977
Cipro XR Tablets 2990
Dapsone Tablets USP 1673
Levaquin (Less than 0.1%) 2384
Levaquin in 5% Dextrose Injection (Less than 0.1%) 2384
Noroxin Tablets 2032
PEG-Intron Powder for Injection (Less than or equal to 1%) 3048
Protonix Tablets (Less than 1%) 3469
Zyrtec Chewable Tablets (Less than 2%) 2594
Zyrtec (Less than 2%) 2594
Zyrtec-D 12 Hour Extended Release Tablets (Less than 2%) 2597

Physical performance, impairment

Adipex-P 1215
Clozaril Tablets 2184
Dilaudid Ampules 440
Dilaudid Non-Sterile Powder 440
Dilaudid Rectal Suppositories 440
Dilaudid Tablets 440
Gris-PEG Tablets (Occasional) 2502
Hycodan 1116
Hycotuss Expectorant Syrup 1117
Kadian Capsules 577
MS Contin Tablets 2701
Percocet Tablets 1131
Percodan Tablets 1132
Phenergan Tablets and Suppositories 3440
Tussionex Pennkinetic Extended-Release Suspension 3327
Tylenol with Codeine Tablets 2391
Vicodin Tablets 535
Vicodin ES Tablets 536
Vicodin HP Tablets 538
Zydone Tablets 1139

Pigmentation

Copaxone for Injection (Infrequent) 3297
Cosmegen for Injection 2459
Cosopt Sterile Ophthalmic Solution 1931
Genotropin Lyophilized Powder (Infrequent) 2638
Risperdal (Frequent) 1676
Risperdal M-Tab Orally Disintegrating Tablets (Frequent) 1676
Solodyn Extended Release Tablets 1890
Timolide Tablets (Less than 1%) 2086
Timoptic Sterile Ophthalmic Solution 2088
Timoptic in Ocudose 2091
Timoptic-XE Sterile Ophthalmic Gel Forming Solution 2092

Pigmentation changes at application site
Clobex Spray (0% to 1%) 1208

Pigmentation disorders
Accutane Capsules 2731
Carbatrol Capsules 3171
Equetro Extended-Release Capsules 3180
Gengraf Capsules (1% to less than 3%) 459
Gleevec Tablets (Infrequent) 2227
Neoral Oral Solution (1% to less than 3%) 2259
Neoral Soft Gelatin Capsules (1% to less than 3%) 2259
Retrovir Capsules 1560
Retrovir IV Infusion 1564
Retrovir 1560
Tegretol/Tegretol-XR 2295
▲ Tri-Luma Cream (2% to 4.04%) 1213
▲ Xalatan Sterile Ophthalmic Solution (5% to 15%) 2649

Pill rolling motion
Thioridazine Hydrochloride Tablets 2163
Thiothixene Capsules 2165

Piloerection
▲ ProAmatine Tablets (13.4%) 3186
▲ Ultram ER Tablets (1% to greater than 5%) 2392

Pituitary apoplexy
Lupron Depot 3.75 mg (Rare) 3260
Lupron Injection Pediatric 3259
Sandostatin Injection (Less than 1%) 2278
Trelstar Depot (Rare) 3394
Trelstar LA Suspension (Rare) 3397
Viadur Implant (Rare) 757

Pituitary tumors
Imitrex Nasal Spray (Rare) 1467

Pituitary unresponsiveness, secondary
Colocort Rectal Suspension, USP (Retention) 100 mg/60 mL 2476
Decadron Tablets 1951
Depo-Medrol Injectable Suspension 2617
Depo-Medrol Single-Dose Vial 2619
Hydrocortone Tablets 1989

Plantar fasciitis
Effexor Tablets (Rare) 3411
Effexor XR Capsules (Rare) 3417
Evoxac Capsules (Less than 1%) 1047

Plasma testosterone level, reduction
Zocor Tablets 2105

Plasminogen, increase
Premarin Tablets 3446
Premphase Tablets 3456
Prempro Tablets 3456

Platelet, decrease
(*see under* Thrombocytopenia)

Platelet, increase
(*see under* Thrombocytosis)

Platelet aggregation decrease
Arthrotec Tablets 3129

Platelet aggregation time, decrease
Menostar Transdermal System 782
Premarin Tablets 3446
Premphase Tablets 3456
Prempro Tablets 3456

Platelet disorder, unspecified
Levaquin (0.1% to 0.9%) 2384
Levaquin in 5% Dextrose Injection (0.1% to 0.9%) 2384
Prevacid NapraPAC 3280
Zelapar Tablets 3372
Zoloft (Rare) 2586

Platelet function, alterations in
Arthrotec Tablets 3129

Pleural disorder, unspecified
Prevacid Delayed-Release Capsules (Less than 1%) 3271
Prevacid for Delayed-Release Oral Suspension (Less than 1%) 3271
Prevacid SoluTab Delayed-Release Orally Disintegrating Tablets (Less than 1%) 3271
Prevacid NapraPAC (Less than 1%) 3280
PREVPAC (Less than 1%) 3284

Pleural effusion
Abelcet Injection 1141
Actiq (Less than 1%) 979
Activase I.V. 1223
Agrylin Capsules 3169
▲ AmBisome for Injection (12.5%) 620
▲ Aredia for Injection (10.7%) 2179
▲ Arranon Injection (1% to 10%) 1357
Avandaryl Tablets 1379
Avandia Tablets 1384
Bexxar 1398
Campath Ampules 811
▲ CellCept Capsules (3% to 34.3%) 2747
▲ CellCept Intravenous (3% to 34.3%) 2747
▲ CellCept Oral Suspension (3% to 34.3%) 2747
▲ CellCept Tablets (3% to 34.3%) 2747
Cipro I.V. (1% or less) 2984
Cipro XR Tablets 2990
Clinoril Tablets (Less than 1 in 100) 1924
▲ Clolar for Intravenous Infusion (10%) 1271
Clozaril Tablets 2184
▲ Cubicin for Injection (5.8%) 1026
▲ Doxil Injection (1% to 10%) 2351
Evoxac Capsules (Less than 1%) 1047
FazaClo Orally Disintegrating Tablets 551
Femara Tablets (Less frequent) 2214
Follistim AQ Cartridge 2338
▲ Gleevec Tablets (3% to 15%) 2227
Herceptin I.V. 1233
▲ Humira Injection (Less than 5%) 466
Invanz for Injection (Greater than 0.1%) 1999
▲ I.V. Busulfex (3%) 2493
Leukine 814
Levaquin (0.1% to 0.9%) 2384
Levaquin in 5% Dextrose Injection (0.1% to 0.9%) 2384
▲ Macugen Injection (1% to 5%) ⊙ 261
Matulane Capsules 3191
Merrem I.V. (Greater than 0.1% to 1%) 686
▲ Neumega for Injection (10%) 3435
Permax Tablets (Rare to infrequent) 3356
▲ Photofrin for Injection (13% to 32%) 702
Prinivil Tablets (0.3% to 1.0%) 2052
Prinzide Tablets 2056
▲ Prograf Capsules and Injection (30% to 36%) 632
▲ Proleukin for Injection (7%) 2266
Proquin XR Tablets 1153
▲ Rapamune Oral Solution and Tablets (3% to 20%) 3475
Remicade for IV Injection (Greater than or equal to 0.2%) 971
ReoPro Vials (1.3%) 1809
Revlimid Capsules (1.4%) 958
Rilutek Tablets (Infrequent) 2930
Rythmol SR Capsules 2727
▲ Sandostatin LAR Depot (1% to 4%) 2280
Sonata Capsules (Rare) 1717
Stalevo Tablets (Rare) 2287
Sular Tablets (Less than or equal to 1%) 3122
Targretin Capsules 1747
Tasmar Tablets (Rare) 3358
▲ Taxotere Injection Concentrate (6%) 2932
Thalomid Capsules 965
▲ Trasylol Injection (7%) 754
▲ Trisenox Injection (20%) 993
▲ Valcyte Tablets (Less than 5%) 2813
Vantin Tablets and Oral Suspension (Less than 1%) 2645
▲ Vesanoid Capsules (20%) 2820
VFEND I.V. (Less than 2%) 2564
VFEND Oral Suspension (Less than 2%) 2564
VFEND Tablets (Less than 2%) 2564
Xeloda Tablets (1% to 2%) 2822
Zelapar Tablets 3372
▲ Zometa for Intravenous Infusion (5% to 10%) 2315
Zosyn (1.3%) 3492

Pleural effusion, exacerbation of
Neumega for Injection 3435

Pleural effusion with pericarditis
Dantrium Capsules (Less frequent) 2694

Pleural thickening
Stalevo Tablets (Rare) 2287

Pleuralgia
▲ Intron A for Injection (Less than 5%) 3024

Pleurisy
▲ Aerobid/Aerobid-M (1% to 3%) 1171
Aricept Tablets (Infrequent) 1094
Aricept ODT Tablets (Infrequent) 1094
Campath Ampules 811
Chantix Tablets (Rare) 2517
Effexor Tablets (Rare) 3411
Effexor XR Capsules (Rare) 3417
Evoxac Capsules (Less than 1%) 1047
Klonopin (Infrequent) 2778
Remicade for IV Injection (Greater than or equal to 0.2%) 971
ReoPro Vials (1.3%) 1809
Requip Tablets (Infrequent) 1555
Trileptal Tablets 2300
Trileptal Oral Suspension 2300

Pleuritis
Amerge Tablets (Rare) 1339
Asacol Delayed-Release Tablets 2692
Permax Tablets (Rare) 3356
Rituxan I.V. 1254

Pneumocystis carinii
Campath Ampules 811
▲ CellCept Capsules (Less than 4%) 2747
▲ CellCept Intravenous (Less than 4%) 2747
CellCept Oral Suspension (Less than 4%) 2747
▲ CellCept Tablets (Less than 4%) 2747
Cutivate Lotion 0.05% (Rare) 2664

Pneumocystis carinii, susceptibility
▲ Doxil Injection (9.2%) 2351
▲ Orthoclone OKT3 Sterile Solution (3.1%) 2360

Pneumocytosis
Remicade for IV Injection 971

Pneumonia
Abilify Oral Solution (Frequent) 882
Abilify Oral Solution (Frequent) 2450
Abilify Discmelt Orally Disintegrating Tablets (Frequent) 882
Abilify Discmelt Orally Disintegrating Tablets (Frequent) 2450
Abilify Tablets (Frequent) 882
Abilify Tablets (Frequent) 2450
Actiq (Less than 1%) 979
▲ Actonel Tablets (0.8% to 3.1%) 2683
▲ Actonel with Calcium Tablets (0.8% to 3.1%) 2688
▲ Advair Diskus 100/50 (1% to 3%) 1308
▲ Advair Diskus 250/50 (1% to 3%) 1308
▲ Advair Diskus 500/50 (1% to 3%) 1308
Advair HFA Inhalation Aerosol 1318
▲ Aerobid/Aerobid-M (1% to 3%) 1171
▲ Agrylin Capsules (1% to 5%) 3169
Ambien Tablets (Rare) 2851
Ambien CR Tablets (Rare) 2855
AmBisome for Injection (Less common) 620
Amerge Tablets (Infrequent) 1339
Amevive 626
Anaprox Tablets (Less than 1%) 2761
Anaprox DS Tablets (Less than 1%) 2761
▲ Aranesp for Injection (27%) 581
▲ Argatroban Injection (3.3%) 1346
Aricept Tablets (Infrequent) 1094
Aricept ODT Tablets (Infrequent) 1094
Arixtra Injection (2.3%) 1351
▲ Arranon Injection (1% to 8%) 1357
Arthrotec Tablets (Rare) 3129
▲ Atripla Tablets (Greater than or equal to 5%) 945
Betaseron for SC Injection 767
▲ Bexxar (0% to 6%) 1398
▲ Boniva Injection (5.9%) 2738
▲ Boniva Tablets (5.9%) 2741
Caduet Tablets (Less than 2%) 2508
▲ Campath Ampules (10% to 16%) 811
Campral Tablets (Infrequent) 1174
▲ Camptosar Injection (1.3% to 3.6%) 2604
Carbatrol Capsules 3171
Celebrex Capsules (0.1% to 1.9%) 3134
Celexa (Infrequent) 1176
▲ CellCept Capsules (3% to less than 20%) 2747
▲ CellCept Intravenous (3% to less than 20%) 2747
▲ CellCept Oral Suspension (3% to less than 20%) 2747
▲ CellCept Tablets (3% to less than 20%) 2747
▲ Clolar for Intravenous Infusion (10%) 1271
Clozaril Tablets (Less than 1%) 2184
Combivent Inhalation Aerosol (1.4%) 847
Comvax 1928
Copaxone for Injection (Infrequent) 3297
▲ Copegus Tablets (3% to 5%) 2754
Crestor Tablets (Greater than or equal to 1%) 678
▲ Cubicin for Injection (3.3%) 1026
▲ Dacogen Injection (22%) 2129
▲ Depacon Injection (1% to 5%) 412
▲ Depakene (1% to 5%) 417
▲ Depakote Sprinkle Capsules (1% to 5%) 422
▲ Depakote Tablets (1% to 5%) 427
Depakote ER Tablets (1%) 434
▲ Doxil Injection (1% to 10%) 2351
DuoNeb Inhalation Solution 1058
EC-Naprosyn Delayed-Release Tablets (Less than 1%) 2761
Effexor Tablets (Infrequent) 3411
Effexor XR Capsules (Infrequent) 3417
Elidel Cream 1% (0.3% to 1.5%) 2200
Elitek (Less than or equal to 1%) 2890
▲ Eloxatin for Injection (2% to 5%) 2892
Enbrel for Injection 584
Equetro Extended-Release Capsules 3180
Evista Tablets (2.6%) 1763
▲ Evoxac Capsules (1% to 3%) 1047
Exubera Inhalation Powder (0.9%) 2524
FazaClo Orally Disintegrating Tablets 551
Ferrlecit Injection 3388
Flovent Diskus 1443
Flovent HFA 1447
Fluarix 1451
Flumist Vaccine 1901
▲ Forteo for Injection (3.9%) 1767
Fortical Nasal Spray (Less than 1%) 3337
Fuzeon Injection (2.7%) 2767
Gabitril Tablets (Frequent) 984
▲ Gengraf Capsules (1% to 6.2%) 459
Geodon Capsules (Infrequent) 2529
▲ Gleevec Tablets (1% to 13%) 2227
▲ Humira Injection (Less than 5%) 466
Hycamtin for Injection (2%) 1458
▲ Imdur Tablets (Less than or equal to 5%) 3018
Intron A for Injection (Rare) 3024
Invanz for Injection (2.1%) 1999
▲ Invirase (Less than 2% to 5.4%) 2772
Ionsys Transdermal System (.1% to less than 1%) 2379
I.V. Busulfex 2493
Kineret Injection 599
Klonopin (Infrequent) 2778
Lamictal (Rare) 1481
▲ Leustatin Injection (6%) 2357
Levaquin (0.1% to 0.9%) 2384
Levaquin in 5% Dextrose Injection (0.1% to 0.9%) 2384
Lexapro Oral Solution (Infrequent) 1190
Lexapro Tablets (Infrequent) 1190
Lipitor Tablets (Less than 2%) 2483
Lofibra Tablets 1219
Lofibra Capsules 1216
Lopressor HCT 50/25 Tablets 2241
Lopressor HCT 100/25 Tablets 2241
Lopressor HCT 100/50 Tablets 2241
Lovenox Injection (0.82%) 2915
Megace ES Oral Suspension (0% to 2%) 2481
Merrem I.V. (Greater than 1%) 686
Miacalcin Nasal Spray (Less than 1%) 2253
Mirapex Tablets (Less than 1% to 2%) 859
Mycamine for Injection 628
▲ Myfortic Tablets (3% to less than 20%) 2255
Myleran Tablets 1525
▲ Mylotarg for Injection (8% to 13%) 3431
Myobloc Injection (Greater than 2%) 3192
▲ Myozyme for Intravenous Infusion (46%) 1279
Namenda (Frequent) 1195
Naprosyn Suspension (Less than 1%) 2761
Naprosyn Tablets (Less than 1%) 2761
▲ Neoral Oral Solution (1% to 6.2%) 2259
▲ Neoral Soft Gelatin Capsules (1% to 6.2%) 2259
Neumega for Injection (Frequent) 3435
Neurontin Capsules (Frequent) 2487
Neurontin Oral Solution (Frequent) 2487
Neurontin Tablets (Frequent) 2487
▲ Nipent for Injection (5%) 1863

NovoSeven (1%) 2331
Omacor Capsules 2725
Omnicef Capsules 511
Omnicef for Oral Suspension 511
▲ Orencia Powder for Intravenous Infusion (0.2% to 5%) 914
Orthoclone OKT3 Sterile Solution 2360
Paxil CR Controlled-Release Tablets (Infrequent) 1538
Paxil (Infrequent) 1530
▲ Pegasys (3% to 5%) 2789
PEG-Intron Powder for Injection 3048
Permax Tablets (Frequent) 3356
Pexeva Tablets (Infrequent) 1694
▲ Photofrin for Injection (18%) 702
Plavix Tablets (1% to 2.5%) 917
Plavix Tablets (1% to 2.5%) 2926
Pletal Tablets (Less than 2%) 2455
Prevacid Delayed-Release Capsules (Less than 1%) 3271
Prevacid for Delayed-Release Oral Suspension (Less than 1%) 3271
Prevacid SoluTab Delayed-Release Orally Disintegrating Tablets (Less than 1%) 3271
Prevacid NapraPAC (Less than 1%) 3280
Prevnar for Injection 3463
PREVPAC (Less than 1%) 3284
Prinivil Tablets (0.3% to 1.0%) 2052
Prinzide Tablets 2056
▲ Prograf Capsules and Injection (3% to 15%) 632
Proleukin for Injection 2266
ProQuad 2064
Protonix I.V. (Less than 1%) 3472
Protonix Tablets (Less than 1%) 3469
Protopic Ointment (1% to 2%) 638
Provigil Tablets (At least 1%) 988
Pulmicort Respules 661
Pulmozyme Inhalation Solution 1248
Quadramet Injection (1.5%) 1040
▲ Rapamune Oral Solution and Tablets (3% to 20%) 3475
Raptiva for Injection 1250
Rebetol 3058
Rebetron Combination Therapy 3063
▲ Refludan for Injection (4.4%) 792
Remicade for IV Injection 971
ReoPro Vials (1.0%) 1809
Rescriptor Tablets 2551
▲ Revlimid Capsules (7.4% to 11.5%) 958
Rilutek Tablets (More than 2%) 2930
Risperdal (Infrequent) 1676
Risperdal Consta Long-Acting Injection (Infrequent) 1682
Risperdal M-Tab Orally Disintegrating Tablets (Infrequent) 1676
RotaTeq (0.2%) 2074
▲ Sandimmune (6.2% to 9.2%) 2275
Sandostatin Injection (Less than 1%) 2278
▲ Sandostatin LAR Depot (1% to 4%) 2280
Seroquel Tablets (Infrequent) 690
▲ Simulect for Injection (3% to 10%) 2284
Singulair (Greater than or equal to 2%) 2077
Sonata Capsules (Infrequent) 1717
Symbyax Capsules (Infrequent) 1819
Synagis (More than 1%) 1897
Tamiflu Capsules (Less than 1%) 2807
Tamiflu Oral Suspension (2%) 2807
Tasmar Tablets (1% or more) 3358
Tegretol/Tegretol-XR 2295
Testim 1% Gel 695
Thalomid Capsules 965
▲ Topamax Sprinkle Capsules (Greater than 1% to 5%) 2404
▲ Topamax Tablets (Greater than 1% to 5%) 2404
Toprol-XL Tablets (Greater than 1%) 668
▲ Trasylol Injection (4%) 754
Tricor Tablets 527
Trileptal Tablets (1% to 2%) 2300
Trileptal Oral Suspension (1% to 2%) 2300
Truvada Tablets 1296
▲ Ultram ER Tablets (1% to greater than 5%) 2392
Uniretic Tablets (Less than 1%) 3100
Vantin Tablets and Oral Suspension (Less than 1%) 2645
Vaprisol (2.7%) 643
Vaqta 2097
Varivax 2100
Vasotec I.V. Injection (1.0%) 2103
▲ Velcade for Injection (10%) 2133
▲ Ventavis Inhalation Solution (4%) 1020
▲ Vesanoid Capsules (14%) 2820
VFEND I.V. (Less than 2%) 2564
VFEND Oral Suspension (Less than 2%) 2564
VFEND Tablets (Less than 2%) 2564
Vicoprofen Tablets (Less than 1%) 539
Virazole for Inhalation Solution 3370
▲ Viread Tablets (2% to 5%) 1301
▲ Visudyne for Injection (1% to 10%) 2305
Vivitrol 995
Voltaren Tablets (Rarely) 2307
Voltaren-XR Tablets (Rarely) 2310
Wellbutrin Tablets (Rare) 1603
Wellbutrin SR Sustained-Release Tablets 1607
Wellbutrin XL Extended-Release Tablets 1613
▲ Xeloda Tablets (Less than 5%) 2822
Xyrem Oral Solution (Infrequent) 1688
Zantac 1624
Zantac Injection 1619
Zantac Injection Pharmacy Bulk Package 1622
Zantac Injection Premixed 1619
Zantac 1624
Zelapar Tablets 3372
▲ Zemplar Capsules (5%) 541
▲ Zemplar Injection (5%) 543
▲ Ziagen (4%) 1626
Zomig Nasal Spray (Rare) 3523
Zyban Sustained-Release Tablets 1644
Zyrtec Chewable Tablets (Less than 2%) 2594
Zyrtec (Less than 2%) 2594
Zyrtec-D 12 Hour Extended Release Tablets (Less than 2%) 2597
Zyvox (0% to 2.8%) 2652

Pneumonia, aspiration
Abilify Oral Solution (Infrequent) 882
Abilify Oral Solution (Infrequent) 2450
Abilify Discmelt Orally Disintegrating Tablets (Infrequent) 882
Abilify Discmelt Orally Disintegrating Tablets (Infrequent) 2450
Abilify Tablets (Infrequent) 882
Abilify Tablets (Infrequent) 2450
Namenda 1195
Neurontin Capsules (Rare) 2487
Neurontin Oral Solution (Rare) 2487
Neurontin Tablets (Rare) 2487

Pneumonia, eosinophilic
▲ Asacol Delayed-Release Tablets (5% or greater) 2692
Eloxatin for Injection 2892
Omnicef Capsules 511
Omnicef for Oral Suspension 511
Prozac Pulvules and Liquid 1801

Pneumonia, fungal
Arranon Injection 1357

Pneumonia, interstitial
Aciphex Tablets 1090
Leukeran Tablets 1504
Norvir (Less than 2%) 503
Omnicef Capsules 511
Omnicef for Oral Suspension 511
Pletal Tablets (Very rare) 2455
Tarceva Tablets 1259
Tarceva Tablets 2444
Taxotere Injection Concentrate 2932

Pneumonia, nosocomial
Zegerid Capsules (1.2%) 2958
Zegerid Powder for Oral Solution (1.2%) 2958

Pneumonia, pneumocystis carinii
Revlimid Capsules 958
Temodar Capsules (Rare) 3073
Thalomid Capsules 965

Pneumonia, tuberculous
Raptiva for Injection 1250

Pneumonia-like symptoms
FazaClo Orally Disintegrating Tablets (Less than 1%) 551

Pneumonitis
Aldoril Tablets 1910
Atacand HCT 651
Attenuvax 1914
Avalide Tablets 888
Avalide Tablets 2874
▲ Campath Ampules (13% to 21%) 811
Carbatrol Capsules 3171
Celexa (Rare) 1176
Clinoril Tablets (Less than 1 in 100) 1924
Cosmegen for Injection 2459
Diovan HCT Tablets 2196
Diuril Oral Suspension 1954
Diuril Sodium Intravenous 2467
Emend Capsules (Greater than 0.5%) 1963
Gantrisin Pediatric Suspension 2770
Herceptin I.V. (Rare) 1233
Hyzaar 50-12.5 Tablets 1990
Hyzaar 100-12.5 Tablets 1990
Hyzaar 100-25 Tablets 1990
Indapamide Tablets 2156
Intron A for Injection (Rare) 3024
Lotensin HCT Tablets 2246
Matulane Capsules 3191
Micardis HCT Tablets 856
M-M-R II 2006
Moduretic Tablets 2028
Orthoclone OKT3 Sterile Solution 2360
PEG-Intron Powder for Injection (Less than or equal to 1%) 3048
Photofrin for Injection 702
Prinzide Tablets 2056
▲ Prometrium Capsules (100 mg, 200 mg) (Less than 5%) 3203
ProQuad 2064
Rapamune Oral Solution and Tablets (Infrequent) 3475
Rebetol 3058
Rebetron Combination Therapy 3063
Revlimid Capsules (1.4%) 958
Rituxan I.V. 1254
Rocephin Injectable Vials, ADD-Vantage, Galaxy, Bulk (Rare) 2800
Tarceva Tablets 1259
Tarceva Tablets 2444
Taxotere Injection Concentrate (Rare) 2932
Tegretol/Tegretol-XR 2295
Teveten HCT Tablets 1737
Timolide Tablets 2086
Uniretic Tablets 3100
Varivax (Less than 1%) 2100

Pneumonitis, allergic
Dyazide Capsules 1423
Equetro Extended-Release Capsules 3180
Levaquin 2384
Levaquin in 5% Dextrose Injection 2384
Rocephin Injectable Vials, ADD-Vantage, Galaxy, Bulk (Rare) 2800
Ticlid Tablets (Rare) 2810

Pneumonitis, eosinophilic
Aceon Tablets (2 mg, 4 mg, 8 mg) 3194
Anaprox Tablets (Less than 1%) 2761
Anaprox DS Tablets (Less than 1%) 2761
Captopril Tablets 2149
EC-Naprosyn Delayed-Release Tablets (Less than 1%) 2761
Lotensin HCT Tablets 2246
Lotrel Capsules 2249
Naprosyn Suspension (Less than 1%) 2761
Naprosyn Tablets (Less than 1%) 2761
Prevacid NapraPAC (Less than 1%) 3280
Prinivil Tablets 2052
Prinzide Tablets 2056
Raptiva for Injection 1250
Uniretic Tablets 3100
Univasc Tablets (Less than 1%) 3104
Vasotec I.V. Injection 2103

Pneumonitis, interstitial
Actimmune (Rare) 1671
Alkeran for Injection 955
Alkeran Tablets 956
Aredia for Injection (One case) 2179
Asacol Delayed-Release Tablets 2692
Cuprimine Capsules (Rare) 1947
Gleevec Tablets (Rare) 2227
Pegasys 2789
PEG-Intron Powder for Injection 3048
Plavix Tablets 917
Plavix Tablets 2926
Raptiva for Injection 1250
Remicade for IV Injection 971
Rituxan I.V. 1254
Soltamox Oral Solution (Very rare) 3527

Pneumonitis, radiation
Tarceva Tablets 1259
Tarceva Tablets 2444

Pneumonitis, hypersensitivity
Pentasa Capsules (Infrequent) 3185

Pneumothorax
Actiq (Less than 1%) 979
Arranon Injection 1357
Campath Ampules 811
▲ CellCept Capsules (3% to less than 20%) 2747
▲ CellCept Intravenous (3% to less than 20%) 2747
▲ CellCept Oral Suspension (3% to less than 20%) 2747
▲ CellCept Tablets (3% to less than 20%) 2747
Doxil Injection (Less than 1%) 2351
Herceptin I.V. (At least one of the 958 patients) 1233
▲ Intron A for Injection (Less than or equal to 5%) 3024
Levaquin (0.1% to 0.9%) 2384
Levaquin in 5% Dextrose Injection (0.1% to 0.9%) 2384
Permax Tablets (Rare) 3356
▲ Prograf Capsules and Injection (3% to 15%) 632
Proleukin for Injection (1%) 2266
Prozac Pulvules and Liquid (Rare) 1801
Pulmozyme Inhalation Solution 1248
Rilutek Tablets (Infrequent) 2930
Sandostatin LAR Depot (Rare) 2280
▲ Trasylol Injection (4%) 754
Virazole for Inhalation Solution 3370
Zegerid Capsules (0.6%) 2958
Zegerid Powder for Oral Solution (0.6%) 2958
Zelapar Tablets 3372
Zosyn (1.3%) 3492

Poliomyelitis
Invirase (Less than 2%) 2772

Pollakiuria
▲ Cymbalta Delayed-Release Capsules (1% to 5%) 1757
Diovan HCT Tablets (Greater than 0.2%) 2196
DynaCirc CR Tablets (0.5% to 1%) 2721
▲ Vaprisol (6%) 643

Polyangitis, microscopic
Fluarix 1451

Polyarteritis nodosa
▲ Intron A for Injection (Less than 5%) 3024
Recombivax HB 2071

Polyarthralgia
Lithobid Tablets 1692
Primaxin I.M. 2045
Primaxin I.V. (Less than 0.2%) 2048
Solodyn Extended Release Tablets 1890

Polyarthralgia, migratory
Cuprimine Capsules (Some patients) 1947

Polyarthritis
Cleocin Vaginal Ovules (Rare) 2616
Invirase (Rare) 2772
Xyrem Oral Solution (Infrequent) 1688

Polycythemia
Androxy Tablets 3335
▲ CellCept Capsules (3% to less than 20%) 2747
▲ CellCept Intravenous (3% to less than 20%) 2747
▲ CellCept Oral Suspension (3% to less than 20%) 2747
▲ CellCept Tablets (3% to less than 20%) 2747
Estratest Tablets 3199
Estratest H.S. Tablets 3199
Geodon Capsules (Rare) 2529
▲ Humira Injection (Less than 5%) 466
Lyrica Capsules (Rare) 2539
Oxandrin Tablets 2962
Permax Tablets (Rare) 3356
Pletal Tablets (Less than 2%) 2455
▲ Prograf Capsules and Injection (3% to 15%) 632
▲ Rapamune Oral Solution and Tablets (3% to 20%) 3475
▲ Simulect for Injection (3% to 10%) 2284
Striant Mucoadhesive 1007
Topamax Sprinkle Capsules (Rare) 2404
Topamax Tablets (Rare) 2404

Polydipsia
Amerge Tablets (Infrequent) 1339
Aricept Tablets (Infrequent) 1094
Aricept ODT Tablets (Infrequent) 1094
Calcijex Injection 411
Clozaril Tablets (Less than 1%) 2184
FazaClo Orally Disintegrating Tablets (Less than 1%) 551
Hectorol Capsules 1275
Hectorol Injection 1278
Imitrex Injection (Rare) 1463

Imitrex Nasal Spray 1467
Imitrex Tablets (Rare) 1471
Lithobid Tablets 1692
Prezista Tablets (Less than 2%) 3306
Risperdal (Frequent) 1676
Risperdal M-Tab Orally Disintegrating Tablets (Frequent) ... 1676
Rocaltrol Capsules 2798
Rocaltrol Oral Solution 2798
Thiothixene Capsules 2165

Polymenorrhea
Sandostatin Injection (Less than 1%) 2278

Polymyalgia rheumatica
Advicor Tablets 1722
Altoprev Extended-Release Tablets (Rare) 3109
Fortical Nasal Spray (Less than 1%) 3337
Lescol Capsules (Rare) 2233
Lescol XL Tablets 2233
Mevacor Tablets (Rare) 2021
Miacalcin Nasal Spray (Less than 1%) 2253
Nexium Delayed-Release Capsules (Less than 1%) 655
Nexium I.V. (Less than 1%) 659
Requip Tablets (Infrequent) 1555
Vytorin 10/10 Tablets 2114
Vytorin 10/10 Tablets 3077
Vytorin 10/20 Tablets 2114
Vytorin 10/20 Tablets 3077
Vytorin 10/40 Tablets 2114
Vytorin 10/40 Tablets 3077
Vytorin 10/80 Tablets 2114
Vytorin 10/80 Tablets 3077
Zocor Tablets (Rare) 2105

Polymyositis
Campath Ampules 811
Cuprimine Capsules (Rare) 1947
Enbrel for Injection (Infrequent) 584

Polyneuritis
Fansidar Tablets 2765
Meruvax II 2019
M-M-R II 2006
Podocon-25 Liquid 2478
ProQuad 2064

Polyneuropathy
▲ Intron A for Injection (Less than 5%) 3024
Meruvax II (Isolated reports) 2019
M-M-R II 2006
Phenytek Capsules 2160
ProQuad 2064
▲ Xeloda Tablets (Less than 5%) 2822

Polyneuropathy, axonal
Avelox 2970
Proquin XR Tablets 1153
Tequin Injection 938
Tequin Injection in 5% Dextrose 938
Tequin Tablets 938

Polyneuropathy, peripheral
Leustatin Injection 2357

Polyphagia
Mirapex Tablets 859

Polyposis, gastric
Lexapro Oral Solution (Infrequent) 1190
Lexapro Tablets (Infrequent) 1190

Polyps, cervical
▲ Menostar Transdermal System (6%) 782

Polyps, fundic gland
Prevacid NapraPAC (Less than 1%) .. 3280

Polyps, gallbladder
Sandostatin Injection (Less than 1%) 2278
Sandostatin LAR Depot (Rare) 2280

Polyps, nasal
▲ Atrovent Nasal Spray 0.03% (3.1%) 837
Pulmozyme Inhalation Solution 1248
Zyrtec Chewable Tablets (Less than 2%) 2594
Zyrtec (Less than 2%) 2594
Zyrtec-D 12 Hour Extended Release Tablets (Less than 2%) 2597

Polyserositis
Avastin IV (Rare) 1227
Biltricide Tablets 2976

Polyuria
Abilify Oral Solution (Rare) 882
Abilify Oral Solution (Rare) 2450
Abilify Discmelt Orally Disintegrating Tablets (Rare) 882
Abilify Discmelt Orally Disintegrating Tablets (Rare) 2450
Abilify Tablets (Rare) 882
Abilify Tablets (Rare) 2450
Aciphex Tablets 1090
Adalat CC Tablets (Less than 1%) 2964
Ambien Tablets (Rare) 2851
Ambien CR Tablets (Rare) 2855
Amerge Tablets (Infrequent) 1339
Anaprox Tablets (Less than 1%) 2761
Anaprox DS Tablets (Less than 1%) .. 2761
Anzemet Injection (Rare) 2859
Anzemet Tablets (Rare) 2862
Arthrotec Tablets (Rare) 3129
Atripla Tablets 945
▲ Avastin IV (3% to 6%) 1227
▲ Betaseron for SC Injection (7%) 767
Caduet Tablets (Less than or equal to 0.1%) 2508
Calcijex Injection 411
Campral Tablets (Rare) 1174
Captopril Tablets (Approximately 1 to 2 of 1000 patients) 2149
Cardene I.V. (1.4%) 2497
Cardizem LA Extended Release Tablets (Less than 2%) 1728
Cardura XL Tablets 2515
Celexa (Frequent) 1176
Chantix Tablets (Frequent) 2517
Cipro (Less than 1%) 2977
Cipro I.V. (1% or less) 2984
Cipro XR Tablets 2990
Colazal Capsules 2838
Coreg Tablets (Greater than 0.1% to 1%) 1414
EC-Naprosyn Delayed-Release Tablets (Less than 1%) 2761
Effexor Tablets (Infrequent) 3411
Effexor XR Capsules (Infrequent) 3417
Elspar for Injection (Low) 2463
Elspar for Injection (Low) 1960
Evoxac Capsules (0.1%) 1047
Exelon Capsules (Infrequent) 2206
Exelon Oral Solution (Infrequent) 2206
Frova Tablets (Infrequent) 1113
Gabitril Tablets (Infrequent) 984
Gengraf Capsules (1% to less than 3%) 459
Geodon Capsules (Infrequent) 2529
Gleevec Tablets (Infrequent) 2227
Hectorol Capsules 1275
Hectorol Injection 1278
▲ Imdur Tablets (Less than or equal to 5%) 3018
Indapamide Tablets (Less than 5%) .. 2156
▲ Intron A for Injection (Less than 5%) 3024
Klonopin (Infrequent) 2778
Lamictal (Infrequent) 1481
Lithobid Tablets 1692
Lofibra Tablets (1%) 1219
Lofibra Capsules (1%) 1216
Lotrel Capsules 2249
Lotronex Tablets (Rare) 1512
Maxalt Tablets (Infrequent) 2008
Maxalt-MLT Orally Disintegrating Tablets (Infrequent) 2008
Midamor Tablets (Less than or equal to 1%) 2026
Moduretic Tablets 2028
Naprosyn Suspension (Less than 1%) 2761
Naprosyn Tablets (Less than 1%) 2761
Neoral Oral Solution (1% to less than 3%) 2259
Neoral Soft Gelatin Capsules (1% to less than 3%) 2259
Neurontin Capsules (Infrequent) 2487
Neurontin Oral Solution (Infrequent) 2487
Neurontin Tablets (Infrequent) 2487
Nexium Delayed-Release Capsules (Less than 1%) 655
Nexium I.V. (Less than 1%) 659
Norvasc Tablets (Less than 0.1%) 2545
Norvir (Less than 2%) 503
OxyContin Tablets (Less than 1%) 2703
Paxil CR Controlled-Release Tablets (Infrequent) 1538
Paxil (Infrequent) 1530
Pexeva Tablets (Infrequent) 1694
Prevacid Delayed-Release Capsules (Less than 1%) 3271
Prevacid for Delayed-Release Oral Suspension (Less than 1%) 3271
Prevacid SoluTab Delayed-Release Orally Disintegrating Tablets (Less than 1%) 3271
Prevacid NapraPAC (Less than 1%) .. 3280
PREVPAC (Less than 1%) 3284
Prezista Tablets (Less than 2%) 3306
Primaxin I.M. 2045
Primaxin I.V. (Less than 0.2%) 2048
Proquin XR Tablets 1153
Prozac Pulvules and Liquid (At least 2%) 1801
▲ Rapamune Oral Solution and Tablets (3% to 20%) 3475
▲ Rebif Prefilled Syringe for Injection (2% to 7%) 3159
Relpax Tablets (Infrequent) 2548
Requip Tablets (Infrequent) 1555
Rescriptor Tablets 2551
Retrovir Capsules 1560
Retrovir IV Infusion 1564
Retrovir 1560
Reyataz Capsules (Less than 3%) 921
Risperdal (Frequent) 1676
Risperdal M-Tab Orally Disintegrating Tablets (Frequent) ... 1676
Rocaltrol Capsules 2798
Rocaltrol Oral Solution 2798
Seroquel Tablets (Rare) 690
Stalevo Tablets 2287
Symbyax Capsules (Infrequent) 1819
Tambocor Tablets (Less than 1%) 1856
Tarka Tablets (Less frequent) 524
Tasmar Tablets (Infrequent) 3358
Teveten Tablets (Less than 1%) 1735
Teveten HCT Tablets (Less than 1%) 1737
Tiazac Capsules (Less than 2%) 1201
Topamax Sprinkle Capsules (Infrequent) 2404
Topamax Tablets (Infrequent) 2404
Tricor Tablets 527
Trileptal Tablets 2300
Trileptal Oral Suspension 2300
Truvada Tablets 1296
Uniretic Tablets (Less than 1%) 3100
▲ Vaprisol (4.9%) 643
Voltaren Tablets (Occasionally) 2307
Voltaren-XR Tablets (Occasionally) 2310
Wellbutrin SR Sustained-Release Tablets (Infrequent) 1607
Wellbutrin XL Extended-Release Tablets (Infrequent) 1613
Xifaxan Tablets (Less than 2%) 2842
Zoloft (Infrequent) 2586
Zomig Tablets (Infrequent) 3519
Zomig Nasal Spray (Infrequent) 3523
Zomig-ZMT Tablets (Infrequent) 3519
Zonegran Capsules (Infrequent) 1101
Zyban Sustained-Release Tablets (Infrequent) 1644
Zyprexa Tablets (Infrequent) 1830
Zyprexa ZYDIS Orally Disintegrating Tablets (Infrequent) 1830
Zyrtec Chewable Tablets (Less than 2%) 2594
Zyrtec (Less than 2%) 2594
Zyrtec-D 12 Hour Extended Release Tablets (Less than 2%) 2597

Porphyria
Arthrotec Tablets (Rare) 3129
Mircette Tablets 1066
NuvaRing 2340
Ortho-Cyclen Tablets 2429
Ortho Evra Transdermal System 2417
Ortho Tri-Cyclen Tablets 2429
Ortho Tri-Cyclen Lo Tablets 2436
Paxil CR Controlled-Release Tablets 1538
Paxil 1530
Pexeva Tablets 1694
Sulfamylon Cream (A single case) 2162
Sulfamylon for 5% Topical Solution .. 2162
Yasmin 28 Tablets 796
Yaz Tablets 803

Porphyria, aggravation of
Angeliq Tablets 762
Climara Transdermal System 771
Climara Pro Transdermal System 776
Enjuvia Tablets 1062
Epogen for Injection (Rare) 591
Estrasorb Topical Emulsion 1147
Estratest Tablets 3199
Estratest H.S. Tablets 3199
Menostar Transdermal System 782
Phenytek Capsules (Isolated reports) 2160
Premarin Intravenous 3442
Premarin Tablets 3446
Premarin Vaginal Cream 3452
Premphase Tablets 3456
Prempro Tablets 3456
Procrit for Injection (Rare) 2364
Zantac (Rare) 1624
Zantac Injection (Rare) 1619
Zantac (Rare) 1624

Porphyria, cutaneous, drug-induced
Photofrin for Injection 702

Porphyria, exacerbation of
Seasonique Tablets 1077

Porphyria, hepatic
Avandaryl Tablets 1379
Duetact Tablets 3226

Porphyria, intermittent, acute
Carbatrol Capsules 3171
Depacon Injection 412
Depakene 417
Depakote Sprinkle Capsules 422
Depakote Tablets 427
Depakote ER Tablets 434
Equetro Extended-Release Capsules 3180
Tegretol/Tegretol-XR 2295

Porphyria cutanea tarda
Anaprox Tablets (Less than 1%) 2761
Anaprox DS Tablets (Less than 1%) .. 2761
Avandaryl Tablets 1379
Duetact Tablets (Less than 1%) 3226
EC-Naprosyn Delayed-Release Tablets (Less than 1%) 2761
Myleran Tablets (Rare) 1525
Naprosyn Suspension (Less than 1%) 2761
Naprosyn Tablets (Less than 1%) 2761

Porphyria cutanea tarda, pseudo
Prevacid NapraPAC (Less than 1%) .. 3280

Potassium loss
(*see under* Hypokalemia)

Potassium retention
(*see under* Hyperkalemia)

Potentia, decrease
Kadian Capsules (Less than 3%) 577

Precocious puberty
Premarin Vaginal Cream 3452

Pregnancy, accidental
Depo-Provera Contraceptive Injection (Less than 1%) 2622
depo-subQ provera 104 Injectable Suspension 2624
Lofibra Tablets 1219
Lofibra Capsules 1216
Tricor Tablets 527
Zomig Nasal Spray (Rare) 3523

Pregnancy, ectopic
Mirena Intrauterine System 787
ParaGard T 380A 1073

Pregnancy, sensation of
Depo-Provera Contraceptive Injection (Less than 1%) 2622

Pregnancy tests, false positive
Thioridazine Hydrochloride Tablets .. 2163
Thiothixene Capsules 2165

Pregnancy, prolonged
Aggrenox Capsules 822
Bayer Aspirin 744
Bayer Aspirin Comprehensive Prescribing Information .... ▣796
Percodan Tablets 1132
St. Joseph 81 mg Aspirin .... ▣688

Premature depolarizations, ventricular
Retavase 2499

Premature ventricular contractions
Imitrex Injection (Infrequent) 1463
Prinivil Tablets (0.3% to 1.0%) 2052
Prinzide Tablets 2056
Tarka Tablets (0.3% or more) 524

Premenstrual-like syndrome
Estratest Tablets 3199
Estratest H.S. Tablets 3199
Lexapro Oral Solution (Infrequent) 1190
Lexapro Tablets (Infrequent) 1190
Mircette Tablets 1066
NuvaRing 2340
Ortho-Cyclen Tablets 2429
Ortho Evra Transdermal System 2417
Ortho Tri-Cyclen Tablets 2429
Ortho Tri-Cyclen Lo Tablets 2436
Premarin Intravenous 3442
Premarin Vaginal Cream 3452

Premphase Tablets 3456
Prempro Tablets 3456
Seasonique Tablets 1077
Yasmin 28 Tablets 796
Yaz Tablets 803
Zyprexa Tablets (2%) 1830
Zyprexa ZYDIS Orally Disintegrating Tablets (2%) 1830

Pressor response, paradoxical
BiDil Tablets 2171

Priapism
Abilify Oral Solution (Rare) 882
Abilify Oral Solution (Rare) 2450
Abilify Discmelt Orally Disintegrating Tablets (Rare) 882
Abilify Discmelt Orally Disintegrating Tablets (Rare) 2450
Abilify Tablets (Rare) 882
Abilify Tablets (Rare) 2450
Androxy Tablets 3335
Bicillin C-R Injectable Suspension 1706
Cardura XL Tablets 2515
▲ Caverject Impulse Injection (4%) 2612
Celexa 1176
Cialis Tablets (Less than 2%) 1838
Clozaril Tablets 2184
Copaxone for Injection (Infrequent) 3297
Coumadin for Injection 898
Coumadin Tablets 898
▲ Edex Injection (Less than 1% to 4%) 3089
Effexor XR Capsules (Rare) 3417
FazaClo Orally Disintegrating Tablets 551
Flomax Capsules (Rare) 850
Geodon for Injection (Up to 1%) 2529
Hytrin Capsules (Rare) 471
Levitra Tablets (Less than 2%) 3034
Lexapro Oral Solution 1190
Lexapro Tablets 1190
Miradon Tablets 3042
Moban Tablets 1119
Oxandrin Tablets 2962
Parcopa Orally Disintegrating Tablets 3097
Paxil CR Controlled-Release Tablets 1538
Paxil 1530
Permax Tablets (Infrequent) 3356
Pexeva Tablets 1694
Prozac Pulvules and Liquid (Rare) 1801
Rilutek Tablets (Infrequent) 2930
Risperdal (Rare) 1676
Risperdal M-Tab Orally Disintegrating Tablets (Rare) 1676
Seroquel Tablets (One case) 690
Stalevo Tablets 2287
Testim 1% Gel (1% or less) 695
Thioridazine Hydrochloride Tablets 2163
Trileptal Tablets 2300
Trileptal Oral Suspension 2300
Uroxatral Tablets 2943
Viagra Tablets 2573
Zoloft (Rare) 2586
Zyprexa Tablets 1830
Zyprexa ZYDIS Orally Disintegrating Tablets 1830

Proctalgia
Remicade for IV Injection (Greater than or equal to 0.2%) 971
Zelnorm Tablets 2312

Proctitis
Aciphex Tablets 1090
Aloprim for Injection (Less than 1%) 2167
Cosmegen for Injection 2459
Doxil Injection (Less than 1%) 2351
Effexor Tablets (Rare) 3411
Effexor XR Capsules (Rare) 3417
▲ Eloxatin for Injection (2% to 5%) 2892
▲ Eulexin Capsules (8%) 3009
Indocin Capsules (Less than 1%) 1995
Indocin I.V. (Less than 1%) 2465
Indocin (Less than 1%) 1995
Lotronex Tablets (Rare) 1512
Neurontin Capsules (Rare) 2487
Neurontin Oral Solution (Rare) 2487
Neurontin Tablets (Rare) 2487
Rilutek Tablets (Rare) 2930
VFEND I.V. (Less than 2%) 2564
VFEND Oral Suspension (Less than 2%) 2564
VFEND Tablets (Less than 2%) 2564
Zoloft (Rare) 2586

Proctitis, ulceration
Doxil Injection (Less than 1%) 2351

Prolactin levels, elevated
(*see under* Hyperprolactinemia)

Prolactinemia
Celexa 1176
Pexeva Tablets 1694

Proptosis
Ortho-Cyclen/Ortho Tri-Cyclen 2429
Ortho Tri-Cyclen Lo Tablets 2436
Premphase Tablets 3456
Prempro Tablets 3456

Prostate disorders, unspecified
▲ AndroGel (3% to 5%) 3329
Atrovent Nasal Spray 0.03% 837
Atrovent Nasal Spray 0.06% 839
Avalide Tablets 888
Avalide Tablets 2874
Avapro Tablets (Less than 1%) 891
Avapro Tablets (Less than 1%) 2871
▲ Betaseron for SC Injection (3%) 767
Caverject Impulse Injection (2%) 2612
Celebrex Capsules (0.1% to 1.9%) 3134
Edex Injection (1%) 3089
Evoxac Capsules (Less than 1%) 1047
Lofibra Tablets 1219
Lofibra Capsules 1216
Mirapex Tablets (Less than 1%) 859
Protonix I.V. (Less than 1%) 3472
Protonix Tablets (Less than 1%) 3469
Requip Tablets (Infrequent) 1555
Tasmar Tablets (Infrequent) 3358
Testim 1% Gel (1%) 695
▲ Travatan Ophthalmic Solution (1% to 5%) 563
Tricor Tablets 527
Viadur Implant (Less than 2%) 757
▲ Visudyne for Injection (1% to 10%) 2305
Wellbutrin SR Sustained-Release Tablets (Infrequent) 1607
Wellbutrin XL Extended-Release Tablets (Infrequent) 1613
Zyban Sustained-Release Tablets 1644

Prostate enlargement
AndroGel (Five patients) 3329
Caverject Impulse Injection (2%) 2612
Effexor Tablets (Frequent) 3411

Prostate specific antigen decrease
▲ Avodart Soft Gelatin Capsules (Approximately 40% to 50%) 1390

Prostate specific antigen increase
Aciphex Tablets 1090
Rythmol SR Capsules 2727
Striant Mucoadhesive 1007
Zelapar Tablets 3372

Prostatic acid phosphatase, decreased
▲ Lupron Depot (Greater than or equal to 5%) 3264

Prostatic acid phosphatase, increased
Vantas (Less than 2%) 3375

Prostatic hypertrophy
Aricept Tablets (Infrequent) 1094
Aricept ODT Tablets (Infrequent) 1094
Caverject Impulse Injection (2%) 2612
Eldepryl Capsules 3208
Invirase (Less than 2%) 2772
Striant Mucoadhesive 1007
Testim 1% Gel (1% or less) 695
▲ Vesanoid Capsules (3%) 2820

Prostatism
Rythmol SR Capsules 2727

Prostatitis
Caverject Impulse Injection (2%) 2612
Effexor Tablets (Frequent) 3411
Effexor XR Capsules (Infrequent) 3417
ReoPro Vials (0.1%) 1809
▲ Strattera Capsules (3%) 1814

Prostration
Bicillin C-R Injectable Suspension 1706

Protein bound iodine, lowered
(*see under* PBI decrease)

Protein catabolism
Depo-Medrol Injectable Suspension 2617
Depo-Medrol Single-Dose Vial 2619
Hydrocortone Tablets 1989

Proteinuria
Accutane Capsules 2731
Aceon Tablets (2 mg, 4 mg, 8 mg) (1.0% to 1.5%) 3194
Aggrenox Capsules 822
Aldara Cream, 5% 1846
Altace Capsules 1702
Anaprox Tablets (Less than 1%) 2761
Anaprox DS Tablets (Less than 1%) 2761
Arthrotec Tablets (Rare) 3129
Atripla Tablets 945
▲ Avastin IV (36%) 1227
Bayer Aspirin 744
Bayer Aspirin Comprehensive Prescribing Information ▣ 796
Bicillin C-R Injectable Suspension 1706
Bumex Tablets (0.3%) 2746
Calcium Disodium Versenate Injection 1851
Captopril Tablets (Approximately 1 of 100 patients) 2149
Cleocin Vaginal Ovules (Rare) 2616
Clinoril Tablets (Less than 1 in 100) 1924
Cubicin for Injection (Less than 1%) 1026
▲ Cuprimine Capsules (6%) 1947
Dolobid Tablets (Less than 1 in 100) 1955
EC-Naprosyn Delayed-Release Tablets (Less than 1%) 2761
Elspar for Injection (Infrequent) 2463
Elspar for Injection (Infrequent) 1960
▲ Emend Capsules (6.8%) 1963
Garamycin Injectable 3014
▲ Gemzar for Injection (2% to 45%) 1771
Gris-PEG Tablets (Rare) 2502
Indocin (Less than 1%) 1995
▲ Intron A for Injection (Less than 5%) 3024
Kepivance (9 patients) 597
Lotensin HCT Tablets 2246
Naprosyn Suspension (Less than 1%) 2761
Naprosyn Tablets (Less than 1%) 2761
Neupogen for Injection (Infrequent) 603
Parcopa Orally Disintegrating Tablets 3097
Percodan Tablets 1132
Prilosec OTC Delayed-Release Tablets (Less than 1%) 2677
Primaxin I.M. 2045
Primaxin I.V. 2048
▲ Proleukin for Injection (12%) 2266
Prozac Pulvules and Liquid 1801
Raniclor Tablets, Chewable 2505
Rescriptor Tablets 2551
Reyataz Capsules (Less than 3%) 921
Rythmol SR Capsules 2727
St. Joseph 81 mg Aspirin Chewable and Enteric Coated Tablets 1869
St. Joseph 81 mg Aspirin ▣ 688
Tarka Tablets (Less frequent) 524
▲ Thiola Tablets (5%) 2141
Truvada Tablets 1296
Vantin Tablets and Oral Suspension (Less than 1%) 2645
Vaqta (Isolated reports) 2097
Voltaren Tablets (Occasionally) 2307
Voltaren-XR Tablets (Occasionally) 2310
Xifaxan Tablets (Less than 2%) 2842
Xyrem Oral Solution (Infrequent) 1688
Zegerid Capsules (Less than 1%) 2958
Zegerid Powder for Oral Solution (Less than 1%) 2958
Zometa for Intravenous Infusion 2315
Zosyn 3492

Proteinuria, increased
Cancidas for Injection (0% to 1.2%) 1918
▲ Chemet Capsules (Up to 3.7%) 2458
Noroxin Tablets (1.0%) 2032
Omnicef Capsules (2%) 511
Omnicef for Oral Suspension (1%) 511

Prothrombin, abnormal
Maxipime for Injection (1.4%) 1105

Prothrombin, decrease
(*see under* Hypoprothrombinemia)

Prothrombin, increase
(*see under* Hyperprothrombinemia)

Prothrombin time, deviation
Avelox (Less than 0.1%) 2970
Bumex Tablets (0.8%) 2746
Maxipime for Injection (1.6%) 1105

Prothrombin time, elevation
Advicor Tablets 1722
Cancidas for Injection (1.3% to 1.5%) 1918
St. Joseph 81 mg Aspirin Chewable and Enteric Coated Tablets 1869

Prothrombin time, increase
(*see under* Prothrombin time prolongation)

Prothrombin time prolongation
Aggrenox Capsules 822
Avelox (0.1% to less than 2%) 2970
Bayer Aspirin 744
Bayer Aspirin Comprehensive Prescribing Information ▣ 796
Biaxin/Biaxin XL (1%) 402
Ceftin 1407
▲ CellCept Capsules (3% to less than 20%) 2747
▲ CellCept Intravenous (3% to less than 20%) 2747
▲ CellCept Oral Suspension (3% to less than 20%) 2747
▲ CellCept Tablets (3% to less than 20%) 2747
Cipro 2977
Cipro I.V. 2984
Cipro XR Tablets 2990
Clinoril Tablets 1924
Colazal Capsules 2838
Cubicin for Injection (Less than 1%) 1026
Elmiron Capsules (Less than or equal to 1%) 2415
Eraxis for Injection (Less than 1% to less than 2%) 2521
Fortaz 1453
Infergen (1% to 3%) 3364
Invanz for Injection (0.3% to 1.2%) 1999
I.V. Busulfex (2%) 2493
Keflex Capsules 549
Levaquin 2384
Levaquin in 5% Dextrose Injection 2384
Mefoxin for Injection 2012
Mefoxin Premixed Intravenous Solution 2016
Merrem I.V. (Greater than 0.2%) 686
Niaspan Extended-Release Tablets 1730
Noroxin Tablets 2032
Oncaspar 1145
Ortho-Cyclen/Ortho Tri-Cyclen 2429
Ortho Tri-Cyclen Lo Tablets 2436
Oxandrin Tablets 2962
Panhematin for Injection 2473
Percodan Tablets 1132
PREVPAC (1%) 3284
Primaxin I.M. 2045
Primaxin I.V. 2048
Proquin XR Tablets 1153
Raniclor Tablets, Chewable 2505
Rescriptor Tablets 2551
Rocephin Injectable Vials, ADD-Vantage, Galaxy, Bulk (Less than 1%) 2800
St. Joseph 81 mg Aspirin ▣ 688
Suprax (Rare) 1843
Testim 1% Gel (1% or less) 695
Timentin ADD-Vantage 1580
Timentin Injection Galaxy Container 1583
Timentin IV Infusion 1577
Timentin Pharmacy Bulk Package 1586
Tygacil for Injection (0% to less than 2%) 3488
Vantin Tablets and Oral Suspension 2645
Zinacef for Injection 1631
Zinacef Injection 1631
Zoloft 2586
Zosyn 3492

Prothrombin time, accelerated
Menostar Transdermal System 782

Prothrombin time, decrease
Cipro 2977
Cipro I.V. 2984
Premarin Tablets 3446
Premphase Tablets 3456
Prempro Tablets 3456

Pruritis, ear
Ciprodex Otic Suspension (1.5%) 559

Pruritus
Abelcet Injection 1141
Abilify Oral Solution (Infrequent) 882
Abilify Oral Solution (Infrequent) 2450
Abilify Discmelt Orally Disintegrating Tablets (Infrequent) 882

Abilify Discmelt Orally Disintegrating Tablets (Infrequent) 2450
Abilify Tablets (Infrequent) 882
Abilify Tablets (Infrequent) 2450
Accolate Tablets 671
Accutane Capsules 2731
Aceon Tablets (2 mg, 4 mg, 8 mg) (0.3% to 1%) 3194
▲ Acetadote Injection (.2% to 20.8%) 1031
Aciphex Tablets 1090
Aclovate Cream (Approximately 2%) 2660
Actiq (Up to 5%) 979
▲ Actonel Tablets (1.9% to 3%) 2683
▲ Actonel with Calcium Tablets (1.9% to 3%) 2688
ADACEL Vaccine (Very rare) 2945
Adalat CC Tablets (Less than 1%) 2964
Advair HFA Inhalation Aerosol 1318
Advate Injection (0.6%) 712
▲ Advicor Tablets (7%) 1722
▲ Aerobid/Aerobid-M (3% to 9%) 1171
Agenerase Capsules 1327
Agenerase Oral Solution (1%) 1332
Aggrenox Capsules (Less than 1%) 822
▲ Agrylin Capsules (5.5%) 3169
Aldara Cream, 5% (0.9%) 1846
Aldurazyme for Intravenous Infusion 1268
Alferon N Injection (2%) 1665
Alinia for Oral Suspension (Less than 1%) 2835
Alinia Tablets (Less than 1%) 2835
Alkeran for Injection 955
Allegra (Rare) 2844
Allegra-D 12 Hour Extended-Release Tablets (Rare) 2846
Allegra-D 24 Hour Extended-Release Tablets (Rare) 2849
Aloprim for Injection (Less than 1%) 2167
Altace Capsules (Less than 1%) 1702
Altoprev Extended-Release Tablets (0.5% to 1%) 3109
Ambien Tablets (Infrequent) 2851
Ambien CR Tablets (Infrequent) 2855
▲ AmBisome for Injection (10.8%) 620
Amerge Tablets (Infrequent) 1339
Amevive (Common) 626
Analpram-HC 1159
▲ Anaprox Tablets (3% to 9%) 2761
▲ Anaprox DS Tablets (3% to 9%) 2761
Angeliq Tablets 762
▲ Anzemet Injection (3.1%) 2859
▲ Anzemet Tablets (3.1%) 2862
Apexicon E Cream 2661
Apidra Injection 2864
Aptivus Capsules (Less than 2%) 826
Aralast (0.1%) 717
▲ Aranesp for Injection (8%) 581
Aricept Tablets (Frequent) 1094
Aricept ODT Tablets (Frequent) 1094
▲ Arimidex Tablets (2% to 5%) 673
Aromasin Tablets (Less frequent) 2600
Arthrotec Tablets (Rare) 3129
▲ Asacol Delayed-Release Tablets (3%) 2692
Astelin Nasal Spray 1904
Atacand Tablets 649
Atacand HCT (0.5% or greater) 651
Atripla Tablets (Greater than or equal to 2%) 945
Augmentin 1360
Augmentin Tablets 1363
Augmentin XR Extended-Release Tablets 1369
Augmentin ES-600 Powder for Oral Suspension 1366
Avalide Tablets 888
Avalide Tablets 2874
Avandaryl Tablets (Less than 1%) 1379
Avapro Tablets (Less than 1%) 891
Avapro Tablets (Less than 1%) 2871
Avelox (0.1% to less than 2%) 2970
Avodart Soft Gelatin Capsules 1390
Axert Tablets (Rare) 2396
Axid Oral Solution (1.7%) 879
Bactroban Cream (Less than 1%) 1394
Bactroban Nasal (1%) 1394
Bactroban Ointment (1%) 1395
Benicar Tablets 1043
Benicar HCT Tablets (Rare) 1044
Bentyl Capsules 697
Bentyl Injection 697
Bentyl Syrup 697
Bentyl Tablets 697
▲ Benzaclin Topical Gel (12%) 2877
Betagan Ophthalmic Solution, USP (Rare) ⊙ 220
Betaseron for SC Injection 767
▲ Bexxar (0% to 10%) 1398
Bicillin C-R Injectable Suspension 1706
Blocadren Tablets (1.1%) 1916
▲ BOTOX Purified Neurotoxin Complex (3% to 10%) 570
Bumex Tablets (0.1% to 2.9%) 2746
Buprenex Injectable (Less than 1%) 2716
Byetta Injection 611
Caduet Tablets (Less than 1% to 2%) 2508
Calcijex Injection 411
▲ Campath Ampules (1% to 24%) 811
▲ Campral Tablets (3% to 4%) 1174
Cancidas for Injection (1.2% to 2.5%) 1918
Captopril Tablets (About 2 of 100 patients) 2149
Carafate Suspension (Less than 0.5%) 701
Carafate Tablets (Less than 0.5%) 701
Cardizem LA Extended Release Tablets (Less than 2%) 1728
▲ Carnitor Injection (3% to 8%) 3188
Catapres Tablets (About 7 in 1,000 patients) 843
▲ Catapres-TTS (51 of 101 patients) 844
Caverject Impulse Injection (Less than 1%) 2612
Ceftin (0.1% to 1%) 1407
Celebrex Capsules (0.1% to 1.9%) 3134
Celexa (Frequent) 1176
▲ CellCept Capsules (3% to less than 20%) 2747
▲ CellCept Intravenous (3% to less than 20%) 2747
▲ CellCept Oral Suspension (3% to less than 20%) 2747
▲ CellCept Tablets (3% to less than 20%) 2747
▲ Cerezyme for Injection (Approximately 6.6%) 1270
Cesamet Capsules 3340
Chantix Tablets (0% to 1%) 2517
▲ Chemet Capsules (2.6% to 11.2%) 2458
Cialis Tablets (Less than 2%) 1838
Cipro (Less than 1%) 2977
Cipro I.V. (1% or less) 2984
Cipro XR Tablets (Less than 1%) 2990
Clarinex Syrup (Rare) 2995
Clarinex Tablets (Rare) 2995
Clarinex Reditabs Tablets (Rare) 2995
Clarinex-D 24-Hour Extended-Release Tablets 2998
Cleocin Vaginal Ovules (Less than 1%) 2616
Climara Transdermal System (0.5% to 6%) 771
Climara Pro Transdermal System 776
Clindagel (0.6%) 1203
Clinoril Tablets (Greater than 1%) 1924
Clobevate Gel (Less than 2%) 3211
Clobex Lotion 1204
Clobex Shampoo (0.5%) 1206
Clorpres Tablets (About 7 in 1,000) 2153
Clozaril Tablets (Less than 1%) 2184
Colazal Capsules 2838
Combivent Inhalation Aerosol 847
Comvax 1928
▲ Copaxone for Injection (18%) 3297
▲ Copegus Tablets (19%) 2754
Coreg Tablets (Greater than 0.1% to 1%) 1414
Cosopt Sterile Ophthalmic Solution 1931
Coumadin for Injection (Infrequent) 898
Coumadin Tablets (Infrequent) 898
Cozaar Tablets (Less than 1%) 1935
Crestor Tablets (Greater than or equal to 1%) 678
▲ Crixivan Capsules (4.2%) 1940
▲ Cubicin for Injection (2.8% to 5.8%) 1026
▲ Cuprimine Capsules (5%) 1947
Cutivate Cream (1.5% to 2.9%) 2662
Cutivate Lotion 0.05% (Less than 1%) 2664
Cutivate Ointment (Less than 1%) 2665
Cymbalta Delayed-Release Capsules (Frequent) 1757
▲ Dacogen Injection (11%) 2129
Dalmane Capsules (Rare) 3342
Dantrium Capsules (Less frequent) 2694
Daranide Tablets 1950
Denavir Cream 2174
▲ Depacon Injection (1% to 5%) 412
▲ Depakene (1% to 5%) 417
▲ Depakote Sprinkle Capsules (1% to 5%) 422
▲ Depakote Tablets (1% to 5%) 427
▲ Depakote ER Tablets (Greater than 1% to 5%) 434
▲ DepoDur Extended-Release Injection (Greater than 10%) 1110
depo-subQ provera 104 Injectable Suspension 2624
Detrol Tablets (1.3%) 2628
Diastat Rectal Delivery System (Less than 1%) 3343
Didronel Tablets 2697
▲ Differin Cream (Less than 1% to 21%) 1210
▲ Differin Gel (10% to 40%) 1211
Dilaudid 440
Dilaudid Non-Sterile Powder 440
Dilaudid Oral Liquid 445
Dilaudid Rectal Suppositories 440
Dilaudid Tablets 440
Dilaudid Tablets - 8 mg 445
Dilaudid-HP (Less frequent) 442
Diovan Tablets 2193
Diovan HCT Tablets (Less frequent) 2196
Diprolene Gel 0.05% (2%) 3001
Diprolene Lotion 0.05% (Infrequent) 3002
Diprolene Ointment 0.05% (2 per 767 patients) 3003
Diprolene AF Cream 0.05% (Infrequent) 3000
Diprosone Cream, USP 0.05% 3004
Dolobid Tablets (Less than 1 in 100) 1955
▲ Doxil Injection (1% to 10%) 2351
Drysol Solution 2507
Duetact Tablets (Less than 1%) 3226
DuoNeb Inhalation Solution (0.3%) 1058
▲ Duragesic Transdermal System (1% to 10%) 2373
DynaCirc CR Tablets (0.5% to 1%) 2721
▲ EC-Naprosyn Delayed-Release Tablets (3% to 9%) 2761
Effexor Tablets (1%) 3411
Effexor XR Capsules (Frequent) 3417
▲ Efudex (Among most frequent) 3363
▲ Elidel Cream 1% (0.6% to 5.5%) 2200
Eligard 22.5 mg (2.6%) 2883
Elmiron Capsules (Less than or equal to 1%) 2415
▲ Elocon Cream 0.1% (1.6% to approximately 7%) 3005
Elocon Lotion 0.1% (1 in 209 patients) 3006
▲ Elocon Ointment 0.1% (4.8% to approximately 7%) 3007
▲ Eloxatin for Injection (2% to 5%) 2892
Emcyt Capsules (2%) 2634
▲ Emtriva Capsules (17% to 30%) 1287
▲ Emtriva Oral Solution (17% to 30%) 1287
Enablex Extended-Release Tablets (Greater than or equal to 1%) 2203
Enbrel for Injection 584
Engerix-B Vaccine (Less than 1%) 1425
Enjuvia Tablets 1062
Epivir 1427
Epivir-HBV 1432
▲ Epogen for Injection (16% to 22%) 591
▲ Equetro Extended-Release Capsules (5% to 8%) 3180
Eraxis for Injection 2521
▲ Erbitux (Less than 1% to 16%) 910
▲ Estrasorb Topical Emulsion (4%) 1147
Estratest Tablets 3199
Estratest H.S. Tablets 3199
Eulexin Capsules 3009
▲ Evoxac Capsules (1% to 3%) 1047
Fabrazyme for Intravenous Infusion 1274
▲ Famvir Tablets (0.9% to 3.7%) 2211
Fansidar Tablets 2765
FazaClo Orally Disintegrating Tablets (Less than 1%) 551
Femara Tablets (1% to 2%) 2214
▲ Ferrlecit Injection (0.5% to 6%) 3388
▲ Finacea Gel (1% to 7%) 1669
Fleet Phospho-soda (Rare) 1166
Fleet Phospho-soda ACCU-PREP (Rare) 1168
Fleet Phospho-soda EZ-PREP (Rare) 1169
Flomax Capsules 850
Flonase Nasal Spray 1440
▲ Flovent Diskus (1% to 6%) 1443
Flovent HFA 1447
▲ Floxin Otic Solution (1% to 4%) 1049
Fluarix 1451
Fluorescite Injection ⊙ 207
Fortaz (2%) 1453
Fortical Nasal Spray (Less than 1%) 3337
Fosamax 1969
Fosamax Plus D Tablets 1977
Fragmin Injection (Rare) 1097
Frova Tablets (Infrequent) 1113
Furosemide Tablets 2154
Fuzeon Injection 2767
Gabitril Tablets (2%) 984
▲ Gammagard Liquid (0.61% to 6.5%) 721
▲ Gamunex Immune Globulin I.V., 10% (4%) 3235
Gantrisin Pediatric Suspension 2770
Garamycin Injectable 3014
▲ Gemzar for Injection (13%) 1771
Gengraf Capsules (1% to less than 3%) 459
▲ Gleevec Tablets (0.8% to 14%) 2227
Havrix Vaccine (Less than 1%) 1456
▲ Hectorol Capsules (8.2%) 1275
▲ Hectorol Injection (8.2%) 1278
Hepsera Tablets (2% or greater) 1292
Humalog-Pen (Less common) 1781
Humalog Mix 50/50-Pen 1783
Humalog Mix 75/25-Pen 1785
▲ Humate-P (6%) 3502
▲ Hyalgan Solution (7%) 2901
▲ Hycamtin for Injection (Rare to 16%) 1458
Hycodan 1116
Hytrin Capsules (At least 1%) 471
Hyzaar 50-12.5 Tablets 1990
Hyzaar 100-12.5 Tablets 1990
Hyzaar 100-25 Tablets 1990
▲ Imdur Tablets (Less than or equal to 5%) 3018
Imitrex Injection (Infrequent) 1463
Imitrex Nasal Spray (Infrequent) 1467
Imitrex Tablets (Infrequent) 1471
Indocin (Less than 1%) 1995
Infanrix Vaccine 1476
Infed Injection 3390
▲ Infergen (11% to 14%) 3364
▲ Intron A for Injection (Up to 11%) 3024
Invanz for Injection (1% to 2%) 1999
▲ Invirase (Greater than or equal to 2% to 3.4%) 2772
▲ Ionsys Transdermal System (6%) 2379
▲ Iressa Tablets (8% to 10%) 684
▲ I.V. Busulfex (28%) 2493
Kadian Capsules (Less than 3%) 577
Kaletra (Less than 2%) 476
▲ Kepivance (35%) 597
Keppra Oral Solution (2%) 3314
Keppra Tablets (2%) 3314
Ketek Tablets (Less than 0.2%) 2903
Klaron Lotion 10% (One of 105 patients) 2909
Klonopin (Infrequent) 2778
Kogenate FS 738
Kogenate FS with Bio-Set (1 case) 740
▲ Lamictal (2% to 3%) 1481
Lamisil Tablets (2.8%) 2232
Lantus Injection 2909
Lariam Tablets (Occasional) 2786
Lescol Capsules 2233
Lescol XL Tablets 2233
▲ Leukine (23%) 814
▲ Leustatin Injection (6%) 2357
Levaquin (0.2% to 1.2%) 2384
Levaquin in 5% Dextrose Injection (0.2% to 1.2%) 2384
Levemir Injection 2320
Levitra Tablets (Less than 2%) 3034
Levothroid Tablets 1186
Levoxyl Tablets 1712
▲ Levulan Kerastick for Topical Solution, 20% (1% to 25%) 1085
Lexapro Oral Solution (Infrequent) 1190
Lexapro Tablets (Infrequent) 1190
▲ Lexiva Tablets (Up to 8%) 1505
Limbrel Capsules (0.011%) 2672
Lipitor Tablets (Less than 2%) 2483
Lithobid Tablets 1692
Locoid Lipocream Cream (Infrequent) 1160
Lofibra Tablets 1219
Lofibra Capsules 1216
▲ Lopressor Injection (5%) 2238
▲ Lopressor Tablets (5%) 2238
Lopressor HCT 50/25 Tablets (Less than 1%) 2241
Lopressor HCT 100/25 Tablets (Less than 1%) 2241
Lopressor HCT 100/50 Tablets (Less than 1%) 2241
Loprox Shampoo (1%) 1888
Lotensin Tablets (Less than 1%) 2243
Lotensin HCT Tablets (0.3% or more) 2246
Lotrimin 3039
Lotrisone 3040
Lovenox Injection 2915
▲ Lunesta Tablets (1% to 4%) 3142
▲ Luxíq Foam (2% to 44%) 1010
Lyrica Capsules (Greater than or equal to 1%) 2539
▲ Malarone Pediatric Tablets (1% to 6%) 1517

▲ Malarone Tablets (1% to 6%) ... 1517
Mavik Tablets (0.3% to 1.0%) ... 486
Maxair Autohaler ... 1852
Maxalt Tablets (Infrequent) ... 2008
Maxalt-MLT Orally Disintegrating Tablets (Infrequent) ... 2008
Maxipime for Injection (Greater than 0.1% to 1%) ... 1105
Mefoxin for Injection ... 2012
Mefoxin Premixed Intravenous Solution ... 2016
▲ Megace ES Oral Suspension (1% to 3%) ... 2481
Menostar Transdermal System ... 782
▲ Mepron Suspension (5%) ... 1521
Meridia Capsules (Greater than or equal to 1%) ... 489
Merrem I.V. (1.2%) ... 686
▲ Metrogel 1% (1.1 to 9.7%) ... 1211
MetroGel-Vaginal Gel (Less than 1%) ... 1855
▲ Mevacor Tablets (0.5% to 5.2%) ... 2021
Miacalcin Nasal Spray (Less than 1%) ... 2253
Micardis Tablets (More than 0.3%) ... 854
Micardis HCT Tablets (Less than 2%) ... 856
Midamor Tablets (Less than or equal to 1%) ... 2026
Migranal Nasal Spray (Infrequent) ... 3348
Mintezol ... 2027
Mirapex Tablets (1% or more) ... 859
Mobic Oral Suspension (0.4% to 2.4%) ... 863
Mobic Tablets (0.4% to 2.4%) ... 863
Moduretic Tablets (Greater than 1%, less than 3%) ... 2028
MS Contin Tablets (Less frequent) ... 2701
Mycamine for Injection (0.7% to 1.2%) ... 628
▲ Myfortic Tablets (3% to less than 20%) ... 2255
▲ Mylotarg for Injection (4% to 10%) ... 3431
Myobloc Injection (Greater than 2%) ... 3192
Myozyme for Intravenous Infusion ... 1279
Nadolol Tablets (1 to 5 of 1000 patients) ... 2159
Naftin Cream (2%) ... 2126
Naftin Gel (1.0%) ... 2126
▲ Nalfon Capsules (4.2%) ... 2502
Namenda (Infrequent) ... 1195
▲ Naprosyn Suspension (3% to 9%) ... 2761
▲ Naprosyn Tablets (3% to 9%) ... 2761
Natrecor for Injection (Greater than or equal to 1%) ... 3127
Neoral Oral Solution (1% to less than 3%) ... 2259
Neoral Soft Gelatin Capsules (1% to less than 3%) ... 2259
Neosporin Ophthalmic Solution Sterile ... ⊙265
Neurontin Capsules (1.3%) ... 2487
Neurontin Oral Solution (1.3%) ... 2487
Neurontin Tablets (1.3%) ... 2487
▲ Nexavar Tablets (0% to 19%) ... 746
▲ Niaspan Extended-Release Tablets (1% to 6%) ... 1730
Nimotop Capsules (Less than 1%) ... 749
▲ Nipent for Injection (10% to 21%) ... 1863
Niravam Orally Disintegrating Tablets ... 3092
Norflex Injection ... 1856
Noroxin Tablets (0.3% to 1.0%) ... 2032
Norvasc Tablets (Less than 1% to 2%) ... 2545
Norvir (Less than 2%) ... 503
NovoLog Injection ... 2326
NovoSeven (1%) ... 2331
Numorphan Injection ... 1120
Olux Foam (Less than 2%) ... 1012
Omacor Capsules ... 2725
Omnicef Capsules (0.2%) ... 511
Omnicef for Oral Suspension (0.2%) ... 511
Oncaspar (Less than 1%) ... 1145
▲ Ontak Vials (20%) ... 1745
▲ Opana Tablets (9%) ... 1122
▲ Opana ER Tablets (0% to 15.2%) ... 1126
Orencia Powder for Intravenous Infusion (Less than 0.1% to 1%) ... 914
Orthoclone OKT3 Sterile Solution ... 2360
OsmoPrep Tablets (Rare) ... 2840
Oxistat (1.6%) ... 2667
▲ Oxsoralen-Ultra Capsules (10%) ... 3353
▲ OxyContin Tablets (13%) ... 2703
OxyFast Oral Concentrate Solution ... 2708
OxyIR Capsules ... 2708
▲ Panretin Gel (4% to 11%) ... 1747
Parcopa Orally Disintegrating Tablets ... 3097
▲ Patanol Ophthalmic Solution (Less than 5%) ... 561
Paxil CR Controlled-Release Tablets (Frequent) ... 1538
Paxil (Frequent) ... 1530
Pediarix Vaccine ... 1548
▲ Pegasys (12%) ... 2789
▲ PEG-Intron Powder for Injection (12%) ... 3048
Pentasa Capsules (Less than 1%) ... 3185
Pepcid Injection (Infrequent) ... 2040
Pepcid (Infrequent) ... 2038
Percocet Tablets ... 1131
Percodan Tablets ... 1132
Permax Tablets (Infrequent) ... 3356
Persantine Tablets ... 868
Pexeva Tablets (Frequent) ... 1694
PhosLo GelCaps (Isolated cases) ... 2169
▲ Photofrin for Injection (4%) ... 702
▲ Plavix Tablets (3.3%) ... 917
▲ Plavix Tablets (3.3%) ... 2926
Pletal Tablets (Very rare) ... 2455
Poly-Pred Ophthalmic Suspension ... ⊙233
Pramosone ... 1161
Premarin Intravenous ... 3442
▲ Premarin Tablets (4% to 5%) ... 3446
Premarin Vaginal Cream ... 3452
▲ Premphase Tablets (5% to 10%) ... 3456
▲ Prempro Tablets (5% to 10%) ... 3456
Prevacid Delayed-Release Capsules (Less than 1%) ... 3271
Prevacid for Delayed-Release Oral Suspension (Less than 1%) ... 3271
Prevacid SoluTab Delayed-Release Orally Disintegrating Tablets (Less than 1%) ... 3271
▲ Prevacid NapraPAC (Less than 1% to 9%) ... 3280
Prevnar for Injection ... 3463
PREVPAC (Less than 1%) ... 3284
Prilosec OTC Delayed-Release Tablets (Less than 1%) ... 2677
Primaxin I.M. ... 2045
Primaxin I.V. (0.3%) ... 2048
Prinivil Tablets (Greater than 1%) ... 2052
Prinzide Tablets (0.3% to 1%) ... 2056
▲ ProAmatine Tablets (12.2%) ... 3186
Prochieve 4% Gel ... 1003
Prochieve 8% Gel ... 1003
▲ Procrit for Injection (14% to 22%) ... 2364
▲ Prograf Capsules and Injection (15% to 36%) ... 632
▲ Proleukin for Injection (24%) ... 2266
Prometrium Capsules (100 mg, 200 mg) ... 3203
ProQuad ... 2064
Proquin XR Tablets (Less than 1%) ... 1153
Proscar Tablets ... 2067
ProSom Tablets (1%) ... 517
ProstaScint Kit ... 1037
▲ Protonix I.V. (4%) ... 3472
Protonix Tablets (Less than 1%) ... 3469
▲ Protopic Ointment (25% to 46%) ... 638
Provigil Tablets (At least 1%) ... 988
▲ Prozac Pulvules and Liquid (3%) ... 1801
▲ Pulmicort Respules (1% to 3%) ... 661
Raniclor Tablets, Chewable (0.5%) ... 2505
▲ Rapamune Oral Solution and Tablets (3% to 20%) ... 3475
▲ Rebetol (12% to 29%) ... 3058
▲ Rebetron Combination Therapy (13% to 21%) ... 3063
Recombivax HB (Less than 1%) ... 2071
ReFacto Vials ... 3484
Refludan for Injection (Uncommon) ... 792
Relpax Tablets (Infrequent) ... 2548
▲ Remicade for IV Injection (7%) ... 971
▲ Renagel Tablets (13.1%) ... 1282
ReoPro Vials (0.3%) ... 1809
Requip Tablets (Infrequent) ... 1555
▲ Rescriptor Tablets (2.2% to 3.1%) ... 2551
▲ Retisert Implant (10% to 35%) ... ⊙258
Retrovir Capsules ... 1560
Retrovir IV Infusion ... 1564
Retrovir ... 1560
▲ Revlimid Capsules (2% to 41.9%) ... 958
Reyataz Capsules (Less than 3%) ... 921
▲ Ribavirin, USP Capsules (12% to 29%) ... 3068
▲ Rilutek Tablets (2.5% to 3.8%) ... 2930
Risperdal (Infrequent to 2%) ... 1676
Risperdal Consta Long-Acting Injection (Infrequent) ... 1682
Risperdal M-Tab Orally Disintegrating Tablets (Infrequent to 2%) ... 1676
▲ Rituxan I.V. (1% to 14%) ... 1254
Rocaltrol Capsules ... 2798
Rocaltrol Oral Solution ... 2798
Rocephin Injectable Vials, ADD-Vantage, Galaxy, Bulk (Less than 1%) ... 2800
Rythmol SR Capsules ... 2727
Sandimmune (Rare) ... 2275
▲ Sandostatin Injection (1% to 4%) ... 2278
▲ Sandostatin LAR Depot (5% to 15%) ... 2280
Seroquel Tablets (Infrequent) ... 690
▲ Simulect for Injection (3% to 10%) ... 2284
Singulair ... 2077
Skelaxin Tablets ... 1716
▲ Solodyn Extended Release Tablets (5%) ... 1890
Soltamox Oral Solution (Infrequently) ... 3527
Sonata Capsules (Frequent) ... 1717
▲ Soriatane Capsules (25% to 50%) ... 1013
Spiriva HandiHaler ... 869
Stalevo Tablets ... 2287
▲ Strattera Capsules (1% or greater) ... 1814
Striant Mucoadhesive ... 1007
▲ Stromectol Tablets (2.8% to 27.5%) ... 2083
Sular Tablets (Less than or equal to 1%) ... 3122
Sulfamylon Cream (2.8%) ... 2162
Sulfamylon for 5% Topical Solution (2.3%) ... 2162
Suprax (Less than 2%) ... 1843
Sustiva Capsules (Less than 1% to 2%) ... 930
Sustiva Tablets (Less than 1% to 2%) ... 930
Symbyax Capsules (Infrequent) ... 1819
Symmetrel Tablets ... 1135
Synera Topical Patch (Less than or equal to 1%) ... 1137
Tambocor Tablets (Less than 1%) ... 1856
▲ Tarceva Tablets (0% to 13%) ... 1259
▲ Tarceva Tablets (0% to 13%) ... 2444
Tarka Tablets (Less frequent) ... 524
Tasmar Tablets (Infrequent) ... 3358
Taxotere Injection Concentrate (0.9% to 11.8%) ... 2932
▲ Temodar Capsules (5% to 8%) ... 3073
Temovate Cream (Less frequent) ... 2668
▲ Temovate Gel (Among most frequent) ... 2669
Temovate Ointment (0.5%) ... 2668
Temovate Scalp Application (1 of 294 patients; infrequent) ... 2670
Temovate E Emollient (Less than 2%) ... 2671
Tequin Injection (Less than 0.1%) ... 938
Tequin Injection in 5% Dextrose (Less than 0.1%) ... 938
Tequin Tablets (Less than 0.1%) ... 938
Tessalon Capsules ... 1199
Tessalon Perles ... 1199
Teveten Tablets (Less than 1%) ... 1735
Teveten HCT Tablets (Less than 1%) ... 1737
▲ Thalomid Capsules (8.3%) ... 965
▲ Thiola Tablets (16.7%) ... 2141
Thiothixene Capsules ... 2165
Thyrogen for Injection ... 1286
Thyrolar Tablets ... 1199
Tiazac Capsules (Less than 2%) ... 1201
Ticlid Tablets (1.3%) ... 2810
Timentin ADD-Vantage ... 1580
Timentin Injection Galaxy Container ... 1583
Timentin IV Infusion ... 1577
Timentin Pharmacy Bulk Package ... 1586
Timolide Tablets ... 2086
Timoptic-XE Sterile Ophthalmic Gel Forming Solution ... 2092
Tindamax Tablets ... 2142
▲ Topamax Sprinkle Capsules (1% to 4%) ... 2404
▲ Topamax Tablets (1% to 4%) ... 2404
▲ Toprol-XL Tablets (About 5 of 100 patients) ... 668
▲ Tracleer Tablets (4%) ... 545
Trasylol Injection ... 754
Trelstar Depot (1.4%) ... 3394
Tricor Tablets ... 527
▲ Tri-Luma Cream (4.22% to 11%) ... 1213
▲ Trisenox Injection (33%) ... 993
Trusopt Sterile Ophthalmic Solution ... 2095
▲ Truvada Tablets (5%) ... 1296
Tussionex Pennkinetic Extended-Release Suspension ... 3327
Twinrix Vaccine (Less than 1%) ... 1595
Tygacil for Injection (2.6%) ... 3488
Tylenol with Codeine Tablets ... 2391
Ultane Liquid for Inhalation (Less than 1%) ... 531
▲ Ultram ER Tablets (6.2% to 11.9%) ... 2392
Uniretic Tablets (Less than 1%) ... 3100
Univasc Tablets (Less than 1%) ... 3104
Uroxatral Tablets ... 2943
▲ Urso 250 Tablets (5%) ... 710
▲ Urso Forte Tablets (5%) ... 710
▲ Valcyte Tablets (Less than 5%) ... 2813
Valtrex Caplets ... 1597
Vancocin HCl Capsules, USP ... 3380
▲ Vandazole Vaginal Gel (6%) ... 3338
Vanos Cream ... 1893
Vantas (Less than 2%) ... 3375
Vaqta (Less than 1%) ... 2097
Varivax (Greater than or equal to 1%) ... 2100
Vasotec I.V. Injection (0.5% to 1.0%) ... 2103
▲ Velcade for Injection (11%) ... 2133
▲ Vesanoid Capsules (20%) ... 2820
VFEND I.V. (1% to 1.1%) ... 2564
VFEND Oral Suspension (1% to 1.1%) ... 2564
VFEND Tablets (1% to 1.1%) ... 2564
Viadur Implant (Less than 2%) ... 757
Viagra Tablets (Less than 2%) ... 2573
Vicodin Tablets ... 535
Vicodin ES Tablets ... 536
Vicodin HP Tablets ... 538
▲ Vicoprofen Tablets (3% to 9%) ... 539
Viracept (Less than 2%) ... 2577
Viramune Oral Suspension ... 873
Viramune Tablets ... 873
▲ Viread Tablets (5% to 18%) ... 1301
Visudyne for Injection ... 2305
Vivitrol ... 995
▲ Voltaren Tablets (1% to 10%) ... 2307
▲ Voltaren-XR Tablets (1% to 10%) ... 2310
Vytorin 10/10 Tablets ... 2114
Vytorin 10/10 Tablets ... 3077
Vytorin 10/20 Tablets ... 2114
Vytorin 10/20 Tablets ... 3077
Vytorin 10/40 Tablets ... 2114
Vytorin 10/40 Tablets ... 3077
Vytorin 10/80 Tablets ... 2114
Vytorin 10/80 Tablets ... 3077
Wellbutrin Tablets (2.2%) ... 1603
▲ Wellbutrin SR Sustained-Release Tablets (2% to 4%) ... 1607
▲ Wellbutrin XL Extended-Release Tablets (2% to 4%) ... 1613
WinRho SDF ... 732
▲ Xeloda Tablets (Less than 5%) ... 2822
Xenical Capsules ... 2831
Xerac AC Solution ... 2507
Xifaxan Tablets ... 2842
Xolair (2%) ... 1266
Xyrem Oral Solution (Frequent) ... 1688
Yasmin 28 Tablets ... 796
Zantac Injection ... 1619
Zegerid Capsules (Less than 1%) ... 2958
Zegerid Powder for Oral Solution (Less than 1%) ... 2958
Zelapar Tablets ... 3372
Zelnorm Tablets (Up to 1%) ... 2312
Zemaira (0.2% to 0.4%) ... 3509
Zemplar Injection ... 543
Zemuron Injection (Less than 1%) ... 2346
Zinacef for Injection (Fewer than 1 in 250 patients) ... 1631
Zinacef Injection (Fewer than 1 in 250 patients) ... 1631
Zmax for Oral Suspension (Less then 1%) ... 2583
Zocor Tablets ... 2105
Zofran Injection (2%) ... 1634
▲ Zofran (5%) ... 1639
▲ Zofran ODT Orally Disintegrating Tablets (5%) ... 1639
Zoloft (Infrequent) ... 2586
Zometa for Intravenous Infusion ... 2315
Zomig Tablets (Infrequent) ... 3519
Zomig Nasal Spray (Infrequent) ... 3523
Zomig-ZMT Tablets (Infrequent) ... 3519
Zonegran Capsules (Frequent) ... 1101
▲ Zosyn (3.1% to 3.2%) ... 3492
Zovirax Capsules ... 1643
Zovirax Cream ... 820
Zovirax Ointment ... 821
Zovirax ... 1643
▲ Zyban Sustained-Release Tablets (3%) ... 1644
Zyflo Tablets (Greater than 1%) ... 1023
Zyprexa Tablets ... 1830
Zyprexa ZYDIS Orally Disintegrating Tablets ... 1830
Zyrtec Chewable Tablets (Less than 2%) ... 2594
Zyrtec (Less than 2%) ... 2594
Zyrtec-D 12 Hour Extended Release Tablets (Less than 2%) ... 2597
Zyvox (0% to 0.4%) ... 2652

Pruritus, ear lobes

Miacalcin Injection ... 2252

Pruritus, exacerbation of

▲ Cutivate Cream (0.8% to 3%) ... 2662

Pruritus, femal genital

Proquin XR Tablets (Less than 1%) ... 1153

Pruritus, genital
Ceftin Tablets (0.1% to 1%) 1407
Cipro (1%) 2977
Cipro I.V. (1%) 2984
Evoxac Capsules (Less than 1%) 1047
Keflex Capsules 549
Levaquin (0.1% to 0.9%) 2384
Levaquin in 5% Dextrose Injection (0.1% to 0.9%) 2384
Neurontin Capsules (Rare) 2487
Neurontin Oral Solution (Rare) 2487
Neurontin Tablets (Rare) 2487
Primaxin I.M. 2045
Primaxin I.V. (Less than 0.2%) 2048
▲ Prochieve 4% Gel (5%) 1003
▲ Prochieve 8% Gel (5%) 1003
ProSom Tablets (Infrequent) 517
Raniclor Tablets, Chewable (1%) 2505
Risperdal (Rare) 1676
Risperdal M-Tab Orally Disintegrating Tablets (Rare) 1676
Suprax (Les than 2%) 1843
Trileptal Tablets 2300
Trileptal Oral Suspension 2300
▲ Vagifem Tablets (6%) 2334
Vantin Tablets and Oral Suspension (Less than 1%) 2645
Zosyn (1.0% or less) 3492

Pruritus, genital, male
Vantas (Less than 2%) 3375

Pruritus, injection site
▲ Alferon N Injection (12%) 1665
Cerezyme for Injection (Less than 1%) 1270
Cipro I.V. (1% or less) 2984
▲ Copaxone for Injection (40%) 3297
▲ Enbrel for Injection (37%) 584
Engerix-B Vaccine (Less than 1%) 1425
▲ Fuzeon Injection (65%) 2767
▲ Gardasil Injection (3.1%) 1984
Humalog-Pen 1781
Humulin 50/50, 100 Units 1791
Humulin 70/30 Pen 1793
Humulin L, 100 Units 1794
Humulin N Pen 1797
▲ Intron A for Injection (Less than 5%) 3024
Invanz for Injection (Greater than 0.5%) 1999
Vaqta (Less than 1%) 2097
▲ Varivax (19.3% to 32.5%) 2100
▲ Vivitrol (6% to 10%) 995
▲ Zostavax Injection (6.6%) 2111

Pruritus, localized
▲ Aldara Cream, 5% (22% to 32%) 1846
Cleocin Vaginal Ovules (Less than 1%) 2616
Mentax Cream (Less than 2%) 2158
▲ Oxytrol Transdermal System (14% to 16.8%) 3392
▲ Polytrim Ophthalmic Solution (Among most frequent) 574
ProctoFoam-HC 3099

Pruritus, ocular
▲ Alphagan P Ophthalmic Solution (Approximately 10% to 20%) 567
▲ Alrex Ophthalmic Suspension 0.2% (5% to 15%) ⊙246
Aredia for Injection (One patient) 2179
Azopt Ophthalmic Suspension (1% to 5%) 557
▲ Betimol Ophthalmic Solution (More than 5%) 3382
▲ Betimol Ophthalmic Solution (More than 5%) ⊙295
Betoptic S Ophthalmic Suspension (Small number of patients) 558
▲ Brimonidine Tartrate Ophthalmic Solution 0.2% (10% to 30%) ⊙248
▲ Carac Cream, 0.5% (5.4%) 2879
▲ Ciloxan Ophthalmic Ointment (Less than 10%) 559
▲ Ciloxan Ophthalmic Solution (Less than 10%) ⊙206
Clorpres Tablets 2153
▲ Cosopt Sterile Ophthalmic Solution (5% to 15%) 1931
▲ Elestat Ophthalmic Solution (1% to 10%) 1669
Imitrex Nasal Spray 1467
▲ Lotemax Ophthalmic Suspension 0.5% (5% to 15%) ⊙251
▲ Lucentis Injection (0% to 13%) 1237
▲ Lumigan Ophthalmic Solution (15% to 45%) 573
Maxalt Tablets (Infrequent) 2008
Maxalt-MLT Orally Disintegrating Tablets (Infrequent) 2008
Neurontin Capsules (Rare) 2487
Neurontin Oral Solution (Rare) 2487
Neurontin Tablets (Rare) 2487
Quixin Ophthalmic Solution (Less than 1%) 3383
▲ Restasis Ophthalmic Emulsion (1% to 5%) 575
▲ Soriatane Capsules (1% to 5%) 1013
Sular Tablets (Less than or equal to 1%) 3122
Timoptic Sterile Ophthalmic Solution 2088
Timoptic in Ocudose 2091
Timoptic-XE Sterile Ophthalmic Gel Forming Solution 2092
TobraDex Ophthalmic Ointment (Less than 4%) 562
TobraDex Ophthalmic Suspension (Less than 4%) 563
Transderm Scōp Transdermal Therapeutic System (Infrequent) 2177
▲ Travatan Ophthalmic Solution (5% to 10%) 563
Vantin Tablets and Oral Suspension (Less than 1%) 2645
Vaqta (Less than 1%) 2097
▲ Vigamox Ophthalmic Solution (1% to 6%) 564
Visine For Contacts Rewetting Drops ⊙289
▲ Visudyne for Injection (1% to 10%) 2305
▲ Voltaren Ophthalmic Solution (Less than or equal to 5%) 2309
▲ Xalatan Sterile Ophthalmic Solution (5% to 15%) 2649
Xopenex Inhalation Solution Concentrate (Less than 2%) 3150

Pruritus, oral
Imitrex Nasal Spray 1467
▲ Nevanac Ophthalmic Suspension 0.1% (1% to 5%) ⊙209

Pruritus, penile
▲ Caverject Impulse Injection (3%) 2612

Pruritus, rhinal
Atrovent Nasal Spray 0.03% (2.0%) 837
▲ Miacalcin Nasal Spray (10.6%) 2253

Pruritus, vaginal
Cipro XR Tablets 2990
FazaClo Orally Disintegrating Tablets (Less than 1%) 551
Invanz for Injection (Greater than 0.1%) 1999
Proquin XR Tablets 1153

Pruritus ani
Arthrotec Tablets (Rare) 3129
Celexa (Rare) 1176
Colazal Capsules 2838
Estring Vaginal Ring 2635
Keflex Capsules 549
Nexium Delayed-Release Capsules (Less than 1%) 655
Nexium I.V. (Less than 1%) 659
Noroxin Tablets (Less frequent) 2032
PREVPAC (Less than 3%) 3284

Pruritus at application site
▲ Clobex Spray (3%) 1208
Evoclin Foam, 1% (1%) 1009
Ionsys Transdermal System (.1% to less than 1%) 2379
Lidoderm Patch 1118

Pseudoaneurysm
ReoPro Vials (0.8%) 1809

Pseudohypoparathyroidism
▲ Rocaltrol Capsules (1 in 3) 2798
▲ Rocaltrol Oral Solution (1 in 3) 2798

Pseudolymphoma
Phenytek Capsules 2160

Pseudomembranous enterocolitis
Rilutek Tablets (Rare) 2930

Pseudoparkinsonism
Thioridazine Hydrochloride Tablets (Infrequent) 2163
Thiothixene Capsules 2165
Wellbutrin Tablets (1.5%) 1603

Pseudotumor cerebri
Accutane Capsules 2731
Depo-Medrol Injectable Suspension 2617
Garamycin Injectable 3014
Hydrocortone Tablets 1989
Levothroid Tablets 1186
Levoxyl Tablets 1712
Solodyn Extended Release Tablets 1890
Soriatane Capsules (Less than 1%) 1013
Synthroid Tablets 520
Tygacil for Injection 3488
Vesanoid Capsules 2820

Psoriasis
Abilify Oral Solution (Infrequent) 882
Abilify Oral Solution (Infrequent) 2450
Abilify Discmelt Orally Disintegrating Tablets (Infrequent) 882
Abilify Discmelt Orally Disintegrating Tablets (Infrequent) 2450
Abilify Tablets (Infrequent) 882
Abilify Tablets (Infrequent) 2450
Aciphex Tablets (Rare) 1090
Asacol Delayed-Release Tablets (Rare) 2692
Campral Tablets (Rare) 1174
Celexa (Infrequent) 1176
Chantix Tablets (Infrequent) 2517
Colazal Capsules 2838
Copaxone for Injection (Infrequent) 3297
Doxil Injection (Less than 1%) 2351
Effexor Tablets (Infrequent) 3411
Effexor XR Capsules (Infrequent) 3417
Gabitril Tablets (Infrequent) 984
▲ Intron A for Injection (Less than 5%) 3024
▲ Limbrel Capsules (Greater than or equal to 2%) 2672
Neurontin Capsules (Rare) 2487
Neurontin Oral Solution (Rare) 2487
Neurontin Tablets (Rare) 2487
Norvir (Less than 2%) 503
Pegasys 2789
Provigil Tablets (At least 1%) 988
Prozac Pulvules and Liquid (Rare) 1801
Raptiva for Injection (0.7%) 1250
Relpax Tablets (Rare) 2548
Requip Tablets (Infrequent) 1555
Rilutek Tablets (Infrequent) 2930
Seroquel Tablets (Rare) 690
Sonata Capsules (Rare) 1717
Symbyax Capsules (Infrequent) 1819
Thalomid Capsules 965
Trileptal Tablets 2300
Trileptal Oral Suspension 2300
Uniretic Tablets (Less than 1%) 3100
VFEND I.V. (Less than 2%) 2564
VFEND Oral Suspension (Less than 2%) 2564
VFEND Tablets (Less than 2%) 2564

Psoriasis, exacerbation of
Cosopt Sterile Ophthalmic Solution 1931
▲ Intron A for Injection (Less than 5%) 3024
Lamisil Tablets 2232
Lithobid Tablets 1692
Neupogen for Injection (Infrequent) 603
Oxsoralen-Ultra Capsules 3353
PEG-Intron Powder for Injection (Less than or equal to 1%) 3048
Risperdal (Rare) 1676
Risperdal M-Tab Orally Disintegrating Tablets (Rare) 1676
Soriatane Capsules (Less than 1%) 1013
Temovate Cream 2668
Temovate Scalp Application (Rare) 2670
Timoptic Sterile Ophthalmic Solution 2088
Timoptic in Ocudose 2091
Timoptic-XE Sterile Ophthalmic Gel Forming Solution 2092
Toprol-XL Tablets 668

Psoriasis, pustular
Cutivate Cream 2662
Cutivate Lotion 0.05% (Rare) 2664
Cutivate Ointment 2665

Psoriasis, worsening of
Enbrel for Injection 584
Lopressor Injection (Very rare) 2238
Lopressor Tablets (Very rare) 2238
Lopressor HCT 50/25 Tablets (Very rare) 2241
Lopressor HCT 100/25 Tablets (Very rare) 2241
Lopressor HCT 100/50 Tablets (Very rare) 2241

Psychiatric disturbances
Accutane Capsules 2731
Advicor Tablets 1722
Aldoril Tablets 1910
Altoprev Extended-Release Tablets 3109
Arthrotec Tablets (Rare) 3129
Clinoril Tablets (Less than 1 in 100) 1924
Cosopt Sterile Ophthalmic Solution 1931
Cuprimine Capsules 1947
Decadron Tablets 1951
Didronel Tablets 2697
▲ Focalin XR Capsules (26% to 46%) 2223
▲ Gengraf Capsules (5.0%) 459
Hydrocortone Tablets 1989
Indocin (Less than 1%) 1995
Infergen 3364
Invirase (Less than 2%) 2772
Lariam Tablets (Occasional) 2786
Lescol Capsules 2233
Lescol XL Tablets 2233
▲ Leukine (15%) 814
Mintezol 2027
Nembutal Sodium Solution, USP (Less than 1%) 2470
Neoral Oral Solution 2259
Neoral Soft Gelatin Capsules 2259
Noroxin Tablets 2032
Pepcid Injection (Infrequent) 2040
Pepcid (Infrequent) 2038
Prilosec OTC Delayed-Release Tablets (Less than 1%) 2677
Primaxin I.M. 2045
Primaxin I.V. (Less than 0.2%) 2048
Pulmicort Respules (Less than 1%) 661
Sandimmune 2275
Thioridazine Hydrochloride Tablets (Extremely rare) 2163
Timoptic Sterile Ophthalmic Solution (Less frequent) 2088
Timoptic in Ocudose (Less frequent) 2091
Timoptic-XE Sterile Ophthalmic Gel Forming Solution 2092
Vytorin 10/10 Tablets 2114
Vytorin 10/10 Tablets 3077
Vytorin 10/20 Tablets 2114
Vytorin 10/20 Tablets 3077
Vytorin 10/40 Tablets 2114
Vytorin 10/40 Tablets 3077
Vytorin 10/80 Tablets 2114
Vytorin 10/80 Tablets 3077
Zegerid Capsules (Less than 1%) 2958
Zegerid Powder for Oral Solution (Less than 1%) 2958
Zocor Tablets 2105

Psychic dependence
(*see under* Dependence, psychological)

Psychomotor retardation
Ambien CR Tablets (2%) 2855
Lithobid Tablets 1692
Sonata Capsules (Rare) 1717
▲ Topamax Sprinkle Capsules (2% to 21%) 2404
▲ Topamax Tablets (2% to 21%) 2404

Psychoses
Abilify Oral Solution 882
Abilify Oral Solution 2450
Abilify Discmelt Orally Disintegrating Tablets 882
Abilify Discmelt Orally Disintegrating Tablets 2450
Abilify Tablets 882
Abilify Tablets 2450
Accutane Capsules 2731
Adderall Tablets (Rare) 3164
Adderall XR Capsules 3166
Adipex-P 1215
Aldoril Tablets 1910
▲ Aredia for Injection (Up to 4%) 2179
Avelox 2970
Azilect Tablets (Infrequent) 3293
Biaxin/Biaxin XL 402
BiDil Tablets 2171
Buprenex Injectable (Less than 1%) 2716
Campral Tablets (Rare) 1174
Celexa (Infrequent) 1176
▲ CellCept Capsules (3% to less than 20%) 2747
▲ CellCept Intravenous (3% to less than 20%) 2747
▲ CellCept Oral Suspension (3% to less than 20%) 2747
▲ CellCept Tablets (3% to less than 20%) 2747
Cesamet Capsules 3340
Chantix Tablets (Rare) 2517
Clinoril Tablets (Less than 1 in 100) 1924
Concerta Extended-Release Tablets 1881
Copegus Tablets (Less than 1%) 2754
Covera-HS Tablets (Less than 2%) 3139
Dapsone Tablets USP 1673

Decadron Tablets 1951
Depacon Injection 412
Depakene 417
Depakote Sprinkle Capsules 422
Depakote Tablets 427
Depakote ER Tablets (Greater than 1%) 434
Desoxyn Tablets, USP (Rare) 2462
Dexedrine (Rare at recommended doses) 1420
DextroStat Tablets (Rare) 3179
Effexor Tablets (Rare) 3411
Effexor XR Capsules (Infrequent) 3417
Exelon Capsules (Infrequent) 2206
Exelon Oral Solution (Infrequent) 2206
Gabitril Tablets (Infrequent) 984
Geodon for Injection (Up to 1%) 2529
Guanidine Hydrochloride Tablets 3016
Hydrocortone Tablets 1989
Indocin (Less than 1%) 1995
Invirase (Less than 2%) 2772
Klonopin 2778
Lamictal (Infrequent) 1481
Lanoxicaps Capsules 1490
Lanoxin Injection 1494
Lanoxin Injection Pediatric 1497
Lariam Tablets (Occasional) 2786
Mirapex Tablets (Less than 1%) 859
Namenda (Infrequent) 1195
Neurontin Capsules (Infrequent) 2487
Neurontin Oral Solution (Infrequent) 2487
Neurontin Tablets (Infrequent) 2487
Noroxin Tablets 2032
Orthoclone OKT3 Sterile Solution 2360
Paxil CR Controlled-Release Tablets (Rare) 1538
Paxil (Rare) 1530
PEG-Intron Powder for Injection (Less than or equal to 1%) 3048
Permax Tablets (2.1%; Frequent) 3356
Pexeva Tablets (rare) 1694
PREVPAC 3284
▲ Prograf Capsules and Injection (3% to 15%) 632
Provigil Tablets 988
Prozac Pulvules and Liquid (Infrequent) 1801
Pulmicort Respules (Less than 1%) 661
Reyataz Capsules (Less than 3%) 921
Rilutek Tablets (Rare) 2930
Ritalin Hydrochloride Tablets 2269
Ritalin LA Capsules 2271
Ritalin-SR Tablets 2269
Rocaltrol Capsules (Rare) 2798
Rocaltrol Oral Solution (Rare) 2798
Seromycin Capsules 1813
Stalevo Tablets 2287
Sustiva Capsules (Less than 2%) 930
Sustiva Tablets (Less than 2%) 930
Symmetrel Tablets (0.1% to 1%) 1135
Tarka Tablets 524
Tasmar Tablets (Infrequent) 3358
Tequin Injection (Less than 0.1%) 938
Tequin Injection in 5% Dextrose (Less than 0.1%) 938
Tequin Tablets (Less than 0.1%) 938
Thalomid Capsules 965
Topamax Sprinkle Capsules (Frequent) 2404
Topamax Tablets (Frequent) 2404
Trecator Tablets 3487
▲ Valcyte Tablets (Less than 5%) 2813
Valtrex Caplets 1597
▲ Velcade for Injection (35%) 2133
Verelan PM Extended-Release Capsules, Controlled-Onset (2% or less) 3106
VFEND I.V. (Less than 2%) 2564
VFEND Oral Suspension (Less than 2%) 2564
VFEND Tablets (Less than 2%) 2564
Wellbutrin Tablets (Infrequent) 1603
Wellbutrin SR Sustained-Release Tablets 1607
Wellbutrin XL Extended-Release Tablets 1613
Zoloft 2586
Zomig Nasal Spray (Rare) 3523
Zovirax 1643
Zyban Sustained-Release Tablets 1644

Psychoses, aggravation
Clozaril Tablets 2184
Decadron Tablets 1951
FazaClo Orally Disintegrating Tablets 551
Hydrocortone Tablets 1989
Seroquel Tablets (Infrequent) 690
Thioridazine Hydrochloride Tablets 2163

Psychoses, toxic
Cesamet Capsules 3340
Cipro 2977
Cipro I.V. (1% or less) 2984
Cipro XR Tablets 2990
Concerta Extended-Release Tablets 1881
Daytrana Transdermal Patch 3174
Focalin Tablets (Rare) 2220
Focalin XR Capsules 2223
Levaquin 2384
Levaquin in 5% Dextrose Injection 2384
Metadate CD Capsules 3323
Proquin XR Tablets 1153
Ritalin Hydrochloride Tablets 2269
Ritalin LA Capsules 2271
Ritalin-SR Tablets 2269

Psychosis, activation
Carbatrol Capsules 3171
FazaClo Orally Disintegrating Tablets 551
Pegasys (Less than 1%) 2789
Risperdal Consta Long-Acting Injection (Frequent) 1682
Tegretol/Tegretol-XR 2295
Wellbutrin SR Sustained-Release Tablets 1607
Wellbutrin XL Extended-Release Tablets 1613
Zyban Sustained-Release Tablets 1644

Psychosis, overt
Calcijex Injection (Rare) 411
Hectorol Capsules 1275
Hectorol Injection (Rare) 1278

Psychosis, unspecified
Atripla Tablets 945
Bicillin C-R Injectable Suspension 1706
Gantrisin Pediatric Suspension 2770
Zelapar Tablets 3372

Psychotic episodes
(*see under* Psychoses)

Psychotic symptoms
DextroStat Tablets 3179
Ritalin Hydrochloride Tablets 2269
Ritalin LA Capsules 2271
Ritalin-SR Tablets 2269

Psychotic symptoms, paradoxical exacerbation
DextroStat Tablets 3179
Thiothixene Capsules 2165

Ptosis
Abilify Oral Solution (Rare) 882
Abilify Oral Solution (Rare) 2450
Abilify Discmelt Orally Disintegrating Tablets (Rare) 882
Abilify Discmelt Orally Disintegrating Tablets (Rare) 2450
Abilify Tablets (Rare) 882
Abilify Tablets (Rare) 2450
Lunesta Tablets (Rare) 3142
Lyrica Capsules (Rare) 2539
Namenda (Infrequent) 1195
Pexeva Tablets (Rare) 1694
Relpax Tablets (Rare) 2548
▲ Retisert Implant (10% to 35%) ⊙258
Topamax Sprinkle Capsules (Infrequent) 2404
Topamax Tablets (Infrequent) 2404

Ptosis, eyelids
Betagan Ophthalmic Solution, USP ⊙220
Betimol Ophthalmic Solution 3382
Betimol Ophthalmic Solution ⊙295
Blephamide Ophthalmic Ointment (Occasional) 568
Blephamide Ophthalmic Suspension 569
Blocadren Tablets 1916
▲ BOTOX Purified Neurotoxin Complex (0.3% to 15.7%) 570
Carteolol Hydrochloride Ophthalmic Solution USP, 1% (Occasional) ⊙249
Celexa (Rare) 1176
Clozaril Tablets (Less than 1%) 2184
Copaxone for Injection (Infrequent) 3297
Cosopt Sterile Ophthalmic Solution 1931
FML Ophthalmic Ointment (Occasional) ⊙228
FML Ophthalmic Suspension (Occasional) ⊙227
FML Forte Ophthalmic Suspension (Occasional) ⊙226
▲ Imdur Tablets (Less than or equal to 5%) 3018
Lamictal (Rare) 1481
Lexapro Oral Solution (Frequent) 1190
Lexapro Tablets (Frequent) 1190
Neurontin Capsules (Infrequent) 2487
Neurontin Oral Solution (Infrequent) 2487
Neurontin Tablets (Infrequent) 2487
Paxil CR Controlled-Release Tablets (Rare) 1538
Paxil (Rare) 1530
Pred Mild Ophthalmic Suspension (Occasional) ⊙238
Pred Forte Ophthalmic Suspension (Occasional) ⊙235
Rythmol SR Capsules 2727
Sonata Capsules (Rare) 1717
Tequin Injection (Less than 0.1%) 938
Tequin Injection in 5% Dextrose (Less than 0.1%) 938
Tequin Tablets (Less than 0.1%) 938
Timolide Tablets 2086
Timoptic Sterile Ophthalmic Solution (Less frequent) 2088
Timoptic in Ocudose (Less frequent) 2091
Timoptic-XE Sterile Ophthalmic Gel Forming Solution 2092
Trileptal Tablets 2300
Trileptal Oral Suspension 2300
Zoloft (Rare) 2586
Zyrtec Chewable Tablets (Less than 2%) 2594
Zyrtec (Less than 2%) 2594
Zyrtec-D 12 Hour Extended Release Tablets (Less than 2%) 2597

Pulmonary allergy, unspecified
▲ Remicade for IV Injection (6%) 971

Pulmonary apoplexy
Sandostatin LAR Depot (Rare) 2280

Pulmonary collapse
Levaquin (0.1% to 0.9%) 2384
Levaquin in 5% Dextrose Injection (0.1% to 0.9%) 2384

Pulmonary complications, unspecified
Follistim AQ Cartridge 2338

Pulmonary congestion
Aldara Cream, 5% (0.5%) 1846
Aricept Tablets (Infrequent) 1094
Aricept ODT Tablets (Infrequent) 1094
Avalide Tablets 888
Avalide Tablets 2874
Avapro Tablets (Less than 1%) 891
Avapro Tablets (Less than 1%) 2871
Evoxac Capsules (Less than 1%) 1047
Prinzide Tablets 2056
▲ Proleukin for Injection (54%) 2266
ProQuad 2064
Rythmol SR Capsules 2727
Vicoprofen Tablets (Less than 1%) 539

Pulmonary disease, chronic obstructive
Campath Ampules 811
Rythmol SR Capsules 2727
Vivitrol 995

Pulmonary disease, chronic obstructive, exacerbation of
▲ Atrovent HFA Inhalation Aerosol (8% to 23%) 841
▲ Orencia Powder for Intravenous Infusion (8%) 914
▲ Zemaira (7 of 30 Patients) 3509

Pulmonary disorder, unspecified
▲ Hycamtin for Injection (17%) 1458
▲ Taxotere Injection Concentrate (21% to 40.9%) 2932

Pulmonary distress
Betoptic S Ophthalmic Suspension (Rare) 558
Follistim AQ Cartridge 2338

Pulmonary edema
(*see under* Edema, pulmonary)

Pulmonary embolism
(*see under* Embolism, pulmonary)

Pulmonary emphysema, interstitial
▲ Infasurf Intratracheal Suspension (7% to 10%) 1184

Pulmonary events, unspecified
▲ Mylotarg for Injection (8% to 10%) 3431

Pulmonary fibrosis
Aceon Tablets (2 mg, 4 mg, 8 mg) (Less than 0.1%) 3194
Agrylin Capsules 3169
Alkeran for Injection 955
Alkeran Tablets 956
Campath Ampules 811
CellCept Capsules (Rare) 2747
CellCept Intravenous (Rare) 2747
CellCept Oral Suspension (Rare) 2747
CellCept Tablets (Rare) 2747
Cuprimine Capsules (Rare) 1947
Eloxatin for Injection 2892
Evoxac Capsules (Less than 1%) 1047
Garamycin Injectable 3014
Gleevec Tablets (Rare) 2227
Herceptin I.V. (Rare) 1233
I.V. Busulfex (Rare) 2493
Leukeran Tablets 1504
Lyrica Capsules (Rare) 2539
Myfortic Tablets (Rare) 2255
Myleran Tablets (Rare) 1525
Paxil CR Controlled-Release Tablets (Rare) 1538
Paxil (Rare) 1530
Pentasa Capsules (One case) 3185
Permax Tablets (Rare) 3356
Pexeva Tablets (Rare) 1694
Rapamune Oral Solution and Tablets 3475
Tarceva Tablets 1259
Tarceva Tablets 2444
Tasmar Tablets (One case) 3358
Taxotere Injection Concentrate (Rare) 2932

Pulmonary function, changes
Eulexin Capsules (Less than 1%) 3009
Intron A for Injection 3024
▲ Leukine (48%) 814
Virazole for Inhalation Solution 3370

Pulmonary function, decreased
Relenza Rotadisk 1552
▲ Rilutek Tablets (13.1% to 16%) 2930

Pulmonary hemorrhage
(*see under* Hemorrhage, pulmonary)

Pulmonary hypersensitivity
Carbatrol Capsules 3171
Equetro Extended-Release Capsules 3180
Tegretol/Tegretol-XR 2295

Pulmonary hypersensitivity, chronic
Timolide Tablets 2086

Pulmonary hypertension
Adipex-P (Rare) 1215
Agrylin Capsules 3169
Bicillin C-R Injectable Suspension 1706
▲ CellCept Capsules (3% to less than 20%) 2747
▲ CellCept Intravenous (3% to less than 20%) 2747
▲ CellCept Oral Suspension (3% to less than 20%) 2747
▲ CellCept Tablets (3% to less than 20%) 2747
Elitek (Less than or equal to 1%) 2890
▲ Indocin I.V. (1% to 3%) 2465
Paxil CR Controlled-Release Tablets 1538
Paxil 1530
Permax Tablets (Rare) 3356
Pexeva Tablets 1694
Prozac Pulvules and Liquid 1801
Revlimid Capsules (1.4%) 958
Sandostatin LAR Depot (Rare) 2280
Trasylol Injection (1% to 2%) 754
▲ Vesanoid Capsules (3%) 2820
Zoloft 2586

Pulmonary infarction
Prinivil Tablets (0.3% to 1.0%) 2052
Prinzide Tablets 2056
Vasotec I.V. Injection (0.5% to 1.0%) 2103

Pulmonary infiltrates
Agrylin Capsules 3169
Campath Ampules 811
Fansidar Tablets 2765
Gantrisin Pediatric Suspension 2770
Herceptin I.V. 1233
▲ Imdur Tablets (Less than or equal to 5%) 3018
Intron A for Injection (Rare) 3024
Leustatin Injection 2357

Pegasys 2789
PEG-Intron Powder for Injection 3048
Pentasa Capsules (Less than 1%) 3185
Prinivil Tablets (0.3% to 1.0%) 2052
Prinzide Tablets 2056
Rebetol 3058
Rebetron Combination Therapy 3063
Rituxan I.V. 1254
Stalevo Tablets (Rare) 2287
Tarceva Tablets 1259
Tarceva Tablets 2444
Thiola Tablets (2%) 2141
Vantin Tablets and Oral Suspension 2645
Vasotec I.V. Injection (0.5% to 1.0%) 2103
▲ Vesanoid Capsules (6%) 2820

Pulmonary insufficiency
Herceptin I.V. 1233

Pulmonary nodule
Sandostatin Injection (Less than 1%) 2278
Sandostatin LAR Depot (Rare) 2280

Pulmonary physical finding
Tygacil for Injection (1.9%) 3488

Pulmonary reembolism
Activase I.V. 1223

Pulmonary symptoms, worsening
Accolate Tablets (Rare) 671
Flovent Diskus 1443
Singulair 2077

Pulmonary toxicity, unspecified
Alkeran for Injection 955
Alkeran Tablets 956
Myleran Tablets 1525

Pulse, fast
Caverject Impulse Injection (Less than 1%) 2612
Humalog-Pen (Less common) 1781
Humalog Mix 50/50-Pen 1783
Humulin 50/50, 100 Units 1791
Humulin 70/30 Pen (Less common) 1793
Humulin L, 100 Units (Less common) 1794
Humulin N Pen (Less common) 1797
Levoxyl Tablets 1712
Children's Motrin Oral Suspension ■ 685
Children's Motrin Non-Staining Dye-Free Oral Suspension ■ 685
Children's Motrin Oral Suspension 1867
Children's Motrin Non-Staining Dye-Free Oral Suspension 1867
Infants' Motrin Concentrated Drops 1867
Infants' Motrin Non-Staining Dye-Free Concentrated Drops 1867
Junior Strength Motrin Caplets and Chewable Tablets 1867
Prosed/DS Tablets 1157

Pulse changes
Clozaril Tablets 2184
Concerta Extended-Release Tablets 1881
Effexor Tablets 3411
Focalin Tablets 2220
Focalin XR Capsules 2223
Imitrex Injection (Rare) 1463
Imitrex Nasal Spray 1467
Mephyton Tablets (Rare) 2018
Metadate CD Capsules 3323
Moban Tablets 1119
Norvasc Tablets (Less than 0.1%) 2545
Plasbumin-5 (Rare) 3251
Plasbumin-20 (Rare) 3252
Plasbumin-25 (Rare) 3253
Risperdal 1676
Risperdal M-Tab Orally Disintegrating Tablets 1676
Ritalin Hydrochloride Tablets 2269
Ritalin LA Capsules 2271
Ritalin-SR Tablets 2269
Rituxan I.V. (Two cases) 1254
Seroquel Tablets (Infrequent) 690

Pulse rate, decreased
Daytrana Transdermal Patch 3174
Focalin XR Capsules 2223

Pulse rate, depression
Lanoxicaps Capsules 1490
Lanoxin Injection 1494
ReoPro Vials (1.0%) 1809

Pulse rate, increased
Agrylin Capsules 3169
Daytrana Transdermal Patch 3174
Focalin XR Capsules 2223
Twinject 0.3 3378
Twinject 0.15 3379

Pulse, irregular
Caduet Tablets (Less than or equal to 0.1%) 2508
Lariam Tablets (Infrequent) 2786
Phenergan Tablets and Suppositories 3440
Rythmol SR Capsules 2727

Pupil enlargement
Cesamet Capsules 3340
Naphcon-A Eye Drops ⊙ 208
Visine-A Eye Allergy Relief Eye Drops ⊙ 289

Purple toes syndrome
Activase I.V. 1223
Coumadin for Injection (Infrequent) 898
Coumadin Tablets (Infrequent) 898
Miradon Tablets 3042

Purpura
Aceon Tablets (2 mg, 4 mg, 8 mg) (0.1%) 3194
Adalat CC Tablets (Rare) 2964
Advicor Tablets 1722
Aggrenox Capsules (1.4%) 822
Aldoril Tablets 1910
Altace Capsules (Less than 1%) 1702
Altoprev Extended-Release Tablets (Rare) 3109
Ambien Tablets (Rare) 2851
Ambien CR Tablets (Rare) 2855
AmBisome for Injection (Less common) 620
Amerge Tablets (Rare) 1339
Anaprox Tablets (Less than 3%) 2761
Anaprox DS Tablets (Less than 3%) 2761
Anzemet Injection (Infrequently) 2859
Anzemet Tablets (Infrequently) 2862
▲ Arixtra Injection (0% to 3.5%) 1351
Arthrotec Tablets (Rare) 3129
Attenuvax (Rare) 1914
Avalide Tablets 888
Avalide Tablets 2874
Azilect Tablets (Rare) 3293
BiDil Tablets 2171
Caduet Tablets (Greater than 0.1% to less than or equal to 1%) 2508
▲ Campath Ampules (8%) 811
Carbatrol Capsules 3171
Cardizem LA Extended Release Tablets (Infrequent) 1728
Cardura XL Tablets 2515
Celexa (Infrequent) 1176
Cipro I.V. (1% or less) 2984
Cipro XR Tablets 2990
Clinoril Tablets (Less than 1 in 100) 1924
Clorpres Tablets (Few) 2153
Comtan Tablets (2%) 2189
▲ Coreg Tablets (Greater than 1% to 3%) 1414
Covera-HS Tablets (Less than 2%) 3139
Dapsone Tablets USP 1673
Diovan HCT Tablets 2196
Diuril Oral Suspension 1954
Diuril Sodium Intravenous 2467
Dyazide Capsules 1423
EC-Naprosyn Delayed-Release Tablets (Less than 3%) 2761
Effexor XR Capsules (Rare) 3417
▲ Eloxatin for Injection (2% to 5%) 2892
Engerix-B Vaccine 1425
Equetro Extended-Release Capsules 3180
Evoxac Capsules (Less than 1%) 1047
Exelon Capsules (Infrequent) 2206
Exelon Oral Solution (Infrequent) 2206
Fansidar Tablets 2765
Frova Tablets (Rare) 1113
Furosemide Tablets 2154
▲ Gamunex Immune Globulin I.V., 10% (40%) 3235
Gantrisin Pediatric Suspension 2770
Garamycin Injectable 3014
Gengraf Capsules (2%) 459
Gleevec Tablets (Infrequent) 2227
Guanidine Hydrochloride Tablets 3016
Hyzaar 50-12.5 Tablets 1990
Hyzaar 100-12.5 Tablets 1990
Hyzaar 100-25 Tablets 1990
▲ Imdur Tablets (Less than or equal to 5%) 3018
Indapamide Tablets 2156
Indocin Capsules (Less than 1%) 1995
Indocin I.V. (Less than 1%) 2465
Indocin (Less than 1%) 1995
Infed Injection 3390
▲ Intron A for Injection (Less than or equal to 5%) 3024
Lescol Capsules (Rare) 2233
Lescol XL Tablets 2233
▲ Leustatin Injection (10%) 2357
Levaquin (0.1% to 0.9%) 2384
Levaquin in 5% Dextrose Injection (0.1% to 0.9%) 2384
Lopressor HCT 50/25 Tablets (1%) 2241
Lopressor HCT 100/25 Tablets (1%) 2241
Lopressor HCT 100/50 Tablets (1%) 2241
Lotensin HCT Tablets 2246
Lovenox Injection 2915
Lyrica Capsules (Rare) 2539
Matulane Capsules 3191
Meruvax II 2019
Mevacor Tablets (Rare) 2021
Micardis HCT Tablets 856
M-M-R II 2006
Mobic Oral Suspension (Less than 2%) 863
Mobic Tablets (Less than 2%) 863
Moduretic Tablets 2028
Mumpsvax (Extremely rare) 2031
Nalfon Capsules (Less than 1%) 2502
Naprosyn Suspension (Less than 3%) 2761
Naprosyn Tablets (Less than 3%) 2761
Neoral Oral Solution (2%) 2259
Neoral Soft Gelatin Capsules (2%) 2259
Neurontin Capsules (Frequent) 2487
Neurontin Oral Solution (Frequent) 2487
Neurontin Tablets (Frequent) 2487
Norvasc Tablets (More than 0.1% to 1%) 2545
NovoSeven (1%) 2331
Oncaspar (Less than 1%) 1145
Paxil CR Controlled-Release Tablets (Infrequent) 1538
Paxil (Infrequent) 1530
Percodan Tablets 1132
Permax Tablets (Rare) 3356
Pexeva Tablets (infrequent) 1694
▲ Plavix Tablets (5.3%) 917
▲ Plavix Tablets (5.3%) 2926
Pletal Tablets (Less than 2%) 2455
Prevacid NapraPAC (Less than 3%) 3280
Prilosec OTC Delayed-Release Tablets 2677
Prinzide Tablets 2056
Prochieve 4% Gel 1003
Prochieve 8% Gel 1003
▲ Proleukin for Injection (4%) 2266
ProQuad 2064
Proquin XR Tablets 1153
ProSom Tablets (Rare) 517
Prozac Pulvules and Liquid (Rare) 1801
▲ Pulmicort Respules (1% to 3%) 661
Quadramet Injection (1%) 1040
Razadyne (Infrequent) 2399
Razadyne ER Extended-Release Capsules (Infrequent) 2399
Relpax Tablets (Rare) 2548
Requip Tablets (Infrequent) 1555
Rescriptor Tablets 2551
Reyataz Capsules (Less than 3%) 921
Rilutek Tablets (Rare) 2930
Risperdal (Infrequent) 1676
Risperdal Consta Long-Acting Injection (Infrequent) 1682
Risperdal M-Tab Orally Disintegrating Tablets (Infrequent) 1676
▲ Simulect for Injection (3% to 10%) 2284
Sonata Capsules (Rare) 1717
▲ Soriatane Capsules (1% to 10%) 1013
Stalevo Tablets (2%) 2287
Symbyax Capsules (Rare) 1819
Tarka Tablets 524
Tegretol/Tegretol-XR 2295
Teveten Tablets (Less than 1%) 1735
Teveten HCT Tablets (Less than 1%) 1737
Thalomid Capsules 965
Tiazac Capsules (Infrequent) 1201
Ticlid Tablets (2.2%) 2810
Timolide Tablets 2086
▲ Topamax Sprinkle Capsules (8%) 2404
▲ Topamax Tablets (8%) 2404
Trecator Tablets (Rare) 3487
Trileptal Tablets (Up to 2%) 2300
Trileptal Oral Suspension (Up to 2%) 2300
Uniretic Tablets 3100
Verelan PM Extended-Release Capsules, Controlled-Onset (2% or less) 3106
VFEND I.V. (Less than 2%) 2564
VFEND Oral Suspension (Less than 2%) 2564
VFEND Tablets (Less than 2%) 2564
Voltaren Tablets (Occasionally) 2307
Voltaren-XR Tablets (Occasionally) 2310
Vytorin 10/10 Tablets 2114
Vytorin 10/10 Tablets 3077
Vytorin 10/20 Tablets 2114
Vytorin 10/20 Tablets 3077
Vytorin 10/40 Tablets 2114
Vytorin 10/40 Tablets 3077
Vytorin 10/80 Tablets 2114
Vytorin 10/80 Tablets 3077
Zegerid Capsules 2958
Zegerid Powder for Oral Solution 2958
Zocor Tablets (Rare) 2105
Zoloft (2%) 2586
Zosyn (1.0% or less) 3492
Zyrtec Chewable Tablets (Less than 2%) 2594
Zyrtec (Less than 2%) 2594
Zyrtec-D 12 Hour Extended Release Tablets (Less than 2%) 2597

Purpura, allergic
Plavix Tablets (Less than 1%) 917
Plavix Tablets (Less than 1%) 2926

Purpura, anaphylactoid
Oracea Capsules 1000
Solodyn Extended Release Tablets 1890

Purpura, nonthrombocytopenic
Blocadren Tablets 1916
Cosopt Sterile Ophthalmic Solution 1931
Edecrin (Rare) 1959
Inderal LA Long-Acting Capsules 3429
InnoPran XL Capsules 2723
Lopressor Injection 2238
Lopressor Tablets 2238
Lopressor HCT 50/25 Tablets 2241
Lopressor HCT 100/25 Tablets 2241
Lopressor HCT 100/50 Tablets 2241
Nadolol Tablets 2159
Timolide Tablets 2086
Timoptic Sterile Ophthalmic Solution 2088
Timoptic in Ocudose 2091
Timoptic-XE Sterile Ophthalmic Gel Forming Solution 2092
Toprol-XL Tablets 668

Purpura, thrombocytopenic
Amoxil Capsules 1343
Amoxil Chewable Tablets 1343
Amoxil Pediatric Drops for Oral Suspension 1343
Amoxil Powder for Oral Suspension 1343
Amoxil Tablets 1343
Augmentin 1360
Augmentin Tablets 1363
Augmentin XR Extended-Release Tablets 1369
Augmentin ES-600 Powder for Oral Suspension 1366
Axid Oral Solution (Rare) 879
Blocadren Tablets 1916
Concerta Extended-Release Tablets 1881
Cosopt Sterile Ophthalmic Solution 1931
Cuprimine Capsules 1947
Daytrana Transdermal Patch 3174
Evoxac Capsules (Less than 1%) 1047
Focalin Tablets 2220
Focalin XR Capsules 2223
Inderal LA Long-Acting Capsules 3429
Indocin Capsules (Less than 1%) 1995
Indocin I.V. (Less than 1%) 2465
Indocin (Less than 1%) 1995
Infanrix Vaccine 1476
InnoPran XL Capsules 2723
▲ Intron A for Injection (Less than 5%) 3024
Lopressor Injection 2238
Lopressor Tablets 2238
Lopressor HCT 50/25 Tablets 2241
Lopressor HCT 100/25 Tablets 2241
Lopressor HCT 100/50 Tablets 2241
Metadate CD Capsules 3323
Nadolol Tablets 2159
Omnicef Capsules 511
Omnicef for Oral Suspension 511
Pediarix Vaccine 1548
PEG-Intron Powder for Injection (Less than or equal to 1%) 3048
PREVPAC 3284
Prograf Capsules and Injection 632
Prozac Pulvules and Liquid 1801
Remicade for IV Injection 971
Ritalin Hydrochloride Tablets 2269

Ritalin LA Capsules ... 2271
Ritalin-SR Tablets ... 2269
Timolide Tablets ... 2086
Timoptic Sterile Ophthalmic Solution ... 2088
Timoptic in Ocudose ... 2091
Timoptic-XE Sterile Ophthalmic Gel Forming Solution ... 2092
Toprol-XL Tablets ... 668
▲ Xeloda Tablets (Less than 5%) ... 2822

Purpura, thrombocytopenic, idiopathic
Pegasys (Less than 1%) ... 2789

Purpura, thrombocytopenic thrombotic
Cuprimine Capsules ... 1947
Levaquin (Rare) ... 2384
Levaquin in 5% Dextrose Injection (Rare) ... 2384
Mycamine for Injection ... 628
Plavix Tablets (Rare) ... 917
Plavix Tablets (Rare) ... 2926
Prevacid Delayed-Release Capsules (Less than 1%) ... 3271
Prevacid for Delayed-Release Oral Suspension (Less than 1%) ... 3271
Prevacid SoluTab Delayed-Release Orally Disintegrating Tablets (Less than 1%) ... 3271
Prevacid NapraPAC ... 3280
Prograf Capsules and Injection ... 632
▲ Rapamune Oral Solution and Tablets (3% to 20%) ... 3475
Remicade for IV Injection ... 971
Risperdal (A single case) ... 1676
Risperdal M-Tab Orally Disintegrating Tablets (A single case) ... 1676
Ticlid Tablets (Rare) ... 2810
Valtrex Caplets ... 1597
VFEND I.V. (Less than 2%) ... 2564
VFEND Oral Suspension (Less than 2%) ... 2564
VFEND Tablets (Less than 2%) ... 2564

Pustules
Cutivate Lotion 0.05% (Less than 1%) ... 2664
▲ Levulan Kerastick for Topical Solution, 20% (4%) ... 1085

Pustules, scalp
Temovate Scalp Application (3 of 294 patients) ... 2670

Pustules, unspecified
Duragesic Transdermal System (Less than 1%) ... 2373
Klonopin (Infrequent) ... 2778

Pustulosis, exanthematous
Augmentin ... 1360
Augmentin Tablets ... 1363
Augmentin XR Extended-Release Tablets ... 1369
Augmentin ES-600 Powder for Oral Suspension ... 1366
Gleevec Tablets (Rare) ... 2227
Lamisil Tablets ... 2232
PREVPAC ... 3284

Pustulosis, provocation
Temovate Scalp Application (Rare) ... 2670

Pyelitis
Amerge Tablets (Rare) ... 1339

Pyelonephritis
Actiq (Less than 1%) ... 979
Ambien Tablets (Rare) ... 2851
Ambien CR Tablets (Rare) ... 2855
Aricept Tablets (Infrequent) ... 1094
Aricept ODT Tablets (Infrequent) ... 1094
Celexa (Rare) ... 1176
▲ CellCept Capsules (3% to less than 20%) ... 2747
▲ CellCept Intravenous (3% to less than 20%) ... 2747
▲ CellCept Oral Suspension (3% to less than 20%) ... 2747
▲ CellCept Tablets (3% to less than 20%) ... 2747
Cleocin Vaginal Ovules (Less than 1%) ... 2616
Copaxone for Injection (Infrequent) ... 3297
▲ Copegus Tablets (3% to 5%) ... 2754
Crixivan Capsules ... 1940
Effexor Tablets (Rare) ... 3411
Effexor XR Capsules (Infrequent) ... 3417
Enbrel for Injection ... 584
Evoxac Capsules (Less than 1%) ... 1047
Fortical Nasal Spray (Less than 1%) ... 3337
Gabitril Tablets (Infrequent) ... 984
Gengraf Capsules (1% to less than 3%) ... 459
Herceptin I.V. (At least one of the 958 patients) ... 1233
▲ Humira Injection (Less than 5%) ... 466
Lunesta Tablets (Rare) ... 3142
Lupron Depot 3.75 mg ... 3260
Lupron Depot–3 Month 11.25 mg ... 3265
Miacalcin Nasal Spray (Less than 1%) ... 2253
Neoral Oral Solution (1% to less than 3%) ... 2259
Neoral Soft Gelatin Capsules (1% to less than 3%) ... 2259
Neurontin Capsules (Rare) ... 2487
Neurontin Oral Solution (Rare) ... 2487
Neurontin Tablets (Rare) ... 2487
Norvir (Less than 2%) ... 503
Orencia Powder for Intravenous Infusion (0.2% to 0.5%) ... 914
▲ Pegasys (3% to 5%) ... 2789
Permax Tablets (Rare) ... 3356
Prinivil Tablets (0.3% to 1.0%) ... 2052
Prinzide Tablets ... 2056
Protonix I.V. (Less than 1%) ... 3472
Protonix Tablets (Less than 1%) ... 3469
▲ Rapamune Oral Solution and Tablets (Less than 20%) ... 3475
Requip Tablets (Rare) ... 1555
Rilutek Tablets (Rare) ... 2930
Uniretic Tablets (Less than 1%) ... 3100
Vandazole Vaginal Gel (Less than 1%) ... 3338
Zoloft (Rare) ... 2586
Zomig Nasal Spray (Rare) ... 3523

Pyloric stenosis
EryPed ... 447
Invanz for Injection (Greater than 0.1%) ... 1999
PCE Dispertab Tablets ... 515

Pyoderma gangrenosum
Asacol Delayed-Release Tablets (Rare) ... 2692

Pyogenic granuloma
Accutane Capsules ... 2731
▲ Soriatane Capsules (1% to 10%) ... 1013

Pyrexia
(*see under* Fever)

Pyrosis
(*see under* Heartburn)

Pyuria
Aricept Tablets (Infrequent) ... 1094
Aricept ODT Tablets (Infrequent) ... 1094
Colazal Capsules ... 2838
Effexor Tablets (Infrequent) ... 3411
Effexor XR Capsules (Infrequent) ... 3417
Evoxac Capsules (Less than 1%) ... 1047
Neurontin Capsules (Rare) ... 2487
Neurontin Oral Solution (Rare) ... 2487
Neurontin Tablets (Rare) ... 2487
▲ Ontak Vials (10%) ... 1745
Paxil CR Controlled-Release Tablets (Rare) ... 1538
Paxil (Rare) ... 1530
Permax Tablets (Infrequent) ... 3356
Pexeva Tablets (Infrequent) ... 1694
Prilosec OTC Delayed-Release Tablets (Less than 1%) ... 2677
▲ Prograf Capsules and Injection (3% to 15%) ... 632
Provigil Tablets (1%) ... 988
▲ Rapamune Oral Solution and Tablets (3% to 20%) ... 3475
Requip Tablets (2%) ... 1555
Rythmol SR Capsules ... 2727
Singulair (1%) ... 2077
Uniretic Tablets (More than 1%) ... 3100
Zegerid Capsules (Less than 1%) ... 2958
Zegerid Powder for Oral Solution (Less than 1%) ... 2958
Zosyn ... 3492
Zyprexa Tablets (Infrequent) ... 1830
Zyprexa ZYDIS Orally Disintegrating Tablets (Infrequent) ... 1830

Q

Quadriplegia
Orthoclone OKT3 Sterile Solution ... 2360
Prograf Capsules and Injection ... 632

Quncke's edema
(*see also under* Angioedema)
Protonix I.V. ... 3472
Protonix Tablets ... 3469

R

Radiation recall syndrome
Taxotere Injection Concentrate ... 2932
▲ Xeloda Tablets (Less than 5%) ... 2822

Radiculoneuropathy
Imitrex Injection ... 1463
Imitrex Tablets (Rare) ... 1471
Pneumovax 23 (Rare) ... 2043
Recombivax HB ... 2071

Rage
Niravam Orally Disintegrating Tablets (Rare) ... 3092
Valium Tablets ... 2819

Rage, paradoxical
Diastat Rectal Delivery System ... 3343

Rales
Adalat CC Tablets (Less than 1%) ... 2964
▲ Aredia for Injection (Up to 6%) ... 2179
Blocadren Tablets (0.6%) ... 1916
▲ Coreg Tablets (4%) ... 1414
Cosopt Sterile Ophthalmic Solution ... 1931
▲ Dacogen Injection (8%) ... 2129
▲ Imdur Tablets (Less than or equal to 5%) ... 3018
Invanz for Injection (0.5% to 1.1%) ... 1999
ReoPro Vials (0.4%) ... 1809
Rythmol SR Capsules (1% to 2%) ... 2727
Sular Tablets (Less than or equal to 1%) ... 3122
Thalomid Capsules ... 965
Timolide Tablets (Less than 1%) ... 2086
Timoptic Sterile Ophthalmic Solution ... 2088
Timoptic in Ocudose ... 2091
Timoptic-XE Sterile Ophthalmic Gel Forming Solution ... 2092
▲ Trisenox Injection (10%) ... 993
▲ Vesanoid Capsules (14%) ... 2820

Rash
▲ Abelcet Injection (4%) ... 1141
▲ Abilify Oral Solution (6%) ... 882
▲ Abilify Oral Solution (6%) ... 2450
▲ Abilify Discmelt Orally Disintegrating Tablets (6%) ... 882
▲ Abilify Discmelt Orally Disintegrating Tablets (6%) ... 2450
▲ Abilify Tablets (6%) ... 882
▲ Abilify Tablets (6%) ... 2450
Accolate Tablets ... 671
Accutane Capsules ... 2731
Aceon Tablets (2 mg, 4 mg, 8 mg) (2.3%) ... 3194
▲ Acetadote Injection (.2% to 20.8%) ... 1031
Aciphex Tablets ... 1090
▲ Actimmune (17%) ... 1671
Actiq (1% to 2%) ... 979
Activase I.V. (Very rare) ... 1223
▲ Actonel Tablets (3.1% to 11.5%) ... 2683
▲ Actonel with Calcium Tablets (3.1% to 7.7%) ... 2688
ADACEL Vaccine (2% to 2.7%) ... 2945
▲ Adalat CC Tablets (3% or less) ... 2964
Adderall Tablets ... 3164
Adderall XR Capsules ... 3166
Advair HFA Inhalation Aerosol (Rare) ... 1318
▲ Advicor Tablets (5%) ... 1722
▲ Aerobid/Aerobid-M (3% to 9%) ... 1171
▲ Agenerase Capsules (20% to 27%) ... 1327
▲ Agenerase Oral Solution (9% to 27%) ... 1332
Aggrastat ... 1907
Aggrenox Capsules ... 822
▲ Agrylin Capsules (8.3%) ... 3169
Albenza Tablets (Rare) ... 1338
Albutein 5%, Albumin (Human) ... 1652
Albutein 25% , Albumin (Human) ... 1653
Aldara Cream, 5% (More than 1%) ... 1846
Aldoril Tablets ... 1910
▲ Aldurazyme for Intravenous Infusion (8%) ... 1268
▲ Alimta for Injection (Up to 22%) ... 1750
Alinia for Oral Suspension (Less than 1%) ... 2835
Alinia Tablets (Less than 1%) ... 2835
Alkeran for Injection ... 955
Alkeran Tablets ... 956
Allegra (Rare) ... 2844
Allegra-D 12 Hour Extended-Release Tablets (Rare) ... 2846
Allegra-D 24 Hour Extended-Release Tablets (Rare) ... 2849
Aloprim for Injection (1.5%) ... 2167
Aloxi Injection (Less than 1%) ... 2127
▲ Alphagan P Ophthalmic Solution (1% to 4%) ... 567
Altace Capsules (Less than 1%) ... 1702
Altoprev Extended-Release Tablets (0.8% to 1.3%) ... 3109
Ambien Tablets (2%) ... 2851
Ambien CR Tablets (1% to frequent) ... 2855
▲ AmBisome for Injection (22.2% to 24.8%) ... 620
Amerge Tablets (Infrequent) ... 1339
Amitiza Capsules (Less than 0.2%) ... 3224
Amoxil Capsules ... 1343
Amoxil Chewable Tablets ... 1343
Amoxil Pediatric Drops for Oral Suspension ... 1343
Amoxil Powder for Oral Suspension ... 1343
Amoxil Tablets ... 1343
▲ Anaprox Tablets (1% to 10%) ... 2761
▲ Anaprox DS Tablets (1% to 10%) ... 2761
Angeliq Tablets ... 762
Anzemet Injection (Rare) ... 2859
Anzemet Tablets (Rare) ... 2862
Apidra Injection ... 2864
Aptivus Capsules (2%) ... 826
Aralast (0.1% to greater than or equal to 0.2%) ... 717
▲ Aranesp for Injection (7%) ... 581
▲ Argatroban Injection (1% to 10%) ... 1346
Aricept Tablets ... 1094
Aricept ODT Tablets ... 1094
▲ Arimidex Tablets (6% to 11%) ... 673
▲ Arixtra Injection (0.6% to 7.5%) ... 1351
Aromasin Tablets (Less frequent) ... 2600
Arthrotec Tablets (Rare) ... 3129
▲ Asacol Delayed-Release Tablets (6%) ... 2692
Astelin Nasal Spray ... 1904
Atacand Tablets (0.5% or greater) ... 649
Atacand HCT (0.5% or greater) ... 651
▲ Atripla Tablets (Greater than or equal to 5%) ... 945
Atrovent HFA Inhalation Aerosol ... 841
Atrovent Nasal Spray 0.03% (Infrequent) ... 837
Atrovent Nasal Spray 0.06% (Rare) ... 839
Attenuvax (Occasional) ... 1914
▲ Augmentin (3%) ... 1360
▲ Augmentin Tablets (3%) ... 1363
Augmentin XR Extended-Release Tablets ... 1369
Augmentin ES-600 Powder for Oral Suspension (1.1%) ... 1366
Avalide Tablets (1% or greater) ... 888
Avalide Tablets (1% or greater) ... 2874
Avapro Tablets (1% or greater) ... 891
Avapro Tablets (1% or greater) ... 2871
Avelox (0.1% to less than 2%) ... 2970
▲ Avinza Capsules (5% to 10%) ... 1741
Avodart Soft Gelatin Capsules ... 1390
Axert Tablets (Rare) ... 2396
Axid Oral Solution (1.9%) ... 879
▲ Azilect Tablets (6%) ... 3293
▲ Azmacort Inhalation Aerosol (1% to 3%) ... 1726
Bactroban Cream (1.1%) ... 1394
Bactroban Nasal (Less than 1%) ... 1394
Bactroban Ointment (Less than 1%) ... 1395
Beconase AQ Nasal Spray (Rare) ... 1396
▲ BeneFix Vials (1.6% to 7.7%) ... 3408
Benicar Tablets (Greater than 0.5%) ... 1043
Benicar HCT Tablets (Greater than 1%) ... 1044
Bentyl Capsules ... 697
Bentyl Injection ... 697
Bentyl Syrup ... 697
Bentyl Tablets ... 697
Betagan Ophthalmic Solution, USP ... ⊙220
▲ Betaseron for SC Injection (24%) ... 767
▲ Betimol Ophthalmic Solution (More than 5%) ... 3382
▲ Betimol Ophthalmic Solution (More than 5%) ... ⊙295
▲ Bexxar (Less than 1% to 17%) ... 1398
▲ Biaxin/Biaxin XL (3%) ... 402
Blocadren Tablets (Less than 1%) ... 1916
Boniva Injection (1.3% to 2.3%) ... 2738
Boniva Tablets (1.3% to 2.3%) ... 2741
Boostrix ... 1404
BOTOX Purified Neurotoxin Complex (7 cases) ... 570
Brimonidine Tartrate Ophthalmic Solution 0.2% ... ⊙248
Bumex Tablets (0.2% to 2.9%) ... 2746
Buprenex Injectable (Infrequent) ... 2716
▲ Caduet Tablets (Less than 1% to 3.9%) ... 2508
▲ Cafcit (8.7%) ... 1886
Calcium Disodium Versenate Injection ... 1851
▲ Campath Ampules (3% to 40%) ... 811

Campral Tablets (Frequent) 1174
▲ Camptosar Injection (0.4% to 14.3%) 2604
Canasa Rectal Suppositories (1.2%) 699
▲ Cancidas for Injection (0% to 6.2%) 1918
▲ Captopril Tablets (About 4 to 7 of 100 patients) 2149
Carafate Suspension (Less than 0.5%) 701
Carafate Tablets (Less than 0.5%) 701
Carbatrol Capsules 3171
▲ Cardizem LA Extended Release Tablets (1% to 4%) 1728
▲ Carnitor Injection (3% to 5%) 3188
Carteolol Hydrochloride Ophthalmic Solution USP, 1% ⊙249
Catapres Tablets (About 1 in 100 patients) 843
Catapres-TTS (0.5% or less) 844
Caverject Impulse Injection (Less than 1%) 2612
Ceftin (0.1% to 1%) 1407
Celebrex Capsules 3134
Celexa (Frequent) 1176
▲ CellCept Capsules (3% to 22.1%) 2747
▲ CellCept Intravenous (3% to 22.1%) 2747
▲ CellCept Oral Suspension (3% to 22.1%) 2747
▲ CellCept Tablets (3% to 22.1%) 2747
▲ Cerezyme for Injection (Approximately 6.5%) 1270
Cesamet Capsules 3340
▲ Chantix Tablets (1% to 3%) 2517
▲ Chemet Capsules (2.6% to 11.2%) 2458
Cialis Tablets (Less than 2%) 1838
Cipro (1% to 1.8%) 2977
Cipro I.V. (Greater than or equal to 1%) 2984
Cipro XR Tablets (Less than 1%) 2990
Clarinex Syrup (Rare) 2995
Clarinex Tablets (Rare) 2995
Clarinex Reditabs Tablets (Rare) 2995
Clarinex-D 24-Hour Extended-Release Tablets 2998
Cleocin Vaginal Ovules (Less than 1%) 2616
Climara Transdermal System 771
Climara Pro Transdermal System (2.4%) 776
▲ Clinoril Tablets (3% to 9%) 1924
Clorpres Tablets (1%) 2153
Clozaril Tablets (2%) 2184
Combivent Inhalation Aerosol (Less than 2%; rare) 847
▲ Combivir Tablets (9%) 1411
Comvax (0.8% to 0.9%) 1928
Concerta Extended-Release Tablets 1881
▲ Copaxone for Injection (18%) 3297
▲ Copegus Tablets (8%) 2754
Cosopt Sterile Ophthalmic Solution (1% to 5%) 1931
Coumadin for Injection (Infrequent) 898
Coumadin Tablets (Infrequent) 898
Covera-HS Tablets (1.2% to 2%) 3139
Cozaar Tablets (Less than 1%) 1935
Crestor Tablets (Greater than or equal to 2%) 678
Crixivan Capsules (1.2%) 1940
▲ Cubicin for Injection (4.3% to 6.7%) 1026
▲ Cuprimine Capsules (5%) 1947
Cutivate Lotion 0.05% (Less than 1%) 2664
Cymbalta Delayed-Release Capsules (Frequent) 1757
▲ Dacogen Injection (19%) 2129
Dalmane Capsules (Rare) 3342
Daytrana Transdermal Patch 3174
Decadron Tablets 1951
Demadex Injection 2759
Demadex Tablets 2759
▲ Depacon Injection (1% to 5%) 412
▲ Depakene (1% to 5%) 417
▲ Depakote Sprinkle Capsules (1% to 5%) 422
▲ Depakote Tablets (1% to 6%) 427
▲ Depakote ER Tablets (Greater than 1% to 5%) 434
▲ Depo-Provera Contraceptive Injection (1% to 5%) 2622
Detrol Tablets (1.9%) 2628
▲ Diastat Rectal Delivery System (3%) 3343
Differin Cream (Less than 1%) 1210
Dilaudid Oral Liquid 445
Dilaudid Tablets - 8 mg 445
Dilaudid-HP (Less frequent) 442
Diovan Tablets (0.2%) 2193
Diovan HCT Tablets (Greater than 0.2%) 2196
▲ Ditropan XL Extended-Release Tablets (2% to less than 5%) 2413
Diuril Oral Suspension 1954
Diuril Sodium Intravenous 2467
▲ Dolobid Tablets (3% to 9%) 1955
▲ Doxil Injection (1% to 28.5%) 2351
DuoNeb Inhalation Solution (0.3%) 1058
Duragesic Transdermal System (1% or greater) 2373
Dyazide Capsules 1423
DynaCirc CR Tablets (1.3% to 2.6%) 2721
Dyrenium Capsules (Rare) 3400
▲ EC-Naprosyn Delayed-Release Tablets (1% to 10%) 2761
Edecrin 1959
▲ Effexor Tablets (3%) 3411
Effexor XR Capsules (Frequent) 3417
▲ Efudex (Among most frequent) 3363
Eldepryl Capsules 3208
▲ Elitek (1% to 13%) 2890
▲ Elmiron Capsules (3%) 2415
▲ Eloxatin for Injection (5% to 9%) 2892
Elspar for Injection 2463
Elspar for Injection 1960
Emcyt Capsules (1%) 2634
Emend Capsules (Greater than 0.5%) 1963
▲ Emsam Transdermal System (4%) 903
▲ Emtriva Capsules (17% to 30%) 1287
▲ Emtriva Oral Solution (17% to 30%) 1287
Enablex Extended-Release Tablets (Greater than or equal to 1%) 2203
▲ Enbrel for Injection (5% to 14%) 584
Engerix-B Vaccine (Less than 1%) 1425
Enjuvia Tablets 1062
▲ Epivir (9%) 1427
▲ Epivir-HBV (5%) 1432
▲ Epogen for Injection (16%) 591
▲ Epzicom Tablets (5%) 1436
▲ Equetro Extended-Release Capsules (13%) 3180
Eraxis for Injection (1%) 2521
Ery-Tab Tablets 449
Estrasorb Topical Emulsion 1147
Estratest Tablets 3199
Estratest H.S. Tablets 3199
▲ Euflexxa (3%) 1162
▲ Eulexin Capsules (3% to 8%) 3009
▲ Evista Tablets (5.5%) 1763
▲ Evoxac Capsules (4.3%) 1047
Exelon Capsules (2% or more) 2206
Exelon Oral Solution (2% or more) 2206
Fabrazyme for Intravenous Infusion 1274
▲ Famvir Tablets (0.4% to 3.3%) 2211
▲ Faslodex Injection (7.3%) 681
FazaClo Orally Disintegrating Tablets (2%) 551
Feiba VH 718
▲ Femara Tablets (4% to 5%) 2214
Ferrlecit Injection 3388
Flebogamma 5%, Immune Globulin Intravenous (Human) 1658
Fleet Phospho-soda (Rare) 1166
Fleet Phospho-soda ACCU-PREP (Rare) 1168
Fleet Phospho-soda EZ-PREP (Rare) 1169
Flomax Capsules 850
Flonase Nasal Spray 1440
▲ Flovent Diskus (8%) 1443
Floxin Otic Solution (1%) 1049
Fluarix 1451
Flumadine (0.3% to 1%) 1183
Flumist Vaccine 1901
Focalin Tablets 2220
Focalin XR Capsules 2223
Follistim AQ Cartridge 2338
Foradil Aerolizer (1.1%) 3010
Fortaz (2%) 1453
▲ Forteo for Injection (4.9%) 1767
Fosamax (Rare) 1969
Fosamax Plus D Tablets 1977
Fragmin Injection (Rare) 1097
Furosemide Tablets 2154
▲ Gabitril Tablets (5%) 984
▲ Gamunex Immune Globulin I.V., 10% (6%) 3235
Gantrisin Pediatric Suspension 2770
Garamycin Injectable 3014
▲ Gemzar for Injection (28% to 30%) 1771
▲ Gengraf Capsules (1% to 8%) 459
Genotropin Lyophilized Powder (Infrequent) 2638
▲ Geodon (4%) 2529
▲ Gleevec Tablets (2.4% to 53%) 2227
GlucaGen 761
Gris-PEG Tablets (Rare) 2502
Guanidine Hydrochloride Tablets 3016
Havrix Vaccine (Less than 1%) 1456
Hepsera Tablets (2% or greater) 1292
▲ Herceptin I.V. (18%) 1233
HibTITER (1 of 1,118 vaccinations) 3426
Humalog-Pen (Less common) 1781
Humalog Mix 50/50-Pen 1783
Humalog Mix 75/25-Pen 1785
Human Albumin Grifols 20%, Albumin (Human) 1651
Human Albumin Grifols 25%, Albumin (Human) 1652
▲ Humate-P (6%) 3502
▲ Humira Injection (Less than 1% to 12%) 466
Humulin 50/50, 100 Units 1791
Humulin 70/30 Pen (Less common) 1793
Humulin L, 100 Units (Less common) 1794
Humulin N Pen (Less common) 1797
▲ Hyalgan Solution (14%) 2901
▲ Hycamtin for Injection (Less than 1% to 16%) 1458
Hycodan 1116
HyperRAB (Rare) 3242
Hyperstat I.V. 3017
Hytrin Capsules (At least 1%) 471
Hyzaar 50-12.5 Tablets (1.4%) 1990
Hyzaar 100-12.5 Tablets (1.4%) 1990
Hyzaar 100-25 Tablets (1.4%) 1990
▲ Imdur Tablets (Less than or equal to 5%) 3018
Imitrex Injection (Infrequent) 1463
Imitrex Nasal Spray (Infrequent) 1467
Imitrex Tablets (Rare to infrequent) 1471
Indocin Capsules (Less than 1%) 1995
Indocin I.V. (Less than 1%) 2465
Indocin (Less than 1%) 1995
Infanrix Vaccine 1476
Infed Injection 3390
▲ Infergen (13%) 3364
▲ Intron A for Injection (Up to 25%) 3024
Invanz for Injection (2.3% to 2.9%) 1999
▲ Invirase (Greater than or equal to 2% to 3.4%) 2772
▲ Ionsys Transdermal System (1% to less than 10%) 2379
▲ Iressa Tablets (44% to 61%) 684
▲ I.V. Busulfex (57%) 2493
Kadian Capsules (Less than 3%) 577
▲ Kaletra (1% to 4%) 476
Keflex Capsules 549
▲ Kepivance (Less than 1% to 62%) 597
Keppra Injection 3320
Keppra Oral Solution (1% to 2%) 3314
Keppra Tablets (1% to 2%) 3314
Ketek Tablets (Greater than or equal to 0.2% to less than 2%) 2903
Klonopin 2778
K-Lor Oral Solution (Rare) 474
Kogenate FS 738
Kogenate FS with Bio-Set 740
K-Tab Tablets (Rare) 475
Kytril Injection (Rare) 2781
▲ Lamictal (5% to 14%) 1481
▲ Lamisil Tablets (5.6%) 2232
Lantus Injection 2909
▲ Lariam Tablets (Among most frequent) 2786
Lescol Capsules (2.3%) 2233
Lescol XL Tablets (1.6%) 2233
Leukeran Tablets (Rare) 1504
▲ Leukine (44% to 70%) 814
▲ Leustatin Injection (10% to 27%) 2357
Levaquin (0.3% to 1.4%) 2384
Levaquin in 5% Dextrose Injection (0.3% to 1.4%) 2384
Levemir Injection 2320
Levitra Tablets (Less than 2%) 3034
Levothroid Tablets 1186
Levoxyl Tablets 1712
Lexapro Oral Solution (Frequent) 1190
Lexapro Tablets (Frequent) 1190
▲ Lexiva Tablets (8% to 35%) 1505
Limbrel Capsules (0.011%) 2672
▲ Lipitor Tablets (1.1% to 3.9%) 2483
Lithobid Tablets 1692
Lofibra Tablets 1219
Lofibra Capsules 1216
▲ Lopressor Injection (5%) 2238
▲ Lopressor Tablets (5%) 2238
Lopressor HCT 50/25 Tablets 2241
Lopressor HCT 100/25 Tablets 2241
Lopressor HCT 100/50 Tablets 2241
Loprox Shampoo 1888
Lotensin Tablets (Less than 1%) 2243
Lotensin HCT Tablets (0.3% to 1%) 2246
Lotrel Capsules 2249
Lotrisone Cream (Less than 1%) 3040
Lotronex Tablets 1512
▲ Lunesta Tablets (3% to 4%) 3142
Lupron Depot 3.75 mg 3260
Lupron Depot 7.5 mg 3264
Lupron Depot–3 Month 11.25 mg 3265
Lupron Depot-PED 7.5 mg, 11.25 mg and 15 mg 3269
Lupron Injection Pediatric (Greater than or equal to 2%) 3259
Malarone Pediatric Tablets 1517
Malarone Tablets 1517
Matulane Capsules 3191
Mavik Tablets (0.3% to 1.0%) 486
Maxair Autohaler 1852
Maxalt Tablets (Infrequent) 2008
Maxalt-MLT Orally Disintegrating Tablets (Infrequent) 2008
▲ Maxipime for Injection (1.1% to 4%) 1105
Mefoxin for Injection 2012
Mefoxin Premixed Intravenous Solution 2016
▲ Megace ES Oral Suspension (2% to 12%) 2481
Menactra Vaccine (1.4% to 1.6%) 2954
Menostar Transdermal System 782
▲ Mepron Suspension (6.3% to 46%) 1521
▲ Meridia Capsules (3.8%) 489
▲ Merrem I.V. (1.6% to 3.1%) 686
Meruvax II 2019
Metadate CD Capsules 3323
MetroGel-Vaginal Gel (Less than 1%) 1855
▲ Mevacor Tablets (0.8% to 5.2%) 2021
Miacalcin Injection 2252
Micardis Tablets (More than 0.3%) 854
Micardis HCT Tablets (2% or greater) 856
Midamor Tablets (Less than or equal to 1%) 2026
Migranal Nasal Spray (Infrequent) 3348
Mintezol 2027
Miradon Tablets 3042
Mirapex Tablets (Greater than or equal to 1%) 859
Mivacron Injection (Less than 1%) 493
M-M-R II (Infrequent) 2006
Moban Tablets 1119
▲ Mobic Oral Suspension (0.3% to 3%) 863
▲ Mobic Tablets (0.3% to 3%) 863
▲ Moduretic Tablets (3% to 8%) 2028
Motrin IB Tablets and Caplets 1866
Children's Motrin Oral Suspension 1867
Children's Motrin Non-Staining Dye-Free Oral Suspension 1867
Children's Motrin Cold Oral Suspension 1867
Infants' Motrin Concentrated Drops 1867
Infants' Motrin Non-Staining Dye-Free Concentrated Drops 1867
Junior Strength Motrin Caplets and Chewable Tablets 1867
MS Contin Tablets (Less frequent) 2701
▲ Mycamine for Injection (1.4% to 3.1%) 628
▲ Myfortic Tablets (3% to less than 20%) 2255
▲ Mylotarg for Injection (18%) 3431
▲ Myozyme for Intravenous Infusion (54%) 1279
Nadolol Tablets (1 to 5 of 1000 patients) 2159
Naftin Gel (0.5%) 2126
▲ Nalfon Capsules (3.7%) 2502
Namenda (Frequent) 1195
▲ Naprosyn Suspension (1% to 10%) 2761
▲ Naprosyn Tablets (1% to 10%) 2761
Natrecor for Injection (Greater than or equal to 1%) 3127
Nembutal Sodium Solution, USP 2470
▲ Neoral Oral Solution (1% to 8%) 2259
▲ Neoral Soft Gelatin Capsules (1% to 8%) 2259
Neulasta Injection 601
▲ Neumega for Injection (25%) 3435
▲ Neupogen for Injection (6% to 12%) 603
Neurontin Capsules (1.2%) 2487
Neurontin Oral Solution (1.2%) 2487
Neurontin Tablets (1.2%) 2487
▲ Nexavar Tablets (0% to 40%) 746
Nexium Delayed-Release Capsules (Less than 1%) 655
Nexium I.V. (Less than 1%) 659
▲ Niaspan Extended-Release Tablets (1% to 5%) 1730
Nicomide Tablets 1088
Nimbex Injection (0.1%) 498
Nimotop Capsules (Up to 2.4%) 749
▲ Nipent for Injection (26% to 43%) 1863
▲ Niravam Orally Disintegrating Tablets (10.8%) 3092
Norditropin Cartridges 2323

Noroxin Tablets (0.3% to 1.0%) 2032
Norvasc Tablets (Less than 1% to 2%) 2545
▲ Norvir (0% to 3.5%) 503
NovoLog Injection 2326
NovoSeven (1%) 2331
Numorphan Injection 1120
NuvaRing 2340
Omacor Capsules (1.8%) 2725
Omnicef Capsules (0.9%) 511
▲ Omnicef for Oral Suspension (3%) 511
▲ Oncaspar (Greater than 5%) 1145
▲ Ontak Vials (34%) 1745
OptiPranolol Metipranolol Ophthalmic Solution 0.3% (A small number of patients) ⊙256
▲ Orencia Powder for Intravenous Infusion (0.1% to 4%) 914
Ortho-Cyclen/Ortho Tri-Cyclen 2429
Ortho Tri-Cyclen Lo Tablets 2436
Orthoclone OKT3 Sterile Solution 2360
OsmoPrep Tablets (Rare) 2840
Oxistat Cream (0.1%) 2667
Oxsoralen-Ultra Capsules 3353
▲ OxyContin Tablets (Between 1% and 5%) 2703
OxyFast Oral Concentrate Solution 2708
OxyIR Capsules 2708
▲ Panretin Gel (25% to 77%) 1747
Parcopa Orally Disintegrating Tablets 3097
Parnate Tablets (Rare) 1527
▲ Paser Granules (Among most common) 1674
▲ Paxil CR Controlled-Release Tablets (2% to 3%) 1538
▲ Paxil (2% to 3%) 1530
▲ Pegasys (5%) 2789
▲ PEG-Intron Powder for Injection (6%) 3048
Penlac Nail Lacquer, Topical Solution, 8% 2924
Pentasa Capsules (1.0% to 1.3%) 3185
Pepcid Injection (Infrequent) 2040
Pepcid (Infrequent) 2038
Percocet Tablets 1131
Percodan Tablets 1132
▲ Permax Tablets (3.2%) 3356
Persantine Tablets (2.3%) 868
▲ Pexeva Tablets (2% to 3%) 1694
Phenergan Tablets and Suppositories 3440
Phenytek Capsules 2160
▲ Photofrin for Injection (7%) 702
▲ Plavix Tablets (4.2%) 917
▲ Plavix Tablets (4.2%) 2926
Pletal Tablets (2% or greater) 2455
Pneumovax 23 (Rare) 2043
Potaba (Infrequent) 1650
Precose Tablets (Rare) 751
Premarin Intravenous 3442
Premarin Tablets 3446
Premarin Vaginal Cream 3452
▲ Premphase Tablets (4% to 6%) 3456
▲ Prempro Tablets (4% to 6%) 3456
Prevacid Delayed-Release Capsules (Less than 1%) 3271
Prevacid for Delayed-Release Oral Suspension (Less than 1%) 3271
Prevacid SoluTab Delayed-Release Orally Disintegrating Tablets (Less than 1%) 3271
Prevacid I.V. for Injection (Less than 1%) 3277
Prevacid NapraPAC (Less than 1%) 3280
PREVPAC (Less than 1%) 3284
Prilosec OTC Delayed-Release Tablets (Less than 1% to 1.5%) 2677
Primaxin I.M. (0.4%) 2045
Primaxin I.V. (1.5%) 2048
Prinivil Tablets (0.3% to 1.7%) 2052
Prinzide Tablets (1.2%) 2056
ProAmatine Tablets (2.4%; Less frequent) 3186
Prochieve 4% Gel 1003
Prochieve 8% Gel 1003
▲ Procrit for Injection (Rare to 16%) 2364
▲ Prograf Capsules and Injection (10% to 24%) 632
Prolastin (Occasional) 3255
Proleukin for Injection (1%) 2266
Propecia Tablets (0.5%) 2060
ProQuad (1.6%) 2064
Proquin XR Tablets (Less than 1%) 1153
Proscar Tablets (0.5%) 2067
ProSom Tablets (Infrequent) 517
ProstaScint Kit 1037
▲ Protonix I.V. (6%) 3472
Protonix Tablets (Less than 1% to 2%) 3469
▲ Protopic Ointment (2% to 5%) 638
Proventil Inhalation Aerosol 3053
Proventil Inhalation Solution 0.083% (Rare) 3055
Proventil HFA Inhalation Aerosol (Less than 3%) 3056
Provigil Tablets (At least 1%) 988
▲ Prozac Pulvules and Liquid (2% to 6%) 1801
▲ Pulmicort Respules (Less than 1% to 4%) 661
▲ Pulmozyme Inhalation Solution (3% to 12%) 1248
Quadramet Injection (1%) 1040
Qvar Inhalation Aerosol (Rare) 3303
Raniclor Tablets, Chewable 2505
▲ Rapamune Oral Solution and Tablets (10% to 20%) 3475
▲ Rebetol (17% to 28%) 3058
▲ Rebetron Combination Therapy (20% to 28%) 3063
Recombivax HB (Less than 1%) 2071
ReFacto Vials 3484
Refludan for Injection (Uncommon) 792
Relpax Tablets (Infrequent) 2548
▲ Remicade for IV Injection (10%) 971
Renagel Tablets 1282
Requip Tablets (Infrequent) 1555
▲ Rescriptor Tablets (13.4% to 19.5%) 2551
▲ Retisert Implant (5% to 15%) ⊙258
▲ Retrovir Capsules (17%) 1560
▲ Retrovir IV Infusion (17%) 1564
▲ Retrovir (17%) 1560
▲ Revlimid Capsules (6.8% to 35.8%) 958
▲ Reyataz Capsules (3% to 21%) 921
▲ Ribavirin, USP Capsules (17% to 28%) 3068
▲ Risperdal (2% to 5%) 1676
Risperdal Consta Long-Acting Injection (Frequent) 1682
▲ Risperdal M-Tab Orally Disintegrating Tablets (2% to 5%) 1676
Ritalin Hydrochloride Tablets 2269
Ritalin LA Capsules 2271
Ritalin-SR Tablets 2269
▲ Rituxan I.V. (1% to 15%) 1254
Rocaltrol Capsules 2798
Rocaltrol Oral Solution 2798
Rocephin Injectable Vials, ADD-Vantage, Galaxy, Bulk (1.7%) 2800
▲ Romazicon Injection (1% to 3%) 2804
Sandostatin Injection (Less than 1%) 2278
▲ Sandostatin LAR Depot (5% to 15%) 2280
▲ Serevent Diskus (Less than 3% to 4%) 1568
Seromycin Capsules 1813
▲ Seroquel Tablets (4%) 690
▲ Simulect for Injection (3% to 10%) 2284
Singulair (1.6% to 2% or greater) 2077
Skelaxin Tablets 1716
Sonata Capsules (Frequent) 1717
▲ Soriatane Capsules (1% to 10%) 1013
▲ Spiriva HandiHaler (2% to 4%) 869
Stromectol Tablets (0.9%) 2083
Sular Tablets (Very rare) 3122
▲ Sulfamylon Cream (4.6%) 2162
▲ Sulfamylon for 5% Topical Solution (4.6%) 2162
Suprax (Less than 2%) 1843
▲ Sustiva Capsules (5% to 46%) 930
▲ Sustiva Tablets (5% to 46%) 930
▲ Sutent Capsules (1% to 38%) 2560
Symmetrel Tablets (0.1% to 1%) 1135
▲ Synagis (25.6%) 1897
▲ Synera Topical Patch (Less than 4%) 1137
Synthroid Tablets 520
▲ Tambocor Tablets (1% to 3%) 1856
Tamiflu Capsules 2807
Tamiflu Oral Suspension 2807
▲ Tarceva Tablets (0% to 69%) 1259
▲ Tarceva Tablets (0% to 69%) 2444
▲ Targretin Capsules (16.7% to 22.6%) 1747
Tarka Tablets (0.3% or more) 524
Tasmar Tablets (Frequent) 3358
▲ Taxotere Injection Concentrate (0.9% to 11.8%) 2932
Tegretol/Tegretol-XR 2295
▲ Temodar Capsules (8% to 13%) 3073
▲ Tequin Injection (0.1% to 3%) 938
▲ Tequin Injection in 5% Dextrose (0.1% to 3%) 938
▲ Tequin Tablets (0.1% to 3%) 938
Teveten Tablets (Less than 1%) 1735
Teveten HCT Tablets (Less than 1%) 1737
▲ Thalomid Capsules (20.8%) 965
Thiothixene Capsules 2165
Thyrogen for Injection 1286
Tiazac Capsules (2%) 1201
▲ Ticlid Tablets (5.1%) 2810
Timentin ADD-Vantage 1580
Timentin Injection Galaxy Container 1583
Timentin IV Infusion 1577
Timentin Pharmacy Bulk Package 1586
Timolide Tablets (Less than 1%) 2086
Timoptic Sterile Ophthalmic Solution (Less frequent) 2088
Timoptic in Ocudose (Less frequent) 2091
Timoptic-XE Sterile Ophthalmic Gel Forming Solution 2092
Tindamax Tablets 2142
TNKase I.V. (Rare) 1264
▲ TOBI Solution for Inhalation (5.4%) 2298
Topamax Sprinkle Capsules (More than 1%) 2404
Topamax Tablets (More than 1%) 2404
▲ Toprol-XL Tablets (About 5 of 100 patients) 668
Transderm Scōp Transdermal Therapeutic System (Infrequent) 2177
Tranxene 2474
Trasylol Injection (2%) 754
Trecator Tablets (Rare) 3487
Trelstar LA Suspension (1.7%) 3397
▲ Tricor Tablets (1.4% to 6%) 527
▲ Trileptal Tablets (2% to 5.3%) 2300
▲ Trileptal Oral Suspension (2% to 5.3%) 2300
▲ Tri-Luma Cream (1% to 5.27%) 1213
▲ Trizivir Tablets (9%) 1589
Trusopt Sterile Ophthalmic Solution (Rare) 2095
▲ Truvada Tablets (5%) 1296
Tussionex Pennkinetic Extended-Release Suspension 3327
Twinrix Vaccine (Less than 1%) 1595
Tygacil for Injection (2.4%) 3488
Tylenol Cough & Sore Throat Daytime Liquid with Cool Burst 1877
Ultane Liquid for Inhalation (Less than 1%) 531
Uniretic Tablets (More than 1%) 3100
Univasc Tablets (Less than 1% to 1.6%) 3104
Uroqid-Acid No. 2 Tablets (Occasional) 760
Urso 250 Tablets (1%) 710
Urso Forte Tablets (1%) 710
Valium Tablets (Infrequent) 2819
▲ Valtrex Caplets (0.4% to 8%) 1597
Vancocin HCl Capsules, USP (Infrequent) 3380
Vandazole Vaginal Gel (1%) 3338
Vantin Tablets and Oral Suspension (Less than 1% to 1.4%) 2645
▲ Vaqta (1% to 4.5%) 2097
Varivax (Greater than or equal to 1%) 2100
Vasotec I.V. Injection (0.5% to 1.4%) 2103
▲ Velcade for Injection (18%) 2133
Ventolin HFA Inhalation Aerosol 1600
Verelan PM Extended-Release Capsules, Controlled-Onset (1.2% to 2%) 3106
▲ Vesanoid Capsules (54%) 2820
▲ VFEND I.V. (1.5% to 5.3%) 2564
▲ VFEND Oral Suspension (1.5% to 5.3%) 2564
▲ VFEND Tablets (1.5% to 5.3%) 2564
Viadur Implant (Less than 2%) 757
Viagra Tablets (2%) 2573
Vicodin Tablets 535
Vicodin ES Tablets 536
Vicodin HP Tablets 538
Vicoprofen Tablets (Less than 1%) 539
▲ Vigamox Ophthalmic Solution (1% to 4%) 564
▲ Viracept (1% to 3%) 2577
▲ Viramune Oral Suspension (8% to 37%) 873
▲ Viramune Tablets (8% to 37%) 873
Virazole for Inhalation Solution 3370
▲ Viread Tablets (5% to 18%) 1301
▲ Visudyne for Injection (10% to 30%) 2305
▲ Vivaglobin (0.2% to 17%) 3506
▲ Vivitrol (5% to 12%) 995
Vivotif 819
VoSpire ER Tablets (Rare) 1052
Vytorin 10/10 Tablets 2114
Vytorin 10/10 Tablets 3077
Vytorin 10/20 Tablets 2114
Vytorin 10/20 Tablets 3077
Vytorin 10/40 Tablets 2114
Vytorin 10/40 Tablets 3077
Vytorin 10/80 Tablets 2114
Vytorin 10/80 Tablets 3077
▲ Wellbutrin Tablets (8.0%) 1603
▲ Wellbutrin SR Sustained-Release Tablets (4% to greater than or equal to 5%) 1607
▲ Wellbutrin XL Extended-Release Tablets (0.9% to 3%) 1613
WinRho SDF 732
Xalatan Sterile Ophthalmic Solution (1% to 2%) 2649
▲ Xenical Capsules (4.3%) 2831
Xifaxan Tablets (Less than 2%) 2842
▲ Xopenex Inhalation Solution (7.5%) 3146
▲ Xopenex Inhalation Solution Concentrate (7.5%) 3150
▲ Xopenex HFA Inhalation Aerosol (7.5%) 3154
Yasmin 28 Tablets 796
Zantac (Rare) 1624
Zantac Injection 1619
Zantac Injection Pharmacy Bulk Package (Rare) 1622
Zantac Injection Premixed 1619
Zantac (Rare) 1624
Zegerid Capsules (Less than 1% to 1.5%) 2958
Zegerid Powder for Oral Solution (Less than 1% to 1.5%) 2958
▲ Zelapar Tablets (4%) 3372
Zelnorm Tablets (1%) 2312
Zemaira (0.4%) 3509
Zemplar Injection 543
Zemuron Injection (Less than 1%) 2346
Zetia Tablets 2120
Zetia Tablets 3083
▲ Ziagen (5% to 7%) 1626
Zinacef for Injection (1 in 125 patients) 1631
Zinacef Injection (1 in 125 patients) 1631
Zmax for Oral Suspension (Less then 1%) 2583
Zofran Injection (Approximately 1%) 1634
Zofran (Approximately 1%) 1639
Zofran ODT Orally Disintegrating Tablets (Approximately 1%) 1639
▲ Zoloft (3%) 2586
Zometa for Intravenous Infusion 2315
Zomig Tablets (Infrequent) 3519
Zomig Nasal Spray (Infrequent) 3523
Zomig-ZMT Tablets (Infrequent) 3519
▲ Zonegran Capsules (3%) 1101
▲ Zosyn (1.3% to 4.2%) 3492
Zovirax Capsules 1643
Zovirax Ointment 821
Zovirax 1643
▲ Zyban Sustained-Release Tablets (3% to 4%) 1644
Zyflo Tablets 1023
Zyprexa Tablets 1830
Zyprexa ZYDIS Orally Disintegrating Tablets 1830
Zyrtec Chewable Tablets (Less than 2%) 2594
Zyrtec (Less than 2%) 2594
Zyrtec-D 12 Hour Extended Release Tablets (Less than 2%) 2597
▲ Zyvox (0.4% to 7%) 2652

Rash, allergic

Mircette Tablets 1066
Ortho-Cyclen Tablets 2429
Ortho Evra Transdermal System 2417
Ortho Tri-Cyclen Tablets 2429
Ortho Tri-Cyclen Lo Tablets 2436
Premphase Tablets 3456
Prempro Tablets 3456
Prometrium Capsules (100 mg, 200 mg) 3203
Seasonique Tablets 1077
Varivax (Greater than or equal to 1%) 2100
Yaz Tablets 803

Rash, bullous

Actonel with Calcium Tablets 2688
Caduet Tablets 2508
Exelon Capsules (Frequent) 2206
Exelon Oral Solution (Frequent) 2206
Lipitor Tablets 2483
Topamax Sprinkle Capsules 2404
Topamax Tablets 2404
▲ Zosyn (4.2%) 3492

Rash, circumocular

Polytrim Ophthalmic Solution (Multiple reports) 574

Rash, diaper

▲ Augmentin ES-600 Powder for Oral Suspension (3.5%) 1366
▲ Ceftin for Oral Suspension (3.4%) 1407
Comvax (0.2% to 0.5%) 1928
▲ Invanz for Injection (4.7%) 1999

▲ Myozyme for Intravenous Infusion (36%) ... 1279

Rash, drug
Nitrolingual Pumpspray ... 3120

Rash, eczematous
Exelon Capsules (Frequent) ... 2206
Exelon Oral Solution (Frequent) ... 2206
▲ Ontak Vials (34%) ... 1745
Thalomid Capsules ... 965

Rash, erythematous
Blocadren Tablets ... 1916
Caduet Tablets (Greater than 0.1% to less than or equal to 1%) ... 2508
▲ Campath Ampules (3% to 40%) ... 811
Carbatrol Capsules ... 3171
Celebrex Capsules (0.1% to 1.9%) ... 3134
Clindagel ... 1203
Colazal Capsules ... 2838
Coreg Tablets (Greater than 0.1% to 1%) ... 1414
Cosopt Sterile Ophthalmic Solution ... 1931
Cymbalta Delayed-Release Capsules (Infrequent) ... 1757
Denavir Cream (0.1%) ... 2174
Duragesic Transdermal System (1% or greater) ... 2373
▲ Eloxatin for Injection (2% to 5%) ... 2892
Equetro Extended-Release Capsules ... 3180
▲ Evoxac Capsules (1% to 3%) ... 1047
Exelon Capsules (Frequent) ... 2206
Exelon Oral Solution (Frequent) ... 2206
▲ Femara Tablets (4% to 5%) ... 2214
Floxin Otic Solution (Single report) ... 1049
▲ Fortical Nasal Spray (1% to 3%) ... 3337
▲ Hycamtin for Injection (Less than 1% to 16%) ... 1458
Inderal LA Long-Acting Capsules ... 3429
InnoPran XL Capsules ... 2723
▲ Intron A for Injection (Less than 5%) ... 3024
Invanz for Injection (Greater than 0.5%) ... 1999
Levaquin (0.1% to 0.9%) ... 2384
Levaquin in 5% Dextrose Injection (0.1% to 0.9%) ... 2384
▲ Miacalcin Nasal Spray (1% to 3%) ... 2253
▲ Mobic Oral Suspension (0.3% to 3%) ... 863
▲ Mobic Tablets (0.3% to 3%) ... 863
Namenda (Infrequent) ... 1195
Nexium Delayed-Release Capsules (Less than 1%) ... 655
Nexium I.V. (Less than 1%) ... 659
Norvasc Tablets (More than 0.1% to 1%) ... 2545
Oracea Capsules ... 1000
Plavix Tablets (Less than 1%) ... 917
Plavix Tablets (Less than 1%) ... 2926
▲ Rebif Prefilled Syringe for Injection (5% to 7%) ... 3159
Remicade for IV Injection (Less than 1%) ... 971
Risperdal Consta Long-Acting Injection (Infrequent) ... 1682
Rocaltrol Capsules ... 2798
Rocaltrol Oral Solution ... 2798
▲ Soriatane Capsules (10% to 25%) ... 1013
Tegretol/Tegretol-XR ... 2295
Thalomid Capsules ... 965
Timolide Tablets ... 2086
Timoptic Sterile Ophthalmic Solution ... 2088
Timoptic in Ocudose ... 2091
Timoptic-XE Sterile Ophthalmic Gel Forming Solution ... 2092
Topamax Sprinkle Capsules (Less than 1% to 2%) ... 2404
Topamax Tablets (Less than 1% to 2%) ... 2404
Trileptal Tablets ... 2300
Trileptal Oral Suspension ... 2300
▲ Xeloda Tablets (Less than 1% to 9%) ... 2822
Zoloft (Infrequent) ... 2586
▲ Zosyn (3.9%) ... 3492
Zyrtec Chewable Tablets (Less than 2%) ... 2594
Zyrtec (Less than 2%) ... 2594
Zyrtec-D 12 Hour Extended Release Tablets (Less than 2%) ... 2597

Rash, erythematous maculopapular
Amoxil Capsules ... 1343
Amoxil Chewable Tablets ... 1343
Amoxil Pediatric Drops for Oral Suspension ... 1343
Amoxil Powder for Oral Suspension ... 1343
Amoxil Tablets ... 1343
PREVPAC ... 3284
▲ Thiola Tablets (16.7%) ... 2141
Viramune Oral Suspension ... 873
Viramune Tablets ... 873

Rash, exfoliative
Exelon Capsules (Frequent) ... 2206
Exelon Oral Solution (Frequent) ... 2206

Rash, follicular
Diprolene Gel 0.05% ... 3001
Floxin Otic Solution (Single report) ... 1049
Zoloft (Rare) ... 2586

Rash, heat
Cubicin for Injection (Less than 1%) ... 1026
Trileptal Tablets ... 2300
Trileptal Oral Suspension ... 2300
▲ Vivitrol (5% to 12%) ... 995

Rash, herpetic
(*see under* Eruptions, herpetic)

Rash, injection site
ProQuad (2.3%) ... 2064

Rash, lichenoid
Permax Tablets (Rare) ... 3356

Rash, lupus erythematosus
Evoxac Capsules (Less than 1%) ... 1047

Rash, macular
Amerge Tablets (Rare) ... 1339
Byetta Injection ... 611
Lithostat Tablets ... 2140
R-Gene 10 for Intravenous Use (One patient) ... 2641

Rash, maculopapular
Abelcet Injection ... 1141
Abilify Oral Solution (Infrequent) ... 882
Abilify Oral Solution (Infrequent) ... 2450
Abilify Discmelt Orally Disintegrating Tablets (Infrequent) ... 882
Abilify Discmelt Orally Disintegrating Tablets (Infrequent) ... 2450
Abilify Tablets (Infrequent) ... 882
Abilify Tablets (Infrequent) ... 2450
Actiq (Less than 1%) ... 979
Agenerase Capsules ... 1327
Agenerase Oral Solution (1%) ... 1332
▲ Atripla Tablets (Greater than or equal to 5%) ... 945
Avelox (0.1% to less than 2%) ... 2970
Caduet Tablets (Greater than 0.1% to less than or equal to 1%) ... 2508
▲ Campath Ampules (3% to 40%) ... 811
Campral Tablets (Infrequent) ... 1174
Capastat Sulfate for Injection ... 1755
Captopril Tablets ... 2149
Catapres-TTS ... 844
Celebrex Capsules (0.1% to 1.9%) ... 3134
Cipro XR Tablets (Less than 1%) ... 2990
▲ Clarinex Syrup (3.1%) ... 2995
Cleocin Vaginal Ovules ... 2616
Copaxone for Injection (Infrequent) ... 3297
Coreg Tablets (Greater than 0.1% to 1%) ... 1414
Depacon Injection (1% or more) ... 412
Depakene (1% or more) ... 417
Depakote Sprinkle Capsules ... 422
▲ Depakote Tablets (1% to 5%) ... 427
Depakote ER Tablets (Greater than 1%) ... 434
Didronel Tablets ... 2697
▲ Doxil Injection (Less than 1% to 10%) ... 2351
Effexor Tablets (Infrequent) ... 3411
Effexor XR Capsules (Infrequent) ... 3417
▲ Emtriva Capsules (17% to 30%) ... 1287
▲ Emtriva Oral Solution (17% to 30%) ... 1287
Epivir ... 1427
Exelon Capsules (Frequent) ... 2206
Exelon Oral Solution (Frequent) ... 2206
▲ Femara Tablets (4% to 5%) ... 2214
Gabitril Tablets (Infrequent) ... 984
Geodon Capsules (Infrequent) ... 2529
▲ Hycamtin for Injection (Less than 1% to 16%) ... 1458
▲ Intron A for Injection (Less than 5%) ... 3024
Invirase (Less than 2%) ... 2772
▲ I.V. Busulfex (8%) ... 2493
Kaletra (Less than 2%) ... 476
Lamictal (Infrequent) ... 1481
Lanoxicaps Capsules (Rare) ... 1490
Lanoxin Injection (Rare) ... 1494
Lanoxin Injection Pediatric (Rare) ... 1497
Lanoxin Tablets (Rare) ... 1500
Levaquin (Less than 0.1%) ... 2384
Levaquin in 5% Dextrose Injection (Less than 0.1%) ... 2384
Lofibra Tablets ... 1219
Lofibra Capsules ... 1216
Lunesta Tablets (Rare) ... 3142
▲ Mobic Oral Suspension (0.3% to 3%) ... 863
▲ Mobic Tablets (0.3% to 3%) ... 863
Neurontin Capsules (Rare) ... 2487
Neurontin Oral Solution (Rare) ... 2487
Neurontin Tablets (Rare) ... 2487
Nexium Delayed-Release Capsules (Less than 1%) ... 655
Nexium I.V. (Less than 1%) ... 659
Norvasc Tablets (More than 0.1% to 1%) ... 2545
Norvir (Less than 2%) ... 503
Omnicef for Oral Suspension (0.2%) ... 511
▲ Ontak Vials (34%) ... 1745
Oracea Capsules ... 1000
Paxil CR Controlled-Release Tablets (Rare) ... 1538
Paxil (Rare) ... 1530
Pexeva Tablets (Rare) ... 1694
Plavix Tablets (Less than 1%) ... 917
Plavix Tablets (Less than 1%) ... 2926
Prevacid Delayed-Release Capsules (Less than 1%) ... 3271
Prevacid for Delayed-Release Oral Suspension (Less than 1%) ... 3271
Prevacid SoluTab Delayed-Release Orally Disintegrating Tablets (Less than 1%) ... 3271
Prevacid NapraPAC (Less than 1%) ... 3280
PREVPAC (Less than 1%) ... 3284
Prezista Tablets (Less than 2%) ... 3306
Protonix I.V. (Less than 1%) ... 3472
Protonix Tablets (Less than 1%) ... 3469
Protopic Ointment (2% to 4%) ... 638
Prozac Pulvules and Liquid (Infrequent) ... 1801
Raptiva for Injection ... 1250
▲ Rebif Prefilled Syringe for Injection (4% to 5%) ... 3159
Relpax Tablets (Rare) ... 2548
Requip Tablets (Infrequent) ... 1555
▲ Rescriptor Tablets (4.5% to 6.6%) ... 2551
Seroquel Tablets (Infrequent) ... 690
Sonata Capsules (Infrequent) ... 1717
Sular Tablets (Less than or equal to 1%) ... 3122
▲ Sustiva Capsules (16.7% to 24.5%) ... 930
▲ Sustiva Tablets (16.7% to 24.5%) ... 930
Symbyax Capsules (Rare) ... 1819
Targretin Capsules ... 1747
Tequin Injection (Less than 0.1%) ... 938
Tequin Injection in 5% Dextrose (Less than 0.1%) ... 938
Tequin Tablets (Less than 0.1%) ... 938
Teveten Tablets (Less than 1%) ... 1735
Teveten HCT Tablets (Less than 1%) ... 1737
▲ Thalomid Capsules (4.2%) ... 965
Ticlid Tablets ... 2810
Tricor Tablets ... 527
Trileptal Tablets (1.3%) ... 2300
Trileptal Oral Suspension (1.3%) ... 2300
Trizivir Tablets ... 1589
▲ Truvada Tablets (5%) ... 1296
Uniretic Tablets (Less than 1%) ... 3100
Vantin Tablets and Oral Suspension (Less than 1%) ... 2645
VFEND I.V. (0.5% to 1.5%) ... 2564
VFEND Oral Suspension (0.5% to 1.5%) ... 2564
VFEND Tablets (0.5% to 1.5%) ... 2564
Viracept (Less than 2%) ... 2577
▲ Viread Tablets (5% to 18%) ... 1301
Wellbutrin SR Sustained-Release Tablets (Rare) ... 1607
Wellbutrin XL Extended-Release Tablets (Rare) ... 1613
Ziagen ... 1626
Zoloft (Infrequent) ... 2586
Zonegran Capsules (Infrequent) ... 1101
▲ Zosyn (4.2%) ... 3492
Zyban Sustained-Release Tablets (Rare) ... 1644
Zyprexa Tablets (Rare) ... 1830
Zyprexa ZYDIS Orally Disintegrating Tablets (Rare) ... 1830
Zyrtec Chewable Tablets (Less than 2%) ... 2594
Zyrtec (Less than 2%) ... 2594
Zyrtec-D 12 Hour Extended Release Tablets (Less than 2%) ... 2597

Rash, measles-like
▲ ProQuad (3%) ... 2064

Rash, morbilliform
▲ Cleocin Vaginal Ovules (Among most frequent) ... 2616
▲ Phenytek Capsules (Among most common) ... 2160
▲ Thiola Tablets (16.7%) ... 2141

Rash, oral
▲ Advair Diskus 100/50 (1% to 3%) ... 1308
▲ Advair Diskus 250/50 (1% to 3%) ... 1308
▲ Advair Diskus 500/50 (1% to 3%) ... 1308

Rash, papular
Aclovate (Approximately 2%) ... 2660
Byetta Injection ... 611
▲ Chemet Capsules (2.6% to 11.2%) ... 2458
Migranal Nasal Spray (Rare) ... 3348
▲ Stromectol Tablets (22.7%) ... 2083
▲ Vivitrol (5% to 12%) ... 995

Rash, papular, neck
Alferon N Injection (1%) ... 1665

Rash, pemphigoid
Nadolol Tablets ... 2159
Stalevo Tablets ... 2287

Rash, penile
Caverject Impulse Injection (1%) ... 2612

Rash, perianal
Mintezol ... 2027

Rash, petechial
Adalat CC Tablets (Less than 1%) ... 2964
Effexor XR Capsules (Rare) ... 3417
Lyrica Capsules (Rare) ... 2539
▲ Ontak Vials (34%) ... 1745
Prozac Pulvules and Liquid (Rare) ... 1801

Rash, pruritic
Amerge Tablets (Rare) ... 1339
▲ Captopril Tablets (About 4 to 7 of 100 patients) ... 2149
Carbatrol Capsules ... 3171
Cymbalta Delayed-Release Capsules (Infrequent) ... 1757
Equetro Extended-Release Capsules ... 3180
Premphase Tablets ... 3456
Prempro Tablets ... 3456
Skelaxin Tablets ... 1716
Tegretol/Tegretol-XR ... 2295

Rash, psoriaform
Coreg Tablets (Less than or equal to 0.1% to 1%) ... 1414
Cosopt Sterile Ophthalmic Solution ... 1931
Exelon Capsules (Frequent) ... 2206
Exelon Oral Solution (Frequent) ... 2206
▲ Femara Tablets (4% to 5%) ... 2214
Inderal LA Long-Acting Capsules (Rare) ... 3429
InnoPran XL Capsules (Rare) ... 2723
Lamisil Tablets ... 2232
Requip Tablets (Infrequent) ... 1555
▲ Soriatane Capsules (1% to 10%) ... 1013
Timoptic Sterile Ophthalmic Solution ... 2088
Timoptic in Ocudose ... 2091
Timoptic-XE Sterile Ophthalmic Gel Forming Solution ... 2092

Rash, purpuric
Avelox (0.1% to less than 2%) ... 2970
Campath Ampules ... 811
Lyrica Capsules (Rare) ... 2539
Phenytek Capsules ... 2160
Prozac Pulvules and Liquid (Rare) ... 1801
Uniretic Tablets (Less than 1%) ... 3100

Rash, pustular
Anaprox Tablets ... 2761
Anaprox DS Tablets ... 2761
▲ Atripla Tablets (Greater than or equal to 5%) ... 945
Avelox (0.1% to less than 2%) ... 2970
Copaxone for Injection (Frequent) ... 3297
Doxil Injection (Less than 1%) ... 2351
EC-Naprosyn Delayed-Release Tablets ... 2761
Effexor Tablets (Rare) ... 3411
Effexor XR Capsules (Rare) ... 3417
▲ Emtriva Capsules (17% to 30%) ... 1287
▲ Emtriva Oral Solution (17% to 30%) ... 1287
Lamictal (Rare) ... 1481
Lyrica Capsules (Rare) ... 2539
Naprosyn Suspension ... 2761
Naprosyn Tablets ... 2761
▲ Protopic Ointment (3% to 8%) ... 638

Prozac Pulvules and Liquid (Rare)..... 1801
▲ Pulmicort Respules (1% to 3%) 661
Sonata Capsules (Rare) 1717
▲ Stromectol Tablets (22.7%) 2083
Sular Tablets (Less than or equal to 1%).............................. 3122
Targretin Capsules.......................... 1747
▲ Truvada Tablets (5%) 1296
▲ Viread Tablets (5% to 18%) 1301
Zoloft (Rare)...................................... 2586
Zonegran Capsules (Infrequent)....... 1101
Zyprexa Tablets (Rare)..................... 1830
Zyprexa ZYDIS Orally Disintegrating Tablets (Rare)......... 1830

Rash, rubella-like
ProQuad (Greater than or equal to 0.2% to less than 1%).................. 2064

Rash, scarlatiniform
Phenytek Capsules.......................... 2160

Rash, unspecified
Dilaudid 440
Dilaudid Non-Sterile Powder 440
Dilaudid Rectal Suppositories 440
Dilaudid Tablets 440
▲ Oxytrol Transdermal System (Greater than 1%) 3392
Uroxatral Tablets 2943
Viramune Oral Suspension (2%) 873
Viramune Tablets (2%) 873
▲ Voltaren Tablets (1% to 10%) 2307
▲ Voltaren-XR Tablets (1% to 10%) 2310

Rash, urticarial
Captopril Tablets (Rare) 2149
▲ Ontak Vials (34%) 1745
Prevnar for Injection (0.4% to 1.4%) 3463
ProNutra Protein Supplement 1668
▲ Stromectol Tablets (22.7%) 2083
Ticlid Tablets 2810
Trizivir Tablets 1589
Ziagen 1626
▲ Zosyn (4.2%) 3492

Rash, varicella-like
ProQuad (2.1%) 2064
▲ Varivax (0.9% to 5.5%) 2100

Rash, vasculitic
Accolate Tablets (Rare) 671
Flovent Diskus 1443
Gleevec Tablets (Rare) 2227
Paxil CR Controlled-Release Tablets 1538
Paxil 1530
Singulair 2077

Rash, vesiculobullous
Abilify Oral Solution (Infrequent) 882
Abilify Oral Solution (Infrequent) 2450
Abilify Discmelt Orally Disintegrating Tablets (Infrequent) 882
Abilify Discmelt Orally Disintegrating Tablets (Infrequent) 2450
Abilify Tablets (Infrequent) 882
Abilify Tablets (Infrequent) 2450
Actiq (Less than 1%) 979
AmBisome for Injection (Less common) 620
▲ Atripla Tablets (Greater than or equal to 5%) 945
Azilect Tablets (Greater than 1%) 3293
Campral Tablets (Infrequent) 1174
▲ CellCept Capsules (3% to less than 20%) 2747
▲ CellCept Intravenous (3% to less than 20%) 2747
▲ CellCept Oral Suspension (3% to less than 20%) 2747
▲ CellCept Tablets (3% to less than 20%) 2747
Cipro XR Tablets (Less than 1%) 2990
Cleocin Vaginal Ovules 2616
Copaxone for Injection (Infrequent) ..3297
Crestor Tablets (Less than 1%) 678
Depakote ER Tablets (Greater than 1%) 434
▲ Doxil Injection (Less than 1% to 10%) 2351
Effexor Tablets (Rare) 3411
Effexor XR Capsules (Rare) 3417
▲ Emtriva Capsules (17% to 30%) 1287
▲ Emtriva Oral Solution (17% to 30%) 1287
Gabitril Tablets (Infrequent) 984
Geodon Capsules (Infrequent) 2529
Ionsys Transdermal System (.1% to less than 1%) 2379
Iressa Tablets (1%) 684
▲ I.V. Busulfex (10%) 2493
Keppra Oral Solution (2%) 3314
Keppra Tablets (2%)......................... 3314
Lamictal (Infrequent)........................ 1481
Lovenox Injection............................. 2915
Lunesta Tablets (Rare)..................... 3142
Lyrica Capsules (0.1% to 1%)........... 2539
▲ Megace ES Oral Suspension (1% to 3%).. 2481
Neurontin Capsules (Infrequent)....... 2487
Neurontin Oral Solution (Infrequent)................................. 2487
Neurontin Tablets (Infrequent).......... 2487
Norvir (Less than 2%)....................... 503
▲ Ontak Vials (34%)........................... 1745
Paxil CR Controlled-Release Tablets (Rare).............................. 1538
Paxil (Rare)...................................... 1530
Permax Tablets (Rare)...................... 3356
Pexeva Tablets (Rare)...................... 1694
▲ Protopic Ointment (2% to 3%) 638
Prozac Pulvules and Liquid (Infrequent)................................. 1801
Rescriptor Tablets 2551
Reyataz Capsules (Less than 3%)..... 921
Sonata Capsules (Infrequent)........... 1717
Symbyax Capsules (Infrequent)......... 1819
Synera Topical Patch (Less than or equal to 1%)............................... 1137
Targretin Capsules........................... 1747
Tequin Injection (Less than 0.1%)...... 938
Tequin Injection in 5% Dextrose (Less than 0.1%).......................... 938
Tequin Tablets (Less than 0.1%)....... 938
Thalomid Capsules........................... 965
▲ Truvada Tablets (5%) 1296
Vantin Tablets and Oral Suspension (Less than 1%)........... 2645
▲ Viread Tablets (5% to 18%) 1301
Zonegran Capsules (Infrequent)....... 1101
Zyprexa Tablets (2%)....................... 1830
Zyprexa ZYDIS Orally Disintegrating Tablets (2%)........... 1830

Rash at injection site
ProQuad.. 2064

Raynaud's phenomenon
Blocadren Tablets............................ 1916
Captopril Tablets (2 to 3 of 1000 patients)....................................... 2149
Catapres Tablets (Rare).................. 843
Catapres-TTS (0.5% or less)........... 844
Clorpres Tablets (Rare)................... 2153
Cosopt Sterile Ophthalmic Solution... 1931
Imitrex Injection (Rare).................... 1463
Imitrex Nasal Spray......................... 1467
Imitrex Tablets................................. 1471
Inderal LA Long-Acting Capsules...... 3429
Nadolol Tablets (2 of 100 patients).. 2159
Sandostatin Injection (Less than 1%).. 2278
Sandostatin LAR Depot (Rare).......... 2280
Strattera Capsules (Very Rare)......... 1814
Thalomid Capsules........................... 965
Timolide Tablets............................... 2086
Timoptic Sterile Ophthalmic Solution... 2088
Timoptic in Ocudose......................... 2091
Timoptic-XE Sterile Ophthalmic Gel Forming Solution......................... 2092
Toprol-XL Tablets (About 1 of 100 patients)....................................... 668
Vasotec I.V. Injection (0.5% to 1.0%)... 2103

Reaction, aggravated
Zomig Nasal Spray (0% to 2%)......... 3523

Reaction, local
Humalog Mix 50/50-Pen.................. 1783
▲ Tygacil for Injection (9%) 3488

Reaction, paranoid
Abilify Oral Solution (Frequent)......... 882
Abilify Oral Solution (Frequent)......... 2450
Abilify Discmelt Orally Disintegrating Tablets (Frequent)... 882
Abilify Discmelt Orally Disintegrating Tablets (Frequent)... 2450
Abilify Tablets (Frequent)................ 882
Abilify Tablets (Frequent)................ 2450
Azilect Tablets (Infrequent).............. 3293
Campral Tablets (Rare).................... 1174
Lyrica Capsules (Rare).................... 2539
Mirapex Tablets (2%)....................... 859
Namenda (Infrequent)...................... 1195
Pexeva Tablets (infrequent).............. 1694
Risperdal Consta Long-Acting Injection (Frequent)...................... 1682
Wellbutrin SR Sustained-Release Tablets... 1607
Wellbutrin XL Extended-Release Tablets... 1613

Reaction, schizophrenic
Abilify Oral Solution (Frequent)......... 882
Abilify Oral Solution (Frequent)......... 2450
Abilify Discmelt Orally Disintegrating Tablets (Frequent)... 882
Abilify Discmelt Orally Disintegrating Tablets (Frequent)... 2450
Abilify Tablets (Frequent)................. 882
Abilify Tablets (Frequent)................. 2450
Lyrica Capsules (Rare)..................... 2539

Reaction at injection site
▲ Aldurazyme for Intravenous Infusion (4%)............................. 1268
Aloxi Injection (Very rare)................ 2127
▲ Amevive (2% to 16%) 626
▲ Apidra Injection (10.3%) 2864
Avelox (0.1% to less than 2%)......... 2970
▲ BeneFix Vials (1.6% to 7.7%) 3408
▲ Betaseron for SC Injection (86%) 767
Byetta Injection................................ 611
Cipro I.V. (Greater than 1%)............. 2984
▲ Copegus Tablets (23%) 2754
▲ Cubicin for Injection (5.8%) 1026
▲ depo-subQ provera 104 Injectable Suspension (5%)........... 2624
▲ Eloxatin for Injection (3% to 11%) 2892
▲ Enbrel for Injection (7% to 37%) 584
▲ Ferrlecit Injection (33.3%) 3388
▲ Follistim AQ Cartridge (5% to 10%).. 2338
Fragmin Injection (Rare).................. 1097
▲ Fuzeon Injection (98%) 2767
▲ Gamunex Immune Globulin I.V., 10% (5%).................................... 3235
Gemzar for Injection (Rare)............. 1771
HibTITER... 3426
Humalog Mix 50/50-Pen.................. 1783
▲ Humira Injection (8% to 20%) 466
▲ Imitrex Injection (59%) 1463
Infanrix Vaccine 1476
Ionsys Transdermal System (.1% to less than 1%)........................... 2379
▲ Kineret Injection (71%) 599
Kogenate FS with Bio-Set (2 cases).. 740
Levaquin (0.2%)............................... 2384
Levaquin in 5% Dextrose Injection (0.2%)... 2384
Levemir Injection............................. 2320
▲ Lupron Depot 7.5 mg (Less than 5%)... 3264
▲ Lupron Depot–3 Month 11.25 mg (Less than 5%)............................ 3265
▲ Lupron Injection Pediatric (Greater than or equal to 5%)........ 3259
▲ Maxipime for Injection (3%) 1105
Merrem I.V. (0.9%).......................... 686
Mivacron Injection (Less than 1%).... 493
Natrecor for Injection (Greater than or equal to 1%)..................... 3127
NeoProfen Injection......................... 2472
Norditropin Cartridges..................... 2323
▲ NovoLog Mix 70/30 (7%) 2328
NovoSeven...................................... 2331
Nutropin for Injection (0.3%)............ 1239
Nutropin AQ Injection (0.3%)............ 1243
Nutropin AQ Pen (0.3%).................. 1243
Nutropin AQ Pen Cartridge (0.3%).... 1243
Pediarix Vaccine 1548
▲ Pegasys (22%) 2789
▲ PEG-Intron Powder for Injection (47%).. 3048
Prevacid I.V. for Injection (1%)......... 3277
ProstaScint Kit (Less than 1%)......... 1037
▲ Rebif Prefilled Syringe for Injection (89% to 92%)................. 3159
▲ Ribavirin, USP Capsules (5% to 58%).. 3068
Risperdal Consta Long-Acting Injection (Infrequent)................... 1682
▲ Somavert Injection (4% to 11%) 2642
▲ Taxotere Injection Concentrate (3% to 4.4%).................................. 2932
▲ Tev-Tropin for Injection (8 out of 164 patients)................................ 1222
Tygacil for Injection (0% to less than 2%)... 3488
Vaqta.. 2097
▲ Vivaglobin (Less than 1% to 49%) 3506
▲ Vivitrol (58% to 88%) 995
▲ Xolair (12% to 45%) 1266
Zemaira (0.2% to 0.4%)................... 3509
▲ Zostavax Injection (17%) 2111
▲ Zyvox (0% to 3.3%) 2652

Reactions, allergic contact
Penlac Nail Lacquer, Topical Solution, 8% (Four subjects).......... 2924

Reactions, infusion site
Eraxis for Injection (Less than 1% to less than 2%).............................. 2521
▲ Gammagard Liquid (0.97% to 13.1%)... 721
▲ Vaprisol (20.2% to 52.5%) 643

Reactions, local, unspecified
Boostrix 1404

Reactive airway disease
▲ Flumist Vaccine (1.4% to 3.1%) 1901

Rectal bleeding
Abilify Oral Solution (Infrequent)........ 882
Abilify Oral Solution (Infrequent)....... 2450
Abilify Discmelt Orally Disintegrating Tablets (Infrequent).................................. 882
Abilify Discmelt Orally Disintegrating Tablets (Infrequent).................................. 2450
Abilify Tablets (Infrequent)................ 882
Abilify Tablets (Infrequent)................ 2450
Accutane Capsules.......................... 2731
Aciphex Tablets.............................. 1090
Actiq (1% or greater)....................... 979
Aggrenox Capsules (1.6%)............... 822
Ambien Tablets (Rare)..................... 2851
Anaprox Tablets (Less than 1%)....... 2761
Anaprox DS Tablets (Less than 1%).. 2761
Arthrotec Tablets (Rare).................. 3129
Asacol Delayed-Release Tablets (2% or greater)............................ 2692
Celexa (Rare).................................. 1176
Clozaril Tablets (Less than 1%)........ 2184
Colazal Capsules (2%)..................... 2838
Colocort Rectal Suspension, USP (Retention) 100 mg/60 mL (Rare)... 2476
Copaxone for Injection (Infrequent)... 3297
Depo-Provera Contraceptive Injection (Less than 1%).............. 2622
▲ Doxil Injection (1% to 10%) 2351
EC-Naprosyn Delayed-Release Tablets (Less than 1%).................. 2761
Effexor Tablets (Infrequent).............. 3411
Effexor XR Capsules (Infrequent)...... 3417
Eldepryl Capsules 3208
▲ Elmiron Capsules (6.3% to 15%) 2415
▲ Eloxatin for Injection (2% to 5%) 2892
▲ Eulexin Capsules (14%) 3009
Evoxac Capsules (Less than 1%)...... 1047
Exelon Capsules (Infrequent)............ 2206
Exelon Oral Solution (Infrequent)...... 2206
FazaClo Orally Disintegrating Tablets (Less than 1%).................. 551
Gabitril Tablets (Infrequent).............. 984
Gengraf Capsules (1%).................... 459
Geodon (Infrequent)........................ 2529
Imitrex Nasal Spray......................... 1467
Indocin Capsules (Less than 1%)...... 1995
Indocin I.V. (Less than 1%).............. 2465
Indocin (Less than 1%)..................... 1995
▲ Intron A for Injection (Less than 5%)... 3024
Invirase (Less than 2%)................... 2772
Lipitor Tablets (Less than 2%).......... 2483
Lofibra Tablets................................ 1219
Lofibra Capsules 1216
Lunesta Tablets (Rare).................... 3142
Naprosyn Suspension (Less than 1%)... 2761
Naprosyn Tablets (Less than 1%)..... 2761
Neoral Oral Solution (1%)................. 2259
Neoral Soft Gelatin Capsules (1%).... 2259
Neurontin Capsules (Rare)............... 2487
Neurontin Oral Solution (Rare).......... 2487
Neurontin Tablets (Rare)................. 2487
Paxil CR Controlled-Release Tablets (Infrequent)...................... 1538
Paxil (Infrequent)............................ 1530
Pentasa Capsules (Less than 1%).... 3185
Pexeva Tablets (infrequent).............. 1694
Pletal Tablets (Less than 2%)........... 2455
Prevacid Delayed-Release Capsules (Less than 1%).............. 3271
Prevacid for Delayed-Release Oral Suspension (Less than 1%).......... 3271
Prevacid SoluTab Delayed-Release Orally Disintegrating Tablets (Less than 1%)........................... 3271
PREVPAC (Less than 1%)................ 3284
▲ Prometrium Capsules (100 mg, 200 mg) (Less than 5%)............... 3203
Protonix I.V. (Greater than or equal to 1%).. 3472
Protonix Tablets (Less than 1%)....... 3469
Razadyne (Infrequent)..................... 2399
Razadyne ER Extended-Release Capsules (Infrequent)................... 2399
▲ Refludan for Injection (5.3%) 792
Requip Tablets (Infrequent).............. 1555
Retrovir Capsules............................ 1560
Retrovir IV Infusion......................... 1564
Retrovir 1560
Revlimid Capsules 958
Rythmol SR Capsules...................... 2727
▲ Sandostatin LAR Depot (1% to 4%)... 2280
Seroquel Tablets (Infrequent)........... 690

Sonata Capsules (Infrequent) 1717
Tequin Injection (Less than 0.1%) 938
Tequin Injection in 5% Dextrose (Less than 0.1%) 938
Tequin Tablets (Less than 0.1%) 938
Tricor Tablets 527
Triglide Tablets 3123
Trileptal Tablets (Up to 2%) 2300
Trileptal Oral Suspension (Up to 2%) 2300
Uniretic Tablets (Less than 1%) 3100
Vantin Tablets and Oral Suspension 2645
VFEND I.V. (Less than 2%) 2564
VFEND Oral Suspension (Less than 2%) 2564
VFEND Tablets (Less than 2%) 2564
Viagra Tablets (Less than 2%) 2573
Voltaren Tablets (Occasionally) 2307
Voltaren-XR Tablets (Occasionally) 2310
Xeloda Tablets 2822
Zelnorm Tablets 2312
Zoloft (Rare) 2586
Zonegran Capsules (Infrequent) 1101
Zyprexa Tablets (Infrequent) 1830
Zyprexa ZYDIS Orally Disintegrating Tablets (Infrequent) 1830
Zyrtec Chewable Tablets (Less than 2%) 2594
Zyrtec (Less than 2%) 2594
Zyrtec-D 12 Hour Extended Release Tablets (Less than 2%) 2597

Rectal discomfort
Fleet Glycerin Laxatives 1165
Fleet Glycerin Suppositories 1165
▲ I.V. Busulfex (24%) 2493
▲ Xenical Capsules (3.3% to 5.2%) 2831

Rectal disorders, unspecified
Actiq (1% or greater) 979
Actonel Tablets (2.2%) 2683
Actonel with Calcium Tablets (2.2%) 2688
Asacol Delayed-Release Tablets (2% or greater) 2692
Avinza Capsules (Less than 5%) 1741
▲ CellCept Capsules (3% to less than 20%) 2747
▲ CellCept Intravenous (3% to less than 20%) 2747
▲ CellCept Oral Suspension (3% to less than 20%) 2747
▲ CellCept Tablets (3% to less than 20%) 2747
▲ Entocort EC Capsules (Less than 5%) 2698
Evoxac Capsules (Less than 1%) 1047
Ferrlecit Injection 3388
▲ I.V. Busulfex (25%) 2493
Lofibra Tablets 1219
Lofibra Capsules 1216
Meridia Capsules (1.2%) 489
Neurontin Capsules (Rare) 2487
Neurontin Oral Solution (Rare) 2487
Neurontin Tablets (Rare) 2487
Nexium Delayed-Release Capsules (Less than 1%) 655
Nexium I.V. (Less than 1%) 659
Norvir (Less than 2%) 503
Prevacid Delayed-Release Capsules (Less than 1%) 3271
Prevacid for Delayed-Release Oral Suspension (Less than 1%) 3271
Prevacid SoluTab Delayed-Release Orally Disintegrating Tablets (Less than 1%) 3271
Prevacid NapraPAC (Less than 1%) .. 3280
PREVPAC (Less than 1%) 3284
▲ Prograf Capsules and Injection (3% to 15%) 632
Protonix I.V. (Greater than or equal to 1%) 3472
Protonix Tablets (Greater than or equal to 1%) 3469
Protopic Ointment (0.2% to less than 1%) 638
Rapamune Oral Solution and Tablets 3475
Relpax Tablets (Rare) 2548
Rescriptor Tablets 2551
Tasmar Tablets (Infrequent) 3358
Tricor Tablets 527
Triglide Tablets 3123
Vantin Tablets and Oral Suspension (Less than 1%) 2645
VFEND I.V. (Less than 2%) 2564
VFEND Oral Suspension (Less than 2%) 2564
VFEND Tablets (Less than 2%) 2564
Wellbutrin Tablets (Rare) 1603

Rectal urgency
(*see under* Defecate, desire to)

Red blood cell, aplasia
Rituxan I.V. (One case) 1254

Red blood cell count, decrease
Aldara Cream, 5% 1846
Neumega for Injection 3435
▲ Norvir (18.6%) 503
Rythmol SR Capsules 2727

Red blood cells excretion, increase
Invanz for Injection (1.1% to 2.5%) ... 1999

"Red man" syndrome
Vancocin HCl Capsules, USP 3380

Redness, local
▲ Havrix Vaccine (16% to 21%) 1456
▲ Menactra Vaccine (0.6% to 14.4%) 2954
Ortho Evra Transdermal System 2417
Striant Mucoadhesive 1007
Regular Strength Tylenol Tablets 1870
Tylenol 8 Hour Extended Release Caplets 1870
Tylenol 1870
Extra Strength Tylenol PM Caplets, Vanilla Caplets, Geltabs, Gelcaps and Liquid 1875
Extra Strength Tylenol Rapid Release Gels 1870
Tylenol Allergy Multi-Symptom Caplets with Cool Burst and Gelcaps 1872
Tylenol Allergy Multi-Symptom Nighttime Caplets with Cool Burst 1872
Tylenol Severe Allergy Caplets 1872
Tylenol Arthritis Pain Extended Release Caplets and Geltabs 1870
Tylenol Chest Congestion Caplets with Cool Burst 1872
Tylenol Chest Congestion Liquid with Cool Burst 1872
Children's Tylenol Suspension Liquid and Meltaways 1878
Children's Tylenol Plus Cold Suspension Liquid 1879
Children's Tylenol Plus Cold & Allergy Suspension Liquid 1878
Children's Tylenol Plus Cough & Runny Nose Suspension Liquid 1879
Children's Tylenol Plus Cough & Sore Throat Suspension Liquid 1879
Children's Tylenol Suspension with Flavor Creator 1878
Children's Tylenol Plus Flu Suspension Liquid 1881
Children's Tylenol Plus Multi-Symptom Cold Suspension Liquid 1879
Tylenol Cold Severe Congestion Non-Drowsy Caplets with Cool Burst 1874
Tylenol Cold Head Congestion Daytime Caplets with Cool Burst ... 1873
Tylenol Cold Head Congestion Nighttime Caplets with Cool Burst 1873
Tylenol Cold Head Congestion Severe Caplets with Cool Burst 1873
Tylenol Cough & Sore Throat Daytime Liquid with Cool Burst 1877
Tylenol Cough & Sore Throat Nighttime Liquid with Cool Burst ... 1877
Concentrated Tylenol Infants' Drops 1878
Concentrated Tylenol Infants' Drops Plus Cold 1879
Concentrated Tylenol Infants' Drops Plus Cold and Cough 1879
Jr. Tylenol Meltaways 1878
Tylenol Sinus Severe Congestion Caplets with Cool Burst 1876
Tylenol Sinus Congestion & Pain Daytime Caplets with Cool Burst and Gelcaps 1876
Tylenol Sinus Congestion & Pain Nighttime Caplets with Cool Burst 1876
Tylenol Sinus Congestion & Pain Severe Caplets with Cool Burst 1876
Tylenol Sore Throat Daytime Liquid with Cool Burst 1877
Tylenol Sore Throat Nighttime Liquid with Cool Burst 1877
Women's Tylenol Menstrual Relief Caplets 1877

Redness, nasal
▲ Fortical Nasal Spray (10.6%) 3337

Redness at injection site
▲ Boostrix (1.7% to 47.7%) 1404
▲ Fluarix (15.9% to 17.5%) 1451
Humalog Mix 50/50-Pen 1783
Symlin Injection 613
Xolair 1266

Reflexes, abnormal
Frova Tablets (Rare) 1113
Neurontin Capsules (Frequent) 2487
Neurontin Oral Solution (Frequent) 2487
Neurontin Tablets (Frequent) 2487

Reflexes, increased
(*see under* Hyperreflexia)

Refraction disorder, unspecified
Caduet Tablets (Less than 2%) 2508
Lofibra Tablets 1219
Lofibra Capsules 1216
Tricor Tablets 527

Regurgitation
Altoprev Extended-Release Tablets (0.5% to 1%) 3109
Amerge Tablets (Rare) 1339
Invanz for Injection (1.1% to 1.6%) ... 1999
Lotronex Tablets (2%) 1512
Maxalt Tablets (Infrequent) 2008
Maxalt-MLT Orally Disintegrating Tablets (Infrequent) 2008
Mevacor Tablets (0.5% to 1.0%) 2021
Zyban Sustained-Release Tablets (Infrequent) 1644

Relaxation
Imitrex Injection (Infrequent) 1463

Renal agenesis, unilateral, neonatal
Leukeran Tablets 1504

Renal calculi
(*see under* Nephrolithiasis)

Renal colic
Crixivan Capsules (Less than 2%) 1940
Daranide Tablets 1950
Noroxin Tablets (Less frequent) 2032
Timolide Tablets (Less than 1%) 2086

Renal disease
Anaprox Tablets (Less than 1%) 2761
Anaprox DS Tablets (Less than 1%) .. 2761
EC-Naprosyn Delayed-Release Tablets (Less than 1%) 2761
Naprosyn Suspension (Less than 1%) 2761
Naprosyn Tablets (Less than 1%) 2761
Prevacid NapraPAC (Less than 1%) .. 3280

Renal disorders, unspecified
Ziagen (Less than 1%) 1626

Renal dysfunction
(*see under* Renal impairment)

Renal failure
▲ Abelcet Injection (5%) 1141
Abilify Oral Solution (Infrequent) 882
Abilify Oral Solution (Infrequent) 2450
Abilify Discmelt Orally Disintegrating Tablets (Infrequent) 882
Abilify Discmelt Orally Disintegrating Tablets (Infrequent) 2450
Abilify Tablets (Infrequent) 882
Abilify Tablets (Infrequent) 2450
Actiq (1% or greater) 979
Aggrenox Capsules (Less than 1%) .. 822
Agrylin Capsules (6 of 551 patients) 3169
Aldoril Tablets 1910
Alimta for Injection (Up to 2%) 1750
Aloprim for Injection (1.2%) 2167
AmBisome for Injection (Less common) 620
Anaprox Tablets (Less than 1%) 2761
Anaprox DS Tablets (Less than 1%) .. 2761
Aricept Tablets (Infrequent) 1094
Aricept ODT Tablets (Infrequent) 1094
Arthrotec Tablets (Rare) 3129
Atacand Tablets 649
Atacand HCT (Very rare) 651
Atripla Tablets 945
Avalide Tablets 888
Avalide Tablets 2874
Bayer Aspirin 744
Bayer Aspirin Comprehensive Prescribing Information .... ▣ 796
Benicar Tablets 1043
Benicar HCT Tablets (Rare) 1044
Bicillin C-R Injectable Suspension 1706
Bumex Tablets (0.1%) 2746
Cafcit (2.2%) 1886
Captopril Tablets (Approximately 1 to 2 of 1000 patients) 2149
Carbatrol Capsules 3171
▲ Carnitor Injection (6%) 3188
▲ CellCept Capsules (3% to less than 20%) 2747
▲ CellCept Intravenous (3% to less than 20%) 2747
▲ CellCept Oral Suspension (3% to less than 20%) 2747
▲ CellCept Tablets (3% to less than 20%) 2747
Cipro (Less than 1%) 2977
Cipro I.V. (1% or less) 2984
Cipro XR Tablets 2990
Clinoril Tablets (Less than 1 in 100) 1924
Crestor Tablets (Less than 1%) 678
▲ Cubicin for Injection (2.2% to 3.3%) 1026
Dacogen Injection 2129
Diovan HCT Tablets 2196
Diuril Oral Suspension 1954
Diuril Sodium Intravenous 2467
Dolobid Tablets (Less than 1 in 100) 1955
Dyrenium Capsules (One case) 3400
EC-Naprosyn Delayed-Release Tablets (Less than 1%) 2761
Effexor Tablets 3411
Effexor XR Capsules 3417
Elitek (Less than or equal to 1%) 2890
Equetro Extended-Release Capsules 3180
Erbitux (2%) 910
Ethyol for Injection (Rare) 1898
Fansidar Tablets 2765
Fleet Prep Kits 1170
Fuzeon Injection 2767
Gabitril Tablets (Infrequent) 984
Gemzar for Injection (Rare) 1771
Gleevec Tablets (Infrequent) 2227
Hepsera Tablets (2% or greater) 1292
Herceptin I.V. (At least one of the 958 patients) 1233
Hyzaar 50-12.5 Tablets 1990
Hyzaar 100-12.5 Tablets 1990
Hyzaar 100-25 Tablets 1990
Indocin (Less than 1%) 1995
Lamictal (Rare) 1481
Merrem I.V. (Greater than 0.1% to 1%) 686
Micardis HCT Tablets 856
Mobic Oral Suspension (Less than 2%) 863
Mobic Tablets (Less than 2%) 863
Moduretic Tablets (Less than or equal to 1%) 2028
Mylotarg for Injection 3431
Nalfon Capsules (Less than 1%) 2502
Namenda 1195
Naprosyn Suspension (Less than 1%) 2761
Naprosyn Tablets (Less than 1%) 2761
NeoProfen Injection (1%) 2472
Neumega for Injection 3435
Nipent for Injection (Less than 3%) ... 1863
Noroxin Tablets 2032
Norvir (Less than 2%) 503
NuvaRing 2340
Oncaspar 1145
Orthoclone OKT3 Sterile Solution 2360
PEG-Intron Powder for Injection 3048
Percodan Tablets 1132
Permax Tablets (Infrequent) 3356
Prevacid NapraPAC (Less than 1%) .. 3280
Prezista Tablets (Less than 2%) 3306
Prinzide Tablets 2056
▲ Prograf Capsules and Injection (3% to 15%) 632
Proquin XR Tablets 1153
Prozac Pulvules and Liquid 1801
Remicade for IV Injection (Greater than or equal to 0.2%) 971
Revlimid Capsules 958
Reyataz Capsules (Less than 3%) 921
Rythmol SR Capsules 2727
Sandostatin LAR Depot (Rare) 2280
Solodyn Extended Release Tablets .. 1890
St. Joseph 81 mg Aspirin Chewable and Enteric Coated Tablets 1869
St. Joseph 81 mg Aspirin .... ▣ 688
Tegretol/Tegretol-XR 2295
Teveten HCT Tablets 1737
Ticlid Tablets (Rare) 2810
Timolide Tablets 2086
Trasylol Injection (1% to 2%) 754

▲ Trisenox Injection (8%) 993
Trizivir Tablets 1589
Truvada Tablets 1296
Valtrex Caplets 1597
Vancocin HCl Capsules, USP (Rare) 3380
Vasotec I.V. Injection (0.5% to 1.0%) 2103
Ventavis Inhalation Solution 1020
Viread Tablets 1301
Voltaren Tablets (Occasionally) 2307
Voltaren-XR Tablets (Occasionally) 2310
▲ Xeloda Tablets (Less than 5%) 2822
Ziagen 1626
Zosyn 3492
Zovirax 1643

Renal failure, acute
Abelcet Injection 1141
Aceon Tablets (2 mg, 4 mg, 8 mg) 3194
Activase I.V. 1223
Albenza Tablets 1338
Altace Capsules (Less than 1%) 1702
Ambien Tablets (Rare) 2851
Ambien CR Tablets (Rare) 2855
AmBisome for Injection (Less common) 620
Anzemet Injection (Rare) 2859
Anzemet Tablets (Rare) 2862
Atripla Tablets 945
Campath Ampules 811
Camptosar Injection (Rare) 2604
Carimune NF 3499
Celebrex Capsules (Less than 0.1%) 3134
Celexa 1176
▲ CellCept Capsules (3% to less than 20%) 2747
▲ CellCept Intravenous (3% to less than 20%) 2747
▲ CellCept Oral Suspension (3% to less than 20%) 2747
▲ CellCept Tablets (3% to less than 20%) 2747
Chantix Tablets (Rare) 2517
Crixivan Capsules 1940
CytoGam Intravenous 1895
Dyazide Capsules 1423
Dyrenium Capsules 3400
Eloxatin for Injection 2892
Elspar for Injection 2463
Elspar for Injection 1960
Exelon Capsules (Infrequent) 2206
Exelon Oral Solution (Infrequent) 2206
Flebogamma 5%, Immune Globulin Intravenous (Human) 1658
Gammagard S/D 724
Gantrisin Pediatric Suspension 2770
Imitrex Injection 1463
Imitrex Nasal Spray 1467
Imitrex Tablets 1471
Indocin I.V. (Less than 1%) 2465
Lamictal (Rare) 1481
Levaquin (0.1% to 0.9%) 2384
Levaquin in 5% Dextrose Injection (0.1% to 0.9%) 2384
Lexapro Oral Solution 1190
Lexapro Tablets 1190
Lipitor Tablets (Rare) 2483
Lotrel Capsules (Rare) 2249
Mefoxin for Injection (Rare) 2012
Mefoxin Premixed Intravenous Solution (Rare) 2016
Mevacor Tablets 2021
Mycamine for Injection 628
Neurontin Capsules (Rare) 2487
Neurontin Oral Solution (Rare) 2487
Neurontin Tablets (Rare) 2487
Nexavar Tablets (Infrequent) 746
Omnicef Capsules 511
Omnicef for Oral Suspension 511
Paxil CR Controlled-Release Tablets 1538
Paxil 1530
Pexeva Tablets 1694
Plavix Tablets (1% to 2.5%) 917
Plavix Tablets (1% to 2.5%) 2926
Primaxin I.M. 2045
Primaxin I.V. (Less than 0.2%) 2048
Prinivil Tablets (0.3% to 1.3%) 2052
Prinzide Tablets 2056
Prograf Capsules and Injection 632
Proleukin for Injection (Less than 1%) 2266
Protopic Ointment 638
Requip Tablets (Rare) 1555
Rescriptor Tablets 2551
Risperdal 1676
Risperdal M-Tab Orally Disintegrating Tablets 1676
Rituxan I.V. 1254
Seroquel Tablets (Rare) 690
Suprax 1843
Thalomid Capsules 965
Trasylol Injection (1% to 2%) 754
Vasotec I.V. Injection (Rare) 2103
▲ Vesanoid Capsules (3%) 2820
VFEND I.V. (0% to 0.4%) 2564
VFEND Oral Suspension (0% to 0.4%) 2564
VFEND Tablets (0% to 0.4%) 2564
Zmax for Oral Suspension 2583
Zocor Tablets (Rare) 2105
Zoloft 2586

Renal failure, aggravated
Vantas (Less than 2%) 3375

Renal failure, neonatal
Aceon Tablets (2 mg, 4 mg, 8 mg) 3194
Altace Capsules 1702
Captopril Tablets 2149
Cozaar Tablets 1935
Hyzaar 50-12.5 Tablets 1990
Hyzaar 100-12.5 Tablets 1990
Hyzaar 100-25 Tablets 1990
Lotrel Capsules 2249
Prinivil Tablets 2052
Prinzide Tablets 2056
Vasotec I.V. Injection 2103

Renal function impairment
(*see under* Renal impairment)

Renal impairment
Abelcet Injection 1141
Agrylin Capsules (10 of 551 patients) 3169
Aldoril Tablets 1910
Aloprim for Injection (Less than 1%) 2167
Altace Capsules (Rare) 1702
▲ Anaprox Tablets (1% to 10%) 2761
▲ Anaprox DS Tablets (1% to 10%) 2761
Aredia for Injection 2179
Argatroban Injection (2.8%) 1346
Asacol Delayed-Release Tablets 2692
Atacand Tablets 649
Atacand HCT (Very rare) 651
Avalide Tablets 888
Avalide Tablets 2874
Benicar HCT Tablets 1044
Campath Ampules 811
Camptosar Injection (Rare) 2604
Ceftin 1407
▲ CellCept Capsules (21.8% to 25.6%) 2747
▲ CellCept Intravenous (21.8% to 25.6%) 2747
▲ CellCept Oral Suspension (21.8% to 25.6%) 2747
▲ CellCept Tablets (21.8% to 25.6%) 2747
Cleocin Vaginal Ovules (Rare) 2616
Clinoril Tablets (Less than 1 in 100) 1924
Cubicin for Injection (Less than 1%) 1026
Diovan Tablets 2193
Diovan HCT Tablets 2196
Diuril Oral Suspension 1954
Diuril Sodium Intravenous 2467
Dolobid Tablets (Less than 1 in 100) 1955
Doxil Injection (Less than 1%) 2351
▲ EC-Naprosyn Delayed-Release Tablets (1% to 10%) 2761
Effexor XR Capsules (Rare) 3417
Evoxac Capsules (Less than 1%) 1047
Fortaz 1453
Garamycin Injectable 3014
▲ Gengraf Capsules (25% to 38%) 459
Hyzaar 50-12.5 Tablets 1990
Hyzaar 100-12.5 Tablets 1990
Hyzaar 100-25 Tablets 1990
▲ Indocin I.V. (41% of infants) 2465
Keflex Capsules 549
Lescol Capsules 2233
Lescol XL Tablets 2233
▲ Leukine (8%) 814
Levaquin (0.1% to 0.9%) 2384
Levaquin in 5% Dextrose Injection (0.1% to 0.9%) 2384
Lofibra Tablets 1219
Lofibra Capsules 1216
Maxipime for Injection 1105
Mefoxin for Injection 2012
Mefoxin Premixed Intravenous Solution 2016
Mepron Suspension 1521
Micardis HCT Tablets 856
Mircette Tablets 1066
Moduretic Tablets (Less than or equal to 1%) 2028
Mycamine for Injection 628
▲ Myfortic Tablets (3% to less than 20%) 2255
Mylotarg for Injection 3431
▲ Naprosyn Suspension (1% to 10%) 2761
▲ Naprosyn Tablets (1% to 10%) 2761
▲ NeoProfen Injection (6%) 2472
▲ Neoral Oral Solution (25% to 38%) 2259
▲ Neoral Soft Gelatin Capsules (25% to 38%) 2259
Nipent for Injection (Less than 3%) 1863
Omnicef Capsules 511
Omnicef for Oral Suspension 511
Oncaspar 1145
Ortho-Cyclen Tablets 2429
Ortho Evra Transdermal System 2417
Ortho Tri-Cyclen Tablets 2429
Ortho Tri-Cyclen Lo Tablets 2436
Panhematin for Injection 2473
Paxil CR Controlled-Release Tablets (Rare) 1538
Paxil (Rare) 1530
Plavix Tablets 917
Plavix Tablets 2926
Prinivil Tablets (0.3% to 1.0%) 2052
Prinzide Tablets 2056
▲ Prograf Capsules and Injection (36% to 40%) 632
Proleukin for Injection (2%) 2266
Protopic Ointment 638
Raniclor Tablets, Chewable 2505
Refludan for Injection (1.8%) 792
ReoPro Vials (0.3%) 1809
▲ Sandimmune (25% to 38%) 2275
Seasonique Tablets 1077
▲ Simulect for Injection (3% to 10%) 2284
Striant Mucoadhesive 1007
Suprax 1843
Tequin Injection 938
Tequin Injection in 5% Dextrose 938
Tequin Tablets 938
Teveten HCT Tablets 1737
Timolide Tablets 2086
Tranxene 2474
▲ Trasylol Injection (5% to 30%) 754
Tricor Tablets 527
▲ Trisenox Injection (8%) 993
▲ Valcyte Tablets (Less than 5%) 2813
▲ Vantas (4.7%) 3375
Vantin Tablets and Oral Suspension 2645
Vasotec I.V. Injection (0.5% to 1.0%) 2103
VFEND I.V. (0.5%) 2564
VFEND Oral Suspension (0.5%) 2564
VFEND Tablets (0.5%) 2564
Viramune Oral Suspension 873
Viramune Tablets 873
Yasmin 28 Tablets 796
Yaz Tablets 803

Renal infarct
BeneFix Vials (1.5%) 3408
Vesanoid Capsules 2820

Renal injury
Capastat Sulfate for Injection 1755

Renal insufficiency
Aggrenox Capsules (Less than 1%) 822
Aloprim for Injection (1.2%) 2167
Aptivus Capsules (Less than 2%) 826
Atripla Tablets 945
Bayer Aspirin 744
Bayer Aspirin Comprehensive Prescribing Information ▣796
Cancidas for Injection (0% to 0.9%) 1918
Capastat Sulfate for Injection (1 patient) 1755
Captopril Tablets (Approximately 1 to 2 of 1000 patients) 2149
▲ Coreg Tablets (Greater than 1% to 3%) 1414
Crixivan Capsules (Some cases) 1940
Elspar for Injection 2463
Elspar for Injection 1960
Emend Capsules (Greater than 0.5%) 1963
Erythrocin Stearate Filmtab Tablets (Isolated reports) 453
Fleet Prep Kits 1170
Fuzeon Injection 2767
Hepsera Tablets (2% or greater) 1292
Indocin Capsules (Less than 1%) 1995
Indocin I.V. (Less than 1%) 2465
Indocin (Less than 1%) 1995
Invanz for Injection (Greater than 0.1%) 1999
Neupogen for Injection (Two events) 603
Nipent for Injection (Less than 3%) 1863
Norvir 503
▲ Ontak Vials (Less than 5%) 1745
Orthoclone OKT3 Sterile Solution 2360
PEG-Intron Powder for Injection 3048
Percodan Tablets 1132
Prezista Tablets (Less than 2%) 3306
Proleukin for Injection 2266
Risperdal (Rare) 1676
Risperdal M-Tab Orally Disintegrating Tablets (Rare) 1676
Sandostatin LAR Depot (Rare) 2280
St. Joseph 81 mg Aspirin Chewable and Enteric Coated Tablets 1869
St. Joseph 81 mg Aspirin ▣688
Taxotere Injection Concentrate 2932
Truvada Tablets 1296
Univasc Tablets (Less than 1%) 3104
▲ Vesanoid Capsules (11%) 2820
Viread Tablets 1301
▲ Voltaren Tablets (1% to 10%) 2307
▲ Voltaren-XR Tablets (1% to 10%) 2310

Renal insufficiency, reversible
Actimmune (Rare) 1671

Renal precipitation
Rocephin Injectable Vials, ADD-Vantage, Galaxy, Bulk 2800

Renal stones
Abilify Oral Solution (Infrequent) 882
Abilify Oral Solution (Infrequent) 2450
Abilify Discmelt Orally Disintegrating Tablets (Infrequent) 882
Abilify Discmelt Orally Disintegrating Tablets (Infrequent) 2450
Abilify Tablets (Infrequent) 882
Abilify Tablets (Infrequent) 2450
Campral Tablets (Rare) 1174
Clinoril Tablets 1924
Enbrel for Injection 584
Fortical Nasal Spray (Less than 1%) 3337
Proquin XR Tablets 1153
▲ Topamax Sprinkle Capsules (0% to 3%) 2404
▲ Topamax Tablets (0% to 3%) 2404
Vantas (Less than 2%) 3375
Zelapar Tablets 3372
▲ Zonegran Capsules (4%) 1101

Renal toxicity
(*see also under* Nephrotoxicity)
Arthrotec Tablets 3129

Rencephalopathy, metabolic
Arranon Injection (1%) 1357

Reproductive disorders, female
Amerge Tablets (Rare) 1339
▲ Hycamtin for Injection (5%) 1458

Resistance mechanism
▲ Aldara Cream, 5% (4.2%) 1846

Resistance mechanism disorders
▲ Copegus Tablets (12%) 2754

Respiration, painful
Amitiza Capsules (Less than 0.2%) 3224
Prinivil Tablets (0.3% to 1.0%) 2052
Prinzide Tablets 2056

Respiratory alkalosis
Aggrenox Capsules 822
AmBisome for Injection (Less common) 620
Campath Ampules 811
Coreg Tablets (Less than or equal to 0.1%) 1414
Geodon Capsules (Rare) 2529
St. Joseph 81 mg Aspirin Chewable and Enteric Coated Tablets 1869

Respiratory arrest
Actiq 979
Arranon Injection 1357
Campath Ampules 811
Cipro I.V. (1% or less) 2984
Cipro XR Tablets 2990
Clozaril Tablets (Rare) 2184
Dacogen Injection 2129
Dilaudid Oral Liquid 445
Dilaudid Tablets - 8 mg 445
Dilaudid-HP 442
Ethyol for Injection (Rare) 1898
Infed Injection 3390
Kadian Capsules 577
Lidoderm Patch 1118

MS Contin Tablets........................ 2701
Orthoclone OKT3 Sterile Solution..... 2360
OxyContin Tablets........................ 2703
Proleukin for Injection (Less than 1%).. 2266
Proquin XR Tablets........................ 1153
Synera Topical Patch...................... 1137

Respiratory congestion, unspecified

Comvax (0.3% to 1.2%).................. 1928
Cozaar Tablets (Less than 1%)......... 1935
▲ Epogen for Injection (15%) 591
Hyzaar 50-12.5 Tablets.................. 1990
Hyzaar 100-12.5 Tablets................ 1990
Hyzaar 100-25 Tablets.................. 1990
Maxalt Tablets (Infrequent).............. 2008
Maxalt-MLT Orally Disintegrating Tablets (Infrequent)..................... 2008
▲ Procrit for Injection (15%) 2364
ProQuad (Greater than or equal to 0.2% to less than 1%)................... 2064
Vaqta (1.6%) 2097

Respiratory depression

Actiq 979
Anaprox Tablets (Less than 1%) 2761
Anaprox DS Tablets (Less than 1%) .. 2761
Arthrotec Tablets (Rare) 3129
Campath Ampules 811
Dantrium Capsules (Less frequent) .. 2694
▲ DepoDur Extended-Release Injection (2% to 5%) 1110
Dilaudid 440
Dilaudid Non-Sterile Powder 440
Dilaudid Oral Liquid 445
Dilaudid Rectal Suppositories 440
Dilaudid Tablets 440
Dilaudid Tablets - 8 mg 445
Dilaudid-HP 442
EC-Naprosyn Delayed-Release Tablets (Less than 1%) 2761
Emend Capsules (Greater than 0.5%) 1963
Garamycin Injectable 3014
Hycodan 1116
Hycotuss Expectorant Syrup 1117
Kadian Capsules 577
Klonopin 2778
Levaquin (0.1% to 0.9%) 2384
Levaquin in 5% Dextrose Injection (0.1% to 0.9%)............................ 2384
Lidoderm Patch 1118
MS Contin Tablets 2701
Naprosyn Suspension (Less than 1%) 2761
Naprosyn Tablets (Less than 1%) 2761
Numorphan Injection 1120
Opana Tablets (Less than 1%) 1122
Opana ER Tablets (Less than 1%) 1126
OxyContin Tablets 2703
OxyFast Oral Concentrate Solution .. 2708
OxyIR Capsules 2708
Percocet Tablets 1131
Phenergan Tablets and Suppositories 3440
ProSom Tablets 517
Synera Topical Patch 1137
Tussionex Pennkinetic Extended-Release Suspension 3327
Tylenol with Codeine Tablets 2391
Vicodin Tablets 535
Vicodin ES Tablets 536
Vicodin HP Tablets 538
Vicoprofen Tablets 539
Voltaren Tablets (Rarely) 2307
Voltaren-XR Tablets (Rarely) 2310
Zydone Tablets 1139

Respiratory depression, postoperative

▲ Advair HFA Inhalation Aerosol (1% to 3%) 1318

Respiratory desaturation

Curosurf Intratracheal Suspension ... 1057

Respiratory difficulty

▲ Abelcet Injection (4%) 1141
Allegra-D 12 Hour Extended-Release Tablets 2846
Allegra-D 24 Hour Extended-Release Tablets 2849
Ambien Tablets 2851
Carafate Suspension 701
Carafate Tablets 701
Cardene I.V. (Rare) 2497
EpiPen 1061
Infed Injection 3390
Invirase (Less than 2%) 2772
Kadian Capsules (Less than 3%) 577
▲ Photofrin for Injection (10%) 702
Rilutek Tablets (More than 2%) 2930
Thyrogen for Injection..................... 1286
▲ Trasylol Injection (3%) 754
Twinject 0.3.................................. 3378
Twinject 0.15 3379
▲ Vesanoid Capsules (26%) 2820
Zyrtec-D 12 Hour Extended Release Tablets 2597

Respiratory discharge, upper, unspecified

Emcyt Capsules (1%)...................... 2634

Respiratory disorders, unspecified

Asmanex Twisthaler (1% to less than 3%)................................. 2966
▲ CellCept Capsules (3% to less than 20%)................................ 2747
▲ CellCept Intravenous (3% to less than 20%)................................ 2747
▲ CellCept Oral Suspension (3% to less than 20%)........................ 2747
▲ CellCept Tablets (3% to less than 20%).. 2747
Chantix Tablets (Frequent).............. 2517
▲ Colazal Capsules (4%) 2838
▲ Enbrel for Injection (5%) 584
Evoxac Capsules (Less than 1%)...... 1047
▲ Focalin XR Capsules (9% to 16%) 2223
Gabitril Tablets (Infrequent)............ 984
▲ Geodon Capsules (8%) 2529
▲ Intron A for Injection (Less than or equal to 5%)................................ 3024
Levaquin (0.1% to 0.9%)................. 2384
Levaquin in 5% Dextrose Injection (0.1% to 0.9%)........................... 2384
▲ Lofibra Tablets (6.2%) 1219
▲ Lofibra Capsules (6.2%) 1216
▲ Lupron Depot 7.5 mg (10.7%) 3264
Lupron Injection Pediatric 3259
Meridia Capsules........................... 489
Merrem I.V. (Greater than 0.1% to 1%)... 686
▲ Paxil CR Controlled-Release Tablets (7%)............................... 1538
▲ Paxil (7%) 1530
Plasbumin-5 (Rare)......................... 3251
Plasbumin-20 (Rare)....................... 3252
Plasbumin-25 (Rare)....................... 3253
Prevacid Delayed-Release Capsules (Less than 1%)............. 3271
Prevacid for Delayed-Release Oral Suspension (Less than 1%)......... 3271
Prevacid SoluTab Delayed-Release Orally Disintegrating Tablets (Less than 1%)......................... 3271
Prevacid NapraPAC (Less than 1%).. 3280
PREVPAC (Less than 1%)................ 3284
▲ Prilosec OTC Delayed-Release Tablets (18.5% to 46.2%)............ 2677
▲ Proleukin for Injection (11%) 2266
▲ Proventil HFA Inhalation Aerosol (6%)... 3056
Relpax Tablets (Infrequent).............. 2548
Rituxan I.V. 1254
▲ Simulect for Injection (3% to 10%) ... 2284
▲ TOBI Solution for Inhalation (31.4%)...................................... 2298
Topamax Sprinkle Capsules (1%)..... 2404
Topamax Tablets (1%).................... 2404
▲ Tricor Tablets (6.2%) 527
▲ Triglide Tablets (6.2%) 3123
VFEND I.V. (Less than 2%)............... 2564
VFEND Oral Suspension (Less than 2%)... 2564
VFEND Tablets (Less than 2%).......... 2564
Wellbutrin SR Sustained-Release Tablets (At least 1%).................. 1607
▲ Wellbutrin XL Extended-Release Tablets (At least 1% to 4%)......... 1613
Xyrem Oral Solution (Infrequent)....... 1688
▲ Zegerid Capsules (18.5% to 46.2%).................................... 2958
▲ Zegerid Powder for Oral Solution (18.5% to 46.2%)...................... 2958
Zostavax Injection (1.1%)................ 2111
Zyrtec-D 12 Hour Extended Release Tablets (Less than 2%)..... 2597

Respiratory distress

▲ Agrylin Capsules (1% to 5%) 3169
Aldoril Tablets............................... 1910
Aloprim for Injection (Less than 1%)... 2167
Aredia for Injection (One case)......... 2179
Atacand HCT 651
Atrovent Inhalation Solution (1.4%)... 835
Blocadren Tablets.......................... 1916
Cipro I.V. (1% or less).................... 2984
Cipro XR Tablets............................ 2990
▲ Clolar for Intravenous Infusion (14%).. 1271
Combivent Inhalation Aerosol (2.5%)... 847
Comvax... 1928
Cosopt Sterile Ophthalmic Solution....................................... 1931
Diovan HCT Tablets........................ 2196
Diuril Oral Suspension.................... 1954
Diuril Sodium Intravenous 2467
Duragesic Transdermal System (Less than 1%)........................... 2373
Dyazide Capsules.......................... 1423
▲ Elitek (3%) 2890
Elspar for Injection......................... 2463
Elspar for Injection......................... 1960
Ethyol for Injection (Rare)................ 1898
Fluarix.. 1451
Fuzeon Injection............................ 2767
Glucagon for Injection Vials and Emergency Kit.............................. 1778
Herceptin I.V................................. 1233
▲ Humatrope Vials and Cartridges (3.13% to 6.67%)........................ 1787
Hyzaar 50-12.5 Tablets................... 1990
Hyzaar 100-12.5 Tablets 1990
Hyzaar 100-25 Tablets 1990
Indapamide Tablets 2156
Inderal LA Long-Acting Capsules 3429
Indocin Capsules (Less than 1%) 1995
Indocin I.V. (Less than 1%) 2465
Indocin (Less than 1%) 1995
InnoPran XL Capsules 2723
Lamictal (More than 1%) 1481
Leukine 814
Levaquin 2384
Levaquin in 5% Dextrose Injection 2384
Lopressor Injection 2238
Lopressor Tablets 2238
Lopressor HCT 50/25 Tablets 2241
Lopressor HCT 100/25 Tablets 2241
Lopressor HCT 100/50 Tablets 2241
Lotensin HCT Tablets 2246
Micardis HCT Tablets 856
Moduretic Tablets 2028
▲ Myozyme for Intravenous Infusion (33%)... 1279
Nadolol Tablets 2159
Opana Tablets (Less than 1%) 1122
Opana ER Tablets (Less than 1%) 1126
Paxil CR Controlled-Release Tablets 1538
Paxil 1530
Prinzide Tablets 2056
▲ Prograf Capsules and Injection (3% to 15%) 632
Proquin XR Tablets 1153
Prozac Pulvules and Liquid 1801
Revlimid Capsules (2%) 958
Rituxan I.V. 1254
Sandimmune 2275
Teveten HCT Tablets 1737
▲ Thiola Tablets (4%) 2141
Timolide Tablets 2086
Timoptic Sterile Ophthalmic Solution (Less frequent) 2088
Timoptic in Ocudose 2091
Timoptic-XE Sterile Ophthalmic Gel Forming Solution 2092
Topamax Sprinkle Capsules (1%) 2404
Topamax Tablets (1%) 2404
Toprol-XL Tablets 668
Uniretic Tablets 3100
Virazole for Inhalation Solution 3370
▲ Xeloda Tablets (Less than 5%) 2822

Respiratory distress, neonatal

Hycodan 1116
Hycotuss Expectorant Syrup 1117

Respiratory distress syndrome

Campath Ampules 811
Carimune NF 3499
Flebogamma 5%, Immune Globulin Intravenous (Human) 1658
Gammagard Liquid 721
Gammagard S/D (Rare) 724
Gamunex Immune Globulin I.V., 10% (Rare) 3235
Levaquin (0.1% to 0.9%) 2384
Levaquin in 5% Dextrose Injection (0.1% to 0.9%)............................ 2384
Neulasta Injection 601
Neupogen for Injection 603
Prograf Capsules and Injection 632
Remicade for IV Injection (Greater than or equal to 0.2%) 971
Tarceva Tablets 1259
Tarceva Tablets 2444
Taxotere Injection Concentrate 2932
Trizivir Tablets 1589
VFEND I.V. (Less than 2%) 2564
VFEND Oral Suspension (Less than 2%) 2564
VFEND Tablets (Less than 2%) 2564
▲ Zegerid Capsules (3.4%) 2958
▲ Zegerid Powder for Oral Solution (3.4%)... 2958
Ziagen.. 1626

Respiratory failure

▲ Abelcet Injection (8%) 1141
Abilify Oral Solution (Rare)............... 882
Abilify Oral Solution (Rare)............... 2450
Abilify Discmelt Orally Disintegrating Tablets (Rare)......... 882
Abilify Discmelt Orally Disintegrating Tablets (Rare)......... 2450
Abilify Tablets (Rare)....................... 882
Abilify Tablets (Rare) 2450
Actiq (Less than 1%) 979
Aloprim for Injection (Less than 1%)... 2167
AmBisome for Injection (Less common)..................................... 620
Betagan Ophthalmic Solution, USP... ⊙220
Betimol Ophthalmic Solution 3382
Betimol Ophthalmic Solution .... ⊙295
Betoptic S Ophthalmic Suspension (Rare)... 558
Carteolol Hydrochloride Ophthalmic Solution USP, 1%....... ⊙249
CellCept Capsules.......................... 2747
CellCept Intravenous...................... 2747
CellCept Oral Suspension 2747
CellCept Tablets 2747
Cosopt Sterile Ophthalmic Solution....................................... 1931
Gemzar for Injection (Very rare)........ 1771
▲ Myozyme for Intravenous Infusion (31%)... 1279
▲ NeoProfen Injection (10%) 2472
Omnicef Capsules.......................... 511
Omnicef for Oral Suspension 511
Orthoclone OKT3 Sterile Solution..... 2360
PEG-Intron Powder for Injection........ 3048
Photofrin for Injection...................... 702
Prograf Capsules and Injection......... 632
▲ Proleukin for Injection (Less than 1% to 9%)................................. 2266
Pulmozyme Inhalation Solution......... 1248
Revlimid Capsules 958
Rythmol SR Capsules...................... 2727
Simulect for Injection...................... 2284
Symmetrel Tablets.......................... 1135
Timoptic Sterile Ophthalmic Solution (Less frequent)................ 2088
Timoptic in Ocudose (Less frequent)..................................... 2091
Timoptic-XE Sterile Ophthalmic Gel Forming Solution 2092
Trizivir Tablets 1589
Ziagen.. 1626

Respiratory insufficiency

Aloprim for Injection (Less than 1%)... 2167
Campath Ampules 811
Emend Capsules (Greater than 0.5%)... 1963
Levaquin (0.1% to 0.9%)................. 2384
Levaquin in 5% Dextrose Injection (0.1% to 0.9%)............................ 2384
Remicade for IV Injection (Greater than or equal to 0.2%).................. 971

Respiratory moniliasis

▲ CellCept Capsules (3% to less than 20%).................................. 2747
▲ CellCept Intravenous (3% to less than 20%)................................. 2747
▲ CellCept Oral Suspension (3% to less than 20%)........................ 2747
▲ CellCept Tablets (3% to less than 20%).. 2747
Rilutek Tablets (Infrequent)............... 2930
Tricor Tablets................................ 527

Respiratory rate, decreased

Opana Tablets (Less than 1%)........... 1122
Opana ER Tablets (Less than 1%)...... 1126

Respiratory rate, increased

Xyrem Oral Solution (Infrequent)....... 1688

Respiratory tract disorders

▲ Exubera Inhalation Powder (6.1% to 7.4%)..................................... 2524

Restless Legs Syndrome

Chantix Tablets (Infrequent).............. 2517
Exelon Capsules (Infrequent)............ 2206
Exelon Oral Solution (Infrequent) 2206
Requip Tablets............................... 1555
Xyrem Oral Solution (Infrequent)....... 1688

Restlessness
(*see under* Dysphoria)

Retching
Amitiza Capsules (Less than 0.2%) .. 3224
Imitrex Injection (Rare) 1463
Imitrex Nasal Spray 1467
Imitrex Tablets 1471
Trileptal Tablets 2300
Trileptal Oral Suspension 2300
Xyrem Oral Solution (Infrequent) 1688

Reticulocytopenia
Cosmegen for Injection 2459
Garamycin Injectable 3014

Reticulocytosis
▲ Dapsone Tablets USP (Almost all patients) 1673
Garamycin Injectable 3014
▲ Lithostat Tablets (5% to 6%) 2140
Percodan Tablets 1132
Ticlid Tablets (Rare) 2810
Virazole for Inhalation Solution 3370

Retinal artery occlusion
Activase I.V. 1223
Imitrex Nasal Spray 1467
Imitrex Tablets 1471
Zelapar Tablets 3372

Retinal atrophy
Clinoril Tablets 1924

Retinal damage
Dapsone Tablets USP 1673
Neurontin Capsules (Rare) 2487
Neurontin Oral Solution (Rare) 2487
Neurontin Tablets (Rare) 2487

Retinal degeneration
Aciphex Tablets 1090
Prevacid Delayed-Release Capsules (Less than 1%) 3271
Prevacid for Delayed-Release Oral Suspension (Less than 1%) 3271
Prevacid SoluTab Delayed-Release Orally Disintegrating Tablets (Less than 1%) 3271
Prevacid NapraPAC (Less than 1%) .. 3280
PREVPAC (Less than 1%) 3284
Uniretic Tablets (Less than 1%) 3100

Retinal detachment
Cymbalta Delayed-Release Capsules (Infrequent) 1757
▲ Lucentis Injection (Less than 0.1% to 11%) 1237
Macugen Injection (Less than 1%) ... ⊙ 261
Namenda (Infrequent) 1195
Permax Tablets (Rare) 3356
Sonata Capsules (Rare) 1717
Sular Tablets (Less than or equal to 1%) 3122
▲ Valcyte Tablets (15%) 2813
Visudyne for Injection (Less than 1%) 2305
Xalatan Sterile Ophthalmic Solution (Extremely rare) 2649
Zelapar Tablets 3372

Retinal disorder, unspecified
Evoxac Capsules (Less than 1%) 1047
Lamisil Tablets 2232
Lotensin HCT Tablets (0.3% or more) 2246
Rythmol SR Capsules 2727

Retinal ischemia
PEG-Intron Powder for Injection (Less than or equal to 1%) 3048

Retinal pigmentation disorders
Ontak Vials 1745

Retinal vascular disorder
Betimol Ophthalmic Solution 3382
Betimol Ophthalmic Solution .... ⊙ 295
Climara Transdermal System 771
Climara Pro Transdermal System 776
Intron A for Injection (Rare) 3024
Lyrica Capsules (0.1% to 1%) 2539
Menostar Transdermal System 782
Permax Tablets 3356
Protonix I.V. (Less than 1%) 3472
Protonix Tablets (Less than 1%) 3469
Viagra Tablets 2573
Virazole for Inhalation Solution 3370
Visudyne for Injection (Less than 1%) 2305

Retinal vein occlusion
Cialis Tablets 1838
Evista Tablets (Very rare) 1763
Levitra Tablets (Rare) 3034

Retinitis
Attenuvax (Infrequent) 1914
▲ Doxil Injection (1% to 5%) 2351
Indocin (Less than 1%) 1995
M-M-R II (Infrequent) 2006
ProQuad 2064
VFEND I.V. (Less than 2%) 2564
VFEND Oral Suspension (Less than 2%) 2564
VFEND Tablets (Less than 2%) 2564

Retinoic-acid-APL syndrome
▲ Vesanoid Capsules (Up to 25%) 2820

Retinopathy
Cardizem LA Extended Release Tablets (Infrequent) 1728
Clinoril Tablets 1924
Exelon Capsules (Infrequent) 2206
Exelon Oral Solution (Infrequent) 2206
Intron A for Injection 3024
Neurontin Capsules (Rare) 2487
Neurontin Oral Solution (Rare) 2487
Neurontin Tablets (Rare) 2487
Nipent for Injection (Less than 3%) ... 1863
Pegasys 2789
PEG-Intron Powder for Injection 3048
Tiazac Capsules (Infrequent) 1201

Retinopathy, pigmentary
Thioridazine Hydrochloride Tablets .. 2163

Retinopathy of prematurity
Cafcit (2.2%) 1886

Retrolental fibroplasia
▲ Indocin I.V. (3% to 9%) 2465

Retroperitoneal fibrosis
Blocadren Tablets 1916
Cosopt Sterile Ophthalmic Solution 1931
Stalevo Tablets (Rare) 2287
Timolide Tablets 2086
Timoptic Sterile Ophthalmic Solution (Less frequent) 2088
Timoptic in Ocudose (Less frequent) 2091
Timoptic-XE Sterile Ophthalmic Gel Forming Solution 2092

Retroperitoneum, redistribution/accumulation of body fat
Retrovir 1560

Reye's Syndrome, potential for development of
Aggrenox Capsules 822
Bayer Aspirin 744
Bayer Aspirin Comprehensive Prescribing Information .... ▣ 796
BC Headache Powder .... ▣ 677
BC Allergy Sinus Cold Powder .... ▣ 677
Arthritis Strength BC Powder .... ▣ 677
BC Sinus Cold Powder .... ▣ 677
Dolobid Tablets 1955
Goody's Body Pain Formula Powder .... ▣ 684
Goody's Extra Strength Headache Powders .... ▣ 611
Goody's Extra Strength Pain Relief Tablets .... ▣ 685
Maalox Maximum Strength Total Stomach Relief Peppermint Liquid (Rare) .... ▣ 660
Maalox Maximum Strength Total Stomach Relief Strawberry Liquid (Rare) .... ▣ 672
Pepto-Bismol Original Liquid, Maximum Strength Liquid, Original and Cherry Tablets, Chewable Tablets and Easy-To-Swallow Caplets (Rare) 2676
Pepto-Bismol Maximum Strength Liquid (Rare) .... ▣ 672
Percodan Tablets 1132
St. Joseph 81 mg Aspirin Chewable and Enteric Coated Tablets 1869
St. Joseph 81 mg Aspirin .... ▣ 688

Rhabdomyolysis
Abilify Oral Solution (Rare) 882
Abilify Oral Solution (Rare) 2450
Abilify Discmelt Orally Disintegrating Tablets (Rare) 882
Abilify Discmelt Orally Disintegrating Tablets (Rare) 2450
Abilify Tablets (Rare) 882
Abilify Tablets (Rare) 2450
Accutane Capsules (Rare) 2731
Aciphex Tablets 1090
Activase I.V. 1223
Advicor Tablets 1722
Aggrenox Capsules 822
Altoprev Extended-Release Tablets ... 3109
Atacand Tablets 649
Atacand HCT (Rare) 651
Avalide Tablets 888
Avalide Tablets 2874
Avapro Tablets (Rare) 891
Avapro Tablets (Rare) 2871
Bayer Aspirin 744
Bayer Aspirin Comprehensive Prescribing Information .... ▣ 796
Benicar Tablets 1043
Benicar HCT Tablets (Rare) 1044
Bicillin C-R Injectable Suspension 1706
Caduet Tablets 2508
Celexa 1176
Clozaril Tablets 2184
Combivir Tablets 1411
Comtan Tablets 2189
Cozaar Tablets (Rare) 1935
Crestor Tablets (Less than 1%) 678
Cubicin for Injection 1026
Diovan Tablets 2193
Diovan HCT Tablets 2196
Effexor Tablets 3411
Effexor XR Capsules 3417
Epivir 1427
Epivir-HBV 1432
Epzicom Tablets 1436
FazaClo Orally Disintegrating Tablets 551
Hyzaar 50-12.5 Tablets (Rare) 1990
Hyzaar 100-12.5 Tablets (Rare) 1990
Lamictal 1481
Lescol Capsules 2233
Lescol XL Tablets 2233
Levaquin (0.1% to 0.9%) 2384
Levaquin in 5% Dextrose Injection (0.1% to 0.9%) 2384
Lexapro Oral Solution 1190
Lexapro Tablets 1190
Lipitor Tablets (Rare) 2483
Lofibra Tablets (Rare) 1219
Lofibra Capsules (Rare) 1216
Mevacor Tablets 2021
Micardis Tablets (Rare) 854
Mirapex Tablets (One case) 859
Omnicef Capsules 511
Omnicef for Oral Suspension 511
PEG-Intron Powder for Injection 3048
Percodan Tablets 1132
Proleukin for Injection 2266
Protonix I.V. 3472
Protonix Tablets 3469
Rescriptor Tablets 2551
Retrovir IV Infusion 1564
Risperdal 1676
Risperdal M-Tab Orally Disintegrating Tablets 1676
Sanctura Tablets 1151
Seroquel Tablets 690
St. Joseph 81 mg Aspirin Chewable and Enteric Coated Tablets 1869
St. Joseph 81 mg Aspirin .... ▣ 688
Stalevo Tablets (Rare) 2287
Tasmar Tablets 3358
Teveten Tablets (Rare) 1735
Tricor Tablets 527
Trizivir Tablets 1589
Vytorin 10/10 Tablets 2114
Vytorin 10/10 Tablets 3077
Vytorin 10/20 Tablets 2114
Vytorin 10/20 Tablets 3077
Vytorin 10/40 Tablets 2114
Vytorin 10/40 Tablets 3077
Vytorin 10/80 Tablets 2114
Vytorin 10/80 Tablets 3077
Wellbutrin Tablets 1603
Wellbutrin SR Sustained-Release Tablets 1607
Wellbutrin XL Extended-Release Tablets 1613
Zetia Tablets (Very rarely) 2120
Zetia Tablets (Very rare) 3083
Zocor Tablets (Rare) 2105
Zyban Sustained-Release Tablets 1644

Rheumatism, articular
▲ Advair Diskus 100/50 (1% to 3%) ... 1308
▲ Advair Diskus 250/50 (1% to 3%) ... 1308
▲ Advair Diskus 500/50 (1% to 3%) ... 1308
▲ Advair HFA Inhalation Aerosol (1% to 3%) 1318
▲ Flovent Diskus (1% to 17%) 1443
Serevent Diskus (1% to less than 3%) 1568

Rheumatoid arthritis
Abilify Oral Solution (Rare) 882
Abilify Oral Solution (Rare) 2450
Abilify Discmelt Orally Disintegrating Tablets (Rare) 882
Abilify Discmelt Orally Disintegrating Tablets (Rare) 2450
Abilify Tablets (Rare) 882
Abilify Tablets (Rare) 2450
Asacol Delayed-Release Tablets 2692
Astelin Nasal Spray (Infrequently) 1904
Campral Tablets (Frequent) 1174
Copegus Tablets (Less than 1%) 2754
Effexor Tablets (Rare) 3411
Effexor XR Capsules (Rare) 3417
Evoxac Capsules (Less than 1%) 1047
Pegasys (Less than 1%) 2789
PEG-Intron Powder for Injection (Less than or equal to 1%) 3048
Prozac Pulvules and Liquid (Rare) 1801
Relpax Tablets (Rare) 2548
Rilutek Tablets (Rare) 2930
Symbyax Capsules (Rare) 1819
Zyprexa Tablets (Infrequent) 1830
Zyprexa ZYDIS Orally Disintegrating Tablets (Infrequent) 1830

Rheumatoid arthritis, worsening of
▲ Kineret Injection (19%) 599

Rheumatoid factor, positive
Aldoril Tablets 1910

Rhinitis
▲ Abilify Oral Solution (4%) 882
▲ Abilify Oral Solution (4%) 2450
▲ Abilify Discmelt Orally Disintegrating Tablets (4%) 882
▲ Abilify Discmelt Orally Disintegrating Tablets (4%) 2450
▲ Abilify Tablets (4%) 882
▲ Abilify Tablets (4%) 2450
▲ Aceon Tablets (2 mg, 4 mg, 8 mg) (4.8%) 3194
Actiq (Less than 1%) 979
▲ Actonel Tablets (2.1% to 5.7%) 2683
▲ Actonel with Calcium Tablets (2.1% to 5.7%) 2688
▲ Adalat CC Tablets (3% or less) 2964
▲ Advair Diskus 100/50 (1% to 3%) ... 1308
▲ Advair Diskus 250/50 (1% to 3%) ... 1308
▲ Advair Diskus 500/50 (1% to 3%) ... 1308
Advair HFA Inhalation Aerosol 1318
Advicor Tablets 1722
▲ Aerobid/Aerobid-M (3% to 9%) 1171
Agrylin Capsules (1% to 5%) 3169
▲ Alamast Ophthalmic Solution (10% to 25%) 3381
▲ Aldara Cream, 5% (3.3%) 1846
Alinia for Oral Suspension (Less than 1%) 2835
Alinia Tablets (Less than 1%) 2835
Alphagan P Ophthalmic Solution (1% to 4%) 567
Ambien Tablets (1%) 2851
Ambien CR Tablets (Infrequent) 2855
▲ AmBisome for Injection (11.1%) 620
Amerge Tablets (Rare) 1339
Aralast (Greater than or equal to 0.2%) 717
▲ Aredia for Injection (Up to 6%) 2179
▲ Arimidex Tablets (2% to 5%) 673
▲ Aromasin Tablets (2% to 5%) 2600
▲ Asacol Delayed-Release Tablets (5% or greater) 2692
▲ Astelin Nasal Spray (2.3% to 17%) 1904
Atacand Tablets (2%) 649
Atacand HCT (0.5% or greater) 651
▲ Atripla Tablets (Greater than or equal to 5%) 945
Atrovent Inhalation Solution (2.3%) ... 835
▲ Atrovent HFA Inhalation Aerosol (4% to 6%) 841
Atrovent Nasal Spray 0.03% (2.0% to 5.1%) 837
Attenuvax 1914
Avalide Tablets (1% or greater) 888
Avalide Tablets (1% or greater) 2874
Avapro Tablets (1% or greater) 891
Avapro Tablets (1% or greater) 2871
Axert Tablets (Infrequent) 2396
▲ Axid Oral Solution (9.8%) 879
▲ Azilect Tablets (3%) 3293
Azopt Ophthalmic Suspension (1% to 5%) 557
▲ Bactroban Nasal (1.0% to 6%) 1394
▲ Bexxar (0% to 10%) 1398
▲ BiDil Tablets (4%) 2171
Caduet Tablets (Greater than or equal to 2%) 2508
▲ Campath Ampules (7%) 811
Campral Tablets (Frequent) 1174

▲ Camptosar Injection (0% to 16%) 2604
Captopril Tablets 2149
Carafate Suspension 701
Carafate Tablets 701
Cardizem LA Extended Release Tablets (Less than 2%) 1728
▲ Carnitor Injection (6% to 11%) 3188
Celebrex Capsules (2%) 3134
▲ Celexa (5%) 1176
▲ CellCept Capsules (3% to less than 20%) 2747
▲ CellCept Intravenous (3% to less than 20%) 2747
▲ CellCept Oral Suspension (3% to less than 20%) 2747
▲ CellCept Tablets (3% to less than 20%) 2747
▲ Cipro (3%) 2977
▲ Cipro I.V. (3%) 2984
▲ Climara Transdermal System (2% to 6%) 771
Colazal Capsules (2%) 2838
Combivent Inhalation Aerosol (1.1%) 847
▲ Concerta Extended-Release Tablets (3%) 1881
▲ Copaxone for Injection (14%) 3297
Cozaar Tablets (Less than 1%) 1935
Crestor Tablets (2.2%) 678
Cutivate Lotion 0.05% (Less than 1%) 2664
Demadex Injection (2.8%) 2759
Demadex Tablets (2.8%) 2759
▲ Depacon Injection (5%) 412
▲ Depakene (5%) 417
▲ Depakote Sprinkle Capsules (5%) 422
▲ Depakote Tablets (1% to 5%) 427
▲ Depakote ER Tablets (Greater than 1% to 5%) 434
Depo-Medrol Single-Dose Vial 2619
Detrol Tablets (1.1%) 2628
Diastat Rectal Delivery System (Greater than or equal to 1%) 3343
Diovan Tablets (More than 1%) 2193
▲ Ditropan XL Extended-Release Tablets (2% to 6%) 2413
▲ Doxil Injection (Less than 1% to 10%) 2351
Duragesic Transdermal System (1% or greater) 2373
Effexor Tablets 3411
▲ Effexor XR Capsules (8%) 3417
▲ Elestat Ophthalmic Solution (1% to 3%) 1669
▲ Elidel Cream 1% (0.4% to 4.4%) 2200
Elmiron Capsules (Less than or equal to 1%) 2415
▲ Eloxatin for Injection (5% to 15%) 2892
Emsam Transdermal System 903
▲ Emtriva Capsules (12% to 18%) 1287
▲ Emtriva Oral Solution (12% to 18%) 1287
Enablex Extended-Release Tablets (Greater than or equal to 1%) 2203
▲ Enbrel for Injection (12% to 16%) 584
▲ Enjuvia Tablets (4% to 7%) 1062
▲ Equetro Extended-Release Capsules (Less than 5%) 3180
▲ Euflexxa (3% to 3.13%) 1162
▲ Evoxac Capsules (11.2%) 1047
▲ Exelon Capsules (4%) 2206
▲ Exelon Oral Solution (4%) 2206
▲ Exubera Inhalation Powder (8.8% to 14.5%) 2524
▲ Fabrazyme for Intravenous Infusion (11%) 1274
▲ Ferrlecit Injection (3% to 9%) 3388
▲ Flomax Capsules (13.1% to 17.9%) 850
▲ Flovent Diskus (3% to 13%) 1443
▲ Flovent HFA (1% to 3%) 1447
Floxin Otic Solution (Single report) 1049
Fluarix 1451
▲ Flumist Vaccine (6.3%) 1901
▲ Fortamet Extended-Release Tablets (4.2%) 3115
▲ Forteo for Injection (9.6%) 1767
▲ Fortical Nasal Spray (12%) 3337
▲ Fosrenol Chewable Tablets (5% to 7%) 3183
Frova Tablets (Frequent) 1113
Gabitril Tablets (1% or more) 984
▲ Gamunex Immune Globulin I.V., 10% (51%) 3235
Gemzar for Injection (Infrequent) 1771
▲ Gengraf Capsules (1% to 5%) 459
▲ Geodon (4%) 2529
▲ Hectorol Capsules (Greater than or equal to 5%) 1275
▲ Herceptin I.V. (14%) 1233
▲ Humatrope Vials and Cartridges (6.25% to 13.5%) 1787
Hytrin Capsules (At least 1% to 1.9%) 471
Hyzaar 50-12.5 Tablets 1990
Hyzaar 100-12.5 Tablets 1990
Hyzaar 100-25 Tablets 1990
▲ Imdur Tablets (Less than or equal to 5%) 3018
▲ Indapamide Tablets (Greater than or equal to 5%) 2156
▲ Infergen (7% to 13%) 3364
▲ Intron A for Injection (Less than 5%) 3024
Invanz for Injection (Greater than 0.5%) 1999
Invirase (Less than 2%) 2772
Ionsys Transdermal System (.1% to less than 1%) 2379
▲ I.V. Busulfex (44%) 2493
Kadian Capsules (Less than 3%) 577
Kaletra (Less than 2%) 476
▲ Keppra Injection (4%) 3320
▲ Keppra Oral Solution (4% to 13%) 3314
▲ Keppra Tablets (4% to 13%) 3314
Klonopin (2%) 2778
Kogenate FS 738
Kogenate FS with Bio-Set (1 case) 740
▲ Lamictal (13.6%) 1481
▲ Lescol Capsules (4.7%) 2233
Lescol XL Tablets (1.5%) 2233
▲ Leukine (11%) 814
Levaquin (1.2%) 2384
Levaquin in 5% Dextrose Injection (1.2%) 2384
▲ Levitra Tablets (9%) 3034
▲ Lexapro Oral Solution (5%) 1190
▲ Lexapro Tablets (5%) 1190
Lipitor Tablets (Greater than or equal to 2%) 2483
Lofibra Tablets (2.3%) 1219
Lofibra Capsules (2.3%) 1216
Lopressor Injection 2238
Lopressor Tablets 2238
Lopressor HCT 50/25 Tablets 2241
Lopressor HCT 100/25 Tablets 2241
Lopressor HCT 100/50 Tablets 2241
▲ Lotemax Ophthalmic Suspension 0.5% (Less than 15%) .... ⊙251
Lotensin HCT Tablets (More than 1%) 2246
Lunesta Tablets 3142
▲ Lupron Depot 3.75 mg (Less than 5%) 3260
Lupron Depot–3 Month 11.25 mg (Less than 5%) 3265
Marinol Capsules (Less than 1%) 3333
▲ Mepron Suspension (5% to 24%) 1521
▲ Meridia Capsules (10.2%) 489
Meruvax II 2019
▲ Miacalcin Nasal Spray (12%) 2253
Micardis Tablets (More than 0.3%) 854
Micardis HCT Tablets 856
▲ Migranal Nasal Spray (26%) 3348
▲ Mirapex Tablets (Greater than or equal to 1% to 3%) 859
M-M-R II 2006
Mumpsvax 2031
▲ Mylotarg for Injection (7% to 10%) 3431
▲ Myobloc Injection (1% to 5%) 3192
Myozyme for Intravenous Infusion 1279
Nasacort AQ Nasal Spray (2% or greater) 2922
Nasonex Nasal Spray (Greater than or equal to 2%) 3043
Neoral Oral Solution (1% to 5%) 2259
▲ Neoral Soft Gelatin Capsules (1% to 5%) 2259
▲ Neumega for Injection (42%) 3435
▲ Neurontin Capsules (4.1%) 2487
▲ Neurontin Oral Solution (4.1%) 2487
▲ Neurontin Tablets (4.1%) 2487
Nexium Delayed-Release Capsules (Less than 1%) 655
Nexium I.V. (Less than 1%) 659
▲ Niaspan Extended-Release Tablets (2% to 5%) 1730
▲ Nipent for Injection (10% to 11%) 1863
Norvasc Tablets (Less than 0.1%) 2545
Norvir (Less than 2%) 503
Omacor Capsules 2725
▲ Ontak Vials (13%) 1745
OptiPranolol Metipranolol Ophthalmic Solution 0.3% (A small number of patients) .... ⊙256
▲ Orencia Powder for Intravenous Infusion (Less than 5%) 914
▲ Patanol Ophthalmic Solution (Less than 5%) 561
Paxil CR Controlled-Release Tablets (Frequent) 1538
Paxil (Frequent) 1530
PEG-Intron Powder for Injection (2%) 3048
▲ Permax Tablets (12.2%) 3356
▲ Pexeva Tablets (3%) 1694
▲ Plavix Tablets (4.2%) 917
▲ Plavix Tablets (4.2%) 2926
▲ Pletal Tablets (7% to 12%) 2455
▲ Premarin Tablets (6% to 10%) 3446
▲ Premphase Tablets (6% to 10%) 3456
▲ Prempro Tablets (6% to 10%) 3456
Prevacid Delayed-Release Capsules (Less than 1%) 3271
Prevacid for Delayed-Release Oral Suspension (Less than 1%) 3271
Prevacid SoluTab Delayed-Release Orally Disintegrating Tablets (Less than 1%) 3271
Prevacid NapraPAC (Less than 1%) 3280
PREVPAC (Less than 1%) 3284
Prilosec OTC Delayed-Release Tablets (2%) 2677
Prinivil Tablets (0.3% to 1.0%) 2052
Prinzide Tablets (0.3% to 1%) 2056
▲ ProAir HFA Inhalation Aerosol (5%) 3300
Prochieve 4% Gel 1003
Prochieve 8% Gel 1003
▲ Prograf Capsules and Injection (3% to 15%) 632
▲ Proleukin for Injection (10%) 2266
ProQuad 2064
ProSom Tablets (Infrequent) 517
Protonix I.V. (Greater than 1%) 3472
Protonix Tablets (Greater than or equal to 1%) 3469
▲ Protopic Ointment (3% to 5%) 638
▲ Proventil HFA Inhalation Aerosol (16%) 3056
▲ Provigil Tablets (7%) 988
Prozac Pulvules and Liquid 1801
▲ Pulmicort Respules (7% to 12%) 661
▲ Pulmozyme Inhalation Solution (30%) 1248
▲ Qvar Inhalation Aerosol (3% to 8%) 3303
▲ Rapamune Oral Solution and Tablets (3% to 20%) 3475
▲ Razadyne (4%) 2399
▲ Razadyne ER Extended-Release Capsules (4%) 2399
▲ Rebetol (6% to 8%) 3058
Recombivax HB (Greater than 1%) 2071
ReFacto Vials 3484
Relpax Tablets (Infrequent) 2548
▲ Remicade for IV Injection (8%) 971
▲ Requip Tablets (4%) 1555
Rescriptor Tablets 2551
Retrovir Capsules 1560
Retrovir IV Infusion 1564
Retrovir 1560
▲ Revatio Tablets (4%) 2557
▲ Revlimid Capsules (6.8%) 958
▲ Ribavirin, USP Capsules (6% to 8%) 3068
▲ Rilutek Tablets (7.8% to 8.9%) 2930
▲ Risperdal (3% to 10%) 1676
▲ Risperdal Consta Long-Acting Injection (4% to 14%) 1682
▲ Risperdal M-Tab Orally Disintegrating Tablets (3% to 10%) 1676
▲ Rituxan I.V. (1% to 12%) 1254
Rythmol SR Capsules 2727
▲ Sandostatin LAR Depot (5% to 15%) 2280
▲ Serevent Diskus (2% to 5%) 1568
▲ Seroquel Tablets (3%) 690
▲ Simulect for Injection (3% to 10%) 2284
Singulair (Greater than or equal to 2%) 2077
▲ Soriatane Capsules (25% to 50%) 1013
▲ Spiriva HandiHaler (3% to 6%) 869
▲ Suboxone Tablets (4.7% to 11%) 2717
▲ Subutex Tablets (9.7% to 11%) 2717
Sular Tablets (Less than or equal to 1%) 3122
▲ Synagis (26.8%) 1897
Targretin Capsules 1747
Tasmar Tablets (Infrequent) 3358
▲ Teveten Tablets (4%) 1735
Teveten HCT Tablets (Less than 1%) 1737
▲ Thalomid Capsules (4.2%) 965
Tiazac Capsules (2%) 1201
▲ TOBI Solution for Inhalation (34.5%) 2298
▲ Topamax Sprinkle Capsules (1% to 7%) 2404
▲ Topamax Tablets (1% to 7%) 2404
Tricor Tablets (2.3%) 527
Triglide Tablets (2.3%) 3123
▲ Trileptal Tablets (2% to 10%) 2300
▲ Trileptal Oral Suspension (2% to 10%) 2300
Truvada Tablets 1296
Uniretic Tablets (More than 1%) 3100
Univasc Tablets (Greater than 1%) 3104
Uroxatral Tablets 2943
Vandazole Vaginal Gel (Less than 1%) 3338
Vantin Tablets and Oral Suspension (Less than 1%) 2645
Verelan PM Extended-Release Capsules, Controlled-Onset (2.7%) 3106
VFEND I.V. (Less than 2%) 2564
VFEND Oral Suspension (Less than 2%) 2564
VFEND Tablets (Less than 2%) 2564
Vicoprofen Tablets (Less than 3%) 539
▲ Vigamox Ophthalmic Solution (1% to 4%) 564
Viracept (Less than 2%) 2577
▲ Voltaren Ophthalmic Solution (Less than or equal to 3%) 2309
▲ WelChol Tablets (3%) 1050
Wellbutrin SR Sustained-Release Tablets (At least 1%) 1607
Wellbutrin XL Extended-Release Tablets (At least 1%) 1613
Xifaxan Tablets (Less than 2%) 2842
▲ Xopenex Inhalation Solution (2.7% to 11.1%) 3146
▲ Xopenex Inhalation Solution Concentrate (2.7% to 11.1%) 3150
▲ Xopenex HFA Inhalation Aerosol (2.7% to 11.1%) 3154
Xyrem Oral Solution (Infrequent) 1688
Yaz Tablets (Greater than 1%) 803
Zegerid Capsules (2%) 2958
Zegerid Powder for Oral Solution (2%) 2958
▲ Zelapar Tablets (7%) 3372
Zemaira (0.5%) 3509
Zoloft (Frequent) 2586
Zomig Nasal Spray (Infrequent) 3523
Zonegran Capsules (2%) 1101
Zostavax Injection (1.4%) 2111
Zosyn (1.2%) 3492
▲ Zyban Sustained-Release Tablets (12%) 1644
▲ Zyprexa Tablets (7% to 10%) 1830
▲ Zyprexa ZYDIS Orally Disintegrating Tablets (7% to 10%) 1830
Zyrtec Chewable Tablets (Less than 2%) 2594
Zyrtec (Less than 2%) 2594
Zyrtec-D 12 Hour Extended Release Tablets (Less than 2%) 2597

Rhinitis, allergic

▲ Asmanex Twisthaler (11% to 20%) 2966
▲ BeneFix Vials (4.6%) 3408
Imitrex Injection 1463
Imitrex Nasal Spray 1467
Lotronex Tablets (2%) 1512
Xyrem Oral Solution (Infrequent) 1688

Rhinitis, ulcerative

Atrovent Nasal Spray 0.03% (2.0%) 837

Rhinorrhea

Aceon Tablets (2 mg, 4 mg, 8 mg) (0.3% to 1%) 3194
Acetadote Injection (1%) 1031
▲ Advair Diskus 100/50 (1% to 3%) 1308
▲ Advair Diskus 250/50 (1% to 3%) 1308
▲ Advair Diskus 500/50 (1% to 3%) 1308
▲ Advair HFA Inhalation Aerosol (1% to 3%) 1318
▲ Aerobid/Aerobid-M (3% to 9%) 1171
▲ Atrovent Nasal Spray 0.03% (3.1%) 837
Beconase AQ Nasal Spray (Fewer than 3 per 100 patients) 1396
Calcijex Injection 411
Chantix Tablets (0% to 1%) 2517
▲ Chemet Capsules (0.7% to 3.7%) 2458
▲ Clarinex Syrup (4.5%) 2995
Clozaril Tablets (Less than 1%) 2184
Colyte with Flavor Packs for Oral Solution (Isolated cases) 3088
Comvax (0.2% to 1.3%) 1928
Elidel Cream 1% (Up to 1.9%) 2200
FazaClo Orally Disintegrating Tablets (Less than 1%) 551
▲ Flebogamma 5%, Immune Globulin Intravenous (Human) (20%) 1658
▲ Flonase Nasal Spray (1% to 3%) 1440
▲ Flovent Diskus (1% to 3%) 1443
▲ Flovent HFA (1% to 3%) 1447
HalfLytely and Bisacodyl Tablets Bowel Prep Kit with Flavors Packs 881
Hectorol Capsules 1275
Hectorol Injection 1278
▲ Indapamide Tablets (Less than 5%) 2156
▲ Intron A for Injection (Less than 5%) 3024
Invanz for Injection (Greater than 0.5%) 1999
Klonopin 2778
Maxalt Tablets (Rare) 2008
Maxalt-MLT Orally Disintegrating Tablets (Rare) 2008

▲ Myozyme for Intravenous Infusion (28%) 1279
Nexavar Tablets (Uncommon) 746
Prinivil Tablets (0.3% to 1.0%) 2052
Prinzide Tablets 2056
ProQuad (Greater than or equal to 0.2% to less than 1%) 2064
Rocaltrol Capsules 2798
Rocaltrol Oral Solution 2798
Singulair (Greater than or equal to 2%) 2077
▲ Strattera Capsules (4%) 1814
Tamiflu Capsules 2807
TriLyte with Flavor Packs for Oral Solution 3100
▲ Ultram ER Tablets (1% to greater than 5%) 2392
▲ Valcyte Tablets (Less than 5%) 2813
▲ Vaqta (5.7%) 2097
Vasotec I.V. Injection (0.5% to 1.0%) 2103
▲ Xeloda Tablets (5%) 2822
Xifaxan Tablets (Less than 2%) 2842

Rhonchi
Acetadote Injection (1%) 1031
Invanz for Injection (0.5% to 1.1%) 1999
Orencia Powder for Intravenous Infusion 914
ReoPro Vials (0.1%) 1809
▲ Trisenox Injection (8%) 993
Zemuron Injection (Less than 1%) 2346

Rigidity
Ambien Tablets (Rare) 2851
▲ Clozaril Tablets (3%) 2184
Ethyol for Injection (Rare) 1898
Famvir Tablets (0.5% to 1.5%) 2211
▲ FazaClo Orally Disintegrating Tablets (3%) 551
Flumadine 1183
Gengraf Capsules (1% to less than 3%) 459
Hyzaar 50-12.5 Tablets 1990
Hyzaar 100-12.5 Tablets 1990
Hyzaar 100-25 Tablets 1990
Imitrex Tablets (Rare) 1471
▲ Infergen (57% to 62%) 3364
▲ Intron A for Injection (Up to 42%) 3024
Moban Tablets 1119
Neoral Oral Solution (1% to less than 3%) 2259
Neoral Soft Gelatin Capsules (1% to less than 3%) 2259
▲ Niravam Orally Disintegrating Tablets (4.2%) 3092
Norvasc Tablets (More than 0.1% to 1%) 2545
▲ Orthoclone OKT3 Sterile Solution (8%) 2360
Proleukin for Injection 2266
Risperdal (Infrequent) 1676
Risperdal M-Tab Orally Disintegrating Tablets (Infrequent) 1676
Romazicon Injection (Less than 1%) 2804
▲ Soriatane Capsules (10% to 25%) 1013
Zoloft (Infrequent) 2586
Zosyn (1.0% or less) 3492
Zyrtec Chewable Tablets (Less than 2%) 2594
Zyrtec (Less than 2%) 2594
Zyrtec-D 12 Hour Extended Release Tablets (Less than 2%) 2597

Rigors
Advate Injection (0.6%) 712
Aldara Cream, 5% (1.4%) 1846
Ambien CR Tablets (Rare) 2855
AmBisome for Injection (Less common) 620
Amitiza Capsules (Less than 0.2%) 3224
▲ Arranon Injection (0% to 8%) 1357
BeneFix Vials (1.6%) 3408
Bexxar 1398
Caduet Tablets (Greater than 0.1% to less than or equal to 1%) 2508
▲ Campath Ampules (16% to 86%) 811
Carimune NF 3499
Celexa (Infrequent) 1176
▲ Clolar for Intravenous Infusion (38%) 1271
▲ Copegus Tablets (25%) 2754
Cubicin for Injection (Less than 1%) 1026
Cymbalta Delayed-Release Capsules (Frequent) 1757
▲ Dacogen Injection (22%) 2129
▲ DepoDur Extended-Release Injection (2% to 5%) 1110
Duragesic Transdermal System (Greater than or less than 1%) 2373
Eligard 22.5 mg (Less than 2%) 2883
Elitek (Less than or equal to 1%) 2890
▲ Eloxatin for Injection (7% to 9%) 2892
Emend Capsules (Greater than 0.5%) 1963
Eraxis for Injection (Less than 1% to less than 2%) 2521
Ethyol for Injection 1898
Evoxac Capsules (1.3%) 1047
Exelon Capsules (Frequent) 2206
Exelon Oral Solution (Frequent) 2206
▲ Fabrazyme for Intravenous Infusion (15%) 1274
Ferrlecit Injection 3388
Flebogamma 5%, Immune Globulin Intravenous (Human) 1658
Frova Tablets (Infrequent) 1113
Gammagard Liquid 721
Gammagard S/D 724
Gamunex Immune Globulin I.V., 10% 3235
Gantrisin Pediatric Suspension 2770
▲ Gengraf Capsules (3%) 459
▲ Gleevec Tablets (0% to 12%) 2227
Herceptin I.V. 1233
▲ Hycamtin for Injection (69%) 1458
▲ Imdur Tablets (Less than or equal to 5%) 3018
▲ Intron A for Injection (2% to 42%) 3024
Levaquin (0.1% to 0.9%) 2384
Levaquin in 5% Dextrose Injection (0.1% to 0.9%) 2384
Migranal Nasal Spray (Infrequent) 3348
▲ MoviPrep Oral Solution (33.7%) 2839
Mycamine for Injection (0.2% to 2.3%) 628
Myozyme for Intravenous Infusion 1279
▲ Neoral Oral Solution (3%) 2259
▲ Neoral Soft Gelatin Capsules (3%) 2259
Nexium Delayed-Release Capsules (Less than 1%) 655
Nexium I.V. (Less than 1%) 659
▲ Pegasys (35%) 2789
▲ PEG-Intron Powder for Injection (23%) 3048
Prezista Tablets (Less than 2%) 3306
Proquin XR Tablets (Less than 1%) 1153
Proventil HFA Inhalation Aerosol (Less than 3%) 3056
▲ Rebetol (25% to 48%) 3058
▲ Rebetron Combination Therapy (32% to 42%) 3063
▲ Rebif Prefilled Syringe for Injection (6% to 13%) 3159
Requip Tablets (1% or more) 1555
▲ Revlimid Capsules (6.1%) 958
▲ Ribavirin, USP Capsules (25% to 48%) 3068
Rituxan I.V. 1254
Romazicon Injection (Less than 1%) 2804
▲ Sandostatin LAR Depot (5% to 15%) 2280
▲ Simulect for Injection (3% to 10%) 2284
▲ Strattera Capsules (3%) 1814
▲ Tarceva Tablets (0% to 12%) 1259
▲ Tarceva Tablets (0% to 12%) 2444
Teveten Tablets (Less than 1%) 1735
Teveten HCT Tablets (Less than 1%) 1737
Topamax Sprinkle Capsules (Less than or equal to 1%) 2404
Topamax Tablets (Less than or equal to 1%) 2404
Trileptal Tablets 2300
Trileptal Oral Suspension 2300
▲ Trisenox Injection (38%) 993
▲ Ultram ER Tablets (0.5% to 3.5%) 2392
▲ Velcade for Injection (11%) 2133
Vivitrol 995
▲ Zometa for Intravenous Infusion (11% to less than 15%) 2315

Romberg test, positive
Neurontin Capsules (Infrequent) 2487
Neurontin Oral Solution (Infrequent) 2487
Neurontin Tablets (Infrequent) 2487

Rosacea
Elocon Cream 0.1% 3005
Elocon Ointment 0.1% 3007
Evoxac Capsules (Less than 1%) 1047
Protopic Ointment 638
Tri-Luma Cream (1%) 1213
Xyrem Oral Solution (Infrequent) 1688

Roseola
Prevnar for Injection 3463

Roughness, unspecified
ProQuad 2064

Rupture, Achilles tendon
Cipro XR Tablets 2990

S

S_3 gallop
(*see under* Ventricular gallop)

Saliva, discoloration
Parcopa Orally Disintegrating Tablets 3097
Stalevo Tablets 2287

Salivary gland enlargement
Aciphex Tablets (Rare) 1090
Alinia for Oral Suspension (Less than 1%) 2835
Alinia Tablets (Less than 1%) 2835
Clozaril Tablets 2184
Copaxone for Injection (Frequent) 3297
▲ Evoxac Capsules (1% to 3%) 1047
FazaClo Orally Disintegrating Tablets 551
Gantrisin Pediatric Suspension 2770
Gengraf Capsules (1% to less than 3%) 459
Imitrex Nasal Spray 1467
Lithobid Tablets 1692
Neoral Oral Solution (1% to less than 3%) 2259
Neoral Soft Gelatin Capsules (1% to less than 3%) 2259
Neurontin Capsules (Rare) 2487
Neurontin Oral Solution (Rare) 2487
Neurontin Tablets (Rare) 2487
Permax Tablets (Infrequent) 3356
Pexeva Tablets (Rare) 1694
Prozac Pulvules and Liquid (Rare) 1801
Rilutek Tablets (Rare) 2930

Salivation
(*see under* Sialism)

Salivation, increase
(*see under* Sialism)

Salpingitis
Amerge Tablets (Rare) 1339
Effexor Tablets (Rare) 3411
Effexor XR Capsules (Rare) 3417
Gabitril Tablets (Infrequent) 984
Permax Tablets (Infrequent) 3356
Pexeva Tablets (Rare) 1694
Vandazole Vaginal Gel (Less than 1%) 3338
Wellbutrin SR Sustained-Release Tablets 1607
Wellbutrin XL Extended-Release Tablets 1613
Zyban Sustained-Release Tablets 1644

Sarcoidosis
Copegus Tablets (Less than 1%) 2754
Enbrel for Injection 584
Intron A for Injection (Very rare) 3024
Pegasys (Less than 1%) 2789
PEG-Intron Powder for Injection 3048
Rebetol 3058
Rebetron Combination Therapy 3063
Risperdal (Rare) 1676
Risperdal M-Tab Orally Disintegrating Tablets (Rare) 1676

Sarcoidosis, exacerbation of
Intron A for Injection (Very rare) 3024
Rebetol 3058
Rebetron Combination Therapy 3063

Sarcoma, bone
Permax Tablets (Infrequent) 3356

Sarcoma, unspecified
▲ Megace ES Oral Suspension (1% to 3%) 2481
Thalomid Capsules 965

Scabbing
▲ Aldara Cream, 5% (Up to 13%) 1846
Levulan Kerastick for Topical Solution, 20% (1% to 2%) 1085
▲ Panretin Gel (1% to 8%) 1747

Scalp, tightness
Temovate Scalp Application (1 of 294 patients) 2670

Scalp hair, loss of
NuvaRing 2340

Scalp hair, thinning
Angeliq Tablets 762
Decadron Tablets 1951
Mircette Tablets 1066
Ortho Evra Transdermal System 2417
Seasonique Tablets 1077
Yaz Tablets 803

Scarring
▲ Efudex (Among most frequent) 3363

Schizophrenia, precipitation
Zyprexa Tablets 1830
Zyprexa ZYDIS Orally Disintegrating Tablets 1830

Sciatica
Ambien Tablets (Rare) 2851
Ambien CR Tablets (Rare) 2855
Arranon Injection (1%) 1357
Atacand HCT (0.5% or greater) 651
Gleevec Tablets (Infrequent) 2227
Rythmol SR Capsules 2727
Wellbutrin Tablets (Rare) 1603

Sclera, discoloration
Ticlid Tablets 2810

Scleral injection
Fansidar Tablets 2765
Gantrisin Pediatric Suspension 2770

Scleral thinning
Pred-G Ophthalmic Ointment ⊙237

Scleritis
Ambien Tablets (Infrequent) 2851
Ambien CR Tablets (Infrequent) 2855
Aredia for Injection (Rare) 2179
Effexor Tablets (Rare) 3411
Effexor XR Capsules (Rare) 3417
Evoxac Capsules (Less than 1%) 1047
Fosamax 1969
Fosamax Plus D Tablets (Rarely) 1977
Prozac Pulvules and Liquid (Rare) 1801
VFEND I.V. (Less than 2%) 2564
VFEND Oral Suspension (Less than 2%) 2564
VFEND Tablets (Less than 2%) 2564

Scleroderma
Depo-Provera Contraceptive Injection (Less than 1%) 2622
depo-subQ provera 104 Injectable Suspension 2624
Evoxac Capsules (Less than 1%) 1047
Soriatane Capsules (Less than 1%) 1013

Sclerosis, multiple
Chantix Tablets (Rare) 2517
Enbrel for Injection 584
Engerix-B Vaccine (Less than 1%) 1425
Evoxac Capsules (Less than 1%) 1047
Havrix Vaccine (Rare) 1456
▲ Humira Injection (Less than 5%) 466
Recombivax HB 2071
Remicade for IV Injection 971
Twinrix Vaccine 1595

Sclerosis, multiple, aggravation
Aldara Cream, 5% 1846

Sclerosis, skin
Parnate Tablets 1527

Scoliosis
▲ Humatrope Vials and Cartridges (18.9%) 1787
Nutropin for Injection (0.2%) 1239
Nutropin AQ Injection (0.2%) 1243
Nutropin AQ Pen (0.2%) 1243
Nutropin AQ Pen Cartridge (0.2%) 1243

Scotoma
▲ Visudyne for Injection (10% to 30%) 2305

Scotomata
Adenoscan (Less than 1%) 619
Amerge Tablets (Rare) 1339
Axert Tablets (Rare) 2396
Lithobid Tablets 1692
ProSom Tablets (Rare) 517
Requip Tablets (Rare) 1555
Sandostatin LAR Depot (Rare) 2280
Topamax Sprinkle Capsules (Infrequent) 2404
Topamax Tablets (Infrequent) 2404
Trileptal Tablets 2300
Trileptal Oral Suspension 2300

Scrotal disorder, unspecified
Caverject Impulse Injection (Less than 1%) 2612

Scrotum, swollen
Neurontin Capsules (Rare) 2487
Neurontin Oral Solution (Rare) 2487
Neurontin Tablets (Rare) 2487

Seborrhea
Abilify Oral Solution (Infrequent) 882
Abilify Oral Solution (Infrequent) 2450

Abilify Discmelt Orally Disintegrating Tablets (Infrequent) 882
Abilify Discmelt Orally Disintegrating Tablets (Infrequent) 2450
Abilify Tablets (Infrequent) 882
Abilify Tablets (Infrequent) 2450
Accutane Capsules 2731
Caduet Tablets (Less than 2%) 2508
Depacon Injection (1% or more) 412
Depakene (1% or more) 417
Depakote Sprinkle Capsules 422
▲ Depakote Tablets (1% to 5%) 427
Depakote ER Tablets (Greater than 1%) 434
Effexor Tablets (Rare) 3411
Effexor XR Capsules (Rare) 3417
Evoxac Capsules (Less than 1%) 1047
Finacea Gel (1% or less) 1669
Floxin Otic Solution (Single report) 1049
Invirase (Less than 2%) 2772
Kaletra (Less than 2%) 476
Lamictal (Rare) 1481
Lipitor Tablets (Less than 2%) 2483
Lupron Depot-PED 7.5 mg, 11.25 mg and 15 mg (2%) 3269
Lupron Injection Pediatric (2%) 3259
Neurontin Capsules (Infrequent) 2487
Neurontin Oral Solution (Infrequent) 2487
Neurontin Tablets (Infrequent) 2487
Norvir (Less than 2%) 503
Paxil CR Controlled-Release Tablets (Rare) 1538
Paxil (Rare) 1530
Permax Tablets (Infrequent) 3356
Pexeva Tablets (Rare) 1694
Prochieve 4% Gel 1003
Prochieve 8% Gel 1003
Protopic Ointment (0.2% to less than 1%) 638
Prozac Pulvules and Liquid (Rare) 1801
Requip Tablets (Infrequent) 1555
Rescriptor Tablets 2551
Reyataz Capsules (Less than 3%) 921
Rilutek Tablets (Infrequent) 2930
Risperdal (Up to 1%) 1676
Risperdal Consta Long-Acting Injection (Infrequent) 1682
Risperdal M-Tab Orally Disintegrating Tablets (Up to 1%) 1676
Seroquel Tablets (Infrequent) 690
▲ Soriatane Capsules (1% to 10%) 1013
Symbyax Capsules (Rare) 1819
Synagis (More than 1%) 1897
Tasmar Tablets (Infrequent) 3358
Thalomid Capsules 965
Topamax Sprinkle Capsules (1%) 2404
Topamax Tablets (1%) 2404
Zelapar Tablets 3372
Zyprexa Tablets (Infrequent) 1830
Zyprexa ZYDIS Orally Disintegrating Tablets (Infrequent) 1830
Zyrtec Chewable Tablets (Less than 2%) 2594
Zyrtec (Less than 2%) 2594
Zyrtec-D 12 Hour Extended Release Tablets (Less than 2%) 2597

Sedation
Aldoril Tablets 1910
Amerge Tablets (Rare) 1339
▲ Buprenex Injectable (Most frequent) 2716
▲ Catapres Tablets (About 10 in 100 patients) 843
Catapres-TTS (3 of 101 patients) 844
▲ Cesamet Capsules (3%) 3340
▲ Clorpres Tablets (About 10%) 2153
▲ Clozaril Tablets (More than 5% to 39%) 2184
Dalmane Capsules 3342
▲ Demser Capsules (Almost all patients) 1953
Depacon Injection 412
Depakene 417
Depakote Tablets 427
Depakote ER Tablets 434
Dilaudid 440
Dilaudid Non-Sterile Powder 440
Dilaudid Oral Liquid 445
Dilaudid Rectal Suppositories 440
Dilaudid Tablets 440
Dilaudid Tablets - 8 mg 445
▲ Dilaudid-HP (Among most frequent) 442
▲ FazaClo Orally Disintegrating Tablets (Greater than 5% to 39%) 551
Hycodan 1116
Hycotuss Expectorant Syrup 1117
▲ Imitrex Injection (3%) 1463
Imitrex Nasal Spray (Infrequent) 1467
Imitrex Tablets 1471
Kadian Capsules (Less than 3%) 577
Lotronex Tablets (Rare) 1512
▲ MS Contin Tablets (Among most frequent) 2701
Nadolol Tablets (6 of 1000 patients) 2159
Niravam Orally Disintegrating Tablets 3092
▲ Opana Tablets (1% to less than 10%) 1122
▲ Opana ER Tablets (5.9% to greater than or equal to 10%) 1126
▲ OxyFast Oral Concentrate Solution (Among most frequent) 2708
▲ OxyIR Capsules (Among most frequent) 2708
▲ Percocet Tablets (Among most frequent) 1131
▲ Percodan Tablets (Among most frequent) 1132
Phenergan Tablets and Suppositories 3440
Sonata Capsules 1717
▲ Strattera Capsules (2% to 4%) 1814
Tessalon Capsules 1199
Tessalon Perles 1199
Thiothixene Capsules 2165
Tussionex Pennkinetic Extended-Release Suspension 3327
▲ Tylenol with Codeine Tablets (Among most frequent) 2391
▲ Ultram ER Tablets (1% to greater than 5%) 2392
Valcyte Tablets 2813
▲ Vicodin Tablets (Among most frequent) 535
▲ Vicodin ES Tablets (Among most frequent) 536
▲ Vicodin HP Tablets (Among most frequent) 538
▲ Vivitrol (4% to 12%) 995
▲ Wellbutrin Tablets (19.8%) 1603
▲ Xeloda Tablets (Less than 5%) 2822
Xyrem Oral Solution (Infrequent) 1688
▲ Zofran Injection (8%) 1634
▲ Zofran (20%) 1639
▲ Zofran ODT Orally Disintegrating Tablets (20%) 1639
▲ Zydone Tablets (Among most frequent) 1139

Sedimentation rate, increased
Zelapar Tablets 3372

Seizure control, loss of
Depakote Sprinkle Capsules 422

Seizures
(*see also under* Convulsions)
Abilify Oral Solution (0.1% to 0.3%) 882
Abilify Oral Solution (0.1% to 0.3%) 2450
Abilify Discmelt Orally Disintegrating Tablets (0.1% to 0.3%) 882
Abilify Discmelt Orally Disintegrating Tablets (0.1% to 0.3%) 2450
Abilify Tablets (0.1% to 0.3%) 882
Abilify Tablets (0.1% to 0.3%) 2450
Accutane Capsules 2731
Actimmune (Rare) 1671
Activase I.V. 1223
Adderall Tablets 3164
Adderall XR Capsules 3166
Agrylin Capsules 3169
Allegra-D 12 Hour Extended-Release Tablets 2846
Allegra-D 24 Hour Extended-Release Tablets 2849
Aloprim for Injection (Less than 1%) 2167
Aranesp for Injection (0.6% to 1%) 581
▲ Aredia for Injection (3% to 4%) 2179
▲ Arranon Injection (0% to 6%) 1357
Attenuvax (Rare) 1914
Bayer Aspirin 744
Bayer Aspirin Comprehensive Prescribing Information ▣ 796
Bicillin C-R Injectable Suspension 1706
Carbatrol Capsules 3171
Carimune NF 3499
Carnitor Injection 3188
Carnitor Tablets and Oral Solution 3190
Ceftin Tablets 1407
Celexa (0.3%) 1176
Cipro XR Tablets 2990
▲ Clozaril Tablets (3% to approximately 5%) 2184
Combivir Tablets 1411
Comvax 1928
Cymbalta Delayed-Release Capsules (Very rare) 1757
Dantrium Capsules (Less frequent) 2694
▲ DepoCyt Injection (6.3%) 1143
Depo-Medrol Single-Dose Vial 2619
DextroStat Tablets 3179
Dilaudid 440
Dilaudid Non-Sterile Powder 440
Dilaudid Oral Liquid 445
Dilaudid Tablets - 8 mg 445
Dilaudid-HP Injection 442
Effexor XR Capsules (Infrequent) 3417
Eldepryl Capsules 3208
Elspar for Injection 2463
Elspar for Injection 1960
Enbrel for Injection 584
Engerix-B Vaccine (Less than 1%) 1425
Epogen for Injection (1.1% to approximately 2.5%) 591
Ery-Tab Tablets (Isolated reports) 449
Erythrocin Stearate Filmtab Tablets (Isolated reports) 453
Erythromycin Base Filmtab Tablets (Isolated reports) 455
Erythromycin Delayed-Release Capsules, USP (Isolated reports) 457
Ethyol for Injection (Rare) 1898
Flebogamma 5%, Immune Globulin Intravenous (Human) 1658
Flumist Vaccine 1901
Focalin XR Capsules 2223
Fortaz 1453
Gammagard Liquid 721
Gammagard S/D 724
Gamunex Immune Globulin I.V., 10% 3235
Geodon Capsules (0.4%) 2529
HibTITER (One case) 3426
Imitrex Nasal Spray (Rare) 1467
Imitrex Tablets (Rare) 1471
Infanrix Vaccine 1476
Infed Injection 3390
Invanz for Injection (Greater than 0.1%) 1999
I.V. Busulfex (2%, One patient) 2493
Keflex Capsules 549
K-Phos Neutral Tablets 760
Lariam Tablets 2786
Leukeran Tablets (Rare) 1504
Levothroid Tablets 1186
Levoxyl Tablets (Rare) 1712
Marinol Capsules 3333
Maxipime for Injection 1105
Mefoxin for Injection 2012
Mefoxin Premixed Intravenous Solution 2016
Meridia Capsules (0.1%) 489
Merrem I.V. (Greater than 0.1% to 1%) 686
MS Contin Tablets (Less frequent) 2701
Myleran Tablets 1525
Nalfon Capsules (Less than 1%) 2502
Niravam Orally Disintegrating Tablets 3092
Noroxin Tablets 2032
Norvir 503
Omnicef Capsules 511
Omnicef for Oral Suspension 511
Orthoclone OKT3 Sterile Solution 2360
OxyContin Tablets (Less than 1%) 2703
Pediarix Vaccine 1548
Liquid PedvaxHIB (Infrequent) 2035
PEG-Intron Powder for Injection 3048
Percodan Tablets 1132
Primaxin I.M. 2045
Primaxin I.V. (0.4%) 2048
Prinzide Tablets 2056
▲ Procrit for Injection (1.1% to 10%) 2364
ProQuad 2064
ProSom Tablets (Infrequent) 517
Protopic Ointment 638
Raniclor Tablets, Chewable 2505
Recombivax HB 2071
Remicade for IV Injection (Rare) 971
Retrovir Capsules (Rare; 0.8%) 1560
Retrovir IV Infusion (Rare; 1%) 1564
Retrovir (Rare; 0.8%) 1560
Risperdal (0.3%) 1676
Risperdal M-Tab Orally Disintegrating Tablets (0.3%) 1676
Ritalin Hydrochloride Tablets 2269
Ritalin LA Capsules 2271
Ritalin-SR Tablets 2269
Rocephin Injectable Vials, ADD-Vantage, Galaxy, Bulk (Rare) 2800
Romazicon Injection 2804
▲ RotaTeq (10% to 33%) 2074
Sandostatin Injection (Less than 1%) 2278
Seromycin Capsules 1813
Seroquel Tablets (0.6%) 690
Singulair (Very rare) 2077
St. Joseph 81 mg Aspirin Chewable and Enteric Coated Tablets 1869
Stromectol Tablets 2083
Suprax 1843
Sutent Capsules (Less than 1%) 2560
Tamiflu Capsules 2807
Tamiflu Oral Suspension 2807
Taxotere Injection Concentrate (Rare) 2932
Tegretol/Tegretol-XR 2295
Thalomid Capsules 965
Thiothixene Capsules 2165
Trizivir Tablets 1589
Ultane Liquid for Inhalation (Less than 1%) 531
Uroqid-Acid No. 2 Tablets 760
Valtrex Caplets 1597
Viagra Tablets 2573
Viracept (Less than 2%) 2577
Wellbutrin Tablets (Frequent) 1603
Wellbutrin SR Sustained-Release Tablets (Approximately 0.1% to 0.4%) 1607
Wellbutrin XL Extended-Release Tablets (Approximately 0.1% to 0.4%) 1613
Zinacef for Injection 1631
Zinacef Injection 1631
Zovirax 1643
Zyban Sustained-Release Tablets 1644
Zyprexa Tablets (0.9%) 1830
Zyprexa ZYDIS Orally Disintegrating Tablets (0.9%) 1830
Zyrtec-D 12 Hour Extended Release Tablets 2597

Seizures, afebrile
Attenuvax 1914
Havrix Vaccine (1 Case) 1456
M-M-R II 2006

Seizures, convulsive
Cipro (Less than 1%) 2977
Cipro I.V. (1% or less) 2984
Phenergan Tablets and Suppositories 3440
Thioridazine Hydrochloride Tablets (Infrequent) 2163
Timentin ADD-Vantage 1580
Timentin Injection Galaxy Container 1583
Timentin IV Infusion 1577
Timentin Pharmacy Bulk Package 1586

Seizures, epileptiform
Lithobid Tablets 1692

Seizures, exacerbation of
Enbrel for Injection (Rare) 584
Lamictal (2.3%) 1481
Topamax Sprinkle Capsules (More than 1%) 2404
Topamax Tablets (More than 1%) 2404

Seizures, febrile
Attenuvax 1914
Comvax 1928
Flumist Vaccine 1901
HibTITER 3426
M-M-R II 2006
Mumpsvax 2031
Prevnar for Injection 3463
Recombivax HB 2071

Seizures, generalized
Leukeran Tablets (Rare) 1504
Noroxin Tablets 2032

Seizures, grand mal
Adenocard Injection 617
Cipro I.V. (1% or less) 2984
Cipro XR Tablets 2990
Pepcid Injection (Infrequent) 2040
Pepcid (Infrequent) 2038
Proleukin for Injection (1%) 2266
Topamax Sprinkle Capsules (1%) 2404
Topamax Tablets (1%) 2404
Zofran Injection (Rare) 1634
Zofran (Rare) 1639
Zofran ODT Orally Disintegrating Tablets (Rare) 1639

Seizures, neonatal
Captopril Tablets 2149

Seizures, non-febrile
Varivax 2100

Sensation, abnormal
(*see under* Paresthesia)

Sensation, abnormal, ocular
▲ Retisert Implant (10% to 35%) ⊙ 258

Sensation, burning
▲ Imitrex Injection (7%) 1463

Sensation, disturbance of temperature
▲ Amerge Tablets (2% to 4%) 1339
▲ Fabrazyme for Intravenous Infusion (5%).......... 1274
▲ Frova Tablets (3%) 1113
▲ Imitrex Injection (10.8%) 1463
Imitrex Nasal Spray (Infrequent).......... 1467
▲ Imitrex Tablets (2% to 3%) 1471
Lidoderm Patch.......... 1118
Maxalt Tablets (Infrequent).......... 2008
Maxalt-MLT Orally Disintegrating Tablets (Infrequent).......... 2008

Sensation, heavy
▲ Amerge Tablets (2% to 4%) 1339
▲ Imitrex Injection (7.3%) 1463
Imitrex Nasal Spray (Infrequent).......... 1467
Imitrex Tablets (Less than 1% to 2%).......... 1471

Sensation, hot
Acetadote Injection (1%).......... 1031
▲ Imitrex Injection (11%) 1463
Prograf Capsules and Injection.......... 632
Xyrem Oral Solution (Infrequent).......... 1688

Sensation, lightness
Imitrex Injection (Infrequent).......... 1463
Imitrex Nasal Spray (Infrequent).......... 1467

Sensation, prickling
Imitrex (Infrequent).......... 1463

Sensation of pressure/tightness
▲ Amerge Tablets (2% to 4%) 1339
▲ Imitrex Injection (5% to 7.1%) 1463
Imitrex Nasal Spray (Infrequent).......... 1467
Imitrex Tablets (Less than 1% to 2%).......... 1471
Maxalt Tablets (Less than 2%).......... 2008
Maxalt-MLT Orally Disintegrating Tablets (Less than 2%).......... 2008
Zomig Nasal Spray (Infrequent).......... 3523

Sensations, numbness
Lidoderm Patch.......... 1118

Sensations, pulsating
Imitrex Injection (Infrequent).......... 1463
Imitrex Nasal Spray.......... 1467
Imitrex Tablets (Infrequent).......... 1471

Senses, altered, unspecified
▲ Quadramet Injection (6%) 1040

Sensitivity, light
Cipro.......... 2977
Cipro XR Tablets.......... 2990
Revatio Tablets.......... 2557
Symmetrel Tablets (0.1% to 1%).......... 1135

Sensitivity, sun
Cipro.......... 2977
Cipro XR Tablets.......... 2990
Dantrium Capsules.......... 2694

Sensitivity reactions
Aldara Cream, 5% (More than 1%).......... 1846
Bactroban Ointment.......... 1395
Betadine 5% Ophthalmic Solution .... ⊙202
Bleph-10 Ophthalmic Solution 10% (Rare).......... ⊙222
Brevoxyl-4 Creamy Wash.......... 3210
Brevoxyl-4 Gel.......... 3210
Brevoxyl-8 Creamy Wash.......... 3210
Brevoxyl-8 Gel.......... 3210
Colocort Rectal Suspension, USP (Retention) 100 mg/60 mL (Rare).......... 2476
Combivir Tablets.......... 1411
Creon 10 Capsules.......... 3198
Creon 20 Capsules.......... 3199
FML-S Ophthalmic Suspension.......... ⊙229
HyperRAB (Occasional).......... 3242
HyperRho S/D Mini-Dose (Extremely rare).......... 3244
HyperRho S/D Full Dose (Extremely rare).......... 3246
HyperTET (Extremely rare).......... 3248
Polytrim Ophthalmic Solution (Rare).......... 574
Prinzide Tablets.......... 2056
Retrovir Capsules (Rare).......... 1560
Retrovir IV Infusion (Rare).......... 1564
Retrovir.......... 1560
Trusopt Sterile Ophthalmic Solution.......... 2095
Tylenol Allergy Multi-Symptom Caplets with Cool Burst and Gelcaps (Rare).......... 1872
Tylenol Severe Allergy Caplets (Rare).......... 1872
Children's Tylenol Suspension Liquid and Meltaways (Rare).......... 1878
Children's Tylenol Suspension with Flavor Creator.......... 1878
Concentrated Tylenol Infants' Drops (Rare).......... 1878
Jr. Tylenol Meltaways (Rare).......... 1878

Sensorium, clouded
Blocadren Tablets.......... 1916
Cosopt Sterile Ophthalmic Solution.......... 1931
Inderal LA Long-Acting Capsules.......... 3429
InnoPran XL Capsules.......... 2723
Lopressor Injection.......... 2238
Lopressor Tablets.......... 2238
Lopressor HCT 50/25 Tablets.......... 2241
Lopressor HCT 100/25 Tablets.......... 2241
Lopressor HCT 100/50 Tablets.......... 2241
Nadolol Tablets.......... 2159
Timolide Tablets.......... 2086
Timoptic Sterile Ophthalmic Solution.......... 2088
Timoptic in Ocudose.......... 2091
Timoptic-XE Sterile Ophthalmic Gel Forming Solution.......... 2092
Toprol-XL Tablets.......... 668

Sensory disturbances
Arranon Injection (1%).......... 1357
▲ Chantix Tablets (Greater than 5%) 2517
Depo-Medrol Single-Dose Vial.......... 2619
▲ Eloxatin for Injection (8%) 2892
Emend Capsules (Less than or equal to 0.5%).......... 1963
Hectorol Capsules.......... 1275
Hectorol Injection.......... 1278
▲ Leukine (6%) 814
Paxil CR Controlled-Release Tablets.......... 1538
Paxil.......... 1530
▲ Prograf Capsules and Injection (Approximately 55%).......... 632
▲ Proleukin for Injection (10%) 2266
Rocaltrol Capsules.......... 2798
Rocaltrol Oral Solution.......... 2798
Topamax Sprinkle Capsules (Greater than 1%).......... 2404
Topamax Tablets (Greater than 1%).......... 2404
▲ Wellbutrin Tablets (4.0%) 1603
▲ Wellbutrin XL Extended-Release Tablets (4%).......... 1613

Sensory loss
Arranon Injection (0% to 2%).......... 1357

Sepsis
▲ Abelcet Injection (7%) 1141
Actiq (1% or greater).......... 979
Aloprim for Injection (Less than 1%).......... 2167
▲ AmBisome for Injection (7.4% to 14%).......... 620
Anaprox Tablets (Less than 1%).......... 2761
Anaprox DS Tablets (Less than 1%).......... 2761
▲ Aranesp for Injection (27%) 581
▲ Argatroban Injection (6%) 1346
Arthrotec Tablets (Rare).......... 3129
Bexxar.......... 1398
▲ Cafcit (4.3%).......... 1886
▲ Campath Ampules (10% to 15%) 811
Camptosar Injection.......... 2604
Cathflo Activase.......... 1231
▲ CellCept Capsules (2% to 27.4%) 2747
▲ CellCept Intravenous (2% to 27.4%).......... 2747
▲ CellCept Oral Suspension (2% to 27.4%).......... 2747
▲ CellCept Tablets (2% to 27.4%) 2747
▲ Clolar for Intravenous Infusion (15%).......... 1271
Clozaril Tablets.......... 2184
▲ Copegus Tablets (3% to 5%) 2754
▲ Cubicin for Injection (5%) 1026
Dacogen Injection.......... 2129
▲ Doxil Injection (Less than 1% to 5%).......... 2351
EC-Naprosyn Delayed-Release Tablets (Less than 1%).......... 2761
▲ Elitek (3%) 2890
Enbrel for Injection.......... 584
Epivir.......... 1427
▲ Erbitux (3%) 910
Evoxac Capsules (Less than 1%).......... 1047
FazaClo Orally Disintegrating Tablets.......... 551
Ferrlecit Injection.......... 3388
Gabitril Tablets (Infrequent).......... 984
Gemzar for Injection (Less than 1%).......... 1771
Gleevec Tablets (Infrequent).......... 2227
▲ Humira Injection (Less than 5%) 466
▲ Hycamtin for Injection (26%) 1458
▲ Infasurf Intratracheal Suspension (20% to 28%).......... 1184
▲ Intron A for Injection (Less than 5%).......... 3024
▲ Leukine (11%) 814
Levaquin (0.1% to 0.9%).......... 2384
Levaquin in 5% Dextrose Injection (0.1% to 0.9%).......... 2384
Merrem I.V. (1.6%).......... 686
Mycamine for Injection.......... 628
Myleran Tablets.......... 1525
▲ Mylotarg for Injection (17% to 28%).......... 3431
Naprosyn Suspension (Less than 1%).......... 2761
Naprosyn Tablets (Less than 1%).......... 2761
▲ NeoProfen Injection (43%) 2472
Neurontin Capsules (Rare) 2487
Neurontin Oral Solution (Rare) 2487
Neurontin Tablets (Rare) 2487
▲ Nipent for Injection (3%) 1863
Oncaspar (Less than 1%) 1145
Orthoclone OKT3 Sterile Solution 2360
Paxil CR Controlled-Release Tablets (Rare) 1538
Paxil (Rare) 1530
▲ Pegasys (3% to 5%) 2789
PEG-Intron Powder for Injection (Less than or equal to 1%) 3048
Permax Tablets (Infrequent) 3356
Photofrin for Injection (Occasional) 702
Prevnar for Injection 3463
▲ Prograf Capsules and Injection (3% to 15%) 632
▲ Proleukin for Injection (23%) 2266
Pulmozyme Inhalation Solution 1248
▲ Rapamune Oral Solution and Tablets (3% to 20%) 3475
Raptiva for Injection 1250
▲ Refludan for Injection (3.5%) 792
Remicade for IV Injection (Greater than or equal to 0.2%) 971
Requip Tablets (Infrequent) 1555
Revlimid Capsules (2.7%) 958
Rilutek Tablets (Infrequent) 2930
Rituxan I.V. 1254
▲ Simulect for Injection (3% to 10%) 2284
▲ Soltamox Oral Solution (6%) 3527
Targretin Capsules 1747
Thalomid Capsules 965
▲ Thymoglobulin for Intravenous Infusion (12.2%) 1284
Ticlid Tablets (Rare) 2810
Trasylol Injection (1% to 2%) 754
▲ Trisenox Injection (5%) 993
▲ Valcyte Tablets (Less than 5%) 2813
VFEND I.V. (Less than 2%) 2564
VFEND Oral Suspension (Less than 2%) 2564
VFEND Tablets (Less than 2%) 2564
Voltaren Tablets (Occasionally) 2307
Voltaren-XR Tablets (Occasionally) 2310
▲ Xeloda Tablets (Less than 5%) 2822
▲ Zegerid Capsules (5.1%) 2958
▲ Zegerid Powder for Oral Solution (5.1%) 2958
▲ Zemplar Capsules (5%) 541
▲ Zemplar Injection (5%) 543
▲ Zinecard for Injection (12% to 17%) 2650
▲ Zyvox (0% to 8%) 2652

Sepsis, neutropenic
▲ Alimta for Injection (6%) 1750
Camptosar Injection 2604
Revlimid Capsules 958
▲ Xeloda Tablets (Less than 5%) 2822

Septic shock
Aloprim for Injection (Less than 1%) 2167
Emend Capsules (Greater than 0.5%) 1963
Enbrel for Injection 584
Invanz for Injection (Greater than 0.1%) 1999
Oncaspar (Less than 1%) 1145
Tygacil for Injection (0% to less than 2%) 3488

Septicemia
Bexxar 1398
▲ Gengraf Capsules (5.3%) 459
Invanz for Injection (Greater than 0.1%) 1999
▲ Leustatin Injection (6%) 2357
▲ Neoral Oral Solution (5.3%) 2259
▲ Neoral Soft Gelatin Capsules (5.3%) 2259
Protopic Ointment 638
▲ Sandimmune (4.8% to 5.3%) 2275
Vesanoid Capsules 2820

Seroma
Invanz for Injection (1.3%).......... 1999

Serositis
Aceon Tablets (2 mg, 4 mg, 8 mg).......... 3194
Vasotec I.V. Injection (0.5% to 1.0%).......... 2103

Serotonin syndrome
Celexa.......... 1176
Effexor Tablets.......... 3411
Effexor XR Capsules.......... 3417
Imitrex Injection.......... 1463
Imitrex Tablets.......... 1471
Lexapro Oral Solution.......... 1190
Lexapro Tablets.......... 1190
Maxalt Tablets.......... 2008
Maxalt-MLT Orally Disintegrating Tablets.......... 2008
Meridia Capsules.......... 489
Paxil CR Controlled-Release Tablets.......... 1538
Paxil.......... 1530
Prozac Pulvules and Liquid 1801
Zoloft 2586
Zomig Tablets 3519
Zomig-ZMT Tablets 3519
Zyvox 2652

Serous drainage
▲ Panretin Gel (1% to 8%) 1747
Targretin Capsules 1747

Serum alkaline phosphatase, abnormal
Invirase 2772
Parcopa Orally Disintegrating Tablets 3097
Vytorin 10/10 Tablets 2114
Vytorin 10/10 Tablets 3077
Vytorin 10/20 Tablets 2114
Vytorin 10/20 Tablets 3077
Vytorin 10/40 Tablets 2114
Vytorin 10/40 Tablets 3077
Vytorin 10/80 Tablets 2114
Vytorin 10/80 Tablets 3077
▲ Zyvox (0.2% to 3.5%) 2652

Serum alkaline phosphatase, elevation
Abelcet Injection 1141
Abilify Oral Solution (Infrequent) 882
Abilify Oral Solution (Infrequent) 2450
Abilify Discmelt Orally Disintegrating Tablets (Infrequent) 882
Abilify Discmelt Orally Disintegrating Tablets (Infrequent) 2450
Abilify Tablets (Infrequent) 882
Abilify Tablets (Infrequent) 2450
Accutane Capsules 2731
Aceon Tablets (2 mg, 4 mg, 8 mg) (0.3% to 1%) 3194
Adalat CC Tablets (Rare) 2964
Advicor Tablets 1722
Altoprev Extended-Release Tablets 3109
Ambien Tablets (Rare) 2851
Ambien CR Tablets (Rare) 2855
▲ AmBisome for Injection (7.1% to 22.2%) 620
▲ Arimidex Tablets (2% to 5%) 673
▲ Aromasin Tablets (13.7% to 15%) 2600
Arthrotec Tablets (Rare) 3129
Asacol Delayed-Release Tablets 2692
Atripla Tablets (1%) 945
Augmentin (Infrequent) 1360
Augmentin Tablets (Infrequent) 1363
Augmentin XR Extended-Release Tablets (Infrequent) 1369
Augmentin ES-600 Powder for Oral Suspension (Infrequently) 1366
Axid Oral Solution (Less common) 879
BeneFix Vials (1.6%) 3408
Biaxin/Biaxin XL (Less than 1%) 402
Campath Ampules 811
Campral Tablets (Rare) 1174
▲ Camptosar Injection (4% to 13%) 2604
▲ Cancidas for Injection (2.9% to 10.5%) 1918
Captopril Tablets 2149
Cardizem LA Extended Release Tablets (Less than 2%) 1728
Ceftin 1407
Celebrex Capsules (0.1% to 1.9%) 3134
Celexa (Infrequent) 1176
▲ CellCept Capsules (3% to less than 20%) 2747
▲ CellCept Intravenous (3% to less than 20%) 2747
▲ CellCept Oral Suspension (3% to less than 20%) 2747
▲ CellCept Tablets (3% to less than 20%) 2747

▲ Chemet Capsules (4.2% to 10.4%) ... 2458
Cipro (0.8%) ... 2977
▲ Cipro I.V. (Among most frequent) ... 2984
Colazal Capsules ... 2838
▲ Coreg Tablets (Greater than 1% to 3%) ... 1414
Covera-HS Tablets ... 3139
Cubicin for Injection (1.7%) ... 1026
Cymbalta Delayed-Release Capsules ... 1757
▲ Dacogen Injection (11%) ... 2129
Depo-Medrol Single-Dose Vial ... 2619
▲ Doxil Injection (1.3% to 7.8%) ... 2351
Effexor Tablets (Infrequent) ... 3411
Effexor XR Capsules (Infrequent) ... 3417
▲ Eloxatin for Injection (0% to 4%) ... 2892
Elspar for Injection ... 2463
Elspar for Injection ... 1960
Emend Capsules (Greater than 0.5%) ... 1963
Eraxis for Injection (1.5%) ... 2521
Evoxac Capsules ... 1047
Exelon Capsules (Infrequent) ... 2206
Exelon Oral Solution (Infrequent) ... 2206
▲ Fortaz (1 in 23) ... 1453
▲ Gemzar for Injection (55% to 77%) ... 1771
Geodon Capsules (Infrequent) ... 2529
▲ Gleevec Tablets (0% to 5.5%) ... 2227
▲ Humira Injection (5%) ... 466
▲ Intron A for Injection (Up to 13%) ... 3024
▲ Invanz for Injection (1.1% to 6.6%) ... 1999
▲ I.V. Busulfex (15%) ... 2493
Keflex Capsules ... 549
Ketek Tablets (Less than 0.2%) ... 2903
Klonopin ... 2778
Lamictal (Infrequent) ... 1481
Lescol Capsules ... 2233
Lescol XL Tablets ... 2233
▲ Leukine (8%) ... 814
Lopressor Injection ... 2238
Lopressor Tablets ... 2238
Lopressor HCT 50/25 Tablets ... 2241
Lopressor HCT 100/25 Tablets ... 2241
Lopressor HCT 100/50 Tablets ... 2241
Lotronex Tablets ... 1512
Maxipime for Injection (Greater than 0.1% to less than 1%) ... 1105
Mefoxin for Injection ... 2012
Mefoxin Premixed Intravenous Solution ... 2016
▲ Mepron Suspension (5% to 8%) ... 1521
Meridia Capsules (1.6%) ... 489
Merrem I.V. (Greater than 0.2%) ... 686
Mevacor Tablets ... 2021
Mycamine for Injection (1.5% to 2%) ... 628
▲ Mylotarg for Injection (5% to 10%) ... 3431
▲ Nabi-HB (4%) ... 2169
Nalfon Capsules (Less than 1%) ... 2502
Namenda (Frequent) ... 1195
▲ Neulasta Injection (9%) ... 601
▲ Neupogen for Injection (21% to 58%) ... 603
Neurontin Capsules (Rare) ... 2487
Neurontin Oral Solution (Rare) ... 2487
Neurontin Tablets (Rare) ... 2487
Nexavar Tablets (Uncommon) ... 746
Nexium Delayed-Release Capsules (Less than 1%) ... 655
Nexium I.V. (Less than 1%) ... 659
Nimotop Capsules (0.2%; rare) ... 749
Noroxin Tablets (1.1%) ... 2032
NovoLog Mix 70/30 ... 2328
Nutropin for Injection ... 1239
Nutropin AQ Injection ... 1243
Nutropin AQ Pen ... 1243
Nutropin AQ Pen Cartridge ... 1243
Omnicef Capsules (0.3%) ... 511
Omnicef for Oral Suspension (1%) ... 511
Oxandrin Tablets ... 2962
Paxil CR Controlled-Release Tablets (Rare) ... 1538
Paxil (Rare) ... 1530
Pentasa Capsules (Less than 1%) ... 3185
Prevacid Delayed-Release Capsules ... 3271
Prevacid for Delayed-Release Oral Suspension ... 3271
Prevacid SoluTab Delayed-Release Orally Disintegrating Tablets ... 3271
Prevacid NapraPAC ... 3280
PREVPAC (Less than 1%) ... 3284
▲ Prezista Tablets (2.8% to 4.6%) ... 3306
Prilosec OTC Delayed-Release Tablets (Rare) ... 2677
Primaxin I.M. ... 2045
Primaxin I.V. ... 2048
▲ Prograf Capsules and Injection (3% to 15%) ... 632
▲ Proleukin for Injection (10%) ... 2266
Protonix I.V. (Less than 1%) ... 3472
Protonix Tablets (Less than 1%) ... 3469
Prozac Pulvules and Liquid (Rare) ... 1801
▲ Rapamune Oral Solution and Tablets (3% to 20%) ... 3475
▲ Raptiva for Injection (4%) ... 1250
Razadyne (Infrequent) ... 2399
Razadyne ER Extended-Release Capsules (Infrequent) ... 2399
Relpax Tablets (Rare) ... 2548
Requip Tablets (Infrequent) ... 1555
Rescriptor Tablets ... 2551
Rilutek Tablets (Infrequent) ... 2930
Rocephin Injectable Vials, ADD-Vantage, Galaxy, Bulk (Less than 1%) ... 2800
▲ Rythmol SR Capsules (3%) ... 2727
Seroquel Tablets (Infrequent) ... 690
Somavert Injection (Minimal) ... 2642
Suprax (Less than 2%) ... 1843
Symmetrel Tablets ... 1135
Tabloid Tablets ... 1575
Tambocor Tablets (Rare) ... 1856
Tarka Tablets (2.8%) ... 524
▲ Taxotere Injection Concentrate (4.3%) ... 2932
Tequin Injection (Less than 0.1%) ... 938
Tequin Injection in 5% Dextrose (Less than 0.1%) ... 938
Tequin Tablets (Less than 0.1%) ... 938
Teveten Tablets ... 1735
Teveten HCT Tablets ... 1737
Thalomid Capsules ... 965
Thiothixene Capsules ... 2165
Tiazac Capsules (Less than 2%) ... 1201
Timentin ADD-Vantage ... 1580
Timentin Injection Galaxy Container ... 1583
Timentin IV Infusion ... 1577
Timentin Pharmacy Bulk Package ... 1586
Topamax Sprinkle Capsules (Infrequent) ... 2404
Topamax Tablets (Infrequent) ... 2404
Toprol-XL Tablets ... 668
Trelstar LA Suspension (1.7%) ... 3397
Truvada Tablets (1%) ... 1296
▲ Tygacil for Injection (3.5%) ... 3488
Ultane Liquid for Inhalation (Less than 1%) ... 531
Uniretic Tablets (Less than 1%) ... 3100
▲ Valtrex Caplets (4%) ... 1597
Vantin Tablets and Oral Suspension ... 2645
▲ Ventavis Inhalation Solution (6%) ... 1020
Verelan PM Extended-Release Capsules, Controlled-Onset ... 3106
▲ VFEND I.V. (3.6% to 22.6%) ... 2564
▲ VFEND Oral Suspension (3.6% to 22.6%) ... 2564
▲ VFEND Tablets (3.6% to 22.6%) ... 2564
Viracept (Less than 2%) ... 2577
Xyrem Oral Solution (Infrequent) ... 1688
Zegerid Capsules (Rare) ... 2958
Zegerid Powder for Oral Solution (Rare) ... 2958
Zinacef for Injection (1 in 50 patients) ... 1631
Zinacef Injection (1 in 50 patients) ... 1631
Zocor Tablets ... 2105
Zomig Tablets (Rare) ... 3519
Zomig-ZMT Tablets (Rare) ... 3519
Zonegran Capsules ... 1101
Zosyn ... 3492
Zyprexa Tablets (Infrequent) ... 1830
Zyprexa ZYDIS Orally Disintegrating Tablets (Infrequent) ... 1830

Serum alkaline phosphatase, changes

Bumex Tablets (0.4%) ... 2746
Oxandrin Tablets ... 2962
▲ Sutent Capsules (4% to 24%) ... 2560

Serum aminotransferase, elevation

Arixtra Injection (1.7% to 2.6%) ... 1351

Serum amylase, abnormal

▲ Sutent Capsules (5% to 17%) ... 2560
Zyvox (0.2% to 2.4%) ... 2652

Serum amylase, elevation

Abelcet Injection ... 1141
AmBisome for Injection (Less common) ... 620
Aptivus Capsules (2.9%) ... 826
▲ Atripla Tablets (7%) ... 945
Avelox (0.1% to less than 2%) ... 2970
▲ Baraclude (2% to 3%) ... 894
Cipro (Less than 1%) ... 2977
Cipro I.V. (1% or less) ... 2984
Cipro XR Tablets ... 2990
Colazal Capsules ... 2838
Crixivan Capsules (2.1%) ... 1940
Cuprimine Capsules (Few cases) ... 1947
▲ Emtriva Capsules (2% to 5%) ... 1287
▲ Emtriva Oral Solution (2% to 5%) ... 1287
▲ Epivir (3% to 4.2%) ... 1427
Epivir-HBV (Less than 1%) ... 1432
Epzicom Tablets ... 1436
Eraxis for Injection (Less than 1% to less than 2%) ... 2521
▲ Evoxac Capsules (1% to 3%) ... 1047
Famvir Tablets (1.5%) ... 2211
Fuzeon Injection ... 2767
▲ Hepsera Tablets (4%) ... 1292
Invirase (1% to 2%) ... 2772
Kadian Capsules ... 577
▲ Kaletra (3% to 8%) ... 476
▲ Kepivance (38% to 62%) ... 597
Malarone Pediatric Tablets ... 1517
Malarone Tablets ... 1517
▲ Mepron Suspension (1% to 8%) ... 1521
▲ Nexavar Tablets (Very Common) ... 746
Niaspan Extended-Release Tablets ... 1730
Omnicef Capsules ... 511
Omnicef for Oral Suspension ... 511
Oncaspar (Less than 1%) ... 1145
Pentasa Capsules (Less than 1%) ... 3185
▲ Prezista Tablets (10.8% to 16.9%) ... 3306
Prograf Capsules and Injection ... 632
Proquin XR Tablets ... 1153
Rescriptor Tablets (2.5% to 2.9%) ... 2551
▲ Sustiva Capsules (10%) ... 930
▲ Sustiva Tablets (10%) ... 930
▲ Sutent Capsules (1% to 5%) ... 2560
Targretin Capsules ... 1747
Tequin Injection (Less than 0.1%) ... 938
Tequin Injection in 5% Dextrose (Less than 0.1%) ... 938
Tequin Tablets (Less than 0.1%) ... 938
Trileptal Tablets ... 2300
▲ Truvada Tablets (7%) ... 1296
▲ Tygacil for Injection (3.1%) ... 3488
Uniretic Tablets (Less than 1%) ... 3100
Viracept (Less than 2%) ... 2577
▲ Viread Tablets (6% to 9%) ... 1301
▲ Ziagen (2% to 4%) ... 1626

Serum bicarbonate, decrease

Cancidas for Injection (0% to 0.9%) ... 1918
▲ Dacogen Injection (5%) ... 2129
Omnicef Capsules (0.6%) ... 511
Omnicef for Oral Suspension (1%) ... 511
▲ Prezista Tablets (3.1% to 3.4%) ... 3306
Zmax for Oral Suspension (Greater than or equal to 1%) ... 2583

Serum bicarbonate, increase

Cubicin for Injection (Less than 1%) ... 1026
▲ Dacogen Injection (6%) ... 2129

Serum bicarbonate content, variations

▲ Bumex Tablets (3.1%) ... 2746
▲ Prograf Capsules and Injection (3% to 15%) ... 632

Serum bilirubin, elevation

(*see under* Hyperbilirubinemia)

Serum bilirubin levels, abnormalities

Amerge Tablets (Rare) ... 1339
Bumex Tablets (0.8%) ... 2746
Emcyt Capsules (1% to 2%) ... 2634
Parcopa Orally Disintegrating Tablets ... 3097
▲ Sutent Capsules (1% to 16%) ... 2560
Vytorin 10/10 Tablets ... 2114
Vytorin 10/10 Tablets ... 3077
Vytorin 10/20 Tablets ... 2114
Vytorin 10/20 Tablets ... 3077
Vytorin 10/40 Tablets ... 2114
Vytorin 10/40 Tablets ... 3077
Vytorin 10/80 Tablets ... 2114
Vytorin 10/80 Tablets ... 3077
▲ Zyvox (0.2% to 6.3%) ... 2652

Serum calcium, depression

(*see under* Hypocalcemia)

Serum calcium content, variations

Bumex Tablets (2.4%) ... 2746

Serum calcium decrease

(*see under* Hypocalcemia)

Serum chloride levels, decreased

▲ Dacogen Injection (6%) ... 2129

Serum cholesterol, increase

(*see under* Hypercholesterolemia)

Serum creatine phosphokinase, elevation

Abilify Oral Solution (Frequent) ... 882
Abilify Oral Solution (Frequent) ... 2450
Abilify Discmelt Orally Disintegrating Tablets (Frequent) ... 882
Abilify Discmelt Orally Disintegrating Tablets (Frequent) ... 2450
Abilify Tablets (Frequent) ... 882
Abilify Tablets (Frequent) ... 2450
Accutane Capsules ... 2731
ActoPlus Met Tablets ... 3214
Aricept Tablets (Infrequent) ... 1094
Aricept ODT Tablets (Infrequent) ... 1094
Arthrotec Tablets (Rare) ... 3129
▲ Atripla Tablets (7%) ... 945
Benicar HCT Tablets (Greater than 1%) ... 1044
Caduet Tablets (Less than 2%) ... 2508
Catapres Tablets (Rare) ... 843
▲ Cipro I.V. (Among most frequent) ... 2984
Clorpres Tablets (Rare) ... 2153
Cymbalta Delayed-Release Capsules ... 1757
Epzicom Tablets ... 1436
FazaClo Orally Disintegrating Tablets ... 551
▲ Fuzeon Injection (2.3% to 5.9%) ... 2767
Geodon Capsules (Infrequent) ... 2529
Gleevec Tablets (Infrequent) ... 2227
Havrix Vaccine (Less than 1%) ... 1456
▲ Invirase (7% to 12%) ... 2772
Lipitor Tablets (Less than 2%) ... 2483
Mirapex Tablets (1% or more) ... 859
▲ Norvir (0.9% to 3.4%) ... 503
Protonix I.V. ... 3472
Protonix Tablets ... 3469
Prozac Pulvules and Liquid (Rare) ... 1801
Relpax Tablets (Infrequent) ... 2548
Requip Tablets (Infrequent) ... 1555
Risperdal (Infrequent) ... 1676
Risperdal M-Tab Orally Disintegrating Tablets (Infrequent) ... 1676
Sular Tablets (Less than or equal to 1%) ... 3122
Symmetrel Tablets (Uncommon) ... 1135
Trasylol Injection (2%) ... 754
▲ Triglide Tablets (3%) ... 3123
Trizivir Tablets ... 1589
▲ Ultram ER Tablets (1% to greater than 5%) ... 2392
Viracept (Less than 2%) ... 2577
Zelnorm Tablets ... 2312
▲ Ziagen (7% to 8%) ... 1626
▲ Zocor Tablets (About 5% of patients) ... 2105
Zyprexa Tablets ... 1830
Zyprexa IntraMuscular (Infrequent) ... 1830
Zyprexa ZYDIS Orally Disintegrating Tablets ... 1830

Serum creatinine, abnormal

▲ Sutent Capsules (1% to 12%) ... 2560
Zyvox (0.4% to 2.4%) ... 2652

Serum creatinine, elevation

▲ Abelcet Injection (11%) ... 1141
Abilify Oral Solution (Infrequent) ... 882
Abilify Oral Solution (Infrequent) ... 2450
Abilify Discmelt Orally Disintegrating Tablets (Infrequent) ... 882
Abilify Discmelt Orally Disintegrating Tablets (Infrequent) ... 2450
Abilify Tablets (Infrequent) ... 882
Abilify Tablets (Infrequent) ... 2450
Aceon Tablets (2 mg, 4 mg, 8 mg) (0.3% to 1%) ... 3194
Aggrenox Capsules ... 822
▲ Alimta for Injection (Up to 16%) ... 1750
Alinia for Oral Suspension (Less than 1%) ... 2835
Alinia Tablets (Less than 1%) ... 2835
Aloprim for Injection (Less than 1%) ... 2167
Altace Capsules (1.2% to 1.5%) ... 1702
▲ AmBisome for Injection (18.5% to 22.4%) ... 620
Anaprox Tablets ... 2761
Anaprox DS Tablets ... 2761
▲ AndroGel (3% to 6%) ... 3329
▲ Aredia for Injection (9.1%) ... 2179
▲ Aromasin Tablets (5.5% to 5.8%) ... 2600
▲ Arranon Injection (0% to 6%) ... 1357
Asacol Delayed-Release Tablets ... 2692
Atacand Tablets (Infrequent) ... 649
Avalide Tablets (Less than 0.7%) ... 888

Avalide Tablets (Less than 0.7%) 2874
Avapro Tablets (Less than 0.7%) 891
Avapro Tablets (Less than 0.7%) 2871
Baraclude (0% to 2%) 894
Bayer Aspirin Comprehensive Prescribing Information 796
Benicar Tablets 1043
Benicar HCT Tablets (Rare) 1044
Biaxin/Biaxin XL (Less than 1%) 402
Bicillin C-R Injectable Suspension 1706
▲ Bumex Tablets (7.4%) 2746
Byetta Injection 611
Campral Tablets (Rare) 1174
▲ Cancidas for Injection (0% to 3.7%) 1918
Capastat Sulfate for Injection (A significant number of patients) 1755
Captopril Tablets 2149
Carimune NF 3499
Caverject Impulse Injection (Less than 1%) 2612
Ceftin 1407
Celebrex Capsules (0.1% to 1.9%) 3134
▲ CellCept Capsules (3% to 39.4%) 2747
▲ CellCept Intravenous (3% to 39.4%) 2747
▲ CellCept Oral Suspension (3% to 39.4%) 2747
▲ CellCept Tablets (3% to 39.4%) 2747
Cipro (1.1%) 2977
▲ Cipro I.V. (Among most frequent) 2984
▲ Clolar for Intravenous Infusion (6%) 1271
▲ Coreg Tablets (Greater than 1% to 3%) 1414
Cozaar Tablets (Less than 0.1%) 1935
Crixivan Capsules 1940
Cymbalta Delayed-Release Capsules (Infrequent) 1757
CytoGam Intravenous 1895
Didronel Tablets 2697
▲ Diovan Tablets (0.6% to 4.2%) 2193
Diovan HCT Tablets (2%) 2196
Doxil Injection (Less than 1%) 2351
Dyazide Capsules 1423
Dyrenium Capsules (Rare) 3400
EC-Naprosyn Delayed-Release Tablets 2761
Effexor Tablets (Infrequent) 3411
Effexor XR Capsules (Infrequent) 3417
▲ Eloxatin for Injection (5% to 10%) 2892
▲ Emend Capsules (3.7%) 1963
Eraxis for Injection (Less than 1% to less than 2%) 2521
Eulexin Capsules 3009
Famvir Tablets (0.2%) 2211
Fansidar Tablets 2765
Flebogamma 5%, Immune Globulin Intravenous (Human) 1658
Fortaz (Occasional) 1453
Gammagard S/D 724
Gantrisin Pediatric Suspension 2770
Garamycin Injectable 3014
▲ Gemzar for Injection (Up to 8%) 1771
▲ Gengraf Capsules (18% to 48%) 459
Geodon Capsules (Rare) 2529
▲ Gleevec Tablets (0% to 3%) 2227
Guanidine Hydrochloride Tablets 3016
▲ Hepsera Tablets (2% to 4%) 1292
Hyzaar 50-12.5 Tablets (0.8%) 1990
Hyzaar 100-12.5 Tablets (0.8%) 1990
Hyzaar 100-25 Tablets (0.8%) 1990
▲ Indapamide Tablets (Less than 5%) 2156
Indocin I.V. 2465
▲ Inspra Tablets (0.2% to 6.5%) 2536
▲ Intron A for Injection (Up to 3%) 3024
Invanz for Injection (0.9% to 1.1%) 1999
▲ I.V. Busulfex (21%) 2493
Keflex Capsules 549
Lamictal (Rare) 1481
▲ Leukine (15%) 814
Lofibra Tablets 1219
Lofibra Capsules 1216
Lotensin Tablets (2%) 2243
Lotensin HCT Tablets 2246
Lotrel Capsules 2249
▲ Lupron Depot 7.5 mg (Greater than or equal to 5%) 3264
▲ Mavik Tablets (1.1% to 4.7%) 486
Maxipime for Injection (Greater than 0.1% to less than 1%) 1105
Mefoxin for Injection 2012
Mefoxin Premixed Intravenous Solution 2016
Mepron Suspension (1%) 1521
Merrem I.V. (Greater than 0.2%) 686
Micardis Tablets 854
Mobic Oral Suspension (Less than 2%) 863
Mobic Tablets (Less than 2%) 863
Mycamine for Injection (0.2% to 0.6%) 628
▲ Myfortic Tablets (3% to less than 20%) 2255
Nabi-HB (2%) 2169
Naprosyn Suspension 2761
Naprosyn Tablets 2761
Natrecor for Injection (Greater than or equal to 1%) 3127
▲ Neoral Oral Solution (18% to 48%) 2259
▲ Neoral Soft Gelatin Capsules (18% to 48%) 2259
▲ Nipent for Injection (3% to 10%) 1863
Noroxin Tablets (Less frequent) 2032
Oncaspar 1145
▲ Ontak Vials (7%) 1745
Oxandrin Tablets 2962
Parcopa Orally Disintegrating Tablets 3097
Plavix Tablets 917
Plavix Tablets 2926
Pletal Tablets (Less than 2%) 2455
Prevacid Delayed-Release Capsules 3271
Prevacid for Delayed-Release Oral Suspension 3271
Prevacid SoluTab Delayed-Release Orally Disintegrating Tablets 3271
Prevacid NapraPAC 3280
PREVPAC (Less than 1%) 3284
Prilosec OTC Delayed-Release Tablets (Less than 1%) 2677
Primaxin I.M. 2045
Primaxin I.V. 2048
▲ Prinivil Tablets (About 2.0% to approximately 11.6%) 2052
Prinzide Tablets 2056
▲ Prograf Capsules and Injection (24% to 45%) 632
▲ Proleukin for Injection (33%) 2266
Protopic Ointment (Greater than or equal to 1%) 638
Ranexa Tablets 1035
Raniclor Tablets, Chewable 2505
▲ Rapamune Oral Solution and Tablets (35% to 40%) 3475
Rescriptor Tablets 2551
Revlimid Capsules 958
▲ Rocaltrol Capsules (1 in 6) 2798
▲ Rocaltrol Oral Solution (1 in 6) 2798
Rocephin Injectable Vials, ADD-Vantage, Galaxy, Bulk (Less than 1%) 2800
Rythmol SR Capsules 2727
Sandimmune 2275
Sandostatin LAR Depot (Rare) 2280
Soltamox Oral Solution (2%) 3527
Sular Tablets (Less than or equal to 1%) 3122
Suprax (Less than 2%) 1843
Sutent Capsules 2560
Symbyax Capsules (Rare) 1819
Symmetrel Tablets 1135
Targretin Capsules 1747
Testim 1% Gel (Less than 1%) 695
Teveten Tablets (1.3%) 1735
Teveten HCT Tablets (0.6%) 1737
Thalomid Capsules 965
Timentin ADD-Vantage 1580
Timentin Injection Galaxy Container 1583
Timentin IV Infusion 1577
Timentin Pharmacy Bulk Package 1586
Topamax Sprinkle Capsules (Rare) 2404
Topamax Tablets (Rare) 2404
▲ Trasylol Injection (18% to 21%) 754
Tricor Tablets 527
Trizivir Tablets 1589
Truvada Tablets 1296
Tygacil for Injection (0% to less than 2%) 3488
Ultane Liquid for Inhalation (Less than 1%) 531
Uniretic Tablets (Less than 1%) 3100
Univasc Tablets (1%) 3104
Urso 250 Tablets (1%) 710
Urso Forte Tablets (1%) 710
Valtrex Caplets (Up to 0.7%) 1597
Vancocin HCl Capsules, USP (Rare) 3380
Vantin Tablets and Oral Suspension 2645
▲ Vasotec I.V. Injection (About 0.2% to 20%) 2103
▲ VFEND I.V. (0% to 21.4%) 2564
▲ VFEND Oral Suspension (0% to 21.4%) 2564
▲ VFEND Tablets (0% to 21.4%) 2564
Viread Tablets 1301
▲ Visudyne for Injection (1% to 10%) 2305
Zantac (Rare) 1624
Zantac Injection 1619
Zantac Injection Pharmacy Bulk Package (Rare) 1622
Zantac Injection Premixed 1619
Zantac (Rare) 1624
Zegerid Capsules (Less than 1%) 2958
Zegerid Powder for Oral Solution (Less than 1%) 2958
Ziagen 1626
Zinacef for Injection 1631
Zinacef Injection 1631
Zometa for Intravenous Infusion (0.4% to 1.3%) 2315
Zonegran Capsules 1101
Zosyn 3492
Zovirax 1643

Serum electrolyte changes
(*see under* Electrolyte imbalance)

Serum folate levels, decreased
Seasonique Tablets 1077

Serum gastrin levels, increased
Nexium Delayed-Release Capsules (Less than 1%) 655
Nexium I.V. (Less than 1%) 659
Prevacid NapraPAC 3280

Serum lipase, abnormal
▲ Sutent Capsules (10% to 25%) 2560
Zyvox (0.4% to 2.3%) 2652

Serum lipase, elevation
Aptivus Capsules (Less than 2%) 826
▲ Atripla Tablets (Up to 3%) 945
▲ Baraclude (7% to 8%) 894
Cipro (Less than 1%) 2977
Cipro I.V. (1% or less) 2984
Cipro XR Tablets 2990
Emtriva Capsules (Less than 1% to 1%) 1287
Emtriva Oral Solution (Less than 1% to 1%) 1287
▲ Epivir-HBV (10%) 1432
Epzicom Tablets 1436
Eraxis for Injection (Less than 1% to less than 2%) 2521
▲ Famvir Tablets (4.9%) 2211
▲ Fuzeon Injection (2.3% to 5.9%) 2767
▲ Kepivance (11% to 28%) 597
▲ Lexiva Tablets (8%) 1505
▲ Nexavar Tablets (Very Common to 41%) 746
Oncaspar 1145
Pentasa Capsules (Less than 1%) 3185
▲ Prezista Tablets (6.2% to 8.5%) 3306
Proquin XR Tablets 1153
Rescriptor Tablets 2551
▲ Sutent Capsules (2% to 16%) 2560
Trileptal Tablets 2300
▲ Truvada Tablets (1% to 12%) 1296

Serum Lipids, changes in
Avandamet Tablets 1373
Avandia Tablets 1384
Reyataz Capsules (Less than 3%) 921
Striant Mucoadhesive 1007

Serum PBI levels, decrease
(*see under* PBI decrease)

Serum phosphorus, elevation
Cubicin for Injection (2.5%) 1026
▲ Lupron Depot 3.75 mg (Approximately 5% to 8%) 3260
▲ Lupron Depot 7.5 mg (Greater than or equal to 5%) 3264
Maxipime for Injection (Greater than 0.1% to less than 1%) 1105
Nutropin for Injection 1239
Nutropin AQ Injection 1243
Nutropin AQ Pen 1243
Nutropin AQ Pen Cartridge 1243
Omnicef Capsules (0.6%) 511
Omnicef for Oral Suspension (0.9%) 511

Serum phosphorus content, variations
▲ Bumex Tablets (4.5%) 2746

Serum potassium, reduction
(*see under* Hypokalemia)

Serum proteins, changes
Bumex Tablets (0.7%) 2746
▲ Cancidas for Injection (Up to 3.1%) 1918
Premarin Tablets 3446
Premphase Tablets 3456
Prempro Tablets 3456

Serum sickness
Amoxil Capsules 1343
Amoxil Chewable Tablets 1343
Amoxil Pediatric Drops for Oral Suspension 1343
Amoxil Powder for Oral Suspension 1343
Amoxil Tablets 1343
Antivenin (Black Widow Spider Antivenin) 1913
Augmentin 1360
Augmentin Tablets 1363
Augmentin XR Extended-Release Tablets 1369
Augmentin ES-600 Powder for Oral Suspension 1366
Axid Oral Solution (Rare) 879
Bexxar 1398
Bicillin C-R Injectable Suspension 1706
Campath Ampules 811
Ceftin 1407
Copaxone for Injection (Infrequent) 3297
Engerix-B Vaccine (Less than 1%) 1425
Fansidar Tablets 2765
Fluarix 1451
Gantrisin Pediatric Suspension 2770
Levaquin (Rare) 2384
Levaquin in 5% Dextrose Injection (Rare) 2384
Levothroid Tablets 1186
Levoxyl Tablets 1712
Mefoxin for Injection 2012
Mefoxin Premixed Intravenous Solution 2016
Oracea Capsules 1000
Orthoclone OKT3 Sterile Solution 2360
Plavix Tablets 917
Pneumovax 23 (Rare) 2043
PREVPAC 3284
Recombivax HB (Less than 1%) 2071
Remicade for IV Injection (Greater than or equal to 0.2%) 971
Rituxan I.V. 1254
Rocephin Injectable Vials, ADD-Vantage, Galaxy, Bulk (Rare) 2800
Suprax (Less than 2%) 1843
Ticlid Tablets (Rare) 2810
Twinrix Vaccine 1595
Vantin Tablets and Oral Suspension 2645
Wellbutrin Tablets 1603
Wellbutrin SR Sustained-Release Tablets 1607
Wellbutrin XL Extended-Release Tablets 1613
Zoloft 2586

Serum sickness-like reaction
Cipro 2977
Cipro I.V. 2984
Cipro XR Tablets 2990
Proquin XR Tablets 1153
Raniclor Tablets, Chewable (Less than or equal to 0.5%) 2505
Raptiva for Injection (1 patient) 1250

Serum transaminase, elevation
Advicor Tablets 1722
Altoprev Extended-Release Tablets 3109
Aricept Tablets (Infrequent) 1094
Aricept ODT Tablets (Infrequent) 1094
▲ Arranon Injection (0% to 12%) 1357
Augmentin (Infrequent) 1360
Augmentin Tablets (Infrequent) 1363
Augmentin XR Extended-Release Tablets (Infrequent) 1369
Augmentin ES-600 Powder for Oral Suspension (Infrequently) 1366
Benicar Tablets 1043
Captopril Tablets 2149
▲ Chemet Capsules (6% to 10%) 2458
Concerta Extended-Release Tablets 1881
Covera-HS Tablets 3139
Daytrana Transdermal Patch 3174
Depacon Injection (Frequent) 412
Depakene (Frequent) 417
Depakote Tablets (Frequent) 427
Depakote ER Tablets (Frequent) 434
Enbrel for Injection 584
Eulexin Capsules 3009
Focalin Tablets 2220
Focalin XR Capsules 2223
Garamycin Injectable 3014
▲ Gemzar for Injection (Approximately two-thirds) 1771
Geodon Capsules (Infrequent) 2529
▲ Gleevec Tablets (3% to 6%) 2227
▲ Intron A for Injection (Less than 5%) 3024
Invirase (Isolated cases) 2772
Iressa Tablets 684
Ketek Tablets (Greater than or equal to 0.2% to less than 2%) 2903
Klonopin 2778

▲ Lariam Tablets (Among most frequent) 2786
Lescol Capsules 2233
Lescol XL Tablets 2233
Leustatin Injection 2357
Lofibra Tablets 1219
Lofibra Capsules 1216
Lopressor Injection 2238
Lopressor Tablets 2238
Lopressor HCT 50/25 Tablets 2241
Lopressor HCT 100/25 Tablets 2241
Lopressor HCT 100/50 Tablets 2241
▲ Lupron Depot–3 Month 11.25 mg (3%) 3265
Marinol Capsules (Less than 1%) 3333
Mavik Tablets (0.8% of patients) 486
Metadate CD Capsules 3323
Mevacor Tablets (1.9%) 2021
Mycamine for Injection (0.2% to 0.8%) 628
Mylotarg for Injection (13 Patients) 3431
▲ Nexavar Tablets (Common) 746
Niaspan Extended-Release Tablets 1730
Norvir 503
▲ Ontak Vials (61%) 1745
Paxil CR Controlled-Release Tablets 1538
Paxil 1530
Precose Tablets 751
▲ Proleukin for Injection (56%) 2266
Prometrium Capsules (100 mg, 200 mg) 3203
Prozac Pulvules and Liquid 1801
Remicade for IV Injection 971
Ritalin Hydrochloride Tablets (Some instances) 2269
Ritalin LA Capsules 2271
Ritalin-SR Tablets (Some instances) 2269
Seromycin Capsules 1813
Somavert Injection 2642
Tambocor Tablets (Rare) 1856
Thiothixene Capsules 2165
Ticlid Tablets (Rare) 2810
Tindamax Tablets 2142
Toprol-XL Tablets 668
▲ Trasylol Injection (5%) 754
Tricor Tablets 527
Trileptal Tablets 2300
Trileptal Oral Suspension 2300
Verelan PM Extended-Release Capsules, Controlled-Onset 3106
▲ Viramune Oral Suspension (8.8%) 873
▲ Viramune Tablets (8.8%) 873
Vytorin 10/10 Tablets 2114
Vytorin 10/10 Tablets 3077
Vytorin 10/20 Tablets 2114
Vytorin 10/20 Tablets 3077
Vytorin 10/40 Tablets 2114
Vytorin 10/40 Tablets 3077
Vytorin 10/80 Tablets 2114
Vytorin 10/80 Tablets 3077
Zelnorm Tablets 2312
Zetia Tablets (0.5%) 2120
Zetia Tablets (0.5%) 3083
Zocor Tablets (1%) 2105
Zofran 1639
Zofran ODT Orally Disintegrating Tablets 1639
Zyflo Tablets 1023
Zyrtec Chewable Tablets (Occasional) 2594
Zyrtec (Occasional) 2594
Zyrtec-D 12 Hour Extended Release Tablets (Occasional) 2597

Serum triglyceride, elevation
(*see under* Hypertriglyceridemia)

Serum vitamin B_{12} levels, subnormal
▲ Avandamet Tablets (7%) 1373

Sex hormone binding globulin, elevated
Menostar Transdermal System 782
Prempro Tablets 3456

Sexual activity, decrease
▲ Catapres Tablets (About 3 in 100 patients) 843
Catapres-TTS (0.5% or less) 844
▲ Clorpres Tablets (About 3%) 2153
Risperdal (Frequent) 1676
Risperdal M-Tab Orally Disintegrating Tablets (Frequent) 1676

Sexual dysfunction
Aceon Tablets (2 mg, 4 mg, 8 mg) (0.3% to 1.4%) 3194
Avalide Tablets 888
Avalide Tablets 2874
Avapro Tablets (Less than 1%) 891
Avapro Tablets (Less than 1%) 2871
Bentyl Capsules 697
Bentyl Injection 697
Bentyl Syrup 697
Bentyl Tablets 697
Caduet Tablets (Greater that 0.1% to 2%) 2508
Campral Tablets (Infrequent) 1174
Cardizem LA Extended Release Tablets (Less than 2%) 1728
Catapres-TTS (2 of 101 patients) 844
Celexa 1176
Chantix Tablets (Rare) 2517
Copaxone for Injection (Infrequent) 3297
Effexor Tablets (2%) 3411
Effexor XR Capsules 3417
Eldepryl Capsules 3208
Evoxac Capsules (Less than 1%) 1047
Geodon Capsules (Infrequent) 2529
Gleevec Tablets (Infrequent) 2227
Lexapro Oral Solution 1190
Lexapro Tablets 1190
Lithobid Tablets 1692
Lotronex Tablets (Rare) 1512
Micardis HCT Tablets 856
Neurontin Capsules (Infrequent) 2487
Neurontin Oral Solution (Infrequent) 2487
Neurontin Tablets (Infrequent) 2487
▲ Nexavar Tablets (Common) 746
▲ Niravam Orally Disintegrating Tablets (7.4%) 3092
Norvasc Tablets (Less than 1% to 2%) 2545
▲ Paxil CR Controlled-Release Tablets (3.7% to 10.0%) 1538
▲ Paxil (3.7% to 10.0%) 1530
Risperdal (Frequent) 1676
Risperdal M-Tab Orally Disintegrating Tablets (Frequent) 1676
▲ Strattera Capsules (3% or greater) 1814
Tiazac Capsules (Less than 2%) 1201
Vantas (Less than 2%) 3375
Viracept (Less than 2%) 2577
Wellbutrin Tablets (Frequent) 1603
Zoloft (Frequent) 2586

Sexual maturity, accelerated
Lupron Depot-PED 7.5 mg, 11.25 mg and 15 mg (Less than 2%) 3269
Lupron Injection Pediatric (Less than 2%) 3259

SGOT changes
(*see under* Aspartate aminotransferase levels, changes in)

SGOT elevation
(*see under* Aspartate aminotransferase levels, elevation of)

SGPT changes
(*see under* Alanine aminotransferase levels, changes in)

SGPT elevation
(*see under* Alanine aminotransferase levels, elevation of)

Shaking
(*see under* Tremors)

Shivering
(*see under* Tremors)

Shock
Abelcet Injection (Rare) 1141
Actiq 979
ADACEL Vaccine 2945
Boostrix (Rarely) 1404
Campral Tablets (Rare) 1174
Coumadin for Injection 898
Coumadin Tablets 898
Dilaudid 440
Dilaudid Non-Sterile Powder 440
Dilaudid Oral Liquid 445
Dilaudid Rectal Suppositories 440
Dilaudid Tablets 440
Dilaudid Tablets - 8 mg 445
Dilaudid-HP 442
Doxil Injection (Less than 1%) 2351
Effexor Tablets 3411
Effexor XR Capsules 3417
Elitek 2890
Ferrlecit Injection 3388
Fluarix 1451
Fluorescite Injection ⊙ 207
Herceptin I.V. (At least one of the 958 patients) 1233
Hyalgan Solution (One case) 2901
Hyperstat I.V. 3017
Imitrex Injection 1463
Imitrex Nasal Spray 1467
Imitrex Tablets 1471
Indocin Capsules (Less than 1%) 1995
Indocin I.V. (Less than 1%) 2465
Indocin (Less than 1%) 1995
Infanrix Vaccine 1476
Infed Injection 3390
Kadian Capsules 577
Lyrica Capsules (Rare) 2539
Merrem I.V. (1.2%) 686
Midamor Tablets 2026
Migranal Nasal Spray (Rare) 3348
Mobic Oral Suspension (Less than 0.1%) 863
Mobic Tablets (Less than 0.1%) 863
Motrin IB Tablets and Caplets 1866
Children's Motrin Oral Suspension ▣ 685
Children's Motrin Non-Staining Dye-Free Oral Suspension ▣ 685
Children's Motrin Oral Suspension 1867
Children's Motrin Non-Staining Dye-Free Oral Suspension 1867
Children's Motrin Cold Oral Suspension 1867
Infants' Motrin Concentrated Drops 1867
Infants' Motrin Non-Staining Dye-Free Concentrated Drops 1867
Junior Strength Motrin Caplets and Chewable Tablets 1867
MS Contin Tablets 2701
Mycamine for Injection 628
▲ Mylotarg for Injection (4%) 3431
Nexium I.V. (Rare) 659
Omnicef Capsules 511
Omnicef for Oral Suspension 511
Orthoclone OKT3 Sterile Solution (Less than 1%) 2360
OxyContin Tablets 2703
Pediarix Vaccine (Rare) 1548
Permax Tablets (Infrequent) 3356
Prevacid NapraPAC (Less than 1%) 3280
Prevnar for Injection 3463
Proleukin for Injection (Less than 1%) 2266
Prozac Pulvules and Liquid (Rare) 1801
Relpax Tablets (Rare) 2548
Rhophylac (Rare) 3505
Rilutek Tablets (Infrequent) 2930
Synera Topical Patch 1137
Trasylol Injection (1% to 2%) 754
Viagra Tablets (Less than 2%) 2573
Zofran Injection (Rare) 1634
Zofran 1639
Zofran ODT Orally Disintegrating Tablets 1639

Shock, anaphylactic
(*see under* Anaphylactic shock)

Shock, cardiogenic
Activase I.V. 1223
▲ Mavik Tablets (3.8%) 486
Retavase 2499
Revlimid Capsules 958
Rituxan I.V. 1254
TNKase I.V. 1264

Shock, hypovolemic
Prevacid Delayed-Release Capsules (Less than 1%) 3271
Prevacid for Delayed-Release Oral Suspension (Less than 1%) 3271
Prevacid SoluTab Delayed-Release Orally Disintegrating Tablets (Less than 1%) 3271
PREVPAC (Less than 1%) 3284

Shortness of breath
▲ Adenocard Injection (12%) 617
Aerobid/Aerobid-M (Less than 1%) 1171
Ceftin Tablets (0.1% to 1%) 1407
Clozaril Tablets (1%) 2184
Coumadin for Injection 898
Coumadin Tablets 898
Cubicin for Injection 1026
Dalmane Capsules (Rare) 3342
▲ Doxil Injection (Approximately 6.8%) 2351
DynaCirc CR Tablets (0.5% to 1%) 2721
Eldepryl Capsules 3208
▲ Epogen for Injection (0.14% to 14%) 591
Flumist Vaccine 1901
Gantrisin Pediatric Suspension 2770
Humalog-Pen (Less common) 1781
Humalog Mix 50/50-Pen 1783
Humalog Mix 75/25-Pen (Less common) 1785
Humulin 50/50, 100 Units 1791
Humulin 70/30 Pen (Less common) 1793
Humulin L, 100 Units (Less common) 1794
Humulin N Pen (Less common) 1797
Imitrex Injection 1463
Imitrex Nasal Spray 1467
Imitrex Tablets 1471
Klonopin 2778
K-Phos Original (Sodium Free) Tablets (Less frequent) 760
K-Phos Neutral Tablets 760
Kytril Injection (Rare) 2781
Kytril (Rare) 2784
▲ Leustatin Injection (7%) 2357
Lexapro Oral Solution (Infrequent) 1190
Lexapro Tablets (Infrequent) 1190
▲ Lopressor Injection (3%) 2238
▲ Lopressor Tablets (3%) 2238
▲ Lopressor HCT 50/25 Tablets (3%) 2241
▲ Lopressor HCT 100/25 Tablets (3%) 2241
▲ Lopressor HCT 100/50 Tablets (3%) 2241
Lupron Depot 7.5 mg 3264
Lupron Depot–3 Month 11.25 mg 3265
Lupron Injection Pediatric 3259
Midamor Tablets (Less than or equal to 1%) 2026
Moduretic Tablets 2028
Children's Motrin Oral Suspension ▣ 685
Children's Motrin Non-Staining Dye-Free Oral Suspension ▣ 685
Children's Motrin Oral Suspension 1867
Children's Motrin Non-Staining Dye-Free Oral Suspension 1867
Infants' Motrin Concentrated Drops 1867
Infants' Motrin Non-Staining Dye-Free Concentrated Drops 1867
Junior Strength Motrin Caplets and Chewable Tablets 1867
Neumega for Injection 3435
Niaspan Extended-Release Tablets 1730
NovoLog Injection 2326
Ortho-Cyclen Tablets 2429
Ortho Evra Transdermal System 2417
Ortho Tri-Cyclen Tablets 2429
Ortho Tri-Cyclen Lo Tablets 2436
Orthoclone OKT3 Sterile Solution (Less than 1%) 2360
▲ Procrit for Injection (0.14% to 14%) 2364
Prosed/DS Tablets 1157
ProstaScint Kit 1037
Retrovir Capsules 1560
Retrovir IV Infusion 1564
Retrovir 1560
Sandostatin Injection (Less than 1%) 2278
Sular Tablets (Very rare) 3122
▲ Thrombate III (1 of 17) 3257
▲ Toprol-XL Tablets (Approximately 3 of 100 patients) 668
▲ Tylenol with Codeine Tablets (Among most frequent) 2391
Uroqid-Acid No. 2 Tablets 760
Wellbutrin Tablets (Infrequent) 1603
Ziagen 1626
Zofran Injection (Rare) 1634
Zofran 1639
Zofran ODT Orally Disintegrating Tablets 1639

SIADH secretion syndrome
(*see under* ADH syndrome, inappropriate)

Sialadenitis
Aldoril Tablets 1910
Amerge Tablets (Rare) 1339
Atacand HCT 651
Avalide Tablets 888
Avalide Tablets 2874
Diovan HCT Tablets 2196
Diuril Oral Suspension 1954
Diuril Sodium Intravenous 2467
Dyazide Capsules 1423
▲ Evoxac Capsules (1% to 3%) 1047
Hyzaar 50-12.5 Tablets 1990
Hyzaar 100-12.5 Tablets 1990
Hyzaar 100-25 Tablets 1990
Indapamide Tablets 2156
Kaletra (Less than 2%) 476
Lopressor HCT 50/25 Tablets 2241
Lopressor HCT 100/25 Tablets 2241
Lopressor HCT 100/50 Tablets 2241
Lotensin HCT Tablets 2246

Micardis HCT Tablets....... 856
Moduretic Tablets....... 2028
Paxil CR Controlled-Release Tablets (Rare)....... 1538
Paxil (Rare)....... 1530
Permax Tablets (Rare)....... 3356
Prinzide Tablets....... 2056
Raptiva for Injection (1 case)....... 1250
Rescriptor Tablets....... 2551
Teveten HCT Tablets....... 1737
Timolide Tablets....... 2086
Trileptal Tablets....... 2300
Trileptal Oral Suspension....... 2300
Uniretic Tablets....... 3100
Zomig Nasal Spray (Rare)....... 3523

Sialism

▲ Abilify Oral Solution (3%)....... 882
▲ Abilify Oral Solution (3%)....... 2450
▲ Abilify Discmelt Orally Disintegrating Tablets (3%)....... 882
▲ Abilify Discmelt Orally Disintegrating Tablets (3%)....... 2450
▲ Abilify Tablets (3%)....... 882
▲ Abilify Tablets (3%)....... 2450
Alferon N Injection (1%)....... 1665
Altace Capsules (Less than 1%)....... 1702
Ambien Tablets (Rare)....... 2851
Ambien CR Tablets (Rare)....... 2855
Aricept Tablets (Infrequent)....... 1094
Aricept ODT Tablets (Infrequent)....... 1094
Axert Tablets (Rare)....... 2396
Campral Tablets (Rare)....... 1174
Camptosar Injection....... 2604
Ceftin for Oral Suspension (0.1% to 1%)....... 1407
Celexa (Frequent)....... 1176
▲ Clozaril Tablets (More than 5% to 48%)....... 2184
Dalmane Capsules (Rare)....... 3342
Doxil Injection (Less than 1%)....... 2351
Effexor Tablets (Rare)....... 3411
Effexor XR Capsules (Rare)....... 3417
Emend Capsules (Greater than 0.5%)....... 1963
Evoxac Capsules (2.2%)....... 1047
Exelon Capsules (Infrequent)....... 2206
Exelon Oral Solution (Infrequent)....... 2206
▲ FazaClo Orally Disintegrating Tablets (Greater than 5% to 48%)....... 551
Frova Tablets (Infrequent)....... 1113
Gabitril Tablets (Infrequent)....... 984
Garamycin Injectable....... 3014
▲ Geodon Capsules (4%)....... 2529
Hyperstat I.V....... 3017
Imitrex Injection....... 1463
Imitrex Nasal Spray....... 1467
▲ Intron A for Injection (Less than 5%)....... 3024
Klonopin....... 2778
Lamictal (Infrequent)....... 1481
Lithobid Tablets....... 1692
▲ Megace ES Oral Suspension (1% to 3%)....... 2481
Meridia Capsules....... 489
Mirapex Tablets (1% or more)....... 859
Moban Tablets (Occasional)....... 1119
Neurontin Capsules (Infrequent)....... 2487
Neurontin Oral Solution (Infrequent)....... 2487
Neurontin Tablets (Infrequent)....... 2487
▲ Niravam Orally Disintegrating Tablets (4.2% to 5.6%)....... 3092
Parcopa Orally Disintegrating Tablets....... 3097
Paxil CR Controlled-Release Tablets (Infrequent)....... 1538
Paxil (Infrequent)....... 1530
Prevacid Delayed-Release Capsules (Less than 1%)....... 3271
Prevacid for Delayed-Release Oral Suspension (Less than 1%)....... 3271
Prevacid SoluTab Delayed-Release Orally Disintegrating Tablets (Less than 1%)....... 3271
Prevacid NapraPAC (Less than 1%)....... 3280
PREVPAC (Less than 1%)....... 3284
Primaxin I.M....... 2045
Primaxin I.V. (Less than 0.2%)....... 2048
Prinivil Tablets (Greater than 1%)....... 2052
Prinzide Tablets....... 2056
Protonix I.V....... 3472
Protonix Tablets....... 3469
Prozac Pulvules and Liquid (Infrequent)....... 1801
Razadyne (Infrequent)....... 2399
Razadyne ER Extended-Release Capsules (Infrequent)....... 2399
Relpax Tablets (Infrequent)....... 2548
Requip Tablets (1% or more)....... 1555
Rescriptor Tablets....... 2551
▲ Risperdal (Up to 2% to 5%)....... 1676
▲ Risperdal Consta Long-Acting Injection (2% to 6%)....... 1682
▲ Risperdal M-Tab Orally Disintegrating Tablets (Up to 2% to 5%)....... 1676
Seroquel Tablets (Infrequent)....... 690
Sonata Capsules (Rare)....... 1717
▲ Soriatane Capsules (1% to 10%)....... 1013
Stalevo Tablets....... 2287
Symbyax Capsules (Frequent)....... 1819
Tasmar Tablets (Infrequent)....... 3358
Thiothixene Capsules (Infrequently)....... 2165
Tindamax Tablets....... 2142
▲ Topamax Sprinkle Capsules (6%)....... 2404
▲ Topamax Tablets (6%)....... 2404
Trecator Tablets....... 3487
▲ Ultane Liquid for Inhalation (2% to 4%)....... 531
Valium Tablets (Infrequent)....... 2819
▲ Wellbutrin Tablets (3.4%)....... 1603
Wellbutrin SR Sustained-Release Tablets (Infrequent)....... 1607
Wellbutrin XL Extended-Release Tablets (Infrequent)....... 1613
Xyrem Oral Solution (Infrequent)....... 1688
Zelapar Tablets....... 3372
Zoloft (Infrequent)....... 2586
Zomig Nasal Spray (Infrequent)....... 3523
Zyban Sustained-Release Tablets....... 1644
▲ Zyprexa Tablets (6%)....... 1830
▲ Zyprexa ZYDIS Orally Disintegrating Tablets (6%)....... 1830
Zyrtec Chewable Tablets (Less than 2%)....... 2594
Zyrtec (Less than 2%)....... 2594
Zyrtec-D 12 Hour Extended Release Tablets (Less than 2%)....... 2597

Sialorrhea

(*see under* Sialism)

Sialosis

(*see under* Sialism)

SICCA syndrome

(*see under* Sjögren's syndrome)

Sickle cell crises

Neupogen for Injection....... 603

Sickle cell disease

Neulasta Injection....... 601

Sinoatrial block

Blocadren Tablets (Less than 1%)....... 1916
Flumadine (Less than 0.3%)....... 1183
Neurontin Capsules (Rare)....... 2487
Neurontin Oral Solution (Rare)....... 2487
Neurontin Tablets (Rare)....... 2487
Rythmol SR Capsules....... 2727
Timoptic in Ocudose (Less frequent)....... 2091
Timoptic-XE Sterile Ophthalmic Gel Forming Solution....... 2092

Sinoatrial node dysfunction

Cardene I.V....... 2497

Sinus arrest

Catapres Tablets (Rare)....... 843
Nipent for Injection (Less than 3%)....... 1863
Rythmol SR Capsules....... 2727
▲ Tambocor Tablets (1% to 3%)....... 1856

Sinus bradycardia

Aciphex Tablets....... 1090
Activase I.V....... 1223
Adenocard Injection....... 617
Adenoscan....... 619
Catapres Tablets (Rare)....... 843
Catapres-TTS (0.5% or less)....... 844
Clorpres Tablets (Rare)....... 2153
Cozaar Tablets (Less than 1%)....... 1935
Eldepryl Capsules....... 3208
Hyzaar 50-12.5 Tablets....... 1990
Hyzaar 100-12.5 Tablets....... 1990
Hyzaar 100-25 Tablets....... 1990
Kytril Injection (Rare)....... 2781
Lanoxicaps Capsules....... 1490
Lanoxin Injection....... 1494
Lanoxin Injection Pediatric....... 1497
Lanoxin Tablets....... 1500
Retavase....... 2499
Rythmol SR Capsules (Greater than 2%)....... 2727
▲ Sandostatin Injection (25%)....... 2278
Sonata Capsules (Rare)....... 1717
Uniretic Tablets (Less than 1%)....... 3100
Zelapar Tablets....... 3372

Sinus congestion

▲ Aerobid/Aerobid-M (3% to 9%)....... 1171
▲ Asmanex Twisthaler (9%)....... 2966
Cardizem LA Extended Release Tablets (1% to 2%)....... 1728
Diovan HCT Tablets (Greater than 0.2%)....... 2196
Elidel Cream 1% (0.6% to 1.1%)....... 2200
Lexapro Oral Solution (Frequent)....... 1190
Lexapro Tablets (Frequent)....... 1190
▲ Myfortic Tablets (3% to less than 20%)....... 2255
▲ Serevent Diskus (9%)....... 1568
▲ Strattera Capsules (2% or greater)....... 1814
Tasmar Tablets (1% to 2%)....... 3358
▲ Ultram ER Tablets (1% to greater than 5%)....... 2392
Vivitrol....... 995
Xyrem Oral Solution (Frequent)....... 1688
Zelnorm Tablets (Up to 1%)....... 2312

Sinus discomfort

▲ Aerobid/Aerobid-M (1% to 3%)....... 1171
Avalide Tablets....... 888
Avalide Tablets....... 2874
Avapro Tablets (1% or greater)....... 891
Avapro Tablets (1% or greater)....... 2871
Cozaar Tablets (1% or greater)....... 1935
Imitrex Injection (2.2%)....... 1463
Imitrex Nasal Spray (0.8% to 2.4%)....... 1467
Maxalt Tablets (Infrequent)....... 2008
Maxalt-MLT Orally Disintegrating Tablets (Infrequent)....... 2008

Sinus disorder

Xyrem Oral Solution (Infrequent)....... 1688

Sinus drainage

▲ Aerobid/Aerobid-M (3% to 9%)....... 1171
Alferon N Injection (2%)....... 1665

Sinus exit block

Adenoscan (Less than 1%)....... 619

Sinus node dysfunction

Cardene I.V....... 2497
Lithobid Tablets....... 1692

Sinus pause

Adenoscan (Less than 1%)....... 619

Sinus syndrome, sick

Exelon Capsules (Infrequent)....... 2206
Exelon Oral Solution (Infrequent)....... 2206
Photofrin for Injection....... 702

Sinus tachycardia

Adenocard Injection....... 617
Aloxi Injection (Less than 1%)....... 2127
▲ Arranon Injection (0% to 8%)....... 1357
▲ Proleukin for Injection (70%)....... 2266
Strattera Capsules....... 1814
Taxotere Injection Concentrate (Rare)....... 2932

Sinusitis

Abilify Oral Solution (Frequent)....... 882
Abilify Oral Solution (Frequent)....... 2450
Abilify Discmelt Orally Disintegrating Tablets (Frequent)....... 882
Abilify Discmelt Orally Disintegrating Tablets (Frequent)....... 2450
Abilify Tablets (Frequent)....... 882
Abilify Tablets (Frequent)....... 2450
▲ Aceon Tablets (2 mg, 4 mg, 8 mg) (0.6% to 5.2%)....... 3194
Actiq (1% or greater)....... 979
▲ Actonel Tablets (4.5% to 4.9%)....... 2683
▲ Actonel with Calcium Tablets (4.5% to 4.6%)....... 2688
▲ ActoPlus Met Tablets (4.4% to 5%)....... 3214
▲ Actos Tablets (6.3%)....... 3219
▲ Advair Diskus 100/50 (3% to 4%)....... 1308
▲ Advair Diskus 250/50 (3% to 4%)....... 1308
▲ Advair Diskus 500/50 (3% To 4%)....... 1308
▲ Aerobid/Aerobid-M (3% to 9%)....... 1171
Agrylin Capsules (1% to 5%)....... 3169
Alamast Ophthalmic Solution (Less than 5%)....... 3381
▲ Aldara Cream, 5% (7.4%)....... 1846
Allegra (2.2%)....... 2844
Alphagan P Ophthalmic Solution (1% to 4%)....... 567
▲ Altoprev Extended-Release Tablets (4%)....... 3109
▲ Ambien Tablets (4%)....... 2851
Ambien CR Tablets (Frequent)....... 2855
AmBisome for Injection (Less common)....... 620
Amerge Tablets (Infrequent)....... 1339
▲ Amitiza Capsules (0% to 4.9%)....... 3224
▲ Angeliq Tablets (5.3%)....... 762
Aralast (Greater than or equal to 0.2%)....... 717
▲ Aredia for Injection (15.6%)....... 2179
▲ Arimidex Tablets (2% to 6%)....... 673
Aromasin Tablets (Less frequent)....... 2600
▲ Arranon Injection (0% to 7%)....... 1357
Asacol Delayed-Release Tablets (2% or greater)....... 2692
▲ Asmanex Twisthaler (5% to 22%)....... 2966
▲ Astelin Nasal Spray (Infrequently to 3.2%)....... 1904
Atacand Tablets (More than 1%)....... 649
Atacand HCT (0.5% or greater)....... 651
▲ Atripla Tablets (4%)....... 945
Atrovent Inhalation Solution (2.3%)....... 835
▲ Atrovent HFA Inhalation Aerosol (1% to 11%)....... 841
▲ Avandia Tablets (1% to 3.2%)....... 1384
Axert Tablets (Infrequent)....... 2396
Axid Oral Solution (2.4%)....... 879
▲ Azmacort Inhalation Aerosol (2% to 9%)....... 1726
▲ Betimol Ophthalmic Solution (1% to 5%)....... 3382
▲ Betimol Ophthalmic Solution (1% to 5%)....... ⊙295
▲ BiDil Tablets (4%)....... 2171
▲ Caduet Tablets (2.5% to 6.4%)....... 2508
Campath Ampules....... 811
Carac Cream, 0.5% (1.6%)....... 2879
▲ Carnitor Injection (2% to 3%)....... 3188
Carteolol Hydrochloride Ophthalmic Solution USP, 1% (Occasional)....... ⊙249
Caverject Impulse Injection (2%)....... 2612
Ceftin for Oral Suspension (0.1% to 1%)....... 1407
▲ Celebrex Capsules (5%)....... 3134
▲ Celexa (3%)....... 1176
▲ CellCept Capsules (3% to 26%)....... 2747
▲ CellCept Intravenous (3% to 26%)....... 2747
▲ CellCept Oral Suspension (3% to 26%)....... 2747
▲ CellCept Tablets (3% to 26%)....... 2747
▲ Climara Transdermal System (4% to 5%)....... 771
▲ Climara Pro Transdermal System (3.8%)....... 776
Colazal Capsules (1%)....... 2838
Combivent Inhalation Aerosol (2.3%)....... 847
▲ Concerta Extended-Release Tablets (3%)....... 1881
Copaxone for Injection (At least 2%)....... 3297
Cosopt Sterile Ophthalmic Solution (1% to 5%)....... 1931
▲ Cozaar Tablets (1% to 6%)....... 1935
Crestor Tablets (2%)....... 678
▲ Dacogen Injection (5%)....... 2129
▲ Depacon Injection (1% to 5%)....... 412
▲ Depakene (1% to 5%)....... 417
▲ Depakote Sprinkle Capsules (1% to 5%)....... 422
▲ Depakote Tablets (1% to 5%)....... 427
▲ Depakote ER Tablets (1% to 5%)....... 434
▲ depo-subQ provera 104 Injectable Suspension (1% to less than 5%)....... 2624
Detrol Tablets (1.1%)....... 2628
Detrol LA Capsules (2%)....... 2631
Diovan Tablets (More than 1%)....... 2193
Diovan HCT Tablets (Greater than 0.2%)....... 2196
▲ Ditropan XL Extended-Release Tablets (2% to less than 5%)....... 2413
▲ Doxil Injection (1% to 10%)....... 2351
DuoNeb Inhalation Solution....... 1058
Duragesic Transdermal System (Greater than or less than 1%)....... 2373
Edex Injection (1%)....... 3089
Effexor XR Capsules (2%)....... 3417
▲ Elestat Ophthalmic Solution (1% to 3%)....... 1669
▲ Elidel Cream 1% (0.6% to 3.3%)....... 2200
▲ Emsam Transdermal System (3%)....... 903
Enablex Extended-Release Tablets (Greater than or equal to 1%)....... 2203
▲ Enbrel for Injection (3% to 5%)....... 584
▲ Enjuvia Tablets (3% to 7%)....... 1062
▲ Equetro Extended-Release Capsules (Less than 5%)....... 3180
▲ Estrasorb Topical Emulsion (6%)....... 1147
▲ Estring Vaginal Ring (4%)....... 2635
▲ Evista Tablets (7.9% to 10.3%)....... 1763
▲ Evoxac Capsules (12.3%)....... 1047
▲ Exubera Inhalation Powder (5.4% to 10.3%)....... 2524
Fabrazyme for Intravenous Infusion (2%)....... 1274
Famvir Tablets (1.3% to 2.6%)....... 2211
▲ Flebogamma 5%, Immune Globulin Intravenous (Human) (39%)....... 1658
▲ Flomax Capsules (2.2% to 3.7%)....... 850
▲ Flovent Diskus (10% to 33%)....... 1443
▲ Flovent HFA (1% to 6%)....... 1447
Floxin Otic Solution (Single report)....... 1049
▲ Flumist Vaccine (4.1%)....... 1901
▲ Follistim AQ Cartridge (5%)....... 2338
Foradil Aerolizer (2.7%)....... 3010
▲ Fortical Nasal Spray (1% to 3%)....... 3337

Frova Tablets (Frequent)........ 1113
▲ Fuzeon Injection (6%) 2767
Gabitril Tablets (1% or more)........ 984
Gengraf Capsules (Less than 1%)..... 459
▲ Gleevec Tablets (0.4% to 11%) 2227
Hepsera Tablets (2% or greater)...... 1292
▲ Herceptin I.V. (9%) 1233
▲ Humira Injection (11%) 466
Hytrin Capsules (2.6%)........ 471
Hyzaar 50-12.5 Tablets (1.2%)........ 1990
Hyzaar 100-12.5 Tablets (1.2%)...... 1990
Hyzaar 100-25 Tablets (1.2%)........ 1990
▲ Imdur Tablets (Less than or equal to 5%)........ 3018
Imitrex Nasal Spray 1467
Indapamide Tablets (Less than 5%).. 2156
▲ Infergen (12% to 17%) 3364
▲ Intron A for Injection (Up to 21%) 3024
Invirase (Less than 2% to 2.7%)...... 2772
Ionsys Transdermal System (.1% to less than 1%)........ 2379
▲ I.V. Busulfex (3%) 2493
Kaletra (Less than 2%) 476
Keppra Injection (2%) 3320
Keppra Oral Solution (2%) 3314
Keppra Tablets (2%) 3314
▲ Kineret Injection (7%) 599
▲ Klonopin (4%) 2778
Lamictal (2%) 1481
Lescol Capsules (2.6%) 2233
▲ Lescol XL Tablets (3.5%) 2233
Levaquin (1.1%) 2384
Levaquin in 5% Dextrose Injection (1.1%) 2384
▲ Levitra Tablets (3%) 3034
▲ Lexapro Oral Solution (3%) 1190
▲ Lexapro Tablets (3%) 1190
▲ Lipitor Tablets (Up to 6.4%) 2483
Lofibra Tablets 1219
Lofibra Capsules 1216
Lotensin Tablets (Less than 1%) 2243
Lotensin HCT Tablets (More than 1%) 2246
▲ Lucentis Injection (2% to 8%) 1237
Marinol Capsules (Less than 1%) 3333
▲ Mepron Suspension (7%) 1521
▲ Meridia Capsules (5%) 489
Metrogel 1% (1.4%) 1211
▲ Miacalcin Nasal Spray (1% to 3%) ... 2253
▲ Micardis Tablets (3%) 854
▲ Micardis HCT Tablets (4%) 856
Migranal Nasal Spray (1%) 3348
Mirapex Tablets (1% or more) 859
▲ Mirena Intrauterine System (5% or more) 787
▲ Myfortic Tablets (3% to less than 20%) 2255
Nasacort AQ Nasal Spray 2922
▲ Nasonex Nasal Spray (4% to 5%) 3043
▲ Neoral Oral Solution (1% to 7%) 2259
▲ Neoral Soft Gelatin Capsules (1% to 7%) 2259
Neurontin Capsules (Infrequent) 2487
Neurontin Oral Solution (Infrequent) 2487
Neurontin Tablets (Infrequent) 2487
▲ Nevanac Ophthalmic Suspension 0.1% (1% to 4%)........ ⊙ 209
Nexium Delayed-Release Capsules (Less than 1%) 655
Nexium I.V. (Less than 1%) 659
▲ Nipent for Injection (6%) 1863
▲ NuvaRing (5% to 14%) 2340
Omacor Capsules 2725
Oracea Capsules (2.6%) 1000
▲ Orencia Powder for Intravenous Infusion (5% to 13%) 914
Patanol Ophthalmic Solution (Less than 5%) 561
▲ Paxil CR Controlled-Release Tablets (Infrequent to 4%) 1538
▲ Paxil (Infrequent to 4%) 1530
▲ PEG-Intron Powder for Injection (7%) 3048
Permax Tablets (Infrequent) 3356
▲ Photofrin for Injection (4%) 702
Plavix Tablets (1% to 2.5%) 917
Plavix Tablets (1% to 2.5%) 2926
Pletal Tablets (Less than 2%) 2455
▲ Premarin Tablets (6% to 11%) 3446
▲ Premphase Tablets (7% to 10%) 3456
▲ Prempro Tablets (7% to 10%) 3456
Prevacid Delayed-Release Capsules (Less than 1%) 3271
Prevacid for Delayed-Release Oral Suspension (Less than 1%) 3271
Prevacid SoluTab Delayed-Release Orally Disintegrating Tablets (Less than 1%) 3271
Prevacid NapraPAC (Less than 1%) .. 3280
PREVPAC (Less than 1%) 3284
Prinivil Tablets (0.3% to 1.0%) 2052
Prinzide Tablets (0.3% to 1%) 2056
Prochieve 4% Gel 1003
Prochieve 8% Gel........ 1003
▲ Prograf Capsules and Injection (3% to 15%)........ 632
▲ Prometrium Capsules (100 mg, 200 mg) (Less than 5%)........ 3203
ProQuad........ 2064
ProSom Tablets (Infrequent)........ 517
Protonix I.V. (Greater than or equal to 1%)........ 3472
Protonix Tablets (Greater than or equal to 1%)........ 3469
▲ Protopic Ointment (2% to 7%) 638
Provigil Tablets (At least 1%)........ 988
▲ Prozac Pulvules and Liquid (1% to 6%)........ 1801
Pulmozyme Inhalation Solution........ 1248
Qvar Inhalation Aerosol (Up to 3%)... 3303
▲ Rapamune Oral Solution and Tablets (3% to 20%)........ 3475
Raptiva for Injection........ 1250
▲ Rebetol (Less than 1% to 12%) 3058
▲ Rebetron Combination Therapy (9% to 12%)........ 3063
ReFacto Vials........ 3484
▲ Relenza Rotadisk (2% to 3%) 1552
Relpax Tablets (Rare)........ 2548
▲ Remicade for IV Injection (14%) 971
▲ Requip Tablets (4%) 1555
▲ Rescriptor Tablets (1.2% to 7.3%) ... 2551
▲ Retisert Implant (5% to 15%) .... ⊙ 258
Retrovir Capsules 1560
Retrovir IV Infusion........ 1564
Retrovir........ 1560
▲ Revatio Tablets (3%) 2557
▲ Revlimid Capsules (8.1%) 958
▲ Ribavirin, USP Capsules (Less than 1% to 12%)........ 3068
Rilutek Tablets (0.4% to 1.6%)........ 2930
▲ Risperdal (1% to 4%) 1676
▲ Risperdal Consta Long-Acting Injection (1% to 3%)........ 1682
▲ Risperdal M-Tab Orally Disintegrating Tablets (1% to 4%)........ 1676
▲ Rituxan I.V. (0% to 6%) 1254
▲ Sandimmune (Less than 1% to 7%)........ 2275
▲ Sandostatin LAR Depot (5% to 15%)........ 2280
▲ Serevent Diskus (2% to greater than or equal to 3%)........ 1568
▲ Simulect for Injection (3% to 10%) ... 2284
Singulair (Greater than or equal to 1%)........ 2077
▲ Somavert Injection (4% to 8%) 2642
▲ Soriatane Capsules (1% to 10%) 1013
▲ Spiriva HandiHaler (3% to 11%) 869
▲ Strattera Capsules (6%) 1814
▲ Sular Tablets (3%) 3122
▲ Symbicort 80/4.5 Inhalation Aerosol (5.8%)........ 3511
▲ Symbicort 160/4.5 Inhalation Aerosol (4.8%)........ 3511
Synagis (More than 1%)........ 1897
Tamiflu Capsules (1.7%)........ 2807
Tamiflu Oral Suspension (2%)........ 2807
Tasmar Tablets (1% or more)........ 3358
▲ Temodar Capsules (6%) 3073
Teveten Tablets (1% or greater)........ 1735
Teveten HCT Tablets........ 1737
▲ Thalomid Capsules (4.2%) 965
▲ TOBI Solution for Inhalation (8.1%) .. 2298
▲ Topamax Sprinkle Capsules (2% to 10%)........ 2404
▲ Topamax Tablets (2% to 10%) 2404
Travatan Ophthalmic Solution (1% to 5%)........ 563
Tricor Tablets........ 527
▲ Trileptal Tablets (2% to 4%) 2300
▲ Trileptal Oral Suspension (2% to 4%)........ 2300
▲ Trisenox Injection (20%) 993
▲ Truvada Tablets (4%) 1296
Twinrix Vaccine........ 1595
▲ Ultram ER Tablets (1% to greater than 5%)........ 2392
Uniretic Tablets (More than 1%)........ 3100
Univasc Tablets (Greater than 1%).... 3104
Uroxatral Tablets (1% to 2%)........ 2943
▲ Vagifem Tablets (3% to 5%) 2334
Vantin Tablets and Oral Suspension (Less than 1%)........ 2645
▲ Verelan PM Extended-Release Capsules, Controlled-Onset (3%)........ 3106
VFEND I.V. (Less than 2%)........ 2564
VFEND Oral Suspension (Less than 2%)........ 2564
VFEND Tablets (Less than 2%)........ 2564
Viagra Tablets (Less than 2%)........ 2573
Vicoprofen Tablets (Less than 1%).... 539
Viracept (Less than 2%)........ 2577
▲ Vivitrol (12% to 13%) 995
Vytorin 10/10 Tablets........ 2114
Vytorin 10/10 Tablets........ 3077
Vytorin 10/20 Tablets........ 2114
Vytorin 10/20 Tablets........ 3077
Vytorin 10/40 Tablets........ 2114
Vytorin 10/40 Tablets........ 3077
Vytorin 10/80 Tablets........ 2114
Vytorin 10/80 Tablets........ 3077
WelChol Tablets (2%)........ 1050
▲ Wellbutrin SR Sustained-Release Tablets (1% to 3%)........ 1607
▲ Wellbutrin XL Extended-Release Tablets (1% to 5%)........ 1613
▲ Xolair (16%) 1266
▲ Xopenex Inhalation Solution (1.4% to 4.2%)........ 3146
▲ Xopenex Inhalation Solution Concentrate (1.4% to 4.2%)........ 3150
▲ Xopenex HFA Inhalation Aerosol (1.4% to 4.2%)........ 3154
Xyrem Oral Solution (Frequent)........ 1688
Yasmin 28 Tablets (Greater than 1%)........ 796
Yaz Tablets (Greater than 1%)........ 803
▲ Zelnorm Tablets (3%) 2312
Zemaira (1.5%)........ 3509
▲ Zetia Tablets (3.5% to 4.6%) 2120
▲ Zetia Tablets (3.6% to 4.6%) 3083
Zoloft (Infrequent to 2%)........ 2586
Zomig Nasal Spray (Infrequent)........ 3523
Zyban Sustained-Release Tablets (2%)........ 1644
Zyrtec Chewable Tablets (Less than 2%)........ 2594
Zyrtec (Less than 2%)........ 2594
Zyrtec-D 12 Hour Extended Release Tablets (Less than 2%)..... 2597

Sinusitis, allergic
Xyrem Oral Solution (Infrequent)....... 1688

Sjögren's syndrome
Mintezol 2027

Skin, anesthesia
(*see under* Numbness, skin)

Skin, burning of
Clobex Lotion........ 1204
▲ Differin Cream (Less than 1% to 24%)........ 1210
▲ Differin Gel (10% to 40%) 1211
▲ Diprolene Gel 0.05% (6%) 3001
Diprolene Lotion 0.05% (1%)........ 3002
Diprolene Ointment 0.05% (Infrequent)........ 3003
Diprolene AF Cream 0.05% (Infrequent)........ 3000
Diprosone Cream, USP 0.05%........ 3004
Drysol Solution........ 2507
▲ Duac Topical Gel (0% to 5%) 3212
Klonopin (Infrequent)........ 2778
Lotrisone (1.6%)........ 3040
▲ Luxíq Foam (2% to 44%) 1010
Oxistat (1.7%)........ 2667
Oxsoralen Lotion 1%........ 3352
Oxsoralen-Ultra Capsules........ 3353
ProctoFoam-HC........ 3099
▲ Protopic Ointment (25% to 58%) 638
▲ Tri-Luma Cream (6.68% to 18%) 1213
Zovirax Cream (Less than 1%)........ 820

Skin, cracking
Clobevate Gel (Less than 2%)........ 3211
Diprolene Gel 0.05%........ 3001
Olux Foam (Less than 2%)........ 1012
▲ Panretin Gel (1% to 8%) 1747
Soriatane Capsules 1013
Temovate Cream (Less frequent)..... 2668
▲ Temovate Gel (Among most frequent)........ 2669
Temovate Ointment (Less frequent)........ 2668
Temovate E Emollient (Less than 2%)........ 2671

Skin, darkening
Claripel Cream (Rare)........ 3211

Skin, dryness of
(*see under* Xerosis cutis)

Skin, eruptions of
▲ Anaprox Tablets (3% to 9%) 2761
▲ Anaprox DS Tablets (3% to 9%) 2761
Biaxin/Biaxin XL........ 402
Cosmegen for Injection........ 2459
Daranide Tablets........ 1950
▲ EC-Naprosyn Delayed-Release Tablets (3% to 9%)........ 2761
E.E.S........ 451
Ery-Tab Tablets........ 449
Erythrocin Stearate Filmtab Tablets........ 453
Erythromycin Delayed-Release Capsules, USP (Rare)........ 457
Fansidar Tablets........ 2765
Imitrex Injection (Infrequent)........ 1463
Imitrex Nasal Spray (Infrequent)....... 1467
▲ Naprosyn Suspension (3% to 9%) 2761
▲ Naprosyn Tablets (3% to 9%) 2761
Norvir........ 503
Paser Granules........ 1674
PCE Dispertab Tablets (Rare)........ 515
PREVPAC........ 3284
Tessalon Capsules........ 1199
Tessalon Perles........ 1199
Thioridazine Hydrochloride Tablets (Infrequent)........ 2163
Trasylol Injection........ 754

Skin, exfoliation
Levaquin (0.1% to 0.9%)........ 2384
Levaquin in 5% Dextrose Injection (0.1% to 0.9%)........ 2384
▲ Panretin Gel (3% to 9%) 1747
▲ Trisenox Injection (5%) 993

Skin, exfoliation, application site
Lidoderm Patch........ 1118

Skin, flakiness
▲ Advair Diskus 100/50 (1% to 3%) ... 1308
▲ Advair Diskus 250/50 (1% to 3%) ... 1308
▲ Advair Diskus 500/50 (1% to 3%) ... 1308
▲ Panretin Gel (3% to 9%) 1747
Zovirax Cream (Less than 1%)........ 820

Skin, fragile
Accutane Capsules........ 2731
Colocort Rectal Suspension, USP (Retention) 100 mg/60 mL........ 2476
Depo-Medrol Injectable Suspension........ 2617
Depo-Medrol Single-Dose Vial........ 2619
Photofrin for Injection........ 702
Soriatane Capsules........ 1013

Skin, fragility
Cuprimine Capsules........ 1947
Decadron Tablets........ 1951
Hydrocortone Tablets........ 1989

Skin, friability of
Thiola Tablets........ 2141

Skin, irritation of
Accuzyme Debriding Ointment (Occasional)........ 1662
Accuzyme SE Spray Emulsion (Occasional)........ 1662
Blocadren Tablets........ 1916
Carac Cream, 0.5% (1.2%)........ 2879
Clobevate Gel (Less than 2%)........ 3211
Clobex Lotion........ 1204
▲ Clobex Shampoo (4.7%) 1206
Cosopt Sterile Ophthalmic Solution........ 1931
▲ Cutivate Cream (0.8% to 4.5%) 2662
Differin Cream (1%)........ 1210
Differin Gel (Approximately 1% or less)........ 1211
Diprolene Gel 0.05%........ 3001
Diprolene Lotion 0.05% (Less than 1%)........ 3002
Diprolene Ointment 0.05% (Infrequent)........ 3003
Diprolene AF Cream 0.05% (Infrequent)........ 3000
Diprosone Cream, USP 0.05%........ 3004
Elocon Cream 0.1% (Infrequent)........ 3005
Elocon Lotion 0.1% (Infrequent)........ 3006
Elocon Ointment 0.1% (Infrequent)... 3007
Lotrimin........ 3039
Lotrisone........ 3040
Luxíq Foam........ 1010
Ovide .5% Lotion........ 3290
Oxistat Cream (0.4%)........ 2667
Panafil Ointment (Occasional)........ 1663
Panafil SE Spray Emulsion (Occasional)........ 1663
ProctoFoam-HC........ 3099
Soriatane Capsules (Less than 1%).. 1013
ThermaCare Heat Wraps........ 2677
Timolide Tablets........ 2086
Timoptic Sterile Ophthalmic Solution........ 2088
Timoptic in Ocudose........ 2091
Timoptic-XE Sterile Ophthalmic Gel Forming Solution........ 2092
Tri-Luma Cream (2%)........ 1213
Xerac AC Solution........ 2507

Skin, lesions non-specific
▲ Dacogen Injection (11%) 2129
Invanz for Injection (Greater than 0.5%)........ 1999
▲ NeoProfen Injection (16%) 2472
Prinivil Tablets (0.3% to 1.0%)........ 2052

Prinzide Tablets 2056
▲ Trisenox Injection (8%) 993

Skin, reddening

Motrin IB Tablets and Caplets 1866
Children's Motrin Oral Suspension 1867
Children's Motrin Non-Staining Dye-Free Oral Suspension 1867
Children's Motrin Cold Oral Suspension 1867
Infants' Motrin Concentrated Drops 1867
Infants' Motrin Non-Staining Dye-Free Concentrated Drops 1867
Junior Strength Motrin Caplets and Chewable Tablets 1867
Rosac Cream with Sunscreens 3213
ThermaCare Heat Wraps 2677

Skin, scaling of

▲ Panretin Gel (25% to 77%) 1747

Skin, tenderness

Efudex 3363
Imitrex Injection (Rare) 1463
Imitrex Nasal Spray 1467
Imitrex Tablets (Infrequent) 1471
Naftin Gel (0.5%) 2126

Skin, tightness of

Diprolene Gel 0.05% 3001

Skin, wrinkling

Ambien CR Tablets (1%) 2855
Amerge Tablets (Rare) 1339
Imitrex Nasal Spray 1467
Imitrex Tablets (Rare) 1471
Photofrin for Injection 702
▲ Thiola Tablets (16.7%) 2141

Skin atrophy

Aclovate Cream (Infrequent) 2660
Analpram-HC 1159
Apexicon E Cream 2661
Clobevate Gel (Less than 2%) 3211
▲ Clobex Lotion (4.2%) 1204
Clobex Shampoo (Infrequent) 1206
Copaxone for Injection (Frequent) 3297
Cutivate Cream (Infrequent) 2662
Cutivate Lotion 0.05% (Rare) 2664
Cutivate Ointment (Infrequent to more frequent) 2665
Diprolene Gel 0.05% 3001
Diprolene Lotion 0.05% (Infrequent) 3002
Diprolene Ointment 0.05% (Infrequent) 3003
Diprolene AF Cream 0.05% (Infrequent) 3000
Diprosone Cream, USP 0.05% 3004
Effexor Tablets (Rare) 3411
Effexor XR Capsules (Rare) 3417
Elocon Cream 0.1% (1.6%) 3005
Elocon Lotion 0.1% (Infrequent) 3006
▲ Elocon Ointment 0.1% (4.8%) 3007
Locoid Lipocream Cream (Infrequent) 1160
Lotrisone 3040
Luxíq Foam 1010
Lyrica Capsules (Rare) 2539
Olux Foam (Less than 2%) 1012
Pramosone 1161
ProctoFoam-HC 3099
Soriatane Capsules 1013
Temovate Cream (Less frequent) 2668
▲ Temovate Gel (Among most frequent) 2669
Temovate Ointment (Less frequent) 2668
Temovate Scalp Application (Infrequent) 2670
Temovate E Emollient (Less than 2%) 2671
Tri-Luma Cream 1213
Vanos Cream 1893

Skin desquamation

Gemzar for Injection (Very rare) 1771
▲ Panretin Gel (3% to 9%) 1747
Revlimid Capsules 958
Taxotere Injection Concentrate (1.8%) 2932

Skin discoloration

Abilify Oral Solution (Infrequent) 882
Abilify Oral Solution (Infrequent) 2450
Abilify Discmelt Orally Disintegrating Tablets (Infrequent) 882
Abilify Discmelt Orally Disintegrating Tablets (Infrequent) 2450
Abilify Tablets (Infrequent) 882
Abilify Tablets (Infrequent) 2450
Aciphex Tablets (Rare) 1090
Actiq (Less than 1%) 979
Altoprev Extended-Release Tablets 3109
AmBisome for Injection (Less common) 620
Aricept Tablets (Infrequent) 1094
Aricept ODT Tablets (Infrequent) 1094
Atripla Tablets 945
▲ Avastin IV (2% to 16%) 1227
Betaseron for SC Injection 767
Caduet Tablets (Less than 0.1%) 2508
Carbatrol Capsules 3171
Celexa (Infrequent) 1176
Denavir Cream 2174
Differin Cream (Less than 1%) 1210
▲ Doxil Injection (Less than 1% to 10%) 2351
Effexor Tablets (Rare) 3411
Effexor XR Capsules (Rare) 3417
Emtriva Capsules 1287
Emtriva Oral Solution 1287
Estratest Tablets 3199
Estratest H.S. Tablets 3199
Evoxac Capsules (Less than 1%) 1047
Ferrlecit Injection 3388
Fluorescite Injection ⊙ 207
Gabitril Tablets (Infrequent) 984
Infed Injection 3390
▲ Intron A for Injection (Less than 5%) 3024
Invirase (Less than 2%) 2772
▲ I.V. Busulfex (8%) 2493
Kaletra (Less than 2%) 476
Keppra Oral Solution (2%) 3314
Keppra Tablets (2%) 3314
Lamictal (Rare) 1481
Lescol Capsules 2233
Lescol XL Tablets 2233
Lunesta Tablets (Infrequent) 3142
Mevacor Tablets 2021
Neumega for Injection 3435
Neurontin Capsules (Rare) 2487
Neurontin Oral Solution (Rare) 2487
Neurontin Tablets (Rare) 2487
Norvasc Tablets (Less than 0.1%) 2545
Oxandrin Tablets 2962
Paxil CR Controlled-Release Tablets (Rare) 1538
Paxil (Rare) 1530
Permax Tablets (Infrequent) 3356
Photofrin for Injection 702
Prochieve 4% Gel 1003
Prochieve 8% Gel 1003
▲ Prograf Capsules and Injection (3% to 15%) 632
Protopic Ointment (Greater than or equal to 1%) 638
Prozac Pulvules and Liquid (Infrequent) 1801
Psoriatec Cream 1089
Relpax Tablets (Rare) 2548
Rescriptor Tablets 2551
Retrovir IV Infusion 1564
Seroquel Tablets (Rare) 690
Sonata Capsules (Rare) 1717
Striant Mucoadhesive 1007
Sular Tablets (Less than or equal to 1%) 3122
Sustiva Capsules 930
Sustiva Tablets 930
▲ Sutent Capsules (0% ro 33%) 2560
Symbyax Capsules (Infrequent) 1819
▲ Synera Topical Patch (Less than 4%) 1137
Tasmar Tablets (Infrequent) 3358
Tegretol/Tegretol-XR 2295
Thalomid Capsules 965
Ticlid Tablets 2810
Topamax Sprinkle Capsules (1%) 2404
Topamax Tablets (1%) 2404
Trasylol Injection (1% to 2%) 754
Truvada Tablets 1296
VFEND I.V. (Less than 2%) 2564
VFEND Oral Suspension (Less than 2%) 2564
VFEND Tablets (Less than 2%) 2564
Vytorin 10/10 Tablets 2114
Vytorin 10/10 Tablets 3077
Vytorin 10/20 Tablets 2114
Vytorin 10/20 Tablets 3077
Vytorin 10/40 Tablets 2114
Vytorin 10/40 Tablets 3077
Vytorin 10/80 Tablets 2114
Vytorin 10/80 Tablets 3077
Zelapar Tablets 3372
Zocor Tablets 2105
Zoloft (Rare) 2586
Zyprexa Tablets (Infrequent) 1830
Zyprexa ZYDIS Orally Disintegrating Tablets (Infrequent) 1830

Skin disorder, unspecified

Advicor Tablets 1722
▲ Agrylin Capsules (1% to 5%) 3169
AmBisome for Injection (Less common) 620
▲ Betaseron for SC Injection (12%) 767
▲ Catapres-TTS (51 of 101 patients) 844
▲ CellCept Capsules (3% to less than 20%) 2747
▲ CellCept Intravenous (3% to less than 20%) 2747
▲ CellCept Oral Suspension (3% to less than 20%) 2747
▲ CellCept Tablets (3% to less than 20%) 2747
Cipro XR Tablets (Less than 1%) 2990
depo-subQ provera 104 Injectable Suspension (1%) 2624
▲ Doxil Injection (1% to 5%) 2351
Edex Injection (1%) 3089
Elocon Lotion 0.1% (1 in 65 patients) 3006
Elocon Ointment 0.1% (1 in 63 patients) 3007
▲ Eloxatin for Injection (2% to 32%) 2892
▲ Epogen for Injection (7% to 29%) 591
▲ Erbitux (4% to 15%) 910
EryPed 447
▲ Evoxac Capsules (1% to 3%) 1047
Invirase (Rare) 2772
Klonopin (Infrequent) 2778
Lamisil Tablets (Isolated reports) 2232
Lanoxicaps Capsules (Rare) 1490
Lanoxin Injection (Rare) 1494
Lanoxin Injection Pediatric (Rare) 1497
▲ Leukine (77%) 814
Levaquin (0.1% to 0.9%) 2384
Levaquin in 5% Dextrose Injection (0.1% to 0.9%) 2384
▲ Levulan Kerastick for Topical Solution, 20% (5% to 12%) 1085
Lofibra Tablets 1219
Lofibra Capsules 1216
Loprox Shampoo 1888
Lupron Depot 3.75 mg (2%) 3260
Lupron Depot 7.5 mg (Less than 5%) 3264
Lupron Depot–3 Month 11.25 mg (2%) 3265
▲ Megace ES Oral Suspension (1% to 3%) 2481
Mirapex Tablets (2%) 859
▲ Mirena Intrauterine System (5% or more) 787
▲ Neoral Oral Solution (1% to 17.6%) 2259
▲ Neoral Soft Gelatin Capsules (1% to 17.6%) 2259
▲ Nipent for Injection (4% to 17%) 1863
Prevacid Delayed-Release Capsules (Less than 1%) 3271
Prevacid for Delayed-Release Oral Suspension (Less than 1%) 3271
Prevacid SoluTab Delayed-Release Orally Disintegrating Tablets (Less than 1%) 3271
Prevacid NapraPAC (Less than 1%) 3280
PREVPAC (Less than 1%) 3284
Prilosec OTC Delayed-Release Tablets (Very rare) 2677
Primaxin I.M. 2045
Primaxin I.V. (Less than 0.2%) 2048
Prinivil Tablets (Rare) 2052
Prinzide Tablets (Rare) 2056
Prochieve 4% Gel 1003
Prochieve 8% Gel 1003
▲ Prograf Capsules and Injection (3% to 15%) 632
Protonix I.V. (Less than 1%) 3472
Protonix Tablets (Less than 1%) 3469
Relpax Tablets (Infrequent) 2548
Rescriptor Tablets 2551
Rilutek Tablets (Infrequent) 2930
Rocaltrol Capsules 2798
Rocaltrol Oral Solution 2798
▲ Romazicon Injection (1% to 3%) 2804
Soriatane Capsules (Less than 1%) 1013
▲ Taxotere Injection Concentrate (0.6% to 54.1%) 2932
Thyrolar Tablets 1199
▲ Topamax Sprinkle Capsules (1% to 3%) 2404
▲ Topamax Tablets (1% to 3%) 2404
Tricor Tablets 527
▲ Vesanoid Capsules (14%) 2820
VFEND I.V. (Less than 2%) 2564
VFEND Oral Suspension (Less than 2%) 2564
VFEND Tablets (Less than 2%) 2564
▲ Vivaglobin (0.1% to 3%) 3506
Xalatan Sterile Ophthalmic Solution (1% to 2%) 2649
Yaz Tablets (Greater than 1%) 803
Zegerid Capsules (Very rare) 2958
Zegerid Powder for Oral Solution (Very rare) 2958
Zinecard for Injection (1%) 2650
Zocor Tablets 2105
Zoloft 2586
Zomig Nasal Spray (Infrequent) 3523
Zostavax Injection (1.1%) 2111
Zyrtec Chewable Tablets (Less than 2%) 2594
Zyrtec (Less than 2%) 2594
Zyrtec-D 12 Hour Extended Release Tablets (Less than 2%) 2597
Zyvox (0.9% to 2%) 2652

Skin eruptions

Bicillin C-R Injectable Suspension 1706
Gantrisin Pediatric Suspension 2770
Guanidine Hydrochloride Tablets 3016
Imitrex Tablets 1471
Librium Capsules 3347
▲ Prevacid NapraPAC (3% to 9%) 3280
Prezista Tablets (Less than 2%) 3306

Skin fissures

▲ Panretin Gel (1% to 8%) 1747

Skin hypertrophy

▲ CellCept Capsules (3% to less than 20%) 2747
▲ CellCept Intravenous (3% to less than 20%) 2747
▲ CellCept Oral Suspension (3% to less than 20%) 2747
▲ CellCept Tablets (3% to less than 20%) 2747
Copaxone for Injection (Infrequent) 3297
Effexor Tablets (Infrequent) 3411
Effexor XR Capsules (Infrequent) 3417
▲ Estring Vaginal Ring (1% to 3%) 2635
Evoxac Capsules (Less than 1%) 1047
Neurontin Capsules (Rare) 2487
Neurontin Oral Solution (Rare) 2487
Neurontin Tablets (Rare) 2487
Olux Foam (One case) 1012
Paxil CR Controlled-Release Tablets (Rare) 1538
Paxil (Rare) 1530
Pletal Tablets (Less than 2%) 2455
Protopic Ointment (0.2% to less than 1%) 638
▲ Rapamune Oral Solution and Tablets (3% to 20%) 3475
Relpax Tablets (Rare) 2548
Rescriptor Tablets 2551
Sonata Capsules (Infrequent) 1717
Soriatane Capsules (Less than 1%) 1013
Zelapar Tablets 3372

Skin nodule

Altoprev Extended-Release Tablets 3109
Celebrex Capsules (0.1% to 1.9%) 3134
Copaxone for Injection (2%) 3297
Doxil Injection (Less than 1%) 2351
Gabitril Tablets (Infrequent) 984
▲ Imdur Tablets (Less than or equal to 5%) 3018
Imitrex Nasal Spray 1467
Imitrex Tablets (Rare) 1471
Invirase (Less than 2%) 2772
Lescol Capsules 2233
Lescol XL Tablets 2233
Lexapro Oral Solution (Infrequent) 1190
Lexapro Tablets (Infrequent) 1190
Lotrel Capsules 2249
Lyrica Capsules (Rare) 2539
Mevacor Tablets 2021
Neurontin Capsules (Rare) 2487
Neurontin Oral Solution (Rare) 2487
Neurontin Tablets (Rare) 2487
Permax Tablets (Rare) 3356
Photofrin for Injection 702
Rescriptor Tablets 2551
Rilutek Tablets (Rare) 2930
Soriatane Capsules (Less than 1%) 1013
Targretin Capsules 1747
Vytorin 10/10 Tablets 2114
Vytorin 10/10 Tablets 3077
Vytorin 10/20 Tablets 2114
Vytorin 10/20 Tablets 3077
Vytorin 10/40 Tablets 2114
Vytorin 10/40 Tablets 3077
Vytorin 10/80 Tablets 2114
Vytorin 10/80 Tablets 3077
Zocor Tablets 2105
Zyrtec Chewable Tablets (Less than 2%) 2594

Zyrtec (Less than 2%).............. 2594
Zyrtec-D 12 Hour Extended Release Tablets (Less than 2%)..... 2597

Skin odor, abnormal
▲ Soriatane Capsules (1% to 10%) 1013

Skin papilloma
▲ Elidel Cream 1% (Up to 3.3%) 2200
▲ Fuzeon Injection (4.2%) 2767

Skin reactions, allergic
Duetact Tablets (Less than 1%)........ 3226
Nexavar (Uncommon).................... 746

Skin reactions, unspecified
Actonel Tablets (Very rare).............. 2683
Actonel with Calcium Tablets (Very rare).............. 2688
Aldara Cream, 5%.......................... 1846
Alphagan P Ophthalmic Solution....... 567
Brimonidine Tartrate Ophthalmic Solution 0.2%.......................... ⊙ 248
Duragesic Transdermal System (1% or greater)........................ 2373
Ethyol for Injection (Rare)................ 1898
Fosamax Plus D Tablets (Rarely)....... 1977
▲ Gengraf Capsules (1% to 17.6%) 459
Inderal LA Long-Acting Capsules...... 3429
▲ Protopic Ointment (1% to 4%) 638
▲ Soltamox Oral Solution (5.6% to 19%).............................. 3527
▲ Tri-Luma Cream (5.45%) 1213
▲ Ultrase MT Capsules (0.2%) 709
Xalatan Sterile Ophthalmic Solution (1% to 2%)..................... 2649

Skin redness
▲ MICRhoGAM Ultra-Filtered (Frequent)............................ 2371
▲ Panretin Gel (25% to 77%) 1747
▲ RhoGAM Ultra-Filtered (Frequent) 2371

Skin test reactions, suppression
Colocort Rectal Suspension, USP (Retention) 100 mg/60 mL........... 2476
Decadron Tablets.......................... 1951
Depo-Medrol Single-Dose Vial........... 2619
Hydrocortone Tablets...................... 1989

Skin trauma
Nasonex Nasal Spray (Greater than or equal to 2%)................... 3043

Skull abnormalities, fetal
Accutane Capsules......................... 2731
Aceon Tablets (2 mg, 4 mg, 8 mg)... 3194
Altace Capsules............................ 1702
Captopril Tablets........................... 2149
Cozaar Tablets............................. 1935
Hyzaar 50-12.5 Tablets.................. 1990
Hyzaar 100-12.5 Tablets................ 1990
Hyzaar 100-25 Tablets.................. 1990
Lotrel Capsules............................. 2249
Prinivil Tablets.............................. 2052
Prinzide Tablets............................ 2056
Vasotec I.V. Injection..................... 2103

Sleep, sudden onset of
Xyrem (Infrequent)......................... 1688

Sleep disturbances
Aceon Tablets (2 mg, 4 mg, 8 mg) (2.5%).................................. 3194
Adalat CC Tablets (Rare)................. 2964
▲ Advair Diskus 100/50 (1% to 3%) ... 1308
▲ Advair Diskus 250/50 (1% to 3%) ... 1308
▲ Advair Diskus 500/50 (1% to 3%) ... 1308
▲ Advair HFA Inhalation Aerosol (1% to 3%)................................ 1318
Allegra-D 12 Hour Extended-Release Tablets (Less than 1%)............................. 2846
Allegra-D 24 Hour Extended-Release Tablets (Less than 1%)............................. 2849
Ambien Tablets (Infrequent)............. 2851
Ambien CR Tablets (Infrequent)......... 2855
Amerge Tablets (Infrequent)............. 1339
Anzemet Injection (Infrequently)........ 2859
Anzemet Tablets (Infrequently).......... 2862
Aptivus Capsules (Less than 2%)....... 826
Astelin Nasal Spray (Infrequent)....... 1904
Avalide Tablets............................. 888
Avalide Tablets............................. 2874
Avapro Tablets (Less than 1%)......... 891
Avapro Tablets (Less than 1%)......... 2871
Avelox (Less than 0.1%)................. 2970
Celexa (At least 2%)...................... 1176
▲ Cesamet Capsules (11%) 3340
▲ Chantix Tablets (2% to greater than 5%)........................ 2517
▲ Clozaril Tablets (4%) 2184
▲ Combivir Tablets (11%) 1411
Copaxone for Injection (At least 2%).................................. 3297
Coreg Tablets (Greater than 0.1% to 1%)............................... 1414
Cozaar Tablets (Less than 1%)......... 1935
Cymbalta Delayed-Release Capsules (Frequent).................. 1757
Depakote ER Tablets (Greater than 1%)................................ 434
Effexor Tablets (Infrequent)............. 3411
Eldepryl Capsules.......................... 3208
▲ Entocort EC Capsules (Less than 5%)................................ 2698
▲ Epivir (11%) 1427
▲ FazaClo Orally Disintegrating Tablets (4%)......................... 551
▲ Flovent Diskus (1% to 3%) 1443
▲ Hectorol Capsules (3.3%) 1275
▲ Hectorol Injection (3.3%) 1278
HibTITER.................................... 3426
Hyzaar 50-12.5 Tablets.................. 1990
Hyzaar 100-12.5 Tablets................ 1990
Hyzaar 100-25 Tablets.................. 1990
Imitrex Injection (Rare).................. 1463
Imitrex Nasal Spray (Infrequent)....... 1467
Imitrex Tablets (Rare to infrequent)... 1471
Klonopin (Infrequent)...................... 2778
Lamictal (1.4%)............................ 1481
▲ Lariam Tablets (Among most frequent).................................. 2786
Levaquin (0.1% to 0.9%)................ 2384
Levaquin in 5% Dextrose Injection (0.1% to 0.9%)........................ 2384
Lopressor Injection........................ 2238
Lopressor Tablets.......................... 2238
▲ Lotronex Tablets (3%) 1512
▲ Lupron Depot 3.75 mg (16%) 3260
Lupron Depot 7.5 mg (Less than 5%)................................... 3264
▲ Lupron Depot–3 Month 11.25 mg (16%)................................. 3265
Lupron Injection Pediatric 3259
Mirapex Tablets (Less than or equal to 1%)........................... 859
▲ MoviPrep Oral Solution (39.1%) 2839
Nadolol Tablets............................. 2159
Namenda (Infrequent)..................... 1195
Nexium Delayed-Release Capsules (Less than 1%)...................... 655
Nexium I.V. (Less than 1%)............. 659
Noroxin Tablets (Less frequent)........ 2032
Numorphan Injection...................... 1120
Ortho Evra Transdermal System...... 2417
▲ Pediarix Vaccine (0.4% to 46.7%) 1548
Prevacid Delayed-Release Capsules (Less than 1%).............. 3271
Prevacid for Delayed-Release Oral Suspension (Less than 1%)........... 3271
Prevacid SoluTab Delayed-Release Orally Disintegrating Tablets (Less than 1%).......................... 3271
Prevacid NapraPAC (Less than 1%).. 3280
▲ Prevnar for Injection (15.3% to 25.2%)............................... 3463
PREVPAC (Less than 1%)................ 3284
Prochieve 4% Gel.......................... 1003
Prochieve 8% Gel.......................... 1003
ProQuad (Greater than or equal to 0.2% to less than 1%)................ 2064
ProSom Tablets (Infrequent)............ 517
Protonix I.V. (Less than 1%)............ 3472
Protonix Tablets (Less than 1%)....... 3469
Provigil Tablets (At least 1%)........... 988
Prozac Pulvules and Liquid (Frequent)............................ 1801
Recombivax HB (Less than 1%)......... 2071
Relpax Tablets (Rare)..................... 2548
Rescriptor Tablets......................... 2551
Reyataz Capsules (Less than 3%)..... 921
Risperdal (Frequent)....................... 1676
Risperdal M-Tab Orally Disintegrating Tablets (Frequent)... 1676
Rythmol SR Capsules..................... 2727
▲ Serevent Diskus (1% to 3%) 1568
Sonata Capsules (Rare).................. 1717
▲ Strattera Capsules (4%) 1814
Symbyax Capsules (1% to 2%)......... 1819
▲ Tasmar Tablets (24% to 25%) 3358
Tricor Tablets............................... 527
▲ Trizivir Tablets (7% to 11%) 1589
▲ Ultram ER Tablets (1% to greater than 5%)................................ 2392
Univasc Tablets (Less than 1%)........ 3104
Valium Tablets.............................. 2819
Varivax (Greater than or equal to 1%)................................... 2100
Viracept (Less than 2%).................. 2577
▲ Visudyne for Injection (1% to 10%) .. 2305
▲ Wellbutrin Tablets (4.0%) 1603
▲ Wellbutrin XL Extended-Release Tablets (4%)......................... 1613
▲ Xenical Capsules (3.9%) 2831
▲ Xyrem Oral Solution (2.9% to 6.1%)................................ 1688
Zelapar Tablets............................. 3372
Zelnorm Tablets............................ 2312
▲ Ziagen (10%) 1626
Zyrtec Chewable Tablets (Less than 2%)................................ 2594
Zyrtec (Less than 2%)..................... 2594
Zyrtec-D 12 Hour Extended Release Tablets (Less than 2%)..... 2597

Sleep disturbances, paradoxical
Diastat Rectal Delivery System (Infrequent)............................ 3343
Niravam Orally Disintegrating Tablets (Rare)......................... 3092

Sleep talking
Sonata Capsules (Rare).................. 1717
Xyrem Oral Solution (Infrequent)...... 1688

Sleep walking
Neurontin Capsules....................... 2487
Neurontin Oral Solution.................. 2487
Neurontin Tablets.......................... 2487
Sonata Capsules (Rare).................. 1717
▲ Xyrem Oral Solution (5.7%) 1688

Sleepiness
(*see under* Drowsiness)

Sleeplessness
(*see under* Insomnia)

SLE-like syndrome
(*see under* Lupus erythematosus, systemic)

Slipped capital femoral epiphysis
Levothroid Tablets......................... 1186
Nutropin for Injection..................... 1239
Nutropin AQ Injection..................... 1243
Nutropin AQ Pen........................... 1243
Nutropin AQ Pen Cartridge............... 1243

Sloughing
Efudex....................................... 3363
Fluorescite Injection...................... ⊙ 207
Ophthetic Ophthalmic Solution........ ⊙ 232

Sloughing at injection site
Depo-Medrol Single-Dose Vial.......... 2619

Sluggishness
Cymbalta Delayed-Release Capsules (Infrequent)................ 1757
Lexapro Oral Solution (Infrequent).... 1190
Lexapro Tablets (Infrequent)............ 1190
Thyrolar Tablets............................ 1199
▲ Vivitrol (12% to 23%) 995
Xyrem Oral Solution (Infrequent)...... 1688

Smell, loss of the sense
(*see under* Anosmia)

Smell disturbances
Amerge Tablets (Infrequent)............ 1339
Astelin Nasal Spray (Infrequently)..... 1904
Beconase AQ Nasal Spray (Rare)..... 1396
Biaxin/Biaxin XL........................... 402
Eligard 7.5 mg (Less than 2%)......... 2880
Flonase Nasal Spray...................... 1440
Imitrex Injection (Rare)................... 1463
Imitrex Nasal Spray (Infrequent)....... 1467
Imitrex Tablets (Infrequent)............. 1471
Lotronex Tablets (Rare).................. 1512
Maxair Autohaler (0.6%)................. 1852
Maxalt Tablets (Rare)..................... 2008
Maxalt-MLT Orally Disintegrating Tablets (Rare)......................... 2008
Migranal Nasal Spray (Infrequent)..... 3348
Nasonex Nasal Spray (Very rare)...... 3043
PREVPAC.................................... 3284
Testim 1% Gel (1% or less)............. 695
Timentin ADD-Vantage.................... 1580
Timentin Injection Galaxy Container.................................. 1583
Timentin IV Infusion...................... 1577
Timentin Pharmacy Bulk Package..... 1586

Smoker's tongue
(*see under* Leukoplakia, oral)

Sneezing
Aceon Tablets (2 mg, 4 mg, 8 mg) (0.3% to 1%)........................... 3194
▲ Advair Diskus 100/50 (1% to 3%) ... 1308
▲ Advair Diskus 250/50 (1% to 3%) ... 1308
▲ Advair Diskus 500/50 (1% to 3%) ... 1308
▲ Aerobid/Aerobid-M (3% to 9%) 1171
▲ Alamast Ophthalmic Solution (Less than 5%)....................... 3381
▲ Astelin Nasal Spray (3.1%) 1904
▲ Atrovent Nasal Spray 0.03% (3.1%).................................. 837
Axert Tablets (Rare)...................... 2396
▲ Beconase AQ Nasal Spray (4%) 1396
Bentyl Capsules........................... 697
Bentyl Injection............................ 697
Bentyl Syrup................................ 697
Bentyl Tablets.............................. 697
Calcium Disodium Versenate Injection................................... 1851
Clozaril Tablets (Less than 1%)........ 2184
Ethyol for Injection........................ 1898
FazaClo Orally Disintegrating Tablets (Less than 1%)............... 551
4-Way Fast Acting Nasal Spray....... ▣ 775
▲ Intron A for Injection (Less than or equal to 5%)........................ 3024
Klonopin (Infrequent)...................... 2778
Maxalt Tablets (Rare)..................... 2008
Maxalt-MLT Orally Disintegrating Tablets (Rare)......................... 2008
ProQuad..................................... 2064
Rituxan I.V.................................. 1254
Simulect for Injection..................... 2284
▲ Ultram ER Tablets (1% to greater than 5%)................................ 2392
Vicks NyQuil LiquiCaps/Liquid Multi-Symptom Cold/Flu Relief..... ▣ 763
Vicks Sinex Nasal Spray and Ultra Fine Mist for Sinus Relief............ 2681
Vicks Vapor Inhaler (Temporary)....... 2682
Zicam Cold Remedy Gel Swabs...... ▣ 766
Zicam Cold Remedy Nasal Gel....... ▣ 766
Zicam Cold Remedy Swabs Kids Size.. ▣ 766
Zicam Extreme Congestion Relief... ▣ 767
Zicam Intense Sinus Relief............ ▣ 767

Snoring
Aricept Tablets (Infrequent)............ 1094
Aricept ODT Tablets (Infrequent)...... 1094
▲ Increlex Injection (Greater than or equal to 5%)........................ 3291
Neurontin Capsules (Rare)............... 2487
Neurontin Oral Solution (Rare)......... 2487
Neurontin Tablets (Rare)................. 2487
Sonata Capsules (Infrequent)........... 1717
Xyrem Oral Solution (Infrequent)...... 1688

Social reaction, anti
(*see under* Sociopathy)

Sociopathy
DextroStat Tablets........................ 3179
Neurontin Capsules (Rare)............... 2487
Neurontin Oral Solution (Rare)......... 2487
Neurontin Tablets (Rare)................. 2487
Paxil CR Controlled-Release Tablets (Rare)......................... 1538
Paxil (Rare)................................. 1530
Zyprexa Tablets (Infrequent)............ 1830
Zyprexa ZYDIS Orally Disintegrating Tablets (Infrequent)........................... 1830

Sodium depletion
(*see under* Hyponatremia)

Sodium loss
(*see under* Hyponatremia)

Sodium retention
Androxy Tablets............................ 3335
Colocort Rectal Suspension, USP (Retention) 100 mg/60 mL........... 2476
Decadron Tablets.......................... 1951
Depo-Medrol Injectable Suspension................................ 2617
Depo-Medrol Single-Dose Vial.......... 2619
▲ Estratest Tablets (Among most common)............................. 3199
▲ Estratest H.S. Tablets (Among most common)....................... 3199
Hydrocortone Tablets...................... 1989
Hyperstat I.V................................ 3017
Kionex Powder............................. 2477
Oxandrin Tablets........................... 2962

Somatization
Zyprexa Tablets (Infrequent)............ 1830
Zyprexa ZYDIS Orally Disintegrating Tablets (Infrequent)........................... 1830

Somnambulism
Ambien Tablets (Rare).................... 2851
Ambien CR Tablets (Rare)............... 2855
Requip Tablets (Infrequent).............. 1555
Zoloft (Rare)................................ 2586

Somnolence
(*see under* Drowsiness)

Sore throat
(*see also under* Throat soreness)
Yaz Tablets (Greater than 1%).......... 803

Soreness, injection site
▲ Alferon N Injection (10%) 1665
▲ Comvax (23.9% to 34.5%) 1928
▲ Engerix-B Vaccine (22%) 1425
▲ Havrix Vaccine (21% to 56%) 1456
HyperRAB 3242
HyperRho S/D Mini-Dose 3244
HyperRho S/D Full Dose 3246
HyperTET 3248
Infed Injection 3390
Pneumovax 23 (Common) 2043
▲ ProQuad (22%) 2064
▲ Vaqta (1.2% to 3.5%) 2097
▲ Varivax (19.3% to 32.5%) 2100
WinRho SDF 732

Soreness, nasal
▲ Fortical Nasal Spray (10.6%) 3337

Soreness at insertion site
▲ Vantas (3.6%) 3375

Spasm, biliary tract
Dilaudid 440
Dilaudid Non-Sterile Powder 440
Dilaudid Oral Liquid 445
Dilaudid Rectal Suppositories 440
Dilaudid Tablets 440
Dilaudid Tablets - 8 mg 445
Dilaudid-HP (Less frequent) 442
MS Contin Tablets (Less frequent) 2701
Numorphan Injection 1120

Spasm, gastrointestinal
Lotronex Tablets (Infrequent) 1512

Spasm, generalized
Colazal Capsules 2838
Gabitril Tablets (Infrequent) 984
Invirase (Less than 2%) 2772
Lyrica Capsules (Rare) 2539
Paxil CR Controlled-Release Tablets (Rare) 1538
Paxil (Rare) 1530
Prinivil Tablets (0.3% to 1.0%) 2052
Prinzide Tablets 2056
▲ Prograf Capsules and Injection (3% to 15%) 632
Symbyax Capsules (Infrequent) 1819
▲ Zyprexa Tablets (2% to 3%) 1830
▲ Zyprexa ZYDIS Orally Disintegrating Tablets (2% to 3%) 1830

Spasm, non-site specific
Amerge Tablets (Rare) 1339
Invanz for Injection (Greater than 0.1%) 1999

Spasm, sphincter of Oddi
Zelnorm Tablets 2312

Spasm, urinary bladder
Eligard 22.5 mg (Less than 2%) 2883

Spasm, vesical sphincters
Hycotuss Expectorant Syrup 1117
Tussionex Pennkinetic Extended-Release Suspension 3327
Vicodin Tablets 535
Vicodin ES Tablets 536
Vicodin HP Tablets 538
Zydone Tablets 1139

Speech, incoherent
Clozaril Tablets (Less than 1%) 2184

Speech, pressure of
Cymbalta Delayed-Release Capsules (Infrequent) 1757

Speech, slurring
Clozaril Tablets (1%) 2184
Dalmane Capsules (Rare) 3342
Diastat Rectal Delivery System (Infrequent) 3343
FazaClo Orally Disintegrating Tablets (1%) 551
Kadian Capsules (Less than 3%) 577
Klonopin 2778
Lithobid Tablets 1692
Matulane Capsules 3191
Nadolol Tablets (1 to 5 of 1000 patients) 2159
Niravam Orally Disintegrating Tablets 3092
▲ Phenytek Capsules (Among most common) 2160
Sonata Capsules (Rare) 1717
Symmetrel Tablets (0.1% to 1%) 1135
Tranxene 2474
Valium Tablets (Infrequent) 2819
Vicoprofen Tablets (Less than 1%) 539

Speech difficulties
Clozaril Tablets (Less than 1%) 2184
▲ Demser Capsules (10%) 1953
FazaClo Orally Disintegrating Tablets (Less than 1%) 551
Geodon for Injection (Up to 2%) 2529
Marinol Capsules (Less than 1%) 3333
▲ Zyprexa Tablets (2% to 7%) 1830
▲ Zyprexa ZYDIS Orally Disintegrating Tablets (2% to 7%) 1830

Speech disorder
Ambien CR Tablets (Infrequent) 2855
Cesamet Capsules 3340
▲ Lyrica Capsules (1% to 7%) 2539
Prograf Capsules and Injection 632

Speech disturbances
Actiq (Less than 1%) 979
▲ Adderall XR Capsules (2% to 4%) 3166
Ambien Tablets (Infrequent) 2851
Arranon Injection (1%) 1357
Avelox (Less than 0.1%) 2970
Bentyl Capsules 697
Bentyl Injection 697
Bentyl Syrup 697
Bentyl Tablets 697
Carbatrol Capsules 3171
Copaxone for Injection (2%) 3297
Dantrium Capsules (Less frequent) .. 2694
▲ Depakote Tablets (1% to 5%) 427
▲ Depakote ER Tablets (1% to 5%) 434
Diastat Rectal Delivery System (Greater than or equal to 1%) 3343
Duragesic Transdermal System (1% or greater) 2373
Effexor Tablets (Infrequent) 3411
Effexor XR Capsules (Infrequent) 3417
Eldepryl Capsules 3208
▲ Equetro Extended-Release Capsules (6%) 3180
Evoxac Capsules (Less than 1%) 1047
Frova Tablets (Infrequent) 1113
▲ Gabitril Tablets (4%) 984
Geodon Capsules (2%) 2529
Imitrex Injection 1463
▲ Intron A for Injection (Less than 5%) 3024
Invirase (Less than 2%) 2772
Lamictal (2.5%) 1481
Levaquin (0.1% to 0.9%) 2384
Levaquin in 5% Dextrose Injection (0.1% to 0.9%) 2384
Meridia Capsules 489
Migranal Nasal Spray (Rare) 3348
Neurontin Capsules (Infrequent) 2487
Neurontin Oral Solution (Infrequent) 2487
Neurontin Tablets (Infrequent) 2487
Ortho-Cyclen Tablets 2429
Ortho Evra Transdermal System 2417
Ortho Tri-Cyclen Tablets 2429
Ortho Tri-Cyclen Lo Tablets 2436
OxyContin Tablets (Less than 1%) 2703
Permax Tablets (1.1%) 3356
Prevacid Delayed-Release Capsules (Less than 1%) 3271
Prevacid for Delayed-Release Oral Suspension (Less than 1%) 3271
Prevacid SoluTab Delayed-Release Orally Disintegrating Tablets (Less than 1%) 3271
Prevacid NapraPAC 3280
PREVPAC 3284
▲ Proleukin for Injection (7%) 2266
▲ Prometrium Capsules (100 mg, 200 mg) (Less than 5%) 3203
Protonix I.V. 3472
Protonix Tablets 3469
Relpax Tablets (Infrequent) 2548
Romazicon Injection (Less than 1%) 2804
Rythmol SR Capsules 2727
Symbyax Capsules (Up to 2%) 1819
Tambocor Tablets (Less than 1%) 1856
Tasmar Tablets (Frequent) 3358
Tegretol/Tegretol-XR 2295
▲ Topamax Sprinkle Capsules (Less than 1% to 13%) 2404
▲ Topamax Tablets (Less than 1% to 13%) 2404
▲ Trileptal Tablets (1% to 3%) 2300
▲ Trileptal Oral Suspension (1% to 3%) 2300
▲ Vesanoid Capsules (3%) 2820
Zomig Nasal Spray (Infrequent) 3523
▲ Zonegran Capsules (5%) 1101
▲ Zyprexa Tablets (2% to 7%) 1830
▲ Zyprexa ZYDIS Orally Disintegrating Tablets (2% to 7%) 1830

Spermatogenesis, defective
Mustargen for Injection 2468

Spermatozoa, changes
Decadron Tablets 1951

Spinal cord, compression
▲ Quadramet Injection (6.5%) 1040

Spinal cord infarction
Activase I.V. 1223

Spinal fracture
Arimidex Tablets (1%) 673
Lupron Depot 3.75 mg 3260
Lupron Depot 7.5 mg 3264
Lupron Depot–3 Month 11.25 mg 3265
Lupron Depot-PED 7.5 mg, 11.25 mg and 15 mg 3269
Lupron Injection Pediatric 3259
Revlimid Capsules 958

Spleen disorder
Rescriptor Tablets 2551
Rythmol SR Capsules 2727

Spleen palpable
Thalomid Capsules 965

Spleenomegaly
BiDil Tablets 2171
VFEND I.V. (Less than 2%) 2564
VFEND Oral Suspension (Less than 2%) 2564
VFEND Tablets (Less than 2%) 2564

Splenic infarction
Campath Ampules 811
Revlimid Capsules 958
Zomig Tablets (Rare) 3519
Zomig Nasal Spray (Very rare) 3523
Zomig-ZMT Tablets (Rare) 3519

Splenic rupture
Neulasta Injection (Rare) 601
Neupogen for Injection (Rare) 603

Splenomegaly
Aloprim for Injection (Less than 1%) 2167
Campath Ampules 811
Chantix Tablets (Rare) 2517
Combivir Tablets 1411
Copaxone for Injection (Infrequent) 3297
Dacogen Injection 2129
Epivir 1427
Epivir-HBV 1432
Epzicom Tablets 1436
Garamycin Injectable 3014
Invirase (Less than 2%) 2772
▲ Neupogen for Injection (Approximately 30%) 603
Orthoclone OKT3 Sterile Solution 2360
Permax Tablets (Rare) 3356
Retrovir IV Infusion 1564
RhoGAM Ultra-Filtered (One patient) 2371
Tabloid Tablets 1575
Trizivir Tablets 1589

Spotting
Angeliq Tablets 762
Climara Transdermal System 771
Climara Pro Transdermal System 776
Enjuvia Tablets 1062
Estrasorb Topical Emulsion 1147
Estratest Tablets 3199
Estratest H.S. Tablets 3199
Lexapro Oral Solution (Infrequent) 1190
Lexapro Tablets (Infrequent) 1190
Menostar Transdermal System 782
Mircette Tablets 1066
NuvaRing 2340
Ortho-Cyclen Tablets 2429
Ortho Evra Transdermal System 2417
Ortho Tri-Cyclen Tablets 2429
Ortho Tri-Cyclen Lo Tablets 2436
Premarin Intravenous 3442
Premarin Tablets 3446
Premarin Vaginal Cream 3452
Premphase Tablets 3456
Prempro Tablets 3456
Prometrium Capsules (100 mg, 200 mg) 3203
Seasonique Tablets 1077
Verelan PM Extended-Release Capsules, Controlled-Onset (2% or less) 3106
Yaz Tablets 803

Spotting, irregular
depo-subQ provera 104 Injectable Suspension 2624

Spotting, oily
▲ Xenical Capsules (4.4% to 26.6%) 2831

Spotting, prolonged
depo-subQ provera 104 Injectable Suspension 2624

Sputum, discoloration
▲ TOBI Solution for Inhalation (21.3%) 2298

Sputum increased
Abilify Oral Solution (Rare) 882
Abilify Oral Solution (Rare) 2450
Abilify Discmelt Orally Disintegrating Tablets (Rare) 882
Abilify Discmelt Orally Disintegrating Tablets (Rare) 2450
Abilify Tablets (Rare) 882
Abilify Tablets (Rare) 2450
Actiq (Less than 1%) 979
▲ Aerobid/Aerobid-M (3% to 9%) 1171
Atrovent Inhalation Solution (1.4%) 835
Celexa (Rare) 1176
▲ CellCept Capsules (3% to less than 20%) 2747
▲ CellCept Intravenous (3% to less than 20%) 2747
▲ CellCept Oral Suspension (3% to less than 20%) 2747
▲ CellCept Tablets (3% to less than 20%) 2747
Combivent Inhalation Aerosol (Less than 2%) 847
▲ Exubera Inhalation Powder (2.8% to 3.9%) 2524
Foradil Aerolizer (1.5%) 3010
▲ Imdur Tablets (Less than or equal to 5%) 3018
Lupron Depot 7.5 mg (Less than 5%) 3264
Paxil CR Controlled-Release Tablets (Rare) 1538
Paxil (Rare) 1530
Proventil Inhalation Solution 0.083% (1.5%) 3055
Pulmozyme Inhalation Solution 1248
Relpax Tablets (Rare) 2548
Rilutek Tablets (More than 2%) 2930
Risperdal (Rare) 1676
Risperdal M-Tab Orally Disintegrating Tablets (Rare) 1676
Sonata Capsules (Rare) 1717
Soriatane Capsules (Less than 1%) .. 1013
▲ TOBI Solution for Inhalation (37.6%) 2298
Ultane Liquid for Inhalation (Less than 1%) 531
Viagra Tablets (Less than 2%) 2573
Zomig Nasal Spray (Rare) 3523
Zyrtec Chewable Tablets (Less than 2%) 2594
Zyrtec (Less than 2%) 2594
Zyrtec-D 12 Hour Extended Release Tablets (Less than 2%) 2597

S-T depressed
Lyrica Capsules (Rare) 2539
Ultane Liquid for Inhalation (Less than 1%) 531

ST section changes
(*see under* EKG changes, ST section)

Standing, difficulty in
Stromectol Tablets 2083

Status asthmaticus
Sandostatin Injection (Less than 1%) 2278
Sandostatin LAR Depot (Rare) 2280

Status epilepticus
Aloprim for Injection (Less than 1%) 2167
Arranon Injection (0% to 1%) 1357
Carbatrol Capsules 3171
Clozaril Tablets 2184
FazaClo Orally Disintegrating Tablets 551
Gabitril Tablets 984
Keppra Oral Solution (2%) 3314
Keppra Tablets (2%) 3314
Oncaspar 1145
Paxil CR Controlled-Release Tablets 1538
Paxil 1530
Tegretol/Tegretol-XR 2295

Steatorrhea
Miradon Tablets 3042
▲ Sandostatin Injection (22% to 35%) 2278

▲ Sandostatin LAR Depot (4% to 6%) 2280

Steatosis, hepatic
Combivir Tablets 1411
Cymbalta Delayed-Release Capsules (Infrequent) 1757
Epivir 1427
Epivir-HBV 1432
Epzicom Tablets 1436
Retrovir Capsules 1560
Retrovir IV Infusion (Rare) 1564
Retrovir 1560
Trizivir Tablets 1589
Viread Tablets 1301
Ziagen 1626

Stenosis, aortic
Argatroban Injection (0.9%) 1346
Tasmar Tablets (Infrequent) 3358

Stenosis, bile duct
Prograf Capsules and Injection 632

Stenosis, intestinal
Azilect Tablets (Rare) 3293
Remicade for IV Injection (Greater than or equal to 0.2%) 971

Stenosis, nasal
▲ Fortical Nasal Spray (10.6%) 3337

Stevens-Johnson syndrome
Aciphex Tablets 1090
Adderall Tablets 3164
Advicor Tablets 1722
Agenerase Capsules (1%) 1327
Agenerase Oral Solution (1%) 1332
Aggrenox Capsules 822
Aldoril Tablets 1910
Altoprev Extended-Release Tablets 3109
Amoxil Capsules 1343
Amoxil Chewable Tablets 1343
Amoxil Pediatric Drops for Oral Suspension 1343
Amoxil Powder for Oral Suspension 1343
Amoxil Tablets 1343
Anaprox Tablets (Less than 1%) 2761
Anaprox DS Tablets (Less than 1%) 2761
Arimidex Tablets (Very rare) 673
Arthrotec Tablets (Rare) 3129
Atacand HCT 651
Atripla Tablets 945
Attenuvax 1914
Augmentin (Rare) 1360
Augmentin Tablets (Rare) 1363
Augmentin XR Extended-Release Tablets (Rare) 1369
Augmentin ES-600 Powder for Oral Suspension 1366
Avalide Tablets 888
Avalide Tablets 2874
Avelox 2970
Betagan Ophthalmic Solution, USP ⊙ 220
Biaxin/Biaxin XL (Rare) 402
Bleph-10 Ophthalmic Solution 10% (Isolated incident) ⊙ 222
▲ Blephamide Ophthalmic Ointment (Among most often) 568
Blephamide Ophthalmic Suspension 569
Caduet Tablets 2508
Captopril Tablets 2149
Carbatrol Capsules (Extremely rare) 3171
Carimune NF 3499
Ceftin 1407
Celebrex Capsules (Less than 0.1%) 3134
Cialis Tablets 1838
Cipro 2977
Cipro I.V. (1% or less) 2984
Cipro XR Tablets 2990
Cleocin Vaginal Ovules 2616
Clinoril Tablets (Less than 1 in 100) 1924
Clozaril Tablets 2184
Combivir Tablets 1411
Comvax 1928
Covera-HS Tablets (Less than 2%) 3139
Crixivan Capsules 1940
Daraprim Tablets 1419
Depacon Injection 412
Depakene 417
Depakote Sprinkle Capsules 422
Depakote Tablets 427
Depakote ER Tablets 434
Didronel Tablets (A single case) 2697
Diovan HCT Tablets 2196
Diuril Oral Suspension 1954
Diuril Sodium Intravenous 2467
Dolobid Tablets (Less than 1 in 100) 1955
EC-Naprosyn Delayed-Release Tablets (Less than 1%) 2761
E.E.S. (Rare) 451
Effexor Tablets 3411
Effexor XR Capsules 3417
Emend Capsules (One patient) 1963
Engerix-B Vaccine 1425
Epzicom Tablets 1436
Equetro Extended-Release Capsules 3180
EryPed (Rare) 447
Erythromycin Delayed-Release Capsules, USP (Rare) 457
Ethyol for Injection (Rare) 1898
Exelon Capsules 2206
Exelon Oral Solution 2206
Fansidar Tablets 2765
FazaClo Orally Disintegrating Tablets 551
Flebogamma 5%, Immune Globulin Intravenous (Human) 1658
Fluarix 1451
FML-S Ophthalmic Suspension (Rare) ⊙ 229
Fortaz 1453
Fosamax (Rare) 1969
Fosamax Plus D Tablets (Rarely) 1977
Gammagard Liquid 721
Gammagard S/D (Rare) 724
Gamunex Immune Globulin I.V., 10% (Rare) 3235
Gantrisin Pediatric Suspension 2770
Gleevec Tablets (Rare) 2227
Hyzaar 50-12.5 Tablets 1990
Hyzaar 100-12.5 Tablets 1990
Hyzaar 100-25 Tablets 1990
Indapamide Tablets 2156
Inderal LA Long-Acting Capsules 3429
Indocin Capsules (Less than 1%) 1995
Indocin I.V. (Less than 1%) 2465
Indocin (Less than 1%) 1995
Invirase (Rare) 2772
Keflex Capsules (Rare) 549
Lamictal (Rare) 1481
Lamisil Tablets (Isolated reports) 2232
Lariam Tablets 2786
Lescol Capsules (Rare) 2233
Lescol XL Tablets 2233
Leukeran Tablets (Rare) 1504
Leustatin Injection (Isolated cases) 2357
Levaquin (Rare) 2384
Levaquin in 5% Dextrose Injection (Rare) 2384
Lexiva Tablets (One case) 1505
Lipitor Tablets 2483
Lofibra Tablets (Rare) 1219
Lofibra Capsules (Rare) 1216
Lopressor HCT 50/25 Tablets 2241
Lopressor HCT 100/25 Tablets 2241
Lopressor HCT 100/50 Tablets 2241
Lotensin Tablets (Less than 1%) 2243
Lotensin HCT Tablets (Rare) 2246
Lotrel Capsules (Rare) 2249
Lyrica Capsules (Rare) 2539
Malarone Pediatric Tablets (One case) 1517
Malarone Tablets (One case) 1517
Maxipime for Injection 1105
Mefoxin for Injection 2012
Mefoxin Premixed Intravenous Solution 2016
Merrem I.V. 686
Meruvax II 2019
Mevacor Tablets (Rare) 2021
Micardis HCT Tablets 856
Mintezol 2027
M-M-R II 2006
Mobic Oral Suspension (Less than 0.1%) 863
Mobic Tablets (Less than 0.1%) 863
Moduretic Tablets 2028
Mumpsvax 2031
Nalfon Capsules (Less than 1%) 2502
Namenda 1195
Naprosyn Suspension (Less than 1%) 2761
Naprosyn Tablets (Less than 1%) 2761
Neurontin Capsules 2487
Neurontin Oral Solution 2487
Neurontin Tablets 2487
Nexium Delayed-Release Capsules (Rare) 655
Nexium I.V. (Rare) 659
Niravam Orally Disintegrating Tablets 3092
Noroxin Tablets 2032
Norvir (Rare) 503
Omnicef Capsules 511
Omnicef for Oral Suspension 511
Orthoclone OKT3 Sterile Solution 2360
PCE Dispertab Tablets (Rare) 515
PEG-Intron Powder for Injection 3048
Phenytek Capsules 2160
Plavix Tablets 917
Plavix Tablets 2926
Pletal Tablets (Very rare) 2455
Prevacid NapraPAC (Less than 1%) 3280
PREVPAC (Rare) 3284
Prezista Tablets (Less than 2%) 3306
Prilosec OTC Delayed-Release Tablets (Very rare) 2677
Primaxin I.M. 2045
Primaxin I.V. 2048
Prinivil Tablets (Rare) 2052
Prinzide Tablets (Rare) 2056
Prograf Capsules and Injection 632
ProQuad 2064
Proquin XR Tablets 1153
ProSom Tablets (Rare) 517
Protonix I.V. 3472
Protonix Tablets 3469
Provigil Tablets (Rare) 988
Prozac Pulvules and Liquid 1801
Raniclor Tablets, Chewable (Rare) 2505
Recombivax HB 2071
Rescriptor Tablets 2551
Retrovir IV Infusion 1564
Reyataz Capsules 921
Rituxan I.V. 1254
Sanctura Tablets 1151
Seroquel Tablets 690
Solodyn Extended Release Tablets 1890
Soltamox Oral Solution (Very rare) 3527
Stromectol Tablets 2083
Suprax (Less than 2%) 1843
Sustiva Capsules (Up to 3.5%) 930
Sustiva Tablets (Up to 3.5%) 930
Tamiflu Capsules (Rare) 2807
Tamiflu Oral Suspension (Rare) 2807
Tarka Tablets 524
Taxotere Injection Concentrate (Rare) 2932
Tegretol/Tegretol-XR (Extremely rare) 2295
Tequin Injection 938
Tequin Injection in 5% Dextrose 938
Tequin Tablets 938
Teveten HCT Tablets 1737
Thalomid Capsules 965
Tiazac Capsules (Less than 2%) 1201
Ticlid Tablets (Rare) 2810
Timentin ADD-Vantage 1580
Timentin Injection Galaxy Container 1583
Timentin IV Infusion 1577
Timentin Pharmacy Bulk Package 1586
Timolide Tablets 2086
Topamax Sprinkle Capsules 2404
Topamax Tablets 2404
Tricor Tablets (Rare) 527
Trileptal Tablets 2300
Trileptal Oral Suspension 2300
Trizivir Tablets 1589
Trusopt Sterile Ophthalmic Solution (Rare) 2095
Twinrix Vaccine 1595
Uniretic Tablets 3100
Vancocin HCl Capsules, USP (Infrequent) 3380
Vantin Tablets and Oral Suspension 2645
Varivax 2100
Vasotec I.V. Injection (0.5% to 1.0%) 2103
Verelan PM Extended-Release Capsules, Controlled-Onset (2% or less) 3106
VFEND I.V. (Rare) 2564
VFEND Oral Suspension (Rare) 2564
VFEND Tablets (Rare) 2564
Viramune Oral Suspension 873
Viramune Tablets 873
Voltaren Tablets (Rarely) 2307
Voltaren-XR Tablets (Rarely) 2310
Vytorin 10/10 Tablets 2114
Vytorin 10/10 Tablets 3077
Vytorin 10/20 Tablets 2114
Vytorin 10/20 Tablets 3077
Vytorin 10/40 Tablets 2114
Vytorin 10/40 Tablets 3077
Vytorin 10/80 Tablets 2114
Vytorin 10/80 Tablets 3077
Wellbutrin Tablets (Rare) 1603
Wellbutrin SR Sustained-Release Tablets (Rare) 1607
Wellbutrin XL Extended-Release Tablets (Rare) 1613
Zegerid Capsules (Very rare) 2958
Zegerid Powder for Oral Solution (Very rare) 2958
Ziagen 1626
Zinacef for Injection (Rare) 1631
Zinacef Injection (Rare) 1631
Zmax for Oral Suspension (Rare) 2583
Zocor Tablets (Rare) 2105
Zoloft 2586
Zonegran Capsules (Rare) 1101
Zosyn (Rare) 3492
Zovirax 1643
Zyban Sustained-Release Tablets 1644

Stiffness, unspecified
Fortical Nasal Spray (Less than 1%) 3337
ProQuad 2064

Stillbirths
Aggrenox Capsules 822
Bayer Aspirin 744
Bayer Aspirin Comprehensive Prescribing Information ■ 796
Percodan Tablets 1132
St. Joseph 81 mg Aspirin Chewable and Enteric Coated Tablets 1869
St. Joseph 81 mg Aspirin ■ 688
Zyrtec-D 12 Hour Extended Release Tablets (Rare) 2597

Stimulation
Dalmane Capsules (Rare) 3342
Parcopa Orally Disintegrating Tablets 3097
Sonata Capsules (Rare) 1717
Stalevo Tablets 2287
Valium Tablets 2819

Stinging
▲ Acular Ophthalmic Solution (Up to 40%) 565
▲ Acular LS Ophthalmic Solution (20% to 40%) 566
Aldara Cream, 5% (More than 1%) 1846
Attenuvax 1914
Bactroban Nasal (2%) 1394
Bactroban Ointment (1.5%) 1395
▲ Betagan Ophthalmic Solution, USP (About 1 in 3 patients) ⊙ 220
▲ Betimol Ophthalmic Solution (1 in 8 patients) 3382
▲ Betimol Ophthalmic Solution (1 in 8 patients) ⊙ 295
Bleph-10 Ophthalmic Solution 10% ⊙ 222
▲ Brimonidine Tartrate Ophthalmic Solution 0.2% (10% to 30%) ⊙ 248
Clobevate Gel (Less than 2%) 3211
Clobex Shampoo 1206
▲ Cosopt Sterile Ophthalmic Solution (Up to 30%) 1931
Cozaar Tablets (Less than 1%) 1935
Cutivate Cream (0.8%) 2662
Cutivate Lotion 0.05% (2%) 2664
▲ Differin Cream (Less than 1% to 24%) 1210
Differin Gel (Approximately 1% or less) 1211
Diprolene AF Cream 0.05% (0.4%) 3000
Doxil Injection 2351
Drysol Solution 2507
▲ Elocon Cream 0.1% (1.6% to approximately 7%) 3005
▲ Elocon Ointment 0.1% (4.8% to approximately 7%) 3007
▲ Finacea Gel (4% to 20%) 1669
FML Ophthalmic Suspension ⊙ 227
FML Forte Ophthalmic Suspension ⊙ 226
Hyzaar 50-12.5 Tablets 1990
Hyzaar 100-12.5 Tablets 1990
Hyzaar 100-25 Tablets 1990
Imitrex Injection (Infrequent) 1463
Klaron Lotion 10% 2909
Lotrimin 3039
Lotrisone (Less than 1%) 3040
▲ Luxiq Foam (2% to 44%) 1010
Mentax Cream (Approximately 1%) 2158
Meruvax II 2019
▲ Metrogel 1% (1.3% to 7.2%) 1211
M-M-R II 2006
Mumpsvax 2031
▲ Naftin Cream (6%) 2126
▲ Naftin Gel (5.0%) 2126
Ocufen Ophthalmic Solution ⊙ 232
Olux Foam (Less than 2%) 1012
Ophthetic Ophthalmic Solution (Occasional) ⊙ 232
Oxistat (0.1%) 2667
▲ Panretin Gel (3% to 22%) 1747
Patanol Ophthalmic Solution (Less than 5%) 561
Polytrim Ophthalmic Solution 574
Pred Mild Ophthalmic Suspension ⊙ 238
Pred Forte Ophthalmic Suspension ⊙ 235

Pred-G Ophthalmic Suspension ... ⊙236
▲ Propine Ophthalmic Solution (6%) ... ⊙239
Temovate Cream (1%) ... 2668
▲ Temovate Gel (Among most frequent) ... 2669
Temovate Ointment (Less frequent) ... 2668
▲ Temovate Scalp Application (29 of 294 patients) ... 2670
▲ Temovate E Emollient (5%) ... 2671
▲ Timoptic Sterile Ophthalmic Solution (Approximately 1 in 8 patients) ... 2088
▲ Timoptic in Ocudose (Approximately 1 in 8 patients) ... 2091
▲ Timoptic-XE Sterile Ophthalmic Gel Forming Solution (1 in 8 patients) ... 2092
▲ Trusopt Sterile Ophthalmic Solution (Approximately one-third of patients) ... 2095
▲ Xalatan Sterile Ophthalmic Solution (5% to 15%) ... 2649
Xerac AC Solution ... 2507
▲ Zovirax Ointment (28.3%) ... 821

Stinging at application site
▲ Diprolene Gel 0.05% (6%) ... 3001
Levulan Kerastick for Topical Solution, 20% ... 1085

Stinging at injection site
Alphanate, Antihemophilic Factor (Human) ... 1654
AlphaNine SD, Coagulation Factor IX (Human) ... 1656
▲ Eligard 45 mg (16%) ... 2888
ProQuad ... 2064
Xolair ... 1266

Stomach, nervous
Clozaril Tablets (Less than 1%) ... 2184
FazaClo Orally Disintegrating Tablets (Less than 1%) ... 551

Stomach atony
Tasmar Tablets (Rare) ... 3358

Stomach complaints
Xyrem Oral Solution (Infrequent) ... 1688

Stomachache
▲ Aerobid/Aerobid-M (10%) ... 1171
Arthrotec Tablets ... 3129
▲ Bayer Aspirin (14.5%) ... 744
Bayer Aspirin Comprehensive Prescribing Information ... ▣796
▲ Chemet Capsules (5.2% to 15.7%) ... 2458
Invirase (Less than 2%) ... 2772
Klonopin (Infrequent) ... 2778
Koāte-DVI (0.7%) ... 3250
K-Phos Original (Sodium Free) Tablets ... 760
K-Phos Neutral Tablets ... 760
Ortho-Cyclen Tablets ... 2429
Ortho Evra Transdermal System ... 2417
Ortho Tri-Cyclen Tablets ... 2429
Ortho Tri-Cyclen Lo Tablets ... 2436
Rocaltrol Capsules ... 2798
Rocaltrol Oral Solution ... 2798
St. Joseph 81 mg Aspirin Chewable and Enteric Coated Tablets ... 1869
Uroqid-Acid No. 2 Tablets ... 760
Zofran Injection (2%) ... 1634

Stomatitis
Abilify Oral Solution (Infrequent) ... 882
Abilify Oral Solution (Infrequent) ... 2450
Abilify Discmelt Orally Disintegrating Tablets (Infrequent) ... 882
Abilify Discmelt Orally Disintegrating Tablets (Infrequent) ... 2450
Abilify Tablets (Infrequent) ... 882
Abilify Tablets (Infrequent) ... 2450
Aciphex Tablets ... 1090
Actiq (1% or greater) ... 979
▲ Alferon N Injection (6%) ... 1665
▲ Alimta for Injection (Up to 28%) ... 1750
AmBisome for Injection (Less common) ... 620
Anaprox Tablets (Less than 3%) ... 2761
Anaprox DS Tablets (Less than 3%) ... 2761
Aredia for Injection (Up to 1%) ... 2179
▲ Arranon Injection (0% to 8%) ... 1357
Arthrotec Tablets (Rare) ... 3129
Asacol Delayed-Release Tablets ... 2692
Augmentin ... 1360
Augmentin Tablets ... 1363
Augmentin XR Extended-Release Tablets ... 1369
Augmentin ES-600 Powder for Oral Suspension ... 1366
▲ Avastin IV (30% to 32%) ... 1227
Avelox (0.1% to less than 2%) ... 2970
Azilect Tablets (Infrequent) ... 3293
Biaxin/Biaxin XL ... 402
Caduet Tablets (Less than 2%) ... 2508
▲ Campath Ampules (1% to 14%) ... 811
▲ Camptosar Injection (1% to 12%) ... 2604
Carbatrol Capsules ... 3171
Celebrex Capsules (0.1% to 1.9%) ... 3134
Celexa (Infrequent) ... 1176
▲ CellCept Capsules (3% to less than 20%) ... 2747
▲ CellCept Intravenous (3% to less than 20%) ... 2747
▲ CellCept Oral Suspension (3% to less than 20%) ... 2747
▲ CellCept Tablets (3% to less than 20%) ... 2747
Clinoril Tablets (Less than 1 in 100) ... 1924
Combivir Tablets ... 1411
Copaxone for Injection (Infrequent) ... 3297
Cubicin for Injection (Less than 1%) ... 1026
▲ Dacogen Injection (12%) ... 2129
Depacon Injection (1% or more) ... 412
Depakene (1% or more) ... 417
Depakote Sprinkle Capsules ... 422
▲ Depakote Tablets (1% to 5%) ... 427
▲ Depakote ER Tablets (1% to 5%) ... 434
Dolobid Tablets (Less than 1 in 100) ... 1955
▲ Doxil Injection (5.2% to 41.4%) ... 2351
EC-Naprosyn Delayed-Release Tablets (Less than 3%) ... 2761
Effexor Tablets (Infrequent) ... 3411
Effexor XR Capsules (Infrequent) ... 3417
Efudex ... 3363
▲ Eloxatin for Injection (3% to 42%) ... 2892
▲ Emend Capsules (5.3%) ... 1963
Epivir ... 1427
Epivir-HBV ... 1432
Epzicom Tablets ... 1436
Equetro Extended-Release Capsules ... 3180
▲ Erbitux (11% to 93%) ... 910
Estratest Tablets ... 3199
Estratest H.S. Tablets ... 3199
Evoxac Capsules (Less than 1%) ... 1047
Fansidar Tablets ... 2765
Flumadine ... 1183
Frova Tablets (Rare) ... 1113
Gabitril Tablets (Frequent) ... 984
Gantrisin Pediatric Suspension ... 2770
Garamycin Injectable ... 3014
▲ Gemzar for Injection (10% to 22%) ... 1771
▲ Gengraf Capsules (6%) ... 459
Herceptin I.V. (At least one of the 958 patients) ... 1233
▲ Hycamtin for Injection (Less than 1% to 24%) ... 1458
▲ Intron A for Injection (Less than 5%) ... 3024
Invanz for Injection (Greater than 0.1%) ... 1999
Invirase (Less than 2%) ... 2772
▲ I.V. Busulfex (26% to 97%) ... 2493
Kaletra (Less than 2%) ... 476
Ketek Tablets (Greater than or equal to 0.2% to less than 2%) ... 2903
Lamictal (Infrequent) ... 1481
▲ Leukine (24% to 62%) ... 814
Levaquin (0.1% to 0.9%) ... 2384
Levaquin in 5% Dextrose Injection (0.1% to 0.9%) ... 2384
Lipitor Tablets (Less than 2%) ... 2483
Lunesta Tablets (Rare) ... 3142
Matulane Capsules ... 3191
Maxair Autohaler ... 1852
▲ Mylotarg for Injection (2% to 29%) ... 3431
Myobloc Injection (Greater than 2%) ... 3192
Naprosyn Suspension (Less than 3%) ... 2761
Naprosyn Tablets (Less than 3%) ... 2761
▲ Neoral Oral Solution (6%) ... 2259
▲ Neoral Soft Gelatin Capsules (6%) ... 2259
▲ Neulasta Injection (15% to 72%) ... 601
▲ Neupogen for Injection (5%) ... 603
Neurontin Capsules (Infrequent) ... 2487
Neurontin Oral Solution (Infrequent) ... 2487
Neurontin Tablets (Infrequent) ... 2487
▲ Nexavar Tablets (Common) ... 746
▲ Nipent for Injection (5% to 12%) ... 1863
Noroxin Tablets ... 2032
Omnicef Capsules ... 511
Omnicef for Oral Suspension ... 511
OxyContin Tablets (Less than 1%) ... 2703
Paxil CR Controlled-Release Tablets (Rare) ... 1538
Paxil (Rare) ... 1530
PEG-Intron Powder for Injection ... 3048
Plavix Tablets ... 917
Prevacid Delayed-Release Capsules (Less than 1%) ... 3271
Prevacid for Delayed-Release Oral Suspension (Less than 1%) ... 3271
Prevacid SoluTab Delayed-Release Orally Disintegrating Tablets (Less than 1%) ... 3271
Prevacid NapraPAC (Less than 3%) ... 3280
▲ PREVPAC (Less than 1% to 3%) ... 3284
▲ Prograf Capsules and Injection (3% to 15%) ... 632
▲ Proleukin for Injection (22%) ... 2266
Protonix I.V. (Less than 1%) ... 3472
Protonix Tablets (Less than 1%) ... 3469
Protopic Ointment (0.2% to less than 1%) ... 638
Prozac Pulvules and Liquid (Infrequent) ... 1801
▲ Rapamune Oral Solution and Tablets (3% to 20%) ... 3475
Relpax Tablets (Rare) ... 2548
Requip Tablets (Infrequent) ... 1555
Rescriptor Tablets ... 2551
Retrovir IV Infusion ... 1564
Rilutek Tablets (0.8% to 1.2%) ... 2930
Risperdal (Infrequent) ... 1676
Risperdal Consta Long-Acting Injection (Infrequent) ... 1682
Risperdal M-Tab Orally Disintegrating Tablets (Infrequent) ... 1676
▲ Sandostatin LAR Depot (1% to 4%) ... 2280
Seroquel Tablets (Infrequent) ... 690
Sonata Capsules (Infrequent) ... 1717
▲ Soriatane Capsules (1% to 10%) ... 1013
▲ Spiriva HandiHaler (1% to 3%) ... 869
Striant Mucoadhesive ... 1007
▲ Sutent Capsules (1% to 53%) ... 2560
Symbyax Capsules (Infrequent) ... 1819
Tabloid Tablets (Less frequent) ... 1575
▲ Tarceva Tablets (0% to 22%) ... 1259
▲ Tarceva Tablets (0% to 22%) ... 2444
▲ Taxotere Injection Concentrate (1.1% to 59.3%) ... 2932
Tegretol/Tegretol-XR ... 2295
▲ Temodar Capsules (1% to 9%) ... 3073
▲ Tequin Injection (0.1% to 3%) ... 938
▲ Tequin Injection in 5% Dextrose (0.1% to 3%) ... 938
▲ Tequin Tablets (0.1% to 3%) ... 938
Thalomid Capsules ... 965
Timentin ADD-Vantage ... 1580
Timentin Injection Galaxy Container ... 1583
Timentin IV Infusion ... 1577
Timentin Pharmacy Bulk Package ... 1586
Tindamax Tablets ... 2142
Topamax Sprinkle Capsules (Infrequent) ... 2404
Topamax Tablets (Infrequent) ... 2404
Trecator Tablets ... 3487
Trileptal Tablets ... 2300
Trileptal Oral Suspension ... 2300
Trizivir Tablets ... 1589
Uniretic Tablets (Less than 1%) ... 3100
Vantin Tablets and Oral Suspension (Less than 1%) ... 2645
Vasotec I.V. Injection (0.5% to 1.0%) ... 2103
VFEND I.V. (Less than 2%) ... 2564
VFEND Oral Suspension (Less than 2%) ... 2564
VFEND Tablets (Less than 2%) ... 2564
Viagra Tablets (Less than 2%) ... 2573
Voltaren Tablets (Occasionally) ... 2307
Voltaren-XR Tablets (Occasionally) ... 2310
Wellbutrin Tablets (Frequent) ... 1603
Wellbutrin SR Sustained-Release Tablets (Infrequent) ... 1607
Wellbutrin XL Extended-Release Tablets (Infrequent) ... 1613
▲ Xeloda Tablets (2% to 25%) ... 2822
▲ Zelapar Tablets (5%) ... 3372
▲ Zinecard for Injection (26% to 34%) ... 2650
Zoloft (Rare) ... 2586
▲ Zometa for Intravenous Infusion (8%) ... 2315
Zomig Nasal Spray (Rare) ... 3523
Zonegran Capsules (Infrequent) ... 1101
Zyban Sustained-Release Tablets (Infrequent) ... 1644
Zyprexa Tablets (Infrequent) ... 1830
Zyprexa ZYDIS Orally Disintegrating Tablets (Infrequent) ... 1830
Zyrtec Chewable Tablets (Less than 2%) ... 2594
Zyrtec (Less than 2%) ... 2594
Zyrtec-D 12 Hour Extended Release Tablets (Less than 2%) ... 2597

Stomatitis, ulcerative
▲ Agrylin Capsules (1% to 5%) ... 3169
AmBisome for Injection (Less common) ... 620
Anaprox Tablets (Less than 1%) ... 2761
Anaprox DS Tablets (Less than 1%) ... 2761
Arthrotec Tablets (Rare) ... 3129
Astelin Nasal Spray (Infrequent) ... 1904
Bactroban Cream (Less than 1%) ... 1394
Caduet Tablets (Less than 2%) ... 2508
▲ Campath Ampules (1% to 14%) ... 811
Colazal Capsules ... 2838
Copaxone for Injection (Frequent) ... 3297
Cosmegen for Injection ... 2459
Cymbalta Delayed-Release Capsules (Infrequent) ... 1757
▲ Doxil Injection (1% to 5%) ... 2351
EC-Naprosyn Delayed-Release Tablets (Less than 1%) ... 2761
▲ Evoxac Capsules (1% to 3%) ... 1047
Exelon Capsules (Infrequent) ... 2206
Exelon Oral Solution (Infrequent) ... 2206
Gabitril Tablets (Infrequent) ... 984
Indocin Capsules (Less than 1%) ... 1995
Indocin I.V. (Less than 1%) ... 2465
Indocin (Less than 1%) ... 1995
▲ Intron A for Injection (Less than 5%) ... 3024
Kaletra (Less than 2%) ... 476
Lipitor Tablets (Less than 2%) ... 2483
Lunesta Tablets (Infrequent) ... 3142
Lyrica Capsules (Rare) ... 2539
Mobic Oral Suspension (Less than 2%) ... 863
Mobic Tablets (Less than 2%) ... 863
Naprosyn Suspension (Less than 1%) ... 2761
Naprosyn Tablets (Less than 1%) ... 2761
Neurontin Capsules (Rare) ... 2487
Neurontin Oral Solution (Rare) ... 2487
Neurontin Tablets (Rare) ... 2487
Nexium Delayed-Release Capsules (Less than 1%) ... 655
Nexium I.V. (Less than 1%) ... 659
Paxil CR Controlled-Release Tablets (Rare to infrequent) ... 1538
Paxil (Rare to infrequent) ... 1530
Permax Tablets (Rare) ... 3356
Prevacid Delayed-Release Capsules (Less than 1%) ... 3271
Prevacid for Delayed-Release Oral Suspension (Less than 1%) ... 3271
Prevacid SoluTab Delayed-Release Orally Disintegrating Tablets (Less than 1%) ... 3271
Prevacid NapraPAC (Less than 1%) ... 3280
PREVPAC (Less than 1%) ... 3284
Protonix I.V. (Less than 1%) ... 3472
Protonix Tablets (Less than 1%) ... 3469
Prozac Pulvules and Liquid (Infrequent) ... 1801
Requip Tablets (Infrequent) ... 1555
Reyataz Capsules (Less than 3%) ... 921
Risperdal Consta Long-Acting Injection (Infrequent) ... 1682
▲ Simulect for Injection (3% to 10%) ... 2284
Sonata Capsules (Rare) ... 1717
▲ Soriatane Capsules (1% to 10%) ... 1013
▲ Spiriva HandiHaler (1% to 3%) ... 869
Symbyax Capsules (Rare) ... 1819
Trileptal Tablets ... 2300
Trileptal Oral Suspension ... 2300
Viramune Oral Suspension ... 873
Viramune Tablets ... 873
Zoloft (Rare) ... 2586
Zonegran Capsules (Infrequent) ... 1101
Zosyn (1.0% or less) ... 3492
Zyprexa Tablets (Infrequent) ... 1830
Zyprexa ZYDIS Orally Disintegrating Tablets (Infrequent) ... 1830
Zyrtec Chewable Tablets (Less than 2%) ... 2594
Zyrtec (Less than 2%) ... 2594
Zyrtec-D 12 Hour Extended Release Tablets (Less than 2%) ... 2597

Stool, bloody
(*see under* Hematochezia)

Stool, color changes
Coumadin for Injection ... 898
Coumadin Tablets ... 898
Invirase (Less than 2%) ... 2772
Lamisil Tablets ... 2232
Ortho-Cyclen/Ortho Tri-Cyclen ... 2429
Ortho Tri-Cyclen Lo Tablets ... 2436
Pepto-Bismol Original Liquid, Maximum Strength Liquid, Original and Cherry Tablets, Chewable Tablets and Easy-To-Swallow Caplets ... 2676

Pepto-Bismol Maximum Strength Liquid 672
Prevacid NapraPAC (Less than 1%) 3280
PREVPAC (Less than 3%) 3284
▲ Sandostatin LAR Depot (4% to 6%) 2280
Tasmar Tablets 3358
Ticlid Tablets 2810

Stool, oily
▲ Xenical Capsules (5.5% to 20%) 2831

Stool frequency, increased
Lexapro Oral Solution (Infrequent) 1190
Lexapro Tablets (Infrequent) 1190

Stools, abnormal
Aciphex Tablets 1090
Asacol Delayed-Release Tablets (2% or greater) 2692
Clozaril Tablets (Less than 1%) 2184
Colazal Capsules (1%) 2838
Effexor Tablets (Rare) 3411
Effexor XR Capsules (Rare) 3417
FazaClo Orally Disintegrating Tablets (Less than 1%) 551
Gabitril Tablets (Infrequent) 984
▲ Kaletra (Up to 6%) 476
Neurontin Capsules (Infrequent) 2487
Neurontin Oral Solution (Infrequent) 2487
Neurontin Tablets (Infrequent) 2487
Nexium Delayed-Release Capsules (Less than 1%) 655
Nexium I.V. (Less than 1%) 659
Norvir (Less than 2%) 503
Omnicef Capsules (0.3%) 511
Omnicef for Oral Suspension (0.2%) 511
Pentasa Capsules (Less than 1%) 3185
▲ Pletal Tablets (12% to 15%) 2455
Prevacid Delayed-Release Capsules (Less than 1%) 3271
Prevacid for Delayed-Release Oral Suspension (Less than 1%) 3271
Prevacid SoluTab Delayed-Release Orally Disintegrating Tablets (Less than 1%) 3271
Prevacid NapraPAC (Less than 1%) 3280
PREVPAC (Less than 1%) 3284
Protonix I.V. (Less than 1%) 3472
Protonix Tablets (Less than 1%) 3469
▲ Sandostatin Injection (Less than 10%) 2278
Tasmar Tablets (Infrequent) 3358
Tygacil for Injection (0% to less than 2%) 3488
Ultrase MT Capsules (1.5%) 709
Vicoprofen Tablets (Less than 1%) 539
Zosyn (1.9% to 2.4%) 3492
Zyban Sustained-Release Tablets 1644

Stools, loose
▲ Agenerase Capsules (28% to 60%) 1327
▲ Agenerase Oral Solution (28% to 56%) 1332
▲ Amitiza Capsules (0% to 3.4%) 3224
▲ Augmentin (9%) 1360
▲ Augmentin Tablets (9%) 1363
Augmentin XR Extended-Release Tablets (1.6%) 1369
▲ Avandamet Tablets (5%) 1373
Caduet Tablets (Less than or equal to 0.1%) 2508
▲ Ceftin (8.6%) 1407
▲ Chemet Capsules (12.0% to 20.9%) 2458
Cialis Tablets (Less than 2%) 1838
▲ Cubicin for Injection (4.2%) 1026
▲ Cymbalta Delayed-Release Capsules (2% to 3%) 1757
▲ Dacogen Injection (7%) 2129
Elidel Cream 1% (Up to 1.2%) 2200
▲ Gleevec Tablets (0% to 12%) 2227
▲ Imdur Tablets (Less than or equal to 5%) 3018
▲ Intron A for Injection (Up to 10%) 3024
Invanz for Injection (2.1%) 1999
Ketek Tablets (Greater than or equal to 0.2% to less than 2%) 2903
▲ Lariam Tablets (Among most frequent) 2786
MetroGel-Vaginal Gel (1%) 1855
▲ Myfortic Tablets (3% to less than 20%) 2255
Noroxin Tablets (0.3% to 1.0%) 2032
Norvasc Tablets (Less than 0.1%) 2545
▲ Revlimid Capsules (6.1%) 958
▲ Sandostatin Injection (34% to 61%) 2278
▲ Suprax (6%) 1843
▲ Sustiva Capsules (39%) 930
▲ Sustiva Tablets (39%) 930
▲ Trisenox Injection (10%) 993
Urocit-K Tablets (Some patients) 2144
▲ Vantin Tablets and Oral Suspension (5.9% to 10.6%) 2645
▲ Vivitrol (12% to 13%) 995
Zmax for Oral Suspension (Less then 1%) 2583
▲ Zoloft (20% to 24%) 2586
Zyvox (1.2% to 2.3%) 2652

Strabismus
Aciphex Tablets 1090
Lamictal (Rare) 1481
Neurontin Capsules (Rare) 2487
Neurontin Oral Solution (Rare) 2487
Neurontin Tablets (Rare) 2487
Prozac Pulvules and Liquid (Rare) 1801
Topamax Sprinkle Capsules (Infrequent) 2404
Topamax Tablets (Infrequent) 2404

Strain, muscle
Xyrem Oral Solution (Infrequent) 1688

Strangury
Evoxac Capsules (Less than 1%) 1047

Stress symptoms, unspecified
Ambien CR Tablets (1%) 2855
Xyrem Oral Solution (Infrequent) 1688

Striae
Aclovate Cream (Infrequent) 2660
Analpram-HC 1159
Apexicon E Cream 2661
Aricept Tablets (Infrequent) 1094
Aricept ODT Tablets (Infrequent) 1094
Clobevate Gel 3211
Clobex Lotion 1204
Clobex Shampoo (Infrequent) 1206
Clobex Spray (Less than 1%) 1208
Copaxone for Injection (Infrequent) 3297
Cutivate Cream (Infrequent) 2662
Cutivate Lotion 0.05% (Rare) 2664
Cutivate Ointment (Infrequent to more frequent) 2665
Decadron Tablets 1951
Diprolene Gel 0.05% 3001
Diprolene Lotion 0.05% (Infrequent) 3002
Diprolene Ointment 0.05% (Infrequent) 3003
Diprolene AF Cream 0.05% (Infrequent) 3000
Diprosone Cream, USP 0.05% 3004
Effexor Tablets (Rare) 3411
Elocon Cream 0.1% (Infrequent) 3005
Elocon Lotion 0.1% (Infrequent) 3006
Elocon Ointment 0.1% (Infrequent) 3007
Entocort EC Capsules (1%) 2698
Locoid Lipocream Cream (Infrequent) 1160
Lotrisone 3040
Lupron Depot-PED 7.5 mg, 11.25 mg and 15 mg (Less than 2%) 3269
Lupron Injection Pediatric (Less than 2%) 3259
Luxíq Foam 1010
Olux Foam 1012
Pramosone 1161
ProctoFoam-HC 3099
Temovate Cream 2668
Temovate Gel (Infrequent) 2669
Temovate Ointment 2668
Temovate Scalp Application (Infrequent) 2670
Temovate E Emollient (Infrequent) 2671
Tri-Luma Cream 1213
Vanos Cream 1893

Stridor
Adalat CC Tablets (Less than 1%) 2964
Advair Diskus 100/50 1308
Advair Diskus 250/50 1308
Advair Diskus 500/50 1308
Advair HFA Inhalation Aerosol 1318
Campath Ampules 811
Fluarix 1451
Fortaz 1453
Paxil CR Controlled-Release Tablets (Rare) 1538
Paxil (Rare) 1530
Photofrin for Injection 702
Prevacid Delayed-Release Capsules (Less than 1%) 3271
Prevacid for Delayed-Release Oral Suspension (Less than 1%) 3271
Prevacid SoluTab Delayed-Release Orally Disintegrating Tablets (Less than 1%) 3271
Prevacid NapraPAC (Less than 1%) 3280
PREVPAC (Less than 1%) 3284
Prozac Pulvules and Liquid (Rare) 1801
▲ Pulmicort Respules (1% to 3%) 661
Refludan for Injection (Common) 792
Rilutek Tablets (Infrequent) 2930
Risperdal (Infrequent) 1676
Risperdal Consta Long-Acting Injection (Infrequent) 1682
Risperdal M-Tab Orally Disintegrating Tablets (Infrequent) 1676
Serevent Diskus (Rare) 1568
Ultane Liquid for Inhalation (Less than 1%) 531
Zofran Injection 1634
Zofran 1639
Zofran ODT Orally Disintegrating Tablets 1639
Zoloft (Rare) 2586
Zyprexa Tablets (Rare) 1830
Zyprexa ZYDIS Orally Disintegrating Tablets (Rare) 1830

Stroke
Abilify Oral Solution 882
Abilify Oral Solution 2450
Abilify Discmelt Orally Disintegrating Tablets 882
Abilify Discmelt Orally Disintegrating Tablets 2450
Abilify Tablets 882
Abilify Tablets 2450
Accutane Capsules 2731
Activase I.V. (0.9%) 1223
Adderall Tablets 3164
Adderall XR Capsules 3166
Aloprim for Injection (Less than 1%) 2167
Amerge Tablets 1339
Angeliq Tablets 762
Aranesp for Injection (1%) 581
Arthrotec Tablets 3129
Cialis Tablets 1838
Climara Transdermal System 771
Climara Pro Transdermal System 776
Dolobid Tablets 1955
DynaCirc CR Tablets (0.5% to 1%) 2721
Enbrel for Injection 584
Enjuvia Tablets 1062
Estrasorb Topical Emulsion 1147
Estratest Tablets 3199
Estratest H.S. Tablets 3199
Fabrazyme for Intravenous Infusion 1274
Imitrex Injection 1463
Imitrex Tablets 1471
Integrilin Injection (0.5%) 3020
▲ Intron A for Injection (Less than 5%) 3024
▲ Mavik Tablets (3.3%) 486
Maxalt Tablets 2008
Maxalt-MLT Orally Disintegrating Tablets 2008
Menostar Transdermal System 782
Mobic Oral Suspension 863
Mobic Tablets 863
Neumega for Injection 3435
Ortho-Cyclen/Ortho Tri-Cyclen 2429
Premarin Intravenous 3442
Premarin Tablets 3446
Premarin Vaginal Cream 3452
Premphase Tablets (1.4%) 3456
Prempro Tablets (1.4%) 3456
Prinivil Tablets (0.3% to 1.0%) 2052
Prinzide Tablets 2056
Proleukin for Injection (Less than 1%) 2266
Quadramet Injection (1%) 1040
Risperdal 1676
Risperdal Consta Long-Acting Injection 1682
Risperdal M-Tab Orally Disintegrating Tablets 1676
Ritalin LA Capsules 2271
Soltamox Oral Solution 3527
Soriatane Capsules 1013
Symbyax Capsules 1819
▲ Vesanoid Capsules (3%) 2820
Wellbutrin SR Sustained-Release Tablets (Infrequent) 1607
Wellbutrin XL Extended-Release Tablets (Infrequent) 1613
Zyban Sustained-Release Tablets (Infrequent) 1644

Stroke, hemorrhagic
Activase I.V. (0.7%) 1223
Femara Tablets (Less than or equal to 2%) 2214
Ortho-Cyclen/Ortho Tri-Cyclen 2429

Stroke, new ischemic
Activase I.V. 1223
Vivitrol 995

Stroke, thrombotic
Ortho-Cyclen/Ortho Tri-Cyclen 2429

Stuffiness, nasal
(*see under* Nasal congestion)

Stupor
Abilify Oral Solution (Infrequent) 882
Abilify Oral Solution (Infrequent) 2450
Abilify Discmelt Orally Disintegrating Tablets (Infrequent) 882
Abilify Discmelt Orally Disintegrating Tablets (Infrequent) 2450
Abilify Tablets (Infrequent) 882
Abilify Tablets (Infrequent) 2450
Ambien Tablets (Infrequent) 2851
Ambien CR Tablets (Infrequent) 2855
Azilect Tablets 3293
Celexa (Rare) 1176
Cesamet Capsules 3340
Copaxone for Injection (Frequent) 3297
Duragesic Transdermal System (Less than 1%) 2373
Effexor Tablets (Infrequent) 3411
Effexor XR Capsules (Infrequent) 3417
Gabitril Tablets (Frequent) 984
▲ Invanz for Injection (3.3% to 5.1%) 1999
Lamictal (Infrequent) 1481
Levaquin (0.1% to 0.9%) 2384
Levaquin in 5% Dextrose Injection (0.1% to 0.9%) 2384
Lithobid Tablets 1692
Lunesta Tablets (Rare) 3142
Lyrica Capsules (Greater than or equal to 1%) 2539
Maxipime for Injection 1105
Migranal Nasal Spray (Rare) 3348
Moduretic Tablets (Less than or equal to 1%) 2028
Namenda (Infrequent) 1195
Neurontin Capsules (Infrequent) 2487
Neurontin Oral Solution (Infrequent) 2487
Neurontin Tablets (Infrequent) 2487
Orthoclone OKT3 Sterile Solution 2360
OxyContin Tablets (Less than 1%) 2703
Paxil CR Controlled-Release Tablets (Rare) 1538
Paxil (Rare) 1530
Percodan Tablets 1132
Permax Tablets (Rare) 3356
PhosLo GelCaps 2169
ProSom Tablets (Infrequent) 517
Prozac Pulvules and Liquid (Rare) 1801
Relpax Tablets (Infrequent) 2548
Requip Tablets (Infrequent) 1555
Rilutek Tablets (Infrequent) 2930
Risperdal (Infrequent) 1676
Risperdal M-Tab Orally Disintegrating Tablets (Infrequent) 1676
Romazicon Injection (Less than 1%) 2804
Seroquel Tablets (Infrequent) 690
Sonata Capsules (Rare) 1717
Stromectol Tablets 2083
Symmetrel Tablets 1135
Tambocor Tablets (Less than 1%) 1856
Topamax Sprinkle Capsules (1% to 2%) 2404
Topamax Tablets (1% to 2%) 2404
Trileptal Tablets 2300
Trileptal Oral Suspension 2300
Zyprexa Tablets (Infrequent) 1830
Zyprexa ZYDIS Orally Disintegrating Tablets (Infrequent) 1830

Stuttering
FazaClo Orally Disintegrating Tablets (Less than 1%) 551
Seroquel Tablets (Rare) 690
Zyprexa Tablets (Infrequent) 1830
Zyprexa ZYDIS Orally Disintegrating Tablets (Infrequent) 1830

Stye
▲ Intron A for Injection (Less than 5%) 3024
Klonopin (Infrequent) 2778
Neurontin Capsules (Infrequent) 2487
Neurontin Oral Solution (Infrequent) 2487
Neurontin Tablets (Infrequent) 2487

Sudden Infant Death Syndrome
Infanrix Vaccine 1476
Pediarix Vaccine 1548

Suicidal ideation
Abilify Oral Solution (Frequent) ... 882
Abilify Oral Solution (Frequent) ... 2450
Abilify Discmelt Orally Disintegrating Tablets (Frequent) ... 882
Abilify Discmelt Orally Disintegrating Tablets (Frequent) ... 2450
Abilify Tablets (Frequent) ... 882
Abilify Tablets (Frequent) ... 2450
Accutane Capsules ... 2731
Ambien Tablets ... 2851
Avelox ... 2970
Betaseron for SC Injection ... 767
Campral Tablets (Infrequent) ... 1174
Chantix Tablets (Rare) ... 2517
Cipro XR Tablets (Rare) ... 2990
Copegus Tablets (Less than 1%) ... 2754
Depakote Tablets ... 427
Effexor Tablets (Rare) ... 3411
Effexor XR Capsules (Rare) ... 3417
Exelon Capsules (Infrequent) ... 2206
Exelon Oral Solution (Infrequent) ... 2206
Infergen ... 3364
Intron A for Injection (Rare) ... 3024
Keppra Oral Solution (Rare) ... 3314
Keppra Tablets (Rare) ... 3314
Klonopin (Infrequent) ... 2778
Lamictal (Rare) ... 1481
Lariam Tablets (Rare) ... 2786
Levaquin (Rare) ... 2384
Levaquin in 5% Dextrose Injection (Rare) ... 2384
Lexapro Oral Solution (Infrequent) ... 1190
Lexapro Tablets (Infrequent) ... 1190
Lupron Depot 3.75 mg (Very rare) ... 3260
Lupron Depot–3 Month 11.25 mg (Very rare) ... 3265
Meridia Capsules ... 489
Neurontin Capsules (Infrequent) ... 2487
Neurontin Oral Solution (Infrequent) ... 2487
Neurontin Tablets (Infrequent) ... 2487
Parcopa Orally Disintegrating Tablets ... 3097
▲ Parnate Tablets (4%) ... 1527
Paxil CR Controlled-Release Tablets ... 1538
Paxil ... 1530
Pegasys (Less than 1%) ... 2789
PEG-Intron Powder for Injection (Less than or equal to 1%) ... 3048
Proquin XR Tablets ... 1153
Prozac Pulvules and Liquid ... 1801
Razadyne (Rare) ... 2399
Rebetron Combination Therapy (Less than 1%) ... 3063
Rebif Prefilled Syringe for Injection ... 3159
Seromycin Capsules ... 1813
Soriatane Capsules ... 1013
Stalevo Tablets ... 2287
Sustiva Capsules (0.7%) ... 930
Sustiva Tablets (0.7%) ... 930
Symbyax Capsules ... 1819
Symmetrel Tablets (Less than 0.1%) ... 1135
VFEND I.V. (Less than 2%) ... 2564
VFEND Oral Suspension (Less than 2%) ... 2564
VFEND Tablets (Less than 2%) ... 2564
Viracept (Less than 2%) ... 2577
Wellbutrin Tablets (Rare) ... 1603
Wellbutrin SR Sustained-Release Tablets (Infrequent) ... 1607
Wellbutrin XL Extended-Release Tablets (Infrequent) ... 1613
Zoloft (Rare) ... 2586
Zyban Sustained-Release Tablets (Infrequent) ... 1644
Zyrtec Chewable Tablets (Rare) ... 2594
Zyrtec (Rare) ... 2594
Zyrtec-D 12 Hour Extended Release Tablets (Rare) ... 2597

Suicidal tendency
Pexeva Tablets ... 1694

Suicidality
Paxil CR Controlled-Release Tablets ... 1538
Paxil ... 1530
Pexeva Tablets ... 1694
Prozac Pulvules and Liquid ... 1801
Symbyax Capsules ... 1819
Zoloft ... 2586

Suicide
Aldara Cream, 5% ... 1846
Atripla Tablets ... 945
Cipro XR Tablets (Less than 1%) ... 2990
Copegus Tablets (Less than 1%) ... 2754
Cymbalta Delayed-Release Capsules (Infrequent) ... 1757
Keppra Injection ... 3320
Lyrica Capsules (Rare) ... 2539
Meridia Capsules ... 489
Omacor Capsules ... 2725
Pegasys (Less than 1%) ... 2789
Proquin XR Tablets ... 1153
Razadyne (Very rare) ... 2399
Zyrtec Chewable Tablets (Rare) ... 2594
Zyrtec (Rare) ... 2594
Zyrtec-D 12 Hour Extended Release Tablets (Rare) ... 2597

Suicide, attempt of
Abilify Oral Solution (Infrequent) ... 882
Abilify Oral Solution (Infrequent) ... 2450
Abilify Discmelt Orally Disintegrating Tablets (Infrequent) ... 882
Abilify Discmelt Orally Disintegrating Tablets (Infrequent) ... 2450
Abilify Tablets (Infrequent) ... 882
Abilify Tablets (Infrequent) ... 2450
Accutane Capsules ... 2731
Ambien Tablets (Rare) ... 2851
Ambien CR Tablets (Rare) ... 2855
Campral Tablets (Frequent) ... 1174
Celexa (Frequent) ... 1176
Copaxone for Injection (Infrequent) ... 3297
Cymbalta Delayed-Release Capsules (Infrequent) ... 1757
Effexor Tablets (Infrequent) ... 3411
Effexor XR Capsules (Infrequent) ... 3417
▲ Equetro Extended-Release Capsules (Less than 5%) ... 3180
Exelon Capsules (Infrequent) ... 2206
Exelon Oral Solution (Infrequent) ... 2206
Fuzeon Injection ... 2767
Gabitril Tablets (Infrequent) ... 984
Imitrex Tablets (Rare) ... 1471
Infergen ... 3364
▲ Intron A for Injection (Rare; less than 5%) ... 3024
Invirase (Rare) ... 2772
Keppra Injection ... 3320
Klonopin (Infrequent) ... 2778
Lamictal (Rare) ... 1481
Lariam Tablets (Rare) ... 2786
Levaquin (Rare) ... 2384
Levaquin in 5% Dextrose Injection (Rare) ... 2384
Lexapro Oral Solution (Infrequent) ... 1190
Lexapro Tablets (Infrequent) ... 1190
Lupron Depot 3.75 mg (Very rare) ... 3260
Lupron Depot–3 Month 11.25 mg (Very rare) ... 3265
Lyrica Capsules (0.1% to 1%) ... 2539
Mirapex Tablets (Less than 1%) ... 859
Namenda (Infrequent) ... 1195
Neurontin Capsules (Infrequent) ... 2487
Neurontin Oral Solution (Infrequent) ... 2487
Neurontin Tablets (Infrequent) ... 2487
▲ Parnate Tablets (4%) ... 1527
Paxil CR Controlled-Release Tablets ... 1538
Paxil ... 1530
PEG-Intron Powder for Injection (Less than or equal to 1%) ... 3048
Proleukin for Injection ... 2266
Prozac Pulvules and Liquid (Infrequent) ... 1801
Rebetron Combination Therapy (Less than 1%) ... 3063
Rebif Prefilled Syringe for Injection ... 3159
Remicade for IV Injection (Greater than or equal to 0.2%) ... 971
Requip Tablets (Rare) ... 1555
Reyataz Capsules (Less than 3%) ... 921
Rilutek Tablets (Infrequent) ... 2930
Risperdal (1.2%) ... 1676
▲ Risperdal Consta Long-Acting Injection (1% to 4%) ... 1682
Risperdal M-Tab Orally Disintegrating Tablets (1.2%) ... 1676
Sandostatin LAR Depot (Rare) ... 2280
Seroquel Tablets (Infrequent) ... 690
Sustiva Capsules (0.5%) ... 930
Sustiva Tablets (0.5%) ... 930
Symbyax Capsules (Infrequent) ... 1819
Symmetrel Tablets (Less than 0.1%) ... 1135
Thalomid Capsules ... 965
Topamax Sprinkle Capsules (Frequent) ... 2404
Topamax Tablets (Frequent) ... 2404
Zoloft ... 2586
Zyprexa Tablets (Infrequent) ... 1830
Zyprexa ZYDIS Orally Disintegrating Tablets (Infrequent) ... 1830

Sulfhemoglobinemia
Eulexin Capsules ... 3009
Gantrisin Pediatric Suspension ... 2770

Sulfite, sensitivity to
Dilaudid Oral Liquid ... 445
Dilaudid Tablets - 8 mg ... 445
EpiPen ... 1061
Garamycin Injectable ... 3014
Moban Tablets ... 1119
Norflex Injection ... 1856
Pred Mild Ophthalmic Suspension ... ⊙ 238
Pred Forte Ophthalmic Suspension ... ⊙ 235
Tylenol with Codeine Tablets (Probably low) ... 2391

Sunburn
Accutane Capsules ... 2731
Benzaclin Topical Gel (1%) ... 2877
Differin Cream (2%) ... 1210
Differin Gel (Approximately 1% or less) ... 1211
Diovan HCT Tablets (Less frequent) ... 2196
▲ Photofrin for Injection (4%) ... 702
ProQuad ... 2064
▲ Protopic Ointment (1% to 4%) ... 638
▲ Soriatane Capsules (1% to 10%) ... 1013
Xifaxan Tablets (Less than 2%) ... 2842

Sunburn, exacerbation of
Imitrex Injection ... 1463
Imitrex Nasal Spray ... 1467
Imitrex Tablets ... 1471

Superinfection
Augmentin ... 1360
Augmentin Tablets ... 1363
Augmentin XR Extended-Release Tablets ... 1369
Ceftin ... 1407
Fortaz ... 1453
Mefoxin for Injection ... 2012
Mefoxin Premixed Intravenous Solution ... 2016
PREVPAC ... 3284
Primaxin I.M. ... 2045
Raniclor Tablets, Chewable ... 2505
Suprax ... 1843
Zinacef for Injection ... 1631
Zinacef Injection ... 1631

Suppuration
Efudex ... 3363

Supraventricular contractions, premature
Paxil CR Controlled-Release Tablets (Rare) ... 1538
Paxil (Rare) ... 1530

Surgery
▲ Humira Injection (Less than 5%) ... 466
Yaz Tablets (Greater than 1%) ... 803

Surgery, cataract
Soltamox Oral Solution ... 3527

Surgical site reaction, unspecified
▲ Arixtra Injection (0.8% to 3.2%) ... 1351

Swallowing, impairment
Captopril Tablets ... 2149
Coumadin for Injection ... 898
Coumadin Tablets ... 898
Cubicin for Injection ... 1026
Dantrium Capsules (Rare) ... 2694
Dantrium Intravenous ... 2695
Emend Capsules (Greater than 0.5%) ... 1963
Gengraf Capsules (Rare) ... 459
Imitrex Injection ... 1463
Imitrex Nasal Spray ... 1467
Levaquin ... 2384
Levaquin in 5% Dextrose Injection ... 2384
Lexapro Oral Solution (Infrequent) ... 1190
Lexapro Tablets (Infrequent) ... 1190
Mavik Tablets ... 486
Neoral Oral Solution (Rare) ... 2259
Neoral Soft Gelatin Capsules (Rare) ... 2259
Orthoclone OKT3 Sterile Solution ... 2360
Prinivil Tablets ... 2052
Prinzide Tablets ... 2056
Sandimmune (Rare) ... 2275
Thioridazine Hydrochloride Tablets ... 2163
Vasotec I.V. Injection ... 2103

Sweat, cold
Cymbalta Delayed-Release Capsules (Infrequent) ... 1757
Xyrem Oral Solution (Infrequent) ... 1688

Sweat discoloration
Parcopa Orally Disintegrating Tablets ... 3097
Stalevo Tablets ... 2287

Sweat gland disorder
▲ Advair Diskus 100/50 (1% to 3%) ... 1308
▲ Advair Diskus 250/50 (1% to 3%) ... 1308
▲ Advair Diskus 500/50 (1% to 3%) ... 1308
Soriatane Capsules (Less than 1%) ... 1013

Sweating
(*see under* Diaphoresis)

Sweating, axillary
depo-subQ provera 104 Injectable Suspension ... 2624

Sweating, decreased
(*see under* Hypohidrosis)

Sweating, increased
Advate Injection (0.6%) ... 712
Ambien CR Tablets (Infrequent) ... 2855
Caduet Tablets (Greater than 0.1% to less than or equal to 1%) ... 2508
Colocort Rectal Suspension, USP (Retention) 100 mg/60 mL ... 2476
▲ Copegus Tablets (6%) ... 2754
▲ Cymbalta Delayed-Release Capsules (6%) ... 1757
Decadron Tablets ... 1951
▲ DepoDur Extended-Release Injection (2% to 5%) ... 1110
Depo-Provera Contraceptive Injection (Less than 1%) ... 2622
Eligard 22.5 mg (Less than 2%) ... 2883
Eraxis for Injection (Less than 1% to less than 2%) ... 2521
Ketek Tablets (Greater than or equal to 0.2% to less than 2%) ... 2903
Levothroid Tablets ... 1186
▲ Lexapro Oral Solution (3% to 8%) ... 1190
▲ Lexapro Tablets (3% to 8%) ... 1190
▲ Nalfon Capsules (4.6%) ... 2502
▲ Norditropin Cartridges (8%) ... 2323
▲ Opana Tablets (1% to less than 10%) ... 1122
▲ Opana ER Tablets (8.6% to greater than or equal to 10%) ... 1126
Parcopa Orally Disintegrating Tablets ... 3097
Percodan Tablets ... 1132
Prochieve 4% Gel ... 1003
Prochieve 8% Gel ... 1003
▲ Revlimid Capsules (1.4% to 6.8%) ... 958
▲ Ribavirin, USP Capsules (7% to 11%) ... 3068
Risperdal Consta Long-Acting Injection (Infrequent) ... 1682
Rythmol SR Capsules ... 2727
Stalevo Tablets (2%) ... 2287
▲ Strattera Capsules (4%) ... 1814
Topamax Sprinkle Capsules (Less than or equal to 1%) ... 2404
Topamax Tablets (Less than or equal to 1%) ... 2404
Toprol-XL Tablets ... 668
▲ Trisenox Injection (13%) ... 993
▲ Ultram ER Tablets (1% to less than 6.4%) ... 2392
Vantas (Less than 2%) ... 3375
Visudyne for Injection ... 2305
Voltaren Tablets (Occasionally) ... 2307
Voltaren-XR Tablets (Occasionally) ... 2310
Xifaxan Tablets (Less than 2%) ... 2842
▲ Zoloft (3% to 11%) ... 2586
Zometa for Intravenous Infusion ... 2315

Sweating, non-axillary
▲ BOTOX Purified Neurotoxin Complex (3% to 10%) ... 570

Sweet's syndrome
Gleevec Tablets (Rare) ... 2227
▲ Vesanoid Capsules (3%) ... 2820

Swelling, axillary
Depo-Provera Contraceptive Injection (Less than 1%) ... 2622

Swelling, edematous, ankles
Estratest Tablets ... 3199
Estratest H.S. Tablets ... 3199
Klonopin (Infrequent) ... 2778
Ortho-Cyclen/Ortho Tri-Cyclen ... 2429
Striant Mucoadhesive ... 1007

Swelling, extremities
Avalide Tablets ... 888
Avalide Tablets ... 2874
Avapro Tablets (Less than 1%) ... 891
Avapro Tablets (Less than 1%) ... 2871
Imitrex Injection (Rare) ... 1463

Imitrex Nasal Spray (Rare)................ 1467
Infanrix Vaccine 1476
Noroxin Tablets (Less frequent)........ 2032
Pediarix Vaccine 1548
Women's Rogaine Hair Regrowth Treatment Topical Solution, Spring Bloom Scent and Original Unscented..................... ▣634

Swelling, facial

Altace Capsules............................... 1702
Arthrotec Tablets 3129
Carafate Suspension 701
Carafate Tablets 701
▲ Dacogen Injection (6%) 2129
▲ Doxil Injection (Approximately 6.8%)... 2351
▲ Entocort EC Capsules (11%) 2698
Fluarix 1451
Imitrex Nasal Spray (Rare)............... 1467
Levaquin... 2384
Levaquin in 5% Dextrose Injection 2384
Motrin IB Tablets and Caplets 1866
Children's Motrin Oral Suspension 1867
Children's Motrin Non-Staining Dye-Free Oral Suspension 1867
Children's Motrin Cold Oral Suspension 1867
Infants' Motrin Concentrated Drops 1867
Infants' Motrin Non-Staining Dye-Free Concentrated Drops 1867
Junior Strength Motrin Caplets and Chewable Tablets 1867
Nadolol Tablets (1 to 5 of 1000 patients) 2159
Proscar Tablets 2067
Tamiflu Capsules 2807
Tamiflu Oral Suspension 2807

Swelling, feet

K-Phos Neutral Tablets 760
▲ Prometrium Capsules (100 mg, 200 mg) (6%) 3203
Women's Rogaine Hair Regrowth Treatment Topical Solution, Spring Bloom Scent and Original Unscented .... ▣634
Uroqid-Acid No. 2 Tablets 760

Swelling, hands

▲ Prometrium Capsules (100 mg, 200 mg) (6%) 3203

Swelling, joint

Advate Injection (0.6%) 712
Ceftin for Oral Suspension (0.1% to 1%) 1407
Cozaar Tablets (Less than 1%) 1935
Euflexxa (1.88%) 1162
Fosamax 1969
Fosamax Plus D Tablets 1977
Gleevec Tablets (Less common) 2227
Hyzaar 50-12.5 Tablets 1990
Hyzaar 100-12.5 Tablets 1990
Hyzaar 100-25 Tablets 1990
Imitrex Injection (Infrequent) 1463
Lunesta Tablets (Infrequent) 3142
Neurontin Capsules (Infrequent) 2487
Neurontin Oral Solution (Infrequent) 2487
Neurontin Tablets (Infrequent) 2487
▲ Ultram ER Tablets (1% to greater than 5%) 2392
Xyrem Oral Solution (Infrequent) 1688

Swelling, knee

▲ Euflexxa (3%) 1162

Swelling, legs

K-Phos Neutral Tablets 760
Uroqid-Acid No. 2 Tablets 760

Swelling, lower legs

(*see under* Swelling, legs)

Swelling, mouth

ADACEL Vaccine 2945
Boostrix (Rarely) 1404
Fluarix 1451
Infanrix Vaccine 1476
Pediarix Vaccine (Rare) 1548
Tambocor Tablets (Less than 1%) 1856

Swelling, non-site specific

▲ Advair Diskus 250/50 (1% to 3%) ... 1308
Amerge Tablets (Infrequent) 1339
Bactroban Ointment (Less than 1%) 1395
Coumadin for Injection 898
Coumadin Tablets 898
▲ Doxil Injection (3.4%) 2351
Efudex 3363
Hyzaar 50-12.5 Tablets (1.3%) 1990
Hyzaar 100-12.5 Tablets (1.3%) 1990
Hyzaar 100-25 Tablets (1.3%)......... 1990
Oncaspar 1145
Oxandrin Tablets............................. 2962
▲ Panretin Gel (3% to 8%) 1747
Recombivax HB (Equal to or greater than 1%)............................. 2071
Serevent Diskus (1% to less than 3%).. 1568
Sulfamylon Cream 2162
Sulfamylon for 5% Topical Solution... 2162
▲ TobraDex Ophthalmic Ointment (Less than 4%)................................ 562
▲ TobraDex Ophthalmic Suspension (Less than 4%)................................ 563
Vaqta (Less than 1%)....................... 2097
Viramune Oral Suspension 873
Viramune Tablets 873

Swelling, oropharyngeal

Cymbalta Delayed-Release Capsules (Infrequent).................... 1757
Xyrem Oral Solution (Infrequent)....... 1688

Swelling, peripheral

▲ Revlimid Capsules (8.1%) 958
▲ Ultram ER Tablets (1% to greater than 5%) 2392

Swelling, unspecified

▲ MICRhoGAM Ultra-Filtered (Frequent)...................................... 2371
Neosporin Ophthalmic Solution Sterile .... ⊙265
▲ Pediarix Vaccine (1% to 22.3%) 1548
ProQuad.. 2064
▲ RhoGAM Ultra-Filtered (Frequent) 2371
ThermaCare Heat Wraps 2677
Regular Strength Tylenol Tablets...... 1870
Tylenol 8 Hour Extended Release Caplets.. 1870
Tylenol.. 1870
Extra Strength Tylenol PM Caplets, Vanilla Caplets, Geltabs, Gelcaps and Liquid 1875
Extra Strength Tylenol Rapid Release Gels 1870
Tylenol Allergy Multi-Symptom Caplets with Cool Burst and Gelcaps... 1872
Tylenol Allergy Multi-Symptom Nighttime Caplets with Cool Burst... 1872
Tylenol Severe Allergy Caplets.......... 1872
Tylenol Arthritis Pain Extended Release Caplets and Geltabs 1870
Tylenol Chest Congestion Caplets with Cool Burst............................ 1872
Tylenol Chest Congestion Liquid with Cool Burst............................ 1872
Children's Tylenol Suspension Liquid and Meltaways.................. 1878
Children's Tylenol Plus Cold Suspension Liquid 1879
Children's Tylenol Plus Cold & Allergy Suspension Liquid............ 1878
Children's Tylenol Plus Cough & Runny Nose Suspension Liquid..... 1879
Children's Tylenol Plus Cough & Sore Throat Suspension Liquid..... 1879
Children's Tylenol Suspension with Flavor Creator 1878
Children's Tylenol Plus Flu Suspension Liquid 1881
Children's Tylenol Plus Multi-Symptom Cold Suspension Liquid 1879
Tylenol Cold Severe Congestion Non-Drowsy Caplets with Cool Burst 1874
Tylenol Cold Head Congestion Daytime Caplets with Cool Burst... 1873
Tylenol Cold Head Congestion Nighttime Caplets with Cool Burst 1873
Tylenol Cold Head Congestion Severe Caplets with Cool Burst..... 1873
Tylenol Cough & Sore Throat Daytime Liquid with Cool Burst...... 1877
Tylenol Cough & Sore Throat Nighttime Liquid with Cool Burst... 1877
Concentrated Tylenol Infants' Drops 1878
Concentrated Tylenol Infants' Drops Plus Cold.............................. 1879
Concentrated Tylenol Infants' Drops Plus Cold and Cough........... 1879
Jr. Tylenol Meltaways 1878
Tylenol Sinus Severe Congestion Caplets with Cool Burst................ 1876
Tylenol Sinus Congestion & Pain Daytime Caplets with Cool Burst and Gelcaps 1876
Tylenol Sinus Congestion & Pain Nighttime Caplets with Cool Burst.. 1876
Tylenol Sinus Congestion & Pain Severe Caplets with Cool Burst..... 1876
Tylenol Sore Throat Daytime Liquid with Cool Burst............................ 1877
Tylenol Sore Throat Nighttime Liquid with Cool Burst................... 1877
Women's Tylenol Menstrual Relief Caplets... 1877

Swelling at injection site

▲ ADACEL Vaccine (2.8% to 21%) 2945
▲ Aredia for Injection (Up to 41%) 2179
Attenuvax 1914
▲ Boostrix (0.5% to 38.9%) 1404
Cerezyme for Injection (Less than 1%)... 1270
Cipro I.V. (1% or less)....................... 2984
▲ Comvax (27.2% to 27.6%) 1928
▲ Dacogen Injection (5%) 2129
DAPTACEL Vaccine.......................... 2950
▲ Enbrel for Injection (37%) 584
▲ Engerix-B Vaccine (1% to 10%) 1425
▲ Fluarix (9.3% to 16.7%) 1451
▲ Gardasil Injection (0.6% to 25.4%) .. 1984
▲ Havrix Vaccine (1% to 10%) 1456
HibTITER (Less than 1% to 1.7%)...... 3426
Humalog-Pen.................................... 1781
Humalog Mix 50/50-Pen.................... 1783
▲ Humira Injection (20%) 466
Humulin 50/50, 100 Units 1791
Humulin 70/30 Pen (Occasional)........ 1793
Humulin L, 100 Units (Occasional) ... 1794
Humulin N Pen (Occasional)............. 1797
Hyalgan Solution (Common)............. 2901
Imitrex Injection.............................. 1463
▲ Infanrix Vaccine (0.7% to 32.9%) 1476
Infed Injection 3390
Invanz for Injection (1.8%)................ 1999
▲ Leustatin Injection (9% to 19%) 2357
▲ Menactra Vaccine (0.5% to12.6%) .. 2954
Merrem I.V. (0.2%)........................... 686
M-M-R II... 2006
Pediarix Vaccine 1548
Liquid PedvaxHIB (0.9% to 2.5%)...... 2035
Pneumovax 23 (Common)................ 2043
▲ ProQuad (8.4%) 2064
Risperdal Consta Long-Acting Injection (1%)................................ 1682
Symlin Injection................................ 613
Timentin ADD-Vantage 1580
Timentin Injection Galaxy Container 1583
Timentin IV Infusion......................... 1577
Timentin Pharmacy Bulk Package 1586
Vaprisol (2.7%)................................. 643
▲ Vaqta (1.3% to 13.8%) 2097
▲ Varivax (19.3% to 32.5%) 2100
▲ Vivitrol (8% to 32%) 995
Zemuron Injection (Less than 1%)..... 2346
▲ Zostavax Injection (24.9%) 2111

Swelling at insertion site

Vantas (0.7%).................................... 3375

Syncope

Accutane Capsules.......................... 2731
Aceon Tablets (2 mg, 4 mg, 8 mg) (0.3% to 1%)................................ 3194
▲ Acetadote Injection (.64% to 3.04%).. 1031
Aciphex Tablets 1090
Actimmune (Rare)............................. 1671
Actonel Tablets (0.6% to 2.1%)........ 2683
Actonel with Calcium Tablets (0.6% to 2.1%).............................. 2688
Adalat CC Tablets (Rare).................. 2964
▲ Advair Diskus 250/50 (1% to 3%) ... 1308
Advicor Tablets................................. 1722
▲ Aerobid/Aerobid-M (1% to 3%) 1171
Aggrenox Capsules (1%).................. 822
▲ Agrylin Capsules (1% to 5%) 3169
Aldara Cream, 5%............................. 1846
Alinia for Oral Suspension (Less than 1%)... 2835
Alinia Tablets (Less than 1%)........... 2835
Altace Capsules (Less than 1% to 2.1%).. 1702
Ambien Tablets (Infrequent)............. 2851
Ambien CR Tablets (Infrequent)........ 2855
Amerge Tablets (Infrequent)............. 1339
Amitiza Capsules (Less than 0.2%).. 3224
Anaprox Tablets (Less than 1%)....... 2761
Anaprox DS Tablets (Less than 1%).. 2761
Anzemet Injection (Rare).................. 2859
Anzemet Tablets (Rare).................... 2862
▲ Aredia for Injection (Up to 6%) 2179
Aricept Tablets (2%)......................... 1094
Aricept ODT Tablets (2%).................. 1094
Arthrotec Tablets (Rare).................... 3129
Attenuvax... 1914
Avalide Tablets................................. 888
Avalide Tablets................................. 2874
Avapro Tablets.................................. 891
Avapro Tablets.................................. 2871
▲ Avastin IV (3%) 1227
Avelox (Less than 0.1%).................... 2970
Avinza Capsules (Less than 5%)....... 1741
Axert Tablets (Rare) 2396
Azilect Tablets (Greater than 1%)...... 3293
Bentyl Capsules................................ 697
Bentyl Injection................................ 697
Bentyl Syrup..................................... 697
Bentyl Tablets................................... 697
Betagan Ophthalmic Solution, USP.. ⊙220
Betimol Ophthalmic Solution........... 3382
Betimol Ophthalmic Solution .... ⊙295
Bicillin C-R Injectable Suspension..... 1706
Blocadren Tablets (0.6%) 1916
Brimonidine Tartrate Ophthalmic Solution 0.2% (Less than 3%) ...... ⊙248
Caduet Tablets (Greater than 0.1% to less than 2%) 2508
Campath Ampules 811
Campral Tablets (Frequent) 1174
Camptosar Injection 2604
Captopril Tablets 2149
Carbatrol Capsules 3171
Cardene I.V. (0.7%) 2497
Cardizem LA Extended Release Tablets (Less than 2%) 1728
Cardura XL Tablets (Less than 1%) ... 2515
Carteolol Hydrochloride Ophthalmic Solution USP, 1% .... ⊙249
Catapres Tablets (Rare) 843
Catapres-TTS (0.5% or less) 844
Celebrex Capsules (Less than 0.1%) 3134
Celexa (Infrequent) 1176
▲ CellCept Capsules (3% to less than 20%) 2747
▲ CellCept Intravenous (3% to less than 20%) 2747
▲ CellCept Oral Suspension (3% to less than 20%) 2747
▲ CellCept Tablets (3% to less than 20%) 2747
Cesamet Capsules 3340
Chantix Tablets (Infrequent) 2517
Cialis Tablets (Less than 2%) 1838
Cipro (Less than 1%) 2977
Cipro I.V. (1% or less) 2984
Cipro XR Tablets (Less than 1%) 2990
Clinoril Tablets (Less than 1%) 1924
▲ Clozaril Tablets (More than 5% to 6%) 2184
Comtan Tablets 2189
Comvax 1928
▲ Copaxone for Injection (5 %) 3297
▲ Coreg Tablets (3% to 8%) 1414
Cosopt Sterile Ophthalmic Solution 1931
Covera-HS Tablets (Less than 2%) 3139
Cozaar Tablets (Less than 1%) 1935
Crestor Tablets (Less than 1%) 678
Dalmane Capsules (Rare) 3342
Decadron Tablets 1951
Demadex Injection 2759
Demadex Tablets 2759
Depo-Provera Contraceptive Injection (Less than 1%) 2622
depo-subQ provera 104 Injectable Suspension 2624
Diastat Rectal Delivery System (Infrequent) 3343
Dilaudid Multiple Dose Vials 440
Dilaudid Oral Liquid 445
Dilaudid Tablets - 8 mg 445
Dilaudid-HP (Less frequent) 442
Diovan Tablets (Less frequent) 2193
Diovan HCT Tablets (Less frequent) 2196
Dolobid Tablets (Rare) 1955
Doxil Injection (Less than 1%) 2351
Duragesic Transdermal System (1% or greater) 2373
DynaCirc CR Tablets (0.5% to 1%) 2721
EC-Naprosyn Delayed-Release Tablets (Less than 1%) 2761
Edex Injection (Less than 1%) 3089
Effexor Tablets (Infrequent) 3411
Effexor XR Capsules (Infrequent) 3417
▲ Eldepryl Capsules (7 of 49 patients) 3208
Eligard 7.5 mg (Less than 2%) 2880
Emend Capsules (Greater than 0.5%) 1963
Engerix-B Vaccine 1425
Equetro Extended-Release Capsules 3180

▲ Estring Vaginal Ring (1% to 3%) 2635
Evoxac Capsules (Less than 1%) 1047
▲ Exelon Capsules (3%) 2206
▲ Exelon Oral Solution (3%) 2206
▲ FazaClo Orally Disintegrating Tablets (Greater than 5% to 6%) 551
▲ Ferrlecit Injection (6%) 3388
Fleet Bisacodyl Laxatives 1165
Flomax Capsules (0.2% to 0.4%) 850
Flumadine (Less than 0.3%) 1183
Fluorescite Injection ⊙ 207
Forteo for Injection (2.6%) 1767
Frova Tablets (Rare) 1113
Gabitril Tablets (Frequent) 984
Gantrisin Pediatric Suspension 2770
Geodon Capsules (0.6%) 2529
Gleevec Tablets (Infrequent) 2227
Havrix Vaccine (Rare) 1456
Herceptin I.V. (At least one of the 958 patients) 1233
▲ Humira Injection (Less than 5%) 466
▲ Hytrin Capsules (0.5% to 21%) 471
Hyzaar 50-12.5 Tablets 1990
Hyzaar 100-12.5 Tablets 1990
Hyzaar 100-25 Tablets 1990
Imdur Tablets 3018
Imitrex Injection (Infrequent) 1463
Imitrex Nasal Spray (Infrequent) 1467
Imitrex Tablets (Rare to infrequent) 1471
Indocin (Less than 1%) 1995
Infed Injection 3390
▲ Intron A for Injection (Less than 5%) 3024
Invanz for Injection (Greater than 0.1%) 1999
Invirase (Less than 2%) 2772
Ionsys Transdermal System (.1% to less than 1%) 2379
Kadian Capsules (Less than 3%) 577
Ketek Tablets 2903
Kytril (Rare) 2784
Lamictal (Infrequent) 1481
Lariam Tablets (Occasional) 2786
Leukine 814
Levaquin (0.1% to 0.9%) 2384
Levaquin in 5% Dextrose Injection (0.1% to 0.9%) 2384
Levitra Tablets (Less than 2%) 3034
Lexapro Oral Solution (Infrequent) 1190
Lexapro Tablets (Infrequent) 1190
Lipitor Tablets (Less than 2%) 2483
Lithobid Tablets 1692
Lotensin Tablets (0.1%) 2243
Lotensin HCT Tablets (0.3% or more) 2246
▲ Lupron Depot 3.75 mg (Among most frequent) 3260
Lupron Depot–3 Month 11.25 mg (Less than 5%) 3265
Lupron Depot-PED 7.5 mg, 11.25 mg and 15 mg (Less than 2%) 3269
Lupron Injection Pediatric (Less than 2%) 3259
Lyrica Capsules (0.1% to 1%) 2539
Matulane Capsules 3191
▲ Mavik Tablets (0.2% to 5.9%) 486
Maxair Autohaler 1852
Maxalt Tablets (Rare) 2008
Maxalt-MLT Orally Disintegrating Tablets (Rare) 2008
Meridia Capsules 489
Merrem I.V. (Greater than 0.1% to 1%) 686
Meruvax II 2019
Micardis Tablets 854
Micardis HCT Tablets 856
Mirapex Tablets (1% or more) 859
Mirena Intrauterine System 787
M-M-R II 2006
Mobic Oral Suspension (Less than 2%) 863
Mobic Tablets (Less than 2%) 863
Moduretic Tablets (Less than or equal to 1%) 2028
MS Contin Tablets (Less frequent) 2701
Mumpsvax 2031
Namenda (Frequent) 1195
Naprosyn Suspension (Less than 1%) 2761
Naprosyn Tablets (Less than 1%) 2761
Nembutal Sodium Solution, USP (Less than 1%) 2470
▲ Neumega for Injection (13%) 3435
Neurontin Capsules (Infrequent) 2487
Neurontin Oral Solution (Infrequent) 2487
Neurontin Tablets (Infrequent) 2487
Niaspan Extended-Release Tablets 1730
Nipent for Injection (Less than 3%) 1863
▲ Niravam Orally Disintegrating Tablets (3% to 3.8%) 3092
▲ Nitro-Dur Transdermal Infusion System (4%) 3046
Norflex Injection 1856
Norvasc Tablets (More than 0.1% to 1%) 2545
Norvir (0.6% to 1.7%) 503
Omacor Capsules 2725
Opana Tablets (Less than 1%) 1122
Opana ER Tablets (Less than 1%) 1126
Ortho-Cyclen Tablets 2429
Ortho Evra Transdermal System 2417
Ortho Tri-Cyclen Tablets 2429
OxyContin Tablets (Less than 1%) 2703
Parcopa Orally Disintegrating Tablets 3097
Paxil CR Controlled-Release Tablets (Frequent) 1538
Paxil (Frequent) 1530
Permax Tablets (2.1%) 3356
Phenergan Tablets and Suppositories 3440
Plavix Tablets (1% to 2.5%) 917
Plavix Tablets (1% to 2.5%) 2926
Pletal Tablets (Less than 2%) 2455
Prevacid Delayed-Release Capsules (Less than 1%) 3271
Prevacid for Delayed-Release Oral Suspension (Less than 1%) 3271
Prevacid SoluTab Delayed-Release Orally Disintegrating Tablets (Less than 1%) 3271
Prevacid NapraPAC (Less than 1%) 3280
PREVPAC (Less than 1%) 3284
Prinivil Tablets (0.3% to 1.0%) 2052
Prinzide Tablets (0.8% to 0.1%) 2056
Prochieve 4% Gel 1003
Prochieve 8% Gel 1003
Prograf Capsules and Injection 632
Proleukin for Injection (Less than 1%) 2266
Prometrium Capsules (100 mg, 200 mg) (Rare) 3203
ProQuad 2064
Proquin XR Tablets 1153
ProSom Tablets (Rare) 517
Protonix I.V. (Less than 1%) 3472
Protonix Tablets (Less than 1%) 3469
Protopic Ointment (0.2% to less than 1%) 638
Provigil Tablets (1%) 988
Prozac Pulvules and Liquid (Infrequent) 1801
Ranexa Tablets (0% to 0.7%) 1035
Raniclor Tablets, Chewable (Rare) 2505
▲ Rapamune Oral Solution and Tablets (3% to 20%) 3475
Razadyne (0.4% to 2.2%) 2399
Razadyne ER Extended-Release Capsules (0.4% to 2.2%) 2399
Recombivax HB 2071
Relpax Tablets (Rare) 2548
Remicade for IV Injection (Greater than or equal to 0.2%) 971
▲ Requip Tablets (3% to 12%) 1555
Retrovir Capsules 1560
Retrovir IV Infusion 1564
Retrovir 1560
Revlimid Capsules (0.9% to 1.4%) 958
Reyataz Capsules (Less than 3%) 921
Rilutek Tablets (Infrequent) 2930
Risperdal (0.2%) 1676
Risperdal Consta Long-Acting Injection (Up to 2%) 1682
Risperdal M-Tab Orally Disintegrating Tablets (0.2%) 1676
Rythmol SR Capsules 2727
Sanctura Tablets 1151
Sandostatin Injection (Less than 1%) 2278
▲ Sandostatin LAR Depot (1% to 4%) 2280
Seroquel Tablets (1%) 690
Sonata Capsules (Infrequent) 1717
Stalevo Tablets (1.2%) 2287
Strattera Capsules (Very Rare) 1814
Sular Tablets (Less than or equal to 1%) 3122
Sustiva Capsules (Less than 2%) 930
Sustiva Tablets (Less than 2%) 930
Tambocor Tablets (1% to 3%) 1856
Targretin Capsules 1747
Tarka Tablets (0.1% to 0.3% or more) 524
▲ Tasmar Tablets (4% to 5%) 3358
Taxotere Injection Concentrate 2932
Tegretol/Tegretol-XR 2295
Tequin Injection 938
Tequin Injection in 5% Dextrose 938
Tequin Tablets 938
Thalomid Capsules 965
Thiothixene Capsules 2165
Tiazac Capsules (Less than 2%) 1201
Timolide Tablets (Less than 1%) 2086
Timoptic Sterile Ophthalmic Solution (Less frequent) 2088
Timoptic in Ocudose (Less frequent) 2091
Timoptic-XE Sterile Ophthalmic Gel Forming Solution 2092
Topamax Sprinkle Capsules (Frequent) 2404
Topamax Tablets (Frequent) 2404
Toprol-XL Tablets (Greater than 1%) 668
Trileptal Tablets 2300
Trileptal Oral Suspension 2300
Twinrix Vaccine (Less than 1%) 1595
Ultane Liquid for Inhalation (Less than 1%) 531
▲ Ultram ER Tablets (1% to greater than 5%) 2392
Uniretic Tablets (Less than 1%) 3100
Univasc Tablets (0.51%) 3104
Uroxatral Tablets (0.2%) 2943
Vantin Tablets and Oral Suspension (Less than 1%) 2645
Vasotec I.V. Injection (0.5% to 2.2%) 2103
▲ Ventavis Inhalation Solution (8%) 1020
Verelan PM Extended-Release Capsules, Controlled-Onset (2% or less) 3106
Viadur Implant (Rare) 757
Viagra Tablets (Less than 2%) 2573
Visudyne for Injection (Less than 1%) 2305
▲ Vivitrol (13% to 16%) 995
Voltaren Tablets (Occasionally) 2307
Voltaren-XR Tablets (Occasionally) 2310
Wellbutrin Tablets (1.2%) 1603
Wellbutrin SR Sustained-Release Tablets (Rare) 1607
Wellbutrin XL Extended-Release Tablets (Rare) 1613
▲ Xeloda Tablets (Less than 5%) 2822
Xifaxan Tablets (Less than 2%) 2842
Xopenex Inhalation Solution 3146
Xopenex Inhalation Solution Concentrate 3150
Xopenex HFA Inhalation Aerosol 3154
Xyrem Oral Solution (Infrequent) 1688
Zelapar Tablets 3372
Zelnorm Tablets 2312
Zmax for Oral Suspension 2583
Zofran Injection (Rare) 1634
Zoloft (Infrequent) 2586
Zomig Tablets (Infrequent) 3519
Zomig Nasal Spray (Infrequent) 3523
Zomig-ZMT Tablets (Infrequent) 3519
Zonegran Capsules (Infrequent) 1101
Zosyn (1.0% or less) 3492
Zyban Sustained-Release Tablets (Rare) 1644
Zyprexa Tablets (0.6%) 1830
Zyprexa IntraMuscular (Infrequent) 1830
Zyprexa ZYDIS Orally Disintegrating Tablets (0.6%) 1830
Zyrtec Chewable Tablets (Less than 2%) 2594
Zyrtec (Less than 2%) 2594
Zyrtec-D 12 Hour Extended Release Tablets (Less than 2%) 2597

Synovitis

Actiq (Less than 1%) 979
Celebrex Capsules (0.1% to 1.9%) 3134
Cuprimine Capsules (Some patients) 1947
Evoxac Capsules (Less than 1%) 1047
▲ Humira Injection (Less than 5%) 466
Levaquin (0.1% to 0.9%) 2384
Levaquin in 5% Dextrose Injection (0.1% to 0.9%) 2384
Limbrel Capsules (0.009%) 2672
Prevacid Delayed-Release Capsules (Less than 1%) 3271
Prevacid for Delayed-Release Oral Suspension (Less than 1%) 3271
Prevacid SoluTab Delayed-Release Orally Disintegrating Tablets (Less than 1%) 3271
Prevacid NapraPAC (Less than 1%) 3280
PREVPAC (Less than 1%) 3284
▲ Stromectol Tablets (9.3%) 2083
Viagra Tablets (Less than 2%) 2573

Systemic inflammatory response syndrome

Clolar for Intravenous Infusion 1271

Systolic blood pressure, decreased

Agrylin Capsules 3169

T

T3, decrease

Estratest Tablets 3199
Estratest H.S. Tablets 3199
Premarin Tablets 3446

T3, increase

Premphase Tablets 3456
Prempro Tablets 3456
Striant Mucoadhesive 1007

T4, decrease

Striant Mucoadhesive 1007

T4, increase

Estratest Tablets 3199
Estratest H.S. Tablets 3199
Menostar Transdermal System 782
Ortho-Cyclen/Ortho Tri-Cyclen 2429
Premarin Tablets 3446
Premphase Tablets 3456
Prempro Tablets 3456
Striant Mucoadhesive 1007

Tachyarrhythmia

Actimmune (Rare) 1671
Amerge Tablets (Infrequent) 1339
Lotronex Tablets (Infrequent) 1512

Tachyarrhythmia, ventricular

Avelox 2970
Frova Tablets 1113
Zmax for Oral Suspension 2583

Tachyarrhythmias, supraventricular

Lanoxicaps Capsules 1490
Lanoxin Injection 1494
Lanoxin Injection Pediatric 1497
Lanoxin Tablets 1500
Revlimid Capsules 958

Tachycardia

Abilify Oral Solution (Frequent) 882
Abilify Oral Solution (Frequent) 2450
Abilify Discmelt Orally Disintegrating Tablets (Frequent) 882
Abilify Discmelt Orally Disintegrating Tablets (Frequent) 2450
Abilify Tablets (Frequent) 882
Abilify Tablets (Frequent) 2450
AccuNeb Inhalation Solution 1055
Accutane Capsules 2731
▲ Acetadote Injection (3% to 5%) 1031
Aciphex Tablets 1090
Actiq (Less than 1%) 979
Adalat CC Tablets (Less than 1%) 2964
Adderall Tablets 3164
▲ Adderall XR Capsules (6%) 3166
Adipex-P 1215
▲ Advair HFA Inhalation Aerosol (1% to 3%) 1318
Advicor Tablets 1722
▲ Aerobid/Aerobid-M (1% to 3%) 1171
Aggrenox Capsules (Less than 1%) 822
▲ Agrylin Capsules (7.5%) 3169
Albutein 5%, Albumin (Human) 1652
Albutein 25% , Albumin (Human) 1653
Aldara Cream, 5% 1846
Alinia for Oral Suspension (Less than 1%) 2835
Alinia Tablets (Less than 1%) 2835
Alkeran for Injection (In some patients) 955
Allegra-D 12 Hour Extended-Release Tablets 2846
Allegra-D 24 Hour Extended-Release Tablets 2849
Aloxi Injection (1%) 2127
Alphagan P Ophthalmic Solution 567
▲ Alupent Inhalation Aerosol (2.5% to 16.6%) 826
Ambien Tablets (Infrequent) 2851
Ambien CR Tablets (Infrequent) 2855
▲ AmBisome for Injection (9.4% to 18.5%) 620
Anaprox Tablets (Less than 1%) 2761
Anaprox DS Tablets (Less than 1%) 2761
▲ Anzemet Injection (2.2% to 3.3%) 2859
▲ Anzemet Tablets (2.2% to 3.3%) 2862
▲ Aredia for Injection (Up to 6%) 2179
Arthrotec Tablets (Rare) 3129
Astelin Nasal Spray (Infrequent) 1904
Atacand Tablets (0.5% or greater) 649
Atacand HCT (0.5% or greater) 651
Atrovent Inhalation Solution (Less than 3%) 835
Atrovent HFA Inhalation Aerosol 841
Atrovent Nasal Spray 0.03% 837
Atrovent Nasal Spray 0.06% (Less than 1%) 839
Avalide Tablets (1%) 888
Avalide Tablets (1%) 2874

Avapro Tablets (1% or greater)......... 891
Avapro Tablets (1% or greater)......... 2871
Avelox (0.1% to less than 2%).......... 2970
▲ Avinza Capsules (Less than 5%) 1741
Axert Tablets (Infrequent)................ 2396
Bayer Aspirin................................ 744
Bayer Aspirin Comprehensive Prescribing Information............... ▣796
Benicar Tablets (Greater than 0.5%).. 1043
Bentyl Capsules............................... 697
Bentyl Injection.............................. 697
Bentyl Syrup.................................. 697
Bentyl Tablets................................ 697
▲ Betaseron for SC Injection (4%) 767
Bicillin C-R Injectable Suspension..... 1706
BiDil Tablets (2%)........................... 2171
Brimonidine Tartrate Ophthalmic Solution 0.2%............................ ⊙248
Buprenex Injectable (Less than 1%).. 2716
Caduet Tablets (Greater than 0.1% to less than or equal to 1%)........... 2508
Cafcit.. 1886
Campral Tablets (Infrequent)............ 1174
Cancidas for Injection (0% to 1.8%)... 1918
Captopril Tablets (Approximately 1 of 100 patients)........................... 2149
▲ Cardene I.V. (3.5%) 2497
Cardizem LA Extended Release Tablets (Less than 2%)................ 1728
Cardura XL Tablets (Less than 1%)... 2515
▲ Carnitor Injection (5% to 9%) 3188
Catapres Tablets (About 5 in 1,000 patients)........................... 843
Catapres-TTS (0.5% or less)............ 844
Ceftin Tablets (0.1% to 1%).............. 1407
Celebrex Capsules (0.1% to 1.9%).... 3134
Celexa (Frequent)........................... 1176
▲ CellCept Capsules (3% to 22%) 2747
▲ CellCept Intravenous (3% to 22%) ... 2747
▲ CellCept Oral Suspension (3% to 22%)... 2747
▲ CellCept Tablets (3% to 22%) 2747
▲ Cerezyme for Injection (Approximately 6.5%).................... 1270
Cesamet Capsules......................... 3340
Chantix Tablets (Infrequent).............. 2517
Cialis Tablets (Less than 2%)............ 1838
Cipro (Less than 1%)........................ 2977
Cipro I.V. (1% or less)...................... 2984
Cipro XR Tablets............................. 2990
Clarinex Syrup............................... 2995
Clarinex Tablets.............................. 2995
Clarinex Reditabs Tablets................. 2995
Clarinex-D 24-Hour Extended-Release Tablets............ 2998
Clinoril Tablets (Less than 1 in 100).. 1924
▲ Clolar for Intravenous Infusion (34%)... 1271
Clorpres Tablets (About 5 in 1,000)...................................... 2153
▲ Clozaril Tablets (More than 5% to 25%)... 2184
Combivent Inhalation Aerosol (Less than 2%)............................ 847
Comvax... 1928
Concerta Extended-Release Tablets... 1881
▲ Copaxone for Injection (5%) 3297
Coreg Tablets (Greater than 0.1% to 1%).. 1414
Cozaar Tablets (Less than 1%).......... 1935
Dacogen Injection (Greater than or equal to 1%)................................ 2129
Dantrium Capsules (Less frequent).. 2694
Dapsone Tablets USP..................... 1673
Daytrana Transdermal Patch............ 3174
Decadron Tablets........................... 1951
Demadex Injection.......................... 2759
Demadex Tablets............................ 2759
▲ Depacon Injection (1% to 5%) 412
▲ Depakene (1% to 5%) 417
▲ Depakote Sprinkle Capsules (1% to 5%)... 422
▲ Depakote Tablets (1% to 5%) 427
▲ Depakote ER Tablets (1% to 5%) 434
▲ DepoDur Extended-Release Injection (5% to 10%).................. 1110
Depo-Provera Contraceptive Injection (Less than 1%)................ 2622
depo-subQ provera 104 Injectable Suspension................................. 2624
Desoxyn Tablets, USP..................... 2462
Detrol Tablets................................ 2628
Detrol LA Capsules......................... 2631
Dexedrine...................................... 1420
DextroStat Tablets.......................... 3179
Dibenzyline Capsules...................... 3399
Dilaudid.. 440
Dilaudid Non-Sterile Powder............. 440
Dilaudid Oral Liquid......................... 445
Dilaudid Rectal Suppositories........... 440
Dilaudid Tablets.............................. 440
Dilaudid Tablets - 8 mg..................... 445
Dilaudid-HP (Less frequent).............. 442
Diovan HCT Tablets (Greater than 0.2%)... 2196
Ditropan XL Extended-Release Tablets (Rare)............................. 2413
Donnatal Extentabs......................... 2493
▲ Doxil Injection (1% to 10%) 2351
Duragesic Transdermal System....... 2373
Dyazide Capsules........................... 1423
DynaCirc CR Tablets (0.5% to 1%).... 2721
EC-Naprosyn Delayed-Release Tablets (Less than 1%)................. 2761
Effexor Tablets (2%)........................ 3411
Effexor XR Capsules (Frequent)........ 3417
Eldepryl Capsules........................... 3208
▲ Eloxatin for Injection (2% to 5%) 2892
Emend Capsules (Greater than 0.5%)... 1963
Engerix-B Vaccine 1425
▲ Entocort EC Capsules (Less than 5%)... 2698
EpiPen 1061
Epogen for Injection (0.31%) 591
Ethyol for Injection 1898
Evoxac Capsules (Less than 1%) 1047
Exelon Capsules (Infrequent) 2206
Exelon Oral Solution (Infrequent) 2206
▲ FazaClo Orally Disintegrating Tablets (Greater than 5% to 25%)... 551
▲ Ferrlecit Injection (5% to 21%) 3388
Flebogamma 5%, Immune Globulin Intravenous (Human) 1658
Floxin Otic Solution (Single report) ... 1049
Fluarix 1451
Flumadine (Less than 0.3%) 1183
▲ Focalin Tablets (Among more frequent) 2220
Focalin XR Capsules 2223
Follistim AQ Cartridge 2338
Foradil Aerolizer 3010
Fortical Nasal Spray (Less than 1%) 3337
Frova Tablets (Infrequent) 1113
Furosemide Tablets 2154
Gabitril Tablets (Frequent) 984
Gantrisin Pediatric Suspension 2770
Geodon (Frequent) 2529
Gleevec Tablets (Infrequent) 2227
GlucaGen 761
Guanidine Hydrochloride Tablets 3016
▲ Herceptin I.V. (5%) 1233
Human Albumin Grifols 20%, Albumin (Human) 1651
Human Albumin Grifols 25%, Albumin (Human) 1652
▲ Humira Injection (Less than 5%) 466
Hytrin Capsules (0.6% to 1.9%) 471
Hyzaar 50-12.5 Tablets 1990
Hyzaar 100-12.5 Tablets 1990
Hyzaar 100-25 Tablets 1990
▲ Imdur Tablets (Less than or equal to 5%) 3018
Imitrex Injection (Infrequent) 1463
Imitrex Nasal Spray (Infrequent) 1467
Imitrex Tablets (Infrequent) 1471
Indocin Capsules (Less than 1%) 1995
Indocin I.V. (Less than 1%) 2465
Indocin (Less than 1%) 1995
Infed Injection 3390
▲ Infergen (4%) 3364
▲ Intron A for Injection (Less than 5%) 3024
Invanz for Injection (1.3% to 1.6%) ... 1999
▲ Ionsys Transdermal System (1% to less than 10%) 2379
▲ I.V. Busulfex (44%) 2493
Kadian Capsules (Less than 3%) 577
K-Phos Neutral Tablets 760
Kytril Injection (Rare) 2781
Lamictal (Infrequent) 1481
Lanoxicaps Capsules 1490
Lanoxin Injection 1494
Lanoxin Injection Pediatric 1497
Lanoxin Tablets 1500
Lariam Tablets (Infrequent) 2786
▲ Leukine (11%) 814
▲ Leustatin Injection (6%) 2357
Levaquin (0.1% to 0.9%) 2384
Levaquin in 5% Dextrose Injection (0.1% to 0.9%) 2384
Levitra Tablets (Less than 2%) 3034
Levothroid Tablets 1186
Levoxyl Tablets 1712
Lexapro Oral Solution (Infrequent) 1190
Lexapro Tablets (Infrequent) 1190
Lofibra Tablets 1219
Lofibra Capsules 1216
Lotensin HCT Tablets (0.3% or more)... 2246
▲ Lupron Depot 3.75 mg (Less than 5%)... 3260
Lupron Depot–3 Month 11.25 mg (Less than 5%)............................ 3265
Marinol Capsules (Greater than 1%)... 3333
Matulane Capsules 3191
Maxair Autohaler (1.2% to 1.3%)...... 1852
Maxalt Tablets (Infrequent).............. 2008
Maxalt-MLT Orally Disintegrating Tablets (Infrequent)..................... 2008
Meridia Capsules (2.6%)................. 489
Merrem I.V. (Greater than 0.1% to 1%)... 686
Metadate CD Capsules 3323
Miacalcin Nasal Spray (Less than 1%)... 2253
Micardis Tablets (More than 0.3%).... 854
Micardis HCT Tablets (Less than 2%)... 856
Migranal Nasal Spray (Infrequent) 3348
▲ Mirapex Tablets (Greater than or equal to 1%) 859
Mivacron Injection (Less than 1%) 493
Moban Tablets 1119
Mobic Oral Suspension (Less than 2%)... 863
Mobic Tablets (Less than 2%) 863
Moduretic Tablets (Less than or equal to 1%) 2028
MS Contin Tablets (Less frequent) 2701
Mycamine for Injection 628
▲ Myfortic Tablets (3% to less than 20%) 2255
▲ Mylotarg for Injection (9% to 11%) ... 3431
▲ Myozyme for Intravenous Infusion (23%) 1279
Nalfon Capsules (Less than 1%) 2502
Namenda 1195
Naprosyn Suspension (Less than 1%) 2761
Naprosyn Tablets (Less than 1%) 2761
Natrecor for Injection (Greater than or equal to 1%) 3127
NeoProfen Injection 2472
▲ Neumega for Injection (20% to 84%) 3435
Neupogen for Injection 603
Neurontin Capsules (Infrequent) 2487
Neurontin Oral Solution (Infrequent) 2487
Neurontin Tablets (Infrequent) 2487
Nexium Delayed-Release Capsules (Less than 1%) 655
Nexium I.V. (Less than 1%) 659
Niaspan Extended-Release Tablets ... 1730
Nimotop Capsules (Up to 1.4%) 749
Nipent for Injection (Less than 3%) ... 1863
▲ Niravam Orally Disintegrating Tablets (7.7% to 15.4%) 3092
Norflex Injection 1856
Norvasc Tablets (More than 0.1% to 1%) 2545
Norvir (Less than 2%) 503
Numorphan Injection 1120
Omacor Capsules 2725
▲ Oncaspar (Greater than 1% but less than 5%) 1145
▲ Ontak Vials (12%) 1745
▲ Opana Tablets (1% to less than 10%) 1122
▲ Opana ER Tablets (1% to less than 10%) 1126
▲ Orthoclone OKT3 Sterile Solution (10%) 2360
Parnate Tablets 1527
Paxil CR Controlled-Release Tablets (Frequent) 1538
Paxil (Frequent) 1530
Percodan Tablets 1132
Permax Tablets (Infrequent) 3356
Persantine Tablets (Rare) 868
Phenergan Tablets and Suppositories 3440
▲ Photofrin for Injection (6%) 702
▲ Pletal Tablets (4%) 2455
Prevacid Delayed-Release Capsules (Less than 1%) 3271
Prevacid for Delayed-Release Oral Suspension (Less than 1%) 3271
Prevacid SoluTab Delayed-Release Orally Disintegrating Tablets (Less than 1%) 3271
Prevacid NapraPAC (Less than 1%) .. 3280
PREVPAC (Less than 1%) 3284
Prezista Tablets (Less than 2%) 3306
Prilosec OTC Delayed-Release Tablets (Less than 1%) 2677
Primaxin I.M. 2045
Primaxin I.V. (1.5%) 2048
Prinzide Tablets 2056
▲ ProAir HFA Inhalation Aerosol (3%) ... 3300
Procrit for Injection (0.31%)............ 2364
▲ Prograf Capsules and Injection (3% to 15%)................................. 632
Prolastin (Occasional).................... 3255
▲ Proleukin for Injection (23%) 2266
Propine Ophthalmic Solution........... ⊙239
Proquin XR Tablets......................... 1153
Protonix I.V. (Less than 1%)............. 3472
Protonix Tablets (Less than 1%)....... 3469
Protopic Ointment (0.2% to less than 1%)...................................... 638
▲ Proventil Inhalation Aerosol (10%) ... 3053
Proventil Inhalation Solution 0.083% (1%)................................ 3055
▲ Proventil HFA Inhalation Aerosol (7%).. 3056
Provigil Tablets (2%)....................... 988
Prozac Pulvules and Liquid (Infrequent)................................ 1801
▲ Rapamune Oral Solution and Tablets (3% to 20%).................... 3475
Recombivax HB............................. 2071
ReFacto Vials................................ 3484
Relpax Tablets (Infrequent).............. 2548
Remicade for IV Injection (Greater than or equal to 0.2%)................ 971
Requip Tablets (2%)........................ 1555
Rhophylac (Rare)............................ 3505
Rilutek Tablets (1.3% to 2.0%)......... 2930
▲ Risperdal (3% to 5%) 1676
Risperdal Consta Long-Acting Injection (Frequent to 2%) 1682
▲ Risperdal M-Tab Orally Disintegrating Tablets (3% to 5%)... 1676
Ritalin Hydrochloride Tablets........... 2269
Ritalin LA Capsules........................ 2271
Ritalin-SR Tablets.......................... 2269
Rituxan I.V. 1254
Romazicon Injection (Less than 1%)... 2804
Sanctura Tablets (Greater than or equal to 0.5%)............................. 1151
Sandimmune.................................. 2275
Sandostatin Injection (Less than 1%)... 2278
▲ Sandostatin LAR Depot (1% to 4%)... 2280
▲ Seroquel Tablets (6%) 690
▲ Simulect for Injection (3% to 10%) ... 2284
Sonata Capsules (Infrequent)........... 1717
Spiriva HandiHaler.......................... 869
St. Joseph 81 mg Aspirin Chewable and Enteric Coated Tablets... 1869
St. Joseph 81 mg Aspirin............... ▣688
▲ Stromectol Tablets (3.5%) 2083
Sular Tablets (Very rare).................. 3122
Sustiva Capsules (Less than 2%)...... 930
Sustiva Tablets (Less than 2%)......... 930
Symbyax Capsules (2%)................... 1819
Symmetrel Tablets.......................... 1135
▲ Tambocor Tablets (1% to 3%) 1856
Targretin Capsules......................... 1747
Tarka Tablets (0.3% or more)........... 524
Tasmar Tablets (Infrequent)............. 3358
Taxotere Injection Concentrate........ 2932
Tequin Injection (Less than 0.1%)..... 938
Tequin Injection in 5% Dextrose (Less than 0.1%).......................... 938
Tequin Tablets (Less than 0.1%)....... 938
Teveten Tablets (Less than 1%)........ 1735
Teveten HCT Tablets (Less than 1%)... 1737
Thalomid Capsules......................... 965
Thiothixene Capsules..................... 2165
▲ Thymoglobulin for Intravenous Infusion (26.8%)............................ 1284
Tiazac Capsules (Less than 2%)....... 1201
Trasylol Injection (2%).................... 754
Tricor Tablets................................. 527
Triglide Tablets.............................. 3123
Trileptal Tablets............................. 2300
Trileptal Oral Suspension................ 2300
▲ Trisenox Injection (55%) 993
Twinrix Vaccine.............................. 1595
Tygacil for Injection (0% to less than 2%)...................................... 3488
▲ Ultane Liquid for Inhalation (2% to 6%)... 531
Uniretic Tablets (Less than 1%)........ 3100
Uroqid-Acid No. 2 Tablets................ 760
Uroxatral Tablets............................ 2943
Valtrex Caplets.............................. 1597
Ventolin HFA Inhalation Aerosol (Less than 3%).............................. 1600
VFEND I.V. (0% to 2.4%)................. 2564
VFEND Oral Suspension (0% to 2.4%)... 2564
VFEND Tablets (0% to 2.4%)............ 2564
Viagra Tablets (Less than 2%).......... 2573
Vicoprofen Tablets (Less than 1%).... 539

Virazole for Inhalation Solution (Infrequent) 3370
▲ Vivaglobin (0.1% to 3%) 3506
Voltaren Tablets (Occasionally) 2307
Voltaren-XR Tablets (Occasionally) 2310
VoSpire ER Tablets (2.7%) 1052
▲ Wellbutrin Tablets (10.8%) 1603
Wellbutrin SR Sustained-Release Tablets (Infrequent) 1607
▲ Wellbutrin XL Extended-Release Tablets (11%) 1613
▲ Xeloda Tablets (Less than 5%) 2822
Xopenex Inhalation Solution (2.7%) 3146
Xopenex Inhalation Solution Concentrate (2.7%) 3150
Xopenex HFA Inhalation Aerosol (2.7%) 3154
Xyrem Oral Solution (Infrequent) 1688
Zantac (Rare) 1624
Zantac Injection (Rare) 1619
Zantac Injection Pharmacy Bulk Package (Rare) 1622
Zantac Injection Premixed (Rare) 1619
Zantac (Rare) 1624
▲ Zegerid Capsules (3.4%) 2958
▲ Zegerid Powder for Oral Solution (3.4%) 2958
Zemuron Injection (Less than 1%) 2346
Zofran Injection (Rare) 1634
Zofran (Rare) 1639
Zofran ODT Orally Disintegrating Tablets (Rare) 1639
Zoloft (Infrequent) 2586
Zomig Tablets (Rare) 3519
Zomig Nasal Spray (Infrequent) 3523
Zomig-ZMT Tablets (Rare) 3519
Zonegran Capsules (Infrequent) 1101
Zosyn (1.0% or less) 3492
Zyban Sustained-Release Tablets (Infrequent) 1644
▲ Zyprexa Tablets (3% to 4%) 1830
Zyprexa IntraMuscular 1830
▲ Zyprexa ZYDIS Orally Disintegrating Tablets (3% to 4%) 1830
Zyrtec Chewable Tablets (Less than 2%) 2594
Zyrtec (Less than 2%) 2594
Zyrtec-D 12 Hour Extended Release Tablets (Less than 2%) 2597

Tachycardia, junctional
▲ Lanoxicaps Capsules (Among most common) 1490
Lanoxin Injection 1494
▲ Lanoxin Injection Pediatric (Among most common) 1497
Lanoxin Tablets 1500
Romazicon Injection (1 of 446 patients) 2804

Tachycardia, supraventricular
Abilify Oral Solution (Frequent) 882
Abilify Oral Solution (Frequent) 2450
Abilify Discmelt Orally Disintegrating Tablets (Frequent) 882
Abilify Discmelt Orally Disintegrating Tablets (Frequent) 2450
Abilify Tablets (Frequent) 882
Abilify Tablets (Frequent) 2450
Aciphex Tablets (Rare) 1090
Advair Diskus 100/50 1308
Advair Diskus 250/50 1308
Advair Diskus 500/50 1308
Advair HFA Inhalation Aerosol 1318
Aggrenox Capsules (Less than 1%) 822
Aricept Tablets (Infrequent) 1094
Aricept ODT Tablets (Infrequent) 1094
Atrovent HFA Inhalation Aerosol 841
Avelox (Less than 0.1%) 2970
▲ Campath Ampules (3% to 11%) 811
Cardene I.V. (0.7%) 2497
▲ CellCept Capsules (3% to less than 20%) 2747
▲ CellCept Intravenous (3% to less than 20%) 2747
▲ CellCept Oral Suspension (3% to less than 20%) 2747
▲ CellCept Tablets (3% to less than 20%) 2747
Dacogen Injection 2129
Effexor Tablets 3411
Effexor XR Capsules 3417
Ethyol for Injection (Rare) 1898
Evoxac Capsules (Less than 1%) 1047
Exelon Capsules (Infrequent) 2206
Exelon Oral Solution (Infrequent) 2206
Hytrin Capsules (Occasional) 471
Levaquin (0.1% to 0.9%) 2384
Levaquin in 5% Dextrose Injection (0.1% to 0.9%) 2384
Meridia Capsules 489
Nalfon Capsules (Less than 1%) 2502
Namenda 1195
Photofrin for Injection 702
Pletal Tablets (Less than 2%) 2455
▲ Proleukin for Injection (12%) 2266
Proventil Inhalation Aerosol 3053
Razadyne (Infrequent) 2399
Razadyne ER Extended-Release Capsules (Infrequent) 2399
ReoPro Vials (1.0%) 1809
Requip Tablets (Infrequent) 1555
Retavase 2499
Rilutek Tablets (Rare) 2930
Rituxan I.V. 1254
Rythmol SR Capsules 2727
Serevent Diskus 1568
Spiriva HandiHaler (Less than 1%) 869
Sular Tablets (Less than or equal to 1%) 3122
▲ Trasylol Injection (4%) 754
Ventavis Inhalation Solution 1020
Ventolin HFA Inhalation Aerosol 1600
VFEND I.V. (Less than 2%) 2564
VFEND Oral Suspension (Less than 2%) 2564
VFEND Tablets (Less than 2%) 2564
▲ Xeloda Tablets (Less than 5%) 2822
Xopenex Inhalation Solution 3146
Xopenex Inhalation Solution Concentrate 3150
Xopenex HFA Inhalation Aerosol 3154
Zelapar Tablets 3372
Zelnorm Tablets 2312
Zofran Injection 1634
Zosyn (1.0% or less to 1.3%) 3492

Tachycardia, ventricular
Abilify Oral Solution (Frequent) 882
Abilify Oral Solution (Frequent) 2450
Abilify Discmelt Orally Disintegrating Tablets (Frequent) 882
Abilify Discmelt Orally Disintegrating Tablets (Frequent) 2450
Abilify Tablets (Frequent) 882
Abilify Tablets (Frequent) 2450
Aciphex Tablets (Rare) 1090
Activase I.V. 1223
Adenocard Injection 617
Adenoscan 619
Advair Diskus 100/50 1308
Advair Diskus 250/50 1308
Advair Diskus 500/50 1308
Advair HFA Inhalation Aerosol 1318
Ambien Tablets (Rare) 2851
Ambien CR Tablets (Rare) 2855
▲ Argatroban Injection (4.8%) 1346
Avelox (Less than 0.1%) 2970
Axid Oral Solution (2 individuals) 879
Azilect Tablets (Infrequent) 3293
Biaxin/Biaxin XL (Rare) 402
▲ BiDil Tablets (4%) 2171
Caduet Tablets (Greater than 0.1% to less than or equal to 1%) 2508
Campath Ampules 811
Cardene I.V. (0.7%) 2497
▲ CellCept Capsules (3% to less than 20%) 2747
▲ CellCept Intravenous (3% to less than 20%) 2747
▲ CellCept Oral Suspension (3% to less than 20%) 2747
▲ CellCept Tablets (3% to less than 20%) 2747
Cozaar Tablets (Less than 1%) 1935
Demadex Injection 2759
Demadex Tablets 2759
E.E.S. (Rare) 451
Effexor Tablets (Rare) 3411
Effexor XR Capsules 3417
EryPed (Rare) 447
Ery-Tab Tablets (Occasional reports) 449
Erythrocin Stearate Filmtab Tablets (Occasional reports) 453
Erythromycin Base Filmtab Tablets (Occasional reports) 455
Erythromycin Delayed-Release Capsules, USP (Occasional reports) 457
Hyperstat I.V. 3017
Hyzaar 50-12.5 Tablets 1990
Hyzaar 100-12.5 Tablets 1990
Hyzaar 100-25 Tablets 1990
▲ Imdur Tablets (Less than or equal to 5%) 3018
Imitrex Injection (Extremely rare) 1463
Imitrex Tablets (Rare) 1471
Invanz for Injection (Greater than 0.1%) 1999
Lanoxicaps Capsules 1490
Lanoxin Injection 1494
Lanoxin Injection Pediatric 1497
Lanoxin Tablets 1500
Levaquin (0.1% to 0.9%) 2384
Levaquin in 5% Dextrose Injection (0.1% to 0.9%) 2384
Lexapro Oral Solution 1190
Lexapro Tablets 1190
Loprox Shampoo 1888
Meridia Capsules 489
▲ Natrecor for Injection (2% to 10%) 3127
Norvasc Tablets (More than 0.1% to 1%) 2545
Paxil CR Controlled-Release Tablets 1538
Paxil 1530
PCE Dispertab Tablets 515
Permax Tablets (Infrequent) 3356
Pletal Tablets (Less than 2%) 2455
PREVPAC (Rare) 3284
Prinivil Tablets (0.3% to 1.0%) 2052
Prinzide Tablets 2056
Prozac Pulvules and Liquid 1801
Razadyne (Infrequent) 2399
Razadyne ER Extended-Release Capsules (Infrequent) 2399
Relpax Tablets (Infrequent) 2548
ReoPro Vials (1.4%) 1809
Requip Tablets (Rare) 1555
Retavase 2499
Rilutek Tablets (Rare) 2930
Risperdal (Rare) 1676
Risperdal M-Tab Orally Disintegrating Tablets (Rare) 1676
Rituxan I.V. 1254
Romazicon Injection (1 of 446 patients) 2804
Sonata Capsules (Rare) 1717
Tambocor Tablets (0.4%) 1856
Thioridazine Hydrochloride Tablets 2163
Toprol-XL Tablets (Greater than 1%) 668
Trasylol Injection (1% to 2%) 754
VFEND I.V. (Less than 2%) 2564
VFEND Oral Suspension (Less than 2%) 2564
VFEND Tablets (Less than 2%) 2564
Zofran Injection 1634
Zoloft 2586
Zomig Tablets 3519
Zomig Nasal Spray 3523
Zomig-ZMT Tablets 3519
Zosyn (1.0% or less) 3492

Tachyphylaxis
▲ Sandostatin Injection (35%) 2278

Tachypnea
Abelcet Injection 1141
Actimmune (Rare) 1671
Aggrenox Capsules 822
Bayer Aspirin 744
Bayer Aspirin Comprehensive Prescribing Information ▣ 796
Cancidas for Injection (0% to 1.3%) 1918
Clolar for Intravenous Infusion 1271
Follistim AQ Cartridge 2338
Maxalt Tablets (Rare) 2008
Maxalt-MLT Orally Disintegrating Tablets (Rare) 2008
▲ Myozyme for Intravenous Infusion (23%) 1279
Orthoclone OKT3 Sterile Solution 2360
Percodan Tablets 1132
▲ Proleukin for Injection (8%) 2266
Retrovir Capsules 1560
Retrovir IV Infusion 1564
Retrovir 1560
Sulfamylon Cream 2162
Sulfamylon for 5% Topical Solution 2162
Symmetrel Tablets 1135
▲ Trisenox Injection (8%) 993

Talkativeness
Carbatrol Capsules 3171
Dalmane Capsules 3342
Equetro Extended-Release Capsules 3180
▲ Niravam Orally Disintegrating Tablets (2.2%) 3092
Tegretol/Tegretol-XR 2295

Tardive dyskinesia
Abilify Oral Solution (Infrequent) 882
Abilify Oral Solution (Infrequent) 2450
Abilify Discmelt Orally Disintegrating Tablets (Infrequent) 882
Abilify Discmelt Orally Disintegrating Tablets (Infrequent) 2450
Abilify Tablets (Infrequent) 882
Abilify Tablets (Infrequent) 2450
Clozaril Tablets 2184
Depacon Injection (1% or more) 412
Depakene (1% or more) 417
Depakote Sprinkle Capsules 422
▲ Depakote Tablets (1% to 5%) 427
Depakote ER Tablets (Greater than 1%) 434
Effexor Tablets 3411
Effexor XR Capsules 3417
Eldepryl Capsules 3208
FazaClo Orally Disintegrating Tablets 551
Geodon Capsules 2529
Moban Tablets 1119
Namenda 1195
Risperdal 1676
Risperdal Consta Long-Acting Injection (Infrequent) 1682
Risperdal M-Tab Orally Disintegrating Tablets 1676
Seroquel Tablets 690
Symbyax Capsules 1819
Thioridazine Hydrochloride Tablets 2163
Thiothixene Capsules 2165
Wellbutrin Tablets 1603
Wellbutrin SR Sustained-Release Tablets 1607
Wellbutrin XL Extended-Release Tablets 1613
Zomig Nasal Spray (Rare) 3523
Zyban Sustained-Release Tablets 1644
Zyprexa Tablets (1% to 2%) 1830
Zyprexa ZYDIS Orally Disintegrating Tablets (1% to 2%) 1830

Tardive dyskinesia, unmasking of
Wellbutrin Tablets 1603

Tardive dystonia
(*see under* Dystonia, tardive)

Taste, altered
Abilify Oral Solution (Infrequent) 882
Abilify Oral Solution (Infrequent) 2450
Abilify Discmelt Orally Disintegrating Tablets (Infrequent) 882
Abilify Discmelt Orally Disintegrating Tablets (Infrequent) 2450
Abilify Tablets (Infrequent) 882
Abilify Tablets (Infrequent) 2450
Actiq (Less than 1%) 979
Adalat CC Tablets (Rare) 2964
▲ Advair Diskus 100/50 (1% to 3%) 1308
▲ Advair Diskus 250/50 (1% to 3%) 1308
▲ Advair Diskus 500/50 (1% to 3%) 1308
▲ Agenerase Capsules (2% to 10%) 1327
▲ Agenerase Oral Solution (2% to 10%) 1332
Alferon N Injection (1%) 1665
Alphagan P Ophthalmic Solution (Less than 1%) 567
Altace Capsules (Less than 1%) 1702
Altoprev Extended-Release Tablets 3109
Ambien Tablets (Infrequent) 2851
Ambien CR Tablets (Infrequent) 2855
Amerge Tablets (Rare) 1339
Anzemet Injection (Infrequently) 2859
Anzemet Tablets (Infrequently) 2862
Arthrotec Tablets (Rare) 3129
Asacol Delayed-Release Tablets 2692
Astelin Nasal Spray (Infrequently) 1904
Atrovent HFA Inhalation Aerosol (0.9%) 841
Atrovent Nasal Spray 0.03% (Less than 2%) 837
Atrovent Nasal Spray 0.06% (Less than 1%) 839
▲ Avastin IV (14% to 21%) 1227
Avelox (0.1% to less than 2%) 2970
▲ Avinza Capsules (Less than 5%) 1741
Axert Tablets (Infrequent) 2396
▲ Bactroban Nasal (0.8% to 3%) 1394
▲ BeneFix Vials (4.6%) 3408
▲ Biaxin/Biaxin XL (3%) 402
Bicillin C-R Injectable Suspension 1706
Brimonidine Tartrate Ophthalmic Solution 0.2% (Less than 3%) ⊙ 248
Caduet Tablets (Less than 2%) 2508
Campral Tablets (Frequent) 1174
Captopril Tablets (Approximately 2 to 4 of 100 patients) 2149
▲ Carnitor Injection (2% to 9%) 3188
Carteolol Hydrochloride Ophthalmic Solution USP, 1% (Occasional) ⊙ 249
Catapres-TTS (1 of 101 patients) 844
Celebrex Capsules (0.1% to 1.9%) 3134
Celexa (Frequent) 1176
Cesamet Capsules 3340
Ciprodex Otic Suspension (0.5%) 559
Cipro XR Tablets (Less than 1%) 2990
Colazal Capsules 2838

Combivent Inhalation Aerosol (Less than 2%) 847
Comtan Tablets (1%) 2189
Copaxone for Injection (At least 2%) 3297
▲ Cosopt Sterile Ophthalmic Solution (Up to 30%) 1931
Coumadin for Injection (Infrequent) 898
Coumadin Tablets (Infrequent) 898
Cozaar Tablets (Less than 1%) 1935
Crixivan Capsules (2.7%) 1940
Cubicin for Injection (Less than 1%) 1026
▲ Cuprimine Capsules (12%) 1947
Dantrium Capsules (Less frequent) 2694
Denavir Cream (0.2%) 2174
▲ Depacon Injection (1% to 5%) 412
▲ Depakene (1% to 5%) 417
▲ Depakote Sprinkle Capsules (1% to 5%) 422
▲ Depakote Tablets (1% to 5%) 427
Depakote ER Tablets (Greater than 1%) 434
Dilaudid 440
Dilaudid Non-Sterile Powder 440
Dilaudid Oral Liquid 445
Dilaudid Rectal Suppositories 440
Dilaudid Tablets 440
Dilaudid Tablets - 8 mg 445
Dilaudid-HP (Less frequent) 442
▲ Doxil Injection (Less than 1% to 10%) 2351
DuoNeb Inhalation Solution 1058
Effexor Tablets (2%) 3411
Effexor XR Capsules (Frequent) 3417
Eldepryl Capsules 3208
Eligard 7.5 mg (Less than 2%) 2880
▲ Eloxatin for Injection (5% to 12%) 2892
Emend Capsules (Greater than 0.5%) 1963
Enbrel for Injection 584
Evoxac Capsules (Less than 1%) 1047
Exelon Capsules (Infrequent) 2206
Exelon Oral Solution (Infrequent) 2206
Flonase Nasal Spray 1440
▲ Floxin Otic Solution (7%) 1049
Flumadine (Less than 0.3%) 1183
FML Ophthalmic Suspension ⊙ 227
FML Forte Ophthalmic Suspension ⊙ 226
Fortical Nasal Spray (Less than 1%) 3337
Fosamax (0.1% to 0.5%) 1969
Fosamax Plus D Tablets (0.1% to 0.5%) 1977
Frova Tablets (Infrequent) 1113
Fuzeon Injection 2767
Gabitril Tablets (Infrequent) 984
Gengraf Capsules (1% to less than 3%) 459
▲ Gleevec Tablets (0% to 15%) 2227
Hyperstat I.V. 3017
Hyzaar 50-12.5 Tablets 1990
Hyzaar 100-12.5 Tablets 1990
Hyzaar 100-25 Tablets 1990
Imitrex Injection (Infrequent) 1463
▲ Imitrex Nasal Spray (13.5% to 24.5%) 1467
Imitrex Tablets 1471
Infed Injection 3390
▲ Infergen (3%) 3364
▲ Intron A for Injection (Up to 24%) 3024
Invanz for Injection (Greater than 0.1%) 1999
Invirase (Greater than or equal to 2%) 2772
Kaletra (Less than 2%) 476
▲ Kepivance (16%) 597
Kogenate FS 738
Kytril Injection (2%) 2781
Lamictal (Infrequent) 1481
Lamisil Tablets (2.8%) 2232
Lescol Capsules 2233
Lescol XL Tablets 2233
Levaquin (0.1% to 0.9%) 2384
Levaquin in 5% Dextrose Injection (0.1% to 0.9%) 2384
Lexapro Oral Solution (Infrequent) 1190
Lexapro Tablets (Infrequent) 1190
Lidoderm Patch 1118
Lipitor Tablets (Less than 2%) 2483
Lithobid Tablets 1692
Lotensin HCT Tablets (0.3% to 1%) 2246
Lotronex Tablets (Rare) 1512
▲ Lupron Depot 3.75 mg (Less than 5%) 3260
▲ Lupron Depot–3 Month 11.25 mg (Less than 5%) 3265
Lyrica Capsules (0.1% to 1%) 2539
Maxair Autohaler (0.6%) 1852
▲ Mepron Suspension (3%) 1521
Meridia Capsules (2.2%) 489
MetroGel-Vaginal Gel (2%) 1855
Mevacor Tablets 2021
Miacalcin Nasal Spray (Less than 1%) 2253
▲ Migranal Nasal Spray (8%) 3348
Mirapex Tablets (Greater than or equal to 1%) 859
Mobic Oral Suspension (Less than 2%) 863
Mobic Tablets (Less than 2%) 863
MS Contin Tablets (Less frequent) 2701
Myobloc Injection (Greater than 2%) 3192
Nasonex Nasal Spray (Very rare) 3043
Neoral Oral Solution (1% to less than 3%) 2259
Neoral Soft Gelatin Capsules (1% to less than 3%) 2259
▲ Neulasta Injection (15% to 72%) 601
Neurontin Capsules (Infrequent) 2487
Neurontin Oral Solution (Infrequent) 2487
Neurontin Tablets (Infrequent) 2487
▲ Nexium Delayed-Release Capsules (Less than 1% to 6.6%) 655
▲ Nexium I.V. (Less than 1% to 6.6%) 659
Nipent for Injection (Less than 3%) 1863
Niravam Orally Disintegrating Tablets 3092
Norvasc Tablets (Less than 0.1%) 2545
▲ Norvir (7% to 11.1%) 503
Omacor Capsules (2.7%) 2725
OxyContin Tablets (Less than 1%) 2703
Parcopa Orally Disintegrating Tablets 3097
▲ Patanol Ophthalmic Solution (Less than 5%) 561
Paxil CR Controlled-Release Tablets (2%) 1538
Paxil (2%) 1530
PEG-Intron Powder for Injection (Less than 1%) 3048
Pepcid Injection (Infrequent) 2040
Pepcid (Infrequent) 2038
Permax Tablets (1.6%) 3356
Plavix Tablets 917
Plavix Tablets 2926
Prevacid Delayed-Release Capsules (Less than 1%) 3271
Prevacid for Delayed-Release Oral Suspension (Less than 1%) 3271
Prevacid SoluTab Delayed-Release Orally Disintegrating Tablets (Less than 1%) 3271
Prevacid I.V. for Injection (Less than 1%) 3277
Prevacid NapraPAC (Less than 1%) 3280
▲ PREVPAC (3% to 5%) 3284
▲ Prilosec OTC Delayed-Release Tablets (Less than 1% to 15%) 2677
Primaxin I.M. 2045
Primaxin I.V. (Less than 0.2%) 2048
Prinivil Tablets 2052
Prinzide Tablets 2056
▲ Proleukin for Injection (7%) 2266
ProSom Tablets (Infrequent) 517
ProstaScint Kit 1037
Protonix I.V. (Less than 1%) 3472
Protonix Tablets (Less than 1%) 3469
Protopic Ointment (Greater than or equal to 1%) 638
Proventil Inhalation Aerosol 3053
▲ Proventil HFA Inhalation Aerosol (4%) 3056
Provigil Tablets (1%) 988
Prozac Pulvules and Liquid (Frequent) 1801
▲ Rebetol (Less than 1% to 9%) 3058
▲ Rebetron Combination Therapy (6% to 8%) 3063
ReFacto Vials 3484
Relpax Tablets (Infrequent) 2548
Rescriptor Tablets 2551
▲ Retrovir Capsules (5%) 1560
▲ Retrovir IV Infusion (5%) 1564
▲ Retrovir (5%) 1560
Reyataz Capsules (Less than 3%) 921
▲ Ribavirin, USP Capsules (Less than 1% to 9%) 3068
▲ Rituxan I.V. (1% to 5%) 1254
▲ Rythmol SR Capsules (6% to 22%) 2727
▲ Sandostatin LAR Depot (1% to 4%) 2280
Seroquel Tablets (Infrequent) 690
Sonata Capsules (Frequent) 1717
▲ Soriatane Capsules (1% to 10%) 1013
Stalevo Tablets (1%) 2287
Striant Mucoadhesive (2.0%) 1007
Sular Tablets (Less than or equal to 1%) 3122
Sustiva Capsules (Less than 2%) 930
Sustiva Tablets (Less than 2%) 930
▲ Sutent Capsules (0% to 43%) 2560
Symbyax Capsules (Frequent) 1819
Tambocor Tablets (Less than 1%) 1856
Tasmar Tablets (1% or more) 3358
▲ Taxotere Injection Concentrate (0.6% to 5.7%) 2932
▲ Temodar Capsules (5%) 3073
▲ Tequin Injection (0.1% to 3%) 938
▲ Tequin Injection in 5% Dextrose (0.1% to 3%) 938
▲ Tequin Tablets (0.1% to 3%) 938
Testim 1% Gel (1%) 695
Thiola Tablets 2141
Timentin ADD-Vantage 1580
Timentin Injection Galaxy Container 1583
Timentin IV Infusion 1577
Timentin Pharmacy Bulk Package 1586
Tindamax Tablets 2142
▲ TOBI Solution for Inhalation (6.6%) 2298
▲ Topamax Sprinkle Capsules (2% to 15%) 2404
▲ Topamax Tablets (2% to 15%) 2404
Toprol-XL Tablets 668
Trileptal Tablets 2300
Trileptal Oral Suspension 2300
Tygacil for Injection (0% to less than 2%) 3488
Ultane Liquid for Inhalation (Less than 1%) 531
Univasc Tablets (Less than 1%) 3104
Vandazole Vaginal Gel 3338
Vantin Tablets and Oral Suspension (Less than 1%) 2645
Vasotec I.V. Injection (0.5% to 1.0%) 2103
VFEND I.V. (Less than 2%) 2564
VFEND Oral Suspension (Less than 2%) 2564
VFEND Tablets (Less than 2%) 2564
VoSpire ER Tablets 1052
Vytorin 10/10 Tablets 2114
Vytorin 10/10 Tablets 3077
Vytorin 10/20 Tablets 2114
Vytorin 10/20 Tablets 3077
Vytorin 10/40 Tablets 2114
Vytorin 10/40 Tablets 3077
Vytorin 10/80 Tablets 2114
Vytorin 10/80 Tablets 3077
▲ Wellbutrin SR Sustained-Release Tablets (2% to 4%) 1607
▲ Wellbutrin XL Extended-Release Tablets (2% to 4%) 1613
▲ Zegerid Capsules (Less than 1% to 15%) 2958
▲ Zegerid Powder for Oral Solution (Less than 1% to 15%) 2958
Zemplar Capsules (Rare) 541
Zemplar Injection (Rare) 543
Zmax for Oral Suspension (Less then 1%) 2583
Zocor Tablets 2105
▲ Zomig Nasal Spray (5% to 21%) 3523
Zonegran Capsules (2%) 1101
Zosyn (1.0% or less) 3492
▲ Zyban Sustained-Release Tablets (2% to 3%) 1644
▲ Zymar Ophthalmic Solution (1% to 4%) 575
Zyprexa Tablets (Infrequent) 1830
Zyprexa ZYDIS Orally Disintegrating Tablets (Infrequent) 1830
Zyrtec Chewable Tablets (Less than 2%) 2594
Zyrtec (Less than 2%) 2594
Zyrtec-D 12 Hour Extended Release Tablets (Less than 2%) 2597
Zyvox (0.9% to 1.8%) 2652

Taste, bad

Alupent Inhalation Aerosol (Less frequent) 826
Aricept Tablets (Infrequent) 1094
Aricept ODT Tablets (Infrequent) 1094
▲ Ciloxan Ophthalmic Ointment (Less than 10%) 559
▲ Ciloxan Ophthalmic Solution (Less than 10%) ⊙ 206
Cipro (Less than 1%) 2977
Cipro I.V. (1% or less) 2984
Fluorescite Injection ⊙ 207
Imitrex Injection 1463
▲ Imitrex Nasal Spray (13.5% to 24.5%) 1467
Imitrex Tablets 1471
Moduretic Tablets (Less than or equal to 1%) 2028
▲ Thrombate III (3 of 17) 3257
Vicoprofen Tablets (Less than 1%) 539

Taste, bitter

▲ Astelin Nasal Spray (8.3% to 19.7%) 1904
▲ Azopt Ophthalmic Suspension (5% to 10%) 557
Ceftin Tablets 1407
Clinoril Tablets (Less than 1 in 100) 1924
Clozaril Tablets (Less than 1%) 2184
▲ Cosopt Sterile Ophthalmic Solution (Up to 30%) 1931
Dalmane Capsules (Rare) 3342
FazaClo Orally Disintegrating Tablets (Less than 1%) 551
Noroxin Tablets (Less frequent) 2032
Risperdal (Rare) 1676
Risperdal M-Tab Orally Disintegrating Tablets (Rare) 1676
▲ Striant Mucoadhesive (4.1%) 1007
▲ Tindamax Tablets (3.7% to 6.3%) 2142
▲ Trusopt Sterile Ophthalmic Solution (Approximately one-quarter of patients) 2095

Taste, changes
(*see under* Taste, altered)

Taste, loss
(*see under* Ageusia)

Taste, metallic

Adenocard Injection (Less than 1%) 617
Adenoscan (Less than 1%) 619
Calcijex Injection 411
▲ Chemet Capsules (12.0% to 20.9%) 2458
Clinoril Tablets (Less than 1 in 100) 1924
Hectorol Capsules 1275
Hectorol Injection 1278
Lexapro Oral Solution (Infrequent) 1190
Lexapro Tablets (Infrequent) 1190
Lidoderm Patch 1118
Lithobid Tablets 1692
Metrogel 1% 1211
Nalfon Capsules (Less than 1%) 2502
Rocaltrol Capsules 2798
Rocaltrol Oral Solution 2798
▲ Tindamax Tablets (3.7% to 6.3%) 2142
Trecator Tablets 3487

Taste, perversion

Levaquin 2384
Levaquin in 5% Dextrose Injection 2384
Zelapar Tablets 3372

Taste, salty

Miacalcin Injection 2252

Taste, unpleasant

Adderall Tablets 3164
Adderall XR Capsules 3166
Adipex-P 1215
▲ Aerobid/Aerobid-M (10%) 1171
▲ Azopt Ophthalmic Suspension (5% to 10%) 557
Beconase AQ Nasal Spray 1396
▲ Ceftin for Oral Suspension (5.0%) 1407
Cipro XR Tablets 2990
Desoxyn Tablets, USP 2462
Dexedrine 1420
DextroStat Tablets 3179
Efudex 3363
Flonase Nasal Spray (Less than 1%) 1440
Kogenate FS with Bio-Set (1 case) 740
▲ Lunesta Tablets (8% to 34%) 3142
Mephyton Tablets 2018

Taste disturbances

Zometa for Intravenous Infusion 2315

Tearing, ocular

▲ Nevanac Ophthalmic Suspension 0.1% (1% to 5%) ⊙ 209

Tearing, unspecified

▲ Taxotere Injection Concentrate (0% to 8.1%) 2932

Teeth, discoloration

Neurontin Capsules (Rare) 2487
Neurontin Oral Solution (Rare) 2487
Neurontin Tablets (Rare) 2487
Primaxin I.M. 2045
Primaxin I.V. (Less than 0.2%) 2048

Teeth, mottling of enamel
(*see under* Teeth, discoloration)

Teeth grinding

Celexa (Infrequent) 1176
Zoloft (Infrequent) 2586

Telangiectasia

Clobevate Gel (Less than 2%) 3211
▲ Clobex Lotion (3.2%) 1204
Clobex Shampoo 1206
Cutivate Ointment 2665

Diprolene Gel 0.05% ... 3001
Diprolene AF Cream 0.05% ... 3000
Efudex ... 3363
Lofibra Tablets (Less than 1%) ... 1219
Lofibra Capsules (Less than 1%) ... 1216
Olux Foam (Less than 2%) ... 1012
▲ Temovate Gel (Among most frequent) ... 2669
Temovate Ointment (Less frequent) ... 2668
Temovate E Emollient (Less than 2%) ... 2671
Tricor Tablets ... 527
▲ Tri-Luma Cream (3%) ... 1213

Telogen effluvium
Lariam Tablets ... 2786

Temperature disturbances, cutaneous
Wellbutrin Tablets (1.9%) ... 1603
Xyrem Oral Solution (Infrequent) ... 1688

Temperature elevation
(*see under* Hyperthermia)

Tenderness
Aldara Cream, 5% (More than 1%) ... 1846
Altoprev Extended-Release Tablets .. 3109
Bactroban Ointment (Less than 1%) ... 1395
▲ Dacogen Injection (11%) ... 2129
Efudex (Infrequent) ... 3363
▲ HibTITER (0.3% to 3.7%) ... 3426
Levulan Kerastick for Topical Solution, 20% (1% to 2%) ... 1085
Mevacor Tablets ... 2021
▲ Miacalcin Nasal Spray (10.6%) ... 2253
M-M-R II ... 2006
Oncaspar ... 1145
Proquin XR Tablets (Less than 1%) ... 1153
Recombivax HB (Equal to or greater than 1%) ... 2071
Tabloid Tablets ... 1575
Temovate Scalp Application (1 of 294 patients) ... 2670
Zocor Tablets ... 2105

Tenderness, elbow
Temovate E Emollient (Less than 2%) ... 2671

Tenderness, knee
Euflexxa (0.63%) ... 1162

Tenderness, nasal
▲ Fortical Nasal Spray (10.6%) ... 3337

Tenderness, right upper quadrant
Arthrotec Tablets ... 3129
Celebrex Capsules ... 3134
Tasmar Tablets ... 3358

Tenderness at injection site
▲ Actimmune (14%) ... 1671
▲ DAPTACEL Vaccine (8% to 10.8%) .. 2950
GamaSTAN ... 3234
HyperHep B S/D ... 3240
▲ Infanrix Vaccine (4.0% to 5.2%) ... 1476
▲ Prevnar for Injection (0.8% to 82.8%) ... 3463
▲ ProQuad (22%) ... 2064
Rhophylac ... 3505
Rocephin Injectable Vials, ADD-Vantage, Galaxy, Bulk (1%) ... 2800
▲ Vaqta (1.7% to 52.7%) ... 2097
▲ Vivitrol (42% to 72%) ... 995
WinRho SDF ... 732
▲ Zostavax Injection (33.4%) ... 2111

Tenderness at insertion site
▲ Vantas (3.6%) ... 3375

Tendinitis
Ambien Tablets (Rare) ... 2851
Ambien CR Tablets (Rare) ... 2855
Celebrex Capsules (0.1% to 1.9%) ... 3134
Cipro ... 2977
Cipro I.V. ... 2984
Cipro XR Tablets ... 2990
Evoxac Capsules (Less than 1%) ... 1047
▲ Intron A for Injection (Less than 5%) ... 3024
Klonopin (Infrequent) ... 2778
Levaquin (0.1% to 0.9%) ... 2384
Levaquin in 5% Dextrose Injection (0.1% to 0.9%) ... 2384
Neurontin Capsules ... 2487
Neurontin Oral Solution (Infrequent) ... 2487
Neurontin Tablets ... 2487
Noroxin Tablets ... 2032
Requip Tablets (Infrequent) ... 1555
Risperdal Consta Long-Acting Injection (Infrequent) ... 1682
Teveten Tablets (Less than 1%) ... 1735
Teveten HCT Tablets (Less than 1%) ... 1737

Tendinous contracture
Caduet Tablets (Less than 2%) ... 2508
Gabitril Tablets (Infrequent) ... 984
Lamictal (Rare) ... 1481
Lipitor Tablets (Less than 2%) ... 2483
Symbyax Capsules (Infrequent) ... 1819

Tendon disorder, unspecified
Actiq (Less than 1%) ... 979
▲ Actonel Tablets (3%) ... 2683
▲ Actonel with Calcium Tablets (3%) ... 2688
Avelox (Less than 0.1%) ... 2970
BiDil Tablets (1% to less than 2%) ... 2171
Cipro I.V. ... 2984
Gengraf Capsules (1% to less than 3%) ... 459
▲ Humira Injection (Less than 5%) ... 466
▲ Imdur Tablets (Less than or equal to 5%) ... 3018
Levaquin ... 2384
Levaquin in 5% Dextrose Injection ... 2384
Neoral Oral Solution (1% to less than 3%) ... 2259
Neoral Soft Gelatin Capsules (1% to less than 3%) ... 2259
Neurontin Capsules (Rare) ... 2487
Neurontin Oral Solution (Rare) ... 2487
Neurontin Tablets (Rare) ... 2487
Omacor Capsules ... 2725
Protopic Ointment (0.2% to less than 1%) ... 638
Remicade for IV Injection (Greater than or equal to 0.2%) ... 971
Rescriptor Tablets ... 2551

Tendon rupture
Avelox ... 2970
Cipro ... 2977
Cipro I.V. ... 2984
Cipro XR Tablets ... 2990
Decadron Tablets ... 1951
Depo-Medrol Single-Dose Vial ... 2619
Effexor Tablets (Rare) ... 3411
Effexor XR Capsules (Rare) ... 3417
Hydrocortone Tablets ... 1989
Levaquin ... 2384
Levaquin in 5% Dextrose Injection ... 2384
Noroxin Tablets ... 2032
Proquin XR Tablets ... 1153
Tequin Injection ... 938
Tequin Injection in 5% Dextrose ... 938
Tequin Tablets ... 938
Viagra Tablets (Less than 2%) ... 2573
Zelapar Tablets ... 3372

Tendonitis
Abilify Oral Solution (Rare) ... 882
Abilify Oral Solution (Rare) ... 2450
Abilify Discmelt Orally Disintegrating Tablets (Rare) ... 882
Abilify Discmelt Orally Disintegrating Tablets (Rare) ... 2450
Abilify Tablets (Rare) ... 882
Abilify Tablets (Rare) ... 2450
Accutane Capsules ... 2731
Euflexxa (1.88%) ... 1162
Proquin XR Tablets ... 1153
Rythmol SR Capsules ... 2727
Soriatane Capsules (Less than 1%) .. 1013
Xenical Capsules (2%) ... 2831
Xyrem Oral Solution (Infrequent) ... 1688

Tendons, calcification of
Accutane Capsules ... 2731

Tenesmus
Ambien Tablets (Rare) ... 2851
Ambien CR Tablets (Rare) ... 2855
Arthrotec Tablets (Rare) ... 3129
Asacol Delayed-Release Tablets (2% or greater) ... 2692
Caduet Tablets (Less than 2%) ... 2508
Celebrex Capsules (0.1% to 1.9%) ... 3134
Colazal Capsules ... 2838
Copaxone for Injection (Infrequent) .. 3297
Doxil Injection (Less than 1%) ... 2351
▲ Eloxatin for Injection (2% to 5%) ... 2892
Evoxac Capsules (Less than 1%) ... 1047
Exelon Capsules (Infrequent) ... 2206
Exelon Oral Solution (Infrequent) ... 2206
Lipitor Tablets (Less than 2%) ... 2483
Norvir (Less than 2%) ... 503
Omacor Capsules ... 2725
Prevacid Delayed-Release Capsules (Less than 1%) ... 3271
Prevacid for Delayed-Release Oral Suspension (Less than 1%) ... 3271
Prevacid SoluTab Delayed-Release Orally Disintegrating Tablets (Less than 1%) ... 3271
Prevacid NapraPAC (Less than 1%) .. 3280
PREVPAC (Less than 1%) ... 3284
Rilutek Tablets (Infrequent) ... 2930
▲ Sandostatin LAR Depot (4% to 6%) ... 2280
Soriatane Capsules (Less than 1%) .. 1013
▲ Xifaxan Tablets (7.2%) ... 2842
Zoloft (Rare) ... 2586

Tenosynovitis
Abilify Oral Solution (Rare) ... 882
Abilify Oral Solution (Rare) ... 2450
Abilify Discmelt Orally Disintegrating Tablets (Rare) ... 882
Abilify Discmelt Orally Disintegrating Tablets (Rare) ... 2450
Abilify Tablets (Rare) ... 882
Abilify Tablets (Rare) ... 2450
▲ Azilect Tablets (3%) ... 3293
▲ Azmacort Inhalation Aerosol (1% to 3%) ... 1726
Caduet Tablets (Less than 2%) ... 2508
Copaxone for Injection (Infrequent) ... 3297
Effexor Tablets (Infrequent) ... 3411
Effexor XR Capsules (Infrequent) ... 3417
Evoxac Capsules (Less than 1%) ... 1047
Geodon Capsules (Infrequent) ... 2529
Lipitor Tablets (Less than 2%) ... 2483
Lofibra Tablets ... 1219
Lofibra Capsules ... 1216
Lupron Depot 3.75 mg ... 3260
Lupron Depot 7.5 mg ... 3264
Lupron Depot–3 Month 11.25 mg ... 3265
Lupron Depot-PED 7.5 mg, 11.25 mg and 15 mg ... 3269
Lupron Injection Pediatric ... 3259
Meridia Capsules (1.2%) ... 489
Paxil CR Controlled-Release Tablets (Rare) ... 1538
Paxil (Rare) ... 1530
Permax Tablets (Infrequent) ... 3356
Protonix I.V. (Less than 1%) ... 3472
Protonix Tablets (Less than 1%) ... 3469
Prozac Pulvules and Liquid (Infrequent) ... 1801
Rescriptor Tablets ... 2551
Sonata Capsules (Infrequent) ... 1717
Sular Tablets (Less than or equal to 1%) ... 3122
Symbyax Capsules (Infrequent) ... 1819
Tasmar Tablets (Infrequent) ... 3358
Tricor Tablets ... 527
Uniretic Tablets (Less than 1%) ... 3100
Viagra Tablets (Less than 2%) ... 2573
Zelapar Tablets ... 3372
Zomig Tablets (Infrequent) ... 3519
Zomig Nasal Spray (Rare) ... 3523
Zomig-ZMT Tablets (Infrequent) ... 3519

Tenseness
Allegra-D 12 Hour Extended-Release Tablets ... 2846
Allegra-D 24 Hour Extended-Release Tablets ... 2849
▲ Indapamide Tablets (Greater than or equal to 5%) ... 2156
Zelnorm Tablets ... 2312
Zyrtec-D 12 Hour Extended Release Tablets ... 2597

Tensosynovitis
Relpax Tablets (Rare) ... 2548

Testicular atrophy
▲ Eligard 7.5 mg (5%) ... 2880
Eligard 22.5 mg (Less than 2%) ... 2883
▲ Eligard 30 mg (4.4%) ... 2885
▲ Lupron Depot 7.5 mg (5.4%) ... 3264
Oxandrin Tablets ... 2962
▲ Viadur Implant (3.8%) ... 757

Testicular disorder, unspecified
▲ AndroGel (Up to 3%) ... 3329
Caverject Impulse Injection (Less than 1%) ... 2612
Prevacid Delayed-Release Capsules (Less than 1%) ... 3271
Prevacid for Delayed-Release Oral Suspension (Less than 1%) ... 3271
Prevacid SoluTab Delayed-Release Orally Disintegrating Tablets (Less than 1%) ... 3271
Prevacid NapraPAC (Less than 1%) .. 3280
PREVPAC (Less than 1%) ... 3284
▲ Rapamune Oral Solution and Tablets (3% to 20%) ... 3475

Testicular function, inhibited
Alkeran for Injection ... 955
Oxandrin Tablets ... 2962

Testicular swelling
Neurontin Capsules (Rare) ... 2487
Neurontin Oral Solution (Rare) ... 2487
Neurontin Tablets (Rare) ... 2487
Wellbutrin Tablets (Infrequent) ... 1603

Testosterone serum levels, transient increase
Avodart Soft Gelatin Capsules ... 1390
Vantas (Less than 2%) ... 3375

Tetany
Ambien Tablets (Rare) ... 2851
Ambien CR Tablets (Rare) ... 2855
Aredia for Injection (Rare) ... 2179
Furosemide Tablets ... 2154
Garamycin Injectable ... 3014
Imitrex Injection ... 1463
Imitrex Nasal Spray (Rare) ... 1467
Imitrex Tablets (Rare) ... 1471
Paxil CR Controlled-Release Tablets (Rare) ... 1538
Paxil (Rare) ... 1530
▲ Rapamune Oral Solution and Tablets (3% to 20%) ... 3475
Rescriptor Tablets ... 2551
Rilutek Tablets (Rare) ... 2930
Risperdal Consta Long-Acting Injection (Infrequent) ... 1682
Trileptal Tablets ... 2300
Trileptal Oral Suspension ... 2300
Zomig Tablets (Rare) ... 3519
Zomig-ZMT Tablets (Rare) ... 3519

Thick feeling, nasal
▲ Fortical Nasal Spray (10.6%) ... 3337

Thickening, facial tissue
Increlex Injection (Several patients) .. 3291

Thinking, slowed
Abilify Oral Solution (Infrequent) ... 882
Abilify Oral Solution (Infrequent) ... 2450
Abilify Discmelt Orally Disintegrating Tablets (Infrequent) ... 882
Abilify Discmelt Orally Disintegrating Tablets (Infrequent) ... 2450
Abilify Tablets (Infrequent) ... 882
Abilify Tablets (Infrequent) ... 2450
Lithobid Tablets ... 1692

Thinking abnormality
Actiq (1% to 2%) ... 979
Ambien Tablets (Rare) ... 2851
Ambien CR Tablets (Rare) ... 2855
AmBisome for Injection (Less common) ... 620
Astelin Nasal Spray (Infrequent) ... 1904
Avelox (Less than 0.1%) ... 2970
Avinza Capsules (Less than 5%) ... 1741
Campath Ampules ... 811
Campral Tablets (Frequent) ... 1174
▲ CellCept Capsules (3% to less than 20%) ... 2747
▲ CellCept Intravenous (3% to less than 20%) ... 2747
▲ CellCept Oral Suspension (3% to less than 20%) ... 2747
▲ CellCept Tablets (3% to less than 20%) ... 2747
Cesamet Capsules ... 3340
Chantix Tablets (Infrequent) ... 2517
Coreg Tablets (Greater than 0.1% to 1%) ... 1414
▲ Depacon Injection (6%) ... 412
▲ Depakene (6%) ... 417
▲ Depakote Sprinkle Capsules (6%) ... 422
▲ Depakote Tablets (1% to 6%) ... 427
▲ Depakote ER Tablets (6%) ... 434
Diastat Rectal Delivery System (Greater than or equal to 1%) ... 3343
Doxil Injection (Less than 1%) ... 2351
Duragesic Transdermal System (1% or greater) ... 2373
Effexor Tablets (2%) ... 3411
Effexor XR Capsules (Frequent) ... 3417
Evoxac Capsules (Less than 1%) ... 1047
Frova Tablets (Infrequent) ... 1113
▲ Gabitril Tablets (6%) ... 984
▲ Infergen (8% to 10%) ... 3364
▲ Intron A for Injection (Less than 5%) ... 3024
Kadian Capsules (Less than 3%) ... 577
Kaletra (Less than 2%) ... 476
Keppra Injection ... 3320
Keppra Oral Solution (1% to 2%) ... 3314
Keppra Tablets (1% to 2%) ... 3314
▲ Lamictal (3%) ... 1481
Lunesta Tablets ... 3142

▲ Lyrica Capsules (1% to 9%) 2539
▲ Marinol Capsules (3% to 10%) 3333
▲ Megace ES Oral Suspension (1% to 3%) 2481
Meridia Capsules (Greater than or equal to 1%) 489
▲ Mirapex Tablets (2% to 3%) 859
Namenda (Infrequent) 1195
Nembutal Sodium Solution, USP (Less than 1%) 2470
Neurontin Capsules (1.7% to 2.7%) 2487
Neurontin Oral Solution (1.7% to 2.7%) 2487
Neurontin Tablets (1.7% to 2.7%) 2487
Nipent for Injection (Less than 3%) 1863
Norvir (0% to 0.9%) 503
▲ OxyContin Tablets (Between 1% and 5%) 2703
Paxil CR Controlled-Release Tablets (Infrequent) 1538
Paxil (Infrequent) 1530
Permax Tablets (Frequent) 3356
Prevacid Delayed-Release Capsules (Less than 1%) 3271
Prevacid for Delayed-Release Oral Suspension (Less than 1%) 3271
Prevacid SoluTab Delayed-Release Orally Disintegrating Tablets (Less than 1%) 3271
Prevacid NapraPAC (Less than 1%) 3280
PREVPAC (Less than 1%) 3284
ProAmatine Tablets (Less frequent) 3186
▲ Prograf Capsules and Injection (3% to 15%) 632
ProSom Tablets (2%) 517
Protonix I.V. (Less than 1%) 3472
Protonix Tablets (Less than 1%) 3469
Protopic Ointment (0.2% to less than 1%) 638
Provigil Tablets (At least 1%) 988
Prozac Pulvules and Liquid (2%) 1801
Relpax Tablets (Infrequent) 2548
ReoPro Vials (2.1%) 1809
Rilutek Tablets (Infrequent) 2930
▲ Risperdal Consta Long-Acting Injection (Up to 3%) 1682
Seroquel Tablets (Infrequent) 690
Sonata Capsules (Frequent) 1717
Sular Tablets (Less than or equal to 1%) 3122
▲ Symbyax Capsules (Greater than or equal to 5% to 6%) 1819
Symmetrel Tablets (0.1% to 1%) 1135
Tasmar Tablets (Infrequent) 3358
Tequin Injection (Less than 0.1%) 938
Tequin Injection in 5% Dextrose (Less than 0.1%) 938
Tequin Tablets (Less than 0.1%) 938
Thalomid Capsules 965
Trileptal Tablets (2%) 2300
Trileptal Oral Suspension (2%) 2300
Vicoprofen Tablets (Less than 3%) 539
Wellbutrin Tablets (Infrequent) 1603
Zelapar Tablets 3372
Zomig Nasal Spray (Infrequent) 3523
Zyban Sustained-Release Tablets (1%) 1644
Zyprexa Tablets 1830
Zyprexa ZYDIS Orally Disintegrating Tablets 1830
Zyrtec Chewable Tablets (Less than 2%) 2594
Zyrtec (Less than 2%) 2594
Zyrtec-D 12 Hour Extended Release Tablets (Less than 2%) 2597

Thirst
(*see also under* Dipsesis)

St. Joseph 81 mg Aspirin ▣ 688

Thoracic disorders, unspecified

▲ Focalin XR (9% to 16%) 2223

Throat, aching

InnoPran XL Capsules 2723
Zomig Nasal Spray (Infrequent) 3523

Throat, burning

Astelin Nasal Spray (Infrequent) 1904
Eldepryl Capsules 3208
Emcyt Capsules (1%) 2634
Rhinocort Aqua Nasal Spray (Rare) 665

Throat, congestion

Bentyl Capsules 697
Bentyl Injection 697
Bentyl Syrup 697
Bentyl Tablets 697

Throat, dryness of

▲ Aerobid/Aerobid-M (1% to 3%) 1171
Ambien CR Tablets (1%) 2855
Asmanex Twisthaler (1% to less than 3%) 2966
Astelin Nasal Spray (Infrequently) 1904
Atrovent Nasal Spray 0.03% (Less than 2%) 837
Atrovent Nasal Spray 0.06% (1.4%) 839
Azmacort Inhalation Aerosol 1726
Beconase AQ Nasal Spray 1396
Catapres-TTS (2 of 101 patients) 844
Cesamet Capsules 3340
Clozaril Tablets (Less than 1%) 2184
FazaClo Orally Disintegrating Tablets (Less than 1%) 551
Flonase Nasal Spray 1440
Maxalt Tablets (Infrequent) 2008
Maxalt-MLT Orally Disintegrating Tablets (Infrequent) 2008
Neurontin Capsules (1.7%) 2487
Neurontin Oral Solution (1.7%) 2487
Neurontin Tablets (1.7%) 2487
Rythmol SR Capsules 2727
Sanctura Tablets (Greater than or equal to 0.5%) 1151
Vantin Tablets and Oral Suspension (Less than 1%) 2645
Xifaxan Tablets (Less than 2%) 2842
Xopenex Inhalation Solution 3146
Xopenex Inhalation Solution Concentrate 3150
Xopenex HFA Inhalation Aerosol 3154
Xyrem Oral Solution (Infrequent) 1688

Throat, presence of hard nodule

Lupron Injection Pediatric 3259

Throat, swelling of

Arthrotec Tablets 3129
Cutivate Lotion 0.05% (Rare) 2664
Fluarix 1451
Fortical Nasal Spray 3337
Miacalcin Injection (A few cases) 2252
Miacalcin Nasal Spray (Few reports) 2253
Rhinocort Aqua Nasal Spray (Rare) 665

Throat irritation

▲ Advair Diskus 100/50 (4% to 8%) 1308
▲ Advair Diskus 250/50 (4% To 8%) 1308
▲ Advair Diskus 500/50 (4% to 8%) 1308
▲ Advair HFA Inhalation Aerosol (7% to 9%) 1318
Aerobid/Aerobid-M (1% to 3%) 1171
Allegra (Greater than 1%) 2844
Allegra-D 12 Hour Extended-Release Tablets (2.3%) 2846
Allegra-D 24 Hour Extended-Release Tablets (2.3%) 2849
Alupent Inhalation Aerosol (1 to 4%) 826
Ambien CR Tablets (1%) 2855
Aredia for Injection (One patient) 2179
Azmacort Inhalation Aerosol 1726
Clozaril Tablets (1%) 2184
Cosopt Sterile Ophthalmic Solution 1931
▲ Epivir-HBV (13%) 1432
Flonase Nasal Spray 1440
▲ Flovent Diskus (10% to 13%) 1443
▲ Flovent HFA (8%) 1447
Norvir (1.7% to 2.8%) 503
Paxil CR Controlled-Release Tablets (2%) 1538
Paxil (2%) 1530
Rhinocort Aqua Nasal Spray (Rare) 665
▲ Rituxan I.V. (0% to 9%) 1254
▲ Soltamox Oral Solution (5%) 3527
Spiriva HandiHaler 869
Trusopt Sterile Ophthalmic Solution 2095
▲ Ventolin HFA Inhalation Aerosol (10%) 1600

Throat soreness

Aceon Tablets (2 mg, 4 mg, 8 mg) 3194
Advair Diskus 100/50 1308
Advair Diskus 250/50 1308
Advair Diskus 500/50 1308
Advair HFA Inhalation Aerosol 1318
▲ Aerobid/Aerobid-M (20%) 1171
Altace Capsules 1702
Aricept Tablets (Frequent) 1094
Aricept ODT Tablets (Frequent) 1094
Blocadren Tablets 1916
Captopril Tablets 2149
Carbatrol Capsules 3171
▲ Chemet Capsules (0.7% to 3.7%) 2458
▲ Clolar for Intravenous Infusion (14%) 1271
Clozaril Tablets 2184
Cosopt Sterile Ophthalmic Solution 1931
Cubicin for Injection (1% to 2%) 1026
Dapsone Tablets USP 1673
Demadex Injection (1.6%) 2759
Demadex Tablets (1.6%) 2759
DuoNeb Inhalation Solution 1058
▲ Elidel Cream 1% (3.4% to 8.1%) 2200
▲ Flebogamma 5%, Immune Globulin Intravenous (Human) (20%) 1658
Flovent Diskus 1443
Flovent HFA 1447
▲ Flumist Vaccine (9.3% to 27.8%) 1901
▲ Gleevec Tablets (Up to 11%) 2227
Guanidine Hydrochloride Tablets 3016
▲ Imitrex Injection (3.3%) 1463
Inderal LA Long-Acting Capsules 3429
InnoPran XL Capsules 2723
Lopressor Injection 2238
Lopressor Tablets 2238
Lopressor HCT 50/25 Tablets 2241
Lopressor HCT 100/25 Tablets 2241
Lopressor HCT 100/50 Tablets 2241
Mavik Tablets (0.3% to 1.0%) 486
Maxair Autohaler 1852
Meruvax II 2019
Miradon Tablets 3042
M-M-R II 2006
▲ Myfortic Tablets (3% to less than 20%) 2255
Nadolol Tablets 2159
▲ Neupogen for Injection (4%) 603
Prinivil Tablets 2052
Prinzide Tablets 2056
ProQuad 2064
Remicade for IV Injection 971
Rythmol SR Capsules 2727
▲ Strattera Capsules (2% or greater) 1814
Tegretol/Tegretol-XR 2295
Ticlid Tablets 2810
Timoptic Sterile Ophthalmic Solution 2088
Timoptic in Ocudose 2091
Timoptic-XE Sterile Ophthalmic Gel Forming Solution 2092
Toprol-XL Tablets 668
▲ Trisenox Injection (35%) 993
▲ Ultram ER Tablets (1% to greater than 5%) 2392
Vasotec I.V. Injection (0.5% to 1.0%) 2103
▲ Vivaglobin (17%) 3506
▲ Xeloda Tablets (2% to 12%) 2822
Zemaira (0.9%) 3509
▲ Zometa for Intravenous Infusion (8%) 2315

Throat tightness

Abilify Oral Solution (Rare) 882
Abilify Oral Solution (Rare) 2450
Abilify Discmelt Orally Disintegrating Tablets (Rare) 882
Abilify Discmelt Orally Disintegrating Tablets (Rare) 2450
Abilify Tablets (Rare) 882
Abilify Tablets (Rare) 2450
Acetadote Injection (1%) 1031
Adenocard Injection (Less than 1%) 617
Alferon N Injection (1%) 1665
Amitiza Capsules (Less than 0.2%) 3224
Campath Ampules 811
▲ Doxil Injection (Approximately 6.8%) 2351
Fleet Phospho-soda (Rare) 1166
Fleet Phospho-soda ACCU-PREP (Rare) 1168
Fleet Phospho-soda EZ-PREP (Rare) 1169
▲ Imitrex Tablets (Less than 1% to 3%) 1471
Levaquin 2384
Levaquin in 5% Dextrose Injection 2384
Maxalt Tablets (Less than 2%) 2008
Maxalt-MLT Orally Disintegrating Tablets (Less than 2%) 2008
Neumega for Injection 3435
OsmoPrep Tablets (Rare) 2840
Paxil CR Controlled-Release Tablets (2%) 1538
Paxil (2%) 1530
Rythmol SR Capsules 2727
Zomig Nasal Spray (0% to 2%) 3523

Throbbing, localized

Catapres-TTS (1 of 101 patients) 844

Thrombocythemia
(*see also under* Thrombocytosis)

▲ Tygacil for Injection (6.1%) 3488

Thrombocytopenia

▲ Abelcet Injection (5%) 1141
Abilify Oral Solution (Infrequent) 882
Abilify Oral Solution (Infrequent) 2450
Abilify Discmelt Orally Disintegrating Tablets (Infrequent) 882
Abilify Discmelt Orally Disintegrating Tablets (Infrequent) 2450
Abilify Tablets (Infrequent) 882
Abilify Tablets (Infrequent) 2450
Accutane Capsules 2731
Aceon Tablets (2 mg, 4 mg, 8 mg) 3194
Aciphex Tablets 1090
Actiq (1% or greater) 979
Adalat CC Tablets (Rare) 2964
Advicor Tablets 1722
Aggrastat 1907
Aggrenox Capsules 822
▲ Agrylin Capsules (1% to 5%) 3169
Albenza Tablets (Rare) 1338
Aldara Cream, 5% 1846
Aldoril Tablets 1910
Aldurazyme for Intravenous Infusion (2%) 1268
▲ Alimta for Injection (Up to 27%) 1750
Alkeran Tablets 956
Aloprim for Injection (Less than 1%) 2167
Altace Capsules (Less than 1%) 1702
Altoprev Extended-Release Tablets (Rare) 3109
AmBisome for Injection (Less common) 620
Amerge Tablets (Rare) 1339
Amoxil Capsules 1343
Amoxil Chewable Tablets 1343
Amoxil Pediatric Drops for Oral Suspension 1343
Amoxil Powder for Oral Suspension 1343
Amoxil Tablets 1343
Anaprox Tablets (Less than 1%) 2761
Anaprox DS Tablets (Less than 1%) 2761
Anzemet Injection (Infrequently) 2859
Anzemet Tablets (Infrequently) 2862
Aptivus Capsules (Less than 2%) 826
▲ Aredia for Injection (14%) 2179
Aricept Tablets (Infrequent) 1094
Aricept ODT Tablets (Infrequent) 1094
Arixtra Injection (2.9%) 1351
▲ Arranon Injection (22% to 88%) 1357
Arthrotec Tablets (Rare) 3129
Asacol Delayed-Release Tablets 2692
Atacand Tablets 649
Atacand HCT 651
Attenuvax (Rare) 1914
Augmentin 1360
Augmentin Tablets 1363
Augmentin XR Extended-Release Tablets 1369
Augmentin ES-600 Powder for Oral Suspension 1366
Avalide Tablets 888
Avalide Tablets 2874
Avandaryl Tablets 1379
▲ Avastin IV (5%) 1227
Avelox (Less than 0.1%) 2970
▲ Avinza Capsules (Less than 5%) 1741
Axid Oral Solution (One patient) 879
Baraclude (Less than 1%) 894
Bayer Aspirin 744
Bayer Aspirin Comprehensive Prescribing Information ▣ 796
Betaseron for SC Injection 767
Bexxar 1398
Bicillin C-R Injectable Suspension 1706
Bumex Tablets (0.2%) 2746
Caduet Tablets (Greater than 0.1% to less than 2%) 2508
▲ Campath Ampules (50% to 72%) 811
Campral Tablets (Infrequent) 1174
▲ Camptosar Injection (1% to 96%) 2604
Canasa Rectal Suppositories (One patient) 699
▲ Cancidas for Injection (1.5% to 3.1%) 1918
Capastat Sulfate for Injection (Rare) 1755
Captopril Tablets 2149
Carbatrol Capsules 3171
Cardene I.V. (Rare) 2497
Cardizem LA Extended Release Tablets (Infrequent) 1728
Cardura XL Tablets 2515
Catapres Tablets (Rare) 843
Cathflo Activase 1231
Ceftin 1407
Celebrex Capsules (0.1% to 1.9%) 3134
Celexa 1176
▲ CellCept Capsules (23.5% to 38.3%) 2747
▲ CellCept Intravenous (23.5% to 38.3%) 2747

▲ CellCept Oral Suspension (23.5% to 38.3%) 2747
▲ CellCept Tablets (23.5% to 38.3%) 2747
Chantix Tablets (Rare) 2517
Cipro (0.1%) 2977
▲ Cipro I.V. (Among most frequent) 2984
Cleocin Vaginal Ovules 2616
Clinoril Tablets (Less than 1 in 100) 1924
Clolar for Intravenous Infusion 1271
Clorpres Tablets 2153
Clozaril Tablets 2184
Combivir Tablets (0.4%) 1411
Comvax 1928
Concerta Extended-Release Tablets 1881
▲ Copegus Tablets (5% to 8%) 2754
▲ Coreg Tablets (1% to 3%) 1414
Cosmegen for Injection 2459
Cozaar Tablets (Rare) 1935
Crestor Tablets (Less than 1%) 678
Crixivan Capsules (0.9%) 1940
Cubicin for Injection (Less than 1%) 1026
▲ Cuprimine Capsules (4%) 1947
Cutivate Lotion 0.05% (Rare) 2664
▲ Dacogen Injection (89%) 2129
Dantrium Capsules (Less frequent) 2694
Daranide Tablets 1950
Daraprim Tablets 1419
Demser Capsules (Rare) 1953
▲ Depacon Injection (1% to 24%) 412
▲ Depakene (24%) 417
▲ Depakote Sprinkle Capsules (1% to 24%) 422
▲ Depakote Tablets (24%) 427
▲ Depakote ER Tablets (24%) 434
▲ DepoCyt Injection (5% to 8%) 1143
Diovan Tablets (Very rare) 2193
Diovan HCT Tablets 2196
Diuril Oral Suspension 1954
Diuril Sodium Intravenous 2467
Dolobid Tablets (Less than 1 in 100) 1955
▲ Doxil Injection (1.3% to 24.2%) 2351
Duetact Tablets 3226
Dyazide Capsules 1423
Dyrenium Capsules (Rare) 3400
EC-Naprosyn Delayed-Release Tablets (Less than 1%) 2761
Edecrin (Rare) 1959
Effexor Tablets (Infrequent) 3411
Efudex 3363
Elmiron Capsules (Less than or equal to 1%) 2415
▲ Eloxatin for Injection (2% to 77%) 2892
Emcyt Capsules (1%) 2634
Emend Capsules (Greater than 0.5%) 1963
Enbrel for Injection 584
Engerix-B Vaccine 1425
Epivir (Up to 0.4%) 1427
▲ Epivir-HBV (4%) 1432
Epzicom Tablets 1436
Equetro Extended-Release Capsules 3180
Eraxis for Injection (Less than 1% to less than 2%) 2521
Eulexin Capsules (1%) 3009
Evoxac Capsules (Less than 1%) 1047
Exelon Capsules (Infrequent) 2206
Exelon Oral Solution (Infrequent) 2206
Fansidar Tablets 2765
FazaClo Orally Disintegrating Tablets 551
Fluarix 1451
Fortaz (Very rare) 1453
Fragmin Injection (Rare) 1097
Furosemide Tablets 2154
Fuzeon Injection 2767
Gabitril Tablets (Infrequent) 984
▲ Gamunex Immune Globulin I.V., 10% (15%) 3235
Gantrisin Pediatric Suspension 2770
Garamycin Injectable 3014
▲ Gemzar for Injection (15% to 78%) 1771
Gengraf Capsules (2% or less) 459
Geodon Capsules (Rare) 2529
▲ Gleevec Tablets (0% to 33%) 2227
Guanidine Hydrochloride Tablets 3016
Humira Injection (Infrequent) 466
▲ Hycamtin for Injection (26% to 69%) 1458
Hyperstat I.V. 3017
Hytrin Capsules 471
Hyzaar 50-12.5 Tablets (Rare) 1990
Hyzaar 100-12.5 Tablets (Rare) 1990
Hyzaar 100-25 Tablets (Rare) 1990
▲ Imdur Tablets (Less than or equal to 5%) 3018
Imitrex Injection 1463
Imitrex Nasal Spray 1467
Imitrex Tablets 1471
Indapamide Tablets 2156
▲ Indocin I.V. (1% to 3%) 2465
Infanrix Vaccine 1476
▲ Infergen (18% to 19%) 3364
Integrilin Injection 3020
▲ Intron A for Injection (Less than 5% to 15%) 3024
Invanz for Injection (1.1% to 1.3%) 1999
Invirase (Less than or equal to 2%) 2772
▲ I.V. Busulfex (100%) 2493
Kadian Capsules (Less than 3%) 577
▲ Kaletra (4%) 476
Keflex Capsules 549
Keppra Injection 3320
Keppra Oral Solution 3314
Keppra Tablets 3314
Klonopin 2778
▲ Kytril (3%) 2784
Lamictal (Rare) 1481
Lamisil Tablets (Rare) 2232
Lariam Tablets (Occasional) 2786
Lescol Capsules (Rare) 2233
Lescol XL Tablets 2233
▲ Leukine (19%) 814
▲ Leustatin Injection (12%) 2357
Levaquin (0.1% to 0.9%) 2384
Levaquin in 5% Dextrose Injection (0.1% to 0.9%) 2384
Lexapro Oral Solution 1190
Lexapro Tablets 1190
Lipitor Tablets (Less than 2%) 2483
Lofibra Tablets (Rare) 1219
Lofibra Capsules (Rare) 1216
Lopressor HCT 50/25 Tablets 2241
Lopressor HCT 100/25 Tablets 2241
Lopressor HCT 100/50 Tablets 2241
Lotensin Tablets (Less than 1%) 2243
Lotensin HCT Tablets (Rare) 2246
Lotrel Capsules (Rare) 2249
Lovenox Injection (1.8% to 2.8%) 2915
Lyrica Capsules (0.1% to 1%) 2539
Matulane Capsules (Frequent) 3191
Mavik Tablets (0.3% to 1.0%) 486
Maxipime for Injection (Greater than 0.1% to less than 1%) 1105
Mefoxin for Injection 2012
Mefoxin Premixed Intravenous Solution 2016
Mepron Suspension 1521
Meridia Capsules 489
Merrem I.V. (Greater than 0.2%) 686
Meruvax II 2019
Mevacor Tablets (Rare) 2021
Micardis HCT Tablets 856
Miradon Tablets 3042
M-M-R II 2006
Mobic Oral Suspension (Less than 2%) 863
Mobic Tablets (Less than 2%) 863
Moduretic Tablets 2028
Mumpsvax 2031
Mustargen for Injection 2468
Mycamine for Injection (0.8% to 1.2%) 628
▲ Myfortic Tablets (3% to less than 20%) 2255
Myleran Tablets 1525
▲ Mylotarg for Injection (49% to 52%) 3431
Nalfon Capsules (Less than 1%) 2502
Namenda (More than one patient) 1195
Naprosyn Suspension (Less than 1%) 2761
Naprosyn Tablets (Less than 1%) 2761
NeoProfen Injection 2472
Neoral Oral Solution (2% or less) 2259
Neoral Soft Gelatin Capsules (2% or less) 2259
▲ Neupogen for Injection (Fewer than 6% to 12%) 603
Neurontin Capsules (Infrequent) 2487
Neurontin Oral Solution (Infrequent) 2487
Neurontin Tablets (Infrequent) 2487
▲ Nexavar Tablets (Common) 746
Nexium Delayed-Release Capsules (Less than 1%) 655
Nexium I.V. (Less than 1%) 659
Niaspan Extended-Release Tablets 1730
Nimotop Capsules (0.3%; rare) 749
▲ Nipent for Injection (6% to 32%) 1863
Noroxin Tablets (1.0%) 2032
Norvasc Tablets (More than 0.1% to 1%) 2545
Norvir (Less than 2%) 503
Omnicef Capsules 511
Omnicef for Oral Suspension 511
▲ Oncaspar (Greater than 1% but less than 5%) 1145
▲ Ontak Vials (8%) 1745
Oracea Capsules 1000
Orthoclone OKT3 Sterile Solution 2360
Panhematin for Injection 2473
Parcopa Orally Disintegrating Tablets 3097
Parnate Tablets 1527
Paser Granules 1674
Paxil CR Controlled-Release Tablets 1538
Paxil 1530
Pediarix Vaccine 1548
Liquid PedvaxHIB (One child) 2035
▲ Pegasys (5% to 52%) 2789
▲ PEG-Intron Powder for Injection (7%) 3048
Pentasa Capsules (Less than 1%) 3185
Pepcid Injection (Rare) 2040
Pepcid (Rare) 2038
Percodan Tablets 1132
Permax Tablets (Infrequent) 3356
Persantine Tablets (Rare) 868
Phenergan Tablets and Suppositories 3440
Phenytek Capsules (Occasional) 2160
Plavix Tablets (1% to 2.5%) 917
Plavix Tablets (1% to 2.5%) 2926
Pletal Tablets (Very rare) 2455
Pneumovax 23 2043
Podocan-25 Liquid 2478
Prevacid Delayed-Release Capsules (Less than 1%) 3271
Prevacid for Delayed-Release Oral Suspension (Less than 1%) 3271
Prevacid SoluTab Delayed-Release Orally Disintegrating Tablets (Less than 1%) 3271
Prevacid NapraPAC (Less than 1%) 3280
PREVPAC 3284
Prilosec OTC Delayed-Release Tablets (Rare) 2677
Primaxin I.M. 2045
Primaxin I.V. (Less than 0.2%) 2048
Prinivil Tablets (Rare) 2052
Prinzide Tablets (Rare) 2056
▲ Prograf Capsules and Injection (3% to 24%) 632
▲ Proleukin for Injection (37%) 2266
ProQuad 2064
Proquin XR Tablets 1153
Protonix I.V. (Less than 1%) 3472
Protonix Tablets (Less than 1%) 3469
Prozac Pulvules and Liquid (Rare) 1801
▲ Quadramet Injection (69.3%) 1040
Raniclor Tablets, Chewable (Rare) 2505
▲ Rapamune Oral Solution and Tablets (13% to 30%) 3475
Raptiva for Injection (0.3%) 1250
Razadyne (Infrequent) 2399
Razadyne ER Extended-Release Capsules (Infrequent) 2399
Rebetol (2%) 3058
▲ Rebif Prefilled Syringe for Injection (2% to 8%) 3159
Recombivax HB 2071
Remicade for IV Injection (Greater than or equal to 0.2%) 971
ReoPro Vials (0.7% to 5.2%) 1809
Requip Tablets (Infrequent) 1555
Rescriptor Tablets 2551
▲ Retrovir Capsules (12%) 1560
▲ Retrovir IV Infusion (12%) 1564
▲ Retrovir (12%) 1560
▲ Revlimid Capsules (50% to 61.5%) 958
R-Gene 10 for Intravenous Use (One patient) 2641
▲ Ribavirin, USP Capsules (2% to 5%) 3068
Risperdal (Rare) 1676
Risperdal Consta Long-Acting Injection (Rare) 1682
Risperdal M-Tab Orally Disintegrating Tablets (Rare) 1676
▲ Rituxan I.V. (2% to 12%) 1254
Rocephin Injectable Vials, ADD-Vantage, Galaxy, Bulk (Less than 1%) 2800
Rythmol SR Capsules 2727
Sandimmune (2% or less; occasional) 2275
Sandostatin LAR Depot (Rare) 2280
Seroquel Tablets (Rare) 690
▲ Simulect for Injection (3% to 10%) 2284
Solodyn Extended Release Tablets 1890
Soltamox Oral Solution (0.7% to 2%) 3527
St. Joseph 81 mg Aspirin Chewable and Enteric Coated Tablets 1869
St. Joseph 81 mg Aspirin ▣ 688
Stalevo Tablets 2287
Suprax (Less than 2%) 1843
▲ Sutent Capsules (0% to 38%) 2560
Tabloid Tablets 1575
Tambocor Tablets (Less than 1%) 1856
Targretin Capsules 1747
Tarka Tablets 524
Tasmar Tablets (Rare) 3358
▲ Taxotere Injection Concentrate (2.8% to 25.5%) 2932
Tegretol/Tegretol-XR 2295
▲ Temodar Capsules (5% to 58%) 3073
Tequin Injection 938
Tequin Injection in 5% Dextrose 938
Tequin Tablets 938
Teveten Tablets (0.3%) 1735
Teveten HCT Tablets 1737
Thalomid Capsules 965
▲ Thiola Tablets (4%) 2141
Thioridazine Hydrochloride Tablets 2163
Thiothixene Capsules 2165
▲ Thymoglobulin for Intravenous Infusion (36.6%) 1284
Tiazac Capsules (Infrequent) 1201
Ticlid Tablets (Rare) 2810
Timentin ADD-Vantage 1580
Timentin Injection Galaxy Container 1583
Timentin IV Infusion 1577
Timentin Pharmacy Bulk Package 1586
Timolide Tablets 2086
Tindamax Tablets (Rare) 2142
Topamax Sprinkle Capsules (Infrequent to 1%) 2404
Topamax Tablets (Infrequent to 1%) 2404
Toprol-XL Tablets 668
Trasylol Injection (2%) 754
Trecator Tablets (Rare) 3487
Tricor Tablets (Rare) 527
Triglide Tablets 3123
Trileptal Tablets 2300
Trileptal Oral Suspension 2300
▲ Trisenox Injection (18%) 993
Trizivir Tablets (0.4%) 1589
Twinrix Vaccine 1595
Tygacil for Injection (0% to less than 2%) 3488
Ultane Liquid for Inhalation (Less than 1%) 531
Uniretic Tablets 3100
Urso 250 Tablets 710
Urso Forte Tablets 710
▲ Valcyte Tablets (Less than 5%) 2813
▲ Valtrex Caplets (0.1% to 3%) 1597
Vancocin HCl Capsules, USP (Rare) 3380
Vantin Tablets and Oral Suspension 2645
Vaqta (Very rare) 2097
Varivax 2100
Vasotec I.V. Injection (Rare) 2103
▲ Velcade for Injection (35%-43%) 2133
VFEND I.V. (Less than 2%) 2564
VFEND Oral Suspension (Less than 2%) 2564
VFEND Tablets (Less than 2%) 2564
Vicodin Tablets 535
Vicodin ES Tablets 536
Vicodin HP Tablets 538
Viracept (Less than 2%) 2577
Viramune Oral Suspension (0.8%) 873
Viramune Tablets (0.8%) 873
Vivitrol 995
Voltaren Tablets (Occasionally) 2307
Voltaren-XR Tablets (Occasionally) 2310
Vytorin 10/10 Tablets 2114
Vytorin 10/10 Tablets 3077
Vytorin 10/20 Tablets 2114
Vytorin 10/20 Tablets 3077
Vytorin 10/40 Tablets 2114
Vytorin 10/40 Tablets 3077
Vytorin 10/80 Tablets 2114
Vytorin 10/80 Tablets 3077
Wellbutrin Tablets 1603
Wellbutrin SR Sustained-Release Tablets 1607
Wellbutrin XL Extended-Release Tablets 1613
▲ Xeloda Tablets (1% to 41%) 2822
Zantac (A few patients) 1624
Zantac Injection (Few patients) 1619
Zantac Injection Pharmacy Bulk Package (Infrequent) 1622
Zantac Injection Premixed (Few patients) 1619
Zantac (A few patients) 1624
Zegerid Capsules (0.1%) 2958
Zegerid Powder for Oral Solution (0.1%) 2958
Zetia Tablets 2120
Zetia Tablets 3083
Ziagen (1%) 1626
Zinacef for Injection (Rare) 1631
Zinacef Injection (Rare) 1631
Zinecard for Injection 2650
Zocor Tablets (Rare) 2105

Zoloft 2586
▲ Zometa for Intravenous Infusion (5% to 10%) 2315
Zomig Tablets (Rare) 3519
Zomig-ZMT Tablets (Rare) 3519
Zonegran Capsules (Rare) 1101
Zosyn 3492
Zovirax 1643
Zyban Sustained-Release Tablets 1644
Zyrtec Chewable Tablets (Rare) 2594
Zyrtec (Rare) 2594
Zyrtec-D 12 Hour Extended Release Tablets (Rare) 2597
▲ Zyvox (0% to 4.7%) 2652

Thrombocytopenia, immune
PEG-Intron Powder for Injection (Less than or equal to 1%) 3048
Ticlid Tablets (Rare) 2810

Thrombocytopenia, immuno-allergic
Eloxatin for Injection 2892

Thrombocytopenia, neonatal
Dyazide Capsules (Rare) 1423
Prinzide Tablets 2056

Thrombocytopenia, autoimmune idiopathic
Campath Ampules 811

Thrombocytopenic purpura
(*see under* Purpura, thrombocytopenic)

Thrombocytosis
Abilify Oral Solution (Rare) 882
Abilify Oral Solution (Rare) 2450
Abilify Discmelt Orally Disintegrating Tablets (Rare) 882
Abilify Discmelt Orally Disintegrating Tablets (Rare) 2450
Abilify Tablets (Rare) 882
Abilify Tablets (Rare) 2450
Accutane Capsules 2731
Aggrenox Capsules 822
Aricept Tablets (Infrequent) 1094
Aricept ODT Tablets (Infrequent) 1094
Arthrotec Tablets (Rare) 3129
Augmentin (Less than 1%) 1360
Augmentin Tablets (Less than 1%) 1363
▲ Augmentin XR Extended-Release Tablets (3.6%) 1369
Avelox (0.1% to less than 2%) 2970
Azilect Tablets (Rare) 3293
Campath Ampules 811
Celebrex Capsules (0.1% to 1.9%) 3134
Chemet Capsules (0.5% to 1.5%) 2458
Cipro (0.1%) 2977
▲ Cipro I.V. (Among most frequent) 2984
Clozaril Tablets 2184
Colazal Capsules 2838
Cubicin for Injection (Less than 1%) 1026
Cuprimine Capsules 1947
▲ Dacogen Injection (5%) 2129
Demser Capsules (Rare) 1953
Effexor Tablets (Infrequent) 3411
Eraxis for Injection (Less than 1% to less than 2%) 2521
Estratest Tablets 3199
Estratest H.S. Tablets 3199
Evoxac Capsules (Less than 1%) 1047
FazaClo Orally Disintegrating Tablets 551
Fortaz (1 in 45) 1453
Geodon Capsules (Rare) 2529
▲ Invanz for Injection (4.3% to 6.5%) 1999
Ketek Tablets (Greater than or equal to 0.2% to less than 2%) 2903
Levaquin 2384
Levaquin in 5% Dextrose Injection 2384
Lovenox Injection 2915
▲ Lupron Depot 7.5 mg (Greater than or equal to 5%) 3264
Lyrica Capsules (Rare) 2539
Merrem I.V. (Greater than 0.2%) 686
Neumega for Injection 3435
Omnicef Capsules (0.2%) 511
Omnicef for Oral Suspension (1%) 511
Paxil CR Controlled-Release Tablets (Rare) 1538
Paxil (Rare) 1530
Pentasa Capsules (Less than 1%) 3185
Permax Tablets (Rare) 3356
Premarin Tablets 3446
Prevacid Delayed-Release Capsules 3271
Prevacid for Delayed-Release Oral Suspension 3271
Prevacid SoluTab Delayed-Release Orally Disintegrating Tablets 3271
Prevacid NapraPAC 3280
PREVPAC 3284
▲ Prezista Tablets (2.8% to 3.1%) 3306
Primaxin I.M. 2045
Primaxin I.V. 2048
Prozac Pulvules and Liquid (Rare) 1801
▲ Rocephin Injectable Vials, ADD-Vantage, Galaxy, Bulk (5.1%) 2800
Symbyax Capsules (Rare) 1819
Targretin Capsules 1747
Ticlid Tablets 2810
Topamax Sprinkle Capsules (Infrequent) 2404
Topamax Tablets (Infrequent) 2404
▲ Tygacil for Injection (6.1%) 3488
Vantin Tablets and Oral Suspension 2645
Vesanoid Capsules 2820
Zosyn (1% or less) 3492
Zyprexa Tablets (Rare) 1830
Zyprexa ZYDIS Orally Disintegrating Tablets (Rare) 1830
Zyvox (0% to 2.8%) 2652

Thromboembolic complications
▲ Arimidex Tablets (2% to 4%) 673
▲ Camptosar Injection (5.4%) 2604
Estratest Tablets 3199
Estratest H.S. Tablets 3199
Faslodex Injection (Less than 1%) 681
Femara Tablets (Less than or equal to 2%) 2214
Follistim AQ Cartridge 2338
NovoSeven 2331
Ortho-Cyclen/Ortho Tri-Cyclen 2429
Ortho Tri-Cyclen Lo Tablets 2436
Premarin Intravenous 3442
Premarin Vaginal Cream 3452
Premphase Tablets 3456
Prempro Tablets 3456
Ticlid Tablets 2810

Thromboembolic disease
(*see under* Thromboembolic complications)

Thromboembolism
Activase I.V. 1223
▲ Aranesp for Injection (5.6%) 581
Aromasin Tablets (0.9%) 2600
Camptosar Injection 2604
Carimune NF 3499
Decadron Tablets 1951
▲ Eloxatin for Injection (2% to 9%) 2892
Equetro Extended-Release Capsules 3180
Estratest Tablets 3199
Estratest H.S. Tablets 3199
Flebogamma 5%, Immune Globulin Intravenous (Human) 1658
Gammagard Liquid 721
Gammagard S/D 724
Gamunex Immune Globulin I.V., 10% 3235
Hydrocortone Tablets 1989
Nexavar Tablets (Infrequent) 746
Ortho-Cyclen/Ortho Tri-Cyclen 2429
Ortho Tri-Cyclen Lo Tablets 2436
Premarin Vaginal Cream 3452
Soriatane Capsules 1013
Tegretol-XR Tablets 2295
Thalomid Capsules 965

Thromboembolism, arterial
▲ Lucentis Injection (2.1% to 3%) 1237
Mircette Tablets 1066
NuvaRing 2340
Ortho-Cyclen Tablets 2429
Ortho Evra Transdermal System 2417
Ortho Tri-Cyclen Tablets 2429
Ortho Tri-Cyclen Lo Tablets 2436
Seasonique Tablets 1077
Yasmin 28 Tablets 796
Yaz Tablets 803

Thromboembolism, venous
Mircette Tablets 1066
Premarin Intravenous 3442
Premphase Tablets 3456
▲ Rapamune Oral Solution and Tablets (3% to less than 20%) 3475

Thrombopenia
(*see under* Thrombocytopenia)

Thrombophlebitis
Abelcet Injection 1141
Abilify Oral Solution (Rare) 882
Abilify Oral Solution (Rare) 2450
Abilify Discmelt Orally Disintegrating Tablets (Rare) 882
Abilify Discmelt Orally Disintegrating Tablets (Rare) 2450
Abilify Tablets (Rare) 882
Abilify Tablets (Rare) 2450
Aciphex Tablets (Rare) 1090
Actiq (Less than 1%) 979
Aloprim for Injection (Less than 1%) 2167
Angeliq Tablets 762
Anzemet Injection (Rare) 2859
Anzemet Tablets (Rare) 2862
▲ Aranesp for Injection (5.6%) 581
▲ Arimidex Tablets (2% to 5%) 673
Campath Ampules 811
Campral Tablets (Rare) 1174
Camptosar Injection (1.3% to 5.3%) 2604
▲ Cancidas for Injection (3.5% to 15.7%) 1918
Carbatrol Capsules 3171
Celebrex Capsules (Less than 0.1%) 3134
Cipro I.V. (1% or less) 2984
Climara Transdermal System 771
Climara Pro Transdermal System 776
Clozaril Tablets (Less than 1%) 2184
Cuprimine Capsules (Rare) 1947
Dantrium Intravenous 2695
Decadron Tablets 1951
Depo-Provera Contraceptive Injection (Less than 1%) 2622
depo-subQ provera 104 Injectable Suspension 2624
▲ Doxil Injection (1% to 10%) 2351
Effexor Tablets (Infrequent) 3411
Effexor XR Capsules (Infrequent) 3417
Elitek (Less than or equal to 1%) 2890
▲ Emcyt Capsules (3%) 2634
Enbrel for Injection (Infrequent) 584
Enjuvia Tablets 1062
Epogen for Injection (Rare) 591
Equetro Extended-Release Capsules 3180
Eraxis for Injection (Less than 1% to less than 2%) 2521
Estrasorb Topical Emulsion 1147
Estratest Tablets 3199
Estratest H.S. Tablets 3199
Estring Vaginal Ring 2635
FazaClo Orally Disintegrating Tablets (Less than 1%) 551
Femara Tablets (Less than or equal to 2%) 2214
Fluorescite Injection ⊙ 207
Fortical Nasal Spray (Less than 1%) 3337
Furosemide Tablets 2154
Gabitril Tablets (Infrequent) 984
Geodon Capsules (Rare) 2529
Imitrex Nasal Spray 1467
Imitrex Tablets 1471
Indocin Capsules (Rare) 1995
Indocin I.V. (Less than 1%) 2465
Indocin (Rare) 1995
Invanz for Injection (1.6% to 1.9%) 1999
Invirase (Rare; up to 1%) 2772
Kaletra (Less than 2%) 476
Klonopin (Infrequent) 2778
Lunesta Tablets (Rare) 3142
Mefoxin for Injection 2012
Mefoxin Premixed Intravenous Solution 2016
Megace ES Oral Suspension 2481
Menostar Transdermal System 782
Merrem I.V. (0.8%) 686
Miacalcin Nasal Spray (Less than 1%) 2253
Mircette Tablets 1066
Mustargen for Injection 2468
Namenda (Infrequent) 1195
Neurontin Capsules (Rare) 2487
Neurontin Oral Solution (Rare) 2487
Neurontin Tablets (Rare) 2487
NovoSeven 2331
NuvaRing 2340
Ortho-Cyclen Tablets 2429
Ortho Evra Transdermal System 2417
Ortho Tri-Cyclen Tablets 2429
Ortho Tri-Cyclen Lo Tablets 2436
Paxil CR Controlled-Release Tablets (Rare) 1538
Paxil (Rare) 1530
Permax Tablets (Infrequent) 3356
Premarin Intravenous 3442
Premarin Tablets 3446
Premarin Vaginal Cream 3452
Premphase Tablets 3456
Prempro Tablets 3456
▲ Primaxin I.V. (3.1%) 2048
Procrit for Injection (Rare) 2364
Protonix I.V. (Less than 1%) 3472
Protonix Tablets (Less than 1%) 3469
Prozac Pulvules and Liquid (Rare) 1801
▲ Rapamune Oral Solution and Tablets (3% to 20%) 3475
ReFacto Vials 3484
Relpax Tablets (Rare) 2548
Remicade for IV Injection (Greater than or equal to 0.2%) 971
ReoPro Vials (0.1%) 1809
Revlimid Capsules 958
Risperdal (Rare) 1676
Risperdal Consta Long-Acting Injection (Rare) 1682
Risperdal M-Tab Orally Disintegrating Tablets (Rare) 1676
▲ Romazicon Injection (1% to 3%) 2804
Sandostatin Injection (Less than 1%) 2278
Seasonique Tablets 1077
Seroquel Tablets (Infrequent) 690
Sonata Capsules (Rare) 1717
Sustiva Capsules (Less than 2%) 930
Sustiva Tablets (Less than 2%) 930
Taxotere Injection Concentrate 2932
Tegretol/Tegretol-XR 2295
Thalomid Capsules 965
Timentin ADD-Vantage 1580
Timentin Injection Galaxy Container 1583
Timentin IV Infusion 1577
Timentin Pharmacy Bulk Package 1586
Trasylol Injection (1% to 2%) 754
Tygacil for Injection (0% to less than 2%) 3488
VFEND I.V. (Less than 2%) 2564
VFEND Oral Suspension (Less than 2%) 2564
VFEND Tablets (Less than 2%) 2564
Yasmin 28 Tablets 796
Yaz Tablets 803
Zinacef for Injection (1 in 60 patients) 1631
Zinacef Injection (1 in 60 patients) 1631
Zomig Tablets (Rare) 3519
Zomig Nasal Spray (Infrequent) 3523
Zomig-ZMT Tablets (Rare) 3519
Zonegran Capsules (Infrequent) 1101
Zosyn (0.2% to 1.3%) 3492

Thrombophlebitis, deep-vein
▲ Avastin IV (6% to 34%) 1227
Azilect Tablets (Infrequent) 3293
Cardene I.V. (Rare) 2497
Effexor Tablets 3411
Effexor XR Capsules 3417
Estratest Tablets 3199
Estratest H.S. Tablets 3199
Evoxac Capsules (Less than 1%) 1047
Exelon Capsules (Infrequent) 2206
Exelon Oral Solution (Infrequent) 2206
Ionsys Transdermal System (.1% to less than 1%) 2379
Lamictal (Rare) 1481
Lithostat Tablets (1 case) 2140
Lyrica Capsules (0.1% to 1%) 2539
Nipent for Injection (Less than 3%) 1863
▲ Prograf Capsules and Injection (3% to 15%) 632
Requip Tablets (Rare) 1555
VFEND I.V. (Less than 2%) 2564
VFEND Oral Suspension (Less than 2%) 2564
VFEND Tablets (Less than 2%) 2564

Thrombophlebitis, leg
Requip Tablets (Rare) 1555

Thromboplastin decrease
Avelox (Less than 0.1%) 2970

Thromboplastin time, increase
▲ CellCept Capsules (3% to less than 20%) 2747
▲ CellCept Intravenous (3% to less than 20%) 2747
▲ CellCept Oral Suspension (3% to less than 20%) 2747
▲ CellCept Tablets (3% to less than 20%) 2747
Elmiron Capsules (Less than or equal to 1%) 2415
Merrem I.V. (Greater than 0.2%) 686
▲ Oncaspar (Greater than 1% but less than 5%) 1145
Panhematin for Injection 2473
▲ Prezista Tablets (0.6% to 3.9%) 3306
Testim 1% Gel (Less than 1%) 695
Viramune Oral Suspension 873
Viramune Tablets 873
Zosyn 3492

Thrombosis
▲ Alimta for Injection (1% to 7%) 1750

AlphaNine SD, Coagulation Factor IX (Human) ... 1656
Ambien Tablets (Rare) ... 2851
Ambien CR Tablets (Rare) ... 2855
▲ Aranesp for Injection (5.6%) ... 581
▲ Avastin IV (15.1%) ... 1227
BeneFix Vials ... 3408
Camptosar Injection ... 2604
Celexa ... 1176
▲ CellCept Capsules (3% to less than 20%) ... 2747
▲ CellCept Intravenous (4%) ... 2747
▲ CellCept Oral Suspension (3% to less than 20%) ... 2747
▲ CellCept Tablets (3% to less than 20%) ... 2747
Chantix Tablets (Infrequent) ... 2517
Colazal Capsules ... 2838
Doxil Injection (Less than 1%) ... 2351
Elitek (Less than or equal to 1%) ... 2890
Emcyt Capsules ... 2634
Estratest Tablets ... 3199
Estratest H.S. Tablets ... 3199
Exelon Capsules (Infrequent) ... 2206
Exelon Oral Solution (Infrequent) ... 2206
▲ Ferrlecit Injection (6%) ... 3388
Gamunex Immune Globulin I.V., 10% ... 3235
Herceptin I.V. (At least one of the 958 patients) ... 1233
Imitrex Nasal Spray ... 1467
Imitrex Tablets (Rare) ... 1471
▲ I.V. Busulfex (33%) ... 2493
Leukine ... 814
Leustatin Injection (2%) ... 2357
Lexapro Oral Solution ... 1190
Lexapro Tablets ... 1190
Lovenox Injection (Rare) ... 2915
Mustargen for Injection ... 2468
NovoSeven (Two patients) ... 2331
▲ Oncaspar (Greater than 1% but less than 5%) ... 1145
Paxil CR Controlled-Release Tablets (Rare) ... 1538
Paxil (Rare) ... 1530
Premarin Intravenous ... 3442
Premarin Vaginal Cream ... 3452
Profilnine SD, Factor IX Complex (Human) ... 1660
Proleukin for Injection (1%) ... 2266
Protonix I.V. (Less than 1%) ... 3472
Protonix Tablets (Less than 1%) ... 3469
Prozac Pulvules and Liquid (Rare) ... 1801
▲ Rapamune Oral Solution and Tablets (3% to 20%) ... 3475
Renagel Tablets ... 1282
Requip Tablets (Rare) ... 1555
Revlimid Capsules ... 958
Rilutek Tablets (Rare) ... 2930
Rythmol SR Capsules ... 2727
▲ Simulect for Injection (3% to 10%) ... 2284
Tasmar Tablets (Rare) ... 3358
Thalomid Capsules ... 965
TNKase I.V. ... 1264
Trasylol Injection (1% to 2%) ... 754

Thrombosis, arterial
Argatroban Injection (1.8%) ... 1346
Azilect Tablets (Rare) ... 3293
NovoSeven ... 2331
Orthoclone OKT3 Sterile Solution ... 2360
Sandostatin LAR Depot (Rare) ... 2280
Trasylol Injection (1% to 2%) ... 754

Thrombosis, cerebral
(*see under* Cerebral thrombosis)

Thrombosis, coronary
(*see under* Coronary thrombosis)

Thrombosis, deep-vein
Angeliq Tablets ... 762
Climara Transdermal System ... 771
Climara Pro Transdermal System ... 776
Depo-Provera Contraceptive Injection (Less than 1%) ... 2622
depo-subQ provera 104 Injectable Suspension ... 2624
Emend Capsules (Greater than 0.5%) ... 1963
Enjuvia Tablets ... 1062
▲ Epogen for Injection (5% to 10%) ... 591
Eraxis for Injection (0.8%) ... 2521
Estrasorb Topical Emulsion ... 1147
FazaClo Orally Disintegrating Tablets ... 551
Menostar Transdermal System ... 782
Mycamine for Injection ... 628
NovoSeven ... 2331
Premarin Intravenous ... 3442
Premarin Tablets ... 3446
Premarin Vaginal Cream ... 3452
Premphase Tablets ... 3456
Prempro Tablets ... 3456
▲ Revlimid Capsules (7.8%) ... 958
Rythmol SR Capsules ... 2727
Soltamox Oral Solution (0.8%) ... 3527
▲ Sutent Capsules (3%) ... 2560
Topamax Sprinkle Capsules (Infrequent) ... 2404
Topamax Tablets (Infrequent) ... 2404
Vivitrol ... 995

Thrombosis, glomerular capillary
Gengraf Capsules ... 459
Neoral Oral Solution ... 2259
Neoral Soft Gelatin Capsules ... 2259
Sandimmune ... 2275

Thrombosis, intraabdominal
▲ Avastin IV (3% to 10%) ... 1227

Thrombosis, leg
▲ Humira Injection (Less than 5%) ... 466

Thrombosis, mesenteric
Estratest Tablets ... 3199
Estratest H.S. Tablets ... 3199
Mircette Tablets ... 1066
NuvaRing ... 2340
Ortho Evra Transdermal System ... 2417
Premarin Intravenous ... 3442
Premarin Vaginal Cream ... 3452
Seasonique Tablets ... 1077
Yasmin 28 Tablets ... 796
Yaz Tablets ... 803

Thrombosis, mesenteric venous
Avastin IV (Rare) ... 1227

Thrombosis, mesenteric arterial
Campral Tablets (Rare) ... 1174
Cosopt Sterile Ophthalmic Solution ... 1931
Nadolol Tablets ... 2159
Timoptic-XE Sterile Ophthalmic Gel Forming Solution ... 2092

Thrombosis, portal vein
Femara Tablets (Less than or equal to 2%) ... 2214

Thrombosis, pulmonary
Estratest Tablets ... 3199
Estratest H.S. Tablets ... 3199
Neurontin Capsules (Rare) ... 2487
Neurontin Oral Solution (Rare) ... 2487
Neurontin Tablets (Rare) ... 2487
Trasylol Injection (1% to 2%) ... 754

Thrombosis, renal artery
Epogen for Injection (Rare) ... 591
Procrit for Injection (Rare) ... 2364

Thrombosis, retinal, unspecified
Mircette Tablets ... 1066
NuvaRing ... 2340

Thrombosis, retinal artery
Seasonique Tablets ... 1077
Yaz Tablets ... 803

Thrombosis, retinal vascular
Angeliq Tablets ... 762
Enjuvia Tablets ... 1062
Epogen for Injection (Rare) ... 591
Estrasorb Topical Emulsion ... 1147
Estratest Tablets ... 3199
Estratest H.S. Tablets ... 3199
Imitrex Tablets ... 1471
Intron A for Injection ... 3024
Neurontin Capsules (Rare) ... 2487
Neurontin Oral Solution (Rare) ... 2487
Neurontin Tablets (Rare) ... 2487
Ortho-Cyclen Tablets ... 2429
Ortho Evra Transdermal System ... 2417
Ortho Tri-Cyclen Tablets ... 2429
Ortho Tri-Cyclen Lo Tablets ... 2436
Pegasys ... 2789
PEG-Intron Powder for Injection (Less than or equal to 1%) ... 3048
Premarin Intravenous ... 3442
Premarin Tablets ... 3446
Premarin Vaginal Cream ... 3452
Premphase Tablets ... 3456
Prempro Tablets ... 3456
Procrit for Injection (Rare) ... 2364
Sandostatin LAR Depot (Rare) ... 2280
Seasonique Tablets ... 1077
Yasmin 28 Tablets ... 796
Yaz Tablets ... 803

Thrombosis, sagittal sinus
Oncaspar ... 1145

Thrombosis, shunt
Demadex Injection ... 2759
Demadex Tablets ... 2759

Thrombosis, venous
Abilify Oral Solution (Infrequent) ... 882
Abilify Oral Solution (Infrequent) ... 2450
Abilify Discmelt Orally Disintegrating Tablets (Infrequent) ... 882
Abilify Discmelt Orally Disintegrating Tablets (Infrequent) ... 2450
Abilify Tablets (Infrequent) ... 882
Abilify Tablets (Infrequent) ... 2450
Actimmune (Rare) ... 1671
Activase I.V. ... 1223
Angeliq Tablets ... 762
▲ Aranesp for Injection (5.6%) ... 581
Aricept Tablets (Infrequent) ... 1094
Aricept ODT Tablets (Infrequent) ... 1094
Betaseron for SC Injection ... 767
Campath Ampules ... 811
Cathflo Activase ... 1231
Climara Transdermal System ... 771
Climara Pro Transdermal System ... 776
Clozaril Tablets ... 2184
Enbrel for Injection (Infrequent) ... 584
Enjuvia Tablets ... 1062
Epogen for Injection (Rare) ... 591
Estrasorb Topical Emulsion ... 1147
Femara Tablets (Less than or equal to 2%) ... 2214
Kaletra (Less than 2%) ... 476
Menostar Transdermal System ... 782
Mircette Tablets ... 1066
Nimotop Capsules (Less than 1%) ... 749
Oncaspar ... 1145
Ortho-Cyclen Tablets ... 2429
Ortho Evra Transdermal System ... 2417
Ortho Tri-Cyclen Tablets ... 2429
Ortho Tri-Cyclen Lo Tablets ... 2436
Orthoclone OKT3 Sterile Solution ... 2360
Premarin Intravenous ... 3442
Premarin Tablets ... 3446
Premarin Vaginal Cream ... 3452
Premphase Tablets ... 3456
Prempro Tablets ... 3456
▲ Procrit for Injection (Up to 10%) ... 2364
Prograf Capsules and Injection ... 632
Retavase ... 2499
Taxotere Injection Concentrate ... 2932
▲ Xeloda Tablets (Less than 1% to 8%) ... 2822
Yasmin 28 Tablets ... 796

Thrombosis at injection site
Mycamine for Injection ... 628

Thrombosis of vascular access
▲ Aranesp for Injection (5.6% to 8%) ... 581
Epogen for Injection (0.25%) ... 591
Furosemide Tablets ... 2154
Procrit for Injection ... 2364

Thrombotic events, cardivascular
Voltaren Tablets ... 2307

Thrombotic events, unspecified
▲ Aranesp for Injection (6.2%) ... 581
Arthrotec Tablets ... 3129
Dolobid Tablets ... 1955
Gammagard S/D ... 724
Mobic Oral Suspension ... 863
Mobic Tablets ... 863
Neumega for Injection ... 3435
▲ Ontak Vials (7%) ... 1745
Procrit for Injection ... 2364

Thrombotic vascular disease
Accutane Capsules ... 2731
Ortho-Cyclen/Ortho Tri-Cyclen ... 2429
Ortho Tri-Cyclen Lo Tablets ... 2436

Thrush, oral
(*see under* Candidiasis, oral)

Thymol turbidity test, positive
Cuprimine Capsules ... 1947

Thymus gland abnormalities, fetal
Accutane Capsules ... 2731

Thyroid adenoma
Permax Tablets (Rare) ... 3356
Relpax Tablets (Rare) ... 2548

Thyroid binding globulin, increase
(*see under* T4, increase)

Thyroid disease, exacerbation
Proleukin for Injection ... 2266

Thyroid disorder, unspecified
Betaseron for SC Injection ... 767
Chantix Tablets (Infrequent) ... 2517
▲ Rebif Prefilled Syringe for Injection (4% to 6%) ... 3159
Solodyn Extended Release Tablets ... 1890
Vytorin 10/10 Tablets ... 2114
Vytorin 10/10 Tablets ... 3077
Vytorin 10/20 Tablets ... 2114
Vytorin 10/20 Tablets ... 3077
Vytorin 10/40 Tablets ... 2114
Vytorin 10/40 Tablets ... 3077
Vytorin 10/80 Tablets ... 2114
Vytorin 10/80 Tablets ... 3077

Thyroid disorders
(*see under* T3, decrease; T4, decrease; T4, increase)

Thyroid function test, abnormal
Altoprev Extended-Release Tablets ... 3109
Depacon Injection ... 412
Depakene ... 417
Depakote Sprinkle Capsules ... 422
Depakote Tablets ... 427
Depakote ER Tablets ... 434
▲ Infergen (4% to 9%) ... 3364
Lescol Capsules ... 2233
Lescol XL Tablets ... 2233
Mevacor Tablets ... 2021
Pegasys ... 2789
Proleukin for Injection ... 2266
Zocor Tablets ... 2105

Thyroid gland discoloration
Solodyn Extended Release Tablets ... 1890

Thyroid hormone, changes
(*see under* T3, decrease; T4, decrease; T4, increase)

Thyroid nodule
Effexor Tablets (Rare) ... 3411
Effexor XR Capsules (Rare) ... 3417
ProSom Tablets (Rare) ... 517

Thyroid stimulating hormone elevation
Aciphex Tablets ... 1090
Avodart Soft Gelatin Capsules ... 1390
WelChol Tablets ... 1050

Thyroiditis
Aldara Cream, 5% ... 1846
Cuprimine Capsules ... 1947
Effexor Tablets (Rare) ... 3411
Effexor XR Capsules (Rare) ... 3417
▲ Ontak Vials (Less than 5%) ... 1745
Paxil CR Controlled-Release Tablets (Rare) ... 1538
Paxil (Rare) ... 1530
Pegasys ... 2789
Relpax Tablets (Rare) ... 2548
Sular Tablets (Less than or equal to 1%) ... 3122

Thyrotoxicosis
▲ Ontak Vials (Less than 5%) ... 1745
Synthroid Tablets ... 520

Thyroxin-binding globulin, decrease
Striant Mucoadhesive ... 1007
Testim 1% Gel ... 695

Tics
▲ Daytrana Transdermal Patch (7%) ... 3174
FazaClo Orally Disintegrating Tablets (Less than 1%) ... 551
Lamictal ... 1481
Lexapro Oral Solution (Infrequent) ... 1190
Lexapro Tablets (Infrequent) ... 1190
Lithobid Tablets ... 1692

Tightness, abdominal
Abilify Oral Solution (Infrequent) ... 882
Abilify Oral Solution (Infrequent) ... 2450
Abilify Discmelt Orally Disintegrating Tablets (Infrequent) ... 882
Abilify Discmelt Orally Disintegrating Tablets (Infrequent) ... 2450
Abilify Tablets (Infrequent) ... 882
Abilify Tablets (Infrequent) ... 2450

Tightness, back
Abilify Oral Solution (Infrequent) ... 882
Abilify Oral Solution (Infrequent) ... 2450

Abilify Discmelt Orally Disintegrating Tablets (Infrequent) ... 882
Abilify Discmelt Orally Disintegrating Tablets (Infrequent) ... 2450
Abilify Tablets (Infrequent) ... 882
Abilify Tablets (Infrequent) ... 2450

Tightness, extremities
Abilify Oral Solution (Infrequent) ... 882
Abilify Oral Solution (Infrequent) ... 2450
Abilify Discmelt Orally Disintegrating Tablets (Infrequent) ... 882
Abilify Discmelt Orally Disintegrating Tablets (Infrequent) ... 2450
Abilify Tablets (Infrequent) ... 882
Abilify Tablets (Infrequent) ... 2450

Tightness, feeling of
▲ Imitrex Injection (5%) ... 1463

Tightness, head
Abilify Oral Solution (Infrequent) ... 882
Abilify Oral Solution (Infrequent) ... 2450
Abilify Discmelt Orally Disintegrating Tablets (Infrequent) ... 882
Abilify Discmelt Orally Disintegrating Tablets (Infrequent) ... 2450
Abilify Tablets (Infrequent) ... 882
Abilify Tablets (Infrequent) ... 2450
Imitrex Injection (2%) ... 1463

Tightness, tongue
Abilify Oral Solution (Infrequent) ... 882
Abilify Oral Solution (Infrequent) ... 2450
Abilify Discmelt Orally Disintegrating Tablets (Infrequent) ... 882
Abilify Discmelt Orally Disintegrating Tablets (Infrequent) ... 2450
Abilify Tablets (Infrequent) ... 882
Abilify Tablets (Infrequent) ... 2450

Tinea pedis
Xyrem Oral Solution (Infrequent) ... 1688

Tingling
Bentyl Capsules ... 697
Bentyl Injection ... 697
Bentyl Syrup ... 697
Bentyl Tablets ... 697
BiDil Tablets ... 2171
Calcium Disodium Versenate Injection ... 1851
Cipro ... 2977
Cipro I.V. ... 2984
DynaCirc CR Tablets (0.5% to 1%) ... 2721
▲ Elocon Ointment 0.1% (4.8%) ... 3007
Engerix-B Vaccine (Less than 1%) ... 1425
▲ Finacea Gel (4% to 20%) ... 1669
Gengraf Capsules (Rare) ... 459
▲ Imitrex Injection (14%) ... 1463
Imitrex Nasal Spray (Infrequent) ... 1467
▲ Imitrex Tablets (4% to 8%) ... 1471
K-Phos Original (Sodium Free) Tablets (Less frequent) ... 760
K-Phos Neutral Tablets ... 760
Levaquin ... 2384
Levaquin in 5% Dextrose Injection ... 2384
Metrogel 1% ... 1211
Neoral Oral Solution (Rare) ... 2259
Neoral Soft Gelatin Capsules (Rare) ... 2259
▲ Niaspan Extended-Release Tablets (Among most common) ... 1730
Noroxin Tablets ... 2032
Oxistat Lotion (0.4%) ... 2667
▲ Panretin Gel (3% to 22%) ... 1747
Profilnine SD, Factor IX Complex (Human) ... 1660
▲ Protopic Ointment (1% to 8%) ... 638
Rescriptor Tablets ... 2551
Sandimmune (Rare) ... 2275
Twinrix Vaccine (Less than 1%) ... 1595

Tingling, ears
Ciprodex Otic Suspension (1 patient) ... 559
Koāte-DVI (0.7%) ... 3250

Tingling, extremities
▲ Indapamide Tablets (Less than 5%) ... 2156

Tingling, feet
Alferon N Injection (1%) ... 1665
Uroqid-Acid No. 2 Tablets ... 760

Tingling, fingers
Noroxin Tablets (0.3% to 1.0%) ... 2032

Tingling, hands
Adenocard Injection (1%) ... 617
Koāte-DVI (0.7%) ... 3250
Uroqid-Acid No. 2 Tablets ... 760

Tingling, legs
Alferon N Injection (1%) ... 1665

Tingling, lips
K-Phos Original (Sodium Free) Tablets (Less frequent) ... 760
K-Phos Neutral Tablets ... 760
Striant Mucoadhesive ... 1007
Uroqid-Acid No. 2 Tablets ... 760

Tingling, scalp
Temovate Scalp Application (2 of 294 patients) ... 2670

Tingling, skin
Garamycin Injectable ... 3014

Tinnitus
Abelcet Injection ... 1141
Abilify Oral Solution (Infrequent) ... 882
Abilify Oral Solution (Infrequent) ... 2450
Abilify Discmelt Orally Disintegrating Tablets (Infrequent) ... 882
Abilify Discmelt Orally Disintegrating Tablets (Infrequent) ... 2450
Abilify Tablets (Infrequent) ... 882
Abilify Tablets (Infrequent) ... 2450
Accutane Capsules ... 2731
Aceon Tablets (2 mg, 4 mg, 8 mg) (1.5%) ... 3194
Aciphex Tablets ... 1090
Actiq (1% or greater) ... 979
▲ Actonel Tablets (3.3%) ... 2683
Adalat CC Tablets (Less than 1%) ... 2964
Aggrenox Capsules (Less than 1%) ... 822
Agrylin Capsules (1% to 5%) ... 3169
Alferon N Injection (One patient) ... 1665
Aloxi Injection (Less than 1%) ... 2127
Altace Capsules (Less than 1%) ... 1702
Ambien Tablets (Infrequent) ... 2851
Ambien CR Tablets (Infrequent to 1%) ... 2855
Amerge Tablets (Infrequent) ... 1339
▲ Anaprox Tablets (3% to 9%) ... 2761
▲ Anaprox DS Tablets (3% to 9%) ... 2761
Anzemet Injection (Infrequently) ... 2859
Anzemet Tablets (Infrequently) ... 2862
Aricept Tablets (Infrequent) ... 1094
Aricept ODT Tablets (Infrequent) ... 1094
Arthrotec Tablets (Rare) ... 3129
Asacol Delayed-Release Tablets ... 2692
Atacand HCT (0.5% or greater) ... 651
Atripla Tablets ... 945
Atrovent Nasal Spray 0.06% (Less than 1%) ... 839
Avelox (Less than 0.1%) ... 2970
Axert Tablets (Rare) ... 2396
Bayer Aspirin ... 744
Bayer Aspirin Comprehensive Prescribing Information ... ⊡796
BC Headache Powder ... ⊡677
BC Allergy Sinus Cold Powder ... ⊡677
Arthritis Strength BC Powder ... ⊡677
BC Sinus Cold Powder ... ⊡677
Biaxin/Biaxin XL ... 402
Bicillin C-R Injectable Suspension ... 1706
Blocadren Tablets (Less than 1%) ... 1916
Buprenex Injectable (Less than 1%) ... 2716
Caduet Tablets (Greater than 0.1% to less than 2%) ... 2508
Campral Tablets (Infrequent) ... 1174
Capastat Sulfate for Injection ... 1755
Carbatrol Capsules ... 3171
Cardene I.V. (Rare) ... 2497
Cardizem LA Extended Release Tablets (Less than 2%) ... 1728
Celebrex Capsules (0.1% to 1.9%) ... 3134
Celexa (Infrequent) ... 1176
▲ CellCept Capsules (3% to less than 20%) ... 2747
▲ CellCept Intravenous (3% to less than 20%) ... 2747
▲ CellCept Oral Suspension (3% to less than 20%) ... 2747
▲ CellCept Tablets (3% to less than 20%) ... 2747
Cesamet Capsules ... 3340
Chantix Tablets (Infrequent) ... 2517
Cipro (Less than 1%) ... 2977
Cipro I.V. (1% or less) ... 2984
Cipro XR Tablets ... 2990
Clinoril Tablets (Greater than 1%) ... 1924
Colazal Capsules ... 2838
Copaxone for Injection (At least 2%) ... 3297
Coreg Tablets (Greater than 0.1% to 1%) ... 1414
Cosopt Sterile Ophthalmic Solution ... 1931
Covera-HS Tablets (Less than 2%) ... 3139
Cozaar Tablets (Less than 1%) ... 1935
Cubicin for Injection (Less than 1%) ... 1026
Cuprimine Capsules (Greater than 1%) ... 1947
Dapsone Tablets USP ... 1673
Daranide Tablets ... 1950
Demadex Injection ... 2759
Demadex Tablets ... 2759
▲ Depacon Injection (1% to 7%) ... 412
▲ Depakene (7%) ... 417
▲ Depakote Sprinkle Capsules (1% to 7%) ... 422
▲ Depakote Tablets (1% to 7%) ... 427
▲ Depakote ER Tablets (Greater than 1% to 7%) ... 434
Diovan HCT Tablets (Greater than 0.2%) ... 2196
Dolobid Tablets (Greater than 1 in 100) ... 1955
Doxil Injection (Less than 1%) ... 2351
▲ EC-Naprosyn Delayed-Release Tablets (3% to 9%) ... 2761
Edecrin ... 1959
Effexor Tablets (2%) ... 3411
Effexor XR Capsules (Frequent) ... 3417
Eldepryl Capsules ... 3208
Elmiron Capsules (Less than or equal to 1%) ... 2415
▲ Emend Capsules (3.7%) ... 1963
Engerix-B Vaccine ... 1425
Equetro Extended-Release Capsules ... 3180
Evoxac Capsules (Less than 1%) ... 1047
Exelon Capsules (Frequent) ... 2206
Exelon Oral Solution (Frequent) ... 2206
Fansidar Tablets ... 2765
Floxin Otic Solution (Single report to 0.3%) ... 1049
Flumadine (0.3% to 1%) ... 1183
Fortical Nasal Spray (Less than 1%) ... 3337
Frova Tablets (Frequent) ... 1113
Furosemide Tablets ... 2154
Gabitril Tablets (Frequent) ... 984
Gantrisin Pediatric Suspension ... 2770
Garamycin Injectable ... 3014
Gengraf Capsules (1% to less than 3%) ... 459
Geodon Capsules (Infrequent) ... 2529
Gleevec Tablets (Infrequent) ... 2227
Hyperstat I.V. ... 3017
Hytrin Capsules (At least 1%) ... 471
Hyzaar 50-12.5 Tablets ... 1990
Hyzaar 100-12.5 Tablets ... 1990
Hyzaar 100-25 Tablets ... 1990
▲ Imdur Tablets (Less than or equal to 5%) ... 3018
Imitrex Nasal Spray ... 1467
Indocin (Greater than 1%) ... 1995
▲ Infergen (4% to 6%) ... 3364
▲ Intron A for Injection (Less than 5%) ... 3024
Invirase (Less than 2%) ... 2772
Kaletra (Less than 2%) ... 476
Lamictal (1.1%) ... 1481
▲ Lariam Tablets (Among most frequent) ... 2786
Levaquin (0.1% to 0.9%) ... 2384
Levaquin in 5% Dextrose Injection (0.1% to 0.9%) ... 2384
Levitra Tablets (Less than 2%) ... 3034
Lexapro Oral Solution (Frequent) ... 1190
Lexapro Tablets (Frequent) ... 1190
Lidoderm Patch ... 1118
Lipitor Tablets (Less than 2%) ... 2483
Lithobid Tablets ... 1692
Lopressor Injection ... 2238
Lopressor Tablets ... 2238
Lopressor HCT 50/25 Tablets (1%) ... 2241
Lopressor HCT 100/25 Tablets (1%) ... 2241
Lopressor HCT 100/50 Tablets (1%) ... 2241
Lotensin HCT Tablets (0.3% to 1%) ... 2246
Lotrel Capsules (Infrequent) ... 2249
Lunesta Tablets (Infrequent) ... 3142
Lyrica Capsules (Greater than or equal to 1%) ... 2539
Maalox Maximum Strength Total Stomach Relief Peppermint Liquid ... ⊡660
Marinol Capsules (Less than 1%) ... 3333
Maxalt Tablets (Infrequent) ... 2008
Maxalt-MLT Orally Disintegrating Tablets (Infrequent) ... 2008
Meridia Capsules ... 489
Miacalcin Nasal Spray (Less than 1%) ... 2253
Micardis Tablets (More than 0.3%) ... 854
Micardis HCT Tablets ... 856
Midamor Tablets (Less than or equal to 1%) ... 2026
Migranal Nasal Spray (Infrequent) ... 3348
Mintezol ... 2027
Mirapex Tablets (Greater than or equal to 1%) ... 859
Mobic Oral Suspension (Less than 2%) ... 863
Mobic Tablets (Less than 2%) ... 863
Moduretic Tablets ... 2028
Mustargen for Injection (Infrequent) ... 2468
Myobloc Injection (Greater than 2%) ... 3192
Nadolol Tablets (1 to 5 of 1000 patients) ... 2159
▲ Nalfon Capsules (4.5%) ... 2502
Namenda (Infrequent) ... 1195
▲ Naprosyn Suspension (3% to 9%) ... 2761
▲ Naprosyn Tablets (3% to 9%) ... 2761
Neoral Oral Solution (1% to less than 3%) ... 2259
Neoral Soft Gelatin Capsules (1% to less than 3%) ... 2259
Neurontin Capsules (Infrequent) ... 2487
Neurontin Oral Solution (Infrequent) ... 2487
Neurontin Tablets (Infrequent) ... 2487
Nexavar Tablets (Uncommon) ... 746
Nexium Delayed-Release Capsules (Less than 1%) ... 655
Nexium I.V. (Less than 1%) ... 659
Nipent for Injection (Less than 3%) ... 1863
▲ Niravam Orally Disintegrating Tablets (6.6%) ... 3092
Noroxin Tablets ... 2032
Norvasc Tablets (More than 0.1% to 1%) ... 2545
Norvir (Less than 2%) ... 503
Orthoclone OKT3 Sterile Solution ... 2360
OxyContin Tablets (Less than 1%) ... 2703
Parnate Tablets ... 1527
Paxil CR Controlled-Release Tablets (Frequent) ... 1538
Paxil (Frequent) ... 1530
Pepcid Injection (Infrequent) ... 2040
Pepcid (Infrequent) ... 2038
Pepto-Bismol Original Liquid, Maximum Strength Liquid, Original and Cherry Tablets, Chewable Tablets and Easy-To-Swallow Caplets ... 2676
Pepto-Bismol Maximum Strength Liquid ... ⊡672
Percodan Tablets ... 1132
Permax Tablets (Infrequent) ... 3356
Phenergan Tablets and Suppositories ... 3440
Pletal Tablets (Less than 2%) ... 2455
Prevacid Delayed-Release Capsules (Less than 1%) ... 3271
Prevacid for Delayed-Release Oral Suspension (Less than 1%) ... 3271
Prevacid SoluTab Delayed-Release Orally Disintegrating Tablets (Less than 1%) ... 3271
▲ Prevacid NapraPAC (Less than 1% to 9%) ... 3280
PREVPAC (Less than 1%) ... 3284
Prilosec OTC Delayed-Release Tablets (Less than 1%) ... 2677
Primaxin I.M. ... 2045
Primaxin I.V. (Less than 0.2%) ... 2048
Prinivil Tablets (0.3% to 1.0%) ... 2052
Prinzide Tablets (0.3% to 1%) ... 2056
▲ Prograf Capsules and Injection (3% to 15%) ... 632
Proquin XR Tablets ... 1153
ProSom Tablets (Infrequent) ... 517
Protonix I.V. (Less than 1%) ... 3472
Protonix Tablets (Less than 1%) ... 3469
Proventil HFA Inhalation Aerosol (Less than 3%) ... 3056
Prozac Pulvules and Liquid (Frequent) ... 1801
Ranexa Tablets (Greater than 0.5% to less than 2%) ... 1035
▲ Rapamune Oral Solution and Tablets (3% to 20%) ... 3475
Razadyne (Infrequent) ... 2399
Recombivax HB (Less than 1%) ... 2071

Relpax Tablets (Infrequent) 2548
Requip Tablets (Infrequent) 1555
Rescriptor Tablets 2551
Reyataz Capsules (Less than 3%) 921
Risperdal (Rare) 1676
Risperdal M-Tab Orally Disintegrating Tablets (Rare) 1676
Romazicon Injection (Less than 1%) 2804
Rythmol SR Capsules 2727
Sandimmune (2% or less) 2275
▲ Sandostatin LAR Depot (1% to 4%) 2280
Seroquel Tablets (Infrequent) 690
Solodyn Extended Release Tablets (2%) 1890
Sonata Capsules (Infrequent) 1717
▲ Soriatane Capsules (Less than 1% to 10%) 1013
St. Joseph 81 mg Aspirin Chewable and Enteric Coated Tablets 1869
St. Joseph 81 mg Aspirin ◘ 688
Sular Tablets (Less than or equal to 1%) 3122
Sustiva Capsules (Less than 2%) 930
Sustiva Tablets (Less than 2%) 930
Symbyax Capsules (Frequent) 1819
Synera Topical Patch 1137
Tambocor Tablets (1% to 3%) 1856
Tarka Tablets (Less frequent) 524
Tasmar Tablets (Frequent) 3358
Tegretol/Tegretol-XR 2295
▲ Tequin Injection (0.1% to 3%) 938
▲ Tequin Injection in 5% Dextrose (0.1% to 3%) 938
▲ Tequin Tablets (0.1% to 3%) 938
Teveten Tablets (Less than 1%) 1735
Teveten HCT Tablets (Less than 1%) 1737
Thalomid Capsules 965
Tiazac Capsules (Less than 2%) 1201
Ticlid Tablets (0.5% to 1.0%) 2810
Timolide Tablets 2086
Timoptic Sterile Ophthalmic Solution 2088
Timoptic in Ocudose 2091
Timoptic-XE Sterile Ophthalmic Gel Forming Solution 2092
▲ TOBI Solution for Inhalation (3%) 2298
Topamax Sprinkle Capsules (Less than 1% to 2%) 2404
Topamax Tablets (Less than 1% to 2%) 2404
Toprol-XL Tablets 668
Tricor Tablets 527
Trileptal Tablets 2300
Trileptal Oral Suspension 2300
▲ Trisenox Injection (5%) 993
Twinrix Vaccine 1595
▲ Ultram ER Tablets (1% to greater than 5%) 2392
Uniretic Tablets (Less than 1%) 3100
Univasc Tablets (Less than 1%) 3104
Vancocin HCl Capsules, USP (Rare) 3380
Vantin Tablets and Oral Suspension (Less than 1%) 2645
Vasotec I.V. Injection (0.5% to 1.0%) 2103
Verelan PM Extended-Release Capsules, Controlled-Onset (2% or less) 3106
VFEND I.V. (Less than 2%) 2564
VFEND Oral Suspension (Less than 2%) 2564
VFEND Tablets (Less than 2%) 2564
Viagra Tablets (Less than 2%) 2573
Vicoprofen Tablets (Less than 3%) 539
▲ Voltaren Tablets (1% to 10%) 2307
▲ Voltaren-XR Tablets (1% to 10%) 2310
Wellbutrin Tablets 1603
▲ Wellbutrin SR Sustained-Release Tablets (5% to 6%) 1607
▲ Wellbutrin XL Extended-Release Tablets (3% to 6%) 1613
Xifaxan Tablets (Less than 2%) 2842
▲ Xyrem Oral Solution (5.9%) 1688
Zegerid Capsules (Less than 1%) 2958
Zegerid Powder for Oral Solution (Less than 1%) 2958
Zelapar Tablets 3372
Zmax for Oral Suspension 2583
Zoloft (Frequent) 2586
Zomig Tablets (Infrequent) 3519
Zomig Nasal Spray (Infrequent) 3523
Zomig-ZMT Tablets (Infrequent) 3519
Zonegran Capsules (Frequent) 1101
Zosyn (1.0% or less) 3492
Zyban Sustained-Release Tablets (1%) 1644
Zyprexa Tablets (Infrequent) 1830
Zyprexa ZYDIS Orally Disintegrating Tablets (Infrequent) 1830
Zyrtec Chewable Tablets (Less than 2%) 2594
Zyrtec (Less than 2%) 2594
Zyrtec-D 12 Hour Extended Release Tablets (Less than 2%) 2597

Tiredness
(*see under* Fatigue)

Tobacco misuse
Zyprexa Tablets (Rare) 1830
Zyprexa ZYDIS Orally Disintegrating Tablets (Rare) 1830

Toenails, ingrown
Crixivan Capsules 1940
Prevnar for Injection 3463

Tolerance
Adderall Tablets 3164
Adipex-P 1215
Astelin Nasal Spray 1904
Carnitor Tablets and Oral Solution 3190
Daytrana Transdermal Patch 3174
DextroStat Tablets 3179
Dilaudid Oral Liquid 445
Dilaudid Tablets - 8 mg 445
Duragesic Transdermal System 2373
Hycodan 1116
Hycotuss Expectorant Syrup 1117
Kadian Capsules (Less than 3%) 577
MS Contin Tablets 2701
Nembutal Sodium Solution, USP 2470
Percocet Tablets 1131
Percodan Tablets 1132
Ritalin Hydrochloride Tablets 2269
Ritalin LA Capsules 2271
Ritalin-SR Tablets 2269
Tylenol with Codeine Tablets 2391
Vicodin Tablets 535
Vicodin HP Tablets 538
Vicoprofen Tablets 539
Xyrem Oral Solution 1688
Zemuron Injection (Rare) 2346

Tolerance, diminished
Symbyax Capsules (Rare) 1819
Timolide Tablets 2086

Tolerance, increased
Ambien CR Tablets (Rare) 2855

Tongue, black "hairy"
(*see under* Glossotrichia)

Tongue, burning
Imitrex Injection 1463
Imitrex Nasal Spray (Infrequent) 1467
Imitrex Tablets 1471
Nalfon Capsules (Less than 1%) 2502
Parcopa Orally Disintegrating Tablets 3097
Stalevo Tablets 2287

Tongue, fine vermicular movements
Lithobid Tablets 1692
Moban Tablets 1119
Thioridazine Hydrochloride Tablets 2163
Thiothixene Capsules 2165

Tongue, furry
Tindamax Tablets (Rare) 2142

Tongue, geographic
Evoxac Capsules (Less than 1%) 1047

Tongue, mucosal atrophy
Prilosec OTC Delayed-Release Tablets (Less than 1%) 2677
Zegerid Capsules (Less than 1%) 2958
Zegerid Powder for Oral Solution (Less than 1%) 2958

Tongue, protrusion
Moban Tablets 1119
Phenergan Tablets and Suppositories 3440
Thioridazine Hydrochloride Tablets 2163
Thiothixene Capsules 2165

Tongue, sore
(*see under* Glossodynia)

Tongue, swelling
(*see under* Glossoncus)

Tongue, thickening of
Cesamet Capsules 3340
▲ Kepivance (17%) 597

Tongue discoloration
Avelox (Less than 0.1%) 2970
Biaxin/Biaxin XL 402
Colazal Capsules 2838
Copaxone for Injection (Infrequent) 3297
Effexor Tablets (Rare) 3411
Effexor XR Capsules (Rare) 3417
Evoxac Capsules (Less than 1%) 1047
▲ Kepivance (17%) 597
Paxil CR Controlled-Release Tablets (Rare) 1538
Paxil (Rare) 1530
Pepto-Bismol Original Liquid, Maximum Strength Liquid, Original and Cherry Tablets, Chewable Tablets and Easy-To-Swallow Caplets 2676
Pepto-Bismol Maximum Strength Liquid ◘ 672
PREVPAC (Less than 3%) 3284
Prilosec OTC Delayed-Release Tablets (2%) 2677
Primaxin I.M. 2045
Primaxin I.V. (Less than 0.2%) 2048
Protonix I.V. (Less than 1%) 3472
Protonix Tablets (Less than 1%) 3469
Rilutek Tablets (Rare) 2930
Risperdal (Rare) 1676
Risperdal M-Tab Orally Disintegrating Tablets (Rare) 1676
Sonata Capsules (Rare) 1717
Thalomid Capsules 965
Tindamax Tablets 2142
Uniretic Tablets (Less than 1%) 3100
Zegerid Capsules (2%) 2958
Zegerid Powder for Oral Solution (2%) 2958
Zyprexa Tablets (Rare) 1830
Zyprexa ZYDIS Orally Disintegrating Tablets (Rare) 1830
Zyrtec Chewable Tablets (Less than 2%) 2594
Zyrtec (Less than 2%) 2594
Zyrtec-D 12 Hour Extended Release Tablets (Less than 2%) 2597
Zyvox (0.2% to 1.1%) 2652

Tongue disorder, unspecified
Evoxac Capsules (Less than 1%) 1047
▲ Flovent Diskus (1% to 3%) 1443
Gengraf Capsules (1% to less than 3%) 459
Neoral Oral Solution (1% to less than 3%) 2259
Neoral Soft Gelatin Capsules (1% to less than 3%) 2259
Neurontin Capsules (Infrequent) 2487
Neurontin Oral Solution (Infrequent) 2487
Neurontin Tablets (Infrequent) 2487
Nexium Delayed-Release Capsules (Less than 1%) 655
Nexium I.V. (Less than 1%) 659
Prevacid NapraPAC (Less than 1%) 3280
PREVPAC (Less than 3%) 3284
Relpax Tablets (Rare) 2548
▲ Soriatane Capsules (1% to 10%) 1013
Tasmar Tablets (Infrequent) 3358

Tongue numbness
(*see under* Numbness, buccal mucosa)

Tonsillitis
Advair HFA Inhalation Aerosol 1318
▲ Elidel Cream 1% (0.4% to 6.3%) 2200
▲ Flovent Diskus (1% to 3%) 1443
Fluarix 1451
Foradil Aerolizer (1.2%) 3010
Gengraf Capsules (1% to less than 3%) 459
Neoral Oral Solution (1% to less than 3%) 2259
Neoral Soft Gelatin Capsules (1% to less than 3%) 2259
Singulair (Greater than or equal to 2%) 2077

Tooth discoloration
Amoxil Capsules (Rare) 1343
Amoxil Chewable Tablets (Rare) 1343
Amoxil Pediatric Drops for Oral Suspension (Rare) 1343
Amoxil Powder for Oral Suspension (Rare) 1343
Amoxil Tablets (Rare) 1343
Augmentin (Rare) 1360
Augmentin Tablets (Rare) 1363
Augmentin XR Extended-Release Tablets (Rare) 1369
Augmentin ES-600 Powder for Oral Suspension (Rare) 1366
Biaxin/Biaxin XL 402
PREVPAC 3284
Solodyn Extended Release Tablets 1890

Tooth disorder
Actiq (Less than 1%) 979
Actonel Tablets (2.1%) 2683
Actonel with Calcium Tablets (2.1%) 2688
▲ ActoPlus Met Tablets (5.3%) 3214
▲ Actos Tablets (5.3%) 3219
▲ Adderall XR Capsules (2% to 4%) 3166
▲ Advair HFA Inhalation Aerosol (1% to 3%) 1318
Axid Oral Solution (1.0%) 879
Boniva Injection (3.5%) 2738
Boniva Tablets (3.5%) 2741
Celebrex Capsules (0.1% to 1.9%) 3134
▲ Depakote ER Tablets (Greater than 1% to 5%) 434
▲ Duetact Tablets (At least 5%) 3226
▲ Entocort EC Capsules (Less than 5%) 2698
▲ Estring Vaginal Ring (1% to 3%) 2635
▲ Evoxac Capsules (1% to 3%) 1047
Flomax Capsules (1.2% to 2.0%) 850
▲ Flovent Diskus (1% to 3%) 1443
Forteo for Injection (2%) 1767
Gengraf Capsules (1% to less than 3%) 459
Geodon for Injection (Up to 1%) 2529
Invirase (Less than 2%) 2772
▲ Lamictal (2% to 3%) 1481
Lescol Capsules (2.1%) 2233
Lescol XL Tablets (1.4%) 2233
Lofibra Tablets 1219
Lofibra Capsules 1216
Lotensin HCT Tablets (0.3% or more) 2246
Meridia Capsules (Greater than or equal to 1%) 489
Mirapex Tablets (1% or more) 859
Myobloc Injection (Greater than 2%) 3192
Neoral Oral Solution (1% to less than 3%) 2259
Neoral Soft Gelatin Capsules (1% to less than 3%) 2259
Neurontin Capsules (Infrequent) 2487
Neurontin Oral Solution (Infrequent) 2487
Neurontin Tablets (Infrequent) 2487
▲ Nipent for Injection (3% to 10%) 1863
Paxil CR Controlled-Release Tablets (Rare) 1538
Paxil (Rare) 1530
Prometrium Capsules (100 mg, 200 mg) 3203
Protopic Ointment (Greater than or equal to 1% to 2%) 638
Provigil Tablets (At least 1%) 988
Relpax Tablets (Rare) 2548
Rescriptor Tablets 2551
Rilutek Tablets (Up to 1.2%) 2930
▲ Risperdal Consta Long-Acting Injection (2% to 4%) 1682
Symbyax Capsules (1% to 2%) 1819
Tasmar Tablets (Frequent) 3358
Thalomid Capsules 965
Topamax Sprinkle Capsules (Greater than 1%) 2404
Topamax Tablets (Greater than 1%) 2404
Tricor Tablets 527
Triglide Tablets 3123
Vantin Tablets and Oral Suspension (Less than 1%) 2645
Wellbutrin SR Sustained-Release Tablets (At least 1%) 1607
Wellbutrin XL Extended-Release Tablets (At least 1%) 1613
▲ Xenical Capsules (2.9% to 4.3%) 2831
Yaz Tablets (Greater than 1%) 803
Zelapar Tablets (2%) 3372
Zyprexa Tablets 1830
Zyprexa ZYDIS Orally Disintegrating Tablets 1830
Zyrtec Chewable Tablets (Less than 2%) 2594
Zyrtec (Less than 2%) 2594
Zyrtec-D 12 Hour Extended Release Tablets (Less than 2%) 2597

Toothache
Aricept Tablets (Infrequent) 1094
Aricept ODT Tablets (Infrequent) 1094
Astelin Nasal Spray (Infrequently) 1904
▲ Azmacort Inhalation Aerosol (1% to 3%) 1726
Elidel Cream 1% (0.4% to 2.6%) 2200
▲ Evoxac Capsules (1% to 3%) 1047
Frova Tablets (Rare) 1113

Klonopin (Infrequent) 2778
Lexapro Oral Solution (2%) 1190
Lexapro Tablets (2%) 1190
Micardis Tablets (More than 0.3%) 854
Micardis HCT Tablets 856
▲ Prochieve 4% Gel (Less than 5%) 1003
▲ Prochieve 8% Gel (Less than 5%) 1003
Requip Tablets (Infrequent) 1555
Rescriptor Tablets 2551
Risperdal (2%) 1676
▲ Risperdal Consta Long-Acting Injection (1% to 3%) 1682
Risperdal M-Tab Orally Disintegrating Tablets (2%) 1676
Striant Mucoadhesive 1007
Teveten Tablets (Less than 1%) 1735
Teveten HCT Tablets (Less than 1%) 1737
Trileptal Tablets (1% to 2%) 2300
Trileptal Oral Suspension (1% to 2%) 2300
▲ Ultram ER Tablets (1% to greater than 5%) 2392
Vantin Tablets and Oral Suspension (Infrequent) 2645
Vivitrol 995
Wellbutrin Tablets (Infrequent) 1603
Xyrem Oral Solution (Frequent) 1688

Torsade de pointes
Adenocard Injection 617
Avelox (Very rare) 2970
Biaxin/Biaxin XL (Rare) 402
Celexa 1176
Cipro 2977
Cipro I.V. 2984
Cipro XR Tablets 2990
E.E.S. (Rare) 451
Effexor Tablets (Rare) 3411
Effexor XR Capsules (Rare) 3417
EryPed (Rare) 447
Erythrocin Stearate Filmtab Tablets (Rare) 453
Erythromycin Base Filmtab Tablets (Rare) 455
Erythromycin Delayed-Release Capsules, USP 457
Geodon 2529
Levaquin 2384
Levaquin in 5% Dextrose Injection 2384
Lexapro Oral Solution 1190
Lexapro Tablets 1190
Meridia Capsules 489
Noroxin Tablets (Rare) 2032
Paxil CR Controlled-Release Tablets 1538
Paxil 1530
PCE Dispertab Tablets 515
Pletal Tablets (Very rare) 2455
PREVPAC (Rare) 3284
Prograf Capsules and Injection 632
Proquin XR Tablets 1153
Razadyne 2399
Razadyne ER Extended-Release Capsules 2399
Tambocor Tablets (Rare) 1856
Tequin Injection 938
Tequin Injection in 5% Dextrose 938
Tequin Tablets 938
Thioridazine Hydrochloride Tablets 2163
VFEND I.V. (Less than 2%) 2564
VFEND Oral Suspension (Less than 2%) 2564
VFEND Tablets (Less than 2%) 2564
Viracept 2577
Zmax for Oral Suspension 2583
Zoloft 2586

Torticollis
Abilify Oral Solution (Frequent) 882
Abilify Oral Solution (Frequent) 2450
Abilify Discmelt Orally Disintegrating Tablets (Frequent) 882
Abilify Discmelt Orally Disintegrating Tablets (Frequent) 2450
Abilify Tablets (Frequent) 882
Abilify Tablets (Frequent) 2450
Aceon Tablets (2 mg, 4 mg, 8 mg) (1.4%) 3194
Actiq (1% or greater) 979
Actonel Tablets (1.2% to 2.7%) 2683
▲ Actonel with Calcium Tablets (1.2% to 5.3%) 2688
Adalat CC Tablets (Less than 1%) 2964
Adenocard Injection (Less than 1%) 617
▲ Agrylin Capsules (1% to 5%) 3169
Ambien CR Tablets (1% to 2%) 2855
AmBisome for Injection (Less common) 620
Amerge Tablets (1% to 2%) 1339
▲ Arimidex Tablets (2% to 5%) 673
Asacol Delayed-Release Tablets 2692
Axert Tablets (Infrequent) 2396
▲ Azilect Tablets (2% to 3%) 3293
▲ Bexxar (1% to 6%) 1398
▲ BOTOX Purified Neurotoxin Complex (3 % to 11%) 570
Caduet Tablets (Less than 2%) 2508
Campral Tablets (Rare) 1174
Cardene I.V. (Rare) 2497
▲ CellCept Capsules (3% to less than 20%) 2747
▲ CellCept Intravenous (3% to less than 20%) 2747
▲ CellCept Oral Suspension (3% to less than 20%) 2747
▲ CellCept Tablets (3% to less than 20%) 2747
Cesamet Capsules 3340
Cialis Tablets (Less than 2%) 1838
Cipro (Less than 1%) 2977
Cipro I.V. (1% or less) 2984
Cipro XR Tablets 2990
Clozaril Tablets (1%) 2184
▲ Copaxone for Injection (8%) 3297
Crestor Tablets (Greater than or equal to 1%) 678
Depacon Injection (1% or more) 412
Depakene (1% or more) 417
Depakote Sprinkle Capsules 422
▲ Depakote Tablets (1% to 5%) 427
Depakote ER Tablets (1% or more) 434
Doxil Injection (Less than 1%) 2351
DynaCirc CR Tablets (0.5% to 1%) 2721
Effexor Tablets (Frequent) 3411
▲ Effexor XR Capsules (3%) 3417
Engerix-B Vaccine (Less than 1%) 1425
FazaClo Orally Disintegrating Tablets (1%) 551
Forteo for Injection (3%) 1767
Gabitril Tablets (Frequent) 984
Geodon Capsules (Rare) 2529
Hytrin Capsules (At least 1%) 471
▲ Imdur Tablets (Less than or equal to 5%) 3018
▲ Imitrex Injection (5%) 1463
▲ Imitrex Tablets (Less than 1% to 3%) 1471
▲ Infergen (8% to 14%) 3364
Ionsys Transdermal System (.1% to less than 1%) 2379
▲ Keppra Oral Solution (2% to 8%) 3314
▲ Keppra Tablets (2% to 8%) 3314
Klonopin (Infrequent) 2778
▲ Lamictal (1% to 5%) 1481
Levitra Tablets (Less than 2%) 3034
▲ Lexapro Oral Solution (3%) 1190
▲ Lexapro Tablets (3%) 1190
Lipitor Tablets (Less than 2%) 2483
Lotensin HCT Tablets (0.3% or more) 2246
Lyrica Capsules (Rare) 2539
Meridia Capsules (1.6%) 489
Mirapex Tablets (Greater than or equal to 1%) 859
Moduretic Tablets 2028
▲ Myobloc Injection (0% to 17%) 3192
Neurontin Capsules (Infrequent) 2487
Neurontin Oral Solution (Infrequent) 2487
Neurontin Tablets (Infrequent) 2487
Norvir (Less than 2%) 503
Omacor Capsules 2725
▲ Orthoclone OKT3 Sterile Solution (14%) 2360
OxyContin Tablets (Less than 1%) 2703
Paxil CR Controlled-Release Tablets (Infrequent) 1538
Paxil (Infrequent) 1530
Permax Tablets (2.7%) 3356
Phenergan Tablets and Suppositories 3440
Prevacid Delayed-Release Capsules (Less than 1%) 3271
Prevacid for Delayed-Release Oral Suspension (Less than 1%) 3271
Prevacid SoluTab Delayed-Release Orally Disintegrating Tablets (Less than 1%) 3271
Prevacid NapraPAC (Less than 1%) 3280
PREVPAC (Less than 1%) 3284
Prinivil Tablets (0.3% to 1.0%) 2052
Prinzide Tablets 2056
ProQuad 2064
Proquin XR Tablets 1153
ProSom Tablets (Infrequent) 517
Protonix I.V. (Greater than or equal to 1%) 3472
Protonix Tablets (Greater than or equal to 1%) 3469
Protopic Ointment (Greater than or equal to 1%) 638
Provigil Tablets (Greater than or equal to 1%) 988
Recombivax HB (Less than 1%) 2071
Requip Tablets (Infrequent) 1555
Revlimid Capsules 958
Risperdal (Rare) 1676
Risperdal Consta Long-Acting Injection (Infrequent) 1682
Risperdal M-Tab Orally Disintegrating Tablets (Rare) 1676
Rythmol SR Capsules 2727
Seroquel Tablets (Infrequent) 690
Sonata Capsules (Infrequent) 1717
Symbyax Capsules (Frequent) 1819
Tasmar Tablets (2%) 3358
Tequin Injection (Less than 0.1%) 938
Tequin Injection in 5% Dextrose (Less than 0.1%) 938
Tequin Tablets (Less than 0.1%) 938
▲ Thalomid Capsules (4.2%) 965
Thioridazine Hydrochloride Tablets 2163
Tiazac Capsules (1%) 1201
▲ Trisenox Injection (13%) 993
▲ Ultram ER Tablets (1% to greater than 5%) 2392
Uniretic Tablets (Less than 1%) 3100
Vantas (Less than 2%) 3375
Wellbutrin SR Sustained-Release Tablets (At least 1%) 1607
Wellbutrin XL Extended-Release Tablets (At least 1%) 1613
Xifaxan Tablets (Less than 2%) 2842
Xyrem Oral Solution (Frequent) 1688
Zelapar Tablets 3372
Zomig Nasal Spray (Infrequent) 3523
Zyban Sustained-Release Tablets (2%) 1644
Zyflo Tablets (Greater than 1%) 1023
▲ Zyprexa Tablets (2% to 3%) 1830
▲ Zyprexa ZYDIS Orally Disintegrating Tablets (2% to 3%) 1830

Total proteins, decrease
(*see under* Hypoproteinemia)

Tourette's syndrome
Adderall Tablets 3164
Adderall XR Capsules 3166
Concerta Extended-Release Tablets (Rare) 1881
Daytrana Transdermal Patch 3174
Desoxyn Tablets, USP 2462
Dexedrine 1420
DextroStat Tablets 3179
Focalin Tablets (Rare) 2220
Focalin XR Capsules 2223
Meridia Capsules 489
Metadate CD Capsules (Rare) 3323
Ritalin Hydrochloride Tablets (Rare) 2269
Ritalin LA Capsules (Rare) 2271
Ritalin-SR Tablets (Rare) 2269

Toxic granulation
Efudex 3363

Toxic shock syndrome
Amevive 626

Toxicity, bone marrow
Pegasys 2789

Toxicity, unspecified
▲ Advair HFA Inhalation Aerosol (1% to 3%) 1318

Toxicity, vascular
Gemzar for Injection (Very rare) 1771

Toxoplasmosis
Doxil Injection 2351

Tracheitis
Advair Diskus 100/50 1308
Advair Diskus 250/50 1308
Advair Diskus 500/50 1308
Advair HFA Inhalation Aerosol 1318
Amerge Tablets (Rare) 1339
Lexapro Oral Solution (Infrequent) 1190
Lexapro Tablets (Infrequent) 1190
Liquid PedvaxHIB (One case) 2035
▲ Serevent Diskus (7%) 1568

Tracheobronchitis
Avalide Tablets 888
Avalide Tablets 2874
Avapro Tablets (Less than 1%) 891
Avapro Tablets (Less than 1%) 2871

Transaminase, elevation
(*see under* Serum transaminase, elevation)

Transfusion reactions
▲ Clolar for Intravenous Infusion (10%) 1271
▲ Dacogen Injection (7%) 2129

Trauma
Ambien CR Tablets (Infrequent) 2855
Caverject Impulse Injection (2%) 2612
▲ Cozaar Tablets (4%) 1935
Exelon Capsules (Frequent) 2206
Exelon Oral Solution (Frequent) 2206
Foradil Aerolizer (1.2%) 3010
▲ Gengraf Capsules (4%) 459
▲ Neoral Oral Solution (4%) 2259
▲ Neoral Soft Gelatin Capsules (4%) 2259
ProQuad 2064
▲ Simulect for Injection (3% to 10%) 2284
Singulair (1%) 2077
Starlix Tablets (2.9%) 2292
▲ Zelnorm Tablets (3%) 2312

Trauma, unspecified
Ambien Tablets (Infrequent) 2851
Effexor Tablets (2%) 3411
Invirase (Less than 2%) 2772
▲ Lescol Capsules (5.1%) 2233
▲ Lescol XL Tablets (4.2%) 2233
Neurontin Capsules (Frequent) 2487
Neurontin Oral Solution (Frequent) 2487
Neurontin Tablets (Frequent) 2487
Paxil CR Controlled-Release Tablets (1.4%) 1538
▲ Paxil (1.4% to 6%) 1530
Prinzide Tablets (0.3% to 1%) 2056
▲ Zyvox (2.8% to 3.3%) 2652

Trembling
(*see under* Tremors)

Tremor, fine hand
Lithobid Tablets 1692

Tremors
▲ Abilify Oral Solution (3% to 9%) 882
▲ Abilify Oral Solution (3% to 9%) 2450
▲ Abilify Discmelt Orally Disintegrating Tablets (3% to 9%) 882
▲ Abilify Discmelt Orally Disintegrating Tablets (3% to 9%) 2450
▲ Abilify Tablets (3% to 9%) 882
▲ Abilify Tablets (3% to 9%) 2450
Aciphex Tablets 1090
Adalat CC Tablets (Rare) 2964
Adderall Tablets 3164
Adderall XR Capsules 3166
Adenoscan (Less than 1%) 619
Adipex-P 1215
▲ Advair Diskus 100/50 (1% to 3%) 1308
▲ Advair Diskus 250/50 (1% to 3%) 1308
▲ Advair Diskus 500/50 (1% to 3%) 1308
Advicor Tablets 1722
▲ Aerobid/Aerobid-M (3% to 9%) 1171
Alferon N Injection (One patient) 1665
Alimta for Injection (Less than 1%) 1750
Alinia for Oral Suspension (Less than 1%) 2835
Alinia Tablets (Less than 1%) 2835
Aloprim for Injection (Less than 1%) 2167
Altace Capsules (Less than 1%) 1702
Altoprev Extended-Release Tablets 3109
▲ Alupent Inhalation Aerosol (About 1 in 20 patients) 826
Ambien Tablets (Infrequent) 2851
Ambien CR Tablets (Infrequent to 1%) 2855
AmBisome for Injection (Less common) 620
Amerge Tablets (Infrequent) 1339
Amitiza Capsules (Less than 0.2%) 3224
Anaprox Tablets (Less than 1%) 2761
Anaprox DS Tablets (Less than 1%) 2761
Anzemet Injection (Infrequently) 2859
Anzemet Tablets (Infrequently) 2862
Aricept Tablets (Frequent) 1094
Aricept ODT Tablets (Frequent) 1094
▲ Arranon Injection (0% to 5%) 1357
Arthrotec Tablets (Rare) 3129
Asacol Delayed-Release Tablets 2692
Atripla Tablets 945
Atrovent Inhalation Solution (0.9%) 835
Avalide Tablets 888
Avalide Tablets 2874
Avapro Tablets (Less than 1%) 891
Avapro Tablets (Less than 1%) 2871
Avelox (0.1% to less than 2%) 2970
▲ Avinza Capsules (Less than 5%) 1741
Axert Tablets (Infrequent) 2396
Azilect Tablets (Frequent) 3293
▲ BeneFix Vials (3.1%) 3408
Biaxin/Biaxin XL 402
Bicillin C-R Injectable Suspension 1706
Buprenex Injectable (Infrequent) 2716
Caduet Tablets (Greater than 0.1% to less than or equal to 1%) 2508

Calcium Disodium Versenate Injection 1851
▲ Campath Ampules (7%) 811
Campral Tablets (Frequent) 1174
Cancidas for Injection (0% to 1.8%) 1918
Cardizem LA Extended Release Tablets (Less than 2%) 1728
Carimune NF 3499
▲ Celexa (8%) 1176
▲ CellCept Capsules (24.2% to 33.9%) 2747
▲ CellCept Intravenous (24.2% to 33.9%) 2747
▲ CellCept Oral Suspension (24.2% to 33.9%) 2747
▲ CellCept Tablets (24.2% to 33.9%) 2747
Cesamet Capsules 3340
Chantix Tablets (Infrequent) 2517
Cipro (Less than 1%) 2977
Cipro I.V. (1% or less) 2984
Cipro XR Tablets (Less than 1%) 2990
▲ Clolar for Intravenous Infusion (10%) 1271
▲ Clozaril Tablets (More than 5% to 6%) 2184
Colazal Capsules 2838
Combivent Inhalation Aerosol (Less than 2%) 847
▲ Copaxone for Injection (7%) 3297
Covera-HS Tablets (Less than 2%) 3139
Cozaar Tablets (Less than 1%) 1935
▲ Cymbalta Delayed-Release Capsules (Up to 5%) 1757
Daranide Tablets 1950
▲ Demser Capsules (10%) 1953
▲ Depacon Injection (0.6% to 57%) 412
▲ Depakene (25% to 57%) 417
▲ Depakote Sprinkle Capsules (19% to 57%) 422
▲ Depakote Tablets (9% to 57%) 427
▲ Depakote ER Tablets (Greater than 1% to 57%) 434
Desoxyn Tablets, USP 2462
Dexedrine 1420
DextroStat Tablets 3179
Dilaudid 440
Dilaudid Non-Sterile Powder 440
Dilaudid Oral Liquid (Less frequent) 445
Dilaudid Rectal Suppositories 440
Dilaudid Tablets 440
Dilaudid Tablets - 8 mg (Less frequent) 445
Dilaudid-HP (Less frequent) 442
Duragesic Transdermal System (1% or greater) 2373
Dyazide Capsules 1423
EC-Naprosyn Delayed-Release Tablets (Less than 1%) 2761
▲ Effexor Tablets (5% to 10.2%) 3411
▲ Effexor XR Capsules (4% to 5%) 3417
Eldepryl Capsules 3208
Eligard 7.5 mg (Less than 2%) 2880
Elspar for Injection 2463
Elspar for Injection 1960
Emend Capsules (Greater than 0.5%) 1963
▲ Entocort EC Capsules (Less than 5%) 2698
EpiPen 1061
▲ Evoxac Capsules (1% to 3%) 1047
▲ Exelon Capsules (4% to 10%) 2206
▲ Exelon Oral Solution (4% to 10%) 2206
▲ FazaClo Orally Disintegrating Tablets (Less than 1% to 6%) 551
Flebogamma 5%, Immune Globulin Intravenous (Human) 1658
Floxin Otic Solution (Single report) 1049
▲ Fluarix (3.3% to 6.9%) 1451
Flumadine (Less than 0.3%) 1183
Foradil Aerolizer (1.9%) 3010
Frova Tablets (Infrequent) 1113
▲ Gabitril Tablets (9%) 984
Gammagard Liquid 721
Gammagard S/D 724
Gamunex Immune Globulin I.V., 10% 3235
▲ Gengraf Capsules (13%) 459
▲ Geodon Capsules (14%) 2529
Guanidine Hydrochloride Tablets 3016
▲ Humira Injection (Less than 5%) 466
Hyzaar 50-12.5 Tablets 1990
Hyzaar 100-12.5 Tablets 1990
Hyzaar 100-25 Tablets 1990
▲ Imdur Tablets (Less than or equal to 5%) 3018
Imitrex Injection (Infrequent) 1463
Imitrex Nasal Spray (Infrequent) 1467
Imitrex Tablets (Rare to infrequent) 1471
Infed Injection 3390
▲ Intron A for Injection (Less than 5%) 3024
Invanz for Injection (Greater than 0.1%) 1999
Invirase (Less than 2%) 2772
Ionsys Transdermal System (.1% to less than 1%) 2379
Kadian Capsules (Less than 3%) 577
Kaletra (Less than 2%) 476
Keppra Injection 3320
Keppra Oral Solution (1% to 2%) 3314
Keppra Tablets (1% to 2%) 3314
Klonopin (Infrequent) 2778
▲ Lamictal (4% to 10%) 1481
Lariam Tablets (Occasional) 2786
Lescol Capsules 2233
Lescol XL Tablets 2233
Leukeran Tablets (Rare) 1504
Levaquin (0.1% to 0.9%) 2384
Levaquin in 5% Dextrose Injection (0.1% to 0.9%) 2384
Levothroid Tablets 1186
Levoxyl Tablets 1712
Lexapro Oral Solution (Infrequent) 1190
Lexapro Tablets (Infrequent) 1190
Lidoderm Patch 1118
Lithobid Tablets 1692
▲ Lithostat Tablets (20%) 2140
Lotrel Capsules 2249
Lotronex Tablets (Rare) 1512
Lunesta Tablets (Rare) 3142
▲ Lyrica Capsules (1% to 11%) 2539
Matulane Capsules 3191
▲ Maxair Autohaler (1.3% to 6.0%) 1852
Maxalt Tablets (Frequent) 2008
Maxalt-MLT Orally Disintegrating Tablets (Frequent) 2008
Meridia Capsules 489
Mevacor Tablets (0.5% to 1.0%) 2021
Midamor Tablets (Less than or equal to 1%) 2026
Migranal Nasal Spray (Infrequent) 3348
Mirapex Tablets (1% or more) 859
Moban Tablets 1119
Mobic Oral Suspension (Less than 2%) 863
Mobic Tablets (Less than 2%) 863
Moduretic Tablets 2028
MS Contin Tablets (Less frequent) 2701
▲ Myfortic Tablets (3% to less than 20%) 2255
Myobloc Injection (Greater than 2%) 3192
Myozyme for Intravenous Infusion 1279
Nalfon Capsules (2.2%) 2502
Namenda (Infrequent) 1195
Naprosyn Suspension (Less than 1%) 2761
Naprosyn Tablets (Less than 1%) 2761
Natrecor for Injection (Greater than or equal to 1%) 3127
▲ Neoral Oral Solution (12% to 55%) 2259
▲ Neoral Soft Gelatin Capsules (12% to 55%) 2259
▲ Neurontin Capsules (1% to 6.8%) 2487
▲ Neurontin Oral Solution (1% to 6.8%) 2487
▲ Neurontin Tablets (1% to 6.8%) 2487
Nexium Delayed-Release Capsules (Less than 1%) 655
Nexium I.V. (Less than 1%) 659
▲ Niravam Orally Disintegrating Tablets (4%) 3092
Norflex Injection 1856
Noroxin Tablets 2032
Norvasc Tablets (More than 0.1% to 1%) 2545
Norvir (Less than 2%) 503
▲ Orthoclone OKT3 Sterile Solution (13%) 2360
OxyContin Tablets (Less than 1%) 2703
Parnate Tablets 1527
▲ Paxil CR Controlled-Release Tablets (5% to 14.7%) 1538
▲ Paxil (1% to 14.7%) 1530
▲ Permax Tablets (4.2%) 3356
Phenergan Tablets and Suppositories 3440
Phenytek Capsules (Rare) 2160
Prevacid Delayed-Release Capsules (Less than 1%) 3271
Prevacid for Delayed-Release Oral Suspension (Less than 1%) 3271
Prevacid SoluTab Delayed-Release Orally Disintegrating Tablets (Less than 1%) 3271
Prevacid NapraPAC (Less than 1%) 3280
PREVPAC (Less than 1%) 3284
Prilosec OTC Delayed-Release Tablets (Less than 1%) 2677
Primatene Mist ▣719
Primaxin I.M. 2045
Primaxin I.V. (Less than 0.2%) 2048
Prinivil Tablets (0.3% to 1.0%) 2052
Prinzide Tablets 2056
ProAir HFA Inhalation Aerosol (Frequent) 3300
Prochieve 4% Gel 1003
Prochieve 8% Gel 1003
▲ Prograf Capsules and Injection (15% to 56%) 632
ProQuad 2064
Proquin XR Tablets 1153
ProSom Tablets (Rare) 517
Protonix I.V. (Less than 1%) 3472
Protonix Tablets (Less than 1%) 3469
▲ Proventil Inhalation Aerosol (Less than 15%) 3053
▲ Proventil Inhalation Solution 0.083% (10.7% to 20%) 3055
▲ Proventil HFA Inhalation Aerosol (7%) 3056
Provigil Tablets (1%) 988
▲ Prozac Pulvules and Liquid (3% to 13%) 1801
Ranexa Tablets (Less than or equal to 0.5%) 1035
▲ Rapamune Oral Solution and Tablets (21% to 31%) 3475
▲ Razadyne (3%) 2399
▲ Razadyne ER Extended-Release Capsules (3%) 2399
Relpax Tablets (Infrequent) 2548
Requip Tablets (1% or more) 1555
Rescriptor Tablets 2551
Restoril Capsules (0.5% to 0.9%) 1860
Retrovir Capsules 1560
Retrovir IV Infusion 1564
Retrovir 1560
▲ Revlimid Capsules (19.7%) 958
Rilutek Tablets (Frequent) 2930
▲ Risperdal (17% to 34%) 1676
▲ Risperdal Consta Long-Acting Injection (Up to 3%) 1682
▲ Risperdal M-Tab Orally Disintegrating Tablets (17% to 34%) 1676
▲ Romazicon Injection (3% to 9%) 2804
Rythmol SR Capsules (2%) 2727
▲ Sandimmune (12% to 55%) 2275
Sandostatin Injection (Less than 1%) 2278
▲ Sandostatin LAR Depot (1% to 4%) 2280
Seromycin Capsules 1813
▲ Simulect for Injection (Greater than or equal to 10%) 2284
Sonata Capsules (2%) 1717
Stalevo Tablets 2287
▲ Strattera Capsules (1% to 4%) 1814
Stromectol Tablets (0.9%) 2083
Sular Tablets (Less than or equal to 1%) 3122
Sustiva Capsules (Less than 2%) 930
Sustiva Tablets (Less than 2%) 930
▲ Symbyax Capsules (Greater than or equal to 5% to 9%) 1819
Symmetrel Tablets 1135
Synera Topical Patch 1137
▲ Tambocor Tablets (4.7%) 1856
Tarka Tablets 524
Tasmar Tablets (Frequent) 3358
▲ Tequin Injection (0.1% to 3%) 938
▲ Tequin Injection in 5% Dextrose (0.1% to 3%) 938
▲ Tequin Tablets (0.1% to 3%) 938
Teveten Tablets (Less than 1%) 1735
Teveten HCT Tablets (Less than 1%) 1737
▲ Thalomid Capsules (4.2%) 965
Thioridazine Hydrochloride Tablets 2163
Thyrolar Tablets 1199
Tiazac Capsules (Less than 2%) 1201
▲ Topamax Sprinkle Capsules (Greater than 1% to 9%) 2404
▲ Topamax Tablets (Greater than 1% to 9%) 2404
Tranxene 2474
▲ Trileptal Tablets (3% to 16%) 2300
▲ Trileptal Oral Suspension (3% to 16%) 2300
▲ Trisenox Injection (13%) 993
Twinject 0.3 3378
Twinject 0.15 3379
▲ Ultane Liquid for Inhalation (6%) 531
▲ Ultram ER Tablets (1% to greater than 5%) 2392
Valium Tablets (Infrequent) 2819
Vantas (Less than 2%) 3375
Vantin Tablets and Oral Suspension (Less than 1%) 2645
Verelan PM Extended-Release Capsules, Controlled-Onset (2% or less) 3106
▲ Vesanoid Capsules (3%) 2820
VFEND I.V. (Less than 2%) 2564
VFEND Oral Suspension (Less than 2%) 2564
VFEND Tablets (Less than 2%) 2564
Viadur Implant (Rare) 757
Viagra Tablets (Less than 2%) 2573
Vicoprofen Tablets (Less than 1%) 539
Voltaren Tablets (Occasionally) 2307
Voltaren-XR Tablets (Occasionally) 2310
▲ VoSpire ER Tablets (24.2%) 1052
Vytorin 10/10 Tablets 2114
Vytorin 10/10 Tablets 3077
Vytorin 10/20 Tablets 2114
Vytorin 10/20 Tablets 3077
Vytorin 10/40 Tablets 2114
Vytorin 10/40 Tablets 3077
Vytorin 10/80 Tablets 2114
Vytorin 10/80 Tablets 3077
▲ Wellbutrin Tablets (21.1%) 1603
▲ Wellbutrin SR Sustained-Release Tablets (3% to 6%) 1607
▲ Wellbutrin XL Extended-Release Tablets (3% to 6%) 1613
▲ Xeloda Tablets (Less than 5%) 2822
▲ Xopenex Inhalation Solution (6.8%) 3146
▲ Xopenex Inhalation Solution Concentrate (6.8%) 3150
▲ Xopenex HFA Inhalation Aerosol (6.8%) 3154
Xyrem Oral Solution (Less than 1%) 1688
Zegerid Capsules (Less than 1%) 2958
Zegerid Powder for Oral Solution (Less than 1%) 2958
▲ Zelapar Tablets (3%) 3372
Zocor Tablets 2105
▲ Zofran Injection (7%) 1634
▲ Zofran (5%) 1639
▲ Zofran ODT Orally Disintegrating Tablets (5%) 1639
▲ Zoloft (Less than 1% to 11%) 2586
Zometa for Intravenous Infusion 2315
Zomig Nasal Spray (Infrequent) 3523
Zonegran Capsules (Frequent) 1101
Zosyn (1.0% or less) 3492
Zovirax 1643
Zyban Sustained-Release Tablets (1% to 2%) 1644
▲ Zyprexa Tablets (5% to 23%) 1830
▲ Zyprexa IntraMuscular (1% to 4%) 1830
▲ Zyprexa ZYDIS Orally Disintegrating Tablets (5% to 23%) 1830
Zyrtec Chewable Tablets (Less than 2%) 2594
Zyrtec (Less than 2%) 2594
Zyrtec-D 12 Hour Extended Release Tablets (Less than 2%) 2597

Tremors, extremities
Abilify Oral Solution (Infrequent) 882
Abilify Oral Solution (Infrequent) 2450
Abilify Discmelt Orally Disintegrating Tablets (Infrequent) 882
Abilify Discmelt Orally Disintegrating Tablets (Infrequent) 2450
Abilify Tablets (Infrequent) 882
Abilify Tablets (Infrequent) 2450

Tremulousness
(*see under* Tremors)

Trigeminal neuralgia
(*see under* Neuralgia, trigeminal)

Trigeminy
Lanoxicaps Capsules 1490
Lanoxin Injection 1494
Lanoxin Injection Pediatric 1497
Lanoxin Tablets 1500
Rituxan I.V. (One case) 1254

Trigger finger
Aromasin Tablets (0.3%) 2600

Triglycerides, increase
(*see under* Hypertriglyceridemia)

Trismus
Ceftin Tablets (0.1% to 1%) 1407
Cymbalta Delayed-Release Capsules (Very rare) 1757
Demser Capsules 1953
Effexor Tablets (Frequent) 3411
Effexor XR Capsules (2%) 3417
Geodon Capsules (Rare) 2529
Lyrica Capsules (Rare) 2539
Parcopa Orally Disintegrating Tablets 3097
Paxil CR Controlled-Release Tablets (Rare) 1538
Paxil (Rare) 1530
Rilutek Tablets (Rare) 2930
Sonata Capsules (Rare) 1717
Stalevo Tablets 2287
Thioridazine Hydrochloride Tablets 2163
▲ Ventavis Inhalation Solution (12%) 1020

Troponin 1, incerased
Revlimid Capsules ... 958

TSH, decrease
Thyrolar Tablets ... 1199

TSH, increase
Sutent Capsules (2%) ... 2560
Thyrolar Tablets ... 1199

Tuberculosis
Campath Ampules ... 811
CellCept Capsules ... 2747
CellCept Intravenous ... 2747
CellCept Oral Suspension ... 2747
CellCept Tablets ... 2747
Enbrel for Injection ... 584
Fuzeon Injection ... 2767
Humira Injection ... 466
Myfortic Tablets ... 2255
Remicade for IV Injection ... 971

Tubulopathy
Atripla Tablets ... 945
Truvada Tablets ... 1296

Tumor, central nervous system
Nutropin for Injection ... 1239
Nutropin AQ Injection ... 1243
Nutropin AQ Pen ... 1243
Nutropin AQ Pen Cartridge ... 1243

Tumor flare
▲ Arimidex Tablets (3%) ... 673
Gengraf Capsules (1% to less than 3%) ... 459
Invirase (Less than 2%) ... 2772
Neoral Oral Solution (1% to less than 3%) ... 2259
Neoral Soft Gelatin Capsules (1% to less than 3%) ... 2259

Tumor lysis syndrome
Aloprim for Injection (Less than 1%) ... 2167
Campath Ampules ... 811
Leustatin Injection (Rare) ... 2357
Mylotarg for Injection ... 3431
Rituxan I.V. ... 1254
Thalomid Capsules ... 965
Velcade for Injection ... 2133

Tumors, solid, non-cutaneous
Raptiva for Injection ... 1250

Tumors, solid, non-malignant
Nutropin for Injection (0.1%) ... 1239
Nutropin AQ Injection (0.1%) ... 1243
Nutropin AQ Pen (0.1%) ... 1243
Nutropin AQ Pen Cartridge (0.1%) ... 1243
Raptiva for Injection ... 1250

T-wave, inverted
Ultane Liquid for Inhalation (Less than 1%) ... 531

T-wave flattening
(*see under* EKG changes, T-wave)

Twitching
Abilify Oral Solution (Infrequent) ... 882
Abilify Oral Solution (Infrequent) ... 2450
Abilify Discmelt Orally Disintegrating Tablets (Infrequent) ... 882
Abilify Discmelt Orally Disintegrating Tablets (Infrequent) ... 2450
Abilify Tablets (Infrequent) ... 882
Abilify Tablets (Infrequent) ... 2450
Aciphex Tablets (Rare) ... 1090
▲ Adderall XR Capsules (2% to 4%) ... 3166
Aloprim for Injection (Less than 1%) ... 2167
Anzemet Injection (Rare) ... 2859
Anzemet Tablets (Rare) ... 2862
Caduet Tablets (Less than or equal to 0.1%) ... 2508
Campral Tablets (Rare) ... 1174
Cesamet Capsules ... 3340
Cipro ... 2977
Cipro I.V. ... 2984
Cipro XR Tablets ... 2990
Clozaril Tablets (Less than 1%) ... 2184
Concerta Extended-Release Tablets (1%) ... 1881
▲ Depacon Injection (1% to 5%) ... 412
▲ Depakene (1% to 5%) ... 417
▲ Depakote Tablets (1% to 5%) ... 427
Depakote ER Tablets (Greater than 1%) ... 434
Desoxyn Tablets, USP ... 2462
Effexor Tablets (1%) ... 3411
Effexor XR Capsules (2%) ... 3417
FazaClo Orally Disintegrating Tablets (Less than 1%) ... 551
Focalin XR Capsules ... 2223
Gabitril Tablets (1% or more) ... 984
▲ Geodon Capsules (14%) ... 2529
Imitrex Tablets (Rare) ... 1471
Klonopin (Infrequent) ... 2778
Lamictal (Infrequent) ... 1481
Lexapro Oral Solution (Infrequent) ... 1190
Lexapro Tablets (Infrequent) ... 1190
Lidoderm Patch ... 1118
Lunesta Tablets (Infrequent) ... 3142
▲ Lyrica Capsules (4% to 5%) ... 2539
Meridia Capsules ... 489
Mirapex Tablets (Greater than or equal to 1% to 2%) ... 859
Neurontin Capsules (1.3%) ... 2487
Neurontin Oral Solution (1.3%) ... 2487
Neurontin Tablets (1.3%) ... 2487
Nipent for Injection (Less than 3%) ... 1863
Norvasc Tablets (Less than 0.1%) ... 2545
Norvir (Less than 2%) ... 503
▲ OxyContin Tablets (Between 1% and 5%) ... 2703
Permax Tablets (1.1%) ... 3356
Phenytek Capsules ... 2160
Proquin XR Tablets ... 1153
ProSom Tablets (Infrequent) ... 517
Relpax Tablets (Rare) ... 2548
Retrovir Capsules ... 1560
Retrovir IV Infusion ... 1564
Retrovir ... 1560
Reyataz Capsules (Less than 3%) ... 921
Seroquel Tablets (Infrequent) ... 690
▲ Symbyax Capsules (2% to 6%) ... 1819
Synera Topical Patch ... 1137
Tambocor Tablets (Less than 1%) ... 1856
Tasmar Tablets (Infrequent) ... 3358
Wellbutrin SR Sustained-Release Tablets (1% to 2%) ... 1607
Wellbutrin XL Extended-Release Tablets (1% to 2%) ... 1613
Zoloft (Infrequent) ... 2586
Zomig Tablets (Rare) ... 3519
Zomig Nasal Spray (Rare) ... 3523
Zomig-ZMT Tablets (Rare) ... 3519
Zonegran Capsules (Infrequent) ... 1101
Zyban Sustained-Release Tablets (Infrequent) ... 1644
▲ Zyprexa Tablets (1% to 5%) ... 1830
▲ Zyprexa IntraMuscular (2% to 4%) ... 1830
▲ Zyprexa ZYDIS Orally Disintegrating Tablets (1% to 5%) ... 1830
Zyrtec Chewable Tablets (Less than 2%) ... 2594
Zyrtec (Less than 2%) ... 2594
Zyrtec-D 12 Hour Extended Release Tablets (Less than 2%) ... 2597

Twitching, lid muscle
Neurontin Capsules (Infrequent) ... 2487
Neurontin Oral Solution (Infrequent) ... 2487
Neurontin Tablets (Infrequent) ... 2487

Tympanic membrane perforation
▲ Imdur Tablets (Less than or equal to 5%) ... 3018
Tamiflu Oral Suspension (1%) ... 2807

Tympanometry, abnormal
▲ Increlex Injection (Greater than or equal to 5%) ... 3291

U

Ulceration
▲ Aldara Cream, 5% (Up to 8%) ... 1846
▲ Efudex (Among most frequent) ... 3363
Eulexin Capsules ... 3009
K-Tab Tablets ... 475
▲ Levulan Kerastick for Topical Solution, 20% (2% to 4%) ... 1085
St. Joseph 81 mg Aspirin ... ▣ 688

Ulceration, bucial mucosa
Invirase (Greater than or equal to 2%) ... 2772
Nalfon Capsules (Less than 1%) ... 2502

Ulceration, lip
▲ Dacogen (5%) ... 2129

Ulceration, tongue
Evoxac Capsules (Less than 1%) ... 1047
▲ Invirase (Up to 3.8%) ... 2772
Rescriptor Tablets ... 2551
Soriatane Capsules (Less than 1%) ... 1013
Zoloft (Rare) ... 2586

Ulcers
Paxil CR Controlled-Release Tablets (Rare) ... 1538
Paxil (Rare) ... 1530
▲ Vesanoid Capsules (3%) ... 2820
Zomig Tablets (Rare) ... 3519
Zomig-ZMT Tablets (Rare) ... 3519

Ulcers, aphthous
Captopril Tablets (About 0.5% to 2%) ... 2149
Cesamet Capsules ... 3340

Ulcers, corneal
Copaxone for Injection (Infrequent) ... 3297
FML Ophthalmic Ointment (Occasional) ... ⊙ 228
FML Ophthalmic Suspension (Occasional) ... ⊙ 227
FML Forte Ophthalmic Suspension (Occasional) ... ⊙ 226
FML-S Ophthalmic Suspension ... ⊙ 229
Lyrica Capsules (Rare) ... 2539
Poly-Pred Ophthalmic Suspension ... ⊙ 233

Ulcers, cutaneous
Actiq (1% or greater) ... 979
AmBisome for Injection (Less common) ... 620
Aricept Tablets (Infrequent) ... 1094
Aricept ODT Tablets (Infrequent) ... 1094
Arthrotec Tablets (Rare) ... 3129
▲ CellCept Capsules (3% to less than 20%) ... 2747
▲ CellCept Intravenous (3% to less than 20%) ... 2747
▲ CellCept Oral Suspension (3% to less than 20%) ... 2747
▲ CellCept Tablets (3% to less than 20%) ... 2747
Colazal Capsules ... 2838
Doxil Injection (Less than 1%) ... 2351
Enbrel for Injection ... 584
Evoxac Capsules (Less than 1%) ... 1047
Exelon Capsules (Infrequent) ... 2206
Exelon Oral Solution (Infrequent) ... 2206
Gabitril Tablets (Infrequent) ... 984
Gengraf Capsules ... 459
Herceptin I.V. (At least one of the 958 patients) ... 1233
Invirase (Less than 2%) ... 2772
Kaletra (Less than 2%) ... 476
Levaquin (0.1% to 0.9%) ... 2384
Levaquin in 5% Dextrose Injection (0.1% to 0.9%) ... 2384
Lipitor Tablets (Less than 2%) ... 2483
Lithobid Tablets ... 1692
Lofibra Tablets ... 1219
Lofibra Capsules ... 1216
Miacalcin Nasal Spray (Less than 1%) ... 2253
Neoral Oral Solution ... 2259
Neoral Soft Gelatin Capsules ... 2259
Neurontin Capsules (Infrequent) ... 2487
Neurontin Oral Solution (Infrequent) ... 2487
Neurontin Tablets (Infrequent) ... 2487
Paxil CR Controlled-Release Tablets (Rare) ... 1538
Paxil (Rare) ... 1530
Permax Tablets (Infrequent) ... 3356
Plavix Tablets (1% to 2.5%) ... 917
Plavix Tablets (1% to 2.5%) ... 2926
▲ Prograf Capsules and Injection (3% to 15%) ... 632
Protonix I.V. (Less than 1%) ... 3472
Protonix Tablets (Less than 1%) ... 3469
Prozac Pulvules and Liquid (Infrequent) ... 1801
▲ Rapamune Oral Solution and Tablets (3% to 20%) ... 3475
Remicade for IV Injection (Greater than or equal to 0.2%) ... 971
Requip Tablets (Infrequent) ... 1555
Rilutek Tablets (Infrequent) ... 2930
Risperdal (Rare) ... 1676
Risperdal M-Tab Orally Disintegrating Tablets (Rare) ... 1676
▲ Simulect for Injection (3% to 10%) ... 2284
▲ Soriatane Capsules (1% to 10%) ... 1013
Sular Tablets (Less than or equal to 1%) ... 3122
Tricor Tablets ... 527
Viagra Tablets (Less than 2%) ... 2573
▲ Xeloda Tablets (Less than 5%) ... 2822
Zyprexa Tablets (Infrequent) ... 1830
Zyprexa ZYDIS Orally Disintegrating Tablets (Infrequent) ... 1830

Ulcers, duodenal
Abilify Oral Solution (Rare) ... 882
Abilify Oral Solution (Rare) ... 2450
Abilify Discmelt Orally Disintegrating Tablets (Rare) ... 882
Abilify Discmelt Orally Disintegrating Tablets (Rare) ... 2450
Abilify Tablets (Rare) ... 882
Abilify Tablets (Rare) ... 2450
Agrylin Capsules ... 3169
▲ Anaprox Tablets (1% to 10%) ... 2761
▲ Anaprox DS Tablets (1% to 10%) ... 2761
Aricept Tablets (Infrequent) ... 1094
Aricept ODT Tablets (Infrequent) ... 1094
Caduet Tablets (Less than 2%) ... 2508
Campath Ampules ... 811
Campral Tablets (Rare) ... 1174
Celexa (Rare) ... 1176
Copaxone for Injection (Infrequent) ... 3297
▲ EC-Naprosyn Delayed-Release Tablets (1% to 10%) ... 2761
Exelon Capsules (Infrequent) ... 2206
Exelon Oral Solution (Infrequent) ... 2206
Fosamax ... 1969
Fosamax Plus D Tablets ... 1977
Indocin Capsules (Less than 1%) ... 1995
Indocin I.V. (Less than 1%) ... 2465
Indocin (Less than 1%) ... 1995
Lipitor Tablets (Less than 2%) ... 2483
Lofibra Tablets ... 1219
Lofibra Capsules ... 1216
Meridia Capsules ... 489
Mobic Oral Suspension (Less than 2%) ... 863
Mobic Tablets (Less than 2%) ... 863
Myfortic Tablets ... 2255
▲ Naprosyn Suspension (1% to 10%) ... 2761
▲ Naprosyn Tablets (1% to 10%) ... 2761
Neurontin Capsules (Rare) ... 2487
Neurontin Oral Solution (Rare) ... 2487
Neurontin Tablets (Rare) ... 2487
Parcopa Orally Disintegrating Tablets ... 3097
Pentasa Capsules (Less than 1%) ... 3185
Pletal Tablets (Less than 2%) ... 2455
Proleukin for Injection (Less than 1%) ... 2266
Prozac Pulvules and Liquid (Rare) ... 1801
Sonata Capsules (Rare) ... 1717
Stalevo Tablets ... 2287
Tasmar Tablets (Rare) ... 3358
Taxotere Injection Concentrate ... 2932
Tricor Tablets ... 527
Triglide Tablets ... 3123
Trileptal Tablets ... 2300
Trileptal Oral Suspension ... 2300
VFEND I.V. (Less than 2%) ... 2564
VFEND Oral Suspension (Less than 2%) ... 2564
VFEND Tablets (Less than 2%) ... 2564
▲ Voltaren Tablets (1% to 10%) ... 2307
▲ Voltaren-XR Tablets (1% to 10%) ... 2310
Zonegran Capsules (Infrequent) ... 1101
Zosyn (1.3%) ... 3492

Ulcers, duodenal, hemorrhagic
Mobic Oral Suspension (Less than 2%) ... 863
Mobic Tablets (Less than 2%) ... 863
Percodan Tablets ... 1132

Ulcers, esophageal
Accutane Capsules ... 2731
Actonel Tablets ... 2683
Copaxone for Injection (Infrequent) ... 3297
Doxil Injection (Less than 1%) ... 2351
Effexor Tablets (Rare) ... 3411
Fosamax (0.1% to 1.5%) ... 1969
Herceptin I.V. (At least one of the 958 patients) ... 1233
Lyrica Capsules (Rare) ... 2539
Namenda (Infrequent) ... 1195
Nexium Delayed-Release Capsules (Less than 1%) ... 655
Nexium I.V. (Less than 1%) ... 659
Pentasa Capsules (Less than 1%) ... 3185
Permax Tablets (Rare) ... 3356
Prevacid NapraPAC (Less than 1%) ... 3280
Prozac Pulvules and Liquid (Rare) ... 1801
Reyataz Capsules (Less than 3%) ... 921
VFEND I.V. (Less than 2%) ... 2564
VFEND Oral Suspension (Less than 2%) ... 2564
VFEND Tablets (Less than 2%) ... 2564
Zyprexa Tablets (Rare) ... 1830
Zyprexa ZYDIS Orally Disintegrating Tablets (Rare) ... 1830

Ulcers, gastric
Actonel Tablets ... 2683
Actonel with Calcium Tablets ... 2688
Agrylin Capsules ... 3169
Amerge Tablets (Rare) ... 1339
▲ Anaprox Tablets (1% to 10%) ... 2761
▲ Anaprox DS Tablets (1% to 10%) ... 2761
Campral Tablets (Rare) ... 1174

Celexa (Rare) ... 1176
Chantix Tablets (Rare) ... 2517
Cymbalta Delayed-Release Capsules (Infrequent) ... 1757
▲ EC-Naprosyn Delayed-Release Tablets (1% to 10%) ... 2761
Evoxac Capsules (Less than 1%) ... 1047
Exelon Capsules (Infrequent) ... 2206
Exelon Oral Solution (Infrequent) ... 2206
FazaClo Orally Disintegrating Tablets (Less than 1%) ... 551
Fosamax (Up to 1.1%) ... 1969
Fosamax Plus D Tablets (0% to 1.1%) ... 1977
Gengraf Capsules (1% to less than 3%) ... 459
Lunesta Tablets (Rare) ... 3142
Meridia Capsules ... 489
Mobic Oral Suspension (Less than 2%) ... 863
Mobic Tablets (Less than 2%) ... 863
Myfortic Tablets ... 2255
▲ Naprosyn Suspension (1% to 10%) ... 2761
▲ Naprosyn Tablets (1% to 10%) ... 2761
Neoral Oral Solution (1% to less than 3%) ... 2259
Neoral Soft Gelatin Capsules (1% to less than 3%) ... 2259
Nexium Delayed-Release Capsules (Less than 1%) ... 655
Nexium I.V. (Less than 1%) ... 659
Plavix Tablets (Less than 1%) ... 917
Plavix Tablets (Less than 1%) ... 2926
Pletal Tablets (Less than 2%) ... 2455
Prograf Capsules and Injection ... 632
Prozac Pulvules and Liquid (Infrequent) ... 1801
Requip Tablets (Infrequent) ... 1555
Risperdal Consta Long-Acting Injection (Infrequent) ... 1682
Sandostatin Injection (Less than 1%) ... 2278
Sandostatin LAR Depot (Rare) ... 2280
Thalomid Capsules ... 965
Trileptal Tablets ... 2300
Trileptal Oral Suspension ... 2300
▲ Voltaren Tablets (1% to 10%) ... 2307
▲ Voltaren-XR Tablets (1% to 10%) ... 2310
Wellbutrin SR Sustained-Release Tablets ... 1607
Wellbutrin XL Extended-Release Tablets ... 1613
Zonegran Capsules (Infrequent) ... 1101

Ulcers, gastrointestinal

Aggrenox Capsules (Less than 1%) ... 822
▲ Anaprox Tablets (1% to 10%) ... 2761
▲ Anaprox DS Tablets (1% to 10%) ... 2761
▲ Arthrotec Tablets (3% to 6%) ... 3129
Bayer Aspirin ... 744
Bayer Aspirin Comprehensive Prescribing Information ... ▣796
CellCept Capsules (Infrequent) ... 2747
CellCept Intravenous (Infrequent) ... 2747
CellCept Oral Suspension (Infrequent) ... 2747
CellCept Tablets (Infrequent) ... 2747
Clinoril Tablets ... 1924
Clozaril Tablets (Less than 1%) ... 2184
Cosmegen for Injection ... 2459
Dolobid Tablets ... 1955
▲ EC-Naprosyn Delayed-Release Tablets (1% to 10%) ... 2761
Effexor Tablets (Infrequent) ... 3411
Effexor XR Capsules (Infrequent) ... 3417
Gleevec Tablets (Infrequent) ... 2227
Indocin Capsules (Less than 1%) ... 1995
Indocin I.V. (Less than 1%) ... 2465
Indocin (Less than 1%) ... 1995
▲ Intron A for Injection (Less than 5%) ... 3024
K-Dur Extended-Relase Tablets ... 3033
K-Tab Tablets ... 475
Kionex Powder ... 2477
Lotronex Tablets ... 1512
Mobic Oral Suspension ... 863
Mobic Tablets ... 863
Nalfon Capsules ... 2502
▲ Naprosyn Suspension (1% to 10%) ... 2761
▲ Naprosyn Tablets (1% to 10%) ... 2761
Paxil CR Controlled-Release Tablets (Rare) ... 1538
Paxil (Rare) ... 1530
▲ Photofrin for Injection (Less than 5%) ... 702
Plavix Tablets (Less than 1%) ... 917
Plavix Tablets (Less than 1%) ... 2926
Prevacid NapraPAC (Less than 1%) .. 3280
Rilutek Tablets (Infrequent) ... 2930
Sandostatin Injection (Less than 1%) ... 2278
Sandostatin LAR Depot (Rare) ... 2280
St. Joseph 81 mg Aspirin Chewable and Enteric Coated Tablets ... 1869
▲ Voltaren Tablets (1% to 10%) ... 2307
▲ Voltaren-XR Tablets (1% to 10%) ... 2310
Wellbutrin Tablets (Rare) ... 1603

Ulcers, intestinal

Neurontin Capsules (Rare) ... 2487
Neurontin Oral Solution (Rare) ... 2487
Neurontin Tablets (Rare) ... 2487
VFEND I.V. (Less than 2%) ... 2564
VFFND Oral Suspension (Less than 2%) ... 2564
VFEND Tablets (Less than 2%) ... 2564

Ulcers, leg

Colazal Capsules ... 2838
Enbrel for Injection ... 584
▲ Imdur Tablets (Less than or equal to 5%) ... 3018
Neurontin Capsules (Rare) ... 2487
Neurontin Oral Solution (Rare) ... 2487
Neurontin Tablets (Rare) ... 2487

Ulcers, oral mucosal

Abilify Oral Solution (Infrequent) ... 882
Abilify Oral Solution (Infrequent) ... 2450
Abilify Discmelt Orally Disintegrating Tablets (Infrequent) ... 882
Abilify Discmelt Orally Disintegrating Tablets (Infrequent) ... 2450
Abilify Tablets (Infrequent) ... 882
Abilify Tablets (Infrequent) ... 2450
Aciphex Tablets ... 1090
Actiq (Less than 1%) ... 979
▲ Advair Diskus 100/50 (1% to 3%) ... 1308
▲ Advair Diskus 250/50 (1% to 3%) ... 1308
▲ Advair Diskus 500/50 (1% to 3%) ... 1308
Alkeran for Injection (Infrequent) ... 955
Alkeran Tablets (Infrequent) ... 956
Asacol Delayed-Release Tablets ... 2692
Caduet Tablets (Less than 2%) ... 2508
Campral Tablets (Rare) ... 1174
Carbatrol Capsules ... 3171
Ceftin Tablets (0.1% to 1%) ... 1407
▲ CellCept Capsules (3% to less than 20%) ... 2747
▲ CellCept Intravenous (3% to less than 20%) ... 2747
▲ CellCept Oral Suspension (3% to less than 20%) ... 2747
▲ CellCept Tablets (3% to less than 20%) ... 2747
Cipro I.V. (1% or less) ... 2984
Cipro XR Tablets ... 2990
Clozaril Tablets ... 2184
Combivent Inhalation Aerosol ... 847
Copaxone for Injection (Infrequent) .. 3297
Cuprimine Capsules (Some patients) ... 1947
Depakote ER Tablets (Greater than 1%) ... 434
▲ Doxil Injection (1% to 5%) ... 2351
Effexor Tablets (Infrequent) ... 3411
Effexor XR Capsules (Infrequent) ... 3417
Elmiron Capsules (Less than or equal to 1%) ... 2415
▲ Enbrel for Injection (2% to 6%) ... 584
▲ Flovent Diskus (1% to 3%) ... 1443
Gabitril Tablets (1%) ... 984
Gleevec Tablets (Less common) ... 2227
▲ Intron A for Injection (Less than 5%) ... 3024
Invanz for Injection (Greater than 0.1%) ... 1999
Iressa Tablets (1%) ... 684
Kaletra (Less than 2%) ... 476
Lamictal (Infrequent) ... 1481
Leukeran Tablets (Infrequent) ... 1504
Lipitor Tablets (Less than 2%) ... 2483
Lunesta Tablets (Infrequent) ... 3142
▲ Malarone Pediatric Tablets (2% to 6%) ... 1517
▲ Malarone Tablets (2% to 6%) ... 1517
Meridia Capsules ... 489
Miradon Tablets ... 3042
Neurontin Capsules (Rare) ... 2487
Neurontin Oral Solution (Rare) ... 2487
Neurontin Tablets (Rare) ... 2487
Noroxin Tablets (Less frequent) ... 2032
Norvir (Less than 2%) ... 503
▲ Ontak Vials (Less than 5%) ... 1745
Paxil CR Controlled-Release Tablets (Infrequent) ... 1538
Paxil (Infrequent) ... 1530
Pentasa Capsules (Less than 1%) ... 3185
Prevacid Delayed-Release Capsules (Less than 1%) ... 3271
Prevacid for Delayed-Release Oral Suspension (Less than 1%) ... 3271
Prevacid SoluTab Delayed-Release Orally Disintegrating Tablets (Less than 1%) ... 3271
Prevacid NapraPAC (Less than 1%) .. 3280
PREVPAC (Less than 1%) ... 3284
ProAmatine Tablets (Rare) ... 3186
Proquin XR Tablets ... 1153
ProSom Tablets (Rare) ... 517
Protonix I.V. (Less than 1%) ... 3472
Protonix Tablets (Less than 1%) ... 3469
Provigil Tablets (1%) ... 988
Prozac Pulvules and Liquid (Infrequent) ... 1801
▲ Rapamune Oral Solution and Tablets (3% to 20%) ... 3475
Rescriptor Tablets ... 2551
Retrovir Capsules ... 1560
Retrovir IV Infusion ... 1564
Retrovir ... 1560
Reyataz Capsules (Less than 3%) ... 921
Rythmol SR Capsules ... 2727
Seroquel Tablets (Infrequent) ... 690
Sonata Capsules (Infrequent) ... 1717
Sular Tablets (Less than or equal to 1%) ... 3122
Tasmar Tablets (Infrequent) ... 3358
Tegretol/Tegretol-XR ... 2295
▲ Tequin Injection (0.1% to 3%) ... 938
▲ Tequin Injection in 5% Dextrose (0.1% to 3%) ... 938
▲ Tequin Tablets (0.1% to 3%) ... 938
▲ Thiola Tablets (16.7%) ... 2141
Trizivir Tablets ... 1589
Vantin Tablets and Oral Suspension (Less than 1%) ... 2645
VFEND I.V. (Less than 2%) ... 2564
VFEND Oral Suspension (Less than 2%) ... 2564
VFEND Tablets (Less than 2%) ... 2564
Vicoprofen Tablets (Less than 3%) ... 539
Viracept (Less than 2%) ... 2577
Wellbutrin SR Sustained-Release Tablets (Infrequent) ... 1607
Wellbutrin XL Extended-Release Tablets (Infrequent) ... 1613
Ziagen ... 1626
Zonegran Capsules (Rare) ... 1101
Zyban Sustained-Release Tablets (2%) ... 1644
Zyprexa Tablets (Infrequent) ... 1830
Zyprexa ZYDIS Orally Disintegrating Tablets (Infrequent) ... 1830

Ulcers, oropharyngeal

Fosamax ... 1969
Fosamax Plus D Tablets (Rarely) ... 1977

Ulcers, peptic

Abilify Oral Solution (Rare) ... 882
Abilify Oral Solution (Rare) ... 2450
Abilify Discmelt Orally Disintegrating Tablets (Rare) ... 882
Abilify Discmelt Orally Disintegrating Tablets (Rare) ... 2450
Abilify Tablets (Rare) ... 882
Abilify Tablets (Rare) ... 2450
Advicor Tablets ... 1722
Aricept Tablets (Infrequent) ... 1094
Aricept ODT Tablets (Infrequent) ... 1094
Arthrotec Tablets (Rare) ... 3129
Caduet Tablets (Less than 2%) ... 2508
Campath Ampules ... 811
Captopril Tablets (About 0.5% to 2%) ... 2149
▲ CellCept Capsules (3% to less than 20%) ... 2747
▲ CellCept Intravenous (3% to less than 20%) ... 2747
▲ CellCept Oral Suspension (3% to less than 20%) ... 2747
▲ CellCept Tablets (3% to less than 20%) ... 2747
Clinoril Tablets (Less than 1 in 100) ... 1924
Copegus Tablets (Less than 1%) ... 2754
Cuprimine Capsules (Less than 1%) ... 1947
Depo-Medrol Single-Dose Vial ... 2619
Dolobid Tablets (Less than 1 in 100) ... 1955
Effexor Tablets (Infrequent) ... 3411
Effexor XR Capsules ... 3417
▲ Euflexxa (3%) ... 1162
Evoxac Capsules (Less than 1%) ... 1047
Frova Tablets (Rare) ... 1113
Gengraf Capsules (1% to less than 3%) ... 459
Hydrocortone Tablets ... 1989
▲ Imdur Tablets (Less than or equal to 5%) ... 3018
Imitrex Injection (Rare) ... 1463
Imitrex Nasal Spray ... 1467
Imitrex Tablets (Rare) ... 1471
Indocin Capsules (Less than 1%) ... 1995
Indocin I.V. (Less than 1%) ... 2465
Indocin (Less than 1%) ... 1995
Lamictal (Rare) ... 1481
Lipitor Tablets (Less than 2%) ... 2483
Lofibra Tablets ... 1219
Lofibra Capsules ... 1216
▲ Lupron Depot 7.5 mg (Less than 5%) ... 3264
Midamor Tablets (Rare) ... 2026
Moduretic Tablets ... 2028
Nalfon Capsules (Less than 1%) ... 2502
Neoral Oral Solution (1% to less than 3%) ... 2259
Neoral Soft Gelatin Capsules (1% to less than 3%) ... 2259
Neurontin Capsules (Rare) ... 2487
Neurontin Oral Solution (Rare) ... 2487
Neurontin Tablets (Rare) ... 2487
Niaspan Extended-Release Tablets ... 1730
Omnicef Capsules ... 511
Omnicef for Oral Suspension ... 511
Paxil CR Controlled-Release Tablets (Rare) ... 1538
Paxil (Rare) ... 1530
Pegasys (Less than 1%) ... 2789
Percodan Tablets ... 1132
Permax Tablets (Rare to infrequent) ... 3356
Pletal Tablets (Less than 2%) ... 2455
Prograf Capsules and Injection ... 632
Protonix I.V. (Less than 1%) ... 3472
Protonix Tablets (Less than 1%) ... 3469
Prozac Pulvules and Liquid (Rare) ... 1801
Requip Tablets (Infrequent) ... 1555
Reyataz Capsules (Less than 3%) ... 921
Rythmol SR Capsules ... 2727
Sandimmune (2% or less) ... 2275
Sandostatin Injection (Less than 1%) ... 2278
Sandostatin LAR Depot (Rare) ... 2280
Sonata Capsules (Rare) ... 1717
Symbyax Capsules (Infrequent) ... 1819
Ticlid Tablets (Rare) ... 2810
Tricor Tablets ... 527
Triglide Tablets ... 3123
Urso 250 Tablets (1%) ... 710
Urso Forte Tablets (1%) ... 710
VFEND I.V. (Less than 2%) ... 2564
VFEND Oral Suspension (Less than 2%) ... 2564
VFEND Tablets (Less than 2%) ... 2564
Zelapar Tablets ... 3372
Zosyn (1.0% or less) ... 3492
Zyban Sustained-Release Tablets ... 1644

Ulcers, peptic, aggravation of

Eldepryl Capsules ... 3208
Niaspan Extended-Release Tablets ... 1730

Ulcers, peptic, hemorrhagic

▲ Imdur Tablets (Less than or equal to 5%) ... 3018
Mobic Oral Suspension (Less than 2%) ... 863
Mobic Tablets (Less than 2%) ... 863
Prozac Pulvules and Liquid (Rare) ... 1801
Tarceva Tablets ... 1259
Tarceva Tablets ... 2444
Zoloft (Rare) ... 2586

Ulcers, peptic, reactivation of

Didronel Tablets (A few patients) ... 2697

Ulcers, peptic with or without perforation

Asacol Delayed-Release Tablets (Rare) ... 2692
Didronel Tablets (One report) ... 2697

Ulcers, peptic with perforation and hemorrhage

▲ Anaprox Tablets (Approximately 1% to 4%) ... 2761
▲ Anaprox DS Tablets (Approximately 1% to 4%) ... 2761
Colocort Rectal Suspension, USP (Retention) 100 mg/60 mL ... 2476
Decadron Tablets ... 1951
Depo-Medrol Injectable Suspension ... 2617
▲ EC-Naprosyn Delayed-Release Tablets (Approximately 1% to 4%) ... 2761
Hydrocortone Tablets ... 1989
Mobic Oral Suspension (Less than 2%) ... 863
Mobic Tablets (Less than 2%) ... 863
▲ Naprosyn Suspension (Approximately 1% to 4%) ... 2761
▲ Naprosyn Tablets (Approximately 1% to 4%) ... 2761

Ulcers, skin

Abilify Oral Solution (Frequent) ... 882

Abilify Oral Solution (Frequent) 2450
Abilify Discmelt Orally Disintegrating Tablets (Frequent)... 882
Abilify Discmelt Orally Disintegrating Tablets (Frequent)... 2450
Abilify Tablets (Frequent) 882
Abilify Tablets (Frequent) 2450
▲ Avastin IV (6%) 1227
Bicillin C-R Injectable Suspension 1706
Caduet Tablets (Less than 2%) 2508
Cymbalta Delayed-Release Capsules (Frequent) 1757
Fortical Nasal Spray (Less than 1%) 3337
Levaquin (0.1% to 0.9%) 2384
Levaquin in 5% Dextrose Injection (0.1% to 0.9%) 2384
Lyrica Capsules (0.1% to 1%) 2539
Merrem I.V. (Greater than 0.1% to 1%) 686
Namenda (Infrequent) 1195
Protopic Ointment (0.2% to less than 1%) 638
Symbyax Capsules (Rare) 1819
Zelapar Tablets 3372

Unconsciousness
(*see under* Consciousness, loss of)

Underventilation
(*see under* Hypoventilation)

Unresponsiveness, unspecified
Proquin XR Tablets 1153

Unsteadiness
▲ Carbatrol Capsules (Among most frequent) 3171
Equetro Extended-Release Capsules 3180
Kadian Capsules 577
Matulane Capsules 3191
Tambocor Tablets 1856
▲ Tegretol/Tegretol-XR (Among most frequent) 2295

Upper respiratory symptoms
▲ Bactroban Nasal (5%) 1394
▲ Brimonidine Tartrate Ophthalmic Solution 0.2% (3% to 9%) .... ⊙248
▲ Chantix Tablets (5% to 7%) 2517
Engerix-B Vaccine (Less than 1%) 1425
▲ Neoral Oral Solution (13%) 2259
▲ Neoral Soft Gelatin Capsules (13%) 2259
Tarka Tablets (2.4%) 524
Varivax (Greater than or equal to 1%) 2100
▲ Vesanoid Capsules (63%) 2820
▲ Wellbutrin Tablets (5.0%) 1603

Uremia
(*see under* Azotemia)

Ureteral spasm
Dilaudid 440
Dilaudid Non-Sterile Powder 440
Dilaudid Rectal Suppositories 440
Dilaudid Tablets 440
Hycodan 1116
Hycotuss Expectorant Syrup 1117
Tussionex Pennkinetic Extended-Release Suspension 3327
Vicodin Tablets 535
Vicodin ES Tablets 536
Vicodin HP Tablets 538
Zydone Tablets 1139

Urethral disorder
Chantix Tablets (Infrequent) 2517
Estring Vaginal Ring 2635
Evoxac Capsules (Less than 1%) 1047

Urethritis
Copaxone for Injection (Infrequent)... 3297
Gabitril Tablets (Infrequent) 984
Imitrex Injection 1463
Imitrex Nasal Spray 1467
Lunesta Tablets (Rare) 3142
Norvir (Less than 2%) 503
Paxil CR Controlled-Release Tablets (Rare to infrequent) 1538
Paxil (Rare to infrequent) 1530
Protonix I.V. (Less than 1%) 3472
Protonix Tablets (Less than 1%) 3469
Sonata Capsules (Rare) 1717

Uric acid, reduction of
Timentin ADD-Vantage 1580
Timentin IV Infusion 1577

Uric acid level, changes in
Elitek 2890

▲ Sutent Capsules (8% to 15%) 2560

Uric acid level, increase
(*see under* Hyperuricemia)

Uric acid stones
Revlimid Capsules 958

Uricaciduria
Permax Tablets (Rare) 3356

Urinary bladder, inflammation of
Amerge Tablets (Infrequent) 1339

Urinary bladder malignancies
Permax Tablets (Rare) 3356

Urinary calculi
Adalat CC Tablets (Less than 1%) 2964

Urinary casts
Garamycin Injectable 3014
Primaxin I.M. 2045
Primaxin I.V. 2048
Rocephin Injectable Vials, ADD-Vantage, Galaxy, Bulk (Less than 1%) 2800
Rythmol SR Capsules 2727
Uniretic Tablets (Less than 1%) 3100

Urinary cytology, abnormal
Orthoclone OKT3 Sterile Solution 2360

Urinary difficulty
(*see under* Micturition, difficulty)

Urinary disorders, unspecified
Enablex Extended-Release Tablets (Greater than or equal to 1%) 2203
Ionsys Transdermal System (.1% to less than 1%) 2379

Urinary disturbances
Avapro Tablets (Less than 1%) 891
Avapro Tablets (Less than 1%) 2871
Eldepryl Capsules 3208
FazaClo Orally Disintegrating Tablets (2%) 551
▲ Lupron Depot 7.5 mg (12.5%) 3264
Lupron Depot–3 Month 11.25 mg 3265
▲ Neoral Oral Solution (24.2%) 2259
▲ Neoral Soft Gelatin Capsules (24.2%) 2259

Urinary findings, abnormal
Capastat Sulfate for Injection 1755
Chantix Tablets (Infrequent) 2517
Clozaril Tablets (2%) 2184
Raniclor Tablets, Chewable 2505

Urinary frequency
(*see under* Polyuria)

Urinary glucose, false-positive
▲ Atripla Tablets (Up to 3%) 945
Augmentin 1360
Augmentin Tablets 1363
Augmentin XR Extended-Release Tablets 1369
Ceftin 1407
Fortaz 1453
Mefoxin for Injection 2012
Mefoxin Premixed Intravenous Solution 2016
Raniclor Tablets, Chewable 2505

Urinary hesitancy
Cymbalta Delayed-Release Capsules (Infrequent) 1757
Dilaudid Oral Liquid 445
Dilaudid Tablets - 8 mg 445
Dilaudid-HP (Less frequent) 442
▲ Ditropan XL Extended-Release Tablets (2% to less than 5%) 2413
Donnatal Extentabs 2493
Eldepryl Capsules 3208
Kadian Capsules (Less than 3%) 577
MS Contin Tablets (Less frequent) 2701
Norflex Injection 1856
Numorphan Injection 1120
▲ Paxil CR Controlled-Release Tablets (3%) 1538
▲ Paxil (3%) 1530
ProSom Tablets (Infrequent) 517
Retrovir Capsules 1560
Retrovir IV Infusion 1564
Retrovir 1560
▲ Strattera Capsules (5% or greater) 1814
Valium Tablets (Infrequent) 2819

Urinary incontinence
Abilify Oral Solution (Frequent) 882
Abilify Oral Solution (Frequent) 2450
Abilify Discmelt Orally Disintegrating Tablets (Frequent)... 882
Abilify Discmelt Orally Disintegrating Tablets (Frequent)... 2450
Abilify Tablets (Frequent) 882
Abilify Tablets (Frequent) 2450
Aciphex Tablets (Rare) 1090
Actiq (Less than 1%) 979
Ambien Tablets (Infrequent) 2851
Ambien CR Tablets (Infrequent) 2855
AmBisome for Injection (Less common) 620
Amerge Tablets (Rare) 1339
Aricept Tablets (Frequent) 1094
Aricept ODT Tablets (Frequent) 1094
Caduet Tablets (Less than 2%) 2508
Campral Tablets (Infrequent) 1174
Celebrex Capsules (0.1% to 1.9%) ... 3134
Celexa (Infrequent) 1176
▲ CellCept Capsules (3% to less than 20%) 2747
▲ CellCept Intravenous (3% to less than 20%) 2747
▲ CellCept Oral Suspension (3% to less than 20%) 2747
▲ CellCept Tablets (3% to less than 20%) 2747
Clozaril Tablets (1%) 2184
Copaxone for Injection (At least 2%) 3297
Cymbalta Delayed-Release Capsules (Infrequent) 1757
Dantrium Capsules (Less frequent) .. 2694
▲ Depacon Injection (1% to 5%) 412
▲ Depakene (1% to 5%) 417
▲ Depakote Sprinkle Capsules (1% to 5%) 422
▲ Depakote Tablets (1% to 5%) 427
Depakote ER Tablets (Greater than 1%) 434
DepoCyt Injection (Less than 3%) 1143
▲ Doxil Injection (1% to 10%) 2351
Effexor Tablets (Infrequent) 3411
Effexor XR Capsules (Infrequent) 3417
Eligard 30 mg (1.1%) 2885
▲ Eloxatin for Injection (2% to 5%) 2892
▲ Estring Vaginal Ring (1% to 3%) 2635
Evoxac Capsules (Less than 1%) 1047
Exelon Capsules (2% or more) 2206
Exelon Oral Solution (2% or more) 2206
FazaClo Orally Disintegrating Tablets (1%) 551
Gabitril Tablets (Frequent) 984
Gengraf Capsules (1% to less than 3%) 459
Hytrin Capsules (At least 1%) 471
▲ Intron A for Injection (Less than 5%) 3024
Klonopin (Infrequent) 2778
Lamictal (Infrequent) 1481
Levaquin (0.1% to 0.9%) 2384
Levaquin in 5% Dextrose Injection (0.1% to 0.9%) 2384
Lipitor Tablets (Less than 2%) 2483
Lithobid Tablets 1692
Lunesta Tablets (Infrequent) 3142
Lupron Depot-PED 7.5 mg, 11.25 mg and 15 mg (Less than 2%) 3269
Lupron Injection Pediatric (Less than 2%) 3259
Lyrica Capsules (1% to 2%) 2539
▲ Megace ES Oral Suspension (1% to 3%) 2481
Merrem I.V. (Greater than 0.1% to 1%) 686
Mirapex Tablets (2%) 859
Neoral Oral Solution (1% to less than 3%) 2259
Neoral Soft Gelatin Capsules (1% to less than 3%) 2259
Neurontin Capsules (Infrequent) 2487
Neurontin Oral Solution (Infrequent) 2487
Neurontin Tablets (Infrequent) 2487
Parcopa Orally Disintegrating Tablets 3097
Parnate Tablets 1527
Paxil CR Controlled-Release Tablets (Infrequent) 1538
Paxil (Infrequent) 1530
Permax Tablets (Frequent) 3356
▲ Prograf Capsules and Injection (3% to 15%) 632
ProSom Tablets (Rare) 517
Prozac Pulvules and Liquid (Infrequent) 1801
▲ Rapamune Oral Solution and Tablets (3% to 20%) 3475
Razadyne (Greater than or equal to 2%) 2399
Razadyne ER Extended-Release Capsules (Greater than or equal to 2%) 2399
▲ Rebif Prefilled Syringe for Injection (2% to 4%) 3159
ReoPro Vials (0.1%) 1809
Requip Tablets (2%) 1555
Rilutek Tablets (Infrequent) 2930
Risperdal (Infrequent) 1676
Risperdal Consta Long-Acting Injection (Frequent) 1682
Risperdal M-Tab Orally Disintegrating Tablets (Infrequent) 1676
Rythmol SR Capsules 2727
Seroquel Tablets (Infrequent) 690
Sonata Capsules (Infrequent) 1717
Stalevo Tablets 2287
Stromectol Tablets 2083
Symbyax Capsules (Frequent) 1819
Targretin Capsules 1747
Tasmar Tablets (Frequent) 3358
▲ Temodar Capsules (8%) 3073
Teveten Tablets (Less than 1%) 1735
Teveten HCT Tablets (Less than 1%) 1737
Thioridazine Hydrochloride Tablets .. 2163
▲ Topamax Sprinkle Capsules (1% to 4%) 2404
▲ Topamax Tablets (1% to 4%) 2404
Travatan Ophthalmic Solution (1% to 5%) 563
▲ Trisenox Injection (5%) 993
VFEND I.V. (Less than 2%) 2564
VFEND Oral Suspension (Less than 2%) 2564
VFEND Tablets (Less than 2%) 2564
Viagra Tablets (Less than 2%) 2573
Vicoprofen Tablets (Less than 1%) ... 539
Wellbutrin Tablets (Rare) 1603
Wellbutrin SR Sustained-Release Tablets 1607
Wellbutrin XL Extended-Release Tablets 1613
▲ Xyrem Oral Solution (Infrequent to 7%) 1688
Zelapar Tablets 3372
Zoloft (Infrequent to 2%) 2586
Zomig Nasal Spray (Rare) 3523
Zonegran Capsules (Infrequent) 1101
Zosyn (1.0% or less) 3492
Zyban Sustained-Release Tablets 1644
Zyprexa Tablets (2%) 1830
Zyprexa ZYDIS Orally Disintegrating Tablets (2%) 1830
Zyrtec Chewable Tablets (Less than 2%) 2594
Zyrtec (Less than 2%) 2594
Zyrtec-D 12 Hour Extended Release Tablets (Less than 2%) 2597

Urinary obstruction
Campath Ampules 811

Urinary retention
Abilify Oral Solution (Infrequent) 882
Abilify Oral Solution (Infrequent) 2450
Abilify Discmelt Orally Disintegrating Tablets (Infrequent) 882
Abilify Discmelt Orally Disintegrating Tablets (Infrequent) 2450
Abilify Tablets (Infrequent) 882
Abilify Tablets (Infrequent) 2450
Aceon Tablets (2 mg, 4 mg, 8 mg) (0.3% to 1%) 3194
Actiq (Less than 1%) 979
Aloxi Injection (Less than 1%) 2127
Ambien Tablets (Rare) 2851
Ambien CR Tablets (Rare) 2855
Anzemet Injection (2%) 2859
Arixtra Injection (Up to 2.9%) 1351
Astelin Nasal Spray 1904
Atrovent Inhalation Solution (Less than 3%) 835
Atrovent HFA Inhalation Aerosol 841
Atrovent Nasal Spray 0.03% 837
Atrovent Nasal Spray 0.06% 839
Avinza Capsules (Less than 5%) 1741
Bentyl Capsules 697
Bentyl Injection 697
Bentyl Syrup 697
Bentyl Tablets 697
Buprenex Injectable (Less than 1%) 2716
Caduet Tablets (Less than 2%) 2508
Campath Ampules 811
Carbatrol Capsules 3171
Catapres Tablets (About 1 in 1,000 patients) 843
Celexa (Infrequent) 1176

▲ CellCept Capsules (3% to less than 20%) 2747
▲ CellCept Intravenous (3% to less than 20%) 2747
▲ CellCept Oral Suspension (3% to less than 20%) 2747
▲ CellCept Tablets (3% to less than 20%) 2747
Cesamet Capsules 3340
Chantix Tablets (Rare) 2517
Cipro (Less than 1%) 2977
Cipro I.V. (1% or less) 2984
Cipro XR Tablets 2990
Clorpres Tablets (About 1 in 1,000) 2153
Clozaril Tablets (1%) 2184
Copaxone for Injection (At least 2%) 3297
Cymbalta Delayed-Release Capsules (Infrequent) 1757
Dantrium Capsules (Less frequent) 2694
▲ DepoDur Extended-Release Injection (Greater than 10%) 1110
Detrol Tablets (1.7%) 2628
Detrol LA Capsules 2631
Diastat Rectal Delivery System (Infrequent) 3343
Dilaudid 440
Dilaudid Non-Sterile Powder 440
Dilaudid Oral Liquid 445
Dilaudid Rectal Suppositories 440
Dilaudid Tablets 440
Dilaudid Tablets - 8 mg 445
Dilaudid-HP (Less frequent) 442
▲ Ditropan XL Extended-Release Tablets (2% to less than 5%) 2413
Donnatal Extentabs 2493
▲ Duragesic Transdermal System (3% to 10%) 2373
Effexor Tablets (1%) 3411
Effexor XR Capsules (Frequent) 3417
Eldepryl Capsules (1 of 49 patients) 3208
Eligard 22.5 mg (Less than 2%) 2883
Enablex Extended-Release Tablets (16 patients) 2203
Equetro Extended-Release Capsules 3180
Evoxac Capsules 1047
Exelon Capsules (Infrequent) 2206
Exelon Oral Solution (Infrequent) 2206
FazaClo Orally Disintegrating Tablets (1%) 551
Gabitril Tablets (Infrequent) 984
Gantrisin Pediatric Suspension 2770
Geodon Capsules (Infrequent) 2529
Hycodan 1116
Hycotuss Expectorant Syrup 1117
Invanz for Injection (Greater than 0.1%) 1999
▲ Ionsys Transdermal System (3%) 2379
Kadian Capsules (Less than 3%) 577
Klonopin (Infrequent) 2778
Lamictal (Infrequent) 1481
Levaquin (0.1% to 0.9%) 2384
Levaquin in 5% Dextrose Injection (0.1% to 0.9%) 2384
Lyrica Capsules (0.1% to 1%) 2539
▲ Macugen Injection (1% to 5%) ⊙ 261
Moban Tablets 1119
MS Contin Tablets (Less frequent) 2701
▲ Myfortic Tablets (3% to less than 20%) 2255
Namenda (Infrequent) 1195
Neurontin Capsules (Infrequent) 2487
Neurontin Oral Solution (Infrequent) 2487
Neurontin Tablets (Infrequent) 2487
Niravam Orally Disintegrating Tablets 3092
Norflex Injection 1856
Norvir (Less than 2%) 503
Numorphan Injection 1120
Opana Tablets (Less than 1%) 1122
Opana ER Tablets (Less than 1%) 1126
OxyContin Tablets (Less than 1%) 2703
Parcopa Orally Disintegrating Tablets 3097
Parnate Tablets 1527
Paxil CR Controlled-Release Tablets (Infrequent) 1538
Paxil (Infrequent) 1530
Percodan Tablets 1132
Permax Tablets (Infrequent) 3356
Prevacid Delayed-Release Capsules (Less than 1%) 3271
Prevacid for Delayed-Release Oral Suspension (Less than 1%) 3271
Prevacid SoluTab Delayed-Release Orally Disintegrating Tablets (Less than 1%) 3271
Prevacid NapraPAC 3280
PREVPAC 3284
▲ ProAmatine Tablets (Among most frequent) 3186
Proleukin for Injection (1%) 2266
Proquin XR Tablets 1153
Prosed/DS Tablets 1157
Provigil Tablets (1%) 988
Prozac Pulvules and Liquid (Infrequent) 1801
▲ Rapamune Oral Solution and Tablets (3% to 20%) 3475
Razadyne (Infrequent) 2399
Razadyne ER Extended-Release Capsules (Infrequent) 2399
ReoPro Vials (0.4%) 1809
Revlimid Capsules 958
Rilutek Tablets (Infrequent) 2930
Risperdal (Rare) 1676
Risperdal Consta Long-Acting Injection (Infrequent) 1682
Risperdal M-Tab Orally Disintegrating Tablets (Rare) 1676
Rythmol SR Capsules 2727
Sanctura Tablets (1.2%) 1151
Seroquel Tablets (Infrequent) 690
▲ Simulect for Injection (3% to 10%) 2284
Sonata Capsules (Rare) 1717
Spiriva HandiHaler (Less than 1%) 869
Stalevo Tablets 2287
▲ Strattera Capsules (0.7% or greater) 1814
Symbyax Capsules (Infrequent) 1819
Symmetrel Tablets (0.1% to 1%) 1135
Tambocor Tablets (Less than 1%) 1856
Tasmar Tablets (Infrequent) 3358
Tegretol/Tegretol-XR 2295
Thioridazine Hydrochloride Tablets 2163
Topamax Sprinkle Capsules (Infrequent) 2404
Topamax Tablets (Infrequent) 2404
▲ Trasylol Injection (3%) 754
Trelstar Depot (1.4%) 3394
Trelstar LA Suspension (1.1%) 3397
Tussionex Pennkinetic Extended-Release Suspension 3327
Ultane Liquid for Inhalation (Less than 1%) 531
▲ Ultram ER Tablets (1% to greater than 5%) 2392
Uniretic Tablets (Less than 1%) 3100
Vantas (Less than 2%) 3375
VESIcare Tablets (0% to 1.4%) 646
VFEND I.V. (Less than 2%) 2564
VFEND Oral Suspension (Less than 2%) 2564
VFEND Tablets (Less than 2%) 2564
Viadur Implant (Less than 2%) 757
Vicodin Tablets 535
Vicodin ES Tablets 536
Vicodin HP Tablets 538
Vicoprofen Tablets (Less than 1%) 539
Wellbutrin Tablets (1.9%) 1603
Wellbutrin SR Sustained-Release Tablets 1607
Wellbutrin XL Extended-Release Tablets 1613
▲ Zofran Injection (3%) 1634
▲ Zofran (5%) 1639
▲ Zofran ODT Orally Disintegrating Tablets (5%) 1639
Zoloft (Infrequent) 2586
Zonegran Capsules (Infrequent) 1101
Zosyn (1.0% or less) 3492
Zyban Sustained-Release Tablets 1644
Zydone Tablets 1139
Zyprexa Tablets (Infrequent) 1830
Zyprexa ZYDIS Orally Disintegrating Tablets (Infrequent) 1830
Zyrtec Chewable Tablets (Less than 2%) 2594
Zyrtec (Less than 2%) 2594
Zyrtec-D 12 Hour Extended Release Tablets (Less than 2%) 2597

Urinary sediment, abnormalities
Capastat Sulfate for Injection 1755
Dyazide Capsules 1423

Urinary tract, burning of
Abilify Oral Solution (Infrequent) 882
Abilify Oral Solution (Infrequent) 2450
Abilify Discmelt Orally Disintegrating Tablets (Infrequent) 882
Abilify Discmelt Orally Disintegrating Tablets (Infrequent) 2450
Abilify Tablets (Infrequent) 882
Abilify Tablets (Infrequent) 2450

Urinary tract disorder, unspecified
▲ CellCept Capsules (3% to less than 20%) 2747
▲ CellCept Intravenous (3% to less than 20%) 2747
▲ CellCept Oral Suspension (3% to less than 20%) 2747
▲ CellCept Tablets (3% to less than 20%) 2747
▲ Leukine (14%) 814
Lupron Depot 3.75 mg 3260
Protonix I.V. (Less than 1%) 3472
Protonix Tablets (Less than 1%) 3469
Relpax Tablets (Infrequent) 2548
Tasmar Tablets (Infrequent) 3358
Zomig Nasal Spray (Rare) 3523
Zyban Sustained-Release Tablets 1644

Urinary urgency
Abilify Oral Solution (Infrequent) 882
Abilify Oral Solution (Infrequent) 2450
Abilify Discmelt Orally Disintegrating Tablets (Infrequent) 882
Abilify Discmelt Orally Disintegrating Tablets (Infrequent) 2450
Abilify Tablets (Infrequent) 882
Abilify Tablets (Infrequent) 2450
Actiq (1% or greater) 979
Adenoscan (Less than 1%) 619
Amerge Tablets (Rare) 1339
Aricept Tablets (Infrequent) 1094
Aricept ODT Tablets (Infrequent) 1094
Asacol Delayed-Release Tablets 2692
▲ Avastin IV (3% to 6%) 1227
▲ Betaseron for SC Injection (13%) 767
Caduet Tablets (Less than 2%) 2508
Campral Tablets (Rare) 1174
Caverject Impulse Injection (Less than 1%) 2612
Clozaril Tablets (1%) 2184
▲ Copaxone for Injection (10%) 3297
Effexor Tablets (Infrequent) 3411
Effexor XR Capsules (Infrequent) 3417
Eligard 22.5 mg (2.6%) 2883
Eligard 30 mg (1.1%) 2885
FazaClo Orally Disintegrating Tablets (1%) 551
Gabitril Tablets (Infrequent) 984
Ionsys Transdermal System (.1% to less than 1%) 2379
Keppra Oral Solution (2%) 3314
Keppra Tablets (2%) 3314
Lexapro Oral Solution (Infrequent) 1190
Lexapro Tablets (Infrequent) 1190
Lipitor Tablets (Less than 2%) 2483
Neurontin Capsules (Rare) 2487
Neurontin Oral Solution (Infrequent) 2487
Neurontin Tablets (Rare) 2487
Paxil CR Controlled-Release Tablets (Infrequent) 1538
Paxil (Infrequent) 1530
Prevacid Delayed-Release Capsules (Less than 1%) 3271
Prevacid for Delayed-Release Oral Suspension (Less than 1%) 3271
Prevacid SoluTab Delayed-Release Orally Disintegrating Tablets (Less than 1%) 3271
Prevacid NapraPAC (Less than 1%) 3280
PREVPAC (Less than 1%) 3284
▲ ProAmatine Tablets (Among most frequent) 3186
ProSom Tablets (Infrequent) 517
Prozac Pulvules and Liquid (Infrequent) 1801
Rilutek Tablets (Infrequent) 2930
Sonata Capsules (Infrequent) 1717
Symbyax Capsules (Infrequent) 1819
Targretin Capsules 1747
Viadur Implant (Less than 2%) 757
Wellbutrin SR Sustained-Release Tablets (Up to 2%) 1607
Wellbutrin XL Extended-Release Tablets (2%) 1613
Zelapar Tablets 3372
Zomig Tablets (Infrequent) 3519
Zomig-ZMT Tablets (Infrequent) 3519
Zyban Sustained-Release Tablets (Infrequent) 1644
Zyprexa Tablets (Infrequent) 1830

Urination, difficult
(*see under* Micturition, difficulty)

Urination, excessive
▲ Demadex Injection (6.7%) 2759
▲ Demadex Tablets (6.7%) 2759

Urination, impaired
Actiq (1% or greater) 979
AndroGel (Fewer than 1%) 3329
Cesamet Capsules 3340
Eligard 22.5 mg (Less than 2%) 2883
Ionsys Transdermal System (.1% to less than 1%) 2379
Prevacid Delayed-Release Capsules (Less than 1%) 3271
Prevacid for Delayed-Release Oral Suspension (Less than 1%) 3271
Prevacid SoluTab Delayed-Release Orally Disintegrating Tablets (Less than 1%) 3271
Prevacid NapraPAC (Less than 1%) 3280
PREVPAC (Less than 1%) 3284
Rescriptor Tablets 2551
Symbyax Capsules (Infrequent) 1819
Ultane Liquid for Inhalation (Less than 1%) 531

Urination, painful
(*see under* Micturition, painful)

Urine, abnormal
Aciphex Tablets 1090
Chantix Tablets (Infrequent) 2517
Evoxac Capsules (Less than 1%) 1047
Frova Tablets (Rare) 1113
Gengraf Capsules (1% to less than 3%) 459
Kaletra (Less than 2%) 476
Keppra Oral Solution (2%) 3314
Keppra Tablets (2%) 3314
Lamictal (Rare) 1481
Neoral Oral Solution (1% to less than 3%) 2259
Neoral Soft Gelatin Capsules (1% to less than 3%) 2259
Neurontin Capsules (Rare) 2487
Neurontin Oral Solution (Rare) 2487
Neurontin Tablets (Rare) 2487
Provigil Tablets (1%) 988
Reyataz Capsules (Less than 3%) 921
Rilutek Tablets (Infrequent) 2930
Rythmol SR Capsules 2727
Soriatane Capsules (Less than 1%) 1013
Ultane Liquid for Inhalation (Less than 1%) 531
Viracept (Less than 2%) 2577
▲ Vivaglobin (0.1% to 3%) 3506

Urine, cells in
Accutane Capsules 2731
Garamycin Injectable 3014
Merrem I.V. (Greater than 0.2%) 686
Parcopa Orally Disintegrating Tablets 3097

Urine, color change
Alinia for Oral Suspension (Less than 1%) 2835
Alinia Tablets (Less than 1%) 2835
Clinoril Tablets (Less than 1%) 1924
▲ Comtan Tablets (10%) 2189
Coumadin for Injection 898
Coumadin Tablets 898
Eulexin Capsules 3009
Fluorescite Injection ⊙ 207
Klonopin (Infrequent) 2778
Lamisil Tablets 2232
MetroGel-Vaginal Gel (Less than 1%) 1855
Ortho-Cyclen Tablets 2429
Ortho Evra Transdermal System 2417
Ortho Tri-Cyclen Tablets 2429
Ortho Tri-Cyclen Lo Tablets 2436
Parcopa Orally Disintegrating Tablets 3097
Primaxin I.M. 2045
Primaxin I.V. (Less than 0.2%) 2048
▲ Stalevo Tablets (5% to 10%) 2287
▲ Tasmar Tablets (2% to 7%) 3358
Ticlid Tablets 2810
Tindamax Tablets 2142

Urine, microscopic deposits
Carbatrol Capsules 3171
Equetro Extended-Release Capsules 3180
Tegretol/Tegretol-XR 2295

Urine, output low
(*see under* Hypouresis)

Urine, presence of RBC's
(*see under* Hematuria)

Urine, presence of urobilinogen
Primaxin I.M. 2045
Primaxin I.V. 2048

Urine analysis abnormal
Xyrem Oral Solution (Infrequent) 1688

Urine flow decreased

Cesamet Capsules 3340
Cymbalta Delayed-Release Capsules (infrequent) 1757
Evoxac Capsules (Less than 1%) 1047

Urine flow increased

Cesamet Capsules 3340

Urine odor, abnormal

Proquin XR Tablets (Less than 1%) 1153

Urolithiasis

Abilify Oral Solution (Rare) 882
Abilify Oral Solution (Rare) 2450
Abilify Discmelt Orally Disintegrating Tablets (Rare) 882
Abilify Discmelt Orally Disintegrating Tablets (Rare) 2450
Abilify Tablets (Rare) 882
Abilify Tablets (Rare) 2450
Cosopt Sterile Ophthalmic Solution (Less than 1%) 1931
▲ Crixivan Capsules (Approximately 12.4%) 1940
Effexor Tablets (Rare) 3411
Effexor XR Capsules (Rare) 3417
Kytril Injection (Rare) 2781
Lofibra Tablets 1219
Lofibra Capsules 1216
Paxil CR Controlled-Release Tablets (Rare) 1538
Paxil (Rare) 1530
Permax Tablets (Infrequent) 3356
Tricor Tablets 527
Trusopt Sterile Ophthalmic Solution (Rare) 2095

Urticaria

Abilify Oral Solution (Infrequent) 882
Abilify Oral Solution (Infrequent) 2450
Abilify Discmelt Orally Disintegrating Tablets (Infrequent) 882
Abilify Discmelt Orally Disintegrating Tablets (Infrequent) 2450
Abilify Tablets (Infrequent) 882
Abilify Tablets (Infrequent) 2450
Accolate Tablets 671
AccuNeb Inhalation Solution (0.9% to 1.7%) 1055
Accutane Capsules 2731
▲ Acetadote Injection (.2% to 20.8%) 1031
Aciphex Tablets 1090
Actiq (Less than 1%) 979
Activase I.V. (Very rare) 1223
ADACEL Vaccine (Very rare) 2945
Adalat CC Tablets (Rare) 2964
Adderall Tablets 3164
Adderall XR Capsules 3166
Adipex-P 1215
▲ Advair Diskus 100/50 (1% to 3%) 1308
▲ Advair Diskus 250/50 (1% to 3%) 1308
▲ Advair Diskus 500/50 (1% to 3%) 1308
Advicor Tablets 1722
▲ Aerobid/Aerobid-M (1% to 3%) 1171
Aggrastat 1907
Aggrenox Capsules (Less than 1%) 822
▲ Agrylin Capsules (8.3%) 3169
Albenza Tablets (Rare) 1338
Aldoril Tablets 1910
Aldurazyme for Intravenous Infusion 1268
Alferon N Injection 1665
Alkeran for Injection 955
Allegra (Rare) 2844
Allegra-D 12 Hour Extended-Release Tablets (Rare) 2846
Allegra-D 24 Hour Extended-Release Tablets (Rare) 2849
Aloprim for Injection (Less than 1%) 2167
Alphanate, Antihemophilic Factor (Human) 1654
Altace Capsules (Less than 1%) 1702
Altoprev Extended-Release Tablets (Rare) 3109
Ambien Tablets (Rare) 2851
Ambien CR Tablets (Rare to 1%) 2855
AmBisome for Injection (Less common) 620
Amerge Tablets (Infrequent) 1339
Amevive (Less than 1%) 626
Aminohippurate Sodium PAH Injection 1913
Amitiza Capsules (Less than 0.2%) 3224
Amoxil Capsules 1343
Amoxil Chewable Tablets 1343
Amoxil Pediatric Drops for Oral Suspension 1343
Amoxil Powder for Oral Suspension 1343
Amoxil Tablets 1343
Anaprox Tablets (Less than 1%) 2761
Anaprox DS Tablets (Less than 1%) 2761
Angeliq Tablets 762
Anzemet Injection (Rare) 2859
Anzemet Tablets (Rare) 2862
Appearex Tablets 2125
Aricept Tablets (Frequent) 1094
Aricept ODT Tablets (Frequent) 1094
Arimidex Tablets (Very rare) 673
Arthrotec Tablets (Rare) 3129
Asacol Delayed-Release Tablets 2692
Atacand Tablets 649
Atacand HCT 651
▲ Atripla Tablets (Greater than or equal to 5%) 945
Atrovent Inhalation Solution (Less than 3%) 835
Atrovent HFA Inhalation Aerosol 841
Atrovent Nasal Spray 0.06% (Rare) 839
Attenuvax (Rare) 1914
▲ Augmentin (3%) 1360
▲ Augmentin Tablets (3%) 1363
Augmentin XR Extended-Release Tablets 1369
Augmentin ES-600 Powder for Oral Suspension 1366
Avalide Tablets (Rare) 888
Avalide Tablets (Rare) 2874
Avandaryl Tablets (Less than 1%) 1379
Avapro Tablets (Rare) 891
Avapro Tablets (Less than 1%) 2871
Avelox (0.1% to less than 2%) 2970
▲ Avinza Capsules (Less than 5%) 1741
Avodart Soft Gelatin Capsules 1390
Axid Oral Solution (More frequent) 879
Azmacort Inhalation Aerosol (Rare) 1726
Azopt Ophthalmic Suspension (Less than 1%) 557
Bactroban Cream (One report) 1394
Bayer Aspirin 744
Beconase AQ Nasal Spray (Rare) 1396
▲ BeneFix Vials (3.1% to 4.8%) 3408
Benicar Tablets 1043
Benicar HCT Tablets (Rare) 1044
Bentyl Capsules 697
Bentyl Injection 697
Bentyl Syrup 697
Bentyl Tablets 697
Betagan Ophthalmic Solution, USP (Rare) ⊙ 220
Betaseron for SC Injection 767
Betimol Ophthalmic Solution 3382
Betimol Ophthalmic Solution ⊙ 295
Betoptic S Ophthalmic Suspension (Rare) 558
Biaxin/Biaxin XL 402
Bicillin C-R Injectable Suspension 1706
Biltricide Tablets (Rare) 2976
Boostrix (Rarely) 1404
Bumex Tablets (0.2% to 2.9%) 2746
Buprenex Injectable (Rare) 2716
Byetta Injection 611
Caduet Tablets (Less than 2%) 2508
▲ Campath Ampules (5% to 30%) 811
Campral Tablets (Infrequent) 1174
Capastat Sulfate for Injection 1755
Carafate Suspension 701
Carafate Tablets 701
Carbatrol Capsules 3171
Cardura XL Tablets 2515
Catapres Tablets (About 5 in 1,000 patients) 843
Catapres-TTS (2 cases of 3,539 patients) 844
Ceftin (0.1% to 1%) 1407
Celebrex Capsules (0.1% to 1.9%) 3134
Celexa (Infrequent) 1176
▲ Cerezyme for Injection (Approximately 6.6%) 1270
Chantix Tablets (Infrequent) 2517
Cialis Tablets 1838
Cipro (Less than 1%) 2977
Cipro I.V. (1% or less) 2984
Cipro XR Tablets (Less than 1%) 2990
Clarinex Syrup (Rare) 2995
Clarinex Tablets (Rare) 2995
Clarinex Reditabs Tablets (Rare) 2995
Clarinex-D 24-Hour Extended-Release Tablets 2998
Cleocin Vaginal Ovules 2616
Climara Transdermal System 771
Climara Pro Transdermal System 776
Clobex Shampoo 1206
Clorpres Tablets (About 5 in 1,000) 2153
Clozaril Tablets (Less than 1%) 2184
Colyte with Flavor Packs for Oral Solution (Isolated cases) 3088
Combivent Inhalation Aerosol (Less than 2%; rare) 847
Combivir Tablets 1411
Comvax 1928
Concerta Extended-Release Tablets 1881
▲ Copaxone for Injection (5%) 3297
Cosopt Sterile Ophthalmic Solution 1931
Coumadin for Injection (Infrequent) 898
Coumadin Tablets (Infrequent) 898
Covera-HS Tablets (Less than 2%) 3139
Cozaar Tablets (Less than 1%) 1935
Crestor Tablets (Less than 1%) 678
Crixivan Capsules (Less than 2%) 1940
Cubicin for Injection 1026
Cuprimine Capsules 1947
Cutivate Lotion 0.05% (Rare) 2664
Cutivate Ointment (Less than 1%) 2665
▲ Dacogen Injection (6%) 2129
Dantrium Capsules (Less frequent) 2694
Dantrium Intravenous (Rare) 2695
Daytrana Transdermal Patch 3174
Decadron Tablets 1951
Demser Capsules (Rare) 1953
Denavir Cream 2174
Depo-Medrol Single-Dose Vial 2619
depo-subQ provera 104 Injectable Suspension 2624
Desoxyn Tablets, USP 2462
Dexedrine 1420
DextroStat Tablets 3179
Diastat Rectal Delivery System (Infrequent) 3343
Didronel Tablets 2697
Dilaudid 440
Dilaudid Non-Sterile Powder 440
Dilaudid Oral Liquid 445
Dilaudid Rectal Suppositories 440
Dilaudid Tablets 440
Dilaudid Tablets - 8 mg 445
Dilaudid-HP (Less frequent) 442
Diovan HCT Tablets 2196
Diuril Oral Suspension 1954
Diuril Sodium Intravenous 2467
Dolobid Tablets (Less than 1 in 100) 1955
Donnatal Extentabs 2493
▲ Doxil Injection (1% to 5%) 2351
Duetact Tablets (Less than 1%) 3226
DuoNeb Inhalation Solution (0.3%) 1058
Dyazide Capsules 1423
DynaCirc CR Tablets (0.5% to 1%) 2721
EC-Naprosyn Delayed-Release Tablets (Less than 1%) 2761
E.E.S. 451
Effexor Tablets (Infrequent) 3411
Effexor XR Capsules 3417
Efudex 3363
Elidel Cream 1% (0.3% to 1.1%) 2200
Elitek 2890
Elmiron Capsules (Less than or equal to 1%) 2415
Eloxatin for Injection (Less than 1%) 2892
Elspar for Injection 2463
Elspar for Injection 1960
▲ Emend Capsules (Greater than 0.5%) 1963
▲ Emtriva Capsules (17% to 30%) 1287
▲ Emtriva Oral Solution (17% to 30%) 1287
Enbrel for Injection 584
Engerix-B Vaccine (Less than 1%) 1425
Enjuvia Tablets 1062
Epivir 1427
Epivir-HBV 1432
Epogen for Injection (Rare) 591
Epzicom Tablets 1436
Equetro Extended-Release Capsules 3180
Eraxis for Injection 2521
Erbitux 910
EryPed 447
Ery-Tab Tablets 449
Erythrocin Stearate Filmtab Tablets 453
Erythromycin Base Filmtab Tablets 455
Erythromycin Delayed-Release Capsules, USP 457
Estrasorb Topical Emulsion 1147
Estratest Tablets 3199
Estratest H.S. Tablets 3199
Ethyol for Injection 1898
Evoxac Capsules (Less than 1%) 1047
Exelon Capsules (Infrequent) 2206
Exelon Oral Solution (Infrequent) 2206
Fabrazyme for Intravenous Infusion 1274
Famvir Tablets (Infrequent) 2211
Fansidar Tablets 2765
Faslodex Injection (Less than 1%) 681
FazaClo Orally Disintegrating Tablets (Less than 1%) 551
Feiba VH 718
Fleet Phospho-soda (Rare) 1166
Fleet Phospho-soda ACCU-PREP (Rare) 1168
Fleet Phospho-soda EZ-PREP (Rare) 1169
Flexbumin I.V. (Occasional) 720
Flomax Capsules 850
Flonase Nasal Spray (Less than 1%) 1440
Flovent Diskus 1443
Flovent HFA (Rare) 1447
Floxin Otic Solution (Single report) 1049
Fluarix 1451
Flumist Vaccine 1901
Fluorescite Injection ⊙ 207
Focalin Tablets 2220
Focalin XR Capsules 2223
Follistim AQ Cartridge 2338
Fortaz 1453
Fosamax 1969
Fosamax Plus D Tablets 1977
Furosemide Tablets 2154
Gabitril Tablets (Infrequent) 984
GamaSTAN 3234
Gammagard Liquid 721
Gammagard S/D (Occasional) 724
▲ Gamunex Immune Globulin I.V., 10% (0.5% to 5%) 3235
Gantrisin Pediatric Suspension 2770
Garamycin Injectable 3014
Gengraf Capsules (1% to less than 3%) 459
Geodon Capsules (Infrequent) 2529
Glucagon for Injection Vials and Emergency Kit 1778
Gris-PEG Tablets 2502
HalfLytely and Bisacodyl Tablets Bowel Prep Kit with Flavors Packs 881
Havrix Vaccine (Less than 1%) 1456
Hemofil M (Extremely rare) 728
HibTITER 3426
Human Albumin Grifols 20%, Albumin (Human) 1651
Human Albumin Grifols 25%, Albumin (Human) 1652
▲ Humate-P (6%) 3502
▲ Hycamtin for Injection (Less than 1% to 16%) 1458
Hydrocortone Tablets 1989
HyperHep B S/D 3240
Hyzaar 50-12.5 Tablets 1990
Hyzaar 100-12.5 Tablets 1990
Hyzaar 100-25 Tablets 1990
Imitrex Injection 1463
Imitrex Nasal Spray 1467
Imitrex Tablets 1471
Inderal LA Long-Acting Capsules 3429
Indocin Capsules (Less than 1%) 1995
Indocin I.V. (Less than 1%) 2465
Indocin (Less than 1%) 1995
Infanrix Vaccine 1476
Infed Injection 3390
▲ Intron A for Injection (Rare; Less than 5%) 3024
Invanz for Injection (Greater than 0.1%) 1999
Invirase (Less than 2%) 2772
Keflex Capsules 549
Ketek Tablets (Less than 0.2%) 2903
Kogenate FS (Rare) 738
Kytril Injection (Rare) 2781
Kytril (Rare) 2784
Lamictal (Infrequent) 1481
Lamisil Tablets (1.1%) 2232
Lescol Capsules (Rare) 2233
Lescol XL Tablets 2233
Leukeran Tablets 1504
Leustatin Injection 2357
Levaquin (0.1% to 0.9%) 2384
Levaquin in 5% Dextrose Injection (0.1% to 0.9%) 2384
Levothroid Tablets 1186
Levoxyl Tablets 1712
Limbrel Capsules (0.003%) 2672
Lipitor Tablets (Less than 2%) 2483
Lofibra Tablets 1219
Lofibra Capsules 1216
Lopressor HCT 50/25 Tablets 2241
Lopressor HCT 100/25 Tablets 2241
Lopressor HCT 100/50 Tablets 2241
Lotensin HCT Tablets 2246
Lotrimin 3039
Lotrisone 3040
Lotronex Tablets (Infrequent) 1512
Lovenox Injection 2915
Lunesta Tablets (Infrequent) 3142
Lupron Depot 3.75 mg 3260
Lupron Depot 7.5 mg 3264

Lupron Depot–3 Month 11.25 mg 3265
Lupron Depot-PED 7.5 mg, 11.25 mg and 15 mg 3269
Lupron Injection Pediatric 3259
Lyrica Capsules (0.1% to 1%) 2539
Malarone Pediatric Tablets 1517
Malarone Tablets 1517
Matulane Capsules 3191
Maxalt Tablets (Infrequent) 2008
Maxalt-MLT Orally Disintegrating Tablets (Infrequent) 2008
Maxipime for Injection (Greater than 0.1% to less than 1%) 1105
Mefoxin for Injection 2012
Mefoxin Premixed Intravenous Solution 2016
Menostar Transdermal System 782
Meridia Capsules 489
Merrem I.V. (Greater than 0.1% to 1%) 686
Meruvax II 2019
Metadate CD Capsules 3323
Mevacor Tablets (Rare) 2021
Micardis Tablets 854
Micardis HCT Tablets 856
Migranal Nasal Spray (Rare) 3348
Miradon Tablets 3042
Mivacron Injection (Less than 1%) 493
M-M-R II 2006
Mobic Oral Suspension (Less than 2%) 863
Mobic Tablets (Less than 2%) 863
Moduretic Tablets 2028
Motrin IB Tablets and Caplets 1866
Children's Motrin Oral Suspension ▣ 685
Children's Motrin Non-Staining Dye-Free Oral Suspension ▣ 685
Children's Motrin Oral Suspension 1867
Children's Motrin Non-Staining Dye-Free Oral Suspension 1867
Children's Motrin Cold Oral Suspension 1867
Infants' Motrin Concentrated Drops 1867
Infants' Motrin Non-Staining Dye-Free Concentrated Drops 1867
Junior Strength Motrin Caplets and Chewable Tablets 1867
MS Contin Tablets (Less frequent) 2701
Mumpsvax (Extremely rare) 2031
Mycamine for Injection 628
Myleran Tablets 1525
▲ Myozyme for Intravenous Infusion (21%) 1279
Nalfon Capsules (Less than 1%) 2502
Namenda (Infrequent) 1195
Naprosyn Suspension (Less than 1%) 2761
Naprosyn Tablets (Less than 1%) 2761
Neoral Oral Solution (1% to less than 3%) 2259
Neoral Soft Gelatin Capsules (1% to less than 3%) 2259
Neulasta Injection 601
Neumega for Injection 3435
Neupogen for Injection 603
Neurontin Capsules (Infrequent) 2487
Neurontin Oral Solution (Infrequent) 2487
Neurontin Tablets (Infrequent) 2487
Nexavar Tablets (Uncommon) 746
Nexium Delayed-Release Capsules (Less than 1%) 655
Nexium I.V. (Less than 1%) 659
Niaspan Extended-Release Tablets 1730
▲ Nipent for Injection (3% to 10%) 1863
Norflex Injection (Rare) 1856
Noroxin Tablets (Less frequent) 2032
Norvasc Tablets (Less than 0.1%) 2545
Norvir (Less than 2%) 503
Numorphan Injection 1120
▲ Oncaspar (Greater than 5%) 1145
Opana Tablets (Less than 1%) 1122
Opana ER Tablets (Less than 1%) 1126
Oracea Capsules 1000
Orencia Powder for Intravenous Infusion (0.1% to 1%) 914
Orthoclone OKT3 Sterile Solution 2360
OsmoPrep Tablets (Rare) 2840
Oxsoralen-Ultra Capsules 3353
ParaGard T 380A Intrauterine Copper Contraceptive 1073
Parcopa Orally Disintegrating Tablets 3097
Parnate Tablets 1527
Paxil CR Controlled-Release Tablets (Infrequent) 1538
Paxil (Infrequent) 1530
PCE Dispertab Tablets 515
Pediarix Vaccine (Rare) 1548
Liquid PedvaxHIB (Two children) 2035
Pegasys 2789
PEG-Intron Powder for Injection (Less than or equal to 1%) 3048
Pentasa Capsules (Less than 1%) 3185
Pepcid Injection (Infrequent) 2040
Pepcid (Infrequent) 2038
Percodan Tablets 1132
Persantine Tablets (Rare) 868
Phenergan Tablets and Suppositories 3440
Plasbumin-5 (Rare) 3251
Plasbumin-20 (Rare) 3252
Plasbumin-25 (Rare) 3253
Plasmanate (Occasional) 3255
Plavix Tablets (Less than 1%) 917
Plavix Tablets (Less than 1%) 2926
Pletal Tablets (Less than 2%) 2455
Pneumovax 23 (Rare) 2043
Premarin Intravenous 3442
Premarin Tablets 3446
Premarin Vaginal Cream 3452
Premphase Tablets 3456
Prempro Tablets 3456
Prevacid Delayed-Release Capsules (Less than 1%) 3271
Prevacid for Delayed-Release Oral Suspension (Less than 1%) 3271
Prevacid SoluTab Delayed-Release Orally Disintegrating Tablets (Less than 1%) 3271
Prevacid NapraPAC (Less than 1%) 3280
PREVPAC (Less than 1%) 3284
Prilosec OTC Delayed-Release Tablets (Less than 1%) 2677
Primaxin I.M. 2045
Primaxin I.V. (0.2%) 2048
Prinivil Tablets (0.3% to 1.0%) 2052
Prinzide Tablets 2056
Prochieve 4% Gel 1003
Prochieve 8% Gel 1003
Procrit for Injection (Rare) 2364
Profilnine SD, Factor IX Complex (Human) 1660
Proleukin for Injection (2%) 2266
Propecia Tablets 2060
Proquin XR Tablets (Less than 1%) 1153
Proscar Tablets 2067
ProSom Tablets (Infrequent) 517
Protonix I.V. (Less than 1%) 3472
Protonix Tablets (Less than 1%) 3469
▲ Protopic Ointment (3% to 5%) 638
Proventil Inhalation Aerosol 3053
Proventil Inhalation Solution 0.083% (Rare) 3055
Proventil HFA Inhalation Aerosol (Rare) 3056
Prozac Pulvules and Liquid 1801
Pulmozyme Inhalation Solution 1248
Qvar Inhalation Aerosol (Rare) 3303
Raniclor Tablets, Chewable (0.5%) 2505
Raptiva for Injection (1%) 1250
Rebetron Combination Therapy 3063
Recombinate (Extremely rare) 729
Recombivax HB (Less than 1%) 2071
ReFacto Vials 3484
Refludan for Injection (Uncommon) 792
Relenza Rotadisk (Less than 1.5%) 1552
Relpax Tablets (Rare) 2548
Remicade for IV Injection (Less than 1%) 971
Requip Tablets (Infrequent) 1555
Rescriptor Tablets 2551
Retrovir Capsules 1560
Retrovir IV Infusion 1564
Retrovir 1560
Reyataz Capsules (Less than 3%) 921
Rilutek Tablets (Infrequent) 2930
Risperdal (Rare) 1676
Risperdal M-Tab Orally Disintegrating Tablets (Rare) 1676
Ritalin Hydrochloride Tablets 2269
Ritalin LA Capsules 2271
Ritalin-SR Tablets 2269
▲ Rituxan I.V. (1% to 8%) 1254
Rocaltrol Capsules 2798
Rocaltrol Oral Solution 2798
Rythmol SR Capsules 2727
Sandostatin Injection (Less than 1%) 2278
▲ Sandostatin LAR Depot (1% to 4%) 2280
Seasonique Tablets 1077
▲ Serevent Diskus (3%) 1568
Singulair (Greater than or equal to 2%) 2077
Solodyn Extended Release Tablets (2%) 1890
Sonata Capsules (Infrequent) 1717
Soriatane Capsules (Less than 1%) 1013
Spiriva HandiHaler 869
St. Joseph 81 mg Aspirin Chewable and Enteric Coated Tablets 1869
St. Joseph 81 mg Aspirin ▣ 688
Stalevo Tablets 2287
Stromectol Tablets (0.9%) 2083
Sular Tablets (Less than or equal to 1%) 3122
Sulfamylon Cream 2162
Sulfamylon for 5% Topical Solution 2162
Suprax (Less than 2%) 1843
Sustiva Capsules (Less than 2%) 930
Sustiva Tablets (Less than 2%) 930
Synera Topical Patch (Less than or equal to 1%) 1137
Synthroid Tablets 520
Tambocor Tablets (Less than 1%) 1856
Tarka Tablets 524
Tasmar Tablets (Infrequent) 3358
Tegretol/Tegretol-XR 2295
Teveten HCT Tablets 1737
Thalomid Capsules 965
▲ Thiola Tablets (16.7%) 2141
Thioridazine Hydrochloride Tablets (Infrequent) 2163
Thiothixene Capsules 2165
▲ Thrombate III (1 of 17) 3257
Thyrogen for Injection 1286
Thyrolar Tablets 1199
Ticlid Tablets (0.5% to 1.0%) 2810
Timentin ADD-Vantage 1580
Timentin Injection Galaxy Container 1583
Timentin IV Infusion 1577
Timentin Pharmacy Bulk Package 1586
Timolide Tablets 2086
Timoptic Sterile Ophthalmic Solution (Less frequent) 2088
Timoptic in Ocudose (Less frequent) 2091
Timoptic-XE Sterile Ophthalmic Gel Forming Solution 2092
Tindamax Tablets 2142
TNKase I.V. (Rare) 1264
Topamax Sprinkle Capsules (Infrequent) 2404
Topamax Tablets (Infrequent) 2404
Toprol-XL Tablets 668
Tricor Tablets (1.1%) 527
TriLyte with Flavor Packs for Oral Solution 3100
▲ Trisenox Injection (8%) 993
Trizivir Tablets 1589
Trusopt Sterile Ophthalmic Solution 2095
▲ Truvada Tablets (Greater than 5%) 1296
Twinrix Vaccine (Less than 1%) 1595
Ultane Liquid for Inhalation (Less than 1%) 531
▲ Ultram ER Tablets (1% to greater than 5%) 2392
Uniretic Tablets (Less than 1%) 3100
Univasc Tablets (Less than 1%) 3104
Uroxatral Tablets 2943
Valtrex Caplets 1597
Vancocin HCl Capsules, USP 3380
Vandazole Vaginal Gel (Less than 1%) 3338
Vantin Tablets and Oral Suspension (Less than 1%) 2645
Vaqta (Less than 1%) 2097
Varivax (Greater than or equal to 1%) 2100
Vasotec I.V. Injection (0.5% to 1.0%) 2103
Ventolin HFA Inhalation Aerosol 1600
Verelan PM Extended-Release Capsules, Controlled-Onset (2% or less) 3106
VFEND I.V. (Less than 2%) 2564
VFEND Oral Suspension (Less than 2%) 2564
VFEND Tablets (Less than 2%) 2564
Viagra Tablets (Less than 2%) 2573
Vicoprofen Tablets (Less than 1%) 539
Viracept (Less than 2%) 2577
Viramune Oral Suspension 873
Viramune Tablets 873
▲ Viread Tablets (5% to 18%) 1301
Visudyne for Injection 2305
Vivitrol 995
Vivotif (Infrequent) 819
Voltaren Tablets (Rarely) 2307
Voltaren-XR Tablets (Rarely) 2310
VoSpire ER Tablets (Rare) 1052
Vytorin 10/10 Tablets 2114
Vytorin 10/10 Tablets 3077
Vytorin 10/20 Tablets 2114
Vytorin 10/20 Tablets 3077
Vytorin 10/40 Tablets 2114
Vytorin 10/40 Tablets 3077
Vytorin 10/80 Tablets 2114
Vytorin 10/80 Tablets 3077
Wellbutrin Tablets 1603
Wellbutrin SR Sustained-Release Tablets (1% to 2%) 1607
Wellbutrin XL Extended-Release Tablets (1% to 2%) 1613
Xenical Capsules 2831
Xifaxan Tablets 2842
Xolair 1266
▲ Xopenex Inhalation Solution (3%) 3146
▲ Xopenex Inhalation Solution Concentrate (3%) 3150
▲ Xopenex HFA Inhalation Aerosol (3%) 3154
Xyrem Oral Solution (Infrequent) 1688
Zegerid Capsules (Less than 1%) 2958
Zegerid Powder for Oral Solution (Less than 1%) 2958
Zelnorm Tablets 2312
Zemplar Injection 543
Zetia Tablets 2120
Zinacef for Injection (Fewer than 1 in 250 patients) 1631
Zinacef Injection (Fewer than 1 in 250 patients) 1631
Zinecard for Injection (2%) 2650
Zmax for Oral Suspension (Less then 1%) 2583
Zocor Tablets (Rare) 2105
Zofran Injection (Rare) 1634
Zofran 1639
Zofran ODT Orally Disintegrating Tablets 1639
Zoloft (Infrequent) 2586
Zomig Tablets (Infrequent) 3519
Zomig-ZMT Tablets (Infrequent) 3519
Zonegran Capsules (Infrequent) 1101
Zovirax 1643
Zyban Sustained-Release Tablets (1% to 2%) 1644
Zyflo Tablets 1023
Zyprexa Tablets (Infrequent) 1830
Zyprexa ZYDIS Orally Disintegrating Tablets (Infrequent) 1830
Zyrtec Chewable Tablets (Less than 2%) 2594
Zyrtec (Less than 2%) 2594
Zyrtec-D 12 Hour Extended Release Tablets (Less than 2%) 2597

Uterine contractions, abnormal

Cervidil Vaginal Insert (2.0% to 4.7%) 1181

Uterine contractions, altered

Proventil Inhalation Solution 0.083% 3055

Uterine disorder, unspecified

Evista Tablets 1763
Zomig Nasal Spray (Rare) 3523

Uterine fibroids

Zomig Nasal Spray (Rare) 3523

Uterine fibroids, enlarged

Symbyax Capsules (Rare) 1819

Uterine fibromyomata, increase in size

Climara Transdermal System 771
Estratest Tablets 3199
Estratest H.S. Tablets 3199
Premarin Intravenous 3442
Premarin Tablets 3446
Premarin Vaginal Cream 3452
Premphase Tablets 3456
Prempro Tablets 3456
Prozac Pulvules and Liquid (Rare) 1801
Zyprexa Tablets (Infrequent) 1830
Zyprexa ZYDIS Orally Disintegrating Tablets (Infrequent) 1830

Uterine inertia

Tasmar Tablets (Infrequent) 3358

Uterine leiomyomata, enlargement

Angeliq Tablets 762
Climara Transdermal System 771
Climara Pro Transdermal System 776
Enjuvia Tablets 1062
Estrasorb Topical Emulsion 1147
Menostar Transdermal System 782
Premarin Vaginal Cream 3452

Uterine rupture

Cervidil Vaginal Insert 1181

Uterine spasm

Effexor Tablets (Rare) 3411
Effexor XR Capsules (Rare) 3417
Paxil CR Controlled-Release Tablets (Rare) 1538
Paxil (Rare) 1530

Uveitis
Actonel Tablets (Very rare) 2683
Actonel with Calcium Tablets (Very rare) 2688
Alrex Ophthalmic Suspension 0.2% (Less than 5%) ⊙ 246
Aredia for Injection (Rare) 2179
Blephamide Ophthalmic Ointment 568
Blephamide Ophthalmic Suspension 569
Effexor Tablets (Rare) 3411
Effexor XR Capsules (Rare) 3417
FML Ophthalmic Ointment ⊙ 228
FML Ophthalmic Suspension ⊙ 227
FML Forte Ophthalmic Suspension ⊙ 226
Fosamax (Rare) 1969
Fosamax Plus D Tablets (Rarely) 1977
Lamictal (Rare) 1481
Lotemax Ophthalmic Suspension 0.5% (Less than 5%) ⊙ 251
Lyrica Capsules (Rare) 2539
Nipent for Injection (Less than 3%) 1863
Norvir (Less than 2%) 503
OptiPranolol Metipranolol Ophthalmic Solution 0.3% ⊙ 256
Pred Mild Ophthalmic Suspension ⊙ 238
Pred Forte Ophthalmic Suspension ⊙ 235
Rituxan I.V. 1254
Stromectol Tablets 2083
VFEND I.V. (Less than 2%) 2564
VFEND Oral Suspension (Less than 2%) 2564
VFEND Tablets (Less than 2%) 2564
▲ Voltaren Ophthalmic Solution (Less than or equal to 5%) 2309
Xalatan Sterile Ophthalmic Solution 2649

V

Vagina, dryness
Arimidex Tablets (1% to 2%) 673
▲ Intron A for Injection (Less than 5%) 3024
Prochieve 4% Gel 1003
Prochieve 8% Gel 1003
Prometrium Capsules (100 mg, 200 mg) (Less than 6%) 3203
Risperdal (Frequent) 1676
Risperdal M-Tab Orally Disintegrating Tablets (Frequent) 1676

Vaginal burning
Vagistat-1 ▣ 804

Vaginal candidiasis
Abilify Oral Solution (Infrequent) 882
Abilify Oral Solution (Infrequent) 2450
Abilify Discmelt Orally Disintegrating Tablets (Infrequent) 882
Abilify Discmelt Orally Disintegrating Tablets (Infrequent) 2450
Abilify Tablets (Infrequent) 882
Abilify Tablets (Infrequent) 2450
Advair Diskus 100/50 1308
Advair Diskus 250/50 1308
Advair Diskus 500/50 1308
Advair HFA Inhalation Aerosol 1318
Angeliq Tablets 762
Ceftin (Less frequent) 1407
Cipro 2977
Cipro I.V. 2984
Cipro XR Tablets 2990
Climara Transdermal System 771
Climara Pro Transdermal System 776
Clozaril Tablets (Less than 1%) 2184
▲ Copaxone for Injection (8%) 3297
Cubicin for Injection (1.7%) 1026
▲ depo-subQ provera 104 Injectable Suspension (1% to less than 5%) 2624
Doxil Injection (Less than 1%) 2351
Estrasorb Topical Emulsion 1147
Estratest Tablets 3199
Estratest H.S. Tablets 3199
Ketek Tablets (Greater than or equal to 0.2% to less than 2%) 2903
Lamictal (Infrequent) 1481
Lofibra Tablets 1219
Lofibra Capsules 1216
Menostar Transdermal System 782
Meridia Capsules (1.2%) 489
Metrogel 1% (0.2%) 1211
▲ MetroGel-Vaginal Gel (10%) 1855
Mircette Tablets 1066
Myobloc Injection (2% or greater) 3192
Neurontin Capsules (Infrequent) 2487
Neurontin Oral Solution (Infrequent) 2487
Neurontin Tablets (Infrequent) 2487
Noroxin Tablets 2032
NuvaRing 2340
▲ Omnicef Capsules (5%) 511
Omnicef for Oral Suspension (0.3%) 511
Oracea Capsules 1000
Ortho-Cyclen Tablets 2429
Ortho Evra Transdermal System 2417
Ortho Tri-Cyclen Tablets 2429
Ortho Tri-Cyclen Lo Tablets 2436
Premarin Tablets 3446
Premarin Vaginal Cream 3452
Premphase Tablets 3456
Prempro Tablets 3456
▲ Prometrium Capsules (100 mg, 200 mg) (Less than 5%) 3203
Protopic Ointment (Greater than or equal to 1%) 638
Seroquel Tablets (Infrequent) 690
Soriatane Capsules 1013
Tricor Tablets 527
▲ Vantin Tablets and Oral Suspension (3.1%) 2645
Yasmin 28 Tablets (Greater than 1%) 796
Yaz Tablets 803
Zinacef for Injection 1631
Zinacef Injection 1631
Zyvox (1% to 1.6%) 2652

Vaginal discharge
▲ Arimidex Tablets (3% to 4%) 673
Ceftin Tablets (0.1% to 1%) 1407
Cleocin Vaginal Ovules (Less than 1%) 2616
Invirase (Less than 2%) 2772
Keflex Capsules 549
Lupron Depot-PED 7.5 mg, 11.25 mg and 15 mg (2%) 3269
Lupron Injection Pediatric (2%) 3259
▲ MetroGel-Vaginal Gel (12%) 1855
▲ NuvaRing (5% to 14%) 2340
▲ Prochieve 4% Gel (7%) 1003
▲ Prochieve 8% Gel (7%) 1003
▲ Prometrium Capsules (100 mg, 200 mg) (10%) 3203
ProSom Tablets (Infrequent) 517
▲ Soltamox Oral Solution (30% to 55%) 3527
Tindamax Tablets 2142

Vaginal perversion
Myobloc Injection (Greater than 2%) 3192

Vaginal pressure
Adenoscan (Less than 1%) 619

Vaginitis
Abilify Oral Solution 882
Abilify Oral Solution 2450
Abilify Discmelt Orally Disintegrating Tablets 882
Abilify Discmelt Orally Disintegrating Tablets 2450
Abilify Tablets 882
Abilify Tablets 2450
Aceon Tablets (2 mg, 4 mg, 8 mg) (0.3% to 1%) 3194
Actiq (1% or greater) 979
Advair Diskus 100/50 1308
Advair Diskus 250/50 1308
Advair Diskus 500/50 1308
Advair HFA Inhalation Aerosol 1318
Ambien Tablets (Infrequent) 2851
Ambien CR Tablets (Infrequent) 2855
Amerge Tablets (Rare) 1339
Angeliq Tablets 762
Aricept Tablets (Infrequent) 1094
Aricept ODT Tablets (Infrequent) 1094
▲ Arimidex Tablets (4%) 673
Augmentin (1%) 1360
Augmentin Tablets (1%) 1363
Augmentin XR Extended-Release Tablets (1%) 1369
Avelox (0.1% to less than 2%) 2970
Campral Tablets (Infrequent) 1174
▲ Ceftin Tablets (0.1% to 5.4%) 1407
Celebrex Capsules (0.1% to 1.9%) 3134
Cipro (Less than 1% to 2%) 2977
Cipro I.V. (1% or less) 2984
Cipro XR Tablets (Less than 1%) 2990
Cleocin Vaginal Ovules (Less than 1%) 2616
Climara Transdermal System 771
Climara Pro Transdermal System (1.9%) 776
Copaxone for Injection (At least 2%) 3297
▲ Depacon Injection (1% to 5%) 412
▲ Depakene (1% to 5%) 417
▲ Depakote Sprinkle Capsules (1% to 5%) 422
▲ Depakote Tablets (1% to 5%) 427
▲ Depakote ER Tablets (Greater than 1% to 5%) 434
▲ Depo-Provera Contraceptive Injection (1% to 5%) 2622
▲ depo-subQ provera 104 Injectable Suspension (1% to less than 5%) 2624
Doxil Injection (Less than 1%) 2351
Effexor Tablets (Frequent) 3411
Effexor XR Capsules (Frequent) 3417
Enablex Extended-Release Tablets (Greater than or equal to 1%) 2203
▲ Enjuvia Tablets (2% to 7%) 1062
Estrasorb Topical Emulsion 1147
▲ Estring Vaginal Ring (5%) 2635
▲ Evista Tablets (4.3%) 1763
▲ Evoxac Capsules (1% to 3%) 1047
Fortaz (Less than 1%) 1453
Gabitril Tablets (Frequent) 984
▲ Infergen (5% to 8%) 3364
▲ Invanz for Injection (1.4% to 3.3%) 1999
Keflex Capsules 549
Ketek Tablets (Greater than or equal to 0.2% to less than 2%) 2903
Klonopin (1%) 2778
▲ Lamictal (4.1%) 1481
Levaquin (0.5% to 1.3%) 2384
Levaquin in 5% Dextrose Injection (0.5% to 1.3%) 2384
Lunesta Tablets (Infrequent) 3142
▲ Lupron Depot 3.75 mg (10%) 3260
▲ Lupron Depot–3 Month 11.25 mg (10%) 3265
Lupron Depot-PED 7.5 mg, 11.25 mg and 15 mg (2%) 3269
Lupron Injection Pediatric (2%) 3259
Maxipime for Injection (Greater than 0.1% to less than 1%) 1105
Mefoxin for Injection 2012
Mefoxin Premixed Intravenous Solution 2016
Menostar Transdermal System 782
Migranal Nasal Spray (Rare) 3348
Mircette Tablets 1066
▲ Mirena Intrauterine System (5% or more) 787
Nexium Delayed-Release Capsules (Less than 1%) 655
Nexium I.V. (Less than 1%) 659
▲ NuvaRing (5% to 14%) 2340
Omnicef Capsules (1%) 511
Omnicef for Oral Suspension (0.3%) 511
Ortho-Cyclen Tablets 2429
Ortho Evra Transdermal System 2417
Ortho Tri-Cyclen Tablets 2429
Ortho Tri-Cyclen Lo Tablets 2436
ParaGard T 380A Intrauterine Copper Contraceptive 1073
Paxil CR Controlled-Release Tablets (Infrequent) 1538
Paxil (Infrequent) 1530
Permax Tablets (Infrequent) 3356
Pletal Tablets (Less than 2%) 2455
▲ Premarin Tablets (5% to 7%) 3446
Premarin Vaginal Cream 3452
▲ Premphase Tablets (4% to 7%) 3456
▲ Prempro Tablets (4% to 7%) 3456
Prevacid Delayed-Release Capsules (Less than 1%) 3271
Prevacid for Delayed-Release Oral Suspension (Less than 1%) 3271
Prevacid SoluTab Delayed-Release Orally Disintegrating Tablets (Less than 1%) 3271
Prevacid NapraPAC (Less than 1%) 3280
PREVPAC (Less than 3%) 3284
▲ Prograf Capsules and Injection (3% to 15%) 632
Prometrium Capsules (100 mg, 200 mg) (Less than 5%) 3203
Proquin XR Tablets (Less than 1%) 1153
Protonix I.V. (Less than 1%) 3472
Protonix Tablets (Less than 1%) 3469
Protopic Ointment (0.2% to less than 1%) 638
Raniclor Tablets, Chewable (1%) 2505
Relpax Tablets (Rare) 2548
Risperdal Consta Long-Acting Injection (Infrequent) 1682
Rocephin Injectable Vials, ADD-Vantage, Galaxy, Bulk (Occasional) 2800
Sandostatin Injection (Less than 1%) 2278
Seasonique Tablets 1077
Seroquel Tablets (Infrequent) 690
Sonata Capsules (Infrequent) 1717
Sular Tablets (Less than or equal to 1%) 3122
Suprax (Less than 2%) 1843
Symbyax Capsules (Infrequent) 1819
Tasmar Tablets (Infrequent) 3358
▲ Tequin Injection (6%) 938
▲ Tequin Injection in 5% Dextrose (6%) 938
▲ Tequin Tablets (6%) 938
Trileptal Tablets (Up to 2%) 2300
Trileptal Oral Suspension (Up to 2%) 2300
Tygacil for Injection (0% to less than 2%) 3488
Uniretic Tablets (Less than 1%) 3100
▲ Vagifem Tablets (3% to 5%) 2334
Vandazole Vaginal Gel (Less than 1%) 3338
Vantin Tablets and Oral Suspension (Less than 1%) 2645
Wellbutrin Tablets (Infrequent) 1603
Wellbutrin SR Sustained-Release Tablets 1607
Wellbutrin XL Extended-Release Tablets 1613
Xenical Capsules (2.6% to 3.8%) 2831
Yasmin 28 Tablets (Greater than 1%) 796
Yaz Tablets (Greater than 1%) 803
Zinacef for Injection 1631
Zinacef Injection 1631
Zmax for Oral Suspension (Less then 1%) 2583
Zomig Nasal Spray (Rare) 3523
Zosyn (1.0% or less) 3492
Zyban Sustained-Release Tablets 1644
Zyflo Tablets (Greater than 1%) 1023
Zyprexa Tablets (2%) 1830
Zyprexa ZYDIS Orally Disintegrating Tablets (2%) 1830
Zyrtec Chewable Tablets (Less than 2%) 2594
Zyrtec (Less than 2%) 2594
Zyrtec-D 12 Hour Extended Release Tablets (Less than 2%) 2597

Vaginitis, atrophic
Evoxac Capsules (Less than 1%) 1047
Exelon Capsules (Infrequent) 2206
Exelon Oral Solution (Infrequent) 2206
▲ Imdur Tablets (Less than or equal to 5%) 3018
Soriatane Capsules (Less than 1%) 1013
Zoloft (Rare) 2586

Vaginitis, bacterial
▲ depo-subQ provera 104 Injectable Suspension (1% to less than 5%) 2624
Proquin XR Tablets (Less than 1%) 1153

Vaginosis, fungal
Ketek Tablets (Greater than or equal to 0.2% to less than 2%) 2903
Proquin XR Tablets (Less than 1%) 1153

Varicella
▲ Clarinex Syrup (3.6%) 2995
Elidel Cream 1% (0.7% to 2.9%) 2200
Singulair (Greater than or equal to 2%) 2077

Varices, esophageal
Myleran Tablets 1525
Nexium Delayed-Release Capsules (Less than 1%) 655
Nexium I.V. (Less than 1%) 659
Tabloid Tablets 1575

Varicose vein
Ambien CR Tablets (Rare) 2855
▲ Limbrel Capsules (Greater than or equal to 2%) 2672

Varicose vein, aggravation of
Seasonique Tablets 1077

Vascular access, clotting
▲ Epogen for Injection (0.25% to 7%) 591
▲ Procrit for Injection (0.25 to 7%) 2364

Vascular collapse
Carimune NF 3499
Flebogamma 5%, Immune Globulin Intravenous (Human) 1658
Gammagard Liquid 721
Gammagard S/D (Rare) 724
Gamunex Immune Globulin I.V., 10% (Rare) 3235

Vascular complications, unspecified
Camptosar Injection 2604
▲ Carnitor Injection (2% to 6%) 3188
▲ Cozaar Tablets (4%) 1935
Follistim AQ Cartridge 2338
▲ Humira Injection (Less than 5%) 466

Lofibra Tablets ... 1219
Lofibra Capsules ... 1216
Ortho-Cyclen/Ortho Tri-Cyclen ... 2429
Ortho Tri-Cyclen Lo Tablets ... 2436
ReoPro Vials (1.8%) ... 1809
▲ Sandostatin LAR Depot (1% to 4%) ... 2280
Tricor Tablets ... 527
Zofran (Rare) ... 1639
Zofran ODT Orally Disintegrating Tablets (Rare) ... 1639
Zomig Nasal Spray (Rare) ... 3523

Vascular insufficiency
Zonegran Capsules (Infrequent) ... 1101

Vascular leak syndrome
▲ Ontak Vials (27%) ... 1745

Vasculitis
Accutane Capsules ... 2731
Aceon Tablets (2 mg, 4 mg, 8 mg) ... 3194
Advair Diskus 100/50 ... 1308
Advair Diskus 250/50 ... 1308
Advair Diskus 500/50 ... 1308
Advicor Tablets ... 1722
Aldoril Tablets ... 1910
Alkeran for Injection ... 955
Alkeran Tablets ... 956
Altace Capsules (Less than 1%) ... 1702
Altoprev Extended-Release Tablets (Rare) ... 3109
Anaprox Tablets (Less than 1%) ... 2761
Anaprox DS Tablets (Less than 1%) .. 2761
Arthrotec Tablets (Rare) ... 3129
Atacand HCT ... 651
Attenuvax ... 1914
Avalide Tablets ... 888
Avalide Tablets ... 2874
Axid Oral Solution (Rare) ... 879
Caduet Tablets (Greater than 0.1% to less than or equal to 1%) ... 2508
Cancidas for Injection (0%) ... 1918
Captopril Tablets ... 2149
Celebrex Capsules (Less than 0.1%) ... 3134
Cipro ... 2977
Cipro I.V. (1% or less) ... 2984
Cipro XR Tablets ... 2990
Clorpres Tablets ... 2153
Clozaril Tablets ... 2184
Combivir Tablets ... 1411
Coumadin for Injection (Infrequent) ... 898
Coumadin Tablets (Infrequent) ... 898
Covera-HS Tablets (Less than 2%) ... 3139
Cozaar Tablets ... 1935
Crixivan Capsules ... 1940
Decadron Tablets ... 1951
Diovan HCT Tablets ... 2196
Diuril Oral Suspension ... 1954
Diuril Sodium Intravenous ... 2467
Dyazide Capsules ... 1423
EC-Naprosyn Delayed-Release Tablets (Less than 1%) ... 2761
Evoxac Capsules (Less than 1%) ... 1047
Exelon Capsules (Infrequent) ... 2206
Exelon Oral Solution (Infrequent) ... 2206
FazaClo Orally Disintegrating Tablets ... 551
Fluarix ... 1451
Furosemide Tablets ... 2154
Gantrisin Pediatric Suspension ... 2770
Gemzar for Injection (Very rare) ... 1771
Hyzaar 50-12.5 Tablets ... 1990
Hyzaar 100-12.5 Tablets ... 1990
Hyzaar 100-25 Tablets ... 1990
Kaletra (Less than 2%) ... 476
Lamictal ... 1481
Lescol Capsules (Rare) ... 2233
Lescol XL Tablets ... 2233
Levaquin (Rare) ... 2384
Levaquin in 5% Dextrose Injection (Rare) ... 2384
Meruvax II ... 2019
Mevacor Tablets (Rare) ... 2021
Micardis HCT Tablets ... 856
M-M-R II ... 2006
Mobic Oral Suspension (Less than 2%) ... 863
Mobic Tablets (Less than 2%) ... 863
Moduretic Tablets ... 2028
Mumpsvax (Rare) ... 2031
Naprosyn Suspension (Less than 1%) ... 2761
Naprosyn Tablets (Less than 1%) ... 2761
Nipent for Injection (Less than 3%) ... 1863
Noroxin Tablets ... 2032
Norvasc Tablets (More than 0.1% to 1%) ... 2545
Orthoclone OKT3 Sterile Solution ... 2360
Paser Granules ... 1674
PEG-Intron Powder for Injection (Less than or equal to 1%) ... 3048
Permax Tablets (Rare) ... 3356
Plavix Tablets ... 917
Plavix Tablets ... 2926
Prevacid NapraPAC (Less than 1%) ... 3280
Prinivil Tablets (0.3% to 1.0%) ... 2052
Prinzide Tablets ... 2056
Proquin XR Tablets ... 1153
Recombivax HB ... 2071
Remicade for IV Injection ... 971
Retrovir Capsules (Rare) ... 1560
Retrovir IV Infusion (Rare) ... 1564
Retrovir (Rare) ... 1560
Ritalin Hydrochloride Tablets ... 2269
Ritalin LA Capsules ... 2271
Ritalin-SR Tablets ... 2269
Rituxan I.V. ... 1254
Tarka Tablets ... 524
Tegretol/Tegretol-XR ... 2295
Teveten HCT Tablets ... 1737
Ticlid Tablets (Rare) ... 2810
Timolide Tablets ... 2086
Trizivir Tablets ... 1589
Vancocin HCl Capsules, USP (Rare) ... 3380
Vasotec I.V. Injection (0.5% to 1.0%) ... 2103
Verelan PM Extended-Release Capsules, Controlled-Onset (2% or less) ... 3106
Vesanoid Capsules ... 2820
Voltaren Tablets (Rarely) ... 2307
Voltaren-XR Tablets (Rarely) ... 2310
Vytorin 10/10 Tablets ... 2114
Vytorin 10/10 Tablets ... 3077
Vytorin 10/20 Tablets ... 2114
Vytorin 10/20 Tablets ... 3077
Vytorin 10/40 Tablets ... 2114
Vytorin 10/40 Tablets ... 3077
Vytorin 10/80 Tablets ... 2114
Vytorin 10/80 Tablets ... 3077
Zantac (Rare) ... 1624
Zantac Injection (Rare) ... 1619
Zantac Injection Pharmacy Bulk Package (Rare) ... 1622
Zantac Injection Premixed (Rare) ... 1619
Zantac (Rare) ... 1624
Zocor Tablets (Rare) ... 2105
Zoloft ... 2586

Vasculitis, allergic
Aggrenox Capsules ... 822
Amoxil Capsules ... 1343
Amoxil Chewable Tablets ... 1343
Amoxil Pediatric Drops for Oral Suspension ... 1343
Amoxil Powder for Oral Suspension ... 1343
Amoxil Tablets ... 1343
Avandaryl Tablets ... 1379
Bicillin C-R Injectable Suspension ... 1706
Duetact Tablets (Less than 1%) ... 3226
Imitrex Nasal Spray ... 1467
Imitrex Tablets ... 1471
Omnicef Capsules ... 511
Omnicef for Oral Suspension ... 511

Vasculitis, central nervous system
Imitrex Nasal Spray ... 1467
Imitrex Tablets ... 1471

Vasculitis, cutaneous
Atacand HCT ... 651
Avalide Tablets ... 888
Avalide Tablets ... 2874
Clorpres Tablets ... 2153
Depacon Injection ... 412
Depakene ... 417
Depakote Sprinkle Capsules ... 422
Depakote Tablets ... 427
Depakote ER Tablets ... 434
Diovan HCT Tablets ... 2196
Diuril Oral Suspension ... 1954
Diuril Sodium Intravenous ... 2467
Enbrel for Injection ... 584
Hyzaar 50-12.5 Tablets ... 1990
Hyzaar 100-12.5 Tablets ... 1990
Hyzaar 100-25 Tablets ... 1990
Micardis HCT Tablets ... 856
Moduretic Tablets ... 2028
Neupogen for Injection (Infrequent) .. 603
Prinzide Tablets ... 2056
Remicade for IV Injection ... 971
Teveten HCT Tablets ... 1737
Timolide Tablets ... 2086

Vasculitis, eosinophilic
Accolate Tablets (Rare) ... 671
Advair HFA Inhalation Aerosol ... 1318

Vasculitis, leukocytoclastic
Rescriptor Tablets ... 2551
Tiazac Capsules ... 1201
Valtrex Caplets ... 1597
Zovirax ... 1643

Vasculitis, necrotizing
Concerta Extended-Release Tablets ... 1881
Daytrana Transdermal Patch ... 3174
Focalin Tablets ... 2220
Focalin XR Capsules ... 2223
Metadate CD Capsules ... 3323

Vasculitis, renal
Cuprimine Capsules (Rare) ... 1947

Vasoconstriction
Invirase (Rare) ... 2772

Vasodilation
Abilify Oral Solution (Infrequent) ... 882
Abilify Oral Solution (Infrequent) ... 2450
Abilify Discmelt Orally Disintegrating Tablets (Infrequent) ... 882
Abilify Discmelt Orally Disintegrating Tablets (Infrequent) ... 2450
Abilify Tablets (Infrequent) ... 882
Abilify Tablets (Infrequent) ... 2450
Aceon Tablets (2 mg, 4 mg, 8 mg) (0.3% to 1%) ... 3194
▲ Acetadote Injection (1.47% to 9.84%) ... 1031
Aciphex Tablets (Rare) ... 1090
Actiq (Up to 2%) ... 979
Actonel Tablets (1.4% to 2.3%) ... 2683
Actonel with Calcium Tablets (1.4% to 2.3%) ... 2688
▲ Agrylin Capsules (1% to 5%) ... 3169
Alphagan P Ophthalmic Solution ... 567
AmBisome for Injection (Less common) ... 620
AndroGel (Fewer than 1%) ... 3329
Aralast (0.1%) ... 717
▲ Argatroban Injection (1% to 10%) ... 1346
Aricept Tablets (Frequent) ... 1094
Aricept ODT Tablets (Frequent) ... 1094
▲ Arimidex Tablets (25% to 41%) ... 673
Asacol Delayed-Release Tablets (2% or greater) ... 2692
Avelox (0.1% to less than 2%) ... 2970
Avinza Capsules (Less than 5%) ... 1741
Axert Tablets (Infrequent) ... 2396
▲ Betaseron for SC Injection (8%) ... 767
▲ Bexxar (0% to 5%) ... 1398
Bicillin C-R Injectable Suspension ... 1706
Brimonidine Tartrate Ophthalmic Solution 0.2% ... ⊙248
Caduet Tablets (Less than 2%) ... 2508
Campral Tablets (Frequent) ... 1174
▲ Camptosar Injection (0% to 11%) ... 2604
Cardene I.V. (0.7%) ... 2497
Caverject Impulse Injection (Less than 1%) ... 2612
▲ CellCept Capsules (3% to less than 20%) ... 2747
▲ CellCept Intravenous (3% to less than 20%) ... 2747
▲ CellCept Oral Suspension (3% to less than 20%) ... 2747
▲ CellCept Tablets (3% to less than 20%) ... 2747
Cipro I.V. (1% or less) ... 2984
▲ Copaxone for Injection (27%) ... 3297
Cosopt Sterile Ophthalmic Solution ... 1931
Crestor Tablets (Greater than or equal to 1%) ... 678
Depacon Injection (0.9%) ... 412
Depakene (1% or more) ... 417
Depakote Sprinkle Capsules ... 422
▲ Depakote Tablets (1% to 5%) ... 427
▲ Depakote ER Tablets (1% to 5%) ... 434
Diastat Rectal Delivery System (1% to 2%) ... 3343
▲ Ditropan XL Extended-Release Tablets (2% to less than 5%) ... 2413
▲ Doxil Injection (1% to 10%) ... 2351
▲ Effexor Tablets (2.3% to 5.6%) ... 3411
▲ Effexor XR Capsules (3% to 5%) ... 3417
Enbrel for Injection ... 584
▲ Faslodex Injection (17.7%) ... 681
Ferrlecit Injection ... 3388
Gabitril Tablets (2%) ... 984
Geodon for Injection (Up to 1%) ... 2529
Humate-P (2%) ... 3502
Hyperstat I.V. ... 3017
Hytrin Capsules (At least 1%) ... 471
Imitrex Injection (Rare) ... 1463
Imitrex Nasal Spray ... 1467
Imitrex Tablets (Rare) ... 1471
Ionsys Transdermal System (.1% to less than 1%) ... 2379
▲ I.V. Busulfex (25%) ... 2493
Kadian Capsules (Less than 3%) ... 577
Lamictal (Infrequent) ... 1481
Levaquin ... 2384
Levaquin in 5% Dextrose Injection ... 2384
Lipitor Tablets (Less than 2%) ... 2483
Lofibra Tablets ... 1219
Lofibra Capsules ... 1216
Lotrel Capsules ... 2249
Lupron Depot-PED 7.5 mg, 11.25 mg and 15 mg (Less than 2%) ... 3269
Lupron Injection Pediatric (Less than 2%) ... 3259
Marinol Capsules (Greater than 1%) ... 3333
Meridia Capsules (2.4%) ... 489
Mirapex Tablets (1% or more) ... 859
Myobloc Injection (Greater than 2%) ... 3192
▲ Neumega for Injection (19%) ... 3435
Neurontin Capsules (1.1%) ... 2487
Neurontin Oral Solution (1.1%) ... 2487
Neurontin Tablets (1.1%) ... 2487
Norvir (1.7%) ... 503
Omacor Capsules ... 2725
▲ Ontak Vials (22%) ... 1745
OxyContin Tablets (Less than 1%) ... 2703
▲ Paxil CR Controlled-Release Tablets (3% to 4%) ... 1538
▲ Paxil (3% to 4%) ... 1530
Pentasa Capsules (Less than 1%) ... 3185
▲ Permax Tablets (3.2%) ... 3356
Pletal Tablets (Less than 2%) ... 2455
Prevacid Delayed-Release Capsules (Less than 1%) ... 3271
Prevacid for Delayed-Release Oral Suspension (Less than 1%) ... 3271
Prevacid SoluTab Delayed-Release Orally Disintegrating Tablets (Less than 1%) ... 3271
Prevacid I.V. for Injection (Less than 1%) ... 3277
Prevacid NapraPAC (Less than 1%) .. 3280
PREVPAC (Less than 1%) ... 3284
ProAmatine Tablets (Less frequent) ... 3186
▲ Proleukin for Injection (13%) ... 2266
Protonix I.V. (Less than 1%) ... 3472
Protonix Tablets (Less than 1%) ... 3469
Protopic Ointment (Greater than or equal to 1%) ... 638
Provigil Tablets (2%) ... 988
▲ Prozac Pulvules and Liquid (1% to 5%) ... 1801
Raniclor Tablets, Chewable (Rare) ... 2505
▲ Rapamune Oral Solution and Tablets (3% to 20%) ... 3475
ReFacto Vials ... 3484
Retrovir Capsules ... 1560
Retrovir IV Infusion ... 1564
Retrovir ... 1560
Reyataz Capsules (Less than 3%) ... 921
Seroquel Tablets (Infrequent) ... 690
Sonata Capsules (Infrequent) ... 1717
▲ Suboxone Tablets (9.30%) ... 2717
▲ Subutex Tablets (3.9%) ... 2717
▲ Sular Tablets (4%) ... 3122
Symbyax Capsules (Frequent) ... 1819
Tasmar Tablets (Infrequent) ... 3358
▲ Tequin Injection (0.1% to 3%) ... 938
▲ Tequin Injection in 5% Dextrose (0.1% to 3%) ... 938
▲ Tequin Tablets (0.1% to 3%) ... 938
Thalomid Capsules ... 965
▲ Tiazac Capsules (4%) ... 1201
Timolide Tablets ... 2086
Timoptic Sterile Ophthalmic Solution ... 2088
Timoptic in Ocudose ... 2091
Timoptic-XE Sterile Ophthalmic Gel Forming Solution ... 2092
Topamax Sprinkle Capsules (Infrequent) ... 2404
Topamax Tablets (Infrequent) ... 2404
Tricor Tablets ... 527
Triglide Tablets ... 3123
Tygacil for Injection (0% to less than 2%) ... 3488
▲ Ultram ER Tablets (1% to greater than 5%) ... 2392
Vantin Tablets and Oral Suspension (Less than 1%) ... 2645
▲ Ventavis Inhalation Solution (27%) ... 1020
VFEND I.V. (1% to 1.5%) ... 2564
VFEND Oral Suspension (1% to 1.5%) ... 2564
VFEND Tablets (1% to 1.5%) ... 2564
▲ Viadur Implant (67.9%) ... 757
Vicoprofen Tablets (Less than 3%) ... 539
Wellbutrin SR Sustained-Release Tablets (Infrequent) ... 1607
Wellbutrin XL Extended-Release Tablets (Infrequent) ... 1613
WinRho SDF ... 732

Zelapar Tablets ... 3372
Zemaira (0.2% to 0.4%) ... 3509
Zoloft (Rare) ... 2586
Zomig Nasal Spray (Rare) ... 3523
Zyban Sustained-Release Tablets (Infrequent) ... 1644
Zyprexa Tablets (Infrequent) ... 1830
Zyprexa ZYDIS Orally Disintegrating Tablets (Infrequent) ... 1830

Vasodilation, peripheral
Aggrenox Capsules ... 822
Persantine Tablets ... 868

Vasomotor disturbances
Aminohippurate Sodium PAH Injection ... 1913
Niravam Orally Disintegrating Tablets (2%) ... 3092

Vasospasm, coronary artery
Amerge Tablets ... 1339
Frova Tablets ... 1113
Imitrex Tablets ... 1471
Migranal Nasal Spray ... 3348
Relpax Tablets (Rare) ... 2548
Zomig Tablets ... 3519
Zomig Nasal Spray ... 3523
Zomig-ZMT Tablets ... 3519

Vasospasm, rebound
Nimotop Capsules (Less than 1%) ... 749

Vasospasm, unspecified
Bicillin C-R Injectable Suspension ... 1706
▲ CellCept Capsules (3% to less than 20%) ... 2747
▲ CellCept Intravenous (3% to less than 20%) ... 2747
▲ CellCept Oral Suspension (3% to less than 20%) ... 2747
▲ CellCept Tablets (3% to less than 20%) ... 2747
Prozac Pulvules and Liquid (Rare) ... 1801
Relpax Tablets (Rare) ... 2548
Topamax Sprinkle Capsules (Rare) ... 2404
Topamax Tablets (Rare) ... 2404

Vasospastic reactions
Imitrex Tablets ... 1471

Vasovagal episode
Abilify Oral Solution (Rare) ... 882
Abilify Oral Solution (Rare) ... 2450
Abilify Discmelt Orally Disintegrating Tablets (Rare) ... 882
Abilify Discmelt Orally Disintegrating Tablets (Rare) ... 2450
Abilify Tablets (Rare) ... 882
Abilify Tablets (Rare) ... 2450
ADACEL Vaccine ... 2945
Aggrastat (2%) ... 1907
Alferon N Injection (2%) ... 1665
Bicillin C-R Injectable Suspension ... 1706
Caverject Impulse Injection (Less than 1%) ... 2612
Exelon Capsules (Infrequent) ... 2206
Exelon Oral Solution (Infrequent) ... 2206
Visudyne for Injection (Less than 1%) ... 2305

Vein, pigmentation of
Aloxi Injection (Less than 1%) ... 2127

Vein disorder, unspecified
▲ Aldurazyme for Intravenous Infusion (3%) ... 1268

Vein distention
Aloxi Injection (Less than 1%) ... 2127

Veins, varicosis
Ambien Tablets (Rare) ... 2851
Amerge Tablets (Rare) ... 1339
Campral Tablets (Infrequent) ... 1174
Copaxone for Injection (Infrequent) ... 3297
Depo-Provera Contraceptive Injection (Less than 1%) ... 2622
▲ Imdur Tablets (Less than or equal to 5%) ... 3018
Kaletra (Less than 2%) ... 476
Lexapro Oral Solution (Infrequent) ... 1190
Lexapro Tablets (Infrequent) ... 1190
Lofibra Tablets ... 1219
Lofibra Capsules ... 1216
Neurontin Capsules (Rare) ... 2487
Neurontin Oral Solution (Rare) ... 2487
Neurontin Tablets (Rare) ... 2487
Paxil CR Controlled-Release Tablets (Rare) ... 1538
Paxil (Rare) ... 1530
Permax Tablets (Infrequent) ... 3356
Pletal Tablets (Less than 2%) ... 2455
Requip Tablets (Infrequent) ... 1555
Tricor Tablets ... 527
Triglide Tablets ... 3123
▲ Visudyne for Injection (1% to 10%) ... 2305

Veno-occlusive disease, unspecified
Eloxatin for Injection ... 2892
▲ Mylotarg for Injection (1% to 20%) ... 3431

Venous infection at injection site
Primaxin I.V. (0.1%) ... 2048

Venous irritation
▲ R-Gene 10 for Intravenous Use (3%) ... 2641

Venous leak
▲ Caverject Impulse Injection (3%) ... 2612

Venous thromboembolism
Arimidex Tablets (1% to 2%) ... 673
Prempro Tablets ... 3456

Venous thrombophlebitis
NuvaRing ... 2340
▲ Xeloda Tablets (Less than 5%) ... 2822

Ventilator dependence
Virazole for Inhalation Solution ... 3370

Ventricular bigeminy
Proquin XR Tablets (Less than 1%) ... 1153

Ventricular contractions, premature
Adenocard Injection ... 617
Amerge Tablets (Infrequent) ... 1339
Arthrotec Tablets (Rare) ... 3129
Clozaril Tablets (Less than 1%) ... 2184
FazaClo Orally Disintegrating Tablets (Less than 1%) ... 551
▲ Indapamide Tablets (Less than 5%) ... 2156
Lanoxin Injection (Less common) ... 1494
Lanoxin Injection Pediatric (Less common) ... 1497
▲ Proleukin for Injection (5%) ... 2266
Zantac (Rare) ... 1624
Zantac Injection (Rare) ... 1619
Zantac Injection Pharmacy Bulk Package (Rare) ... 1622
Zantac Injection Premixed (Rare) ... 1619
Zantac (Rare) ... 1624
Zofran Injection ... 1634

Ventricular contractions, premature, multifocal
Lanoxicaps Capsules (Common) ... 1490
Lanoxin Injection ... 1494
Lanoxin Injection Pediatric (Less common) ... 1497
▲ Lanoxin Tablets (Among most common) ... 1500

Ventricular contractions, premature, unifocal
Lanoxicaps Capsules (Common) ... 1490
Lanoxin Injection ... 1494
Lanoxin Injection Pediatric (Less common) ... 1497
▲ Lanoxin Tablets (Among most common) ... 1500

Ventricular dilation, left-side
Retrovir Capsules (0.8%) ... 1560
Retrovir IV Infusion (1%) ... 1564
Retrovir (0.8%) ... 1560

Ventricular dysfunction
Herceptin I.V. ... 1233
Prograf Capsules and Injection (Rare) ... 632
Revlimid Capsules ... 958
Taxotere Injection Concentrate ... 2932

Ventricular ectopic beats
Cipro (Less than 1%) ... 2977
Cipro I.V. (1% or less) ... 2984
Cipro XR Tablets ... 2990
Digibind for Injection ... 1421
Imitrex Tablets ... 1471
Kytril Injection (Rare) ... 2781

Ventricular extrasystoles
Aceon Tablets (2 mg, 4 mg, 8 mg) (0.3% to 1%) ... 3194
Cardene I.V. (1.4%) ... 2497
Cardizem LA Extended Release Tablets (Less than 2%) ... 1728
▲ CellCept Capsules (3% to less than 20%) ... 2747
▲ CellCept Intravenous (3% to less than 20%) ... 2747
▲ CellCept Oral Suspension (3% to less than 20%) ... 2747
▲ CellCept Tablets (3% to less than 20%) ... 2747
Chantix Tablets (Infrequent) ... 2517
Effexor Tablets ... 3411
Effexor XR Capsules ... 3417
Eraxis for Injection (Less than 1% to less than 2%) ... 2521
I.V. Busulfex (2%) ... 2493
Lanoxicaps Capsules ... 1490
Lanoxin Injection ... 1494
Lanoxin Injection Pediatric ... 1497
Lanoxin Tablets ... 1500
Lofibra Tablets ... 1219
Lofibra Capsules ... 1216
Lotrel Capsules (Infrequent) ... 2249
▲ Natrecor for Injection (3% to 4%) ... 3127
Neurontin Capsules (Rare) ... 2487
Neurontin Oral Solution (Rare) ... 2487
Neurontin Tablets (Rare) ... 2487
Nipent for Injection (Less than 3%) ... 1863
Paxil CR Controlled-Release Tablets (Rare) ... 1538
Paxil (Rare) ... 1530
Permax Tablets (Infrequent) ... 3356
Pletal Tablets (Less than 2%) ... 2455
Prograf Capsules and Injection ... 632
Proleukin for Injection (Less than 1%) ... 2266
Provigil Tablets (At least 1%) ... 988
Prozac Pulvules and Liquid (Rare) ... 1801
Rilutek Tablets (Infrequent) ... 2930
Risperdal (Rare) ... 1676
Risperdal M-Tab Orally Disintegrating Tablets (Rare) ... 1676
Romazicon Injection (Less than 1%) ... 2804
Rythmol SR Capsules ... 2727
Sonata Capsules (Infrequent) ... 1717
Sular Tablets (Less than or equal to 1%) ... 3122
Tiazac Capsules (Less than 2%) ... 1201
▲ Trasylol Injection (6%) ... 754
Tricor Tablets ... 527
Ultane Liquid for Inhalation (Less than 1%) ... 531
Uniretic Tablets (Less than 1%) ... 3100
Vantas (Less than 2%) ... 3375
▲ Xeloda Tablets (Less than 5%) ... 2822
Zonegran Capsules (Rare) ... 1101
Zyprexa Tablets (Infrequent) ... 1830
Zyprexa ZYDIS Orally Disintegrating Tablets (Infrequent) ... 1830

Ventricular gallop
Herceptin I.V. ... 1233
Retrovir Capsules (0.8%) ... 1560
Retrovir IV Infusion (1%) ... 1564
Retrovir (0.8%) ... 1560

Ventricular hypertrophy
Rythmol SR Capsules ... 2727

Ventricular irritation
Timolide Tablets ... 2086

Ventricular response, rapid
Verelan PM Extended-Release Capsules, Controlled-Onset ... 3106

Verruca
Aldara Cream, 5% (0.5%) ... 1846
Copaxone for Injection (Frequent) ... 3297
Evoxac Capsules (Less than 1%) ... 1047
Invirase (Greater than or equal to 2%) ... 2772
▲ Prometrium Capsules (100 mg, 200 mg) (Less than 5%) ... 3203
Rescriptor Tablets ... 2551
Risperdal (Rare) ... 1676
Risperdal M-Tab Orally Disintegrating Tablets (Rare) ... 1676
Soriatane Capsules (Less than 1%) ... 1013
▲ Thiola Tablets (16.7%) ... 2141

Vertebral compression fractures
Colocort Rectal Suspension, USP (Retention) 100 mg/60 mL ... 2476
Depo-Medrol Injectable Suspension ... 2617
Revlimid Capsules ... 958

Vertical deviation
▲ BOTOX Purified Neurotoxin Complex (2.1% to 16.9%) ... 570

Vertigo
Abelcet Injection ... 1141
Abilify Oral Solution (Infrequent) ... 882
Abilify Oral Solution (Infrequent) ... 2450
Abilify Discmelt Orally Disintegrating Tablets (Infrequent) ... 882
Abilify Discmelt Orally Disintegrating Tablets (Infrequent) ... 2450
Abilify Tablets (Infrequent) ... 882
Abilify Tablets (Infrequent) ... 2450
Aceon Tablets (2 mg, 4 mg, 8 mg) (0.3% to 1%) ... 3194
Aciphex Tablets ... 1090
Actiq (Up to 1%) ... 979
▲ Actonel Tablets (1.6% to 3.3%) ... 2683
▲ Actonel with Calcium Tablets (1.6% to 3.3%) ... 2688
▲ Adalat CC Tablets (3% or less) ... 2964
Advicor Tablets ... 1722
Aerobid/Aerobid-M (1% to 3%) ... 1171
Albenza Tablets (Less than 1.0% to 1.2%) ... 1338
Aldoril Tablets ... 1910
Altace Capsules (Less than 1% to 1.5%) ... 1702
Altoprev Extended-Release Tablets ... 3109
Ambien Tablets (Frequent) ... 2851
Ambien CR Tablets (2% to frequent) ... 2855
Amerge Tablets (Frequent) ... 1339
Amitiza Capsules (Less than 0.2%) ... 3224
Anaprox Tablets (Less than 3%) ... 2761
Anaprox DS Tablets (Less than 3%) ... 2761
Anzemet Injection (Infrequently) ... 2859
Anzemet Tablets (Infrequently) ... 2862
Aricept Tablets (Frequent) ... 1094
Aricept ODT Tablets (Frequent) ... 1094
Arthrotec Tablets (Rare) ... 3129
Asacol Delayed-Release Tablets ... 2692
Astelin Nasal Spray (Infrequent) ... 1904
Atacand Tablets (0.5% or greater) ... 649
Atacand HCT (0.5% or greater) ... 651
Avalide Tablets ... 888
Avalide Tablets ... 2874
Avapro Tablets ... 891
Avapro Tablets ... 2871
Avelox (0.1% to less than 2%) ... 2970
▲ Avinza Capsules (Less than 5%) ... 1741
Axert Tablets (Infrequent) ... 2396
Azilect Tablets (2%) ... 3293
Benicar Tablets (Greater than 0.5%) ... 1043
Benicar HCT Tablets (Greater than 1%) ... 1044
Betoptic S Ophthalmic Suspension (Rare) ... 558
Biaxin/Biaxin XL ... 402
Biltricide Tablets ... 2976
Blocadren Tablets (0.6%) ... 1916
▲ Boniva Injection (3%) ... 2738
▲ Boniva Tablets (3%) ... 2741
Bumex Tablets (0.1%) ... 2746
▲ Buprenex Injectable (5% to 10%) ... 2716
Caduet Tablets (Greater than 0.1% to less than or equal to 1%) ... 2508
Campral Tablets (Infrequent) ... 1174
Camptosar Injection ... 2604
Capastat Sulfate for Injection ... 1755
Carafate Suspension (Less than 0.5%) ... 701
Carafate Tablets (Less than 0.5%) ... 701
Cardura XL Tablets (1.5%) ... 2515
▲ Carnitor Injection (2% to 6%) ... 3188
Celebrex Capsules (0.1% to 1.9%) ... 3134
Celexa (Infrequent) ... 1176
▲ CellCept Capsules (3% to less than 20%) ... 2747
▲ CellCept Intravenous (3% to less than 20%) ... 2747
▲ CellCept Oral Suspension (3% to less than 20%) ... 2747
▲ CellCept Tablets (3% to less than 20%) ... 2747
▲ Cesamet Capsules (52% to 59%) ... 3340
Chantix Tablets (Infrequent) ... 2517
Cialis Tablets (Less than 2%) ... 1838
Cipro XR Tablets (Less than 1%) ... 2990
Clinoril Tablets (Less than 1 in 100) ... 1924
Clorpres Tablets ... 2153
▲ Clozaril Tablets (More than 5% to 27%) ... 2184
Colocort Rectal Suspension, USP (Retention) 100 mg/60 mL ... 2476
▲ Copaxone for Injection (6%) ... 3297
▲ Coreg Tablets (Greater than 1% to 3%) ... 1414
Cosopt Sterile Ophthalmic Solution ... 1931
Cozaar Tablets (Less than 1%) ... 1935
Crestor Tablets (Greater than or equal to 1%) ... 678
Cubicin for Injection (Less than 1%) ... 1026

Albalon Ophthalmic Solution ⊙ 218
Aldoril Tablets 1910
▲ Alferon N Injection (3% to 6%) 1665
▲ Alphagan P Ophthalmic Solution (1% to 4%) 567
▲ Alrex Ophthalmic Suspension 0.2% (5% to 15%) ⊙ 246
Altoprev Extended-Release Tablets (0.9% to 1.2%) 3109
Ambien CR Tablets (2%) 2855
Amerge Tablets (Infrequent) 1339
Anaprox Tablets (Less than 1%) 2761
Anaprox DS Tablets (Less than 1%) 2761
Aricept Tablets (Frequent) 1094
Aricept ODT Tablets (Frequent) 1094
▲ Arranon Injection (4%) 1357
Arthrotec Tablets (Rare) 3129
Asacol Delayed-Release Tablets 2692
Atacand HCT 651
Atrovent Nasal Spray 0.03% (Less than 2%) 837
Atrovent Nasal Spray 0.06% (Less than 1%) 839
Avalide Tablets 888
Avalide Tablets 2874
Avandaryl Tablets 1379
▲ Azopt Ophthalmic Suspension (5% to 10%) 557
▲ Bentyl Capsules (27%) 697
▲ Bentyl Injection (27%) 697
▲ Bentyl Syrup (27%) 697
▲ Bentyl Tablets (27%) 697
Betimol Ophthalmic Solution (1% to 5%) 3382
Betimol Ophthalmic Solution (1% to 5%) ⊙ 295
Betoptic S Ophthalmic Suspension (Small number of patients) 558
Bicillin C-R Injectable Suspension 1706
▲ Brimonidine Tartrate Ophthalmic Solution 0.2% (10% to 30%) ⊙ 248
Captopril Tablets 2149
Carbatrol Capsules 3171
Cardura XL Tablets 2515
Carteolol Hydrochloride Ophthalmic Solution USP, 1% (Occasional) ⊙ 249
Catapres Tablets 843
Catapres-TTS (0.5% or less) 844
Celebrex Capsules (0.1% to 1.9%) 3134
Chantix Tablets (Infrequent) 2517
Cialis Tablets (Less than 2%) 1838
Ciloxan Ophthalmic Ointment (Less than 1%) 559
Ciloxan Ophthalmic Solution (Less than 1%) ⊙ 206
Cipro (Less than 1%) 2977
Cipro I.V. (1% or less) 2984
Cipro XR Tablets 2990
Clinoril Tablets (Less than 1 in 100) 1924
Clorpres Tablets 2153
Combivent Inhalation Aerosol 847
Concerta Extended-Release Tablets 1881
▲ Copegus Tablets (5%) 2754
▲ Coreg Tablets (Greater than 1% to 3%) 1414
▲ Cosopt Sterile Ophthalmic Solution (5% to 15%) 1931
Covera-HS Tablets (Less than 2%) 3139
Cozaar Tablets (Less than 1%) 1935
Cubicin for Injection (Less than 1%) 1026
Cutivate Lotion 0.05% (Rare) 2664
▲ Cymbalta Delayed-Release Capsules (4%) 1757
▲ Dacogen Injection (6%) 2129
Dalmane Capsules (Rare) 3342
Dapsone Tablets USP 1673
Daytrana Transdermal Patch 3174
▲ Depacon Injection (8% to 12%) 412
▲ Depakene (8% to 12%) 417
▲ Depakote Sprinkle Capsules (4% to 12%) 422
▲ Depakote Tablets (8% to 12%) 427
▲ Depakote ER Tablets (12%) 434
Detrol Tablets 2628
Detrol LA Capsules 2631
Dilaudid 440
Dilaudid Non-Sterile Powder 440
Dilaudid Oral Liquid (Less frequent) 445
Dilaudid Rectal Suppositories 440
Dilaudid Tablets 440
Dilaudid Tablets - 8 mg (Less frequent) 445
Dilaudid-HP (Less frequent) 442
Diovan HCT Tablets (Less frequent) 2196
▲ Ditropan XL Extended-Release Tablets (1% to 8%) 2413
Diuril Oral Suspension 1954
Diuril Sodium Intravenous 2467
Dolobid Tablets (Less than 1 in 100) 1955
Donnatal Extentabs 2493
Duetact Tablets (Less than 1%) 3226
DuoNeb Inhalation Solution 1058
Duragesic Transdermal System 2373
Dyazide Capsules 1423
EC-Naprosyn Delayed-Release Tablets (Less than 1%) 2761
Edecrin 1959
▲ Effexor Tablets (6%) 3411
▲ Effexor XR Capsules (4% to 8%) 3417
Eldepryl Capsules 3208
Equetro Extended-Release Capsules 3180
Eraxis for Injection (Less than 1% to less than 2%) 2521
Exelon Capsules (Infrequent) 2206
Exelon Oral Solution (Infrequent) 2206
Femara Tablets (Less than 1%) 2214
Flonase Nasal Spray 1440
FML Ophthalmic Suspension ⊙ 227
FML Forte Ophthalmic Suspension ⊙ 226
Focalin Tablets 2220
Focalin XR Capsules 2223
Fortical Nasal Spray (Less than 1%) 3337
Furosemide Tablets 2154
Gleevec Tablets (Less common) 2227
Hycotuss Expectorant Syrup 1117
Hyperstat I.V. 3017
Hytrin Capsules (0.6% to 1.6%) 471
Hyzaar 50-12.5 Tablets 1990
Hyzaar 100-12.5 Tablets 1990
Hyzaar 100-25 Tablets 1990
Indocin (Less than 1%) 1995
▲ Intron A for Injection (Less than 5%) 3024
Ionsys Transdermal System (.1% to less than 1%) 2379
Kadian Capsules (Less than 3%) 577
Ketek Tablets (Greater than or equal to 0.2% to less than 2%) 2903
Klonopin (1%) 2778
Koāte-DVI (0.7%) 3250
Lacrisert Sterile Ophthalmic Insert 2005
▲ Lamictal (4% to 25%) 1481
Lanoxicaps Capsules 1490
Lanoxin Injection 1494
Lanoxin Injection Pediatric 1497
Lanoxin Tablets 1500
Levitra Tablets (Less than 2%) 3034
Lexapro Oral Solution (Frequent) 1190
Lexapro Tablets (Frequent) 1190
Lidoderm Patch 1118
Lithobid Tablets 1692
Lofibra Tablets 1219
Lofibra Capsules 1216
Lopressor Injection 2238
Lopressor Tablets 2238
Lopressor HCT 50/25 Tablets (1%) 2241
Lopressor HCT 100/25 Tablets (1%) 2241
Lopressor HCT 100/50 Tablets (1%) 2241
▲ Lotemax Ophthalmic Suspension 0.5% (5% to 15%) ⊙ 251
Lotensin HCT Tablets 2246
▲ Lucentis Injection (4% to 17%) 1237
▲ Lyrica Capsules (1% to 12%) 2539
▲ Macugen Injection (10% to 40%) ⊙ 261
Maxalt Tablets (Infrequent) 2008
Maxalt-MLT Orally Disintegrating Tablets (Infrequent) 2008
Meridia Capsules 489
Metadate CD Capsules 3323
Mevacor Tablets (0.9% to 1.5%) 2021
Miacalcin Nasal Spray (Less than 1%) 2253
Micardis HCT Tablets 856
Mintezol 2027
Miradon Tablets 3042
Moban Tablets (Occasional) 1119
Moduretic Tablets 2028
MS Contin Tablets (Less frequent) 2701
▲ Myfortic Tablets (3% to less than 20%) 2255
Nadolol Tablets (1 to 5 of 1000 patients) 2159
Nalfon Capsules (2.2%) 2502
Namenda (Infrequent) 1195
Naprosyn Suspension (Less than 1%) 2761
Naprosyn Tablets (Less than 1%) 2761
Neumega for Injection 3435
Neurontin Capsules (2.7%) 2487
Neurontin Oral Solution (2.7%) 2487
Neurontin Tablets (2.7%) 2487
Nexium I.V. (Rare) 659
Nicomide Tablets 1088
▲ Niravam Orally Disintegrating Tablets (6.2% to 21%) 3092
Norflex Injection 1856
Noroxin Tablets (Less frequent) 2032
Norvir (Less than 2%) 503
Opana Tablets (Less than 1%) 1122
Opana ER Tablets (Less than 1%) 1126
OptiPranolol Metipranolol Ophthalmic Solution 0.3% (A small number of patients) ⊙ 256
Orthoclone OKT3 Sterile Solution 2360
Parcopa Orally Disintegrating Tablets 3097
Parnate Tablets 1527
▲ Patanol Ophthalmic Solution (Less than 5%) 561
▲ Paxil CR Controlled-Release Tablets (2.0% to 7.8%) 1538
▲ Paxil (2.0% to 7.8%) 1530
▲ Pegasys (4%) 2789
PEG-Intron Powder for Injection (2%) 3048
Phenergan Tablets and Suppositories 3440
Pred Forte Ophthalmic Suspension ⊙ 235
Prevacid NapraPAC (Less than 1%) 3280
Prilosec OTC Delayed-Release Tablets (Less than 1%) 2677
Prinivil Tablets (0.3% to 1.0%) 2052
Prinzide Tablets (0.3% to 1%) 2056
Propine Ophthalmic Solution ⊙ 239
Proquin XR Tablets 1153
Prosed/DS Tablets 1157
Protonix I.V. 3472
Protonix Tablets 3469
Ranexa Tablets (Less than or equal to 0.5%) 1035
▲ Rebetol (5% to 6%) 3058
Rescriptor Tablets 2551
▲ Restasis Ophthalmic Emulsion (1% to 5%) 575
Restoril Capsules (1.3%) 1860
▲ Retisert Implant (10% to 35%) ⊙ 258
Revatio Tablets 2557
▲ Revlimid Capsules (14.7%) 958
▲ Ribavirin, USP Capsules (5% to 6%) 3068
Ritalin Hydrochloride Tablets 2269
Ritalin LA Capsules 2271
Ritalin-SR Tablets 2269
▲ Romazicon Injection (1% to 9%) 2804
▲ Rythmol SR Capsules (1% to 6%) 2727
Sanctura Tablets (Greater than or equal to 0.5%) 1151
▲ Sandostatin Injection (1% to 4%) 2278
▲ Soriatane Capsules (1% to 10%) 1013
Stalevo Tablets 2287
Synera Topical Patch 1137
Tambocor Tablets 1856
Tarka Tablets (Less frequent) 524
Tasmar Tablets (1% or more) 3358
Tegretol/Tegretol-XR 2295
▲ Temodar Capsules (8%) 3073
Teveten HCT Tablets 1737
Thioridazine Hydrochloride Tablets 2163
Thiothixene Capsules (Infrequently) 2165
Timolide Tablets 2086
Timoptic-XE Sterile Ophthalmic Gel Forming Solution 2092
▲ Topamax Sprinkle Capsules (2% to 4%) 2404
▲ Topamax Tablets (2% to 4%) 2404
Toprol-XL Tablets 668
Transderm Scōp Transdermal Therapeutic System 2177
Tranxene (Less common) 2474
▲ Travatan Ophthalmic Solution (1% to 4%) 563
Trecator Tablets 3487
▲ Trisenox Injection (10%) 993
▲ Trusopt Sterile Ophthalmic Solution (Approximately 1% to 5%) 2095
▲ Ultram ER Tablets (1% to greater than 5%) 2392
Uniretic Tablets 3100
Valium Tablets (Infrequent) 2819
Vasotec I.V. Injection (0.5% to 1.0%) 2103
▲ Velcade for Injection (11%) 2133
Verelan PM Extended-Release Capsules, Controlled-Onset (2% or less) 3106
▲ VESIcare Tablets (3.8% to 4.8%) 646
▲ VFEND I.V. (Approximately 30%) 2564
▲ VFEND Oral Suspension (Approximately 30%) 2564
▲ VFEND Tablets (Approximately 30%) 2564
▲ Viagra Tablets (3%) 2573
Visine For Contacts Rewetting Drops ⊙ 289
▲ Visudyne for Injection (10% to 30%) 2305
▲ Voltaren Ophthalmic Solution (Less than or equal to 5%) 2309
Voltaren Tablets (Occasionally) 2307
Voltaren-XR Tablets (Occasionally) 2310
▲ Wellbutrin Tablets (14.6%) 1603
▲ Xalatan Sterile Ophthalmic Solution (5% to 15%) 2649
▲ Xyrem Oral Solution (Less than 1% to 5.9%) 1688
Zantac (Rare) 1624
Zantac Injection (Rare) 1619
Zantac Injection Pharmacy Bulk Package (Rare) 1622
Zantac Injection Premixed (Rare) 1619
Zantac (Rare) 1624
Zegerid Capsules (Less than 1%) 2958
Zegerid Powder for Oral Solution (Less than 1%) 2958
Zofran Injection 1634
Zometa for Intravenous Infusion 2315

Vision, changes
(*see under* Visual disturbances)

Vision, color tinge to
▲ Viagra Tablets (3%) 2573

Vision, complete loss
Ortho-Cyclen/Ortho Tri-Cyclen 2429
Ortho Tri-Cyclen Lo Tablets 2436
Premphase Tablets 3456
Prempro Tablets 3456

Vision, double
(*see under* Diplopia)

Vision, loss of
Imitrex Injection 1463
Imitrex Nasal Spray 1467
Imitrex Tablets 1471
Intron A for Injection 3024
Levitra Tablets (Rare) 3034
Nipent for Injection (Less than 3%) 1863
Ontak Vials 1745
Ortho Evra Transdermal System 2417
Pegasys 2789
PEG-Intron Powder for Injection 3048
Prinivil Tablets (0.3% to 1.0%) 2052
Prinzide Tablets 2056
Sutent Capsules 2560
Viagra Tablets 2573
▲ Visudyne for Injection (1% to 10%) 2305
Zyvox 2652

Vision, loss of color
Cipro (Less than 1%) 2977
Cipro I.V. (1% or less) 2984
Cipro XR Tablets 2990
Ontak Vials 1745

Vision, partial loss
Imitrex Tablets 1471
Mintezol 2027
Ortho-Cyclen/Ortho Tri-Cyclen 2429
Ortho Tri-Cyclen Lo Tablets 2436
Premphase Tablets 3456
Prempro Tablets 3456

Vision, temporary loss of
Sular Tablets (Less than or equal to 1%) 3122
Viagra Tablets 2573

Vision abnormalities
(*see under* Visual disturbances)

Visual acuity, decreased
Avandaryl Tablets (Very rare) 1379
Emend Capsules (Less than or equal to 0.5%) 1963
Ketek Tablets (Greater than or equal to 0.2% to less than 2%) 2903
Levitra Tablets (Rare) 3034
▲ Lucentis Injection (4% to 17%) 1237
▲ Macugen Injection (10% to 40%) ⊙ 261
Namenda (Infrequent) 1195
▲ Nevanac Ophthalmic Suspension 0.1% (5% to 10%) ⊙ 209
Proquin XR Tablets 1153
▲ Retisert Implant (10% to 35%) ⊙ 258
Rythmol SR Capsules 2727
▲ Vigamox Ophthalmic Solution (1% to 6%) 564

Visual acuity, defects
Alphagan P Ophthalmic Solution (1% to 4%) 567
Alrex Ophthalmic Suspension 0.2% ⊙ 246
Betoptic S Ophthalmic Suspension (Small number of patients) 558
Blephamide Ophthalmic Ointment 568

Blephamide Ophthalmic Suspension 569
Cipro (Less than 1%) 2977
Cipro I.V. (1% or less) 2984
Cozaar Tablets (Less than 1%) 1935
Eloxatin for Injection 2892
FML Ophthalmic Ointment ⊙ 228
FML Ophthalmic Suspension ⊙ 227
FML Forte Ophthalmic Suspension ⊙ 226
FML-S Ophthalmic Suspension ⊙ 229
Hyzaar 50-12.5 Tablets 1990
Hyzaar 100-12.5 Tablets 1990
Hyzaar 100-25 Tablets 1990
Intron A for Injection 3024
Lotemax Ophthalmic Suspension 0.5% ⊙ 251
PEG-Intron Powder for Injection (Less than or equal to 1%) 3048
Pred Mild Ophthalmic Suspension ⊙ 238
Pred Forte Ophthalmic Suspension ⊙ 235
Pred-G Ophthalmic Ointment ⊙ 237
Pred-G Ophthalmic Suspension ⊙ 236
Retisert Implant ⊙ 258
Symmetrel Tablets (0.1% to 1%) 1135
TobraDex Ophthalmic Ointment 562
TobraDex Ophthalmic Suspension 563
▲ Travatan Ophthalmic Solution (5% to 10%) 563
▲ Vesanoid Capsules (6%) 2820
▲ Vigamox Ophthalmic Solution (1% to 6%) ⊙ 215
Visine For Contacts Rewetting Drops ⊙ 289
▲ Visudyne for Injection (10% to 30%) 2305
▲ Zymar Ophthalmic Solution (1% to 4%) 575

Visual depth perception, altered

Ambien CR Tablets (1%) 2855
Cesamet Capsules 3340

Visual disturbances

Accutane Capsules 2731
Aciphex Tablets 1090
Actiq (1% to 2%) 979
Acular Ophthalmic Solution (Rare) 565
Adalat CC Tablets (Less than 1%) 2964
▲ Agrylin Capsules (1% to 5%) 3169
Alferon N Injection (1%) 1665
▲ Alphagan P Ophthalmic Solution (Approximately 5% to 9%) 567
▲ Alrex Ophthalmic Suspension 0.2% (5% to 15%) ⊙ 246
Altace Capsules (Less than 1%) 1702
Ambien Tablets (Frequent) 2851
▲ Ambien CR Tablets (3% to frequent) 2855
Anaprox Tablets (Less than 3%) 2761
Anaprox DS Tablets (Less than 3%) 2761
Anzemet Injection (Infrequently) 2859
Anzemet Tablets (Infrequently) 2862
Aralast (0.1%) 717
▲ Aromasin Tablets (5%) 2600
Arthrotec Tablets (Rare) 3129
Asacol Delayed-Release Tablets (2% or greater) 2692
Astelin Nasal Spray 1904
Atripla Tablets 945
Avalide Tablets 888
Avalide Tablets 2874
Avapro Tablets (Less than 1%) 891
Avapro Tablets (Less than 1%) 2871
Avelox (Less than 0.1%) 2970
BeneFix Vials (1.5%) 3408
Betagan Ophthalmic Solution, USP ⊙ 220
▲ Betimol Ophthalmic Solution (More than 5%) 3382
▲ Betimol Ophthalmic Solution (More than 5%) ⊙ 295
Blephamide Ophthalmic Suspension 569
Blocadren Tablets 1916
▲ Brimonidine Tartrate Ophthalmic Solution 0.2% (3% to 9%) ⊙ 248
Buprenex Injectable (Less than 1%) 2716
Caduet Tablets (Greater than 0.1% to less than or equal to 1%) 2508
Campral Tablets (Frequent) 1174
Carteolol Hydrochloride Ophthalmic Solution USP, 1% (Occasional) ⊙ 249
Celexa (At least 2%) 1176
▲ CellCept Capsules (3% to less than 20%) 2747
▲ CellCept Intravenous (3% to less than 20%) 2747
▲ CellCept Oral Suspension (3% to less than 20%) 2747
▲ CellCept Tablets (3% to less than 20%) 2747
▲ Cesamet Capsules (13%) 3340
Chantix Tablets (Infrequent) 2517
Cipro (Less than 1%) 2977
Cipro I.V. (1% or less) 2984
Cipro XR Tablets 2990
Clinoril Tablets (Less than 1 in 100) 1924
▲ Clozaril Tablets (5% or more) 2184
Colazal Capsules 2838
Comvax 1928
Concerta Extended-Release Tablets 1881
Copaxone for Injection (At least 2%) 3297
▲ Coreg Tablets (5%) 1414
Cosopt Sterile Ophthalmic Solution 1931
Cuprimine Capsules 1947
Dantrium Capsules (Less frequent) 2694
Daytrana Transdermal Patch 3174
▲ Depacon Injection (1% to 5%) 412
▲ Depakene (1% to 5%) 417
▲ Depakote Sprinkle Capsules (1% to 5%) 422
▲ Depakote Tablets (1% to 5%) 427
▲ Depakote ER Tablets (1% to 5%) 434
DepoCyt Injection 1143
▲ Detrol Tablets (4.7%) 2628
Detrol LA Capsules (1%) 2631
DextroStat Tablets 3179
Dilaudid 440
Dilaudid Non-Sterile Powder 440
Dilaudid Oral Liquid (Less frequent) 445
Dilaudid Rectal Suppositories 440
Dilaudid Tablets 440
Dilaudid Tablets - 8 mg (Less frequent) 445
Dilaudid-HP (Less frequent) 442
Diovan HCT Tablets (Greater than 0.2%) 2196
Dolobid Tablets (Less than 1 in 100) 1955
Doxil Injection (Less than 1%) 2351
DynaCirc CR Tablets (0.5% to 1%) 2721
EC-Naprosyn Delayed-Release Tablets (Less than 3%) 2761
Edex Injection (1%) 3089
Effexor Tablets (Frequent) 3411
▲ Effexor XR Capsules (4% to 5%) 3417
Eloxatin for Injection 2892
Enablex Extended-Release Tablets (Greater than or equal to 1%) 2203
Engerix-B Vaccine 1425
▲ Entocort EC Capsules (Less than 5%) 2698
Eraxis for Injection (Less than 1% to less than 2%) 2521
Estratest Tablets 3199
Estratest H.S. Tablets 3199
Estring Vaginal Ring 2635
▲ Evoxac Capsules (1% to 3%) 1047
▲ FazaClo Orally Disintegrating Tablets (Greater than 5%) 551
Ferrlecit Injection 3388
FML Ophthalmic Suspension ⊙ 227
FML Forte Ophthalmic Suspension ⊙ 226
FML-S Ophthalmic Suspension ⊙ 229
Focalin Tablets (Rare) 2220
Focalin XR Capsules 2223
Frova Tablets (Frequent) 1113
Gabitril Tablets (Frequent) 984
Garamycin Injectable 3014
Gengraf Capsules (1% to less than 3%) 459
Genotropin Lyophilized Powder (A small number of patients) 2638
▲ Geodon Capsules (3% to 6%) 2529
Humatrope Vials and Cartridges 1787
▲ Hycamtin for Injection (5%) 1458
Hytrin Capsules (At least 1%) 471
▲ Imdur Tablets (Less than or equal to 5%) 3018
Imitrex Injection (Frequent) 1463
Imitrex Nasal Spray (Infrequent) 1467
▲ Imitrex Tablets (Up to 3%) 1471
Increlex Injection 3291
Inderal LA Long-Acting Capsules 3429
▲ Infergen (3% to 5%) 3364
InnoPran XL Capsules 2723
▲ Intron A for Injection (Less than 5%) 3024
Invirase (Less than 2%) 2772
Ionsys Transdermal System (.1% to less than 1%) 2379
Kaletra (Less than 2%) 476
Ketek Tablets 2903
Klonopin (Infrequent) 2778
▲ Lamictal (2% to 3%) 1481
Lamisil Tablets (1.1%) 2232
Lanoxicaps Capsules 1490
Lanoxin Injection 1494
Lanoxin Injection Pediatric 1497
Lanoxin Tablets 1500
Lariam Tablets 2786
Levaquin (0.1% to 0.9%) 2384
Levaquin in 5% Dextrose Injection (0.1% to 0.9%) 2384
Levitra Tablets (Less than 2%) 3034
Lexapro Oral Solution (Infrequent) 1190
Lexapro Tablets (Infrequent) 1190
Lidoderm Patch 1118
Lofibra Tablets 1219
Lofibra Capsules 1216
Lopressor Injection 2238
Lopressor Tablets 2238
Lopressor HCT 50/25 Tablets 2241
Lopressor HCT 100/25 Tablets 2241
Lopressor HCT 100/50 Tablets 2241
▲ Lotemax Ophthalmic Suspension 0.5% (5% to 15%) ⊙ 251
Lotensin HCT Tablets (0.3% or more) 2246
▲ Lucentis Injection (0% to 14%) 1237
▲ Lumigan Ophthalmic Solution (3% to 10%) 573
Lupron Injection Pediatric 3259
▲ Lyrica Capsules (1% to 5%) 2539
▲ Macugen Injection (10% to 40%) ⊙ 261
Malarone Pediatric Tablets (2%) 1517
Malarone Tablets (2%) 1517
Marinol Capsules (Less than 1%) 3333
Meridia Capsules 489
Metadate CD Capsules 3323
Micardis Tablets (More than 0.3%) 854
Micardis HCT Tablets 856
Midamor Tablets (Less than or equal to 1%) 2026
Migranal Nasal Spray (Infrequent) 3348
▲ Mirapex Tablets (3%) 859
Mobic Oral Suspension (Less than 2%) 863
Mobic Tablets (Less than 2%) 863
Moduretic Tablets (Less than or equal to 1%) 2028
MS Contin Tablets (Less frequent) 2701
Myobloc Injection (Greater than 2%) 3192
Nadolol Tablets 2159
Naprosyn Suspension (Less than 3%) 2761
Naprosyn Tablets (Less than 3%) 2761
Neoral Oral Solution (1% to less than 3%) 2259
Neoral Soft Gelatin Capsules (1% to less than 3%) 2259
Neumega for Injection 3435
Neurontin Capsules (Frequent) 2487
Neurontin Oral Solution (Frequent) 2487
Neurontin Tablets (Frequent) 2487
Nexium Delayed-Release Capsules (Less than 1%) 655
Nexium I.V. (Less than 1%) 659
Nipent for Injection (Less than 3%) 1863
Norditropin Cartridges (Small number of patients) 2323
Noroxin Tablets 2032
Norvasc Tablets (More than 0.1% to 1%) 2545
Norvir (Less than 2%) 503
Nutropin for Injection (A small number of patients) 1239
Nutropin AQ Injection (A small number of patients) 1243
Nutropin AQ Pen (A small number of patients) 1243
Nutropin AQ Pen Cartridge (A small number of patients) 1243
Ontak Vials 1745
Opana Tablets (Less than 1%) 1122
Opana ER Tablets (Less than 1%) 1126
OptiPranolol Metipranolol Ophthalmic Solution 0.3% (A small number of patients) ⊙ 256
Ortho-Cyclen Tablets 2429
Ortho Evra Transdermal System 2417
Ortho Tri-Cyclen Tablets 2429
Ortho Tri-Cyclen Lo Tablets 2436
OxyContin Tablets (Less than 1%) 2703
Oxytrol Transdermal System (2.5%) 3392
▲ Paxil CR Controlled-Release Tablets (2% to 4%) 1538
▲ Paxil (2% to 4%) 1530
Pegasys 2789
PEG-Intron Powder for Injection 3048
Percodan Tablets 1132
▲ Permax Tablets (5.8%) 3356
Photofrin for Injection 702
Pred Forte Ophthalmic Suspension ⊙ 235
Premarin Tablets 3446
Premphase Tablets 3456
Prempro Tablets 3456
Prevacid Delayed-Release Capsules (Less than 1%) 3271
Prevacid for Delayed-Release Oral Suspension (Less than 1%) 3271
Prevacid SoluTab Delayed-Release Orally Disintegrating Tablets (Less than 1%) 3271
Prevacid NapraPAC (Less than 3%) 3280
PREVPAC (Less than 1%) 3284
▲ Prograf Capsules and Injection (3% to 15%) 632
▲ Proleukin for Injection (7%) 2266
Prometrium Capsules (100 mg, 200 mg) (Less than 5%) 3203
Proquin XR Tablets 1153
ProSom Tablets (Infrequent) 517
Protonix I.V. (Less than 1%) 3472
Protonix Tablets (Less than 1%) 3469
Protopic Ointment (0.2% to less than 1%) 638
Provigil Tablets (1%) 988
Prozac Pulvules and Liquid (2%) 1801
▲ Quixin Ophthalmic Solution (1% to 3%) 3383
▲ Rapamune Oral Solution and Tablets (3% to 20%) 3475
▲ Rebif Prefilled Syringe for Injection (7% to 13%) 3159
Recombivax HB (Less than 1%) 2071
ReFacto Vials 3484
Relpax Tablets (Infrequent) 2548
ReoPro Vials (0.7%) 1809
▲ Requip Tablets (6%) 1555
▲ Restasis Ophthalmic Emulsion (1% to 5%) 575
▲ Retisert Implant (5% to 9%) ⊙ 258
▲ Risperdal (1% to 6%) 1676
▲ Risperdal Consta Long-Acting Injection (2% to 3%) 1682
▲ Risperdal M-Tab Orally Disintegrating Tablets (1% to 6%) 1676
Ritalin Hydrochloride Tablets (Rare) 2269
Ritalin LA Capsules 2271
Ritalin-SR Tablets 2269
▲ Romazicon Injection (1% to 9%) 2804
Sanctura Tablets 1151
Sandimmune (Rare) 2275
▲ Sandostatin Injection (1% to 4%) 2278
▲ Sandostatin LAR Depot (1% to 4%) 2280
Seroquel Tablets (Infrequent) 690
▲ Simulect for Injection (3% to 10%) 2284
Sonata Capsules (Less than 1% to 2%) 1717
▲ Soriatane Capsules (1% to 10%) 1013
Sular Tablets (Less than or equal to 1%) 3122
Sustiva Capsules 930
Sustiva Tablets 930
Symbyax Capsules (Frequent) 1819
Symmetrel Tablets (0.1% to 1%) 1135
▲ Tambocor Tablets (15.9%) 1856
Taxotere Injection Concentrate (Rare) 2932
▲ Temodar Capsules (5%) 3073
▲ Tequin Injection (0.1% to 3%) 938
▲ Tequin Injection in 5% Dextrose (0.1% to 3%) 938
▲ Tequin Tablets (0.1% to 3%) 938
Teveten Tablets (Less than 1%) 1735
Teveten HCT Tablets (Less than 1%) 1737
Tev-Tropin for Injection (Small number of patients) 1222
Timolide Tablets 2086
Timoptic Sterile Ophthalmic Solution (Less frequent) 2088
Timoptic in Ocudose (Less frequent) 2091
Timoptic-XE Sterile Ophthalmic Gel Forming Solution 2092
▲ Topamax Sprinkle Capsules (1% to 13%) 2404
▲ Topamax Tablets (1% to 13%) 2404
▲ Travatan Ophthalmic Solution (1% to 4%) 563
Tricor Tablets 527
▲ Trileptal Tablets (2% to 14%) 2300
▲ Trileptal Oral Suspension (2% to 14%) 2300
Twinrix Vaccine 1595
Uniretic Tablets (Less than 1%) 3100
Valtrex Caplets 1597
▲ Vesanoid Capsules (17%) 2820
▲ VFEND I.V. (13.5% to 21%) 2564
▲ VFEND Oral Suspension (13.5% to 21%) 2564
▲ VFEND Tablets (13.5% to 21%) 2564
▲ Viagra Tablets (3%) 2573
Vicoprofen Tablets (Less than 1%) 539
Visine For Contacts Rewetting Drops ⊙ 289

▲ Visudyne for Injection (10% to 30%) 2305
▲ Voltaren Ophthalmic Solution (Less than or equal to 5%) 2309
Wellbutrin Tablets (Infrequent) 1603
▲ Xeloda Tablets (5%) 2822
Zelapar Tablets 3372
Zelnorm Tablets 2312
▲ Zoloft (4%) 2586
Zovirax 1643
Zyprexa Tablets (2%) 1830
Zyprexa ZYDIS Orally Disintegrating Tablets (2%) 1830

Visual disturbances, flashing lights

Cipro XR Tablets 2990
▲ Visudyne for Injection (10% to 30%) 2305

Visual field defect

▲ Agrylin Capsules (1% to 5%) 3169
▲ Alphagan P Ophthalmic Solution (1% to 4%) 567
Alrex Ophthalmic Suspension 0.2% .... ⊙246
Blephamide Ophthalmic Ointment 568
Blephamide Ophthalmic Suspension 569
Cesamet Capsules 3340
Chantix Tablets (Rare) 2517
Cialis Tablets 1838
▲ Cosopt Sterile Ophthalmic Solution (1% to 5%) 1931
Doxil Injection (Less than 1%) 2351
Effexor Tablets (Infrequent) 3411
Effexor XR Capsules (Infrequent) 3417
FML Ophthalmic Ointment .... ⊙228
FML Ophthalmic Suspension .... ⊙227
FML Forte Ophthalmic Suspension .... ⊙226
FML-S Ophthalmic Suspension .... ⊙229
Gabitril Tablets (Infrequent) 984
Geodon Capsules (Rare) 2529
Intron A for Injection 3024
Klonopin (Infrequent) 2778
Levitra Tablets (Rare) 3034
Lotemax Ophthalmic Suspension 0.5% .... ⊙251
Lyrica Capsules (Greater than or equal to 2%) 2539
Neurontin Capsules (Infrequent) 2487
Neurontin Oral Solution (Infrequent) 2487
Neurontin Tablets (Infrequent) 2487
Nexium Delayed-Release Capsules (Less than 1%) 655
Nexium I.V. (Less than 1%) 659
Norvir (Less than 2%) 503
Paxil CR Controlled-Release Tablets (Infrequent) 1538
Paxil (Infrequent) 1530
Permax Tablets (Infrequent) 3356
Pred Mild Ophthalmic Suspension .... ⊙238
Pred Forte Ophthalmic Suspension .... ⊙235
Pred-G Ophthalmic Suspension .... ⊙236
Prevacid Delayed-Release Capsules (Less than 1%) 3271
Prevacid for Delayed-Release Oral Suspension (Less than 1%) 3271
Prevacid SoluTab Delayed-Release Orally Disintegrating Tablets (Less than 1%) 3271
Prevacid NapraPAC (Less than 1%) 3280
PREVPAC (Less than 1%) 3284
ProAmatine Tablets (Rare) 3186
Prozac Pulvules and Liquid (Rare) 1801
Retisert Implant .... ⊙258
▲ Romazicon Injection (1% to 3%) 2804
Sandostatin LAR Depot (Rare) 2280
Sonata Capsules (Rare) 1717
Targretin Capsules 1747
TobraDex Ophthalmic Ointment 562
TobraDex Ophthalmic Suspension 563
Topamax Sprinkle Capsules (Infrequent) 2404
Topamax Tablets (Infrequent) 2404
▲ Vesanoid Capsules (3%) 2820
VFEND I.V. (Less than 2%) 2564
VFEND Oral Suspension (Less than 2%) 2564
VFEND Tablets (Less than 2%) 2564
▲ Visudyne for Injection (10% to 30%) 2305
Zoloft (Rare) 2586
Zomig Nasal Spray (Rare) 3523
Zonegran Capsules (Infrequent) 1101
Zyrtec Chewable Tablets (Less than 2%) 2594
Zyrtec (Less than 2%) 2594
Zyrtec-D 12 Hour Extended Release Tablets (Less than 2%) 2597

Visual impairment

Abelcet Injection 1141
Ciloxan Ophthalmic Ointment (Less than 1%) 559
Ciloxan Ophthalmic Solution (Less than 1%) .... ⊙206
Cipro XR Tablets 2990
Depo-Medrol Single-Dose Vial 2619
Ortho-Cyclen/Ortho Tri-Cyclen (Rare) 2429
Ortho Tri-Cyclen Lo Tablets 2436

Vitamin B12 deficiency

Nexium Delayed-Release Capsules (Less than 1%) 655
Nexium I.V. (Less than 1%) 659

Vitiligo

▲ Intron A for Injection (Less than 5%) 3024
Proleukin for Injection 2266
Trileptal Tablets 2300
Trileptal Oral Suspension 2300

Vitreous detachment

▲ Alphagan P Ophthalmic Solution (1% to 4%) 567
▲ Cosopt Sterile Ophthalmic Solution (1% to 5%) 1931
Evoxac Capsules (Less than 1%) 1047
▲ Nevanac Ophthalmic Suspension 0.1% (1% to 5%) .... ⊙209
Viagra Tablets 2573

Vitreous disorder, unspecified

▲ Macugen Injection (6% to 10%) .... ⊙261

Vitreous floaters

▲ Alphagan P Ophthalmic Solution (1% to 4%) 567
Chantix Tablets (Rare) 2517
Fortical Nasal Spray (Less than 1%) 3337
▲ Lucentis Injection (3% to 32%) 1237
▲ Macugen Injection (10% to 40%) .... ⊙261
Miacalcin Nasal Spray (Less than 1%) 2253
▲ Retisert Implant (10% to 35%) .... ⊙258
Sular Tablets (Less than or equal to 1%) 3122

Vitreous opacity

▲ Macugen Injection (10% to 40%) .... ⊙261
▲ Retisert Implant (5% to 9%) .... ⊙258

Voice, deepening of

▲ Androxy Tablets (Most Common) 3335
Estratest Tablets 3199
Estratest H.S. Tablets 3199
Oxandrin Tablets 2962

Voice, hoarseness

Estratest Tablets 3199
Estratest H.S. Tablets 3199

Voice, loss of
(*see under* Aphonia)

Voice alteration

Accutane Capsules 2731
Actiq (Less than 1%) 979
▲ Avastin IV (6% to 9%) 1227
▲ Avinza Capsules (Less than 5%) 1741
▲ Azmacort Inhalation Aerosol (1% to 3%) 1726
▲ CellCept Capsules (3% to less than 20%) 2747
▲ CellCept Intravenous (3% to less than 20%) 2747
▲ CellCept Oral Suspension (3% to less than 20%) 2747
▲ CellCept Tablets (3% to less than 20%) 2747
Cesamet Capsules 3340
Copaxone for Injection (Infrequent) 3297
Doxil Injection (Less than 1%) 2351
DuoNeb Inhalation Solution (More than 1%) 1058
Effexor Tablets (Infrequent) 3411
Effexor XR Capsules (Infrequent) 3417
Emend Capsules (Greater than 0.5%) 1963
Flonase Nasal Spray 1440
Gabitril Tablets (Infrequent) 984
Imitrex Injection 1463
Imitrex Nasal Spray (Rare) 1467
Imitrex Tablets (Rare) 1471
Invanz for Injection (Greater than 0.1%) 1999
Kadian Capsules (Less than 3%) 577
Lotensin HCT Tablets 2246
▲ Mirapex Tablets (Greater than or equal to 1%) 859
Neurontin Capsules (Rare) 2487
Neurontin Oral Solution (Rare) 2487
Neurontin Tablets (Rare) 2487
OxyContin Tablets (Less than 1%) 2703
Paxil CR Controlled-Release Tablets (Infrequent) 1538
Paxil (Infrequent) 1530
Permax Tablets (Infrequent) 3356
▲ Prograf Capsules and Injection (3% to 15%) 632
Protonix I.V. (Less than 1%) 3472
Protonix Tablets (Less than 1%) 3469
▲ Pulmozyme Inhalation Solution (12% to 18%) 1248
Relpax Tablets (Infrequent) 2548
Sonata Capsules (Infrequent) 1717
Symbyax Capsules (Infrequent) 1819
Thalomid Capsules 965
▲ TOBI Solution for Inhalation (13%) 2298
Uniretic Tablets (Less than 1%) 3100
VFEND I.V. (Less than 2%) 2564
VFEND Oral Suspension (Less than 2%) 2564
VFEND Tablets (Less than 2%) 2564
Zelapar Tablets 3372
Zomig Tablets (Rare) 3519
Zomig Nasal Spray (Infrequent) 3523
Zomig-ZMT Tablets (Rare) 3519
Zyprexa Tablets (Infrequent) 1830
Zyprexa ZYDIS Orally Disintegrating Tablets (Infrequent) 1830

Voice disorders

Exubera Inhalation Powder (0.1% to 1.3%) 2524

Vomiting

▲ Abelcet Injection (3% to 8%) 1141
▲ Abilify Oral Solution (Frequent to 11%) 882
▲ Abilify Oral Solution (Frequent to 11%) 2450
▲ Abilify Discmelt Orally Disintegrating Tablets (Frequent to 11%) 882
▲ Abilify Discmelt Orally Disintegrating Tablets (Frequent to 11%) 2450
▲ Abilify Tablets (Frequent to 11%) 882
▲ Abilify Tablets (Frequent to 11%) 2450
Accolate Tablets (1.5%) 671
Accutane Capsules 2731
Aceon Tablets (2 mg, 4 mg, 8 mg) (1.5%) 3194
▲ Acetadote Injection (9% to 12%) 1031
Aciphex Tablets 1090
▲ Actimmune (13%) 1671
▲ Actiq (6% to 15%) 979
Activase I.V. 1223
Actonel Tablets (1.9% to 2.5%) 2683
Actonel with Calcium Tablets (1.9% to 2.5%) 2688
▲ ADACEL Vaccine (0.5% to 4.6%) 2945
Adalat CC Tablets (Less than 1%) 2964
▲ Adderall XR Capsules (7%) 3166
▲ Advair Diskus 100/50 (4% to 5%) 1308
▲ Advair Diskus 250/50 (4% To 5%) 1308
▲ Advair Diskus 500/50 (4% to 5%) 1308
▲ Advair HFA Inhalation Aerosol (3% to 5%) 1318
▲ Advicor Tablets (3%) 1722
▲ Aerobid/Aerobid-M (25%) 1171
▲ Agenerase Capsules (9% to 34%) 1327
▲ Agenerase Oral Solution (9% to 34%) 1332
▲ Aggrenox Capsules (8.4%) 822
▲ Agrylin Capsules (9.7%) 3169
▲ Albenza Tablets (3.7% to 6.2%) 1338
Albutein 5%, Albumin (Human) 1652
Albutein 25% , Albumin (Human) 1653
Aldara Cream, 5% (1.4%) 1846
Aldoril Tablets 1910
▲ Alferon N Injection (3% to 29%) 1665
▲ Alimta for Injection (Up to 58%) 1750
Alinia for Oral Suspension (1.1%) 2835
Alinia Tablets (1.1%) 2835
Alkeran for Injection (Infrequent) 955
Alkeran Tablets (Infrequent) 956
Aloprim for Injection (1.2%) 2167
Alphanate, Antihemophilic Factor (Human) 1654
Altace Capsules (Less than 1% to 2%) 1702
Altoprev Extended-Release Tablets (0.5% to 1%) 3109
Alupent Inhalation Aerosol (Approximately 1 in 300 patients) 826
Ambien Tablets (1%) 2851
Ambien CR Tablets (Infrequent to 1%) 2855
▲ AmBisome for Injection (22.4% to 31.8%) 620
Amerge Tablets (Frequent) 1339
Aminohippurate Sodium PAH Injection 1913
▲ Amitiza Capsules (0% to 4.6%) 3224
Amoxil Capsules 1343
Amoxil Chewable Tablets 1343
Amoxil Pediatric Drops for Oral Suspension 1343
Amoxil Powder for Oral Suspension 1343
Amoxil Tablets 1343
▲ Anaprox Tablets (1% to 10%) 2761
▲ Anaprox DS Tablets (1% to 10%) 2761
Angeliq Tablets 762
▲ Aptivus Capsules (3.4%) 826
▲ Aranesp for Injection (15%) 581
▲ Aredia for Injection (35.7%) 2179
▲ Argatroban Injection (4.2% to 6.3%) 1346
▲ Aricept Tablets (3% to 8%) 1094
▲ Aricept ODT Tablets (3% to 8%) 1094
▲ Arimidex Tablets (8% to 11%) 673
▲ Arixtra Injection (0.6% to 5.9%) 1351
▲ Aromasin Tablets (7%) 2600
▲ Arranon Injection (0% to 22%) 1357
Arthrotec Tablets (Rare) 3129
▲ Asacol Delayed-Release Tablets (5%) 2692
Asmanex Twisthaler (1% to less than 3%) 2966
Astelin Nasal Spray (Infrequent) 1904
Atacand Tablets (More than 1%) 649
Atacand HCT (0.5% or greater) 651
Atripla Tablets (1%) 945
Augmentin (1%) 1360
Augmentin Tablets (1%) 1363
Augmentin XR Extended-Release Tablets 1369
Augmentin ES-600 Powder for Oral Suspension (2.2%) 1366
▲ Avalide Tablets (3%) 888
▲ Avalide Tablets (3%) 2874
▲ Avandamet Tablets (16%) 1373
Avandaryl Tablets (Less than 1%) 1379
▲ Avandia Tablets (3%) 1384
Avapro Tablets (1% or greater) 891
Avapro Tablets (1% or greater) 2871
▲ Avastin IV (47% to 52%) 1227
Avelox (0.1% to less than 2%) 2970
▲ Avinza Capsules (Greater than 10%) 1741
Axert Tablets (Infrequent) 2396
▲ Axid Oral Solution (1.2% to 3.6%) 879
▲ Azilect Tablets (7%) 3293
▲ Azmacort Inhalation Aerosol (1% to 3%) 1726
Baraclude (Less than 1%) 894
Bayer Aspirin (2.1%) 744
Bayer Aspirin Comprehensive Prescribing Information .... ▣796
BeneFix Vials (1.5%) 3408
Benicar Tablets 1043
Benicar HCT Tablets (Rare) 1044
Bentyl Capsules 697
Bentyl Injection 697
Bentyl Syrup 697
Bentyl Tablets 697
Betaseron for SC Injection 767
▲ Bexxar (1% to 15%) 1398
▲ Biaxin/Biaxin XL (6%) 402
Bicillin C-R Injectable Suspension 1706
▲ BiDil Tablets (4%) 2171
Biltricide Tablets 2976
Blocadren Tablets (Less than 1%) 1916
Boniva Injection (2.7%) 2738
Boniva Tablets (2.7%) 2741
▲ Boostrix (3% to 26%) 1404
Bumex Tablets (0.2% to 2.9%) 2746
▲ Buprenex Injectable (1% to 5%) 2716
▲ Byetta Injection (13%) 611
Caduet Tablets (Greater than 0.1% to less than 2%) 2508
Calcijex Injection 411
Calcium Disodium Versenate Injection 1851
▲ Campath Ampules (4% to 41%) 811
Campral Tablets 1174
▲ Camptosar Injection (12% to 67%) 2604
▲ Cancidas for Injection (1.2% to 3.5%) 1918
Captopril Tablets (About 0.5% to 2%) 2149
Carafate Suspension (Less than 0.5%) 701
Carafate Tablets (Less than 0.5%) 701
▲ Carbatrol Capsules (Among most frequent) 3171
▲ Cardene I.V. (4.9%) 2497
Cardura XL Tablets 2515
▲ Carnitor Injection (9% to 12%) 3188
Carnitor Tablets and Oral Solution 3190
▲ Catapres Tablets (About 5 in 100 patients) 843
Catapres-TTS (0.5% or less) 844

Ceftin (2.6%) 1407
Celebrex Capsules (0.1% to 1.9%) 3134
▲ Celexa (4%) 1176
▲ CellCept Capsules (32.9% to 33.9%) 2747
▲ CellCept Intravenous (32.9% to 33.9%) 2747
▲ CellCept Oral Suspension (32.9% to 33.9%) 2747
▲ CellCept Tablets (32.9% to 33.9%) 2747
▲ Cerezyme for Injection (Approximately 6.5%) 1270
Cervidil Vaginal Insert (Less than 1%) 1181
Cesamet Capsules 3340
▲ Chantix Tablets (1% to greater than 5%) 2517
▲ Chemet Capsules (12.0% to 20.9%) 2458
Cialis Tablets (Less than 2%) 1838
▲ Cipro (1% to 4.8%) 2977
▲ Cipro I.V. (1% to 4.8%) 2984
Cipro XR Tablets (1% to 2%) 2990
▲ Clarinex Syrup (6.1%) 2995
Cleocin Vaginal Ovules (Less than 1%) 2616
Climara Transdermal System 771
Climara Pro Transdermal System 776
Clinoril Tablets (Greater than 1%) 1924
▲ Clolar for Intravenous Infusion (83%) 1271
▲ Clorpres Tablets (About 5%) 2153
▲ Clozaril Tablets (3% to 17%) 2184
▲ Colazal Capsules (4%) 2838
Colyte with Flavor Packs for Oral Solution (Less frequent) 3088
Combivent Inhalation Aerosol (Less than 2%) 847
▲ Combivir Tablets (13%) 1411
▲ Comtan Tablets (4%) 2189
Comvax (1.0% to 2.5%) 1928
▲ Concerta Extended-Release Tablets (3% to 4%) 1881
▲ Copaxone for Injection (6%) 3297
▲ Copegus Tablets (25%) 2754
▲ Coreg Tablets (1% to 6%) 1414
Cosmegen for Injection (Common) 2459
▲ Cosopt Sterile Ophthalmic Solution (1% to 5%) 1931
Coumadin for Injection (Infrequent) 898
Coumadin Tablets (Infrequent) 898
Cozaar Tablets (Less than 1%) 1935
▲ Creon 5 Capsules (Among most frequent) 3198
▲ Creon 10 Capsules (Among most frequent) 3198
▲ Creon 20 Capsules (Among most frequent) 3199
Crestor Tablets (Greater than or equal to 1%) 678
▲ Crixivan Capsules (8.4%) 1940
▲ Cubicin for Injection (3.2% to 11.7%) 1026
Cuprimine Capsules (Greater than 1%) 1947
Cutivate Lotion 0.05% (1%) 2664
▲ Cymbalta Delayed-Release Capsules (5% to 6%) 1757
CytoGam Intravenous (Less than 5.0%) 1895
▲ Dacogen Injection (25%) 2129
Dalmane Capsules 3342
Dantrium Capsules (Rare) 2694
Dapsone Tablets USP 1673
▲ DAPTACEL Vaccine (4.3% to 6.9%) 2950
▲ Daranide Tablets (Among the most common effects) 1950
Daraprim Tablets 1419
▲ Daytrana Transdermal Patch (10%) 3174
Demadex Injection 2759
Demadex Tablets 2759
Demser Capsules (Infrequent) 1953
▲ Depacon Injection (1.3% to 27%) 412
▲ Depakene (23% to 27%) 417
▲ Depakote Sprinkle Capsules (15% to 27%) 422
▲ Depakote Tablets (11% to 27%) 427
▲ Depakote ER Tablets (7% to 27%) 434
▲ DepoCyt Injection (3% to 12%) 1143
▲ DepoDur Extended-Release Injection (Greater than 10%) 1110
▲ Detrol Tablets (4.2%) 2628
Diastat Rectal Delivery System (Less than 1%) 3343
Dilaudid (Infrequent) 440
Dilaudid Non-Sterile Powder (Infrequent) 440
Dilaudid Oral Liquid 445
Dilaudid Rectal Suppositories (Infrequent) 440
Dilaudid Tablets (Infrequent) 440
Dilaudid Tablets - 8 mg 445
▲ Dilaudid-HP (Among most frequent) 442
Diovan Tablets (Less frequent) 2193
Diovan HCT Tablets (Greater than 0.2%) 2196
Diuril Oral Suspension 1954
Diuril Sodium Intravenous 2467
Dolobid Tablets (Greater than 1 in 100) 1955
Donnatal Extentabs 2493
▲ Doxil Injection (7.8% to 32.6%) 2351
Duetact Tablets (Less than 1%) 3226
▲ Duragesic Transdermal System (Greater than 10% to 33%) 2373
Dyazide Capsules 1423
DynaCirc CR Tablets (0.5% to 1%) 2721
Dyrenium Capsules (Rare) 3400
▲ EC-Naprosyn Delayed-Release Tablets (1% to 10%) 2761
Edecrin 1959
▲ E.E.S. (Among most frequent) 451
▲ Effexor Tablets (6% to 7.9%) 3411
▲ Effexor XR Capsules (3% to 5%) 3417
Eldepryl Capsules 3208
▲ Elidel Cream 1% (0.6% to 8%) 2200
▲ Elitek (50%) 2890
Elmiron Capsules (Less than or equal to 1%) 2415
▲ Eloxatin for Injection (6% to 47%) 2892
Elspar for Injection 2463
Elspar for Injection 1960
Emcyt Capsules (1%) 2634
▲ Emend Capsules (7.5%) 1963
▲ Emtriva Capsules (9%) 1287
▲ Emtriva Oral Solution (9%) 1287
Enablex Extended-Release Tablets (Greater than or equal to 1%) 2203
▲ Enbrel for Injection (3% to 5%) 584
Engerix-B Vaccine (Less than 1%) 1425
Enjuvia Tablets 1062
▲ Entocort EC Capsules (6%) 2698
EpiPen 1061
▲ Epivir (13%) 1427
▲ Epivir-HBV (15%) 1432
▲ Epogen for Injection (0.26% to 29%) 591
▲ Equetro Extended-Release Capsules (18%) 3180
Eraxis for Injection (0.7%) 2521
▲ Erbitux (Less than 1% to 41%) 910
▲ EryPed (Among most frequent) 447
▲ Ery-Tab Tablets (Among most frequent) 449
▲ Erythrocin Stearate Filmtab Tablets (Among most frequent) 453
▲ Erythromycin Base Filmtab Tablets (Among most frequent) 455
▲ Erythromycin Delayed-Release Capsules, USP (Among most frequent) 457
Estrasorb Topical Emulsion 1147
Estratest Tablets 3199
Estratest H.S. Tablets 3199
Estring Vaginal Ring 2635
▲ Ethyol for Injection (8% to 96%) 1898
▲ Eulexin Capsules (11%) 3009
▲ Evista Tablets (3.4% to 4.8%) 1763
▲ Evoxac Capsules (4.6%) 1047
▲ Exelon Capsules (17% to 31%) 2206
▲ Exelon Oral Solution (17% to 31%) 2206
Fabrazyme for Intravenous Infusion 1274
▲ Famvir Tablets (1.3% to 4.8%) 2211
Fansidar Tablets 2765
▲ Faslodex Injection (13%) 681
▲ FazaClo Orally Disintegrating Tablets (3% to 17%) 551
▲ Femara Tablets (7%) 2214
▲ Ferrlecit Injection (2% to 35%) 3388
Flomax Capsules (Infrequent) 850
▲ Flonase Nasal Spray (2.6% to 4.8%) 1440
▲ Flovent Diskus (4% to 9%) 1443
Floxin Otic Solution (0.3%) 1049
Fluarix (1.4%) 1451
Flumadine (1.7%) 1183
▲ Flumist Vaccine (4.7% to 5.6%) 1901
Fluorescite Injection ⊙207
Focalin Tablets 2220
Follistim AQ Cartridge 2338
Fortaz (1 in 500 patients) 1453
▲ Forteo for Injection (3%) 1767
Fortical Nasal Spray (Less than 1%) 3337
Fosamax (0.2% to 1%) 1969
Fosamax Plus D Tablets (0.2% to 1%) 1977
▲ Fosrenol Chewable Tablets (9% to 26%) 3183
Frova Tablets (Frequent) 1113
Furosemide Tablets 2154
▲ Gabitril Tablets (7%) 984
▲ Gammagard Liquid (1.21% to 14.8%) 721
Gammagard S/D (Occasional) 724
▲ Gamunex Immune Globulin I.V., 10% (13% to 21%) 3235
Gantrisin Pediatric Suspension 2770
Garamycin Injectable 3014
Gardasil Injection (2.4%) 1984
▲ Gemzar for Injection (58% to 71%) 1771
▲ Gengraf Capsules (2% to 10%) 459
Genotropin Lyophilized Powder (A small number of patients) 2638
▲ Geodon (5%) 2529
▲ Gleevec Tablets (1.5% to 58%) 2227
GlucaGen (Occassional) 761
Glucagon for Injection Vials and Emergency Kit (Occasional) 1778
Gris-PEG Tablets (Occassional) 2502
▲ HalfLytely and Bisacodyl Tablets Bowel Prep Kit with Flavors Packs (5.9%) 881
Havrix Vaccine (Less than 1%) 1456
▲ Hectorol Capsules (21.3%) 1275
▲ Hectorol Injection (21.3%) 1278
Hepsera Tablets (2% or greater) 1292
▲ Herceptin I.V. (8% to 23%) 1233
HibTITER (9 of 1,118 vaccinations) 3426
Human Albumin Grifols 20%, Albumin (Human) 1651
Human Albumin Grifols 25%, Albumin (Human) 1652
Humatrope Vials and Cartridges 1787
▲ Humira Injection (Less than 5%) 466
▲ Hycamtin for Injection (Less than 1% to 58%) 1458
Hycodan 1116
Hycotuss Expectorant Syrup 1117
▲ Hyperstat I.V. (4%) 3017
Hytrin Capsules (At least 1%) 471
Hyzaar 50-12.5 Tablets 1990
Hyzaar 100-12.5 Tablets 1990
Hyzaar 100-25 Tablets 1990
▲ Imdur Tablets (Less than or equal to 5%) 3018
▲ Imitrex Injection (4%) 1463
▲ Imitrex Nasal Spray (11% to 13.5%) 1467
Imitrex Tablets (Greater than 1%) 1471
▲ Increlex Injection (Greater than or equal to 5%) 3291
▲ Indapamide Tablets (Less than 5%) 2156
Inderal LA Long-Acting Capsules 3429
▲ Indocin I.V. (1% to 3%) 2465
▲ Infanrix Vaccine (3.3% to 6.6.%) 1476
Infed Injection 3390
▲ Infergen (12% to 13%) 3364
InnoPran XL Capsules 2723
▲ Intron A for Injection (1% to 66%) 3024
▲ Invanz for Injection (3.7% to 10.2%) 1999
▲ Invirase (Less than 2% to 7.4%) 2772
▲ Ionsys Transdermal System (12%) 2379
▲ Iressa Tablets (10% to 12%) 684
▲ I.V. Busulfex (43% to 95%) 2493
Kadian Capsules (Less than 3%) 577
▲ Kaletra (2% to 6%) 476
K-Dur Extended-Relase Tablets 3033
Keflex Capsules (Rare) 549
Keppra Injection 3320
▲ Keppra Oral Solution (1% to 15%) 3314
▲ Keppra Tablets (1% to 15%) 3314
Ketek Tablets (2.4% to 2.9%) 2903
▲ K-Lor Oral Solution (Among most common) 474
K-Phos Original (Sodium Free) Tablets 760
K-Phos Neutral Tablets 760
Kristalose for Oral Solution 1034
▲ K-Tab Tablets (Most common) 475
Kionex Powder 2477
▲ Kytril (9% to 12%) 2784
▲ Lamictal (5% to 20%) 1481
Lamisil Tablets 2232
Lanoxicaps Capsules (Common) 1490
Lanoxin Injection (Common) 1494
Lanoxin Injection Pediatric 1497
Lanoxin Tablets (Common) 1500
▲ Lariam Tablets (Among most frequent) 2786
Lescol Capsules 2233
Lescol XL Tablets 2233
Leukeran Tablets (Infrequent) 1504
▲ Leukine (46% to 85%) 814
▲ Leustatin Injection (13%) 2357
Levaquin (0.3% to 2.4%) 2384
Levaquin in 5% Dextrose Injection (0.3% to 2.4%) 2384
Levitra Tablets (Less than 2%) 3034
Levothroid Tablets 1186
Levoxyl Tablets 1712
▲ Lexapro Oral Solution (3%) 1190
▲ Lexapro Tablets (3%) 1190
▲ Lexiva Tablets (2% to 20%) 1505
Lidoderm Patch 1118
Limbrel Capsules (0.011%) 2672
Lipitor Tablets (Less than 2%) 2483
Lithobid Tablets 1692
▲ Lithostat Tablets (20% to 25%) 2140
Lofibra Tablets 1219
Lofibra Capsules 1216
Lopressor Injection 2238
Lopressor Tablets 2238
Lopressor HCT 50/25 Tablets (1%) 2241
Lopressor HCT 100/25 Tablets (1%) 2241
Lopressor HCT 100/50 Tablets (1%) 2241
Lotensin Tablets (Less than 1%) 2243
Lotensin HCT Tablets (0.3% to 1%) 2246
▲ Lunesta Tablets (0% to 3%) 3142
▲ Lupron Depot 3.75 mg (13%) 3260
▲ Lupron Depot–3 Month 11.25 mg (13%) 3265
Lupron Depot-PED 7.5 mg, 11.25 mg and 15 mg (Less than 2%) 3269
Lupron Injection Pediatric (Less than 2%) 3259
▲ Lyrica Capsules (1% to 3%) 2539
▲ Macugen Injection (1% to 5%) ⊙261
▲ Malarone Pediatric Tablets (Less than 1% to 19%) 1517
▲ Malarone Tablets (Less than 1% to 19%) 1517
▲ Marinol Capsules (3% to 10%) 3333
▲ Matulane Capsules (Among most frequent) 3191
Mavik Tablets (0.3% to 1.0%) 486
Maxair Autohaler 1852
Maxalt Tablets (Frequent) 2008
Maxalt-MLT Orally Disintegrating Tablets (Frequent) 2008
Maxipime for Injection (Greater than 0.1% to 1%) 1105
Mefoxin for Injection (Rare) 2012
Mefoxin Premixed Intravenous Solution (Rarely) 2016
▲ Megace ES Oral Suspension (0% to 6%) 2481
Menactra Vaccine (0.2% to 2.3%) 2954
Menostar Transdermal System 782
▲ Mepron Suspension (1.3% to 22%) 1521
Meridia Capsules (1.5%) 489
▲ Merrem I.V. (0.8% to 3.6%) 686
Meruvax II 2019
▲ MetroGel-Vaginal Gel (4%) 1855
Mevacor Tablets (0.5% to 1.0%) 2021
▲ Miacalcin Injection (About 10%) 2252
Miacalcin Nasal Spray (Less than 1% to 1.8%) 2253
Micardis Tablets (More than 0.3%) 854
Micardis HCT Tablets (Less than 2%) 856
▲ Midamor Tablets (3% to 8%) 2026
▲ Migranal Nasal Spray (4%) 3348
Mintezol 2027
Miradon Tablets 3042
Mirapex Tablets (1% or more) 859
Mircette Tablets 1066
M-M-R II 2006
Mobic Oral Suspension (0.6% to 1.8%) 863
Mobic Tablets (0.6% to 1.8%) 863
Moduretic Tablets (Less than or equal to 1%) 2028
▲ MoviPrep Oral Solution (7.8%) 2839
▲ MS Contin Tablets (Among most frequent) 2701
Mustargen for Injection 2468
Mycamine for Injection (1.2% to 2.4%) 628
▲ Myfortic Tablets (3% to 23%) 2255
Myleran Tablets 1525
▲ Mylotarg for Injection (53% to 66%) 3431
Myobloc Injection (Greater than 2%) 3192
▲ Myozyme for Intravenous Infusion (49%) 1279
Nadolol Tablets (1 to 5 of 1000 patients) 2159
Nalfon Capsules (2.6%) 2502
▲ Namenda (3%) 1195
▲ Naprosyn Suspension (1% to 10%) 2761
▲ Naprosyn Tablets (1% to 10%) 2761
Nasacort AQ Nasal Spray 2922
▲ Nasonex Nasal Spray (1% to 5%) 3043
▲ Natrecor for Injection (1% to 4%) 3127
Nembutal Sodium Solution, USP (Less than 1%) 2470
▲ Neoral Oral Solution (2% to 10%) 2259
▲ Neoral Soft Gelatin Capsules (2% to 10%) 2259
▲ Neulasta Injection (15% to 72%) 601
▲ Neumega for Injection (77%) 3435
▲ Neupogen for Injection (7% to 57%) 603

▲ Neurontin Capsules (1% to 8.4%) 2487
▲ Neurontin Oral Solution (1% to 8.4%) 2487
▲ Neurontin Tablets (1% to 8.4%) 2487
▲ Nevanac Ophthalmic Suspension 0.1% (1% to 4%) ⊙209
▲ Nexavar Tablets (0% to 16%) 746
Nexium Delayed-Release Capsules (Less than 1%) 655
Nexium I.V. (Less than 1%) 659
Nicomide Tablets 1088
Nimotop Capsules (Less than 1%) 749
▲ Nipent for Injection (53% to 63%) 1863
▲ Niravam Orally Disintegrating Tablets (9.6% to 22%) 3092
Nitrolingual Pumpspray (Uncommon) 3120
Norditropin Cartridges (Small number of patients) 2323
Norflex Injection 1856
Noroxin Tablets (0.3 to 1.0%) 2032
Norvasc Tablets (More than 0.1% to 1%) 2545
▲ Norvir (13.7% to 17.4%) 503
NovoSeven (1%) 2331
Numorphan Injection 1120
Nutropin for Injection (A small number of patients) 1239
Nutropin AQ Injection (A small number of patients) 1243
Nutropin AQ Pen (A small number of patients) 1243
Nutropin AQ Pen Cartridge (A small number of patients) 1243
NuvaRing 2340
Omacor Capsules 2725
Omnicef Capsules (0.7%) 511
Omnicef for Oral Suspension (1%) 511
▲ Oncaspar (Greater than 5%) 1145
▲ Ontak Vials (64%) 1745
▲ Opana Tablets (6.8%) 1122
▲ Opana ER Tablets (0% to 15.6%) 1126
Oracea Capsules 1000
Ortho-Cyclen Tablets 2429
Ortho Evra Transdermal System (1% to 2.4%) 2417
Ortho Tri-Cyclen Tablets 2429
Ortho Tri-Cyclen Lo Tablets 2436
▲ Orthoclone OKT3 Sterile Solution (19%) 2360
▲ OsmoPrep Tablets (4% to 10%) 2840
Oxandrin Tablets 2962
▲ OxyContin Tablets (Less than 1% to 12%) 2703
▲ OxyFast Oral Concentrate Solution (Among most frequent) 2708
▲ OxyIR Capsules (Among most frequent) 2708
Paddock Nystatin USP for Oral Suspension 2478
▲ Pancrease MT Capsules (Among most frequent) 1885
Parcopa Orally Disintegrating Tablets 3097
▲ Paser Granules (Among most common) 1674
▲ Paxil CR Controlled-Release Tablets (1% to 3%) 1538
▲ Paxil (1% to 3%) 1530
▲ PCE Dispertab Tablets (Among most frequent) 515
Pediarix Vaccine 1548
▲ Pegasys (24%) 2789
▲ PEG-Intron Powder for Injection (7%) 3048
Pentasa Capsules (1.5%) 3185
Pepcid Injection (Infrequent) 2040
Pepcid (Infrequent) 2038
▲ Percocet Tablets (Among most frequent) 1131
▲ Percodan Tablets (Among most frequent) 1132
Permax Tablets (2.7%; Frequent) 3356
Persantine Tablets 868
Phenergan Tablets and Suppositories 3440
Phenytek Capsules 2160
PhosLo GelCaps 2169
▲ Photofrin for Injection (17% to 34%) 702
▲ Plan B Tablets (5.6%) 1076
Plavix Tablets (1% to 2.5%) 917
Plavix Tablets (1% to 2.5%) 2926
Pletal Tablets (2% or greater) 2455
Pneumovax 23 2043
Premarin Intravenous 3442
Premarin Tablets 3446
Premarin Vaginal Cream 3452
Premphase Tablets 3456
Prempro Tablets 3456
Prevacid Delayed-Release Capsules (Less than 1%) 3271
Prevacid for Delayed-Release Oral Suspension (Less than 1%) 3271
Prevacid SoluTab Delayed-Release Orally Disintegrating Tablets (Less than 1%) 3271
Prevacid I.V. for Injection (Less than 1%) 3277
Prevacid NapraPAC (Less than 1%) 3280
▲ Prevnar for Injection (4.9% to 16.8%) 3463
▲ PREVPAC (3% to 6%) 3284
Prezista Tablets (1.5% to 2.4%) 3306
▲ Prilosec OTC Delayed-Release Tablets (1.5% to 3.2%) 2677
Primaxin I.M. (0.3%) 2045
Primaxin I.V. (Up to 1.5%) 2048
Prinivil Tablets (0.3% to 1.0%) 2052
Prinzide Tablets (1.4%) 2056
▲ Prochieve 4% Gel (5%) 1003
▲ Prochieve 8% Gel (5%) 1003
▲ Procrit for Injection (0.26% to 29%) 2364
Profilnine SD, Factor IX Complex (Human) 1660
▲ Prograf Capsules and Injection (14% to 29%) 632
▲ Proleukin for Injection (50%) 2266
▲ Prometrium Capsules (100 mg, 200 mg) (5% to 8%) 3203
ProQuad (Greater than or equal to 0.2% to less than 1%) 2064
Proquin XR Tablets (Less than 1%) 1153
Prosed/DS Tablets 1157
ProSom Tablets (Infrequent) 517
Protonix I.V. (Greater than 1%) 3472
Protonix Tablets (2%) 3469
▲ Protopic Ointment (1% to 5%) 638
Proventil Inhalation Aerosol 3053
▲ Proventil HFA Inhalation Aerosol (7%) 3056
Provigil Tablets (Greater than or equal to 1%) 988
▲ Prozac Pulvules and Liquid (3%) 1801
▲ Pulmicort Respules (2% to 4%) 661
▲ Quadramet Injection (32.7%) 1040
Ranexa Tablets (Greater than 0.5% to less than 2%) 1035
Raniclor Tablets, Chewable (Rare) 2505
▲ Rapamune Oral Solution and Tablets (19% to 25%) 3475
▲ Razadyne (6% to 13%) 2399
▲ Razadyne ER Extended-Release Capsules (6% to 13%) 2399
▲ Rebetol (9% to 42%) 3058
▲ Rebetron Combination Therapy (9% to 12%) 3063
Recombivax HB (Less to greater than 1%) 2071
ReFacto Vials 3484
Relenza Rotadisk (1% to 2%) 1552
▲ Renagel Tablets (22.2%) 1282
▲ ReoPro Vials (11.4%) 1809
▲ Requip Tablets (7% to 12%) 1555
▲ Rescriptor Tablets (2.5% to 6.5%) 2551
Restoril Capsules (0.5% to 0.9%) 1860
Retavase 2499
▲ Retisert Implant (5% to 15%) ⊙258
▲ Retrovir Capsules (4.8% to 25%) 1560
▲ Retrovir IV Infusion (6% to 25%) 1564
▲ Retrovir (4.8% to 25%) 1560
▲ Revlimid Capsules (1.4% to 10.1%) 958
▲ Reyataz Capsules (6% to 8%) 921
▲ R-Gene 10 for Intravenous Use (3%) 2641
Rhophylac (Rare) 3505
▲ Ribavirin, USP Capsules (9% to 42%) 3068
▲ Rilutek Tablets (4.2% to 4.5%) 2930
▲ Risperdal (5% to 7%) 1676
Risperdal Consta Long-Acting Injection (Frequent) 1682
▲ Risperdal M-Tab Orally Disintegrating Tablets (5% to 7%) 1676
▲ Rituxan I.V. (1% to 10%) 1254
Rocaltrol Capsules 2798
Rocaltrol Oral Solution 2798
Rocephin Injectable Vials, ADD-Vantage, Galaxy, Bulk (Less than 1%) 2800
▲ Romazicon Injection (11%) 2804
▲ RotaTeq (2.9% to 15.2%) 2074
▲ Rythmol SR Capsules (1% to 6%) 2727
Sanctura Tablets (Greater than or equal to 0.5%) 1151
▲ Sandimmune (2% to 10%) 2275
▲ Sandostatin Injection (Less than 10% to 35%) 2278
▲ Sandostatin LAR Depot (6.5%) 2280
Seasonique Tablets 1077
▲ Sensipar Tablets (27%) 608
▲ Serevent Diskus (3%) 1568
▲ Seroquel Tablets (6%) 690
▲ Simulect for Injection (Greater than or equal to 10%) 2284
Singulair 2077
▲ Skelaxin Tablets (Most frequent) 1716
Soriatane Capsules 1013
▲ Spiriva HandiHaler (1% to 4%) 869
St. Joseph 81 mg Aspirin Chewable and Enteric Coated Tablets 1869
St. Joseph 81 mg Aspirin ■688
▲ Stalevo Tablets (4%) 2287
▲ Strattera Capsules (0.5% to 15%) 1814
Striant Mucoadhesive 1007
Stromectol Tablets (0.9%) 2083
▲ Suboxone Tablets (5% to 7.5%) 2717
▲ Subutex Tablets (5% to 7.8%) 2717
Suprax (Less than 2%) 1843
▲ Sustiva Capsules (3% to 16%) 930
▲ Sustiva Tablets (3% to 16%) 930
▲ Sutent Capsules (2% to 37%) 2560
Symbicort 80/4.5 Inhalation Aerosol (1.4%) 3511
▲ Symbicort 160/4.5 Inhalation Aerosol (3.2%) 3511
Symbyax Capsules (Infrequent) 1819
▲ Symlin Injection (7% to 11%) 613
Symmetrel Tablets (0.1% to 1%) 1135
Synagis (More than 1%) 1897
Synera Topical Patch (Less than or equal to 1%) 1137
Tabloid Tablets (Less frequent) 1575
▲ Tambocor Tablets (1% to 3%) 1856
▲ Tamiflu Capsules (2% to 15%) 2807
▲ Tamiflu Oral Suspension (2% to 15%) 2807
▲ Tarceva Tablets (Less than 1% to 42%) 1259
▲ Tarceva Tablets (Less than 1% to 42%) 2444
▲ Targretin Capsules (3.6% to 13.2%) 1747
▲ Tasmar Tablets (8% to 10%) 3358
▲ Taxotere Injection Concentrate (2.8% to 66.5%) 2932
▲ Tegretol/Tegretol-XR (Among most frequent) 2295
▲ Temodar Capsules (29% to 51%) 3073
▲ Tequin Injection (0.1% to 3%) 938
▲ Tequin Injection in 5% Dextrose (0.1% to 3%) 938
▲ Tequin Tablets (0.1% to 3%) 938
Teveten Tablets (Less than 1%) 1735
Teveten HCT Tablets (Less than 1%) 1737
Tev-Tropin for Injection (Small number of patients) 1222
Thalomid Capsules 965
▲ Thiola Tablets (16.7%) 2141
Thioridazine Hydrochloride Tablets 2163
Thiothixene Capsules 2165
Thyrogen for Injection (2.1%) 1286
Tiazac Capsules (Less than 2%) 1201
Ticlid Tablets (1.9%) 2810
Timentin ADD-Vantage 1580
Timentin Injection Galaxy Container 1583
Timentin IV Infusion 1577
Timentin Pharmacy Bulk Package 1586
Timolide Tablets 2086
Timoptic Sterile Ophthalmic Solution 2088
Timoptic in Ocudose 2091
Timoptic-XE Sterile Ophthalmic Gel Forming Solution 2092
Tindamax Tablets (0.9% to 1.5%) 2142
TNKase I.V. 1264
▲ TOBI Solution for Inhalation (14%) 2298
▲ Topamax Sprinkle Capsules (1% to 3%) 2404
▲ Topamax Tablets (1% to 3%) 2404
Toprol-XL Tablets 668
Tracleer Tablets 545
Transderm Scōp Transdermal Therapeutic System (Few patients) 2177
▲ Trasylol Injection (3%) 754
Trecator Tablets 3487
Trelstar Depot (2.1%) 3394
Tricor Tablets 527
Triglide Tablets 3123
▲ Trileptal Tablets (5% to 36%) 2300
▲ Trileptal Oral Suspension (5% to 36%) 2300
TriLyte with Flavor Packs for Oral Solution 3100
▲ Trisenox Injection (58%) 993
▲ Trizivir Tablets (12% to 30%) 1589
Truvada Tablets (1%) 1296
Tussionex Pennkinetic Extended-Release Suspension 3327
Twinject 0.3 3378
Twinject 0.15 3379
Twinrix Vaccine (Up to 1%) 1595
▲ Tygacil for Injection (19.5% to 20%) 3488
▲ Tylenol with Codeine Tablets (Among most frequent) 2391
▲ Ultane Liquid for Inhalation (18%) 531
▲ Ultram ER Tablets (5% to 9.4%) 2392
Uniphyl Tablets 2710
Uniretic Tablets (Less than 1%) 3100
Univasc Tablets (Less than 1%) 3104
Urocit-K Tablets (Some patients) 2144
Uroqid-Acid No. 2 Tablets 760
Urso 250 Tablets 710
Urso Forte Tablets 710
▲ Valcyte Tablets (21%) 2813
▲ Valtrex Caplets (Less than 1% to 6%) 1597
Vandazole Vaginal Gel (Less than 1%) 3338
Vantin Tablets and Oral Suspension (1%) 2645
▲ Vaprisol (6.6%) 643
▲ Vaqta (1% to 4%) 2097
Varivax (Greater than or equal to 1%) 2100
Vasotec I.V. Injection (1.3%) 2103
▲ Velcade for Injection (35%) 2133
▲ Ventavis Inhalation Solution (7%) 1020
▲ Vesanoid Capsules (57%) 2820
VESIcare Tablets (0.2% to 1.1%) 646
▲ VFEND I.V. (1% to 4.4%) 2564
▲ VFEND Oral Suspension (1% to 4.4%) 2564
▲ VFEND Tablets (1% to 4.4%) 2564
Viadur Implant (Rare) 757
Viagra Tablets (Less than 2%) 2573
▲ Vicodin Tablets (Among most frequent) 535
▲ Vicodin ES Tablets (Among most frequent) 536
▲ Vicodin HP Tablets (Among most frequent) 538
▲ Vicoprofen Tablets (3% to 9%) 539
Viracept (Less than 2%) 2577
▲ Viramune Oral Suspension (2% to 15%) 873
▲ Viramune Tablets (2% to 15%) 873
▲ Viread Tablets (4% to 7%) 1301
▲ Vivitrol (10% to 14%) 995
Vivotif (Infrequent) 819
▲ Voltaren Ophthalmic Solution (Less than or equal to 3%) 2309
▲ Voltaren Tablets (1% to 10%) 2307
▲ Voltaren-XR Tablets (1% to 10%) 2310
▲ VoSpire ER Tablets (4.2%) 1052
Vytorin 10/10 Tablets 2114
Vytorin 10/10 Tablets 3077
Vytorin 10/20 Tablets 2114
Vytorin 10/20 Tablets 3077
Vytorin 10/40 Tablets 2114
Vytorin 10/40 Tablets 3077
Vytorin 10/80 Tablets 2114
Vytorin 10/80 Tablets 3077
▲ Wellbutrin Tablets (22.9%) 1603
▲ Wellbutrin SR Sustained-Release Tablets (2% to 4%) 1607
▲ Wellbutrin XL Extended-Release Tablets (2% to 4%) 1613
WinRho SDF 732
▲ Xeloda Tablets (4% to 27%) 2822
▲ Xenical Capsules (3.8%) 2831
Xifaxan Tablets (2.2%) 2842
Xopenex Inhalation Solution 3146
Xopenex Inhalation Solution Concentrate 3150
Xopenex HFA Inhalation Aerosol 3154
▲ Xyrem Oral Solution (1% to 22.9%) 1688
Yasmin 28 Tablets (Greater than 1%) 796
Yaz Tablets (Greater than 1%) 803
Zantac 1624
Zantac Injection 1619
Zantac Injection Pharmacy Bulk Package (Frequent) 1622
Zantac Injection Premixed 1619
Zantac 1624
▲ Zegerid Capsules (1.5% to 3.2%) 2958
▲ Zegerid Powder for Oral Solution (1.5% to 3.2%) 2958
▲ Zelapar Tablets (3%) 3372
Zelnorm Tablets (1% to 2%) 2312
▲ Zemplar Capsules (8%) 541
▲ Zemplar Injection (8%) 543
Zemuron Injection (Less than 1%) 2346
▲ Ziagen (2% to 10%) 1626
Zinacef for Injection 1631
Zinacef Injection 1631
▲ Zinecard for Injection (42% to 59%) 2650
Zmax for Oral Suspension (1.1%) 2583
Zocor Tablets 2105
▲ Zoloft (4%) 2586
▲ Zometa for Intravenous Infusion (14% to 32%) 2315
Zomig Nasal Spray (1% to less than 2%) 3523
Zonegran Capsules (Frequent) 1101
▲ Zosyn (2.6% to 3.3%) 3492
Zovirax (2.7%) 1643
Zyban Sustained-Release Tablets (Frequent) 1644

▲ Zydone Tablets (Among most frequent) ... 1139
Zyflo Tablets (Greater than 1%) ... 1023
▲ Zyprexa Tablets (4%) ... 1830
▲ Zyprexa ZYDIS Orally Disintegrating Tablets (4%) ... 1830
Zyrtec Chewable Tablets (2.3% to 2.5%) ... 2594
Zyrtec (2.3% to 2.5%) ... 2594
Zyrtec-D 12 Hour Extended Release Tablets (2.3% to 2.5%) ... 2597
▲ Zyvox (0.9% to 9.4%) ... 2652

Vulva, dryness
(*see under* Vagina, dryness)

Vulvar disorder
Estring Vaginal Ring ... 2635

Vulvitis
Zovirax Ointment (0.3%) ... 821

Vulvovaginal disorder, unspecified
▲ Cleocin Vaginal Ovules (3.4%) ... 2616
Vandazole Vaginal Gel (Less than 1%) ... 3338

Vulvovaginitis
Advair Diskus 100/50 ... 1308
Advair Diskus 250/50 ... 1308
Advair Diskus 500/50 ... 1308
Advair HFA Inhalation Aerosol ... 1318
▲ Arimidex Tablets (4% to 6%) ... 673
Invanz for Injection (Greater than 0.1%) ... 1999
Seroquel Tablets (Infrequent) ... 690

W

Walking disorders
Cesamet Capsules ... 3340
Imitrex Nasal Spray (Rare) ... 1467

Warm sensation
▲ Imitrex Injection (11%) ... 1463
▲ Imitrex Tablets (2% to 3%) ... 1471
ProQuad ... 2064
▲ Zomig Tablets (Common) ... 3519
▲ Zomig-ZMT Tablets (Common) ... 3519

Warm to touch
ProQuad ... 2064

Warmth
Aceon Tablets (2 mg, 4 mg, 8 mg) (0.3% to 1%) ... 3194
▲ Adalat CC Tablets (4%) ... 2964
Bicillin C-R Injectable Suspension ... 1706
Buprenex Injectable (Less than 1%) ... 2716
Cancidas for Injection (0% to 1.5%) ... 1918
Ethyol for Injection ... 1898
Hyperstat I.V. ... 3017
▲ Imitrex Injection (11%) ... 1463
Imitrex Nasal Spray (Infrequent) ... 1467
Miacalcin Injection ... 2252
▲ Niaspan Extended-Release Tablets (Among most common) ... 1730
Niravam Orally Disintegrating Tablets (1.3%) ... 3092
Recombivax HB (Less than 1%) ... 2071
▲ Zomig Nasal Spray (0% to 4%) ... 3523

Warmth at injection site
Boostrix ... 1404
Fluarix ... 1451
HibTITER (Less than 1% to 1.8%) ... 3426
Hyalgan Solution ... 2901
Pneumovax 23 (Common) ... 2043
Rocephin Injectable Vials, ADD-Vantage, Galaxy, Bulk ... 2800
▲ Vaqta (0.6% to 17.4%) ... 2097
Xolair ... 1266
Zostavax Injection (1.5%) ... 2111

Warts
(*see under* Verruca)

Wasting syndrome
Invirase (Less than 2%) ... 2772

Water intoxication
Aloprim for Injection (Less than 1%) ... 2167
Carbatrol Capsules ... 3171
Equetro Extended-Release Capsules ... 3180
Seroquel Tablets (Infrequent) ... 690
Tegretol/Tegretol-XR ... 2295
Zyprexa Tablets (Rare) ... 1830
Zyprexa ZYDIS Orally Disintegrating Tablets (Rare) ... 1830

Water retention
(*see also under* Edema)
Androxy Tablets ... 3335
Hyperstat I.V. ... 3017
Prochieve 4% Gel ... 1003
Prochieve 8% Gel ... 1003

WBC, immature
Cipro I.V. (Infrequent) ... 2984
▲ Clozaril Tablets (3%) ... 2184
Lupron Depot 3.75 mg ... 3260
Lupron Depot–3 Month 11.25 mg ... 3265
Merrem I.V. (Greater than 0.2%) ... 686
Neurontin Capsules (1.1%) ... 2487
Neurontin Oral Solution (Rare) ... 2487
Neurontin Tablets (1.1%) ... 2487

WBC counts, fluctuation
Aciphex Tablets ... 1090
Effexor Tablets (Infrequent) ... 3411
Invanz for Injection (0.8% to 1.5%) ... 1999
Levaquin (0.1% to 0.9%) ... 2384
Levaquin in 5% Dextrose Injection (0.1% to 0.9%) ... 2384
▲ Lupron Depot 3.75 mg (Approximately 5% to 8%) ... 3260
Neurontin Capsules (Rare) ... 2487
Neurontin Oral Solution (1.1%) ... 2487
Neurontin Tablets (Rare) ... 2487
Noroxin Tablets (1.3% to 1.4%) ... 2032
Prevacid Delayed-Release Capsules ... 3271
Prevacid for Delayed-Release Oral Suspension ... 3271
Prevacid SoluTab Delayed-Release Orally Disintegrating Tablets ... 3271
Prevacid NapraPAC ... 3280
PREVPAC ... 3284
Primaxin I.M. ... 2045
Uniretic Tablets (Less than 1%) ... 3100
▲ Visudyne for Injection (1% to 10%) ... 2305

Weakness
(*see under* Asthenia)

Weakness, feet
K-Phos Original (Sodium Free) Tablets (Less frequent) ... 760
K-Phos Neutral Tablets ... 760
Uroqid-Acid No. 2 Tablets ... 760

Weakness, hands
K-Phos Original (Sodium Free) Tablets (Less frequent) ... 760
K-Phos Neutral Tablets ... 760
Uroqid-Acid No. 2 Tablets ... 760

Weakness, legs
Dantrium Intravenous ... 2695
K-Phos Original (Sodium Free) Tablets (Less frequent) ... 760
K-Phos Neutral Tablets ... 760
Uroqid-Acid No. 2 Tablets ... 760
▲ Vesanoid Capsules (3%) ... 2820

Weakness, local
Cosopt Sterile Ophthalmic Solution ... 1931
Timoptic Sterile Ophthalmic Solution ... 2088
Timoptic in Ocudose (Less frequent) ... 2091
Timoptic-XE Sterile Ophthalmic Gel Forming Solution ... 2092

Weakness, musculoskeletal
Niravam Orally Disintegrating Tablets ... 3092

Weeping, skin
Aldara Cream, 5% ... 1846

Weight change, unspecified
Anaprox Tablets (Less than 1%) ... 2761
Anaprox DS Tablets (Less than 1%) ... 2761
Arthrotec Tablets (Rare) ... 3129
▲ Depo-Provera Contraceptive Injection (Greater than 5%) ... 2622
EC-Naprosyn Delayed-Release Tablets (Less than 1%) ... 2761
Focalin XR Capsules ... 2223
▲ Lupron Depot 3.75 mg (6%) ... 3260
▲ Lupron Depot–3 Month 11.25 mg (6%) ... 3265
Naprosyn Suspension (Less than 1%) ... 2761
Naprosyn Tablets (Less than 1%) ... 2761
Univasc Tablets (Less than 1%) ... 3104
Voltaren Tablets (Occasionally) ... 2307
Voltaren-XR Tablets (Occasionally) ... 2310

Weight changes, increase or decrease
▲ Avastin IV (15% to 16%) ... 1227
Climara Transdermal System ... 771
▲ Clolar for Intravenous Infusion (15%) ... 1271
Estrasorb Topical Emulsion ... 1147
Estratest Tablets ... 3199
Estratest H.S. Tablets ... 3199
Klonopin (Infrequent) ... 2778
Moban Tablets ... 1119
Ortho-Cyclen Tablets ... 2429
Ortho Evra Transdermal System ... 2417
Ortho Tri-Cyclen Tablets ... 2429
Ortho Tri-Cyclen Lo Tablets ... 2436
Premphase Tablets ... 3456
Prempro Tablets ... 3456
Prometrium Capsules (100 mg, 200 mg) ... 3203
Rescriptor Tablets ... 2551
Seasonique Tablets ... 1077
Yasmin 28 Tablets ... 796
Yaz Tablets ... 803

Weight decrease
(*see under* Weight loss)

Weight gain
▲ Abilify Oral Solution (5.1% to 30%) ... 882
▲ Abilify Oral Solution (5.1% to 30%) ... 2450
▲ Abilify Discmelt Orally Disintegrating Tablets (5.1% to 30%) ... 882
▲ Abilify Discmelt Orally Disintegrating Tablets (5.1% to 30%) ... 2450
▲ Abilify Tablets (5.1% to 30%) ... 882
▲ Abilify Tablets (5.1% to 30%) ... 2450
Aciphex Tablets ... 1090
▲ ActoPlus Met Tablets (2.9% to 6.7%) ... 3214
▲ Actos Tablets (0.9% to 3.6%) ... 3219
Advair Diskus 100/50 ... 1308
Advair Diskus 250/50 ... 1308
Advair Diskus 500/50 ... 1308
▲ Advair HFA Inhalation Aerosol (1% to 3%) ... 1318
Aerobid/Aerobid-M (1% to 3%) ... 1171
Aldoril Tablets ... 1910
Altace Capsules (Less than 1%) ... 1702
Amitiza Capsules (0% to 1%) ... 3224
Angeliq Tablets ... 762
Aricept Tablets (Infrequent) ... 1094
Aricept ODT Tablets (Infrequent) ... 1094
▲ Arimidex Tablets (2% to 13%) ... 673
Astelin Nasal Spray (2.0%) ... 1904
Avandamet Tablets ... 1373
Avandaryl Tablets ... 1379
Avandia Tablets ... 1384
▲ Azmacort Inhalation Aerosol (1% to 3%) ... 1726
Betaseron for SC Injection ... 767
Caduet Tablets (Greater than 0.1% to less than 2%) ... 2508
Campral Tablets (Frequent) ... 1174
Cardizem LA Extended Release Tablets (Less than 2%) ... 1728
▲ Carnitor Injection (2% to 6%) ... 3188
Catapres Tablets (About 1 in 100 patients) ... 843
Catapres-TTS (0.5% or less) ... 844
Celebrex Capsules (0.1% to 1.9%) ... 3134
Celexa (Frequent) ... 1176
▲ CellCept Capsules (3% to less than 20%) ... 2747
▲ CellCept Intravenous (3% to less than 20%) ... 2747
▲ CellCept Oral Suspension (3% to less than 20%) ... 2747
▲ CellCept Tablets (3% to less than 20%) ... 2747
Chantix Tablets (Frequent) ... 2517
Climara Pro Transdermal System (2.8%) ... 776
Clorpres Tablets (About 1%) ... 2153
▲ Clozaril Tablets (4% to 31%) ... 2184
Colazal Capsules ... 2838
▲ Copaxone for Injection (3%) ... 3297
▲ Coreg Tablets (10% to 12%) ... 1414
▲ Cozaar Tablets (4%) ... 1935
Cymbalta Delayed-Release Capsules (Frequent) ... 1757
Decadron Tablets ... 1951
▲ Depacon Injection (4% to 9%) ... 412
▲ Depakene (9%) ... 417
▲ Depakote Sprinkle Capsules (4% to 9%) ... 422
▲ Depakote Tablets (8% to 9%) ... 427
▲ Depakote ER Tablets (Greater than 1% to 9%) ... 434
▲ depo-subQ provera 104 Injectable Suspension (6%) ... 2624
Detrol Tablets (1%) ... 2628
Doxil Injection (Less than 1%) ... 2351
Duetact Tablets (Less than 1%) ... 3226
DynaCirc CR Tablets (0.5% to 1%) ... 2721
Effexor Tablets (Frequent) ... 3411
Effexor XR Capsules (Frequent) ... 3417
Eligard 7.5 mg (Less than 2%) ... 2880
▲ Eloxatin for Injection (10%) ... 2892
Emsam Transdermal System (2.1%) ... 903
Enablex Extended-Release Tablets (Greater than or equal to 1%) ... 2203
Enbrel for Injection ... 584
Enjuvia Tablets ... 1062
▲ Entocort EC Capsules (Less than 5%) ... 2698
Estring Vaginal Ring ... 2635
▲ Evista Tablets (8.8%) ... 1763
Evoxac Capsules (Less than 1%) ... 1047
▲ FazaClo Orally Disintegrating Tablets (4% to 31%) ... 551
Femara Tablets (2%) ... 2214
▲ Flovent Diskus (1% to 3%) ... 1443
Flovent HFA ... 1447
Follistim AQ Cartridge ... 2338
Fortical Nasal Spray (Less than 1%) ... 3337
Gabitril Tablets (Frequent) ... 984
Gengraf Capsules (1% to less than 3%) ... 459
▲ Geodon Capsules (10%) ... 2529
▲ Gleevec Tablets (1% to 32%) ... 2227
▲ Hectorol Capsules (4.9%) ... 1275
▲ Hectorol Injection (4.9%) ... 1278
▲ Hycamtin for Injection (69%) ... 1458
Hydrocortone Tablets ... 1989
Hytrin Capsules (0.5%) ... 471
Imitrex Injection ... 1463
Imitrex Nasal Spray ... 1467
Imitrex Tablets (Rare) ... 1471
Indocin Capsules (Less than 1%) ... 1995
Indocin I.V. (Less than 1%) ... 2465
Indocin (Less than 1%) ... 1995
▲ Intron A for Injection (Less than or equal to 5%) ... 3024
Invirase (Less than 2%) ... 2772
▲ I.V. Busulfex (8%) ... 2493
Kaletra (Less than 2%) ... 476
Keppra Injection ... 3320
Keppra Oral Solution (1% or more) ... 3314
Keppra Tablets (1% or more) ... 3314
K-Phos Neutral Tablets ... 760
Lamictal (Frequent) ... 1481
▲ Leukine (8%) ... 814
Levemir Injection ... 2320
Lexapro Oral Solution (Frequent) ... 1190
Lexapro Tablets (Frequent) ... 1190
Lipitor Tablets (Less than 2%) ... 2483
Lithobid Tablets ... 1692
Lofibra Tablets ... 1219
Lofibra Capsules ... 1216
Lopressor Injection (Very rare) ... 2238
Lopressor Tablets (Very rare) ... 2238
Lopressor HCT 50/25 Tablets (Very rare) ... 2241
Lopressor HCT 100/25 Tablets (Very rare) ... 2241
Lopressor HCT 100/50 Tablets (Very rare) ... 2241
Lunesta Tablets (Infrequent) ... 3142
Lupron Depot-PED 7.5 mg, 11.25 mg and 15 mg (Less than 2%) ... 3269
Lupron Injection Pediatric (Less than 2%) ... 3259
▲ Lyrica Capsules (4% to 16%) ... 2539
Maxair Autohaler ... 1852
Menostar Transdermal System ... 782
Miacalcin Nasal Spray (Less than 1%) ... 2253
Mirapex Tablets ... 859
Mircette Tablets ... 1066
▲ Mirena Intrauterine System (5% or more) ... 787
Mobic Oral Suspension (Less than 2%) ... 863
Mobic Tablets (Less than 2%) ... 863
▲ Myfortic Tablets (3% to less than 20%) ... 2255
Nadolol Tablets (1 to 5 of 1000 patients) ... 2159
Neoral Oral Solution (1% to less than 3%) ... 2259
Neoral Soft Gelatin Capsules (1% to less than 3%) ... 2259
▲ Neurontin Capsules (1.8% to 3.4%) ... 2487
▲ Neurontin Oral Solution (1.8 to 3.4%) ... 2487
▲ Neurontin Tablets (1.8% to 3.4%) ... 2487
Nexium Delayed-Release Capsules (Less than 1%) ... 655
Nexium I.V. (Less than 1%) ... 659
▲ Niravam Orally Disintegrating Tablets (2.7% to 27.2%) ... 3092
Norvasc Tablets (More than 0.1% to 1%) ... 2545
▲ NuvaRing (5% to 14%) ... 2340

Ortho Micronor Tablets (Rare) 2426
Parcopa Orally Disintegrating Tablets 3097
Paxil CR Controlled-Release Tablets (Frequent) 1538
Paxil (Frequent) 1530
Permax Tablets (1.6%; Frequent) 3356
Premarin Intravenous 3442
Premarin Tablets 3446
Premarin Vaginal Cream 3452
Prevacid Delayed-Release Capsules (Less than 1%) 3271
Prevacid for Delayed-Release Oral Suspension (Less than 1%) 3271
Prevacid SoluTab Delayed-Release Orally Disintegrating Tablets (Less than 1%) 3271
Prevacid NapraPAC (Less than 1%) 3280
PREVPAC (Less than 1%) 3284
Prilosec OTC Delayed-Release Tablets (Less than 1%) 2677
Prinivil Tablets (0.3% to 1.0%) 2052
Prinzide Tablets 2056
▲ Prograf Capsules and Injection (3% to 15%) 632
▲ Proleukin for Injection (16%) 2266
ProSom Tablets (Rare) 517
Protonix I.V. (Less than 1%) 3472
Protonix Tablets (Less than 1%) 3469
Provigil Tablets (At least 1%) 988
Prozac Pulvules and Liquid (Frequent) 1801
▲ Rapamune Oral Solution and Tablets (8% to 21%) 3475
Relpax Tablets (Rare) 2548
Requip Tablets (Infrequent) 1555
Rescriptor Tablets 2551
Reyataz Capsules (Less than 3%) 921
Rilutek Tablets (Infrequent) 2930
▲ Risperdal (2% to 18%) 1676
▲ Risperdal Consta Long-Acting Injection (4% to 9%) 1682
▲ Risperdal M-Tab Orally Disintegrating Tablets (2% to 18%) 1676
Women's Rogaine Hair Regrowth Treatment Topical Solution, Spring Bloom Scent and Original Unscented ▣ 634
Rythmol SR Capsules 2727
▲ Seroquel Tablets (5% to 23%) 690
▲ Simulect for Injection (3% to 10%) 2284
Somavert Injection 2642
Sonata Capsules (Infrequent) 1717
Soriatane Capsules (Less than 1%) 1013
Stalevo Tablets 2287
Sular Tablets (Less than or equal to 1%) 3122
▲ Symbyax Capsules (Up to 21%) 1819
Targretin Capsules 1747
Taxotere Injection Concentrate 2932
▲ Temodar Capsules (5%) 3073
Thalomid Capsules 965
Thioridazine Hydrochloride Tablets 2163
Thiothixene Capsules 2165
Thyrolar Tablets 1199
Tiazac Capsules (Less than 2%) 1201
Topamax Sprinkle Capsules (1%) 2404
Topamax Tablets (1%) 2404
Tricor Tablets 527
Triglide Tablets 3123
Trileptal Tablets (1% to 2%) 2300
Trileptal Oral Suspension (1% to 2%) 2300
▲ Trisenox Injection (13%) 993
Uniretic Tablets (Less than 1%) 3100
Uroqid-Acid No. 2 Tablets 760
Vantas (2.3%) 3375
Vantin Tablets and Oral Suspension (Less than 1%) 2645
▲ Vesanoid Capsules (23%) 2820
Viadur Implant (2.3%) 757
▲ Wellbutrin Tablets (9.4% to 13.6%) 1603
▲ Wellbutrin SR Sustained-Release Tablets (2% to 3%) 1607
▲ Wellbutrin XL Extended-Release Tablets (11%) 1613
Yaz Tablets (Greater than 1%) 803
Zegerid Capsules (Less than 1%) 2958
Zegerid Powder for Oral Solution (Less than 1%) 2958
Zoloft (Frequent) 2586
Zometa for Intravenous Infusion 2315
Zomig Nasal Spray (Rare) 3523
Zonegran Capsules (Infrequent) 1101
Zyban Sustained-Release Tablets (Infrequent) 1644
▲ Zyprexa Tablets (5% to 56%) 1830
▲ Zyprexa ZYDIS Orally Disintegrating Tablets (5% to 56%) 1830
Zyrtec Chewable Tablets (Less than 2%) 2594
Zyrtec (Less than 2%) 2594
Zyrtec-D 12 Hour Extended Release Tablets (Less than 2%) 2597

Weight gain, delayed

Elocon Cream 0.1% 3005
Elocon Lotion 0.1% 3006
Elocon Ointment 0.1% 3007
▲ Sandostatin Injection (32%) 2278

Weight loss

Abelcet Injection 1141
Abilify Oral Solution (Frequent) 882
Abilify Oral Solution (Frequent) 2450
Abilify Discmelt Orally Disintegrating Tablets (Frequent) 882
Abilify Discmelt Orally Disintegrating Tablets (Frequent) 2450
Abilify Tablets (Frequent) 882
Abilify Tablets (Frequent) 2450
Accutane Capsules 2731
Aciphex Tablets 1090
▲ Actimmune (6%) 1671
Actiq (Less than 1%) 979
Adalat CC Tablets (Less than 1%) 2964
Adderall Tablets 3164
▲ Adderall XR Capsules (1.2% to 11%) 3166
Alferon N Injection (1%) 1665
Alkeran for Injection 955
Alkeran Tablets 956
Ambien Tablets (Rare) 2851
Ambien CR Tablets (Rare) 2855
Angeliq Tablets 762
Aptivus Capsules (Less than 2%) 826
▲ Aricept Tablets (3%) 1094
▲ Aricept ODT Tablets (3%) 1094
▲ Avinza Capsules (Less than 5%) 1741
▲ Azilect Tablets (9%) 3293
▲ Bexxar (Less than 1% to 6%) 1398
Blocadren Tablets 1916
Caduet Tablets (Greater than 0.1% to less than or equal to 1%) 2508
Calcijex Injection 411
Campral Tablets (Infrequent) 1174
▲ Camptosar Injection (1% to 30%) 2604
Captopril Tablets 2149
▲ Carnitor Injection (3% to 8%) 3188
Celexa (Frequent) 1176
▲ CellCept Capsules (3% to less than 20%) 2747
▲ CellCept Intravenous (3% to less than 20%) 2747
▲ CellCept Oral Suspension (3% to less than 20%) 2747
▲ CellCept Tablets (3% to less than 20%) 2747
Climara Pro Transdermal System 776
Clozaril Tablets 2184
Colazal Capsules 2838
Concerta Extended-Release Tablets 1881
Copaxone for Injection (Infrequent) 3297
▲ Copegus Tablets (10% to 16%) 2754
▲ Coreg Tablets (Greater than 1% to 3%) 1414
Cosopt Sterile Ophthalmic Solution 1931
Cymbalta Delayed-Release Capsules (2%) 1757
Daranide Tablets 1950
▲ Daytrana Transdermal Patch (9%) 3174
▲ Depacon Injection (6%) 412
▲ Depakene (6%) 417
▲ Depakote Sprinkle Capsules (6%) 422
▲ Depakote Tablets (6%) 427
▲ Depakote ER Tablets (6%) 434
Dexedrine 1420
DextroStat Tablets 3179
▲ Doxil Injection (1% to 10%) 2351
Duragesic Transdermal System 2373
Effexor Tablets (1%) 3411
▲ Effexor XR Capsules (3% to 4%) 3417
Eldepryl Capsules (1 of 49 patients) 3208
▲ Eloxatin for Injection (2% to 5%) 2892
Elspar for Injection 2463
Elspar for Injection 1960
Emend Capsules (Greater than 0.5%) 1963
▲ Emsam Transdermal System (5%) 903
Enjuvia Tablets 1062
▲ Erbitux (1% to 84%) 910
Estring Vaginal Ring 2635
Evoxac Capsules (Less than 1%) 1047
▲ Exelon Capsules (3%) 2206
▲ Exelon Oral Solution (3%) 2206
FazaClo Orally Disintegrating Tablets 551
▲ Femara Tablets (7%) 2214
▲ Focalin Tablets (Among more frequent) 2220
Focalin XR Capsules 2223
▲ Fuzeon Injection (6.6%) 2767
Gabitril Tablets (Frequent) 984
Garamycin Injectable 3014
Gengraf Capsules (1% to less than 3%) 459
Gleevec Tablets (Infrequent) 2227
Hectorol Capsules 1275
Hectorol Injection 1278
Herceptin I.V. (At least one of the 958 patients) 1233
▲ Hycamtin for Injection (69%) 1458
Imitrex Injection 1463
Imitrex Nasal Spray (Rare) 1467
Imitrex Tablets (Rare) 1471
▲ Indapamide Tablets (Less than 5%) 2156
▲ Infergen (5%) 3364
▲ Intron A for Injection (Less than 1% to 10%) 3024
Invanz for Injection (Greater than 0.1%) 1999
Invirase (Less than 2%) 2772
▲ Iressa Tablets (3% to 6%) 684
▲ Kaletra (Up to 3%) 476
Keppra Injection 3320
Keppra Oral Solution 3314
Keppra Tablets 3314
Lamictal (Infrequent) 1481
Lamisil Tablets 2232
▲ Leukine (37%) 814
Levaquin (0.1% to 0.9%) 2384
Levaquin in 5% Dextrose Injection (0.1% to 0.9%) 2384
Levothroid Tablets 1186
Levoxyl Tablets 1712
Lexapro Oral Solution (Infrequent) 1190
Lexapro Tablets (Infrequent) 1190
Lithobid Tablets 1692
Lofibra Tablets 1219
Lofibra Capsules 1216
Lunesta Tablets (Infrequent) 3142
Menostar Transdermal System 782
Metadate CD Capsules 3323
Mirapex Tablets (2%) 859
Mircette Tablets 1066
Mobic Oral Suspension (Less than 2%) 863
Mobic Tablets (Less than 2%) 863
Myleran Tablets 1525
Namenda (Frequent) 1195
Neoral Oral Solution (1% to less than 3%) 2259
Neoral Soft Gelatin Capsules (1% to less than 3%) 2259
Neurontin Capsules (Infrequent) 2487
Neurontin Oral Solution (Infrequent) 2487
Neurontin Tablets (Infrequent) 2487
Nexavar Tablets (0% to 10%) 746
Nexium Delayed-Release Capsules (Less than 1%) 655
Nexium I.V. (Less than 1%) 659
▲ Niravam Orally Disintegrating Tablets (2.3% to 22.6%) 3092
Norvir (0 to 2.4%) 503
Oncaspar (Less than 1%) 1145
▲ Ontak Vials (14%) 1745
Opana Tablets (Less than 1%) 1122
Opana ER Tablets (Less than 1%) 1126
Parcopa Orally Disintegrating Tablets 3097
Paxil CR Controlled-Release Tablets (Frequent) 1538
Paxil (Frequent) 1530
▲ Pegasys (4%) 2789
▲ PEG-Intron Powder for Injection (11%) 3048
Permax Tablets (Frequent) 3356
Pexeva Tablets 1694
▲ Photofrin for Injection (6% to 9%) 702
Premarin Intravenous 3442
Premarin Tablets 3446
Premarin Vaginal Cream 3452
Prevacid Delayed-Release Capsules (Less than 1%) 3271
Prevacid for Delayed-Release Oral Suspension (Less than 1%) 3271
Prevacid SoluTab Delayed-Release Orally Disintegrating Tablets (Less than 1%) 3271
Prevacid NapraPAC (Less than 1%) 3280
PREVPAC (Less than 1%) 3284
Prinivil Tablets (0.3% to 1.0%) 2052
Prinzide Tablets 2056
Prograf Capsules and Injection 632
▲ Proleukin for Injection (5%) 2266
ProSom Tablets (Rare) 517
Protonix I.V. (Less than 1%) 3472
Protonix Tablets (Less than 1%) 3469
Provigil Tablets (Greater than or equal to 1%) 988
Prozac Pulvules and Liquid (1.4% to 2%) 1801
Pulmozyme Inhalation Solution 1248
▲ Rapamune Oral Solution and Tablets (3% to 20%) 3475
▲ Razadyne (5% to 7%) 2399
▲ Razadyne ER Extended-Release Capsules (5% to 7%) 2399
▲ Rebetol (20% to 29%) 3058
Relpax Tablets (Rare) 2548
Requip Tablets (1% or more) 1555
Rescriptor Tablets 2551
Retrovir Capsules (0.8%) 1560
Retrovir IV Infusion (1%) 1564
Retrovir (0.8%) 1560
▲ Revlimid Capsules (18.2%) 958
Reyataz Capsules (Less than 3%) 921
▲ Ribavirin, USP Capsules (20% to 29%) 3068
▲ Rilutek Tablets (3.7% to 4.6%) 2930
Risperdal (Infrequent) 1676
▲ Risperdal Consta Long-Acting Injection (1% to 4%) 1682
Risperdal M-Tab Orally Disintegrating Tablets (Infrequent) 1676
Ritalin Hydrochloride Tablets 2269
Ritalin LA Capsules 2271
Ritalin-SR Tablets 2269
Rocaltrol Capsules 2798
Rocaltrol Oral Solution 2798
Rythmol SR Capsules 2727
Sandimmune (Rare) 2275
Sandostatin Injection (Less than 1%) 2278
▲ Sandostatin LAR Depot (5% to 15%) 2280
Seroquel Tablets (Infrequent) 690
▲ Soltamox Oral Solution (23%) 3527
Sonata Capsules (Rare) 1717
Stalevo Tablets 2287
Strattera Capsules (2%) 1814
Sular Tablets (Less than or equal to 1%) 3122
Symbyax Capsules (Frequent) 1819
▲ Tarceva Tablets (0% to 39%) 1259
▲ Tarceva Tablets (0% to 39%) 2444
Targretin Capsules 1747
Timolide Tablets 2086
Timoptic Sterile Ophthalmic Solution 2088
Timoptic in Ocudose 2091
Timoptic-XE Sterile Ophthalmic Gel Forming Solution 2092
▲ TOBI Solution for Inhalation (10.1%) 2298
▲ Topamax Sprinkle Capsules (4% to 21%) 2404
▲ Topamax Tablets (4% to 21%) 2404
Trecator Tablets 3487
Tricor Tablets 527
Triglide Tablets 3123
Trileptal Tablets 2300
Trileptal Oral Suspension 2300
▲ Trisenox Injection (8%) 993
Truvada Tablets 1296
▲ Ultram ER Tablets (1% to greater than 5%) 2392
Vantas (Less than 2%) 3375
▲ Vesanoid Capsules (17%) 2820
Vicoprofen Tablets (Less than 1%) 539
▲ Viread Tablets (2% to 4%) 1301
Vivitrol 995
▲ Wellbutrin Tablets (23.2% to 28%) 1603
▲ Wellbutrin SR Sustained-Release Tablets (14% to 19%) 1607
▲ Wellbutrin XL Extended-Release Tablets (23%) 1613
▲ Xeloda Tablets (Up to 7%) 2822
Xifaxan Tablets (Less than 2%) 2842
Xyrem Oral Solution (Frequent) 1688
Zoloft 2586
▲ Zometa for Intravenous Infusion (16%) 2315
▲ Zonegran Capsules (3%) 1101
Zyprexa Tablets (Frequent) 1830
Zyprexa ZYDIS Orally Disintegrating Tablets (Frequent) 1830

Wenckebach block

Buprenex Injectable (Less than 1%) 2716
Lanoxin Injection 1494
Lanoxin Injection Pediatric 1497
Lanoxin Tablets 1500

Wenckebach's period

(*see under* A-V conduction, prolongation)

Wheal at injection site

ProQuad 2064

Wheals

Attenuvax (Rare) 1914
Dilaudid-HP (Less frequent) 442

▲ Levulan Kerastick for Topical Solution, 20% (1% to 7%)............. 1085
Meruvax II....................................... 2019
M-M-R II... 2006
Mumpsvax (Extremely rare)............. 2031

Wheezing

Abelcet Injection............................. 1141
▲ Advair Diskus 100/50 (1% to 3%) ... 1308
▲ Advair Diskus 250/50 (1% to 3%) ... 1308
▲ Advair Diskus 500/50 (1% to 3%) ... 1308
Advair HFA Inhalation Aerosol........... 1318
▲ Aerobid/Aerobid-M (3% to 9%) 1171
Alferon N Injection.......................... 1665
Aricept Tablets (Infrequent)............. 1094
Aricept ODT Tablets (Infrequent)....... 1094
▲ Arranon Injection (0% to 5%) 1357
Avalide Tablets................................. 888
Avalide Tablets................................. 2874
Avapro Tablets (Less than 1%).......... 891
Avapro Tablets (Less than 1%).......... 2871
Azmacort Inhalation Aerosol............. 1726
Beconase AQ Nasal Spray (Rare)..... 1396
Cesamet Capsules........................... 3340
Clozaril Tablets (Less than 1%)......... 2184
Combivent Inhalation Aerosol........... 847
Combivir Tablets............................... 1411
▲ CytoGam Intravenous (Less than 5%).. 1895
DuoNeb Inhalation Solution.............. 1058
Elidel Cream 1% (Up to 1.2%).......... 2200
Emend Capsules (Less than or equal to 0.5%)............................ 1963
Epivir.. 1427
Epivir-HBV... 1432
Epzicom Tablets............................... 1436
FazaClo Orally Disintegrating Tablets (Less than 1%)................. 551
▲ Flebogamma 5%, Immune Globulin Intravenous (Human) (18%).. 1658
Flonase Nasal Spray......................... 1440
Flovent Diskus.................................. 1443
Flovent HFA...................................... 1447
Flumist Vaccine................................ 1901
Gammagard Liquid........................... 721
Humalog-Pen (Less common).......... 1781
Humalog Mix 50/50-Pen.................. 1783
Humalog Mix 75/25-Pen (Less common)... 1785
Humulin 50/50, 100 Units............... 1791
Humulin 70/30 Pen (Less common)... 1793
Humulin L, 100 Units (Less common)... 1794
Humulin N Pen (Less common)........ 1797
Imitrex Tablets................................. 1471
Infed Injection.................................. 3390
▲ Intron A for Injection (Less than or equal to 5%)............................... 3024
Invanz for Injection (1%).................. 1999
Levothroid Tablets............................ 1186
Levoxyl Tablets................................. 1712
Lopressor Injection (1%).................. 2238
Lopressor Tablets (1%).................... 2238
Lopressor HCT 50/25 Tablets (Less than 1%)............................. 2241
Lopressor HCT 100/25 Tablets (Less than 1%)............................. 2241
Lopressor HCT 100/50 Tablets (Less than 1%)............................. 2241
Maxair Autohaler.............................. 1852
Maxalt Tablets.................................. 2008
Maxalt-MLT Orally Disintegrating Tablets... 2008
Mivacron Injection (Less than 1%).... 493
Motrin IB Tablets and Caplets........... 1866
Children's Motrin Oral Suspension.... 1867
Children's Motrin Non-Staining Dye-Free Oral Suspension............ 1867
Children's Motrin Cold Oral Suspension..................................... 1867
Infants' Motrin Concentrated Drops.. 1867
Infants' Motrin Non-Staining Dye-Free Concentrated Drops....... 1867
Junior Strength Motrin Caplets and Chewable Tablets......................... 1867
Myozyme for Intravenous Infusion.... 1279
Nasonex Nasal Spray (Greater than or equal to 2%)..................... 3043
Neumega for Injection...................... 3435
Neupogen for Injection..................... 603
Nimotop Capsules (Less than 1%).... 749
NovoLog Injection............................ 2326
Orencia Powder for Intravenous Infusion (0.1% to 1%)................... 914
▲ Orthoclone OKT3 Sterile Solution (13%).. 2360
Prevnar for Injection........................ 3463
Prinivil Tablets (0.3% to 1.0%)......... 2052
Prinzide Tablets............................... 2056
▲ Proleukin for Injection (6%) 2266
ProQuad.. 2064
Proventil Inhalation Solution 0.083% (1% to 1.5%).................. 3055
Pulmozyme Inhalation Solution......... 1248
Revlimid Capsules........................... 958
Rhinocort Aqua Nasal Spray (Rare)... 665
Rythmol SR Capsules (2%)............... 2727
Sandimmune.................................... 2275
Simulect for Injection....................... 2284
Singulair (Greater than or equal to 2%).. 2077
Sular Tablets (Less than or equal to 1%)... 3122
Synagis (More than 1%).................. 1897
Toprol-XL Tablets (About 1 of 100 patients)....................................... 668
▲ Trisenox Injection (13%) 993
Trizivir Tablets................................. 1589
Ultane Liquid for Inhalation (Less than 1%)..................................... 531
Vancocin HCl Capsules, USP 3380
Vantin Tablets and Oral Suspension (Less than 1%) 2645
Vaqta (Less than 1%) 2097
▲ Vesanoid Capsules (14%) 2820
Xopenex Inhalation Solution 3146
Xopenex Inhalation Solution Concentrate 3150
Xopenex HFA Inhalation Aerosol 3154
Zemuron Injection (Less than 1%) 2346

White blood cell count, decreased

Lupron Depot 7.5 mg 3264
Lupron Depot-PED 7.5 mg, 11.25 mg and 15 mg 3269
Lupron Injection Pediatric 3259
Mycamine for Injection 628
Zyflo Tablets (1%) 1023

Withdrawal reactions

Ambien Tablets (Rare) 2851
Aricept Tablets (Infrequent) 1094
Aricept ODT Tablets (Infrequent) 1094
Avinza Capsules (Less than 5%) 1741
Catapres Tablets 843
Catapres-TTS (0.5% or less) 844
Celexa 1176
Cesamet Capsules 3340
Chantix Tablets 2517
Concerta Extended-Release Tablets 1881
Dexedrine.. 1420
Dilaudid 440
Dilaudid Non-Sterile Powder 440
Dilaudid Rectal Suppositories 440
Dilaudid Tablets 440
Effexor Tablets (Rare) 3411
Effexor XR Capsules (Infrequent) 3417
Kadian Capsules (Less than 3%) 577
Klonopin 2778
Levaquin (0.1% to 0.9%) 2384
Levaquin in 5% Dextrose Injection (0.1% to 0.9%) 2384
MS Contin Tablets 2701
Nembutal Sodium Solution, USP 2470
OxyContin Tablets (Less than 1%) 2703
Paxil CR Controlled-Release Tablets (Rare) 1538
Paxil (Rare) 1530
ProSom Tablets 517
Risperdal (Rare) 1676
Risperdal M-Tab Orally Disintegrating Tablets (Rare) 1676
▲ Suboxone Tablets (22% to 25.2%) .. 2717
▲ Subutex Tablets (18.4% to 22%) 2717
Tranxene 2474
Valium Tablets 2819
Zoloft (Rare) 2586
Zyprexa Tablets (Infrequent) 1830
Zyprexa ZYDIS Orally Disintegrating Tablets (Infrequent) 1830

Withdrawal syndrome

Adderall Tablets 3164
Campral Tablets (Infrequent) 1174
Daytrana Transdermal Patch 3174
Symbyax Capsules (Rare) 1819
Transderm Scōp Transdermal Therapeutic System 2177
▲ Ultram ER Tablets (1% to greater than 5%) 2392
Vivitrol 995

Worsening of underlying illness

Regular Strength Tylenol Tablets 1870
Tylenol 8 Hour Extended Release Caplets 1870
Tylenol 1870
Extra Strength Tylenol PM Caplets, Vanilla Caplets, Geltabs, Gelcaps and Liquid 1875
Extra Strength Tylenol Rapid Release Gels 1870
Tylenol Allergy Multi-Symptom Caplets with Cool Burst and Gelcaps... 1872
Tylenol Allergy Multi-Symptom Nighttime Caplets with Cool Burst... 1872
Tylenol Severe Allergy Caplets......... 1872
Tylenol Arthritis Pain Extended Release Caplets and Geltabs........ 1870
Tylenol Chest Congestion Caplets with Cool Burst............................ 1872
Tylenol Chest Congestion Liquid with Cool Burst............................ 1872
Children's Tylenol Suspension Liquid and Meltaways................... 1878
Children's Tylenol Plus Cold Suspension Liquid 1879
Children's Tylenol Plus Cold & Allergy Suspension Liquid 1878
Children's Tylenol Plus Cough & Runny Nose Suspension Liquid 1879
Children's Tylenol Plus Cough & Sore Throat Suspension Liquid 1879
Children's Tylenol Suspension with Flavor Creator 1878
Children's Tylenol Plus Flu Suspension Liquid 1881
Children's Tylenol Plus Multi-Symptom Cold Suspension Liquid 1879
Tylenol Cold Severe Congestion Non-Drowsy Caplets with Cool Burst 1874
Tylenol Cold Head Congestion Daytime Caplets with Cool Burst ... 1873
Tylenol Cold Head Congestion Nighttime Caplets with Cool Burst 1873
Tylenol Cold Head Congestion Severe Caplets with Cool Burst 1873
Tylenol Cough & Sore Throat Daytime Liquid with Cool Burst 1877
Tylenol Cough & Sore Throat Nighttime Liquid with Cool Burst ... 1877
Concentrated Tylenol Infants' Drops 1878
Concentrated Tylenol Infants' Drops Plus Cold 1879
Concentrated Tylenol Infants' Drops Plus Cold and Cough 1879
Jr. Tylenol Meltaways 1878
Tylenol Sinus Severe Congestion Caplets with Cool Burst 1876
Tylenol Sinus Congestion & Pain Daytime Caplets with Cool Burst and Gelcaps 1876
Tylenol Sinus Congestion & Pain Nighttime Caplets with Cool Burst 1876
Tylenol Sinus Congestion & Pain Severe Caplets with Cool Burst 1876
Tylenol Sore Throat Daytime Liquid with Cool Burst 1877
Tylenol Sore Throat Nighttime Liquid with Cool Burst 1877
Women's Tylenol Menstrual Relief Caplets 1877

Wound, nasal

▲ Fortical Nasal Spray (10.6%) 3337

Wound complication

Invanz for Injection (2.9%) 1999

Wound dehiscence

Emend Capsules (Greater than 0.5%) 1963
Invanz for Injection (1.3%) 1999
▲ Valcyte Tablets (Less than 5%) 2813

Wound drainage, increased

▲ Arixtra Injection (0.6% to 4.5%) 1351
▲ Valcyte Tablets (Less than 5%) 2813

Wound healing, impaired

Blephamide Ophthalmic Ointment (Infrequent) 568
Blephamide Ophthalmic Suspension 569
Colocort Rectal Suspension, USP (Retention) 100 mg/60 mL 2476
Decadron Tablets 1951
Depo-Medrol Injectable Suspension 2617
Depo-Medrol Single-Dose Vial 2619
FML Ophthalmic Ointment (Infrequent) .... ⊙228
FML Ophthalmic Suspension .... ⊙227
FML Forte Ophthalmic Suspension (Infrequent) .... ⊙226
FML-S Ophthalmic Suspension .... ⊙229
Hydrocortone Tablets...................... 1989
Ocufen Ophthalmic Solution............ ⊙232
Poly-Pred Ophthalmic Suspension... ⊙233
Pred Mild Ophthalmic Suspension (Infrequent)................................ ⊙238
Pred Forte Ophthalmic Suspension.................................. ⊙235
Pred-G Ophthalmic Ointment............ ⊙237
Pred-G Ophthalmic Suspension....... ⊙236
▲ Rapamune Oral Solution and Tablets (3% to less than 20%)....... 3475
Retisert Implant............................... ⊙258
TobraDex Ophthalmic Ointment......... 562
TobraDex Ophthalmic Suspension.... 563
▲ Zofran (28%) 1639
▲ Zofran ODT Orally Disintegrating Tablets (28%)................................ 1639

Wound infection

▲ Arixtra Injection (4.9%) 1351
Enbrel for Injection.......................... 584
▲ Gengraf Capsules (7%) 459
▲ Infergen (3% to 4%) 3364
▲ Invanz for Injection (6.5%) 1999
▲ Myfortic Tablets (3% to less than 20%) 2255
▲ Neoral Oral Solution (7.0%) 2259
▲ Neoral Soft Gelatin Capsules (7.0%) 2259
▲ Sandimmune (7.0% to 10.1%) 2275
▲ Valcyte Tablets (Less than 5%) 2813

Wound secretion

Invanz for Injection (1.9%) 1999

Wrist fracture

Arimidex Tablets (2%) 673

Wrist-drop

Azilect Tablets (Rare) 3293
Rilutek Tablets (Rare) 2930

X

Xanthomas, eruptive

Accutane Capsules 2731

Xanthopsia

Aldoril Tablets 1910
Atacand HCT 651
Avalide Tablets 888
Avalide Tablets 2874
Clorpres Tablets 2153
Diovan HCT Tablets 2196
Diuril Oral Suspension 1954
Diuril Sodium Intravenous 2467
Dyazide Capsules 1423
Furosemide Tablets 2154
Hyzaar 50-12.5 Tablets (One subject) 1990
Hyzaar 100-12.5 Tablets (One subject) 1990
Hyzaar 100-25 Tablets (One subject) 1990
Indapamide Tablets 2156
Lanoxicaps Capsules 1490
Lanoxin Injection 1494
Lanoxin Injection Pediatric 1497
Lanoxin Tablets 1500
Lopressor HCT 50/25 Tablets 2241
Lopressor HCT 100/25 Tablets 2241
Lopressor HCT 100/50 Tablets 2241
Lotensin HCT Tablets 2246
Micardis HCT Tablets 856
Mintezol 2027
Moduretic Tablets 2028
Prinzide Tablets 2056
Teveten HCT Tablets 1737
Timolide Tablets 2086
Uniretic Tablets 3100

Xerochilia

Invirase (2%) 2772
Lexapro Oral Solution (Infrequent) 1190
Lexapro Tablets (Infrequent) 1190
Xifaxan Tablets (Less than 2%) 2842
Zovirax Cream (Less than 1%) 820

Xeroderma

(*see under* Xerosis cutis)

Xeromycteria

Accutane Capsules 2731
▲ Advair HFA Inhalation Aerosol (1% to 3%) 1318
Alphagan P Ophthalmic Solution (Less than 1%) 567
AmBisome for Injection (Less common) 620
▲ Atrovent Nasal Spray 0.03% (5.1%) 837
▲ Atrovent Nasal Spray 0.06% (4.8%) 839
Beconase AQ Nasal Spray 1396

Brimonidine Tartrate Ophthalmic Solution 0.2% (Less than 3%) ⊙ 248
Catapres Tablets 843
Cesamet Capsules 3340
Clorpres Tablets 2153
▲ Ditropan XL Extended-Release Tablets (2% to less than 5%) 2413
Flonase Nasal Spray (Less than 1%) 1440
▲ Fortical Nasal Spray (10.6%) 3337
Maxalt Tablets (Infrequent) 2008
Maxalt-MLT Orally Disintegrating Tablets (Infrequent) 2008
▲ Miacalcin Nasal Spray (10.6%) 2253
Protopic Ointment (0.2% to less than 1%) 638
▲ Symmetrel Tablets (1% to 5%) 1135

Xerophthalmia

Abilify Oral Solution (Infrequent) 882
Abilify Oral Solution (Infrequent) 2450
Abilify Discmelt Orally Disintegrating Tablets (Infrequent) 882
Abilify Discmelt Orally Disintegrating Tablets (Infrequent) 2450
Abilify Tablets (Infrequent) 882
Abilify Tablets (Infrequent) 2450
Accutane Capsules 2731
Aciphex Tablets 1090
▲ Actonel Tablets (3.3%) 2683
Acular Ophthalmic Solution (Rare) 565
▲ Advair Diskus 250/50 (1% to 3%) 1308
Alamast Ophthalmic Solution (Less than 5%) 3381
Alphagan P Ophthalmic Solution (1% to 4%) 567
▲ Alrex Ophthalmic Suspension 0.2% (5% to 15%) ⊙ 246
AmBisome for Injection (Less common) 620
Amerge Tablets (Rare) 1339
Aricept Tablets (Infrequent) 1094
Aricept ODT Tablets (Infrequent) 1094
Astelin Nasal Spray 1904
Axert Tablets (Rare) 2396
Azopt Ophthalmic Suspension (1% to 5%) 557
▲ Betimol Ophthalmic Solution (More than 5%) 3382
▲ Betimol Ophthalmic Solution (More than 5%) ⊙ 295
Betoptic S Ophthalmic Suspension (Small number of patients) 558
Blocadren Tablets 1916
BOTOX Purified Neurotoxin Complex 570
▲ Brimonidine Tartrate Ophthalmic Solution 0.2% (3% to 9%) ⊙ 248
Caduet Tablets (Less than 2%) 2508
Catapres Tablets 843
Catapres-TTS (0.5% or less) 844
Celexa (Infrequent) 1176
Cesamet Capsules 3340
Chantix Tablets (Infrequent) 2517
Ciloxan Ophthalmic Ointment (Less than 1%) 559
Clorpres Tablets 2153
Copaxone for Injection (Infrequent) 3297
▲ Cosopt Sterile Ophthalmic Solution (1% to 5%) 1931
Depacon Injection (1% or more) 412
Depakene (1% or more) 417
Depakote Sprinkle Capsules 422
▲ Depakote Tablets (1% to 5%) 427
Depakote ER Tablets (Greater than 1%) 434
▲ Detrol Tablets (3%) 2628
▲ Detrol LA Capsules (3%) 2631
▲ Ditropan XL Extended-Release Tablets (3% to 6%) 2413
▲ Doxil Injection (1% to 10%) 2351
Effexor Tablets (Infrequent) 3411
Effexor XR Capsules (Infrequent) 3417
Enablex Extended-Release Tablets (1.5% to 2.1%) 2203
Enbrel for Injection 584
▲ Evoxac Capsules (1% to 3%) 1047
Flonase Nasal Spray 1440
Geodon Capsules (Infrequent) 2529
Gleevec Tablets (Infrequent) 2227
Inderal LA Long-Acting Capsules (Rare) 3429
InnoPran XL Capsules (Rare) 2723
▲ Intron A for Injection (Less than 5%) 3024
Invirase (Less than 2%) 2772
Klonopin (Infrequent) 2778
Lamictal (Infrequent) 1481
Lexapro Oral Solution (Infrequent) 1190
Lexapro Tablets (Infrequent) 1190
Lipitor Tablets (Less than 2%) 2483
Lopressor Injection (Rare) 2238
Lopressor Tablets (Rare) 2238
▲ Lotemax Ophthalmic Suspension 0.5% (5% to 15%) ⊙ 251
▲ Lucentis Injection (3% to 10%) 1237
▲ Lumigan Ophthalmic Solution (3% to 10%) 573
Lunesta Tablets (Infrequent) 3142
Lyrica Capsules (0.1% to 1%) 2539
Maxalt Tablets (Infrequent) 2008
Maxalt-MLT Orally Disintegrating Tablets (Infrequent) 2008
Meridia Capsules 489
Mintezol 2027
Nadolol Tablets (1 to 5 of 1000 patients) 2159
Namenda (Infrequent) 1195
Neurontin Capsules (Infrequent) 2487
Neurontin Oral Solution (Infrequent) 2487
Neurontin Tablets (Infrequent) 2487
▲ Nevanac Ophthalmic Suspension 0.1% (1% to 5%) ⊙ 209
Nipent for Injection (Less than 3%) 1863
Norvasc Tablets (Less than 0.1%) 2545
Patanol Ophthalmic Solution (Less than 5%) 561
Prevacid Delayed-Release Capsules (Less than 1%) 3271
Prevacid for Delayed-Release Oral Suspension (Less than 1%) 3271
Prevacid SoluTab Delayed-Release Orally Disintegrating Tablets (Less than 1%) 3271
Prevacid NapraPAC (Less than 1%) 3280
PREVPAC (Less than 1%) 3284
Prilosec OTC Delayed-Release Tablets (Less than 1%) 2677
Prochieve 4% Gel 1003
Prochieve 8% Gel 1003
Protopic Ointment (0.2% to less than 1%) 638
Prozac Pulvules and Liquid (Infrequent) 1801
Quixin Ophthalmic Solution (Less than 1%) 3383
▲ Rebif Prefilled Syringe for Injection (1% to 3%) 3159
Relpax Tablets (Rare) 2548
Requip Tablets (2%) 1555
Rescriptor Tablets 2551
▲ Retisert Implant (10 % to 35%) ⊙ 258
Risperdal (Infrequent) 1676
Risperdal M-Tab Orally Disintegrating Tablets (Infrequent) 1676
Sanctura Tablets (1.2%) 1151
Seroquel Tablets (Infrequent) 690
Sonata Capsules (Infrequent) 1717
▲ Soriatane Capsules (10% to 25%) 1013
Symbyax Capsules (Infrequent) 1819
Targretin Capsules 1747
Teveten Tablets (Less than 1%) 1735
Teveten HCT Tablets (Less than 1%) 1737
Timolide Tablets 2086
Timoptic Sterile Ophthalmic Solution 2088
Timoptic in Ocudose 2091
Timoptic-XE Sterile Ophthalmic Gel Forming Solution 2092
Topamax Sprinkle Capsules (Infrequent) 2404
Topamax Tablets (Infrequent) 2404
Toprol-XL Tablets (Rare) 668
Transderm Scōp Transdermal Therapeutic System (Infrequent) 2177
Travatan Ophthalmic Solution (1% to 4%) 563
Trileptal Tablets 2300
Trileptal Oral Suspension 2300
▲ Trisenox Injection (8%) 993
Trusopt Sterile Ophthalmic Solution (Approximately 1% to 5%) 2095
Vasotec I.V. Injection (0.5% to 1.0%) 2103
VESIcare Tablets (0.3% to 1.6%) 646
VFEND I.V. (Less than 2%) 2564
VFEND Oral Suspension (Less than 2%) 2564
VFEND Tablets (Less than 2%) 2564
Viagra Tablets (Less than 2%) 2573
Vicoprofen Tablets (Less than 1%) 539
▲ Vigamox Ophthalmic Solution (1% to 6%) 564
Visine For Contacts Rewetting Drops ⊙ 289
▲ Visudyne for Injection (1% to 10%) 2305
Wellbutrin SR Sustained-Release Tablets (Infrequent) 1607
Wellbutrin XL Extended-Release Tablets (Infrequent) 1613
Xalatan Sterile Ophthalmic Solution (1% to 4%) 2649
Zegerid Capsules (Less than 1%) 2958
Zegerid Powder for Oral Solution (Less than 1%) 2958
Zelapar Tablets 3372
Zoloft (Rare) 2586
Zomig Tablets (Infrequent) 3519
Zomig Nasal Spray (Rare) 3523
Zomig-ZMT Tablets (Infrequent) 3519
Zyban Sustained-Release Tablets (Infrequent) 1644
▲ Zymar Ophthalmic Solution (1% to 4%) 575
Zyprexa Tablets (Infrequent) 1830
Zyprexa ZYDIS Orally Disintegrating Tablets (Infrequent) 1830
Zyrtec Chewable Tablets (Less than 2%) 2594
Zyrtec (Less than 2%) 2594
Zyrtec-D 12 Hour Extended Release Tablets (Less than 2%) 2597

Xerosis cutis

Abilify Oral Solution (Frequent) 882
Abilify Oral Solution (Frequent) 2450
Abilify Discmelt Orally Disintegrating Tablets (Frequent) 882
Abilify Discmelt Orally Disintegrating Tablets (Frequent) 2450
Abilify Tablets (Frequent) 882
Abilify Tablets (Frequent) 2450
Accutane Capsules 2731
Aceon Tablets (2 mg, 4 mg, 8 mg) (0.3% to 1%) 3194
Aciphex Tablets (Rare) 1090
Advicor Tablets 1722
Aldara Cream, 5% 1846
Altoprev Extended-Release Tablets 3109
AmBisome for Injection (Less common) 620
Amerge Tablets (Rare) 1339
AndroGel (Fewer than 1%) 3329
Asacol Delayed-Release Tablets 2692
▲ Avastin IV (7% to 20%) 1227
Avinza Capsules (Less than 5%) 1741
Bactroban Cream (One report) 1394
Bactroban Ointment (Less than 1%) 1395
▲ Benzaclin Topical Gel (3%) 2877
Caduet Tablets (Less than 0.1%) 2508
Cafcit (2.2%) 1886
Campral Tablets (Infrequent) 1174
▲ Carac Cream, 0.5% (83.4%) 2879
Celebrex Capsules (0.1% to 1.9%) 3134
Celexa (Infrequent) 1176
Chantix Tablets (Infrequent) 2517
Cipro XR Tablets (Less than 1%) 2990
Clindagel 1203
Clobevate Gel 3211
Clobex Lotion (1%) 1204
Clobex Shampoo 1206
▲ Clolar for Intravenous Infusion (10%) 1271
Copaxone for Injection (Infrequent) 3297
▲ Copegus Tablets (10%) 2754
Cozaar Tablets (Less than 1%) 1935
Crixivan Capsules 1940
Cutivate Cream (0.8%) 2662
▲ Cutivate Lotion 0.05% (7%) 2664
Decadron Tablets 1951
▲ Depacon Injection (1% to 5%) 412
▲ Depakene (1% to 5%) 417
▲ Depakote Sprinkle Capsules (1% to 5%) 422
▲ Depakote Tablets (1% to 5%) 427
Depakote ER Tablets (Greater than 1%) 434
Depo-Provera Contraceptive Injection (Less than 1%) 2622
depo-subQ provera 104 Injectable Suspension 2624
Detrol Tablets (1%) 2628
▲ Differin Cream (Less than 1% to 38%) 1210
▲ Differin Gel (10% to 40%) 1211
▲ Diprolene Gel 0.05% (4%) 3001
Diprolene Lotion 0.05% (Infrequent) 3002
Diprolene Ointment 0.05% (Infrequent) 3003
Diprolene AF Cream 0.05% (Infrequent) 3000
Diprosone Cream, USP 0.05% 3004
▲ Ditropan XL Extended-Release Tablets (2% to less than 5%) 2413
▲ Doxil Injection (1% to 10%) 2351
▲ Duac Topical Gel (3%) 3212
Effexor Tablets (Infrequent) 3411
Effexor XR Capsules (Infrequent) 3417
Elocon Cream 0.1% (Infrequent) 3005
Elocon Ointment 0.1% (Infrequent) 3007
▲ Eloxatin for Injection (2% to 5%) 2892
Emcyt Capsules (2%) 2634
Enablex Extended-Release Tablets (Greater than or equal to 1%) 2203
Evoxac Capsules (Less than 1%) 1047
▲ Finacea Gel (1% to 6%) 1669
Follistim AQ Cartridge 2338
Gabitril Tablets (Frequent) 984
Gengraf Capsules (1% to less than 3%) 459
Gleevec Tablets (Less common) 2227
Guanidine Hydrochloride Tablets 3016
Hyzaar 50-12.5 Tablets 1990
Hyzaar 100-12.5 Tablets 1990
Hyzaar 100-25 Tablets 1990
Imitrex Injection 1463
Imitrex Nasal Spray 1467
Imitrex Tablets (Rare) 1471
▲ Infergen (2% to 6%) 3364
▲ Intron A for Injection (Up to 10%) 3024
Invirase (Less than or equal to 2%) 2772
▲ Iressa Tablets (13% to 30%) 684
Kaletra (Less than 2%) 476
Klonopin (Infrequent) 2778
▲ Lamictal (2% to 5%) 1481
Lescol Capsules 2233
Lescol XL Tablets 2233
Levaquin (0.1% to 0.9%) 2384
Levaquin in 5% Dextrose Injection (0.1% to 0.9%) 2384
Lexapro Oral Solution (Infrequent) 1190
Lexapro Tablets (Infrequent) 1190
Lipitor Tablets (Less than 2%) 2483
Lithobid Tablets 1692
Lotrisone (1.6%) 3040
Lunesta Tablets (Infrequent) 3142
Luxíq Foam 1010
Lyrica Capsules (0.1% to 1%) 2539
▲ Metrogel 1% (0.6% to 17.1%) 1211
Mevacor Tablets 2021
Myleran Tablets (Rare) 1525
Neoral Oral Solution (1% to less than 3%) 2259
Neoral Soft Gelatin Capsules (1% to less than 3%) 2259
Neurontin Capsules (Infrequent) 2487
Neurontin Oral Solution (Infrequent) 2487
Neurontin Tablets (Infrequent) 2487
▲ Nexavar Tablets (0% to 11%) 746
Niaspan Extended-Release Tablets 1730
▲ Nipent for Injection (3% to 10%) 1863
Norvasc Tablets (Less than 0.1%) 2545
Norvir (Less than 2%) 503
Olux Foam (One case) 1012
OxyContin Tablets (Less than 1%) 2703
Paxil CR Controlled-Release Tablets (Infrequent) 1538
Paxil (Infrequent) 1530
▲ Pegasys (4%) 2789
▲ PEG-Intron Powder for Injection (11%) 3048
Pentasa Capsules (Less than 1%) 3185
Pepcid Injection (Infrequent) 2040
Pepcid (Infrequent) 2038
Permax Tablets (Infrequent) 3356
Pletal Tablets (Less than 2%) 2455
Prevacid Delayed-Release Capsules (Less than 1%) 3271
Prevacid for Delayed-Release Oral Suspension (Less than 1%) 3271
Prevacid SoluTab Delayed-Release Orally Disintegrating Tablets (Less than 1%) 3271
Prevacid NapraPAC (Less than 1%) 3280
PREVPAC (Less than 1%) 3284
Prilosec OTC Delayed-Release Tablets (Less than 1%) 2677
ProAmatine Tablets (Rare) 3186
ProctoFoam-HC 3099
▲ Proleukin for Injection (15%) 2266
ProSom Tablets (Rare) 517
Protonix Tablets (Less than 1%) 3469
▲ Protopic Ointment (Up to 3%) 638
Provigil Tablets (1%) 988
▲ Rebetol (23% to 24%) 3058
Relpax Tablets 2548
Rescriptor Tablets 2551
▲ Revlimid Capsules (14.2%) 958
Reyataz Capsules (Less than 3%) 921
▲ Ribavirin, USP Capsules (23% to 24%) 3068
▲ Risperdal (2% to 4%) 1676
Risperdal Consta Long-Acting Injection (Up to 2%) 1682
▲ Risperdal M-Tab Orally Disintegrating Tablets (2% to 4%) 1676
Rythmol SR Capsules 2727
Sanctura Tablets (Greater than or equal to 0.5%) 1151

Sonata Capsules (Infrequent) 1717
▲ Soriatane Capsules (25% to 50%) 1013
Sular Tablets (Less than or equal to 1%) 3122
▲ Sutent Capsules (0% to 17%) 2560
Symbyax Capsules (Infrequent) 1819
▲ Tarceva Tablets (0% to 12%) 1259
▲ Tarceva Tablets (0% to 12%) 2444
▲ Targretin Capsules (9.4% to 10.7%) 1747
Taxotere Injection Concentrate 2932
▲ Temodar Capsules (5%) 3073
Tequin Injection (Less than 0.1%) 938
Tequin Injection in 5% Dextrose (Less than 0.1%) 938
Tequin Tablets (Less than 0.1%) 938
Thalomid Capsules 965
Topamax Sprinkle Capsules (Infrequent) 2404
Topamax Tablets (Infrequent) 2404
Triaz 1892
Triaz Pads 1892
▲ Tri-Luma Cream (8.08% to 14%) 1213
▲ Trisenox Injection (15%) 993
Uniretic Tablets (Less than 1%) 3100
Varivax (Greater than or equal to 1%) 2100
▲ Vesanoid Capsules (77%) 2820
VFEND I.V. (Less than 2%) 2564
VFEND Oral Suspension (Less than 2%) 2564
VFEND Tablets (Less than 2%) 2564
Vytorin 10/10 Tablets 2114
Vytorin 10/10 Tablets 3077
Vytorin 10/20 Tablets 2114
Vytorin 10/20 Tablets 3077
Vytorin 10/40 Tablets 2114
Vytorin 10/40 Tablets 3077
Vytorin 10/80 Tablets 2114
Vytorin 10/80 Tablets 3077
Wellbutrin Tablets (Infrequent) 1603
Xenical Capsules (2.1%) 2831
Zegerid Capsules (Less than 1%) 2958
Zegerid Powder for Oral Solution (Less than 1%) 2958
Zelapar Tablets 3372
Zocor Tablets 2105
Zoloft (Infrequent) 2586
Zonegran Capsules (Infrequent) 1101
Zovirax Cream (Less than 1%) 820
Zyban Sustained-Release Tablets (2%) 1644
Zyprexa Tablets (Infrequent) 1830
Zyprexa ZYDIS Orally Disintegrating Tablets (Infrequent) 1830
Zyrtec Chewable Tablets (Less than 2%) 2594
Zyrtec (Less than 2%) 2594
Zyrtec-D 12 Hour Extended Release Tablets (Less than 2%) 2597

Xerostomia

Abilify Oral Solution 882
Abilify Oral Solution 2450
Abilify Discmelt Orally Disintegrating Tablets 882
Abilify Discmelt Orally Disintegrating Tablets 2450
Abilify Tablets 882
Abilify Tablets 2450
Accutane Capsules 2731
Aceon Tablets (2 mg, 4 mg, 8 mg) (0.3% to 1%) 3194
Aciphex Tablets 1090
Actiq (1% to 2%) 979
Actonel Tablets (1.4% to 2.5%) 2683
Actonel with Calcium Tablets (1.4% to 2.5%) 2688
Adalat CC Tablets (Less than 1%) 2964
Adderall Tablets 3164
▲ Adderall XR Capsules (35%) 3166
Adenoscan (Less than 1%) 619
Adipex-P 1215
Advair Diskus 100/50 1308
Advair Diskus 250/50 1308
Advair Diskus 500/50 1308
Advair HFA Inhalation Aerosol 1318
Advicor Tablets 1722
Aldoril Tablets 1910
Alferon N Injection (One patient) 1665
Alimta for Injection (Less than 1%) 1750
Allegra-D 12 Hour Extended-Release Tablets (2.8%) 2846
Allegra-D 24 Hour Extended-Release Tablets (2.8%) 2849
Aloxi Injection (Less than 1%) 2127
▲ Alphagan P Ophthalmic Solution (Approximately 5% to 9%) 567
Altace Capsules (Less than 1%) 1702
Altoprev Extended-Release Tablets (0.5% to 1%) 3109
▲ Ambien Tablets (3%) 2851
Ambien CR Tablets (Frequent) 2855
AmBisome for Injection (Less common) 620
Amitiza Capsules (0% to 1.5%) 3224
Anaprox Tablets (Less than 1%) 2761
Anaprox DS Tablets (Less than 1%) 2761
Aricept Tablets (Infrequent) 1094
Aricept ODT Tablets (Infrequent) 1094
▲ Arimidex Tablets (4% to 6%) 673
Arthrotec Tablets (Rare) 3129
Asacol Delayed-Release Tablets 2692
Astelin Nasal Spray (2.8%) 1904
▲ Atrovent Inhalation Solution (3.2%) 835
▲ Atrovent HFA Inhalation Aerosol (1.6% to 4%) 841
Atrovent Nasal Spray 0.03% (Less than 2%) 837
Atrovent Nasal Spray 0.06% (1.4%) 839
Avalide Tablets 888
Avalide Tablets 2874
▲ Avastin IV (4% to 7%) 1227
Avelox (0.1% to less than 2%) 2970
▲ Avinza Capsules (5% to 10%) 1741
Axert Tablets (1%) 2396
Axid Oral Solution (1.4%) 879
▲ Azilect Tablets (6%) 3293
▲ Azmacort Inhalation Aerosol (1% to 3%) 1726
Azopt Ophthalmic Suspension (Less than 1%) 557
Bactroban Nasal (Less than 1%) 1394
▲ Bentyl Capsules (33%) 697
▲ Bentyl Injection (33%) 697
▲ Bentyl Syrup (33%) 697
▲ Bentyl Tablets (33%) 697
▲ Betimol Ophthalmic Solution (More than 5%) 3382
▲ Betimol Ophthalmic Solution (More than 5%) ⊙ 295
▲ Brimonidine Tartrate Ophthalmic Solution 0.2% (10% to 30%) ⊙ 248
Bumex Tablets (0.1%) 2746
Caduet Tablets (Greater than 0.1 to less than 2%) 2508
Calcijex Injection 411
▲ Campral Tablets (1% to 3%) 1174
Captopril Tablets (About 0.5% to 2%) 2149
Carafate Suspension (Less than 0.5%) 701
Carafate Tablets (Less than 0.5%) 701
Carbatrol Capsules 3171
Cardizem LA Extended Release Tablets (Less than 2%) 1728
▲ Catapres Tablets (40 of 100 patients) 843
▲ Catapres-TTS (25 of 101 patients) 844
Caverject Impulse Injection (Less than 1%) 2612
Celebrex Capsules (0.1% to 1.9%) 3134
▲ Celexa (20%) 1176
▲ CellCept Capsules (3% to less than 20%) 2747
▲ CellCept Intravenous (3% to less than 20%) 2747
▲ CellCept Oral Suspension (3% to less than 20%) 2747
▲ CellCept Tablets (3% to less than 20%) 2747
▲ Cesamet Capsules (22% to 36%) 3340
▲ Chantix Tablets (4% to 6%) 2517
Cialis Tablets (Less than 2%) 1838
Cipro I.V. (1% or less) 2984
Cipro XR Tablets (Less than 1%) 2990
▲ Clarinex Tablets (3%) 2995
▲ Clarinex Reditabs Tablets (3%) 2995
▲ Clarinex-D 24-Hour Extended-Release Tablets (8%) 2998
Clinoril Tablets (Less than 1%) 1924
▲ Clorpres Tablets (40%) 2153
▲ Clozaril Tablets (More than 5% to 6%) 2184
Colazal Capsules (1%) 2838
Combivent Inhalation Aerosol (Less than 2%) 847
▲ Comtan Tablets (3%) 2189
Copaxone for Injection (At least 2%) 3297
▲ Copegus Tablets (4%) 2754
Coreg Tablets (Greater than 0.1% to 1%) 1414
Cosopt Sterile Ophthalmic Solution (Less than 1%) 1931
Covera-HS Tablets (Less than 2%) 3139
Cozaar Tablets (Less than 1%) 1935
Cubicin for Injection (Less than 1%) 1026
▲ Cymbalta Delayed-Release Capsules (5% to 20%) 1757
Dalmane Capsules (Rare) 3342
Demadex Injection 2759
Demadex Tablets 2759
Demser Capsules (Infrequent) 1953
Depacon Injection (1% or more) 412
Depakene (1% or more) 417
Depakote Sprinkle Capsules 422
▲ Depakote Tablets (1% to 5%) 427
▲ Depakote ER Tablets (Greater than 1% to 5%) 434
Desoxyn Tablets, USP 2462
▲ Detrol Tablets (35%) 2628
▲ Detrol LA Capsules (23.4%) 2631
Dexedrine 1420
DextroStat Tablets 3179
Dilaudid 440
Dilaudid Non-Sterile Powder 440
Dilaudid Oral Liquid 445
Dilaudid Rectal Suppositories 440
Dilaudid Tablets 440
Dilaudid Tablets - 8 mg 445
Dilaudid-HP (Less frequent) 442
Diovan Tablets 2193
Diovan HCT Tablets (Greater than 0.2%) 2196
▲ Ditropan XL Extended-Release Tablets (29% to 61%) 2413
Diuril Sodium Intravenous 2467
Donnatal Extentabs 2493
▲ Doxil Injection (1% to 10%) 2351
▲ Duragesic Transdermal System (10% or more) 2373
Dyazide Capsules 1423
DynaCirc CR Tablets (0.5% to 1%) 2721
Dyrenium Capsules (Rare) 3400
EC-Naprosyn Delayed-Release Tablets (Less than 1%) 2761
▲ Effexor Tablets (2% to 22%) 3411
▲ Effexor XR Capsules (5% to 17%) 3417
▲ Eldepryl Capsules (3 of 49 patients) 3208
Elocon Lotion 0.1% (1 in 65 patients) 3006
▲ Eloxatin for Injection (2% to 5%) 2892
Emend Capsules (Greater than 0.5%) 1963
▲ Emsam Transdermal System (8%) 903
▲ Enablex Extended-Release Tablets (18.7% to 35.3%) 2203
Enbrel for Injection 584
▲ Equetro Extended-Release Capsules (8%) 3180
▲ Erbitux (5% to 72%) 910
▲ Evoxac Capsules (1% to 3%) 1047
Exelon Capsules (Infrequent) 2206
Exelon Oral Solution (Infrequent) 2206
Exubera Inhalation Powder (2.4%) 2524
▲ FazaClo Orally Disintegrating Tablets (Greater than 5% to 6%) 551
Ferrlecit Injection (Two or more patients) 3388
Floxin Otic Solution (0.5%) 1049
Flumadine (1.5%) 1183
▲ Focalin XR Capsules (7% to 20%) 2223
Foradil Aerolizer (1.2%) 3010
Fortical Nasal Spray (Less than 1%) 3337
▲ Frova Tablets (3%) 1113
Furosemide Tablets 2154
Fuzeon Injection (2.1%) 2767
Gabitril Tablets (1% or more) 984
Gengraf Capsules (1% to less than 3%) 459
▲ Geodon (4% to 5%) 2529
Guanidine Hydrochloride Tablets 3016
Hectorol Capsules 1275
Hectorol Injection 1278
Hyperstat I.V. 3017
Hytrin Capsules (At least 1%) 471
Hyzaar 50-12.5 Tablets 1990
Hyzaar 100-12.5 Tablets 1990
Hyzaar 100-25 Tablets 1990
▲ Imdur Tablets (Less than or equal to 5%) 3018
Imitrex Injection 1463
Imitrex Nasal Spray (Infrequent) 1467
Imitrex Tablets 1471
▲ Infergen (4% to 6%) 3364
▲ Intron A for Injection (Up to 28%) 3024
Invirase (Less than 2%) 2772
Ionsys Transdermal System (.1% to less than 1%) 2379
▲ I.V. Busulfex (26%) 2493
Kadian Capsules (Less than 3%) 577
Kaletra (Less than 2%) 476
Ketek Tablets (Greater than or equal to 0.2% to less than 2%) 2903
Klonopin 2778
▲ Lamictal (2% to 6%) 1481
Levaquin (0.2%) 2384
Levaquin in 5% Dextrose Injection (0.2%) 2384
Levitra Tablets (Less than 2%) 3034
▲ Lexapro Oral Solution (4% to 9%) 1190
▲ Lexapro Tablets (4% to 9%) 1190
Lipitor Tablets (Less than 2%) 2483
Lithobid Tablets 1692
Lofibra Tablets 1219
Lofibra Capsules 1216
Lopressor Injection (1%) 2238
Lopressor Tablets (1%) 2238
Lopressor HCT 50/25 Tablets (1%) 2241
Lopressor HCT 100/25 Tablets (1%) 2241
Lopressor HCT 100/50 Tablets (1%) 2241
Lotensin HCT Tablets (0.3% to 1%) 2246
Lotrel Capsules 2249
▲ Lunesta Tablets (3% to 7%) 3142
▲ Lupron Depot 3.75 mg (Less than 5%) 3260
Lupron Depot–3 Month 11.25 mg (Less than 5%) 3265
▲ Lyrica Capsules (3% to 15%) 2539
Matulane Capsules 3191
Maxair Autohaler (1.3%) 1852
▲ Maxalt Tablets (3%) 2008
▲ Maxalt-MLT Orally Disintegrating Tablets (3%) 2008
▲ Megace ES Oral Suspension (1% to 3%) 2481
▲ Meridia Capsules (17.2%) 489
MetroGel-Vaginal Gel (Less than 1%) 1855
Mevacor Tablets (0.5% to 1.0%) 2021
Miacalcin Nasal Spray (Less than 1%) 2253
Micardis Tablets (More than 0.3%) 854
Micardis HCT Tablets 856
Midamor Tablets (Less than or equal to 1%) 2026
Migranal Nasal Spray (1%) 3348
Mintezol 2027
▲ Mirapex Tablets (Greater than or equal to 1% to 7%) 859
Moban Tablets (Occasional) 1119
Mobic Oral Suspension (Less than 2%) 863
Mobic Tablets (Less than 2%) 863
Moduretic Tablets 2028
MS Contin Tablets (Less frequent) 2701
▲ Myobloc Injection (3% to 34%) 3192
Nadolol Tablets (1 to 5 of 1000 patients) 2159
Nalfon Capsules (Less than 1%) 2502
Naprosyn Suspension (Less than 1%) 2761
Naprosyn Tablets (Less than 1%) 2761
Neoral Oral Solution (1% to less than 3%) 2259
Neoral Soft Gelatin Capsules (1% to less than 3%) 2259
▲ Neurontin Capsules (1.7% to 4.8%) 2487
▲ Neurontin Oral Solution (1.7% to 4.8%) 2487
▲ Neurontin Tablets (1.7% to 4.8%) 2487
▲ Nexavar Tablets (Common) 746
Nexium Delayed-Release Capsules (Greater than or equal to 1%) 655
Nexium I.V. (Greater than or equal to 1%) 659
Niaspan Extended-Release Tablets 1730
▲ Niravam Orally Disintegrating Tablets (14.7%) 3092
Norflex Injection 1856
Noroxin Tablets (0.3 to 1.0%) 2032
Norvasc Tablets (More than 0.1% to 1%) 2545
Norvir (Less than 2%) 503
Numorphan Injection 1120
Omacor Capsules 2725
Omnicef Capsules (0.3%) 511
▲ Opana Tablets (1% to less than 10%) 1122
▲ Opana ER Tablets (1% to less than 10%) 1126
Oracea Capsules (1.1%) 1000
▲ OxyContin Tablets (6%) 2703
▲ Oxytrol Transdermal System (4.1% to 9.6%) 3392
Parcopa Orally Disintegrating Tablets 3097
Parnate Tablets 1527
▲ Paxil CR Controlled-Release Tablets (1.0% to 20.6%) 1538
▲ Paxil (1.0% to 20.6%) 1530
▲ Pegasys (6%) 2789
▲ PEG-Intron Powder for Injection (6%) 3048
Pepcid Injection (Infrequent) 2040
Pepcid (Infrequent) 2038
Percodan Tablets 1132
▲ Permax Tablets (3.7%; Frequent) 3356
Phenergan Tablets and Suppositories 3440
Prevacid Delayed-Release Capsules (Less than 1%) 3271
Prevacid for Delayed-Release Oral Suspension (Less than 1%) 3271

Prevacid SoluTab Delayed-Release Orally Disintegrating Tablets (Less than 1%) 3271
Prevacid NapraPAC (Less than 1%) 3280
PREVPAC (Less than 1% to 3%) 3284
Prezista Tablets (Less than 2%) 3306
Prilosec OTC Delayed-Release Tablets (Less than 1%) 2677
Prinivil Tablets (0.3% to 1.0%) 2052
Prinzide Tablets (0.3% to 1%) 2056
ProAmatine Tablets (Less frequent) 3186
Prochieve 4% Gel 1003
Prochieve 8% Gel 1003
▲ Prometrium Capsules (100 mg, 200 mg) (Less than 5%) 3203
Proquin XR Tablets 1153
Prosed/DS Tablets 1157
ProSom Tablets (Frequent) 517
Protonix I.V. (Less than 1%) 3472
Protonix Tablets (Less than 1%) 3469
Protopic Ointment (0.2% to less than 1%) 638
Proventil HFA Inhalation Aerosol (Less than 3%) 3056
▲ Provigil Tablets (4%) 988
▲ Prozac Pulvules and Liquid (4% to 12%) 1801
Ranexa Tablets (Greater than 0.5% to less than 2%) 1035
Razadyne (Infrequent) 2399
Razadyne ER Extended-Release Capsules (Infrequent) 2399
▲ Rebetol (8% to 12%) 3058
▲ Rebif Prefilled Syringe for Injection (1% to 5%) 3159
▲ Relpax Tablets (2% to 4%) 2548
ReoPro Vials (0.1%) 1809
▲ Requip Tablets (3% to 5%) 1555
Rescriptor Tablets 2551
Restoril Capsules (1.7%) 1860
▲ Revlimid Capsules (6.8%) 958
▲ Ribavirin, USP Capsules (8% to 12%) 3068
▲ Rilutek Tablets (2.0% to 3.0%) 2930
▲ Risperdal (3%) 1676
▲ Risperdal Consta Long-Acting Injection (Up to 7%) 1682
▲ Risperdal M-Tab Orally Disintegrating Tablets (3%) 1676
Rocaltrol Capsules 2798
Rocaltrol Oral Solution 2798
▲ Romazicon Injection (3% to 9%) 2804
▲ Rythmol SR Capsules (1% to 4%) 2727
▲ Sanctura Tablets (20.1%) 1151
▲ Sandostatin LAR Depot (1% to 4%) 2280
▲ Seroquel Tablets (9%) 690
Solodyn Extended Release Tablets (1%) 1890
Sonata Capsules (Frequent) 1717
▲ Spiriva HandiHaler (12% to 16%) 869
▲ Stalevo Tablets (3%) 2287
▲ Strattera Capsules (21%) 1814
Striant Mucoadhesive 1007
Sular Tablets (Less than or equal to 1%) 3122
▲ Symbyax Capsules (11% to 16%) 1819
▲ Symmetrel Tablets (1% to 5%) 1135
Tambocor Tablets (Less than 1%) 1856
Targretin Capsules 1747
Tarka Tablets (0.3% or more) 524
▲ Tasmar Tablets (5% to 6%) 3358
Tegretol/Tegretol-XR 2295
Teveten Tablets (Less than 1%) 1735
Teveten HCT Tablets (Less than 1%) 1737
▲ Thalomid Capsules (8.3% to 9.4%) 965
Thioridazine Hydrochloride Tablets 2163
Thiothixene Capsules 2165
Tiazac Capsules (Less than 2%) 1201
Timoptic Sterile Ophthalmic Solution (Less frequent) 2088
Timoptic in Ocudose (Less frequent) 2091
Timoptic-XE Sterile Ophthalmic Gel Forming Solution 2092
Tindamax Tablets 2142
▲ Topamax Sprinkle Capsules (2% to 5%) 2404
▲ Topamax Tablets (2% to 5%) 2404
Toprol-XL Tablets (About 1 of 100 patients) 668
▲ Transderm Scōp Transdermal Therapeutic System (29% to about two-thirds) 2177
Tranxene (Less common) 2474
Tricor Tablets 527
▲ Trileptal Tablets (Up to 3%) 2300
▲ Trileptal Oral Suspension (Up to 3%) 2300
Tri-Luma Cream (1%) 1213
▲ Trisenox Injection (8%) 993
Trusopt Sterile Ophthalmic Solution 2095
Tygacil for Injection (0% to less than 2%) 3488
Ultane Liquid for Inhalation (Less than 1%) 531
Uniretic Tablets (Less than 1%) 3100
Univasc Tablets (Less than 1%) 3104
Vantin Tablets and Oral Suspension (Less than 1%) 2645
▲ Vaprisol (3.8%) 643
Vasotec I.V. Injection (0.5% to 1.0%) 2103
Verelan PM Extended-Release Capsules, Controlled-Onset (2% or less) 3106
▲ VESIcare Tablets (10.9% to 27.6%) 646
VFEND I.V. (Less than 2%) 2564
VFEND Oral Suspension (Less than 2%) 2564
VFEND Tablets (Less than 2%) 2564
Viadur Implant (Less than 2%) 757
Viagra Tablets (Less than 2%) 2573
▲ Vicoprofen Tablets (3% to 9%) 539
▲ Vivitrol (4% to 24%) 995
Voltaren Tablets (Occasionally) 2307
Voltaren-XR Tablets (Occasionally) 2310
▲ Wellbutrin Tablets (27.6%) 1603
▲ Wellbutrin SR Sustained-Release Tablets (5% to 24%) 1607
▲ Wellbutrin XL Extended-Release Tablets (5% to 26%) 1613
▲ Xeloda Tablets (Less than 1% to 6%) 2822
Xopenex Inhalation Solution 3146
Xopenex Inhalation Solution Concentrate 3150
Xopenex HFA Inhalation Aerosol 3154
Zegerid Capsules (Less than 1%) 2958
Zegerid Powder for Oral Solution (Less than 1%) 2958
▲ Zelapar Tablets (4%) 3372
▲ Zemplar Capsules (3%) 541
▲ Zemplar Injection (3%) 543
Zofran (1% to 2%) 1639
Zofran ODT Orally Disintegrating Tablets (1% to 2%) 1639
▲ Zoloft (6% to 16%) 2586
Zometa for Intravenous Infusion 2315
▲ Zomig Nasal Spray (1% to 3%) 3523
Zonegran Capsules (2%) 1101
▲ Zyban Sustained-Release Tablets (10% to 11%) 1644
▲ Zyprexa Tablets (2% to 32%) 1830
▲ Zyprexa ZYDIS Orally Disintegrating Tablets (2% to 32%) 1830
▲ Zyrtec Chewable Tablets (Less than 2% to 5%) 2594
▲ Zyrtec (Less than 2% to 5%) 2594
▲ Zyrtec-D 12 Hour Extended Release Tablets (3.6% to 5%) 2597

Y

Yawning

Ambien Tablets (Rare) 2851
Ambien CR Tablets (Rare) 2855
Celexa (2%) 1176
▲ Effexor Tablets (3% to 8%) 3411
▲ Effexor XR Capsules (3% to 5%) 3417
Evoxac Capsules 1047
Imitrex Injection (Rare) 1463
Imitrex Nasal Spray 1467
Imitrex Tablets 1471
Klonopin (Infrequent) 2778
Lamictal (Infrequent) 1481
Lexapro Oral Solution (2%) 1190
Lexapro Tablets (2%) 1190
Lyrica Capsules (Rare) 2539
Maxalt Tablets (Infrequent) 2008
Maxalt-MLT Orally Disintegrating Tablets (Infrequent) 2008
Meridia Capsules 489
Migranal Nasal Spray (Rare) 3348
▲ Paxil CR Controlled-Release Tablets (4%) 1538
▲ Paxil (4%) 1530
▲ Prozac Pulvules and Liquid (3%) 1801
Relpax Tablets (Infrequent) 2548
▲ Requip Tablets (3%) 1555
Rilutek Tablets (Infrequent) 2930
Risperdal (Rare) 1676
Risperdal M-Tab Orally Disintegrating Tablets (Rare) 1676
Symbyax Capsules (Infrequent) 1819
▲ Ultram ER Tablets (1% to greater than 5%) 2392
Zoloft (Frequent) 2586
Zomig Tablets (Infrequent) 3519
Zomig Nasal Spray (Rare) 3523
Zomig-ZMT Tablets (Infrequent) 3519

Z

Zinc deficiency

Calcium Disodium Versenate Injection 1851

Zollinger-Ellison syndrome

Zegerid Capsules (Less than 1%) 2958
Zegerid Powder for Oral Solution (Less than 1%) 2958

SECTION 4

INDICATIONS INDEX

This section lists in alphabetical order every indication cited in *PDR®* and its companion volumes, with cross-references to each product entry in which the indication is found. For easy comparison, each listing includes the product's brand name, generic ingredients, and manufacturer. Page numbers refer to the 2007 editions of *PDR®*, *PDR for Ophthalmic Medicines™* and the *PDR for Nonprescription Drugs, Dietary Supplements and Herbs™*, which is published later each year. A key to the symbols denoting the companion volumes appears in the bottom margin.

Because *PDR®* publishes only official product labeling, only approved indications are cited here. No unapproved uses are listed.

This index is intended to assist you in identifying the extent and nature of your prescribing alternatives as quickly and easily as possible. However, it is by its nature only an extract of the official labeling as it appears in *PDR®*. For more definitive information, always consult the underlying *PDR®* text.

A

A. baumanii infections
Zosyn (Piperacillin Sodium, Tazobactam Sodium) Wyeth **3492**

Abrasions, pain associated with
(*see under* Pain, topical relief of)

Abrasions, skin
(*see under* Infections, skin, bacterial, minor)

Abscess, cutaneous
(*see also under* Infections, skin and skin structure)
Levaquin (Levofloxacin) Ortho-McNeil **2384**
Levaquin in 5% Dextrose Injection (Levofloxacin) Ortho-McNeil **2384**
Zosyn (Piperacillin Sodium, Tazobactam Sodium) Wyeth **3492**

Abscess, hepatic
(*see under* Infections, intra-abdominal)

Abscess, intra-abdominal
(*see also under* Infections, intra-abdominal)
Cancidas for Injection (Caspofungin acetate) Merck **1918**
Cleocin Vaginal Ovules (Clindamycin Hydrochloride) Pharmacia & Upjohn **2616**
Mefoxin for Injection (Cefoxitin Sodium) Merck **2012**
Mefoxin Premixed Intravenous Solution (Cefoxitin Sodium) Merck **2016**

Abscess, lung
(*see also under* Infections, lower respiratory tract)
Cleocin Vaginal Ovules (Clindamycin Hydrochloride) Pharmacia & Upjohn **2616**
Mefoxin for Injection (Cefoxitin Sodium) Merck **2012**
Mefoxin Premixed Intravenous Solution (Cefoxitin Sodium) Merck **2016**

Abscess, tubo-ovarian
(*see under* Infections, gynecologic)

Acetaminophen overdose, management of
Acetadote Injection (Acetylcysteine) Cumberland **1031**

Aches
(*see under* Pain, general)

Aches, muscular
(*see under* Pain, muscular, temporary relief of)

Aches due to common cold
(*see under* Pain associated with upper respiratory infection)

Acid alpha glucosidase, deficiency of
Myozyme for Intravenous Infusion (Alglucosidase alfa) Genzyme........ **1279**

Acid indigestion
(*see under* Hyperacidity, gastric, symptomatic relief of)

Acinetobacter calcoaceticus infections
Primaxin I.M. (Cilastatin Sodium, Imipenem) Merck **2045**
Rocephin Injectable Vials, ADD-Vantage, Galaxy, Bulk (Ceftriaxone Sodium) Roche......... **2800**

Acinetobacter calcoaceticus infections, ocular
Quixin Ophthalmic Solution (Levofloxacin) Vistakon.......................... **3383**
TobraDex Ophthalmic Ointment (Dexamethasone, Tobramycin) Alcon.. **562**
TobraDex Ophthalmic Suspension (Dexamethasone, Tobramycin) Alcon.. **563**

Acinetobacter calcoaceticus skin and skin structure infections
Primaxin I.M. (Cilastatin Sodium, Imipenem) Merck **2045**

Acinetobacter iwoffi
Vigamox Ophthalmic Solution (Moxifloxacin Hydrochloride) Alcon.. **564**

Acinetobacter species infections
Primaxin I.M. (Cilastatin Sodium, Imipenem) Merck **2045**
Primaxin I.V. (Cilastatin Sodium, Imipenem) Merck **2048**

Acinetobacter species lower respiratory tract infection
Primaxin I.V. (Cilastatin Sodium, Imipenem) Merck **2048**

Acinetobacter species skin and skin structure infections
Primaxin I.M. (Cilastatin Sodium, Imipenem) Merck **2045**
Primaxin I.V. (Cilastatin Sodium, Imipenem) Merck **2048**
Rocephin Injectable Vials, ADD-Vantage, Galaxy, Bulk (Ceftriaxone Sodium) Roche.......... **2800**

Acne, cystic, severe recalcitrant
Accutane Capsules (Isotretinoin) Roche.. **2731**

Acne rosacea
Avar Cleanser (Sodium Sulfacetamide, Sulfur) Dusa **1085**
Avar Gel (Sodium Sulfacetamide, Sulfur) Dusa................................ **1085**
Avar Green Gel (Sodium Sulfacetamide, Sulfur) Dusa **1085**
Avar-e Emollient Cream (Sodium Sulfacetamide, Sulfur) Dusa **1085**
Avar-e Green Cream (Sodium Sulfacetamide, Sulfur) Dusa................ **1085**
Nicomide Tablets (Folic Acid, Nicotinamide, Zinc Oxide) Dusa **1088**
Plexion (Sodium Sulfacetamide, Sulfur) Medicis **1889**
Rosac Cream with Sunscreens (Sodium Sulfacetamide, Sulfur) Stiefel... **3213**

Acne vulgaris
Avar Cleanser (Sodium Sulfacetamide, Sulfur) Dusa **1085**
Avar Gel (Sodium Sulfacetamide, Sulfur) Dusa................................ **1085**
Avar Green Gel (Sodium Sulfacetamide, Sulfur) Dusa **1085**
Avar-e Emollient Cream (Sodium Sulfacetamide, Sulfur) Dusa **1085**
Avar-e Green Cream (Sodium Sulfacetamide, Sulfur) Dusa................ **1085**
Benzaclin Topical Gel (Benzoyl Peroxide, Clindamycin Phosphate) sanofi-aventis **2877**
Brevoxyl-4 Creamy Wash (Benzoyl Peroxide) Stiefel **3210**
Brevoxyl-4 Gel (Benzoyl Peroxide) Stiefel... **3210**
Brevoxyl-8 Creamy Wash (Benzoyl Peroxide) Stiefel **3210**
Brevoxyl-8 Gel (Benzoyl Peroxide) Stiefel... **3210**
Clindagel (Clindamycin Phosphate) Galderma.................................... **1203**
Differin Cream (Adapalene) Galderma.................................... **1210**

Differin Gel (Adapalene) Galderma 1211
Duac Topical Gel (Benzoyl Peroxide, Clindamycin) Stiefel 3212
Evoclin Foam, 1% (Clindamycin Phosphate) Connetics 1009
Klaron Lotion 10% (Sulfacetamide Sodium) sanofi-aventis 2909
Nicomide Tablets (Folic Acid, Nicotinamide, Zinc Oxide) Dusa 1088
Ortho Tri-Cyclen Tablets (Ethinyl Estradiol, Norgestimate) Ortho Women's Health & Urology........... 2429
Plexion (Sodium Sulfacetamide, Sulfur) Medicis 1889
Rosac Cream with Sunscreens (Sodium Sulfacetamide, Sulfur) Stiefel.. 3213
Solodyn Extended Release Tablets (Minocycline Hydrochloride) Medicis.. 1890
Triaz (Benzoyl Peroxide) Medicis 1892
Triaz Pads (Benzoyl Peroxide) Medicis 1892

Acquired immunodeficiency syndrome
(*see under* Infections, human immunodeficiency virus)

Acromegaly
Sandostatin Injection (Octreotide Acetate) Novartis 2278
Sandostatin LAR Depot (Octreotide Acetate) Novartis 2280
Somavert Injection (Pegvisomant) Pharmacia & Upjohn 2642

Actinic keratoses, topical treatment of
Levulan Kerastick for Topical Solution, 20% (Aminolevulinic Acid Hydrochloride) Dusa 1085

Addison's disease
(*see under* Adrenocortical insufficiency)

Adenocarcinoma, cervical, prevention of
Gardasil Injection (Quadrivalent Human Papillomavirus (Types 6, 11, 16, 18) Recombinant Vaccine) Merck 1984

Adenomatous polyposis, familial
Celebrex Capsules (Celecoxib) Searle 3134

Adenosine deaminase, enzyme replacement therapy for
Flebogamma 5%, Immune Globulin Intravenous (Human) (Globulin, Immune (Human)) Grifols 1658
Gamunex Immune Globulin I.V., 10% (Immune Globulin Intravenous (Human)) Talecris 3235

ADHD
(*see under* Attention Deficit Hyperactivity Disorder)

Adrenal hyperplasia, congenital
Decadron Tablets (Dexamethasone) Merck 1951
Depo-Medrol Injectable Suspension (Methylprednisolone Acetate) Pharmacia & Upjohn 2617
Depo-Medrol Single-Dose Vial (Methylprednisolone Acetate) Pharmacia & Upjohn 2619
Hydrocortone Tablets (Hydrocortisone) Merck 1989

Adrenocortical hyperfunction, diagnostic testing of
Decadron Tablets (Dexamethasone) Merck 1951

Adrenocortical insufficiency
Depo-Medrol Injectable Suspension (Methylprednisolone Acetate) Pharmacia & Upjohn 2617
Depo-Medrol Single-Dose Vial (Methylprednisolone Acetate) Pharmacia & Upjohn 2619
Hydrocortone Tablets (Hydrocortisone) Merck 1989

Aerobacter aerogenes infections
(*see under* Enterobacter aerogenes infections)

Agammaglobulinemias, congenital
Gammagard Liquid (Immune Globulin Intravenous (Human)) Baxter Healthcare 721
Gammagard S/D (Immune Globulin Intravenous (Human)) Baxter Healthcare 724
Gamunex Immune Globulin I.V., 10% (Immune Globulin Intravenous (Human)) Talecris................. 3235

AIDS
(*see under* Infections, human immunodeficiency virus)

AIDS related complex
(*see under* Infections, acquired immunodeficiency syndrome-related complex)

Airway obstruction disorders
(*see under* Bronchial asthma; Emphysema)

Albinism
(*see under* Hypopigmentation, skin)

Alcohol dependence
Vivitrol (Naltrexone) Cephalon 995

Alcohol withdrawal, acute, symptomatic relief of
Librium Capsules (Chlordiazepoxide Hydrochloride) Valeant 3347
Tranxene (Clorazepate Dipotassium) Ovation 2474
Valium Tablets (Diazepam) Roche 2819

Alcoholism, chronic, an aid in the management of
Campral Tablets (Acamprosate Calcium) Forest 1174

Allergic reactions, drug-induced
(*see under* Hypersensitivity reactions, drug-induced)

Allergic reactions, general
Decadron Tablets (Dexamethasone) Merck 1951
Depo-Medrol Injectable Suspension (Methylprednisolone Acetate) Pharmacia & Upjohn 2617
EpiPen (Epinephrine) Dey 1061
Hydrocortone Tablets (Hydrocortisone) Merck 1989
Twinject 0.3 (Epinephrine) Verus 3378
Twinject 0.15 (Epinephrine) Verus 3379

Allergic reactions associated with blood or plasma
Phenergan Tablets and Suppositories (Promethazine Hydrochloride) Wyeth 3440

Allergic rhinitis
(*see under* Rhinitis, allergic)

Allergies, respiratory
Advil Allergy Sinus Caplets (Chlorpheniramine Maleate, Ibuprofen, Pseudoephedrine Hydrochloride) Wyeth ....▣770
Advil Multi-Symptom Cold Caplets (Chlorpheniramine Maleate, Ibuprofen, Pseudoephedrine Hydrochloride) Wyeth ....▣770
Alavert Allergy & Sinus D-12 Hour Tablets (Loratadine, Pseudoephedrine Sulfate) Wyeth ....▣771
Claritin Non-Drowsy 24 Hour Tablets (Loratadine) Schering-Plough ....▣772
Claritin Reditabs 24 Hour Non-Drowsy Tablets (Loratadine) Schering-Plough ....▣772
Claritin-D Non-Drowsy 12 Hour Tablets (Loratadine, Pseudoephedrine Sulfate) Schering-Plough ....▣772
Claritin-D Non-Drowsy 24 Hour Tablets (Loratadine, Pseudoephedrine Sulfate) Schering-Plough ....▣772
Children's Dimetapp Cold & Allergy Elixir (Brompheniramine Maleate, Phenylephrine Hydrochloride) Wyeth ....▣730
Children's Dimetapp Cold & Allergy Chewable Tablets (Brompheniramine Maleate, Phenylephrine Hydrochloride) Wyeth ....▣730
Children's Dimetapp DM Cold & Cough Elixir (Brompheniramine Maleate, Dextromethorphan Hydrobromide, Phenylephrine Hydrochloride) Wyeth ....▣731
Toddler's Dimetapp Cold and Cough Drops (Dextromethorphan Hydrobromide, Phenylephrine Hydrochloride) Wyeth ....▣732
4-Way Menthol Nasal Spray (Phenylephrine Hydrochloride) Novartis Consumer ....▣775
Robitussin Cough & Cold Long-Acting Liquid (Chlorpheniramine Maleate, Dextromethorphan Hydrobromide) Wyeth ....▣735
Robitussin Cough & Allergy Syrup (Chlorpheniramine Maleate, Dextromethorphan Hydrobromide, Phenylephrine Hydrochloride) Wyeth ....▣736
Robitussin Cough & Cold Nighttime Liquid (Chlorpheniramine Maleate, Dextromethorphan Hydrobromide, Phenylephrine Hydrochloride) Wyeth ....▣736
Robitussin Cough, Cold & Flu Nighttime Liquid (Acetaminophen, Chlorpheniramine Maleate, Dextromethorphan Hydrobromide, Phenylephrine Hydrochloride) Wyeth ....▣738
Robitussin Pediatric Cough & Cold Long-Acting Liquid (Chlorpheniramine Maleate, Dextromethorphan Hydrobromide) Wyeth ....▣735
Robitussin Pediatric Cough & Cold Nighttime Liquid (Chlorpheniramine Maleate, Dextromethorphan Hydrobromide, Phenylephrine Hydrochloride) Wyeth ....▣736
TheraFlu Cold & Cough Hot Liquid (Dextromethorphan Hydrobromide, Pheniramine Maleate, Phenylephrine Hydrochloride) Novartis Consumer ....▣740
TheraFlu Cold & Sore Throat Hot Liquid (Acetaminophen, Pheniramine Maleate, Phenylephrine Hydrochloride) Novartis Consumer ....▣741
TheraFlu Flu & Sore Throat Hot Liquid (Acetaminophen, Pheniramine Maleate, Phenylephrine Hydrochloride) Novartis Consumer ....▣742
TheraFlu Nighttime Severe Cold Hot Liquid (Acetaminophen, Pheniramine Maleate, Phenylephrine Hydrochloride) Novartis Consumer ....▣740
Children's Tylenol Plus Cold & Allergy Oral Suspension (Acetaminophen, Diphenhydramine Hydrochloride, Phenylephrine Hydrochloride) McNeil Consumer .▣716
Tylenol Allergy Multi-Symptom Caplets with Cool Burst and Gelcaps (Acetaminophen, Chlorpheniramine Maleate, Phenylephrine Hydrochloride) McNeil Consumer 1872
Tylenol Allergy Multi-Symptom Nighttime Caplets with Cool Burst (Acetaminophen, Diphenhydramine Hydrochloride, Phenylephrine Hydrochloride) McNeil Consumer 1872
Tylenol Severe Allergy Caplets (Acetaminophen, Diphenhydramine Hydrochloride) McNeil Consumer 1872
Children's Tylenol Plus Cold & Allergy Suspension Liquid (Acetaminophen, Diphenhydramine Hydrochloride, Phenylephrine Hydrochloride) McNeil Consumer ..1878
Tylenol Sinus Congestion & Pain Daytime Caplets with Cool Burst and Gelcaps (Acetaminophen, Phenylephrine Hydrochloride) McNeil Consumer 1876
Vicks Sinex Nasal Spray and Ultra Fine Mist for Sinus Relief (Oxymetazoline Hydrochloride) Procter & Gamble........................ 2681
Vicks Sinex 12-Hour Nasal Spray and Ultra Fine Mist for Sinus Relief (Oxymetazoline Hydrochloride) Procter & Gamble 2681
Vicks Vapor Inhaler (Levmetamfetamine) Procter & Gamble............ 2682
Zicam Allergy Relief (Histanium Hydrochloricum, Luffa operculata, Galphimia Glauca, Sulfur) Matrixx.. ▣774
Zicam Extreme Congestion Relief (Oxymetazoline Hydrochloride) Matrixx.. ▣767
Zicam Intense Sinus Relief (Oxymetazoline Hydrochloride) Matrixx.. ▣767

Allergy, insect stings, immunotherapy of
Twinject 0.3 (Epinephrine) Verus 3378
Twinject 0.15 (Epinephrine) Verus 3379

Allergy, unspecified, immunotherapy of
Twinject 0.3 (Epinephrine) Verus 3378
Twinject 0.15 (Epinephrine) Verus 3379

Alopecia, androgenetic
Propecia Tablets (Finasteride) Merck 2060

Alopecia areata
Depo-Medrol Single-Dose Vial (Methylprednisolone Acetate) Pharmacia & Upjohn 2619

Alpha1-Proteinase inhibitor deficiency
Zemaira (Alpha$_1$-Proteinase Inhibitor (Human)) ZLB Behring............. 3509

Alzheimer's disease
(*see under* Dementia, Alzheimer's type)

Amebiasis, acute intestinal
E.E.S. (Erythromycin Ethylsuccinate) Abbott...................................... 451
EryPed (Erythromycin Ethylsuccinate) Abbott....................................... 447
Ery-Tab Tablets (Erythromycin) Abbott 449
Erythrocin Stearate Filmtab Tablets (Erythromycin Stearate) Abbott 453
Erythromycin Base Filmtab Tablets (Erythromycin) Abbott 455
Erythromycin Delayed-Release Capsules, USP (Erythromycin) Abbott 457
PCE Dispertab Tablets (Erythromycin) Abbott....................................... 515

Amebiasis, intestinal
Tindamax (Tinidazole) Mission 2142

Amebic liver abscess
Tindamax Tablets (Tinidazole) Mission... 2142

Amenorrhea, secondary
Prochieve 4% Gel (Progesterone) Columbia 1003
Prochieve 8% Gel (Progesterone) Columbia 1003
Prometrium Capsules (100 mg, 200 mg) (Progesterone) Solvay 3203

Amyotrophic lateral sclerosis
Rilutek Tablets (Riluzole) sanofi-aventis................................ 2930

Analgesia
(*see under* Pain, general)

Anaphylactic reactions, adjunctive therapy in
Phenergan Tablets and Suppositories (Promethazine Hydrochloride) Wyeth.................... 3440

Anaphylactic shock, due to insect bite
Twinject 0.3 (Epinephrine) Verus 3378
Twinject 0.15 (Epinephrine) Verus 3379

Anaphylactoid reactions
EpiPen (Epinephrine) Dey 1061

Anaphylactoid reactions, contrast media-induced
Twinject 0.3 (Epinephrine) Verus 3378
Twinject 0.15 (Epinephrine) Verus 3379

Anaphylaxis, idiopathic
EpiPen (Epinephrine) Dey 1061
Twinject 0.3 (Epinephrine) Verus 3378
Twinject 0.15 (Epinephrine) Verus 3379

Anaphylaxis, treatment of
EpiPen (Epinephrine) Dey 1061
Twinject 0.3 (Epinephrine) Verus 3378
Twinject 0.15 (Epinephrine) Verus 3379

Ancylostoma duodenale infections
Mintezol (Thiabendazole) Merck........ 2027

Androgen, absence or deficiency of
AndroGel (Testosterone) Unimed 3329
Androxy Tablets (Fluoxymesterone) Upsher-Smith 3335
Striant Mucoadhesive (Testosterone) Columbia 1007
Testim 1% Gel (Testosterone) Auxilium.. 695

Anemia, AZT-treated HIV-infected patients, treatment of
Epogen for Injection (Epoetin Alfa) Amgen 591
Procrit for Injection (Epoetin Alfa) Ortho Biotech 2364

Anemia, chemotherapy-induced in cancer patients
Aranesp for Injection (Darbepoetin alfa) Amgen 581
Epogen for Injection (Epoetin Alfa) Amgen 591
Procrit for Injection (Epoetin Alfa) Ortho Biotech 2364

Anemia, hemolytic, acquired
Decadron Tablets (Dexamethasone) Merck 1951
Depo-Medrol Injectable Suspension (Methylprednisolone Acetate) Pharmacia & Upjohn 2617
Depo-Medrol Single-Dose Vial (Methylprednisolone Acetate) Pharmacia & Upjohn 2619
Hydrocortone Tablets (Hydrocortisone) Merck 1989

Anemia, hypoplastic, congenital
Decadron Tablets (Dexamethasone) Merck 1951
Depo-Medrol Injectable Suspension (Methylprednisolone Acetate) Pharmacia & Upjohn 2617
Depo-Medrol Single-Dose Vial (Methylprednisolone Acetate) Pharmacia & Upjohn 2619
Hydrocortone Tablets (Hydrocortisone) Merck 1989

Anemia, iron deficiency
Ferrlecit Injection (Sodium Ferric Gluconate) Watson 3388
Nu-Iron 150 Capsules (Polysaccharide Iron Complex) Merz 2127
Slow Fe Iron Tablets (Ferrous Sulfate) Novartis Consumer ....■818
Slow Fe with Folic Acid Tablets (Ferrous Sulfate, Folic Acid) Novartis Consumer ....■819

Anemia, myelodysplastic syndrome associated
Revlimid Capsules (Lenalidomide) Celgene 958

Anemia, RBC
(*see under* Erythroblastopenia)

Anemia, surgical procedure-induced, to reduce the need for allogeneic blood transfusions
Epogen for Injection (Epoetin Alfa) Amgen 591
Procrit for Injection (Epoetin Alfa) Ortho Biotech 2364

Anemia associated with chronic renal failure
Aranesp for Injection (Darbepoetin alfa) Amgen 581
Epogen for Injection (Epoetin Alfa) Amgen 591
Procrit for Injection (Epoetin Alfa) Ortho Biotech 2364

Anesthesia, general
Ultane Liquid for Inhalation (Sevoflurane) Abbott.............................. 531

Anesthesia, general, adjunct in
Mivacron Injection (Mivacurium Chloride) Abbott............................ 493
Nembutal Sodium Solution, USP (Pentobarbital Sodium) Ovation 2470
Nimbex Injection (Cisatracurium Besylate) Abbott 498
Numorphan Injection (Oxymorphone Hydrochloride) Endo Labs... 1120
Phenergan Tablets and Suppositories (Promethazine Hydrochloride) Wyeth.................. 3440
Zemuron Injection (Rocuronium Bromide) Organon USA 2346

Anesthesia, general, supplement to
(*see under* Anesthesia, general, adjunct in)

Anesthesia, local
Hurricaine Topical Anesthetic Spray, 2 oz. Wild Cherry (Benzocaine) Beutlich ....■712
Hurricaine Topical Anesthetic Gel, 1 oz. Wild Cherry, Pina Colada, Watermelon, and Fresh Mint, 5.25 g. Wild Cherry (Benzocaine) Beutlich ....■712
Hurricaine Topical Anesthetic Liquid, 1 oz. Wild Cherry, Pina Colada, 0.005 fl. oz. Snap-n-Go Swabs Wild Cherry (Benzocaine) Beutlich ....■712
Hurricaine Topical Anesthetic Spray Extension Tubes (200) (Benzocaine) Beutlich ....■712
Hurricaine Topical Anesthetic Spray Kit, 2 oz. Wild Cherry with disposable Extension Tubes (200) (Benzocaine) Beutlich ....■712
Synera Topical Patch (Lidocaine, Tetracaine) Endo Labs 1137

Anesthesia, local, ocular
Ophthetic Ophthalmic Solution (Proparacaine Hydrochloride) Allergan ....⊙232

Anesthesia, local, oral cavity
Hurricaine Topical Anesthetic Spray, 2 oz. Wild Cherry (Benzocaine) Beutlich ....■712
Hurricaine Topical Anesthetic Gel, 1 oz. Wild Cherry, Pina Colada, Watermelon, and Fresh Mint, 5.25 g. Wild Cherry (Benzocaine) Beutlich ....■712
Hurricaine Topical Anesthetic Liquid, 1 oz. Wild Cherry, Pina Colada, 0.005 fl. oz. Snap-n-Go Swabs Wild Cherry (Benzocaine) Beutlich ....■712
Hurricaine Topical Anesthetic Spray Extension Tubes (200) (Benzocaine) Beutlich ....■712
Hurricaine Topical Anesthetic Spray Kit, 2 oz. Wild Cherry with disposable Extension Tubes (200) (Benzocaine) Beutlich ....■712

Anesthesia, local, pharyngeal
Hurricaine Topical Anesthetic Spray, 2 oz. Wild Cherry (Benzocaine) Beutlich ....■712
Hurricaine Topical Anesthetic Gel, 1 oz. Wild Cherry, Pina Colada, Watermelon, and Fresh Mint, 5.25 g. Wild Cherry (Benzocaine) Beutlich ....■712
Hurricaine Topical Anesthetic Liquid, 1 oz. Wild Cherry, Pina Colada, 0.005 fl. oz. Snap-n-Go Swabs Wild Cherry (Benzocaine) Beutlich ....■712
Hurricaine Topical Anesthetic Spray Extension Tubes (200) (Benzocaine) Beutlich ....■712
Hurricaine Topical Anesthetic Spray Kit, 2 oz. Wild Cherry with disposable Extension Tubes (200) (Benzocaine) Beutlich ....■712

Angina
(*see under* Angina pectoris)

Angina, chronic
Ranexa Tablets (Ranolazine) CV Therapeutics................................ 1035

Angina, chronic stable
Caduet Tablets (Amlodipine Besylate, Atorvastatin Calcium) Pfizer... 2508
Norvasc Tablets (Amlodipine Besylate) Pfizer 2545
Tiazac Capsules (Diltiazem Hydrochloride) Forest 1201

Angina, classic effort-associated
(*see under* Angina, chronic stable)

Angina, crescendo
(*see under* Angina, unstable)

Angina, pre-infarction
(*see under* Angina, unstable)

Angina, Prinzmetal's
Caduet Tablets (Amlodipine Besylate, Atorvastatin Calcium) Pfizer... 2508
Norvasc Tablets (Amlodipine Besylate) Pfizer 2545

Angina, unstable
Bayer Aspirin (Aspirin) Bayer Healthcare LLC 744
Fragmin Injection (Dalteparin Sodium) Eisai 1097
Mevacor Tablets (Lovastatin) Merck . 2021

Angina, unstable, adjuvant therapy for
ReoPro Vials (Abciximab) Lilly.......... 1809

Angina, variant
(*see under* Angina, Prinzmetal's)

Angina, vasospastic
(*see under* Angina, Prinzmetal's)

Angina pectoris
Covera-HS Tablets (Verapamil Hydrochloride) Searle 3139
Imdur Tablets (Isosorbide Mononitrate) Schering.............................. 3018
Inderal LA Long-Acting Capsules (Propranolol Hydrochloride) Wyeth.. 3429
Lopressor Injection (Metoprolol Tartrate) Novartis............................ 2238
Lopressor Tablets (Metoprolol Tartrate) Novartis 2238
Nitro-Dur Transdermal Infusion System (Nitroglycerin) Schering 3046
Nitrolingual Pumpspray (Nitroglycerin) Sciele 3120
Toprol-XL Tablets (Metoprolol Succinate) AstraZeneca LP 668

Angina pectoris, acute, prophylaxis
Nitrolingual Pumpspray (Nitroglycerin) Sciele 3120

Angina pectoris, reduce complications from
Bayer Aspirin (Aspirin) Bayer Healthcare LLC............................ 744

Angioedema, adjunctive therapy in
Phenergan Tablets and Suppositories (Promethazine Hydrochloride) Wyeth.................. 3440

Angiography, fluorescein, fundus
Fluorescite (Fluorescein Sodium) Alcon.. ⊙207

Angiography, fluorescein, iris vasculature
Fluorescite (Fluorescein Sodium) Alcon.. ⊙207

Ankylosing spondylitis
Anaprox Tablets (Naproxen Sodium) Roche.................................. 2761
Anaprox DS Tablets (Naproxen Sodium) Roche 2761
Bayer Aspirin (Aspirin) Bayer Healthcare LLC............................ 744
Celebrex Capsules (Celecoxib) Searle 3134
Clinoril Tablets (Sulindac) Merck....... 1924
Decadron Tablets (Dexamethasone) Merck.. 1951
Depo-Medrol Injectable Suspension (Methylprednisolone Acetate) Pharmacia & Upjohn 2617
Depo-Medrol Single-Dose Vial (Methylprednisolone Acetate) Pharmacia & Upjohn 2619
EC-Naprosyn Delayed-Release Tablets (Naproxen) Roche 2761
Enbrel for Injection (Etanercept) Amgen.. 584
Hydrocortone Tablets (Hydrocortisone) Merck 1989
Indocin (Indomethacin) Merck........... 1995
Naprosyn Suspension (Naproxen) Roche.. 2761
Naprosyn Tablets (Naproxen) Roche.. 2761
Remicade for IV Injection (Infliximab) Centocor 971
Traumeel Injection Solution (Homeopathic Formulations) Heel........... 1664
Voltaren Tablets (Diclofenac Sodium) Novartis.................................. 2307

Anorexia associated with weight loss, AIDS-induced
Marinol Capsules (Dronabinol) Unimed.. 3333
Megace ES Oral Suspension (Megestrol Acetate) Par 2481

Anterior segment inflammation
(*see under* Inflammation, anterior segment)

Anthrax
(*see under* B. anthracis infections)

Antithrombin III deficiency, hereditary
Thrombate III (Antithrombin III) Talecris... 3257

Anxiety, preoperative
Librium Capsules (Chlordiazepoxide Hydrochloride) Valeant............ 3347

Anxiety, short-term symptomatic relief of
Effexor XR Capsules (Venlafaxine Hydrochloride) Wyeth.................. 3417
Hyland's Nerve Tonic Tablets and Caplets (Homeopathic Formulations) Standard Homeopathic ...... ■829
Librium Capsules (Chlordiazepoxide Hydrochloride) Valeant............ 3347
Tranxene (Clorazepate Dipotassium) Ovation 2474
Valium Tablets (Diazepam) Roche..... 2819

Anxiety disorder, generalized
Lexapro Oral Solution (Escitalopram Oxalate) Forest 1190
Lexapro Tablets (Escitalopram Oxalate) Forest................................ 1190
Paxil (Paroxetine Hydrochloride) GlaxoSmithKline.............................. 1530

Anxiety disorder, social
Effexor XR Capsules (Venlafaxine Hydrochloride) Wyeth.................. 3417
Paxil CR Controlled-Release Tablets (Paroxetine Hydrochloride) GlaxoSmithKline.......................... 1538
Paxil (Paroxetine Hydrochloride) GlaxoSmithKline.............................. 1530
Zoloft (Sertraline Hydrochloride) Pfizer.. 2586

Anxiety disorders, management of
Librium Capsules (Chlordiazepoxide Hydrochloride) Valeant............ 3347
Niravam Orally Disintegrating Tablets (Alprazolam) Schwarz........ 3092
Phenergan Tablets and Suppositories (Promethazine Hydrochloride) Wyeth.................. 3440
Tranxene (Clorazepate Dipotassium) Ovation 2474
Valium Tablets (Diazepam) Roche..... 2819

Aplasia, pure red cell
Decadron Tablets (Dexamethasone) Merck.. 1951

Apnea of prematurity
Cafcit (Caffeine Citrate) Mead Johnson... 1886

Appendicitis, gangrenous
Primaxin I.M. (Cilastatin Sodium, Imipenem) Merck 2045

Appendicitis, perforated
Primaxin I.M. (Cilastatin Sodium, Imipenem) Merck 2045

Appendicitis with peritonitis
Merrem I.V. (Meropenem) AstraZeneca Pharmaceuticals 686
Primaxin I.M. (Cilastatin Sodium, Imipenem) Merck 2045

Zosyn (Piperacillin Sodium, Tazobactam Sodium) Wyeth ... 3492

Appetite, suppression of
(*see under* Obesity, exogenous)

Apprehension
(*see under* Anxiety disorders, management of)

ARC
(*see under* Infections, acquired immunodeficiency syndrome-related complex)

Arrhythmias, ventricular
Tambocor (Flecainide Acetate) 3M ... 1856

Arrhythmias, ventricular, life-threatening
Tambocor (Flecainide Acetate) 3M ... 1856

Arteritis, temporal
Decadron Tablets (Dexamethasone) Merck ... 1951

Arthralgia, topical relief of
(*see under* Pain, topical relief of)

Arthritis
(*see also under* Arthritis, rheumatoid; Osteoarthritis)
Goody's Body Pain Formula Powder (Acetaminophen, Aspirin, Acetaminophen, Aspirin) GlaxoSmithKline ... ▣ 684
Motrin IB Tablets and Caplets (Ibuprofen) McNeil Consumer ... 1866
ThermaCare Heat Wraps (Device) Procter & Gamble ... 2677

Arthritis, acute, gouty
Clinoril Tablets (Sulindac) Merck ... 1924
Decadron Tablets (Dexamethasone) Merck ... 1951
Depo-Medrol Injectable Suspension (Methylprednisolone Acetate) Pharmacia & Upjohn ... 2617
Depo-Medrol Single-Dose Vial (Methylprednisolone Acetate) Pharmacia & Upjohn ... 2619
Hydrocortone Tablets (Hydrocortisone) Merck ... 1989
Indocin (Indomethacin) Merck ... 1995
Traumeel Injection Solution (Homeopathic Formulations) Heel ... 1664

Arthritis, juvenile
Anaprox Tablets (Naproxen Sodium) Roche ... 2761
Anaprox DS Tablets (Naproxen Sodium) Roche ... 2761
EC-Naprosyn Delayed-Release Tablets (Naproxen) Roche ... 2761
Naprosyn Suspension (Naproxen) Roche ... 2761
Naprosyn Tablets (Naproxen) Roche ... 2761

Arthritis, osteo-
(*see under* Osteoarthritis)

Arthritis, psoriatic
Bayer Aspirin (Aspirin) Bayer Healthcare LLC ... 744
Decadron Tablets (Dexamethasone) Merck ... 1951
Depo-Medrol Injectable Suspension (Methylprednisolone Acetate) Pharmacia & Upjohn ... 2617
Depo-Medrol Single-Dose Vial (Methylprednisolone Acetate) Pharmacia & Upjohn ... 2619
Enbrel for Injection (Etanercept) Amgen ... 584
Hydrocortone Tablets (Hydrocortisone) Merck ... 1989
Remicade for IV Injection (Infliximab) Centocor ... 971

Arthritis, rheumatoid
Anaprox Tablets (Naproxen Sodium) Roche ... 2761
Anaprox DS Tablets (Naproxen Sodium) Roche ... 2761
Arthrotec Tablets (Diclofenac Sodium, Misoprostol) Searle ... 3129
Bayer Aspirin (Aspirin) Bayer Healthcare LLC ... 744
Bayer Aspirin Comprehensive Prescribing Information (Aspirin) Bayer Healthcare ... ▣ 796
Celebrex Capsules (Celecoxib) Searle ... 3134
Clinoril Tablets (Sulindac) Merck ... 1924
Cuprimine Capsules (Penicillamine) Merck ... 1947
Decadron Tablets (Dexamethasone) Merck ... 1951
Depo-Medrol Injectable Suspension (Methylprednisolone Acetate) Pharmacia & Upjohn ... 2617
Depo-Medrol Single-Dose Vial (Methylprednisolone Acetate) Pharmacia & Upjohn ... 2619
Dolobid Tablets (Diflunisal) Merck ... 1955
EC-Naprosyn Delayed-Release Tablets (Naproxen) Roche ... 2761
Enbrel for Injection (Etanercept) Amgen ... 584
Gengraf Capsules (Cyclosporine) Abbott ... 459
Humira Injection (Adalimumab) Abbott ... 466
Hydrocortone Tablets (Hydrocortisone) Merck ... 1989
Indocin (Indomethacin) Merck ... 1995
Kineret Injection (Anakinra) Amgen ... 599
Mobic Oral Suspension (Meloxicam) Boehringer Ingelheim ... 863
Mobic Tablets (Meloxicam) Boehringer Ingelheim ... 863
Nalfon Capsules (Fenoprofen Calcium) Pedinol ... 2502
Naprosyn Suspension (Naproxen) Roche ... 2761
Naprosyn Tablets (Naproxen) Roche ... 2761
Neoral Oral Solution (Cyclosporine) Novartis ... 2259
Neoral Soft Gelatin Capsules (Cyclosporine) Novartis ... 2259
Orencia Powder for Intravenous Infusion (Abatacept) Bristol-Myers Squibb ... 914
Remicade for IV Injection (Infliximab) Centocor ... 971
Rituxan I.V. (Rituximab) Genentech ... 1254
Voltaren Tablets (Diclofenac Sodium) Novartis ... 2307
Voltaren-XR Tablets (Diclofenac Sodium) Novartis ... 2310

Arthritis, topical adjunct to
Thera-Gesic Creme (Menthol, Methyl Salicylate) Mission ... ▣ 691

Arthritis, unspecified
Bufferin Extra Strength Tablets (Aspirin Buffered) Novartis Consumer ... ▣ 678
Bufferin Regular Strength Tablets (Aspirin Buffered) Novartis Consumer ... ▣ 678
Excedrin Extra Strength Caplets/Tablets/Geltabs (Acetaminophen, Aspirin, Caffeine) Novartis Consumer ... ▣ 684
Mineral Ice (Menthol) Novartis Consumer ... ▣ 685

Ascariasis, as secondary therapy in
Mintezol (Thiabendazole) Merck ... 2027

Aspergillosis
Abelcet Injection (Amphotericin B Lipid Complex) Enzon ... 1141
AmBisome for Injection (Amphotericin B, liposomal) Astellas ... 620
Cancidas for Injection (Caspofungin acetate) Merck ... 1918
VFEND I.V. (Voriconazole) Pfizer ... 2564
VFEND Oral Suspension (Voriconazole) Pfizer ... 2564
VFEND Tablets (Voriconazole) Pfizer ... 2564

Aspergillus fumigatus infections
(*see under* Aspergillosis)

Asthma, allergen induced
Xolair (Omalizumab) Genentech ... 1266

Asthma, bronchial
(*see under* Bronchial asthma)

Asthma, nocturnal
Serevent Diskus (Salmeterol Xinafoate) GlaxoSmithKline ... 1568

Astrocytoma, anaplastic
Temodar Capsules (Temozolomide) Schering ... 3073

Athetosis, adjunctive therapy in
Valium Tablets (Diazepam) Roche ... 2819

Athlete's foot
(*see under* Tinea pedis infections)

Atrial fibrillation
Lanoxicaps Capsules (Digoxin) GlaxoSmithKline ... 1490
Lanoxin Injection (Digoxin) GlaxoSmithKline ... 1494
Lanoxin Injection Pediatric (Digoxin) GlaxoSmithKline ... 1497
Lanoxin Tablets (Digoxin) GlaxoSmithKline ... 1500
Rythmol SR Capsules (Propafenone Hydrochloride) Reliant ... 2727

Atrial fibrillation, paroxysmal
Tambocor Tablets (Flecainide Acetate) 3M ... 1856

Atrial fibrillation with embolism
Coumadin for Injection (Warfarin Sodium) Bristol-Myers Squibb ... 898
Coumadin Tablets (Warfarin Sodium) Bristol-Myers Squibb ... 898
Miradon Tablets (Anisindione) Schering ... 3042

Attention Deficit Hyperactivity Disorder
Adderall Tablets (Amphetamine Aspartate, Amphetamine Sulfate, Dextroamphetamine Saccharate, Dextroamphetamine Sulfate) Shire US ... 3164
Adderall XR Capsules (Amphetamine Aspartate, Amphetamine Sulfate, Dextroamphetamine Saccharate, Dextroamphetamine Sulfate) Shire US ... 3166
Concerta Extended-Release Tablets (Methylphenidate Hydrochloride) McNeil Pediatrics ... 1881
Daytrana Transdermal Patch (Methylphenidate) Shire US ... 3174
Desoxyn Tablets, USP (Methamphetamine Hydrochloride) Ovation ... 2462
Dexedrine (Dextroamphetamine Sulfate) GlaxoSmithKline ... 1420
DextroStat Tablets (Dextroamphetamine Sulfate) Shire US ... 3179
Focalin Tablets (Dexmethylphenidate Hydrochloride) Novartis ... 2220
Focalin XR Capsules (Dexmethylphenidate Hydrochloride) Novartis ... 2223
Metadate CD Capsules (Methylphenidate Hydrochloride) UCB ... 3323
Ritalin Hydrochloride Tablets (Methylphenidate Hydrochloride) Novartis ... 2269
Ritalin LA Capsules (Methylphenidate Hydrochloride) Novartis ... 2271
Ritalin-SR Tablets (Methylphenidate Hydrochloride) Novartis ... 2269
Strattera Capsules (Atomoxetine Hydrochloride) Lilly ... 1814

B

B. anthracis infections
Cipro (Ciprofloxacin) Schering ... 2977
Levaquin (Levofloxacin) Ortho-McNeil ... 2384
Levaquin in 5% Dextrose Injection (Levofloxacin) Ortho-McNeil ... 2384

B. distasonis infections
Invanz for Injection (Ertapenem) Merck ... 1999
Primaxin I.M. (Cilastatin Sodium, Imipenem) Merck ... 2045

B. distasonis intra-abdominal infections
Invanz for Injection (Ertapenem) Merck ... 1999
Primaxin I.M. (Cilastatin Sodium, Imipenem) Merck ... 2045

B. fragilis endomyometritis
Invanz for Injection (Ertapenem) Merck ... 1999

B. fragilis gynecologic infections
Mefoxin for Injection (Cefoxitin Sodium) Merck ... 2012
Mefoxin Premixed Intravenous Solution (Cefoxitin Sodium) Merck ... 2016
Primaxin I.V. (Cilastatin Sodium, Imipenem) Merck ... 2048

B. fragilis infections
Avelox (Moxifloxacin Hydrochloride) Schering ... 2970
Cipro (Ciprofloxacin) Schering ... 2977
Cipro I.V. (Ciprofloxacin) Schering ... 2984
Invanz for Injection (Ertapenem) Merck ... 1999
Mefoxin for Injection (Cefoxitin Sodium) Merck ... 2012
Mefoxin Premixed Intravenous Solution (Cefoxitin Sodium) Merck ... 2016
Merrem I.V. (Meropenem) AstraZeneca Pharmaceuticals ... 686
Primaxin I.M. (Cilastatin Sodium, Imipenem) Merck ... 2045
Primaxin I.V. (Cilastatin Sodium, Imipenem) Merck ... 2048
Rocephin Injectable Vials, ADD-Vantage, Galaxy, Bulk (Ceftriaxone Sodium) Roche ... 2800
Timentin ADD-Vantage (Clavulanate Potassium, Ticarcillin Disodium) GlaxoSmithKline ... 1580
Timentin Injection Galaxy Container (Clavulanate Potassium, Ticarcillin Disodium) GlaxoSmithKline ... 1583
Timentin IV Infusion (Clavulanate Potassium, Ticarcillin Disodium) GlaxoSmithKline ... 1577
Timentin Pharmacy Bulk Package (Clavulanate Potassium, Ticarcillin Disodium) GlaxoSmithKline ... 1586
Tygacil for Injection (Tigecycline) Wyeth ... 3488
Zosyn (Piperacillin Sodium, Tazobactam Sodium) Wyeth ... 3492

B. fragilis intra-abdominal infections
Avelox (Moxifloxacin Hydrochloride) Schering ... 2970
Cipro (Ciprofloxacin) Schering ... 2977
Cipro I.V. (Ciprofloxacin) Schering ... 2984
Fortaz (Ceftazidime) GlaxoSmithKline ... 1453
Invanz for Injection (Ertapenem) Merck ... 1999
Maxipime for Injection (Cefepime Hydrochloride) Elan ... 1105
Mefoxin for Injection (Cefoxitin Sodium) Merck ... 2012
Mefoxin Premixed Intravenous Solution (Cefoxitin Sodium) Merck ... 2016
Merrem I.V. (Meropenem) AstraZeneca Pharmaceuticals ... 686
Primaxin I.M. (Cilastatin Sodium, Imipenem) Merck ... 2045
Primaxin I.V. (Cilastatin Sodium, Imipenem) Merck ... 2048
Rocephin Injectable Vials, ADD-Vantage, Galaxy, Bulk (Ceftriaxone Sodium) Roche ... 2800
Timentin ADD-Vantage (Clavulanate Potassium, Ticarcillin Disodium) GlaxoSmithKline ... 1580
Timentin Injection Galaxy Container (Clavulanate Potassium, Ticarcillin Disodium) GlaxoSmithKline ... 1583
Timentin IV Infusion (Clavulanate Potassium, Ticarcillin Disodium) GlaxoSmithKline ... 1577
Timentin Pharmacy Bulk Package (Clavulanate Potassium, Ticarcillin Disodium) GlaxoSmithKline ... 1586
Tygacil for Injection (Tigecycline) Wyeth ... 3488

B. fragilis peritonitis
Mefoxin for Injection (Cefoxitin Sodium) Merck ... 2012
Mefoxin Premixed Intravenous Solution (Cefoxitin Sodium) Merck ... 2016
Merrem I.V. (Meropenem) AstraZeneca Pharmaceuticals ... 686
Timentin ADD-Vantage (Clavulanate Potassium, Ticarcillin Disodium) GlaxoSmithKline ... 1580
Timentin Injection Galaxy Container (Clavulanate Potassium, Ticarcillin Disodium) GlaxoSmithKline ... 1583
Timentin IV Infusion (Clavulanate Potassium, Ticarcillin Disodium) GlaxoSmithKline ... 1577
Timentin Pharmacy Bulk Package (Clavulanate Potassium, Ticarcillin Disodium) GlaxoSmithKline ... 1586

Zosyn (Piperacillin Sodium, Tazobactam Sodium) Wyeth 3492

B. fragilis septicemia
Mefoxin for Injection (Cefoxitin Sodium) Merck 2012
Mefoxin Premixed Intravenous Solution (Cefoxitin Sodium) Merck 2016
Primaxin I.V. (Cilastatin Sodium, Imipenem) Merck 2048

B. fragilis skin and skin structure infections
Invanz for Injection (Ertapenem) Merck 1999
Mefoxin for Injection (Cefoxitin Sodium) Merck 2012
Mefoxin Premixed Intravenous Solution (Cefoxitin Sodium) Merck 2016
Merrem I.V. (Meropenem) AstraZeneca Pharmaceuticals 686
Primaxin I.M. (Cilastatin Sodium, Imipenem) Merck 2045
Primaxin I.V. (Cilastatin Sodium, Imipenem) Merck 2048
Rocephin Injectable Vials, ADD-Vantage, Galaxy, Bulk (Ceftriaxone Sodium) Roche 2800
Tygacil for Injection (Tigecycline) Wyeth 3488

B. intermedius infections
Primaxin I.M. (Cilastatin Sodium, Imipenem) Merck 2045

B. intermedius intra-abdominal infections
Primaxin I.M. (Cilastatin Sodium, Imipenem) Merck 2045

B. melaninogenicus endometritis
Timentin ADD-Vantage (Clavulanate Potassium, Ticarcillin Disodium) GlaxoSmithKline 1580
Timentin Injection Galaxy Container (Clavulanate Potassium, Ticarcillin Disodium) GlaxoSmithKline 1583
Timentin IV Infusion (Clavulanate Potassium, Ticarcillin Disodium) GlaxoSmithKline 1577
Timentin Pharmacy Bulk Package (Clavulanate Potassium, Ticarcillin Disodium) GlaxoSmithKline 1586

B. melaninogenicus infections
Timentin ADD-Vantage (Clavulanate Potassium, Ticarcillin Disodium) GlaxoSmithKline 1580
Timentin Injection Galaxy Container (Clavulanate Potassium, Ticarcillin Disodium) GlaxoSmithKline 1583
Timentin IV Infusion (Clavulanate Potassium, Ticarcillin Disodium) GlaxoSmithKline 1577
Timentin Pharmacy Bulk Package (Clavulanate Potassium, Ticarcillin Disodium) GlaxoSmithKline 1586

B. ovatus infections
Zosyn (Piperacillin Sodium, Tazobactam Sodium) Wyeth 3492

B. ovatus peritonitis
Zosyn (Piperacillin Sodium, Tazobactam Sodium) Wyeth 3492

B. pertussis infections
E.E.S. (Erythromycin Ethylsuccinate) Abbott 451
EryPed (Erythromycin Ethylsuccinate) Abbott 447
Ery-Tab Tablets (Erythromycin) Abbott 449
Erythrocin Stearate Filmtab Tablets (Erythromycin Stearate) Abbott 453
Erythromycin Base Filmtab Tablets (Erythromycin) Abbott 455
Erythromycin Delayed-Release Capsules, USP (Erythromycin) Abbott 457
PCE Dispertab Tablets (Erythromycin) Abbott 515

B. pertussis respiratory tract infections
E.E.S. (Erythromycin Ethylsuccinate) Abbott 451
EryPed (Erythromycin Ethylsuccinate) Abbott 447
Ery-Tab Tablets (Erythromycin) Abbott 449
Erythrocin Stearate Filmtab Tablets (Erythromycin Stearate) Abbott 453
Erythromycin Base Filmtab Tablets (Erythromycin) Abbott 455
Erythromycin Delayed-Release Capsules, USP (Erythromycin) Abbott 457
PCE Dispertab Tablets (Erythromycin) Abbott 515

B. thetaiotaomicron infections
Avelox (Moxifloxacin Hydrochloride) Schering 2970
Merrem I.V. (Meropenem) AstraZeneca Pharmaceuticals 686
Primaxin I.M. (Cilastatin Sodium, Imipenem) Merck 2045
Tygacil for Injection (Tigecycline) Wyeth 3488
Zosyn (Piperacillin Sodium, Tazobactam Sodium) Wyeth 3492

B. thetaiotaomicron intra-abdominal infections
Avelox (Moxifloxacin Hydrochloride) Schering 2970
Merrem I.V. (Meropenem) AstraZeneca Pharmaceuticals 686
Primaxin I.M. (Cilastatin Sodium, Imipenem) Merck 2045
Tygacil for Injection (Tigecycline) Wyeth 3488

B. thetaiotaomicron peritonitis
Merrem I.V. (Meropenem) AstraZeneca Pharmaceuticals 686
Zosyn (Piperacillin Sodium, Tazobactam Sodium) Wyeth 3492

B. uniformis infections
Tygacil (Tigecycline) Wyeth 3488

B. vulgatus infections
Zosyn (Piperacillin Sodium, Tazobactam Sodium) Wyeth 3492

B. vulgatus intra-abdominal infections
Tygacil for Injection (Tigecycline) Wyeth 3488

B. vulgatus peritonitis
Zosyn (Piperacillin Sodium, Tazobactam Sodium) Wyeth 3492

Backache
Aleve Caplets (Naproxen Sodium) Bayer Healthcare LLC 742
Aleve Gelcaps (Naproxen Sodium) Bayer Healthcare LLC 743
Aleve Tablets (Naproxen Sodium) Bayer Healthcare LLC 743
Hyland's BackAche with Arnica Caplets (Homeopathic Formulations) Standard Homeopathic .... ▣828
Mineral Ice (Menthol) Novartis Consumer .... ▣685
Motrin IB Tablets and Caplets (Ibuprofen) McNeil Consumer 1866
Thera-Gesic Creme (Menthol, Methyl Salicylate) Mission 2141
Extra Strength Tylenol Rapid Release Gels (Acetaminophen) McNeil Consumer 1870
Women's Tylenol Menstrual Relief Caplets (Acetaminophen, Pamabrom) McNeil Consumer 1877

Backache, systemic, symptomatic relief of
Advil (Ibuprofen) Wyeth .... ▣674
Goody's Extra Strength Headache Powders (Acetaminophen, Aspirin, Caffeine) GlaxoSmithKline .... ▣611
Goody's Extra Strength Pain Relief Tablets (Acetaminophen, Aspirin, Caffeine) GlaxoSmithKline .... ▣685
Traumeel Injection Solution (Homeopathic Formulations) Heel 1664
Regular Strength Tylenol Tablets (Acetaminophen) McNeil Consumer 1870
Tylenol 8 Hour Extended Release Caplets (Acetaminophen) McNeil Consumer 1870
Tylenol (Acetaminophen) McNeil Consumer 1870

Backache, temporary relief of
(*see under* Pain, topical relief of)

Bacteremia
(*see under* Septicemia, bacterial)

Bacteriuria associated with cystitis, elimination or suppression of
(*see also under* Infections, urinary tract)
Uroqid-Acid No. 2 Tablets (Methenamine Mandelate, Sodium Acid Phosphate) Beach 760

Bacteriuria associated with polynephritis, elimination or suppression of
(*see under* Infections, urinary tract)

Bacteroides distasonis infections
(*see under* B. distasonis infections)

Bacteroides fragilis infections
(*see under* B. fragilis infections)

Bacteroides ovatus infections
(*see under* B. ovatus infections)

Bacteroides species gynecologic infections
Mefoxin for Injection (Cefoxitin Sodium) Merck 2012
Mefoxin Premixed Intravenous Solution (Cefoxitin Sodium) Merck 2016
Primaxin I.M. (Cilastatin Sodium, Imipenem) Merck 2045
Primaxin I.V. (Cilastatin Sodium, Imipenem) Merck 2048

Bacteroides species infections
(*see also under* B. distasonis infections; B. fragilis infections; B. ovatus infections; B. thetaiotaomicron infections; B. vulgatus infections)
Fortaz (Ceftazidime) GlaxoSmithKline 1453
Invanz for Injection (Ertapenem) Merck 1999
Mefoxin for Injection (Cefoxitin Sodium) Merck 2012
Mefoxin Premixed Intravenous Solution (Cefoxitin Sodium) Merck 2016
Primaxin I.M. (Cilastatin Sodium, Imipenem) Merck 2045
Primaxin I.V. (Cilastatin Sodium, Imipenem) Merck 2048
Tygacil for Injection (Tigecycline) Wyeth 3488

Bacteroides species intra-abdominal infections
Fortaz (Ceftazidime) GlaxoSmithKline 1453
Invanz for Injection (Ertapenem) Merck 1999
Mefoxin for Injection (Cefoxitin Sodium) Merck 2012
Mefoxin Premixed Intravenous Solution (Cefoxitin Sodium) Merck 2016
Primaxin I.M. (Cilastatin Sodium, Imipenem) Merck 2045
Primaxin I.V. (Cilastatin Sodium, Imipenem) Merck 2048

Bacteroides species lower respiratory tract infections
Mefoxin for Injection (Cefoxitin Sodium) Merck 2012
Mefoxin Premixed Intravenous Solution (Cefoxitin Sodium) Merck 2016

Bacteroides species lung abscess
Mefoxin for Injection (Cefoxitin Sodium) Merck 2012
Mefoxin Premixed Intravenous Solution (Cefoxitin Sodium) Merck 2016

Bacteroides species peritonitis
Mefoxin for Injection (Cefoxitin Sodium) Merck 2012
Mefoxin Premixed Intravenous Solution (Cefoxitin Sodium) Merck 2016
Primaxin I.M. (Cilastatin Sodium, Imipenem) Merck 2045

Bacteroides species pneumonia
Mefoxin for Injection (Cefoxitin Sodium) Merck 2012
Mefoxin Premixed Intravenous Solution (Cefoxitin Sodium) Merck 2016

Bacteroides species septicemia
Mefoxin for Injection (Cefoxitin Sodium) Merck 2012
Mefoxin Premixed Intravenous Solution (Cefoxitin Sodium) Merck 2016
Primaxin I.V. (Cilastatin Sodium, Imipenem) Merck 2048

Bacteroides species skin and skin structure infections
Mefoxin for Injection (Cefoxitin Sodium) Merck 2012
Mefoxin Premixed Intravenous Solution (Cefoxitin Sodium) Merck 2016
Primaxin I.M. (Cilastatin Sodium, Imipenem) Merck 2045
Primaxin I.V. (Cilastatin Sodium, Imipenem) Merck 2048

Bacteroides thetaiotaomicron infections
(*see under* B. thetaiotaomicron infections)

Bacteroides vulgatus infections
(*see under* B. vulgatus infections)

Baldness, male pattern of vertex of scalp
Propecia Tablets (Finasteride) Merck 2060
Men's Rogaine Extra Strength Hair Regrowth Treatment Topical Solution, Ocean Rush Scent and Original Unscented (Minoxidil) Pfizer Consumer Healthcare .... ▣633

Barber's itch
(*see under* Folliculitis barbae)

Barrett's esophagus
Photofrin for Injection (Porfimer Sodium) Axcan Scandipharm 702

Bedsores
(*see under* Ulcers, decubitus, adjunctive therapy in)

Benzodiazepine overdose, management of
Romazicon Injection (Flumazenil) Roche 2804

Berylliosis
Decadron Tablets (Dexamethasone) Merck 1951
Depo-Medrol Injectable Suspension (Methylprednisolone Acetate) Pharmacia & Upjohn 2617
Depo-Medrol Single-Dose Vial (Methylprednisolone Acetate) Pharmacia & Upjohn 2619
Hydrocortone Tablets (Hydrocortisone) Merck 1989

Bifidobacterium species gynecologic infections
Primaxin I.V. (Cilastatin Sodium, Imipenem) Merck 2048

Bifidobacterium species infections
Primaxin I.V. (Cilastatin Sodium, Imipenem) Merck 2048

Bifidobacterium species intra-abdominal infections
Primaxin I.V. (Cilastatin Sodium, Imipenem) Merck 2048

Biotin, deficiency of
Appearex Tablets (Biotin) Merz 2125

Bipolar disorder
Lamictal (Lamotrigine) GlaxoSmithKline 1481

Bipolar disorder, acute mixed
Abilify Oral Solution (Aripiprazole) Bristol-Myers Squibb 882
Abilify Oral Solution (Aripiprazole) Otsuka America 2450
Abilify Discmelt Orally Disintegrating Tablets (Aripiprazole) Bristol-Myers Squibb 882
Abilify Discmelt Orally Disintegrating Tablets (Aripiprazole) Otsuka America 2450
Abilify Tablets (Aripiprazole) Bristol-Myers Squibb 882
Abilify Tablets (Aripiprazole) Otsuka America 2450
Depakote ER Tablets (Divalproex Sodium) Abbott 434
Equetro Extended-Release Capsules (Carbamazepine) Shire US 3180
Risperdal (Risperidone) Janssen 1676

Risperdal M-Tab Orally Disintegrating Tablets (Risperidone) Janssen ... 1676
Zyprexa Tablets (Olanzapine) Lilly ... 1830
Zyprexa ZYDIS Orally Disintegrating Tablets (Olanzapine) Lilly ... 1830

Bipolar disorder, manic episodes
(*see also under* Manic episodes associated with bipolar disorder)
Abilify Oral Solution (Aripiprazole) Bristol-Myers Squibb ... 882
Abilify Discmelt Orally Disintegrating Tablets (Aripiprazole) Bristol-Myers Squibb ... 882
Abilify Tablets (Aripiprazole) Bristol-Myers Squibb ... 882
Depakote Tablets (Divalproex Sodium) Abbott ... 427
Depakote ER Tablets (Divalproex Sodium) Abbott ... 434
Equetro Extended-Release Capsules (Carbamazepine) Shire US ... 3180
Lithobid Tablets (Lithium Carbonate) JDS ... 1692
Risperdal (Risperidone) Janssen ... 1676
Risperdal M-Tab Orally Disintegrating Tablets (Risperidone) Janssen ... 1676
Zyprexa Tablets (Olanzapine) Lilly ... 1830
Zyprexa ZYDIS Orally Disintegrating Tablets (Olanzapine) Lilly ... 1830

Bites, black widow spider
Antivenin (Black Widow Spider Antivenin) (Black Widow Spider Antivenin (Equine)) Merck ... 1913

Bites, crotalidae
(*see under* Envenomation, pit viper)

Bites, insect
EpiPen (Epinephrine) Dey ... 1061

Bites, pit vipers
(*see under* Envenomation, pit viper)

Bleeding, upper gastrointestinal, in critically ill
Zegerid Capsules (Omeprazole) Santarus ... 2958
Zegerid Powder for Oral Solution (Omeprazole) Santarus ... 2958

Bleeding associated with congenital hemophiliacs
NovoSeven (Antihemophilic Factor (Recombinant)) Novo Nordisk ... 2331

Bleeding associated with hemophilia A
Advate Injection (Antihemophilic Factor (Recombinant)) Baxter Healthcare ... 712
Alphanate, Antihemophilic Factor (Human) (Antihemophilic Factor (Human), Factor VIII (AHF, AHG)) Grifols ... 1654
Feiba VH (Anti-Inhibitor Coagulant Complex) Baxter Healthcare ... 718
Humate-P (Antihemophilic Factor (Human), von Willebrand Factor (Human)) ZLB Behring ... 3502
NovoSeven (Antihemophilic Factor (Recombinant)) Novo Nordisk ... 2331

Bleeding associated with hemophilia B
Feiba VH (Anti-Inhibitor Coagulant Complex) Baxter Healthcare ... 718
NovoSeven (Antihemophilic Factor (Recombinant)) Novo Nordisk ... 2331
Profilnine SD, Factor IX Complex (Human) (Factor IX Complex) Grifols ... 1660

Blepharitis
Pred Mild Ophthalmic Suspension (Prednisolone Acetate) Allergan ... ⊙238

Blepharitis, fungal
Natacyn Antifungal Ophthalmic Suspension (Natamycin) Alcon ... ⊙208

Blepharoconjunctivitis
Polytrim Ophthalmic Solution (Polymyxin B Sulfate, Trimethoprim Sulfate) Allergan ... 574

Blepharospasm
BOTOX Purified Neurotoxin Complex (Botulinum Toxin Type A) Allergan ... 570

Blood loss, perioperative, reduction of
Trasylol Injection (Aprotinin) Bayer ... 754

Body aches
(*see under* Pain, general)

Boils, symptomatic relief of
(*see under* Furunculosis, symptomatic relief of)

Bone disease, metabolic, with chronic renal failure
(*see under* Osteodystrophy, renal)

Bone marrow transplantation, allogeneic or autologous, delayed or failed
Leukine (Sargramostim) Berlex ... 814

Bone mass, loss of
(*see under* Osteoporosis)

Bone metastases of solid tumors
Zometa for Intravenous Infusion (Zoledronic acid) Novartis ... 2315

Bordetella pertussis
(*see under* B. pertussis infections)

Bordetella pertussis, immunization against
(*see also under* Immunization, diphtheria, tetanus and pertussis)
ADACEL Vaccine (Diphtheria & Tetanus Toxoids and Acellular Pertussis Vaccine Adsorbed) Sanofi Pasteur ... 2945
Boostrix (Diphtheria & Tetanus Toxoids and Acellular Pertussis Vaccine Adsorbed) GlaxoSmithKline ... 1404
DAPTACEL Vaccine (Diphtheria & Tetanus Toxoids and Acellular Pertussis Vaccine Adsorbed) Sanofi Pasteur ... 2950
Infanrix Vaccine (Diphtheria & Tetanus Toxoids and Acellular Pertussis Vaccine Adsorbed) GlaxoSmithKline ... 1476
Pediarix Vaccine (Diphtheria & Tetanus Toxoids and Pertussis Vaccine Adsorbed, Hepatitis B Vaccine, Recombinant, Poliovirus Vaccine Inactivated, Trivalent Types 1,2,3) GlaxoSmithKline ... 1548

Borrelia burgdorferi infection
Ceftin Tablets (Cefuroxime Axetil) GlaxoSmithKline ... 1407

Bowel, evacuation of
Colyte with Flavor Packs for Oral Solution (Polyethylene Glycol, Potassium Chloride, Sodium Bicarbonate, Sodium Chloride, Sodium Sulfate) Schwarz ... 3088
Fleet Bisacodyl Laxatives (Bisacodyl) Fleet ... 1165
Fleet Enema (Sodium Phosphate) Fleet ... 1165
Fleet Mineral Oil Enema (Mineral Oil) Fleet ... 1166
Fleet Phospho-soda (Sodium Phosphate) Fleet ... 1166
Fleet Phospho-soda ACCU-PREP (Glycerin, Pramoxine Hydrochloride, Sodium Phosphate) Fleet ... 1168
Fleet Phospho-soda EZ-PREP (Glycerin, Pramoxine Hydrochloride, Sodium Phosphate) Fleet ... 1169
Fleet Prep Kits (Bisacodyl, Sodium Phosphate) Fleet ... 1170
HalfLytely and Bisacodyl Tablets Bowel Prep Kit with Flavors Packs (Bisacodyl, Polyethylene Glycol, Potassium Chloride, Sodium Bicarbonate, Sodium Chloride) Braintree ... 881
MoviPrep Oral Solution (Ascorbic Acid, PEG-3350, Potassium Chloride, Sodium Ascorbate, Sodium Chloride, Sodium Sulfate) Salix ... 2839
OsmoPrep Tablets (Sodium Phosphate) Salix ... 2840
TriLyte with Flavor Packs for Oral Solution (PEG-3350, Potassium Chloride, Sodium Bicarbonate, Sodium Chloride) Schwarz ... 3100

Bowel, irritable, syndrome
Bentyl Capsules (Dicyclomine Hydrochloride) Axcan Scandipharm ... 697
Bentyl Injection (Dicyclomine Hydrochloride) Axcan Scandipharm ... 697
Bentyl Syrup (Dicyclomine Hydrochloride) Axcan Scandipharm ... 697
Bentyl Tablets (Dicyclomine Hydrochloride) Axcan Scandipharm ... 697
Citrucel Orange Flavor Powder (Methylcellulose) GlaxoSmithKline ... ▣647
Citrucel Sugar Free Orange Flavor Powder (Methylcellulose) GlaxoSmithKline ... ▣648
Donnatal Extentabs (Atropine Sulfate, Hyoscyamine Sulfate, Phenobarbital, Scopolamine Hydrobromide) PBM ... 2493
Lotronex Tablets (Alosetron Hydrochloride) GlaxoSmithKline ... 1512
Metamucil Capsules (Psyllium Preparations) Procter & Gamble ... 2675
Metamucil (Psyllium Preparations) Procter & Gamble ... 2675
Zelnorm Tablets (Tegaserod maleate) Novartis ... 2312

Branhamella catarrhalis
(*see under* M. catarrhalis infections)

Breast cancer
(*see under* Carcinoma, breast)

Breast carcinoma
(*see under* Carcinoma, breast)

Bromhidrosis, topical relief of
(*see under* Hyperhidrosis, topical relief of)

Bronchial airway hyperreactivity, diagnosis of
Provocholine Powder for Inhalation (Methacholine Chloride) Methapharm ... 2127

Bronchial asthma
Accolate Tablets (Zafirlukast) AstraZeneca Pharmaceuticals ... 671
AccuNeb Inhalation Solution (Albuterol Sulfate) Dey ... 1055
Advair Diskus 100/50 (Fluticasone Propionate, Salmeterol Xinafoate) GlaxoSmithKline ... 1308
Advair Diskus 250/50 (Fluticasone Propionate, Salmeterol Xinafoate) GlaxoSmithKline ... 1308
Advair Diskus 500/50 (Fluticasone Propionate, Salmeterol Xinafoate) GlaxoSmithKline ... 1308
Advair HFA Inhalation Aerosol (Fluticasone Propionate, Salmeterol Xinafoate) GlaxoSmithKline ... 1318
Aerobid/Aerobid-M (Flunisolide) Forest ... 1171
Alupent Inhalation Aerosol (Metaproterenol Sulfate) Boehringer Ingelheim ... 826
Asmanex Twisthaler (Mometasone Furoate) Schering ... 2966
Atrovent HFA Inhalation Aerosol (Ipratropium Bromide) Boehringer Ingelheim ... 841
Azmacort Inhalation Aerosol (Triamcinolone Acetonide) Kos ... 1726
Combivent Inhalation Aerosol (Albuterol Sulfate, Ipratropium Bromide) Boehringer Ingelheim ... 847
Decadron Tablets (Dexamethasone) Merck ... 1951
Depo-Medrol Injectable Suspension (Methylprednisolone Acetate) Pharmacia & Upjohn ... 2617
Depo-Medrol Single-Dose Vial (Methylprednisolone Acetate) Pharmacia & Upjohn ... 2619
DuoNeb Inhalation Solution (Albuterol Sulfate, Ipratropium Bromide) Dey ... 1058
Flovent Diskus (Fluticasone Propionate) GlaxoSmithKline ... 1443
Flovent HFA (Fluticasone Propionate HFA) GlaxoSmithKline ... 1447
Foradil Aerolizer (Formoterol Fumarate) Schering ... 3010
Hydrocortone Tablets (Hydrocortisone) Merck ... 1989
Maxair Autohaler (Pirbuterol Acetate) 3M ... 1852
Primatene Mist (Epinephrine) Wyeth ... ▣719
Proventil Inhalation Aerosol (Albuterol) Schering ... 3053
Proventil Inhalation Solution 0.083% (Albuterol Sulfate) Schering ... 3055
Pulmicort Respules (Budesonide) AstraZeneca LP ... 661
Qvar Inhalation Aerosol (Beclomethasone Dipropionate) Teva Specialty ... 3303
Serevent Diskus (Salmeterol Xinafoate) GlaxoSmithKline ... 1568
Singulair (Montelukast Sodium) Merck ... 2077
Uniphyl Tablets (Theophylline Anhydrous) Purdue Pharmaceutical ... 2710
Ventolin HFA Inhalation Aerosol (Albuterol Sulfate) GlaxoSmithKline ... 1600
Xopenex Inhalation Solution (Levalbuterol Hydrochloride) Sepracor ... 3146
Xopenex Inhalation Solution Concentrate (Levalbuterol Hydrochloride) Sepracor ... 3150
Xopenex HFA Inhalation Aerosol (Levalbuterol Tartrate) Sepracor ... 3154
Zyflo Tablets (Zileuton) Critical ... 1023

Bronchial asthma, maintenance treatment of
Symbicort 80/4.5 Inhalation Aerosol (Budesonide, Formoterol fumarate dihydrate) AstraZeneca LP ... 3511
Symbicort 160/4.5 Inhalation Aerosol (Budesonide, Formoterol fumarate dihydrate) AstraZeneca LP ... 3511

Bronchial asthma, prophylactic therapy
Zyflo Tablets (Zileuton) Critical ... 1023

Bronchial congestion
Mucinex Extended-Release Bi-Layer Tablets (Guaifenesin) Adams ... ▣720
Mucinex D Extended-Release Bi-Layer Tablets (Guaifenesin, Pseudoephedrine Hydrochloride) Adams ... ▣776
Mucinex DM Extended-Release Bi-Layer Tablets (Dextromethorphan Hydrobromide, Guaifenesin) Adams ... ▣720
Robitussin Chest Congestion Liquid (Guaifenesin) Wyeth ... ▣721
Robitussin Cough & Cold CF Liquid (Dextromethorphan Hydrobromide, Guaifenesin, Pseudoephedrine Hydrochloride) Wyeth ... ▣735
Robitussin Cough & Cold Pediatric Drops (Dextromethorphan Hydrobromide, Guaifenesin, Pseudoephedrine Hydrochloride) Wyeth ... ▣735
Robitussin Cough & Congestion Liquid (Dextromethorphan Hydrobromide, Guaifenesin) Wyeth ... ▣738
Robitussin Cough DM Syrup (Dextromethorphan Hydrobromide, Guaifenesin) Wyeth ... ▣738
Robitussin Cough DM Infant Drops (Dextromethorphan Hydrobromide, Guaifenesin) Wyeth ... ▣738
Robitussin Head & Chest Congestion PE Syrup (Guaifenesin, Phenylephrine Hydrochloride) Wyeth ... ▣739
Robitussin Sugar Free Cough (Dextromethorphan Hydrobromide, Guaifenesin) Wyeth ... ▣738
TheraFlu Flu & Chest Congestion Hot Liquid (Acetaminophen, Guaifenesin) Novartis Consumer ... ▣741
Triaminic Chest & Nasal Congestion Liquid (Guaifenesin, Phenylephrine Hydrochloride) Novartis Consumer ... ▣746

Tylenol Cold Head Congestion Severe Caplets with Cool Burst (Acetaminophen, Dextromethorphan Hydrobromide, Guaifenesin, Phenylephrine Hydrochloride) McNeil Consumer ▣750
Tylenol Cold Multi-Symptom Severe Daytime Liquid (Acetaminophen, Dextromethorphan Hydrobromide, Guaifenesin, Phenylephrine Hydrochloride) McNeil Consumer ▣752

Bronchial irritation, symptomatic relief of
Triaminic Cough & Runny Nose Softchews (Chlorpheniramine Maleate, Dextromethorphan Hydrobromide) Novartis Consumer ▣748

Bronchial secretions, thinning of
Humibid Extended-Release Bi-Layer Tablets (Guaifenesin) Adams ▣720
Refenesen 400 Caplets (Guaifenesin) Reese ▣721
Refenesen DM Caplets (Dextromethorphan Hydrobromide, Guaifenesin) Reese ▣721
Refenesen PE Caplets (Guaifenesin, Phenylephrine Hydrochloride) Reese ▣721
Robitussin Cough & Congestion Liquid (Dextromethorphan Hydrobromide, Guaifenesin) Wyeth ▣738
Robitussin Cough DM Syrup (Dextromethorphan Hydrobromide, Guaifenesin) Wyeth ▣738
Robitussin Cough DM Infant Drops (Dextromethorphan Hydrobromide, Guaifenesin) Wyeth ▣738
Robitussin Head & Chest Congestion PE Syrup (Guaifenesin, Phenylephrine Hydrochloride) Wyeth ▣739
Robitussin Sugar Free Cough (Dextromethorphan Hydrobromide, Guaifenesin) Wyeth ▣738
Triaminic Chest & Nasal Congestion Liquid (Guaifenesin, Phenylephrine Hydrochloride) Novartis Consumer ▣746
Tylenol Chest Congestion Caplets with Cool Burst (Acetaminophen, Guaifenesin) McNeil Consumer ▣722
Tylenol Chest Congestion Liquid with Cool Burst (Acetaminophen, Guaifenesin) McNeil Consumer ▣722
Tylenol Cold Multi-Symptom Severe Caplets with Cool Burst (Acetaminophen, Dextromethorphan Hydrobromide, Guaifenesin, Phenylephrine Hydrochloride) McNeil Consumer ▣752
Tylenol Sinus Severe Congestion Caplets with Cool Burst (Acetaminophen, Guaifenesin, Pseudoephedrine Hydrochloride) McNeil Consumer ▣778
Tylenol Chest Congestion Caplets with Cool Burst (Acetaminophen, Guaifenesin) McNeil Consumer 1872
Tylenol Chest Congestion Liquid with Cool Burst (Acetaminophen, Guaifenesin) McNeil Consumer 1872
Tylenol Cold Severe Congestion Non-Drowsy Caplets with Cool Burst (Acetaminophen, Dextromethorphan Hydrobromide, Guaifenesin, Pseudoephedrine Hydrochloride) McNeil Consumer 1874
Tylenol Cold Head Congestion Severe Caplets with Cool Burst (Acetaminophen, Dextromethorphan Hydrobromide, Guaifenesin, Phenylephrine Hydrochloride) McNeil Consumer 1873
Tylenol Cold Multi-Symptom Severe Caplets with Cool Burst (Acetaminophen, Dextromethorphan Hydrobromide, Guaifenesin, Phenylephrine Hydrochloride) McNeil Consumer 1874
Tylenol Cold Multi-Symptom Severe Daytime Liquid with Citrus Burst (Acetaminophen, Dextromethorphan Hydrobromide, Guaifenesin, Phenylephrine Hydrochloride) McNeil Consumer 1874
Tylenol Sinus Severe Congestion Caplets with Cool Burst (Acetaminophen, Guaifenesin, Pseudoephedrine Hydrochloride) McNeil Consumer 1876
Tylenol Sinus Congestion & Pain Severe Caplets with Cool Burst (Acetaminophen, Guaifenesin, Phenylephrine Hydrochloride) McNeil Consumer 1876
Vicks 44E Cough & Chest Congestion Relief Liquid (Dextromethorphan Hydrobromide, Guaifenesin) Procter & Gamble 2679
Pediatric Vicks 44e Cough & Chest Congestion Relief Liquid (Dextromethorphan Hydrobromide, Guaifenesin) Procter & Gamble 2676

Bronchitis, acute
Omnicef Capsules (Cefdinir) Abbott 511
Omnicef for Oral Suspension (Cefdinir) Abbott 511
Suprax (Cefixime) Lupin 1843

Bronchitis, chronic
Advair Diskus 250/50 (Fluticasone Propionate, Salmeterol Xinafoate) GlaxoSmithKline 1308
Atrovent HFA Inhalation Aerosol (Ipratropium Bromide) Boehringer Ingelheim 841
Serevent Diskus (Salmeterol Xinafoate) GlaxoSmithKline 1568
Spiriva HandiHaler (Tiotropium bromide) Boehringer Ingelheim 869
Uniphyl Tablets (Theophylline Anhydrous) Purdue Pharmaceutical 2710

Bronchitis, chronic, acute exacerbation of
Avelox (Moxifloxacin Hydrochloride) Schering 2970
Biaxin/Biaxin XL (Clarithromycin) Abbott 402
Ceftin Tablets (Cefuroxime Axetil) GlaxoSmithKline 1407
Cipro (Ciprofloxacin) Schering 2977
Ketek Tablets (Telithromycin) sanofi-aventis 2903
Levaquin (Levofloxacin) Ortho-McNeil 2384
Levaquin in 5% Dextrose Injection (Levofloxacin) Ortho-McNeil 2384
Omnicef Capsules (Cefdinir) Abbott 511
Omnicef for Oral Suspension (Cefdinir) Abbott 511
Primaxin I.M. (Cilastatin Sodium, Imipenem) Merck 2045
Suprax (Cefixime) Lupin 1843
Tequin Injection (Gatifloxacin) Bristol-Myers Squibb 938
Tequin Injection in 5% Dextrose (Gatifloxacin) Bristol-Myers Squibb 938
Tequin Tablets (Gatifloxacin) Bristol-Myers Squibb 938
Vantin Tablets and Oral Suspension (Cefpodoxime Proxetil) Pharmacia & Upjohn 2645

Bronchospasm, exercise-induced
Foradil Aerolizer (Formoterol Fumarate) Schering 3010
ProAir HFA Inhalation Aerosol (Albuterol Sulfate) Teva Specialty 3300
Proventil Inhalation Aerosol (Albuterol) Schering 3053
Proventil HFA Inhalation Aerosol (Albuterol Sulfate) Schering 3056
Serevent Diskus (Salmeterol Xinafoate) GlaxoSmithKline 1568

Bronchospasm, prevention and relief of
Xopenex Inhalation Solution (Levalbuterol Hydrochloride) Sepracor 3146
Xopenex Inhalation Solution Concentrate (Levalbuterol Hydrochloride) Sepracor 3150
Xopenex HFA Inhalation Aerosol (Levalbuterol Tartrate) Sepracor 3154

Bronchospasm, reversible
(*see also under* Bronchial asthma)
AccuNeb Inhalation Solution (Albuterol Sulfate) Dey 1055
Alupent Inhalation Aerosol (Metaproterenol Sulfate) Boehringer Ingelheim 826
Atrovent Inhalation Solution (Ipratropium Bromide) Boehringer Ingelheim 835
Atrovent HFA Inhalation Aerosol (Ipratropium Bromide) Boehringer Ingelheim 841
Proventil Inhalation Aerosol (Albuterol) Schering 3053
Proventil Inhalation Solution 0.083% (Albuterol Sulfate) Schering 3055
Proventil HFA Inhalation Aerosol (Albuterol Sulfate) Schering 3056
Uniphyl Tablets (Theophylline Anhydrous) Purdue Pharmaceutical 2710
Ventolin HFA Inhalation Aerosol (Albuterol Sulfate) GlaxoSmithKline 1600
Xopenex Inhalation Solution (Levalbuterol Hydrochloride) Sepracor 3146
Xopenex Inhalation Solution Concentrate (Levalbuterol Hydrochloride) Sepracor 3150
Xopenex HFA Inhalation Aerosol (Levalbuterol Tartrate) Sepracor 3154

Bronchospasm associated with chronic obstructive pulmonary disease
Alupent Inhalation Aerosol (Metaproterenol Sulfate) Boehringer Ingelheim 826
Atrovent Inhalation Solution (Ipratropium Bromide) Boehringer Ingelheim 835
Atrovent HFA Inhalation Aerosol (Ipratropium Bromide) Boehringer Ingelheim 841
Foradil Aerolizer (Formoterol Fumarate) Schering 3010
Maxair Autohaler (Pirbuterol Acetate) 3M 1852
Serevent Diskus (Salmeterol Xinafoate) GlaxoSmithKline 1568
Spiriva HandiHaler (Tiotropium bromide) Boehringer Ingelheim 869
Uniphyl Tablets (Theophylline Anhydrous) Purdue Pharmaceutical 2710

Bronchospasm associated with reversible obstructive airways disease
Foradil Aerolizer (Formoterol Fumarate) Schering 3010
ProAir HFA Inhalation Aerosol (Albuterol Sulfate) Teva Specialty 3300
Serevent Diskus (Salmeterol Xinafoate) GlaxoSmithKline 1568
VoSpire ER Tablets (Albuterol Sulfate) Dava Pharmaceuticals 1052
Xopenex Inhalation Solution (Levalbuterol Hydrochloride) Sepracor 3146
Xopenex Inhalation Solution Concentrate (Levalbuterol Hydrochloride) Sepracor 3150
Xopenex HFA Inhalation Aerosol (Levalbuterol Tartrate) Sepracor 3154

Bruises
Mineral Ice (Menthol) Novartis Consumer ▣685
Thera-Gesic Creme (Menthol, Methyl Salicylate) Mission ▣691

Bruises, topical relief of
(*see under* Pain, topical relief of)

Bubble boy disease
(*see under* Adenosine deaminase, enzyme replacement therapy for)

Bulbar conjunctiva inflammation
Blephamide Ophthalmic Suspension (Prednisolone Acetate, Sulfacetamide Sodium) Allergan 569
FML Ophthalmic Ointment (Fluorometholone) Allergan ⊙228
FML Ophthalmic Suspension (Fluorometholone) Allergan ⊙227
FML Forte Ophthalmic Suspension (Fluorometholone) Allergan ⊙226
FML-S Ophthalmic Suspension (Fluorometholone, Sulfacetamide Sodium) Allergan ⊙229
Lotemax Ophthalmic Suspension 0.5% (Loteprednol Etabonate) Bausch & Lomb ⊙251
Poly-Pred Ophthalmic Suspension (Neomycin Sulfate, Polymyxin B Sulfate, Prednisolone Acetate) Allergan ⊙233
Pred Forte Ophthalmic Suspension (Prednisolone Acetate) Allergan ⊙235
Pred-G Ophthalmic Ointment (Gentamicin Sulfate, Prednisolone Acetate) Allergan ⊙237
Pred-G Ophthalmic Suspension (Gentamicin Sulfate, Prednisolone Acetate) Allergan ⊙236
TobraDex Ophthalmic Ointment (Dexamethasone, Tobramycin) Alcon 562
TobraDex Ophthalmic Suspension (Dexamethasone, Tobramycin) Alcon 563

Bulimia nervosa
Prozac Pulvules and Liquid (Fluoxetine Hydrochloride) Lilly 1801

Burn wound infections
(*see under* Infections, burn wound)

Burning, vaginal
Estring Vaginal Ring (Estradiol) Pharmacia & Upjohn 2635

Burns, adjunctive therapy in
Accuzyme SE Spray Emulsion (Papain, Urea) Healthpoint 1662
Flexbumin I.V. (Albumin (human)) Baxter Healthcare 720
Panafil Ointment (Chlorophyllin Copper Complex Sodium, Papain, Urea) Healthpoint 1663
Panafil SE Spray Emulsion (Chlorophyllin Copper Complex Sodium, Papain, Urea) Healthpoint 1663

Burns, maintenance of electrolyte balance
Plasbumin-5 (Albumin (human)) Talecris 3251
Plasbumin-20 (Albumin (human)) Talecris 3252
Plasbumin-25 (Albumin (human)) Talecris 3253

Burns, minor
Neosporin Antibiotic Ointment (Bacitracin, Neomycin, Polymyxin B Sulfate) Pfizer Consumer Healthcare ▣643
Neosporin + Pain Relief Antibiotic Cream and Ointment (Maximum Strength) (Neomycin, Polymyxin B Sulfate, Pramoxine Hydrochloride) Pfizer Consumer Healthcare ▣643
Polysporin First Aid Antibiotic Ointment (Bacitracin, Polymyxin B Sulfate) Pfizer Consumer Healthcare ▣643

Burns, pain associated with
(*see under* Pain, topical relief of)

Burns, second- and third-degree, adjunctive therapy in
Sulfamylon for 5% Topical Solution (Mafenide Acetate) Mylan 2162

Burns, to prevent hemoconcentration
Plasbumin-5 (Albumin (human)) Talecris 3251
Plasbumin-20 (Albumin (human)) Talecris 3252
Plasbumin-25 (Albumin (human)) Talecris 3253

Bursitis
Anaprox Tablets (Naproxen Sodium) Roche 2761
Anaprox DS Tablets (Naproxen Sodium) Roche 2761
Depo-Medrol Injectable Suspension (Methylprednisolone Acetate) Pharmacia & Upjohn 2617
Depo-Medrol Single-Dose Vial (Methylprednisolone Acetate) Pharmacia & Upjohn 2619
Hydrocortone Tablets (Hydrocortisone) Merck 1989
Indocin (Indomethacin) Merck 1995

Naprosyn Suspension (Naproxen) Roche 2761
Naprosyn Tablets (Naproxen) Roche 2761
Traumeel Injection Solution (Homeopathic Formulations) Heel 1664

Bursitis, subacromial, acute, symptomatic relief of
Clinoril Tablets (Sulindac) Merck 1924
Indocin (Indomethacin) Merck 1995

C

C. difficile infection
(*see under* Colitis, pseudomembranous, antibiotic-associated)

C. diphtheriae infections
E.E.S. (Erythromycin Ethylsuccinate) Abbott 451
EryPed (Erythromycin Ethylsuccinate) Abbott 447
Ery-Tab Tablets (Erythromycin) Abbott 449
Erythrocin Stearate Filmtab Tablets (Erythromycin Stearate) Abbott 453
Erythromycin Base Filmtab Tablets (Erythromycin) Abbott 455
Erythromycin Delayed-Release Capsules, USP (Erythromycin) Abbott 457
PCE Dispertab Tablets (Erythromycin) Abbott 515

C. minutissimum infections
E.E.S. (Erythromycin Ethylsuccinate) Abbott 451
EryPed (Erythromycin Ethylsuccinate) Abbott 447
Ery-Tab Tablets (Erythromycin) Abbott 449
Erythrocin Stearate Filmtab Tablets (Erythromycin Stearate) Abbott 453
Erythromycin Base Filmtab Tablets (Erythromycin) Abbott 455
Erythromycin Delayed-Release Capsules, USP (Erythromycin) Abbott 457
PCE Dispertab Tablets (Erythromycin) Abbott 515

C. perfringens infections
Avelox (Moxifloxacin Hydrochloride) Schering 2970
Tygacil for Injection (Tigecycline) Wyeth 3488

C. perfringens intra-abdominal infections
Avelox (Moxifloxacin Hydrochloride) Schering 2970
Tygacil for Injection (Tigecycline) Wyeth 3488

Cachexia associated with weight loss, AIDS-induced
Megace ES Oral Suspension (Megestrol Acetate) Par 2481

Calcium deficiency
(*see under* Hypocalcemia)

Campylobacter jejuni infectious diarrhea
Cipro (Ciprofloxacin) Schering 2977

Cancer, prostatic
(*see under* Carcinoma, prostate, palliative treatment of)

Candida albicans infections
Eraxis for Injection (Anidulafungin) Pfizer 2521
Lotrimin (Clotrimazole) Schering 3039
Nystop Topical Powder USP (Nystatin) Paddock 2478
Paddock Nystatin USP for Oral Suspension (Nystatin) Paddock 2478

Candida infections, abdomen
Eraxis for Injection (Anidulafungin) Pfizer 2521
VFEND I.V. (Voriconazole) Pfizer 2564
VFEND Oral Suspension (Voriconazole) Pfizer 2564
VFEND Tablets (Voriconazole) Pfizer 2564

Candida infections, bladder wall
VFEND I.V. (Voriconazole) Pfizer 2564
VFEND Oral Suspension (Voriconazole) Pfizer 2564
VFEND Tablets (Voriconazole) Pfizer 2564

Candida infections, disseminated, skin
VFEND I.V. (Voriconazole) Pfizer 2564
VFEND Oral Suspension (Voriconazole) Pfizer 2564
VFEND Tablets (Voriconazole) Pfizer 2564

Candida infections, kidney
VFEND I.V. (Voriconazole) Pfizer 2564
VFEND Oral Suspension (Voriconazole) Pfizer 2564
VFEND Tablets (Voriconazole) Pfizer 2564

Candida infections, prophylaxis in hematopoietic stem cell transplantation
Mycamine for Injection (Micafungin Sodium) Astellas 628

Candida infections, wounds
VFEND I.V. (Voriconazole) Pfizer 2564
VFEND Oral Suspension (Voriconazole) Pfizer 2564
VFEND Tablets (Voriconazole) Pfizer 2564

Candidemia
Cancidas for Injection (Caspofungin acetate) Merck 1918
Eraxis for Injection (Anidulafungin) Pfizer 2521

Candidemia, non-neutropenic patients
VFEND I.V. (Voriconazole) Pfizer 2564
VFEND Oral Suspension (Voriconazole) Pfizer 2564
VFEND Tablets (Voriconazole) Pfizer 2564

Candidiasis, cutaneous
Lotrimin (Clotrimazole) Schering 3039
Nystop Topical Powder USP (Nystatin) Paddock 2478

Candidiasis, esophageal
Cancidas for Injection (Caspofungin acetate) Merck 1918
Eraxis for Injection (Anidulafungin) Pfizer 2521
Mycamine for Injection (Micafungin Sodium) Astellas 628
VFEND I.V. (Voriconazole) Pfizer 2564
VFEND Oral Suspension (Voriconazole) Pfizer 2564
VFEND Tablets (Voriconazole) Pfizer 2564

Candidiasis, intestinal
Paddock Nystatin USP for Oral Suspension (Nystatin) Paddock 4278

Candidiasis, oral cavity
Paddock Nystatin USP for Oral Suspension (Nystatin) Paddock 4278

Candidiasis, systemic
Abelcet Injection (Amphotericin B Lipid Complex) Enzon 1141
AmBisome for Injection (Amphotericin B, liposomal) Astellas 620

Candidiasis, vaginal
Vagistat-1 (Tioconazole) Novartis Consumer .... ▣804

Carbuncles
(*see under* Furunculosis, symptomatic relief of)

Carbuncles, adjunctive therapy in
Accuzyme SE Spray Emulsion (Papain, Urea) Healthpoint 1662
Panafil Ointment (Chlorophyllin Copper Complex Sodium, Papain, Urea) Healthpoint 1663

Carcinoma, advanced renal cell, treatment of
Nexavar Tablets (Sorafenib) Bayer 746

Carcinoma, breast
Arimidex Tablets (Anastrozole) AstraZeneca Pharmaceuticals 673
Aromasin Tablets (Exemestane) Pharmacia & Upjohn 2600
Faslodex Injection (Fulvestrant) AstraZeneca Pharmaceuticals 681
Femara Tablets (Letrozole) Novartis 2214
Taxotere Injection Concentrate (Docetaxel) sanofi-aventis 2932
Xeloda Tablets (Capecitabine) Roche 2822

Carcinoma, breast, adjunctive therapy in
Femara Tablets (Letrozole) Novartis 2214
Soltamox Oral Solution (Tamoxifen Citrate) Cytogen 3527

Carcinoma, breast, metastatic, resistant, treatment of (Monotherapy)
Xeloda Tablets (Capecitabine) Roche 2822

Carcinoma, breast, metastatic, treatment of
Faslodex Injection (Fulvestrant) AstraZeneca Pharmaceuticals 681
Gemzar for Injection (Gemcitabine Hydrochloride) Lilly 1771
Herceptin I.V. (Trastuzumab) Genentech 1233
Soltamox Oral Solution (Tamoxifen Citrate) Cytogen 3527
Taxotere Injection Concentrate (Docetaxel) sanofi-aventis 2932
Xeloda Tablets (Capecitabine) Roche 2822

Carcinoma, breast, osteolytic bone metastases of
Aredia for Injection (Pamidronate Disodium) Novartis 2179

Carcinoma, breast, palliative therapy in
Premarin Tablets (Estrogens, Conjugated) Wyeth 3446

Carcinoma, breast, to reduce the incidence of
Soltamox Oral Solution (Tamoxifen Citrate) Cytogen 3527

Carcinoma, bronchogenic
Mustargen for Injection (Mechlorethamine Hydrochloride) Ovation 2468

Carcinoma, cervical, prevention of
Gardasil Injection (Quadrivalent Human Papillomavirus (Types 6, 11, 16, 18) Recombinant Vaccine) Merck 1984

Carcinoma, colon, Dukes' stage C, adjunctive treatment in
Xeloda Tablets (Capecitabine) Roche 2822

Carcinoma, colon, metastatic
Camptosar Injection (Irinotecan Hydrochloride) Pharmacia & Upjohn 2604
Xeloda Tablets (Capecitabine) Roche 2822

Carcinoma, colorectal
Eloxatin for Injection (Oxaliplatin) sanofi-aventis 2892
Erbitux (Cetuximab) Bristol-Myers Squibb 910
Xeloda Tablets (Capecitabine) Roche 2822

Carcinoma, colorectal, adjunctive therapy in
Avastin IV (Bevacizumab) Genentech 1227
Erbitux (Cetuximab) Bristol-Myers Squibb 910

Carcinoma, ductual, in-situ
Soltamox Oral Solution (Tamoxifen Citrate) Cytogen 3527

Carcinoma, esophageal, obstructing, palliative treatment of
Photofrin for Injection (Porfimer Sodium) Axcan Scandipharm 702

Carcinoma, gastric
Taxotere (Docetaxel) sanofi-aventis 2932

Carcinoma, gastric adjunctive therapy in
Taxotere (Docetaxel) sanofi-aventis 2932

Carcinoma, gastroesophageal junction, adjunctive therapy in
Taxotere (Docetaxel) sanofi-aventis 2932

Carcinoma, head and neck
Erbitux (Cetuximab) Bristol-Myers Squibb 910

Carcinoma, head and neck, adjunct in
Erbitux (Cetuximab) Bristol-Myers Squibb 910

Carcinoma, lung, non-small cell
Alimta for Injection (Pemetrexed) Lilly 1750
Gemzar for Injection (Gemcitabine Hydrochloride) Lilly 1771
Iressa Tablets (Gefitinib) AstraZeneca Pharmaceuticals 684
Photofrin for Injection (Porfimer Sodium) Axcan Scandipharm 702
Tarceva Tablets (Erlotinib) Genentech 1259
Tarceva Tablets (Erlotinib) OSI 2444
Taxotere Injection Concentrate (Docetaxel) sanofi-aventis 2932

Carcinoma, lung, small cell
Hycamtin for Injection (Topotecan Hydrochloride) GlaxoSmithKline 1458

Carcinoma, mammary, metastatic, postmenopausal
Androxy Tablets (Fluoxymesterone) Upsher-Smith 3335

Carcinoma, metastatic, palliative treatment of
Mustargen for Injection (Mechlorethamine Hydrochloride) Ovation 2468

Carcinoma, ovary
Alkeran Tablets (Melphalan) Celgene 956
Doxil Injection (Doxorubicin Hydrochloride Liposome) Ortho Biotech 2351
Gemzar for Injection (Gemcitabine Hydrochloride) Lilly 1771
Hycamtin for Injection (Topotecan Hydrochloride) GlaxoSmithKline 1458

Carcinoma, pancreas
Gemzar for Injection (Gemcitabine Hydrochloride) Lilly 1771
Tarceva Tablets (Erlotinib) Genentech 1259
Tarceva Tablets (Erlotinib) OSI 2444

Carcinoma, prostate
Eulexin Capsules (Flutamide) Schering 3009
Taxotere Injection Concentrate (Docetaxel) sanofi-aventis 2932

Carcinoma, prostate, adjunctive therapy in
Eulexin Capsules (Flutamide) Schering 3009

Carcinoma, prostate, diagnostic agent in
ProstaScint Kit (Capromab Pendetide) Cytogen 1037

Carcinoma, prostate, palliative treatment of
Eligard 7.5 mg (Leuprolide Acetate) sanofi-aventis 2880
Eligard 22.5 mg (Leuprolide Acetate) sanofi-aventis 2883
Eligard 30 mg (Leuprolide Acetate) sanofi-aventis 2885
Eligard 45 mg (Leuprolide Acetate) sanofi-aventis 2888
Emcyt Capsules (Estramustine Phosphate Sodium) Pharmacia & Upjohn 2634
Lupron Depot 7.5 mg (Leuprolide Acetate) TAP 3264
Premarin Tablets (Estrogens, Conjugated) Wyeth 3446
Trelstar Depot (Triptorelin Pamoate) Watson 3394
Trelstar LA Suspension (Triptorelin Pamoate) Watson 3397
Vantas (Histrelin Acetate) Valera 3375
Viadur Implant (Leuprolide Acetate) Bayer 757

Carcinoma, rectal, metastatic
Camptosar Injection (Irinotecan Hydrochloride) Pharmacia & Upjohn 2604

Carcinoma, renal cell
Sutent Capsules (Sunitinib malate) Pfizer 2560

Carcinoma, renal cell, metastatic, in adults
Proleukin for Injection (Aldesleukin) Novartis 2266

Carcinoma, superficial basal cell
Efudex (Fluorouracil) Valeant North America 3363

Carcinoma, testis, advanced
Cosmegen for Injection (Dactinomycin) Ovation 2459

Carcinoma, thyroid
Cytomel Tablets (Liothyronine Sodium) King 1710
Levothroid Tablets (Levothyroxine Sodium) Forest 1186
Levoxyl Tablets (Levothyroxine Sodium) King 1712
Naturethroid Tablets (Levothyroxine, Liothyronine) Western Research 3401
Synthroid Tablets (Levothyroxine Sodium) Abbott 520
Thyrolar Tablets (Liotrix) Forest 1199
Westhroid Tablets (Levothyroxine Sodium, Liothyronine Sodium) Western Research 3403

Carcinoma, thyroid, adjunctive diagnostic tool for serum thyroglobulin testing
Thyrogen for Injection (Thyrotropin alfa) Genzyme 1286

Cardiac failure
(*see under* Congestive heart failure, adjunct in)

Cardiac ischemic complications, acute, prevention of, adjunct to PTCA
ReoPro Vials (Abciximab) Lilly 1809

Cardiomyopathy, doxorubicin-induced, to reduce the incidence and severity of
Zinecard for Injection (Dexrazoxane) Pharmacia & Upjohn 2650

Cardiopulmonary bypass surgery, adjunct in
Albutein 5%, Albumin (Human) (Albumin (human)) Grifols 1652
Albutein 25% , Albumin (Human) (Albumin (human)) Grifols 1653
Flexbumin I.V. (Albumin (human)) Baxter Healthcare 720
Human Albumin Grifols 20%, Albumin (Human) (Albumin (human)) Grifols 1651
Human Albumin Grifols 25%, Albumin (Human) (Albumin (human)) Grifols 1652
Plasbumin-5 (Albumin (human)) Talecris 3251
Plasbumin-20 (Albumin (human)) Talecris 3252
Plasbumin-25 (Albumin (human)) Talecris 3253

Cardiovascular disease, prevention of
Caduet Tablets (Amlodipine Besylate, Atorvastatin Calcium) Pfizer .. 2508
Lipitor Tablets (Atorvastatin Calcium) Parke-Davis 2483

Cardiovascular mortality, reduction of, post-MI
Bayer Aspirin Comprehensive Prescribing Information (Aspirin) Bayer Healthcare .... ▣796
Diovan Tablets (Valsartan) Novartis .. 2193
Lopressor Injection (Metoprolol Tartrate) Novartis 2238
Lopressor Tablets (Metoprolol Tartrate) Novartis 2238

Carnitine, deficiency of
Carnitor Injection (Levocarnitine) Sigma-Tau 3188
Carnitor Tablets and Oral Solution (Levocarnitine) Sigma-Tau 3190

Catabolic or tissue depleting processes, adjunctive therapy
Oxandrin Tablets (Oxandrolone) Savient 2962

Cataplexy
Xyrem Oral Solution (Sodium Oxybate) Jazz Pharmaceuticals 1688

Cataract surgery, treatment adjunct
Nevanac Ophthalmic Suspension 0.1% (Nepafenac) Alcon .... ⊙209

Cellulitis
Levaquin (Levofloxacin) Ortho-McNeil 2384
Levaquin in 5% Dextrose Injection (Levofloxacin) Ortho-McNeil 2384

Cellulitis, adjunctive therapy
Plasbumin-20 (Albumin (human)) Talecris 3252

Cellulitis, pelvic
(*see under* Pelvic cellulitis)

Cephalalgia, histaminic
Imitrex Injection (Sumatriptan Succinate) GlaxoSmithKline 1463

Cerebral edema
(*see under* Edema, cerebral)

Cerumen, removal of
Debrox Drops (Carbamide Peroxide) GlaxoSmithKline .... ▣715

Cervix, ripening of, in pregnant women at or near term
Cervidil Vaginal Insert (Dinoprostone) Forest 1181

Chancroid
Gantrisin Pediatric Suspension (Acetyl Sulfisoxazole) Roche 2770

Chickenpox
(*see under* Varicella, acute, treatment of)

Chlamydia pneumoniae infections
Avelox (Moxifloxacin Hydrochloride) Schering 2970
Biaxin/Biaxin XL (Clarithromycin) Abbott 402
Levaquin (Levofloxacin) Ortho-McNeil 2384
Levaquin in 5% Dextrose Injection (Levofloxacin) Ortho-McNeil 2384
Tequin Injection (Gatifloxacin) Bristol-Myers Squibb 938
Tequin Injection in 5% Dextrose (Gatifloxacin) Bristol-Myers Squibb 938
Tequin Tablets (Gatifloxacin) Bristol-Myers Squibb 938
Zmax for Oral Suspension (Azithromycin) Pfizer 2583

Chlamydia pneumoniae lower respiratory tract infections
Avelox (Moxifloxacin Hydrochloride) Schering 2970
Biaxin/Biaxin XL (Clarithromycin) Abbott 402
Ketek Tablets (Telithromycin) sanofi-aventis 2903
Levaquin (Levofloxacin) Ortho-McNeil 2384
Levaquin in 5% Dextrose Injection (Levofloxacin) Ortho-McNeil 2384
Tequin Injection (Gatifloxacin) Bristol-Myers Squibb 938
Tequin Injection in 5% Dextrose (Gatifloxacin) Bristol-Myers Squibb 938
Tequin Tablets (Gatifloxacin) Bristol-Myers Squibb 938
Zmax for Oral Suspension (Azithromycin) Pfizer 2583

Chlamydia trachomatis conjunctivitis of the newborn
E.E.S. (Erythromycin Ethylsuccinate) Abbott 451
EryPed (Erythromycin Ethylsuccinate) Abbott 447
Ery-Tab Tablets (Erythromycin) Abbott 449
Erythrocin Stearate Filmtab Tablets (Erythromycin Stearate) Abbott 453
Erythromycin Base Filmtab Tablets (Erythromycin) Abbott 455
Erythromycin Delayed-Release Capsules, USP (Erythromycin) Abbott 457
PCE Dispertab Tablets (Erythromycin) Abbott 515

Chlamydia trachomatis endocervical infections
E.E.S. (Erythromycin Ethylsuccinate) Abbott 451
EryPed (Erythromycin Ethylsuccinate) Abbott 447
Ery-Tab Tablets (Erythromycin) Abbott 449
Erythrocin Stearate Filmtab Tablets (Erythromycin Stearate) Abbott 453
Erythromycin Base Filmtab Tablets (Erythromycin) Abbott 455
Erythromycin Delayed-Release Capsules, USP (Erythromycin) Abbott 457
PCE Dispertab Tablets (Erythromycin) Abbott 515

Chlamydia trachomatis infections
E.E.S. (Erythromycin Ethylsuccinate) Abbott 451
EryPed (Erythromycin Ethylsuccinate) Abbott 447
Ery-Tab Tablets (Erythromycin) Abbott 449
Erythrocin Stearate Filmtab Tablets (Erythromycin Stearate) Abbott 453
Erythromycin Base Filmtab Tablets (Erythromycin) Abbott 455
Erythromycin Delayed-Release Capsules, USP (Erythromycin) Abbott 457
PCE Dispertab Tablets (Erythromycin) Abbott 515
Vigamox Ophthalmic Solution (Moxifloxacin Hydrochloride) Alcon 564

Chlamydia trachomatis infections, ocular
(*see under* Trachoma)

Chlamydia trachomatis pneumonia of infancy
E.E.S. (Erythromycin Ethylsuccinate) Abbott 451
EryPed (Erythromycin Ethylsuccinate) Abbott 447
Ery-Tab Tablets (Erythromycin) Abbott 449
Erythrocin Stearate Filmtab Tablets (Erythromycin Stearate) Abbott 453
Erythromycin Base Filmtab Tablets (Erythromycin) Abbott 455
Erythromycin Delayed-Release Capsules, USP (Erythromycin) Abbott 457
PCE Dispertab Tablets (Erythromycin) Abbott 515

Chlamydia trachomatis rectal infections
E.E.S. (Erythromycin Ethylsuccinate) Abbott 451
EryPed (Erythromycin Ethylsuccinate) Abbott 447
Ery-Tab Tablets (Erythromycin) Abbott 449
Erythrocin Stearate Filmtab Tablets (Erythromycin Stearate) Abbott 453
Erythromycin Base Filmtab Tablets (Erythromycin) Abbott 455
Erythromycin Delayed-Release Capsules, USP (Erythromycin) Abbott 457
PCE Dispertab Tablets (Erythromycin) Abbott 515

Chlamydia trachomatis urethral infections
E.E.S. (Erythromycin Ethylsuccinate) Abbott 451
EryPed (Erythromycin Ethylsuccinate) Abbott 447
Ery-Tab Tablets (Erythromycin) Abbott 449
Erythrocin Stearate Filmtab Tablets (Erythromycin Stearate) Abbott 453
Erythromycin Base Filmtab Tablets (Erythromycin) Abbott 455
Erythromycin Delayed-Release Capsules, USP (Erythromycin) Abbott 457
PCE Dispertab Tablets (Erythromycin) Abbott 515

Chlamydia trachomatis urogenital infections during pregnancy
E.E.S. (Erythromycin Ethylsuccinate) Abbott 451
EryPed (Erythromycin Ethylsuccinate) Abbott 447
Ery-Tab Tablets (Erythromycin) Abbott 449
Erythrocin Stearate Filmtab Tablets (Erythromycin Stearate) Abbott 453
Erythromycin Base Filmtab Tablets (Erythromycin) Abbott 455
Erythromycin Delayed-Release Capsules, USP (Erythromycin) Abbott 457
PCE Dispertab Tablets (Erythromycin) Abbott 515

Chloasma
(*see under* Hyperpigmentation, skin, bleaching of)

Cholangitis
(*see under* Infections, intra-abdominal)

Cholecystitis, acute
(*see under* Infections, intra-abdominal)

Cholesterol levels, elevated
(*see under* Hypercholesterolemia, primary, adjunct to diet)

Chorioretinitis
Depo-Medrol Injectable Suspension (Methylprednisolone Acetate) Pharmacia & Upjohn 2617
Hydrocortone Tablets (Hydrocortisone) Merck 1989

Choroidal neovascularization, secondary to macular degeneration
Visudyne for Injection (Verteporfin) Novartis 2305

Choroiditis
Depo-Medrol Injectable Suspension (Methylprednisolone Acetate) Pharmacia & Upjohn 2617
Hydrocortone Tablets (Hydrocortisone) Merck 1989

Christmas disease
(*see under* Hemophilia B)

Cirrhosis, biliary
Urso 250 Tablets (Ursodiol) Axcan Scandipharm 710
Urso Forte Tablets (Ursodiol) Axcan Scandipharm 710

Citrobacter diversus infections
Cipro (Ciprofloxacin) Schering 2977
Cipro I.V. (Ciprofloxacin) Schering 2984

Citrobacter diversus urinary tract infections
Cipro (Ciprofloxacin) Schering 2977
Cipro I.V. (Ciprofloxacin) Schering 2984

Citrobacter freundii infections
Cipro (Ciprofloxacin) Schering 2977
Cipro I.V. (Ciprofloxacin) Schering 2984
Noroxin Tablets (Norfloxacin) Merck . 2032
Tygacil (Tigecycline) Wyeth 3488

Citrobacter freundii intra-abdominal infections
Tygacil for injection (Tigecycline) Wyeth 3488

Citrobacter freundii skin and skin structure infections
Cipro (Ciprofloxacin) Schering 2977
Cipro I.V. (Ciprofloxacin) Schering 2984

Citrobacter freundii urinary tract infections
Cipro (Ciprofloxacin) Schering 2977
Cipro I.V. (Ciprofloxacin) Schering 2984
Noroxin Tablets (Norfloxacin) Merck . 2032

Citrobacter species infections
Fortaz (Ceftazidime) GlaxoSmithKline 1453
Garamycin Injectable (Gentamicin Sulfate) Schering 3014
Primaxin I.M. (Cilastatin Sodium, Imipenem) Merck 2045
Primaxin I.V. (Cilastatin Sodium, Imipenem) Merck 2048

Timentin ADD-Vantage (Clavulanate Potassium, Ticarcillin Disodium) GlaxoSmithKline ... 1580
Timentin Injection Galaxy Container (Clavulanate Potassium, Ticarcillin Disodium) GlaxoSmithKline ... 1583
Timentin IV Infusion (Clavulanate Potassium, Ticarcillin Disodium) GlaxoSmithKline ... 1577
Timentin Pharmacy Bulk Package (Clavulanate Potassium, Ticarcillin Disodium) GlaxoSmithKline ... 1586

Citrobacter species intra-abdominal infections
Primaxin I.V. (Cilastatin Sodium, Imipenem) Merck ... 2048

Citrobacter species lower respiratory tract infections
Fortaz (Ceftazidime) GlaxoSmithKline ... 1453

Citrobacter species skin and skin structure infections
Primaxin I.M. (Cilastatin Sodium, Imipenem) Merck ... 2045
Primaxin I.V. (Cilastatin Sodium, Imipenem) Merck ... 2048

Citrobacter species urinary tract infections
Timentin ADD-Vantage (Clavulanate Potassium, Ticarcillin Disodium) GlaxoSmithKline ... 1580
Timentin Injection Galaxy Container (Clavulanate Potassium, Ticarcillin Disodium) GlaxoSmithKline ... 1583
Timentin IV Infusion (Clavulanate Potassium, Ticarcillin Disodium) GlaxoSmithKline ... 1577
Timentin Pharmacy Bulk Package (Clavulanate Potassium, Ticarcillin Disodium) GlaxoSmithKline ... 1586

Claudication, intermittent
Pletal Tablets (Cilostazol) Otsuka America ... 2455

Clonorchiasis
Biltricide (Praziquantel) Schering ... 2976

Clororchis sinensis/Cloisthorchis viverrini infections
Biltricide (Praziquantel) Schering ... 2976

Clostridium species gynecologic infections
Mefoxin for Injection (Cefoxitin Sodium) Merck ... 2012
Mefoxin Premixed Intravenous Solution (Cefoxitin Sodium) Merck ... 2016

Clostridium species infections
Mefoxin for Injection (Cefoxitin Sodium) Merck ... 2012
Mefoxin Premixed Intravenous Solution (Cefoxitin Sodium) Merck ... 2016
Primaxin I.V. (Cilastatin Sodium, Imipenem) Merck ... 2048
Rocephin Injectable Vials, ADD-Vantage, Galaxy, Bulk (Ceftriaxone Sodium) Roche ... 2800

Clostridium species intra-abdominal infections
Invanz for Injection (Ertapenem) Merck ... 1999
Mefoxin for Injection (Cefoxitin Sodium) Merck ... 2012
Mefoxin Premixed Intravenous Solution (Cefoxitin Sodium) Merck ... 2016
Primaxin I.V. (Cilastatin Sodium, Imipenem) Merck ... 2048
Rocephin Injectable Vials, ADD-Vantage, Galaxy, Bulk (Ceftriaxone Sodium) Roche ... 2800

Clostridium species peritonitis
Mefoxin for Injection (Cefoxitin Sodium) Merck ... 2012
Mefoxin Premixed Intravenous Solution (Cefoxitin Sodium) Merck ... 2016

Clostridium species skin and skin structure infections
Mefoxin for Injection (Cefoxitin Sodium) Merck ... 2012
Mefoxin Premixed Intravenous Solution (Cefoxitin Sodium) Merck ... 2016

Clostridium tetani, immunization against
(*see also under* Immunization, diphtheria, tetanus and pertussis; Immunization, tetanus)
ADACEL Vaccine (Diphtheria & Tetanus Toxoids and Acellular Pertussis Vaccine Adsorbed) Sanofi Pasteur ... 2945
Boostrix (Diphtheria & Tetanus Toxoids and Acellular Pertussis Vaccine Adsorbed) GlaxoSmithKline ... 1404
DAPTACEL Vaccine (Diphtheria & Tetanus Toxoids and Acellular Pertussis Vaccine Adsorbed) Sanofi Pasteur ... 2950
HyperTET (Tetanus Immune Globulin (Human)) Talecris ... 3248
Infanrix Vaccine (Diphtheria & Tetanus Toxoids and Acellular Pertussis Vaccine Adsorbed) GlaxoSmithKline ... 1476
Pediarix Vaccine (Diphtheria & Tetanus Toxoids and Pertussis Vaccine Adsorbed, Hepatitis B Vaccine, Recombinant, Poliovirus Vaccine Inactivated, Trivalent Types 1,2,3) GlaxoSmithKline ... 1548

Cold, common, symptomatic relief of
(*see also under* Influenza syndrome, symptomatic relief of)
Advil Allergy Sinus Caplets (Chlorpheniramine Maleate, Ibuprofen, Pseudoephedrine Hydrochloride) Wyeth ... ▣770
Advil Caplets (Ibuprofen) Wyeth ... ▣674
Children's Advil Oral Suspension (Ibuprofen) Wyeth ... ▣603
Children's Advil Chewable Tablets (Ibuprofen) Wyeth ... ▣603
Advil Cold & Sinus (Ibuprofen, Pseudoephedrine Hydrochloride) Wyeth ... ▣723
Advil Gel Caplets (Ibuprofen) Wyeth ... ▣674
Infants' Advil Concentrated Drops (Ibuprofen) Wyeth ... ▣604
Infants' Advil Concentrated Drops - White Grape (Dye-Free) (Ibuprofen) Wyeth ... ▣604
Junior Strength Advil Swallow Tablets (Ibuprofen) Wyeth ... ▣605
Advil Liqui-Gels (Ibuprofen) Wyeth ... ▣674
Advil Multi-Symptom Cold Caplets (Chlorpheniramine Maleate, Ibuprofen, Pseudoephedrine Hydrochloride) Wyeth ... ▣770
Advil Tablets (Ibuprofen) Wyeth ... ▣674
Alavert Allergy & Sinus D-12 Hour Tablets (Loratadine, Pseudoephedrine Sulfate) Wyeth ... ▣771
Aleve Caplets (Naproxen Sodium) Bayer Healthcare LLC ... 742
Aleve Gelcaps (Naproxen Sodium) Bayer Healthcare LLC ... 743
Aleve Tablets (Naproxen Sodium) Bayer Healthcare LLC ... 743
BC Cold Powder (Aspirin, Chlorpheniramine Maleate, Pseudoephedrine Hydrochloride) GlaxoSmithKline ... ▣677
Contac Cold and Flu Maximum Strength Caplets (Acetaminophen, Chlorpheniramine Maleate, Phenylephrine Hydrochloride) GlaxoSmithKline ... ▣728
Contac Cold and Flu Day and Night Caplets (Day Formulation Only) (Acetaminophen, Phenylephrine Hydrochloride) GlaxoSmithKline ... ▣727
Contac Cold and Flu Day and Night Caplets (Night Formulation Only) (Acetaminophen, Chlorpheniramine Maleate, Phenylephrine Hydrochloride) GlaxoSmithKline ... ▣727
Contac Cold and Flu Non-Drowsy Caplets (Acetaminophen, Phenylephrine Hydrochloride) GlaxoSmithKline ... ▣728
Delsym Extended-Release Suspension 12 Hour Cough Suppressant (Dextromethorphan Polistirex) UCB ... ▣611
Children's Dimetapp DM Cold & Cough Elixir (Brompheniramine Maleate, Dextromethorphan Hydrobromide, Phenylephrine Hydrochloride) Wyeth ... ▣731
Toddler's Dimetapp Cold and Cough Drops (Dextromethorphan Hydrobromide, Phenylephrine Hydrochloride) Wyeth ... ▣732
Excedrin Extra Strength Caplets/Tablets/Geltabs (Acetaminophen, Aspirin, Caffeine) Novartis Consumer ... ▣684
4-Way Menthol Nasal Spray (Phenylephrine Hydrochloride) Novartis Consumer ... ▣775
Hyland's Complete Flu Care 4 Kids Tablets (Dietary Supplement) Standard Homeopathic ... ▣732
Hyland's Sniffles 'N Sneezes 4 Kids Tablets (Dietary Supplement) Standard Homeopathic ... ▣732
Children's Motrin Oral Suspension (Ibuprofen) McNeil Consumer ... ▣685
Children's Motrin Non-Staining Dye-Free Oral Suspension (Ibuprofen) McNeil Consumer ... ▣685
Children's Motrin Cold Oral Suspension (Ibuprofen, Pseudoephedrine Hydrochloride) McNeil Consumer ... ▣733
Mucinex Extended-Release Bi-Layer Tablets (Guaifenesin) Adams ... ▣720
Mucinex DM Extended-Release Bi-Layer Tablets (Dextromethorphan Hydrobromide, Guaifenesin) Adams ... ▣720
Robitussin Chest Congestion Liquid (Guaifenesin) Wyeth ... ▣721
Robitussin Cough & Cold CF Liquid (Dextromethorphan Hydrobromide, Guaifenesin, Pseudoephedrine Hydrochloride) Wyeth ... ▣735
Robitussin Cough & Cold Long-Acting Liquid (Chlorpheniramine Maleate, Dextromethorphan Hydrobromide) Wyeth ... ▣735
Robitussin Cough & Cold Nighttime Liquid (Chlorpheniramine Maleate, Dextromethorphan Hydrobromide, Phenylephrine Hydrochloride) Wyeth ... ▣736
Robitussin Cough & Cold Pediatric Drops (Dextromethorphan Hydrobromide, Guaifenesin, Pseudoephedrine Hydrochloride) Wyeth ... ▣735
Robitussin Cough, Cold & Flu Nighttime Liquid (Acetaminophen, Chlorpheniramine Maleate, Dextromethorphan Hydrobromide, Phenylephrine Hydrochloride) Wyeth ... ▣738
Robitussin Cough & Congestion Liquid (Dextromethorphan Hydrobromide, Guaifenesin) Wyeth ... ▣738
Robitussin Cough Long Acting Liquid (Dextromethorphan Hydrobromide) Wyeth ... ▣739
Robitussin Cough DM Syrup (Dextromethorphan Hydrobromide, Guaifenesin) Wyeth ... ▣738
Robitussin Cough DM Infant Drops (Dextromethorphan Hydrobromide, Guaifenesin) Wyeth ... ▣738
Robitussin Cough Drops Menthol, Cherry, and Honey-Lemon (Menthol) Wyeth ... ▣737
Robitussin Honey Cough Drops (Menthol) Wyeth ... ▣737
Robitussin Sugar Free Throat Drops (Menthol) Wyeth ... ▣737
Robitussin Head & Chest Congestion PE Syrup (Guaifenesin, Phenylephrine Hydrochloride) Wyeth ... ▣739
Robitussin Pediatric Cough Long Acting Liquid (Dextromethorphan Hydrobromide) Wyeth ... ▣739
Robitussin Pediatric Cough & Cold Long-Acting Liquid (Chlorpheniramine Maleate, Dextromethorphan Hydrobromide) Wyeth ... ▣735
Robitussin Pediatric Cough & Cold Nighttime Liquid (Chlorpheniramine Maleate, Dextromethorphan Hydrobromide, Phenylephrine Hydrochloride) Wyeth ... ▣736
Robitussin Sugar Free Cough (Dextromethorphan Hydrobromide, Guaifenesin) Wyeth ... ▣738
TheraFlu Cold & Cough Hot Liquid (Dextromethorphan Hydrobromide, Pheniramine Maleate, Phenylephrine Hydrochloride) Novartis Consumer ... ▣740
TheraFlu Cold & Sore Throat Hot Liquid (Acetaminophen, Pheniramine Maleate, Phenylephrine Hydrochloride) Novartis Consumer ... ▣741
TheraFlu Flu & Chest Congestion Hot Liquid (Acetaminophen, Guaifenesin) Novartis Consumer ... ▣741
TheraFlu Flu & Sore Throat Hot Liquid (Acetaminophen, Pheniramine Maleate, Phenylephrine Hydrochloride) Novartis Consumer ... ▣742
TheraFlu Daytime Severe Cold Hot Liquid (Acetaminophen, Phenylephrine Hydrochloride) Novartis Consumer ... ▣742
TheraFlu Nighttime Severe Cold Hot Liquid (Acetaminophen, Pheniramine Maleate, Phenylephrine Hydrochloride) Novartis Consumer ... ▣740
TheraFlu Thin Strips Multi Symptom (Diphenhydramine Hydrochloride) Novartis Consumer ... ▣744
Triaminic Chest & Nasal Congestion Liquid (Guaifenesin, Phenylephrine Hydrochloride) Novartis Consumer ... ▣746
Children's Tylenol Suspension Liquid and Meltaways (Acetaminophen) McNeil Consumer ... ▣679
Children's Tylenol with Flavor Creator (Acetaminophen) McNeil Consumer ... ▣679
Children's Tylenol Plus Cough & Runny Nose Suspension Liquid (Acetaminophen, Chlorpheniramine Maleate, Dextromethorphan Hydrobromide) McNeil Consumer ... ▣754
Children's Tylenol Plus Cough & Sore Throat Suspension Liquid (Acetaminophen, Dextromethorphan Hydrobromide) McNeil Consumer ... ▣754
Children's Tylenol Plus Cold Suspension Liquid (Acetaminophen, Chlorpheniramine Maleate, Phenylephrine Hydrochloride) McNeil Consumer ... ▣754
Children's Tylenol Plus Multi-Symptom Cold Suspension Liquid (Acetaminophen, Chlorpheniramine Maleate, Dextromethorphan Hydrobromide, Phenylephrine Hydrochloride) McNeil Consumer ... ▣754
Children's Tylenol Plus Cold & Allergy Oral Suspension (Acetaminophen, Diphenhydramine Hydrochloride, Phenylephrine Hydrochloride) McNeil Consumer ... ▣716
Children's Tylenol Plus Flu Oral Suspension (Acetaminophen, Chlorpheniramine Maleate, Dextromethorphan Hydrobromide, Phenylephrine Hydrochloride) McNeil Consumer ... ▣749
Concentrated Tylenol Infants' Drops (Acetaminophen) McNeil Consumer ... ▣679
Concentrated Tylenol Infants' Drops Plus Cold (Acetaminophen, Phenylephrine Hydrochloride) McNeil Consumer ... ▣754
Concentrated Tylenol Infants' Drops Plus Cold & Cough (Acetaminophen, Dextromethorphan Hydrobromide, Phenylephrine Hydrochloride) McNeil Consumer ... ▣754
Jr. Tylenol Meltaways (Acetaminophen) McNeil Consumer ... ▣679
Tylenol Chest Congestion Caplets with Cool Burst (Acetaminophen, Guaifenesin) McNeil Consumer ... 1872
Tylenol Chest Congestion Liquid with Cool Burst (Acetaminophen, Guaifenesin) McNeil Consumer ... 1872
Children's Tylenol Suspension Liquid and Meltaways (Acetaminophen) McNeil Consumer ... 1878

Children's Tylenol Plus Cold Suspension Liquid (Acetaminophen, Chlorpheniramine Maleate, Phenylephrine Hydrochloride) McNeil Consumer ... 1879
Children's Tylenol Plus Cold & Allergy Suspension Liquid (Acetaminophen, Diphenhydramine Hydrochloride, Phenylephrine Hydrochloride) McNeil Consumer ... 1878
Children's Tylenol Plus Cough & Runny Nose Suspension Liquid (Acetaminophen, Chlorpheniramine Maleate, Dextromethorphan Hydrobromide) McNeil Consumer ... 1879
Children's Tylenol Plus Cough & Sore Throat Suspension Liquid (Acetaminophen, Dextromethorphan Hydrobromide) McNeil Consumer ... 1879
Children's Tylenol Suspension with Flavor Creator (Acetaminophen) McNeil Consumer ... 1878
Children's Tylenol Plus Flu Suspension Liquid (Acetaminophen, Chlorpheniramine Maleate, Dextromethorphan Hydrobromide, Phenylephrine Hydrochloride) McNeil Consumer ... 1881
Children's Tylenol Plus Multi-Symptom Cold Suspension Liquid (Acetaminophen, Chlorpheniramine Maleate, Dextromethorphan Hydrobromide, Phenylephrine Hydrochloride) McNeil Consumer ... 1879
Tylenol Cold Head Congestion Daytime Caplets with Cool Burst (Acetaminophen, Dextromethorphan Hydrobromide, Phenylephrine Hydrochloride) McNeil Consumer ... 1873
Tylenol Cold Head Congestion Nighttime Caplets with Cool Burst (Acetaminophen, Chlorpheniramine Maleate, Dextromethorphan Hydrobromide, Phenylephrine Hydrochloride) McNeil Consumer ... 1873
Tylenol Cold Head Congestion Severe Caplets with Cool Burst (Acetaminophen, Dextromethorphan Hydrobromide, Guaifenesin, Phenylephrine Hydrochloride) McNeil Consumer ... 1873
Tylenol Cold Multi-Symptom Daytime Caplets with Cool Burst and Gelcaps (Acetaminophen, Dextromethorphan Hydrobromide, Phenylephrine Hydrochloride) McNeil Consumer ... 1874
Tylenol Cold Multi-Symptom Daytime Liquid with Citrus Burst (Acetaminophen, Dextromethorphan Hydrobromide, Phenylephrine Hydrochloride) McNeil Consumer ... 1874
Tylenol Cold Multi-Symptom Nighttime Caplets with Cool Burst (Acetaminophen, Chlorpheniramine Maleate, Dextromethorphan Hydrobromide, Phenylephrine Hydrochloride) McNeil Consumer ... 1874
Tylenol Cold Multi-Symptom Nighttime Liquid with Cool Burst (Acetaminophen, Dextromethorphan Hydrobromide, Doxylamine Succinate, Phenylephrine Hydrochloride) McNeil Consumer ... 1874
Tylenol Cold Multi-Symptom Severe Caplets with Cool Burst (Acetaminophen, Dextromethorphan Hydrobromide, Guaifenesin, Phenylephrine Hydrochloride) McNeil Consumer ... 1874
Tylenol Cold Multi-Symptom Severe Daytime Liquid with Citrus Burst (Acetaminophen, Dextromethorphan Hydrobromide, Guaifenesin, Phenylephrine Hydrochloride) McNeil Consumer ... 1874
Tylenol Cough & Sore Throat Daytime Liquid with Cool Burst (Acetaminophen, Dextromethorphan Hydrobromide) McNeil Consumer ... 1877
Tylenol Cough & Sore Throat Nighttime Liquid with Cool Burst (Acetaminophen, Dextromethorphan Hydrobromide, Doxylamine Succinate) McNeil Consumer ... 1877
Concentrated Tylenol Infants' Drops (Acetaminophen) McNeil Consumer ... 1878
Concentrated Tylenol Infants' Drops Plus Cold (Acetaminophen) McNeil Consumer ... 1879
Concentrated Tylenol Infants' Drops Plus Cold and Cough (Acetaminophen, Dextromethorphan Hydrobromide) McNeil Consumer ... 1879
Jr. Tylenol Meltaways (Acetaminophen) McNeil Consumer ... 1878
Tylenol Sore Throat Daytime Liquid with Cool Burst (Acetaminophen) McNeil Consumer ... 1877
Vicks 44 Cough Relief Liquid (Dextromethorphan Hydrobromide) Procter & Gamble ... 2679
Vicks 44D Cough & Head Congestion Relief Liquid (Dextromethorphan Hydrobromide, Pseudoephedrine Hydrochloride) Procter & Gamble ... 2679
Vicks 44E Cough & Chest Congestion Relief Liquid (Dextromethorphan Hydrobromide, Guaifenesin) Procter & Gamble ... 2679
Pediatric Vicks 44e Cough & Chest Congestion Relief Liquid (Dextromethorphan Hydrobromide, Guaifenesin) Procter & Gamble ... 2676
Vicks 44M Cough, Cold & Flu Relief Liquid (Acetaminophen, Chlorpheniramine Maleate, Dextromethorphan Hydrobromide, Pseudoephedrine Hydrochloride) Procter & Gamble ... 2680
Pediatric Vicks 44m Cough & Cold Relief Liquid (Chlorpheniramine Maleate, Dextromethorphan Hydrobromide) Procter & Gamble ... 2676
Vicks Cough Drops, Menthol & Cherry Flavors (Menthol) Procter & Gamble ... 2678
Vicks DayQuil Multi-Symptom Cold/Flu Relief Liquid (Acetaminophen, Dextromethorphan Hydrobromide, Pseudoephedrine Hydrochloride) Procter & Gamble ... 2678
Vicks DayQuil Multi-Symptom Cold/Flu Relief LiquiCaps (Acetaminophen, Dextromethorphan Hydrobromide, Pseudoephedrine Hydrochloride) Procter & Gamble ... 2678
Vicks NyQuil LiquiCaps/Liquid Multi-Symptom Cold/Flu Relief (Acetaminophen, Dextromethorphan Hydrobromide, Doxylamine Succinate) Procter & Gamble ... ▣ 763
Vicks NyQuil Cough Liquid (Dextromethorphan Hydrobromide, Doxylamine Succinate) Procter & Gamble ... 2680
Children's Vicks NyQuil Cold/Cough Relief Liquid (Chlorpheniramine Maleate, Dextromethorphan Hydrobromide, Pseudoephedrine Hydrochloride) Procter & Gamble ... 2680
Vicks Sinex Nasal Spray and Ultra Fine Mist for Sinus Relief (Oxymetazoline Hydrochloride) Procter & Gamble ... 2681
Vicks Vapor Inhaler (Levmetamfetamine) Procter & Gamble ... 2682
Vicks VapoRub Cream (Camphor, Menthol) Procter & Gamble ... 2682
Vicks VapoRub Ointment (Camphor, Eucalyptus, Oil of, Menthol) Procter & Gamble ... 2682
Vicks VapoSteam (Camphor) Procter & Gamble ... 2682
Zicam Cold Remedy Chewables (Zincum Aceticum, Zincum Gluconicum) Matrixx ... ▣ 766
Zicam Cold Remedy ChewCaps (Zincum Aceticum, Zincum Gluconicum) Matrixx ... ▣ 766
Zicam Cold Remedy Gel Swabs (Zincum Gluconicum) Matrixx ... ▣ 766
Zicam Cold Remedy Nasal Gel (Zincum Gluconicum) Matrixx ... ▣ 766
Zicam Cold Remedy Oral Mist (Zincum Aceticum, Zincum Gluconicum) Matrixx ... ▣ 766
Zicam Cold Remedy RapidMelts (Zincum Aceticum, Zincum Gluconicum) Matrixx ... ▣ 766
Zicam Cold Remedy RapidMelts with Vitamin C (Zincum Aceticum, Zincum Gluconicum) Matrixx ... ▣ 766
Zicam Cold Remedy Swabs Kids Size (Zincum Gluconicum) Matrixx ... ▣ 766
Zicam Cough Plus D Cough Spray (Dextromethorphan Hydrobromide, Phenylephrine Hydrochloride) Matrixx ... ▣ 767
Zicam Extreme Congestion Relief (Oxymetazoline Hydrochloride) Matrixx ... ▣ 767
Zicam Maximum Strength Flu Daytime (Acetaminophen, Chlorpheniramine Maleate, Dextromethorphan Hydrobromide) Matrixx ... ▣ 768
Zicam Maximum Strength Flu Nighttime (Acetaminophen, Dextromethorphan Hydrobromide, Doxylamine Succinate) Matrixx ... ▣ 768
Zicam Intense Sinus Relief (Oxymetazoline Hydrochloride) Matrixx ... ▣ 767

Cold sores
(*see under* Herpetic manifestations, oral, symptomatic relief of)

Colitis, distal ulcerative
Colocort Rectal Suspension, USP (Retention) 100 mg/60 mL (Hydrocortisone) Paddock ... 2476

Colitis, mucous
(*see under* Bowel, irritable, syndrome)

Colitis, pseudomembranous, antibiotic-associated
Vancocin HCl Capsules, USP (Vancomycin Hydrochloride) ViroPharma ... 3380

Colitis, ulcerative
Asacol Delayed-Release Tablets (Mesalamine) Procter & Gamble Pharmaceuticals ... 2692
Colazal Capsules (Balsalazide Disodium) Salix ... 2838
Colocort Rectal Suspension, USP (Retention) 100 mg/60 mL (Hydrocortisone) Paddock ... 2476
Decadron Tablets (Dexamethasone) Merck ... 1951
Depo-Medrol Injectable Suspension (Methylprednisolone Acetate) Pharmacia & Upjohn ... 2617
Depo-Medrol Single-Dose Vial (Methylprednisolone Acetate) Pharmacia & Upjohn ... 2619
Hydrocortone Tablets (Hydrocortisone) Merck ... 1989
Pentasa Capsules (Mesalamine) Shire US ... 3185
Remicade for IV Injection (Infliximab) Centocor ... 971

Collagen disease
Depo-Medrol Injectable Suspension (Methylprednisolone Acetate) Pharmacia & Upjohn ... 2617
Hydrocortone Tablets (Hydrocortisone) Merck ... 1989

Colon, irritable
(*see under* Bowel, irritable, syndrome)

Colon, spastic
(*see under* Bowel, irritable, syndrome)

Colorectal polyps, adenomatous
Celebrex Capsules (Celecoxib) Searle ... 3134

Condylomata acuminata
Aldara Cream, 5% (Imiquimod) 3M ... 1846
Alferon N Injection (Interferon alfa-N3 (Human Leukocyte Derived)) Hemispherx ... 1665
Intron A for Injection (Interferon alfa-2b, Recombinant) Schering ... 3024
Podocon-25 Liquid (Podophyllin, Tincture of Benzoin) Paddock ... 2478

Condylomata acuminata, prevention of
Gardasil Injection (Quadrivalent Human Papillomavirus (Types 6, 11, 16, 18) Recombinant Vaccine) Merck ... 1984

Congestive heart failure, adjunct in
(*see also under* Edema, adjunctive therapy in)
BiDil Tablets (Hydralazine Hydrochloride, Isosorbide Dinitrate) Nitromed ... 2171
Captopril Tablets (Captopril) Mylan ... 2149
Coreg Tablets (Carvedilol) GlaxoSmithKline ... 1414
Demadex Tablets (Torsemide) Roche ... 2759
Diuril Oral Suspension (Chlorothiazide) Merck ... 1954
Diuril Sodium Intravenous (Chlorothiazide Sodium) Ovation ... 2467
Dyrenium Capsules (Triamterene) WellSpring ... 3400
Edecrin (Ethacrynic Acid) Merck ... 1959
Furosemide Tablets (Furosemide) Mylan ... 2154
Indapamide Tablets (Indapamide) Mylan ... 2156
Lanoxicaps Capsules (Digoxin) GlaxoSmithKline ... 1490
Lanoxin Injection (Digoxin) GlaxoSmithKline ... 1494
Lanoxin Injection Pediatric (Digoxin) GlaxoSmithKline ... 1497
Lanoxin Tablets (Digoxin) GlaxoSmithKline ... 1500
Midamor Tablets (Amiloride Hydrochloride) Merck ... 2026
Moduretic Tablets (Amiloride Hydrochloride, Hydrochlorothiazide) Merck ... 2028
Natrecor for Injection (Nesiritide) Scios Inc. ... 3127
Prinivil Tablets (Lisinopril) Merck ... 2052

Congestive heart failure, post-myocardial infarction
Altace Capsules (Ramipril) King ... 1702
Inspra Tablets (Eplerenone) Pfizer ... 2536
Mavik Tablets (Trandolapril) Abbott ... 486

Conjunctival inflammation, bulbar, steroid-responsive
Blephamide (Prednisolone Acetate, Sulfacetamide Sodium) Allergan ... 568

Conjunctival inflammation, palpebral, steroid-responsive
Blephamide (Prednisolone Acetate, Sulfacetamide Sodium) Allergan ... 568

Conjunctivitis, allergic
Alamast Ophthalmic Solution (Pemirolast Potassium) Vistakon ... 3381
Alrex Ophthalmic Suspension 0.2% (Loteprednol Etabonate) Bausch & Lomb ... ⊙ 246
Depo-Medrol Injectable Suspension (Methylprednisolone Acetate) Pharmacia & Upjohn ... 2617
Elestat Ophthalmic Solution (Epinastine Hydrochloride) Inspire ... 1669
Hydrocortone Tablets (Hydrocortisone) Merck ... 1989
Patanol Ophthalmic Solution (Olopatadine Hydrochloride) Alcon ... 561
Phenergan Tablets and Suppositories (Promethazine Hydrochloride) Wyeth ... 3440

Conjunctivitis, bacterial
Ciloxan Ophthalmic Ointment (Ciprofloxacin Hydrochloride) Alcon ... 559
Ciloxan Ophthalmic Solution (Ciprofloxacin Hydrochloride) Alcon ... ⊙ 206
Polytrim Ophthalmic Solution (Polymyxin B Sulfate, Trimethoprim Sulfate) Allergan ... 574
Quixin Ophthalmic Solution (Levofloxacin) Vistakon ... 3383
Vigamox Ophthalmic Solution (Moxifloxacin Hydrochloride) Alcon ... 564

Conjunctivitis, fungal
Natacyn Antifungal Ophthalmic Suspension (Natamycin) Alcon ... ⊙ 208

Conjunctivitis, granular
(*see under* Trachoma)

Conjunctivitis, inclusion
Gantrisin Pediatric Suspension (Acetyl Sulfisoxazole) Roche 2770

Conjunctivitis, infective
Blephamide Ophthalmic Ointment (Prednisolone Acetate, Sulfacetamide Sodium) Allergan 568
Blephamide Ophthalmic Suspension (Prednisolone Acetate, Sulfacetamide Sodium) Allergan 569
FML-S Ophthalmic Suspension (Fluorometholone, Sulfacetamide Sodium) Allergan .... ⊙229
Poly-Pred Ophthalmic Suspension (Neomycin Sulfate, Polymyxin B Sulfate, Prednisolone Acetate) Allergan .... ⊙233
Pred-G Ophthalmic Ointment (Gentamicin Sulfate, Prednisolone Acetate) Allergan .... ⊙237
Pred-G Ophthalmic Suspension (Gentamicin Sulfate, Prednisolone Acetate) Allergan .... ⊙236
TobraDex Ophthalmic Ointment (Dexamethasone, Tobramycin) Alcon 562
TobraDex Ophthalmic Suspension (Dexamethasone, Tobramycin) Alcon 563

Conjunctivitis, neonatal
Ery-Tab Tablets (Erythromycin) Abbott 449
Erythrocin Stearate Filmtab Tablets (Erythromycin Stearate) Abbott 453
Erythromycin Base Filmtab Tablets (Erythromycin) Abbott 455
Erythromycin Delayed-Release Capsules, USP (Erythromycin) Abbott 457
PCE Dispertab Tablets (Erythromycin) Abbott 515

Conjunctivitis, unspecified
Bleph-10 Ophthalmic Solution 10% (Sulfacetamide Sodium) Allergan .. ⊙222
Pred Mild Ophthalmic Suspension (Prednisolone Acetate) Allergan .... ⊙238

Constipation
Dulcolax Stool Softener (Docusate Sodium) Boehringer Ingelheim ..... ■648
Metamucil Capsules (Psyllium Preparations) Procter & Gamble .. ■652

Constipation, chronic
Kristalose for Oral Solution (Lactulose) Cumberland 1034
Metamucil Capsules (Psyllium Preparations) Procter & Gamble ... 2675
Metamucil (Psyllium Preparations) Procter & Gamble 2675

Constipation, chronic idiopathic
Amitiza Capsules (Lubiprostone) Takeda 3224
Zelnorm Tablets (Tegaserod maleate) Novartis 2312

Constipation, temporary
Citrucel Caplets (Methylcellulose) GlaxoSmithKline .... ■647
Citrucel Orange Flavor Powder (Methylcellulose) GlaxoSmithKline .... ■647
Citrucel Sugar Free Orange Flavor Powder (Methylcellulose) GlaxoSmithKline .... ■648
Dulcolax Suppositories (Bisacodyl) Boehringer Ingelheim .... ■648
Dulcolax Tablets (Bisacodyl) Boehringer Ingelheim .... ■649
Ex•Lax Chocolated Laxative Pieces (Sennosides) Novartis Consumer .... ■649
Ex•Lax Regular Strength Pills (Sennosides) Novartis Consumer . ■649
Ex•Lax Maximum Strength Pills (Sennosides) Novartis Consumer . ■649
FiberCon Caplets (Calcium Polycarbophil) Wyeth .... ■650
Fleet Bisacodyl Laxatives (Bisacodyl) Fleet 1165
Fleet Enema (Sodium Phosphate) Fleet 1165
Fleet Glycerin Laxatives (Glycerin) Fleet 1165
Fleet Glycerin Suppositories (Glycerin) Fleet 1165
Fleet Mineral Oil Enema (Mineral Oil) Fleet 1166
Fleet Phospho-soda (Sodium Phosphate) Fleet 1166

Contact lenses, fitting of, adjunct in
Fluor-I-Strip A.T. Ophthalmic Strips 1 mg (Fluorescein Sodium) Bausch & Lomb .... ⊙250

Contraception
(*see under* Pregnancy, prevention of)

Convulsive disorders, adjunctive therapy in
Valium Tablets (Diazepam) Roche 2819

Convulsive episodes, control of
Nembutal Sodium Solution, USP (Pentobarbital Sodium) Ovation 2470

Corneal erosions, recurrent
Lacrisert Sterile Ophthalmic Insert (Hydroxypropyl Cellulose) Merck.... 2005

Corneal inflammation, steroid-responsive
Blephamide Ophthalmic Ointment (Prednisolone Acetate, Sulfacetamide Sodium) Allergan 568
Blephamide Ophthalmic Suspension (Prednisolone Acetate, Sulfacetamide Sodium) Allergan 569
FML Ophthalmic Ointment (Fluorometholone) Allergan .... ⊙228
FML Ophthalmic Suspension (Fluorometholone) Allergan .... ⊙227
FML Forte Ophthalmic Suspension (Fluorometholone) Allergan .... ⊙226
FML-S Ophthalmic Suspension (Fluorometholone, Sulfacetamide Sodium) Allergan .... ⊙229
Lotemax Ophthalmic Suspension 0.5% (Loteprednol Etabonate) Bausch & Lomb .... ⊙251
Poly-Pred Ophthalmic Suspension (Neomycin Sulfate, Polymyxin B Sulfate, Prednisolone Acetate) Allergan .... ⊙233
Pred Forte Ophthalmic Suspension (Prednisolone Acetate) Allergan .... ⊙235
Pred-G Ophthalmic Ointment (Gentamicin Sulfate, Prednisolone Acetate) Allergan .... ⊙237
Pred-G Ophthalmic Suspension (Gentamicin Sulfate, Prednisolone Acetate) Allergan .... ⊙236
TobraDex Ophthalmic Ointment (Dexamethasone, Tobramycin) Alcon 562
TobraDex Ophthalmic Suspension (Dexamethasone, Tobramycin) Alcon 563

Corneal injury, chemical
Blephamide Ophthalmic Ointment (Prednisolone Acetate, Sulfacetamide Sodium) Allergan 568
Blephamide Ophthalmic Suspension (Prednisolone Acetate, Sulfacetamide Sodium) Allergan 569
FML-S Ophthalmic Suspension (Fluorometholone, Sulfacetamide Sodium) Allergan .... ⊙229
Poly-Pred Ophthalmic Suspension (Neomycin Sulfate, Polymyxin B Sulfate, Prednisolone Acetate) Allergan .... ⊙233
Pred Mild Ophthalmic Suspension (Prednisolone Acetate) Allergan .... ⊙238
Pred-G Ophthalmic Ointment (Gentamicin Sulfate, Prednisolone Acetate) Allergan .... ⊙237
Pred-G Ophthalmic Suspension (Gentamicin Sulfate, Prednisolone Acetate) Allergan .... ⊙236
TobraDex Ophthalmic Ointment (Dexamethasone, Tobramycin) Alcon 562
TobraDex Ophthalmic Suspension (Dexamethasone, Tobramycin) Alcon 563

Corneal injury, foreign bodies
Blephamide Ophthalmic Ointment (Prednisolone Acetate, Sulfacetamide Sodium) Allergan 568
Blephamide Ophthalmic Suspension (Prednisolone Acetate, Sulfacetamide Sodium) Allergan 569
FML-S Ophthalmic Suspension (Fluorometholone, Sulfacetamide Sodium) Allergan .... ⊙229
Poly-Pred Ophthalmic Suspension (Neomycin Sulfate, Polymyxin B Sulfate, Prednisolone Acetate) Allergan .... ⊙233
Pred-G Ophthalmic Ointment (Gentamicin Sulfate, Prednisolone Acetate) Allergan .... ⊙237
Pred-G Ophthalmic Suspension (Gentamicin Sulfate, Prednisolone Acetate) Allergan .... ⊙236
TobraDex Ophthalmic Ointment (Dexamethasone, Tobramycin) Alcon 562
TobraDex Ophthalmic Suspension (Dexamethasone, Tobramycin) Alcon 563

Corneal injury, radiation
Blephamide Ophthalmic Ointment (Prednisolone Acetate, Sulfacetamide Sodium) Allergan 568
Blephamide Ophthalmic Suspension (Prednisolone Acetate, Sulfacetamide Sodium) Allergan 569
FML-S Ophthalmic Suspension (Fluorometholone, Sulfacetamide Sodium) Allergan .... ⊙229
Poly-Pred Ophthalmic Suspension (Neomycin Sulfate, Polymyxin B Sulfate, Prednisolone Acetate) Allergan .... ⊙233
Pred-G Ophthalmic Ointment (Gentamicin Sulfate, Prednisolone Acetate) Allergan .... ⊙237
Pred-G Ophthalmic Suspension (Gentamicin Sulfate, Prednisolone Acetate) Allergan .... ⊙236
TobraDex Ophthalmic Ointment (Dexamethasone, Tobramycin) Alcon 562
TobraDex Ophthalmic Suspension (Dexamethasone, Tobramycin) Alcon 563

Corneal injury, thermal burns
Blephamide Ophthalmic Ointment (Prednisolone Acetate, Sulfacetamide Sodium) Allergan 568
Blephamide Ophthalmic Suspension (Prednisolone Acetate, Sulfacetamide Sodium) Allergan 569
FML-S Ophthalmic Suspension (Fluorometholone, Sulfacetamide Sodium) Allergan .... ⊙229
Poly-Pred Ophthalmic Suspension (Neomycin Sulfate, Polymyxin B Sulfate, Prednisolone Acetate) Allergan .... ⊙233
Pred Mild Ophthalmic Suspension (Prednisolone Acetate) Allergan .... ⊙238
Pred-G Ophthalmic Ointment (Gentamicin Sulfate, Prednisolone Acetate) Allergan .... ⊙237
Pred-G Ophthalmic Suspension (Gentamicin Sulfate, Prednisolone Acetate) Allergan .... ⊙236
TobraDex Ophthalmic Ointment (Dexamethasone, Tobramycin) Alcon 562
TobraDex Ophthalmic Suspension (Dexamethasone, Tobramycin) Alcon 563

Corneal marginal ulcers, allergic
Depo-Medrol Injectable Suspension (Methylprednisolone Acetate) Pharmacia & Upjohn 2617
Hydrocortone Tablets (Hydrocortisone) Merck 1989

Corneal sensitivity, decreased
Lacrisert Sterile Ophthalmic Insert (Hydroxypropyl Cellulose) Merck ... 2005

Corneal ulcers
Bleph-10 Ophthalmic Solution 10% (Sulfacetamide Sodium) Allergan .. ⊙222
Ciloxan Ophthalmic Ointment (Ciprofloxacin Hydrochloride) Alcon 559
Ciloxan Ophthalmic Solution (Ciprofloxacin Hydrochloride) Alcon .... ⊙206

Coronary artery disease, angiographically documented
Caduet Tablets (Amlodipine Besylate, Atorvastatin Calcium) Pfizer... 2508
Norvasc Tablets (Amlodipine Besylate) Pfizer 2545

Coronary artery disease, reducing the risk of
Aceon Tablets (2 mg, 4 mg, 8 mg) (Perindopril Erbumine) Solvay.......... 3194
Altoprev Extended-Release Tablets (Lovastatin) Sciele 3109
Caduet Tablets (Amlodipine Besylate, Atorvastatin Calcium) Pfizer... 2508
Metamucil Dietary Fiber Supplement (Psyllium Preparations) Procter & Gamble .... ■650
Mevacor Tablets (Lovastatin) Merck . 2021
Norvasc Tablets (Amlodipine Besylate) Pfizer 2545
Zocor Tablets (Simvastatin) Merck ...2105

Coronary atherosclerosis, to slow the progression of
(*see also under* Coronary artery disease, reducing the risk of)
Altoprev Extended-Release Tablets (Lovastatin) Sciele 3109
Lescol Capsules (Fluvastatin Sodium) Novartis 2233
Lescol XL Tablets (Fluvastatin Sodium) Novartis 2233
Mevacor Tablets (Lovastatin) Merck .2021
Niaspan Extended-Release Tablets (Niacin) Kos 1730

Coronary syndrome, acute
(*see also under* Cardiac ischemic complications, acute, prevention of, adjunct to PTCA)
Aggrastat (Tirofiban Hydrochloride) Merck 1907
Integrilin Injection (Eptifibatide) Schering 3020
Lovenox Injection (Enoxaparin Sodium) sanofi-aventis 2915
Plavix Tablets (Clopidogrel Bisulfate) Bristol-Myers Squibb 917
Plavix Tablets (Clopidogrel Bisulfate) sanofi-aventis 2926

Corynebacterium diphtheriae
(*see under* C. diphtheriae infections)

Corynebacterium diphtheriae, immunization against
(*see also under* Immunization, diphtheria, tetanus and pertussis)
ADACEL Vaccine (Diphtheria & Tetanus Toxoids and Acellular Pertussis Vaccine Adsorbed) Sanofi Pasteur 2945
Boostrix (Diphtheria & Tetanus Toxoids and Acellular Pertussis Vaccine Adsorbed) GlaxoSmithKline 1404
DAPTACEL Vaccine (Diphtheria & Tetanus Toxoids and Acellular Pertussis Vaccine Adsorbed) Sanofi Pasteur 2950
Infanrix Vaccine (Diphtheria & Tetanus Toxoids and Acellular Pertussis Vaccine Adsorbed) GlaxoSmithKline 1476
Pediarix Vaccine (Diphtheria & Tetanus Toxoids and Pertussis Vaccine Adsorbed, Hepatitis B Vaccine, Recombinant, Poliovirus Vaccine Inactivated, Trivalent Types 1,2,3) GlaxoSmithKline 1548

Corynebacterium infections, ocular
Vigamox Ophthalmic Solution (Moxifloxacin Hydrochloride) Alcon 564

Corynebacterium infections, unspecified
Vigamox Ophthalmic Solution (Moxifloxacin Hydrochloride) Alcon .... ⊙215

Corynebacterium minutissimum
(*see under* C. minutissimum infections)

Corynebacterium vaginitis

Coryza, acute

(*see under* Cold, common, symptomatic relief of)

Cough, symptomatic relief of

Concentrated Tylenol Infants' Drops Plus Cold and Cough (Acetaminophen, Dextromethorphan Hydrobromide) McNeil Consumer 1879
Vicks 44 Cough Relief Liquid (Dextromethorphan Hydrobromide) Procter & Gamble 2679
Vicks 44D Cough & Head Congestion Relief Liquid (Dextromethorphan Hydrobromide, Pseudoephedrine Hydrochloride) Procter & Gamble 2679
Vicks 44E Cough & Chest Congestion Relief Liquid (Dextromethorphan Hydrobromide, Guaifenesin) Procter & Gamble 2679
Pediatric Vicks 44e Cough & Chest Congestion Relief Liquid (Dextromethorphan Hydrobromide, Guaifenesin) Procter & Gamble 2676
Vicks 44D Cough & Head Congestion Relief Liquid (Dextromethorphan Hydrobromide, Phenylephrine Hydrochloride) Procter & Gamble ▣ 760
Pediatric Vicks 44m Cough & Cold Relief Liquid (Chlorpheniramine Maleate, Dextromethorphan Hydrobromide) Procter & Gamble 2676
Vicks 44M Cough, Cold & Flu Relief Liquid (Acetaminophen, Chlorpheniramine Maleate, Dextromethorphan Hydrobromide) Procter & Gamble ▣ 760
Vicks DayQuil LiquiCaps/Liquid Multi-Symptom Cold/Flu Relief (Acetaminophen, Dextromethorphan Hydrobromide, Phenylephrine Hydrochloride) Procter & Gamble ▣ 761
Vicks Cough Drops, Menthol & Cherry Flavors (Menthol) Procter & Gamble 2678
Vicks DayQuil Multi-Symptom Cold/Flu Relief LiquiCaps (Acetaminophen, Dextromethorphan Hydrobromide, Pseudoephedrine Hydrochloride) Procter & Gamble 2678
Vicks DayQuil Multi-Symptom Cold/Flu Relief Liquid (Acetaminophen, Dextromethorphan Hydrobromide, Pseudoephedrine Hydrochloride) Procter & Gamble 2678
Vicks NyQuil Multi-Symptom Cold/Flu Relief Liquid (Acetaminophen, Dextromethorphan Hydrobromide, Doxylamine Succinate, Pseudoephedrine Hydrochloride) Procter & Gamble 2681
Vicks NyQuil Multi-Symptom Cold/Flu Relief LiquiCaps (Acetaminophen, Dextromethorphan Hydrobromide, Doxylamine Succinate, Pseudoephedrine Hydrochloride) Procter & Gamble 2681
Vicks NyQuil LiquiCaps/Liquid Multi-Symptom Cold/Flu Relief (Acetaminophen, Dextromethorphan Hydrobromide, Doxylamine Succinate) Procter & Gamble ▣ 763
Vicks NyQuil Cough Liquid (Dextromethorphan Hydrobromide, Doxylamine Succinate) Procter & Gamble 2680
Children's Vicks NyQuil Cold/Cough Relief Liquid (Chlorpheniramine Maleate, Dextromethorphan Hydrobromide, Pseudoephedrine Hydrochloride) Procter & Gamble 2680
Vicks VapoRub Cream (Camphor, Menthol) Procter & Gamble 2682
Vicks VapoRub Ointment (Camphor, Eucalyptus, Oil of, Menthol) Procter & Gamble 2682
Vicks VapoSteam (Camphor) Procter & Gamble 2682
Zicam Cold Remedy Chewables (Zincum Aceticum, Zincum Gluconicum) Matrixx ▣ 766
Zicam Cold Remedy ChewCaps (Zincum Aceticum, Zincum Gluconicum) Matrixx ▣ 766
Zicam Cold Remedy Gel Swabs (Zincum Gluconicum) Matrixx ▣ 766
Zicam Cold Remedy Nasal Gel (Zincum Gluconicum) Matrixx ▣ 766
Zicam Cold Remedy Oral Mist (Zincum Aceticum, Zincum Gluconicum) Matrixx ▣ 766
Zicam Cold Remedy RapidMelts (Zincum Aceticum, Zincum Gluconicum) Matrixx ▣ 766
Zicam Cold Remedy RapidMelts with Vitamin C (Zincum Aceticum, Zincum Gluconicum) Matrixx ▣ 766
Zicam Cold Remedy Swabs Kids Size (Zincum Gluconicum) Matrixx ▣ 766
Zicam Cough Max Nighttime Cough Spray (Dextromethorphan Hydrobromide) Matrixx ▣ 767
Zicam Cough Max Cough Spray (Dextromethorphan Hydrobromide) Matrixx ▣ 767
Zicam Cough Max Cough Melts (Dextromethorphan Hydrobromide) Matrixx ▣ 767
Zicam Cough Plus D Cough Spray (Dextromethorphan Hydrobromide, Phenylephrine Hydrochloride) Matrixx ▣ 767
Zicam Cough Relief Cough Spray (Dextromethorphan Hydrobromide) Matrixx ▣ 767
Zicam Maximum Strength Flu Daytime (Acetaminophen, Chlorpheniramine Maleate, Dextromethorphan Hydrobromide) Matrixx ▣ 768
Zicam Maximum Strength Flu Nighttime (Acetaminophen, Dextromethorphan Hydrobromide, Doxylamine Succinate) Matrixx ▣ 768

Cough, whooping
(*see under* Pertussis)

Cradle cap
(*see under* Dermatitis, seborrheic)

Creeping eruptions
(*see under* Larva migrans, cutaneous)

Cretinism
(*see under* Hypothyroidism, replacement or supplemental therapy in)

Crohn's disease
Entocort EC Capsules (Budesonide) Prometheus 2698
Remicade for IV Injection (Infliximab) Centocor 971

Cryptococcosis
Abelcet Injection (Amphotericin B Lipid Complex) Enzon 1141
AmBisome for Injection (Amphotericin B, liposomal) Astellas 620

Cushing's syndrome, diagnosis of
(*see under* Adrenocortical hyperfunction, diagnostic testing of)

Cuts, minor, infection from
(*see under* Infections, skin, bacterial, minor)

Cuts, minor, pain associated with
(*see under* Pain, topical relief of)

Cystic fibrosis, adjunctive therapy in
Pulmozyme Inhalation Solution (Dornase Alfa) Genentech 1248
TOBI Solution for Inhalation (Tobramycin) Novartis 2298

Cystic tumors
Depo-Medrol Single-Dose Vial (Methylprednisolone Acetate) Pharmacia & Upjohn 2619

Cystinuria
Cuprimine Capsules (Penicillamine) Merck 1947

Cystitis
Cipro (Ciprofloxacin) Schering 2977
Cipro XR Tablets (Ciprofloxacin) Schering 2990
Gantrisin Pediatric Suspension (Acetyl Sulfisoxazole) Roche 2770
Noroxin Tablets (Norfloxacin) Merck 2032
Proquin XR Tablets (Ciprofloxacin Hydrochloride) Esprit 1153
Prosed/DS Tablets (Benzoic Acid, Hyoscyamine Sulfate, Methenamine, Methylene Blue, Phenyl Salicylate) Esprit 1157
Raniclor Tablets, Chewable (Cefaclor Monohydrate) Pedinol 2505
Tequin Injection (Gatifloxacin) Bristol-Myers Squibb 938
Tequin Injection in 5% Dextrose (Gatifloxacin) Bristol-Myers Squibb 938
Tequin Tablets (Gatifloxacin) Bristol-Myers Squibb 938
Uroqid-Acid No. 2 Tablets (Methenamine Mandelate, Sodium Acid Phosphate) Beach 760
Vantin Tablets and Oral Suspension (Cefpodoxime Proxetil) Pharmacia & Upjohn 2645

Cystitis, interstitial, symptomatic relief of
Elmiron Capsules (Pentosan Polysulfate Sodium) Ortho Women's Health & Urology 2415

Cytomegalovirus disease associated with renal transplantation, prophylaxis of
CytoGam Intravenous (Cytomegalovirus Immune Globulin) MedImmune 1895

D

Dandruff
(*see also under* Dermatitis, seborrheic)
Nizoral A-D Shampoo, 1% (Ketoconazole) McNeil Consumer 1868

Dementia, Alzheimer's type
Aricept Tablets (Donepezil Hydrochloride) Eisai 1094
Aricept ODT Tablets (Donepezil Hydrochloride) Eisai 1094
Exelon Capsules (Rivastigmine Tartrate) Novartis 2206
Exelon Oral Solution (Rivastigmine Tartrate) Novartis 2206
Namenda (Memantine Hydrochloride) Forest 1195
Razadyne (Galantamine Hydrobromide) Ortho-McNeil Neurologics 2399
Razadyne ER Extended-Release Capsules (Galantamine Hydrobromide) Ortho-McNeil Neurologics 2399

Dementia, Parkinson's disease, associated with
Exelon Capsules (Rivastigmine Tartrate) Novartis 2206
Exelon Oral Solution (Rivastigmine Tartrate) Novartis 2206

Depression, bipolar
(*see under* Depression, manic-depressive)

Depression, major, without melancholia
Parnate Tablets (Tranylcypromine Sulfate) GlaxoSmithKline 1527

Depression, manic-depressive
(*see also under* Mania, bipolar)
Symbyax Capsules (Fluoxetine Hydrochloride, Olanzapine) Lilly 1819

Depression, treatment of
Celexa (Citalopram Hydrobromide) Forest 1176
Cymbalta Delayed-Release Capsules (Duloxetine Hydrochloride) Lilly 1757
Effexor Tablets (Venlafaxine Hydrochloride) Wyeth 3411
Effexor XR Capsules (Venlafaxine Hydrochloride) Wyeth 3417
Emsam Transdermal System (Selegiline) Bristol-Myers Squibb 903
Lexapro Oral Solution (Escitalopram Oxalate) Forest 1190
Lexapro Tablets (Escitalopram Oxalate) Forest 1190
Paxil CR Controlled-Release Tablets (Paroxetine Hydrochloride) GlaxoSmithKline 1538
Paxil (Paroxetine Hydrochloride) GlaxoSmithKline 1530
Pexeva Tablets (Paroxetine Mesylate) JDS 1694
Prozac Pulvules and Liquid (Fluoxetine Hydrochloride) Lilly 1801
Wellbutrin Tablets (Bupropion Hydrochloride) GlaxoSmithKline 1603
Wellbutrin SR Sustained-Release Tablets (Bupropion Hydrochloride) GlaxoSmithKline 1607
Wellbutrin XL Extended-Release Tablets (Bupropion Hydrochloride) GlaxoSmithKline 1613
Zoloft (Sertraline Hydrochloride) Pfizer 2586

Dermatitis, allergic
MimyX Cream (Glycerin) Stiefel 3213

Dermatitis, atopic
Cutivate Lotion 0.05% (Fluticasone Propionate) Pharmaderm 2664
Decadron Tablets (Dexamethasone) Merck 1951
Depo-Medrol Injectable Suspension (Methylprednisolone Acetate) Pharmacia & Upjohn 2617
Depo-Medrol Single-Dose Vial (Methylprednisolone Acetate) Pharmacia & Upjohn 2619
Elidel Cream 1% (Pimecrolimus) Novartis 2200
Hydrocortone Tablets (Hydrocortisone) Merck 1989
MimyX Cream (Glycerin) Stiefel 3213
Protopic Ointment (Tacrolimus) Astellas 638

Dermatitis, contact
(*see also under* Dermatoses, corticosteroid-responsive)
Decadron Tablets (Dexamethasone) Merck 1951
Depo-Medrol Injectable Suspension (Methylprednisolone Acetate) Pharmacia & Upjohn 2617
Depo-Medrol Single-Dose Vial (Methylprednisolone Acetate) Pharmacia & Upjohn 2619
Hydrocortone Tablets (Hydrocortisone) Merck 1989

Dermatitis, corticosteroid-responsive, anal region
Analpram-HC (Hydrocortisone Acetate, Pramoxine Hydrochloride) Ferndale 1159

Dermatitis, exfoliative
Depo-Medrol Injectable Suspension (Methylprednisolone Acetate) Pharmacia & Upjohn 2617
Depo-Medrol Single-Dose Vial (Methylprednisolone Acetate) Pharmacia & Upjohn 2619
Hydrocortone Tablets (Hydrocortisone) Merck 1989

Dermatitis, herpetiformis
Dapsone Tablets USP (Dapsone) Jacobus 1673

Dermatitis, herpetiformis bullous
Decadron Tablets (Dexamethasone) Merck 1951
Depo-Medrol Injectable Suspension (Methylprednisolone Acetate) Pharmacia & Upjohn 2617
Depo-Medrol Single-Dose Vial (Methylprednisolone Acetate) Pharmacia & Upjohn 2619
Hydrocortone Tablets (Hydrocortisone) Merck 1989

Dermatitis, radiation
MimyX Cream (Glycerin) Stiefel 3213

Dermatitis, seborrheic
Avar Cleanser (Sodium Sulfacetamide, Sulfur) Dusa 1085
Avar Gel (Sodium Sulfacetamide, Sulfur) Dusa 1085
Avar Green Gel (Sodium Sulfacetamide, Sulfur) Dusa 1085
Avar-e Emollient Cream (Sodium Sulfacetamide, Sulfur) Dusa 1085
Avar-e Green Cream (Sodium Sulfacetamide, Sulfur) Dusa 1085
Head & Shoulders Intensive Solutions (Pyrithione Zinc) Procter & Gamble ▣ 638
Head & Shoulders Intensive Solutions Dandruff Shampoo (Pyrithione Zinc) Procter & Gamble 2674

Loprox Shampoo (Ciclopirox) Medicis 1888
Plexion (Sodium Sulfacetamide, Sulfur) Medicis 1889
Rosac Cream with Sunscreens (Sodium Sulfacetamide, Sulfur) Stiefel 3213

Dermatitis, seborrheic, severe
Depo-Medrol Injectable Suspension (Methylprednisolone Acetate) Pharmacia & Upjohn 2617
Depo-Medrol Single-Dose Vial (Methylprednisolone Acetate) Pharmacia & Upjohn 2619
Hydrocortone Tablets (Hydrocortisone) Merck 1989

Dermatomycosis, systemic
Decadron Tablets (Dexamethasone) Merck 1951

Dermatomyositis, possibly effective in
Potaba (Aminobenzoate Potassium) Glenwood 1650

Dermatomyositis, systemic
Depo-Medrol Injectable Suspension (Methylprednisolone Acetate) Pharmacia & Upjohn 2617
Depo-Medrol Single-Dose Vial (Methylprednisolone Acetate) Pharmacia & Upjohn 2619
Hydrocortone Tablets (Hydrocortisone) Merck 1989

Dermatoses, corticosteroid-responsive
(*see also under* Skin, inflammatory conditions)
Aclovate (Alclometasone Dipropionate) Pharmaderm 2660
Apexicon E Cream (Diflorasone Diacetate) Pharmaderm 2661
Clobevate Gel (Clobetasol Propionate) Stiefel 3211
Clobex Lotion (Clobetasol Propionate) Galderma 1204
Cutivate Cream (Fluticasone Propionate) Pharmaderm 2662
Cutivate Ointment (Fluticasone Propionate) Pharmaderm 2665
Diprolene Ointment 0.05% (Betamethasone Dipropionate) Schering 3003
Diprolene AF Cream 0.05% (Betamethasone Dipropionate) Schering 3000
Diprosone Cream, USP 0.05% (Betamethasone Dipropionate) Schering 3004
Elocon Cream 0.1% (Mometasone Furoate) Schering 3005
Elocon Lotion 0.1% (Mometasone Furoate) Schering 3006
Elocon Ointment 0.1% (Mometasone Furoate) Schering 3007
Locoid Lipocream Cream (Hydrocortisone Butyrate) Ferndale 1160
Luxíq Foam (Betamethasone Valerate) Connetics 1010
Olux Foam (Clobetasol Propionate) Connetics 1012
Pramosone (Hydrocortisone Acetate, Pramoxine Hydrochloride) Ferndale 1161
ProctoFoam-HC (Hydrocortisone Acetate, Pramoxine Hydrochloride) Schwarz 3099
Temovate Cream (Clobetasol Propionate) Pharmaderm 2668
Temovate Gel (Clobetasol Propionate) Pharmaderm 2669
Temovate Ointment (Clobetasol Propionate) Pharmaderm 2668
Temovate Scalp Application (Clobetasol Propionate) Pharmaderm 2670
Temovate E Emollient (Clobetasol Propionate) Pharmaderm 2671

Dermographism
Phenergan Tablets and Suppositories (Promethazine Hydrochloride) Wyeth 3440

Detrusor overactivity
Ditropan XL Extended-Release Tablets (Oxybutynin Chloride) Ortho Women's Health & Urology 2413

Diabetes mellitus
(*see under* Hyperglycemia, control of, adjunct to diet)

Diabetes mellitus, insulin-dependent
Exubera Inhalation Powder (Insulin, Human (rDNA origin)) Pfizer 2524
Humalog-Pen (Insulin Lispro, Human) Lilly 1781
Humalog Mix 50/50-Pen (Insulin Lispro, Human, Insulin Lispro Protamine, Human) Lilly 1783
Humalog Mix 75/25-Pen (Insulin Lispro, Human, Insulin Lispro Protamine, Human) Lilly 1785
Humulin 50/50, 100 Units (Insulin, Human Regular and Human NPH Mixture) Lilly 1791
Humulin 70/30 Pen (Insulin, Human Regular and Human NPH Mixture) Lilly 1793
Humulin L, 100 Units (Insulin, Human, Zinc Suspension) Lilly 1794
Humulin N, 100 Units (Insulin, Human NPH) Lilly 1795
Humulin N Pen (Insulin, Human NPH) Lilly 1797
Humulin R, 100 Units (Insulin, Human Regular) Lilly 1798
Humulin U, 100 Units (Insulin, Human, Zinc Suspension) Lilly 1800
Lantus Injection (Insulin glargine) sanofi-aventis 2909
NovoLog Injection (Insulin Aspart, Human Regular) Novo Nordisk 2326
NovoLog Mix 70/30 (Insulin Aspart, Human, Insulin Aspart Protamine, Human) Novo Nordisk 2328
Symlin Injection (Pramlintide Acetate) Amylin 613

Diabetes mellitus, non-insulin-dependent
ActoPlus Met Tablets (Metformin Hydrochloride, Pioglitazone Hydrochloride) Takeda 3214
Actos Tablets (Pioglitazone Hydrochloride) Takeda 3219
Avandamet Tablets (Rosiglitazone Maleate, Metformin Hydrochloride) GlaxoSmithKline 1373
Avandaryl Tablets (Rosiglitazone Maleate, Glimepiride) GlaxoSmithKline 1379
Avandia Tablets (Rosiglitazone Maleate) GlaxoSmithKline 1384
Byetta Injection (Exenatide) Amylin 611
Lantus Injection (Insulin glargine) sanofi-aventis 2909
Precose Tablets (Acarbose) Bayer 751
Starlix Tablets (Nateglinide) Novartis 2292

Diabetes mellitus, type 1
Exubera Inhalation Powder (Insulin, Human (rDNA origin)) Pfizer 2524
Lantus Injection (Insulin glargine) sanofi-aventis 2909
Levemir Injection (Insulin Detemir (rDNA Origin)) Novo Nordisk 2320

Diabetes mellitus, type 2
Duetact Tablets (Glimepiride, Pioglitazone Hydrochloride) Takeda 3226
Exubera Inhalation Powder (Insulin, Human (rDNA origin)) Pfizer 2524
Fortamet Extended-Release Tablets (Metformin Hydrochloride) Sciele 3115
Lantus Injection (Insulin glargine) sanofi-aventis 2909
Levemir Injection (Insulin Detemir (rDNA Origin)) Novo Nordisk 2320

Diabetic nephropathy
(*see under* Nephropathy, diabetic)

Diarrhea
Maalox Maximum Strength Total Stomach Relief Strawberry Liquid (Bismuth Subsalicylate) Novartis Consumer .... ■ 672

Diarrhea, adjunctive therapy in
Imodium Advanced Caplets and Chewable Tablets (Loperamide Hydrochloride, Simethicone) McNeil Consumer 1866

Diarrhea, bacterial
(*see under* Diarrhea, infectious)

Diarrhea, cryptosporidium parvum-induced
Alinia for Oral Suspension (Nitazoxanide) Romark 2835
Alinia Tablets (Nitazoxanide) Romark 2835

Diarrhea, E. coli-induced
Cipro (Ciprofloxacin) Schering 2977

Diarrhea, giardia lamblia-induced
Alinia for Oral Suspension (Nitazoxanide) Romark 2835
Alinia Tablets (Nitazoxanide) Romark 2835

Diarrhea, infectious
Alinia for Oral Suspension (Nitazoxanide) Romark 2835
Alinia Tablets (Nitazoxanide) Romark 2835
Cipro (Ciprofloxacin) Schering 2977

Diarrhea, protozoal
(*see under* Diarrhea, infectious)

Diarrhea, symptomatic relief of
Imodium A-D Liquid and Caplets (Loperamide Hydrochloride) McNeil Consumer 1865
Imodium Advanced Caplets and Chewable Tablets (Loperamide Hydrochloride, Simethicone) McNeil Consumer 1866
Pepto-Bismol Original Liquid, Maximum Strength Liquid, Original and Cherry Tablets, Chewable Tablets and Easy-To-Swallow Caplets (Bismuth Subsalicylate) Procter & Gamble 2676
Pepto-Bismol Maximum Strength Liquid (Bismuth Subsalicylate) Procter & Gamble .... ■ 672

Diarrhea, traveler's
Xifaxan Tablets (Rifaximin) Salix 2842

Diarrhea associated with vasoactive intestinal peptide tumors
Sandostatin Injection (Octreotide Acetate) Novartis 2278
Sandostatin LAR Depot (Octreotide Acetate) Novartis 2280

Diet, supplementation of
Active Calcium Tablets (Calcium Citrate, Vitamin D) Usana 3339
Ambrotose AO Capsules (Herbals with Vitamins) Mannatech .... ■ 826
Ambrotose Capsules (Herbals, Multiple) Mannatech .... ■ 826
Ambrotose Powder (Glucosamine Hydrochloride, Herbals, Multiple) Mannatech .... ■ 826
Ambrotose with Lecithin Capsules (Lecithin, Herbals, Multiple) Mannatech .... ■ 826
Animi-3 Capsules (Docosahexaenoic Acid (DHA), EPA (Eicosapentaenoic Acid), Folic Acid, Vitamin B_6, Vitamin B_{12}) PBM 2492
Authia Cream (Thiamine Disulfide, Vitamin B_{12}) Westlake 3404
Awareness Clear Capsules (Herbals, Multiple) Awareness Corporation/AwarenessLife .... ■ 827
Bausch & Lomb PreserVision AREDS Tablets (Vitamins with Minerals) Bausch & Lomb .... ⊙ 254
Bausch & Lomb Ocuvite Adult Eye Vitamin and Mineral Supplement Soft Gels (Lutein, Copper, Omega-3 Acids, Vitamin C, Vitamin E, Zinc Oxide) Bausch & Lomb .... ■ 706
Bausch & Lomb Ocuvite Adult 50+ Eye Vitamin and Mineral Supplement Soft Gels (Lutein, Copper, Omega-3 Acids, Vitamin C, Vitamin E, Zinc Oxide) Bausch & Lomb .... ■ 706
Bausch & Lomb PreserVision Eye Vitamin and Mineral Supplement Original Tablets Bausch & Lomb .... ■ 806
Beelith Tablets (Magnesium Oxide, Vitamin B_6) Beach 759
Benefiber Fiber Supplement Caplets (Fiber, dietary) Novartis Consumer .... ■ 808
Benefiber Fiber Supplement Powder (Fiber, dietary) Novartis Consumer .... ■ 807
Benefiber Fiber Supplement Chewable Tablets (Fiber, dietary) Novartis Consumer .... ■ 808
Bevitamel Tablets (Folic Acid, Melatonin, Vitamin B_{12}) Westlake 3404
BioLean Accelerator Tablets (Amino Acid Preparations, Herbals, Multiple) Wellness International .... ■ 631
BioLean Free Tablets (Amino Acid Preparations, Ginkgo biloba, Herbals with Vitamins & Minerals, Ginseng) Wellness International .... ■ 631
BioLean II Tablets (Amino Acid Preparations, Herbals, Multiple) Wellness International .... ■ 808
BioLean LipoTrim Capsules (Herbals with Minerals) Wellness International .... ■ 631
BioLean ProXtreme Dietary Supplement (Amino Acid Preparations, Protein Preparations, Vitamins with Minerals) Wellness International .... ■ 808
Bios Life Drink Mix (Fiber, Vitamins with Minerals) Unicity 3328
Calcet Tablets (Calcium Carbonate, Calcium Gluconate, Calcium Lactate, Cholecalciferol) Mission 2138
Caltrate 600 PLUS (Calcium Carbonate, Minerals, Multiple, Vitamin D) Wyeth .... ■ 809
Caltrate 600 + D Tablets (Calcium Carbonate, Vitamin D) Wyeth .... ■ 809
Cardio Essentials Capsules (Coenzyme Q-10) Unicity 3328
Centrum Tablets (Vitamins with Minerals) Wyeth .... ■ 809
Centrum Kids Complete Children's Chewables (Vitamins with Minerals) Wyeth .... ■ 810
Centrum Performance Multivitamin/Multimineral Supplement (Ginkgo biloba, Herbals with Vitamins & Minerals, Ginseng, Vitamins with Minerals) Wyeth .... ■ 811
Centrum Silver Tablets (Vitamins with Minerals) Wyeth .... ■ 811
Chelated Mineral Tablets (Minerals, Multiple) Usana 3339
Citracal Caplets (Calcium Citrate) Mission .... ■ 703
Citracal Lemon Cream Creamy Bites (Calcium Citrate) Mission 2139
Citracal Prenatal + DHA Tablets and Capsules (Calcium Citrate, Docosahexaenoic Acid (DHA), Multivitamins with Minerals) Mission 2139
COLD-fX Capsules (Dietary Supplement) Cold-FX 1000
CoQuinone Capsules (Coenzyme Q-10, Lipoic Acid) Usana 3339
CordyMax Cs-4 Capsules (Herbals, Multiple) Pharmanex 2672
Daily Complete Liquid (Aloe vera, Amino Acid Preparations, Herbals with Vitamins & Minerals, Antioxidants) Awareness Corporation/AwarenessLife .... ■ 827
DHEA Plus Capsules (Dihydroepiandrosterone (DHEA), Ginkgo biloba) Wellness International .... ■ 827
Experience Capsules (Psyllium Preparations, Herbals, Multiple) Awareness Corporation/AwarenessLife .... ■ 828
Flintstones Complete with Choline Tablets (Vitamins with Minerals) Bayer Healthcare .... ■ 813
Flintstones Gummies (Vitamins, Multiple) Bayer Healthcare .... ■ 813
Folgard RX Tablets (Folic Acid, Vitamin B_6, Vitamin B_{12}) Upsher-Smith 3337
Food for Thought Dietary Supplement (Amino Acid Preparations, Vitamins with Minerals) Wellness International .... ■ 814
Hyland's Complete Flu Care Tablets (Herbals, Multiple) Standard Homeopathic .... ■ 828
Hyland's Earache Drops (Herbals, Multiple) Standard Homeopathic .... ■ 828

immune^{26} BALANCE Powder Shake Mix (Egg product, hyperimmune) Legacy for Life ■ 815
immune^{26} COMPLETE Support Powder Shake Mix (Egg product, hyperimmune) Legacy for Life ■ 815
immune^{26} Powder, Capsules and Chewable Tablets (Egg product, hyperimmune) Legacy for Life ■ 815
immune^{26} Power Chews Children's Chewable Tablets (Egg product, hyperimmune) Legacy for Life ■ 815
Immunocal Powder Sachets (Whey Protein Isolate) Immunotec 1668
Intelectol Tablets (Vinpocetine) Memory Secret ■ 830
Lifepak Capsules (Vitamins with Minerals) Pharmanex 2672
L-Tryptophan Capsules (L-Tryptophan) Montiff 2145
MarineOmega Softgel Capsules (Fatty Acids, Vitamin E) Pharmanex 2672
Mass Appeal Tablets (Amino Acid Preparations, Minerals) Wellness International ■ 830
MDR Vital Factors (Vitamins with Minerals) MDR 1886
Mega Antioxidant Tablets (Vitamins, Multiple) Usana 3339
Metamucil Dietary Fiber Supplement (Psyllium Preparations) Procter & Gamble ■ 650
My First Flintstones Multivitamin Tablets (Vitamins, Multiple) Bayer Healthcare ■ 814
Natural Joint Capsules (Dietary Supplement) Greek Island Labs ■ 831
Ocuvite Adult Vitamin and Mineral Supplement (Lutein, Copper, Omega-3 Acids, Vitamin C, Vitamin E, Vitamins with Minerals, Zinc Oxide) Bausch & Lomb ⊙ 253
Ocuvite Adult 50+ Vitamin and Mineral Supplement (Lutein, Copper, Omega-3 Acids, Vitamin C, Vitamin E, Vitamins with Minerals, Zinc Oxide) Bausch & Lomb ⊙ 253
Ocuvite Lutein Vitamin and Mineral Supplement Bausch & Lomb ■ 707
One-A-Day Cholesterol Plus Tablets (Multivitamins with Minerals) Bayer Healthcare ■ 815
One-A-Day Men's Health Formula Tablets (Fish Oils, Multivitamins with Minerals, Soy-containing dietary supplements) Bayer Healthcare ■ 815
One-A-Day Weight Smart Tablets (Herbals with Vitamins & Minerals, Green Tea Extract, Vitamins with Minerals) Bayer Healthcare ■ 816
One-A-Day Women's Tablets (Vitamins with Minerals) Bayer Healthcare ■ 816
Peridin-C Vitamin C Supplement (Bioflavonoids, Hesperidin Complex, Hesperidin Methyl Chalcone, Vitamin C) Beutlich ■ 818
Phyto-Vite Tablets (Bioflavonoids, Ginkgo biloba, Herbals with Vitamins & Minerals, Antioxidants) Wellness International ■ 831
PLUS with Ambrotose Complex Caplets (Amino Acid Preparations) Mannatech ■ 831
PremCal Light, Regular, and Extra Strength Tablets (Calcium Carbonate, Magnesium Oxide, Vitamin D_3) Danmarie ■ 818
Procosa II Tablets (Glucosamine Sulfate) Usana 3339
Proflavanol 90 Tablets (Dietary Supplement) Usana 3339
PureTrim Mediterranean Wellness Shake (Fatty Acids, Rice Protein, Antioxidants) Awareness Corporation/AwarenessLife ■ 818
Reishimax Capsules (Ganoderma lucinum mushroom extract) Pharmanex 2672
Satiete Tablets (Amino Acid Preparations, Ginkgo biloba, Herbals with Vitamins & Minerals, Hypericum) Wellness International ■ 832
Sen-Sei-Ro Liquid (Dietary Supplement) Kyowa 1740
Sen-Sei-Ro Powder Gold (Dietary Supplement) Kyowa 1741
Sleep-Tite Caplets (Valeriana officinalis, Herbals, Multiple, Kava-Kava) Wellness International ■ 832
SON Formula Tablets (Amino Acid Preparations) International Nutrition Research 1673
StePHan Clarity Capsules (Amino Acid Preparations, Ginkgo biloba, Herbals with Vitamins) Wellness International ■ 819
StePHan Elasticity Capsules (Amino Acid Preparations, Herbals with Vitamins & Minerals) Wellness International ■ 819
StePHan Elixir Capsules (Amino Acid Preparations, Ginkgo biloba, Herbals with Vitamins & Minerals) Wellness International ■ 814
StePHan Essential Capsules (Amino Acid Preparations, Herbals with Vitamins & Minerals, Vitamins with Minerals) Wellness International ■ 820
StePHan Feminine Capsules (Amino Acid Preparations, Vitamins with Minerals) Wellness International ■ 833
StePHan Flexibility Capsules (Amino Acid Preparations, Vitamins with Minerals) Wellness International ■ 820
StePHan Lovpil Capsules (Amino Acid Preparations, Herbals with Vitamins & Minerals) Wellness International ■ 820
StePHan Masculine Capsules (Amino Acid Preparations, Herbals with Minerals) Wellness International ■ 821
StePHan Protector Capsules (Amino Acid Preparations, Astragalus, Herbals, Multiple) Wellness International ■ 821
StePHan Relief Capsules (Amino Acid Preparations, Psyllium Preparations, Herbals with Vitamins) Wellness International ■ 821
StePHan Tranquility Capsules (Amino Acid Preparations, Valeriana officinalis, Herbals with Vitamins & Minerals) Wellness International ■ 821
Sure2Endure Tablets (Herbals with Vitamins & Minerals, Glucosamine Hydrochloride) Wellness International ■ 821
SynergyDefense Capsules (Herbals, Multiple) Awareness Corporation/AwarenessLife ■ 833
Tahitian Noni Liquid (Dietary Supplement) Tahitian Noni International ■ 834
Tēgreen 97 Capsules (Camellia sinensis) Pharmanex 2672
4Life Transfer Factor Plus Advanced Formula (Amino Acid Preparations) 4Life ■ 835
Vemma Nutrition Program - Essential Minerals (Minerals, Multiple) Vemma ■ 835
Vemma Nutrition Program - Mangosteen Plus (Aloe vera, Phytonutrients, Folic Acid, Herbals with Vitamins, Vitamins, Multiple) Vemma ■ 835
Vibe Liquid Multi-Nutrient Supplement (Herbals with Vitamins & Minerals, Vitamins with Minerals) Eniva ■ 822
Visutein Capsules (Lutein, Acetylcysteine, Carotenoids, Vitamin A, Vitamin B_2, Zinc) Unicity 3329
Winrgy Dietary Supplement (Amino Acid Preparations, Caffeine, Vitamins with Minerals) Wellness International ■ 823
Wobenzym Tablets (Dietary Supplement) Marlyn 1862
Zavita Liquid Herbal Supplement (Herbals, Multiple) Zavita ■ 823
Zinc-220 Capsules (Zinc Sulfate) Alto 580

Digestive disorders, symptomatic relief of
DDS-Acidophilus Capsules, Tablets, and Powder (Lactobacillus Acidophilus) UAS Labs ■ 812
Gas-X with Maalox (Calcium Carbonate, Simethicone) Novartis Consumer ■ 656
Maalox Max Maximum Strength Antacid/Anti-Gas Liquid (Aluminum Hydroxide, Magnesium Hydroxide, Simethicone) Novartis Consumer ■ 659
Maalox Maximum Strength Total Stomach Relief Peppermint Liquid (Bismuth Subsalicylate) Novartis Consumer ■ 660
Maalox Maximum Strength Total Stomach Relief Strawberry Liquid (Bismuth Subsalicylate) Novartis Consumer ■ 672
Maalox Max Maximum Strength Chewable Tablets (Calcium Carbonate, Simethicone) Novartis Consumer ■ 660

Digoxin intoxication, life-threatening
Digibind for Injection (Digoxin Immune Fab (Ovine)) GlaxoSmithKline 1421

Diphtheria
(*see under* C. diphtheriae infections)

Diphtheria, tetanus, pertussis vaccine
(*see also under* Immunization, diphtheria, tetanus and pertussis)
ADACEL Vaccine (Diphtheria & Tetanus Toxoids and Acellular Pertussis Vaccine Adsorbed) Sanofi Pasteur 2945
Boostrix (Diphtheria & Tetanus Toxoids and Acellular Pertussis Vaccine Adsorbed) GlaxoSmithKline 1404
DAPTACEL Vaccine (Diphtheria & Tetanus Toxoids and Acellular Pertussis Vaccine Adsorbed) Sanofi Pasteur 2950
Infanrix Vaccine (Diphtheria & Tetanus Toxoids and Acellular Pertussis Vaccine Adsorbed) GlaxoSmithKline 1476
Pediarix Vaccine (Diphtheria & Tetanus Toxoids and Pertussis Vaccine Adsorbed, Hepatitis B Vaccine, Recombinant, Poliovirus Vaccine Inactivated, Trivalent Types 1,2,3) GlaxoSmithKline 1548

Diplococcus pneumoniae infections
(*see under* S. pneumoniae infections)

Discomfort, anorectal
Fleet Phospho-soda ACCU-PREP (Glycerin, Pramoxine Hydrochloride, Sodium Phosphate) Fleet 1168
Fleet Phospho-soda EZ-PREP (Glycerin, Pramoxine Hydrochloride, Sodium Phosphate) Fleet 1169

Diuresis, induction of in edema due to lupus erythematosus
Decadron Tablets (Dexamethasone) Merck 1951
Depo-Medrol Injectable Suspension (Methylprednisolone Acetate) Pharmacia & Upjohn 2617
Hydrocortone Tablets (Hydrocortisone) Merck 1989

Diuresis, induction of in nephrotic syndrome
Decadron Tablets (Dexamethasone) Merck 1951
Depo-Medrol Injectable Suspension (Methylprednisolone Acetate) Pharmacia & Upjohn 2617
Depo-Medrol Single-Dose Vial (Methylprednisolone Acetate) Pharmacia & Upjohn 2619
Hydrocortone Tablets (Hydrocortisone) Merck 1989

Drowsiness, symptomatic relief of
Vivarin (Caffeine) GlaxoSmithKline ■ 602

Dryness, vaginal
Estring Vaginal Ring (Estradiol) Pharmacia & Upjohn 2635

Ductus arteriosus, patent, palliative maintenance
Indocin I.V. (Indomethacin Sodium Trihydrate) Ovation 2465
NeoProfen Injection (Ibuprofen Lysine) Ovation 2472

Dukes' stage C colon cancer
(*see under* Carcinoma, colon, Dukes' stage C, adjunctive treatment in)

Duodenal ulcer and H. pylori infection, adjunct in
Aciphex Tablets (Rabeprazole Sodium) Eisai 1090
Amoxil Capsules (Amoxicillin) GlaxoSmithKline 1343
Amoxil Chewable Tablets (Amoxicillin) GlaxoSmithKline 1343
Amoxil Pediatric Drops for Oral Suspension (Amoxicillin) GlaxoSmithKline 1343
Amoxil Powder for Oral Suspension (Amoxicillin) GlaxoSmithKline 1343
Amoxil Tablets (Amoxicillin) GlaxoSmithKline 1343
Biaxin/Biaxin XL (Clarithromycin) Abbott 402
Prevacid Delayed-Release Capsules (Lansoprazole) TAP 3271
Prevacid for Delayed-Release Oral Suspension (Lansoprazole) TAP 3271
Prevacid SoluTab Delayed-Release Orally Disintegrating Tablets (Lansoprazole) TAP 3271
PREVPAC (Amoxicillin, Clarithromycin, Lansoprazole) TAP 3284

Duodenal ulcers, active, short-term treatment of
Aciphex Tablets (Rabeprazole Sodium) Eisai 1090
Axid Oral Solution (Nizatidine) Braintree 879
Carafate Suspension (Sucralfate) Axcan Scandipharm 701
Carafate Tablets (Sucralfate) Axcan Scandipharm 701
Pepcid Injection (Famotidine) Merck 2040
Pepcid (Famotidine) Merck 2038
Prevacid Delayed-Release Capsules (Lansoprazole) TAP 3271
Prevacid for Delayed-Release Oral Suspension (Lansoprazole) TAP 3271
Prevacid SoluTab Delayed-Release Orally Disintegrating Tablets (Lansoprazole) TAP 3271
Zantac (Ranitidine Hydrochloride) GlaxoSmithKline 1624
Zantac Injection (Ranitidine Hydrochloride) GlaxoSmithKline 1619
Zantac Injection Pharmacy Bulk Package (Ranitidine Hydrochloride) GlaxoSmithKline 1622
Zantac Injection Premixed (Ranitidine Hydrochloride) GlaxoSmithKline 1619
Zantac (Ranitidine Hydrochloride) GlaxoSmithKline 1624
Zegerid Capsules (Omeprazole) Santarus 2958
Zegerid Powder for Oral Solution (Omeprazole) Santarus 2958

Duodenal ulcers, adjunctive therapy for
Donnatal Extentabs (Atropine Sulfate, Hyoscyamine Sulfate, Phenobarbital, Scopolamine Hydrobromide) PBM 2493

Duodenal ulcers, maintenance therapy for
Axid Oral Solution (Nizatidine) Braintree 879
Carafate Tablets (Sucralfate) Axcan Scandipharm 701
Pepcid Injection (Famotidine) Merck 2040
Pepcid (Famotidine) Merck 2038
Prevacid Delayed-Release Capsules (Lansoprazole) TAP 3271
Prevacid for Delayed-Release Oral Suspension (Lansoprazole) TAP 3271
Prevacid SoluTab Delayed-Release Orally Disintegrating Tablets (Lansoprazole) TAP 3271

Primaxin I.V. (Cilastatin Sodium, Imipenem) Merck 2048
Rocephin Injectable Vials, ADD-Vantage, Galaxy, Bulk (Ceftriaxone Sodium) Roche 2800
Timentin ADD-Vantage (Clavulanate Potassium, Ticarcillin Disodium) GlaxoSmithKline 1580
Timentin Injection Galaxy Container (Clavulanate Potassium, Ticarcillin Disodium) GlaxoSmithKline 1583
Timentin IV Infusion (Clavulanate Potassium, Ticarcillin Disodium) GlaxoSmithKline 1577
Timentin Pharmacy Bulk Package (Clavulanate Potassium, Ticarcillin Disodium) GlaxoSmithKline 1586
Tygacil for Injection (Tigecycline) Wyeth 3488
Zinacef for Injection (Cefuroxime) GlaxoSmithKline 1631
Zinacef Injection (Cefuroxime) GlaxoSmithKline 1631

E. coli urinary tract infections
Augmentin (Amoxicillin, Clavulanate Potassium) GlaxoSmithKline 1360
Augmentin Tablets (Amoxicillin, Clavulanate Potassium) GlaxoSmithKline 1363
Ceftin Tablets (Cefuroxime Axetil) GlaxoSmithKline 1407
Cipro (Ciprofloxacin) Schering 2977
Cipro I.V. (Ciprofloxacin) Schering 2984
Cipro XR Tablets (Ciprofloxacin) Schering 2990
Fortaz (Ceftazidime) GlaxoSmithKline 1453
Gantrisin Pediatric Suspension (Acetyl Sulfisoxazole) Roche 2770
Invanz for Injection (Ertapenem) Merck 1999
Keflex Capsules (Cephalexin) Advancis 549
Levaquin (Levofloxacin) Ortho-McNeil 2384
Levaquin in 5% Dextrose Injection (Levofloxacin) Ortho-McNeil 2384
Maxipime for Injection (Cefepime Hydrochloride) Elan 1105
Mefoxin for Injection (Cefoxitin Sodium) Merck 2012
Mefoxin Premixed Intravenous Solution (Cefoxitin Sodium) Merck 2016
Noroxin Tablets (Norfloxacin) Merck 2032
Primaxin I.V. (Cilastatin Sodium, Imipenem) Merck 2048
Proquin XR Tablets (Ciprofloxacin Hydrochloride) Esprit 1153
Raniclor Tablets, Chewable (Cefaclor Monohydrate) Pedinol 2505
Rocephin Injectable Vials, ADD-Vantage, Galaxy, Bulk (Ceftriaxone Sodium) Roche 2800
Seromycin Capsules (Cycloserine) Lilly 1813
Suprax (Cefixime) Lupin 1843
Tequin Injection (Gatifloxacin) Bristol-Myers Squibb 938
Tequin Injection in 5% Dextrose (Gatifloxacin) Bristol-Myers Squibb 938
Tequin Tablets (Gatifloxacin) Bristol-Myers Squibb 938
Timentin ADD-Vantage (Clavulanate Potassium, Ticarcillin Disodium) GlaxoSmithKline 1580
Timentin Injection Galaxy Container (Clavulanate Potassium, Ticarcillin Disodium) GlaxoSmithKline 1583
Timentin IV Infusion (Clavulanate Potassium, Ticarcillin Disodium) GlaxoSmithKline 1577
Timentin Pharmacy Bulk Package (Clavulanate Potassium, Ticarcillin Disodium) GlaxoSmithKline 1586
Vantin Tablets and Oral Suspension (Cefpodoxime Proxetil) Pharmacia & Upjohn 2645
Zinacef for Injection (Cefuroxime) GlaxoSmithKline 1631
Zinacef Injection (Cefuroxime) GlaxoSmithKline 1631

E. coli-induced diarrhea
(*see under* Diarrhea, E. coli-induced)

E. faecalis (vancomycin susceptible strains) intra-abdominal infections
Tygacil (Tigecycline) Wyeth 3488

E. faecalis (vancomycin susceptible strains) skin and skin structure infections
Cubicin for Injection (Daptomycin) Cubist 1026
Tygacil (Tigecycline) Wyeth 3488

E. faecalis infections
Avelox (Moxifloxacin Hydrochloride) Schering 2970
Merrem I.V. (Meropenem) AstraZeneca Pharmaceuticals 686
Tygacil for Injection (Tigecycline) Wyeth 3488

E. faecalis intra-abdominal infections
Avelox (Moxifloxacin Hydrochloride) Schering 2970

E. faecalis prostatitis
Levaquin (Levofloxacin) Ortho-McNeil 2384
Levaquin in 5% Dextrose Injection (Levofloxacin) Ortho-McNeil 2384

E. faecalis skin and skin structure infections
Levaquin (Levofloxacin) Ortho-McNeil 2384
Levaquin in 5% Dextrose Injection (Levofloxacin) Ortho-McNeil 2384
Merrem I.V. (Meropenem) AstraZeneca Pharmaceuticals 686

E. faecalis urinary tract infections
Cipro XR Tablets (Ciprofloxacin) Schering 2990
Levaquin (Levofloxacin) Ortho-McNeil 2384
Levaquin in 5% Dextrose Injection (Levofloxacin) Ortho-McNeil 2384

Ear, infection
(*see under* Otitis externa; Otitis media, acute)

Eaton-Lambert syndrome, symptomatic relief of
Guanidine Hydrochloride Tablets (Guanidine Hydrochloride) Schering 3016

Echinococcus granulosus infections
Albenza Tablets (Albendazole) GlaxoSmithKline 1338

Eczema, unspecified
(*see under* Skin, inflammatory conditions)

Edema, adjunctive therapy in
Demadex Tablets (Torsemide) Roche 2759
Diuril Oral Suspension (Chlorothiazide) Merck 1954
Diuril Sodium Intravenous (Chlorothiazide Sodium) Ovation 2467
Dyazide Capsules (Hydrochlorothiazide, Triamterene) GlaxoSmithKline 1423
Dyrenium Capsules (Triamterene) WellSpring 3400
Edecrin (Ethacrynic Acid) Merck 1959
Furosemide Tablets (Furosemide) Mylan 2154
Indapamide Tablets (Indapamide) Mylan 2156

Edema, cerebral
Decadron Tablets (Dexamethasone) Merck 1951

Edema, congestive heart failure-induced, treatment of
Bumex Tablets (Bumetanide) Roche 2746
Demadex Injection (Torsemide) Roche 2759

Edema, corneal, temporary relief of
Muro 128 Ophthalmic Ointment (Sodium Chloride) Bausch & Lomb .... ⊙ 253
Muro 128 Ophthalmic Solution 2% and 5% (Sodium Chloride) Bausch & Lomb .... ⊙ 252

Edema, hepatic disease-induced, treatment of
Bumex Tablets (Bumetanide) Roche 2746
Demadex Injection (Torsemide) Roche 2759

Edema, renal disease-induced, treatment of
Bumex Tablets (Bumetanide) Roche 2746
Demadex Injection (Torsemide) Roche 2759

Embolism, atrial fibrillation with
(*see under* Atrial fibrillation with embolism)

Embolism, pulmonary
Activase I.V. (Alteplase) Genentech 1223
Arixtra Injection (Fondaparinux Sodium) GlaxoSmithKline 1351
Coumadin for Injection (Warfarin Sodium) Bristol-Myers Squibb 898
Coumadin Tablets (Warfarin Sodium) Bristol-Myers Squibb 898
Lovenox Injection (Enoxaparin Sodium) sanofi-aventis 2915
Miradon Tablets (Anisindione) Schering 3042

Embolism, pulmonary, acute, lysis of
Activase I.V. (Alteplase) Genentech 1223

Embolism, pulmonary, prophylaxis of
Coumadin for Injection (Warfarin Sodium) Bristol-Myers Squibb 898
Coumadin Tablets (Warfarin Sodium) Bristol-Myers Squibb 898
Miradon Tablets (Anisindione) Schering 3042

Embolism, systemic, post-myocardial infarction, prophylaxis
Coumadin for Injection (Warfarin Sodium) Bristol-Myers Squibb 898
Coumadin Tablets (Warfarin Sodium) Bristol-Myers Squibb 898

Emotionalism
Hyland's Calm Forte 4 Kids Tablets (Homeopathic Formulations, Sulfur) Standard Homeopathic .... ◘ 828

Emphysema
Atrovent HFA Inhalation Aerosol (Ipratropium Bromide) Boehringer Ingelheim 841
Serevent Diskus (Salmeterol Xinafoate) GlaxoSmithKline 1568
Spiriva HandiHaler (Tiotropium bromide) Boehringer Ingelheim 869
Uniphyl Tablets (Theophylline Anhydrous) Purdue Pharmaceutical 2710
Zemaira (Alpha$_1$-Proteinase Inhibitor (Human)) ZLB Behring 3509

Emphysema, panacinar, due to congenital Alpha1-antitrypsin deficiency
Aralast (Alpha$_1$-Proteinase Inhibitor (Human)) Baxter Healthcare 717
Prolastin (Alpha$_1$-Proteinase Inhibitor (Human)) Talecris 3255

Empyema
Bicillin C-R Injectable Suspension (Penicillin G Benzathine, Penicillin G Procaine) King 1706
Cleocin Vaginal Ovules (Clindamycin Hydrochloride) Pharmacia & Upjohn 2616

Endocarditis, bacterial
Garamycin Injectable (Gentamicin Sulfate) Schering 3014
Primaxin I.V. (Cilastatin Sodium, Imipenem) Merck 2048

Endocarditis, bacterial, prophylaxis
Erythrocin Stearate Filmtab Tablets (Erythromycin Stearate) Abbott 453
Erythromycin Base Filmtab Tablets (Erythromycin) Abbott 455
Erythromycin Delayed-Release Capsules, USP (Erythromycin) Abbott 457

Endocrine adenomas, multiple
(*see also under* Hypersecretory conditions, pathological)
Pepcid Injection (Famotidine) Merck 2040
Pepcid (Famotidine) Merck 2038

Endocrine disorders
Decadron Tablets (Dexamethasone) Merck 1951
Depo-Medrol Injectable Suspension (Methylprednisolone Acetate) Pharmacia & Upjohn 2617
Hydrocortone Tablets (Hydrocortisone) Merck 1989

Endometrial hyperplasia, prevention of
Prometrium Capsules (100 mg, 200 mg) (Progesterone) Solvay 3203

Endometriosis
Lupron Depot 3.75 mg (Leuprolide Acetate) TAP 3260
Lupron Depot–3 Month 11.25 mg (Leuprolide Acetate) TAP 3265

Endometritis
(*see also under* Infections, gynecologic)
Cleocin Vaginal Ovules (Clindamycin Hydrochloride) Pharmacia & Upjohn 2616
Fortaz (Ceftazidime) GlaxoSmithKline 1453
Mefoxin for Injection (Cefoxitin Sodium) Merck 2012
Mefoxin Premixed Intravenous Solution (Cefoxitin Sodium) Merck 2016
Timentin ADD-Vantage (Clavulanate Potassium, Ticarcillin Disodium) GlaxoSmithKline 1580
Timentin Injection Galaxy Container (Clavulanate Potassium, Ticarcillin Disodium) GlaxoSmithKline 1583
Timentin IV Infusion (Clavulanate Potassium, Ticarcillin Disodium) GlaxoSmithKline 1577
Timentin Pharmacy Bulk Package (Clavulanate Potassium, Ticarcillin Disodium) GlaxoSmithKline 1586

Endomyometritis
Invanz for Injection (Ertapenem) Merck 1999
Primaxin I.M. (Cilastatin Sodium, Imipenem) Merck 2045

Entamoeba histolytica
(*see under* Amebiasis, acute intestinal)

Enteritis, regional, systemic therapy for
Decadron Tablets (Dexamethasone) Merck 1951
Depo-Medrol Injectable Suspension (Methylprednisolone Acetate) Pharmacia & Upjohn 2617
Depo-Medrol Single-Dose Vial (Methylprednisolone Acetate) Pharmacia & Upjohn 2619
Hydrocortone Tablets (Hydrocortisone) Merck 1989

Enterobacter aerogenes infections
Noroxin Tablets (Norfloxacin) Merck 2032
Rocephin Injectable Vials, ADD-Vantage, Galaxy, Bulk (Ceftriaxone Sodium) Roche 2800

Enterobacter aerogenes infections, ocular
Pred-G Ophthalmic Ointment (Gentamicin Sulfate, Prednisolone Acetate) Allergan .... ⊙ 237
Pred-G Ophthalmic Suspension (Gentamicin Sulfate, Prednisolone Acetate) Allergan .... ⊙ 236
TobraDex Ophthalmic Ointment (Dexamethasone, Tobramycin) Alcon 562
TobraDex Ophthalmic Suspension (Dexamethasone, Tobramycin) Alcon 563

Enterobacter aerogenes lower respiratory tract infections
Rocephin Injectable Vials, ADD-Vantage, Galaxy, Bulk (Ceftriaxone Sodium) Roche 2800

Enterobacter aerogenes urinary tract infections
Noroxin Tablets (Norfloxacin) Merck 2032

Enterobacter cloacae bone and joint infections
Cipro (Ciprofloxacin) Schering 2977
Cipro I.V. (Ciprofloxacin) Schering 2984

Enterobacter cloacae infections
Cipro (Ciprofloxacin) Schering 2977
Cipro I.V. (Ciprofloxacin) Schering 2984

Levaquin (Levofloxacin) Ortho-McNeil ... 2384
Levaquin in 5% Dextrose Injection (Levofloxacin) Ortho-McNeil ... 2384
Noroxin Tablets (Norfloxacin) Merck . 2032
Primaxin I.M. (Cilastatin Sodium, Imipenem) Merck ... 2045
Rocephin Injectable Vials, ADD-Vantage, Galaxy, Bulk (Ceftriaxone Sodium) Roche ... 2800
Timentin ADD-Vantage (Clavulanate Potassium, Ticarcillin Disodium) GlaxoSmithKline ... 1580
Timentin Injection Galaxy Container (Clavulanate Potassium, Ticarcillin Disodium) GlaxoSmithKline ... 1583
Timentin IV Infusion (Clavulanate Potassium, Ticarcillin Disodium) GlaxoSmithKline ... 1577
Timentin Pharmacy Bulk Package (Clavulanate Potassium, Ticarcillin Disodium) GlaxoSmithKline ... 1586
Tygacil for Injection (Tigecycline) Wyeth ... 3488

Enterobacter cloacae infections, ocular
Neosporin Ophthalmic Solution Sterile (Gramicidin, Neomycin Sulfate, Polymyxin B Sulfate) King ... ⊙ 265

Enterobacter cloacae intra-abdominal infections
Tygacil for Injection (Tigecycline) Wyeth ... 3488

Enterobacter cloacae lower respiratory tract infections
Cipro (Ciprofloxacin) Schering ... 2977
Cipro I.V. (Ciprofloxacin) Schering ... 2984

Enterobacter cloacae skin and skin structure infections
Cipro (Ciprofloxacin) Schering ... 2977
Cipro I.V. (Ciprofloxacin) Schering ... 2984
Primaxin I.M. (Cilastatin Sodium, Imipenem) Merck ... 2045
Rocephin Injectable Vials, ADD-Vantage, Galaxy, Bulk (Ceftriaxone Sodium) Roche ... 2800

Enterobacter cloacae urinary tract infections
Cipro (Ciprofloxacin) Schering ... 2977
Cipro I.V. (Ciprofloxacin) Schering ... 2984
Levaquin (Levofloxacin) Ortho-McNeil ... 2384
Levaquin in 5% Dextrose Injection (Levofloxacin) Ortho-McNeil ... 2384
Noroxin Tablets (Norfloxacin) Merck . 2032
Timentin ADD-Vantage (Clavulanate Potassium, Ticarcillin Disodium) GlaxoSmithKline ... 1580
Timentin Injection Galaxy Container (Clavulanate Potassium, Ticarcillin Disodium) GlaxoSmithKline ... 1583
Timentin IV Infusion (Clavulanate Potassium, Ticarcillin Disodium) GlaxoSmithKline ... 1577
Timentin Pharmacy Bulk Package (Clavulanate Potassium, Ticarcillin Disodium) GlaxoSmithKline ... 1586

Enterobacter species bone and joint infections
Fortaz (Ceftazidime) GlaxoSmithKline ... 1453
Primaxin I.V. (Cilastatin Sodium, Imipenem) Merck ... 2048
Rocephin Injectable Vials, ADD-Vantage, Galaxy, Bulk (Ceftriaxone Sodium) Roche ... 2800

Enterobacter species gynecologic infections
Primaxin I.V. (Cilastatin Sodium, Imipenem) Merck ... 2048
Timentin ADD-Vantage (Clavulanate Potassium, Ticarcillin Disodium) GlaxoSmithKline ... 1580
Timentin Injection Galaxy Container (Clavulanate Potassium, Ticarcillin Disodium) GlaxoSmithKline ... 1583
Timentin IV Infusion (Clavulanate Potassium, Ticarcillin Disodium) GlaxoSmithKline ... 1577
Timentin Pharmacy Bulk Package (Clavulanate Potassium, Ticarcillin Disodium) GlaxoSmithKline ... 1586

Enterobacter species infections
Augmentin (Amoxicillin, Clavulanate Potassium) GlaxoSmithKline ... 1360
Augmentin Tablets (Amoxicillin, Clavulanate Potassium) GlaxoSmithKline ... 1363
Fortaz (Ceftazidime) GlaxoSmithKline ... 1453
Garamycin Injectable (Gentamicin Sulfate) Schering ... 3014
Primaxin I.V. (Cilastatin Sodium, Imipenem) Merck ... 2048
Rocephin Injectable Vials, ADD-Vantage, Galaxy, Bulk (Ceftriaxone Sodium) Roche ... 2800
Seromycin Capsules (Cycloserine) Lilly ... 1813
Timentin ADD-Vantage (Clavulanate Potassium, Ticarcillin Disodium) GlaxoSmithKline ... 1580
Timentin Injection Galaxy Container (Clavulanate Potassium, Ticarcillin Disodium) GlaxoSmithKline ... 1583
Timentin IV Infusion (Clavulanate Potassium, Ticarcillin Disodium) GlaxoSmithKline ... 1577
Timentin Pharmacy Bulk Package (Clavulanate Potassium, Ticarcillin Disodium) GlaxoSmithKline ... 1586
Zinacef for Injection (Cefuroxime) GlaxoSmithKline ... 1631
Zinacef Injection (Cefuroxime) GlaxoSmithKline ... 1631

Enterobacter species infections, ocular
Pred-G Ophthalmic Ointment (Gentamicin Sulfate, Prednisolone Acetate) Allergan ... ⊙ 237

Enterobacter species intra-abdominal infections
Maxipime for Injection (Cefepime Hydrochloride) Elan ... 1105
Primaxin I.V. (Cilastatin Sodium, Imipenem) Merck ... 2048

Enterobacter species lower respiratory tract infections
Fortaz (Ceftazidime) GlaxoSmithKline ... 1453
Maxipime for Injection (Cefepime Hydrochloride) Elan ... 1105
Primaxin I.V. (Cilastatin Sodium, Imipenem) Merck ... 2048

Enterobacter species septicemia
Primaxin I.V. (Cilastatin Sodium, Imipenem) Merck ... 2048

Enterobacter species skin and skin structure infections
Fortaz (Ceftazidime) GlaxoSmithKline ... 1453
Primaxin I.V. (Cilastatin Sodium, Imipenem) Merck ... 2048
Zinacef for Injection (Cefuroxime) GlaxoSmithKline ... 1631
Zinacef Injection (Cefuroxime) GlaxoSmithKline ... 1631

Enterobacter species urinary tract infections
Augmentin (Amoxicillin, Clavulanate Potassium) GlaxoSmithKline ... 1360
Augmentin Tablets (Amoxicillin, Clavulanate Potassium) GlaxoSmithKline ... 1363
Fortaz (Ceftazidime) GlaxoSmithKline ... 1453
Primaxin I.V. (Cilastatin Sodium, Imipenem) Merck ... 2048
Seromycin Capsules (Cycloserine) Lilly ... 1813

Enterobiasis
Reese's Pinworm Treatments (Pyrantel Pamoate) Reese ... ▣ 670

Enterococci infections
(*see under* Streptococci group D infections)

Enterococcus faecium, vancomycin-resistant bacteremia
Zyvox (Linezolid) Pharmacia & Upjohn ... 2652

Enterococcus faecium, vancomycin-resistant infections
Zyvox (Linezolid) Pharmacia & Upjohn ... 2652

Enterocolitis, acute
Donnatal Extentabs (Atropine Sulfate, Hyoscyamine Sulfate, Phenobarbital, Scopolamine Hydrobromide) PBM ... 2493

Enterocolitis, staphylococcal
Vancocin HCl Capsules, USP (Vancomycin Hydrochloride) ViroPharma ... 3380

Envenomation, Micrurus fulvius
Antivenin (Micrurus fulvius) (Antivenin (Micrurus Fulvius)) Wyeth ... 3407

Envenomation, pit viper
Antivenin Polyvalent (Antivenin (Crotalidae) Polyvalent) Wyeth ... 3405

Epicondylitis
Depo-Medrol Injectable Suspension (Methylprednisolone Acetate) Pharmacia & Upjohn ... 2617
Depo-Medrol Single-Dose Vial (Methylprednisolone Acetate) Pharmacia & Upjohn ... 2619
Hydrocortone Tablets (Hydrocortisone) Merck ... 1989
Traumeel Injection Solution (Homeopathic Formulations) Heel ... 1664

Epidermophyton floccosum infections
Gris-PEG Tablets (Griseofulvin) Pedinol ... 2502
Lotrimin (Clotrimazole) Schering ... 3039
Lotrisone (Betamethasone Dipropionate, Clotrimazole) Schering ... 3040
Naftin Cream (Naftifine Hydrochloride) Merz ... 2126
Naftin Gel (Naftifine Hydrochloride) Merz ... 2126
Oxistat (Oxiconazole Nitrate) Pharmaderm ... 2667

Epilepsy
Depakote Tablets (Divalproex Sodium) Abbott ... 427
Lamictal (Lamotrigine) GlaxoSmithKline ... 1481

Epilepsy, generalized
(*see under* Seizures, generalized, tonic-clonic)

Epilepsy, grand mal
(*see under* Seizures, generalized, tonic-clonic)

Epilepsy, petit mal
(*see under* Seizures, generalized, absence)

Epilepticus, status
Nembutal Sodium Solution, USP (Pentobarbital Sodium) Ovation ... 2470

Episiotomy, topical debriding in
(*see under* Wounds, debridement of)

Erectile dysfunction
Caverject Impulse Injection (Alprostadil) Pharmacia & Upjohn ... 2612
Cialis Tablets (Tadalafil) Lilly ICOS ... 1838
Edex Injection (Alprostadil) Schwarz . 3089
Levitra Tablets (Vardenafil Hydrochloride) Schering ... 3034
Viagra Tablets (Sildenafil Citrate) Pfizer ... 2573

Erectile dysfunction, diagnosis of
Caverject Impulse Injection (Alprostadil) Pharmacia & Upjohn ... 2612

Erysipelas
Bicillin C-R Injectable Suspension (Penicillin G Benzathine, Penicillin G Procaine) King ... 1706

Erythema multiforme, severe
(*see under* Stevens-Johnson syndrome)

Erythema nodosum leprosum
Thalomid Capsules (Thalidomide) Celgene ... 965

Erythrasma
E.E.S. (Erythromycin Ethylsuccinate) Abbott ... 451
EryPed (Erythromycin Ethylsuccinate) Abbott ... 447
Ery-Tab Tablets (Erythromycin) Abbott ... 449
Erythrocin Stearate Filmtab Tablets (Erythromycin Stearate) Abbott ... 453
Erythromycin Base Filmtab Tablets (Erythromycin) Abbott ... 455
Erythromycin Delayed-Release Capsules, USP (Erythromycin) Abbott ... 457
PCE Dispertab Tablets (Erythromycin) Abbott ... 515

Erythroblastopenia
Depo-Medrol Injectable Suspension (Methylprednisolone Acetate) Pharmacia & Upjohn ... 2617
Depo-Medrol Single-Dose Vial (Methylprednisolone Acetate) Pharmacia & Upjohn ... 2619
Hydrocortone Tablets (Hydrocortisone) Merck ... 1989

Erythroblastosis fetalis, prevention of
HyperRho S/D Full Dose (Rh_0 (D) Immune Globulin (Human)) Talecris ... 3246

Erythrocyle, resuspension
Plasbumin-20 (Albumin (human)) Talecris ... 3252

Erythroderma, exfoliative
Decadron Tablets (Dexamethasone) Merck ... 1951

Escherichia coli
(*see under* E. coli infections)

Esophagitis, erosive
(*see also under* Gastroesophageal reflux disease)
Axid Oral Solution (Nizatidine) Braintree ... 879
Nexium Delayed-Release Capsules (Esomeprazole Magnesium) AstraZeneca LP ... 655
Nexium I.V. (Esomeprazole Sodium) AstraZeneca LP ... 659
Prevacid Delayed-Release Capsules (Lansoprazole) TAP ... 3271
Prevacid for Delayed-Release Oral Suspension (Lansoprazole) TAP ... 3271
Prevacid SoluTab Delayed-Release Orally Disintegrating Tablets (Lansoprazole) TAP ... 3271
Prevacid I.V. for Injection (Lansoprazole) TAP ... 3277
Protonix I.V. (Pantoprazole Sodium) Wyeth ... 3472
Protonix Tablets (Pantoprazole Sodium) Wyeth ... 3469
Zantac (Ranitidine Hydrochloride) GlaxoSmithKline ... 1624
Zegerid Capsules (Omeprazole) Santarus ... 2958
Zegerid Powder for Oral Solution (Omeprazole) Santarus ... 2958

Esophagitis, ulcerative
Axid Oral Solution (Nizatidine) Braintree ... 879

Estrogen, deficiency
(*see under* Hypoestrogenism)

Eubacterium species infections
Invanz for Injection (Ertapenem) Merck ... 1999
Primaxin I.V. (Cilastatin Sodium, Imipenem) Merck ... 2048

Eubacterium species intra-abdominal infections
Invanz for Injection (Ertapenem) Merck ... 1999
Primaxin I.V. (Cilastatin Sodium, Imipenem) Merck ... 2048

Ewing's sarcoma, palliative treatment of
Cosmegen for Injection (Dactinomycin) Ovation ... 2459

Extrapyramidal reactions, drug-induced
Symmetrel Tablets (Amantadine Hydrochloride) Endo Labs ... 1135

Eyes, anterior segment, staining of
Fluor-I-Strip A.T. Ophthalmic Strips 1 mg (Fluorescein Sodium) Bausch & Lomb ... ⊙ 250

Eye, anterior segment Inflammation
(*see under* Inflammation, anterior segment)

Eyes, burning, reduction of
Acular LS Ophthalmic Solution (Ketorolac Tromethamine) Allergan ... 566
Refresh Endura Lubricant Eye Drops (Glycerin, Polysorbate 80) Allergan ... ⊙ 240
Refresh Liquigel Lubricant Eye Drops (Carboxymethylcellulose Sodium) Allergan ... ⊙ 241
Refresh Tears Lubricant Eye Drops (Carboxymethylcellulose Sodium) Allergan ... ⊙ 241
Systane Lubricant Eye Drops (Polyethylene Glycol, Propylene Glycol) Alcon ... 562
Visine A.C. Seasonal Itching and Redness Relief Drops (Tetrahydrozoline Hydrochloride, Zinc Sulfate) Pfizer Consumer ... ⊙ 289
Visine Pure Tears Eye Drops Single Drop Dispenser (Hypromellose, Glycerin, Polyethylene Glycol) Pfizer Consumer ... ⊙ 291

Eyes, diagnostic procedures, adjunct in
Fluor-I-Strip A.T. Ophthalmic Strips 1 mg (Fluorescein Sodium) Bausch & Lomb ... ⊙ 250

Eyes, dry
(*see under* Keratoconjunctivitis sicca)

Eyes, inflammation
(*see under* Ocular inflammation)

Eyes, irrigation of
Betadine 5% Ophthalmic Solution (Povidone Iodine) Alcon ... ⊙ 202

Eyes, irritation, symptomatic relief of
Refresh Endura Lubricant Eye Drops (Glycerin, Polysorbate 80) Allergan ... ⊙ 240
Refresh Liquigel Lubricant Eye Drops (Carboxymethylcellulose Sodium) Allergan ... ⊙ 241
Refresh Tears Lubricant Eye Drops (Carboxymethylcellulose Sodium) Allergan ... ⊙ 241
Systane Lubricant Eye Drops (Polyethylene Glycol, Propylene Glycol) Alcon ... 562
Triaminic Thin Strips Cough & Runny Nose (Diphenhydramine Hydrochloride) Novartis Consumer ... ▣ 749
Visine Original Eye Drops (Tetrahydrozoline Hydrochloride) Pfizer Consumer ... ⊙ 290
Visine A.C. Seasonal Itching and Redness Relief Drops (Tetrahydrozoline Hydrochloride, Zinc Sulfate) Pfizer Consumer ... ⊙ 289
Advanced Relief Visine Eye Drops (Dextran 70, Polyethylene Glycol, Povidone, Tetrahydrozoline Hydrochloride) Pfizer Consumer ... ⊙ 288
Visine For Contacts Rewetting Drops (Glycerin, Hydroxypropyl Methylcellulose) Pfizer Consumer ... ⊙ 289
Visine L.R. Long Lasting Eye Drops (Oxymetazoline Hydrochloride) Pfizer Consumer ... ⊙ 290
Visine Tears Eye Drops (Hypromellose, Glycerin, Polyethylene Glycol) Pfizer Consumer ... ⊙ 290
Visine Pure Tears Eye Drops Single Drop Dispenser (Hypromellose, Glycerin, Polyethylene Glycol) Pfizer Consumer ... ⊙ 291
Visine Pure Tears Portables (Hypromellose, Glycerin, Polyethylene Glycol) Pfizer Consumer ... ⊙ 291
VIVA Lubricating Eye Drops (Polysorbate 80) Vision Pharmaceuticals ... ⊙ 293
Zicam Allergy Relief (Histanium Hydrochloricum, Luffa operculata, Galphimia Glauca, Sulfur) Matrixx ... ▣ 774

Eyes, lubrication of
(*see also under* Keratoconjunctivitis sicca)
Restasis Ophthalmic Emulsion (Cyclosporine) Allergan ... 575

Eyes, surgery, adjunct to
Acular LS Ophthalmic Solution (Ketorolac Tromethamine) Allergan ... 566

Eyes, watery
(*see under* Lacrimation, symptomatic relief of)

F

Fabry disease
Fabrazyme for Intravenous Infusion (Agalsidase beta) Genzyme ... 1274

Factor IX, deficiency of, hemophilia B caused
AlphaNine SD, Coagulation Factor IX (Human) (Factor IX (Human)) Grifols ... 1656
Profilnine SD, Factor IX Complex (Human) (Factor IX Complex) Grifols ... 1660

Fatigue, symptomatic relief of
Vivarin (Caffeine) GlaxoSmithKline ... ▣ 602

Female castration
(*see under* Ovaries, castration of)

Fever, reduction of
Advil Caplets (Ibuprofen) Wyeth ... ▣ 674
Children's Advil Oral Suspension (Ibuprofen) Wyeth ... ▣ 603
Children's Advil Chewable Tablets (Ibuprofen) Wyeth ... ▣ 603
Advil Gel Caplets (Ibuprofen) Wyeth ... ▣ 674
Infants' Advil Concentrated Drops (Ibuprofen) Wyeth ... ▣ 604
Infants' Advil Concentrated Drops - White Grape (Dye-Free) (Ibuprofen) Wyeth ... ▣ 604
Junior Strength Advil Swallow Tablets (Ibuprofen) Wyeth ... ▣ 605
Advil (Ibuprofen) Wyeth ... ▣ 674
Aleve Caplets (Naproxen Sodium) Bayer Healthcare LLC ... 742
Aleve Gelcaps (Naproxen Sodium) Bayer Healthcare LLC ... 743
Aleve Cold & Sinus Caplets (Naproxen Sodium, Pseudoephedrine Hydrochloride) Bayer Healthcare LLC ... 744
Aleve Tablets (Naproxen Sodium) Bayer Healthcare LLC ... 743
Aleve Cold & Sinus Caplets (Naproxen Sodium, Pseudoephedrine Hydrochloride) Bayer Healthcare ... ▣ 724
BC Headache Powder (Aspirin, Caffeine, Salicylamide) GlaxoSmithKline ... ▣ 677
Bufferin Extra Strength Tablets (Aspirin Buffered) Novartis Consumer ... ▣ 678
Bufferin Regular Strength Tablets (Aspirin Buffered) Novartis Consumer ... ▣ 678
Comtrex Maximum Strength Cold & Cough Day/Night Caplets - Day Formulation (Acetaminophen, Dextromethorphan Hydrobromide, Pseudoephedrine Hydrochloride) Novartis Consumer ... ▣ 726
Comtrex Maximum Strength Cold & Cough Day/Night Caplets - Night Formulation (Acetaminophen, Chlorpheniramine Maleate, Dextromethorphan Hydrobromide, Pseudoephedrine Hydrochloride) Novartis Consumer ... ▣ 726
Comtrex Maximum Strength Non-Drowsy Cold & Cough Caplets (Acetaminophen, Dextromethorphan Hydrobromide, Phenylephrine Hydrochloride) Novartis Consumer ... ▣ 725
Contac Cold and Flu Maximum Strength Caplets (Acetaminophen, Chlorpheniramine Maleate, Phenylephrine Hydrochloride) GlaxoSmithKline ... ▣ 728
Contac Cold and Flu Day and Night Caplets (Day Formulation Only) (Acetaminophen, Phenylephrine Hydrochloride) GlaxoSmithKline ... ▣ 727
Contac Cold and Flu Day and Night Caplets (Night Formulation Only) (Acetaminophen, Chlorpheniramine Maleate, Phenylephrine Hydrochloride) GlaxoSmithKline ... ▣ 727
Contac Cold and Flu Non-Drowsy Caplets (Acetaminophen, Phenylephrine Hydrochloride) GlaxoSmithKline ... ▣ 728
Goody's Extra Strength Headache Powders (Acetaminophen, Aspirin, Caffeine) GlaxoSmithKline ... ▣ 611
Goody's Extra Strength Pain Relief Tablets (Acetaminophen, Aspirin, Caffeine) GlaxoSmithKline ... ▣ 685
Motrin IB Tablets and Caplets (Ibuprofen) McNeil Consumer ... 1866
Children's Motrin Oral Suspension (Ibuprofen) McNeil Consumer ... ▣ 685
Children's Motrin Non-Staining Dye-Free Oral Suspension (Ibuprofen) McNeil Consumer ... ▣ 685
Children's Motrin Oral Suspension (Ibuprofen) McNeil Consumer ... 1867
Children's Motrin Non-Staining Dye-Free Oral Suspension (Ibuprofen) McNeil Consumer ... 1867
Infants' Motrin Concentrated Drops (Ibuprofen) McNeil Consumer ... 1867
Infants' Motrin Non-Staining Dye-Free Concentrated Drops (Ibuprofen) McNeil Consumer ... 1867
Junior Strength Motrin Caplets and Chewable Tablets (Ibuprofen) McNeil Consumer ... 1867
TheraFlu Cold & Sore Throat Hot Liquid (Acetaminophen, Pheniramine Maleate, Phenylephrine Hydrochloride) Novartis Consumer ... ▣ 741
TheraFlu Flu & Chest Congestion Hot Liquid (Acetaminophen, Guaifenesin) Novartis Consumer ... ▣ 741
TheraFlu Flu & Sore Throat Hot Liquid (Acetaminophen, Pheniramine Maleate, Phenylephrine Hydrochloride) Novartis Consumer ... ▣ 742
TheraFlu Daytime Severe Cold Hot Liquid (Acetaminophen, Phenylephrine Hydrochloride) Novartis Consumer ... ▣ 742
TheraFlu Nighttime Severe Cold Hot Liquid (Acetaminophen, Pheniramine Maleate, Phenylephrine Hydrochloride) Novartis Consumer ... ▣ 740
TheraFlu Warming Relief Daytime Severe Cold (Acetaminophen, Dextromethorphan Hydrobromide, Phenylephrine Hydrochloride) Novartis Consumer ... ▣ 743
TheraFlu Warming Relief Nighttime Severe Cold (Acetaminophen, Diphenhydramine Hydrochloride, Phenylephrine Hydrochloride) Novartis Consumer ... ▣ 743
Regular Strength Tylenol Tablets (Acetaminophen) McNeil Consumer ... 1870
Tylenol 8 Hour Extended Release Caplets (Acetaminophen) McNeil Consumer ... ▣ 695
Tylenol Chest Congestion Caplets with Cool Burst (Acetaminophen, Guaifenesin) McNeil Consumer ... ▣ 722
Tylenol Chest Congestion Liquid with Cool Burst (Acetaminophen, Guaifenesin) McNeil Consumer ... ▣ 722
Children's Tylenol Suspension Liquid and Meltaways (Acetaminophen) McNeil Consumer ... ▣ 679
Children's Tylenol with Flavor Creator (Acetaminophen) McNeil Consumer ... ▣ 679
Children's Tylenol Plus Cough & Runny Nose Suspension Liquid (Acetaminophen, Chlorpheniramine Maleate, Dextromethorphan Hydrobromide) McNeil Consumer ... ▣ 754
Children's Tylenol Plus Cough & Sore Throat Suspension Liquid (Acetaminophen, Dextromethorphan Hydrobromide) McNeil Consumer ... ▣ 754
Children's Tylenol Plus Cold Suspension Liquid (Acetaminophen, Chlorpheniramine Maleate, Phenylephrine Hydrochloride) McNeil Consumer ... ▣ 754
Children's Tylenol Plus Multi-Symptom Cold Suspension Liquid (Acetaminophen, Chlorpheniramine Maleate, Dextromethorphan Hydrobromide, Phenylephrine Hydrochloride) McNeil Consumer ... ▣ 754
Children's Tylenol Plus Cold & Allergy Oral Suspension (Acetaminophen, Diphenhydramine Hydrochloride, Phenylephrine Hydrochloride) McNeil Consumer ... ▣ 716
Tylenol Cold Head Congestion Severe Caplets with Cool Burst (Acetaminophen, Dextromethorphan Hydrobromide, Guaifenesin, Phenylephrine Hydrochloride) McNeil Consumer ... ▣ 750
Tylenol Cold Multi-Symptom Daytime Caplets with Cool Burst and Gelcaps (Acetaminophen, Dextromethorphan Hydrobromide, Phenylephrine Hydrochloride) McNeil Consumer ... ▣ 752
Tylenol Cold Multi-Symptom NightTime Liquid with Cool Burst (Acetaminophen, Dextromethorphan Hydrobromide, Doxylamine Succinate, Phenylephrine Hydrochloride) McNeil Consumer ... ▣ 752
Tylenol Cold Multi-Symptom Severe Caplets with Cool Burst (Acetaminophen, Dextromethorphan Hydrobromide, Guaifenesin, Phenylephrine Hydrochloride) McNeil Consumer ... ▣ 752
Tylenol Cold Multi-Symptom Severe Daytime Liquid (Acetaminophen, Dextromethorphan Hydrobromide, Guaifenesin, Phenylephrine Hydrochloride) McNeil Consumer ... ▣ 752
Tylenol Cough & Sore Throat Daytime Liquid with Cool Burst (Acetaminophen, Dextromethorphan Hydrobromide) McNeil Consumer ... ▣ 790
Tylenol Cough & Sore Throat Nighttime Liquid with Cool Burst (Acetaminophen, Dextromethorphan Hydrobromide, Doxylamine Succinate) McNeil Consumer ... ▣ 790
Tylenol 8 Hour Extended Release Caplets (Acetaminophen) McNeil Consumer ... 1870
Tylenol (Acetaminophen) McNeil Consumer ... 1870
Extra Strength Tylenol Rapid Release Gels (Acetaminophen) McNeil Consumer ... 1870
Concentrated Tylenol Infants' Drops (Acetaminophen) McNeil Consumer ... ▣ 679
Concentrated Tylenol Infants' Drops Plus Cold (Acetaminophen, Phenylephrine Hydrochloride) McNeil Consumer ... ▣ 754
Concentrated Tylenol Infants' Drops Plus Cold & Cough (Acetaminophen, Dextromethorphan Hydrobromide, Phenylephrine Hydrochloride) McNeil Consumer ... ▣ 754
Jr. Tylenol Meltaways (Acetaminophen) McNeil Consumer ... ▣ 679

Tylenol Sore Throat Daytime Liquid with Cool Burst (Acetaminophen) McNeil Consumer .... ▣ 790
Tylenol Sore Throat Nighttime Liquid with Cool Burst (Acetaminophen, Diphenhydramine Hydrochloride) McNeil Consumer. ▣ 790
Tylenol Chest Congestion Caplets with Cool Burst (Acetaminophen, Guaifenesin) McNeil Consumer 1872
Tylenol Chest Congestion Liquid with Cool Burst (Acetaminophen, Guaifenesin) McNeil Consumer 1872
Children's Tylenol Suspension Liquid and Meltaways (Acetaminophen) McNeil Consumer 1878
Children's Tylenol Plus Cold Suspension Liquid (Acetaminophen, Chlorpheniramine Maleate, Phenylephrine Hydrochloride) McNeil Consumer 1879
Children's Tylenol Plus Cold & Allergy Suspension Liquid (Acetaminophen, Diphenhydramine Hydrochloride, Phenylephrine Hydrochloride) McNeil Consumer .. 1878
Children's Tylenol Plus Cough & Runny Nose Suspension Liquid (Acetaminophen, Chlorpheniramine Maleate, Dextromethorphan Hydrobromide) McNeil Consumer .. 1879
Children's Tylenol Plus Cough & Sore Throat Suspension Liquid (Acetaminophen, Dextromethorphan Hydrobromide) McNeil Consumer 1879
Children's Tylenol Suspension with Flavor Creator (Acetaminophen) McNeil Consumer 1878
Children's Tylenol Plus Flu Suspension Liquid (Acetaminophen, Chlorpheniramine Maleate, Dextromethorphan Hydrobromide, Phenylephrine Hydrochloride) McNeil Consumer 1881
Children's Tylenol Plus Multi-Symptom Cold Suspension Liquid (Acetaminophen, Chlorpheniramine Maleate, Dextromethorphan Hydrobromide, Phenylephrine Hydrochloride) McNeil Consumer 1879
Tylenol Cold Severe Congestion Non-Drowsy Caplets with Cool Burst (Acetaminophen, Dextromethorphan Hydrobromide, Guaifenesin, Pseudoephedrine Hydrochloride) McNeil Consumer .. 1874
Tylenol Cold Head Congestion Severe Caplets with Cool Burst (Acetaminophen, Dextromethorphan Hydrobromide, Guaifenesin, Phenylephrine Hydrochloride) McNeil Consumer 1873
Tylenol Cold Multi-Symptom Daytime Caplets with Cool Burst and Gelcaps (Acetaminophen, Dextromethorphan Hydrobromide, Phenylephrine Hydrochloride) McNeil Consumer 1874
Tylenol Cold Multi-Symptom Daytime Liquid with Citrus Burst (Acetaminophen, Dextromethorphan Hydrobromide, Phenylephrine Hydrochloride) McNeil Consumer 1874
Tylenol Cold Multi-Symptom Nighttime Caplets with Cool Burst (Acetaminophen, Chlorpheniramine Maleate, Dextromethorphan Hydrobromide, Phenylephrine Hydrochloride) McNeil Consumer 1874
Tylenol Cold Multi-Symptom Nighttime Liquid with Cool Burst (Acetaminophen, Dextromethorphan Hydrobromide, Doxylamine Succinate, Phenylephrine Hydrochloride) McNeil Consumer 1874
Tylenol Cold Multi-Symptom Severe Caplets with Cool Burst (Acetaminophen, Dextromethorphan Hydrobromide, Guaifenesin, Phenylephrine Hydrochloride) McNeil Consumer 1874
Tylenol Cold Multi-Symptom Severe Daytime Liquid with Citrus Burst (Acetaminophen, Dextromethorphan Hydrobromide, Guaifenesin, Phenylephrine Hydrochloride) McNeil Consumer 1874
Concentrated Tylenol Infants' Drops (Acetaminophen) McNeil Consumer 1878
Concentrated Tylenol Infants' Drops Plus Cold (Acetaminophen) McNeil Consumer 1879
Concentrated Tylenol Infants' Drops Plus Cold and Cough (Acetaminophen, Dextromethorphan Hydrobromide) McNeil Consumer.................................... 1879
Jr. Tylenol Meltaways (Acetaminophen) McNeil Consumer 1878
Tylenol Sore Throat Daytime Liquid with Cool Burst (Acetaminophen) McNeil Consumer 1877
Tylenol Sore Throat Nighttime Liquid with Cool Burst (Acetaminophen, Diphenhydramine) McNeil Consumer 1877
Vicks 44M Cough, Cold & Flu Relief Liquid (Acetaminophen, Chlorpheniramine Maleate, Dextromethorphan Hydrobromide, Pseudoephedrine Hydrochloride) Procter & Gamble 2680
Vicks DayQuil LiquiCaps/Liquid Multi-Symptom Cold/Flu Relief (Acetaminophen, Dextromethorphan Hydrobromide, Phenylephrine Hydrochloride) Procter & Gamble .... ▣ 761
Vicks DayQuil Multi-Symptom Cold/Flu Relief Liquid (Acetaminophen, Dextromethorphan Hydrobromide, Pseudoephedrine Hydrochloride) Procter & Gamble .. 2678
Vicks DayQuil Multi-Symptom Cold/Flu Relief LiquiCaps (Acetaminophen, Dextromethorphan Hydrobromide, Pseudoephedrine Hydrochloride) Procter & Gamble .. 2678
Zicam Maximum Strength Flu Daytime (Acetaminophen, Chlorpheniramine Maleate, Dextromethorphan Hydrobromide) Matrixx .... ▣ 768
Zicam Maximum Strength Flu Nighttime (Acetaminophen, Dextromethorphan Hydrobromide, Doxylamine Succinate) Matrixx .... ▣ 768

Fever associated with common cold
Advil Allergy Sinus Caplets (Chlorpheniramine Maleate, Ibuprofen, Pseudoephedrine Hydrochloride) Wyeth .... ▣ 770
Advil Cold & Sinus (Ibuprofen, Pseudoephedrine Hydrochloride) Wyeth .... ▣ 723
Advil Multi-Symptom Cold Caplets (Chlorpheniramine Maleate, Ibuprofen, Pseudoephedrine Hydrochloride) Wyeth .... ▣ 770
BC Cold Powder (Aspirin, Chlorpheniramine Maleate, Pseudoephedrine Hydrochloride) GlaxoSmithKline .... ▣ 677
Children's Motrin Cold Oral Suspension (Ibuprofen, Pseudoephedrine Hydrochloride) McNeil Consumer 1867
Triaminic Cough & Sore Throat Liquid (Acetaminophen, Dextromethorphan Hydrobromide) Novartis Consumer .... ▣ 747
Children's Tylenol Plus Cold Suspension Liquid (Acetaminophen, Chlorpheniramine Maleate, Phenylephrine Hydrochloride) McNeil Consumer 1879
Tylenol Cold Multi-Symptom Daytime Liquid with Citrus Burst (Acetaminophen, Dextromethorphan Hydrobromide, Phenylephrine Hydrochloride) McNeil Consumer 1874
Tylenol Cold Multi-Symptom Nighttime Liquid with Cool Burst (Acetaminophen, Dextromethorphan Hydrobromide, Doxylamine Succinate, Phenylephrine Hydrochloride) McNeil Consumer 1874
Tylenol Cold Multi-Symptom Severe Caplets with Cool Burst (Acetaminophen, Dextromethorphan Hydrobromide, Guaifenesin, Phenylephrine Hydrochloride) McNeil Consumer 1874
Tylenol Cold Multi-Symptom Severe Daytime Liquid with Citrus Burst (Acetaminophen, Dextromethorphan Hydrobromide, Guaifenesin, Phenylephrine Hydrochloride) McNeil Consumer 1874
Concentrated Tylenol Infants' Drops Plus Cold (Acetaminophen) McNeil Consumer 1879
Concentrated Tylenol Infants' Drops Plus Cold and Cough (Acetaminophen, Dextromethorphan Hydrobromide) McNeil Consumer.................................... 1879
Vicks NyQuil LiquiCaps/Liquid Multi-Symptom Cold/Flu Relief (Acetaminophen, Dextromethorphan Hydrobromide, Doxylamine Succinate) Procter & Gamble ...... ▣ 763

Fever blisters
(*see under* Herpetic manifestations, oral, symptomatic relief of)

Fiber, deficiency of
Metamucil Dietary Fiber Supplement (Psyllium Preparations) Procter & Gamble .... ▣ 650

Flatulence, relief of
Gas-X Extra Strength (Simethicone) Novartis Consumer .... ▣ 656
Gas-X Maximum Strength Softgels (Simethicone) Novartis Consumer .... ▣ 656
Gas-X with Maalox (Calcium Carbonate, Simethicone) Novartis Consumer .... ▣ 656
Gas-X Regular Strength Chewable Tablets (Simethicone) Novartis Consumer .... ▣ 656
Maalox Regular Strength Antacid/Antigas Liquid (Aluminum Hydroxide, Magnesium Hydroxide, Simethicone) Novartis Consumer 2175
Maalox Max Maximum Strength Antacid/Anti-Gas Liquid (Aluminum Hydroxide, Magnesium Hydroxide, Simethicone) Novartis Consumer 2176
Phazyme-125 mg Quick Dissolve Chewable Tablets (Simethicone) GlaxoSmithKline .... ▣ 657
Phazyme-180 mg Ultra Strength Softgels (Simethicone) GlaxoSmithKline .... ▣ 657

Flu symptoms
(*see under* Influenza syndrome, symptomatic relief of)

Folic acid deficiency, prevention of
Slow Fe with Folic Acid Tablets (Ferrous Sulfate, Folic Acid) Novartis Consumer .... ▣ 819

Folliculitis barbae
Gris-PEG Tablets (Griseofulvin) Pedinol 2502

Fungal infections, skin
(*see under* Infections, mycotic, cutaneous)

Furunculosis
Levaquin (Levofloxacin) Ortho-McNeil 2384
Levaquin in 5% Dextrose Injection (Levofloxacin) Ortho-McNeil 2384

Furunculosis, symptomatic relief of
Panafil Ointment (Chlorophyllin Copper Complex Sodium, Papain, Urea) Healthpoint 1663
Panafil SE Spray Emulsion (Chlorophyllin Copper Complex Sodium, Papain, Urea) Healthpoint 1663

Fusarium solani infections
VFEND I.V. (Voriconazole) Pfizer 2564
VFEND Oral Suspension (Voriconazole) Pfizer 2564
VFEND Tablets (Voriconazole) Pfizer 2564

Fusobacterium species infections
Primaxin I.M. (Cilastatin Sodium, Imipenem) Merck 2045
Primaxin I.V. (Cilastatin Sodium, Imipenem) Merck 2048

Fusobacterium species intra-abdominal infections
Primaxin I.M. (Cilastatin Sodium, Imipenem) Merck 2045

Fusobacterium species skin and skin structure infections
Primaxin I.V. (Cilastatin Sodium, Imipenem) Merck 2048

G

Gag reflex, suppression
Cetacaine Topical Anesthetic (Benzocaine, Butyl Aminobenzoate, Tetracaine Hydrochloride) Cetylite 999

Gardnerella vaginalis infections
MetroGel-Vaginal Gel (Metronidazole) 3M 1855
Primaxin I.V. (Cilastatin Sodium, Imipenem) Merck 2048

Gardnerella vaginalis vaginitis
(*see under* H. vaginalis vaginitis)

Gas
Gas-X Extra Strength Thin Strips (Simethicone) Novartis Consumer .... ▣ 657
Imodium Advanced Caplets and Chewable Tablets McNeil Consumer .... ▣ 655
Maalox Regular Strength Antacid/Anti-Gas Liquid (Aluminum Hydroxide, Magnesium Hydroxide, Simethicone) Novartis Consumer .... ▣ 660
Maalox Max Maximum Strength Antacid/Anti-Gas Liquid (Aluminum Hydroxide, Magnesium Hydroxide, Simethicone) Novartis Consumer .... ▣ 659
Maalox Maximum Strength Total Stomach Relief Strawberry Liquid (Bismuth Subsalicylate) Novartis Consumer .... ▣ 672
Maalox Max Maximum Strength Chewable Tablets (Calcium Carbonate, Simethicone) Novartis Consumer .... ▣ 660

Gastric ulcer, nonsteroidal anti-inflammatory drug induced
Prevacid Delayed-Release Capsules (Lansoprazole) TAP 3271
Prevacid for Delayed-Release Oral Suspension (Lansoprazole) TAP..... 3271
Prevacid SoluTab Delayed-Release Orally Disintegrating Tablets (Lansoprazole) TAP 3271

Gastric ulcer, NSAID-associated, risk reductions
Nexium Delayed-Release Capsules (Esomeprazole Magnesium) AstraZeneca LP 655

Gastric ulcers, active, benign, short-term treatment of
Axid Oral Solution (Nizatidine) Braintree 879
Pepcid Injection (Famotidine) Merck . 2040
Pepcid (Famotidine) Merck............... 2038
Prevacid Delayed-Release Capsules (Lansoprazole) TAP 3271
Prevacid for Delayed-Release Oral Suspension (Lansoprazole) TAP..... 3271
Prevacid SoluTab Delayed-Release Orally Disintegrating Tablets (Lansoprazole) TAP 3271
Zantac (Ranitidine Hydrochloride) GlaxoSmithKline 1624
Zegerid Capsules (Omeprazole) Santarus.. 2958
Zegerid Powder for Oral Solution (Omeprazole) Santarus 2958

Gastric ulcers, nonsteroidal anti-inflammatory drug-induced, prevention of
Prevacid NapraPAC (Lansoprazole, Naproxen) TAP................................ 3280

Gastroenteritis, rotavirus, prevention of
RotaTeq (Rotavirus vaccine, live, oral, pentavalent) Merck ... 2074

Gastroesophageal reflux, symptomatic
Zegerid Capsules (Omeprazole) Santarus ... 2958
Zegerid Powder for Oral Solution (Omeprazole) Santarus ... 2958

Gastroesophageal reflux disease
Aciphex Tablets (Rabeprazole Sodium) Eisai ... 1090
Axid Oral Solution (Nizatidine) Braintree ... 879
Nexium Delayed-Release Capsules (Esomeprazole Magnesium) AstraZeneca LP ... 655
Nexium I.V. (Esomeprazole Sodium) AstraZeneca LP ... 659
Pepcid Injection (Famotidine) Merck . 2040
Pepcid (Famotidine) Merck ... 2038
Prevacid Delayed-Release Capsules (Lansoprazole) TAP ... 3271
Prevacid for Delayed-Release Oral Suspension (Lansoprazole) TAP ... 3271
Prevacid SoluTab Delayed-Release Orally Disintegrating Tablets (Lansoprazole) TAP ... 3271
Protonix I.V. (Pantoprazole Sodium) Wyeth ... 3472
Protonix Tablets (Pantoprazole Sodium) Wyeth ... 3469
Zantac (Ranitidine Hydrochloride) GlaxoSmithKline ... 1624
Zegerid Capsules (Omeprazole) Santarus ... 2958
Zegerid Powder for Oral Solution (Omeprazole) Santarus ... 2958

Gastrointestinal stromal tumors
(*see under* Tumors, gastrointestinal stromal)

Gaucher disease, Type 1
Cerezyme for Injection (Imiglucerase) Genzyme ... 1270

Gelineau's syndrome
(*see under* Narcolepsy)

Genital warts
(*see under* Condylomata acuminata)

GERD
(*see under* Gastroesophageal reflux disease)

German measles
(*see under* Rubella, prophylaxis)

Gestational trophoblastic neoplasia
Cosmegen for Injection (Dactinomycin) Ovation ... 2459

Giardiasis
Tindamax Tablets (Tinidazole) Mission ... 2142

GIST
(*see under* Tumors, gastrointestinal stromal)

Glaucoma, angle-closure, acute
Daranide Tablets (Dichlorphenamide) Merck ... 1950

Glaucoma, chronic open-angle
Betagan Ophthalmic Solution, USP (Levobunolol Hydrochloride) Allergan ... ⊙220
Betoptic S Ophthalmic Suspension (Betaxolol Hydrochloride) Alcon ... 558
Carteolol Hydrochloride Ophthalmic Solution USP, 1% (Carteolol Hydrochloride) Bausch & Lomb ... ⊙249
Daranide Tablets (Dichlorphenamide) Merck ... 1950
OptiPranolol Metipranolol Ophthalmic Solution 0.3% (Metipranolol) Bausch & Lomb ... ⊙256
Propine Ophthalmic Solution (Dipivefrin Hydrochloride) Allergan ... ⊙239
Timoptic Sterile Ophthalmic Solution (Timolol Maleate) Merck ... 2088
Timoptic in Ocudose (Timolol Maleate) Merck ... 2091
Timoptic-XE Sterile Ophthalmic Gel Forming Solution (Timolol Maleate) Merck ... 2092

Glaucoma, open-angle
Alphagan P Ophthalmic Solution (Brimonidine Tartrate) Allergan ... 567
Azopt Ophthalmic Suspension (Brinzolamide) Alcon ... 557
Brimonidine Tartrate Ophthalmic Solution 0.2% (Brimonidine Tartrate) Bausch & Lomb ... ⊙248
Cosopt Sterile Ophthalmic Solution (Dorzolamide Hydrochloride, Timolol Maleate) Merck ... 1931
Lumigan Ophthalmic Solution (Bimatoprost) Allergan ... 573
Travatan Ophthalmic Solution (Travoprost) Alcon ... 563
Trusopt Sterile Ophthalmic Solution (Dorzolamide Hydrochloride) Merck ... 2095
Xalatan Sterile Ophthalmic Solution (Latanoprost) Pharmacia & Upjohn ... 2649

Glaucoma, secondary
Daranide Tablets (Dichlorphenamide) Merck ... 1950

Glioblastoma multiforme
Temodar Capsules (Temozolomide) Schering ... 3073

Goiter, euthyroid, treatment or prevention of
Naturethroid Tablets (Levothyroxine, Liothyronine) Western Research ... 3401
Synthroid Tablets (Levothyroxine Sodium) Abbott ... 520
Thyrolar Tablets (Liotrix) Forest ... 1199
Westhroid Tablets (Levothyroxine Sodium, Liothyronine Sodium) Western Research ... 3403

Goiter, suppression of pituitary TSH in
Cytomel Tablets (Liothyronine Sodium) King ... 1710
Levothroid Tablets (Levothyroxine Sodium) Forest ... 1186
Levoxyl Tablets (Levothyroxine Sodium) King ... 1712
Naturethroid Tablets (Levothyroxine, Liothyronine) Western Research ... 3401
Synthroid Tablets (Levothyroxine Sodium) Abbott ... 520
Thyrolar Tablets (Liotrix) Forest ... 1199
Westhroid Tablets (Levothyroxine Sodium, Liothyronine Sodium) Western Research ... 3403

Gonococcal infections, uncomplicated
Rocephin Injectable Vials, ADD-Vantage, Galaxy, Bulk (Ceftriaxone Sodium) Roche ... 2800
Vantin Tablets and Oral Suspension (Cefpodoxime Proxetil) Pharmacia & Upjohn ... 2645
Zinacef for Injection (Cefuroxime) GlaxoSmithKline ... 1631
Zinacef Injection (Cefuroxime) GlaxoSmithKline ... 1631

Gonorrhea
(*see also under* N. gonorrhoeae infections)
Amoxil Capsules (Amoxicillin) GlaxoSmithKline ... 1343
Amoxil Chewable Tablets (Amoxicillin) GlaxoSmithKline ... 1343
Amoxil Pediatric Drops for Oral Suspension (Amoxicillin) GlaxoSmithKline ... 1343
Amoxil Powder for Oral Suspension (Amoxicillin) GlaxoSmithKline ... 1343
Amoxil Tablets (Amoxicillin) GlaxoSmithKline ... 1343
Rocephin Injectable Vials, ADD-Vantage, Galaxy, Bulk (Ceftriaxone Sodium) Roche ... 2800
Zinacef for Injection (Cefuroxime) GlaxoSmithKline ... 1631
Zinacef Injection (Cefuroxime) GlaxoSmithKline ... 1631

Gonorrhea, cervical/urethral
Cipro (Ciprofloxacin) Schering ... 2977
Noroxin Tablets (Norfloxacin) Merck . 2032
Rocephin Injectable Vials, ADD-Vantage, Galaxy, Bulk (Ceftriaxone Sodium) Roche ... 2800
Vantin Tablets and Oral Suspension (Cefpodoxime Proxetil) Pharmacia & Upjohn ... 2645

Gonorrhea, pharyngeal
Rocephin (Ceftriaxone Sodium) Roche ... 2800

Gonorrhea, rectal
Rocephin Injectable Vials, ADD-Vantage, Galaxy, Bulk (Ceftriaxone Sodium) Roche ... 2800

Gonorrhea, uncomplicated
Ceftin Tablets (Cefuroxime Axetil) GlaxoSmithKline ... 1407
Cipro (Ciprofloxacin) Schering ... 2977
Noroxin Tablets (Norfloxacin) Merck . 2032
Rocephin Injectable Vials, ADD-Vantage, Galaxy, Bulk (Ceftriaxone Sodium) Roche ... 2800

Gout, acute
Anaprox Tablets (Naproxen Sodium) Roche ... 2761
Anaprox DS Tablets (Naproxen Sodium) Roche ... 2761
Naprosyn Suspension (Naproxen) Roche ... 2761
Naprosyn Tablets (Naproxen) Roche ... 2761

Grand mal epilepsy
(*see under* Seizures, generalized, tonic-clonic)

Granuloma annulare, infiltrated inflammatory lesions of
Depo-Medrol Single-Dose Vial (Methylprednisolone Acetate) Pharmacia & Upjohn ... 2619

Granulomatous disease, chronic
Actimmune (Interferon Gamma-1B) InterMune ... 1671

Growth, in children, stimulation of
Increlex Injection (Mecasermin [rDNA origin]) Tercica ... 3291

Growth failure, chronic renal insufficiency-induced in children
Nutropin for Injection (Somatropin) Genentech ... 1239
Nutropin AQ Injection (Somatropin) Genentech ... 1243
Nutropin AQ Pen (Somatropin) Genentech ... 1243
Nutropin AQ Pen Cartridge (Somatropin) Genentech ... 1243

Growth hormone secretion, evaluation of the secreting capability of
R-Gene 10 for Intravenous Use (Arginine Hydrochloride) Pharmacia & Upjohn ... 2641

Growth hormone secretion, inadequate
Genotropin Lyophilized Powder (Somatropin) Pharmacia & Upjohn ... 2638
Humatrope Vials and Cartridges (Somatropin) Lilly ... 1787
Norditropin Cartridges (Somatropin) Novo Nordisk ... 2323
Nutropin for Injection (Somatropin) Genentech ... 1239
Nutropin AQ Injection (Somatropin) Genentech ... 1243
Nutropin AQ Pen (Somatropin) Genentech ... 1243
Nutropin AQ Pen Cartridge (Somatropin) Genentech ... 1243
Tev-Tropin for Injection (Somatropin (rDNA Origin)) Gate ... 1222

Gums, sore
(*see under* Pain, dental)

H

H. aegypticus infections, ocular
TobraDex Ophthalmic Ointment (Dexamethasone, Tobramycin) Alcon ... 562
TobraDex Ophthalmic Suspension (Dexamethasone, Tobramycin) Alcon ... 563

H. influenzae, central nervous system infections
Fortaz (Ceftazidime) GlaxoSmithKline ... 1453

H. influenzae bronchitis
Avelox (Moxifloxacin Hydrochloride) Schering ... 2970
Biaxin/Biaxin XL (Clarithromycin) Abbott ... 402
Ceftin Tablets (Cefuroxime Axetil) GlaxoSmithKline ... 1407
Ketek Tablets (Telithromycin) sanofi-aventis ... 2903
Levaquin (Levofloxacin) Ortho-McNeil ... 2384
Levaquin in 5% Dextrose Injection (Levofloxacin) Ortho-McNeil ... 2384
Omnicef Capsules (Cefdinir) Abbott .. 511
Omnicef for Oral Suspension (Cefdinir) Abbott ... 511
Tequin Injection (Gatifloxacin) Bristol-Myers Squibb ... 938
Tequin Injection in 5% Dextrose (Gatifloxacin) Bristol-Myers Squibb ... 938
Tequin Tablets (Gatifloxacin) Bristol-Myers Squibb ... 938
Vantin Tablets and Oral Suspension (Cefpodoxime Proxetil) Pharmacia & Upjohn ... 2645

H. influenzae infections
Amoxil Capsules (Amoxicillin) GlaxoSmithKline ... 1343
Amoxil Chewable Tablets (Amoxicillin) GlaxoSmithKline ... 1343
Amoxil Pediatric Drops for Oral Suspension (Amoxicillin) GlaxoSmithKline ... 1343
Amoxil Powder for Oral Suspension (Amoxicillin) GlaxoSmithKline ... 1343
Amoxil Tablets (Amoxicillin) GlaxoSmithKline ... 1343
Augmentin (Amoxicillin, Clavulanate Potassium) GlaxoSmithKline ... 1360
Augmentin Tablets (Amoxicillin, Clavulanate Potassium) GlaxoSmithKline ... 1363
Augmentin XR Extended-Release Tablets (Amoxicillin, Clavulanate Potassium) GlaxoSmithKline ... 1369
Augmentin ES-600 Powder for Oral Suspension (Amoxicillin, Clavulanate Potassium) GlaxoSmithKline ... 1366
Avelox (Moxifloxacin Hydrochloride) Schering ... 2970
Biaxin/Biaxin XL (Clarithromycin) Abbott ... 402
Ceftin (Cefuroxime Axetil) GlaxoSmithKline ... 1407
Cipro (Ciprofloxacin) Schering ... 2977
Cipro I.V. (Ciprofloxacin) Schering ... 2984
E.E.S. (Erythromycin Ethylsuccinate) Abbott ... 451
EryPed (Erythromycin Ethylsuccinate) Abbott ... 447
Ery-Tab Tablets (Erythromycin) Abbott ... 449
Erythrocin Stearate Filmtab Tablets (Erythromycin Stearate) Abbott ... 453
Erythromycin Base Filmtab Tablets (Erythromycin) Abbott ... 455
Erythromycin Delayed-Release Capsules, USP (Erythromycin) Abbott ... 457
Fortaz (Ceftazidime) GlaxoSmithKline ... 1453
Invanz for Injection (Ertapenem) Merck ... 1999
Levaquin (Levofloxacin) Ortho-McNeil ... 2384
Levaquin in 5% Dextrose Injection (Levofloxacin) Ortho-McNeil ... 2384

Headache, cluster

Headache, migraine

Headache, migraine, prophylaxis of

Headache, sinus, symptomatic relief of

Headache, vascular

Headache accompanied by insomnia

Headache associated with common cold

Heart, allogeneic transplants, prophylaxis of organ rejection in
CellCept Capsules (Mycophenolate Mofetil) Roche 2747
CellCept Intravenous (Mycophenolate Mofetil Hydrochloride) Roche .. 2747
CellCept Oral Suspension (Mycophenolate Mofetil) Roche 2747
CellCept Tablets (Mycophenolate Mofetil) Roche 2747
Gengraf Capsules (Cyclosporine) Abbott 459
Neoral Oral Solution (Cyclosporine) Novartis 2259
Neoral Soft Gelatin Capsules (Cyclosporine) Novartis 2259
Orthoclone OKT3 Sterile Solution (Muromonab-CD3) Ortho Biotech ... 2360
Prograf Capsules and Injection (Tacrolimus) Astellas 632
Sandimmune (Cyclosporine) Novartis 2275

Heart failure
(*see under* Congestive heart failure, adjunct in)

Heart failure, congestive
(*see under* Congestive heart failure, adjunct in)

Heart failure, NYHA Class II - IV
Atacand Tablets (Candesartan Cilexetil) AstraZeneca LP 649
Diovan Tablets (Valsartan) Novartis .. 2193
Toprol-XL Tablets (Metoprolol Succinate) AstraZeneca LP 668

Heartburn
(*see under* Hyperacidity, gastric, symptomatic relief of)

Hematopoietic progenitor cells, mobilization of
Neupogen for Injection (Filgrastim) Amgen 603

Hemodialysis, adjunct in
Albutein 5%, Albumin (Human) (Albumin (human)) Grifols 1652
Albutein 25% , Albumin (Human) (Albumin (human)) Grifols 1653

Hemolytic disease, newborn
Flexbumin I.V. (Albumin (human)) Baxter Healthcare 720
Plasbumin-20 (Albumin (human)) Talecris 3252

Hemolytic disease, Rh, prevention of
(*see under* Erythroblastosis fetalis, prevention of)

Hemolytic disease, unspecified
Plasbumin-20 (Albumin (human)) Talecris 3252
Plasbumin-25 (Albumin (human)) Talecris 3253

Hemophilia A
Advate Injection (Antihemophilic Factor (Recombinant)) Baxter Healthcare 712
Hemofil M (Antihemophilic Factor (Human)) Baxter Healthcare 728
Koāte-DVI (Antihemophilic Factor (Human)) Talecris 3250
Kogenate FS (Antihemophilic Factor (Recombinant)) Bayer Healthcare LLC 738
Kogenate FS with Bio-Set (Antihemophilic Factor (Recombinant)) Bayer Healthcare LLC 740
Recombinate (Antihemophilic Factor (Recombinant)) Baxter Healthcare 729
ReFacto Vials (Antihemophilic Factor (Recombinant)) Wyeth 3484

Hemophilia A, perioperative management of
Advate Injection (Antihemophilic Factor (Recombinant)) Baxter Healthcare 712

Hemophilia A with Factor VIII inhibitors
Alphanate, Antihemophilic Factor (Human) (Antihemophilic Factor (Human), Factor VIII (AHF, AHG)) Grifols 1654

Hemophilia B
BeneFix Vials (Antihemophilic Factor (Recombinant)) Wyeth 3408
NovoSeven (Antihemophilic Factor (Recombinant)) Novo Nordisk 2331

Hemorrhage, subarachnoid, resulting in neurological deficits
Nimotop Capsules (Nimodipine) Bayer 749

Hemorrhoids
Preparation H Maximum Strength Cream (Glycerin, Petrolatum, Phenylephrine Hydrochloride, Pramoxine Hydrochloride) Wyeth . ■ 666
Preparation H Cooling Gel (Phenylephrine Hydrochloride) Wyeth ...... ■ 666
Preparation H (Mineral Oil, Petrolatum, Phenylephrine Hydrochloride, Shark Liver Oil) Wyeth .... ■ 666
Preparation H Medicated Wipes (Witch Hazel) Wyeth .... ■ 667

Hemostasis, an aid in
Trasylol Injection (Aprotinin) Bayer 754

Hepatitis A, prophylaxis
GamaSTAN (Globulin, Immune (Human)) Talecris 3234

Hepatitis A virus, immunization against
(*see also under* Hepatitis A virus vaccine; Immunization, hepatitis A and B virus; Immunization, hepatitis A virus)
Havrix Vaccine (Hepatitis A Vaccine, Inactivated) GlaxoSmithKline 1456
Twinrix Vaccine (Hepatitis A Vaccine, Inactivated, Hepatitis B Vaccine, Recombinant) GlaxoSmithKline 1595
Vaqta (Hepatitis A Vaccine, Inactivated) Merck 2097

Hepatitis A virus vaccine
(*see also under* Hepatitis A virus, immunization against; Immunization, hepatitis A and B virus; Immunization, hepatitis A virus)
Havrix Vaccine (Hepatitis A Vaccine, Inactivated) GlaxoSmithKline 1456
Twinrix Vaccine (Hepatitis A Vaccine, Inactivated, Hepatitis B Vaccine, Recombinant) GlaxoSmithKline 1595
Vaqta (Hepatitis A Vaccine, Inactivated) Merck 2097

Hepatitis B, chronic
Baraclude (Entecavir) Bristol-Myers Squibb 894
Epivir-HBV (Lamivudine) GlaxoSmithKline 1432
Hepsera Tablets (Adefovir dipivoxil) Gilead 1292
Intron A for Injection (Interferon alfa-2b, Recombinant) Schering 3024
Pegasys (Peginterferon alfa-2a) Roche 2789

Hepatitis B virus, immunization against
(*see also under* Immunization, haemophilus influenzae type B and hepatitis B virus; Immunization, hepatitis A and B virus)
Comvax (Haemophilus B Conjugate Vaccine, Hepatitis B Vaccine, Recombinant) Merck 1928
Engerix-B Vaccine (Hepatitis B Vaccine, Recombinant) GlaxoSmithKline 1425
Pediarix Vaccine (Diphtheria & Tetanus Toxoids and Pertussis Vaccine Adsorbed, Hepatitis B Vaccine, Recombinant, Poliovirus Vaccine Inactivated, Trivalent Types 1,2,3) GlaxoSmithKline 1548
Recombivax HB (Hepatitis B Vaccine, Recombinant) Merck 2071
Twinrix Vaccine (Hepatitis A Vaccine, Inactivated, Hepatitis B Vaccine, Recombinant) GlaxoSmithKline 1595

Hepatitis B virus, postexposure prophylaxis
HyperHep B S/D (Hepatitis B Immune Globulin (Human)) Talecris 3240
Nabi-HB (Hepatitis B Immune Globulin (Human)) Nabi 2169

Hepatitis B virus vaccine
(*see also under* Haemophilus influenzae type b, immunization against; Haemophilus influenzae type b vaccine; Hepatitis B virus, immunization against; Immunization, haemophilus influenzae type B and hepatitis B virus; Immunization, hepatitis A and B virus; Immunization, hepatitis B virus)
Comvax (Haemophilus B Conjugate Vaccine, Hepatitis B Vaccine, Recombinant) Merck 1928
Engerix-B Vaccine (Hepatitis B Vaccine, Recombinant) GlaxoSmithKline 1425
Pediarix Vaccine (Diphtheria & Tetanus Toxoids and Pertussis Vaccine Adsorbed, Hepatitis B Vaccine, Recombinant, Poliovirus Vaccine Inactivated, Trivalent Types 1,2,3) GlaxoSmithKline 1548
Recombivax HB (Hepatitis B Vaccine, Recombinant) Merck 2071
Twinrix Vaccine (Hepatitis A Vaccine, Inactivated, Hepatitis B Vaccine, Recombinant) GlaxoSmithKline 1595

Hepatitis C, chronic
Copegus Tablets (Ribavirin) Roche ... 2754
Infergen (Interferon Alfacon-1) Valeant North America 3364
Intron A for Injection (Interferon alfa-2b, Recombinant) Schering 3024
Pegasys (Peginterferon alfa-2a) Roche 2789
PEG-Intron Powder for Injection (Peginterferon Alfa-2b) Schering 3048
Rebetol (Ribavirin) Schering 3058
Rebetron Combination Therapy (Interferon alfa-2b, Recombinant, Ribavirin) Schering 3063
Ribavirin, USP Capsules (Ribavirin) Schering 3068

Hepatitis C, chronic, HIV co-infection
Copegus Tablets (Ribavirin) Roche ... 2754

Herellea vaginicola
(*see under* Acinetobacter calcoaceticus infections, ocular)

Herpes, genital, initial and recurrent episodes
Famvir Tablets (Famciclovir) Novartis 2211
Zovirax (Acyclovir) GlaxoSmithKline .. 1643

Herpes genitalis
Valtrex Caplets (Valacyclovir Hydrochloride) GlaxoSmithKline 1597
Zovirax Capsules (Acyclovir) GlaxoSmithKline 1643
Zovirax Cream (Acyclovir) Biovail 820
Zovirax Ointment (Acyclovir) Biovail .. 821
Zovirax (Acyclovir) GlaxoSmithKline .. 1643

Herpes labialis
Valtrex Caplets (Valacyclovir Hydrochloride) GlaxoSmithKline 1597

Herpes labialis, recurrent
Famvir Tablets (Famciclovir) Novartis 2211
Zovirax Cream (Acyclovir) Biovail 820

Herpes simplex keratitis
Viroptic Ophthalmic Solution (Trifluridine) King .... ⊙ 266

Herpes simplex virus infections
Denavir Cream (Penciclovir) Novartis Consumer 2174
Famvir Tablets (Famciclovir) Novartis 2211
Zovirax Cream (Acyclovir) Biovail 820
Zovirax Ointment (Acyclovir) Biovail .. 821

Herpes simplex virus mucocutaneous infection
Famvir Tablets (Famciclovir) Novartis 2211
Zovirax Cream (Acyclovir) Biovail 820
Zovirax Ointment (Acyclovir) Biovail .. 821

Herpes zoster, prevention of
Zostavax Injection (Zoster Vaccine Live) Merck 2111

Herpes zoster infections
Famvir Tablets (Famciclovir) Novartis 2211
Valtrex Caplets (Valacyclovir Hydrochloride) GlaxoSmithKline 1597
Zovirax (Acyclovir) GlaxoSmithKline .. 1643

Herpes zoster ophthalmicus
Depo-Medrol Injectable Suspension (Methylprednisolone Acetate) Pharmacia & Upjohn 2617
Hydrocortone Tablets (Hydrocortisone) Merck 1989

Herpetic manifestations, oral, symptomatic relief of
(*see also under* Herpes simplex virus infections)
Abreva Cream (Docosanol) GlaxoSmithKline .... ■ 710
Anbesol Cold Sore Therapy Ointment (Allantoin, Benzocaine, Camphor, Petrolatum, White) Wyeth .... ■ 710
Denavir Cream (Penciclovir) Novartis Consumer 2174
Valtrex Caplets (Valacyclovir Hydrochloride) GlaxoSmithKline 1597

HIV Infection
(*see under* Infections, human immunodeficiency virus)

Hodgkin's disease
Leukeran Tablets (Chlorambucil) GlaxoSmithKline 1504

Hodgkin's disease, adjunctive therapy in
Leukine (Sargramostim) Berlex 814

Hodgkin's disease, stages III and IV, palliative treatment of
Matulane Capsules (Procarbazine Hydrochloride) Sigma-Tau 3191
Mustargen for Injection (Mechlorethamine Hydrochloride) Ovation ... 2468

Hookworm, American
(*see under* Necator americanus infections)

Hookworm infections
(*see under* Ancylostoma duodenale infections)

Horton's headache
(*see under* Cephalalgia, histaminic)

Hot flashes
Peridin-C Vitamin C Supplement (Bioflavonoids, Hesperidin Complex, Hesperidin Methyl Chalcone, Vitamin C) Beutlich .... ■ 818

Human papillomavirus vaccine
Gardasil Injection (Quadrivalent Human Papillomavirus (Types 6, 11, 16, 18) Recombinant Vaccine) Merck 1984

Hydatid disease, cystic
Albenza Tablets (Albendazole) GlaxoSmithKline 1338

Hyperacidity, gastric, symptomatic relief of
- Gas-X with Maalox (Calcium Carbonate, Simethicone) Novartis Consumer ■ 656
- Gaviscon Regular Strength Liquid (Aluminum Hydroxide, Magnesium Carbonate) GlaxoSmithKline ■ 658
- Gaviscon Regular Strength Tablets (Aluminum Hydroxide, Magnesium Trisilicate) GlaxoSmithKline ■ 658
- Gaviscon Extra Strength Liquid (Aluminum Hydroxide, Magnesium Carbonate) GlaxoSmithKline ■ 658
- Gaviscon Extra Strength Tablets (Aluminum Hydroxide, Magnesium Carbonate) GlaxoSmithKline ■ 658
- Maalox Regular Strength Antacid/Anti-Gas Liquid (Aluminum Hydroxide, Magnesium Hydroxide, Simethicone) Novartis Consumer ■ 660
- Maalox Regular Strength Antacid/Antigas Liquid (Aluminum Hydroxide, Magnesium Hydroxide, Simethicone) Novartis Consumer 2175
- Maalox Regular Strength Antacid Chewable Tablets (Calcium Carbonate) Novartis Consumer 2177
- Maalox Max Maximum Strength Antacid/Anti-Gas Liquid (Aluminum Hydroxide, Magnesium Hydroxide, Simethicone) Novartis Consumer ■ 659
- Maalox Maximum Strength Total Stomach Relief Peppermint Liquid (Bismuth Subsalicylate) Novartis Consumer ■ 660
- Maalox Maximum Strength Total Stomach Relief Strawberry Liquid (Bismuth Subsalicylate) Novartis Consumer ■ 672
- Maalox Regular Strength Antacid Chewable Tablets Novartis Consumer ■ 659
- Maalox Max Maximum Strength Antacid/Antigas Chewable Tablets (Calcium Carbonate) Novartis Consumer 2176
- Maalox Max Maximum Strength Chewable Tablets (Calcium Carbonate, Simethicone) Novartis Consumer ■ 660
- Maalox Max Maximum Strength Antacid/Anti-Gas Liquid (Aluminum Hydroxide, Magnesium Hydroxide, Simethicone) Novartis Consumer 2176
- Nexium Delayed-Release Capsules (Esomeprazole Magnesium) AstraZeneca LP 655
- Pepcid AC Tablets and Gelcaps (Famotidine) J&J – Merck ■ 661
- Maximum Strength Pepcid AC Tablets (Famotidine) J&J – Merck ■ 661
- Pepcid Complete Chewable Tablets (Calcium Carbonate, Famotidine, Magnesium Hydroxide) J&J – Merck ■ 662
- Pepcid AC Gelcaps (Famotidine) J&J – Merck 1701
- Pepcid AC Tablets (Famotidine) J&J – Merck 1701
- Maximum Strength Pepcid AC Tablets (Famotidine) J&J – Merck 1701
- Pepcid Complete Chewable Tablets (Calcium Carbonate, Famotidine, Magnesium Hydroxide) J&J – Merck 1701
- Children's Pepto (Calcium Carbonate) Procter & Gamble 2674
- Prilosec OTC Delayed-Release Tablets (Omeprazole magnesium) Procter & Gamble 2677
- Tagamet HB 200 Tablets (Cimetidine) GlaxoSmithKline ■ 664
- Tums (Calcium Carbonate) GlaxoSmithKline ■ 664

Hyperbetalipoproteinemia
(*see under* Hyperlipoproteinemia, types IIa and IIb, adjunct to diet)

Hyperbilirubinemia, neonatal
- Albutein 25% , Albumin (Human) (Albumin (human)) Grifols 1653
- Human Albumin Grifols 20%, Albumin (Human) (Albumin (human)) Grifols 1651
- Human Albumin Grifols 25%, Albumin (Human) (Albumin (human)) Grifols 1652

Hypercalcemia associated with cancer
- Aredia for Injection (Pamidronate Disodium) Novartis 2179
- Decadron Tablets (Dexamethasone) Merck 1951
- Depo-Medrol Injectable Suspension (Methylprednisolone Acetate) Pharmacia & Upjohn 2617
- Depo-Medrol Single-Dose Vial (Methylprednisolone Acetate) Pharmacia & Upjohn 2619
- Hydrocortone Tablets (Hydrocortisone) Merck 1989
- Sensipar Tablets (Cinacalcet Hydrochloride) Amgen 608
- Zometa for Intravenous Infusion (Zoledronic acid) Novartis 2315

Hypercalcemic emergencies, adjunct in
- Miacalcin Injection (Calcitonin-Salmon) Novartis 2252

Hypercholesterolemia
- Niaspan Extended-Release Tablets (Niacin) Kos 1730
- Zetia Tablets (Ezetimibe) Merck/Schering Plough 2120
- Zetia Tablets (Ezetimibe) Schering 3083

Hypercholesterolemia, homozygous, familial, adjunct to other agents
- Crestor Tablets (Rosuvastatin Calcium) AstraZeneca Pharmaceuticals 678
- Vytorin 10/10 Tablets (Ezetimibe, Simvastatin) Merck/Schering Plough 2114
- Vytorin 10/10 Tablets (Ezetimibe, Simvastatin) Schering 3077
- Vytorin 10/20 Tablets (Ezetimibe, Simvastatin) Merck/Schering Plough 2114
- Vytorin 10/20 Tablets (Ezetimibe, Simvastatin) Schering 3077
- Vytorin 10/40 Tablets (Ezetimibe, Simvastatin) Merck/Schering Plough 2114
- Vytorin 10/40 Tablets (Ezetimibe, Simvastatin) Schering 3077
- Vytorin 10/80 Tablets (Ezetimibe, Simvastatin) Merck/Schering Plough 2114
- Vytorin 10/80 Tablets (Ezetimibe, Simvastatin) Schering 3077
- Zetia Tablets (Ezetimibe) Merck/Schering Plough 2120
- Zetia Tablets (Ezetimibe) Schering 3083

Hypercholesterolemia, primary, adjunct to diet
- Advicor Tablets (Lovastatin, Niacin) Kos 1722
- Altoprev Extended-Release Tablets (Lovastatin) Sciele 3109
- Caduet Tablets (Amlodipine Besylate, Atorvastatin Calcium) Pfizer 2508
- Crestor Tablets (Rosuvastatin Calcium) AstraZeneca Pharmaceuticals 678
- Lescol Capsules (Fluvastatin Sodium) Novartis 2233
- Lescol XL Tablets (Fluvastatin Sodium) Novartis 2233
- Lipitor Tablets (Atorvastatin Calcium) Parke-Davis 2483
- Lofibra Tablets (Fenofibrate) Gate 1219
- Lofibra Capsules (Fenofibrate) Gate 1216
- Mevacor Tablets (Lovastatin) Merck 2021
- Niaspan Extended-Release Tablets (Niacin) Kos 1730
- Tricor Tablets (Fenofibrate) Abbott 527
- Triglide Tablets (Fenofibrate) Sciele 3123
- Vytorin 10/10 Tablets (Ezetimibe, Simvastatin) Merck/Schering Plough 2114
- Vytorin 10/10 Tablets (Ezetimibe, Simvastatin) Schering 3077
- Vytorin 10/20 Tablets (Ezetimibe, Simvastatin) Merck/Schering Plough 2114
- Vytorin 10/20 Tablets (Ezetimibe, Simvastatin) Schering 3077
- Vytorin 10/40 Tablets (Ezetimibe, Simvastatin) Merck/Schering Plough 2114
- Vytorin 10/40 Tablets (Ezetimibe, Simvastatin) Schering 3077
- Vytorin 10/80 Tablets (Ezetimibe, Simvastatin) Merck/Schering Plough 2114
- Vytorin 10/80 Tablets (Ezetimibe, Simvastatin) Schering 3077
- WelChol Tablets (Colesevelam Hydrochloride) Daiichi Sankyo 1050
- Zetia Tablets (Ezetimibe) Merck/Schering Plough 2120
- Zetia Tablets (Ezetimibe) Schering 3083
- Zocor Tablets (Simvastatin) Merck 2105

Hyperglycemia, control of, adjunct to diet
(*see also under* Diabetes mellitus, insulin-dependent; Diabetes mellitus, non-insulin-dependent)
- ActoPlus Met Tablets (Metformin Hydrochloride, Pioglitazone Hydrochloride) Takeda 3214
- Actos Tablets (Pioglitazone Hydrochloride) Takeda 3219
- Apidra Injection (Insulin Glulisine) sanofi-aventis 2864
- Avandamet Tablets (Rosiglitazone Maleate, Metformin Hydrochloride) GlaxoSmithKline 1373
- Avandaryl Tablets (Rosiglitazone Maleate, Glimepiride) GlaxoSmithKline 1379
- Avandia Tablets (Rosiglitazone Maleate) GlaxoSmithKline 1384
- Byetta Injection (Exenatide) Amylin 611
- Exubera Inhalation Powder (Insulin, Human (rDNA origin)) Pfizer 2524
- Fortamet Extended-Release Tablets (Metformin Hydrochloride) Sciele 3115
- Precose Tablets (Acarbose) Bayer 751
- Starlix Tablets (Nateglinide) Novartis 2292

Hyperhidrosis
- BOTOX Purified Neurotoxin Complex (Botulinum Toxin Type A) Allergan 570

Hyperhidrosis, topical relief of
- Drysol Solution (Aluminum Chloride) Person & Covey 2507
- Xerac AC Solution (Aluminum Chloride) Person & Covey 2507

Hyperkalemia
- Kionex Powder (Sodium Polystyrene Sulfonate) Paddock 2477

Hyperlipoproteinemia, type III, adjunct to diet
- Zocor Tablets (Simvastatin) Merck 2105

Hyperlipoproteinemia, types IIa and IIb, adjunct to diet
- Advicor Tablets (Lovastatin, Niacin) Kos 1722
- Altoprev Extended-Release Tablets (Lovastatin) Sciele 3109
- Caduet Tablets (Amlodipine Besylate, Atorvastatin Calcium) Pfizer 2508
- Crestor Tablets (Rosuvastatin Calcium) AstraZeneca Pharmaceuticals 678
- Lescol Capsules (Fluvastatin Sodium) Novartis 2233
- Lescol XL Tablets (Fluvastatin Sodium) Novartis 2233
- Lipitor Tablets (Atorvastatin Calcium) Parke-Davis 2483
- Mevacor Tablets (Lovastatin) Merck 2021
- Niaspan Extended-Release Tablets (Niacin) Kos 1730
- Triglide Tablets (Fenofibrate) Sciele 3123
- Zetia Tablets (Ezetimibe) Schering 3083
- Zocor Tablets (Simvastatin) Merck 2105

Hyperlipoproteinemia, types IV and V, adjunct to diet
- Lofibra Tablets (Fenofibrate) Gate 1219
- Lofibra Capsules (Fenofibrate) Gate 1216
- Niaspan Extended-Release Tablets (Niacin) Kos 1730
- Tricor Tablets (Fenofibrate) Abbott 527
- Triglide Tablets (Fenofibrate) Sciele 3123

Hyperparathyroidism, secondary
- Hectorol Capsules (Doxercalciferol) Genzyme 1275
- Hectorol Injection (Doxercalciferol) Genzyme 1278
- Rocaltrol Capsules (Calcitriol) Roche 2798
- Rocaltrol Oral Solution (Calcitriol) Roche 2798
- Sensipar Tablets (Cinacalcet Hydrochloride) Amgen 608
- Zemplar Capsules (Paricalcitol) Abbott 541
- Zemplar Injection (Paricalcitol) Abbott 543

Hyperphosphatemia
- Fosrenol Chewable Tablets (Lanthanum Carbonate) Shire US 3183
- PhosLo GelCaps (Calcium Acetate) Nabi 2169
- Renagel Tablets (Sevelamer Hydrochloride) Genzyme 1282

Hyperpigmentation, skin, bleaching of
- Claripel Cream (Hydroquinone) Stiefel 3211
- Lustra Cream (Hydroquinone) TaroPharma 3289
- Lustra-AF Cream (Hydroquinone) TaroPharma 3289
- Lustra-Ultra Cream (Hydroquinone) TaroPharma 3289
- Pure Gardens Cream (Herbals with Vitamins) Awareness Corporation/AwarenessLife ■ 832
- Tri-Luma Cream (Fluocinolone Acetonide, Hydroquinone, Tretinoin) Galderma 1213

Hypersecretory conditions, pathological
- Aciphex Tablets (Rabeprazole Sodium) Eisai 1090
- Pepcid Injection (Famotidine) Merck 2040
- Pepcid (Famotidine) Merck 2038
- Prevacid Delayed-Release Capsules (Lansoprazole) TAP 3271
- Prevacid for Delayed-Release Oral Suspension (Lansoprazole) TAP 3271
- Prevacid SoluTab Delayed-Release Orally Disintegrating Tablets (Lansoprazole) TAP 3271
- Protonix I.V. (Pantoprazole Sodium) Wyeth 3472
- Protonix Tablets (Pantoprazole Sodium) Wyeth 3469
- Zantac (Ranitidine Hydrochloride) GlaxoSmithKline 1624
- Zantac Injection (Ranitidine Hydrochloride) GlaxoSmithKline 1619
- Zantac Injection Pharmacy Bulk Package (Ranitidine Hydrochloride) GlaxoSmithKline 1622
- Zantac Injection Premixed (Ranitidine Hydrochloride) GlaxoSmithKline 1619
- Zantac (Ranitidine Hydrochloride) GlaxoSmithKline 1624

Hypersensitivity reactions, drug-induced
- Decadron Tablets (Dexamethasone) Merck 1951
- Depo-Medrol Injectable Suspension (Methylprednisolone Acetate) Pharmacia & Upjohn 2617
- Depo-Medrol Single-Dose Vial (Methylprednisolone Acetate) Pharmacia & Upjohn 2619
- EpiPen (Epinephrine) Dey 1061
- Hydrocortone Tablets (Hydrocortisone) Merck 1989
- Twinject 0.3 (Epinephrine) Verus 3378
- Twinject 0.15 (Epinephrine) Verus 3379

Hypersensitivity reactions, general
- HibTITER (Haemophilus B Conjugate Vaccine) Wyeth 3426

Hypersensitivity to asparaginase
- Oncaspar (Pegaspargase) Enzon 1145

Hypertension
- Aceon Tablets (2 mg, 4 mg, 8 mg) (Perindopril Erbumine) Solvay 3194
- Adalat CC Tablets (Nifedipine) Schering 2964
- Aldoril Tablets (Hydrochlorothiazide, Methyldopa) Merck 1910
- Altace Capsules (Ramipril) King 1702

Atacand Tablets (Candesartan Cilexetil) AstraZeneca LP 649
Atacand HCT (Hydrochlorothiazide, Candesartan Cilexetil) AstraZeneca LP 651
Avalide Tablets (Irbesartan, Hydrochlorothiazide) Bristol-Myers Squibb 888
Avalide Tablets (Irbesartan, Hydrochlorothiazide) sanofi-aventis 2874
Avapro Tablets (Irbesartan) Bristol-Myers Squibb 891
Avapro Tablets (Irbesartan) sanofi-aventis 2871
Benicar Tablets (Olmesartan Medoxomil) Daiichi Sankyo 1043
Benicar HCT Tablets (Olmesartan Medoxomil, Hydrochlorothiazide) Daiichi Sankyo 1044
Blocadren Tablets (Timolol Maleate) Merck 1916
Caduet Tablets (Amlodipine Besylate, Atorvastatin Calcium) Pfizer 2508
Captopril Tablets (Captopril) Mylan 2149
Cardene I.V. (Nicardipine Hydrochloride) PDL 2497
Cardizem LA Extended Release Tablets (Diltiazem Hydrochloride) Kos 1728
Catapres Tablets (Clonidine Hydrochloride) Boehringer Ingelheim 843
Catapres-TTS (Clonidine) Boehringer Ingelheim 844
Clorpres Tablets (Chlorthalidone, Clonidine Hydrochloride) Mylan 2153
Coreg Tablets (Carvedilol) GlaxoSmithKline 1414
Covera-HS Tablets (Verapamil Hydrochloride) Searle 3139
Cozaar Tablets (Losartan Potassium) Merck 1935
Demadex Injection (Torsemide) Roche 2759
Demadex Tablets (Torsemide) Roche 2759
Diovan Tablets (Valsartan) Novartis 2193
Diovan HCT Tablets (Hydrochlorothiazide, Valsartan) Novartis 2196
Diuril Oral Suspension (Chlorothiazide) Merck 1954
Dyazide Capsules (Hydrochlorothiazide, Triamterene) GlaxoSmithKline 1423
DynaCirc CR Tablets (Isradipine) Reliant 2721
Furosemide Tablets (Furosemide) Mylan 2154
Hytrin Capsules (Terazosin Hydrochloride) Abbott 471
Hyzaar 50-12.5 Tablets (Hydrochlorothiazide, Losartan Potassium) Merck 1990
Hyzaar 100-12.5 Tablets (Hydrochlorothiazide, Losartan Potassium) Merck 1990
Hyzaar 100-25 Tablets (Hydrochlorothiazide, Losartan Potassium) Merck 1990
Indapamide Tablets (Indapamide) Mylan 2156
Inderal LA Long-Acting Capsules (Propranolol Hydrochloride) Wyeth 3429
InnoPran XL Capsules (Propranolol Hydrochloride) Reliant 2723
Inspra Tablets (Eplerenone) Pfizer 2536
Lopressor Injection (Metoprolol Tartrate) Novartis 2238
Lopressor Tablets (Metoprolol Tartrate) Novartis 2238
Lopressor HCT 50/25 Tablets (Hydrochlorothiazide, Metoprolol Tartrate) Novartis 2241
Lopressor HCT 100/25 Tablets (Hydrochlorothiazide, Metoprolol Tartrate) Novartis 2241
Lopressor HCT 100/50 Tablets (Hydrochlorothiazide, Metoprolol Tartrate) Novartis 2241
Lotensin Tablets (Benazepril Hydrochloride) Novartis 2243
Lotensin HCT Tablets (Benazepril Hydrochloride, Hydrochlorothiazide) Novartis 2246
Lotrel Capsules (Amlodipine Besylate, Benazepril Hydrochloride) Novartis 2249
Mavik Tablets (Trandolapril) Abbott 486
Micardis Tablets (Telmisartan) Boehringer Ingelheim 854
Micardis HCT Tablets (Hydrochlorothiazide, Telmisartan) Boehringer Ingelheim 856
Midamor Tablets (Amiloride Hydrochloride) Merck 2026
Moduretic Tablets (Amiloride Hydrochloride, Hydrochlorothiazide) Merck 2028
Nadolol Tablets (Nadolol) Mylan 2159
Norvasc Tablets (Amlodipine Besylate) Pfizer 2545
Prinivil Tablets (Lisinopril) Merck 2052
Prinzide Tablets (Hydrochlorothiazide, Lisinopril) Merck 2056
Sular Tablets (Nisoldipine) Sciele 3122
Tarka Tablets (Trandolapril, Verapamil Hydrochloride) Abbott 524
Teveten Tablets (Eprosartan Mesylate) Kos 1735
Teveten HCT Tablets (Eprosartan Mesylate, Hydrochlorothiazide) Kos 1737
Tiazac Capsules (Diltiazem Hydrochloride) Forest 1201
Timolide Tablets (Hydrochlorothiazide, Timolol Maleate) Merck 2086
Toprol-XL Tablets (Metoprolol Succinate) AstraZeneca LP 668
Uniretic Tablets (Hydrochlorothiazide, Moexipril Hydrochloride) Schwarz 3100
Univasc Tablets (Moexipril Hydrochloride) Schwarz 3104
Vasotec I.V. Injection (Enalapril Maleate) Merck 2103
Verelan PM Extended-Release Capsules, Controlled-Onset (Verapamil Hydrochloride) Schwarz 3106

Hypertension, adjunctive treatment
Micardis Tablets (Telmisartan) Boehringer Ingelheim 854

Hypertension, essential
(*see under* Hypertension)

Hypertension, malignant
Hyperstat I.V. (Diazoxide) Schering 3017

Hypertension, non-malignant
Hyperstat I.V. (Diazoxide) Schering 3017

Hypertension, ocular
(*see also under* Glaucoma, chronic open-angle; Glaucoma, secondary)
Alphagan P Ophthalmic Solution (Brimonidine Tartrate) Allergan 567
Azopt Ophthalmic Suspension (Brinzolamide) Alcon 557
Betagan Ophthalmic Solution, USP (Levobunolol Hydrochloride) Allergan .... ⊙220
Betimol Ophthalmic Solution (Timolol Hemihydrate) Vistakon 3382
Betimol Ophthalmic Solution (Timolol Hemihydrate) Vistakon .... ⊙295
Betoptic S Ophthalmic Suspension (Betaxolol Hydrochloride) Alcon 558
Brimonidine Tartrate Ophthalmic Solution 0.2% (Brimonidine Tartrate) Bausch & Lomb .... ⊙248
Carteolol Hydrochloride Ophthalmic Solution USP, 1% (Carteolol Hydrochloride) Bausch & Lomb .... ⊙249
Cosopt Sterile Ophthalmic Solution (Dorzolamide Hydrochloride, Timolol Maleate) Merck 1931
Lumigan Ophthalmic Solution (Bimatoprost) Allergan 573
OptiPranolol Metipranolol Ophthalmic Solution 0.3% (Metipranolol) Bausch & Lomb .... ⊙256
Timoptic Sterile Ophthalmic Solution (Timolol Maleate) Merck 2088
Timoptic in Ocudose (Timolol Maleate) Merck 2091
Timoptic-XE Sterile Ophthalmic Gel Forming Solution (Timolol Maleate) Merck 2092
Travatan Ophthalmic Solution (Travoprost) Alcon 563
Trusopt Sterile Ophthalmic Solution (Dorzolamide Hydrochloride) Merck 2095
Xalatan Sterile Ophthalmic Solution (Latanoprost) Pharmacia & Upjohn 2649

Hypertension, pulmonary
Tracleer Tablets (Bosentan) Actelion 545

Hypertension, pulmonary arterial
Revatio Tablets (Sildenafil Citrate) Pfizer 2557
Ventavis Inhalation Solution (Iloprost) Cotherix 1020

Hypertension, severe
Hyperstat I.V. (Diazoxide) Schering 3017

Hypertensive crises
(*see under* Hypertension)

Hypertensive episodes, control of, in pheochromocytoma
(*see also under* Pheochromocytoma, adjunctive therapy)
Dibenzyline Capsules (Phenoxybenzamine Hydrochloride) WellSpring 3399

Hyperthermia, malignant, prophylaxis
Dantrium Capsules (Dantrolene Sodium) Procter & Gamble Pharmaceuticals 2694
Dantrium Intravenous (Dantrolene Sodium) Procter & Gamble Pharmaceuticals 2695

Hypertherma, malignant, treatment adjunct
Dantrium Intravenous (Dantrolene Sodium) Procter & Gamble Pharmaceuticals 2694

Hypertriglyceridemia, adjunct to diet
(*see also under* Dysbetalipoproteinemia)
Caduet Tablets (Amlodipine Besylate, Atorvastatin Calcium) Pfizer 2508
Crestor Tablets (Rosuvastatin Calcium) AstraZeneca Pharmaceuticals 678
Lescol Capsules (Fluvastatin Sodium) Novartis 2233
Lescol XL Tablets (Fluvastatin Sodium) Novartis 2233
Lipitor Tablets (Atorvastatin Calcium) Parke-Davis 2483
Lofibra Tablets (Fenofibrate) Gate 1219
Lofibra Capsules (Fenofibrate) Gate 1216
Omacor Capsules (Omega-3-acid ethyl esters) Reliant 2725
Tricor Tablets (Fenofibrate) Abbott 527
Triglide Tablets (Fenofibrate) Sciele 3123
Zocor Tablets (Simvastatin) Merck 2105

Hyperuricemia
Elitek (Rasburicase) sanofi-aventis 2890

Hypnotic
(*see under* Sleep, induction of)

Hypoalbuminemia
Albutein 5%, Albumin (Human) (Albumin (human)) Grifols 1652
Flexbumin I.V. (Albumin (human)) Baxter Healthcare 720

Hypocalcemia
Os-Cal Chewable Tablets (Calcium Carbonate) GlaxoSmithKline .... ▣818
Os-Cal 500 Tablets (Calcium) GlaxoSmithKline .... ▣817
Rocaltrol Capsules (Calcitriol) Roche 2798
Rocaltrol Oral Solution (Calcitriol) Roche 2798

Hypocalcemia associated with chronic renal failure
Calcijex Injection (Calcitriol) Abbott 411
Rocaltrol Capsules (Calcitriol) Roche 2798
Rocaltrol Oral Solution (Calcitriol) Roche 2798

Hypocalcemia associated with idiopathic hypoparathyroidism
Rocaltrol Capsules (Calcitriol) Roche 2798
Rocaltrol Oral Solution (Calcitriol) Roche 2798

Hypocalcemia associated with postsurgical hypoparathyroidism
Rocaltrol Capsules (Calcitriol) Roche 2798
Rocaltrol Oral Solution (Calcitriol) Roche 2798

Hypocalcemia associated with pseudohypoparathyroidism
Rocaltrol Capsules (Calcitriol) Roche 2798
Rocaltrol Oral Solution (Calcitriol) Roche 2798

Hypocalcemia with vitamin D, deficiency of
Caltrate 600 PLUS (Calcium Carbonate, Minerals, Multiple, Vitamin D) Wyeth .... ▣809
Caltrate 600 + D Tablets (Calcium Carbonate, Vitamin D) Wyeth .... ▣809
Os-Cal 250 + D Tablets (Calcium, Vitamin D) GlaxoSmithKline .... ▣817
Os-Cal 500 + D Tablets (Calcium, Vitamin D) GlaxoSmithKline .... ▣817

Hypoestrogenism
Climara Transdermal System (Estradiol) Berlex 771
Premarin Intravenous (Estrogens, Conjugated) Wyeth 3442
Premarin Tablets (Estrogens, Conjugated) Wyeth 3446

Hypoglycemia
GlucaGen (Glucagon) Bedford 761
Glucagon for Injection Vials and Emergency Kit (Glucagon) Lilly 1778

Hypogonadism, hypogonadotropic, in males
AndroGel (Testosterone) Unimed 3329
Androxy Tablets (Fluoxymesterone) Upsher-Smith 3335
Striant Mucoadhesive (Testosterone) Columbia 1007
Testim 1% Gel (Testosterone) Auxilium 695

Hypogonadism, male, primary
AndroGel (Testosterone) Unimed 3329
Androxy Tablets (Fluoxymesterone) Upsher-Smith 3335
Striant Mucoadhesive (Testosterone) Columbia 1007
Testim 1% Gel (Testosterone) Auxilium 695

Hypokalemia
K-Dur Extended-Release Tablets (Potassium Chloride) Schering 3033
K-Lor Oral Solution (Potassium Chloride) Abbott 474
K-Tab Tablets (Potassium Chloride) Abbott 475

Hyponatremia, euvolemic
Vaprisol (Conivaptan Hydrochloride) Astellas 643

Hypophosphatemia
K-Phos Neutral Tablets (Potassium Phosphate, Sodium Phosphate) Beach 760

Hypopigmentation, skin
Oxsoralen Lotion 1% (Methoxsalen) Valeant 3352

Hypoproteinemia
Plasbumin-20 (Albumin (human)) Talecris 3252
Plasbumin-25 (Albumin (human)) Talecris 3253

Hypoprothrombinemia, drug-induced
Mephyton (Vitamin K_1) Merck 2018

Hypoprothrombinemia, salicylate-induced
Mephyton (Vitamin K_1) Merck 2018

Hypoprothrombinemia, secondary factors-induced
Mephyton (Vitamin K_1) Merck 2018

Hypotension, orthostatic
ProAmatine Tablets (Midodrine Hydrochloride) Shire US 3186

Hypothyroidism, ordinary
(*see under* Hypothyroidism, replacement or supplemental therapy in)

Hypothyroidism, primary
(*see under* Hypothyroidism, replacement or supplemental therapy in)

Hypothyroidism, replacement or supplemental therapy in
Cytomel Tablets (Liothyronine Sodium) King 1710
Levothroid Tablets (Levothyroxine Sodium) Forest 1186
Levoxyl Tablets (Levothyroxine Sodium) King 1712

Naturethroid Tablets (Levothyroxine, Liothyronine) Western Research ... 3401
Synthroid Tablets (Levothyroxine Sodium) Abbott ... 520
Thyrolar Tablets (Liotrix) Forest ... 1199
Westhroid Tablets (Levothyroxine Sodium, Liothyronine Sodium) Western Research ... 3403

Hypothyroidism, secondary
(*see under* Hypothyroidism, replacement or supplemental therapy in)

Hypothyroidism, tertiary
(*see under* Hypothyroidism, replacement or supplemental therapy in)

Hypovolemia
Flexbumin I.V. (Albumin (human)) Baxter Healthcare ... 720
Plasbumin-5 (Albumin (human)) Talecris ... 3251

Hypovolemic shock
Albutein 5%, Albumin (Human) (Albumin (human)) Grifols ... 1652
Albutein 25% , Albumin (Human) (Albumin (human)) Grifols ... 1653
Human Albumin Grifols 20%, Albumin (Human) (Albumin (human)) Grifols ... 1651
Human Albumin Grifols 25%, Albumin (Human) (Albumin (human)) Grifols ... 1652

I

Idiopathic thrombocytopenic purpura
(*see under* Purpura, idiopathic thrombocytopenic)

Immune deficiency, primary
Vivaglobin (Immune Globulin Subcutaneous (Human)) ZLB Behring ... 3506

Immunization, diphtheria, tetanus and pertussis
ADACEL Vaccine (Diphtheria & Tetanus Toxoids and Acellular Pertussis Vaccine Adsorbed) Sanofi Pasteur ... 2945
Boostrix (Diphtheria & Tetanus Toxoids and Acellular Pertussis Vaccine Adsorbed) GlaxoSmithKline ... 1404
DAPTACEL Vaccine (Diphtheria & Tetanus Toxoids and Acellular Pertussis Vaccine Adsorbed) Sanofi Pasteur ... 2950
Infanrix Vaccine (Diphtheria & Tetanus Toxoids and Acellular Pertussis Vaccine Adsorbed) GlaxoSmithKline ... 1476
Pediarix Vaccine (Diphtheria & Tetanus Toxoids and Pertussis Vaccine Adsorbed, Hepatitis B Vaccine, Recombinant, Poliovirus Vaccine Inactivated, Trivalent Types 1,2,3) GlaxoSmithKline ... 1548

Immunization, haemophilus influenzae type b
HibTITER (Haemophilus B Conjugate Vaccine) Wyeth ... 3426
Liquid PedvaxHIB (Haemophilus B Conjugate Vaccine) Merck ... 2035

Immunization, haemophilus influenzae type B and hepatitis B virus
Comvax (Haemophilus B Conjugate Vaccine, Hepatitis B Vaccine, Recombinant) Merck ... 1928

Immunization, hepatitis A and B virus
Twinrix Vaccine (Hepatitis A Vaccine, Inactivated, Hepatitis B Vaccine, Recombinant) GlaxoSmithKline ... 1595

Immunization, hepatitis A virus
Havrix Vaccine (Hepatitis A Vaccine, Inactivated) GlaxoSmithKline ... 1456
Vaqta (Hepatitis A Vaccine, Inactivated) Merck ... 2097

Immunization, hepatitis B virus
Engerix-B Vaccine (Hepatitis B Vaccine, Recombinant) GlaxoSmithKline ... 1425
Pediarix Vaccine (Diphtheria & Tetanus Toxoids and Pertussis Vaccine Adsorbed, Hepatitis B Vaccine, Recombinant, Poliovirus Vaccine Inactivated, Trivalent Types 1,2,3) GlaxoSmithKline ... 1548
Recombivax HB (Hepatitis B Vaccine, Recombinant) Merck ... 2071

Immunization, human papillomavirus
Gardasil Injection (Quadrivalent Human Papillomavirus (Types 6, 11, 16, 18) Recombinant Vaccine) Merck ... 1984

Immunization, influenza virus, types A and B
Fluarix (Influenza Virus Vaccine) GlaxoSmithKline ... 1451
Flumist Vaccine (Influenza Virus Vaccine) Medimmune ... 1901

Immunization, meningococcal
Menactra Vaccine (Meningococcal Polysaccharide Diphtheria Toxoid Conjugate Vaccine) Sanofi Pasteur ... 2954

Immunization, pneumococcal disease
(*see also under* Pneumococcal disease, immunization against)
Pneumovax 23 (Pneumococcal Vaccine, Polyvalent) Merck ... 2043
Prevnar for Injection (Pneumococcal vaccine, diphtheria conjugate) Wyeth ... 3463

Immunization, poliovirus 1, 2, and 3
Pediarix Vaccine (Diphtheria & Tetanus Toxoids and Pertussis Vaccine Adsorbed, Hepatitis B Vaccine, Recombinant, Poliovirus Vaccine Inactivated, Trivalent Types 1,2,3) GlaxoSmithKline ... 1548

Immunization, tetanus
HyperTET (Tetanus Immune Globulin (Human)) Talecris ... 3248

Immunization, typhoid fever
Vivotif (Typhoid Vaccine Live Oral TY21a) Berna ... 819

Immunization, varicella
Varivax (Varicella Virus Vaccine Live) Merck ... 2100

Immunodeficiencies
Carimune NF (Immune Globulin Intravenous (Human)) ZLB Behring ... 3499
GamaSTAN (Globulin, Immune (Human)) Talecris ... 3234
Gammagard Liquid (Immune Globulin Intravenous (Human)) Baxter Healthcare ... 721
Gammagard S/D (Immune Globulin Intravenous (Human)) Baxter Healthcare ... 724
Gamunex Immune Globulin I.V., 10% (Immune Globulin Intravenous (Human)) Talecris ... 3235

Immunodeficiency, common variable
Flebogamma 5%, Immune Globulin Intravenous (Human) (Globulin, Immune (Human)) Grifols ... 1658
Gammagard S/D (Immune Globulin Intravenous (Human)) Baxter Healthcare ... 724
Gamunex Immune Globulin I.V., 10% (Immune Globulin Intravenous (Human)) Talecris ... 3235

Immunodeficiency, unspecified
(*see under* Infection, tendency to)

Immunodeficiency disease, severe combined
(*see under* Adenosine deaminase, enzyme replacement therapy for)

Impetigo contagiosa
Bactroban Ointment (Mupirocin) GlaxoSmithKline ... 1395
Ceftin for Oral Suspension (Cefuroxime Axetil) GlaxoSmithKline ... 1407
Levaquin (Levofloxacin) Ortho-McNeil ... 2384
Levaquin in 5% Dextrose Injection (Levofloxacin) Ortho-McNeil ... 2384

Impotence, male
(*see under* Erectile dysfunction)

Infection, tendency to
Carimune NF (Immune Globulin Intravenous (Human)) ZLB Behring ... 3499

Infection, urinary, chronic urea-splitting
Lithostat Tablets (Acetohydroxamic Acid) Mission ... 2140

Infections, acquired immunodeficiency syndrome-related complex
AmBisome for Injection (Amphotericin B, liposomal) Astellas ... 620
Biaxin/Biaxin XL (Clarithromycin) Abbott ... 402
Famvir Tablets (Famciclovir) Novartis ... 2211
Intron A for Injection (Interferon alfa-2b, Recombinant) Schering ... 3024
Marinol Capsules (Dronabinol) Unimed ... 3333
Retrovir IV Infusion (Zidovudine) GlaxoSmithKline ... 1564
Valcyte Tablets (Valganciclovir Hydrochloride) Roche ... 2813
WinRho SDF (Rh_0 (D) Immune Globulin (Human)) Baxter Healthcare ... 732

Infections, aerobic organisms
Fortaz (Ceftazidime) GlaxoSmithKline ... 1453
Mefoxin for Injection (Cefoxitin Sodium) Merck ... 2012
Mefoxin Premixed Intravenous Solution (Cefoxitin Sodium) Merck ... 2016

Infections, anaerobic organisms
Cleocin Vaginal Ovules (Clindamycin Hydrochloride) Pharmacia & Upjohn ... 2616
Fortaz (Ceftazidime) GlaxoSmithKline ... 1453
Garamycin Injectable (Gentamicin Sulfate) Schering ... 3014
Mefoxin for Injection (Cefoxitin Sodium) Merck ... 2012
Mefoxin Premixed Intravenous Solution (Cefoxitin Sodium) Merck ... 2016
Primaxin I.V. (Cilastatin Sodium, Imipenem) Merck ... 2048

Infections, beta-lactamase producing organisms
Augmentin (Amoxicillin, Clavulanate Potassium) GlaxoSmithKline ... 1360
Augmentin Tablets (Amoxicillin, Clavulanate Potassium) GlaxoSmithKline ... 1363
Augmentin XR Extended-Release Tablets (Amoxicillin, Clavulanate Potassium) GlaxoSmithKline ... 1369
Ceftin (Cefuroxime Axetil) GlaxoSmithKline ... 1407
Merrem I.V. (Meropenem) AstraZeneca Pharmaceuticals ... 686
Vantin Tablets and Oral Suspension (Cefpodoxime Proxetil) Pharmacia & Upjohn ... 2645
Zosyn (Piperacillin Sodium, Tazobactam Sodium) Wyeth ... 3492

Infections, bone and joint
Cipro (Ciprofloxacin) Schering ... 2977
Cipro I.V. (Ciprofloxacin) Schering ... 2984
Fortaz (Ceftazidime) GlaxoSmithKline ... 1453
Garamycin Injectable (Gentamicin Sulfate) Schering ... 3014
Mefoxin for Injection (Cefoxitin Sodium) Merck ... 2012
Mefoxin Premixed Intravenous Solution (Cefoxitin Sodium) Merck ... 2016
Primaxin I.V. (Cilastatin Sodium, Imipenem) Merck ... 2048
Rocephin Injectable Vials, ADD-Vantage, Galaxy, Bulk (Ceftriaxone Sodium) Roche ... 2800
Timentin ADD-Vantage (Clavulanate Potassium, Ticarcillin Disodium) GlaxoSmithKline ... 1580
Timentin Injection Galaxy Container (Clavulanate Potassium, Ticarcillin Disodium) GlaxoSmithKline ... 1583
Timentin IV Infusion (Clavulanate Potassium, Ticarcillin Disodium) GlaxoSmithKline ... 1577
Timentin Pharmacy Bulk Package (Clavulanate Potassium, Ticarcillin Disodium) GlaxoSmithKline ... 1586
Zinacef for Injection (Cefuroxime) GlaxoSmithKline ... 1631
Zinacef Injection (Cefuroxime) GlaxoSmithKline ... 1631

Infections, burn wound
(*see also under* Infections, skin, bacterial, minor)
Garamycin Injectable (Gentamicin Sulfate) Schering ... 3014
Sulfamylon Cream (Mafenide Acetate) Mylan ... 2162

Infections, central nervous system
Fortaz (Ceftazidime) GlaxoSmithKline ... 1453
Garamycin Injectable (Gentamicin Sulfate) Schering ... 3014

Infections, ear, nose and throat
Amoxil Capsules (Amoxicillin) GlaxoSmithKline ... 1343
Amoxil Chewable Tablets (Amoxicillin) GlaxoSmithKline ... 1343
Amoxil Pediatric Drops for Oral Suspension (Amoxicillin) GlaxoSmithKline ... 1343
Amoxil Powder for Oral Suspension (Amoxicillin) GlaxoSmithKline ... 1343
Amoxil Tablets (Amoxicillin) GlaxoSmithKline ... 1343

Infections, fungal, systemic
Abelcet Injection (Amphotericin B Lipid Complex) Enzon ... 1141

Infections, genitourinary tract
Amoxil Capsules (Amoxicillin) GlaxoSmithKline ... 1343
Amoxil Chewable Tablets (Amoxicillin) GlaxoSmithKline ... 1343
Amoxil Pediatric Drops for Oral Suspension (Amoxicillin) GlaxoSmithKline ... 1343
Amoxil Powder for Oral Suspension (Amoxicillin) GlaxoSmithKline ... 1343
Amoxil Tablets (Amoxicillin) GlaxoSmithKline ... 1343

Infections, gram-negative bacteria
Amoxil Capsules (Amoxicillin) GlaxoSmithKline ... 1343
Amoxil Chewable Tablets (Amoxicillin) GlaxoSmithKline ... 1343
Amoxil Pediatric Drops for Oral Suspension (Amoxicillin) GlaxoSmithKline ... 1343
Amoxil Powder for Oral Suspension (Amoxicillin) GlaxoSmithKline ... 1343
Amoxil Tablets (Amoxicillin) GlaxoSmithKline ... 1343
Garamycin Injectable (Gentamicin Sulfate) Schering ... 3014
Mefoxin for Injection (Cefoxitin Sodium) Merck ... 2012
Mefoxin Premixed Intravenous Solution (Cefoxitin Sodium) Merck ... 2016
Primaxin I.V. (Cilastatin Sodium, Imipenem) Merck ... 2048
Seromycin Capsules (Cycloserine) Lilly ... 1813

Infections, gram-positive anaerobic cocci
Mefoxin for Injection (Cefoxitin Sodium) Merck ... 2012
Mefoxin Premixed Intravenous Solution (Cefoxitin Sodium) Merck ... 2016

Infections, gram-positive bacteria
Amoxil Capsules (Amoxicillin) GlaxoSmithKline 1343
Amoxil Chewable Tablets (Amoxicillin) GlaxoSmithKline 1343
Amoxil Pediatric Drops for Oral Suspension (Amoxicillin) GlaxoSmithKline 1343
Amoxil Powder for Oral Suspension (Amoxicillin) GlaxoSmithKline 1343
Amoxil Tablets (Amoxicillin) GlaxoSmithKline 1343
Primaxin I.V. (Cilastatin Sodium, Imipenem) Merck 2048
Seromycin Capsules (Cycloserine) Lilly 1813

Infections, gynecologic
Cleocin Vaginal Ovules (Clindamycin Hydrochloride) Pharmacia & Upjohn 2616
Ery-Tab Tablets (Erythromycin) Abbott 449
Erythrocin Stearate Filmtab Tablets (Erythromycin Stearate) Abbott 453
Erythromycin Base Filmtab Tablets (Erythromycin) Abbott 455
Erythromycin Delayed-Release Capsules, USP (Erythromycin) Abbott 457
Fortaz (Ceftazidime) GlaxoSmithKline 1453
Mefoxin for Injection (Cefoxitin Sodium) Merck 2012
Mefoxin Premixed Intravenous Solution (Cefoxitin Sodium) Merck 2016
PCE Dispertab Tablets (Erythromycin) Abbott 515
Primaxin I.M. (Cilastatin Sodium, Imipenem) Merck 2045
Primaxin I.V. (Cilastatin Sodium, Imipenem) Merck 2048
Timentin ADD-Vantage (Clavulanate Potassium, Ticarcillin Disodium) GlaxoSmithKline 1580
Timentin Injection Galaxy Container (Clavulanate Potassium, Ticarcillin Disodium) GlaxoSmithKline 1583
Timentin IV Infusion (Clavulanate Potassium, Ticarcillin Disodium) GlaxoSmithKline 1577
Timentin Pharmacy Bulk Package (Clavulanate Potassium, Ticarcillin Disodium) GlaxoSmithKline 1586
Vantin Tablets and Oral Suspension (Cefpodoxime Proxetil) Pharmacia & Upjohn 2645
Zosyn (Piperacillin Sodium, Tazobactam Sodium) Wyeth 3492

Infections, human immunodeficiency virus
Agenerase Capsules (Amprenavir) GlaxoSmithKline 1327
Agenerase Oral Solution (Amprenavir) GlaxoSmithKline 1332
Aptivus Capsules (Tipranavir) Boehringer Ingelheim 826
Atripla Tablets (Tenofovir Disoproxil Fumarate, Efavirenz, Emtricitabine) Bristol-Myers Squibb Company & Gilead Sciences 945
Combivir Tablets (Lamivudine, Zidovudine) GlaxoSmithKline 1411
Crixivan Capsules (Indinavir Sulfate) Merck 1940
Emtriva Capsules (Emtricitabine) Gilead 1287
Emtriva Oral Solution (Emtricitabine) Gilead 1287
Epivir (Lamivudine) GlaxoSmithKline 1427
Epzicom Tablets (Lamivudine, Abacavir Sulfate) GlaxoSmithKline 1436
Fuzeon Injection (Enfuvirtide) Roche 2767
Invirase (Saquinavir Mesylate) Roche 2772
Kaletra (Lopinavir, Ritonavir) Abbott 476
Lexiva Tablets (Fosamprenavir Calcium) GlaxoSmithKline 1505
Norvir (Ritonavir) Abbott 503
Prezista Tablets (Darunavir) Tibotec 3306
Retrovir Capsules (Zidovudine) GlaxoSmithKline 1560
Retrovir IV Infusion (Zidovudine) GlaxoSmithKline 1564
Retrovir (Zidovudine) GlaxoSmithKline 1560
Reyataz Capsules (Atazanavir sulfate) Bristol-Myers Squibb 921
Sustiva Capsules (Efavirenz) Bristol-Myers Squibb 930
Sustiva Tablets (Efavirenz) Bristol-Myers Squibb 930
Trizivir Tablets (Lamivudine, Abacavir Sulfate, Zidovudine) GlaxoSmithKline 1589
Truvada Tablets (Tenofovir Disoproxil Fumarate, Emtricitabine) Gilead 1296
Viracept (Nelfinavir Mesylate) Pfizer 2577
Viramune Oral Suspension (Nevirapine) Boehringer Ingelheim 873
Viramune Tablets (Nevirapine) Boehringer Ingelheim 873
Viread Tablets (Tenofovir Disoproxil Fumarate) Gilead 1301
Ziagen (Abacavir Sulfate) GlaxoSmithKline 1626

Infections, human immunodeficiency virus, adjunct
Prezista Tablets (Darunavir) Tibotec 3306
Rescriptor Tablets (Delavirdine Mesylate) Pfizer 2551

Infections, human immunodeficiency virus, in combination with ritonavir
Prezista Tablets (Darunavir) Tibotec 3306

Infections, human immunodeficiency virus, in combination with zidovudine
Aptivus Capsules (Tipranavir) Boehringer Ingelheim 826

Infections, intra-abdominal
Avelox (Moxifloxacin Hydrochloride) Schering 2970
Cipro (Ciprofloxacin) Schering 2977
Cipro I.V. (Ciprofloxacin) Schering 2984
Cleocin Vaginal Ovules (Clindamycin Hydrochloride) Pharmacia & Upjohn 2616
Fortaz (Ceftazidime) GlaxoSmithKline 1453
Garamycin Injectable (Gentamicin Sulfate) Schering 3014
Invanz for Injection (Ertapenem) Merck 1999
Maxipime for Injection (Cefepime Hydrochloride) Elan 1105
Mefoxin for Injection (Cefoxitin Sodium) Merck 2012
Mefoxin Premixed Intravenous Solution (Cefoxitin Sodium) Merck 2016
Merrem I.V. (Meropenem) AstraZeneca Pharmaceuticals 686
Primaxin I.M. (Cilastatin Sodium, Imipenem) Merck 2045
Primaxin I.V. (Cilastatin Sodium, Imipenem) Merck 2048
Rocephin Injectable Vials, ADD-Vantage, Galaxy, Bulk (Ceftriaxone Sodium) Roche 2800
Timentin ADD-Vantage (Clavulanate Potassium, Ticarcillin Disodium) GlaxoSmithKline 1580
Timentin Injection Galaxy Container (Clavulanate Potassium, Ticarcillin Disodium) GlaxoSmithKline 1583
Timentin IV Infusion (Clavulanate Potassium, Ticarcillin Disodium) GlaxoSmithKline 1577
Timentin Pharmacy Bulk Package (Clavulanate Potassium, Ticarcillin Disodium) GlaxoSmithKline 1586

Infections, liver flukes
(*see under* Clonorchiasis)

Infections, lower respiratory tract
Amoxil Capsules (Amoxicillin) GlaxoSmithKline 1343
Amoxil Chewable Tablets (Amoxicillin) GlaxoSmithKline 1343
Amoxil Pediatric Drops for Oral Suspension (Amoxicillin) GlaxoSmithKline 1343
Amoxil Powder for Oral Suspension (Amoxicillin) GlaxoSmithKline 1343
Amoxil Tablets (Amoxicillin) GlaxoSmithKline 1343
Augmentin (Amoxicillin, Clavulanate Potassium) GlaxoSmithKline 1360
Augmentin Tablets (Amoxicillin, Clavulanate Potassium) GlaxoSmithKline 1363
Augmentin XR Extended-Release Tablets (Amoxicillin, Clavulanate Potassium) GlaxoSmithKline 1369
Avelox (Moxifloxacin Hydrochloride) Schering 2970
Biaxin/Biaxin XL (Clarithromycin) Abbott 402
Cipro (Ciprofloxacin) Schering 2977
Cipro I.V. (Ciprofloxacin) Schering 2984
Cleocin Vaginal Ovules (Clindamycin Hydrochloride) Pharmacia & Upjohn 2616
E.E.S. (Erythromycin Ethylsuccinate) Abbott 451
EryPed (Erythromycin Ethylsuccinate) Abbott 447
Ery-Tab Tablets (Erythromycin) Abbott 449
Erythrocin Stearate Filmtab Tablets (Erythromycin Stearate) Abbott 453
Erythromycin Base Filmtab Tablets (Erythromycin) Abbott 455
Erythromycin Delayed-Release Capsules, USP (Erythromycin) Abbott 457
Fortaz (Ceftazidime) GlaxoSmithKline 1453
Invanz for Injection (Ertapenem) Merck 1999
Levaquin (Levofloxacin) Ortho-McNeil 2384
Levaquin in 5% Dextrose Injection (Levofloxacin) Ortho-McNeil 2384
Mefoxin for Injection (Cefoxitin Sodium) Merck 2012
Mefoxin Premixed Intravenous Solution (Cefoxitin Sodium) Merck 2016
Omnicef Capsules (Cefdinir) Abbott 511
Omnicef for Oral Suspension (Cefdinir) Abbott 511
PCE Dispertab Tablets (Erythromycin) Abbott 515
Primaxin I.M. (Cilastatin Sodium, Imipenem) Merck 2045
Primaxin I.V. (Cilastatin Sodium, Imipenem) Merck 2048
Rocephin Injectable Vials, ADD-Vantage, Galaxy, Bulk (Ceftriaxone Sodium) Roche 2800
Tequin Injection (Gatifloxacin) Bristol-Myers Squibb 938
Tequin Injection in 5% Dextrose (Gatifloxacin) Bristol-Myers Squibb 938
Tequin Tablets (Gatifloxacin) Bristol-Myers Squibb 938
Timentin ADD-Vantage (Clavulanate Potassium, Ticarcillin Disodium) GlaxoSmithKline 1580
Timentin Injection Galaxy Container (Clavulanate Potassium, Ticarcillin Disodium) GlaxoSmithKline 1583
Timentin IV Infusion (Clavulanate Potassium, Ticarcillin Disodium) GlaxoSmithKline 1577
Timentin Pharmacy Bulk Package (Clavulanate Potassium, Ticarcillin Disodium) GlaxoSmithKline 1586
Vantin Tablets and Oral Suspension (Cefpodoxime Proxetil) Pharmacia & Upjohn 2645
Zinacef for Injection (Cefuroxime) GlaxoSmithKline 1631
Zinacef Injection (Cefuroxime) GlaxoSmithKline 1631
Zosyn (Piperacillin Sodium, Tazobactam Sodium) Wyeth 3492

Infections, lower respiratory tract, RSV-induced
Virazole for Inhalation Solution (Ribavirin) Valeant North America 3370

Infections, lower respiratory tract, RSV-induced, prevention of
Synagis (Palivizumab) MedImmune 1897

Infections, manifested by febrile neutropenia, to decrease incidence of
Maxipime for Injection (Cefepime Hydrochloride) Elan 1105

Infections, mycotic, cutaneous
Nystop (Nystatin) Paddock 2478

Infections, mycotic, mucocutaneous
Nystop (Nystatin) Paddock 2478

Infections, ocular, bacterial
Bleph-10 Ophthalmic Solution 10% (Sulfacetamide Sodium) Allergan ⊙222
Polytrim Ophthalmic Solution (Polymyxin B Sulfate, Trimethoprim Sulfate) Allergan 574
Quixin Ophthalmic Solution (Levofloxacin) Vistakon 3383

Infections, perioperative, reduction of the incidence of
Rocephin Injectable Vials, ADD-Vantage, Galaxy, Bulk (Ceftriaxone Sodium) Roche 2800
Zinacef for Injection (Cefuroxime) GlaxoSmithKline 1631
Zinacef Injection (Cefuroxime) GlaxoSmithKline 1631

Infections, polymicrobic
Fortaz (Ceftazidime) GlaxoSmithKline 1453
Primaxin I.V. (Cilastatin Sodium, Imipenem) Merck 2048

Infections, respiratory tract, unspecified
E.E.S. (Erythromycin Ethylsuccinate) Abbott 451
EryPed (Erythromycin Ethylsuccinate) Abbott 447
Erythrocin Stearate Filmtab Tablets (Erythromycin Stearate) Abbott 453
Erythromycin Base Filmtab Tablets (Erythromycin) Abbott 455
Erythromycin Delayed-Release Capsules, USP (Erythromycin) Abbott 457
Garamycin Injectable (Gentamicin Sulfate) Schering 3014
Omnicef Capsules (Cefdinir) Abbott 511
Omnicef for Oral Suspension (Cefdinir) Abbott 511
PCE Dispertab Tablets (Erythromycin) Abbott 515

Infections, skin, bacterial, minor
Bactroban Ointment (Mupirocin) GlaxoSmithKline 1395
Clorpactin WCS-90 (Sodium Oxychlorosene) Guardian 1662
Garamycin Injectable (Gentamicin Sulfate) Schering 3014
Neosporin Antibiotic Ointment (Bacitracin, Neomycin, Polymyxin B Sulfate) Pfizer Consumer Healthcare ■643
Neosporin + Pain Relief Antibiotic Cream and Ointment (Maximum Strength) (Neomycin, Polymyxin B Sulfate, Pramoxine Hydrochloride) Pfizer Consumer Healthcare ■643
Polysporin First Aid Antibiotic Ointment (Bacitracin, Polymyxin B Sulfate) Pfizer Consumer Healthcare ■643

Infections, skin and skin structure
Amoxil Capsules (Amoxicillin) GlaxoSmithKline 1343
Amoxil Chewable Tablets (Amoxicillin) GlaxoSmithKline 1343
Amoxil Pediatric Drops for Oral Suspension (Amoxicillin) GlaxoSmithKline 1343
Amoxil Powder for Oral Suspension (Amoxicillin) GlaxoSmithKline 1343
Amoxil Tablets (Amoxicillin) GlaxoSmithKline 1343
Augmentin (Amoxicillin, Clavulanate Potassium) GlaxoSmithKline 1360
Augmentin Tablets (Amoxicillin, Clavulanate Potassium) GlaxoSmithKline 1363
Avelox (Moxifloxacin Hydrochloride) Schering 2970
Bactroban Cream (Mupirocin Calcium) GlaxoSmithKline 1394
Biaxin/Biaxin XL (Clarithromycin) Abbott 402
Ceftin Tablets (Cefuroxime Axetil) GlaxoSmithKline 1407
Cipro (Ciprofloxacin) Schering 2977
Cipro I.V. (Ciprofloxacin) Schering 2984
Cleocin Vaginal Ovules (Clindamycin Hydrochloride) Pharmacia & Upjohn 2616

E.E.S. (Erythromycin Ethylsuccinate) Abbott ... 451
EryPed (Erythromycin Ethylsuccinate) Abbott ... 447
Ery-Tab Tablets (Erythromycin) Abbott ... 449
Erythrocin Stearate Filmtab Tablets (Erythromycin Stearate) Abbott ... 453
Erythromycin Base Filmtab Tablets (Erythromycin) Abbott ... 455
Erythromycin Delayed-Release Capsules, USP (Erythromycin) Abbott ... 457
Fortaz (Ceftazidime) GlaxoSmithKline ... 1453
Garamycin Injectable (Gentamicin Sulfate) Schering ... 3014
Invanz for Injection (Ertapenem) Merck ... 1999
Levaquin (Levofloxacin) Ortho-McNeil ... 2384
Levaquin in 5% Dextrose Injection (Levofloxacin) Ortho-McNeil ... 2384
Maxipime for Injection (Cefepime Hydrochloride) Elan ... 1105
Mefoxin for Injection (Cefoxitin Sodium) Merck ... 2012
Mefoxin Premixed Intravenous Solution (Cefoxitin Sodium) Merck ... 2016
Merrem I.V. (Meropenem) AstraZeneca Pharmaceuticals ... 686
Omnicef Capsules (Cefdinir) Abbott ... 511
Omnicef for Oral Suspension (Cefdinir) Abbott ... 511
PCE Dispertab Tablets (Erythromycin) Abbott ... 515
Primaxin I.M. (Cilastatin Sodium, Imipenem) Merck ... 2045
Primaxin I.V. (Cilastatin Sodium, Imipenem) Merck ... 2048
Rocephin Injectable Vials, ADD-Vantage, Galaxy, Bulk (Ceftriaxone Sodium) Roche ... 2800
Tequin Injection (Gatifloxacin) Bristol-Myers Squibb ... 938
Tequin Injection in 5% Dextrose (Gatifloxacin) Bristol-Myers Squibb ... 938
Tequin Tablets (Gatifloxacin) Bristol-Myers Squibb ... 938
Timentin ADD-Vantage (Clavulanate Potassium, Ticarcillin Disodium) GlaxoSmithKline ... 1580
Timentin Injection Galaxy Container (Clavulanate Potassium, Ticarcillin Disodium) GlaxoSmithKline ... 1583
Timentin IV Infusion (Clavulanate Potassium, Ticarcillin Disodium) GlaxoSmithKline ... 1577
Timentin Pharmacy Bulk Package (Clavulanate Potassium, Ticarcillin Disodium) GlaxoSmithKline ... 1586
Vantin Tablets and Oral Suspension (Cefpodoxime Proxetil) Pharmacia & Upjohn ... 2645
Zinacef for Injection (Cefuroxime) GlaxoSmithKline ... 1631
Zinacef Injection (Cefuroxime) GlaxoSmithKline ... 1631
Zosyn (Piperacillin Sodium, Tazobactam Sodium) Wyeth ... 3492
Zyvox (Linezolid) Pharmacia & Upjohn ... 2652

Infections, soft tissues
(*see under* Infections, skin and skin structure)

Infections, superficial, external auditory canal
(*see under* Otitis externa)

Infections, surgical, colorectal, prevention of
Invanz for Injection (Ertapenem) Merck ... 1999

Infections, surgical, ophthalmic, prevention of
Betadine 5% Ophthalmic Solution (Povidone Iodine) Alcon ... ⊙ 202

Infections, tapeworm
Albenza Tablets (Albendazole) GlaxoSmithKline ... 1338

Infections, upper respiratory tract
Amoxil Capsules (Amoxicillin) GlaxoSmithKline ... 1343
Amoxil Chewable Tablets (Amoxicillin) GlaxoSmithKline ... 1343
Amoxil Pediatric Drops for Oral Suspension (Amoxicillin) GlaxoSmithKline ... 1343
Amoxil Powder for Oral Suspension (Amoxicillin) GlaxoSmithKline ... 1343
Amoxil Tablets (Amoxicillin) GlaxoSmithKline ... 1343
Avelox (Moxifloxacin Hydrochloride) Schering ... 2970
Biaxin/Biaxin XL (Clarithromycin) Abbott ... 402
Bicillin C-R Injectable Suspension (Penicillin G Benzathine, Penicillin G Procaine) King ... 1706
E.E.S. (Erythromycin Ethylsuccinate) Abbott ... 451
EryPed (Erythromycin Ethylsuccinate) Abbott ... 447
Ery-Tab Tablets (Erythromycin) Abbott ... 449
Erythrocin Stearate Filmtab Tablets (Erythromycin Stearate) Abbott ... 453
Erythromycin Base Filmtab Tablets (Erythromycin) Abbott ... 455
Erythromycin Delayed-Release Capsules, USP (Erythromycin) Abbott ... 457
Omnicef Capsules (Cefdinir) Abbott ... 511
Omnicef for Oral Suspension (Cefdinir) Abbott ... 511
PCE Dispertab Tablets (Erythromycin) Abbott ... 515
Suprax (Cefixime) Lupin ... 1843
Tequin Injection (Gatifloxacin) Bristol-Myers Squibb ... 938
Tequin Injection in 5% Dextrose (Gatifloxacin) Bristol-Myers Squibb ... 938
Tequin Tablets (Gatifloxacin) Bristol-Myers Squibb ... 938
Vantin Tablets and Oral Suspension (Cefpodoxime Proxetil) Pharmacia & Upjohn ... 2645

Infections, urinary tract
Amoxil Capsules (Amoxicillin) GlaxoSmithKline ... 1343
Amoxil Chewable Tablets (Amoxicillin) GlaxoSmithKline ... 1343
Amoxil Pediatric Drops for Oral Suspension (Amoxicillin) GlaxoSmithKline ... 1343
Amoxil Powder for Oral Suspension (Amoxicillin) GlaxoSmithKline ... 1343
Amoxil Tablets (Amoxicillin) GlaxoSmithKline ... 1343
Augmentin (Amoxicillin, Clavulanate Potassium) GlaxoSmithKline ... 1360
Augmentin Tablets (Amoxicillin, Clavulanate Potassium) GlaxoSmithKline ... 1363
Ceftin Tablets (Cefuroxime Axetil) GlaxoSmithKline ... 1407
Cipro (Ciprofloxacin) Schering ... 2977
Cipro I.V. (Ciprofloxacin) Schering ... 2984
Cipro XR Tablets (Ciprofloxacin) Schering ... 2990
Fortaz (Ceftazidime) GlaxoSmithKline ... 1453
Gantrisin Pediatric Suspension (Acetyl Sulfisoxazole) Roche ... 2770
Garamycin Injectable (Gentamicin Sulfate) Schering ... 3014
Invanz for Injection (Ertapenem) Merck ... 1999
Levaquin (Levofloxacin) Ortho-McNeil ... 2384
Levaquin in 5% Dextrose Injection (Levofloxacin) Ortho-McNeil ... 2384
Maxipime for Injection (Cefepime Hydrochloride) Elan ... 1105
Mefoxin for Injection (Cefoxitin Sodium) Merck ... 2012
Mefoxin Premixed Intravenous Solution (Cefoxitin Sodium) Merck ... 2016
Noroxin Tablets (Norfloxacin) Merck ... 2032
Primaxin I.V. (Cilastatin Sodium, Imipenem) Merck ... 2048
Proquin XR Tablets (Ciprofloxacin Hydrochloride) Esprit ... 1153
Rocephin Injectable Vials, ADD-Vantage, Galaxy, Bulk (Ceftriaxone Sodium) Roche ... 2800
Seromycin Capsules (Cycloserine) Lilly ... 1813
Suprax (Cefixime) Lupin ... 1843
Tequin Injection (Gatifloxacin) Bristol-Myers Squibb ... 938
Tequin Injection in 5% Dextrose (Gatifloxacin) Bristol-Myers Squibb ... 938
Tequin Tablets (Gatifloxacin) Bristol-Myers Squibb ... 938
Timentin ADD-Vantage (Clavulanate Potassium, Ticarcillin Disodium) GlaxoSmithKline ... 1580
Timentin Injection Galaxy Container (Clavulanate Potassium, Ticarcillin Disodium) GlaxoSmithKline ... 1583
Timentin IV Infusion (Clavulanate Potassium, Ticarcillin Disodium) GlaxoSmithKline ... 1577
Timentin Pharmacy Bulk Package (Clavulanate Potassium, Ticarcillin Disodium) GlaxoSmithKline ... 1586
Uroqid-Acid No. 2 Tablets (Methenamine Mandelate, Sodium Acid Phosphate) Beach ... 760
Vantin Tablets and Oral Suspension (Cefpodoxime Proxetil) Pharmacia & Upjohn ... 2645
Zinacef for Injection (Cefuroxime) GlaxoSmithKline ... 1631
Zinacef Injection (Cefuroxime) GlaxoSmithKline ... 1631

Infections, vaginal cuff, post-surgical
Cleocin Vaginal Ovules (Clindamycin Hydrochloride) Pharmacia & Upjohn ... 2616

Infections, venereal
(*see under* Gonorrhea)

Infectious diarrhea
(*see under* Diarrhea, infectious)

Infertility, progesterone deficiency-induced
Prochieve 8% Gel (Progesterone) Columbia ... 1003

Inflammation, anorectal
Analpram-HC (Hydrocortisone Acetate, Pramoxine Hydrochloride) Ferndale ... 1159
ProctoFoam-HC (Hydrocortisone Acetate, Pramoxine Hydrochloride) Schwarz ... 3099

Inflammation, anterior segment
Blephamide Ophthalmic Ointment (Prednisolone Acetate, Sulfacetamide Sodium) Allergan ... 568
Blephamide Ophthalmic Suspension (Prednisolone Acetate, Sulfacetamide Sodium) Allergan ... 569
Depo-Medrol Injectable Suspension (Methylprednisolone Acetate) Pharmacia & Upjohn ... 2617
FML Ophthalmic Ointment (Fluorometholone) Allergan ... ⊙ 228
FML Ophthalmic Suspension (Fluorometholone) Allergan ... ⊙ 227
FML Forte Ophthalmic Suspension (Fluorometholone) Allergan ... ⊙ 226
FML-S Ophthalmic Suspension (Fluorometholone, Sulfacetamide Sodium) Allergan ... ⊙ 229
Hydrocortone Tablets (Hydrocortisone) Merck ... 1989
Lotemax Ophthalmic Suspension 0.5% (Loteprednol Etabonate) Bausch & Lomb ... ⊙ 251
Poly-Pred Ophthalmic Suspension (Neomycin Sulfate, Polymyxin B Sulfate, Prednisolone Acetate) Allergan ... ⊙ 233
Pred Forte Ophthalmic Suspension (Prednisolone Acetate) Allergan ... ⊙ 235
Pred-G Ophthalmic Ointment (Gentamicin Sulfate, Prednisolone Acetate) Allergan ... ⊙ 237
Pred-G Ophthalmic Suspension (Gentamicin Sulfate, Prednisolone Acetate) Allergan ... ⊙ 236
TobraDex Ophthalmic Ointment (Dexamethasone, Tobramycin) Alcon ... 562
TobraDex Ophthalmic Suspension (Dexamethasone, Tobramycin) Alcon ... 563

Influenza, prophylaxis of
Relenza Rotadisk (Zanamivir) GlaxoSmithKline ... 1552

Influenza, symptomatic relief of
Contac Cold and Flu Maximum Strength Caplets (Acetaminophen, Chlorpheniramine Maleate, Phenylephrine Hydrochloride) GlaxoSmithKline ... [■] 728
Contac Cold and Flu Day and Night Caplets (Day Formulation Only) (Acetaminophen, Phenylephrine Hydrochloride) GlaxoSmithKline ... [■] 727
Contac Cold and Flu Day and Night Caplets (Night Formulation Only) (Acetaminophen, Chlorpheniramine Maleate, Phenylephrine Hydrochloride) GlaxoSmithKline ... [■] 727
Children's Tylenol Plus Cough & Runny Nose Suspension Liquid (Acetaminophen, Chlorpheniramine Maleate, Dextromethorphan Hydrobromide) McNeil Consumer ... [■] 754
Children's Tylenol Plus Cough & Sore Throat Suspension Liquid (Acetaminophen, Dextromethorphan Hydrobromide) McNeil Consumer ... [■] 754
Children's Tylenol Plus Cold Suspension Liquid (Acetaminophen, Chlorpheniramine Maleate, Phenylephrine Hydrochloride) McNeil Consumer ... [■] 754
Children's Tylenol Plus Multi-Symptom Cold Suspension Liquid (Acetaminophen, Chlorpheniramine Maleate, Dextromethorphan Hydrobromide, Phenylephrine Hydrochloride) McNeil Consumer ... [■] 754
Tylenol Cold Head Congestion Severe Caplets with Cool Burst (Acetaminophen, Dextromethorphan Hydrobromide, Guaifenesin, Phenylephrine Hydrochloride) McNeil Consumer ... [■] 750
Children's Tylenol Plus Cold Suspension Liquid (Acetaminophen, Chlorpheniramine Maleate, Phenylephrine Hydrochloride) McNeil Consumer ... 1879
Children's Tylenol Plus Cough & Runny Nose Suspension Liquid (Acetaminophen, Chlorpheniramine Maleate, Dextromethorphan Hydrobromide) McNeil Consumer ... 1879
Children's Tylenol Plus Cough & Sore Throat Suspension Liquid (Acetaminophen, Dextromethorphan Hydrobromide) McNeil Consumer ... 1879
Children's Tylenol Suspension with Flavor Creator (Acetaminophen) McNeil Consumer ... 1878
Children's Tylenol Plus Multi-Symptom Cold Suspension Liquid (Acetaminophen, Chlorpheniramine Maleate, Dextromethorphan Hydrobromide, Phenylephrine Hydrochloride) McNeil Consumer ... 1879
Tylenol Cold Head Congestion Severe Caplets with Cool Burst (Acetaminophen, Dextromethorphan Hydrobromide, Guaifenesin, Phenylephrine Hydrochloride) McNeil Consumer ... 1873
Concentrated Tylenol Infants' Drops Plus Cold and Cough (Acetaminophen, Dextromethorphan Hydrobromide) McNeil Consumer ... 1879

Influenza A virus, acute illness, treatment of
Relenza Rotadisk (Zanamivir) GlaxoSmithKline ... 1552
Tamiflu Capsules (Oseltamivir Phosphate) Roche ... 2807
Tamiflu Oral Suspension (Oseltamivir Phosphate) Roche ... 2807

Influenza A virus, respiratory tract illness, chemoprophylaxis of
Flumadine (Rimantadine Hydrochloride) Forest ... 1183
Symmetrel Tablets (Amantadine Hydrochloride) Endo Labs ... 1135

Tamiflu Capsules (Oseltamivir Phosphate) Roche 2807
Tamiflu Oral Suspension (Oseltamivir Phosphate) Roche 2807

Influenza A virus, respiratory tract illness, treatment of
Flumadine (Rimantadine Hydrochloride) Forest 1183
Symmetrel Tablets (Amantadine Hydrochloride) Endo Labs 1135

Influenza syndrome, symptomatic relief of
Advil Cold & Sinus (Ibuprofen, Pseudoephedrine Hydrochloride) Wyeth .... ▣723
Bufferin Extra Strength Tablets (Aspirin Buffered) Novartis Consumer .... ▣678
Bufferin Regular Strength Tablets (Aspirin Buffered) Novartis Consumer .... ▣678
Hyland's Complete Flu Care 4 Kids Tablets (Dietary Supplement) Standard Homeopathic .... ▣732
Children's Motrin Cold Oral Suspension (Ibuprofen, Pseudoephedrine Hydrochloride) McNeil Consumer 1867
Robitussin Cough & Allergy Syrup (Chlorpheniramine Maleate, Dextromethorphan Hydrobromide, Phenylephrine Hydrochloride) Wyeth .... ▣736
Robitussin Cough & Cold Nighttime Liquid (Chlorpheniramine Maleate, Dextromethorphan Hydrobromide, Phenylephrine Hydrochloride) Wyeth .... ▣736
Robitussin Cough, Cold & Flu Nighttime Liquid (Acetaminophen, Chlorpheniramine Maleate, Dextromethorphan Hydrobromide, Phenylephrine Hydrochloride) Wyeth .... ▣738
Robitussin Pediatric Cough & Cold Nighttime Liquid (Chlorpheniramine Maleate, Dextromethorphan Hydrobromide, Phenylephrine Hydrochloride) Wyeth .... ▣736
TheraFlu Cold & Sore Throat Hot Liquid (Acetaminophen, Pheniramine Maleate, Phenylephrine Hydrochloride) Novartis Consumer .... ▣741
TheraFlu Flu & Chest Congestion Hot Liquid (Acetaminophen, Guaifenesin) Novartis Consumer .. ▣741
TheraFlu Flu & Sore Throat Hot Liquid (Acetaminophen, Pheniramine Maleate, Phenylephrine Hydrochloride) Novartis Consumer .... ▣742
TheraFlu Nighttime Severe Cold Hot Liquid (Acetaminophen, Pheniramine Maleate, Phenylephrine Hydrochloride) Novartis Consumer .... ▣740
Tussionex Pennkinetic Extended-Release Suspension (Chlorpheniramine Polistirex, Hydrocodone Polistirex) UCB 3327
Children's Tylenol with Flavor Creator (Acetaminophen) McNeil Consumer .... ▣679
Tylenol Cold Head Congestion Severe Caplets with Cool Burst (Acetaminophen, Dextromethorphan Hydrobromide, Guaifenesin, Phenylephrine Hydrochloride) McNeil Consumer .... ▣750
Children's Tylenol Suspension Liquid and Meltaways (Acetaminophen) McNeil Consumer 1878
Concentrated Tylenol Infants' Drops (Acetaminophen) McNeil Consumer 1878
Jr. Tylenol Meltaways (Acetaminophen) McNeil Consumer 1878
Vicks NyQuil Multi-Symptom Cold/Flu Relief Liquid (Acetaminophen, Dextromethorphan Hydrobromide, Doxylamine Succinate, Pseudoephedrine Hydrochloride) Procter & Gamble 2681
Vicks NyQuil Multi-Symptom Cold/Flu Relief LiquiCaps (Acetaminophen, Dextromethorphan Hydrobromide, Doxylamine Succinate, Pseudoephedrine Hydrochloride) Procter & Gamble 2681
Vicks NyQuil LiquiCaps/Liquid Multi-Symptom Cold/Flu Relief (Acetaminophen, Dextromethorphan Hydrobromide, Doxylamine Succinate) Procter & Gamble .... ▣763
Zicam Maximum Strength Flu Daytime (Acetaminophen, Chlorpheniramine Maleate, Dextromethorphan Hydrobromide) Matrixx .... ▣768
Zicam Maximum Strength Flu Nighttime (Acetaminophen, Dextromethorphan Hydrobromide, Doxylamine Succinate) Matrixx .... ▣768

Influenza virus type A and B, immunization against
(*see also under* Immunization, influenza virus, types A and B)
Fluarix (Influenza Virus Vaccine) GlaxoSmithKline 1451
Flumist Vaccine (Influenza Virus Vaccine) Medimmune 1901

Influenza virus type A and B vaccine
(*see also under* Immunization, influenza virus, types A and B)
Fluarix (Influenza Virus Vaccine) GlaxoSmithKline 1451
Flumist Vaccine (Influenza Virus Vaccine) Medimmune 1901

Insect bites, pain due to
(*see under* Pain, topical relief of)

Insomnia
(*see also under* Sleep, induction of)
Advil PM Caplets (Diphenhydramine Citrate, Ibuprofen) Wyeth .... ▣615
Hyland's Calm Forte 4 Kids Tablets (Homeopathic Formulations, Sulfur) Standard Homeopathic .... ▣828

Intermittent claudication
(*see under* Claudication, intermittent)

Intertrigo
(*see under* Skin, inflammatory conditions)

Intraocular pressure, elevation
(*see under* Hypertension, ocular)

Intravascular device, maintenance of patency
Cathflo Activase (Alteplase) Genentech 1231

Intubation, endotracheal
Mivacron Injection (Mivacurium Chloride) Abbott 493
Nimbex Injection (Cisatracurium Besylate) Abbott 498
Zemuron Injection (Rocuronium Bromide) Organon USA 2346

Iridocyclitis
Depo-Medrol Injectable Suspension (Methylprednisolone Acetate) Pharmacia & Upjohn 2617
Hydrocortone Tablets (Hydrocortisone) Merck 1989

Iritis
Depo-Medrol Injectable Suspension (Methylprednisolone Acetate) Pharmacia & Upjohn 2617
Hydrocortone Tablets (Hydrocortisone) Merck 1989

Iron deficiency
Infed Injection (Iron Dextran) Watson 3390
Slow Fe Iron Tablets (Ferrous Sulfate) Novartis Consumer .... ▣818

Irritable bowel syndrome
(*see under* Bowel, irritable, syndrome)

Ischemic attacks, transient
Bayer Aspirin (Aspirin) Bayer Healthcare LLC 744

Ischemic attacks, transient, reduce risk of
Bayer Aspirin (Aspirin) Bayer Healthcare LLC 744

Isoimmunization, prevention of in Rho(D) negative individuals
HyperRho S/D Full Dose (Rh_o (D) Immune Globulin (Human)) Talecris 3246
Rhophylac (Rh_o (D) Immune Globulin (Human)) ZLB Behring 3505

Isoimmunization, prevention of in Rho(D) negative women
HyperRho S/D Mini-Dose (Rh_o (D) Immune Globulin (Human)) Talecris 3244
MICRhoGAM Ultra-Filtered (Rh_o (D) Immune Globulin (Human)) Ortho-Clinical 2371
RhoGAM Ultra-Filtered (Rh_o (D) Immune Globulin (Human)) Ortho-Clinical 2371
Rhophylac (Rh_o (D) Immune Globulin (Human)) ZLB Behring 3505

Itching, eye, reduction of
Advil Allergy Sinus Caplets (Chlorpheniramine Maleate, Ibuprofen, Pseudoephedrine Hydrochloride) Wyeth .... ▣770
Advil Multi-Symptom Cold Caplets (Chlorpheniramine Maleate, Ibuprofen, Pseudoephedrine Hydrochloride) Wyeth .... ▣770
Children's Claritin Allergy Oral Solution (Loratadine) Schering-Plough .... ▣771
Claritin Non-Drowsy 24 Hour Tablets (Loratadine) Schering-Plough .... ▣772
Claritin-D Non-Drowsy 12 Hour Tablets (Loratadine, Pseudoephedrine Sulfate) Schering-Plough .... ▣772
Claritin-D Non-Drowsy 24 Hour Tablets (Loratadine, Pseudoephedrine Sulfate) Schering-Plough .... ▣772
Children's Dimetapp Long Acting Cough Plus Cold Syrup (Chlorpheniramine Maleate, Dextromethorphan Hydrobromide) Wyeth .... ▣731
TheraFlu Cold & Cough Hot Liquid (Dextromethorphan Hydrobromide, Pheniramine Maleate, Phenylephrine Hydrochloride) Novartis Consumer .... ▣740
TheraFlu Cold & Sore Throat Hot Liquid (Acetaminophen, Pheniramine Maleate, Phenylephrine Hydrochloride) Novartis Consumer .... ▣741
TheraFlu Flu & Sore Throat Hot Liquid (Acetaminophen, Pheniramine Maleate, Phenylephrine Hydrochloride) Novartis Consumer .... ▣742
TheraFlu Nighttime Severe Cold Hot Liquid (Acetaminophen, Pheniramine Maleate, Phenylephrine Hydrochloride) Novartis Consumer .... ▣740
TheraFlu Thin Strips Multi Symptom (Diphenhydramine Hydrochloride) Novartis Consumer .... ▣744
Triaminic Cold & Allergy Liquid (Chlorpheniramine Maleate, Phenylephrine Hydrochloride) Novartis Consumer .... ▣746
Triaminic Nighttime Cold & Cough Liquid (Diphenhydramine Hydrochloride, Phenylephrine Hydrochloride) Novartis Consumer .... ▣746
Triaminic Cough & Runny Nose Softchews (Chlorpheniramine Maleate, Dextromethorphan Hydrobromide) Novartis Consumer .... ▣748
Tylenol Allergy Multi-Symptom Caplets with Cool Burst and Gelcaps (Acetaminophen, Chlorpheniramine Maleate, Phenylephrine Hydrochloride) McNeil Consumer 1872
Tylenol Allergy Multi-Symptom Nighttime Caplets with Cool Burst (Acetaminophen, Diphenhydramine Hydrochloride, Phenylephrine Hydrochloride) McNeil Consumer 1872
Tylenol Severe Allergy Caplets (Acetaminophen, Diphenhydramine Hydrochloride) McNeil Consumer 1872
Children's Tylenol Plus Cold & Allergy Suspension Liquid (Acetaminophen, Diphenhydramine Hydrochloride, Phenylephrine Hydrochloride) McNeil Consumer .. 1878
Visine A.C. Seasonal Itching and Redness Relief Drops (Tetrahydrozoline Hydrochloride, Zinc Sulfate) Pfizer Consumer .... ⊙289

Itching, skin
(*see under* Pruritus, topical relief of)

Itching, sunburn
(*see under* Pruritus, topical relief of)

J

Jock itch
(*see under* Tinea cruris infections)

Joint pain
(*see under* Pain, arthritic, minor)

K

K. pneumoniae bacteremia
Rocephin (Ceftriaxone Sodium) Roche 2800

K. pneumoniae bone and joint infections
Rocephin (Ceftriaxone Sodium) Roche 2800

K. pneumoniae gynecologic infections
Primaxin I.M. (Cilastatin Sodium, Imipenem) Merck 2045
Timentin ADD-Vantage (Clavulanate Potassium, Ticarcillin Disodium) GlaxoSmithKline 1580
Timentin Injection Galaxy Container (Clavulanate Potassium, Ticarcillin Disodium) GlaxoSmithKline 1583
Timentin IV Infusion (Clavulanate Potassium, Ticarcillin Disodium) GlaxoSmithKline 1577
Timentin Pharmacy Bulk Package (Clavulanate Potassium, Ticarcillin Disodium) GlaxoSmithKline 1586

K. pneumoniae infections
Augmentin XR Extended-Release Tablets (Amoxicillin, Clavulanate Potassium) GlaxoSmithKline 1369
Avelox (Moxifloxacin Hydrochloride) Schering 2970
Ceftin Tablets (Cefuroxime Axetil) GlaxoSmithKline 1407
Cipro (Ciprofloxacin) Schering 2977
Cipro I.V. (Ciprofloxacin) Schering 2984
Invanz for Injection (Ertapenem) Merck 1999
Levaquin (Levofloxacin) Ortho-McNeil 2384
Levaquin in 5% Dextrose Injection (Levofloxacin) Ortho-McNeil 2384
Merrem I.V. (Meropenem) AstraZeneca Pharmaceuticals 686
Noroxin Tablets (Norfloxacin) Merck . 2032
Primaxin I.M. (Cilastatin Sodium, Imipenem) Merck 2045
Proquin XR Tablets (Ciprofloxacin Hydrochloride) Esprit 1153
Rocephin Injectable Vials, ADD-Vantage, Galaxy, Bulk (Ceftriaxone Sodium) Roche 2800
Suprax (Cefixime) Lupin 1843
Tequin Injection (Gatifloxacin) Bristol-Myers Squibb 938
Tequin Injection in 5% Dextrose (Gatifloxacin) Bristol-Myers Squibb 938
Tequin Tablets (Gatifloxacin) Bristol-Myers Squibb 938
Timentin ADD-Vantage (Clavulanate Potassium, Ticarcillin Disodium) GlaxoSmithKline 1580
Timentin Injection Galaxy Container (Clavulanate Potassium, Ticarcillin Disodium) GlaxoSmithKline 1583
Timentin IV Infusion (Clavulanate Potassium, Ticarcillin Disodium) GlaxoSmithKline 1577
Timentin Pharmacy Bulk Package (Clavulanate Potassium, Ticarcillin Disodium) GlaxoSmithKline 1586
Tygacil for Injection (Tigecycline) Wyeth 3488

Timentin ADD-Vantage (Clavulanate Potassium, Ticarcillin Disodium) GlaxoSmithKline 1580
Timentin Injection Galaxy Container (Clavulanate Potassium, Ticarcillin Disodium) GlaxoSmithKline 1583
Timentin IV Infusion (Clavulanate Potassium, Ticarcillin Disodium) GlaxoSmithKline 1577
Timentin Pharmacy Bulk Package (Clavulanate Potassium, Ticarcillin Disodium) GlaxoSmithKline 1586
Zinacef for Injection (Cefuroxime) GlaxoSmithKline 1631
Zinacef Injection (Cefuroxime) GlaxoSmithKline 1631

Klebsiella-Enterobacter species infections, ocular

Blephamide Ophthalmic Ointment (Prednisolone Acetate, Sulfacetamide Sodium) Allergan 568
Blephamide Ophthalmic Suspension (Prednisolone Acetate, Sulfacetamide Sodium) Allergan 569
FML-S Ophthalmic Suspension (Fluorometholone, Sulfacetamide Sodium) Allergan .... ⊙229
Poly-Pred Ophthalmic Suspension (Neomycin Sulfate, Polymyxin B Sulfate, Prednisolone Acetate) Allergan .... ⊙233
Pred-G Ophthalmic Suspension (Gentamicin Sulfate, Prednisolone Acetate) Allergan .... ⊙236
TobraDex Ophthalmic Ointment (Dexamethasone, Tobramycin) Alcon 562
TobraDex Ophthalmic Suspension (Dexamethasone, Tobramycin) Alcon 563

Koch-Weeks bacillus infections, ocular

(*see under* H. aegypticus infections, ocular)

L

Lacrimation, symptomatic relief of

Advil Allergy Sinus Caplets (Chlorpheniramine Maleate, Ibuprofen, Pseudoephedrine Hydrochloride) Wyeth .... ▣770
Advil Multi-Symptom Cold Caplets (Chlorpheniramine Maleate, Ibuprofen, Pseudoephedrine Hydrochloride) Wyeth .... ▣770
Alavert Allergy & Sinus D-12 Hour Tablets (Loratadine, Pseudoephedrine Sulfate) Wyeth .... ▣771
Alavert (Loratadine) Wyeth .... ▣771
Allegra-D 12 Hour Extended-Release Tablets (Fexofenadine Hydrochloride, Pseudoephedrine Hydrochloride) sanofi-aventis 2846
Children's Claritin Allergy Oral Solution (Loratadine) Schering-Plough .... ▣771
Claritin Non-Drowsy 24 Hour Tablets (Loratadine) Schering-Plough .... ▣772
Claritin Reditabs 24 Hour Non-Drowsy Tablets (Loratadine) Schering-Plough .... ▣772
Claritin-D Non-Drowsy 12 Hour Tablets (Loratadine, Pseudoephedrine Sulfate) Schering-Plough .... ▣772
Claritin-D Non-Drowsy 24 Hour Tablets (Loratadine, Pseudoephedrine Sulfate) Schering-Plough .... ▣772
Children's Dimetapp Cold & Allergy Elixir (Brompheniramine Maleate, Phenylephrine Hydrochloride) Wyeth .... ▣730
Children's Dimetapp Cold & Allergy Chewable Tablets (Brompheniramine Maleate, Phenylephrine Hydrochloride) Wyeth .... ▣730
Children's Dimetapp Long Acting Cough Plus Cold Syrup (Chlorpheniramine Maleate, Dextromethorphan Hydrobromide) Wyeth .... ▣731
Robitussin Cough & Cold Long-Acting Liquid (Chlorpheniramine Maleate, Dextromethorphan Hydrobromide) Wyeth .... ▣735
Robitussin Cough & Allergy Syrup (Chlorpheniramine Maleate, Dextromethorphan Hydrobromide, Phenylephrine Hydrochloride) Wyeth .... ▣736
Robitussin Cough & Cold Nighttime Liquid (Chlorpheniramine Maleate, Dextromethorphan Hydrobromide, Phenylephrine Hydrochloride) Wyeth .... ▣736
Robitussin Cough, Cold & Flu Nighttime Liquid (Acetaminophen, Chlorpheniramine Maleate, Dextromethorphan Hydrobromide, Phenylephrine Hydrochloride) Wyeth .... ▣738
Robitussin Pediatric Cough & Cold Long-Acting Liquid (Chlorpheniramine Maleate, Dextromethorphan Hydrobromide) Wyeth .... ▣735
Robitussin Pediatric Cough & Cold Nighttime Liquid (Chlorpheniramine Maleate, Dextromethorphan Hydrobromide, Phenylephrine Hydrochloride) Wyeth .... ▣736
TheraFlu Cold & Cough Hot Liquid (Dextromethorphan Hydrobromide, Pheniramine Maleate, Phenylephrine Hydrochloride) Novartis Consumer .... ▣740
TheraFlu Cold & Sore Throat Hot Liquid (Acetaminophen, Pheniramine Maleate, Phenylephrine Hydrochloride) Novartis Consumer .... ▣741
TheraFlu Flu & Sore Throat Hot Liquid (Acetaminophen, Pheniramine Maleate, Phenylephrine Hydrochloride) Novartis Consumer .... ▣742
TheraFlu Nighttime Severe Cold Hot Liquid (Acetaminophen, Pheniramine Maleate, Phenylephrine Hydrochloride) Novartis Consumer .... ▣740
TheraFlu Warming Relief Nighttime Severe Cold (Acetaminophen, Diphenhydramine Hydrochloride, Phenylephrine Hydrochloride) Novartis Consumer .... ▣743
TheraFlu Thin Strips Multi Symptom (Diphenhydramine Hydrochloride) Novartis Consumer .... ▣744
Triaminic Cold & Allergy Liquid (Chlorpheniramine Maleate, Phenylephrine Hydrochloride) Novartis Consumer .... ▣746
Triaminic Nighttime Cold & Cough Liquid (Diphenhydramine Hydrochloride, Phenylephrine Hydrochloride) Novartis Consumer .... ▣746
Triaminic Cough & Runny Nose Softchews (Chlorpheniramine Maleate, Dextromethorphan Hydrobromide) Novartis Consumer .... ▣748
Triaminic Thin Strips Cough & Runny Nose (Diphenhydramine Hydrochloride) Novartis Consumer .... ▣749
Children's Tylenol Plus Cold & Allergy Oral Suspension (Acetaminophen, Diphenhydramine Hydrochloride, Phenylephrine Hydrochloride) McNeil Consumer .... ▣716
Tylenol Allergy Multi-Symptom Caplets with Cool Burst and Gelcaps (Acetaminophen, Chlorpheniramine Maleate, Phenylephrine Hydrochloride) McNeil Consumer 1872
Tylenol Allergy Multi-Symptom Nighttime Caplets with Cool Burst (Acetaminophen, Diphenhydramine Hydrochloride, Phenylephrine Hydrochloride) McNeil Consumer 1872
Tylenol Severe Allergy Caplets (Acetaminophen, Diphenhydramine Hydrochloride) McNeil Consumer 1872
Children's Tylenol Plus Cold & Allergy Suspension Liquid (Acetaminophen, Diphenhydramine Hydrochloride, Phenylephrine Hydrochloride) McNeil Consumer 1878
Visine A.C. Seasonal Itching and Redness Relief Drops (Tetrahydrozoline Hydrochloride, Zinc Sulfate) Pfizer Consumer .... ⊙289
Zicam Allergy Relief (Histanium Hydrochloricum, Luffa operculata, Galphimia Glauca, Sulfur) Matrixx .... ▣774
Zicam Maximum Strength Flu Daytime (Acetaminophen, Chlorpheniramine Maleate, Dextromethorphan Hydrobromide) Matrixx .... ▣768
Zicam Maximum Strength Flu Nighttime (Acetaminophen, Dextromethorphan Hydrobromide, Doxylamine Succinate) Matrixx .... ▣768

Lactobacillus acidophilus, deficiency of

DDS-Acidophilus Capsules, Tablets, and Powder (Lactobacillus Acidophilus) UAS Labs .... ▣812

Lactose intolerance

Lactaid Original Strength Caplets (Lactase (beta-d-Galactosidase)) McNeil Nutritionals, LLC 1881
Lactaid Fast Act Caplets and Chewable Tablets (Lactase (beta-d-Galactosidase)) McNeil Nutritionals, LLC 1881
Lactaid Fast Act Caplets and Chewable Tablets (Lactase (beta-d-Galactosidase)) McNeil Consumer .... ▣668

Larva migrans, cutaneous

Mintezol (Thiabendazole) Merck 2027

Laryngeal edema, acute noninfectious, adjunctive therapy in

Depo-Medrol Injectable Suspension (Methylprednisolone Acetate) Pharmacia & Upjohn 2617
Depo-Medrol Single-Dose Vial (Methylprednisolone Acetate) Pharmacia & Upjohn 2619

LDL cholesterol, elevation

(*see under* Hyperlipoproteinemia, types IIa and IIb, adjunct to diet)

Lead encephalopathy

Calcium Disodium Versenate (Calcium Disodium Edetate) 3M 1851

Lead poisoning

Chemet Capsules (Succimer) Ovation 2458

Leg muscle cramps

Hyland's Leg Cramps with Quinine Tablets and Caplets (Homeopathic Formulations) Standard Homeopathic .... ▣829

Legionella pneumophila infections

(*see under* Legionnaires' disease)

Legionnaires' disease

E.E.S. (Erythromycin Ethylsuccinate) Abbott 451
EryPed (Erythromycin Ethylsuccinate) Abbott 447
Ery-Tab Tablets (Erythromycin) Abbott 449
Erythrocin Stearate Filmtab Tablets (Erythromycin Stearate) Abbott 453
Erythromycin Base Filmtab Tablets (Erythromycin) Abbott 455
Erythromycin Delayed-Release Capsules, USP (Erythromycin) Abbott 457
Levaquin (Levofloxacin) Ortho-McNeil 2384
Levaquin in 5% Dextrose Injection (Levofloxacin) Ortho-McNeil 2384
PCE Dispertab Tablets (Erythromycin) Abbott 515
Tequin Injection (Gatifloxacin) Bristol-Myers Squibb 938
Tequin Injection in 5% Dextrose (Gatifloxacin) Bristol-Myers Squibb 938
Tequin Tablets (Gatifloxacin) Bristol-Myers Squibb 938

Lennox-Gastaut syndrome

Klonopin (Clonazepam) Roche 2778
Lamictal (Lamotrigine) GlaxoSmithKline 1481
Topamax Sprinkle Capsules (Topiramate) Ortho-McNeil Neurologics 2404
Topamax Tablets (Topiramate) Ortho-McNeil Neurologics 2404

Leprosy

Dapsone Tablets USP (Dapsone) Jacobus 1673

Lesions, inflammatory, rosacea associated

Oracea Capsules (Doxycycline Monohydrate) CollaGenex 1000

Leukemia, acute, palliative management of in childhood

Depo-Medrol Single-Dose Vial (Methylprednisolone Acetate) Pharmacia & Upjohn 2619
Hydrocortone Tablets (Hydrocortisone) Merck 1989

Leukemia, acute, promyelocytic

Trisenox Injection (Arsenic Trioxide) Cephalon 993
Vesanoid Capsules (Tretinoin) Roche 2820

Leukemia, acute lymphoblastic

Arranon Injection (Nelarabine) GlaxoSmithKline 1357
Clolar for Intravenous Infusion (Clofarabine) Genzyme 1271
Oncaspar (Pegaspargase) Enzon 1145

Leukemia, acute lymphocytic

Elspar for Injection (Asparaginase) Ovation 2463
Elspar for Injection (Asparaginase) Merck 1960

Leukemia, acute myelogenous

Leukine (Sargramostim) Berlex 814

Leukemia, acute myeloid, adjunctive therapy in

Neupogen for Injection (Filgrastim) Amgen 603

Leukemia, acute myeloid, CD33 positive

Mylotarg for Injection (Gemtuzumab Ozogamicin) Wyeth 3431

Leukemia, acute nonlymphocytic

Tabloid Tablets (Thioguanine) GlaxoSmithKline 1575

Leukemia, adjunctive therapy in

Aloprim for Injection (Allopurinol Sodium) Nabi 2167
Elitek (Rasburicase) sanofi-aventis 2890

Leukemia, chronic lymphocytic

Leukeran Tablets (Chlorambucil) GlaxoSmithKline 1504
Mustargen for Injection (Mechlorethamine Hydrochloride) Ovation 2468

Leukemia, chronic lymphocytic, B-cell

Campath Ampules (Alemtuzumab) Berlex 811

Leukemia, chronic lymphocytic, B-cell, prevention of bacterial infection in

Gammagard S/D (Immune Globulin Intravenous (Human)) Baxter Healthcare 724

Leukemia, chronic myeloid

Gleevec Tablets (Imatinib Mesylate) Novartis 2227
I.V. Busulfex (Busulfan) PDL 2493
Mustargen for Injection (Mechlorethamine Hydrochloride) Ovation 2468
Myleran Tablets (Busulfan) GlaxoSmithKline 1525

Leukemia, hairy cell

Intron A for Injection (Interferon alfa-2b, Recombinant) Schering 3024
Leustatin Injection (Cladribine) Ortho Biotech 2357

Leukemia, hairy cell, alpha-interferon-refractory
Nipent for Injection (Pentostatin) Mayne 1863

Leukemia, lymphoblastic, adjunctive therapy in
Leukine (Sargramostim) Berlex 814

Leukemias, palliative management of
Decadron Tablets (Dexamethasone) Merck 1951
Depo-Medrol Injectable Suspension (Methylprednisolone Acetate) Pharmacia & Upjohn 2617
Depo-Medrol Single-Dose Vial (Methylprednisolone Acetate) Pharmacia & Upjohn 2619
Hydrocortone Tablets (Hydrocortisone) Merck 1989

Lice, body
(*see under* Pediculosis, human)

Lice, head
(*see under* Pediculosis, human)

Lice, pubic
(*see under* Pediculosis, human)

Lichen planus
Depo-Medrol Single-Dose Vial (Methylprednisolone Acetate) Pharmacia & Upjohn 2619

Lichen simplex chronicus
Depo-Medrol Single-Dose Vial (Methylprednisolone Acetate) Pharmacia & Upjohn 2619

Listeria monocytogenes infections
E.E.S. (Erythromycin Ethylsuccinate) Abbott 451
EryPed (Erythromycin Ethylsuccinate) Abbott 447
Ery-Tab Tablets (Erythromycin) Abbott 449
Erythrocin Stearate Filmtab Tablets (Erythromycin Stearate) Abbott 453
Erythromycin Base Filmtab Tablets (Erythromycin) Abbott 455
Erythromycin Delayed-Release Capsules, USP (Erythromycin) Abbott 457
PCE Dispertab Tablets (Erythromycin) Abbott 515

Listeriosis
E.E.S. (Erythromycin Ethylsuccinate) Abbott 451
EryPed (Erythromycin Ethylsuccinate) Abbott 447
Erythromycin Delayed-Release Capsules, USP (Erythromycin) Abbott 457
PCE Dispertab Tablets (Erythromycin) Abbott 515

Liver, allogeneic transplants, prophylaxis of organ rejection in
CellCept Capsules (Mycophenolate Mofetil) Roche 2747
CellCept Intravenous (Mycophenolate Mofetil Hydrochloride) Roche .. 2747
CellCept Oral Suspension (Mycophenolate Mofetil) Roche 2747
CellCept Tablets (Mycophenolate Mofetil) Roche 2747
Gengraf Capsules (Cyclosporine) Abbott 459
Neoral Oral Solution (Cyclosporine) Novartis 2259
Neoral Soft Gelatin Capsules (Cyclosporine) Novartis 2259
Orthoclone OKT3 Sterile Solution (Muromonab-CD3) Ortho Biotech ... 2360
Prograf Capsules and Injection (Tacrolimus) Astellas 632
Sandimmune (Cyclosporine) Novartis 2275

Liver abscess, amebic
(*see under* Amebic liver abscess)

Liver failure, acute
Plasbumin-5 (Albumin (human)) Talecris 3251
Plasbumin-20 (Albumin (human)) Talecris 3252
Plasbumin-25 (Albumin (human)) Talecris 3253

Locoregional solid malignancies
Cosmegen for Injection (Dactinomycin) Ovation 2459

Loeffler's syndrome
Depo-Medrol Injectable Suspension (Methylprednisolone Acetate) Pharmacia & Upjohn 2617
Depo-Medrol Single-Dose Vial (Methylprednisolone Acetate) Pharmacia & Upjohn 2619
Hydrocortone Tablets (Hydrocortisone) Merck 1989

Lou Gehrig's disease
(*see under* Amyotrophic lateral sclerosis)

Lung abscess
(*see under* Abscess, lung)

Lupus erythematosus, systemic
Bayer Aspirin (Aspirin) Bayer Healthcare LLC 744
Decadron Tablets (Dexamethasone) Merck 1951
Depo-Medrol Injectable Suspension (Methylprednisolone Acetate) Pharmacia & Upjohn 2617
Depo-Medrol Single-Dose Vial (Methylprednisolone Acetate) Pharmacia & Upjohn 2619
Hydrocortone Tablets (Hydrocortisone) Merck 1989

Lupus erythematosus discoides
Depo-Medrol Single-Dose Vial (Methylprednisolone Acetate) Pharmacia & Upjohn 2619

Lyme disease
(*see under* Borrelia burgdorferi infection)

Lymphoma, cutaneous T-cell
Ontak Vials (Denileukin Diftitox) Ligand 1745
Targretin Capsules (Bexarotene) Ligand 1747

Lymphoma, lymphoblastic
Arranon Injection (Nelarabine) GlaxoSmithKline 1357

Lymphoma, non-Hodgkin's, follicular
Bexxar (Iodine I 131 Tositumomab, Tositumomab) GlaxoSmithKline 1398
Intron A for Injection (Interferon alfa-2b, Recombinant) Schering 3024

Lymphoma, unspecified, adjunctive therapy in
Aloprim for Injection (Allopurinol Sodium) Nabi 2167
Elitek (Rasburicase) sanofi-aventis 2890

Lymphomas, giant follicular
Leukeran Tablets (Chlorambucil) GlaxoSmithKline 1504

Lymphomas, Hodgkin's
(*see under* Hodgkin's disease)

Lymphomas, malignant
Leukeran Tablets (Chlorambucil) GlaxoSmithKline 1504

Lymphomas, non-Hodgkin's
Bexxar (Iodine I 131 Tositumomab, Tositumomab) GlaxoSmithKline 1398
Leukeran Tablets (Chlorambucil) GlaxoSmithKline 1504
Rituxan I.V. (Rituximab) Genentech 1254

Lymphomas, non-Hodgkin's, adjunctive therapy in
Leukine (Sargramostim) Berlex 814

Lymphomas, non-Hodgkin's, refractory
Bexxar (Iodine I 131 Tositumomab, Tositumomab) GlaxoSmithKline 1398

Lymphomas, palliative management of
Decadron Tablets (Dexamethasone) Merck 1951

Lymphomas, palliative management of in adults
Depo-Medrol Injectable Suspension (Methylprednisolone Acetate) Pharmacia & Upjohn 2617
Depo-Medrol Single-Dose Vial (Methylprednisolone Acetate) Pharmacia & Upjohn 2619
Hydrocortone Tablets (Hydrocortisone) Merck 1989

Lymphomatous meningitis
DepoCyt Injection (Cytarabine Liposome) Enzon 1143

Lymphosarcoma
(*see under* Lymphomas, non-Hodgkin's)

M

M. catarrhalis, otitis media
Augmentin (Amoxicillin, Clavulanate Potassium) GlaxoSmithKline 1360
Augmentin Tablets (Amoxicillin, Clavulanate Potassium) GlaxoSmithKline 1363
Augmentin ES-600 Powder for Oral Suspension (Amoxicillin, Clavulanate Potassium) GlaxoSmithKline 1366
Biaxin/Biaxin XL (Clarithromycin) Abbott 402
Ceftin (Cefuroxime Axetil) GlaxoSmithKline 1407
Floxin Otic Solution (Ofloxacin) Daiichi Sankyo 1049
Keflex Capsules (Cephalexin) Advancis 549
Omnicef Capsules (Cefdinir) Abbott .. 511
Omnicef for Oral Suspension (Cefdinir) Abbott 511
Rocephin Injectable Vials, ADD-Vantage, Galaxy, Bulk (Ceftriaxone Sodium) Roche 2800
Suprax (Cefixime) Lupin 1843
Vantin Tablets and Oral Suspension (Cefpodoxime Proxetil) Pharmacia & Upjohn 2645

M. catarrhalis bronchitis
Ketek Tablets (Telithromycin) sanofi-aventis 2903
Levaquin (Levofloxacin) Ortho-McNeil 2384
Levaquin in 5% Dextrose Injection (Levofloxacin) Ortho-McNeil 2384

M. catarrhalis infections
Augmentin (Amoxicillin, Clavulanate Potassium) GlaxoSmithKline 1360
Augmentin Tablets (Amoxicillin, Clavulanate Potassium) GlaxoSmithKline 1363
Augmentin XR Extended-Release Tablets (Amoxicillin, Clavulanate Potassium) GlaxoSmithKline 1369
Augmentin ES-600 Powder for Oral Suspension (Amoxicillin, Clavulanate Potassium) GlaxoSmithKline 1366
Avelox (Moxifloxacin Hydrochloride) Schering 2970
Biaxin/Biaxin XL (Clarithromycin) Abbott 402
Ceftin (Cefuroxime Axetil) GlaxoSmithKline 1407
Cipro (Ciprofloxacin) Schering 2977
Invanz for Injection (Ertapenem) Merck 1999
Levaquin (Levofloxacin) Ortho-McNeil 2384
Levaquin in 5% Dextrose Injection (Levofloxacin) Ortho-McNeil 2384
Omnicef Capsules (Cefdinir) Abbott .. 511
Omnicef for Oral Suspension (Cefdinir) Abbott 511
Suprax (Cefixime) Lupin 1843
Tequin Injection (Gatifloxacin) Bristol-Myers Squibb 938
Tequin Injection in 5% Dextrose (Gatifloxacin) Bristol-Myers Squibb 938
Tequin Tablets (Gatifloxacin) Bristol-Myers Squibb 938
Vantin Tablets and Oral Suspension (Cefpodoxime Proxetil) Pharmacia & Upjohn 2645
Zmax for Oral Suspension (Azithromycin) Pfizer 2583

M. catarrhalis lower respiratory tract infections
Augmentin (Amoxicillin, Clavulanate Potassium) GlaxoSmithKline 1360
Augmentin Tablets (Amoxicillin, Clavulanate Potassium) GlaxoSmithKline 1363
Augmentin XR Extended-Release Tablets (Amoxicillin, Clavulanate Potassium) GlaxoSmithKline 1369
Avelox (Moxifloxacin Hydrochloride) Schering 2970
Biaxin/Biaxin XL (Clarithromycin) Abbott 402
Cipro (Ciprofloxacin) Schering 2977
Invanz for Injection (Ertapenem) Merck 1999
Levaquin (Levofloxacin) Ortho-McNeil 2384
Levaquin in 5% Dextrose Injection (Levofloxacin) Ortho-McNeil 2384
Omnicef Capsules (Cefdinir) Abbott .. 511
Omnicef for Oral Suspension (Cefdinir) Abbott 511
Tequin Injection (Gatifloxacin) Bristol-Myers Squibb 938
Tequin Injection in 5% Dextrose (Gatifloxacin) Bristol-Myers Squibb 938
Tequin Tablets (Gatifloxacin) Bristol-Myers Squibb 938
Vantin Tablets and Oral Suspension (Cefpodoxime Proxetil) Pharmacia & Upjohn 2645

M. catarrhalis pneumonia
Avelox (Moxifloxacin Hydrochloride) Schering 2970
Invanz for Injection (Ertapenem) Merck 1999
Ketek Tablets (Telithromycin) sanofi-aventis 2903
Omnicef Capsules (Cefdinir) Abbott .. 511
Omnicef for Oral Suspension (Cefdinir) Abbott 511
Tequin Injection (Gatifloxacin) Bristol-Myers Squibb 938
Tequin Injection in 5% Dextrose (Gatifloxacin) Bristol-Myers Squibb 938
Tequin Tablets (Gatifloxacin) Bristol-Myers Squibb 938

M. catarrhalis sinusitis
Augmentin (Amoxicillin, Clavulanate Potassium) GlaxoSmithKline 1360
Augmentin Tablets (Amoxicillin, Clavulanate Potassium) GlaxoSmithKline 1363
Augmentin XR Extended-Release Tablets (Amoxicillin, Clavulanate Potassium) GlaxoSmithKline 1369
Avelox (Moxifloxacin Hydrochloride) Schering 2970
Biaxin/Biaxin XL (Clarithromycin) Abbott 402
Cipro (Ciprofloxacin) Schering 2977
Cipro I.V. (Ciprofloxacin) Schering 2984
Ketek Tablets (Telithromycin) sanofi-aventis 2903
Levaquin (Levofloxacin) Ortho-McNeil 2384
Levaquin in 5% Dextrose Injection (Levofloxacin) Ortho-McNeil 2384
Vantin Tablets and Oral Suspension (Cefpodoxime Proxetil) Pharmacia & Upjohn 2645
Zmax for Oral Suspension (Azithromycin) Pfizer 2583

Macular degeneration
Macugen (Pegaptanib sodium, Pegaptinab) EyeTech .... ⊙261

Macular degeneration, age-related, neovascular
Lucentis Injection (Ranibizumab) Genentech 1237

Major depressive disorder
Emsam Transdermal System (Selegiline) Bristol-Myers Squibb 903
Pexeva Tablets (Paroxetine Mesylate) JDS 1694

Malaria
(*see under* P. falciparum infections; P. malariae infections; P. ovale infections; P. vivax infections)

Malaria, prophylaxis of
Daraprim Tablets (Pyrimethamine) GlaxoSmithKline ... 1419
Lariam Tablets (Mefloquine Hydrochloride) Roche ... 2786
Malarone Pediatric Tablets (Atovaquone, Proguanil Hydrochloride) GlaxoSmithKline ... 1517
Malarone Tablets (Atovaquone, Proguanil Hydrochloride) GlaxoSmithKline ... 1517

Malaria, treatment or prophylaxis of
Fansidar Tablets (Pyrimethamine, Sulfadoxine) Roche ... 2765

Malassezia furfur
(*see under* Pityrosporon orbiculare infections)

Mania, bipolar
Abilify Oral Solution (Aripiprazole) Bristol-Myers Squibb ... 882
Abilify Discmelt Orally Disintegrating Tablets (Aripiprazole) Bristol-Myers Squibb ... 882
Abilify Tablets (Aripiprazole) Bristol-Myers Squibb ... 882
Depakote Tablets (Divalproex Sodium) Abbott ... 427
Geodon (Ziprasidone Hydrochloride) Pfizer ... 2529
Zyprexa Tablets (Olanzapine) Lilly ... 1830
Zyprexa IntraMuscular (Olanzapine) Lilly ... 1830
Zyprexa ZYDIS Orally Disintegrating Tablets (Olanzapine) Lilly ... 1830

Manic episodes associated with bipolar disorder
Depakote Tablets (Divalproex Sodium) Abbott ... 427
Seroquel Tablets (Quetiapine Fumarate) AstraZeneca Pharmaceuticals ... 690

Mastocytosis, systemic
Zantac (Ranitidine Hydrochloride) GlaxoSmithKline ... 1624

Measles, prevention or modification of
GamaSTAN (Globulin, Immune (Human)) Talecris ... 3234

Measles, prophylaxis
Attenuvax (Measles Virus Vaccine Live) Merck ... 1914
M-M-R II (Measles, Mumps & Rubella Virus Vaccine, Live) Merck ... 2006
ProQuad (Measles, Mumps, Rubella and Varicella Virus Vaccine Live) Merck ... 2064

Mediastinitis, adjunctive therapy
Plasbumin-20 (Albumin (human)) Talecris ... 3252

Melanin hyperpigmentation
(*see under* Hyperpigmentation, skin, bleaching of)

Melanoma
Intron A for Injection (Interferon alfa-2b, Recombinant) Schering ... 3024
Proleukin for Injection (Aldesleukin) Novartis ... 2266

Melasma
(*see under* Hyperpigmentation, skin, bleaching of)

Membranes, swollen, shrinkage of
Excedrin Sinus Headache Caplets/Tablets (Acetaminophen, Phenylephrine Hydrochloride) Novartis Consumer ... ▣610
Refenesen PE Caplets (Guaifenesin, Phenylephrine Hydrochloride) Reese ... ▣721

Meningitis
Bicillin C-R Injectable Suspension (Penicillin G Benzathine, Penicillin G Procaine) King ... 1706
Fortaz (Ceftazidime) GlaxoSmithKline ... 1453
Garamycin Injectable (Gentamicin Sulfate) Schering ... 3014
Merrem I.V. (Meropenem) AstraZeneca Pharmaceuticals ... 686
Rocephin Injectable Vials, ADD-Vantage, Galaxy, Bulk (Ceftriaxone Sodium) Roche ... 2800
Zinacef for Injection (Cefuroxime) GlaxoSmithKline ... 1631
Zinacef Injection (Cefuroxime) GlaxoSmithKline ... 1631

Meningitis, meningococcal, prophylaxis of
Gantrisin Pediatric (Acetyl Sulfisoxazole) Roche ... 2770

Meningitis, meningococcal, treatment of
Gantrisin Pediatric (Acetyl Sulfisoxazole) Roche ... 2770

Meningitis, tuberculous
Decadron Tablets (Dexamethasone) Merck ... 1951
Depo-Medrol Injectable Suspension (Methylprednisolone Acetate) Pharmacia & Upjohn ... 2617
Depo-Medrol Single-Dose Vial (Methylprednisolone Acetate) Pharmacia & Upjohn ... 2619
Hydrocortone Tablets (Hydrocortisone) Merck ... 1989

Meningococcal vaccine
(*see also under* Immunization, meningococcal)
Menactra Vaccine (Meningoccal Polysaccharide Diphtheria Toxoid Conjugate Vaccine) Sanofi Pasteur ... 2954

Menopause, vasomotor symptoms of
Angeliq Tablets (Estradiol, Drospirenone) Berlex ... 762
Climara Transdermal System (Estradiol) Berlex ... 771
Climara Pro Transdermal System (Estradiol, Levonorgestrel) Berlex ... 776
Enjuvia Tablets (Estrogens, Conjugated, Synthetic B) Duramed ... 1062
Estrasorb Topical Emulsion (Estradiol) Esprit ... 1147
Estratest Tablets (Estrogens, Esterified, Methyltestosterone) Solvay ... 3199
Estratest H.S. Tablets (Estrogens, Esterified, Methyltestosterone) Solvay ... 3199
Premarin Tablets (Estrogens, Conjugated) Wyeth ... 3446
Premphase Tablets (Estrogens, Conjugated, Medroxyprogesterone Acetate) Wyeth ... 3456
Prempro Tablets (Estrogens, Conjugated, Medroxyprogesterone Acetate) Wyeth ... 3456

Menstrual cramps
(*see under* Pain, menstrual)

Micrococcus luteus
Vigamox Ophthalmic Solution (Moxifloxacin Hydrochloride) Alcon ... 564

Microsporum audouinii infections
Gris-PEG (Griseofulvin) Pedinol ... 2502

Microsporum canis infections
Lotrimin (Clotrimazole) Schering ... 3039

Microsporum gypseum infections
Gris-PEG Tablets (Griseofulvin) Pedinol ... 2502

Migraine headache
(*see under* Headache, migraine; Headache, migraine, prophylaxis of)

Mima-Herellea species infections
(*see under* Acinetobacter species infections)

Miosis, intraoperative, inhibition of
Ocufen Ophthalmic Solution (Flurbiprofen Sodium) Allergan ... ⊙232

Moraxella catarrhalis
(*see under* M. catarrhalis infections)

Moraxella lacunata infections, ocular
TobraDex Ophthalmic Ointment (Dexamethasone, Tobramycin) Alcon ... 562
TobraDex Ophthalmic Suspension (Dexamethasone, Tobramycin) Alcon ... 563

Morganella morganii infections
Cipro (Ciprofloxacin) Schering ... 2977
Cipro I.V. (Ciprofloxacin) Schering ... 2984
Fortaz (Ceftazidime) GlaxoSmithKline ... 1453
Mefoxin for Injection (Cefoxitin Sodium) Merck ... 2012
Mefoxin Premixed Intravenous Solution (Cefoxitin Sodium) Merck ... 2016
Primaxin I.V. (Cilastatin Sodium, Imipenem) Merck ... 2048
Rocephin Injectable Vials, ADD-Vantage, Galaxy, Bulk (Ceftriaxone Sodium) Roche ... 2800

Morganella morganii infections, ocular
TobraDex Ophthalmic Ointment (Dexamethasone, Tobramycin) Alcon ... 562
TobraDex Ophthalmic Suspension (Dexamethasone, Tobramycin) Alcon ... 563

Morganella morganii skin and skin structure infections
Cipro (Ciprofloxacin) Schering ... 2977
Cipro I.V. (Ciprofloxacin) Schering ... 2984
Primaxin I.V. (Cilastatin Sodium, Imipenem) Merck ... 2048
Rocephin Injectable Vials, ADD-Vantage, Galaxy, Bulk (Ceftriaxone Sodium) Roche ... 2800

Morganella morganii urinary tract infections
Cipro (Ciprofloxacin) Schering ... 2977
Cipro I.V. (Ciprofloxacin) Schering ... 2984
Mefoxin for Injection (Cefoxitin Sodium) Merck ... 2012
Mefoxin Premixed Intravenous Solution (Cefoxitin Sodium) Merck ... 2016
Primaxin I.V. (Cilastatin Sodium, Imipenem) Merck ... 2048
Rocephin Injectable Vials, ADD-Vantage, Galaxy, Bulk (Ceftriaxone Sodium) Roche ... 2800

Morphea, possibly effective in
Potaba (Aminobenzoate Potassium) Glenwood ... 1650

Motion sickness
Phenergan Tablets and Suppositories (Promethazine Hydrochloride) Wyeth ... 3440
Transderm Scōp Transdermal Therapeutic System (Scopolamine) Novartis Consumer ... 2177

Mouth, sore, pain
Robitussin Cough Drops Menthol, Cherry, and Honey-Lemon (Menthol) Wyeth ... ▣737
Robitussin Honey Cough Drops (Menthol) Wyeth ... ▣737
Robitussin Sugar Free Throat Drops (Menthol) Wyeth ... ▣737

Mucopolysaccharidosis
Aldurazyme for Intravenous Infusion (Laronidase) Genzyme ... 1268

Mucormycosis
(*see under* Zygomycosis)

Mucositis
Kepivance (Palifermin) Amgen ... 597

Multiple sclerosis, acute exacerbations
Copaxone for Injection (Glatiramer Acetate) Teva Neuroscience ... 3297
Decadron Tablets (Dexamethasone) Merck ... 1951
Depo-Medrol Injectable Suspension (Methylprednisolone Acetate) Pharmacia & Upjohn ... 2617
Depo-Medrol Single-Dose Vial (Methylprednisolone Acetate) Pharmacia & Upjohn ... 2619

Multiple sclerosis, alleviation of signs and symptoms
Dantrium Capsules (Dantrolene Sodium) Procter & Gamble Pharmaceuticals ... 2694

Multiple sclerosis, relapsing-remitting
Betaseron for SC Injection (Interferon Beta-1b) Berlex ... 767
Copaxone for Injection (Glatiramer Acetate) Teva Neuroscience ... 3297
Rebif Prefilled Syringe for Injection (Interferon Beta-1a) Serono ... 3159

Mumps, prophylaxis
M-M-R II (Measles, Mumps & Rubella Virus Vaccine, Live) Merck ... 2006
Mumpsvax (Mumps Virus Vaccine, Live) Merck ... 2031
ProQuad (Measles, Mumps, Rubella and Varicella Virus Vaccine Live) Merck ... 2064

Muscles, skeletal, relaxation, preoperative
Mivacron Injection (Mivacurium Chloride) Abbott ... 493
Nimbex Injection (Cisatracurium Besylate) Abbott ... 498
Zemuron Injection (Rocuronium Bromide) Organon USA ... 2346

Musculo-skeletal discomfort, adjunct in
Norflex Injection (Orphenadrine Citrate) 3M ... 1856
Skelaxin Tablets (Metaxalone) King ... 1716

Myalgia
(*see under* Pain, muscular, temporary relief of)

Myalgia, topical relief of
(*see under* Pain, topical relief of)

Mycobacterium avium complex (MAC) disease, disseminated
Biaxin/Biaxin XL (Clarithromycin) Abbott ... 402

Mycobacterium intracellulare infections
Biaxin/Biaxin XL (Clarithromycin) Abbott ... 402

Mycobacterium leprae infections
(*see under* Leprosy)

Mycobacterium tuberculosis infection, pulmonary
Capastat Sulfate for Injection (Capreomycin Sulfate) Lilly ... 1755

Mycoplasma pneumoniae infection
Avelox (Moxifloxacin Hydrochloride) Schering ... 2970
Biaxin/Biaxin XL (Clarithromycin) Abbott ... 402
E.E.S. (Erythromycin Ethylsuccinate) Abbott ... 451
EryPed (Erythromycin Ethylsuccinate) Abbott ... 447
Ery-Tab Tablets (Erythromycin) Abbott ... 449
Erythrocin Stearate Filmtab Tablets (Erythromycin Stearate) Abbott ... 453
Erythromycin Base Filmtab Tablets (Erythromycin) Abbott ... 455
Erythromycin Delayed-Release Capsules, USP (Erythromycin) Abbott ... 457
Levaquin (Levofloxacin) Ortho-McNeil ... 2384
Levaquin in 5% Dextrose Injection (Levofloxacin) Ortho-McNeil ... 2384
PCE Dispertab Tablets (Erythromycin) Abbott ... 515
Tequin Injection (Gatifloxacin) Bristol-Myers Squibb ... 938
Tequin Injection in 5% Dextrose (Gatifloxacin) Bristol-Myers Squibb ... 938
Tequin Tablets (Gatifloxacin) Bristol-Myers Squibb ... 938

Mycoplasma pneumoniae respiratory tract infections
Biaxin/Biaxin XL (Clarithromycin) Abbott 402
E.E.S. (Erythromycin Ethylsuccinate) Abbott 451
EryPed (Erythromycin Ethylsuccinate) Abbott 447
Ery-Tab Tablets (Erythromycin) Abbott 449
Erythrocin Stearate Filmtab Tablets (Erythromycin Stearate) Abbott 453
Erythromycin Base Filmtab Tablets (Erythromycin) Abbott 455
Erythromycin Delayed-Release Capsules, USP (Erythromycin) Abbott 457
Ketek Tablets (Telithromycin) sanofi-aventis 2903
Levaquin (Levofloxacin) Ortho-McNeil 2384
Levaquin in 5% Dextrose Injection (Levofloxacin) Ortho-McNeil 2384
PCE Dispertab Tablets (Erythromycin) Abbott 515

Mycosis fungoides
Decadron Tablets (Dexamethasone) Merck 1951
Depo-Medrol Injectable Suspension (Methylprednisolone Acetate) Pharmacia & Upjohn 2617
Depo-Medrol Single-Dose Vial (Methylprednisolone Acetate) Pharmacia & Upjohn 2619
Hydrocortone Tablets (Hydrocortisone) Merck 1989
Mustargen for Injection (Mechlorethamine Hydrochloride) Ovation 2468

Myelodysplastic syndrome
Dacogen Injection (Decitabine) MGI 2129

Myeloid recovery, acceleration of
Leukine (Sargramostim) Berlex 814

Myeloma, multiple
Alkeran Tablets (Melphalan) Celgene 956
Velcade for Injection (Bortezomib) Millennium 2133
Zometa for Intravenous Infusion (Zoledronic acid) Novartis 2315

Myeloma, multiple, adjunct in
Alkeran for Injection (Melphalan Hydrochloride) Celgene 955
Aredia for Injection (Pamidronate Disodium) Novartis 2179
Revlimid Capsules (Lenalidomide) Celgene 958
Thalomid Capsules (Thalidomide) Celgene 965

Myocardial infarction, acute
Activase I.V. (Alteplase) Genentech 1223
Bayer Aspirin (Aspirin) Bayer Healthcare LLC 744
Integrilin Injection (Eptifibatide) Schering 3020
Plavix Tablets (Clopidogrel Bisulfate) Bristol-Myers Squibb 917
Plavix Tablets (Clopidogrel Bisulfate) sanofi-aventis 2926
Retavase (Reteplase) PDL 2499
TNKase I.V. (Tenecteplase) Genentech 1264

Myocardial infarction, non-Q-wave
Aggrastat (Tirofiban Hydrochloride) Merck 1907
Fragmin Injection (Dalteparin Sodium) Eisai 1097
Integrilin Injection (Eptifibatide) Schering 3020
Lovenox Injection (Enoxaparin Sodium) sanofi-aventis 2915

Myocardial infarction, post, left ventricular dysfunction
Captopril Tablets (Captopril) Mylan 2149
Coreg Tablets (Carvedilol) GlaxoSmithKline 1414
Mavik Tablets (Trandolapril) Abbott 486

Myocardial infarction, prophylaxis, adjunct in
Altoprev Extended-Release Tablets (Lovastatin) Sciele 3109
Mevacor Tablets (Lovastatin) Merck 2021

Myocardial infarction, to reduce the risk of
Altace Capsules (Ramipril) King 1702
Bayer Aspirin (Aspirin) Bayer Healthcare LLC 744
Bayer Aspirin Comprehensive Prescribing Information (Aspirin) Bayer Healthcare ▣796
Niaspan Extended-Release Tablets (Niacin) Kos 1730
Zocor Tablets (Simvastatin) Merck 2105

Myocardial infarction, treatment adjunct
Altace Capsules (Ramipril) King 1702
Mavik Tablets (Trandolapril) Abbott 486
Prinivil Tablets (Lisinopril) Merck 2052

Myocardial perfusion imaging, thallium, adjunct in
Adenoscan (Adenosine) Astellas 619

Myocardial reinfarction, prophylaxis
Bayer Aspirin (Aspirin) Bayer Healthcare LLC 744
Blocadren Tablets (Timolol Maleate) Merck 1916
Coumadin for Injection (Warfarin Sodium) Bristol-Myers Squibb 898
Coumadin Tablets (Warfarin Sodium) Bristol-Myers Squibb 898
Plavix Tablets (Clopidogrel Bisulfate) Bristol-Myers Squibb 917
Plavix Tablets (Clopidogrel Bisulfate) sanofi-aventis 2926

Myocardial revascularization procedures, to reduce the risk of
Bayer Aspirin (Aspirin) Bayer Healthcare LLC 744
Bayer Aspirin Comprehensive Prescribing Information (Aspirin) Bayer Healthcare ▣796
Lescol Capsules (Fluvastatin Sodium) Novartis 2233
Lescol XL Tablets (Fluvastatin Sodium) Novartis 2233
Mevacor Tablets (Lovastatin) Merck 2021
Zocor Tablets (Simvastatin) Merck 2105

Myxedema
(*see under* Hypothyroidism, replacement or supplemental therapy in)

Myxedema coma/precoma
(*see under* Hypothyroidism, replacement or supplemental therapy in)

N

N. gonorrhoeae endocervical infections
Ceftin Tablets (Cefuroxime Axetil) GlaxoSmithKline 1407
Cipro (Ciprofloxacin) Schering 2977
Noroxin Tablets (Norfloxacin) Merck 2032
Rocephin Injectable Vials, ADD-Vantage, Galaxy, Bulk (Ceftriaxone Sodium) Roche 2800
Vantin Tablets and Oral Suspension (Cefpodoxime Proxetil) Pharmacia & Upjohn 2645

N. gonorrhoeae gynecologic infections
Erythrocin Stearate Filmtab Tablets (Erythromycin Stearate) Abbott 453
Erythromycin Base Filmtab Tablets (Erythromycin) Abbott 455
Erythromycin Delayed-Release Capsules, USP (Erythromycin) Abbott 457
Mefoxin for Injection (Cefoxitin Sodium) Merck 2012
Mefoxin Premixed Intravenous Solution (Cefoxitin Sodium) Merck 2016
Noroxin Tablets (Norfloxacin) Merck 2032
PCE Dispertab Tablets (Erythromycin) Abbott 515

N. gonorrhoeae infections
Amoxil Capsules (Amoxicillin) GlaxoSmithKline 1343
Amoxil Chewable Tablets (Amoxicillin) GlaxoSmithKline 1343
Amoxil Pediatric Drops for Oral Suspension (Amoxicillin) GlaxoSmithKline 1343
Amoxil Powder for Oral Suspension (Amoxicillin) GlaxoSmithKline 1343
Amoxil Tablets (Amoxicillin) GlaxoSmithKline 1343
Ceftin Tablets (Cefuroxime Axetil) GlaxoSmithKline 1407
Cipro (Ciprofloxacin) Schering 2977
E.E.S. (Erythromycin Ethylsuccinate) Abbott 451
EryPed (Erythromycin Ethylsuccinate) Abbott 447
Ery-Tab Tablets (Erythromycin) Abbott 449
Erythrocin Stearate Filmtab Tablets (Erythromycin Stearate) Abbott 453
Erythromycin Base Filmtab Tablets (Erythromycin) Abbott 455
Erythromycin Delayed-Release Capsules, USP (Erythromycin) Abbott 457
Fortaz (Ceftazidime) GlaxoSmithKline 1453
Mefoxin for Injection (Cefoxitin Sodium) Merck 2012
Mefoxin Premixed Intravenous Solution (Cefoxitin Sodium) Merck 2016
Noroxin Tablets (Norfloxacin) Merck 2032
PCE Dispertab Tablets (Erythromycin) Abbott 515
Rocephin Injectable Vials, ADD-Vantage, Galaxy, Bulk (Ceftriaxone Sodium) Roche 2800
Tequin Injection (Gatifloxacin) Bristol-Myers Squibb 938
Tequin Injection in 5% Dextrose (Gatifloxacin) Bristol-Myers Squibb 938
Tequin Tablets (Gatifloxacin) Bristol-Myers Squibb 938
Vantin Tablets and Oral Suspension (Cefpodoxime Proxetil) Pharmacia & Upjohn 2645
Zinacef for Injection (Cefuroxime) GlaxoSmithKline 1631
Zinacef Injection (Cefuroxime) GlaxoSmithKline 1631

N. gonorrhoeae infections, ocular
Pred-G Ophthalmic Ointment (Gentamicin Sulfate, Prednisolone Acetate) Allergan ⊙237
Pred-G Ophthalmic Suspension (Gentamicin Sulfate, Prednisolone Acetate) Allergan ⊙236

N. gonorrhoeae pelvic inflammatory disease
E.E.S. (Erythromycin Ethylsuccinate) Abbott 451
EryPed (Erythromycin Ethylsuccinate) Abbott 447
Ery-Tab Tablets (Erythromycin) Abbott 449
Erythromycin Delayed-Release Capsules, USP (Erythromycin) Abbott 457
Mefoxin for Injection (Cefoxitin Sodium) Merck 2012
Mefoxin Premixed Intravenous Solution (Cefoxitin Sodium) Merck 2016
Rocephin (Ceftriaxone Sodium) Roche 2800

N. gonorrhoeae pharyngeal infections
Rocephin (Ceftriaxone Sodium) Roche 2800

N. gonorrhoeae rectal infections
Ceftin Tablets (Cefuroxime Axetil) GlaxoSmithKline 1407
Rocephin Injectable Vials, ADD-Vantage, Galaxy, Bulk (Ceftriaxone Sodium) Roche 2800
Vantin Tablets and Oral Suspension (Cefpodoxime Proxetil) Pharmacia & Upjohn 2645

N. gonorrhoeae urethral infections
Ceftin Tablets (Cefuroxime Axetil) GlaxoSmithKline 1407
Cipro (Ciprofloxacin) Schering 2977
Noroxin Tablets (Norfloxacin) Merck 2032
Rocephin Injectable Vials, ADD-Vantage, Galaxy, Bulk (Ceftriaxone Sodium) Roche 2800
Tequin Injection (Gatifloxacin) Bristol-Myers Squibb 938
Tequin Injection in 5% Dextrose (Gatifloxacin) Bristol-Myers Squibb 938
Tequin Tablets (Gatifloxacin) Bristol-Myers Squibb 938
Vantin Tablets and Oral Suspension (Cefpodoxime Proxetil) Pharmacia & Upjohn 2645

N. meningitidis infections
Fortaz (Ceftazidime) GlaxoSmithKline 1453
Merrem I.V. (Meropenem) AstraZeneca Pharmaceuticals 686
Rocephin Injectable Vials, ADD-Vantage, Galaxy, Bulk (Ceftriaxone Sodium) Roche 2800
Zinacef for Injection (Cefuroxime) GlaxoSmithKline 1631
Zinacef Injection (Cefuroxime) GlaxoSmithKline 1631

N. meningitidis meningitis
Fortaz (Ceftazidime) GlaxoSmithKline 1453
Merrem I.V. (Meropenem) AstraZeneca Pharmaceuticals 686
Rocephin Injectable Vials, ADD-Vantage, Galaxy, Bulk (Ceftriaxone Sodium) Roche 2800
Zinacef for Injection (Cefuroxime) GlaxoSmithKline 1631
Zinacef Injection (Cefuroxime) GlaxoSmithKline 1631

N. meningitidis serogroups A, C, Y, and W-135, immunization against
(*see also under* Immunization, meningococcal)
Menactra Vaccine (Meningoccal Polysaccharide Diphtheria Toxoid Conjugate Vaccine) Sanofi Pasteur 2954

Nail, dry brittle
Appearex Tablets (Biotin) Merz 2125

Narcolepsy
Adderall Tablets (Amphetamine Aspartate, Amphetamine Sulfate, Dextroamphetamine Saccharate, Dextroamphetamine Sulfate) Shire US 3164
Dexedrine (Dextroamphetamine Sulfate) GlaxoSmithKline 1420
DextroStat Tablets (Dextroamphetamine Sulfate) Shire US 3179
Provigil Tablets (Modafinil) Cephalon 988
Ritalin Hydrochloride Tablets (Methylphenidate Hydrochloride) Novartis 2269
Ritalin-SR Tablets (Methylphenidate Hydrochloride) Novartis 2269

Nasal congestion, symptomatic relief of
Advil Allergy Sinus Caplets (Chlorpheniramine Maleate, Ibuprofen, Pseudoephedrine Hydrochloride) Wyeth ▣770
Advil Cold & Sinus (Ibuprofen, Pseudoephedrine Hydrochloride) Wyeth ▣723
Advil Multi-Symptom Cold Caplets (Chlorpheniramine Maleate, Ibuprofen, Pseudoephedrine Hydrochloride) Wyeth ▣770
Alavert Allergy & Sinus D-12 Hour Tablets (Loratadine, Pseudoephedrine Sulfate) Wyeth ▣771
Aleve Cold & Sinus Caplets (Naproxen Sodium, Pseudoephedrine Hydrochloride) Bayer Healthcare LLC 744
Allegra-D 12 Hour Extended-Release Tablets (Fexofenadine Hydrochloride, Pseudoephedrine Hydrochloride) sanofi-aventis 2846
Allegra-D 24 Hour Extended-Release Tablets (Fexofenadine Hydrochloride, Pseudoephedrine Hydrochloride) sanofi-aventis 2849
BC Cold Powder (Aspirin, Chlorpheniramine Maleate, Pseudoephedrine Hydrochloride) GlaxoSmithKline ▣677

Tylenol Sinus Congestion & Pain Daytime Caplets with Cool Burst and Gelcaps (Acetaminophen, Phenylephrine Hydrochloride) McNeil Consumer 1876
Tylenol Sinus Congestion & Pain Nighttime Caplets with Cool Burst (Acetaminophen, Chlorpheniramine Maleate, Phenylephrine Hydrochloride) McNeil Consumer 1876
Tylenol Sinus Congestion & Pain Severe Caplets with Cool Burst (Acetaminophen, Guaifenesin, Phenylephrine Hydrochloride) McNeil Consumer 1876
Vicks 44D Cough & Head Congestion Relief Liquid (Dextromethorphan Hydrobromide, Pseudoephedrine Hydrochloride) Procter & Gamble 2679
Vicks 44M Cough, Cold & Flu Relief Liquid (Acetaminophen, Chlorpheniramine Maleate, Dextromethorphan Hydrobromide, Pseudoephedrine Hydrochloride) Procter & Gamble 2680
Vicks 44D Cough & Head Congestion Relief Liquid (Dextromethorphan Hydrobromide, Phenylephrine Hydrochloride) Procter & Gamble .... ▣ 760
Vicks DayQuil LiquiCaps/Liquid Multi-Symptom Cold/Flu Relief (Acetaminophen, Dextromethorphan Hydrobromide, Phenylephrine Hydrochloride) Procter & Gamble .... ▣ 761
Vicks DayQuil Multi-Symptom Cold/Flu Relief LiquiCaps (Acetaminophen, Dextromethorphan Hydrobromide, Pseudoephedrine Hydrochloride) Procter & Gamble ..2678
Vicks DayQuil Multi-Symptom Cold/Flu Relief Liquid (Acetaminophen, Dextromethorphan Hydrobromide, Pseudoephedrine Hydrochloride) Procter & Gamble ..2678
Vicks NyQuil Multi-Symptom Cold/Flu Relief Liquid (Acetaminophen, Dextromethorphan Hydrobromide, Doxylamine Succinate, Pseudoephedrine Hydrochloride) Procter & Gamble 2681
Vicks NyQuil Multi-Symptom Cold/Flu Relief LiquiCaps (Acetaminophen, Dextromethorphan Hydrobromide, Doxylamine Succinate, Pseudoephedrine Hydrochloride) Procter & Gamble 2681
Vicks NyQuil LiquiCaps/Liquid Multi-Symptom Cold/Flu Relief (Acetaminophen, Dextromethorphan Hydrobromide, Doxylamine Succinate) Procter & Gamble .... ▣ 763
Children's Vicks NyQuil Cold/Cough Relief Liquid (Chlorpheniramine Maleate, Dextromethorphan Hydrobromide, Pseudoephedrine Hydrochloride) Procter & Gamble ..2680
Vicks Sinex Nasal Spray and Ultra Fine Mist for Sinus Relief (Oxymetazoline Hydrochloride) Procter & Gamble 2681
Vicks Sinex 12-Hour Nasal Spray and Ultra Fine Mist for Sinus Relief (Oxymetazoline Hydrochloride) Procter & Gamble 2681
Vicks Vapor Inhaler (Levmetamfetamine) Procter & Gamble 2682
Zicam Allergy Relief (Histanium Hydrochloricum, Luffa operculata, Galphimia Glauca, Sulfur) Matrixx .... ▣ 774
Zicam Cold Remedy Chewables (Zincum Aceticum, Zincum Gluconicum) Matrixx .... ▣ 766
Zicam Cold Remedy ChewCaps (Zincum Aceticum, Zincum Gluconicum) Matrixx .... ▣ 766
Zicam Cold Remedy Gel Swabs (Zincum Gluconicum) Matrixx .... ▣ 766
Zicam Cold Remedy Nasal Gel (Zincum Gluconicum) Matrixx .... ▣ 766
Zicam Cold Remedy Oral Mist (Zincum Aceticum, Zincum Gluconicum) Matrixx .... ▣ 766
Zicam Cold Remedy RapidMelts (Zincum Aceticum, Zincum Gluconicum) Matrixx .... ▣ 766
Zicam Cold Remedy RapidMelts with Vitamin C (Zincum Aceticum, Zincum Gluconicum) Matrixx .... ▣ 766
Zicam Cold Remedy Swabs Kids Size (Zincum Gluconicum) Matrixx .... ▣ 766
Zicam Cough Plus D Cough Spray (Dextromethorphan Hydrobromide, Phenylephrine Hydrochloride) Matrixx .... ▣ 767
Zicam Extreme Congestion Relief (Oxymetazoline Hydrochloride) Matrixx .... ▣ 767
Zicam Intense Sinus Relief (Oxymetazoline Hydrochloride) Matrixx .... ▣ 767

Nasal dryness
4-Way Saline Nasal Spray (Dietary Supplement) Novartis Consumer . ▣ 775
Nasal Comfort Moisture Therapy Sprays - Scented and Unscented (Sodium Chloride) Matrixx .... ▣ 733

Nasal irritation, symptomatic relief of
4-Way Saline Nasal Spray (Dietary Supplement) Novartis Consumer . ▣ 775

Nausea
(*see also under* Motion sickness)
Maalox Maximum Strength Total Stomach Relief Peppermint Liquid (Bismuth Subsalicylate) Novartis Consumer .... ▣ 660
Maalox Maximum Strength Total Stomach Relief Strawberry Liquid (Bismuth Subsalicylate) Novartis Consumer .... ▣ 672

Nausea, emetogenic, cancer chemotherapy-induced
Aloxi Injection (Palonosetron Hydrochloride) MGI 2127
Anzemet Injection (Dolasetron Mesylate) sanofi-aventis 2859
Anzemet Tablets (Dolasetron Mesylate) sanofi-aventis 2862
Cesamet Capsules (Nabilone) Valeant 3340
Emend Capsules (Aprepitant) Merck 1963
Kytril Injection (Granisetron Hydrochloride) Roche 2781
Kytril (Granisetron Hydrochloride) Roche 2784
Marinol Capsules (Dronabinol) Unimed 3333
Zofran Injection (Ondansetron Hydrochloride) GlaxoSmithKline 1634
Zofran (Ondansetron Hydrochloride) GlaxoSmithKline 1639
Zofran ODT Orally Disintegrating Tablets (Ondansetron) GlaxoSmithKline 1639

Nausea, emetogenic, cancer chemotherapy-induced, adjunct in
Emend Capsules (Aprepitant) Merck 1963

Nausea, emetogenic, radiation therapy-induced
Kytril (Granisetron Hydrochloride) Roche 2784
Zofran (Ondansetron Hydrochloride) GlaxoSmithKline 1639
Zofran ODT Orally Disintegrating Tablets (Ondansetron) GlaxoSmithKline 1639

Nausea, postoperative
Anzemet Injection (Dolasetron Mesylate) sanofi-aventis 2859
Anzemet Tablets (Dolasetron Mesylate) sanofi-aventis 2862
Emend Capsules (Aprepitant) Merck 1963
Kytril Injection (Granisetron Hydrochloride) Roche 2781
Phenergan Tablets and Suppositories (Promethazine Hydrochloride) Wyeth 3440
Zofran Injection (Ondansetron Hydrochloride) GlaxoSmithKline 1634
Zofran (Ondansetron Hydrochloride) GlaxoSmithKline 1639
Zofran ODT Orally Disintegrating Tablets (Ondansetron) GlaxoSmithKline 1639

Necator americanus infections
Mintezol (Thiabendazole) Merck 2027

Necrobiosis lipoidica diabeticorum
Depo-Medrol Single-Dose Vial (Methylprednisolone Acetate) Pharmacia & Upjohn 2619

Necrotic tissue, debridement of
Accuzyme SE Spray Emulsion (Papain, Urea) Healthpoint 1662
Panafil Ointment (Chlorophyllin Copper Complex Sodium, Papain, Urea) Healthpoint 1663
Panafil SE Spray Emulsion (Chlorophyllin Copper Complex Sodium, Papain, Urea) Healthpoint 1663

Neisseria gonorrhoeae
(*see under* N. gonorrhoeae infections)

Neisseria meningitidis
(*see under* N. gonorrhoeae infections)

Neisseria species infections, ocular
Neosporin Ophthalmic Solution Sterile (Gramicidin, Neomycin Sulfate, Polymyxin B Sulfate) King .... ⊙ 265
Poly-Pred Ophthalmic Suspension (Neomycin Sulfate, Polymyxin B Sulfate, Prednisolone Acetate) Allergan .... ⊙ 233
Pred-G Ophthalmic Suspension (Gentamicin Sulfate, Prednisolone Acetate) Allergan .... ⊙ 236
TobraDex Ophthalmic Ointment (Dexamethasone, Tobramycin) Alcon 562
TobraDex Ophthalmic Suspension (Dexamethasone, Tobramycin) Alcon 563

Neoplasia, cervical intraepithelial, prevention of
Gardasil (Quadrivalent Human Papillomavirus (Types 6, 11, 16, 18) Recombinant Vaccine) Merck 1984

Neoplasia, vaginal intraepithelial, prevention of
Gardasil (Quadrivalent Human Papillomavirus (Types 6, 11, 16, 18) Recombinant Vaccine) Merck 1984

Neoplasia, vulvar intraepithelial, prevention of
Gardasil (Quadrivalent Human Papillomavirus (Types 6, 11, 16, 18) Recombinant Vaccine) Merck 1984

Nephroblastoma
(*see under* Wilms' tumor)

Nephrolithiasis, calcium
Urocit-K Tablets (Potassium Citrate) Mission 2144

Nephropathy, diabetic
Avapro Tablets (Irbesartan) Bristol-Myers Squibb 891
Avapro Tablets (Irbesartan) sanofi-aventis 2871
Cozaar Tablets (Losartan Potassium) Merck 1935

Nephrosis, acute, adjunctive therapy
Flexbumin I.V. (Albumin (human)) Baxter Healthcare 720
Human Albumin Grifols 20%, Albumin (Human) (Albumin (human)) Grifols 1651
Human Albumin Grifols 25%, Albumin (Human) (Albumin (human)) Grifols 1652
Plasbumin-20 (Albumin (human)) Talecris 3252
Plasbumin-25 (Albumin (human)) Talecris 3253

Neuralgia
(*see under* Pain, neurogenic)

Neuralgia, glossopharyngeal
Carbatrol Capsules (Carbamazepine) Shire US 3171
Tegretol/Tegretol-XR (Carbamazepine) Novartis 2295

Neuralgia, postherpetic
Lidoderm Patch (Lidocaine) Endo Labs 1118
Lyrica Capsules (Pregabalin) Pfizer... 2539
Neurontin Capsules (Gabapentin) Parke-Davis 2487
Neurontin Oral Solution (Gabapentin) Parke-Davis 2487
Neurontin Tablets (Gabapentin) Parke-Davis 2487

Neuralgia, trigeminal
Carbatrol Capsules (Carbamazepine) Shire US 3171
Tegretol/Tegretol-XR (Carbamazepine) Novartis 2295

Neuritis, peripheral, acute
(*see under* Pain, neurogenic)

Neurocysticercosis
Albenza Tablets (Albendazole) GlaxoSmithKline 1338

Neurodermatitis
(*see under* Lichen simplex chronicus)

Neurological deficits, post-SAH, improvement of
Nimotop Capsules (Nimodipine) Bayer 749

Neutropenia, chemotherapy-induced
Neulasta Injection (Pegfilgrastim) Amgen 601
Neupogen for Injection (Filgrastim) Amgen 603

Neutropenia, febrile, to decrease the incidence of infection
AmBisome for Injection (Amphotericin B, liposomal) Astellas 620
Cipro I.V. (Ciprofloxacin) Schering 2984
Neulasta Injection (Pegfilgrastim) Amgen 601
Neupogen (Filgrastim) Amgen 603

Neutropenia, post-bone marrow transplant
Neupogen (Filgrastam) Amgen 603

Neutropenia-related clinical sequelae, post-bone marrow transplant
Neupogen for Injection (Filgrastim) Amgen 603

Night-terrors
Hyland's Calm Forte 4 Kids Tablets (Homeopathic Formulations, Sulfur) Standard Homeopathic .... ▣ 828

Nocardia asteroides infections
(*see under* Nocardiosis)

Nocardiosis
Gantrisin Pediatric Suspension (Acetyl Sulfisoxazole) Roche 2770

Nose, itchy
(*see under* Pruritus, rhinopharyngeal, symptomatic relief of)

Nose, runny
(*see also under* Rhinorrhea)
Comtrex Maximum Strength Cold & Cough Day/Night Caplets - Night Formulation (Acetaminophen, Chlorpheniramine Maleate, Dextromethorphan Hydrobromide, Pseudoephedrine Hydrochloride) Novartis Consumer .... ▣ 726

Nutrients, deficiency of
Folgard RX Tablets (Folic Acid, Vitamin B_6, Vitamin B_{12}) Upsher-Smith 3337
Marlyn Formula 50 Capsules (Amino Acid Preparations, Vitamin B_6) Marlyn 1862
ProNutra Protein Supplement (Vitamins with Minerals, Whey Protein Isolate) Immunotec 1668

Nutrients, deficiency of, stress-induced
(*see under* Nutrients, deficiency of)

Nutrients, deficiency of, surgery-induced
(*see under* Nutrients, deficiency of)

O

Obesity, exogenous
- Adipex-P (Phentermine Hydrochloride) Gate 1215
- Desoxyn Tablets, USP (Methamphetamine Hydrochloride) Ovation 2462
- Meridia Capsules (Sibutramine Hydrochloride Monohydrate) Abbott 489
- Xenical Capsules (Orlistat) Roche 2831

Obsessive compulsive disorder
- Paxil (Paroxetine Hydrochloride) GlaxoSmithKline 1530
- Pexeva Tablets (Paroxetine Mesylate) JDS 1694
- Prozac Pulvules and Liquid (Fluoxetine Hydrochloride) Lilly 1801
- Zoloft (Sertraline Hydrochloride) Pfizer 2586

Ocular congestion, symptomatic relief of
- Albalon Ophthalmic Solution (Naphazoline Hydrochloride) Allergan .... ⊙218

Ocular health, maintenance
- Bausch & Lomb PreserVision AREDS Softgels (Vitamins with Minerals) Bausch & Lomb .... ⊙247
- Bausch & Lomb PreserVision Lutein Softgels (Lutein, Vitamins with Minerals) Bausch & Lomb .... ⊙247
- Bausch & Lomb PreserVision AREDS Eye Vitamin and Mineral Supplement Soft Gels (Vitamins with Minerals) Bausch & Lomb .... ▣806
- Bausch & Lomb PreserVision Lutein Eye Vitamin and Mineral Supplement Soft Gels (Lutein, Vitamins with Minerals) Bausch & Lomb .... ▣807

Ocular inflammation
- Decadron Tablets (Dexamethasone) Merck 1951
- Poly-Pred Ophthalmic Suspension (Neomycin Sulfate, Polymyxin B Sulfate, Prednisolone Acetate) Allergan .... ⊙233
- Pred Mild Ophthalmic Suspension (Prednisolone Acetate) Allergan .... ⊙238

Ocular inflammation, postoperative
- Acular Ophthalmic Solution (Ketorolac Tromethamine) Allergan 565
- Voltaren Ophthalmic Solution (Diclofenac Sodium) Novartis 2309

Ocular inflammation, steroid-responsive
- FML Ophthalmic Suspension (Fluorometholone) Allergan .... ⊙227
- Lotemax Ophthalmic Suspension 0.5% (Loteprednol Etabonate) Bausch & Lomb .... ⊙251
- Pred Forte Ophthalmic Suspension (Prednisolone Acetate) Allergan .... ⊙235

Ocular inflammation with bacterial infection, steroid-responsive
- Blephamide Ophthalmic Ointment (Prednisolone Acetate, Sulfacetamide Sodium) Allergan 568
- Blephamide Ophthalmic Suspension (Prednisolone Acetate, Sulfacetamide Sodium) Allergan 569
- FML-S Ophthalmic Suspension (Fluorometholone, Sulfacetamide Sodium) Allergan .... ⊙229
- Poly-Pred Ophthalmic Suspension (Neomycin Sulfate, Polymyxin B Sulfate, Prednisolone Acetate) Allergan .... ⊙233
- Pred-G Ophthalmic Ointment (Gentamicin Sulfate, Prednisolone Acetate) Allergan .... ⊙237
- Pred-G Ophthalmic Suspension (Gentamicin Sulfate, Prednisolone Acetate) Allergan .... ⊙236
- TobraDex Ophthalmic Ointment (Dexamethasone, Tobramycin) Alcon 562
- TobraDex Ophthalmic Suspension (Dexamethasone, Tobramycin) Alcon 563

Ocular redness
- Naphcon-A Eye Drops (Naphazoline Hydrochloride, Pheniramine Maleate) Alcon .... ⊙208
- Visine Original Eye Drops (Tetrahydrozoline Hydrochloride) Pfizer Consumer .... ⊙290
- Visine A.C. Seasonal Itching and Redness Relief Drops (Tetrahydrozoline Hydrochloride, Zinc Sulfate) Pfizer Consumer .... ⊙289
- Advanced Relief Visine Eye Drops (Dextran 70, Polyethylene Glycol, Povidone, Tetrahydrozoline Hydrochloride) Pfizer Consumer .... ⊙288
- Visine L.R. Long Lasting Eye Drops (Oxymetazoline Hydrochloride) Pfizer Consumer .... ⊙290
- Visine-A Eye Allergy Relief Eye Drops (Naphazoline Hydrochloride, Pheniramine Maleate) Pfizer Consumer .... ⊙289

Onchocerciasis
- Stromectol Tablets (Ivermectin) Merck 2083

Onychomycosis
(*see under* Tinea unguium infections)

Ophthalmia, Egyptian
(*see under* Trachoma)

Ophthalmia, sympathetic
- Decadron Tablets (Dexamethasone) Merck 1951
- Depo-Medrol Injectable Suspension (Methylprednisolone Acetate) Pharmacia & Upjohn 2617
- Hydrocortone Tablets (Hydrocortisone) Merck 1989

Ophthalmic disorders
- Depo-Medrol Single-Dose Vial (Methylprednisolone Acetate) Pharmacia & Upjohn 2619

Opioid dependence, treatment of
- Suboxone Tablets (Buprenorphine Hydrochloride, Naloxone Hydrochloride) Reckitt Benckiser 2717
- Subutex Tablets (Buprenorphine Hydrochloride) Reckitt Benckiser 2717

Optic neuritis
- Depo-Medrol Injectable Suspension (Methylprednisolone Acetate) Pharmacia & Upjohn 2617
- Hydrocortone Tablets (Hydrocortisone) Merck 1989

Ossification, heterotopic
- Didronel Tablets (Etidronate Disodium) Procter & Gamble Pharmaceuticals 2697

Osteitis deformans
(*see under* Paget's disease of bone)

Osteoarthritis
- Anaprox Tablets (Naproxen Sodium) Roche 2761
- Anaprox DS Tablets (Naproxen Sodium) Roche 2761
- Arthrotec Tablets (Diclofenac Sodium, Misoprostol) Searle 3129
- Bayer Aspirin (Aspirin) Bayer Healthcare LLC 744
- Bayer Aspirin Comprehensive Prescribing Information (Aspirin) Bayer Healthcare .... ▣796
- Bayer Aspirin (Aspirin) Bayer Healthcare LLC 744
- Celebrex Capsules (Celecoxib) Searle 3134
- Clinoril Tablets (Sulindac) Merck 1924
- CM Plex (Cetyl Myristate, Cetyl Myristoleate, Fatty Acids) Unicity 3329
- Dolobid Tablets (Diflunisal) Merck 1955
- EC-Naprosyn Delayed-Release Tablets (Naproxen) Roche 2761
- Euflexxa (Sodium Hyaluronate) Ferring 1162
- Hyalgan Solution (Sodium Hyaluronate) sanofi-aventis 2901
- Indocin (Indomethacin) Merck 1995
- Limbrel Capsules (Flavocoxid) Primus 2672
- Mobic Oral Suspension (Meloxicam) Boehringer Ingelheim 863
- Mobic Tablets (Meloxicam) Boehringer Ingelheim 863
- Nalfon Capsules (Fenoprofen Calcium) Pedinol 2502
- Naprosyn Suspension (Naproxen) Roche 2761
- Naprosyn Tablets (Naproxen) Roche 2761
- Traumeel Injection Solution (Homeopathic Formulations) Heel 1664
- Tylenol 8 Hour Extended Release Caplets (Acetaminophen) McNeil Consumer .... ▣695
- Tylenol Arthritis Pain Extended Release Caplets and Geltabs (Acetaminophen) McNeil Consumer 1870
- Voltaren Tablets (Diclofenac Sodium) Novartis 2307
- Voltaren-XR Tablets (Diclofenac Sodium) Novartis 2310

Osteoarthritis, post-traumatic
- Depo-Medrol Injectable Suspension (Methylprednisolone Acetate) Pharmacia & Upjohn 2617
- Depo-Medrol Single-Dose Vial (Methylprednisolone Acetate) Pharmacia & Upjohn 2619
- Hydrocortone Tablets (Hydrocortisone) Merck 1989

Osteoarthritis, symptoms of
- Zeel Solution (Arnica montana, Sulfur, Herbals, Multiple) Heel 1665

Osteoarthritis, synovitis of
- Depo-Medrol Injectable Suspension (Methylprednisolone Acetate) Pharmacia & Upjohn 2617
- Depo-Medrol Single-Dose Vial (Methylprednisolone Acetate) Pharmacia & Upjohn 2619
- Hydrocortone Tablets (Hydrocortisone) Merck 1989

Osteodystrophy, renal
- Calcijex Injection (Calcitriol) Abbott 411

Osteolytic bone lesions, multiple myeloma-induced
- Aredia for Injection (Pamidronate Disodium) Novartis 2179

Osteoporosis
- Boniva Injection (Ibandronate Sodium) Roche 2738
- Boniva Tablets (Ibandronate Sodium) Roche 2741
- Evista Tablets (Raloxifene Hydrochloride) Lilly 1763
- Forteo for Injection (Teriparatide) Lilly 1767
- Fosamax (Alendronate Sodium) Merck 1969
- Fosamax Plus D Tablets (Alendronate Sodium, Cholecalciferol) Merck 1977
- Premphase Tablets (Estrogens, Conjugated, Medroxyprogesterone Acetate) Wyeth 3456
- Prempro Tablets (Estrogens, Conjugated, Medroxyprogesterone Acetate) Wyeth 3456

Osteoporosis, corticosteroid-induced
- Actonel Tablets (Risedronate Sodium) Procter & Gamble Pharmaceuticals 2683
- Fosamax (Alendronate Sodium) Merck 1969

Osteoporosis, postmenopausal, prevention of
- Actonel Tablets (Risedronate Sodium) Procter & Gamble Pharmaceuticals 2683
- Actonel with Calcium Tablets (Risedronate Sodium, Calcium Carbonate) Procter & Gamble Pharmaceuticals 2688
- Boniva Injection (Ibandronate Sodium) Roche 2738
- Boniva Tablets (Ibandronate Sodium) Roche 2741
- Climara Transdermal System (Estradiol) Berlex 771
- Climara Pro Transdermal System (Estradiol, Levonorgestrel) Berlex 776
- Menostar Transdermal System (Estradiol) Berlex 782
- Premphase Tablets (Estrogens, Conjugated, Medroxyprogesterone Acetate) Wyeth 3456
- Prempro Tablets (Estrogens, Conjugated, Medroxyprogesterone Acetate) Wyeth 3456

Osteoporosis, postmenopausal, treatment adjunct
- Fortical Nasal Spray (Calcitonin-Salmon) Upsher-Smith 3337
- Miacalcin Injection (Calcitonin-Salmon) Novartis 2252
- Miacalcin Nasal Spray (Calcitonin-Salmon) Novartis 2253
- Premarin Tablets (Estrogens, Conjugated) Wyeth 3446

Osteoporosis, postmenopausal, treatment of
- Actonel Tablets (Risedronate Sodium) Procter & Gamble Pharmaceuticals 2683
- Actonel with Calcium Tablets (Risedronate Sodium, Calcium Carbonate) Procter & Gamble Pharmaceuticals 2688
- Miacalcin Nasal Spray (Calcitonin-Salmon) Novartis 2253

Osteoporosis in men
- Actonel Tablets (Risedronate Sodium) Procter & Gamble Pharmaceuticals 2683

Otitis externa
- Floxin Otic Solution (Ofloxacin) Daiichi Sankyo 1049

Otitis externa, acute
- Ciprodex Otic Suspension (Ciprofloxacin, Dexamethasone) Alcon 559

Otitis media
- Bicillin C-R Injectable Suspension (Penicillin G Benzathine, Penicillin G Procaine) King 1706

Otitis media, acute
- Amoxil Capsules (Amoxicillin) GlaxoSmithKline 1343
- Amoxil Chewable Tablets (Amoxicillin) GlaxoSmithKline 1343
- Amoxil Pediatric Drops for Oral Suspension (Amoxicillin) GlaxoSmithKline 1343
- Amoxil Powder for Oral Suspension (Amoxicillin) GlaxoSmithKline 1343
- Amoxil Tablets (Amoxicillin) GlaxoSmithKline 1343
- Augmentin (Amoxicillin, Clavulanate Potassium) GlaxoSmithKline 1360
- Augmentin Tablets (Amoxicillin, Clavulanate Potassium) GlaxoSmithKline 1363
- Augmentin XR Extended-Release Tablets (Amoxicillin, Clavulanate Potassium) GlaxoSmithKline 1369
- Augmentin ES-600 Powder for Oral Suspension (Amoxicillin, Clavulanate Potassium) GlaxoSmithKline 1366
- Biaxin/Biaxin XL (Clarithromycin) Abbott 402
- Ceftin (Cefuroxime Axetil) GlaxoSmithKline 1407
- Ciprodex Otic Suspension (Ciprofloxacin, Dexamethasone) Alcon 559
- Floxin Otic Solution (Ofloxacin) Daiichi Sankyo 1049
- Omnicef Capsules (Cefdinir) Abbott 511
- Omnicef for Oral Suspension (Cefdinir) Abbott 511
- Rocephin Injectable Vials, ADD-Vantage, Galaxy, Bulk (Ceftriaxone Sodium) Roche 2800
- Suprax (Cefixime) Lupin 1843
- Vantin Tablets and Oral Suspension (Cefpodoxime Proxetil) Pharmacia & Upjohn 2645

Otitis media, adjunctive therapy
- Hyland's Earache Tablets (Homeopathic Formulations) Standard Homeopathic .... ▣829

Otitis media, chronic suppurative
- Floxin Otic Solution (Ofloxacin) Daiichi Sankyo 1049

Tylenol Cold Head Congestion Daytime Caplets with Cool Burst (Acetaminophen, Dextromethorphan Hydrobromide, Phenylephrine Hydrochloride) McNeil Consumer 1873
Tylenol Cold Head Congestion Nighttime Caplets with Cool Burst (Acetaminophen, Chlorpheniramine Maleate, Dextromethorphan Hydrobromide, Phenylephrine Hydrochloride) McNeil Consumer 1873
Tylenol Cold Head Congestion Severe Caplets with Cool Burst (Acetaminophen, Dextromethorphan Hydrobromide, Guaifenesin, Phenylephrine Hydrochloride) McNeil Consumer 1873
Tylenol Cough & Sore Throat Daytime Liquid with Cool Burst (Acetaminophen, Dextromethorphan Hydrobromide) McNeil Consumer 1877
Tylenol Cough & Sore Throat Nighttime Liquid with Cool Burst (Acetaminophen, Dextromethorphan Hydrobromide, Doxylamine Succinate) McNeil Consumer 1877
Concentrated Tylenol Infants' Drops Plus Cold (Acetaminophen) McNeil Consumer 1879
Concentrated Tylenol Infants' Drops Plus Cold and Cough (Acetaminophen, Dextromethorphan Hydrobromide) McNeil Consumer 1879
Tylenol Sinus Severe Congestion Caplets with Cool Burst (Acetaminophen, Guaifenesin, Pseudoéphedrine Hydrochloride) McNeil Consumer 1876
Tylenol Sinus Congestion & Pain Daytime Caplets with Cool Burst and Gelcaps (Acetaminophen, Phenylephrine Hydrochloride) McNeil Consumer 1876
Tylenol Sinus Congestion & Pain Severe Caplets with Cool Burst (Acetaminophen, Guaifenesin, Phenylephrine Hydrochloride) McNeil Consumer 1876
Tylenol Sore Throat Daytime Liquid with Cool Burst (Acetaminophen) McNeil Consumer 1877
Tylenol Sore Throat Nighttime Liquid with Cool Burst (Acetaminophen, Diphenhydramine) McNeil Consumer 1877
Women's Tylenol Menstrual Relief Caplets (Acetaminophen, Pamabrom) McNeil Consumer 1877
Vicks DayQuil LiquiCaps/Liquid Multi-Symptom Cold/Flu Relief (Acetaminophen, Dextromethorphan Hydrobromide, Phenylephrine Hydrochloride) Procter & Gamble 761
Vicks VapoRub Cream (Camphor, Menthol) Procter & Gamble 2682
Vicks VapoRub Ointment (Camphor, Eucalyptus, Oil of, Menthol) Procter & Gamble 2682

Pain, intractable chronic
(*see under* Pain, severe)

Pain, joint

Biofreeze Pain Relieving Roll on/Gel and Cryospray (Menthol) Performance Health 678
Mineral Ice (Menthol) Novartis Consumer 685

Pain, major surgical

DepoDur Extended-Release Injection (Morphine sulfate, liposomal) Endo Labs 1110

Pain, menstrual

Advil (Ibuprofen) Wyeth 674
Aleve Caplets (Naproxen Sodium) Bayer Healthcare LLC 742
Aleve Gelcaps (Naproxen Sodium) Bayer Healthcare LLC 743
Aleve Tablets (Naproxen Sodium) Bayer Healthcare LLC 743
BC Headache Powder (Aspirin, Caffeine, Salicylamide) GlaxoSmithKline 677
Bufferin Extra Strength Tablets (Aspirin Buffered) Novartis Consumer 678
Bufferin Regular Strength Tablets (Aspirin Buffered) Novartis Consumer 678
Excedrin Extra Strength Caplets/Tablets/Geltabs (Acetaminophen, Aspirin, Caffeine) Novartis Consumer 684
Goody's Extra Strength Pain Relief Tablets (Acetaminophen, Aspirin, Caffeine) GlaxoSmithKline 685
Motrin IB Tablets and Caplets (Ibuprofen) McNeil Consumer 1866
ThermaCare Heat Wraps (Device) Procter & Gamble 2677
Regular Strength Tylenol Tablets (Acetaminophen) McNeil Consumer 1870
Tylenol 8 Hour Extended Release Caplets (Acetaminophen) McNeil Consumer 1870
Tylenol (Acetaminophen) McNeil Consumer 1870
Extra Strength Tylenol Rapid Release Gels (Acetaminophen) McNeil Consumer 1870
Tylenol Arthritis Pain Extended Release Caplets and Geltabs (Acetaminophen) McNeil Consumer 1870
Women's Tylenol Menstrual Relief Caplets (Acetaminophen, Pamabrom) McNeil Consumer 1877

Pain, mild

Advil Caplets (Ibuprofen) Wyeth 674
Children's Advil Oral Suspension (Ibuprofen) Wyeth 603
Children's Advil Chewable Tablets (Ibuprofen) Wyeth 603
Advil Gel Caplets (Ibuprofen) Wyeth 674
Infants' Advil Concentrated Drops (Ibuprofen) Wyeth 604
Infants' Advil Concentrated Drops - White Grape (Dye-Free) (Ibuprofen) Wyeth 604
Junior Strength Advil Swallow Tablets (Ibuprofen) Wyeth 605
Advil (Ibuprofen) Wyeth 674
Goody's Body Pain Formula Powder (Acetaminophen, Aspirin, Acetaminophen, Aspirin) GlaxoSmithKline 684
Goody's Extra Strength Headache Powders (Acetaminophen, Aspirin, Caffeine) GlaxoSmithKline 611
Goody's Extra Strength Pain Relief Tablets (Acetaminophen, Aspirin, Caffeine) GlaxoSmithKline 685
Goody's PM Powder for Pain with Sleeplessness (Acetaminophen, Diphenhydramine Citrate) GlaxoSmithKline 612
Junior Strength Motrin Caplets and Chewable Tablets (Ibuprofen) McNeil Consumer 1867
Regular Strength Tylenol Tablets (Acetaminophen) McNeil Consumer 1870
Tylenol 8 Hour Extended Release Caplets (Acetaminophen) McNeil Consumer 1870
Extra Strength Tylenol Caplets, Cool Caplets, Go Tabs and EZ Tabs (Acetaminophen) McNeil Consumer 1870
Extra Strength Tylenol Rapid Release Gels (Acetaminophen) McNeil Consumer 1870
Concentrated Tylenol Infants' Drops Plus Cold & Cough (Acetaminophen, Dextromethorphan Hydrobromide, Phenylephrine Hydrochloride) McNeil Consumer 754

Pain, mild to moderate

Anaprox Tablets (Naproxen Sodium) Roche 2761
Anaprox DS Tablets (Naproxen Sodium) Roche 2761
Dolobid Tablets (Diflunisal) Merck 1955
Nalfon Capsules (Fenoprofen Calcium) Pedinol 2502
Naprosyn Suspension (Naproxen) Roche 2761
Naprosyn Tablets (Naproxen) Roche 2761

Pain, mild to moderate, acute musculo-skeletal

Biofreeze Pain Relieving Roll on/Gel and Cryospray (Menthol) Performance Health 678

Pain, moderate

Opana Tablets (Oxymorphone Hydrochloride) Endo Labs 1122
Opana ER Tablets (Oxymorphone Hydrochloride) Endo Labs 1126

Pain, moderate to moderately severe

OxyFast Oral Concentrate Solution (Oxycodone Hydrochloride) Purdue Pharma 2708
OxyIR Capsules (Oxycodone Hydrochloride) Purdue Pharma 2708
Percocet Tablets (Acetaminophen, Oxycodone Hydrochloride) Endo Labs 1131
Percodan Tablets (Aspirin, Oxycodone Hydrochloride) Endo Labs 1132
Tylenol with Codeine Tablets (Acetaminophen, Codeine Phosphate) Ortho-McNeil 2391
Vicodin Tablets (Acetaminophen, Hydrocodone Bitartrate) Abbott 535
Vicodin ES Tablets (Acetaminophen, Hydrocodone Bitartrate) Abbott 536
Vicodin HP Tablets (Acetaminophen, Hydrocodone Bitartrate) Abbott 538
Zydone Tablets (Acetaminophen, Hydrocodone Bitartrate) Endo Labs 1139

Pain, moderate to severe

Avinza Capsules (Morphine Sulfate) Ligand 1741
Buprenex Injectable (Buprenorphine Hydrochloride) Reckitt Benckiser 2716
Celebrex Capsules (Celecoxib) Searle 3134
Dilaudid (Hydromorphone Hydrochloride) Abbott 440
Dilaudid Non-Sterile Powder (Hydromorphone Hydrochloride) Abbott 440
Dilaudid Oral Liquid (Hydromorphone Hydrochloride) Abbott 445
Dilaudid Rectal Suppositories (Hydromorphone Hydrochloride) Abbott 440
Dilaudid Tablets (Hydromorphone Hydrochloride) Abbott 440
Dilaudid Tablets - 8 mg (Hydromorphone Hydrochloride) Abbott 445
Dilaudid-HP (Hydromorphone Hydrochloride) Abbott 442
Duragesic Transdermal System (Fentanyl) Ortho-McNeil 2373
Kadian Capsules (Morphine Sulfate) Alpharma Branded Products 577
MS Contin Tablets (Morphine Sulfate) Purdue Pharma 2701
Numorphan Injection (Oxymorphone Hydrochloride) Endo Labs 1120
Opana Tablets (Oxymorphone Hydrochloride) Endo Labs 1122
Opana ER Tablets (Oxymorphone Hydrochloride) Endo Labs 1126
OxyContin Tablets (Oxycodone Hydrochloride) Purdue Pharma 2703
Vicoprofen Tablets (Hydrocodone Bitartrate, Ibuprofen) Abbott 539

Pain, muscular, temporary relief of

Aleve Caplets (Naproxen Sodium) Bayer Healthcare LLC 742
Aleve Gelcaps (Naproxen Sodium) Bayer Healthcare LLC 743
Aleve Tablets (Naproxen Sodium) Bayer Healthcare LLC 743
Bayer Aspirin Comprehensive Prescribing Information (Aspirin) Bayer Healthcare 796
Bufferin Extra Strength Tablets (Aspirin Buffered) Novartis Consumer 678
Bufferin Regular Strength Tablets (Aspirin Buffered) Novartis Consumer 678
Excedrin Extra Strength Caplets/Tablets/Geltabs (Acetaminophen, Aspirin, Caffeine) Novartis Consumer 684
Excedrin Tension Headache Caplets/Tablets/Geltabs (Acetaminophen, Caffeine) Novartis Consumer 611
Goody's Body Pain Formula Powder (Acetaminophen, Aspirin, Acetaminophen, Aspirin) GlaxoSmithKline 684
Motrin IB Tablets and Caplets (Ibuprofen) McNeil Consumer 1866
Thera-Gesic Creme (Menthol, Methyl Salicylate) Mission 2141
ThermaCare Heat Wraps (Device) Procter & Gamble 2677
Traumeel Injection Solution (Homeopathic Formulations) Heel 1664
Regular Strength Tylenol Tablets (Acetaminophen) McNeil Consumer 1870
Tylenol 8 Hour Extended Release Caplets (Acetaminophen) McNeil Consumer 695
Tylenol Cough & Sore Throat Daytime Liquid with Cool Burst (Acetaminophen, Dextromethorphan Hydrobromide) McNeil Consumer 790
Tylenol 8 Hour Extended Release Caplets (Acetaminophen) McNeil Consumer 1870
Tylenol (Acetaminophen) McNeil Consumer 1870
Extra Strength Tylenol Rapid Release Gels (Acetaminophen) McNeil Consumer 1870
Tylenol Sore Throat Daytime Liquid with Cool Burst (Acetaminophen) McNeil Consumer 790
Tylenol Arthritis Pain Extended Release Caplets and Geltabs (Acetaminophen) McNeil Consumer 1870
Tylenol Sore Throat Daytime Liquid with Cool Burst (Acetaminophen) McNeil Consumer 1877
Vicks DayQuil Multi-Symptom Cold/Flu Relief Liquid (Acetaminophen, Dextromethorphan Hydrobromide, Pseudoephedrine Hydrochloride) Procter & Gamble 2678
Vicks DayQuil Multi-Symptom Cold/Flu Relief LiquiCaps (Acetaminophen, Dextromethorphan Hydrobromide, Pseudoephedrine Hydrochloride) Procter & Gamble 2678
Zicam Maximum Strength Flu Daytime (Acetaminophen, Chlorpheniramine Maleate, Dextromethorphan Hydrobromide) Matrixx 768
Zicam Maximum Strength Flu Nighttime (Acetaminophen, Dextromethorphan Hydrobromide, Doxylamine Succinate) Matrixx 768

Pain, neurogenic

BC Headache Powder (Aspirin, Caffeine, Salicylamide) GlaxoSmithKline 677
Arthritis Strength BC Powder (Aspirin, Caffeine, Salicylamide) GlaxoSmithKline 677
Tegretol/Tegretol-XR (Carbamazepine) Novartis 2295

Pain, neuropathic, associated with diabetic peripheral neuropathy

Cymbalta Delayed-Release Capsules (Duloxetine Hydrochloride) Lilly 1757
Lyrica Capsules (Pregabalin) Pfizer 2539

Pain, ocular

Acular LS Ophthalmic Solution (Ketorolac Tromethamine) Allergan 566

Pain, oral

Hurricaine Topical Anesthetic Spray, 2 oz. Wild Cherry (Benzocaine) Beutlich 712
Hurricaine Topical Anesthetic Gel, 1 oz. Wild Cherry, Pina Colada, Watermelon, and Fresh Mint, 5.25 g. Wild Cherry (Benzocaine) Beutlich 712
Hurricaine Topical Anesthetic Liquid, 1 oz. Wild Cherry, Pina Colada, 0.005 fl. oz. Snap-n-Go Swabs Wild Cherry (Benzocaine) Beutlich 712

Children's Tylenol Plus Cough & Sore Throat Suspension Liquid (Acetaminophen, Dextromethorphan Hydrobromide) McNeil Consumer 1879
Children's Tylenol Suspension with Flavor Creator (Acetaminophen) McNeil Consumer 1878
Children's Tylenol Plus Multi-Symptom Cold Suspension Liquid (Acetaminophen, Chlorpheniramine Maleate, Dextromethorphan Hydrobromide, Phenylephrine Hydrochloride) McNeil Consumer 1879
Tylenol Cold Head Congestion Daytime Caplets with Cool Burst (Acetaminophen, Dextromethorphan Hydrobromide, Phenylephrine Hydrochloride) McNeil Consumer 1873
Tylenol Cold Head Congestion Nighttime Caplets with Cool Burst (Acetaminophen, Chlorpheniramine Maleate, Dextromethorphan Hydrobromide, Phenylephrine Hydrochloride) McNeil Consumer 1873
Tylenol Cold Head Congestion Severe Caplets with Cool Burst (Acetaminophen, Dextromethorphan Hydrobromide, Guaifenesin, Phenylephrine Hydrochloride) McNeil Consumer 1873
Tylenol Cold Multi-Symptom Daytime Caplets with Cool Burst and Gelcaps (Acetaminophen, Dextromethorphan Hydrobromide, Phenylephrine Hydrochloride) McNeil Consumer 1874
Tylenol Cold Multi-Symptom Daytime Liquid with Citrus Burst (Acetaminophen, Dextromethorphan Hydrobromide, Phenylephrine Hydrochloride) McNeil Consumer 1874
Tylenol Cold Multi-Symptom Nighttime Caplets with Cool Burst (Acetaminophen, Chlorpheniramine Maleate, Dextromethorphan Hydrobromide, Phenylephrine Hydrochloride) McNeil Consumer 1874
Tylenol Cold Multi-Symptom Nighttime Liquid with Cool Burst (Acetaminophen, Dextromethorphan Hydrobromide, Doxylamine Succinate, Phenylephrine Hydrochloride) McNeil Consumer 1874
Tylenol Cold Multi-Symptom Severe Caplets with Cool Burst (Acetaminophen, Dextromethorphan Hydrobromide, Guaifenesin, Phenylephrine Hydrochloride) McNeil Consumer 1874
Tylenol Cold Multi-Symptom Severe Daytime Liquid with Citrus Burst (Acetaminophen, Dextromethorphan Hydrobromide, Guaifenesin, Phenylephrine Hydrochloride) McNeil Consumer 1874
Concentrated Tylenol Infants' Drops (Acetaminophen) McNeil Consumer 1878
Concentrated Tylenol Infants' Drops Plus Cold (Acetaminophen) McNeil Consumer 1879
Concentrated Tylenol Infants' Drops Plus Cold and Cough (Acetaminophen, Dextromethorphan Hydrobromide) McNeil Consumer 1879
Jr. Tylenol Meltaways (Acetaminophen) McNeil Consumer 1878
Tylenol Sore Throat Daytime Liquid with Cool Burst (Acetaminophen) McNeil Consumer 1877
Vicks DayQuil Multi-Symptom Cold/Flu Relief LiquiCaps (Acetaminophen, Dextromethorphan Hydrobromide, Pseudoephedrine Hydrochloride) Procter & Gamble 2678
Vicks DayQuil Multi-Symptom Cold/Flu Relief Liquid (Acetaminophen, Dextromethorphan Hydrobromide, Pseudoephedrine Hydrochloride) Procter & Gamble 2678
Vicks NyQuil LiquiCaps/Liquid Multi-Symptom Cold/Flu Relief (Acetaminophen, Dextromethorphan Hydrobromide, Doxylamine Succinate) Procter & Gamble ..... ▣763
Zicam Maximum Strength Flu Daytime (Acetaminophen, Chlorpheniramine Maleate, Dextromethorphan Hydrobromide) Matrixx ..... ▣768
Zicam Maximum Strength Flu Nighttime (Acetaminophen, Dextromethorphan Hydrobromide, Doxylamine Succinate) Matrixx ..... ▣768

Pain due to common cold
(*see under* Pain associated with upper respiratory infection)

Palpebral conjunctiva inflammation
Blephamide Ophthalmic Suspension (Prednisolone Acetate, Sulfacetamide Sodium) Allergan 569
FML Ophthalmic Ointment (Fluorometholone) Allergan ..... ⊙228
FML Ophthalmic Suspension (Fluorometholone) Allergan ..... ⊙227
FML Forte Ophthalmic Suspension (Fluorometholone) Allergan ..... ⊙226
FML-S Ophthalmic Suspension (Fluorometholone, Sulfacetamide Sodium) Allergan ..... ⊙229
Lotemax Ophthalmic Suspension 0.5% (Loteprednol Etabonate) Bausch & Lomb ..... ⊙251
Poly-Pred Ophthalmic Suspension (Neomycin Sulfate, Polymyxin B Sulfate, Prednisolone Acetate) Allergan ..... ⊙233
Pred Forte Ophthalmic Suspension (Prednisolone Acetate) Allergan ..... ⊙235
Pred-G Ophthalmic Ointment (Gentamicin Sulfate, Prednisolone Acetate) Allergan ..... ⊙237
Pred-G Ophthalmic Suspension (Gentamicin Sulfate, Prednisolone Acetate) Allergan ..... ⊙236
TobraDex Ophthalmic Ointment (Dexamethasone, Tobramycin) Alcon 562
TobraDex Ophthalmic Suspension (Dexamethasone, Tobramycin) Alcon 563

Pancreas, disseminated adenocarcinoma
(*see under* Carcinoma, pancreas)

Pancreatic cystic fibrosis
Pancrease MT Capsules (Pancrelipase) McNeil Pediatrics 1885
Viokase (Pancrelipase) Axcan Scandipharm 711

Pancreatic insufficiency
Creon 5 Capsules (Pancrelipase) Solvay 3198
Creon 10 Capsules (Pancrelipase) Solvay 3198
Creon 20 Capsules (Pancrelipase) Solvay 3199
Pancrease MT Capsules (Pancrelipase) McNeil Pediatrics 1885
Ultrase Capsules (Pancrelipase) Axcan Scandipharm 708
Ultrase MT Capsules (Pancrelipase) Axcan Scandipharm 709
Viokase (Pancrelipase) Axcan Scandipharm 711

Pancreatitis, adjunctive therapy
Plasbumin-5 (Albumin (human)) Talecris 3251
Plasbumin-20 (Albumin (human)) Talecris 3252
Plasbumin-25 (Albumin (human)) Talecris 3253

Panic disorder
Klonopin (Clonazepam) Roche 2778
Niravam Orally Disintegrating Tablets (Alprazolam) Schwarz 3092
Paxil CR Controlled-Release Tablets (Paroxetine Hydrochloride) GlaxoSmithKline 1538
Paxil (Paroxetine Hydrochloride) GlaxoSmithKline 1530
Pexeva Tablets (Paroxetine Mesylate) JDS 1694
Prozac Pulvules and Liquid (Fluoxetine Hydrochloride) Lilly 1801
Zoloft (Sertraline Hydrochloride) Pfizer 2586

Papillitis
(*see under* Optic neuritis)

Paralysis agitans
(*see under* Parkinson's disease)

Parkinsonism
Parcopa Orally Disintegrating Tablets (Carbidopa, Levodopa) Schwarz 3097

Parkinson's disease
Azilect Tablets (Rasagiline mesylate) Teva Neuroscience 3293
Comtan Tablets (Entacapone) Novartis 2189
Eldepryl Capsules (Selegiline Hydrochloride) Somerset 3208
Mirapex Tablets (Pramipexole Dihydrochloride) Boehringer Ingelheim 859
Parcopa Orally Disintegrating Tablets (Carbidopa, Levodopa) Schwarz 3097
Permax Tablets (Pergolide Mesylate) Valeant 3356
Requip Tablets (Ropinirole Hydrochloride) GlaxoSmithKline 1555
Stalevo Tablets (Carbidopa, Levodopa, Entacapone) Novartis 2287
Symmetrel Tablets (Amantadine Hydrochloride) Endo Labs 1135

Parkinson's disease, adjunct to levodopa/carbidopa therapy in the management of
Azilect Tablets (Rasagiline mesylate) Teva Neuroscience 3293
Tasmar Tablets (Tolcapone) Valeant 3358
Zelapar Tablets (Selegiline Hydrochloride) Valeant North America 3372

Parkinson's disease, idiopathic
Azilect Tablets (Rasagiline mesylate) Teva Neuroscience 3293
Tasmar Tablets (Tolcapone) Valeant 3358

PCP
(*see under* Pneumocystis carinii pneumonia)

Pediculosis, human
Ovide .5% Lotion (Malathion) TaroPharma 3290

Pediculosis capitis infestation
Permethrin Lotion (Permethrin) Actavis ..... ▣641

Pelvic cellulitis
(*see also under* Infections, gynecologic)
Cleocin Vaginal Ovules (Clindamycin Hydrochloride) Pharmacia & Upjohn 2616
Fortaz (Ceftazidime) GlaxoSmithKline 1453
Mefoxin for Injection (Cefoxitin Sodium) Merck 2012
Mefoxin Premixed Intravenous Solution (Cefoxitin Sodium) Merck 2016

Pelvic inflammatory disease
(*see also under* Infections, gynecologic)
E.E.S. (Erythromycin Ethylsuccinate) Abbott 451
EryPed (Erythromycin Ethylsuccinate) Abbott 447
Mefoxin for Injection (Cefoxitin Sodium) Merck 2012
Mefoxin Premixed Intravenous Solution (Cefoxitin Sodium) Merck 2016
PCE Dispertab Tablets (Erythromycin) Abbott 515
Rocephin Injectable Vials, ADD-Vantage, Galaxy, Bulk (Ceftriaxone Sodium) Roche 2800

Pemphigus
Decadron Tablets (Dexamethasone) Merck 1951
Depo-Medrol Injectable Suspension (Methylprednisolone Acetate) Pharmacia & Upjohn 2617
Depo-Medrol Single-Dose Vial (Methylprednisolone Acetate) Pharmacia & Upjohn 2619
Hydrocortone Tablets (Hydrocortisone) Merck 1989

Pemphigus, possibly effective in
Potaba (Aminobenzoate Potassium) Glenwood 1650

Penicillin therapy, an adjuvant to
E.E.S. (Erythromycin Ethylsuccinate) Abbott 451
EryPed (Erythromycin Ethylsuccinate) Abbott 447
PCE Dispertab Tablets (Erythromycin) Abbott 515

Peptococcus niger infections
Mefoxin Premixed IV (Cefoxitin Sodium) Merck 2016

Peptococcus niger skin and skin structure infections
Mefoxin Premixed IV (Cefoxitin Sodium) Merck 2016

Peptococcus niger gynecologic infections
Mefoxin Premixed IV (Cefoxitin Sodium) Merck 2016

Peptococcus species gynecologic infections
Primaxin I.V. (Cilastatin Sodium, Imipenem) Merck 2048

Peptococcus species intra-abdominal infections
Primaxin I.M. (Cilastatin Sodium, Imipenem) Merck 2045
Primaxin I.V. (Cilastatin Sodium, Imipenem) Merck 2048

Peptostreptococcus species endometritis
Mefoxin for Injection (Cefoxitin Sodium) Merck 2012
Mefoxin Premixed Intravenous Solution (Cefoxitin Sodium) Merck 2016

Peptostreptococcus species endomyometritis
Invanz for Injection (Ertapenem) Merck 1999

Peptostreptococcus species gynecologic infections
Mefoxin for Injection (Cefoxitin Sodium) Merck 2012
Mefoxin Premixed Intravenous Solution (Cefoxitin Sodium) Merck 2016
Primaxin I.M. (Cilastatin Sodium, Imipenem) Merck 2045
Primaxin I.V. (Cilastatin Sodium, Imipenem) Merck 2048

Peptostreptococcus species infections
Avelox (Moxifloxacin Hydrochloride) Schering 2970
Invanz for Injection (Ertapenem) Merck 1999
Mefoxin for Injection (Cefoxitin Sodium) Merck 2012
Mefoxin Premixed Intravenous Solution (Cefoxitin Sodium) Merck 2016
Merrem I.V. (Meropenem) AstraZeneca Pharmaceuticals 686
Primaxin I.M. (Cilastatin Sodium, Imipenem) Merck 2045
Primaxin I.V. (Cilastatin Sodium, Imipenem) Merck 2048
Rocephin Injectable Vials, ADD-Vantage, Galaxy, Bulk (Ceftriaxone Sodium) Roche 2800
Tygacil for Injection (Tigecycline) Wyeth 3488

Peptostreptococcus species intra-abdominal infections
Avelox (Moxifloxacin Hydrochloride) Schering 2970
Invanz for Injection (Ertapenem) Merck 1999
Merrem I.V. (Meropenem) AstraZeneca Pharmaceuticals 686
Primaxin I.M. (Cilastatin Sodium, Imipenem) Merck 2045
Primaxin I.V. (Cilastatin Sodium, Imipenem) Merck 2048

Rocephin Injectable Vials, ADD-Vantage, Galaxy, Bulk (Ceftriaxone Sodium) Roche 2800
Tygacil for Injection (Tigecycline) Wyeth 3488

Peptostreptococcus species peritonitis
Merrem I.V. (Meropenem) AstraZeneca Pharmaceuticals 686

Peptostreptococcus species skin and skin structure infections
Invanz for Injection (Ertapenem) Merck 1999
Mefoxin for Injection (Cefoxitin Sodium) Merck 2012
Mefoxin Premixed Intravenous Solution (Cefoxitin Sodium) Merck 2016
Merrem I.V. (Meropenem) AstraZeneca Pharmaceuticals 686
Primaxin I.V. (Cilastatin Sodium, Imipenem) Merck 2048
Rocephin Injectable Vials, ADD-Vantage, Galaxy, Bulk (Ceftriaxone Sodium) Roche 2800

Percutaneous coronary intervention, adjunct in
ReoPro Vials (Abciximab) Lilly 1809

Pericarditis, bacterial
Bicillin C-R Injectable Suspension (Penicillin G Benzathine, Penicillin G Procaine) King 1706

Peripheral blood progenitor cell transplantation
(*see under* Hematopoietic progenitor cells, mobilization of)

Peripheral vascular disease
Plavix Tablets (Clopidogrel Bisulfate) Bristol-Myers Squibb 917

Peritonitis
(*see also under* Infections, intra-abdominal)
Bicillin C-R Injectable Suspension (Penicillin G Benzathine, Penicillin G Procaine) King 1706
Cleocin Vaginal Ovules (Clindamycin Hydrochloride) Pharmacia & Upjohn 2616
Fortaz (Ceftazidime) GlaxoSmithKline 1453
Garamycin Injectable (Gentamicin Sulfate) Schering 3014
Mefoxin for Injection (Cefoxitin Sodium) Merck 2012
Mefoxin Premixed Intravenous Solution (Cefoxitin Sodium) Merck 2016
Timentin ADD-Vantage (Clavulanate Potassium, Ticarcillin Disodium) GlaxoSmithKline 1580
Timentin Injection Galaxy Container (Clavulanate Potassium, Ticarcillin Disodium) GlaxoSmithKline 1583
Timentin IV Infusion (Clavulanate Potassium, Ticarcillin Disodium) GlaxoSmithKline 1577
Timentin Pharmacy Bulk Package (Clavulanate Potassium, Ticarcillin Disodium) GlaxoSmithKline 1586

Peritonitis, adjunctive therapy
Plasbumin-5 (Albumin (human)) Talecris 3251
Plasbumin-20 (Albumin (human)) Talecris 3252
Plasbumin-25 (Albumin (human)) Talecris 3253

Peritonitis, candidal
Cancidas for Injection (Caspofungin acetate) Merck 1918
Eraxis for Injection (Anidulafungin) Pfizer 2521

Pertussis
E.E.S. (Erythromycin Ethylsuccinate) Abbott 451
EryPed (Erythromycin Ethylsuccinate) Abbott 447
Ery-Tab Tablets (Erythromycin) Abbott 449
Erythrocin Stearate Filmtab Tablets (Erythromycin Stearate) Abbott 453
Erythromycin Base Filmtab Tablets (Erythromycin) Abbott 455
Erythromycin Delayed-Release Capsules, USP (Erythromycin) Abbott 457
PCE Dispertab Tablets (Erythromycin) Abbott 515

Petit mal epilepsy
(*see under* Seizures, generalized, absence)

Peyronie's disease, possibly effective in
Potaba (Aminobenzoate Potassium) Glenwood 1650

Pharyngitis, symptomatic relief of
Advil Caplets (Ibuprofen) Wyeth .... ■674
Children's Advil Oral Suspension (Ibuprofen) Wyeth .... ■603
Children's Advil Chewable Tablets (Ibuprofen) Wyeth .... ■603
Advil Cold & Sinus (Ibuprofen, Pseudoephedrine Hydrochloride) Wyeth .... ■723
Advil Gel Caplets (Ibuprofen) Wyeth .... ■674
Infants' Advil Concentrated Drops (Ibuprofen) Wyeth .... ■604
Infants' Advil Concentrated Drops - White Grape (Dye-Free) (Ibuprofen) Wyeth .... ■604
Advil (Ibuprofen) Wyeth .... ■674
Hurricaine Topical Anesthetic Gel, 1 oz. Wild Cherry, Pina Colada, Watermelon, and Fresh Mint, 5.25 g. Wild Cherry (Benzocaine) Beutlich .... ■712
Hurricaine Topical Anesthetic Liquid, 1 oz. Wild Cherry, Pina Colada, 0.005 fl. oz. Snap-n-Go Swabs Wild Cherry (Benzocaine) Beutlich .... ■712
Hurricaine Topical Anesthetic Spray, 2 oz. Wild Cherry (Benzocaine) Beutlich .... ■712
Hurricaine Topical Anesthetic Spray Extension Tubes (200) (Benzocaine) Beutlich .... ■712
Hurricaine Topical Anesthetic Spray Kit, 2 oz. Wild Cherry with disposable Extension Tubes (200) (Benzocaine) Beutlich .... ■712
Junior Strength Motrin Caplets and Chewable Tablets (Ibuprofen) McNeil Consumer 1867
Robitussin Cough Drops Menthol, Cherry, and Honey-Lemon (Menthol) Wyeth .... ■737
Robitussin Honey Cough Drops (Menthol) Wyeth .... ■737
Robitussin Sugar Free Throat Drops (Menthol) Wyeth .... ■737
TheraFlu Cold & Sore Throat Hot Liquid (Acetaminophen, Pheniramine Maleate, Phenylephrine Hydrochloride) Novartis Consumer .... ■741
TheraFlu Flu & Chest Congestion Hot Liquid (Acetaminophen, Guaifenesin) Novartis Consumer .... ■741
TheraFlu Flu & Sore Throat Hot Liquid (Acetaminophen, Pheniramine Maleate, Phenylephrine Hydrochloride) Novartis Consumer .... ■742
TheraFlu Daytime Severe Cold Hot Liquid (Acetaminophen, Phenylephrine Hydrochloride) Novartis Consumer .... ■742
TheraFlu Nighttime Severe Cold Hot Liquid (Acetaminophen, Pheniramine Maleate, Phenylephrine Hydrochloride) Novartis Consumer .... ■740

Pharyngitis, treatment of
Amoxil Capsules (Amoxicillin) GlaxoSmithKline 1343
Amoxil Chewable Tablets (Amoxicillin) GlaxoSmithKline 1343
Amoxil Pediatric Drops for Oral Suspension (Amoxicillin) GlaxoSmithKline 1343
Amoxil Powder for Oral Suspension (Amoxicillin) GlaxoSmithKline 1343
Amoxil Tablets (Amoxicillin) GlaxoSmithKline 1343
Biaxin/Biaxin XL (Clarithromycin) Abbott 402
Ceftin (Cefuroxime Axetil) GlaxoSmithKline 1407
E.E.S. (Erythromycin Ethylsuccinate) Abbott 451
EryPed (Erythromycin Ethylsuccinate) Abbott 447
Ery-Tab Tablets (Erythromycin) Abbott 449
Erythrocin Stearate Filmtab Tablets (Erythromycin Stearate) Abbott 453
Erythromycin Base Filmtab Tablets (Erythromycin) Abbott 455
Erythromycin Delayed-Release Capsules, USP (Erythromycin) Abbott 457
Omnicef Capsules (Cefdinir) Abbott 511
Omnicef for Oral Suspension (Cefdinir) Abbott 511
PCE Dispertab Tablets (Erythromycin) Abbott 515
Suprax (Cefixime) Lupin 1843
Vantin Tablets and Oral Suspension (Cefpodoxime Proxetil) Pharmacia & Upjohn 2645

Pheochromocytoma
Demser Capsules (Metyrosine) Merck 1953
Dibenzyline Capsules (Phenoxybenzamine Hydrochloride) WellSpring 3399

Pheochromocytoma, adjunctive therapy
Demser Capsules (Metyrosine) Merck 1953

Phlegm, loosen
Tylenol Chest Congestion Caplets with Cool Burst (Acetaminophen, Guaifenesin) McNeil Consumer 1872
Tylenol Chest Congestion Liquid with Cool Burst (Acetaminophen, Guaifenesin) McNeil Consumer 1872
Tylenol Cold Severe Congestion Non-Drowsy Caplets with Cool Burst (Acetaminophen, Dextromethorphan Hydrobromide, Guaifenesin, Pseudoephedrine Hydrochloride) McNeil Consumer 1874
Tylenol Cold Head Congestion Severe Caplets with Cool Burst (Acetaminophen, Dextromethorphan Hydrobromide, Guaifenesin, Phenylephrine Hydrochloride) McNeil Consumer 1873
Tylenol Cold Multi-Symptom Severe Caplets with Cool Burst (Acetaminophen, Dextromethorphan Hydrobromide, Guaifenesin, Phenylephrine Hydrochloride) McNeil Consumer 1874
Tylenol Cold Multi-Symptom Severe Daytime Liquid with Citrus Burst (Acetaminophen, Dextromethorphan Hydrobromide, Guaifenesin, Phenylephrine Hydrochloride) McNeil Consumer 1874
Tylenol Sinus Congestion & Pain Severe Caplets with Cool Burst (Acetaminophen, Guaifenesin, Phenylephrine Hydrochloride) McNeil Consumer 1876

Phosphorus deficiency
(*see under* Hypophosphatemia)

Photophobia
Voltaren Ophthalmic Solution (Diclofenac Sodium) Novartis 2309

Phycomycosis
(*see under* Zygomycosis)

Pityrosporon orbiculare infections
Lotrimin (Clotrimazole) Schering 3039
Mentax Cream (Butenafine Hydrochloride) Mylan 2158
Oxistat (Oxiconazole Nitrate) Pharmaderm 2667

Plasmodium infection
(*see under* P. falciparum infections; P. malariae infections; P. ovale infections; P. vivax infections)

Platelet transfusions, reduction of the need for
Neumega for Injection (Oprelvekin) Wyeth 3435

Pleural effusion, malignant
Alimta for Injection (Pemetrexed) Lilly 1750

PMDD
(*see under* Dysphoric disorder, premenstrual)

Pneumococcal disease, immunization against
Pneumovax 23 (Pneumococcal Vaccine, Polyvalent) Merck 2043
Prevnar for Injection (Pneumococcal vaccine, diphtheria conjugate) Wyeth 3463

Pneumocystis carinii pneumonia
Mepron Suspension (Atovaquone) GlaxoSmithKline 1521

Pneumonia
(*see also under* Infections, lower respiratory tract)
Avelox (Moxifloxacin Hydrochloride) Schering 2970
Biaxin/Biaxin XL (Clarithromycin) Abbott 402
Bicillin C-R Injectable Suspension (Penicillin G Benzathine, Penicillin G Procaine) King 1706
Cleocin Vaginal Ovules (Clindamycin Hydrochloride) Pharmacia & Upjohn 2616
Ery-Tab Tablets (Erythromycin) Abbott 449
Erythrocin Stearate Filmtab Tablets (Erythromycin Stearate) Abbott 453
Erythromycin Base Filmtab Tablets (Erythromycin) Abbott 455
Fortaz (Ceftazidime) GlaxoSmithKline 1453
Invanz for Injection (Ertapenem) Merck 1999
Ketek Tablets (Telithromycin) sanofi-aventis 2903
Levaquin (Levofloxacin) Ortho-McNeil 2384
Levaquin in 5% Dextrose Injection (Levofloxacin) Ortho-McNeil 2384
Maxipime for Injection (Cefepime Hydrochloride) Elan 1105
Mefoxin for Injection (Cefoxitin Sodium) Merck 2012
Mefoxin Premixed Intravenous Solution (Cefoxitin Sodium) Merck 2016
Omnicef Capsules (Cefdinir) Abbott 511
Omnicef for Oral Suspension (Cefdinir) Abbott 511
Vantin Tablets and Oral Suspension (Cefpodoxime Proxetil) Pharmacia & Upjohn 2645
Zinacef for Injection (Cefuroxime) GlaxoSmithKline 1631
Zinacef Injection (Cefuroxime) GlaxoSmithKline 1631
Zmax for Oral Suspension (Azithromycin) Pfizer 2583
Zyvox (Linezolid) Pharmacia & Upjohn 2652

Pneumonia, community-acquired
Augmentin XR Extended-Release Tablets (Amoxicillin, Clavulanate Potassium) GlaxoSmithKline 1369
Avelox (Moxifloxacin Hydrochloride) Schering 2970
Invanz for Injection (Ertapenem) Merck 1999
Ketek Tablets (Telithromycin) sanofi-aventis 2903
Levaquin (Levofloxacin) Ortho-McNeil 2384
Levaquin in 5% Dextrose Injection (Levofloxacin) Ortho-McNeil 2384
Tequin Injection (Gatifloxacin) Bristol-Myers Squibb 938
Tequin Injection in 5% Dextrose (Gatifloxacin) Bristol-Myers Squibb 938
Tequin Tablets (Gatifloxacin) Bristol-Myers Squibb 938

Vantin Tablets and Oral Suspension (Cefpodoxime Proxetil) Pharmacia & Upjohn 2645
Zmax for Oral Suspension (Azithromycin) Pfizer.................................. 2583
Zosyn (Piperacillin Sodium, Tazobactam Sodium) Wyeth................ 3492
Zyvox (Linezolid) Pharmacia & Upjohn... 2652

Pneumonia, idiopathic eosinophilic
Decadron Tablets (Dexamethasone) Merck.. 1951

Pneumonia, nosocomial
(*see also under* Infections, lower respiratory tract)
Cipro I.V. (Ciprofloxacin) Schering 2984
Levaquin (Levofloxacin) Ortho-McNeil................................ 2384
Levaquin in 5% Dextrose Injection (Levofloxacin) Ortho-McNeil........... 2384
Zosyn (Piperacillin Sodium, Tazobactam Sodium) Wyeth................ 3492
Zyvox (Linezolid) Pharmacia & Upjohn... 2652

Pneumonia, pneumocystis carinii
(*see under* Pneumocystis carinii pneumonia)

Pneumonitis, aspiration
Depo-Medrol Injectable Suspension (Methylprednisolone Acetate) Pharmacia & Upjohn 2617
Depo-Medrol Single-Dose Vial (Methylprednisolone Acetate) Pharmacia & Upjohn 2619
Hydrocortone Tablets (Hydrocortisone) Merck 1989

Pneumonococcal septic arthritis, acute
Bicillin C-R Injectable Suspension (Penicillin G Benzathine, Penicillin G Procaine) King.......................... 1706

Poison Ivy
(*see under* Dermatitis, contact)

Poison Oak
(*see under* Dermatitis, contact)

Poison Sumac
(*see under* Dermatitis, contact)

Poliomyelitis, prevention of
(*see under* Immunization, poliovirus 1, 2, and 3)

Poliovirus types 1, 2, and 3 vaccine
(*see also under* Immunization, poliovirus 1, 2, and 3)
Pediarix (Diphtheria & Tetanus Toxoids and Pertussis Vaccine Adsorbed, Hepatitis B Vaccine, Recombinant, Poliovirus Vaccine Inactivated, Trivalent Types 1,2,3) GlaxoSmithKline 1548

Pollinosis
(*see also under* Rhinitis, seasonal allergic)
Advil Allergy Sinus Caplets (Chlorpheniramine Maleate, Ibuprofen, Pseudoephedrine Hydrochloride) Wyeth .... ■ 770
Advil Multi-Symptom Cold Caplets (Chlorpheniramine Maleate, Ibuprofen, Pseudoephedrine Hydrochloride) Wyeth .... ■ 770
Alavert Allergy & Sinus D-12 Hour Tablets (Loratadine, Pseudoephedrine Sulfate) Wyeth .... ■ 771
Alavert (Loratadine) Wyeth............. ■ 771
Claritin Reditabs 24 Hour Non-Drowsy Tablets (Loratadine) Schering-Plough .... ■ 772
Children's Dimetapp Cold & Allergy Elixir (Brompheniramine Maleate, Phenylephrine Hydrochloride) Wyeth .... ■ 730
Children's Dimetapp Cold & Allergy Chewable Tablets (Brompheniramine Maleate, Phenylephrine Hydrochloride) Wyeth .... ■ 730
Toddler's Dimetapp Cold and Cough Drops (Dextromethorphan Hydrobromide, Phenylephrine Hydrochloride) Wyeth .... ■ 732
4-Way Menthol Nasal Spray (Phenylephrine Hydrochloride) Novartis Consumer .... ■ 775
Robitussin Cough & Cold Long-Acting Liquid (Chlorpheniramine Maleate, Dextromethorphan Hydrobromide) Wyeth .... ■ 735
Robitussin Cough & Allergy Syrup (Chlorpheniramine Maleate, Dextromethorphan Hydrobromide, Phenylephrine Hydrochloride) Wyeth .... ■ 736
Robitussin Cough & Cold Nighttime Liquid (Chlorpheniramine Maleate, Dextromethorphan Hydrobromide, Phenylephrine Hydrochloride) Wyeth .... ■ 736
Robitussin Cough, Cold & Flu Nighttime Liquid (Acetaminophen, Chlorpheniramine Maleate, Dextromethorphan Hydrobromide, Phenylephrine Hydrochloride) Wyeth .... ■ 738
Robitussin Pediatric Cough & Cold Long-Acting Liquid (Chlorpheniramine Maleate, Dextromethorphan Hydrobromide) Wyeth .... ■ 735
Robitussin Pediatric Cough & Cold Nighttime Liquid (Chlorpheniramine Maleate, Dextromethorphan Hydrobromide, Phenylephrine Hydrochloride) Wyeth .... ■ 736
TheraFlu Thin Strips Multi Symptom (Diphenhydramine Hydrochloride) Novartis Consumer .... ■ 744
Tylenol Allergy Multi-Symptom Caplets with Cool Burst and Gelcaps (Acetaminophen, Chlorpheniramine Maleate, Phenylephrine Hydrochloride) McNeil Consumer.................................. 1872
Tylenol Allergy Multi-Symptom Nighttime Caplets with Cool Burst (Acetaminophen, Diphenhydramine Hydrochloride, Phenylephrine Hydrochloride) McNeil Consumer.................................. 1872
Tylenol Severe Allergy Caplets (Acetaminophen, Diphenhydramine Hydrochloride) McNeil Consumer.................................. 1872
Vicks Sinex 12-Hour Nasal Spray and Ultra Fine Mist for Sinus Relief (Oxymetazoline Hydrochloride) Procter & Gamble................ 2681
Vicks Vapor Inhaler (Levmetamfetamine) Procter & Gamble........... ■ 764
Zicam Allergy Relief (Histanium Hydrochloricum, Luffa operculata, Galphimia Glauca, Sulfur) Matrixx.. ■ 774
Zicam Extreme Congestion Relief (Oxymetazoline Hydrochloride) Matrixx.. ■ 767
Zicam Intense Sinus Relief (Oxymetazoline Hydrochloride) Matrixx.. ■ 767

Polycythemia vera
Mustargen for Injection (Mechlorethamine Hydrochloride) Ovation... 2468

Polymyositis
(*see under* Dermatomyositis, systemic)

Polyps, nasal, prevention of recurrence
Beconase AQ Nasal Spray (Beclomethasone Dipropionate Monohydrate) GlaxoSmithKline 1396

Polyps, nasal, treatment of
Nasonex Nasal Spray (Mometasone Furoate Monohydrate) Schering.. 3043

Pompe disease
Myozyme for Intravenous Infusion (Alglucosidase alfa) Genzyme........ 1279

Porphyria, acute intermittent, amelioration of recurrent attacks of
Panhematin (Hemin) Ovation............ 2473

Porphyria, variegata
Panhematin (Hemin) Ovation............ 2473

Porphyromonas asaccharolytica endomyometritis
Invanz (Ertapenem) Merck................ 1999

Porphyromonas asaccharolytica skin and skin structure infections
Invanz (Ertapenem) Merck................ 1999

Postnasal drip
(*see under* Cold, common, symptomatic relief of)

Post-traumatic stress disorder
(*see under* Stress disorder, post-traumatic)

Prader-Willi syndrome
Genotropin Lyophilized Powder (Somatropin) Pharmacia & Upjohn... 2638

Pregnancy, prevention of
Depo-Provera Contraceptive Injection (Medroxyprogesterone Acetate) Pharmacia & Upjohn....... 2622
depo-subQ provera 104 Injectable Suspension (Medroxyprogesterone Acetate) Pharmacia & Upjohn... 2624
Mircette Tablets (Desogestrel, Ethinyl Estradiol) Duramed................. 1066
Mirena Intrauterine System (Levonorgestrel) Berlex 787
NuvaRing (Etonogestrel, Ethinyl Estradiol) Organon USA................ 2340
Ortho-Cyclen Tablets (Ethinyl Estradiol, Norgestimate) Ortho Women's Health & Urology........... 2429
Ortho Evra Transdermal System (Norelgestromin, Ethinyl Estradiol) Ortho Women's Health & Urology 2417
Ortho Micronor Tablets (Norethindrone) Ortho Women's Health & Urology 2426
Ortho Tri-Cyclen Tablets (Ethinyl Estradiol, Norgestimate) Ortho Women's Health & Urology........... 2429
Ortho Tri-Cyclen Lo Tablets (Ethinyl Estradiol, Norgestimate) Ortho Women's Health & Urology........... 2436
ParaGard T 380A Intrauterine Copper Contraceptive (Copper, Intrauterine) Duramed 1073
Plan B Tablets (Levonorgestrel) Duramed 1076
Seasonique Tablets (Ethinyl Estradiol, Levonorgestrel) Duramed......... 1077
Yasmin 28 Tablets (Ethinyl Estradiol, Drospirenone) Berlex.............. 796
Yaz Tablets (Ethinyl Estradiol, Drospirenone) Berlex......................... 803

Pregnancy, vitamin supplement for
(*see under* Vitamin deficiency, postpartum; Vitamin deficiency, prenatal)

Premenstrual dysphoric disorder
(*see under* Dysphoric disorder, premenstrual)

Premenstrual syndrome, management of
(*see under* Dysphoric disorder, premenstrual)

Prevotella bivia endomyometritis
Invanz (Ertapenem) Merck............... 1999

Prevotella melaninogenica, endometritis
Timentin ADD-Vantage (Clavulanate Potassium, Ticarcillin Disodium) GlaxoSmithKline........................... 1580
Timentin IV Infusion (Clavulanate Potassium, Ticarcillin Disodium) GlaxoSmithKline........................... 1577

Prevotella melaninogenica, infections
Timentin ADD-Vantage (Clavulanate Potassium, Ticarcillin Disodium) GlaxoSmithKline........................... 1580
Timentin IV Infusion (Clavulanate Potassium, Ticarcillin Disodium) GlaxoSmithKline........................... 1577

Prinzmetal's angina
(*see under* Angina, Prinzmetal's)

Proctitis, ulcerative
Canasa Rectal Suppositories (Mesalamine) Axcan Scandipharm 699
Colocort (Hydrocortisone) Paddock.. 2476

Proctosigmoiditis, ulcerative
Colocort (Hydrocortisone) Paddock.. 2476

Promote the natural immune system of the body
Ambrotose AO Capsules (Herbals with Vitamins) Mannatech .... ■ 826
immune[26] BALANCE Powder Shake Mix (Egg product, hyperimmune) Legacy for Life .... ■ 815
immune[26] COMPLETE Support Powder Shake Mix (Egg product, hyperimmune) Legacy for Life.. ■ 815
immune[26] Powder, Capsules and Chewable Tablets (Egg product, hyperimmune) Legacy for Life..... ■ 815
immune[26] Power Chews Children's Chewable Tablets (Egg product, hyperimmune) Legacy for Life..... ■ 815
SynergyDefense Capsules (Herbals, Multiple) Awareness Corporation/AwarenessLife .... ■ 833

Propionibacterium species gynecologic infections
Primaxin I.V. (Cilastatin Sodium, Imipenem) Merck 2048

Propionibacterium species infections
Primaxin I.V. (Cilastatin Sodium, Imipenem) Merck 2048

Propionibacterium species intra-abdominal infections
Primaxin I.V. (Cilastatin Sodium, Imipenem) Merck 2048

Prostatic cancer
(*see under* Carcinoma, prostate)

Prostatic cancer, palliative treatment of
(*see under* Carcinoma, prostate, palliative treatment of)

Prostatic hyperplasia, benign, symptomatic treatment
Avodart Soft Gelatin Capsules (Dutasteride) GlaxoSmithKline........ 1390
Cardura XL Tablets (Doxazosin Mesylate) Pfizer 2515
Flomax Capsules (Tamsulosin Hydrochloride) Boehringer Ingelheim.. 850
Hytrin Capsules (Terazosin Hydrochloride) Abbott 471
Proscar Tablets (Finasteride) Merck.. 2067
Uroxatral Tablets (Alfuzosin Hydrochloride) sanofi-aventis................. 2943

Prostatitis
Cipro (Ciprofloxacin) Schering 2977
Cipro I.V. (Ciprofloxacin) Schering 2984
Levaquin (Levofloxacin) Ortho-McNeil.................................. 2384
Levaquin in 5% Dextrose Injection (Levofloxacin) Ortho-McNeil........... 2384
Noroxin Tablets (Norfloxacin) Merck . 2032

Proteinuria, remission of in lupus erythematosus
Decadron Tablets (Dexamethasone) Merck.. 1951

Proteinuria, remission of in nephrotic syndrome
Depo-Medrol Injectable Suspension (Methylprednisolone Acetate) Pharmacia & Upjohn 2617
Depo-Medrol Single-Dose Vial (Methylprednisolone Acetate) Pharmacia & Upjohn 2619
Hydrocortone Tablets (Hydrocortisone) Merck 1989

Proteus, indole-positive, infections
(*see under* Morganella morganii infections)

Proteus mirabilis
(*see under* P. mirabilis infections)

Proteus species gynecologic infections
Primaxin I.V. (Cilastatin Sodium, Imipenem) Merck 2048

Proteus species infections
Fortaz (Ceftazidime) GlaxoSmithKline.......................... 1453
Garamycin Injectable (Gentamicin Sulfate) Schering 3014
Primaxin I.V. (Cilastatin Sodium, Imipenem) Merck 2048

Proteus species infections, ocular, indole-negative
Pred-G Ophthalmic Suspension (Gentamicin Sulfate, Prednisolone Acetate) Allergan ⊙236

Proteus species intra-abdominal infections
Primaxin I.V. (Cilastatin Sodium, Imipenem) Merck 2048

Proteus species skin and skin structure infections
Fortaz (Ceftazidime) GlaxoSmithKline 1453

Proteus species urinary tract infections
Gantrisin Pediatric Suspension (Acetyl Sulfisoxazole) Roche 2770

Proteus vulgaris
(*see under* P. vulgaris infections)

Prothrombin deficiency, anticoagulant-induced
Mephyton Tablets (Vitamin K_1) Merck 2018

Providencia rettgeri infections
Cipro (Ciprofloxacin) Schering 2977
Cipro I.V. (Ciprofloxacin) Schering 2984
Mefoxin for Injection (Cefoxitin Sodium) Merck 2012
Mefoxin Premixed Intravenous Solution (Cefoxitin Sodium) Merck 2016
Primaxin I.V. (Cilastatin Sodium, Imipenem) Merck 2048

Providencia rettgeri skin and skin structure infections
Primaxin I.V. (Cilastatin Sodium, Imipenem) Merck 2048

Providencia rettgeri urinary tract infections
Cipro (Ciprofloxacin) Schering 2977
Cipro I.V. (Ciprofloxacin) Schering 2984
Mefoxin for Injection (Cefoxitin Sodium) Merck 2012
Mefoxin Premixed Intravenous Solution (Cefoxitin Sodium) Merck 2016
Primaxin I.V. (Cilastatin Sodium, Imipenem) Merck 2048

Providencia species infections
Mefoxin for Injection (Cefoxitin Sodium) Merck 2012
Mefoxin Premixed Intravenous Solution (Cefoxitin Sodium) Merck 2016

Providencia species urinary tract infections
Mefoxin for Injection (Cefoxitin Sodium) Merck 2012
Mefoxin Premixed Intravenous Solution (Cefoxitin Sodium) Merck 2016

Providencia stuartii infections
Cipro (Ciprofloxacin) Schering 2977
Cipro I.V. (Ciprofloxacin) Schering 2984

Providencia stuartii skin and skin structure infections
Cipro (Ciprofloxacin) Schering 2977
Cipro I.V. (Ciprofloxacin) Schering 2984

Pruritus
Hyland's Restful Legs Tablets (Dietary Supplement) Standard Homeopathic ▣829

Pruritus, anogenital
Analpram-HC (Hydrocortisone Acetate, Pramoxine Hydrochloride) Ferndale 1159
Preparation H Maximum Strength Cream (Glycerin, Petrolatum, Phenylephrine Hydrochloride, Pramoxine Hydrochloride) Wyeth ▣666
Preparation H Cooling Gel (Phenylephrine Hydrochloride) Wyeth ▣666
Preparation H Hydrocortisone Cream (Hydrocortisone) Wyeth ▣646
Preparation H (Mineral Oil, Petrolatum, Phenylephrine Hydrochloride, Shark Liver Oil) Wyeth ▣666
Preparation H Medicated Wipes (Witch Hazel) Wyeth ▣667
ProctoFoam-HC (Hydrocortisone Acetate, Pramoxine Hydrochloride) Schwarz 3099

Pruritus, ocular
Acular Ophthalmic Solution (Ketorolac Tromethamine) Allergan 565
Naphcon-A Eye Drops (Naphazoline Hydrochloride, Pheniramine Maleate) Alcon ⊙208
Visine-A Eye Allergy Relief Eye Drops (Naphazoline Hydrochloride, Pheniramine Maleate) Pfizer Consumer ⊙289

Pruritus, rhinopharyngeal, symptomatic relief of
Advil Allergy Sinus Caplets (Chlorpheniramine Maleate, Ibuprofen, Pseudoephedrine Hydrochloride) Wyeth ▣770
Advil Multi-Symptom Cold Caplets (Chlorpheniramine Maleate, Ibuprofen, Pseudoephedrine Hydrochloride) Wyeth ▣770
Alavert Allergy & Sinus D-12 Hour Tablets (Loratadine, Pseudoephedrine Sulfate) Wyeth ▣771
Alavert (Loratadine) Wyeth ▣771
Allegra-D 12 Hour Extended-Release Tablets (Fexofenadine Hydrochloride, Pseudoephedrine Hydrochloride) sanofi-aventis 2846
Children's Claritin Allergy Oral Solution (Loratadine) Schering-Plough ▣771
Claritin Non-Drowsy 24 Hour Tablets (Loratadine) Schering-Plough ▣772
Claritin Reditabs 24 Hour Non-Drowsy Tablets (Loratadine) Schering-Plough ▣772
Claritin-D Non-Drowsy 12 Hour Tablets (Loratadine, Pseudoephedrine Sulfate) Schering-Plough ▣772
Claritin-D Non-Drowsy 24 Hour Tablets (Loratadine, Pseudoephedrine Sulfate) Schering-Plough ▣772
Children's Dimetapp Cold & Allergy Elixir (Brompheniramine Maleate, Phenylephrine Hydrochloride) Wyeth ▣730
Children's Dimetapp Cold & Allergy Chewable Tablets (Brompheniramine Maleate, Phenylephrine Hydrochloride) Wyeth ▣730
Children's Dimetapp Long Acting Cough Plus Cold Syrup (Chlorpheniramine Maleate, Dextromethorphan Hydrobromide) Wyeth ▣731
Robitussin Cough & Cold Long-Acting Liquid (Chlorpheniramine Maleate, Dextromethorphan Hydrobromide) Wyeth ▣735
Robitussin Cough & Allergy Syrup (Chlorpheniramine Maleate, Dextromethorphan Hydrobromide, Phenylephrine Hydrochloride) Wyeth ▣736
Robitussin Cough & Cold Nighttime Liquid (Chlorpheniramine Maleate, Dextromethorphan Hydrobromide, Phenylephrine Hydrochloride) Wyeth ▣736
Robitussin Cough, Cold & Flu Nighttime Liquid (Acetaminophen, Chlorpheniramine Maleate, Dextromethorphan Hydrobromide, Phenylephrine Hydrochloride) Wyeth ▣738
Robitussin Pediatric Cough & Cold Long-Acting Liquid (Chlorpheniramine Maleate, Dextromethorphan Hydrobromide) Wyeth ▣735
Robitussin Pediatric Cough & Cold Nighttime Liquid (Chlorpheniramine Maleate, Dextromethorphan Hydrobromide, Phenylephrine Hydrochloride) Wyeth ▣736
TheraFlu Cold & Cough Hot Liquid (Dextromethorphan Hydrobromide, Pheniramine Maleate, Phenylephrine Hydrochloride) Novartis Consumer ▣740
TheraFlu Cold & Sore Throat Hot Liquid (Acetaminophen, Pheniramine Maleate, Phenylephrine Hydrochloride) Novartis Consumer ▣741
TheraFlu Flu & Sore Throat Hot Liquid (Acetaminophen, Pheniramine Maleate, Phenylephrine Hydrochloride) Novartis Consumer ▣742
TheraFlu Nighttime Severe Cold Hot Liquid (Acetaminophen, Pheniramine Maleate, Phenylephrine Hydrochloride) Novartis Consumer ▣740
TheraFlu Warming Relief Nighttime Severe Cold (Acetaminophen, Diphenhydramine Hydrochloride, Phenylephrine Hydrochloride) Novartis Consumer ▣743
TheraFlu Thin Strips Multi Symptom (Diphenhydramine Hydrochloride) Novartis Consumer ▣744
Triaminic Cold & Allergy Liquid (Chlorpheniramine Maleate, Phenylephrine Hydrochloride) Novartis Consumer ▣746
Triaminic Nighttime Cold & Cough Liquid (Diphenhydramine Hydrochloride, Phenylephrine Hydrochloride) Novartis Consumer ▣746
Triaminic Cough & Runny Nose Softchews (Chlorpheniramine Maleate, Dextromethorphan Hydrobromide) Novartis Consumer ▣748
Triaminic Thin Strips Cough & Runny Nose (Diphenhydramine Hydrochloride) Novartis Consumer ▣749
Tylenol Allergy Multi-Symptom Caplets with Cool Burst and Gelcaps (Acetaminophen, Chlorpheniramine Maleate, Phenylephrine Hydrochloride) McNeil Consumer 1872
Tylenol Allergy Multi-Symptom Nighttime Caplets with Cool Burst (Acetaminophen, Diphenhydramine Hydrochloride, Phenylephrine Hydrochloride) McNeil Consumer 1872
Tylenol Severe Allergy Caplets (Acetaminophen, Diphenhydramine Hydrochloride) McNeil Consumer 1872

Pruritus, topical relief of
Aclovate (Alclometasone Dipropionate) Pharmaderm 2660
Apexicon E Cream (Diflorasone Diacetate) Pharmaderm 2661
Clobevate Gel (Clobetasol Propionate) Stiefel 3211
Cutivate Cream (Fluticasone Propionate) Pharmaderm 2662
Cutivate Lotion 0.05% (Fluticasone Propionate) Pharmaderm 2664
Cutivate Ointment (Fluticasone Propionate) Pharmaderm 2665
Diprolene Gel 0.05% (Betamethasone Dipropionate) Schering 3001
Diprolene Lotion 0.05% (Betamethasone Dipropionate) Schering 3002
Diprolene Ointment 0.05% (Betamethasone Dipropionate) Schering 3003
Diprolene AF Cream 0.05% (Betamethasone Dipropionate) Schering 3000
Diprosone Cream, USP 0.05% (Betamethasone Dipropionate) Schering 3004
Elocon Cream 0.1% (Mometasone Furoate) Schering 3005
Elocon Lotion 0.1% (Mometasone Furoate) Schering 3006
Elocon Ointment 0.1% (Mometasone Furoate) Schering 3007
Locoid Lipocream Cream (Hydrocortisone Butyrate) Ferndale 1160
Luxíq Foam (Betamethasone Valerate) Connetics 1010
Olux Foam (Clobetasol Propionate) Connetics 1012
Pramosone (Hydrocortisone Acetate, Pramoxine Hydrochloride) Ferndale 1161
Preparation H Hydrocortisone Cream (Hydrocortisone) Wyeth ▣646
Temovate Gel (Clobetasol Propionate) Pharmaderm 2669
Temovate Scalp Application (Clobetasol Propionate) Pharmaderm 2670

Pruritus, vaginal
Estring Vaginal Ring (Estradiol) Pharmacia & Upjohn 2635

Pruritus ani
(*see under* Pruritus, anogenital)

Pseudomonas aeruginosa infections
(*see under* P. aeruginosa infections)

Pseudomonas species infections
Fortaz (Ceftazidime) GlaxoSmithKline 1453

Pseudomonas species infections, ocular
Blephamide Ophthalmic Suspension (Prednisolone Acetate, Sulfacetamide Sodium) Allergan 569
Neosporin Ophthalmic Solution Sterile (Gramicidin, Neomycin Sulfate, Polymyxin B Sulfate) King ⊙265

Pseudomonas species septicemia
Timentin ADD-Vantage (Clavulanate Potassium, Ticarcillin Disodium) GlaxoSmithKline 1580
Timentin Injection Galaxy Container (Clavulanate Potassium, Ticarcillin Disodium) GlaxoSmithKline 1583
Timentin IV Infusion (Clavulanate Potassium, Ticarcillin Disodium) GlaxoSmithKline 1577
Timentin Pharmacy Bulk Package (Clavulanate Potassium, Ticarcillin Disodium) GlaxoSmithKline 1586

Pseudomonas species urinary tract infections
Timentin ADD-Vantage (Clavulanate Potassium, Ticarcillin Disodium) GlaxoSmithKline 1580
Timentin Injection Galaxy Container (Clavulanate Potassium, Ticarcillin Disodium) GlaxoSmithKline 1583
Timentin IV Infusion (Clavulanate Potassium, Ticarcillin Disodium) GlaxoSmithKline 1577
Timentin Pharmacy Bulk Package (Clavulanate Potassium, Ticarcillin Disodium) GlaxoSmithKline 1586

Psoriasis
Amevive (Alefacept) Astellas 626
Olux Foam (Clobetasol Propionate) Connetics 1012
Oxsoralen-Ultra Capsules (Methoxsalen) Valeant 3353
Psoriatec Cream (Anthralin) Dusa 1089
Raptiva for Injection (Efalizumab) Genentech 1250

Psoriasis, erythrodermic
Soriatane (Acitretin) Connetics 1013

Psoriasis, scalp
Clobex Shampoo (Clobetasol Propionate) Galderma 1206

Psoriasis, plaque-type
Enbrel for Injection (Etanercept) Amgen 584
Vanos Cream (Fluocinonide) Medicis 1893

Psoriasis, pustulaf
Soriatane (Acitretin) Connetics 1013

Psoriasis, severe
Depo-Medrol Injectable Suspension (Methylprednisolone Acetate) Pharmacia & Upjohn 2617
Depo-Medrol Single-Dose Vial (Methylprednisolone Acetate) Pharmacia & Upjohn 2619
Enbrel for Injection (Etanercept) Amgen 584
Hydrocortone Tablets (Hydrocortisone) Merck 1989

Psoriasis, severe recalcitrant
Gengraf Capsules (Cyclosporine) Abbott 459
Neoral Oral Solution (Cyclosporine) Novartis 2259
Neoral Soft Gelatin Capsules (Cyclosporine) Novartis 2259

Psoriatic arthritis
(*see under* Arthritis, psoriatic)

Psoriatic plaques
Amevive (Alefacept) Astellas............ 626
Clobex Lotion (Clobetasol Propionate) Galderma.......................... 1204
Clobex Spray (Clobetasol Propionate) Galderma.......................... 1208
Depo-Medrol Injectable Suspension (Methylprednisolone Acetate) Pharmacia & Upjohn 2617
Depo-Medrol Single-Dose Vial (Methylprednisolone Acetate) Pharmacia & Upjohn 2619
Enbrel for Injection (Etanercept) Amgen.. 584
Gengraf Capsules (Cyclosporine) Abbott 459
Neoral Oral Solution (Cyclosporine) Novartis 2259
Neoral Soft Gelatin Capsules (Cyclosporine) Novartis................ 2259
Raptiva for Injection (Efalizumab) Genentech.................................. 1250

Psychotic disorders, management of the manifestations of
(*see under* Schizophrenia)

Puberty, central precocious
Lupron Depot-PED 7.5 mg, 11.25 mg and 15 mg (Leuprolide Acetate) TAP 3269
Lupron Injection Pediatric (Leuprolide Acetate) TAP 3259

Puberty, delayed
Androxy Tablets (Fluoxymesterone) Upsher-Smith 3335

Pulmonary emphysema
(*see under* Emphysema)

Purpura, idiopathic thrombocytopenic
Carimune NF (Immune Globulin Intravenous (Human)) ZLB Behring 3499
Decadron Tablets (Dexamethasone) Merck 1951
Depo-Medrol Injectable Suspension (Methylprednisolone Acetate) Pharmacia & Upjohn 2617
Gammagard S/D (Immune Globulin Intravenous (Human)) Baxter Healthcare 724
Gamunex Immune Globulin I.V., 10% (Immune Globulin Intravenous (Human)) Talecris 3235
Hydrocortone Tablets (Hydrocortisone) Merck 1989
WinRho SDF (Rh_0 (D) Immune Globulin (Human)) Baxter Healthcare 732

Pyelitis
Gantrisin Pediatric Suspension (Acetyl Sulfisoxazole) Roche 2770
Uroqid-Acid No. 2 Tablets (Methenamine Mandelate, Sodium Acid Phosphate) Beach 760

Pyelonephritis
Cipro (Ciprofloxacin) Schering 2977
Cipro I.V. (Ciprofloxacin) Schering 2984
Cipro XR Tablets (Ciprofloxacin) Schering 2990
Gantrisin Pediatric Suspension (Acetyl Sulfisoxazole) Roche 2770
Levaquin (Levofloxacin) Ortho-McNeil 2384
Levaquin in 5% Dextrose Injection (Levofloxacin) Ortho-McNeil 2384
Maxipime for Injection (Cefepime Hydrochloride) Elan 1105
Raniclor Tablets, Chewable (Cefaclor Monohydrate) Pedinol 2505
Tequin Injection (Gatifloxacin) Bristol-Myers Squibb 938
Tequin Injection in 5% Dextrose (Gatifloxacin) Bristol-Myers Squibb 938
Tequin Tablets (Gatifloxacin) Bristol-Myers Squibb 938
Uroqid-Acid No. 2 Tablets (Methenamine Mandelate, Sodium Acid Phosphate) Beach 760

Pyoderma gangrenosum
Levaquin (Levofloxacin) Ortho-McNeil 2384
Levaquin in 5% Dextrose Injection (Levofloxacin) Ortho-McNeil 2384

R

Rabies, postexposure prophylaxis
HyperRAB (Rabies Immune Globulin (Human)) Talecris 3242

Radiography, gastrointestinal tract, adjunct in
GlucaGen (Glucagon) Bedford........... 761
Glucagon for Injection Vials and Emergency Kit (Glucagon) Lilly 1778

Rash, drug
(*see under* Hypersensitivity reactions, drug-induced)

Rash, unspecified
(*see under* Skin, inflammatory conditions)

RDS
(*see under* Respiratory distress syndrome)

Reiter's syndrome
Bayer Aspirin (Aspirin) Bayer Healthcare LLC 744

Renal allogeneic transplants, prophylaxis of organ rejection in
CellCept Capsules (Mycophenolate Mofetil) Roche 2747
CellCept Intravenous (Mycophenolate Mofetil Hydrochloride) Roche .. 2747
CellCept Oral Suspension (Mycophenolate Mofetil) Roche.............. 2747
CellCept Tablets (Mycophenolate Mofetil) Roche 2747

Renal allograft transplants, acute rejection in
Orthoclone OKT3 Sterile Solution (Muromonab-CD3) Ortho Biotech ... 2360

Renal allograft transplants, prophylaxis of organ rejection
Myfortic Tablets (Mycophenolic Acid) Novartis.............................. 2255

Renal calculi, homozygous cystinuria caused
Thiola Tablets (Tiopronin) Mission 2141

Renal dialysis, adjunctive therapy
Plasbumin-20 (Albumin (human)) Talecris... 3252
Plasbumin-25 (Albumin (human)) Talecris... 3253

Renal plasma flow, estimation of
Aminohippurate Sodium PAH Injection (Aminohippurate Sodium) Merck 1913

Renal toxicity, cumulative, cisplatin-induced
Ethyol for Injection (Amifostine) MedImmune Oncology 1898

Renal transplantation, prevention of rejection in
CellCept Capsules (Mycophenolate Mofetil) Roche 2747
CellCept Intravenous (Mycophenolate Mofetil Hydrochloride) Roche .. 2747
CellCept Oral Suspension (Mycophenolate Mofetil) Roche.............. 2747
CellCept Tablets (Mycophenolate Mofetil) Roche 2747
Gengraf Capsules (Cyclosporine) Abbott 459
Neoral Oral Solution (Cyclosporine) Novartis 2259
Neoral Soft Gelatin Capsules (Cyclosporine) Novartis................ 2259
Prograf Capsules and Injection (Tacrolimus) Astellas 632
Rapamune Oral Solution and Tablets (Sirolimus) Wyeth 3475
Sandimmune (Cyclosporine) Novartis 2275
Simulect for Injection (Basiliximab) Novartis 2284
Thymoglobulin for Intravenous Infusion (Anti-thymocyte Globulin) Genzyme 1284

Renal tubular acidosis, management of
Urocit-K Tablets (Potassium Citrate) Mission....................................... 2144

Renal tubular secretory mechanism, measurement of the functional capacity of
Aminohippurate Sodium PAH Injection (Aminohippurate Sodium) Merck 1913

Respiratory distress syndrome
Curosurf Intratracheal Suspension (Poractant alfa) Dey 1057
Flexbumin I.V. (Albumin (human)) Baxter Healthcare 720
Infasurf Intratracheal Suspension (Calfactant) Forest 1184
Plasbumin-20 (Albumin (human)) Talecris... 3252
Plasbumin-25 (Albumin (human)) Talecris... 3253

Respiratory symptoms, upper, relief of
(*see under* Influenza syndrome, symptomatic relief of)

Respiratory syncytial virus (RSV) infections
(*see under* Infections, lower respiratory tract, RSV-induced)

Restless leg syndrome
Hyland's Restful Legs Tablets (Dietary Supplement) Standard Homeopathic .... ▣829

Restless legs syndrome
Requip Tablets (Ropinirole Hydrochloride) GlaxoSmithKline............. 1555

Retinitis, cytomegalovirus
Valcyte Tablets (Valganciclovir Hydrochloride) Roche.................. 2813

Rhabdomyosarcoma
Cosmegen for Injection (Dactinomycin) Ovation............................ 2459

Rheumatic carditis, acute
Decadron Tablets (Dexamethasone) Merck.. 1951
Depo-Medrol Injectable Suspension (Methylprednisolone Acetate) Pharmacia & Upjohn 2617
Depo-Medrol Single-Dose Vial (Methylprednisolone Acetate) Pharmacia & Upjohn 2619
Hydrocortone Tablets (Hydrocortisone) Merck 1989

Rheumatic fever, prophylaxis of
E.E.S. (Erythromycin Ethylsuccinate) Abbott................................ 451
EryPed (Erythromycin Ethylsuccinate) Abbott................................ 447
Erythromycin Base Filmtab Tablets (Erythromycin) Abbott 455
Erythromycin Delayed-Release Capsules, USP (Erythromycin) Abbott 457
PCE Dispertab Tablets (Erythromycin) Abbott................................ 515

Rheumatoid arthritis, juvenile
Bayer Aspirin (Aspirin) Bayer Healthcare LLC 744
Bayer Aspirin Comprehensive Prescribing Information (Aspirin) Bayer Healthcare .... ▣796
Decadron Tablets (Dexamethasone) Merck.. 1951
Depo-Medrol Injectable Suspension (Methylprednisolone Acetate) Pharmacia & Upjohn 2617
Enbrel for Injection (Etanercept) Amgen.. 584
Hydrocortone Tablets (Hydrocortisone) Merck 1989
Mobic Oral Suspension (Meloxicam) Boehringer Ingelheim........... 863
Mobic Tablets (Meloxicam) Boehringer Ingelheim 863

Rhinitis
Advil Caplets (Ibuprofen) Wyeth ...... ▣674
Children's Advil Oral Suspension (Ibuprofen) Wyeth .... ▣603
Children's Advil Chewable Tablets (Ibuprofen) Wyeth .... ▣603
Advil Cold & Sinus (Ibuprofen, Pseudoephedrine Hydrochloride) Wyeth .... ▣723
Advil (Ibuprofen) Wyeth .... ▣674
Contac-D Cold Non-Drowsy Tablets (Phenylephrine Hydrochloride) GlaxoSmithKline .... ▣729
TheraFlu Daytime Severe Cold Hot Liquid (Acetaminophen, Phenylephrine Hydrochloride) Novartis Consumer .... ▣742

Rhinitis, allergic
Atrovent Nasal Spray 0.03% (Ipratropium Bromide) Boehringer Ingelheim... 837
Children's Dimetapp Cold & Allergy Elixir (Brompheniramine Maleate, Phenylephrine Hydrochloride) Wyeth .... ▣730
Children's Dimetapp Cold & Allergy Chewable Tablets (Brompheniramine Maleate, Phenylephrine Hydrochloride) Wyeth .... ▣730
Phenergan Tablets and Suppositories (Promethazine Hydrochloride) Wyeth 3440

Rhinitis, perennial allergic
Atrovent Nasal Spray 0.03% (Ipratropium Bromide) Boehringer Ingelheim 837
Beconase AQ Nasal Spray (Beclomethasone Dipropionate Monohydrate) GlaxoSmithKline 1396
Clarinex Syrup (Desloratadine) Schering 2995
Clarinex Tablets (Desloratadine) Schering 2995
Clarinex Reditabs Tablets (Desloratadine) Schering 2995
Decadron Tablets (Dexamethasone) Merck 1951
Depo-Medrol Injectable Suspension (Methylprednisolone Acetate) Pharmacia & Upjohn 2617
Depo-Medrol Single-Dose Vial (Methylprednisolone Acetate) Pharmacia & Upjohn 2619
Flonase Nasal Spray (Fluticasone Propionate) GlaxoSmithKline 1440
Hydrocortone Tablets (Hydrocortisone) Merck 1989
Nasacort AQ Nasal Spray (Triamcinolone Acetonide) sanofi-aventis 2922
Nasonex Nasal Spray (Mometasone Furoate Monohydrate) Schering 3043
Rhinocort Aqua Nasal Spray (Budesonide) AstraZeneca LP 665
Singulair (Montelukast Sodium) Merck 2077
Zyrtec Chewable Tablets (Cetirizine Hydrochloride) Pfizer 2594
Zyrtec (Cetirizine Hydrochloride) Pfizer 2594
Zyrtec-D 12 Hour Extended Release Tablets (Cetirizine Hydrochloride, Pseudoephedrine Hydrochloride) Pfizer 2597

Rhinitis, seasonal allergic
Allegra (Fexofenadine Hydrochloride) sanofi-aventis 2844
Allegra-D 12 Hour Extended-Release Tablets (Fexofenadine Hydrochloride, Pseudoephedrine Hydrochloride) sanofi-aventis 2846
Allegra-D 24 Hour Extended-Release Tablets (Fexofenadine Hydrochloride, Pseudoephedrine Hydrochloride) sanofi-aventis 2849
Astelin Nasal Spray (Azelastine Hydrochloride) MedPointe 1904
Beconase AQ Nasal Spray (Beclomethasone Dipropionate Monohydrate) GlaxoSmithKline 1396
Clarinex Syrup (Desloratadine) Schering 2995
Clarinex Tablets (Desloratadine) Schering 2995
Clarinex Reditabs Tablets (Desloratadine) Schering 2995
Clarinex-D 24-Hour Extended-Release Tablets (Desloratadine, Pseudoephedrine Sulfate) Schering 2998

Rhinitis, vasomotor

Rhinorrhea

Ringworm infections of the body

(*see under* Tinea corporis infections)

Ringworm infections of the feet

(*see under* Tinea pedis infections)

Ringworm infections of the groin

(*see under* Tinea cruris infections)

Ringworm infections of the nails

(*see under* Tinea unguium infections)

Ringworm infections of the scalp

(*see under* Tinea capitis infections)

Rosacea

Rubella, prophylaxis

S

Erythromycin Base Filmtab Tablets (Erythromycin) Abbott 455
Erythromycin Delayed-Release Capsules, USP (Erythromycin) Abbott 457
Fortaz (Ceftazidime) GlaxoSmithKline 1453
Invanz for Injection (Ertapenem) Merck 1999
Keflex Capsules (Cephalexin) Advancis 549
Levaquin (Levofloxacin) Ortho-McNeil 2384
Levaquin in 5% Dextrose Injection (Levofloxacin) Ortho-McNeil 2384
Maxipime for Injection (Cefepime Hydrochloride) Elan 1105
Mefoxin for Injection (Cefoxitin Sodium) Merck 2012
Mefoxin Premixed Intravenous Solution (Cefoxitin Sodium) Merck 2016
Merrem I.V. (Meropenem) AstraZeneca Pharmaceuticals 686
Omnicef Capsules (Cefdinir) Abbott 511
Omnicef for Oral Suspension (Cefdinir) Abbott 511
PCE Dispertab Tablets (Erythromycin) Abbott 515
Primaxin I.M. (Cilastatin Sodium, Imipenem) Merck 2045
Primaxin I.V. (Cilastatin Sodium, Imipenem) Merck 2048
Raniclor Tablets, Chewable (Cefaclor Monohydrate) Pedinol 2505
Rocephin Injectable Vials, ADD-Vantage, Galaxy, Bulk (Ceftriaxone Sodium) Roche 2800
Tequin Injection (Gatifloxacin) Bristol-Myers Squibb 938
Tequin Injection in 5% Dextrose (Gatifloxacin) Bristol-Myers Squibb 938
Tequin Tablets (Gatifloxacin) Bristol-Myers Squibb 938
Tygacil for Injection (Tigecycline) Wyeth 3488
Vantin Tablets and Oral Suspension (Cefpodoxime Proxetil) Pharmacia & Upjohn 2645
Zinacef for Injection (Cefuroxime) GlaxoSmithKline 1631
Zinacef Injection (Cefuroxime) GlaxoSmithKline 1631
Zyvox (Linezolid) Pharmacia & Upjohn 2652

S. pyogenes tonsillitis
Biaxin/Biaxin XL (Clarithromycin) Abbott 402
Ceftin (Cefuroxime Axetil) GlaxoSmithKline 1407
Omnicef Capsules (Cefdinir) Abbott 511
Omnicef for Oral Suspension (Cefdinir) Abbott 511
Raniclor Tablets, Chewable (Cefaclor Monohydrate) Pedinol 2505
Suprax (Cefixime) Lupin 1843
Vantin Tablets and Oral Suspension (Cefpodoxime Proxetil) Pharmacia & Upjohn 2645

S. pyogenes upper respiratory tract infections
Biaxin/Biaxin XL (Clarithromycin) Abbott 402
E.E.S. (Erythromycin Ethylsuccinate) Abbott 451
EryPed (Erythromycin Ethylsuccinate) Abbott 447
Ery-Tab Tablets (Erythromycin) Abbott 449
Erythrocin Stearate Filmtab Tablets (Erythromycin Stearate) Abbott 453
Erythromycin Base Filmtab Tablets (Erythromycin) Abbott 455
Erythromycin Delayed-Release Capsules, USP (Erythromycin) Abbott 457
Omnicef Capsules (Cefdinir) Abbott 511
Omnicef for Oral Suspension (Cefdinir) Abbott 511
PCE Dispertab Tablets (Erythromycin) Abbott 515
Suprax (Cefixime) Lupin 1843

S. saprophyticus urinary tract infections
Cipro (Ciprofloxacin) Schering 2977
Cipro XR Tablets (Ciprofloxacin) Schering 2990
Noroxin Tablets (Norfloxacin) Merck 2032
Vantin Tablets and Oral Suspension (Cefpodoxime Proxetil) Pharmacia & Upjohn 2645

S. viridans endocarditis
Erythrocin Stearate Filmtab Tablets (Erythromycin Stearate) Abbott 453
Erythromycin Base Filmtab Tablets (Erythromycin) Abbott 455

S. viridans skin and skin structure infections
Merrem I.V. (Meropenem) AstraZeneca Pharmaceuticals 686

S. warnerii infections, ocular
Vigamox Ophthalmic Solution (Moxifloxacin Hydrochloride) Alcon 564

SAH
(*see under* Hemorrhage, subarachnoid, resulting in neurological deficits)

Salmonella typhi, immunization against
(*see also under* Immunization, typhoid fever)
Vivotif (Typhoid Vaccine Live Oral TY21a) Berna 819

Salmonella typhi infections
Cipro (Ciprofloxacin) Schering 2977

Sarcoidosis, symptomatic
Decadron Tablets (Dexamethasone) Merck 1951
Depo-Medrol Injectable Suspension (Methylprednisolone Acetate) Pharmacia & Upjohn 2617
Depo-Medrol Single-Dose Vial (Methylprednisolone Acetate) Pharmacia & Upjohn 2619
Hydrocortone Tablets (Hydrocortisone) Merck 1989

Sarcoma botryoides
Cosmegen for Injection (Dactinomycin) Ovation 2459

Scar tissue
Mederma Topical Gel (Allantoin, Allium cepa) Merz 2126
Mederma for Kids Topical Gel (Allantoin, Allium cepa) Merz 2126

Scarlatina
Bicillin C-R Injectable Suspension (Penicillin G Benzathine, Penicillin G Procaine) King 1706

Scarlet fever
(*see under* Scarlatina)

Scedosporium apiospermum infections
VFEND I.V. (Voriconazole) Pfizer 2564
VFEND Oral Suspension (Voriconazole) Pfizer 2564
VFEND Tablets (Voriconazole) Pfizer 2564

Schistosoma haematobium infections
Biltricide (Praziquantel) Schering 2976

Schistosoma japonicum infections
Biltricide (Praziquantel) Schering 2976

Schistosoma mansoni infections
Biltricide (Praziquantel) Schering 2976

Schistosoma mekongi infections
Biltricide (Praziquantel) Schering 2976

Schizophrenia
Abilify Oral Solution (Aripiprazole) Bristol-Myers Squibb 882
Abilify Oral Solution (Aripiprazole) Otsuka America 2450
Abilify Discmelt Orally Disintegrating Tablets (Aripiprazole) Bristol-Myers Squibb 882
Abilify Discmelt Orally Disintegrating Tablets (Aripiprazole) Otsuka America 2450
Abilify Tablets (Aripiprazole) Bristol-Myers Squibb 882
Abilify Tablets (Aripiprazole) Otsuka America 2450
Clozaril Tablets (Clozapine) Novartis 2184
FazaClo Orally Disintegrating Tablets (Clozapine) Alamo 551
Geodon (Ziprasidone Hydrochloride) Pfizer 2529
Moban Tablets (Molindone Hydrochloride) Endo Labs 1119
Risperdal (Risperidone) Janssen 1676
Risperdal Consta Long-Acting Injection (Risperidone) Janssen 1682
Risperdal M-Tab Orally Disintegrating Tablets (Risperidone) Janssen 1676
Seroquel Tablets (Quetiapine Fumarate) AstraZeneca Pharmaceuticals 690
Thioridazine Hydrochloride Tablets (Thioridazine Hydrochloride) Mylan 2163
Thiothixene Capsules (Thiothixene) Mylan 2165
Zyprexa Tablets (Olanzapine) Lilly 1830
Zyprexa IntraMuscular (Olanzapine) Lilly 1830
Zyprexa ZYDIS Orally Disintegrating Tablets (Olanzapine) Lilly 1830

Schizophrenia, treatment-resistant
FazaClo Orally Disintegrating Tablets (Clozapine) Alamo 551

Sciatica, temporary relief of
BC Headache Powder (Aspirin, Caffeine, Salicylamide) GlaxoSmithKline .... ▣ 677
Arthritis Strength BC Powder (Aspirin, Caffeine, Salicylamide) GlaxoSmithKline .... ▣ 677

Scleroderma, linear, possibly effective in
Potaba (Aminobenzoate Potassium) Glenwood 1650

Scleroderma, possibly effective in
Potaba (Aminobenzoate Potassium) Glenwood 1650

Seasonal Affective Disorder
Wellbutrin XL Extended-Release Tablets (Bupropion Hydrochloride) GlaxoSmithKline 1613

Seborrhea
(*see under* Dandruff)

Sedation
(*see also under* Sleep, induction of)
Nembutal Sodium Solution, USP (Pentobarbital Sodium) Ovation 2470
Phenergan Tablets and Suppositories (Promethazine Hydrochloride) Wyeth 3440

Sedation, benzodiazepine-induced, complete or partial reversal of
Romazicon Injection (Flumazenil) Roche 2804

Sedation, daytime
Xyrem Oral Solution (Sodium Oxybate) Jazz Pharmaceuticals 1688

Sedation, obstetric
Phenergan Tablets and Suppositories (Promethazine Hydrochloride) Wyeth 3440

Seizures, absence, adjunctive therapy in
Depacon Injection (Valproate Sodium) Abbott 412
Depakene (Valproic Acid) Abbott 417
Depakote Sprinkle Capsules (Divalproex Sodium) Abbott 422
Depakote Tablets (Divalproex Sodium) Abbott 427
Depakote ER Tablets (Divalproex Sodium) Abbott 434

Seizures, akinetic
Klonopin (Clonazepam) Roche 2778

Seizures, centrencephalic
(*see under* Seizures, generalized, absence; Seizures, generalized, tonic-clonic)

Seizures, focal
Carbatrol Capsules (Carbamazepine) Shire US 3171
Depacon Injection (Valproate Sodium) Abbott 412
Depakene (Valproic Acid) Abbott 417
Depakote Sprinkle Capsules (Divalproex Sodium) Abbott 422
Depakote Tablets (Divalproex Sodium) Abbott 427
Depakote ER Tablets (Divalproex Sodium) Abbott 434
Lamictal (Lamotrigine) GlaxoSmithKline 1481
Lyrica Capsules (Pregabalin) Pfizer 2539
Phenytek Capsules (Phenytoin Sodium) Mylan 2160
Tegretol/Tegretol-XR (Carbamazepine) Novartis 2295
Tranxene T-TAB Tablets (Clorazepate Dipotassium) Ovation 2474
Trileptal Tablets (Oxcarbazepine) Novartis 2300
Trileptal Oral Suspension (Oxcarbazepine) Novartis 2300

Seizures, focal, adjunctive therapy in
Depakote Sprinkle Capsules (Divalproex Sodium) Abbott 422
Keppra Oral Solution (Levetiracetam) UCB 3314
Keppra Tablets (Levetiracetam) UCB 3314
Neurontin Capsules (Gabapentin) Parke-Davis 2487
Neurontin Oral Solution (Gabapentin) Parke-Davis 2487
Neurontin Tablets (Gabapentin) Parke-Davis 2487
Topamax Sprinkle Capsules (Topiramate) Ortho-McNeil Neurologics 2404
Topamax Tablets (Topiramate) Ortho-McNeil Neurologics 2404
Tranxene (Clorazepate Dipotassium) Ovation 2474
Trileptal Tablets (Oxcarbazepine) Novartis 2300
Trileptal Oral Suspension (Oxcarbazepine) Novartis 2300

Seizures, generalized, absence
Depacon Injection (Valproate Sodium) Abbott 412
Depakene (Valproic Acid) Abbott 417
Depakote Sprinkle Capsules (Divalproex Sodium) Abbott 422
Depakote Tablets (Divalproex Sodium) Abbott 427
Depakote ER Tablets (Divalproex Sodium) Abbott 434
Klonopin (Clonazepam) Roche 2778

Seizures, generalized, tonic-clonic
Carbatrol Capsules (Carbamazepine) Shire US 3171
Phenytek Capsules (Phenytoin Sodium) Mylan 2160
Tegretol/Tegretol-XR (Carbamazepine) Novartis 2295
Topamax Sprinkle Capsules (Topiramate) Ortho-McNeil Neurologics 2404
Topamax Tablets (Topiramate) Ortho-McNeil Neurologics 2404

Seizures, multiple, adjunctive therapy in
Depacon Injection (Valproate Sodium) Abbott 412
Depakene (Valproic Acid) Abbott 417
Depakote Tablets (Divalproex Sodium) Abbott 427
Depakote ER Tablets (Divalproex Sodium) Abbott 434

Seizures, myoclonic
Keppra Oral Solution (Levetiracetam) UCB 3314
Keppra Tablets (Levetiracetam) UCB 3314
Klonopin (Clonazepam) Roche 2778

Seizures, myoclonic, adjunctive therapy in
Keppra Oral Solution (Levetiracetam) UCB 3314
Keppra Tablets (Levetiracetam) UCB 3314

Seizures, neurosurgery-induced
Phenytek Capsules (Phenytoin Sodium) Mylan 2160

Seizures, partial
(*see under* Seizures, focal)

Seizures, partial, adjunctive therapy in
Depacon Injection (Valproate Sodium) Abbott 412
Depakene (Valproic Acid) Abbott 417

Depakote Sprinkle Capsules (Divalproex Sodium) Abbott 422
Depakote Tablets (Divalproex Sodium) Abbott 427
Depakote ER Tablets (Divalproex Sodium) Abbott 434
Gabitril Tablets (Tiagabine Hydrochloride) Cephalon 984
Keppra Injection (Levetiracetam) UCB 3320
Keppra Oral Solution (Levetiracetam) UCB 3314
Keppra Tablets (Levetiracetam) UCB 3314
Lamictal (Lamotrigine) GlaxoSmithKline 1481
Trileptal Tablets (Oxcarbazepine) Novartis 2300
Trileptal Oral Suspension (Oxcarbazepine) Novartis 2300
Zonegran Capsules (Zonisamide) Eisai 1101

Seizures, psychomotor
Carbatrol Capsules (Carbamazepine) Shire US 3171
Phenytek Capsules (Phenytoin Sodium) Mylan 2160
Tegretol-XR Tablets (Carbamazepine) Novartis 2295

Seizures, unspecified, adjunctive therapy in
Diastat Rectal Delivery System (Diazepam) Valeant 3343

Senile lentigines
(*see under* Hyperpigmentation, skin, bleaching of)

Sepsis
Zinacef for Injection (Cefuroxime) GlaxoSmithKline 1631
Zinacef Injection (Cefuroxime) GlaxoSmithKline 1631

Sepsis, bacterial, neonatal
Garamycin Injectable (Gentamicin Sulfate) Schering 3014

Sepsis, severe
Xigris Powder for Intravenous Infusion (Drotrecogin alfa (activated)) Lilly 1828

Septicemia, bacterial
Bicillin C-R Injectable Suspension (Penicillin G Benzathine, Penicillin G Procaine) King 1706
Cipro I.V. (Ciprofloxacin) Schering 2984
Cleocin Vaginal Ovules (Clindamycin Hydrochloride) Pharmacia & Upjohn 2616
Fortaz (Ceftazidime) GlaxoSmithKline 1453
Garamycin Injectable (Gentamicin Sulfate) Schering 3014
Invanz for Injection (Ertapenem) Merck 1999
Mefoxin for Injection (Cefoxitin Sodium) Merck 2012
Mefoxin Premixed Intravenous Solution (Cefoxitin Sodium) Merck 2016
Primaxin I.V. (Cilastatin Sodium, Imipenem) Merck 2048
Rocephin Injectable Vials, ADD-Vantage, Galaxy, Bulk (Ceftriaxone Sodium) Roche 2800
Timentin ADD-Vantage (Clavulanate Potassium, Ticarcillin Disodium) GlaxoSmithKline 1580
Timentin Injection Galaxy Container (Clavulanate Potassium, Ticarcillin Disodium) GlaxoSmithKline 1583
Timentin IV Infusion (Clavulanate Potassium, Ticarcillin Disodium) GlaxoSmithKline 1577
Timentin Pharmacy Bulk Package (Clavulanate Potassium, Ticarcillin Disodium) GlaxoSmithKline 1586
Zinacef for Injection (Cefuroxime) GlaxoSmithKline 1631
Zinacef Injection (Cefuroxime) GlaxoSmithKline 1631
Zyvox (Linezolid) Pharmacia & Upjohn 2652

Serratia marcescens bone and joint infections
Cipro (Ciprofloxacin) Schering 2977
Cipro I.V. (Ciprofloxacin) Schering 2984

Serratia marcescens infections
Cipro (Ciprofloxacin) Schering 2977
Cipro I.V. (Ciprofloxacin) Schering 2984
Noroxin Tablets (Norfloxacin) Merck 2032
Primaxin I.V. (Cilastatin Sodium, Imipenem) Merck 2048
Rocephin Injectable Vials, ADD-Vantage, Galaxy, Bulk (Ceftriaxone Sodium) Roche 2800
Timentin ADD-Vantage (Clavulanate Potassium, Ticarcillin Disodium) GlaxoSmithKline 1580
Timentin Injection Galaxy Container (Clavulanate Potassium, Ticarcillin Disodium) GlaxoSmithKline 1583
Timentin IV Infusion (Clavulanate Potassium, Ticarcillin Disodium) GlaxoSmithKline 1577
Timentin Pharmacy Bulk Package (Clavulanate Potassium, Ticarcillin Disodium) GlaxoSmithKline 1586

Serratia marcescens infections, ocular
Ciloxan Ophthalmic Ointment (Ciprofloxacin Hydrochloride) Alcon 559
Ciloxan Ophthalmic Solution (Ciprofloxacin Hydrochloride) Alcon .... ⊙ 206
Pred-G Ophthalmic Ointment (Gentamicin Sulfate, Prednisolone Acetate) Allergan .... ⊙ 237
Pred-G Ophthalmic Suspension (Gentamicin Sulfate, Prednisolone Acetate) Allergan .... ⊙ 236
Quixin Ophthalmic Solution (Levofloxacin) Vistakon 3383

Serratia marcescens lower respiratory tract infections
Levaquin (Levofloxacin) Ortho-McNeil 2384
Levaquin in 5% Dextrose Injection (Levofloxacin) Ortho-McNeil 2384
Primaxin I.V. (Cilastatin Sodium, Imipenem) Merck 2048
Rocephin Injectable Vials, ADD-Vantage, Galaxy, Bulk (Ceftriaxone Sodium) Roche 2800

Serratia marcescens skin and skin structure infections
Rocephin Injectable Vials, ADD-Vantage, Galaxy, Bulk (Ceftriaxone Sodium) Roche 2800

Serratia marcescens urinary tract infections
Cipro (Ciprofloxacin) Schering 2977
Cipro I.V. (Ciprofloxacin) Schering 2984
Noroxin Tablets (Norfloxacin) Merck 2032
Timentin ADD-Vantage (Clavulanate Potassium, Ticarcillin Disodium) GlaxoSmithKline 1580
Timentin Injection Galaxy Container (Clavulanate Potassium, Ticarcillin Disodium) GlaxoSmithKline 1583
Timentin IV Infusion (Clavulanate Potassium, Ticarcillin Disodium) GlaxoSmithKline 1577
Timentin Pharmacy Bulk Package (Clavulanate Potassium, Ticarcillin Disodium) GlaxoSmithKline 1586

Serratia species infections
Fortaz (Ceftazidime) GlaxoSmithKline 1453
Garamycin Injectable (Gentamicin Sulfate) Schering 3014
Primaxin I.V. (Cilastatin Sodium, Imipenem) Merck 2048

Serratia species lower respiratory tract infections
Fortaz (Ceftazidime) GlaxoSmithKline 1453

Serratia species septicemia
Primaxin I.V. (Cilastatin Sodium, Imipenem) Merck 2048

Serratia species skin and skin structure infections
Fortaz (Ceftazidime) GlaxoSmithKline 1453
Primaxin I.V. (Cilastatin Sodium, Imipenem) Merck 2048

Serum sickness
Decadron Tablets (Dexamethasone) Merck 1951
Depo-Medrol Injectable Suspension (Methylprednisolone Acetate) Pharmacia & Upjohn 2617
Depo-Medrol Single-Dose Vial (Methylprednisolone Acetate) Pharmacia & Upjohn 2619
Hydrocortone Tablets (Hydrocortisone) Merck 1989

Shigella flexneri infectious diarrhea
Cipro (Ciprofloxacin) Schering 2977

Shigella sonnei infectious diarrhea
Cipro (Ciprofloxacin) Schering 2977

Shingles
(*see under* Herpes zoster infections)

Shock, emergency treatment of
Plasbumin-5 (Albumin (human)) Talecris 3251
Plasbumin-20 (Albumin (human)) Talecris 3252
Plasbumin-25 (Albumin (human)) Talecris 3253
Plasmanate (Plasma Protein Fraction (Human)) Talecris 3255

Short stature, children
Nutropin for Injection (Somatropin) Genentech 1239
Nutropin AQ Injection (Somatropin) Genentech 1243
Nutropin AQ Pen (Somatropin) Genentech 1243
Nutropin AQ Pen Cartridge (Somatropin) Genentech 1243

Short stature, idiopathic
Humatrope Vials and Cartridges (Somatropin) Lilly 1787
Nutropin for Injection (Somatropin) Genentech 1239
Nutropin AQ Injection (Somatropin) Genentech 1243
Nutropin AQ Pen (Somatropin) Genentech 1243
Nutropin AQ Pen Cartridge (Somatropin) Genentech 1243

Shoulder, acute painful
(*see under* Bursitis, subacromial, acute, symptomatic relief of)

Sinus congestion, symptomatic relief of
Advil Allergy Sinus Caplets (Chlorpheniramine Maleate, Ibuprofen, Pseudoephedrine Hydrochloride) Wyeth .... ▣ 770
Advil Multi-Symptom Cold Caplets (Chlorpheniramine Maleate, Ibuprofen, Pseudoephedrine Hydrochloride) Wyeth .... ▣ 770
Alavert Allergy & Sinus D-12 Hour Tablets (Loratadine, Pseudoephedrine Sulfate) Wyeth .... ▣ 771
Aleve Cold & Sinus Caplets (Naproxen Sodium, Pseudoephedrine Hydrochloride) Bayer Healthcare LLC 744
Claritin-D Non-Drowsy 12 Hour Tablets (Loratadine, Pseudoephedrine Sulfate) Schering-Plough .... ▣ 772
Claritin-D Non-Drowsy 24 Hour Tablets (Loratadine, Pseudoephedrine Sulfate) Schering-Plough .... ▣ 772
Comtrex Maximum Strength Day/Night Severe Cold & Sinus Caplets - Day Formulation (Acetaminophen, Phenylephrine Hydrochloride) Novartis Consumer .... ▣ 725
Comtrex Maximum Strength Day/Night Severe Cold & Sinus Caplets - Night Formulation (Acetaminophen, Chlorpheniramine Maleate, Phenylephrine Hydrochloride) Novartis Consumer .... ▣ 725
Contac Cold and Flu Day and Night Caplets (Day Formulation Only) (Acetaminophen, Phenylephrine Hydrochloride) GlaxoSmithKline .... ▣ 727
Contac Cold and Flu Non-Drowsy Caplets (Acetaminophen, Phenylephrine Hydrochloride) GlaxoSmithKline .... ▣ 728
Contac-D Cold Non-Drowsy Tablets (Phenylephrine Hydrochloride) GlaxoSmithKline .... ▣ 729
Children's Dimetapp Cold & Allergy Elixir (Brompheniramine Maleate, Phenylephrine Hydrochloride) Wyeth .... ▣ 730
Excedrin Sinus Headache Caplets/Tablets (Acetaminophen, Phenylephrine Hydrochloride) Novartis Consumer .... ▣ 610
Children's Motrin Cold Oral Suspension (Ibuprofen, Pseudoephedrine Hydrochloride) McNeil Consumer .... ▣ 733
Mucinex D Extended-Release Bi-Layer Tablets (Guaifenesin, Pseudoephedrine Hydrochloride) Adams .... ▣ 776
TheraFlu Cold & Cough Hot Liquid (Dextromethorphan Hydrobromide, Pheniramine Maleate, Phenylephrine Hydrochloride) Novartis Consumer .... ▣ 740
TheraFlu Daytime Severe Cold Hot Liquid (Acetaminophen, Phenylephrine Hydrochloride) Novartis Consumer .... ▣ 742
TheraFlu Warming Relief Nighttime Severe Cold (Acetaminophen, Diphenhydramine Hydrochloride, Phenylephrine Hydrochloride) Novartis Consumer .... ▣ 743
Triaminic Chest & Nasal Congestion Liquid (Guaifenesin, Phenylephrine Hydrochloride) Novartis Consumer .... ▣ 746
Triaminic Cold & Allergy Liquid (Chlorpheniramine Maleate, Phenylephrine Hydrochloride) Novartis Consumer .... ▣ 746
Triaminic Daytime Cold & Cough Liquid (Dextromethorphan Hydrobromide, Phenylephrine Hydrochloride) Novartis Consumer .... ▣ 745
Triaminic Nighttime Cold & Cough Liquid (Diphenhydramine Hydrochloride, Phenylephrine Hydrochloride) Novartis Consumer .... ▣ 746
Triaminic Thin Strips Cold (Phenylephrine Hydrochloride) Novartis Consumer .... ▣ 748
Triaminic Thin Strips Cold & Cough (Dextromethorphan Hydrobromide, Phenylephrine Hydrochloride) Novartis Consumer .... ▣ 778
Triaminic Infant Thin Strips Decongestant (Phenylephrine Hydrochloride) Novartis Consumer .... ▣ 747
Triaminic Infant Thin Strips Decongestant Plus Cough (Dextromethorphan Hydrobromide, Phenylephrine Hydrochloride) Novartis Consumer .... ▣ 747
Tylenol Cold Head Congestion Daytime Caplets with Cool Burst and Gelcaps (Acetaminophen, Dextromethorphan Hydrobromide, Phenylephrine Hydrochloride) McNeil Consumer .... ▣ 750
Tylenol Cold Head Congestion Nighttime Caplets with Cool Burst (Acetaminophen, Chlorpheniramine Maleate, Dextromethorphan Hydrobromide, Phenylephrine Hydrochloride) McNeil Consumer .... ▣ 750
Tylenol Cold Multi-Symptom Daytime Liquid (Acetaminophen, Dextromethorphan Hydrobromide, Phenylephrine Hydrochloride) McNeil Consumer .... ▣ 752
Tylenol Allergy Multi-Symptom Caplets with Cool Burst and Gelcaps (Acetaminophen, Chlorpheniramine Maleate, Phenylephrine Hydrochloride) McNeil Consumer 1872
Tylenol Allergy Multi-Symptom Nighttime Caplets with Cool Burst (Acetaminophen, Diphenhydramine Hydrochloride, Phenylephrine Hydrochloride) McNeil Consumer 1872

Tylenol Chest Congestion Caplets with Cool Burst (Acetaminophen, Guaifenesin) McNeil Consumer...... 1872
Tylenol Chest Congestion Liquid with Cool Burst (Acetaminophen, Guaifenesin) McNeil Consumer...... 1872
Tylenol Cold Head Congestion Daytime Caplets with Cool Burst (Acetaminophen, Dextromethorphan Hydrobromide, Phenylephrine Hydrochloride) McNeil Consumer.................................... 1873
Tylenol Cold Head Congestion Nighttime Caplets with Cool Burst (Acetaminophen, Chlorpheniramine Maleate, Dextromethorphan Hydrobromide, Phenylephrine Hydrochloride) McNeil Consumer.................................... 1873
Tylenol Cold Multi-Symptom Daytime Liquid with Citrus Burst (Acetaminophen, Dextromethorphan Hydrobromide, Phenylephrine Hydrochloride) McNeil Consumer 1874
Tylenol Cold Multi-Symptom Severe Daytime Liquid with Citrus Burst (Acetaminophen, Dextromethorphan Hydrobromide, Guaifenesin, Phenylephrine Hydrochloride) McNeil Consumer 1874
Tylenol Sinus Congestion & Pain Daytime Caplets with Cool Burst and Gelcaps (Acetaminophen, Phenylephrine Hydrochloride) McNeil Consumer 1876
Tylenol Sinus Congestion & Pain Nighttime Caplets with Cool Burst (Acetaminophen, Chlorpheniramine Maleate, Phenylephrine Hydrochloride) McNeil Consumer 1876
Tylenol Sinus Congestion & Pain Severe Caplets with Cool Burst (Acetaminophen, Guaifenesin, Phenylephrine Hydrochloride) McNeil Consumer 1876
Vicks Sinex 12-Hour Nasal Spray and Ultra Fine Mist for Sinus Relief (Oxymetazoline Hydrochloride) Procter & Gamble 2681
Zicam Allergy Relief (Histanium Hydrochloricum, Luffa operculata, Galphimia Glauca, Sulfur) Matrixx .... ■ 774
Zicam Cold Remedy ChewCaps (Zincum Aceticum, Zincum Gluconicum) Matrixx .... ■ 766
Zicam Cold Remedy RapidMelts (Zincum Aceticum, Zincum Gluconicum) Matrixx .... ■ 766
Zicam Cold Remedy RapidMelts with Vitamin C (Zincum Aceticum, Zincum Gluconicum) Matrixx .... ■ 766
Zicam Extreme Congestion Relief (Oxymetazoline Hydrochloride) Matrixx .... ■ 767
Zicam Intense Sinus Relief (Oxymetazoline Hydrochloride) Matrixx .... ■ 767

Sinus headache

Aleve Cold & Sinus Caplets (Naproxen Sodium, Pseudoephedrine Hydrochloride) Bayer Healthcare LLC 744
Contac Cold and Flu Day and Night Caplets (Day Formulation Only) (Acetaminophen, Phenylephrine Hydrochloride) GlaxoSmithKline .... ■ 727
Robitussin Cough, Cold & Flu Nighttime Liquid (Acetaminophen, Chlorpheniramine Maleate, Dextromethorphan Hydrobromide, Phenylephrine Hydrochloride) Wyeth .... ■ 738
Tylenol Sinus Severe Congestion Caplets with Cool Burst (Acetaminophen, Guaifenesin, Pseudoephedrine Hydrochloride) McNeil Consumer 1876
Tylenol Sinus Congestion & Pain Daytime Caplets with Cool Burst and Gelcaps (Acetaminophen, Phenylephrine Hydrochloride) McNeil Consumer 1876

Vicks NyQuil LiquiCaps/Liquid Multi-Symptom Cold/Flu Relief (Acetaminophen, Dextromethorphan Hydrobromide, Doxylamine Succinate) Procter & Gamble ...... ■ 763

Sinusitis

Contac-D Cold Non-Drowsy Tablets (Phenylephrine Hydrochloride) GlaxoSmithKline .... ■ 729
Excedrin Extra Strength Caplets/Tablets/Geltabs (Acetaminophen, Aspirin, Caffeine) Novartis Consumer .... ■ 684
Zicam Extreme Congestion Relief (Oxymetazoline Hydrochloride) Matrixx...................................... ■ 767
Zicam Intense Sinus Relief (Oxymetazoline Hydrochloride) Matrixx...................................... ■ 767
Zmax for Oral Suspension (Azithromycin) Pfizer.................................... 2583

Sinusitis, adjunctive therapy

Advil Caplets (Ibuprofen) Wyeth ...... ■ 674
Children's Advil Oral Suspension (Ibuprofen) Wyeth .... ■ 603
Children's Advil Chewable Tablets (Ibuprofen) Wyeth .... ■ 603
Advil Cold & Sinus (Ibuprofen, Pseudoephedrine Hydrochloride) Wyeth .... ■ 723
Advil Gel Caplets (Ibuprofen) Wyeth .... ■ 674
Infants' Advil Concentrated Drops (Ibuprofen) Wyeth .... ■ 604
Infants' Advil Concentrated Drops - White Grape (Dye-Free) (Ibuprofen) Wyeth .... ■ 604
Advil (Ibuprofen) Wyeth .... ■ 674
Children's Dimetapp DM Cold & Cough Elixir (Brompheniramine Maleate, Dextromethorphan Hydrobromide, Phenylephrine Hydrochloride) Wyeth .... ■ 731
Toddler's Dimetapp Cold and Cough Drops (Dextromethorphan Hydrobromide, Phenylephrine Hydrochloride) Wyeth .... ■ 732
Children's Motrin Cold Oral Suspension (Ibuprofen, Pseudoephedrine Hydrochloride) McNeil Consumer 1867
TheraFlu Daytime Severe Cold Hot Liquid (Acetaminophen, Phenylephrine Hydrochloride) Novartis Consumer .... ■ 742
Triaminic Chest & Nasal Congestion Liquid (Guaifenesin, Phenylephrine Hydrochloride) Novartis Consumer .... ■ 746
Vicks Sinex 12-Hour Nasal Spray and Ultra Fine Mist for Sinus Relief (Oxymetazoline Hydrochloride) Procter & Gamble 2681
Vicks Vapor Inhaler (Levmetamfetamine) Procter & Gamble .... ■ 764

Sinusitis, treatment of

Amoxil Capsules (Amoxicillin) GlaxoSmithKline 1343
Amoxil Chewable Tablets (Amoxicillin) GlaxoSmithKline 1343
Amoxil Pediatric Drops for Oral Suspension (Amoxicillin) GlaxoSmithKline 1343
Amoxil Powder for Oral Suspension (Amoxicillin) GlaxoSmithKline 1343
Amoxil Tablets (Amoxicillin) GlaxoSmithKline 1343
Augmentin (Amoxicillin, Clavulanate Potassium) GlaxoSmithKline 1360
Augmentin Tablets (Amoxicillin, Clavulanate Potassium) GlaxoSmithKline 1363
Augmentin XR Extended-Release Tablets (Amoxicillin, Clavulanate Potassium) GlaxoSmithKline 1369
Avelox (Moxifloxacin Hydrochloride) Schering 2970
Biaxin/Biaxin XL (Clarithromycin) Abbott 402
Ceftin Tablets (Cefuroxime Axetil) GlaxoSmithKline 1407
Cipro (Ciprofloxacin) Schering 2977
Cipro I.V. (Ciprofloxacin) Schering 2984
E.E.S. (Erythromycin Ethylsuccinate) Abbott 451
EryPed (Erythromycin Ethylsuccinate) Abbott 447
Ery-Tab Tablets (Erythromycin) Abbott 449
Erythrocin Stearate Filmtab Tablets (Erythromycin Stearate) Abbott 453
Erythromycin Base Filmtab Tablets (Erythromycin) Abbott 455
Erythromycin Delayed-Release Capsules, USP (Erythromycin) Abbott 457
Ketek Tablets (Telithromycin) sanofi-aventis 2903
Levaquin (Levofloxacin) Ortho-McNeil...................................... 2384
Levaquin in 5% Dextrose Injection (Levofloxacin) Ortho-McNeil 2384
Omnicef Capsules (Cefdinir) Abbott .. 511
Omnicef for Oral Suspension (Cefdinir) Abbott.................................... 511
PCE Dispertab Tablets (Erythromycin) Abbott.. 515
Tequin Injection (Gatifloxacin) Bristol-Myers Squibb 938
Tequin Injection in 5% Dextrose (Gatifloxacin) Bristol-Myers Squibb 938
Tequin Tablets (Gatifloxacin) Bristol-Myers Squibb 938
Tylenol Sinus Severe Congestion Caplets with Cool Burst (Acetaminophen, Guaifenesin, Pseudoephedrine Hydrochloride) McNeil Consumer.................................... 1876
Vantin Tablets and Oral Suspension (Cefpodoxime Proxetil) Pharmacia & Upjohn 2645

Sitosterolemia

Zetia Tablets (Ezetimibe) Merck/Schering Plough................ 2120
Zetia Tablets (Ezetimibe) Schering.... 3083

Sjogren's syndrome

Evoxac Capsules (Cevimeline Hydrochloride) Daiichi Sankyo 1047

Skin, dry, moisturization of

MimyX Cream (Glycerin) Stiefel 3213
Pure Gardens Cream (Herbals with Vitamins) Awareness Corporation/AwarenessLife .... ■ 832
Tahitian Noni Seed Oil (Herbal Medicines, unspecified) Tahitian Noni International .... ■ 834

Skin, fine wrinkles, mitigation of

Athena 7 Minute Lift Cream (Herbals, Multiple) Greek Island Labs ... ■ 827
Pure Gardens Cream (Herbals with Vitamins) Awareness Corporation/AwarenessLife .... ■ 832

Skin, hyperpigmentation
(*see under* Hyperpigmentation, skin, bleaching of)

Skin, inflammatory conditions
(*see also under* Dermatitis, contact; Dermatoses, corticosteroid-responsive)

Apexicon E Cream (Diflorasone Diacetate) Pharmaderm 2661
Cutivate Cream (Fluticasone Propionate) Pharmaderm 2662
Cutivate Lotion 0.05% (Fluticasone Propionate) Pharmaderm 2664
Cutivate Ointment (Fluticasone Propionate) Pharmaderm 2665
Diprolene Gel 0.05% (Betamethasone Dipropionate) Schering 3001
Diprolene Lotion 0.05% (Betamethasone Dipropionate) Schering.................................... 3002

Skin, irritation, minor, pain associated with
(*see under* Pain, topical relief of)

Skin, irritation, minor, temporary relief of

Smile's Prid Salve (Homeopathic Formulations) Standard Homeopathic .... ■ 833

Skin abscesses
(*see under* Infections, skin and skin structure)

Skin and skin structure disorders

Levaquin (Levofloxacin) Ortho-McNeil.............................. 2384
Levaquin in 5% Dextrose Injection (Levofloxacin) Ortho-McNeil........... 2384

Skin infections, bacterial, minor
(*see under* Infections, skin, bacterial, minor)

Skin lacerations, infected
(*see under* Infections, skin and skin structure)

Skin sagginess, reduction of

Athena 7 Minute Lift Cream (Herbals, Multiple) Greek Island Labs ... ■ 827

Skin ulcers, venous insufficiency-induced, non-infected

ProNutra Protein Supplement (Vitamins with Minerals, Whey Protein Isolate) Immunotec 1668

Sleep, induction of
(*see also under* Sedation)

Ambien Tablets (Zolpidem Tartrate) sanofi-aventis.............................. 2851
Ambien CR Tablets (Zolpidem Tartrate) sanofi-aventis...................... 2855
Dalmane Capsules (Flurazepam Hydrochloride) Valeant 3342
Hyland's Calms Forté Tablets and Caplets (Homeopathic Formulations) Standard Homeopathic ...... ■ 828
Lunesta Tablets (Eszopiclone) Sepracor 3142
Nembutal Sodium Solution, USP (Pentobarbital Sodium) Ovation 2470
Nytol QuickCaps Caplets (Diphenhydramine Hydrochloride) GlaxoSmithKline .... ■ 615
Nytol QuickGels Softgels Maximum Strength (Diphenhydramine Hydrochloride) GlaxoSmithKline .... ■ 616
ProSom Tablets (Estazolam) Abbott . 517
Restoril Capsules (Temazepam) Mallinckrodt....................................... 1860
Rozerem Tablets (Ramelteon) Takeda 3231
Simply Sleep Caplets (Diphenhydramine Hydrochloride) McNeil Consumer.................................... 1868
Sleep-Tite Caplets (Valeriana officinalis, Herbals, Multiple, Kava-Kava) Wellness International .... ■ 832
Sominex Original Formula Tablets (Diphenhydramine Hydrochloride) GlaxoSmithKline .... ■ 616
Sonata Capsules (Zaleplon) King 1717

Sleep disorders

Provigil Tablets (Modafinil) Cephalon 988

Slough, liquefaction of

Accuzyme SE Spray Emulsion (Papain, Urea) Healthpoint............ 1662

Smoking cessation, temporary aid to

Chantix Tablets (Varenicline Tartrate) Pfizer 2517
NicoDerm CQ Clear Patch (Nicotine) GlaxoSmithKline.................. ■ 622
Zyban Sustained-Release Tablets (Bupropion Hydrochloride) GlaxoSmithKline.......................... 1644

Sneezing

Advil Allergy Sinus Caplets (Chlorpheniramine Maleate, Ibuprofen, Pseudoephedrine Hydrochloride) Wyeth .... ■ 770
Advil Multi-Symptom Cold Caplets (Chlorpheniramine Maleate, Ibuprofen, Pseudoephedrine Hydrochloride) Wyeth .... ■ 770
Alavert Allergy & Sinus D-12 Hour Tablets (Loratadine, Pseudoephedrine Sulfate) Wyeth .... ■ 771
Alavert (Loratadine) Wyeth............. ■ 771

Social phobia
(*see under* Anxiety disorder, social)

Solar lentigines
(*see under* Hyperpigmentation, skin, bleaching of)

Somatotropin deficiency syndrome

Sore throat

Sour stomach
(*see under* Hyperacidity, gastric, symptomatic relief of)

Spasm, skeletal muscle

Spasticity, cerebral palsy-induced
(*see under* Spasticity, upper motor neuron disorder-induced)

Spasticity, multiple sclerosis-induced
(*see under* Spasticity, upper motor neuron disorder-induced)

Spasticity, spinal cord injury-induced
(*see under* Spasticity, upper motor neuron disorder-induced)

Spasticity, stroke-induced
(*see under* Spasticity, upper motor neuron disorder-induced)

Spasticity, upper motor neuron disorder-induced

Spondyloarthropathy

Sprains, topical relief of
(*see under* Pain, topical relief of)

Staphylococcal enterocolitis
(*see under* Enterocolitis, staphylococcal)

Staphylococci, coagulase-negative, infections, ocular

TobraDex Ophthalmic Ointment (Dexamethasone, Tobramycin) Alcon ... 562
TobraDex Ophthalmic Suspension (Dexamethasone, Tobramycin) Alcon ... 563

Staphylococci, coagulase-positive, infections, ocular
Pred-G Ophthalmic Suspension (Gentamicin Sulfate, Prednisolone Acetate) Allergan ... ⊙236
TobraDex Ophthalmic Ointment (Dexamethasone, Tobramycin) Alcon ... 562
TobraDex Ophthalmic Suspension (Dexamethasone, Tobramycin) Alcon ... 563

Staphylococci, nonpenicillinase-producing, infections
Amoxil Capsules (Amoxicillin) GlaxoSmithKline ... 1343
Amoxil Chewable Tablets (Amoxicillin) GlaxoSmithKline ... 1343
Amoxil Pediatric Drops for Oral Suspension (Amoxicillin) GlaxoSmithKline ... 1343
Amoxil Powder for Oral Suspension (Amoxicillin) GlaxoSmithKline ... 1343
Amoxil Tablets (Amoxicillin) GlaxoSmithKline ... 1343

Staphylococci otitis media
Raniclor (Cefactor Monohydrate) Pedinol ... 2505

Staphylococci, penicillinase-producing, infections
Mefoxin for Injection (Cefoxitin Sodium) Merck ... 2012
Mefoxin Premixed Intravenous Solution (Cefoxitin Sodium) Merck ... 2016

Staphylococci, urinary tract infections
Gantrisin Pediatric Suspension (Acetyl Sulfisoxazole) Roche ... 2770
Raniclor (Cefaclor Monohydrate) Pedinol ... 2505

Staphylococcus aureus
(*see under* S. aureus infections)

Staphylococcus epidermidis
(*see under* S. epidermis infections)

Staphylococcus species infections
Garamycin (Gentamicin Sulfate) Schering ... 3014

Staphylococcus species, coagulase-negative, infections
Garamycin (Gentamicin Sulfate) Schering ... 3014

Status epilepticus
(*see under* Epilepticus, status)

Steatorrhea, adjunctive therapy in
Ultrase MT Capsules (Pancrelipase) Axcan Scandipharm ... 709

Stenosis, hypertrophic subaortic
Inderal LA Long-Acting Capsules (Propranolol Hydrochloride) Wyeth ... 3429

Stevens-Johnson syndrome
Decadron Tablets (Dexamethasone) Merck ... 1951
Depo-Medrol Injectable Suspension (Methylprednisolone Acetate) Pharmacia & Upjohn ... 2617
Depo-Medrol Single-Dose Vial (Methylprednisolone Acetate) Pharmacia & Upjohn ... 2619
Hydrocortone Tablets (Hydrocortisone) Merck ... 1989

Stiff-man syndrome, adjunctive therapy in
Valium Tablets (Diazepam) Roche ... 2819

Stomach, sour
(*see under* Hyperacidity, gastric, symptomatic relief of)

Stomatitis, recurrent aphthous, symptomatic relief of
Gly-Oxide Liquid (Carbamide Peroxide) GlaxoSmithKline ... ▣709

Hurricaine Topical Anesthetic Gel, 1 oz. Wild Cherry, Pina Colada, Watermelon, and Fresh Mint, 5.25 g. Wild Cherry (Benzocaine) Beutlich ... ▣712
Hurricaine Topical Anesthetic Liquid, 1 oz. Wild Cherry, Pina Colada, 0.005 fl. oz. Snap-n-Go Swabs Wild Cherry (Benzocaine) Beutlich ... ▣712
Hurricaine Topical Anesthetic Spray, 2 oz. Wild Cherry (Benzocaine) Beutlich ... ▣712
Hurricaine Topical Anesthetic Spray Extension Tubes (200) (Benzocaine) Beutlich ... ▣712
Hurricaine Topical Anesthetic Spray Kit, 2 oz. Wild Cherry with disposable Extension Tubes (200) (Benzocaine) Beutlich ... ▣712

Strabismus
BOTOX Purified Neurotoxin Complex (Botulinum Toxin Type A) Allergan ... 570

Strep throat
(*see under* Streptococci species upper respiratory tract infections)

Streptococcal pharyngitis
E.E.S. (Erythromycin Ethylsuccinate) Abbott ... 451
Omnicef Capsules (Cefdinir) Abbott ... 511
Omnicef for Oral Suspension (Cefdinir) Abbott ... 511
Suprax (Cefixime) Lupin ... 1843

Streptococci group A beta-hemolytic infections
(*see also under* Erysipelas)
Primaxin I.V. (Cilastatin Sodium, Imipenem) Merck ... 2048

Streptococci group A beta-hemolytic skin and skin structure infections
Fortaz (Ceftazidime) GlaxoSmithKline ... 1453
Primaxin I.V. (Cilastatin Sodium, Imipenem) Merck ... 2048

Streptococci group A beta-hemolytic species infections, ocular
Pred-G Ophthalmic Ointment (Gentamicin Sulfate, Prednisolone Acetate) Allergan ... ⊙237
Pred-G Ophthalmic Suspension (Gentamicin Sulfate, Prednisolone Acetate) Allergan ... ⊙236
TobraDex Ophthalmic Ointment (Dexamethasone, Tobramycin) Alcon ... 562
TobraDex Ophthalmic Suspension (Dexamethasone, Tobramycin) Alcon ... 563

Streptococci group A beta-hemolytic upper respiratory tract infections
PCE Dispertab Tablets (Erythromycin) Abbott ... 515

Streptococci group B infections
Mefoxin for Injection (Cefoxitin Sodium) Merck ... 2012
Mefoxin Premixed Intravenous Solution (Cefoxitin Sodium) Merck ... 2016
Primaxin I.V. (Cilastatin Sodium, Imipenem) Merck ... 2048

Streptococci group D bone and joint infections
Primaxin I.V. (Cilastatin Sodium, Imipenem) Merck ... 2048

Streptococci group D endocarditis, adjunct in
Garamycin Injectable (Gentamicin Sulfate) Schering ... 3014

Streptococci group D genitourinary tract infections
Primaxin I.V. (Cilastatin Sodium, Imipenem) Merck ... 2048

Streptococci group D gynecologic infections
Primaxin I.M. (Cilastatin Sodium, Imipenem) Merck ... 2045

Streptococci group D infections
Garamycin Injectable (Gentamicin Sulfate) Schering ... 3014
Primaxin I.V. (Cilastatin Sodium, Imipenem) Merck ... 2048

Streptococci group D intra-abdominal infections
Primaxin I.M. (Cilastatin Sodium, Imipenem) Merck ... 2045
Primaxin I.V. (Cilastatin Sodium, Imipenem) Merck ... 2048

Streptococci group D septicemia
Primaxin I.V. (Cilastatin Sodium, Imipenem) Merck ... 2048

Streptococci group D skin and skin structure infections
Primaxin I.M. (Cilastatin Sodium, Imipenem) Merck ... 2045
Primaxin I.V. (Cilastatin Sodium, Imipenem) Merck ... 2048

Streptococci infections, ocular
Neosporin Ophthalmic Solution Sterile (Gramicidin, Neomycin Sulfate, Polymyxin B Sulfate) King ... ⊙265
Quixin Ophthalmic Solution (Levofloxacin) Vistakon ... 3383
TobraDex Ophthalmic Ointment (Dexamethasone, Tobramycin) Alcon ... 562
TobraDex Ophthalmic Suspension (Dexamethasone, Tobramycin) Alcon ... 563

Streptococci non-hemolytic species infections, ocular
Pred-G Ophthalmic Suspension (Gentamicin Sulfate, Prednisolone Acetate) Allergan ... ⊙236
TobraDex Ophthalmic Ointment (Dexamethasone, Tobramycin) Alcon ... 562
TobraDex Ophthalmic Suspension (Dexamethasone, Tobramycin) Alcon ... 563

Streptococci skin and skin structure infections
Bicillin C-R Injectable Suspension (Penicillin G Benzathine, Penicillin G Procaine) King ... 1706
Mefoxin for Injection (Cefoxitin Sodium) Merck ... 2012
Mefoxin Premixed Intravenous Solution (Cefoxitin Sodium) Merck ... 2016

Streptococci species infections
Bicillin C-R Injectable Suspension (Penicillin G Benzathine, Penicillin G Procaine) King ... 1706

Streptococci species upper respiratory tract infections
Ceftin (Cefuroxime Axetil) GlaxoSmithKline ... 1407
Omnicef Capsules (Cefdinir) Abbott ... 511
Omnicef for Oral Suspension (Cefdinir) Abbott ... 511
Suprax (Cefixime) Lupin ... 1843

Streptococci (viridans group) infections, ocular
Blephamide Ophthalmic Suspension (Prednisolone Acetate, Sulfacetamide Sodium) Allergan ... 569
Ciloxan Ophthalmic Ointment (Ciprofloxacin Hydrochloride) Alcon ... 559
Ciloxan Ophthalmic Solution (Ciprofloxacin Hydrochloride) Alcon ... ⊙206
FML-S Ophthalmic Suspension (Fluorometholone, Sulfacetamide Sodium) Allergan ... ⊙229
Polytrim Ophthalmic Solution (Polymyxin B Sulfate, Trimethoprim Sulfate) Allergan ... 574
Quixin Ophthalmic Solution (Levofloxacin) Vistakon ... 3383

Streptococci (viridans group) intra-abdominal infections
Maxipime for Injection (Cefepime Hydrochloride) Elan ... 1105

Streptococcus agalactiae infections
(*see under* S. agalactiae infections)

Streptococcus faecalis
(*see under* S. faecalis infections)

Streptococcus pneumoniae
(*see under* S. pneumoniae infections)

Streptococcus pneumoniae, immunization against
(*see also under* Pneumococcal disease, immunization against)
Pneumovax 23 (Pneumococcal Vaccine, Polyvalent) Merck ... 2043
Prevnar for Injection (Pneumococcal vaccine, diphtheria conjugate) Wyeth ... 3463

Streptococcus pneumoniae infections, ocular
Neosporin Ophthalmic Solution Sterile (Gramicidin, Neomycin Sulfate, Polymyxin B Sulfate) King ... ⊙265

Streptococcus pyogenes
(*see under* S. pyogenes infections)

Streptococcus species infections
Amoxil Capsules (Amoxicillin) GlaxoSmithKline ... 1343
Amoxil Chewable Tablets (Amoxicillin) GlaxoSmithKline ... 1343
Amoxil Pediatric Drops for Oral Suspension (Amoxicillin) GlaxoSmithKline ... 1343
Amoxil Powder for Oral Suspension (Amoxicillin) GlaxoSmithKline ... 1343
Amoxil Tablets (Amoxicillin) GlaxoSmithKline ... 1343
Bactroban Ointment (Mupirocin) GlaxoSmithKline ... 1395
Cleocin Vaginal Ovules (Clindamycin Hydrochloride) Pharmacia & Upjohn ... 2616
Garamycin Injectable (Gentamicin Sulfate) Schering ... 3014
Omnicef Capsules (Cefdinir) Abbott ... 511
Omnicef for Oral Suspension (Cefdinir) Abbott ... 511
Suprax (Cefixime) Lupin ... 1843

Streptococcus species lower respiratory tract infections
Mefoxin for Injection (Cefoxitin Sodium) Merck ... 2012
Mefoxin Premixed Intravenous Solution (Cefoxitin Sodium) Merck ... 2016

Streptococcus species respiratory tract infections
Cleocin Vaginal Ovules (Clindamycin Hydrochloride) Pharmacia & Upjohn ... 2616

Streptococcus tonsillitis
(*see under* Streptococci species upper respiratory tract infections)

Streptococcus viridans group infections
Blephamide Ophthalmic Ointment (Prednisolone Acetate, Sulfacetamide Sodium) Allergan ... 568
Merrem I.V. (Meropenem) AstraZeneca Pharmaceuticals ... 686
Primaxin I.M. (Cilastatin Sodium, Imipenem) Merck ... 2045
Rocephin Injectable Vials, ADD-Vantage, Galaxy, Bulk (Ceftriaxone Sodium) Roche ... 2800
Vigamox Ophthalmic Solution (Moxifloxacin Hydrochloride) Alcon ... 564

Stress disorder, post-traumatic
Paxil (Paroxetine Hydrochloride) GlaxoSmithKline ... 1530
Zoloft (Sertraline Hydrochloride) Pfizer ... 2586

Stroke, ischemic
Activase I.V. (Alteplase) Genentech ... 1223

Stroke, to reduce the risk of
Aggrenox Capsules (Aspirin, Dipyridamole) Boehringer Ingelheim 822
Altace Capsules (Ramipril) King 1702
Bayer Aspirin (Aspirin) Bayer Healthcare LLC 744
Bayer Aspirin Comprehensive Prescribing Information (Aspirin) Bayer Healthcare .... ▣796
Coumadin for Injection (Warfarin Sodium) Bristol-Myers Squibb 898
Coumadin Tablets (Warfarin Sodium) Bristol-Myers Squibb 898
Cozaar Tablets (Losartan Potassium) Merck 1935
Hyzaar 50-12.5 Tablets (Hydrochlorothiazide, Losartan Potassium) Merck 1990
Hyzaar 100-12.5 Tablets (Hydrochlorothiazide, Losartan Potassium) Merck 1990
Hyzaar 100-25 Tablets (Hydrochlorothiazide, Losartan Potassium) Merck 1990
Plavix Tablets (Clopidogrel Bisulfate) Bristol-Myers Squibb 917
Plavix Tablets (Clopidogrel Bisulfate) sanofi-aventis 2926
Ticlid Tablets (Ticlopidine Hydrochloride) Roche 2810
Zocor Tablets (Simvastatin) Merck 2105

Strongyloidiasis
Mintezol (Thiabendazole) Merck 2027
Stromectol Tablets (Ivermectin) Merck 2083

Suicidal behavior, recurrent, in schizoaffective disorder
Clozaril (Clozapine) Novartis 2184

Suicidal behavior, recurrent, in schizophrenia
Clozaril (Clozapine) Novartis 2184

Sunburn, pain associated with
(*see under* Pain, topical relief of)

Swelling, unspecified
Tylenol Sinus Congestion & Pain Daytime Caplets with Cool Burst and Gelcaps (Acetaminophen, Phenylephrine Hydrochloride) McNeil Consumer 1876

Sympathetic ophthalmia
(*see under* Ophthalmia, sympathetic)

Syphilis
Erythromycin Delayed-Release Capsules, USP (Erythromycin) Abbott 457

T

T. pallidum infections
E.E.S. (Erythromycin Ethylsuccinate) Abbott 451
EryPed (Erythromycin Ethylsuccinate) Abbott 447
Ery-Tab Tablets (Erythromycin) Abbott 449
Erythrocin Stearate Filmtab Tablets (Erythromycin Stearate) Abbott 453
Erythromycin Base Filmtab Tablets (Erythromycin) Abbott 455
Erythromycin Delayed-Release Capsules, USP (Erythromycin) Abbott 457
PCE Dispertab Tablets (Erythromycin) Abbott 515

T. vaginalis infections
Tindamax Tablets (Tinidazole) Mission 2142

Tachycardia, paroxysmal supraventricular
Adenocard Injection (Adenosine) Astellas 617
Tambocor Tablets (Flecainide Acetate) 3M 1856

Tachycardia, paroxysmal supraventricular associated with Wolff-Parkinson-White syndrome
(*see under* Wolff-Parkinson-White syndrome)

Tachycardia, supraventricular
Tambocor Tablets (Flecainide Acetate) 3M 1856

Tachycardia, ventricular
Tambocor Tablets (Flecainide Acetate) 3M 1856

Tachycardia, ventricular, sustained
Tambocor Tablets (Flecainide Acetate) 3M 1856

Tachycardias, paroxysmal atrial
(*see under* Tachycardia, paroxysmal supraventricular)

Taenia solium infections
Albenza Tablets (Albendazole) GlaxoSmithKline 1338

Tapeworm infections
(*see under* Infections, tapeworm)

Tendonitis
Anaprox Tablets (Naproxen Sodium) Roche 2761
Anaprox DS Tablets (Naproxen Sodium) Roche 2761
Clinoril Tablets (Sulindac) Merck 1924
Indocin (Indomethacin) Merck 1995
Naprosyn Suspension (Naproxen) Roche 2761
Naprosyn Tablets (Naproxen) Roche 2761
Traumeel Injection Solution (Homeopathic Formulations) Heel 1664

Tenosynovitis, acute nonspecific
Depo-Medrol Injectable Suspension (Methylprednisolone Acetate) Pharmacia & Upjohn 2617
Depo-Medrol Single-Dose Vial (Methylprednisolone Acetate) Pharmacia & Upjohn 2619
Hydrocortone Tablets (Hydrocortisone) Merck 1989

Testis, advanced carcinoma of
(*see under* Carcinoma, testis, advanced)

Testosterone, deficiency of
(*see under* Androgen, absence or deficiency of)

Tetanus vaccine
(*see also under* Immunization, tetanus)
HyperTET (Tetanus Immune Globulin (Human)) Talecris 3248

Threadworm infestations
(*see under* Strongyloidiasis)

Throat, itchy
(*see under* Pruritus, rhinopharyngeal, symptomatic relief of)

Throat, sore
(*see under* Pharyngitis, symptomatic relief of)

Thrombocythemia
Agrylin Capsules (Anagrelide Hydrochloride) Shire US 3169

Thrombocytopenia, heparin-induced
Argatroban Injection (Argatroban) GlaxoSmithKline 1346
Refludan for Injection (Lepirudin) Berlex 792

Thrombocytopenia, prevention of
Neumega for Injection (Oprelvekin) Wyeth 3435

Thrombocytopenia, secondary
Decadron Tablets (Dexamethasone) Merck 1951
Depo-Medrol Injectable Suspension (Methylprednisolone Acetate) Pharmacia & Upjohn 2617
Depo-Medrol Single-Dose Vial (Methylprednisolone Acetate) Pharmacia & Upjohn 2619
Hydrocortone Tablets (Hydrocortisone) Merck 1989

Thromboembolic complications
Coumadin for Injection (Warfarin Sodium) Bristol-Myers Squibb 898
Coumadin Tablets (Warfarin Sodium) Bristol-Myers Squibb 898
Fragmin Injection (Dalteparin Sodium) Eisai 1097
Refludan for Injection (Lepirudin) Berlex 792

Thromboembolism, postoperative, adjunct in
Persantine Tablets (Dipyridamole) Boehringer Ingelheim 868

Thrombosis, deep venous, prophylaxis of
Arixtra Injection (Fondaparinux Sodium) GlaxoSmithKline 1351
Fragmin Injection (Dalteparin Sodium) Eisai 1097

Thrombosis, deep venous, treatment of
Arixtra Injection (Fondaparinux Sodium) GlaxoSmithKline 1351

Thrombosis, venous
Coumadin for Injection (Warfarin Sodium) Bristol-Myers Squibb 898
Coumadin Tablets (Warfarin Sodium) Bristol-Myers Squibb 898
Miradon Tablets (Anisindione) Schering 3042

Thrombosis, venous, prophylaxis of
Coumadin for Injection (Warfarin Sodium) Bristol-Myers Squibb 898
Coumadin Tablets (Warfarin Sodium) Bristol-Myers Squibb 898
Lovenox Injection (Enoxaparin Sodium) sanofi-aventis 2915
Miradon Tablets (Anisindione) Schering 3042

Thyroid function, aid in the diagnosis of
Cytomel Tablets (Liothyronine Sodium) King 1710
Levothroid Tablets (Levothyroxine Sodium) Forest 1186
Levoxyl Tablets (Levothyroxine Sodium) King 1712
Naturethroid Tablets (Levothyroxine, Liothyronine) Western Research 3401
Synthroid Tablets (Levothyroxine Sodium) Abbott 520
Thyrolar Tablets (Liotrix) Forest 1199
Westhroid Tablets (Levothyroxine Sodium, Liothyronine Sodium) Western Research 3403

Thyroiditis, chronic lymphocytic
(*see under* Hashimoto's thyroiditis)

Thyroiditis, nonsuppurative
Decadron Tablets (Dexamethasone) Merck 1951
Depo-Medrol Injectable Suspension (Methylprednisolone Acetate) Pharmacia & Upjohn 2617
Depo-Medrol Single-Dose Vial (Methylprednisolone Acetate) Pharmacia & Upjohn 2619
Hydrocortone Tablets (Hydrocortisone) Merck 1989

Tinea barbae
(*see under* Folliculitis barbae)

Tinea capitis infections
Gris-PEG Tablets (Griseofulvin) Pedinol 2502

Tinea corporis infections
Desenex Athlete's Foot Cream (Clotrimazole) Novartis Consumer .... ▣635
Desenex Athlete's Foot Spray Powder (Miconazole Nitrate) Novartis Consumer .... ▣635
Desenex Jock Itch Spray Powder (Miconazole Nitrate) Novartis Consumer .... ▣635
Gris-PEG Tablets (Griseofulvin) Pedinol 2502
Lamisil AF Defense Powders (Shake & Spray) (Tolnaftate) Novartis Consumer .... ▣636
Lotrimin (Clotrimazole) Schering 3039
Lotrisone (Betamethasone Dipropionate, Clotrimazole) Schering 3040
Naftin Cream (Naftifine Hydrochloride) Merz 2126
Naftin Gel (Naftifine Hydrochloride) Merz 2126
Oxistat (Oxiconazole Nitrate) Pharmaderm 2667

Tinea cruris infections
Desenex Athlete's Foot Cream (Clotrimazole) Novartis Consumer .... ▣635
Desenex Athlete's Foot Liquid Spray (Miconazole Nitrate) Novartis Consumer .... ▣635
Gris-PEG Tablets (Griseofulvin) Pedinol 2502
Lotrimin (Clotrimazole) Schering 3039
Lotrisone (Betamethasone Dipropionate, Clotrimazole) Schering 3040
Naftin Cream (Naftifine Hydrochloride) Merz 2126
Naftin Gel (Naftifine Hydrochloride) Merz 2126
Oxistat (Oxiconazole Nitrate) Pharmaderm 2667

Tinea pedis infections
Desenex Athlete's Foot Cream (Clotrimazole) Novartis Consumer .... ▣635
Desenex (Miconazole Nitrate) Novartis Consumer .... ▣635
Desenex Jock Itch Spray Powder (Miconazole Nitrate) Novartis Consumer .... ▣635
Gordochom Solution (Chloroxylenol, Undecylenic Acid) Gordon 1650
Gris-PEG Tablets (Griseofulvin) Pedinol 2502
Lamisil AT Creams (Athlete's Foot & Jock Itch) (Terbinafine Hydrochloride) Novartis Consumer .... ▣636
Lamisil AF Defense Powders (Shake & Spray) (Tolnaftate) Novartis Consumer .... ▣636
Lotrimin (Clotrimazole) Schering 3039
Lotrisone (Betamethasone Dipropionate, Clotrimazole) Schering 3040
Naftin Cream (Naftifine Hydrochloride) Merz 2126
Naftin Gel (Naftifine Hydrochloride) Merz 2126
Oxistat (Oxiconazole Nitrate) Pharmaderm 2667

Tinea unguium infections
Gris-PEG Tablets (Griseofulvin) Pedinol 2502
Lamisil Tablets (Terbinafine Hydrochloride) Novartis 2232
Penlac Nail Lacquer, Topical Solution, 8% (Ciclopirox) sanofi-aventis 2924

Tinea versicolor infections
(*see under* Pityrosporon orbiculare infections)

Tonsillitis
Amoxil Capsules (Amoxicillin) GlaxoSmithKline 1343
Amoxil Chewable Tablets (Amoxicillin) GlaxoSmithKline 1343
Amoxil Pediatric Drops for Oral Suspension (Amoxicillin) GlaxoSmithKline 1343
Amoxil Powder for Oral Suspension (Amoxicillin) GlaxoSmithKline 1343
Amoxil Tablets (Amoxicillin) GlaxoSmithKline 1343
Biaxin/Biaxin XL (Clarithromycin) Abbott 402
Ceftin (Cefuroxime Axetil) GlaxoSmithKline 1407
E.E.S. (Erythromycin Ethylsuccinate) Abbott 451
EryPed (Erythromycin Ethylsuccinate) Abbott 447
Ery-Tab Tablets (Erythromycin) Abbott 449
Erythrocin Stearate Filmtab Tablets (Erythromycin Stearate) Abbott 453
Erythromycin Base Filmtab Tablets (Erythromycin) Abbott 455
Erythromycin Delayed-Release Capsules, USP (Erythromycin) Abbott 457
Omnicef Capsules (Cefdinir) Abbott .. 511

Omnicef for Oral Suspension (Cefdinir) Abbott 511
PCE Dispertab Tablets (Erythromycin) Abbott 515
Suprax (Cefixime) Lupin 1843
Vantin Tablets and Oral Suspension (Cefpodoxime Proxetil) Pharmacia & Upjohn 2645

Tooth, hypersensitivity of
Sensodyne Original Flavor (Potassium Nitrate, Sodium Fluoride) GlaxoSmithKline .... ▣ 711
Sensodyne Cool Gel (Potassium Nitrate, Sodium Fluoride) GlaxoSmithKline .... ▣ 711
Sensodyne Extra Whitening (Potassium Nitrate, Sodium Monofluorophosphate) GlaxoSmithKline .... ▣ 711
Sensodyne Fresh Impact (Potassium Nitrate, Sodium Fluoride) GlaxoSmithKline .... ▣ 711
Sensodyne Fresh Mint (Potassium Nitrate, Sodium Fluoride) GlaxoSmithKline .... ▣ 711
Sensodyne Tartar Control (Potassium Nitrate, Sodium Fluoride) GlaxoSmithKline .... ▣ 711
Sensodyne Tartar Control Plus Whitening (Potassium Nitrate, Sodium Fluoride) GlaxoSmithKline .... ▣ 711
Sensodyne with Baking Soda (Potassium Nitrate, Sodium Fluoride) GlaxoSmithKline .... ▣ 711

Torulosis
(*see under* Cryptococcosis)

Toxoplasmosis, adjunctive therapy in
Daraprim Tablets (Pyrimethamine) GlaxoSmithKline 1419
Gantrisin Pediatric Suspension (Acetyl Sulfisoxazole) Roche 2770

Trachoma
Gantrisin Pediatric Suspension (Acetyl Sulfisoxazole) Roche 2770

Trachoma, adjunct in
Bleph-10 Ophthalmic Solution 10% (Sulfacetamide Sodium) Allergan .. ⊙ 222

Treponema pallidum
(*see under* T. pallidum infections)

Trichinosis
Mintezol (Thiabendazole) Merck 2027

Trichinosis with myocardial involvement
Decadron Tablets (Dexamethasone) Merck 1951
Depo-Medrol Injectable Suspension (Methylprednisolone Acetate) Pharmacia & Upjohn 2617
Depo-Medrol Single-Dose Vial (Methylprednisolone Acetate) Pharmacia & Upjohn 2619
Hydrocortone Tablets (Hydrocortisone) Merck 1989

Trichinosis with neurologic involvement
Decadron Tablets (Dexamethasone) Merck 1951
Depo-Medrol Injectable Suspension (Methylprednisolone Acetate) Pharmacia & Upjohn 2617
Hydrocortone Tablets (Hydrocortisone) Merck 1989

Trichomoniasis, asymptomatic
Tindamax (Tinidazole) Mission 2142

Trichomoniasis, symptomatic
Tindamax (Tinidazole) Mission 2142

Trichophyton crateriform infections
Gris-PEG (Griseofulvin) Pedinol 2502

Trichophyton gallinae infections
Gris-PEG (Griseofulvin) Pedinol 2502

Trichophyton interdigitalis infections
Gris-PEG (Griseofulvin) Pedinol 2502

Trichophyton megnini infections
Gris-PEG (Griseofulvin) Pedinol 2502

Trichophyton mentagrophytes infections
Lotrimin (Clotrimazole) Schering 3039
Lotrisone (Betamethasone Dipropionate, Clotrimazole) Schering 3040
Naftin Cream (Naftifine Hydrochloride) Merz 2126
Naftin Gel (Naftifine Hydrochloride) Merz 2126
Oxistat (Oxiconazole Nitrate) Pharmaderm 2667

Trichophyton rubrum infections
Gris-PEG Tablets (Griseofulvin) Pedinol 2502
Lotrimin (Clotrimazole) Schering 3039
Lotrisone (Betamethasone Dipropionate, Clotrimazole) Schering 3040
Naftin Cream (Naftifine Hydrochloride) Merz 2126
Naftin Gel (Naftifine Hydrochloride) Merz 2126
Oxistat (Oxiconazole Nitrate) Pharmaderm 2667
Penlac Nail Lacquer, Topical Solution, 8% (Ciclopirox) sanofi-aventis 2924

Trichophyton schoenleini infections
Gris-PEG (Griseofulvin) Pedinol 2502

Trichophyton sulfureum infections
Gris-PEG (Griseofulvin) Pedinol 2502

Trichophyton tonsurans infections
Naftin Gel (Naftifine Hydrochloride) Merz 2126

Trichophyton verrucosum infections
Gris-PEG Tablets (Griseofulvin) Pedinol 2502

Trichuriasis, as secondary therapy
Mintezol (Thiabendazole) Merck 2027

Triglyceride levels, elevated
(*see under* Hypertriglyceridemia, adjunct to diet)

Trigonitis
Prosed/DS Tablets (Benzoic Acid, Hyoscyamine Sulfate, Methenamine, Methylene Blue, Phenyl Salicylate) Esprit 1157

Tuberculosis, pulmonary
Seromycin Capsules (Cycloserine) Lilly 1813

Tuberculosis, pulmonary, disseminated
Decadron Tablets (Dexamethasone) Merck 1951
Depo-Medrol Injectable Suspension (Methylprednisolone Acetate) Pharmacia & Upjohn 2617
Depo-Medrol Single-Dose Vial (Methylprednisolone Acetate) Pharmacia & Upjohn 2619
Hydrocortone Tablets (Hydrocortisone) Merck 1989

Tuberculosis, pulmonary, fulminating
Decadron Tablets (Dexamethasone) Merck 1951
Depo-Medrol Injectable Suspension (Methylprednisolone Acetate) Pharmacia & Upjohn 2617
Depo-Medrol Single-Dose Vial (Methylprednisolone Acetate) Pharmacia & Upjohn 2619
Hydrocortone Tablets (Hydrocortisone) Merck 1989

Tuberculosis, resistant, treatment of
Trecator Tablets (Ethionamide) Wyeth 3487

Tuberculosis, treatment
Seromycin Capsules (Cycloserine) Lilly 1813

Tuberculosis, treatment adjunct
Capastat Sulfate for Injection (Capreomycin Sulfate) Lilly 1755
Paser Granules (Aminosalicylic Acid) Jacobus 1674

Tuberculosis meningitis, adjunctive therapy in
(*see under* Meningitis, tuberculous)

Tumor therapy adjuntive
Elitek (Rasburicase) sanofi-aventis 2890

Tumors, carcinoid, symptomatic relief of
Sandostatin Injection (Octreotide Acetate) Novartis 2278
Sandostatin LAR Depot (Octreotide Acetate) Novartis 2280

Tumors, gastrointestinal stromal
Gleevec Tablets (Imatinib Mesylate) Novartis 2227
Sutent Capsules (Sunitinib malate) Pfizer 2560

Turner's syndrome
Humatrope Vials and Cartridges (Somatropin) Lilly 1787

Typhoid fever
Cipro (Ciprofloxacin) Schering 2977

Typhoid fever vaccine
(*see also under* Immunization, typhoid fever)
Vivotif (Typhoid Vaccine Live Oral TY21a) Berna 819

U

Ulcerative colitis
(*see under* Colitis, ulcerative)

Ulcerative colitis, adjunctive therapy in
Colocort (Hydrocortisone) Paddock 2476

Ulcerative colitis, left sided
Colocort (Hydrocortisone) Paddock 2476

Ulcers, decubitus, adjunctive therapy in
Panafil Ointment (Chlorophyllin Copper Complex Sodium, Papain, Urea) Healthpoint 1663
Panafil SE Spray Emulsion (Chlorophyllin Copper Complex Sodium, Papain, Urea) Healthpoint 1663

Ulcers, dermal
Accuzyme SE Spray Emulsion (Papain, Urea) Healthpoint 1662
Primaxin I.M. (Cilastatin Sodium, Imipenem) Merck 2045

Ulcers, diabetic, adjunctive therapy in
Accuzyme Debriding Ointment (Papain, Urea) Healthpoint 1662
Accuzyme SE Spray Emulsion (Papain, Urea) Healthpoint 1662
Panafil Ointment (Chlorophyllin Copper Complex Sodium, Papain, Urea) Healthpoint 1663
Panafil SE Spray Emulsion (Chlorophyllin Copper Complex Sodium, Papain, Urea) Healthpoint 1663

Ulcers, varicose, adjunctive therapy in
Accuzyme Debriding Ointment (Papain, Urea) Healthpoint 1662
Accuzyme SE Spray Emulsion (Papain, Urea) Healthpoint 1662
Panafil Ointment (Chlorophyllin Copper Complex Sodium, Papain, Urea) Healthpoint 1663
Panafil SE Spray Emulsion (Chlorophyllin Copper Complex Sodium, Papain, Urea) Healthpoint 1663

Uncinariasis, as secondary therapy
Mintezol (Thiabendazole) Merck 2027

Ureaplasma urealyticum infections
Erythromycin Delayed-Release Capsules, USP (Erythromycin) Abbott 457

Ureaplasma urealyticum urethritis
E.E.S. (Erythromycin Ethylsuccinate) Abbott 451

Ureaplasma urealyticum urethritis, nongonococcal
EryPed (Erythromycin Ethylsuccinate) Abbott 447
PCE Dispertab Tablets (Erythromycin) Abbott 515

Urethritis
E.E.S. Granules (Erythromycin Ethylsuccinate) Abbott 451
Prosed/DS Tablets (Benzoic Acid, Hyoscyamine Sulfate, Methenamine, Methylene Blue, Phenyl Salicylate) Esprit 1157

Urethritis, nongonococcal
E.E.S. (Erythromycin Ethylsuccinate) Abbott 451
EryPed (Erythromycin Ethylsuccinate) Abbott 447
PCE Dispertab Tablets (Erythromycin) Abbott 515

Uric acid lithiasis
(*see under* Urolithiasis, management of)

Urinary bladder, overactive
Detrol Tablets (Tolterodine Tartrate) Pharmacia & Upjohn 2628
Detrol LA Capsules (Tolterodine Tartrate) Pharmacia & Upjohn 2631
Ditropan XL Extended-Release Tablets (Oxybutynin Chloride) Ortho Women's Health & Urology .. 2413
Enablex Extended-Release Tablets (Darifenacin) Novartis 2203
Oxytrol Transdermal System (Oxybutynin) Watson 3392
Sanctura Tablets (Trospium Chloride) Esprit 1151
VESIcare Tablets (Solifenacin Succinate) Astellas 646

Urinary frequency, symptomatic relief of
Detrol (Tolterodine Tartrate) Pharmacia & Upjohn 2628

Urinary incontinence
Detrol (Tolterodine Tartrate) Pharmacia & Upjohn 2628

Urinary tract, lower, hypermotility disorders
Prosed/DS Tablets (Benzoic Acid, Hyoscyamine Sulfate, Methenamine, Methylene Blue, Phenyl Salicylate) Esprit 1157

Urinary urgency, symptomatic relief of
Detrol Tablets (Tolterodine Tartrate) Pharmacia & Upjohn 2628
Estring Vaginal Ring (Estradiol) Pharmacia & Upjohn 2635

Urine, acidification of
K-Phos Original (Sodium Free) Tablets (Potassium Acid Phosphate) Beach 760

Urolithiasis, management of
Urocit-K Tablets (Potassium Citrate) Mission 2144

Urticaria, chronic
(*see also under* Urticarial manifestations, relief of)
Allegra (Fexofenadine Hydrochloride) sanofi-aventis 2844
Clarinex Syrup (Desloratadine) Schering 2995
Clarinex Tablets (Desloratadine) Schering 2995
Clarinex Reditabs Tablets (Desloratadine) Schering 2995
Zyrtec Chewable Tablets (Cetirizine Hydrochloride) Pfizer 2594
Zyrtec (Cetirizine Hydrochloride) Pfizer 2594

Urticarial manifestations, relief of
(*see also under* Urticaria, chronic)
Phenergan Tablets and Suppositories (Promethazine Hydrochloride) Wyeth 3440

Urticarial transfusion reactions
Depo-Medrol Single-Dose Vial (Methylprednisolone Acetate) Pharmacia & Upjohn 2619

Uterine bleeding, abnormal
Premarin Intravenous (Estrogens, Conjugated) Wyeth 3442

Uterine leiomymata
Lupron Depot 3.75 mg (Leuprolide Acetate) TAP 3260
Lupron Depot–3 Month 11.25 mg (Leuprolide Acetate) TAP 3265

Uveitis
Decadron Tablets (Dexamethasone) Merck 1951

Uveitis, chronic anterior, steroid-responsive
Blephamide Ophthalmic Ointment (Prednisolone Acetate, Sulfacetamide Sodium) Allergan 568
Blephamide Ophthalmic Suspension (Prednisolone Acetate, Sulfacetamide Sodium) Allergan 569
FML-S Ophthalmic Suspension (Fluorometholone, Sulfacetamide Sodium) Allergan .... ⊙229
Poly-Pred Ophthalmic Suspension (Neomycin Sulfate, Polymyxin B Sulfate, Prednisolone Acetate) Allergan .... ⊙233
Pred-G Ophthalmic Ointment (Gentamicin Sulfate, Prednisolone Acetate) Allergan .... ⊙237
Pred-G Ophthalmic Suspension (Gentamicin Sulfate, Prednisolone Acetate) Allergan .... ⊙236
TobraDex Ophthalmic Ointment (Dexamethasone, Tobramycin) Alcon 562
TobraDex Ophthalmic Suspension (Dexamethasone, Tobramycin) Alcon 563

Uveitis, diffuse posterior
Depo-Medrol Injectable Suspension (Methylprednisolone Acetate) Pharmacia & Upjohn 2617
Hydrocortone Tablets (Hydrocortisone) Merck 1989

Uveitis, non-infectious, chronic posterior
Retisert Implant (Fluocinolone Acetonide) Bausch & Lomb .... ⊙258

V

Vagina, cleansing of
Massengill Feminine Cleansing Wash (Cleanser) GlaxoSmithKline .... ▣801

Vaginal and anogenital areas, external, cleansing of
Massengill Baby Powder Scent Soft Cloth Towelette (Lactic Acid, Potassium Sorbate, Sodium Lactate) GlaxoSmithKline .... ▣801
Preparation H Medicated Wipes (Witch Hazel) Wyeth .... ▣667

Vaginal atrophy
Angeliq Tablets (Estradiol, Drospirenone) Berlex 762
Climara Transdermal System (Estradiol) Berlex 771
Premarin Tablets (Estrogens, Conjugated) Wyeth 3446
Premphase Tablets (Estrogens, Conjugated, Medroxyprogesterone Acetate) Wyeth 3456
Prempro Tablets (Estrogens, Conjugated, Medroxyprogesterone Acetate) Wyeth 3456

Vaginal atrophy, postmenopausal
Estring Vaginal Ring (Estradiol) Pharmacia & Upjohn 2635

Vaginitis
(*see under* Vaginosis, bacterial)

Vaginitis, atrophic
Premarin Vaginal Cream (Estrogens, Conjugated) Wyeth 3452
Vagifem Tablets (Estradiol) Novo Nordisk 2334

Vaginosis, bacterial
Cleocin Vaginal Ovules (Clindamycin Hydrochloride) Pharmacia & Upjohn 2616
MetroGel-Vaginal Gel (Metronidazole) 3M 1855
Vandazole Vaginal Gel (Metronidazole) Upsher-Smith 3338

Varicella, acute, treatment of
Zovirax (Acyclovir) GlaxoSmithKline 1643

Varicella, prevention or modification of
GamaSTAN (Globulin, Immune (Human)) Talecris 3234

Varicella vaccine
(*see also under* Immunization, varicella)
ProQuad (Measles, Mumps, Rubella and Varicella Virus Vaccine Live) Merck 2064
Varivax (Varicella Virus Vaccine Live) Merck 2100

Varicella virus, immunization against
Varivax (Varicella Virus Vaccine Live) Merck 2100

Ventilation, mechanical, facilitation of
Mivacron Injection (Mivacurium Chloride) Abbott 493
Nimbex Injection (Cisatracurium Besylate) Abbott 498
Zemuron Injection (Rocuronium Bromide) Organon USA 2346

Ventricular arrhythmias
(*see under* Arrhythmias, ventricular)

Ventricular dysfunction, left, asymptomatic
(*see under* Myocardial infarction, post, left ventricular dysfunction)

Ventricular tachycardia, sustained
(*see under* Tachycardia, ventricular, sustained)

Ventriculitis
(*see under* Infections, central nervous system)

VIPomas diarrhea
(*see under* Diarrhea associated with vasoactive intestinal peptide tumors)

Vitamin, multiple, deficiency of
Hep-Forte Capsules (Vitamins with Minerals) Marlyn 1862
Mega Antioxidant Tablets (Vitamins, Multiple) Usana 3339

Vitamin and mineral, multiple, deficiency of
Centrum Tablets (Vitamins with Minerals) Wyeth .... ▣809
Centrum Kids Complete Children's Chewables (Vitamins with Minerals) Wyeth .... ▣810
Centrum Performance Multivitamin/Multimineral Supplement (Ginkgo biloba, Herbals with Vitamins & Minerals, Ginseng, Vitamins with Minerals) Wyeth .... ▣811
Centrum Silver Tablets (Vitamins with Minerals) Wyeth .... ▣811
MDR Fitness Tabs for Men and Women (Vitamins with Minerals) MDR 1886
Ocuvite Lutein Vitamin and Mineral Supplement (Lutein, Vitamins with Minerals) Bausch & Lomb .... ⊙254
Vibe Liquid Multi-Nutrient Supplement (Herbals with Vitamins & Minerals, Vitamins with Minerals) Eniva .... ▣822

Vitamin B complex, deficiency of
Eldertonic (Vitamins with Minerals) Merz 2126

Vitamin deficiency, postpartum
Citracal Prenatal Rx Tablets (Vitamins, Prenatal) Mission 2139
Prenate Elite Tablets (Vitamins, Prenatal) Sciele 3121

Vitamin deficiency, prenatal
Animi-3 Capsules (Docosahexaenoic Acid (DHA), EPA (Eicosapentaenoic Acid), Folic Acid, Vitamin B_6, Vitamin B_{12}) PBM 2492
Citracal Prenatal Rx Tablets (Vitamins, Prenatal) Mission 2139
Prenate Elite Tablets (Vitamins, Prenatal) Sciele 3121

Vitamin multiple, deficiency of
Hep-Forte (Liver Preparations, Vitamins with Minerals) Maryln 1862
Mega Antioxidant (Dietary Supplement; Vitamins, Multiple) Usana 3339

Vitiligo
(*see under* Hypopigmentation, skin)

Vomiting
(*see under* Motion sickness)

Vomiting, emetogenic, cancer chemotherapy-induced
Aloxi Injection (Palonosetron Hydrochloride) MGI 2127
Anzemet Injection (Dolasetron Mesylate) sanofi-aventis 2859
Anzemet Tablets (Dolasetron Mesylate) sanofi-aventis 2862
Cesamet Capsules (Nabilone) Valeant 3340
Kytril Injection (Granisetron Hydrochloride) Roche 2781
Kytril (Granisetron Hydrochloride) Roche 2784
Marinol Capsules (Dronabinol) Unimed 3333
Zofran Injection (Ondansetron Hydrochloride) GlaxoSmithKline 1634
Zofran (Ondansetron Hydrochloride) GlaxoSmithKline 1639
Zofran ODT Orally Disintegrating Tablets (Ondansetron) GlaxoSmithKline 1639

Vomiting, emetogenic, cancer chemotherapy-induced, adjunct in
Emend Capsules (Aprepitant) Merck 1963

Vomiting, emetogenic, radiation therapy-induced
Kytril (Granisetron Hydrochloride) Roche 2784
Zofran (Ondansetron Hydrochloride) GlaxoSmithKline 1639
Zofran ODT Orally Disintegrating Tablets (Ondansetron) GlaxoSmithKline 1639

Vomiting, postoperative
Anzemet Injection (Dolasetron Mesylate) sanofi-aventis 2859
Anzemet Tablets (Dolasetron Mesylate) sanofi-aventis 2862
Emend Capsules (Aprepitant) Merck 1963
Kytril Injection (Granisetron Hydrochloride) Roche 2781
Phenergan Tablets and Suppositories (Promethazine Hydrochloride) Wyeth 3440
Zofran Injection (Ondansetron Hydrochloride) GlaxoSmithKline 1634
Zofran (Ondansetron Hydrochloride) GlaxoSmithKline 1639
Zofran ODT Orally Disintegrating Tablets (Ondansetron) GlaxoSmithKline 1639

von Willebrand's disease
Humate-P (Antihemophilic Factor (Human), von Willebrand Factor (Human)) ZLB Behring 3502

Vulvae, kraurosis
Premarin Vaginal Cream (Estrogens, Conjugated) Wyeth 3452

Vulvar atrophy
Angeliq Tablets (Estradiol, Drospirenone) Berlex 762
Climara Transdermal System (Estradiol) Berlex 771
Premarin Tablets (Estrogens, Conjugated) Wyeth 3446
Premphase Tablets (Estrogens, Conjugated, Medroxyprogesterone Acetate) Wyeth 3456
Prempro Tablets (Estrogens, Conjugated, Medroxyprogesterone Acetate) Wyeth 3456

W

Warts, genital
(*see under* Condylomata acuminata)

Warts, veneral
Podocon-25 Liquid (Podophyllin, Tincture of Benzoin) Paddock 2478

Weight, body, management of
Oxandrin Tablets (Oxandrolone) Savient 2962

Wheezing, symptomatic relief of
(*see also under* Bronchial asthma)
Primatene Mist (Epinephrine) Wyeth .... ▣719

Whooping cough
(*see under* Pertussis)

Wilms' tumor
Cosmegen for Injection (Dactinomycin) Ovation 2459

Wilson's disease
Cuprimine Capsules (Penicillamine) Merck 1947
Syprine Capsules (Trientine Hydrochloride) Merck 2085

Wiskott-Aldrich syndrome
Flebogamma 5%, Immune Globulin Intravenous (Human) (Globulin, Immune (Human)) Grifols 1658
Gammagard Liquid (Immune Globulin Intravenous (Human)) Baxter Healthcare 721
Gammagard S/D (Immune Globulin Intravenous (Human)) Baxter Healthcare 724
Gamunex Immune Globulin I.V., 10% (Immune Globulin Intravenous (Human)) Talecris 3235

Wolff-Parkinson-White syndrome
Adenocard Injection (Adenosine) Astellas 617

Wound care, adjunctive therapy in
Panafil Ointment (Chlorophyllin Copper Complex Sodium, Papain, Urea) Healthpoint 1663
Preparation H Medicated Wipes (Witch Hazel) Wyeth .... ▣667
Xenaderm Ointment (Balsam Peru, Castor Oil, Trypsin) Healthpoint 1664

Wounds, debridement of
Accuzyme Debriding Ointment (Papain, Urea) Healthpoint 1662
Accuzyme SE Spray Emulsion (Papain, Urea) Healthpoint 1662
Panafil Ointment (Chlorophyllin Copper Complex Sodium, Papain, Urea) Healthpoint 1663
Panafil SE Spray Emulsion (Chlorophyllin Copper Complex Sodium, Papain, Urea) Healthpoint 1663

Wounds, infected, adjunctive therapy in
Accuzyme SE Spray Emulsion (Papain, Urea) Healthpoint 1662
Panafil Ointment (Chlorophyllin Copper Complex Sodium, Papain, Urea) Healthpoint 1663
Panafil SE Spray Emulsion (Chlorophyllin Copper Complex Sodium, Papain, Urea) Healthpoint 1663

Wounds, pilonidal cyst, adjunctive therapy in
Accuzyme SE Spray Emulsion (Papain, Urea) Healthpoint 1662
Panafil Ointment (Chlorophyllin Copper Complex Sodium, Papain, Urea) Healthpoint 1663
Panafil SE Spray Emulsion (Chlorophyllin Copper Complex Sodium, Papain, Urea) Healthpoint 1663

Wounds, postoperative, adjunctive therapy in
Accuzyme SE Spray Emulsion (Papain, Urea) Healthpoint 1662
Panafil Ointment (Chlorophyllin Copper Complex Sodium, Papain, Urea) Healthpoint 1663
Panafil SE Spray Emulsion (Chlorophyllin Copper Complex Sodium, Papain, Urea) Healthpoint 1663

Wounds, removal of exudates, aids in
Panafil Ointment (Chlorophyllin Copper Complex Sodium, Papain, Urea) Healthpoint 1663

Wounds, superficial
Levaquin (Levofloxacin) Ortho-McNeil 2384

Levaquin in 5% Dextrose Injection (Levofloxacin) Ortho-McNeil 2384

Wounds, traumatic, adjunctive therapy in

Accuzyme SE Spray Emulsion (Papain, Urea) Healthpoint 1662

Panafil Ointment (Chlorophyllin Copper Complex Sodium, Papain, Urea) Healthpoint 1663

Panafil SE Spray Emulsion (Chlorophyllin Copper Complex Sodium, Papain, Urea) Healthpoint 1663

X

Xerostomia, radiotherapy-induced

Ethyol for Injection (Amifostine) MedImmune Oncology 1898

X-linked agammaglobulinemia

Flebogamma 5%, Immune Globulin Intravenous (Human) (Globulin, Immune (Human)) Grifols 1658

X-linked immunodeficiency with hyper IgM

Gamunex Immune Globulin I.V., 10% (Immune Globulin Intravenous (Human)) Talecris 3235

XO syndrome
(*see under* Turner's syndrome)

Z

Zollinger-Ellison syndrome

Aciphex Tablets (Rabeprazole Sodium) Eisai 1090

Pepcid Injection (Famotidine) Merck . 2040

Pepcid (Famotidine) Merck 2038

Protonix I.V. (Pantoprazole Sodium) Wyeth 3472

Protonix Tablets (Pantoprazole Sodium) Wyeth 3469

Zantac (Ranitidine Hydrochloride) GlaxoSmithKline 1624

Zygomycosis

Abelcet Injection (Amphotericin B Lipid Complex) Enzon 1141

SECTION 5

CONTRAINDICATIONS INDEX

This section lists in alphabetical order every medical condition cited as a contraindication in *PDR®* and its companion volumes, with cross-references to all product entries in which the contraindication is found. Page numbers refer to the 2007 editions of *PDR®*, *PDR For Ophthalmic Medicines™* and the *PDR For Nonprescription Drugs, Dietary Supplements and Herbs™*, which is published later in the year. A key to the symbols denoting the companion volumes appears in the bottom margin.

These listings will enable you to quickly identify drugs that generally threaten to be inappropriate in the presence of a given complication. However, a drug's suitability is sometimes affected by the severity of the complicating condition, the age or gender of the patient, and the drug's route of administration. In ambiguous situations, a quick review of the underlying *PDR®* text may therefore prove helpful.

Note, too, that the index does not list other drugs and dietary items whose use would present a contraindication. Contraindicated combinations can be found in the Interactions Index and the Food Interactions Cross-Reference. Hypersensitivity to the product's ingredients—an almost universal contraindication—also has not been indexed here. If the clinical picture includes the risk of allergic reaction, be sure to check individual product labeling for additional information.

A

Abdominal adhesions
Zelnorm Tablets....2312

Abortion, infected
Mirena Intrauterine System.... 787

Abortion, missed
Prochieve 4% Gel....1003
Prochieve 8% Gel....1003
Prometrium Capsules (100 mg, 200 mg)....3203

Abortion, threatened
Coumadin for Injection.... 898
Coumadin Tablets.... 898
Miradon Tablets....3042

Achalasia, esophageal
Fosamax....1969
Fosamax Plus D Tablets....1977

Acid base imbalance, uncorrected
(*see under* Acidosis, hyperchloremic; Acidosis, metabolic, unspecified; Ketoacidosis, diabetic)

Acidosis, hyperchloremic
Daranide Tablets....1950

Acidosis, metabolic, unspecified
(*see also under* Ketoacidosis, diabetic)
ActoPlus Met Tablets....3214
Avandamet Tablets....1373
Fortamet Extended-Release Tablets....3115

Acquired immune deficiency syndrome
(*see also under* Human immunodeficiency virus)
Attenuvax....1914
Flumist Vaccine....1901
Meruvax II....2019
M-M-R II....2006
Mumpsvax....2031
Varivax....2100
Zostavax Injection....2111

Actinomycosis, genital
Mirena Intrauterine System.... 787

Adenoma, hepatic
Mircette Tablets....1066
NuvaRing....2340
Ortho-Cyclen Tablets....2429
Ortho Evra Transdermal System....2417
Ortho Tri-Cyclen Tablets....2429
Ortho Tri-Cyclen Lo Tablets....2436
Yasmin 28 Tablets.... 796

Adrenal cortical insufficiency
(*see under* Adrenal insufficiency, uncorrected; Adrenal insufficiency, unspecified)

Adrenal cortical insufficiency, uncorrected
Naturethroid Tablets....3401
Thyrolar Tablets....1199
Westhroid Tablets....3403

Adrenal dysfunction, uncontrolled
Follistim AQ Cartridge....2338

Adrenal dysfunction, uncorrected
(*see under* Adrenal insufficiency, uncorrected)

Adrenal gland failure
(*see under* Adrenal insufficiency, unspecified)

Adrenal insufficiency, uncorrected
Cytomel Tablets....1710
Levothroid Tablets....1186
Levoxyl Tablets....1712
Synthroid Tablets.... 520

Adrenal insufficiency, unspecified
Angeliq Tablets.... 762
Daranide Tablets....1950
Urocit-K Tablets....2144
Yasmin 28 Tablets.... 796
Yaz Tablets.... 803

Adrenocortical insufficiency
(*see under* Adrenal insufficiency, uncorrected; Adrenal insufficiency, unspecified)

Agammaglobulinemia
Flumist Vaccine....1901

Agitated states
(*see under* Agitation)

Agitation
Adderall Tablets....3164
Adderall XR Capsules....3166
Adipex-P....1215
Concerta Extended-Release Tablets....1881
Daytrana Transdermal Patch....3174
Desoxyn Tablets, USP....2462
Dexedrine....1420
DextroStat Tablets....3179
Focalin Tablets....2220
Focalin XR Capsules....2223
Metadate CD Capsules....3323
Ritalin Hydrochloride Tablets....2269
Ritalin LA Capsules....2271
Ritalin-SR Tablets....2269

Agranulocytosis, history of
Clozaril Tablets....2184
Cuprimine Capsules....1947
FazaClo Orally Disintegrating Tablets.... 551
Thiola Tablets....2141

AIDS
(*see under* Acquired immune deficiency syndrome)

Albinism
Oxsoralen-Ultra Capsules....3353

Alcohol discontinuation, abrupt
Zyban Sustained-Release Tablets....1644

Alcoholism
Seromycin Capsules....1813

Alcoholism, unsupervised
Coumadin for Injection.... 898
Coumadin Tablets.... 898

Allergic reaction, history of
Oncaspar....1145

Allergic reaction to aspirin
Anaprox Tablets....2761
Anaprox DS Tablets....2761
Clinoril Tablets....1924
EC-Naprosyn Delayed-Release Tablets....2761
Naprosyn Suspension....2761
Naprosyn Tablets....2761

Prevacid NapraPAC 3280
Voltaren Tablets 2307
Zomig Nasal Spray 3523

Allergic reaction to non-steroidal anti-inflammatory drugs
Anaprox Tablets 2761
Anaprox DS Tablets 2761
Clinoril Tablets 1924
EC-Naprosyn Delayed-Release Tablets 2761
Naprosyn Suspension 2761
Naprosyn Tablets 2761
Prevacid NapraPAC 3280
Voltaren Tablets 2307
Zomig Nasal Spray 3523

Allergic reaction to sulfonamides
Micardis HCT Tablets 856

Allograft
(*see under* Organ allograft)

Amino acid metabolism disorders
(*see under* Electrolyte imbalance, uncorrected)

Amniocentesis, genetic
MICRhoGAM Ultra-Filtered 2371

Anastomosis, unspecified
(*see under* Ileocolostomy)

Anemia, aplastic, history of
Cuprimine Capsules 1947
Thiola Tablets 2141
Ticlid Tablets 2810

Anemia, hemolytic, history of
Elitek 2890
Skelaxin Tablets 1716

Anemia, megaloblastic, unspecified
Daraprim Tablets 1419
Fansidar Tablets 2765

Anemia, non-iron deficiency, unspecified
Ferrlecit Injection 3388
Infed Injection 3390

Anemia, sickle cell
Caverject Impulse Injection 2612

Anemia, unspecified
Albutein 5%, Albumin (Human) 1652
Albutein 25% , Albumin (Human) 1653
Flexbumin I.V. 720
Human Albumin Grifols 20%, Albumin (Human) 1651
Human Albumin Grifols 25%, Albumin (Human) 1652
Plasbumin-5 3251
Plasbumin-20 3252
Plasbumin-25 3253
Plasmanate 3255

Anemia, unspecified, history of
Plasbumin-20 3252
Skelaxin Tablets 1716

Anesthesia, general
Parnate Tablets 1527

Anesthesia, local
(*see also under* Anesthesia, major regional lumbar block)
Parnate Tablets 1527

Anesthesia, major regional lumbar block
Coumadin for Injection 898
Coumadin Tablets 898

Aneurysm
(*see also under* Cerebrovascular accident)
Activase I.V. 1223
Aggrastat 1907
Coumadin for Injection 898
Coumadin Tablets 898
Miradon Tablets 3042
ReoPro Vials 1809
Retavase 2499
TNKase I.V. 1264

Angina pectoris
Amerge Tablets 1339
Axert Tablets 2396
Frova Tablets 1113
Imitrex Injection 1463
Imitrex Nasal Spray 1467
Imitrex Tablets 1471
Maxalt Tablets 2008
Maxalt-MLT Orally Disintegrating Tablets 2008
Migranal Nasal Spray 3348
Relpax Tablets 2548
Zomig Tablets 3519
Zomig Nasal Spray 3523
Zomig-ZMT Tablets 3519

Angina, Prinzmetal's
Amerge Tablets 1339
Axert Tablets 2396
Frova Tablets 1113
Imitrex Injection 1463
Imitrex Nasal Spray 1467
Imitrex Tablets 1471
Maxalt Tablets 2008
Maxalt-MLT Orally Disintegrating Tablets 2008
Migranal Nasal Spray 3348
Relpax Tablets 2548
Zomig Tablets 3519
Zomig Nasal Spray 3523
Zomig-ZMT Tablets 3519

Angina, unspecified, history of
Proleukin for Injection 2266

Angioedema, hereditary
Prinivil Tablets 2052
Prinzide Tablets 2056
Vasotec I.V. Injection 2103

Angioedema, idiopathic
Prinivil Tablets 2052
Prinzide Tablets 2056
Vasotec I.V. Injection 2103

Angulation, penile
Caverject Impulse Injection 2612
Edex Injection 3089

Anorexia nervosa
Meridia Capsules 489
Wellbutrin Tablets 1603
Wellbutrin SR Sustained-Release Tablets 1607
Wellbutrin XL Extended-Release Tablets 1613
Zyban Sustained-Release Tablets 1644

Antepartum prophylaxis
MICRhoGAM Ultra-Filtered 2371

Anuria
Aldoril Tablets 1910
Atacand HCT 651
Avalide Tablets 888
Avalide Tablets 2874
Benicar HCT Tablets 1044
Bumex Tablets 2746
Calcium Disodium Versenate Injection 1851
Clorpres Tablets 2153
Demadex Injection 2759
Demadex Tablets 2759
Diovan HCT Tablets 2196
Diuril Oral Suspension 1954
Diuril Sodium Intravenous 2467
Dyazide Capsules 1423
Dyrenium Capsules 3400
Edecrin 1959
Furosemide Tablets 2154
Hyzaar 50-12.5 Tablets 1990
Hyzaar 100-12.5 Tablets 1990
Hyzaar 100-25 Tablets 1990
Indapamide Tablets 2156
Lopressor HCT 50/25 Tablets 2241
Lopressor HCT 100/25 Tablets 2241
Lopressor HCT 100/50 Tablets 2241
Lotensin HCT Tablets 2246
Micardis HCT Tablets 856
Midamor Tablets 2026
Moduretic Tablets 2028
Prinzide Tablets 2056
Teveten HCT Tablets 1737
Timolide Tablets 2086
Uniretic Tablets 3100

Anxiety
Concerta Extended-Release Tablets 1881
Daytrana Transdermal Patch 3174
Focalin Tablets 2220
Focalin XR Capsules 2223
Metadate CD Capsules 3323
Ritalin Hydrochloride Tablets 2269
Ritalin LA Capsules 2271
Ritalin-SR Tablets 2269
Seromycin Capsules 1813

Aortic coarctation
(*see under* Stenosis, aortic)

Aortic dissection
Aggrastat 1907

Aortic stenosis
(*see under* Stenosis, aortic)

Aphakia
Oxsoralen-Ultra Capsules 3353

Apoplexy, cerebral
(*see under* Cerebrovascular accident)

Appendicitis
Dulcolax Suppositories ▣ 648

Arrhythmia, cardiac, history of
Proleukin for Injection 2266
Thioridazine Hydrochloride Tablets 2163

Arrhythmia, cardiac, unspecified
(*see also under* Bradycardia, sinus; Bradycardia, unspecified; Fibrillation, atrial; Fibrillation, ventricular; Flutter, atrial; Heart block, greater than first degree; Heart block, unspecified; Lown-Ganong-Levine syndrome; Q-T interval prolongation; Sick sinus syndrome; Sinus node dysfunction, unspecified; Tachycardia, unspecified; Tachycardia, ventricular, history of; Wolff-Parkinson-White syndrome)
Rythmol SR Capsules 2727

Arrhythmia, ventricular, unspecified
(*see under* Fibrillation, ventricular; Tachycardia, ventricular, history of; Ventricular dysfunction, left)

Arterial disease, unspecified
(*see under* Angina pectoris; Angina, Prinzmetal's; Arteriosclerosis, unspecified; Arteriovenous malformation; Coronary artery disease; Coronary artery disease, history of; Coronary artery vasospasm; Stenosis, aortic)

Arteriosclerosis, advanced
Adderall XR Capsules 3166

Arteriosclerosis, unspecified
(*see also under* Coronary artery disease; Stenosis, aortic)
Adderall Tablets 3164
Adderall XR Capsules 3166
Adipex-P 1215
Desoxyn Tablets, USP 2462
Dexedrine 1420
DextroStat Tablets 3179

Arteriovenous malformation
Activase I.V. 1223
Aggrastat 1907
ReoPro Vials 1809
Retavase 2499
TNKase I.V. 1264

As primary therapy in patients with cardiogenic shock
Natrecor for Injection 3127

Asthma, acute
(*see also under* Status asthmaticus)
Advair Diskus 100/50 1308
Advair Diskus 250/50 1308
Advair Diskus 500/50 1308
Advair HFA Inhalation Aerosol 1318
Asmanex Twisthaler 2966
Avinza Capsules 1741
Azmacort Inhalation Aerosol 1726
DepoDur Extended-Release Injection 1110
Duragesic Transdermal System 2373
Flovent Diskus 1443
InnoPran XL Capsules 2723
Kadian Capsules 577
MS Contin Tablets 2701
OxyContin Tablets 2703
OxyFast Oral Concentrate Solution 2708
OxyIR Capsules 2708
Pulmicort Respules 661
Qvar Inhalation Aerosol 3303
Symbicort 80/4.5 Inhalation Aerosol 3511
Symbicort 160/4.5 Inhalation Aerosol 3511

Asthma, history of
Betagan Ophthalmic Solution, USP ⊙ 220
Betimol Ophthalmic Solution 3382
Betimol Ophthalmic Solution ⊙ 295
Blocadren Tablets 1916
Carteolol Hydrochloride Ophthalmic Solution USP, 1% ⊙ 249
Cosopt Sterile Ophthalmic Solution 1931
Duragesic Transdermal System 2373
InnoPran XL Capsules 2723
OptiPranolol Metipranolol Ophthalmic Solution 0.3% ⊙ 256
Timolide Tablets 2086
Timoptic Sterile Ophthalmic Solution 2088
Timoptic in Ocudose 2091
Timoptic-XE Sterile Ophthalmic Gel Forming Solution 2092

Asthma, unspecified
Adenoscan 619
Avinza Capsules 1741
Betagan Ophthalmic Solution, USP ⊙ 220
Betimol Ophthalmic Solution 3382
Betimol Ophthalmic Solution ⊙ 295
Blocadren Tablets 1916
Carteolol Hydrochloride Ophthalmic Solution USP, 1% ⊙ 249
Coreg Tablets 1414
Cosopt Sterile Ophthalmic Solution 1931
DepoDur Extended-Release Injection 1110
Inderal LA Long-Acting Capsules 3429
InnoPran XL Capsules 2723
Kadian Capsules 577
MS Contin Tablets 2701
Nadolol Tablets 2159
Opana ER Tablets 1126
OptiPranolol Metipranolol Ophthalmic Solution 0.3% ⊙ 256
OxyContin Tablets 2703
OxyFast Oral Concentrate Solution 2708
OxyIR Capsules 2708
Phenergan Tablets and Suppositories 3440
Timolide Tablets 2086
Timoptic Sterile Ophthalmic Solution 2088
Timoptic in Ocudose 2091
Timoptic-XE Sterile Ophthalmic Gel Forming Solution 2092

Asthmatic attack
(*see under* Asthma, acute)

Atony, intestinal
Donnatal Extentabs 2493

Atresia, pulmonary
Indocin I.V. 2465
NeoProfen Injection 2472

Atrial fibrillation
(*see under* Fibrillation, atrial)

Atrial flutter
(*see under* Flutter, atrial)

Atrioventricular block
(*see under* Heart block, greater than first degree; Heart block, unspecified)

AV block
(*see under* Heart block, greater than first degree; Heart block, unspecified)

Azotemia
Edecrin 1959

B

Bacterial endocarditis
(*see under* Endocarditis, bacterial)

Birthmarks
Podocon-25 Liquid 2478

Bladder neck obstruction
(*see under* Obstruction, bladder neck)

Bleeding, abnormal, unspecified
Indocin I.V. 2465

Bleeding, arterial
Advicor Tablets 1722
Niaspan Extended-Release Tablets 1730

Bleeding, cerebrovascular
(*see under* Bleeding, intracranial; Cerebrovascular accident)

Bleeding, gastrointestinal
Indocin I.V. 2465
NeoProfen Injection 2472
Plavix Tablets 917
Plavix Tablets 2926
ReoPro Vials 1809
Ticlid Tablets 2810

Bleeding, gastrointestinal, history of
Proleukin for Injection 2266

Bleeding, genital, abnormal
(*see also under* Bleeding, genitourinary)
Angeliq Tablets 762
Cervidil Vaginal Insert 1181
Climara Transdermal System 771
Climara Pro Transdermal System 776
Depo-Provera Contraceptive Injection 2622
depo-subQ provera 104 Injectable Suspension 2624
Enjuvia Tablets 1062
Estrasorb Topical Emulsion 1147
Estratest Tablets 3199
Estratest H.S. Tablets 3199
Estring Vaginal Ring 2635
Follistim AQ Cartridge 2338
Lupron Depot 3.75 mg 3260
Lupron Depot–3 Month 11.25 mg 3265
Menostar Transdermal System 782
Mircette Tablets 1066
Mirena Intrauterine System 787
NuvaRing 2340
Ortho-Cyclen Tablets 2429
Ortho Evra Transdermal System 2417
Ortho Micronor Tablets 2426
Ortho Tri-Cyclen Tablets 2429
Ortho Tri-Cyclen Lo Tablets 2436
ParaGard T 380A Intrauterine Copper Contraceptive 1073
Plan B Tablets 1076
Premarin Intravenous 3442
Premarin Tablets 3446
Premarin Vaginal Cream 3452
Premphase Tablets 3456
Prempro Tablets 3456
Prochieve 4% Gel 1003
Prochieve 8% Gel 1003
Prometrium Capsules (100 mg, 200 mg) 3203
Vagifem Tablets 2334
Yasmin 28 Tablets 796

Bleeding, genitourinary
(*see also under* Bleeding, genital, abnormal)
Estrasorb Topical Emulsion 1147
ReoPro Vials 1809

Bleeding, history of
Aggrastat 1907
Integrilin Injection 3020
Oncaspar 1145

Bleeding, internal, unspecified
Activase I.V. 1223
NeoProfen Injection 2472
ReoPro Vials 1809
Retavase 2499
TNKase I.V. 1264
Xigris Powder for Intravenous Infusion 1828

Bleeding, intracranial
(*see also under* Cerebrovascular accident)
Activase I.V. 1223
Aggrastat 1907
Coumadin for Injection 898
Coumadin Tablets 898
Indocin I.V. 2465
Miradon Tablets 3042
NeoProfen Injection 2472
Plavix Tablets 917
Plavix Tablets 2926
Pletal Tablets 2455
Ticlid Tablets 2810

Bleeding, rectal
Dulcolax Suppositories ■ 648
Indocin Suppositories 1995

Bleeding, ulcer, peptic
Plavix Tablets 917
Pletal Tablets 2455

Bleeding, unspecified
(*see also under* Bleeding, internal, unspecified)
Argatroban Injection 1346
Arixtra Injection 1351
Coumadin for Injection 898
Coumadin Tablets 898
Lovenox Injection 2915
Miradon Tablets 3042
Ticlid Tablets 2810

Bleeding, uterine
(*see under* Bleeding, genital, abnormal)

Bleeding, vaginal, abnormal
(*see under* Bleeding, genital, abnormal)

Bleeding, vaginal, undiagnosed
Seasonique Tablets 1077
Yaz Tablets 803

Bleeding disorders, unspecified
(*see also under* Bleeding tendencies; Hemophilia; Thrombocytopenia, unspecified)
Indocin I.V. 2465
Ticlid Tablets 2810

Bleeding tendencies
Activase I.V. 1223
Aggrastat 1907
Coumadin for Injection 898
Coumadin Tablets 898
Fragmin Injection 1097
Miradon Tablets 3042
ReoPro Vials 1809
Retavase 2499
TNKase I.V. 1264

Blood circulation, poor
Podocon-25 Liquid 2478

Blood disorders, unspecified
NeoProfen Injection 2472

Blood dyscrasias, unspecified
(*see also under* Agranulocytosis, history of; Anemia, aplastic, history of; Anemia, hemolytic, history of; Anemia, megaloblastic, unspecified; Anemia, non-iron deficiency, unspecified; Anemia, sickle cell; Anemia, unspecified; Anemia, unspecified, history of; Bleeding disorders, unspecified; Granulocytopenia, history of; Hemophilia; Neutropenia; Thrombocytopenia, unspecified)
Attenuvax 1914
Coumadin for Injection 898
Coumadin Tablets 898
Fansidar Tablets 2765
Meruvax II 2019
Miradon Tablets 3042
M-M-R II 2006
Mumpsvax 2031
ProQuad 2064
Thiothixene Capsules 2165
Ticlid Tablets 2810
Varivax 2100

Blood vessel, major, tumors eroding into
Photofrin for Injection 702

Body weight less than 50 kg
Arixtra Injection 1351

Bone marrow aplasia
(*see under* Bone marrow depression)

Bone marrow damage
(*see under* Bone marrow depression)

Bone marrow depression
Hycamtin for Injection 1458

Bone marrow depression, history of
Carbatrol Capsules 3171
Equetro Extended-Release Capsules 3180
Tegretol/Tegretol-XR 2295

Bone marrow function impairment
(*see under* Bone marrow depression)

Bone marrow hypoplasia
(*see under* Bone marrow depression)

Bone marrow reserve, inadequate
Matulane Capsules 3191

Bowel disease, inflammatory
(*see under* Inflammation, gastrointestinal tract)

Bowel ischemia, history of
Amerge Tablets 1339
Frova Tablets 1113
Imitrex Nasal Spray 1467
Imitrex Tablets 1471
Kionex Powder 2477
Lotronex Tablets 1512
Proleukin for Injection 2266
Relpax Tablets 2548

Bowel obstruction
(*see under* Bowel ischemia, history of; Obstruction, gastrointestinal tract)

Bowel perforation
(*see under* Perforation, gastrointestinal tract)

Bowel perforation, history of
(*see under* Perforation, gastrointestinal tract, history of)

Bradycardia, sinus
Adenocard Injection 617
Adenoscan 619
Betagan Ophthalmic Solution, USP ⊙ 220
Betimol Ophthalmic Solution 3382
Betimol Ophthalmic Solution ⊙ 295
Betoptic S Ophthalmic Suspension 558
Blocadren Tablets 1916
Inderal LA Long-Acting Capsules 3429
InnoPran XL Capsules 2723
Lopressor Injection 2238
Lopressor Tablets 2238
Lopressor HCT 50/25 Tablets 2241
Lopressor HCT 100/25 Tablets 2241
Lopressor HCT 100/50 Tablets 2241
Nadolol Tablets 2159
OptiPranolol Metipranolol Ophthalmic Solution 0.3% ⊙ 256
Timolide Tablets 2086
Timoptic Sterile Ophthalmic Solution 2088
Timoptic in Ocudose 2091
Timoptic-XE Sterile Ophthalmic Gel Forming Solution 2092
Toprol-XL Tablets 668

Bradycardia, unspecified
Coreg Tablets 1414
Rythmol SR Capsules 2727

Brain tumor
(*see under* Tumor, pituitary, unspecified)

Breast cancer
(*see also under* Carcinoma, breast, history of; Carcinoma, breast, male; Carcinoma, breast, unspecified)
NuvaRing 2340
Seasonique Tablets 1077
Yaz Tablets 803

Breastfeeding
Advicor Tablets 1722
Altoprev Extended-Release Tablets 3109
Bentyl Capsules 697
Bentyl Injection 697
Bentyl Syrup 697
Bentyl Tablets 697
Caduet Tablets 2508
Crestor Tablets 678
Cuprimine Capsules 1947
Doxil Injection 2351
Estratest Tablets 3199
Estratest H.S. Tablets 3199
Evista Tablets 1763
Fansidar Tablets 2765
Gantrisin Pediatric Suspension 2770
Hycamtin for Injection 1458
Lescol Capsules 2233
Lescol XL Tablets 2233
Lipitor Tablets 2483
Lupron Depot 3.75 mg 3260
Lupron Depot–3 Month 11.25 mg 3265
Mevacor Tablets 2021
Migranal Nasal Spray 3348
Orthoclone OKT3 Sterile Solution 2360
Podocon-25 Liquid 2478
Testim 1% Gel 695
Vytorin 10/10 Tablets 2114
Vytorin 10/10 Tablets 3077
Vytorin 10/20 Tablets 2114
Vytorin 10/20 Tablets 3077
Vytorin 10/40 Tablets 2114
Vytorin 10/40 Tablets 3077
Vytorin 10/80 Tablets 2114
Vytorin 10/80 Tablets 3077
Zetia Tablets 2120
Zocor Tablets 2105

Breathing problems, unspecified
(*see under* Pulmonary disorders, unspecified; Respiratory illness, febrile)

Bronchial asthma
(*see under* Asthma, acute; Asthma, history of; Asthma, unspecified)

Bronchoesophageal, fistula, existence of
Photofrin for Injection 702

Bronchospastic disorders, unspecified
(*see also under* Asthma, acute; Asthma, history of; Asthma, unspecified)
Adenoscan 619
Coreg Tablets 1414
Rythmol SR Capsules 2727

Bulimia
Meridia Capsules 489
Wellbutrin Tablets 1603
Wellbutrin SR Sustained-Release Tablets 1607
Wellbutrin XL Extended-Release Tablets 1613
Zyban Sustained-Release Tablets 1644

Bundle branch block
(*see under* Heart block, unspecified)

C

CAD
(*see under* Coronary artery disease)

Cancer
(*see under* Carcinoma, breast, history of; Carcinoma, breast, male; Carcinoma, breast, unspecified; Carcinoma, cervical; Carcinoma, endometrium; Carcinoma, female reproductive organs; Carcinoma, genital, unspecified; Carcinoma, hepatic; Carcinoma, prostate; Carcinoma, skin, unspecified; Carcinoma, uterine; Malignancy, generalized; Neoplasm, bone marrow system, malignant; Neoplasm, lymphatic system, malignant)

Carcinoma, breast, history of
Angeliq Tablets 762
Estring Vaginal Ring 2635
Mircette Tablets 1066
NuvaRing 2340
Premphase Tablets 3456
Prempro Tablets 3456

Carcinoma, breast, male
(*see also under* Carcinoma, breast, unspecified)
AndroGel 3329
Androxy Tablets 3335
Oxandrin Tablets 2962
Striant Mucoadhesive 1007
Testim 1% Gel 695

Carcinoma, breast, unspecified
(*see also under* Carcinoma, breast, history of; Carcinoma, breast, male; Neoplasm, estrogen dependent)
Climara Transdermal System 771
Climara Pro Transdermal System 776
Depo-Provera Contraceptive Injection 2622
depo-subQ provera 104 Injectable Suspension 2624
Enjuvia Tablets 1062
Estrasorb Topical Emulsion 1147
Estratest Tablets 3199
Estratest H.S. Tablets 3199
Menostar Transdermal System 782
Mirena Intrauterine System 787
Ortho-Cyclen Tablets 2429
Ortho Evra Transdermal System 2417
Ortho Micronor Tablets 2426
Ortho Tri-Cyclen Tablets 2429
Ortho Tri-Cyclen Lo Tablets 2436
Oxandrin Tablets 2962
Premarin Intravenous 3442
Premarin Tablets 3446
Premarin Vaginal Cream 3452
Premphase Tablets 3456
Prempro Tablets 3456
Prochieve 4% Gel 1003
Prochieve 8% Gel 1003
Prometrium Capsules (100 mg, 200 mg) 3203
Vagifem Tablets 2334
Yasmin 28 Tablets 796

Carcinoma, cervical
(*see also under* Carcinoma, female reproductive organs; Carcinoma, genital, unspecified)
Mirena Intrauterine System 787

Carcinoma, endometrium
(*see also under* Carcinoma, female reproductive organs; Carcinoma, uterine)
Mircette Tablets 1066
NuvaRing 2340
Ortho-Cyclen Tablets 2429
Ortho Evra Transdermal System 2417
Ortho Tri-Cyclen Tablets 2429
Ortho Tri-Cyclen Lo Tablets 2436
Seasonique Tablets 1077
Yasmin 28 Tablets 796
Yaz Tablets 803

Carcinoma, female reproductive organs
(*see under* Carcinoma, cervical; Carcinoma, endometrium; Carcinoma, genital, unspecified; Carcinoma, uterine)

Carcinoma, genital, unspecified
(*see also under* Carcinoma, cervical; Carcinoma, female reproductive organs; Carcinoma, prostate)
Prochieve 4% Gel 1003
Prochieve 8% Gel 1003

Carcinoma, hepatic
Mircette Tablets 1066
Mirena Intrauterine System 787
NuvaRing 2340
Ortho-Cyclen Tablets 2429
Ortho Evra Transdermal System 2417
Ortho Micronor Tablets 2426
Ortho Tri-Cyclen Tablets 2429
Ortho Tri-Cyclen Lo Tablets 2436
Seasonique Tablets 1077
Yasmin 28 Tablets 796
Yaz Tablets 803

Carcinoma, ovarian
(*see under* Carcinoma, female reproductive organs)

Carcinoma, prostate
(*see also under* Carcinoma, genital, unspecified)
AndroGel 3329
Androxy Tablets 3335
Oxandrin Tablets 2962
Striant Mucoadhesive 1007
Testim 1% Gel 695

Carcinoma, skin, unspecified
(*see also under* Melanoma, history of)
Oxsoralen Lotion 1% 3352

Carcinoma, squamous cell, unspecified
Oxsoralen-Ultra Capsules 3353

Carcinoma, uterine
(*see also under* Carcinoma, endometrium; Carcinoma, female reproductive organs)
Mirena Intrauterine System 787

Carcinoma, visceral
Miradon Tablets 3042

Cardiac arrhythmia
(*see under* Arrhythmia, cardiac, unspecified)

Cardiac decompensation
(*see under* Heart failure, unspecified)

Cardiac dilation
Daranide Tablets 1950

Cardiac disease
(*see under* Cardiovascular disorders, unspecified)

Cardiac dysfunction
(*see under* Cardiovascular disorders, unspecified)

Cardiac failure
(*see under* Heart failure, unspecified)

Cardiac failure, NYHA class IV decompensated
Coreg Tablets 1414
Toprol-XL Tablets 668

Cardiac insufficiency
(*see under* Cardiovascular disorders, unspecified)

Cardiac rhythm disturbances, unspecified
(*see under* Arrhythmia, cardiac, unspecified)

Cardiogenic shock
Betagan Ophthalmic Solution, USP ⊙ 220
Betimol Ophthalmic Solution 3382
Betimol Ophthalmic Solution ⊙ 295
Betoptic S Ophthalmic Suspension 558
Blocadren Tablets 1916
Carteolol Hydrochloride Ophthalmic Solution USP, 1% ⊙ 249
Coreg Tablets 1414
Cosopt Sterile Ophthalmic Solution 1931
Covera-HS Tablets 3139
Inderal LA Long-Acting Capsules 3429
InnoPran XL Capsules 2723
Lopressor Injection 2238
Lopressor Tablets 2238
Lopressor HCT 50/25 Tablets 2241
Lopressor HCT 100/25 Tablets 2241
Lopressor HCT 100/50 Tablets 2241
Nadolol Tablets 2159
OptiPranolol Metipranolol Ophthalmic Solution 0.3% ⊙ 256
Rythmol SR Capsules 2727
Tambocor Tablets 1856
Tarka Tablets 524
Timolide Tablets 2086
Timoptic Sterile Ophthalmic Solution 2088
Timoptic in Ocudose 2091
Timoptic-XE Sterile Ophthalmic Gel Forming Solution 2092
Toprol-XL Tablets 668

Cardiopulmonary bypass
Plasmanate 3255

Cardiospasm
Norflex Injection 1856

Cardiovascular collapse
(*see under* Shock, unspecified)

Cardiovascular disorders, unspecified
(*see also under* Angina pectoris; Angina, Prinzmetal's; Arrhythmia, cardiac, unspecified; Cardiogenic shock; Cardiospasm; Congestive heart failure, uncontrolled; Congestive heart failure, unspecified; Coronary artery disease; Coronary artery disease, history of; ECG changes, history of; Endocarditis, bacterial; Heart disease, ischemic; Heart failure, unspecified; Hypertension, unspecified; Myocardial infarction; Myocardial infarction, history of; Pericardial effusion)
Adderall Tablets 3164
Adderall XR Capsules 3166
Adipex-P 1215
Amerge Tablets 1339
Desoxyn Tablets, USP 2462
Dexedrine 1420
DextroStat Tablets 3179
Imitrex Injection 1463
Indocin I.V. 2465
Parnate Tablets 1527
Relpax Tablets 2548
Zomig Tablets 3519
Zomig-ZMT Tablets 3519

Cardiovascular status, unstable in acute hemorrhage
Bentyl Capsules 697
Bentyl Injection 697
Bentyl Syrup 697
Bentyl Tablets 697
Donnatal Extentabs 2493

Cavernosal fibrosis
(*see under* Fibrosis, cavernosal)

Cellular immune deficiency
(*see under* Immunodeficiency, unspecified)

Central nervous system depression
Clozaril Tablets 2184
FazaClo Orally Disintegrating Tablets 551
Moban Tablets 1119
Thioridazine Hydrochloride Tablets 2163
Thiothixene Capsules 2165

Cephalopelvic disproportion
Cervidil Vaginal Insert 1181

Cerebral apoplexy
(*see under* Cerebrovascular accident)

Cerebral herniation
Xigris Powder for Intravenous Infusion 1828

Cerebral vascular accident
(*see under* Cerebrovascular accident)

Cerebral vascular disease
(*see also under* Bleeding, intracranial; Cerebrovascular accident)
Depo-Provera Contraceptive Injection 2622
depo-subQ provera 104 Injectable Suspension 2624
Mircette Tablets 1066
NuvaRing 2340
Ortho-Cyclen Tablets 2429
Ortho Evra Transdermal System 2417
Ortho Tri-Cyclen Tablets 2429
Ortho Tri-Cyclen Lo Tablets 2436
Parnate Tablets 1527
Seasonique Tablets 1077
Yasmin 28 Tablets 796
Yaz Tablets 803

Cerebral vascular disease, history of
(*see also under* Cerebrovascular accident, history of)
Depo-Provera Contraceptive Injection 2622
depo-subQ provera 104 Injectable Suspension 2624
NuvaRing 2340
Seasonique Tablets 1077
Yaz Tablets 803

Cerebrovascular accident
(*see also under* Bleeding, intracranial)
Amerge Tablets 1339
Estratest H.S. Tablets 3199
Frova Tablets 1113
Imitrex Injection 1463
Imitrex Nasal Spray 1467
Imitrex Tablets 1471
Premphase Tablets 3456
Prempro Tablets 3456
Prometrium Capsules (100 mg, 200 mg) 3203
Relpax Tablets 2548
ReoPro Vials 1809

Cerebrovascular accident, history of
Activase I.V. 1223
Aggrastat 1907
Estratest H.S. Tablets 3199
Integrilin Injection 3020
Prempro Tablets 3456
Prometrium Capsules (100 mg, 200 mg) 3203
ReoPro Vials 1809
Retavase 2499
TNKase I.V. 1264

Cerebrovascular defects
(*see under* Cerebral vascular disease)

Cerebrovascular disorders, unspecified
(*see under* Cerebral vascular disease; Neurological disorders, unspecified)

Cerebrovascular hemorrhage
(*see under* Bleeding, intracranial; Cerebrovascular accident)

Cerebrovascular syndrome
Amerge Tablets ... 1339
Imitrex Nasal Spray ... 1467
Imitrex Tablets ... 1471
Relpax Tablets ... 2548
Zomig Nasal Spray ... 3523

Cervicitis, mucopurulent
ParaGard T 380A Intrauterine Copper Contraceptive ... 1073

Cervicitis, untreated
Mirena Intrauterine System ... 787

Cesarean section, history of
Cervidil Vaginal Insert ... 1181

Chest pain, unspecified, history of
(*see also under* Angina, unspecified, history of)
Proleukin for Injection ... 2266

CHF
(*see under* Congestive heart failure, uncontrolled; Congestive heart failure, unspecified)

Chicken pox
(*see under* Varicella)

Children
Avodart Soft Gelatin Capsules ... 1390
Edex Injection ... 3089
Eligard 22.5 mg ... 2883
Eligard 30 mg ... 2885
Vantas ... 3375

Children below the age of 4 years
Agenerase Capsules ... 1327
Agenerase Oral Solution ... 1332

Cholestasis
Xenical Capsules ... 2831

Chronic obstructive pulmonary disease
(*see also under* Asthma, history of; Asthma, unspecified)
Betagan Ophthalmic Solution, USP ... ⊙220
Betimol Ophthalmic Solution ... 3382
Betimol Ophthalmic Solution ... ⊙295
Blocadren Tablets ... 1916
Carteolol Hydrochloride Ophthalmic Solution USP, 1% ... ⊙249
Cosopt Sterile Ophthalmic Solution ... 1931
OptiPranolol Metipranolol Ophthalmic Solution 0.3% ... ⊙256
Timolide Tablets ... 2086
Timoptic Sterile Ophthalmic Solution ... 2088
Timoptic in Ocudose ... 2091
Timoptic-XE Sterile Ophthalmic Gel Forming Solution ... 2092

Chronic obstructive pulmonary disease, acute
Advair Diskus 100/50 ... 1308
Advair Diskus 250/50 ... 1308
Advair Diskus 500/50 ... 1308

Circulatory collapse
(*see under* Shock, unspecified)

Cirrhosis, primary biliary
Lofibra Tablets ... 1219
Lofibra Capsules ... 1216
Tricor Tablets ... 527
Triglide Tablets ... 3123

Cirrhosis, unspecified
Aldoril Tablets ... 1910
Dantrium Capsules ... 2694
Precose Tablets ... 751

Coagulation disorders
(*see under* Bleeding disorders, unspecified; Hemophilia)

Colitis, antibiotic-associated
Cleocin Vaginal Ovules ... 2616
Duac Topical Gel ... 3212
Evoclin Foam, 1% ... 1009

Colitis, ischemic, history of
Lotronex Tablets ... 1512

Colitis, pseudomembranous
Duac Topical Gel ... 3212

Colitis, toxic
Colyte with Flavor Packs for Oral Solution ... 3088
HalfLytely and Bisacodyl Tablets Bowel Prep Kit with Flavors Packs ... 881
TriLyte with Flavor Packs for Oral Solution ... 3100

Colitis, ulcerative
Bentyl Capsules ... 697
Bentyl Injection ... 697
Bentyl Syrup ... 697
Bentyl Tablets ... 697
Cleocin Vaginal Ovules ... 2616
Donnatal Extentabs ... 2493
Evoclin Foam, 1% ... 1009
Lotronex Tablets ... 1512
Miradon Tablets ... 3042
Precose Tablets ... 751

Colitis, ulcerative, history of
Benzaclin Topical Gel ... 2877
Clindagel ... 1203
Duac Topical Gel ... 3212
Lotronex Tablets ... 1512

Colitis, unspecified
(*see under* Colitis, ulcerative; Enterocolitis, necrotizing)

Colitis, unspecified, history of
Benzaclin Topical Gel ... 2877
Clindagel ... 1203

Collagen diseases, unspecified
(*see under* Lupus erythematosus)

Colonic ulceration
(*see under* Colitis, ulcerative)

Coma, diabetic
Avandamet Tablets ... 1373
FazaClo Orally Disintegrating Tablets ... 551

Coma, hepatic
Bumex Tablets ... 2746
FazaClo Orally Disintegrating Tablets ... 551

Coma, unspecified
Clozaril Tablets ... 2184
FazaClo Orally Disintegrating Tablets ... 551
Moban Tablets ... 1119
Phenergan Tablets and Suppositories ... 3440
Thioridazine Hydrochloride Tablets ... 2163
Thiothixene Capsules ... 2165

Coma, unspecified, history of
Proleukin for Injection ... 2266

Comatose states
(*see under* Coma, diabetic; Coma, hepatic; Coma, unspecified)

Conduction disorders, cardiac
(*see under* Arrhythmia, cardiac, unspecified)

Conduction disturbances
(*see under* Arrhythmia, cardiac, unspecified)

Confusion, drug-induced
Tasmar Tablets ... 3358

Congestive heart failure, uncontrolled
Rythmol SR Capsules ... 2727

Congestive heart failure, unspecified
Fortamet Extended-Release Tablets ... 3115
Inderal LA Long-Acting Capsules ... 3429
Plasbumin-5 ... 3251
Plasbumin-20 ... 3252
Plasbumin-25 ... 3253
Plasmanate ... 3255
Pletal Tablets ... 2455
Remicade for IV Injection ... 971

Constipation
Lotronex Tablets ... 1512

Constipation, severe chronic
Lotronex Tablets ... 1512

Convulsions, history of
(*see under* Seizure disorders, history of)

Convulsive disorders
(*see under* Seizure disorders, unspecified)

Convulsive disorders, history of
(*see under* Seizure disorders, history of)

COPD
(*see under* Chronic obstructive pulmonary disease)

Corneal foreign body removal
Blephamide Ophthalmic Suspension ... 569
Poly-Pred Ophthalmic Suspension ... ⊙233
TobraDex Ophthalmic Ointment ... 562
TobraDex Ophthalmic Suspension ... 563

Coronary artery disease
(*see also under* Coronary artery vasospasm; Stenosis, aortic)
Allegra-D 24 Hour Extended-Release Tablets ... 2849
Mircette Tablets ... 1066
NuvaRing ... 2340
Ortho-Cyclen Tablets ... 2429
Ortho Evra Transdermal System ... 2417
Ortho Tri-Cyclen Tablets ... 2429
Ortho Tri-Cyclen Lo Tablets ... 2436
Seasonique Tablets ... 1077
Yasmin 28 Tablets ... 796
Yaz Tablets ... 803
Zyrtec-D 12 Hour Extended Release Tablets ... 2597

Coronary artery disease, history of
NuvaRing ... 2340
Seasonique Tablets ... 1077
Yaz Tablets ... 803

Coronary artery disease, severe
Allegra-D 12 Hour Extended-Release Tablets ... 2846
Clarinex-D 24-Hour Extended-Release Tablets ... 2998

Coronary artery vasospasm
(*see also under* Angina pectoris; Angina, Prinzmetal's)
Axert Tablets ... 2396
Frova Tablets ... 1113
Imitrex Injection ... 1463
Maxalt Tablets ... 2008
Maxalt-MLT Orally Disintegrating Tablets ... 2008
Migranal Nasal Spray ... 3348
Zomig Tablets ... 3519
Zomig Nasal Spray ... 3523
Zomig-ZMT Tablets ... 3519

Coronary heart disease
(*see under* Cardiovascular disorders, unspecified)

Coronary insufficiency
(*see under* Cardiovascular disorders, unspecified)

Coronary occlusion
(*see under* Myocardial infarction)

Creatinine clearance, abnormal
(*see under* Renal dysfunction)

Critical illness, acute
Genotropin Lyophilized Powder ... 2638
Humatrope Vials and Cartridges ... 1787
Norditropin Cartridges ... 2323
Nutropin for Injection ... 1239
Nutropin AQ Injection ... 1243
Nutropin AQ Pen ... 1243
Nutropin AQ Pen Cartridge ... 1243
Tev-Tropin for Injection ... 1222

Crohn's disease
Lotronex Tablets ... 1512

Cysticercosis, ocular
Biltricide Tablets ... 2976

Cysts, ovarian
Follistim AQ Cartridge ... 2338

D

Deep vein thrombophlebitis, history of
(*see under* Thrombophlebitis, history of)

Deep vein thrombosis
Climara Transdermal System ... 771
Climara Pro Transdermal System ... 776
Enjuvia Tablets ... 1062
Estrasorb Topical Emulsion ... 1147
Estratest Tablets ... 3199
Estratest H.S. Tablets ... 3199
Menostar Transdermal System ... 782
Premarin Intravenous ... 3442
Premarin Tablets ... 3446
Premarin Vaginal Cream ... 3452
Prempro Tablets ... 3456
Prometrium Capsules (100 mg, 200 mg) ... 3203

Deep vein thrombosis, history of
Climara Transdermal System ... 771
Climara Pro Transdermal System ... 776
Enjuvia Tablets ... 1062
Estrasorb Topical Emulsion ... 1147
Estratest Tablets ... 3199
Estratest H.S. Tablets ... 3199
Menostar Transdermal System ... 782
Premarin Intravenous ... 3442
Premarin Tablets ... 3446
Premarin Vaginal Cream ... 3452
Premphase Tablets ... 3456
Prempro Tablets ... 3456
Prometrium Capsules (100 mg, 200 mg) ... 3203
Soltamox Oral Solution ... 3527

Dehydration, unspecified
Urocit-K Tablets ... 2144
Uroqid-Acid No. 2 Tablets ... 760

Delivery, unspecified
Dilaudid Oral Liquid ... 445
Dilaudid Tablets - 8 mg ... 445
Dilaudid-HP ... 442

Dendritic keratitis
(*see under* Herpes simplex keratitis)

Depression, mental
Seromycin Capsules ... 1813

Diabetes, type 2, with microalbuminuria
Inspra Tablets ... 2536

Diabetes, unspecified
Podocon-25 Liquid ... 2478

Diabetes mellitus
Tequin Injection ... 938
Tequin Injection in 5% Dextrose ... 938
Tequin Tablets ... 938
Urocit-K Tablets ... 2144

Diabetes mellitus, type 1, sole therapy
Starlix Tablets ... 2292

Diabetes with vascular involvement
NuvaRing ... 2340
Ortho Evra Transdermal System ... 2417
Ortho Tri-Cyclen Lo Tablets ... 2436
Seasonique Tablets ... 1077
Yaz Tablets ... 803

Diabetic gastroparesis
(*see under* Gastroparesis, diabetic)

Diabetic ketoacidosis
(*see under* Ketoacidosis, diabetic)

Diabetic nephropathy
(*see under* Nephropathy, diabetic)

Diarrhea, severe
Edecrin ... 1959

Dihydropyrimidine Dehydrogenase (DPD) Deficiency
Carac Cream, 0.5% ... 2879
Efudex ... 3363
Xeloda Tablets ... 2822

Disease, infectious, unspecified
Mustargen for Injection ... 2468

Dissecting aorta
Coumadin for Injection ... 898
Coumadin Tablets ... 898

Diverticulitis
Lotronex Tablets ... 1512
Miradon Tablets ... 3042

Drug abuse, history of
Adderall Tablets ... 3164
Adderall XR Capsules ... 3166
Adipex-P ... 1215
Desoxyn Tablets, USP ... 2462
Dexedrine ... 1420
DextroStat Tablets ... 3179

Dysgammaglobulinemia
Attenuvax ... 1914
Meruvax II ... 2019
M-M-R II ... 2006
Mumpsvax ... 2031
ProQuad ... 2064
Varivax ... 2100

E

ECG, QT syndrome, long
Thioridazine Hydrochloride Tablets ... 2163

ECG changes, history of
Proleukin for Injection ... 2266

Eclampsia
Coumadin for Injection ... 898
Coumadin Tablets ... 898
Miradon Tablets ... 3042

Effusion, pericardial
(*see under* Pericardial effusion)

Electrocardiogram changes
(*see under* ECG changes, history of)

Electrocardiographic alterations, QTc prolongation
Ranexa Tablets ... 1035

Electrolyte depletion
(*see under* Electrolyte imbalance, uncorrected)

Electrolyte disturbances
(*see under* Electrolyte imbalance, uncorrected)

Electrolyte imbalance, uncorrected
(*see also under* Hypercalcemia; Hyperkalemia; Hyperphosphatemia; Hypocalcemia; Hypokalemia; Hyponatremia)
Bumex Tablets ... 2746
Edecrin ... 1959
Rythmol SR Capsules ... 2727

Emaciation
Miradon Tablets ... 3042

Encephalopathy, history of
ADACEL Vaccine ... 2945
Boostrix ... 1404
DAPTACEL Vaccine ... 2950
Infanrix Vaccine ... 1476
Pediarix Vaccine ... 1548

Endocarditis, bacterial
Arixtra Injection ... 1351
Coumadin for Injection ... 898
Coumadin Tablets ... 898
Miradon Tablets ... 3042

Endometrial cancer
(*see under* Carcinoma, endometrium)

Endometritis, postpartum
Mirena Intrauterine System ... 787
ParaGard T 380A Intrauterine Copper Contraceptive ... 1073

Enteritis, history of
Benzaclin Topical Gel ... 2877
Cleocin Vaginal Ovules ... 2616
Clindagel ... 1203
Duac Topical Gel ... 3212
Evoclin Foam, 1% ... 1009

Enterobiasis, prophylactic treatment for
Mintezol ... 2027

Enterocolitis, necrotizing
Indocin I.V. ... 2465
NeoProfen Injection ... 2472

Epidural catheter, presence of
Xigris Powder for Intravenous Infusion ... 1828

Epilepsy
Seromycin Capsules ... 1813

Epilepsy, uncontrolled
(*see also under* Status epilepticus)
ADACEL Vaccine ... 2945
Boostrix ... 1404
Clozaril Tablets ... 2184
FazaClo Orally Disintegrating Tablets ... 551
Infanrix Vaccine ... 1476
Pediarix Vaccine ... 1548

Epiphyses, closed
Genotropin Lyophilized Powder ... 2638
Humatrope Vials and Cartridges ... 1787
Increlex Injection ... 3291
Norditropin Cartridges ... 2323
Nutropin for Injection ... 1239
Nutropin AQ Injection ... 1243
Nutropin AQ Pen ... 1243
Nutropin AQ Pen Cartridge ... 1243
Tev-Tropin for Injection ... 1222

Epiphyses, fused
(*see under* Epiphyses, closed)

Epithelial herpes simplex keratitis
(*see under* Herpes simplex keratitis)

Esophageal abnormalities, unspecified
(*see also under* Achalasia, esophageal; Esophageal compression; Esophagitis, reflux; Stricture, esophageal)
Fosamax ... 1969
Fosamax Plus D Tablets ... 1977

Esophageal achalasia
(*see under* Achalasia, esophageal)

Esophageal compression
K-Dur Extended-Relase Tablets ... 3033

Esophageal stricture
(*see under* Stricture, esophageal)

Esophageal ulcers less than 1 cm
Photofrin for Injection ... 702

Esophageal varices
Photofrin for Injection ... 702

Esophagitis, reflux
Bentyl Capsules ... 697
Bentyl Injection ... 697
Bentyl Syrup ... 697
Bentyl Tablets ... 697

Exercise, strenuous physical
Urocit-K Tablets ... 2144

Eye infection
(*see under* Cysticercosis, ocular; Infection, ophthalmic, fungal; Infection, ophthalmic, mycobacterial; Infection, ophthalmic, viral; Iritis, acute)

Eye surgery
(*see under* Surgery, ophthalmic)

F

Fallot's tetralogy
(*see under* Tetralogy of Fallot)

Febrile illness
(*see under* Fever; Infection, febrile; Respiratory illness, febrile)

Fecal impaction
Citrucel Orange Flavor Powder ... ▣ 647
Citrucel Sugar Free Orange Flavor Powder ... ▣ 648

Fetal distress, non-imminent delivery
Cervidil Vaginal Insert ... 1181

Fever
(*see also under* Infection, febrile; Respiratory illness, febrile)
DAPTACEL Vaccine ... 2950
ProQuad ... 2064
Tasmar Tablets ... 3358

Fibrillation, atrial
Covera-HS Tablets ... 3139
Verelan PM Extended-Release Capsules, Controlled-Onset ... 3106

Fibrillation, ventricular
Lanoxicaps Capsules ... 1490
Lanoxin Injection ... 1494
Lanoxin Injection Pediatric ... 1497
Lanoxin Tablets ... 1500

Fibrosis, cavernosal
Caverject Impulse Injection ... 2612
Edex Injection ... 3089

Fibrosis, unspecified
(*see under* Fibrosis, cavernosal)

Fibrotic processes
(*see under* Fibrosis, cavernosal)

Fluid overload
Orthoclone OKT3 Sterile Solution ... 2360

Flutter, atrial
Covera-HS Tablets ... 3139
Verelan PM Extended-Release Capsules, Controlled-Onset ... 3106

Fungal disease, ophthalmic
Retisert Implant ... ⊙ 258

Fungal infections
(*see under* Actinomycosis, genital; Infection, ophthalmic, fungal; Infection, systemic, fungal)

G

Gallbladder disease, unspecified
Lofibra Tablets ... 1219
Lofibra Capsules ... 1216
Tricor Tablets ... 527
Triglide Tablets ... 3123
Zelnorm Tablets ... 2312

Gastric retention
Colyte with Flavor Packs for Oral Solution ... 3088
Detrol Tablets ... 2628
Detrol LA Capsules ... 2631
Ditropan XL Extended-Release Tablets ... 2413
Enablex Extended-Release Tablets ... 2203
HalfLytely and Bisacodyl Tablets Bowel Prep Kit with Flavors Packs ... 881
Oxytrol Transdermal System ... 3392
Sanctura Tablets ... 1151
TriLyte with Flavor Packs for Oral Solution ... 3100
VESIcare Tablets ... 646

Gastric varices
Photofrin for Injection ... 702

Gastroenteritis
Dulcolax Suppositories ... ▣ 648

Gastrointestinal adhesion, history of
Lotronex Tablets ... 1512

Gastrointestinal disorders
(*see under* Bleeding, gastrointestinal; Esophageal abnormalities, unspecified; Gastric retention; Gastroparesis, diabetic; Hernia, hiatal; Inflammation, gastrointestinal tract; Intestinal disorders, unspecified; Obstruction, gastrointestinal tract; Perforation, gastrointestinal tract; Ulcer, gastrointestinal)

Gastrointestinal obstruction
(*see under* Obstruction, gastrointestinal tract)

Gastrointestinal perforation
(*see under* Perforation, gastrointestinal tract)

Gastroparesis
Symlin Injection ... 613

Gastroparesis, diabetic
K-Tab Tablets ... 475

General anesthesia
(*see under* Anesthesia, general)

Genital bleeding
(*see under* Bleeding, genital, abnormal)

Glaucoma, narrow-angle, uncontrolled
Detrol Tablets ... 2628
Detrol LA Capsules ... 2631
Enablex Extended-Release Tablets ... 2203
Sanctura Tablets ... 1151
VESIcare Tablets ... 646

Glaucoma, angle closure
Albalon Ophthalmic Solution ... ⊙ 218
Allegra-D 12 Hour Extended-Release Tablets ... 2846
Allegra-D 24 Hour Extended-Release Tablets ... 2849
Clarinex-D 24-Hour Extended-Release Tablets ... 2998
Cymbalta Delayed-Release Capsules ... 1757
Diastat Rectal Delivery System ... 3343
Ditropan XL Extended-Release Tablets ... 2413
Evoxac Capsules ... 1047
Klonopin ... 2778
Niravam Orally Disintegrating Tablets ... 3092
Oxytrol Transdermal System ... 3392
Parcopa Orally Disintegrating Tablets ... 3097
Stalevo Tablets ... 2287
Strattera Capsules ... 1814
Transderm Scōp Transdermal Therapeutic System ... 2177
Tranxene ... 2474
Valium Tablets ... 2819
Zyrtec-D 12 Hour Extended Release Tablets ... 2597

Glaucoma, narrow angle
(*see under* Glaucoma, angle closure)

Glaucoma, open angle, untreated
Klonopin 2778
Niravam Orally Disintegrating Tablets 3092
Valium Tablets 2819

Glaucoma, unspecified
Adderall Tablets 3164
Adderall XR Capsules 3166
Adipex-P 1215
Bentyl Capsules 697
Bentyl Injection 697
Bentyl Syrup 697
Bentyl Tablets 697
Concerta Extended-Release Tablets 1881
Daytrana Transdermal Patch 3174
Desoxyn Tablets, USP 2462
Dexedrine 1420
DextroStat Tablets 3179
Donnatal Extentabs 2493
Focalin Tablets 2220
Focalin XR Capsules 2223
Metadate CD Capsules 3323
Norflex Injection 1856
Ritalin Hydrochloride Tablets 2269
Ritalin LA Capsules 2271
Ritalin-SR Tablets 2269

Glucose-6-phosphate dehydrogenase
Elitek 2890

Granulocytopenia, history of
Clozaril Tablets 2184
FazaClo Orally Disintegrating Tablets 551

Guillain-Barre syndrome, history of
Flumist Vaccine 1901
Menactra Vaccine 2954

H

Head injury
(*see also under* Trauma, intracranial)
DepoDur Extended-Release Injection 1110

Headache
(*see under* Headache, history of; Migraine, basilar; Migraine, hemiplegic)

Headache, history of
Parnate Tablets 1527

Headaches with focal neurological symptoms
NuvaRing 2340
Ortho-Cyclen Tablets 2429
Ortho Evra Transdermal System 2417
Ortho Tri-Cyclen Tablets 2429
Ortho Tri-Cyclen Lo Tablets 2436
Seasonique Tablets 1077
Yasmin 28 Tablets 796
Yaz Tablets 803

Heart attack
(*see under* Myocardial infarction)

Heart block, first degree, significant
Lopressor Injection 2238
Lopressor Tablets 2238

Heart block, greater than first degree
Adenocard Injection 617
Adenoscan 619
Betagan Ophthalmic Solution, USP ⊙ 220
Betimol Ophthalmic Solution 3382
Betimol Ophthalmic Solution ⊙ 295
Betoptic S Ophthalmic Suspension 558
Blocadren Tablets 1916
Cardizem LA Extended Release Tablets 1728
Carteolol Hydrochloride Ophthalmic Solution USP, 1% ⊙ 249
Coreg Tablets 1414
Covera-HS Tablets 3139
Inderal LA Long-Acting Capsules 3429
InnoPran XL Capsules 2723
Lopressor Injection 2238
Lopressor Tablets 2238
Lopressor HCT 50/25 Tablets 2241
Lopressor HCT 100/25 Tablets 2241
Lopressor HCT 100/50 Tablets 2241
Nadolol Tablets 2159
OptiPranolol Metipranolol Ophthalmic Solution 0.3% ⊙ 256
Tambocor Tablets 1856
Tarka Tablets 524
Tiazac Capsules 1201
Timolide Tablets 2086
Timoptic Sterile Ophthalmic Solution 2088
Timoptic in Ocudose 2091
Timoptic-XE Sterile Ophthalmic Gel Forming Solution 2092
Toprol-XL Tablets 668
Verelan PM Extended-Release Capsules, Controlled-Onset 3106

Heart block, second degree
Lopressor Injection 2238
Lopressor Tablets 2238

Heart block, third degree
Lopressor Injection 2238
Lopressor Tablets 2238

Heart block, unspecified
Primaxin I.M. 2045
Tambocor Tablets 1856

Heart damage
(*see under* Cardiovascular disorders, unspecified)

Heart disease, ischemic
(*see also under* Angina pectoris; Ischemia, silent; Myocardial infarction)
Amerge Tablets 1339
Axert Tablets 2396
Frova Tablets 1113
Imitrex Injection 1463
Imitrex Nasal Spray 1467
Imitrex Tablets 1471
Maxalt Tablets 2008
Maxalt-MLT Orally Disintegrating Tablets 2008
Migranal Nasal Spray 3348
Relpax Tablets 2548
Zomig Tablets 3519
Zomig Nasal Spray 3523
Zomig-ZMT Tablets 3519

Heart disease, severe organic
ProAmatine Tablets 3186

Heart disease, unspecified
(*see under* Cardiovascular disorders, unspecified)

Heart disease, valvular
NuvaRing 2340
Yasmin 28 Tablets 796

Heart failure, intravascular volume, increased
Albutein 5%, Albumin (Human) 1652
Albutein 25% , Albumin (Human) 1653

Heart failure, moderate
Lopressor Injection 2238
Lopressor Tablets 2238

Heart failure, severe
Lopressor Injection 2238
Lopressor Tablets 2238

Heart failure, unspecified
(*see also under* Congestive heart failure, unspecified)
Albutein 5%, Albumin (Human) 1652
Albutein 25% , Albumin (Human) 1653
Betagan Ophthalmic Solution, USP ⊙ 220
Betimol Ophthalmic Solution 3382
Betimol Ophthalmic Solution ⊙ 295
Betoptic S Ophthalmic Suspension 558
Blocadren Tablets 1916
Carteolol Hydrochloride Ophthalmic Solution USP, 1% ⊙ 249
Cosopt Sterile Ophthalmic Solution 1931
Flexbumin I.V. 720
Geodon 2529
Human Albumin Grifols 20%, Albumin (Human) 1651
Human Albumin Grifols 25%, Albumin (Human) 1652
Lopressor Injection 2238
Lopressor Tablets 2238
Lopressor HCT 50/25 Tablets 2241
Lopressor HCT 100/25 Tablets 2241
Lopressor HCT 100/50 Tablets 2241
Nadolol Tablets 2159
OptiPranolol Metipranolol Ophthalmic Solution 0.3% ⊙ 256
Orthoclone OKT3 Sterile Solution 2360
Timolide Tablets 2086
Timoptic Sterile Ophthalmic Solution 2088
Timoptic in Ocudose 2091
Timoptic-XE Sterile Ophthalmic Gel Forming Solution 2092
Toprol-XL Tablets 668

Heart rate less than 45 beats per minute
Lopressor Injection 2238
Lopressor Tablets 2238

Hematologic disorders
(*see under* Bleeding disorders, unspecified; Blood dyscrasias, unspecified)

Hematopoietic disorders
(*see under* Blood dyscrasias, unspecified; Bone marrow depression)

Hemoglobinopathies
Copegus Tablets 2754
Rebetol 3058
Ribavirin, USP Capsules 3068

Hemophilia
Percodan Tablets 1132

Hemorrhage
(*see under* Bleeding disorders, unspecified; Bleeding tendencies; Bleeding, abnormal, unspecified; Bleeding, gastrointestinal; Bleeding, gastrointestinal, history of; Bleeding, genital, abnormal; Bleeding, genitourinary; Bleeding, history of; Bleeding, internal, unspecified; Bleeding, intracranial; Bleeding, rectal; Bleeding, unspecified; Cardiovascular status, unstable in acute hemorrhage)

Hemorrhagic diathesis
(*see under* Bleeding tendencies)

Hemorrhagic stroke
(*see under* Stroke, hemorrhagic)

Hemostatic disorders
(*see under* Bleeding disorders, unspecified)

Hepatic adenoma
(*see under* Adenoma, hepatic)

Hepatic cancer
(*see under* Carcinoma, hepatic)

Hepatic coma
(*see under* Coma, hepatic)

Hepatic damage
(*see under* Liver dysfunction)

Hepatic decompensation
Copegus Tablets 2754
Infergen 3364
Pegasys 2789

Hepatic disease
(*see under* Liver disease, unspecified)

Hepatic dysfunction
(*see also under* Liver dysfunction)
Triglide Tablets 3123
Yaz Tablets 803

Hepatic failure
(*see under* Liver failure)

Hepatic impairment
(*see under* Liver dysfunction)

Hepatic impairment, moderate
Aptivus Capsules 826
Opana Tablets 1122

Hepatic impairment, severe
Agrylin Capsules 3169
Amerge Tablets 1339
Aptivus Capsules 826
Miradon Tablets 3042
Opana Tablets 1122
Trecator Tablets 3487

Hepatic injury
(*see under* Liver dysfunction)

Hepatic insufficiency
(*see under* Liver dysfunction)

Hepatitis
Aldoril Tablets 1910
Calcium Disodium Versenate Injection 1851
Dantrium Capsules 2694

Hepatitis, autoimmune
Copegus Tablets 2754
Infergen 3364
Pegasys 2789
PEG-Intron Powder for Injection 3048
Rebetron Combination Therapy 3063
Ribavirin, USP Capsules 3068

Hepatitis, history of
Ketek Tablets 2903

Hepatocellular failure
(*see under* Liver failure)

Hernia, hiatal
Donnatal Extentabs 2493

Herpes simplex keratitis
Alrex Ophthalmic Suspension 0.2% ⊙ 246
Blephamide Ophthalmic Ointment 568
Blephamide Ophthalmic Suspension 569
FML Ophthalmic Ointment ⊙ 228
FML Ophthalmic Suspension ⊙ 227
FML Forte Ophthalmic Suspension ⊙ 226
FML-S Ophthalmic Suspension ⊙ 229
Lotemax Ophthalmic Suspension 0.5% ⊙ 251
Poly-Pred Ophthalmic Suspension ⊙ 233
Pred Mild Ophthalmic Suspension ⊙ 238
Pred Forte Ophthalmic Suspension ⊙ 235
Pred-G Ophthalmic Ointment ⊙ 237
Pred-G Ophthalmic Suspension ⊙ 236
TobraDex Ophthalmic Ointment 562
TobraDex Ophthalmic Suspension 563

Herpes zoster
Cosmegen for Injection 2459

Hiatal hernia
(*see under* Hernia, hiatal)

HIV
(*see under* Human immunodeficiency virus)

Human Immunodeficiency Syndrome
Zostavax Injection 2111

Human immunodeficiency virus
(*see also under* Acquired immune deficiency syndrome)
Amevive 626
Attenuvax 1914
Flumist Vaccine 1901
Infanrix Vaccine 1476
Mumpsvax 2031
Pediarix Vaccine 1548
ProQuad 2064
Varivax 2100

Hypercalcemia
Actonel with Calcium Tablets 2688
Calcijex Injection 411

Hectorol Capsules 1275
Hectorol Injection 1278
Oxandrin Tablets 2962
PhosLo GelCaps 2169
Rocaltrol Capsules 2798
Rocaltrol Oral Solution 2798
Zemplar Capsules 541
Zemplar Injection 543

Hypercarbia
Opana ER Tablets 1126
OxyContin Tablets 2703
OxyFast Oral Concentrate Solution 2708
OxyIR Capsules 2708
Percodan Tablets 1132

Hypercoagulable state, history of
Lotronex Tablets 1512

Hyperkalemia
Dyazide Capsules 1423
Dyrenium Capsules 3400
Inspra Tablets 2536
K-Dur Extended-Relase Tablets 3033
K-Lor Oral Solution 474
K-Phos Original (Sodium Free) Tablets 760
K-Tab Tablets 475
Midamor Tablets 2026
Moduretic Tablets 2028
Urocit-K Tablets 2144

Hyperphosphatemia
K-Phos Original (Sodium Free) Tablets 760
K-Phos Neutral Tablets 760
Uroqid-Acid No. 2 Tablets 760

Hypersensitivity to benzyl alcohol
Lovenox Injection 2915
Nutropin for Injection 1239

Hypersensitivity to pork products
Lovenox Injection 2915

Hypertension, compensatory
Hyperstat I.V. 3017

Hypertension, excessive supine
ProAmatine Tablets 3186

Hypertension, malignant
Coumadin for Injection 898
Coumadin Tablets 898
Miradon Tablets 3042

Hypertension, moderate
Adderall XR Capsules 3166
DextroStat Tablets 3179

Hypertension, severe
Adderall XR Capsules 3166
Allegra-D 12 Hour Extended-Release Tablets 2846
Clarinex-D 24-Hour Extended-Release Tablets 2998
DextroStat Tablets 3179
Miradon Tablets 3042
NuvaRing 2340
Seasonique Tablets 1077
Yaz Tablets 803

Hypertension, uncontrolled
Activase I.V. 1223
Aggrastat 1907
Amerge Tablets 1339
Aranesp for Injection 581
Axert Tablets 2396
Epogen for Injection 591
Frova Tablets 1113
Gengraf Capsules 459
Imitrex Nasal Spray 1467
Imitrex Tablets 1471
Integrilin Injection 3020
Maxalt Tablets 2008
Maxalt-MLT Orally Disintegrating Tablets 2008
Migranal Nasal Spray 3348
Neoral Oral Solution 2259
Neoral Soft Gelatin Capsules 2259
Orthoclone OKT3 Sterile Solution 2360
Procrit for Injection 2364
Relpax Tablets 2548
ReoPro Vials 1809
Retavase 2499
TNKase I.V. 1264
Zomig Tablets 3519
Zomig Nasal Spray 3523
Zomig-ZMT Tablets 3519

Hypertension, unspecified
Adderall Tablets 3164
Adipex-P 1215
Allegra-D 24 Hour Extended-Release Tablets 2849
Desoxyn Tablets, USP 2462
Dexedrine 1420
DextroStat Tablets 3179
Imitrex Injection 1463
Ortho Evra Transdermal System 2417
Ortho Tri-Cyclen Lo Tablets 2436
Parnate Tablets 1527
Yasmin 28 Tablets 796
Zyrtec-D 12 Hour Extended Release Tablets 2597

Hyperthermia, malignant, susceptibility to
Ultane Liquid for Inhalation 531

Hyperthyroidism
(*see also under* Thyrotoxicosis; Thyrotoxicosis, untreated)
Adderall Tablets 3164
Adderall XR Capsules 3166
Adipex-P 1215
Desoxyn Tablets, USP 2462
Dexedrine 1420
DextroStat Tablets 3179

Hypervitaminosis D
(*see under* Toxicity, vitamin D)

Hypervolemia
Plasmanate 3255

Hypocalcemia
Actonel Tablets 2683
Actonel with Calcium Tablets 2688
Boniva Injection 2738
Boniva Tablets 2741
Fosamax 1969
Fosamax Plus D Tablets 1977

Hypogammaglobulinemia
(*see also under* Immunodeficiency, unspecified)
Attenuvax 1914
Meruvax II 2019
M-M-R II 2006
Mumpsvax 2031
ProQuad 2064
Varivax 2100

Hypoglycemia, unspecified
Apidra Injection 2864
Humalog-Pen 1781
Humalog Mix 50/50-Pen 1783
Humulin R, 100 Units 1798
NovoLog Injection 2326
NovoLog Mix 70/30 2328
Symlin Injection 613

Hypokalemia
Daranide Tablets 1950

Hypomotility syndrome, neonates
Kionex Powder 2477

Hyponatremia
Daranide Tablets 1950
Kionex Powder 2477

Hyponatremia, hypovolemic
Vaprisol 643

Hypophosphatemia
Renagel Tablets 1282

Hypotension, history of
Mivacron Injection 493

Hypotension, unspecified
Cardizem LA Extended Release Tablets 1728
Covera-HS Tablets 3139
Rythmol SR Capsules 2727
Tarka Tablets 524
Tiazac Capsules 1201
Verelan PM Extended-Release Capsules, Controlled-Onset 3106

Hypovolemia
(*see under* Shock, unspecified)

I

IgA deficiencies, selective
(*see under* Immunoglobulin A deficiency)

Ileocolostomy
Activase I.V. 1223
Colocort Rectal Suspension, USP (Retention) 100 mg/60 mL 2476

Ileus, paralytic
Avinza Capsules 1741
DepoDur Extended-Release Injection 1110
Donnatal Extentabs 2493
Duragesic Transdermal System 2373
FazaClo Orally Disintegrating Tablets 551
Kadian Capsules 577
MS Contin Tablets 2701
Opana Tablets 1122
Opana ER Tablets 1126
OxyContin Tablets 2703
OxyFast Oral Concentrate Solution 2708
OxyIR Capsules 2708
Percodan Tablets 1132

Ileus, unspecified
(*see also under* Ileus, paralytic)
Colyte with Flavor Packs for Oral Solution 3088
HalfLytely and Bisacodyl Tablets Bowel Prep Kit with Flavors Packs 881
TriLyte with Flavor Packs for Oral Solution 3100

Immunodeficiency, family history of
Meruvax II 2019
M-M-R II 2006
Mumpsvax 2031
ProQuad 2064

Immunodeficiency, history of
Attenuvax 1914
ProQuad 2064
Varivax 2100
Zostavax Injection 2111

Immunodeficiency, unspecified
(*see also under* Acquired immune deficiency syndrome; Dysgammaglobulinemia; Human immunodeficiency virus; Hypogammaglobulinemia; Immunodeficiency, family history of; Immunodeficiency, history of; Immunoglobulin A deficiency; Immunosuppression)
Attenuvax 1914
Flumist Vaccine 1901
Meruvax II 2019
M-M-R II 2006
Mumpsvax 2031
ProQuad 2064
Varivax 2100
Vivotif 819

Immunodeficient state
(*see under* Immunodeficiency, unspecified)

Immunoglobulin A deficiency
Aralast 717
CytoGam Intravenous 1895
Flebogamma 5%, Immune Globulin Intravenous (Human) 1658
GamaSTAN 3234
Gammagard S/D 724
Vivaglobin 3506

Immunosuppression
Attenuvax 1914
Flumist Vaccine 1901
Meruvax II 2019
M-M-R II 2006
Mumpsvax 2031
ProQuad 2064
Varivax 2100
Vivotif 819

Impulse generation disorders
(*see under* Arrhythmia, cardiac, unspecified)

Inability to stand or sit upright for at least 30 minutes
Actonel Tablets 2683
Actonel with Calcium Tablets 2688
Fosamax 1969
Fosamax Plus D Tablets 1977

Inability to stand or sit upright for at least 60 minutes
Boniva Tablets 2741

Increased intracranial pressure
(*see under* Intracranial pressure, increased)

Infants
Agenerase Capsules 1327
Agenerase Oral Solution 1332
Bentyl Capsules 697
Bentyl Injection 697
Bentyl Syrup 697
Bentyl Tablets 697
Caverject Impulse Injection 2612
Fansidar Tablets 2765
Gantrisin Pediatric Suspension 2770
Ovide .5% Lotion 3290
Pegasys 2789
WinRho SDF 732

Infection, bacterial, unspecified
(*see under* Endocarditis, bacterial)

Infection, febrile
Attenuvax 1914
DAPTACEL Vaccine 2950
Meruvax II 2019
M-M-R II 2006
Mumpsvax 2031
ProQuad 2064
Varivax 2100

Infection, fungal
(*see under* Actinomycosis, genital; Infection, ophthalmic, fungal; Infection, systemic, fungal)

Infection, fungal, unspecified
(*see under* Actinomycosis, genital)

Infection, injection site
BOTOX Purified Neurotoxin Complex 570
Euflexxa 1162
Hyalgan Solution 2901

Infection, knee joint
Euflexxa 1162

Infection, mycobacterial
(*see under* Infection, ophthalmic, mycobacterial)

Infection, ocular
Lucentis Injection 1237
Macugen Injection ⊙261

Infection, ophthalmic, active
Restasis Ophthalmic Emulsion 575

Infection, ophthalmic, cysticercosis
(*see under* Cysticercosis, ocular)

Infection, ophthalmic, fungal
Alrex Ophthalmic Suspension 0.2% ⊙246
Blephamide Ophthalmic Ointment 568
Blephamide Ophthalmic Suspension 569
FML Ophthalmic Ointment ⊙228
FML Ophthalmic Suspension ⊙227
FML Forte Ophthalmic Suspension ⊙226
FML-S Ophthalmic Suspension ⊙229
Lotemax Ophthalmic Suspension 0.5% ⊙251
Poly-Pred Ophthalmic Suspension ⊙233
Pred Mild Ophthalmic Suspension ⊙238
Pred Forte Ophthalmic Suspension ⊙235
Pred-G Ophthalmic Ointment ⊙237
Pred-G Ophthalmic Suspension ⊙236
TobraDex Ophthalmic Ointment 562
TobraDex Ophthalmic Suspension 563

Infection, ophthalmic, mycobacterial
Alrex Ophthalmic Suspension 0.2% ⊙246
Blephamide Ophthalmic Ointment 568
Blephamide Ophthalmic Suspension 569
FML Ophthalmic Ointment ⊙228
FML Ophthalmic Suspension ⊙227
FML Forte Ophthalmic Suspension ⊙226

FML-S Ophthalmic Suspension ⊙ 229
Lotemax Ophthalmic Suspension 0.5% ⊙ 251
Poly-Pred Ophthalmic Suspension ⊙ 233
Pred Mild Ophthalmic Suspension ⊙ 238
Pred Forte Ophthalmic Suspension ⊙ 235
Pred-G Ophthalmic Ointment ⊙ 237
Pred-G Ophthalmic Suspension ⊙ 236
TobraDex Ophthalmic Ointment 562
TobraDex Ophthalmic Suspension 563

Infection, ophthalmic, unspecified
(*see under* Cysticercosis, ocular; Iritis, acute)

Infection, ophthalmic, untreated
Pred Mild Ophthalmic Suspension ⊙ 238
Pred Forte Ophthalmic Suspension ⊙ 235

Infection, ophthalmic, viral
(*see also under* Herpes simplex keratitis)
Blephamide Ophthalmic Ointment 568
Blephamide Ophthalmic Suspension 569
FML Ophthalmic Ointment ⊙ 228
FML Ophthalmic Suspension ⊙ 227
FML Forte Ophthalmic Suspension ⊙ 226
Lotemax Ophthalmic Suspension 0.5% ⊙ 251
Poly-Pred Ophthalmic Suspension ⊙ 233
Pred Mild Ophthalmic Suspension ⊙ 238
Pred Forte Ophthalmic Suspension ⊙ 235
Pred-G Ophthalmic Ointment ⊙ 237
Pred-G Ophthalmic Suspension ⊙ 236
TobraDex Ophthalmic Ointment 562
TobraDex Ophthalmic Suspension 563

Infection, periocular
Lucentis Injection 1237
Macugen Injection ⊙ 261

Infection, respiratory
(*see under* Respiratory illness, febrile)

Infection, scalp
Temovate Scalp Application 2670

Infection, systemic, fungal
Colocort Rectal Suspension, USP (Retention) 100 mg/60 mL 2476
Decadron Tablets 1951
Depo-Medrol Injectable Suspension 2617
Depo-Medrol Single-Dose Vial 2619
Hydrocortone Tablets 1989

Infection, untreated
(*see also under* Infection, ophthalmic, untreated)
Indocin I.V. 2465
NeoProfen Injection 2472

Infection, vaginal
(*see under* Cervicitis, untreated; Vaginitis, untreated; Vaginosis, bacterial, untreated)

Infection, viral
(*see also under* Herpes simplex keratitis; Herpes zoster; Human immunodeficiency virus; Infection, ophthalmic, viral; Varicella)
Bayer Aspirin 744
Bayer Aspirin Comprehensive Prescribing Information ▣ 796
Percodan Tablets 1132

Infection, viral, external canal
Ciprodex Otic Suspension 559

Infertility, treatment of
Synthroid Tablets 520

Inflammation, gastrointestinal tract
(*see also under* Colitis, toxic; Colitis, ulcerative; Colitis, ulcerative, history of; Colitis, unspecified, history of; Diverticulitis; Enteritis, history of; Enterocolitis, necrotizing; Esophagitis, reflux; Gastroenteritis; Ulcer, gastrointestinal)
Precose Tablets 751

Inflammatory bowel disease
(*see under* Inflammation, gastrointestinal tract)

Intestinal atony
(*see under* Atony, intestinal)

Intestinal circulation, impaired
Lotronex Tablets 1512

Intestinal disorders, unspecified
(*see also under* Atony, intestinal; Bowel ischemia, history of; Inflammation, gastrointestinal tract; Megacolon, toxic; Obstruction, gastrointestinal tract; Perforation, gastrointestinal tract)
Precose Tablets 751

Intestinal obstruction
(*see under* Obstruction, gastrointestinal tract)

Intoxication, unspecified
Ultram ER 2392

Intracranial pressure, increased
DepoDur Extended-Release Injection 1110
Hycotuss Expectorant Syrup 1117
Romazicon Injection 2804

Intracranial trauma
(*see under* Trauma, intracranial)

Intrathecal administration
Depo-Medrol Single-Dose Vial 2619

Intravenous administration
Increlex Injection 3291

Intubation, history of
Proleukin for Injection 2266

Iritis, acute
Evoxac Capsules 1047

Iron overload, evidence of
Ferrlecit Injection 3388

Ischemia, silent
Amerge Tablets 1339
Axert Tablets 2396
Frova Tablets 1113
Imitrex Injection 1463
Imitrex Nasal Spray 1467
Imitrex Tablets 1471
Maxalt Tablets 2008
Maxalt-MLT Orally Disintegrating Tablets 2008
Migranal Nasal Spray 3348
Relpax Tablets 2548
Zomig Tablets 3519
Zomig Nasal Spray 3523
Zomig-ZMT Tablets 3519

Ischemia, unspecified
Imitrex Injection 1463

Ischemic attacks, transient
Amerge Tablets 1339
Frova Tablets 1113
Imitrex Injection 1463
Imitrex Nasal Spray 1467
Imitrex Tablets 1471
Relpax Tablets 2548
Zomig Nasal Spray 3523

Ischemic heart disease
(*see under* Heart disease, ischemic)

Ischemic myocardial disease
(*see under* Heart disease, ischemic)

J

Jaundice, cholestatic of pregnancy, history of
Mircette Tablets 1066
NuvaRing 2340
Ortho-Cyclen Tablets 2429
Ortho Evra Transdermal System 2417
Ortho Tri-Cyclen Tablets 2429
Ortho Tri-Cyclen Lo Tablets 2436
Seasonique Tablets 1077
Yasmin 28 Tablets 796
Yaz Tablets 803

Jaundice, history of
Augmentin 1360
Augmentin Tablets 1363
Augmentin XR Extended-Release Tablets 1369
Augmentin ES-600 Powder for Oral Suspension 1366
Ketek Tablets 2903
Mircette Tablets 1066
Ortho-Cyclen Tablets 2429
Ortho Evra Transdermal System 2417
Ortho Tri-Cyclen Tablets 2429
Ortho Tri-Cyclen Lo Tablets 2436
Seasonique Tablets 1077
Yasmin 28 Tablets 796
Yaz Tablets 803

K

Keratitis, dendritic
(*see under* Herpes simplex keratitis)

Ketoacidosis, diabetic
ActoPlus Met Tablets 3214
Avandamet Tablets 1373
Avandaryl Tablets 1379
Duetact Tablets 3226
Precose Tablets 751
Starlix Tablets 2292

Kidney damage
(*see under* Renal dysfunction)

Kidney disease
(*see under* Renal disease, unspecified)

Kidney failure
(*see under* Renal failure)

L

Labor
Dilaudid Oral Liquid 445
Dilaudid Tablets - 8 mg 445
Dilaudid-HP 442

Lactation
(*see under* Breastfeeding)

Left ventricular dysfunction
(*see under* Ventricular dysfunction, left)

Lesions, gastrointestinal, unspecified
(*see under* Colitis, ulcerative; Colitis, ulcerative, history of; Ulcer, gastrointestinal)

Lesions, intracranial, unspecified
(*see also under* Tumor, intracranial, unspecified; Tumor, pituitary, unspecified)
Genotropin Lyophilized Powder 2638
Hycotuss Expectorant Syrup 1117
Tev-Tropin for Injection 1222

Lesions, malignant, unspecified
(*see under* Carcinoma, breast, history of; Carcinoma, breast, male; Carcinoma, breast, unspecified; Carcinoma, cervical; Carcinoma, endometrium; Carcinoma, female reproductive organs; Carcinoma, genital, unspecified; Carcinoma, hepatic; Carcinoma, prostate; Carcinoma, skin, unspecified; Carcinoma, squamous cell, unspecified; Melanoma, history of; Melanoma, unspecified; Neoplasm, bone marrow system, malignant; Neoplasm, lymphatic system, malignant)

Lesions, skin, unspecified
(*see also under* Melanoma, unspecified)
Parcopa Orally Disintegrating Tablets 3097
Stalevo Tablets 2287

Lesions, skin, viral
(*see under* Herpes zoster; Varicella)

Leukemia, acute
Zostavax Injection 2111

Leukemia, chronic myelogenous, without definitive diagnosis
Myleran Tablets 1525

Leukemia, unspecified
Attenuvax 1914
Caverject Impulse Injection 2612
Flumist Vaccine 1901
Meruvax II 2019
Miradon Tablets 3042
M-M-R II 2006
Mumpsvax 2031
ProQuad 2064
Varivax 2100

Liver adenoma
(*see under* Adenoma, hepatic)

Liver cancer
(*see under* Carcinoma, hepatic)

Liver damage
(*see under* Liver dysfunction)

Liver disease, active
NuvaRing 2340
Seasonique Tablets 1077
Yaz Tablets 803
Zetia Tablets 2120
Zyflo Tablets 1023

Liver disease, decompensated
PEG-Intron Powder for Injection 3048

Liver disease, history of
(*see under* Hepatitis, history of; Liver dysfunction, history of)

Liver disease, unspecified
(*see also under* Cirrhosis, primary biliary; Cirrhosis, unspecified; Hepatitis; Liver dysfunction)
Advicor Tablets 1722
Aldoril Tablets 1910
Altoprev Extended-Release Tablets 3109
Caduet Tablets 2508
Climara Transdermal System 771
Climara Pro Transdermal System 776
Crestor Tablets 678
Dantrium Capsules 2694
Depacon Injection 412
Depakene 417
Depakote Sprinkle Capsules 422
Depakote Tablets 427
Depakote ER Tablets 434
Depo-Provera Contraceptive Injection 2622
depo-subQ provera 104 Injectable Suspension 2624
Dyrenium Capsules 3400

Enjuvia Tablets 1062
Estratest Tablets 3199
Estratest H.S. Tablets 3199
Klonopin 2778
Lescol Capsules 2233
Lescol XL Tablets 2233
Lipitor Tablets 2483
Menostar Transdermal System 782
Mevacor Tablets 2021
Mirena Intrauterine System 787
Ortho Micronor Tablets 2426
Premarin Intravenous 3442
Premarin Tablets 3446
Premarin Vaginal Cream 3452
Premphase Tablets 3456
Prempro Tablets 3456
Prochieve 4% Gel 1003
Prochieve 8% Gel 1003
Prometrium Capsules (100 mg, 200 mg) 3203
Tasmar Tablets 3358
Uroqid-Acid No. 2 Tablets 760
Vytorin 10/10 Tablets 2114
Vytorin 10/10 Tablets 3077
Vytorin 10/20 Tablets 2114
Vytorin 10/20 Tablets 3077
Vytorin 10/40 Tablets 2114
Vytorin 10/40 Tablets 3077
Vytorin 10/80 Tablets 2114
Vytorin 10/80 Tablets 3077
Ziagen Tablets 1626
Zocor Tablets 2105

Liver disorders, history of
Aldoril Tablets 1910
Augmentin 1360
Augmentin ES-600 Powder for Oral Suspension 1366
Felbatol Oral Suspension

Liver disorders, unspecified
(*see under* Liver dysfunction)

Liver dysfunction
(*see also under* Jaundice, cholestatic of pregnancy, history of; Jaundice, history of; Liver disease, unspecified; Liver failure; Serum transaminase elevation)
Advicor Tablets 1722
Angeliq Tablets 762
Climara Transdermal System 771
Climara Pro Transdermal System 776
Coreg Tablets 1414
Daranide Tablets 1950
Depacon Injection 412
Depakene 417
Depakote Sprinkle Capsules 422
Depakote Tablets 427
Depo-Provera Contraceptive Injection 2622
depo-subQ provera 104 Injectable Suspension 2624
Enjuvia Tablets 1062
Epzicom Tablets 1436
Estrasorb Topical Emulsion 1147
Estratest Tablets 3199
Estratest H.S. Tablets 3199
Imitrex Injection 1463
Imitrex Tablets 1471
Lofibra Tablets 1219
Lofibra Capsules 1216
Menostar Transdermal System 782
Niaspan Extended-Release Tablets 1730
Opana ER Tablets 1126
Premarin Intravenous 3442
Premarin Tablets 3446
Premarin Vaginal Cream 3452
Premphase Tablets 3456
Prempro Tablets 3456
Prochieve 4% Gel 1003
Prochieve 8% Gel 1003
Prometrium Capsules (100 mg, 200 mg) 3203
Ranexa Tablets 1035
Relpax Tablets 2548
Seasonique Tablets 1077
Skelaxin Tablets 1716
Tasmar Tablets 3358
Ticlid Tablets 2810
Tricor Tablets 527
Trizivir Tablets 1589
Uroxatral Tablets 2943
Yasmin 28 Tablets 796
Yaz Tablets 803
Zelnorm Tablets 2312
Ziagen 1626

Liver dysfunction, history of
Augmentin Tablets 1363
Augmentin XR Extended-Release Tablets 1369

Liver dysfunction, severe
(*see under* Hepatic impairment, severe)

Liver failure
(*see also under* Coma, hepatic; Liver dysfunction)
Agenerase Capsules 1327
Agenerase Oral Solution 1332
Fansidar Tablets 2765
Gris-PEG Tablets 2502
Ortho-Cyclen/Ortho Tri-Cyclen 2429
Soriatane Capsules 1013

Liver function tests, abnormal
(*see under* Serum transaminase elevation)

Liver insufficiency
(*see under* Liver dysfunction)

Liver tumor
(*see under* Adenoma, hepatic; Carcinoma, hepatic; Tumor, liver, benign)

Local anesthesia
(*see under* Anesthesia, local)

Lown-Ganong-Levine syndrome
Covera-HS Tablets 3139
Tarka Tablets 524
Verelan PM Extended-Release Capsules, Controlled-Onset 3106

Lung disease, unspecified
(*see under* Pulmonary disorders, unspecified)

Lupus erythematosus
Oxsoralen Lotion 1% 3352
Oxsoralen-Ultra Capsules 3353

Lymphoma
(*see also under* Neoplasm, lymphatic system, malignant)
Attenuvax 1914
Flumist Vaccine 1901
Meruvax II 2019
M-M-R II 2006
Mumpsvax 2031
ProQuad 2064
Varivax 2100
Zostavax Injection 2111

M

Malabsorption syndrome
Xenical Capsules 2831

Malignancies, unspecified
Gengraf Capsules 459
Neoral Oral Solution 2259
Neoral Soft Gelatin Capsules 2259
Nutropin for Injection 1239
Nutropin AQ Injection 1243
Nutropin AQ Pen 1243
Nutropin AQ Pen Cartridge 1243

Malignancy
(*see under* Carcinoma, breast, history of; Carcinoma, breast, male; Carcinoma, breast, unspecified; Carcinoma, endometrium; Carcinoma, hepatic; Carcinoma, prostate; Carcinoma, skin, unspecified; Hypertension, malignant; Leukemia, unspecified; Lymphoma; Malignancy, generalized; Melanoma, history of; Melanoma, unspecified; Neoplasm, bone marrow system, malignant; Neoplasm, lymphatic system, malignant)

Malignancy, cervical
ParaGard T 380A Intrauterine Copper Contraceptive 1073

Malignancy, generalized
Flumist Vaccine 1901
Norditropin Cartridges 2323

Malignancy, uterine
ParaGard T 380A Intrauterine Copper Contraceptive 1073

Malnutrition
Miradon Tablets 3042

Mechanical disorders of ventilation
(*see under* Asthma, acute; Asthma, history of; Asthma, unspecified; Obstruction, respiratory tract)

Megacolon, toxic
Colyte with Flavor Packs for Oral Solution 3088
HalfLytely and Bisacodyl Tablets Bowel Prep Kit with Flavors Packs 881
Lotronex Tablets 1512
TriLyte with Flavor Packs for Oral Solution 3100

Megaloblastic anemia
(*see under* Anemia, megaloblastic, unspecified)

Melanoma, history of
Oxsoralen Lotion 1% 3352
Oxsoralen-Ultra Capsules 3353
Parcopa Orally Disintegrating Tablets 3097
Stalevo Tablets 2287

Melanoma, unspecified
Oxsoralen Lotion 1% 3352
Oxsoralen-Ultra Capsules 3353

Mental depression
(*see under* Depression, mental)

Metabolic acidosis
(*see under* Acidosis, hyperchloremic; Acidosis, metabolic, unspecified; Ketoacidosis, diabetic)

Migraine, basilar
Amerge Tablets 1339
Axert Tablets 2396
Frova Tablets 1113
Imitrex Injection 1463
Imitrex Nasal Spray 1467
Imitrex Tablets 1471
Maxalt Tablets 2008
Maxalt-MLT Orally Disintegrating Tablets 2008
Migranal Nasal Spray 3348
Relpax Tablets 2548
Zomig Tablets 3519
Zomig Nasal Spray 3523
Zomig-ZMT Tablets 3519

Migraine, hemiplegic
Amerge Tablets 1339
Axert Tablets 2396
Frova Tablets 1113
Imitrex Injection 1463
Imitrex Nasal Spray 1467
Imitrex Tablets 1471
Maxalt Tablets 2008
Maxalt-MLT Orally Disintegrating Tablets 2008
Migranal Nasal Spray 3348
Relpax Tablets 2548
Zomig Tablets 3519
Zomig Nasal Spray 3523
Zomig-ZMT Tablets 3519

Moles
Podocon-25 Liquid 2478

Multipara, unspecified
Cervidil Vaginal Insert 1181

Myasthenia gravis
Bentyl Capsules 697
Bentyl Injection 697
Bentyl Syrup 697
Bentyl Tablets 697
Donnatal Extentabs 2493
Norflex Injection 1856

Mycobacterial infection
(*see under* Infection, ophthalmic, mycobacterial)

Mycobacterial infections, ophthalmic
Retisert Implant ⊙258

Myeloid blasts, leukemic
Leukine 814

Myeloma, multiple
Caverject Impulse Injection 2612

Myeloproliferative disorders
(*see also under* Leukemia, acute; Leukemia, unspecified; Myeloma, multiple)
Clozaril Tablets 2184
FazaClo Orally Disintegrating Tablets 551

Myelosuppression
(*see under* Bone marrow depression)

Myocardial damage
(*see under* Cardiovascular disorders, unspecified)

Myocardial disease
(*see under* Cardiovascular disorders, unspecified)

Myocardial infarction
Cardizem LA Extended Release Tablets 1728
Cytomel Tablets 1710
Estrasorb Topical Emulsion 1147
Estratest Tablets 3199
Estratest H.S. Tablets 3199
Geodon 2529
Levothroid Tablets 1186
Levoxyl Tablets 1712
Premphase Tablets 3456
Prempro Tablets 3456
Prometrium Capsules (100 mg, 200 mg) 3203
Tiazac Capsules 1201
Zomig-ZMT Tablets 3519

Myocardial infarction, history of
Amerge Tablets 1339
Axert Tablets 2396
Estrasorb Topical Emulsion 1147
Estratest Tablets 3199
Estratest H.S. Tablets 3199
Frova Tablets 1113
Imitrex Injection 1463
Imitrex Nasal Spray 1467
Imitrex Tablets 1471
Maxalt Tablets 2008
Maxalt-MLT Orally Disintegrating Tablets 2008
Migranal Nasal Spray 3348
Proleukin for Injection 2266
Prometrium Capsules (100 mg, 200 mg) 3203
Relpax Tablets 2548
Zomig Tablets 3519
Zomig Nasal Spray 3523

N

Naloxone challenge test, failed
Vivitrol 995

Narcotic dependence
Vivitrol 995

Narcotic withdrawal, acute
Vivitrol 995

Narrow angle glaucoma
(*see under* Glaucoma, angle closure)

Narrow angles
Propine Ophthalmic Solution ⊙239

Necrosis
(*see also under* Enterocolitis, necrotizing)
Urocit-K Tablets 2144

Neonates
(*see under* Infants)
Ovide .5% Lotion 3290
Pegasys 2789

Neoplasia, unspecified
Increlex Injection 3291
Norditropin Cartridges 2323

Neoplasia, estrogen dependent
(*see under* Neoplasm, estrogen dependent)

Neoplasia, hepatic
(*see under* Adenoma, hepatic; Carcinoma, hepatic; Tumor, liver, benign)

Neoplasia, unspecified
(*see under* Neoplasm, unspecified)

Neoplasm, androgen dependent
(*see under* Carcinoma, prostate)

Neoplasm, bone marrow system, malignant
(*see also under* Myeloid blasts, leukemic; Myeloma, multiple)
Attenuvax 1914
Meruvax II 2019
M-M-R II 2006
Mumpsvax 2031
ProQuad 2064
Varivax 2100
Zostavax Injection 2111

Neoplasm, estrogen dependent
(*see also under* Carcinoma, breast, male; Carcinoma, breast, unspecified)
Angeliq Tablets 762
Climara Transdermal System 771
Climara Pro Transdermal System 776
Enjuvia Tablets 1062
Estrasorb Topical Emulsion 1147
Estratest Tablets 3199
Estratest H.S. Tablets 3199
Estring Vaginal Ring 2635
Menostar Transdermal System 782
Mircette Tablets 1066
NuvaRing 2340
Ortho-Cyclen Tablets 2429
Ortho Evra Transdermal System 2417
Ortho Tri-Cyclen Tablets 2429
Ortho Tri-Cyclen Lo Tablets 2436
Premarin Intravenous 3442
Premarin Tablets 3446
Premarin Vaginal Cream 3452
Premphase Tablets 3456
Prempro Tablets 3456
Seasonique Tablets 1077
Vagifem Tablets 2334
Yasmin 28 Tablets 796
Yaz Tablets 803

Neoplasm, estrogen dependent, history of
(*see under* Carcinoma, breast, history of)

Neoplasm, hepatic, unspecified
(*see under* Adenoma, hepatic; Carcinoma, hepatic; Tumor, liver, benign)

Neoplasm, intracranial
(*see under* Tumor, intracranial, unspecified)

Neoplasm, lymphatic system, malignant
(*see also under* Lymphoma)
Attenuvax 1914
Meruvax II 2019
M-M-R II 2006
Mumpsvax 2031
ProQuad 2064
Varivax 2100

Neoplasm, ovarian
(*see under* Cysts, ovarian)

Neoplasm, unspecified
Nutropin for Injection 1239
Nutropin AQ Injection 1243
Nutropin AQ Pen 1243
Nutropin AQ Pen Cartridge 1243

Neoplastic activity, unspecified
(*see under* Neoplasm, unspecified; Tumor activity, unspecified)

Nephropathy, diabetic
Midamor Tablets 2026
Moduretic Tablets 2028

Nephrosis
Oxandrin Tablets 2962

Neurological disorders, unspecified
(*see also under* Central nervous system depression; Cerebral vascular disease; Cerebral vascular disease, history of; Cerebrovascular accident; Cerebrovascular accident, history of; Depression, mental; Encephalopathy, history of; Epilepsy; Epilepsy, uncontrolled; Guillain-Barre syndrome, history of; Intracranial pressure, increased; Myasthenia gravis; Psychosis; Psychosis, toxic, history of; Psychosis, unsupervised; Seizure disorders, history of; Seizure disorders, unspecified; Senility, unsupervised; Tourette's syndrome)
ADACEL Vaccine 2945
Boostrix 1404
Infanrix Vaccine 1476
Pediarix Vaccine 1548

Neutropenia
Taxotere Injection Concentrate 2932
Ticlid Tablets 2810

Nursing mothers
(*see under* Breastfeeding)

O

Obesity, therapy of
Synthroid Tablets 520

Obstetrics
(*see under* Delivery, unspecified; Labor)

Obstruction, biliary tract
(*see under* Jaundice, cholestatic of pregnancy, history of; Jaundice, history of)

Obstruction, bladder neck
(*see also under* Obstruction, urinary tract)
Norflex Injection 1856

Obstruction, gastrointestinal tract
(*see also under* Achalasia, esophageal; Bowel ischemia, history of; Fecal impaction; Ileus, paralytic; Ileus, unspecified; Stenosis, pyloroduodenal; Stricture, esophageal)
Amitiza Capsules 3224
Bentyl Capsules 697
Bentyl Injection 697
Bentyl Syrup 697
Bentyl Tablets 697
Citrucel Orange Flavor Powder .... ■□ 647
Citrucel Sugar Free Orange Flavor Powder .... ■□ 648
Colyte with Flavor Packs for Oral Solution 3088
Ditropan XL Extended-Release Tablets 2413
Donnatal Extentabs 2493
Dulcolax Suppositories .... ■□ 648
HalfLytely and Bisacodyl Tablets Bowel Prep Kit with Flavors Packs 881
Kionex Powder 2477
Lotronex Tablets 1512
Norflex Injection 1856
Precose Tablets 751
Renagel Tablets 1282
TriLyte with Flavor Packs for Oral Solution 3100
WelChol Tablets 1050
Zelnorm Tablets 2312

Obstruction, pulmonary
Daranide Tablets 1950

Obstruction, respiratory tract
(*see also under* Obstruction, pulmonary)
Daranide Tablets 1950
DepoDur Extended-Release Injection 1110

Obstruction, urinary tract
(*see also under* Obstruction, bladder neck; Prostatic hypertrophy; Urinary retention)
Bentyl Capsules 697
Bentyl Injection 697
Bentyl Syrup 697
Bentyl Tablets 697
Donnatal Extentabs 2493

Obstruction, urogenital tract
(*see under* Obstruction, urinary tract)

Obstructive uropathy
(*see under* Obstruction, urinary tract)

Ocular herpes simplex
(*see under* Herpes simplex keratitis)

Oliguria
Edecrin 1959

Opioid dependence
(*see under* Narcotic dependence)

Opioid intolerance
Duragesic Transdermal System 2373

Opioid urine screen, positive
Vivitrol 995

Opioid withdrawal
(*see under* Narcotic withdrawal, acute)

Oral administration, neonates
Kionex Powder 2477

Organ allograft
Proleukin for Injection 2266

Organic heart disease
(*see under* Cardiovascular disorders, unspecified; Heart disease, ischemic)

Ovarian failure, primary
Follistim AQ Cartridge 2338

Overt cardiac failure
(*see under* Heart failure, unspecified)

P

Pain, acute
Actiq 979
Duragesic Transdermal System 2373

Pain, intermittent
Actiq 979
Duragesic Transdermal System 2373

Pain, mild
Actiq 979
Duragesic Transdermal System 2373
Opana ER Tablets 1126

Pain, peri-operative, associated with coronary artery bypass graft surgery
Celebrex Capsules 3134
Indocin 1995

Pain, peri-operative, coronary artery bypass graft surgery
Anaprox Tablets 2761
Anaprox DS Tablets 2761
Arthrotec Tablets 3129
Clinoril Tablets 1924
Dolobid Tablets 1955
EC-Naprosyn Delayed-Release Tablets 2761
Mobic Oral Suspension 863
Mobic Tablets 863
Naprosyn Suspension 2761
Naprosyn Tablets 2761
Voltaren Tablets 2307
Voltaren-XR Tablets 2310

Pain, post operative
Actiq 979
Duragesic Transdermal System 2373
Opana ER Tablets 1126

Pancreatic diseases, unspecified
Ultrase Capsules 708
Ultrase MT Capsules 709

Pancreatitis
Creon 5 Capsules 3198
Creon 10 Capsules 3198
Creon 20 Capsules 3199
Elspar for Injection 2463
Elspar for Injection 1960
Ultrase Capsules 708
Ultrase MT Capsules 709

Pancreatitis, history of
Elspar for Injection 2463
Elspar for Injection 1960
Oncaspar 1145

Paralytic ileus
(*see under* Ileus, paralytic)

Pediatric patients 18 years of age and younger
Anzemet Injection 2859
Anzemet Tablets 2862

Pediatric patients less than 2 years of age
Phenergan Tablets and Suppositories 3440

Pelvic inflammatory disease
Mirena Intrauterine System 787
ParaGard T 380A Intrauterine Copper Contraceptive 1073

Pelvic inflammatory disease, history of
ParaGard T 380A Intrauterine Copper Contraceptive 1073

Penile deformation
(*see under* Angulation, penile; Fibrosis, cavernosal; Peyronie's disease)

Peptic ulcer
(*see under* Ulcer, peptic)

Perforation, gastrointestinal tract
(*see also under* Ulcer, gastrointestinal)
Colyte with Flavor Packs for Oral Solution 3088
HalfLytely and Bisacodyl Tablets Bowel Prep Kit with Flavors Packs 881
TriLyte with Flavor Packs for Oral Solution 3100

Perforation, gastrointestinal tract, history of
Lotronex Tablets 1512
Proleukin for Injection 2266

Perforation, intestinal
(*see under* Perforation, gastrointestinal tract)

Pericardial effusion
Coumadin for Injection 898
Coumadin Tablets 898

Pericardial tamponade, history of
Proleukin for Injection 2266

Pericarditis, acute
Aggrastat 1907

Pericarditis, unspecified
Coumadin for Injection 898
Coumadin Tablets 898
Miradon Tablets 3042

Peripheral arterial disease
(*see under* Peripheral vascular disease)

Peripheral vascular disease
(*see also under* Arteriosclerosis, unspecified; Thrombophlebitis)
Amerge Tablets 1339
Frova Tablets 1113

Imitrex Injection 1463
Imitrex Nasal Spray 1467
Imitrex Tablets 1471
Relpax Tablets 2548

Peripheral vascular disease, severe
Lopressor Injection 2238
Lopressor Tablets 2238
Lopressor HCT 50/25 Tablets 2241
Lopressor HCT 100/25 Tablets 2241
Lopressor HCT 100/50 Tablets 2241

Peripheral vascular insufficiency
(*see under* Peripheral vascular disease)

Peyronie's disease
Caverject Impulse Injection 2612
Edex Injection 3089

Pheochromocytoma
Azilect Tablets 3293
Emsam Transdermal System 903
GlucaGen 761
Glucagon for Injection Vials and Emergency Kit 1778
Lopressor Injection 2238
Lopressor Tablets 2238
Lopressor HCT 50/25 Tablets 2241
Lopressor HCT 100/25 Tablets 2241
Lopressor HCT 100/50 Tablets 2241
Parnate Tablets 1527
ProAmatine Tablets 3186

Phlebitis
(*see under* Thrombophlebitis)

Phosphate stones, infected
K-Phos Original (Sodium Free) Tablets 760
K-Phos Neutral Tablets 760

Photosensitivity diseases, unspecified
(*see also under* Albinism; Lupus erythematosus; Porphyria cutanea tarda; Porphyria, acute; Porphyria, erythropoietic; Porphyria, unspecified; Xeroderma pigmentosum)
Oxsoralen Lotion 1% 3352
Oxsoralen-Ultra Capsules 3353

Photosensitivity, cutaneous
Levulan Kerastick for Topical Solution, 20% 1085

Poly-arthritis
Miradon Tablets 3042

Polycythemia
Miradon Tablets 3042

Poor nutritional state
(*see under* Electrolyte imbalance, uncorrected; Malnutrition)

Porphyria cutanea tarda
Oxsoralen-Ultra Capsules 3353

Porphyria, acute
Donnatal Extentabs 2493

Porphyria, erythropoietic
Oxsoralen-Ultra Capsules 3353

Porphyria, unspecified
Gris-PEG Tablets 2502
Nembutal Sodium Solution, USP 2470
Oxsoralen Lotion 1% 3352
Photofrin for Injection 702
Vagifem Tablets 2334
Visudyne for Injection 2305

Porphyria, variegate
Oxsoralen-Ultra Capsules 3353

Prader-Willi Syndrome
Humatrope Vials and Cartridges 1787
Norditropin Cartridges 2323
Nutropin for Injection 1239
Nutropin AQ Injection 1243
Nutropin AQ Pen 1243
Nutropin AQ Pen Cartridge 1243
Tev-Tropin for Injection 1222

Preeclampsia
Coumadin for Injection 898
Coumadin Tablets 898
Miradon Tablets 3042

Pregnancy
Accutane Capsules 2731
Advicor Tablets 1722
Agenerase Capsules 1327
Agenerase Oral Solution 1332
Altoprev Extended-Release Tablets 3109
Androxy Tablets 3335
Arthrotec Tablets 3129
Attenuvax 1914
Caduet Tablets 2508
Carac Cream, 0.5% 2879
Climara Transdermal System 771
Climara Pro Transdermal System 776
Copegus Tablets 2754
Coumadin for Injection 898
Coumadin Tablets 898
Crestor Tablets 678
Cuprimine Capsules 1947
Dalmane Capsules 3342
Depo-Provera Contraceptive Injection 2622
depo-subQ provera 104 Injectable Suspension 2624
Efudex 3363
Eligard 7.5 mg 2880
Eligard 22.5 mg 2883
Eligard 30 mg 2885
Eligard 45 mg 2888
Enjuvia Tablets 1062
Estrasorb Topical Emulsion 1147
Estratest Tablets 3199
Estratest H.S. Tablets 3199
Estring Vaginal Ring 2635
Evista Tablets 1763
Fansidar Tablets 2765
Faslodex Injection 681
Follistim AQ Cartridge 2338
Gantrisin Pediatric Suspension 2770
Gris-PEG Tablets 2502
Hycamtin for Injection 1458
Lescol Capsules 2233
Lescol XL Tablets 2233
Lipitor Tablets 2483
Lithostat Tablets 2140
Lupron Depot 3.75 mg 3260
Lupron Depot 7.5 mg 3264
Lupron Depot–3 Month 11.25 mg 3265
Lupron Depot-PED 7.5 mg, 11.25 mg and 15 mg 3269
Lupron Injection Pediatric 3259
Menostar Transdermal System 782
Meruvax II 2019
Mevacor Tablets 2021
Migranal Nasal Spray 3348
Miradon Tablets 3042
Mircette Tablets 1066
Mirena Intrauterine System 787
M-M-R II 2006
Mumpsvax 2031
NuvaRing 2340
Ortho-Cyclen Tablets 2429
Ortho Evra Transdermal System 2417
Ortho Micronor Tablets 2426
Ortho Tri-Cyclen Tablets 2429
Ortho Tri-Cyclen Lo Tablets 2436
Orthoclone OKT3 Sterile Solution 2360
Oxandrin Tablets 2962
ParaGard T 380A Intrauterine Copper Contraceptive 1073
Plan B Tablets 1076
Podocon-25 Liquid 2478
Premarin Intravenous 3442
Premarin Tablets 3446
Premarin Vaginal Cream 3452
Premphase Tablets 3456
Prempro Tablets 3456
Prometrium Capsules (100 mg, 200 mg) 3203
Propecia Tablets 2060
ProQuad 2064
Proscar Tablets 2067
ProSom Tablets 517
Rebetol 3058
Rebetron Combination Therapy 3063
Restoril Capsules 1860
Revlimid Capsules 958
Ribavirin, USP Capsules 3068
Seasonique Tablets 1077
Soriatane Capsules 1013
Targretin Capsules 1747
Testim 1% Gel 695
Thalomid Capsules 965
Tindamax Tablets 2142
Tracleer Tablets 545
Travatan Ophthalmic Solution 563
Trelstar Depot 3394
Trelstar LA Suspension 3397
Vagifem Tablets 2334
Varivax 2100
Viadur Implant 757
Virazole for Inhalation Solution 3370
Vytorin 10/10 Tablets 2114
Vytorin 10/10 Tablets 3077
Vytorin 10/20 Tablets 2114
Vytorin 10/20 Tablets 3077
Vytorin 10/40 Tablets 2114
Vytorin 10/40 Tablets 3077
Vytorin 10/80 Tablets 2114
Vytorin 10/80 Tablets 3077
Yasmin 28 Tablets 796
Yaz Tablets 803
Zetia Tablets 2120
Zocor Tablets 2105
Zostavax Injection 2111

Pregnancy, diagnostic test for
Prometrium Capsules (100 mg, 200 mg) 3203

Priapism, predisposition to
Edex Injection 3089

Proctitis, history of
Indocin Suppositories 1995

Prolactinoma, pituitary
(*see under* Tumor, intracranial, unspecified)

Prostate enlargement
(*see under* Prostatic hypertrophy)

Prostatic hypertrophy
Norflex Injection 1856

Protoporphyria
(*see under* Porphyria, erythropoietic)

Psoriasis, acute
Psoriatec Cream 1089

Psoriatic eruptions, acute
(*see under* Psoriasis, acute)

Psychic disturbances
(*see under* Psychosis)

Psychosis
Seromycin Capsules 1813

Psychosis, toxic, history of
Proleukin for Injection 2266

Psychosis, unsupervised
Coumadin for Injection 898
Coumadin Tablets 898

Pulmonary atresia
(*see under* Atresia, pulmonary)

Pulmonary congestion
Cardizem LA Extended Release Tablets 1728
Tiazac Capsules 1201

Pulmonary disorders, unspecified
(*see also under* Asthma, acute; Asthma, unspecified; Atresia, pulmonary; Chronic obstructive pulmonary disease; Obstruction, pulmonary; Pulmonary congestion; Pulmonary function test, abnormal; Respiratory tract conditions, lower)
Exubera Inhalation Powder 2524

Pulmonary embolism
Angeliq Tablets 762
Climara Transdermal System 771
Climara Pro Transdermal System 776
Enjuvia Tablets 1062
Estrasorb Topical Emulsion 1147
Estratest Tablets 3199
Estratest H.S. Tablets 3199
Evista Tablets 1763
Menostar Transdermal System 782
Premarin Intravenous 3442
Premarin Tablets 3446
Premarin Vaginal Cream 3452
Premphase Tablets 3456
Prempro Tablets 3456
Prometrium Capsules (100 mg, 200 mg) 3203

Pulmonary embolism, history of
Climara Transdermal System 771
Climara Pro Transdermal System 776
Enjuvia Tablets 1062
Estrasorb Topical Emulsion 1147
Estratest Tablets 3199
Estratest H.S. Tablets 3199
Menostar Transdermal System 782
Premarin Intravenous 3442
Premarin Tablets 3446
Premarin Vaginal Cream 3452
Premphase Tablets 3456
Prempro Tablets 3456
Prometrium Capsules (100 mg, 200 mg) 3203
Soltamox Oral Solution 3527

Pulmonary function test, abnormal
Proleukin for Injection 2266

Pyloroduodenal stenosis
(*see under* Stenosis, pyloroduodenal)

Q

Q-T interval prolongation
Geodon 2529

R

Radiation therapy
Flumist Vaccine 1901
Gengraf Capsules 459
Leukine 814
Neoral Oral Solution 2259
Neoral Soft Gelatin Capsules 2259

Radiotherapy
(*see under* Radiation therapy)

Rectal bleeding
(*see under* Bleeding, rectal)

Renal decompensation
(*see under* Renal failure)

Renal dialysis
Augmentin XR Extended-Release Tablets 1369
Integrilin Injection 3020

Renal disease, unspecified
(*see also under* Nephropathy, diabetic; Nephrosis; Renal dysfunction)
ActoPlus Met Tablets 3214
Avandamet Tablets 1373
Avar Cleanser 1085
Avar Gel 1085
Avar Green Gel 1085
Avar-e Emollient Cream 1085
Avar-e Green Cream 1085
Calcium Disodium Versenate Injection 1851
Dyrenium Capsules 3400
Fortamet Extended-Release Tablets 3115
Paser Granules 1674
ProAmatine Tablets 3186
Rosac Cream with Sunscreens 3213

Renal dysfunction
(*see also under* Anuria; Oliguria; Renal disease, unspecified; Renal failure)
ActoPlus Met Tablets 3214
Angeliq Tablets 762
Augmentin XR Extended-Release Tablets 1369
Avandamet Tablets 1373
Cuprimine Capsules 1947
Dyazide Capsules 1423
Dyrenium Capsules 3400
Fortamet Extended-Release Tablets 3115
Gengraf Capsules 459
Indocin I.V. 2465
Inspra Tablets 2536
Integrilin Injection 3020
K-Phos Original (Sodium Free) Tablets 760
K-Phos Neutral Tablets 760
Midamor Tablets 2026
Moduretic Tablets 2028
Nalfon Capsules 2502
NeoProfen Injection 2472
Neoral Oral Solution 2259
Neoral Soft Gelatin Capsules 2259
Plasbumin-5 3251
Plasbumin-20 3252

Plasbumin-25 3253
Seromycin Capsules 1813
Skelaxin Tablets 1716
Tricor Tablets 527
Uroqid-Acid No. 2 Tablets 760
Xeloda Tablets 2822
Yasmin 28 Tablets 796
Yaz Tablets 803
Zelnorm Tablets 2312

Renal dysfunction, history of
Cuprimine Capsules 1947
Lithostat Tablets 2140
Proleukin for Injection 2266

Renal dysfunction, severe
Lofibra Tablets 1219
Lofibra Capsules 1216
Malarone Pediatric Tablets 1517
Malarone Tablets 1517
Miradon Tablets 3042
Triglide Tablets 3123

Renal excretory function impairment
(*see under* Renal dysfunction)

Renal failure
(*see also under* Renal dysfunction)
Agenerase Capsules 1327
Agenerase Oral Solution 1332
Daranide Tablets 1950
Fansidar Tablets 2765
Soriatane Capsules 1013
Urocit-K Tablets 2144

Renal impairment
(*see under* Renal dysfunction)

Renal insufficiency
(*see under* Renal dysfunction)

Respiratory depression
Avinza Capsules 1741
DepoDur Extended-Release Injection 1110
Dilaudid 440
Dilaudid Non-Sterile Powder 440
Dilaudid Oral Liquid 445
Dilaudid Rectal Suppositories 440
Dilaudid Tablets 440
Dilaudid Tablets - 8 mg 445
Dilaudid-HP 442
Duragesic Transdermal System 2373
Hycotuss Expectorant Syrup 1117
Kadian Capsules 577
MS Contin Tablets 2701
Opana Tablets 1122
Opana ER Tablets 1126
OxyContin Tablets 2703
OxyFast Oral Concentrate Solution 2708
OxyIR Capsules 2708

Respiratory depression, in absence of resuscitative equipment
Percodan Tablets 1132

Respiratory depression, history of
Mivacron Injection 493

Respiratory disease, unspecified
(*see under* Respiratory illness, febrile)

Respiratory disorders
(*see under* Bronchospastic disorders, unspecified; Obstruction, respiratory tract; Pulmonary disorders, unspecified; Respiratory depression; Respiratory tract conditions, lower)

Respiratory distress
(*see under* Asthma, acute; Respiratory depression)

Respiratory distress, acute, caused by obstructing endobronchial lesion
Photofrin for Injection 702

Respiratory failure
Norditropin Cartridges 2323

Respiratory illness, febrile
Attenuvax 1914
Meruvax II 2019
M-M-R II 2006
Mumpsvax 2031
Varivax 2100

Respiratory illness, unspecified
(*see under* Pulmonary disorders, unspecified; Respiratory illness, febrile)

Respiratory insufficiency, unspecified
(*see also under* Obstruction, respiratory tract; Pulmonary disorders, unspecified; Respiratory illness, febrile)
Humatrope Vials and Cartridges 1787

Respiratory obstruction
(*see under* Obstruction, respiratory tract)

Respiratory tract conditions, lower
(*see also under* Pulmonary disorders, unspecified)
Phenergan Tablets and Suppositories 3440

Retinopathy, diabetic
Norditropin Cartridges 2323
Nutropin for Injection 1239
Nutropin AQ Injection 1243
Nutropin AQ Pen 1243
Nutropin AQ Pen Cartridge 1243

Rhabdomyolysis, non-traumatic, history of
Tasmar Tablets 3358

S

Seizure disorders, history of
Orthoclone OKT3 Sterile Solution 2360
Proleukin for Injection 2266

Seizure disorders, unspecified
(*see also under* Epilepsy; Epilepsy, uncontrolled; Status epilepticus)
Wellbutrin Tablets 1603
Wellbutrin SR Sustained-Release Tablets 1607
Wellbutrin XL Extended-Release Tablets 1613
Zyban Sustained-Release Tablets 1644

Seizure disorders, untreated
(*see under* Epilepsy, uncontrolled)

Seizures, history of
(*see under* Seizure disorders, history of)

Senility, unsupervised
Coumadin for Injection 898
Coumadin Tablets 898

Sepsis
(*see under* Toxemia)

Serum creatinine, elevated
Inspra Tablets 2536

Serum transaminase elevation
(*see also under* Liver dysfunction)
Advicor Tablets 1722
Altoprev Extended-Release Tablets 3109
Caduet Tablets 2508
Crestor Tablets 678
Lescol Capsules 2233
Lescol XL Tablets 2233
Lipitor Tablets 2483
Mevacor Tablets 2021
Vytorin 10/10 Tablets 2114
Vytorin 10/10 Tablets 3077
Vytorin 10/20 Tablets 2114
Vytorin 10/20 Tablets 3077
Vytorin 10/40 Tablets 2114
Vytorin 10/40 Tablets 3077
Vytorin 10/80 Tablets 2114
Vytorin 10/80 Tablets 3077
Zetia Tablets 2120
Zocor Tablets 2105

Zyflo Tablets 1023

Severe left ventricular dysfunction
(*see under* Ventricular dysfunction, left)

Shingles
(*see under* Herpes zoster)

Shock, cardiogenic
(*see under* Cardiogenic shock)

Shock, circulatory
DepoDur Extended-Release Injection 1110

Shock, unspecified
(*see also under* Cardiogenic shock)
Primaxin I.M. 2045
Thiothixene Capsules 2165

Sick sinus node syndrome
(*see under* Sick sinus syndrome)

Sick sinus syndrome
Adenocard Injection 617
Adenoscan 619
Cardizem LA Extended Release Tablets 1728
Coreg Tablets 1414
Covera-HS Tablets 3139
Lopressor Injection 2238
Lopressor Tablets 2238
Lopressor HCT 50/25 Tablets 2241
Lopressor HCT 100/25 Tablets 2241
Lopressor HCT 100/50 Tablets 2241
Rythmol SR Capsules 2727
Tarka Tablets 524
Tiazac Capsules 1201
Toprol-XL Tablets 668
Verelan PM Extended-Release Capsules, Controlled-Onset 3106

Sickle cell anemia
(*see under* Anemia, sickle cell)

Sino-atrial block
(*see under* Heart block, greater than first degree; Heart block, unspecified)

Sinus node disease
(*see under* Bradycardia, sinus; Sick sinus syndrome; Sinus node dysfunction, unspecified)

Sinus node dysfunction, unspecified
Adenocard Injection 617
Adenoscan 619

Skin disease at injection site
Euflexxa 1162

Skin disorders, unspecified
(*see under* Lesions, skin, unspecified; Melanoma, history of; Melanoma, unspecified; Psoriasis, acute; Skin, denuded; Xeroderma pigmentosum)

Skin lesions
(*see under* Lesions, skin, unspecified)

Skin, denuded
ThermaCare Heat Wraps 2677

Smoking
Exubera Inhalation Powder 2524

Smoking, heavy
NuvaRing 2340
Yasmin 28 Tablets 796
Yaz Tablets 803

Sodium depletion
(*see under* Hyponatremia)

Spasms, infantile, history of
Infanrix Vaccine 1476
Pediarix Vaccine 1548

Sphincter of Oddi dysfunction
Zelnorm Tablets 2312

Spinal puncture
Coumadin for Injection 898
Coumadin Tablets 898

Status asthmaticus
Advair Diskus 100/50 1308
Advair Diskus 250/50 1308
Advair Diskus 500/50 1308
Advair HFA Inhalation Aerosol 1318
Aerobid/Aerobid-M 1171
Asmanex Twisthaler 2966
Azmacort Inhalation Aerosol 1726
Dilaudid 440
Dilaudid Non-Sterile Powder 440
Dilaudid Oral Liquid 445
Dilaudid Rectal Suppositories 440
Dilaudid Tablets 440
Dilaudid Tablets - 8 mg 445
Dilaudid-HP 442
Flovent HFA 1447
Pulmicort Respules 661
Qvar Inhalation Aerosol 3303
Symbicort 80/4.5 Inhalation Aerosol 3511
Symbicort 160/4.5 Inhalation Aerosol 3511

Status epilepticus
Romazicon Injection 2804

Stenosis, aortic
Cardene I.V. 2497
Indocin I.V. 2465
NeoProfen Injection 2472

Stenosis, pyloric
(*see under* Stenosis, pyloroduodenal)

Stenosis, pyloroduodenal
Norflex Injection 1856

Stress test, abnormal
Proleukin for Injection 2266

Stricture, esophageal
Fosamax 1969
Fosamax Plus D Tablets 1977

Stroke
(*see under* Cerebrovascular accident)

Stroke, hemorrhagic
Aggrastat 1907
Xigris Powder for Intravenous Infusion 1828

Stroke, history of
(*see under* Cerebrovascular accident, history of)

Succinic semialdehyde dehydrogenase deficiency
Xyrem Oral Solution 1688

Superficial herpes simplex keratitis
(*see under* Herpes simplex keratitis)

Surgery, abdominal
Dulcolax Suppositories ▣ 648

Surgery, central nervous system
(*see also under* Surgery, intracranial; Surgery, intraspinal)
Coumadin for Injection 898
Coumadin Tablets 898
Miradon Tablets 3042

Surgery, elective
Parnate Tablets 1527

Surgery, intracranial
Activase I.V. 1223
Retavase 2499
TNKase I.V. 1264
Xigris Powder for Intravenous Infusion 1828

Surgery, intraspinal
Activase I.V. 1223
Miradon Tablets 3042
Retavase 2499
Xigris Powder for Intravenous Infusion 1828

Surgery, major, with prolonged immobilization
NuvaRing 2340
Ortho Evra Transdermal System 2417

Ortho Tri-Cyclen Lo Tablets 2436
Seasonique Tablets 1077
Yaz Tablets 803

Surgery, ophthalmic
Coumadin for Injection............898
Coumadin Tablets............898
Miradon Tablets............3042

Surgery, traumatic
Coumadin for Injection............898
Coumadin Tablets............898
Miradon Tablets............3042

Surgery, unspecified
Integrilin Injection............3020
ReoPro Vials............1809

Surgery, uterine, history of
(*see also under* Cesarean section, history of)
Cervidil Vaginal Insert............1181

Surgical abdomen
(*see under* Surgery, abdominal)

Systemic lupus erythematosus
(*see under* Lupus erythematosus)

Systolic blood pressure less than 90 mm Hg
Natrecor for Injection............3127

Systolic blood pressure less than 100 mm Hg
Lopressor Injection............2238
Lopressor Tablets............2238

T

Tachyarrhythmia
(*see under* Arrhythmia, cardiac, unspecified; Tachycardia, unspecified)

Tachycardia, unspecified
Alupent Inhalation Aerosol............826

Tachycardia, ventricular, history of
Proleukin for Injection............2266

Tendinitis, history of
Noroxin Tablets............2032

Tendon rupture, history of
Noroxin Tablets............2032

Tension
Concerta Extended-Release Tablets............1881
Daytrana Transdermal Patch............3174
Focalin Tablets............2220
Focalin XR Capsules............2223
Metadate CD Capsules............3323
Ritalin Hydrochloride Tablets............2269
Ritalin LA Capsules............2271
Ritalin-SR Tablets............2269

Tetralogy of Fallot
Indocin I.V. 2465
NeoProfen Injection............2472

Thallium stress test, abnormal
(*see under* Stress test, abnormal)

Thrombocytopathy, unspecified
(*see under* Thrombocytopenia, unspecified)

Thrombocytopenia, unspecified
Aggrastat............1907
Arixtra Injection............1351
Fragmin Injection............1097
Indocin I.V. 2465
Integrilin Injection............3020
Lovenox Injection............2915
NeoProfen Injection............2472
ReoPro Vials............1809
Thiola Tablets............2141
Ticlid Tablets............2810

Thromboembolic disorders
(*see also under* Cerebrovascular accident)
Climara Transdermal System............771
Climara Pro Transdermal System............776
Depo-Provera Contraceptive Injection............2622
depo-subQ provera 104 Injectable Suspension............2624
Emcyt Capsules............2634
Enjuvia Tablets............1062
Estrasorb Topical Emulsion............1147
Estratest Tablets............3199
Estratest H.S. Tablets............3199
Menostar Transdermal System............782
Mircette Tablets............1066
NuvaRing............2340
Ortho-Cyclen Tablets............2429
Ortho Evra Transdermal System............2417
Ortho Tri-Cyclen Tablets............2429
Ortho Tri-Cyclen Lo Tablets............2436
Premarin Intravenous............3442
Premarin Tablets............3446
Premarin Vaginal Cream............3452
Premphase Tablets............3456
Prempro Tablets............3456
Prochieve 4% Gel............1003
Prochieve 8% Gel............1003
Prometrium Capsules (100 mg, 200 mg)............3203
Seasonique Tablets............1077
Yasmin 28 Tablets............796
Yaz Tablets............803

Thromboembolic disorders, arterial
Angeliq Tablets............762

Thromboembolic disorders, history of
(*see also under* Cerebrovascular accident, history of)
Depo-Provera Contraceptive Injection............2622
depo-subQ provera 104 Injectable Suspension............2624
Estrasorb Topical Emulsion............1147
Estratest Tablets............3199
Estratest H.S. Tablets............3199
Evista Tablets............1763
Menostar Transdermal System............782
Mircette Tablets............1066
NuvaRing............2340
Ortho-Cyclen Tablets............2429
Ortho Evra Transdermal System............2417
Ortho Tri-Cyclen Tablets............2429
Ortho Tri-Cyclen Lo Tablets............2436
Premarin Intravenous............3442
Premarin Vaginal Cream............3452
Premphase Tablets............3456
Prempro Tablets............3456
Prochieve 4% Gel............1003
Prochieve 8% Gel............1003
Prometrium Capsules (100 mg, 200 mg)............3203
Seasonique Tablets............1077
Vagifem Tablets............2334
Yasmin 28 Tablets............796
Yaz Tablets............803

Thrombogenic valvulopathies
Seasonique Tablets............1077
Yaz Tablets............803

Thrombophlebitis
Depo-Provera Contraceptive Injection............2622
depo-subQ provera 104 Injectable Suspension............2624
Emcyt Capsules............2634
Mircette Tablets............1066
NuvaRing............2340
Ortho-Cyclen Tablets............2429
Ortho Evra Transdermal System............2417
Ortho Tri-Cyclen Tablets............2429
Ortho Tri-Cyclen Lo Tablets............2436
Prochieve 4% Gel............1003
Prochieve 8% Gel............1003
Seasonique Tablets............1077
Vagifem Tablets............2334
Yasmin 28 Tablets............796
Yaz Tablets............803

Thrombophlebitis, history of
Lotronex Tablets............1512
Mircette Tablets............1066
NuvaRing............2340
Ortho-Cyclen Tablets............2429
Ortho Evra Transdermal System............2417
Ortho Tri-Cyclen Tablets............2429
Ortho Tri-Cyclen Lo Tablets............2436
Prochieve 4% Gel............1003
Prochieve 8% Gel............1003
Seasonique Tablets............1077
Yasmin 28 Tablets............796
Yaz Tablets............803

Thrombosis, deep vein
Angeliq Tablets............762
Premphase Tablets............3456

Thrombosis, history of
Angeliq Tablets............762
Estratest Tablets............3199
Estratest H.S. Tablets............3199
Evista Tablets............1763
Oncaspar............1145
Premarin Intravenous............3442
Premarin Vaginal Cream............3452

Thrombotic thrombocytopenic purpura, history of
Ticlid Tablets............2810

Thymic abnormalities
Flumist Vaccine............1901

Thyroid dysfunction, uncontrolled
Follistim AQ Cartridge............2338

Thyrotoxicosis
ProAmatine Tablets............3186

Thyrotoxicosis, untreated
Cytomel Tablets............1710
Levothroid Tablets............1186
Levoxyl Tablets............1712
Naturethroid Tablets............3401
Synthroid Tablets............520
Thyrolar Tablets............1199
Westhroid Tablets............3403

Tics, motor
Concerta Extended-Release Tablets............1881
Daytrana Transdermal Patch............3174
Focalin Tablets............2220
Focalin XR Capsules............2223
Metadate CD Capsules............3323
Ritalin Hydrochloride Tablets............2269
Ritalin LA Capsules............2271
Ritalin-SR Tablets............2269

Tissue breakdown
(*see under* Necrosis)

Tourette's syndrome
Concerta Extended-Release Tablets............1881
Daytrana Transdermal Patch............3174
Focalin Tablets............2220
Focalin XR Capsules............2223
Metadate CD Capsules............3323
Ritalin Hydrochloride Tablets............2269
Ritalin LA Capsules............2271
Ritalin-SR Tablets............2269

Tourette's syndrome, history of
Concerta Extended-Release Tablets............1881
Daytrana Transdermal Patch............3174
Focalin Tablets............2220
Focalin XR Capsules............2223
Metadate CD Capsules............3323
Ritalin Hydrochloride Tablets............2269
Ritalin LA Capsules............2271
Ritalin-SR Tablets............2269

Toxemia
Enbrel for Injection............584

Toxic megacolon
(*see under* Megacolon, toxic)

Toxicity, vitamin D
Calcijex Injection............411
Hectorol Capsules............1275
Hectorol Injection............1278
Rocaltrol Capsules............2798
Rocaltrol Oral Solution............2798
Zemplar Capsules............541
Zemplar Injection............543

Tracheoesophageal fistula, existence of
Photofrin for Injection............702

Transaminases elevation, serum
(*see under* Serum transaminase elevation)

Transplant
(*see under* Organ allograft)

Trauma, intracranial
(*see also under* Cerebrovascular accident; Head injury)
Activase I.V. 1223
Retavase............2499
TNKase I.V. 1264

Trauma, intracranial, unspecified
TNKase I.V. 1264
Xigris Powder for Intravenous Infusion............1828

Trauma, intraspinal
Activase I.V. 1223
Retavase............2499
TNKase I.V. 1264

Trauma, unspecified
ReoPro Vials............1809

Tuberculosis, unspecified
(*see under* Infection, ophthalmic, mycobacterial)

Tuberculosis, untreated
Attenuvax............1914
Meruvax II............2019
M-M-R II............2006
Mumpsvax............2031
ProQuad............2064
Varivax............2100
Zostavax Injection............2111

Tumor, adrenal
(*see under* Pheochromocytoma)

Tumor, breast
Follistim AQ Cartridge............2338

Tumor, breast, malignant
(*see under* Carcinoma, breast, history of; Carcinoma, breast, male; Carcinoma, breast, unspecified)

Tumor, hepatic
(*see under* Adenoma, hepatic; Carcinoma, hepatic; Tumor, liver, benign)

Tumor, hormone dependent
(*see under* Neoplasm, estrogen dependent)

Tumor, hypothalamus
Follistim AQ Cartridge............2338

Tumor, intracranial, unspecified
(*see also under* Lesions, intracranial, unspecified; Tumor, pituitary, unspecified)
Activase I.V. 1223
Aggrastat............1907
Nutropin for Injection............1239
Nutropin AQ Injection............1243
Nutropin AQ Pen............1243
Nutropin AQ Pen Cartridge............1243
ReoPro Vials............1809
Retavase............2499
TNKase I.V. 1264
Xigris Powder for Intravenous Infusion............1828

Tumor, liver, benign
Mirena Intrauterine System............787
Seasonique Tablets............1077
Yaz Tablets............803

Tumor, liver, malignant
(*see under* Carcinoma, hepatic)

Tumor, ovarian
Follistim AQ Cartridge........2338

Tumor, pituitary, unspecified
(*see also under* Tumor, intracranial, unspecified)
Follistim AQ Cartridge........2338

Tumor, unspecified
(*see under* Neoplasm, unspecified)

Tumor activity, unspecified
Genotropin Lyophilized Powder........2638
Humatrope Vials and Cartridges........1787

Tumors, intracranial, in hypopituitary children
Norditropin Cartridges........2323

U

Ulcer, gastrointestinal
(*see also under* Perforation, gastrointestinal tract; Ulcer, peptic)
Miradon Tablets........3042

Ulcer, peptic
Advicor Tablets........1722
Niaspan Extended-Release Tablets........1730
Norflex Injection........1856

Ulcer, unspecified
(*see under* Ulceration, unspecified)

Ulceration, unspecified
Coumadin for Injection........898
Coumadin Tablets........898
Miradon Tablets........3042

Ulcerative colitis
(*see under* Colitis, ulcerative)

Unstable cardiovascular status in acute hemorrhage
(*see under* Cardiovascular status, unstable in acute hemorrhage)

Urea cycle disorders
Depacon Injection........412
Depakene........417
Depakote Sprinkle Capsules........422
Depakote Tablets........427
Depakote ER Tablets........434

Uremia
(*see under* Azotemia)

Urinary obstruction
(*see under* Obstruction, urinary tract)

Urinary retention
(*see also under* Obstruction, urinary tract; Prostatic hypertrophy)
Allegra-D 12 Hour Extended-Release Tablets........2846
Allegra-D 24 Hour Extended-Release Tablets........2849
Clarinex-D 24-Hour Extended-Release Tablets........2998
Detrol Tablets........2628
Detrol LA Capsules........2631
Ditropan XL Extended-Release Tablets........2413
Enablex Extended-Release Tablets........2203
Oxytrol Transdermal System........3392
ProAmatine Tablets........3186
Sanctura Tablets........1151
VESIcare Tablets........646
Zyrtec-D 12 Hour Extended Release Tablets........2597

Urinary tract disorders
(*see under* Obstruction, urinary tract; Renal disease, unspecified; Renal dysfunction)

Uropathy, obstructive
(*see under* Obstruction, urinary tract)

Uterine abnormalities, unspecified
Mirena Intrauterine System........787

Uterine cavity distortion
ParaGard T 380A Intrauterine Copper Contraceptive........1073

V

Vaccinia
Alrex Ophthalmic Suspension 0.2%........⊙ 246
Blephamide Ophthalmic Ointment........568
Blephamide Ophthalmic Suspension........569
FML Ophthalmic Ointment........⊙ 228
FML Ophthalmic Suspension........⊙ 227
FML Forte Ophthalmic Suspension........⊙ 226
FML-S Ophthalmic Suspension........⊙ 229
Lotemax Ophthalmic Suspension 0.5%........⊙ 251
Poly-Pred Ophthalmic Suspension........⊙ 233
Pred Mild Ophthalmic Suspension........⊙ 238
Pred Forte Ophthalmic Suspension........⊙ 235
Pred-G Ophthalmic Ointment........⊙ 237
Pred-G Ophthalmic Suspension........⊙ 236
TobraDex Ophthalmic Ointment........562
TobraDex Ophthalmic Suspension........563

Vaginal bleeding, abnormal
(*see under* Bleeding, genital, abnormal)

Vaginitis, untreated
Mirena Intrauterine System........787

Vaginosis, bacterial, untreated
Mirena Intrauterine System........787

Varicella
Alrex Ophthalmic Suspension 0.2%........⊙ 246
Blephamide Ophthalmic Ointment........568
Blephamide Ophthalmic Suspension........569
Cosmegen for Injection........2459
FML Ophthalmic Ointment........⊙ 228
FML Ophthalmic Suspension........⊙ 227
FML Forte Ophthalmic Suspension........⊙ 226
FML-S Ophthalmic Suspension........⊙ 229
Lotemax Ophthalmic Suspension 0.5%........⊙ 251
Poly-Pred Ophthalmic Suspension........⊙ 233
Pred Mild Ophthalmic Suspension........⊙ 238
Pred Forte Ophthalmic Suspension........⊙ 235
Pred-G Ophthalmic Ointment........⊙ 237
Pred-G Ophthalmic Suspension........⊙ 236
TobraDex Ophthalmic Ointment........562
TobraDex Ophthalmic Suspension........563

Vascular impairment of extremities
(*see also under* Peripheral vascular disease)
Yasmin 28 Tablets........796

Vasculitis, history of
ReoPro Vials........1809

Vasospasm, coronary artery
(*see under* Coronary artery vasospasm)

Ventilatory function depression
(*see under* Respiratory depression)

Ventricular dysfunction, left
Covera-HS Tablets........3139
Tarka Tablets........524
Verelan PM Extended-Release Capsules, Controlled-Onset........3106

Ventricular fibrillation
(*see under* Fibrillation, ventricular)

Viral disease, conjunctiva
Retisert Implant........⊙ 258

Viral disease, cornea
Retisert Implant........⊙ 258

Viral illnesses, acute
Thymoglobulin for Intravenous Infusion........1284

Viral infections
(*see under* Herpes simplex keratitis; Herpes zoster; Human immunodeficiency virus; Infection, ophthalmic, viral; Varicella)

Vitamin C, deficiency of
Miradon Tablets........3042

Vitamin D toxicity
(*see under* Toxicity, vitamin D)

Vitamin K, deficiency of
Miradon Tablets........3042

W

Warts, atypical
Podocon-25 Liquid........2478

Warts, bleeding
Podocon-25 Liquid........2478

Wilson's disease
Nicomide Tablets........1088
ParaGard T 380A Intrauterine Copper Contraceptive........1073

Wolff-Parkinson-White syndrome
Covera-HS Tablets........3139
Tarka Tablets........524
Verelan PM Extended-Release Capsules, Controlled-Onset........3106

Women
Avodart Soft Gelatin Capsules........1390
Edex Injection........3089
Eligard 22.5 mg........2883
Eligard 30 mg........2885
Eligard 45 mg........2888
Striant Mucoadhesive........1007
Vantas........3375

X

Xeroderma pigmentosum
Oxsoralen Lotion 1%........3352
Oxsoralen-Ultra Capsules........3353

SECTION 6

INTERNATIONAL DRUG NAME INDEX

This section names the *PDR®* equivalents of over 33,000 foreign pharmaceutical products. Organized alphabetically by overseas trade name, it shows the country (or countries) in which the name is used, gives the product's closest U.S. generic equivalent, and lists the associated brand-name prescription drugs described by *PDR®*, together with the page on which they are found.

Products from the following nations are included:

Argentina	France	Malaysia	Sweden
Australia	Germany	Mexico	Switzerland
Austria	Greece	Monaco	Thailand
Belgium	Hong Kong	New Zealand	The Netherlands
Brazil	Hungary	Norway	United Arab Emirates
Canada	India	Portugal	United Kingdom
Chile	Irish Republic	Russia	Venezuela
Czech Republic	Israel	Singapore	
Denmark	Italy	South Africa	
Finland	Japan	Spain	

Page numbers refer to the 2007 editions of *PDR®* and the *PDR for Ophthalmic Medicines™*. The symbol denoting an entry in *PDR for Ophthalmic Medicines™* appears in the bottom margin.

These entries are intended only as an aid in approximating the contents of a foreign prescription. For proper dosing guidelines, indications, contraindications, warnings, and precautions of its U.S. equivalents, always consult the underlying *PDR®* text. Foreign trade names are courtesy of *PDR*'s affiliate, MICROMEDEX, Inc.

3A OFTENO (Chile, Mexico)
DICLOFENAC SODIUM
Voltaren Tablets 2307
Voltaren-XR Tablets 2310

3TC (Argentina, Australia, Canada, Hong Kong, Malaysia, Mexico, New Zealand, South Africa, Switzerland)
LAMIVUDINE
Epivir Oral Solution 1427
Epivir Tablets 1427
Epivir-HBV Oral Solution 1432
Epivir-HBV Tablets 1432

3TC COMPLEX (Argentina)
LAMIVUDINE
Epivir Oral Solution 1427
Epivir Tablets 1427
Epivir-HBV Oral Solution 1432
Epivir-HBV Tablets 1432

3TC/AZT (Argentina)
LAMIVUDINE
Epivir Oral Solution 1427
Epivir Tablets 1427
Epivir-HBV Oral Solution 1432
Epivir-HBV Tablets 1432

3TC/EPIVIR (Chile)
LAMIVUDINE
Epivir Oral Solution 1427
Epivir Tablets 1427
Epivir-HBV Oral Solution 1432
Epivir-HBV Tablets 1432

5-MONO (India)
ISOSORBIDE MONONITRATE
Imdur Tablets 3018

9PM (India)
LATANOPROST
Xalatan Ophthalmic Solution . . . . ⊙291

A ACIDO (Argentina)
TRETINOIN
Vesanoid Capsules 2820

A Z OFTENO (Mexico)
AZELASTINE HYDROCHLORIDE
Astelin Nasal Spray 1904

ABAGLIN (Argentina)
GABAPENTIN
Neurontin Capsules 2487

ABAMUNE (India)
ABACAVIR SULFATE
Ziagen Oral Solution 1626
Ziagen Tablets 1626

ABBOCALCIJEX (Greece)
CALCITRIOL
Calcijex Injection 411
Rocaltrol Capsules 2798
Rocaltrol Oral Solution 2798

ABBONIDAZOLE (South Africa)
METRONIDAZOLE
MetroGel-Vaginal Gel 1855

ABBOSYNAGIS (Israel)
PALIVIZUMAB
Synagis Intramuscular Powder 1897

ABENTEL (Thailand)
ALBENDAZOLE
Albenza Tablets 1338

ABEREL (France)
TRETINOIN
Vesanoid Capsules 2820

ABERELA (Norway, Sweden)
TRETINOIN
Vesanoid Capsules 2820

ABERTEN (Greece)
THEOPHYLLINE
Uniphyl Tablets 2710

ABIOLEX (Chile)
AMOXICILLIN
Amoxil Pediatric Drops for Oral Suspension 1343
Amoxil Tablets 1343

ABIOTYL (Argentina)
AMOXICILLIN
Amoxil Pediatric Drops for Oral Suspension 1343
Amoxil Tablets 1343

ABITREN (Hong Kong, Israel, Thailand)
DICLOFENAC SODIUM
Voltaren Tablets 2307
Voltaren-XR Tablets 2310

ABRILAR (Argentina)
SALMETEROL XINAFOATE
Serevent Diskus 1568

ABSORLENT (Spain)
ESTRADIOL
Climara Transdermal System 771
Estring Vaginal Ring 2635

ABTRIM (United Kingdom)
CLOTRIMAZOLE
Lotrimin Cream 3039
Lotrimin Lotion 1% 3039
Lotrimin Topical Solution 1% 3039

ABUTIROI (Mexico)
LEVOTHYROXINE SODIUM
Levothroid Tablets 1186
Levoxyl Tablets 1712
Synthroid Tablets 520

AC VASCULAR (Argentina)
NIMODIPINE
Nimotop Capsules 749

ACALIX (Argentina, Venezuela)
DILTIAZEM HYDROCHLORIDE
Cardizem LA Extended Release Tablets . . . 1728
Tiazac Capsules 1201

ACALKA (Brazil, Chile, Portugal, Spain)
POTASSIUM CITRATE
Urocit-K Tablets 2144

ACANTEX (Chile)
CEFTRIAXONE SODIUM
Rocephin Injectable Vials, ADD-Vantage, Galaxy, Bulk 2800

ACARBAY (India)
ACARBOSE
Precose Tablets 751

ACASMUL (Chile)
DILTIAZEM HYDROCHLORIDE
Cardizem LA Extended Release Tablets . . . 1728
Tiazac Capsules 1201

ACCOLATE (Argentina, Australia, Belgium, Brazil, Canada, Chile, Czech Republic, Finland, Hong Kong, Hungary, Irish Republic, Israel, Mexico, Portugal, Russia, Singapore, South Africa, Spain, Switzerland, Thailand, United Kingdom, Venezuela)
ZAFIRLUKAST
Accolate Tablets 671

ACCOLEIT (Italy)
ZAFIRLUKAST
Accolate Tablets 671

ACCURAN (Greece)
ISOTRETINOIN
Accutane Capsules 2731

ACCURE (Australia)
ISOTRETINOIN
Accutane Capsules 2731

ACCUSITE (United Kingdom)
FLUOROURACIL
Efudex Topical Cream 3363
Efudex Topical Solutions 3363

ACCUTANE (Canada)
ISOTRETINOIN
Accutane Capsules 2731

ACCUTIN (Denmark)
ISOTRETINOIN
Accutane Capsules 2731

ACEA (United Kingdom)
METRONIDAZOLE
MetroGel-Vaginal Gel 1855

ACECOMB (Austria)
HYDROCHLOROTHIAZIDE/LISINOPRIL
Prinzide Tablets 2056

ACE-HEMMER COMP (Germany)
CAPTOPRIL
Captopril Tablets 2149

ACEMEDROX (Brazil)
MEDROXYPROGESTERONE ACETATE
Depo-Medrol Single-Dose Vial 2619

ACEMIN (Austria)
LISINOPRIL
Prinivil Tablets 2052

ACENORM (Australia, Germany)
CAPTOPRIL
Captopril Tablets 2149

ACENORM HCT (Germany)
CAPTOPRIL
Captopril Tablets 2149

ACEOMEL (Hungary, Irish Republic)
CAPTOPRIL
Captopril Tablets 2149

ACEOTO (Spain)
CIPROFLOXACIN
Cipro Oral Suspension 2977

ACEPRAN (Chile)
CLONAZEPAM
Klonopin Tablets 2778

ACEPRESS (Italy)
CAPTOPRIL
Captopril Tablets 2149

ACEPRIL (Denmark, Hong Kong, Hungary, Switzerland, United Kingdom)
LISINOPRIL
Prinivil Tablets 2052

ACEPRILEX (Italy)
CAPTOPRIL
Captopril Tablets 2149

ACERCOMP (Finland)
HYDROCHLOROTHIAZIDE/LISINOPRIL
Prinzide Tablets 2056

ACERDIL (Chile)
LISINOPRIL
Prinivil Tablets 2052

ACERDIL-D (Chile)
HYDROCHLOROTHIAZIDE/LISINOPRIL
Prinzide Tablets 2056

ACEREN (Denmark)
ENALAPRIL MALEATE
Vasotec I.V. Injection 2103

ACERIL (Israel)
CAPTOPRIL
Captopril Tablets 2149

ACETAN (Austria)
LISINOPRIL
Prinivil Tablets 2052

ACETEC (Malaysia)
ENALAPRIL MALEATE
Vasotec I.V. Injection 2103

ACETEN (India, Russia, South Africa)
CAPTOPRIL
Captopril Tablets 2149

ACETENSIL (Czech Republic, Spain)
ENALAPRIL MALEATE
Vasotec I.V. Injection 2103

ACETOFLUX (Brazil)
MEDROXYPROGESTERONE ACETATE
Depo-Medrol Single-Dose Vial 2619

ACETOPT (Australia, New Zealand)
SULFACETAMIDE SODIUM
Klaron Lotion 10% 2909

ACETOXYL (Canada, United Kingdom)
BENZOYL PEROXIDE
Brevoxyl-4 Creamy Wash 3210
Brevoxyl-4 Gel 3210
Brevoxyl-8 Creamy Wash 3210
Brevoxyl-8 Gel 3210
Triaz Cleanser 1892
Triaz Gel 1892

ACID A VIT (Belgium, The Netherlands)
TRETINOIN
Vesanoid Capsules 2820

ACID HALT (Canada)
FAMOTIDINE
Pepcid Injection 2040
Pepcid Injection Premixed 2040
Pepcid Tablets 2038
Pepcid for Oral Suspension 2038

ACIDINE (Malaysia)
FAMOTIDINE
Pepcid Injection 2040
Pepcid Injection Premixed 2040
Pepcid Tablets 2038
Pepcid for Oral Suspension 2038

ACIFLUX (Chile)
RANITIDINE HYDROCHLORIDE
Zantac 25 EFFERdose Tablets 1624
Zantac 150 EFFERdose Tablets 1624
Zantac 150 Tablets 1624
Zantac 300 Tablets 1624
Zantac Injection 1619
Zantac Injection Premixed 1619
Zantac Syrup 1624

ACILAC (Canada)
LACTULOSE
Kristalose for Oral Solution 1034

ACILOC (India, Thailand)
RANITIDINE HYDROCHLORIDE
Zantac 25 EFFERdose Tablets 1624
Zantac 150 EFFERdose Tablets 1624
Zantac 150 Tablets 1624
Zantac 300 Tablets 1624
Zantac Injection 1619
Zantac Injection Premixed 1619
Zantac Syrup 1624

ACILOC RD (India)
RANITIDINE HYDROCHLORIDE
Zantac 25 EFFERdose Tablets 1624
Zantac 150 EFFERdose Tablets 1624
Zantac 150 Tablets 1624
Zantac 300 Tablets 1624
Zantac Injection 1619
Zantac Injection Premixed 1619
Zantac Syrup 1624

ACIVAL (Argentina)
NIMODIPINE
Nimotop Capsules 749

ACLAREX (Greece)
CELECOXIB
Celebrex Capsules 3134

ACLAV (Argentina)
AMOXICILLIN
Amoxil Pediatric Drops for Oral Suspension 1343
Amoxil Tablets 1343

ACLENE (India)
ADAPALENE
Differin Gel 1211

ACLIN (Australia, Hong Kong)
SULINDAC
Clinoril Tablets 1924

ACLINDA (Germany)
CLINDAMYCIN HYDROCHLORIDE
Cleocin Vaginal Ovules 2616

ACLONIUM (Italy)
GABAPENTIN
Neurontin Capsules 2487

ACLORAL (Mexico)
RANITIDINE HYDROCHLORIDE
Zantac 25 EFFERdose Tablets 1624
Zantac 150 EFFERdose Tablets 1624
Zantac 150 Tablets 1624
Zantac 300 Tablets 1624
Zantac Injection 1619
Zantac Injection Premixed 1619
Zantac Syrup 1624

ACLOSAN (Argentina)
TAMSULOSIN HYDROCHLORIDE
Flomax Capsules 850

ACLOSONE (France, South Africa, The Netherlands)
ALCLOMETASONE DIPROPIONATE
Aclovate Cream 2660
Aclovate Ointment 2660

ACNACYL (Australia, Hong Kong, Singapore)
BENZOYL PEROXIDE
Brevoxyl-4 Creamy Wash 3210
Brevoxyl-4 Gel 3210
Brevoxyl-8 Creamy Wash 3210
Brevoxyl-8 Gel 3210
Triaz Cleanser 1892
Triaz Gel 1892

ACNE DERM (Israel)
BENZOYL PEROXIDE
Brevoxyl-4 Creamy Wash 3210
Brevoxyl-4 Gel 3210
Brevoxyl-8 Creamy Wash 3210
Brevoxyl-8 Gel 3210
Triaz Cleanser 1892
Triaz Gel 1892

ACNE HERMAL (Greece)
ERYTHROMYCIN
Ery-Tab Tablets 449
Erythromycin Base Filmtab Tablets 455
Erythromycin Delayed-Release Capsules, USP 457
PCE Dispertab Tablets 515

ACNE MASK (Israel)
BENZOYL PEROXIDE
Brevoxyl-4 Creamy Wash 3210
Brevoxyl-4 Gel 3210
Brevoxyl-8 Creamy Wash 3210
Brevoxyl-8 Gel 3210
Triaz Cleanser 1892
Triaz Gel 1892

ACNE-AID (Spain)
BENZOYL PEROXIDE
Brevoxyl-4 Creamy Wash 3210
Brevoxyl-4 Gel 3210
Brevoxyl-8 Creamy Wash 3210
Brevoxyl-8 Gel 3210
Triaz Cleanser 1892
Triaz Gel 1892

ACNECIDE (Irish Republic, United Kingdom)
BENZOYL PEROXIDE
Brevoxyl-4 Creamy Wash 3210
Brevoxyl-4 Gel 3210
Brevoxyl-8 Creamy Wash 3210
Brevoxyl-8 Gel 3210
Triaz Cleanser 1892
Triaz Gel 1892

ACNECLEAR (Hong Kong)
BENZOYL PEROXIDE
Brevoxyl-4 Creamy Wash 3210
Brevoxyl-4 Gel 3210
Brevoxyl-8 Creamy Wash 3210
Brevoxyl-8 Gel 3210
Triaz Cleanser 1892
Triaz Gel 1892

ACNECOLOR (Switzerland)
CLOTRIMAZOLE
Lotrimin Cream 3039
Lotrimin Lotion 1% 3039
Lotrimin Topical Solution 1% 3039

ACNEFUGE (Switzerland)
BENZOYL PEROXIDE
Brevoxyl-4 Creamy Wash 3210
Brevoxyl-4 Gel 3210
Brevoxyl-8 Creamy Wash 3210
Brevoxyl-8 Gel 3210
Triaz Cleanser 1892
Triaz Gel 1892

ACNEGEL (United Kingdom)
BENZOYL PEROXIDE
Brevoxyl-4 Creamy Wash 3210
Brevoxyl-4 Gel 3210
Brevoxyl-8 Creamy Wash 3210
Brevoxyl-8 Gel 3210
Triaz Cleanser 1892
Triaz Gel 1892

ACNE-MED (Hungary)
BENZOYL PEROXIDE
Brevoxyl-4 Creamy Wash 3210
Brevoxyl-4 Gel 3210
Brevoxyl-8 Creamy Wash 3210
Brevoxyl-8 Gel 3210
Triaz Cleanser 1892
Triaz Gel 1892

ACNEMIN (Spain)
ISOTRETINOIN
Accutane Capsules 2731

ACNEPAS (Argentina)
BENZOYL PEROXIDE
Brevoxyl-4 Creamy Wash 3210
Brevoxyl-4 Gel 3210
Brevoxyl-8 Creamy Wash 3210
Brevoxyl-8 Gel 3210
Triaz Cleanser 1892
Triaz Gel 1892

ACNEPAS E (Argentina)
BENZOYL PEROXIDE
Brevoxyl-4 Creamy Wash 3210
Brevoxyl-4 Gel 3210
Brevoxyl-8 Creamy Wash 3210
Brevoxyl-8 Gel 3210
Triaz Cleanser 1892
Triaz Gel 1892

ACNERYNE (Belgium)
ERYTHROMYCIN
Ery-Tab Tablets 449
Erythromycin Base Filmtab Tablets 455
Erythromycin Delayed-Release Capsules, USP 457
PCE Dispertab Tablets 515

ACNESAN (Argentina, Brazil)
BENZOYL PEROXIDE
Brevoxyl-4 Creamy Wash 3210
Brevoxyl-4 Gel 3210
Brevoxyl-8 Creamy Wash 3210
Brevoxyl-8 Gel 3210
Triaz Cleanser 1892
Triaz Gel 1892

ACNESOL (India)
ERYTHROMYCIN
Ery-Tab Tablets 449
Erythromycin Base Filmtab Tablets 455
Erythromycin Delayed-Release Capsules, USP 457
PCE Dispertab Tablets 515

ACNETANE (South Africa)
ISOTRETINOIN
Accutane Capsules 2731

ACNETRIM (Israel)
ERYTHROMYCIN
Ery-Tab Tablets 449
Erythromycin Base Filmtab Tablets 455
Erythromycin Delayed-Release Capsules, USP 457
PCE Dispertab Tablets 515

ACNEX (Venezuela)
BENZOYL PEROXIDE
Brevoxyl-4 Creamy Wash 3210
Brevoxyl-4 Gel 3210
Brevoxyl-8 Creamy Wash 3210
Brevoxyl-8 Gel 3210
Triaz Cleanser 1892
Triaz Gel 1892

ACNEXYL (Thailand)
BENZOYL PEROXIDE
Brevoxyl-4 Creamy Wash 3210
Brevoxyl-4 Gel 3210
Brevoxyl-8 Creamy Wash 3210
Brevoxyl-8 Gel 3210
Triaz Cleanser 1892
Triaz Gel 1892

ACNIL (Mexico)
TRETINOIN
Vesanoid Capsules 2820

ACNOTIN (Chile, Hong Kong)
ISOTRETINOIN
Accutane Capsules 2731

A-CNOTREN (Greece)
ISOTRETINOIN
Accutane Capsules 2731

ACOFLAM (United Kingdom)
DICLOFENAC SODIUM
Voltaren Tablets 2307
Voltaren-XR Tablets 2310

ACONEX (Austria)
NAPHAZOLINE HYDROCHLORIDE
Albalon Ophthalmic Solution . . . . . ⊙218

ACOVIL (Spain)
RAMIPRIL
Altace Capsules 1702

ACREL (Spain)
RISEDRONATE SODIUM
Actonel Tablets 2683

ACRIDILOLE (Russia)
CARVEDILOL
Coreg Tablets 1414

ACRILANS (Russia)
LANSOPRAZOLE
Prevacid Delayed-Release Capsules 3271

ACSACEA (Austria)
METRONIDAZOLE
MetroGel-Vaginal Gel 1855

ACTA (Hong Kong, Singapore)
TRETINOIN
Vesanoid Capsules 2820

ACTICIN (United Kingdom)
TRETINOIN
Vesanoid Capsules 2820

ACTIDINE (Hong Kong)
FAMOTIDINE
Pepcid Injection 2040
Pepcid Injection Premixed 2040
Pepcid Tablets 2038
Pepcid for Oral Suspension 2038

ACTILAX (Australia)
LACTULOSE
Kristalose for Oral Solution 1034

ACTIMAX (Argentina)
ALENDRONATE SODIUM
Fosamax Tablets 1969

ACTIMOL (India)
DICLOFENAC SODIUM
Voltaren Tablets 2307
Voltaren-XR Tablets 2310

ACTINERVAL (Argentina)
CARBAMAZEPINE
Carbatrol Capsules 3171
Tegretol Chewable Tablets 2295
Tegretol Suspension 2295
Tegretol Tablets 2295
Tegretol-XR Tablets 2295

ACTINO-HERMAL (Germany)
FLUOROURACIL
Efudex Topical Cream 3363
Efudex Topical Solutions 3363

ACTIPRAM (Chile)
CITALOPRAM HYDROBROMIDE
Celexa Tablets 1176

ACTIQ (Australia, Denmark, Finland, France, Germany, Greece, Irish Republic, Norway, Spain, Sweden, United Kingdom)
FENTANYL CITRATE
Actiq 979

ACTIQUIM (Mexico)
NAPROXEN
EC-Naprosyn Delayed-Release Tablets 2761
Naprosyn Suspension 2761
Naprosyn Tablets 2761

ACTISKENAN (France)
MORPHINE SULFATE
Kadian Capsules 577
MS Contin Tablets 2701

ACTISON (Argentina)
AMANTADINE HYDROCHLORIDE
Symmetrel Tablets 1135

ACTIVELLE (Argentina, Brazil, Czech Republic, France, Hong Kong, Hungary, Irish Republic, Israel, Malaysia, Portugal, South Africa, Spain, Thailand, The Netherlands)
ESTRADIOL
Climara Transdermal System 771
Estring Vaginal Ring 2635

ACTONEL (Argentina, Australia, Austria, Belgium, Brazil, Canada, Chile, Czech Republic, France, Greece, Hong Kong, Hungary, Irish Republic, Israel, Italy, Mexico, Portugal, Singapore, South Africa, Spain, Switzerland, Thailand, The Netherlands, Venezuela)
RISEDRONATE SODIUM
Actonel Tablets 2683

ACTOPRIL (Irish Republic)
CAPTOPRIL
Captopril Tablets 2149

ACTOS (Argentina, Australia, Austria, Belgium, Brazil, Canada, Chile, Czech Republic, Denmark, Finland, France, Germany, Greece, Hong Kong, Italy, Japan, New Zealand, Norway, Portugal, Russia, South Africa, Spain, Sweden, Switzerland, Thailand, United Kingdom)
PIOGLITAZONE HYDROCHLORIDE
Actos Tablets 3219

ACUGESIC (Hong Kong)
TRAMADOL HYDROCHLORIDE
Ultram ER Tablets 2392

ACUMOD (South Africa)
AMILORIDE HYDROCHLORIDE/HYDROCHLOROTHIAZIDE
Moduretic Tablets 2028

ACURA (Norway, Sweden)
CETIRIZINE HYDROCHLORIDE
Zyrtec Syrup 2594
Zyrtec Tablets 2594

ACUSPRAIN (South Africa)
NAPROXEN
EC-Naprosyn Delayed-Release Tablets 2761
Naprosyn Suspension 2761
Naprosyn Tablets 2761

ACUTRET (India)
ISOTRETINOIN
Accutane Capsules 2731

ACUZOLE (South Africa)
METRONIDAZOLE
MetroGel-Vaginal Gel 1855

ADAFERIN (Greece, India, Israel, Mexico)
ADAPALENE
Differin Gel 1211

ADALAT (Argentina, Australia, Austria, Belgium, Brazil, Canada, Chile, Czech Republic, Denmark, Finland, Germany, Greece, Hong Kong, Hungary, Irish Republic, Italy, Japan, Malaysia, Mexico, New Zealand, Norway, Portugal, Russia, Singapore, South Africa, Spain, Sweden, Switzerland, Thailand, The Netherlands, United Kingdom, Venezuela)
NIFEDIPINE
Adalat CC Tablets 2964

ADALATE (France)
NIFEDIPINE
Adalat CC Tablets 2964

ADALEX (Brazil)
NIFEDIPINE
Adalat CC Tablets 2964

ADALKEN (Mexico)
PENICILLAMINE
Cuprimine Capsules 1947

ADAMON (Argentina, Austria, Hungary)
TRAMADOL HYDROCHLORIDE
Ultram ER Tablets 2392

ADANA (Argentina)
IRBESARTAN
Avapro Tablets 891

ADANT (France, Israel)
SODIUM HYALURONATE
Hyalgan Solution 2901

ADAPINE (Australia)
NIFEDIPINE
Adalat CC Tablets 2964

ADAPRESS (Switzerland)
NIFEDIPINE
Adalat CC Tablets 2964

ADCO-AMOCLAV (South Africa)
AMOXICILLIN
Amoxil Pediatric Drops for Oral Suspension 1343
Amoxil Tablets 1343

ADCO-CIPRIN (South Africa)
CIPROFLOXACIN
Cipro Oral Suspension 2977

ADCO-LIQUILAX (South Africa)
LACTULOSE
Kristalose for Oral Solution 1034

ADCOR (Brazil)
NIFEDIPINE
Adalat CC Tablets 2964

ADCO-RETIC (South Africa)
AMILORIDE HYDROCHLORIDE/HYDROCHLOROTHIAZIDE
Moduretic Tablets 2028

ADCORTYL (Irish Republic, Israel, United Kingdom)
TRIAMCINOLONE ACETONIDE
Azmacort Inhalation Aerosol 1726
Nasacort AQ Nasal Spray 2922

ADCORTYL IN ORABASE (Irish Republic, United Kingdom)
TRIAMCINOLONE ACETONIDE
Azmacort Inhalation Aerosol 1726
Nasacort AQ Nasal Spray 2922

ADDI-K (Hong Kong, Singapore, Thailand)
POTASSIUM CHLORIDE
K-Dur Extended-Relase Tablets 3033
K-Lor Oral Solution 474
K-Tab Tablets 475

ADECUR (Mexico)
TERAZOSIN HYDROCHLORIDE
Hytrin Capsules 471

ADEFIN (Australia)
NIFEDIPINE
Adalat CC Tablets 2964

ADEKIN (Germany)
AMANTADINE HYDROCHLORIDE
Symmetrel Tablets 1135

ADEL (Mexico)
CLARITHROMYCIN
Biaxin Filmtab Tablets 402
Biaxin Granules 402

ADENOCARD (Brazil, Canada)
ADENOSINE
Adenocard Injection 617
Adenoscan 619

ADENOCOR (Australia, Belgium, Czech Republic, Denmark, Finland, Greece, Hungary, Irish Republic, Israel, Malaysia, New Zealand, Norway, Portugal, Singapore, South Africa, Spain, Sweden, Thailand, The Netherlands, United Kingdom, Venezuela)
ADENOSINE
Adenocard Injection 617
Adenoscan 619

ADENOJECT (India)
ADENOSINE
Adenocard Injection 617
Adenoscan 619

ADENOSCAN (Australia, Austria, Czech Republic, Finland, France, Germany, Hong Kong, Italy, Japan, Spain, The Netherlands, United Kingdom)
ADENOSINE
Adenocard Injection 617
Adenoscan 619

ADEPRIL (Mexico)
CARBAMAZEPINE
Carbatrol Capsules 3171
Tegretol Chewable Tablets 2295
Tegretol Suspension 2295
Tegretol Tablets 2295
Tegretol-XR Tablets 2295

ADERAN (Argentina)
SIBUTRAMINE HYDROCHLORIDE
Meridia Capsules 489

ADESIPRESS-TTS (Italy)
CLONIDINE
Catapres-TTS 844

ADEXONE (Israel)
DEXAMETHASONE
Decadron Tablets 1951

ADEZAN (Greece)
DIPYRIDAMOLE
Persantine Tablets 868

ADEZIO (Hong Kong, Malaysia, Singapore)
CETIRIZINE HYDROCHLORIDE
Zyrtec Syrup 2594
Zyrtec Tablets 2594

ADGYN ESTRO (United Kingdom)
ESTRADIOL
Climara Transdermal System 771
Estring Vaginal Ring 2635

ADGYN MEDRO (United Kingdom)
MEDROXYPROGESTERONE ACETATE
Depo-Medrol Single-Dose Vial 2619

ADIATIN (Mexico)
FAMOTIDINE
Pepcid Injection 2040
Pepcid Injection Premixed 2040
Pepcid Tablets 2038
Pepcid for Oral Suspension 2038

ADICANIL (Greece)
LISINOPRIL
Prinivil Tablets 2052

ADICLAIR (Germany)
NYSTATIN
Nystop Topical Powder USP 2478
Paddock Nystatin USP for Oral Suspension 2478

ADIFEN (Malaysia)
NIFEDIPINE
Adalat CC Tablets 2964

ADIFF (India)
ADAPALENE
Differin Gel 1211

ADIPINE (United Kingdom)
NIFEDIPINE
Adalat CC Tablets 2964

ADIPROST (Greece)
FLUTAMIDE
Eulexin Capsules 3009

ADIPUR (Switzerland)
SIMVASTATIN
Zocor Tablets 2105

ADISAR (Chile)
SIBUTRAMINE HYDROCHLORIDE
Meridia Capsules 489

ADIZEM (Irish Republic, Israel, United Kingdom)
DILTIAZEM HYDROCHLORIDE
Cardizem LA Extended Release Tablets 1728
Tiazac Capsules 1201

ADMON (Spain)
NIMODIPINE
Nimotop Capsules 749

ADOCOMP (Germany)
CAPTOPRIL
Captopril Tablets 2149

ADOCOR (Germany)
CAPTOPRIL
Captopril Tablets 2149

ADOLONTA (Spain)
TRAMADOL HYDROCHLORIDE
Ultram ER Tablets 2392

ADOMAL (Italy)
DIFLUNISAL
Dolobid Tablets 1955

ADRECORT (Mexico)
DEXAMETHASONE
Decadron Tablets 1951

ADREKAR (Austria, Germany)
ADENOSINE
Adenocard Injection 617
Adenoscan 619

ADREXAN (France)
PROPRANOLOL HYDROCHLORIDE
Inderal LA Long-Acting Capsules 3429

ADRONAT (Italy, Portugal)
ALENDRONATE SODIUM
Fosamax Tablets 1969

ADRUCIL (Canada)
FLUOROURACIL
Efudex Topical Cream 3363
Efudex Topical Solutions 3363

ADUCIN (Denmark)
RANITIDINE HYDROCHLORIDE
Zantac 25 EFFERdose Tablets 1624
Zantac 150 EFFERdose Tablets 1624
Zantac 150 Tablets 1624
Zantac 300 Tablets 1624
Zantac Injection 1619
Zantac Injection Premixed 1619
Zantac Syrup 1624

AERFLU (Italy)
FLUNISOLIDE
Aerobid Inhaler System 1171
Aerobid-M Inhaler System 1171

AEROCEF (Austria)
CEFIXIME
Suprax 1843

AERODAN (Chile)
FEXOFENADINE HYDROCHLORIDE
Allegra Capsules 2844

AERODIOL (Argentina, Australia, Austria, Belgium, Brazil, Denmark, France, Germany, Greece, Hong Kong, Irish Republic, Italy, New Zealand, Switzerland, The Netherlands, United Kingdom, Venezuela)
ESTRADIOL
Climara Transdermal System **771**
Estring Vaginal Ring **2635**

AEROLID (Italy)
FLUNISOLIDE
Aerobid Inhaler System............. **1171**
Aerobid-M Inhaler System **1171**

AEROMAX (Germany)
SALMETEROL XINAFOATE
Serevent Diskus **1568**

AERONIX (Spain)
ZAFIRLUKAST
Accolate Tablets **671**

AEROTROP (Argentina)
IPRATROPIUM BROMIDE
Atrovent Inhalation Solution **835**
Atrovent Nasal Spray 0.03%........... **837**
Atrovent Nasal Spray 0.06%........... **839**

AEROVENT (Israel)
IPRATROPIUM BROMIDE
Atrovent Inhalation Solution **835**
Atrovent Nasal Spray 0.03%........... **837**
Atrovent Nasal Spray 0.06%........... **839**

AEROXINA (Argentina)
CLARITHROMYCIN
Biaxin Filmtab Tablets............... **402**
Biaxin Granules................... **402**

AFAZOL (Mexico)
NAPHAZOLINE HYDROCHLORIDE
Albalon Ophthalmic Solution .... **⊙218**

AFENEXIL (Argentina)
PAROXETINE HYDROCHLORIDE
Paxil Oral Suspension.............. **1530**
Paxil Tablets.................... **1530**

AFENIL (Greece)
TRANDOLAPRIL
Mavik Tablets **486**

AFENOXIN (Greece)
CIPROFLOXACIN HYDROCHLORIDE
Ciloxan Ophthalmic Ointment .... **⊙204, 559**
Ciloxan Ophthalmic Solution .... **⊙206**
Cipro Tablets **2977**

AFLODAC (Italy)
SULINDAC
Clinoril Tablets **1924**

AFLODERM (Czech Republic)
ALCLOMETASONE DIPROPIONATE
Aclovate Cream **2660**
Aclovate Ointment................ **2660**

AFLORIX (Argentina)
CLOTRIMAZOLE
Lotrimin Cream.................. **3039**
Lotrimin Lotion 1%................ **3039**
Lotrimin Topical Solution 1% **3039**

AFLUON (Greece, Spain)
AZELASTINE HYDROCHLORIDE
Astelin Nasal Spray **1904**

AFLUTA (Austria)
FLUTAMIDE
Eulexin Capsules................. **3009**

AFONILUM (Austria, Czech Republic, Germany)
THEOPHYLLINE
Uniphyl Tablets **2710**

AFPRED-THEO (Germany)
THEOPHYLLINE
Uniphyl Tablets **2710**

AFTAB (Finland, Germany, Italy)
TRIAMCINOLONE ACETONIDE
Azmacort Inhalation Aerosol.......... **1726**
Nasacort AQ Nasal Spray **2922**

AFTACH (Hong Kong, Japan, Portugal)
TRIAMCINOLONE ACETONIDE
Azmacort Inhalation Aerosol.......... **1726**
Nasacort AQ Nasal Spray **2922**

AFTER BURN (Israel)
LIDOCAINE
Lidoderm Patch **1118**

AGELAN (Hong Kong, Irish Republic)
INDAPAMIDE
Indapamide Tablets **2156**

AGELMIN (Greece, Singapore)
CETIRIZINE HYDROCHLORIDE
Zyrtec Syrup **2594**
Zyrtec Tablets **2594**

AGENERASE (Argentina, Australia, Austria, Belgium, Brazil, Canada, Chile, Denmark, Finland, France, Germany, Greece, Irish Republic, Israel, Italy, Mexico, New Zealand, Norway, Portugal, Russia, Spain, Sweden, Switzerland, United Kingdom, Venezuela)
AMPRENAVIR
Agenerase Capsules **1327**
Agenerase Oral Solution **1332**

AGGRASTAT (Australia, Austria, Belgium, Canada, Czech Republic, Denmark, Finland, Germany, Greece, Hong Kong, Hungary, Irish Republic, Israel, Italy, Malaysia, New Zealand, Norway, Singapore, Sweden, Switzerland, Thailand, The Netherlands, United Kingdom)
TIROFIBAN HYDROCHLORIDE
Aggrastat Injection................ **1907**
Aggrastat Injection Premixed **1907**

AGGRASTET (South Africa)
TIROFIBAN HYDROCHLORIDE
Aggrastat Injection................ **1907**
Aggrastat Injection Premixed **1907**

AGGRENOX (Belgium, Canada, Czech Republic, Germany, Hong Kong, Portugal, Thailand)
DIPYRIDAMOLE
Persantine Tablets **868**

AGILOMED (Austria)
DICLOFENAC SODIUM
Voltaren Tablets **2307**
Voltaren-XR Tablets **2310**

AGIOTEN (Greece)
ENALAPRIL MALEATE
Vasotec I.V. Injection **2103**

AGISTEN (Israel)
CLOTRIMAZOLE
Lotrimin Cream.................. **3039**
Lotrimin Lotion 1%................ **3039**
Lotrimin Topical Solution 1% **3039**

AGOFENAC (Switzerland)
DICLOFENAC SODIUM
Voltaren Tablets **2307**
Voltaren-XR Tablets **2310**

AGOPTON (Austria, Germany, Switzerland)
LANSOPRAZOLE
Prevacid Delayed-Release Capsules **3271**

AGOREX (Switzerland)
AMILORIDE HYDROCHLORIDE/HYDROCHLOROTHIAZIDE
Moduretic Tablets **2028**

AGRASTAT (Argentina, Brazil, Chile, France, Mexico, Spain, Venezuela)
TIROFIBAN HYDROCHLORIDE
Aggrastat Injection................ **1907**
Aggrastat Injection Premixed **1907**

AGREDAMOL (Belgium)
DIPYRIDAMOLE
Persantine Tablets **868**

AGREGAMINA (Portugal)
TICLOPIDINE HYDROCHLORIDE
Ticlid Tablets **2810**

AGREMOL (Thailand)
DIPYRIDAMOLE
Persantine Tablets **868**

AGRENOX (Argentina)
DIPYRIDAMOLE
Persantine Tablets **868**

AGRYLIN (Australia, Brazil, Canada, Greece, Israel, South Africa)
ANAGRELIDE HYDROCHLORIDE
Agrylin Capsules................. **3169**

AGUFAM (Thailand)
FAMOTIDINE
Pepcid Injection **2040**
Pepcid Injection Premixed **2040**
Pepcid Tablets **2038**
Pepcid for Oral Suspension **2038**

AGYR (Austria)
CIPROFLOXACIN HYDROCHLORIDE
Ciloxan Ophthalmic Ointment .... **⊙204, 559**
Ciloxan Ophthalmic Solution .... **⊙206**
Cipro Tablets **2977**

AIRBRONAL (Argentina)
THEOPHYLLINE
Uniphyl Tablets **2710**

AIRCLIN (Brazil)
TRIAMCINOLONE ACETONIDE
Azmacort Inhalation Aerosol.......... **1726**
Nasacort AQ Nasal Spray **2922**

AIROL (Australia, Austria, Czech Republic, Germany, Greece, Israel, Italy, Mexico, Norway, South Africa, Switzerland)
TRETINOIN
Vesanoid Capsules................ **2820**

AK-CIDE (Canada)
PREDNISOLONE ACETATE/SULFACETAMIDE SODIUM
Blephamide Ophthalmic Ointment........ **568**
Blephamide Ophthalmic Suspension **569**

AK-CON (Canada)
NAPHAZOLINE HYDROCHLORIDE
Albalon Ophthalmic Solution .... **⊙218**

AK-FLUOR (Canada)
FLUORESCEIN SODIUM
Fluorescite Injection .... **⊙207**

AKILEN (Hong Kong, Malaysia)
VERAPAMIL HYDROCHLORIDE
Covera-HS Tablets................ **3139**
Verelan PM Extended-Release Capsules, Controlled-Onset **3106**

AKNE CORDES (Austria, Germany)
ERYTHROMYCIN
Ery-Tab Tablets.................. **449**
Erythromycin Base Filmtab Tablets....... **455**
Erythromycin Delayed-Release Capsules, USP **457**
PCE Dispertab Tablets **515**

AKNE-AID-LOTION MILD (Germany)
BENZOYL PEROXIDE
Brevoxyl-4 Creamy Wash............ **3210**
Brevoxyl-4 Gel **3210**
Brevoxyl-8 Creamy Wash............ **3210**
Brevoxyl-8 Gel **3210**
Triaz Cleanser **1892**
Triaz Gel...................... **1892**

AKNECIDE (Czech Republic)
BENZOYL PEROXIDE
Brevoxyl-4 Creamy Wash............ **3210**
Brevoxyl-4 Gel **3210**
Brevoxyl-8 Creamy Wash............ **3210**
Brevoxyl-8 Gel **3210**
Triaz Cleanser **1892**
Triaz Gel...................... **1892**

AKNECOLOR (Czech Republic)
CLOTRIMAZOLE
Lotrimin Cream.................. **3039**
Lotrimin Lotion 1%................ **3039**
Lotrimin Topical Solution 1% **3039**

AKNEDERM ERY (Germany)
ERYTHROMYCIN
Ery-Tab Tablets.................. **449**
Erythromycin Base Filmtab Tablets....... **455**
Erythromycin Delayed-Release Capsules, USP **457**
PCE Dispertab Tablets **515**

AKNEDERM OXID (Germany)
BENZOYL PEROXIDE
Brevoxyl-4 Creamy Wash............ **3210**
Brevoxyl-4 Gel **3210**
Brevoxyl-8 Creamy Wash............ **3210**
Brevoxyl-8 Gel **3210**
Triaz Cleanser **1892**
Triaz Gel...................... **1892**

AKNEFUG (Czech Republic)
ESTRADIOL
Climara Transdermal System **771**
Estring Vaginal Ring **2635**

AKNEFUG ISO (Germany)
ISOTRETINOIN
Accutane Capsules **2731**

AKNEFUG-EL (Czech Republic, Germany, Hungary)
ERYTHROMYCIN
Ery-Tab Tablets.................. **449**
Erythromycin Base Filmtab Tablets....... **455**
Erythromycin Delayed-Release Capsules, USP **457**
PCE Dispertab Tablets **515**

AKNEFUG-OXID (Czech Republic, Germany, Hungary)
BENZOYL PEROXIDE
Brevoxyl-4 Creamy Wash............ **3210**
Brevoxyl-4 Gel **3210**
Brevoxyl-8 Creamy Wash............ **3210**
Brevoxyl-8 Gel **3210**
Triaz Cleanser **1892**
Triaz Gel...................... **1892**

AKNEMAGO (Germany)
ERYTHROMYCIN
Ery-Tab Tablets.................. **449**
Erythromycin Base Filmtab Tablets....... **455**
Erythromycin Delayed-Release Capsules, USP **457**
PCE Dispertab Tablets **515**

AKNEMYCIN (Austria, Belgium, Czech Republic, Germany, Hong Kong, Hungary, Israel, Singapore, Switzerland, The Netherlands)
ERYTHROMYCIN
Ery-Tab Tablets.................. **449**
Erythromycin Base Filmtab Tablets....... **455**
Erythromycin Delayed-Release Capsules, USP **457**
PCE Dispertab Tablets **515**

AKNE-MYCIN (Portugal)
ERYTHROMYCIN
Ery-Tab Tablets.................. **449**
Erythromycin Base Filmtab Tablets....... **455**
Erythromycin Delayed-Release Capsules, USP **457**
PCE Dispertab Tablets **515**

AKNEMYCIN (Malaysia)
ERYTHROMYCIN
Ery-Tab Tablets.................. **449**
Erythromycin Base Filmtab Tablets....... **455**
Erythromycin Delayed-Release Capsules, USP **457**
PCE Dispertab Tablets **515**

AKNEMYCIN PLUS (Germany, Israel, Malaysia, Singapore, United Kingdom)
ERYTHROMYCIN
Ery-Tab Tablets.................. **449**
Erythromycin Base Filmtab Tablets....... **455**
Erythromycin Delayed-Release Capsules, USP **457**
PCE Dispertab Tablets **515**

AKNENORMIN (Germany)
ISOTRETINOIN
Accutane Capsules **2731**

AKNEROXID (Austria, Belgium, Czech Republic, Germany, Hungary, Malaysia, Singapore, Switzerland, The Netherlands)
BENZOYL PEROXIDE
Brevoxyl-4 Creamy Wash............ **3210**
Brevoxyl-4 Gel **3210**
Brevoxyl-8 Creamy Wash............ **3210**
Brevoxyl-8 Gel **3210**
Triaz Cleanser **1892**
Triaz Gel...................... **1892**

AKNESIL (Greece)
ISOTRETINOIN
Accutane Capsules **2731**

AKNEX (Switzerland)
BENZOYL PEROXIDE
Brevoxyl-4 Creamy Wash............ **3210**
Brevoxyl-4 Gel **3210**
Brevoxyl-8 Creamy Wash............ **3210**
Brevoxyl-8 Gel **3210**
Triaz Cleanser **1892**
Triaz Gel...................... **1892**

AKNILOX (Switzerland)
ERYTHROMYCIN
Ery-Tab Tablets.................. **449**
Erythromycin Base Filmtab Tablets....... **455**
Erythromycin Delayed-Release Capsules, USP **457**
PCE Dispertab Tablets **515**

AKNIN (Germany)
ERYTHROMYCIN
Ery-Tab Tablets.................. **449**

Erythromycin Base Filmtab Tablets....... 455
Erythromycin Delayed-Release Capsules, USP 457
PCE Dispertab Tablets 515

AKRIPAMIDE (Russia)
INDAPAMIDE
Indapamide Tablets 2156

AK-SULF (Canada)
SULFACETAMIDE SODIUM
Klaron Lotion 10%........ 2909

AKTIOSAN (Argentina)
DICLOFENAC SODIUM
Voltaren Tablets 2307
Voltaren-XR Tablets 2310

AKUDOL (Italy)
NAPROXEN SODIUM
Anaprox DS Tablets 2761
Anaprox Tablets 2761

ALACOR (Denmark)
ENALAPRIL MALEATE
Vasotec I.V. Injection 2103

ALAGER (Argentina)
AZELASTINE HYDROCHLORIDE
Astelin Nasal Spray 1904

ALAMIL (Brazil)
TERBINAFINE HYDROCHLORIDE
Lamisil Tablets 2232

ALANDIEM (Portugal)
DILTIAZEM HYDROCHLORIDE
Cardizem LA Extended Release Tablets... 1728
Tiazac Capsules 1201

ALAPREN (South Africa)
ENALAPRIL MALEATE
Vasotec I.V. Injection 2103

ALAPRIL (Austria, Italy)
ENALAPRIL MALEATE
Vasotec I.V. Injection 2103

ALBA-3 (Brazil)
ALBENDAZOLE
Albenza Tablets........ 1338

ALBALON (Australia, Belgium, Canada, Hong Kong, Irish Republic, Malaysia, New Zealand, South Africa, Switzerland, Thailand, The Netherlands)
NAPHAZOLINE HYDROCHLORIDE
Albalon Ophthalmic Solution .... ⊙218

ALBALON-A (Australia)
NAPHAZOLINE HYDROCHLORIDE
Albalon Ophthalmic Solution .... ⊙218

ALBASOL (Chile)
NAPHAZOLINE HYDROCHLORIDE
Albalon Ophthalmic Solution .... ⊙218

ALBATEL (Thailand)
ALBENDAZOLE
Albenza Tablets........ 1338

ALBEC (Mexico)
ENALAPRIL MALEATE
Vasotec I.V. Injection 2103

ALBEN (Brazil, Thailand)
ALBENDAZOLE
Albenza Tablets........ 1338

ALBENDA (Thailand, United Arab Emirates)
ALBENDAZOLE
Albenza Tablets........ 1338

ALBENDOL (Malaysia)
ALBENDAZOLE
Albenza Tablets........ 1338

ALBENDROX (Brazil)
ALBENDAZOLE
Albenza Tablets........ 1338

ALBENDY (Brazil)
ALBENDAZOLE
Albenza Tablets........ 1338

ALBENIX (Brazil)
ALBENDAZOLE
Albenza Tablets........ 1338

ALBENSIL (Mexico)
ALBENDAZOLE
Albenza Tablets........ 1338

ALBENTEL (Brazil)
ALBENDAZOLE
Albenza Tablets........ 1338

ALBENZONIL (Brazil)
ALBENDAZOLE
Albenza Tablets........ 1338

ALBEOLER (Chile)
FLUTICASONE PROPIONATE
Cutivate Cream........ 2662
Cutivate Ointment 2665
Flonase Nasal Spray 1440

ALBESINE BIOTIC (Argentina)
AMOXICILLIN
Amoxil Pediatric Drops for Oral Suspension........ 1343
Amoxil Tablets 1343

ALBEZIN (Brazil)
ALBENDAZOLE
Albenza Tablets........ 1338

ALBEZOLE (India)
ALBENDAZOLE
Albenza Tablets........ 1338

ALBICAR (Argentina, Venezuela)
LEVOCARNITINE
Carnitor Injection........ 3188
Carnitor Tablets and Oral Solution 3190

ALBICORT (Belgium, The Netherlands)
TRIAMCINOLONE ACETONIDE
Azmacort Inhalation Aerosol........ 1726
Nasacort AQ Nasal Spray 2922

ALBISTIN (Brazil)
NYSTATIN
Nystop Topical Powder USP........ 2478
Paddock Nystatin USP for Oral Suspension........ 2478

ALBORAL (Mexico)
DIAZEPAM
Diastat Rectal Delivery System 3343
Valium Tablets 2819

ALBUCID (Germany, India, South Africa, United Kingdom)
SULFACETAMIDE SODIUM
Klaron Lotion 10%........ 2909

ALCIS (Spain)
ESTRADIOL
Climara Transdermal System 771
Estring Vaginal Ring 2635

ALCOMICIN (Belgium, Canada, Spain)
GENTAMICIN SULFATE
Garamycin Injectable 3014

ALCOPHYLLIN (South Africa)
THEOPHYLLINE
Uniphyl Tablets 2710

ALDA (Thailand)
ALBENDAZOLE
Albenza Tablets........ 1338

ALDAR (Mexico)
NIFEDIPINE
Adalat CC Tablets 2964

ALDARA (Argentina, Australia, Belgium, Brazil, Canada, Chile, Czech Republic, Denmark, Finland, France, Germany, Greece, Hong Kong, Irish Republic, Israel, Italy, Malaysia, Mexico, New Zealand, Norway, Singapore, South Africa, Spain, Sweden, Switzerland, Thailand, The Netherlands, United Kingdom)
IMIQUIMOD
Aldara Cream, 5%........ 1846

ALDAZINE (Australia, New Zealand)
THIORIDAZINE HYDROCHLORIDE
Thioridazine Hydrochloride Tablets...... 2163

ALDIC (Thailand)
FUROSEMIDE
Furosemide Tablets 2154

ALDIPIN (Switzerland)
NIFEDIPINE
Adalat CC Tablets 2964

ALDIZEM (Czech Republic)
DILTIAZEM HYDROCHLORIDE
Cardizem LA Extended Release Tablets... 1728
Tiazac Capsules 1201

ALDOACNE (Spain)
BENZOYL PEROXIDE
Brevoxyl-4 Creamy Wash 3210
Brevoxyl-4 Gel 3210
Brevoxyl-8 Creamy Wash........ 3210
Brevoxyl-8 Gel 3210
Triaz Cleanser 1892
Triaz Gel........ 1892

ALDOCUMAR (Spain)
WARFARIN SODIUM
Coumadin Tablets 898
Coumadin for Injection 898

ALDORETIC (Portugal)
AMILORIDE HYDROCHLORIDE/HYDROCHLOROTHIAZIDE
Moduretic Tablets 2028

ALDORIL (Canada)
HYDROCHLOROTHIAZIDE/METHYLDOPA
Aldoril Tablets........ 1910

ALDORON NF (Argentina)
DICLOFENAC SODIUM
Voltaren Tablets 2307
Voltaren-XR Tablets 2310

ALDOTRIDE (Italy)
HYDROCHLOROTHIAZIDE/METHYLDOPA
Aldoril Tablets........ 1910

ALDROX (Chile)
ALENDRONATE SODIUM
Fosamax Tablets........ 1969

ALENATO (Argentina)
ALENDRONATE SODIUM
Fosamax Tablets........ 1969

ALENBIT (Greece)
NORFLOXACIN
Noroxin Tablets........ 2032

ALENDIL (Brazil)
ALENDRONATE SODIUM
Fosamax Tablets 1969

ALENDROS (Italy)
ALENDRONATE SODIUM
Fosamax Tablets 1969

ALENSTRAN (Greece)
CETIRIZINE HYDROCHLORIDE
Zyrtec Syrup 2594
Zyrtec Tablets 2594

ALERCINA (Spain)
CETIRIZINE HYDROCHLORIDE
Zyrtec Syrup 2594
Zyrtec Tablets 2594

ALERCORTIL (Argentina)
HYDROCORTISONE
Hydrocortone Tablets........ 1989

ALERDUAL (France)
AZELASTINE HYDROCHLORIDE
Astelin Nasal Spray 1904

ALERFEDINE (Argentina)
FEXOFENADINE HYDROCHLORIDE
Allegra Capsules........ 2844

ALERGI (Argentina)
DEXAMETHASONE
Decadron Tablets 1951

ALERGIDERM (Brazil)
PROMETHAZINE HYDROCHLORIDE
Phenergan Tablets and Suppositories 3440

ALERID (Czech Republic, Germany, India, Sweden)
CETIRIZINE HYDROCHLORIDE
Zyrtec Syrup 2594
Zyrtec Tablets 2594

ALERION (Argentina)
CLONAZEPAM
Klonopin Tablets 2778

ALERLISIN (Spain)
CETIRIZINE HYDROCHLORIDE
Zyrtec Syrup 2594
Zyrtec Tablets 2594

ALERNEX (India)
FEXOFENADINE HYDROCHLORIDE
Allegra Capsules........ 2844

ALERTEC (Canada)
MODAFINIL
Provigil Tablets 988

ALERTOP (Chile)
CETIRIZINE HYDROCHLORIDE
Zyrtec Syrup 2594
Zyrtec Tablets 2594

ALERTOP-D (Chile)
CETIRIZINE HYDROCHLORIDE
Zyrtec Syrup 2594
Zyrtec Tablets 2594

ALETIR (Brazil)
CETIRIZINE HYDROCHLORIDE
Zyrtec Syrup 2594
Zyrtec Tablets 2594

ALEVE (Argentina, Australia, Austria, Belgium, Czech Republic, France, Germany, Hungary, Italy, South Africa, Spain, Switzerland, The Netherlands)
NAPROXEN SODIUM
Anaprox DS Tablets 2761
Anaprox Tablets 2761

ALEXIA (Chile)
FEXOFENADINE HYDROCHLORIDE
Allegra Capsules........ 2844

ALEXIN (Portugal)
LANSOPRAZOLE
Prevacid Delayed-Release Capsules 3271

ALFACORT (Argentina, United Arab Emirates)
HYDROCORTISONE
Hydrocortone Tablets........ 1989

ALFAKEN (Mexico)
LISINOPRIL
Prinivil Tablets 2052

ALFAPROST (Spain)
TERAZOSIN HYDROCHLORIDE
Hytrin Capsules........ 471

ALFASIN (Brazil)
FINASTERIDE
Propecia Tablets........ 2060
Proscar Tablets........ 2067

ALFASON (Germany)
HYDROCORTISONE BUTYRATE
Locoid Lipocream Cream 1160

ALFAZOL (Mexico)
ALBENDAZOLE
Albenza Tablets........ 1338

ALFEROS (Spain)
AZELASTINE HYDROCHLORIDE
Astelin Nasal Spray 1904

ALFIN (Chile)
SILDENAFIL CITRATE
Viagra Tablets 2573

ALFUCA (Thailand)
ALBENDAZOLE
Albenza Tablets........ 1338

ALGEDOL (Argentina)
MORPHINE SULFATE
Kadian Capsules 577
MS Contin Tablets 2701

ALGEFIT (Austria)
DICLOFENAC SODIUM
Voltaren Tablets 2307
Voltaren-XR Tablets 2310

ALGICORTIS (Italy)
HYDROCORTISONE
Hydrocortone Tablets........ 1989

ALGIDERM (Argentina)
ERYTHROMYCIN
Ery-Tab Tablets 449
Erythromycin Base Filmtab Tablets....... 455
Erythromycin Delayed-Release Capsules, USP 457
PCE Dispertab Tablets 515

ALGIOPRUX (Argentina)
NAPROXEN
EC-Naprosyn Delayed-Release Tablets.... 2761
Naprosyn Suspension........ 2761
Naprosyn Tablets 2761

ALGIREM (Russia)
RIMANTADINE HYDROCHLORIDE
Flumadine Syrup 1183
Flumadine Tablets 1183

ALGOCETIL (Italy)
SULINDAC
Clinoril Tablets 1924

ALGONAPRIL (Italy)
NAPROXEN
EC-Naprosyn Delayed-Release Tablets.... 2761

(⊙ Described in PDR For Ophthalmic Medicines™)

Naprosyn Suspension 2761
Naprosyn Tablets 2761

ALGOSENAC (Italy)
DICLOFENAC SODIUM
Voltaren Tablets 2307
Voltaren-XR Tablets 2310

ALGYBREX (Argentina)
CELECOXIB
Celebrex Capsules 3134

ALIB (Brazil)
ALBENDAZOLE
Albenza Tablets 1338

ALIDASE (Argentina)
NAPROXEN
EC-Naprosyn Delayed-Release Tablets 2761
Naprosyn Suspension 2761
Naprosyn Tablets 2761

ALIFLUS (Italy)
SALMETEROL XINAFOATE
Serevent Diskus 1568

ALIN (Brazil)
ALBENDAZOLE
Albenza Tablets 1338

ALIOT (Venezuela)
ALENDRONATE SODIUM
Fosamax Tablets 1969

ALIPASE (France)
PANCRELIPASE
Ultrase Capsules 708
Ultrase MT Capsules 709

ALISEUM (Italy)
DIAZEPAM
Diastat Rectal Delivery System 3343
Valium Tablets 2819

ALIVIOMAS (Spain)
NAPROXEN
EC-Naprosyn Delayed-Release Tablets 2761
Naprosyn Suspension 2761
Naprosyn Tablets 2761

ALKADIL (Czech Republic)
CAPTOPRIL
Captopril Tablets 2149

ALKALIT (Czech Republic)
POTASSIUM CITRATE
Urocit-K Tablets 2144

ALKERAN (Australia, Austria, Belgium, Brazil, Canada, Chile, Czech Republic, Denmark, Finland, France, Germany, Hong Kong, India, Irish Republic, Israel, Italy, Malaysia, Mexico, New Zealand, Norway, Portugal, Russia, Singapore, South Africa, Switzerland, Thailand, The Netherlands)
MELPHALAN
Alkeran Tablets 956
Alkeran for Injection 955

ALKERANA (Argentina)
MELPHALAN
Alkeran Tablets 956
Alkeran for Injection 955

ALL CLEAR (Hong Kong)
NAPHAZOLINE HYDROCHLORIDE
Albalon Ophthalmic Solution ⊙218

ALLECET (South Africa)
CETIRIZINE HYDROCHLORIDE
Zyrtec Syrup 2594
Zyrtec Tablets 2594

ALLEGRA (Argentina, Brazil, Canada, Chile, India, Mexico, Venezuela)
FEXOFENADINE HYDROCHLORIDE
Allegra Capsules 2844

ALLEGRA-D (Canada, Chile, Venezuela)
FEXOFENADINE HYDROCHLORIDE/PSEUDOEPHEDRINE HYDROCHLORIDE
Allegra-D 12 Hour Extended-Release Tablets 2846

ALLEGRO (Israel)
FLUTICASONE PROPIONATE
Cutivate Cream 2662
Cutivate Ointment 2665
Flonase Nasal Spray 1440

ALLER-EZE (United Kingdom)
AZELASTINE HYDROCHLORIDE
Astelin Nasal Spray 1904

ALLERFEN (Italy)
PROMETHAZINE HYDROCHLORIDE
Phenergan Tablets and Suppositories 3440

ALLERGODIL (Argentina, Austria, Belgium, Chile, Czech Republic, Denmark, France, Germany, Hungary, Italy, Portugal, Russia, Switzerland, The Netherlands, Venezuela)
AZELASTINE HYDROCHLORIDE
Astelin Nasal Spray 1904

ALLERGY DROPS (Canada)
NAPHAZOLINE HYDROCHLORIDE
Albalon Ophthalmic Solution ⊙218

ALLERGY RELIEF (Canada)
CETIRIZINE HYDROCHLORIDE
Zyrtec Syrup 2594
Zyrtec Tablets 2594

ALLERMAX (Australia)
MOMETASONE FUROATE
Elocon Cream 0.1% 3005
Elocon Lotion 0.1% 3006
Elocon Ointment 0.1% 3007
Nasonex Nasal Spray 3043

ALLERTEC (Russia, Singapore)
CETIRIZINE HYDROCHLORIDE
Zyrtec Syrup 2594
Zyrtec Tablets 2594

ALLVORAN (Germany)
DICLOFENAC SODIUM
Voltaren Tablets 2307
Voltaren-XR Tablets 2310

ALMARION (Thailand)
THEOPHYLLINE
Uniphyl Tablets 2710

ALMARYTM (Italy)
FLECAINIDE ACETATE
Tambocor Tablets 1856

ALMIRAL (Hong Kong, Russia)
DICLOFENAC SODIUM
Voltaren Tablets 2307
Voltaren-XR Tablets 2310

ALMODAN (United Kingdom)
AMOXICILLIN
Amoxil Pediatric Drops for Oral Suspension 1343
Amoxil Tablets 1343

ALNA (Austria, Germany)
TAMSULOSIN HYDROCHLORIDE
Flomax Capsules 850

ALNOK (Denmark)
CETIRIZINE HYDROCHLORIDE
Zyrtec Syrup 2594
Zyrtec Tablets 2594

ALOPRESIN (Spain)
CAPTOPRIL
Captopril Tablets 2149

ALOVENT (Venezuela)
IPRATROPIUM BROMIDE
Atrovent Inhalation Solution 835
Atrovent Nasal Spray 0.03% 837
Atrovent Nasal Spray 0.06% 839

ALPERTAN (Argentina)
VALSARTAN
Diovan Tablets 2193

ALPHADERM (Belgium, United Kingdom)
HYDROCORTISONE
Hydrocortone Tablets 1989

ALPHADINAL (Mexico)
NAPHAZOLINE HYDROCHLORIDE
Albalon Ophthalmic Solution ⊙218

ALPHADINE (Greece)
RANITIDINE HYDROCHLORIDE
Zantac 25 EFFERdose Tablets 1624
Zantac 150 EFFERdose Tablets 1624
Zantac 150 Tablets 1624
Zantac 300 Tablets 1624
Zantac Injection 1619
Zantac Injection Premixed 1619
Zantac Syrup 1624

ALPHA-LAC (Canada)
LACTULOSE
Kristalose for Oral Solution 1034

ALPHAPRIL (Australia)
ENALAPRIL MALEATE
Vasotec I.V. Injection 2103

ALPOXEN (Denmark, Finland, Norway, Sweden)
NAPROXEN
EC-Naprosyn Delayed-Release Tablets 2761
Naprosyn Suspension 2761
Naprosyn Tablets 2761

ALPROFEN (Spain)
NAPROXEN
EC-Naprosyn Delayed-Release Tablets 2761
Naprosyn Suspension 2761
Naprosyn Tablets 2761

ALPROSTAN (Czech Republic)
ALPROSTADIL
Edex Injection 3089

ALPROSTAPINT (Austria, Czech Republic, Hungary, Israel)
ALPROSTADIL
Edex Injection 3089

ALQUEN (Spain)
RANITIDINE HYDROCHLORIDE
Zantac 25 EFFERdose Tablets 1624
Zantac 150 EFFERdose Tablets 1624
Zantac 150 Tablets 1624
Zantac 300 Tablets 1624
Zantac Injection 1619
Zantac Injection Premixed 1619
Zantac Syrup 1624

ALSARTAN (India)
LOSARTAN POTASSIUM
Cozaar Tablets 1935

ALSARTAN-AM (India)
LOSARTAN POTASSIUM
Cozaar Tablets 1935

ALSARTAN-H (India)
LOSARTAN POTASSIUM
Cozaar Tablets 1935

ALSIDEXTEN (Mexico)
DICLOFENAC SODIUM
Voltaren Tablets 2307
Voltaren-XR Tablets 2310

ALSUCRAL (Finland, Malaysia, Singapore)
SUCRALFATE
Carafate Suspension 701
Carafate Tablets 701

ALTACE (Canada, Venezuela)
RAMIPRIL
Altace Capsules 1702

ALTACEF (India)
CEFUROXIME AXETIL
Ceftin Tablets 1407
Ceftin for Oral Suspension 1407

ALTEMOL (Mexico)
INTERFERON ALFA-N3
Alferon N Injection 1665

ALTEN (Hong Kong, Malaysia, Singapore)
TRETINOIN
Vesanoid Capsules 2820

ALTERCOR (The Netherlands)
SIMVASTATIN
Zocor Tablets 2105

ALTERGEN (Italy)
SODIUM HYALURONATE
Hyalgan Solution 2901

ALTER-H2 (Mexico)
RANITIDINE HYDROCHLORIDE
Zantac 25 EFFERdose Tablets 1624
Zantac 150 EFFERdose Tablets 1624
Zantac 150 Tablets 1624
Zantac 300 Tablets 1624
Zantac Injection 1619
Zantac Injection Premixed 1619
Zantac Syrup 1624

ALTIAZEM (Hong Kong, Italy, Russia, Singapore, Thailand)
DILTIAZEM HYDROCHLORIDE
Cardizem LA Extended Release Tablets 1728
Tiazac Capsules 1201

ALTICORT (Chile)
CLOBETASOL PROPIONATE
Temovate Cream 2668
Temovate E Emollient 2671
Temovate Gel 2669
Temovate Ointment 2668
Temovate Scalp Application 2670

ALTI-MPA (Canada)
MEDROXYPROGESTERONE ACETATE
Depo-Medrol Single-Dose Vial 2619

ALTISBEN (Spain)
SERTRALINE HYDROCHLORIDE
Zoloft Tablets 2586

ALTIVER (Mexico)
CAPTOPRIL
Captopril Tablets 2149

ALTOSONE (Italy)
MOMETASONE FUROATE
Elocon Cream 0.1% 3005
Elocon Lotion 0.1% 3006
Elocon Ointment 0.1% 3007
Nasonex Nasal Spray 3043

ALTRAZ (India)
ANASTROZOLE
Arimidex Tablets 673

ALTRICAL (Mexico)
CALCITRIOL
Calcijex Injection 411
Rocaltrol Capsules 2798
Rocaltrol Oral Solution 2798

ALTROL (Mexico)
CALCITRIOL
Calcijex Injection 411
Rocaltrol Capsules 2798
Rocaltrol Oral Solution 2798

ALTRULINE (Chile, Mexico)
SERTRALINE HYDROCHLORIDE
Zoloft Tablets 2586

ALUDROX AC (Argentina)
RANITIDINE HYDROCHLORIDE
Zantac 25 EFFERdose Tablets 1624
Zantac 150 EFFERdose Tablets 1624
Zantac 150 Tablets 1624
Zantac 300 Tablets 1624
Zantac Injection 1619
Zantac Injection Premixed 1619
Zantac Syrup 1624

ALUPRAM (United Kingdom)
DIAZEPAM
Diastat Rectal Delivery System 3343
Valium Tablets 2819

ALUSULIN (Hungary)
SUCRALFATE
Carafate Suspension 701
Carafate Tablets 701

ALUTAN (Switzerland)
CITALOPRAM HYDROBROMIDE
Celexa Tablets 1176

ALUZINE (United Kingdom)
FUROSEMIDE
Furosemide Tablets 2154

ALVENT (Brazil)
IPRATROPIUM BROMIDE
Atrovent Inhalation Solution 835
Atrovent Nasal Spray 0.03% 837
Atrovent Nasal Spray 0.06% 839

ALVIDINA (Mexico)
RANITIDINE HYDROCHLORIDE
Zantac 25 EFFERdose Tablets 1624
Zantac 150 EFFERdose Tablets 1624
Zantac 150 Tablets 1624
Zantac 300 Tablets 1624
Zantac Injection 1619
Zantac Injection Premixed 1619
Zantac Syrup 1624

ALVI-TEC (Mexico)
AMOXICILLIN
Amoxil Pediatric Drops for Oral Suspension 1343
Amoxil Tablets 1343

ALXEN (Mexico)
NAPROXEN
EC-Naprosyn Delayed-Release Tablets 2761
Naprosyn Suspension 2761
Naprosyn Tablets 2761

ALZAIMAX (Argentina)
DONEPEZIL HYDROCHLORIDE
Aricept Tablets 1094

ALZEN (Portugal)
QUETIAPINE FUMARATE
Seroquel Tablets 690

ALZENTAL (Singapore)
ALBENDAZOLE
Albenza Tablets. 1338

ALZOBEN (Brazil)
ALBENDAZOLE
Albenza Tablets. 1338

ALZOL (Thailand)
ALBENDAZOLE
Albenza Tablets. 1338

ALZOMED-F (Mexico)
BENZONATATE
Tessalon Perles 1199

ALZYR (Finland)
CETIRIZINE HYDROCHLORIDE
Zyrtec Syrup 2594
Zyrtec Tablets 2594

ALZYTEC (Singapore)
CETIRIZINE HYDROCHLORIDE
Zyrtec Syrup 2594
Zyrtec Tablets 2594

AMANTA (Germany)
AMANTADINE HYDROCHLORIDE
Symmetrel Tablets. 1135

AMANTAGAMMA (Germany)
AMANTADINE HYDROCHLORIDE
Symmetrel Tablets. 1135

AMANTAN (Belgium)
AMANTADINE HYDROCHLORIDE
Symmetrel Tablets. 1135

AMATINE (Canada)
MIDODRINE HYDROCHLORIDE
ProAmatine Tablets 3186

AMBAMIDA (Argentina)
ERYTHROMYCIN
Ery-Tab Tablets 449
Erythromycin Base Filmtab Tablets. 455
Erythromycin Delayed-Release Capsules, USP 457
PCE Dispertab Tablets 515

AMBERIN (Sweden)
HYDROCORTISONE
Hydrocortone Tablets 1989

AMBONEURAL (Austria)
SELEGILINE HYDROCHLORIDE
Eldepryl Capsules 3208

AMBRAL (South Africa)
METRONIDAZOLE
MetroGel-Vaginal Gel 1855

AMBROSIL (Brazil)
METRONIDAZOLE
MetroGel-Vaginal Gel 1855

AMCEF (Mexico)
CEFTRIAXONE SODIUM
Rocephin Injectable Vials, ADD-Vantage, Galaxy, Bulk 2800

AMCOLD (India)
CETIRIZINE HYDROCHLORIDE
Zyrtec Syrup 2594
Zyrtec Tablets 2594

AMEBIL (Brazil)
METRONIDAZOLE
MetroGel-Vaginal Gel 1855

AMERGE (Canada)
NARATRIPTAN HYDROCHLORIDE
Amerge Tablets. 1339

AMERIDE (Spain)
AMILORIDE HYDROCHLORIDE/HYDROCHLOROTHIAZIDE
Moduretic Tablets 2028

AMFAMOX (Australia)
FAMOTIDINE
Pepcid Injection 2040
Pepcid Injection Premixed 2040
Pepcid Tablets 2038
Pepcid for Oral Suspension 2038

AMIAS (United Kingdom)
CANDESARTAN CILEXETIL
Atacand Tablets 649

AMICLARAN (Czech Republic)
AMILORIDE HYDROCHLORIDE
Midamor Tablets 2026

AMICLOTON (Czech Republic)
AMILORIDE HYDROCHLORIDE
Midamor Tablets 2026

AMICROBIN (Spain)
NORFLOXACIN
Noroxin Tablets. 2032

AMIDAL (Australia)
AMILORIDE HYDROCHLORIDE
Midamor Tablets 2026

AMIDURET (Germany)
AMILORIDE HYDROCHLORIDE/HYDROCHLOROTHIAZIDE
Moduretic Tablets 2028

AMIGRENIN (Russia)
SUMATRIPTAN SUCCINATE
Imitrex Injection 1463
Imitrex Tablets 1471

AMI-HYDROTRIDE (Malaysia)
AMILORIDE HYDROCHLORIDE
Midamor Tablets 2026

AMIKAL (Denmark, Sweden)
AMILORIDE HYDROCHLORIDE
Midamor Tablets 2026

AMILAMONT (United Kingdom)
AMILORIDE HYDROCHLORIDE
Midamor Tablets 2026

AMILCO (Denmark, Hong Kong, Irish Republic)
AMILORIDE HYDROCHLORIDE/HYDROCHLOROTHIAZIDE
Moduretic Tablets 2028

AMIL-CO (United Kingdom)
AMILORIDE HYDROCHLORIDE/HYDROCHLOROTHIAZIDE
Moduretic Tablets 2028

AMILENE (Chile)
ONDANSETRON
Zofran ODT Orally Disintegrating Tablets . . 1639

AMILIDE (Thailand)
AMILORIDE HYDROCHLORIDE/HYDROCHLOROTHIAZIDE
Moduretic Tablets 2028

AMILMAXCO (United Kingdom)
AMILORIDE HYDROCHLORIDE/HYDROCHLOROTHIAZIDE
Moduretic Tablets 2028

AMILO-BASAN (Switzerland)
AMILORIDE HYDROCHLORIDE/HYDROCHLOROTHIAZIDE
Moduretic Tablets 2028

AMILOCOMP BETA (Germany)
AMILORIDE HYDROCHLORIDE/HYDROCHLOROTHIAZIDE
Moduretic Tablets 2028

AMILOFERM (Sweden)
AMILORIDE HYDROCHLORIDE/HYDROCHLOROTHIAZIDE
Moduretic Tablets 2028

AMILO-OPT (Germany)
AMILORIDE HYDROCHLORIDE/HYDROCHLOROTHIAZIDE
Moduretic Tablets 2028

AMILORAL/HCT (Austria)
AMILORIDE HYDROCHLORIDE/HYDROCHLOROTHIAZIDE
Moduretic Tablets 2028

AMILORETIC (South Africa)
AMILORIDE HYDROCHLORIDE/HYDROCHLOROTHIAZIDE
Moduretic Tablets 2028

AMILORETIK (Austria, Germany)
AMILORIDE HYDROCHLORIDE/HYDROCHLOROTHIAZIDE
Moduretic Tablets 2028

AMILORID COMP (Austria, Switzerland)
AMILORIDE HYDROCHLORIDE/HYDROCHLOROTHIAZIDE
Moduretic Tablets 2028

AMILORID/HCT (Austria, Czech Republic)
AMILORIDE HYDROCHLORIDE/HYDROCHLOROTHIAZIDE
Moduretic Tablets 2028

AMILORIDE COMPOSTO (Portugal)
AMILORIDE HYDROCHLORIDE/HYDROCHLOROTHIAZIDE
Moduretic Tablets 2028

AMILORIDE/HCTZ (Switzerland)
AMILORIDE HYDROCHLORIDE
Midamor Tablets 2026

AMILOSPARE (United Kingdom)
AMILORIDE HYDROCHLORIDE
Midamor Tablets 2026

AMILOSTAD HCT (Austria)
AMILORIDE HYDROCHLORIDE/HYDROCHLOROTHIAZIDE
Moduretic Tablets 2028

AMILOTHIAZID (Germany)
AMILORIDE HYDROCHLORIDE/HYDROCHLOROTHIAZIDE
Moduretic Tablets 2028

AMILOZID (Germany)
AMILORIDE HYDROCHLORIDE/HYDROCHLOROTHIAZIDE
Moduretic Tablets 2028

AMILOZID-B (Hungary)
AMILORIDE HYDROCHLORIDE
Midamor Tablets 2026

AMIMOX (Norway)
AMOXICILLIN
Amoxil Pediatric Drops for Oral Suspension. 1343
Amoxil Tablets 1343

AMINDAN (Germany)
SELEGILINE HYDROCHLORIDE
Eldepryl Capsules 3208

AMINOFILIN (Argentina)
THEOPHYLLINE
Uniphyl Tablets 2710

AMINOMAL (Italy)
THEOPHYLLINE
Uniphyl Tablets 2710

AMINOMUX (Argentina, Chile, Venezuela)
PAMIDRONATE DISODIUM
Aredia for Injection 2179

AMIPHOS (India)
AMIFOSTINE
Ethyol for Injection. 1898

AMIRETIC (Brazil)
AMILORIDE HYDROCHLORIDE/HYDROCHLOROTHIAZIDE
Moduretic Tablets 2028

AMITHIAZIDE (Hong Kong)
AMILORIDE HYDROCHLORIDE/HYDROCHLOROTHIAZIDE
Moduretic Tablets 2028

AMITRID (Finland)
AMILORIDE HYDROCHLORIDE/HYDROCHLOROTHIAZIDE
Moduretic Tablets 2028

AMIXEN (Argentina)
AMOXICILLIN
Amoxil Pediatric Drops for Oral Suspension. 1343
Amoxil Tablets 1343

AMIXX (Germany)
AMANTADINE HYDROCHLORIDE
Symmetrel Tablets. 1135

AMIYODAZOL (Mexico)
METRONIDAZOLE
MetroGel-Vaginal Gel 1855

AMIZIDE (Australia, Irish Republic, New Zealand, South Africa)
AMILORIDE HYDROCHLORIDE/HYDROCHLOROTHIAZIDE
Moduretic Tablets 2028

AMMINAC (Thailand)
DICLOFENAC SODIUM
Voltaren Tablets 2307
Voltaren-XR Tablets 2310

AMMITRAM (Thailand)
TRAMADOL HYDROCHLORIDE
Ultram ER Tablets 2392

AMMI-VOTARA (Thailand)
DICLOFENAC SODIUM
Voltaren Tablets 2307
Voltaren-XR Tablets 2310

AMO VITRAX (Australia, New Zealand, Singapore, South Africa, Sweden, Switzerland, Thailand)
SODIUM HYALURONATE
Hyalgan Solution 2901

AMOBIOTIC (Chile)
AMOXICILLIN
Amoxil Pediatric Drops for Oral Suspension. 1343
Amoxil Tablets 1343

AMOFAT (Mexico)
FAMOTIDINE
Pepcid Injection 2040
Pepcid Injection Premixed 2040
Pepcid Tablets 2038
Pepcid for Oral Suspension 2038

AMOPEN (United Kingdom)
AMOXICILLIN
Amoxil Pediatric Drops for Oral Suspension. 1343
Amoxil Tablets 1343

AMOSPES (Greece)
AMOXICILLIN
Amoxil Pediatric Drops for Oral Suspension. 1343
Amoxil Tablets 1343

AMOTEIN (Spain)
METRONIDAZOLE
MetroGel-Vaginal Gel 1855

AMOVAL (Chile)
AMOXICILLIN
Amoxil Pediatric Drops for Oral Suspension. 1343
Amoxil Tablets 1343

AMOVAL DUO (Chile)
AMOXICILLIN
Amoxil Pediatric Drops for Oral Suspension. 1343
Amoxil Tablets 1343

AMOX (Brazil)
AMOXICILLIN
Amoxil Pediatric Drops for Oral Suspension. 1343
Amoxil Tablets 1343

AMOXAL (Venezuela)
AMOXICILLIN
Amoxil Pediatric Drops for Oral Suspension. 1343
Amoxil Tablets 1343

AMOXAPEN (Hong Kong, Singapore)
AMOXICILLIN
Amoxil Pediatric Drops for Oral Suspension. 1343
Amoxil Tablets 1343

AMOXCILLIN (Thailand)
AMOXICILLIN
Amoxil Pediatric Drops for Oral Suspension. 1343
Amoxil Tablets 1343

AMOX-G (Argentina)
AMOXICILLIN
Amoxil Pediatric Drops for Oral Suspension. 1343
Amoxil Tablets 1343

AMOX-G BRONQUIAL (Argentina)
AMOXICILLIN
Amoxil Pediatric Drops for Oral Suspension. 1343
Amoxil Tablets 1343

AMOXI (Argentina)
AMOXICILLIN
Amoxil Pediatric Drops for Oral Suspension. 1343
Amoxil Tablets 1343

AMOXI RESPIRATORIO (Argentina)
AMOXICILLIN
Amoxil Pediatric Drops for Oral Suspension. 1343
Amoxil Tablets 1343

AMOXI-BASAN (Switzerland)
AMOXICILLIN
Amoxil Pediatric Drops for Oral Suspension. 1343
Amoxil Tablets 1343

AMOXIBIOCIN (Germany)
AMOXICILLIN
Amoxil Pediatric Drops for Oral Suspension. 1343
Amoxil Tablets 1343

AMOXIBIOT (Argentina)
AMOXICILLIN
Amoxil Pediatric Drops for Oral Suspension . . . 1343
Amoxil Tablets . . . 1343

AMOXIBRON (Brazil)
AMOXICILLIN
Amoxil Pediatric Drops for Oral Suspension . . . 1343
Amoxil Tablets . . . 1343

AMOXICAP (Brazil)
AMOXICILLIN
Amoxil Pediatric Drops for Oral Suspension . . . 1343
Amoxil Tablets . . . 1343

AMOXICINA (Argentina)
AMOXICILLIN
Amoxil Pediatric Drops for Oral Suspension . . . 1343
Amoxil Tablets . . . 1343

AMOXICOM (Brazil)
AMOXICILLIN
Amoxil Pediatric Drops for Oral Suspension . . . 1343
Amoxil Tablets . . . 1343

AMOXIDAL (Argentina)
AMOXICILLIN
Amoxil Pediatric Drops for Oral Suspension . . . 1343
Amoxil Tablets . . . 1343

AMOXIDENT (United Kingdom)
AMOXICILLIN
Amoxil Pediatric Drops for Oral Suspension . . . 1343
Amoxil Tablets . . . 1343

AMOXIDUO (Venezuela)
AMOXICILLIN
Amoxil Pediatric Drops for Oral Suspension . . . 1343
Amoxil Tablets . . . 1343

AMOXIFAR BALSAMICO (Brazil)
AMOXICILLIN
Amoxil Pediatric Drops for Oral Suspension . . . 1343
Amoxil Tablets . . . 1343

AMOXIGA (Venezuela)
AMOXICILLIN
Amoxil Pediatric Drops for Oral Suspension . . . 1343
Amoxil Tablets . . . 1343

AMOXIGRAND (Argentina)
AMOXICILLIN
Amoxil Pediatric Drops for Oral Suspension . . . 1343
Amoxil Tablets . . . 1343

AMOXIGRAND BRONQUIAL (Argentina)
AMOXICILLIN
Amoxil Pediatric Drops for Oral Suspension . . . 1343
Amoxil Tablets . . . 1343

AMOXIGRAND COMPUESTO (Argentina)
AMOXICILLIN
Amoxil Pediatric Drops for Oral Suspension . . . 1343
Amoxil Tablets . . . 1343

AMOXIL (Hong Kong, Singapore)
AMOXICILLIN
Amoxil Pediatric Drops for Oral Suspension . . . 1343
Amoxil Tablets . . . 1343

AMOXIMED (Brazil)
AMOXICILLIN
Amoxil Pediatric Drops for Oral Suspension . . . 1343
Amoxil Tablets . . . 1343

AMOXINA (Brazil)
AMOXICILLIN
Amoxil Pediatric Drops for Oral Suspension . . . 1343
Amoxil Tablets . . . 1343

AMOXI-PED (Brazil)
AMOXICILLIN
Amoxil Pediatric Drops for Oral Suspension . . . 1343
Amoxil Tablets . . . 1343

AMOXIPOTEN (Argentina)
AMOXICILLIN
Amoxil Pediatric Drops for Oral Suspension . . . 1343
Amoxil Tablets . . . 1343

AMOXITAN (Brazil)
AMOXICILLIN
Amoxil Pediatric Drops for Oral Suspension . . . 1343
Amoxil Tablets . . . 1343

AMOXITENK (Argentina)
AMOXICILLIN
Amoxil Pediatric Drops for Oral Suspension . . . 1343
Amoxil Tablets . . . 1343

AMOXITENK PLUS (Argentina)
AMOXICILLIN
Amoxil Pediatric Drops for Oral Suspension . . . 1343
Amoxil Tablets . . . 1343

AMOXITENK RESPIRATORIO (Argentina)
AMOXICILLIN
Amoxil Pediatric Drops for Oral Suspension . . . 1343
Amoxil Tablets . . . 1343

AMOXIVAN (India)
AMOXICILLIN
Amoxil Pediatric Drops for Oral Suspension . . . 1343
Amoxil Tablets . . . 1343

AMOXOL (Argentina)
AMOXICILLIN
Amoxil Pediatric Drops for Oral Suspension . . . 1343
Amoxil Tablets . . . 1343

AMPINA (Argentina)
NIMODIPINE
Nimotop Capsules . . . 749

AMPLAL (Brazil)
AMOXICILLIN
Amoxil Pediatric Drops for Oral Suspension . . . 1343
Amoxil Tablets . . . 1343

AMPLEXOL (Portugal)
ISOSORBIDE MONONITRATE
Imdur Tablets . . . 3018

AMPLIAR (Argentina)
ATORVASTATIN CALCIUM
Lipitor Tablets . . . 2483

AMPLOMICINA (Brazil)
GENTAMICIN SULFATE
Garamycin Injectable . . . 3014

AMPLOSPEC (Brazil)
CEFTRIAXONE SODIUM
Rocephin Injectable Vials, ADD-Vantage, Galaxy, Bulk . . . 2800

AMPLOZOL (Brazil)
ALBENDAZOLE
Albenza Tablets . . . 1338

AMPRACE (Australia)
ENALAPRIL MALEATE
Vasotec I.V. Injection . . . 2103

AMVISC (Austria, Canada, Israel, Norway, South Africa, Sweden)
SODIUM HYALURONATE
Hyalgan Solution . . . 2901

AMX (Mexico)
AMOXICILLIN
Amoxil Pediatric Drops for Oral Suspension . . . 1343
Amoxil Tablets . . . 1343

AMYCLON (Russia)
CLOTRIMAZOLE
Lotrimin Cream . . . 3039
Lotrimin Lotion 1% . . . 3039
Lotrimin Topical Solution 1% . . . 3039

ANABACT (Irish Republic, Singapore, Thailand, United Kingdom)
METRONIDAZOLE
MetroGel-Vaginal Gel . . . 1855

ANABET (Portugal)
NADOLOL
Nadolol Tablets . . . 2159

ANADOL (Thailand)
TRAMADOL HYDROCHLORIDE
Ultram ER Tablets . . . 2392

ANAEROBEX (Austria)
METRONIDAZOLE
MetroGel-Vaginal Gel . . . 1855

ANAEROBYL (South Africa)
METRONIDAZOLE
MetroGel-Vaginal Gel . . . 1855

ANAEROMET (Belgium, The Netherlands)
METRONIDAZOLE
MetroGel-Vaginal Gel . . . 1855

ANA-FLEX (Brazil)
DICLOFENAC SODIUM
Voltaren Tablets . . . 2307
Voltaren-XR Tablets . . . 2310

ANAFLIN (Mexico)
NAPROXEN
EC-Naprosyn Delayed-Release Tablets . . . 2761
Naprosyn Suspension . . . 2761
Naprosyn Tablets . . . 2761

ANAGREGAL (Italy)
TICLOPIDINE HYDROCHLORIDE
Ticlid Tablets . . . 2810

ANALAB (Malaysia, Thailand)
TRAMADOL HYDROCHLORIDE
Ultram ER Tablets . . . 2392

ANALEPT (Greece)
ENALAPRIL MALEATE
Vasotec I.V. Injection . . . 2103

ANALERGIN (Russia)
CETIRIZINE HYDROCHLORIDE
Zyrtec Syrup . . . 2594
Zyrtec Tablets . . . 2594

ANALERIC (Greece)
DIFLUNISAL
Dolobid Tablets . . . 1955

ANALFIN (Mexico)
MORPHINE SULFATE
Kadian Capsules . . . 577
MS Contin Tablets . . . 2701

ANALPAN (Hong Kong)
DICLOFENAC SODIUM
Voltaren Tablets . . . 2307
Voltaren-XR Tablets . . . 2310

ANAMORPH (Australia)
MORPHINE SULFATE
Kadian Capsules . . . 577
MS Contin Tablets . . . 2701

ANANGOR (Brazil)
TRAMADOL HYDROCHLORIDE
Ultram ER Tablets . . . 2392

ANAPRIL (Hong Kong, Singapore, Thailand)
ENALAPRIL MALEATE
Vasotec I.V. Injection . . . 2103

ANAPROX (Australia, Canada, Greece, Spain)
NAPROXEN SODIUM
Anaprox DS Tablets . . . 2761
Anaprox Tablets . . . 2761

ANAPSYL (Mexico)
NAPROXEN SODIUM
Anaprox DS Tablets . . . 2761
Anaprox Tablets . . . 2761

ANAPTIVAN (Greece)
CEFUROXIME SODIUM
Zinacef Injection . . . 1631

ANAREX (Malaysia)
ORPHENADRINE CITRATE
Norflex Injection . . . 1856

ANASKEBIR (Argentina)
ANASTROZOLE
Arimidex Tablets . . . 673

ANASMOL (Venezuela)
WARFARIN SODIUM
Coumadin Tablets . . . 898
Coumadin for Injection . . . 898

ANASTRAZE (Argentina)
ANASTROZOLE
Arimidex Tablets . . . 673

ANATINE (Argentina)
FINASTERIDE
Propecia Tablets . . . 2060
Proscar Tablets . . . 2067

ANAUS (Argentina)
SILDENAFIL CITRATE
Viagra Tablets . . . 2573

ANAX (Singapore)
NAPROXEN SODIUM
Anaprox DS Tablets . . . 2761
Anaprox Tablets . . . 2761

ANDAPSIN (Sweden)
SUCRALFATE
Carafate Suspension . . . 701
Carafate Tablets . . . 701

ANDRAXAN (Czech Republic)
FLUTAMIDE
Eulexin Capsules . . . 3009

ANDREGEN (India)
GENTAMICIN SULFATE
Garamycin Injectable . . . 3014

ANDRIN (Argentina)
TERAZOSIN HYDROCHLORIDE
Hytrin Capsules . . . 471

ANDROBLOC (Austria)
FLUTAMIDE
Eulexin Capsules . . . 3009

ANDRODOR (Chile)
FLUTAMIDE
Eulexin Capsules . . . 3009

ANDROFLOXIN (Brazil)
NORFLOXACIN
Noroxin Tablets . . . 2032

ANDROLIP (Brazil)
SIMVASTATIN
Zocor Tablets . . . 2105

ANDROPEL (Argentina)
FINASTERIDE
Propecia Tablets . . . 2060
Proscar Tablets . . . 2067

ANDROSTAT (Irish Republic)
FLUTAMIDE
Eulexin Capsules . . . 3009

ANDROTIN (Mexico)
FAMOTIDINE
Pepcid Injection . . . 2040
Pepcid Injection Premixed . . . 2040
Pepcid Tablets . . . 2038
Pepcid for Oral Suspension . . . 2038

ANEMUL MONO (Germany)
DEXAMETHASONE
Decadron Tablets . . . 1951

ANEUROL (Spain)
DIAZEPAM
Diastat Rectal Delivery System . . . 3343
Valium Tablets . . . 2819

ANEXATE (Australia, Austria, Belgium, Canada, Czech Republic, France, Germany, Greece, Hong Kong, Hungary, Irish Republic, Israel, Italy, New Zealand, Norway, Portugal, Singapore, South Africa, Spain, Switzerland, Thailand, The Netherlands, United Kingdom)
FLUMAZENIL
Romazicon Injection . . . 2804

ANFENAX (New Zealand, South Africa)
DICLOFENAC SODIUM
Voltaren Tablets . . . 2307
Voltaren-XR Tablets . . . 2310

ANFLAM (United Kingdom)
HYDROCORTISONE
Hydrocortone Tablets . . . 1989

ANFOZAN (Greece)
ETIDRONATE DISODIUM
Didronel Tablets . . . 2697

ANGELIQ (Argentina, Australia, Greece, South Africa, The Netherlands, United Kingdom)
ESTRADIOL
Climara Transdermal System . . . 771
Estring Vaginal Ring . . . 2635

ANGEZE (United Kingdom)
ISOSORBIDE MONONITRATE
Imdur Tablets . . . 3018

ANGIACT (Denmark)
DILTIAZEM HYDROCHLORIDE
Cardizem LA Extended Release Tablets . . . 1728

Tiazac Capsules 1201

ANGICONTIN (Denmark)
DILTIAZEM HYDROCHLORIDE
Cardizem LA Extended Release Tablets. . . 1728
Tiazac Capsules 1201

ANGIDIL (Italy)
DILTIAZEM HYDROCHLORIDE
Cardizem LA Extended Release Tablets. . . 1728
Tiazac Capsules 1201

ANGILOL (Hong Kong, New Zealand, United Kingdom)
PROPRANOLOL HYDROCHLORIDE
Inderal LA Long-Acting Capsules 3429

ANGIMON (United Kingdom)
VERAPAMIL HYDROCHLORIDE
Covera-HS Tablets 3139
Verelan PM Extended-Release Capsules, Controlled-Onset 3106

ANGINAMIDE (Belgium)
SULFACETAMIDE SODIUM
Klaron Lotion 10%. 2909

ANGINOR (South Africa)
NIFEDIPINE
Adalat CC Tablets 2964

ANGIODROX (Spain)
DILTIAZEM HYDROCHLORIDE
Cardizem LA Extended Release Tablets. . . 1728
Tiazac Capsules 1201

ANGIOFLUOR (Argentina)
FLUORESCEIN SODIUM
Fluorescite Injection . . . . ⊙207

ANGIOLONG (Brazil)
DILTIAZEM HYDROCHLORIDE
Cardizem LA Extended Release Tablets. . . 1728
Tiazac Capsules 1201

ANGIOPINE (United Kingdom)
NIFEDIPINE
Adalat CC Tablets 2964

ANGIOPRIL (Brazil)
ENALAPRIL MALEATE
Vasotec I.V. Injection 2103

ANGIOSAN (Austria)
VALSARTAN
Diovan Tablets 2193

ANGIOTROFIN (Mexico)
DILTIAZEM HYDROCHLORIDE
Cardizem LA Extended Release Tablets. . . 1728
Tiazac Capsules 1201

ANGIOVAL (Greece)
ISOSORBIDE MONONITRATE
Imdur Tablets 3018

ANGIOZEM (United Kingdom)
DILTIAZEM HYDROCHLORIDE
Cardizem LA Extended Release Tablets. . . 1728
Tiazac Capsules 1201

ANGIPRESS (Italy)
DILTIAZEM HYDROCHLORIDE
Cardizem LA Extended Release Tablets. . . 1728
Tiazac Capsules 1201

ANGITIL (United Kingdom)
DILTIAZEM HYDROCHLORIDE
Cardizem LA Extended Release Tablets. . . 1728
Tiazac Capsules 1201

ANGITRATE (South Africa)
ISOSORBIDE MONONITRATE
Imdur Tablets 3018

ANGIZEM (Italy, Singapore, Thailand)
DILTIAZEM HYDROCHLORIDE
Cardizem LA Extended Release Tablets. . . 1728
Tiazac Capsules 1201

ANIDUV (Argentina)
NIMODIPINE
Nimotop Capsules 749

ANIFED (Italy)
NIFEDIPINE
Adalat CC Tablets 2964

ANISTAL (Mexico)
RANITIDINE HYDROCHLORIDE
Zantac 25 EFFERdose Tablets 1624
Zantac 150 EFFERdose Tablets. 1624
Zantac 150 Tablets 1624
Zantac 300 Tablets 1624
Zantac Injection 1619
Zantac Injection Premixed 1619
Zantac Syrup 1624

ANNOXEN (Thailand)
NAPROXEN SODIUM
Anaprox DS Tablets 2761
Anaprox Tablets 2761

ANORFIN (Denmark)
BUPRENORPHINE HYDROCHLORIDE
Buprenex Injectable 2716

ANPEC (Australia)
VERAPAMIL HYDROCHLORIDE
Covera-HS Tablets 3139
Verelan PM Extended-Release Capsules, Controlled-Onset 3106

ANPINE (Australia)
NIFEDIPINE
Adalat CC Tablets 2964

ANSENTRON (Brazil)
ONDANSETRON HYDROCHLORIDE
Zofran Injection. 1634
Zofran Injection Premixed 1634
Zofran Oral Solution. 1639
Zofran Tablets 1639

ANSILAN (Greece)
FAMOTIDINE
Pepcid Injection 2040
Pepcid Injection Premixed 2040
Pepcid Tablets 2038
Pepcid for Oral Suspension 2038

ANSILIVE (Brazil)
DIAZEPAM
Diastat Rectal Delivery System 3343
Valium Tablets 2819

ANSIOLIN (Italy)
DIAZEPAM
Diastat Rectal Delivery System 3343
Valium Tablets 2819

ANSIUM (Spain)
DIAZEPAM
Diastat Rectal Delivery System 3343
Valium Tablets 2819

ANTADINE (Australia, South Africa)
AMANTADINE HYDROCHLORIDE
Symmetrel Tablets. 1135

ANTAFIT (Thailand)
CARBAMAZEPINE
Carbatrol Capsules 3171
Tegretol Chewable Tablets 2295
Tegretol Suspension. 2295
Tegretol Tablets 2295
Tegretol-XR Tablets 2295

ANTAGON (Brazil)
RANITIDINE HYDROCHLORIDE
Zantac 25 EFFERdose Tablets 1624
Zantac 150 EFFERdose Tablets. 1624
Zantac 150 Tablets 1624
Zantac 300 Tablets 1624
Zantac Injection 1619
Zantac Injection Premixed 1619
Zantac Syrup 1624

ANTAGOSAN (France, Germany, Italy)
APROTININ
Trasylol Injection 754

ANTAK (Brazil)
RANITIDINE HYDROCHLORIDE
Zantac 25 EFFERdose Tablets 1624
Zantac 150 EFFERdose Tablets. 1624
Zantac 150 Tablets 1624
Zantac 300 Tablets 1624
Zantac Injection 1619
Zantac Injection Premixed 1619
Zantac Syrup 1624

ANTALGIN (Spain)
NAPROXEN SODIUM
Anaprox DS Tablets 2761
Anaprox Tablets 2761

ANTAMEX (Switzerland)
NIFEDIPINE
Adalat CC Tablets 2964

ANTAROL (Hong Kong, Irish Republic)
PROPRANOLOL HYDROCHLORIDE
Inderal LA Long-Acting Capsules 3429

ANTASTEN (Argentina)
CAPTOPRIL
Captopril Tablets. 2149

ANTEBOR (Belgium, France, Switzerland)
SULFACETAMIDE SODIUM
Klaron Lotion 10% 2909

ANTELEPSIN (Czech Republic, Germany)
CLONAZEPAM
Klonopin Tablets 2778

ANTENEX (Australia)
DIAZEPAM
Diastat Rectal Delivery System 3343
Valium Tablets 2819

ANTEPSIN (Argentina, Brazil, Denmark, Finland, Irish Republic, Italy, Norway)
SUCRALFATE
Carafate Suspension 701
Carafate Tablets 701

ANTHEL (Thailand)
ALBENDAZOLE
Albenza Tablets. 1338

ANTHRAXITON (Greece)
DICLOFENAC SODIUM
Voltaren Tablets 2307
Voltaren-XR Tablets 2310

ANTI CD3 (Brazil)
MUROMONAB-CD3
Orthoclone OKT3 Sterile Solution 2360

ANTIBACIN (Greece)
CEFTRIAXONE SODIUM
Rocephin Injectable Vials, ADD-Vantage, Galaxy, Bulk 2800

ANTIBIOCILINA (Argentina)
AMOXICILLIN
Amoxil Pediatric Drops for Oral Suspension. 1343
Amoxil Tablets 1343

ANTIBIOPTAL (Argentina)
TOBRAMYCIN
TOBI Solution for Inhalation 2298

ANTIBIOTREX (France)
ISOTRETINOIN
Accutane Capsules 2731

ANTIBLUT (Greece)
NIFEDIPINE
Adalat CC Tablets 2964

ANTICHOL (Greece)
SIMVASTATIN
Zocor Tablets. 2105

ANTIDIN (Brazil)
RANITIDINE HYDROCHLORIDE
Zantac 25 EFFERdose Tablets 1624
Zantac 150 EFFERdose Tablets. 1624
Zantac 150 Tablets 1624
Zantac 300 Tablets 1624
Zantac Injection 1619
Zantac Injection Premixed 1619
Zantac Syrup 1624

ANTIFUNGOL (Germany, Russia)
CLOTRIMAZOLE
Lotrimin Cream. 3039
Lotrimin Lotion 1%. 3039
Lotrimin Topical Solution 1% 3039

ANTIGREG (Italy, Malaysia, Singapore)
TICLOPIDINE HYDROCHLORIDE
Ticlid Tablets 2810

ANTILYSIN (Czech Republic)
APROTININ
Trasylol Injection 754

ANTIMED (Mexico)
CIPROFLOXACIN
Cipro Oral Suspension 2977

ANTIMICOTICO (Italy)
CLOTRIMAZOLE
Lotrimin Cream. 3039
Lotrimin Lotion 1%. 3039
Lotrimin Topical Solution 1% 3039

ANTIMICOTICO MARTEL (Brazil)
CLOTRIMAZOLE
Lotrimin Cream. 3039
Lotrimin Lotion 1%. 3039
Lotrimin Topical Solution 1% 3039

ANTIMIGRIN (Austria)
NARATRIPTAN HYDROCHLORIDE
Amerge Tablets. 1339

ANTIMYK (Germany)
CLOTRIMAZOLE
Lotrimin Cream. 3039
Lotrimin Lotion 1%. 3039
Lotrimin Topical Solution 1% 3039

ANTIOBIOCILINA (Argentina)
AMOXICILLIN
Amoxil Pediatric Drops for Oral Suspension. 1343
Amoxil Tablets 1343

ANTIPARKIN (Germany)
SELEGILINE HYDROCHLORIDE
Eldepryl Capsules 3208

ANTIPLAQ (Argentina)
CLOPIDOGREL BISULFATE
Plavix Tablets 917, 2926

ANTIPREX (Greece)
ENALAPRIL MALEATE
Vasotec I.V. Injection 2103

ANTITENSIN (Brazil)
PROPRANOLOL HYDROCHLORIDE
Inderal LA Long-Acting Capsules 3429

ANTOPAR (Czech Republic, Hong Kong)
BENZOYL PEROXIDE
Brevoxyl-4 Creamy Wash. 3210
Brevoxyl-4 Gel 3210
Brevoxyl-8 Creamy Wash. 3210
Brevoxyl-8 Gel 3210
Triaz Cleanser 1892
Triaz Gel. 1892

ANTRAL (Mexico)
METRONIDAZOLE
MetroGel-Vaginal Gel 1855

ANULBET (Chile)
FAMOTIDINE
Pepcid Injection 2040
Pepcid Injection Premixed 2040
Pepcid Tablets 2038
Pepcid for Oral Suspension 2038

ANXICALM (Irish Republic)
DIAZEPAM
Diastat Rectal Delivery System 3343
Valium Tablets 2819

ANZEM (South Africa)
DILTIAZEM HYDROCHLORIDE
Cardizem LA Extended Release Tablets. . . 1728
Tiazac Capsules 1201

ANZOPROL (Brazil)
LANSOPRAZOLE
Prevacid Delayed-Release Capsules 3271

AORTEN (Brazil)
CAPTOPRIL
Captopril Tablets. 2149

AOVA (Greece)
RANITIDINE HYDROCHLORIDE
Zantac 25 EFFERdose Tablets 1624
Zantac 150 EFFERdose Tablets. 1624
Zantac 150 Tablets 1624
Zantac 300 Tablets 1624
Zantac Injection 1619
Zantac Injection Premixed 1619
Zantac Syrup 1624

AP INYECT CLORURO POTASICO (Spain)
POTASSIUM CHLORIDE
K-Dur Extended-Relase Tablets 3033
K-Lor Oral Solution. 474
K-Tab Tablets 475

APARO (Austria)
PAROXETINE HYDROCHLORIDE
Paxil Oral Suspension. 1530
Paxil Tablets. 1530

APAURIN (Czech Republic, Russia)
DIAZEPAM
Diastat Rectal Delivery System 3343
Valium Tablets 2819

APECITAB (Argentina)
CAPECITABINE
Xeloda Tablets 2822

APEPLUS (Chile)
FINASTERIDE
Propecia Tablets 2060
Proscar Tablets. 2067

APILCAV (Brazil)
ALPROSTADIL
Edex Injection. 3089

APIMID (Germany)
FLUTAMIDE
Eulexin Capsules 3009

APIROL (Israel)
NORFLOXACIN
Noroxin Tablets 2032

APLAKET (Czech Republic, Hong Kong, Italy, Malaysia, Portugal, Singapore, Thailand)
TICLOPIDINE HYDROCHLORIDE
Ticlid Tablets 2810

APLATIC (Hungary)
TICLOPIDINE HYDROCHLORIDE
Ticlid Tablets 2810

A-PLEX (Mexico)
TRETINOIN
Vesanoid Capsules 2820

APOACOR (Israel)
VERAPAMIL HYDROCHLORIDE
Covera-HS Tablets 3139
Verelan PM Extended-Release Capsules, Controlled-Onset 3106

APO-AMILZIDE (Canada, Czech Republic, Hong Kong, Malaysia, Singapore)
AMILORIDE HYDROCHLORIDE/HYDROCHLOROTHIAZIDE
Moduretic Tablets 2028

APO-AMOXI (Hong Kong)
AMOXICILLIN
Amoxil Pediatric Drops for Oral Suspension 1343
Amoxil Tablets 1343

APOBACE (Mexico)
CARBAMAZEPINE
Carbatrol Capsules 3171
Tegretol Chewable Tablets 2295
Tegretol Suspension 2295
Tegretol Tablets 2295
Tegretol-XR Tablets 2295

APOCANDA (Germany)
CLOTRIMAZOLE
Lotrimin Cream 3039
Lotrimin Lotion 1% 3039
Lotrimin Topical Solution 1% 3039

APOCAPEN (Israel)
CAPTOPRIL
Captopril Tablets 2149

APO-CAPTO (Canada, Czech Republic, Hong Kong, Malaysia, Russia, Singapore)
CAPTOPRIL
Captopril Tablets 2149

APOCARD (Portugal, Spain)
FLECAINIDE ACETATE
Tambocor Tablets 1856

APO-DICLO (Czech Republic, Malaysia, New Zealand, Russia)
DICLOFENAC SODIUM
Voltaren Tablets 2307
Voltaren-XR Tablets 2310

APO-DILTIAZ (Canada, Hong Kong)
DILTIAZEM HYDROCHLORIDE
Cardizem LA Extended Release Tablets 1728
Tiazac Capsules 1201

APO-ERYTHRO (Hong Kong)
ERYTHROMYCIN
Ery-Tab Tablets 449
Erythromycin Base Filmtab Tablets 455
Erythromycin Delayed-Release Capsules, USP 457
PCE Dispertab Tablets 515

APO-FEDIPISAL (Mexico)
NIFEDIPINE
Adalat CC Tablets 2964

APO-FENO (Canada, Czech Republic)
FENOFIBRATE
Tricor Tablets 527

APO-FENO-MICRO (Hong Kong, Malaysia)
FENOFIBRATE
Tricor Tablets 527

APOFLOX (Mexico)
CIPROFLOXACIN
Cipro Oral Suspension 2977

APOGASTINE (Israel)
FAMOTIDINE
Pepcid Injection 2040
Pepcid Injection Premixed 2040
Pepcid Tablets 2038
Pepcid for Oral Suspension 2038

APO-IPRAVENT (Canada, New Zealand)
IPRATROPIUM BROMIDE
Atrovent Inhalation Solution 835
Atrovent Nasal Spray 0.03% 837
Atrovent Nasal Spray 0.06% 839

APO-K (Canada, Hong Kong, Malaysia)
POTASSIUM CHLORIDE
K-Dur Extended-Relase Tablets 3033
K-Lor Oral Solution 474
K-Tab Tablets 475

APOLLONSET (Greece)
DIAZEPAM
Diastat Rectal Delivery System 3343
Valium Tablets 2819

APO-MEDROXY (Canada)
MEDROXYPROGESTERONE ACETATE
Depo-Medrol Single-Dose Vial 2619

APO-METHAZIDE (Canada)
HYDROCHLOROTHIAZIDE/METHYLDOPA
Aldoril Tablets 1910

APOMEX (Israel)
SELEGILINE HYDROCHLORIDE
Eldepryl Capsules 3208

APOMOXYN (Israel)
AMOXICILLIN
Amoxil Pediatric Drops for Oral Suspension 1343
Amoxil Tablets 1343

APONACIN (Israel)
NAPROXEN
EC-Naprosyn Delayed-Release Tablets 2761
Naprosyn Suspension 2761
Naprosyn Tablets 2761

APO-NADOL (Canada, Hong Kong)
NADOLOL
Nadolol Tablets 2159

APO-NAPRO-NA (Canada, Hong Kong, Malaysia, Singapore)
NAPROXEN SODIUM
Anaprox DS Tablets 2761
Anaprox Tablets 2761

APO-NIFED (Canada, Singapore)
NIFEDIPINE
Adalat CC Tablets 2964

APONISTAN V (Mexico)
NYSTATIN
Nystop Topical Powder USP 2478
Paddock Nystatin USP for Oral Suspension 2478

APO-NORFLOX (Canada)
NORFLOXACIN
Noroxin Tablets 2032

APO-OFLOX (Canada, Malaysia)
OFLOXACIN
Floxin Otic Solution 1049

A-POR (South Africa)
CLOTRIMAZOLE
Lotrimin Cream 3039
Lotrimin Lotion 1% 3039
Lotrimin Topical Solution 1% 3039

APO-SELEG (Czech Republic)
SELEGILINE HYDROCHLORIDE
Eldepryl Capsules 3208

APO-SULIN (Canada, Malaysia)
SULINDAC
Clinoril Tablets 1924

APOTEOPROL (Mexico)
THEOPHYLLINE
Uniphyl Tablets 2710

APO-THEO (Canada, Hong Kong, Malaysia, Singapore)
THEOPHYLLINE
Uniphyl Tablets 2710

APO-TIC (Czech Republic)
TICLOPIDINE HYDROCHLORIDE
Ticlid Tablets 2810

APOTIL (Israel)
TIMOLOL MALEATE
Blocadren Tablets 1916
Timoptic Sterile Ophthalmic Solution 2088
Timoptic in Ocudose 2091
Timoptic-XE Sterile Ophthalmic Gel Forming Solution 2092

APO-TIMOL (Canada, New Zealand)
TIMOLOL MALEATE
Blocadren Tablets 1916
Timoptic Sterile Ophthalmic Solution 2088
Timoptic in Ocudose 2091
Timoptic-XE Sterile Ophthalmic Gel Forming Solution 2092

APO-TIMOP (Canada, Hong Kong, New Zealand)
TIMOLOL MALEATE
Blocadren Tablets 1916
Timoptic Sterile Ophthalmic Solution 2088
Timoptic in Ocudose 2091
Timoptic-XE Sterile Ophthalmic Gel Forming Solution 2092

APO-TRIAZIDE (Hong Kong, Russia, Singapore)
HYDROCHLOROTHIAZIDE/TRIAMTERENE
Dyazide Capsules 1423

APO-TRINA (Mexico)
ERYTHROMYCIN
Ery-Tab Tablets 449
Erythromycin Base Filmtab Tablets 455
Erythromycin Delayed-Release Capsules, USP 457
PCE Dispertab Tablets 515

APOVEN (Australia)
IPRATROPIUM BROMIDE
Atrovent Inhalation Solution 835
Atrovent Nasal Spray 0.03% 837
Atrovent Nasal Spray 0.06% 839

APOVENT (Israel)
IPRATROPIUM BROMIDE
Atrovent Inhalation Solution 835
Atrovent Nasal Spray 0.03% 837
Atrovent Nasal Spray 0.06% 839

APO-VERAP (Canada, Czech Republic)
VERAPAMIL HYDROCHLORIDE
Covera-HS Tablets 3139
Verelan PM Extended-Release Capsules, Controlled-Onset 3106

APOZAN (Israel)
RANITIDINE HYDROCHLORIDE
Zantac 25 EFFERdose Tablets 1624
Zantac 150 EFFERdose Tablets 1624
Zantac 150 Tablets 1624
Zantac 300 Tablets 1624
Zantac Injection 1619
Zantac Injection Premixed 1619
Zantac Syrup 1624

APOZEPAM (Denmark, Sweden)
DIAZEPAM
Diastat Rectal Delivery System 3343
Valium Tablets 2819

APRACUR BIOTIC (Argentina)
AMOXICILLIN
Amoxil Pediatric Drops for Oral Suspension 1343
Amoxil Tablets 1343

APRA-GEL (Belgium)
NAPROXEN
EC-Naprosyn Delayed-Release Tablets 2761
Naprosyn Suspension 2761
Naprosyn Tablets 2761

APRANAX (Belgium, France, Hungary, Switzerland, Venezuela)
NAPROXEN SODIUM
Anaprox DS Tablets 2761
Anaprox Tablets 2761

APRICAL (Czech Republic, Germany, Israel)
NIFEDIPINE
Adalat CC Tablets 2964

APROTEX (Russia)
APROTININ
Trasylol Injection 754

APROVEL (Argentina, Belgium, Brazil, Chile, Czech Republic, Denmark, France, Germany, Greece, Hong Kong, Hungary, Irish Republic, Italy, Malaysia, Mexico, Russia, Singapore, South Africa, Spain, Thailand, Venezuela)
IRBESARTAN
Avapro Tablets 891

APROVEL HCT (Hong Kong, Thailand)
IRBESARTAN
Avapro Tablets 891

APROZIDE (Brazil)
IRBESARTAN
Avapro Tablets 891

APSOLOL (United Kingdom)
PROPRANOLOL HYDROCHLORIDE
Inderal LA Long-Acting Capsules 3429

APUZIN (Malaysia)
CAPTOPRIL
Captopril Tablets 2149

AQUACORT (Canada)
HYDROCORTISONE
Hydrocortone Tablets 1989

AQUANIL (Denmark, Finland, Norway, Sweden)
TIMOLOL MALEATE
Blocadren Tablets 1916
Timoptic Sterile Ophthalmic Solution 2088
Timoptic in Ocudose 2091
Timoptic-XE Sterile Ophthalmic Gel Forming Solution 2092

AQUANIL HC (Chile, Mexico)
HYDROCORTISONE
Hydrocortone Tablets 1989

AQUARETIC (Germany)
AMILORIDE HYDROCHLORIDE/HYDROCHLOROTHIAZIDE
Moduretic Tablets 2028

AQUARID (South Africa)
FUROSEMIDE
Furosemide Tablets 2154

AQUEDUX (Portugal)
FUROSEMIDE
Furosemide Tablets 2154

ARADOIS (Brazil)
LOSARTAN POTASSIUM
Cozaar Tablets 1935

ARADOIS H (Brazil)
LOSARTAN POTASSIUM
Cozaar Tablets 1935

ARAGEST (Israel)
MEDROXYPROGESTERONE ACETATE
Depo-Medrol Single-Dose Vial 2619

ARATAN (Chile)
LOSARTAN POTASSIUM
Cozaar Tablets 1935

ARATAN D (Chile)
HYDROCHLOROTHIAZIDE/LOSARTAN POTASSIUM
Hyzaar 100-25 Tablets 1990
Hyzaar 50-12.5 Tablets 1990

ARBIL (United Kingdom)
CARBAMAZEPINE
Carbatrol Capsules 3171
Tegretol Chewable Tablets 2295
Tegretol Suspension 2295
Tegretol Tablets 2295
Tegretol-XR Tablets 2295

ARBRALENE (United Kingdom)
METOPROLOL TARTRATE
Lopressor Tablets 2238

ARCANAFENAC (South Africa)
DICLOFENAC SODIUM
Voltaren Tablets 2307
Voltaren-XR Tablets 2310

ARCANAMIDE (South Africa)
FUROSEMIDE
Furosemide Tablets 2154

ARCANARETIC (South Africa)
AMILORIDE HYDROCHLORIDE/HYDROCHLOROTHIAZIDE
Moduretic Tablets 2028

ARCID (Spain)
RANITIDINE HYDROCHLORIDE
Zantac 25 EFFERdose Tablets **1624**
Zantac 150 EFFERdose Tablets. **1624**
Zantac 150 Tablets **1624**
Zantac 300 Tablets **1624**
Zantac Injection **1619**
Zantac Injection Premixed **1619**
Zantac Syrup **1624**

ARCLONAC (Thailand)
DICLOFENAC SODIUM
Voltaren Tablets **2307**
Voltaren-XR Tablets **2310**

ARCOIRAN (Spain)
SUMATRIPTAN SUCCINATE
Imitrex Injection **1463**
Imitrex Tablets **1471**

ARDORAL (Spain)
RANITIDINE HYDROCHLORIDE
Zantac 25 EFFERdose Tablets **1624**
Zantac 150 EFFERdose Tablets. **1624**
Zantac 150 Tablets **1624**
Zantac 300 Tablets **1624**
Zantac Injection **1619**
Zantac Injection Premixed **1619**
Zantac Syrup **1624**

AREDIA (Australia, Austria, Belgium, Brazil, Canada, Chile, Czech Republic, Denmark, Finland, France, Germany, Greece, Hong Kong, Hungary, Irish Republic, Israel, Italy, Malaysia, Mexico, New Zealand, Norway, Portugal, Russia, Singapore, South Africa, Spain, Sweden, Switzerland, Thailand, The Netherlands, United Kingdom, Venezuela)
PAMIDRONATE DISODIUM
Aredia for Injection **2179**

AREDRONET (India)
PAMIDRONATE DISODIUM
Aredia for Injection **2179**

AREMIS (Spain)
SERTRALINE HYDROCHLORIDE
Zoloft Tablets **2586**

ARENDAL (Argentina, Chile)
ALENDRONATE SODIUM
Fosamax Tablets **1969**

ARETENSIN (Germany)
RAMIPRIL
Altace Capsules **1702**

ARFLOXINA (Mexico)
CIPROFLOXACIN
Cipro Oral Suspension **2977**

ARGEFLOX (Argentina)
CIPROFLOXACIN HYDROCHLORIDE
Ciloxan Ophthalmic Ointment . . . . ⊙**204, 559**
Ciloxan Ophthalmic Solution . . . . ⊙**206**
Cipro Tablets **2977**

ARIAL (Italy)
SALMETEROL XINAFOATE
Serevent Diskus **1568**

ARICEPT (Australia, Austria, Belgium, Canada, Czech Republic, Denmark, Finland, France, Greece, Hong Kong, Hungary, Irish Republic, Israel, Italy, Japan, Malaysia, New Zealand, Norway, Portugal, Singapore, South Africa, Spain, Sweden, Switzerland, Thailand, United Kingdom)
DONEPEZIL HYDROCHLORIDE
Aricept Tablets **1094**

ARIDIL (United Kingdom)
FUROSEMIDE
Furosemide Tablets **2154**

ARIFON (Russia)
INDAPAMIDE
Indapamide Tablets **2156**

ARILIN (Germany, Switzerland)
METRONIDAZOLE
MetroGel-Vaginal Gel **1855**

ARILINE (Austria)
METRONIDAZOLE
MetroGel-Vaginal Gel **1855**

ARIMIDEX (Argentina, Australia, Austria, Belgium, Brazil, Canada, Chile, Czech Republic, Denmark, Finland, France, Germany, Greece, Hong Kong, Hungary, Irish Republic, Israel, Italy, Malaysia, Mexico, New Zealand, Norway, Portugal, Russia, Singapore, South Africa, Spain, Sweden, Switzerland, Thailand, The Netherlands, United Kingdom, Venezuela)
ANASTROZOLE
Arimidex Tablets **673**

ARISTIN-C (Greece)
CIPROFLOXACIN
Cipro Oral Suspension **2977**

ARISTOCOR (Austria)
FLECAINIDE ACETATE
Tambocor Tablets **1856**

ARISTOCORT (Australia, Hong Kong, New Zealand, Thailand)
TRIAMCINOLONE ACETONIDE
Azmacort Inhalation Aerosol. **1726**
Nasacort AQ Nasal Spray **2922**

ARISTOGYL (India)
METRONIDAZOLE
MetroGel-Vaginal Gel **1855**

ARISTOGYL-F (India)
METRONIDAZOLE
MetroGel-Vaginal Gel **1855**

ARISTROL (India)
CALCITRIOL
Calcijex Injection **411**
Rocaltrol Capsules. **2798**
Rocaltrol Oral Solution **2798**

ARISTROL FORTE (India)
CALCITRIOL
Calcijex Injection **411**
Rocaltrol Capsules. **2798**
Rocaltrol Oral Solution **2798**

ARKAMIN (India)
CLONIDINE HYDROCHLORIDE
Catapres Tablets **843**

ARKAMIN-H (India)
CLONIDINE HYDROCHLORIDE
Catapres Tablets **843**

ARMAMENT (Greece)
BETAXOLOL HYDROCHLORIDE
Betoptic S Ophthalmic Suspension. ⊙**203, 558**

ARMISTOR (Mexico)
ESTRADIOL
Climara Transdermal System **771**
Estring Vaginal Ring **2635**

ARMONIL (Italy)
ESTRADIOL
Estring Vaginal Ring **2635**
Climara Transdermal System **771**

ARMOPHYLLINE (France)
THEOPHYLLINE
Uniphyl Tablets **2710**

ARMOTRAZ (India)
ANASTROZOLE
Arimidex Tablets **673**

ARMOXIN (Mexico)
AMOXICILLIN
Amoxil Pediatric Drops for Oral Suspension. **1343**
Amoxil Tablets **1343**

ARNELA (Chile)
CLOTRIMAZOLE
Lotrimin Cream. **3039**
Lotrimin Lotion 1%. **3039**
Lotrimin Topical Solution 1% **3039**

ARNETIN (Czech Republic, Malaysia)
RANITIDINE HYDROCHLORIDE
Zantac 25 EFFERdose Tablets **1624**
Zantac 150 EFFERdose Tablets. **1624**
Zantac 150 Tablets **1624**
Zantac 300 Tablets **1624**
Zantac Injection **1619**
Zantac Injection Premixed **1619**
Zantac Syrup **1624**

AROMENAL (Argentina)
ANASTROZOLE
Arimidex Tablets **673**

AROPAX (Argentina, Australia, Belgium, Brazil, Mexico, New Zealand, South Africa, Spain)
PAROXETINE HYDROCHLORIDE
Paxil Oral Suspension. **1530**
Paxil Tablets. **1530**

AROXAT (Chile)
PAROXETINE HYDROCHLORIDE
Paxil Oral Suspension. **1530**
Paxil Tablets. **1530**

ARPAMYL LP (France)
VERAPAMIL HYDROCHLORIDE
Covera-HS Tablets **3139**
Verelan PM Extended-Release Capsules, Controlled-Onset **3106**

ARRETIN (Mexico)
TRETINOIN
Vesanoid Capsules. **2820**

ARSENAL (Mexico)
NAPROXEN
EC-Naprosyn Delayed-Release Tablets. . . . **2761**
Naprosyn Suspension **2761**
Naprosyn Tablets **2761**

ARSENAL COMPUESTO (Mexico)
NAPROXEN SODIUM
Anaprox DS Tablets **2761**
Anaprox Tablets **2761**

ARSORB (Australia)
ISOSORBIDE MONONITRATE
Imdur Tablets **3018**

ARTAGEN (India, Thailand)
NAPROXEN
EC-Naprosyn Delayed-Release Tablets. . . . **2761**
Naprosyn Suspension. **2761**
Naprosyn Tablets **2761**

ARTAMIN (Austria, Malaysia, Singapore)
PENICILLAMINE
Cuprimine Capsules **1947**

ARTEROSAN (Chile)
SIMVASTATIN
Zocor Tablets. **2105**

ARTESOL (Chile)
CILOSTAZOL
Pletal Tablets **2455**

ARTFLEX (Argentina)
SODIUM HYALURONATE
Hyalgan Solution **2901**

ARTHREASE (Germany, Israel, United Kingdom)
SODIUM HYALURONATE
Hyalgan Solution **2901**

ARTHREX (Germany)
DICLOFENAC SODIUM
Voltaren Tablets **2307**
Voltaren-XR Tablets **2310**

ARTHREX DUO (Germany)
DICLOFENAC SODIUM
Voltaren Tablets **2307**
Voltaren-XR Tablets **2310**

ARTHROCINE (France)
SULINDAC
Clinoril Tablets **1924**

ARTHROSIN (United Kingdom)
NAPROXEN
EC-Naprosyn Delayed-Release Tablets. . . . **2761**
Naprosyn Suspension. **2761**
Naprosyn Tablets **2761**

ARTHROTEC (Australia, Austria, Belgium, Canada, Czech Republic, Denmark, Finland, Greece, Hong Kong, Irish Republic, Israel, Norway, Portugal, Russia, Singapore, South Africa, Sweden, Switzerland, Thailand, The Netherlands, United Kingdom, Venezuela)
DICLOFENAC SODIUM
Voltaren Tablets **2307**
Voltaren-XR Tablets **2310**

ARTHROXEN (United Kingdom)
NAPROXEN
EC-Naprosyn Delayed-Release Tablets. . . . **2761**
Naprosyn Suspension. **2761**
Naprosyn Tablets **2761**

ARTHRU-DERM (South Africa)
DICLOFENAC SODIUM
Voltaren Tablets **2307**
Voltaren-XR Tablets **2310**

ARTHRUM H (France)
SODIUM HYALURONATE
Hyalgan Solution **2901**

ARTILOG (Italy)
CELECOXIB
Celebrex Capsules. **3134**

ARTONIL (Sweden)
RANITIDINE HYDROCHLORIDE
Zantac 25 EFFERdose Tablets **1624**
Zantac 150 EFFERdose Tablets. **1624**
Zantac 150 Tablets **1624**
Zantac 300 Tablets **1624**
Zantac Injection **1619**
Zantac Injection Premixed **1619**
Zantac Syrup **1624**

ARTOTEC (France)
DICLOFENAC SODIUM
Voltaren Tablets **2307**
Voltaren-XR Tablets **2310**

ARTREN (Brazil)
DICLOFENAC SODIUM
Voltaren Tablets **2307**
Voltaren-XR Tablets **2310**

ARTRENAC (Mexico)
DICLOFENAC SODIUM
Voltaren Tablets **2307**
Voltaren-XR Tablets **2310**

ARTRENAC PRO (Mexico)
DICLOFENAC SODIUM
Voltaren Tablets **2307**
Voltaren-XR Tablets **2310**

ARTRENE (Mexico)
DICLOFENAC SODIUM
Voltaren Tablets **2307**
Voltaren-XR Tablets **2310**

ARTRIBID (Portugal)
SULINDAC
Clinoril Tablets **1924**

ARTRODOL (Italy)
DIFLUNISAL
Dolobid Tablets. **1955**

ARTROFENAC (Italy)
DICLOFENAC SODIUM
Voltaren Tablets **2307**
Voltaren-XR Tablets **2310**

ARTRON (Mexico)
NAPROXEN
EC-Naprosyn Delayed-Release Tablets. . . . **2761**
Naprosyn Suspension. **2761**
Naprosyn Tablets **2761**

ARTROSONE (Spain)
DEXAMETHASONE
Decadron Tablets **1951**

ARTROTEC (Italy, Mexico, Spain)
DICLOFENAC SODIUM
Voltaren Tablets **2307**
Voltaren-XR Tablets **2310**

ARTROXEN (Italy)
NAPROXEN
EC-Naprosyn Delayed-Release Tablets. . . . **2761**
Naprosyn Suspension. **2761**
Naprosyn Tablets **2761**

ARTZ (Denmark, Italy)
SODIUM HYALURONATE
Hyalgan Solution **2901**

ARTZAL (Austria, Finland, Sweden)
SODIUM HYALURONATE
Hyalgan Solution **2901**

ARU C (Germany)
CLOTRIMAZOLE
Lotrimin Cream. **3039**
Lotrimin Lotion 1%. **3039**
Lotrimin Topical Solution 1% **3039**

ARUCLONIN (Czech Republic, Germany, Hungary)
CLONIDINE HYDROCHLORIDE
Catapres Tablets **843**

ARUDEL (Spain)
SIMVASTATIN
Zocor Tablets. **2105**

ARUTIMOL (Czech Republic, Germany, Hungary, Russia)
TIMOLOL MALEATE
Blocadren Tablets **1916**

Timoptic Sterile Ophthalmic Solution 2088
Timoptic in Ocudose 2091
Timoptic-XE Sterile Ophthalmic Gel Forming Solution 2092

ARUTRIN (Germany)
TRIAMCINOLONE ACETONIDE
Azmacort Inhalation Aerosol.......... 1726
Nasacort AQ Nasal Spray 2922

ARUTROPID (Germany)
IPRATROPIUM BROMIDE
Atrovent Inhalation Solution 835
Atrovent Nasal Spray 0.03%........... 837
Atrovent Nasal Spray 0.06%........... 839

ARXEN (Mexico)
NAPROXEN
EC-Naprosyn Delayed-Release Tablets.... 2761
Naprosyn Suspension............. 2761
Naprosyn Tablets 2761

ARXEN COMPOSITUM (Mexico)
NAPROXEN
EC-Naprosyn Delayed-Release Tablets.... 2761
Naprosyn Suspension............. 2761
Naprosyn Tablets 2761

ARYTHMOL (Irish Republic, United Kingdom)
PROPAFENONE HYDROCHLORIDE
Rythmol SR Capsules.............. 2727

ARZEDYN (Greece)
CETIRIZINE HYDROCHLORIDE
Zyrtec Syrup 2594
Zyrtec Tablets 2594

ARZEPAM (Mexico)
DIAZEPAM
Diastat Rectal Delivery System........ 3343
Valium Tablets 2819

ASASANTIN (Australia, Austria, Denmark, Finland, Hungary, Mexico, Sweden, The Netherlands)
DIPYRIDAMOLE
Persantine Tablets 868

ASASANTINE (France)
DIPYRIDAMOLE
Persantine Tablets 868

ASAX (Chile)
FUROSEMIDE
Furosemide Tablets 2154

ASENTA (Israel)
DONEPEZIL HYDROCHLORIDE
Aricept Tablets 1094

ASENTRA (Russia, The Netherlands)
SERTRALINE HYDROCHLORIDE
Zoloft Tablets.................. 2586

ASIAZOLE (Thailand)
METRONIDAZOLE
MetroGel-Vaginal Gel 1855

ASIOLEX (Argentina)
ANASTROZOLE
Arimidex Tablets 673

ASMABIOL (Argentina)
THEOPHYLLINE
Uniphyl Tablets 2710

ASMAFLU (Italy)
FLUNISOLIDE
Aerobid Inhaler System............ 1171
Aerobid-M Inhaler System 1171

ASMANEX (Austria, Brazil, Czech Republic, Denmark, Finland, Germany, Greece, Irish Republic, New Zealand, Spain, Sweden, The Netherlands, United Kingdom)
MOMETASONE FUROATE
Elocon Cream 0.1%.............. 3005
Elocon Lotion 0.1%.............. 3006
Elocon Ointment 0.1% 3007
Nasonex Nasal Spray............. 3043

ASMATIL (Portugal)
FLUTICASONE PROPIONATE
Cutivate Cream................. 2662
Cutivate Ointment 2665
Flonase Nasal Spray 1440

ASMO (Spain)
THEOPHYLLINE
Uniphyl Tablets 2710

ASMO-LAVI (Portugal)
FLUTICASONE PROPIONATE
Cutivate Cream.................. 2662
Cutivate Ointment 2665
Flonase Nasal Spray 1440

ASODOCEL (Argentina)
DOCETAXEL
Taxotere Injection Concentrate 2932

ASOFLUT (Argentina)
FLUTAMIDE
Eulexin Capsules................ 3009

ASONACOR (Austria)
PROPAFENONE HYDROCHLORIDE
Rythmol SR Capsules.............. 2727

ASPASERINE B6 TRANQ (Spain)
DIAZEPAM
Diastat Rectal Delivery System........ 3343
Valium Tablets 2819

ASPENIL (Italy)
AMOXICILLIN
Amoxil Pediatric Drops for Oral Suspension.................. 1343
Amoxil Tablets 1343

ASPITRATE (India)
ISOSORBIDE MONONITRATE
Imdur Tablets................... 3018

ASSIVAL (Israel)
DIAZEPAM
Diastat Rectal Delivery System........ 3343
Valium Tablets 2819

ASTELIN (Mexico)
AZELASTINE HYDROCHLORIDE
Astelin Nasal Spray 1904

ASTERGYL (Brazil)
METRONIDAZOLE
MetroGel-Vaginal Gel 1855

ASTHMA T (Israel)
THEOPHYLLINE
Uniphyl Tablets.................. 2710

ASTRAMORPH (Brazil)
MORPHINE SULFATE
Kadian Capsules 577
MS Contin Tablets 2701

ASUCROSE (India)
ACARBOSE
Precose Tablets 751

ASYTEC (Denmark)
CETIRIZINE HYDROCHLORIDE
Zyrtec Syrup 2594
Zyrtec Tablets 2594

ATAC (Chile)
NAPROXEN SODIUM
Anaprox DS Tablets 2761
Anaprox Tablets 2761

ATACAND (Argentina, Australia, Austria, Belgium, Brazil, Canada, Chile, Czech Republic, Denmark, Finland, France, Greece, Hungary, Irish Republic, Israel, Malaysia, Mexico, New Zealand, Norway, Portugal, Russia, Singapore, South Africa, Spain, Sweden, Switzerland, The Netherlands)
CANDESARTAN CILEXETIL
Atacand Tablets 649

ATACAND PLUS (Australia, Belgium, Canada, Czech Republic, Hungary, Israel, Malaysia, Mexico, Norway, Singapore, South Africa, Spain, Switzerland, The Netherlands)
CANDESARTAN CILEXETIL
Atacand Tablets 649

ATACAND-D (Argentina)
CANDESARTAN CILEXETIL
Atacand Tablets 649

ATACANDZID (Denmark)
CANDESARTAN CILEXETIL
Atacand Tablets 649

ATAMIR (Denmark)
PENICILLAMINE
Cuprimine Capsules............... 1947

ATARIN (Finland)
AMANTADINE HYDROCHLORIDE
Symmetrel Tablets................ 1135

ATARVA (Argentina)
ATORVASTATIN CALCIUM
Lipitor Tablets 2483

ATARVITON (Greece)
DIAZEPAM
Diastat Rectal Delivery System........ 3343
Valium Tablets 2819

ATAZID (Denmark)
CANDESARTAN CILEXETIL
Atacand Tablets 649

ATEM (Italy)
IPRATROPIUM BROMIDE
Atrovent Inhalation Solution 835
Atrovent Nasal Spray 0.03%........... 837
Atrovent Nasal Spray 0.06%........... 839

ATEMUR (Germany)
FLUTICASONE PROPIONATE
Cutivate Cream.................. 2662
Cutivate Ointment 2665
Flonase Nasal Spray 1440

ATENFAR (Chile)
ATORVASTATIN CALCIUM
Lipitor Tablets 2483

ATENIX (Chile)
SIBUTRAMINE HYDROCHLORIDE
Meridia Capsules................. 489

ATENS (Brazil)
ENALAPRIL MALEATE
Vasotec I.V. Injection 2103

ATENSES (Mexico)
NIFEDIPINE
Adalat CC Tablets 2964

ATENSIN (Thailand)
PROPRANOLOL HYDROCHLORIDE
Inderal LA Long-Acting Capsules 3429

ATENSINA (Brazil)
CLONIDINE HYDROCHLORIDE
Catapres Tablets................. 843

ATENSINE (Irish Republic, United Kingdom)
DIAZEPAM
Diastat Rectal Delivery System........ 3343
Valium Tablets 2819

ATERKEY (Spain)
LOVASTATIN
Mevacor Tablets 2021

ATEROCLAR (Argentina, Chile)
ATORVASTATIN CALCIUM
Lipitor Tablets 2483

ATHLETES FOOT CREAM (United Kingdom)
CLOTRIMAZOLE
Lotrimin Cream.................. 3039
Lotrimin Lotion 1%.............. 3039
Lotrimin Topical Solution 1% 3039

ATHROFEN (Switzerland)
DICLOFENAC SODIUM
Voltaren Tablets 2307
Voltaren-XR Tablets 2310

ATIBAX C (Argentina)
CIPROFLOXACIN
Cipro Oral Suspension 2977

ATIFLAN (Mexico)
NAPROXEN
EC-Naprosyn Delayed-Release Tablets.... 2761
Naprosyn Suspension............. 2761
Naprosyn Tablets 2761

A-TINIC (Thailand)
TRETINOIN
Vesanoid Capsules............... 2820

ATLACNE (Argentina)
ISOTRETINOIN
Accutane Capsules 2731

ATLAMICIN (Argentina)
ERYTHROMYCIN
Ery-Tab Tablets 449
Erythromycin Base Filmtab Tablets....... 455
Erythromycin Delayed-Release Capsules, USP 457
PCE Dispertab Tablets 515

ATORLIP (Chile, India)
ATORVASTATIN CALCIUM
Lipitor Tablets 2483

ATORVA (India)
ATORVASTATIN CALCIUM
Lipitor Tablets 2483

ATOSIL (Germany)
PROMETHAZINE HYDROCHLORIDE
Phenergan Tablets and Suppositories.... 3440

ATRISER (Mexico)
SULINDAC
Clinoril Tablets 1924

ATRISOL (Mexico)
CAPTOPRIL
Captopril Tablets................. 2149

ATRIVAL (Argentina)
AMOXICILLIN
Amoxil Pediatric Drops for Oral Suspension.................. 1343
Amoxil Tablets 1343

ATROMBIN (Finland)
DIPYRIDAMOLE
Persantine Tablets 868

ATRONASE (Austria, Belgium, South Africa)
IPRATROPIUM BROMIDE
Atrovent Inhalation Solution 835
Atrovent Nasal Spray 0.03%........... 837
Atrovent Nasal Spray 0.06%........... 839

ATROVENT (Argentina, Australia, Austria, Belgium, Brazil, Canada, Chile, Czech Republic, Denmark, Finland, France, Germany, Greece, Hong Kong, Hungary, Irish Republic, Israel, Italy, Japan, Malaysia, Mexico, New Zealand, Norway, Portugal, Russia, Singapore, South Africa, Spain, Sweden, Switzerland, Thailand, The Netherlands, United Kingdom)
IPRATROPIUM BROMIDE
Atrovent Inhalation Solution 835
Atrovent Nasal Spray 0.03%........... 837
Atrovent Nasal Spray 0.06%........... 839

ATTENTA (Australia)
METHYLPHENIDATE HYDROCHLORIDE
Ritalin Hydrochloride Tablets.......... 2269
Ritalin-SR Tablets................ 2269

ATTOR (India)
ATORVASTATIN CALCIUM
Lipitor Tablets 2483

AT-V (Mexico)
DIAZEPAM
Diastat Rectal Delivery System........ 3343
Valium Tablets 2819

AUDOCAINA (Venezuela)
LIDOCAINE
Lidoderm Patch 1118

AUGELIT (Brazil)
DICLOFENAC SODIUM
Voltaren Tablets 2307
Voltaren-XR Tablets 2310

AUGMENTIN (Venezuela)
AMOXICILLIN
Amoxil Pediatric Drops for Oral Suspension.................. 1343
Amoxil Tablets 1343

AUGMENTIN BID (Venezuela)
AMOXICILLIN
Amoxil Pediatric Drops for Oral Suspension.................. 1343
Amoxil Tablets 1343

AUGMEX (Singapore)
AMOXICILLIN
Amoxil Pediatric Drops for Oral Suspension.................. 1343
Amoxil Tablets 1343

AURODIPINE (Greece)
NIMODIPINE
Nimotop Capsules 749

AUROFOX (Mexico)
CEFTRIAXONE SODIUM
Rocephin Injectable Vials, ADD-Vantage, Galaxy, Bulk 2800

AUROSTATIN (Greece)
LOVASTATIN
Mevacor Tablets 2021

AUSCARD (Australia)
DILTIAZEM HYDROCHLORIDE
Cardizem LA Extended Release Tablets... 1728
Tiazac Capsules 1201

AUSFAM (Australia)
FAMOTIDINE
Pepcid Injection 2040
Pepcid Injection Premixed 2040

Pepcid Tablets . . . 2038
Pepcid for Oral Suspension . . . 2038

AUSPRIL (Australia)
ENALAPRIL MALEATE
Vasotec I.V. Injection . . . 2103

AUSRAN (Australia)
RANITIDINE HYDROCHLORIDE
Zantac 25 EFFERdose Tablets . . . 1624
Zantac 150 EFFERdose Tablets . . . 1624
Zantac 150 Tablets . . . 1624
Zantac 300 Tablets . . . 1624
Zantac Injection . . . 1619
Zantac Injection Premixed . . . 1619
Zantac Syrup . . . 1624

AUSTYN (Australia, Singapore)
THEOPHYLLINE
Uniphyl Tablets . . . 2710

AUTDOL (Chile)
DICLOFENAC SODIUM
Voltaren Tablets . . . 2307
Voltaren-XR Tablets . . . 2310

AUXXIL (Chile)
LEVOFLOXACIN
Levaquin Injection . . . 2384
Levaquin Tablets . . . 2384

AVALIDE (Mexico)
IRBESARTAN
Avapro Tablets . . . 891

AVANDAMET (Argentina, Canada, Chile, Denmark, Finland, France, Greece, Irish Republic, Malaysia, Mexico, Singapore, Sweden, United Kingdom)
ROSIGLITAZONE MALEATE
Avandia Tablets . . . 1384

AVANDIA (Argentina, Australia, Belgium, Brazil, Canada, Chile, Czech Republic, Denmark, Finland, France, Germany, Greece, Hong Kong, Hungary, Irish Republic, Israel, Italy, Malaysia, Mexico, New Zealand, Norway, Portugal, Singapore, South Africa, Spain, Sweden, Switzerland, Thailand, The Netherlands, United Kingdom, Venezuela)
ROSIGLITAZONE MALEATE
Avandia Tablets . . . 1384

AVAPRO (Argentina, Australia, Brazil, Mexico)
IRBESARTAN
Avapro Tablets . . . 891

AVAPRO HCT (Argentina, Australia)
IRBESARTAN
Avapro Tablets . . . 891

AVEPTOL (Greece)
LEVOCARNITINE
Carnitor Injection . . . 3188
Carnitor Tablets and Oral Solution . . . 3190

AVERTEX (Argentina)
FINASTERIDE
Propecia Tablets . . . 2060
Proscar Tablets . . . 2067

AVICIS (Brazil)
ESTRADIOL
Climara Transdermal System . . . 771
Estring Vaginal Ring . . . 2635

AVILAC (Israel)
LACTULOSE
Kristalose for Oral Solution . . . 1034

AVITCID (Finland)
TRETINOIN
Vesanoid Capsules . . . 2820

AVLOCARDYL (France)
PROPRANOLOL HYDROCHLORIDE
Inderal LA Long-Acting Capsules . . . 3429

AVLOSULFON (Canada, Israel)
DAPSONE
Dapsone Tablets USP . . . 1673

AVUXILAN (Mexico)
AMOXICILLIN
Amoxil Pediatric Drops for Oral Suspension . . . 1343
Amoxil Tablets . . . 1343

AXACEF (Denmark, Sweden)
CEFUROXIME SODIUM
Zinacef Injection . . . 1631

AXANT (Chile)
LACTULOSE
Kristalose for Oral Solution . . . 1034

AXASOL (Chile)
CLOTRIMAZOLE
Lotrimin Cream . . . 3039
Lotrimin Lotion 1% . . . 3039
Lotrimin Topical Solution 1% . . . 3039

AXCIL (Mexico)
AMOXICILLIN
Amoxil Pediatric Drops for Oral Suspension . . . 1343
Amoxil Tablets . . . 1343

AXELVIN (Greece)
LISINOPRIL
Prinivil Tablets . . . 2052

AXEPIM (France)
CEFEPIME HYDROCHLORIDE
Maxipime for Injection . . . 1105

AXER (Italy)
NAPROXEN SODIUM
Anaprox DS Tablets . . . 2761
Anaprox Tablets . . . 2761

AXETINE (Belgium, Czech Republic, Hong Kong, Russia, Thailand)
CEFUROXIME AXETIL
Ceftin Tablets . . . 1407
Ceftin for Oral Suspension . . . 1407

AXONE (India)
CEFTRIAXONE SODIUM
Rocephin Injectable Vials, ADD-Vantage, Galaxy, Bulk . . . 2800

AXOTIDE (Switzerland)
FLUTICASONE PROPIONATE
Cutivate Cream . . . 2662
Cutivate Ointment . . . 2665
Flonase Nasal Spray . . . 1440

AXTAR (Mexico)
CEFTRIAXONE SODIUM
Rocephin Injectable Vials, ADD-Vantage, Galaxy, Bulk . . . 2800

AXUROCEF (Thailand)
CEFUROXIME AXETIL
Ceftin Tablets . . . 1407
Ceftin for Oral Suspension . . . 1407

AZ (Venezuela)
AZELASTINE HYDROCHLORIDE
Astelin Nasal Spray . . . 1904

AZ OFTENO (Chile)
AZELASTINE HYDROCHLORIDE
Astelin Nasal Spray . . . 1904

AZANTAC (France, Mexico)
RANITIDINE HYDROCHLORIDE
Zantac 25 EFFERdose Tablets . . . 1624
Zantac 150 EFFERdose Tablets . . . 1624
Zantac 150 Tablets . . . 1624
Zantac 300 Tablets . . . 1624
Zantac Injection . . . 1619
Zantac Injection Premixed . . . 1619
Zantac Syrup . . . 1624

AZATYL (Greece)
CEFTRIAXONE SODIUM
Rocephin Injectable Vials, ADD-Vantage, Galaxy, Bulk . . . 2800

AZELAST (Brazil)
AZELASTINE HYDROCHLORIDE
Astelin Nasal Spray . . . 1904

AZELVIN (Sweden)
AZELASTINE HYDROCHLORIDE
Astelin Nasal Spray . . . 1904

AZEP (Australia, Hong Kong, India, Malaysia, Portugal, Singapore, Thailand)
AZELASTINE HYDROCHLORIDE
Astelin Nasal Spray . . . 1904

AZEPAL (Hungary)
CARBAMAZEPINE
Carbatrol Capsules . . . 3171
Tegretol Chewable Tablets . . . 2295
Tegretol Suspension . . . 2295
Tegretol Tablets . . . 2295
Tegretol-XR Tablets . . . 2295

AZEPAM (Thailand)
DIAZEPAM
Diastat Rectal Delivery System . . . 3343
Valium Tablets . . . 2819

AZEPTIN (Japan)
AZELASTINE HYDROCHLORIDE
Astelin Nasal Spray . . . 1904

AZETAVIR (Mexico)
ZIDOVUDINE
Retrovir Capsules . . . 1560
Retrovir IV Infusion . . . 1564
Retrovir Syrup . . . 1560
Retrovir Tablets . . . 1560

AZIDE (Australia)
CHLOROTHIAZIDE
Diuril Oral Suspension . . . 1954

AZILIV (Brazil)
RANITIDINE HYDROCHLORIDE
Zantac 25 EFFERdose Tablets . . . 1624
Zantac 150 EFFERdose Tablets . . . 1624
Zantac 150 Tablets . . . 1624
Zantac 300 Tablets . . . 1624
Zantac Injection . . . 1619
Zantac Injection Premixed . . . 1619
Zantac Syrup . . . 1624

AZIMAX (Spain)
ZAFIRLUKAST
Accolate Tablets . . . 671

AZMACORT (Brazil, Canada, Czech Republic)
TRIAMCINOLONE ACETONIDE
Azmacort Inhalation Aerosol . . . 1726
Nasacort AQ Nasal Spray . . . 2922

AZOAZOL (Argentina)
ZIDOVUDINE
Retrovir Capsules . . . 1560
Retrovir IV Infusion . . . 1564
Retrovir Syrup . . . 1560
Retrovir Tablets . . . 1560

AZONA (Mexico)
DEXAMETHASONE
Decadron Tablets . . . 1951

AZOPT (Argentina, Australia, Austria, Belgium, Brazil, Canada, Chile, Czech Republic, Denmark, Finland, France, Germany, Greece, Hong Kong, Hungary, Irish Republic, Israel, Italy, Malaysia, Mexico, New Zealand, Norway, Portugal, Russia, Singapore, Spain, Sweden, Switzerland, Thailand, United Kingdom, Venezuela)
BRINZOLAMIDE
Azopt Ophthalmic Suspension . . . ⊙201, 557

AZOPTIC (South Africa)
BRINZOLAMIDE
Azopt Ophthalmic Suspension . . . ⊙201, 557

AZOTINE (Argentina)
ZIDOVUDINE
Retrovir Capsules . . . 1560
Retrovir IV Infusion . . . 1564
Retrovir Syrup . . . 1560
Retrovir Tablets . . . 1560

AZUMETOP (Germany)
METOPROLOL TARTRATE
Lopressor Tablets . . . 2238

AZUMETOP HCT (Germany)
HYDROCHLOROTHIAZIDE/METOPROLOL TARTRATE
Lopressor HCT 100/25 Tablets . . . 2241

AZUPAMIL (Germany)
VERAPAMIL HYDROCHLORIDE
Covera-HS Tablets . . . 3139
Verelan PM Extended-Release Capsules, Controlled-Onset . . . 3106

AZURANIT (Germany)
RANITIDINE HYDROCHLORIDE
Zantac 25 EFFERdose Tablets . . . 1624
Zantac 150 EFFERdose Tablets . . . 1624
Zantac 150 Tablets . . . 1624
Zantac 300 Tablets . . . 1624
Zantac Injection . . . 1619
Zantac Injection Premixed . . . 1619
Zantac Syrup . . . 1624

AZUTRIMAZOL (Germany)
CLOTRIMAZOLE
Lotrimin Cream . . . 3039
Lotrimin Lotion 1% . . . 3039
Lotrimin Topical Solution 1% . . . 3039

B DEXOL (Thailand)
DEXAMETHASONE
Decadron Tablets . . . 1951

BABY AGISTEN (Israel)
CLOTRIMAZOLE
Lotrimin Cream . . . 3039
Lotrimin Lotion 1% . . . 3039
Lotrimin Topical Solution 1% . . . 3039

BACCIDAL (Japan, Spain)
NORFLOXACIN
Noroxin Tablets . . . 2032

BACDA-B (Thailand)
CLOTRIMAZOLE
Lotrimin Cream . . . 3039
Lotrimin Lotion 1% . . . 3039
Lotrimin Topical Solution 1% . . . 3039

BACIGYL (India)
NORFLOXACIN
Noroxin Tablets . . . 2032

BACIGYL-N (India)
NORFLOXACIN
Noroxin Tablets . . . 2032

BACIPRO (Venezuela)
CIPROFLOXACIN
Cipro Oral Suspension . . . 2977

BACPROIN (Mexico)
CIPROFLOXACIN HYDROCHLORIDE
Ciloxan Ophthalmic Ointment . . . ⊙204, 559
Ciloxan Ophthalmic Solution . . . ⊙206
Cipro Tablets . . . 2977

BACROCIN (Brazil)
MUPIROCIN
Bactroban Ointment . . . 1395

BACTIFLOX (Malaysia)
CIPROFLOXACIN HYDROCHLORIDE
Ciloxan Ophthalmic Ointment . . . ⊙204, 559
Ciloxan Ophthalmic Solution . . . ⊙206
Cipro Tablets . . . 2977

BACTIO RHIN (Argentina)
NAPHAZOLINE HYDROCHLORIDE
Albalon Ophthalmic Solution . . . ⊙218

BACTIO RHIN PREDNISOLONA (Argentina)
NAPHAZOLINE HYDROCHLORIDE
Albalon Ophthalmic Solution . . . ⊙218

BACTOCIN (Mexico)
OFLOXACIN
Floxin Otic Solution . . . 1049

BACTODERM (Israel)
MUPIROCIN
Bactroban Ointment . . . 1395

BACTOFLOX (Portugal)
OFLOXACIN
Floxin Otic Solution . . . 1049

BACTOQUIN (India)
CIPROFLOXACIN HYDROCHLORIDE
Ciloxan Ophthalmic Ointment . . . ⊙204, 559
Ciloxan Ophthalmic Solution . . . ⊙206
Cipro Tablets . . . 2977

BACTRACID (Germany)
NORFLOXACIN
Noroxin Tablets . . . 2032

BACTRIZOL (Venezuela)
METRONIDAZOLE
MetroGel-Vaginal Gel . . . 1855

BACTROBAN (Argentina, Australia, Belgium, Brazil, Chile, Czech Republic, France, Greece, Hong Kong, Hungary, India, Japan, Malaysia, Mexico, New Zealand, Portugal, Russia, Singapore, South Africa, Spain, Thailand, United Kingdom, Venezuela)
MUPIROCIN
Bactroban Ointment . . . 1395

BACTROBANDOS (Venezuela)
MUPIROCIN CALCIUM
Bactroban Cream . . . 1394
Bactroban Nasal . . . 1394

BACTRONEO (Brazil)
MUPIROCIN
Bactroban Ointment . . . 1395

BAC-ZIDIM (Mexico)
CEFTAZIDIME
Fortaz for Injection . . . 1453

BAFLOX (Venezuela)
CIPROFLOXACIN
Cipro Oral Suspension . . . 2977

BAJATEN (Argentina, Chile)
INDAPAMIDE
Indapamide Tablets 2156

B-ALCERIN (Greece)
RANITIDINE HYDROCHLORIDE
Zantac 25 EFFERdose Tablets 1624
Zantac 150 EFFERdose Tablets 1624
Zantac 150 Tablets 1624
Zantac 300 Tablets 1624
Zantac Injection 1619
Zantac Injection Premixed 1619
Zantac Syrup 1624

BALCOR (Brazil, Portugal)
DILTIAZEM HYDROCHLORIDE
Cardizem LA Extended Release Tablets 1728
Tiazac Capsules 1201

BALEPTON (Greece)
CIPROFLOXACIN HYDROCHLORIDE
Ciloxan Ophthalmic Ointment ⊙204, 559
Ciloxan Ophthalmic Solution ⊙206
Cipro Tablets 2977

BALPRIL (Portugal)
ENALAPRIL MALEATE
Vasotec I.V. Injection 2103

BALSULPH (Canada)
SULFACETAMIDE SODIUM
Klaron Lotion 10% 2909

BAMALITE (Spain)
LANSOPRAZOLE
Prevacid Delayed-Release Capsules 3271

BANAN (Hong Kong, Japan, Thailand)
CEFPODOXIME PROXETIL
Vantin Tablets and Oral Suspension 2645

BANATIN (Greece)
FAMOTIDINE
Pepcid Injection 2040
Pepcid Injection Premixed 2040
Pepcid Tablets 2038
Pepcid for Oral Suspension 2038

BANTIX (Chile)
MUPIROCIN
Bactroban Ointment 1395

BARAZAN (Germany)
NORFLOXACIN
Noroxin Tablets 2032

BARCLYD (France)
CLONIDINE HYDROCHLORIDE
Catapres Tablets 843

BARIPRIL (Spain)
ENALAPRIL MALEATE
Vasotec I.V. Injection 2103

BARMICIL (Mexico)
GENTAMICIN SULFATE
Garamycin Injectable 3014

BAROXAL (Greece)
RANITIDINE HYDROCHLORIDE
Zantac 25 EFFERdose Tablets 1624
Zantac 150 EFFERdose Tablets 1624
Zantac 150 Tablets 1624
Zantac 300 Tablets 1624
Zantac Injection 1619
Zantac Injection Premixed 1619
Zantac Syrup 1624

BARRIERE-HC (Canada)
HYDROCORTISONE
Hydrocortone Tablets 1989

BASIRON (Denmark, Finland, Norway, Russia, Sweden, Switzerland, The Netherlands)
BENZOYL PEROXIDE
Brevoxyl-4 Creamy Wash 3210
Brevoxyl-4 Gel 3210
Brevoxyl-8 Creamy Wash 3210
Brevoxyl-8 Gel 3210
Triaz Cleanser 1892
Triaz Gel 1892

BAXAMED (Mexico)
NORFLOXACIN
Noroxin Tablets 2032

BAYCUTEN (Brazil, Chile, Czech Republic, Mexico, Portugal)
CLOTRIMAZOLE
Lotrimin Cream 3039
Lotrimin Lotion 1% 3039
Lotrimin Topical Solution 1% 3039

BAYCUTEN HC (Germany)
CLOTRIMAZOLE
Lotrimin Cream 3039
Lotrimin Lotion 1% 3039
Lotrimin Topical Solution 1% 3039

BAYCUTEN N (Malaysia)
CLOTRIMAZOLE
Lotrimin Cream 3039
Lotrimin Lotion 1% 3039
Lotrimin Topical Solution 1% 3039

BAYCUTEN SD (Germany)
CLOTRIMAZOLE
Lotrimin Cream 3039
Lotrimin Lotion 1% 3039
Lotrimin Topical Solution 1% 3039

BAYMYCARD (Germany, Hungary)
NISOLDIPINE
Sular Tablets 3122

BEACON K (Malaysia)
POTASSIUM CHLORIDE
K-Dur Extended-Release Tablets 3033
K-Lor Oral Solution 474
K-Tab Tablets 475

BEAGENTA (Malaysia)
GENTAMICIN SULFATE
Garamycin Injectable 3014

BEAMOKEN A (Mexico)
DEXAMETHASONE
Decadron Tablets 1951

BEATIZEM (Singapore)
DILTIAZEM HYDROCHLORIDE
Cardizem LA Extended Release Tablets 1728
Tiazac Capsules 1201

BEATROLOL (Malaysia)
METOPROLOL TARTRATE
Lopressor Tablets 2238

BECABIL (Spain)
AMOXICILLIN
Amoxil Pediatric Drops for Oral Suspension 1343
Amoxil Tablets 1343

BECACORT (Malaysia)
HYDROCORTISONE
Hydrocortone Tablets 1989

BECARDIN (Hong Kong)
PROPRANOLOL HYDROCHLORIDE
Inderal LA Long-Acting Capsules 3429

BECONASE ALLERGY (Australia)
FLUTICASONE PROPIONATE
Cutivate Cream 2662
Cutivate Ointment 2665
Flonase Nasal Spray 1440

BECTAM (Chile)
PAROXETINE HYDROCHLORIDE
Paxil Oral Suspension 1530
Paxil Tablets 1530

BEDOL (United Kingdom)
ESTRADIOL
Climara Transdermal System 771
Estring Vaginal Ring 2635

BEDRANOL (Switzerland, United Kingdom)
PROPRANOLOL HYDROCHLORIDE
Inderal LA Long-Acting Capsules 3429

BEFAR (Hong Kong)
ALPROSTADIL
Edex Injection 3089

BEFARIN (Thailand)
WARFARIN SODIUM
Coumadin Tablets 898
Coumadin for Injection 898

BEFIMAT (Greece)
NIMODIPINE
Nimotop Capsules 749

BEGLAN (Spain)
SALMETEROL XINAFOATE
Serevent Diskus 1568

BEILANDE (Hong Kong)
FAMOTIDINE
Pepcid Injection 2040
Pepcid Injection Premixed 2040
Pepcid Tablets 2038
Pepcid for Oral Suspension 2038

BEKNOL (Mexico)
BENZONATATE
Tessalon Perles 1199

BEL (Germany)
SIMVASTATIN
Zocor Tablets 2105

BELIDRAL (Belgium)
AMILORIDE HYDROCHLORIDE/HYDROCHLOROTHIAZIDE
Moduretic Tablets 2028

BELIVON (Austria, Italy)
RISPERIDONE
Risperdal Oral Solution 1676
Risperdal Tablets 1676

BELMACINA (Spain)
CIPROFLOXACIN HYDROCHLORIDE
Ciloxan Ophthalmic Ointment ⊙204, 559
Ciloxan Ophthalmic Solution ⊙206
Cipro Tablets 2977

BELMALAX (Spain)
LACTULOSE
Kristalose for Oral Solution 1034

BELMALIP (Spain)
SIMVASTATIN
Zocor Tablets 2105

BELOC (Argentina, Austria, Switzerland)
METOPROLOL TARTRATE
Lopressor Tablets 2238

BELOC COMP (Austria, Germany)
HYDROCHLOROTHIAZIDE/METOPROLOL TARTRATE
Lopressor HCT 100/25 Tablets 2241

BELOC COR (Switzerland)
METOPROLOL TARTRATE
Lopressor Tablets 2238

BELOC-ZOK (Switzerland)
METOPROLOL SUCCINATE
Toprol-XL Tablets 668

BELOKEN (Spain)
METOPROLOL SUCCINATE
Toprol-XL Tablets 668

BELOZOK (Argentina)
METOPROLOL SUCCINATE
Toprol-XL Tablets 668

BEMAZ (Chile)
BETAXOLOL HYDROCHLORIDE
Betoptic S Ophthalmic Suspension ⊙203, 558

BEMETRAZOLE (South Africa)
METRONIDAZOLE
MetroGel-Vaginal Gel 1855

BEMPLAS (Argentina)
CLONIDINE HYDROCHLORIDE
Catapres Tablets 843

BENACE (India)
BENAZEPRIL HYDROCHLORIDE
Lotensin Tablets 2243

BENACNE (Portugal)
BENZOYL PEROXIDE
Brevoxyl-4 Creamy Wash 3210
Brevoxyl-4 Gel 3210
Brevoxyl-8 Creamy Wash 3210
Brevoxyl-8 Gel 3210
Triaz Cleanser 1892
Triaz Gel 1892

BENADAY (Denmark)
CETIRIZINE HYDROCHLORIDE
Zyrtec Syrup 2594
Zyrtec Tablets 2594

BENADRYL ALLERGY ORAL SOLUTION (United Kingdom)
CETIRIZINE HYDROCHLORIDE
Zyrtec Syrup 2594
Zyrtec Tablets 2594

BENADRYL ONE A DAY (United Kingdom)
CETIRIZINE HYDROCHLORIDE
Zyrtec Syrup 2594
Zyrtec Tablets 2594

BENALAPRIL (Germany)
ENALAPRIL MALEATE
Vasotec I.V. Injection 2103

BENAPROST (Argentina)
TERAZOSIN HYDROCHLORIDE
Hytrin Capsules 471

BENAXONA (Mexico)
CEFTRIAXONE SODIUM
Rocephin Injectable Vials, ADD-Vantage, Galaxy, Bulk 2800

BENDAPAR (Mexico)
ALBENDAZOLE
Albenza Tablets 1338

BENDEX (India, South Africa)
ALBENDAZOLE
Albenza Tablets 1338

BENECUT (Austria)
NAFTIFINE HYDROCHLORIDE
Naftin Cream 2126
Naftin Gel 2126

BENET (Japan)
RISEDRONATE SODIUM
Actonel Tablets 2683

BENFOFEN (Germany)
DICLOFENAC SODIUM
Voltaren Tablets 2307
Voltaren-XR Tablets 2310

BENITROM (Mexico)
ERYTHROMYCIN
Ery-Tab Tablets 449
Erythromycin Base Filmtab Tablets 455
Erythromycin Delayed-Release Capsules, USP 457
PCE Dispertab Tablets 515

BENOXID (Italy)
BENZOYL PEROXIDE
Brevoxyl-4 Creamy Wash 3210
Brevoxyl-4 Gel 3210
Brevoxyl-8 Creamy Wash 3210
Brevoxyl-8 Gel 3210
Triaz Cleanser 1892
Triaz Gel 1892

BENOXYGEL (Portugal, Spain)
BENZOYL PEROXIDE
Brevoxyl-4 Creamy Wash 3210
Brevoxyl-4 Gel 3210
Brevoxyl-8 Creamy Wash 3210
Brevoxyl-8 Gel 3210
Triaz Cleanser 1892
Triaz Gel 1892

BENOXYL (Australia, Canada, Irish Republic, Mexico, New Zealand, South Africa, United Kingdom, Venezuela)
BENZOYL PEROXIDE
Brevoxyl-4 Creamy Wash 3210
Brevoxyl-4 Gel 3210
Brevoxyl-8 Creamy Wash 3210
Brevoxyl-8 Gel 3210
Triaz Cleanser 1892
Triaz Gel 1892

BENPH (Irish Republic)
TERAZOSIN HYDROCHLORIDE
Hytrin Capsules 471

BENPINE (Malaysia, Singapore, Thailand)
CHLORDIAZEPOXIDE HYDROCHLORIDE
Librium Capsules 3347

BENTIAMIN (Brazil)
ALBENDAZOLE
Albenza Tablets 1338

BENZAC (Australia, Belgium, Brazil, Canada, Italy, New Zealand, Portugal, Singapore, Switzerland, Thailand, The Netherlands)
BENZOYL PEROXIDE
Brevoxyl-4 Creamy Wash 3210
Brevoxyl-4 Gel 3210
Brevoxyl-8 Creamy Wash 3210
Brevoxyl-8 Gel 3210
Triaz Cleanser 1892
Triaz Gel 1892

BENZAC AC (India, Mexico, Venezuela)
BENZOYL PEROXIDE
Brevoxyl-4 Creamy Wash 3210
Brevoxyl-4 Gel 3210
Brevoxyl-8 Creamy Wash 3210
Brevoxyl-8 Gel 3210
Triaz Cleanser 1892
Triaz Gel 1892

BENZAC ERITROMICINA (Brazil)
ERYTHROMYCIN
Ery-Tab Tablets 449
Erythromycin Base Filmtab Tablets 455
Erythromycin Delayed-Release Capsules, USP 457
PCE Dispertab Tablets 515

BENZAC PLUS (Chile, Mexico)
BENZOYL PEROXIDE
Brevoxyl-4 Creamy Wash 3210

(⊙ Described in PDR For Ophthalmic Medicines™)

Brevoxyl-4 Gel **3210**
Brevoxyl-8 Creamy Wash **3210**
Brevoxyl-8 Gel **3210**
Triaz Cleanser **1892**
Triaz Gel **1892**

BENZAC-AC (Brazil, Hong Kong, Israel, Malaysia, South Africa)
BENZOYL PEROXIDE
Brevoxyl-4 Creamy Wash **3210**
Brevoxyl-4 Gel **3210**
Brevoxyl-8 Creamy Wash **3210**
Brevoxyl-8 Gel **3210**
Triaz Cleanser **1892**
Triaz Gel **1892**

BENZAC-W (Greece)
BENZOYL PEROXIDE
Brevoxyl-4 Creamy Wash **3210**
Brevoxyl-4 Gel **3210**
Brevoxyl-8 Creamy Wash **3210**
Brevoxyl-8 Gel **3210**
Triaz Cleanser **1892**
Triaz Gel **1892**

BENZADERM (Mexico)
BENZOYL PEROXIDE
Brevoxyl-4 Creamy Wash **3210**
Brevoxyl-4 Gel **3210**
Brevoxyl-8 Creamy Wash **3210**
Brevoxyl-8 Gel **3210**
Triaz Cleanser **1892**
Triaz Gel **1892**

BENZAGEL (Brazil, France, United Kingdom)
BENZOYL PEROXIDE
Brevoxyl-4 Creamy Wash **3210**
Brevoxyl-4 Gel **3210**
Brevoxyl-8 Creamy Wash **3210**
Brevoxyl-8 Gel **3210**
Triaz Cleanser **1892**
Triaz Gel **1892**

BENZAKNEN (Austria, Germany)
BENZOYL PEROXIDE
Brevoxyl-4 Creamy Wash **3210**
Brevoxyl-4 Gel **3210**
Brevoxyl-8 Creamy Wash **3210**
Brevoxyl-8 Gel **3210**
Triaz Cleanser **1892**
Triaz Gel **1892**

BENZAMYCIN (Argentina, Belgium, Canada, Chile, Hong Kong, Israel, Mexico, United Kingdom)
BENZOYL PEROXIDE
Brevoxyl-4 Creamy Wash **3210**
Brevoxyl-4 Gel **3210**
Brevoxyl-8 Creamy Wash **3210**
Brevoxyl-8 Gel **3210**
Triaz Cleanser **1892**
Triaz Gel **1892**

BENZAMYCINE (South Africa)
BENZOYL PEROXIDE
Brevoxyl-4 Creamy Wash **3210**
Brevoxyl-4 Gel **3210**
Brevoxyl-8 Creamy Wash **3210**
Brevoxyl-8 Gel **3210**
Triaz Cleanser **1892**
Triaz Gel **1892**

BENZEVIT (Brazil)
NYSTATIN
Nystop Topical Powder USP **2478**
Paddock Nystatin USP for Oral Suspension **2478**

BENZIHEX (Argentina)
BENZOYL PEROXIDE
Brevoxyl-4 Creamy Wash **3210**
Brevoxyl-4 Gel **3210**
Brevoxyl-8 Creamy Wash **3210**
Brevoxyl-8 Gel **3210**
Triaz Cleanser **1892**
Triaz Gel **1892**

BENZODERM MYCO (Germany)
CLOTRIMAZOLE
Lotrimin Cream **3039**
Lotrimin Lotion 1% **3039**
Lotrimin Topical Solution 1% **3039**

BENZODIAPIN (Italy)
CHLORDIAZEPOXIDE HYDROCHLORIDE
Librium Capsules **3347**

BENZOL (Brazil)
ALBENDAZOLE
Albenza Tablets **1338**

BENZOMIX (Italy)
BENZOYL PEROXIDE
Brevoxyl-4 Creamy Wash **3210**
Brevoxyl-4 Gel **3210**
Brevoxyl-8 Creamy Wash **3210**
Brevoxyl-8 Gel **3210**
Triaz Cleanser **1892**
Triaz Gel **1892**

BENZONAL (Mexico)
BENZONATATE
Tessalon Perles **1199**

BENZOPIN (South Africa)
DIAZEPAM
Diastat Rectal Delivery System **3343**
Valium Tablets **2819**

BENZOYT (Germany)
BENZOYL PEROXIDE
Brevoxyl-4 Creamy Wash **3210**
Brevoxyl-4 Gel **3210**
Brevoxyl-8 Creamy Wash **3210**
Brevoxyl-8 Gel **3210**
Triaz Cleanser **1892**
Triaz Gel **1892**

BENZPEROX (Germany)
BENZOYL PEROXIDE
Brevoxyl-4 Creamy Wash **3210**
Brevoxyl-4 Gel **3210**
Brevoxyl-8 Creamy Wash **3210**
Brevoxyl-8 Gel **3210**
Triaz Cleanser **1892**
Triaz Gel **1892**

BENZYME (Mexico)
DIAZEPAM
Diastat Rectal Delivery System **3343**
Valium Tablets **2819**

BEOCID PUROPTAL (Austria)
SULFACETAMIDE SODIUM
Klaron Lotion 10% **2909**

BEOF (Chile)
BETAXOLOL HYDROCHLORIDE
Betoptic S Ophthalmic Suspension . ⊙**203, 558**

BEPRANE (France)
PROPRANOLOL HYDROCHLORIDE
Inderal LA Long-Acting Capsules **3429**

BEPROLO (Italy)
METOPROLOL TARTRATE
Lopressor Tablets **2238**

BEPTAZINE (India)
PROPRANOLOL HYDROCHLORIDE
Inderal LA Long-Acting Capsules **3429**

BERAMICINA (Mexico)
GENTAMICIN SULFATE
Garamycin Injectable **3014**

BERAZOLE (South Africa)
METRONIDAZOLE
MetroGel-Vaginal Gel **1855**

BERKATENS (Irish Republic, United Kingdom)
VERAPAMIL HYDROCHLORIDE
Covera-HS Tablets **3139**
Verelan PM Extended-Release Capsules, Controlled-Onset **3106**

BERKOLOL (Hong Kong, Irish Republic, United Kingdom)
PROPRANOLOL HYDROCHLORIDE
Inderal LA Long-Acting Capsules **3429**

BERLEX (Argentina)
ALENDRONATE SODIUM
Fosamax Tablets **1969**

BERLIPRIL (Czech Republic, Russia)
ENALAPRIL MALEATE
Vasotec I.V. Injection **2103**

BERLTHYROX (Germany)
LEVOTHYROXINE SODIUM
Levothroid Tablets **1186**
Levoxyl Tablets **1712**
Synthroid Tablets **520**

BERMACIA (Brazil)
THEOPHYLLINE
Uniphyl Tablets **2710**

BERTOCIL (Portugal)
BETAXOLOL HYDROCHLORIDE
Betoptic S Ophthalmic Suspension . ⊙**203, 558**

BESITRAN (Spain)
SERTRALINE HYDROCHLORIDE
Zoloft Tablets **2586**

BESTATIN (Thailand)
SIMVASTATIN
Zocor Tablets **2105**

BETABIOT (Mexico)
AMOXICILLIN
Amoxil Pediatric Drops for Oral Suspension **1343**
Amoxil Tablets **1343**

BETABLOC (India)
PROPRANOLOL HYDROCHLORIDE
Inderal LA Long-Acting Capsules **3429**

BETAC (Russia)
BETAXOLOL HYDROCHLORIDE
Betoptic S Ophthalmic Suspension . ⊙**203, 558**

BETACAINE (Canada, Mexico)
LIDOCAINE
Lidoderm Patch **1118**

BETACEF (Italy)
CEFOXITIN SODIUM
Mefoxin Premixed Intravenous Solution . . . **2016**
Mefoxin for Injection **2012**

BETACLAV (Brazil)
AMOXICILLIN
Amoxil Pediatric Drops for Oral Suspension **1343**
Amoxil Tablets **1343**

BETADIUR (Switzerland)
AMILORIDE HYDROCHLORIDE/HYDROCHLOROTHIAZIDE
Moduretic Tablets **2028**

BETADUR CR (United Kingdom)
PROPRANOLOL HYDROCHLORIDE
Inderal LA Long-Acting Capsules **3429**

BETAFERON (Argentina, Australia, Austria, Belgium, Brazil, Chile, Czech Republic, Denmark, Finland, France, Germany, Hong Kong, Hungary, Irish Republic, Israel, Italy, Malaysia, Mexico, New Zealand, Norway, Portugal, Russia, Singapore, South Africa, Spain, Sweden, Switzerland, Thailand, The Netherlands, United Kingdom)
INTERFERON BETA-1B
Betaseron for SC Injection **767**

BETALOC (Australia, Canada, Czech Republic, Hungary, India, Irish Republic, Malaysia, New Zealand, Thailand, United Kingdom)
METOPROLOL TARTRATE
Lopressor Tablets **2238**

BETALOC COMP (Hong Kong)
HYDROCHLOROTHIAZIDE/METOPROLOL TARTRATE
Lopressor HCT 100/25 Tablets **2241**

BETALOC ZOK (Russia)
METOPROLOL SUCCINATE
Toprol-XL Tablets **668**

BETALOL (Thailand)
PROPRANOLOL HYDROCHLORIDE
Inderal LA Long-Acting Capsules **3429**

BETAMICAN (Spain)
SALMETEROL XINAFOATE
Serevent Diskus **1568**

BETAPAM (South Africa)
DIAZEPAM
Diastat Rectal Delivery System **3343**
Valium Tablets **2819**

BETAPLEX (Chile)
CARVEDILOL
Coreg Tablets **1414**

BETAPRESS (Thailand)
PROPRANOLOL HYDROCHLORIDE
Inderal LA Long-Acting Capsules **3429**

BETA-PROGRANE (United Kingdom)
PROPRANOLOL HYDROCHLORIDE
Inderal LA Long-Acting Capsules **3429**

BETAPROL (Switzerland)
PROPRANOLOL HYDROCHLORIDE
Inderal LA Long-Acting Capsules **3429**

BETAREN (Israel)
DICLOFENAC SODIUM
Voltaren Tablets **2307**
Voltaren-XR Tablets **2310**

BETARETIC (South Africa)
AMILORIDE HYDROCHLORIDE/HYDROCHLOROTHIAZIDE
Moduretic Tablets **2028**

BETARRETIN (Venezuela)
TRETINOIN
Vesanoid Capsules **2820**

BETASEL (Argentina)
BETAXOLOL HYDROCHLORIDE
Betoptic S Ophthalmic Suspension . ⊙**203, 558**

BETASERON (Canada)
INTERFERON BETA-1B
Betaseron for SC Injection **767**

BETASOL (Malaysia, Thailand)
CLOBETASOL PROPIONATE
Temovate Cream **2668**
Temovate E Emollient **2671**
Temovate Gel **2669**
Temovate Ointment **2668**
Temovate Scalp Application **2670**

BETASPAN (India)
PROPRANOLOL HYDROCHLORIDE
Inderal LA Long-Acting Capsules **3429**

BETA-TABLINEN (Germany)
PROPRANOLOL HYDROCHLORIDE
Inderal LA Long-Acting Capsules **3429**

BETA-TIM (Canada)
TIMOLOL MALEATE
Blocadren Tablets **1916**
Timoptic Sterile Ophthalmic Solution **2088**
Timoptic in Ocudose **2091**
Timoptic-XE Sterile Ophthalmic Gel Forming Solution **2092**

BETA-TIMELETS (Germany)
PROPRANOLOL HYDROCHLORIDE
Inderal LA Long-Acting Capsules **3429**

BETAXOL (Venezuela)
BETAXOLOL HYDROCHLORIDE
Betoptic S Ophthalmic Suspension . ⊙**203, 558**

BETAZOK (Irish Republic)
METOPROLOL SUCCINATE
Toprol-XL Tablets **668**

BETIM (Irish Republic, Norway, United Kingdom)
TIMOLOL MALEATE
Blocadren Tablets **1916**
Timoptic Sterile Ophthalmic Solution **2088**
Timoptic in Ocudose **2091**
Timoptic-XE Sterile Ophthalmic Gel Forming Solution **2092**

BETOPTIC (Australia, Austria, Belgium, Brazil, Canada, Chile, Czech Republic, Denmark, Finland, France, Greece, Hong Kong, Hungary, Irish Republic, Italy, Malaysia, Mexico, New Zealand, Norway, Portugal, Russia, Singapore, South Africa, Spain, Sweden, Thailand, The Netherlands, United Kingdom)
BETAXOLOL HYDROCHLORIDE
Betoptic S Ophthalmic Suspension . ⊙**203, 558**

BETOPTIC S (Israel, Switzerland)
BETAXOLOL HYDROCHLORIDE
Betoptic S Ophthalmic Suspension . ⊙**203, 558**

BETOPTICS (Venezuela)
BETAXOLOL HYDROCHLORIDE
Betoptic S Ophthalmic Suspension . ⊙**203, 558**

BETOPTIMA (Germany)
BETAXOLOL HYDROCHLORIDE
Betoptic S Ophthalmic Suspension . ⊙**203, 558**

BETOQUIN (Australia)
BETAXOLOL HYDROCHLORIDE
Betoptic S Ophthalmic Suspension . ⊙**203, 558**

BETULAC (Sweden)
LACTULOSE
Kristalose for Oral Solution **1034**

BEURISES (South Africa)
FUROSEMIDE
Furosemide Tablets **2154**

BEVINDAZOL (Venezuela)
ALBENDAZOLE
Albenza Tablets **1338**

BEXID (Sweden)
BENZOYL PEROXIDE
Brevoxyl-4 Creamy Wash **3210**
Brevoxyl-4 Gel **3210**
Brevoxyl-8 Creamy Wash **3210**
Brevoxyl-8 Gel **3210**

Triaz Cleanser 1892
Triaz Gel 1892

BEXINE (Mexico)
DEXAMETHASONE
Decadron Tablets 1951

BEXINOR (Singapore)
NORFLOXACIN
Noroxin Tablets 2032

BEXON (Argentina)
METRONIDAZOLE
MetroGel-Vaginal Gel 1855

BGB NORFLOX (Thailand)
NORFLOXACIN
Noroxin Tablets 2032

BI PRETERAX (Belgium)
PERINDOPRIL ERBUMINE
Aceon Tablets (2 mg, 4 mg, 8 mg) 3194

BIALZEPAM (Portugal)
DIAZEPAM
Diastat Rectal Delivery System 3343
Valium Tablets 2819

BIAMOTIL (Brazil)
CIPROFLOXACIN HYDROCHLORIDE
Ciloxan Ophthalmic Ointment . . . . ⊙204, 559
Ciloxan Ophthalmic Solution . . . . ⊙206
Cipro Tablets 2977

BIARTAC (Belgium)
DIFLUNISAL
Dolobid Tablets 1955

BIAXIN (Canada, Germany)
CLARITHROMYCIN
Biaxin Filmtab Tablets 402
Biaxin Granules 402

BICLAR (Belgium)
CLARITHROMYCIN
Biaxin Filmtab Tablets 402
Biaxin Granules 402

BICLOPAN (Singapore)
DICLOFENAC SODIUM
Voltaren Tablets 2307
Voltaren-XR Tablets 2310

BIDECAR (Argentina)
CARVEDILOL
Coreg Tablets 1414

BIDOFLOX (India)
OFLOXACIN
Floxin Otic Solution 1049

BIDOFLOX-OZ (India)
OFLOXACIN
Floxin Otic Solution 1049

BIDURET (India)
AMILORIDE HYDROCHLORIDE
Midamor Tablets 2026

BIFARDOL (Mexico)
NAPROXEN SODIUM
Anaprox DS Tablets 2761
Anaprox Tablets 2761

BIFINORMA (Germany)
LACTULOSE
Kristalose for Oral Solution 1034

BIFITERAL (Austria, Belgium, Germany)
LACTULOSE
Kristalose for Oral Solution 1034

BIFORT (Argentina)
SILDENAFIL CITRATE
Viagra Tablets 2573

BIFOSA (India)
ALENDRONATE SODIUM
Fosamax Tablets 1969

BILATEN (Chile)
CANDESARTAN CILEXETIL
Atacand Tablets 649

BILATEN-D (Chile)
CANDESARTAN CILEXETIL
Atacand Tablets 649

BILDURETIC (Thailand)
AMILORIDE HYDROCHLORIDE
Midamor Tablets 2026

BILORDYL (Germany)
THEOPHYLLINE
Uniphyl Tablets 2710

BILTRICIDE (Australia, Canada, France, Germany, Greece, Hong Kong, Israel, South Africa, Thailand, The Netherlands)
PRAZIQUANTEL
Biltricide Tablets 2976

BIMOXIN (Brazil)
AMOXICILLIN
Amoxil Pediatric Drops for Oral Suspension 1343
Amoxil Tablets 1343

BINDAZAC (Greece)
RANITIDINE HYDROCHLORIDE
Zantac 25 EFFERdose Tablets 1624
Zantac 150 EFFERdose Tablets 1624
Zantac 150 Tablets 1624
Zantac 300 Tablets 1624
Zantac Injection 1619
Zantac Injection Premixed 1619
Zantac Syrup 1624

BIO CABAL (Argentina)
DEXAMETHASONE
Decadron Tablets 1951

BIO TARBUN (Argentina)
NORFLOXACIN
Noroxin Tablets 2032

BIO-AMOKSICLAV (South Africa)
AMOXICILLIN
Amoxil Pediatric Drops for Oral Suspension 1343
Amoxil Tablets 1343

BIOCARD (Irish Republic)
CARVEDILOL
Coreg Tablets 1414

BIOCARN (Germany)
LEVOCARNITINE
Carnitor Injection 3188
Carnitor Tablets and Oral Solution 3190

BIOCEF (Austria)
CEFPODOXIME PROXETIL
Vantin Tablets and Oral Suspension 2645

BIO-CEST (Mexico)
PRAZIQUANTEL
Biltricide Tablets 2976

BIOCICLIN (Italy)
CEFUROXIME SODIUM
Zinacef Injection 1631

BIOCIP (India)
CIPROFLOXACIN
Cipro Oral Suspension 2977

BIOCIPRO (Greece)
CIPROFLOXACIN
Cipro Oral Suspension 2977

BIOCIP-TZ (India)
CIPROFLOXACIN
Cipro Oral Suspension 2977

BIOCLAR (India)
CLARITHROMYCIN
Biaxin Filmtab Tablets 402
Biaxin Granules 402

BIOCORD (Brazil)
NIFEDIPINE
Adalat CC Tablets 2964

BIOCORTIN (Argentina)
HYDROCORTISONE
Hydrocortone Tablets 1989

BIO-DAC (Mexico)
SULINDAC
Clinoril Tablets 1924

BIODALGIC (France)
TRAMADOL HYDROCHLORIDE
Ultram ER Tablets 2392

BIODEZIL (Mexico)
CAPTOPRIL
Captopril Tablets 2149

BIODOL (Irish Republic)
TRAMADOL HYDROCHLORIDE
Ultram ER Tablets 2392

BIODROP (Argentina)
DORZOLAMIDE HYDROCHLORIDE
Trusopt Sterile Ophthalmic Solution 2095

BIOFANAL (Germany)
NYSTATIN
Nystop Topical Powder USP 2478
Paddock Nystatin USP for Oral Suspension 2478

BIOFERON (Thailand)
INTERFERON ALFA-2B
Intron A for Injection 3024

BIOFF (India)
OFLOXACIN
Floxin Otic Solution 1049

BIOFLOX (Mexico)
CIPROFLOXACIN
Cipro Oral Suspension 2977

BIOFLOXIN (India)
NORFLOXACIN
Noroxin Tablets 2032

BIOFLOX-TZ (India)
NORFLOXACIN
Noroxin Tablets 2032

BIOFUREX (Italy)
CEFUROXIME SODIUM
Zinacef Injection 1631

BIOGARACIN (India)
GENTAMICIN SULFATE
Garamycin Injectable 3014

BIOGEN (Spain)
GENTAMICIN SULFATE
Garamycin Injectable 3014

BIOGYL (Thailand)
METRONIDAZOLE
MetroGel-Vaginal Gel 1855

BIOLAC (Italy)
LACTULOSE
Kristalose for Oral Solution 1034

BIOLAN (Germany)
SODIUM HYALURONATE
Hyalgan Solution 2901

BIOLON (Brazil, Canada, Chile, Germany, Israel, Italy, Mexico, Switzerland)
SODIUM HYALURONATE
Hyalgan Solution 2901

BIOLONE (South Africa)
SODIUM HYALURONATE
Hyalgan Solution 2901

BIOMARGEN (Spain)
GENTAMICIN SULFATE
Garamycin Injectable 3014

BIOMIDA (Brazil)
FLUTAMIDE
Eulexin Capsules 3009

BIOMISEN (Mexico)
FUROSEMIDE
Furosemide Tablets 2154

BIOMONA (Mexico)
METRONIDAZOLE
MetroGel-Vaginal Gel 1855

BIOMOX (Thailand)
AMOXICILLIN
Amoxil Pediatric Drops for Oral Suspension 1343
Amoxil Tablets 1343

BIOMOXIL (India)
AMOXICILLIN
Amoxil Pediatric Drops for Oral Suspension 1343
Amoxil Tablets 1343

BIOMOXIL-LB (India)
AMOXICILLIN
Amoxil Pediatric Drops for Oral Suspension 1343
Amoxil Tablets 1343

BIONEURYL (Mexico)
CARBAMAZEPINE
Carbatrol Capsules 3171
Tegretol Chewable Tablets 2295
Tegretol Suspension 2295
Tegretol Tablets 2295
Tegretol-XR Tablets 2295

BIONIF (Italy)
NIFEDIPINE
Adalat CC Tablets 2964

BIOPHYLLIN (South Africa)
THEOPHYLLINE
Uniphyl Tablets 2710

BIOPIME (India)
CEFEPIME HYDROCHLORIDE
Maxipime for Injection 1105

BIOPLASMA FDP (South Africa)
PLASMA PROTEIN FRACTION
Plasmanate 3255

BIOPRIL (India)
LISINOPRIL
Prinivil Tablets 2052

BIOPRIL-AM (India)
LISINOPRIL
Prinivil Tablets 2052

BIOPTIC (Argentina)
TOBRAMYCIN
TOBI Solution for Inhalation 2298

BIOPTIC DX (Argentina)
TOBRAMYCIN
TOBI Solution for Inhalation 2298

BIOQUIL (Portugal)
OFLOXACIN
Floxin Otic Solution 1049

BIOREUNIL (Mexico)
CARBAMAZEPINE
Carbatrol Capsules 3171
Tegretol Chewable Tablets 2295
Tegretol Suspension 2295
Tegretol Tablets 2295
Tegretol-XR Tablets 2295

BIOSEMIDA (Venezuela)
FUROSEMIDE
Furosemide Tablets 2154

BIOSETRON (Greece)
ONDANSETRON
Zofran ODT Orally Disintegrating Tablets . . 1639

BIOSIM (India)
SIMVASTATIN
Zocor Tablets 2105

BIOTAX-O (India)
CEFIXIME
Suprax 1843

BIOTAZOL (Mexico)
METRONIDAZOLE
MetroGel-Vaginal Gel 1855

BIOTECAN (Argentina)
IRINOTECAN HYDROCHLORIDE
Camptosar Injection 2604

BIOTIC (Argentina)
CIPROFLOXACIN HYDROCHLORIDE
Ciloxan Ophthalmic Ointment . . . . ⊙204, 559
Ciloxan Ophthalmic Solution . . . . ⊙206
Cipro Tablets 2977

BIOTREDINE (Greece)
ETIDRONATE DISODIUM
Didronel Tablets 2697

BIOTRIL (Mexico)
ERYTHROMYCIN
Ery-Tab Tablets 449
Erythromycin Base Filmtab Tablets 455
Erythromycin Delayed-Release Capsules, USP 457
PCE Dispertab Tablets 515

BIOVANCOMIN (Brazil)
VANCOMYCIN HYDROCHLORIDE
Vancocin HCl Capsules, USP 3380

BIOVIR (Brazil)
LAMIVUDINE
Epivir Oral Solution 1427
Epivir Tablets 1427
Epivir-HBV Oral Solution 1432
Epivir-HBV Tablets 1432

BIOXAN (Mexico)
NAPROXEN
EC-Naprosyn Delayed-Release Tablets 2761
Naprosyn Suspension 2761
Naprosyn Tablets 2761

BIOXILINA (Argentina)
AMOXICILLIN
Amoxil Pediatric Drops for Oral Suspension 1343
Amoxil Tablets 1343

BIOXILINA PLUS (Argentina)
AMOXICILLIN
Amoxil Pediatric Drops for Oral Suspension 1343

Amoxil Tablets . . . 1343

BIOXIMA (Italy)
CEFUROXIME SODIUM
Zinacef Injection . . . 1631

BIOZIDIMA (Venezuela)
CEFTAZIDIME
Fortaz for Injection . . . 1453

BIPREDONIUM (Spain)
INDAPAMIDE
Indapamide Tablets . . . 2156

BIPRETERAX (Argentina)
PERINDOPRIL ERBUMINE
Aceon Tablets (2 mg, 4 mg, 8 mg) . . . 3194

BIPRONYL (Singapore)
NAPROXEN
EC-Naprosyn Delayed-Release Tablets . . . 2761
Naprosyn Suspension . . . 2761
Naprosyn Tablets . . . 2761

BIRVAC (Argentina)
LAMIVUDINE
Epivir Oral Solution . . . 1427
Epivir Tablets . . . 1427
Epivir-HBV Oral Solution . . . 1432
Epivir-HBV Tablets . . . 1432

BISEKO (Czech Republic)
PLASMA PROTEIN FRACTION
Plasmanate . . . 3255

BISTATIN V (Mexico)
NYSTATIN
Nystop Topical Powder USP . . . 2478
Paddock Nystatin USP for Oral Suspension . . . 2478

BISTON (Czech Republic)
CARBAMAZEPINE
Carbatrol Capsules . . . 3171
Tegretol Chewable Tablets . . . 2295
Tegretol Suspension . . . 2295
Tegretol Tablets . . . 2295
Tegretol-XR Tablets . . . 2295

BITENSIL (Spain)
ENALAPRIL MALEATE
Vasotec I.V. Injection . . . 2103

BI-TILDIEM (France)
DILTIAZEM HYDROCHLORIDE
Cardizem LA Extended Release Tablets . . . 1728
Tiazac Capsules . . . 1201

BIVORILAN (Greece)
CIPROFLOXACIN HYDROCHLORIDE
Ciloxan Ophthalmic Ointment . . . ⊙204, 559
Ciloxan Ophthalmic Solution . . . ⊙206
Cipro Tablets . . . 2977

BK HC (New Zealand)
HYDROCORTISONE
Hydrocortone Tablets . . . 1989

BLADER (Argentina)
CIPROFLOXACIN
Cipro Oral Suspension . . . 2977

BLEF-10 (Mexico)
SULFACETAMIDE SODIUM
Klaron Lotion 10% . . . 2909

BLEFAMIDE (Chile)
PREDNISOLONE ACETATE/SULFACETAMIDE SODIUM
Blephamide Ophthalmic Ointment . . . 568
Blephamide Ophthalmic Suspension . . . 569

BLENOX (Spain)
AMOXICILLIN
Amoxil Pediatric Drops for Oral Suspension . . . 1343
Amoxil Tablets . . . 1343

BLEPH-10 (Australia, Canada, Hong Kong, Irish Republic, New Zealand, South Africa, Thailand)
SULFACETAMIDE SODIUM
Klaron Lotion 10% . . . 2909

BLEPHAMIDE (Switzerland)
PREDNISOLONE ACETATE/SULFACETAMIDE SODIUM
Blephamide Ophthalmic Ointment . . . 568
Blephamide Ophthalmic Suspension . . . 569

BLEPHASULF (Austria)
SULFACETAMIDE SODIUM
Klaron Lotion 10% . . . 2909

BLEZAMONT (Greece)
CETIRIZINE HYDROCHLORIDE
Zyrtec Syrup . . . 2594
Zyrtec Tablets . . . 2594

BLOCACID (India, Mexico, Singapore)
FAMOTIDINE
Pepcid Injection . . . 2040
Pepcid Injection Premixed . . . 2040
Pepcid Tablets . . . 2038
Pepcid for Oral Suspension . . . 2038

BLOCADREN (Australia, Austria, Belgium, Canada, Hong Kong, Irish Republic, Italy, Mexico, Norway, Portugal, South Africa, Spain, Sweden, Switzerland, The Netherlands, United Kingdom)
TIMOLOL MALEATE
Blocadren Tablets . . . 1916
Timoptic Sterile Ophthalmic Solution . . . 2088
Timoptic in Ocudose . . . 2091
Timoptic-XE Sterile Ophthalmic Gel Forming Solution . . . 2092

BLOCALCIN (Czech Republic, Hungary, Russia)
DILTIAZEM HYDROCHLORIDE
Cardizem LA Extended Release Tablets . . . 1728
Tiazac Capsules . . . 1201

BLOCANOL (Finland)
TIMOLOL MALEATE
Blocadren Tablets . . . 1916
Timoptic Sterile Ophthalmic Solution . . . 2088
Timoptic in Ocudose . . . 2091
Timoptic-XE Sterile Ophthalmic Gel Forming Solution . . . 2092

BLOCAR (Chile)
CARVEDILOL
Coreg Tablets . . . 1414

BLOKIUM FLEX (Argentina)
DICLOFENAC SODIUM
Voltaren Tablets . . . 2307
Voltaren-XR Tablets . . . 2310

BLOKTUS (Mexico)
BENZONATATE
Tessalon Perles . . . 1199

BLOOTEC (Brazil)
ENALAPRIL MALEATE
Vasotec I.V. Injection . . . 2103

BLOPRESID (Italy)
CANDESARTAN CILEXETIL
Atacand Tablets . . . 649

BLOPRESS (Austria, Brazil, Chile, Czech Republic, Germany, Hong Kong, Italy, Japan, Malaysia, Mexico, Portugal, Spain, Switzerland, Thailand, Venezuela)
CANDESARTAN CILEXETIL
Atacand Tablets . . . 649

BLOPRESS 16 MG + 12,5 MG (Portugal)
CANDESARTAN CILEXETIL
Atacand Tablets . . . 649

BLOPRESS PLUS (Germany, Mexico, Switzerland)
CANDESARTAN CILEXETIL
Atacand Tablets . . . 649

B-LOVATIN (Greece)
LOVASTATIN
Mevacor Tablets . . . 2021

BLOX (Chile)
CANDESARTAN CILEXETIL
Atacand Tablets . . . 649

BLUMOL (Greece)
RANITIDINE HYDROCHLORIDE
Zantac 25 EFFERdose Tablets . . . 1624
Zantac 150 EFFERdose Tablets . . . 1624
Zantac 150 Tablets . . . 1624
Zantac 300 Tablets . . . 1624
Zantac Injection . . . 1619
Zantac Injection Premixed . . . 1619
Zantac Syrup . . . 1624

BOCATRIOL (Austria, Denmark, Germany, Switzerland)
CALCITRIOL
Calcijex Injection . . . 411
Rocaltrol Capsules . . . 2798
Rocaltrol Oral Solution . . . 2798

BOLBAMOX (Mexico)
AMOXICILLIN
Amoxil Pediatric Drops for Oral Suspension . . . 1343
Amoxil Tablets . . . 1343

BONALEN (Brazil)
ALENDRONATE SODIUM
Fosamax Tablets . . . 1969

BONCEUR (South Africa)
VERAPAMIL HYDROCHLORIDE
Covera-HS Tablets . . . 3139
Verelan PM Extended-Release Capsules, Controlled-Onset . . . 3106

BONCORDIN (Argentina)
BENAZEPRIL HYDROCHLORIDE
Lotensin Tablets . . . 2243

BONDIL (Norway, Sweden)
ALPROSTADIL
Edex Injection . . . 3089

BONEMASS (Brazil)
ETIDRONATE DISODIUM
Didronel Tablets . . . 2697

BONJELA TEETHING GEL (United Kingdom)
LIDOCAINE
Lidoderm Patch . . . 1118

BONMAX (India)
RALOXIFENE HYDROCHLORIDE
Evista Tablets . . . 1763

BONOCEF (Portugal)
CEFIXIME
Suprax . . . 1843

BONYL (Denmark)
NAPROXEN
EC-Naprosyn Delayed-Release Tablets . . . 2761
Naprosyn Suspension . . . 2761
Naprosyn Tablets . . . 2761

BONZOL (Mexico)
LANSOPRAZOLE
Prevacid Delayed-Release Capsules . . . 3271

BQL (India)
ENALAPRIL MALEATE
Vasotec I.V. Injection . . . 2103

BRADELMIN (Mexico)
ALBENDAZOLE
Albenza Tablets . . . 1338

BRAINAL (Chile, Czech Republic, Russia, Spain)
NIMODIPINE
Nimotop Capsules . . . 749

BREK (Argentina)
ALENDRONATE SODIUM
Fosamax Tablets . . . 1969

BREMON (Spain)
CLARITHROMYCIN
Biaxin Filmtab Tablets . . . 402
Biaxin Granules . . . 402

BRENOXIL (Mexico)
AMOXICILLIN
Amoxil Pediatric Drops for Oral Suspension . . . 1343
Amoxil Tablets . . . 1343

BRESEC (Greece)
CEFTRIAXONE SODIUM
Rocephin Injectable Vials, ADD-Vantage, Galaxy, Bulk . . . 2800

BREVOXYL (Australia, Austria, Finland, France, Germany, Greece, Hong Kong, Irish Republic, Malaysia, New Zealand, Norway, Singapore, South Africa, Sweden, Thailand, United Kingdom)
BENZOYL PEROXIDE
Brevoxyl-4 Creamy Wash . . . 3210
Brevoxyl-4 Gel . . . 3210
Brevoxyl-8 Creamy Wash . . . 3210
Brevoxyl-8 Gel . . . 3210
Triaz Cleanser . . . 1892
Triaz Gel . . . 1892

BREXONASE (Chile)
FLUTICASONE PROPIONATE
Cutivate Cream . . . 2662
Cutivate Ointment . . . 2665
Flonase Nasal Spray . . . 1440

BREXOVENT (Chile)
FLUTICASONE PROPIONATE
Cutivate Cream . . . 2662
Cutivate Ointment . . . 2665
Flonase Nasal Spray . . . 1440

BRIAZIDE (France)
BENAZEPRIL HYDROCHLORIDE/HYDROCHLOROTHIAZIDE
Lotensin HCT Tablets . . . 2246

BRIEM (France)
BENAZEPRIL HYDROCHLORIDE
Lotensin Tablets . . . 2243

BRINAF (Czech Republic)
TERBINAFINE HYDROCHLORIDE
Lamisil Tablets . . . 2232

BRINTENAL (Argentina)
SELEGILINE HYDROCHLORIDE
Eldepryl Capsules . . . 3208

BRISOVENT (Portugal)
FLUTICASONE PROPIONATE
Cutivate Cream . . . 2662
Cutivate Ointment . . . 2665
Flonase Nasal Spray . . . 1440

BRISTAMOX (Sweden)
AMOXICILLIN
Amoxil Pediatric Drops for Oral Suspension . . . 1343
Amoxil Tablets . . . 1343

BRITIAZIM (United Kingdom)
DILTIAZEM HYDROCHLORIDE
Cardizem LA Extended Release Tablets . . . 1728
Tiazac Capsules . . . 1201

BRIXIA (Argentina, Chile, Venezuela)
AZELASTINE HYDROCHLORIDE
Astelin Nasal Spray . . . 1904

BRIXORAL (Greece)
RANITIDINE HYDROCHLORIDE
Zantac 25 EFFERdose Tablets . . . 1624
Zantac 150 EFFERdose Tablets . . . 1624
Zantac 150 Tablets . . . 1624
Zantac 300 Tablets . . . 1624
Zantac Injection . . . 1619
Zantac Injection Premixed . . . 1619
Zantac Syrup . . . 1624

BROLIN (Spain)
FAMOTIDINE
Pepcid Injection . . . 2040
Pepcid Injection Premixed . . . 2040
Pepcid Tablets . . . 2038
Pepcid for Oral Suspension . . . 2038

BRONALIDE (Canada, Germany, Greece)
FLUNISOLIDE
Aerobid Inhaler System . . . 1171
Aerobid-M Inhaler System . . . 1171

BRONCHOPHEN (South Africa)
THEOPHYLLINE
Uniphyl Tablets . . . 2710

BRONCHOPHYLLINE (Israel)
THEOPHYLLINE
Uniphyl Tablets . . . 2710

BRONCHORETARD (Germany)
THEOPHYLLINE
Uniphyl Tablets . . . 2710

BRONCOFOL (India)
THEOPHYLLINE
Uniphyl Tablets . . . 2710

BRONCOFOL-P (India)
THEOPHYLLINE
Uniphyl Tablets . . . 2710

BRONCONEX (New Zealand)
MOMETASONE FUROATE
Elocon Cream 0.1% . . . 3005
Elocon Lotion 0.1% . . . 3006
Elocon Ointment 0.1% . . . 3007
Nasonex Nasal Spray . . . 3043

BRONCORT (Belgium, Switzerland)
FLUNISOLIDE
Aerobid Inhaler System . . . 1171
Aerobid-M Inhaler System . . . 1171

BRONILIDE (Czech Republic, France, Switzerland)
FLUNISOLIDE
Aerobid Inhaler System . . . 1171
Aerobid-M Inhaler System . . . 1171

BRONKASMA (Argentina)
THEOPHYLLINE
Uniphyl Tablets . . . 2710

BRONPAX (Mexico)
BENZONATATE
Tessalon Perles . . . 1199

BRONQUIASMA (Brazil)
THEOPHYLLINE
Uniphyl Tablets . . . 2710

BROVAFLAMP (South Africa)
DICLOFENAC SODIUM
Voltaren Tablets . . . 2307
Voltaren-XR Tablets . . . 2310

BROVICARPINE (Greece)
VERAPAMIL HYDROCHLORIDE
Covera-HS Tablets . . . 3139
Verelan PM Extended-Release Capsules, Controlled-Onset . . . 3106

BROXOLIM-AM (Mexico)
AMOXICILLIN
Amoxil Pediatric Drops for Oral Suspension . . . 1343
Amoxil Tablets . . . 1343

BRUCAP (Mexico)
CAPTOPRIL
Captopril Tablets . . . 2149

BRULAMYCIN (Czech Republic)
TOBRAMYCIN
TOBI Solution for Inhalation . . . 2298

BRUNAZINE (South Africa)
PROMETHAZINE HYDROCHLORIDE
Phenergan Tablets and Suppositories . . . 3440

BTX-HA OFTENO (Mexico)
BETAXOLOL HYDROCHLORIDE
Betoptic S Ophthalmic Suspension . ⊙203, 558

BUCONIF (Austria)
NIFEDIPINE
Adalat CC Tablets . . . 2964

BUCORT (Finland)
HYDROCORTISONE BUTYRATE
Locoid Lipocream Cream . . . 1160

BUGAZON (Mexico)
CAPTOPRIL
Captopril Tablets . . . 2149

BUMAFLEX N (Argentina)
NAPROXEN
EC-Naprosyn Delayed-Release Tablets . . . 2761
Naprosyn Suspension . . . 2761
Naprosyn Tablets . . . 2761

BUPREN (Hungary)
BUPRENORPHINE HYDROCHLORIDE
Buprenex Injectable . . . 2716

BUPREX (Portugal, Spain)
BUPRENORPHINE HYDROCHLORIDE
Buprenex Injectable . . . 2716

BUPRINE (Thailand)
BUPRENORPHINE HYDROCHLORIDE
Buprenex Injectable . . . 2716

BURAM (Irish Republic)
AMILORIDE HYDROCHLORIDE
Midamor Tablets . . . 2026

BUROFIX (Hungary)
CALCIUM ACETATE
PhosLo GelCaps . . . 2169

BUSILVEX (Denmark, Greece, Spain, Sweden, United Kingdom)
BUSULFAN
Myleran Tablets . . . 1525

BUSULFEX (Canada, Hong Kong, Israel)
BUSULFAN
Myleran Tablets . . . 1525

BUTAVATE (Greece)
CLOBETASOL PROPIONATE
Temovate Cream . . . 2668
Temovate E Emollient . . . 2671
Temovate Gel . . . 2669
Temovate Ointment . . . 2668
Temovate Scalp Application . . . 2670

BUTISEL (Mexico)
DEXAMETHASONE
Decadron Tablets . . . 1951

BUTOP (India)
BUTENAFINE HYDROCHLORIDE
Mentax Cream . . . 2158

BUTOSALI (Mexico)
FUROSEMIDE
Furosemide Tablets . . . 2154

BUXON (Chile)
BUPROPION HYDROCHLORIDE
Wellbutrin SR Sustained-Release Tablets . . 1607
Wellbutrin Tablets . . . 1603
Zyban Sustained-Release Tablets . . . 1644

BYANODINE (Hungary)
PENICILLAMINE
Cuprimine Capsules . . . 1947

BY-MADOL (Irish Republic)
TRAMADOL HYDROCHLORIDE
Ultram ER Tablets . . . 2392

CABAL (Argentina)
CETIRIZINE HYDROCHLORIDE
Zyrtec Syrup . . . 2594
Zyrtec Tablets . . . 2594

CABIOTEN (Brazil)
CAPTOPRIL
Captopril Tablets . . . 2149

CAGINAL (Thailand)
CLOTRIMAZOLE
Lotrimin Cream . . . 3039
Lotrimin Lotion 1% . . . 3039
Lotrimin Topical Solution 1% . . . 3039

CALANIF (United Kingdom)
NIFEDIPINE
Adalat CC Tablets . . . 2964

CAL-ANTAGON (Portugal)
DILTIAZEM HYDROCHLORIDE
Cardizem LA Extended Release Tablets . . . 1728
Tiazac Capsules . . . 1201

CALAPTIN (India)
VERAPAMIL HYDROCHLORIDE
Covera-HS Tablets . . . 3139
Verelan PM Extended-Release Capsules, Controlled-Onset . . . 3106

CALAZEM (United Kingdom)
DILTIAZEM HYDROCHLORIDE
Cardizem LA Extended Release Tablets . . . 1728
Tiazac Capsules . . . 1201

CALCETAT (Italy)
CALCIUM ACETATE
PhosLo GelCaps . . . 2169

CALCHAN (United Kingdom)
NIFEDIPINE
Adalat CC Tablets . . . 2964

CALCICARD (South Africa, United Kingdom)
VERAPAMIL HYDROCHLORIDE
Covera-HS Tablets . . . 3139
Verelan PM Extended-Release Capsules, Controlled-Onset . . . 3106

CALCIGARD (India, Thailand)
NIFEDIPINE
Adalat CC Tablets . . . 2964

CALCIJEX (Australia, Austria, Brazil, Canada, Czech Republic, Finland, Hong Kong, Hungary, Irish Republic, Israel, Italy, Malaysia, Mexico, Norway, Singapore, Spain, Sweden, Switzerland, United Kingdom)
CALCITRIOL
Calcijex Injection . . . 411
Rocaltrol Capsules . . . 2798
Rocaltrol Oral Solution . . . 2798

CALCILAT (United Kingdom)
NIFEDIPINE
Adalat CC Tablets . . . 2964

CALFATE (Portugal)
SUCRALFATE
Carafate Suspension . . . 701
Carafate Tablets . . . 701

CALIDIOL (Hungary)
ESTRADIOL
Climara Transdermal System . . . 771
Estring Vaginal Ring . . . 2635

CALMADOR (Argentina)
TRAMADOL HYDROCHLORIDE
Ultram ER Tablets . . . 2392

CALMANTE DE DENTICION (Chile)
LIDOCAINE
Lidoderm Patch . . . 1118

CALMARIL (Thailand)
THIORIDAZINE HYDROCHLORIDE
Thioridazine Hydrochloride Tablets . . . 2163

CALMAVEN (Spain)
DIAZEPAM
Diastat Rectal Delivery System . . . 3343
Valium Tablets . . . 2819

CALMICORT (France)
HYDROCORTISONE
Hydrocortone Tablets . . . 1989

CALMIDAN (Spain)
SUCRALFATE
Carafate Suspension . . . 701
Carafate Tablets . . . 701

CALMIGEN (Irish Republic)
DIAZEPAM
Diastat Rectal Delivery System . . . 3343
Valium Tablets . . . 2819

CALMOCITENO (Brazil)
DIAZEPAM
Diastat Rectal Delivery System . . . 3343
Valium Tablets . . . 2819

CALMOSERPIN (Germany)
HYDROCHLOROTHIAZIDE/TRIAMTERENE
Dyazide Capsules . . . 1423

CALMPOSE (India, South Africa)
DIAZEPAM
Diastat Rectal Delivery System . . . 3343
Valium Tablets . . . 2819

CALMURID (Chile)
HYDROCORTISONE
Hydrocortone Tablets . . . 1989

CALNIF (India)
NIFEDIPINE
Adalat CC Tablets . . . 2964

CALNIT (Spain)
NIMODIPINE
Nimotop Capsules . . . 749

CALZEM (Brazil)
DILTIAZEM HYDROCHLORIDE
Cardizem LA Extended Release Tablets . . . 1728
Tiazac Capsules . . . 1201

CAMOXIN (Brazil)
AMOXICILLIN
Amoxil Pediatric Drops for Oral Suspension . . . 1343
Amoxil Tablets . . . 1343

CAMPTO (Austria, Belgium, Czech Republic, Denmark, Finland, France, Germany, Greece, Hong Kong, Hungary, Irish Republic, Israel, Italy, Malaysia, Norway, Portugal, Russia, Singapore, South Africa, Spain, Sweden, Switzerland, Thailand, The Netherlands, United Kingdom)
IRINOTECAN HYDROCHLORIDE
Camptosar Injection . . . 2604

CAMPTOSAR (Argentina, Australia, Brazil, Canada, Chile, Mexico, New Zealand, Venezuela)
IRINOTECAN HYDROCHLORIDE
Camptosar Injection . . . 2604

CANADINE (Thailand)
CLOTRIMAZOLE
Lotrimin Cream . . . 3039
Lotrimin Lotion 1% . . . 3039
Lotrimin Topical Solution 1% . . . 3039

CANALBA (South Africa)
CLOTRIMAZOLE
Lotrimin Cream . . . 3039
Lotrimin Lotion 1% . . . 3039
Lotrimin Topical Solution 1% . . . 3039

CANAZOL (Denmark, Thailand)
CLOTRIMAZOLE
Lotrimin Cream . . . 3039
Lotrimin Lotion 1% . . . 3039
Lotrimin Topical Solution 1% . . . 3039

CANDACIDE (South Africa)
NYSTATIN
Nystop Topical Powder USP . . . 2478
Paddock Nystatin USP for Oral Suspension . . . 2478

CANDACORT (Malaysia, Singapore)
CLOTRIMAZOLE
Lotrimin Cream . . . 3039
Lotrimin Lotion 1% . . . 3039
Lotrimin Topical Solution 1% . . . 3039

CANDASPOR (South Africa)
CLOTRIMAZOLE
Lotrimin Cream . . . 3039
Lotrimin Lotion 1% . . . 3039
Lotrimin Topical Solution 1% . . . 3039

CANDAZOL (Germany)
CLOTRIMAZOLE
Lotrimin Cream . . . 3039
Lotrimin Lotion 1% . . . 3039
Lotrimin Topical Solution 1% . . . 3039

CANDAZOLE (Malaysia, Singapore)
CLOTRIMAZOLE
Lotrimin Cream . . . 3039
Lotrimin Lotion 1% . . . 3039
Lotrimin Topical Solution 1% . . . 3039

CANDERME (Brazil)
METRONIDAZOLE
MetroGel-Vaginal Gel . . . 1855

CANDERMIL (Argentina)
NYSTATIN
Nystop Topical Powder USP . . . 2478
Paddock Nystatin USP for Oral Suspension . . . 2478

CANDIBENE (Austria, Czech Republic, Hungary, Russia)
CLOTRIMAZOLE
Lotrimin Cream . . . 3039
Lotrimin Lotion 1% . . . 3039
Lotrimin Topical Solution 1% . . . 3039

CANDID (India, Malaysia, Portugal, Russia, Thailand)
CLOTRIMAZOLE
Lotrimin Cream . . . 3039
Lotrimin Lotion 1% . . . 3039
Lotrimin Topical Solution 1% . . . 3039

CANDID B (India)
CLOTRIMAZOLE
Lotrimin Cream . . . 3039
Lotrimin Lotion 1% . . . 3039
Lotrimin Topical Solution 1% . . . 3039

CANDID EAR DROPS (India)
CLOTRIMAZOLE
Lotrimin Cream . . . 3039
Lotrimin Lotion 1% . . . 3039
Lotrimin Topical Solution 1% . . . 3039

CANDID V6 (Russia)
CLOTRIMAZOLE
Lotrimin Cream . . . 3039
Lotrimin Lotion 1% . . . 3039
Lotrimin Topical Solution 1% . . . 3039

CANDIDA-LOKALICID (Germany)
NYSTATIN
Nystop Topical Powder USP . . . 2478
Paddock Nystatin USP for Oral Suspension . . . 2478

CANDIDEN (United Kingdom)
CLOTRIMAZOLE
Lotrimin Cream . . . 3039
Lotrimin Lotion 1% . . . 3039
Lotrimin Topical Solution 1% . . . 3039

CANDIDIAS (Argentina)
NYSTATIN
Nystop Topical Powder USP . . . 2478
Paddock Nystatin USP for Oral Suspension . . . 2478

CANDID-TV (India)
CLOTRIMAZOLE
Lotrimin Cream . . . 3039
Lotrimin Lotion 1% . . . 3039
Lotrimin Topical Solution 1% . . . 3039

CANDIMON (Mexico)
CLOTRIMAZOLE
Lotrimin Cream . . . 3039
Lotrimin Lotion 1% . . . 3039
Lotrimin Topical Solution 1% . . . 3039

CANDINOX (Thailand)
CLOTRIMAZOLE
Lotrimin Cream . . . 3039
Lotrimin Lotion 1% . . . 3039
Lotrimin Topical Solution 1% . . . 3039

CANDIO (Austria, Germany, Switzerland)
NYSTATIN
Nystop Topical Powder USP . . . 2478
Paddock Nystatin USP for Oral Suspension . . . 2478

CANDIPHEN (Mexico)
CLOTRIMAZOLE
Lotrimin Cream . . . 3039
Lotrimin Lotion 1% . . . 3039

Lotrimin Topical Solution 1% 3039

CANDISTATIN (Brazil, Canada)
NYSTATIN
Nystop Topical Powder USP 2478
Paddock Nystatin USP for Oral Suspension 2478

CANDIZOLE (South Africa)
CLOTRIMAZOLE
Lotrimin Cream.................. 3039
Lotrimin Lotion 1%................ 3039
Lotrimin Topical Solution 1% 3039

CANEF (Denmark, Finland, Mexico, Norway, Portugal, Sweden, The Netherlands)
FLUVASTATIN SODIUM
Lescol Capsules 2233

CANESTEN (Australia, Austria, Brazil, Canada, Chile, Denmark, Finland, Germany, Greece, Hong Kong, Hungary, Irish Republic, Italy, Malaysia, Mexico, New Zealand, Norway, Portugal, Singapore, South Africa, Spain, Sweden, Thailand, The Netherlands, United Kingdom, Venezuela)
CLOTRIMAZOLE
Lotrimin Cream.................. 3039
Lotrimin Lotion 1%................ 3039
Lotrimin Topical Solution 1% 3039

CANESTEN COMBI (United Kingdom)
CLOTRIMAZOLE
Lotrimin Cream.................. 3039
Lotrimin Lotion 1%................ 3039
Lotrimin Topical Solution 1% 3039

CANESTEN HC (Germany, Hong Kong, United Kingdom)
CLOTRIMAZOLE
Lotrimin Cream.................. 3039
Lotrimin Lotion 1%................ 3039
Lotrimin Topical Solution 1% 3039

CANESTENE (Belgium, Switzerland)
CLOTRIMAZOLE
Lotrimin Cream.................. 3039
Lotrimin Lotion 1%................ 3039
Lotrimin Topical Solution 1% 3039

CANEX (South Africa)
CLOTRIMAZOLE
Lotrimin Cream.................. 3039
Lotrimin Lotion 1%................ 3039
Lotrimin Topical Solution 1% 3039

CANIFUG (Czech Republic, Germany, Hungary)
CLOTRIMAZOLE
Lotrimin Cream.................. 3039
Lotrimin Lotion 1%................ 3039
Lotrimin Topical Solution 1% 3039

CANSTAT (South Africa)
NYSTATIN
Nystop Topical Powder USP 2478
Paddock Nystatin USP for Oral Suspension 2478

CANTANIDIN (Austria)
CLONIDINE HYDROCHLORIDE
Catapres Tablets 843

CAPACE (Australia, Austria, India, South Africa)
CAPTOPRIL
Captopril Tablets 2149

CAPIN (Hungary)
CAPTOPRIL
Captopril Tablets 2149

CAPOCARD (Hong Kong)
CAPTOPRIL
Captopril Tablets 2149

CAPOSTAD (Austria)
CAPTOPRIL
Captopril Tablets 2149

CAPOTEN (Australia, Belgium, Brazil, Canada, Chile, Czech Republic, Denmark, Finland, Greece, Hong Kong, Irish Republic, Italy, Malaysia, New Zealand, Norway, Portugal, Singapore, South Africa, Spain, Sweden, Thailand, The Netherlands, United Kingdom, Venezuela)
CAPTOPRIL
Captopril Tablets 2149

CAPOTENA (Mexico)
CAPTOPRIL
Captopril Tablets 2149

CAPOTRIL (Brazil)
CAPTOPRIL
Captopril Tablets 2149

CAPOX (Brazil)
CAPTOPRIL
Captopril Tablets 2149

CAPOX H (Brazil)
CAPTOPRIL
Captopril Tablets 2149

CAPOZID (Denmark)
CAPTOPRIL
Captopril Tablets 2149

CAPOZIDE (Germany, Mexico, New Zealand, South Africa, United Kingdom, Venezuela)
CAPTOPRIL
Captopril Tablets 2149

CAPRIL (Brazil, Hong Kong)
CAPTOPRIL
Captopril Tablets 2149

CAPROS (Germany)
MORPHINE SULFATE
Kadian Capsules 577
MS Contin Tablets 2701

CAPRYSIN (Finland)
CLONIDINE HYDROCHLORIDE
Catapres Tablets 843

CAPSICOF (Mexico)
BENZONATATE
Tessalon Perles 1199

CAPTI (Israel)
CAPTOPRIL
Captopril Tablets 2149

CAPTIL (Brazil)
CAPTOPRIL
Captopril Tablets 2149

CAPTIREX (France)
CAPTOPRIL
Captopril Tablets 2149

CAPTO PLUS (Germany)
CAPTOPRIL
Captopril Tablets 2149

CAPTO-BASAN (Switzerland)
CAPTOPRIL
Captopril Tablets 2149

CAPTOBEL (Brazil)
CAPTOPRIL
Captopril Tablets 2149

CAPTOBETA (Germany)
CAPTOPRIL
Captopril Tablets 2149

CAPTOBETA COMP (Germany)
CAPTOPRIL
Captopril Tablets 2149

CAPTO-CO (United Kingdom)
CAPTOPRIL
Captopril Tablets 2149

CAPTOCORD (Brazil)
CAPTOPRIL
Captopril Tablets 2149

CAPTODAN (Denmark)
CAPTOPRIL
Captopril Tablets 2149

CAPTODOC (Germany)
CAPTOPRIL
Captopril Tablets 2149

CAPTODOC COMP (Germany)
CAPTOPRIL
Captopril Tablets 2149

CAPTO-DURA COR (Germany)
CAPTOPRIL
Captopril Tablets 2149

CAPTO-DURA M (Germany)
CAPTOPRIL
Captopril Tablets 2149

CAPTOFLUX (Germany)
CAPTOPRIL
Captopril Tablets 2149

CAPTOGAMMA (Germany, Hungary)
CAPTOPRIL
Captopril Tablets 2149

CAPTOGAMMA HCT (Germany)
CAPTOPRIL
Captopril Tablets 2149

CAPTOHEXAL (Australia, Germany, New Zealand, South Africa)
CAPTOPRIL
Captopril Tablets 2149

CAPTOHEXAL COMP (Austria, Czech Republic, Germany)
CAPTOPRIL
Captopril Tablets 2149

CAPTOL (Denmark)
CAPTOPRIL
Captopril Tablets 2149

CAPTOLAB (Brazil)
CAPTOPRIL
Captopril Tablets 2149

CAPTOLANE (France)
CAPTOPRIL
Captopril Tablets 2149

CAPTOLIN (Brazil)
CAPTOPRIL
Captopril Tablets 2149

CAPTOMAX (South Africa)
CAPTOPRIL
Captopril Tablets 2149

CAPTOMED (Austria, Brazil)
CAPTOPRIL
Captopril Tablets 2149

CAPTOMERCK (Germany)
CAPTOPRIL
Captopril Tablets 2149

CAPTOMIN (Finland)
CAPTOPRIL
Captopril Tablets 2149

CAPTON (Brazil)
CAPTOPRIL
Captopril Tablets 2149

CAPTOPHAR (United Arab Emirates)
CAPTOPRIL
Captopril Tablets 2149

CAPTOPIRIL (Brazil)
CAPTOPRIL
Captopril Tablets 2149

CAPTOPLUS (Austria)
CAPTOPRIL
Captopril Tablets 2149

CAPTOPRESS (Germany)
CAPTOPRIL
Captopril Tablets 2149

CAPTOPRIL HCT (Austria)
CAPTOPRIL
Captopril Tablets 2149

CAPTOPRIL PLUS (Germany)
CAPTOPRIL
Captopril Tablets 2149

CAPTOPRON (Brazil)
CAPTOPRIL
Captopril Tablets 2149

CAPTOR (Austria, Irish Republic)
CAPTOPRIL
Captopril Tablets 2149

CAPTOREAL (Germany)
CAPTOPRIL
Captopril Tablets 2149

CAPTORETIC (South Africa)
CAPTOPRIL
Captopril Tablets 2149

CAPTOR-HCT (Irish Republic)
CAPTOPRIL
Captopril Tablets 2149

CAPTOSEN (Brazil)
CAPTOPRIL
Captopril Tablets 2149

CAPTOSER (Mexico)
CAPTOPRIL
Captopril Tablets 2149

CAPTOSIF (Brazil)
CAPTOPRIL
Captopril Tablets 2149

CAPTOSINA (Spain)
CAPTOPRIL
Captopril Tablets 2149

CAPTOSOL (Switzerland)
CAPTOPRIL
Captopril Tablets 2149

CAPTOSOL COMP (Switzerland)
CAPTOPRIL
Captopril Tablets 2149

CAPTOSTAD (Finland)
CAPTOPRIL
Captopril Tablets 2149

CAPTOTEC (Brazil)
CAPTOPRIL
Captopril Tablets 2149

CAPTOTEC + HCT (Brazil)
CAPTOPRIL
Captopril Tablets 2149

CAPTOTYROL (Austria)
CAPTOPRIL
Captopril Tablets 2149

CAPTOZEN (Brazil)
CAPTOPRIL
Captopril Tablets 2149

CAPTRAL (Mexico)
CAPTOPRIL
Captopril Tablets 2149

CAPTRIL (Canada)
CAPTOPRIL
Captopril Tablets 2149

CAPTRIZIN (Brazil)
CAPTOPRIL
Captopril Tablets 2149

CARACE (Irish Republic, United Kingdom)
LISINOPRIL
Prinivil Tablets 2052

CARACE PLUS (Irish Republic, United Kingdom)
HYDROCHLOROTHIAZIDE/LISINOPRIL
Prinzide Tablets 2056

CARAFATE (Australia, New Zealand)
SUCRALFATE
Carafate Suspension 701
Carafate Tablets 701

CARALPHA (United Kingdom)
LISINOPRIL
Prinivil Tablets 2052

CARASEL (Spain)
RAMIPRIL
Altace Capsules 1702

CARBABETA (Germany)
CARBAMAZEPINE
Carbatrol Capsules 3171
Tegretol Chewable Tablets 2295
Tegretol Suspension.............. 2295
Tegretol Tablets 2295
Tegretol-XR Tablets 2295

CARBACTOL RETARD (Chile)
CARBAMAZEPINE
Carbatrol Capsules 3171
Tegretol Chewable Tablets 2295
Tegretol Suspension.............. 2295
Tegretol Tablets 2295
Tegretol-XR Tablets 2295

CARBADURA (Germany)
CARBAMAZEPINE
Carbatrol Capsules 3171
Tegretol Chewable Tablets 2295
Tegretol Suspension.............. 2295
Tegretol Tablets 2295
Tegretol-XR Tablets 2295

CARBAFLUX (Germany)
CARBAMAZEPINE
Carbatrol Capsules 3171
Tegretol Chewable Tablets 2295
Tegretol Suspension.............. 2295
Tegretol Tablets 2295
Tegretol-XR Tablets 2295

CARBAGAMMA (Germany)
CARBAMAZEPINE
Carbatrol Capsules 3171

Tegretol Chewable Tablets 2295
Tegretol Suspension 2295
Tegretol Tablets 2295
Tegretol-XR Tablets 2295

CARBAGEN (United Kingdom)
CARBAMAZEPINE
Carbatrol Capsules 3171
Tegretol Chewable Tablets 2295
Tegretol Suspension 2295
Tegretol Tablets 2295
Tegretol-XR Tablets 2295

CARBAGRAMON (Argentina)
CARBAMAZEPINE
Carbatrol Capsules 3171
Tegretol Chewable Tablets 2295
Tegretol Suspension 2295
Tegretol Tablets 2295
Tegretol-XR Tablets 2295

CARBALAN (Mexico)
CARBAMAZEPINE
Carbatrol Capsules 3171
Tegretol Chewable Tablets 2295
Tegretol Suspension 2295
Tegretol Tablets 2295
Tegretol-XR Tablets 2295

CARBAMAT (Argentina)
CARBAMAZEPINE
Carbatrol Capsules 3171
Tegretol Chewable Tablets 2295
Tegretol Suspension 2295
Tegretol Tablets 2295
Tegretol-XR Tablets 2295

CARBAPIN (Russia)
CARBAMAZEPINE
Carbatrol Capsules 3171
Tegretol Chewable Tablets 2295
Tegretol Suspension 2295
Tegretol Tablets 2295
Tegretol-XR Tablets 2295

CARBASAL (Mexico)
CARBAMAZEPINE
Carbatrol Capsules 3171
Tegretol Chewable Tablets 2295
Tegretol Suspension 2295
Tegretol Tablets 2295
Tegretol-XR Tablets 2295

CARBATOL (Thailand)
CARBAMAZEPINE
Carbatrol Capsules 3171
Tegretol Chewable Tablets 2295
Tegretol Suspension 2295
Tegretol Tablets 2295
Tegretol-XR Tablets 2295

CARBAVAL (Mexico)
CARBAMAZEPINE
Carbatrol Capsules 3171
Tegretol Chewable Tablets 2295
Tegretol Suspension 2295
Tegretol Tablets 2295
Tegretol-XR Tablets 2295

CARBAZENE (Thailand)
CARBAMAZEPINE
Carbatrol Capsules 3171
Tegretol Chewable Tablets 2295
Tegretol Suspension 2295
Tegretol Tablets 2295
Tegretol-XR Tablets 2295

CARBAZEP (Mexico)
CARBAMAZEPINE
Carbatrol Capsules 3171
Tegretol Chewable Tablets 2295
Tegretol Suspension 2295
Tegretol Tablets 2295
Tegretol-XR Tablets 2295

CARBAZINA (Mexico)
CARBAMAZEPINE
Carbatrol Capsules 3171
Tegretol Chewable Tablets 2295
Tegretol Suspension 2295
Tegretol Tablets 2295
Tegretol-XR Tablets 2295

CARBI (Israel)
CARBAMAZEPINE
Carbatrol Capsules 3171
Tegretol Chewable Tablets 2295
Tegretol Suspension 2295
Tegretol Tablets 2295
Tegretol-XR Tablets 2295

CARBIUM (Australia, Germany)
CARBAMAZEPINE
Carbatrol Capsules 3171
Tegretol Chewable Tablets 2295
Tegretol Suspension 2295
Tegretol Tablets 2295
Tegretol-XR Tablets 2295

CARBLOC (Chile)
NIFEDIPINE
Adalat CC Tablets 2964

CARBRITAL (Australia)
PENTOBARBITAL SODIUM
Nembutal Sodium Solution, USP 2470

CARDACE (Finland, India)
RAMIPRIL
Altace Capsules 1702

CARDACE COMP (Finland)
RAMIPRIL
Altace Capsules 1702

CARDALIN (Brazil)
NIFEDIPINE
Adalat CC Tablets 2964

CARDCAL (Australia)
DILTIAZEM HYDROCHLORIDE
Cardizem LA Extended Release Tablets 1728
Tiazac Capsules 1201

CARDCOR (Brazil)
DIGOXIN
Lanoxicaps Capsules 1490
Lanoxin Injection 1494
Lanoxin Injection Pediatric 1497
Lanoxin Tablets 1500

CARDELOC (Thailand)
METOPROLOL TARTRATE
Lopressor Tablets 2238

CARDENOL (Thailand)
PROPRANOLOL HYDROCHLORIDE
Inderal LA Long-Acting Capsules 3429

CARDIACE (South Africa)
CAPTOPRIL
Captopril Tablets 2149

CARDIACTON (Austria)
DILTIAZEM HYDROCHLORIDE
Cardizem LA Extended Release Tablets 1728
Tiazac Capsules 1201

CARDIAGEN (Germany)
CAPTOPRIL
Captopril Tablets 2149

CARDIAGEN HCT (Germany)
CAPTOPRIL
Captopril Tablets 2149

CARDIAGUTT (Germany)
VERAPAMIL HYDROCHLORIDE
Covera-HS Tablets 3139
Verelan PM Extended-Release Capsules, Controlled-Onset 3106

CARDIBELTIN (Germany)
VERAPAMIL HYDROCHLORIDE
Covera-HS Tablets 3139
Verelan PM Extended-Release Capsules, Controlled-Onset 3106

CARDIBLOK (South Africa)
PROPRANOLOL HYDROCHLORIDE
Inderal LA Long-Acting Capsules 3429

CARDICON (Chile)
NIFEDIPINE
Adalat CC Tablets 2964

CARDIFEN (South Africa)
NIFEDIPINE
Adalat CC Tablets 2964

CARDIL (Denmark, Greece, Malaysia, Russia, Singapore, Thailand)
DILTIAZEM HYDROCHLORIDE
Cardizem LA Extended Release Tablets 1728
Tiazac Capsules 1201

CARDILAT (South Africa)
NIFEDIPINE
Adalat CC Tablets 2964

CARDILATE MR (Hong Kong, United Kingdom)
NIFEDIPINE
Adalat CC Tablets 2964

CARDILOL (Brazil, United Arab Emirates)
CARVEDILOL
Coreg Tablets 1414

CARDILOM (Brazil)
CAPTOPRIL
Captopril Tablets 2149

CARDINOL (Australia, New Zealand, United Kingdom)
PROPRANOLOL HYDROCHLORIDE
Inderal LA Long-Acting Capsules 3429

CARDINORM (Italy)
VERAPAMIL HYDROCHLORIDE
Covera-HS Tablets 3139
Verelan PM Extended-Release Capsules, Controlled-Onset 3106

CARDIOBIL (Italy)
LEVOCARNITINE
Carnitor Injection 3188
Carnitor Tablets and Oral Solution 3190

CARDIOBRON (Argentina)
ALPROSTADIL
Edex Injection 3089

CARDIOFENONE (Italy)
PROPAFENONE HYDROCHLORIDE
Rythmol SR Capsules 2727

CARDIOGEN (Italy)
LEVOCARNITINE
Carnitor Injection 3188
Carnitor Tablets and Oral Solution 3190

CARDIOGOXIN (Argentina)
DIGOXIN
Lanoxicaps Capsules 1490
Lanoxin Injection 1494
Lanoxin Injection Pediatric 1497
Lanoxin Tablets 1500

CARDIOL (Finland, Portugal)
CARVEDILOL
Coreg Tablets 1414

CARDIOLEN (Chile)
VERAPAMIL HYDROCHLORIDE
Covera-HS Tablets 3139
Verelan PM Extended-Release Capsules, Controlled-Onset 3106

CARDIONIL (Brazil, Spain)
ISOSORBIDE MONONITRATE
Imdur Tablets 3018

CARDIOPINA (Brazil)
NIFEDIPINE
Adalat CC Tablets 2964

CARDIOPINE (United Arab Emirates)
NIFEDIPINE
Adalat CC Tablets 2964

CARDIOPRANOL (Brazil)
PROPRANOLOL HYDROCHLORIDE
Inderal LA Long-Acting Capsules 3429

CARDIOPROTECT (Germany)
VERAPAMIL HYDROCHLORIDE
Covera-HS Tablets 3139
Verelan PM Extended-Release Capsules, Controlled-Onset 3106

CARDIOREG (Italy)
DIGOXIN
Lanoxicaps Capsules 1490
Lanoxin Injection 1494
Lanoxin Injection Pediatric 1497
Lanoxin Tablets 1500

CARDIOSTATIN (Russia)
LOVASTATIN
Mevacor Tablets 2021

CARDIOVAS (Spain)
ISOSORBIDE MONONITRATE
Imdur Tablets 3018

CARDIOXIN (India)
DIGOXIN
Lanoxicaps Capsules 1490
Lanoxin Injection 1494
Lanoxin Injection Pediatric 1497
Lanoxin Tablets 1500

CARDIPIN (Switzerland)
NIFEDIPINE
Adalat CC Tablets 2964

CARDIPRIL (Mexico)
CAPTOPRIL
Captopril Tablets 2149

CARDISER (Spain)
DILTIAZEM HYDROCHLORIDE
Cardizem LA Extended Release Tablets 1728
Tiazac Capsules 1201

CARDISORB (Hungary)
ISOSORBIDE MONONITRATE
Imdur Tablets 3018

CARDISPAN (Mexico)
LEVOCARNITINE
Carnitor Injection 3188
Carnitor Tablets and Oral Solution 3190

CARDISPARE (South Africa)
PROPRANOLOL HYDROCHLORIDE
Inderal LA Long-Acting Capsules 3429

CARDITRIL (Brazil)
CAPTOPRIL
Captopril Tablets 2149

CARDIUM (Hong Kong, Singapore)
DILTIAZEM HYDROCHLORIDE
Cardizem LA Extended Release Tablets 1728
Tiazac Capsules 1201

CARDIVAS (Russia)
CARVEDILOL
Coreg Tablets 1414

CARDIZEM (Australia, Brazil, Canada, Denmark, Finland, New Zealand, Norway, Sweden)
DILTIAZEM HYDROCHLORIDE
Cardizem LA Extended Release Tablets 1728
Tiazac Capsules 1201

CARDOXIN (Israel)
DIPYRIDAMOLE
Persantine Tablets 868

CARDOXONE (Thailand)
METOPROLOL TARTRATE
Lopressor Tablets 2238

CARDULES (India)
NIFEDIPINE
Adalat CC Tablets 2964

CARDYL (Spain)
ATORVASTATIN CALCIUM
Lipitor Tablets 2483

CAREFLU (Italy)
FLUNISOLIDE
Aerobid Inhaler System 1171
Aerobid-M Inhaler System 1171

CARENCIL (Portugal)
CAPTOPRIL
Captopril Tablets 2149

CARLOC (India, South Africa)
CARVEDILOL
Coreg Tablets 1414

CARMAPINE (Thailand)
CARBAMAZEPINE
Carbatrol Capsules 3171
Tegretol Chewable Tablets 2295
Tegretol Suspension 2295
Tegretol Tablets 2295
Tegretol-XR Tablets 2295

CARMAZIN (Brazil)
CARBAMAZEPINE
Carbatrol Capsules 3171
Tegretol Chewable Tablets 2295
Tegretol Suspension 2295
Tegretol Tablets 2295
Tegretol-XR Tablets 2295

CARMICINA (Portugal)
CIPROFLOXACIN HYDROCHLORIDE
Ciloxan Ophthalmic Ointment ⊙204, 559
Ciloxan Ophthalmic Solution ⊙206
Cipro Tablets 2977

CARNICOR (Chile, Italy)
LEVOCARNITINE
Carnitor Injection 3188
Carnitor Tablets and Oral Solution 3190

CARNIDOSE (Greece)
LEVOCARNITINE
Carnitor Injection 3188
Carnitor Tablets and Oral Solution 3190

CARNIL (Greece)
LEVOCARNITINE
Carnitor Injection 3188
Carnitor Tablets and Oral Solution 3190

CARNISIN (Venezuela)
LEVOCARNITINE
Carnitor Injection 3188
Carnitor Tablets and Oral Solution 3190

CARNITENE (Hong Kong, Italy)
LEVOCARNITINE
Carnitor Injection **3188**
Carnitor Tablets and Oral Solution **3190**

CARNITOP (Italy)
LEVOCARNITINE
Carnitor Injection **3188**
Carnitor Tablets and Oral Solution **3190**

CARNITOR (Canada, Hong Kong, United Kingdom)
LEVOCARNITINE
Carnitor Injection **3188**
Carnitor Tablets and Oral Solution **3190**

CARNOVIS (Italy)
LEVOCARNITINE
Carnitor Injection **3188**
Carnitor Tablets and Oral Solution **3190**

CARNUM (Italy)
LEVOCARNITINE
Carnitor Injection **3188**
Carnitor Tablets and Oral Solution **3190**

CARPAZ (South Africa)
CARBAMAZEPINE
Carbatrol Capsules **3171**
Tegretol Chewable Tablets **2295**
Tegretol Suspension **2295**
Tegretol Tablets **2295**
Tegretol-XR Tablets **2295**

CARPIN (Mexico)
CARBAMAZEPINE
Carbatrol Capsules **3171**
Tegretol Chewable Tablets **2295**
Tegretol Suspension **2295**
Tegretol Tablets **2295**
Tegretol-XR Tablets **2295**

CARPINE (Thailand)
CARBAMAZEPINE
Carbatrol Capsules **3171**
Tegretol Chewable Tablets **2295**
Tegretol Suspension **2295**
Tegretol Tablets **2295**
Tegretol-XR Tablets **2295**

CARRELDON (Spain)
DILTIAZEM HYDROCHLORIDE
Cardizem LA Extended Release Tablets . . . **1728**
Tiazac Capsules **1201**

CARRIER (Italy)
LEVOCARNITINE
Carnitor Injection **3188**
Carnitor Tablets and Oral Solution **3190**

CARTAZID (Venezuela)
CAPTOPRIL
Captopril Tablets **2149**

CARVEDEXXON (Israel)
CARVEDILOL
Coreg Tablets **1414**

CARVEDIL (Argentina)
CARVEDILOL
Coreg Tablets **1414**

CARVEL (Argentina)
CARVEDILOL
Coreg Tablets **1414**

CARVETONE (Denmark)
CARVEDILOL
Coreg Tablets **1414**

CARVIL (India)
CARVEDILOL
Coreg Tablets **1414**

CARVIPRESS (Italy)
CARVEDILOL
Coreg Tablets **1414**

CARZEM (Italy)
DILTIAZEM HYDROCHLORIDE
Cardizem LA Extended Release Tablets . . . **1728**
Tiazac Capsules **1201**

CARZEPINE (Thailand)
CARBAMAZEPINE
Carbatrol Capsules **3171**
Tegretol Chewable Tablets **2295**
Tegretol Suspension **2295**
Tegretol Tablets **2295**
Tegretol-XR Tablets **2295**

CASBAME (Mexico)
LOVASTATIN
Mevacor Tablets **2021**

CASBOL (Spain)
PAROXETINE HYDROCHLORIDE
Paxil Oral Suspension **1530**
Paxil Tablets **1530**

CASCOR (Malaysia, Thailand)
DILTIAZEM HYDROCHLORIDE
Cardizem LA Extended Release Tablets . . . **1728**
Tiazac Capsules **1201**

CATALIP (Portugal)
FENOFIBRATE
Tricor Tablets **527**

CATAPRES (Australia, Canada, Hong Kong, India, Irish Republic, Japan, New Zealand, South Africa, Thailand, United Kingdom)
CLONIDINE HYDROCHLORIDE
Catapres Tablets **843**

CATAPRES DIU (India)
CLONIDINE HYDROCHLORIDE
Catapres Tablets **843**

CATAPRESAN (Austria, Chile, Czech Republic, Denmark, Finland, Germany, Greece, Mexico, Norway, Portugal, Spain, Sweden, Switzerland, The Netherlands, Venezuela)
CLONIDINE HYDROCHLORIDE
Catapres Tablets **843**

CATAPRESSAN (Belgium, France)
CLONIDINE HYDROCHLORIDE
Catapres Tablets **843**

CATEX (Spain)
CIPROFLOXACIN HYDROCHLORIDE
Ciloxan Ophthalmic Ointment . . . . ⊙**204, 559**
Ciloxan Ophthalmic Solution . . . . ⊙**206**
Cipro Tablets **2977**

CATEXAN (South Africa)
INDAPAMIDE
Indapamide Tablets **2156**

CATONA (Mexico)
CAPTOPRIL
Captopril Tablets **2149**

CATONET (Denmark)
CAPTOPRIL
Captopril Tablets **2149**

CATOPLIN (Singapore)
CAPTOPRIL
Captopril Tablets **2149**

CATOPROL (Brazil)
CAPTOPRIL
Captopril Tablets **2149**

CAUSALON PRO (Argentina)
NAPROXEN
EC-Naprosyn Delayed-Release Tablets **2761**
Naprosyn Suspension **2761**
Naprosyn Tablets **2761**

CAVERIL (Thailand)
VERAPAMIL HYDROCHLORIDE
Covera-HS Tablets **3139**
Verelan PM Extended-Release Capsules, Controlled-Onset **3106**

CAVERJECT (Argentina, Australia, Austria, Belgium, Brazil, Canada, Chile, Czech Republic, Denmark, Finland, France, Germany, Greece, Hong Kong, Hungary, Irish Republic, Israel, Italy, Malaysia, Mexico, New Zealand, Norway, Portugal, Russia, Singapore, South Africa, Spain, Sweden, Switzerland, Thailand, The Netherlands, United Kingdom, Venezuela)
ALPROSTADIL
Edex Injection **3089**

CAVERTA (India)
SILDENAFIL CITRATE
Viagra Tablets **2573**

C-BILDZ (Austria)
CIPROFLOXACIN HYDROCHLORIDE
Ciloxan Ophthalmic Ointment . . . . ⊙**204, 559**
Ciloxan Ophthalmic Solution . . . . ⊙**206**
Cipro Tablets **2977**

CEBRALAT (Brazil)
CILOSTAZOL
Pletal Tablets **2455**

CEBRILIN (Brazil)
PAROXETINE HYDROCHLORIDE
Paxil Oral Suspension **1530**
Paxil Tablets **1530**

CEBROCAL (Argentina)
DONEPEZIL HYDROCHLORIDE
Aricept Tablets **1094**

CEBROFORT (Argentina)
NIMODIPINE
Nimotop Capsules **749**

CECNOIN (Brazil)
ISOTRETINOIN
Accutane Capsules **2731**

CECURAL (Greece)
LOVASTATIN
Mevacor Tablets **2021**

CEDETRIN-T (Czech Republic)
MUROMONAB-CD3
Orthoclone OKT3 Sterile Solution **2360**

CEF-3 (Thailand)
CEFTRIAXONE SODIUM
Rocephin Injectable Vials, ADD-Vantage, Galaxy, Bulk **2800**

CEF-4 (Thailand)
CEFTAZIDIME
Fortaz for Injection **1453**

CEFAMAR (Italy, Thailand)
CEFUROXIME SODIUM
Zinacef Injection **1631**

CEFASYN (India)
CEFUROXIME AXETIL
Ceftin Tablets **1407**
Ceftin for Oral Suspension **1407**

CEFAXICINA (Spain)
CEFOXITIN SODIUM
Mefoxin Premixed Intravenous Solution . . . **2016**
Mefoxin for Injection **2012**

CEFAXONA (Mexico)
CEFTRIAXONE SODIUM
Rocephin Injectable Vials, ADD-Vantage, Galaxy, Bulk **2800**

CEFAXONE (Czech Republic, Malaysia, Singapore)
CEFTRIAXONE SODIUM
Rocephin Injectable Vials, ADD-Vantage, Galaxy, Bulk **2800**

CEFAZID (India)
CEFTAZIDIME
Fortaz for Injection **1453**

CEFAZIMA (Brazil)
CEFTAZIDIME
Fortaz for Injection **1453**

CEFAZIME (Singapore)
CEFTAZIDIME
Fortaz for Injection **1453**

CEFEPEN (Brazil)
CEFEPIME HYDROCHLORIDE
Maxipime for Injection **1105**

CEFGRAM (Venezuela)
CEFTAZIDIME
Fortaz for Injection **1453**

CEFICAD (India)
CEFEPIME HYDROCHLORIDE
Maxipime for Injection **1105**

CEFIMEN-K (Argentina)
CEFEPIME HYDROCHLORIDE
Maxipime for Injection **1105**

CEFIMIX (Portugal)
CEFIXIME
Suprax **1843**

CEFIN (Singapore)
CEFTRIAXONE SODIUM
Rocephin Injectable Vials, ADD-Vantage, Galaxy, Bulk **2800**

CEFINE (Thailand)
CEFTRIAXONE SODIUM
Rocephin Injectable Vials, ADD-Vantage, Galaxy, Bulk **2800**

CEFIRAX (Chile)
CEFPODOXIME PROXETIL
Vantin Tablets and Oral Suspension **2645**

CEFITON (Portugal)
CEFIXIME
Suprax **1843**

CEFIX (India, Venezuela)
CEFIXIME
Suprax **1843**

CEFIX LB (India)
CEFIXIME
Suprax **1843**

CEFIXDURA (Germany)
CEFIXIME
Suprax **1843**

CEFIXORAL (Italy)
CEFIXIME
Suprax **1843**

CEFLOUR (Malaysia)
CEFUROXIME SODIUM
Zinacef Injection **1631**

CEFNAX (Brazil)
CEFIXIME
Suprax **1843**

CEFOCEF (India)
CEFTRIAXONE SODIUM
Rocephin Injectable Vials, ADD-Vantage, Galaxy, Bulk **2800**

CEFOCEF-LB (India)
CEFIXIME
Suprax **1843**

CEFOCICLIN (Italy)
CEFOXITIN SODIUM
Mefoxin Premixed Intravenous Solution . . . **2016**
Mefoxin for Injection **2012**

CEFODIME (Thailand)
CEFTAZIDIME
Fortaz for Injection **1453**

CEFODOX (France, Irish Republic, Italy)
CEFPODOXIME PROXETIL
Vantin Tablets and Oral Suspension **2645**

CEFOFIX (Portugal)
CEFUROXIME SODIUM
Zinacef Injection **1631**

CEFOGEN (India, Thailand)
CEFUROXIME SODIUM
Zinacef Injection **1631**

CEFOMAX (Argentina)
CEFTRIAXONE SODIUM
Rocephin Injectable Vials, ADD-Vantage, Galaxy, Bulk **2800**

CEFOPRIM (Greece, Italy)
CEFUROXIME SODIUM
Zinacef Injection **1631**

CEFOPROX (India)
CEFPODOXIME PROXETIL
Vantin Tablets and Oral Suspension **2645**

CEFORTAM (Portugal)
CEFTAZIDIME SODIUM
Fortaz for Injection **1453**

CEFOTRIX (Denmark, Hungary)
CEFTRIAXONE SODIUM
Rocephin Injectable Vials, ADD-Vantage, Galaxy, Bulk **2800**

CEFOXIM (India)
CEFUROXIME AXETIL
Ceftin Tablets **1407**
Ceftin for Oral Suspension **1407**

CEFOXIN (Brazil, Thailand)
CEFOXITIN SODIUM
Mefoxin Premixed Intravenous Solution . . . **2016**
Mefoxin for Injection **2012**

CEFRADEN (Mexico)
CEFTRIAXONE SODIUM
Rocephin Injectable Vials, ADD-Vantage, Galaxy, Bulk **2800**

CEFSPAN (Chile, Japan, Thailand)
CEFIXIME
Suprax **1843**

CEFT (Brazil)
CEFTRIAXONE SODIUM
Rocephin Injectable Vials, ADD-Vantage, Galaxy, Bulk **2800**

CEFTANORTH (Brazil)
CEFTAZIDIME
Fortaz for Injection **1453**

CEFTARIDEM (Greece)
CEFTAZIDIME
Fortaz for Injection **1453**

(⊙ Described in PDR For Ophthalmic Medicines™)

CEFTAZ (India)
CEFTAZIDIME
Fortaz for Injection 1453

CEFTAZIDON (Brazil)
CEFTAZIDIME
Fortaz for Injection 1453

CEFTEN (Brazil)
CEFTAZIDIME
Fortaz for Injection 1453

CEFTIDIN (India)
CEFTAZIDIME
Fortaz for Injection 1453

CEFTIM (Italy)
CEFTAZIDIME
Fortaz for Injection 1453

CEFTIN (Canada)
CEFUROXIME AXETIL
Ceftin Tablets 1407
Ceftin for Oral Suspension 1407

CEFTON (Brazil)
CEFOXITIN SODIUM
Mefoxin Premixed Intravenous Solution . . . 2016
Mefoxin for Injection 2012

CEFTORAL (Greece)
CEFIXIME
Suprax 1843

CEFTREX (Malaysia, Mexico, Thailand)
CEFTRIAXONE SODIUM
Rocephin Injectable Vials, ADD-Vantage, Galaxy, Bulk 2800

CEFTRILEM (Mexico)
CEFTRIAXONE SODIUM
Rocephin Injectable Vials, ADD-Vantage, Galaxy, Bulk 2800

CEFTRINAL (Greece)
RANITIDINE HYDROCHLORIDE
Zantac 25 EFFERdose Tablets 1624
Zantac 150 EFFERdose Tablets 1624
Zantac 150 Tablets 1624
Zantac 300 Tablets 1624
Zantac Injection 1619
Zantac Injection Premixed 1619
Zantac Syrup 1624

CEFTRIPHIN (Thailand)
CEFTRIAXONE SODIUM
Rocephin Injectable Vials, ADD-Vantage, Galaxy, Bulk 2800

CEFUDURA (Germany)
CEFUROXIME AXETIL
Ceftin Tablets 1407
Ceftin for Oral Suspension 1407

CEFUHEXAL (Germany)
CEFUROXIME AXETIL
Ceftin Tablets 1407
Ceftin for Oral Suspension 1407

CEFUMAX (Italy)
CEFUROXIME SODIUM
Zinacef Injection 1631

CEFUR (Italy)
CEFUROXIME SODIUM
Zinacef Injection 1631

CEFURACET (Mexico)
CEFUROXIME AXETIL
Ceftin Tablets 1407
Ceftin for Oral Suspension 1407

CEFURAX (Germany)
CEFUROXIME AXETIL
Ceftin Tablets 1407
Ceftin for Oral Suspension 1407

CEFUREX (Italy)
CEFUROXIME SODIUM
Zinacef Injection 1631

CEFURIN (Italy)
CEFUROXIME SODIUM
Zinacef Injection 1631

CEFURO-PUREN (Germany)
CEFUROXIME AXETIL
Ceftin Tablets 1407
Ceftin for Oral Suspension 1407

CEFUROX (Argentina)
CEFUROXIME AXETIL
Ceftin Tablets 1407
Ceftin for Oral Suspension 1407

CEFUROX-REU (Germany)
CEFUROXIME SODIUM
Zinacef Injection 1631

CEFUROX-WOLFF (Germany)
CEFUROXIME AXETIL
Ceftin Tablets 1407
Ceftin for Oral Suspension 1407

CEFUZIME (United Arab Emirates)
CEFUROXIME AXETIL
Ceftin Tablets 1407
Ceftin for Oral Suspension 1407

CEFXITIN (Thailand)
CEFOXITIN SODIUM
Mefoxin Premixed Intravenous Solution . . . 2016
Mefoxin for Injection 2012

CEFZON (Japan)
CEFDINIR
Omnicef Capsules 511
Omnicef for Oral Suspension 511

CELAPRAM (Australia, New Zealand)
CITALOPRAM HYDROBROMIDE
Celexa Tablets 1176

CELCOX (Israel)
CELECOXIB
Celebrex Capsules 3134

CELEBRA (Brazil, Chile, Denmark, Finland, Israel)
CELECOXIB
Celebrex Capsules 3134

CELEBREX (Argentina, Australia, Austria, Belgium, Canada, Czech Republic, France, Germany, Greece, Hungary, Irish Republic, Italy, Malaysia, Mexico, New Zealand, Portugal, Russia, Singapore, South Africa, Spain, Switzerland, Thailand, The Netherlands, United Kingdom, Venezuela)
CELECOXIB
Celebrex Capsules 3134

CELEDOL (India)
CELECOXIB
Celebrex Capsules 3134

CELEFER (Spain)
MUPIROCIN
Bactroban Ointment 1395

CELEMAX (Argentina)
CELECOXIB
Celebrex Capsules 3134

CELEXA (Canada)
CITALOPRAM HYDROBROMIDE
Celexa Tablets 1176

CELIB (India)
CELECOXIB
Celebrex Capsules 3134

CELLCEPT (Argentina, Belgium, Brazil, Chile, Czech Republic, Denmark, Finland, France, Greece, Hong Kong, Hungary, Israel, Italy, Japan, Mexico, New Zealand, Norway, Singapore, South Africa, Spain, Sweden, Switzerland, Thailand, The Netherlands, Venezuela)
MYCOPHENOLATE MOFETIL
CellCept Capsules 2747
CellCept Oral Suspension 2747
CellCept Tablets 2747

CELLMUNE (India)
MYCOPHENOLATE MOFETIL
CellCept Capsules 2747
CellCept Oral Suspension 2747
CellCept Tablets 2747

CELLOIDS PC 73 (Australia)
POTASSIUM CHLORIDE
K-Dur Extended-Relase Tablets 3033
K-Lor Oral Solution 474
K-Tab Tablets 475

CELUNAF (Mexico)
NAPHAZOLINE HYDROCHLORIDE
Albalon Ophthalmic Solution . . . . ⊙218

CELVISTA (Thailand)
RALOXIFENE HYDROCHLORIDE
Evista Tablets 1763

CEMAX (Brazil)
CEFEPIME HYDROCHLORIDE
Maxipime for Injection 1105

CENLIDAC (Thailand)
SULINDAC
Clinoril Tablets 1924

CENPIDINE (Thailand)
TICLOPIDINE HYDROCHLORIDE
Ticlid Tablets 2810

CENTOCORT (Thailand)
TRIAMCINOLONE ACETONIDE
Azmacort Inhalation Aerosol 1726
Nasacort AQ Nasal Spray 2922

CENTRAPRYL (United Kingdom)
SELEGILINE HYDROCHLORIDE
Eldepryl Capsules 3208

CENTROMICINA (Argentina)
CLARITHROMYCIN
Biaxin Filmtab Tablets 402
Biaxin Granules 402

CEPAL (Greece)
FAMOTIDINE
Pepcid Injection 2040
Pepcid Injection Premixed 2040
Pepcid Tablets 2038
Pepcid for Oral Suspension 2038

CEPARIDIN (Spain)
TRAMADOL HYDROCHLORIDE
Ultram ER Tablets 2392

CEPAZINE (France)
CEFUROXIME AXETIL
Ceftin Tablets 1407
Ceftin for Oral Suspension 1407

CEPHORAL (Germany, Switzerland)
CEFIXIME
Suprax 1843

CEPHULAC (Canada)
LACTULOSE
Kristalose for Oral Solution 1034

CEPIM (Italy)
CEFEPIME HYDROCHLORIDE
Maxipime for Injection 1105

CEPIMEX (Italy)
CEFEPIME HYDROCHLORIDE
Maxipime for Injection 1105

CEPLON (Venezuela)
CAPTOPRIL
Captopril Tablets 2149

CEPODEM (India, South Africa)
CEFPODOXIME PROXETIL
Vantin Tablets and Oral Suspension 2645

CEPRAZOL (Chile)
ALBENDAZOLE
Albenza Tablets 1338

CEPRIMAX (Spain)
CIPROFLOXACIN HYDROCHLORIDE
Ciloxan Ophthalmic Ointment . . . . ⊙204, 559
Ciloxan Ophthalmic Solution . . . . ⊙206
Cipro Tablets 2977

CEPTAZ (Canada)
CEFTAZIDIME
Fortaz for Injection 1453

CERCON (Mexico)
PRAZIQUANTEL
Biltricide Tablets 2976

CEREBRAMED (Germany)
AMANTADINE HYDROCHLORIDE
Symmetrel Tablets 1135

CEREBROVASE (United Kingdom)
DIPYRIDAMOLE
Persantine Tablets 868

CERELLA (Germany)
ESTRADIOL
Climara Transdermal System 771
Estring Vaginal Ring 2635

CERELUC (Argentina)
PIOGLITAZONE HYDROCHLORIDE
Actos Tablets 3219

CEREX (Czech Republic)
CETIRIZINE HYDROCHLORIDE
Zyrtec Syrup 2594
Zyrtec Tablets 2594

CEREZYME (Australia, Austria, Canada, Czech Republic, Denmark, France, Germany, Hong Kong, Israel, Italy, Japan, New Zealand, Norway, Portugal, South Africa, Spain, Sweden, Switzerland, United Kingdom)
IMIGLUCERASE
Cerezyme for Injection 1270

CERINA (Switzerland)
ESTRADIOL
Climara Transdermal System 771
Estring Vaginal Ring 2635

CEROFENE (Greece)
CEFUROXIME SODIUM
Zinacef Injection 1631

CEROXIM (Hungary, South Africa)
CEFUROXIME AXETIL
Ceftin Tablets 1407
Ceftin for Oral Suspension 1407

CERTALAC (Belgium)
LACTULOSE
Kristalose for Oral Solution 1034

CERUXIM (Greece)
CEFUROXIME SODIUM
Zinacef Injection 1631

CERVIDIL (Australia, Canada, New Zealand)
DINOPROSTONE
Cervidil Vaginal Insert 1181

CERVIPRIME (India)
DINOPROSTONE
Cervidil Vaginal Insert 1181

CERVIPROST (Austria, Germany, Norway, Sweden, Switzerland, The Netherlands)
DINOPROSTONE
Cervidil Vaginal Insert 1181

CESOL (Chile, Germany, Mexico)
PRAZIQUANTEL
Biltricide Tablets 2976

CESPLON (Spain)
CAPTOPRIL
Captopril Tablets 2149

CESTOP (Chile)
CLOTRIMAZOLE
Lotrimin Cream 3039
Lotrimin Lotion 1% 3039
Lotrimin Topical Solution 1% 3039

CESTOX (Brazil)
PRAZIQUANTEL
Biltricide Tablets 2976

CETA SULFA (Mexico)
SULFACETAMIDE SODIUM
Klaron Lotion 10% 2909

CETALERG (Germany)
CETIRIZINE HYDROCHLORIDE
Zyrtec Syrup 2594
Zyrtec Tablets 2594

CETALLERG (Switzerland)
CETIRIZINE HYDROCHLORIDE
Zyrtec Syrup 2594
Zyrtec Tablets 2594

CETAMIDE (Canada)
SULFACETAMIDE SODIUM
Klaron Lotion 10% 2909

CETAMPRIL (Portugal)
ENALAPRIL MALEATE
Vasotec I.V. Injection 2103

CETAPRED (Belgium)
PREDNISOLONE ACETATE/SULFACETAMIDE SODIUM
Blephamide Ophthalmic Ointment 568
Blephamide Ophthalmic Suspension 569

CETASIL (Thailand)
SULFACETAMIDE SODIUM
Klaron Lotion 10% 2909

CETAXIM (Argentina)
CEFIXIME
Suprax 1843

CETAZ (Brazil)
CEFTAZIDIME
Fortaz for Injection 1453

CETAZIME (Hungary)
CEFTAZIDIME
Fortaz for Injection 1453

CETAZIN (Austria)
SULFACETAMIDE SODIUM
Klaron Lotion 10% 2909

CETCIP (India)
CETIRIZINE HYDROCHLORIDE
Zyrtec Syrup 2594

Zyrtec Tablets **2594**

CETERIFUG (Germany)
CETIRIZINE HYDROCHLORIDE
Zyrtec Syrup **2594**
Zyrtec Tablets **2594**

CETI (Germany)
CETIRIZINE HYDROCHLORIDE
Zyrtec Syrup **2594**
Zyrtec Tablets **2594**

CETIDERM (Germany)
CETIRIZINE HYDROCHLORIDE
Zyrtec Syrup **2594**
Zyrtec Tablets **2594**

CETIDURA (Germany)
CETIRIZINE HYDROCHLORIDE
Zyrtec Syrup **2594**
Zyrtec Tablets **2594**

CETIHEXAL (Brazil)
CETIRIZINE HYDROCHLORIDE
Zyrtec Syrup **2594**
Zyrtec Tablets **2594**

CETIHIS (Thailand)
CETIRIZINE HYDROCHLORIDE
Zyrtec Syrup **2594**
Zyrtec Tablets **2594**

CETIL (Germany)
CETIRIZINE HYDROCHLORIDE
Zyrtec Syrup **2594**
Zyrtec Tablets **2594**

CETILICH (Germany)
CETIRIZINE HYDROCHLORIDE
Zyrtec Syrup **2594**
Zyrtec Tablets **2594**

CETIRAM (Greece)
CETIRIZINE HYDROCHLORIDE
Zyrtec Syrup **2594**
Zyrtec Tablets **2594**

CETIRHEXAL (Austria)
CETIRIZINE HYDROCHLORIDE
Zyrtec Syrup **2594**
Zyrtec Tablets **2594**

CETIRIGAMMA (Germany)
CETIRIZINE HYDROCHLORIDE
Zyrtec Syrup **2594**
Zyrtec Tablets **2594**

CETIRISTAD (Austria)
CETIRIZINE HYDROCHLORIDE
Zyrtec Syrup **2594**
Zyrtec Tablets **2594**

CETIRLAN (Germany)
CETIRIZINE HYDROCHLORIDE
Zyrtec Syrup **2594**
Zyrtec Tablets **2594**

CETIROCOL (United Kingdom)
CETIRIZINE HYDROCHLORIDE
Zyrtec Syrup **2594**
Zyrtec Tablets **2594**

CETIZINE (Argentina)
CETIRIZINE HYDROCHLORIDE
Zyrtec Syrup **2594**
Zyrtec Tablets **2594**

CETRALON (United Arab Emirates)
CETIRIZINE HYDROCHLORIDE
Zyrtec Syrup **2594**
Zyrtec Tablets **2594**

CETRAPHYLLINE (France)
THEOPHYLLINE
Uniphyl Tablets **2710**

CETRAXAL PLUS (Spain)
CIPROFLOXACIN
Cipro Oral Suspension **2977**

CETRILER (Argentina)
CETIRIZINE HYDROCHLORIDE
Zyrtec Syrup **2594**
Zyrtec Tablets **2594**

CETRIMED (Thailand)
CETIRIZINE HYDROCHLORIDE
Zyrtec Syrup **2594**
Zyrtec Tablets **2594**

CETRINE (Russia, Singapore, Thailand, Venezuela)
CETIRIZINE HYDROCHLORIDE
Zyrtec Syrup **2594**
Zyrtec Tablets **2594**

CETRIWAL (India)
CETIRIZINE HYDROCHLORIDE
Zyrtec Syrup **2594**
Zyrtec Tablets **2594**

CETRIZET (India, Thailand)
CETIRIZINE HYDROCHLORIDE
Zyrtec Syrup **2594**
Zyrtec Tablets **2594**

CETRIZIN (Brazil, Thailand)
CETIRIZINE HYDROCHLORIDE
Zyrtec Syrup **2594**
Zyrtec Tablets **2594**

CETRON (Argentina)
ONDANSETRON
Zofran ODT Orally Disintegrating Tablets . . **1639**

CETYROL (Austria)
CETIRIZINE HYDROCHLORIDE
Zyrtec Syrup **2594**
Zyrtec Tablets **2594**

CEVAS (India)
CARVEDILOL
Coreg Tablets **1414**

CEXIDAL OTICO (Spain)
CIPROFLOXACIN
Cipro Oral Suspension **2977**

CEXIM (Hungary)
CEFUROXIME SODIUM
Zinacef Injection **1631**

CEZA (Thailand)
CETIRIZINE HYDROCHLORIDE
Zyrtec Syrup **2594**
Zyrtec Tablets **2594**

C-FLOX (Australia)
CIPROFLOXACIN HYDROCHLORIDE
Ciloxan Ophthalmic Ointment . . . . **⊙204, 559**
Ciloxan Ophthalmic Solution . . . . **⊙206**
Cipro Tablets **2977**

C-FLOXACIN (Thailand)
CIPROFLOXACIN HYDROCHLORIDE
Ciloxan Ophthalmic Ointment . . . . **⊙204, 559**
Ciloxan Ophthalmic Solution . . . . **⊙206**
Cipro Tablets **2977**

C-G (Argentina)
SULFACETAMIDE SODIUM
Klaron Lotion 10% **2909**

CHAMPS D-WORMS (Malaysia)
ALBENDAZOLE
Albenza Tablets **1338**

CHANTALINE (Spain)
THEOPHYLLINE
Uniphyl Tablets **2710**

CHEMISTS OWN CLOZOLE (Australia)
CLOTRIMAZOLE
Lotrimin Cream **3039**
Lotrimin Lotion 1% **3039**
Lotrimin Topical Solution 1% **3039**

CHEMISTS OWN PERIOD PAIN TABLETS (Australia)
NAPROXEN SODIUM
Anaprox DS Tablets **2761**
Anaprox Tablets **2761**

CHEMYDUR (United Kingdom)
ISOSORBIDE MONONITRATE
Imdur Tablets **3018**

CHEXID (India)
LANSOPRAZOLE
Prevacid Delayed-Release Capsules **3271**

CHIBRETICO (Portugal)
AMILORIDE HYDROCHLORIDE/HYDROCHLOROTHIAZIDE
Moduretic Tablets **2028**

CHIBRO-PROSCAR (France)
FINASTERIDE
Propecia Tablets **2060**
Proscar Tablets **2067**

CHIBRO-TIMOPTOL (Germany)
TIMOLOL MALEATE
Blocadren Tablets **1916**
Timoptic Sterile Ophthalmic Solution **2088**
Timoptic in Ocudose **2091**
Timoptic-XE Sterile Ophthalmic Gel Forming Solution **2092**

CHIBROXIN (Argentina, Brazil, Chile, Germany, Hong Kong, Israel, Malaysia, Singapore, Spain, Venezuela)
NORFLOXACIN
Noroxin Tablets **2032**

CHIBROXINE (France)
NORFLOXACIN
Noroxin Tablets **2032**

CHIBROXOL (Belgium, Portugal, Switzerland, The Netherlands)
NORFLOXACIN
Noroxin Tablets **2032**

CHIMAX (United Kingdom)
FLUTAMIDE
Eulexin Capsules **3009**

CHINGAZOL (Thailand)
CLOTRIMAZOLE
Lotrimin Cream **3039**
Lotrimin Lotion 1% **3039**
Lotrimin Topical Solution 1% **3039**

CHINOPAMIL (Hungary)
VERAPAMIL HYDROCHLORIDE
Covera-HS Tablets **3139**
Verelan PM Extended-Release Capsules, Controlled-Onset **3106**

CHIRON IL-2 (South Africa)
ALDESLEUKIN
Proleukin for Injection **2266**

CHLORAMINOPHENE (Monaco)
CHLORAMBUCIL
Leukeran Tablets **1504**

CHLOROPOTASSURIL (Belgium)
POTASSIUM CHLORIDE
K-Dur Extended-Relase Tablets **3033**
K-Lor Oral Solution **474**
K-Tab Tablets **475**

CHLORVESCENT (New Zealand)
POTASSIUM CHLORIDE
K-Dur Extended-Relase Tablets **3033**
K-Lor Oral Solution **474**
K-Tab Tablets **475**

CHLORZIDE (Singapore)
CHLOROTHIAZIDE
Diuril Oral Suspension **1954**

CHLOTRIDE (Australia, Denmark, The Netherlands)
CHLOROTHIAZIDE
Diuril Oral Suspension **1954**

CHRISTATIN (Greece)
SIMVASTATIN
Zocor Tablets **2105**

CHRONADALATE (France)
NIFEDIPINE
Adalat CC Tablets **2964**

CHRONOPHYLLIN (South Africa)
THEOPHYLLINE
Uniphyl Tablets **2710**

CHRONOVERA (Austria, Canada, The Netherlands)
VERAPAMIL HYDROCHLORIDE
Covera-HS Tablets **3139**
Verelan PM Extended-Release Capsules, Controlled-Onset **3106**

CHRONULAC (Canada)
LACTULOSE
Kristalose for Oral Solution **1034**

CIAZIL (Australia)
CITALOPRAM HYDROBROMIDE
Celexa Tablets **1176**

CIBACE (South Africa)
BENAZEPRIL HYDROCHLORIDE
Lotensin Tablets **2243**

CIBACEN (Austria, Belgium, Denmark, Germany, Greece, Irish Republic, Israel, Italy, New Zealand, Spain, Switzerland, The Netherlands)
BENAZEPRIL HYDROCHLORIDE
Lotensin Tablets **2243**

CIBACENE (France)
BENAZEPRIL HYDROCHLORIDE
Lotensin Tablets **2243**

CIBADREX (Austria, Denmark, France, Germany, Greece, Italy, South Africa, Spain, Sweden, Switzerland, The Netherlands)
BENAZEPRIL HYDROCHLORIDE/HYDROCHLOROTHIAZIDE
Lotensin HCT Tablets **2246**

CIBRAL (United Kingdom)
ISOSORBIDE MONONITRATE
Imdur Tablets **3018**

CIBRAMICINA (Brazil)
AMOXICILLIN
Amoxil Pediatric Drops for Oral Suspension **1343**
Amoxil Tablets **1343**

CIBROGAN (Argentina)
CILOSTAZOL
Pletal Tablets **2455**

CICLOTAL (Mexico, Russia)
MEDROXYPROGESTERONE ACETATE
Depo-Medrol Single-Dose Vial **2619**

CICLOTRAN (Argentina)
RALOXIFENE HYDROCHLORIDE
Evista Tablets **1763**

CICLOX (Argentina)
CLONAZEPAM
Klonopin Tablets **2778**

CIDANAMOX (Spain)
AMOXICILLIN
Amoxil Pediatric Drops for Oral Suspension **1343**
Amoxil Tablets **1343**

CIDOMYCIN (Australia, Canada, Irish Republic, Israel, South Africa)
GENTAMICIN SULFATE
Garamycin Injectable **3014**

CIDRON (Denmark, Finland, Sweden)
CETIRIZINE HYDROCHLORIDE
Zyrtec Syrup **2594**
Zyrtec Tablets **2594**

CIDROPS (Greece)
CIPROFLOXACIN
Cipro Oral Suspension **2977**

CIFIN (Denmark)
CIPROFLOXACIN HYDROCHLORIDE
Ciloxan Ophthalmic Ointment . . . . **⊙204, 559**
Ciloxan Ophthalmic Solution . . . . **⊙206**
Cipro Tablets **2977**

CIFLAN (Portugal)
CIPROFLOXACIN HYDROCHLORIDE
Ciloxan Ophthalmic Ointment . . . . **⊙204, 559**
Ciloxan Ophthalmic Solution . . . . **⊙206**
Cipro Tablets **2977**

CIFLOC (South Africa)
CIPROFLOXACIN
Cipro Oral Suspension **2977**

CIFLOCINA (Brazil)
CIPROFLOXACIN
Cipro Oral Suspension **2977**

CIFLOLAN (Thailand)
CIPROFLOXACIN
Cipro Oral Suspension **2977**

CIFLOX (Austria, Brazil, Italy, Venezuela)
CIPROFLOXACIN HYDROCHLORIDE
Ciloxan Ophthalmic Ointment . . . . **⊙204, 559**
Ciloxan Ophthalmic Solution . . . . **⊙206**
Cipro Tablets **2977**

CIFLOXAN (Brazil)
CIPROFLOXACIN
Cipro Oral Suspension **2977**

CIFLOXIN (Chile)
CIPROFLOXACIN
Cipro Oral Suspension **2977**

CIFLOXINAL (Czech Republic, Russia)
CIPROFLOXACIN HYDROCHLORIDE
Ciloxan Ophthalmic Ointment . . . . **⊙204, 559**
Ciloxan Ophthalmic Solution . . . . **⊙206**
Cipro Tablets **2977**

CIFLOXTRON (Brazil)
CIPROFLOXACIN HYDROCHLORIDE
Ciloxan Ophthalmic Ointment . . . . **⊙204, 559**
Ciloxan Ophthalmic Solution . . . . **⊙206**
Cipro Tablets **2977**

CIFRAN (Czech Republic, Hungary, Malaysia, South Africa)
CIPROFLOXACIN HYDROCHLORIDE
Ciloxan Ophthalmic Ointment . . . . **⊙204, 559**
Ciloxan Ophthalmic Solution . . . . **⊙206**
Cipro Tablets **2977**

CIFRANTIL (Brazil)
ERYTHROMYCIN
Ery-Tab Tablets 449
Erythromycin Base Filmtab Tablets 455
Erythromycin Delayed-Release Capsules, USP 457
PCE Dispertab Tablets 515

CIL (Germany)
FENOFIBRATE
Tricor Tablets 527

CILAB (Thailand)
CIPROFLOXACIN
Cipro Oral Suspension 2977

CILAMIN (India)
PENICILLAMINE
Cuprimine Capsules 1947

CILATRON (Argentina)
ISOSORBIDE MONONITRATE
Imdur Tablets 3018

CILEX (Germany)
CITALOPRAM HYDROBROMIDE
Celexa Tablets 1176

CILIFT (South Africa)
CITALOPRAM HYDROBROMIDE
Celexa Tablets 1176

CILODEX (Chile, Mexico)
CIPROFLOXACIN HYDROCHLORIDE
Ciloxan Ophthalmic Ointment . . . . ⊙204, 559
Ciloxan Ophthalmic Solution . . . . ⊙206
Cipro Tablets 2977

CILOQUIN (Australia)
CIPROFLOXACIN HYDROCHLORIDE
Ciloxan Ophthalmic Ointment . . . . ⊙204, 559
Ciloxan Ophthalmic Solution . . . . ⊙206
Cipro Tablets 2977

CILOSTAL (Argentina)
CILOSTAZOL
Pletal Tablets 2455

CILOVAS (Argentina)
CILOSTAZOL
Pletal Tablets 2455

CILOX (Norway)
CIPROFLOXACIN HYDROCHLORIDE
Ciloxan Ophthalmic Ointment . . . . ⊙204, 559
Ciloxan Ophthalmic Solution . . . . ⊙206
Cipro Tablets 2977

CILOXACIN (Chile)
CIPROFLOXACIN HYDROCHLORIDE
Ciloxan Ophthalmic Ointment . . . . ⊙204, 559
Ciloxan Ophthalmic Solution . . . . ⊙206
Cipro Tablets 2977

CILOXADEX (Argentina)
CIPROFLOXACIN HYDROCHLORIDE
Ciloxan Ophthalmic Ointment . . . . ⊙204, 559
Ciloxan Ophthalmic Solution . . . . ⊙206
Cipro Tablets 2977

CILOXAN (Argentina, Australia, Austria, Belgium, Brazil, Canada, Czech Republic, Denmark, France, Germany, Greece, Hong Kong, Hungary, Israel, Malaysia, Mexico, New Zealand, Russia, Singapore, South Africa, Sweden, Switzerland, Thailand, The Netherlands, United Kingdom, Venezuela)
CIPROFLOXACIN HYDROCHLORIDE
Ciloxan Ophthalmic Ointment . . . . ⊙204, 559
Ciloxan Ophthalmic Solution . . . . ⊙206
Cipro Tablets 2977

CIMAL (Chile)
CITALOPRAM HYDROBROMIDE
Celexa Tablets 1176

CIMECARD (Brazil)
DIGOXIN
Lanoxicaps Capsules 1490
Lanoxin Injection 1494
Lanoxin Injection Pediatric 1497
Lanoxin Tablets 1500

CIMOGAL (Mexico)
CIPROFLOXACIN HYDROCHLORIDE
Ciloxan Ophthalmic Ointment . . . . ⊙204, 559
Ciloxan Ophthalmic Solution . . . . ⊙206
Cipro Tablets 2977

CINABEL (Mexico)
CLOTRIMAZOLE
Lotrimin Cream 3039
Lotrimin Lotion 1% 3039
Lotrimin Topical Solution 1% 3039

CINCO-FU (Argentina)
FLUOROURACIL
Efudex Topical Cream 3363
Efudex Topical Solutions 3363

CINCORDIL (Brazil)
ISOSORBIDE MONONITRATE
Imdur Tablets 3018

CINFLOXINE (Thailand)
CIPROFLOXACIN HYDROCHLORIDE
Ciloxan Ophthalmic Ointment . . . . ⊙204, 559
Ciloxan Ophthalmic Solution . . . . ⊙206
Cipro Tablets 2977

CINKEF-U (Portugal)
FLUOROURACIL
Efudex Topical Cream 3363
Efudex Topical Solutions 3363

CINOFLAX (Brazil)
CIPROFLOXACIN HYDROCHLORIDE
Ciloxan Ophthalmic Ointment . . . . ⊙204, 559
Ciloxan Ophthalmic Solution . . . . ⊙206
Cipro Tablets 2977

CINTSU (Malaysia)
VERAPAMIL HYDROCHLORIDE
Covera-HS Tablets 3139
Verelan PM Extended-Release Capsules, Controlled-Onset 3106

CIP ECO (Switzerland)
CIPROFLOXACIN HYDROCHLORIDE
Ciloxan Ophthalmic Ointment . . . . ⊙204, 559
Ciloxan Ophthalmic Solution . . . . ⊙206
Cipro Tablets 2977

CIPALAT (South Africa)
NIFEDIPINE
Adalat CC Tablets 2964

CIPCORLIN (India)
HYDROCORTISONE
Hydrocortone Tablets 1989

CIPFLOCIN (Thailand)
CIPROFLOXACIN
Cipro Oral Suspension 2977

CIPFLOX (New Zealand)
CIPROFLOXACIN
Cipro Oral Suspension 2977

CIPGEN (India)
CIPROFLOXACIN
Cipro Oral Suspension 2977

CIPGEN TZ (India)
CIPROFLOXACIN
Cipro Oral Suspension 2977

CIPHIN (Czech Republic)
CIPROFLOXACIN
Cipro Oral Suspension 2977

CIPIDE (Hong Kong)
CIPROFLOXACIN HYDROCHLORIDE
Ciloxan Ophthalmic Ointment . . . . ⊙204, 559
Ciloxan Ophthalmic Solution . . . . ⊙206
Cipro Tablets 2977

CIPLACEF (India)
CEFTRIAXONE SODIUM
Rocephin Injectable Vials, ADD-Vantage, Galaxy, Bulk 2800

CIPLAR (India)
PROPRANOLOL HYDROCHLORIDE
Inderal LA Long-Acting Capsules 3429

CIPLAR-H (India)
PROPRANOLOL HYDROCHLORIDE
Inderal LA Long-Acting Capsules 3429

CIPLATEC (South Africa)
ENALAPRIL MALEATE
Vasotec I.V. Injection 2103

CIPLOX (Israel, Portugal)
CIPROFLOXACIN
Cipro Oral Suspension 2977

CIPLOX D (India)
CIPROFLOXACIN
Cipro Oral Suspension 2977

CIPLOX TZ (India)
CIPROFLOXACIN
Cipro Oral Suspension 2977

CIPLOXX (South Africa)
CIPROFLOXACIN HYDROCHLORIDE
Ciloxan Ophthalmic Ointment . . . . ⊙204, 559
Ciloxan Ophthalmic Solution . . . . ⊙206
Cipro Tablets 2977

CIPOBACTER (Spain)
CIPROFLOXACIN HYDROCHLORIDE
Ciloxan Ophthalmic Ointment . . . . ⊙204, 559
Ciloxan Ophthalmic Solution . . . . ⊙206
Cipro Tablets 2977

CIPOFIX (South Africa)
CEFUROXIME SODIUM
Zinacef Injection 1631

CIPRAGER (Irish Republic)
CITALOPRAM HYDROBROMIDE
Celexa Tablets 1176

CIPRAIN (Mexico)
CIPROFLOXACIN
Cipro Oral Suspension 2977

CIPRAM (Hong Kong, Malaysia, Singapore, Thailand)
CITALOPRAM HYDROBROMIDE
Celexa Tablets 1176

CIPRAMIL (Australia, Chile, Germany, Israel, New Zealand, Norway, Russia, South Africa)
CITALOPRAM HYDROBROMIDE
Celexa Tablets 1176

CIPRAPINE (Irish Republic, The Netherlands)
CITALOPRAM HYDROBROMIDE
Celexa Tablets 1176

CIPRENIT OTICO (Spain)
CIPROFLOXACIN HYDROCHLORIDE
Ciloxan Ophthalmic Ointment . . . . ⊙204, 559
Ciloxan Ophthalmic Solution . . . . ⊙206
Cipro Tablets 2977

CIPREX (Brazil)
CIPROFLOXACIN HYDROCHLORIDE
Ciloxan Ophthalmic Ointment . . . . ⊙204, 559
Ciloxan Ophthalmic Solution . . . . ⊙206
Cipro Tablets 2977

CIPRIL (India)
LISINOPRIL
Prinivil Tablets 2052

CIPRIL-H (India)
LISINOPRIL
Prinivil Tablets 2052

CIPRIVAX (Venezuela)
CIPROFLOXACIN
Cipro Oral Suspension 2977

CIPRO HC (Argentina, Brazil, Hong Kong)
CIPROFLOXACIN HYDROCHLORIDE
Ciloxan Ophthalmic Ointment . . . . ⊙204, 559
Ciloxan Ophthalmic Solution . . . . ⊙206
Cipro Tablets 2977

CIPROANT (Brazil)
CIPROFLOXACIN
Cipro Oral Suspension 2977

CIPROBAY (Czech Republic, Greece, Hungary)
CIPROFLOXACIN
Cipro Oral Suspension 2977

CIPROBAY HC (Singapore, South Africa)
CIPROFLOXACIN
Cipro Oral Suspension 2977

CIPROBAY HC OTIC (Czech Republic)
CIPROFLOXACIN HYDROCHLORIDE
Ciloxan Ophthalmic Ointment . . . . ⊙204, 559
Ciloxan Ophthalmic Solution . . . . ⊙206
Cipro Tablets 2977

CIPROBETA (Germany)
CIPROFLOXACIN HYDROCHLORIDE
Ciloxan Ophthalmic Ointment . . . . ⊙204, 559
Ciloxan Ophthalmic Solution . . . . ⊙206
Cipro Tablets 2977

CIPROBID (Czech Republic, Thailand)
CIPROFLOXACIN HYDROCHLORIDE
Ciloxan Ophthalmic Ointment . . . . ⊙204, 559
Ciloxan Ophthalmic Solution . . . . ⊙206
Cipro Tablets 2977

CIPROBIOT (Brazil)
CIPROFLOXACIN HYDROCHLORIDE
Ciloxan Ophthalmic Ointment . . . . ⊙204, 559
Ciloxan Ophthalmic Solution . . . . ⊙206
Cipro Tablets 2977

CIPROBIOTIC (Mexico)
CIPROFLOXACIN HYDROCHLORIDE
Ciloxan Ophthalmic Ointment . . . . ⊙204, 559
Ciloxan Ophthalmic Solution . . . . ⊙206
Cipro Tablets 2977

CIPRO-CENT (India)
CIPROFLOXACIN HYDROCHLORIDE
Ciloxan Ophthalmic Ointment . . . . ⊙204, 559
Ciloxan Ophthalmic Solution . . . . ⊙206
Cipro Tablets 2977

CIPROCEP (Thailand)
CIPROFLOXACIN
Cipro Oral Suspension 2977

CIPROCIN (Brazil)
CIPROFLOXACIN
Cipro Oral Suspension 2977

CIPROCINA (Brazil)
CIPROFLOXACIN
Cipro Oral Suspension 2977

CIPROCTAL (Spain)
CIPROFLOXACIN HYDROCHLORIDE
Ciloxan Ophthalmic Ointment . . . . ⊙204, 559
Ciloxan Ophthalmic Solution . . . . ⊙206
Cipro Tablets 2977

CIPRODEX (Israel)
CIPROFLOXACIN HYDROCHLORIDE
Ciloxan Ophthalmic Ointment . . . . ⊙204, 559
Ciloxan Ophthalmic Solution . . . . ⊙206
Cipro Tablets 2977

CIPRODINE (Brazil)
CIPROFLOXACIN HYDROCHLORIDE
Ciloxan Ophthalmic Ointment . . . . ⊙204, 559
Ciloxan Ophthalmic Solution . . . . ⊙206
Cipro Tablets 2977

CIPRODURA (Germany)
CIPROFLOXACIN HYDROCHLORIDE
Ciloxan Ophthalmic Ointment . . . . ⊙204, 559
Ciloxan Ophthalmic Solution . . . . ⊙206
Cipro Tablets 2977

CIPROFAL (Greece)
CIPROFLOXACIN
Cipro Oral Suspension 2977

CIPROFAR (Brazil)
CIPROFLOXACIN HYDROCHLORIDE
Ciloxan Ophthalmic Ointment . . . . ⊙204, 559
Ciloxan Ophthalmic Solution . . . . ⊙206
Cipro Tablets 2977

CIPROFIN (Thailand)
CIPROFLOXACIN
Cipro Oral Suspension 2977

CIPROFLONAX (Brazil)
CIPROFLOXACIN
Cipro Oral Suspension 2977

CIPROFLOX (Brazil, Germany, Switzerland, Venezuela)
CIPROFLOXACIN
Cipro Oral Suspension 2977

CIPROFLOXIL (Brazil)
CIPROFLOXACIN
Cipro Oral Suspension 2977

CIPROFUR (Mexico)
CIPROFLOXACIN HYDROCHLORIDE
Ciloxan Ophthalmic Ointment . . . . ⊙204, 559
Ciloxan Ophthalmic Solution . . . . ⊙206
Cipro Tablets 2977

CIPROGAMMA (Germany)
CIPROFLOXACIN HYDROCHLORIDE
Ciloxan Ophthalmic Ointment . . . . ⊙204, 559
Ciloxan Ophthalmic Solution . . . . ⊙206
Cipro Tablets 2977

CIPROGEN (South Africa, Thailand)
CIPROFLOXACIN
Cipro Oral Suspension 2977

CIPROGIS (Israel)
CIPROFLOXACIN
Cipro Oral Suspension 2977

CIPROGLEN (Thailand)
CIPROFLOXACIN
Cipro Oral Suspension 2977

CIPROHEXAL (Mexico)
CIPROFLOXACIN HYDROCHLORIDE
Ciloxan Ophthalmic Ointment . . . . ⊙204, 559

Ciloxan Ophthalmic Solution . . . . ⊙206
Cipro Tablets 2977

CIPRO-HEXAL (South Africa)
CIPROFLOXACIN
Cipro Oral Suspension 2977

CIPROK (Spain)
CIPROFLOXACIN HYDROCHLORIDE
Ciloxan Ophthalmic Ointment . . . . ⊙204, 559
Ciloxan Ophthalmic Solution . . . . ⊙206
Cipro Tablets 2977

CIPROL (Australia)
CIPROFLOXACIN HYDROCHLORIDE
Ciloxan Ophthalmic Ointment . . . . ⊙204, 559
Ciloxan Ophthalmic Solution . . . . ⊙206
Cipro Tablets 2977

CIPROLET (Russia, Singapore, Venezuela)
CIPROFLOXACIN HYDROCHLORIDE
Ciloxan Ophthalmic Ointment . . . . ⊙204, 559
Ciloxan Ophthalmic Solution . . . . ⊙206
Cipro Tablets 2977

CIPRO-LICH (Germany)
CIPROFLOXACIN HYDROCHLORIDE
Ciloxan Ophthalmic Ointment . . . . ⊙204, 559
Ciloxan Ophthalmic Solution . . . . ⊙206
Cipro Tablets 2977

CIPROLONE (Russia)
CIPROFLOXACIN HYDROCHLORIDE
Ciloxan Ophthalmic Ointment . . . . ⊙204, 559
Ciloxan Ophthalmic Solution . . . . ⊙206
Cipro Tablets 2977

CIPROMED (Austria, Finland, Russia)
CIPROFLOXACIN HYDROCHLORIDE
Ciloxan Ophthalmic Ointment . . . . ⊙204, 559
Ciloxan Ophthalmic Solution . . . . ⊙206
Cipro Tablets 2977

CIPRO-MED (Switzerland)
CIPROFLOXACIN HYDROCHLORIDE
Ciloxan Ophthalmic Ointment . . . . ⊙204, 559
Ciloxan Ophthalmic Solution . . . . ⊙206
Cipro Tablets 2977

CIPROMIZIN (Brazil)
CIPROFLOXACIN
Cipro Oral Suspension 2977

CIPROMYCIN (Greece)
CIPROFLOXACIN HYDROCHLORIDE
Ciloxan Ophthalmic Ointment . . . . ⊙204, 559
Ciloxan Ophthalmic Solution . . . . ⊙206
Cipro Tablets 2977

CIPRONAL (Brazil)
CIPROFLOXACIN HYDROCHLORIDE
Ciloxan Ophthalmic Ointment . . . . ⊙204, 559
Ciloxan Ophthalmic Solution . . . . ⊙206
Cipro Tablets 2977

CIPRONOM (Brazil)
CIPROFLOXACIN
Cipro Oral Suspension 2977

CIPRO-OTICO (Argentina)
CIPROFLOXACIN HYDROCHLORIDE
Ciloxan Ophthalmic Ointment . . . . ⊙204, 559
Ciloxan Ophthalmic Solution . . . . ⊙206
Cipro Tablets 2977

CIPROQUINOL (Portugal)
CIPROFLOXACIN
Cipro Oral Suspension 2977

CIPRO-SAAR (Germany)
CIPROFLOXACIN HYDROCHLORIDE
Ciloxan Ophthalmic Ointment . . . . ⊙204, 559
Ciloxan Ophthalmic Solution . . . . ⊙206
Cipro Tablets 2977

CIPROSER (Mexico)
CIPROFLOXACIN
Cipro Oral Suspension 2977

CIPROSPES (Greece)
CIPROFLOXACIN HYDROCHLORIDE
Ciloxan Ophthalmic Ointment . . . . ⊙204, 559
Ciloxan Ophthalmic Solution . . . . ⊙206
Cipro Tablets 2977

CIPROSTAD (Austria)
CIPROFLOXACIN HYDROCHLORIDE
Ciloxan Ophthalmic Ointment . . . . ⊙204, 559
Ciloxan Ophthalmic Solution . . . . ⊙206
Cipro Tablets 2977

CIPROSUN (Russia, Thailand)
CIPROFLOXACIN
Cipro Oral Suspension 2977

CIPROVAL (Chile)
CIPROFLOXACIN
Cipro Oral Suspension 2977

CIPROWIN (India)
CIPROFLOXACIN
Cipro Oral Suspension 2977

CIPRO-WOLFF (Germany)
CIPROFLOXACIN HYDROCHLORIDE
Ciloxan Ophthalmic Ointment . . . . ⊙204, 559
Ciloxan Ophthalmic Solution . . . . ⊙206
Cipro Tablets 2977

CIPROX (Germany)
CIPROFLOXACIN HYDROCHLORIDE
Ciloxan Ophthalmic Ointment . . . . ⊙204, 559
Ciloxan Ophthalmic Solution . . . . ⊙206
Cipro Tablets 2977

CIPROXAN (Brazil, Thailand)
CIPROFLOXACIN
Cipro Oral Suspension 2977

CIPROXEN (Brazil)
CIPROFLOXACIN
Cipro Oral Suspension 2977

CIPROXIL (Brazil)
CIPROFLOXACIN HYDROCHLORIDE
Ciloxan Ophthalmic Ointment . . . . ⊙204, 559
Ciloxan Ophthalmic Solution . . . . ⊙206
Cipro Tablets 2977

CIPROXIN (Israel)
CIPROFLOXACIN
Cipro Oral Suspension 2977

CIPROXIN HC (Australia, Israel, New Zealand, Switzerland)
CIPROFLOXACIN HYDROCHLORIDE
Ciloxan Ophthalmic Ointment . . . . ⊙204, 559
Ciloxan Ophthalmic Solution . . . . ⊙206
Cipro Tablets 2977

CIPROXINA (Portugal, Venezuela)
CIPROFLOXACIN HYDROCHLORIDE
Ciloxan Ophthalmic Ointment . . . . ⊙204, 559
Ciloxan Ophthalmic Solution . . . . ⊙206
Cipro Tablets 2977

CIPROXINA HC (Mexico)
CIPROFLOXACIN
Cipro Oral Suspension 2977

CIPROXINA SIMPLE (Spain)
CIPROFLOXACIN HYDROCHLORIDE
Ciloxan Ophthalmic Ointment . . . . ⊙204, 559
Ciloxan Ophthalmic Solution . . . . ⊙206
Cipro Tablets 2977

CIPROXINE (Belgium)
CIPROFLOXACIN
Cipro Oral Suspension 2977

CIPROXINO (Chile)
CIPROFLOXACIN
Cipro Oral Suspension 2977

CIPROXYL (Hong Kong, Thailand)
CIPROFLOXACIN
Cipro Oral Suspension 2977

CIPTINI (India)
CIPROFLOXACIN
Cipro Oral Suspension 2977

CIQFADIN (Mexico)
CIPROFLOXACIN
Cipro Oral Suspension 2977

CIRCUVIT (Argentina)
WARFARIN SODIUM
Coumadin Tablets 898
Coumadin for Injection 898

CIRFLOX-G (Argentina)
CIPROFLOXACIN
Cipro Oral Suspension 2977

CIRIAX (Argentina)
CIPROFLOXACIN
Cipro Oral Suspension 2977

CIRIAX OTIC (Argentina)
CIPROFLOXACIN HYDROCHLORIDE
Ciloxan Ophthalmic Ointment . . . . ⊙204, 559
Ciloxan Ophthalmic Solution . . . . ⊙206
Cipro Tablets 2977

CIRIZINE (Greece)
CETIRIZINE HYDROCHLORIDE
Zyrtec Syrup 2594
Zyrtec Tablets 2594

CIROK (Singapore)
CIPROFLOXACIN HYDROCHLORIDE
Ciloxan Ophthalmic Ointment . . . . ⊙204, 559
Ciloxan Ophthalmic Solution . . . . ⊙206
Cipro Tablets 2977

CIROXIN (Singapore)
CIPROFLOXACIN HYDROCHLORIDE
Ciloxan Ophthalmic Ointment . . . . ⊙204, 559
Ciloxan Ophthalmic Solution . . . . ⊙206
Cipro Tablets 2977

CISCUTAN (Austria)
ISOTRETINOIN
Accutane Capsules 2731

CISDAY (Germany)
NIFEDIPINE
Adalat CC Tablets 2964

CI-SONS (Mexico)
CIPROFLOXACIN HYDROCHLORIDE
Ciloxan Ophthalmic Ointment . . . . ⊙204, 559
Ciloxan Ophthalmic Solution . . . . ⊙206
Cipro Tablets 2977

CISTAMINE (Thailand)
CETIRIZINE HYDROCHLORIDE
Zyrtec Syrup 2594
Zyrtec Tablets 2594

CISTICID (Brazil, Chile, Mexico, Venezuela)
PRAZIQUANTEL
Biltricide Tablets 2976

CITADEP (India)
CITALOPRAM HYDROBROMIDE
Celexa Tablets 1176

CITADUR (Denmark)
CITALOPRAM HYDROBROMIDE
Celexa Tablets 1176

CITADURA (Germany)
CITALOPRAM HYDROBROMIDE
Celexa Tablets 1176

CITAHAM (Denmark)
CITALOPRAM HYDROBROMIDE
Celexa Tablets 1176

CITALEC (Czech Republic)
CITALOPRAM HYDROBROMIDE
Celexa Tablets 1176

CITALHEXAL (Austria)
CITALOPRAM HYDROBROMIDE
Celexa Tablets 1176

CITALON (Austria)
CITALOPRAM HYDROBROMIDE
Celexa Tablets 1176

CITARCANA (Austria)
CITALOPRAM HYDROBROMIDE
Celexa Tablets 1176

CITAVIE (Sweden)
CITALOPRAM HYDROBROMIDE
Celexa Tablets 1176

CITIDOL (Italy)
DIFLUNISAL
Dolobid Tablets 1955

CITIFLUX (Italy)
FLUNISOLIDE
Aerobid Inhaler System 1171
Aerobid-M Inhaler System 1171

CITILAT (Italy)
NIFEDIPINE
Adalat CC Tablets 2964

CITIREUMA (Italy)
SULINDAC
Clinoril Tablets 1924

CITIZEM (Italy)
DILTIAZEM HYDROCHLORIDE
Cardizem LA Extended Release Tablets . . . 1728
Tiazac Capsules 1201

CITIZOL (India)
CIPROFLOXACIN
Cipro Oral Suspension 2977

CITOGEL (Austria, Italy)
SUCRALFATE
Carafate Suspension 701
Carafate Tablets 701

CITOR (Austria)
CITALOPRAM HYDROBROMIDE
Celexa Tablets 1176

CITRIHEXAL (Australia)
CALCITRIOL
Calcijex Injection 411
Rocaltrol Capsules 2798
Rocaltrol Oral Solution 2798

CITROL (Irish Republic)
CITALOPRAM HYDROBROMIDE
Celexa Tablets 1176

CITROVENOT (Greece)
CIPROFLOXACIN HYDROCHLORIDE
Ciloxan Ophthalmic Ointment . . . . ⊙204, 559
Ciloxan Ophthalmic Solution . . . . ⊙206
Cipro Tablets 2977

CIVICOR (New Zealand, Singapore)
VERAPAMIL HYDROCHLORIDE
Covera-HS Tablets 3139
Verelan PM Extended-Release Capsules, Controlled-Onset 3106

CIZETOL (India)
CARBAMAZEPINE
Carbatrol Capsules 3171
Tegretol Chewable Tablets 2295
Tegretol Suspension 2295
Tegretol Tablets 2295
Tegretol-XR Tablets 2295

CLACIN (Hong Kong)
CLARITHROMYCIN
Biaxin Filmtab Tablets 402
Biaxin Granules 402

CLACINA (Portugal)
CLARITHROMYCIN
Biaxin Filmtab Tablets 402
Biaxin Granules 402

CLAMENTIN (South Africa)
AMOXICILLIN
Amoxil Pediatric Drops for Oral Suspension 1343
Amoxil Tablets 1343

CLAMICIN (Brazil)
CLARITHROMYCIN
Biaxin Filmtab Tablets 402
Biaxin Granules 402

CLAMYCIN (United Arab Emirates)
CLARITHROMYCIN
Biaxin Filmtab Tablets 402
Biaxin Granules 402

CLARAC (Australia)
CLARITHROMYCIN
Biaxin Filmtab Tablets 402
Biaxin Granules 402

CLARASOL (Venezuela)
NAPHAZOLINE HYDROCHLORIDE
Albalon Ophthalmic Solution . . . . ⊙218

CLARBACT (India)
CLARITHROMYCIN
Biaxin Filmtab Tablets 402
Biaxin Granules 402

CLARELUX (United Kingdom)
CLOBETASOL PROPIONATE
Temovate Cream 2668
Temovate E Emollient 2671
Temovate Gel 2669
Temovate Ointment 2668
Temovate Scalp Application 2670

CLARIBID (India)
CLARITHROMYCIN
Biaxin Filmtab Tablets 402
Biaxin Granules 402

CLARIBIOTIC (Argentina)
CLARITHROMYCIN
Biaxin Filmtab Tablets 402
Biaxin Granules 402

CLARICINA (Brazil)
CLARITHROMYCIN
Biaxin Filmtab Tablets 402
Biaxin Granules 402

CLARICIP (India)
CLARITHROMYCIN
Biaxin Filmtab Tablets 402
Biaxin Granules 402

CLARIMAC (India)
CLARITHROMYCIN
Biaxin Filmtab Tablets 402
Biaxin Granules 402

CLARIMAX (Brazil, Chile)
CLARITHROMYCIN
Biaxin Filmtab Tablets 402
Biaxin Granules 402

CLARIMID (Argentina)
CLARITHROMYCIN
Biaxin Filmtab Tablets 402

Biaxin Granules 402

CLARIMIR (Chile)
NAPHAZOLINE HYDROCHLORIDE
Albalon Ophthalmic Solution . . . . . . ⊙218

CLARINEO (Brazil)
CLARITHROMYCIN
Biaxin Filmtab Tablets 402
Biaxin Granules 402

CLARIPEN (Greece, Singapore)
CLARITHROMYCIN
Biaxin Filmtab Tablets 402
Biaxin Granules 402

CLARITAB (Brazil)
CLARITHROMYCIN
Biaxin Filmtab Tablets 402
Biaxin Granules 402

CLARITH (Japan, Thailand)
CLARITHROMYCIN
Biaxin Filmtab Tablets 402
Biaxin Granules 402

CLARITIN SKIN ITCH RELIEF (Canada)
HYDROCORTISONE
Hydrocortone Tablets 1989

CLARITROMAX (Brazil)
CLARITHROMYCIN
Biaxin Filmtab Tablets 402
Biaxin Granules 402

CLARITRON (Brazil)
CLARITHROMYCIN
Biaxin Filmtab Tablets 402
Biaxin Granules 402

CLARITUR (Spain)
CLARITHROMYCIN
Biaxin Filmtab Tablets 402
Biaxin Granules 402

CLAROFT (Brazil)
NAPHAZOLINE HYDROCHLORIDE
Albalon Ophthalmic Solution . . . . . . ⊙218

CLAROMYCIN (Greece)
CLARITHROMYCIN
Biaxin Filmtab Tablets 402
Biaxin Granules 402

CLARON (Thailand)
CLARITHROMYCIN
Biaxin Filmtab Tablets 402
Biaxin Granules 402

CLAROPRAM (Switzerland)
CITALOPRAM HYDROBROMIDE
Celexa Tablets 1176

CLAROSIP (United Kingdom)
CLARITHROMYCIN
Biaxin Filmtab Tablets 402
Biaxin Granules 402

CLAROVIL (Argentina)
CLARITHROMYCIN
Biaxin Filmtab Tablets 402
Biaxin Granules 402

CLATIC (Chile)
CLARITHROMYCIN
Biaxin Filmtab Tablets 402
Biaxin Granules 402

CLATORIN (Brazil)
CLARITHROMYCIN
Biaxin Filmtab Tablets 402
Biaxin Granules 402

CLATROCIN (Mexico)
CLARITHROMYCIN
Biaxin Filmtab Tablets 402
Biaxin Granules 402

CLATROMICIN (Argentina)
CLARITHROMYCIN
Biaxin Filmtab Tablets 402
Biaxin Granules 402

CLAV-AIR (Brazil)
AMOXICILLIN
Amoxil Pediatric Drops for Oral Suspension 1343
Amoxil Tablets 1343

CLEAN & CLEAR CONTINUOUS CONTROL (Canada)
BENZOYL PEROXIDE
Brevoxyl-4 Creamy Wash 3210
Brevoxyl-4 Gel 3210
Brevoxyl-8 Creamy Wash 3210
Brevoxyl-8 Gel 3210
Triaz Cleanser 1892
Triaz Gel 1892

CLEAN & CLEAR PERSA GEL (Canada)
BENZOYL PEROXIDE
Brevoxyl-4 Creamy Wash 3210
Brevoxyl-4 Gel 3210
Brevoxyl-8 Creamy Wash 3210
Brevoxyl-8 Gel 3210
Triaz Cleanser 1892
Triaz Gel 1892

CLEAR EYES (Australia, Canada, New Zealand)
NAPHAZOLINE HYDROCHLORIDE
Albalon Ophthalmic Solution . . . . . . ⊙218

CLEAR EYES ACR (New Zealand)
NAPHAZOLINE HYDROCHLORIDE
Albalon Ophthalmic Solution . . . . . . ⊙218

CLEARAMED (Spain, Sweden)
BENZOYL PEROXIDE
Brevoxyl-4 Creamy Wash 3210
Brevoxyl-4 Gel 3210
Brevoxyl-8 Creamy Wash 3210
Brevoxyl-8 Gel 3210
Triaz Cleanser 1892
Triaz Gel 1892

CLEARASIL B.P. PLUS (Canada)
BENZOYL PEROXIDE
Brevoxyl-4 Creamy Wash 3210
Brevoxyl-4 Gel 3210
Brevoxyl-8 Creamy Wash 3210
Brevoxyl-8 Gel 3210
Triaz Cleanser 1892
Triaz Gel 1892

CLEARASIL BENZOYL P (South Africa)
BENZOYL PEROXIDE
Brevoxyl-4 Creamy Wash 3210
Brevoxyl-4 Gel 3210
Brevoxyl-8 Creamy Wash 3210
Brevoxyl-8 Gel 3210
Triaz Cleanser 1892
Triaz Gel 1892

CLEARASIL EXTRA STRENGTH (Australia)
BENZOYL PEROXIDE
Brevoxyl-4 Creamy Wash 3210
Brevoxyl-4 Gel 3210
Brevoxyl-8 Creamy Wash 3210
Brevoxyl-8 Gel 3210
Triaz Cleanser 1892
Triaz Gel 1892

CLEARASIL MAX 10 (United Kingdom)
BENZOYL PEROXIDE
Brevoxyl-4 Creamy Wash 3210
Brevoxyl-4 Gel 3210
Brevoxyl-8 Creamy Wash 3210
Brevoxyl-8 Gel 3210
Triaz Cleanser 1892
Triaz Gel 1892

CLEARASIL PLUS (Mexico)
BENZOYL PEROXIDE
Brevoxyl-4 Creamy Wash 3210
Brevoxyl-4 Gel 3210
Brevoxyl-8 Creamy Wash 3210
Brevoxyl-8 Gel 3210
Triaz Cleanser 1892
Triaz Gel 1892

CLEARASIL ULTRA (Australia, Italy, New Zealand)
BENZOYL PEROXIDE
Brevoxyl-4 Creamy Wash 3210
Brevoxyl-4 Gel 3210
Brevoxyl-8 Creamy Wash 3210
Brevoxyl-8 Gel 3210
Triaz Cleanser 1892
Triaz Gel 1892

CLEAREX COVER UP (Israel)
BENZOYL PEROXIDE
Brevoxyl-4 Creamy Wash 3210
Brevoxyl-4 Gel 3210
Brevoxyl-8 Creamy Wash 3210
Brevoxyl-8 Gel 3210
Triaz Cleanser 1892
Triaz Gel 1892

CLEARINE (India)
NAPHAZOLINE HYDROCHLORIDE
Albalon Ophthalmic Solution . . . . . . ⊙218

CLEARIZE (Venezuela)
NAPHAZOLINE HYDROCHLORIDE
Albalon Ophthalmic Solution . . . . . . ⊙218

CLEOCIN (Australia, Austria)
CLINDAMYCIN HYDROCHLORIDE
Cleocin Vaginal Ovules 2616

CLERIDIUM (France)
DIPYRIDAMOLE
Persantine Tablets 868

CLERON (Hong Kong)
CLARITHROMYCIN
Biaxin Filmtab Tablets 402
Biaxin Granules 402

CLETONOL (Argentina)
NIMODIPINE
Nimotop Capsules 749

CLEVERON (Brazil)
ALENDRONATE SODIUM
Fosamax Tablets 1969

CLEXANE (Argentina, Australia, Belgium, Brazil, Chile, Czech Republic, Germany, Greece, Hong Kong, Hungary, India, Irish Republic, Israel, Italy, Malaysia, Mexico, New Zealand, Russia, Singapore, South Africa, Spain, Switzerland, Thailand, The Netherlands, United Kingdom, Venezuela)
ENOXAPARIN SODIUM
Lovenox Injection 2915

CLIANE (Brazil, New Zealand, Venezuela)
ESTRADIOL
Climara Transdermal System 771
Estring Vaginal Ring 2635

CLIARVAS (Argentina)
LOSARTAN POTASSIUM
Cozaar Tablets 1935

CLIDAM (Austria)
CLINDAMYCIN HYDROCHLORIDE
Cleocin Vaginal Ovules 2616

CLIMADAN (Singapore)
CLINDAMYCIN HYDROCHLORIDE
Cleocin Vaginal Ovules 2616

CLIMADERM (Argentina, Brazil, Chile, Mexico, Venezuela)
ESTRADIOL
Climara Transdermal System 771
Estring Vaginal Ring 2635

CLIMANOR (United Kingdom)
MEDROXYPROGESTERONE ACETATE
Depo-Medrol Single-Dose Vial 2619

CLIMARA (Australia, Austria, Belgium, Canada, Czech Republic, Denmark, Finland, France, Irish Republic, Israel, Italy, New Zealand, Norway, Portugal, Russia, South Africa, Sweden, Switzerland, Thailand, The Netherlands)
ESTRADIOL
Climara Transdermal System 771
Estring Vaginal Ring 2635

CLIMASTON (France)
ESTRADIOL
Climara Transdermal System 771
Estring Vaginal Ring 2635

CLINAC (Portugal)
ERYTHROMYCIN
Ery-Tab Tablets 449
Erythromycin Base Filmtab Tablets 455
Erythromycin Delayed-Release Capsules, USP 457
PCE Dispertab Tablets 515

CLINAZOLE (South Africa)
METRONIDAZOLE
MetroGel-Vaginal Gel 1855

CLINDABETA (Germany)
CLINDAMYCIN HYDROCHLORIDE
Cleocin Vaginal Ovules 2616

CLINDAC (Austria)
CLINDAMYCIN HYDROCHLORIDE
Cleocin Vaginal Ovules 2616

CLINDAHEXAL (South Africa)
CLINDAMYCIN HYDROCHLORIDE
Cleocin Vaginal Ovules 2616

CLINDAL (Austria)
CLINDAMYCIN HYDROCHLORIDE
Cleocin Vaginal Ovules 2616

CLINDALAF (Argentina)
CLINDAMYCIN HYDROCHLORIDE
Cleocin Vaginal Ovules 2616

CLINDAMIN C (Brazil)
CLINDAMYCIN HYDROCHLORIDE
Cleocin Vaginal Ovules 2616

CLINDASTAD (Germany)
CLINDAMYCIN HYDROCHLORIDE
Cleocin Vaginal Ovules 2616

CLINDATECH (Australia, Hong Kong, Singapore)
CLINDAMYCIN HYDROCHLORIDE
Cleocin Vaginal Ovules 2616

CLINDOXYL (Argentina)
BENZOYL PEROXIDE
Brevoxyl-4 Creamy Wash 3210
Brevoxyl-4 Gel 3210
Brevoxyl-8 Creamy Wash 3210
Brevoxyl-8 Gel 3210
Triaz Cleanser 1892
Triaz Gel 1892

CLINFAR (Brazil)
SIMVASTATIN
Zocor Tablets 2105

CLINIFLAM (South Africa)
DICLOFENAC SODIUM
Voltaren Tablets 2307
Voltaren-XR Tablets 2310

CLINIRETIC (South Africa)
AMILORIDE HYDROCHLORIDE/HYDROCHLOROTHIAZIDE
Moduretic Tablets 2028

CLINODERM (Thailand)
CLOBETASOL PROPIONATE
Temovate Cream 2668
Temovate E Emollient 2671
Temovate Gel 2669
Temovate Ointment 2668
Temovate Scalp Application 2670

CLINOFEM (Germany)
MEDROXYPROGESTERONE ACETATE
Depo-Medrol Single-Dose Vial 2619

CLINOFUG GEL (Germany)
ERYTHROMYCIN
Ery-Tab Tablets 449
Erythromycin Base Filmtab Tablets 455
Erythromycin Delayed-Release Capsules, USP 457
PCE Dispertab Tablets 515

CLINOLAT (South Africa)
NIFEDIPINE
Adalat CC Tablets 2964

CLINORIL (Australia, Austria, Belgium, Canada, Czech Republic, Denmark, Hong Kong, Irish Republic, Italy, Malaysia, Mexico, New Zealand, Norway, South Africa, Sweden, Switzerland, Thailand, The Netherlands, United Kingdom, Venezuela)
SULINDAC
Clinoril Tablets 1924

CLINOSYN (South Africa)
NAPROXEN
EC-Naprosyn Delayed-Release Tablets 2761
Naprosyn Suspension 2761
Naprosyn Tablets 2761

CLINOTT (Thailand)
CLINDAMYCIN HYDROCHLORIDE
Cleocin Vaginal Ovules 2616

CLINOVIR (Germany)
MEDROXYPROGESTERONE ACETATE
Depo-Medrol Single-Dose Vial 2619

CLIN-SANORANIA (Germany)
CLINDAMYCIN HYDROCHLORIDE
Cleocin Vaginal Ovules 2616

CLINTOPIC (Argentina)
CLINDAMYCIN HYDROCHLORIDE
Cleocin Vaginal Ovules 2616

CLIOGAN (Spain)
ESTRADIOL
Climara Transdermal System 771

Estring Vaginal Ring 2635

CLIPTO (Spain)
ENALAPRIL MALEATE
Vasotec I.V. Injection 2103

CLISON (Mexico)
SULINDAC
Clinoril Tablets 1924

CLISUNDAC (Italy)
SULINDAC
Clinoril Tablets 1924

CLIVOTEN (Italy)
ISRADIPINE
DynaCirc CR Tablets. 2721

CLOBASOL (Hong Kong)
CLOBETASOL PROPIONATE
Temovate Cream. 2668
Temovate E Emollient. 2671
Temovate Gel. 2669
Temovate Ointment 2668
Temovate Scalp Application 2670

CLOBASONE (Thailand)
CLOBETASOL PROPIONATE
Temovate Cream. 2668
Temovate E Emollient. 2671
Temovate Gel. 2669
Temovate Ointment 2668
Temovate Scalp Application 2670

CLOBEGALEN (Germany)
CLOBETASOL PROPIONATE
Temovate Cream. 2668
Temovate E Emollient. 2671
Temovate Gel. 2669
Temovate Ointment 2668
Temovate Scalp Application 2670

CLOBENDIAN (Spain)
DILTIAZEM HYDROCHLORIDE
Cardizem LA Extended Release Tablets. . . 1728
Tiazac Capsules 1201

CLOBEPLUS (Argentina)
CLOBETASOL PROPIONATE
Temovate Cream. 2668
Temovate E Emollient. 2671
Temovate Gel. 2669
Temovate Ointment 2668
Temovate Scalp Application 2670

CLOBESOL (Argentina, Brazil, Italy, Mexico)
CLOBETASOL PROPIONATE
Temovate Cream. 2668
Temovate E Emollient. 2671
Temovate Gel. 2669
Temovate Ointment 2668
Temovate Scalp Application 2670

CLOBESOL LA (Argentina)
CLOBETASOL PROPIONATE
Temovate Cream. 2668
Temovate E Emollient. 2671
Temovate Gel. 2669
Temovate Ointment 2668
Temovate Scalp Application 2670

CLOBESON (Singapore)
CLOBETASOL PROPIONATE
Temovate Cream. 2668
Temovate E Emollient. 2671
Temovate Gel. 2669
Temovate Ointment 2668
Temovate Scalp Application 2670

CLOBET (Malaysia, Thailand)
CLOBETASOL PROPIONATE
Temovate Cream. 2668
Temovate E Emollient. 2671
Temovate Gel. 2669
Temovate Ointment 2668
Temovate Scalp Application 2670

CLOBETATE (Thailand)
CLOBETASOL PROPIONATE
Temovate Cream. 2668
Temovate E Emollient. 2671
Temovate Gel. 2669
Temovate Ointment 2668
Temovate Scalp Application 2670

CLOBEX (Argentina)
CLOBETASOL PROPIONATE
Temovate Cream. 2668
Temovate E Emollient. 2671
Temovate Gel. 2669
Temovate Ointment 2668
Temovate Scalp Application 2670

CLOB-X (Brazil, Chile)
CLOBETASOL PROPIONATE
Temovate Cream. 2668
Temovate E Emollient. 2671
Temovate Gel. 2669
Temovate Ointment 2668
Temovate Scalp Application 2670

CLOCAN (Mexico)
CLOTRIMAZOLE
Lotrimin Cream. 3039
Lotrimin Lotion 1%. 3039
Lotrimin Topical Solution 1% 3039

CLOCIM (Switzerland)
CLOTRIMAZOLE
Lotrimin Cream. 3039
Lotrimin Lotion 1%. 3039
Lotrimin Topical Solution 1% 3039

CLOCIP (India)
CLOTRIMAZOLE
Lotrimin Cream. 3039
Lotrimin Lotion 1%. 3039
Lotrimin Topical Solution 1% 3039

CLOCIP B (India)
CLOTRIMAZOLE
Lotrimin Cream. 3039
Lotrimin Lotion 1%. 3039
Lotrimin Topical Solution 1% 3039

CLOCREME (Hong Kong, New Zealand)
CLOTRIMAZOLE
Lotrimin Cream. 3039
Lotrimin Lotion 1%. 3039
Lotrimin Topical Solution 1% 3039

CLODAVAN (Chile)
CLOBETASOL PROPIONATE
Temovate Cream. 2668
Temovate E Emollient. 2671
Temovate Gel. 2669
Temovate Ointment 2668
Temovate Scalp Application 2670

CLODERM (Germany, India, Malaysia, Singapore)
CLOBETASOL PROPIONATE
Temovate Cream. 2668
Temovate E Emollient. 2671
Temovate Gel. 2669
Temovate Ointment 2668
Temovate Scalp Application 2670

CLODIAN (Argentina)
CLOPIDOGREL BISULFATE
Plavix Tablets 917, 2926

CLODREL (Argentina)
CLOPIDOGREL BISULFATE
Plavix Tablets 917, 2926

CLOFAMOX (Argentina)
AMOXICILLIN
Amoxil Pediatric Drops for Oral Suspension. 1343
Amoxil Tablets 1343

CLOFEC (Hong Kong, Malaysia, Singapore, Thailand)
DICLOFENAC SODIUM
Voltaren Tablets 2307
Voltaren-XR Tablets 2310

CLOFEME (Australia)
CLOTRIMAZOLE
Lotrimin Cream. 3039
Lotrimin Lotion 1%. 3039
Lotrimin Topical Solution 1% 3039

CLOFENAC (Hong Kong, Malaysia, Singapore)
DICLOFENAC SODIUM
Voltaren Tablets 2307
Voltaren-XR Tablets 2310

CLOFENID (Brazil)
DICLOFENAC SODIUM
Voltaren Tablets 2307
Voltaren-XR Tablets 2310

CLOFLOW (India)
CLOPIDOGREL BISULFATE
Plavix Tablets 917, 2926

CLOFLOW PLUS (India)
CLOPIDOGREL BISULFATE
Plavix Tablets 917, 2926

CLOFON (Thailand)
DICLOFENAC SODIUM
Voltaren Tablets 2307
Voltaren-XR Tablets 2310

CLOGEN (Brazil)
CLOTRIMAZOLE
Lotrimin Cream. 3039
Lotrimin Lotion 1%. 3039
Lotrimin Topical Solution 1% 3039

CLOMADERM (South Africa)
CLOTRIMAZOLE
Lotrimin Cream. 3039
Lotrimin Lotion 1%. 3039
Lotrimin Topical Solution 1% 3039

CLOMAZEN (Brazil)
CLOTRIMAZOLE
Lotrimin Cream. 3039
Lotrimin Lotion 1%. 3039
Lotrimin Topical Solution 1% 3039

CLOMAZOL (Brazil, New Zealand)
CLOTRIMAZOLE
Lotrimin Cream. 3039
Lotrimin Lotion 1%. 3039
Lotrimin Topical Solution 1% 3039

CLOMENT (South Africa)
CLOZAPINE
Clozaril Tablets 2184

CLOMYCIN (India)
CLOTRIMAZOLE
Lotrimin Cream. 3039
Lotrimin Lotion 1%. 3039
Lotrimin Topical Solution 1% 3039

CLONAC (Australia, Greece)
DICLOFENAC SODIUM
Voltaren Tablets 2307
Voltaren-XR Tablets 2310

CLONAGIN (Argentina)
CLONAZEPAM
Klonopin Tablets 2778

CLONAPAM (Canada, Chile, Hungary)
CLONAZEPAM
Klonopin Tablets 2778

CLONASTEN (Brazil)
CLOTRIMAZOLE
Lotrimin Cream. 3039
Lotrimin Lotion 1%. 3039
Lotrimin Topical Solution 1% 3039

CLONAX (Argentina)
CLONAZEPAM
Klonopin Tablets 2778

CLONDEPRYL (Irish Republic)
SELEGILINE HYDROCHLORIDE
Eldepryl Capsules 3208

CLONEA (Australia)
CLOTRIMAZOLE
Lotrimin Cream. 3039
Lotrimin Lotion 1%. 3039
Lotrimin Topical Solution 1% 3039

CLONER (Argentina)
CLONAZEPAM
Klonopin Tablets 2778

CLONESINA (Brazil)
CLONIDINE HYDROCHLORIDE
Catapres Tablets 843

CLONEX (Chile, Israel)
CLONAZEPAM
Klonopin Tablets 2778

CLONID-OPHTAL (Germany)
CLONIDINE HYDROCHLORIDE
Catapres Tablets 843

CLONIDURAL (Argentina)
CLONIDINE
Catapres-TTS 844

CLONILIX (Irish Republic)
INDAPAMIDE
Indapamide Tablets 2156

CLONIPRES (Venezuela)
CLONIDINE HYDROCHLORIDE
Catapres Tablets 843

CLONISTADA (Germany)
CLONIDINE HYDROCHLORIDE
Catapres Tablets 843

CLONNIRIT (Israel)
CLONIDINE HYDROCHLORIDE
Catapres Tablets 843

CLONODIFEN (Mexico)
DICLOFENAC SODIUM
Voltaren Tablets 2307
Voltaren-XR Tablets 2310

CLONOGAL (Hungary)
CLONAZEPAM
Klonopin Tablets 2778

CLONOTRIL (Brazil)
CLONAZEPAM
Klonopin Tablets 2778

CLONOVATE (Thailand)
CLOBETASOL PROPIONATE
Temovate Cream. 2668
Temovate E Emollient. 2671
Temovate Gel. 2669
Temovate Ointment 2668
Temovate Scalp Application 2670

CLONT (Germany)
METRONIDAZOLE
MetroGel-Vaginal Gel 1855

CLONURETIC (Irish Republic)
AMILORIDE HYDROCHLORIDE/HYDROCHLOROTHIAZIDE
Moduretic Tablets 2028

CLOPACT (India)
CLOPIDOGREL BISULFATE
Plavix Tablets 917, 2926

CLOPACT A (India)
CLOPIDOGREL BISULFATE
Plavix Tablets 917, 2926

CLOPINE (Australia, New Zealand)
CLOZAPINE
Clozaril Tablets. 2184

CLOPIVAS (India)
CLOPIDOGREL BISULFATE
Plavix Tablets 917, 2926

CLOPIVAS AP (India)
CLOPIDOGREL BISULFATE
Plavix Tablets 917, 2926

CLOPOD (India)
CLOPIDOGREL BISULFATE
Plavix Tablets 917, 2926

CLOPOD-A (India)
CLOPIDOGREL BISULFATE
Plavix Tablets 917, 2926

CLOPSINE (Mexico)
CLOZAPINE
Clozaril Tablets. 2184

CLORADEX (Italy)
DEXAMETHASONE
Decadron Tablets 1951

CLOR-K-ZAF (Mexico)
POTASSIUM CHLORIDE
K-Dur Extended-Relase Tablets 3033
K-Lor Oral Solution. 474
K-Tab Tablets 475

CLORPAX (Australia)
BUPROPION HYDROCHLORIDE
Wellbutrin SR Sustained-Release Tablets . . 1607
Wellbutrin Tablets 1603
Zyban Sustained-Release Tablets. 1644

CLORTILEN (Venezuela)
CLOTRIMAZOLE
Lotrimin Cream. 3039
Lotrimin Lotion 1%. 3039
Lotrimin Topical Solution 1% 3039

CLOSCRIPT (South Africa)
CLOTRIMAZOLE
Lotrimin Cream. 3039
Lotrimin Lotion 1%. 3039
Lotrimin Topical Solution 1% 3039

CLOSIN (Germany)
PROMETHAZINE HYDROCHLORIDE
Phenergan Tablets and Suppositories 3440

CLOSINA (Australia)
CYCLOSERINE
Seromycin Capsules. 1813

CLOSTEDAL (Mexico)
CARBAMAZEPINE
Carbatrol Capsules 3171
Tegretol Chewable Tablets. 2295
Tegretol Suspension. 2295
Tegretol Tablets 2295
Tegretol-XR Tablets 2295

CLOTASSIO (Brazil)
POTASSIUM CHLORIDE
K-Dur Extended-Relase Tablets 3033
K-Lor Oral Solution. 474

K-Tab Tablets 475

CLOT-BASAN (Switzerland)
CLOTRIMAZOLE
Lotrimin Cream 3039
Lotrimin Lotion 1% 3039
Lotrimin Topical Solution 1% 3039

CLOTIGEN (Brazil)
CLOTRIMAZOLE
Lotrimin Cream 3039
Lotrimin Lotion 1% 3039
Lotrimin Topical Solution 1% 3039

CLOTREME (Australia)
CLOTRIMAZOLE
Lotrimin Cream 3039
Lotrimin Lotion 1% 3039
Lotrimin Topical Solution 1% 3039

CLOTREN (Brazil)
CLOTRIMAZOLE
Lotrimin Cream 3039
Lotrimin Lotion 1% 3039
Lotrimin Topical Solution 1% 3039

CLOTRI (Thailand)
CLOTRIMAZOLE
Lotrimin Cream 3039
Lotrimin Lotion 1% 3039
Lotrimin Topical Solution 1% 3039

CLOTRI OPT (Germany)
CLOTRIMAZOLE
Lotrimin Cream 3039
Lotrimin Lotion 1% 3039
Lotrimin Topical Solution 1% 3039

CLOTRICIN (Thailand)
CLOTRIMAZOLE
Lotrimin Cream 3039
Lotrimin Lotion 1% 3039
Lotrimin Topical Solution 1% 3039

CLOTRI-DENK (Hong Kong)
CLOTRIMAZOLE
Lotrimin Cream 3039
Lotrimin Lotion 1% 3039
Lotrimin Topical Solution 1% 3039

CLOTRIDERM (Brazil)
CLOTRIMAZOLE
Lotrimin Cream 3039
Lotrimin Lotion 1% 3039
Lotrimin Topical Solution 1% 3039

CLOTRIFERM (Sweden)
CLOTRIMAZOLE
Lotrimin Cream 3039
Lotrimin Lotion 1% 3039
Lotrimin Topical Solution 1% 3039

CLOTRIFUG (Germany)
CLOTRIMAZOLE
Lotrimin Cream 3039
Lotrimin Lotion 1% 3039
Lotrimin Topical Solution 1% 3039

CLOTRIGALEN (Germany)
CLOTRIMAZOLE
Lotrimin Cream 3039
Lotrimin Lotion 1% 3039
Lotrimin Topical Solution 1% 3039

CLOTRIHEXAL (New Zealand)
CLOTRIMAZOLE
Lotrimin Cream 3039
Lotrimin Lotion 1% 3039
Lotrimin Topical Solution 1% 3039

CLOTRIMADERM (Canada, Israel, New Zealand)
CLOTRIMAZOLE
Lotrimin Cream 3039
Lotrimin Lotion 1% 3039
Lotrimin Topical Solution 1% 3039

CLOTRIMIN (Chile)
CLOTRIMAZOLE
Lotrimin Cream 3039
Lotrimin Lotion 1% 3039
Lotrimin Topical Solution 1% 3039

CLOTRIMIX (Brazil)
CLOTRIMAZOLE
Lotrimin Cream 3039
Lotrimin Lotion 1% 3039
Lotrimin Topical Solution 1% 3039

CLOTRINOLON (Hong Kong)
CLOTRIMAZOLE
Lotrimin Cream 3039
Lotrimin Lotion 1% 3039
Lotrimin Topical Solution 1% 3039

CLOTRIZAN (Brazil)
CLOTRIMAZOLE
Lotrimin Cream 3039
Lotrimin Lotion 1% 3039
Lotrimin Topical Solution 1% 3039

CLOTRIZOL (Venezuela)
CLOTRIMAZOLE
Lotrimin Cream 3039
Lotrimin Lotion 1% 3039
Lotrimin Topical Solution 1% 3039

CLOVATE (Spain)
CLOBETASOL PROPIONATE
Temovate Cream 2668
Temovate E Emollient 2671
Temovate Gel 2669
Temovate Ointment 2668
Temovate Scalp Application 2670

CLOX (Italy)
TICLOPIDINE HYDROCHLORIDE
Ticlid Tablets 2810

CLOXIB (Argentina)
CELECOXIB
Celebrex Capsules 3134

CLOZANIL (Chile)
CLONAZEPAM
Klonopin Tablets 2778

CLOZARIL (Australia, Canada, Hong Kong, Irish Republic, Malaysia, New Zealand, Singapore, Thailand, United Kingdom)
CLOZAPINE
Clozaril Tablets 2184

CLOZOL (India)
CLOTRIMAZOLE
Lotrimin Cream 3039
Lotrimin Lotion 1% 3039
Lotrimin Topical Solution 1% 3039

CLOZOLE (Australia, Hong Kong, Singapore)
CLOTRIMAZOLE
Lotrimin Cream 3039
Lotrimin Lotion 1% 3039
Lotrimin Topical Solution 1% 3039

CLUSINOL (Australia)
SULINDAC
Clinoril Tablets 1924

CMP (Argentina)
CARBAMAZEPINE
Carbatrol Capsules 3171
Tegretol Chewable Tablets 2295
Tegretol Suspension 2295
Tegretol Tablets 2295
Tegretol-XR Tablets 2295

CO-ACEPRIL (Switzerland)
ENALAPRIL MALEATE
Vasotec I.V. Injection 2103

CO-ACETAN (Austria)
HYDROCHLOROTHIAZIDE/LISINOPRIL
Prinzide Tablets 2056

CO-AMILORID (Switzerland)
AMILORIDE HYDROCHLORIDE/HYDROCHLOROTHIAZIDE
Moduretic Tablets 2028

CO-AMOXYCLAV (South Africa)
AMOXICILLIN
Amoxil Pediatric Drops for Oral Suspension 1343
Amoxil Tablets 1343

COAPROVEL (Argentina, Belgium, Chile, Czech Republic, Denmark, Germany, Hong Kong, Hungary, Irish Republic, Italy, Malaysia, Mexico, Singapore, South Africa, Spain, Thailand, Venezuela)
IRBESARTAN
Avapro Tablets 891

COBADEX (United Kingdom)
HYDROCORTISONE
Hydrocortone Tablets 1989

COBAY (Thailand)
CIPROFLOXACIN HYDROCHLORIDE
Ciloxan Ophthalmic Ointment . . . . ⊙204, 559
Ciloxan Ophthalmic Solution . . . . ⊙206
Cipro Tablets 2977

CO-BETALOC (Irish Republic, United Kingdom)
HYDROCHLOROTHIAZIDE/METOPROLOL TARTRATE
Lopressor HCT 100/25 Tablets 2241

COBIX (India)
CELECOXIB
Celebrex Capsules 3134

CO-CAPTOPRIL (Austria)
CAPTOPRIL
Captopril Tablets 2149

CO-CAPTOTYROL (Austria)
CAPTOPRIL
Captopril Tablets 2149

CO-CAPTRAL (Mexico)
CAPTOPRIL
Captopril Tablets 2149

CO-DIOVAN (Austria, Czech Republic, Germany, Hong Kong, Irish Republic, Israel, Malaysia, Mexico, Portugal, Russia, Singapore, South Africa, Spain, Switzerland, Thailand, The Netherlands, United Kingdom)
HYDROCHLOROTHIAZIDE/VALSARTAN
Diovan HCT Tablets 2196

CO-DIOVANE (Belgium)
HYDROCHLOROTHIAZIDE/VALSARTAN
Diovan HCT Tablets 2196

CODRINAN (Brazil)
THEOPHYLLINE
Uniphyl Tablets 2710

CO-ENAC (Austria)
ENALAPRIL MALEATE
Vasotec I.V. Injection 2103

CO-ENALAPRIL (Austria, Belgium)
ENALAPRIL MALEATE
Vasotec I.V. Injection 2103

CO-ENARAN (Austria)
ENALAPRIL MALEATE
Vasotec I.V. Injection 2103

CO-ENATEC (Switzerland)
ENALAPRIL MALEATE
Vasotec I.V. Injection 2103

CO-ENATYROL (Austria)
ENALAPRIL MALEATE
Vasotec I.V. Injection 2103

CO-EPRIL (Switzerland)
ENALAPRIL MALEATE
Vasotec I.V. Injection 2103

COFENAC (India)
DICLOFENAC SODIUM
Voltaren Tablets 2307
Voltaren-XR Tablets 2310

COGNITIV (Austria, Czech Republic, Russia)
SELEGILINE HYDROCHLORIDE
Eldepryl Capsules 3208

COLATAN (Spain)
NARATRIPTAN HYDROCHLORIDE
Amerge Tablets 1339

COLDAN (Austria, Greece)
NAPHAZOLINE HYDROCHLORIDE
Albalon Ophthalmic Solution . . . . ⊙218

COLEDIS (Argentina)
SIMVASTATIN
Zocor Tablets 2105

COLEMIN (Spain)
SIMVASTATIN
Zocor Tablets 2105

COLESVIR (Spain)
LOVASTATIN
Mevacor Tablets 2021

COLEVIX (Chile)
LOVASTATIN
Mevacor Tablets 2021

COLIFOSSIM (Italy)
CEFUROXIME SODIUM
Zinacef Injection 1631

COLIRIOCILINA GENTAM (Spain)
GENTAMICIN SULFATE
Garamycin Injectable 3014

COLITROMIN (Mexico)
ERYTHROMYCIN
Ery-Tab Tablets 449
Erythromycin Base Filmtab Tablets 455
Erythromycin Delayed-Release Capsules, USP 457
PCE Dispertab Tablets 515

COLLICORT (Mexico)
HYDROCORTISONE
Hydrocortone Tablets 1989

COLPISTAR (Brazil)
METRONIDAZOLE
MetroGel-Vaginal Gel 1855

COLPOCIN-T (Greece)
METRONIDAZOLE
MetroGel-Vaginal Gel 1855

COLPROSTERONE (Spain)
PROGESTERONE
Prometrium Capsules (100 mg, 200 mg) . 3203

COLSANAC (Portugal)
LACTULOSE
Kristalose for Oral Solution 1034

COLTHER (Greece)
TOBRAMYCIN
TOBI Solution for Inhalation 2298

COMALOSE-R (Canada)
LACTULOSE
Kristalose for Oral Solution 1034

COMAT (Thailand)
CLOTRIMAZOLE
Lotrimin Cream 3039
Lotrimin Lotion 1% 3039
Lotrimin Topical Solution 1% 3039

COMBAREN (Venezuela)
DICLOFENAC SODIUM
Voltaren Tablets 2307
Voltaren-XR Tablets 2310

COMBID (Thailand)
LAMIVUDINE
Epivir Oral Solution 1427
Epivir Tablets 1427
Epivir-HBV Oral Solution 1432
Epivir-HBV Tablets 1432

COMBINED (Argentina)
OLANZAPINE
Zyprexa Tablets 1830

COMBIPROTECT (Germany)
AMILORIDE HYDROCHLORIDE/HYDROCHLOROTHIAZIDE
Moduretic Tablets 2028

COMBIREX (India)
LAMIVUDINE
Epivir Oral Solution 1427
Epivir Tablets 1427
Epivir-HBV Oral Solution 1432
Epivir-HBV Tablets 1432

COMBISARTAN (Italy)
HYDROCHLOROTHIAZIDE/VALSARTAN
Diovan HCT Tablets 2196

COMBIVENT (Argentina, Australia, Brazil, Malaysia, Venezuela)
IPRATROPIUM BROMIDE
Atrovent Inhalation Solution 835
Atrovent Nasal Spray 0.03% 837
Atrovent Nasal Spray 0.06% 839

COMBIVIR (Australia, Austria, Belgium, Brazil, Canada, Chile, Czech Republic, Denmark, Finland, France, Germany, Greece, Hong Kong, Irish Republic, Israel, Italy, Malaysia, Mexico, New Zealand, Norway, Portugal, Russia, Singapore, South Africa, Spain, Sweden, Switzerland, The Netherlands, United Kingdom, Venezuela)
LAMIVUDINE
Epivir Oral Solution 1427
Epivir Tablets 1427
Epivir-HBV Oral Solution 1432
Epivir-HBV Tablets 1432

CO-MICARDIS (South Africa)
TELMISARTAN
Micardis Tablets 854

COMILORID (Switzerland)
AMILORIDE HYDROCHLORIDE/HYDROCHLOROTHIAZIDE
Moduretic Tablets 2028

COMPAZ (Brazil)
DIAZEPAM
Diastat Rectal Delivery System 3343

Valium Tablets 2819

COMPLUTINE (Spain)
DIAZEPAM
Diastat Rectal Delivery System 3343
Valium Tablets 2819

CONCERTA (Argentina, Australia, Austria, Belgium, Brazil, Canada, Finland, France, Germany, Greece, Hong Kong, Irish Republic, Israel, Mexico, New Zealand, Norway, Portugal, Singapore, Spain, Sweden, Switzerland, The Netherlands, United Kingdom)
METHYLPHENIDATE HYDROCHLORIDE
Ritalin Hydrochloride Tablets. 2269
Ritalin-SR Tablets. 2269

CONDROTEC (United Kingdom)
NAPROXEN
EC-Naprosyn Delayed-Release Tablets. . . . 2761
Naprosyn Suspension. 2761
Naprosyn Tablets 2761

CONDUCIL (Venezuela)
NIFEDIPINE
Adalat CC Tablets 2964

CONEF (Argentina)
FINASTERIDE
Propecia Tablets 2060
Proscar Tablets. 2067

CONEXINE (Venezuela)
SERTRALINE HYDROCHLORIDE
Zoloft Tablets 2586

CONFOBOS (Spain)
FAMOTIDINE
Pepcid Injection 2040
Pepcid Injection Premixed 2040
Pepcid Tablets 2038
Pepcid for Oral Suspension 2038

CONFORMAL (Argentina)
CARBAMAZEPINE
Carbatrol Capsules 3171
Tegretol Chewable Tablets 2295
Tegretol Suspension. 2295
Tegretol Tablets 2295
Tegretol-XR Tablets 2295

CONGEX (Argentina)
NAPROXEN
EC-Naprosyn Delayed-Release Tablets. . . . 2761
Naprosyn Suspension. 2761
Naprosyn Tablets 2761

CONJUNCTIN-S (Austria)
NEOMYCIN SULFATE/POLYMYXIN B SULFATE/PREDNISOLONE ACETATE
Poly-Pred Ophthalmic Suspension . . . . . . ⊙233

CONNETTIVINA (Austria, Hong Kong, Italy, Thailand)
SODIUM HYALURONATE
Hyalgan Solution 2901

CONPIN (Germany)
ISOSORBIDE MONONITRATE
Imdur Tablets 3018

CONPRES (Hungary)
LISINOPRIL
Prinivil Tablets 2052

CONSEC (India)
RANITIDINE HYDROCHLORIDE
Zantac 25 EFFERdose Tablets 1624
Zantac 150 EFFERdose Tablets. 1624
Zantac 150 Tablets 1624
Zantac 300 Tablets 1624
Zantac Injection 1619
Zantac Injection Premixed 1619
Zantac Syrup 1624

CONSTILAX (Greece)
NORFLOXACIN
Noroxin Tablets. 2032

CONTALGIN (Denmark)
MORPHINE SULFATE
Kadian Capsules 577
MS Contin Tablets 2701

CONTIPHYLLIN (Germany)
THEOPHYLLINE
Uniphyl Tablets 2710

CONTRACEP (Brazil, Thailand)
MEDROXYPROGESTERONE ACETATE
Depo-Medrol Single-Dose Vial 2619

CONTRACNE (France)
ISOTRETINOIN
Accutane Capsules 2731

CONTRAFUNGIN (Germany)
CLOTRIMAZOLE
Lotrimin Cream. 3039
Lotrimin Lotion 1%. 3039
Lotrimin Topical Solution 1% 3039

CONTRAMAL (Belgium, France, India, Italy)
TRAMADOL HYDROCHLORIDE
Ultram ER Tablets 2392

CONTROL K (Argentina)
POTASSIUM CHLORIDE
K-Dur Extended-Release Tablets 3033
K-Lor Oral Solution. 474
K-Tab Tablets 475

CONTROLIP (Mexico)
FENOFIBRATE
Tricor Tablets 527

CONTROLPROS (Argentina)
TAMSULOSIN HYDROCHLORIDE
Flomax Capsules 850

CONTROLVAS (Spain)
ENALAPRIL MALEATE
Vasotec I.V. Injection 2103

CONTRYKAL (Russia)
APROTININ
Trasylol Injection 754

CONVADEN (Czech Republic)
ESTRADIOL
Climara Transdermal System 771
Estring Vaginal Ring 2635

CONVECTAL (Spain)
DILTIAZEM HYDROCHLORIDE
Cardizem LA Extended Release Tablets. . . 1728
Tiazac Capsules 1201

CONVERTAL (Portugal)
CAPTOPRIL
Captopril Tablets 2149

CONVERTEN (Italy)
ENALAPRIL MALEATE
Vasotec I.V. Injection 2103

CONVERTIN (Israel)
ENALAPRIL MALEATE
Vasotec I.V. Injection 2103

CONVULEX (Belgium, Czech Republic, Hungary, Russia, Singapore, United Kingdom, Venezuela)
VALPROIC ACID
Depakene Capsules 417
Depakene Oral Solution. 417

CONVULSAN (Brazil)
CARBAMAZEPINE
Carbatrol Capsules 3171
Tegretol Chewable Tablets. 2295
Tegretol Suspension. 2295
Tegretol Tablets 2295
Tegretol-XR Tablets 2295

COOLIPS (Chile)
CETIRIZINE HYDROCHLORIDE
Zyrtec Syrup 2594
Zyrtec Tablets 2594

COPAL (Mexico)
SULINDAC
Clinoril Tablets 1924

COPAXONE (Argentina, Australia, Austria, Belgium, Brazil, Canada, Czech Republic, Denmark, Finland, France, Greece, Hungary, Irish Republic, Israel, Italy, New Zealand, Norway, Portugal, Russia, Spain, Sweden, Switzerland, The Netherlands)
GLATIRAMER ACETATE
Copaxone for Injection 3297

COPEGUS (Argentina, Austria, Belgium, Denmark, Finland, France, Germany, Greece, Hong Kong, Irish Republic, Israel, Italy, New Zealand, Norway, Portugal, Spain, Sweden, Switzerland, The Netherlands, United Kingdom)
RIBAVIRIN
Virazole for Inhalation Solution 3370

COPHADYL (Singapore)
PROMETHAZINE HYDROCHLORIDE
Phenergan Tablets and Suppositories 3440

COPOVAN (Italy)
VANCOMYCIN HYDROCHLORIDE
Vancocin HCl Capsules, USP 3380

CO-PRESSOLESS (Brazil)
ENALAPRIL MALEATE
Vasotec I.V. Injection 2103

CO-PRESSOTEC (Brazil)
ENALAPRIL MALEATE
Vasotec I.V. Injection 2103

COR TENSOBON (Germany)
CAPTOPRIL
Captopril Tablets 2149

CORACTEN (Greece, Hong Kong, Thailand, United Kingdom)
NIFEDIPINE
Adalat CC Tablets 2964

CORAGOXINE (France)
DIGOXIN
Lanoxicaps Capsules 1490
Lanoxin Injection 1494
Lanoxin Injection Pediatric 1497
Lanoxin Tablets. 1500

CORAL (Italy, Mexico)
NIFEDIPINE
Adalat CC Tablets 2964

CORALEN (Spain)
RANITIDINE HYDROCHLORIDE
Zantac 25 EFFERdose Tablets 1624
Zantac 150 EFFERdose Tablets. 1624
Zantac 150 Tablets 1624
Zantac 300 Tablets 1624
Zantac Injection 1619
Zantac Injection Premixed 1619
Zantac Syrup 1624

CORAMIL (Sweden)
DILTIAZEM HYDROCHLORIDE
Cardizem LA Extended Release Tablets. . . 1728
Tiazac Capsules 1201

CORANGIN (Austria, Germany, Hong Kong, New Zealand)
ISOSORBIDE MONONITRATE
Imdur Tablets 3018

CORANGINE (Switzerland)
ISOSORBIDE MONONITRATE
Imdur Tablets 3018

CORAS (Australia)
DILTIAZEM HYDROCHLORIDE
Cardizem LA Extended Release Tablets. . . 1728
Tiazac Capsules 1201

CORAZEM (Austria, Venezuela)
DILTIAZEM HYDROCHLORIDE
Cardizem LA Extended Release Tablets. . . 1728
Tiazac Capsules 1201

CORAZET (Germany)
DILTIAZEM HYDROCHLORIDE
Cardizem LA Extended Release Tablets. . . 1728
Tiazac Capsules 1201

CORBETA (India)
PROPRANOLOL HYDROCHLORIDE
Inderal LA Long-Acting Capsules 3429

CORDAFEN (Czech Republic, Russia)
NIFEDIPINE
Adalat CC Tablets 2964

CORDAFLEX (Hungary, Russia)
NIFEDIPINE
Adalat CC Tablets 2964

CORDES BPO (Germany)
BENZOYL PEROXIDE
Brevoxyl-4 Creamy Wash. 3210
Brevoxyl-4 Gel 3210
Brevoxyl-8 Creamy Wash. 3210
Brevoxyl-8 Gel 3210
Triaz Cleanser 1892
Triaz Gel. 1892

CORDES NYSTATIN SOFT (Germany)
NYSTATIN
Nystop Topical Powder USP. 2478
Paddock Nystatin USP for Oral Suspension. 2478

CORDES VAS (Germany)
TRETINOIN
Vesanoid Capsules. 2820

CORDICANT (Germany)
NIFEDIPINE
Adalat CC Tablets 2964

CORDILAN (Spain)
NIFEDIPINE
Adalat CC Tablets 2964

CORDILAT (Brazil, Mexico)
VERAPAMIL HYDROCHLORIDE
Covera-HS Tablets 3139
Verelan PM Extended-Release Capsules, Controlled-Onset 3106

CORDILOX (Australia, United Kingdom)
VERAPAMIL HYDROCHLORIDE
Covera-HS Tablets 3139
Verelan PM Extended-Release Capsules, Controlled-Onset 3106

CORDIPIN (Czech Republic, Hungary, Russia, Singapore)
NIFEDIPINE
Adalat CC Tablets 2964

CORDIRON (Brazil)
SIMVASTATIN
Zocor Tablets. 2105

COREG (Brazil, Canada)
CARVEDILOL
Coreg Tablets. 1414

CORENISTAD (Austria)
ENALAPRIL MALEATE
Vasotec I.V. Injection 2103

CO-RENITEC (Argentina, Hungary, Venezuela)
ENALAPRIL MALEATE
Vasotec I.V. Injection 2103

CORFLENE (Spain)
FLECAINIDE ACETATE
Tambocor Tablets 1856

CORGARD (Argentina, Belgium, Brazil, Canada, Chile, France, Hong Kong, Irish Republic, Italy, Malaysia, Mexico, New Zealand, South Africa, Spain, Switzerland, United Kingdom, Venezuela)
NADOLOL
Nadolol Tablets. 2159

CORGARETIC (Mexico, United Kingdom)
NADOLOL
Nadolol Tablets. 2159

CORIBON (Italy)
DIPYRIDAMOLE
Persantine Tablets 868

CORIC (Germany)
LISINOPRIL
Prinivil Tablets 2052

CORIC PLUS (Germany)
HYDROCHLOROTHIAZIDE/LISINOPRIL
Prinzide Tablets 2056

CORIDIL (Switzerland)
DILTIAZEM HYDROCHLORIDE
Cardizem LA Extended Release Tablets. . . 1728
Tiazac Capsules 1201

CORIFINA (Spain)
AZELASTINE HYDROCHLORIDE
Astelin Nasal Spray 1904

CORILAX (Thailand)
ORPHENADRINE CITRATE
Norflex Injection 1856

CORINFAR (Czech Republic, Germany, Hungary, Russia)
NIFEDIPINE
Adalat CC Tablets 2964

CORIODAL (Chile)
PROPRANOLOL HYDROCHLORIDE
Inderal LA Long-Acting Capsules 3429

CORISOL (Switzerland)
CLOTRIMAZOLE
Lotrimin Cream. 3039
Lotrimin Lotion 1%. 3039
Lotrimin Topical Solution 1% 3039

CORITENSIL (Argentina)
CARVEDILOL
Coreg Tablets. 1414

(⊙ Described in PDR For Ophthalmic Medicines™)

CORIXA (Argentina)
CLARITHROMYCIN
Biaxin Filmtab Tablets 402
Biaxin Granules 402

CORNEL (Spain)
NISOLDIPINE
Sular Tablets 3122

CORODAY (United Kingdom)
NIFEDIPINE
Adalat CC Tablets 2964

CORODIL (Denmark)
ENALAPRIL MALEATE
Vasotec I.V. Injection 2103

CORODIN (Chile)
LOSARTAN POTASSIUM
Cozaar Tablets 1935

CORODIN D (Chile)
HYDROCHLOROTHIAZIDE/LOSARTAN POTASSIUM
Hyzaar 100-25 Tablets 1990
Hyzaar 50-12.5 Tablets 1990

COROGAL (Mexico)
NIFEDIPINE
Adalat CC Tablets 2964

COROLATER (Spain)
DILTIAZEM HYDROCHLORIDE
Cardizem LA Extended Release Tablets 1728
Tiazac Capsules 1201

COROLIN (Finland)
SIMVASTATIN
Zocor Tablets 2105

CORONAR (Brazil)
ISOSORBIDE MONONITRATE
Imdur Tablets 3018

CORONARINE (France)
DIPYRIDAMOLE
Persantine Tablets 868

CORONORM (Germany)
CAPTOPRIL
Captopril Tablets 2149

CORONOVO (Chile)
NIFEDIPINE
Adalat CC Tablets 2964

CORONUR (Spain)
ISOSORBIDE MONONITRATE
Imdur Tablets 3018

COROPRES (Spain)
CARVEDILOL
Coreg Tablets 1414

COROSAN (Italy)
DIPYRIDAMOLE
Persantine Tablets 868

COROTREND (Germany, Mexico, Switzerland)
NIFEDIPINE
Adalat CC Tablets 2964

COROXIN (Italy)
DIPYRIDAMOLE
Persantine Tablets 868

COROZELL (Austria)
POTASSIUM CHLORIDE
K-Dur Extended-Release Tablets 3033
K-Lor Oral Solution 474
K-Tab Tablets 475

CORPAMIL (Switzerland)
VERAPAMIL HYDROCHLORIDE
Covera-HS Tablets 3139
Verelan PM Extended-Release Capsules, Controlled-Onset 3106

CORPENDOL (Portugal)
PROPRANOLOL HYDROCHLORIDE
Inderal LA Long-Acting Capsules 3429

CORPRIL (Thailand)
RAMIPRIL
Altace Capsules 1702

CORPRILOR (Singapore, Spain)
ENALAPRIL MALEATE
Vasotec I.V. Injection 2103

CORTALEN C (Brazil)
CLOBETASOL PROPIONATE
Temovate Cream 2668
Temovate E Emollient 2671
Temovate Gel 2669
Temovate Ointment 2668
Temovate Scalp Application 2670

CORTALER NOVO (Argentina)
DEXAMETHASONE
Decadron Tablets 1951

CORTAPAISYL (France)
HYDROCORTISONE
Hydrocortone Tablets 1989

CORTEF (Hungary, Russia)
HYDROCORTISONE
Hydrocortone Tablets 1989

CORTENEM (Argentina)
HYDROCORTISONE
Hydrocortone Tablets 1989

CORTENEMA (Canada, United Kingdom)
HYDROCORTISONE
Hydrocortone Tablets 1989

CORTICIN (Hong Kong)
HYDROCORTISONE
Hydrocortone Tablets 1989

CORTICINA (Venezuela)
HYDROCORTISONE
Hydrocortone Tablets 1989

CORTICOSAN (Argentina)
LOSARTAN POTASSIUM
Cozaar Tablets 1935

CORTICOTHERAPIQUE (Switzerland)
TRIAMCINOLONE ACETONIDE
Azmacort Inhalation Aerosol 1726
Nasacort AQ Nasal Spray 2922

CORTIDEX (Brazil, Mexico)
DEXAMETHASONE
Decadron Tablets 1951

CORTIDEXASON (Germany)
DEXAMETHASONE
Decadron Tablets 1951

CORTISEDERMYL (France)
HYDROCORTISONE
Hydrocortone Tablets 1989

CORTISUMMAN (Germany)
DEXAMETHASONE
Decadron Tablets 1951

CORTIZONE (Israel)
HYDROCORTISONE
Hydrocortone Tablets 1989

CORTODERM (Canada)
HYDROCORTISONE
Hydrocortone Tablets 1989

CORTOLA-M (India)
SULFACETAMIDE SODIUM
Klaron Lotion 10% 2909

CORTOPIC (Chile)
CLOBETASOL PROPIONATE
Temovate Cream 2668
Temovate E Emollient 2671
Temovate Gel 2669
Temovate Ointment 2668
Temovate Scalp Application 2670

CORTOPIN (Irish Republic, United Kingdom)
HYDROCORTISONE
Hydrocortone Tablets 1989

CORTRAN (Chile)
CITALOPRAM HYDROBROMIDE
Celexa Tablets 1176

CORTRIL (Finland)
HYDROCORTISONE
Hydrocortone Tablets 1989

CORTROPIN (United Kingdom)
HYDROCORTISONE
Hydrocortone Tablets 1989

CORUBIN (Argentina, Greece)
CARVEDILOL
Coreg Tablets 1414

CORUS (Brazil)
LOSARTAN POTASSIUM
Cozaar Tablets 1935

CORUS H (Brazil)
LOSARTAN POTASSIUM
Cozaar Tablets 1935

CORVASAL (Germany)
ISOSORBIDE MONONITRATE
Imdur Tablets 3018

CORVITOL (Czech Republic, Russia)
METOPROLOL TARTRATE
Lopressor Tablets 2238

CORVO (Germany)
ENALAPRIL MALEATE
Vasotec I.V. Injection 2103

CORZIDE (Canada)
NADOLOL
Nadolol Tablets 2159

COSAAR (Austria, Switzerland)
LOSARTAN POTASSIUM
Cozaar Tablets 1935

COSAAR PLUS (Austria, Switzerland)
HYDROCHLOROTHIAZIDE/LOSARTAN POTASSIUM
Hyzaar 100-25 Tablets 1990
Hyzaar 50-12.5 Tablets 1990

CO-SALT (Argentina)
POTASSIUM CHLORIDE
K-Dur Extended-Release Tablets 3033
K-Lor Oral Solution 474
K-Tab Tablets 475

COSIL (Venezuela)
ENALAPRIL MALEATE
Vasotec I.V. Injection 2103

COSMOFER (Denmark, Germany, Greece, Irish Republic, Norway, Thailand, United Kingdom)
IRON DEXTRAN
Infed Injection 3390

COSMOPRIL (Greece)
SELEGILINE HYDROCHLORIDE
Eldepryl Capsules 3208

COSOPT (Argentina, Australia, Brazil, Chile, Czech Republic, Greece, Hong Kong, Hungary, Irish Republic, New Zealand, Portugal, Singapore, Thailand, The Netherlands, Venezuela)
DORZOLAMIDE HYDROCHLORIDE
Trusopt Sterile Ophthalmic Solution 2095

COTAREG (Brazil, France, Italy)
VALSARTAN
Diovan Tablets 2193

CO-TAREG (Portugal)
VALSARTAN
Diovan Tablets 2193

COTAZYM (Canada, New Zealand)
PANCRELIPASE
Ultrase Capsules 708
Ultrase MT Capsules 709

COTAZYM S FORTE (Australia)
PANCRELIPASE
Ultrase Capsules 708
Ultrase MT Capsules 709

COTAZYM-S (The Netherlands)
PANCRELIPASE
Ultrase Capsules 708
Ultrase MT Capsules 709

COTREN (Hong Kong, Malaysia, Singapore, Thailand)
CLOTRIMAZOLE
Lotrimin Cream 3039
Lotrimin Lotion 1% 3039
Lotrimin Topical Solution 1% 3039

COTRISAN (Chile)
CLOTRIMAZOLE
Lotrimin Cream 3039
Lotrimin Lotion 1% 3039
Lotrimin Topical Solution 1% 3039

COULERGIN (Spain)
CETIRIZINE HYDROCHLORIDE
Zyrtec Syrup 2594
Zyrtec Tablets 2594

COUMADIN (Argentina, Australia, Brazil, Canada, Chile, Germany, Israel, Italy, Malaysia, Mexico, New Zealand, Singapore, South Africa, Venezuela)
WARFARIN SODIUM
Coumadin Tablets 898
Coumadin for Injection 898

COUMADINE (France)
WARFARIN SODIUM
Coumadin Tablets 898
Coumadin for Injection 898

CO-VALS (Spain)
HYDROCHLOROTHIAZIDE/VALSARTAN
Diovan HCT Tablets 2196

COVANCE (India)
LOSARTAN POTASSIUM
Cozaar Tablets 1935

CO-VASOCOR (Switzerland)
ENALAPRIL MALEATE
Vasotec I.V. Injection 2103

COVASTIN (Hong Kong, Malaysia, Singapore)
SIMVASTATIN
Zocor Tablets 2105

COVERENE (Argentina)
PERINDOPRIL ERBUMINE
Aceon Tablets (2 mg, 4 mg, 8 mg) 3194

COVEREX (Hungary, The Netherlands)
PERINDOPRIL ERBUMINE
Aceon Tablets (2 mg, 4 mg, 8 mg) 3194

COVEREX KOMB (Hungary)
PERINDOPRIL ERBUMINE
Aceon Tablets (2 mg, 4 mg, 8 mg) 3194

COVERSUM (Austria, Germany, Switzerland)
PERINDOPRIL ERBUMINE
Aceon Tablets (2 mg, 4 mg, 8 mg) 3194

COVERSUM COMBI (Germany, Switzerland)
PERINDOPRIL ERBUMINE
Aceon Tablets (2 mg, 4 mg, 8 mg) 3194

COVERSYL (Australia, Belgium, Brazil, Canada, Chile, Denmark, Finland, France, Greece, India, Irish Republic, Italy, Japan, Malaysia, Mexico, New Zealand, Portugal, Singapore, South Africa, Spain, Thailand, The Netherlands, United Kingdom, Venezuela)
PERINDOPRIL ERBUMINE
Aceon Tablets (2 mg, 4 mg, 8 mg) 3194

COVERSYL COMP (Denmark, Finland)
PERINDOPRIL ERBUMINE
Aceon Tablets (2 mg, 4 mg, 8 mg) 3194

COVERSYL PLUS (Australia, Belgium, Canada, India, Irish Republic, Malaysia, New Zealand, South Africa, The Netherlands, United Kingdom)
PERINDOPRIL ERBUMINE
Aceon Tablets (2 mg, 4 mg, 8 mg) 3194

COVOCEF-N (Greece)
CEFIXIME
Suprax 1843

COVOCORT (South Africa)
HYDROCORTISONE
Hydrocortone Tablets 1989

COVOSPOR (South Africa)
CLOTRIMAZOLE
Lotrimin Cream 3039
Lotrimin Lotion 1% 3039
Lotrimin Topical Solution 1% 3039

COVOSULF (South Africa)
SULFACETAMIDE SODIUM
Klaron Lotion 10% 2909

COXEL (Argentina)
CELECOXIB
Celebrex Capsules 3134

COXTENK (Argentina)
CELECOXIB
Celebrex Capsules 3134

COZAAR (Australia, Belgium, Brazil, Canada, Chile, Czech Republic, Denmark, Finland, France, Greece, Hong Kong, Hungary, Irish Republic, Malaysia, Mexico, New Zealand, Norway, Portugal, Russia, Singapore, South Africa, Spain, Sweden, Thailand, The Netherlands, United Kingdom, Venezuela)
LOSARTAN POTASSIUM
Cozaar Tablets 1935

COZAAR COMP (Denmark, Finland, Irish Republic, Norway, South Africa, Sweden, United Kingdom)
HYDROCHLOROTHIAZIDE/LOSARTAN POTASSIUM
Hyzaar 100-25 Tablets **1990**
Hyzaar 50-12.5 Tablets. **1990**

COZAAR PLUS (Belgium, Portugal, Spain, The Netherlands)
HYDROCHLOROTHIAZIDE/LOSARTAN POTASSIUM
Hyzaar 100-25 Tablets **1990**
Hyzaar 50-12.5 Tablets. **1990**

COZAAREX (Argentina)
LOSARTAN POTASSIUM
Cozaar Tablets **1935**

COZAAREX D (Argentina)
LOSARTAN POTASSIUM
Cozaar Tablets **1935**

COZEP (Thailand)
CHLORDIAZEPOXIDE HYDROCHLORIDE
Librium Capsules. **3347**

CP-CARBA (Hong Kong)
CARBAMAZEPINE
Carbatrol Capsules **3171**
Tegretol Chewable Tablets **2295**
Tegretol Suspension. **2295**
Tegretol Tablets **2295**
Tegretol-XR Tablets **2295**

CP-FURO (Hong Kong)
FUROSEMIDE
Furosemide Tablets **2154**

CP-METOLOL (Hong Kong)
METOPROLOL TARTRATE
Lopressor Tablets **2238**

CP-METOLOL CO (Hong Kong)
METOPROLOL TARTRATE
Lopressor Tablets **2238**

CP-THEO (Hong Kong)
THEOPHYLLINE
Uniphyl Tablets **2710**

CRAFILM (Italy)
SUCRALFATE
Carafate Suspension **701**
Carafate Tablets **701**

CRALSANIC (South Africa)
SUCRALFATE
Carafate Suspension **701**
Carafate Tablets **701**

CRANOC (Germany)
FLUVASTATIN SODIUM
Lescol Capsules **2233**

CRASNITIN (Germany, Italy, The Netherlands)
ASPARAGINASE
Elspar for Injection **2463**

CRASNITINE (Switzerland)
ASPARAGINASE
Elspar for Injection **2463**

CRAVERIL (Argentina)
FENOFIBRATE
Tricor Tablets **527**

CRAVIT (Hong Kong, Japan, Malaysia, Singapore)
LEVOFLOXACIN
Levaquin Injection **2384**
Levaquin Tablets **2384**

CREDAXOL (Mexico)
RANITIDINE HYDROCHLORIDE
Zantac 25 EFFERdose Tablets **1624**
Zantac 150 EFFERdose Tablets. **1624**
Zantac 150 Tablets **1624**
Zantac 300 Tablets **1624**
Zantac Injection **1619**
Zantac Injection Premixed **1619**
Zantac Syrup **1624**

CREMICORT-H (Belgium)
HYDROCORTISONE
Hydrocortone Tablets. **1989**

CREMINEM (Chile)
CLOTRIMAZOLE
Lotrimin Cream. **3039**
Lotrimin Lotion 1%. **3039**
Lotrimin Topical Solution 1% **3039**

CRIMA (Argentina)
CEFTAZIDIME
Fortaz for Injection **1453**

CRINONE (Argentina, Brazil, Canada, Chile, Denmark, Finland, Germany, Greece, Hong Kong, Irish Republic, Israel, Italy, Malaysia, Mexico, New Zealand, Norway, Portugal, Singapore, Spain, Sweden, Switzerland, Thailand, United Kingdom, Venezuela)
PROGESTERONE
Prometrium Capsules (100 mg, 200 mg) . **3203**

CRINOREN (Spain)
ENALAPRIL MALEATE
Vasotec I.V. Injection **2103**

CRISACIDE (Argentina)
CIPROFLOXACIN
Cipro Oral Suspension **2977**

CRISASMA (Argentina)
THEOPHYLLINE
Uniphyl Tablets **2710**

CRISAZET (Argentina)
ZIDOVUDINE
Retrovir Capsules **1560**
Retrovir IV Infusion. **1564**
Retrovir Syrup **1560**
Retrovir Tablets. **1560**

CRISMOL (Chile)
CLONAZEPAM
Klonopin Tablets **2778**

CRISOMET (Spain)
LAMOTRIGINE
Lamictal Chewable Dispersible Tablets . . . **1481**
Lamictal Tablets **1481**

CRISTACLAR (Argentina)
DONEPEZIL HYDROCHLORIDE
Aricept Tablets **1094**

CRISTAN (Singapore)
CLOTRIMAZOLE
Lotrimin Cream. **3039**
Lotrimin Lotion 1%. **3039**
Lotrimin Topical Solution 1% **3039**

CRISTERONA (Argentina)
ESTRADIOL
Climara Transdermal System **771**
Estring Vaginal Ring **2635**

CRIXAN (Malaysia, Singapore, Thailand)
CLARITHROMYCIN
Biaxin Filmtab Tablets **402**
Biaxin Granules **402**

CRIXIVAN (Argentina, Australia, Austria, Belgium, Brazil, Canada, Chile, Czech Republic, Denmark, Finland, France, Germany, Greece, Hong Kong, Irish Republic, Israel, Italy, Malaysia, Mexico, New Zealand, Norway, Portugal, Russia, Singapore, South Africa, Spain, Sweden, Switzerland, Thailand, The Netherlands, United Kingdom, Venezuela)
INDINAVIR SULFATE
Crixivan Capsules **1940**

CROMIDIN (Chile)
TACROLIMUS
Prograf Capsules and Injection **632**

CROMYCIN (Austria)
TOBRAMYCIN
TOBI Solution for Inhalation **2298**

CRONASMA (Germany)
THEOPHYLLINE
Uniphyl Tablets **2710**

CRONOCOL (Portugal)
GENTAMICIN SULFATE
Garamycin Injectable **3014**

CRONODINE (Spain)
DILTIAZEM HYDROCHLORIDE
Cardizem LA Extended Release Tablets. . . **1728**
Tiazac Capsules **1201**

CRONOL (Spain)
FAMOTIDINE
Pepcid Injection **2040**
Pepcid Injection Premixed **2040**
Pepcid Tablets **2038**
Pepcid for Oral Suspension **2038**

CRONOVERA (Brazil, Mexico, Venezuela)
VERAPAMIL HYDROCHLORIDE
Covera-HS Tablets **3139**
Verelan PM Extended-Release Capsules, Controlled-Onset **3106**

CROTAMITON H (Malaysia)
HYDROCORTISONE
Hydrocortone Tablets **1989**

CRYOMETASONA (Mexico)
DEXAMETHASONE
Decadron Tablets **1951**

CRYOPRIL (Mexico)
CAPTOPRIL
Captopril Tablets. **2149**

CRYOVAL (Mexico)
VALPROIC ACID
Depakene Capsules **417**
Depakene Oral Solution. **417**

CRYOZOL (Mexico)
METRONIDAZOLE
MetroGel-Vaginal Gel **1855**

CRYSANAL (Australia)
NAPROXEN SODIUM
Anaprox DS Tablets **2761**
Anaprox Tablets **2761**

CRYSTACIT (South Africa)
POTASSIUM CITRATE
Urocit-K Tablets. **2144**

CST (Thailand)
CLOTRIMAZOLE
Lotrimin Cream. **3039**
Lotrimin Lotion 1%. **3039**
Lotrimin Topical Solution 1% **3039**

CUADEL (Argentina)
DIAZEPAM
Diastat Rectal Delivery System **3343**
Valium Tablets **2819**

CUANTIN (Spain)
FAMOTIDINE
Pepcid Injection **2040**
Pepcid Injection Premixed **2040**
Pepcid Tablets **2038**
Pepcid for Oral Suspension **2038**

CUERPO AMARILLO FUERTE (Mexico)
PROGESTERONE
Prometrium Capsules (100 mg, 200 mg) . **3203**

CUNESIN (Spain)
CIPROFLOXACIN HYDROCHLORIDE
Ciloxan Ophthalmic Ointment . . . . ⊙**204, 559**
Ciloxan Ophthalmic Solution . . . . ⊙**206**
Cipro Tablets **2977**

CUPAX (Greece)
CEFUROXIME AXETIL
Ceftin Tablets **1407**
Ceftin for Oral Suspension **1407**

CUPRIMINE (Argentina, Brazil, Canada, Hong Kong, Israel, Norway, Sweden, Thailand, The Netherlands)
PENICILLAMINE
Cuprimine Capsules **1947**

CUPRIPEN (Argentina, Greece, Spain)
PENICILLAMINE
Cuprimine Capsules **1947**

CURACNE (France)
ISOTRETINOIN
Accutane Capsules **2731**

CURAM (Hong Kong, Malaysia, Venezuela)
AMOXICILLIN
Amoxil Pediatric Drops for Oral Suspension. **1343**
Amoxil Tablets **1343**

CURANTYL (Russia)
DIPYRIDAMOLE
Persantine Tablets **868**

CURANTYL N (Czech Republic, Germany)
DIPYRIDAMOLE
Persantine Tablets **868**

CURATANE (Israel)
ISOTRETINOIN
Accutane Capsules **2731**

CURBAN (Greece)
NIMODIPINE
Nimotop Capsules **749**

CURIOSIN (Czech Republic)
SODIUM HYALURONATE
Hyalgan Solution **2901**

CUROCEF (Austria, Chile)
CEFUROXIME SODIUM
Zinacef Injection **1631**

CUROXIM (Italy)
CEFUROXIME SODIUM
Zinacef Injection **1631**

CUROXIMA (Spain)
CEFUROXIME SODIUM
Zinacef Injection **1631**

CUROXIME (Portugal)
CEFUROXIME SODIUM
Zinacef Injection **1631**

CUSIMICINA (Spain)
ERYTHROMYCIN STEARATE
Erythrocin Stearate Filmtab Tablets **453**

CUSIMOLOL (Hong Kong, Hungary, Italy, Malaysia, Mexico, Portugal, Spain)
TIMOLOL MALEATE
Blocadren Tablets **1916**
Timoptic Sterile Ophthalmic Solution **2088**
Timoptic in Ocudose **2091**
Timoptic-XE Sterile Ophthalmic Gel Forming Solution **2092**

CUTACNYL (France)
BENZOYL PEROXIDE
Brevoxyl-4 Creamy Wash. **3210**
Brevoxyl-4 Gel **3210**
Brevoxyl-8 Creamy Wash. **3210**
Brevoxyl-8 Gel **3210**
Triaz Cleanser **1892**
Triaz Gel. **1892**

CUTADERM (South Africa)
HYDROCORTISONE
Hydrocortone Tablets. **1989**

CUTANUM (Germany)
ESTRADIOL
Climara Transdermal System **771**
Estring Vaginal Ring **2635**

CUTENOX (Brazil)
ENOXAPARIN SODIUM
Lovenox Injection **2915**

CUTIFITOL (Spain)
PROGESTERONE
Prometrium Capsules (100 mg, 200 mg) . **3203**

CUTISTAD (Germany, Switzerland)
CLOTRIMAZOLE
Lotrimin Cream. **3039**
Lotrimin Lotion 1%. **3039**
Lotrimin Topical Solution 1% **3039**

CUTIVAT (Denmark)
FLUTICASONE PROPIONATE
Cutivate Cream. **2662**
Cutivate Ointment **2665**
Flonase Nasal Spray **1440**

CUTIVATE (Argentina, Austria, Belgium, Czech Republic, Hong Kong, Hungary, Israel, Malaysia, Mexico, Portugal, Russia, Singapore, South Africa, Spain, Switzerland, The Netherlands, United Kingdom, Venezuela)
FLUTICASONE PROPIONATE
Cutivate Cream. **2662**
Cutivate Ointment **2665**
Flonase Nasal Spray **1440**

CUXAFENON (Germany)
PROPAFENONE HYDROCHLORIDE
Rythmol SR Capsules **2727**

CYCIN (Singapore)
CIPROFLOXACIN HYDROCHLORIDE
Ciloxan Ophthalmic Ointment . . . . ⊙**204, 559**
Ciloxan Ophthalmic Solution . . . . ⊙**206**
Cipro Tablets **2977**

CYCLOBIOL (Chile)
ESTRADIOL
Climara Transdermal System **771**
Estring Vaginal Ring **2635**

CYCLODERM (Austria)
ESTRADIOL
Climara Transdermal System **771**
Estring Vaginal Ring **2635**

(⊙ Described in PDR For Ophthalmic Medicines™)

CYCLOGEST (Hong Kong, Malaysia, Singapore, South Africa, Thailand, United Kingdom)
PROGESTERONE
Prometrium Capsules (100 mg, 200 mg) . 3203

CYCLORINE (India)
CYCLOSERINE
Seromycin Capsules. 1813

CYCLOSERINE (TM) (United Kingdom)
CYCLOSERINE
Seromycin Capsules. 1813

CYCRIN (Argentina, Brazil, Mexico)
MEDROXYPROGESTERONE ACETATE
Depo-Medrol Single-Dose Vial 2619

CYFLOX (Thailand)
CIPROFLOXACIN
Cipro Oral Suspension 2977

CYFLOXIN (Hong Kong)
CIPROFLOXACIN HYDROCHLORIDE
Ciloxan Ophthalmic Ointment . . . . ⊙204, 559
Ciloxan Ophthalmic Solution . . . . . ⊙206
Cipro Tablets 2977

CYKRINA (Finland, Sweden)
MEDROXYPROGESTERONE ACETATE
Depo-Medrol Single-Dose Vial 2619

CYLLIND (Germany)
CLARITHROMYCIN
Biaxin Filmtab Tablets. 402
Biaxin Granules 402

CYLOCORT (Brazil)
CIPROFLOXACIN HYDROCHLORIDE
Ciloxan Ophthalmic Ointment . . . . ⊙204, 559
Ciloxan Ophthalmic Solution . . . . . ⊙206
Cipro Tablets 2977

CYMALON CRANBERRY (United Kingdom)
POTASSIUM CITRATE
Urocit-K Tablets. 2144

CYNOMEL (Brazil, France, Greece, Mexico)
LIOTHYRONINE SODIUM
Cytomel Tablets 1710

CYPRAL (Venezuela)
CIPROFLOXACIN
Cipro Oral Suspension 2977

CYSTICIDE (Germany, South Africa)
PRAZIQUANTEL
Biltricide Tablets 2976

CYSTISTAT (Canada, United Kingdom)
SODIUM HYALURONATE
Hyalgan Solution 2901

CYSTOPURIN (Irish Republic, United Kingdom)
POTASSIUM CITRATE
Urocit-K Tablets. 2144

CYTAMID (Hungary)
FLUTAMIDE
Eulexin Capsules. 3009

CYTOMEL (Belgium, Canada, The Netherlands)
LIOTHYRONINE SODIUM
Cytomel Tablets 1710

CYTOMID (India)
FLUTAMIDE
Eulexin Capsules. 3009

CYTOSAFE (Germany)
FLUOROURACIL
Efudex Topical Cream. 3363
Efudex Topical Solutions 3363

CYZINE (Thailand)
CETIRIZINE HYDROCHLORIDE
Zyrtec Syrup 2594
Zyrtec Tablets 2594

DABENZOL (Mexico)
ALBENDAZOLE
Albenza Tablets. 1338

DABONAL (Spain)
ENALAPRIL MALEATE
Vasotec I.V. Injection 2103

DABROSON (Greece)
GENTAMICIN SULFATE
Garamycin Injectable 3014

DACALA (Spain)
AMOXICILLIN
Amoxil Pediatric Drops for Oral Suspension. 1343
Amoxil Tablets 1343

DACIN-F (Thailand)
CLINDAMYCIN HYDROCHLORIDE
Cleocin Vaginal Ovules 2616

DACLIN (New Zealand)
SULINDAC
Clinoril Tablets 1924

DACTEN (Argentina)
CANDESARTAN CILEXETIL
Atacand Tablets 649

DACTEN D (Argentina)
CANDESARTAN CILEXETIL
Atacand Tablets 649

DAFEX (Argentina)
LAMOTRIGINE
Lamictal Chewable Dispersible Tablets . . . 1481
Lamictal Tablets 1481

DAFLOXEN (Mexico)
NAPROXEN SODIUM
Anaprox DS Tablets 2761
Anaprox Tablets 2761

DAFLOXEN-F (Mexico)
NAPROXEN SODIUM
Anaprox DS Tablets 2761
Anaprox Tablets 2761

DAGOTIL (Chile)
RISPERIDONE
Risperdal Oral Solution 1676
Risperdal Tablets. 1676

DAIV (Argentina)
DIAZEPAM
Diastat Rectal Delivery System 3343
Valium Tablets 2819

DAKAR (Belgium)
LANSOPRAZOLE
Prevacid Delayed-Release Capsules 3271

DALACIN (Venezuela)
CLINDAMYCIN HYDROCHLORIDE
Cleocin Vaginal Ovules 2616

DALACIN C (Australia, Brazil, Czech Republic, Irish Republic, Malaysia, New Zealand, Russia)
CLINDAMYCIN HYDROCHLORIDE
Cleocin Vaginal Ovules 2616

DALACIN V (Brazil)
CLINDAMYCIN HYDROCHLORIDE
Cleocin Vaginal Ovules 2616

DALCAP (India)
CLINDAMYCIN HYDROCHLORIDE
Cleocin Vaginal Ovules 2616

DALGEX (Brazil)
ORPHENADRINE CITRATE
Norflex Injection 1856

DALMADORM (Brazil, Hong Kong, Singapore, Switzerland, The Netherlands)
FLURAZEPAM HYDROCHLORIDE
Dalmane Capsules. 3342

DALMANE (Canada, Irish Republic)
FLURAZEPAM HYDROCHLORIDE
Dalmane Capsules. 3342

DALTROID (Mexico)
LEVOTHYROXINE SODIUM
Levothroid Tablets 1186
Levoxyl Tablets 1712
Synthroid Tablets. 520

DALZAD (Greece)
VALSARTAN
Diovan Tablets 2193

DALZOLSTON (Brazil)
METRONIDAZOLE
MetroGel-Vaginal Gel 1855

DAMIDE (Italy)
INDAPAMIDE
Indapamide Tablets 2156

DAMOSAL (Mexico)
DIPYRIDAMOLE
Persantine Tablets 868

DANILAX (Denmark, Hong Kong)
LACTULOSE
Kristalose for Oral Solution 1034

DANILON (Venezuela)
NORFLOXACIN
Noroxin Tablets. 2032

DANKIT (Greece)
ERYTHROMYCIN
Ery-Tab Tablets 449
Erythromycin Base Filmtab Tablets. 455
Erythromycin Delayed-Release Capsules, USP 457
PCE Dispertab Tablets 515

DANLENE (Italy)
DANTROLENE SODIUM
Dantrium Capsules 2694
Dantrium Intravenous 2695

DANSSAN (Hong Kong)
ENALAPRIL MALEATE
Vasotec I.V. Injection 2103

DANTAMACRIN (Austria, Germany, Switzerland)
DANTROLENE SODIUM
Dantrium Capsules 2694
Dantrium Intravenous 2695

DANTENK (Argentina)
ONDANSETRON HYDROCHLORIDE
Zofran Injection. 1634
Zofran Injection Premixed 1634
Zofran Oral Solution. 1639
Zofran Tablets 1639

DANTRALEN (Spain)
DANTROLENE SODIUM
Dantrium Capsules 2694
Dantrium Intravenous 2695

DANTRIUM (Australia, Belgium, Canada, Chile, Denmark, France, Greece, Hong Kong, Irish Republic, Israel, Italy, New Zealand, Portugal, South Africa, The Netherlands, United Kingdom)
DANTROLENE SODIUM
Dantrium Capsules 2694
Dantrium Intravenous 2695

DANTROLEN (Brazil, Greece)
DANTROLENE SODIUM
Dantrium Capsules 2694
Dantrium Intravenous 2695

DANTRON (PREPARATION) (Thailand)
ONDANSETRON
Zofran ODT Orally Disintegrating Tablets . . 1639

DAPAMAX (South Africa)
INDAPAMIDE
Indapamide Tablets 2156

DAPA-TABS (Australia, Hong Kong)
INDAPAMIDE
Indapamide Tablets 2156

DAPRIL (Czech Republic, Russia, Singapore)
LISINOPRIL
Prinivil Tablets 2052

DAPROX (Denmark)
NAPROXEN
EC-Naprosyn Delayed-Release Tablets. . . . 2761
Naprosyn Suspension. 2761
Naprosyn Tablets 2761

DAPS (Argentina)
DAPSONE
Dapsone Tablets USP. 1673

DAPSODERM-X (Mexico)
DAPSONE
Dapsone Tablets USP. 1673

DAPTRIL (South Africa)
INDAPAMIDE
Indapamide Tablets 2156

DARALIX (South Africa)
PROMETHAZINE HYDROCHLORIDE
Phenergan Tablets and Suppositories 3440

DARAPRIM (Argentina, Australia, Austria, Belgium, Brazil, Canada, Chile, Germany, Irish Republic, Israel, Mexico, South Africa, Spain, Sweden, Switzerland, Thailand, The Netherlands, United Kingdom)
PYRIMETHAMINE
Daraprim Tablets. 1419

DARAPRIN (Brazil)
PYRIMETHAMINE
Daraprim Tablets. 1419

DARDEX (Spain)
CAPTOPRIL
Captopril Tablets. 2149

DAREN (Singapore)
ENALAPRIL MALEATE
Vasotec I.V. Injection 2103

DARI (Spain)
NIFEDIPINE
Adalat CC Tablets 2964

DARIC (Argentina)
FINASTERIDE
Propecia Tablets 2060
Proscar Tablets. 2067

DARMOL LACTULOSE (Austria)
LACTULOSE
Kristalose for Oral Solution 1034

DARSTIN (Spain)
PROGESTERONE
Prometrium Capsules (100 mg, 200 mg) . 3203

DARTROX (Mexico)
NAPROXEN
EC-Naprosyn Delayed-Release Tablets. . . . 2761
Naprosyn Suspension. 2761
Naprosyn Tablets 2761

DARZITIL (Argentina)
AMOXICILLIN
Amoxil Pediatric Drops for Oral Suspension. 1343
Amoxil Tablets 1343

DARZITIL SB (Argentina)
AMOXICILLIN
Amoxil Pediatric Drops for Oral Suspension. 1343
Amoxil Tablets 1343

DASKIL (Austria, Italy)
TERBINAFINE HYDROCHLORIDE
Lamisil Tablets 2232

DASKYL (Portugal)
TERBINAFINE HYDROCHLORIDE
Lamisil Tablets 2232

DASMETROL (Mexico)
METRONIDAZOLE
MetroGel-Vaginal Gel 1855

DASOLIN (Mexico)
METRONIDAZOLE
MetroGel-Vaginal Gel 1855

DATEVAN (Argentina)
PAROXETINE HYDROCHLORIDE
Paxil Oral Suspension. 1530
Paxil Tablets. 1530

DATRON (Spain)
ONDANSETRON HYDROCHLORIDE
Zofran Injection. 1634
Zofran Injection Premixed 1634
Zofran Oral Solution. 1639
Zofran Tablets 1639

DAVIXOLOL (Portugal)
BETAXOLOL HYDROCHLORIDE
Betoptic S Ophthalmic Suspension. ⊙203, 558

DAXOTEL (India, Thailand)
DOCETAXEL
Taxotere Injection Concentrate 2932

DAZID (Thailand)
TRIAMTERENE
Dyrenium Capsules 3400

DAZINE (Thailand)
THIORIDAZINE HYDROCHLORIDE
Thioridazine Hydrochloride Tablets. 2163

DAZOCAN (Mexico)
ALBENDAZOLE
Albenza Tablets. 1338

DAZOL (Brazil)
ALBENDAZOLE
Albenza Tablets. 1338

DAZOLIN (Argentina, Chile, Mexico)
NAPHAZOLINE HYDROCHLORIDE
Albalon Ophthalmic Solution . . . . . ⊙218

DAZOTRON (Argentina)
METRONIDAZOLE
MetroGel-Vaginal Gel 1855

(⊙ Described in PDR For Ophthalmic Medicines™)

D-CYCLOSERIN (Greece)
CYCLOSERINE
Seromycin Capsules. . . . 1813

DEALGIC (Italy)
DICLOFENAC SODIUM
Voltaren Tablets 2307
Voltaren-XR Tablets 2310

DEBAX (Austria)
CAPTOPRIL
Captopril Tablets. . . . 2149

DEBRIL (Argentina)
NAPROXEN
EC-Naprosyn Delayed-Release Tablets. . . . 2761
Naprosyn Suspension. . . . 2761
Naprosyn Tablets 2761

DECADRON (Brazil, Canada, France, Greece, Hong Kong, Irish Republic, Malaysia, Mexico, South Africa, Switzerland, Thailand, The Netherlands, United Kingdom, Venezuela)
DEXAMETHASONE
Decadron Tablets 1951

DECADRON CON CIPROFLOXINA (Argentina)
DEXAMETHASONE
Decadron Tablets 1951

DECADRON CON NISTATINA (Mexico)
DEXAMETHASONE
Decadron Tablets 1951

DECADRON CON TOBRAMICINA (Argentina)
DEXAMETHASONE
Decadron Tablets 1951

DECAN (Malaysia)
DEXAMETHASONE
Decadron Tablets 1951

DECDAN (India)
DEXAMETHASONE
Decadron Tablets 1951

DECIPAR (Spain)
ENOXAPARIN SODIUM
Lovenox Injection 2915

DECLOBAN (Spain)
CLOBETASOL PROPIONATE
Temovate Cream. . . . 2668
Temovate E Emollient. . . . 2671
Temovate Gel. . . . 2669
Temovate Ointment 2668
Temovate Scalp Application 2670

DECLOFON (Greece)
DICLOFENAC SODIUM
Voltaren Tablets 2307
Voltaren-XR Tablets 2310

DECOBEL (Venezuela)
DEXAMETHASONE
Decadron Tablets 1951

DECOFLUOR (Italy)
DEXAMETHASONE
Decadron Tablets 1951

DECOSIL (Mexico)
NAPROXEN SODIUM
Anaprox DS Tablets 2761
Anaprox Tablets 2761

DECOSTRIOL (Germany)
CALCITRIOL
Calcijex Injection 411
Rocaltrol Capsules. . . . 2798
Rocaltrol Oral Solution 2798

DEDILE (Argentina)
FLUTAMIDE
Eulexin Capsules. . . . 3009

DEDOLOR (Austria)
DICLOFENAC SODIUM
Voltaren Tablets 2307
Voltaren-XR Tablets 2310

DEFANAC (United Kingdom)
DICLOFENAC SODIUM
Voltaren Tablets 2307
Voltaren-XR Tablets 2310

DEFLAMAT (Austria, Italy, Switzerland)
DICLOFENAC SODIUM
Voltaren Tablets 2307
Voltaren-XR Tablets 2310

DEFLAMM (Austria)
DICLOFENAC SODIUM
Voltaren Tablets 2307
Voltaren-XR Tablets 2310

DEFLAMON (Czech Republic, Italy)
METRONIDAZOLE
MetroGel-Vaginal Gel 1855

DEFLAMOX (Mexico)
NAPROXEN SODIUM
Anaprox DS Tablets 2761
Anaprox Tablets 2761

DEFLAREN (Brazil)
DEXAMETHASONE
Decadron Tablets 1951

DEFLOX (Spain)
TERAZOSIN HYDROCHLORIDE
Hytrin Capsules. . . . 471

DEFLUIN (Argentina)
ENALAPRIL MALEATE
Vasotec I.V. Injection 2103

DEFLUIN PLUS (Argentina)
ENALAPRIL MALEATE
Vasotec I.V. Injection 2103

DEFUNGO (Thailand)
CLOTRIMAZOLE
Lotrimin Cream. . . . 3039
Lotrimin Lotion 1%. . . . 3039
Lotrimin Topical Solution 1% 3039

DEGEST 2 (Canada)
NAPHAZOLINE HYDROCHLORIDE
Albalon Ophthalmic Solution . . . . ⊙218

DEGRANOL (South Africa)
CARBAMAZEPINE
Carbatrol Capsules 3171
Tegretol Chewable Tablets. . . . 2295
Tegretol Suspension. . . . 2295
Tegretol Tablets 2295
Tegretol-XR Tablets 2295

DELEPTIN (Austria)
CARBAMAZEPINE
Carbatrol Capsules 3171
Tegretol Chewable Tablets. . . . 2295
Tegretol Suspension. . . . 2295
Tegretol Tablets 2295
Tegretol-XR Tablets 2295

DELIDOSE (France)
ESTRADIOL
Climara Transdermal System 771
Estring Vaginal Ring. . . . 2635

DELIMON (Greece)
DICLOFENAC SODIUM
Voltaren Tablets 2307
Voltaren-XR Tablets 2310

DELIX (Germany)
RAMIPRIL
Altace Capsules 1702

DELONAL (Germany, Switzerland)
ALCLOMETASONE DIPROPIONATE
Aclovate Cream 2660
Aclovate Ointment. . . . 2660

DELPHI (Belgium, The Netherlands)
TRIAMCINOLONE ACETONIDE
Azmacort Inhalation Aerosol. . . . 1726
Nasacort AQ Nasal Spray 2922

DELPHIMIX 1 (Germany)
DICLOFENAC SODIUM
Voltaren Tablets 2307
Voltaren-XR Tablets 2310

DELPHINAC (Germany)
DICLOFENAC SODIUM
Voltaren Tablets 2307
Voltaren-XR Tablets 2310

DELTA 80 (Italy)
BENZOYL PEROXIDE
Brevoxyl-4 Creamy Wash. . . . 3210
Brevoxyl-4 Gel 3210
Brevoxyl-8 Creamy Wash. . . . 3210
Brevoxyl-8 Gel 3210
Triaz Cleanser 1892
Triaz Gel. . . . 1892

DELTACEF (Italy)
CEFUROXIME SODIUM
Zinacef Injection 1631

DELTASORALEN (Irish Republic)
METHOXSALEN
Oxsoralen Lotion 1% 3352
Oxsoralen-Ultra Capsules. . . . 3353

DELTAZEN (France)
DILTIAZEM HYDROCHLORIDE
Cardizem LA Extended Release Tablets. . . 1728
Tiazac Capsules 1201

DELVAS (United Kingdom)
AMILORIDE HYDROCHLORIDE/HYDROCHLOROTHIAZIDE
Moduretic Tablets 2028

DEMIDERM (Venezuela)
ALCLOMETASONE DIPROPIONATE
Aclovate Cream 2660
Aclovate Ointment. . . . 2660

DEMSIL (Greece)
TERBINAFINE HYDROCHLORIDE
Lamisil Tablets 2232

DENACLOF (Greece)
DICLOFENAC SODIUM
Voltaren Tablets 2307
Voltaren-XR Tablets 2310

DENAN (Germany)
SIMVASTATIN
Zocor Tablets. . . . 2105

DENAPRIL (Portugal)
ENALAPRIL MALEATE
Vasotec I.V. Injection 2103

DENAXPREN (Spain)
NAPROXEN
EC-Naprosyn Delayed-Release Tablets. . . . 2761
Naprosyn Suspension. . . . 2761
Naprosyn Tablets 2761

DENAZOX (Thailand)
DILTIAZEM HYDROCHLORIDE
Cardizem LA Extended Release Tablets. . . 1728
Tiazac Capsules 1201

DENCORUB ANTI-INFLAMMATORY (Australia)
DICLOFENAC SODIUM
Voltaren Tablets 2307
Voltaren-XR Tablets 2310

DENERVAL (Portugal)
PAROXETINE HYDROCHLORIDE
Paxil Oral Suspension. . . . 1530
Paxil Tablets. . . . 1530

DENEX (Hong Kong, Malaysia, Singapore, Thailand)
METOPROLOL TARTRATE
Lopressor Tablets 2238

DENIREN (Mexico)
AMOXICILLIN
Amoxil Pediatric Drops for Oral Suspension. . . . 1343
Amoxil Tablets 1343

DENKACORT (Hong Kong)
TRIAMCINOLONE ACETONIDE
Azmacort Inhalation Aerosol. . . . 1726
Nasacort AQ Nasal Spray 2922

DENTOMYCIN (Germany)
CLINDAMYCIN HYDROCHLORIDE
Cleocin Vaginal Ovules 2616

DENULCER (Spain)
RANITIDINE HYDROCHLORIDE
Zantac 25 EFFERdose Tablets 1624
Zantac 150 EFFERdose Tablets. . . . 1624
Zantac 150 Tablets 1624
Zantac 300 Tablets 1624
Zantac Injection 1619
Zantac Injection Premixed 1619
Zantac Syrup 1624

DENVAR (Mexico, Spain)
CEFIXIME
Suprax 1843

DENZAPINE (United Kingdom)
CLOZAPINE
Clozaril Tablets. . . . 2184

DEPAKENE (Argentina, Brazil, Canada, Chile)
VALPROIC ACID
Depakene Capsules 417
Depakene Oral Solution. . . . 417

DEPAKINE ZUUR (The Netherlands)
VALPROIC ACID
Depakene Capsules 417
Depakene Oral Solution. . . . 417

DEPEN (Canada)
PENICILLAMINE
Cuprimine Capsules 1947

DEPESERT (Spain)
SERTRALINE HYDROCHLORIDE
Zoloft Tablets 2586

DEPICOR (India)
NIFEDIPINE
Adalat CC Tablets 2964

DEPIN (India)
NIFEDIPINE
Adalat CC Tablets 2964

DEPIN-E (Russia)
NIFEDIPINE
Adalat CC Tablets 2964

DEPO MODERIN (Spain)
METHYLPREDNISOLONE ACETATE
Depo-Medrol Injectable Suspension 2617

DEPO-CLINOVIR (Germany)
MEDROXYPROGESTERONE ACETATE
Depo-Medrol Single-Dose Vial 2619

DEPOCON (Austria)
MEDROXYPROGESTERONE ACETATE
Depo-Medrol Single-Dose Vial 2619

DEPO-GESTIN (Thailand)
MEDROXYPROGESTERONE ACETATE
Depo-Medrol Single-Dose Vial 2619

DEPO-MEDRATE (Germany)
METHYLPREDNISOLONE ACETATE
Depo-Medrol Injectable Suspension 2617

DEPO-MEDROL (Australia, Austria, Belgium, Brazil, Canada, Chile, Czech Republic, Denmark, Finland, France, Greece, Hong Kong, Hungary, India, Israel, Italy, Malaysia, Mexico, New Zealand, Norway, Portugal, Russia, South Africa, Sweden, Switzerland, Thailand, The Netherlands, Venezuela)
METHYLPREDNISOLONE ACETATE
Depo-Medrol Injectable Suspension 2617

DEPO-MEDRONE (Greece, Irish Republic, Sweden, United Kingdom)
METHYLPREDNISOLONE ACETATE
Depo-Medrol Injectable Suspension 2617

DEPO-NISOLONE (Australia)
METHYLPREDNISOLONE ACETATE
Depo-Medrol Injectable Suspension 2617

DEPO-PRODASONE (Chile, France)
MEDROXYPROGESTERONE ACETATE
Depo-Medrol Single-Dose Vial 2619

DEPO-PROGESNO (Thailand)
MEDROXYPROGESTERONE ACETATE
Depo-Medrol Single-Dose Vial 2619

DEPO-PROGESTA (Thailand)
MEDROXYPROGESTERONE ACETATE
Depo-Medrol Single-Dose Vial 2619

DEPO-PROGEVERA (Spain)
MEDROXYPROGESTERONE ACETATE
Depo-Medrol Single-Dose Vial 2619

DEPO-PROVERA (Argentina, Australia, Austria, Belgium, Brazil, Canada, Czech Republic, Denmark, Finland, France, Greece, Hong Kong, Hungary, India, Irish Republic, Israel, Italy, Malaysia, Mexico, New Zealand, Norway, Portugal, Russia, Singapore, South Africa, Sweden, Switzerland, Thailand, The Netherlands, United Kingdom, Venezuela)
MEDROXYPROGESTERONE ACETATE
Depo-Medrol Single-Dose Vial 2619

DEPO-RALOVERA (Australia)
MEDROXYPROGESTERONE ACETATE
Depo-Medrol Single-Dose Vial 2619

DEPRENYL (France, Germany)
SELEGILINE HYDROCHLORIDE
Eldepryl Capsules 3208

DEPRILAN (Brazil)
SELEGILINE HYDROCHLORIDE
Eldepryl Capsules 3208

DEPROCID (Chile)
METRONIDAZOLE
MetroGel-Vaginal Gel 1855

DEPUROL (Chile)
VENLAFAXINE HYDROCHLORIDE
Effexor Tablets ... 3411
Effexor XR Capsules ... 3417

DERALIN (Australia, Israel)
PROPRANOLOL HYDROCHLORIDE
Inderal LA Long-Acting Capsules ... 3429

DERCOME (Germany)
BENZOYL PEROXIDE
Brevoxyl-4 Creamy Wash ... 3210
Brevoxyl-4 Gel ... 3210
Brevoxyl-8 Creamy Wash ... 3210
Brevoxyl-8 Gel ... 3210
Triaz Cleanser ... 1892
Triaz Gel ... 1892

DERCUTANE (Spain)
ISOTRETINOIN
Accutane Capsules ... 2731

DERICIP (India)
THEOPHYLLINE
Uniphyl Tablets ... 2710

DERICIP PLUS (India)
THEOPHYLLINE
Uniphyl Tablets ... 2710

DERIPIL (Spain)
ERYTHROMYCIN
Ery-Tab Tablets ... 449
Erythromycin Base Filmtab Tablets ... 455
Erythromycin Delayed-Release Capsules, USP ... 457
PCE Dispertab Tablets ... 515

DERIVA (India)
ADAPALENE
Differin Gel ... 1211

DERIVA-C (India)
ADAPALENE
Differin Gel ... 1211

DERMABAZ (Hong Kong)
TRETINOIN
Vesanoid Capsules ... 2820

DERMACARE (Brazil)
CLOBETASOL PROPIONATE
Temovate Cream ... 2668
Temovate E Emollient ... 2671
Temovate Gel ... 2669
Temovate Ointment ... 2668
Temovate Scalp Application ... 2670

DERMACNE (Canada)
BENZOYL PEROXIDE
Brevoxyl-4 Creamy Wash ... 3210
Brevoxyl-4 Gel ... 3210
Brevoxyl-8 Creamy Wash ... 3210
Brevoxyl-8 Gel ... 3210
Triaz Cleanser ... 1892
Triaz Gel ... 1892

DERMACOM (Chile)
BUTENAFINE HYDROCHLORIDE
Mentax Cream ... 2158

DERMACORT (Finland, Hong Kong, Malaysia, Singapore, United Kingdom)
HYDROCORTISONE
Hydrocortone Tablets ... 1989

DERMADEX (Argentina)
CLOBETASOL PROPIONATE
Temovate Cream ... 2668
Temovate E Emollient ... 2671
Temovate Gel ... 2669
Temovate Ointment ... 2668
Temovate Scalp Application ... 2670

DERM-AID (Australia, Hong Kong, Malaysia, New Zealand, Singapore)
HYDROCORTISONE
Hydrocortone Tablets ... 1989

DERMAIROL (Sweden)
TRETINOIN
Vesanoid Capsules ... 2820

DERMALLERG (Germany)
HYDROCORTISONE
Hydrocortone Tablets ... 1989

DERMANCE (Canada)
BENZOYL PEROXIDE
Brevoxyl-4 Creamy Wash ... 3210
Brevoxyl-4 Gel ... 3210
Brevoxyl-8 Creamy Wash ... 3210
Brevoxyl-8 Gel ... 3210
Triaz Cleanser ... 1892
Triaz Gel ... 1892

DERMAORAL (Denmark)
ISOTRETINOIN
Accutane Capsules ... 2731

DERMAREST DRICORT ANTI-ITCH (Canada)
HYDROCORTISONE
Hydrocortone Tablets ... 1989

DERMASIL (Thailand)
CLOBETASOL PROPIONATE
Temovate Cream ... 2668
Temovate E Emollient ... 2671
Temovate Gel ... 2669
Temovate Ointment ... 2668
Temovate Scalp Application ... 2670

DERMASONE (Canada, Hong Kong)
CLOBETASOL PROPIONATE
Temovate Cream ... 2668
Temovate E Emollient ... 2671
Temovate Gel ... 2669
Temovate Ointment ... 2668
Temovate Scalp Application ... 2670

DERMASPRAY DEMANGEAISON (France)
HYDROCORTISONE
Hydrocortone Tablets ... 1989

DERMASTEN (Mexico)
CLOTRIMAZOLE
Lotrimin Cream ... 3039
Lotrimin Lotion 1% ... 3039
Lotrimin Topical Solution 1% ... 3039

DERMATEN (Thailand)
CLOTRIMAZOLE
Lotrimin Cream ... 3039
Lotrimin Lotion 1% ... 3039
Lotrimin Topical Solution 1% ... 3039

DERMATOVATE (Mexico)
CLOBETASOL PROPIONATE
Temovate Cream ... 2668
Temovate E Emollient ... 2671
Temovate Gel ... 2669
Temovate Ointment ... 2668
Temovate Scalp Application ... 2670

DERMATRANS (Chile)
ESTRADIOL
Climara Transdermal System ... 771
Estring Vaginal Ring ... 2635

DERMENET (Chile)
MOMETASONE FUROATE
Elocon Cream 0.1% ... 3005
Elocon Lotion 0.1% ... 3006
Elocon Ointment 0.1% ... 3007
Nasonex Nasal Spray ... 3043

DERMESTRIL (Australia, Austria, Belgium, Czech Republic, Finland, France, Germany, Greece, Hong Kong, Hungary, Irish Republic, Italy, Portugal, Spain, Switzerland, The Netherlands, United Kingdom)
ESTRADIOL
Climara Transdermal System ... 771
Estring Vaginal Ring ... 2635

DERMEXANE (Argentina)
CLOBETASOL PROPIONATE
Temovate Cream ... 2668
Temovate E Emollient ... 2671
Temovate Gel ... 2669
Temovate Ointment ... 2668
Temovate Scalp Application ... 2670

DERMIL (Denmark)
HYDROCORTISONE
Hydrocortone Tablets ... 1989

DERMIMADE HIDROCORTISONA (Portugal)
HYDROCORTISONE
Hydrocortone Tablets ... 1989

DERMINOIN (Greece)
ISOTRETINOIN
Accutane Capsules ... 2731

DERMO (Hong Kong)
CLOBETASOL PROPIONATE
Temovate Cream ... 2668
Temovate E Emollient ... 2671
Temovate Gel ... 2669
Temovate Ointment ... 2668
Temovate Scalp Application ... 2670

DERMO POSTERISAN (Germany)
HYDROCORTISONE
Hydrocortone Tablets ... 1989

DERMOBENE (Brazil)
CLOTRIMAZOLE
Lotrimin Cream ... 3039
Lotrimin Lotion 1% ... 3039
Lotrimin Topical Solution 1% ... 3039

DERMOCORTAL (Italy)
HYDROCORTISONE
Hydrocortone Tablets ... 1989

DERMODAN (Chile)
TRETINOIN
Vesanoid Capsules ... 2820

DERMOFENAC (France)
HYDROCORTISONE
Hydrocortone Tablets ... 1989

DERMOJUVENTUS (Spain)
TRETINOIN
Vesanoid Capsules ... 2820

DERMOL (New Zealand)
CLOBETASOL PROPIONATE
Temovate Cream ... 2668
Temovate E Emollient ... 2671
Temovate Gel ... 2669
Temovate Ointment ... 2668
Temovate Scalp Application ... 2670

DERMOPERATIVE (Argentina)
HYDROCORTISONE
Hydrocortone Tablets ... 1989

DERMORETIN (Brazil)
TRETINOIN
Vesanoid Capsules ... 2820

DERMOSOL (Malaysia, Singapore)
CLOBETASOL PROPIONATE
Temovate Cream ... 2668
Temovate E Emollient ... 2671
Temovate Gel ... 2669
Temovate Ointment ... 2668
Temovate Scalp Application ... 2670

DERMOSONA (Chile)
MOMETASONE FUROATE
Elocon Cream 0.1% ... 3005
Elocon Lotion 0.1% ... 3006
Elocon Ointment 0.1% ... 3007
Nasonex Nasal Spray ... 3043

DERMOVAGISIL (Spain)
LIDOCAINE
Lidoderm Patch ... 1118

DERMOVAL (France)
CLOBETASOL PROPIONATE
Temovate Cream ... 2668
Temovate E Emollient ... 2671
Temovate Gel ... 2669
Temovate Ointment ... 2668
Temovate Scalp Application ... 2670

DERMOVAT (Denmark, Finland, Norway, Sweden)
CLOBETASOL PROPIONATE
Temovate Cream ... 2668
Temovate E Emollient ... 2671
Temovate Gel ... 2669
Temovate Ointment ... 2668
Temovate Scalp Application ... 2670

DERMOVATE (Austria, Belgium, Canada, Chile, Czech Republic, Hong Kong, Hungary, Irish Republic, Israel, Malaysia, New Zealand, Portugal, Russia, Singapore, South Africa, Switzerland, Thailand, The Netherlands, United Kingdom, Venezuela)
CLOBETASOL PROPIONATE
Temovate Cream ... 2668
Temovate E Emollient ... 2671
Temovate Gel ... 2669
Temovate Ointment ... 2668
Temovate Scalp Application ... 2670

DERMOX (Mexico)
METHOXSALEN
Oxsoralen Lotion 1% ... 3352
Oxsoralen-Ultra Capsules ... 3353

DERMOXIN (Germany)
CLOBETASOL PROPIONATE
Temovate Cream ... 2668
Temovate E Emollient ... 2671
Temovate Gel ... 2669
Temovate Ointment ... 2668
Temovate Scalp Application ... 2670

DERMOXINALE (Germany)
CLOBETASOL PROPIONATE
Temovate Cream ... 2668
Temovate E Emollient ... 2671
Temovate Gel ... 2669
Temovate Ointment ... 2668
Temovate Scalp Application ... 2670

DERMOXYL (Canada, Chile)
BENZOYL PEROXIDE
Brevoxyl-4 Creamy Wash ... 3210
Brevoxyl-4 Gel ... 3210
Brevoxyl-8 Creamy Wash ... 3210
Brevoxyl-8 Gel ... 3210
Triaz Cleanser ... 1892
Triaz Gel ... 1892

DERONGA HEILPASTE (Germany)
NATAMYCIN
Natacyn Antifungal Ophthalmic Suspension ... ⊙208

DERONIL (Canada)
DEXAMETHASONE
Decadron Tablets ... 1951

DEROXAT (France, Switzerland)
PAROXETINE HYDROCHLORIDE
Paxil Oral Suspension ... 1530
Paxil Tablets ... 1530

DESALARK (Italy)
DEXAMETHASONE
Decadron Tablets ... 1951

DESAMIN SAME (Italy)
NAPHAZOLINE HYDROCHLORIDE
Albalon Ophthalmic Solution ... ⊙218

DESANDEN (Switzerland)
BENZOYL PEROXIDE
Brevoxyl-4 Creamy Wash ... 3210
Brevoxyl-4 Gel ... 3210
Brevoxyl-8 Creamy Wash ... 3210
Brevoxyl-8 Gel ... 3210
Triaz Cleanser ... 1892
Triaz Gel ... 1892

DESERONIL (Italy)
DEXAMETHASONE
Decadron Tablets ... 1951

DESIKEN (Mexico)
RIBAVIRIN
Virazole for Inhalation Solution ... 3370

DESINFLAM (Argentina)
DICLOFENAC SODIUM
Voltaren Tablets ... 2307
Voltaren-XR Tablets ... 2310

DESITAL (Norway)
CITALOPRAM HYDROBROMIDE
Celexa Tablets ... 1176

DESITICLOPIDIN (Germany)
TICLOPIDINE HYDROCHLORIDE
Ticlid Tablets ... 2810

DESQUAM-X (Canada)
BENZOYL PEROXIDE
Brevoxyl-4 Creamy Wash ... 3210
Brevoxyl-4 Gel ... 3210
Brevoxyl-8 Creamy Wash ... 3210
Brevoxyl-8 Gel ... 3210
Triaz Cleanser ... 1892
Triaz Gel ... 1892

DETENSOL (Canada)
PROPRANOLOL HYDROCHLORIDE
Inderal LA Long-Acting Capsules ... 3429

DETIDRON (Austria)
ETIDRONATE DISODIUM
Didronel Tablets ... 2697

DETROL (Canada)
TOLTERODINE TARTRATE
Detrol Tablets ... 2628

DETRUSITOL (Argentina, Austria, Belgium, Brazil, Chile, Czech Republic, Denmark, Finland, France, Germany, Greece, Hong Kong, Hungary, India, Irish Republic, Israel, Italy, Malaysia, Mexico, New Zealand, Norway, Portugal, Russia, Singapore, South Africa, Spain, Sweden, Switzerland, Thailand, The Netherlands, United Kingdom, Venezuela)
TOLTERODINE TARTRATE
Detrol Tablets ... 2628

DETSEL (Austria, The Netherlands)
TOLTERODINE TARTRATE
Detrol Tablets ... 2628

DEUCOVAL (Chile)
NAPROXEN SODIUM
Anaprox DS Tablets 2761
Anaprox Tablets 2761

DEXA TEOSONA (Argentina)
THEOPHYLLINE
Uniphyl Tablets 2710

DEXACAP (Hong Kong)
CAPTOPRIL
Captopril Tablets 2149

DEXACIP (India)
DEXAMETHASONE
Decadron Tablets 1951

DEXACLOR (Brazil)
DEXAMETHASONE
Decadron Tablets 1951

DEXACORT (Brazil)
DEXAMETHASONE
Decadron Tablets 1951

DEXACORTAL (Sweden)
DEXAMETHASONE
Decadron Tablets 1951

DEXACORTIN-K (Switzerland)
DEXAMETHASONE
Decadron Tablets 1951

DEXADEN (Brazil)
DEXAMETHASONE
Decadron Tablets 1951

DEXADUTIL (Mexico)
DEXAMETHASONE
Decadron Tablets 1951

DEXAFLAM (Germany)
DEXAMETHASONE
Decadron Tablets 1951

DEXAFLAN (Brazil)
DEXAMETHASONE
Decadron Tablets 1951

DEXAGALEN (Germany)
DEXAMETHASONE
Decadron Tablets 1951

DEXA-GENTAMICIN (Czech Republic)
DEXAMETHASONE
Decadron Tablets 1951

DEXAGREEN (Brazil)
DEXAMETHASONE
Decadron Tablets 1951

DEXAGRIN (Mexico)
DEXAMETHASONE
Decadron Tablets 1951

DEXAL (Mexico)
DEXAMETHASONE
Decadron Tablets 1951

DEXALOCAL (Hong Kong, Switzerland)
DEXAMETHASONE
Decadron Tablets 1951

DEXALTIN (Czech Republic, Malaysia, Singapore, Thailand)
DEXAMETHASONE
Decadron Tablets 1951

DEXAMED (Hong Kong, Russia, Singapore)
DEXAMETHASONE
Decadron Tablets 1951

DEXAMERAL (Argentina)
DEXAMETHASONE
Decadron Tablets 1951

DEXAMETAX (Brazil)
DEXAMETHASONE
Decadron Tablets 1951

DEXAMETONAL (Brazil)
DEXAMETHASONE
Decadron Tablets 1951

DEXAMETRAT (Brazil)
DEXAMETHASONE
Decadron Tablets 1951

DEXAMEX (Brazil)
DEXAMETHASONE
Decadron Tablets 1951

DEXAMILAN (Mexico)
DEXAMETHASONE
Decadron Tablets 1951

DEXAMINOR (Brazil)
DEXAMETHASONE
Decadron Tablets 1951

DEXAMISO (Spain)
DEXAMETHASONE
Decadron Tablets 1951

DEXAMONOZON (Germany)
DEXAMETHASONE
Decadron Tablets 1951

DEXAMONOZON N (Germany)
DEXAMETHASONE
Decadron Tablets 1951

DEXAMYCIN (Greece)
DEXAMETHASONE
Decadron Tablets 1951

DEXAMYTREX (Brazil, Greece)
GENTAMICIN SULFATE
Garamycin Injectable 3014

DEXANEOL (Venezuela)
DEXAMETHASONE
Decadron Tablets 1951

DEXANO (Thailand)
DEXAMETHASONE
Decadron Tablets 1951

DEXAPLAST (Spain)
DEXAMETHASONE
Decadron Tablets 1951

DEXAPOSTAFEN (Venezuela)
DEXAMETHASONE
Decadron Tablets 1951

DEXASONE (Canada, Hong Kong, India, Malaysia)
DEXAMETHASONE
Decadron Tablets 1951

DEXATAM (Mexico)
DEXAMETHASONE
Decadron Tablets 1951

DEXATOTAL (Argentina)
DEXAMETHASONE
Decadron Tablets 1951

DEXICAR (Mexico)
DEXAMETHASONE
Decadron Tablets 1951

DEXIRON (Canada)
IRON DEXTRAN
Infed Injection 3390

DEXIVEN (Argentina)
CALCITRIOL
Calcijex Injection 411
Rocaltrol Capsules 2798
Rocaltrol Oral Solution 2798

DEXMENE (Brazil)
DEXAMETHASONE
Decadron Tablets 1951

DEXMETHSONE (Australia, Hong Kong)
DEXAMETHASONE
Decadron Tablets 1951

DEXNE (Mexico)
DEXAMETHASONE
Decadron Tablets 1951

DEXNON (Spain)
LEVOTHYROXINE SODIUM
Levothroid Tablets 1186
Levoxyl Tablets 1712
Synthroid Tablets 520

DEXOLAN (Switzerland)
DEXAMETHASONE
Decadron Tablets 1951

DEXOMON (United Kingdom)
DICLOFENAC SODIUM
Voltaren Tablets 2307
Voltaren-XR Tablets 2310

DEXONA (Czech Republic, India, Mexico)
DEXAMETHASONE
Decadron Tablets 1951

DEXONA-D (Russia)
DEXAMETHASONE
Decadron Tablets 1951

DEXTONE (Mexico)
DEXAMETHASONE
Decadron Tablets 1951

DEZABIL (Mexico)
ALBENDAZOLE
Albenza Tablets 1338

DEZEPAN (Argentina)
DIAZEPAM
Diastat Rectal Delivery System 3343
Valium Tablets 2819

DHABESOL (Hong Kong, Malaysia, Singapore)
CLOBETASOL PROPIONATE
Temovate Cream 2668
Temovate E Emollient 2671
Temovate Gel 2669
Temovate Ointment 2668
Temovate Scalp Application 2670

DHACTULOSE (Singapore)
LACTULOSE
Kristalose for Oral Solution 1034

DI RETARD (Spain)
DICLOFENAC SODIUM
Voltaren Tablets 2307
Voltaren-XR Tablets 2310

DIABEN (Argentina)
ROSIGLITAZONE MALEATE
Avandia Tablets 1384

DIABESTAT (Chile)
PIOGLITAZONE HYDROCHLORIDE
Actos Tablets 3219

DIACARDIN (Italy)
DILTIAZEM HYDROCHLORIDE
Cardizem LA Extended Release Tablets . . . 1728
Tiazac Capsules 1201

DIACEPAM (Mexico)
DIAZEPAM
Diastat Rectal Delivery System 3343
Valium Tablets 2819

DIACEPLEX (Spain)
DIAZEPAM
Diastat Rectal Delivery System 3343
Valium Tablets 2819

DIACEPLEX SIMPLE (Spain)
DIAZEPAM
Diastat Rectal Delivery System 3343
Valium Tablets 2819

DIA-COLON (Italy)
LACTULOSE
Kristalose for Oral Solution 1034

DIACOR (France)
DILTIAZEM HYDROCHLORIDE
Cardizem LA Extended Release Tablets . . . 1728
Tiazac Capsules 1201

DIACORDIN (Czech Republic)
DILTIAZEM HYDROCHLORIDE
Cardizem LA Extended Release Tablets . . . 1728
Tiazac Capsules 1201

DIACTAL (Argentina)
DIAZEPAM
Diastat Rectal Delivery System 3343
Valium Tablets 2819

DIAGLIT (India)
PIOGLITAZONE HYDROCHLORIDE
Actos Tablets 3219

DIALAR (United Kingdom)
DIAZEPAM
Diastat Rectal Delivery System 3343
Valium Tablets 2819

DIANO (Thailand)
DIAZEPAM
Diastat Rectal Delivery System 3343
Valium Tablets 2819

DIAPAM (Finland, Thailand)
DIAZEPAM
Diastat Rectal Delivery System 3343
Valium Tablets 2819

DIAPANIL (Mexico)
DIAZEPAM
Diastat Rectal Delivery System 3343
Valium Tablets 2819

DIAPINE (Malaysia, Singapore, Thailand)
DIAZEPAM
Diastat Rectal Delivery System 3343
Valium Tablets 2819

DIAPO (Malaysia)
DIAZEPAM
Diastat Rectal Delivery System 3343
Valium Tablets 2819

DIAQUEL (South Africa)
DIAZEPAM
Diastat Rectal Delivery System 3343
Valium Tablets 2819

DIASTAT (Canada)
DIAZEPAM
Diastat Rectal Delivery System 3343
Valium Tablets 2819

DIASTONE (Argentina)
DICLOFENAC SODIUM
Voltaren Tablets 2307
Voltaren-XR Tablets 2310

DIATEX (Mexico)
DIAZEPAM
Diastat Rectal Delivery System 3343
Valium Tablets 2819

DIATIL (South Africa)
DILTIAZEM HYDROCHLORIDE
Cardizem LA Extended Release Tablets . . . 1728
Tiazac Capsules 1201

DIATRACIN (Spain)
VANCOMYCIN HYDROCHLORIDE
Vancocin HCl Capsules, USP 3380

DIAZ (Israel)
DIAZEPAM
Diastat Rectal Delivery System 3343
Valium Tablets 2819

DIAZEFAST (Brazil)
DIAZEPAM
Diastat Rectal Delivery System 3343
Valium Tablets 2819

DIAZELONG (Brazil)
DIAZEPAM
Diastat Rectal Delivery System 3343
Valium Tablets 2819

DIAZEM (Russia)
DILTIAZEM HYDROCHLORIDE
Cardizem LA Extended Release Tablets . . . 1728
Tiazac Capsules 1201

DIAZEMULS (Australia, Canada, Germany, Hong Kong, Irish Republic, Italy, The Netherlands, United Kingdom)
DIAZEPAM
Diastat Rectal Delivery System 3343
Valium Tablets 2819

DIAZEPAN (Brazil)
DIAZEPAM
Diastat Rectal Delivery System 3343
Valium Tablets 2819

DIBUTASONA (Mexico)
DEXAMETHASONE
Decadron Tablets 1951

DICEPIN B6 (Spain)
DIAZEPAM
Diastat Rectal Delivery System 3343
Valium Tablets 2819

DICIL (Chile)
TERBINAFINE HYDROCHLORIDE
Lamisil Tablets 2232

DICLAC (Australia, Austria, Brazil, Germany, Hungary, Irish Republic, Mexico, Switzerland)
DICLOFENAC SODIUM
Voltaren Tablets 2307
Voltaren-XR Tablets 2310

DICLAX (New Zealand)
DICLOFENAC SODIUM
Voltaren Tablets 2307
Voltaren-XR Tablets 2310

DICLAXOL (Austria)
DICLOFENAC SODIUM
Voltaren Tablets 2307
Voltaren-XR Tablets 2310

DICLO (Irish Republic, Switzerland)
DICLOFENAC SODIUM
Voltaren Tablets 2307
Voltaren-XR Tablets 2310

DICLO-ATTRITIN (Germany)
DICLOFENAC SODIUM
Voltaren Tablets 2307
Voltaren-XR Tablets 2310

DICLO-BASAN (Switzerland)
DICLOFENAC SODIUM
Voltaren Tablets 2307

Voltaren-XR Tablets 2310

DICLOBENE (Russia)
DICLOFENAC SODIUM
Voltaren Tablets 2307
Voltaren-XR Tablets 2310

DICLOBERL (Germany, Russia)
DICLOFENAC SODIUM
Voltaren Tablets 2307
Voltaren-XR Tablets 2310

DICLOCULAR (Italy)
DICLOFENAC SODIUM
Voltaren Tablets 2307
Voltaren-XR Tablets 2310

DICLO-DENK (Hong Kong, Singapore)
DICLOFENAC SODIUM
Voltaren Tablets 2307
Voltaren-XR Tablets 2310

DICLO-DIVIDO (Germany)
DICLOFENAC SODIUM
Voltaren Tablets 2307
Voltaren-XR Tablets 2310

DICLODOC (Germany)
DICLOFENAC SODIUM
Voltaren Tablets 2307
Voltaren-XR Tablets 2310

DICLODOL (Italy)
DICLOFENAC SODIUM
Voltaren Tablets 2307
Voltaren-XR Tablets 2310

DICLO-F (Russia)
DICLOFENAC SODIUM
Voltaren Tablets 2307
Voltaren-XR Tablets 2310

DICLOFAN (Italy)
DICLOFENAC SODIUM
Voltaren Tablets 2307
Voltaren-XR Tablets 2310

DICLOFEN (Czech Republic, Thailand)
DICLOFENAC SODIUM
Voltaren Tablets 2307
Voltaren-XR Tablets 2310

DICLOFENBETA (Germany)
DICLOFENAC SODIUM
Voltaren Tablets 2307
Voltaren-XR Tablets 2310

DICLOFLAM (South Africa)
DICLOFENAC SODIUM
Voltaren Tablets 2307
Voltaren-XR Tablets 2310

DICLOFLEX (United Kingdom)
DICLOFENAC SODIUM
Voltaren Tablets 2307
Voltaren-XR Tablets 2310

DICLOFTAL (Portugal)
DICLOFENAC SODIUM
Voltaren Tablets 2307
Voltaren-XR Tablets 2310

DICLOFTIL (Italy)
DICLOFENAC SODIUM
Voltaren Tablets 2307
Voltaren-XR Tablets 2310

DICLOGEA (Denmark)
DICLOFENAC SODIUM
Voltaren Tablets 2307
Voltaren-XR Tablets 2310

DICLO-GEL (Germany)
DICLOFENAC SODIUM
Voltaren Tablets 2307
Voltaren-XR Tablets 2310

DICLOGENOM (Brazil)
DICLOFENAC SODIUM
Voltaren Tablets 2307
Voltaren-XR Tablets 2310

DICLOGENTA (India)
DICLOFENAC SODIUM
Voltaren Tablets 2307
Voltaren-XR Tablets 2310

DICLOGESIC (Hong Kong)
DICLOFENAC SODIUM
Voltaren Tablets 2307
Voltaren-XR Tablets 2310

DICLOGESIC RELAX (Argentina)
DICLOFENAC SODIUM
Voltaren Tablets 2307
Voltaren-XR Tablets 2310

DICLOGRUN (Germany)
DICLOFENAC SODIUM
Voltaren Tablets 2307
Voltaren-XR Tablets 2310

DICLOHEXAL (Australia, New Zealand)
DICLOFENAC SODIUM
Voltaren Tablets 2307
Voltaren-XR Tablets 2310

DICLOLAN (Thailand)
DICLOFENAC SODIUM
Voltaren Tablets 2307
Voltaren-XR Tablets 2310

DICLOMAX (Irish Republic, United Kingdom)
DICLOFENAC SODIUM
Voltaren Tablets 2307
Voltaren-XR Tablets 2310

DICLOMEL (Hungary, Irish Republic)
DICLOFENAC SODIUM
Voltaren Tablets 2307
Voltaren-XR Tablets 2310

DICLOMELAN (Austria)
DICLOFENAC SODIUM
Voltaren Tablets 2307
Voltaren-XR Tablets 2310

DICLOMERCK (Germany)
DICLOFENAC SODIUM
Voltaren Tablets 2307
Voltaren-XR Tablets 2310

DICLOMETIN (Finland)
DICLOFENAC SODIUM
Voltaren Tablets 2307
Voltaren-XR Tablets 2310

DICLOMOL (India)
DICLOFENAC SODIUM
Voltaren Tablets 2307
Voltaren-XR Tablets 2310

DICLON (Denmark)
DICLOFENAC SODIUM
Voltaren Tablets 2307
Voltaren-XR Tablets 2310

DICLONAC (India)
DICLOFENAC SODIUM
Voltaren Tablets 2307
Voltaren-XR Tablets 2310

DICLONACO (Brazil)
DICLOFENAC SODIUM
Voltaren Tablets 2307
Voltaren-XR Tablets 2310

DICLONAT (Russia)
DICLOFENAC SODIUM
Voltaren Tablets 2307
Voltaren-XR Tablets 2310

DICLONATRIUM (Brazil)
DICLOFENAC SODIUM
Voltaren Tablets 2307
Voltaren-XR Tablets 2310

DICLO-OPT (Germany)
DICLOFENAC SODIUM
Voltaren Tablets 2307
Voltaren-XR Tablets 2310

DICLOPHLOGONT (Germany, Greece)
DICLOFENAC SODIUM
Voltaren Tablets 2307
Voltaren-XR Tablets 2310

DICLO-PUREN (Germany)
DICLOFENAC SODIUM
Voltaren Tablets 2307
Voltaren-XR Tablets 2310

DICLORAN (Mexico)
DICLOFENAC SODIUM
Voltaren Tablets 2307
Voltaren-XR Tablets 2310

DICLORAN-A (India)
DICLOFENAC SODIUM
Voltaren Tablets 2307
Voltaren-XR Tablets 2310

DICLOREKTAL (Germany)
DICLOFENAC SODIUM
Voltaren Tablets 2307
Voltaren-XR Tablets 2310

DICLORENGEL (Israel)
DICLOFENAC SODIUM
Voltaren Tablets 2307
Voltaren-XR Tablets 2310

DICLOREUM (Czech Republic)
DICLOFENAC SODIUM
Voltaren Tablets 2307
Voltaren-XR Tablets 2310

DICLO-SAAR (Germany)
DICLOFENAC SODIUM
Voltaren Tablets 2307
Voltaren-XR Tablets 2310

DICLOSIAN (Thailand)
DICLOFENAC SODIUM
Voltaren Tablets 2307
Voltaren-XR Tablets 2310

DICLOSIFAR (Switzerland)
DICLOFENAC SODIUM
Voltaren Tablets 2307
Voltaren-XR Tablets 2310

DICLOSOD (Brazil)
DICLOFENAC SODIUM
Voltaren Tablets 2307
Voltaren-XR Tablets 2310

DICLOSODICO (Brazil)
DICLOFENAC SODIUM
Voltaren Tablets 2307
Voltaren-XR Tablets 2310

DICLO-SPONDYRIL (Germany)
DICLOFENAC SODIUM
Voltaren Tablets 2307
Voltaren-XR Tablets 2310

DICLOSTAD (Austria)
DICLOFENAC SODIUM
Voltaren Tablets 2307
Voltaren-XR Tablets 2310

DICLOSTAN (Venezuela)
DICLOFENAC SODIUM
Voltaren Tablets 2307
Voltaren-XR Tablets 2310

DICLOSYL (Austria)
DICLOFENAC SODIUM
Voltaren Tablets 2307
Voltaren-XR Tablets 2310

DICLO-TABLINEN (Germany)
DICLOFENAC SODIUM
Voltaren Tablets 2307
Voltaren-XR Tablets 2310

DICLOTARD (United Kingdom)
DICLOFENAC SODIUM
Voltaren Tablets 2307
Voltaren-XR Tablets 2310

DICLOTAREN (Chile)
DICLOFENAC SODIUM
Voltaren Tablets 2307
Voltaren-XR Tablets 2310

DICLOTEARS (Italy)
DICLOFENAC SODIUM
Voltaren Tablets 2307
Voltaren-XR Tablets 2310

DICLOTEC (Canada, Portugal)
DICLOFENAC SODIUM
Voltaren Tablets 2307
Voltaren-XR Tablets 2310

DICLOVIT (Russia)
DICLOFENAC SODIUM
Voltaren Tablets 2307
Voltaren-XR Tablets 2310

DICLOVOL (United Kingdom)
DICLOFENAC SODIUM
Voltaren Tablets 2307
Voltaren-XR Tablets 2310

DICLOWAL (Hong Kong, Singapore)
DICLOFENAC SODIUM
Voltaren Tablets 2307
Voltaren-XR Tablets 2310

DICLOZIP (United Kingdom)
DICLOFENAC SODIUM
Voltaren Tablets 2307
Voltaren-XR Tablets 2310

DIDAMOL (Belgium)
DIPYRIDAMOLE
Persantine Tablets 868

DIDRONATE (Denmark, Finland, Norway, Sweden)
ETIDRONATE DISODIUM
Didronel Tablets 2697

DIDRONEL (Australia, Austria, Belgium, Canada, France, Germany, Hong Kong, Irish Republic, Israel, Italy, Japan, New Zealand, Portugal, South Africa, Switzerland, The Netherlands, United Kingdom)
ETIDRONATE DISODIUM
Didronel Tablets 2697

DIENPAX (Brazil)
DIAZEPAM
Diastat Rectal Delivery System 3343
Valium Tablets 2819

DIFEN (Thailand)
DICLOFENAC SODIUM
Voltaren Tablets 2307
Voltaren-XR Tablets 2310

DIFENA (Hong Kong)
DICLOFENAC SODIUM
Voltaren Tablets 2307
Voltaren-XR Tablets 2310

DIFENAC (Argentina, Hong Kong, Singapore, South Africa, Thailand, Venezuela)
DICLOFENAC SODIUM
Voltaren Tablets 2307
Voltaren-XR Tablets 2310

DIFENAN (Brazil)
DICLOFENAC SODIUM
Voltaren Tablets 2307
Voltaren-XR Tablets 2310

DIFEND (Greece)
DICLOFENAC SODIUM
Voltaren Tablets 2307
Voltaren-XR Tablets 2310

DIFENE (Austria, Irish Republic)
DICLOFENAC SODIUM
Voltaren Tablets 2307
Voltaren-XR Tablets 2310

DIFENET (Denmark)
DICLOFENAC SODIUM
Voltaren Tablets 2307
Voltaren-XR Tablets 2310

DIFENO (Thailand)
DICLOFENAC SODIUM
Voltaren Tablets 2307
Voltaren-XR Tablets 2310

DIFENOL (Hong Kong)
DICLOFENAC SODIUM
Voltaren Tablets 2307
Voltaren-XR Tablets 2310

DIFERBEST (Mexico)
NAPROXEN SODIUM
Anaprox DS Tablets 2761
Anaprox Tablets 2761

DIFFERIN (Argentina, Australia, Austria, Belgium, Brazil, Canada, Chile, Finland, Germany, Hong Kong, Hungary, Irish Republic, Italy, Malaysia, New Zealand, Norway, Portugal, Russia, Singapore, South Africa, Sweden, Switzerland, Thailand, United Kingdom, Venezuela)
ADAPALENE
Differin Gel 1211

DIFFERINE (Czech Republic, France, Spain)
ADAPALENE
Differin Gel 1211

DIFFU-K (France)
POTASSIUM CHLORIDE
K-Dur Extended-Release Tablets 3033
K-Lor Oral Solution. 474
K-Tab Tablets 475

DIFFUMAL (Italy)
THEOPHYLLINE
Uniphyl Tablets 2710

DIFIX (Italy)
CALCITRIOL
Calcijex Injection 411
Rocaltrol Capsules. 2798
Rocaltrol Oral Solution 2798

DIFLERIX (Hong Kong, Malaysia)
INDAPAMIDE
Indapamide Tablets 2156

DIFLONID (Denmark, Norway, Sweden)
DIFLUNISAL
Dolobid Tablets 1955

DIFLUDOL (Italy)
DIFLUNISAL
Dolobid Tablets 1955

DIFLUNIL (Italy)
DIFLUNISAL
Dolobid Tablets 1955

DIFLUSAL (Belgium)
DIFLUNISAL
Dolobid Tablets 1955

DIFLUSAN (Italy)
DIFLUNISAL
Dolobid Tablets 1955

DIFNAL (Singapore)
DICLOFENAC SODIUM
Voltaren Tablets 2307
Voltaren-XR Tablets 2310

DIFOSFEN (Argentina, Singapore, Spain)
ETIDRONATE DISODIUM
Didronel Tablets 2697

DIFOXACIL (Mexico)
NORFLOXACIN
Noroxin Tablets 2032

DIGACIN (Germany)
DIGOXIN
Lanoxicaps Capsules 1490
Lanoxin Injection 1494
Lanoxin Injection Pediatric 1497
Lanoxin Tablets 1500

DIGAOL (France)
TIMOLOL MALEATE
Blocadren Tablets 1916
Timoptic Sterile Ophthalmic Solution 2088
Timoptic in Ocudose 2091
Timoptic-XE Sterile Ophthalmic Gel Forming Solution 2092

DIGARIL (Spain)
FLUVASTATIN SODIUM
Lescol Capsules 2233

DIGENAC (United Kingdom)
DICLOFENAC SODIUM
Voltaren Tablets 2307
Voltaren-XR Tablets 2310

DIGERVIN (Spain)
FAMOTIDINE
Pepcid Injection 2040
Pepcid Injection Premixed 2040
Pepcid Tablets 2038
Pepcid for Oral Suspension 2038

DIGESS (Canada)
PANCRELIPASE
Ultrase Capsules 708
Ultrase MT Capsules 709

DIGESTOSAN (Austria)
RANITIDINE HYDROCHLORIDE
Zantac 25 EFFERdose Tablets 1624
Zantac 150 EFFERdose Tablets 1624
Zantac 150 Tablets 1624
Zantac 300 Tablets 1624
Zantac Injection 1619
Zantac Injection Premixed 1619
Zantac Syrup 1624

DIGEZANOL (Mexico)
ALBENDAZOLE
Albenza Tablets 1338

DIGITAX (Brazil)
DIGOXIN
Lanoxicaps Capsules 1490
Lanoxin Injection 1494
Lanoxin Injection Pediatric 1497
Lanoxin Tablets 1500

DIGIXINA (Brazil)
DIGOXIN
Lanoxicaps Capsules 1490
Lanoxin Injection 1494
Lanoxin Injection Pediatric 1497
Lanoxin Tablets 1500

DIGNOFENAC (Chile, Germany)
DICLOFENAC SODIUM
Voltaren Tablets 2307
Voltaren-XR Tablets 2310

DIGNOKONSTANT (Germany)
NIFEDIPINE
Adalat CC Tablets 2964

DIGNOMETOPROL (Germany)
METOPROLOL TARTRATE
Lopressor Tablets 2238

DIGNORETIK (Germany)
AMILORIDE HYDROCHLORIDE/HYDROCHLOROTHIAZIDE
Moduretic Tablets 2028

DIGNOTRIMAZOL (Germany)
CLOTRIMAZOLE
Lotrimin Cream 3039
Lotrimin Lotion 1% 3039
Lotrimin Topical Solution 1% 3039

DIGNOVER (Germany)
VERAPAMIL HYDROCHLORIDE
Covera-HS Tablets 3139
Verelan PM Extended-Release Capsules, Controlled-Onset 3106

DIGOCARD-G (Argentina)
DIGOXIN
Lanoxicaps Capsules 1490
Lanoxin Injection 1494
Lanoxin Injection Pediatric 1497
Lanoxin Tablets 1500

DIGOMAL (Italy)
DIGOXIN
Lanoxicaps Capsules 1490
Lanoxin Injection 1494
Lanoxin Injection Pediatric 1497
Lanoxin Tablets 1500

DIGOREGEN (Germany)
DIGOXIN
Lanoxicaps Capsules 1490
Lanoxin Injection 1494
Lanoxin Injection Pediatric 1497
Lanoxin Tablets 1500

DIGOSIN (Japan)
DIGOXIN
Lanoxicaps Capsules 1490
Lanoxin Injection 1494
Lanoxin Injection Pediatric 1497
Lanoxin Tablets 1500

DIGOX (Brazil)
DIGOXIN
Lanoxicaps Capsules 1490
Lanoxin Injection 1494
Lanoxin Injection Pediatric 1497
Lanoxin Tablets 1500

DIGOXAN (Brazil)
DIGOXIN
Lanoxicaps Capsules 1490
Lanoxin Injection 1494
Lanoxin Injection Pediatric 1497
Lanoxin Tablets 1500

DIGOXEN (Brazil)
DIGOXIN
Lanoxicaps Capsules 1490
Lanoxin Injection 1494
Lanoxin Injection Pediatric 1497
Lanoxin Tablets 1500

DIGOXIL (Brazil)
DIGOXIN
Lanoxicaps Capsules 1490
Lanoxin Injection 1494
Lanoxin Injection Pediatric 1497
Lanoxin Tablets 1500

DILABAR (Spain)
CAPTOPRIL
Captopril Tablets 2149

DILACARD (Brazil)
VERAPAMIL HYDROCHLORIDE
Covera-HS Tablets 3139
Verelan PM Extended-Release Capsules, Controlled-Onset 3106

DILACLAN (Spain)
DILTIAZEM HYDROCHLORIDE
Cardizem LA Extended Release Tablets . . . 1728
Tiazac Capsules 1201

DILACOR (Brazil)
VERAPAMIL HYDROCHLORIDE
Covera-HS Tablets 3139
Verelan PM Extended-Release Capsules, Controlled-Onset 3106

DILACORAN (Mexico)
VERAPAMIL HYDROCHLORIDE
Covera-HS Tablets 3139
Verelan PM Extended-Release Capsules, Controlled-Onset 3106

DILACORON (Brazil)
VERAPAMIL HYDROCHLORIDE
Covera-HS Tablets 3139
Verelan PM Extended-Release Capsules, Controlled-Onset 3106

DILADEL (Italy)
DILTIAZEM HYDROCHLORIDE
Cardizem LA Extended Release Tablets . . . 1728
Tiazac Capsules 1201

DILAFLUX (Brazil)
NIFEDIPINE
Adalat CC Tablets 2964

DILAHIM (Argentina)
DILTIAZEM HYDROCHLORIDE
Cardizem LA Extended Release Tablets . . . 1728
Tiazac Capsules 1201

DILAMAX (Portugal)
SALMETEROL XINAFOATE
Serevent Diskus 1568

DILANACIN (Germany)
DIGOXIN
Lanoxicaps Capsules 1490
Lanoxin Injection 1494
Lanoxin Injection Pediatric 1497
Lanoxin Tablets 1500

DILAPLUS (Austria)
CARVEDILOL
Coreg Tablets 1414

DILATAM (Israel, South Africa, Thailand)
DILTIAZEM HYDROCHLORIDE
Cardizem LA Extended Release Tablets . . . 1728
Tiazac Capsules 1201

DILATAME (Austria)
DILTIAZEM HYDROCHLORIDE
Cardizem LA Extended Release Tablets . . . 1728
Tiazac Capsules 1201

DILATOL (Portugal)
ISRADIPINE
DynaCirc CR Tablets 2721

DILATREND (Argentina, Australia, Austria, Brazil, Chile, Czech Republic, Germany, Greece, Hong Kong, Hungary, Italy, Mexico, New Zealand, Norway, Singapore, South Africa, Switzerland, Thailand, Venezuela)
CARVEDILOL
Coreg Tablets 1414

DILAUDID (Australia, Austria, Canada, Germany, Irish Republic, New Zealand)
HYDROMORPHONE HYDROCHLORIDE
Dilaudid Ampules 440
Dilaudid Multiple Dose Vials 440
Dilaudid Non-Sterile Powder 440
Dilaudid Oral Liquid 445
Dilaudid Rectal Suppositories 440
Dilaudid Tablets 440
Dilaudid Tablets - 8 mg 445
Dilaudid-HP Injection 442
Dilaudid-HP Lyophilized Powder 250 mg . . . 442

DILBLOC (Portugal)
CARVEDILOL
Coreg Tablets 1414

DILCARD (New Zealand)
DILTIAZEM HYDROCHLORIDE
Cardizem LA Extended Release Tablets . . . 1728
Tiazac Capsules 1201

DILCARDIA (India, Russia, United Kingdom)
DILTIAZEM HYDROCHLORIDE
Cardizem LA Extended Release Tablets . . . 1728
Tiazac Capsules 1201

DILCEREN (Czech Republic)
NIMODIPINE
Nimotop Capsules 749

DILCONTIN (India)
DILTIAZEM HYDROCHLORIDE
Cardizem LA Extended Release Tablets . . . 1728
Tiazac Capsules 1201

DILCOR (Denmark, Spain)
DILTIAZEM HYDROCHLORIDE
Cardizem LA Extended Release Tablets . . . 1728
Tiazac Capsules 1201

DILEM (Hong Kong, Italy, Malaysia)
DILTIAZEM HYDROCHLORIDE
Cardizem LA Extended Release Tablets . . . 1728
Tiazac Capsules 1201

DILETAN (Portugal)
SUMATRIPTAN SUCCINATE
Imitrex Injection 1463
Imitrex Tablets 1471

DILFAR (Portugal)
DILTIAZEM HYDROCHLORIDE
Cardizem LA Extended Release Tablets . . . 1728
Tiazac Capsules 1201

DILGARD (India)
DILTIAZEM HYDROCHLORIDE
Cardizem LA Extended Release Tablets . . . 1728
Tiazac Capsules 1201

DILITER (Italy)
DILTIAZEM HYDROCHLORIDE
Cardizem LA Extended Release Tablets . . . 1728
Tiazac Capsules 1201

DILIZEM (Singapore, Thailand)
DILTIAZEM HYDROCHLORIDE
Cardizem LA Extended Release Tablets . . . 1728
Tiazac Capsules 1201

DILMIN (Finland)
DILTIAZEM HYDROCHLORIDE
Cardizem LA Extended Release Tablets . . . 1728
Tiazac Capsules 1201

DILOC (The Netherlands)
DILTIAZEM HYDROCHLORIDE
Cardizem LA Extended Release Tablets . . . 1728
Tiazac Capsules 1201

DILONGO (Portugal)
DILTIAZEM HYDROCHLORIDE
Cardizem LA Extended Release Tablets . . . 1728
Tiazac Capsules 1201

DILPRAL (Finland)
DILTIAZEM HYDROCHLORIDE
Cardizem LA Extended Release Tablets . . . 1728
Tiazac Capsules 1201

DILRENE (France, Hungary)
DILTIAZEM HYDROCHLORIDE
Cardizem LA Extended Release Tablets . . . 1728
Tiazac Capsules 1201

DILSAL (Germany)
DILTIAZEM HYDROCHLORIDE
Cardizem LA Extended Release Tablets . . . 1728
Tiazac Capsules 1201

DIL-SANORANIA (Germany)
DILTIAZEM HYDROCHLORIDE
Cardizem LA Extended Release Tablets . . . 1728
Tiazac Capsules 1201

DILTABETA (Germany)
DILTIAZEM HYDROCHLORIDE
Cardizem LA Extended Release Tablets . . . 1728
Tiazac Capsules 1201

DILTAHEXAL (Australia, Austria, Germany, New Zealand)
DILTIAZEM HYDROCHLORIDE
Cardizem LA Extended Release Tablets . . . 1728
Tiazac Capsules 1201

DILTAM (Irish Republic)
DILTIAZEM HYDROCHLORIDE
Cardizem LA Extended Release Tablets . . . 1728
Tiazac Capsules 1201

DILTAN (Hong Kong, Hungary, Thailand)
DILTIAZEM HYDROCHLORIDE
Cardizem LA Extended Release Tablets . . . 1728
Tiazac Capsules 1201

DILTAPHAM (Germany)
DILTIAZEM HYDROCHLORIDE
Cardizem LA Extended Release Tablets . . . 1728
Tiazac Capsules 1201

DILTARETARD (Germany)
DILTIAZEM HYDROCHLORIDE
Cardizem LA Extended Release Tablets . . . 1728
Tiazac Capsules 1201

DILTEC (Thailand)
DILTIAZEM HYDROCHLORIDE
Cardizem LA Extended Release Tablets . . . 1728
Tiazac Capsules 1201

DILTEM (Greece)
DILTIAZEM HYDROCHLORIDE
Cardizem LA Extended Release Tablets . . . 1728
Tiazac Capsules 1201

DILTI (Germany)
DILTIAZEM HYDROCHLORIDE
Cardizem LA Extended Release Tablets . . . 1728

Tiazac Capsules 1201

DILTIACOR (Argentina, Brazil)
DILTIAZEM HYDROCHLORIDE
Cardizem LA Extended Release Tablets . . . 1728
Tiazac Capsules 1201

DILTIAGAMMA (Germany)
DILTIAZEM HYDROCHLORIDE
Cardizem LA Extended Release Tablets . . . 1728
Tiazac Capsules 1201

DILTIAMAX (Australia)
DILTIAZEM HYDROCHLORIDE
Cardizem LA Extended Release Tablets . . . 1728
Tiazac Capsules 1201

DILTIAMERCK (Germany)
DILTIAZEM HYDROCHLORIDE
Cardizem LA Extended Release Tablets . . . 1728
Tiazac Capsules 1201

DILTIANGINA (Portugal)
DILTIAZEM HYDROCHLORIDE
Cardizem LA Extended Release Tablets . . . 1728
Tiazac Capsules 1201

DILTIASTAD (Austria)
DILTIAZEM HYDROCHLORIDE
Cardizem LA Extended Release Tablets . . . 1728
Tiazac Capsules 1201

DILTIEM (Portugal)
DILTIAZEM HYDROCHLORIDE
Cardizem LA Extended Release Tablets . . . 1728
Tiazac Capsules 1201

DILTI-ESSEX (Germany)
DILTIAZEM HYDROCHLORIDE
Cardizem LA Extended Release Tablets . . . 1728
Tiazac Capsules 1201

DILTIKARD (Norway)
DILTIAZEM HYDROCHLORIDE
Cardizem LA Extended Release Tablets . . . 1728
Tiazac Capsules 1201

DILTIPRESS (Brazil)
DILTIAZEM HYDROCHLORIDE
Cardizem LA Extended Release Tablets . . . 1728
Tiazac Capsules 1201

DILTIUC (Germany)
DILTIAZEM HYDROCHLORIDE
Cardizem LA Extended Release Tablets . . . 1728
Tiazac Capsules 1201

DILTIWAS (Spain)
DILTIAZEM HYDROCHLORIDE
Cardizem LA Extended Release Tablets . . . 1728
Tiazac Capsules 1201

DILTIZEM (Brazil)
DILTIAZEM HYDROCHLORIDE
Cardizem LA Extended Release Tablets . . . 1728
Tiazac Capsules 1201

DILTOR (Brazil)
DILTIAZEM HYDROCHLORIDE
Cardizem LA Extended Release Tablets . . . 1728
Tiazac Capsules 1201

DILUCID (Mexico)
LOVASTATIN
Mevacor Tablets 2021

DILUTOL (Argentina)
ENOXAPARIN SODIUM
Lovenox Injection 2915

DILVAS (India)
ENALAPRIL MALEATE
Vasotec I.V. Injection 2103

DILVAS AM (India)
ENALAPRIL MALEATE
Vasotec I.V. Injection 2103

DILZATYROL (Austria)
DILTIAZEM HYDROCHLORIDE
Cardizem LA Extended Release Tablets . . . 1728
Tiazac Capsules 1201

DILZEM (Australia, Austria, Czech Republic, Finland, Germany, Hong Kong, Hungary, India, Irish Republic, New Zealand, Switzerland, Thailand, United Kingdom)
DILTIAZEM HYDROCHLORIDE
Cardizem LA Extended Release Tablets . . . 1728
Tiazac Capsules 1201

DILZENE (Italy)
DILTIAZEM HYDROCHLORIDE
Cardizem LA Extended Release Tablets . . . 1728
Tiazac Capsules 1201

DILZEREAL (Germany)
DILTIAZEM HYDROCHLORIDE
Cardizem LA Extended Release Tablets . . . 1728
Tiazac Capsules 1201

DILZICARDIN (Germany)
DILTIAZEM HYDROCHLORIDE
Cardizem LA Extended Release Tablets . . . 1728
Tiazac Capsules 1201

DIMALOSIO (Italy)
LACTULOSE
Kristalose for Oral Solution 1034

DIMENFORMON (The Netherlands)
ESTRADIOL
Climara Transdermal System 771
Estring Vaginal Ring 2635

DIMITONE (Belgium, Denmark, Israel)
CARVEDILOL
Coreg Tablets 1414

DIMORF (Brazil)
MORPHINE SULFATE
Kadian Capsules 577
MS Contin Tablets 2701

DINAC (Australia)
DICLOFENAC SODIUM
Voltaren Tablets 2307
Voltaren-XR Tablets 2310

DINACLON (Greece)
DICLOFENAC SODIUM
Voltaren Tablets 2307
Voltaren-XR Tablets 2310

DINAFLOX (Mexico)
CIPROFLOXACIN HYDROCHLORIDE
Ciloxan Ophthalmic Ointment . . . . ⊙204, 559
Ciloxan Ophthalmic Solution . . . . ⊙206
Cipro Tablets 2977

DINAVIR (Brazil)
INDINAVIR SULFATE
Crixivan Capsules 1940

DINAXIN (Mexico)
RANITIDINE HYDROCHLORIDE
Zantac 25 EFFERdose Tablets 1624
Zantac 150 EFFERdose Tablets 1624
Zantac 150 Tablets 1624
Zantac 300 Tablets 1624
Zantac Injection 1619
Zantac Injection Premixed 1619
Zantac Syrup 1624

DINAZIDE (Thailand)
HYDROCHLOROTHIAZIDE/TRIAMTERENE
Dyazide Capsules 1423

DINEURIN (Chile)
GABAPENTIN
Neurontin Capsules 2487

DINILL-D (Mexico)
CIPROFLOXACIN HYDROCHLORIDE
Ciloxan Ophthalmic Ointment . . . . ⊙204, 559
Ciloxan Ophthalmic Solution . . . . ⊙206
Cipro Tablets 2977

DINISOR (Spain)
DILTIAZEM HYDROCHLORIDE
Cardizem LA Extended Release Tablets . . . 1728
Tiazac Capsules 1201

DINUL (Portugal)
FAMOTIDINE
Pepcid Injection 2040
Pepcid Injection Premixed 2040
Pepcid Tablets 2038
Pepcid for Oral Suspension 2038

DIOCAM (Argentina)
CLONAZEPAM
Klonopin Tablets 2778

DIODERM (Irish Republic, United Kingdom)
HYDROCORTISONE
Hydrocortone Tablets 1989

DIOFLUOR (Canada)
FLUORESCEIN SODIUM
Fluorescite Injection . . . . ⊙207

DIOGENT (Canada)
GENTAMICIN SULFATE
Garamycin Injectable 3014

DIOMICETE (Portugal)
CLOTRIMAZOLE
Lotrimin Cream 3039
Lotrimin Lotion 1% 3039
Lotrimin Topical Solution 1% 3039

DIOMYCIN (Canada)
ERYTHROMYCIN
Ery-Tab Tablets 449
Erythromycin Base Filmtab Tablets 455
Erythromycin Delayed-Release Capsules, USP 457
PCE Dispertab Tablets 515

DIOPTICON (Canada)
NAPHAZOLINE HYDROCHLORIDE
Albalon Ophthalmic Solution . . . . ⊙218

DIOSULF (Canada)
SULFACETAMIDE SODIUM
Klaron Lotion 10% 2909

DIOVAN (Argentina, Austria, Brazil, Canada, Czech Republic, Denmark, Finland, Germany, Greece, Hong Kong, Hungary, India, Irish Republic, Israel, Malaysia, Mexico, New Zealand, Norway, Portugal, Russia, Singapore, South Africa, Spain, Sweden, Switzerland, Thailand, The Netherlands, United Kingdom, Venezuela)
VALSARTAN
Diovan Tablets 2193

DIOVAN COMP (Denmark, Finland, Norway, Sweden)
HYDROCHLOROTHIAZIDE/VALSARTAN
Diovan HCT Tablets 2196

DIOVAN D (Argentina)
VALSARTAN
Diovan Tablets 2193

DIOVAN HCT (Brazil, Canada, Hungary, Mexico, Venezuela)
VALSARTAN
Diovan Tablets 2193

DIOVANE (Belgium)
VALSARTAN
Diovan Tablets 2193

DIOXAFLEX (Brazil)
DICLOFENAC SODIUM
Voltaren Tablets 2307
Voltaren-XR Tablets 2310

DIOXAFLEX FORTE (Argentina)
DICLOFENAC SODIUM
Voltaren Tablets 2307
Voltaren-XR Tablets 2310

DIOXAFLEX PLUS (Argentina)
DICLOFENAC SODIUM
Voltaren Tablets 2307
Voltaren-XR Tablets 2310

DIP (Venezuela)
SUCRALFATE
Carafate Suspension 701
Carafate Tablets 701

DIPARENE (Belgium)
NAPROXEN
EC-Naprosyn Delayed-Release Tablets 2761
Naprosyn Suspension 2761
Naprosyn Tablets 2761

DIPEDYNE (Mexico)
ZIDOVUDINE
Retrovir Capsules 1560
Retrovir IV Infusion 1564
Retrovir Syrup 1560
Retrovir Tablets 1560

DIPEZONA (Argentina)
DIAZEPAM
Diastat Rectal Delivery System 3343
Valium Tablets 2819

DIPHAR (France)
DIPYRIDAMOLE
Persantine Tablets 868

DIPHOS (Germany)
ETIDRONATE DISODIUM
Didronel Tablets 2697

DIPINAL (Brazil)
NIFEDIPINE
Adalat CC Tablets 2964

DIPNI (Argentina)
NYSTATIN
Nystop Topical Powder USP 2478
Paddock Nystatin USP for Oral Suspension 2478

DIPRES (Mexico)
DIPYRIDAMOLE
Persantine Tablets 868

DI-PROMAL (Austria)
IPRATROPIUM BROMIDE
Atrovent Inhalation Solution 835
Atrovent Nasal Spray 0.03% 837
Atrovent Nasal Spray 0.06% 839

DIPROX (Brazil)
LANSOPRAZOLE
Prevacid Delayed-Release Capsules 3271

DIPSIN (Portugal)
FAMOTIDINE
Pepcid Injection 2040
Pepcid Injection Premixed 2040
Pepcid Tablets 2038
Pepcid for Oral Suspension 2038

DIPYRIDAN (Belgium)
DIPYRIDAMOLE
Persantine Tablets 868

DIPYRIN (Finland)
DIPYRIDAMOLE
Persantine Tablets 868

DIPYROL (South Africa)
DIPYRIDAMOLE
Persantine Tablets 868

DIRALON (Venezuela)
DICLOFENAC SODIUM
Voltaren Tablets 2307
Voltaren-XR Tablets 2310

DIRINE (Malaysia, Singapore, Thailand)
FUROSEMIDE
Furosemide Tablets 2154

DIRINOL (Mexico)
DIPYRIDAMOLE
Persantine Tablets 868

DIROTON (Czech Republic, Russia)
LISINOPRIL
Prinivil Tablets 2052

DIRRET (Mexico)
DICLOFENAC SODIUM
Voltaren Tablets 2307
Voltaren-XR Tablets 2310

DIRUNEZ (Greece)
NORFLOXACIN
Noroxin Tablets 2032

DISCOID (Germany)
FUROSEMIDE
Furosemide Tablets 2154

DISEL (Argentina)
NAPHAZOLINE HYDROCHLORIDE
Albalon Ophthalmic Solution . . . . ⊙218

DISEL HIDROCORTISONA (Argentina)
NAPHAZOLINE HYDROCHLORIDE
Albalon Ophthalmic Solution . . . . ⊙218

DISEQUENS (Argentina)
ESTRADIOL
Climara Transdermal System 771
Estring Vaginal Ring 2635

DISIPAN (Argentina)
DICLOFENAC SODIUM
Voltaren Tablets 2307
Voltaren-XR Tablets 2310

DISLIPIN (Venezuela)
LOVASTATIN
Mevacor Tablets 2021

DISLIPINA (Portugal)
SIMVASTATIN
Zocor Tablets 2105

DISLIPOR (Chile)
ATORVASTATIN CALCIUM
Lipitor Tablets 2483

DISMAM (Chile)
LACTULOSE
Kristalose for Oral Solution 1034

DISMOLAN (Argentina)
ONDANSETRON HYDROCHLORIDE
Zofran Injection 1634

(⊙ Described in PDR For Ophthalmic Medicines™)

Zofran Injection Premixed 1634
Zofran Oral Solution. 1639
Zofran Tablets 1639

DISNE ASMOL (Spain)
IPRATROPIUM BROMIDE
Atrovent Inhalation Solution 835
Atrovent Nasal Spray 0.03%. 837
Atrovent Nasal Spray 0.06%. 839

DISOGRAM (United Kingdom)
DILTIAZEM HYDROCHLORIDE
Cardizem LA Extended Release Tablets. . . 1728
Tiazac Capsules 1201

DISOPAM (Israel)
DIAZEPAM
Diastat Rectal Delivery System 3343
Valium Tablets 2819

DISPACLONIDIN (Germany)
CLONIDINE HYDROCHLORIDE
Catapres Tablets 843

DISPAGENT (Germany)
GENTAMICIN SULFATE
Garamycin Injectable 3014

DISPASAN (Germany)
SODIUM HYALURONATE
Hyalgan Solution 2901

DISPATIM (Austria, Germany)
TIMOLOL MALEATE
Blocadren Tablets 1916
Timoptic Sterile Ophthalmic Solution 2088
Timoptic in Ocudose 2091
Timoptic-XE Sterile Ophthalmic Gel Forming Solution 2092

DISPROMIL (Spain)
FAMOTIDINE
Pepcid Injection 2040
Pepcid Injection Premixed 2040
Pepcid Tablets 2038
Pepcid for Oral Suspension 2038

DISTALENE (Argentina)
ANASTROZOLE
Arimidex Tablets 673

DISTAMINE (Austria, Irish Republic, New Zealand, The Netherlands, United Kingdom)
PENICILLAMINE
Cuprimine Capsules 1947

DISTOBRAM (Portugal)
TOBRAMYCIN
TOBI Solution for Inhalation 2298

DITENATE N (Germany)
THEOPHYLLINE
Uniphyl Tablets 2710

DITENSOR (Spain)
ENALAPRIL MALEATE
Vasotec I.V. Injection 2103

DITIZEM (Thailand)
DILTIAZEM HYDROCHLORIDE
Cardizem LA Extended Release Tablets. . . 1728
Tiazac Capsules 1201

DIUBELOC (Argentina)
METOPROLOL TARTRATE
Lopressor Tablets 2238

DIUMIDE-K CONTINUS (United Kingdom)
FUROSEMIDE
Furosemide Tablets 2154

DIURAL (Denmark, Norway, Sweden)
FUROSEMIDE
Furosemide Tablets 2154

DIURAMIN (Finland)
AMILORIDE HYDROCHLORIDE/HYDROCHLOROTHIAZIDE
Moduretic Tablets 2028

DIURAPID (Germany)
FUROSEMIDE
Furosemide Tablets 2154

DIUREMIDA (Brazil)
FUROSEMIDE
Furosemide Tablets 2154

DIURENE (Portugal)
AMILORIDE HYDROCHLORIDE/HYDROCHLOROTHIAZIDE
Moduretic Tablets 2028

DIURESAL (Switzerland)
FUROSEMIDE
Furosemide Tablets 2154

DIURET (Brazil)
FUROSEMIDE
Furosemide Tablets 2154

DIURETIKUM VERLA (Germany)
HYDROCHLOROTHIAZIDE/TRIAMTERENE
Dyazide Capsules 1423

DIUREX (Brazil, Finland)
FUROSEMIDE
Furosemide Tablets 2154

DIUREX A (Argentina)
AMILORIDE HYDROCHLORIDE
Midamor Tablets 2026

DIURID (Austria)
HYDROCHLOROTHIAZIDE/TRIAMTERENE
Dyazide Capsules 1423

DIURIN (New Zealand)
FUROSEMIDE
Furosemide Tablets 2154

DIURIT (Brazil)
FUROSEMIDE
Furosemide Tablets 2154

DIURIX (Brazil, Switzerland)
FUROSEMIDE
Furosemide Tablets 2154

DIUROLAN (Mexico)
FUROSEMIDE
Furosemide Tablets 2154

DIUROLASA (Spain)
FUROSEMIDE
Furosemide Tablets 2154

DIURSAN (Germany)
AMILORIDE HYDROCHLORIDE/HYDROCHLOROTHIAZIDE
Moduretic Tablets 2028

DIUTEC (South Africa)
AMILORIDE HYDROCHLORIDE/HYDROCHLOROTHIAZIDE
Moduretic Tablets 2028

DIUTENSAT (Germany)
HYDROCHLOROTHIAZIDE/TRIAMTERENE
Dyazide Capsules 1423

DIU-TONOLYTRIL (Germany)
HYDROCHLOROTHIAZIDE/TRIAMTERENE
Dyazide Capsules 1423

DIUZINE (Spain)
AMILORIDE HYDROCHLORIDE/HYDROCHLOROTHIAZIDE
Moduretic Tablets 2028

DIVAL (Venezuela)
DICLOFENAC SODIUM
Voltaren Tablets 2307
Voltaren-XR Tablets 2310

DIVELOL (Brazil)
CARVEDILOL
Coreg Tablets. 1414

DIVIGEL (Czech Republic, Denmark, Finland, Hungary, Irish Republic, Malaysia, Singapore, Sweden, Switzerland, Thailand)
ESTRADIOL
Climara Transdermal System 771
Estring Vaginal Ring 2635

DIXAMID (Greece)
INDAPAMIDE
Indapamide Tablets 2156

DIXARIT (Australia, Belgium, Canada, Germany, Hong Kong, Irish Republic, Malaysia, New Zealand, Singapore, South Africa, The Netherlands, United Kingdom)
CLONIDINE HYDROCHLORIDE
Catapres Tablets 843

DIZAN (Thailand)
DIAZEPAM
Diastat Rectal Delivery System 3343
Valium Tablets 2819

DIZEPAM (Thailand)
DIAZEPAM
Diastat Rectal Delivery System 3343
Valium Tablets 2819

DNAREN (Brazil)
DICLOFENAC SODIUM
Voltaren Tablets 2307
Voltaren-XR Tablets 2310

DOBET (Venezuela)
DORZOLAMIDE HYDROCHLORIDE
Trusopt Sterile Ophthalmic Solution 2095

DOBUPAL (Spain)
VENLAFAXINE HYDROCHLORIDE
Effexor Tablets 3411
Effexor XR Capsules 3417

DOCEKEBIR (Argentina)
DOCETAXEL
Taxotere Injection Concentrate 2932

DOCETAX (India)
DOCETAXEL
Taxotere Injection Concentrate 2932

DOCITON (Germany)
PROPRANOLOL HYDROCHLORIDE
Inderal LA Long-Acting Capsules 3429

DOCITRAL (Venezuela)
PROPRANOLOL HYDROCHLORIDE
Inderal LA Long-Acting Capsules 3429

DOCLIS (Spain)
DILTIAZEM HYDROCHLORIDE
Cardizem LA Extended Release Tablets. . . 1728
Tiazac Capsules 1201

DOFEN (Mexico)
DICLOFENAC SODIUM
Voltaren Tablets 2307
Voltaren-XR Tablets 2310

DOFLEX (India)
DICLOFENAC SODIUM
Voltaren Tablets 2307
Voltaren-XR Tablets 2310

DOGOXINE (Mexico)
DIGOXIN
Lanoxicaps Capsules 1490
Lanoxin Injection 1494
Lanoxin Injection Pediatric 1497
Lanoxin Tablets. 1500

DOLAK (Spain)
ISOSORBIDE MONONITRATE
Imdur Tablets 3018

DOLAUT (Italy)
DICLOFENAC SODIUM
Voltaren Tablets 2307
Voltaren-XR Tablets 2310

DOLCONTIN (Finland, Norway, Sweden)
MORPHINE SULFATE
Kadian Capsules 577
MS Contin Tablets 2701

DOLECTRAN (Argentina)
DOCETAXEL
Taxotere Injection Concentrate 2932

DOLFLAM (Mexico)
DICLOFENAC SODIUM
Voltaren Tablets 2307
Voltaren-XR Tablets 2310

DOLGIT-DICLO (Germany)
DICLOFENAC SODIUM
Voltaren Tablets 2307
Voltaren-XR Tablets 2310

DOLILUX (Italy)
RANITIDINE HYDROCHLORIDE
Zantac 25 EFFERdose Tablets 1624
Zantac 150 EFFERdose Tablets. 1624
Zantac 150 Tablets 1624
Zantac 300 Tablets 1624
Zantac Injection 1619
Zantac Injection Premixed 1619
Zantac Syrup 1624

DOLISAL (Italy)
DIFLUNISAL
Dolobid Tablets. 1955

DOLMIGRAL (Spain)
SUMATRIPTAN SUCCINATE
Imitrex Injection 1463
Imitrex Tablets 1471

DOLMINA (Czech Republic)
DICLOFENAC SODIUM
Voltaren Tablets 2307
Voltaren-XR Tablets 2310

DOLNAXEN (Mexico)
NAPROXEN
EC-Naprosyn Delayed-Release Tablets. . . . 2761
Naprosyn Suspension. 2761
Naprosyn Tablets 2761

DOLO NERVOBION (Spain)
DICLOFENAC SODIUM
Voltaren Tablets 2307
Voltaren-XR Tablets 2310

DOLOATRIXEN (Mexico)
NAPROXEN
EC-Naprosyn Delayed-Release Tablets. . . . 2761
Naprosyn Suspension. 2761
Naprosyn Tablets 2761

DOLOBASAN (Germany)
DICLOFENAC SODIUM
Voltaren Tablets 2307
Voltaren-XR Tablets 2310

DOLOBID (Australia, Canada, Hong Kong, Irish Republic, Israel, Italy, Mexico, Portugal, South Africa, Spain, Thailand, United Kingdom, Venezuela)
DIFLUNISAL
Dolobid Tablets. 1955

DOLOBIS (France)
DIFLUNISAL
Dolobid Tablets. 1955

DOLOCID (The Netherlands)
DIFLUNISAL
Dolobid Tablets. 1955

DOLODOL (Spain)
TRAMADOL HYDROCHLORIDE
Ultram ER Tablets 2392

DOLOL (Austria, Denmark)
TRAMADOL HYDROCHLORIDE
Ultram ER Tablets 2392

DOLONOVAG (Argentina)
HYDROMORPHONE HYDROCHLORIDE
Dilaudid Ampules. 440
Dilaudid Multiple Dose Vials 440
Dilaudid Non-Sterile Powder 440
Dilaudid Oral Liquid 445
Dilaudid Rectal Suppositories 440
Dilaudid Tablets. 440
Dilaudid Tablets - 8 mg 445
Dilaudid-HP Injection. 442
Dilaudid-HP Lyophilized Powder 250 mg . . . 442

DOLORMIN MIT NAPROXEN (Germany)
NAPROXEN
EC-Naprosyn Delayed-Release Tablets. . . . 2761
Naprosyn Suspension. 2761
Naprosyn Tablets 2761

DOLOTANDAX (Mexico)
NAPROXEN SODIUM
Anaprox DS Tablets 2761
Anaprox Tablets 2761

DOLOTRAMINE (Switzerland)
TRAMADOL HYDROCHLORIDE
Ultram ER Tablets 2392

DOLOVISANO DICLO (Germany)
DICLOFENAC SODIUM
Voltaren Tablets 2307
Voltaren-XR Tablets 2310

DOLO-VOLTAREN (Spain)
DICLOFENAC SODIUM
Voltaren Tablets 2307
Voltaren-XR Tablets 2310

DOLPASSE (Austria)
DICLOFENAC SODIUM
Voltaren Tablets 2307
Voltaren-XR Tablets 2310

DOLTARD (Czech Republic, Denmark)
MORPHINE SULFATE
Kadian Capsules 577
MS Contin Tablets 2701

DOLVAN (Argentina)
DICLOFENAC SODIUM
Voltaren Tablets 2307
Voltaren-XR Tablets 2310

DOLXEN (Mexico)
NAPROXEN
EC-Naprosyn Delayed-Release Tablets. . . . 2761

Naprosyn Suspension 2761
Naprosyn Tablets 2761

DOLZAM (Belgium)
TRAMADOL HYDROCHLORIDE
Ultram ER Tablets 2392

DOMNAMID (Denmark)
ESTAZOLAM
ProSom Tablets 517

DONAPROX (Mexico)
NAPROXEN
EC-Naprosyn Delayed-Release Tablets 2761
Naprosyn Suspension 2761
Naprosyn Tablets 2761

DONATAXEL (Argentina)
DOCETAXEL
Taxotere Injection Concentrate 2932

DONAZ (India)
DONEPEZIL HYDROCHLORIDE
Aricept Tablets 1094

DONECEPT (India)
DONEPEZIL HYDROCHLORIDE
Aricept Tablets 1094

DONEKA (Spain)
LISINOPRIL
Prinivil Tablets 2052

DONEKA PLUS (Spain)
HYDROCHLOROTHIAZIDE/LISINOPRIL
Prinzide Tablets 2056

DONICER (Spain)
AMILORIDE HYDROCHLORIDE/HYDROCHLOROTHIAZIDE
Moduretic Tablets 2028

DONOBID (Denmark, Finland, Norway, Sweden)
DIFLUNISAL
Dolobid Tablets 1955

DOPSAN (Thailand)
DAPSONE
Dapsone Tablets USP 1673

DORANOL (Spain)
ERYTHROMYCIN STEARATE
Erythrocin Stearate Filmtab Tablets 453

DORBID (Brazil)
DIFLUNISAL
Dolobid Tablets 1955

DORCALOR (Portugal)
DICLOFENAC SODIUM
Voltaren Tablets 2307
Voltaren-XR Tablets 2310

DORGEN (Brazil)
DICLOFENAC SODIUM
Voltaren Tablets 2307
Voltaren-XR Tablets 2310

DORICOFLU (Italy)
FLUNISOLIDE
Aerobid Inhaler System 1171
Aerobid-M Inhaler System 1171

DORIMAN (Spain)
CIPROFLOXACIN HYDROCHLORIDE
Ciloxan Ophthalmic Ointment . . . . ⊙204, 559
Ciloxan Ophthalmic Solution . . . . . ⊙206
Cipro Tablets 2977

DORLAMIDA (Argentina)
DORZOLAMIDE HYDROCHLORIDE
Trusopt Sterile Ophthalmic Solution 2095

DORLAMIDA T (Argentina)
DORZOLAMIDE HYDROCHLORIDE
Trusopt Sterile Ophthalmic Solution 2095

DORMODOR (Spain)
FLURAZEPAM HYDROCHLORIDE
Dalmane Capsules 3342

DOROXAN (Italy)
DICLOFENAC SODIUM
Voltaren Tablets 2307
Voltaren-XR Tablets 2310

DORPANE (Thailand)
ORPHENADRINE CITRATE
Norflex Injection 1856

DORPIEL (Argentina)
TRETINOIN
Vesanoid Capsules 2820

DORSOF T (Chile)
DORZOLAMIDE HYDROCHLORIDE/TIMOLOL MALEATE
Cosopt Sterile Ophthalmic Solution . . . . . ⊙268, 1931

DORZOFLAX (Argentina)
DORZOLAMIDE HYDROCHLORIDE
Trusopt Sterile Ophthalmic Solution 2095

DORZOL (Venezuela)
DORZOLAMIDE HYDROCHLORIDE
Trusopt Sterile Ophthalmic Solution 2095

DORZONE (Brazil)
ORPHENADRINE CITRATE
Norflex Injection 1856

DORZOX (India)
DORZOLAMIDE HYDROCHLORIDE
Trusopt Sterile Ophthalmic Solution 2095

DOSIER (Argentina, Chile)
TICLOPIDINE HYDROCHLORIDE
Ticlid Tablets 2810

DOVAL (South Africa)
DIAZEPAM
Diastat Rectal Delivery System 3343
Valium Tablets 2819

DOVATE (South Africa)
CLOBETASOL PROPIONATE
Temovate Cream 2668
Temovate E Emollient 2671
Temovate Gel 2669
Temovate Ointment 2668
Temovate Scalp Application 2670

DOXAPRIL (Argentina)
LISINOPRIL
Prinivil Tablets 2052

DOXETAL (Argentina)
DOCETAXEL
Taxotere Injection Concentrate 2932

DOXMIL (Argentina)
DOCETAXEL
Taxotere Injection Concentrate 2932

DOXTRAN FLEX (Argentina)
DICLOFENAC SODIUM
Voltaren Tablets 2307
Voltaren-XR Tablets 2310

DOZIC (Argentina)
RISPERIDONE
Risperdal Oral Solution 1676
Risperdal Tablets 1676

DP GESIC (India)
DICLOFENAC SODIUM
Voltaren Tablets 2307
Voltaren-XR Tablets 2310

DP HYDROCORTISONE (New Zealand)
HYDROCORTISONE
Hydrocortone Tablets 1989

D-PAM (New Zealand)
DIAZEPAM
Diastat Rectal Delivery System 3343
Valium Tablets 2819

D-PENAMINE (Australia, New Zealand)
PENICILLAMINE
Cuprimine Capsules 1947

DRALEN (Greece)
ETIDRONATE DISODIUM
Didronel Tablets 2697

DRAXON (Portugal)
FLUTAMIDE
Eulexin Capsules 3009

DRENIAN (Spain)
DIAZEPAM
Diastat Rectal Delivery System 3343
Valium Tablets 2819

DRIKEN (Mexico)
IRON DEXTRAN
Infed Injection 3390

DRILYNA (Argentina)
THEOPHYLLINE
Uniphyl Tablets 2710

DROGENIL (Chile, Irish Republic, Italy, The Netherlands, United Kingdom)
FLUTAMIDE
Eulexin Capsules 3009

DROLASONA (Spain)
FLUTICASONE PROPIONATE
Cutivate Cream 2662
Cutivate Ointment 2665
Flonase Nasal Spray 1440

DROMADOL (United Kingdom)
TRAMADOL HYDROCHLORIDE
Ultram ER Tablets 2392

DRONAL (Italy)
ALENDRONATE SODIUM
Fosamax Tablets 1969

DRONATE-OS (India)
ETIDRONATE DISODIUM
Didronel Tablets 2697

DROPICINE (Argentina)
RISPERIDONE
Risperdal Oral Solution 1676
Risperdal Tablets 1676

DROPSTAR (Argentina, Italy)
SODIUM HYALURONATE
Hyalgan Solution 2901

DROPTIMOL (Italy)
TIMOLOL MALEATE
Blocadren Tablets 1916
Timoptic Sterile Ophthalmic Solution 2088
Timoptic in Ocudose 2091
Timoptic-XE Sterile Ophthalmic Gel Forming Solution 2092

DROSTEAKARD (Germany)
VERAPAMIL HYDROCHLORIDE
Covera-HS Tablets 3139
Verelan PM Extended-Release Capsules, Controlled-Onset 3106

DRY & CLEAR (South Africa)
BENZOYL PEROXIDE
Brevoxyl-4 Creamy Wash 3210
Brevoxyl-4 Gel 3210
Brevoxyl-8 Creamy Wash 3210
Brevoxyl-8 Gel 3210
Triaz Cleanser 1892
Triaz Gel 1892

DRYPTAL (Czech Republic, Hong Kong, Irish Republic, United Kingdom)
FUROSEMIDE
Furosemide Tablets 2154

D-TATO (Mexico)
BENZONATATE
Tessalon Perles 1199

D-TRIOL (Greece)
CALCITRIOL
Calcijex Injection 411
Rocaltrol Capsules 2798
Rocaltrol Oral Solution 2798

DUAC (Australia)
BENZOYL PEROXIDE
Brevoxyl-4 Creamy Wash 3210
Brevoxyl-4 Gel 3210
Brevoxyl-8 Creamy Wash 3210
Brevoxyl-8 Gel 3210
Triaz Cleanser 1892
Triaz Gel 1892

DUAC ONCE DAILY (United Kingdom)
BENZOYL PEROXIDE
Brevoxyl-4 Creamy Wash 3210
Brevoxyl-4 Gel 3210
Brevoxyl-8 Creamy Wash 3210
Brevoxyl-8 Gel 3210
Triaz Cleanser 1892
Triaz Gel 1892

DUALIZOL (Mexico)
METRONIDAZOLE
MetroGel-Vaginal Gel 1855

DUALTEN (Chile)
CARVEDILOL
Coreg Tablets 1414

DUBAGEST (India)
PROGESTERONE
Prometrium Capsules (100 mg, 200 mg) . 3203

DUBE (Singapore)
LIDOCAINE
Lidoderm Patch 1118

DUCENE (Australia)
DIAZEPAM
Diastat Rectal Delivery System 3343
Valium Tablets 2819

DUCTOCINA (Brazil)
CIPROFLOXACIN
Cipro Oral Suspension 2977

DUCTONAR (Argentina)
RISEDRONATE SODIUM
Actonel Tablets 2683

DUCTOPRIL (Brazil)
CAPTOPRIL
Captopril Tablets 2149

DULAX (Irish Republic)
LACTULOSE
Kristalose for Oral Solution 1034

DUMOZOL (Portugal)
METRONIDAZOLE
MetroGel-Vaginal Gel 1855

DUNOX (Argentina)
AMOXICILLIN
Amoxil Pediatric Drops for Oral Suspension 1343
Amoxil Tablets 1343

DUOBLOC (Argentina)
CARVEDILOL
Coreg Tablets 1414

DUOFLEX (Mexico)
DICLOFENAC SODIUM
Voltaren Tablets 2307
Voltaren-XR Tablets 2310

DUOKLIMAN (Austria)
ESTRADIOL
Climara Transdermal System 771
Estring Vaginal Ring 2635

DUOLAX (Spain)
LACTULOSE
Kristalose for Oral Solution 1034

DUOLIN (New Zealand)
IPRATROPIUM BROMIDE
Atrovent Inhalation Solution 835
Atrovent Nasal Spray 0.03% 837
Atrovent Nasal Spray 0.06% 839

DUONASE (India)
AZELASTINE HYDROCHLORIDE
Astelin Nasal Spray 1904

DUOPRIL (Brazil)
ENALAPRIL MALEATE
Vasotec I.V. Injection 2103

DUORAN (Italy)
RANITIDINE HYDROCHLORIDE
Zantac 25 EFFERdose Tablets 1624
Zantac 150 EFFERdose Tablets 1624
Zantac 150 Tablets 1624
Zantac 300 Tablets 1624
Zantac Injection 1619
Zantac Injection Premixed 1619
Zantac Syrup 1624

DUOVIR (Brazil, India, South Africa)
LAMIVUDINE
Epivir Oral Solution 1427
Epivir Tablets 1427
Epivir-HBV Oral Solution 1432
Epivir-HBV Tablets 1432

DUOVIR N (India)
LAMIVUDINE
Epivir Oral Solution 1427
Epivir Tablets 1427
Epivir-HBV Oral Solution 1432
Epivir-HBV Tablets 1432

DUPHALAC (Australia, Austria, Belgium, Canada, Chile, Czech Republic, Finland, France, Greece, Hong Kong, Hungary, India, Irish Republic, Italy, Malaysia, New Zealand, Norway, Portugal, Russia, Singapore, South Africa, Spain, Sweden, Switzerland, Thailand, The Netherlands, United Kingdom)
LACTULOSE
Kristalose for Oral Solution 1034

DUPLAMIN (Italy)
PROMETHAZINE HYDROCHLORIDE
Phenergan Tablets and Suppositories 3440

DURACRALFAT (Germany)
SUCRALFATE
Carafate Suspension 701
Carafate Tablets 701

DURADIAZEPAM (Germany)
DIAZEPAM
Diastat Rectal Delivery System 3343

Valium Tablets 2819

DURADIURET (Germany)
HYDROCHLOROTHIAZIDE/TRIAMTERENE
Dyazide Capsules 1423

DURAERYTHROMYCIN (Germany)
ERYTHROMYCIN STEARATE
Erythrocin Stearate Filmtab Tablets 453

DURAFENAT (Germany)
FENOFIBRATE
Tricor Tablets 527

DURAFUNGOL (Germany)
CLOTRIMAZOLE
Lotrimin Cream. 3039
Lotrimin Lotion 1%. 3039
Lotrimin Topical Solution 1% 3039

DURAFURID (Germany)
FUROSEMIDE
Furosemide Tablets 2154

DURAGENTAM (Germany)
GENTAMICIN SULFATE
Garamycin Injectable 3014

DURAGENTAMICIN (Germany)
GENTAMICIN SULFATE
Garamycin Injectable 3014

DURAGESIC (Canada)
FENTANYL
Duragesic Transdermal System. 2373

DURALGIN (Denmark)
MORPHINE SULFATE
Kadian Capsules 577
MS Contin Tablets 2701

DURALMOR (Mexico)
MORPHINE SULFATE
Kadian Capsules 577
MS Contin Tablets 2701

DURAMONITAT (Germany)
ISOSORBIDE MONONITRATE
Imdur Tablets 3018

DURAMORPH (Argentina)
MORPHINE SULFATE
Kadian Capsules 577
MS Contin Tablets 2701

DURANIFIN (Germany)
NIFEDIPINE
Adalat CC Tablets 2964

DURANIFIN SALI (Germany)
NIFEDIPINE
Adalat CC Tablets 2964

DURANOL (Irish Republic)
PROPRANOLOL HYDROCHLORIDE
Inderal LA Long-Acting Capsules 3429

DURAPHYLLIN (Germany)
THEOPHYLLINE
Uniphyl Tablets 2710

DURARESE (Germany)
AMILORIDE HYDROCHLORIDE/HYDROCHLOROTHIAZIDE
Moduretic Tablets 2028

DURASOPTIN (Germany)
VERAPAMIL HYDROCHLORIDE
Covera-HS Tablets 3139
Verelan PM Extended-Release Capsules, Controlled-Onset 3106

DURATER (Mexico)
FAMOTIDINE
Pepcid Injection 2040
Pepcid Injection Premixed 2040
Pepcid Tablets 2038
Pepcid for Oral Suspension 2038

DURATIMOL (Germany)
TIMOLOL MALEATE
Blocadren Tablets 1916
Timoptic Sterile Ophthalmic Solution 2088
Timoptic in Ocudose 2091
Timoptic-XE Sterile Ophthalmic Gel Forming Solution 2092

DURAVOLTEN (Germany)
DICLOFENAC SODIUM
Voltaren Tablets 2307
Voltaren-XR Tablets 2310

DURA-ZOK (Denmark)
METOPROLOL SUCCINATE
Toprol-XL Tablets 668

DUREKAL (Finland)
POTASSIUM CHLORIDE
K-Dur Extended-Relase Tablets 3033
K-Lor Oral Solution. 474
K-Tab Tablets 475

DUREMID (Argentina)
INDAPAMIDE
Indapamide Tablets 2156

DURIDE (Australia, New Zealand)
ISOSORBIDE MONONITRATE
Imdur Tablets 3018

DUROGESIC (Argentina, Australia, Austria, Belgium, Brazil, Chile, Czech Republic, Denmark, Finland, France, Germany, Greece, Hong Kong, Hungary, India, Irish Republic, Israel, Italy, Malaysia, Mexico, New Zealand, Norway, Portugal, Russia, Singapore, South Africa, Spain, Sweden, Switzerland, Thailand, The Netherlands, United Kingdom, Venezuela)
FENTANYL
Duragesic Transdermal System. 2373

DURO-K (Australia)
POTASSIUM CHLORIDE
K-Dur Extended-Relase Tablets 3033
K-Lor Oral Solution. 474
K-Tab Tablets 475

DURONITRIN (Italy)
ISOSORBIDE MONONITRATE
Imdur Tablets 3018

DUXIMA (Italy)
CEFUROXIME SODIUM
Zinacef Injection 1631

DUZIMICIN (Brazil)
AMOXICILLIN
Amoxil Pediatric Drops for Oral Suspension. 1343
Amoxil Tablets 1343

DYAZIDE (Canada, Hong Kong, Irish Republic, Mexico, New Zealand, Portugal, Singapore, South Africa, Switzerland)
HYDROCHLOROTHIAZIDE/TRIAMTERENE
Dyazide Capsules 1423

DYNABLOK (South Africa)
PROPRANOLOL HYDROCHLORIDE
Inderal LA Long-Acting Capsules 3429

DYNACIRC (Argentina, Canada, Chile, Hong Kong, Malaysia, Mexico, New Zealand, Singapore, South Africa, Thailand, Venezuela)
ISRADIPINE
DynaCirc CR Tablets. 2721

DYNAFLOC (South Africa)
CIPROFLOXACIN
Cipro Oral Suspension 2977

DYNAMETRON (South Africa)
METRONIDAZOLE
MetroGel-Vaginal Gel 1855

DYNAMIN (United Kingdom)
ISOSORBIDE MONONITRATE
Imdur Tablets 3018

DYNAPAM (South Africa)
DIAZEPAM
Diastat Rectal Delivery System 3343
Valium Tablets 2819

DYNASPOR (South Africa)
CLOTRIMAZOLE
Lotrimin Cream. 3039
Lotrimin Lotion 1%. 3039
Lotrimin Topical Solution 1% 3039

DYRENIUM (Canada, Switzerland)
TRIAMTERENE
Dyrenium Capsules 3400

DYSALFA (France)
TERAZOSIN HYDROCHLORIDE
Hytrin Capsules. 471

DYSMENALGIT (Germany)
NAPROXEN
EC-Naprosyn Delayed-Release Tablets. . . . 2761
Naprosyn Suspension. 2761
Naprosyn Tablets 2761

DYTAC (Australia, Belgium, Irish Republic, The Netherlands, United Kingdom)
TRIAMTERENE
Dyrenium Capsules 3400

DYTA-URESE (Belgium, The Netherlands)
TRIAMTERENE
Dyrenium Capsules 3400

DYTENZIDE (Belgium, The Netherlands)
TRIAMTERENE
Dyrenium Capsules 3400

DYTERENE (Thailand)
HYDROCHLOROTHIAZIDE/TRIAMTERENE
Dyazide Capsules 1423

DYTIDE H (Austria, Germany)
HYDROCHLOROTHIAZIDE/TRIAMTERENE
Dyazide Capsules 1423

EASY DAYZ (India)
NAPROXEN SODIUM
Anaprox DS Tablets 2761
Anaprox Tablets 2761

EBOREN (The Netherlands)
ERYTHROMYCIN
Ery-Tab Tablets 449
Erythromycin Base Filmtab Tablets. 455
Erythromycin Delayed-Release Capsules, USP 457
PCE Dispertab Tablets 515

ECAMAIS (Portugal)
LISINOPRIL
Prinivil Tablets 2052

ECAPRESAN (Mexico)
CAPTOPRIL
Captopril Tablets. 2149

ECAPRIL (Mexico, Portugal)
CAPTOPRIL
Captopril Tablets. 2149

ECATEN (Mexico)
CAPTOPRIL
Captopril Tablets. 2149

ECLARAN (Argentina, Czech Republic, France, Portugal)
BENZOYL PEROXIDE
Brevoxyl-4 Creamy Wash. 3210
Brevoxyl-4 Gel 3210
Brevoxyl-8 Creamy Wash. 3210
Brevoxyl-8 Gel 3210
Triaz Cleanser 1892
Triaz Gel. 1892

ECNAGEL PB (Argentina)
BENZOYL PEROXIDE
Brevoxyl-4 Creamy Wash. 3210
Brevoxyl-4 Gel 3210
Brevoxyl-8 Creamy Wash. 3210
Brevoxyl-8 Gel 3210
Triaz Cleanser 1892
Triaz Gel. 1892

ECODIPINE (Switzerland)
NIFEDIPINE
Adalat CC Tablets 2964

ECODOLOR (Switzerland)
TRAMADOL HYDROCHLORIDE
Ultram ER Tablets 2392

ECODUREX (Switzerland)
AMILORIDE HYDROCHLORIDE/HYDROCHLOROTHIAZIDE
Moduretic Tablets 2028

ECOFENAC (Switzerland)
DICLOFENAC SODIUM
Voltaren Tablets 2307
Voltaren-XR Tablets 2310

ECOLINE (Greece)
CEFUROXIME AXETIL
Ceftin Tablets. 1407
Ceftin for Oral Suspension. 1407

ECONAC (United Kingdom)
DICLOFENAC SODIUM
Voltaren Tablets 2307
Voltaren-XR Tablets 2310

ECOPACE (United Kingdom)
CAPTOPRIL
Captopril Tablets. 2149

E-COR (Czech Republic)
ENALAPRIL MALEATE
Vasotec I.V. Injection 2103

ECRINAL (Spain)
FLECAINIDE ACETATE
Tambocor Tablets 1856

ECTIVA (Italy, Mexico)
SIBUTRAMINE HYDROCHLORIDE
Meridia Capsules. 489

ECUADERM (Venezuela)
BENZOYL PEROXIDE
Brevoxyl-4 Creamy Wash. 3210
Brevoxyl-4 Gel 3210
Brevoxyl-8 Creamy Wash. 3210
Brevoxyl-8 Gel 3210
Triaz Cleanser 1892
Triaz Gel. 1892

ECURAL (Germany)
MOMETASONE FUROATE
Elocon Cream 0.1%. 3005
Elocon Lotion 0.1% 3006
Elocon Ointment 0.1% 3007
Nasonex Nasal Spray. 3043

EDALEN (Argentina)
RISPERIDONE
Risperdal Oral Solution 1676
Risperdal Tablets. 1676

EDEM (Mexico)
NAPROXEN SODIUM
Anaprox DS Tablets 2761
Anaprox Tablets 2761

EDEMID (Venezuela)
FUROSEMIDE
Furosemide Tablets 2154

EDENOL (Mexico)
FUROSEMIDE
Furosemide Tablets 2154

EDEX (France, Greece)
ALPROSTADIL
Edex Injection. 3089

EDICIN (Czech Republic, Hungary, Russia, Thailand)
VANCOMYCIN HYDROCHLORIDE
Vancocin HCl Capsules, USP 3380

EDICTUM (Argentina)
CLONAZEPAM
Klonopin Tablets 2778

EDIP (India)
NIFEDIPINE
Adalat CC Tablets 2964

EDISTOL (Spain)
ISOSORBIDE MONONITRATE
Imdur Tablets. 3018

EDNYT (Czech Republic, Hungary, Irish Republic, Russia, United Kingdom)
ENALAPRIL MALEATE
Vasotec I.V. Injection 2103

EDOLGLAU (Portugal)
CLONIDINE HYDROCHLORIDE
Catapres Tablets 843

EFAVILEA (Argentina)
EFAVIRENZ
Sustiva Capsules. 930

EFAVIR (India)
EFAVIRENZ
Sustiva Capsules. 930

EFCORLIN (India)
HYDROCORTISONE
Hydrocortone Tablets 1989

EFCORTELAN (United Kingdom)
HYDROCORTISONE
Hydrocortone Tablets 1989

EFECTIN (Austria, Czech Republic, Hungary)
VENLAFAXINE HYDROCHLORIDE
Effexor Tablets 3411
Effexor XR Capsules 3417

EFEKTOLOL (Germany)
PROPRANOLOL HYDROCHLORIDE
Inderal LA Long-Acting Capsules 3429

EFEMOLINA (Argentina)
FLUOROMETHOLONE
FML Ophthalmic Ointment. . . . . ⊙228

EFEROX (Germany)
LEVOTHYROXINE SODIUM
Levothroid Tablets 1186

Levoxyl Tablets 1712
Synthroid Tablets 520

EFEROX JOD (Germany)
LEVOTHYROXINE SODIUM
Levothroid Tablets 1186
Levoxyl Tablets 1712
Synthroid Tablets 520

EFEXOR (Argentina, Australia, Austria, Belgium, Brazil, Chile, Denmark, Finland, Greece, Hong Kong, Irish Republic, Israel, Italy, Malaysia, Mexico, New Zealand, Norway, Portugal, Singapore, South Africa, Switzerland, Thailand, The Netherlands, United Kingdom, Venezuela)
VENLAFAXINE HYDROCHLORIDE
Effexor Tablets 3411
Effexor XR Capsules 3417

EFFACNE (France, Switzerland)
BENZOYL PEROXIDE
Brevoxyl-4 Creamy Wash 3210
Brevoxyl-4 Gel 3210
Brevoxyl-8 Creamy Wash 3210
Brevoxyl-8 Gel 3210
Triaz Cleanser 1892
Triaz Gel 1892

EFFECTSAL (Singapore)
NORFLOXACIN
Noroxin Tablets 2032

EFFEDERM (France)
TRETINOIN
Vesanoid Capsules 2820

EFFEKTON (Germany)
DICLOFENAC SODIUM
Voltaren Tablets 2307
Voltaren-XR Tablets 2310

EFFEXOR (Canada)
VENLAFAXINE HYDROCHLORIDE
Effexor Tablets 3411
Effexor XR Capsules 3417

EFFLUMIDEX (Czech Republic, Germany, Hungary)
FLUOROMETHOLONE
FML Ophthalmic Ointment ⊙228

EFFOX (Czech Republic, Russia)
ISOSORBIDE MONONITRATE
Imdur Tablets 3018

EFIXANO (Argentina)
IRINOTECAN HYDROCHLORIDE
Camptosar Injection 2604

EFLORAN (Czech Republic, Russia)
METRONIDAZOLE
MetroGel-Vaginal Gel 1855

EFTRIVAL (Venezuela)
CEFTRIAXONE SODIUM
Rocephin Injectable Vials, ADD-Vantage, Galaxy, Bulk 2800

EFUDEX (Canada)
FLUOROURACIL
Efudex Topical Cream 3363
Efudex Topical Solutions 3363

EFUDIX (Argentina, Australia, Belgium, Chile, France, Germany, Hong Kong, Hungary, Irish Republic, Israel, Italy, Mexico, New Zealand, Singapore, South Africa, Spain, Switzerland, Thailand, The Netherlands, United Kingdom)
FLUOROURACIL
Efudex Topical Cream 3363
Efudex Topical Solutions 3363

EFURIX (Brazil)
FLUOROURACIL
Efudex Topical Cream 3363
Efudex Topical Solutions 3363

EGERY (France)
ERYTHROMYCIN
Ery-Tab Tablets 449
Erythromycin Base Filmtab Tablets 455
Erythromycin Delayed-Release Capsules, USP 457
PCE Dispertab Tablets 515

EGIBREN (Italy)
SELEGILINE HYDROCHLORIDE
Eldepryl Capsules 3208

EGIFILIN (Hungary)
THEOPHYLLINE
Uniphyl Tablets 2710

EGILOK (Czech Republic)
METOPROLOL TARTRATE
Lopressor Tablets 2238

EGLANDIN (Singapore)
ALPROSTADIL
Edex Injection 3089

EGLIDON (Argentina)
TERAZOSIN HYDROCHLORIDE
Hytrin Capsules 471

EGOCORT (Australia, Hong Kong, Malaysia, New Zealand, Singapore)
HYDROCORTISONE
Hydrocortone Tablets 1989

EHLITEN (Mexico)
PRAZIQUANTEL
Biltricide Tablets 2976

EHLIXACIN (Mexico)
CIPROFLOXACIN
Cipro Oral Suspension 2977

EIFEL (Greece)
BETAXOLOL HYDROCHLORIDE
Betoptic S Ophthalmic Suspension ⊙203, 558

EINALAT (Austria)
NIFEDIPINE
Adalat CC Tablets 2964

EISMYCIN (Germany)
MUPIROCIN
Bactroban Ointment 1395

EK-3 (Mexico)
ENALAPRIL MALEATE
Vasotec I.V. Injection 2103

ELAFAX (Argentina)
VENLAFAXINE HYDROCHLORIDE
Effexor Tablets 3411
Effexor XR Capsules 3417

ELAN (Italy)
ISOSORBIDE MONONITRATE
Imdur Tablets 3018

ELANDUR (Argentina)
ALENDRONATE SODIUM
Fosamax Tablets 1969

ELANTAN (Austria, Germany, Hong Kong, Irish Republic, Malaysia, Mexico, South Africa, Switzerland, Thailand, United Kingdom, Venezuela)
ISOSORBIDE MONONITRATE
Imdur Tablets 3018

ELANVER (Greece)
VERAPAMIL HYDROCHLORIDE
Covera-HS Tablets 3139
Verelan PM Extended-Release Capsules, Controlled-Onset 3106

ELBAT (Greece)
FLUTAMIDE
Eulexin Capsules 3009

ELBROL (Germany)
PROPRANOLOL HYDROCHLORIDE
Inderal LA Long-Acting Capsules 3429

ELCAR (Russia)
LEVOCARNITINE
Carnitor Injection 3188
Carnitor Tablets and Oral Solution 3190

ELCION (India)
DIAZEPAM
Diastat Rectal Delivery System 3343
Valium Tablets 2819

ELDEPRINE (France)
SELEGILINE HYDROCHLORIDE
Eldepryl Capsules 3208

ELDEPRYL (Australia, Belgium, Canada, Denmark, Finland, Irish Republic, New Zealand, Norway, South Africa, Sweden, The Netherlands, United Kingdom)
SELEGILINE HYDROCHLORIDE
Eldepryl Capsules 3208

ELEGELIN (Singapore, Thailand)
SELEGILINE HYDROCHLORIDE
Eldepryl Capsules 3208

ELEM (Chile)
METHYLPHENIDATE HYDROCHLORIDE
Ritalin Hydrochloride Tablets 2269
Ritalin-SR Tablets 2269

ELEQUINE (Mexico)
LEVOFLOXACIN
Levaquin Injection 2384
Levaquin Tablets 2384

ELEVAT (South Africa)
DRONABINOL
Marinol Capsules 3333

ELFAXONE (The Netherlands)
CEFTRIAXONE SODIUM
Rocephin Injectable Vials, ADD-Vantage, Galaxy, Bulk 2800

ELICA (Mexico, South Africa, Spain)
MOMETASONE FUROATE
Elocon Cream 0.1% 3005
Elocon Lotion 0.1% 3006
Elocon Ointment 0.1% 3007
Nasonex Nasal Spray 3043

ELIUR (Argentina)
FUROSEMIDE
Furosemide Tablets 2154

ELIXIFILIN (Spain)
THEOPHYLLINE
Uniphyl Tablets 2710

ELIXINE (Chile)
THEOPHYLLINE
Uniphyl Tablets 2710

ELIXOFILINA (Mexico)
THEOPHYLLINE
Uniphyl Tablets 2710

ELIXOPHYLLIN (Australia, Canada)
THEOPHYLLINE
Uniphyl Tablets 2710

ELLANCO (Hong Kong)
LOVASTATIN
Mevacor Tablets 2021

ELLECI (Italy)
LEVOCARNITINE
Carnitor Injection 3188
Carnitor Tablets and Oral Solution 3190

ELLESTE (Czech Republic)
ESTRADIOL
Climara Transdermal System 771
Estring Vaginal Ring 2635

ELLESTE-SOLO (United Kingdom)
ESTRADIOL
Climara Transdermal System 771
Estring Vaginal Ring 2635

ELMENDOS (Australia, Germany)
LAMOTRIGINE
Lamictal Chewable Dispersible Tablets 1481
Lamictal Tablets 1481

ELMIRON (Argentina, Australia, Canada, Hong Kong)
PENTOSAN POLYSULFATE SODIUM
Elmiron Capsules 2415

ELOCIN (Thailand)
ERYTHROMYCIN STEARATE
Erythrocin Stearate Filmtab Tablets 453

ELOCOM (Belgium, Brazil, Canada, Chile, Czech Republic, Hungary, Israel, Portugal, Russia, Spain, Switzerland)
MOMETASONE FUROATE
Elocon Cream 0.1% 3005
Elocon Lotion 0.1% 3006
Elocon Ointment 0.1% 3007
Nasonex Nasal Spray 3043

ELOCON (Argentina, Australia, Austria, Denmark, Finland, Greece, India, Irish Republic, Italy, New Zealand, Norway, South Africa, Sweden, The Netherlands, United Kingdom, Venezuela)
MOMETASONE FUROATE
Elocon Cream 0.1% 3005
Elocon Lotion 0.1% 3006
Elocon Ointment 0.1% 3007
Nasonex Nasal Spray 3043

ELOCONEX (Venezuela)
MOMETASONE FUROATE
Elocon Cream 0.1% 3005
Elocon Lotion 0.1% 3006
Elocon Ointment 0.1% 3007
Nasonex Nasal Spray 3043

ELOCOR (Mexico)
NIFEDIPINE
Adalat CC Tablets 2964

ELOCORT (Brazil)
HYDROCORTISONE
Hydrocortone Tablets 1989

ELOMET (Hong Kong, Malaysia, Mexico, Singapore, Thailand, Venezuela)
MOMETASONE FUROATE
Elocon Cream 0.1% 3005
Elocon Lotion 0.1% 3006
Elocon Ointment 0.1% 3007
Nasonex Nasal Spray 3043

ELONGAL (Chile)
DIAZEPAM
Diastat Rectal Delivery System 3343
Valium Tablets 2819

ELOSALIC (Argentina, Austria, Brazil, Hong Kong, South Africa, Sweden, Thailand, Venezuela)
MOMETASONE FUROATE
Elocon Cream 0.1% 3005
Elocon Lotion 0.1% 3006
Elocon Ointment 0.1% 3007
Nasonex Nasal Spray 3043

ELOVENT (Austria, Greece, The Netherlands)
MOMETASONE FUROATE
Elocon Cream 0.1% 3005
Elocon Lotion 0.1% 3006
Elocon Ointment 0.1% 3007
Nasonex Nasal Spray 3043

ELPRADIL (Switzerland)
ENALAPRIL MALEATE
Vasotec I.V. Injection 2103

ELPRADIL HCT (Switzerland)
ENALAPRIL MALEATE
Vasotec I.V. Injection 2103

ELSPAR (Brazil, Hong Kong)
ASPARAGINASE
Elspar for Injection 2463

ELSTATIN (Singapore)
LOVASTATIN
Mevacor Tablets 2021

ELTHYRONE (Belgium)
LEVOTHYROXINE SODIUM
Levothroid Tablets 1186
Levoxyl Tablets 1712
Synthroid Tablets 520

ELTOCIN (India)
ERYTHROMYCIN
Ery-Tab Tablets 449
Erythromycin Base Filmtab Tablets 455
Erythromycin Delayed-Release Capsules, USP 457
PCE Dispertab Tablets 515

ELTROXIN (Canada, Czech Republic, Denmark, Hong Kong, India, Irish Republic, Israel, New Zealand, Singapore, South Africa, Thailand, The Netherlands, United Kingdom)
LEVOTHYROXINE SODIUM
Levothroid Tablets 1186
Levoxyl Tablets 1712
Synthroid Tablets 520

ELTROXINE (Switzerland)
LEVOTHYROXINE SODIUM
Levothroid Tablets 1186
Levoxyl Tablets 1712
Synthroid Tablets 520

ELUTIT-NATRIUM (Germany)
SODIUM POLYSTYRENE SULFONATE
Kionex Powder 2477

ELVENAVIR (Argentina)
INDINAVIR SULFATE
Crixivan Capsules 1940

ELYZOL (Finland, Hong Kong, Mexico, Singapore, Thailand, The Netherlands)
METRONIDAZOLE
MetroGel-Vaginal Gel 1855

EMANTHAL (India)
ALBENDAZOLE
Albenza Tablets 1338

EMEDAL (Greece)
METRONIDAZOLE
MetroGel-Vaginal Gel . . . 1855

EMESET (Czech Republic, India, Thailand)
ONDANSETRON HYDROCHLORIDE
Zofran Injection . . . 1634
Zofran Injection Premixed . . . 1634
Zofran Oral Solution . . . 1639
Zofran Tablets . . . 1639

EMESTID (France)
ERYTHROMYCIN STEARATE
Erythrocin Stearate Filmtab Tablets . . . 453

EMETRON (Czech Republic, Hungary, Russia)
ONDANSETRON HYDROCHLORIDE
Zofran Injection . . . 1634
Zofran Injection Premixed . . . 1634
Zofran Oral Solution . . . 1639
Zofran Tablets . . . 1639

EMFORAL (Thailand)
PROPRANOLOL HYDROCHLORIDE
Inderal LA Long-Acting Capsules . . . 3429

EMISGENTA (Brazil)
GENTAMICIN SULFATE
Garamycin Injectable . . . 3014

EMIVOX (Argentina)
ONDANSETRON
Zofran ODT Orally Disintegrating Tablets . . 1639

EMLA (Czech Republic, Finland, United Kingdom)
LIDOCAINE
Lidoderm Patch . . . 1118

EMOCAL (Finland)
CITALOPRAM HYDROBROMIDE
Celexa Tablets . . . 1176

EMO-CORT (Canada)
HYDROCORTISONE
Hydrocortone Tablets . . . 1989

EMPECID (Argentina)
CLOTRIMAZOLE
Lotrimin Cream . . . 3039
Lotrimin Lotion 1% . . . 3039
Lotrimin Topical Solution 1% . . . 3039

EMPECID CORT (Argentina)
CLOTRIMAZOLE
Lotrimin Cream . . . 3039
Lotrimin Lotion 1% . . . 3039
Lotrimin Topical Solution 1% . . . 3039

EMU-V (Australia, Czech Republic, South Africa)
ERYTHROMYCIN
Ery-Tab Tablets . . . 449
Erythromycin Base Filmtab Tablets . . . 455
Erythromycin Delayed-Release Capsules, USP . . . 457
PCE Dispertab Tablets . . . 515

EMUVIN (Austria)
ERYTHROMYCIN
Ery-Tab Tablets . . . 449
Erythromycin Base Filmtab Tablets . . . 455
Erythromycin Delayed-Release Capsules, USP . . . 457
PCE Dispertab Tablets . . . 515

E-MYCIN (Canada, Hong Kong, Israel, Singapore)
ERYTHROMYCIN
Ery-Tab Tablets . . . 449
Erythromycin Base Filmtab Tablets . . . 455
Erythromycin Delayed-Release Capsules, USP . . . 457
PCE Dispertab Tablets . . . 515

ENA-BASAN (Switzerland)
ENALAPRIL MALEATE
Vasotec I.V. Injection . . . 2103

ENABETA (Germany)
ENALAPRIL MALEATE
Vasotec I.V. Injection . . . 2103

ENABETA COMP (Germany)
ENALAPRIL MALEATE
Vasotec I.V. Injection . . . 2103

ENAC (Austria)
ENALAPRIL MALEATE
Vasotec I.V. Injection . . . 2103

ENACARD (United Kingdom)
ENALAPRIL MALEATE
Vasotec I.V. Injection . . . 2103

ENACE (India)
ENALAPRIL MALEATE
Vasotec I.V. Injection . . . 2103

ENACE-D (India)
ENALAPRIL MALEATE
Vasotec I.V. Injection . . . 2103

ENACODAN (Denmark)
ENALAPRIL MALEATE
Vasotec I.V. Injection . . . 2103

ENACOSTAD (Austria, The Netherlands)
ENALAPRIL MALEATE
Vasotec I.V. Injection . . . 2103

ENACOZID (Denmark)
ENALAPRIL MALEATE
Vasotec I.V. Injection . . . 2103

ENADIL (Denmark)
ENALAPRIL MALEATE
Vasotec I.V. Injection . . . 2103

ENADIOL NETA (Chile)
ESTRADIOL
Climara Transdermal System . . . 771
Estring Vaginal Ring . . . 2635

ENADURA (Germany)
ENALAPRIL MALEATE
Vasotec I.V. Injection . . . 2103

ENAFARM (Russia)
ENALAPRIL MALEATE
Vasotec I.V. Injection . . . 2103

ENAHEXAL (Australia, Germany, New Zealand)
ENALAPRIL MALEATE
Vasotec I.V. Injection . . . 2103

ENAHEXAL COMP (Germany)
ENALAPRIL MALEATE
Vasotec I.V. Injection . . . 2103

ENAL (Germany)
ENALAPRIL MALEATE
Vasotec I.V. Injection . . . 2103

ENALABAL (Brazil)
ENALAPRIL MALEATE
Vasotec I.V. Injection . . . 2103

ENALABENE (Austria)
ENALAPRIL MALEATE
Vasotec I.V. Injection . . . 2103

ENALADEX (Israel)
ENALAPRIL MALEATE
Vasotec I.V. Injection . . . 2103

ENALADIL (Mexico)
ENALAPRIL MALEATE
Vasotec I.V. Injection . . . 2103

ENALAFEL (Argentina)
ENALAPRIL MALEATE
Vasotec I.V. Injection . . . 2103

ENALAGAMMA (Germany)
ENALAPRIL MALEATE
Vasotec I.V. Injection . . . 2103

ENALAPRIL PLUS (Germany)
ENALAPRIL MALEATE
Vasotec I.V. Injection . . . 2103

ENALDUN (Hong Kong)
ENALAPRIL MALEATE
Vasotec I.V. Injection . . . 2103

ENALICH (Germany)
ENALAPRIL MALEATE
Vasotec I.V. Injection . . . 2103

ENALIND (Germany)
ENALAPRIL MALEATE
Vasotec I.V. Injection . . . 2103

ENALOC (Finland)
ENALAPRIL MALEATE
Vasotec I.V. Injection . . . 2103

ENALPRIN (Brazil)
ENALAPRIL MALEATE
Vasotec I.V. Injection . . . 2103

ENALTEN (Chile)
ENALAPRIL MALEATE
Vasotec I.V. Injection . . . 2103

ENAM (Russia, Thailand, Venezuela)
ENALAPRIL MALEATE
Vasotec I.V. Injection . . . 2103

ENAP (Czech Republic, Hungary, Irish Republic, Russia, Singapore, South Africa)
ENALAPRIL MALEATE
Vasotec I.V. Injection . . . 2103

ENAP-CO (South Africa)
ENALAPRIL MALEATE
Vasotec I.V. Injection . . . 2103

ENAP-H (Czech Republic)
ENALAPRIL MALEATE
Vasotec I.V. Injection . . . 2103

ENAP-HL (Czech Republic, Hungary, Singapore)
ENALAPRIL MALEATE
Vasotec I.V. Injection . . . 2103

ENAPIREX (Czech Republic)
ENALAPRIL MALEATE
Vasotec I.V. Injection . . . 2103

ENAPREN (Italy)
ENALAPRIL MALEATE
Vasotec I.V. Injection . . . 2103

ENAPRESS (Finland)
ENALAPRIL MALEATE
Vasotec I.V. Injection . . . 2103

ENAPRIL (Austria, Brazil, Czech Republic, Hungary, Thailand)
ENALAPRIL MALEATE
Vasotec I.V. Injection . . . 2103

ENAPRIVAL (Venezuela)
ENALAPRIL MALEATE
Vasotec I.V. Injection . . . 2103

ENAPROTEC (Brazil)
ENALAPRIL MALEATE
Vasotec I.V. Injection . . . 2103

ENA-PUREN (Germany)
ENALAPRIL MALEATE
Vasotec I.V. Injection . . . 2103

ENARAN (Austria)
ENALAPRIL MALEATE
Vasotec I.V. Injection . . . 2103

ENARENAL (Russia)
ENALAPRIL MALEATE
Vasotec I.V. Injection . . . 2103

ENARIL (Singapore, Thailand)
ENALAPRIL MALEATE
Vasotec I.V. Injection . . . 2103

ENASIFAR (Switzerland)
ENALAPRIL MALEATE
Vasotec I.V. Injection . . . 2103

ENATEC (Brazil, Switzerland)
ENALAPRIL MALEATE
Vasotec I.V. Injection . . . 2103

ENATEC F (Brazil)
ENALAPRIL MALEATE
Vasotec I.V. Injection . . . 2103

ENATRIAL (Argentina)
ENALAPRIL MALEATE
Vasotec I.V. Injection . . . 2103

ENATYROL (Austria)
ENALAPRIL MALEATE
Vasotec I.V. Injection . . . 2103

ENAZIL (Russia)
ENALAPRIL MALEATE
Vasotec I.V. Injection . . . 2103

ENBREL (Argentina, Australia, Belgium, Brazil, Canada, Chile, Czech Republic, Denmark, Finland, France, Germany, Greece, Hong Kong, Hungary, Irish Republic, Israel, Italy, Mexico, New Zealand, Norway, Portugal, Spain, Sweden, Switzerland, Thailand, United Kingdom)
ETANERCEPT
Enbrel for Injection . . . 584

ENDANTADINE (Canada)
AMANTADINE HYDROCHLORIDE
Symmetrel Tablets . . . 1135

ENDOCLAR (Argentina)
DONEPEZIL HYDROCHLORIDE
Aricept Tablets . . . 1094

ENDOERITRIN (Spain)
ERYTHROMYCIN
Ery-Tab Tablets . . . 449
Erythromycin Base Filmtab Tablets . . . 455
Erythromycin Delayed-Release Capsules, USP . . . 457
PCE Dispertab Tablets . . . 515

ENDOMETRIN (Hong Kong, Israel)
PROGESTERONE
Prometrium Capsules (100 mg, 200 mg) . 3203

ENDOMINA (Spain)
ESTRADIOL
Climara Transdermal System . . . 771
Estring Vaginal Ring . . . 2635

ENDONE (Australia)
OXYCODONE HYDROCHLORIDE
OxyContin Tablets . . . 2703
OxyFast Oral Concentrate Solution . . . 2708
OxyIR Capsules . . . 2708

ENDRONAX (Brazil)
ALENDRONATE SODIUM
Fosamax Tablets . . . 1969

ENEAS (Germany, Greece, Spain)
ENALAPRIL MALEATE
Vasotec I.V. Injection . . . 2103

ENECAL (Venezuela)
ENALAPRIL MALEATE
Vasotec I.V. Injection . . . 2103

ENI (Mexico)
CIPROFLOXACIN HYDROCHLORIDE
Ciloxan Ophthalmic Ointment . . . ⊙204, 559
Ciloxan Ophthalmic Solution . . . ⊙206
Cipro Tablets . . . 2977

ENIT (Spain)
ENALAPRIL MALEATE
Vasotec I.V. Injection . . . 2103

ENLACE (Mexico)
CAPTOPRIL
Captopril Tablets . . . 2149

ENOXIN (Malaysia)
CIPROFLOXACIN HYDROCHLORIDE
Ciloxan Ophthalmic Ointment . . . ⊙204, 559
Ciloxan Ophthalmic Solution . . . ⊙206
Cipro Tablets . . . 2977

ENPER (Argentina)
ZIDOVUDINE
Retrovir Capsules . . . 1560
Retrovir IV Infusion . . . 1564
Retrovir Syrup . . . 1560
Retrovir Tablets . . . 1560

ENPOTT (Thailand)
POTASSIUM CHLORIDE
K-Dur Extended-Relase Tablets . . . 3033
K-Lor Oral Solution . . . 474
K-Tab Tablets . . . 475

ENROMIC (Argentina)
LOSARTAN POTASSIUM
Cozaar Tablets . . . 1935

ENSIAL (Greece)
LEVOCARNITINE
Carnitor Injection . . . 3188
Carnitor Tablets and Oral Solution . . . 3190

ENTIZOL (Czech Republic)
METRONIDAZOLE
MetroGel-Vaginal Gel . . . 1855

ENTOPLUS (Mexico)
ALBENDAZOLE
Albenza Tablets . . . 1338

ENTRYDIL (Irish Republic)
DILTIAZEM HYDROCHLORIDE
Cardizem LA Extended Release Tablets . . . 1728
Tiazac Capsules . . . 1201

ENULID (Italy)
MOEXIPRIL HYDROCHLORIDE
Univasc Tablets . . . 3104

ENVAS (India, Thailand)
ENALAPRIL MALEATE
Vasotec I.V. Injection . . . 2103

ENZACE (Australia)
CAPTOPRIL
Captopril Tablets . . . 2149

ENZIPAN (Italy)
PANCRELIPASE
Ultrase Capsules . . . 708
Ultrase MT Capsules . . . 709

EPADOREN (Greece)
RANITIDINE HYDROCHLORIDE
Zantac 25 EFFERdose Tablets . . . 1624

Zantac 150 EFFERdose Tablets 1624
Zantac 150 Tablets 1624
Zantac 300 Tablets 1624
Zantac Injection 1619
Zantac Injection Premixed 1619
Zantac Syrup 1624

EPALAT EPS (Italy)
LACTULOSE
Kristalose for Oral Solution 1034

EPALFEN (Italy)
LACTULOSE
Kristalose for Oral Solution 1034

EPAQ (Argentina, Mexico)
METRONIDAZOLE
MetroGel-Vaginal Gel 1855

EPHELIA (Germany, Italy)
ESTRADIOL
Climara Transdermal System 771
Estring Vaginal Ring 2635

EPI-ABEREL (Germany)
TRETINOIN
Vesanoid Capsules 2820

EPICLODINA (Mexico)
CLONIDINE
Catapres-TTS 844

EPICORDIN (Austria, Germany)
ISOSORBIDE MONONITRATE
Imdur Tablets 3018

EPIESTROL (Chile, Irish Republic, Italy, Switzerland)
ESTRADIOL
Climara Transdermal System 771
Estring Vaginal Ring 2635

EPIFON (Venezuela)
LAMOTRIGINE
Lamictal Chewable Dispersible Tablets 1481
Lamictal Tablets 1481

EPILENIL (Brazil)
VALPROIC ACID
Depakene Capsules 417
Depakene Oral Solution 417

EPILEPAX (Argentina)
LAMOTRIGINE
Lamictal Chewable Dispersible Tablets 1481
Lamictal Tablets 1481

EPIMAZ (United Kingdom)
CARBAMAZEPINE
Carbatrol Capsules 3171
Tegretol Chewable Tablets 2295
Tegretol Suspension 2295
Tegretol Tablets 2295
Tegretol-XR Tablets 2295

EPIMORPH (Canada)
MORPHINE SULFATE
Kadian Capsules 577
MS Contin Tablets 2701

EPITOMAX (France)
TOPIRAMATE
Topamax Sprinkle Capsules 2404
Topamax Tablets 2404

EPITREL (Mexico)
TRETINOIN
Vesanoid Capsules 2820

EPITRIAM (The Netherlands)
TRIAMTERENE
Dyrenium Capsules 3400

EPITRIL (India)
CLONAZEPAM
Klonopin Tablets 2778

EPIVIR (Austria, Belgium, Brazil, Czech Republic, Denmark, Finland, France, Germany, Greece, Irish Republic, Israel, Italy, Japan, Norway, Portugal, Russia, Singapore, Spain, Sweden, Thailand, The Netherlands, United Kingdom, Venezuela)
LAMIVUDINE
Epivir Oral Solution 1427
Epivir Tablets 1427
Epivir-HBV Oral Solution 1432
Epivir-HBV Tablets 1432

EPIZAM (India)
CLONAZEPAM
Klonopin Tablets 2778

EPOGEN (Argentina)
EPOETIN ALFA
Epogen for Injection 591
Procrit for Injection 2364

EPOPEN (Spain)
EPOETIN ALFA
Epogen for Injection 591
Procrit for Injection 2364

EPOSAL (Chile)
CARBAMAZEPINE
Carbatrol Capsules 3171
Tegretol Chewable Tablets 2295
Tegretol Suspension 2295
Tegretol Tablets 2295
Tegretol-XR Tablets 2295

EPOXIDE (Thailand)
CHLORDIAZEPOXIDE HYDROCHLORIDE
Librium Capsules 3347

EPOXITIN (Italy)
EPOETIN ALFA
Epogen for Injection 591
Procrit for Injection 2364

EPREX (Argentina, Australia, Belgium, Brazil, Canada, Chile, Czech Republic, Denmark, Finland, France, Germany, Greece, Hong Kong, Hungary, Irish Republic, Israel, Italy, Malaysia, Mexico, New Zealand, Norway, Russia, Singapore, South Africa, Spain, Sweden, Switzerland, Thailand, The Netherlands, United Kingdom, Venezuela)
EPOETIN ALFA
Epogen for Injection 591
Procrit for Injection 2364

EPRIL (Switzerland)
ENALAPRIL MALEATE
Vasotec I.V. Injection 2103

EPSITRON (Hong Kong, Thailand)
CAPTOPRIL
Captopril Tablets 2149

EQUASYM (Denmark, Germany, Irish Republic, The Netherlands, United Kingdom)
METHYLPHENIDATE HYDROCHLORIDE
Ritalin Hydrochloride Tablets 2269
Ritalin-SR Tablets 2269

EQUIPAX (Spain)
GABAPENTIN
Neurontin Capsules 2487

ERADIX (Austria)
FAMOTIDINE
Pepcid Injection 2040
Pepcid Injection Premixed 2040
Pepcid Tablets 2038
Pepcid for Oral Suspension 2038

ERANZ (Argentina, Brazil, Chile, Mexico, Venezuela)
DONEPEZIL HYDROCHLORIDE
Aricept Tablets 1094

ERI (Argentina)
ERYTHROMYCIN
Ery-Tab Tablets 449
Erythromycin Base Filmtab Tablets 455
Erythromycin Delayed-Release Capsules, USP 457
PCE Dispertab Tablets 515

ERIBEC (Mexico)
ERYTHROMYCIN
Ery-Tab Tablets 449
Erythromycin Base Filmtab Tablets 455
Erythromycin Delayed-Release Capsules, USP 457
PCE Dispertab Tablets 515

ERIBER (Mexico)
ERYTHROMYCIN
Ery-Tab Tablets 449
Erythromycin Base Filmtab Tablets 455
Erythromycin Delayed-Release Capsules, USP 457
PCE Dispertab Tablets 515

ERIBUS (Mexico)
ERYTHROMYCIN
Ery-Tab Tablets 449
Erythromycin Base Filmtab Tablets 455
Erythromycin Delayed-Release Capsules, USP 457
PCE Dispertab Tablets 515

ERICIN (Thailand)
ERYTHROMYCIN STEARATE
Erythrocin Stearate Filmtab Tablets 453

ERICOSOL (Switzerland)
ERYTHROMYCIN STEARATE
Erythrocin Stearate Filmtab Tablets 453

ERIDAN (Italy)
DIAZEPAM
Diastat Rectal Delivery System 3343
Valium Tablets 2819

ERIDOSIS (Spain)
ERYTHROMYCIN
Ery-Tab Tablets 449
Erythromycin Base Filmtab Tablets 455
Erythromycin Delayed-Release Capsules, USP 457
PCE Dispertab Tablets 515

ERIFOSTINE (Argentina)
AMIFOSTINE
Ethyol for Injection 1898

ERIGRAND (Argentina)
ERYTHROMYCIN
Ery-Tab Tablets 449
Erythromycin Base Filmtab Tablets 455
Erythromycin Delayed-Release Capsules, USP 457
PCE Dispertab Tablets 515

ERIMICIN (Argentina)
BENZOYL PEROXIDE
Brevoxyl-4 Creamy Wash 3210
Brevoxyl-4 Gel 3210
Brevoxyl-8 Creamy Wash 3210
Brevoxyl-8 Gel 3210
Triaz Cleanser 1892
Triaz Gel 1892

ERIMICINA (Brazil, Mexico)
ERYTHROMYCIN
Ery-Tab Tablets 449
Erythromycin Base Filmtab Tablets 455
Erythromycin Delayed-Release Capsules, USP 457
PCE Dispertab Tablets 515

ERIPRODIN (Spain)
ERYTHROMYCIN
Ery-Tab Tablets 449
Erythromycin Base Filmtab Tablets 455
Erythromycin Delayed-Release Capsules, USP 457
PCE Dispertab Tablets 515

ERISOL (Argentina)
ERYTHROMYCIN
Ery-Tab Tablets 449
Erythromycin Base Filmtab Tablets 455
Erythromycin Delayed-Release Capsules, USP 457
PCE Dispertab Tablets 515

ERISUSPEN (Mexico)
ERYTHROMYCIN
Ery-Tab Tablets 449
Erythromycin Base Filmtab Tablets 455
Erythromycin Delayed-Release Capsules, USP 457
PCE Dispertab Tablets 515

ERIT (Argentina)
ERYTHROMYCIN
Ery-Tab Tablets 449
Erythromycin Base Filmtab Tablets 455
Erythromycin Delayed-Release Capsules, USP 457
PCE Dispertab Tablets 515

ERITIMIX (Venezuela)
ERYTHROMYCIN
Ery-Tab Tablets 449
Erythromycin Base Filmtab Tablets 455
Erythromycin Delayed-Release Capsules, USP 457
PCE Dispertab Tablets 515

ERITINA (Brazil)
EPOETIN ALFA
Epogen for Injection 591
Procrit for Injection 2364

ERITOLAT (Mexico)
ERYTHROMYCIN
Ery-Tab Tablets 449
Erythromycin Base Filmtab Tablets 455
Erythromycin Delayed-Release Capsules, USP 457
PCE Dispertab Tablets 515

ERITRERBA (Mexico)
ERYTHROMYCIN
Ery-Tab Tablets 449
Erythromycin Base Filmtab Tablets 455
Erythromycin Delayed-Release Capsules, USP 457
PCE Dispertab Tablets 515

ERITREX A (Brazil)
ERYTHROMYCIN
Ery-Tab Tablets 449
Erythromycin Base Filmtab Tablets 455
Erythromycin Delayed-Release Capsules, USP 457
PCE Dispertab Tablets 515

ERITRIL (Brazil)
ERYTHROMYCIN
Ery-Tab Tablets 449
Erythromycin Base Filmtab Tablets 455
Erythromycin Delayed-Release Capsules, USP 457
PCE Dispertab Tablets 515

ERITRODERM (Argentina)
ERYTHROMYCIN
Ery-Tab Tablets 449
Erythromycin Base Filmtab Tablets 455
Erythromycin Delayed-Release Capsules, USP 457
PCE Dispertab Tablets 515

ERITROFARMIN (Mexico)
ERYTHROMYCIN
Ery-Tab Tablets 449
Erythromycin Base Filmtab Tablets 455
Erythromycin Delayed-Release Capsules, USP 457
PCE Dispertab Tablets 515

ERITROLAT (Mexico)
ERYTHROMYCIN
Ery-Tab Tablets 449
Erythromycin Base Filmtab Tablets 455
Erythromycin Delayed-Release Capsules, USP 457
PCE Dispertab Tablets 515

ERITROMED (Argentina)
ERYTHROMYCIN
Ery-Tab Tablets 449
Erythromycin Base Filmtab Tablets 455
Erythromycin Delayed-Release Capsules, USP 457
PCE Dispertab Tablets 515

ERITROQUIM (Mexico)
ERYTHROMYCIN
Ery-Tab Tablets 449
Erythromycin Base Filmtab Tablets 455
Erythromycin Delayed-Release Capsules, USP 457
PCE Dispertab Tablets 515

ERITROSOL (Mexico)
ERYTHROMYCIN
Ery-Tab Tablets 449
Erythromycin Base Filmtab Tablets 455
Erythromycin Delayed-Release Capsules, USP 457
PCE Dispertab Tablets 515

ERITROVIT (Brazil)
ERYTHROMYCIN
Ery-Tab Tablets 449
Erythromycin Base Filmtab Tablets 455
Erythromycin Delayed-Release Capsules, USP 457
PCE Dispertab Tablets 515

ERITROWEL (Mexico)
ERYTHROMYCIN
Ery-Tab Tablets 449
Erythromycin Base Filmtab Tablets 455
Erythromycin Delayed-Release Capsules, USP 457
PCE Dispertab Tablets 515

ERIWEST (Mexico)
ERYTHROMYCIN STEARATE
Erythrocin Stearate Filmtab Tablets 453

ERLADEXONE (Singapore)
DEXAMETHASONE
Decadron Tablets 1951

ERMOFAN (Greece)
OFLOXACIN
Floxin Otic Solution 1049

ERMYCIN (Singapore)
ERYTHROMYCIN STEARATE
Erythrocin Stearate Filmtab Tablets 453

EROMEL (South Africa)
ERYTHROMYCIN STEARATE
Erythrocin Stearate Filmtab Tablets 453

EROTAB (Malaysia, Singapore)
ERYTHROMYCIN STEARATE
Erythrocin Stearate Filmtab Tablets 453

ERROLON (Argentina)
FUROSEMIDE
Furosemide Tablets . . . 2154

ERWINASE (Greece)
ASPARAGINASE
Elspar for Injection . . . 2463

ERXETILAN (Greece)
ENALAPRIL MALEATE
Vasotec I.V. Injection . . . 2103

ERY (Germany)
ERYTHROMYCIN STEARATE
Erythrocin Stearate Filmtab Tablets . . . 453

ERYACNE (Argentina, Australia, France, Greece, Hong Kong, Italy, New Zealand, Singapore, Thailand, The Netherlands, United Kingdom, Venezuela)
ERYTHROMYCIN
Ery-Tab Tablets . . . 449
Erythromycin Base Filmtab Tablets . . . 455
Erythromycin Delayed-Release Capsules, USP . . . 457
PCE Dispertab Tablets . . . 515

ERYACNEN (Brazil, Chile, Mexico)
ERYTHROMYCIN
Ery-Tab Tablets . . . 449
Erythromycin Base Filmtab Tablets . . . 455
Erythromycin Delayed-Release Capsules, USP . . . 457
PCE Dispertab Tablets . . . 515

ERYAKNEN (Austria, Germany, Switzerland)
ERYTHROMYCIN
Ery-Tab Tablets . . . 449
Erythromycin Base Filmtab Tablets . . . 455
Erythromycin Delayed-Release Capsules, USP . . . 457
PCE Dispertab Tablets . . . 515

ERYBID (Canada)
ERYTHROMYCIN
Ery-Tab Tablets . . . 449
Erythromycin Base Filmtab Tablets . . . 455
Erythromycin Delayed-Release Capsules, USP . . . 457
PCE Dispertab Tablets . . . 515

ERYC (Australia, Canada, Hong Kong, Hungary, Israel, New Zealand, The Netherlands)
ERYTHROMYCIN
Ery-Tab Tablets . . . 449
Erythromycin Base Filmtab Tablets . . . 455
Erythromycin Delayed-Release Capsules, USP . . . 457
PCE Dispertab Tablets . . . 515

ERYCEN (United Kingdom)
ERYTHROMYCIN
Ery-Tab Tablets . . . 449
Erythromycin Base Filmtab Tablets . . . 455
Erythromycin Delayed-Release Capsules, USP . . . 457
PCE Dispertab Tablets . . . 515

ERYCETTE (South Africa)
ERYTHROMYCIN
Ery-Tab Tablets . . . 449
Erythromycin Base Filmtab Tablets . . . 455
Erythromycin Delayed-Release Capsules, USP . . . 457
PCE Dispertab Tablets . . . 515

ERYCIN (India, Thailand)
ERYTHROMYCIN
Ery-Tab Tablets . . . 449
Erythromycin Base Filmtab Tablets . . . 455
Erythromycin Delayed-Release Capsules, USP . . . 457
PCE Dispertab Tablets . . . 515

ERYCINUM (Austria)
ERYTHROMYCIN
Ery-Tab Tablets . . . 449
Erythromycin Base Filmtab Tablets . . . 455
Erythromycin Delayed-Release Capsules, USP . . . 457
PCE Dispertab Tablets . . . 515

ERYCIP (India)
ERYTHROMYCIN STEARATE
Erythrocin Stearate Filmtab Tablets . . . 453

ERYCREAM (Greece)
ERYTHROMYCIN
Ery-Tab Tablets . . . 449
Erythromycin Base Filmtab Tablets . . . 455
Erythromycin Delayed-Release Capsules, USP . . . 457
PCE Dispertab Tablets . . . 515

ERYDERM (Belgium, Israel, Malaysia, Mexico, Singapore, South Africa, Switzerland, The Netherlands)
ERYTHROMYCIN
Ery-Tab Tablets . . . 449
Erythromycin Base Filmtab Tablets . . . 455
Erythromycin Delayed-Release Capsules, USP . . . 457
PCE Dispertab Tablets . . . 515

ERYDERMEC (Germany)
ERYTHROMYCIN
Ery-Tab Tablets . . . 449
Erythromycin Base Filmtab Tablets . . . 455
Erythromycin Delayed-Release Capsules, USP . . . 457
PCE Dispertab Tablets . . . 515

ERYFLUID (Argentina, Czech Republic, France, Portugal)
ERYTHROMYCIN
Ery-Tab Tablets . . . 449
Erythromycin Base Filmtab Tablets . . . 455
Erythromycin Delayed-Release Capsules, USP . . . 457
PCE Dispertab Tablets . . . 515

ERYGEL (Greece)
ERYTHROMYCIN
Ery-Tab Tablets . . . 449
Erythromycin Base Filmtab Tablets . . . 455
Erythromycin Delayed-Release Capsules, USP . . . 457
PCE Dispertab Tablets . . . 515

ERYLAR (Mexico)
ERYTHROMYCIN
Ery-Tab Tablets . . . 449
Erythromycin Base Filmtab Tablets . . . 455
Erythromycin Delayed-Release Capsules, USP . . . 457
PCE Dispertab Tablets . . . 515

ERYLIK (France, Hong Kong)
ERYTHROMYCIN
Ery-Tab Tablets . . . 449
Erythromycin Base Filmtab Tablets . . . 455
Erythromycin Delayed-Release Capsules, USP . . . 457
PCE Dispertab Tablets . . . 515

ERYMAX (Irish Republic, South Africa, Switzerland, United Kingdom)
ERYTHROMYCIN
Ery-Tab Tablets . . . 449
Erythromycin Base Filmtab Tablets . . . 455
Erythromycin Delayed-Release Capsules, USP . . . 457
PCE Dispertab Tablets . . . 515

ERY-MAX (Spain)
ERYTHROMYCIN
Ery-Tab Tablets . . . 449
Erythromycin Base Filmtab Tablets . . . 455
Erythromycin Delayed-Release Capsules, USP . . . 457
PCE Dispertab Tablets . . . 515

ERYPARK (Chile)
ERYTHROMYCIN
Ery-Tab Tablets . . . 449
Erythromycin Base Filmtab Tablets . . . 455
Erythromycin Delayed-Release Capsules, USP . . . 457
PCE Dispertab Tablets . . . 515

ERYPO (Austria, Germany)
EPOETIN ALFA
Epogen for Injection . . . 591
Procrit for Injection . . . 2364

ERYSAFE (India)
ERYTHROMYCIN
Ery-Tab Tablets . . . 449
Erythromycin Base Filmtab Tablets . . . 455
Erythromycin Delayed-Release Capsules, USP . . . 457
PCE Dispertab Tablets . . . 515

ERYSOL (Canada)
ERYTHROMYCIN
Ery-Tab Tablets . . . 449
Erythromycin Base Filmtab Tablets . . . 455
Erythromycin Delayed-Release Capsules, USP . . . 457
PCE Dispertab Tablets . . . 515

ERYSTAD (Austria)
ERYTHROMYCIN STEARATE
Erythrocin Stearate Filmtab Tablets . . . 453

ERYTAB (Israel)
ERYTHROMYCIN
Ery-Tab Tablets . . . 449
Erythromycin Base Filmtab Tablets . . . 455
Erythromycin Delayed-Release Capsules, USP . . . 457
PCE Dispertab Tablets . . . 515

ERY-TAB (Thailand)
ERYTHROMYCIN
Ery-Tab Tablets . . . 449
Erythromycin Base Filmtab Tablets . . . 455
Erythromycin Delayed-Release Capsules, USP . . . 457
PCE Dispertab Tablets . . . 515

ERYTAB-S (Singapore)
ERYTHROMYCIN STEARATE
Erythrocin Stearate Filmtab Tablets . . . 453

ERYTHROCIN (India, United Kingdom)
ERYTHROMYCIN
Ery-Tab Tablets . . . 449
Erythromycin Base Filmtab Tablets . . . 455
Erythromycin Delayed-Release Capsules, USP . . . 457
PCE Dispertab Tablets . . . 515

ERYTHRODERM (Israel)
ERYTHROMYCIN
Ery-Tab Tablets . . . 449
Erythromycin Base Filmtab Tablets . . . 455
Erythromycin Delayed-Release Capsules, USP . . . 457
PCE Dispertab Tablets . . . 515

ERYTHROGEL (France, Greece)
ERYTHROMYCIN
Ery-Tab Tablets . . . 449
Erythromycin Base Filmtab Tablets . . . 455
Erythromycin Delayed-Release Capsules, USP . . . 457
PCE Dispertab Tablets . . . 515

ERYTHROMID (Canada, Irish Republic, South Africa, United Kingdom)
ERYTHROMYCIN
Ery-Tab Tablets . . . 449
Erythromycin Base Filmtab Tablets . . . 455
Erythromycin Delayed-Release Capsules, USP . . . 457
PCE Dispertab Tablets . . . 515

ERYTHROSKID (Czech Republic)
ERYTHROMYCIN
Ery-Tab Tablets . . . 449
Erythromycin Base Filmtab Tablets . . . 455
Erythromycin Delayed-Release Capsules, USP . . . 457
PCE Dispertab Tablets . . . 515

ERYTOP (Germany)
ERYTHROMYCIN
Ery-Tab Tablets . . . 449
Erythromycin Base Filmtab Tablets . . . 455
Erythromycin Delayed-Release Capsules, USP . . . 457
PCE Dispertab Tablets . . . 515

ERYTRAN (Switzerland)
ERYTHROMYCIN STEARATE
Erythrocin Stearate Filmtab Tablets . . . 453

ERYTROCICLIN (Italy)
ERYTHROMYCIN STEARATE
Erythrocin Stearate Filmtab Tablets . . . 453

ESALDOX (Chile)
LEVOTHYROXINE SODIUM
Levothroid Tablets . . . 1186
Levoxyl Tablets . . . 1712
Synthroid Tablets . . . 520

ESALFON (Chile)
ENALAPRIL MALEATE
Vasotec I.V. Injection . . . 2103

ESCLEBIN (Spain)
NORFLOXACIN
Noroxin Tablets . . . 2032

ESCLIMA (Italy)
ESTRADIOL
Climara Transdermal System . . . 771
Estring Vaginal Ring . . . 2635

ESCORETIC (Switzerland)
AMILORIDE HYDROCHLORIDE/HYDROCHLOROTHIAZIDE
Moduretic Tablets . . . 2028

ESCOZEM (Switzerland)
DILTIAZEM HYDROCHLORIDE
Cardizem LA Extended Release Tablets . . . 1728
Tiazac Capsules . . . 1201

ESCUDO (Italy)
SUCRALFATE
Carafate Suspension . . . 701
Carafate Tablets . . . 701

ESGIPYRIN (India)
DICLOFENAC SODIUM
Voltaren Tablets . . . 2307
Voltaren-XR Tablets . . . 2310

ESGIPYRIN DS (India)
DICLOFENAC SODIUM
Voltaren Tablets . . . 2307
Voltaren-XR Tablets . . . 2310

ESILGAN (Italy)
ESTAZOLAM
ProSom Tablets . . . 517

ESITEREN (Germany)
HYDROCHLOROTHIAZIDE/TRIAMTERENE
Dyazide Capsules . . . 1423

ESKAZOLE (Australia, Austria, France, Germany, Greece, Israel, Mexico, Spain, The Netherlands, United Kingdom)
ALBENDAZOLE
Albenza Tablets . . . 1338

ESMERON (Australia, Austria, Belgium, Brazil, Chile, Czech Republic, Denmark, Finland, France, Germany, Greece, Hong Kong, Hungary, Irish Republic, Israel, Italy, Malaysia, Mexico, New Zealand, Norway, Portugal, Russia, Singapore, South Africa, Spain, Sweden, Switzerland, Thailand, The Netherlands, United Kingdom, Venezuela)
ROCURONIUM BROMIDE
Zemuron Injection . . . 2346

ESOFEX (Finland)
RANITIDINE HYDROCHLORIDE
Zantac 25 EFFERdose Tablets . . . 1624
Zantac 150 EFFERdose Tablets . . . 1624
Zantac 150 Tablets . . . 1624
Zantac 300 Tablets . . . 1624
Zantac Injection . . . 1619
Zantac Injection Premixed . . . 1619
Zantac Syrup . . . 1624

ESOLUT (Italy)
PROGESTERONE
Prometrium Capsules (100 mg, 200 mg) . . . 3203

ESOTRAN (Spain)
ESTRADIOL
Climara Transdermal System . . . 771
Estring Vaginal Ring . . . 2635

ESPA-LEPSIN (Germany)
CARBAMAZEPINE
Carbatrol Capsules . . . 3171
Tegretol Chewable Tablets . . . 2295
Tegretol Suspension . . . 2295
Tegretol Tablets . . . 2295
Tegretol-XR Tablets . . . 2295

ESPARIL (Germany)
CAPTOPRIL
Captopril Tablets . . . 2149

ESPASEVIT (Argentina)
ONDANSETRON
Zofran ODT Orally Disintegrating Tablets . . . 1639

ESPEDEN (Spain)
NORFLOXACIN
Noroxin Tablets . . . 2032

ESPO (Japan)
EPOETIN ALFA
Epogen for Injection . . . 591
Procrit for Injection . . . 2364

ESPONTAL (Argentina)
TAMSULOSIN HYDROCHLORIDE
Flomax Capsules . . . 850

ESPRASONE (Spain)
ESTRADIOL
Climara Transdermal System . . . 771
Estring Vaginal Ring . . . 2635

ESRADIN (Italy)
ISRADIPINE
DynaCirc CR Tablets . . . 2721

ESSELDON (Greece)
FAMOTIDINE
Pepcid Injection . . . 2040

Pepcid Injection Premixed 2040
Pepcid Tablets 2038
Pepcid for Oral Suspension 2038

ESSVENTIA (Mexico)
ESTRADIOL
Climara Transdermal System 771
Estring Vaginal Ring 2635

ESTALIS (Argentina, Austria, Brazil, Canada, Czech Republic, Irish Republic, Norway, Portugal, Spain, Switzerland)
ESTRADIOL
Climara Transdermal System 771
Estring Vaginal Ring 2635

ESTALIS CONTINUOUS (Australia)
ESTRADIOL
Climara Transdermal System 771
Estring Vaginal Ring 2635

ESTAVAM (Mexico)
VANCOMYCIN HYDROCHLORIDE
Vancocin HCl Capsules, USP 3380

ESTEROMICIN (Mexico)
ERYTHROMYCIN
Ery-Tab Tablets 449
Erythromycin Base Filmtab Tablets 455
Erythromycin Delayed-Release Capsules, USP 457
PCE Dispertab Tablets 515

ESTILOMICIN (Argentina)
METRONIDAZOLE
MetroGel-Vaginal Gel 1855

ESTIMA (France)
PROGESTERONE
Prometrium Capsules (100 mg, 200 mg) 3203

ESTOMIL (Spain)
LANSOPRAZOLE
Prevacid Delayed-Release Capsules 3271

ESTRABETA (Germany)
ESTRADIOL
Climara Transdermal System 771
Estring Vaginal Ring 2635

ESTRACE (Canada, Czech Republic)
ESTRADIOL
Climara Transdermal System 771
Estring Vaginal Ring 2635

ESTRACE-C (Czech Republic)
ESTRADIOL
Climara Transdermal System 771
Estring Vaginal Ring 2635

ESTRACUTAN (Austria)
ESTRADIOL
Climara Transdermal System 771
Estring Vaginal Ring 2635

ESTRADELLE (Brazil)
ESTRADIOL
Climara Transdermal System 771
Estring Vaginal Ring 2635

ESTRADERM (Argentina, Australia, Austria, Belgium, Brazil, Canada, Czech Republic, Denmark, Finland, France, Germany, Hong Kong, Hungary, India, Irish Republic, Israel, Italy, Mexico, New Zealand, Norway, Portugal, Singapore, South Africa, Spain, Sweden, Switzerland, The Netherlands, United Kingdom, Venezuela)
ESTRADIOL
Climara Transdermal System 771
Estring Vaginal Ring 2635

ESTRADERM TTS (Greece)
ESTRADIOL
Climara Transdermal System 771
Estring Vaginal Ring 2635

ESTRADOT (Argentina, Australia, Austria, Brazil, Canada, Finland, Germany, Greece, Hungary, Irish Republic, Norway, Portugal, Spain, Sweden, Switzerland, The Netherlands, United Kingdom)
ESTRADIOL
Climara Transdermal System 771
Estring Vaginal Ring 2635

ESTRAGEST (Argentina, Brazil, Czech Republic, Hungary, Venezuela)
ESTRADIOL
Climara Transdermal System 771
Estring Vaginal Ring 2635

ESTRAHEXAL (Czech Republic)
ESTRADIOL
Climara Transdermal System 771
Estring Vaginal Ring 2635

ESTRAMON (Austria, Germany, Greece, Hungary, Irish Republic, Mexico, Switzerland)
ESTRADIOL
Climara Transdermal System 771
Estring Vaginal Ring 2635

ESTRAPATCH (France)
ESTRADIOL
Climara Transdermal System 771
Estring Vaginal Ring 2635

ESTRENA (Finland)
ESTRADIOL
Climara Transdermal System 771
Estring Vaginal Ring 2635

ESTREVA (Argentina, Belgium, Brazil, Chile, Czech Republic, Germany, Hong Kong, Mexico, Monaco, Singapore, Switzerland)
ESTRADIOL
Climara Transdermal System 771
Estring Vaginal Ring 2635

ESTRIFAM (Germany)
ESTRADIOL
Climara Transdermal System 771
Estring Vaginal Ring 2635

ESTRIMAX (Czech Republic, Hungary, Russia)
ESTRADIOL
Climara Transdermal System 771
Estring Vaginal Ring 2635

ESTRING (Argentina, Australia, Austria, Canada, Czech Republic, Denmark, Finland, Germany, Greece, New Zealand, Norway, South Africa, Switzerland, The Netherlands, United Kingdom)
ESTRADIOL
Climara Transdermal System 771
Estring Vaginal Ring 2635

ESTROACT (India)
RALOXIFENE HYDROCHLORIDE
Evista Tablets 1763

ESTROCLIM (Italy)
ESTRADIOL
Climara Transdermal System 771
Estring Vaginal Ring 2635

ESTRODOSE (Italy)
ESTRADIOL
Climara Transdermal System 771
Estring Vaginal Ring 2635

ESTROFEM (Argentina, Australia, Austria, Belgium, Brazil, Czech Republic, Denmark, Finland, France, Greece, Hong Kong, Hungary, Irish Republic, Israel, Italy, Malaysia, New Zealand, Portugal, Russia, Singapore, South Africa, Thailand, The Netherlands)
ESTRADIOL
Climara Transdermal System 771
Estring Vaginal Ring 2635

ESTROFEM N (Switzerland)
ESTRADIOL
Climara Transdermal System 771
Estring Vaginal Ring 2635

ESTROFFIK (Spain)
ESTRADIOL
Climara Transdermal System 771
Estring Vaginal Ring 2635

ESTROGEL (Austria, Canada, Denmark, Finland, Greece)
ESTRADIOL
Climara Transdermal System 771
Estring Vaginal Ring 2635

ESTRONAR (Portugal)
ESTRADIOL
Climara Transdermal System 771
Estring Vaginal Ring 2635

ESTRONORM (Germany)
ESTRADIOL
Climara Transdermal System 771
Estring Vaginal Ring 2635

ETACONIL (Chile)
FLUTAMIDE
Eulexin Capsules 3009

ETAMUCIN (Austria)
SODIUM HYALURONATE
Hyalgan Solution 2901

ETHEOPHYL (Germany)
THEOPHYLLINE
Uniphyl Tablets 2710

ETHIMIL (United Kingdom)
VERAPAMIL HYDROCHLORIDE
Covera-HS Tablets 3139
Verelan PM Extended-Release Capsules, Controlled-Onset 3106

ETHIMYCIN (South Africa)
ERYTHROMYCIN STEARATE
Erythrocin Stearate Filmtab Tablets 453

ETHIPAM (South Africa)
DIAZEPAM
Diastat Rectal Delivery System 3343
Valium Tablets 2819

ETHYOL (Argentina, Australia, Belgium, Brazil, Canada, Chile, Czech Republic, Denmark, Finland, France, Germany, Greece, Hong Kong, Hungary, Israel, Italy, Malaysia, Mexico, New Zealand, Portugal, Singapore, South Africa, Spain, Sweden, Switzerland, Thailand, The Netherlands, United Kingdom, Venezuela)
AMIFOSTINE
Ethyol for Injection 1898

ETIDRATE (New Zealand)
ETIDRONATE DISODIUM
Didronel Tablets 2697

ETIDRON (Greece, Italy)
ETIDRONATE DISODIUM
Didronel Tablets 2697

ETIMONIS (Switzerland)
ISOSORBIDE MONONITRATE
Imdur Tablets 3018

ETIPLUS (Greece)
ETIDRONATE DISODIUM
Didronel Tablets 2697

ETISUX (Argentina)
ERYTHROMYCIN
Ery-Tab Tablets 449
Erythromycin Base Filmtab Tablets 455
Erythromycin Delayed-Release Capsules, USP 457
PCE Dispertab Tablets 515

ETIZEM (Czech Republic, Portugal)
DILTIAZEM HYDROCHLORIDE
Cardizem LA Extended Release Tablets 1728
Tiazac Capsules 1201

E-TROCIMA-P (Mexico)
ERYTHROMYCIN
Ery-Tab Tablets 449
Erythromycin Base Filmtab Tablets 455
Erythromycin Delayed-Release Capsules, USP 457
PCE Dispertab Tablets 515

ETRONIL (Argentina)
METRONIDAZOLE
MetroGel-Vaginal Gel 1855

ETYOFIL (India)
THEOPHYLLINE
Uniphyl Tablets 2710

ETYZEM (Italy)
DILTIAZEM HYDROCHLORIDE
Cardizem LA Extended Release Tablets 1728
Tiazac Capsules 1201

EUBINE (France)
OXYCODONE HYDROCHLORIDE
OxyContin Tablets 2703
OxyFast Oral Concentrate Solution 2708
OxyIR Capsules 2708

EUBORAL (Spain)
NAPHAZOLINE HYDROCHLORIDE
Albalon Ophthalmic Solution ⊙218

EUCARDIC (Irish Republic, Sweden, The Netherlands, United Kingdom)
CARVEDILOL
Coreg Tablets 1414

EUCARNIL (Italy)
LEVOCARNITINE
Carnitor Injection 3188
Carnitor Tablets and Oral Solution 3190

EUCOPROST (Spain)
FINASTERIDE
Propecia Tablets 2060
Proscar Tablets 2067

EUCOR (Thailand)
SIMVASTATIN
Zocor Tablets 2105

EUDEMINE (Greece, Irish Republic, United Kingdom)
DIAZOXIDE
Hyperstat I.V. 3017

EUDIGOX (Italy)
DIGOXIN
Lanoxicaps Capsules 1490
Lanoxin Injection 1494
Lanoxin Injection Pediatric 1497
Lanoxin Tablets 1500

EUDYNA (Austria, Germany, Hong Kong, India, Mexico, Singapore)
TRETINOIN
Vesanoid Capsules 2820

EUFATIN (Mexico)
FAMOTIDINE
Pepcid Injection 2040
Pepcid Injection Premixed 2040
Pepcid Tablets 2038
Pepcid for Oral Suspension 2038

EUFILINA (Portugal, Spain)
THEOPHYLLINE
Uniphyl Tablets 2710

EUFLEX (Canada)
FLUTAMIDE
Eulexin Capsules 3009

EUFLOXIN (Mexico)
CIPROFLOXACIN
Cipro Oral Suspension 2977

EUGALAC (Austria, Germany)
LACTULOSE
Kristalose for Oral Solution 1034

EUGERIAL (Argentina, Brazil)
NIMODIPINE
Nimotop Capsules 749

EUKODAL (Germany)
OXYCODONE HYDROCHLORIDE
OxyContin Tablets 2703
OxyFast Oral Concentrate Solution 2708
OxyIR Capsules 2708

EULEXIN (Argentina, Australia, Belgium, Brazil, Denmark, Finland, Israel, Italy, Mexico, New Zealand, Norway, Portugal, South Africa, Spain, Sweden, The Netherlands, Venezuela)
FLUTAMIDE
Eulexin Capsules 3009

EULEXINE (France)
FLUTAMIDE
Eulexin Capsules 3009

EUPHYLLIN (Belgium, Czech Republic, Finland, Germany, Norway, South Africa)
THEOPHYLLINE
Uniphyl Tablets 2710

EUPHYLLIN 200 (Germany)
THEOPHYLLINE
Uniphyl Tablets 2710

EUPHYLLINA (Italy)
THEOPHYLLINE
Uniphyl Tablets 2710

EUPHYLLINE (France)
THEOPHYLLINE
Uniphyl Tablets 2710

EUPHYLONG (Czech Republic, Germany, Hong Kong, Hungary, Sweden, Switzerland, The Netherlands)
THEOPHYLLINE
Uniphyl Tablets 2710

EUPRESSIN (Brazil)
ENALAPRIL MALEATE
Vasotec I.V. Injection 2103

(⊙ Described in PDR For Ophthalmic Medicines™)

EURALBEN (Mexico)
ALBENDAZOLE
Albenza Tablets **1338**

EURITSIN (Argentina)
ADENOSINE
Adenocard Injection **617**
Adenoscan. **619**

EURODERM (Mexico)
CLOTRIMAZOLE
Lotrimin Cream. **3039**
Lotrimin Lotion 1%. **3039**
Lotrimin Topical Solution 1% **3039**

EURODIN (Japan)
ESTAZOLAM
ProSom Tablets **517**

EUROFLU (Italy)
FLUNISOLIDE
Aerobid Inhaler System. **1171**
Aerobid-M Inhaler System **1171**

EUROGESIC (Chile)
NAPROXEN
EC-Naprosyn Delayed-Release Tablets. . . . **2761**
Naprosyn Suspension. **2761**
Naprosyn Tablets **2761**

EUROMICINA (Chile)
CLARITHROMYCIN
Biaxin Filmtab Tablets **402**
Biaxin Granules **402**

EUROSAN (Switzerland)
CLOTRIMAZOLE
Lotrimin Cream. **3039**
Lotrimin Lotion 1%. **3039**
Lotrimin Topical Solution 1% **3039**

EUROTRETIN (Argentina)
TRETINOIN
Vesanoid Capsules. **2820**

EUSEDON MONO (Germany)
PROMETHAZINE HYDROCHLORIDE
Phenergan Tablets and Suppositories **3440**

EUSKIN (Spain)
ERYTHROMYCIN
Ery-Tab Tablets **449**
Erythromycin Base Filmtab Tablets. **455**
Erythromycin Delayed-Release Capsules, USP **457**
PCE Dispertab Tablets **515**

EUSTIDIL (Portugal)
FLUTICASONE PROPIONATE
Cutivate Cream. **2662**
Cutivate Ointment **2665**
Flonase Nasal Spray **1440**

EUTHYROX (Argentina, Austria, Belgium, Brazil, Czech Republic, Germany, Hungary, Russia, Singapore, Sweden, Switzerland, Thailand, The Netherlands, Venezuela)
LEVOTHYROXINE SODIUM
Levothroid Tablets. **1186**
Levoxyl Tablets. **1712**
Synthroid Tablets. **520**

EUTIMIL (Italy)
PAROXETINE HYDROCHLORIDE
Paxil Oral Suspension. **1530**
Paxil Tablets. **1530**

EUTIROX (Chile, Italy, Mexico, Spain)
LEVOTHYROXINE SODIUM
Levothroid Tablets. **1186**
Levoxyl Tablets. **1712**
Synthroid Tablets. **520**

EUTIZ (Argentina)
FINASTERIDE
Propecia Tablets **2060**
Proscar Tablets. **2067**

EUTROXSIG (Australia)
LEVOTHYROXINE SODIUM
Levothroid Tablets. **1186**
Levoxyl Tablets. **1712**
Synthroid Tablets. **520**

EUXAT (Italy)
NIFEDIPINE
Adalat CC Tablets **2964**

EVACALM (United Kingdom)
DIAZEPAM
Diastat Rectal Delivery System **3343**
Valium Tablets **2819**

EVADOL (Mexico)
DICLOFENAC SODIUM
Voltaren Tablets **2307**
Voltaren-XR Tablets **2310**

EVAFILM (France)
ESTRADIOL
Climara Transdermal System **771**
Estring Vaginal Ring **2635**

EVAPAUSE (France)
PROGESTERONE
Prometrium Capsules (100 mg, 200 mg) . **3203**

EVIANTRINA (Spain)
FAMOTIDINE
Pepcid Injection **2040**
Pepcid Injection Premixed **2040**
Pepcid Tablets **2038**
Pepcid for Oral Suspension **2038**

EVIMAL (Chile)
DONEPEZIL HYDROCHLORIDE
Aricept Tablets **1094**

EVINOPON (Greece)
DICLOFENAC SODIUM
Voltaren Tablets **2307**
Voltaren-XR Tablets **2310**

EVISTA (Argentina, Australia, Austria, Belgium, Brazil, Canada, Chile, Czech Republic, Denmark, Finland, France, Germany, Greece, Hong Kong, Hungary, Irish Republic, Israel, Italy, Malaysia, Mexico, New Zealand, Norway, Portugal, Singapore, South Africa, Spain, Sweden, Switzerland, The Netherlands, United Kingdom, Venezuela)
RALOXIFENE HYDROCHLORIDE
Evista Tablets. **1763**

EVOPAD (Spain)
ESTRADIOL
Climara Transdermal System **771**
Estring Vaginal Ring. **2635**

EVOREL (Argentina, Denmark, Finland, Germany, Irish Republic, Israel, Mexico, Norway, South Africa, Sweden, United Kingdom)
ESTRADIOL
Climara Transdermal System **771**
Estring Vaginal Ring. **2635**

EVOREL CONTI (Argentina, Irish Republic, Israel, Mexico, United Kingdom)
ESTRADIOL
Climara Transdermal System **771**
Estring Vaginal Ring. **2635**

EXAMICYN (Mexico)
ERYTHROMYCIN
Ery-Tab Tablets **449**
Erythromycin Base Filmtab Tablets. **455**
Erythromycin Delayed-Release Capsules, USP **457**
PCE Dispertab Tablets **515**

EXAMIDA (Mexico)
SULFACETAMIDE SODIUM
Klaron Lotion 10%. **2909**

EXAMYCIN (Mexico)
ERYTHROMYCIN
Ery-Tab Tablets **449**
Erythromycin Base Filmtab Tablets. **455**
Erythromycin Delayed-Release Capsules, USP **457**
PCE Dispertab Tablets **515**

EXE-CORT (United Kingdom)
HYDROCORTISONE
Hydrocortone Tablets **1989**

EXERTIAL (Argentina)
CIPROFLOXACIN
Cipro Oral Suspension **2977**

EXFOLIUM (Argentina)
TRIAMCINOLONE ACETONIDE
Azmacort Inhalation Aerosol. **1726**
Nasacort AQ Nasal Spray **2922**

EXIBRAL (Argentina)
VALPROIC ACID
Depakene Capsules **417**
Depakene Oral Solution. **417**

EXIFINE (Malaysia, Russia)
TERBINAFINE HYDROCHLORIDE
Lamisil Tablets **2232**

EXIMIUS (Argentina)
CLOTRIMAZOLE
Lotrimin Cream. **3039**
Lotrimin Lotion 1%. **3039**
Lotrimin Topical Solution 1% **3039**

EXINOL (Venezuela)
SUCRALFATE
Carafate Suspension **701**
Carafate Tablets **701**

EXIREL (Austria)
PIRBUTEROL ACETATE
Maxair Autohaler. **1852**

EXOCIN (Denmark, Finland, Greece, Irish Republic, Italy, Portugal, South Africa, Spain, United Kingdom)
OFLOXACIN
Floxin Otic Solution **1049**

EXOCINE (France)
OFLOXACIN
Floxin Otic Solution **1049**

EXODERIL (Austria, Czech Republic, Germany, Hong Kong, Hungary, Israel, Malaysia, Singapore, Switzerland)
NAFTIFINE HYDROCHLORIDE
Naftin Cream **2126**
Naftin Gel **2126**

EXOGRAN (The Netherlands)
CEFTRIAXONE SODIUM
Rocephin Injectable Vials, ADD-Vantage, Galaxy, Bulk **2800**

EXOVIR (Argentina)
ZIDOVUDINE
Retrovir Capsules **1560**
Retrovir IV Infusion. **1564**
Retrovir Syrup **1560**
Retrovir Tablets. **1560**

EXPIT (Argentina)
SILDENAFIL CITRATE
Viagra Tablets **2573**

EXPLANER (Argentina)
NIMODIPINE
Nimotop Capsules **749**

EXPROS (Finland)
TAMSULOSIN HYDROCHLORIDE
Flomax Capsules **850**

EXTISER-Q (Mexico)
PRAZIQUANTEL
Biltricide Tablets **2976**

EXTRACORT (Germany)
TRIAMCINOLONE ACETONIDE
Azmacort Inhalation Aerosol. **1726**
Nasacort AQ Nasal Spray **2922**

EXTUR (Spain)
INDAPAMIDE
Indapamide Tablets **2156**

EYEBREX (Greece)
TOBRAMYCIN
TOBI Solution for Inhalation **2298**

EYEBREX-DEXA (Greece)
DEXAMETHASONE/TOBRAMYCIN
TobraDex Ophthalmic Ointment . . . **562**, ⊙**212**
TobraDex Ophthalmic Suspension . **563**, ⊙**211**

EYECLOF (Greece)
DICLOFENAC SODIUM
Voltaren Tablets **2307**
Voltaren-XR Tablets **2310**

EYECON (Israel)
SODIUM HYALURONATE
Hyalgan Solution **2901**

EYESTIL (Canada)
SODIUM HYALURONATE
Hyalgan Solution **2901**

EYETOBRIN (Greece)
TOBRAMYCIN
TOBI Solution for Inhalation **2298**

EYEZEP (New Zealand)
AZELASTINE HYDROCHLORIDE
Astelin Nasal Spray **1904**

EZOPTA (Greece)
RANITIDINE HYDROCHLORIDE
Zantac 25 EFFERdose Tablets **1624**
Zantac 150 EFFERdose Tablets. **1624**
Zantac 150 Tablets **1624**
Zantac 300 Tablets **1624**
Zantac Injection **1619**
Zantac Injection Premixed **1619**
Zantac Syrup **1624**

EZOSINA (Italy)
TERAZOSIN HYDROCHLORIDE
Hytrin Capsules. **471**

EZUMYCIN (Greece)
CLARITHROMYCIN
Biaxin Filmtab Tablets **402**
Biaxin Granules **402**

FABAMOX (Argentina)
AMOXICILLIN
Amoxil Pediatric Drops for Oral Suspension. **1343**
Amoxil Tablets **1343**

FABOFUROX (Argentina)
FUROSEMIDE
Furosemide Tablets **2154**

FABOTRANIL (Argentina)
DIAZEPAM
Diastat Rectal Delivery System **3343**
Valium Tablets **2819**

FABRALGINA (Argentina)
NAPROXEN
EC-Naprosyn Delayed-Release Tablets. . . . **2761**
Naprosyn Suspension. **2761**
Naprosyn Tablets **2761**

FABUTIN (Mexico)
FAMOTIDINE
Pepcid Injection **2040**
Pepcid Injection Premixed **2040**
Pepcid Tablets **2038**
Pepcid for Oral Suspension **2038**

FACORT (Thailand)
TRIAMCINOLONE ACETONIDE
Azmacort Inhalation Aerosol. **1726**
Nasacort AQ Nasal Spray **2922**

FACTODIN (Greece)
CLOTRIMAZOLE
Lotrimin Cream. **3039**
Lotrimin Lotion 1%. **3039**
Lotrimin Topical Solution 1% **3039**

FADAFLUMAZ (Argentina)
FLUMAZENIL
Romazicon Injection **2804**

FADALIVIO (Argentina)
NAPROXEN
EC-Naprosyn Delayed-Release Tablets. . . . **2761**
Naprosyn Suspension. **2761**
Naprosyn Tablets **2761**

FADAMETASONA (Argentina)
DEXAMETHASONE
Decadron Tablets **1951**

FADINE (Hong Kong, India, Malaysia, Thailand)
FAMOTIDINE
Pepcid Injection **2040**
Pepcid Injection Premixed **2040**
Pepcid Tablets **2038**
Pepcid for Oral Suspension **2038**

FADIPINA (Venezuela)
FAMOTIDINE
Pepcid Injection **2040**
Pepcid Injection Premixed **2040**
Pepcid Tablets **2038**
Pepcid for Oral Suspension **2038**

FADUL (Germany)
FAMOTIDINE
Pepcid Injection **2040**
Pepcid Injection Premixed **2040**
Pepcid Tablets **2038**
Pepcid for Oral Suspension **2038**

FAGASTRIL (Spain)
FAMOTIDINE
Pepcid Injection **2040**
Pepcid Injection Premixed **2040**
Pepcid Tablets **2038**
Pepcid for Oral Suspension **2038**

FAGATRIM (Mexico)
FAMOTIDINE
Pepcid Injection **2040**
Pepcid Injection Premixed **2040**
Pepcid Tablets **2038**
Pepcid for Oral Suspension **2038**

FAGIZOL (Mexico)
METRONIDAZOLE
MetroGel-Vaginal Gel **1855**

FAGUS (Spain)
RANITIDINE HYDROCHLORIDE
Zantac 25 EFFERdose Tablets **1624**

Zantac 150 EFFERdose Tablets........ 1624
Zantac 150 Tablets 1624
Zantac 300 Tablets 1624
Zantac Injection 1619
Zantac Injection Premixed 1619
Zantac Syrup 1624

FALICARD (Germany)
VERAPAMIL HYDROCHLORIDE
Covera-HS Tablets 3139
Verelan PM Extended-Release Capsules, Controlled-Onset 3106

FAMILY MEDICATED SUNBURN RELIEF (Canada)
LIDOCAINE
Lidoderm Patch 1118

FAMINE (Hong Kong)
FAMOTIDINE
Pepcid Injection 2040
Pepcid Injection Premixed 2040
Pepcid Tablets 2038
Pepcid for Oral Suspension 2038

FAMO (Israel)
FAMOTIDINE
Pepcid Injection 2040
Pepcid Injection Premixed 2040
Pepcid Tablets 2038
Pepcid for Oral Suspension 2038

FAMOBETA (Germany)
FAMOTIDINE
Pepcid Injection 2040
Pepcid Injection Premixed 2040
Pepcid Tablets 2038
Pepcid for Oral Suspension 2038

FAMOC (Singapore, Thailand)
FAMOTIDINE
Pepcid Injection 2040
Pepcid Injection Premixed 2040
Pepcid Tablets 2038
Pepcid for Oral Suspension 2038

FAMOCID (Russia, Singapore, Thailand)
FAMOTIDINE
Pepcid Injection 2040
Pepcid Injection Premixed 2040
Pepcid Tablets 2038
Pepcid for Oral Suspension 2038

FAMODIL (Italy)
FAMOTIDINE
Pepcid Injection 2040
Pepcid Injection Premixed 2040
Pepcid Tablets 2038
Pepcid for Oral Suspension 2038

FAMODIN (India)
FAMOTIDINE
Pepcid Injection 2040
Pepcid Injection Premixed 2040
Pepcid Tablets 2038
Pepcid for Oral Suspension 2038

FAMODINE (Brazil, Hong Kong)
FAMOTIDINE
Pepcid Injection 2040
Pepcid Injection Premixed 2040
Pepcid Tablets 2038
Pepcid for Oral Suspension 2038

FAMOGEL (Venezuela)
FAMOTIDINE
Pepcid Injection 2040
Pepcid Injection Premixed 2040
Pepcid Tablets 2038
Pepcid for Oral Suspension 2038

FAMOHEXAL (Australia)
FAMOTIDINE
Pepcid Injection 2040
Pepcid Injection Premixed 2040
Pepcid Tablets 2038
Pepcid for Oral Suspension 2038

FAMOKEY (Spain)
FAMOTIDINE
Pepcid Injection 2040
Pepcid Injection Premixed 2040
Pepcid Tablets 2038
Pepcid for Oral Suspension 2038

FAMOLTA (Hong Kong)
FAMOTIDINE
Pepcid Injection 2040
Pepcid Injection Premixed 2040
Pepcid Tablets 2038
Pepcid for Oral Suspension 2038

FAMONERTON (Germany)
FAMOTIDINE
Pepcid Injection 2040
Pepcid Injection Premixed 2040
Pepcid Tablets 2038
Pepcid for Oral Suspension 2038

FAMONIT (Russia)
FAMOTIDINE
Pepcid Injection 2040
Pepcid Injection Premixed 2040
Pepcid Tablets 2038
Pepcid for Oral Suspension 2038

FAMONOX (Thailand)
FAMOTIDINE
Pepcid Injection 2040
Pepcid Injection Premixed 2040
Pepcid Tablets 2038
Pepcid for Oral Suspension 2038

FAMOPRIL (Singapore)
FAMOTIDINE
Pepcid Injection 2040
Pepcid Injection Premixed 2040
Pepcid Tablets 2038
Pepcid for Oral Suspension 2038

FAMOPSIN (Hong Kong, Malaysia, Singapore, Thailand)
FAMOTIDINE
Pepcid Injection 2040
Pepcid Injection Premixed 2040
Pepcid Tablets 2038
Pepcid for Oral Suspension 2038

FAMOSAN (Czech Republic, Russia)
FAMOTIDINE
Pepcid Injection 2040
Pepcid Injection Premixed 2040
Pepcid Tablets 2038
Pepcid for Oral Suspension 2038

FAMOSET (Brazil)
FAMOTIDINE
Pepcid Injection 2040
Pepcid Injection Premixed 2040
Pepcid Tablets 2038
Pepcid for Oral Suspension 2038

FAMOSIA (Thailand)
FAMOTIDINE
Pepcid Injection 2040
Pepcid Injection Premixed 2040
Pepcid Tablets 2038
Pepcid for Oral Suspension 2038

FAMOSIN (Austria)
FAMOTIDINE
Pepcid Injection 2040
Pepcid Injection Premixed 2040
Pepcid Tablets 2038
Pepcid for Oral Suspension 2038

FAMOTAB (Thailand)
FAMOTIDINE
Pepcid Injection 2040
Pepcid Injection Premixed 2040
Pepcid Tablets 2038
Pepcid for Oral Suspension 2038

FAMOTAL (Norway)
FAMOTIDINE
Pepcid Injection 2040
Pepcid Injection Premixed 2040
Pepcid Tablets 2038
Pepcid for Oral Suspension 2038

FAMOTEC (United Arab Emirates)
FAMOTIDINE
Pepcid Injection 2040
Pepcid Injection Premixed 2040
Pepcid Tablets 2038
Pepcid for Oral Suspension 2038

FAMOTID (Brazil)
FAMOTIDINE
Pepcid Injection 2040
Pepcid Injection Premixed 2040
Pepcid Tablets 2038
Pepcid for Oral Suspension 2038

FAMOTIL (Brazil)
FAMOTIDINE
Pepcid Injection 2040
Pepcid Injection Premixed 2040
Pepcid Tablets 2038
Pepcid for Oral Suspension 2038

FAMOTIN (Hong Kong, Singapore, Thailand)
FAMOTIDINE
Pepcid Injection 2040
Pepcid Injection Premixed 2040
Pepcid Tablets 2038
Pepcid for Oral Suspension 2038

FAMOWAL (India)
FAMOTIDINE
Pepcid Injection 2040
Pepcid Injection Premixed 2040
Pepcid Tablets 2038
Pepcid for Oral Suspension 2038

FAMOX (Brazil, Hong Kong, New Zealand)
FAMOTIDINE
Pepcid Injection 2040
Pepcid Injection Premixed 2040
Pepcid Tablets 2038
Pepcid for Oral Suspension 2038

FAMOXAL (Mexico)
FAMOTIDINE
Pepcid Injection 2040
Pepcid Injection Premixed 2040
Pepcid Tablets 2038
Pepcid for Oral Suspension 2038

FAMOXIL (Brazil)
FAMOTIDINE
Pepcid Injection 2040
Pepcid Injection Premixed 2040
Pepcid Tablets 2038
Pepcid for Oral Suspension 2038

FAMTAC (India)
FAMOTIDINE
Pepcid Injection 2040
Pepcid Injection Premixed 2040
Pepcid Tablets 2038
Pepcid for Oral Suspension 2038

FAMULCER (Spain, Venezuela)
FAMOTIDINE
Pepcid Injection 2040
Pepcid Injection Premixed 2040
Pepcid Tablets 2038
Pepcid for Oral Suspension 2038

FANOSIN (Spain)
FAMOTIDINE
Pepcid Injection 2040
Pepcid Injection Premixed 2040
Pepcid Tablets 2038
Pepcid for Oral Suspension 2038

FANOX (Spain)
FAMOTIDINE
Pepcid Injection 2040
Pepcid Injection Premixed 2040
Pepcid Tablets 2038
Pepcid for Oral Suspension 2038

FARAXEN (Mexico)
NAPROXEN
EC-Naprosyn Delayed-Release Tablets.... 2761
Naprosyn Suspension............... 2761
Naprosyn Tablets 2761

FARCEF (Greece)
CEFTRIAXONE SODIUM
Rocephin Injectable Vials, ADD-Vantage, Galaxy, Bulk 2800

FARGANESSE (Italy)
PROMETHAZINE HYDROCHLORIDE
Phenergan Tablets and Suppositories 3440

FARGO (Australia)
LIDOCAINE
Lidoderm Patch 1118

FARLAC (Brazil)
LACTULOSE
Kristalose for Oral Solution 1034

FARLUTAL (Australia, Austria, Belgium, Brazil, Chile, Finland, France, Germany, Greece, Hong Kong, Italy, Malaysia, Mexico, New Zealand, Norway, Singapore, South Africa, Spain, Sweden, Switzerland, Thailand, The Netherlands, United Kingdom, Venezuela)
MEDROXYPROGESTERONE ACETATE
Depo-Medrol Single-Dose Vial 2619

FARLUTALE (Argentina)
MEDROXYPROGESTERONE ACETATE
Depo-Medrol Single-Dose Vial 2619

FARMACICLIN (Italy)
VANCOMYCIN HYDROCHLORIDE
Vancocin HCl Capsules, USP 3380

FARMIN (Mexico)
DIAZEPAM
Diastat Rectal Delivery System 3343
Valium Tablets 2819

FARMOTEX (Mexico)
FAMOTIDINE
Pepcid Injection 2040
Pepcid Injection Premixed 2040
Pepcid Tablets 2038
Pepcid for Oral Suspension 2038

FARM-X DUO (Argentina)
METRONIDAZOLE
MetroGel-Vaginal Gel 1855

FARM-X GINECOLOGICO (Argentina)
METRONIDAZOLE
MetroGel-Vaginal Gel 1855

FARNITIN (Italy)
LEVOCARNITINE
Carnitor Injection................. 3188
Carnitor Tablets and Oral Solution 3190

FARPRESSE (Portugal)
LISINOPRIL
Prinivil Tablets 2052

FARXEN (Mexico)
NAPROXEN
EC-Naprosyn Delayed-Release Tablets.... 2761
Naprosyn Suspension............... 2761
Naprosyn Tablets 2761

FASE (Italy)
APROTININ
Trasylol Injection 754

FASELUT (Argentina)
PROGESTERONE
Prometrium Capsules (100 mg, 200 mg) . 3203

FASIDINE (Thailand)
FAMOTIDINE
Pepcid Injection 2040
Pepcid Injection Premixed 2040
Pepcid Tablets 2038
Pepcid for Oral Suspension 2038

FASTIN (Canada)
PHENTERMINE HYDROCHLORIDE
Adipex-P Capsules 1215
Adipex-P Tablets 1215

FATEC (Thailand)
CETIRIZINE HYDROCHLORIDE
Zyrtec Syrup 2594
Zyrtec Tablets 2594

FATIDIN (Portugal)
FAMOTIDINE
Pepcid Injection 2040
Pepcid Injection Premixed 2040
Pepcid Tablets 2038
Pepcid for Oral Suspension 2038

FATORIL (Mexico)
FAMOTIDINE
Pepcid Injection 2040
Pepcid Injection Premixed 2040
Pepcid Tablets 2038
Pepcid for Oral Suspension 2038

FAULTENOCAN (Portugal)
IRINOTECAN HYDROCHLORIDE
Camptosar Injection............... 2604

FAUSTAN (Germany)
DIAZEPAM
Diastat Rectal Delivery System 3343
Valium Tablets 2819

FAWODIN (Mexico)
FAMOTIDINE
Pepcid Injection 2040
Pepcid Injection Premixed 2040
Pepcid Tablets 2038
Pepcid for Oral Suspension 2038

FAXINE (Italy)
VENLAFAXINE HYDROCHLORIDE
Effexor Tablets 3411
Effexor XR Capsules 3417

FEACEF (Greece)
CEFUROXIME AXETIL
Ceftin Tablets 1407
Ceftin for Oral Suspension........... 1407

FEBRAX (Mexico)
NAPROXEN SODIUM
Anaprox DS Tablets 2761
Anaprox Tablets 2761

FEDILEX (Venezuela)
NIFEDIPINE
Adalat CC Tablets 2964

FEDIP (Austria, Switzerland)
NIFEDIPINE
Adalat CC Tablets 2964

FEGENOR (France)
FENOFIBRATE
Tricor Tablets 527

FELANOR (Argentina)
CLONAZEPAM
Klonopin Tablets 2778

FELIBERAL (Mexico)
ENALAPRIL MALEATE
Vasotec I.V. Injection 2103

FELISELIN (Greece)
SELEGILINE HYDROCHLORIDE
Eldepryl Capsules 3208

FELIXENE (Spain)
CIPROFLOXACIN HYDROCHLORIDE
Ciloxan Ophthalmic Ointment .... ⊙204, 559
Ciloxan Ophthalmic Solution .... ⊙206
Cipro Tablets 2977

FELORAN (Czech Republic)
DICLOFENAC SODIUM
Voltaren Tablets 2307
Voltaren-XR Tablets 2310

FEM 7 (Argentina, Brazil, Chile, Czech Republic, Germany, Hong Kong, Mexico, Singapore, Switzerland, The Netherlands)
ESTRADIOL
Climara Transdermal System 771
Estring Vaginal Ring 2635

FEMALON (Chile)
ESTRADIOL
Climara Transdermal System 771
Estring Vaginal Ring 2635

FEMANEST (Denmark, Sweden)
ESTRADIOL
Climara Transdermal System 771
Estring Vaginal Ring 2635

FEMATAB (Irish Republic)
ESTRADIOL
Climara Transdermal System 771
Estring Vaginal Ring 2635

FEMATRIX (Irish Republic, United Kingdom)
ESTRADIOL
Climara Transdermal System 771
Estring Vaginal Ring 2635

FEMEX (The Netherlands)
NAPROXEN SODIUM
Anaprox DS Tablets 2761
Anaprox Tablets 2761

FEMIDERM (Chile)
ESTRADIOL
Climara Transdermal System 771
Estring Vaginal Ring 2635

FEMIDOTT (Chile)
ESTRADIOL
Climara Transdermal System 771
Estring Vaginal Ring 2635

FEMIGEL (South Africa)
ESTRADIOL
Climara Transdermal System 771
Estring Vaginal Ring 2635

FEMINOFLEX (Greece)
ETIDRONATE DISODIUM
Didronel Tablets 2697

FEMINOVA (Belgium)
ESTRADIOL
Climara Transdermal System 771
Estring Vaginal Ring 2635

FEMIPRES (Italy)
MOEXIPRIL HYDROCHLORIDE
Univasc Tablets 3104

FEMIPRES PLUS (Italy)
HYDROCHLOROTHIAZIDE/MOEXIPRIL HYDROCHLORIDE
Uniretic Tablets 3100

FEMIZOL (Australia)
CLOTRIMAZOLE
Lotrimin Cream 3039
Lotrimin Lotion 1% 3039
Lotrimin Topical Solution 1% 3039

FEMME FREE (Australia)
NAPROXEN
EC-Naprosyn Delayed-Release Tablets 2761
Naprosyn Suspension 2761
Naprosyn Tablets 2761

FEM-MONO (Denmark, Sweden)
ISOSORBIDE MONONITRATE
Imdur Tablets 3018

FEMOSTON 1/5 (Portugal)
ESTRADIOL
Climara Transdermal System 771
Estring Vaginal Ring 2635

FEMOSTON CONTI (Austria, Belgium, Brazil, Chile, Finland, Germany, Italy, Switzerland, United Kingdom)
ESTRADIOL
Climara Transdermal System 771
Estring Vaginal Ring 2635

FEMOSTON MONO (Germany)
ESTRADIOL
Climara Transdermal System 771
Estring Vaginal Ring 2635

FEMPHASCYL CONTI (Austria)
ESTRADIOL
Climara Transdermal System 771
Estring Vaginal Ring 2635

FEMPRESS (Austria, Germany, Switzerland)
MOEXIPRIL HYDROCHLORIDE
Univasc Tablets 3104

FEMPRESS PLUS (Austria, Germany)
HYDROCHLOROTHIAZIDE/MOEXIPRIL HYDROCHLORIDE
Uniretic Tablets 3100

FEMSEPT (France)
ESTRADIOL
Climara Transdermal System 771
Estring Vaginal Ring 2635

FEMSEVEN (Austria, Denmark, Finland, Italy, Sweden, Switzerland, United Kingdom, Venezuela)
ESTRADIOL
Climara Transdermal System 771
Estring Vaginal Ring 2635

FEMSEVEN CONTI (United Kingdom)
ESTRADIOL
Climara Transdermal System 771
Estring Vaginal Ring 2635

FEMSIEBEN (Austria)
ESTRADIOL
Climara Transdermal System 771
Estring Vaginal Ring 2635

FEMTAB CONTINUOUS (United Kingdom)
ESTRADIOL
Climara Transdermal System 771
Estring Vaginal Ring 2635

FEMTRAN (Australia, New Zealand)
ESTRADIOL
Climara Transdermal System 771
Estring Vaginal Ring 2635

FENAC (Australia)
DICLOFENAC SODIUM
Voltaren Tablets 2307
Voltaren-XR Tablets 2310

FENACTOL (United Kingdom)
DICLOFENAC SODIUM
Voltaren Tablets 2307
Voltaren-XR Tablets 2310

FENADIUM (Malaysia)
DICLOFENAC SODIUM
Voltaren Tablets 2307
Voltaren-XR Tablets 2310

FENADOL (Italy)
DICLOFENAC SODIUM
Voltaren Tablets 2307
Voltaren-XR Tablets 2310

FENAMON (Hong Kong, Malaysia, Russia, Singapore, Thailand)
NIFEDIPINE
Adalat CC Tablets 2964

FENAPLUS (India)
DICLOFENAC SODIUM
Voltaren Tablets 2307
Voltaren-XR Tablets 2310

FENAREN (Austria)
DICLOFENAC SODIUM
Voltaren Tablets 2307
Voltaren-XR Tablets 2310

FENAX (Chile)
FEXOFENADINE HYDROCHLORIDE
Allegra Capsules 2844

FENAZIL (Italy)
PROMETHAZINE HYDROCHLORIDE
Phenergan Tablets and Suppositories 3440

FENBURIL (Brazil)
DICLOFENAC SODIUM
Voltaren Tablets 2307
Voltaren-XR Tablets 2310

FENDER (Italy)
DICLOFENAC SODIUM
Voltaren Tablets 2307
Voltaren-XR Tablets 2310

FENERGAN (Argentina, Portugal, Venezuela)
PROMETHAZINE HYDROCHLORIDE
Phenergan Tablets and Suppositories 3440

FENIDINA (Italy)
NIFEDIPINE
Adalat CC Tablets 2964

FENIKEN (Mexico)
NIFEDIPINE
Adalat CC Tablets 2964

FENIL-V (Portugal)
DICLOFENAC SODIUM
Voltaren Tablets 2307
Voltaren-XR Tablets 2310

FENOBETA (Germany)
FENOFIBRATE
Tricor Tablets 527

FENOBRAT (Hungary)
FENOFIBRATE
Tricor Tablets 527

FENOBRATE (Argentina)
FENOFIBRATE
Tricor Tablets 527

FENOCLOF (Greece)
DICLOFENAC SODIUM
Voltaren Tablets 2307
Voltaren-XR Tablets 2310

FENODID (Mexico)
FENTANYL CITRATE
Actiq 979

FENOGAL (Belgium, United Kingdom)
FENOFIBRATE
Tricor Tablets 527

FENOGAL LIDOSE (Singapore)
FENOFIBRATE
Tricor Tablets 527

FENOLIP (Argentina, Austria, India)
FENOFIBRATE
Tricor Tablets 527

FENORIT (Italy)
PROPAFENONE HYDROCHLORIDE
Rythmol SR Capsules 2727

FENSAIDE (India)
DICLOFENAC SODIUM
Voltaren Tablets 2307
Voltaren-XR Tablets 2310

FENSAIDE-P (India)
DICLOFENAC SODIUM
Voltaren Tablets 2307
Voltaren-XR Tablets 2310

FENSARTAN (Argentina)
LOSARTAN POTASSIUM
Cozaar Tablets 1935

FENSARTAN D (Argentina)
LOSARTAN POTASSIUM
Cozaar Tablets 1935

FENTABBOTT (Brazil)
FENTANYL CITRATE
Actiq 979

FENTANEST (Brazil, Italy, Mexico, Spain)
FENTANYL CITRATE
Actiq 979

FENTATIL (Brazil)
FENTANYL
Duragesic Transdermal System 2373

FENTAX (Argentina)
FENTANYL CITRATE
Actiq 979

FERCAYL (Belgium)
IRON DEXTRAN
Infed Injection 3390

FERLEX (Mexico)
AMOXICILLIN
Amoxil Pediatric Drops for Oral Suspension 1343
Amoxil Tablets 1343

FERMATHRON (Australia, Germany, United Kingdom)
SODIUM HYALURONATE
Hyalgan Solution 2901

FERMAVISC (Switzerland)
SODIUM HYALURONATE
Hyalgan Solution 2901

FERMENTMYCIN (South Africa)
GENTAMICIN SULFATE
Garamycin Injectable 3014

FERROCEL (Mexico)
IRON DEXTRAN
Infed Injection 3390

FERROIN (Mexico)
IRON DEXTRAN
Infed Injection 3390

FERVEX (Mexico)
DICLOFENAC SODIUM
Voltaren Tablets 2307
Voltaren-XR Tablets 2310

FESTAL REFORMULADO (Venezuela)
AMYLASE/LIPASE/PROTEASE
Creon 10 Capsules 3198
Creon 20 Capsules 3199
Creon 5 Capsules 3198
Pancrease MT Capsules 1885
Ultrase Capsules 708
Ultrase MT Capsules 709
Viokase Powder 711
Viokase Tablets 711

FEXADIN (Russia)
FEXOFENADINE HYDROCHLORIDE
Allegra Capsules 2844

FEXIGRA (India)
FEXOFENADINE HYDROCHLORIDE
Allegra Capsules 2844

FEXIRON (Argentina)
IRON DEXTRAN
Infed Injection 3390

FEXOFEN (Argentina, India)
FEXOFENADINE HYDROCHLORIDE
Allegra Capsules 2844

FEXOTABS (Australia)
FEXOFENADINE HYDROCHLORIDE
Allegra Capsules 2844

FEXOVA (India)
FEXOFENADINE HYDROCHLORIDE
Allegra Capsules 2844

FIAGRA (India)
SILDENAFIL CITRATE
Viagra Tablets 2573

FIBONEL (Chile, Spain)
FAMOTIDINE
Pepcid Injection 2040
Pepcid Injection Premixed 2040
Pepcid Tablets 2038
Pepcid for Oral Suspension 2038

FIBRAMOX (Venezuela)
AMOXICILLIN
Amoxil Pediatric Drops for Oral Suspension 1343
Amoxil Tablets 1343

FIBRASE (Italy)
PENTOSAN POLYSULFATE SODIUM
Elmiron Capsules 2415

FIBREZYM (Germany)
PENTOSAN POLYSULFATE SODIUM
Elmiron Capsules 2415

FIBROCARD (Belgium)
VERAPAMIL HYDROCHLORIDE
Covera-HS Tablets 3139

Verelan PM Extended-Release Capsules, Controlled-Onset . . . 3106

FIBROCID (Spain)
PENTOSAN POLYSULFATE SODIUM
Elmiron Capsules . . . 2415

FIBROCIDE (Portugal)
PENTOSAN POLYSULFATE SODIUM
Elmiron Capsules . . . 2415

FIBROXYN (South Africa)
NAPROXEN
EC-Naprosyn Delayed-Release Tablets . . . 2761
Naprosyn Suspension . . . 2761
Naprosyn Tablets . . . 2761

FIBSOL (Australia)
LISINOPRIL
Prinivil Tablets . . . 2052

FIDECAINA (Argentina)
LIDOCAINE
Lidoderm Patch . . . 1118

FIGOZANT (Greece)
NIMODIPINE
Nimotop Capsules . . . 749

FIGREL (Greece)
DICLOFENAC SODIUM
Voltaren Tablets . . . 2307
Voltaren-XR Tablets . . . 2310

FILE (Argentina)
SILDENAFIL CITRATE
Viagra Tablets . . . 2573

FILGINASE (Argentina)
EFAVIRENZ
Sustiva Capsules . . . 930

FILTEN (Argentina)
CARVEDILOL
Coreg Tablets . . . 1414

FINABER (Argentina)
ONDANSETRON
Zofran ODT Orally Disintegrating Tablets . . . 1639

FINACILEN (Argentina)
NIMODIPINE
Nimotop Capsules . . . 749

FINALOP (Brazil)
FINASTERIDE
Propecia Tablets . . . 2060
Proscar Tablets . . . 2067

FINAP (Chile)
CITALOPRAM HYDROBROMIDE
Celexa Tablets . . . 1176

FINASEPT (Argentina)
CLARITHROMYCIN
Biaxin Filmtab Tablets . . . 402
Biaxin Granules . . . 402

FINAST (Russia, Venezuela)
FINASTERIDE
Propecia Tablets . . . 2060
Proscar Tablets . . . 2067

FINASTEC (Brazil)
FINASTERIDE
Propecia Tablets . . . 2060
Proscar Tablets . . . 2067

FINASTERIN (Argentina)
FINASTERIDE
Propecia Tablets . . . 2060
Proscar Tablets . . . 2067

FINASTID (Italy)
FINASTERIDE
Propecia Tablets . . . 2060
Proscar Tablets . . . 2067

FINASTIL (Brazil)
FINASTERIDE
Propecia Tablets . . . 2060
Proscar Tablets . . . 2067

FINCAR (India)
FINASTERIDE
Propecia Tablets . . . 2060
Proscar Tablets . . . 2067

FINDALER (Chile)
CETIRIZINE HYDROCHLORIDE
Zyrtec Syrup . . . 2594
Zyrtec Tablets . . . 2594

FINDECLIN (Argentina)
ALENDRONATE SODIUM
Fosamax Tablets . . . 1969

FINEX (Brazil, Czech Republic)
TERBINAFINE HYDROCHLORIDE
Lamisil Tablets . . . 2232

FINIBRON (Italy)
BUPRENORPHINE HYDROCHLORIDE
Buprenex Injectable . . . 2716

FINLEPSIN (Germany, Hungary, Russia)
CARBAMAZEPINE
Carbatrol Capsules . . . 3171
Tegretol Chewable Tablets . . . 2295
Tegretol Suspension . . . 2295
Tegretol Tablets . . . 2295
Tegretol-XR Tablets . . . 2295

FINOPTIN (Russia)
VERAPAMIL HYDROCHLORIDE
Covera-HS Tablets . . . 3139
Verelan PM Extended-Release Capsules, Controlled-Onset . . . 3106

FINOXI (Argentina)
ONDANSETRON
Zofran ODT Orally Disintegrating Tablets . . . 1639

FINPECIA (India)
FINASTERIDE
Propecia Tablets . . . 2060
Proscar Tablets . . . 2067

FINPROSTAT (Argentina)
FINASTERIDE
Propecia Tablets . . . 2060
Proscar Tablets . . . 2067

FINTOP (India)
BUTENAFINE HYDROCHLORIDE
Mentax Cream . . . 2158

FIRIN (Germany)
NORFLOXACIN
Noroxin Tablets . . . 2032

FIRMALONE (Italy)
DEXAMETHASONE
Decadron Tablets . . . 1951

FITAXAL (France)
LACTULOSE
Kristalose for Oral Solution . . . 1034

FITZECALM (United Arab Emirates)
CARBAMAZEPINE
Carbatrol Capsules . . . 3171
Tegretol Chewable Tablets . . . 2295
Tegretol Suspension . . . 2295
Tegretol Tablets . . . 2295
Tegretol-XR Tablets . . . 2295

FIVEFLURO (India)
FLUOROURACIL
Efudex Topical Cream . . . 3363
Efudex Topical Solutions . . . 3363

FIVEROCIL (Mexico)
FLUOROURACIL
Efudex Topical Cream . . . 3363
Efudex Topical Solutions . . . 3363

FIVOFLU (Thailand, Venezuela)
FLUOROURACIL
Efudex Topical Cream . . . 3363
Efudex Topical Solutions . . . 3363

FIXCA (Spain)
ONDANSETRON HYDROCHLORIDE
Zofran Injection . . . 1634
Zofran Injection Premixed . . . 1634
Zofran Oral Solution . . . 1639
Zofran Tablets . . . 1639

FIXIM (The Netherlands)
CEFIXIME
Suprax . . . 1843

FIXIME (South Africa)
CEFIXIME
Suprax . . . 1843

FIXOPAN (Venezuela)
ALENDRONATE SODIUM
Fosamax Tablets . . . 1969

FIXX (India)
CEFIXIME
Suprax . . . 1843

FLADEX (Singapore)
METRONIDAZOLE
MetroGel-Vaginal Gel . . . 1855

FLADON (Brazil)
DICLOFENAC SODIUM
Voltaren Tablets . . . 2307
Voltaren-XR Tablets . . . 2310

FLAGEPAT (Mexico)
METRONIDAZOLE
MetroGel-Vaginal Gel . . . 1855

FLAGINAZOL (Mexico)
METRONIDAZOLE
MetroGel-Vaginal Gel . . . 1855

FLAGYL (Argentina, Australia, Austria, Belgium, Brazil, Canada, Finland, Germany, Hong Kong, India, Israel, Italy, Malaysia, Mexico, Portugal, Russia, Singapore, South Africa, Switzerland)
METRONIDAZOLE
MetroGel-Vaginal Gel . . . 1855

FLAGYL COMP (Finland)
METRONIDAZOLE
MetroGel-Vaginal Gel . . . 1855

FLAGYL NISTATINA (Brazil)
METRONIDAZOLE
MetroGel-Vaginal Gel . . . 1855

FLAGYSTATIN (Argentina)
METRONIDAZOLE
MetroGel-Vaginal Gel . . . 1855

FLAGYSTATIN V (Mexico)
METRONIDAZOLE
MetroGel-Vaginal Gel . . . 1855

FLAMALGEN (Brazil)
DICLOFENAC SODIUM
Voltaren Tablets . . . 2307
Voltaren-XR Tablets . . . 2310

FLAMATAK (United Kingdom)
DICLOFENAC SODIUM
Voltaren Tablets . . . 2307
Voltaren-XR Tablets . . . 2310

FLAMIN (Mexico)
METRONIDAZOLE
MetroGel-Vaginal Gel . . . 1855

FLAMIN 400 (Mexico)
METRONIDAZOLE
MetroGel-Vaginal Gel . . . 1855

FLAMON (Switzerland)
VERAPAMIL HYDROCHLORIDE
Covera-HS Tablets . . . 3139
Verelan PM Extended-Release Capsules, Controlled-Onset . . . 3106

FLAMRASE (United Kingdom)
DICLOFENAC SODIUM
Voltaren Tablets . . . 2307
Voltaren-XR Tablets . . . 2310

FLANAREN (Brazil)
DICLOFENAC SODIUM
Voltaren Tablets . . . 2307
Voltaren-XR Tablets . . . 2310

FLANAX (Brazil, Mexico)
NAPROXEN SODIUM
Anaprox DS Tablets . . . 2761
Anaprox Tablets . . . 2761

FLANIZOL (Brazil)
METRONIDAZOLE
MetroGel-Vaginal Gel . . . 1855

FLANKOL (Mexico)
DICLOFENAC SODIUM
Voltaren Tablets . . . 2307
Voltaren-XR Tablets . . . 2310

FLATEZOL (Mexico)
ALBENDAZOLE
Albenza Tablets . . . 1338

FLAVIX (India)
VENLAFAXINE HYDROCHLORIDE
Effexor Tablets . . . 3411
Effexor XR Capsules . . . 3417

FLAVOXEN (Mexico)
NAPROXEN
EC-Naprosyn Delayed-Release Tablets . . . 2761
Naprosyn Suspension . . . 2761
Naprosyn Tablets . . . 2761

FLAXENDOL (Mexico)
NAPROXEN SODIUM
Anaprox DS Tablets . . . 2761
Anaprox Tablets . . . 2761

FLAXIN (Brazil)
FINASTERIDE
Propecia Tablets . . . 2060
Proscar Tablets . . . 2067

FLAXTEC (Mexico)
METRONIDAZOLE
MetroGel-Vaginal Gel . . . 1855

FLAXVAN (Argentina)
NAPROXEN
EC-Naprosyn Delayed-Release Tablets . . . 2761
Naprosyn Suspension . . . 2761
Naprosyn Tablets . . . 2761

FLECADURA (Germany)
FLECAINIDE ACETATE
Tambocor Tablets . . . 1856

FLECAINE (France)
FLECAINIDE ACETATE
Tambocor Tablets . . . 1856

FLECATAB (Australia)
FLECAINIDE ACETATE
Tambocor Tablets . . . 1856

FLECOR-N (Greece)
NIFEDIPINE
Adalat CC Tablets . . . 2964

FLEGYL (Venezuela)
METRONIDAZOLE
MetroGel-Vaginal Gel . . . 1855

FLEMOXIN (Greece, New Zealand, Russia, Switzerland)
AMOXICILLIN
Amoxil Pediatric Drops for Oral Suspension . . . 1343
Amoxil Tablets . . . 1343

FLEXAGEN (South Africa)
DICLOFENAC SODIUM
Voltaren Tablets . . . 2307
Voltaren-XR Tablets . . . 2310

FLEXAMINA (Brazil)
DICLOFENAC SODIUM
Voltaren Tablets . . . 2307
Voltaren-XR Tablets . . . 2310

FLEXEN (Mexico)
NAPROXEN
EC-Naprosyn Delayed-Release Tablets . . . 2761
Naprosyn Suspension . . . 2761
Naprosyn Tablets . . . 2761

FLEXIN (Israel)
ORPHENADRINE CITRATE
Norflex Injection . . . 1856

FLEXOTARD (United Kingdom)
DICLOFENAC SODIUM
Voltaren Tablets . . . 2307
Voltaren-XR Tablets . . . 2310

FLEXRESAN (Spain)
ISOTRETINOIN
Accutane Capsules . . . 2731

FLIXODERM (Italy)
FLUTICASONE PROPIONATE
Cutivate Cream . . . 2662
Cutivate Ointment . . . 2665
Flonase Nasal Spray . . . 1440

FLIXONASE (Argentina, Australia, Austria, Belgium, Brazil, Chile, Czech Republic, Denmark, Finland, France, Greece, Hong Kong, Hungary, Irish Republic, Israel, Italy, Malaysia, Mexico, New Zealand, Russia, Singapore, South Africa, Spain, Thailand, The Netherlands, United Kingdom, Venezuela)
FLUTICASONE PROPIONATE
Cutivate Cream . . . 2662
Cutivate Ointment . . . 2665
Flonase Nasal Spray . . . 1440

FLIXOTAIDE (Portugal)
FLUTICASONE PROPIONATE
Cutivate Cream . . . 2662
Cutivate Ointment . . . 2665
Flonase Nasal Spray . . . 1440

FLIXOTIDE (Argentina, Australia, Austria, Belgium, Brazil, Chile, Czech Republic, Denmark, Finland, France, Greece, Hong Kong, Hungary, Irish Republic, Israel, Italy, Malaysia, Mexico, New Zealand, Russia, Singapore, South Africa, Spain, Thailand, The Netherlands, United Kingdom, Venezuela)
FLUTICASONE PROPIONATE
Cutivate Cream . . . 2662

Cutivate Ointment ... 2665
Flonase Nasal Spray ... 1440

FLIXOVATE (France)
FLUTICASONE PROPIONATE
Cutivate Cream ... 2662
Cutivate Ointment ... 2665
Flonase Nasal Spray ... 1440

FLOBAC (Brazil)
CIPROFLOXACIN
Cipro Oral Suspension ... 2977

FLOBACIN (Italy)
OFLOXACIN
Floxin Otic Solution ... 1049

FLOCIPRIN (Greece)
CIPROFLOXACIN HYDROCHLORIDE
Ciloxan Ophthalmic Ointment ... ⊙204, 559
Ciloxan Ophthalmic Solution ... ⊙206
Cipro Tablets ... 2977

FLOGAREN (Venezuela)
DICLOFENAC SODIUM
Voltaren Tablets ... 2307
Voltaren-XR Tablets ... 2310

FLOGEN (Mexico)
NAPROXEN SODIUM
Anaprox DS Tablets ... 2761
Anaprox Tablets ... 2761

FLOGENAC (Argentina)
DICLOFENAC SODIUM
Voltaren Tablets ... 2307
Voltaren-XR Tablets ... 2310

FLOGESIC (Brazil)
DICLOFENAC SODIUM
Voltaren Tablets ... 2307
Voltaren-XR Tablets ... 2310

FLOGINAX (Italy)
NAPROXEN
EC-Naprosyn Delayed-Release Tablets ... 2761
Naprosyn Suspension ... 2761
Naprosyn Tablets ... 2761

FLOGOCEFAL (Argentina)
NAPROXEN
EC-Naprosyn Delayed-Release Tablets ... 2761
Naprosyn Suspension ... 2761
Naprosyn Tablets ... 2761

FLOGOCORT (Chile)
MOMETASONE FUROATE
Elocon Cream 0.1% ... 3005
Elocon Lotion 0.1% ... 3006
Elocon Ointment 0.1% ... 3007
Nasonex Nasal Spray ... 3043

FLOGOGIN (Italy)
NAPROXEN SODIUM
Anaprox DS Tablets ... 2761
Anaprox Tablets ... 2761

FLOGOLISIN (Argentina)
DICLOFENAC SODIUM
Voltaren Tablets ... 2307
Voltaren-XR Tablets ... 2310

FLOHALE (India)
FLUTICASONE PROPIONATE
Cutivate Cream ... 2662
Cutivate Ointment ... 2665
Flonase Nasal Spray ... 1440

FLOMAX (Australia, Canada, New Zealand, South Africa, United Kingdom)
TAMSULOSIN HYDROCHLORIDE
Flomax Capsules ... 850

FLOMAXTRA (United Kingdom)
TAMSULOSIN HYDROCHLORIDE
Flomax Capsules ... 850

FLOMEX (India)
FLUOROMETHOLONE
FML Ophthalmic Ointment ... ⊙228

FLOMEX N (India)
FLUOROMETHOLONE
FML Ophthalmic Ointment ... ⊙228

FLOMIST (India)
FLUTICASONE PROPIONATE
Cutivate Cream ... 2662
Cutivate Ointment ... 2665
Flonase Nasal Spray ... 1440

FLONACIN (Mexico)
OFLOXACIN
Floxin Otic Solution ... 1049

FLONASE (Canada)
FLUTICASONE PROPIONATE
Cutivate Cream ... 2662
Cutivate Ointment ... 2665
Flonase Nasal Spray ... 1440

FLORAC (India)
FLUOROURACIL
Efudex Topical Cream ... 3363
Efudex Topical Solutions ... 3363

FLORALAC (Austria)
LACTULOSE
Kristalose for Oral Solution ... 1034

FLORAXINA (Argentina)
CIPROFLOXACIN HYDROCHLORIDE
Ciloxan Ophthalmic Ointment ... ⊙204, 559
Ciloxan Ophthalmic Solution ... ⊙206
Cipro Tablets ... 2977

FLORAZOLE (Canada)
METRONIDAZOLE
MetroGel-Vaginal Gel ... 1855

FLOSEF (India)
FLUOROMETHOLONE
FML Ophthalmic Ointment ... ⊙228

FLOSSAC (Italy)
NORFLOXACIN
Noroxin Tablets ... 2032

FLOTRIN (Germany)
TERAZOSIN HYDROCHLORIDE
Hytrin Capsules ... 471

FLOVENT (Canada)
FLUTICASONE PROPIONATE
Cutivate Cream ... 2662
Cutivate Ointment ... 2665
Flonase Nasal Spray ... 1440

FLOVID (Hong Kong, Malaysia)
OFLOXACIN
Floxin Otic Solution ... 1049

FLOX (Brazil)
NORFLOXACIN
Noroxin Tablets ... 2032

FLOXACIN (Austria, Brazil, Mexico)
NORFLOXACIN
Noroxin Tablets ... 2032

FLOXACIPRON (Portugal)
CIPROFLOXACIN
Cipro Oral Suspension ... 2977

FLOXAGER (Mexico)
CIPROFLOXACIN HYDROCHLORIDE
Ciloxan Ophthalmic Ointment ... ⊙204, 559
Ciloxan Ophthalmic Solution ... ⊙206
Cipro Tablets ... 2977

FLOXAKIN (Mexico)
CIPROFLOXACIN
Cipro Oral Suspension ... 2977

FLOXAL (Austria, Czech Republic, Germany, Hungary, Russia, Switzerland)
OFLOXACIN
Floxin Otic Solution ... 1049

FLOXALIN (Italy)
NAPROXEN SODIUM
Anaprox DS Tablets ... 2761
Anaprox Tablets ... 2761

FLOXAMICIN (Argentina)
NORFLOXACIN
Noroxin Tablets ... 2032

FLOXAN (Brazil)
CIPROFLOXACIN
Cipro Oral Suspension ... 2977

FLOXANOR (Brazil)
NORFLOXACIN
Noroxin Tablets ... 2032

FLOXANTINA (Mexico)
CIPROFLOXACIN HYDROCHLORIDE
Ciloxan Ophthalmic Ointment ... ⊙204, 559
Ciloxan Ophthalmic Solution ... ⊙206
Cipro Tablets ... 2977

FLOXATOM (Brazil)
NORFLOXACIN
Noroxin Tablets ... 2032

FLOXATRAL (Argentina)
NORFLOXACIN
Noroxin Tablets ... 2032

FLOXATRAT (Brazil)
NORFLOXACIN
Noroxin Tablets ... 2032

FLOXEDOL (Portugal)
OFLOXACIN
Floxin Otic Solution ... 1049

FLOXELENA (Mexico)
CIPROFLOXACIN
Cipro Oral Suspension ... 2977

FLOXEN (Hong Kong)
NORFLOXACIN
Noroxin Tablets ... 2032

FLOXENOR (Thailand)
NORFLOXACIN
Noroxin Tablets ... 2032

FLOXIL (Argentina, Mexico)
OFLOXACIN
Floxin Otic Solution ... 1049

FLOXILIN (Brazil)
NORFLOXACIN
Noroxin Tablets ... 2032

FLOXIN (Canada, South Africa)
OFLOXACIN
Floxin Otic Solution ... 1049

FLOXINA (Brazil)
OFLOXACIN
Floxin Otic Solution ... 1049

FLOXINOL (Brazil)
NORFLOXACIN
Noroxin Tablets ... 2032

FLOXLEVO (Argentina)
LEVOFLOXACIN
Levaquin Injection ... 2384
Levaquin Tablets ... 2384

FLOXSTAT (Brazil, Mexico, Venezuela)
OFLOXACIN
Floxin Otic Solution ... 1049

FLOXUR (India)
OFLOXACIN
Floxin Otic Solution ... 1049

FLOXY (Thailand)
OFLOXACIN
Floxin Otic Solution ... 1049

FLU OPH (Thailand)
FLUOROMETHOLONE
FML Ophthalmic Ointment ... ⊙228

FLUATON (Italy)
FLUOROMETHOLONE
FML Ophthalmic Ointment ... ⊙228

FLUCINOM (Czech Republic, Greece)
FLUTAMIDE
Eulexin Capsules ... 3009

FLUCINOME (Switzerland)
FLUTAMIDE
Eulexin Capsules ... 3009

FLUCOL (Mexico)
NAPROXEN
EC-Naprosyn Delayed-Release Tablets ... 2761
Naprosyn Suspension ... 2761
Naprosyn Tablets ... 2761

FLUCON (Australia, Belgium, Czech Republic, France, Greece, Hong Kong, Hungary, New Zealand, South Africa, Switzerland, Thailand, The Netherlands)
FLUOROMETHOLONE
FML Ophthalmic Ointment ... ⊙228

FLUDAPAMIDE (Switzerland)
INDAPAMIDE
Indapamide Tablets ... 2156

FLUDEX (Austria, Belgium, Denmark, France, Greece, Portugal, Switzerland, The Netherlands)
INDAPAMIDE
Indapamide Tablets ... 2156

FLUFORTE (Chile, Mexico)
FLUOROMETHOLONE
FML Ophthalmic Ointment ... ⊙228

FLUFORTE N (Mexico)
FLUOROMETHOLONE
FML Ophthalmic Ointment ... ⊙228

FLUGEN (Spain)
FLUOROMETHOLONE
FML Ophthalmic Ointment ... ⊙228

FLUIDEMA (Portugal)
INDAPAMIDE
Indapamide Tablets ... 2156

FLUILAST (Italy)
TICLOPIDINE HYDROCHLORIDE
Ticlid Tablets ... 2810

FLUINOL (Spain)
FLUTICASONE PROPIONATE
Cutivate Cream ... 2662
Cutivate Ointment ... 2665
Flonase Nasal Spray ... 1440

FLUI-THEOPHYLLINE (Germany)
THEOPHYLLINE
Uniphyl Tablets ... 2710

FLUKEN (Mexico)
FLUTAMIDE
Eulexin Capsules ... 3009

FLULEM (Chile, Mexico)
FLUTAMIDE
Eulexin Capsules ... 3009

FLUMADINE (Israel)
RIMANTADINE HYDROCHLORIDE
Flumadine Syrup ... 1183
Flumadine Tablets ... 1183

FLUMAGE (Argentina)
FLUMAZENIL
Romazicon Injection ... 2804

FLUMANOVAG (Argentina)
FLUMAZENIL
Romazicon Injection ... 2804

FLUMARC (Argentina)
TERAZOSIN HYDROCHLORIDE
Hytrin Capsules ... 471

FLUMAZEN (Argentina)
FLUMAZENIL
Romazicon Injection ... 2804

FLUMAZIL (Brazil)
FLUMAZENIL
Romazicon Injection ... 2804

FLUMETHOLON (Hong Kong)
FLUOROMETHOLONE
FML Ophthalmic Ointment ... ⊙228

FLUMETOL (Greece, Venezuela)
TIMOLOL MALEATE
Blocadren Tablets ... 1916
Timoptic Sterile Ophthalmic Solution ... 2088
Timoptic in Ocudose ... 2091
Timoptic-XE Sterile Ophthalmic Gel Forming Solution ... 2092

FLUMETOL S (Czech Republic)
FLUOROMETHOLONE
FML Ophthalmic Ointment ... ⊙228

FLUMETOL SEMPLICE (Italy)
FLUOROMETHOLONE
FML Ophthalmic Ointment ... ⊙228

FLUMEX (Brazil)
FLUOROMETHOLONE
FML Ophthalmic Ointment ... ⊙228

FLUMID (Germany)
FLUTAMIDE
Eulexin Capsules ... 3009

FLUMINEX (Italy)
FLUNISOLIDE
Aerobid Inhaler System ... 1171
Aerobid-M Inhaler System ... 1171

FLUMOX (South Africa)
AMOXICILLIN
Amoxil Pediatric Drops for Oral Suspension ... 1343
Amoxil Tablets ... 1343

FLUNASE (Israel)
FLUNISOLIDE
Aerobid Inhaler System ... 1171
Aerobid-M Inhaler System ... 1171

FLUNIDOR (Portugal)
DIFLUNISAL
Dolobid Tablets ... 1955

FLUNIGAR (Italy)
FLUNISOLIDE
Aerobid Inhaler System ... 1171
Aerobid-M Inhaler System ... 1171

FLUNIGET (Austria, Germany)
DIFLUNISAL
Dolobid Tablets ... 1955

FLUNITEC (Argentina, Brazil, Denmark, Norway)
FLUNISOLIDE
Aerobid Inhaler System **1171**
Aerobid-M Inhaler System **1171**

FLUNITOP (Italy)
FLUNISOLIDE
Aerobid Inhaler System **1171**
Aerobid-M Inhaler System **1171**

FLUODONIL (Italy)
DIFLUNISAL
Dolobid Tablets **1955**

FLUOFTAL (Austria)
FLUORESCEIN SODIUM
Fluorescite Injection . . . . ⊙**207**

FLUORACILO (Chile)
FLUOROURACIL
Efudex Topical Cream **3363**
Efudex Topical Solutions **3363**

FLUORALFA (Italy)
FLUORESCEIN SODIUM
Fluorescite Injection . . . . ⊙**207**

FLUOR-AMPS (United Kingdom)
FLUORESCEIN SODIUM
Fluorescite Injection . . . . ⊙**207**

FLUORE STAIN STRIPS (India)
FLUORESCEIN SODIUM
Fluorescite Injection . . . . ⊙**207**

FLUORES (South Africa)
FLUORESCEIN SODIUM
Fluorescite Injection . . . . ⊙**207**

FLUORESCITE (Argentina, Australia, Canada, Czech Republic, Hong Kong, Malaysia, New Zealand, Singapore, South Africa, Thailand)
FLUORESCEIN SODIUM
Fluorescite Injection . . . . ⊙**207**

FLUORETS (Australia, Canada, Hong Kong, Irish Republic, New Zealand, Singapore, South Africa)
FLUORESCEIN SODIUM
Fluorescite Injection . . . . ⊙**207**

FLUOR-I-STRIP AT (Canada)
FLUORESCEIN SODIUM
Fluorescite Injection . . . . ⊙**207**

FLUOROMETIL (Mexico)
FLUOROMETHOLONE
FML Ophthalmic Ointment . . . . ⊙**228**

FLUORO-OPHTAL (Germany)
FLUOROMETHOLONE
FML Ophthalmic Ointment . . . . ⊙**228**

FLUOROPLEX (Australia, Canada)
FLUOROURACIL
Efudex Topical Cream **3363**
Efudex Topical Solutions **3363**

FLUOROPOS (Czech Republic, Germany)
FLUOROMETHOLONE
FML Ophthalmic Ointment . . . . ⊙**228**

FLUPID (Italy)
TICLOPIDINE HYDROCHLORIDE
Ticlid Tablets **2810**

FLUPROSIN (Denmark)
FLUTAMIDE
Eulexin Capsules **3009**

FLUPROST (Italy)
FLUTAMIDE
Eulexin Capsules **3009**

FLURABLASTIN (Denmark, Finland, Norway)
FLUOROURACIL
Efudex Topical Cream **3363**
Efudex Topical Solutions **3363**

FLURACEDYL (Israel, Malaysia, Norway)
FLUOROURACIL
Efudex Topical Cream **3363**
Efudex Topical Solutions **3363**

FLURACIL (India)
FLUOROURACIL
Efudex Topical Cream **3363**
Efudex Topical Solutions **3363**

FLURESS (Australia)
FLUORESCEIN SODIUM
Fluorescite Injection . . . . ⊙**207**

FLUROBLASTIN (Australia, Germany, South Africa)
FLUOROURACIL
Efudex Topical Cream **3363**
Efudex Topical Solutions **3363**

FLUROBLASTINE (Switzerland)
FLUOROURACIL
Efudex Topical Cream **3363**
Efudex Topical Solutions **3363**

FLUROLON (Denmark)
FLUOROMETHOLONE
FML Ophthalmic Ointment . . . . ⊙**228**

FLUROP (Portugal)
FLUOROMETHOLONE
FML Ophthalmic Ointment . . . . ⊙**228**

FLUROX (Mexico, Russia, Thailand)
FLUOROURACIL
Efudex Topical Cream **3363**
Efudex Topical Solutions **3363**

FLUSEMINAL (Greece)
NORFLOXACIN
Noroxin Tablets **2032**

FLUSONAL (Spain)
FLUTICASONE PROPIONATE
Cutivate Cream **2662**
Cutivate Ointment **2665**
Flonase Nasal Spray **1440**

FLUSPIRAL (Italy)
FLUTICASONE PROPIONATE
Cutivate Cream **2662**
Cutivate Ointment **2665**
Flonase Nasal Spray **1440**

FLUSTAR (Italy)
DIFLUNISAL
Dolobid Tablets **1955**

FLUTABENE (Austria)
FLUTAMIDE
Eulexin Capsules **3009**

FLUTACAN (Czech Republic, Denmark, Sweden)
FLUTAMIDE
Eulexin Capsules **3009**

FLUTAHEXAL (Austria, South Africa)
FLUTAMIDE
Eulexin Capsules **3009**

FLUTAIDE (Portugal)
FLUTICASONE PROPIONATE
Cutivate Cream **2662**
Cutivate Ointment **2665**
Flonase Nasal Spray **1440**

FLUTAM (Hungary)
FLUTAMIDE
Eulexin Capsules **3009**

FLUTAMEX (Germany)
FLUTAMIDE
Eulexin Capsules **3009**

FLUTAMID (Russia)
FLUTAMIDE
Eulexin Capsules **3009**

FLUTAMIN (Australia, New Zealand)
FLUTAMIDE
Eulexin Capsules **3009**

FLUTAN (Hong Kong, Malaysia, Thailand)
FLUTAMIDE
Eulexin Capsules **3009**

FLUTANDRONA (Spain)
FLUTAMIDE
Eulexin Capsules **3009**

FLUTAPLEX (Argentina, Belgium, Denmark, Greece, Malaysia, Russia, South Africa, Spain)
FLUTAMIDE
Eulexin Capsules **3009**

FLUTASTAD (Austria)
FLUTAMIDE
Eulexin Capsules **3009**

FLUTAX (Argentina)
FLUTAMIDE
Eulexin Capsules **3009**

FLUTEPAN (Argentina)
FLUTAMIDE
Eulexin Capsules **3009**

FLUTIAMIK (Argentina)
FINASTERIDE
Propecia Tablets **2060**
Proscar Tablets **2067**

FLUTICAPS (Brazil)
FLUTICASONE PROPIONATE
Cutivate Cream **2662**
Cutivate Ointment **2665**
Flonase Nasal Spray **1440**

FLUTICORT (Argentina)
FLUTICASONE PROPIONATE
Cutivate Cream **2662**
Cutivate Ointment **2665**
Flonase Nasal Spray **1440**

FLUTIDE (Norway, Sweden)
FLUTICASONE PROPIONATE
Cutivate Cream **2662**
Cutivate Ointment **2665**
Flonase Nasal Spray **1440**

FLUTI-K (Argentina)
FLUTICASONE PROPIONATE
Cutivate Cream **2662**
Cutivate Ointment **2665**
Flonase Nasal Spray **1440**

FLUTINASE (Switzerland)
FLUTICASONE PROPIONATE
Cutivate Cream **2662**
Cutivate Ointment **2665**
Flonase Nasal Spray **1440**

FLUTIVATE (Brazil, Chile, Germany, Norway, Sweden)
FLUTICASONE PROPIONATE
Cutivate Cream **2662**
Cutivate Ointment **2665**
Flonase Nasal Spray **1440**

FLUTIVENT (Argentina)
FLUTICASONE PROPIONATE
Cutivate Cream **2662**
Cutivate Ointment **2665**
Flonase Nasal Spray **1440**

FLUTOL (New Zealand)
FLUTAMIDE
Eulexin Capsules **3009**

FLUTRAX (Argentina)
FLUTAMIDE
Eulexin Capsules **3009**

FLUXIDIN (Italy)
TICLOPIDINE HYDROCHLORIDE
Ticlid Tablets **2810**

FLUXIFARM (Argentina)
FLUMAZENIL
Romazicon Injection **2804**

FLUXIL (Brazil)
FUROSEMIDE
Furosemide Tablets **2154**

FLUXINAM (Greece)
FLUOROMETHOLONE
FML Ophthalmic Ointment . . . . ⊙**228**

FLUXOCOR (Brazil)
DIPYRIDAMOLE
Persantine Tablets **868**

FLUXPIREN (Argentina)
DICLOFENAC SODIUM
Voltaren Tablets **2307**
Voltaren-XR Tablets **2310**

FML (Argentina, Australia, Belgium, Canada, Finland, Greece, Hong Kong, Irish Republic, Israel, Malaysia, Mexico, New Zealand, Portugal, Singapore, South Africa, Spain, Switzerland, Thailand, The Netherlands, United Kingdom)
FLUOROMETHOLONE
FML Ophthalmic Ointment . . . . ⊙**228**

FML NEO (Argentina)
FLUOROMETHOLONE
FML Ophthalmic Ointment . . . . ⊙**228**

FOILLE INSETTI (Italy)
HYDROCORTISONE
Hydrocortone Tablets **1989**

FOKALEPSIN (Germany)
CARBAMAZEPINE
Carbatrol Capsules **3171**
Tegretol Chewable Tablets **2295**
Tegretol Suspension **2295**
Tegretol Tablets **2295**
Tegretol-XR Tablets **2295**

FOLCRES (Argentina)
FINASTERIDE
Propecia Tablets **2060**
Proscar Tablets **2067**

FOLITABS (Spain)
FINASTERIDE
Propecia Tablets **2060**
Proscar Tablets **2067**

FONX (France)
OXICONAZOLE NITRATE
Oxistat Cream **2667**
Oxistat Lotion **2667**

FORDRIM (Argentina)
FLURAZEPAM HYDROCHLORIDE
Dalmane Capsules **3342**

FOREXIN (Thailand)
CIPROFLOXACIN
Cipro Oral Suspension **2977**

FORMAT (Argentina)
METRONIDAZOLE
MetroGel-Vaginal Gel **1855**

FORMISTIN (Italy)
CETIRIZINE HYDROCHLORIDE
Zyrtec Syrup **2594**
Zyrtec Tablets **2594**

FORPAR (India)
CEFEPIME HYDROCHLORIDE
Maxipime for Injection **1105**

FORTAM (Spain, Switzerland)
CEFTAZIDIME
Fortaz for Injection **1453**

FORTAZ (Brazil, Canada)
CEFTAZIDIME
Fortaz for Injection **1453**

FORTECORTIN (Czech Republic, Spain)
DEXAMETHASONE
Decadron Tablets **1951**

FORTENAC (Switzerland)
DICLOFENAC SODIUM
Voltaren Tablets **2307**
Voltaren-XR Tablets **2310**

FORTERRA (Greece)
CIPROFLOXACIN HYDROCHLORIDE
Ciloxan Ophthalmic Ointment . . . . ⊙**204, 559**
Ciloxan Ophthalmic Solution . . . . ⊙**206**
Cipro Tablets **2977**

FORTFEN (South Africa)
DICLOFENAC SODIUM
Voltaren Tablets **2307**
Voltaren-XR Tablets **2310**

FORTIMAX (Spain)
NORFLOXACIN
Noroxin Tablets **2032**

FORTIPINE (United Kingdom)
NIFEDIPINE
Adalat CC Tablets **2964**

FORTRADOL (Italy)
TRAMADOL HYDROCHLORIDE
Ultram ER Tablets **2392**

FORTUM (Argentina, Australia, Austria, Chile, Czech Republic, Denmark, France, Hong Kong, Hungary, India, Irish Republic, Israel, Malaysia, Mexico, New Zealand, Norway, Russia, Singapore, South Africa, Sweden, Thailand, The Netherlands, United Kingdom, Venezuela)
CEFTAZIDIME
Fortaz for Injection **1453**

FORTUMSET (France)
CEFTAZIDIME
Fortaz for Injection **1453**

FORTZAAR (Denmark, France, Malaysia, Portugal, South Africa, Spain, Thailand, The Netherlands)
LOSARTAN POTASSIUM
Cozaar Tablets **1935**

FORZAAR (Italy)
LOSARTAN POTASSIUM
Cozaar Tablets **1935**

FORZID (Thailand)
CEFTAZIDIME
Fortaz for Injection 1453

FOSALAN (Israel)
ALENDRONATE SODIUM
Fosamax Tablets 1969

FOSALEN (Greece)
ALENDRONATE SODIUM
Fosamax Tablets 1969

FOSAMAX (Argentina, Australia, Austria, Belgium, Brazil, Canada, Chile, Czech Republic, Denmark, Finland, France, Germany, Greece, Hong Kong, Hungary, Irish Republic, Italy, Malaysia, Mexico, New Zealand, Norway, Portugal, Russia, Singapore, South Africa, Spain, Sweden, Switzerland, Thailand, The Netherlands, United Kingdom, Venezuela)
ALENDRONATE SODIUM
Fosamax Tablets 1969

FOSSYOL (Germany)
METRONIDAZOLE
MetroGel-Vaginal Gel 1855

FOSVAL (Chile)
ALENDRONATE SODIUM
Fosamax Tablets 1969

FOTADEX (Argentina)
TOBRAMYCIN
TOBI Solution for Inhalation 2298

FOTEX (Argentina)
TOBRAMYCIN
TOBI Solution for Inhalation 2298

FOUCACILLIN (Greece)
CEFUROXIME AXETIL
Ceftin Tablets 1407
Ceftin for Oral Suspension 1407

FOURNOX (Thailand)
CEFTAZIDIME
Fortaz for Injection 1453

FOXIN (Thailand)
NORFLOXACIN
Noroxin Tablets 2032

FOXINON (Thailand)
NORFLOXACIN
Noroxin Tablets 2032

FOXTIL (Brazil)
CEFOXITIN SODIUM
Mefoxin Premixed Intravenous Solution . . . 2016
Mefoxin for Injection 2012

FP TAB (Japan)
SELEGILINE HYDROCHLORIDE
Eldepryl Capsules 3208

FRACTAL (France)
FLUVASTATIN SODIUM
Lescol Capsules 2233

FRANOL (Thailand)
THEOPHYLLINE
Uniphyl Tablets 2710

FRAXIDOL (Italy)
TRAMADOL HYDROCHLORIDE
Ultram ER Tablets 2392

FRECUENTAL (Argentina)
FUROSEMIDE
Furosemide Tablets 2154

FREDYR (Greece)
CEFUROXIME SODIUM
Zinacef Injection 1631

FRESENIZOL (Mexico)
METRONIDAZOLE
MetroGel-Vaginal Gel 1855

FREUDAL (Mexico)
DIAZEPAM
Diastat Rectal Delivery System 3343
Valium Tablets 2819

FRIDALIT (Argentina)
HYDROCORTISONE
Hydrocortone Tablets 1989

FRINOVA (Spain)
PROMETHAZINE HYDROCHLORIDE
Phenergan Tablets and Suppositories 3440

FRIVENT (Italy)
THEOPHYLLINE
Uniphyl Tablets 2710

FROIDIR (Finland)
CLOZAPINE
Clozaril Tablets 2184

FROLICIN (Greece)
AMOXICILLIN
Amoxil Pediatric Drops for Oral Suspension 1343
Amoxil Tablets 1343

FROMIL (Venezuela)
FUROSEMIDE
Furosemide Tablets 2154

FROMILID (Czech Republic, Hungary, Russia)
CLARITHROMYCIN
Biaxin Filmtab Tablets 402
Biaxin Granules 402

FROOP (United Kingdom)
FUROSEMIDE
Furosemide Tablets 2154

FROSINOR (Spain)
PAROXETINE HYDROCHLORIDE
Paxil Oral Suspension 1530
Paxil Tablets 1530

FROTIN (Malaysia)
METRONIDAZOLE
MetroGel-Vaginal Gel 1855

FROXAL (Mexico)
CEFUROXIME SODIUM
Zinacef Injection 1631

FRUDEMISAN (Mexico)
FUROSEMIDE
Furosemide Tablets 2154

FRUMAX (United Kingdom)
FUROSEMIDE
Furosemide Tablets 2154

FRUMERON (Hong Kong, Thailand)
INDAPAMIDE
Indapamide Tablets 2156

FRUMIL (Greece)
FUROSEMIDE
Furosemide Tablets 2154

FRUSEHEXAL (Australia)
FUROSEMIDE
Furosemide Tablets 2154

FRUSEMIX (India)
FUROSEMIDE
Furosemide Tablets 2154

FRUSENE (Irish Republic, United Kingdom)
FUROSEMIDE
Furosemide Tablets 2154

FRUSENEX (India)
FUROSEMIDE
Furosemide Tablets 2154

FRUSETIC (United Kingdom)
FUROSEMIDE
Furosemide Tablets 2154

FRUSID (Australia, Hong Kong, New Zealand, Singapore, United Kingdom)
FUROSEMIDE
Furosemide Tablets 2154

FRUSIDE (Irish Republic)
FUROSEMIDE
Furosemide Tablets 2154

FRUSIX (India)
FUROSEMIDE
Furosemide Tablets 2154

FRUSOL (United Kingdom)
FUROSEMIDE
Furosemide Tablets 2154

FRUTENOR (Greece)
LEVOCARNITINE
Carnitor Injection 3188
Carnitor Tablets and Oral Solution 3190

FTAZIDIME (Greece)
CEFTAZIDIME
Fortaz for Injection 1453

FTDA (Argentina)
FLUTAMIDE
Eulexin Capsules 3009

FTONAVIL (Greece)
CAPTOPRIL
Captopril Tablets 2149

FTOROCORT (Hungary, Russia, Thailand)
TRIAMCINOLONE ACETONIDE
Azmacort Inhalation Aerosol 1726
Nasacort AQ Nasal Spray 2922

FUCEROX (Mexico)
CEFUROXIME SODIUM
Zinacef Injection 1631

FUDERMEX (Chile)
LANSOPRAZOLE
Prevacid Delayed-Release Capsules 3271

FUDIRINE (Thailand)
FUROSEMIDE
Furosemide Tablets 2154

FUDONE (India)
FAMOTIDINE
Pepcid Injection 2040
Pepcid Injection Premixed 2040
Pepcid Tablets 2038
Pepcid for Oral Suspension 2038

FUGEREL (Australia, Austria, Germany, Hong Kong, Hungary, Malaysia, Singapore, Thailand)
FLUTAMIDE
Eulexin Capsules 3009

FUGOLIN (Venezuela)
CLOTRIMAZOLE
Lotrimin Cream 3039
Lotrimin Lotion 1% 3039
Lotrimin Topical Solution 1% 3039

FULCRO (Italy)
FENOFIBRATE
Tricor Tablets 527

FUL-GLO (Australia, New Zealand)
FLUORESCEIN SODIUM
Fluorescite Injection . . . . . ⊙207

FULGRAM (Chile, Italy, Venezuela)
NORFLOXACIN
Noroxin Tablets 2032

FUMARENID (Germany)
FUROSEMIDE
Furosemide Tablets 2154

FUNDUSCEIN (Canada)
FLUORESCEIN SODIUM
Fluorescite Injection . . . . . ⊙207

FUNGEDERM (United Kingdom)
CLOTRIMAZOLE
Lotrimin Cream 3039
Lotrimin Lotion 1% 3039
Lotrimin Topical Solution 1% 3039

FUNGICIDIN (Czech Republic)
NYSTATIN
Nystop Topical Powder USP 2478
Paddock Nystatin USP for Oral Suspension 2478

FUNGICON (Thailand)
CLOTRIMAZOLE
Lotrimin Cream 3039
Lotrimin Lotion 1% 3039
Lotrimin Topical Solution 1% 3039

FUNGIDERM (Germany, Thailand)
CLOTRIMAZOLE
Lotrimin Cream 3039
Lotrimin Lotion 1% 3039
Lotrimin Topical Solution 1% 3039

FUNGIDERMO (Spain)
CLOTRIMAZOLE
Lotrimin Cream 3039
Lotrimin Lotion 1% 3039
Lotrimin Topical Solution 1% 3039

FUNGIMAX (Brazil)
METRONIDAZOLE
MetroGel-Vaginal Gel 1855

FUNGIREDUCT (Germany)
NYSTATIN
Nystop Topical Powder USP 2478
Paddock Nystatin USP for Oral Suspension 2478

FUNGISPOR (South Africa)
CLOTRIMAZOLE
Lotrimin Cream 3039
Lotrimin Lotion 1% 3039
Lotrimin Topical Solution 1% 3039

FUNGISTEN (Norway)
CLOTRIMAZOLE
Lotrimin Cream 3039
Lotrimin Lotion 1% 3039
Lotrimin Topical Solution 1% 3039

FUNGIZID (Germany, Hong Kong, New Zealand)
CLOTRIMAZOLE
Lotrimin Cream 3039
Lotrimin Lotion 1% 3039
Lotrimin Topical Solution 1% 3039

FUNGOTERBINE (Russia)
TERBINAFINE HYDROCHLORIDE
Lamisil Tablets 2232

FUNGOTOX (Switzerland)
CLOTRIMAZOLE
Lotrimin Cream 3039
Lotrimin Lotion 1% 3039
Lotrimin Topical Solution 1% 3039

FUNTOPIC (Venezuela)
TERBINAFINE HYDROCHLORIDE
Lamisil Tablets 2232

FUNTYL (Brazil)
TERBINAFINE HYDROCHLORIDE
Lamisil Tablets 2232

FUNZAL (Chile)
CLOTRIMAZOLE
Lotrimin Cream 3039
Lotrimin Lotion 1% 3039
Lotrimin Topical Solution 1% 3039

FURAGRAND (Argentina)
FUROSEMIDE
Furosemide Tablets 2154

FURAL (Austria)
FUROSEMIDE
Furosemide Tablets 2154

FURANTHRIL (Czech Republic, Germany)
FUROSEMIDE
Furosemide Tablets 2154

FURAXIL (Greece)
CEFUROXIME AXETIL
Ceftin Tablets 1407
Ceftin for Oral Suspension 1407

FURAZOLON (Brazil)
HYDROCORTISONE
Hydrocortone Tablets 1989

FURDIUREN (Venezuela)
FUROSEMIDE
Furosemide Tablets 2154

FURESE (Denmark)
FUROSEMIDE
Furosemide Tablets 2154

FURESIN (Brazil)
FUROSEMIDE
Furosemide Tablets 2154

FURESIS (Finland)
FUROSEMIDE
Furosemide Tablets 2154

FURESIS COMP (Finland)
FUROSEMIDE
Furosemide Tablets 2154

FURETIC (Thailand)
FUROSEMIDE
Furosemide Tablets 2154

FURIDE (Thailand)
FUROSEMIDE
Furosemide Tablets 2154

FURINE (Thailand)
FUROSEMIDE
Furosemide Tablets 2154

FURITAL (Argentina)
FUROSEMIDE
Furosemide Tablets 2154

FURIX (Argentina, Denmark, Norway, Sweden)
FUROSEMIDE
Furosemide Tablets 2154

FURMIDAL (Mexico)
FUROSEMIDE
Furosemide Tablets 2154

FURMIDE (Malaysia)
FUROSEMIDE
Furosemide Tablets 2154

FURO-BASAN (Switzerland)
FUROSEMIDE
Furosemide Tablets 2154

FURO-BASF (Germany)
FUROSEMIDE
Furosemide Tablets 2154

FUROBETA (Germany)
FUROSEMIDE
Furosemide Tablets 2154

FUROGAMMA (Germany)
FUROSEMIDE
Furosemide Tablets 2154

FUROHEXAL (Austria)
FUROSEMIDE
Furosemide Tablets 2154

FUROMED (Germany)
FUROSEMIDE
Furosemide Tablets 2154

FUROMIL (Mexico)
FUROSEMIDE
Furosemide Tablets 2154

FUROMIN (Finland)
FUROSEMIDE
Furosemide Tablets 2154

FURON (Czech Republic, Hungary)
FUROSEMIDE
Furosemide Tablets 2154

FURONET (Denmark)
FUROSEMIDE
Furosemide Tablets 2154

FURONEX (Mexico)
FUROSEMIDE
Furosemide Tablets 2154

FURO-PUREN (Germany)
FUROSEMIDE
Furosemide Tablets 2154

FURORESE (Czech Republic)
FUROSEMIDE
Furosemide Tablets 2154

FUROSAL (Germany)
FUROSEMIDE
Furosemide Tablets 2154

FUROSAN (Brazil, Mexico)
FUROSEMIDE
Furosemide Tablets 2154

FUROSCAND (Sweden)
FUROSEMIDE
Furosemide Tablets 2154

FUROSECORD (Brazil)
FUROSEMIDE
Furosemide Tablets 2154

FUROSEM (Brazil)
FUROSEMIDE
Furosemide Tablets 2154

FUROSEMIX (France)
FUROSEMIDE
Furosemide Tablets 2154

FUROSEN (Brazil)
FUROSEMIDE
Furosemide Tablets 2154

FUROSETRON (Brazil)
FUROSEMIDE
Furosemide Tablets 2154

FUROSIFAR (Switzerland)
FUROSEMIDE
Furosemide Tablets 2154

FUROSIX (Brazil)
FUROSEMIDE
Furosemide Tablets 2154

FUROSTAD (Austria)
FUROSEMIDE
Furosemide Tablets 2154

FUROTER (Mexico)
FUROSEMIDE
Furosemide Tablets 2154

FUROTYROL (Austria)
FUROSEMIDE
Furosemide Tablets 2154

FUROVITE (Israel)
FUROSEMIDE
Furosemide Tablets 2154

FUROXIM (Austria)
CEFUROXIME AXETIL
Ceftin Tablets 1407
Ceftin for Oral Suspension 1407

FUROZIX (Brazil)
FUROSEMIDE
Furosemide Tablets 2154

FURSEMIDA (Brazil)
FUROSEMIDE
Furosemide Tablets 2154

FURSOL (Switzerland)
FUROSEMIDE
Furosemide Tablets 2154

FURTENK (Argentina)
FUROSEMIDE
Furosemide Tablets 2154

FUSANIDAZOL (Mexico)
METRONIDAZOLE
MetroGel-Vaginal Gel 1855

FUSEPINA (Mexico)
NIFEDIPINE
Adalat CC Tablets 2964

FUSERIDE (Thailand)
FUROSEMIDE
Furosemide Tablets 2154

FUSID (Israel, The Netherlands)
FUROSEMIDE
Furosemide Tablets 2154

FUSTAREN (Mexico)
DICLOFENAC SODIUM
Voltaren Tablets 2307
Voltaren-XR Tablets 2310

FUXEN (Mexico)
NAPROXEN
EC-Naprosyn Delayed-Release Tablets 2761
Naprosyn Suspension 2761
Naprosyn Tablets 2761

G-80 (India)
GENTAMICIN SULFATE
Garamycin Injectable 3014

GABAMERCK (Spain)
GABAPENTIN
Neurontin Capsules 2487

GABAMOX (Portugal)
GABAPENTIN
Neurontin Capsules 2487

GABATAL (Austria)
GABAPENTIN
Neurontin Capsules 2487

GABATRIL (Mexico)
TIAGABINE HYDROCHLORIDE
Gabitril Tablets 984

GABATUR (Spain)
GABAPENTIN
Neurontin Capsules 2487

GABEX (Chile)
GABAPENTIN
Neurontin Capsules 2487

GABIROL (Mexico)
RIMANTADINE HYDROCHLORIDE
Flumadine Syrup 1183
Flumadine Tablets 1183

GABITRIL (Australia, Austria, Belgium, Brazil, Czech Republic, Denmark, Finland, France, Germany, Greece, Hungary, Irish Republic, Italy, Portugal, Spain, Switzerland, United Kingdom)
TIAGABINE HYDROCHLORIDE
Gabitril Tablets 984

GABOX (Venezuela)
CARBAMAZEPINE
Carbatrol Capsules 3171
Tegretol Chewable Tablets 2295
Tegretol Suspension 2295
Tegretol Tablets 2295
Tegretol-XR Tablets 2295

GADOPRIL (Argentina)
ENALAPRIL MALEATE
Vasotec I.V. Injection 2103

GADOPRIL D (Argentina)
ENALAPRIL MALEATE
Vasotec I.V. Injection 2103

GALEBIRON (Greece)
RANITIDINE HYDROCHLORIDE
Zantac 25 EFFERdose Tablets 1624
Zantac 150 EFFERdose Tablets 1624
Zantac 150 Tablets 1624
Zantac 300 Tablets 1624
Zantac Injection 1619
Zantac Injection Premixed 1619
Zantac Syrup 1624

GALEDOL (Mexico)
DICLOFENAC SODIUM
Voltaren Tablets 2307
Voltaren-XR Tablets 2310

GALEMIN (Greece)
CEFUROXIME SODIUM
Zinacef Injection 1631

GALENTROMICINA (Mexico)
ERYTHROMYCIN
Ery-Tab Tablets 449
Erythromycin Base Filmtab Tablets 455
Erythromycin Delayed-Release Capsules, USP 457
PCE Dispertab Tablets 515

GALIDRIN (Mexico)
RANITIDINE HYDROCHLORIDE
Zantac 25 EFFERdose Tablets 1624
Zantac 150 EFFERdose Tablets 1624
Zantac 150 Tablets 1624
Zantac 300 Tablets 1624
Zantac Injection 1619
Zantac Injection Premixed 1619
Zantac Syrup 1624

GAMACEF (Brazil)
CEFOXITIN SODIUM
Mefoxin Premixed Intravenous Solution 2016
Mefoxin for Injection 2012

GAMAVATE (United Arab Emirates)
CLOBETASOL PROPIONATE
Temovate Cream 2668
Temovate E Emollient 2671
Temovate Gel 2669
Temovate Ointment 2668
Temovate Scalp Application 2670

GAMMAKINE (Italy)
INTERFERON GAMMA-1B
Actimmune 1671

GANAVAX (Argentina)
VENLAFAXINE HYDROCHLORIDE
Effexor Tablets 3411
Effexor XR Capsules 3417

GANOR (Germany)
FAMOTIDINE
Pepcid Injection 2040
Pepcid Injection Premixed 2040
Pepcid Tablets 2038
Pepcid for Oral Suspension 2038

GANTIN (Australia)
GABAPENTIN
Neurontin Capsules 2487

GANVIREL (Argentina)
LAMIVUDINE
Epivir Oral Solution 1427
Epivir Tablets 1427
Epivir-HBV Oral Solution 1432
Epivir-HBV Tablets 1432

GANVIREL DUO (Argentina)
LAMIVUDINE
Epivir Oral Solution 1427
Epivir Tablets 1427
Epivir-HBV Oral Solution 1432
Epivir-HBV Tablets 1432

GAOPTOL (Monaco)
TIMOLOL MALEATE
Blocadren Tablets 1916
Timoptic Sterile Ophthalmic Solution 2088
Timoptic in Ocudose 2091
Timoptic-XE Sterile Ophthalmic Gel Forming Solution 2092

GAPROXEN (Greece)
RANITIDINE HYDROCHLORIDE
Zantac 25 EFFERdose Tablets 1624
Zantac 150 EFFERdose Tablets 1624
Zantac 150 Tablets 1624
Zantac 300 Tablets 1624
Zantac Injection 1619
Zantac Injection Premixed 1619
Zantac Syrup 1624

GARABET (Venezuela)
GENTAMICIN SULFATE
Garamycin Injectable 3014

GARACIN (Brazil)
GENTAMICIN SULFATE
Garamycin Injectable 3014

GARACOL (The Netherlands)
GENTAMICIN SULFATE
Garamycin Injectable 3014

GARACOLL (Mexico, South Africa)
GENTAMICIN SULFATE
Garamycin Injectable 3014

GARALEN (Mexico)
GENTAMICIN SULFATE
Garamycin Injectable 3014

GARALONE (Portugal)
GENTAMICIN SULFATE
Garamycin Injectable 3014

GARAMYCIN (Australia, Austria, Canada, Czech Republic, Denmark, Greece, Hong Kong, Hungary, Israel, Malaysia, Norway, Singapore, South Africa, Sweden, Switzerland, Thailand, The Netherlands, United Kingdom)
GENTAMICIN SULFATE
Garamycin Injectable 3014

GARANIL (Spain)
CAPTOPRIL
Captopril Tablets 2149

GARASONE (Czech Republic, Hungary, Venezuela)
GENTAMICIN SULFATE
Garamycin Injectable 3014

GARATEC (Canada)
GENTAMICIN SULFATE
Garamycin Injectable 3014

GARDEX (Denmark, Finland)
CETIRIZINE HYDROCHLORIDE
Zyrtec Syrup 2594
Zyrtec Tablets 2594

GARDOTON (Chile)
ONDANSETRON
Zofran ODT Orally Disintegrating Tablets 1639

GARIA (Spain)
CEFPODOXIME PROXETIL
Vantin Tablets and Oral Suspension 2645

GARRANIL (Spain)
CAPTOPRIL
Captopril Tablets 2149

GASCOP (Mexico)
ALBENDAZOLE
Albenza Tablets 1338

GASTENIN (Spain)
FAMOTIDINE
Pepcid Injection 2040
Pepcid Injection Premixed 2040
Pepcid Tablets 2038
Pepcid for Oral Suspension 2038

GASTER (Japan)
FAMOTIDINE
Pepcid Injection 2040
Pepcid Injection Premixed 2040
Pepcid Tablets 2038
Pepcid for Oral Suspension 2038

GASTEROGEN (Greece)
FAMOTIDINE
Pepcid Injection 2040
Pepcid Injection Premixed 2040
Pepcid Tablets 2038
Pepcid for Oral Suspension 2038

GASTOPRIDE (Portugal)
FAMOTIDINE
Pepcid Injection 2040
Pepcid Injection Premixed 2040
Pepcid Tablets 2038
Pepcid for Oral Suspension 2038

GASTRAL (Spain)
SUCRALFATE
Carafate Suspension 701
Carafate Tablets 701

GASTRAZOL (Venezuela)
LANSOPRAZOLE
Prevacid Delayed-Release Capsules 3271

GASTREX (Portugal)
LANSOPRAZOLE
Prevacid Delayed-Release Capsules 3271

GASTRIDE (Chile)
LANSOPRAZOLE
Prevacid Delayed-Release Capsules 3271

GASTRIDIN (Italy, Mexico)
FAMOTIDINE
Pepcid Injection 2040

Pepcid Injection Premixed **2040**
Pepcid Tablets **2038**
Pepcid for Oral Suspension **2038**

GASTRIDINA (Portugal)
RANITIDINE HYDROCHLORIDE
Zantac 25 EFFERdose Tablets **1624**
Zantac 150 EFFERdose Tablets. **1624**
Zantac 150 Tablets **1624**
Zantac 300 Tablets **1624**
Zantac Injection **1619**
Zantac Injection Premixed **1619**
Zantac Syrup **1624**

GASTRIFAM (Portugal)
FAMOTIDINE
Pepcid Injection **2040**
Pepcid Injection Premixed **2040**
Pepcid Tablets **2038**
Pepcid for Oral Suspension **2038**

GASTRIL (Hong Kong)
RANITIDINE HYDROCHLORIDE
Zantac 25 EFFERdose Tablets **1624**
Zantac 150 EFFERdose Tablets. **1624**
Zantac 150 Tablets **1624**
Zantac 300 Tablets **1624**
Zantac Injection **1619**
Zantac Injection Premixed **1619**
Zantac Syrup **1624**

GASTRION (Spain)
FAMOTIDINE
Pepcid Injection **2040**
Pepcid Injection Premixed **2040**
Pepcid Tablets **2038**
Pepcid for Oral Suspension **2038**

GASTRIUM (Chile)
FAMOTIDINE
Pepcid Injection **2040**
Pepcid Injection Premixed **2040**
Pepcid Tablets **2038**
Pepcid for Oral Suspension **2038**

GASTRO (Israel)
FAMOTIDINE
Pepcid Injection **2040**
Pepcid Injection Premixed **2040**
Pepcid Tablets **2038**
Pepcid for Oral Suspension **2038**

GASTROCOL (Chile)
SUCRALFATE
Carafate Suspension **701**
Carafate Tablets **701**

GASTRODOMINA (Hong Kong, Spain)
FAMOTIDINE
Pepcid Injection **2040**
Pepcid Injection Premixed **2040**
Pepcid Tablets **2038**
Pepcid for Oral Suspension **2038**

GASTROGEL (Italy, Switzerland)
SUCRALFATE
Carafate Suspension **701**
Carafate Tablets **701**

GASTROLAV (Portugal)
RANITIDINE HYDROCHLORIDE
Zantac 25 EFFERdose Tablets **1624**
Zantac 150 EFFERdose Tablets. **1624**
Zantac 150 Tablets **1624**
Zantac 300 Tablets **1624**
Zantac Injection **1619**
Zantac Injection Premixed **1619**
Zantac Syrup **1624**

GASTROLETS (Argentina)
RANITIDINE HYDROCHLORIDE
Zantac 25 EFFERdose Tablets **1624**
Zantac 150 EFFERdose Tablets. **1624**
Zantac 150 Tablets **1624**
Zantac 300 Tablets **1624**
Zantac Injection **1619**
Zantac Injection Premixed **1619**
Zantac Syrup **1624**

GASTROLIBER (Portugal)
LANSOPRAZOLE
Prevacid Delayed-Release Capsules **3271**

GASTROPEN (Spain)
FAMOTIDINE
Pepcid Injection **2040**
Pepcid Injection Premixed **2040**
Pepcid Tablets **2038**
Pepcid for Oral Suspension **2038**

GASTROSEDOL (Argentina)
RANITIDINE HYDROCHLORIDE
Zantac 25 EFFERdose Tablets **1624**
Zantac 150 EFFERdose Tablets. **1624**
Zantac 150 Tablets **1624**
Zantac 300 Tablets **1624**
Zantac Injection **1619**
Zantac Injection Premixed **1619**
Zantac Syrup **1624**

GASTROSIDIN (Russia)
FAMOTIDINE
Pepcid Injection **2040**
Pepcid Injection Premixed **2040**
Pepcid Tablets **2038**
Pepcid for Oral Suspension **2038**

GASTRULCER (Portugal)
RANITIDINE HYDROCHLORIDE
Zantac 25 EFFERdose Tablets **1624**
Zantac 150 EFFERdose Tablets. **1624**
Zantac 150 Tablets **1624**
Zantac 300 Tablets **1624**
Zantac Injection **1619**
Zantac Injection Premixed **1619**
Zantac Syrup **1624**

GATINAR (Spain, Switzerland)
LACTULOSE
Kristalose for Oral Solution **1034**

GAVILAST (United Kingdom)
RANITIDINE HYDROCHLORIDE
Zantac 25 EFFERdose Tablets **1624**
Zantac 150 EFFERdose Tablets. **1624**
Zantac 150 Tablets **1624**
Zantac 300 Tablets **1624**
Zantac Injection **1619**
Zantac Injection Premixed **1619**
Zantac Syrup **1624**

G-DIL (Greece)
ISOSORBIDE MONONITRATE
Imdur Tablets **3018**

GEABATAN (Finland)
GABAPENTIN
Neurontin Capsules **2487**

GEANGIN (Denmark, Norway, The Netherlands, United Kingdom)
VERAPAMIL HYDROCHLORIDE
Covera-HS Tablets **3139**
Verelan PM Extended-Release Capsules, Controlled-Onset **3106**

GEFINA (Finland)
FINASTERIDE
Propecia Tablets **2060**
Proscar Tablets. **2067**

GELCAIN (Chile)
LIDOCAINE
Lidoderm Patch **1118**

GELERIT (Chile)
ERYTHROMYCIN
Ery-Tab Tablets **449**
Erythromycin Base Filmtab Tablets. **455**
Erythromycin Delayed-Release Capsules, USP **457**
PCE Dispertab Tablets **515**

GELESTRA (Italy)
ESTRADIOL
Climara Transdermal System **771**
Estring Vaginal Ring **2635**

GEL-LIDO (Brazil)
LIDOCAINE
Lidoderm Patch **1118**

GELMICIN (Mexico)
CLOTRIMAZOLE
Lotrimin Cream. **3039**
Lotrimin Lotion 1%. **3039**
Lotrimin Topical Solution 1% **3039**

GELODERM (Chile)
METRONIDAZOLE
MetroGel-Vaginal Gel **1855**

GEL-OSE (Canada)
LACTULOSE
Kristalose for Oral Solution **1034**

GEMCITE (India)
GEMCITABINE HYDROCHLORIDE
Gemzar for Injection. **1771**

GEMISTATIN (Argentina)
SIMVASTATIN
Zocor Tablets **2105**

GEMTRO (Argentina)
GEMCITABINE HYDROCHLORIDE
Gemzar for Injection. **1771**

GEMZAR (Australia, Austria, Belgium, Brazil, Canada, Chile, Czech Republic, Denmark, Finland, France, Germany, Greece, Hong Kong, Hungary, Irish Republic, Israel, Italy, Malaysia, Mexico, New Zealand, Norway, Portugal, Russia, Singapore, South Africa, Spain, Sweden, Switzerland, Thailand, The Netherlands, United Kingdom, Venezuela)
GEMCITABINE HYDROCHLORIDE
Gemzar for Injection. **1771**

GEMZIL (Thailand)
CAPTOPRIL
Captopril Tablets **2149**

GENALEN (Italy)
ALENDRONATE SODIUM
Fosamax Tablets **1969**

GENALGEN (Mexico)
NAPROXEN
EC-Naprosyn Delayed-Release Tablets. . . . **2761**
Naprosyn Suspension. **2761**
Naprosyn Tablets **2761**

GENAPROST (Italy)
FINASTERIDE
Propecia Tablets **2060**
Proscar Tablets. **2067**

GENCIN (Germany, South Africa)
GENTAMICIN SULFATE
Garamycin Injectable **3014**

GENDAZEL (Thailand)
ALBENDAZOLE
Albenza Tablets. **1338**

GENEMICIN (Mexico)
GENTAMICIN SULFATE
Garamycin Injectable **3014**

GENEPHOXAL (Greece)
CEFUROXIME AXETIL
Ceftin Tablets. **1407**
Ceftin for Oral Suspension. **1407**

GENERLOG (Thailand)
TRIAMCINOLONE ACETONIDE
Azmacort Inhalation Aerosol. **1726**
Nasacort AQ Nasal Spray **2922**

GENFLOX (India)
OFLOXACIN
Floxin Otic Solution **1049**

GENFLOX TZ (India)
OFLOXACIN
Floxin Otic Solution **1049**

GENGIGEL (Portugal)
SODIUM HYALURONATE
Hyalgan Solution **2901**

GENITOFLOX (Brazil)
NORFLOXACIN
Noroxin Tablets. **2032**

GENKOVA (Mexico)
GENTAMICIN SULFATE
Garamycin Injectable **3014**

GENLAC (Australia)
LACTULOSE
Kristalose for Oral Solution **1034**

GEN-LAC (Canada)
LACTULOSE
Kristalose for Oral Solution **1034**

GEN-MEDROXY (Canada)
MEDROXYPROGESTERONE ACETATE
Depo-Medrol Single-Dose Vial **2619**

GENMOX (India)
AMOXICILLIN
Amoxil Pediatric Drops for Oral Suspension. **1343**
Amoxil Tablets **1343**

GENOCOLAN (Argentina)
LACTULOSE
Kristalose for Oral Solution **1034**

GENOPTIC (Australia, Belgium, Hong Kong, New Zealand, Singapore, South Africa, Spain)
GENTAMICIN SULFATE
Garamycin Injectable **3014**

GENOVOX (Greece)
NIMODIPINE
Nimotop Capsules **749**

GENOXEN (Hong Kong, Irish Republic)
NAPROXEN
EC-Naprosyn Delayed-Release Tablets. . . . **2761**
Naprosyn Suspension. **2761**
Naprosyn Tablets **2761**

GENPROL (Spain)
CITALOPRAM HYDROBROMIDE
Celexa Tablets **1176**

GENREX (Mexico)
GENTAMICIN SULFATE
Garamycin Injectable **3014**

GENSER (Mexico)
GENTAMICIN SULFATE
Garamycin Injectable **3014**

GENSUMYCIN (Denmark, Finland, Norway, Sweden)
GENTAMICIN SULFATE
Garamycin Injectable **3014**

GENTA (Germany, Mexico)
GENTAMICIN SULFATE
Garamycin Injectable **3014**

GENTA GOBENS (Portugal, Spain)
GENTAMICIN SULFATE
Garamycin Injectable **3014**

GENTABILLES (France)
GENTAMICIN SULFATE
Garamycin Injectable **3014**

GENTAC (Brazil, Thailand)
GENTAMICIN SULFATE
Garamycin Injectable **3014**

GENTACIDIN (Canada)
GENTAMICIN SULFATE
Garamycin Injectable **3014**

GENTACIN (Mexico, Thailand)
GENTAMICIN SULFATE
Garamycin Injectable **3014**

GENTACOLL (Denmark, Finland)
GENTAMICIN SULFATE
Garamycin Injectable **3014**

GENTACORT (Italy)
GENTAMICIN SULFATE
Garamycin Injectable **3014**

GENTADERM (Argentina)
GENTAMICIN SULFATE
Garamycin Injectable **3014**

GENTAGRAN (Brazil)
GENTAMICIN SULFATE
Garamycin Injectable **3014**

GENTAL (Thailand, United Arab Emirates)
GENTAMICIN SULFATE
Garamycin Injectable **3014**

GENTALLINE (France)
GENTAMICIN SULFATE
Garamycin Injectable **3014**

GENTALLORENS (Spain)
GENTAMICIN SULFATE
Garamycin Injectable **3014**

GENTALODINA (Spain)
GENTAMICIN SULFATE
Garamycin Injectable **3014**

GENTALYN (Chile, Italy, Venezuela)
GENTAMICIN SULFATE
Garamycin Injectable **3014**

GENTAMEDICAL (Spain)
GENTAMICIN SULFATE
Garamycin Injectable **3014**

GENTAMEN (Italy)
GENTAMICIN SULFATE
Garamycin Injectable **3014**

GENTAMICIL (Venezuela)
GENTAMICIN SULFATE
Garamycin Injectable **3014**

GENTAMIL (Brazil, Mexico)
GENTAMICIN SULFATE
Garamycin Injectable **3014**

GENTAMILAN (Venezuela)
GENTAMICIN SULFATE
Garamycin Injectable **3014**

GENTAMIN (Spain)
GENTAMICIN SULFATE
Garamycin Injectable **3014**

GENTAMINA (Argentina)
GENTAMICIN SULFATE
Garamycin Injectable 3014

GENTAMIVAL (Spain)
GENTAMICIN SULFATE
Garamycin Injectable 3014

GENTAMIX (Germany)
GENTAMICIN SULFATE
Garamycin Injectable 3014

GENTAMORGENS (Spain)
GENTAMICIN SULFATE
Garamycin Injectable 3014

GENTAMYTREX (Belgium, Germany, Malaysia, Singapore, The Netherlands)
GENTAMICIN SULFATE
Garamycin Injectable 3014

GENTA-OPH (Thailand)
GENTAMICIN SULFATE
Garamycin Injectable 3014

GENTAPLUS (Brazil)
GENTAMICIN SULFATE
Garamycin Injectable 3014

GENTAREN (Argentina)
GENTAMICIN SULFATE
Garamycin Injectable 3014

GENTARIM (Mexico)
GENTAMICIN SULFATE
Garamycin Injectable 3014

GENTARON (Brazil)
GENTAMICIN SULFATE
Garamycin Injectable 3014

GENTASPORIN (India)
GENTAMICIN SULFATE
Garamycin Injectable 3014

GENTATENK (Argentina)
GENTAMICIN SULFATE
Garamycin Injectable 3014

GENTATRIM (Israel)
GENTAMICIN SULFATE
Garamycin Injectable 3014

GENTAX (Austria, Brazil)
GENTAMICIN SULFATE
Garamycin Injectable 3014

GENTAZAF Z (Mexico)
GENTAMICIN SULFATE
Garamycin Injectable 3014

GENTIBIOPTAL (Italy)
GENTAMICIN SULFATE
Garamycin Injectable 3014

GENTICIN (Irish Republic, United Kingdom)
GENTAMICIN SULFATE
Garamycin Injectable 3014

GENTICINA (Spain)
GENTAMICIN SULFATE
Garamycin Injectable 3014

GENTICOL (Argentina, Italy)
GENTAMICIN SULFATE
Garamycin Injectable 3014

GENTICYN (India)
GENTAMICIN SULFATE
Garamycin Injectable 3014

GENTICYN EYE/EAR (India)
GENTAMICIN SULFATE
Garamycin Injectable 3014

GENTICYN HC (India)
GENTAMICIN SULFATE
Garamycin Injectable 3014

GEN-TIMOLOL (New Zealand)
TIMOLOL MALEATE
Blocadren Tablets 1916
Timoptic Sterile Ophthalmic Solution 2088
Timoptic in Ocudose 2091
Timoptic-XE Sterile Ophthalmic Gel Forming Solution 2092

GENTIRAN (Greece)
CETIRIZINE HYDROCHLORIDE
Zyrtec Syrup 2594
Zyrtec Tablets 2594

GENTISUL (Venezuela)
GENTAMICIN SULFATE
Garamycin Injectable 3014

GENTISUM (Spain)
GENTAMICIN SULFATE
Garamycin Injectable 3014

GENTOCIL (Portugal)
GENTAMICIN SULFATE
Garamycin Injectable 3014

GENTOGRAM (France, The Netherlands)
GENTAMICIN SULFATE
Garamycin Injectable 3014

GENTOLER (Argentina)
GENTAMICIN SULFATE
Garamycin Injectable 3014

GENTOMIL (Italy)
GENTAMICIN SULFATE
Garamycin Injectable 3014

GENT-OPHTAL (Germany)
GENTAMICIN SULFATE
Garamycin Injectable 3014

GENTOPTINE (Monaco)
GENTAMICIN SULFATE
Garamycin Injectable 3014

GENTRALAY (Spain)
GENTAMICIN SULFATE
Garamycin Injectable 3014

GENTRASUL (Canada)
GENTAMICIN SULFATE
Garamycin Injectable 3014

GEOMYCINE (Belgium)
GENTAMICIN SULFATE
Garamycin Injectable 3014

GEPROMI (Mexico)
PROGESTERONE
Prometrium Capsules (100 mg, 200 mg) . 3203

GERELAX (Irish Republic, Israel)
LACTULOSE
Kristalose for Oral Solution 1034

GERICARB (Irish Republic)
CARBAMAZEPINE
Carbatrol Capsules 3171
Tegretol Chewable Tablets 2295
Tegretol Suspension. 2295
Tegretol Tablets 2295
Tegretol-XR Tablets 2295

GERINAP (Irish Republic)
NAPROXEN
EC-Naprosyn Delayed-Release Tablets. . . . 2761
Naprosyn Suspension. 2761
Naprosyn Tablets 2761

GERIPROST (Argentina)
TERAZOSIN HYDROCHLORIDE
Hytrin Capsules. 471

GERODYL (The Netherlands)
PENICILLAMINE
Cuprimine Capsules 1947

GEROTEN (Irish Republic)
CAPTOPRIL
Captopril Tablets. 2149

GEROXALEN (Denmark, Hungary, Norway, The Netherlands)
METHOXSALEN
Oxsoralen Lotion 1% 3352
Oxsoralen-Ultra Capsules. 3353

GERTAC (Irish Republic)
RANITIDINE HYDROCHLORIDE
Zantac 25 EFFERdose Tablets 1624
Zantac 150 EFFERdose Tablets. 1624
Zantac 150 Tablets 1624
Zantac 300 Tablets 1624
Zantac Injection 1619
Zantac Injection Premixed 1619
Zantac Syrup 1624

GERTOCALM (Greece)
RANITIDINE HYDROCHLORIDE
Zantac 25 EFFERdose Tablets 1624
Zantac 150 EFFERdose Tablets. 1624
Zantac 150 Tablets 1624
Zantac 300 Tablets 1624
Zantac Injection 1619
Zantac Injection Premixed 1619
Zantac Syrup 1624

GERVAKEN (Mexico)
CLARITHROMYCIN
Biaxin Filmtab Tablets 402
Biaxin Granules 402

GERXIDIN (Venezuela)
CIPROFLOXACIN
Cipro Oral Suspension 2977

GESICAIN (India)
LIDOCAINE
Lidoderm Patch 1118

GESIPROX (Singapore)
NAPROXEN SODIUM
Anaprox DS Tablets 2761
Anaprox Tablets 2761

GESLUTIN (Mexico)
PROGESTERONE
Prometrium Capsules (100 mg, 200 mg) . 3203

GESTAPOLAR (Germany)
MEDROXYPROGESTERONE ACETATE
Depo-Medrol Single-Dose Vial 2619

GESTAPURAN (Finland, Sweden)
MEDROXYPROGESTERONE ACETATE
Depo-Medrol Single-Dose Vial 2619

GESTER (Argentina)
PROGESTERONE
Prometrium Capsules (100 mg, 200 mg) . 3203

GESTEROL (Canada)
PROGESTERONE
Prometrium Capsules (100 mg, 200 mg) . 3203

GESTONE (Israel, New Zealand, Thailand, United Kingdom)
PROGESTERONE
Prometrium Capsules (100 mg, 200 mg) . 3203

GESTORAL (France, Greece)
MEDROXYPROGESTERONE ACETATE
Depo-Medrol Single-Dose Vial 2619

GEVRAMYCIN (Spain)
GENTAMICIN SULFATE
Garamycin Injectable 3014

GEVRAMYCIN TOPICA (Spain)
GENTAMICIN SULFATE
Garamycin Injectable 3014

GEWACALM (Austria)
DIAZEPAM
Diastat Rectal Delivery System 3343
Valium Tablets 2819

GEWADILAT (Austria)
NIFEDIPINE
Adalat CC Tablets 2964

GEWAZEM (Austria)
DILTIAZEM HYDROCHLORIDE
Cardizem LA Extended Release Tablets. . . 1728
Tiazac Capsules 1201

GEZT (Argentina)
GEMCITABINE HYDROCHLORIDE
Gemzar for Injection. 1771

G-FARLUTAL (Germany)
MEDROXYPROGESTERONE ACETATE
Depo-Medrol Single-Dose Vial 2619

GI (Mexico)
GENTAMICIN SULFATE
Garamycin Injectable 3014

GIARDYL (India)
METRONIDAZOLE
MetroGel-Vaginal Gel 1855

GIBAC (Mexico)
CIPROFLOXACIN
Cipro Oral Suspension 2977

GIBICEF (Italy)
CEFUROXIME SODIUM
Zinacef Injection 1631

GIBIFLU (Italy)
FLUNISOLIDE
Aerobid Inhaler System. 1171
Aerobid-M Inhaler System 1171

GIBINAP (Italy)
NAPROXEN SODIUM
Anaprox DS Tablets 2761
Anaprox Tablets 2761

GIBIXEN (Italy)
NAPROXEN
EC-Naprosyn Delayed-Release Tablets. . . . 2761
Naprosyn Suspension. 2761
Naprosyn Tablets 2761

GILT (Germany)
CLOTRIMAZOLE
Lotrimin Cream. 3039
Lotrimin Lotion 1%. 3039
Lotrimin Topical Solution 1% 3039

GIMABROL (Mexico)
AMOXICILLIN
Amoxil Pediatric Drops for Oral Suspension. 1343
Amoxil Tablets 1343

GINAIKOS (Italy)
ESTRADIOL
Climara Transdermal System 771
Estring Vaginal Ring 2635

GINATEX (Argentina)
ESTRADIOL
Climara Transdermal System 771
Estring Vaginal Ring 2635

GINE CANESTEN (Spain)
CLOTRIMAZOLE
Lotrimin Cream. 3039
Lotrimin Lotion 1%. 3039
Lotrimin Topical Solution 1% 3039

GINECOSID (Venezuela)
PROGESTERONE
Prometrium Capsules (100 mg, 200 mg) . 3203

GINECOSIDE (Brazil)
PROGESTERONE
Prometrium Capsules (100 mg, 200 mg) . 3203

GINEDISC (Brazil, Mexico)
ESTRADIOL
Climara Transdermal System 771
Estring Vaginal Ring 2635

GINEFLAVIR (Italy)
METRONIDAZOLE
MetroGel-Vaginal Gel 1855

GINEFOLIN (Chile)
ESTRADIOL
Climara Transdermal System 771
Estring Vaginal Ring 2635

GINKAN (Argentina)
METRONIDAZOLE
MetroGel-Vaginal Gel 1855

GINO CIRIAX (Argentina)
CIPROFLOXACIN HYDROCHLORIDE
Ciloxan Ophthalmic Ointment . . . . ⊙204, 559
Ciloxan Ophthalmic Solution . . . . ⊙206
Cipro Tablets 2977

GINO CLOTRIMIX (Brazil)
CLOTRIMAZOLE
Lotrimin Cream. 3039
Lotrimin Lotion 1%. 3039
Lotrimin Topical Solution 1% 3039

GINO-CANESTEN (Brazil, Portugal)
CLOTRIMAZOLE
Lotrimin Cream. 3039
Lotrimin Lotion 1%. 3039
Lotrimin Topical Solution 1% 3039

GINODERM (Chile)
ESTRADIOL
Climara Transdermal System 771
Estring Vaginal Ring 2635

GINO-LOTREMINE (Portugal)
CLOTRIMAZOLE
Lotrimin Cream. 3039
Lotrimin Lotion 1%. 3039
Lotrimin Topical Solution 1% 3039

GINOLOTRICOMB (Venezuela)
CLOTRIMAZOLE
Lotrimin Cream. 3039
Lotrimin Lotion 1%. 3039
Lotrimin Topical Solution 1% 3039

GINORECTOL (Greece, Singapore)
CIPROFLOXACIN HYDROCHLORIDE
Ciloxan Ophthalmic Ointment . . . . ⊙204, 559
Ciloxan Ophthalmic Solution . . . . ⊙206
Cipro Tablets 2977

GINOVAGIN (Brazil)
METRONIDAZOLE
MetroGel-Vaginal Gel 1855

GIROFLOX (Portugal, Spain)
CIPROFLOXACIN
Cipro Oral Suspension 2977

GI-TAK (South Africa)
RANITIDINE HYDROCHLORIDE
Zantac 25 EFFERdose Tablets 1624

Zantac 150 EFFERdose Tablets........ **1624**
Zantac 150 Tablets **1624**
Zantac 300 Tablets **1624**
Zantac Injection **1619**
Zantac Injection Premixed **1619**
Zantac Syrup **1624**

GIVAIR (Italy)
FLUNISOLIDE
Aerobid Inhaler System............. **1171**
Aerobid-M Inhaler System **1171**

GLADEM (Austria, Germany, Switzerland)
SERTRALINE HYDROCHLORIDE
Zoloft Tablets.................... **2586**

GLADIUS (Greece)
CEFTRIAXONE SODIUM
Rocephin Injectable Vials, ADD-Vantage, Galaxy, Bulk **2800**

GLAFEMAK (Greece)
TIMOLOL MALEATE
Blocadren Tablets **1916**
Timoptic Sterile Ophthalmic Solution **2088**
Timoptic in Ocudose **2091**
Timoptic-XE Sterile Ophthalmic Gel Forming Solution **2092**

GLATIM (Argentina)
TIMOLOL MALEATE
Blocadren Tablets **1916**
Timoptic Sterile Ophthalmic Solution **2088**
Timoptic in Ocudose **2091**
Timoptic-XE Sterile Ophthalmic Gel Forming Solution **2092**

GLAUCOL (United Kingdom)
TIMOLOL MALEATE
Blocadren Tablets **1916**
Timoptic Sterile Ophthalmic Solution **2088**
Timoptic in Ocudose **2091**
Timoptic-XE Sterile Ophthalmic Gel Forming Solution **2092**

GLAUCO-OPH (Hong Kong, Thailand)
TIMOLOL MALEATE
Blocadren Tablets **1916**
Timoptic Sterile Ophthalmic Solution **2088**
Timoptic in Ocudose **2091**
Timoptic-XE Sterile Ophthalmic Gel Forming Solution **2092**

GLAUCOSAN (South Africa)
TIMOLOL MALEATE
Blocadren Tablets **1916**
Timoptic Sterile Ophthalmic Solution **2088**
Timoptic in Ocudose **2091**
Timoptic-XE Sterile Ophthalmic Gel Forming Solution **2092**

GLAUCOSTAT (Argentina)
LATANOPROST
Xalatan Ophthalmic Solution .... **⊙291**

GLAUCOTENSIL (Chile)
DORZOLAMIDE HYDROCHLORIDE
Trusopt Sterile Ophthalmic Solution **2095**

GLAUCOTENSIL T (Chile)
DORZOLAMIDE HYDROCHLORIDE/TIMOLOL MALEATE
Cosopt Sterile Ophthalmic Solution .... **⊙268, 1931**

GLAUSINE (Austria)
CLONIDINE HYDROCHLORIDE
Catapres Tablets.................. **843**

GLAUSOLETS (Chile)
TIMOLOL MALEATE
Blocadren Tablets **1916**
Timoptic Sterile Ophthalmic Solution **2088**
Timoptic in Ocudose **2091**
Timoptic-XE Sterile Ophthalmic Gel Forming Solution **2092**

GLAUTIMOL (Brazil)
TIMOLOL MALEATE
Blocadren Tablets **1916**
Timoptic Sterile Ophthalmic Solution **2088**
Timoptic in Ocudose **2091**
Timoptic-XE Sterile Ophthalmic Gel Forming Solution **2092**

GLAZIDIM (Belgium, Finland, Italy)
CEFTAZIDIME
Fortaz for Injection **1453**

GLEVO (India)
LEVOFLOXACIN
Levaquin Injection **2384**
Levaquin Tablets **2384**

GLEVOMICINA (Argentina)
GENTAMICIN SULFATE
Garamycin Injectable **3014**

GLICEMIN (Brazil)
DIAZOXIDE
Hyperstat I.V.................... **3017**

GLICOBASE (Italy)
ACARBOSE
Precose Tablets **751**

GLIFAPEN (Argentina)
AMOXICILLIN
Amoxil Pediatric Drops for Oral Suspension................... **1343**
Amoxil Tablets **1343**

GLIMIDE (Argentina)
ROSIGLITAZONE MALEATE
Avandia Tablets.................. **1384**

GLIOSARTAN (Argentina)
TELMISARTAN
Micardis Tablets **854**

GLIOSARTAN PLUS (Argentina)
TELMISARTAN
Micardis Tablets **854**

GLIOTEN (Argentina, Brazil, Chile, Mexico)
ENALAPRIL MALEATE
Vasotec I.V. Injection **2103**

GLIOTENZIDE (Argentina, Brazil, Mexico)
ENALAPRIL MALEATE
Vasotec I.V. Injection **2103**

GLITA (India)
PIOGLITAZONE HYDROCHLORIDE
Actos Tablets.................... **3219**

GLOBUCE (Spain)
CIPROFLOXACIN HYDROCHLORIDE
Ciloxan Ophthalmic Ointment .... **⊙204, 559**
Ciloxan Ophthalmic Solution .... **⊙206**
Cipro Tablets **2977**

GLOBUREN (Italy)
EPOETIN ALFA
Epogen for Injection............... **591**
Procrit for Injection **2364**

GLOPIR (Greece)
NIFEDIPINE
Adalat CC Tablets **2964**

GLORIXONE (Greece)
CEFTRIAXONE SODIUM
Rocephin Injectable Vials, ADD-Vantage, Galaxy, Bulk **2800**

GLOSSYFIN (Greece)
CIPROFLOXACIN HYDROCHLORIDE
Ciloxan Ophthalmic Ointment .... **⊙204, 559**
Ciloxan Ophthalmic Solution .... **⊙206**
Cipro Tablets **2977**

GLUBOSE (India)
ACARBOSE
Precose Tablets **751**

GLUCAGEN (Argentina, Australia, Austria, Belgium, Czech Republic, Denmark, Finland, France, Germany, Greece, Hong Kong, Hungary, India, Irish Republic, Israel, Italy, Malaysia, New Zealand, Portugal, Russia, Singapore, South Africa, Spain, Switzerland, Thailand, United Kingdom)
GLUCAGON HYDROCHLORIDE
Glucagon for Injection Vials and Emergency Kit................. **1778**

GLUCAR (India)
ACARBOSE
Precose Tablets **751**

GLUCOBAY (Argentina, Australia, Austria, Belgium, Brazil, Chile, Czech Republic, Denmark, Finland, Greece, Hong Kong, Hungary, India, Irish Republic, Italy, Malaysia, Mexico, New Zealand, Norway, Portugal, Russia, Singapore, South Africa, Spain, Sweden, Switzerland, Thailand, The Netherlands, United Kingdom, Venezuela)
ACARBOSE
Precose Tablets **751**

GLUCOMOL (India)
TIMOLOL MALEATE
Blocadren Tablets **1916**
Timoptic Sterile Ophthalmic Solution **2088**
Timoptic in Ocudose **2091**
Timoptic-XE Sterile Ophthalmic Gel Forming Solution **2092**

GLUCOR (France)
ACARBOSE
Precose Tablets **751**

GLUCOSULMID (Germany)
SULFACETAMIDE SODIUM
Klaron Lotion 10%................ **2909**

GLUCOTIM (India)
TIMOLOL MALEATE
Blocadren Tablets **1916**
Timoptic Sterile Ophthalmic Solution **2088**
Timoptic in Ocudose **2091**
Timoptic-XE Sterile Ophthalmic Gel Forming Solution **2092**

GLUDEX (Argentina)
ROSIGLITAZONE MALEATE
Avandia Tablets.................. **1384**

GLUMIDA (Spain)
ACARBOSE
Precose Tablets **751**

GLUTASEDAN (Argentina)
DIAZEPAM
Diastat Rectal Delivery System **3343**
Valium Tablets **2819**

GLUTASEY (Spain)
SIMVASTATIN
Zocor Tablets.................... **2105**

GLYMOL (Russia)
TIMOLOL MALEATE
Blocadren Tablets **1916**
Timoptic Sterile Ophthalmic Solution **2088**
Timoptic in Ocudose **2091**
Timoptic-XE Sterile Ophthalmic Gel Forming Solution **2092**

GLYTOP (Argentina)
TRIAMCINOLONE ACETONIDE
Azmacort Inhalation Aerosol.......... **1726**
Nasacort AQ Nasal Spray **2922**

GNOSTOCARDIN (Greece)
ENALAPRIL MALEATE
Vasotec I.V. Injection **2103**

GNOSTOL (Greece)
METRONIDAZOLE
MetroGel-Vaginal Gel **1855**

GNOSTOVAL (Greece)
LISINOPRIL
Prinivil Tablets **2052**

GOBANAL (Spain)
DIAZEPAM
Diastat Rectal Delivery System **3343**
Valium Tablets **2819**

GOBBICAINA (Argentina)
LIDOCAINE
Lidoderm Patch **1118**

GODAFILIN (Spain)
THEOPHYLLINE
Uniphyl Tablets **2710**

GOLAN (Mexico)
FUROSEMIDE
Furosemide Tablets **2154**

GOLD CROSS ANTIHISTAMINE ELIXIR (Australia)
PROMETHAZINE HYDROCHLORIDE
Phenergan Tablets and Suppositories **3440**

GOLDASTATIN (Greece)
SIMVASTATIN
Zocor Tablets.................... **2105**

GONDONAR (Argentina)
ANASTROZOLE
Arimidex Tablets **673**

GONIF (Greece)
CEFUROXIME SODIUM
Zinacef Injection **1631**

GONNING (Hong Kong)
CIPROFLOXACIN
Cipro Oral Suspension **2977**

GONORCIN (Thailand)
NORFLOXACIN
Noroxin Tablets.................. **2032**

GOODNIGHT (New Zealand)
PROMETHAZINE HYDROCHLORIDE
Phenergan Tablets and Suppositories **3440**

GO-ON (Germany, Hong Kong, Italy, Malaysia)
SODIUM HYALURONATE
Hyalgan Solution **2901**

GOPTEN (Australia, Austria, Brazil, Denmark, Finland, France, Germany, Hungary, Irish Republic, Italy, Mexico, New Zealand, Norway, Portugal, South Africa, Spain, Sweden, Switzerland, The Netherlands, United Kingdom)
TRANDOLAPRIL
Mavik Tablets **486**

GORDOX (Czech Republic, Hungary, Russia)
APROTININ
Trasylol Injection **754**

GOTABIOTIC (Argentina)
TOBRAMYCIN
TOBI Solution for Inhalation **2298**

GOTABIOTIC F (Argentina)
TOBRAMYCIN
TOBI Solution for Inhalation **2298**

GOTADEX (Mexico)
DEXAMETHASONE
Decadron Tablets **1951**

GOTAS OTOLOGICAS (Chile)
LIDOCAINE
Lidoderm Patch **1118**

GOTELY (Chile)
TAMSULOSIN HYDROCHLORIDE
Flomax Capsules.................. **850**

GOTINAL (Argentina, Mexico)
NAPHAZOLINE HYDROCHLORIDE
Albalon Ophthalmic Solution .... **⊙218**

GOVAL (Chile)
RISPERIDONE
Risperdal Oral Solution **1676**
Risperdal Tablets................. **1676**

GRAMMICIN (Thailand)
GENTAMICIN SULFATE
Garamycin Injectable **3014**

GRAMMIXIN (Thailand)
GENTAMICIN SULFATE
Garamycin Injectable **3014**

GRATEN (Mexico)
MORPHINE SULFATE
Kadian Capsules **577**
MS Contin Tablets **2701**

GRAVIDEX (Spain)
DINOPROSTONE
Cervidil Vaginal Insert............. **1181**

GRAY-F (Argentina)
FENTANYL CITRATE
Actiq **979**

GRENIS (Greece)
NORFLOXACIN
Noroxin Tablets.................. **2032**

GRENIS-CIPRO (Greece)
CIPROFLOXACIN HYDROCHLORIDE
Ciloxan Ophthalmic Ointment .... **⊙204, 559**
Ciloxan Ophthalmic Solution .... **⊙206**
Cipro Tablets **2977**

GRENIS-OFLO (Greece)
OFLOXACIN
Floxin Otic Solution **1049**

GREPIFLOX (Argentina)
LEVOFLOXACIN
Levaquin Injection **2384**
Levaquin Tablets **2384**

GREXIN (Thailand)
DIGOXIN
Lanoxicaps Capsules **1490**
Lanoxin Injection **1494**
Lanoxin Injection Pediatric **1497**
Lanoxin Tablets.................. **1500**

GRIFOCIPROX (Chile)
CIPROFLOXACIN
Cipro Oral Suspension **2977**

GRIFODILZEM (Chile)
DILTIAZEM HYDROCHLORIDE
Cardizem LA Extended Release Tablets... **1728**

Tiazac Capsules 1201

GRIFONIMOD (Chile)
NIMODIPINE
Nimotop Capsules 749

GRIFOPRIL (Chile)
ENALAPRIL MALEATE
Vasotec I.V. Injection 2103

GRIFOTRIAXONA (Chile)
CEFTRIAXONE SODIUM
Rocephin Injectable Vials, ADD-Vantage, Galaxy, Bulk 2800

GRISETIN (Spain)
FLUTAMIDE
Eulexin Capsules 3009

GROFENAC (Hong Kong, Switzerland)
DICLOFENAC SODIUM
Voltaren Tablets 2307
Voltaren-XR Tablets 2310

GROFIBRAT (Czech Republic)
FENOFIBRATE
Tricor Tablets 527

GROMAZOL (Switzerland)
CLOTRIMAZOLE
Lotrimin Cream 3039
Lotrimin Lotion 1% 3039
Lotrimin Topical Solution 1% 3039

GROWART (Greece)
LEVOCARNITINE
Carnitor Injection 3188
Carnitor Tablets and Oral Solution 3190

GUTRON (Austria, Chile, Czech Republic, France, Germany, Hong Kong, Hungary, Israel, Italy, Mexico, New Zealand, Portugal, Russia, Singapore, Switzerland, Thailand)
MIDODRINE HYDROCHLORIDE
ProAmatine Tablets 3186

GYNEBO (Thailand)
CLOTRIMAZOLE
Lotrimin Cream 3039
Lotrimin Lotion 1% 3039
Lotrimin Topical Solution 1% 3039

GYNE-LOTREMIN (Hong Kong, Malaysia, Singapore)
CLOTRIMAZOLE
Lotrimin Cream 3039
Lotrimin Lotion 1% 3039
Lotrimin Topical Solution 1% 3039

GYNE-LOTRIMIN (Australia)
CLOTRIMAZOLE
Lotrimin Cream 3039
Lotrimin Lotion 1% 3039
Lotrimin Topical Solution 1% 3039

GYNESTEN-B (Thailand)
CLOTRIMAZOLE
Lotrimin Cream 3039
Lotrimin Lotion 1% 3039
Lotrimin Topical Solution 1% 3039

GYNESTREL (Italy)
NAPROXEN SODIUM
Anaprox DS Tablets 2761
Anaprox Tablets 2761

GYNEZOL (South Africa)
CLOTRIMAZOLE
Lotrimin Cream 3039
Lotrimin Lotion 1% 3039
Lotrimin Topical Solution 1% 3039

GYNO CANESTEN (Venezuela)
CLOTRIMAZOLE
Lotrimin Cream 3039
Lotrimin Lotion 1% 3039
Lotrimin Topical Solution 1% 3039

GYNO OCERAL (Austria)
OXICONAZOLE NITRATE
Oxistat Cream 2667
Oxistat Lotion 2667

GYNOCANESTEN (Chile)
CLOTRIMAZOLE
Lotrimin Cream 3039
Lotrimin Lotion 1% 3039
Lotrimin Topical Solution 1% 3039

GYNO-CANESTEN (Germany, Italy)
CLOTRIMAZOLE
Lotrimin Cream 3039
Lotrimin Lotion 1% 3039
Lotrimin Topical Solution 1% 3039

GYNO-CANESTENE (Belgium, Switzerland)
CLOTRIMAZOLE
Lotrimin Cream 3039
Lotrimin Lotion 1% 3039
Lotrimin Topical Solution 1% 3039

GYNO-LIDERMAN (Austria)
OXICONAZOLE NITRATE
Oxistat Cream 2667
Oxistat Lotion 2667

GYNO-MYFUNGAR (Czech Republic, Mexico, Switzerland)
OXICONAZOLE NITRATE
Oxistat Cream 2667
Oxistat Lotion 2667

GYNOPLIX (Hong Kong)
METRONIDAZOLE
MetroGel-Vaginal Gel 1855

GYNOSTATUM (Malaysia)
CLOTRIMAZOLE
Lotrimin Cream 3039
Lotrimin Lotion 1% 3039
Lotrimin Topical Solution 1% 3039

GYNO-TRIMAZE (South Africa)
CLOTRIMAZOLE
Lotrimin Cream 3039
Lotrimin Lotion 1% 3039
Lotrimin Topical Solution 1% 3039

GYNPOLAR (Germany)
ESTRADIOL
Climara Transdermal System 771
Estring Vaginal Ring 2635

GYRABLOCK (Czech Republic, Russia, Singapore, Thailand)
NORFLOXACIN
Noroxin Tablets 2032

GYROFLOX (Germany)
OFLOXACIN
Floxin Otic Solution 1049

GY-SOL (Mexico)
GENTAMICIN SULFATE
Garamycin Injectable 3014

H2 OXYL (Germany)
BENZOYL PEROXIDE
Brevoxyl-4 Creamy Wash 3210
Brevoxyl-4 Gel 3210
Brevoxyl-8 Creamy Wash 3210
Brevoxyl-8 Gel 3210
Triaz Cleanser 1892
Triaz Gel 1892

H2OXYL (Canada, Switzerland)
BENZOYL PEROXIDE
Brevoxyl-4 Creamy Wash 3210
Brevoxyl-4 Gel 3210
Brevoxyl-8 Creamy Wash 3210
Brevoxyl-8 Gel 3210
Triaz Cleanser 1892
Triaz Gel 1892

HAEMITON (Germany, Russia)
CLONIDINE HYDROCHLORIDE
Catapres Tablets 843

HAEMITON-AUGENTROPFEN (Germany)
CLONIDINE HYDROCHLORIDE
Catapres Tablets 843

HAIMASERUM (Italy)
PLASMA PROTEIN FRACTION
Plasmanate 3255

HALDID (Denmark)
FENTANYL CITRATE
Actiq 979

HALF BETADUR CR (United Kingdom)
PROPRANOLOL HYDROCHLORIDE
Inderal LA Long-Acting Capsules 3429

HALF BETA-PROGRANE (United Kingdom)
PROPRANOLOL HYDROCHLORIDE
Inderal LA Long-Acting Capsules 3429

HALF CAPOZIDE (Irish Republic)
CAPTOPRIL
Captopril Tablets 2149

HALF INDERAL (Irish Republic, United Kingdom)
PROPRANOLOL HYDROCHLORIDE
Inderal LA Long-Acting Capsules 3429

HALF SECURON (United Kingdom)
VERAPAMIL HYDROCHLORIDE
Covera-HS Tablets 3139
Verelan PM Extended-Release Capsules, Controlled-Onset 3106

HALONIX (India)
SODIUM HYALURONATE
Hyalgan Solution 2901

HAMOXILLIN (Hong Kong)
AMOXICILLIN
Amoxil Pediatric Drops for Oral Suspension 1343
Amoxil Tablets 1343

HARNAL (Hong Kong, Japan, Thailand)
TAMSULOSIN HYDROCHLORIDE
Flomax Capsules 850

HART (Argentina)
DILTIAZEM HYDROCHLORIDE
Cardizem LA Extended Release Tablets . . . 1728
Tiazac Capsules 1201

HAWKMIDE (Thailand)
FUROSEMIDE
Furosemide Tablets 2154

HAYFEVER & ALLERGY RELIEF (United Kingdom)
CETIRIZINE HYDROCHLORIDE
Zyrtec Syrup 2594
Zyrtec Tablets 2594

HAYFEVER RELIEF (United Kingdom)
CETIRIZINE HYDROCHLORIDE
Zyrtec Syrup 2594
Zyrtec Tablets 2594

HEALON (Australia, Belgium, Brazil, Canada, Chile, Czech Republic, Finland, France, Germany, Hong Kong, Hungary, Israel, Italy, Malaysia, New Zealand, Norway, Russia, Singapore, South Africa, Sweden, Switzerland, Thailand, The Netherlands, Venezuela)
SODIUM HYALURONATE
Hyalgan Solution 2901

HEALONID (Austria, France, Irish Republic, United Kingdom)
SODIUM HYALURONATE
Hyalgan Solution 2901

HEARTBURN RELIEF (Australia)
RANITIDINE HYDROCHLORIDE
Zantac 25 EFFERdose Tablets 1624
Zantac 150 EFFERdose Tablets 1624
Zantac 150 Tablets 1624
Zantac 300 Tablets 1624
Zantac Injection 1619
Zantac Injection Premixed 1619
Zantac Syrup 1624

HEINIX (Finland)
CETIRIZINE HYDROCHLORIDE
Zyrtec Syrup 2594
Zyrtec Tablets 2594

HEITRIN (Germany)
TERAZOSIN HYDROCHLORIDE
Hytrin Capsules 471

HEKTULOSE (Germany)
LACTULOSE
Kristalose for Oral Solution 1034

HELAL (Venezuela)
ALBENDAZOLE
Albenza Tablets 1338

HELICLAR (Belgium)
CLARITHROMYCIN
Biaxin Filmtab Tablets 402
Biaxin Granules 402

HELICODID (Brazil)
CLARITHROMYCIN
Biaxin Filmtab Tablets 402
Biaxin Granules 402

HELIMOX (Italy)
AMOXICILLIN
Amoxil Pediatric Drops for Oral Suspension 1343
Amoxil Tablets 1343

HELIPAC (India)
AMOXICILLIN
Amoxil Pediatric Drops for Oral Suspension 1343
Amoxil Tablets 1343

HELMINE (Spain)
ONDANSETRON HYDROCHLORIDE
Zofran Injection 1634
Zofran Injection Premixed 1634
Zofran Oral Solution 1639
Zofran Tablets 1639

HELMINTAL (Brazil)
ALBENDAZOLE
Albenza Tablets 1338

HELMISONS (Mexico)
ALBENDAZOLE
Albenza Tablets 1338

HELMIZOL (Brazil)
METRONIDAZOLE
MetroGel-Vaginal Gel 1855

HEMAX (Thailand)
EPOETIN ALFA
Epogen for Injection 591
Procrit for Injection 2364

HEMIGOXINE NATIVELLE (France)
DIGOXIN
Lanoxicaps Capsules 1490
Lanoxin Injection 1494
Lanoxin Injection Pediatric 1497
Lanoxin Tablets 1500

HEMIPRALON (France)
PROPRANOLOL HYDROCHLORIDE
Inderal LA Long-Acting Capsules 3429

HENEXAL (Mexico)
FUROSEMIDE
Furosemide Tablets 2154

HEPALAC (Thailand)
LACTULOSE
Kristalose for Oral Solution 1034

HEPA-MERZ LACT (Germany)
LACTULOSE
Kristalose for Oral Solution 1034

HEPATICUM-LAC-MEDICE (Germany)
LACTULOSE
Kristalose for Oral Solution 1034

HEPRONE (Spain)
SUCRALFATE
Carafate Suspension 701
Carafate Tablets 701

HEPTODINE (Argentina, Venezuela)
LAMIVUDINE
Epivir Oral Solution 1427
Epivir Tablets 1427
Epivir-HBV Oral Solution 1432
Epivir-HBV Tablets 1432

HEPTOVIR (Canada)
LAMIVUDINE
Epivir Oral Solution 1427
Epivir Tablets 1427
Epivir-HBV Oral Solution 1432
Epivir-HBV Tablets 1432

HERBESSER (Hong Kong, Japan, Malaysia, Portugal, Singapore, Thailand)
DILTIAZEM HYDROCHLORIDE
Cardizem LA Extended Release Tablets . . . 1728
Tiazac Capsules 1201

HERCEPTIN (Argentina, Australia, Belgium, Brazil, Canada, Chile, Czech Republic, Denmark, Finland, France, Germany, Greece, Hong Kong, Hungary, Irish Republic, Israel, Italy, Mexico, New Zealand, Norway, Portugal, Singapore, South Africa, Spain, Sweden, Switzerland, Thailand, United Kingdom, Venezuela)
TRASTUZUMAB
Herceptin I.V. 1233

HERMOLEPSIN (Sweden)
CARBAMAZEPINE
Carbatrol Capsules 3171
Tegretol Chewable Tablets 2295
Tegretol Suspension 2295
Tegretol Tablets 2295

Tegretol-XR Tablets 2295

HERTEN (Spain)
ENALAPRIL MALEATE
Vasotec I.V. Injection 2103

HETACLOXACIN (Greece)
OFLOXACIN
Floxin Otic Solution 1049

HEVRONAZ (Greece)
MUPIROCIN
Bactroban Ointment 1395

HEXABOTIN (Denmark)
ERYTHROMYCIN STEARATE
Erythrocin Stearate Filmtab Tablets 453

HEXADILAT (Denmark)
NIFEDIPINE
Adalat CC Tablets 2964

HEXADROL (Canada)
DEXAMETHASONE
Decadron Tablets 1951

HEXAGASTRON (Denmark)
SUCRALFATE
Carafate Suspension 701
Carafate Tablets 701

HEXALID (Denmark)
DIAZEPAM
Diastat Rectal Delivery System 3343
Valium Tablets 2819

HEXAMYCIN (Denmark)
GENTAMICIN SULFATE
Garamycin Injectable 3014

HEXASOPTIN (Denmark)
VERAPAMIL HYDROCHLORIDE
Covera-HS Tablets 3139
Verelan PM Extended-Release Capsules, Controlled-Onset 3106

HIALID (Hong Kong, Singapore, Thailand)
SODIUM HYALURONATE
Hyalgan Solution 2901

HIALUDORF (Argentina)
SODIUM HYALURONATE
Hyalgan Solution 2901

HICONCIL (The Netherlands)
AMOXICILLIN
Amoxil Pediatric Drops for Oral Suspension 1343
Amoxil Tablets 1343

HIDALONE (Portugal)
HYDROCORTISONE
Hydrocortone Tablets 1989

HIDERM (Australia)
CLOTRIMAZOLE
Lotrimin Cream 3039
Lotrimin Lotion 1% 3039
Lotrimin Topical Solution 1% 3039

HIDEX (Mexico)
IRON DEXTRAN
Infed Injection 3390

HIDRASAL (Mexico)
FUROSEMIDE
Furosemide Tablets 2154

HIDROALTESONA (Spain)
HYDROCORTISONE
Hydrocortone Tablets 1989

HIDROCOL (Brazil)
HYDROCORTISONE
Hydrocortone Tablets 1989

HIDROCORTIN (Argentina)
HYDROCORTISONE
Hydrocortone Tablets 1989

HIDROFENIL (Mexico)
HYDROCORTISONE
Hydrocortone Tablets 1989

HIDROPRIL (Brazil)
CAPTOPRIL
Captopril Tablets 2149

HIDRORONOL T (Chile)
HYDROCHLOROTHIAZIDE/TRIAMTERENE
Dyazide Capsules 1423

HIDROTIAZIDA (Brazil)
NYSTATIN
Nystop Topical Powder USP 2478
Paddock Nystatin USP for Oral Suspension 2478

HIDROTISONA (Argentina)
HYDROCORTISONE
Hydrocortone Tablets 1989

HINCOMOX (Brazil)
AMOXICILLIN
Amoxil Pediatric Drops for Oral Suspension 1343
Amoxil Tablets 1343

HIPEN (India)
AMOXICILLIN
Amoxil Pediatric Drops for Oral Suspension 1343
Amoxil Tablets 1343

HIPERSON (Chile)
ENALAPRIL MALEATE
Vasotec I.V. Injection 2103

HIPERTAN (Argentina)
ENALAPRIL MALEATE
Vasotec I.V. Injection 2103

HIPERTEX (Mexico)
CAPTOPRIL
Captopril Tablets 2149

HIPERTIL (Portugal)
CAPTOPRIL
Captopril Tablets 2149

HIPERTIN (Brazil)
ENALAPRIL MALEATE
Vasotec I.V. Injection 2103

HIPOARTEL (Chile, Spain)
ENALAPRIL MALEATE
Vasotec I.V. Injection 2103

HIPOCATRIL (Brazil)
CAPTOPRIL
Captopril Tablets 2149

HIPOGLOS CON HIDROCORTISONA (Venezuela)
HYDROCORTISONE
Hydrocortone Tablets 1989

HIPOSTEROL (Chile)
LOVASTATIN
Mevacor Tablets 2021

HIPOTEN (Brazil)
CAPTOPRIL
Captopril Tablets 2149

HIPOTENSIL (Portugal)
CAPTOPRIL
Captopril Tablets 2149

HIPOVASTIN (Argentina)
LOVASTATIN
Mevacor Tablets 2021

HIPRANOL (South Africa)
PROPRANOLOL HYDROCHLORIDE
Inderal LA Long-Acting Capsules 3429

HIPRESS (Brazil)
LOSARTAN POTASSIUM
Cozaar Tablets 1935

HIPTEN (Portugal)
ENALAPRIL MALEATE
Vasotec I.V. Injection 2103

HISPLENIL (Venezuela)
SIMVASTATIN
Zocor Tablets 2105

HISTAC (Czech Republic, Hungary, India, Malaysia, Russia, Singapore, Thailand)
RANITIDINE HYDROCHLORIDE
Zantac 25 EFFERdose Tablets 1624
Zantac 150 EFFERdose Tablets 1624
Zantac 150 Tablets 1624
Zantac 300 Tablets 1624
Zantac Injection 1619
Zantac Injection Premixed 1619
Zantac Syrup 1624

HISTAFILIN (Spain)
THEOPHYLLINE
Uniphyl Tablets 2710

HISTAFREN (Greece)
CETIRIZINE HYDROCHLORIDE
Zyrtec Syrup 2594
Zyrtec Tablets 2594

HISTAK (South Africa)
RANITIDINE HYDROCHLORIDE
Zantac 25 EFFERdose Tablets 1624
Zantac 150 EFFERdose Tablets 1624
Zantac 150 Tablets 1624
Zantac 300 Tablets 1624
Zantac Injection 1619
Zantac Injection Premixed 1619
Zantac Syrup 1624

HISTALEN D (Chile)
CETIRIZINE HYDROCHLORIDE
Zyrtec Syrup 2594
Zyrtec Tablets 2594

HISTALOC (United Arab Emirates)
PROMETHAZINE HYDROCHLORIDE
Phenergan Tablets and Suppositories 3440

HISTANTIL (Canada)
PROMETHAZINE HYDROCHLORIDE
Phenergan Tablets and Suppositories 3440

HISTATEC (Switzerland)
CETIRIZINE HYDROCHLORIDE
Zyrtec Syrup 2594
Zyrtec Tablets 2594

HISTAX (Chile)
CETIRIZINE HYDROCHLORIDE
Zyrtec Syrup 2594
Zyrtec Tablets 2594

HISTAZINE (Hong Kong)
CETIRIZINE HYDROCHLORIDE
Zyrtec Syrup 2594
Zyrtec Tablets 2594

HISTEC (Finland)
CETIRIZINE HYDROCHLORIDE
Zyrtec Syrup 2594
Zyrtec Tablets 2594

HISTEK (Irish Republic)
CETIRIZINE HYDROCHLORIDE
Zyrtec Syrup 2594
Zyrtec Tablets 2594

HISTICA (Thailand)
CETIRIZINE HYDROCHLORIDE
Zyrtec Syrup 2594
Zyrtec Tablets 2594

HISTOP (Spain)
SIMVASTATIN
Zocor Tablets 2105

HIVIRUX (Argentina)
LAMIVUDINE
Epivir Oral Solution 1427
Epivir Tablets 1427
Epivir-HBV Oral Solution 1432
Epivir-HBV Tablets 1432

HIVIRUX COMPLEX (Argentina)
LAMIVUDINE
Epivir Oral Solution 1427
Epivir Tablets 1427
Epivir-HBV Oral Solution 1432
Epivir-HBV Tablets 1432

HIZAAR (Italy)
HYDROCHLOROTHIAZIDE/LOSARTAN POTASSIUM
Hyzaar 100-25 Tablets 1990
Hyzaar 50-12.5 Tablets 1990

H-MIDE (Thailand)
FUROSEMIDE
Furosemide Tablets 2154

HOFCOMANT (Greece)
AMANTADINE HYDROCHLORIDE
Symmetrel Tablets 1135

HOLADREN (Chile)
ALENDRONATE SODIUM
Fosamax Tablets 1969

HOLETAR (Czech Republic, Russia)
LOVASTATIN
Mevacor Tablets 2021

HOLFUNGIN (Germany)
CLOTRIMAZOLE
Lotrimin Cream 3039
Lotrimin Lotion 1% 3039
Lotrimin Topical Solution 1% 3039

HOPECARD (India)
RAMIPRIL
Altace Capsules 1702

HOPRANOLOL (Hong Kong)
PROPRANOLOL HYDROCHLORIDE
Inderal LA Long-Acting Capsules 3429

HOREX (Mexico)
TIMOLOL MALEATE
Blocadren Tablets 1916
Timoptic Sterile Ophthalmic Solution 2088
Timoptic in Ocudose 2091
Timoptic-XE Sterile Ophthalmic Gel Forming Solution 2092

HORIZEM (United Kingdom)
DILTIAZEM HYDROCHLORIDE
Cardizem LA Extended Release Tablets . . . 1728
Tiazac Capsules 1201

HORMODIOL (Argentina)
ESTRADIOL
Climara Transdermal System 771
Estring Vaginal Ring 2635

HORMODOSE (Brazil)
ESTRADIOL
Climara Transdermal System 771
Estring Vaginal Ring 2635

HORMORAL (Chile)
PROGESTERONE
Prometrium Capsules (100 mg, 200 mg) . 3203

HOSBOCIN (Spain)
CEFTRIAXONE SODIUM
Rocephin Injectable Vials, ADD-Vantage, Galaxy, Bulk 2800

HOSBOGEN (Spain)
GENTAMICIN SULFATE
Garamycin Injectable 3014

HPB (Argentina)
FINASTERIDE
Propecia Tablets 2060
Proscar Tablets 2067

HUBERDINA (Spain)
FAMOTIDINE
Pepcid Injection 2040
Pepcid Injection Premixed 2040
Pepcid Tablets 2038
Pepcid for Oral Suspension 2038

HUBERPLEX (Spain)
CHLORDIAZEPOXIDE HYDROCHLORIDE
Librium Capsules 3347

HUMA-CAPTORIL (Hungary)
CAPTOPRIL
Captopril Tablets 2149

HUMA-DIFENAC (Hungary)
DICLOFENAC SODIUM
Voltaren Tablets 2307
Voltaren-XR Tablets 2310

HUMA-METOPROL (Hungary)
METOPROLOL TARTRATE
Lopressor Tablets 2238

HUMA-PRONOL (Hungary)
PROPRANOLOL HYDROCHLORIDE
Inderal LA Long-Acting Capsules 3429

HUMA-RANIDINE (Hungary)
RANITIDINE HYDROCHLORIDE
Zantac 25 EFFERdose Tablets 1624
Zantac 150 EFFERdose Tablets 1624
Zantac 150 Tablets 1624
Zantac 300 Tablets 1624
Zantac Injection 1619
Zantac Injection Premixed 1619
Zantac Syrup 1624

HUMA-SEMIDE (Hungary)
FUROSEMIDE
Furosemide Tablets 2154

HUMORAP (Argentina)
CITALOPRAM HYDROBROMIDE
Celexa Tablets 1176

HYABAK (Italy)
SODIUM HYALURONATE
Hyalgan Solution 2901

HYA-JECT (Germany)
SODIUM HYALURONATE
Hyalgan Solution 2901

HYAL (Malaysia)
SODIUM HYALURONATE
Hyalgan Solution 2901

HYALART (Argentina, Greece, Italy, Portugal)
SODIUM HYALURONATE
Hyalgan Solution 2901

HYAL-DROP (France, Switzerland)
SODIUM HYALURONATE
Hyalgan Solution 2901

HYALEIN (Japan)
SODIUM HYALURONATE
Hyalgan Solution 2901

HYALGAN (Austria, Canada, Chile, Czech Republic, Denmark, Finland, France, Hong Kong, Hungary, Irish Republic, Italy, Singapore, Spain, Sweden, United Kingdom, Venezuela)
SODIUM HYALURONATE
Hyalgan Solution 2901

HYALISTIL (Italy)
SODIUM HYALURONATE
Hyalgan Solution 2901

HYAL-SYSTEM (Germany)
SODIUM HYALURONATE
Hyalgan Solution 2901

HYALUBRIX (Germany)
SODIUM HYALURONATE
Hyalgan Solution 2901

HYALUDERMIN (Brazil)
SODIUM HYALURONATE
Hyalgan Solution 2901

HYANAC (Argentina)
DICLOFENAC SODIUM
Voltaren Tablets 2307
Voltaren-XR Tablets 2310

HYA-OPHTAL (Germany)
SODIUM HYALURONATE
Hyalgan Solution 2901

HYASOL (Argentina, Mexico)
SODIUM HYALURONATE
Hyalgan Solution 2901

HYBRIDIL (Austria)
CARVEDILOL
Coreg Tablets 1414

HYCAMTIN (Argentina, Australia, Austria, Belgium, Brazil, Canada, Chile, Czech Republic, Denmark, Finland, France, Germany, Greece, Hong Kong, Hungary, Irish Republic, Israel, Italy, Norway, Portugal, Russia, Singapore, South Africa, Spain, Sweden, Switzerland, Thailand, The Netherlands, United Kingdom, Venezuela)
TOPOTECAN HYDROCHLORIDE
Hycamtin for Injection 1458

HYCOR (Australia)
HYDROCORTISONE
Hydrocortone Tablets 1989

HYCORT (Canada)
HYDROCORTISONE
Hydrocortone Tablets 1989

HYCORTIN (Hong Kong)
HYDROCORTISONE
Hydrocortone Tablets 1989

HYDAL (Austria)
HYDROMORPHONE HYDROCHLORIDE
Dilaudid Ampules 440
Dilaudid Multiple Dose Vials 440
Dilaudid Non-Sterile Powder 440
Dilaudid Oral Liquid 445
Dilaudid Rectal Suppositories 440
Dilaudid Tablets 440
Dilaudid Tablets - 8 mg 445
Dilaudid-HP Injection 442
Dilaudid-HP Lyophilized Powder 250 mg . . . 442

HYDOFTAL SINE NEOMYCINO (Austria)
HYDROCORTISONE
Hydrocortone Tablets 1989

HYDRACORT (France)
HYDROCORTISONE
Hydrocortone Tablets 1989

HYDRENE (Australia)
TRIAMTERENE
Dyrenium Capsules 3400

HYDREX (South Africa)
FUROSEMIDE
Furosemide Tablets 2154

HYDROCOMP (Germany)
AMILORIDE HYDROCHLORIDE/HYDROCHLOROTHIAZIDE
Moduretic Tablets 2028

HYDROCORT MILD (Germany)
HYDROCORTISONE
Hydrocortone Tablets 1989

HYDROCORTISON MED TERRAMYCIN (Denmark)
HYDROCORTISONE
Hydrocortone Tablets 1989

HYDROCORTISYL (Irish Republic, United Kingdom)
HYDROCORTISONE
Hydrocortone Tablets 1989

HYDROCORTONE (Austria, Irish Republic, Switzerland, United Kingdom)
HYDROCORTISONE
Hydrocortone Tablets 1989

HYDROCUTAN MILD (Germany)
HYDROCORTISONE
Hydrocortone Tablets 1989

HYDRODERM (Austria)
HYDROCORTISONE
Hydrocortone Tablets 1989

HYDRODERM HC (Germany)
HYDROCORTISONE
Hydrocortone Tablets 1989

HYDRODERMED (Germany)
ERYTHROMYCIN
Ery-Tab Tablets 449
Erythromycin Base Filmtab Tablets 455
Erythromycin Delayed-Release Capsules, USP 457
PCE Dispertab Tablets 515

HYDROFLUX (Greece)
FUROSEMIDE
Furosemide Tablets 2154

HYDROFORM (Australia)
HYDROCORTISONE
Hydrocortone Tablets 1989

HYDROGALEN (Germany)
HYDROCORTISONE
Hydrocortone Tablets 1989

HYDRO-LESS (South Africa)
INDAPAMIDE
Indapamide Tablets 2156

HYDROLID (Switzerland)
AMILORIDE HYDROCHLORIDE/HYDROCHLOROTHIAZIDE
Moduretic Tablets 2028

HYDROMET (Irish Republic)
HYDROCHLOROTHIAZIDE/METHYLDOPA
Aldoril Tablets 1910

HYDROMORPH (Canada)
HYDROMORPHONE HYDROCHLORIDE
Dilaudid Ampules 440
Dilaudid Multiple Dose Vials 440
Dilaudid Non-Sterile Powder 440
Dilaudid Oral Liquid 445
Dilaudid Rectal Suppositories 440
Dilaudid Tablets 440
Dilaudid Tablets - 8 mg 445
Dilaudid-HP Injection 442
Dilaudid-HP Lyophilized Powder 250 mg . . . 442

HYDRONET (Denmark)
AMILORIDE HYDROCHLORIDE/HYDROCHLOROTHIAZIDE
Moduretic Tablets 2028

HY-DROP (Italy)
SODIUM HYALURONATE
Hyalgan Solution 2901

HYDRO-RAPID (Germany)
FUROSEMIDE
Furosemide Tablets 2154

HYDRO-RAPID-TABLINEN (Switzerland)
FUROSEMIDE
Furosemide Tablets 2154

HYDROSONE (Canada)
HYDROCORTISONE
Hydrocortone Tablets 1989

HYDRO-WOLFF (Germany)
HYDROCORTISONE
Hydrocortone Tablets 1989

HYDROZIDE (Hong Kong)
AMILORIDE HYDROCHLORIDE/HYDROCHLOROTHIAZIDE
Moduretic Tablets 2028

HYDROZIDE PLUS (Thailand)
AMILORIDE HYDROCHLORIDE/HYDROCHLOROTHIAZIDE
Moduretic Tablets 2028

HYDROZOLE (Australia)
HYDROCORTISONE
Hydrocortone Tablets 1989

HYFLOX (Thailand)
OFLOXACIN
Floxin Otic Solution 1049

HY-GAG (Germany)
SODIUM HYALURONATE
Hyalgan Solution 2901

HYLAN (Germany)
SODIUM HYALURONATE
Hyalgan Solution 2901

HYLO-COMOD (France, Germany, Israel, Italy, Portugal, Switzerland)
SODIUM HYALURONATE
Hyalgan Solution 2901

HYLUPROTECT (France, Italy)
SODIUM HYALURONATE
Hyalgan Solution 2901

HYPACE (South Africa)
ENALAPRIL MALEATE
Vasotec I.V. Injection 2103

HYPAN (Belgium)
NIFEDIPINE
Adalat CC Tablets 2964

HYPERMOL (New Zealand)
TIMOLOL MALEATE
Blocadren Tablets 1916
Timoptic Sterile Ophthalmic Solution 2088
Timoptic in Ocudose 2091
Timoptic-XE Sterile Ophthalmic Gel Forming Solution 2092

HYPERRETIC (Thailand)
AMILORIDE HYDROCHLORIDE/HYDROCHLOROTHIAZIDE
Moduretic Tablets 2028

HYPERSTAT (Australia, Belgium, Canada, France, Greece, Italy, Mexico, South Africa, Spain, Sweden, Switzerland, The Netherlands)
DIAZOXIDE
Hyperstat I.V. 3017

HYPERTANE (United Kingdom)
AMILORIDE HYDROCHLORIDE/HYDROCHLOROTHIAZIDE
Moduretic Tablets 2028

HYPERTONALUM (Germany)
DIAZOXIDE
Hyperstat I.V. 3017

HYPERTORR (Germany)
HYDROCHLOROTHIAZIDE/TRIAMTERENE
Dyazide Capsules 1423

HYPODINE (Thailand)
CLONIDINE HYDROCHLORIDE
Catapres Tablets 843

HYPOLAR RETARD (United Kingdom)
NIFEDIPINE
Adalat CC Tablets 2964

HYPOLIP (Czech Republic)
FENOFIBRATE
Tricor Tablets 527

HYPOMED (Austria)
LISINOPRIL
Prinivil Tablets 2052

HYPOTENSOR (Greece)
CAPTOPRIL
Captopril Tablets 2149

HYPREN (Austria)
RAMIPRIL
Altace Capsules 1702

HYRON (Hungary)
TERAZOSIN HYDROCHLORIDE
Hytrin Capsules 471

HYRUAN (Hong Kong)
SODIUM HYALURONATE
Hyalgan Solution 2901

HYSAN (Germany)
SODIUM HYALURONATE
Hyalgan Solution 2901

HYSONE (Australia)
HYDROCORTISONE
Hydrocortone Tablets 1989

HYTACAND (Portugal)
CANDESARTAN CILEXETIL
Atacand Tablets 649

HYTENEZE (United Kingdom)
CAPTOPRIL
Captopril Tablets 2149

HYTISONE (Hong Kong)
HYDROCORTISONE
Hydrocortone Tablets 1989

HYTRIN (Australia, Belgium, Brazil, Canada, Chile, Czech Republic, Greece, Hong Kong, Hungary, India, Irish Republic, Israel, Malaysia, Mexico, New Zealand, Portugal, Russia, Singapore, South Africa, Thailand, The Netherlands, United Kingdom, Venezuela)
TERAZOSIN HYDROCHLORIDE
Hytrin Capsules 471

HYTRIN BPH (Switzerland)
TERAZOSIN HYDROCHLORIDE
Hytrin Capsules 471

HYTRINE (France)
TERAZOSIN HYDROCHLORIDE
Hytrin Capsules 471

HYTRINEX (Sweden)
TERAZOSIN HYDROCHLORIDE
Hytrin Capsules 471

HYZAAR (Brazil, Canada, Chile, Czech Republic, France, Greece, Hong Kong, Hungary, Malaysia, Mexico, New Zealand, Russia, Singapore, Thailand, The Netherlands, Venezuela)
LOSARTAN POTASSIUM
Cozaar Tablets 1935

HYZAAR PLUS (Venezuela)
LOSARTAN POTASSIUM
Cozaar Tablets 1935

HYZAN (Hong Kong, Malaysia, Singapore)
RANITIDINE HYDROCHLORIDE
Zantac 25 EFFERdose Tablets 1624
Zantac 150 EFFERdose Tablets 1624
Zantac 150 Tablets 1624
Zantac 300 Tablets 1624
Zantac Injection 1619
Zantac Injection Premixed 1619
Zantac Syrup 1624

IAL (Hong Kong, Hungary, Italy, Switzerland)
SODIUM HYALURONATE
Hyalgan Solution 2901

IALECT (Italy)
SODIUM HYALURONATE
Hyalgan Solution 2901

IALUGEN (Switzerland)
SODIUM HYALURONATE
Hyalgan Solution 2901

IALUGEN PLUS (Czech Republic, Hungary)
SODIUM HYALURONATE
Hyalgan Solution 2901

IALUM (Italy)
SODIUM HYALURONATE
Hyalgan Solution 2901

IALUREX (Italy)
SODIUM HYALURONATE
Hyalgan Solution 2901

IALUSET (France)
SODIUM HYALURONATE
Hyalgan Solution 2901

IBAMOXIL (Brazil)
AMOXICILLIN
Amoxil Pediatric Drops for Oral Suspension 1343
Amoxil Tablets 1343

IBIAMOX (Thailand)
AMOXICILLIN
Amoxil Pediatric Drops for Oral Suspension 1343
Amoxil Tablets 1343

IBIPROVIR (Italy)
TERAZOSIN HYDROCHLORIDE
Hytrin Capsules 471

ICAZ (France)
ISRADIPINE
DynaCirc CR Tablets 2721

ICHTHOCORTIN (Germany)
HYDROCORTISONE
Hydrocortone Tablets 1989

ICORAN (Greece)
LISINOPRIL
Prinivil Tablets 2052

ICORSAN (Mexico)
HYDROCORTISONE
Hydrocortone Tablets 1989

ICTAN (Spain)
CLOTRIMAZOLE
Lotrimin Cream 3039
Lotrimin Lotion 1% 3039
Lotrimin Topical Solution 1% 3039

ICTUS (Brazil)
CARVEDILOL
Coreg Tablets 1414

IDENONA (Argentina)
HYDROCORTISONE
Hydrocortone Tablets 1989

IDRIL N SINE (Germany)
NAPHAZOLINE HYDROCHLORIDE
Albalon Ophthalmic Solution . . . . . ⊙218

IDROLAC (Italy)
LACTULOSE
Kristalose for Oral Solution 1034

IDUVO (Argentina)
ZIDOVUDINE
Retrovir Capsules 1560
Retrovir IV Infusion 1564
Retrovir Syrup 1560
Retrovir Tablets 1560

IECATEC (Spain, Thailand)
ENALAPRIL MALEATE
Vasotec I.V. Injection 2103

IFA REDUCCING (Mexico)
PHENTERMINE HYDROCHLORIDE
Adipex-P Capsules 1215
Adipex-P Tablets 1215

IFACIL (Mexico)
FLUOROURACIL
Efudex Topical Cream 3363
Efudex Topical Solutions 3363

IFADA (Spain)
FAMOTIDINE
Pepcid Injection 2040
Pepcid Injection Premixed 2040
Pepcid Tablets 2038
Pepcid for Oral Suspension 2038

IFAVAC (Mexico)
VANCOMYCIN HYDROCHLORIDE
Vancocin HCl Capsules, USP 3380

IFICIPRO (Russia)
CIPROFLOXACIN
Cipro Oral Suspension 2977

IFISTATIN (Singapore)
SIMVASTATIN
Zocor Tablets 2105

IFOCID (Argentina)
FLUOROURACIL
Efudex Topical Cream 3363
Efudex Topical Solutions 3363

IFOS (Chile)
OFLOXACIN
Floxin Otic Solution 1049

I-GESIC (India)
DICLOFENAC SODIUM
Voltaren Tablets 2307
Voltaren-XR Tablets 2310

IGUASSINA (Brazil)
HYDROCHLOROTHIAZIDE/TRIAMTERENE
Dyazide Capsules 1423

IHD (India)
ISOSORBIDE MONONITRATE
Imdur Tablets 3018

IKACOR (Israel)
VERAPAMIL HYDROCHLORIDE
Covera-HS Tablets 3139
Verelan PM Extended-Release Capsules, Controlled-Onset 3106

IKAPRESS (Israel)
VERAPAMIL HYDROCHLORIDE
Covera-HS Tablets 3139
Verelan PM Extended-Release Capsules, Controlled-Onset 3106

IKATIN (Mexico)
GENTAMICIN SULFATE
Garamycin Injectable 3014

IKOBEL (Greece)
TOBRAMYCIN
TOBI Solution for Inhalation 2298

IKOLAN (Argentina)
CLOTRIMAZOLE
Lotrimin Cream 3039
Lotrimin Lotion 1% 3039
Lotrimin Topical Solution 1% 3039

IKTORIVIL (Sweden)
CLONAZEPAM
Klonopin Tablets 2778

ILACEN (Spain)
DIFLUNISAL
Dolobid Tablets 1955

ILAGANE (Spain)
NAPROXEN
EC-Naprosyn Delayed-Release Tablets 2761
Naprosyn Suspension 2761
Naprosyn Tablets 2761

ILOCAP (Australia)
ERYTHROMYCIN
Ery-Tab Tablets 449
Erythromycin Base Filmtab Tablets 455
Erythromycin Delayed-Release Capsules, USP 457
PCE Dispertab Tablets 515

ILOPAR (Greece)
LOVASTATIN
Mevacor Tablets 2021

ILOSIN (Mexico)
ERYTHROMYCIN
Ery-Tab Tablets 449
Erythromycin Base Filmtab Tablets 455
Erythromycin Delayed-Release Capsules, USP 457
PCE Dispertab Tablets 515

ILOTICINA (Argentina, Spain, Venezuela)
ERYTHROMYCIN
Ery-Tab Tablets 449
Erythromycin Base Filmtab Tablets 455
Erythromycin Delayed-Release Capsules, USP 457
PCE Dispertab Tablets 515

ILOTICINA ANTI ACNE (Spain)
ERYTHROMYCIN
Ery-Tab Tablets 449
Erythromycin Base Filmtab Tablets 455
Erythromycin Delayed-Release Capsules, USP 457
PCE Dispertab Tablets 515

ILOTREX (Brazil)
ERYTHROMYCIN STEARATE
Erythrocin Stearate Filmtab Tablets 453

ILOTYCIN TS (South Africa)
ERYTHROMYCIN
Ery-Tab Tablets 449
Erythromycin Base Filmtab Tablets 455
Erythromycin Delayed-Release Capsules, USP 457
PCE Dispertab Tablets 515

ILOTYCIN-A (South Africa)
TRETINOIN
Vesanoid Capsules 2820

ILSATEC (Argentina, Brazil, Mexico, Venezuela)
LANSOPRAZOLE
Prevacid Delayed-Release Capsules 3271

IMACILLIN (Denmark)
AMOXICILLIN
Amoxil Pediatric Drops for Oral Suspension 1343
Amoxil Tablets 1343

IMAVERMIL (Brazil)
ALBENDAZOLE
Albenza Tablets 1338

IMAZOL (Czech Republic, Germany, Switzerland, Venezuela)
CLOTRIMAZOLE
Lotrimin Cream 3039
Lotrimin Lotion 1% 3039
Lotrimin Topical Solution 1% 3039

IMAZOL PLUS (Czech Republic)
CLOTRIMAZOLE
Lotrimin Cream 3039
Lotrimin Lotion 1% 3039
Lotrimin Topical Solution 1% 3039

IMBISTAD (Mexico)
SIMVASTATIN
Zocor Tablets 2105

IMDEX (Malaysia, Singapore)
ISOSORBIDE MONONITRATE
Imdur Tablets 3018

IMDUR (Australia, Austria, Canada, Czech Republic, Denmark, Finland, Greece, Hong Kong, Irish Republic, Malaysia, Mexico, New Zealand, Norway, Portugal, Singapore, South Africa, Spain, Sweden, Switzerland, Thailand, United Kingdom)
ISOSORBIDE MONONITRATE
Imdur Tablets 3018

IMEPAS (Mexico)
DIAZEPAM
Diastat Rectal Delivery System 3343
Valium Tablets 2819

IMFERDEX (Switzerland)
IRON DEXTRAN
Infed Injection 3390

IMFERON (Australia, Belgium, Canada, India, Mexico, South Africa, Spain, The Netherlands, United Kingdom)
IRON DEXTRAN
Infed Injection 3390

IMFLAC (Australia)
DICLOFENAC SODIUM
Voltaren Tablets 2307
Voltaren-XR Tablets 2310

IMIDEX (Mexico)
LANSOPRAZOLE
Prevacid Delayed-Release Capsules 3271

IMIDIL (India)
CLOTRIMAZOLE
Lotrimin Cream 3039
Lotrimin Lotion 1% 3039
Lotrimin Topical Solution 1% 3039

IMIGRAN (Argentina, Australia, Brazil, Chile, Czech Republic, Germany, Greece, Hong Kong, Hungary, Irish Republic, Malaysia, New Zealand, Norway, Portugal, Russia, Singapore, South Africa, Spain, Thailand, United Kingdom, Venezuela)
SUMATRIPTAN SUCCINATE
Imitrex Injection 1463
Imitrex Tablets 1471

IMIJECT (France)
SUMATRIPTAN SUCCINATE
Imitrex Injection 1463
Imitrex Tablets 1471

IMIMORE (Argentina)
IMIQUIMOD
Aldara Cream, 5% 1846

IMIPEM (Italy)
CILASTATIN SODIUM/IMIPENEM
Primaxin I.M. 2045
Primaxin I.V. 2048

IMITREX (Argentina, Israel)
SUMATRIPTAN
Imitrex Nasal Spray 1467

IMMUKIN (Hong Kong, Irish Republic)
INTERFERON GAMMA-1B
Actimmune 1671

IMMUKINE (The Netherlands)
INTERFERON GAMMA-1B
Actimmune 1671

IMOT (Mexico, Venezuela)
TIMOLOL MALEATE
Blocadren Tablets 1916
Timoptic Sterile Ophthalmic Solution 2088
Timoptic in Ocudose 2091
Timoptic-XE Sterile Ophthalmic Gel Forming Solution 2092

IMPOSERGON (Greece)
FAMOTIDINE
Pepcid Injection 2040
Pepcid Injection Premixed 2040
Pepcid Tablets 2038
Pepcid for Oral Suspension 2038

IMPUGAN (Denmark, Sweden, Switzerland, Thailand)
FUROSEMIDE
Furosemide Tablets 2154

IMTRATE (Australia, New Zealand)
ISOSORBIDE MONONITRATE
Imdur Tablets 3018

IMUFOR (Argentina, Austria)
INTERFERON GAMMA-1B
Actimmune 1671

IMUKIN (Austria, Denmark, Finland, France, Germany, Italy, Norway, Portugal, Spain, Sweden)
INTERFERON GAMMA-1B
Actimmune 1671

IMUNOXA (Argentina)
LAMIVUDINE
Epivir Oral Solution 1427
Epivir Tablets 1427
Epivir-HBV Oral Solution 1432
Epivir-HBV Tablets 1432

IMUNOXA COMPLEX (Argentina)
LAMIVUDINE
Epivir Oral Solution 1427
Epivir Tablets 1427
Epivir-HBV Oral Solution 1432
Epivir-HBV Tablets 1432

IMUXGEN (Argentina)
MYCOPHENOLATE MOFETIL
CellCept Capsules 2747
CellCept Oral Suspension 2747
CellCept Tablets 2747

INAC (Singapore)
DICLOFENAC SODIUM
Voltaren Tablets 2307
Voltaren-XR Tablets 2310

INALACOR (Spain)
FLUTICASONE PROPIONATE
Cutivate Cream 2662
Cutivate Ointment 2665
Flonase Nasal Spray 1440

INALCORT (Italy)
FLUNISOLIDE
Aerobid Inhaler System 1171
Aerobid-M Inhaler System 1171

INAMIDE (Irish Republic)
INDAPAMIDE
Indapamide Tablets 2156

INASPIR (Spain)
SALMETEROL XINAFOATE
Serevent Diskus 1568

INASTMOL (Argentina)
THEOPHYLLINE
Uniphyl Tablets 2710

INCIDAL-OD (Thailand)
CETIRIZINE HYDROCHLORIDE
Zyrtec Syrup 2594
Zyrtec Tablets 2594

INCLENS (Venezuela)
FUROSEMIDE
Furosemide Tablets 2154

INCORIL (Argentina, Brazil, Chile)
DILTIAZEM HYDROCHLORIDE
Cardizem LA Extended Release Tablets 1728
Tiazac Capsules 1201

INDACAR (Denmark)
INDAPAMIDE
Indapamide Tablets 2156

INDAFLEX (Italy)
INDAPAMIDE
Indapamide Tablets 2156

INDAHEXAL (Australia)
INDAPAMIDE
Indapamide Tablets 2156

INDALIX (Hong Kong, South Africa)
INDAPAMIDE
Indapamide Tablets 2156

INDAMOL (Italy)
INDAPAMIDE
Indapamide Tablets **2156**

INDANORM (United Arab Emirates)
INDAPAMIDE
Indapamide Tablets **2156**

INDAP (Czech Republic, Russia)
INDAPAMIDE
Indapamide Tablets **2156**

INDAPEN (Brazil)
INDAPAMIDE
Indapamide Tablets **2156**

INDAPRESS (Chile)
INDAPAMIDE
Indapamide Tablets **2156**

INDA-PUREN (Germany)
INDAPAMIDE
Indapamide Tablets **2156**

INDARZONA-N (Mexico)
DEXAMETHASONE
Decadron Tablets **1951**

INDERAL (Argentina, Australia, Austria, Belgium, Brazil, Canada, Denmark, Finland, Hong Kong, India, Irish Republic, Israel, Italy, Malaysia, New Zealand, Norway, Portugal, Singapore, South Africa, Sweden, Switzerland, Thailand, The Netherlands, United Kingdom, Venezuela)
PROPRANOLOL HYDROCHLORIDE
Inderal LA Long-Acting Capsules **3429**

INDERALICI (Mexico)
PROPRANOLOL HYDROCHLORIDE
Inderal LA Long-Acting Capsules **3429**

INDERM (Belgium, Germany, Switzerland, The Netherlands, Venezuela)
ERYTHROMYCIN
Ery-Tab Tablets **449**
Erythromycin Base Filmtab Tablets **455**
Erythromycin Delayed-Release Capsules, USP **457**
PCE Dispertab Tablets **515**

INDICONTIN (India)
INDAPAMIDE
Indapamide Tablets **2156**

INDITOR (India)
INDAPAMIDE
Indapamide Tablets **2156**

INDIVAN (India)
INDINAVIR SULFATE
Crixivan Capsules **1940**

INDOBLOC (Germany)
PROPRANOLOL HYDROCHLORIDE
Inderal LA Long-Acting Capsules **3429**

INDOBLOK (South Africa)
PROPRANOLOL HYDROCHLORIDE
Inderal LA Long-Acting Capsules **3429**

INDOLIN (Italy)
INDAPAMIDE
Indapamide Tablets **2156**

INDUZEPAM (Argentina)
CLONAZEPAM
Klonopin Tablets **2778**

INESTOM (Greece)
LEVOCARNITINE
Carnitor Injection **3188**
Carnitor Tablets and Oral Solution **3190**

INF (Argentina)
INTERFERON ALFA-2B
Intron A for Injection **3024**

INFASURF (Israel)
CALFACTANT
Infasurf Intratracheal Suspension **1184**

INFECTOCIN (South Africa)
ERYTHROMYCIN STEARATE
Erythrocin Stearate Filmtab Tablets **453**

INFECTOCLONT (Germany)
METRONIDAZOLE
MetroGel-Vaginal Gel **1855**

INFECTOFLAM (Brazil, Czech Republic, Malaysia)
FLUOROMETHOLONE
FML Ophthalmic Ointment . . . . ⊙**228**

INFECTOFLU (Germany)
AMANTADINE HYDROCHLORIDE
Symmetrel Tablets **1135**

INFECTOMOX (Germany)
AMOXICILLIN
Amoxil Pediatric Drops for Oral Suspension **1343**
Amoxil Tablets **1343**

INFECTOPYODERM (Germany)
MUPIROCIN
Bactroban Ointment **1395**

INFECTOSS (Brazil)
ERYTHROMYCIN
Ery-Tab Tablets **449**
Erythromycin Base Filmtab Tablets **455**
Erythromycin Delayed-Release Capsules, USP **457**
PCE Dispertab Tablets **515**

INFERAX (Germany)
INTERFERON ALFACON-1
Infergen **3364**

INFERGEN (Belgium, Canada, Czech Republic, France, Greece, Hungary, Italy, The Netherlands)
INTERFERON ALFACON-1
Infergen **3364**

INFESTAT (United Kingdom)
NYSTATIN
Nystop Topical Powder USP **2478**
Paddock Nystatin USP for Oral Suspension **2478**

INFLA-BAN (South Africa)
DICLOFENAC SODIUM
Voltaren Tablets **2307**
Voltaren-XR Tablets **2310**

INFLAMAC (Switzerland)
DICLOFENAC SODIUM
Voltaren Tablets **2307**
Voltaren-XR Tablets **2310**

INFLAMAX (Brazil)
DICLOFENAC SODIUM
Voltaren Tablets **2307**
Voltaren-XR Tablets **2310**

INFLANAC (Hong Kong, Singapore, Thailand)
DICLOFENAC SODIUM
Voltaren Tablets **2307**
Voltaren-XR Tablets **2310**

INFLANOX (Mexico)
NAPROXEN
EC-Naprosyn Delayed-Release Tablets **2761**
Naprosyn Suspension **2761**
Naprosyn Tablets **2761**

INFLOXA (Mexico)
CIPROFLOXACIN
Cipro Oral Suspension **2977**

INFLU-A (Israel)
AMANTADINE HYDROCHLORIDE
Symmetrel Tablets **1135**

INFUFER (Canada)
IRON DEXTRAN
Infed Injection **3390**

INGASTRI (Spain)
FAMOTIDINE
Pepcid Injection **2040**
Pepcid Injection Premixed **2040**
Pepcid Tablets **2038**
Pepcid for Oral Suspension **2038**

INHACORT (Germany)
FLUNISOLIDE
Aerobid Inhaler System **1171**
Aerobid-M Inhaler System **1171**

INHALEX (Thailand)
IPRATROPIUM BROMIDE
Atrovent Inhalation Solution **835**
Atrovent Nasal Spray 0.03% **837**
Atrovent Nasal Spray 0.06% **839**

INHIBACE (Israel)
CAPTOPRIL
Captopril Tablets **2149**

INIBIL (Italy)
APROTININ
Trasylol Injection **754**

INIPROL (Belgium, France, Italy)
APROTININ
Trasylol Injection **754**

INKAMIL (Spain)
CIPROFLOXACIN HYDROCHLORIDE
Ciloxan Ophthalmic Ointment . . . . ⊙**204, 559**
Ciloxan Ophthalmic Solution . . . . ⊙**206**
Cipro Tablets **2977**

INNOMEL (Irish Republic)
ENALAPRIL MALEATE
Vasotec I.V. Injection **2103**

INNOVACE (Irish Republic, United Kingdom)
ENALAPRIL MALEATE
Vasotec I.V. Injection **2103**

INOFLOX (Malaysia, Singapore)
OFLOXACIN
Floxin Otic Solution **1049**

INOFUNGIN (Brazil)
NYSTATIN
Nystop Topical Powder USP **2478**
Paddock Nystatin USP for Oral Suspension **2478**

INOSERT (India)
SERTRALINE HYDROCHLORIDE
Zoloft Tablets **2586**

INOTRIN (Greece)
ISOTRETINOIN
Accutane Capsules **2731**

INOVAL (Brazil)
FENTANYL CITRATE
Actiq **979**

INPAMIDE (Thailand)
INDAPAMIDE
Indapamide Tablets **2156**

INPANOL (Hong Kong, Singapore)
PROPRANOLOL HYDROCHLORIDE
Inderal LA Long-Acting Capsules **3429**

INSENSYE (Australia)
NORFLOXACIN
Noroxin Tablets **2032**

INSERTEC (Argentina)
SERTRALINE HYDROCHLORIDE
Zoloft Tablets **2586**

INSIDE (Sweden)
RANITIDINE HYDROCHLORIDE
Zantac 25 EFFERdose Tablets **1624**
Zantac 150 EFFERdose Tablets **1624**
Zantac 150 Tablets **1624**
Zantac 300 Tablets **1624**
Zantac Injection **1619**
Zantac Injection Premixed **1619**
Zantac Syrup **1624**

INSIDE BRUS (Finland, Norway)
RANITIDINE HYDROCHLORIDE
Zantac 25 EFFERdose Tablets **1624**
Zantac 150 EFFERdose Tablets **1624**
Zantac 150 Tablets **1624**
Zantac 300 Tablets **1624**
Zantac Injection **1619**
Zantac Injection Premixed **1619**
Zantac Syrup **1624**

INSIG (Australia)
INDAPAMIDE
Indapamide Tablets **2156**

INSOMN-EZE (Australia)
PROMETHAZINE HYDROCHLORIDE
Phenergan Tablets and Suppositories **3440**

INSTANA (Spain)
CEFPODOXIME PROXETIL
Vantin Tablets and Oral Suspension **2645**

INSUP (Spain)
ENALAPRIL MALEATE
Vasotec I.V. Injection **2103**

INTEGRILIN (Australia, Belgium, Brazil, Canada, Chile, Czech Republic, Denmark, Finland, France, Germany, Greece, Hong Kong, Hungary, Irish Republic, Israel, Italy, Malaysia, New Zealand, Norway, Portugal, Russia, Singapore, South Africa, Spain, Sweden, Switzerland, Thailand, The Netherlands, United Kingdom)
EPTIFIBATIDE
Integrilin Injection **3020**

INTELECTA (Greece)
LEVOCARNITINE
Carnitor Injection **3188**
Carnitor Tablets and Oral Solution **3190**

INTER 2-B (Argentina)
INTERFERON ALFA-2B
Intron A for Injection **3024**

INTERBERIN (Austria)
SARGRAMOSTIM
Leukine **814**

INTERBION (Greece)
CEFUROXIME AXETIL
Ceftin Tablets **1407**
Ceftin for Oral Suspension **1407**

INTERMIGRAN (Germany)
PROPRANOLOL HYDROCHLORIDE
Inderal LA Long-Acting Capsules **3429**

INTOCEL (Argentina)
CLADRIBINE
Leustatin Injection **2357**

INTRACEF (Brazil, South Africa)
CEFTAZIDIME
Fortaz for Injection **1453**

INTRON (Venezuela)
INTERFERON ALFA-2B
Intron A for Injection **3024**

INTRON A (Canada, Czech Republic, Hong Kong, Hungary, Israel, Malaysia, Mexico, Portugal, Singapore, South Africa, Spain, Switzerland, The Netherlands, Venezuela)
INTERFERON ALFA-2B
Intron A for Injection **3024**

INTRONA (Austria, Denmark, Finland, France, Irish Republic, Norway, Sweden, Thailand)
INTERFERON ALFA-2B
Intron A for Injection **3024**

INVEOXEL (Chile)
NAPROXEN
EC-Naprosyn Delayed-Release Tablets **2761**
Naprosyn Suspension **2761**
Naprosyn Tablets **2761**

INVIGAN (Spain)
FAMOTIDINE
Pepcid Injection **2040**
Pepcid Injection Premixed **2040**
Pepcid Tablets **2038**
Pepcid for Oral Suspension **2038**

INVORIL (Czech Republic, Hungary, Malaysia, Russia, Singapore, Thailand)
ENALAPRIL MALEATE
Vasotec I.V. Injection **2103**

INVOZIDE (India)
ENALAPRIL MALEATE
Vasotec I.V. Injection **2103**

INZA (Australia, Hong Kong)
NAPROXEN
EC-Naprosyn Delayed-Release Tablets **2761**
Naprosyn Suspension **2761**
Naprosyn Tablets **2761**

IOR T3 (Chile, Mexico)
MUROMONAB-CD3
Orthoclone OKT3 Sterile Solution **2360**

IPACEF (Italy)
CEFUROXIME SODIUM
Zinacef Injection **1631**

IPAGASTRIL (Italy)
SUCRALFATE
Carafate Suspension **701**
Carafate Tablets **701**

IPALAT (Venezuela)
CLOTRIMAZOLE
Lotrimin Cream **3039**
Lotrimin Lotion 1% **3039**
Lotrimin Topical Solution 1% **3039**

IPAMIX (Italy)
INDAPAMIDE
Indapamide Tablets **2156**

IPATON (Czech Republic, Hungary)
TICLOPIDINE HYDROCHLORIDE
Ticlid Tablets **2810**

IPOMEX (Argentina)
SIBUTRAMINE HYDROCHLORIDE
Meridia Capsules **489**

IPOTENSIUM (Italy)
CLONIDINE HYDROCHLORIDE
Catapres Tablets **843**

IPRA (New Zealand)
IPRATROPIUM BROMIDE
Atrovent Inhalation Solution 835
Atrovent Nasal Spray 0.03%. 837
Atrovent Nasal Spray 0.06%. 839

IPRABON (Brazil)
IPRATROPIUM BROMIDE
Atrovent Inhalation Solution 835
Atrovent Nasal Spray 0.03%. 837
Atrovent Nasal Spray 0.06%. 839

IPRABRON (Argentina)
IPRATROPIUM BROMIDE
Atrovent Inhalation Solution 835
Atrovent Nasal Spray 0.03%. 837
Atrovent Nasal Spray 0.06%. 839

IPRADUAL (Argentina)
IPRATROPIUM BROMIDE
Atrovent Inhalation Solution 835
Atrovent Nasal Spray 0.03%. 837
Atrovent Nasal Spray 0.06%. 839

IPRAMID (Greece)
SIMVASTATIN
Zocor Tablets 2105

IPRAMOL (United Kingdom)
IPRATROPIUM BROMIDE
Atrovent Inhalation Solution 835
Atrovent Nasal Spray 0.03%. 837
Atrovent Nasal Spray 0.06%. 839

IPRANASE (India)
IPRATROPIUM BROMIDE
Atrovent Inhalation Solution 835
Atrovent Nasal Spray 0.03%. 837
Atrovent Nasal Spray 0.06%. 839

IPRANEO (Brazil)
IPRATROPIUM BROMIDE
Atrovent Inhalation Solution 835
Atrovent Nasal Spray 0.03%. 837
Atrovent Nasal Spray 0.06%. 839

IPRASALB (Argentina)
IPRATROPIUM BROMIDE
Atrovent Inhalation Solution 835
Atrovent Nasal Spray 0.03%. 837
Atrovent Nasal Spray 0.06%. 839

IPRATRIN (Australia)
IPRATROPIUM BROMIDE
Atrovent Inhalation Solution 835
Atrovent Nasal Spray 0.03%. 837
Atrovent Nasal Spray 0.06%. 839

IPRAVENT (Australia, Hong Kong, India)
IPRATROPIUM BROMIDE
Atrovent Inhalation Solution 835
Atrovent Nasal Spray 0.03%. 837
Atrovent Nasal Spray 0.06%. 839

IPROXIN (Venezuela)
CIPROFLOXACIN
Cipro Oral Suspension 2977

IPVENT (South Africa)
IPRATROPIUM BROMIDE
Atrovent Inhalation Solution 835
Atrovent Nasal Spray 0.03%. 837
Atrovent Nasal Spray 0.06%. 839

IQFADINA (Mexico)
RANITIDINE HYDROCHLORIDE
Zantac 25 EFFERdose Tablets 1624
Zantac 150 EFFERdose Tablets. 1624
Zantac 150 Tablets 1624
Zantac 300 Tablets 1624
Zantac Injection 1619
Zantac Injection Premixed 1619
Zantac Syrup 1624

IQFAMICINA (Mexico)
ERYTHROMYCIN
Ery-Tab Tablets 449
Erythromycin Base Filmtab Tablets. 455
Erythromycin Delayed-Release Capsules, USP 457
PCE Dispertab Tablets 515

IQFASOL (Mexico)
NAPROXEN
EC-Naprosyn Delayed-Release Tablets. . . . 2761
Naprosyn Suspension. 2761
Naprosyn Tablets 2761

IRBAN (Israel)
IRBESARTAN
Avapro Tablets 891

IRBAN PLUS (Israel)
IRBESARTAN
Avapro Tablets 891

IRENAX (Argentina, Brazil)
IRINOTECAN HYDROCHLORIDE
Camptosar Injection 2604

IRICIL (Spain)
LISINOPRIL
Prinivil Tablets 2052

IRICIL PLUS (Spain)
LISINOPRIL
Prinivil Tablets 2052

IRIDINA DUE (Italy)
NAPHAZOLINE HYDROCHLORIDE
Albalon Ophthalmic Solution . . . . ⊙218

IRILENS (Italy)
SODIUM HYALURONATE
Hyalgan Solution 2901

IRINOGEN (Argentina)
IRINOTECAN HYDROCHLORIDE
Camptosar Injection 2604

IRINOTEL (Thailand)
IRINOTECAN HYDROCHLORIDE
Camptosar Injection 2604

IRONDEX (Mexico)
IRON DEXTRAN
Infed Injection 3390

IROVEL (India)
IRBESARTAN
Avapro Tablets 891

IRRADIAL (Argentina)
SERTRALINE HYDROCHLORIDE
Zoloft Tablets 2586

IRUMED (Czech Republic)
LISINOPRIL
Prinivil Tablets 2052

IS 5 MONO (Germany)
ISOSORBIDE MONONITRATE
Imdur Tablets 3018

ISADOL (Mexico)
ZIDOVUDINE
Retrovir Capsules 1560
Retrovir IV Infusion. 1564
Retrovir Syrup 1560
Retrovir Tablets. 1560

ISANGINA (Finland)
ISOSORBIDE MONONITRATE
Imdur Tablets 3018

ISAXION (Portugal)
TICLOPIDINE HYDROCHLORIDE
Ticlid Tablets 2810

ISCLOFEN (United Kingdom)
DICLOFENAC SODIUM
Voltaren Tablets 2307
Voltaren-XR Tablets 2310

ISCOVER (Argentina, Australia, Brazil, Germany, Greece, Italy, Mexico, Portugal, Spain, Switzerland)
CLOPIDOGREL BISULFATE
Plavix Tablets 917, 2926

ISDINIUM (Spain)
HYDROCORTISONE
Hydrocortone Tablets 1989

ISET (Argentina)
CLARITHROMYCIN
Biaxin Filmtab Tablets 402
Biaxin Granules 402

ISIB (United Kingdom)
ISOSORBIDE MONONITRATE
Imdur Tablets 3018

ISIMOXIN (Italy)
AMOXICILLIN
Amoxil Pediatric Drops for Oral Suspension. 1343
Amoxil Tablets 1343

ISMEXIN (Finland)
ISOSORBIDE MONONITRATE
Imdur Tablets 3018

ISMO (Canada, Chile, Denmark, Germany, Hong Kong, India, Israel, Italy, New Zealand, Norway, Portugal, Singapore, South Africa, Spain, Sweden, Switzerland, Thailand, The Netherlands, United Kingdom, Venezuela)
ISOSORBIDE MONONITRATE
Imdur Tablets 3018

ISMOX (Finland)
ISOSORBIDE MONONITRATE
Imdur Tablets 3018

ISO ESTEDI (Spain)
ISOTRETINOIN
Accutane Capsules 2731

ISOACNE (Brazil)
ISOTRETINOIN
Accutane Capsules 2731

ISOBLOC (Argentina)
CARVEDILOL
Coreg Tablets. 1414

ISO-CARD (South Africa)
VERAPAMIL HYDROCHLORIDE
Covera-HS Tablets 3139
Verelan PM Extended-Release Capsules, Controlled-Onset 3106

ISOCUTAN (Austria)
ISOTRETINOIN
Accutane Capsules 2731

ISODERM (Germany)
ISOTRETINOIN
Accutane Capsules 2731

ISODERMAL (Greece)
ISOTRETINOIN
Accutane Capsules 2731

ISODUR (Denmark, Sweden, United Kingdom)
ISOSORBIDE MONONITRATE
Imdur Tablets 3018

ISOFACE (Mexico)
ISOTRETINOIN
Accutane Capsules 2731

ISOFTAL (Austria)
NAPHAZOLINE HYDROCHLORIDE
Albalon Ophthalmic Solution . . . . ⊙218

ISOGERIL (Greece)
ISOTRETINOIN
Accutane Capsules 2731

ISOGLAUCON (Austria, Germany, Italy, Spain)
CLONIDINE HYDROCHLORIDE
Catapres Tablets 843

ISOHEXAL (Australia)
ISOTRETINOIN
Accutane Capsules 2731

ISOLAN (Argentina)
ISOSORBIDE MONONITRATE
Imdur Tablets 3018

ISOMEL (Irish Republic)
ISOSORBIDE MONONITRATE
Imdur Tablets 3018

ISOMIN (India)
ISOSORBIDE MONONITRATE
Imdur Tablets 3018

ISOMINA (Venezuela)
FAMOTIDINE
Pepcid Injection 2040
Pepcid Injection Premixed 2040
Pepcid Tablets 2038
Pepcid for Oral Suspension 2038

ISOMON (Greece)
ISOSORBIDE MONONITRATE
Imdur Tablets 3018

ISOMONAT (Austria)
ISOSORBIDE MONONITRATE
Imdur Tablets 3018

ISOMONIT (Australia, Denmark, Germany, Irish Republic)
ISOSORBIDE MONONITRATE
Imdur Tablets 3018

ISOMONOREAL (Germany)
ISOSORBIDE MONONITRATE
Imdur Tablets 3018

ISONITRIL (Spain)
ISOSORBIDE MONONITRATE
Imdur Tablets 3018

ISONTYN (Argentina)
TERAZOSIN HYDROCHLORIDE
Hytrin Capsules. 471

ISOPAMIL (Thailand)
VERAPAMIL HYDROCHLORIDE
Covera-HS Tablets 3139
Verelan PM Extended-Release Capsules, Controlled-Onset 3106

ISOPEN (Thailand)
ISOSORBIDE MONONITRATE
Imdur Tablets 3018

ISOPTIN (Australia, Austria, Canada, Czech Republic, Denmark, Finland, Germany, Greece, Hong Kong, Hungary, Irish Republic, Italy, Malaysia, New Zealand, Norway, Portugal, Russia, Singapore, South Africa, Sweden, Switzerland, Thailand, The Netherlands)
VERAPAMIL HYDROCHLORIDE
Covera-HS Tablets 3139
Verelan PM Extended-Release Capsules, Controlled-Onset 3106

ISOPTINE (Belgium, France)
VERAPAMIL HYDROCHLORIDE
Covera-HS Tablets 3139
Verelan PM Extended-Release Capsules, Controlled-Onset 3106

ISOPTO CETAMIDE (Belgium, Canada)
SULFACETAMIDE SODIUM
Klaron Lotion 10%. 2909

ISOPTO CETAPRED (Belgium, Canada, Greece)
PREDNISOLONE ACETATE/SULFACETAMIDE SODIUM
Blephamide Ophthalmic Ointment. 568
Blephamide Ophthalmic Suspension 569

ISOPTO DEX (Germany)
DEXAMETHASONE
Decadron Tablets 1951

ISOPTO FLUCON (Germany, Spain)
FLUOROMETHOLONE
FML Ophthalmic Ointment. . . . . ⊙228

ISOPTO MAXIDEX (Argentina, Norway, Sweden)
DEXAMETHASONE
Decadron Tablets 1951

ISOSKIN (Greece)
ISOTRETINOIN
Accutane Capsules 2731

ISOSOL (Austria)
ISOTRETINOIN
Accutane Capsules 2731

ISOSPAN (Hungary)
ISOSORBIDE MONONITRATE
Imdur Tablets 3018

ISOTANE (New Zealand, Thailand)
ISOTRETINOIN
Accutane Capsules 2731

ISOTARD (United Kingdom)
ISOSORBIDE MONONITRATE
Imdur Tablets 3018

ISOTRATE (Hong Kong, Singapore, United Kingdom)
ISOSORBIDE MONONITRATE
Imdur Tablets 3018

ISOTRET (Germany)
ISOTRETINOIN
Accutane Capsules 2731

ISOTREX (Argentina, Australia, Austria, Brazil, Canada, Chile, Czech Republic, Denmark, France, Germany, Hong Kong, Hungary, Irish Republic, Israel, Italy, Malaysia, Mexico, New Zealand, Portugal, Singapore, South Africa, Spain, Thailand, United Kingdom, Venezuela)
ISOTRETINOIN
Accutane Capsules 2731

ISOTREX ERITROMICINA (Spain)
ISOTRETINOIN
Accutane Capsules 2731

ISOTREXIN (Austria, Brazil, Germany, Irish Republic, Italy, Portugal, Singapore, Thailand, United Kingdom)
ISOTRETINOIN
Accutane Capsules 2731

ISOTROIN (Greece, India)
ISOTRETINOIN
Accutane Capsules 2731

(⊙ Described in PDR For Ophthalmic Medicines™)

ISTOPRIL (Thailand)
ENALAPRIL MALEATE
Vasotec I.V. Injection . . . 2103

ITALNIK (Mexico)
CIPROFLOXACIN
Cipro Oral Suspension . . . 2977

ITOREX (Italy)
CEFUROXIME SODIUM
Zinacef Injection . . . 1631

ITRIN (Italy)
TERAZOSIN HYDROCHLORIDE
Hytrin Capsules . . . 471

ITROP (Austria, Czech Republic, Germany, Switzerland)
IPRATROPIUM BROMIDE
Atrovent Inhalation Solution . . . 835
Atrovent Nasal Spray 0.03% . . . 837
Atrovent Nasal Spray 0.06% . . . 839

IVERMEC (Brazil)
IVERMECTIN
Stromectol Tablets . . . 2083

IVEXTERM (Mexico)
IVERMECTIN
Stromectol Tablets . . . 2083

IVIDOL (Greece)
AMILORIDE HYDROCHLORIDE/HYDROCHLOROTHIAZIDE
Moduretic Tablets . . . 2028

IZADIMA (Mexico)
CEFTAZIDIME
Fortaz for Injection . . . 1453

JABASTATINA (Portugal)
SIMVASTATIN
Zocor Tablets . . . 2105

JANACIN (Hong Kong, Malaysia, Thailand)
NORFLOXACIN
Noroxin Tablets . . . 2032

JATROPUR (Germany)
TRIAMTERENE
Dyrenium Capsules . . . 3400

JATROSOM N (Germany)
TRANYLCYPROMINE SULFATE
Parnate Tablets . . . 1527

JEDIPIN (Germany, Thailand)
NIFEDIPINE
Adalat CC Tablets . . . 2964

JENAFENAC (Germany)
DICLOFENAC SODIUM
Voltaren Tablets . . . 2307
Voltaren-XR Tablets . . . 2310

JENAMAZOL (Czech Republic, Germany)
CLOTRIMAZOLE
Lotrimin Cream . . . 3039
Lotrimin Lotion 1% . . . 3039
Lotrimin Topical Solution 1% . . . 3039

JENAPAMIL (Germany)
VERAPAMIL HYDROCHLORIDE
Covera-HS Tablets . . . 3139
Verelan PM Extended-Release Capsules, Controlled-Onset . . . 3106

JENATEREN COMP (Germany)
HYDROCHLOROTHIAZIDE/TRIAMTERENE
Dyazide Capsules . . . 1423

JENOQUINE (United Arab Emirates)
LEVOFLOXACIN
Levaquin Injection . . . 2384
Levaquin Tablets . . . 2384

JEPROLOL (Germany)
METOPROLOL TARTRATE
Lopressor Tablets . . . 2238

JODTHYROX (Czech Republic)
LEVOTHYROXINE SODIUM
Levothroid Tablets . . . 1186
Levoxyl Tablets . . . 1712
Synthroid Tablets . . . 520

JOHNSONS CLEAN & CLEAR PERSA GEL (Canada)
BENZOYL PEROXIDE
Brevoxyl-4 Creamy Wash . . . 3210
Brevoxyl-4 Gel . . . 3210
Brevoxyl-8 Creamy Wash . . . 3210
Brevoxyl-8 Gel . . . 3210
Triaz Cleanser . . . 1892
Triaz Gel . . . 1892

JOSIR (France)
TAMSULOSIN HYDROCHLORIDE
Flomax Capsules . . . 850

JOSKEN (Mexico)
SIMVASTATIN
Zocor Tablets . . . 2105

JOSSALIND (Germany)
SODIUM HYALURONATE
Hyalgan Solution . . . 2901

JOYZOL (India)
OLANZAPINE
Zyprexa Tablets . . . 1830

JUAN (India)
SILDENAFIL CITRATE
Viagra Tablets . . . 2573

JULAB (Hong Kong, Thailand)
SELEGILINE HYDROCHLORIDE
Eldepryl Capsules . . . 3208

JUMEX (Argentina, Austria, Czech Republic, Hong Kong, Hungary, Israel, Italy, Malaysia, Portugal, Singapore, Thailand, Venezuela)
SELEGILINE HYDROCHLORIDE
Eldepryl Capsules . . . 3208

JUMEXAL (Switzerland)
SELEGILINE HYDROCHLORIDE
Eldepryl Capsules . . . 3208

JUMEXIL (Brazil)
SELEGILINE HYDROCHLORIDE
Eldepryl Capsules . . . 3208

JUNGLE FORMULA STING RELIEF CREAM (United Kingdom)
HYDROCORTISONE
Hydrocortone Tablets . . . 1989

JUNO (Argentina)
LEVOTHYROXINE SODIUM
Levothroid Tablets . . . 1186
Levoxyl Tablets . . . 1712
Synthroid Tablets . . . 520

K-10 (Canada)
POTASSIUM CHLORIDE
K-Dur Extended-Relase Tablets . . . 3033
K-Lor Oral Solution . . . 474
K-Tab Tablets . . . 475

KAARMEPAKKAUS (Finland)
DEXAMETHASONE
Decadron Tablets . . . 1951

KABIZOL (Chile)
METRONIDAZOLE
MetroGel-Vaginal Gel . . . 1855

KADALEX (Italy)
POTASSIUM CHLORIDE
K-Dur Extended-Relase Tablets . . . 3033
K-Lor Oral Solution . . . 474
K-Tab Tablets . . . 475

KADEFUNGIN (Germany)
CLOTRIMAZOLE
Lotrimin Cream . . . 3039
Lotrimin Lotion 1% . . . 3039
Lotrimin Topical Solution 1% . . . 3039

KADIAN (Canada)
MORPHINE SULFATE
Kadian Capsules . . . 577
MS Contin Tablets . . . 2701

KAILASA (Argentina)
CLARITHROMYCIN
Biaxin Filmtab Tablets . . . 402
Biaxin Granules . . . 402

KAINEVER (Portugal)
ESTAZOLAM
ProSom Tablets . . . 517

KAION RETARD (Chile)
POTASSIUM CHLORIDE
K-Dur Extended-Relase Tablets . . . 3033
K-Lor Oral Solution . . . 474
K-Tab Tablets . . . 475

KAIZEM (India)
DILTIAZEM HYDROCHLORIDE
Cardizem LA Extended Release Tablets . . . 1728
Tiazac Capsules . . . 1201

KAJOS (Norway, Sweden)
POTASSIUM CITRATE
Urocit-K Tablets . . . 2144

KALDYUM (Czech Republic, Hungary)
POTASSIUM CHLORIDE
K-Dur Extended-Relase Tablets . . . 3033
K-Lor Oral Solution . . . 474
K-Tab Tablets . . . 475

KALEORID (Denmark, France, Norway, Sweden)
POTASSIUM CHLORIDE
K-Dur Extended-Relase Tablets . . . 3033
K-Lor Oral Solution . . . 474
K-Tab Tablets . . . 475

KALICET (Italy)
FEXOFENADINE HYDROCHLORIDE
Allegra Capsules . . . 2844

KALIGLUTOL (Switzerland)
POTASSIUM CHLORIDE
K-Dur Extended-Relase Tablets . . . 3033
K-Lor Oral Solution . . . 474
K-Tab Tablets . . . 475

KALIJECT (Thailand)
POTASSIUM CHLORIDE
K-Dur Extended-Relase Tablets . . . 3033
K-Lor Oral Solution . . . 474
K-Tab Tablets . . . 475

KALILENTE (Norway, Sweden)
POTASSIUM CHLORIDE
K-Dur Extended-Relase Tablets . . . 3033
K-Lor Oral Solution . . . 474
K-Tab Tablets . . . 475

KALINORM (Denmark, Finland, Norway)
POTASSIUM CHLORIDE
K-Dur Extended-Relase Tablets . . . 3033
K-Lor Oral Solution . . . 474
K-Tab Tablets . . . 475

KALINOR-RETARD P (Germany)
POTASSIUM CHLORIDE
K-Dur Extended-Relase Tablets . . . 3033
K-Lor Oral Solution . . . 474
K-Tab Tablets . . . 475

KALIOLITE (Mexico)
POTASSIUM CHLORIDE
K-Dur Extended-Relase Tablets . . . 3033
K-Lor Oral Solution . . . 474
K-Tab Tablets . . . 475

KALIPOR (Sweden)
POTASSIUM CHLORIDE
K-Dur Extended-Relase Tablets . . . 3033
K-Lor Oral Solution . . . 474
K-Tab Tablets . . . 475

KALISOL (Finland)
POTASSIUM CHLORIDE
K-Dur Extended-Relase Tablets . . . 3033
K-Lor Oral Solution . . . 474
K-Tab Tablets . . . 475

KALISTERIL (Finland)
POTASSIUM CHLORIDE
K-Dur Extended-Relase Tablets . . . 3033
K-Lor Oral Solution . . . 474
K-Tab Tablets . . . 475

KALI-STEROP (Belgium)
POTASSIUM CHLORIDE
K-Dur Extended-Relase Tablets . . . 3033
K-Lor Oral Solution . . . 474
K-Tab Tablets . . . 475

KALITABS (Sweden)
POTASSIUM CHLORIDE
K-Dur Extended-Relase Tablets . . . 3033
K-Lor Oral Solution . . . 474
K-Tab Tablets . . . 475

KALITRANS RETARD (Germany)
POTASSIUM CHLORIDE
K-Dur Extended-Relase Tablets . . . 3033
K-Lor Oral Solution . . . 474
K-Tab Tablets . . . 475

KALIUM (Germany, Hong Kong)
POTASSIUM CITRATE
Urocit-K Tablets . . . 2144

KALIUM DURETTER (Finland, Sweden)
POTASSIUM CHLORIDE
K-Dur Extended-Relase Tablets . . . 3033
K-Lor Oral Solution . . . 474
K-Tab Tablets . . . 475

KALIUM DURETTES (Belgium, The Netherlands)
POTASSIUM CHLORIDE
K-Dur Extended-Relase Tablets . . . 3033
K-Lor Oral Solution . . . 474
K-Tab Tablets . . . 475

KALIUM DURULES (Canada, Hungary, Singapore)
POTASSIUM CHLORIDE
K-Dur Extended-Relase Tablets . . . 3033
K-Lor Oral Solution . . . 474
K-Tab Tablets . . . 475

KALIUM RETARD (Sweden)
POTASSIUM CHLORIDE
K-Dur Extended-Relase Tablets . . . 3033
K-Lor Oral Solution . . . 474
K-Tab Tablets . . . 475

KALIUM-DURILES (Germany)
POTASSIUM CHLORIDE
K-Dur Extended-Relase Tablets . . . 3033
K-Lor Oral Solution . . . 474
K-Tab Tablets . . . 475

KALIUM-R (Hungary)
POTASSIUM CHLORIDE
K-Dur Extended-Relase Tablets . . . 3033
K-Lor Oral Solution . . . 474
K-Tab Tablets . . . 475

KALIXOCIN (Australia)
CLARITHROMYCIN
Biaxin Filmtab Tablets . . . 402
Biaxin Granules . . . 402

KALNORMIN (Czech Republic)
POTASSIUM CHLORIDE
K-Dur Extended-Relase Tablets . . . 3033
K-Lor Oral Solution . . . 474
K-Tab Tablets . . . 475

KALPIREN (Russia)
ENALAPRIL MALEATE
Vasotec I.V. Injection . . . 2103

KALPRESS (Spain)
VALSARTAN
Diovan Tablets . . . 2193

KALPRESS PLUS (Spain)
VALSARTAN
Diovan Tablets . . . 2193

KALTIN MF (India)
METRONIDAZOLE
MetroGel-Vaginal Gel . . . 1855

KALURIL (Australia, Israel)
AMILORIDE HYDROCHLORIDE
Midamor Tablets . . . 2026

KAMICIN (Hong Kong)
CLOTRIMAZOLE
Lotrimin Cream . . . 3039
Lotrimin Lotion 1% . . . 3039
Lotrimin Topical Solution 1% . . . 3039

KANDISTAT (Brazil)
NYSTATIN
Nystop Topical Powder USP . . . 2478
Paddock Nystatin USP for Oral Suspension . . . 2478

KANEZIN (Thailand)
CLOTRIMAZOLE
Lotrimin Cream . . . 3039
Lotrimin Lotion 1% . . . 3039
Lotrimin Topical Solution 1% . . . 3039

KANOLONE (Thailand)
TRIAMCINOLONE ACETONIDE
Azmacort Inhalation Aerosol . . . 1726
Nasacort AQ Nasal Spray . . . 2922

KAOCHLOR (Canada)
POTASSIUM CHLORIDE
K-Dur Extended-Relase Tablets . . . 3033
K-Lor Oral Solution . . . 474
K-Tab Tablets . . . 475

KAPABLOC (Austria)
MORPHINE SULFATE
Kadian Capsules . . . 577
MS Contin Tablets . . . 2701

KAPANOL (Australia, Austria, Belgium, Denmark, France, Germany, Israel, Mexico, New Zealand, Norway, Switzerland, The Netherlands)
MORPHINE SULFATE
Kadian Capsules . . . 577
MS Contin Tablets . . . 2701

KAPARLON-S (Greece)
ENALAPRIL MALEATE
Vasotec I.V. Injection . . . 2103

KAPLON (United Kingdom)
CAPTOPRIL
Captopril Tablets **2149**

KARBAC (Brazil)
CARBAMAZEPINE
Carbatrol Capsules **3171**
Tegretol Chewable Tablets **2295**
Tegretol Suspension **2295**
Tegretol Tablets **2295**
Tegretol-XR Tablets **2295**

KARDIL (Norway)
DILTIAZEM HYDROCHLORIDE
Cardizem LA Extended Release Tablets . . . **1728**
Tiazac Capsules **1201**

KARIN (Israel)
CLARITHROMYCIN
Biaxin Filmtab Tablets **402**
Biaxin Granules **402**

KARISON (Germany)
CLOBETASOL PROPIONATE
Temovate Cream **2668**
Temovate E Emollient **2671**
Temovate Gel **2669**
Temovate Ointment **2668**
Temovate Scalp Application **2670**

KARON (Czech Republic)
ALPROSTADIL
Edex Injection **3089**

KARRER (Italy)
LEVOCARNITINE
Carnitor Injection **3188**
Carnitor Tablets and Oral Solution **3190**

KARVEA (Australia, Germany, Greece, Italy, Spain)
IRBESARTAN
Avapro Tablets **891**

KARVEZIDE (Australia, Germany, Italy, Spain)
IRBESARTAN
Avapro Tablets **891**

KASELE (Mexico)
POTASSIUM CHLORIDE
K-Dur Extended-Relase Tablets **3033**
K-Lor Oral Solution **474**
K-Tab Tablets **475**

KATA (Italy)
VERAPAMIL HYDROCHLORIDE
Covera-HS Tablets **3139**
Verelan PM Extended-Release Capsules, Controlled-Onset **3106**

KATION (Italy)
POTASSIUM CITRATE
Urocit-K Tablets **2144**

KATOPIL (Czech Republic)
CAPTOPRIL
Captopril Tablets **2149**

KATOPRIL (Singapore)
CAPTOPRIL
Captopril Tablets **2149**

KATTWILACT (Germany)
LACTULOSE
Kristalose for Oral Solution **1034**

KAVELOR (Venezuela)
SIMVASTATIN
Zocor Tablets **2105**

KAY CIEL (Australia, Canada)
POTASSIUM CHLORIDE
K-Dur Extended-Relase Tablets **3033**
K-Lor Oral Solution **474**
K-Tab Tablets **475**

KAY-CEE-L (Irish Republic, United Kingdom)
POTASSIUM CHLORIDE
K-Dur Extended-Relase Tablets **3033**
K-Lor Oral Solution **474**
K-Tab Tablets **475**

KAYEXALATE (Canada, France, Greece, Israel, Italy, Thailand, Venezuela)
SODIUM POLYSTYRENE SULFONATE
Kionex Powder **2477**

K-CITRA (Canada)
POTASSIUM CITRATE
Urocit-K Tablets **2144**

KCL-RETARD (Austria, Germany)
POTASSIUM CHLORIDE
K-Dur Extended-Relase Tablets **3033**
K-Lor Oral Solution **474**
K-Tab Tablets **475**

K-DUR (Canada, Mexico)
POTASSIUM CHLORIDE
K-Dur Extended-Relase Tablets **3033**
K-Lor Oral Solution **474**
K-Tab Tablets **475**

KEAL (France)
SUCRALFATE
Carafate Suspension **701**
Carafate Tablets **701**

KEBIRTECAN (Argentina)
IRINOTECAN HYDROCHLORIDE
Camptosar Injection **2604**

KECIFLOX (Germany)
CIPROFLOXACIN
Cipro Oral Suspension **2977**

KEEFLOXIN (Portugal)
CIPROFLOXACIN HYDROCHLORIDE
Ciloxan Ophthalmic Ointment . . . . ⊙**204, 559**
Ciloxan Ophthalmic Solution . . . . ⊙**206**
Cipro Tablets **2977**

KEFADIM (Belgium, Brazil, Czech Republic, Thailand, United Kingdom)
CEFTAZIDIME
Fortaz for Injection **1453**

KEFAMIN (Spain)
CEFTAZIDIME
Fortaz for Injection **1453**

KEFAZIM (Austria)
CEFTAZIDIME
Fortaz for Injection **1453**

KEFNIR (India)
CEFDINIR
Omnicef Capsules **511**
Omnicef for Oral Suspension **511**

KEFOX (Italy)
CEFUROXIME SODIUM
Zinacef Injection **1631**

KEFPOD (India)
CEFPODOXIME PROXETIL
Vantin Tablets and Oral Suspension **2645**

KEFTRAGARD (India)
CEFTRIAXONE SODIUM
Rocephin Injectable Vials, ADD-Vantage, Galaxy, Bulk **2800**

KEFTRIAXON (Israel)
CEFTRIAXONE SODIUM
Rocephin Injectable Vials, ADD-Vantage, Galaxy, Bulk **2800**

KEFURIM (Israel)
CEFUROXIME SODIUM
Zinacef Injection **1631**

KEFURION (Finland)
CEFUROXIME SODIUM
Zinacef Injection **1631**

KEFUROX (Belgium, Canada)
CEFUROXIME SODIUM
Zinacef Injection **1631**

KEFZIM (Chile, South Africa)
CEFTAZIDIME
Fortaz for Injection **1453**

KELA (Thailand)
TRIAMCINOLONE ACETONIDE
Azmacort Inhalation Aerosol **1726**
Nasacort AQ Nasal Spray **2922**

KELATIN (Belgium, The Netherlands)
PENICILLAMINE
Cuprimine Capsules **1947**

KELATINE (Portugal)
PENICILLAMINE
Cuprimine Capsules **1947**

KELBIUM (Spain)
CEFPODOXIME PROXETIL
Vantin Tablets and Oral Suspension **2645**

KELEFUSIN (Mexico)
POTASSIUM CHLORIDE
K-Dur Extended-Relase Tablets **3033**
K-Lor Oral Solution **474**
K-Tab Tablets **475**

KEMZID (Hong Kong, Singapore, Thailand)
TRIAMCINOLONE ACETONIDE
Azmacort Inhalation Aerosol **1726**
Nasacort AQ Nasal Spray **2922**

KENACORT (Belgium, France, Italy, Thailand)
TRIAMCINOLONE ACETONIDE
Azmacort Inhalation Aerosol **1726**
Nasacort AQ Nasal Spray **2922**

KENACORT-A (Argentina, Australia, Belgium, Chile, Greece, Hong Kong, Irish Republic, Malaysia, New Zealand, Singapore, Switzerland, The Netherlands)
TRIAMCINOLONE ACETONIDE
Azmacort Inhalation Aerosol **1726**
Nasacort AQ Nasal Spray **2922**

KENACORT-T (Finland, Norway, Sweden)
TRIAMCINOLONE ACETONIDE
Azmacort Inhalation Aerosol **1726**
Nasacort AQ Nasal Spray **2922**

KENALIN (Mexico)
SULINDAC
Clinoril Tablets **1924**

KENALOG (Canada, Czech Republic, Denmark, Germany, Hungary, Irish Republic, Israel, United Kingdom, Venezuela)
TRIAMCINOLONE ACETONIDE
Azmacort Inhalation Aerosol **1726**
Nasacort AQ Nasal Spray **2922**

KENALOG IN ORABASE (Australia, Canada, Hong Kong, Israel, Malaysia, New Zealand, Singapore, South Africa, Spain, Thailand)
TRIAMCINOLONE ACETONIDE
Azmacort Inhalation Aerosol **1726**
Nasacort AQ Nasal Spray **2922**

KENALONE (Australia)
TRIAMCINOLONE ACETONIDE
Azmacort Inhalation Aerosol **1726**
Nasacort AQ Nasal Spray **2922**

KENAPRIL (Mexico)
CAPTOPRIL
Captopril Tablets **2149**

KENAPROL (Mexico)
METOPROLOL TARTRATE
Lopressor Tablets **2238**

KENAPROX (Mexico)
NAPROXEN
EC-Naprosyn Delayed-Release Tablets **2761**
Naprosyn Suspension **2761**
Naprosyn Tablets **2761**

KENBRID (Mexico)
ISOSORBIDE MONONITRATE
Imdur Tablets **3018**

KENERGON (Switzerland)
LIDOCAINE
Lidoderm Patch **1118**

KENESIL (Spain)
NIMODIPINE
Nimotop Capsules **749**

KENICET (Mexico)
CETIRIZINE HYDROCHLORIDE
Zyrtec Syrup **2594**
Zyrtec Tablets **2594**

KENO (Thailand)
TRIAMCINOLONE ACETONIDE
Azmacort Inhalation Aerosol **1726**
Nasacort AQ Nasal Spray **2922**

KENOIDAL (Belgium)
TRIAMCINOLONE ACETONIDE
Azmacort Inhalation Aerosol **1726**
Nasacort AQ Nasal Spray **2922**

KENOKET (Mexico)
CLONAZEPAM
Klonopin Tablets **2778**

KENOLAN (Mexico)
CAPTOPRIL
Captopril Tablets **2149**

KENOPRIL (Mexico)
ENALAPRIL MALEATE
Vasotec I.V. Injection **2103**

KENSEDAL (Mexico)
NAPROXEN
EC-Naprosyn Delayed-Release Tablets **2761**
Naprosyn Suspension **2761**
Naprosyn Tablets **2761**

KENZEN (France)
CANDESARTAN CILEXETIL
Atacand Tablets **649**

KENZOFLEX (Mexico)
CIPROFLOXACIN HYDROCHLORIDE
Ciloxan Ophthalmic Ointment . . . . ⊙**204, 559**
Ciloxan Ophthalmic Solution . . . . ⊙**206**
Cipro Tablets **2977**

KENZOLOL (Mexico)
NIMODIPINE
Nimotop Capsules **749**

KERLOCAL (France)
TRETINOIN
Vesanoid Capsules **2820**

KERLON (Denmark, Finland, Italy, Sweden, Switzerland, The Netherlands)
BETAXOLOL HYDROCHLORIDE
Betoptic S Ophthalmic Suspension . ⊙**203, 558**

KERLONE (Austria, Belgium, France, Germany, Greece, Hong Kong, Israel, Malaysia, Singapore, Spain, Thailand, United Kingdom)
BETAXOLOL HYDROCHLORIDE
Betoptic S Ophthalmic Suspension . ⊙**203, 558**

KERLONG (Japan)
BETAXOLOL HYDROCHLORIDE
Betoptic S Ophthalmic Suspension . ⊙**203, 558**

KERNIT (Italy)
LEVOCARNITINE
Carnitor Injection **3188**
Carnitor Tablets and Oral Solution **3190**

KESINT (Italy)
CEFUROXIME SODIUM
Zinacef Injection **1631**

KESS (Argentina)
LAMIVUDINE
Epivir Oral Solution **1427**
Epivir Tablets **1427**
Epivir-HBV Oral Solution **1432**
Epivir-HBV Tablets **1432**

KESS COMPLEX (Argentina)
LAMIVUDINE
Epivir Oral Solution **1427**
Epivir Tablets **1427**
Epivir-HBV Oral Solution **1432**
Epivir-HBV Tablets **1432**

KESTERINA (Venezuela)
CEFTAZIDIME
Fortaz for Injection **1453**

KETANINE (Singapore)
CAPTOPRIL
Captopril Tablets **2149**

KETIDIN (Argentina)
RALOXIFENE HYDROCHLORIDE
Evista Tablets **1763**

KETOCEF (Russia)
CEFUROXIME SODIUM
Zinacef Injection **1631**

KETREL (France, Portugal)
TRETINOIN
Vesanoid Capsules **2820**

KEVAL (Mexico)
LANSOPRAZOLE
Prevacid Delayed-Release Capsules **3271**

KEXELATE (South Africa)
SODIUM POLYSTYRENE SULFONATE
Kionex Powder **2477**

K-EXIT (Canada)
SODIUM POLYSTYRENE SULFONATE
Kionex Powder **2477**

KEYERPRIL (Mexico)
CAPTOPRIL
Captopril Tablets **2149**

KEYLYTE (India)
POTASSIUM CHLORIDE
K-Dur Extended-Relase Tablets **3033**
K-Lor Oral Solution **474**
K-Tab Tablets **475**

KEZEPIN (Mexico)
CARBAMAZEPINE
Carbatrol Capsules **3171**

Tegretol Chewable Tablets . . . 2295
Tegretol Suspension . . . 2295
Tegretol Tablets . . . 2295
Tegretol-XR Tablets . . . 2295

KIATRIUM (Brazil)
DIAZEPAM
Diastat Rectal Delivery System . . . 3343
Valium Tablets . . . 2819

KIDROLASE (Argentina, Canada, Czech Republic, France, Israel)
ASPARAGINASE
Elspar for Injection . . . 2463

KILLIT (Brazil)
FLUOROURACIL
Efudex Topical Cream . . . 3363
Efudex Topical Solutions . . . 3363

KIMAFAN (Hong Kong)
CAPTOPRIL
Captopril Tablets . . . 2149

KINABIDE (Argentina)
SELEGILINE HYDROCHLORIDE
Eldepryl Capsules . . . 3208

KINASTEN (Brazil)
CLOTRIMAZOLE
Lotrimin Cream . . . 3039
Lotrimin Lotion 1% . . . 3039
Lotrimin Topical Solution 1% . . . 3039

KINDAREN (Brazil)
DICLOFENAC SODIUM
Voltaren Tablets . . . 2307
Voltaren-XR Tablets . . . 2310

KINESTREL (Mexico)
AMANTADINE HYDROCHLORIDE
Symmetrel Tablets . . . 1135

KINFIL D (Argentina)
ENALAPRIL MALEATE
Vasotec I.V. Injection . . . 2103

KINLINE (Thailand)
SELEGILINE HYDROCHLORIDE
Eldepryl Capsules . . . 3208

KINZAL (Switzerland)
TELMISARTAN
Micardis Tablets . . . 854

KINZALKOMB (Belgium, Denmark, Finland, Germany, Sweden)
TELMISARTAN
Micardis Tablets . . . 854

KINZALMONO (Belgium, Denmark, Finland, Germany, Sweden)
TELMISARTAN
Micardis Tablets . . . 854

KINZALPLUS (Switzerland)
TELMISARTAN
Micardis Tablets . . . 854

KIPRES (Japan)
MONTELUKAST SODIUM
Singulair Chewable Tablets . . . 2077
Singulair Tablets . . . 2077

KIR RICHTER (Italy)
APROTININ
Trasylol Injection . . . 754

KITACNE (Argentina)
ERYTHROMYCIN
Ery-Tab Tablets . . . 449
Erythromycin Base Filmtab Tablets . . . 455
Erythromycin Delayed-Release Capsules, USP . . . 457
PCE Dispertab Tablets . . . 515

KITACNE AR (Argentina)
ERYTHROMYCIN
Ery-Tab Tablets . . . 449
Erythromycin Base Filmtab Tablets . . . 455
Erythromycin Delayed-Release Capsules, USP . . . 457
PCE Dispertab Tablets . . . 515

KITACNE PB (Argentina)
ERYTHROMYCIN
Ery-Tab Tablets . . . 449
Erythromycin Base Filmtab Tablets . . . 455
Erythromycin Delayed-Release Capsules, USP . . . 457
PCE Dispertab Tablets . . . 515

KITON (Italy)
ISOSORBIDE MONONITRATE
Imdur Tablets . . . 3018

KLABAX (Russia)
CLARITHROMYCIN
Biaxin Filmtab Tablets . . . 402
Biaxin Granules . . . 402

KLABET (Mexico)
CLARITHROMYCIN
Biaxin Filmtab Tablets . . . 402
Biaxin Granules . . . 402

KLACID (Australia, Czech Republic, Denmark, Finland, Germany, Hungary, Irish Republic, Israel, Italy, Malaysia, New Zealand, Norway, Portugal, Russia, Singapore, South Africa, Spain, Sweden, Thailand, The Netherlands)
CLARITHROMYCIN
Biaxin Filmtab Tablets . . . 402
Biaxin Granules . . . 402

KLACIPED (Switzerland)
CLARITHROMYCIN
Biaxin Filmtab Tablets . . . 402
Biaxin Granules . . . 402

KLAMACIN (Thailand)
CLOTRIMAZOLE
Lotrimin Cream . . . 3039
Lotrimin Lotion 1% . . . 3039
Lotrimin Topical Solution 1% . . . 3039

KLAMIRAN (Hungary)
CLARITHROMYCIN
Biaxin Filmtab Tablets . . . 402
Biaxin Granules . . . 402

KLARI (Hungary)
CLARITHROMYCIN
Biaxin Filmtab Tablets . . . 402
Biaxin Granules . . . 402

KLARICID (Argentina, Brazil, Chile, Greece, The Netherlands, United Kingdom, Venezuela)
CLARITHROMYCIN
Biaxin Filmtab Tablets . . . 402
Biaxin Granules . . . 402

KLARIDEX (Israel)
CLARITHROMYCIN
Biaxin Filmtab Tablets . . . 402
Biaxin Granules . . . 402

KLARIFAR (Greece)
CLARITHROMYCIN
Biaxin Filmtab Tablets . . . 402
Biaxin Granules . . . 402

KLARITHRIN (Greece)
CLARITHROMYCIN
Biaxin Filmtab Tablets . . . 402
Biaxin Granules . . . 402

KLARITRIL (Brazil)
CLARITHROMYCIN
Biaxin Filmtab Tablets . . . 402
Biaxin Granules . . . 402

KLARIX (Mexico)
CLARITHROMYCIN
Biaxin Filmtab Tablets . . . 402
Biaxin Granules . . . 402

KLARMYN (Mexico)
CLARITHROMYCIN
Biaxin Filmtab Tablets . . . 402
Biaxin Granules . . . 402

KLARON (Israel)
SULFACETAMIDE SODIUM
Klaron Lotion 10% . . . 2909

KLARPHARMA (Mexico)
CLARITHROMYCIN
Biaxin Filmtab Tablets . . . 402
Biaxin Granules . . . 402

KLEREN (Venezuela)
NIMODIPINE
Nimotop Capsules . . . 749

KLERIMED (Hong Kong, Russia, Singapore)
CLARITHROMYCIN
Biaxin Filmtab Tablets . . . 402
Biaxin Granules . . . 402

KLEXANE (Denmark, Finland, Norway, Sweden)
ENOXAPARIN SODIUM
Lovenox Injection . . . 2915

KLIANE (Czech Republic)
ESTRADIOL
Climara Transdermal System . . . 771
Estring Vaginal Ring . . . 2635

KLICINA (Venezuela)
CIPROFLOXACIN
Cipro Oral Suspension . . . 2977

KLIMAPUR (Austria)
ESTRADIOL
Climara Transdermal System . . . 771
Estring Vaginal Ring . . . 2635

KLIMAREDUCT (Austria)
ESTRADIOL
Climara Transdermal System . . . 771
Estring Vaginal Ring . . . 2635

KLIMICIN (Czech Republic, Hungary)
CLINDAMYCIN HYDROCHLORIDE
Cleocin Vaginal Ovules . . . 2616

KLINOTAL (Venezuela)
FAMOTIDINE
Pepcid Injection . . . 2040
Pepcid Injection Premixed . . . 2040
Pepcid Tablets . . . 2038
Pepcid for Oral Suspension . . . 2038

KLINOXID (Germany)
BENZOYL PEROXIDE
Brevoxyl-4 Creamy Wash . . . 3210
Brevoxyl-4 Gel . . . 3210
Brevoxyl-8 Creamy Wash . . . 3210
Brevoxyl-8 Gel . . . 3210
Triaz Cleanser . . . 1892
Triaz Gel . . . 1892

KLIOFEM (United Kingdom)
ESTRADIOL
Climara Transdermal System . . . 771
Estring Vaginal Ring . . . 2635

KLIOGEST (Argentina, Australia, Belgium, Brazil, Czech Republic, Hungary, Malaysia, New Zealand)
ESTRADIOL
Climara Transdermal System . . . 771
Estring Vaginal Ring . . . 2635

KLION (Czech Republic, Hungary, Russia, Thailand)
METRONIDAZOLE
MetroGel-Vaginal Gel . . . 1855

KLION-D (Czech Republic, Hungary)
METRONIDAZOLE
MetroGel-Vaginal Gel . . . 1855

KLIOVANCE (Australia, New Zealand)
ESTRADIOL
Climara Transdermal System . . . 771
Estring Vaginal Ring . . . 2635

KLODIN (Italy)
TICLOPIDINE HYDROCHLORIDE
Ticlid Tablets . . . 2810

KLODIPIN (Portugal)
TICLOPIDINE HYDROCHLORIDE
Ticlid Tablets . . . 2810

KLOMAZOLE (Argentina)
CLOTRIMAZOLE
Lotrimin Cream . . . 3039
Lotrimin Lotion 1% . . . 3039
Lotrimin Topical Solution 1% . . . 3039

KLONACID (Argentina)
CLARITHROMYCIN
Biaxin Filmtab Tablets . . . 402
Biaxin Granules . . . 402

KLONALFLOX (Argentina)
OFLOXACIN
Floxin Otic Solution . . . 1049

KLONALMOX (Argentina)
AMOXICILLIN
Amoxil Pediatric Drops for Oral Suspension . . . 1343
Amoxil Tablets . . . 1343

KLONAMICIN (Argentina)
TOBRAMYCIN
TOBI Solution for Inhalation . . . 2298

KLONAMICIN COMPUESTO (Argentina)
TOBRAMYCIN
TOBI Solution for Inhalation . . . 2298

KLONAPROST (Argentina)
LATANOPROST
Xalatan Ophthalmic Solution . . . ⊙291

KLONASTIN (Argentina)
SIMVASTATIN
Zocor Tablets . . . 2105

K-LONG (Canada)
POTASSIUM CHLORIDE
K-Dur Extended-Relase Tablets . . . 3033
K-Lor Oral Solution . . . 474
K-Tab Tablets . . . 475

KLONT (Thailand)
METRONIDAZOLE
MetroGel Vaginal Gel . . . 1855

K-LOR (Canada)
POTASSIUM CHLORIDE
K-Dur Extended-Relase Tablets . . . 3033
K-Lor Oral Solution . . . 474
K-Tab Tablets . . . 475

KLOREN (Brazil)
POTASSIUM CHLORIDE
K-Dur Extended-Relase Tablets . . . 3033
K-Lor Oral Solution . . . 474
K-Tab Tablets . . . 475

KLORPO (Singapore)
CHLORDIAZEPOXIDE HYDROCHLORIDE
Librium Capsules . . . 3347

KLOSARTAN D (Argentina)
LOSARTAN POTASSIUM
Cozaar Tablets . . . 1935

KLOTRICID (Finland)
CLOTRIMAZOLE
Lotrimin Cream . . . 3039
Lotrimin Lotion 1% . . . 3039
Lotrimin Topical Solution 1% . . . 3039

K-LYTE (Canada)
POTASSIUM CITRATE
Urocit-K Tablets . . . 2144

K-LYTE/CL (Canada)
POTASSIUM CHLORIDE
K-Dur Extended-Relase Tablets . . . 3033
K-Lor Oral Solution . . . 474
K-Tab Tablets . . . 475

K-MED 900 (Canada)
POTASSIUM CHLORIDE
K-Dur Extended-Relase Tablets . . . 3033
K-Lor Oral Solution . . . 474
K-Tab Tablets . . . 475

K-MIC (Sweden)
POTASSIUM CHLORIDE
K-Dur Extended-Relase Tablets . . . 3033
K-Lor Oral Solution . . . 474
K-Tab Tablets . . . 475

KODAKON (Mexico)
DEXAMETHASONE
Decadron Tablets . . . 1951

KOFRON (Spain)
CLARITHROMYCIN
Biaxin Filmtab Tablets . . . 402
Biaxin Granules . . . 402

KOLKIN (Argentina)
FUROSEMIDE
Furosemide Tablets . . . 2154

KOLPAZOL (Brazil)
NYSTATIN
Nystop Topical Powder USP . . . 2478
Paddock Nystatin USP for Oral Suspension . . . 2478

KOLPOVENT (Chile)
SALMETEROL XINAFOATE
Serevent Diskus . . . 1568

KONIFUNGIL (Chile)
CLOTRIMAZOLE
Lotrimin Cream . . . 3039
Lotrimin Lotion 1% . . . 3039
Lotrimin Topical Solution 1% . . . 3039

KONOVID (Thailand)
OFLOXACIN
Floxin Otic Solution . . . 1049

KONTIC (Greece)
ENALAPRIL MALEATE
Vasotec I.V. Injection . . . 2103

KOPTILAN (Greece)
LEVOCARNITINE
Carnitor Injection . . . 3188
Carnitor Tablets and Oral Solution . . . 3190

KORANDIL (Singapore, Thailand)
ENALAPRIL MALEATE
Vasotec I.V. Injection . . . 2103

(⊙ Described in PDR For Ophthalmic Medicines™)

KORNAM (Czech Republic, Hungary, Russia)
TERAZOSIN HYDROCHLORIDE
Hytrin Capsules . . . 471

KORTIKOID-RATIOPHARM (Germany)
TRIAMCINOLONE ACETONIDE
Azmacort Inhalation Aerosol . . . 1726
Nasacort AQ Nasal Spray . . . 2922

KOSTEO (Australia)
CALCITRIOL
Calcijex Injection . . . 411
Rocaltrol Capsules . . . 2798
Rocaltrol Oral Solution . . . 2798

KRATIUM (Hong Kong)
DIAZEPAM
Diastat Rectal Delivery System . . . 3343
Valium Tablets . . . 2819

KRAUTIN (Greece)
SELEGILINE HYDROCHLORIDE
Eldepryl Capsules . . . 3208

KREBSILASI (Italy)
PANCRELIPASE
Ultrase Capsules . . . 708
Ultrase MT Capsules . . . 709

KREDEX (Australia, Belgium, France, Italy, Norway, Portugal, Spain, Sweden)
CARVEDILOL
Coreg Tablets . . . 1414

KRENOSIN (France, Italy, Mexico)
ADENOSINE
Adenocard Injection . . . 617
Adenoscan . . . 619

KRENOSINE (Switzerland)
ADENOSINE
Adenocard Injection . . . 617
Adenoscan . . . 619

KRIADEX (Mexico)
CLONAZEPAM
Klonopin Tablets . . . 2778

KROBICIN (Mexico)
CLARITHROMYCIN
Biaxin Filmtab Tablets . . . 402
Biaxin Granules . . . 402

K-SAN (Australia)
POTASSIUM CHLORIDE
K-Dur Extended-Relase Tablets . . . 3033
K-Lor Oral Solution . . . 474
K-Tab Tablets . . . 475

KSR (Australia, Hong Kong)
POTASSIUM CHLORIDE
K-Dur Extended-Relase Tablets . . . 3033
K-Lor Oral Solution . . . 474
K-Tab Tablets . . . 475

K-SR (New Zealand)
POTASSIUM CHLORIDE
K-Dur Extended-Relase Tablets . . . 3033
K-Lor Oral Solution . . . 474
K-Tab Tablets . . . 475

KURACID (Denmark)
RANITIDINE HYDROCHLORIDE
Zantac 25 EFFERdose Tablets . . . 1624
Zantac 150 EFFERdose Tablets . . . 1624
Zantac 150 Tablets . . . 1624
Zantac 300 Tablets . . . 1624
Zantac Injection . . . 1619
Zantac Injection Premixed . . . 1619
Zantac Syrup . . . 1624

KYMAZOL (Greece)
SIMVASTATIN
Zocor Tablets . . . 2105

KYYPAKKAUS (Finland)
HYDROCORTISONE
Hydrocortone Tablets . . . 1989

LA MORPH (New Zealand)
MORPHINE SULFATE
Kadian Capsules . . . 577
MS Contin Tablets . . . 2701

LABEL (Brazil)
RANITIDINE HYDROCHLORIDE
Zantac 25 EFFERdose Tablets . . . 1624
Zantac 150 EFFERdose Tablets . . . 1624
Zantac 150 Tablets . . . 1624
Zantac 300 Tablets . . . 1624
Zantac Injection . . . 1619
Zantac Injection Premixed . . . 1619
Zantac Syrup . . . 1624

LABENDA (Thailand)
ALBENDAZOLE
Albenza Tablets . . . 1338

LABENTROL (Greece)
CIPROFLOXACIN HYDROCHLORIDE
Ciloxan Ophthalmic Ointment . . . ⊙204, 559
Ciloxan Ophthalmic Solution . . . ⊙206
Cipro Tablets . . . 2977

LABILENO (Spain)
LAMOTRIGINE
Lamictal Chewable Dispersible Tablets . . . 1481
Lamictal Tablets . . . 1481

LABILEX (Greece)
CEFTRIAXONE SODIUM
Rocephin Injectable Vials, ADD-Vantage, Galaxy, Bulk . . . 2800

LABISTATIN (Argentina)
SIMVASTATIN
Zocor Tablets . . . 2105

LABITRIX (Mexico)
METRONIDAZOLE
MetroGel-Vaginal Gel . . . 1855

LABOCNE (Chile)
ERYTHROMYCIN
Ery-Tab Tablets . . . 449
Erythromycin Base Filmtab Tablets . . . 455
Erythromycin Delayed-Release Capsules, USP . . . 457
PCE Dispertab Tablets . . . 515

LABODREX (Spain)
BENAZEPRIL HYDROCHLORIDE
Lotensin Tablets . . . 2243

LABOPAL (Spain)
BENAZEPRIL HYDROCHLORIDE
Lotensin Tablets . . . 2243

LABOTEROL (Chile)
CLOTRIMAZOLE
Lotrimin Cream . . . 3039
Lotrimin Lotion 1% . . . 3039
Lotrimin Topical Solution 1% . . . 3039

LAC-DOL (Australia)
LACTULOSE
Kristalose for Oral Solution . . . 1034

LACEROL (Spain)
DILTIAZEM HYDROCHLORIDE
Cardizem LA Extended Release Tablets . . . 1728
Tiazac Capsules . . . 1201

LACIN (Thailand)
CLINDAMYCIN HYDROCHLORIDE
Cleocin Vaginal Ovules . . . 2616

LACRIPHARMA (Argentina)
SODIUM HYALURONATE
Hyalgan Solution . . . 2901

LACROMYCIN (Israel)
GENTAMICIN SULFATE
Garamycin Injectable . . . 3014

LACSON (South Africa)
LACTULOSE
Kristalose for Oral Solution . . . 1034

LACTICARE-HC (Chile, Hong Kong, Mexico, Venezuela)
HYDROCORTISONE
Hydrocortone Tablets . . . 1989

LACTID HC (Argentina)
HYDROCORTISONE
Hydrocortone Tablets . . . 1989

LACTISONA (Portugal, Spain)
HYDROCORTISONE
Hydrocortone Tablets . . . 1989

LACTOCUR (Australia, Germany)
LACTULOSE
Kristalose for Oral Solution . . . 1034

LACTOFALK (Germany)
LACTULOSE
Kristalose for Oral Solution . . . 1034

LACTOGER (Italy)
LACTULOSE
Kristalose for Oral Solution . . . 1034

LACTUFLOR (Germany)
LACTULOSE
Kristalose for Oral Solution . . . 1034

LACTUGAL (United Kingdom)
LACTULOSE
Kristalose for Oral Solution . . . 1034

LACTUL (Malaysia)
LACTULOSE
Kristalose for Oral Solution . . . 1034

LACTULAX (Canada, Israel, Mexico)
LACTULOSE
Kristalose for Oral Solution . . . 1034

LACTULON (Argentina)
LACTULOSE
Kristalose for Oral Solution . . . 1034

LACTULONA (Brazil, Venezuela)
LACTULOSE
Kristalose for Oral Solution . . . 1034

LACTUMED (Malaysia)
LACTULOSE
Kristalose for Oral Solution . . . 1034

LACTUS (Singapore)
LACTULOSE
Kristalose for Oral Solution . . . 1034

LACTUVERLAN (Germany)
LACTULOSE
Kristalose for Oral Solution . . . 1034

LACTYL (Italy)
LACTULOSE
Kristalose for Oral Solution . . . 1034

LADIWIN (India)
LAMIVUDINE
Epivir Oral Solution . . . 1427
Epivir Tablets . . . 1427
Epivir-HBV Oral Solution . . . 1432
Epivir-HBV Tablets . . . 1432

LAEVILAC S (Germany)
LACTULOSE
Kristalose for Oral Solution . . . 1034

LAEVOLAC (Austria, Czech Republic, Hong Kong, Hungary, Israel, Italy, New Zealand, Portugal, South Africa, Switzerland, Thailand)
LACTULOSE
Kristalose for Oral Solution . . . 1034

LAFEDAM (Argentina)
ALENDRONATE SODIUM
Fosamax Tablets . . . 1969

LAFELAX (Argentina)
LACTULOSE
Kristalose for Oral Solution . . . 1034

LAFIN (Mexico)
LANSOPRAZOLE
Prevacid Delayed-Release Capsules . . . 3271

LA-FU (Czech Republic)
FLUOROURACIL
Efudex Topical Cream . . . 3363
Efudex Topical Solutions . . . 3363

LAFUREX (Italy)
CEFUROXIME SODIUM
Zinacef Injection . . . 1631

LAGARMICIN (Spain)
ERYTHROMYCIN STEARATE
Erythrocin Stearate Filmtab Tablets . . . 453

LAGOTRAN (Argentina)
LAMOTRIGINE
Lamictal Chewable Dispersible Tablets . . . 1481
Lamictal Tablets . . . 1481

LAGRICEL (Mexico)
SODIUM HYALURONATE
Hyalgan Solution . . . 2901

LAGRICEL OFTENO (Chile)
SODIUM HYALURONATE
Hyalgan Solution . . . 2901

LAGUR (Brazil)
CLARITHROMYCIN
Biaxin Filmtab Tablets . . . 402
Biaxin Granules . . . 402

LAGYLAN (Mexico)
METRONIDAZOLE
MetroGel-Vaginal Gel . . . 1855

LAKE (Spain)
RANITIDINE HYDROCHLORIDE
Zantac 25 EFFERdose Tablets . . . 1624
Zantac 150 EFFERdose Tablets . . . 1624
Zantac 150 Tablets . . . 1624
Zantac 300 Tablets . . . 1624
Zantac Injection . . . 1619
Zantac Injection Premixed . . . 1619
Zantac Syrup . . . 1624

LAKTIPEX (Sweden)
LACTULOSE
Kristalose for Oral Solution . . . 1034

LAKTULAX (Austria)
LACTULOSE
Kristalose for Oral Solution . . . 1034

LAMBLIT (Mexico)
METRONIDAZOLE
MetroGel-Vaginal Gel . . . 1855

LAMDA (India)
LAMIVUDINE
Epivir Oral Solution . . . 1427
Epivir Tablets . . . 1427
Epivir-HBV Oral Solution . . . 1432
Epivir-HBV Tablets . . . 1432

LAMDA-Z (India)
LAMIVUDINE
Epivir Oral Solution . . . 1427
Epivir Tablets . . . 1427
Epivir-HBV Oral Solution . . . 1432
Epivir-HBV Tablets . . . 1432

LAMEPIL (India)
LAMOTRIGINE
Lamictal Chewable Dispersible Tablets . . . 1481
Lamictal Tablets . . . 1481

LAMETEC (India)
LAMOTRIGINE
Lamictal Chewable Dispersible Tablets . . . 1481
Lamictal Tablets . . . 1481

LAMI (Brazil)
LAMIVUDINE
Epivir Oral Solution . . . 1427
Epivir Tablets . . . 1427
Epivir-HBV Oral Solution . . . 1432
Epivir-HBV Tablets . . . 1432

LAMIBERGEN (Argentina)
LAMIVUDINE
Epivir Oral Solution . . . 1427
Epivir Tablets . . . 1427
Epivir-HBV Oral Solution . . . 1432
Epivir-HBV Tablets . . . 1432

LAMICSTART (France)
LAMOTRIGINE
Lamictal Chewable Dispersible Tablets . . . 1481
Lamictal Tablets . . . 1481

LAMICTAL (Argentina, Australia, Austria, Belgium, Brazil, Canada, Chile, Czech Republic, Denmark, Finland, France, Germany, Greece, Hong Kong, Hungary, Irish Republic, Israel, Italy, Malaysia, Mexico, New Zealand, Norway, Portugal, Russia, Singapore, Spain, Sweden, Switzerland, Thailand, The Netherlands, United Kingdom, Venezuela)
LAMOTRIGINE
Lamictal Chewable Dispersible Tablets . . . 1481
Lamictal Tablets . . . 1481

LAMICTIN (South Africa)
LAMOTRIGINE
Lamictal Chewable Dispersible Tablets . . . 1481
Lamictal Tablets . . . 1481

LAMIDAC (India)
LAMIVUDINE
Epivir Oral Solution . . . 1427
Epivir Tablets . . . 1427
Epivir-HBV Oral Solution . . . 1432
Epivir-HBV Tablets . . . 1432

LAMIDEN (Brazil)
LAMIVUDINE
Epivir Oral Solution . . . 1427
Epivir Tablets . . . 1427
Epivir-HBV Oral Solution . . . 1432
Epivir-HBV Tablets . . . 1432

LAMILEA (Argentina)
LAMIVUDINE
Epivir Oral Solution . . . 1427
Epivir Tablets . . . 1427
Epivir-HBV Oral Solution . . . 1432
Epivir-HBV Tablets . . . 1432

LAMIRAX (Argentina)
LAMOTRIGINE
Lamictal Chewable Dispersible Tablets . . . 1481

Lamictal Tablets ... 1481

LAMIREX (India)
LAMIVUDINE
Epivir Oral Solution ... 1427
Epivir Tablets ... 1427
Epivir-HBV Oral Solution ... 1432
Epivir-HBV Tablets ... 1432

LAMISIL (Argentina, Belgium, Canada, Czech Republic, Denmark, Finland, France, Germany, Hong Kong, India, Irish Republic, Italy, Mexico, New Zealand, Portugal, Singapore, South Africa, Spain, Thailand, The Netherlands, United Kingdom)
TERBINAFINE HYDROCHLORIDE
Lamisil Tablets ... 2232

LAMITOR (Brazil, The Netherlands)
LAMOTRIGINE
Lamictal Chewable Dispersible Tablets ... 1481
Lamictal Tablets ... 1481

LAMITRIN (Australia)
LAMOTRIGINE
Lamictal Chewable Dispersible Tablets ... 1481
Lamictal Tablets ... 1481

LAMIVIR (India)
LAMIVUDINE
Epivir Oral Solution ... 1427
Epivir Tablets ... 1427
Epivir-HBV Oral Solution ... 1432
Epivir-HBV Tablets ... 1432

LAMIVIR S (India)
LAMIVUDINE
Epivir Oral Solution ... 1427
Epivir Tablets ... 1427
Epivir-HBV Oral Solution ... 1432
Epivir-HBV Tablets ... 1432

LAMODEX (Israel)
LAMOTRIGINE
Lamictal Chewable Dispersible Tablets ... 1481
Lamictal Tablets ... 1481

LAMOGINE (Israel)
LAMOTRIGINE
Lamictal Chewable Dispersible Tablets ... 1481
Lamictal Tablets ... 1481

LAMPOSPORIN (Italy)
CEFUROXIME SODIUM
Zinacef Injection ... 1631

LAMRA (Germany)
DIAZEPAM
Diastat Rectal Delivery System ... 3343
Valium Tablets ... 2819

LAMUZID (India)
LAMIVUDINE
Epivir Oral Solution ... 1427
Epivir Tablets ... 1427
Epivir-HBV Oral Solution ... 1432
Epivir-HBV Tablets ... 1432

LANACARD (Germany)
DIGOXIN
Lanoxicaps Capsules ... 1490
Lanoxin Injection ... 1494
Lanoxin Injection Pediatric ... 1497
Lanoxin Tablets ... 1500

LANACORDIN (Spain)
DIGOXIN
Lanoxicaps Capsules ... 1490
Lanoxin Injection ... 1494
Lanoxin Injection Pediatric ... 1497
Lanoxin Tablets ... 1500

LANACRIST (Sweden)
DIGOXIN
Lanoxicaps Capsules ... 1490
Lanoxin Injection ... 1494
Lanoxin Injection Pediatric ... 1497
Lanoxin Tablets ... 1500

LANALGET (Austria)
TRAMADOL HYDROCHLORIDE
Ultram ER Tablets ... 2392

LANATIN (Denmark)
LISINOPRIL
Prinivil Tablets ... 2052

LANCUS (India)
LANSOPRAZOLE
Prevacid Delayed-Release Capsules ... 3271

LANDOLAXIN (Greece)
LISINOPRIL
Prinivil Tablets ... 2052

LANDROLEN (Mexico)
ALENDRONATE SODIUM
Fosamax Tablets ... 1969

LANEXAT (Argentina, Brazil, Chile, Denmark, Finland, Mexico, Sweden, Venezuela)
FLUMAZENIL
Romazicon Injection ... 2804

LANFAST (United Arab Emirates)
LANSOPRAZOLE
Prevacid Delayed-Release Capsules ... 3271

LANICOR (Argentina, Austria, Germany, Italy, The Netherlands, Venezuela)
DIGOXIN
Lanoxicaps Capsules ... 1490
Lanoxin Injection ... 1494
Lanoxin Injection Pediatric ... 1497
Lanoxin Tablets ... 1500

LANITOP (Venezuela)
DIGOXIN
Lanoxicaps Capsules ... 1490
Lanoxin Injection ... 1494
Lanoxin Injection Pediatric ... 1497
Lanoxin Tablets ... 1500

LANOC (Austria)
METOPROLOL TARTRATE
Lopressor Tablets ... 2238

LANODIZOL (Mexico)
LANSOPRAZOLE
Prevacid Delayed-Release Capsules ... 3271

LANOGASTRO (Brazil)
LANSOPRAZOLE
Prevacid Delayed-Release Capsules ... 3271

LANOLEPT (Austria)
CLOZAPINE
Clozaril Tablets ... 2184

LANOXICAPS (The Netherlands)
DIGOXIN
Lanoxicaps Capsules ... 1490
Lanoxin Injection ... 1494
Lanoxin Injection Pediatric ... 1497
Lanoxin Tablets ... 1500

LANOXIN (Argentina, Australia, Belgium, Brazil, Canada, Hong Kong, India, Irish Republic, Israel, Italy, Malaysia, Mexico, New Zealand, Norway, Portugal, Singapore, South Africa, Sweden, Switzerland, Thailand, The Netherlands, United Kingdom)
DIGOXIN
Lanoxicaps Capsules ... 1490
Lanoxin Injection ... 1494
Lanoxin Injection Pediatric ... 1497
Lanoxin Tablets ... 1500

LANSONE (Czech Republic, Hungary)
LANSOPRAZOLE
Prevacid Delayed-Release Capsules ... 3271

LANSOPRID (Brazil)
LANSOPRAZOLE
Prevacid Delayed-Release Capsules ... 3271

LANSOVAX (Venezuela)
LANSOPRAZOLE
Prevacid Delayed-Release Capsules ... 3271

LANSOX (Italy, Portugal)
LANSOPRAZOLE
Prevacid Delayed-Release Capsules ... 3271

LANTOGENT (Spain)
GENTAMICIN SULFATE
Garamycin Injectable ... 3014

LANTON (Israel)
LANSOPRAZOLE
Prevacid Delayed-Release Capsules ... 3271

LANURETIC (Austria)
AMILORIDE HYDROCHLORIDE/HYDROCHLOROTHIAZIDE
Moduretic Tablets ... 2028

LANZ (Brazil)
LANSOPRAZOLE
Prevacid Delayed-Release Capsules ... 3271

LANZAP (Russia, Venezuela)
LANSOPRAZOLE
Prevacid Delayed-Release Capsules ... 3271

LANZO (Denmark, Norway, Sweden)
LANSOPRAZOLE
Prevacid Delayed-Release Capsules ... 3271

LANZOGASTRO (Portugal)
LANSOPRAZOLE
Prevacid Delayed-Release Capsules ... 3271

LANZOL (Brazil, India, Spain, Venezuela)
LANSOPRAZOLE
Prevacid Delayed-Release Capsules ... 3271

LANZOPEPT (Brazil)
LANSOPRAZOLE
Prevacid Delayed-Release Capsules ... 3271

LANZOPRAL (Argentina, Chile, Venezuela)
LANSOPRAZOLE
Prevacid Delayed-Release Capsules ... 3271

LANZOR (France, Germany, South Africa)
LANSOPRAZOLE
Prevacid Delayed-Release Capsules ... 3271

LANZUL (Czech Republic)
LANSOPRAZOLE
Prevacid Delayed-Release Capsules ... 3271

LAPENAX (Argentina)
CLOZAPINE
Clozaril Tablets ... 2184

LAPOL (Portugal)
LANSOPRAZOLE
Prevacid Delayed-Release Capsules ... 3271

LAPRAZOL (Greece)
LANSOPRAZOLE
Prevacid Delayed-Release Capsules ... 3271

LAPRIL (Hong Kong, Thailand, Venezuela)
ENALAPRIL MALEATE
Vasotec I.V. Injection ... 2103

LAPROST (Venezuela)
LATANOPROST
Xalatan Ophthalmic Solution ... ⊙291

LARAFLEX (United Kingdom)
NAPROXEN
EC-Naprosyn Delayed-Release Tablets ... 2761
Naprosyn Suspension ... 2761
Naprosyn Tablets ... 2761

LARIAM (Australia, Austria, Belgium, Canada, Chile, Czech Republic, Denmark, Finland, France, Germany, Greece, Hong Kong, Hungary, Irish Republic, Israel, Italy, New Zealand, Norway, Singapore, South Africa, Sweden, Switzerland, The Netherlands, United Kingdom)
MEFLOQUINE HYDROCHLORIDE
Lariam Tablets ... 2786

LARIMEF (India)
MEFLOQUINE HYDROCHLORIDE
Lariam Tablets ... 2786

LARJANCAINA (Argentina)
LIDOCAINE
Lidoderm Patch ... 1118

LARSEN (Argentina)
TOBRAMYCIN
TOBI Solution for Inhalation ... 2298

LARSIMAL (Argentina)
FLUOROMETHOLONE
FML Ophthalmic Ointment ... ⊙228

LASER (Italy)
NAPROXEN
EC-Naprosyn Delayed-Release Tablets ... 2761
Naprosyn Suspension ... 2761
Naprosyn Tablets ... 2761

LASERVIS (Germany, Malaysia, Switzerland)
SODIUM HYALURONATE
Hyalgan Solution ... 2901

LASIKAL (United Kingdom)
FUROSEMIDE
Furosemide Tablets ... 2154

LASILACTON (Mexico)
FUROSEMIDE
Furosemide Tablets ... 2154

LASILACTONE (United Kingdom)
FUROSEMIDE
Furosemide Tablets ... 2154

LASILETTEN (The Netherlands)
FUROSEMIDE
Furosemide Tablets ... 2154

LASILIX (France)
FUROSEMIDE
Furosemide Tablets ... 2154

LASIPRESSIN (United Kingdom)
FUROSEMIDE
Furosemide Tablets ... 2154

LASIX (Argentina, Australia, Belgium, Brazil, Canada, Czech Republic, Denmark, Finland, Hong Kong, India, Irish Republic, Israel, Malaysia, Mexico, New Zealand, Norway, Portugal, Russia, Singapore, South Africa, Sweden, Thailand, The Netherlands, United Kingdom, Venezuela)
FUROSEMIDE
Furosemide Tablets ... 2154

LASMA (Irish Republic, United Kingdom)
THEOPHYLLINE
Uniphyl Tablets ... 2710

LASORIDE (United Kingdom)
FUROSEMIDE
Furosemide Tablets ... 2154

L-ASP (Argentina)
ASPARAGINASE
Elspar for Injection ... 2463

LASPAR (South Africa)
ASPARAGINASE
Elspar for Injection ... 2463

LASSIFAR (Italy)
LACTULOSE
Kristalose for Oral Solution ... 1034

LASTICOM (Austria, Italy)
AZELASTINE HYDROCHLORIDE
Astelin Nasal Spray ... 1904

LASTIN (Finland, Norway, Sweden)
AZELASTINE HYDROCHLORIDE
Astelin Nasal Spray ... 1904

LATANOPRESS (Venezuela)
LATANOPROST
Xalatan Ophthalmic Solution ... ⊙291

LATICORT (Czech Republic, Germany, Hungary, Russia)
HYDROCORTISONE BUTYRATE
Locoid Lipocream Cream ... 1160

LATOF (Chile)
LATANOPROST
Xalatan Ophthalmic Solution ... ⊙291

LATOTRYD (Mexico)
ERYTHROMYCIN
Ery-Tab Tablets ... 449
Erythromycin Base Filmtab Tablets ... 455
Erythromycin Delayed-Release Capsules, USP ... 457
PCE Dispertab Tablets ... 515

LATTUBIO (Italy)
LACTULOSE
Kristalose for Oral Solution ... 1034

LATTULAC (Italy)
LACTULOSE
Kristalose for Oral Solution ... 1034

LAURIMICINA (Mexico)
ERYTHROMYCIN
Ery-Tab Tablets ... 449
Erythromycin Base Filmtab Tablets ... 455
Erythromycin Delayed-Release Capsules, USP ... 457
PCE Dispertab Tablets ... 515

LAVER (Thailand)
TRIAMCINOLONE ACETONIDE
Azmacort Inhalation Aerosol ... 1726
Nasacort AQ Nasal Spray ... 2922

LAXARON (France)
LACTULOSE
Kristalose for Oral Solution ... 1034

LAXEERSIROOP (The Netherlands)
LACTULOSE
Kristalose for Oral Solution ... 1034

LAXETTE (South Africa)
LACTULOSE
Kristalose for Oral Solution **1034**

LAXILOSE (Canada)
LACTULOSE
Kristalose for Oral Solution **1034**

LAXOMUNDIN (Germany)
LACTULOSE
Kristalose for Oral Solution **1034**

LAXOSE (Irish Republic, United Kingdom)
LACTULOSE
Kristalose for Oral Solution **1034**

LAXULAC (Italy)
LACTULOSE
Kristalose for Oral Solution **1034**

LAXYL (Mexico)
DIAZEPAM
Diastat Rectal Delivery System **3343**
Valium Tablets **2819**

L-CARN (Germany)
LEVOCARNITINE
Carnitor Injection................ **3188**
Carnitor Tablets and Oral Solution **3190**

LECIBIS (Venezuela)
CLOTRIMAZOLE
Lotrimin Cream.................. **3039**
Lotrimin Lotion 1%................ **3039**
Lotrimin Topical Solution 1% **3039**

LEDERCORT (Argentina, Sweden)
TRIAMCINOLONE ACETONIDE
Azmacort Inhalation Aerosol.......... **1726**
Nasacort AQ Nasal Spray **2922**

LEDERCORT CON NEOMICINA (Argentina)
TRIAMCINOLONE ACETONIDE
Azmacort Inhalation Aerosol.......... **1726**
Nasacort AQ Nasal Spray **2922**

LEDERCORT-N (India)
TRIAMCINOLONE ACETONIDE
Azmacort Inhalation Aerosol.......... **1726**
Nasacort AQ Nasal Spray **2922**

LEDERLIND (Germany)
NYSTATIN
Nystop Topical Powder USP.......... **2478**
Paddock Nystatin USP for Oral Suspension.................. **2478**

LEDERPAX (Argentina, Mexico, Spain)
ERYTHROMYCIN
Ery-Tab Tablets **449**
Erythromycin Base Filmtab Tablets....... **455**
Erythromycin Delayed-Release Capsules, USP **457**
PCE Dispertab Tablets **515**

LEDOX (Norway)
NAPROXEN
EC-Naprosyn Delayed-Release Tablets.... **2761**
Naprosyn Suspension............. **2761**
Naprosyn Tablets **2761**

LEDOXID ACNE (Switzerland)
BENZOYL PEROXIDE
Brevoxyl-4 Creamy Wash............ **3210**
Brevoxyl-4 Gel **3210**
Brevoxyl-8 Creamy Wash............ **3210**
Brevoxyl-8 Gel **3210**
Triaz Cleanser **1892**
Triaz Gel...................... **1892**

LEFCAR (Italy)
LEVOCARNITINE
Carnitor Injection................ **3188**
Carnitor Tablets and Oral Solution **3190**

LEGEDERM (Denmark, Finland, Italy, Sweden)
ALCLOMETASONE DIPROPIONATE
Aclovate Cream **2660**
Aclovate Ointment................ **2660**

LEGENDAL (Switzerland, The Netherlands)
LACTULOSE
Kristalose for Oral Solution **1034**

LEGIL (Greece)
SELEGILINE HYDROCHLORIDE
Eldepryl Capsules **3208**

LEGIS (Spain)
IPRATROPIUM BROMIDE
Atrovent Inhalation Solution **835**
Atrovent Nasal Spray 0.03%........... **837**
Atrovent Nasal Spray 0.06%........... **839**

LEICESTER (Italy)
ISOSORBIDE MONONITRATE
Imdur Tablets **3018**

LEKOKLAR (Czech Republic)
CLARITHROMYCIN
Biaxin Filmtab Tablets **402**
Biaxin Granules.................. **402**

LEKOPTIN (Czech Republic, Russia)
VERAPAMIL HYDROCHLORIDE
Covera-HS Tablets **3139**
Verelan PM Extended-Release Capsules, Controlled-Onset **3106**

LELONG CONTUSIONS (France)
PENTOSAN POLYSULFATE SODIUM
Elmiron Capsules **2415**

LEMBROL (Argentina)
DIAZEPAM
Diastat Rectal Delivery System **3343**
Valium Tablets **2819**

LEMERON (Mexico)
INTERFERON ALFA-2B
Intron A for Injection.............. **3024**

LEMLAX (United Kingdom)
LACTULOSE
Kristalose for Oral Solution **1034**

LEMNIS FATTY CREAM HC (New Zealand)
HYDROCORTISONE
Hydrocortone Tablets **1989**

LEMORCAN (Greece)
NORFLOXACIN
Noroxin Tablets.................. **2032**

LEMOXOL (Greece)
CEFTAZIDIME
Fortaz for Injection **1453**

LEMTOSID (Mexico)
BENZONATATE
Tessalon Perles **1199**

LEMYTRIOL (Mexico)
CALCITRIOL
Calcijex Injection.................. **411**
Rocaltrol Capsules................ **2798**
Rocaltrol Oral Solution **2798**

LENAZINE (South Africa)
PROMETHAZINE HYDROCHLORIDE
Phenergan Tablets and Suppositories **3440**

LENDACIN (Czech Republic, Hungary, Russia)
CEFTRIAXONE SODIUM
Rocephin Injectable Vials, ADD-Vantage, Galaxy, Bulk **2800**

LENDRONAL (Argentina)
ALENDRONATE SODIUM
Fosamax Tablets................. **1969**

LENIARTRIL (Italy)
NAPROXEN
EC-Naprosyn Delayed-Release Tablets.... **2761**
Naprosyn Suspension............. **2761**
Naprosyn Tablets **2761**

LENITIL (Argentina)
DICLOFENAC SODIUM
Voltaren Tablets **2307**
Voltaren-XR Tablets **2310**

LENOXICAPS (Germany)
DIGOXIN
Lanoxicaps Capsules **1490**
Lanoxin Injection **1494**
Lanoxin Injection Pediatric **1497**
Lanoxin Tablets.................. **1500**

LENOXIN (Germany)
DIGOXIN
Lanoxicaps Capsules **1490**
Lanoxin Injection **1494**
Lanoxin Injection Pediatric **1497**
Lanoxin Tablets.................. **1500**

LENPRYL (Mexico)
CAPTOPRIL
Captopril Tablets................. **2149**

LENTO-KALIUM (Italy)
POTASSIUM CHLORIDE
K-Dur Extended-Relase Tablets **3033**
K-Lor Oral Solution................ **474**
K-Tab Tablets **475**

LEO K (Irish Republic, United Kingdom)
POTASSIUM CHLORIDE
K-Dur Extended-Relase Tablets **3033**
K-Lor Oral Solution................ **474**
K-Tab Tablets **475**

LEO-400 (Thailand)
ALBENDAZOLE
Albenza Tablets.................. **1338**

LEODRIN (Chile)
ALENDRONATE SODIUM
Fosamax Tablets................. **1969**

LEOVINEZAL (Greece)
ENALAPRIL MALEATE
Vasotec I.V. Injection **2103**

LEPHIN (Thailand)
CEFTRIAXONE SODIUM
Rocephin Injectable Vials, ADD-Vantage, Galaxy, Bulk **2800**

LEPOBRON (Portugal)
THEOPHYLLINE
Uniphyl Tablets **2710**

LEPONEX (Austria, Belgium, Brazil, Chile, Czech Republic, Denmark, Finland, France, Germany, Greece, Hungary, Israel, Italy, Mexico, Norway, Portugal, Russia, South Africa, Spain, Sweden, Switzerland, The Netherlands, Venezuela)
CLOZAPINE
Clozaril Tablets................. **2184**

LEPROFEN (Argentina)
ANASTROZOLE
Arimidex Tablets **673**

LEPTANAL (Norway, Sweden)
FENTANYL CITRATE
Actiq **979**

LEPTANAL COMP (Sweden)
FENTANYL CITRATE
Actiq **979**

LEPTIC (Argentina)
CLONAZEPAM
Klonopin Tablets **2778**

LEPUR (Greece)
SIMVASTATIN
Zocor Tablets................... **2105**

LERGIGAN (Sweden)
PROMETHAZINE HYDROCHLORIDE
Phenergan Tablets and Suppositories **3440**

LERGOSIN (Mexico)
DEXAMETHASONE
Decadron Tablets **1951**

LERGOSIN A (Mexico)
DEXAMETHASONE
Decadron Tablets **1951**

LERSA (Spain)
SULFACETAMIDE SODIUM
Klaron Lotion 10%............... **2909**

LERTUS CD (Mexico)
DICLOFENAC SODIUM
Voltaren Tablets **2307**
Voltaren-XR Tablets **2310**

LERUZE (Greece)
LISINOPRIL
Prinivil Tablets **2052**

LESCOL (Argentina, Australia, Austria, Belgium, Brazil, Canada, Czech Republic, Denmark, Finland, France, Greece, Hong Kong, Hungary, Irish Republic, Israel, Italy, Malaysia, Mexico, New Zealand, Norway, Portugal, Russia, Singapore, South Africa, Spain, Sweden, Switzerland, Thailand, The Netherlands, United Kingdom, Venezuela)
FLUVASTATIN SODIUM
Lescol Capsules **2233**

LESTRIC (Malaysia)
LOVASTATIN
Mevacor Tablets **2021**

LETANSIL (Brazil)
DIAZEPAM
Diastat Rectal Delivery System **3343**
Valium Tablets **2819**

LETEQUATRO (Portugal)
LEVOTHYROXINE SODIUM
Levothroid Tablets................ **1186**
Levoxyl Tablets.................. **1712**
Synthroid Tablets................. **520**

LETIZEN (Czech Republic, Russia)
CETIRIZINE HYDROCHLORIDE
Zyrtec Syrup **2594**
Zyrtec Tablets **2594**

LETROX (Czech Republic, Hungary)
LEVOTHYROXINE SODIUM
Levothroid Tablets................ **1186**
Levoxyl Tablets.................. **1712**
Synthroid Tablets................. **520**

LETTER (Portugal)
LEVOTHYROXINE SODIUM
Levothroid Tablets................ **1186**
Levoxyl Tablets.................. **1712**
Synthroid Tablets................. **520**

LEUCOGEN (Spain)
ASPARAGINASE
Elspar for Injection **2463**

LEUKAST (Chile)
MONTELUKAST SODIUM
Singulair Chewable Tablets **2077**
Singulair Tablets **2077**

LEUKERAN (Argentina, Australia, Austria, Belgium, Brazil, Canada, Chile, Czech Republic, Denmark, Finland, Germany, Greece, Hong Kong, India, Irish Republic, Israel, Italy, Malaysia, Mexico, New Zealand, Norway, Portugal, Russia, Singapore, South Africa, Spain, Sweden, Switzerland, Thailand, The Netherlands, United Kingdom)
CHLORAMBUCIL
Leukeran Tablets................. **1504**

LEUNASE (Hong Kong, India, Japan, Malaysia, Mexico, Singapore, Thailand)
ASPARAGINASE
Elspar for Injection **2463**

LEUSTAT (Argentina, United Kingdom)
CLADRIBINE
Leustatin Injection **2357**

LEUSTATIN (Australia, Austria, Belgium, Brazil, Canada, Czech Republic, Denmark, Finland, Germany, Greece, Hong Kong, Israel, Italy, New Zealand, Norway, South Africa, Spain, Sweden, Switzerland, Thailand, The Netherlands)
CLADRIBINE
Leustatin Injection **2357**

LEUSTATINE (France)
CLADRIBINE
Leustatin Injection **2357**

LEVAMIN (Greece)
LEVOCARNITINE
Carnitor Tablets and Oral Solution **3190**
Carnitor Injection................ **3188**

LEVAQUIN (Argentina, Brazil, Canada, Venezuela)
LEVOFLOXACIN
Levaquin Injection **2384**
Levaquin Tablets **2384**

LEVAXIN (Norway, Sweden)
LEVOTHYROXINE SODIUM
Levothroid Tablets................ **1186**
Levoxyl Tablets.................. **1712**
Synthroid Tablets................. **520**

LEVEDAD (Argentina)
DICLOFENAC SODIUM
Voltaren Tablets **2307**
Voltaren-XR Tablets **2310**

LEVIOGEL (Italy)
DICLOFENAC SODIUM
Voltaren Tablets **2307**
Voltaren-XR Tablets **2310**

LEVISTAN (Venezuela)
LOVASTATIN
Mevacor Tablets **2021**

LEVO (Israel)
LEVOFLOXACIN
Levaquin Injection **2384**

Levaquin Tablets 2384

LEVOCARNIL (France, Greece)
LEVOCARNITINE
Carnitor Injection. 3188
Carnitor Tablets and Oral Solution 3190

LEVOCARVIT (Italy)
LEVOCARNITINE
Carnitor Injection. 3188
Carnitor Tablets and Oral Solution 3190

LEVOCIDE (India)
LEVOFLOXACIN
Levaquin Injection 2384
Levaquin Tablets 2384

LEVODEX (Israel)
DILTIAZEM HYDROCHLORIDE
Cardizem LA Extended Release Tablets. . . 1728
Tiazac Capsules 1201

LEVOFF (India)
LEVOFLOXACIN
Levaquin Injection 2384
Levaquin Tablets 2384

LEVOFLOX (India)
LEVOFLOXACIN
Levaquin Injection 2384
Levaquin Tablets 2384

LEVOFLOX OZ KIT (India)
LEVOFLOXACIN
Levaquin Injection 2384
Levaquin Tablets 2384

LEVOLAC (Finland, Norway)
LACTULOSE
Kristalose for Oral Solution 1034

LEVONIS (Italy)
FLUNISOLIDE
Aerobid Inhaler System. 1171
Aerobid-M Inhaler System 1171

LEVO-T (Canada)
LEVOTHYROXINE SODIUM
Levothroid Tablets 1186
Levoxyl Tablets. 1712
Synthroid Tablets. 520

LEVOTAC (Brazil)
LEVOFLOXACIN
Levaquin Injection 2384
Levaquin Tablets 2384

LEVOTEC (Canada)
LEVOTHYROXINE SODIUM
Levothroid Tablets 1186
Levoxyl Tablets. 1712
Synthroid Tablets. 520

LEVOTHROID (Greece, Spain)
LEVOTHYROXINE SODIUM
Levothroid Tablets 1186
Levoxyl Tablets. 1712
Synthroid Tablets. 520

LEVOTHYROX (France)
LEVOTHYROXINE SODIUM
Levothroid Tablets 1186
Levoxyl Tablets. 1712
Synthroid Tablets. 520

LEVOTIROX (Italy)
LEVOTHYROXINE SODIUM
Levothroid Tablets 1186
Levoxyl Tablets. 1712
Synthroid Tablets. 520

LEVOTRIN (Argentina)
LIOTHYRONINE SODIUM
Cytomel Tablets 1710

LEVOVANOX (Italy)
VANCOMYCIN HYDROCHLORIDE
Vancocin HCl Capsules, USP 3380

LEVOXACIN (Italy)
LEVOFLOXACIN
Levaquin Injection 2384
Levaquin Tablets 2384

LEVOXIN (Brazil)
LEVOFLOXACIN
Levaquin Injection 2384
Levaquin Tablets 2384

LEXEMIN (Hong Kong, Singapore, Thailand)
FENOFIBRATE
Tricor Tablets 527

LEXFOR (Thailand)
NORFLOXACIN
Noroxin Tablets. 2032

LEXIFLOX (Hong Kong)
NORFLOXACIN
Noroxin Tablets. 2032

LEXINOR (Finland, Hong Kong, Malaysia, Singapore, Sweden, Thailand)
NORFLOXACIN
Noroxin Tablets. 2032

LEXOBENE (Germany)
DICLOFENAC SODIUM
Voltaren Tablets 2307
Voltaren-XR Tablets 2310

LEZIDIM (Mexico)
CEFTAZIDIME
Fortaz for Injection 1453

LEZOLE (Argentina)
ANASTROZOLE
Arimidex Tablets 673

LGHYAL (India)
SODIUM HYALURONATE
Hyalgan Solution. 2901

LIBERALGIUM (Spain)
DICLOFENAC SODIUM
Voltaren Tablets 2307
Voltaren-XR Tablets 2310

LIBERAXIM (Mexico)
HYDROMORPHONE HYDROCHLORIDE
Dilaudid Ampules. 440
Dilaudid Multiple Dose Vials 440
Dilaudid Non-Sterile Powder 440
Dilaudid Oral Liquid 445
Dilaudid Rectal Suppositories 440
Dilaudid Tablets. 440
Dilaudid Tablets - 8 mg 445
Dilaudid-HP Injection. 442
Dilaudid-HP Lyophilized Powder 250 mg . . . 442

LIBRIUM (Canada, Italy, United Kingdom)
CHLORDIAZEPOXIDE HYDROCHLORIDE
Librium Capsules. 3347

LICUAGEN (Argentina)
CILOSTAZOL
Pletal Tablets 2455

LIDERMA (Switzerland)
ISOTRETINOIN
Accutane Capsules 2731

LIDERMAN (Austria)
OXICONAZOLE NITRATE
Oxistat Cream 2667
Oxistat Lotion. 2667

LIDIAL (Brazil)
LIDOCAINE
Lidoderm Patch 1118

LIDOCAINA SPRAY (Italy)
LIDOCAINE
Lidoderm Patch 1118

LIDONOSTRUM (Portugal)
LIDOCAINE
Lidoderm Patch 1118

LIDOPOSTERINE (Germany)
LIDOCAINE
Lidoderm Patch 1118

LIDOSPRAY (Brazil)
LIDOCAINE
Lidoderm Patch 1118

LIDOSTON (Brazil)
LIDOCAINE
Lidoderm Patch 1118

LIFAMOX (Brazil)
AMOXICILLIN
Amoxil Pediatric Drops for Oral Suspension. 1343
Amoxil Tablets 1343

LIFENAC (Mexico)
DICLOFENAC SODIUM
Voltaren Tablets 2307
Voltaren-XR Tablets 2310

LIFERXINA (Mexico)
CIPROFLOXACIN
Cipro Oral Suspension 2977

LIFERZIT (Greece)
LOVASTATIN
Mevacor Tablets 2021

LIFERZOL (Mexico)
CLOTRIMAZOLE
Lotrimin Cream. 3039
Lotrimin Lotion 1%. 3039
Lotrimin Topical Solution 1% 3039

LIFTER (Chile)
SILDENAFIL CITRATE
Viagra Tablets 2573

LIFUROM (South Africa)
CEFUROXIME SODIUM
Zinacef Injection 1631

LIFUROX (Czech Republic, Denmark, Finland, Norway, Spain, Sweden, Venezuela)
CEFUROXIME SODIUM
Zinacef Injection 1631

LIGNOSPAN SPECIAL (South Africa)
LIDOCAINE
Lidoderm Patch 1118

LIKENIL (Spain)
LISINOPRIL
Prinivil Tablets 2052

LIMOX (Greece)
CIPROFLOXACIN
Cipro Oral Suspension 2977

LIMOXIN (Mexico)
AMOXICILLIN
Amoxil Pediatric Drops for Oral Suspension. 1343
Amoxil Tablets 1343

LIMPIDEX (Italy)
LANSOPRAZOLE
Prevacid Delayed-Release Capsules 3271

LINATECAN (Chile)
IRINOTECAN HYDROCHLORIDE
Camptosar Injection 2604

LINATIL (Finland, Norway, Sweden)
ENALAPRIL MALEATE
Vasotec I.V. Injection 2103

LINDACIL (Mexico)
CLINDAMYCIN HYDROCHLORIDE
Cleocin Vaginal Ovules 2616

LINDISC (Argentina, Brazil)
ESTRADIOL
Climara Transdermal System 771
Estring Vaginal Ring. 2635

LINFOL (Argentina)
METRONIDAZOLE
MetroGel-Vaginal Gel 1855

LINFOLYSIN (Italy)
CHLORAMBUCIL
Leukeran Tablets. 1504

LINOLADIOL (Austria)
ESTRADIOL
Climara Transdermal System 771
Estring Vaginal Ring. 2635

LINOLADIOL N (Czech Republic, Germany, Hungary)
ESTRADIOL
Climara Transdermal System 771
Estring Vaginal Ring. 2635

LINOLADIOL-H N (Czech Republic, Germany, Hungary)
ESTRADIOL
Climara Transdermal System 771
Estring Vaginal Ring. 2635

LINOPRIL (Brazil)
LISINOPRIL
Prinivil Tablets 2052

LINORIL (India)
LISINOPRIL
Prinivil Tablets 2052

LINOTEN (Spain)
PAMIDRONATE DISODIUM
Aredia for Injection 2179

LINVAS (India)
LISINOPRIL
Prinivil Tablets 2052

LIOCORT (Venezuela)
HYDROCORTISONE
Hydrocortone Tablets 1989

LIOTREX (Chile)
SUMATRIPTAN SUCCINATE
Imitrex Injection 1463
Imitrex Tablets 1471

LIPANON (Brazil)
FENOFIBRATE
Tricor Tablets 527

LIPANTHYL (Belgium, Finland, France, Germany, Greece, Hong Kong, Hungary, Italy, Malaysia, Portugal, Russia, Singapore, Sweden, Switzerland, Thailand)
FENOFIBRATE
Tricor Tablets 527

LIPANTIL (Irish Republic, United Kingdom)
FENOFIBRATE
Tricor Tablets 527

LIPAREX (Argentina)
ATORVASTATIN CALCIUM
Lipitor Tablets 2483

LIPARISON (Spain)
FENOFIBRATE
Tricor Tablets 527

LIPAXAN (Italy)
FLUVASTATIN SODIUM
Lescol Capsules 2233

LIPAZ (Portugal)
SIMVASTATIN
Zocor Tablets. 2105

LIPCOR (Austria)
FENOFIBRATE
Tricor Tablets 527

LIPCUT (Finland)
SIMVASTATIN
Zocor Tablets. 2105

LIPDAUNE (Portugal)
LOVASTATIN
Mevacor Tablets 2021

LIPEROL (Mexico)
LOVASTATIN
Mevacor Tablets 2021

LIPEX (Australia, New Zealand)
SIMVASTATIN
Zocor Tablets. 2105

LIPIBEC (Argentina)
ATORVASTATIN CALCIUM
Lipitor Tablets 2483

LIPICARD (India)
FENOFIBRATE
Tricor Tablets 527

LIPIDAX (Italy)
FENOFIBRATE
Tricor Tablets 527

LIPIDIL (Argentina, Australia, Brazil, Canada, Chile, Germany, Greece, Hungary, Mexico)
FENOFIBRATE
Tricor Tablets 527

LIPIDLESS (Greece)
LOVASTATIN
Mevacor Tablets 2021

LIPIL (Italy)
FENOFIBRATE
Tricor Tablets 527

LIPIREX (Czech Republic, France)
FENOFIBRATE
Tricor Tablets 527

LIPITOR (Argentina, Australia, Belgium, Brazil, Canada, Chile, Finland, Greece, Hong Kong, Irish Republic, Israel, Italy, Japan, Malaysia, Mexico, New Zealand, Norway, Singapore, South Africa, Sweden, Thailand, The Netherlands, United Kingdom, Venezuela)
ATORVASTATIN CALCIUM
Lipitor Tablets 2483

LIPIVAS (Denmark)
LOVASTATIN
Mevacor Tablets 2021

LIPLE (Japan)
ALPROSTADIL
Edex Injection. 3089

LIPO RED (Spain)
FENOFIBRATE
Tricor Tablets 527

LIPOCAMBI (Argentina)
ATORVASTATIN CALCIUM
Lipitor Tablets 2483

LIPOCIDEN (Spain)
SIMVASTATIN
Zocor Tablets 2105

LIPOCLAR (Italy)
FENOFIBRATE
Tricor Tablets 527

LIPOFEN (Portugal)
FENOFIBRATE
Tricor Tablets 527

LIPOFENE (Italy)
FENOFIBRATE
Tricor Tablets 527

LIPOFIN (Argentina)
ATORVASTATIN CALCIUM
Lipitor Tablets 2483

LIPOFREN (Spain)
LOVASTATIN
Mevacor Tablets 2021

LIPONORM (Argentina, Italy)
ATORVASTATIN CALCIUM
Lipitor Tablets 2483

LIPOPLASMIN (Argentina)
FENOFIBRATE
Tricor Tablets 527

LIPOREST (India)
ATORVASTATIN CALCIUM
Lipitor Tablets 2483

LIPOREX (Greece)
SIMVASTATIN
Zocor Tablets 2105

LIPOSCLER (Spain)
LOVASTATIN
Mevacor Tablets 2021

LIPOSIT (Italy, Spain)
FENOFIBRATE
Tricor Tablets 527

LIPOVAS (Spain)
FENOFIBRATE
Tricor Tablets 527

LIPRACE (Australia)
LISINOPRIL
Prinivil Tablets 2052

LIPREREN (Chile)
LISINOPRIL
Prinivil Tablets 2052

LIPRIL (India, Portugal)
LISINOPRIL
Prinivil Tablets 2052

LIPRIMAR (Hungary, Russia)
ATORVASTATIN CALCIUM
Lipitor Tablets 2483

LIPSIN (Austria, France, Italy, South Africa)
FENOFIBRATE
Tricor Tablets 527

LIPUS (Portugal)
LOVASTATIN
Mevacor Tablets 2021

LIROKEN (Mexico)
DICLOFENAC SODIUM
Voltaren Tablets 2307
Voltaren-XR Tablets 2310

LIS (Italy)
LACTULOSE
Kristalose for Oral Solution 1034

LISAC (Argentina)
SIMVASTATIN
Zocor Tablets 2105

LISACNE (Chile)
ISOTRETINOIN
Accutane Capsules 2731

LISDENE (Singapore)
LISINOPRIL
Prinivil Tablets 2052

LISEFOR (Greece)
LEVOCARNITINE
Carnitor Injection 3188
Carnitor Tablets and Oral Solution 3190

LISI LICH (Germany)
LISINOPRIL
Prinivil Tablets 2052

LISIBETA (Germany)
LISINOPRIL
Prinivil Tablets 2052

LISICOSTAD (United Kingdom)
LISINOPRIL
Prinivil Tablets 2052

LISIFLEN (Italy)
DICLOFENAC SODIUM
Voltaren Tablets 2307
Voltaren-XR Tablets 2310

LISIGAMMA (Germany)
LISINOPRIL
Prinivil Tablets 2052

LISIHEXAL (Austria, Germany)
LISINOPRIL
Prinivil Tablets 2052

LISIKEN (Mexico)
CLINDAMYCIN HYDROCHLORIDE
Cleocin Vaginal Ovules 2616

LISILET (Venezuela)
LISINOPRIL
Prinivil Tablets 2052

LISINAL (Argentina)
LISINOPRIL
Prinivil Tablets 2052

LISINOBELL (Australia)
LISINOPRIL
Prinivil Tablets 2052

LISINOGEN (Denmark)
LISINOPRIL
Prinivil Tablets 2052

LISINORETIC (Brazil)
LISINOPRIL
Prinivil Tablets 2052

LISINOSPES (Greece)
LISINOPRIL
Prinivil Tablets 2052

LISINOSTAD (Austria)
LISINOPRIL
Prinivil Tablets 2052

LISINOTYROL (Austria)
LISINOPRIL
Prinivil Tablets 2052

LISIPRIL (Finland)
LISINOPRIL
Prinivil Tablets 2052

LISIPRIL COMP (Finland)
HYDROCHLOROTHIAZIDE/LISINOPRIL
Prinzide Tablets 2056

LISI-PUREN (Germany)
LISINOPRIL
Prinivil Tablets 2052

LISITRIL (Switzerland)
LISINOPRIL
Prinivil Tablets 2052

LISOCLOR (Brazil)
LISINOPRIL
Prinivil Tablets 2052

LISODER (Chile)
MOMETASONE FUROATE
Elocon Cream 0.1% 3005
Elocon Lotion 0.1% 3006
Elocon Ointment 0.1% 3007
Nasonex Nasal Spray 3043

LISODUR (Australia)
LISINOPRIL
Prinivil Tablets 2052

LISODURA (Germany)
LISINOPRIL
Prinivil Tablets 2052

LISONOTEC (Brazil)
LISINOPRIL
Prinivil Tablets 2052

LISOPRESS (Hungary, Irish Republic)
LISINOPRIL
Prinivil Tablets 2052

LISOPRIL (Switzerland)
LISINOPRIL
Prinivil Tablets 2052

LISORIL (India, Russia, Singapore)
LISINOPRIL
Prinivil Tablets 2052

LISORIL-5HT (India)
LISINOPRIL
Prinivil Tablets 2052

LISOTRAN (Brazil)
ERYTHROMYCIN
Ery-Tab Tablets 449
Erythromycin Base Filmtab Tablets 455
Erythromycin Delayed-Release Capsules, USP 457
PCE Dispertab Tablets 515

LISOTREX (Brazil)
ERYTHROMYCIN
Ery-Tab Tablets 449
Erythromycin Base Filmtab Tablets 455
Erythromycin Delayed-Release Capsules, USP 457
PCE Dispertab Tablets 515

LISPOR (Chile)
LOVASTATIN
Mevacor Tablets 2021

LISPRIL (Irish Republic, Thailand)
LISINOPRIL
Prinivil Tablets 2052

LISPRIL-HYDROCHLOROTHIAZIDE (Irish Republic)
LISINOPRIL
Prinivil Tablets 2052

LISTRIL (Brazil, Czech Republic)
LISINOPRIL
Prinivil Tablets 2052

LITAK (Australia, France, Israel, Switzerland)
CLADRIBINE
Leustatin Injection 2357

LITHIMOLE (Greece)
TIMOLOL MALEATE
Blocadren Tablets 1916
Timoptic Sterile Ophthalmic Solution 2088
Timoptic in Ocudose 2091
Timoptic-XE Sterile Ophthalmic Gel Forming Solution 2092

LITOCIT (Brazil)
POTASSIUM CITRATE
Urocit-K Tablets 2144

LIVESAN (France)
FENOFIBRATE
Tricor Tablets 527

LIVO LUK (India)
LACTULOSE
Kristalose for Oral Solution 1034

LIVOMONIL (Argentina)
CLOTRIMAZOLE
Lotrimin Cream 3039
Lotrimin Lotion 1% 3039
Lotrimin Topical Solution 1% 3039

LIXAMIDE (South Africa)
INDAPAMIDE
Indapamide Tablets 2156

LIXI (Venezuela)
LEVOCARNITINE
Carnitor Injection 3188
Carnitor Tablets and Oral Solution 3190

LIXOGAN (Mexico)
NAPROXEN
EC-Naprosyn Delayed-Release Tablets 2761
Naprosyn Suspension 2761
Naprosyn Tablets 2761

LIZUL (Portugal)
LANSOPRAZOLE
Prevacid Delayed-Release Capsules 3271

LOBATE (India)
CLOBETASOL PROPIONATE
Temovate Cream 2668
Temovate E Emollient 2671
Temovate Gel 2669
Temovate Ointment 2668
Temovate Scalp Application 2670

LOBATE-G (India)
CLOBETASOL PROPIONATE
Temovate Cream 2668
Temovate E Emollient 2671
Temovate Gel 2669
Temovate Ointment 2668
Temovate Scalp Application 2670

LOBATE-M (India)
CLOBETASOL PROPIONATE
Temovate Cream 2668
Temovate E Emollient 2671
Temovate Gel 2669
Temovate Ointment 2668
Temovate Scalp Application 2670

LOBESOL (Malaysia)
CLOBETASOL PROPIONATE
Temovate Cream 2668
Temovate E Emollient 2671
Temovate Gel 2669
Temovate Ointment 2668
Temovate Scalp Application 2670

LOBEVAT (Chile, Mexico)
CLOBETASOL PROPIONATE
Temovate Cream 2668
Temovate E Emollient 2671
Temovate Gel 2669
Temovate Ointment 2668
Temovate Scalp Application 2670

LOCACID (Argentina, Czech Republic, France, Hong Kong, Israel, Portugal)
TRETINOIN
Vesanoid Capsules 2820

LOCASYN (Denmark)
FLUNISOLIDE
Aerobid Inhaler System 1171
Aerobid-M Inhaler System 1171

LOCEPTIN (Sweden)
MORPHINE SULFATE
Kadian Capsules 577
MS Contin Tablets 2701

LOCHOL (Hungary, Thailand)
FLUVASTATIN SODIUM
Lescol Capsules 2233

LOCOID (Belgium, Brazil, Chile, Czech Republic, Denmark, Finland, France, Hungary, Irish Republic, Mexico, Norway, Portugal, Russia, South Africa, Sweden, Switzerland, The Netherlands, United Kingdom)
HYDROCORTISONE BUTYRATE
Locoid Lipocream Cream 1160

LOCOID CRELO (Sweden)
HYDROCORTISONE BUTYRATE
Locoid Lipocream Cream 1160

LOCOIDON (Austria, Italy)
HYDROCORTISONE BUTYRATE
Locoid Lipocream Cream 1160

LOCOL (Germany)
FLUVASTATIN SODIUM
Lescol Capsules 2233

LOCTENK (Argentina)
LOSARTAN POTASSIUM
Cozaar Tablets 1935

LOCULA (India)
SULFACETAMIDE SODIUM
Klaron Lotion 10% 2909

LODALES (France)
SIMVASTATIN
Zocor Tablets 2105

LODIMOL (Mexico)
DIPYRIDAMOLE
Persantine Tablets 868

LODIPRES (Chile)
CARVEDILOL
Coreg Tablets 1414

LODIXAL (Belgium)
VERAPAMIL HYDROCHLORIDE
Covera-HS Tablets 3139
Verelan PM Extended-Release Capsules, Controlled-Onset 3106

LODYFEN (Mexico)
DICLOFENAC SODIUM
Voltaren Tablets 2307
Voltaren-XR Tablets 2310

LOFACOL (Hong Kong)
LOVASTATIN
Mevacor Tablets 2021

LOFENSAID (United Kingdom)
DICLOFENAC SODIUM
Voltaren Tablets 2307
Voltaren-XR Tablets 2310

LOFOSTIN (Greece)
LEVOCARNITINE
Carnitor Injection 3188
Carnitor Tablets and Oral Solution 3190

LOFOTO (Greece)
DEXAMETHASONE/TOBRAMYCIN
TobraDex Ophthalmic Ointment . . . 562, ⊙212
TobraDex Ophthalmic Suspension . 563, ⊙211

LOGAT (Brazil)
RANITIDINE HYDROCHLORIDE
Zantac 25 EFFERdose Tablets 1624
Zantac 150 EFFERdose Tablets 1624
Zantac 150 Tablets 1624
Zantac 300 Tablets 1624
Zantac Injection 1619
Zantac Injection Premixed 1619
Zantac Syrup 1624

LOGECINE (France)
ERYTHROMYCIN
Ery-Tab Tablets 449
Erythromycin Base Filmtab Tablets 455
Erythromycin Delayed-Release Capsules, USP 457
PCE Dispertab Tablets 515

LOGESIC (Mexico)
DICLOFENAC SODIUM
Voltaren Tablets 2307
Voltaren-XR Tablets 2310

LOGISTIC (Argentina)
GABAPENTIN
Neurontin Capsules 2487

LOGODERM (Australia, Chile, Mexico, New Zealand)
ALCLOMETASONE DIPROPIONATE
Aclovate Cream 2660
Aclovate Ointment 2660

LOGOMED AKNE-GEL (Germany)
BENZOYL PEROXIDE
Brevoxyl-4 Creamy Wash 3210
Brevoxyl-4 Gel 3210
Brevoxyl-8 Creamy Wash 3210
Brevoxyl-8 Gel 3210
Triaz Cleanser 1892
Triaz Gel 1892

LOGOMED HAUTPILZ-SALBE (Germany)
CLOTRIMAZOLE
Lotrimin Cream 3039
Lotrimin Lotion 1% 3039
Lotrimin Topical Solution 1% 3039

LOGROTON (Belgium, Malaysia)
METOPROLOL TARTRATE
Lopressor Tablets 2238

LOKALICID (Germany)
CLOTRIMAZOLE
Lotrimin Cream 3039
Lotrimin Lotion 1% 3039
Lotrimin Topical Solution 1% 3039

LOKALISON-F (Germany)
DEXAMETHASONE
Decadron Tablets 1951

LOKALISON-UNIVERSALE (Germany)
DEXAMETHASONE
Decadron Tablets 1951

LOKILAN (Norway)
FLUNISOLIDE
Aerobid Inhaler System 1171
Aerobid-M Inhaler System 1171

LOKILAN NASAL (Sweden)
FLUNISOLIDE
Aerobid Inhaler System 1171
Aerobid-M Inhaler System 1171

LOKREN (Czech Republic, Hungary, Russia)
BETAXOLOL HYDROCHLORIDE
Betoptic S Ophthalmic Suspension . ⊙203, 558

LOMADRYL (Greece)
RANITIDINE HYDROCHLORIDE
Zantac 25 EFFERdose Tablets 1624
Zantac 150 EFFERdose Tablets 1624
Zantac 150 Tablets 1624
Zantac 300 Tablets 1624
Zantac Injection 1619
Zantac Injection Premixed 1619
Zantac Syrup 1624

LOMAR (Hong Kong)
LOVASTATIN
Mevacor Tablets 2021

LOMECAN V (Mexico)
CLOTRIMAZOLE
Lotrimin Cream 3039
Lotrimin Lotion 1% 3039
Lotrimin Topical Solution 1% 3039

LOMESONE (Greece)
ALCLOMETASONE DIPROPIONATE
Aclovate Cream 2660
Aclovate Ointment 2660

LOMIR (Austria, Belgium, Brazil, Czech Republic, Denmark, Finland, Germany, Greece, Hungary, Italy, Norway, Portugal, Russia, Spain, Sweden, Switzerland, The Netherlands)
ISRADIPINE
DynaCirc CR Tablets 2721

LONAVAR (Australia, Israel)
OXANDROLONE
Oxandrin Tablets 2962

LONCORD (Brazil)
NIFEDIPINE
Adalat CC Tablets 2964

LONESTIN (Mexico)
CLOTRIMAZOLE
Lotrimin Cream 3039
Lotrimin Lotion 1% 3039
Lotrimin Topical Solution 1% 3039

LONGACEF (Venezuela)
CEFIXIME
Suprax 1843

LONGACEPH (Czech Republic)
CEFTRIAXONE SODIUM
Rocephin Injectable Vials, ADD-Vantage, Galaxy, Bulk 2800

LONGAZEM (Italy)
DILTIAZEM HYDROCHLORIDE
Cardizem LA Extended Release Tablets . . . 1728
Tiazac Capsules 1201

LONTAX (The Netherlands)
CITALOPRAM HYDROBROMIDE
Celexa Tablets 1176

LOORTAN (Belgium)
LOSARTAN POTASSIUM
Cozaar Tablets 1935

LOORTAN PLUS (Belgium)
HYDROCHLOROTHIAZIDE/LOSARTAN POTASSIUM
Hyzaar 100-25 Tablets 1990
Hyzaar 50-12.5 Tablets 1990

LO-P-CAPS (Thailand)
CALCIUM ACETATE
PhosLo GelCaps 2169

LOPIRETIC (Portugal)
CAPTOPRIL
Captopril Tablets 2149

LOPIRIN (Austria, Germany, Switzerland)
CAPTOPRIL
Captopril Tablets 2149

LOPLAC (Argentina)
LOSARTAN POTASSIUM
Cozaar Tablets 1935

LOPLAC-D (Argentina)
LOSARTAN POTASSIUM
Cozaar Tablets 1935

LOPRANOL LA (United Kingdom)
PROPRANOLOL HYDROCHLORIDE
Inderal LA Long-Acting Capsules 3429

LOPRATIN (The Netherlands)
CEFTRIAXONE SODIUM
Rocephin Injectable Vials, ADD-Vantage, Galaxy, Bulk 2800

LOPRESOR (Argentina, Australia, Austria, Belgium, Canada, Germany, Greece, Irish Republic, Italy, Mexico, New Zealand, Portugal, South Africa, Spain, United Kingdom, Venezuela)
METOPROLOL TARTRATE
Lopressor Tablets 2238

LOPRESSOR (Brazil, France)
METOPROLOL TARTRATE
Lopressor Tablets 2238

LOPRIL (Brazil, Finland, France)
CAPTOPRIL
Captopril Tablets 2149

LOPTOMIT (The Netherlands)
TIMOLOL MALEATE
Blocadren Tablets 1916
Timoptic Sterile Ophthalmic Solution 2088
Timoptic in Ocudose 2091
Timoptic-XE Sterile Ophthalmic Gel Forming Solution 2092

LORADUR (Austria, Czech Republic)
AMILORIDE HYDROCHLORIDE/HYDROCHLOROTHIAZIDE
Moduretic Tablets 2028

LORAGA (Finland, Sweden)
LACTULOSE
Kristalose for Oral Solution 1034

LORBIFLOXACINA (Argentina)
CIPROFLOXACIN
Cipro Oral Suspension 2977

LORBINAFIL (Argentina)
SILDENAFIL CITRATE
Viagra Tablets 2573

LORCAMIN (Greece)
NORFLOXACIN
Noroxin Tablets 2032

LORENTIN (Australia)
METHYLPHENIDATE HYDROCHLORIDE
Ritalin Hydrochloride Tablets 2269
Ritalin-SR Tablets 2269

LORETIC (South Africa)
HYDROCHLOROTHIAZIDE/TRIAMTERENE
Dyazide Capsules 1423

LOREXEN (Mexico)
NAPROXEN
EC-Naprosyn Delayed-Release Tablets 2761
Naprosyn Suspension 2761
Naprosyn Tablets 2761

LOREXIL M (Mexico)
AMOXICILLIN
Amoxil Pediatric Drops for Oral Suspension 1343
Amoxil Tablets 1343

LORISTA (Czech Republic)
LOSARTAN POTASSIUM
Cozaar Tablets 1935

LORITER (Argentina)
LOVASTATIN
Mevacor Tablets 2021

LOROXIDE (Canada)
BENZOYL PEROXIDE
Brevoxyl-4 Creamy Wash 3210
Brevoxyl-4 Gel 3210
Brevoxyl-8 Creamy Wash 3210
Brevoxyl-8 Gel 3210
Triaz Cleanser 1892
Triaz Gel 1892

LORSACOR (Brazil)
LOSARTAN POTASSIUM
Cozaar Tablets 1935

LORSAR + HCT (Brazil)
LOSARTAN POTASSIUM
Cozaar Tablets 1935

LORTAAN (Italy, Portugal)
LOSARTAN POTASSIUM
Cozaar Tablets 1935

LORTAAN PLUS (Portugal)
HYDROCHLOROTHIAZIDE/LOSARTAN POTASSIUM
Hyzaar 100-25 Tablets 1990
Hyzaar 50-12.5 Tablets 1990

LORVAS (India, Thailand)
INDAPAMIDE
Indapamide Tablets 2156

LORZAAR (Germany)
LOSARTAN POTASSIUM
Cozaar Tablets 1935

LORZAAR PLUS (Germany)
HYDROCHLOROTHIAZIDE/LOSARTAN POTASSIUM
Hyzaar 100-25 Tablets 1990
Hyzaar 50-12.5 Tablets 1990

LOSACAR (India)
LOSARTAN POTASSIUM
Cozaar Tablets 1935

LOSACAR-H (India)
LOSARTAN POTASSIUM
Cozaar Tablets 1935

LOSACOR (Argentina)
LOSARTAN POTASSIUM
Cozaar Tablets 1935

LOSACOR D (Argentina)
LOSARTAN POTASSIUM
Cozaar Tablets 1935

LOSANORM (India)
LOSARTAN POTASSIUM
Cozaar Tablets 1935

LOSAPRES (Chile)
LOSARTAN POTASSIUM
Cozaar Tablets 1935

LOSAPRES-D (Chile)
HYDROCHLOROTHIAZIDE/LOSARTAN POTASSIUM
Hyzaar 100-25 Tablets 1990
Hyzaar 50-12.5 Tablets 1990

LOSAPREX (Italy)
LOSARTAN POTASSIUM
Cozaar Tablets 1935

LOSARTEC (Brazil)
LOSARTAN POTASSIUM
Cozaar Tablets 1935

LOSATAL (Brazil)
LOSARTAN POTASSIUM
Cozaar Tablets 1935

LOSAZID (Italy)
HYDROCHLOROTHIAZIDE/LOSARTAN POTASSIUM
Hyzaar 100-25 Tablets 1990
Hyzaar 50-12.5 Tablets 1990

LOSE.LAX (Austria)
LACTULOSE
Kristalose for Oral Solution 1034

LOSIL-T (Mexico)
TERBINAFINE HYDROCHLORIDE
Lamisil Tablets 2232

LOSIUM (India)
LOSARTAN POTASSIUM
Cozaar Tablets 1935

LOSTAPRES (Argentina)
RAMIPRIL
Altace Capsules 1702

LOSTATIN (Malaysia, Singapore, Venezuela)
LOVASTATIN
Mevacor Tablets 2021

LOTENSIN (Brazil, Canada, Hungary, Mexico, Russia, Venezuela)
BENAZEPRIL HYDROCHLORIDE
Lotensin Tablets 2243

LOTENSIN H (Brazil)
BENAZEPRIL HYDROCHLORIDE/HYDROCHLOROTHIAZIDE
Lotensin HCT Tablets 2246

LOTENSIN HCT (Hungary)
BENAZEPRIL HYDROCHLORIDE
Lotensin Tablets 2243

LOTIOBLANC (Argentina)
TRETINOIN
Vesanoid Capsules 2820

LOTREMIN (Australia, Hong Kong, Malaysia, Singapore)
CLOTRIMAZOLE
Lotrimin Cream 3039
Lotrimin Lotion 1% 3039
Lotrimin Topical Solution 1% 3039

LOTREMINE (Portugal)
CLOTRIMAZOLE
Lotrimin Cream 3039
Lotrimin Lotion 1% 3039
Lotrimin Topical Solution 1% 3039

LOTRIAL (Chile)
ENALAPRIL MALEATE
Vasotec I.V. Injection 2103

(⊙ Described in PDR For Ophthalmic Medicines™)

LOTRIAL D (Argentina)
ENALAPRIL MALEATE
Vasotec I.V. Injection 2103

LOTRIMIN (Mexico)
CLOTRIMAZOLE
Lotrimin Cream. 3039
Lotrimin Lotion 1%. 3039
Lotrimin Topical Solution 1% 3039

LOTRIX (Argentina)
ENALAPRIL MALEATE
Vasotec I.V. Injection 2103

LOUTEN (Argentina, Chile)
LATANOPROST
Xalatan Ophthalmic Solution . . . . ⊙291

LOUTEN T (Argentina)
LATANOPROST
Xalatan Ophthalmic Solution . . . . ⊙291

LOVA (Germany)
LOVASTATIN
Mevacor Tablets 2021

LOVABETA (Germany)
LOVASTATIN
Mevacor Tablets 2021

LOVACARD (Czech Republic, India)
LOVASTATIN
Mevacor Tablets 2021

LOVACODAN (Denmark)
LOVASTATIN
Mevacor Tablets 2021

LOVACOL (Chile, Finland)
LOVASTATIN
Mevacor Tablets 2021

LOVACOR (Brazil)
SIMVASTATIN
Zocor Tablets. 2105

LOVADRUG (Greece)
LOVASTATIN
Mevacor Tablets 2021

LOVADURA (Germany)
LOVASTATIN
Mevacor Tablets 2021

LOVAGAMMA (Germany)
LOVASTATIN
Mevacor Tablets 2021

LOVAHEXAL (Germany)
LOVASTATIN
Mevacor Tablets 2021

LOVALIP (Israel)
LOVASTATIN
Mevacor Tablets 2021

LOVANIL (Venezuela)
LOVASTATIN
Mevacor Tablets 2021

LOVAPEN (Greece)
LOVASTATIN
Mevacor Tablets 2021

LOVAS (Venezuela)
LOVASTATIN
Mevacor Tablets 2021

LOVASC (Brazil)
LOVASTATIN
Mevacor Tablets 2021

LOVAST (Brazil)
LOVASTATIN
Mevacor Tablets 2021

LOVASTEN (Greece)
LOVASTATIN
Mevacor Tablets 2021

LOVASTEROL (Russia)
LOVASTATIN
Mevacor Tablets 2021

LOVASTIN (Malaysia)
LOVASTATIN
Mevacor Tablets 2021

LOVATEX (Greece)
LOVASTATIN
Mevacor Tablets 2021

LOVATON (Brazil)
LOVASTATIN
Mevacor Tablets 2021

LOVATOP (Greece)
LOVASTATIN
Mevacor Tablets 2021

LOVAX (Brazil)
LOVASTATIN
Mevacor Tablets 2021

LOVENOX (Austria, Canada, France, Portugal, Switzerland)
ENOXAPARIN SODIUM
Lovenox Injection 2915

LOVERAL (Mexico)
ALBENDAZOLE
Albenza Tablets. 1338

LOWCHOLID (Greece)
SIMVASTATIN
Zocor Tablets. 2105

LOWFIN (Chile)
SERTRALINE HYDROCHLORIDE
Zoloft Tablets 2586

LOWLIPID (Greece)
LOVASTATIN
Mevacor Tablets 2021

LOWPRE (Mexico)
CAPTOPRIL
Captopril Tablets. 2149

LOWPRES (Venezuela)
CLONIDINE HYDROCHLORIDE
Catapres Tablets 843

LOWPRESS (Brazil)
ENALAPRIL MALEATE
Vasotec I.V. Injection 2103

LOXIFEN (Argentina)
RALOXIFENE HYDROCHLORIDE
Evista Tablets. 1763

LOXIN (Germany)
AZELASTINE HYDROCHLORIDE
Astelin Nasal Spray 1904

LOZAP (Czech Republic)
LOSARTAN POTASSIUM
Cozaar Tablets 1935

LOZAPIN (India)
CLOZAPINE
Clozaril Tablets. 2184

LOZAPINE (Israel)
CLOZAPINE
Clozaril Tablets. 2184

LOZIDE (Canada)
INDAPAMIDE
Indapamide Tablets 2156

LOZITAN (India)
LOSARTAN POTASSIUM
Cozaar Tablets 1935

L-THYROX (Germany)
LEVOTHYROXINE SODIUM
Levothroid Tablets. 1186
Levoxyl Tablets. 1712
Synthroid Tablets. 520

L-TINE (India)
LEVOCARNITINE
Carnitor Injection. 3188
Carnitor Tablets and Oral Solution 3190

LTK250 (Argentina)
POTASSIUM CITRATE
Urocit-K Tablets. 2144

LUASE (Spain)
DICLOFENAC SODIUM
Voltaren Tablets 2307
Voltaren-XR Tablets 2310

LUBEXYL (Hungary, Switzerland)
BENZOYL PEROXIDE
Brevoxyl-4 Creamy Wash. 3210
Brevoxyl-4 Gel 3210
Brevoxyl-8 Creamy Wash. 3210
Brevoxyl-8 Gel 3210
Triaz Cleanser 1892
Triaz Gel 1892

LUFAC-Z (Mexico)
DICLOFENAC SODIUM
Voltaren Tablets 2307
Voltaren-XR Tablets 2310

LUFI (India)
LEVOFLOXACIN
Levaquin Injection 2384
Levaquin Tablets 2384

LUGACIN (United Kingdom)
GENTAMICIN SULFATE
Garamycin Injectable 3014

LUGESTERON (Finland)
PROGESTERONE
Prometrium Capsules (100 mg, 200 mg) . 3203

LUITASE (Italy)
PANCRELIPASE
Ultrase Capsules. 708
Ultrase MT Capsules 709

LUKAIR (Argentina)
MONTELUKAST SODIUM
Singulair Chewable Tablets 2077
Singulair Tablets 2077

LUKASM (Italy)
MONTELUKAST SODIUM
Singulair Chewable Tablets 2077
Singulair Tablets 2077

LUMAREN (Greece, Singapore)
RANITIDINE HYDROCHLORIDE
Zantac 25 EFFERdose Tablets 1624
Zantac 150 EFFERdose Tablets. 1624
Zantac 150 Tablets 1624
Zantac 300 Tablets 1624
Zantac Injection 1619
Zantac Injection Premixed 1619
Zantac Syrup 1624

LUMIX (Argentina)
SILDENAFIL CITRATE
Viagra Tablets 2573

LUMOX (Mexico)
AMOXICILLIN
Amoxil Pediatric Drops for Oral Suspension. 1343
Amoxil Tablets 1343

LUMOXBRON S (Mexico)
AMOXICILLIN
Amoxil Pediatric Drops for Oral Suspension. 1343
Amoxil Tablets 1343

LUNDIRAN (Spain)
NAPROXEN
EC-Naprosyn Delayed-Release Tablets. . . . 2761
Naprosyn Suspension. 2761
Naprosyn Tablets 2761

LUNIBRON (Italy)
FLUNISOLIDE
Aerobid Inhaler System. 1171
Aerobid-M Inhaler System 1171

LUNIS (Italy)
FLUNISOLIDE
Aerobid Inhaler System. 1171
Aerobid-M Inhaler System 1171

LUPAREN (Brazil)
DICLOFENAC SODIUM
Voltaren Tablets 2307
Voltaren-XR Tablets 2310

LURDEX (Mexico)
ALBENDAZOLE
Albenza Tablets. 1338

LUSTRAL (Irish Republic, Israel, United Kingdom)
SERTRALINE HYDROCHLORIDE
Zoloft Tablets 2586

LUTOGIN (Italy)
PROGESTERONE
Prometrium Capsules (100 mg, 200 mg) . 3203

LUTOPOLAR (Finland)
MEDROXYPROGESTERONE ACETATE
Depo-Medrol Single-Dose Vial 2619

LUTORAL (Italy)
MEDROXYPROGESTERONE ACETATE
Depo-Medrol Single-Dose Vial 2619

LUXAZONE (Italy)
DEXAMETHASONE
Decadron Tablets 1951

LYCEFT (India)
CEFTRIAXONE SODIUM
Rocephin Injectable Vials, ADD-Vantage, Galaxy, Bulk 2800

LYMETEL (Spain)
FLUVASTATIN SODIUM
Lescol Capsules 2233

LYNDAK (Italy)
SULINDAC
Clinoril Tablets 1924

LYOTRET (Greece)
ISOTRETINOIN
Accutane Capsules 2731

LYPHOCIN (Hong Kong)
VANCOMYCIN HYDROCHLORIDE
Vancocin HCl Capsules, USP 3380

LYSOVIR (United Kingdom)
AMANTADINE HYDROCHLORIDE
Symmetrel Tablets. 1135

LYSTIN (Hong Kong, Thailand)
NYSTATIN
Nystop Topical Powder USP. 2478
Paddock Nystatin USP for Oral Suspension. 2478

MAALOX H2 ACID CONTROLLER (Canada)
FAMOTIDINE
Pepcid Injection 2040
Pepcid Injection Premixed 2040
Pepcid Tablets 2038
Pepcid for Oral Suspension 2038

MABICROL (Mexico)
CLARITHROMYCIN
Biaxin Filmtab Tablets 402
Biaxin Granules 402

MABRON (Czech Republic, Hong Kong, Malaysia, Russia, Singapore, Thailand, United Kingdom)
TRAMADOL HYDROCHLORIDE
Ultram ER Tablets 2392

MABTHERA (Argentina, Australia, Austria, Belgium, Brazil, Chile, Czech Republic, Denmark, Finland, France, Germany, Greece, Hong Kong, Hungary, Irish Republic, Israel, Italy, Mexico, New Zealand, Norway, Portugal, Singapore, South Africa, Spain, Sweden, Switzerland, Thailand, The Netherlands, United Kingdom, Venezuela)
RITUXIMAB
Rituxan I.V. 1254

MACLADIN (Italy)
CLARITHROMYCIN
Biaxin Filmtab Tablets 402
Biaxin Granules 402

MACLAR (Austria, Belgium, India, Portugal)
CLARITHROMYCIN
Biaxin Filmtab Tablets 402
Biaxin Granules 402

MACOBAL (Argentina)
NIMODIPINE
Nimotop Capsules 749

MACOREL (Greece)
NIFEDIPINE
Adalat CC Tablets 2964

MACROLIN (France)
ALDESLEUKIN
Proleukin for Injection 2266

MACROMICINA (Argentina)
CLARITHROMYCIN
Biaxin Filmtab Tablets 402
Biaxin Granules 402

MACSORALEN (India)
METHOXSALEN
Oxsoralen Lotion 1% 3352
Oxsoralen-Ultra Capsules. 3353

MADAPROX (Spain)
NAPROXEN
EC-Naprosyn Delayed-Release Tablets. . . . 2761
Naprosyn Suspension. 2761
Naprosyn Tablets 2761

MADOL (Thailand)
TRAMADOL HYDROCHLORIDE
Ultram ER Tablets 2392

MADOLA (Thailand)
TRAMADOL HYDROCHLORIDE
Ultram ER Tablets 2392

MAFEL (Argentina)
PROGESTERONE
Prometrium Capsules (100 mg, 200 mg) . 3203

MAFENA (Mexico)
DICLOFENAC SODIUM
Voltaren Tablets ... 2307
Voltaren-XR Tablets ... 2310

MAFORAN (Thailand)
WARFARIN SODIUM
Coumadin Tablets ... 898
Coumadin for Injection ... 898

MAGLUPHEN (Austria)
DICLOFENAC SODIUM
Voltaren Tablets ... 2307
Voltaren-XR Tablets ... 2310

MAGNASPOR (Thailand)
CEFUROXIME AXETIL
Ceftin Tablets ... 1407
Ceftin for Oral Suspension ... 1407

MAGNITON-R (Greece)
INDAPAMIDE
Indapamide Tablets ... 2156

MAGNOGEN (Argentina)
BUPRENORPHINE HYDROCHLORIDE
Buprenex Injectable ... 2716

MAGNUROL (Spain)
TERAZOSIN HYDROCHLORIDE
Hytrin Capsules ... 471

MAGNUS (Argentina)
SILDENAFIL CITRATE
Viagra Tablets ... 2573

MAJOLAT (Austria)
NIFEDIPINE
Adalat CC Tablets ... 2964

MALANIL (South Africa)
ATOVAQUONE
Mepron Suspension ... 1521

MALARONE (Australia, Brazil, Israel, Italy, New Zealand, Norway, Spain, The Netherlands, United Kingdom)
ATOVAQUONE
Mepron Suspension ... 1521

MALASTOP (Belgium)
PYRIMETHAMINE
Daraprim Tablets ... 1419

MALEAPRIL (Brazil)
ENALAPRIL MALEATE
Vasotec I.V. Injection ... 2103

MALEDROL (Greece)
LEVOCARNITINE
Carnitor Injection ... 3188
Carnitor Tablets and Oral Solution ... 3190

MALEN (Portugal)
ENALAPRIL MALEATE
Vasotec I.V. Injection ... 2103

MALEXIN (Germany)
NAPROXEN
EC-Naprosyn Delayed-Release Tablets ... 2761
Naprosyn Suspension ... 2761
Naprosyn Tablets ... 2761

MALFIN (Denmark)
MORPHINE SULFATE
Kadian Capsules ... 577
MS Contin Tablets ... 2701

MALOCEF (Greece)
CEFTAZIDIME
Fortaz for Injection ... 1453

MALOCIDE (France)
PYRIMETHAMINE
Daraprim Tablets ... 1419

MALOCIN (Thailand)
ERYTHROMYCIN STEARATE
Erythrocin Stearate Filmtab Tablets ... 453

MALOPRIM (Belgium, Irish Republic)
PYRIMETHAMINE
Daraprim Tablets ... 1419

MANDOLGIN (Denmark)
TRAMADOL HYDROCHLORIDE
Ultram ER Tablets ... 2392

MANDROLAX LACTU (Germany)
LACTULOSE
Kristalose for Oral Solution ... 1034

MANDRO-ZEP (Germany)
DIAZEPAM
Diastat Rectal Delivery System ... 3343
Valium Tablets ... 2819

MANIDON (Spain, Venezuela)
VERAPAMIL HYDROCHLORIDE
Covera-HS Tablets ... 3139
Verelan PM Extended-Release Capsules, Controlled-Onset ... 3106

MANODEPO (Thailand)
MEDROXYPROGESTERONE ACETATE
Depo-Medrol Single-Dose Vial ... 2619

MANOFLOX (Thailand)
NORFLOXACIN
Noroxin Tablets ... 2032

MANOLONE (Thailand)
TRIAMCINOLONE ACETONIDE
Azmacort Inhalation Aerosol ... 1726
Nasacort AQ Nasal Spray ... 2922

MANOMAZOLE (Thailand)
CLOTRIMAZOLE
Lotrimin Cream ... 3039
Lotrimin Lotion 1% ... 3039
Lotrimin Topical Solution 1% ... 3039

MANTADAN (Italy)
AMANTADINE HYDROCHLORIDE
Symmetrel Tablets ... 1135

MANTADINE (United Kingdom)
AMANTADINE HYDROCHLORIDE
Symmetrel Tablets ... 1135

MANTADIX (Belgium, France)
AMANTADINE HYDROCHLORIDE
Symmetrel Tablets ... 1135

MANTIDAN (Brazil)
AMANTADINE HYDROCHLORIDE
Symmetrel Tablets ... 1135

MAOTIL (Germany)
SELEGILINE HYDROCHLORIDE
Eldepryl Capsules ... 3208

MAP AN (Argentina)
MEDROXYPROGESTERONE ACETATE
Depo-Medrol Single-Dose Vial ... 2619

MAPELOR (The Netherlands)
TAMSULOSIN HYDROCHLORIDE
Flomax Capsules ... 850

MAPEZINE (Thailand)
CARBAMAZEPINE
Carbatrol Capsules ... 3171
Tegretol Chewable Tablets ... 2295
Tegretol Suspension ... 2295
Tegretol Tablets ... 2295
Tegretol-XR Tablets ... 2295

MAPLUXIN (Mexico)
DIGOXIN
Lanoxicaps Capsules ... 1490
Lanoxin Injection ... 1494
Lanoxin Injection Pediatric ... 1497
Lanoxin Tablets ... 1500

MARADEX (Venezuela)
DEXAMETHASONE
Decadron Tablets ... 1951

MARDUK (Germany)
BENZOYL PEROXIDE
Brevoxyl-4 Creamy Wash ... 3210
Brevoxyl-4 Gel ... 3210
Brevoxyl-8 Creamy Wash ... 3210
Brevoxyl-8 Gel ... 3210
Triaz Cleanser ... 1892
Triaz Gel ... 1892

MAREVAN (Australia, Belgium, Brazil, Denmark, Finland, Greece, New Zealand, Norway, Singapore, United Kingdom)
WARFARIN SODIUM
Coumadin Tablets ... 898
Coumadin for Injection ... 898

MARFLOXACIN (Hong Kong)
OFLOXACIN
Floxin Otic Solution ... 1049

MARINOL (Canada)
DRONABINOL
Marinol Capsules ... 3333

MARMODINE (Hong Kong)
FAMOTIDINE
Pepcid Injection ... 2040
Pepcid Injection Premixed ... 2040
Pepcid Tablets ... 2038
Pepcid for Oral Suspension ... 2038

MARPHAZOLE (Hong Kong)
METRONIDAZOLE
MetroGel-Vaginal Gel ... 1855

MARTIGENTA (France)
GENTAMICIN SULFATE
Garamycin Injectable ... 3014

MARTULOSE (Hong Kong)
LACTULOSE
Kristalose for Oral Solution ... 1034

MARVIL (Argentina)
ALENDRONATE SODIUM
Fosamax Tablets ... 1969

MASAWORM (Thailand)
ALBENDAZOLE
Albenza Tablets ... 1338

MASDIL (Spain)
DILTIAZEM HYDROCHLORIDE
Cardizem LA Extended Release Tablets ... 1728
Tiazac Capsules ... 1201

MASNODERM (United Kingdom)
CLOTRIMAZOLE
Lotrimin Cream ... 3039
Lotrimin Lotion 1% ... 3039
Lotrimin Topical Solution 1% ... 3039

MATIGEL (Venezuela)
TIMOLOL MALEATE
Blocadren Tablets ... 1916
Timoptic Sterile Ophthalmic Solution ... 2088
Timoptic in Ocudose ... 2091
Timoptic-XE Sterile Ophthalmic Gel Forming Solution ... 2092

MATILOL (Venezuela)
TIMOLOL MALEATE
Blocadren Tablets ... 1916
Timoptic Sterile Ophthalmic Solution ... 2088
Timoptic in Ocudose ... 2091
Timoptic-XE Sterile Ophthalmic Gel Forming Solution ... 2092

MATULANE (Canada)
PROCARBAZINE HYDROCHLORIDE
Matulane Capsules ... 3191

MAURAN (Italy)
RANITIDINE HYDROCHLORIDE
Zantac 25 EFFERdose Tablets ... 1624
Zantac 150 EFFERdose Tablets ... 1624
Zantac 150 Tablets ... 1624
Zantac 300 Tablets ... 1624
Zantac Injection ... 1619
Zantac Injection Premixed ... 1619
Zantac Syrup ... 1624

MAVID (Germany)
CLARITHROMYCIN
Biaxin Filmtab Tablets ... 402
Biaxin Granules ... 402

MAVIFLOX (Mexico)
CIPROFLOXACIN
Cipro Oral Suspension ... 2977

MAVIK (Canada, South Africa)
TRANDOLAPRIL
Mavik Tablets ... 486

MAVILAN (Mexico)
LANSOPRAZOLE
Prevacid Delayed-Release Capsules ... 3271

MAXAIR (France, Switzerland)
PIRBUTEROL ACETATE
Maxair Autohaler ... 1852

MAXALT (Argentina, Austria, Belgium, Brazil, Canada, Chile, Czech Republic, Denmark, Finland, Germany, Greece, Hungary, Italy, Mexico, New Zealand, Norway, Portugal, South Africa, Spain, Sweden, Switzerland, The Netherlands, United Kingdom, Venezuela)
RIZATRIPTAN BENZOATE
Maxalt Tablets ... 2008
Maxalt-MLT Orally Disintegrating Tablets ... 2008

MAXCEF (Argentina, Brazil, Israel)
CEFEPIME HYDROCHLORIDE
Maxipime for Injection ... 1105

MAXDOSA (Argentina)
SILDENAFIL CITRATE
Viagra Tablets ... 2573

MAXIBONE (Israel)
ALENDRONATE SODIUM
Fosamax Tablets ... 1969

MAXIBRAL (Greece)
ETIDRONATE DISODIUM
Didronel Tablets ... 2697

MAXICARDIL (Argentina)
DIPYRIDAMOLE
Persantine Tablets ... 868

MAXIDEX (Australia, Belgium, Brazil, Canada, Chile, Denmark, France, Greece, Hong Kong, Hungary, Irish Republic, Israel, Malaysia, Mexico, New Zealand, Russia, Singapore, South Africa, Spain, Switzerland, The Netherlands, United Kingdom)
DEXAMETHASONE
Decadron Tablets ... 1951

MAXIDON (Sweden)
MORPHINE SULFATE
Kadian Capsules ... 577
MS Contin Tablets ... 2701

MAXIFLOX (Brazil)
CIPROFLOXACIN HYDROCHLORIDE
Ciloxan Ophthalmic Ointment ... ⊙204, 559
Ciloxan Ophthalmic Solution ... ⊙206
Cipro Tablets ... 2977

MAXIFLOX D (Brazil)
CIPROFLOXACIN HYDROCHLORIDE
Ciloxan Ophthalmic Ointment ... ⊙204, 559
Ciloxan Ophthalmic Solution ... ⊙206
Cipro Tablets ... 2977

MAXIL (Brazil)
CEFEPIME HYDROCHLORIDE
Maxipime for Injection ... 1105

MAXILERG (Brazil)
DICLOFENAC SODIUM
Voltaren Tablets ... 2307
Voltaren-XR Tablets ... 2310

MAXIMO (Argentina)
SILDENAFIL CITRATE
Viagra Tablets ... 2573

MAXINT (Mexico)
AMOXICILLIN
Amoxil Pediatric Drops for Oral Suspension ... 1343
Amoxil Tablets ... 1343

MAXIOSTENIL (Argentina)
SODIUM HYALURONATE
Hyalgan Solution ... 2901

MAXIPIME (Australia, Austria, Belgium, Canada, Chile, Czech Republic, Denmark, Finland, Germany, Greece, Hong Kong, Hungary, Irish Republic, Italy, Malaysia, Mexico, New Zealand, Portugal, Russia, Singapore, South Africa, Spain, Sweden, Switzerland, Thailand, The Netherlands, Venezuela)
CEFEPIME HYDROCHLORIDE
Maxipime for Injection ... 1105

MAXIPRIL (Italy)
CAPTOPRIL
Captopril Tablets ... 2149

MAXIVANIL (Italy)
VANCOMYCIN HYDROCHLORIDE
Vancocin HCl Capsules, USP ... 3380

MAXTRAL (Argentina)
ALENDRONATE SODIUM
Fosamax Tablets ... 1969

MAXZIDE (Belgium)
TRIAMTERENE
Dyrenium Capsules ... 3400

MAZEPINE (Canada)
CARBAMAZEPINE
Carbatrol Capsules ... 3171
Tegretol Chewable Tablets ... 2295
Tegretol Suspension ... 2295
Tegretol Tablets ... 2295
Tegretol-XR Tablets ... 2295

MAZETOL (India)
CARBAMAZEPINE
Carbatrol Capsules ... 3171
Tegretol Chewable Tablets ... 2295
Tegretol Suspension ... 2295
Tegretol Tablets ... 2295
Tegretol-XR Tablets ... 2295

M-BETA (Germany)
MORPHINE SULFATE
Kadian Capsules ... 577

(⊙ Described in PDR For Ophthalmic Medicines™)

MS Contin Tablets 2701

MCR (Israel)
MORPHINE SULFATE
Kadian Capsules 577
MS Contin Tablets 2701

MCR-50 (United Kingdom)
ISOSORBIDE MONONITRATE
Imdur Tablets 3018

MDILTIWAS (Spain)
DILTIAZEM HYDROCHLORIDE
Cardizem LA Extended Release Tablets . . . 1728
Tiazac Capsules 1201

M-DOLOR (Austria, Germany)
MORPHINE SULFATE
Kadian Capsules 577
MS Contin Tablets 2701

MEBENIX (Brazil)
ALBENDAZOLE
Albenza Tablets 1338

MECTIZAN (France)
IVERMECTIN
Stromectol Tablets 2083

MEDALIN (Venezuela)
FAMOTIDINE
Pepcid Injection 2040
Pepcid Injection Premixed 2040
Pepcid Tablets 2038
Pepcid for Oral Suspension 2038

MEDAMET (South Africa)
METRONIDAZOLE
MetroGel-Vaginal Gel 1855

MEDAMOR (Finland)
AMILORIDE HYDROCHLORIDE
Midamor Tablets 2026

MEDAREN (Thailand)
DICLOFENAC SODIUM
Voltaren Tablets 2307
Voltaren-XR Tablets 2310

MEDASPOR (South Africa)
CLOTRIMAZOLE
Lotrimin Cream 3039
Lotrimin Lotion 1% 3039
Lotrimin Topical Solution 1% 3039

MEDAXONE (Russia)
CEFTRIAXONE SODIUM
Rocephin Injectable Vials, ADD-Vantage, Galaxy, Bulk 2800

MEDAZOL (Chile, Czech Republic, Mexico)
METRONIDAZOLE
MetroGel-Vaginal Gel 1855

MEDAZYL (Thailand)
METRONIDAZOLE
MetroGel-Vaginal Gel 1855

MEDETON (Thailand)
MEDROXYPROGESTERONE ACETATE
Depo-Medrol Single-Dose Vial 2619

MEDGESIC (Thailand)
ORPHENADRINE CITRATE
Norflex Injection 1856

MEDIBIOX (Chile)
LEVOFLOXACIN
Levaquin Injection 2384
Levaquin Tablets 2384

MEDICLEAR (United Kingdom)
BENZOYL PEROXIDE
Brevoxyl-4 Creamy Wash 3210
Brevoxyl-4 Gel 3210
Brevoxyl-8 Creamy Wash 3210
Brevoxyl-8 Gel 3210
Triaz Cleanser 1892
Triaz Gel 1892

MEDIFUNGOL (Argentina)
CLOTRIMAZOLE
Lotrimin Cream 3039
Lotrimin Lotion 1% 3039
Lotrimin Topical Solution 1% 3039

MEDIKINET (Germany)
METHYLPHENIDATE HYDROCHLORIDE
Ritalin Hydrochloride Tablets 2269
Ritalin-SR Tablets 2269

MEDILAX (Denmark)
LACTULOSE
Kristalose for Oral Solution 1034

MEDILET (Austria, Germany)
LACTULOSE
Kristalose for Oral Solution 1034

MEDILIUM (Canada)
CHLORDIAZEPOXIDE HYDROCHLORIDE
Librium Capsules 3347

MEDINOX MONO (Germany)
PENTOBARBITAL SODIUM
Nembutal Sodium Solution, USP 2470

MEDIPAM (Finland)
DIAZEPAM
Diastat Rectal Delivery System 3343
Valium Tablets 2819

MEDIPHYLLIN CHRONO (Greece)
THEOPHYLLINE
Uniphyl Tablets 2710

MEDIPINA (Portugal)
NIFEDIPINE
Adalat CC Tablets 2964

MEDIPO (Italy)
SIMVASTATIN
Zocor Tablets 2105

MEDIPRIM (Mexico)
LANSOPRAZOLE
Prevacid Delayed-Release Capsules 3271

MEDISPORT ATHLETE'S FOOT (United Kingdom)
CLOTRIMAZOLE
Lotrimin Cream 3039
Lotrimin Lotion 1% 3039
Lotrimin Topical Solution 1% 3039

MEDIURESIX (Thailand)
FUROSEMIDE
Furosemide Tablets 2154

MEDIXIL (Chile)
SIBUTRAMINE HYDROCHLORIDE
Meridia Capsules 489

MEDIXIN (Argentina)
LACTULOSE
Kristalose for Oral Solution 1034

MEDIZOL (Mexico)
METRONIDAZOLE
MetroGel-Vaginal Gel 1855

MEDOCARNITIN (Italy)
LEVOCARNITINE
Carnitor Injection 3188
Carnitor Tablets and Oral Solution 3190

MEDOCIPRIN (Hong Kong, Russia, Thailand)
CIPROFLOXACIN HYDROCHLORIDE
Ciloxan Ophthalmic Ointment . . . . ⊙204, 559
Ciloxan Ophthalmic Solution . . . . ⊙206
Cipro Tablets 2977

MEDOCOR (Argentina)
ISOSORBIDE MONONITRATE
Imdur Tablets 3018

MEDODERMONE (Hong Kong, Singapore, Thailand)
CLOBETASOL PROPIONATE
Temovate Cream 2668
Temovate E Emollient 2671
Temovate Gel 2669
Temovate Ointment 2668
Temovate Scalp Application 2670

MEDOFLOXINE (Malaysia)
OFLOXACIN
Floxin Otic Solution 1049

MEDOSTATIN (Czech Republic, Hong Kong, Malaysia, Russia, Singapore)
LOVASTATIN
Mevacor Tablets 2021

MEDOVASCIN (Greece)
LOVASTATIN
Mevacor Tablets 2021

MEDOXEM (Greece)
CEFUROXIME SODIUM
Zinacef Injection 1631

MEDOXIM (Italy)
CEFUROXIME SODIUM
Zinacef Injection 1631

MEDOXONUM (Hong Kong)
CEFTRIAXONE SODIUM
Rocephin Injectable Vials, ADD-Vantage, Galaxy, Bulk 2800

MEDOZEM (Thailand)
DILTIAZEM HYDROCHLORIDE
Cardizem LA Extended Release Tablets . . . 1728
Tiazac Capsules 1201

MEDOZIDE (Italy)
HYDROCHLOROTHIAZIDE/METHYLDOPA
Aldoril Tablets 1910

MED-PHYLLINE (Thailand)
THEOPHYLLINE
Uniphyl Tablets 2710

MEDROCIL (Argentina)
HYDROCORTISONE
Hydrocortone Tablets 1989

MEDROL VERIDERM (Canada, Italy)
METHYLPREDNISOLONE ACETATE
Depo-Medrol Injectable Suspension 2617

MEDROSTERONA (Argentina)
MEDROXYPROGESTERONE ACETATE
Depo-Medrol Single-Dose Vial 2619

MEDROXITEST (Brazil)
MEDROXYPROGESTERONE ACETATE
Depo-Medrol Single-Dose Vial 2619

MEDROXYHEXAL (Australia)
MEDROXYPROGESTERONE ACETATE
Depo-Medrol Single-Dose Vial 2619

MED-TRICOCIDE (Thailand)
METRONIDAZOLE
MetroGel-Vaginal Gel 1855

MEFIRON (Thailand)
METRONIDAZOLE
MetroGel-Vaginal Gel 1855

MEFLIAM (India, South Africa)
MEFLOQUINE HYDROCHLORIDE
Lariam Tablets 2786

MEFLOC (India)
MEFLOQUINE HYDROCHLORIDE
Lariam Tablets 2786

MEFOXIL (Greece)
CEFOXITIN SODIUM
Mefoxin Premixed Intravenous Solution . . . 2016
Mefoxin for Injection 2012

MEFOXIN (Argentina, Australia, Belgium, Brazil, Canada, Czech Republic, Finland, France, Hong Kong, Irish Republic, Italy, New Zealand, Portugal, South Africa, The Netherlands, United Kingdom)
CEFOXITIN SODIUM
Mefoxin Premixed Intravenous Solution . . . 2016
Mefoxin for Injection 2012

MEFOXITIN (Austria, Germany, Norway, Spain, Sweden, Switzerland, Venezuela)
CEFOXITIN SODIUM
Mefoxin Premixed Intravenous Solution . . . 2016
Mefoxin for Injection 2012

MEGACINA (Portugal)
OFLOXACIN
Floxin Otic Solution 1049

MEGAFLOX (Portugal)
CIPROFLOXACIN HYDROCHLORIDE
Ciloxan Ophthalmic Ointment . . . . ⊙204, 559
Ciloxan Ophthalmic Solution . . . . ⊙206
Cipro Tablets 2977

MEGALAT (Israel)
NIFEDIPINE
Adalat CC Tablets 2964

MEGALEX (Argentina)
RANITIDINE HYDROCHLORIDE
Zantac 25 EFFERdose Tablets 1624
Zantac 150 EFFERdose Tablets 1624
Zantac 150 Tablets 1624
Zantac 300 Tablets 1624
Zantac Injection 1619
Zantac Injection Premixed 1619
Zantac Syrup 1624

MEGALIS (Venezuela)
DIPYRIDAMOLE
Persantine Tablets 868

MEGAPRESS (Greece)
ENALAPRIL MALEATE
Vasotec I.V. Injection 2103

MEGASIN (Portugal)
OFLOXACIN
Floxin Otic Solution 1049

MEGAVIS (Italy)
LEVOCARNITINE
Carnitor Injection 3188
Carnitor Tablets and Oral Solution 3190

MEGENTAL (Czech Republic)
GENTAMICIN SULFATE
Garamycin Injectable 3014

MEGENTAL PEDIATRICO (Italy)
GENTAMICIN SULFATE
Garamycin Injectable 3014

MEGION (Hungary, Mexico, Venezuela)
CEFTRIAXONE SODIUM
Rocephin Injectable Vials, ADD-Vantage, Galaxy, Bulk 2800

MELADININA (Mexico)
METHOXSALEN
Oxsoralen Lotion 1% 3352
Oxsoralen-Ultra Capsules 3353

MELADININE (France, Germany, Malaysia, Switzerland, Thailand, The Netherlands)
METHOXSALEN
Oxsoralen Lotion 1% 3352
Oxsoralen-Ultra Capsules 3353

MELANOCYL (India)
METHOXSALEN
Oxsoralen Lotion 1% 3352
Oxsoralen-Ultra Capsules 3353

MELAOLINE (Greece)
METHOXSALEN
Oxsoralen Lotion 1% 3352
Oxsoralen-Ultra Capsules 3353

MELAXOSE (France)
LACTULOSE
Kristalose for Oral Solution 1034

MELERIL (Spain, Venezuela)
THIORIDAZINE HYDROCHLORIDE
Thioridazine Hydrochloride Tablets 2163

MELGAR (Argentina)
NAPROXEN
EC-Naprosyn Delayed-Release Tablets 2761
Naprosyn Suspension 2761
Naprosyn Tablets 2761

MELLERETTEN (Germany, The Netherlands)
THIORIDAZINE HYDROCHLORIDE
Thioridazine Hydrochloride Tablets 2163

MELLERETTES (Switzerland)
THIORIDAZINE HYDROCHLORIDE
Thioridazine Hydrochloride Tablets 2163

MELLERIL (Austria, Belgium, Brazil, Denmark, Finland, Greece, Hong Kong, Hungary, Irish Republic, Israel, Italy, Malaysia, New Zealand, Norway, Portugal, South Africa, Switzerland, The Netherlands)
THIORIDAZINE HYDROCHLORIDE
Thioridazine Hydrochloride Tablets 2163

MELOL (Thailand)
METOPROLOL TARTRATE
Lopressor Tablets 2238

MELZINE (Irish Republic)
THIORIDAZINE HYDROCHLORIDE
Thioridazine Hydrochloride Tablets 2163

MEMAC (Italy)
DONEPEZIL HYDROCHLORIDE
Aricept Tablets 1094

MEMENTO NF (Argentina)
NORFLOXACIN
Noroxin Tablets 2032

MENAELLE (Monaco)
PROGESTERONE
Prometrium Capsules (100 mg, 200 mg) . 3203

MENISOLE (Thailand)
METRONIDAZOLE
MetroGel-Vaginal Gel 1855

MENIZOL (Venezuela)
METRONIDAZOLE
MetroGel-Vaginal Gel 1855

MENOGRAINE (South Africa)
CLONIDINE HYDROCHLORIDE
Catapres Tablets 843

MENO-IMPLANT (Belgium, The Netherlands)
ESTRADIOL
Climara Transdermal System 771
Estring Vaginal Ring 2635

MENO-PATCH (Israel)
ESTRADIOL
Climara Transdermal System 771
Estring Vaginal Ring 2635

MENOREST (Australia, Austria, Brazil, Czech Republic, Denmark, Finland, France, Germany, Greece, Irish Republic, Italy, Norway, Portugal, South Africa, Spain, Sweden, Switzerland, The Netherlands, United Kingdom)
ESTRADIOL
Climara Transdermal System 771
Estring Vaginal Ring 2635

MENSOMA (Portugal)
FAMOTIDINE
Pepcid Injection 2040
Pepcid Injection Premixed 2040
Pepcid Tablets 2038
Pepcid for Oral Suspension 2038

MENTAX (Brazil, Israel, Japan)
BUTENAFINE HYDROCHLORIDE
Mentax Cream 2158

MENTIX (Chile)
MODAFINIL
Provigil Tablets 988

MEPAGYL (Thailand)
METRONIDAZOLE
MetroGel-Vaginal Gel 1855

MEPASTAT (Finland)
MEDROXYPROGESTERONE ACETATE
Depo-Medrol Single-Dose Vial 2619

MEPHAQUIN (Brazil, Czech Republic, Hong Kong, Israel, Malaysia, Portugal, Singapore, Thailand)
MEFLOQUINE HYDROCHLORIDE
Lariam Tablets 2786

MEPHAQUINE (Switzerland)
MEFLOQUINE HYDROCHLORIDE
Lariam Tablets 2786

MEPLAR (Argentina)
PAROXETINE HYDROCHLORIDE
Paxil Oral Suspension 1530
Paxil Tablets 1530

MEPRANIX (United Kingdom)
METOPROLOL TARTRATE
Lopressor Tablets 2238

MEPRATE (India)
MEDROXYPROGESTERONE ACETATE
Depo-Medrol Single-Dose Vial 2619

MEPRIL (Austria)
ENALAPRIL MALEATE
Vasotec I.V. Injection 2103

MEPROLOL (Germany)
METOPROLOL TARTRATE
Lopressor Tablets 2238

MEPROLOL COMP (Germany)
METOPROLOL TARTRATE
Lopressor Tablets 2238

MEPRON (Canada)
ATOVAQUONE
Mepron Suspension 1521

MEPRONET (Denmark)
METOPROLOL TARTRATE
Lopressor Tablets 2238

MEQUIN (Thailand)
MEFLOQUINE HYDROCHLORIDE
Lariam Tablets 2786

MERANOL (Venezuela)
DIPYRIDAMOLE
Persantine Tablets 868

MERAPRIL (Italy)
CAPTOPRIL
Captopril Tablets 2149

MERCAPTYL (Switzerland)
PENICILLAMINE
Cuprimine Capsules 1947

MEREDAZOL (Mexico)
METRONIDAZOLE
MetroGel-Vaginal Gel 1855

MEREPRINE (Portugal)
CAPTOPRIL
Captopril Tablets 2149

MERIDIA (Austria, Canada, Russia)
SIBUTRAMINE HYDROCHLORIDE
Meridia Capsules 489

MERLIT (Greece)
LEVOCARNITINE
Carnitor Injection 3188
Carnitor Tablets and Oral Solution 3190

MERONEM (Belgium, Brazil, Chile, Czech Republic, Denmark, Finland, Germany, Greece, Hong Kong, Hungary, Irish Republic, Israel, Malaysia, Norway, Portugal, Russia, Singapore, South Africa, Spain, Sweden, Switzerland, Thailand, The Netherlands, United Kingdom, Venezuela)
MEROPENEM
Merrem I.V. 686

MEROPEN (Japan)
MEROPENEM
Merrem I.V. 686

MEROXIL (Brazil)
MEROPENEM
Merrem I.V. 686

MEROZEN (Argentina)
MEROPENEM
Merrem I.V. 686

MERREM (Australia, Canada, Italy, Mexico, New Zealand)
MEROPENEM
Merrem I.V. 686

MERTAN (Austria)
NAPHAZOLINE HYDROCHLORIDE
Albalon Ophthalmic Solution . . . . ⊙218

MERXIL (Mexico)
DICLOFENAC SODIUM
Voltaren Tablets 2307
Voltaren-XR Tablets 2310

MESACTOL (Argentina)
LANSOPRAZOLE
Prevacid Delayed-Release Capsules 3271

MESIN (Thailand)
ALBENDAZOLE
Albenza Tablets 1338

M-ESLON (Canada, Chile, Czech Republic, Hong Kong, Hungary, New Zealand)
MORPHINE SULFATE
Kadian Capsules 577
MS Contin Tablets 2701

MESOLEX (Thailand)
METRONIDAZOLE
MetroGel-Vaginal Gel 1855

MESPORIN (Hong Kong, Portugal)
CEFTRIAXONE SODIUM
Rocephin Injectable Vials, ADD-Vantage, Galaxy, Bulk 2800

META (Thailand)
PROMETHAZINE HYDROCHLORIDE
Phenergan Tablets and Suppositories 3440

METADATE (Israel)
METHYLPHENIDATE HYDROCHLORIDE
Ritalin Hydrochloride Tablets 2269
Ritalin-SR Tablets 2269

METAFLEX PLUS NF (Argentina)
DICLOFENAC SODIUM
Voltaren Tablets 2307
Voltaren-XR Tablets 2310

METAGYL (South Africa)
METRONIDAZOLE
MetroGel-Vaginal Gel 1855

METALCAPTASE (Czech Republic, Germany, Japan, South Africa)
PENICILLAMINE
Cuprimine Capsules 1947

METAMIDOL (Portugal)
DIAZEPAM
Diastat Rectal Delivery System 3343
Valium Tablets 2819

METAPTYL (Greece)
CEFOXITIN SODIUM
Mefoxin Premixed Intravenous Solution . . . 2016
Mefoxin for Injection 2012

METASON (Argentina)
MOMETASONE FUROATE
Elocon Cream 0.1% 3005
Elocon Lotion 0.1% 3006
Elocon Ointment 0.1% 3007
Nasonex Nasal Spray 3043

METASPRAY (India)
MOMETASONE FUROATE
Elocon Cream 0.1% 3005
Elocon Lotion 0.1% 3006
Elocon Ointment 0.1% 3007
Nasonex Nasal Spray 3043

METAZEM (Hong Kong, Singapore, Thailand, United Kingdom)
DILTIAZEM HYDROCHLORIDE
Cardizem LA Extended Release Tablets . . . 1728
Tiazac Capsules 1201

METAZOL (South Africa)
METRONIDAZOLE
MetroGel-Vaginal Gel 1855

METBLOCK (Finland)
METOPROLOL TARTRATE
Lopressor Tablets 2238

METHYLIN (Argentina)
METHYLPHENIDATE HYDROCHLORIDE
Ritalin Hydrochloride Tablets 2269
Ritalin-SR Tablets 2269

METICEL (Spain)
RANITIDINE HYDROCHLORIDE
Zantac 25 EFFERdose Tablets 1624
Zantac 150 EFFERdose Tablets 1624
Zantac 150 Tablets 1624
Zantac 300 Tablets 1624
Zantac Injection 1619
Zantac Injection Premixed 1619
Zantac Syrup 1624

METILBETASONE SOLUBILE (Italy)
METHYLPREDNISOLONE ACETATE
Depo-Medrol Injectable Suspension 2617

METIMYD (Canada, Sweden)
PREDNISOLONE ACETATE/SULFACETAMIDE SODIUM
Blephamide Ophthalmic Ointment 568
Blephamide Ophthalmic Suspension 569

METLIGINE (Japan)
MIDODRINE HYDROCHLORIDE
ProAmatine Tablets 3186

METO COMP (Germany)
HYDROCHLOROTHIAZIDE/METOPROLOL TARTRATE
Lopressor HCT 100/25 Tablets 2241

METOBETA (Germany)
METOPROLOL TARTRATE
Lopressor Tablets 2238

METOBETA COMP (Germany)
HYDROCHLOROTHIAZIDE/METOPROLOL TARTRATE
Lopressor HCT 100/25 Tablets 2241

METOBLOCK (Thailand)
METOPROLOL TARTRATE
Lopressor Tablets 2238

METOCAR (Denmark)
METOPROLOL TARTRATE
Lopressor Tablets 2238

METO-COMP (Germany)
HYDROCHLOROTHIAZIDE/METOPROLOL TARTRATE
Lopressor HCT 100/25 Tablets 2241

METOCOR (Irish Republic)
METOPROLOL TARTRATE
Lopressor Tablets 2238

METODOC (Germany)
METOPROLOL TARTRATE
Lopressor Tablets 2238

METODURA (Germany)
METOPROLOL TARTRATE
Lopressor Tablets 2238

METODURA COMP (Germany)
HYDROCHLOROTHIAZIDE/METOPROLOL TARTRATE
Lopressor HCT 100/25 Tablets 2241

METOHEXAL (Australia, Austria, Czech Republic, Germany)
METOPROLOL TARTRATE
Lopressor Tablets 2238

METOHEXAL COMP (Germany)
HYDROCHLOROTHIAZIDE/METOPROLOL TARTRATE
Lopressor HCT 100/25 Tablets 2241

METO-ISIS COMP (Germany)
METOPROLOL TARTRATE
Lopressor Tablets 2238

METOK (Germany)
METOPROLOL TARTRATE
Lopressor Tablets 2238

METOLAR (India)
METOPROLOL TARTRATE
Lopressor Tablets 2238

METOLAR-H (India)
METOPROLOL TARTRATE
Lopressor Tablets 2238

METOLE (Hong Kong)
METRONIDAZOLE
MetroGel-Vaginal Gel 1855

METOLOL (Australia, Austria, Thailand)
METOPROLOL TARTRATE
Lopressor Tablets 2238

METOLOL COMPOSITUM (Austria)
HYDROCHLOROTHIAZIDE/METOPROLOL TARTRATE
Lopressor HCT 100/25 Tablets 2241

METOMED (Austria)
METOPROLOL TARTRATE
Lopressor Tablets 2238

METOMERCK (Germany)
METOPROLOL TARTRATE
Lopressor Tablets 2238

METOP (Irish Republic)
METOPROLOL TARTRATE
Lopressor Tablets 2238

METOPAL (Austria)
METOPROLOL TARTRATE
Lopressor Tablets 2238

METOPRESS (Israel, Switzerland)
METOPROLOL TARTRATE
Lopressor Tablets 2238

METOPROFERM (Sweden)
METOPROLOL TARTRATE
Lopressor Tablets 2238

METOPROGAMMA (Germany)
METOPROLOL TARTRATE
Lopressor Tablets 2238

METOPROLIN (Finland)
METOPROLOL TARTRATE
Lopressor Tablets 2238

METOPROLOL COMP (Germany)
METOPROLOL TARTRATE
Lopressor Tablets 2238

METOPROLOL COMPOSITUM (Austria)
METOPROLOL TARTRATE
Lopressor Tablets 2238

METORAL (Thailand)
TRIAMCINOLONE ACETONIDE
Azmacort Inhalation Aerosol 1726
Nasacort AQ Nasal Spray 2922

METOSAN (Mexico)
METRONIDAZOLE
MetroGel-Vaginal Gel 1855

METOSTAD COMP (Germany)
HYDROCHLOROTHIAZIDE/METOPROLOL TARTRATE
Lopressor HCT 100/25 Tablets 2241

METO-TABLINEN (Germany)
METOPROLOL TARTRATE
Lopressor Tablets 2238

METO-THIAZID (Germany)
HYDROCHLOROTHIAZIDE/METOPROLOL TARTRATE
Lopressor HCT 100/25 Tablets 2241
METOTYROL (Austria)
METOPROLOL TARTRATE
Lopressor Tablets 2238
METOZOC (Denmark, Finland, Norway)
METOPROLOL TARTRATE
Lopressor Tablets 2238
METRACIN (Mexico)
DICLOFENAC SODIUM
Voltaren Tablets 2307
Voltaren-XR Tablets 2310
METRAL (Argentina)
METRONIDAZOLE
MetroGel-Vaginal Gel 1855
METRAZOLE (South Africa, Thailand)
METRONIDAZOLE
MetroGel-Vaginal Gel 1855
METREN (Venezuela)
METRONIDAZOLE
MetroGel-Vaginal Gel 1855
METRICOM (Mexico)
METRONIDAZOLE
MetroGel-Vaginal Gel 1855
METRIS (Venezuela)
METRONIDAZOLE
MetroGel-Vaginal Gel 1855
METRIZOL (Brazil, Mexico, Switzerland)
METRONIDAZOLE
MetroGel-Vaginal Gel 1855
METROCEV (Argentina)
METRONIDAZOLE
MetroGel-Vaginal Gel 1855
METROCIDE (Thailand)
METRONIDAZOLE
MetroGel-Vaginal Gel 1855
METROCREAM (Canada, Chile, Mexico)
METRONIDAZOLE
MetroGel-Vaginal Gel 1855
METROCREME (Germany)
METRONIDAZOLE
MetroGel-Vaginal Gel 1855
METRODAX (Brazil)
METRONIDAZOLE
MetroGel-Vaginal Gel 1855
METRODERME (Portugal)
METRONIDAZOLE
MetroGel-Vaginal Gel 1855
METROFUR (Mexico)
METRONIDAZOLE
MetroGel-Vaginal Gel 1855
METROGEL (Canada, Chile, Denmark, Germany, Irish Republic, Mexico, The Netherlands, United Kingdom)
METRONIDAZOLE
MetroGel-Vaginal Gel 1855
METROGYL (Australia, Brazil, Greece, Hong Kong, India, Israel, Russia)
METRONIDAZOLE
MetroGel-Vaginal Gel 1855
METROL (Australia)
METOPROLOL TARTRATE
Lopressor Tablets 2238
METROLEX (Thailand)
METRONIDAZOLE
MetroGel-Vaginal Gel 1855
METROLYL (United Kingdom)
METRONIDAZOLE
MetroGel-Vaginal Gel 1855
METRONIB (Brazil)
METRONIDAZOLE
MetroGel-Vaginal Gel 1855
METRONIDE (Australia, Brazil, Irish Republic)
METRONIDAZOLE
MetroGel-Vaginal Gel 1855
METRONID-PUREN (Germany)
METRONIDAZOLE
MetroGel-Vaginal Gel 1855
METRONIFLEX (Brazil)
METRONIDAZOLE
MetroGel-Vaginal Gel 1855
METRONIMERCK (Germany)
METRONIDAZOLE
MetroGel-Vaginal Gel 1855
METRONIN (Brazil)
METRONIDAZOLE
MetroGel-Vaginal Gel 1855
METRONIX (Brazil)
METRONIDAZOLE
MetroGel-Vaginal Gel 1855
METRONOM (Austria)
PROPAFENONE HYDROCHLORIDE
Rythmol SR Capsules 2727
METRONOUR (Germany)
METRONIDAZOLE
MetroGel-Vaginal Gel 1855
METRONT (Germany)
METRONIDAZOLE
MetroGel-Vaginal Gel 1855
METROPAST (Chile)
METRONIDAZOLE
MetroGel-Vaginal Gel 1855
METROSA (United Kingdom)
METRONIDAZOLE
MetroGel-Vaginal Gel 1855
METROSON (Mexico)
METRONIDAZOLE
MetroGel-Vaginal Gel 1855
METROSTAT (South Africa)
METRONIDAZOLE
MetroGel-Vaginal Gel 1855
METROTIX (Brazil)
METRONIDAZOLE
MetroGel-Vaginal Gel 1855
METROTOP (Irish Republic, United Kingdom)
METRONIDAZOLE
MetroGel-Vaginal Gel 1855
METROVAL (Brazil)
METRONIDAZOLE
MetroGel-Vaginal Gel 1855
METROVAX (Venezuela)
METRONIDAZOLE
MetroGel-Vaginal Gel 1855
METROVIFORM (Mexico)
METRONIDAZOLE
MetroGel-Vaginal Gel 1855
METROZINE (Australia, Hong Kong)
METRONIDAZOLE
MetroGel-Vaginal Gel 1855
METROZOL (Brazil, United Kingdom)
METRONIDAZOLE
MetroGel-Vaginal Gel 1855
METROZOLE (Singapore)
METRONIDAZOLE
MetroGel-Vaginal Gel 1855
METRYL (South Africa)
METRONIDAZOLE
MetroGel-Vaginal Gel 1855
MEVACOR (Austria, Brazil, Canada, Chile, Czech Republic, Denmark, Finland, Greece, Hong Kong, Hungary, Malaysia, Mexico, Norway, Spain, Venezuela)
LOVASTATIN
Mevacor Tablets 2021
MEVAL (Canada)
DIAZEPAM
Diastat Rectal Delivery System 3343
Valium Tablets 2819
MEVAMYST (Greece)
LEVOCARNITINE
Carnitor Injection 3188
Carnitor Tablets and Oral Solution 3190
MEVASTEROL (Spain)
LOVASTATIN
Mevacor Tablets 2021
MEVASTIN (Greece)
LOVASTATIN
Mevacor Tablets 2021
MEVECAN (Greece)
CEFUROXIME AXETIL
Ceftin Tablets 1407
Ceftin for Oral Suspension 1407
MEVINACOR (Germany, Portugal)
LOVASTATIN
Mevacor Tablets 2021
MEVINOL (Greece)
LOVASTATIN
Mevacor Tablets 2021
MEVLOR (Argentina, Portugal)
LOVASTATIN
Mevacor Tablets 2021
MEXASONE (Singapore)
DEXAMETHASONE
Decadron Tablets 1951
MEXCYN (Mexico)
ERYTHROMYCIN
Ery-Tab Tablets 449
Erythromycin Base Filmtab Tablets 455
Erythromycin Delayed-Release Capsules, USP 457
PCE Dispertab Tablets 515
MEXONA (Mexico)
DEXAMETHASONE
Decadron Tablets 1951
M-FLOX (Thailand)
NORFLOXACIN
Noroxin Tablets 2032
MIBAZOL (Mexico)
METRONIDAZOLE
MetroGel-Vaginal Gel 1855
MIBESAN-S (Mexico)
NYSTATIN
Nystop Topical Powder USP 2478
Paddock Nystatin USP for Oral Suspension 2478
MICARDIS (Argentina, Australia, Austria, Belgium, Brazil, Canada, Chile, Czech Republic, Denmark, Finland, France, Germany, Greece, Hong Kong, Hungary, Irish Republic, Italy, Japan, Malaysia, Mexico, Norway, Portugal, Russia, Singapore, South Africa, Spain, Sweden, Switzerland, Thailand, The Netherlands, United Kingdom)
TELMISARTAN
Micardis Tablets 854
MICARDIS HCT (Brazil)
TELMISARTAN
Micardis Tablets 854
MICARDIS PLUS (Australia, Canada, Greece, Hong Kong, Italy, Malaysia, Mexico, Portugal, Singapore, Spain, Sweden, The Netherlands)
TELMISARTAN
Micardis Tablets 854
MICARDISPLUS (Austria, Belgium, Denmark, Finland, France, Germany, Irish Republic, Norway, Switzerland, United Kingdom)
TELMISARTAN
Micardis Tablets 854
MICITREX (Mexico)
TOBRAMYCIN
TOBI Solution for Inhalation 2298
MICLONAZOL (Brazil)
CLOTRIMAZOLE
Lotrimin Cream 3039
Lotrimin Lotion 1% 3039
Lotrimin Topical Solution 1% 3039
MICOBAN (Greece)
MUPIROCIN
Bactroban Ointment 1395
MICOCLIN (Argentina)
CLOTRIMAZOLE
Lotrimin Cream 3039
Lotrimin Lotion 1% 3039
Lotrimin Topical Solution 1% 3039
MICOMAX (Argentina)
CLOTRIMAZOLE
Lotrimin Cream 3039
Lotrimin Lotion 1% 3039
Lotrimin Topical Solution 1% 3039
MICOMAZOL (Argentina)
CLOTRIMAZOLE
Lotrimin Cream 3039
Lotrimin Lotion 1% 3039
Lotrimin Topical Solution 1% 3039
MICOMAZOL B (Argentina)
CLOTRIMAZOLE
Lotrimin Cream 3039
Lotrimin Lotion 1% 3039
Lotrimin Topical Solution 1% 3039
MICOMAZOL DEO (Argentina)
CLOTRIMAZOLE
Lotrimin Cream 3039
Lotrimin Lotion 1% 3039
Lotrimin Topical Solution 1% 3039
MICOMISAN (South Africa, Spain)
CLOTRIMAZOLE
Lotrimin Cream 3039
Lotrimin Lotion 1% 3039
Lotrimin Topical Solution 1% 3039
MICONACINA (Mexico)
NATAMYCIN
Natacyn Antifungal Ophthalmic Suspension .... ⊙208
MICOSEP (Argentina)
CLOTRIMAZOLE
Lotrimin Cream 3039
Lotrimin Lotion 1% 3039
Lotrimin Topical Solution 1% 3039
MICOSEP B (Argentina)
CLOTRIMAZOLE
Lotrimin Cream 3039
Lotrimin Lotion 1% 3039
Lotrimin Topical Solution 1% 3039
MICOSET (Chile)
TERBINAFINE HYDROCHLORIDE
Lamisil Tablets 2232
MICOSIL (Brazil)
TERBINAFINE HYDROCHLORIDE
Lamisil Tablets 2232
MICOSONA (Spain)
NAFTIFINE HYDROCHLORIDE
Naftin Cream 2126
Naftin Gel 2126
MICOSTAL (Brazil)
NYSTATIN
Nystop Topical Powder USP 2478
Paddock Nystatin USP for Oral Suspension 2478
MICOSTALAB (Brazil)
NYSTATIN
Nystop Topical Powder USP 2478
Paddock Nystatin USP for Oral Suspension 2478
MICOSTATIN (Argentina, Brazil, Chile, Mexico, Venezuela)
NYSTATIN
Nystop Topical Powder USP 2478
Paddock Nystatin USP for Oral Suspension 2478
MICOSTATIN BABY (Mexico)
NYSTATIN
Nystop Topical Powder USP 2478
Paddock Nystatin USP for Oral Suspension 2478
MICOSTEN (Brazil)
CLOTRIMAZOLE
Lotrimin Cream 3039
Lotrimin Lotion 1% 3039
Lotrimin Topical Solution 1% 3039
MICOSTOP (Chile)
TERBINAFINE HYDROCHLORIDE
Lamisil Tablets 2232
MICOTER (Malaysia, Spain)
CLOTRIMAZOLE
Lotrimin Cream 3039
Lotrimin Lotion 1% 3039
Lotrimin Topical Solution 1% 3039
MICOTRAT (Brazil)
CLOTRIMAZOLE
Lotrimin Cream 3039
Lotrimin Lotion 1% 3039
Lotrimin Topical Solution 1% 3039
MICOTRIM (Argentina)
CLOTRIMAZOLE
Lotrimin Cream 3039

Lotrimin Lotion 1%. 3039
Lotrimin Topical Solution 1% 3039

MICOTRIZOL (Brazil)
CLOTRIMAZOLE
Lotrimin Cream. 3039
Lotrimin Lotion 1%. 3039
Lotrimin Topical Solution 1% 3039

MICRANIL (Argentina)
SUMATRIPTAN SUCCINATE
Imitrex Injection 1463
Imitrex Tablets 1471

MICRODIT (Mexico)
RANITIDINE HYDROCHLORIDE
Zantac 25 EFFERdose Tablets 1624
Zantac 150 EFFERdose Tablets. 1624
Zantac 150 Tablets 1624
Zantac 300 Tablets 1624
Zantac Injection 1619
Zantac Injection Premixed 1619
Zantac Syrup 1624

MICRO-K (Canada, South Africa)
POTASSIUM CHLORIDE
K-Dur Extended-Relase Tablets 3033
K-Lor Oral Solution. 474
K-Tab Tablets 475

MICROKALEORID (France)
POTASSIUM CHLORIDE
K-Dur Extended-Relase Tablets 3033
K-Lor Oral Solution. 474
K-Tab Tablets 475

MICRO-KALIUM (Austria)
POTASSIUM CHLORIDE
K-Dur Extended-Relase Tablets 3033
K-Lor Oral Solution. 474
K-Tab Tablets 475

MICRONOAN (Italy)
DIAZEPAM
Diastat Rectal Delivery System 3343
Valium Tablets 2819

MICROPHYLLIN (South Africa)
THEOPHYLLINE
Uniphyl Tablets 2710

MICRORGAN (Mexico)
CIPROFLOXACIN HYDROCHLORIDE
Ciloxan Ophthalmic Ointment . . . . ⊙204, 559
Ciloxan Ophthalmic Solution . . . . ⊙206
Cipro Tablets 2977

MICROSONA (Argentina, Mexico)
HYDROCORTISONE
Hydrocortone Tablets 1989

MICROSONA OTICA (Argentina)
HYDROCORTISONE
Hydrocortone Tablets 1989

MICROSULF (Argentina)
CIPROFLOXACIN HYDROCHLORIDE
Ciloxan Ophthalmic Ointment . . . . ⊙204, 559
Ciloxan Ophthalmic Solution . . . . ⊙206
Cipro Tablets 2977

MICROXIN (Mexico)
NORFLOXACIN
Noroxin Tablets. 2032

MICTASOL (Mexico)
NORFLOXACIN
Noroxin Tablets. 2032

MIDAMOR (Australia, Austria, Canada, Hong Kong, New Zealand, Norway, Sweden, Switzerland, The Netherlands, United Kingdom)
AMILORIDE HYDROCHLORIDE
Midamor Tablets 2026

MIDAVEN (Mexico)
RANITIDINE HYDROCHLORIDE
Zantac 25 EFFERdose Tablets 1624
Zantac 150 EFFERdose Tablets. 1624
Zantac 150 Tablets 1624
Zantac 300 Tablets 1624
Zantac Injection 1619
Zantac Injection Premixed 1619
Zantac Syrup 1624

MIDAX (Argentina)
OLANZAPINE
Zyprexa Tablets 1830

MIDON (Irish Republic)
MIDODRINE HYDROCHLORIDE
ProAmatine Tablets 3186

MIDORIDE (Australia)
AMILORIDE HYDROCHLORIDE
Midamor Tablets 2026

MIDRAN (Italy, South Africa)
APROTININ
Trasylol Injection 754

MIDRAT (Mexico)
CAPTOPRIL
Captopril Tablets 2149

MIDURET (Thailand)
AMILORIDE HYDROCHLORIDE/HYDROCHLOROTHIAZIDE
Moduretic Tablets 2028

MIELUCIN (Brazil)
BUSULFAN
Myleran Tablets. 1525

MIGRADEXAN (Mexico)
DEXAMETHASONE
Decadron Tablets 1951

MIGRAVAL (Venezuela)
SUMATRIPTAN
Imitrex Nasal Spray 1467

MIGRIL (Brazil)
SUMATRIPTAN SUCCINATE
Imitrex Injection 1463
Imitrex Tablets 1471

MIKOSTAT (United Arab Emirates)
NYSTATIN
Nystop Topical Powder USP. 2478
Paddock Nystatin USP for Oral Suspension. 2478

MIKOSTAT BABY OINTMENT (United Arab Emirates)
NYSTATIN
Nystop Topical Powder USP. 2478
Paddock Nystatin USP for Oral Suspension. 2478

MILANIDAZOLE (Thailand)
METRONIDAZOLE
MetroGel-Vaginal Gel 1855

MILANOLONE (Thailand)
TRIAMCINOLONE ACETONIDE
Azmacort Inhalation Aerosol. 1726
Nasacort AQ Nasal Spray 2922

MILDISON (Denmark, Finland, Irish Republic, Norway, Sweden, The Netherlands, United Kingdom)
HYDROCORTISONE
Hydrocortone Tablets 1989

MILEZZOL (Mexico)
METRONIDAZOLE
MetroGel-Vaginal Gel 1855

MILICAL (Chile)
SIBUTRAMINE HYDROCHLORIDE
Meridia Capsules. 489

MILLIBAR (Hong Kong, Italy, Singapore)
INDAPAMIDE
Indapamide Tablets 2156

MILLICORTENE (Switzerland)
DEXAMETHASONE
Decadron Tablets 1951

MILLICORTENOL (India)
DEXAMETHASONE
Decadron Tablets 1951

MILODERME (Portugal)
ALCLOMETASONE DIPROPIONATE
Aclovate Cream 2660
Aclovate Ointment 2660

MILOREX (Thailand)
AMILORIDE HYDROCHLORIDE/HYDROCHLOROTHIAZIDE
Moduretic Tablets 2028

MILORIDE (Finland)
AMILORIDE HYDROCHLORIDE/HYDROCHLOROTHIAZIDE
Moduretic Tablets 2028

MINARTINE (Greece)
LEVOCARNITINE
Carnitor Injection. 3188
Carnitor Tablets and Oral Solution 3190

MINAX (Australia, Hong Kong, Thailand)
METOPROLOL TARTRATE
Lopressor Tablets 2238

MINEGYL (Brazil)
METRONIDAZOLE
MetroGel-Vaginal Gel 1855

MINEGYL C/NISTATINA (Brazil)
METRONIDAZOLE
MetroGel-Vaginal Gel 1855

MINIDEX (Brazil)
DEXAMETHASONE
Decadron Tablets 1951

MINIDOL (Chile)
TRAMADOL HYDROCHLORIDE
Ultram ER Tablets 2392

MINIOSTENIL (Argentina)
SODIUM HYALURONATE
Hyalgan Solution 2901

MINOA (Greece)
LEVOCARNITINE
Carnitor Injection. 3188
Carnitor Tablets and Oral Solution 3190

MINOBESE (South Africa)
PHENTERMINE HYDROCHLORIDE
Adipex-P Capsules 1215
Adipex-P Tablets 1215

MINOR (Brazil)
LOVASTATIN
Mevacor Tablets 2021

MINOREMED (Germany)
AMILORIDE HYDROCHLORIDE/HYDROCHLOROTHIAZIDE
Moduretic Tablets 2028

MINPROG (Austria, Germany)
ALPROSTADIL
Edex Injection. 3089

MINPROSTIN (Denmark, Finland, Greece, Norway, Sweden)
DINOPROSTONE
Cervidil Vaginal Insert. 1181

MINPROSTIN E2 (Germany)
DINOPROSTONE
Cervidil Vaginal Insert. 1181

MINUSLIP (Argentina)
FENOFIBRATE
Tricor Tablets 527

MINUSORB (Brazil)
ALENDRONATE SODIUM
Fosamax Tablets 1969

MIOCALM (Argentina)
DICLOFENAC SODIUM
Voltaren Tablets 2307
Voltaren-XR Tablets 2310

MIOCAP (Mexico)
CAPTOPRIL
Captopril Tablets 2149

MIOCARDIN (Italy)
LEVOCARNITINE
Carnitor Injection. 3188
Carnitor Tablets and Oral Solution 3190

MIOCOR (Italy)
LEVOCARNITINE
Carnitor Injection. 3188
Carnitor Tablets and Oral Solution 3190

MIOPOTASIO (Spain)
POTASSIUM CHLORIDE
K-Dur Extended-Relase Tablets 3033
K-Lor Oral Solution. 474
K-Tab Tablets 475

MIOSEN (Spain)
DIPYRIDAMOLE
Persantine Tablets 868

MIOTONAL (Italy)
LEVOCARNITINE
Carnitor Injection. 3188
Carnitor Tablets and Oral Solution 3190

MIO-VIROBRON NF (Argentina)
DICLOFENAC SODIUM
Voltaren Tablets 2307
Voltaren-XR Tablets 2310

MIPHAR (Israel)
FUROSEMIDE
Furosemide Tablets 2154

MIQUIMOD (Argentina)
IMIQUIMOD
Aldara Cream, 5% 1846

MIR (Israel)
MORPHINE SULFATE
Kadian Capsules 577
MS Contin Tablets 2701

MIRACLAR (Spain)
NAPHAZOLINE HYDROCHLORIDE
Albalon Ophthalmic Solution . . . . ⊙218

MIRAMYCIN (Hong Kong, Malaysia, Singapore, Thailand)
GENTAMICIN SULFATE
Garamycin Injectable 3014

MIRANAX (Austria, Denmark, Finland, Sweden)
NAPROXEN SODIUM
Anaprox DS Tablets 2761
Anaprox Tablets 2761

MIRASAN (Argentina)
NAPHAZOLINE HYDROCHLORIDE
Albalon Ophthalmic Solution . . . . ⊙218

MIRETIC (Thailand)
AMILORIDE HYDROCHLORIDE/HYDROCHLOROTHIAZIDE
Moduretic Tablets 2028

MIRFAT (Germany)
CLONIDINE HYDROCHLORIDE
Catapres Tablets 843

MIRUS (Mexico)
NAPHAZOLINE HYDROCHLORIDE
Albalon Ophthalmic Solution . . . . ⊙218

MIRUS-S (Argentina)
NAPHAZOLINE HYDROCHLORIDE
Albalon Ophthalmic Solution . . . . ⊙218

MISODOMIN (Greece)
LOVASTATIN
Mevacor Tablets 2021

MISOFENAC (Italy)
DICLOFENAC SODIUM
Voltaren Tablets 2307
Voltaren-XR Tablets 2310

MISORDIL (Argentina)
ISOSORBIDE MONONITRATE
Imdur Tablets 3018

MISULBAN (Italy, Monaco)
BUSULFAN
Myleran Tablets. 1525

MITEN (Spain)
VALSARTAN
Diovan Tablets 2193

MITEN PLUS (Spain)
VALSARTAN
Diovan Tablets 2193

MITOCORTYL (France)
HYDROCORTISONE
Hydrocortone Tablets 1989

MITROKEN (Mexico)
CIPROFLOXACIN HYDROCHLORIDE
Ciloxan Ophthalmic Ointment . . . . ⊙204, 559
Ciloxan Ophthalmic Solution . . . . ⊙206
Cipro Tablets 2977

MIVACRON (Argentina, Australia, Austria, Belgium, Brazil, Canada, Chile, Czech Republic, Denmark, Finland, France, Germany, Greece, Hong Kong, Hungary, Irish Republic, Israel, Italy, Malaysia, Mexico, New Zealand, Norway, Portugal, Singapore, South Africa, Spain, Sweden, Switzerland, Thailand, The Netherlands, United Kingdom)
MIVACURIUM CHLORIDE
Mivacron Injection 493

MIVALEN (Brazil)
SIMVASTATIN
Zocor Tablets. 2105

MIXCILIN (Argentina)
AMOXICILLIN
Amoxil Pediatric Drops for Oral Suspension. 1343
Amoxil Tablets 1343

M-LONG (Austria, Germany)
MORPHINE SULFATE
Kadian Capsules 577
MS Contin Tablets 2701

MND (Singapore)
METRONIDAZOLE
MetroGel-Vaginal Gel 1855

(⊙ Described in PDR For Ophthalmic Medicines™)

MOBAN (Hong Kong)
MOLINDONE HYDROCHLORIDE
Moban Tablets 1119

MOCIMED (Mexico)
AMOXICILLIN
Amoxil Pediatric Drops for Oral Suspension 1343
Amoxil Tablets 1343

MODAMIDE (France)
AMILORIDE HYDROCHLORIDE
Midamor Tablets 2026

MODAPLATE (United Kingdom)
DIPYRIDAMOLE
Persantine Tablets 868

MODASOMIL (Austria, Switzerland)
MODAFINIL
Provigil Tablets 988

MODAVIGIL (Australia, New Zealand)
MODAFINIL
Provigil Tablets 988

MODERAN (Venezuela)
LACTULOSE
Kristalose for Oral Solution 1034

MODIFENAC (Denmark, Norway, Sweden)
DICLOFENAC SODIUM
Voltaren Tablets 2307
Voltaren-XR Tablets 2310

MODIFICAL (Brazil)
ONDANSETRON HYDROCHLORIDE
Zofran Injection 1634
Zofran Injection Premixed 1634
Zofran Oral Solution 1639
Zofran Tablets 1639

MODINA (Portugal)
NIMODIPINE
Nimotop Capsules 749

MODINOL (Greece)
RIZATRIPTAN BENZOATE
Maxalt Tablets 2008
Maxalt-MLT Orally Disintegrating Tablets . . 2008

MODIODAL (Denmark, France, Greece, Mexico, Norway, Portugal, Spain, Sweden, The Netherlands)
MODAFINIL
Provigil Tablets 988

MODISAL (Switzerland, United Kingdom)
ISOSORBIDE MONONITRATE
Imdur Tablets 3018

MODIZIDE (Australia)
AMILORIDE HYDROCHLORIDE/HYDROCHLOROTHIAZIDE
Moduretic Tablets 2028

MODRADERM (Belgium)
ALCLOMETASONE DIPROPIONATE
Aclovate Cream 2660
Aclovate Ointment 2660

MODRASONE (Irish Republic, United Kingdom)
ALCLOMETASONE DIPROPIONATE
Aclovate Cream 2660
Aclovate Ointment 2660

MODUCREN (United Kingdom)
AMILORIDE HYDROCHLORIDE/HYDROCHLOROTHIAZIDE
Moduretic Tablets 2028

MODULAN (Thailand)
AMILORIDE HYDROCHLORIDE
Midamor Tablets 2026

MODU-PUREN (Germany)
AMILORIDE HYDROCHLORIDE/HYDROCHLOROTHIAZIDE
Moduretic Tablets 2028

MODURET (Canada, Irish Republic, United Kingdom)
AMILORIDE HYDROCHLORIDE/HYDROCHLOROTHIAZIDE
Moduretic Tablets 2028

MODURETIC (Argentina, Australia, Austria, Belgium, Brazil, Czech Republic, Denmark, Finland, France, Greece, Hong Kong, Irish Republic, Italy, Malaysia, Mexico, New Zealand, Norway, Portugal, South Africa, Sweden, Switzerland, Thailand, The Netherlands, United Kingdom, Venezuela)
AMILORIDE HYDROCHLORIDE
Midamor Tablets 2026

MODURETIK (Germany)
AMILORIDE HYDROCHLORIDE/HYDROCHLOROTHIAZIDE
Moduretic Tablets 2028

MODUS (Spain)
NIMODIPINE
Nimotop Capsules 749

MOEX (Czech Republic, Denmark, France, Hong Kong, Russia)
MOEXIPRIL HYDROCHLORIDE
Univasc Tablets 3104

MOGETIC (Germany)
MORPHINE SULFATE
Kadian Capsules 577
MS Contin Tablets 2701

MOKCAN (India)
AMOXICILLIN
Amoxil Pediatric Drops for Oral Suspension 1343
Amoxil Tablets 1343

MOMATE (India)
MOMETASONE FUROATE
Elocon Cream 0.1% 3005
Elocon Lotion 0.1% 3006
Elocon Ointment 0.1% 3007
Nasonex Nasal Spray 3043

MOMATE-S (India)
MOMETASONE FUROATE
Elocon Cream 0.1% 3005
Elocon Lotion 0.1% 3006
Elocon Ointment 0.1% 3007
Nasonex Nasal Spray 3043

MOMELAB (Chile)
MOMETASONE FUROATE
Elocon Cream 0.1% 3005
Elocon Lotion 0.1% 3006
Elocon Ointment 0.1% 3007
Nasonex Nasal Spray 3043

MOMEN (Spain)
NAPROXEN
EC-Naprosyn Delayed-Release Tablets 2761
Naprosyn Suspension 2761
Naprosyn Tablets 2761

MOMENDOL (Italy, Portugal)
NAPROXEN SODIUM
Anaprox DS Tablets 2761
Anaprox Tablets 2761

MONARIT (Argentina)
NAPROXEN SODIUM
Anaprox DS Tablets 2761
Anaprox Tablets 2761

MONASIN (Switzerland)
METRONIDAZOLE
MetroGel-Vaginal Gel 1855

MONAXIN (Belgium)
CLARITHROMYCIN
Biaxin Filmtab Tablets 402
Biaxin Granules 402

MONDRIAN (Chile)
BUPROPION HYDROCHLORIDE
Wellbutrin SR Sustained-Release Tablets . . 1607
Wellbutrin Tablets 1603
Zyban Sustained-Release Tablets 1644

MONICOR (France, India)
ISOSORBIDE MONONITRATE
Imdur Tablets 3018

MONIGEN (United Kingdom)
ISOSORBIDE MONONITRATE
Imdur Tablets 3018

MONILAC (Japan)
LACTULOSE
Kristalose for Oral Solution 1034

MONI-SANORANIA (Germany)
ISOSORBIDE MONONITRATE
Imdur Tablets 3018

MONISOL (Russia)
ISOSORBIDE MONONITRATE
Imdur Tablets 3018

MONIT (United Kingdom)
ISOSORBIDE MONONITRATE
Imdur Tablets 3018

MONIT-PUREN (Germany)
ISOSORBIDE MONONITRATE
Imdur Tablets 3018

MONIZOLE (India)
METRONIDAZOLE
MetroGel-Vaginal Gel 1855

MONO ACIS (Germany)
ISOSORBIDE MONONITRATE
Imdur Tablets 3018

MONO BAYCUTEN (Germany)
CLOTRIMAZOLE
Lotrimin Cream 3039
Lotrimin Lotion 1% 3039
Lotrimin Topical Solution 1% 3039

MONO CORAX (Germany)
ISOSORBIDE MONONITRATE
Imdur Tablets 3018

MONO MACK (Austria, Chile, Czech Republic, Germany, Hong Kong, Hungary, Mexico, Singapore, South Africa, Thailand, The Netherlands)
ISOSORBIDE MONONITRATE
Imdur Tablets 3018

MONO WOLFF (Germany)
ISOSORBIDE MONONITRATE
Imdur Tablets 3018

MONO-A (India)
ISOSORBIDE MONONITRATE
Imdur Tablets 3018

MONOBETA (Germany)
ISOSORBIDE MONONITRATE
Imdur Tablets 3018

MONOBRACIN (Greece)
TOBRAMYCIN
TOBI Solution for Inhalation 2298

MONO-CEDOCARD (United Kingdom)
ISOSORBIDE MONONITRATE
Imdur Tablets 3018

MONOCEF (India)
CEFTRIAXONE SODIUM
Rocephin Injectable Vials, ADD-Vantage, Galaxy, Bulk 2800

MONOCEF-O (India)
CEFPODOXIME PROXETIL
Vantin Tablets and Oral Suspension 2645

MONOCID (Austria)
CLARITHROMYCIN
Biaxin Filmtab Tablets 402
Biaxin Granules 402

MONOCINQUE (Hong Kong, Italy, Russia)
ISOSORBIDE MONONITRATE
Imdur Tablets 3018

MONOCLAIR (Germany)
ISOSORBIDE MONONITRATE
Imdur Tablets 3018

MONOCONTIN (India)
ISOSORBIDE MONONITRATE
Imdur Tablets 3018

MONOCORAT (Mexico)
ISOSORBIDE MONONITRATE
Imdur Tablets 3018

MONOCORD (Israel)
ISOSORBIDE MONONITRATE
Imdur Tablets 3018

MONOCORDIL (Brazil)
ISOSORBIDE MONONITRATE
Imdur Tablets 3018

MONOCRIXO (France)
TRAMADOL HYDROCHLORIDE
Ultram ER Tablets 2392

MONODUR (Australia)
ISOSORBIDE MONONITRATE
Imdur Tablets 3018

MONOFLAM (Germany)
DICLOFENAC SODIUM
Voltaren Tablets 2307
Voltaren-XR Tablets 2310

MONOFLOCET (France)
OFLOXACIN
Floxin Otic Solution 1049

MONOGINAL (Greece)
ISOSORBIDE MONONITRATE
Imdur Tablets 3018

MONOKET (Argentina, Austria, Greece, Italy, Norway, Portugal, Sweden)
ISOSORBIDE MONONITRATE
Imdur Tablets 3018

MONOLIN (Thailand)
ISOSORBIDE MONONITRATE
Imdur Tablets 3018

MONOLITUM (Portugal, Spain)
LANSOPRAZOLE
Prevacid Delayed-Release Capsules 3271

MONOLONG (Germany, Israel, Russia)
ISOSORBIDE MONONITRATE
Imdur Tablets 3018

MONOMACK (Venezuela)
ISOSORBIDE MONONITRATE
Imdur Tablets 3018

MONOMAX (United Kingdom)
ISOSORBIDE MONONITRATE
Imdur Tablets 3018

MONOMIL (United Kingdom)
ISOSORBIDE MONONITRATE
Imdur Tablets 3018

MONONAXY (France)
CLARITHROMYCIN
Biaxin Filmtab Tablets 402
Biaxin Granules 402

MONONIT (Israel)
ISOSORBIDE MONONITRATE
Imdur Tablets 3018

MONONITRAT (Germany)
ISOSORBIDE MONONITRATE
Imdur Tablets 3018

MONONITRIL (Portugal)
ISOSORBIDE MONONITRATE
Imdur Tablets 3018

MONOPRONT (Portugal)
ISOSORBIDE MONONITRATE
Imdur Tablets 3018

MONOPUR (Germany)
ISOSORBIDE MONONITRATE
Imdur Tablets 3018

MONORYTHM (Greece)
ISOSORBIDE MONONITRATE
Imdur Tablets 3018

MONOSAN (Czech Republic, Russia)
ISOSORBIDE MONONITRATE
Imdur Tablets 3018

MONOSORB (France, United Kingdom)
ISOSORBIDE MONONITRATE
Imdur Tablets 3018

MONOSORBITRATE (India)
ISOSORBIDE MONONITRATE
Imdur Tablets 3018

MONOSORDIL (Greece)
ISOSORBIDE MONONITRATE
Imdur Tablets 3018

MONOSTENASE (Germany)
ISOSORBIDE MONONITRATE
Imdur Tablets 3018

MONOTAX (India)
CEFTRIAXONE SODIUM
Rocephin Injectable Vials, ADD-Vantage, Galaxy, Bulk 2800

MONOTAX-O (India)
CEFPODOXIME PROXETIL
Vantin Tablets and Oral Suspension 2645

MONO-TILDIEM (France, Malaysia, Singapore, Thailand)
DILTIAZEM HYDROCHLORIDE
Cardizem LA Extended Release Tablets . . . 1728

Tiazac Capsules 1201

MONOTOBRIN (Greece)
TOBRAMYCIN
TOBI Solution for Inhalation 2298

MONOTRATE (India, Singapore, Thailand)
ISOSORBIDE MONONITRATE
Imdur Tablets 3018

MONOTRIN (Argentina)
ISOSORBIDE MONONITRATE
Imdur Tablets 3018

MONOZECLAR (France)
CLARITHROMYCIN
Biaxin Filmtab Tablets 402
Biaxin Granules 402

MONOZOL (Brazil)
ALBENDAZOLE
Albenza Tablets 1338

MONSALIC (Czech Republic)
MOMETASONE FUROATE
Elocon Cream 0.1% 3005
Elocon Lotion 0.1% 3006
Elocon Ointment 0.1% 3007
Nasonex Nasal Spray 3043

MONTAIR (India)
MONTELUKAST SODIUM
Singulair Chewable Tablets 2077
Singulair Tablets 2077

MONTAIR PLUS (India)
MONTELUKAST SODIUM
Singulair Chewable Tablets 2077
Singulair Tablets 2077

MONTEGEN (Italy)
MONTELUKAST SODIUM
Singulair Chewable Tablets 2077
Singulair Tablets 2077

MOPSORALEN (Belgium)
METHOXSALEN
Oxsoralen Lotion 1% 3352
Oxsoralen-Ultra Capsules 3353

MORAPID (Austria)
MORPHINE SULFATE
Kadian Capsules 577
MS Contin Tablets 2701

MORAXEN (United Kingdom)
MORPHINE SULFATE
Kadian Capsules 577
MS Contin Tablets 2701

MORCAP (United Kingdom)
MORPHINE SULFATE
Kadian Capsules 577
MS Contin Tablets 2701

MORCONTIN (India)
MORPHINE SULFATE
Kadian Capsules 577
MS Contin Tablets 2701

MORETAL (Hungary)
MORPHINE SULFATE
Kadian Capsules 577
MS Contin Tablets 2701

MORFEX (Portugal)
FLURAZEPAM HYDROCHLORIDE
Dalmane Capsules 3342

MORONAL (Germany)
NYSTATIN
Nystop Topical Powder USP 2478
Paddock Nystatin USP for Oral Suspension 2478

MORPH (Germany)
MORPHINE SULFATE
Kadian Capsules 577
MS Contin Tablets 2701

MORPHGESIC (United Kingdom)
MORPHINE SULFATE
Kadian Capsules 577
MS Contin Tablets 2701

MORSTEL (Irish Republic)
MORPHINE SULFATE
Kadian Capsules 577
MS Contin Tablets 2701

MOSALAN (Greece)
CEFUROXIME AXETIL
Ceftin Tablets 1407
Ceftin for Oral Suspension 1407

MOSCONTIN (France)
MORPHINE SULFATE
Kadian Capsules 577
MS Contin Tablets 2701

MOSTRELAN (Greece)
FAMOTIDINE
Pepcid Injection 2040
Pepcid Injection Premixed 2040
Pepcid Tablets 2038
Pepcid for Oral Suspension 2038

MOTIAX (Italy)
FAMOTIDINE
Pepcid Injection 2040
Pepcid Injection Premixed 2040
Pepcid Tablets 2038
Pepcid for Oral Suspension 2038

MOTIDIN (Hungary)
FAMOTIDINE
Pepcid Injection 2040
Pepcid Injection Premixed 2040
Pepcid Tablets 2038
Pepcid for Oral Suspension 2038

MOTIDINE (Hong Kong, Singapore, Thailand)
FAMOTIDINE
Pepcid Injection 2040
Pepcid Injection Premixed 2040
Pepcid Tablets 2038
Pepcid for Oral Suspension 2038

MOTIFENE (Belgium, Finland, United Kingdom)
DICLOFENAC SODIUM
Voltaren Tablets 2307
Voltaren-XR Tablets 2310

MOTIRON (Denmark)
METHYLPHENIDATE HYDROCHLORIDE
Ritalin Hydrochloride Tablets 2269
Ritalin-SR Tablets 2269

MOTIVAN (Spain)
PAROXETINE HYDROCHLORIDE
Paxil Oral Suspension 1530
Paxil Tablets 1530

MOVERGAN (Germany)
SELEGILINE HYDROCHLORIDE
Eldepryl Capsules 3208

MOVESAN (Greece)
MOMETASONE FUROATE
Elocon Cream 0.1% 3005
Elocon Lotion 0.1% 3006
Elocon Ointment 0.1% 3007
Nasonex Nasal Spray 3043

MOVEX (Mexico)
NAPROXEN
EC-Naprosyn Delayed-Release Tablets 2761
Naprosyn Suspension 2761
Naprosyn Tablets 2761

MOVIN (Portugal)
TICLOPIDINE HYDROCHLORIDE
Ticlid Tablets 2810

MOX (India)
AMOXICILLIN
Amoxil Pediatric Drops for Oral Suspension 1343
Amoxil Tablets 1343

MOXADENT (Portugal)
AMOXICILLIN
Amoxil Pediatric Drops for Oral Suspension 1343
Amoxil Tablets 1343

MOXAN (South Africa)
AMOXICILLIN
Amoxil Pediatric Drops for Oral Suspension 1343
Amoxil Tablets 1343

MOXICEL (Mexico)
AMOXICILLIN
Amoxil Pediatric Drops for Oral Suspension 1343
Amoxil Tablets 1343

MOXICLINA (Mexico)
AMOXICILLIN
Amoxil Pediatric Drops for Oral Suspension 1343
Amoxil Tablets 1343

MOXIPEN (Portugal, Singapore)
AMOXICILLIN
Amoxil Pediatric Drops for Oral Suspension 1343
Amoxil Tablets 1343

MOXITRAL (Argentina)
AMOXICILLIN
Amoxil Pediatric Drops for Oral Suspension 1343
Amoxil Tablets 1343

MOXLIN CLV (Mexico)
AMOXICILLIN
Amoxil Pediatric Drops for Oral Suspension 1343
Amoxil Tablets 1343

MOXYCARB (India)
AMOXICILLIN
Amoxil Pediatric Drops for Oral Suspension 1343
Amoxil Tablets 1343

MOXYCLAV (South Africa)
AMOXICILLIN
Amoxil Pediatric Drops for Oral Suspension 1343
Amoxil Tablets 1343

MOXYMAX (South Africa)
AMOXICILLIN
Amoxil Pediatric Drops for Oral Suspension 1343
Amoxil Tablets 1343

MPA (Germany)
MEDROXYPROGESTERONE ACETATE
Depo-Medrol Single-Dose Vial 2619

MPA GYN (Germany)
MEDROXYPROGESTERONE ACETATE
Depo-Medrol Single-Dose Vial 2619

MPA-BETA (Germany)
MEDROXYPROGESTERONE ACETATE
Depo-Medrol Single-Dose Vial 2619

MPA-NOURY (Germany)
MEDROXYPROGESTERONE ACETATE
Depo-Medrol Single-Dose Vial 2619

MS CONTIN (Australia, Belgium, Canada, Italy, The Netherlands)
MORPHINE SULFATE
Kadian Capsules 577
MS Contin Tablets 2701

MS DIRECT (Belgium)
MORPHINE SULFATE
Kadian Capsules 577
MS Contin Tablets 2701

MS MONO (Australia)
MORPHINE SULFATE
Kadian Capsules 577
MS Contin Tablets 2701

MSI (Germany)
MORPHINE SULFATE
Kadian Capsules 577
MS Contin Tablets 2701

MSIR (Canada)
MORPHINE SULFATE
Kadian Capsules 577
MS Contin Tablets 2701

MS-LONG (Brazil)
MORPHINE SULFATE
Kadian Capsules 577
MS Contin Tablets 2701

MSP (Israel)
MORPHINE SULFATE
Kadian Capsules 577
MS Contin Tablets 2701

MSR (Germany)
MORPHINE SULFATE
Kadian Capsules 577
MS Contin Tablets 2701

MST (Portugal)
MORPHINE SULFATE
Kadian Capsules 577
MS Contin Tablets 2701

MST CONTINUS (Argentina, Brazil, Hong Kong, Irish Republic, Mexico, New Zealand, Singapore, South Africa, Spain, Switzerland, United Kingdom)
MORPHINE SULFATE
Kadian Capsules 577
MS Contin Tablets 2701

MST MONO (New Zealand)
MORPHINE SULFATE
Kadian Capsules 577
MS Contin Tablets 2701

MST UNICONTINUS (Spain)
MORPHINE SULFATE
Kadian Capsules 577
MS Contin Tablets 2701

MST UNO (Czech Republic)
MORPHINE SULFATE
Kadian Capsules 577
MS Contin Tablets 2701

MUCLOX (Spain)
FAMOTIDINE
Pepcid Injection 2040
Pepcid Injection Premixed 2040
Pepcid Tablets 2038
Pepcid for Oral Suspension 2038

MULCATEL (Chile)
SUCRALFATE
Carafate Suspension 701
Carafate Tablets 701

MULTICOR (Brazil)
VERAPAMIL HYDROCHLORIDE
Covera-HS Tablets 3139
Verelan PM Extended-Release Capsules, Controlled-Onset 3106

MULTILIND (Germany, United Kingdom)
NYSTATIN
Nystop Topical Powder USP 2478
Paddock Nystatin USP for Oral Suspension 2478

MULTIPRESSIM (Brazil)
ENALAPRIL MALEATE
Vasotec I.V. Injection 2103

MULTISORO (Brazil)
NAPHAZOLINE HYDROCHLORIDE
Albalon Ophthalmic Solution . . . . ⊙218

MUNDIDOL (Austria)
MORPHINE SULFATE
Kadian Capsules 577
MS Contin Tablets 2701

MUNDIL (Germany)
CAPTOPRIL
Captopril Tablets 2149

MUNITREN H (Germany)
HYDROCORTISONE
Hydrocortone Tablets 1989

MUNOTRAS (Argentina)
MYCOPHENOLATE MOFETIL
CellCept Capsules 2747
CellCept Oral Suspension 2747
CellCept Tablets 2747

MUPAX (Argentina)
MUPIROCIN
Bactroban Ointment 1395

MUPIDERM (France)
MUPIROCIN
Bactroban Ointment 1395

MUPIRAN (Greece)
MUPIROCIN
Bactroban Ointment 1395

MUPIROX (Argentina)
MUPIROCIN
Bactroban Ointment 1395

MUPORIN (Thailand)
MUPIROCIN
Bactroban Ointment 1395

MURINE (Portugal, United Kingdom)
NAPHAZOLINE HYDROCHLORIDE
Albalon Ophthalmic Solution . . . . ⊙218

MURINE CLEAR EYES (South Africa)
NAPHAZOLINE HYDROCHLORIDE
Albalon Ophthalmic Solution . . . . ⊙218

MUS (Chile)
CLARITHROMYCIN
Biaxin Filmtab Tablets 402
Biaxin Granules 402

(⊙ Described in PDR For Ophthalmic Medicines™)

MUSE (Australia, Austria, Brazil, Canada, Czech Republic, Denmark, Finland, France, Germany, Hong Kong, Irish Republic, Israel, Mexico, New Zealand, Singapore, South Africa, Spain, Switzerland, Thailand, United Kingdom)
ALPROSTADIL
Edex Injection. 3089

MUSTOPIC (India)
TACROLIMUS
Prograf Capsules and Injection 632

MUVIDINA (Argentina)
ZIDOVUDINE
Retrovir Capsules 1560
Retrovir IV Infusion. 1564
Retrovir Syrup 1560
Retrovir Tablets. 1560

MXL (Irish Republic, Portugal, United Kingdom)
MORPHINE SULFATE
Kadian Capsules 577
MS Contin Tablets 2701

MYCANDEN (Argentina)
CLOTRIMAZOLE
Lotrimin Cream. 3039
Lotrimin Lotion 1%. 3039
Lotrimin Topical Solution 1% 3039

MYCARZEM (Greece)
DILTIAZEM HYDROCHLORIDE
Cardizem LA Extended Release Tablets. . . 1728
Tiazac Capsules 1201

MYCEPT (India)
MYCOPHENOLATE MOFETIL
CellCept Capsules 2747
CellCept Oral Suspension 2747
CellCept Tablets 2747

MYCIL GOLD (United Kingdom)
CLOTRIMAZOLE
Lotrimin Cream. 3039
Lotrimin Lotion 1%. 3039
Lotrimin Topical Solution 1% 3039

MYCINOPRED (Switzerland)
NEOMYCIN SULFATE/POLYMYXIN B SULFATE/PREDNISOLONE ACETATE
Poly-Pred Ophthalmic Suspension . . . . . . ⊙233

MYCLO-DERM (Canada)
CLOTRIMAZOLE
Lotrimin Cream. 3039
Lotrimin Lotion 1%. 3039
Lotrimin Topical Solution 1% 3039

MYCLO-GYNE (Canada)
CLOTRIMAZOLE
Lotrimin Cream. 3039
Lotrimin Lotion 1%. 3039
Lotrimin Topical Solution 1% 3039

MYCOBAN (South Africa)
CLOTRIMAZOLE
Lotrimin Cream. 3039
Lotrimin Lotion 1%. 3039
Lotrimin Topical Solution 1% 3039

MYCOCID (India)
CLOTRIMAZOLE
Lotrimin Cream. 3039
Lotrimin Lotion 1%. 3039
Lotrimin Topical Solution 1% 3039

MYCODERM-C (India)
CLOTRIMAZOLE
Lotrimin Cream. 3039
Lotrimin Lotion 1%. 3039
Lotrimin Topical Solution 1% 3039

MYCOFUG (Austria, Germany)
CLOTRIMAZOLE
Lotrimin Cream. 3039
Lotrimin Lotion 1%. 3039
Lotrimin Topical Solution 1% 3039

MYCOHAUG C (Germany)
CLOTRIMAZOLE
Lotrimin Cream. 3039
Lotrimin Lotion 1%. 3039
Lotrimin Topical Solution 1% 3039

MYCO-HERMAL (Israel, Singapore)
CLOTRIMAZOLE
Lotrimin Cream. 3039
Lotrimin Lotion 1%. 3039
Lotrimin Topical Solution 1% 3039

MYCOHEXAL (South Africa)
CLOTRIMAZOLE
Lotrimin Cream. 3039
Lotrimin Lotion 1%. 3039
Lotrimin Topical Solution 1% 3039

MYCO-INTRADERMI (Germany)
NYSTATIN
Nystop Topical Powder USP. 2478
Paddock Nystatin USP for Oral Suspension. 2478

MYCORIL (Hong Kong, Singapore)
CLOTRIMAZOLE
Lotrimin Cream. 3039
Lotrimin Lotion 1%. 3039
Lotrimin Topical Solution 1% 3039

MYCOSTATIN (Australia, Austria, Denmark, Finland, Greece, Hong Kong, India, Irish Republic, Italy, Malaysia, New Zealand, Norway, Portugal, Singapore, South Africa, Spain, Sweden, Thailand)
NYSTATIN
Nystop Topical Powder USP. 2478
Paddock Nystatin USP for Oral Suspension. 2478

MYCOSTATINE (France, Switzerland)
NYSTATIN
Nystop Topical Powder USP. 2478
Paddock Nystatin USP for Oral Suspension. 2478

MYCOTEL (Thailand)
ALBENDAZOLE
Albenza Tablets. 1338

MYCOTRICIDE (Thailand)
PRAZIQUANTEL
Biltricide Tablets 2976

MYCOZOLE (Thailand)
CLOTRIMAZOLE
Lotrimin Cream. 3039
Lotrimin Lotion 1%. 3039
Lotrimin Topical Solution 1% 3039

MYDA-B (Thailand)
CLOTRIMAZOLE
Lotrimin Cream. 3039
Lotrimin Lotion 1%. 3039
Lotrimin Topical Solution 1% 3039

MYFLOXIN (Thailand)
NORFLOXACIN
Noroxin Tablets. 2032

MYFUNGAR (Czech Republic, Germany, Mexico, Russia, Switzerland)
OXICONAZOLE NITRATE
Oxistat Cream 2667
Oxistat Lotion. 2667

MYKO CORDES (Austria, Germany)
CLOTRIMAZOLE
Lotrimin Cream. 3039
Lotrimin Lotion 1%. 3039
Lotrimin Topical Solution 1% 3039

MYKODERM HEILSALBE (Germany)
NYSTATIN
Nystop Topical Powder USP. 2478
Paddock Nystatin USP for Oral Suspension. 2478

MYKOFUNGIN (Germany)
CLOTRIMAZOLE
Lotrimin Cream. 3039
Lotrimin Lotion 1%. 3039
Lotrimin Topical Solution 1% 3039

MYKOHAUG (Germany)
CLOTRIMAZOLE
Lotrimin Cream. 3039
Lotrimin Lotion 1%. 3039
Lotrimin Topical Solution 1% 3039

MYKOPOSTERINE N (Germany)
NYSTATIN
Nystop Topical Powder USP. 2478
Paddock Nystatin USP for Oral Suspension. 2478

MYKUNDEX (Germany)
NYSTATIN
Nystop Topical Powder USP. 2478
Paddock Nystatin USP for Oral Suspension. 2478

MYKUNDEX HEILSALBE (Germany)
NYSTATIN
Nystop Topical Powder USP. 2478
Paddock Nystatin USP for Oral Suspension. 2478

MYKUNDEX MONO (Germany)
NYSTATIN
Nystop Topical Powder USP. 2478
Paddock Nystatin USP for Oral Suspension. 2478

MYKUNDEX OVULA (Germany)
NYSTATIN
Nystop Topical Powder USP. 2478
Paddock Nystatin USP for Oral Suspension. 2478

MYLERAN (Argentina, Australia, Austria, Belgium, Brazil, Canada, Chile, Czech Republic, France, Germany, Greece, Hong Kong, India, Irish Republic, Israel, Italy, Malaysia, Mexico, New Zealand, Norway, Portugal, Russia, Singapore, South Africa, Sweden, Switzerland, Thailand, The Netherlands, United Kingdom)
BUSULFAN
Myleran Tablets. 1525

MYLPROIN (Germany)
VALPROIC ACID
Depakene Capsules 417
Depakene Oral Solution. 417

MYOCARDON MONO (Austria)
ISOSORBIDE MONONITRATE
Imdur Tablets 3018

MYOCARDON N (Germany)
THEOPHYLLINE
Uniphyl Tablets 2710

MYODIPINE (Greece)
NIMODIPINE
Nimotop Capsules 749

MYOGARD (India)
NIFEDIPINE
Adalat CC Tablets 2964

MYOGIT (Czech Republic, Germany)
DICLOFENAC SODIUM
Voltaren Tablets 2307
Voltaren-XR Tablets 2310

MYONIL (Denmark)
DILTIAZEM HYDROCHLORIDE
Cardizem LA Extended Release Tablets. . . 1728
Tiazac Capsules 1201

MYOPRIL (Russia)
ENALAPRIL MALEATE
Vasotec I.V. Injection 2103

MYOSPA (Thailand)
ORPHENADRINE CITRATE
Norflex Injection 1856

MYTOLAC (Sweden)
BENZOYL PEROXIDE
Brevoxyl-4 Creamy Wash. 3210
Brevoxyl-4 Gel 3210
Brevoxyl-8 Creamy Wash. 3210
Brevoxyl-8 Gel 3210
Triaz Cleanser 1892
Triaz Gel. 1892

NABACT (South Africa)
METRONIDAZOLE
MetroGel-Vaginal Gel 1855

NABESAC (Thailand)
ORPHENADRINE CITRATE
Norflex Injection 1856

NABICORTIN (Greece)
LOVASTATIN
Mevacor Tablets 2021

NABOREL (Greece)
NIMODIPINE
Nimotop Capsules 749

NABRATIN (Argentina)
CLOPIDOGREL BISULFATE
Plavix Tablets 917, 2926

NAC (India)
DICLOFENAC SODIUM
Voltaren Tablets 2307
Voltaren-XR Tablets 2310

NACLODIN (Venezuela)
CLONIDINE HYDROCHLORIDE
Catapres Tablets 843

NACLOF (Austria, Czech Republic, Norway, Russia, South Africa, Sweden, Thailand, The Netherlands)
DICLOFENAC SODIUM
Voltaren Tablets 2307
Voltaren-XR Tablets 2310

NACOR (Spain)
ENALAPRIL MALEATE
Vasotec I.V. Injection 2103

NACTOL (Mexico)
BENZONATATE
Tessalon Perles 1199

NACUA (Venezuela)
FUROSEMIDE
Furosemide Tablets 2154

NADIPINIA (Hong Kong)
NIFEDIPINE
Adalat CC Tablets 2964

NADOSTINE (Canada, Hong Kong)
NYSTATIN
Nystop Topical Powder USP. 2478
Paddock Nystatin USP for Oral Suspension. 2478

NAFASOL (South Africa)
NAPROXEN
EC-Naprosyn Delayed-Release Tablets. . . . 2761
Naprosyn Suspension. 2761
Naprosyn Tablets 2761

NAFLAPEN (Mexico)
NAPROXEN
EC-Naprosyn Delayed-Release Tablets. . . . 2761
Naprosyn Suspension. 2761
Naprosyn Tablets 2761

NAFLUVENT (Argentina)
FENTANYL
Duragesic Transdermal System. 2373

NAFORDYL (Greece)
LISINOPRIL
Prinivil Tablets 2052

NAFTAZOLINA (Italy)
NAPHAZOLINE HYDROCHLORIDE
Albalon Ophthalmic Solution . . . . ⊙218

NAFTIN (Canada)
NAFTIFINE HYDROCHLORIDE
Naftin Cream 2126
Naftin Gel 2126

NAKLOFEN (Czech Republic, Russia)
DICLOFENAC SODIUM
Voltaren Tablets 2307
Voltaren-XR Tablets 2310

NAKLOFEN DUO (Russia)
DICLOFENAC SODIUM
Voltaren Tablets 2307
Voltaren-XR Tablets 2310

NALABEST (Mexico)
ENALAPRIL MALEATE
Vasotec I.V. Injection 2103

NALAPRES (Italy)
HYDROCHLOROTHIAZIDE/LISINOPRIL
Prinzide Tablets 2056

NALAPRIX (Brazil)
ENALAPRIL MALEATE
Vasotec I.V. Injection 2103

NALGESIN (Czech Republic, Russia)
NAPROXEN SODIUM
Anaprox DS Tablets 2761
Anaprox Tablets 2761

NALGISA (Italy)
DIFLUNISAL
Dolobid Tablets. 1955

NALION (Spain)
NORFLOXACIN
Noroxin Tablets. 2032

NALOPRIL (Thailand)
ENALAPRIL MALEATE
Vasotec I.V. Injection 2103

NALOX (Argentina)
METRONIDAZOLE
MetroGel-Vaginal Gel 1855

NAPAMIDE (Australia, Hong Kong, Malaysia, New Zealand, Singapore)
INDAPAMIDE
Indapamide Tablets 2156

NAPFLAM (South Africa)
NAPROXEN
EC-Naprosyn Delayed-Release Tablets. . . . 2761

Naprosyn Suspension 2761
Naprosyn Tablets 2761

NAPHACEL (Mexico)
NAPHAZOLINE HYDROCHLORIDE
Albalon Ophthalmic Solution . . . . ⊙218

NAPHASAL (Israel)
NAPHAZOLINE HYDROCHLORIDE
Albalon Ophthalmic Solution . . . . ⊙218

NAPHCON (Australia, Belgium, Greece, Hungary, New Zealand, Thailand, Venezuela)
NAPHAZOLINE HYDROCHLORIDE
Albalon Ophthalmic Solution . . . . ⊙218

NAPHCON FORTE (Canada, Israel)
NAPHAZOLINE HYDROCHLORIDE
Albalon Ophthalmic Solution . . . . ⊙218

NAPHCON-A (Australia, Malaysia)
NAPHAZOLINE HYDROCHLORIDE
Albalon Ophthalmic Solution . . . . ⊙218

NAPLIN (New Zealand)
INDAPAMIDE
Indapamide Tablets 2156

NAPMEL (Hungary, Irish Republic)
NAPROXEN
EC-Naprosyn Delayed-Release Tablets. . . . 2761
Naprosyn Suspension. 2761
Naprosyn Tablets 2761

NAPRATEC (United Kingdom)
NAPROXEN
EC-Naprosyn Delayed-Release Tablets. . . . 2761
Naprosyn Suspension. 2761
Naprosyn Tablets 2761

NAPREL (South Africa)
NAPROXEN
EC-Naprosyn Delayed-Release Tablets. . . . 2761
Naprosyn Suspension. 2761
Naprosyn Tablets 2761

NAPRELAN (Sweden)
NAPROXEN SODIUM
Anaprox DS Tablets 2761
Anaprox Tablets 2761

NAPREN (Norway)
NAPROXEN
EC-Naprosyn Delayed-Release Tablets. . . . 2761
Naprosyn Suspension. 2761
Naprosyn Tablets 2761

NAPREX (Irish Republic, Israel)
NAPROXEN
EC-Naprosyn Delayed-Release Tablets. . . . 2761
Naprosyn Suspension. 2761
Naprosyn Tablets 2761

NAPRILENE (Italy, Spain)
ENALAPRIL MALEATE
Vasotec I.V. Injection 2103

NAPRIUM (Italy)
NAPROXEN
EC-Naprosyn Delayed-Release Tablets. . . . 2761
Naprosyn Suspension. 2761
Naprosyn Tablets 2761

NAPRIUS (Italy)
NAPROXEN
EC-Naprosyn Delayed-Release Tablets. . . . 2761
Naprosyn Suspension. 2761
Naprosyn Tablets 2761

NAPRIX (Brazil)
RAMIPRIL
Altace Capsules 1702

NAPRIX A (Brazil)
RAMIPRIL
Altace Capsules 1702

NAPRIX D (Brazil)
RAMIPRIL
Altace Capsules 1702

NAPRIZIDE (Israel)
ENALAPRIL MALEATE
Vasotec I.V. Injection 2103

NAPROBENE (Austria, Czech Republic)
NAPROXEN
EC-Naprosyn Delayed-Release Tablets. . . . 2761
Naprosyn Suspension. 2761
Naprosyn Tablets 2761

NAPROCOAT (The Netherlands)
NAPROXEN
EC-Naprosyn Delayed-Release Tablets. . . . 2761
Naprosyn Suspension. 2761
Naprosyn Tablets 2761

NAPRODIL (Mexico)
NAPROXEN
EC-Naprosyn Delayed-Release Tablets. . . . 2761
Naprosyn Suspension. 2761
Naprosyn Tablets 2761

NAPRODIL PLUS (Mexico)
NAPROXEN SODIUM
Anaprox DS Tablets 2761
Anaprox Tablets 2761

NAPRODOL (Italy)
NAPROXEN SODIUM
Anaprox DS Tablets 2761
Anaprox Tablets 2761

NAPRO-DORSCH (Germany)
NAPROXEN
EC-Naprosyn Delayed-Release Tablets. . . . 2761
Naprosyn Suspension. 2761
Naprosyn Tablets 2761

NAPROFIDEX (Argentina)
NAPROXEN
EC-Naprosyn Delayed-Release Tablets. . . . 2761
Naprosyn Suspension. 2761
Naprosyn Tablets 2761

NAPROGEN (Argentina)
NAPROXEN
EC-Naprosyn Delayed-Release Tablets. . . . 2761
Naprosyn Suspension. 2761
Naprosyn Tablets 2761

NAPROGESIC (Australia, Chile, New Zealand)
NAPROXEN SODIUM
Anaprox DS Tablets 2761
Anaprox Tablets 2761

NAPROKES (Spain)
NAPROXEN
EC-Naprosyn Delayed-Release Tablets. . . . 2761
Naprosyn Suspension. 2761
Naprosyn Tablets 2761

NAPROLAG (Switzerland)
NAPROXEN
EC-Naprosyn Delayed-Release Tablets. . . . 2761
Naprosyn Suspension. 2761
Naprosyn Tablets 2761

NAPROMETIN (Finland)
NAPROXEN
EC-Naprosyn Delayed-Release Tablets. . . . 2761
Naprosyn Suspension. 2761
Naprosyn Tablets 2761

NAPROMEX (Finland)
NAPROXEN
EC-Naprosyn Delayed-Release Tablets. . . . 2761
Naprosyn Suspension. 2761
Naprosyn Tablets 2761

NAPRONAX (Brazil)
NAPROXEN SODIUM
Anaprox DS Tablets 2761
Anaprox Tablets 2761

NAPRONET (Denmark)
NAPROXEN
EC-Naprosyn Delayed-Release Tablets. . . . 2761
Naprosyn Suspension. 2761
Naprosyn Tablets 2761

NAPRONTAG (Argentina)
NAPROXEN
EC-Naprosyn Delayed-Release Tablets. . . . 2761
Naprosyn Suspension. 2761
Naprosyn Tablets 2761

NAPRONTAG FLEX (Argentina)
NAPROXEN
EC-Naprosyn Delayed-Release Tablets. . . . 2761
Naprosyn Suspension. 2761
Naprosyn Tablets 2761

NAPROREX (Hong Kong, Italy)
NAPROXEN
EC-Naprosyn Delayed-Release Tablets. . . . 2761
Naprosyn Suspension. 2761
Naprosyn Tablets 2761

NAPROSCRIPT (South Africa)
NAPROXEN
EC-Naprosyn Delayed-Release Tablets. . . . 2761
Naprosyn Suspension. 2761
Naprosyn Tablets 2761

NAPROSIAN (Thailand)
NAPROXEN
EC-Naprosyn Delayed-Release Tablets. . . . 2761
Naprosyn Suspension. 2761
Naprosyn Tablets 2761

NAPROSO (Thailand)
NAPROXEN SODIUM
Anaprox DS Tablets 2761
Anaprox Tablets 2761

NAPROSYN (Australia, Brazil, Canada, Czech Republic, Denmark, Finland, Greece, Hong Kong, Hungary, India, Irish Republic, Italy, New Zealand, Norway, Portugal, Singapore, South Africa, Spain, Sweden, Switzerland, Thailand, United Kingdom)
NAPROXEN
EC-Naprosyn Delayed-Release Tablets. . . . 2761
Naprosyn Suspension. 2761
Naprosyn Tablets 2761

NAPROSYNE (Belgium, France, The Netherlands)
NAPROXEN
EC-Naprosyn Delayed-Release Tablets. . . . 2761
Naprosyn Suspension. 2761
Naprosyn Tablets 2761

NAPROVAL (Spain)
NAPROXEN
EC-Naprosyn Delayed-Release Tablets. . . . 2761
Naprosyn Suspension. 2761
Naprosyn Tablets 2761

NAPROVITE (The Netherlands)
NAPROXEN SODIUM
Anaprox DS Tablets 2761
Anaprox Tablets 2761

NAPROX (Brazil)
NAPROXEN
EC-Naprosyn Delayed-Release Tablets. . . . 2761
Naprosyn Suspension. 2761
Naprosyn Tablets 2761

NAPROXI (Israel)
NAPROXEN
EC-Naprosyn Delayed-Release Tablets. . . . 2761
Naprosyn Suspension. 2761
Naprosyn Tablets 2761

NAPRUX (Argentina)
NAPROXEN
EC-Naprosyn Delayed-Release Tablets. . . . 2761
Naprosyn Suspension. 2761
Naprosyn Tablets 2761

NAPSEN (Thailand)
NAPROXEN
EC-Naprosyn Delayed-Release Tablets. . . . 2761
Naprosyn Suspension. 2761
Naprosyn Tablets 2761

NAPSYN (Czech Republic)
NAPROXEN
EC-Naprosyn Delayed-Release Tablets. . . . 2761
Naprosyn Suspension. 2761
Naprosyn Tablets 2761

NAPXEN (Hong Kong, Thailand)
NAPROXEN
EC-Naprosyn Delayed-Release Tablets. . . . 2761
Naprosyn Suspension. 2761
Naprosyn Tablets 2761

NAQUA (Portugal)
FUROSEMIDE
Furosemide Tablets 2154

NARAGRAN (Denmark)
NARATRIPTAN HYDROCHLORIDE
Amerge Tablets. 1339

NARAMIG (Argentina, Australia, Austria, Belgium, Brazil, Chile, Czech Republic, Finland, France, Greece, Hungary, Israel, Mexico, New Zealand, Norway, Portugal, Russia, Singapore, South Africa, Spain, Sweden, Switzerland, Thailand, The Netherlands, United Kingdom)
NARATRIPTAN HYDROCHLORIDE
Amerge Tablets. 1339

NARAPRIL (United Arab Emirates)
ENALAPRIL MALEATE
Vasotec I.V. Injection 2103

NARIAL (Brazil)
NAPHAZOLINE HYDROCHLORIDE
Albalon Ophthalmic Solution . . . . ⊙218

NARIDE (Australia)
INDAPAMIDE
Indapamide Tablets 2156

NARIDEX (Brazil)
NAPHAZOLINE HYDROCHLORIDE
Albalon Ophthalmic Solution . . . . ⊙218

NARIGEN (Greece)
RANITIDINE HYDROCHLORIDE
Zantac 25 EFFERdose Tablets 1624
Zantac 150 EFFERdose Tablets. 1624
Zantac 150 Tablets 1624
Zantac 300 Tablets 1624
Zantac Injection 1619
Zantac Injection Premixed 1619
Zantac Syrup 1624

NARILET (Spain)
IPRATROPIUM BROMIDE
Atrovent Inhalation Solution 835
Atrovent Nasal Spray 0.03%. 837
Atrovent Nasal Spray 0.06%. 839

NARITEC (Thailand)
ENALAPRIL MALEATE
Vasotec I.V. Injection 2103

NAROBIC (South Africa)
METRONIDAZOLE
MetroGel-Vaginal Gel 1855

NAROCIN (Israel)
NAPROXEN SODIUM
Anaprox DS Tablets 2761
Anaprox Tablets 2761

NARZEN (Thailand)
NAPROXEN
EC-Naprosyn Delayed-Release Tablets. . . . 2761
Naprosyn Suspension. 2761
Naprosyn Tablets 2761

NASACOR (South Africa)
TRIAMCINOLONE ACETONIDE
Azmacort Inhalation Aerosol. 1726
Nasacort AQ Nasal Spray 2922

NASACORT (Argentina, Austria, Brazil, Canada, Chile, Czech Republic, Denmark, Finland, France, Germany, Greece, Hong Kong, Irish Republic, Italy, Mexico, New Zealand, Norway, Singapore, Spain, Sweden, Switzerland, Thailand, The Netherlands, United Kingdom, Venezuela)
TRIAMCINOLONE ACETONIDE
Azmacort Inhalation Aerosol. 1726
Nasacort AQ Nasal Spray 2922

NASACORT AQ (Australia, Malaysia)
TRIAMCINOLONE ACETONIDE
Azmacort Inhalation Aerosol. 1726
Nasacort AQ Nasal Spray 2922

NASALIDE (France)
FLUNISOLIDE
Aerobid Inhaler System. 1171
Aerobid-M Inhaler System 1171

NASOCAN (Mexico)
NAPROXEN SODIUM
Anaprox DS Tablets 2761
Anaprox Tablets 2761

NASOFAN (United Kingdom)
FLUTICASONE PROPIONATE
Cutivate Cream. 2662
Cutivate Ointment 2665
Flonase Nasal Spray 1440

NASOMET (Portugal)
MOMETASONE FUROATE
Elocon Cream 0.1%. 3005
Elocon Lotion 0.1% 3006
Elocon Ointment 0.1% 3007
Nasonex Nasal Spray. 3043

NASONEX (Argentina, Australia, Austria, Belgium, Brazil, Canada, Chile, Czech Republic, Denmark, Finland, France, Germany, Greece, Hong Kong, Hungary, Irish Republic, Israel, Italy, Malaysia, Norway, Russia, Singapore, South Africa, Spain, Sweden, Switzerland, Thailand, The Netherlands, United Kingdom, Venezuela)
MOMETASONE FUROATE
Elocon Cream 0.1%. 3005
Elocon Lotion 0.1% 3006
Elocon Ointment 0.1% 3007
Nasonex Nasal Spray. 3043

NASTERID (Brazil)
FINASTERIDE
Propecia Tablets 2060
Proscar Tablets 2067

NASTERID A (Brazil)
FINASTERIDE
Propecia Tablets 2060
Proscar Tablets 2067

NASTERIL (Argentina)
FINASTERIDE
Propecia Tablets 2060
Proscar Tablets 2067

NASTEROL (Venezuela)
FINASTERIDE
Propecia Tablets 2060
Proscar Tablets 2067

NATACYN (Argentina, Singapore, South Africa, Thailand)
NATAMYCIN
Natacyn Antifungal Ophthalmic Suspension ⊙208

NATADROPS (India)
NATAMYCIN
Natacyn Antifungal Ophthalmic Suspension ⊙208

NATAFUCIN (Italy)
NATAMYCIN
Natacyn Antifungal Ophthalmic Suspension ⊙208

NATIFA (Brazil)
ESTRADIOL
Climara Transdermal System 771
Estring Vaginal Ring 2635

NATIFA PRO (Brazil)
ESTRADIOL
Climara Transdermal System 771
Estring Vaginal Ring 2635

NATRAMID (United Kingdom)
INDAPAMIDE
Indapamide Tablets 2156

NATRILIX (Argentina, Australia, Brazil, Chile, Denmark, Finland, Germany, Hong Kong, India, Irish Republic, Italy, Malaysia, Mexico, New Zealand, Singapore, South Africa, Thailand, United Kingdom, Venezuela)
INDAPAMIDE
Indapamide Tablets 2156

NATRIOXEN (Italy)
NAPROXEN SODIUM
Anaprox DS Tablets 2761
Anaprox Tablets 2761

NATULAN (Australia, Austria, Belgium, Canada, France, Germany, Greece, Hungary, Israel, Italy, Mexico, New Zealand, Norway, South Africa, Spain, Switzerland, The Netherlands, United Kingdom)
PROCARBAZINE HYDROCHLORIDE
Matulane Capsules 3191

NATULANAR (Brazil, Sweden)
PROCARBAZINE HYDROCHLORIDE
Matulane Capsules 3191

NATULAX (Germany)
LACTULOSE
Kristalose for Oral Solution 1034

NATURA FENAC (Argentina)
DICLOFENAC SODIUM
Voltaren Tablets 2307
Voltaren-XR Tablets 2310

NATUROGEST (India)
PROGESTERONE
Prometrium Capsules (100 mg, 200 mg) 3203

NATYL (Switzerland)
DIPYRIDAMOLE
Persantine Tablets 868

NAUSEDRON (Brazil)
ONDANSETRON HYDROCHLORIDE
Zofran Injection 1634
Zofran Injection Premixed 1634
Zofran Oral Solution 1639
Zofran Tablets 1639

NAVIXEN (Mexico)
NAPROXEN
EC-Naprosyn Delayed-Release Tablets 2761
Naprosyn Suspension 2761
Naprosyn Tablets 2761

NAXEN (Australia, Canada, Mexico, New Zealand, South Africa)
NAPROXEN
EC-Naprosyn Delayed-Release Tablets 2761
Naprosyn Suspension 2761
Naprosyn Tablets 2761

NAXIL (Mexico)
NAPROXEN
EC-Naprosyn Delayed-Release Tablets 2761
Naprosyn Suspension 2761
Naprosyn Tablets 2761

NAXODOL (Mexico)
NAPROXEN
EC-Naprosyn Delayed-Release Tablets 2761
Naprosyn Suspension 2761
Naprosyn Tablets 2761

NAXOPAAR (Mexico)
NAPROXEN
EC-Naprosyn Delayed-Release Tablets 2761
Naprosyn Suspension 2761
Naprosyn Tablets 2761

NAXOPREN (Finland)
NAPROXEN
EC-Naprosyn Delayed-Release Tablets 2761
Naprosyn Suspension 2761
Naprosyn Tablets 2761

NAXY (France)
CLARITHROMYCIN
Biaxin Filmtab Tablets 402
Biaxin Granules 402

NAXYN (Israel)
NAPROXEN
EC-Naprosyn Delayed-Release Tablets 2761
Naprosyn Suspension 2761
Naprosyn Tablets 2761

NAZICOL (Brazil)
NAPHAZOLINE HYDROCHLORIDE
Albalon Ophthalmic Solution ⊙218

NAZOBIO (Brazil)
NAPHAZOLINE HYDROCHLORIDE
Albalon Ophthalmic Solution ⊙218

NEBAPUL (Chile)
METHYLPHENIDATE HYDROCHLORIDE
Ritalin Hydrochloride Tablets 2269
Ritalin-SR Tablets 2269

NEBULCORT (Italy)
FLUNISOLIDE
Aerobid Inhaler System 1171
Aerobid-M Inhaler System 1171

NECOPEN (Spain)
CEFIXIME
Suprax 1843

NEDICLON (Mexico)
DICLOFENAC SODIUM
Voltaren Tablets 2307
Voltaren-XR Tablets 2310

NEDOXAL (Mexico)
NAPROXEN SODIUM
Anaprox DS Tablets 2761
Anaprox Tablets 2761

NEFAZAN (Argentina)
CLOPIDOGREL BISULFATE
Plavix Tablets 917, 2926

NEFELID (Greece)
NIFEDIPINE
Adalat CC Tablets 2964

NEFOBEN (Argentina)
THEOPHYLLINE
Uniphyl Tablets 2710

NEFROCARNIT (Germany)
LEVOCARNITINE
Carnitor Injection 3188
Carnitor Tablets and Oral Solution 3190

NEFROTAL (Venezuela)
LOSARTAN POTASSIUM
Cozaar Tablets 1935

NEFROTAL H (Venezuela)
LOSARTAN POTASSIUM
Cozaar Tablets 1935

NEGACEF (United Arab Emirates)
CEFTAZIDIME
Fortaz for Injection 1453

NEGAFLOX (Russia)
NORFLOXACIN
Noroxin Tablets 2032

NELABOCIN (Greece)
CEFUROXIME AXETIL
Ceftin Tablets 1407
Ceftin for Oral Suspension 1407

NELAPINE (Thailand)
NIFEDIPINE
Adalat CC Tablets 2964

NELBINEX (Greece)
NIMODIPINE
Nimotop Capsules 749

NEMBUTAL (Australia, Canada, Hong Kong, Thailand)
PENTOBARBITAL SODIUM
Nembutal Sodium Solution, USP 2470

NEMODINE (Venezuela)
NIMODIPINE
Nimotop Capsules 749

NEMOTAN (Russia)
NIMODIPINE
Nimotop Capsules 749

NEMOXIL (Brazil)
AMOXICILLIN
Amoxil Pediatric Drops for Oral Suspension 1343
Amoxil Tablets 1343

NEMOZOLE (India, Russia)
ALBENDAZOLE
Albenza Tablets 1338

NEO BENDAZOL (Brazil)
ALBENDAZOLE
Albenza Tablets 1338

NEO CARDIOL (Italy)
LEVOCARNITINE
Carnitor Injection 3188
Carnitor Tablets and Oral Solution 3190

NEO CEFIX (Brazil)
CEFIXIME
Suprax 1843

NEO CLODIL (Brazil)
CLONIDINE HYDROCHLORIDE
Catapres Tablets 843

NEO CLOTRIMAZYL (Brazil)
CLOTRIMAZOLE
Lotrimin Cream 3039
Lotrimin Lotion 1% 3039
Lotrimin Topical Solution 1% 3039

NEO EBLIMON (Italy)
NAPROXEN
EC-Naprosyn Delayed-Release Tablets 2761
Naprosyn Suspension 2761
Naprosyn Tablets 2761

NEO ELIXIFILIN (Spain)
THEOPHYLLINE
Uniphyl Tablets 2710

NEO FEDIPINA (Brazil)
NIFEDIPINE
Adalat CC Tablets 2964

NEO METRODAZOL (Brazil)
METRONIDAZOLE
MetroGel-Vaginal Gel 1855

NEO MISTATIN (Brazil)
NYSTATIN
Nystop Topical Powder USP 2478
Paddock Nystatin USP for Oral Suspension 2478

NEO PROPRANOL (Brazil)
PROPRANOLOL HYDROCHLORIDE
Inderal LA Long-Acting Capsules 3429

NEO STRATA ASTRINGENT ACNE TREATMENT (Canada)
BENZOYL PEROXIDE
Brevoxyl-4 Creamy Wash 3210

NEO STRATA BLEMISH SPOT (Canada)
BENZOYL PEROXIDE
Brevoxyl-4 Creamy Wash 3210
Brevoxyl-4 Gel 3210
Brevoxyl-8 Creamy Wash 3210
Brevoxyl-8 Gel 3210
Triaz Cleanser 1892
Triaz Gel 1892

NEO VERPAMIL (Brazil)
VERAPAMIL HYDROCHLORIDE
Covera-HS Tablets 3139
Verelan PM Extended-Release Capsules, Controlled-Onset 3106

NEOBLOC (Israel)
METOPROLOL TARTRATE
Lopressor Tablets 2238

NEOCEF (Portugal)
CEFIXIME
Suprax 1843

NEOCEFTRIONA (Brazil)
CEFTRIAXONE SODIUM
Rocephin Injectable Vials, ADD-Vantage, Galaxy, Bulk 2800

NEOCEL (Argentina)
DOCETAXEL
Taxotere Injection Concentrate 2932

NEOCIP (India)
CIPROFLOXACIN
Cipro Oral Suspension 2977

NEOCIP M (India)
CIPROFLOXACIN
Cipro Oral Suspension 2977

NEOCOLPOBEN (Argentina)
METRONIDAZOLE
MetroGel-Vaginal Gel 1855

NEOCORTIGAMMA (Italy)
HYDROCORTISONE
Hydrocortone Tablets 1989

NEO-CURRINO (Argentina)
NAPHAZOLINE HYDROCHLORIDE
Albalon Ophthalmic Solution ⊙218

NEODEX (Thailand)
DEXAMETHASONE
Decadron Tablets 1951

NEO-DISTERIN (Greece)
FENOFIBRATE
Tricor Tablets 527

NEODOLPASSE (Czech Republic, Hungary)
DICLOFENAC SODIUM
Voltaren Tablets 2307
Voltaren-XR Tablets 2310

NEOFLOXIN (Brazil, Singapore)
NORFLOXACIN
Noroxin Tablets 2032

NEOFLUOR (Germany)
FLUOROURACIL
Efudex Topical Cream 3363
Efudex Topical Solutions 3363

NEO-IPERTAS (Greece)
CAPTOPRIL
Captopril Tablets 2149

NEOLAPRIL (Brazil)
ENALAPRIL MALEATE
Vasotec I.V. Injection 2103

NEOLIPID (Brazil)
LOVASTATIN
Mevacor Tablets 2021

NEO-LOTAN (Italy)
LOSARTAN POTASSIUM
Cozaar Tablets 1935

NEO-LOTAN PLUS (Italy)
HYDROCHLOROTHIAZIDE/LOSARTAN POTASSIUM
Hyzaar 100-25 Tablets 1990
Hyzaar 50-12.5 Tablets 1990

NEO-METRIC (Canada)
METRONIDAZOLE
MetroGel-Vaginal Gel 1855

NEONAXIL (Mexico)
NAPROXEN
EC-Naprosyn Delayed-Release Tablets 2761
Naprosyn Suspension 2761
Naprosyn Tablets 2761

NEO-PENOTRAN (Singapore)
METRONIDAZOLE
MetroGel-Vaginal Gel 1855

NEO-PREOCIL (Portugal)
FLUOROMETHOLONE
FML Ophthalmic Ointment ⊙228

NEOPRESS (Brazil)
LOSARTAN POTASSIUM
Cozaar Tablets 1935

NEO-PYRAZON (Malaysia, Singapore)
DICLOFENAC SODIUM
Voltaren Tablets 2307
Voltaren-XR Tablets 2310

NEORINOL (Chile)
IPRATROPIUM BROMIDE
Atrovent Inhalation Solution 835
Atrovent Nasal Spray 0.03%. 837
Atrovent Nasal Spray 0.06%. 839

NEORPAN PLUS (Mexico)
NAPROXEN SODIUM
Anaprox DS Tablets 2761
Anaprox Tablets 2761

NEOSAC (Brazil)
RANITIDINE HYDROCHLORIDE
Zantac 25 EFFERdose Tablets 1624
Zantac 150 EFFERdose Tablets. 1624
Zantac 150 Tablets 1624
Zantac 300 Tablets 1624
Zantac Injection 1619
Zantac Injection Premixed 1619
Zantac Syrup 1624

NEOSEMID (Brazil)
FUROSEMIDE
Furosemide Tablets 2154

NEOSORO (Brazil)
NAPHAZOLINE HYDROCHLORIDE
Albalon Ophthalmic Solution . . . . ⊙218

NEOSTATIN (Brazil)
NYSTATIN
Nystop Topical Powder USP. 2478
Paddock Nystatin USP for Oral Suspension. 2478

NEOTAREN (Brazil)
DICLOFENAC SODIUM
Voltaren Tablets 2307
Voltaren-XR Tablets 2310

NEOTENSIN (Spain)
ENALAPRIL MALEATE
Vasotec I.V. Injection 2103

NEOTIGASON (Argentina, Australia, Austria, Belgium, Brazil, Chile, Czech Republic, Denmark, Finland, Germany, Greece, Hong Kong, Hungary, Irish Republic, Israel, Italy, Mexico, New Zealand, Norway, Portugal, Singapore, South Africa, Spain, Sweden, Switzerland, Thailand, The Netherlands, United Kingdom, Venezuela)
ACITRETIN
Soriatane Capsules 1013

NEO-TIROIMADE (Portugal)
LIOTHYRONINE SODIUM
Cytomel Tablets 1710

NEOTRETIN (Argentina)
TRETINOIN
Vesanoid Capsules. 2820

NEOTREX (Mexico)
ISOTRETINOIN
Accutane Capsules 2731

NEOTUL (Spain)
FAMOTIDINE
Pepcid Injection 2040
Pepcid Injection Premixed 2040
Pepcid Tablets 2038
Pepcid for Oral Suspension 2038

NEOVISC (Canada)
SODIUM HYALURONATE
Hyalgan Solution 2901

NEOZOL (Brazil)
LANSOPRAZOLE
Prevacid Delayed-Release Capsules 3271

NEO-ZOL (Canada)
CLOTRIMAZOLE
Lotrimin Cream. 3039
Lotrimin Lotion 1%. 3039
Lotrimin Topical Solution 1% 3039

NEPHRAL (Germany)
HYDROCHLOROTHIAZIDE/TRIAMTERENE
Dyazide Capsules 1423

NEPHREX (Australia, Hong Kong)
CALCIUM ACETATE
PhosLo GelCaps 2169

NEREFLUN (Italy)
FLUNISOLIDE
Aerobid Inhaler System. 1171
Aerobid-M Inhaler System 1171

NERGADAN (Spain)
LOVASTATIN
Mevacor Tablets 2021

NERICUR (United Kingdom)
BENZOYL PEROXIDE
Brevoxyl-4 Creamy Wash. 3210
Brevoxyl-4 Gel 3210
Brevoxyl-8 Creamy Wash. 3210
Brevoxyl-8 Gel 3210
Triaz Cleanser 1892
Triaz Gel. 1892

NEROLID (Mexico)
DIAZEPAM
Diastat Rectal Delivery System 3343
Valium Tablets 2819

NERVIX (Chile)
VENLAFAXINE HYDROCHLORIDE
Effexor Tablets 3411
Effexor XR Capsules 3417

NESBILER (Argentina)
FLUOROMETHOLONE
FML Ophthalmic Ointment. . . . . ⊙228

NESTIC (Thailand)
CLOTRIMAZOLE
Lotrimin Cream. 3039
Lotrimin Lotion 1%. 3039
Lotrimin Topical Solution 1% 3039

NETAZON (Brazil)
DEXAMETHASONE
Decadron Tablets 1951

NETUNAL (Argentina)
SUCRALFATE
Carafate Suspension 701
Carafate Tablets 701

NEUGAL (Mexico)
RANITIDINE HYDROCHLORIDE
Zantac 25 EFFERdose Tablets 1624
Zantac 150 EFFERdose Tablets. 1624
Zantac 150 Tablets 1624
Zantac 300 Tablets 1624
Zantac Injection 1619
Zantac Injection Premixed 1619
Zantac Syrup 1624

NEUGERON (Mexico)
CARBAMAZEPINE
Carbatrol Capsules 3171
Tegretol Chewable Tablets. 2295
Tegretol Suspension. 2295
Tegretol Tablets 2295
Tegretol-XR Tablets 2295

NEUMEGA (Argentina, Brazil, Chile, Mexico)
OPRELVEKIN
Neumega for Injection 3435

NEURAL (Brazil)
LAMOTRIGINE
Lamictal Chewable Dispersible Tablets . . . 1481
Lamictal Tablets 1481

NEURALPRONA (Argentina)
NAPROXEN
EC-Naprosyn Delayed-Release Tablets. . . . 2761
Naprosyn Suspension. 2761
Naprosyn Tablets 2761

NEURIL (Denmark, Finland)
GABAPENTIN
Neurontin Capsules 2487

NEURIUM (Brazil)
LAMOTRIGINE
Lamictal Chewable Dispersible Tablets . . . 1481
Lamictal Tablets 1481

NEUROCEFAL TRANQUI (Spain)
DIAZEPAM
Diastat Rectal Delivery System. 3343
Valium Tablets 2819

NEURODOL TISSUGEL (Switzerland)
LIDOCAINE
Lidoderm Patch 1118

NEUROGERON (Chile)
NIMODIPINE
Nimotop Capsules 749

NEUROLEP (Mexico)
CARBAMAZEPINE
Carbatrol Capsules 3171
Tegretol Chewable Tablets. 2295
Tegretol Suspension. 2295
Tegretol Tablets 2295
Tegretol-XR Tablets 2295

NEUROLYTRIL (Germany)
DIAZEPAM
Diastat Rectal Delivery System 3343
Valium Tablets 2819

NEURON (Brazil)
NIMODIPINE
Nimotop Capsules 749

NEURONTIN (Argentina, Australia, Austria, Belgium, Brazil, Canada, Czech Republic, Finland, France, Greece, Hong Kong, Hungary, India, Irish Republic, Israel, Italy, Malaysia, Mexico, New Zealand, Norway, Portugal, Russia, Singapore, South Africa, Spain, Sweden, Switzerland, Thailand, The Netherlands, United Kingdom, Venezuela)
GABAPENTIN
Neurontin Capsules 2487

NEUROSTIL (Irish Republic)
GABAPENTIN
Neurontin Capsules 2487

NEUROTOL (Finland)
CARBAMAZEPINE
Carbatrol Capsules 3171
Tegretol Chewable Tablets. 2295
Tegretol Suspension. 2295
Tegretol Tablets 2295
Tegretol-XR Tablets 2295

NEUROTOP (Austria, Czech Republic, Hungary, Singapore, Switzerland)
CARBAMAZEPINE
Carbatrol Capsules 3171
Tegretol Chewable Tablets. 2295
Tegretol Suspension. 2295
Tegretol Tablets 2295
Tegretol-XR Tablets 2295

NEURYL (Argentina, Chile)
CLONAZEPAM
Klonopin Tablets 2778

NEUTOP (Argentina)
TOPIRAMATE
Topamax Sprinkle Capsules 2404
Topamax Tablets 2404

NEUTROGENA ACNE MASK (Australia, Canada)
BENZOYL PEROXIDE
Brevoxyl-4 Creamy Wash. 3210
Brevoxyl-4 Gel 3210
Brevoxyl-8 Creamy Wash. 3210
Brevoxyl-8 Gel 3210
Triaz Cleanser 1892
Triaz Gel. 1892

NEUTROGENA ON THE SPOT ACNE TREATMENT (Canada)
BENZOYL PEROXIDE
Brevoxyl-4 Creamy Wash. 3210
Brevoxyl-4 Gel 3210
Brevoxyl-8 Creamy Wash. 3210
Brevoxyl-8 Gel 3210
Triaz Cleanser 1892
Triaz Gel. 1892

NEWFLOX (Argentina)
OFLOXACIN
Floxin Otic Solution 1049

NEXADRON (Argentina)
DEXAMETHASONE
Decadron Tablets 1951

NEXADRON COMPUESTO (Argentina)
DEXAMETHASONE
Decadron Tablets 1951

NIACEL (Mexico)
METRONIDAZOLE
MetroGel-Vaginal Gel 1855

NIAR (Brazil, Mexico)
SELEGILINE HYDROCHLORIDE
Eldepryl Capsules 3208

NICARDIA (India, Russia)
NIFEDIPINE
Adalat CC Tablets 2964

NICHOGENCIN (Germany)
GENTAMICIN SULFATE
Garamycin Injectable 3014

NICOSTAT (Brazil)
NYSTATIN
Nystop Topical Powder USP. 2478
Paddock Nystatin USP for Oral Suspension. 2478

NICOTEX (India)
BUPROPION HYDROCHLORIDE
Wellbutrin SR Sustained-Release Tablets . . 1607
Wellbutrin Tablets 1603
Zyban Sustained-Release Tablets 1644

NIDAGEL (Canada)
METRONIDAZOLE
MetroGel-Vaginal Gel 1855

NIDATRON (South Africa)
METRONIDAZOLE
MetroGel-Vaginal Gel 1855

NIDAZOL (United Kingdom)
METRONIDAZOLE
MetroGel-Vaginal Gel 1855

NIDAZOLEM (Mexico)
METRONIDAZOLE
MetroGel-Vaginal Gel 1855

NIDAZOLIN (Brazil)
NYSTATIN
Nystop Topical Powder USP. 2478
Paddock Nystatin USP for Oral Suspension. 2478

NIDRALON-V (Mexico)
METRONIDAZOLE
MetroGel-Vaginal Gel 1855

NIFADIL (Brazil)
NIFEDIPINE
Adalat CC Tablets 2964

NIFAL (Austria, Venezuela)
NIFEDIPINE
Adalat CC Tablets 2964

NIFANGIN (Finland)
NIFEDIPINE
Adalat CC Tablets 2964

NIFATIN (Brazil)
NYSTATIN
Nystop Topical Powder USP. 2478
Paddock Nystatin USP for Oral Suspension. 2478

NIFDEMIN (Finland)
NIFEDIPINE
Adalat CC Tablets 2964

NIFE UNO (Germany)
NIFEDIPINE
Adalat CC Tablets 2964

NIFE-BASAN (Switzerland)
NIFEDIPINE
Adalat CC Tablets 2964

NIFEBENE (Austria)
NIFEDIPINE
Adalat CC Tablets 2964

NIFECARD (Australia, Austria, Czech Republic, Hong Kong, Hungary, Russia, Singapore, Thailand)
NIFEDIPINE
Adalat CC Tablets 2964

NIFECLAIR (Germany)
NIFEDIPINE
Adalat CC Tablets 2964

NIFECODAN (Denmark)
NIFEDIPINE
Adalat CC Tablets 2964

NIFECOR (Argentina, Finland, Germany)
NIFEDIPINE
Adalat CC Tablets 2964

NIFED (Irish Republic)
NIFEDIPINE
Adalat CC Tablets 2964

NIFED SOL (Argentina)
NIFEDIPINE
Adalat CC Tablets 2964

NIFEDALAT (South Africa)
NIFEDIPINE
Adalat CC Tablets 2964

NIFEDAX (Brazil)
NIFEDIPINE
Adalat CC Tablets 2964

NIFEDEL (Argentina)
NIFEDIPINE
Adalat CC Tablets 2964

NIFEDICOR (Greece, Italy, Switzerland)
NIFEDIPINE
Adalat CC Tablets 2964

NIFEDICRON (Italy)
NIFEDIPINE
Adalat CC Tablets 2964

NIFEDI-DENK (Singapore)
NIFEDIPINE
Adalat CC Tablets 2964

NIFEDIGEL (Mexico)
NIFEDIPINE
Adalat CC Tablets 2964

NIFEDIN (Brazil, Italy)
NIFEDIPINE
Adalat CC Tablets 2964

NIFEDINE (India)
NIFEDIPINE
Adalat CC Tablets 2964

NIFEDIPAT (Germany, Greece)
NIFEDIPINE
Adalat CC Tablets 2964

NIFEDIPRES (Mexico)
NIFEDIPINE
Adalat CC Tablets 2964

NIFEDIPRESS (United Kingdom)
NIFEDIPINE
Adalat CC Tablets 2964

NIFEDOTARD (United Kingdom)
NIFEDIPINE
Adalat CC Tablets 2964

NIFEHEXAL (Australia, Austria, Brazil, Czech Republic, Germany)
NIFEDIPINE
Adalat CC Tablets 2964

NIFEHEXAL SALI (Germany)
NIFEDIPINE
Adalat CC Tablets 2964

NIFELAT (Argentina, Brazil, Germany, India, Singapore, Thailand)
NIFEDIPINE
Adalat CC Tablets 2964

NIFELATE (France)
NIFEDIPINE
Adalat CC Tablets 2964

NIFELEASE (Irish Republic, United Kingdom)
NIFEDIPINE
Adalat CC Tablets 2964

NIFENSAR (Irish Republic)
NIFEDIPINE
Adalat CC Tablets 2964

NIFENSAR XL (United Kingdom)
NIFEDIPINE
Adalat CC Tablets 2964

NIFESAL (Italy)
NIFEDIPINE
Adalat CC Tablets 2964

NIFEZZARD (Mexico)
NIFEDIPINE
Adalat CC Tablets 2964

NIFICAL (Germany)
NIFEDIPINE
Adalat CC Tablets 2964

NIFICARD (Thailand)
NIFEDIPINE
Adalat CC Tablets 2964

NIFIDINE (South Africa)
NIFEDIPINE
Adalat CC Tablets 2964

NIFIRAN (Thailand)
NIFEDIPINE
Adalat CC Tablets 2964

NIFLAM (Argentina)
CELECOXIB
Celebrex Capsules. 3134

NIFOPRESS (United Kingdom)
NIFEDIPINE
Adalat CC Tablets 2964

NIFREAL (Germany)
NIFEDIPINE
Adalat CC Tablets 2964

NIFSER (Mexico)
NIFEDIPINE
Adalat CC Tablets 2964

NIJ-TEROL (Chile)
LOVASTATIN
Mevacor Tablets 2021

NIKION (Argentina)
ENALAPRIL MALEATE
Vasotec I.V. Injection 2103

NILPERIDOL (Brazil)
FENTANYL CITRATE
Actiq 979

NILSTAT (Australia, Belgium, Canada, New Zealand)
NYSTATIN
Nystop Topical Powder USP. 2478
Paddock Nystatin USP for Oral Suspension. 2478

NIM (Germany)
NIMODIPINE
Nimotop Capsules 749

NIMEGEN (Singapore)
ISOTRETINOIN
Accutane Capsules 2731

NIMICOR (Chile)
SIMVASTATIN
Zocor Tablets. 2105

NIMODIL (Greece)
NIMODIPINE
Nimotop Capsules 749

NIMODILAT (Argentina)
NIMODIPINE
Nimotop Capsules 749

NIMODILAT PLUS (Argentina)
NIMODIPINE
Nimotop Capsules 749

NIMODREL (United Kingdom)
NIFEDIPINE
Adalat CC Tablets 2964

NIMOPAX (Brazil)
NIMODIPINE
Nimotop Capsules 749

NIMOREAGIN (Argentina)
NIMODIPINE
Nimotop Capsules 749

NIMOTOP (Argentina, Australia, Austria, Belgium, Brazil, Canada, Chile, Czech Republic, Denmark, Finland, France, Germany, Greece, Hong Kong, Hungary, Irish Republic, Israel, Italy, Malaysia, Mexico, New Zealand, Norway, Portugal, Russia, Singapore, South Africa, Spain, Sweden, Switzerland, Thailand, The Netherlands, United Kingdom, Venezuela)
NIMODIPINE
Nimotop Capsules 749

NIMOVAS (Brazil)
NIMODIPINE
Nimotop Capsules 749

NINDAXA (United Kingdom)
INDAPAMIDE
Indapamide Tablets 2156

NIPENT (Belgium, Canada, France, Germany, Greece, Italy, Portugal, Spain, United Kingdom)
PENTOSTATIN
Nipent for Injection 1863

NIPIN (Italy, Singapore)
NIFEDIPINE
Adalat CC Tablets 2964

NIPODUR (Greece)
RANITIDINE HYDROCHLORIDE
Zantac 25 EFFERdose Tablets 1624
Zantac 150 EFFERdose Tablets. 1624
Zantac 150 Tablets 1624
Zantac 300 Tablets 1624
Zantac Injection 1619
Zantac Injection Premixed 1619
Zantac Syrup 1624

NIPOGALIN (Greece)
CEFUROXIME SODIUM
Zinacef Injection 1631

NIPRESS (Chile)
NIFEDIPINE
Adalat CC Tablets 2964

NIRULID (Denmark)
AMILORIDE HYDROCHLORIDE
Midamor Tablets 2026

NISIS (France)
VALSARTAN
Diovan Tablets 2193

NISISCO (France)
HYDROCHLOROTHIAZIDE/VALSARTAN
Diovan HCT Tablets 2196

NISODIPEN (Argentina)
NISOLDIPINE
Sular Tablets 3122

NISOLID (Italy)
FLUNISOLIDE
Aerobid Inhaler System. 1171
Aerobid-M Inhaler System 1171

NISPIL (Mexico)
DEXAMETHASONE
Decadron Tablets 1951

NISTAFESA (Venezuela)
NYSTATIN
Nystop Topical Powder USP. 2478
Paddock Nystatin USP for Oral Suspension. 2478

NISTAGEN (Brazil)
NYSTATIN
Nystop Topical Powder USP. 2478
Paddock Nystatin USP for Oral Suspension. 2478

NISTAGRAND (Argentina)
NYSTATIN
Nystop Topical Powder USP. 2478
Paddock Nystatin USP for Oral Suspension. 2478

NISTAGYN (Brazil)
NYSTATIN
Nystop Topical Powder USP. 2478
Paddock Nystatin USP for Oral Suspension. 2478

NISTAKEN (Mexico)
PROPAFENONE HYDROCHLORIDE
Rythmol SR Capsules 2727

NISTAN (Mexico)
NYSTATIN
Nystop Topical Powder USP. 2478
Paddock Nystatin USP for Oral Suspension. 2478

NISTANIL (Brazil)
NYSTATIN
Nystop Topical Powder USP. 2478
Paddock Nystatin USP for Oral Suspension. 2478

NISTAQUIM (Mexico)
NYSTATIN
Nystop Topical Powder USP. 2478
Paddock Nystatin USP for Oral Suspension. 2478

NISTAT (Argentina)
NYSTATIN
Nystop Topical Powder USP. 2478
Paddock Nystatin USP for Oral Suspension. 2478

NISTATIN (Brazil)
NYSTATIN
Nystop Topical Powder USP. 2478
Paddock Nystatin USP for Oral Suspension. 2478

NISTAVAL (Brazil)
NYSTATIN
Nystop Topical Powder USP. 2478
Paddock Nystatin USP for Oral Suspension. 2478

NISTAX (Brazil)
NYSTATIN
Nystop Topical Powder USP. 2478
Paddock Nystatin USP for Oral Suspension. 2478

NISTINOL (Argentina)
NYSTATIN
Nystop Topical Powder USP. 2478
Paddock Nystatin USP for Oral Suspension. 2478

NISTORAL (Chile)
NYSTATIN
Nystop Topical Powder USP. 2478
Paddock Nystatin USP for Oral Suspension. 2478

NITASTIN (Greece)
SIMVASTATIN
Zocor Tablets. 2105

NITEN (Argentina)
LOSARTAN POTASSIUM
Cozaar Tablets 1935

NITEN D (Argentina)
LOSARTAN POTASSIUM
Cozaar Tablets 1935

NITEREY (Argentina)
TRETINOIN
Vesanoid Capsules. 2820

NITISED (Greece)
RANITIDINE HYDROCHLORIDE
Zantac 25 EFFERdose Tablets 1624
Zantac 150 EFFERdose Tablets. 1624
Zantac 150 Tablets 1624
Zantac 300 Tablets 1624
Zantac Injection 1619
Zantac Injection Premixed 1619
Zantac Syrup 1624

NITRAMIN (Greece)
ISOSORBIDE MONONITRATE
Imdur Tablets 3018

NITREX (Italy)
ISOSORBIDE MONONITRATE
Imdur Tablets 3018

NITRILAN (Greece)
ISOSORBIDE MONONITRATE
Imdur Tablets 3018

NITROCIT (South Africa)
POTASSIUM CITRATE
Urocit-K Tablets. 2144

NITROLERG (Brazil)
HYDROCORTISONE
Hydrocortone Tablets 1989

NITROMIDAGER (Mexico)
METRONIDAZOLE
MetroGel-Vaginal Gel 1855

NIVADOR (Spain)
CEFUROXIME AXETIL
Ceftin Tablets 1407
Ceftin for Oral Suspension. 1407

NIVAS (Argentina, Chile)
NIMODIPINE
Nimotop Capsules 749

NIVAS PLUS (Argentina)
NIMODIPINE
Nimotop Capsules 749

NIVATEN (United Kingdom)
NIFEDIPINE
Adalat CC Tablets 2964

NIVELIPOL (Argentina)
SIMVASTATIN
Zocor Tablets. 2105

NIVOFLOX (Mexico)
CIPROFLOXACIN HYDROCHLORIDE
Ciloxan Ophthalmic Ointment . . . . ⊙204, 559
Ciloxan Ophthalmic Solution . . . . ⊙206
Cipro Tablets 2977

NIXAL (Mexico)
NAPROXEN SODIUM
Anaprox DS Tablets 2761
Anaprox Tablets 2761

NIXIN (Brazil, Portugal)
CIPROFLOXACIN HYDROCHLORIDE
Ciloxan Ophthalmic Ointment . . . . ⊙204, 559
Ciloxan Ophthalmic Solution . . . . ⊙206
Cipro Tablets 2977

NIZIN-V (Mexico)
NYSTATIN
Nystop Topical Powder USP. 2478

(⊙ Described in PDR For Ophthalmic Medicines™)

Paddock Nystatin USP for Oral Suspension.................... 2478

NIZOLE (Singapore)
METRONIDAZOLE
MetroGel-Vaginal Gel 1855

NM POWDER (India)
NORFLOXACIN
Noroxin Tablets.................. 2032

NOALDOL (Italy)
DIFLUNISAL
Dolobid Tablets.................. 1955

NOAN (Brazil, Italy)
DIAZEPAM
Diastat Rectal Delivery System 3343
Valium Tablets 2819

NOBLIGAN (Argentina, Austria, Denmark, Mexico, Norway, Sweden)
TRAMADOL HYDROCHLORIDE
Ultram ER Tablets 2392

NOCEPTIN (The Netherlands)
MORPHINE SULFATE
Kadian Capsules 577
MS Contin Tablets 2701

NOCTAL (Brazil)
ESTAZOLAM
ProSom Tablets 517

NODOL (Italy)
RANITIDINE HYDROCHLORIDE
Zantac 25 EFFERdose Tablets 1624
Zantac 150 EFFERdose Tablets........ 1624
Zantac 150 Tablets 1624
Zantac 300 Tablets 1624
Zantac Injection 1619
Zantac Injection Premixed 1619
Zantac Syrup 1624

NOFLAM (New Zealand)
NAPROXEN
EC-Naprosyn Delayed-Release Tablets.... 2761
Naprosyn Suspension............... 2761
Naprosyn Tablets 2761

NOFLAM-N (Hong Kong)
NAPROXEN SODIUM
Anaprox DS Tablets 2761
Anaprox Tablets 2761

NOFLOROX (Mexico)
NORFLOXACIN
Noroxin Tablets.................. 2032

NOITRON (Greece)
ISOTRETINOIN
Accutane Capsules 2731

NOKLOT (India)
CLOPIDOGREL BISULFATE
Plavix Tablets 917, 2926

NOKTONE (Norway)
RANITIDINE HYDROCHLORIDE
Zantac 25 EFFERdose Tablets 1624
Zantac 150 EFFERdose Tablets........ 1624
Zantac 150 Tablets 1624
Zantac 300 Tablets 1624
Zantac Injection 1619
Zantac Injection Premixed 1619
Zantac Syrup 1624

NOLICIN (Czech Republic, Hungary, Russia)
NORFLOXACIN
Noroxin Tablets.................. 2032

NOLIPAX (Italy)
FENOFIBRATE
Tricor Tablets 527

NOLIPREL (Czech Republic, Hungary)
PERINDOPRIL ERBUMINE
Aceon Tablets (2 mg, 4 mg, 8 mg) 3194

NOLOL (South Africa)
PROPRANOLOL HYDROCHLORIDE
Inderal LA Long-Acting Capsules 3429

NOODIPINA (Brazil)
NIMODIPINE
Nimotop Capsules 749

NOPAN (Russia)
BUPRENORPHINE HYDROCHLORIDE
Buprenex Injectable 2716

NOR 2 (Argentina)
NORFLOXACIN
Noroxin Tablets.................. 2032

NOR T (India)
NORFLOXACIN
Noroxin Tablets.................. 2032

NORACIN (Brazil, Thailand)
NORFLOXACIN
Noroxin Tablets.................. 2032

NORANAT (Argentina)
INDAPAMIDE
Indapamide Tablets 2156

NORAXIN (Thailand)
NORFLOXACIN
Noroxin Tablets.................. 2032

NORBACTIN (India, Malaysia, Russia, Singapore, Thailand)
NORFLOXACIN
Noroxin Tablets.................. 2032

NORDOTOL (Denmark)
CARBAMAZEPINE
Carbatrol Capsules 3171
Tegretol Chewable Tablets........... 2295
Tegretol Suspension............... 2295
Tegretol Tablets 2295
Tegretol-XR Tablets 2295

NORFCIN (Thailand)
NORFLOXACIN
Noroxin Tablets.................. 2032

NORFENON (Mexico)
PROPAFENONE HYDROCHLORIDE
Rythmol SR Capsules.............. 2727

NORFLAMIN (Brazil)
NORFLOXACIN
Noroxin Tablets.................. 2032

NORFLEX (Australia, Austria, Belgium, Canada, Denmark, Finland, Germany, Greece, Malaysia, Mexico, New Zealand, Portugal, Singapore, South Africa, Sweden, Switzerland, Thailand, United Kingdom, Venezuela)
ORPHENADRINE CITRATE
Norflex Injection 1856

NORFLO (Thailand)
NORFLOXACIN
Noroxin Tablets.................. 2032

NORFLOCIN (Thailand)
NORFLOXACIN
Noroxin Tablets.................. 2032

NORFLOCINE (Switzerland)
NORFLOXACIN
Noroxin Tablets.................. 2032

NORFLOHEXAL (Australia, Germany)
NORFLOXACIN
Noroxin Tablets.................. 2032

NORFLOK (Spain)
NORFLOXACIN
Noroxin Tablets.................. 2032

NORFLOL (Argentina)
NORFLOXACIN
Noroxin Tablets.................. 2032

NORFLOSAL (Germany)
NORFLOXACIN
Noroxin Tablets.................. 2032

NORFLOSAN (Venezuela)
NORFLOXACIN
Noroxin Tablets.................. 2032

NORFLOSTAD (Austria)
NORFLOXACIN
Noroxin Tablets.................. 2032

NORFLOVAL (Venezuela)
NORFLOXACIN
Noroxin Tablets.................. 2032

NORFLOX (Brazil, India)
NORFLOXACIN
Noroxin Tablets.................. 2032

NORFLOX TZ (India)
NORFLOXACIN
Noroxin Tablets.................. 2032

NORFLOXASAN (Brazil)
NORFLOXACIN
Noroxin Tablets.................. 2032

NORFLOX-AZU (Germany)
NORFLOXACIN
Noroxin Tablets.................. 2032

NORFLOXBETA (Germany)
NORFLOXACIN
Noroxin Tablets.................. 2032

NORFLOXIL (Brazil)
NORFLOXACIN
Noroxin Tablets.................. 2032

NORFLOXIN (Thailand)
NORFLOXACIN
Noroxin Tablets.................. 2032

NORFLOXINOR (Malaysia)
NORFLOXACIN
Noroxin Tablets.................. 2032

NORFLOXMED (Brazil)
NORFLOXACIN
Noroxin Tablets.................. 2032

NORFLOX-PUREN (Germany)
NORFLOXACIN
Noroxin Tablets.................. 2032

NORGESIC (Australia, Malaysia, Venezuela)
ORPHENADRINE CITRATE
Norflex Injection 1856

NORILET (Russia, Venezuela)
NORFLOXACIN
Noroxin Tablets.................. 2032

NORIMOX (South Africa)
AMOXICILLIN
Amoxil Pediatric Drops for Oral Suspension.................... 1343
Amoxil Tablets 1343

NORIPLEX (Hungary)
INDAPAMIDE
Indapamide Tablets 2156

NORITATE (Argentina, Canada, Chile, Hong Kong, Israel, United Kingdom)
METRONIDAZOLE
MetroGel-Vaginal Gel 1855

NORLAMINE (Venezuela)
OFLOXACIN
Floxin Otic Solution 1049

NORMAFENAC (Greece)
CEFUROXIME SODIUM
Zinacef Injection 1631

NORMALIP PRO (Germany)
FENOFIBRATE
Tricor Tablets 527

NORMAPRIL (Brazil)
CAPTOPRIL
Captopril Tablets 2149

NORMASE (Italy)
LACTULOSE
Kristalose for Oral Solution 1034

NORMATENSIL (Argentina)
HYDROCHLOROTHIAZIDE/METHYLDOPA
Aldoril Tablets.................. 1910

NORMATOL (Chile)
GABAPENTIN
Neurontin Capsules 2487

NORMAX (India, Russia)
NORFLOXACIN
Noroxin Tablets.................. 2032

NORMAX TZ (India)
NORFLOXACIN
Noroxin Tablets.................. 2032

NORMETIC (United Kingdom)
AMILORIDE HYDROCHLORIDE/HYDROCHLOROTHIAZIDE
Moduretic Tablets 2028

NORMOLOSE (Greece)
CAPTOPRIL
Captopril Tablets 2149

NORMOLOSE-H (Greece)
CAPTOPRIL
Captopril Tablets 2149

NORMOMENSIL (Brazil)
PROGESTERONE
Prometrium Capsules (100 mg, 200 mg) . 3203

NORMOPRES (Brazil)
NIFEDIPINE
Adalat CC Tablets 2964

NORMOPRESAN (Israel)
CLONIDINE HYDROCHLORIDE
Catapres Tablets 843

NORMOPRIL (India)
LISINOPRIL
Prinivil Tablets 2052

NORMORIX (Norway, Sweden)
AMILORIDE HYDROCHLORIDE/HYDROCHLOROTHIAZIDE
Moduretic Tablets 2028

NORMORYTMIN (Argentina, Irish Republic)
PROPAFENONE HYDROCHLORIDE
Rythmol SR Capsules.............. 2727

NORMOSPOR (South Africa)
CLOTRIMAZOLE
Lotrimin Cream................... 3039
Lotrimin Lotion 1%................ 3039
Lotrimin Topical Solution 1% 3039

NORMOTENSOR (Brazil)
FUROSEMIDE
Furosemide Tablets 2154

NORMOTHERIN (Greece)
SIMVASTATIN
Zocor Tablets.................... 2105

NORMOTIL (Portugal)
CAPTOPRIL
Captopril Tablets 2149

NORMPRESS (Thailand)
PROPRANOLOL HYDROCHLORIDE
Inderal LA Long-Acting Capsules 3429

NORMULEN (Spain)
DICLOFENAC SODIUM
Voltaren Tablets 2307
Voltaren-XR Tablets 2310

NOROCIN (Greece)
NORFLOXACIN
Noroxin Tablets.................. 2032

NOROXIN (Argentina, Australia, Canada, Chile, Finland, Italy, Mexico, New Zealand, Portugal, South Africa, Spain, Switzerland, The Netherlands, United Kingdom, Venezuela)
NORFLOXACIN
Noroxin Tablets.................. 2032

NOROXINE (France)
NORFLOXACIN
Noroxin Tablets.................. 2032

NORPHIN (India)
BUPRENORPHINE HYDROCHLORIDE
Buprenex Injectable 2716

NORPRIL (Mexico)
ENALAPRIL MALEATE
Vasotec I.V. Injection 2103

NORPRO (South Africa)
PROPRANOLOL HYDROCHLORIDE
Inderal LA Long-Acting Capsules 3429

NORQUINOL (Mexico)
NORFLOXACIN
Noroxin Tablets.................. 2032

NORSA (Thailand)
NORFLOXACIN
Noroxin Tablets.................. 2032

NORSOL (Argentina, Switzerland)
NORFLOXACIN
Noroxin Tablets.................. 2032

NORTENSIN (Argentina)
TRANDOLAPRIL
Mavik Tablets 486

NORTOLAN (Greece)
NIMODIPINE
Nimotop Capsules 749

NORTON (Brazil)
NIMODIPINE
Nimotop Capsules 749

NORVIR (Australia, Belgium, Canada, Chile, Czech Republic, Denmark, Finland, France, Germany, Greece, Hong Kong, Hungary, Irish Republic, Israel, Italy, Japan, Malaysia, Mexico, New Zealand, Norway, Portugal, Russia, South Africa, Spain, Sweden, Switzerland, Thailand, The Netherlands, United Kingdom, Venezuela)
RITONAVIR
Norvir Oral Solution 503
Norvir Soft Gelatin Capsules. 503

NORXACIN (Brazil, Thailand)
NORFLOXACIN
Noroxin Tablets. 2032

NORXIA (Thailand)
NORFLOXACIN
Noroxin Tablets. 2032

NORXIN (Brazil)
NORFLOXACIN
Noroxin Tablets. 2032

NOS (Spain)
FAMOTIDINE
Pepcid Injection 2040
Pepcid Injection Premixed 2040
Pepcid Tablets 2038
Pepcid for Oral Suspension 2038

NOSTEROL (Argentina)
SIMVASTATIN
Zocor Tablets. 2105

NOVA (Canada)
PENTOBARBITAL SODIUM
Nembutal Sodium Solution, USP 2470

NOVA RECTAL (Canada)
PENTOBARBITAL SODIUM
Nembutal Sodium Solution, USP 2470

NOVACEF (Argentina, Mexico)
CEFIXIME
Suprax 1843

NOVACETOL (Chile)
CLOTRIMAZOLE
Lotrimin Cream. 3039
Lotrimin Lotion 1%. 3039
Lotrimin Topical Solution 1% 3039

NOVACIL (Brazil)
AMOXICILLIN
Amoxil Pediatric Drops for Oral Suspension. 1343
Amoxil Tablets 1343

NOVACILINA (Chile)
LEVOFLOXACIN
Levaquin Injection 2384
Levaquin Tablets 2384

NOVACLAV (India)
AMOXICILLIN
Amoxil Pediatric Drops for Oral Suspension. 1343
Amoxil Tablets 1343

NOVACLOX LB (India)
AMOXICILLIN
Amoxil Pediatric Drops for Oral Suspension. 1343
Amoxil Tablets 1343

NOVACRIUM (Austria)
MIVACURIUM CHLORIDE
Mivacron Injection 493

NOVADEX (Mexico)
NAPROXEN
EC-Naprosyn Delayed-Release Tablets. . . . 2761
Naprosyn Suspension. 2761
Naprosyn Tablets 2761

NOVAL (Greece)
TIMOLOL MALEATE
Blocadren Tablets 1916
Timoptic Sterile Ophthalmic Solution 2088
Timoptic in Ocudose 2091
Timoptic-XE Sterile Ophthalmic Gel Forming Solution 2092

NOVAMILOR (Canada)
AMILORIDE HYDROCHLORIDE/HYDROCHLOROTHIAZIDE
Moduretic Tablets 2028

NOVAMOX (India)
AMOXICILLIN
Amoxil Pediatric Drops for Oral Suspension. 1343
Amoxil Tablets 1343

NOVAMOX AX (India)
AMOXICILLIN
Amoxil Pediatric Drops for Oral Suspension. 1343
Amoxil Tablets 1343

NOVAMOX LB (India)
AMOXICILLIN
Amoxil Pediatric Drops for Oral Suspension. 1343
Amoxil Tablets 1343

NOVAPAM (New Zealand)
CHLORDIAZEPOXIDE HYDROCHLORIDE
Librium Capsules. 3347

NOVAPAMYL (France)
VERAPAMIL HYDROCHLORIDE
Covera-HS Tablets 3139
Verelan PM Extended-Release Capsules, Controlled-Onset 3106

NOVAPHYLLINE (Greece)
THEOPHYLLINE
Uniphyl Tablets 2710

NOVAPIRINA (Italy)
DICLOFENAC SODIUM
Voltaren Tablets 2307
Voltaren-XR Tablets 2310

NOVAPRES (Mexico)
CAPTOPRIL
Captopril Tablets. 2149

NOVAPSYL (Mexico)
BENZONATATE
Tessalon Perles 1199

NOVASONE (Argentina, Australia)
MOMETASONE FUROATE
Elocon Cream 0.1%. 3005
Elocon Lotion 0.1% 3006
Elocon Ointment 0.1% 3007
Nasonex Nasal Spray. 3043

NOVASULFON (Mexico)
DAPSONE
Dapsone Tablets USP. 1673

NOVATEC (Belgium, The Netherlands)
LISINOPRIL
Prinivil Tablets 2052

NOVATIV (Brazil)
SERTRALINE HYDROCHLORIDE
Zoloft Tablets. 2586

NOVAVIR (Mexico)
ZIDOVUDINE
Retrovir Capsules 1560
Retrovir IV Infusion. 1564
Retrovir Syrup 1560
Retrovir Tablets. 1560

NOVAXEN (Mexico)
NAPROXEN
EC-Naprosyn Delayed-Release Tablets. . . . 2761
Naprosyn Suspension. 2761
Naprosyn Tablets 2761

NOVAZAM (France)
DIAZEPAM
Diastat Rectal Delivery System 3343
Valium Tablets 2819

NOVAZYD (Belgium, The Netherlands)
LISINOPRIL
Prinivil Tablets 2052

NOVELIAN (Spain)
SUMATRIPTAN SUCCINATE
Imitrex Injection 1463
Imitrex Tablets 1471

NOVIDAT (Argentina)
CIPROFLOXACIN HYDROCHLORIDE
Ciloxan Ophthalmic Ointment . . . . ⊙204, 559
Ciloxan Ophthalmic Solution . . . . ⊙206
Cipro Tablets 2977

NOVO RINO (Brazil)
NAPHAZOLINE HYDROCHLORIDE
Albalon Ophthalmic Solution . . . . ⊙218

NOVO-AZT (Canada)
ZIDOVUDINE
Retrovir Capsules 1560
Retrovir IV Infusion. 1564
Retrovir Syrup 1560
Retrovir Tablets. 1560

NOVO-CAPTORIL (Canada, Hong Kong)
CAPTOPRIL
Captopril Tablets. 2149

NOVOCAR (Chile)
CARVEDILOL
Coreg Tablets. 1414

NOVO-CARBAMAZ (Canada)
CARBAMAZEPINE
Carbatrol Capsules 3171
Tegretol Chewable Tablets 2295
Tegretol Suspension. 2295
Tegretol Tablets 2295
Tegretol-XR Tablets 2295

NOVOCRAL (Greece)
CEFTAZIDIME
Fortaz for Injection 1453

NOVO-DIFENAC (Hong Kong)
DICLOFENAC SODIUM
Voltaren Tablets 2307
Voltaren-XR Tablets 2310

NOVODIL (Italy)
DIPYRIDAMOLE
Persantine Tablets 868

NOVO-DILTAZEM (Canada)
DILTIAZEM HYDROCHLORIDE
Cardizem LA Extended Release Tablets. . . 1728
Tiazac Capsules 1201

NOVO-DIPAM (Canada)
DIAZEPAM
Diastat Rectal Delivery System 3343
Valium Tablets 2819

NOVO-DIPIRADOL (Canada)
DIPYRIDAMOLE
Persantine Tablets 868

NOVO-FLUPAM (Canada)
FLURAZEPAM HYDROCHLORIDE
Dalmane Capsules. 3342

NOVO-HYDROCORT (Canada)
HYDROCORTISONE
Hydrocortone Tablets 1989

NOVO-IPRAMIDE (Canada)
IPRATROPIUM BROMIDE
Atrovent Inhalation Solution 835
Atrovent Nasal Spray 0.03%. 837
Atrovent Nasal Spray 0.06%. 839

NOVOLENTE-K (Canada)
POTASSIUM CHLORIDE
K-Dur Extended-Relase Tablets 3033
K-Lor Oral Solution. 474
K-Tab Tablets 475

NOVO-MEDRONE (Canada)
MEDROXYPROGESTERONE ACETATE
Depo-Medrol Single-Dose Vial 2619

NOVO-METOPROL (Canada, Hong Kong)
METOPROLOL TARTRATE
Lopressor Tablets 2238

NOVO-NAPROX (Canada)
NAPROXEN
EC-Naprosyn Delayed-Release Tablets. . . . 2761
Naprosyn Suspension. 2761
Naprosyn Tablets 2761

NOVO-NIDAZOL (Canada)
METRONIDAZOLE
MetroGel-Vaginal Gel 1855

NOVO-NIFEDIN (Canada)
NIFEDIPINE
Adalat CC Tablets 2964

NOVO-POXIDE (Canada)
CHLORDIAZEPOXIDE HYDROCHLORIDE
Librium Capsules. 3347

NOVO-PRANOL (Canada)
PROPRANOLOL HYDROCHLORIDE
Inderal LA Long-Acting Capsules 3429

NOVOQUIN (Mexico)
CIPROFLOXACIN HYDROCHLORIDE
Ciloxan Ophthalmic Ointment . . . . ⊙204, 559
Ciloxan Ophthalmic Solution . . . . ⊙206
Cipro Tablets 2977

NOVO-RANIDINE (Canada, Hong Kong)
RANITIDINE HYDROCHLORIDE
Zantac 25 EFFERdose Tablets 1624
Zantac 150 EFFERdose Tablets. 1624
Zantac 150 Tablets 1624
Zantac 300 Tablets 1624
Zantac Injection 1619
Zantac Injection Premixed 1619
Zantac Syrup 1624

NOVO-RIDAZINE (Canada)
THIORIDAZINE HYDROCHLORIDE
Thioridazine Hydrochloride Tablets 2163

NOVO-RYTHRO (Canada)
ERYTHROMYCIN
Ery-Tab Tablets 449
Erythromycin Base Filmtab Tablets. 455
Erythromycin Delayed-Release Capsules, USP 457
PCE Dispertab Tablets 515

NOVOSEF (Czech Republic)
CEFTRIAXONE SODIUM
Rocephin Injectable Vials, ADD-Vantage, Galaxy, Bulk 2800

NOVO-SEMIDE (Canada)
FUROSEMIDE
Furosemide Tablets 2154

NOVO-SUCRALATE (Canada)
SUCRALFATE
Carafate Suspension 701
Carafate Tablets 701

NOVO-SUNDAC (Canada)
SULINDAC
Clinoril Tablets 1924

NOVO-THEOPHYL (Canada, Hong Kong)
THEOPHYLLINE
Uniphyl Tablets 2710

NOVOTHYRAL (Czech Republic)
LIOTHYRONINE SODIUM
Cytomel Tablets 1710

NOVO-TIMOL (Canada)
TIMOLOL MALEATE
Blocadren Tablets 1916
Timoptic Sterile Ophthalmic Solution 2088
Timoptic in Ocudose 2091
Timoptic-XE Sterile Ophthalmic Gel Forming Solution 2092

NOVO-TRIAMZIDE (Canada)
HYDROCHLOROTHIAZIDE/TRIAMTERENE
Dyazide Capsules 1423

NOVO-VERAMIL (Canada)
VERAPAMIL HYDROCHLORIDE
Covera-HS Tablets 3139
Verelan PM Extended-Release Capsules, Controlled-Onset 3106

NOVOXIL (Brazil)
AMOXICILLIN
Amoxil Pediatric Drops for Oral Suspension. 1343
Amoxil Tablets 1343

NOVRAL (Brazil)
LISINOPRIL
Prinivil Tablets 2052

NOXINE (Thailand)
NORFLOXACIN
Noroxin Tablets. 2032

NOXINOR (Thailand)
NORFLOXACIN
Noroxin Tablets. 2032

NOXUFEN (Switzerland)
NORFLOXACIN
Noroxin Tablets. 2032

N-STATIN (Australia)
NYSTATIN
Nystop Topical Powder USP. 2478
Paddock Nystatin USP for Oral Suspension. 2478

NU-CAPTO (Canada)
CAPTOPRIL
Captopril Tablets. 2149

NUCLOGEN (Spain)
GENTAMICIN SULFATE
Garamycin Injectable 3014

NUCTALON (France)
ESTAZOLAM
ProSom Tablets 517

NU-DICLO (Canada)
DICLOFENAC SODIUM
Voltaren Tablets 2307

Voltaren-XR Tablets 2310

NU-DILTIAZ (Canada)
DILTIAZEM HYDROCHLORIDE
Cardizem LA Extended Release Tablets. . . 1728
Tiazac Capsules 1201

NUELIN (Australia, Denmark, Finland, Hong Kong, Malaysia, New Zealand, Norway, Singapore, South Africa, Thailand, United Kingdom, Venezuela)
THEOPHYLLINE
Uniphyl Tablets 2710

NUFLOXIB (Australia)
NORFLOXACIN
Noroxin Tablets. 2032

NU-K (United Kingdom)
POTASSIUM CHLORIDE
K-Dur Extended-Relase Tablets 3033
K-Lor Oral Solution. 474
K-Tab Tablets 475

NULCERIN (Spain)
FAMOTIDINE
Pepcid Injection 2040
Pepcid Injection Premixed 2040
Pepcid Tablets 2038
Pepcid for Oral Suspension 2038

NU-LOTAN (Japan)
LOSARTAN POTASSIUM
Cozaar Tablets 1935

NUMEN (Spain)
CIPROFLOXACIN HYDROCHLORIDE
Ciloxan Ophthalmic Ointment . . . . ⊙204, 559
Ciloxan Ophthalmic Solution . . . . ⊙206
Cipro Tablets 2977

NU-METOP (Canada)
METOPROLOL TARTRATE
Lopressor Tablets 2238

NUMORPHAN (Canada)
OXYMORPHONE HYDROCHLORIDE
Numorphan Injection 1120

NU-NAPROX (Canada)
NAPROXEN
EC-Naprosyn Delayed-Release Tablets. . . . 2761
Naprosyn Suspension. 2761
Naprosyn Tablets 2761

NU-NIFED (Canada)
NIFEDIPINE
Adalat CC Tablets 2964

NUPENTIN (Australia)
GABAPENTIN
Neurontin Capsules 2487

NUPRAFEN (Singapore)
NAPROXEN
EC-Naprosyn Delayed-Release Tablets. . . . 2761
Naprosyn Suspension. 2761
Naprosyn Tablets 2761

NU-RANIT (Canada)
RANITIDINE HYDROCHLORIDE
Zantac 25 EFFERdose Tablets 1624
Zantac 150 EFFERdose Tablets. 1624
Zantac 150 Tablets 1624
Zantac 300 Tablets 1624
Zantac Injection 1619
Zantac Injection Premixed 1619
Zantac Syrup 1624

NURIL (India)
ENALAPRIL MALEATE
Vasotec I.V. Injection 2103

NUROCAIN (New Zealand)
LIDOCAINE
Lidoderm Patch 1118

NUROLASTS (Australia)
NAPROXEN SODIUM
Anaprox DS Tablets 2761
Anaprox Tablets 2761

NU-ROX (Chile)
ENOXAPARIN SODIUM
Lovenox Injection 2915

NUTRACORT (Brazil, Greece, Mexico, Venezuela)
HYDROCORTISONE
Hydrocortone Tablets 1989

NUTRALONA (Chile)
HYDROCORTISONE
Hydrocortone Tablets 1989

NU-TRIAZIDE (Canada)
HYDROCHLOROTHIAZIDE/TRIAMTERENE
Dyazide Capsules 1423

NU-VERAP (Canada)
VERAPAMIL HYDROCHLORIDE
Covera-HS Tablets 3139
Verelan PM Extended-Release Capsules, Controlled-Onset 3106

NYADERM (Canada)
NYSTATIN
Nystop Topical Powder USP. 2478
Paddock Nystatin USP for Oral Suspension. 2478

NYAL PLUS+ ALLERGY RELIEF (Australia)
PROMETHAZINE HYDROCHLORIDE
Phenergan Tablets and Suppositories 3440

NYCODOL (Austria)
TRAMADOL HYDROCHLORIDE
Ultram ER Tablets 2392

NYCOPIN (Denmark, Norway)
NIFEDIPINE
Adalat CC Tablets 2964

NYCOPREN (Austria, Belgium, Denmark, Finland, Greece, Switzerland, The Netherlands, United Kingdom)
NAPROXEN
EC-Naprosyn Delayed-Release Tablets. . . . 2761
Naprosyn Suspension. 2761
Naprosyn Tablets 2761

NYEFAX (Australia, New Zealand)
NIFEDIPINE
Adalat CC Tablets 2964

NYOGEL (Australia, France, Germany, Greece, Irish Republic, Italy, New Zealand, Portugal, South Africa, United Kingdom)
TIMOLOL MALEATE
Blocadren Tablets 1916
Timoptic Sterile Ophthalmic Solution 2088
Timoptic in Ocudose 2091
Timoptic-XE Sterile Ophthalmic Gel Forming Solution 2092

NYOLOL (Brazil, Chile, France, Greece, Hong Kong, Israel, Malaysia, Mexico, Portugal, Singapore, Spain, Switzerland, Thailand, Venezuela)
TIMOLOL MALEATE
Blocadren Tablets 1916
Timoptic Sterile Ophthalmic Solution 2088
Timoptic in Ocudose 2091
Timoptic-XE Sterile Ophthalmic Gel Forming Solution 2092

NYPINE (Australia)
NIFEDIPINE
Adalat CC Tablets 2964

NYSPES (United Kingdom)
NYSTATIN
Nystop Topical Powder USP. 2478
Paddock Nystatin USP for Oral Suspension. 2478

NYSTACID (South Africa)
NYSTATIN
Nystop Topical Powder USP. 2478
Paddock Nystatin USP for Oral Suspension. 2478

NYSTADERM (Austria, Germany)
NYSTATIN
Nystop Topical Powder USP. 2478
Paddock Nystatin USP for Oral Suspension. 2478

NYSTADERMAL (United Kingdom)
NYSTATIN
Nystop Topical Powder USP. 2478
Paddock Nystatin USP for Oral Suspension. 2478

NYSTAFORM (United Kingdom)
NYSTATIN
Nystop Topical Powder USP. 2478
Paddock Nystatin USP for Oral Suspension. 2478

NYSTAMONT (Greece, United Kingdom)
NYSTATIN
Nystop Topical Powder USP. 2478
Paddock Nystatin USP for Oral Suspension. 2478

NYSTAN (United Kingdom)
NYSTATIN
Nystop Topical Powder USP. 2478
Paddock Nystatin USP for Oral Suspension. 2478

NYSTASAN (Mexico)
NYSTATIN
Nystop Topical Powder USP. 2478
Paddock Nystatin USP for Oral Suspension. 2478

NYSTATIN-DOME (United Kingdom)
NYSTATIN
Nystop Topical Powder USP. 2478
Paddock Nystatin USP for Oral Suspension. 2478

NYSTAVESCENT (United Kingdom)
NYSTATIN
Nystop Topical Powder USP. 2478
Paddock Nystatin USP for Oral Suspension. 2478

NYZOC (Austria)
SIMVASTATIN
Zocor Tablets 2105

OASIL (Greece)
CHLORDIAZEPOXIDE HYDROCHLORIDE
Librium Capsules. 3347

OBESTAT (India)
SIBUTRAMINE HYDROCHLORIDE
Meridia Capsules. 489

O-BIOTIC (Greece)
TOBRAMYCIN
TOBI Solution for Inhalation 2298

OBLIOSER (Italy, Spain)
MORPHINE SULFATE
Kadian Capsules 577
MS Contin Tablets 2701

OBRY (Mexico)
TOBRAMYCIN
TOBI Solution for Inhalation 2298

OBRYPRE (Mexico)
TOBRAMYCIN
TOBI Solution for Inhalation 2298

OBSIDAN (Germany, Russia)
PROPRANOLOL HYDROCHLORIDE
Inderal LA Long-Acting Capsules 3429

OCCIDAL (Thailand)
OFLOXACIN
Floxin Otic Solution 1049

OCEFAX (Argentina)
CIPROFLOXACIN
Cipro Oral Suspension 2977

OCERAL (Austria, Brazil, Switzerland)
OXICONAZOLE NITRATE
Oxistat Cream 2667
Oxistat Lotion. 2667

OCERAL GB (Germany)
OXICONAZOLE NITRATE
Oxistat Cream 2667
Oxistat Lotion. 2667

OCLOVIR (Argentina)
RIMANTADINE HYDROCHLORIDE
Flumadine Syrup 1183
Flumadine Tablets 1183

OCM (Argentina)
CHLORDIAZEPOXIDE HYDROCHLORIDE
Librium Capsules. 3347

OCSAAR (Israel)
LOSARTAN POTASSIUM
Cozaar Tablets 1935

OCSAAR PLUS (Israel)
HYDROCHLOROTHIAZIDE/LOSARTAN POTASSIUM
Hyzaar 100-25 Tablets 1990
Hyzaar 50-12.5 Tablets. 1990

OCTIL (Israel)
TIMOLOL MALEATE
Blocadren Tablets 1916
Timoptic Sterile Ophthalmic Solution 2088
Timoptic in Ocudose 2091
Timoptic-XE Sterile Ophthalmic Gel Forming Solution 2092

OCTIN (South Africa)
OFLOXACIN
Floxin Otic Solution 1049

OCTODIOL (Czech Republic)
ESTRADIOL
Climara Transdermal System 771
Estring Vaginal Ring 2635

OCTORAX (Greece)
ENALAPRIL MALEATE
Vasotec I.V. Injection 2103

OCUBRAX (Belgium, Hungary, Spain)
DICLOFENAC SODIUM
Voltaren Tablets 2307
Voltaren-XR Tablets 2310

OCUFLOX (Australia, Canada, Mexico)
OFLOXACIN
Floxin Otic Solution 1049

OCUGRAM (Canada)
GENTAMICIN SULFATE
Garamycin Injectable 3014

OCULASTIN (Austria, Switzerland)
AZELASTINE HYDROCHLORIDE
Astelin Nasal Spray 1904

OCUMED (Russia)
TIMOLOL MALEATE
Blocadren Tablets 1916
Timoptic Sterile Ophthalmic Solution 2088
Timoptic in Ocudose 2091
Timoptic-XE Sterile Ophthalmic Gel Forming Solution 2092

OCUPROST (Argentina)
LATANOPROST
Xalatan Ophthalmic Solution . . . . ⊙291

OCUSOL (United Kingdom)
SULFACETAMIDE SODIUM
Klaron Lotion 10%. 2909

OCUSTIL (Italy)
SODIUM HYALURONATE
Hyalgan Solution. 2901

OCUSTRESS (India)
NAPHAZOLINE HYDROCHLORIDE
Albalon Ophthalmic Solution . . . . ⊙218

OCU-SULF (India)
SULFACETAMIDE SODIUM
Klaron Lotion 10%. 2909

OCUTIM (India)
TIMOLOL MALEATE
Blocadren Tablets 1916
Timoptic Sterile Ophthalmic Solution 2088
Timoptic in Ocudose 2091
Timoptic-XE Sterile Ophthalmic Gel Forming Solution 2092

OCUTOB (India)
TOBRAMYCIN
TOBI Solution for Inhalation 2298

OCUTOB-D (India)
TOBRAMYCIN
TOBI Solution for Inhalation 2298

ODANET (Greece)
RANITIDINE HYDROCHLORIDE
Zantac 25 EFFERdose Tablets 1624
Zantac 150 EFFERdose Tablets. 1624
Zantac 150 Tablets 1624
Zantac 300 Tablets 1624
Zantac Injection 1619
Zantac Injection Premixed 1619
Zantac Syrup 1624

ODANEX (Chile)
ONDANSETRON
Zofran ODT Orally Disintegrating Tablets . . 1639

ODEMASE (Germany)
FUROSEMIDE
Furosemide Tablets 2154

ODIFEX (India)
FEXOFENADINE HYDROCHLORIDE
Allegra Capsules. 2844

ODIVIR KIT (India)
EFAVIRENZ
Sustiva Capsules. 930

ODRIC (Japan)
TRANDOLAPRIL
Mavik Tablets 486

(⊙ Described in PDR For Ophthalmic Medicines™)

ODRIK (Australia, Brazil, Denmark, France, Greece, Irish Republic, New Zealand, Portugal, Spain, United Kingdom)
TRANDOLAPRIL
Mavik Tablets **486**

ODUPRIL (Greece)
CAPTOPRIL
Captopril Tablets **2149**

OECOZOL (Austria)
METRONIDAZOLE
MetroGel-Vaginal Gel **1855**

OEDEMEX (Switzerland)
FUROSEMIDE
Furosemide Tablets **2154**

OESCLIM (Austria, Brazil, Canada, Chile, Czech Republic, France, Greece, Hungary, Sweden)
ESTRADIOL
Climara Transdermal System **771**
Estring Vaginal Ring **2635**

OESTRACLIN (Spain)
ESTRADIOL
Climara Transdermal System **771**
Estring Vaginal Ring **2635**

OESTRING (Sweden)
ESTRADIOL
Climara Transdermal System **771**
Estring Vaginal Ring **2635**

OESTRO GEL (Argentina)
ESTRADIOL
Climara Transdermal System **771**
Estring Vaginal Ring **2635**

OESTRODOSE (France, Israel, Spain)
ESTRADIOL
Climara Transdermal System **771**
Estring Vaginal Ring **2635**

OESTROGEL (Belgium, Brazil, Czech Republic, France, Greece, Hong Kong, Hungary, Irish Republic, Israel, Malaysia, Mexico, Russia, Singapore, Switzerland, Thailand, United Kingdom)
ESTRADIOL
Climara Transdermal System **771**
Estring Vaginal Ring **2635**

OFAL (Argentina)
TIMOLOL MALEATE
Blocadren Tablets **1916**
Timoptic Sterile Ophthalmic Solution **2088**
Timoptic in Ocudose **2091**
Timoptic-XE Sterile Ophthalmic Gel Forming Solution **2092**

OFAL P (Argentina)
TIMOLOL MALEATE
Blocadren Tablets **1916**
Timoptic Sterile Ophthalmic Solution **2088**
Timoptic in Ocudose **2091**
Timoptic-XE Sterile Ophthalmic Gel Forming Solution **2092**

OFAMIX (Venezuela)
AMOXICILLIN
Amoxil Pediatric Drops for Oral Suspension **1343**
Amoxil Tablets **1343**

OFCIN (Malaysia, Singapore)
OFLOXACIN
Floxin Otic Solution **1049**

OFF-TEN (Chile)
CARVEDILOL
Coreg Tablets **1414**

OFLER (India)
OFLOXACIN
Floxin Otic Solution **1049**

OFLER-TZ (India)
OFLOXACIN
Floxin Otic Solution **1049**

OFLIN (India)
OFLOXACIN
Floxin Otic Solution **1049**

OFLO (Germany, Russia)
OFLOXACIN
Floxin Otic Solution **1049**

OFLOCEE (Thailand)
OFLOXACIN
Floxin Otic Solution **1049**

OFLOCET (Australia, France, New Zealand)
OFLOXACIN
Floxin Otic Solution **1049**

OFLOCIN (Greece, Italy)
ETIDRONATE DISODIUM
Didronel Tablets **2697**

OFLODEX (Israel)
OFLOXACIN
Floxin Otic Solution **1049**

OFLODURA (Germany)
OFLOXACIN
Floxin Otic Solution **1049**

OFLOHEXAL (Germany)
OFLOXACIN
Floxin Otic Solution **1049**

OFLONO (Chile)
CIPROFLOXACIN HYDROCHLORIDE
Ciloxan Ophthalmic Ointment . . . . ⊙**204, 559**
Ciloxan Ophthalmic Solution . . . . ⊙**206**
Cipro Tablets **2977**

OFLOVIR (Spain)
OFLOXACIN
Floxin Otic Solution **1049**

OFLOX (Argentina, Austria, Brazil, Chile, India, Israel, Venezuela)
OFLOXACIN
Floxin Otic Solution **1049**

O-FLOX (Thailand)
OFLOXACIN
Floxin Otic Solution **1049**

OFLOX D (India)
OFLOXACIN
Floxin Otic Solution **1049**

OFLOX TZ (India)
OFLOXACIN
Floxin Otic Solution **1049**

OFLOXA (Thailand)
OFLOXACIN
Floxin Otic Solution **1049**

OFLOXAN (Brazil)
OFLOXACIN
Floxin Otic Solution **1049**

OFLOXBETA (Germany)
OFLOXACIN
Floxin Otic Solution **1049**

OFLOXCIN (Thailand)
OFLOXACIN
Floxin Otic Solution **1049**

OFLOXIN (Brazil, Czech Republic, Russia)
OFLOXACIN
Floxin Otic Solution **1049**

O-FLUOR (Germany)
FLUOROURACIL
Efudex Topical Cream **3363**
Efudex Topical Solutions **3363**

OFNIFENIL (Greece)
ENALAPRIL MALEATE
Vasotec I.V. Injection **2103**

OFOXIN (Brazil)
CIPROFLOXACIN HYDROCHLORIDE
Ciloxan Ophthalmic Ointment . . . . ⊙**204, 559**
Ciloxan Ophthalmic Solution . . . . ⊙**206**
Cipro Tablets **2977**

OFRAMAX (Czech Republic, India, Russia, Singapore, South Africa, Thailand)
CEFTRIAXONE SODIUM
Rocephin Injectable Vials, ADD-Vantage, Galaxy, Bulk **2800**

OFTACILOX (Italy, Portugal, Spain)
CIPROFLOXACIN HYDROCHLORIDE
Ciloxan Ophthalmic Ointment . . . . ⊙**204, 559**
Ciloxan Ophthalmic Solution . . . . ⊙**206**
Cipro Tablets **2977**

OFTACIPROX (Chile)
CIPROFLOXACIN HYDROCHLORIDE
Ciloxan Ophthalmic Ointment . . . . ⊙**204, 559**
Ciloxan Ophthalmic Solution . . . . ⊙**206**
Cipro Tablets **2977**

OFTAGEN (Chile)
GENTAMICIN SULFATE
Garamycin Injectable **3014**

OFTALBRAX (Argentina)
TOBRAMYCIN
TOBI Solution for Inhalation **2298**

OFTALMOLOSA CUSI (Malaysia)
ERYTHROMYCIN
Ery-Tab Tablets **449**
Erythromycin Base Filmtab Tablets **455**
Erythromycin Delayed-Release Capsules, USP **457**
PCE Dispertab Tablets **515**

OFTAMOLOL (Denmark, Norway)
TIMOLOL MALEATE
Blocadren Tablets **1916**
Timoptic Sterile Ophthalmic Solution **2088**
Timoptic in Ocudose **2091**
Timoptic-XE Sterile Ophthalmic Gel Forming Solution **2092**

OFTAN (Hong Kong, Israel, Norway, Switzerland, Thailand)
TIMOLOL MALEATE
Blocadren Tablets **1916**
Timoptic Sterile Ophthalmic Solution **2088**
Timoptic in Ocudose **2091**
Timoptic-XE Sterile Ophthalmic Gel Forming Solution **2092**

OFTAN DEXAMETHASON (Russia)
DEXAMETHASONE
Decadron Tablets **1951**

OFTAN TIMOLOL (Russia)
TIMOLOL MALEATE
Blocadren Tablets **1916**
Timoptic Sterile Ophthalmic Solution **2088**
Timoptic in Ocudose **2091**
Timoptic-XE Sterile Ophthalmic Gel Forming Solution **2092**

OFTAQUIN (Mexico)
CIPROFLOXACIN
Cipro Oral Suspension **2977**

OFTAQUIX (Denmark, Finland, Germany, Sweden, The Netherlands, United Kingdom)
LEVOFLOXACIN
Levaquin Injection **2384**
Levaquin Tablets **2384**

OFTENSIN (Czech Republic)
TIMOLOL MALEATE
Blocadren Tablets **1916**
Timoptic Sterile Ophthalmic Solution **2088**
Timoptic in Ocudose **2091**
Timoptic-XE Sterile Ophthalmic Gel Forming Solution **2092**

OFTIC (Chile)
DICLOFENAC SODIUM
Voltaren Tablets **2307**
Voltaren-XR Tablets **2310**

OFTIMOLO (Italy)
TIMOLOL MALEATE
Blocadren Tablets **1916**
Timoptic Sterile Ophthalmic Solution **2088**
Timoptic in Ocudose **2091**
Timoptic-XE Sterile Ophthalmic Gel Forming Solution **2092**

OFUS (Hong Kong)
OFLOXACIN
Floxin Otic Solution **1049**

OGAST (France)
LANSOPRAZOLE
Prevacid Delayed-Release Capsules **3271**

OGASTO (Argentina, Chile, Portugal)
LANSOPRAZOLE
Prevacid Delayed-Release Capsules **3271**

OGASTORO (France)
LANSOPRAZOLE
Prevacid Delayed-Release Capsules **3271**

OGASTRO (Brazil, Mexico, Venezuela)
LANSOPRAZOLE
Prevacid Delayed-Release Capsules **3271**

OKAFLOX M (India)
OFLOXACIN
Floxin Otic Solution **1049**

OKALAN D (India)
LANSOPRAZOLE
Prevacid Delayed-Release Capsules **3271**

OKAMYCIN (India)
ERYTHROMYCIN
Ery-Tab Tablets **449**
Erythromycin Base Filmtab Tablets **455**
Erythromycin Delayed-Release Capsules, USP **457**
PCE Dispertab Tablets **515**

OKLARICID (Greece)
CLARITHROMYCIN
Biaxin Filmtab Tablets **402**
Biaxin Granules **402**

OLAN (Mexico)
LANSOPRAZOLE
Prevacid Delayed-Release Capsules **3271**

OLBENDITAL (Mexico)
ALBENDAZOLE
Albenza Tablets **1338**

OLDINOT (Argentina)
DONEPEZIL HYDROCHLORIDE
Aricept Tablets **1094**

OLEXAR (India)
OLANZAPINE
Zyprexa Tablets **1830**

OLFEN (Brazil, Czech Republic, Hong Kong, Hungary, Israel, Malaysia, Portugal, Singapore, Thailand)
DICLOFENAC SODIUM
Voltaren Tablets **2307**
Voltaren-XR Tablets **2310**

OLFI (India)
OFLOXACIN
Floxin Otic Solution **1049**

OLFI TZ (India)
OFLOXACIN
Floxin Otic Solution **1049**

OLICARD (Czech Republic, Germany, Hungary, Spain, Switzerland)
ISOSORBIDE MONONITRATE
Imdur Tablets **3018**

OLICARD RETARD (Russia)
ISOSORBIDE MONONITRATE
Imdur Tablets **3018**

OLICARDIN (Austria)
ISOSORBIDE MONONITRATE
Imdur Tablets **3018**

OLIMER (Argentina)
CLONAZEPAM
Klonopin Tablets **2778**

OLIVIN (Chile)
OLANZAPINE
Zyprexa Tablets **1830**

OLMORAN (Spain)
ZAFIRLUKAST
Accolate Tablets **671**

OLTENS (France)
CAPTOPRIL
Captopril Tablets **2149**

OLTER (Argentina)
FLUTAMIDE
Eulexin Capsules **3009**

OLUX (The Netherlands)
CLOBETASOL PROPIONATE
Temovate Cream **2668**
Temovate E Emollient **2671**
Temovate Gel **2669**
Temovate Ointment **2668**
Temovate Scalp Application **2670**

OLWORM (India)
ALBENDAZOLE
Albenza Tablets **1338**

OLYSTER (India)
TERAZOSIN HYDROCHLORIDE
Hytrin Capsules **471**

OMAFLAXINA (Argentina)
CIPROFLOXACIN
Cipro Oral Suspension **2977**

OMCILON A ORABASE (Brazil)
TRIAMCINOLONE ACETONIDE
Azmacort Inhalation Aerosol **1726**
Nasacort AQ Nasal Spray **2922**

OMIC (Belgium)
TAMSULOSIN HYDROCHLORIDE
Flomax Capsules **850**

OMINOL (Mexico)
PROGESTERONE
Prometrium Capsules (100 mg, 200 mg) . **3203**

(⊙ Described in PDR For Ophthalmic Medicines™)

OMIX (Austria, France)
TAMSULOSIN HYDROCHLORIDE
Flomax Capsules ... 850

OMNALIO (Spain)
CHLORDIAZEPOXIDE HYDROCHLORIDE
Librium Capsules ... 3347

OMNIC (Argentina, Brazil, Chile, Czech Republic, Denmark, Finland, Germany, Greece, Hungary, Irish Republic, Israel, Italy, Norway, Portugal, Russia, Spain, The Netherlands)
TAMSULOSIN HYDROCHLORIDE
Flomax Capsules ... 850

OMNICEF (Austria, Thailand)
CEFDINIR
Omnicef Capsules ... 511
Omnicef for Oral Suspension ... 511

ONAPAN (Mexico)
DIAZEPAM
Diastat Rectal Delivery System ... 3343
Valium Tablets ... 2819

ONCASPAR (Argentina, Canada, Germany, Russia)
PEGASPARGASE
Oncaspar ... 1145

ONCLAST (Japan)
ALENDRONATE SODIUM
Fosamax Tablets ... 1969

ONCOFU (Argentina)
FLUOROURACIL
Efudex Topical Cream ... 3363
Efudex Topical Solutions ... 3363

ONCOGEM (India)
GEMCITABINE HYDROCHLORIDE
Gemzar for Injection ... 1771

ONCOSAL (Spain)
FLUTAMIDE
Eulexin Capsules ... 3009

ONDAREN (Greece)
ONDANSETRON
Zofran ODT Orally Disintegrating Tablets ... 1639

ONDAZ (Australia)
ONDANSETRON
Zofran ODT Orally Disintegrating Tablets ... 1639

ONDEMET (Czech Republic)
ONDANSETRON HYDROCHLORIDE
Zofran Injection ... 1634
Zofran Injection Premixed ... 1634
Zofran Oral Solution ... 1639
Zofran Tablets ... 1639

ONEXMOL (Mexico)
NAPROXEN SODIUM
Anaprox DS Tablets ... 2761
Anaprox Tablets ... 2761

ONKOFLUOR (Germany)
FLUOROURACIL
Efudex Topical Cream ... 3363
Efudex Topical Solutions ... 3363

ONKOMORPHIN (Germany)
MORPHINE SULFATE
Kadian Capsules ... 577
MS Contin Tablets ... 2701

ONSENAL (France, Spain)
CELECOXIB
Celebrex Capsules ... 3134

ONSIA (Thailand)
ONDANSETRON HYDROCHLORIDE
Zofran Injection ... 1634
Zofran Injection Premixed ... 1634
Zofran Oral Solution ... 1639
Zofran Tablets ... 1639

ONTRAX (Brazil)
ONDANSETRON HYDROCHLORIDE
Zofran Injection ... 1634
Zofran Injection Premixed ... 1634
Zofran Oral Solution ... 1639
Zofran Tablets ... 1639

ONYCHON (Czech Republic)
TERBINAFINE HYDROCHLORIDE
Lamisil Tablets ... 2232

ONYMYKEN (Germany)
CLOTRIMAZOLE
Lotrimin Cream ... 3039
Lotrimin Lotion 1% ... 3039
Lotrimin Topical Solution 1% ... 3039

OPATANOL (Belgium, Denmark, Finland, France, Germany, Greece, Irish Republic, Italy, Norway, Portugal, Spain, Sweden, Switzerland, United Kingdom)
OLOPATADINE HYDROCHLORIDE
Patanol Ophthalmic Solution ... 561, ⊙210

OPCON (Canada)
NAPHAZOLINE HYDROCHLORIDE
Albalon Ophthalmic Solution ... ⊙218

OPCON-A (Mexico)
NAPHAZOLINE HYDROCHLORIDE
Albalon Ophthalmic Solution ... ⊙218

OPHTAGRAM (Czech Republic, France, Germany, Portugal, Singapore, Switzerland)
GENTAMICIN SULFATE
Garamycin Injectable ... 3014

OPHTALIN (Italy)
SODIUM HYALURONATE
Hyalgan Solution ... 2901

OPHTHALIN (Australia, Hong Kong, Hungary, Irish Republic, Israel, New Zealand, Singapore, Thailand, United Kingdom)
SODIUM HYALURONATE
Hyalgan Solution ... 2901

OPHTHO-SULF (Canada)
SULFACETAMIDE SODIUM
Klaron Lotion 10% ... 2909

OPHTILAN (Austria)
TIMOLOL MALEATE
Blocadren Tablets ... 1916
Timoptic Sterile Ophthalmic Solution ... 2088
Timoptic in Ocudose ... 2091
Timoptic-XE Sterile Ophthalmic Gel Forming Solution ... 2092

OPHTIM (France)
TIMOLOL MALEATE
Blocadren Tablets ... 1916
Timoptic Sterile Ophthalmic Solution ... 2088
Timoptic in Ocudose ... 2091
Timoptic-XE Sterile Ophthalmic Gel Forming Solution ... 2092

OPIDOL (Denmark, Finland, Sweden)
HYDROMORPHONE HYDROCHLORIDE
Dilaudid Ampules ... 440
Dilaudid Multiple Dose Vials ... 440
Dilaudid Non-Sterile Powder ... 440
Dilaudid Oral Liquid ... 445
Dilaudid Rectal Suppositories ... 440
Dilaudid Tablets ... 440
Dilaudid Tablets - 8 mg ... 445
Dilaudid-HP Injection ... 442
Dilaudid-HP Lyophilized Powder 250 mg ... 442

OPIREN (Spain)
LANSOPRAZOLE
Prevacid Delayed-Release Capsules ... 3271

OPRIDAN (Greece)
ISOTRETINOIN
Accutane Capsules ... 2731

OPSAR (Thailand)
SULFACETAMIDE SODIUM
Klaron Lotion 10% ... 2909

OPTAL (Thailand)
SULFACETAMIDE SODIUM
Klaron Lotion 10% ... 2909

OPTAMAX (Brazil)
DICLOFENAC SODIUM
Voltaren Tablets ... 2307
Voltaren-XR Tablets ... 2310

OPTAMID (Italy)
SULFACETAMIDE SODIUM
Klaron Lotion 10% ... 2909

OPTAMIDE (Australia)
SULFACETAMIDE SODIUM
Klaron Lotion 10% ... 2909

OPTAZINE (Australia)
NAPHAZOLINE HYDROCHLORIDE
Albalon Ophthalmic Solution ... ⊙218

OPTERON (Italy)
TICLOPIDINE HYDROCHLORIDE
Ticlid Tablets ... 2810

OPTHAFLOX (Mexico)
CIPROFLOXACIN HYDROCHLORIDE
Ciloxan Ophthalmic Ointment ... ⊙204, 559
Ciloxan Ophthalmic Solution ... ⊙206
Cipro Tablets ... 2977

OPTICET (South Africa)
SULFACETAMIDE SODIUM
Klaron Lotion 10% ... 2909

OPTICIDE (Thailand)
PRAZIQUANTEL
Biltricide Tablets ... 2976

OPTIFLUOR (Mexico)
FLUORESCEIN SODIUM
Fluorescite Injection ... ⊙207

OPTIGEN (Hong Kong)
GENTAMICIN SULFATE
Garamycin Injectable ... 3014

OPTI-GENTA (Israel)
GENTAMICIN SULFATE
Garamycin Injectable ... 3014

OPTIL (United Kingdom)
DILTIAZEM HYDROCHLORIDE
Cardizem LA Extended Release Tablets ... 1728
Tiazac Capsules ... 1201

OPTILAST (Israel, United Kingdom)
AZELASTINE HYDROCHLORIDE
Astelin Nasal Spray ... 1904

OPTIMOL (Australia, Denmark, Hong Kong, Russia, Sweden)
TIMOLOL MALEATE
Blocadren Tablets ... 1916
Timoptic Sterile Ophthalmic Solution ... 2088
Timoptic in Ocudose ... 2091
Timoptic-XE Sterile Ophthalmic Gel Forming Solution ... 2092

OPTINATE (Finland, Italy, Norway, Sweden)
RISEDRONATE SODIUM
Actonel Tablets ... 2683

OPTINEM (Austria)
MEROPENEM
Merrem I.V. ... 686

OPTIPAR (Finland)
PAROXETINE HYDROCHLORIDE
Paxil Oral Suspension ... 1530
Paxil Tablets ... 1530

OPTIPRES (India)
BETAXOLOL HYDROCHLORIDE
Betoptic S Ophthalmic Suspension ... ⊙203, 558

OPTISOL (Israel)
SULFACETAMIDE SODIUM
Klaron Lotion 10% ... 2909

OPTOBET (Greece)
DICLOFENAC SODIUM
Voltaren Tablets ... 2307
Voltaren-XR Tablets ... 2310

OPTOMICIN (Mexico)
ERYTHROMYCIN STEARATE
Erythrocin Stearate Filmtab Tablets ... 453

OPTROL (Australia)
SALMETEROL XINAFOATE
Serevent Diskus ... 1568

OPTRUMA (Austria, Finland, France, Germany, Italy, Portugal, Spain)
RALOXIFENE HYDROCHLORIDE
Evista Tablets ... 1763

OPUMIDE (United Kingdom)
INDAPAMIDE
Indapamide Tablets ... 2156

ORABIOT UD (Argentina)
CLARITHROMYCIN
Biaxin Filmtab Tablets ... 402
Biaxin Granules ... 402

ORACORT (Canada, Israel, New Zealand, Thailand)
TRIAMCINOLONE ACETONIDE
Azmacort Inhalation Aerosol ... 1726
Nasacort AQ Nasal Spray ... 2922

ORADEXON (Belgium, Chile, Portugal, United Kingdom)
DEXAMETHASONE
Decadron Tablets ... 1951

ORAKIT (Argentina)
POTASSIUM CHLORIDE
K-Dur Extended-Relase Tablets ... 3033
K-Lor Oral Solution ... 474
K-Tab Tablets ... 475

ORALMUV (Argentina)
LAMIVUDINE
Epivir Oral Solution ... 1427
Epivir Tablets ... 1427
Epivir-HBV Oral Solution ... 1432
Epivir-HBV Tablets ... 1432

ORAL-T (Thailand)
TRIAMCINOLONE ACETONIDE
Azmacort Inhalation Aerosol ... 1726
Nasacort AQ Nasal Spray ... 2922

ORALTEN TROCHE (Israel)
CLOTRIMAZOLE
Lotrimin Cream ... 3039
Lotrimin Lotion 1% ... 3039
Lotrimin Topical Solution 1% ... 3039

ORAMEDY (Singapore)
TRIAMCINOLONE ACETONIDE
Azmacort Inhalation Aerosol ... 1726
Nasacort AQ Nasal Spray ... 2922

ORAMINAX (Portugal)
AMOXICILLIN
Amoxil Pediatric Drops for Oral Suspension ... 1343
Amoxil Tablets ... 1343

ORAMORPH (Austria, Canada, Czech Republic, Irish Republic, Italy, Spain, Sweden, The Netherlands, United Kingdom)
MORPHINE SULFATE
Kadian Capsules ... 577
MS Contin Tablets ... 2701

ORANOR (Mexico)
NORFLOXACIN
Noroxin Tablets ... 2032

ORAQIX (Sweden, United Kingdom)
LIDOCAINE
Lidoderm Patch ... 1118

ORA-SED LOTION (Australia)
LIDOCAINE
Lidoderm Patch ... 1118

ORASORBIL (Germany, Italy, Portugal)
ISOSORBIDE MONONITRATE
Imdur Tablets ... 3018

ORATANE (Australia, Hong Kong, Malaysia, Mexico, New Zealand, Singapore, South Africa)
ISOTRETINOIN
Accutane Capsules ... 2731

ORAXIM (Italy)
CEFUROXIME AXETIL
Ceftin Tablets ... 1407
Ceftin for Oral Suspension ... 1407

ORCILONE (Thailand)
TRIAMCINOLONE ACETONIDE
Azmacort Inhalation Aerosol ... 1726
Nasacort AQ Nasal Spray ... 2922

ORELOX (Australia, Brazil, Czech Republic, Denmark, France, Germany, Italy, Mexico, South Africa, Spain, Sweden, Switzerland, The Netherlands, United Kingdom)
CEFPODOXIME PROXETIL
Vantin Tablets and Oral Suspension ... 2645

ORFARIN (Malaysia, Singapore, Thailand)
WARFARIN SODIUM
Coumadin Tablets ... 898
Coumadin for Injection ... 898

ORFENACE (Canada)
ORPHENADRINE CITRATE
Norflex Injection ... 1856

ORIVAN (Finland)
VANCOMYCIN HYDROCHLORIDE
Vancocin HCl Capsules, USP ... 3380

ORLAMIX (Brazil)
DEXAMETHASONE
Decadron Tablets ... 1951

ORMOX (Finland)
ISOSORBIDE MONONITRATE
Imdur Tablets ... 3018

OROKEN (France)
CEFIXIME
Suprax ... 1843

OROMONE (France)
ESTRADIOL
Climara Transdermal System 771
Estring Vaginal Ring 2635

OROTREX (Portugal)
ISOTRETINOIN
Accutane Capsules 2731

OROXINE (Australia, Malaysia, Singapore)
LEVOTHYROXINE SODIUM
Levothroid Tablets 1186
Levoxyl Tablets 1712
Synthroid Tablets 520

ORPHENADOL (Malaysia, Singapore)
ORPHENADRINE CITRATE
Norflex Injection 1856

ORPHENGESIC (Thailand)
ORPHENADRINE CITRATE
Norflex Injection 1856

ORPIC (South Africa)
CIPROFLOXACIN HYDROCHLORIDE
Ciloxan Ophthalmic Ointment . . . . ⊙204, 559
Ciloxan Ophthalmic Solution . . . . ⊙206
Cipro Tablets 2977

ORREPASTE (Malaysia, Singapore)
TRIAMCINOLONE ACETONIDE
Azmacort Inhalation Aerosol 1726
Nasacort AQ Nasal Spray 2922

ORTHOCEL (India)
CELECOXIB
Celebrex Capsules 3134

ORTHOCLONE (Greece, South Africa)
MUROMONAB-CD3
Orthoclone OKT3 Sterile Solution 2360

ORTHOCLONE OKT3 (Australia, Belgium, Brazil, Canada, Czech Republic, Finland, France, Germany, Hong Kong, Israel, Italy, Malaysia, Mexico, New Zealand, Norway, Sweden, Switzerland, Thailand, The Netherlands)
MUROMONAB-CD3
Orthoclone OKT3 Sterile Solution 2360

ORTHOVISC (Canada, Germany, Israel, United Kingdom)
SODIUM HYALURONATE
Hyalgan Solution 2901

ORTOCICLINA (Brazil)
ERYTHROMYCIN
Ery-Tab Tablets 449
Erythromycin Base Filmtab Tablets 455
Erythromycin Delayed-Release Capsules, USP 457
PCE Dispertab Tablets 515

ORTOFLAN (Brazil)
DICLOFENAC SODIUM
Voltaren Tablets 2307
Voltaren-XR Tablets 2310

ORTOPSIQUE (Mexico)
DIAZEPAM
Diastat Rectal Delivery System 3343
Valium Tablets 2819

ORTRIZOL (Mexico)
METRONIDAZOLE
MetroGel-Vaginal Gel 1855

OSDRON (Brazil)
ALENDRONATE SODIUM
Fosamax Tablets 1969

OSEMIN (Mexico)
FUROSEMIDE
Furosemide Tablets 2154

OSEOTENK (Argentina)
ALENDRONATE SODIUM
Fosamax Tablets 1969

OSFO (Greece)
ETIDRONATE DISODIUM
Didronel Tablets 2697

OSKANA (Greece)
LEVOCARNITINE
Carnitor Injection 3188
Carnitor Tablets and Oral Solution 3190

OSMO-ADALAT (Israel)
NIFEDIPINE
Adalat CC Tablets 2964

OSMOLAC (Italy)
LACTULOSE
Kristalose for Oral Solution 1034

OSPAMOX (Greece, Hungary, Portugal)
AMOXICILLIN
Amoxil Pediatric Drops for Oral Suspension 1343
Amoxil Tablets 1343

OSPOCARD (Austria)
NIFEDIPINE
Adalat CC Tablets 2964

OSSOMAX (Brazil)
ALENDRONATE SODIUM
Fosamax Tablets 1969

OSTALERT (Greece)
ALENDRONATE SODIUM
Fosamax Tablets 1969

OSTAREN (Thailand)
DICLOFENAC SODIUM
Voltaren Tablets 2307
Voltaren-XR Tablets 2310

OSTEDRON (Greece)
ETIDRONATE DISODIUM
Didronel Tablets 2697

OSTENAN (Brazil)
ALENDRONATE SODIUM
Fosamax Tablets 1969

OSTENIL (France, Germany, Switzerland, United Kingdom)
SODIUM HYALURONATE
Hyalgan Solution 2901

OSTEO D (Israel)
CALCITRIOL
Calcijex Injection 411
Rocaltrol Capsules 2798
Rocaltrol Oral Solution 2798

OSTEODIDRONEL (Belgium)
ETIDRONATE DISODIUM
Didronel Tablets 2697

OSTEODRUG (Greece)
ETIDRONATE DISODIUM
Didronel Tablets 2697

OSTEOFAR (Brazil)
ALENDRONATE SODIUM
Fosamax Tablets 1969

OSTEOFEM (Chile)
ALENDRONATE SODIUM
Fosamax Tablets 1969

OSTEOFENE (Argentina)
ALENDRONATE SODIUM
Fosamax Tablets 1969

OSTEOFORM (Brazil)
ALENDRONATE SODIUM
Fosamax Tablets 1969

OSTEOFOS (India)
ALENDRONATE SODIUM
Fosamax Tablets 1969

OSTEONATE (Argentina)
ALENDRONATE SODIUM
Fosamax Tablets 1969

OSTEORAL (Brazil)
ALENDRONATE SODIUM
Fosamax Tablets 1969

OSTEOSAN (Chile)
ALENDRONATE SODIUM
Fosamax Tablets 1969

OSTEOTON (Greece)
ETIDRONATE DISODIUM
Didronel Tablets 2697

OSTEOTOP (Chile)
ETIDRONATE DISODIUM
Didronel Tablets 2697

OSTEOTRAT (Brazil)
ALENDRONATE SODIUM
Fosamax Tablets 1969

OSTEOTRIOL (Germany, Russia)
CALCITRIOL
Calcijex Injection 411
Rocaltrol Capsules 2798
Rocaltrol Oral Solution 2798

OSTEPAM (France)
PAMIDRONATE DISODIUM
Aredia for Injection 2179

OSTEUM (Spain)
ETIDRONATE DISODIUM
Didronel Tablets 2697

OSTOGENE (Greece)
ETIDRONATE DISODIUM
Didronel Tablets 2697

OSTOPOR (Greece)
ETIDRONATE DISODIUM
Didronel Tablets 2697

OSTRIOL (Brazil)
CALCITRIOL
Calcijex Injection 411
Rocaltrol Capsules 2798
Rocaltrol Oral Solution 2798

OTARI (Greece)
CALCITRIOL
Calcijex Injection 411
Rocaltrol Capsules 2798
Rocaltrol Oral Solution 2798

OTEX HC (Argentina)
CIPROFLOXACIN HYDROCHLORIDE
Ciloxan Ophthalmic Ointment . . . . ⊙204, 559
Ciloxan Ophthalmic Solution . . . . ⊙206
Cipro Tablets 2977

OTO BIOTAER (Argentina)
CIPROFLOXACIN
Cipro Oral Suspension 2977

OTOBACID N (Czech Republic)
DEXAMETHASONE
Decadron Tablets 1951

OTOCIPRIN (Spain)
CIPROFLOXACIN HYDROCHLORIDE
Ciloxan Ophthalmic Ointment . . . . ⊙204, 559
Ciloxan Ophthalmic Solution . . . . ⊙206
Cipro Tablets 2977

OTOCIPRO (Argentina)
HYDROCORTISONE
Hydrocortone Tablets 1989

OTODON (Venezuela)
LIDOCAINE
Lidoderm Patch 1118

OTOFLOX (Argentina)
OFLOXACIN
Floxin Otic Solution 1049

OTOIAL (Italy)
SODIUM HYALURONATE
Hyalgan Solution 2901

OTOSAT (Spain)
CIPROFLOXACIN HYDROCHLORIDE
Ciloxan Ophthalmic Ointment . . . . ⊙204, 559
Ciloxan Ophthalmic Solution . . . . ⊙206
Cipro Tablets 2977

OTOSPORIN C CIPROFLOXACINA (Argentina)
CIPROFLOXACIN HYDROCHLORIDE
Ciloxan Ophthalmic Ointment . . . . ⊙204, 559
Ciloxan Ophthalmic Solution . . . . ⊙206
Cipro Tablets 2977

OTRASEL (France)
SELEGILINE HYDROCHLORIDE
Eldepryl Capsules 3208

OTREON (Austria, Italy, Spain)
CEFPODOXIME PROXETIL
Vantin Tablets and Oral Suspension 2645

OTRIVIN NEUSALLERGIE AZELASTINE (The Netherlands)
AZELASTINE HYDROCHLORIDE
Astelin Nasal Spray 1904

OTRIVIN RHUME DES FOINS (Switzerland)
AZELASTINE HYDROCHLORIDE
Astelin Nasal Spray 1904

OTRIVINE ANTI-ALLERGIE (Belgium)
AZELASTINE HYDROCHLORIDE
Astelin Nasal Spray 1904

OTROZOL (Mexico)
METRONIDAZOLE
MetroGel-Vaginal Gel 1855

OVAZOL-V (Mexico)
METRONIDAZOLE
MetroGel-Vaginal Gel 1855

OVINOL (Greece)
NORFLOXACIN
Noroxin Tablets 2032

OVIS NEU (Germany)
CLOTRIMAZOLE
Lotrimin Cream 3039
Lotrimin Lotion 1% 3039
Lotrimin Topical Solution 1% 3039

OXA FORTE (Argentina)
DICLOFENAC SODIUM
Voltaren Tablets 2307
Voltaren-XR Tablets 2310

OXAL (Mexico)
ALBENDAZOLE
Albenza Tablets 1338

OXALGIN (India)
DICLOFENAC SODIUM
Voltaren Tablets 2307
Voltaren-XR Tablets 2310

OXALGIN-DP (India)
DICLOFENAC SODIUM
Voltaren Tablets 2307
Voltaren-XR Tablets 2310

OXANDRIN (Australia)
OXANDROLONE
Oxandrin Tablets 2962

OXANEST (Finland)
OXYCODONE HYDROCHLORIDE
OxyContin Tablets 2703
OxyFast Oral Concentrate Solution 2708
OxyIR Capsules 2708

OXAPROST (Argentina)
DICLOFENAC SODIUM
Voltaren Tablets 2307
Voltaren-XR Tablets 2310

OXCORD (Brazil)
NIFEDIPINE
Adalat CC Tablets 2964

OXEPAR (Portugal)
PAROXETINE HYDROCHLORIDE
Paxil Oral Suspension 1530
Paxil Tablets 1530

OXET (Germany)
PAROXETINE HYDROCHLORIDE
Paxil Oral Suspension 1530
Paxil Tablets 1530

OXETINE (Australia, Denmark)
PAROXETINE HYDROCHLORIDE
Paxil Oral Suspension 1530
Paxil Tablets 1530

OXIDERMA (Spain)
BENZOYL PEROXIDE
Brevoxyl-4 Creamy Wash 3210
Brevoxyl-4 Gel 3210
Brevoxyl-8 Creamy Wash 3210
Brevoxyl-8 Gel 3210
Triaz Cleanser 1892
Triaz Gel 1892

OXIGEN (Brazil)
NIMODIPINE
Nimotop Capsules 749

OXINOVAG (Argentina)
OXYCODONE HYDROCHLORIDE
OxyContin Tablets 2703
OxyFast Oral Concentrate Solution 2708
OxyIR Capsules 2708

OXINOVAG COMPLEX (Argentina)
OXYCODONE HYDROCHLORIDE
OxyContin Tablets 2703
OxyFast Oral Concentrate Solution 2708
OxyIR Capsules 2708

OXISOL (Venezuela)
CLOTRIMAZOLE
Lotrimin Cream 3039
Lotrimin Lotion 1% 3039
Lotrimin Topical Solution 1% 3039

OXISTAT (Argentina, Mexico)
OXICONAZOLE NITRATE
Oxistat Cream 2667
Oxistat Lotion 2667

OXITRAT (Brazil)
OXICONAZOLE NITRATE
Oxistat Cream 2667
Oxistat Lotion 2667

OXIZOLE (Canada)
OXICONAZOLE NITRATE
Oxistat Cream 2667
Oxistat Lotion 2667

OXKEN (Mexico)
OFLOXACIN
Floxin Otic Solution 1049

(⊙ Described in PDR For Ophthalmic Medicines™)

OXODAL (Spain)
BETAXOLOL HYDROCHLORIDE
Betoptic S Ophthalmic Suspension . ⊙203, 558

OXSORALEN (Australia, Austria, Brazil, Canada, Chile, Czech Republic, Hong Kong, Israel, Italy, Japan, Malaysia, Mexico, New Zealand, Singapore, South Africa, Spain, The Netherlands)
METHOXSALEN
Oxsoralen Lotion 1% . . . 3352
Oxsoralen-Ultra Capsules . . . 3353

OXSORALON (Belgium)
METHOXSALEN
Oxsoralen Lotion 1% . . . 3352
Oxsoralen-Ultra Capsules . . . 3353

OXY (Australia, Canada, Czech Republic, Germany, Hong Kong, Israel, Mexico, United Kingdom)
BENZOYL PEROXIDE
Brevoxyl-4 Creamy Wash . . . 3210
Brevoxyl-4 Gel . . . 3210
Brevoxyl-8 Creamy Wash . . . 3210
Brevoxyl-8 Gel . . . 3210
Triaz Cleanser . . . 1892
Triaz Gel . . . 1892

OXY IR (Canada)
OXYCODONE HYDROCHLORIDE
OxyContin Tablets . . . 2703
OxyFast Oral Concentrate Solution . . . 2708
OxyIR Capsules . . . 2708

OXY SENSITIVE (Israel)
BENZOYL PEROXIDE
Brevoxyl-4 Creamy Wash . . . 3210
Brevoxyl-4 Gel . . . 3210
Brevoxyl-8 Creamy Wash . . . 3210
Brevoxyl-8 Gel . . . 3210
Triaz Cleanser . . . 1892
Triaz Gel . . . 1892

OXYCARDIN (France)
ISOSORBIDE MONONITRATE
Imdur Tablets . . . 3018

OXYCOD (Israel)
OXYCODONE HYDROCHLORIDE
OxyContin Tablets . . . 2703
OxyFast Oral Concentrate Solution . . . 2708
OxyIR Capsules . . . 2708

OXYCONTIN (Argentina, Australia, Brazil, Canada, Chile, Czech Republic, Denmark, Finland, France, Irish Republic, Israel, Mexico, New Zealand, Norway, Spain, Sweden, Switzerland, The Netherlands, United Kingdom)
OXYCODONE HYDROCHLORIDE
OxyContin Tablets . . . 2703
OxyFast Oral Concentrate Solution . . . 2708
OxyIR Capsules . . . 2708

OXYDERM (Canada)
BENZOYL PEROXIDE
Brevoxyl-4 Creamy Wash . . . 3210
Brevoxyl-4 Gel . . . 3210
Brevoxyl-8 Creamy Wash . . . 3210
Brevoxyl-8 Gel . . . 3210
Triaz Cleanser . . . 1892
Triaz Gel . . . 1892

OXYGESIC (Germany)
OXYCODONE HYDROCHLORIDE
OxyContin Tablets . . . 2703
OxyFast Oral Concentrate Solution . . . 2708
OxyIR Capsules . . . 2708

OXYNORM (Australia, Denmark, Finland, France, Irish Republic, New Zealand, Norway, Sweden, Switzerland, The Netherlands, United Kingdom)
OXYCODONE HYDROCHLORIDE
OxyContin Tablets . . . 2703
OxyFast Oral Concentrate Solution . . . 2708
OxyIR Capsules . . . 2708

OXYTOKO (Spain)
BENZOYL PEROXIDE
Brevoxyl-4 Creamy Wash . . . 3210
Brevoxyl-4 Gel . . . 3210
Brevoxyl-8 Creamy Wash . . . 3210
Brevoxyl-8 Gel . . . 3210
Triaz Cleanser . . . 1892
Triaz Gel . . . 1892

OZAPIN (India)
OLANZAPINE
Zyprexa Tablets . . . 1830

OZEPAM (India)
CLONAZEPAM
Klonopin Tablets . . . 2778

PABALAT (Chile)
NIFEDIPINE
Adalat CC Tablets . . . 2964

PACEUM (Switzerland)
DIAZEPAM
Diastat Rectal Delivery System . . . 3343
Valium Tablets . . . 2819

PACINAX (Chile)
DIAZEPAM
Diastat Rectal Delivery System . . . 3343
Valium Tablets . . . 2819

PACIUM (Spain)
DIAZEPAM
Diastat Rectal Delivery System . . . 3343
Valium Tablets . . . 2819

PACTENS (Mexico)
NAPROXEN SODIUM
Anaprox DS Tablets . . . 2761
Anaprox Tablets . . . 2761

PADET (Argentina)
METRONIDAZOLE
MetroGel-Vaginal Gel . . . 1855

PADIKEN (Mexico)
AMANTADINE HYDROCHLORIDE
Symmetrel Tablets . . . 1135

PAFTEC (Portugal)
FLUNISOLIDE
Aerobid Inhaler System . . . 1171
Aerobid-M Inhaler System . . . 1171

PAHTLISAN (Mexico)
CHLOROTHIAZIDE
Diuril Oral Suspension . . . 1954

PAINDOL (Thailand)
TRAMADOL HYDROCHLORIDE
Ultram ER Tablets . . . 2392

PAINEX (Portugal)
DICLOFENAC SODIUM
Voltaren Tablets . . . 2307
Voltaren-XR Tablets . . . 2310

PALANE (Mexico)
ENALAPRIL MALEATE
Vasotec I.V. Injection . . . 2103

PALATRIN (Mexico)
LANSOPRAZOLE
Prevacid Delayed-Release Capsules . . . 3271

PALDAR (Argentina)
MUPIROCIN
Bactroban Ointment . . . 1395

PALIATIN (Spain)
CHLORDIAZEPOXIDE HYDROCHLORIDE
Librium Capsules . . . 3347

PALISTOP (Greece)
FLUTAMIDE
Eulexin Capsules . . . 3009

PALLADON (Germany, Switzerland, The Netherlands)
HYDROMORPHONE HYDROCHLORIDE
Dilaudid Ampules . . . 440
Dilaudid Multiple Dose Vials . . . 440
Dilaudid Non-Sterile Powder . . . 440
Dilaudid Oral Liquid . . . 445
Dilaudid Rectal Suppositories . . . 440
Dilaudid Tablets . . . 440
Dilaudid Tablets - 8 mg . . . 445
Dilaudid-HP Injection . . . 442
Dilaudid-HP Lyophilized Powder 250 mg . . . 442

PALLADONE (Irish Republic, Israel, United Kingdom)
HYDROMORPHONE HYDROCHLORIDE
Dilaudid Ampules . . . 440
Dilaudid Multiple Dose Vials . . . 440
Dilaudid Non-Sterile Powder . . . 440
Dilaudid Oral Liquid . . . 445
Dilaudid Rectal Suppositories . . . 440
Dilaudid Tablets . . . 440
Dilaudid Tablets - 8 mg . . . 445
Dilaudid-HP Injection . . . 442
Dilaudid-HP Lyophilized Powder 250 mg . . . 442

PALON (Hong Kong, Thailand)
PROPRANOLOL HYDROCHLORIDE
Inderal LA Long-Acting Capsules . . . 3429

PALUX (Japan)
ALPROSTADIL
Edex Injection . . . 3089

PALUXETIL (Austria)
PAROXETINE HYDROCHLORIDE
Paxil Oral Suspension . . . 1530
Paxil Tablets . . . 1530

PAMDOSA (Argentina)
PAMIDRONATE DISODIUM
Aredia for Injection . . . 2179

PAMERGAN (Brazil)
PROMETHAZINE HYDROCHLORIDE
Phenergan Tablets and Suppositories . . . 3440

PAMID (Israel)
INDAPAMIDE
Indapamide Tablets . . . 2156

PAMIDRAN (Portugal)
PAMIDRONATE DISODIUM
Aredia for Injection . . . 2179

PAMIDRIA (India)
PAMIDRONATE DISODIUM
Aredia for Injection . . . 2179

PAMIFOS (India)
PAMIDRONATE DISODIUM
Aredia for Injection . . . 2179

PAMISOL (Australia, Hong Kong, Malaysia, Mexico, New Zealand, Singapore, Thailand)
PAMIDRONATE DISODIUM
Aredia for Injection . . . 2179

PAMITOR (Austria, Hungary)
PAMIDRONATE DISODIUM
Aredia for Injection . . . 2179

PAMPE (Portugal)
LANSOPRAZOLE
Prevacid Delayed-Release Capsules . . . 3271

PANALBA (Greece)
FAMOTIDINE
Pepcid Injection . . . 2040
Pepcid Injection Premixed . . . 2040
Pepcid Tablets . . . 2038
Pepcid for Oral Suspension . . . 2038

PANALDINE (Japan)
TICLOPIDINE HYDROCHLORIDE
Ticlid Tablets . . . 2810

PANALENE (Argentina)
ADAPALENE
Differin Gel . . . 1211

PANBESY (Belgium, Hong Kong, Singapore, Thailand)
PHENTERMINE HYDROCHLORIDE
Adipex-P Capsules . . . 1215
Adipex-P Tablets . . . 1215

PANCARDIOL (Spain)
ISOSORBIDE MONONITRATE
Imdur Tablets . . . 3018

PANCLOFLEX (Argentina)
DICLOFENAC SODIUM
Voltaren Tablets . . . 2307
Voltaren-XR Tablets . . . 2310

PANCREASE (Australia, Belgium, Brazil, Canada, Denmark, Finland, Israel, Italy, Mexico, New Zealand, Norway, Spain, Sweden, The Netherlands, United Kingdom, Venezuela)
PANCRELIPASE
Ultrase Capsules . . . 708
Ultrase MT Capsules . . . 709

PANDERMIL (Portugal)
HYDROCORTISONE
Hydrocortone Tablets . . . 1989

PANDERMIN CICATRIZANTE (Spain)
SODIUM HYALURONATE
Hyalgan Solution . . . 2901

PANDRAT (Argentina)
PAMIDRONATE DISODIUM
Aredia for Injection . . . 2179

PAN-FUNGEX (Portugal)
CLOTRIMAZOLE
Lotrimin Cream . . . 3039
Lotrimin Lotion 1% . . . 3039
Lotrimin Topical Solution 1% . . . 3039

PANGEL (Belgium)
BENZOYL PEROXIDE
Brevoxyl-4 Creamy Wash . . . 3210
Brevoxyl-4 Gel . . . 3210
Brevoxyl-8 Creamy Wash . . . 3210
Brevoxyl-8 Gel . . . 3210
Triaz Cleanser . . . 1892
Triaz Gel . . . 1892

PANGRAF (India)
TACROLIMUS
Prograf Capsules and Injection . . . 632

PANITOL (Thailand)
CARBAMAZEPINE
Carbatrol Capsules . . . 3171
Tegretol Chewable Tablets . . . 2295
Tegretol Suspension . . . 2295
Tegretol Tablets . . . 2295
Tegretol-XR Tablets . . . 2295

PANKREADEN (Italy)
PANCRELIPASE
Ultrase Capsules . . . 708
Ultrase MT Capsules . . . 709

PANKREASE (South Africa)
PANCRELIPASE
Ultrase Capsules . . . 708
Ultrase MT Capsules . . . 709

PANMICOL (Argentina)
CLOTRIMAZOLE
Lotrimin Cream . . . 3039
Lotrimin Lotion 1% . . . 3039
Lotrimin Topical Solution 1% . . . 3039

PANNOGEL (France)
BENZOYL PEROXIDE
Brevoxyl-4 Creamy Wash . . . 3210
Brevoxyl-4 Gel . . . 3210
Brevoxyl-8 Creamy Wash . . . 3210
Brevoxyl-8 Gel . . . 3210
Triaz Cleanser . . . 1892
Triaz Gel . . . 1892

PANOTILE CIPRO (Germany)
CIPROFLOXACIN HYDROCHLORIDE
Ciloxan Ophthalmic Ointment . . . ⊙204, 559
Ciloxan Ophthalmic Solution . . . ⊙206
Cipro Tablets . . . 2977

PANOXYL (Australia, Austria, Brazil, Canada, Finland, France, Germany, Hong Kong, Irish Republic, Israel, Italy, Malaysia, Mexico, New Zealand, Norway, Portugal, Singapore, South Africa, Spain, Switzerland, Thailand, United Kingdom, Venezuela)
BENZOYL PEROXIDE
Brevoxyl-4 Creamy Wash . . . 3210
Brevoxyl-4 Gel . . . 3210
Brevoxyl-8 Creamy Wash . . . 3210
Brevoxyl-8 Gel . . . 3210
Triaz Cleanser . . . 1892
Triaz Gel . . . 1892

PANQUIL (Australia)
PROMETHAZINE HYDROCHLORIDE
Phenergan Tablets and Suppositories . . . 3440

PANSULFOX (Chile)
BENZOYL PEROXIDE
Brevoxyl-4 Creamy Wash . . . 3210
Brevoxyl-4 Gel . . . 3210
Brevoxyl-8 Creamy Wash . . . 3210
Brevoxyl-8 Gel . . . 3210
Triaz Cleanser . . . 1892
Triaz Gel . . . 1892

PANTASOL (Italy)
FLUNISOLIDE
Aerobid Inhaler System . . . 1171
Aerobid-M Inhaler System . . . 1171

PANTESTONE (Argentina)
ANASTROZOLE
Arimidex Tablets . . . 673

PANTINOL (Austria)
APROTININ
Trasylol Injection . . . 754

PANTOCORT (Venezuela)
HYDROCORTISONE
Hydrocortone Tablets . . . 1989

PANTODRIN (Spain)
ERYTHROMYCIN
Ery-Tab Tablets . . . 449
Erythromycin Base Filmtab Tablets . . . 455
Erythromycin Delayed-Release Capsules, USP . . . 457
PCE Dispertab Tablets . . . 515

PANTOK (Spain)
SIMVASTATIN
Zocor Tablets . . . 2105

(⊙ Described in PDR For Ophthalmic Medicines™)

PANTOMICINA (Argentina, Brazil, Venezuela)
ERYTHROMYCIN
Ery-Tab Tablets 449
Erythromycin Base Filmtab Tablets 455
Erythromycin Delayed-Release Capsules, USP 457
PCE Dispertab Tablets 515

PANTOSTIN (Germany)
ESTRADIOL
Climara Transdermal System 771
Estring Vaginal Ring 2635

PANTYSON (Finland)
HYDROCORTISONE
Hydrocortone Tablets 1989

PANWARFIN (Greece)
WARFARIN SODIUM
Coumadin Tablets 898
Coumadin for Injection 898

PANZID (Italy)
CEFTAZIDIME
Fortaz for Injection 1453

PANZYTRAT (Australia, New Zealand)
PANCRELIPASE
Ultrase Capsules 708
Ultrase MT Capsules 709

PAPASINE (Argentina)
NAPROXEN
EC-Naprosyn Delayed-Release Tablets 2761
Naprosyn Suspension 2761
Naprosyn Tablets 2761

PARABACT (India)
NORFLOXACIN
Noroxin Tablets 2032

PARACEFAN (Belgium)
CLONIDINE HYDROCHLORIDE
Catapres Tablets 843

PARACNE (Argentina)
BENZOYL PEROXIDE
Brevoxyl-4 Creamy Wash 3210
Brevoxyl-4 Gel 3210
Brevoxyl-8 Creamy Wash 3210
Brevoxyl-8 Gel 3210
Triaz Cleanser 1892
Triaz Gel 1892

PARANTHIL (South Africa)
ALBENDAZOLE
Albenza Tablets 1338

PARAPRES (Spain)
CANDESARTAN CILEXETIL
Atacand Tablets 649

PARAPRES PLUS (Spain)
CANDESARTAN CILEXETIL
Atacand Tablets 649

PARAQUEIMOL (Brazil)
SULFACETAMIDE SODIUM
Klaron Lotion 10% 2909

PARASIN (Brazil)
ALBENDAZOLE
Albenza Tablets 1338

PARASTHMAN (Germany)
THEOPHYLLINE
Uniphyl Tablets 2710

PARATONINA (Spain)
PAROXETINE HYDROCHLORIDE
Paxil Oral Suspension 1530
Paxil Tablets 1530

PARCETIN (Argentina)
NORFLOXACIN
Noroxin Tablets 2032

PARDEX (Mexico)
DEXAMETHASONE
Decadron Tablets 1951

PAREXAT (Switzerland)
PAROXETINE HYDROCHLORIDE
Paxil Oral Suspension 1530
Paxil Tablets 1530

PARI (India)
PAROXETINE HYDROCHLORIDE
Paxil Oral Suspension 1530
Paxil Tablets 1530

PARITREL (Israel)
AMANTADINE HYDROCHLORIDE
Symmetrel Tablets 1135

PARKADINA (Portugal)
AMANTADINE HYDROCHLORIDE
Symmetrel Tablets 1135

PARKEXIN (Brazil)
SELEGILINE HYDROCHLORIDE
Eldepryl Capsules 3208

PARLAZIN (Hungary)
CETIRIZINE HYDROCHLORIDE
Zyrtec Syrup 2594
Zyrtec Tablets 2594

PARNATE (Argentina, Australia, Brazil, Canada, Czech Republic, Germany, Irish Republic, New Zealand, South Africa, Spain)
TRANYLCYPROMINE SULFATE
Parnate Tablets 1527

PAROCETAN (Austria)
PAROXETINE HYDROCHLORIDE
Paxil Oral Suspension 1530
Paxil Tablets 1530

PAROLICH (Germany)
PAROXETINE HYDROCHLORIDE
Paxil Oral Suspension 1530
Paxil Tablets 1530

PARONAL (Belgium)
ASPARAGINASE
Elspar for Injection 2463

PAROSER (Irish Republic)
PAROXETINE HYDROCHLORIDE
Paxil Oral Suspension 1530
Paxil Tablets 1530

PAROTIN (India)
PAROXETINE HYDROCHLORIDE
Paxil Oral Suspension 1530
Paxil Tablets 1530

PAROTUR (Spain)
PAROXETINE HYDROCHLORIDE
Paxil Oral Suspension 1530
Paxil Tablets 1530

PAROX (Irish Republic)
PAROXETINE HYDROCHLORIDE
Paxil Oral Suspension 1530
Paxil Tablets 1530

PAROXAT (Austria, Germany, Hungary)
PAROXETINE HYDROCHLORIDE
Paxil Oral Suspension 1530
Paxil Tablets 1530

PAROXEDURA (Germany)
PAROXETINE HYDROCHLORIDE
Paxil Oral Suspension 1530
Paxil Tablets 1530

PAROXIFLEX (Sweden)
PAROXETINE HYDROCHLORIDE
Paxil Oral Suspension 1530
Paxil Tablets 1530

PARSILID (Italy)
TICLOPIDINE HYDROCHLORIDE
Ticlid Tablets 2810

PARVEMAXOL (The Netherlands)
CLOTRIMAZOLE
Lotrimin Cream 3039
Lotrimin Lotion 1% 3039
Lotrimin Topical Solution 1% 3039

PARVEN (Mexico)
BENZONATATE
Tessalon Perles 1199

PATANOL (Argentina, Australia, Brazil, Canada, Chile, Hong Kong, Malaysia, Mexico, New Zealand, Singapore, South Africa, Thailand, Venezuela)
OLOPATADINE HYDROCHLORIDE
Patanol Ophthalmic Solution . . . . . 561, ⊙210

PATOX (Mexico)
CIPROFLOXACIN HYDROCHLORIDE
Ciloxan Ophthalmic Ointment . . . . ⊙204, 559
Ciloxan Ophthalmic Solution . . . . ⊙206
Cipro Tablets 2977

PATXEN (Mexico)
NAPROXEN
EC-Naprosyn Delayed-Release Tablets 2761
Naprosyn Suspension 2761
Naprosyn Tablets 2761

PAUSOGEST (Czech Republic, Hungary)
ESTRADIOL
Climara Transdermal System 771
Estring Vaginal Ring 2635

PAX (South Africa)
DIAZEPAM
Diastat Rectal Delivery System 3343
Valium Tablets 2819

PAXAM (Australia, New Zealand)
CLONAZEPAM
Klonopin Tablets 2778

PAXATE (Mexico)
DIAZEPAM
Diastat Rectal Delivery System 3343
Valium Tablets 2819

PAXETIL (Portugal)
PAROXETINE HYDROCHLORIDE
Paxil Oral Suspension 1530
Paxil Tablets 1530

PAXIL (Argentina, Canada, Mexico, Russia, Venezuela)
PAROXETINE HYDROCHLORIDE
Paxil Oral Suspension 1530
Paxil Tablets 1530

PAXILFAR (Portugal)
TRAMADOL HYDROCHLORIDE
Ultram ER Tablets 2392

PAXON (Argentina)
LOSARTAN POTASSIUM
Cozaar Tablets 1935

PAXON-D (Argentina)
LOSARTAN POTASSIUM
Cozaar Tablets 1935

PAXTINE (Australia)
PAROXETINE HYDROCHLORIDE
Paxil Oral Suspension 1530
Paxil Tablets 1530

PAXUM (India)
DIAZEPAM
Diastat Rectal Delivery System 3343
Valium Tablets 2819

PAXXET (Israel)
PAROXETINE HYDROCHLORIDE
Paxil Oral Suspension 1530
Paxil Tablets 1530

PAZOLINI (Brazil)
DIAZEPAM
Diastat Rectal Delivery System 3343
Valium Tablets 2819

PB GEL (Argentina)
BENZOYL PEROXIDE
Brevoxyl-4 Creamy Wash 3210
Brevoxyl-4 Gel 3210
Brevoxyl-8 Creamy Wash 3210
Brevoxyl-8 Gel 3210
Triaz Cleanser 1892
Triaz Gel 1892

PCE (Canada, Hong Kong)
ERYTHROMYCIN
Ery-Tab Tablets 449
Erythromycin Base Filmtab Tablets 455
Erythromycin Delayed-Release Capsules, USP 457
PCE Dispertab Tablets 515

PEAULINE (The Netherlands)
BENZOYL PEROXIDE
Brevoxyl-4 Creamy Wash 3210
Brevoxyl-4 Gel 3210
Brevoxyl-8 Creamy Wash 3210
Brevoxyl-8 Gel 3210
Triaz Cleanser 1892
Triaz Gel 1892

PEBEGAL (Mexico)
BENZONATATE
Tessalon Perles 1199

PEDIAPHYLLIN PL (The Netherlands)
THEOPHYLLINE
Uniphyl Tablets 2710

PEDIKUROL (Austria)
CLOTRIMAZOLE
Lotrimin Cream 3039
Lotrimin Lotion 1% 3039
Lotrimin Topical Solution 1% 3039

PEDISAFE (Germany)
CLOTRIMAZOLE
Lotrimin Cream 3039
Lotrimin Lotion 1% 3039
Lotrimin Topical Solution 1% 3039

PEKTROL (Russia)
ISOSORBIDE MONONITRATE
Imdur Tablets 3018

PELICREP (Argentina)
FINASTERIDE
Propecia Tablets 2060
Proscar Tablets 2067

PELVICILLIN NF (Argentina)
METRONIDAZOLE
MetroGel-Vaginal Gel 1855

PENDINE (Australia)
GABAPENTIN
Neurontin Capsules 2487

PENDRAMINE (United Kingdom)
PENICILLAMINE
Cuprimine Capsules 1947

PENEGRA (India)
SILDENAFIL CITRATE
Viagra Tablets 2573

PENESTER (Czech Republic)
FINASTERIDE
Propecia Tablets 2060
Proscar Tablets 2067

PENGESIC (Malaysia, Singapore)
TRAMADOL HYDROCHLORIDE
Ultram ER Tablets 2392

PENGON (Greece)
DICLOFENAC SODIUM
Voltaren Tablets 2307
Voltaren-XR Tablets 2310

PENLES (Japan)
LIDOCAINE
Lidoderm Patch 1118

PENMOX (South Africa)
AMOXICILLIN
Amoxil Pediatric Drops for Oral Suspension 1343
Amoxil Tablets 1343

PENNSAID (Canada, Italy, Portugal, United Kingdom)
DICLOFENAC SODIUM
Voltaren Tablets 2307
Voltaren-XR Tablets 2310

PENSODIL (Mexico)
NAPROXEN SODIUM
Anaprox DS Tablets 2761
Anaprox Tablets 2761

PENTACARD (Belgium, Thailand)
ISOSORBIDE MONONITRATE
Imdur Tablets 3018

PENTALAC (Brazil)
LACTULOSE
Kristalose for Oral Solution 1034

PENTICLOX (Mexico)
AMOXICILLIN
Amoxil Pediatric Drops for Oral Suspension 1343
Amoxil Tablets 1343

PENTILZENO (Portugal)
DILTIAZEM HYDROCHLORIDE
Cardizem LA Extended Release Tablets . . . 1728
Tiazac Capsules 1201

PENTOCLAVE (Argentina)
ERYTHROMYCIN
Ery-Tab Tablets 449
Erythromycin Base Filmtab Tablets 455
Erythromycin Delayed-Release Capsules, USP 457
PCE Dispertab Tablets 515

PENTOREL (India)
BUPRENORPHINE HYDROCHLORIDE
Buprenex Injectable 2716

PENVICILIN (Brazil)
AMOXICILLIN
Amoxil Pediatric Drops for Oral Suspension 1343
Amoxil Tablets 1343

PEPAR (India)
PIOGLITAZONE HYDROCHLORIDE
Actos Tablets 3219

PEPCID (Australia, Austria, Finland, Germany, Hong Kong, Irish Republic, New Zealand, Norway, South Africa, Spain, Sweden, Switzerland, The Netherlands)
FAMOTIDINE
Pepcid Injection 2040
Pepcid Injection Premixed 2040
Pepcid Tablets 2038
Pepcid for Oral Suspension 2038

PEPCIDAC (France)
FAMOTIDINE
Pepcid Injection 2040
Pepcid Injection Premixed 2040
Pepcid Tablets 2038
Pepcid for Oral Suspension 2038

PEPCIDIN (Denmark, Finland, Norway, Sweden, The Netherlands)
FAMOTIDINE
Pepcid Injection 2040
Pepcid Injection Premixed 2040
Pepcid Tablets 2038
Pepcid for Oral Suspension 2038

PEPCIDINA (Portugal)
FAMOTIDINE
Pepcid Injection 2040
Pepcid Injection Premixed 2040
Pepcid Tablets 2038
Pepcid for Oral Suspension 2038

PEPCIDINE (Australia, Austria, Belgium, Hong Kong, Malaysia, Mexico, New Zealand, Singapore, Switzerland, Thailand, Venezuela)
FAMOTIDINE
Pepcid Injection 2040
Pepcid Injection Premixed 2040
Pepcid Tablets 2038
Pepcid for Oral Suspension 2038

PEPCINE (Thailand)
FAMOTIDINE
Pepcid Injection 2040
Pepcid Injection Premixed 2040
Pepcid Tablets 2038
Pepcid for Oral Suspension 2038

PEPDENAL (Thailand)
FAMOTIDINE
Pepcid Injection 2040
Pepcid Injection Premixed 2040
Pepcid Tablets 2038
Pepcid for Oral Suspension 2038

PEPDINE (France)
FAMOTIDINE
Pepcid Injection 2040
Pepcid Injection Premixed 2040
Pepcid Tablets 2038
Pepcid for Oral Suspension 2038

PEPDUL (Germany)
FAMOTIDINE
Pepcid Injection 2040
Pepcid Injection Premixed 2040
Pepcid Tablets 2038
Pepcid for Oral Suspension 2038

PEPFAMIN (Thailand)
FAMOTIDINE
Pepcid Injection 2040
Pepcid Injection Premixed 2040
Pepcid Tablets 2038
Pepcid for Oral Suspension 2038

PEP-RANI (Portugal)
RANITIDINE HYDROCHLORIDE
Zantac 25 EFFERdose Tablets 1624
Zantac 150 EFFERdose Tablets. 1624
Zantac 150 Tablets 1624
Zantac 300 Tablets 1624
Zantac Injection 1619
Zantac Injection Premixed 1619
Zantac Syrup 1624

PEPTAB (Portugal)
RANITIDINE HYDROCHLORIDE
Zantac 25 EFFERdose Tablets 1624
Zantac 150 EFFERdose Tablets. 1624
Zantac 150 Tablets 1624
Zantac 300 Tablets 1624
Zantac Injection 1619
Zantac Injection Premixed 1619
Zantac Syrup 1624

PEPTAN (Greece)
FAMOTIDINE
Pepcid Injection 2040
Pepcid Injection Premixed 2040
Pepcid Tablets 2038
Pepcid for Oral Suspension 2038

PEPTIC GUARD (Canada)
FAMOTIDINE
Pepcid Injection 2040
Pepcid Injection Premixed 2040
Pepcid Tablets 2038
Pepcid for Oral Suspension 2038

PEPTIC RELIEF (Canada)
RANITIDINE HYDROCHLORIDE
Zantac 25 EFFERdose Tablets 1624
Zantac 150 EFFERdose Tablets. 1624
Zantac 150 Tablets 1624
Zantac 300 Tablets 1624
Zantac Injection 1619
Zantac Injection Premixed 1619
Zantac Syrup 1624

PEPTIFAR (Portugal)
RANITIDINE HYDROCHLORIDE
Zantac 25 EFFERdose Tablets 1624
Zantac 150 EFFERdose Tablets. 1624
Zantac 150 Tablets 1624
Zantac 300 Tablets 1624
Zantac Injection 1619
Zantac Injection Premixed 1619
Zantac Syrup 1624

PEPTIGAL (Hungary)
FAMOTIDINE
Pepcid Injection 2040
Pepcid Injection Premixed 2040
Pepcid Tablets 2038
Pepcid for Oral Suspension 2038

PEPTOCI (Thailand)
FAMOTIDINE
Pepcid Injection 2040
Pepcid Injection Premixed 2040
Pepcid Tablets 2038
Pepcid for Oral Suspension 2038

PEPTONORM (Greece)
SUCRALFATE
Carafate Suspension 701
Carafate Tablets 701

PEPZAN (Australia, Hong Kong, Malaysia, New Zealand, Singapore)
FAMOTIDINE
Pepcid Injection 2040
Pepcid Injection Premixed 2040
Pepcid Tablets 2038
Pepcid for Oral Suspension 2038

PEPZOL (Portugal)
LANSOPRAZOLE
Prevacid Delayed-Release Capsules 3271

PERASTHMAN N (Germany)
THEOPHYLLINE
Uniphyl Tablets 2710

PERCLODIN (Irish Republic)
DIPYRIDAMOLE
Persantine Tablets 868

PERCORINA (Spain)
ISOSORBIDE MONONITRATE
Imdur Tablets 3018

PERDERM (Hong Kong, Hungary, Malaysia, Singapore)
ALCLOMETASONE DIPROPIONATE
Aclovate Cream 2660
Aclovate Ointment 2660

PERDIX (Denmark, Finland, Irish Republic, Israel, South Africa, Sweden, United Kingdom)
MOEXIPRIL HYDROCHLORIDE
Univasc Tablets. 3104

PERENAL (Greece)
LISINOPRIL
Prinivil Tablets 2052

PERICHOL (Denmark)
SIMVASTATIN
Zocor Tablets. 2105

PERILOX (Switzerland)
METRONIDAZOLE
MetroGel-Vaginal Gel 1855

PERINAL (United Kingdom)
HYDROCORTISONE
Hydrocortone Tablets. 1989

PERIPLUM (Italy)
NIMODIPINE
Nimotop Capsules 749

PERISET (India)
ONDANSETRON HYDROCHLORIDE
Zofran Injection. 1634
Zofran Injection Premixed 1634
Zofran Oral Solution. 1639
Zofran Tablets 1639

PERKOD (France)
DIPYRIDAMOLE
Persantine Tablets 868

PERLOL (Thailand)
PROPRANOLOL HYDROCHLORIDE
Inderal LA Long-Acting Capsules 3429

PERLUTEX (Denmark, Norway)
MEDROXYPROGESTERONE ACETATE
Depo-Medrol Single-Dose Vial 2619

PEROXACNE (Spain)
BENZOYL PEROXIDE
Brevoxyl-4 Creamy Wash. 3210
Brevoxyl-4 Gel 3210
Brevoxyl-8 Creamy Wash. 3210
Brevoxyl-8 Gel 3210
Triaz Cleanser 1892
Triaz Gel. 1892

PEROXIBEN (Spain)
BENZOYL PEROXIDE
Brevoxyl-4 Creamy Wash. 3210
Brevoxyl-4 Gel 3210
Brevoxyl-8 Creamy Wash. 3210
Brevoxyl-8 Gel 3210
Triaz Cleanser 1892
Triaz Gel. 1892

PEROXIBEN PLUS (Chile)
BENZOYL PEROXIDE
Brevoxyl-4 Creamy Wash. 3210
Brevoxyl-4 Gel 3210
Brevoxyl-8 Creamy Wash. 3210
Brevoxyl-8 Gel 3210
Triaz Cleanser 1892
Triaz Gel. 1892

PEROXIMICINA (Argentina)
BENZOYL PEROXIDE
Brevoxyl-4 Creamy Wash. 3210
Brevoxyl-4 Gel 3210
Brevoxyl-8 Creamy Wash. 3210
Brevoxyl-8 Gel 3210
Triaz Cleanser 1892
Triaz Gel. 1892

PERSA-GEL W (Australia)
BENZOYL PEROXIDE
Brevoxyl-4 Creamy Wash. 3210
Brevoxyl-4 Gel 3210
Brevoxyl-8 Creamy Wash. 3210
Brevoxyl-8 Gel 3210
Triaz Cleanser 1892
Triaz Gel. 1892

PERSANTIN (Argentina, Australia, Austria, Brazil, Chile, Czech Republic, Denmark, Finland, Germany, Hong Kong, India, Irish Republic, Italy, Japan, Malaysia, Mexico, New Zealand, Norway, Portugal, Russia, Singapore, South Africa, Sweden, Thailand, The Netherlands, United Kingdom, Venezuela)
DIPYRIDAMOLE
Persantine Tablets 868

PERSANTIN PLUS (Hong Kong)
DIPYRIDAMOLE
Persantine Tablets 868

PERSANTIN S (Brazil)
DIPYRIDAMOLE
Persantine Tablets 868

PERSANTINE (Belgium, Canada, France, Switzerland)
DIPYRIDAMOLE
Persantine Tablets 868

PERSOL (India)
BENZOYL PEROXIDE
Brevoxyl-4 Creamy Wash. 3210
Brevoxyl-4 Gel 3210
Brevoxyl-8 Creamy Wash. 3210
Brevoxyl-8 Gel 3210
Triaz Cleanser 1892
Triaz Gel. 1892

PERSOL FORTE (India)
BENZOYL PEROXIDE
Brevoxyl-4 Creamy Wash. 3210
Brevoxyl-4 Gel 3210
Brevoxyl-8 Creamy Wash. 3210
Brevoxyl-8 Gel 3210
Triaz Cleanser 1892
Triaz Gel. 1892

PERTACILON (Greece, Singapore)
CAPTOPRIL
Captopril Tablets 2149

PERTAXOL (Greece)
BETAXOLOL HYDROCHLORIDE
Betoptic S Ophthalmic Suspension . ⊙203, 558

PERTENSAL (Spain)
NIFEDIPINE
Adalat CC Tablets 2964

PERTENSO (Argentina)
CLONIDINE
Catapres-TTS 844

PERTIL (Spain)
ISOSORBIDE MONONITRATE
Imdur Tablets 3018

PETOGEN (South Africa)
MEDROXYPROGESTERONE ACETATE
Depo-Medrol Single-Dose Vial 2619

PETSIX (India)
FUROSEMIDE
Furosemide Tablets 2154

P-GLITZ (India)
PIOGLITAZONE HYDROCHLORIDE
Actos Tablets 3219

PHACOVIT (Greece)
LEVOCARNITINE
Carnitor Injection. 3188
Carnitor Tablets and Oral Solution 3190

PHAMOPRIL (Germany)
CAPTOPRIL
Captopril Tablets 2149

PHAMORANIT (Germany)
RANITIDINE HYDROCHLORIDE
Zantac 25 EFFERdose Tablets 1624
Zantac 150 EFFERdose Tablets. 1624
Zantac 150 Tablets 1624
Zantac 300 Tablets 1624
Zantac Injection 1619
Zantac Injection Premixed 1619
Zantac Syrup 1624

PHARCINA (Mexico)
CIPROFLOXACIN HYDROCHLORIDE
Ciloxan Ophthalmic Ointment . . . . ⊙204, 559
Ciloxan Ophthalmic Solution . . . . ⊙206
Cipro Tablets 2977

PHARMADOL (Thailand)
TRAMADOL HYDROCHLORIDE
Ultram ER Tablets 2392

PHARMAFIL (Mexico)
THEOPHYLLINE
Uniphyl Tablets 2710

PHARMAFLAM (South Africa)
DICLOFENAC SODIUM
Voltaren Tablets 2307
Voltaren-XR Tablets 2310

PHARMAFLEX (Belgium)
METRONIDAZOLE
MetroGel-Vaginal Gel 1855

PHARMALOSE (Canada)
LACTULOSE
Kristalose for Oral Solution 1034

PHARMAMOX (Switzerland)
AMOXICILLIN
Amoxil Pediatric Drops for Oral Suspension. 1343
Amoxil Tablets 1343

PHARMAPRESS (South Africa)
ENALAPRIL MALEATE
Vasotec I.V. Injection 2103

PHARMAPRESS CO (South Africa)
ENALAPRIL MALEATE
Vasotec I.V. Injection 2103

PHARMOTIDINE (Thailand)
FAMOTIDINE
Pepcid Injection 2040
Pepcid Injection Premixed 2040
Pepcid Tablets 2038
Pepcid for Oral Suspension 2038

PHARMOX (Brazil)
AMOXICILLIN
Amoxil Pediatric Drops for Oral Suspension 1343
Amoxil Tablets 1343

PHARPHYLLINE (The Netherlands)
THEOPHYLLINE
Uniphyl Tablets 2710

PHARYNGOCIN (Germany)
ERYTHROMYCIN
Ery-Tab Tablets 449
Erythromycin Base Filmtab Tablets 455
Erythromycin Delayed-Release Capsules, USP 457
PCE Dispertab Tablets 515

PHENEDRINE (Hong Kong)
THEOPHYLLINE
Uniphyl Tablets 2710

PHENERGAN (Australia, Belgium, Denmark, Hong Kong, India, Irish Republic, New Zealand, Norway, Singapore, South Africa, Thailand, The Netherlands, United Kingdom)
PROMETHAZINE HYDROCHLORIDE
Phenergan Tablets and Suppositories 3440

PHENHALAL (United Kingdom)
PROMETHAZINE HYDROCHLORIDE
Phenergan Tablets and Suppositories 3440

PHENSEDYL (Malaysia)
PROMETHAZINE HYDROCHLORIDE
Phenergan Tablets and Suppositories 3440

PHOS-EX (Austria, Denmark, Finland, Germany, Norway, Sweden, United Kingdom)
CALCIUM ACETATE
PhosLo GelCaps 2169

PHOSFORID (India)
CALCIUM ACETATE
PhosLo GelCaps 2169

PHOSLO (Chile)
CALCIUM ACETATE
PhosLo GelCaps 2169

PHOSTARAC (Argentina)
ALENDRONATE SODIUM
Fosamax Tablets 1969

PHYLOBID (India)
THEOPHYLLINE
Uniphyl Tablets 2710

PHYLODAY (India)
THEOPHYLLINE
Uniphyl Tablets 2710

PHYZIDINE (Hong Kong)
FAMOTIDINE
Pepcid Injection 2040
Pepcid Injection Premixed 2040
Pepcid Tablets 2038
Pepcid for Oral Suspension 2038

PIAMFUCIN (Russia)
NATAMYCIN
Natacyn Antifungal Ophthalmic Suspension . . . . . ⊙208

PIDILAT (Germany)
NIFEDIPINE
Adalat CC Tablets 2964

PILOTIM (Argentina)
TIMOLOL MALEATE
Blocadren Tablets 1916
Timoptic Sterile Ophthalmic Solution 2088
Timoptic in Ocudose 2091
Timoptic-XE Sterile Ophthalmic Gel Forming Solution 2092

PIMA BICIRON N (Germany)
NATAMYCIN
Natacyn Antifungal Ophthalmic Suspension . . . . . ⊙208

PIMAFUCIN (Belgium, Czech Republic, Finland, Germany, Hungary, Russia, United Kingdom)
NATAMYCIN
Natacyn Antifungal Ophthalmic Suspension . . . . . ⊙208

PINAMOX (Irish Republic)
AMOXICILLIN
Amoxil Pediatric Drops for Oral Suspension 1343
Amoxil Tablets 1343

PINIFED (Irish Republic)
NIFEDIPINE
Adalat CC Tablets 2964

PINIOL (Germany)
NAPHAZOLINE HYDROCHLORIDE
Albalon Ophthalmic Solution . . . . . ⊙218

PINIOL NASENSPRAY (Germany)
NAPHAZOLINE HYDROCHLORIDE
Albalon Ophthalmic Solution . . . . . ⊙218

PIOGLIT (Argentina)
PIOGLITAZONE HYDROCHLORIDE
Actos Tablets 3219

PIOMED (India)
PIOGLITAZONE HYDROCHLORIDE
Actos Tablets 3219

PIOSAFE (India)
PIOGLITAZONE HYDROCHLORIDE
Actos Tablets 3219

PIOZULIN (India)
PIOGLITAZONE HYDROCHLORIDE
Actos Tablets 3219

PIPLEX (Chile)
ISOTRETINOIN
Accutane Capsules 2731

PIPOLPHEN (Hungary, Russia)
PROMETHAZINE HYDROCHLORIDE
Phenergan Tablets and Suppositories 3440

PIPROL (Spain)
CIPROFLOXACIN HYDROCHLORIDE
Ciloxan Ophthalmic Ointment . . . . ⊙204, 559
Ciloxan Ophthalmic Solution . . . . . ⊙206
Cipro Tablets 2977

PIREXYL (Chile)
DICLOFENAC SODIUM
Voltaren Tablets 2307
Voltaren-XR Tablets 2310

PIRIDASMIN (Spain)
THEOPHYLLINE
Uniphyl Tablets 2710

PIRIMECIDAN (Spain)
PYRIMETHAMINE
Daraprim Tablets 1419

PIRITEZE (United Kingdom)
CETIRIZINE HYDROCHLORIDE
Zyrtec Syrup 2594
Zyrtec Tablets 2594

PIROBAC (Chile)
BENZOYL PEROXIDE
Brevoxyl-4 Creamy Wash 3210
Brevoxyl-4 Gel 3210
Brevoxyl-8 Creamy Wash 3210
Brevoxyl-8 Gel 3210
Triaz Cleanser 1892
Triaz Gel 1892

PISTOFIL (Greece)
NORFLOXACIN
Noroxin Tablets 2032

PLACIDOX (India)
DIAZEPAM
Diastat Rectal Delivery System 3343
Valium Tablets 2819

PLAKET (Brazil)
TICLOPIDINE HYDROCHLORIDE
Ticlid Tablets 2810

PLAKETAR (Brazil)
TICLOPIDINE HYDROCHLORIDE
Ticlid Tablets 2810

PLAN (Argentina)
ATORVASTATIN CALCIUM
Lipitor Tablets 2483

PLANITRIX (Greece)
FENOFIBRATE
Tricor Tablets 527

PLANIZOL (Mexico)
METRONIDAZOLE
MetroGel-Vaginal Gel 1855

PLAQUETAL (Portugal)
TICLOPIDINE HYDROCHLORIDE
Ticlid Tablets 2810

PLAQUETIL (Chile)
TICLOPIDINE HYDROCHLORIDE
Ticlid Tablets 2810

PLASIMINE (Spain)
MUPIROCIN
Bactroban Ointment 1395

PLASMANATE (Brazil, Malaysia)
PLASMA PROTEIN FRACTION
Plasmanate 3255

PLASMATEIN (United Kingdom)
PLASMA PROTEIN FRACTION
Plasmanate 3255

PLASMAVIRAL (Italy)
PLASMA PROTEIN FRACTION
Plasmanate 3255

PLATELET (Italy)
DIPYRIDAMOLE
Persantine Tablets 868

PLATIGREN (Czech Republic)
TICLOPIDINE HYDROCHLORIDE
Ticlid Tablets 2810

PLATO (South Africa)
DIPYRIDAMOLE
Persantine Tablets 868

PLAUCINA (Spain)
ENOXAPARIN SODIUM
Lovenox Injection 2915

PLAVIX (Argentina, Australia, Austria, Belgium, Brazil, Chile, Czech Republic, Denmark, Germany, Greece, Hungary, Israel, Italy, Mexico, New Zealand, Portugal, Russia, South Africa, Spain, Thailand, Venezuela)
CLOPIDOGREL BISULFATE
Plavix Tablets 917, 2926

PLENACTOL (Chile)
ORPHENADRINE CITRATE
Norflex Injection 1856

PLENAX (Brazil)
CEFIXIME
Suprax 1843

PLENISH-K (South Africa)
POTASSIUM CHLORIDE
K-Dur Extended-Relase Tablets 3033
K-Lor Oral Solution 474
K-Tab Tablets 475

PLENOLYT (Spain)
CIPROFLOXACIN HYDROCHLORIDE
Ciloxan Ophthalmic Ointment . . . . ⊙204, 559
Ciloxan Ophthalmic Solution . . . . . ⊙206
Cipro Tablets 2977

PLENOMICINA (Brazil)
ERYTHROMYCIN STEARATE
Erythrocin Stearate Filmtab Tablets 453

PLENTY (Brazil)
SIBUTRAMINE HYDROCHLORIDE
Meridia Capsules 489

PLETAAL (Argentina, Hong Kong, Japan, Thailand)
CILOSTAZOL
Pletal Tablets 2455

PLETAL (United Kingdom)
CILOSTAZOL
Pletal Tablets 2455

PLETOZ (India)
CILOSTAZOL
Pletal Tablets 2455

PLEXXO (The Netherlands)
LAMOTRIGINE
Lamictal Chewable Dispersible Tablets . . . 1481
Lamictal Tablets 1481

PLEYAR (Argentina)
CLOPIDOGREL BISULFATE
Plavix Tablets 917, 2926

PLIDAN (Argentina)
DIAZEPAM
Diastat Rectal Delivery System 3343
Valium Tablets 2819

PLIDEX (Argentina)
DIAZEPAM
Diastat Rectal Delivery System 3343
Valium Tablets 2819

PLIMYCOL (Czech Republic)
CLOTRIMAZOLE
Lotrimin Cream 3039
Lotrimin Lotion 1% 3039
Lotrimin Topical Solution 1% 3039

PLOSTIM (Argentina)
TIMOLOL MALEATE
Blocadren Tablets 1916
Timoptic Sterile Ophthalmic Solution 2088
Timoptic in Ocudose 2091
Timoptic-XE Sterile Ophthalmic Gel Forming Solution 2092

PLURAIR (Brazil)
FLUTICASONE PROPIONATE
Cutivate Cream 2662
Cutivate Ointment 2665
Flonase Nasal Spray 1440

PLURICEFO (Argentina)
CEFOXITIN SODIUM
Mefoxin Premixed Intravenous Solution . . . 2016
Mefoxin for Injection 2012

PLURIMEN (Spain)
SELEGILINE HYDROCHLORIDE
Eldepryl Capsules 3208

PLUS KALIUM RETARD (Switzerland)
POTASSIUM CHLORIDE
K-Dur Extended-Relase Tablets 3033
K-Lor Oral Solution 474
K-Tab Tablets 475

PLUSGIN (Argentina)
CIPROFLOXACIN
Cipro Oral Suspension 2977

PLUSTAXANO (Argentina)
DOCETAXEL
Taxotere Injection Concentrate 2932

PMS-DOPAZIDE (Canada)
HYDROCHLOROTHIAZIDE/METHYLDOPA
Aldoril Tablets 1910

POCIN (Thailand)
ERYTHROMYCIN STEARATE
Erythrocin Stearate Filmtab Tablets 453

PODIUM (Spain)
DIAZEPAM
Diastat Rectal Delivery System 3343
Valium Tablets 2819

PODOMEXEF (Germany, Switzerland)
CEFPODOXIME PROXETIL
Vantin Tablets and Oral Suspension 2645

POENFLOX (Chile, Venezuela)
OFLOXACIN
Floxin Otic Solution 1049

POENTIMOL (Argentina)
TIMOLOL MALEATE
Blocadren Tablets 1916
Timoptic Sterile Ophthalmic Solution 2088
Timoptic in Ocudose 2091
Timoptic-XE Sterile Ophthalmic Gel Forming Solution 2092

POENTOBRAL (Venezuela)
TOBRAMYCIN
TOBI Solution for Inhalation 2298

POENTOBRAL PLUS (Chile, Venezuela)
DEXAMETHASONE/TOBRAMYCIN
TobraDex Ophthalmic Ointment . . . 562, ⊙212
TobraDex Ophthalmic Suspension . 563, ⊙211

POINT (Israel)
NAPROXEN SODIUM
Anaprox DS Tablets 2761
Anaprox Tablets 2761

POLET (Mexico)
NAPROXEN
EC-Naprosyn Delayed-Release Tablets 2761
Naprosyn Suspension 2761
Naprosyn Tablets 2761

POLIBAC (Brazil)
AMOXICILLIN
Amoxil Pediatric Drops for Oral Suspension 1343
Amoxil Tablets 1343

POLICANO (Greece)
ISOTRETINOIN
Accutane Capsules 2731

POLI-CIFLOXIN (Thailand)
CIPROFLOXACIN
Cipro Oral Suspension 2977

POLICOR (Argentina)
CILOSTAZOL
Pletal Tablets 2455

POLIDELTAXIN NF (Mexico)
DEXAMETHASONE
Decadron Tablets 1951

POLIK (Venezuela)
CLOTRIMAZOLE
Lotrimin Cream. 3039
Lotrimin Lotion 1%. 3039
Lotrimin Topical Solution 1% 3039

POLIOFTAL (Argentina)
TOBRAMYCIN
TOBI Solution for Inhalation 2298

POLIREUMIN (Brazil)
SODIUM HYALURONATE
Hyalgan Solution 2901

POLI-URETIC (Thailand)
AMILORIDE HYDROCHLORIDE/HYDROCHLOROTHIAZIDE
Moduretic Tablets 2028

POLIXIMA (Italy)
CEFUROXIME SODIUM
Zinacef Injection 1631

POLTAX (Brazil)
DICLOFENAC SODIUM
Voltaren Tablets 2307
Voltaren-XR Tablets 2310

POLY PRED (Spain)
NEOMYCIN SULFATE/POLYMYXIN B SULFATE/PREDNISOLONE ACETATE
Poly-Pred Ophthalmic Suspension . . . . . . ⊙233

POLYANION (Austria)
PENTOSAN POLYSULFATE SODIUM
Elmiron Capsules 2415

POLYCITRA-K (Canada)
POTASSIUM CITRATE
Urocit-K Tablets. 2144

POLY-COF (Thailand)
PROMETHAZINE HYDROCHLORIDE
Phenergan Tablets and Suppositories 3440

POLYFLAM (Belgium)
DICLOFENAC SODIUM
Voltaren Tablets 2307
Voltaren-XR Tablets 2310

POLYTRIM (Canada)
POLYMYXIN B SULFATE/TRIMETHOPRIM SULFATE
Polytrim Ophthalmic Solution 574

POLYXEN (Thailand)
NAPROXEN
EC-Naprosyn Delayed-Release Tablets. . . . 2761
Naprosyn Suspension. 2761
Naprosyn Tablets 2761

PONDERA (Brazil)
PAROXETINE HYDROCHLORIDE
Paxil Oral Suspension. 1530
Paxil Tablets. 1530

PONDTROXIN (Thailand)
LEVOTHYROXINE SODIUM
Levothroid Tablets 1186
Levoxyl Tablets 1712
Synthroid Tablets 520

PONTALSIC (Spain)
TRAMADOL HYDROCHLORIDE
Ultram ER Tablets 2392

POROSAL (Venezuela)
ALENDRONATE SODIUM
Fosamax Tablets 1969

PORPHYROCIN (Hong Kong)
ERYTHROMYCIN STEARATE
Erythrocin Stearate Filmtab Tablets 453

PORUXIN (Greece)
FINASTERIDE
Propecia Tablets 2060
Proscar Tablets. 2067

POSANIN (Thailand)
DIPYRIDAMOLE
Persantine Tablets 868

POSIVYL (Chile)
PAROXETINE HYDROCHLORIDE
Paxil Oral Suspension. 1530
Paxil Tablets. 1530

POSNAC (Thailand)
DICLOFENAC SODIUM
Voltaren Tablets 2307
Voltaren-XR Tablets 2310

POTASIO C (Argentina)
POTASSIUM CHLORIDE
K-Dur Extended-Relase Tablets 3033
K-Lor Oral Solution. 474
K-Tab Tablets 475

POTASION (Spain)
POTASSIUM CHLORIDE
K-Dur Extended-Relase Tablets 3033
K-Lor Oral Solution. 474
K-Tab Tablets 475

POTASSRIDE (Thailand)
POTASSIUM CHLORIDE
K-Dur Extended-Relase Tablets 3033
K-Lor Oral Solution. 474
K-Tab Tablets 475

POTCIT (Malaysia)
POTASSIUM CITRATE
Urocit-K Tablets. 2144

POTENCORT (United Arab Emirates)
FLUTICASONE PROPIONATE
Cutivate Cream. 2662
Cutivate Ointment 2665
Flonase Nasal Spray 1440

POTENDAL (Spain)
CEFTAZIDIME
Fortaz for Injection 1453

POTKLOR (India)
POTASSIUM CHLORIDE
K-Dur Extended-Relase Tablets 3033
K-Lor Oral Solution. 474
K-Tab Tablets 475

POWERCEF (India)
CEFTRIAXONE SODIUM
Rocephin Injectable Vials, ADD-Vantage, Galaxy, Bulk 2800

POWERGYL (India)
NORFLOXACIN
Noroxin Tablets. 2032

PPS (Italy)
PLASMA PROTEIN FRACTION
Plasmanate 3255

PRACAP (Brazil)
FINASTERIDE
Propecia Tablets 2060
Proscar Tablets. 2067

PRACEM (Mexico)
DIPYRIDAMOLE
Persantine Tablets 868

PRADIF (Greece, Italy, Portugal, Switzerland)
TAMSULOSIN HYDROCHLORIDE
Flomax Capsules 850

PRADINOLOL (Brazil)
PROPRANOLOL HYDROCHLORIDE
Inderal LA Long-Acting Capsules 3429

PRAECICOR (Germany)
VERAPAMIL HYDROCHLORIDE
Covera-HS Tablets 3139
Verelan PM Extended-Release Capsules, Controlled-Onset 3106

PRALENAL (United Kingdom)
ENALAPRIL MALEATE
Vasotec I.V. Injection 2103

PRALOL (Thailand)
PROPRANOLOL HYDROCHLORIDE
Inderal LA Long-Acting Capsules 3429

PRAM (Austria)
CITALOPRAM HYDROBROMIDE
Celexa Tablets 1176

PRAMACE (Irish Republic, Sweden)
RAMIPRIL
Altace Capsules 1702

PRAMCIL (Chile)
CITALOPRAM HYDROBROMIDE
Celexa Tablets 1176

PRANADOX (Mexico)
ZIDOVUDINE
Retrovir Capsules 1560
Retrovir IV Infusion. 1564
Retrovir Syrup 1560
Retrovir Tablets. 1560

PRANDASE (Canada, Israel)
ACARBOSE
Precose Tablets 751

PRANDIN E2 (South Africa)
DINOPROSTONE
Cervidil Vaginal Insert. 1181

PRANDIOL (France)
DIPYRIDAMOLE
Persantine Tablets 868

PRANIX (Mexico)
LANSOPRAZOLE
Prevacid Delayed-Release Capsules 3271

PRANOLAL (Brazil)
PROPRANOLOL HYDROCHLORIDE
Inderal LA Long-Acting Capsules 3429

PRANOLOL (Norway)
PROPRANOLOL HYDROCHLORIDE
Inderal LA Long-Acting Capsules 3429

PRANOXEN (South Africa)
NAPROXEN
EC-Naprosyn Delayed-Release Tablets. . . . 2761
Naprosyn Suspension. 2761
Naprosyn Tablets 2761

PRANOXEN CONTINUS (United Kingdom)
NAPROXEN
EC-Naprosyn Delayed-Release Tablets. . . . 2761
Naprosyn Suspension. 2761
Naprosyn Tablets 2761

PRAQUANTEL (Thailand)
PRAZIQUANTEL
Biltricide Tablets 2976

PRASIKON (Thailand)
PRAZIQUANTEL
Biltricide Tablets 2976

PRAXEDOL (Mexico)
NAPROXEN
EC-Naprosyn Delayed-Release Tablets. . . . 2761
Naprosyn Suspension. 2761
Naprosyn Tablets 2761

PRAYANOL (Chile)
AMANTADINE HYDROCHLORIDE
Symmetrel Tablets. 1135

PRAZITE (Thailand)
PRAZIQUANTEL
Biltricide Tablets 2976

PRAZITRAL (Argentina)
PRAZIQUANTEL
Biltricide Tablets 2976

PRAZOL (Brazil)
LANSOPRAZOLE
Prevacid Delayed-Release Capsules 3271

PRECAPTIL (Mexico)
CAPTOPRIL
Captopril Tablets 2149

PRECAR (Venezuela)
DIPYRIDAMOLE
Persantine Tablets 868

PRE-CLAR (Chile)
CLARITHROMYCIN
Biaxin Filmtab Tablets 402
Biaxin Granules 402

PREDALGIC (France)
TRAMADOL HYDROCHLORIDE
Ultram ER Tablets 2392

PREDMYCIN (Thailand)
NEOMYCIN SULFATE/POLYMYXIN B SULFATE/PREDNISOLONE ACETATE
Poly-Pred Ophthalmic Suspension . . . . . . ⊙233

PREDMYCIN P (Belgium)
NEOMYCIN SULFATE/POLYMYXIN B SULFATE/PREDNISOLONE ACETATE
Poly-Pred Ophthalmic Suspension . . . . . . ⊙233

PREDMYCIN-P (Singapore)
NEOMYCIN SULFATE/POLYMYXIN B SULFATE/PREDNISOLONE ACETATE
Poly-Pred Ophthalmic Suspension . . . . . . ⊙233

PREDMYCIN-P LIQUIFILM (The Netherlands)
NEOMYCIN SULFATE/POLYMYXIN B SULFATE/PREDNISOLONE ACETATE
Poly-Pred Ophthalmic Suspension . . . . . . ⊙233

PREDNI-F-TABLINEN (Germany)
DEXAMETHASONE
Decadron Tablets 1951

PREDONIUM (Austria, Hong Kong, New Zealand, Portugal, The Netherlands)
PERINDOPRIL ERBUMINE
Aceon Tablets (2 mg, 4 mg, 8 mg) 3194

PREDXAL (Mexico)
TELMISARTAN
Micardis Tablets 854

PREDXAL PLUS (Mexico)
TELMISARTAN
Micardis Tablets 854

PREFACE (India)
RAMIPRIL
Altace Capsules 1702

PREFEST (Brazil)
ESTRADIOL
Climara Transdermal System 771
Estring Vaginal Ring 2635

PREFIN (Spain)
BUPRENORPHINE HYDROCHLORIDE
Buprenex Injectable 2716

PRELECTAL (Italy)
PERINDOPRIL ERBUMINE
Aceon Tablets (2 mg, 4 mg, 8 mg) 3194

PRELIS (Germany)
METOPROLOL TARTRATE
Lopressor Tablets 2238

PREMASTAN (Mexico)
PROGESTERONE
Prometrium Capsules (100 mg, 200 mg) . 3203

PREMJACT (United Kingdom)
LIDOCAINE
Lidoderm Patch 1118

PREPIDIL (Austria, Belgium, Canada, Czech Republic, France, Germany, Hong Kong, Hungary, Irish Republic, Israel, Italy, Mexico, New Zealand, Russia, South Africa, Spain, Switzerland, The Netherlands, United Kingdom)
DINOPROSTONE
Cervidil Vaginal Insert. 1181

PRERAN (Japan)
TRANDOLAPRIL
Mavik Tablets 486

PRES (Germany)
ENALAPRIL MALEATE
Vasotec I.V. Injection 2103

PRESCAL (Irish Republic, United Kingdom)
ISRADIPINE
DynaCirc CR Tablets. 2721

PRESI REGUL (Argentina)
ENALAPRIL MALEATE
Vasotec I.V. Injection 2103

PRESI REGUL D (Argentina)
ENALAPRIL MALEATE
Vasotec I.V. Injection 2103

PRESINOR (Argentina)
LOSARTAN POTASSIUM
Cozaar Tablets 1935

PRESINOR D (Argentina)
LOSARTAN POTASSIUM
Cozaar Tablets 1935

PRESMIN (Brazil)
BETAXOLOL HYDROCHLORIDE
Betoptic S Ophthalmic Suspension . ⊙203, 558

PRESOCOR (Chile)
VERAPAMIL HYDROCHLORIDE
Covera-HS Tablets 3139
Verelan PM Extended-Release Capsules, Controlled-Onset 3106

PRESOKIN (Chile)
LISINOPRIL
Prinivil Tablets 2052

PRESOQUIN (Venezuela)
DILTIAZEM HYDROCHLORIDE
Cardizem LA Extended Release Tablets. . . 1728
Tiazac Capsules 1201

PRESS-12 (Greece)
LISINOPRIL
Prinivil Tablets 2052

PRESSANOL (South Africa)
PROPRANOLOL HYDROCHLORIDE
Inderal LA Long-Acting Capsules 3429

PRESSEL (Brazil)
ENALAPRIL MALEATE
Vasotec I.V. Injection 2103

PRESSITAN (Spain)
ENALAPRIL MALEATE
Vasotec I.V. Injection 2103

PRESSOLAT (Israel)
NIFEDIPINE
Adalat CC Tablets 2964

PRESSOMAX (Brazil)
CAPTOPRIL
Captopril Tablets................. 2149

PRESSOTEC (Brazil)
ENALAPRIL MALEATE
Vasotec I.V. Injection 2103

PRESSURAL (Italy)
INDAPAMIDE
Indapamide Tablets 2156

PRESSURIL (Greece)
LISINOPRIL
Prinivil Tablets 2052

PRESTARIUM (Czech Republic)
PERINDOPRIL ERBUMINE
Aceon Tablets (2 mg, 4 mg, 8 mg) 3194

PRESTOLE (France)
HYDROCHLOROTHIAZIDE/TRIAMTERENE
Dyazide Capsules 1423

PRESYNDRAL (Spain)
ENALAPRIL MALEATE
Vasotec I.V. Injection 2103

PRETANIX (Hungary)
INDAPAMIDE
Indapamide Tablets 2156

PRETERAX (Argentina, Austria, Belgium, Brazil, Canada, Germany, Greece, Irish Republic, Italy, Mexico, Portugal, Singapore, South Africa, Spain, The Netherlands, Venezuela)
PERINDOPRIL ERBUMINE
Aceon Tablets (2 mg, 4 mg, 8 mg) 3194

PREVACID (Canada, Japan, Malaysia, Singapore, Thailand)
LANSOPRAZOLE
Prevacid Delayed-Release Capsules 3271

PREVENCOR (Spain)
ATORVASTATIN CALCIUM
Lipitor Tablets 2483

PREVEX HC (Canada, Thailand)
HYDROCORTISONE
Hydrocortone Tablets 1989

PREXAN (Italy)
NAPROXEN
EC-Naprosyn Delayed-Release Tablets.... 2761
Naprosyn Suspension.............. 2761
Naprosyn Tablets 2761

PREXUM (South Africa)
PERINDOPRIL ERBUMINE
Aceon Tablets (2 mg, 4 mg, 8 mg) 3194

PREZAL (The Netherlands)
LANSOPRAZOLE
Prevacid Delayed-Release Capsules 3271

PRILACE (Italy, Venezuela)
RAMIPRIL
Altace Capsules 1702

PRILAN (Portugal)
ENALAPRIL MALEATE
Vasotec I.V. Injection 2103

PRILOSIN (South Africa)
LISINOPRIL
Prinivil Tablets 2052

PRILOVASE (Portugal)
CAPTOPRIL
Captopril Tablets................. 2149

PRILPRESSIN (Brazil)
CAPTOPRIL
Captopril Tablets................. 2149

PRILTENK (Argentina)
ENALAPRIL MALEATE
Vasotec I.V. Injection 2103

PRIMAQUIN (Chile)
ESTRADIOL
Climara Transdermal System 771
Estring Vaginal Ring............... 2635

PRIMAXIN (Canada, Greece, United Kingdom)
CILASTATIN SODIUM/IMIPENEM
Primaxin I.M. 2045
Primaxin I.V.................... 2048

PRIMERAL (Italy)
NAPROXEN SODIUM
Anaprox DS Tablets 2761
Anaprox Tablets 2761

PRIMESIN (Italy)
FLUVASTATIN SODIUM
Lescol Capsules 2233

PRIMIPROST (India)
DINOPROSTONE
Cervidil Vaginal Insert............. 1181

PRIMOCID (Greece)
CLARITHROMYCIN
Biaxin Filmtab Tablets............... 402
Biaxin Granules 402

PRIMOFENAC (Switzerland)
DICLOFENAC SODIUM
Voltaren Tablets 2307
Voltaren-XR Tablets 2310

PRIMOSON-F (Mexico)
PROGESTERONE
Prometrium Capsules (100 mg, 200 mg) . 3203

PRIMOXIL (Italy)
MOEXIPRIL HYDROCHLORIDE
Univasc Tablets.................. 3104

PRIMULEX (Hungary)
SELEGILINE HYDROCHLORIDE
Eldepryl Capsules 3208

PRINARTEN (Mexico)
CAPTOPRIL
Captopril Tablets................. 2149

PRINCESS PROLIB (Spain)
FLUVASTATIN SODIUM
Lescol Capsules 2233

PRINCIPROX (Switzerland)
CIPROFLOXACIN HYDROCHLORIDE
Ciloxan Ophthalmic Ointment .... ⊙204, 559
Ciloxan Ophthalmic Solution .... ⊙206
Cipro Tablets 2977

PRINIL (Switzerland)
LISINOPRIL
Prinivil Tablets 2052

PRINISER (Mexico)
LISINOPRIL
Prinivil Tablets 2052

PRINIVIL (Australia, Austria, Brazil, Canada, Czech Republic, France, Greece, Hong Kong, Italy, Malaysia, Mexico, New Zealand, Portugal, Singapore, South Africa, Spain, Venezuela)
LISINOPRIL
Prinivil Tablets 2052

PRINIVIL PLUS (Spain)
HYDROCHLOROTHIAZIDE/LISINOPRIL
Prinzide Tablets 2056

PRINZIDE (Austria, Brazil, Canada, France, Italy, Mexico, New Zealand, Portugal, Switzerland)
HYDROCHLOROTHIAZIDE/LISINOPRIL
Prinzide Tablets 2056

PRIRETIC (Venezuela)
ENALAPRIL MALEATE
Vasotec I.V. Injection 2103

PRISDAL (Spain)
CITALOPRAM HYDROBROMIDE
Celexa Tablets 1176

PRISMA (Chile)
CITALOPRAM HYDROBROMIDE
Celexa Tablets 1176

PRITOR (Argentina, Australia, Brazil, Czech Republic, France, Greece, Hungary, Italy, Portugal, Russia, Spain, Venezuela)
TELMISARTAN
Micardis Tablets 854

PRITOR HCT (Brazil)
TELMISARTAN
Micardis Tablets 854

PRITOR PLUS (Greece, Portugal, Spain)
TELMISARTAN
Micardis Tablets 854

PRITORAL (Chile)
TELMISARTAN
Micardis Tablets 854

PRITORPLUS (France, Hungary, Italy)
TELMISARTAN
Micardis Tablets 854

PRIVACOM (United Kingdom)
CLOTRIMAZOLE
Lotrimin Cream.................. 3039
Lotrimin Lotion 1%................ 3039
Lotrimin Topical Solution 1% 3039

PRIVINE (Canada)
NAPHAZOLINE HYDROCHLORIDE
Albalon Ophthalmic Solution .... ⊙218

PRIXAR (Italy)
LEVOFLOXACIN
Levaquin Injection 2384
Levaquin Tablets 2384

PRIZEM (Mexico)
DIAZEPAM
Diastat Rectal Delivery System 3343
Valium Tablets 2819

PRO ULCO (Spain)
LANSOPRAZOLE
Prevacid Delayed-Release Capsules 3271

PROAIR (Argentina)
FLUTICASONE PROPIONATE
Cutivate Cream................... 2662
Cutivate Ointment 2665
Flonase Nasal Spray 1440

PROBETA LA (United Kingdom)
PROPRANOLOL HYDROCHLORIDE
Inderal LA Long-Acting Capsules 3429

PROCAPTAN (Italy)
PERINDOPRIL ERBUMINE
Aceon Tablets (2 mg, 4 mg, 8 mg) 3194

PROCARDIN (Singapore)
DIPYRIDAMOLE
Persantine Tablets 868

PROCARDOL (Greece)
ISOSORBIDE MONONITRATE
Imdur Tablets................... 3018

PROCETOKEN (Argentina)
FENOFIBRATE
Tricor Tablets................... 527

PROCIN (Brazil)
CIPROFLOXACIN
Cipro Oral Suspension 2977

PROCIP (India)
CIPROFLOXACIN
Cipro Oral Suspension 2977

PROCLIM (Canada)
MEDROXYPROGESTERONE ACETATE
Depo-Medrol Single-Dose Vial 2619

PROCOR (Brazil)
DIPYRIDAMOLE
Persantine Tablets................. 868

PROCOR S (Brazil)
DIPYRIDAMOLE
Persantine Tablets................. 868

PROCTOCREM (Argentina)
LIDOCAINE
Lidoderm Patch 1118

PROCULIN (Czech Republic, Germany, Hungary)
NAPHAZOLINE HYDROCHLORIDE
Albalon Ophthalmic Solution .... ⊙218

PRO-CURE (Israel)
FINASTERIDE
Propecia Tablets................. 2060
Proscar Tablets.................. 2067

PROCUTA (France)
ISOTRETINOIN
Accutane Capsules 2731

PROCUTAN (South Africa)
HYDROCORTISONE
Hydrocortone Tablets.............. 1989

PROCYTHOL (Greece)
SELEGILINE HYDROCHLORIDE
Eldepryl Capsules 3208

PRODAFEM (Austria, Switzerland)
MEDROXYPROGESTERONE ACETATE
Depo-Medrol Single-Dose Vial 2619

PRODASONE (Chile, France)
MEDROXYPROGESTERONE ACETATE
Depo-Medrol Single-Dose Vial 2619

PRODOLOR (Germany)
NAPROXEN
EC-Naprosyn Delayed-Release Tablets.... 2761
Naprosyn Suspension............... 2761
Naprosyn Tablets 2761

PRODOPINA (Brazil)
NIFEDIPINE
Adalat CC Tablets 2964

PRODOPRESSIN (Brazil)
ENALAPRIL MALEATE
Vasotec I.V. Injection 2103

PRODOROL (South Africa)
PROPRANOLOL HYDROCHLORIDE
Inderal LA Long-Acting Capsules 3429

PRODOXIN (Brazil)
CEFTRIAXONE SODIUM
Rocephin Injectable Vials, ADD-Vantage, Galaxy, Bulk 2800

PRODUVIR (Brazil)
ZIDOVUDINE
Retrovir Capsules 1560
Retrovir IV Infusion............... 1564
Retrovir Syrup 1560
Retrovir Tablets.................. 1560

PROFAMID (Denmark, Finland)
FLUTAMIDE
Eulexin Capsules................. 3009

PROFENAC (India)
DICLOFENAC SODIUM
Voltaren Tablets 2307
Voltaren-XR Tablets 2310

PROFERGAN (Brazil)
PROMETHAZINE HYDROCHLORIDE
Phenergan Tablets and Suppositories 3440

PROFEX (Israel)
PROPAFENONE HYDROCHLORIDE
Rythmol SR Capsules.............. 2727

PROFINE (India)
PROGESTERONE
Prometrium Capsules (100 mg, 200 mg) . 3203

PROFLAG (Mexico)
METRONIDAZOLE
MetroGel-Vaginal Gel 1855

PROFLAX (Argentina)
TIMOLOL MALEATE
Blocadren Tablets 1916
Timoptic Sterile Ophthalmic Solution 2088
Timoptic in Ocudose 2091
Timoptic-XE Sterile Ophthalmic Gel Forming Solution 2092

PROFLOX (Brazil, Thailand)
CIPROFLOXACIN
Cipro Oral Suspension 2977

PROFLOXIN (Australia)
CIPROFLOXACIN HYDROCHLORIDE
Ciloxan Ophthalmic Ointment .... ⊙204, 559
Ciloxan Ophthalmic Solution .... ⊙206
Cipro Tablets 2977

PROGAN (Australia)
PROMETHAZINE HYDROCHLORIDE
Phenergan Tablets and Suppositories 3440

PROGEFFIK (Italy, Spain)
PROGESTERONE
Prometrium Capsules (100 mg, 200 mg) . 3203

PROGENAR (Portugal)
PROGESTERONE
Prometrium Capsules (100 mg, 200 mg) . 3203

PROGENDO (Chile)
PROGESTERONE
Prometrium Capsules (100 mg, 200 mg) . 3203

PROGERING (Chile)
PROGESTERONE
Prometrium Capsules (100 mg, 200 mg) . 3203

PROGESAN (Brazil)
MEDROXYPROGESTERONE ACETATE
Depo-Medrol Single-Dose Vial **2619**

PROGEST (Argentina, India)
PROGESTERONE
Prometrium Capsules (100 mg, 200 mg) . **3203**

PROGESTAN (The Netherlands)
PROGESTERONE
Prometrium Capsules (100 mg, 200 mg) . **3203**

PROGESTASERT (Canada, France)
PROGESTERONE
Prometrium Capsules (100 mg, 200 mg) . **3203**

PROGESTERONE IMPLANTS (United Kingdom)
PROGESTERONE
Prometrium Capsules (100 mg, 200 mg) . **3203**

PROGESTOGEL (Belgium, France, Hong Kong, Italy, Portugal, Russia, Spain, Switzerland, Thailand)
PROGESTERONE
Prometrium Capsules (100 mg, 200 mg) . **3203**

PROGESTOL (Italy)
PROGESTERONE
Prometrium Capsules (100 mg, 200 mg) . **3203**

PROGESTOSOL (France, Spain, Switzerland)
PROGESTERONE
Prometrium Capsules (100 mg, 200 mg) . **3203**

PROGEVERA (Greece, Spain)
MEDROXYPROGESTERONE ACETATE
Depo-Medrol Single-Dose Vial **2619**

PROGEVERA 250 (Spain)
MEDROXYPROGESTERONE ACETATE
Depo-Medrol Single-Dose Vial **2619**

PROGLICEM (Argentina, France, Germany, Italy, Switzerland, The Netherlands)
DIAZOXIDE
Hyperstat I.V. **3017**

PROGLYCEM (Canada, Greece)
DIAZOXIDE
Hyperstat I.V. **3017**

PROGOR (Belgium)
DILTIAZEM HYDROCHLORIDE
Cardizem LA Extended Release Tablets . . . **1728**
Tiazac Capsules **1201**

PROGRAF (Argentina, Australia, Austria, Brazil, Canada, Chile, Czech Republic, Denmark, Finland, France, Germany, Greece, Hong Kong, Hungary, Irish Republic, Israel, Italy, Japan, Malaysia, Mexico, New Zealand, Norway, Portugal, Singapore, South Africa, Spain, Sweden, Switzerland, Thailand, United Kingdom)
TACROLIMUS
Prograf Capsules and Injection **632**

PROGRAFT (Belgium, The Netherlands)
TACROLIMUS
Prograf Capsules and Injection **632**

PROGRESSE (Brazil)
GABAPENTIN
Neurontin Capsules **2487**

PROGYNOVA (United Kingdom)
ESTRADIOL
Climara Transdermal System **771**
Estring Vaginal Ring **2635**

PROHAIR (Brazil, Chile)
FINASTERIDE
Propecia Tablets **2060**
Proscar Tablets. **2067**

PRO-HDL (India)
LOVASTATIN
Mevacor Tablets **2021**

PROHIST (South Africa)
PROMETHAZINE HYDROCHLORIDE
Phenergan Tablets and Suppositories **3440**

PROKEN M (Mexico)
METOPROLOL TARTRATE
Lopressor Tablets **2238**

PROLAKEN (Mexico)
METOPROLOL TARTRATE
Lopressor Tablets **2238**

PROLDIN (Mexico)
CAPTOPRIL
Captopril Tablets **2149**

PROLEKOFEN (Czech Republic)
PROPAFENONE HYDROCHLORIDE
Rythmol SR Capsules **2727**

PROLEUKIN (Argentina, Australia, Austria, Belgium, Brazil, Canada, Czech Republic, Denmark, France, Germany, Greece, Hong Kong, Hungary, Israel, Italy, Mexico, New Zealand, Portugal, Singapore, Spain, Switzerland, The Netherlands, United Kingdom)
ALDESLEUKIN
Proleukin for Injection **2266**

PROLIDON (Mexico)
PROGESTERONE
Prometrium Capsules (100 mg, 200 mg) . **3203**

PROLIPASE (Argentina, Austria, Switzerland)
PANCRELIPASE
Ultrase Capsules **708**
Ultrase MT Capsules **709**

PROLISINA E2 (Argentina)
DINOPROSTONE
Cervidil Vaginal Insert **1181**

PROLISINA VR (Argentina)
ALPROSTADIL
Edex Injection. **3089**

PROLOL (Hong Kong, Israel, Thailand)
PROPRANOLOL HYDROCHLORIDE
Inderal LA Long-Acting Capsules **3429**

PROLONG (Chile)
LIDOCAINE
Lidoderm Patch **1118**

PROLUTON (Argentina, Australia, Italy, Thailand)
PROGESTERONE
Prometrium Capsules (100 mg, 200 mg) . **3203**

PROMAHIST (South Africa)
PROMETHAZINE HYDROCHLORIDE
Phenergan Tablets and Suppositories **3440**

PROMAL (Austria)
ATOVAQUONE
Mepron Suspension **1521**

PROMETRIUM (Canada, Italy)
PROGESTERONE
Prometrium Capsules (100 mg, 200 mg) . **3203**

PROMIBASOL (Mexico)
METRONIDAZOLE
MetroGel-Vaginal Gel **1855**

PROMICIN (Mexico)
ERYTHROMYCIN
Ery-Tab Tablets **449**
Erythromycin Base Filmtab Tablets. **455**
Erythromycin Delayed-Release Capsules, USP **457**
PCE Dispertab Tablets **515**

PROMKIDDI (Germany)
PROMETHAZINE HYDROCHLORIDE
Phenergan Tablets and Suppositories **3440**

PROMOCARD (Belgium, The Netherlands)
ISOSORBIDE MONONITRATE
Imdur Tablets **3018**

PRONASTERON (Brazil)
FINASTERIDE
Propecia Tablets **2060**
Proscar Tablets. **2067**

PRONAT (Mexico)
NAPROXEN
EC-Naprosyn Delayed-Release Tablets. . . . **2761**
Naprosyn Suspension. **2761**
Naprosyn Tablets **2761**

PRONAXEN (Finland, Sweden)
NAPROXEN
EC-Naprosyn Delayed-Release Tablets. . . . **2761**
Naprosyn Suspension. **2761**
Naprosyn Tablets **2761**

PRONAXIL (Mexico)
NAPROXEN
EC-Naprosyn Delayed-Release Tablets. . . . **2761**
Naprosyn Suspension. **2761**
Naprosyn Tablets **2761**

PRONAX-P (Mexico)
NAPROXEN SODIUM
Anaprox DS Tablets **2761**
Anaprox Tablets **2761**

PRONEURIN (Germany)
PROMETHAZINE HYDROCHLORIDE
Phenergan Tablets and Suppositories **3440**

PRONOSIL (Thailand)
PROPRANOLOL HYDROCHLORIDE
Inderal LA Long-Acting Capsules **3429**

PRONOVAN (Norway)
PROPRANOLOL HYDROCHLORIDE
Inderal LA Long-Acting Capsules **3429**

PRONOXEN (Mexico)
NAPROXEN
EC-Naprosyn Delayed-Release Tablets. . . . **2761**
Naprosyn Suspension. **2761**
Naprosyn Tablets **2761**

PRONTALGIN (Italy)
TRAMADOL HYDROCHLORIDE
Ultram ER Tablets **2392**

PRONTAMID (Italy)
SULFACETAMIDE SODIUM
Klaron Lotion 10%. **2909**

PRONTOFORT (Mexico)
TRAMADOL HYDROCHLORIDE
Ultram ER Tablets **2392**

PRONTOGEST (Italy)
PROGESTERONE
Prometrium Capsules (100 mg, 200 mg) . **3203**

PROPABLOC (Germany)
PROPRANOLOL HYDROCHLORIDE
Inderal LA Long-Acting Capsules **3429**

PROPACOR (Brazil)
PROPRANOLOL HYDROCHLORIDE
Inderal LA Long-Acting Capsules **3429**

PROPAFEN (Germany)
PROPAFENONE HYDROCHLORIDE
Rythmol SR Capsules **2727**

PROPAL (Denmark)
PROPRANOLOL HYDROCHLORIDE
Inderal LA Long-Acting Capsules **3429**

PROPALEM (Mexico)
PROPRANOLOL HYDROCHLORIDE
Inderal LA Long-Acting Capsules **3429**

PROPALOL (Brazil)
PROPRANOLOL HYDROCHLORIDE
Inderal LA Long-Acting Capsules **3429**

PROPALONG (Argentina)
PROPRANOLOL HYDROCHLORIDE
Inderal LA Long-Acting Capsules **3429**

PROPAM (New Zealand)
DIAZEPAM
Diastat Rectal Delivery System **3343**
Valium Tablets **2819**

PRO-PAM (Australia)
DIAZEPAM
Diastat Rectal Delivery System **3343**
Valium Tablets **2819**

PROPAMERCK (Germany)
PROPAFENONE HYDROCHLORIDE
Rythmol SR Capsules **2727**

PROPANIX (United Kingdom)
PROPRANOLOL HYDROCHLORIDE
Inderal LA Long-Acting Capsules **3429**

PROPANOL (Malaysia)
PROPRANOLOL HYDROCHLORIDE
Inderal LA Long-Acting Capsules **3429**

PROPANORM (Czech Republic, Russia)
PROPAFENONE HYDROCHLORIDE
Rythmol SR Capsules **2727**

PROPANOX (Brazil)
PROPRANOLOL HYDROCHLORIDE
Inderal LA Long-Acting Capsules **3429**

PROPA-ORAMON (Germany)
PROPAFENONE HYDROCHLORIDE
Rythmol SR Capsules **2727**

PROPARIL (Brazil)
PROPRANOLOL HYDROCHLORIDE
Inderal LA Long-Acting Capsules **3429**

PROPASTAD (Germany)
PROPAFENONE HYDROCHLORIDE
Rythmol SR Capsules **2727**

PROPA-TABLETTEN (Czech Republic)
PROPAFENONE HYDROCHLORIDE
Rythmol SR Capsules **2727**

PROPAYERST (Argentina)
PROPRANOLOL HYDROCHLORIDE
Inderal LA Long-Acting Capsules **3429**

PROPAYERST PLUS (Argentina)
PROPRANOLOL HYDROCHLORIDE
Inderal LA Long-Acting Capsules **3429**

PROPECIA (Argentina, Australia, Austria, Brazil, Canada, Czech Republic, Denmark, Finland, France, Germany, Greece, Hong Kong, Israel, Italy, Malaysia, New Zealand, Portugal, Singapore, South Africa, Spain, Sweden, Switzerland, Thailand, The Netherlands, United Kingdom, Venezuela)
FINASTERIDE
Propecia Tablets **2060**
Proscar Tablets. **2067**

PROPERIL (Chile)
CAPTOPRIL
Captopril Tablets **2149**

PROPESHIA (Mexico)
FINASTERIDE
Propecia Tablets **2060**
Proscar Tablets. **2067**

PROPESS (Argentina, Austria, Czech Republic, Denmark, Finland, France, Germany, Greece, Hong Kong, Hungary, Irish Republic, Israel, Italy, Mexico, Portugal, South Africa, Spain, Sweden, Switzerland, The Netherlands, United Kingdom)
DINOPROSTONE
Cervidil Vaginal Insert **1181**

PROPHYLUX (Germany)
PROPRANOLOL HYDROCHLORIDE
Inderal LA Long-Acting Capsules **3429**

PROPIONAL (Mexico)
NAPROXEN
EC-Naprosyn Delayed-Release Tablets. . . . **2761**
Naprosyn Suspension. **2761**
Naprosyn Tablets **2761**

PROPIOSOL (Brazil)
CLOBETASOL PROPIONATE
Temovate Cream. **2668**
Temovate E Emollient. **2671**
Temovate Gel. **2669**
Temovate Ointment **2668**
Temovate Scalp Application **2670**

PROPOTEN (Brazil)
CEFOXITIN SODIUM
Mefoxin Premixed Intravenous Solution . . . **2016**
Mefoxin for Injection. **2012**

PROPRA (Germany)
PROPRANOLOL HYDROCHLORIDE
Inderal LA Long-Acting Capsules **3429**

PROPRAHEXAL (Austria)
PROPRANOLOL HYDROCHLORIDE
Inderal LA Long-Acting Capsules **3429**

PROPRAL (Finland)
PROPRANOLOL HYDROCHLORIDE
Inderal LA Long-Acting Capsules **3429**

PROPRANET (Denmark)
PROPRANOLOL HYDROCHLORIDE
Inderal LA Long-Acting Capsules **3429**

PROPRANOL (Brazil)
PROPRANOLOL HYDROCHLORIDE
Inderal LA Long-Acting Capsules **3429**

PROPRANOLIL (Brazil)
PROPRANOLOL HYDROCHLORIDE
Inderal LA Long-Acting Capsules **3429**

PROPRANOLUM (Brazil)
PROPRANOLOL HYDROCHLORIDE
Inderal LA Long-Acting Capsules **3429**

PROPRANUR (Germany)
PROPRANOLOL HYDROCHLORIDE
Inderal LA Long-Acting Capsules **3429**

PROQUIN (Australia)
CIPROFLOXACIN HYDROCHLORIDE
Ciloxan Ophthalmic Ointment .... ⊙204, 559
Ciloxan Ophthalmic Solution .... ⊙206
Cipro Tablets 2977

PRORYNORM (Germany)
PROPAFENONE HYDROCHLORIDE
Rythmol SR Capsules 2727

PROSAID (United Kingdom)
NAPROXEN
EC-Naprosyn Delayed-Release Tablets.... 2761
Naprosyn Suspension 2761
Naprosyn Tablets 2761

PROSCAR (Argentina, Australia, Austria, Belgium, Brazil, Canada, Chile, Czech Republic, Denmark, Finland, Germany, Greece, Hong Kong, Hungary, Irish Republic, Italy, Malaysia, Mexico, New Zealand, Norway, Portugal, Russia, Singapore, South Africa, Spain, Sweden, Switzerland, Thailand, The Netherlands, United Kingdom, Venezuela)
FINASTERIDE
Propecia Tablets 2060
Proscar Tablets 2067

PROSDINA (Venezuela)
FINASTERIDE
Propecia Tablets 2060
Proscar Tablets 2067

PROSERINE (Thailand)
CYCLOSERINE
Seromycin Capsules 1813

PROSMIN (Argentina)
FINASTERIDE
Propecia Tablets 2060
Proscar Tablets 2067

PROSOM (Canada)
ESTAZOLAM
ProSom Tablets 517

PROSTACUR (Spain)
FLUTAMIDE
Eulexin Capsules 3009

PROSTADIREX (France)
FLUTAMIDE
Eulexin Capsules 3009

PROSTALL (Chile)
TAMSULOSIN HYDROCHLORIDE
Flomax Capsules 850

PROSTAMID (India)
FLUTAMIDE
Eulexin Capsules 3009

PROSTAMIDE (Greece)
FLUTAMIDE
Eulexin Capsules 3009

PROSTANDRIL (Czech Republic)
FLUTAMIDE
Eulexin Capsules 3009

PROSTANIL (Argentina)
FINASTERIDE
Propecia Tablets 2060
Proscar Tablets 2067

PROSTANOVAG (Argentina)
FINASTERIDE
Propecia Tablets 2060
Proscar Tablets 2067

PROSTATIL (Italy)
TERAZOSIN HYDROCHLORIDE
Hytrin Capsules 471

PROSTENE (Argentina)
FINASTERIDE
Propecia Tablets 2060
Proscar Tablets 2067

PROSTERID (Hungary)
FINASTERIDE
Propecia Tablets 2060
Proscar Tablets 2067

PROSTICA (Germany)
FLUTAMIDE
Eulexin Capsules 3009

PROSTIDE (Brazil, Italy)
FINASTERIDE
Propecia Tablets 2060
Proscar Tablets 2067

PROSTIN E2 (Australia, Austria, Belgium, Canada, Czech Republic, Greece, Hong Kong, Hungary, Irish Republic, Israel, Italy, Malaysia, New Zealand, Portugal, Russia, Singapore, South Africa, Switzerland, Thailand, The Netherlands, United Kingdom)
DINOPROSTONE
Cervidil Vaginal Insert 1181

PROSTIN PEDIATRICO (Chile)
ALPROSTADIL
Edex Injection 3089

PROSTIN VR (Australia, Belgium, Canada, Czech Republic, Greece, Hong Kong, Hungary, India, Israel, Italy, Malaysia, New Zealand, Portugal, South Africa, Switzerland, Thailand, The Netherlands, United Kingdom)
ALPROSTADIL
Edex Injection 3089

PROSTINE E2 (France)
DINOPROSTONE
Cervidil Vaginal Insert 1181

PROSTINE VR (France)
ALPROSTADIL
Edex Injection 3089

PROSTIVAS (Denmark, Finland, Norway, Sweden)
ALPROSTADIL
Edex Injection 3089

PROSTOGENAT (Germany)
FLUTAMIDE
Eulexin Capsules 3009

PROTANGIX (France)
DIPYRIDAMOLE
Persantine Tablets 868

PROTENATE (Hong Kong)
PLASMA PROTEIN FRACTION
Plasmanate 3255

PROTEVAL (Mexico)
VALPROIC ACID
Depakene Capsules 417
Depakene Oral Solution 417

PROTEVIS (Argentina)
TIMOLOL MALEATE
Blocadren Tablets 1916
Timoptic Sterile Ophthalmic Solution 2088
Timoptic in Ocudose 2091
Timoptic-XE Sterile Ophthalmic Gel Forming Solution 2092

PROTEXIN (Spain)
AMANTADINE HYDROCHLORIDE
Symmetrel Tablets 1135

PROTHAZINE (Australia, Malaysia)
PROMETHAZINE HYDROCHLORIDE
Phenergan Tablets and Suppositories 3440

PROTHIAZINE (Israel)
PROMETHAZINE HYDROCHLORIDE
Phenergan Tablets and Suppositories 3440

PROTININ (Mexico)
APROTININ
Trasylol Injection 754

PROTOGYL (Hong Kong, Malaysia, Singapore)
METRONIDAZOLE
MetroGel-Vaginal Gel 1855

PROTOPIC (Argentina, Austria, Belgium, Canada, Denmark, Finland, France, Germany, Greece, Hong Kong, Irish Republic, Israel, Italy, Japan, Norway, Portugal, Spain, Sweden, Switzerland, United Kingdom)
TACROLIMUS
Prograf Capsules and Injection 632

PROTOSOL (Israel)
APROTININ
Trasylol Injection 754

PROTOSTAT (Australia)
METRONIDAZOLE
MetroGel-Vaginal Gel 1855

PROTRADON (Czech Republic)
TRAMADOL HYDROCHLORIDE
Ultram ER Tablets 2392

PROVAMES (France)
ESTRADIOL
Climara Transdermal System 771
Estring Vaginal Ring 2635

PRO-VENT (Irish Republic, United Kingdom)
THEOPHYLLINE
Uniphyl Tablets 2710

PROVERA (Australia, Austria, Belgium, Brazil, Canada, Chile, Czech Republic, Denmark, Finland, Greece, Hong Kong, Hungary, Irish Republic, Israel, Italy, Malaysia, Mexico, New Zealand, Norway, Portugal, Singapore, South Africa, Sweden, Switzerland, Thailand, The Netherlands, United Kingdom, Venezuela)
MEDROXYPROGESTERONE ACETATE
Depo-Medrol Single-Dose Vial 2619

PROVETAL (Mexico)
VALPROIC ACID
Depakene Capsules 417
Depakene Oral Solution 417

PROVICAR (Mexico, Venezuela)
LEVOCARNITINE
Carnitor Injection 3188
Carnitor Tablets and Oral Solution 3190

PROVIGIL (Belgium, Irish Republic, Israel, Italy, South Africa, United Kingdom)
MODAFINIL
Provigil Tablets 988

PROVISC (Argentina, Australia, Austria, Belgium, France, Germany, Hong Kong, Hungary, Irish Republic, Italy, Malaysia, New Zealand, Norway, Singapore, South Africa, Thailand, United Kingdom, Venezuela)
SODIUM HYALURONATE
Hyalgan Solution 2901

PROVISUAL (Argentina)
GENTAMICIN SULFATE
Garamycin Injectable 3014

PROXACIN (Brazil)
CIPROFLOXACIN HYDROCHLORIDE
Ciloxan Ophthalmic Ointment .... ⊙204, 559
Ciloxan Ophthalmic Solution .... ⊙206
Cipro Tablets 2977

PROXALIN (Mexico)
NAPROXEN
EC-Naprosyn Delayed-Release Tablets.... 2761
Naprosyn Suspension 2761
Naprosyn Tablets 2761

PROXALIN PLUS (Mexico)
NAPROXEN
EC-Naprosyn Delayed-Release Tablets.... 2761
Naprosyn Suspension 2761
Naprosyn Tablets 2761

PROXATAN (Argentina)
TERAZOSIN HYDROCHLORIDE
Hytrin Capsules 471

PROXEM (Mexico)
NAPROXEN
EC-Naprosyn Delayed-Release Tablets.... 2761
Naprosyn Suspension 2761
Naprosyn Tablets 2761

PROXEN (Australia, Austria, Hong Kong, South Africa, Switzerland, Thailand)
NAPROXEN
EC-Naprosyn Delayed-Release Tablets.... 2761
Naprosyn Suspension 2761
Naprosyn Tablets 2761

PROXINE (Italy)
NAPROXEN
EC-Naprosyn Delayed-Release Tablets.... 2761
Naprosyn Suspension 2761
Naprosyn Tablets 2761

PROXINOR (Thailand)
NORFLOXACIN
Noroxin Tablets 2032

PROXITEC (Mexico)
CIPROFLOXACIN
Cipro Oral Suspension 2977

PROZINE (South Africa)
CARBAMAZEPINE
Carbatrol Capsules 3171
Tegretol Chewable Tablets 2295
Tegretol Suspension 2295
Tegretol Tablets 2295
Tegretol-XR Tablets 2295

PROZITEL (Mexico)
PRAZIQUANTEL
Biltricide Tablets 2976

PRUDENCIAL (Argentina)
NIFEDIPINE
Adalat CC Tablets 2964

PSICOASTEN (Argentina)
PAROXETINE HYDROCHLORIDE
Paxil Oral Suspension 1530
Paxil Tablets 1530

PSICOFAR (Italy)
CHLORDIAZEPOXIDE HYDROCHLORIDE
Librium Capsules 3347

PSICONOR (Argentina)
CITALOPRAM HYDROBROMIDE
Celexa Tablets 1176

PSICOTERINA (Italy)
CHLORDIAZEPOXIDE HYDROCHLORIDE
Librium Capsules 3347

PSOREX (Brazil)
CLOBETASOL PROPIONATE
Temovate Cream 2668
Temovate E Emollient 2671
Temovate Gel 2669
Temovate Ointment 2668
Temovate Scalp Application 2670

PSORIN (Brazil)
CLOBETASOL PROPIONATE
Temovate Cream 2668
Temovate E Emollient 2671
Temovate Gel 2669
Temovate Ointment 2668
Temovate Scalp Application 2670

PSYCHOLANZ (India)
OLANZAPINE
Zyprexa Tablets 1830

PSYCHOPAX (Austria, Switzerland)
DIAZEPAM
Diastat Rectal Delivery System 3343
Valium Tablets 2819

PTINOLIN (Greece)
RANITIDINE HYDROCHLORIDE
Zantac 25 EFFERdose Tablets 1624
Zantac 150 EFFERdose Tablets 1624
Zantac 150 Tablets 1624
Zantac 300 Tablets 1624
Zantac Injection 1619
Zantac Injection Premixed 1619
Zantac Syrup 1624

PUIRITOL (Hong Kong)
OFLOXACIN
Floxin Otic Solution 1049

PULMENO (Spain)
THEOPHYLLINE
Uniphyl Tablets 2710

PULMIDUR (Austria)
THEOPHYLLINE
Uniphyl Tablets 2710

PULMILIDE (Austria)
FLUNISOLIDE
Aerobid Inhaler System 1171
Aerobid-M Inhaler System 1171

PULMIST (Italy)
FLUNISOLIDE
Aerobid Inhaler System 1171
Aerobid-M Inhaler System 1171

PULMOPHYLLIN (South Africa)
THEOPHYLLINE
Uniphyl Tablets 2710

PULMOPHYLLINE (Canada)
THEOPHYLLINE
Uniphyl Tablets 2710

PULMO-TIMELETS (Denmark, Germany)
THEOPHYLLINE
Uniphyl Tablets 2710

PULSOL (Mexico)
ENALAPRIL MALEATE
Vasotec I.V. Injection 2103

PURAN T4 (Brazil)
LEVOTHYROXINE SODIUM
Levothroid Tablets 1186

(⊙ Described in PDR For Ophthalmic Medicines™)

Levoxyl Tablets 1712
Synthroid Tablets 520

PUR-BLOKA (South Africa)
PROPRANOLOL HYDROCHLORIDE
Inderal LA Long-Acting Capsules 3429

PURESIS (South Africa)
FUROSEMIDE
Furosemide Tablets 2154

PURGOLAC (Greece)
LACTULOSE
Kristalose for Oral Solution 1034

PURGOXIN (South Africa)
DIGOXIN
Lanoxicaps Capsules 1490
Lanoxin Injection 1494
Lanoxin Injection Pediatric 1497
Lanoxin Tablets 1500

PUTAREN (Thailand)
DICLOFENAC SODIUM
Voltaren Tablets 2307
Voltaren-XR Tablets 2310

PUVASORALEN (United Kingdom)
METHOXSALEN
Oxsoralen Lotion 1% 3352
Oxsoralen-Ultra Capsules 3353

P-VATE (Thailand)
CLOBETASOL PROPIONATE
Temovate Cream 2668
Temovate E Emollient 2671
Temovate Gel 2669
Temovate Ointment 2668
Temovate Scalp Application 2670

PYLOKIT (India)
LANSOPRAZOLE
Prevacid Delayed-Release Capsules 3271

PYRALFIN (India)
PYRIMETHAMINE
Daraprim Tablets 1419

PYRAMET (India)
PYRIMETHAMINE
Daraprim Tablets 1419

PYRIDAMEL (Irish Republic)
DIPYRIDAMOLE
Persantine Tablets 868

PYRIMON (India)
DEXAMETHASONE
Decadron Tablets 1951

PYTAZEN (New Zealand)
DIPYRIDAMOLE
Persantine Tablets 868

Q-MAZINE (United Kingdom)
PROMETHAZINE HYDROCHLORIDE
Phenergan Tablets and Suppositories 3440

QUAGU-TEST (Argentina)
APROTININ
Trasylol Injection 754

QUALECON (Argentina)
FENOFIBRATE
Tricor Tablets 527

QUAMATEL (Czech Republic, Hong Kong, Hungary, Russia)
FAMOTIDINE
Pepcid Injection 2040
Pepcid Injection Premixed 2040
Pepcid Tablets 2038
Pepcid for Oral Suspension 2038

QUARDIN (Portugal)
RANITIDINE HYDROCHLORIDE
Zantac 25 EFFERdose Tablets 1624
Zantac 150 EFFERdose Tablets 1624
Zantac 150 Tablets 1624
Zantac 300 Tablets 1624
Zantac Injection 1619
Zantac Injection Premixed 1619
Zantac Syrup 1624

QUARK (Italy)
RAMIPRIL
Altace Capsules 1702

QUASAR (Italy)
VERAPAMIL HYDROCHLORIDE
Covera-HS Tablets 3139
Verelan PM Extended-Release Capsules, Controlled-Onset 3106

QUEDOX (Mexico)
CLARITHROMYCIN
Biaxin Filmtab Tablets 402
Biaxin Granules 402

QUEIMALIVE (Brazil)
SULFACETAMIDE SODIUM
Klaron Lotion 10% 2909

QUEL (India)
QUETIAPINE FUMARATE
Seroquel Tablets 690

QUERATAL (Mexico)
TRETINOIN
Vesanoid Capsules 2820

QUERTO (Germany)
CARVEDILOL
Coreg Tablets 1414

QUIBRON (Thailand)
THEOPHYLLINE
Uniphyl Tablets 2710

QUIBRON-T (Canada)
THEOPHYLLINE
Uniphyl Tablets 2710

QUIDEX (Argentina)
CIPROFLOXACIN
Cipro Oral Suspension 2977

QUIFLOX (Brazil)
CIPROFLOXACIN HYDROCHLORIDE
Ciloxan Ophthalmic Ointment . . . . ⊙204, 559
Ciloxan Ophthalmic Solution . . . . ⊙206
Cipro Tablets 2977

QUIFLOXONA (Mexico)
CIPROFLOXACIN
Cipro Oral Suspension 2977

QUIFLURAL (Mexico)
OFLOXACIN
Floxin Otic Solution 1049

QUILAGEN (Mexico)
GENTAMICIN SULFATE
Garamycin Injectable 3014

QUIMALAN (Mexico)
ENALAPRIL MALEATE
Vasotec I.V. Injection 2103

QUIMOBROM (Mexico)
ERYTHROMYCIN
Ery-Tab Tablets 449
Erythromycin Base Filmtab Tablets 455
Erythromycin Delayed-Release Capsules, USP 457
PCE Dispertab Tablets 515

QUIMOLAURIL (Mexico)
ERYTHROMYCIN
Ery-Tab Tablets 449
Erythromycin Base Filmtab Tablets 455
Erythromycin Delayed-Release Capsules, USP 457
PCE Dispertab Tablets 515

QUINOBACT (India)
CIPROFLOXACIN
Cipro Oral Suspension 2977

QUINOBIOT (Chile)
LEVOFLOXACIN
Levaquin Injection 2384
Levaquin Tablets 2384

QUINOFLEX (Portugal)
NORFLOXACIN
Noroxin Tablets 2032

QUINOFLOX (Mexico)
CIPROFLOXACIN HYDROCHLORIDE
Ciloxan Ophthalmic Ointment . . . . ⊙204, 559
Ciloxan Ophthalmic Solution . . . . ⊙206
Cipro Tablets 2977

QUINOFORM (Brazil)
NORFLOXACIN
Noroxin Tablets 2032

QUINOFTAL (Venezuela)
CIPROFLOXACIN
Cipro Oral Suspension 2977

QUINOMED (Argentina)
OFLOXACIN
Floxin Otic Solution 1049

QUINOX (Portugal)
CIPROFLOXACIN
Cipro Oral Suspension 2977

QUINOXAN (Brazil)
OFLOXACIN
Floxin Otic Solution 1049

QUINTAMICINA (Spain)
GENTAMICIN SULFATE
Garamycin Injectable 3014

QUINTOR (Czech Republic)
CIPROFLOXACIN HYDROCHLORIDE
Ciloxan Ophthalmic Ointment . . . . ⊙204, 559
Ciloxan Ophthalmic Solution . . . . ⊙206
Cipro Tablets 2977

QUIPRO (Czech Republic, Spain)
CIPROFLOXACIN HYDROCHLORIDE
Ciloxan Ophthalmic Ointment . . . . ⊙204, 559
Ciloxan Ophthalmic Solution . . . . ⊙206
Cipro Tablets 2977

QUISEGEN (Argentina)
CIPROFLOXACIN HYDROCHLORIDE
Ciloxan Ophthalmic Ointment . . . . ⊙204, 559
Ciloxan Ophthalmic Solution . . . . ⊙206
Cipro Tablets 2977

QUOMEM (Austria, Italy, Spain, Thailand)
BUPROPION HYDROCHLORIDE
Wellbutrin SR Sustained-Release Tablets 1607
Wellbutrin Tablets 1603
Zyban Sustained-Release Tablets 1644

RABIODINA (Brazil)
RANITIDINE HYDROCHLORIDE
Zantac 25 EFFERdose Tablets 1624
Zantac 150 EFFERdose Tablets 1624
Zantac 150 Tablets 1624
Zantac 300 Tablets 1624
Zantac Injection 1619
Zantac Injection Premixed 1619
Zantac Syrup 1624

RABLAS (Greece)
ENALAPRIL MALEATE
Vasotec I.V. Injection 2103

RADAN (Brazil)
RANITIDINE HYDROCHLORIDE
Zantac 25 EFFERdose Tablets 1624
Zantac 150 EFFERdose Tablets 1624
Zantac 150 Tablets 1624
Zantac 300 Tablets 1624
Zantac Injection 1619
Zantac Injection Premixed 1619
Zantac Syrup 1624

RADICACINE (Argentina)
CELECOXIB
Celebrex Capsules 3134

RADIGEN (Chile)
RISPERIDONE
Risperdal Oral Solution 1676
Risperdal Tablets 1676

RADIKAL (Germany)
CLOTRIMAZOLE
Lotrimin Cream 3039
Lotrimin Lotion 1% 3039
Lotrimin Topical Solution 1% 3039

RADILEM (Mexico)
METHYLPREDNISOLONE ACETATE
Depo-Medrol Injectable Suspension 2617

RADIN (Hong Kong)
RANITIDINE HYDROCHLORIDE
Zantac 25 EFFERdose Tablets 1624
Zantac 150 EFFERdose Tablets 1624
Zantac 150 Tablets 1624
Zantac 300 Tablets 1624
Zantac Injection 1619
Zantac Injection Premixed 1619
Zantac Syrup 1624

RADINA (Argentina)
TOBRAMYCIN
TOBI Solution for Inhalation 2298

RADINA DEX (Argentina)
TOBRAMYCIN
TOBI Solution for Inhalation 2298

RADINE (Thailand)
RANITIDINE HYDROCHLORIDE
Zantac 25 EFFERdose Tablets 1624
Zantac 150 EFFERdose Tablets 1624
Zantac 150 Tablets 1624
Zantac 300 Tablets 1624
Zantac Injection 1619
Zantac Injection Premixed 1619
Zantac Syrup 1624

RADUCTIL (Argentina, Mexico)
SIBUTRAMINE HYDROCHLORIDE
Meridia Capsules 489

RAFFONIN (Chile)
FLUTICASONE PROPIONATE
Cutivate Cream 2662
Cutivate Ointment 2665
Flonase Nasal Spray 1440

RAFOCILINA (Argentina)
OFLOXACIN
Floxin Otic Solution 1049

RALISTA (India)
RALOXIFENE HYDROCHLORIDE
Evista Tablets 1763

RALIZON (Greece)
CETIRIZINE HYDROCHLORIDE
Zyrtec Syrup 2594
Zyrtec Tablets 2594

RALOVERA (Australia)
MEDROXYPROGESTERONE ACETATE
Depo-Medrol Single-Dose Vial 2619

RAMACE (Australia, Belgium, Denmark, Finland, Mexico, South Africa)
RAMIPRIL
Altace Capsules 1702

RAMCOR (India)
RAMIPRIL
Altace Capsules 1702

RAMCOR H (India)
RAMIPRIL
Altace Capsules 1702

RAMIPRES (Chile, India)
RAMIPRIL
Altace Capsules 1702

RAMIPRES H (India)
RAMIPRIL
Altace Capsules 1702

RAN (Italy, Portugal)
RANITIDINE HYDROCHLORIDE
Zantac 25 EFFERdose Tablets 1624
Zantac 150 EFFERdose Tablets 1624
Zantac 150 Tablets 1624
Zantac 300 Tablets 1624
Zantac Injection 1619
Zantac Injection Premixed 1619
Zantac Syrup 1624

RAN H2 (Spain)
RANITIDINE HYDROCHLORIDE
Zantac 25 EFFERdose Tablets 1624
Zantac 150 EFFERdose Tablets 1624
Zantac 150 Tablets 1624
Zantac 300 Tablets 1624
Zantac Injection 1619
Zantac Injection Premixed 1619
Zantac Syrup 1624

RAN LICH (Germany)
RANITIDINE HYDROCHLORIDE
Zantac 25 EFFERdose Tablets 1624
Zantac 150 EFFERdose Tablets 1624
Zantac 150 Tablets 1624
Zantac 300 Tablets 1624
Zantac Injection 1619
Zantac Injection Premixed 1619
Zantac Syrup 1624

RANACID (Norway)
RANITIDINE HYDROCHLORIDE
Zantac 25 EFFERdose Tablets 1624
Zantac 150 EFFERdose Tablets 1624
Zantac 150 Tablets 1624
Zantac 300 Tablets 1624
Zantac Injection 1619
Zantac Injection Premixed 1619
Zantac Syrup 1624

RANAPS (United Kingdom)
RANITIDINE HYDROCHLORIDE
Zantac 25 EFFERdose Tablets 1624
Zantac 150 EFFERdose Tablets 1624
Zantac 150 Tablets 1624
Zantac 300 Tablets 1624
Zantac Injection 1619
Zantac Injection Premixed 1619
Zantac Syrup 1624

RANCLAV (Thailand)
AMOXICILLIN
Amoxil Pediatric Drops for Oral Suspension 1343
Amoxil Tablets 1343

RANGIN (Hungary)
ISOSORBIDE MONONITRATE
Imdur Tablets 3018

RANI (Singapore)
RANITIDINE HYDROCHLORIDE
Zantac 25 EFFERdose Tablets 1624

Zantac 150 EFFERdose Tablets. **1624**
Zantac 150 Tablets **1624**
Zantac 300 Tablets **1624**
Zantac Injection **1619**
Zantac Injection Premixed **1619**
Zantac Syrup **1624**

RANI 2 (Australia)
RANITIDINE HYDROCHLORIDE
Zantac 25 EFFERdose Tablets **1624**
Zantac 150 EFFERdose Tablets. **1624**
Zantac 150 Tablets **1624**
Zantac 300 Tablets **1624**
Zantac Injection **1619**
Zantac Injection Premixed **1619**
Zantac Syrup **1624**

RANIBEN (Italy)
RANITIDINE HYDROCHLORIDE
Zantac 25 EFFERdose Tablets **1624**
Zantac 150 EFFERdose Tablets. **1624**
Zantac 150 Tablets **1624**
Zantac 300 Tablets **1624**
Zantac Injection **1619**
Zantac Injection Premixed **1619**
Zantac Syrup **1624**

RANIBERL (Czech Republic, Germany)
RANITIDINE HYDROCHLORIDE
Zantac 25 EFFERdose Tablets **1624**
Zantac 150 EFFERdose Tablets. **1624**
Zantac 150 Tablets **1624**
Zantac 300 Tablets **1624**
Zantac Injection **1619**
Zantac Injection Premixed **1619**
Zantac Syrup **1624**

RANIBETA (Germany)
RANITIDINE HYDROCHLORIDE
Zantac 25 EFFERdose Tablets **1624**
Zantac 150 EFFERdose Tablets. **1624**
Zantac 150 Tablets **1624**
Zantac 300 Tablets **1624**
Zantac Injection **1619**
Zantac Injection Premixed **1619**
Zantac Syrup **1624**

RANIBLOC (Germany, Italy, Venezuela)
RANITIDINE HYDROCHLORIDE
Zantac 25 EFFERdose Tablets **1624**
Zantac 150 EFFERdose Tablets. **1624**
Zantac 150 Tablets **1624**
Zantac 300 Tablets **1624**
Zantac Injection **1619**
Zantac Injection Premixed **1619**
Zantac Syrup **1624**

RANIC (Austria, Belgium)
RANITIDINE HYDROCHLORIDE
Zantac 25 EFFERdose Tablets **1624**
Zantac 150 EFFERdose Tablets. **1624**
Zantac 150 Tablets **1624**
Zantac 300 Tablets **1624**
Zantac Injection **1619**
Zantac Injection Premixed **1619**
Zantac Syrup **1624**

RANICEL (Chile)
RANITIDINE HYDROCHLORIDE
Zantac 25 EFFERdose Tablets **1624**
Zantac 150 EFFERdose Tablets. **1624**
Zantac 150 Tablets **1624**
Zantac 300 Tablets **1624**
Zantac Injection **1619**
Zantac Injection Premixed **1619**
Zantac Syrup **1624**

RANICID (Thailand)
RANITIDINE HYDROCHLORIDE
Zantac 25 EFFERdose Tablets **1624**
Zantac 150 EFFERdose Tablets. **1624**
Zantac 150 Tablets **1624**
Zantac 300 Tablets **1624**
Zantac Injection **1619**
Zantac Injection Premixed **1619**
Zantac Syrup **1624**

RANICLON (Greece)
RANITIDINE HYDROCHLORIDE
Zantac 25 EFFERdose Tablets **1624**
Zantac 150 EFFERdose Tablets. **1624**
Zantac 150 Tablets **1624**
Zantac 300 Tablets **1624**
Zantac Injection **1619**
Zantac Injection Premixed **1619**
Zantac Syrup **1624**

RANICLOR (Brazil)
RANITIDINE HYDROCHLORIDE
Zantac 25 EFFERdose Tablets **1624**
Zantac 150 EFFERdose Tablets. **1624**

Zantac 150 Tablets **1624**
Zantac 300 Tablets **1624**
Zantac Injection **1619**
Zantac Injection Premixed **1619**
Zantac Syrup **1624**

RANICODAN (Denmark)
RANITIDINE HYDROCHLORIDE
Zantac 25 EFFERdose Tablets **1624**
Zantac 150 EFFERdose Tablets. **1624**
Zantac 150 Tablets **1624**
Zantac 300 Tablets **1624**
Zantac Injection **1619**
Zantac Injection Premixed **1619**
Zantac Syrup **1624**

RANICUR (Finland)
RANITIDINE HYDROCHLORIDE
Zantac 25 EFFERdose Tablets **1624**
Zantac 150 EFFERdose Tablets. **1624**
Zantac 150 Tablets **1624**
Zantac 300 Tablets **1624**
Zantac Injection **1619**
Zantac Injection Premixed **1619**
Zantac Syrup **1624**

RANICUX (Germany)
RANITIDINE HYDROCHLORIDE
Zantac 25 EFFERdose Tablets **1624**
Zantac 150 EFFERdose Tablets. **1624**
Zantac 150 Tablets **1624**
Zantac 300 Tablets **1624**
Zantac Injection **1619**
Zantac Injection Premixed **1619**
Zantac Syrup **1624**

RANIDIL (Italy)
RANITIDINE HYDROCHLORIDE
Zantac 25 EFFERdose Tablets **1624**
Zantac 150 EFFERdose Tablets. **1624**
Zantac 150 Tablets **1624**
Zantac 300 Tablets **1624**
Zantac Injection **1619**
Zantac Injection Premixed **1619**
Zantac Syrup **1624**

RANIDIN (Brazil, Spain)
RANITIDINE HYDROCHLORIDE
Zantac 25 EFFERdose Tablets **1624**
Zantac 150 EFFERdose Tablets. **1624**
Zantac 150 Tablets **1624**
Zantac 300 Tablets **1624**
Zantac Injection **1619**
Zantac Injection Premixed **1619**
Zantac Syrup **1624**

RANIDINA (Brazil)
RANITIDINE HYDROCHLORIDE
Zantac 25 EFFERdose Tablets **1624**
Zantac 150 EFFERdose Tablets. **1624**
Zantac 150 Tablets **1624**
Zantac 300 Tablets **1624**
Zantac Injection **1619**
Zantac Injection Premixed **1619**
Zantac Syrup **1624**

RANIDURA T (Germany)
RANITIDINE HYDROCHLORIDE
Zantac 25 EFFERdose Tablets **1624**
Zantac 150 EFFERdose Tablets. **1624**
Zantac 150 Tablets **1624**
Zantac 300 Tablets **1624**
Zantac Injection **1619**
Zantac Injection Premixed **1619**
Zantac Syrup **1624**

RANIFESA (Venezuela)
RANITIDINE HYDROCHLORIDE
Zantac 25 EFFERdose Tablets **1624**
Zantac 150 EFFERdose Tablets. **1624**
Zantac 150 Tablets **1624**
Zantac 300 Tablets **1624**
Zantac Injection **1619**
Zantac Injection Premixed **1619**
Zantac Syrup **1624**

RANIFLEX (Brazil)
RANITIDINE HYDROCHLORIDE
Zantac 25 EFFERdose Tablets **1624**
Zantac 150 EFFERdose Tablets. **1624**
Zantac 150 Tablets **1624**
Zantac 300 Tablets **1624**
Zantac Injection **1619**
Zantac Injection Premixed **1619**
Zantac Syrup **1624**

RANIGAST (Russia)
RANITIDINE HYDROCHLORIDE
Zantac 25 EFFERdose Tablets **1624**
Zantac 150 EFFERdose Tablets. **1624**
Zantac 150 Tablets **1624**
Zantac 300 Tablets **1624**
Zantac Injection **1619**
Zantac Injection Premixed **1619**

Zantac Syrup **1624**

RANIHEXAL (Australia, South Africa)
RANITIDINE HYDROCHLORIDE
Zantac 25 EFFERdose Tablets **1624**
Zantac 150 EFFERdose Tablets. **1624**
Zantac 150 Tablets **1624**
Zantac 300 Tablets **1624**
Zantac Injection **1619**
Zantac Injection Premixed **1619**
Zantac Syrup **1624**

RANIL (Finland)
RANITIDINE HYDROCHLORIDE
Zantac 25 EFFERdose Tablets **1624**
Zantac 150 EFFERdose Tablets. **1624**
Zantac 150 Tablets **1624**
Zantac 300 Tablets **1624**
Zantac Injection **1619**
Zantac Injection Premixed **1619**
Zantac Syrup **1624**

RANILONGA (Spain)
RANITIDINE HYDROCHLORIDE
Zantac 25 EFFERdose Tablets **1624**
Zantac 150 EFFERdose Tablets. **1624**
Zantac 150 Tablets **1624**
Zantac 300 Tablets **1624**
Zantac Injection **1619**
Zantac Injection Premixed **1619**
Zantac Syrup **1624**

RANIMED (Argentina, Switzerland)
RANITIDINE HYDROCHLORIDE
Zantac 25 EFFERdose Tablets **1624**
Zantac 150 EFFERdose Tablets. **1624**
Zantac 150 Tablets **1624**
Zantac 300 Tablets **1624**
Zantac Injection **1619**
Zantac Injection Premixed **1619**
Zantac Syrup **1624**

RANIMERCK (Germany)
RANITIDINE HYDROCHLORIDE
Zantac 25 EFFERdose Tablets **1624**
Zantac 150 EFFERdose Tablets. **1624**
Zantac 150 Tablets **1624**
Zantac 300 Tablets **1624**
Zantac Injection **1619**
Zantac Injection Premixed **1619**
Zantac Syrup **1624**

RANIMEX (Finland)
RANITIDINE HYDROCHLORIDE
Zantac 25 EFFERdose Tablets **1624**
Zantac 150 EFFERdose Tablets. **1624**
Zantac 150 Tablets **1624**
Zantac 300 Tablets **1624**
Zantac Injection **1619**
Zantac Injection Premixed **1619**
Zantac Syrup **1624**

RANI-NERTON (Germany)
RANITIDINE HYDROCHLORIDE
Zantac 25 EFFERdose Tablets **1624**
Zantac 150 EFFERdose Tablets. **1624**
Zantac 150 Tablets **1624**
Zantac 300 Tablets **1624**
Zantac Injection **1619**
Zantac Injection Premixed **1619**
Zantac Syrup **1624**

RANINORM (Austria)
RANITIDINE HYDROCHLORIDE
Zantac 25 EFFERdose Tablets **1624**
Zantac 150 EFFERdose Tablets. **1624**
Zantac 150 Tablets **1624**
Zantac 300 Tablets **1624**
Zantac Injection **1619**
Zantac Syrup **1624**

RANIPLEX (France)
RANITIDINE HYDROCHLORIDE
Zantac 25 EFFERdose Tablets **1624**
Zantac 150 EFFERdose Tablets. **1624**
Zantac 150 Tablets **1624**
Zantac 300 Tablets **1624**
Zantac Injection **1619**
Zantac Injection Premixed **1619**
Zantac Syrup **1624**

RANIPROTECT (Germany)
RANITIDINE HYDROCHLORIDE
Zantac 25 EFFERdose Tablets **1624**
Zantac 150 EFFERdose Tablets. **1624**
Zantac 150 Tablets **1624**
Zantac 300 Tablets **1624**
Zantac Injection **1619**
Zantac Injection Premixed **1619**
Zantac Syrup **1624**

RANI-Q (Sweden)
RANITIDINE HYDROCHLORIDE
Zantac 25 EFFERdose Tablets **1624**

Zantac 150 EFFERdose Tablets. **1624**
Zantac 150 Tablets **1624**
Zantac 300 Tablets **1624**
Zantac Injection **1619**
Zantac Injection Premixed **1619**
Zantac Syrup **1624**

RANISAN (Czech Republic, Russia)
RANITIDINE HYDROCHLORIDE
Zantac 25 EFFERdose Tablets **1624**
Zantac 150 EFFERdose Tablets. **1624**
Zantac 150 Tablets **1624**
Zantac 300 Tablets **1624**
Zantac Injection **1619**
Zantac Injection Premixed **1619**
Zantac Syrup **1624**

RANISEN (Mexico)
RANITIDINE HYDROCHLORIDE
Zantac 25 EFFERdose Tablets **1624**
Zantac 150 EFFERdose Tablets. **1624**
Zantac 150 Tablets **1624**
Zantac 300 Tablets **1624**
Zantac Injection **1619**
Zantac Injection Premixed **1619**
Zantac Syrup **1624**

RANISIFAR (Switzerland)
RANITIDINE HYDROCHLORIDE
Zantac 25 EFFERdose Tablets **1624**
Zantac 150 EFFERdose Tablets. **1624**
Zantac 150 Tablets **1624**
Zantac 300 Tablets **1624**
Zantac Injection **1619**
Zantac Injection Premixed **1619**
Zantac Syrup **1624**

RANITAB (Germany)
RANITIDINE HYDROCHLORIDE
Zantac 25 EFFERdose Tablets **1624**
Zantac 150 EFFERdose Tablets. **1624**
Zantac 150 Tablets **1624**
Zantac 300 Tablets **1624**
Zantac Injection **1619**
Zantac Injection Premixed **1619**
Zantac Syrup **1624**

RANITAK (Brazil)
RANITIDINE HYDROCHLORIDE
Zantac 25 EFFERdose Tablets **1624**
Zantac 150 EFFERdose Tablets. **1624**
Zantac 150 Tablets **1624**
Zantac 300 Tablets **1624**
Zantac Injection **1619**
Zantac Injection Premixed **1619**
Zantac Syrup **1624**

RANITAL (Czech Republic)
RANITIDINE HYDROCHLORIDE
Zantac 25 EFFERdose Tablets **1624**
Zantac 150 EFFERdose Tablets. **1624**
Zantac 150 Tablets **1624**
Zantac 300 Tablets **1624**
Zantac Injection **1619**
Zantac Injection Premixed **1619**
Zantac Syrup **1624**

RANITIC (Argentina, Australia, Germany, Hungary, Irish Republic, United Kingdom)
RANITIDINE HYDROCHLORIDE
Zantac 25 EFFERdose Tablets **1624**
Zantac 150 EFFERdose Tablets. **1624**
Zantac 150 Tablets **1624**
Zantac 300 Tablets **1624**
Zantac Injection **1619**
Zantac Injection Premixed **1619**
Zantac Syrup **1624**

RANITIDOC (Germany)
RANITIDINE HYDROCHLORIDE
Zantac 25 EFFERdose Tablets **1624**
Zantac 150 EFFERdose Tablets. **1624**
Zantac 150 Tablets **1624**
Zantac 300 Tablets **1624**
Zantac Injection **1619**
Zantac Injection Premixed **1619**
Zantac Syrup **1624**

RANITIL (Brazil, United Kingdom)
RANITIDINE HYDROCHLORIDE
Zantac 25 EFFERdose Tablets **1624**
Zantac 150 EFFERdose Tablets. **1624**
Zantac 150 Tablets **1624**
Zantac 300 Tablets **1624**
Zantac Injection **1619**
Zantac Syrup **1624**

RANITIN (Brazil, Czech Republic)
RANITIDINE HYDROCHLORIDE
Zantac 25 EFFERdose Tablets **1624**
Zantac 150 EFFERdose Tablets. **1624**

Zantac 150 Tablets 1624
Zantac 300 Tablets 1624
Zantac Injection 1619
Zantac Injection Premixed 1619
Zantac Syrup 1624

RANITINE (Portugal)
RANITIDINE HYDROCHLORIDE
Zantac 25 EFFERdose Tablets 1624
Zantac 150 EFFERdose Tablets. 1624
Zantac 150 Tablets 1624
Zantac 300 Tablets 1624
Zantac Injection 1619
Zantac Injection Premixed 1619
Zantac Syrup 1624

RANITINOL (Brazil)
RANITIDINE HYDROCHLORIDE
Zantac 25 EFFERdose Tablets 1624
Zantac 150 EFFERdose Tablets. 1624
Zantac 150 Tablets 1624
Zantac 300 Tablets 1624
Zantac Injection 1619
Zantac Injection Premixed 1619
Zantac Syrup 1624

RANITION (Brazil)
RANITIDINE HYDROCHLORIDE
Zantac 25 EFFERdose Tablets 1624
Zantac 150 EFFERdose Tablets. 1624
Zantac 150 Tablets 1624
Zantac 300 Tablets 1624
Zantac Injection 1619
Zantac Injection Premixed 1619
Zantac Syrup 1624

RANITRAL (Argentina)
RANITIDINE HYDROCHLORIDE
Zantac 25 EFFERdose Tablets 1624
Zantac 150 EFFERdose Tablets. 1624
Zantac 150 Tablets 1624
Zantac 300 Tablets 1624
Zantac Injection 1619
Zantac Injection Premixed 1619
Zantac Syrup 1624

RANITRAT (Brazil)
RANITIDINE HYDROCHLORIDE
Zantac 25 EFFERdose Tablets 1624
Zantac 150 EFFERdose Tablets. 1624
Zantac 150 Tablets 1624
Zantac 300 Tablets 1624
Zantac Injection 1619
Zantac Injection Premixed 1619
Zantac Syrup 1624

RANITYROL (Austria)
RANITIDINE HYDROCHLORIDE
Zantac 25 EFFERdose Tablets 1624
Zantac 150 EFFERdose Tablets. 1624
Zantac 150 Tablets 1624
Zantac 300 Tablets 1624
Zantac Injection 1619
Zantac Injection Premixed 1619
Zantac Syrup 1624

RANIVEL (Spain)
RANITIDINE HYDROCHLORIDE
Zantac 25 EFFERdose Tablets 1624
Zantac 150 EFFERdose Tablets. 1624
Zantac 150 Tablets 1624
Zantac 300 Tablets 1624
Zantac Injection 1619
Zantac Injection Premixed 1619
Zantac Syrup 1624

RANIX (Spain, Venezuela)
RANITIDINE HYDROCHLORIDE
Zantac 25 EFFERdose Tablets 1624
Zantac 150 EFFERdose Tablets. 1624
Zantac 150 Tablets 1624
Zantac 300 Tablets 1624
Zantac Injection 1619
Zantac Injection Premixed 1619
Zantac Syrup 1624

RANIXAL (Finland)
RANITIDINE HYDROCHLORIDE
Zantac 25 EFFERdose Tablets 1624
Zantac 150 EFFERdose Tablets. 1624
Zantac 150 Tablets 1624
Zantac 300 Tablets 1624
Zantac Injection 1619
Zantac Injection Premixed 1619
Zantac Syrup 1624

RANIZAC (Greece)
RANITIDINE HYDROCHLORIDE
Zantac 25 EFFERdose Tablets 1624
Zantac 150 EFFERdose Tablets. 1624
Zantac 150 Tablets 1624
Zantac 300 Tablets 1624
Zantac Injection 1619
Zantac Injection Premixed 1619

Zantac Syrup 1624

RANIZAN (Venezuela)
RANITIDINE HYDROCHLORIDE
Zantac 25 EFFERdose Tablets 1624
Zantac 150 EFFERdose Tablets. 1624
Zantac 150 Tablets 1624
Zantac 300 Tablets 1624
Zantac Injection 1619
Zantac Injection Premixed 1619
Zantac Syrup 1624

RANOLTA (Hong Kong)
RANITIDINE HYDROCHLORIDE
Zantac 25 EFFERdose Tablets 1624
Zantac 150 EFFERdose Tablets. 1624
Zantac 150 Tablets 1624
Zantac 300 Tablets 1624
Zantac Injection 1619
Zantac Injection Premixed 1619
Zantac Syrup 1624

RANOPINE (Irish Republic)
RANITIDINE HYDROCHLORIDE
Zantac 25 EFFERdose Tablets 1624
Zantac 150 EFFERdose Tablets. 1624
Zantac 150 Tablets 1624
Zantac 300 Tablets 1624
Zantac Injection 1619
Zantac Injection Premixed 1619
Zantac Syrup 1624

RANOPRIL (Malaysia)
LISINOPRIL
Prinivil Tablets 2052

RANOPRIN (Finland)
PROPRANOLOL HYDROCHLORIDE
Inderal LA Long-Acting Capsules 3429

RANOXYL (Australia)
RANITIDINE HYDROCHLORIDE
Zantac 25 EFFERdose Tablets 1624
Zantac 150 EFFERdose Tablets. 1624
Zantac 150 Tablets 1624
Zantac 300 Tablets 1624
Zantac Injection 1619
Zantac Injection Premixed 1619
Zantac Syrup 1624

RANTAC (India, Russia)
RANITIDINE HYDROCHLORIDE
Zantac 25 EFFERdose Tablets 1624
Zantac 150 EFFERdose Tablets. 1624
Zantac 150 Tablets 1624
Zantac 300 Tablets 1624
Zantac Injection 1619
Zantac Injection Premixed 1619
Zantac Syrup 1624

RANTAG (United Arab Emirates)
RANITIDINE HYDROCHLORIDE
Zantac 25 EFFERdose Tablets 1624
Zantac 150 EFFERdose Tablets. 1624
Zantac 150 Tablets 1624
Zantac 300 Tablets 1624
Zantac Injection 1619
Zantac Injection Premixed 1619
Zantac Syrup 1624

RANTEC (United Kingdom)
RANITIDINE HYDROCHLORIDE
Zantac 25 EFFERdose Tablets 1624
Zantac 150 EFFERdose Tablets. 1624
Zantac 150 Tablets 1624
Zantac 300 Tablets 1624
Zantac Injection 1619
Zantac Injection Premixed 1619
Zantac Syrup 1624

RANTEEN (South Africa)
RANITIDINE HYDROCHLORIDE
Zantac 25 EFFERdose Tablets 1624
Zantac 150 EFFERdose Tablets. 1624
Zantac 150 Tablets 1624
Zantac 300 Tablets 1624
Zantac Injection 1619
Zantac Injection Premixed 1619
Zantac Syrup 1624

RANTEX (Venezuela)
LISINOPRIL
Prinivil Tablets 2052

RANUBER (Spain)
RANITIDINE HYDROCHLORIDE
Zantac 25 EFFERdose Tablets 1624
Zantac 150 EFFERdose Tablets. 1624
Zantac 150 Tablets 1624
Zantac 300 Tablets 1624
Zantac Injection 1619
Zantac Injection Premixed 1619
Zantac Syrup 1624

RANZAC (United Kingdom)
RANITIDINE HYDROCHLORIDE
Zantac 25 EFFERdose Tablets 1624

Zantac 150 EFFERdose Tablets. 1624
Zantac 150 Tablets 1624
Zantac 300 Tablets 1624
Zantac Injection 1619
Zantac Injection Premixed 1619
Zantac Syrup 1624

RAPICLAV (India)
AMOXICILLIN
Amoxil Pediatric Drops for Oral
Suspension. 1343
Amoxil Tablets 1343

RASITOL (Malaysia)
FUROSEMIDE
Furosemide Tablets 2154

RATACAND (Italy)
CANDESARTAN CILEXETIL
Atacand Tablets 649

RATACAND PLUS (Italy)
CANDESARTAN CILEXETIL
Atacand Tablets 649

RATHIMED (Germany)
METRONIDAZOLE
MetroGel-Vaginal Gel 1855

RATHIMED N (Germany)
METRONIDAZOLE
MetroGel-Vaginal Gel 1855

RATIC (Singapore)
RANITIDINE HYDROCHLORIDE
Zantac 25 EFFERdose Tablets 1624
Zantac 150 EFFERdose Tablets. 1624
Zantac 150 Tablets 1624
Zantac 300 Tablets 1624
Zantac Injection 1619
Zantac Injection Premixed 1619
Zantac Syrup 1624

RATICINA (Argentina)
RANITIDINE HYDROCHLORIDE
Zantac 25 EFFERdose Tablets 1624
Zantac 150 EFFERdose Tablets. 1624
Zantac 150 Tablets 1624
Zantac 300 Tablets 1624
Zantac Injection 1619
Zantac Injection Premixed 1619
Zantac Syrup 1624

RATIOALLERG (Austria, Germany)
CETIRIZINE HYDROCHLORIDE
Zyrtec Syrup 2594
Zyrtec Tablets 2594

RATIO-IPRA SAL UDV (Canada)
IPRATROPIUM BROMIDE
Atrovent Inhalation Solution 835
Atrovent Nasal Spray 0.03%. 837
Atrovent Nasal Spray 0.06%. 839

RATIO-MPA (Canada)
MEDROXYPROGESTERONE ACETATE
Depo-Medrol Single-Dose Vial 2619

RAUDIL (Mexico)
RANITIDINE HYDROCHLORIDE
Zantac 25 EFFERdose Tablets 1624
Zantac 150 EFFERdose Tablets. 1624
Zantac 150 Tablets 1624
Zantac 300 Tablets 1624
Zantac Injection 1619
Zantac Injection Premixed 1619
Zantac Syrup 1624

RAVALTON (Greece)
CIPROFLOXACIN HYDROCHLORIDE
Ciloxan Ophthalmic Ointment ⊙204, 559
Ciloxan Ophthalmic Solution ⊙206
Cipro Tablets 2977

RAVAMIL (South Africa)
VERAPAMIL HYDROCHLORIDE
Covera-HS Tablets 3139
Verelan PM Extended-Release Capsules,
Controlled-Onset 3106

RAVOTAF (Mexico)
AMOXICILLIN
Amoxil Pediatric Drops for Oral
Suspension. 1343
Amoxil Tablets 1343

RAVOTRIL (Chile)
CLONAZEPAM
Klonopin Tablets 2778

RAXENOL (Mexico)
NAPROXEN
EC-Naprosyn Delayed-Release Tablets. . . . 2761
Naprosyn Suspension. 2761
Naprosyn Tablets 2761

RAYNE (Mexico)
DIAZEPAM
Diastat Rectal Delivery System 3343
Valium Tablets 2819

RAZENE (New Zealand)
CETIRIZINE HYDROCHLORIDE
Zyrtec Syrup 2594
Zyrtec Tablets 2594

REACEL-A (Mexico)
TRETINOIN
Vesanoid Capsules. 2820

REACTINE (Belgium, Canada,
France, Germany, Norway, Spain,
Sweden, The Netherlands)
CETIRIZINE HYDROCHLORIDE
Zyrtec Syrup 2594
Zyrtec Tablets 2594

REACUR (Argentina)
HYDROCORTISONE
Hydrocortone Tablets 1989

REALDIRON (Russia)
INTERFERON ALFA-2B
Intron A for Injection. 3024

REBATEN (Brazil)
PROPRANOLOL HYDROCHLORIDE
Inderal LA Long-Acting Capsules 3429

REBETOL (Austria, Belgium, Brazil,
Chile, Czech Republic, Denmark,
Finland, France, Germany, Greece,
Hong Kong, Hungary, Irish Republic,
Israel, Italy, Malaysia, Norway,
Portugal, Singapore, Spain, Sweden,
Switzerland, Thailand, The
Netherlands, United Kingdom,
Venezuela)
RIBAVIRIN
Virazole for Inhalation Solution 3370

REBETRON (South Africa)
INTERFERON ALFA-2B
Intron A for Injection. 3024

RECA (Spain)
ENALAPRIL MALEATE
Vasotec I.V. Injection 2103

RECAMICINA (Chile)
LEVOFLOXACIN
Levaquin Injection 2384
Levaquin Tablets 2384

REC-DZ (India)
DIAZEPAM
Diastat Rectal Delivery System 3343
Valium Tablets 2819

RECEANT (Greece)
CEFUROXIME SODIUM
Zinacef Injection 1631

RECEPTOZINE (South Africa)
PROMETHAZINE HYDROCHLORIDE
Phenergan Tablets and Suppositories 3440

RECITAL (Israel)
CITALOPRAM HYDROBROMIDE
Celexa Tablets 1176

RECO (Argentina)
RANITIDINE HYDROCHLORIDE
Zantac 25 EFFERdose Tablets 1624
Zantac 150 EFFERdose Tablets. 1624
Zantac 150 Tablets 1624
Zantac 300 Tablets 1624
Zantac Injection 1619
Zantac Injection Premixed 1619
Zantac Syrup 1624

RED AWAY (Canada)
NAPHAZOLINE HYDROCHLORIDE
Albalon Ophthalmic Solution ⊙218

REDAP (Denmark)
ADAPALENE
Differin Gel 1211

REDUCOL (Brazil)
LOVASTATIN
Mevacor Tablets 2021

REDUCTEL (Mexico)
CAPTOPRIL
Captopril Tablets 2149

(⊙ Described in PDR For Ophthalmic Medicines™)

REDUCTIL (Australia, Austria, Belgium, Brazil, Chile, Denmark, Finland, Germany, Greece, Hong Kong, Hungary, Irish Republic, Israel, Italy, Malaysia, New Zealand, Norway, Portugal, Singapore, South Africa, Spain, Sweden, Switzerland, Thailand, The Netherlands, United Kingdom, Venezuela)
SIBUTRAMINE HYDROCHLORIDE
Meridia Capsules **489**

REDUPRES (Spain)
VERAPAMIL HYDROCHLORIDE
Covera-HS Tablets **3139**
Verelan PM Extended-Release Capsules, Controlled-Onset **3106**

REDUPRESS (Brazil)
LOSARTAN POTASSIUM
Cozaar Tablets **1935**

REDUSA (Hong Kong)
PHENTERMINE HYDROCHLORIDE
Adipex-P Capsules **1215**
Adipex-P Tablets **1215**

REDUSCAR (Brazil)
FINASTERIDE
Propecia Tablets **2060**
Proscar Tablets **2067**

REDUSTEROL (Argentina)
SIMVASTATIN
Zocor Tablets **2105**

REDUTEN (Chile)
SIBUTRAMINE HYDROCHLORIDE
Meridia Capsules **489**

REDUTENSIL (Argentina)
VALSARTAN
Diovan Tablets **2193**

REDUXADE (Italy)
SIBUTRAMINE HYDROCHLORIDE
Meridia Capsules **489**

REFENAX COLIRIO (Argentina)
NAPHAZOLINE HYDROCHLORIDE
Albalon Ophthalmic Solution . . . . ⊙**218**

REFOBACIN (Austria, Venezuela)
GENTAMICIN SULFATE
Garamycin Injectable **3014**

REFRAT (Brazil)
MYCOPHENOLATE MOFETIL
CellCept Capsules **2747**
CellCept Oral Suspension **2747**
CellCept Tablets **2747**

REGENESIS (Argentina)
ALENDRONATE SODIUM
Fosamax Tablets **1969**

REGENTAL (Chile)
NIMODIPINE
Nimotop Capsules **749**

REGEPAR (Austria, Switzerland)
SELEGILINE HYDROCHLORIDE
Eldepryl Capsules **3208**

REGIOCAINA (Argentina)
LIDOCAINE
Lidoderm Patch **1118**

REGOMED (Austria)
ENALAPRIL MALEATE
Vasotec I.V. Injection **2103**

REGULACT (Mexico)
LACTULOSE
Kristalose for Oral Solution **1034**

REGULOSE (United Kingdom)
LACTULOSE
Kristalose for Oral Solution **1034**

REJUVA-A (Canada)
TRETINOIN
Vesanoid Capsules **2820**

REKAWAN (Austria, Germany)
POTASSIUM CHLORIDE
K-Dur Extended-Release Tablets **3033**
K-Lor Oral Solution **474**
K-Tab Tablets **475**

RELANIUM (Russia)
DIAZEPAM
Diastat Rectal Delivery System **3343**
Valium Tablets **2819**

RELASAN (Mexico)
DIAZEPAM
Diastat Rectal Delivery System **3343**
Valium Tablets **2819**

RELASTEF (Italy)
TRETINOIN
Vesanoid Capsules **2820**

RELAXYL (India)
DICLOFENAC SODIUM
Voltaren-XR Tablets **2310**
Voltaren Tablets **2307**

RELAXYL PLUS (India)
DICLOFENAC SODIUM
Voltaren Tablets **2307**
Voltaren-XR Tablets **2310**

RELAZEPAM (Mexico)
DIAZEPAM
Diastat Rectal Delivery System **3343**
Valium Tablets **2819**

RELIBERAN (Italy)
CHLORDIAZEPOXIDE HYDROCHLORIDE
Librium Capsules **3347**

RELIPAIN (Greece, Italy)
DICLOFENAC SODIUM
Voltaren Tablets **2307**
Voltaren-XR Tablets **2310**

RELIUM (Russia)
DIAZEPAM
Diastat Rectal Delivery System **3343**
Valium Tablets **2819**

RELOXYL (Italy)
BENZOYL PEROXIDE
Brevoxyl-4 Creamy Wash **3210**
Brevoxyl-4 Gel **3210**
Brevoxyl-8 Creamy Wash **3210**
Brevoxyl-8 Gel **3210**
Triaz Cleanser **1892**
Triaz Gel **1892**

REMAFEN (Hong Kong, Malaysia, Singapore)
DICLOFENAC SODIUM
Voltaren Tablets **2307**
Voltaren-XR Tablets **2310**

REMEDERM HC (Germany)
HYDROCORTISONE
Hydrocortone Tablets **1989**

REMENA (Greece)
CIPROFLOXACIN HYDROCHLORIDE
Ciloxan Ophthalmic Ointment . . . . ⊙**204, 559**
Ciloxan Ophthalmic Solution . . . . ⊙**206**
Cipro Tablets **2977**

REMETHAN (Hong Kong, Malaysia)
DICLOFENAC SODIUM
Voltaren Tablets **2307**
Voltaren-XR Tablets **2310**

REMICADE (Argentina, Australia, Belgium, Brazil, Canada, Chile, Czech Republic, Denmark, Finland, France, Germany, Greece, Hong Kong, Hungary, Irish Republic, Israel, Italy, Japan, Mexico, New Zealand, Norway, Portugal, Russia, Singapore, Spain, Sweden, Switzerland, The Netherlands, United Kingdom, Venezuela)
INFLIXIMAB
Remicade for IV Injection **971**

REMIK (The Netherlands)
RAMIPRIL
Altace Capsules **1702**

REMINAL (Venezuela)
ENALAPRIL MALEATE
Vasotec I.V. Injection **2103**

REMINALET (Venezuela)
ENALAPRIL MALEATE
Vasotec I.V. Injection **2103**

REMITEX (Chile)
CETIRIZINE HYDROCHLORIDE
Zyrtec Syrup **2594**
Zyrtec Tablets **2594**

REMONTAL (Spain)
NIMODIPINE
Nimotop Capsules **749**

RENACIDIN (Argentina)
FINASTERIDE
Propecia Tablets **2060**
Proscar Tablets **2067**

RENALAPRIL (Brazil)
ENALAPRIL MALEATE
Vasotec I.V. Injection **2103**

RENASE (Thailand)
AMILORIDE HYDROCHLORIDE/HYDROCHLOROTHIAZIDE
Moduretic Tablets **2028**

RENATON (Singapore)
ENALAPRIL MALEATE
Vasotec I.V. Injection **2103**

RENCEF (Chile)
LACTULOSE
Kristalose for Oral Solution **1034**

RENEZIDE (South Africa)
HYDROCHLOROTHIAZIDE/TRIAMTERENE
Dyazide Capsules **1423**

RENIDAC (Mexico)
SULINDAC
Clinoril Tablets **1924**

RENIPRESS (Brazil)
ENALAPRIL MALEATE
Vasotec I.V. Injection **2103**

RENIPRIL (Portugal)
ENALAPRIL MALEATE
Vasotec I.V. Injection **2103**

RENIPRIL PLUS (Portugal)
ENALAPRIL MALEATE
Vasotec I.V. Injection **2103**

RENISTAD (Austria)
ENALAPRIL MALEATE
Vasotec I.V. Injection **2103**

RENITEC (Argentina, Australia, Belgium, Czech Republic, Denmark, France, Greece, Hong Kong, Hungary, Malaysia, Mexico, New Zealand, Portugal, Russia, Singapore, South Africa, Thailand, The Netherlands, Venezuela)
ENALAPRIL MALEATE
Vasotec I.V. Injection **2103**

RENITEC PLUS (Australia, Hungary)
ENALAPRIL MALEATE
Vasotec I.V. Injection **2103**

RENOTENS (South Africa)
LISINOPRIL
Prinivil Tablets **2052**

RENOVA (Canada, Malaysia, South Africa, Thailand)
TRETINOIN
Vesanoid Capsules **2820**

RENOXACIN (Italy)
NORFLOXACIN
Noroxin Tablets **2032**

REOPRO (Argentina, Australia, Austria, Belgium, Brazil, Canada, Chile, Czech Republic, Denmark, Finland, France, Germany, Greece, Hong Kong, India, Irish Republic, Israel, Italy, Malaysia, Mexico, New Zealand, Norway, Russia, Singapore, South Africa, Spain, Sweden, Switzerland, Thailand, The Netherlands, United Kingdom)
ABCIXIMAB
ReoPro Vials **1809**

REPLASYN (Argentina)
ESTRADIOL
Climara Transdermal System **771**
Estring Vaginal Ring **2635**

REPLIGEN (Argentina)
METRONIDAZOLE
MetroGel-Vaginal Gel **1855**

REPRIADOL (Denmark)
MORPHINE SULFATE
Kadian Capsules **577**
MS Contin Tablets **2701**

REPROST (Chile)
NAPROXEN
EC-Naprosyn Delayed-Release Tablets **2761**
Naprosyn Suspension **2761**
Naprosyn Tablets **2761**

REQUIP (Argentina, Austria, Belgium, Canada, Chile, Czech Republic, Denmark, Finland, France, Germany, Greece, Hong Kong, Hungary, Irish Republic, Israel, Italy, Malaysia, New Zealand, Norway, Portugal, Singapore, South Africa, Spain, Sweden, Switzerland, The Netherlands, United Kingdom)
ROPINIROLE HYDROCHLORIDE
Requip Tablets **1555**

RESIMIDA (Venezuela)
FUROSEMIDE
Furosemide Tablets **2154**

RESINSODIO (Singapore, Spain)
SODIUM POLYSTYRENE SULFONATE
Kionex Powder **2477**

RESMA (Belgium)
ZAFIRLUKAST
Accolate Tablets **671**

RESONIUM (Denmark, Finland, Portugal, Sweden)
SODIUM POLYSTYRENE SULFONATE
Kionex Powder **2477**

RESONIUM A (Australia, Austria, Germany, Hong Kong, Hungary, Irish Republic, Malaysia, New Zealand, Switzerland, Thailand, The Netherlands, United Kingdom)
SODIUM POLYSTYRENE SULFONATE
Kionex Powder **2477**

RESOSTYL (Greece)
SELEGILINE HYDROCHLORIDE
Eldepryl Capsules **3208**

RESPEXIL (Brazil)
NORFLOXACIN
Noroxin Tablets **2032**

RESPICORT (Switzerland)
TRIAMCINOLONE ACETONIDE
Azmacort Inhalation Aerosol **1726**
Nasacort AQ Nasal Spray **2922**

RESPICUR (Austria, Italy)
THEOPHYLLINE
Uniphyl Tablets **2710**

RESPIDUAL (Venezuela)
IPRATROPIUM BROMIDE
Atrovent Inhalation Solution **835**
Atrovent Nasal Spray 0.03% **837**
Atrovent Nasal Spray 0.06% **839**

RESPONTIN (Norway, United Kingdom)
IPRATROPIUM BROMIDE
Atrovent Inhalation Solution **835**
Atrovent Nasal Spray 0.03% **837**
Atrovent Nasal Spray 0.06% **839**

RESTELEA (Argentina)
RISPERIDONE
Risperdal Oral Solution **1676**
Risperdal Tablets **1676**

RESTOPON (Greece)
RANITIDINE HYDROCHLORIDE
Zantac 25 EFFERdose Tablets **1624**
Zantac 150 EFFERdose Tablets **1624**
Zantac 150 Tablets **1624**
Zantac 300 Tablets **1624**
Zantac Injection **1619**
Zantac Injection Premixed **1619**
Zantac Syrup **1624**

RETACNYL (Argentina, Brazil, Chile, France, Hong Kong, Malaysia, Mexico, Singapore, South Africa, Thailand, Venezuela)
TRETINOIN
Vesanoid Capsules **2820**

RETAFYLLIN (Finland, Hungary, Malaysia, Singapore, Thailand)
THEOPHYLLINE
Uniphyl Tablets **2710**

RETALZEM (Hong Kong)
DILTIAZEM HYDROCHLORIDE
Cardizem LA Extended Release Tablets . . . **1728**
Tiazac Capsules **1201**

RETAMIN (Venezuela)
RANITIDINE HYDROCHLORIDE
Zantac 25 EFFERdose Tablets **1624**

Zantac 150 EFFERdose Tablets. 1624
Zantac 150 Tablets 1624
Zantac 300 Tablets 1624
Zantac Injection 1619
Zantac Injection Premixed 1619
Zantac Syrup 1624

RET-A-PRES (Mexico)
TRETINOIN
Vesanoid Capsules. 2820

RETAVIT (Israel)
TRETINOIN
Vesanoid Capsules. 2820

RETCIN (United Kingdom)
ERYTHROMYCIN
Ery-Tab Tablets 449
Erythromycin Base Filmtab Tablets. 455
Erythromycin Delayed-Release Capsules, USP 457
PCE Dispertab Tablets 515

RETEP (Argentina)
FUROSEMIDE
Furosemide Tablets 2154

RETICNE (Argentina)
TRETINOIN
Vesanoid Capsules. 2820

RETIN-A (Argentina, Australia, Austria, Brazil, Canada, Chile, Czech Republic, France, Hong Kong, Irish Republic, Israel, Italy, Malaysia, Mexico, New Zealand, Portugal, Singapore, South Africa, Switzerland, Thailand, United Kingdom)
TRETINOIN
Vesanoid Capsules. 2820

RETINEI (Venezuela)
TRETINOIN
Vesanoid Capsules. 2820

RETINIDE (Argentina)
ISOTRETINOIN
Accutane Capsules 2731

RETINOVA (Belgium, Brazil, Denmark, France, New Zealand, Singapore, Spain, Sweden, United Kingdom)
TRETINOIN
Vesanoid Capsules. 2820

RETIRIDES (Spain)
TRETINOIN
Vesanoid Capsules. 2820

RETISOL-A (Canada)
TRETINOIN
Vesanoid Capsules. 2820

RETITOP (France)
TRETINOIN
Vesanoid Capsules. 2820

RETOFAR (Mexico)
METRONIDAZOLE
MetroGel-Vaginal Gel 1855

RETRIEVE (Australia, Hong Kong)
TRETINOIN
Vesanoid Capsules. 2820

RETROVIR (Argentina, Australia, Austria, Belgium, Brazil, Canada, Chile, Czech Republic, Denmark, Finland, France, Germany, Greece, Hong Kong, India, Irish Republic, Israel, Italy, Malaysia, Mexico, New Zealand, Norway, Portugal, Russia, Singapore, South Africa, Spain, Sweden, Switzerland, Thailand, The Netherlands, United Kingdom, Venezuela)
ZIDOVUDINE
Retrovir Capsules 1560
Retrovir IV Infusion. 1564
Retrovir Syrup 1560
Retrovir Tablets. 1560

REUCORTIL (Mexico)
NAPROXEN
EC-Naprosyn Delayed-Release Tablets. . . . 2761
Naprosyn Suspension. 2761
Naprosyn Tablets 2761

REUFLOS (Italy)
DIFLUNISAL
Dolobid Tablets. 1955

REUMAREN (Brazil)
DICLOFENAC SODIUM
Voltaren Tablets 2307
Voltaren-XR Tablets 2310

REUMYL (Italy)
SULINDAC
Clinoril Tablets 1924

REUSAN (Mexico)
DEXAMETHASONE
Decadron Tablets 1951

REUXEN (Portugal)
NAPROXEN
EC-Naprosyn Delayed-Release Tablets. . . . 2761
Naprosyn Suspension. 2761
Naprosyn Tablets 2761

REVALINTABS (The Netherlands)
CETIRIZINE HYDROCHLORIDE
Zyrtec Syrup 2594
Zyrtec Tablets 2594

REVANGE (Brazil)
ISOSORBIDE MONONITRATE
Imdur Tablets 3018

REVASTIN (Brazil)
SIMVASTATIN
Zocor Tablets 2105

REVATIO (United Kingdom)
SILDENAFIL CITRATE
Viagra Tablets 2573

REVECTINA (Brazil)
IVERMECTIN
Stromectol Tablets. 2083

REVELLEX (Argentina, South Africa)
INFLIXIMAB
Remicade for IV Injection. 971

REVELOL (India)
METOPROLOL SUCCINATE
Toprol-XL Tablets 668

REVION (Greece)
CIPROFLOXACIN HYDROCHLORIDE
Ciloxan Ophthalmic Ointment . . . . ⊙204, 559
Ciloxan Ophthalmic Solution . . . . ⊙206
Cipro Tablets 2977

REVIRAX (Brazil)
ZIDOVUDINE
Retrovir Capsules 1560
Retrovir IV Infusion. 1564
Retrovir Syrup 1560
Retrovir Tablets. 1560

REWODINA (Czech Republic, Germany)
DICLOFENAC SODIUM
Voltaren Tablets 2307
Voltaren-XR Tablets 2310

REXACIN (Hong Kong, Thailand)
NORFLOXACIN
Noroxin Tablets. 2032

REXAMAT (Argentina)
CALCITRIOL
Calcijex Injection 411
Rocaltrol Capsules. 2798
Rocaltrol Oral Solution 2798

REXETIN (Russia)
PAROXETINE HYDROCHLORIDE
Paxil Oral Suspension. 1530
Paxil Tablets. 1530

REXGENTA (Spain)
GENTAMICIN SULFATE
Garamycin Injectable 3014

REXIGEN (South Africa)
PROPRANOLOL HYDROCHLORIDE
Inderal LA Long-Acting Capsules 3429

REXNER (Argentina)
CIPROFLOXACIN HYDROCHLORIDE
Ciloxan Ophthalmic Ointment . . . . ⊙204, 559
Ciloxan Ophthalmic Solution . . . . ⊙206
Cipro Tablets 2977

REZAMID (Argentina)
TRIAMCINOLONE ACETONIDE
Azmacort Inhalation Aerosol. 1726
Nasacort AQ Nasal Spray 2922

REZAMID D, REZAMID F, REZAMID M (Argentina)
TRIAMCINOLONE ACETONIDE
Azmacort Inhalation Aerosol. 1726
Nasacort AQ Nasal Spray 2922

REZULT (India)
ROSIGLITAZONE MALEATE
Avandia Tablets. 1384

RFG-KIT (Argentina)
FLUORESCEIN SODIUM
Fluorescite Injection . . . . ⊙207

R-FLEX (South Africa)
SULINDAC
Clinoril Tablets 1924

RHEFLUIN (Czech Republic, Germany, Switzerland)
AMILORIDE HYDROCHLORIDE
Midamor Tablets 2026

RHEMOFENAX (Hong Kong)
DICLOFENAC SODIUM
Voltaren Tablets 2307
Voltaren-XR Tablets 2310

RHEUFENAC (Switzerland)
DICLOFENAC SODIUM
Voltaren Tablets 2307
Voltaren-XR Tablets 2310

RHEUFLEX (United Kingdom)
NAPROXEN
EC-Naprosyn Delayed-Release Tablets. . . . 2761
Naprosyn Suspension. 2761
Naprosyn Tablets 2761

RHEUMABENE (Austria)
DICLOFENAC SODIUM
Voltaren Tablets 2307
Voltaren-XR Tablets 2310

RHEUMASAN D (Germany)
DICLOFENAC SODIUM
Voltaren Tablets 2307
Voltaren-XR Tablets 2310

RHEUMATAC (United Kingdom)
DICLOFENAC SODIUM
Voltaren Tablets 2307
Voltaren-XR Tablets 2310

RHEUMAVEK (Greece)
DICLOFENAC SODIUM
Voltaren Tablets 2307
Voltaren-XR Tablets 2310

RHEWLIN (Malaysia)
DICLOFENAC SODIUM
Voltaren Tablets 2307
Voltaren-XR Tablets 2310

RHINALAR (Australia, Canada, Hong Kong)
FLUNISOLIDE
Aerobid Inhaler System. 1171
Aerobid-M Inhaler System 1171

RHINARIS-F (Canada)
FLUNISOLIDE
Aerobid Inhaler System. 1171
Aerobid-M Inhaler System 1171

RHINEX (Germany)
NAPHAZOLINE HYDROCHLORIDE
Albalon Ophthalmic Solution . . . . ⊙218

RHINISAN (Germany)
TRIAMCINOLONE ACETONIDE
Azmacort Inhalation Aerosol. 1726
Nasacort AQ Nasal Spray 2922

RHINOGEN (Switzerland)
SODIUM HYALURONATE
Hyalgan Solution 2901

RHINOLAST (Irish Republic, Israel, New Zealand, South Africa, United Kingdom)
AZELASTINE HYDROCHLORIDE
Astelin Nasal Spray 1904

RHINO-MEX-N (Canada)
NAPHAZOLINE HYDROCHLORIDE
Albalon Ophthalmic Solution . . . . ⊙218

RHINON (Austria)
NAPHAZOLINE HYDROCHLORIDE
Albalon Ophthalmic Solution . . . . ⊙218

RHINOPERD (Austria)
NAPHAZOLINE HYDROCHLORIDE
Albalon Ophthalmic Solution . . . . ⊙218

RHINOVENT (Switzerland)
IPRATROPIUM BROMIDE
Atrovent Inhalation Solution 835
Atrovent Nasal Spray 0.03%. 837
Atrovent Nasal Spray 0.06%. 839

RHIZIN (Singapore)
CETIRIZINE HYDROCHLORIDE
Zyrtec Syrup 2594
Zyrtec Tablets 2594

RHODIALAX (Canada)
LACTULOSE
Kristalose for Oral Solution 1034

RHODIALOSE (Canada)
LACTULOSE
Kristalose for Oral Solution 1034

RHODIAPROX (Canada)
NAPROXEN
EC-Naprosyn Delayed-Release Tablets. . . . 2761
Naprosyn Suspension. 2761
Naprosyn Tablets 2761

RHONURACIL (Mexico)
FLUOROURACIL
Efudex Topical Cream. 3363
Efudex Topical Solutions 3363

RHOTARD (United Kingdom)
MORPHINE SULFATE
Kadian Capsules 577
MS Contin Tablets 2701

RHUMALGAN (Switzerland, United Kingdom)
DICLOFENAC SODIUM
Voltaren Tablets 2307
Voltaren-XR Tablets 2310

RHUMANTIN (Denmark)
PENICILLAMINE
Cuprimine Capsules 1947

RHYTHMOCOR (Austria)
PROPAFENONE HYDROCHLORIDE
Rythmol SR Capsules 2727

RIATUL (Argentina)
RISPERIDONE
Risperdal Oral Solution 1676
Risperdal Tablets. 1676

RIBASTAMIN (Argentina)
RISEDRONATE SODIUM
Actonel Tablets 2683

RIBATRA (Argentina)
CLOBETASOL PROPIONATE
Temovate Cream. 2668
Temovate E Emollient. 2671
Temovate Gel. 2669
Temovate Ointment 2668
Temovate Scalp Application 2670

RIBAV (Brazil)
RIBAVIRIN
Virazole for Inhalation Solution 3370

RIBAVIN (India)
RIBAVIRIN
Virazole for Inhalation Solution 3370

RIBAVIRON C (Brazil)
RIBAVIRIN
Virazole for Inhalation Solution 3370

RIBEX FLU (Italy)
DICLOFENAC SODIUM
Voltaren Tablets 2307
Voltaren-XR Tablets 2310

RIBOFLUOR (Germany)
FLUOROURACIL
Efudex Topical Cream. 3363
Efudex Topical Solutions 3363

RIBOLIN (Greece)
RANITIDINE HYDROCHLORIDE
Zantac 25 EFFERdose Tablets 1624
Zantac 150 EFFERdose Tablets. 1624
Zantac 150 Tablets 1624
Zantac 300 Tablets 1624
Zantac Injection 1619
Zantac Injection Premixed 1619
Zantac Syrup 1624

RIBOMICIN (Italy)
GENTAMICIN SULFATE
Garamycin Injectable 3014

RIDAL (Venezuela)
RISPERIDONE
Risperdal Oral Solution 1676
Risperdal Tablets. 1676

RIDAZIN (Israel)
THIORIDAZINE HYDROCHLORIDE
Thioridazine Hydrochloride Tablets. 2163

RIDAZINE (South Africa, Thailand)
THIORIDAZINE HYDROCHLORIDE
Thioridazine Hydrochloride Tablets **2163**

RIDRON (Argentina)
RISEDRONATE SODIUM
Actonel Tablets **2683**

RIDRON PACK (Argentina)
RISEDRONATE SODIUM
Actonel Tablets **2683**

RIFAXI (Argentina)
RITONAVIR
Norvir Oral Solution **503**
Norvir Soft Gelatin Capsules **503**

RIGIX (Austria)
CETIRIZINE HYDROCHLORIDE
Zyrtec Syrup **2594**
Zyrtec Tablets **2594**

RILATINE (Belgium)
METHYLPHENIDATE HYDROCHLORIDE
Ritalin Hydrochloride Tablets **2269**
Ritalin-SR Tablets **2269**

RILCAPTON (Hong Kong, Russia, Singapore)
CAPTOPRIL
Captopril Tablets **2149**

RILUTEK (Argentina, Australia, Austria, Belgium, Brazil, Canada, Chile, Czech Republic, Denmark, Finland, France, Germany, Greece, Hong Kong, Hungary, Irish Republic, Israel, Italy, Japan, Mexico, Norway, Portugal, Singapore, South Africa, Spain, Sweden, Switzerland, Thailand, The Netherlands, United Kingdom, Venezuela)
RILUZOLE
Rilutek Tablets **2930**

RIMAPAM (United Kingdom)
DIAZEPAM
Diastat Rectal Delivery System **3343**
Valium Tablets **2819**

RIMIDOL (Sweden)
NAPHAZOLINE HYDROCHLORIDE
Albalon Ophthalmic Solution . . . . **⊙218**

RIMOXYN (United Kingdom)
NAPROXEN
EC-Naprosyn Delayed-Release Tablets **2761**
Naprosyn Suspension **2761**
Naprosyn Tablets **2761**

RINALIX (Malaysia, Singapore)
INDAPAMIDE
Indapamide Tablets **2156**

RINATEC (Irish Republic, United Kingdom)
IPRATROPIUM BROMIDE
Atrovent Inhalation Solution **835**
Atrovent Nasal Spray 0.03% **837**
Atrovent Nasal Spray 0.06% **839**

RINELON (Italy, Mexico, South Africa, Spain, Thailand)
MOMETASONE FUROATE
Elocon Cream 0.1% **3005**
Elocon Lotion 0.1% **3006**
Elocon Ointment 0.1% **3007**
Nasonex Nasal Spray **3043**

RINIDYL DN (Mexico)
DEXAMETHASONE
Decadron Tablets **1951**

RINISONA (Argentina)
FLUTICASONE PROPIONATE
Cutivate Cream **2662**
Cutivate Ointment **2665**
Flonase Nasal Spray **1440**

RINO NAFTAZOLINA (Italy)
NAPHAZOLINE HYDROCHLORIDE
Albalon Ophthalmic Solution . . . . **⊙218**

RINO-AZETIN (Brazil)
AZELASTINE HYDROCHLORIDE
Astelin Nasal Spray **1904**

RINOBEREN (Spain)
IPRATROPIUM BROMIDE
Atrovent Inhalation Solution **835**
Atrovent Nasal Spray 0.03% **837**
Atrovent Nasal Spray 0.06% **839**

RINO-LASTIN (Brazil)
AZELASTINE HYDROCHLORIDE
Astelin Nasal Spray **1904**

RINOS-A (Brazil)
NAPHAZOLINE HYDROCHLORIDE
Albalon Ophthalmic Solution . . . . **⊙218**

RINOSONE (Spain)
FLUTICASONE PROPIONATE
Cutivate Cream **2662**
Cutivate Ointment **2665**
Flonase Nasal Spray **1440**

RINOVAGOS (Italy)
IPRATROPIUM BROMIDE
Atrovent Inhalation Solution **835**
Atrovent Nasal Spray 0.03% **837**
Atrovent Nasal Spray 0.06% **839**

RINOVAL (Chile)
MOMETASONE FUROATE
Elocon Cream 0.1% **3005**
Elocon Lotion 0.1% **3006**
Elocon Ointment 0.1% **3007**
Nasonex Nasal Spray **3043**

RINSTEAD TEETHING GEL (United Kingdom)
LIDOCAINE
Lidoderm Patch **1118**

RIPHENIDATE (Canada)
METHYLPHENIDATE HYDROCHLORIDE
Ritalin Hydrochloride Tablets **2269**
Ritalin-SR Tablets **2269**

RISEDON (Argentina)
RISEDRONATE SODIUM
Actonel Tablets **2683**

RISELLE (Brazil, Czech Republic)
ESTRADIOL
Climara Transdermal System **771**
Estring Vaginal Ring **2635**

RISNIA (India)
RISPERIDONE
Risperdal Oral Solution **1676**
Risperdal Tablets **1676**

RISOFOS (India)
RISEDRONATE SODIUM
Actonel Tablets **2683**

RISPEN (Czech Republic)
RISPERIDONE
Risperdal Oral Solution **1676**
Risperdal Tablets **1676**

RISPER (Argentina)
RISPERIDONE
Risperdal Oral Solution **1676**
Risperdal Tablets **1676**

RISPERDAL (Argentina, Australia, Austria, Belgium, Brazil, Chile, Czech Republic, Denmark, Finland, Greece, Hong Kong, Hungary, India, Irish Republic, Israel, Italy, Japan, Malaysia, Mexico, New Zealand, Norway, Portugal, Singapore, South Africa, Spain, Switzerland, Thailand, The Netherlands, United Kingdom, Venezuela)
RISPERIDONE
Risperdal Oral Solution **1676**
Risperdal Tablets **1676**

RISPERID (Venezuela)
RISPERIDONE
Risperdal Oral Solution **1676**
Risperdal Tablets **1676**

RISPERIN (Argentina)
RISPERIDONE
Risperdal Oral Solution **1676**
Risperdal Tablets **1676**

RISPEX (Argentina)
RISPERIDONE
Risperdal Oral Solution **1676**
Risperdal Tablets **1676**

RISPID (India)
RISPERIDONE
Risperdal Oral Solution **1676**
Risperdal Tablets **1676**

RISPOLEPT (Russia)
RISPERIDONE
Risperdal Oral Solution **1676**
Risperdal Tablets **1676**

RISPOLIN (Austria)
RISPERIDONE
Risperdal Oral Solution **1676**
Risperdal Tablets **1676**

RISTALEN (Spain)
ENALAPRIL MALEATE
Vasotec I.V. Injection **2103**

RISTO (Thailand)
TRIAMCINOLONE ACETONIDE
Azmacort Inhalation Aerosol **1726**
Nasacort AQ Nasal Spray **2922**

RITALIN (Australia, Austria, Canada, Chile, Czech Republic, Denmark, Germany, Hong Kong, Hungary, Irish Republic, Israel, Malaysia, Mexico, New Zealand, Norway, Singapore, South Africa, The Netherlands, United Kingdom, Venezuela)
METHYLPHENIDATE HYDROCHLORIDE
Ritalin Hydrochloride Tablets **2269**
Ritalin-SR Tablets **2269**

RITALINA (Argentina, Brazil, Portugal)
METHYLPHENIDATE HYDROCHLORIDE
Ritalin Hydrochloride Tablets **2269**
Ritalin-SR Tablets **2269**

RITALINE (France, Greece, Switzerland)
METHYLPHENIDATE HYDROCHLORIDE
Ritalin Hydrochloride Tablets **2269**
Ritalin-SR Tablets **2269**

RITAPHEN (South Africa)
METHYLPHENIDATE HYDROCHLORIDE
Ritalin Hydrochloride Tablets **2269**
Ritalin-SR Tablets **2269**

RITECHOL (Irish Republic)
SIMVASTATIN
Zocor Tablets **2105**

RITHROPROL (Greece)
CLARITHROMYCIN
Biaxin Filmtab Tablets **402**
Biaxin Granules **402**

RITMENAL (Chile)
GABAPENTIN
Neurontin Capsules **2487**

RITMETOL (Hungary)
METOPROLOL TARTRATE
Lopressor Tablets **2238**

RITMOCOR (Chile)
PROPAFENONE HYDROCHLORIDE
Rythmol SR Capsules **2727**

RITMOLOL (Mexico)
METOPROLOL TARTRATE
Lopressor Tablets **2238**

RITMONORM (Brazil)
PROPAFENONE HYDROCHLORIDE
Rythmol SR Capsules **2727**

RITOMUNE (India)
RITONAVIR
Norvir Oral Solution **503**
Norvir Soft Gelatin Capsules **503**

RITOVIR (Brazil)
RITONAVIR
Norvir Oral Solution **503**
Norvir Soft Gelatin Capsules **503**

RITROCEL (Chile)
METHYLPHENIDATE HYDROCHLORIDE
Ritalin Hydrochloride Tablets **2269**
Ritalin-SR Tablets **2269**

RITROMINE (Argentina)
NORFLOXACIN
Noroxin Tablets **2032**

RITUXAN (Canada, Japan)
RITUXIMAB
Rituxan I.V. **1254**

RIUCLONAZ (Argentina)
CLONAZEPAM
Klonopin Tablets **2778**

RIVATRIL (Finland)
CLONAZEPAM
Klonopin Tablets **2778**

RIVAZOL (Mexico)
ALBENDAZOLE
Albenza Tablets **1338**

RIVERVAN (Argentina)
VANCOMYCIN HYDROCHLORIDE
Vancocin HCl Capsules, USP **3380**

RIVILINA (Argentina)
APROTININ
Trasylol Injection **754**

RIVOSTATIN (Switzerland)
NYSTATIN
Nystop Topical Powder USP **2478**
Paddock Nystatin USP for Oral Suspension **2478**

RIVOTRIL (Argentina, Australia, Austria, Belgium, Brazil, Canada, Czech Republic, Denmark, France, Germany, Hong Kong, Hungary, Irish Republic, Israel, Italy, Mexico, New Zealand, Norway, Portugal, Singapore, South Africa, Spain, Switzerland, Thailand, The Netherlands, United Kingdom, Venezuela)
CLONAZEPAM
Klonopin Tablets **2778**

RIVOXICILLIN (Switzerland)
AMOXICILLIN
Amoxil Pediatric Drops for Oral Suspension **1343**
Amoxil Tablets **1343**

RIZACT (India)
RIZATRIPTAN BENZOATE
Maxalt Tablets **2008**
Maxalt-MLT Orally Disintegrating Tablets . . **2008**

RIZALIEF (Austria)
RIZATRIPTAN BENZOATE
Maxalt Tablets **2008**
Maxalt-MLT Orally Disintegrating Tablets . . **2008**

RIZALIV (Italy)
RIZATRIPTAN BENZOATE
Maxalt Tablets **2008**
Maxalt-MLT Orally Disintegrating Tablets . . **2008**

R-LOC (India)
RANITIDINE HYDROCHLORIDE
Zantac 25 EFFERdose Tablets **1624**
Zantac 150 EFFERdose Tablets **1624**
Zantac 150 Tablets **1624**
Zantac 300 Tablets **1624**
Zantac Injection **1619**
Zantac Injection Premixed **1619**
Zantac Syrup **1624**

RMS (New Zealand)
MORPHINE SULFATE
Kadian Capsules **577**
MS Contin Tablets **2701**

ROACCUTAN (Argentina, Austria, Denmark, Finland, Germany, Hungary, Italy, Mexico, Portugal, Venezuela)
ISOTRETINOIN
Accutane Capsules **2731**

ROACCUTANE (Australia, Belgium, Czech Republic, France, Greece, Hong Kong, Irish Republic, Israel, New Zealand, Singapore, South Africa, Switzerland, Thailand, The Netherlands, United Kingdom)
ISOTRETINOIN
Accutane Capsules **2731**

ROACNETAN (Chile)
ISOTRETINOIN
Accutane Capsules **2731**

ROACUTAN (Brazil, Spain)
ISOTRETINOIN
Accutane Capsules **2731**

ROBAZ (Greece, Thailand)
METRONIDAZOLE
MetroGel-Vaginal Gel **1855**

ROCALTROL (Australia, Austria, Belgium, Brazil, Canada, Chile, Czech Republic, Denmark, France, Germany, Hong Kong, Hungary, Irish Republic, Italy, Japan, Mexico, New Zealand, Norway, Portugal, Singapore, South Africa, Spain, Sweden, Switzerland, Thailand, The Netherlands, United Kingdom, Venezuela)
CALCITRIOL
Calcijex Injection **411**
Rocaltrol Capsules **2798**
Rocaltrol Oral Solution **2798**

ROCEFALIN (Spain)
CEFTRIAXONE SODIUM
Rocephin Injectable Vials, ADD-Vantage, Galaxy, Bulk . . . 2800

ROCEFIN (Brazil, Italy)
CEFTRIAXONE SODIUM
Rocephin Injectable Vials, ADD-Vantage, Galaxy, Bulk . . . 2800

ROCEPHALIN (Denmark, Finland, Norway, Sweden)
CEFTRIAXONE SODIUM
Rocephin Injectable Vials, ADD-Vantage, Galaxy, Bulk . . . 2800

ROCEPHIN (Australia, Austria, Canada, Czech Republic, Germany, Greece, Hong Kong, Hungary, Irish Republic, Israel, Japan, Mexico, New Zealand, Portugal, Singapore, South Africa, Thailand, The Netherlands, United Kingdom, Venezuela)
CEFTRIAXONE SODIUM
Rocephin Injectable Vials, ADD-Vantage, Galaxy, Bulk . . . 2800

ROCEPHINE (Belgium, France, Switzerland)
CEFTRIAXONE SODIUM
Rocephin Injectable Vials, ADD-Vantage, Galaxy, Bulk . . . 2800

ROCHE (Canada)
NAPROXEN SODIUM
Anaprox DS Tablets . . . 2761
Anaprox Tablets . . . 2761

RODERMIL (Portugal)
METRONIDAZOLE
MetroGel-Vaginal Gel . . . 1855

RODINAC BIOTIC (Argentina)
AMOXICILLIN
Amoxil Pediatric Drops for Oral Suspension . . . 1343
Amoxil Tablets . . . 1343

ROFANTEN (Spain)
NAPROXEN
EC-Naprosyn Delayed-Release Tablets . . . 2761
Naprosyn Suspension . . . 2761
Naprosyn Tablets . . . 2761

ROFLUAL (France)
RIMANTADINE HYDROCHLORIDE
Flumadine Syrup . . . 1183
Flumadine Tablets . . . 1183

ROFOXIN (Brazil)
CEFTRIAXONE SODIUM
Rocephin Injectable Vials, ADD-Vantage, Galaxy, Bulk . . . 2800

ROFY (Thailand)
TRAMADOL HYDROCHLORIDE
Ultram ER Tablets . . . 2392

ROGASTI (Israel)
FAMOTIDINE
Pepcid Injection . . . 2040
Pepcid Injection Premixed . . . 2040
Pepcid Tablets . . . 2038
Pepcid for Oral Suspension . . . 2038

RO-GENTYCIN (Canada)
GENTAMICIN SULFATE
Garamycin Injectable . . . 3014

ROGLIN (India)
ROSIGLITAZONE MALEATE
Avandia Tablets . . . 1384

ROGLIN-M (India)
ROSIGLITAZONE MALEATE
Avandia Tablets . . . 1384

ROICAL (Malaysia, Singapore)
CALCITRIOL
Calcijex Injection . . . 411
Rocaltrol Capsules . . . 2798
Rocaltrol Oral Solution . . . 2798

ROLAB-AMOCLAV (South Africa)
AMOXICILLIN
Amoxil Pediatric Drops for Oral Suspension . . . 1343
Amoxil Tablets . . . 1343

ROLICYTIN (Mexico)
CLARITHROMYCIN
Biaxin Filmtab Tablets . . . 402
Biaxin Granules . . . 402

ROLSICAL (India)
CALCITRIOL
Calcijex Injection . . . 411
Rocaltrol Capsules . . . 2798
Rocaltrol Oral Solution . . . 2798

ROMAKEN (Mexico)
TERAZOSIN HYDROCHLORIDE
Hytrin Capsules . . . 471

ROMALINA (Venezuela)
NYSTATIN
Nystop Topical Powder USP . . . 2478
Paddock Nystatin USP for Oral Suspension . . . 2478

ROMESA (Mexico)
WARFARIN SODIUM
Coumadin Tablets . . . 898
Coumadin for Injection . . . 898

ROMIR (Mexico)
CAPTOPRIL
Captopril Tablets . . . 2149

ROMMIX (United Kingdom)
ERYTHROMYCIN
Ery-Tab Tablets . . . 449
Erythromycin Base Filmtab Tablets . . . 455
Erythromycin Delayed-Release Capsules, USP . . . 457
PCE Dispertab Tablets . . . 515

RONABIN (Israel)
DRONABINOL
Marinol Capsules . . . 3333

RO-NAPHZ (Canada)
NAPHAZOLINE HYDROCHLORIDE
Albalon Ophthalmic Solution . . . ⊙218

RONIC (Portugal)
DEXAMETHASONE
Decadron Tablets . . . 1951

RONMIX (United Kingdom)
ERYTHROMYCIN
Ery-Tab Tablets . . . 449
Erythromycin Base Filmtab Tablets . . . 455
Erythromycin Delayed-Release Capsules, USP . . . 457
PCE Dispertab Tablets . . . 515

RONTAGEL (Argentina)
ESTRADIOL
Climara Transdermal System . . . 771
Estring Vaginal Ring . . . 2635

RONTILONA (Portugal, Spain)
FLUTICASONE PROPIONATE
Cutivate Cream . . . 2662
Cutivate Ointment . . . 2665
Flonase Nasal Spray . . . 1440

ROPRIL (Hong Kong)
CAPTOPRIL
Captopril Tablets . . . 2149

ROPSIL (Chile)
CLONAZEPAM
Klonopin Tablets . . . 2778

ROSAGENUS (Greece)
FAMOTIDINE
Pepcid Injection . . . 2040
Pepcid Injection Premixed . . . 2040
Pepcid Tablets . . . 2038
Pepcid for Oral Suspension . . . 2038

ROSALOX (Czech Republic, Switzerland)
METRONIDAZOLE
MetroGel-Vaginal Gel . . . 1855

ROSAMET (Russia)
METRONIDAZOLE
MetroGel-Vaginal Gel . . . 1855

ROSASED (Italy)
METRONIDAZOLE
MetroGel-Vaginal Gel . . . 1855

ROSASOL (Canada)
METRONIDAZOLE
MetroGel-Vaginal Gel . . . 1855

ROSAZOL (Finland)
METRONIDAZOLE
MetroGel-Vaginal Gel . . . 1855

ROSICED (France, The Netherlands)
METRONIDAZOLE
MetroGel-Vaginal Gel . . . 1855

ROSICON (India)
ROSIGLITAZONE MALEATE
Avandia Tablets . . . 1384

ROSICON MF (India)
ROSIGLITAZONE MALEATE
Avandia Tablets . . . 1384

ROSIL (Thailand)
CLINDAMYCIN HYDROCHLORIDE
Cleocin Vaginal Ovules . . . 2616

ROSITAL (Greece)
NIMODIPINE
Nimotop Capsules . . . 749

ROTHONAL (Greece)
RANITIDINE HYDROCHLORIDE
Zantac 25 EFFERdose Tablets . . . 1624
Zantac 150 EFFERdose Tablets . . . 1624
Zantac 150 Tablets . . . 1624
Zantac 300 Tablets . . . 1624
Zantac Injection . . . 1619
Zantac Injection Premixed . . . 1619
Zantac Syrup . . . 1624

ROTIAZ (Argentina)
TERAZOSIN HYDROCHLORIDE
Hytrin Capsules . . . 471

ROUG-MYCIN (Greece)
ERYTHROMYCIN STEARATE
Erythrocin Stearate Filmtab Tablets . . . 453

ROVACOR (India, Russia, Singapore)
LOVASTATIN
Mevacor Tablets . . . 2021

ROWESTIN (Venezuela)
SIMVASTATIN
Zocor Tablets . . . 2105

ROXATINE (Australia)
PAROXETINE HYDROCHLORIDE
Paxil Oral Suspension . . . 1530
Paxil Tablets . . . 1530

ROXEN (Thailand)
NAPROXEN
EC-Naprosyn Delayed-Release Tablets . . . 2761
Naprosyn Suspension . . . 2761
Naprosyn Tablets . . . 2761

ROXIN (Australia)
NORFLOXACIN
Noroxin Tablets . . . 2032

ROYCEFAX (Brazil)
CEFTAZIDIME
Fortaz for Injection . . . 1453

ROYCHLOR (Canada)
POTASSIUM CHLORIDE
K-Dur Extended-Relase Tablets . . . 3033
K-Lor Oral Solution . . . 474
K-Tab Tablets . . . 475

ROYEN (Argentina, Spain)
CALCIUM ACETATE
PhosLo GelCaps . . . 2169

ROZACREME (France)
METRONIDAZOLE
MetroGel-Vaginal Gel . . . 1855

ROZAGEL (France)
METRONIDAZOLE
MetroGel-Vaginal Gel . . . 1855

ROZEK (Venezuela)
METRONIDAZOLE
MetroGel-Vaginal Gel . . . 1855

ROZEX (Argentina, Australia, Austria, Belgium, Brazil, Czech Republic, Denmark, Finland, France, Hong Kong, Irish Republic, Israel, Italy, Malaysia, New Zealand, Norway, Singapore, South Africa, Spain, Sweden, Switzerland, The Netherlands, United Kingdom)
METRONIDAZOLE
MetroGel-Vaginal Gel . . . 1855

R-PRIL (India)
RAMIPRIL
Altace Capsules . . . 1702

RUBACINA (Spain)
FAMOTIDINE
Pepcid Injection . . . 2040
Pepcid Injection Premixed . . . 2040
Pepcid Tablets . . . 2038
Pepcid for Oral Suspension . . . 2038

RUBIFEN (Argentina, New Zealand, Singapore, Spain, The Netherlands)
METHYLPHENIDATE HYDROCHLORIDE
Ritalin Hydrochloride Tablets . . . 2269
Ritalin-SR Tablets . . . 2269

RUBIMYCIN (South Africa)
ERYTHROMYCIN STEARATE
Erythrocin Stearate Filmtab Tablets . . . 453

RUBIULCER (Spain)
RANITIDINE HYDROCHLORIDE
Zantac 25 EFFERdose Tablets . . . 1624
Zantac 150 EFFERdose Tablets . . . 1624
Zantac 150 Tablets . . . 1624
Zantac 300 Tablets . . . 1624
Zantac Injection . . . 1619
Zantac Injection Premixed . . . 1619
Zantac Syrup . . . 1624

RUBOCORT (Greece)
CLOBETASOL PROPIONATE
Temovate Cream . . . 2668
Temovate E Emollient . . . 2671
Temovate Gel . . . 2669
Temovate Ointment . . . 2668
Temovate Scalp Application . . . 2670

RUBROMICIN (Brazil)
ERYTHROMYCIN
Ery-Tab Tablets . . . 449
Erythromycin Base Filmtab Tablets . . . 455
Erythromycin Delayed-Release Capsules, USP . . . 457
PCE Dispertab Tablets . . . 515

RUCAINA (Mexico)
LIDOCAINE
Lidoderm Patch . . . 1118

RUDOLAC (Switzerland)
LACTULOSE
Kristalose for Oral Solution . . . 1034

RUDOPRAM (Switzerland)
CITALOPRAM HYDROBROMIDE
Celexa Tablets . . . 1176

RUMATAB (Thailand)
DICLOFENAC SODIUM
Voltaren Tablets . . . 2307
Voltaren-XR Tablets . . . 2310

RUPEDEX (Argentina)
DEXAMETHASONE
Decadron Tablets . . . 1951

RUPEDIZ (Argentina)
DIAZEPAM
Diastat Rectal Delivery System . . . 3343
Valium Tablets . . . 2819

RUSSEDYL (Malaysia)
PROMETHAZINE HYDROCHLORIDE
Phenergan Tablets and Suppositories . . . 3440

RUSYDE (United Kingdom)
FUROSEMIDE
Furosemide Tablets . . . 2154

RUVOMINOX (Greece)
DICLOFENAC SODIUM
Voltaren Tablets . . . 2307
Voltaren-XR Tablets . . . 2310

RYTHMEX (Israel)
PROPAFENONE HYDROCHLORIDE
Rythmol SR Capsules . . . 2727

RYTHMOL (Canada, France, South Africa)
PROPAFENONE HYDROCHLORIDE
Rythmol SR Capsules . . . 2727

RYTHMONORM (Greece)
PROPAFENONE HYDROCHLORIDE
Rythmol SR Capsules . . . 2727

RYTHOCIN (Thailand)
ERYTHROMYCIN
Ery-Tab Tablets . . . 449
Erythromycin Base Filmtab Tablets . . . 455
Erythromycin Delayed-Release Capsules, USP . . . 457
PCE Dispertab Tablets . . . 515

RYTMOGENAT (Germany)
PROPAFENONE HYDROCHLORIDE
Rythmol SR Capsules . . . 2727

RYTMONORM (Belgium, Chile, Denmark, Finland, Germany, Hong Kong, Hungary, Italy, Malaysia, New Zealand, Portugal, Russia, Singapore, Spain, Sweden, Switzerland, Thailand, The Netherlands, Venezuela)
PROPAFENONE HYDROCHLORIDE
Rythmol SR Capsules . . . 2727

RYTMONORMA (Austria)
PROPAFENONE HYDROCHLORIDE
Rythmol SR Capsules 2727

RYTMO-PUREN (Germany)
PROPAFENONE HYDROCHLORIDE
Rythmol SR Capsules 2727

RYVEL (Hong Kong)
CETIRIZINE HYDROCHLORIDE
Zyrtec Syrup 2594
Zyrtec Tablets 2594

SABAX GENTAMIX (South Africa)
GENTAMICIN SULFATE
Garamycin Injectable 3014

SABIDAL RECTIOL (Italy)
THEOPHYLLINE
Uniphyl Tablets 2710

SAB-PENTASONE (Canada)
GENTAMICIN SULFATE
Garamycin Injectable 3014

SAGITTOL (Germany)
PROPRANOLOL HYDROCHLORIDE
Inderal LA Long-Acting Capsules 3429

SAL DIETETICA (Chile)
POTASSIUM CHLORIDE
K-Dur Extended-Relase Tablets 3033
K-Lor Oral Solution 474
K-Tab Tablets 475

SALAC (Argentina)
CLOBETASOL PROPIONATE
Temovate Cream 2668
Temovate E Emollient 2671
Temovate Gel 2669
Temovate Ointment 2668
Temovate Scalp Application 2670

SALCA (Venezuela)
FUROSEMIDE
Furosemide Tablets 2154

SALDAC (Australia, New Zealand)
SULINDAC
Clinoril Tablets 1924

SALI-ADALAT (Germany)
NIFEDIPINE
Adalat CC Tablets 2964

SALICORT (Argentina)
TRIAMCINOLONE ACETONIDE
Azmacort Inhalation Aerosol 1726
Nasacort AQ Nasal Spray 2922

SALI-PUREN (Germany)
HYDROCHLOROTHIAZIDE/TRIAMTERENE
Dyazide Capsules 1423

SALMETEDUR (Italy)
SALMETEROL XINAFOATE
Serevent Diskus 1568

SALMETER (Venezuela)
SALMETEROL XINAFOATE
Serevent Diskus 1568

SALODIUR (Austria)
HYDROCHLOROTHIAZIDE/TRIAMTERENE
Dyazide Capsules 1423

SALONGO (Spain)
OXICONAZOLE NITRATE
Oxistat Cream 2667
Oxistat Lotion 2667

SALTERMOX (South Africa)
AMOXICILLIN
Amoxil Pediatric Drops for Oral Suspension 1343
Amoxil Tablets 1343

SALUPRAN (Mexico)
NAPROXEN
EC-Naprosyn Delayed-Release Tablets 2761
Naprosyn Suspension 2761
Naprosyn Tablets 2761

SALURIC (Irish Republic, United Kingdom)
CHLOROTHIAZIDE
Diuril Oral Suspension 1954

SALURIN (United Arab Emirates)
FUROSEMIDE
Furosemide Tablets 2154

SALVALERG (Argentina)
CETIRIZINE HYDROCHLORIDE
Zyrtec Syrup 2594
Zyrtec Tablets 2594

SAMERTAN (Chile)
TELMISARTAN
Micardis Tablets 854

SAMIL-O2 (Italy)
BENZOYL PEROXIDE
Brevoxyl-4 Creamy Wash 3210
Brevoxyl-4 Gel 3210
Brevoxyl-8 Creamy Wash 3210
Brevoxyl-8 Gel 3210
Triaz Cleanser 1892
Triaz Gel 1892

SAMONIL (Mexico)
METRONIDAZOLE
MetroGel-Vaginal Gel 1855

SAMOX (Thailand)
AMOXICILLIN
Amoxil Pediatric Drops for Oral Suspension 1343
Amoxil Tablets 1343

SAMOXIN (Thailand)
AMOXICILLIN
Amoxil Pediatric Drops for Oral Suspension 1343
Amoxil Tablets 1343

SANALER (Chile)
CETIRIZINE HYDROCHLORIDE
Zyrtec Syrup 2594
Zyrtec Tablets 2594

SANATISON MONO (Germany)
HYDROCORTISONE
Hydrocortone Tablets 1989

SANCAP (Greece)
CAPTOPRIL
Captopril Tablets 2149

SANCIPRO (Denmark)
CIPROFLOXACIN HYDROCHLORIDE
Ciloxan Ophthalmic Ointment . . . . ⊙204, 559
Ciloxan Ophthalmic Solution . . . . . ⊙206
Cipro Tablets 2977

SANDOSTATIN (Canada, Finland, Germany, Irish Republic, Singapore, United Kingdom)
OCTREOTIDE ACETATE
Sandostatin LAR Depot 2280

SANDOSTATINE (France, Switzerland, The Netherlands)
OCTREOTIDE ACETATE
Sandostatin LAR Depot 2280

SANDOZ K (South Africa)
POTASSIUM CHLORIDE
K-Dur Extended-Relase Tablets 3033
K-Lor Oral Solution 474
K-Tab Tablets 475

SANDRENA (Australia, Austria, Brazil, Chile, Denmark, Germany, Italy, Mexico, New Zealand, Switzerland, The Netherlands, United Kingdom)
ESTRADIOL
Climara Transdermal System 771
Estring Vaginal Ring 2635

SANELOR (Chile)
LOVASTATIN
Mevacor Tablets 2021

SANIPRESIN (Chile)
LOSARTAN POTASSIUM
Cozaar Tablets 1935

SANIPRESIN-D (Chile)
HYDROCHLOROTHIAZIDE/LOSARTAN POTASSIUM
Hyzaar 100-25 Tablets 1990
Hyzaar 50-12.5 Tablets 1990

SANIPROSTOL (Chile)
FINASTERIDE
Propecia Tablets 2060
Proscar Tablets 2067

SANOXIT (Germany)
BENZOYL PEROXIDE
Brevoxyl-4 Creamy Wash 3210
Brevoxyl-4 Gel 3210
Brevoxyl-8 Creamy Wash 3210
Brevoxyl-8 Gel 3210
Triaz Cleanser 1892
Triaz Gel 1892

SANPRONOL (Brazil)
PROPRANOLOL HYDROCHLORIDE
Inderal LA Long-Acting Capsules 3429

SANSACNE (Mexico)
ERYTHROMYCIN
Ery-Tab Tablets 449
Erythromycin Base Filmtab Tablets 455
Erythromycin Delayed-Release Capsules, USP 457
PCE Dispertab Tablets 515

SANSANAL (Germany)
CAPTOPRIL
Captopril Tablets 2149

SANVAPRESS (Brazil)
ENALAPRIL MALEATE
Vasotec I.V. Injection 2103

SARF (United Arab Emirates)
CIPROFLOXACIN HYDROCHLORIDE
Ciloxan Ophthalmic Ointment . . . . ⊙204, 559
Ciloxan Ophthalmic Solution . . . . . ⊙206
Cipro Tablets 2977

SARNA HC (Canada)
HYDROCORTISONE
Hydrocortone Tablets 1989

SAROMET (Argentina)
DIAZEPAM
Diastat Rectal Delivery System 3343
Valium Tablets 2819

SARTON (Czech Republic)
VALSARTAN
Diovan Tablets 2193

SASTID ANTI-FUNGAL (Singapore)
CLOTRIMAZOLE
Lotrimin Cream 3039
Lotrimin Lotion 1% 3039
Lotrimin Topical Solution 1% 3039

SATIGENE (Argentina)
IRINOTECAN HYDROCHLORIDE
Camptosar Injection 2604

SATIL (Venezuela)
SERTRALINE HYDROCHLORIDE
Zoloft Tablets 2586

SAUBASIN (Greece)
DILTIAZEM HYDROCHLORIDE
Cardizem LA Extended Release Tablets . . . 1728
Tiazac Capsules 1201

SAYOMOL (Spain)
PROMETHAZINE HYDROCHLORIDE
Phenergan Tablets and Suppositories 3440

SCALPICIN (Italy)
HYDROCORTISONE
Hydrocortone Tablets 1989

SCALPICIN CAPILAR (Spain)
HYDROCORTISONE
Hydrocortone Tablets 1989

SCF (Australia)
SUCRALFATE
Carafate Suspension 701
Carafate Tablets 701

SCHEINPHARM TRIAMCINE-A (Canada)
TRIAMCINOLONE ACETONIDE
Azmacort Inhalation Aerosol 1726
Nasacort AQ Nasal Spray 2922

SCHERICUR (Argentina, Austria, Germany, Spain)
HYDROCORTISONE
Hydrocortone Tablets 1989

SCHERITONIN (Argentina)
ISOTRETINOIN
Accutane Capsules 2731

SCHEROGEL (Austria, Belgium, Germany, Italy, Spain)
BENZOYL PEROXIDE
Brevoxyl-4 Creamy Wash 3210
Brevoxyl-4 Gel 3210
Brevoxyl-8 Creamy Wash 3210
Brevoxyl-8 Gel 3210
Triaz Cleanser 1892
Triaz Gel 1892

SCHOLL ATHLETE'S FOOT (Canada)
BUTENAFINE HYDROCHLORIDE
Mentax Cream 2158

SCLERIL (Italy)
FENOFIBRATE
Tricor Tablets 527

SCLEROFIN (Argentina)
FENOFIBRATE
Tricor Tablets 527

SCRIPTOPAM (South Africa)
DIAZEPAM
Diastat Rectal Delivery System 3343
Valium Tablets 2819

SD-HERMAL (Germany)
CLOTRIMAZOLE
Lotrimin Cream 3039
Lotrimin Lotion 1% 3039
Lotrimin Topical Solution 1% 3039

SEALDIN (Spain)
SERTRALINE HYDROCHLORIDE
Zoloft Tablets 2586

SEBERCIM (Italy)
NORFLOXACIN
Noroxin Tablets 2032

SECALIP (France, Spain)
FENOFIBRATE
Tricor Tablets 527

SECOTEX (Argentina, Brazil, Chile, Mexico, Venezuela)
TAMSULOSIN HYDROCHLORIDE
Flomax Capsules 850

SECUBAR (Spain)
LISINOPRIL
Prinivil Tablets 2052

SECUBAR DIU (Spain)
HYDROCHLOROTHIAZIDE/LISINOPRIL
Prinzide Tablets 2056

SECURO (Argentina)
IVERMECTIN
Stromectol Tablets 2083

SECURON (United Kingdom)
VERAPAMIL HYDROCHLORIDE
Covera-HS Tablets 3139
Verelan PM Extended-Release Capsules, Controlled-Onset 3106

SEDACRIS (Argentina)
THEOPHYLLINE
Uniphyl Tablets 2710

SEDALIN (Thailand)
CEFTRIAXONE SODIUM
Rocephin Injectable Vials, ADD-Vantage, Galaxy, Bulk 2800

SEDANIUM-R (Greece)
FAMOTIDINE
Pepcid Injection 2040
Pepcid Injection Premixed 2040
Pepcid Tablets 2038
Pepcid for Oral Suspension 2038

SEDESTEROL (Argentina)
DEXAMETHASONE
Decadron Tablets 1951

SEDILIX (Malaysia)
PROMETHAZINE HYDROCHLORIDE
Phenergan Tablets and Suppositories 3440

SEDIVER (Mexico)
DIAZEPAM
Diastat Rectal Delivery System 3343
Valium Tablets 2819

SEDONERVIL COMPLEX (Spain)
DIAZEPAM
Diastat Rectal Delivery System 3343
Valium Tablets 2819

SEDOPAN (Greece)
CEFUROXIME AXETIL
Ceftin Tablets 1407
Ceftin for Oral Suspension 1407

SEDOTENSIL (Argentina)
LISINOPRIL
Prinivil Tablets 2052

SEDOVANON (Argentina)
CLONAZEPAM
Klonopin Tablets 2778

SEDUXEN (Czech Republic, Hungary, Russia)
DIAZEPAM
Diastat Rectal Delivery System 3343
Valium Tablets 2819

SEDUXEN RG (Czech Republic)
DIAZEPAM
Diastat Rectal Delivery System 3343

Valium Tablets 2819

SEFARETIC (Hong Kong, Thailand)
AMILORIDE HYDROCHLORIDE
Midamor Tablets 2026

SEFDIN (India)
CEFDINIR
Omnicef Capsules 511
Omnicef for Oral Suspension 511

SEFLOC (Hong Kong)
METOPROLOL TARTRATE
Lopressor Tablets 2238

SEFMAL (Hong Kong, Singapore, Thailand)
TRAMADOL HYDROCHLORIDE
Ultram ER Tablets 2392

SEFMEX (Hong Kong, Thailand)
SELEGILINE HYDROCHLORIDE
Eldepryl Capsules 3208

SEFNOR (Singapore)
NORFLOXACIN
Noroxin Tablets 2032

SEFULKEN (Mexico)
DIAZOXIDE
Hyperstat I.V. 3017

SEGALIN (Czech Republic)
SELEGILINE HYDROCHLORIDE
Eldepryl Capsules 3208

SEGAN (Russia)
SELEGILINE HYDROCHLORIDE
Eldepryl Capsules 3208

SEGUREX (Argentina)
SILDENAFIL CITRATE
Viagra Tablets 2573

SEGURIL (Spain)
FUROSEMIDE
Furosemide Tablets 2154

SELADIN (Malaysia, Singapore)
NAPROXEN
EC-Naprosyn Delayed-Release Tablets 2761
Naprosyn Suspension 2761
Naprosyn Tablets 2761

SELAN (Spain)
CEFUROXIME AXETIL
Ceftin Tablets 1407
Ceftin for Oral Suspension 1407

SELECIM (Switzerland)
SELEGILINE HYDROCHLORIDE
Eldepryl Capsules 3208

SELECOM (Italy)
SELEGILINE HYDROCHLORIDE
Eldepryl Capsules 3208

SELECTADRIL (Mexico)
METOPROLOL TARTRATE
Lopressor Tablets 2238

SELECTOFEN (Mexico)
DICLOFENAC SODIUM
Voltaren Tablets 2307
Voltaren-XR Tablets 2310

SELECTOFUR (Mexico)
FUROSEMIDE
Furosemide Tablets 2154

SELEDAT (Italy)
SELEGILINE HYDROCHLORIDE
Eldepryl Capsules 3208

SELEGAM (Germany)
SELEGILINE HYDROCHLORIDE
Eldepryl Capsules 3208

SELEGOS (Hong Kong, Malaysia, Russia, Singapore)
SELEGILINE HYDROCHLORIDE
Eldepryl Capsules 3208

SELEMERCK (Germany)
SELEGILINE HYDROCHLORIDE
Eldepryl Capsules 3208

SELEPARK (Germany)
SELEGILINE HYDROCHLORIDE
Eldepryl Capsules 3208

SELER (Chile)
SILDENAFIL CITRATE
Viagra Tablets 2573

SELERIN (India)
SELEGILINE HYDROCHLORIDE
Eldepryl Capsules 3208

SELGENE (Australia, New Zealand, Thailand)
SELEGILINE HYDROCHLORIDE
Eldepryl Capsules 3208

SELGIMED (Germany)
SELEGILINE HYDROCHLORIDE
Eldepryl Capsules 3208

SELGIN (India)
SELEGILINE HYDROCHLORIDE
Eldepryl Capsules 3208

SELGINA (Chile)
SELEGILINE HYDROCHLORIDE
Eldepryl Capsules 3208

SELINE (Thailand)
SELEGILINE HYDROCHLORIDE
Eldepryl Capsules 3208

SELOKEN (Austria, Belgium, Brazil, Denmark, Finland, France, Italy, Japan, Mexico, Norway, Spain, Sweden)
METOPROLOL SUCCINATE
Toprol-XL Tablets 668

SELOKEN ZOC (Finland, Sweden)
METOPROLOL SUCCINATE
Toprol-XL Tablets 668

SELOPRAL (Finland)
METOPROLOL TARTRATE
Lopressor Tablets 2238

SELOPRES (India)
METOPROLOL TARTRATE
Lopressor Tablets 2238

SELOPRESIN (Spain)
HYDROCHLOROTHIAZIDE/METOPROLOL TARTRATE
Lopressor HCT 100/25 Tablets 2241

SELOZIDE (Belgium, Italy)
HYDROCHLOROTHIAZIDE/METOPROLOL TARTRATE
Lopressor HCT 100/25 Tablets 2241

SELOZOK (France)
METOPROLOL SUCCINATE
Toprol-XL Tablets 668

SELO-ZOK (Belgium, Brazil, Denmark, Norway)
METOPROLOL SUCCINATE
Toprol-XL Tablets 668

SELPAR (Italy)
SELEGILINE HYDROCHLORIDE
Eldepryl Capsules 3208

SEMUELE (Greece)
RANITIDINE HYDROCHLORIDE
Zantac 25 EFFERdose Tablets 1624
Zantac 150 EFFERdose Tablets. 1624
Zantac 150 Tablets 1624
Zantac 300 Tablets 1624
Zantac Injection 1619
Zantac Injection Premixed 1619
Zantac Syrup 1624

SENRO (Spain)
NORFLOXACIN
Noroxin Tablets 2032

SENSATON (Argentina)
CLONAZEPAM
Klonopin Tablets 2778

SENSIGARD (Italy)
RANITIDINE HYDROCHLORIDE
Zantac 25 EFFERdose Tablets 1624
Zantac 150 EFFERdose Tablets. 1624
Zantac 150 Tablets 1624
Zantac 300 Tablets 1624
Zantac Injection 1619
Zantac Injection Premixed 1619
Zantac Syrup 1624

SENSIPHARMA (Mexico)
LIDOCAINE
Lidoderm Patch 1118

SENSITRAM (Brazil)
TRAMADOL HYDROCHLORIDE
Ultram ER Tablets 2392

SENTAPEN (Venezuela)
AMOXICILLIN
Amoxil Pediatric Drops for Oral Suspension. 1343
Amoxil Tablets 1343

SENTIAL HYDROCORTISONE (Belgium)
HYDROCORTISONE
Hydrocortone Tablets 1989

SEPATREM (Czech Republic)
SELEGILINE HYDROCHLORIDE
Eldepryl Capsules 3208

SEPCEN (Spain)
CIPROFLOXACIN HYDROCHLORIDE
Ciloxan Ophthalmic Ointment . . . . ⊙204, 559
Ciloxan Ophthalmic Solution . . . . ⊙206
Cipro Tablets 2977

SEPIBEST (Mexico)
CARBAMAZEPINE
Carbatrol Capsules 3171
Tegretol Chewable Tablets 2295
Tegretol Suspension. 2295
Tegretol Tablets 2295
Tegretol-XR Tablets 2295

SEPRAFILM (United Kingdom)
SODIUM HYALURONATE
Hyalgan Solution 2901

SEPRAM (Finland, Germany)
CITALOPRAM HYDROBROMIDE
Celexa Tablets 1176

SEPTICIDE (Argentina)
CIPROFLOXACIN HYDROCHLORIDE
Ciloxan Ophthalmic Ointment . . . . ⊙204, 559
Ciloxan Ophthalmic Solution . . . . ⊙206
Cipro Tablets 2977

SEPTOPAL (Australia, Malaysia)
GENTAMICIN SULFATE
Garamycin Injectable 3014

SEQUAX (Argentina)
CLOZAPINE
Clozaril Tablets 2184

SEQUINAN (Argentina)
RISPERIDONE
Risperdal Oral Solution 1676
Risperdal Tablets 1676

SERACIN (Thailand)
OFLOXACIN
Floxin Otic Solution 1049

SERAD (Italy)
SERTRALINE HYDROCHLORIDE
Zoloft Tablets 2586

SERALGAN (Austria)
CITALOPRAM HYDROBROMIDE
Celexa Tablets 1176

SERASA (Mexico)
ASPARAGINASE
Elspar for Injection 2463

SERBENDAZOL (Mexico)
ALBENDAZOLE
Albenza Tablets. 1338

SERCERIN (Brazil)
SERTRALINE HYDROCHLORIDE
Zoloft Tablets 2586

SERDEP (India)
SERTRALINE HYDROCHLORIDE
Zoloft Tablets 2586

SEREDYN (Mexico)
DIAZEPAM
Diastat Rectal Delivery System 3343
Valium Tablets 2819

SEREN (Italy)
CHLORDIAZEPOXIDE HYDROCHLORIDE
Librium Capsules. 3347

SEREN VITA (Italy)
CHLORDIAZEPOXIDE HYDROCHLORIDE
Librium Capsules. 3347

SERENATA (Brazil)
SERTRALINE HYDROCHLORIDE
Zoloft Tablets 2586

SERETIDE (Argentina, Australia, Belgium, Czech Republic, Hong Kong, Hungary, India, Malaysia, New Zealand, Russia, Venezuela)
SALMETEROL XINAFOATE
Serevent Diskus 1568

SERETRAN (Chile)
PAROXETINE HYDROCHLORIDE
Paxil Oral Suspension. 1530
Paxil Tablets. 1530

SEREUPIN (Italy)
PAROXETINE HYDROCHLORIDE
Paxil Oral Suspension. 1530
Paxil Tablets. 1530

SEREVENT (Argentina, Australia, Austria, Belgium, Brazil, Canada, Chile, Czech Republic, Denmark, Finland, France, Greece, Hong Kong, Hungary, Irish Republic, Israel, Italy, Malaysia, Mexico, New Zealand, Norway, Portugal, Russia, Singapore, South Africa, Spain, Sweden, Switzerland, Thailand, The Netherlands, United Kingdom, Venezuela)
SALMETEROL XINAFOATE
Serevent Diskus 1568

SERITAL (Germany)
CITALOPRAM HYDROBROMIDE
Celexa Tablets 1176

SERIVO (Chile)
SERTRALINE HYDROCHLORIDE
Zoloft Tablets 2586

SERLAIN (Belgium)
SERTRALINE HYDROCHLORIDE
Zoloft Tablets 2586

SERLIFE (South Africa)
SERTRALINE HYDROCHLORIDE
Zoloft Tablets 2586

SERLIFT (Czech Republic, Malaysia)
SERTRALINE HYDROCHLORIDE
Zoloft Tablets 2586

SERLINA (Argentina)
SERTRALINE HYDROCHLORIDE
Zoloft Tablets 2586

SERMOXOL (Mexico)
AMOXICILLIN
Amoxil Pediatric Drops for Oral Suspension. 1343
Amoxil Tablets 1343

SEROBID (India)
SALMETEROL XINAFOATE
Serevent Diskus 1568

SERODUR (Denmark)
PAROXETINE HYDROCHLORIDE
Paxil Oral Suspension. 1530
Paxil Tablets. 1530

SEROMYCIN (Canada, Hong Kong)
CYCLOSERINE
Seromycin Capsules. 1813

SERONEX (Chile)
SERTRALINE HYDROCHLORIDE
Zoloft Tablets 2586

SERONIP (Brazil)
SERTRALINE HYDROCHLORIDE
Zoloft Tablets 2586

SEROPRAM (Argentina, Hungary, Mexico, Spain)
CITALOPRAM HYDROBROMIDE
Celexa Tablets 1176

SEROQUEL (Argentina, Australia, Austria, Belgium, Brazil, Canada, Chile, Czech Republic, Denmark, Finland, Germany, Greece, Hong Kong, Hungary, Irish Republic, Israel, Italy, Japan, Malaysia, Mexico, New Zealand, Norway, Portugal, Russia, Singapore, South Africa, Spain, Sweden, Switzerland, Thailand, The Netherlands, United Kingdom, Venezuela)
QUETIAPINE FUMARATE
Seroquel Tablets 690

SEROQUIN (India)
QUETIAPINE FUMARATE
Seroquel Tablets 690

SEROVIDINA (Mexico)
ZIDOVUDINE
Retrovir Capsules 1560
Retrovir IV Infusion. 1564
Retrovir Syrup 1560
Retrovir Tablets. 1560

SEROXAT (Austria, Belgium, Czech Republic, Denmark, Finland, Germany, Greece, Hong Kong, Hungary, Irish Republic, Israel, Italy, Malaysia, Norway, Portugal, Singapore, Spain, Sweden, Thailand, The Netherlands, United Kingdom)
PAROXETINE HYDROCHLORIDE
Paxil Oral Suspension. 1530

(⊙ Described in PDR For Ophthalmic Medicines™)

Paxil Tablets . . . 1530

SERTA (India)
SERTRALINE HYDROCHLORIDE
Zoloft Tablets . . . 2586

SERTEX (Mexico)
SERTRALINE HYDROCHLORIDE
Zoloft Tablets . . . 2586

SERTIDINE (Mexico)
FAMOTIDINE
Pepcid Injection . . . 2040
Pepcid Injection Premixed . . . 2040
Pepcid Tablets . . . 2038
Pepcid for Oral Suspension . . . 2038

SERTINAL (Argentina)
SIBUTRAMINE HYDROCHLORIDE
Meridia Capsules . . . 489

SERTRIXEN (Mexico)
NAPROXEN
EC-Naprosyn Delayed-Release Tablets . . . 2761
Naprosyn Suspension . . . 2761
Naprosyn Tablets . . . 2761

SERVANOLOL (Switzerland)
PROPRANOLOL HYDROCHLORIDE
Inderal LA Long-Acting Capsules . . . 3429

SERVIDIPINE (Switzerland)
NIFEDIPINE
Adalat CC Tablets . . . 2964

SERVIFLOX (Singapore, Thailand)
CIPROFLOXACIN HYDROCHLORIDE
Ciloxan Ophthalmic Ointment . . . ⊙204, 559
Ciloxan Ophthalmic Solution . . . ⊙206
Cipro Tablets . . . 2977

SERVIGENTA (Mexico, Switzerland)
GENTAMICIN SULFATE
Garamycin Injectable . . . 3014

SERVINAPROX (Switzerland)
NAPROXEN
EC-Naprosyn Delayed-Release Tablets . . . 2761
Naprosyn Suspension . . . 2761
Naprosyn Tablets . . . 2761

SERVIPEP (Hong Kong, Hungary, Singapore)
FAMOTIDINE
Pepcid Injection . . . 2040
Pepcid Injection Premixed . . . 2040
Pepcid Tablets . . . 2038
Pepcid for Oral Suspension . . . 2038

SERVIRADINE (Mexico)
RANITIDINE HYDROCHLORIDE
Zantac 25 EFFERdose Tablets . . . 1624
Zantac 150 EFFERdose Tablets . . . 1624
Zantac 150 Tablets . . . 1624
Zantac 300 Tablets . . . 1624
Zantac Injection . . . 1619
Zantac Injection Premixed . . . 1619
Zantac Syrup . . . 1624

SERVIZOL (Singapore)
METRONIDAZOLE
MetroGel-Vaginal Gel . . . 1855

SESAREN (Argentina)
VENLAFAXINE HYDROCHLORIDE
Effexor Tablets . . . 3411
Effexor XR Capsules . . . 3417

SETANOL (Greece)
NORFLOXACIN
Noroxin Tablets . . . 2032

SETEGIS (Hungary)
TERAZOSIN HYDROCHLORIDE
Hytrin Capsules . . . 471

SETIN (Thailand)
CETIRIZINE HYDROCHLORIDE
Zyrtec Syrup . . . 2594
Zyrtec Tablets . . . 2594

SETRON (Czech Republic)
ONDANSETRON HYDROCHLORIDE
Zofran Injection . . . 1634
Zofran Injection Premixed . . . 1634
Zofran Oral Solution . . . 1639
Zofran Tablets . . . 1639

SETRONIL (Chile)
CITALOPRAM HYDROBROMIDE
Celexa Tablets . . . 1176

SETROZOLE (Malaysia)
METRONIDAZOLE
MetroGel-Vaginal Gel . . . 1855

SEVACOL (Argentina)
SIMVASTATIN
Zocor Tablets . . . 2105

SEVREDOL (Czech Republic, France, Germany, Irish Republic, New Zealand, Portugal, Spain, Switzerland, The Netherlands, United Kingdom)
MORPHINE SULFATE
Kadian Capsules . . . 577
MS Contin Tablets . . . 2701

SEVRE-LONG (Switzerland)
MORPHINE SULFATE
Kadian Capsules . . . 577
MS Contin Tablets . . . 2701

SFINAC (Greece)
DICLOFENAC SODIUM
Voltaren Tablets . . . 2307
Voltaren-XR Tablets . . . 2310

SHEMOL (Mexico)
TIMOLOL MALEATE
Blocadren Tablets . . . 1916
Timoptic Sterile Ophthalmic Solution . . . 2088
Timoptic in Ocudose . . . 2091
Timoptic-XE Sterile Ophthalmic Gel Forming Solution . . . 2092

SHINCEF (Singapore)
CEFUROXIME SODIUM
Zinacef Injection . . . 1631

SHINCORT (Malaysia, Singapore, Thailand)
TRIAMCINOLONE ACETONIDE
Azmacort Inhalation Aerosol . . . 1726
Nasacort AQ Nasal Spray . . . 2922

SIAFIL (Chile)
SILDENAFIL CITRATE
Viagra Tablets . . . 2573

SIBUNAR (Denmark)
CIPROFLOXACIN HYDROCHLORIDE
Ciloxan Ophthalmic Ointment . . . ⊙204, 559
Ciloxan Ophthalmic Solution . . . ⊙206
Cipro Tablets . . . 2977

SIBUTRAL (France)
SIBUTRAMINE HYDROCHLORIDE
Meridia Capsules . . . 489

SIBU-TRATOBES (Argentina)
SIBUTRAMINE HYDROCHLORIDE
Meridia Capsules . . . 489

SICADENTOL PLUS (Argentina)
NAPROXEN
EC-Naprosyn Delayed-Release Tablets . . . 2761
Naprosyn Suspension . . . 2761
Naprosyn Tablets . . . 2761

SICCO (Germany)
INDAPAMIDE
Indapamide Tablets . . . 2156

SICLOT (Thailand)
TICLOPIDINE HYDROCHLORIDE
Ticlid Tablets . . . 2810

SICO RELAX (Spain)
DIAZEPAM
Diastat Rectal Delivery System . . . 3343
Valium Tablets . . . 2819

SICOR (Hungary)
SIMVASTATIN
Zocor Tablets . . . 2105

SICRIT (Chile)
MEDROXYPROGESTERONE ACETATE
Depo-Medrol Single-Dose Vial . . . 2619

SIFLOKS (Russia)
CIPROFLOXACIN HYDROCHLORIDE
Ciloxan Ophthalmic Ointment . . . ⊙204, 559
Ciloxan Ophthalmic Solution . . . ⊙206
Cipro Tablets . . . 2977

SIFLOXAN (Brazil)
CIPROFLOXACIN
Cipro Oral Suspension . . . 2977

SIFTREX (Brazil)
ERYTHROMYCIN
Ery-Tab Tablets . . . 449
Erythromycin Base Filmtab Tablets . . . 455
Erythromycin Delayed-Release Capsules, USP . . . 457
PCE Dispertab Tablets . . . 515

SIGACAP COR (Germany)
CAPTOPRIL
Captopril Tablets . . . 2149

SIGACORA (Germany)
ISOSORBIDE MONONITRATE
Imdur Tablets . . . 3018

SIGAFAM (Mexico)
FAMOTIDINE
Pepcid Injection . . . 2040
Pepcid Injection Premixed . . . 2040
Pepcid Tablets . . . 2038
Pepcid for Oral Suspension . . . 2038

SIGAFENAC (Germany)
DICLOFENAC SODIUM
Voltaren Tablets . . . 2307
Voltaren-XR Tablets . . . 2310

SIGAMOPEN (Switzerland)
AMOXICILLIN
Amoxil Pediatric Drops for Oral Suspension . . . 1343
Amoxil Tablets . . . 1343

SIGAPAEDIL (Germany)
ERYTHROMYCIN
Ery-Tab Tablets . . . 449
Erythromycin Base Filmtab Tablets . . . 455
Erythromycin Delayed-Release Capsules, USP . . . 457
PCE Dispertab Tablets . . . 515

SIGAPROLOL (Germany)
METOPROLOL TARTRATE
Lopressor Tablets . . . 2238

SIGASALUR (Germany)
FUROSEMIDE
Furosemide Tablets . . . 2154

SIGMA CLAV (Brazil)
AMOXICILLIN
Amoxil Pediatric Drops for Oral Suspension . . . 1343
Amoxil Tablets . . . 1343

SIGMATRIOL (Brazil)
CALCITRIOL
Calcijex Injection . . . 411
Rocaltrol Capsules . . . 2798
Rocaltrol Oral Solution . . . 2798

SIGMAXIN (Australia)
DIGOXIN
Lanoxicaps Capsules . . . 1490
Lanoxin Injection . . . 1494
Lanoxin Injection Pediatric . . . 1497
Lanoxin Tablets . . . 1500

SILAGRA (India)
SILDENAFIL CITRATE
Viagra Tablets . . . 2573

SILCOR (Argentina)
CALCITRIOL
Calcijex Injection . . . 411
Rocaltrol Capsules . . . 2798
Rocaltrol Oral Solution . . . 2798

SILDEFIL (Argentina)
SILDENAFIL CITRATE
Viagra Tablets . . . 2573

SILFOX (Argentina)
DICLOFENAC SODIUM
Voltaren Tablets . . . 2307
Voltaren-XR Tablets . . . 2310

SILFOX FLEX (Argentina)
DICLOFENAC SODIUM
Voltaren Tablets . . . 2307
Voltaren-XR Tablets . . . 2310

SILIDRAL (Argentina)
ALENDRONATE SODIUM
Fosamax Tablets . . . 1969

SILINO (Germany)
DICLOFENAC SODIUM
Voltaren Tablets . . . 2307
Voltaren-XR Tablets . . . 2310

SILKIS (Austria, Belgium, Brazil, Chile, Finland, France, Germany, Greece, Irish Republic, Mexico, Norway, Portugal, Singapore, Spain, Switzerland, The Netherlands, United Kingdom, Venezuela)
CALCITRIOL
Calcijex Injection . . . 411
Rocaltrol Capsules . . . 2798
Rocaltrol Oral Solution . . . 2798

SIMATOR (Irish Republic)
SIMVASTATIN
Zocor Tablets . . . 2105

SIMCARD (India)
SIMVASTATIN
Zocor Tablets . . . 2105

SIMCHOL (India)
SIMVASTATIN
Zocor Tablets . . . 2105

SIMCORA (Switzerland)
SIMVASTATIN
Zocor Tablets . . . 2105

SIMCORHEXAL (Austria)
SIMVASTATIN
Zocor Tablets . . . 2105

SIMETAC (Hong Kong)
RANITIDINE HYDROCHLORIDE
Zantac 25 EFFERdose Tablets . . . 1624
Zantac 150 EFFERdose Tablets . . . 1624
Zantac 150 Tablets . . . 1624
Zantac 300 Tablets . . . 1624
Zantac Injection . . . 1619
Zantac Injection Premixed . . . 1619
Zantac Syrup . . . 1624

SIMGAL (Russia)
SIMVASTATIN
Zocor Tablets . . . 2105

SIMIREX (Czech Republic)
SIMVASTATIN
Zocor Tablets . . . 2105

SIMLO (India, Russia)
SIMVASTATIN
Zocor Tablets . . . 2105

SIMOVIL (Israel)
SIMVASTATIN
Zocor Tablets . . . 2105

SIMPERTEN (Chile)
LOSARTAN POTASSIUM
Cozaar Tablets . . . 1935

SIMPERTEN-D (Chile)
HYDROCHLOROTHIAZIDE/LOSARTAN POTASSIUM
Hyzaar 100-25 Tablets . . . 1990
Hyzaar 50-12.5 Tablets . . . 1990

SIMPLAQOR (Mexico)
SIMVASTATIN
Zocor Tablets . . . 2105

SIMSTIN (Austria)
SIMVASTATIN
Zocor Tablets . . . 2105

SIMTAN (Irish Republic)
SIMVASTATIN
Zocor Tablets . . . 2105

SIMTEC (Malaysia)
CETIRIZINE HYDROCHLORIDE
Zyrtec Syrup . . . 2594
Zyrtec Tablets . . . 2594

SIMTIN (Hong Kong, Singapore)
SIMVASTATIN
Zocor Tablets . . . 2105

SIMULECT (Argentina, Australia, Belgium, Brazil, Canada, Chile, Czech Republic, Denmark, Finland, France, Germany, Greece, Hong Kong, Irish Republic, Israel, Italy, Malaysia, Mexico, New Zealand, Norway, Portugal, Russia, Singapore, South Africa, Spain, Sweden, Switzerland, Thailand, The Netherlands, United Kingdom)
BASILIXIMAB
Simulect for Injection . . . 2284

SIMULTAN (Argentina, Chile)
VALSARTAN
Diovan Tablets . . . 2193

SIMULTAN D (Argentina)
VALSARTAN
Diovan Tablets . . . 2193

SIMULTEC (Venezuela)
BASILIXIMAB
Simulect for Injection . . . 2284

SIMVAAPS (Germany)
SIMVASTATIN
Zocor Tablets . . . 2105

SIMVABELL (Australia)
SIMVASTATIN
Zocor Tablets . . . 2105

SIMVABETA (Germany)
SIMVASTATIN
Zocor Tablets 2105

SIMVACARD (Czech Republic, Germany, Russia)
SIMVASTATIN
Zocor Tablets 2105

SIMVACHOL (Greece)
SIMVASTATIN
Zocor Tablets 2105

SIMVACOL (Hungary, Portugal)
SIMVASTATIN
Zocor Tablets 2105

SIMVACOR (Germany, Greece, Israel, Malaysia, Singapore, South Africa)
SIMVASTATIN
Zocor Tablets 2105

SIMVADOR (United Kingdom)
SIMVASTATIN
Zocor Tablets 2105

SIMVADURA (Germany)
SIMVASTATIN
Zocor Tablets 2105

SIMVAGAMMA (Germany)
SIMVASTATIN
Zocor Tablets 2105

SIMVAHEXAL (Australia)
SIMVASTATIN
Zocor Tablets 2105

SIMVAPROL (Greece)
SIMVASTATIN
Zocor Tablets 2105

SIMVAR (Australia)
SIMVASTATIN
Zocor Tablets 2105

SIMVASINE (Switzerland)
SIMVASTATIN
Zocor Tablets 2105

SIMVASS (Chile)
SIMVASTATIN
Zocor Tablets 2105

SIMVAST (Switzerland)
SIMVASTATIN
Zocor Tablets 2105

SIMVASTAD (Austria)
SIMVASTATIN
Zocor Tablets 2105

SIMVASTEN (Spain)
SIMVASTATIN
Zocor Tablets 2105

SIMVASTIN (Switzerland)
SIMVASTATIN
Zocor Tablets 2105

SIMVASTOL (Russia)
SIMVASTATIN
Zocor Tablets 2105

SIMVASTUR (Spain)
SIMVASTATIN
Zocor Tablets 2105

SIMVATIN (Austria, Greece)
SIMVASTATIN
Zocor Tablets 2105

SIMVAX (Czech Republic)
SIMVASTATIN
Zocor Tablets 2105

SIMVOR (Czech Republic, Hungary, Malaysia, Russia, Singapore, Thailand)
SIMVASTATIN
Zocor Tablets 2105

SIMVOTIN (India, South Africa)
SIMVASTATIN
Zocor Tablets 2105

SIMZOR (Irish Republic)
SIMVASTATIN
Zocor Tablets 2105

SINALFA (Denmark, Norway, Sweden)
TERAZOSIN HYDROCHLORIDE
Hytrin Capsules 471

SINCERCK (Mexico)
PRAZIQUANTEL
Biltricide Tablets 2976

SINCROSA (Mexico)
ACARBOSE
Precose Tablets 751

SINFEXINA (Mexico)
CIPROFLOXACIN
Cipro Oral Suspension 2977

SINFRACT (Mexico)
ALENDRONATE SODIUM
Fosamax Tablets 1969

SINGULAIR (Argentina, Australia, Austria, Belgium, Brazil, Canada, Chile, Czech Republic, Denmark, Finland, France, Germany, Greece, Hong Kong, Hungary, Irish Republic, Israel, Italy, Malaysia, Mexico, New Zealand, Norway, Portugal, Singapore, South Africa, Spain, Sweden, Switzerland, Thailand, The Netherlands, United Kingdom, Venezuela)
MONTELUKAST SODIUM
Singulair Chewable Tablets 2077
Singulair Tablets 2077

SINOBID (Greece)
NORFLOXACIN
Noroxin Tablets 2032

SINOPREN (South Africa)
LISINOPRIL
Prinivil Tablets 2052

SINOPRIL (Russia)
LISINOPRIL
Prinivil Tablets 2052

SINOVIAL (France)
SODIUM HYALURONATE
Hyalgan Solution 2901

SINPEBAC (Mexico)
MUPIROCIN
Bactroban Ointment 1395

SINPET (Mexico)
PHENTERMINE HYDROCHLORIDE
Adipex-P Capsules 1215
Adipex-P Tablets 1215

SINPOR (Portugal)
SIMVASTATIN
Zocor Tablets 2105

SINTENYL (Switzerland)
FENTANYL CITRATE
Actiq 979

SINTOFENAC (Brazil)
DICLOFENAC SODIUM
Voltaren Tablets 2307
Voltaren-XR Tablets 2310

SINTOLATT (Italy)
LACTULOSE
Kristalose for Oral Solution 1034

SINVACOR (Italy)
SIMVASTATIN
Zocor Tablets 2105

SINVALIP (Brazil)
SIMVASTATIN
Zocor Tablets 2105

SINVASCOR (Brazil)
SIMVASTATIN
Zocor Tablets 2105

SINVASTACOR (Brazil)
SIMVASTATIN
Zocor Tablets 2105

SINVASTAMED (Brazil)
SIMVASTATIN
Zocor Tablets 2105

SINVASTIL (Portugal)
SIMVASTATIN
Zocor Tablets 2105

SINVASTIN (Brazil)
SIMVASTATIN
Zocor Tablets 2105

SINVATROX (Brazil)
SIMVASTATIN
Zocor Tablets 2105

SINVAX (Brazil)
SIMVASTATIN
Zocor Tablets 2105

SINVAZ (Brazil)
SIMVASTATIN
Zocor Tablets 2105

SIPAM (Thailand)
DIAZEPAM
Diastat Rectal Delivery System 3343
Valium Tablets 2819

SIPRION (Finland)
CIPROFLOXACIN HYDROCHLORIDE
Ciloxan Ophthalmic Ointment ⊙204, 559
Ciloxan Ophthalmic Solution ⊙206
Cipro Tablets 2977

SIROLAX (Israel)
LACTULOSE
Kristalose for Oral Solution 1034

SIROTAMICIN HC (Argentina)
HYDROCORTISONE
Hydrocortone Tablets 1989

SIRTAL (Austria, Germany)
CARBAMAZEPINE
Carbatrol Capsules 3171
Tegretol Chewable Tablets 2295
Tegretol Suspension 2295
Tegretol Tablets 2295
Tegretol-XR Tablets 2295

SISARE MONO (Germany)
ESTRADIOL
Climara Transdermal System 771
Estring Vaginal Ring 2635

SITERIN (Finland)
CETIRIZINE HYDROCHLORIDE
Zyrtec Syrup 2594
Zyrtec Tablets 2594

SITRIOL (Australia)
CALCITRIOL
Calcijex Injection 411
Rocaltrol Capsules 2798
Rocaltrol Oral Solution 2798

SIVASTIN (Brazil, Italy)
SIMVASTATIN
Zocor Tablets 2105

SIVATIN (Irish Republic)
SIMVASTATIN
Zocor Tablets 2105

SIVLOR (Argentina)
LOVASTATIN
Mevacor Tablets 2021

SIZOPIN (India)
CLOZAPINE
Clozaril Tablets 2184

SIZORISP (India)
RISPERIDONE
Risperdal Oral Solution 1676
Risperdal Tablets 1676

SKENAN (Belgium, Czech Republic, France, Italy, Portugal, Spain, The Netherlands)
MORPHINE SULFATE
Kadian Capsules 577
MS Contin Tablets 2701

SKEZIDE (Thailand)
HYDROCHLOROTHIAZIDE/TRIAMTERENE
Dyazide Capsules 1423

SKID E (Germany)
ERYTHROMYCIN
Ery-Tab Tablets 449
Erythromycin Base Filmtab Tablets 455
Erythromycin Delayed-Release Capsules, USP 457
PCE Dispertab Tablets 515

SKINCALM (South Africa)
HYDROCORTISONE
Hydrocortone Tablets 1989

SKINFECT (Thailand)
GENTAMICIN SULFATE
Garamycin Injectable 3014

SKITZ (Australia)
BENZOYL PEROXIDE
Brevoxyl-4 Creamy Wash 3210
Brevoxyl-4 Gel 3210
Brevoxyl-8 Creamy Wash 3210
Brevoxyl-8 Gel 3210
Triaz Cleanser 1892
Triaz Gel 1892

SLIMIN (Germany)
HYDROCHLOROTHIAZIDE/TRIAMTERENE
Dyazide Capsules 1423

SLO-BID (Australia, Canada, Hong Kong, Mexico)
THEOPHYLLINE
Uniphyl Tablets 2710

SLOFEDIPINE (United Kingdom)
NIFEDIPINE
Adalat CC Tablets 2964

SLOFENAC (United Kingdom)
DICLOFENAC SODIUM
Voltaren Tablets 2307
Voltaren-XR Tablets 2310

SLO-MORPH (Irish Republic)
MORPHINE SULFATE
Kadian Capsules 577
MS Contin Tablets 2701

SLO-PHYLLIN (Irish Republic, Italy, United Kingdom)
THEOPHYLLINE
Uniphyl Tablets 2710

SLO-PRO (United Kingdom)
PROPRANOLOL HYDROCHLORIDE
Inderal LA Long-Acting Capsules 3429

SLOPROLOL (United Kingdom)
PROPRANOLOL HYDROCHLORIDE
Inderal LA Long-Acting Capsules 3429

SLO-THEO (Hong Kong)
THEOPHYLLINE
Uniphyl Tablets 2710

SLOVALGIN (Czech Republic)
MORPHINE SULFATE
Kadian Capsules 577
MS Contin Tablets 2701

SLOW DERALIN (Israel)
PROPRANOLOL HYDROCHLORIDE
Inderal LA Long-Acting Capsules 3429

SLOW-K (Australia, Brazil, Canada, Chile, Hong Kong, Irish Republic, Israel, Malaysia, New Zealand, South Africa, The Netherlands)
POTASSIUM CHLORIDE
K-Dur Extended-Relase Tablets 3033
K-Lor Oral Solution 474
K-Tab Tablets 475

SLOW-LOPRESOR (Belgium, New Zealand)
METOPROLOL TARTRATE
Lopressor Tablets 2238

SLOZEM (United Kingdom)
DILTIAZEM HYDROCHLORIDE
Cardizem LA Extended Release Tablets 1728
Tiazac Capsules 1201

SMARIL (Greece)
RANITIDINE HYDROCHLORIDE
Zantac 25 EFFERdose Tablets 1624
Zantac 150 EFFERdose Tablets 1624
Zantac 150 Tablets 1624
Zantac 300 Tablets 1624
Zantac Injection 1619
Zantac Injection Premixed 1619
Zantac Syrup 1624

SNOFFOCIN (Thailand)
NORFLOXACIN
Noroxin Tablets 2032

SOBREPINA (Portugal)
NIMODIPINE
Nimotop Capsules 749

SOBRONIL (Spain)
NAPROXEN
EC-Naprosyn Delayed-Release Tablets 2761
Naprosyn Suspension 2761
Naprosyn Tablets 2761

SOCALM (India)
QUETIAPINE FUMARATE
Seroquel Tablets 690

SODEN (Hong Kong, Singapore)
NAPROXEN SODIUM
Anaprox DS Tablets 2761
Anaprox Tablets 2761

SODEXX FAMOTIDINE (Austria)
FAMOTIDINE
Pepcid Injection 2040
Pepcid Injection Premixed 2040
Pepcid Tablets 2038
Pepcid for Oral Suspension 2038

SODICLO (South Africa)
DICLOFENAC SODIUM
Voltaren Tablets 2307
Voltaren-XR Tablets 2310

SODIP-PHYLLINE (Switzerland)
THEOPHYLLINE
Uniphyl Tablets 2710

SODIUM SULAMYD (Canada)
SULFACETAMIDE SODIUM
Klaron Lotion 10% 2909

SODIXEN (Mexico)
NAPROXEN SODIUM
Anaprox DS Tablets 2761
Anaprox Tablets 2761

SOFASIN (Greece)
NORFLOXACIN
Noroxin Tablets 2032

SOFLAX (United Arab Emirates)
LACTULOSE
Kristalose for Oral Solution 1034

SOKARAL (Germany)
DEXAMETHASONE
Decadron Tablets 1951

SOLARAZE (Denmark, Finland, France, Germany, Irish Republic, Italy, Sweden, United Kingdom)
DICLOFENAC SODIUM
Voltaren Tablets 2307
Voltaren-XR Tablets 2310

SOLARCAINE (Switzerland)
LIDOCAINE
Lidoderm Patch 1118

SOLEXA (Austria, Italy, Portugal, The Netherlands)
CELECOXIB
Celebrex Capsules 3134

SOLFIDIN (Argentina)
CLONAZEPAM
Klonopin Tablets 2778

SOLGENTA (Venezuela)
GENTAMICIN SULFATE
Garamycin Injectable 3014

SOLGERETIK (Germany)
NADOLOL
Nadolol Tablets 2159

SOLGOL (Austria, Germany, Spain)
NADOLOL
Nadolol Tablets 2159

SOLIS (United Kingdom)
DIAZEPAM
Diastat Rectal Delivery System 3343
Valium Tablets 2819

SOLIUM (Canada)
CHLORDIAZEPOXIDE HYDROCHLORIDE
Librium Capsules 3347

SOLOSIN (Germany)
THEOPHYLLINE
Uniphyl Tablets 2710

SOLOSPRIN (India)
ISOSORBIDE MONONITRATE
Imdur Tablets 3018

SOLSOLONA (Mexico)
METHYLPREDNISOLONE ACETATE
Depo-Medrol Injectable Suspension 2617

SOLUCEL (Spain)
BENZOYL PEROXIDE
Brevoxyl-4 Creamy Wash 3210
Brevoxyl-4 Gel 3210
Brevoxyl-8 Creamy Wash 3210
Brevoxyl-8 Gel 3210
Triaz Cleanser 1892
Triaz Gel 1892

SOLUDAMIN (Greece)
LEVOCARNITINE
Carnitor Injection 3188
Carnitor Tablets and Oral Solution 3190

SOLUGEL (Argentina, Brazil, Canada, Chile, Mexico, Venezuela)
BENZOYL PEROXIDE
Brevoxyl-4 Creamy Wash 3210
Brevoxyl-4 Gel 3210
Brevoxyl-8 Creamy Wash 3210
Brevoxyl-8 Gel 3210
Triaz Cleanser 1892
Triaz Gel 1892

SOLUMIDAZOL (Mexico)
METRONIDAZOLE
MetroGel-Vaginal Gel 1855

SOLUTIO CORDES DEXA N (Germany)
DEXAMETHASONE
Decadron Tablets 1951

SOLVETAN (Greece)
CEFTAZIDIME
Fortaz for Injection 1453

SOMAFLEX (Greece)
ETIDRONATE DISODIUM
Didronel Tablets 2697

SOMALGESIC (Mexico)
NAPROXEN
EC-Naprosyn Delayed-Release Tablets 2761
Naprosyn Suspension 2761
Naprosyn Tablets 2761

SOMAPLUS (Brazil)
DIAZEPAM
Diastat Rectal Delivery System 3343
Valium Tablets 2819

SOMATRAN (Chile)
SUMATRIPTAN
Imitrex Nasal Spray 1467

SOMINEX (United Kingdom)
PROMETHAZINE HYDROCHLORIDE
Phenergan Tablets and Suppositories 3440

SOMNATROL (Argentina)
ESTAZOLAM
ProSom Tablets 517

SOMOFILLINA (Italy)
THEOPHYLLINE
Uniphyl Tablets 2710

SOMOPHYLLIN (Canada, South Africa)
THEOPHYLLINE
Uniphyl Tablets 2710

SONAP (Thailand)
NAPROXEN SODIUM
Anaprox DS Tablets 2761
Anaprox Tablets 2761

SOPENTAL (South Africa)
PENTOBARBITAL SODIUM
Nembutal Sodium Solution, USP 2470

SOPHIDONE (France)
HYDROMORPHONE HYDROCHLORIDE
Dilaudid Ampules 440
Dilaudid Multiple Dose Vials 440
Dilaudid Non-Sterile Powder 440
Dilaudid Oral Liquid 445
Dilaudid Rectal Suppositories 440
Dilaudid Tablets 440
Dilaudid Tablets - 8 mg 445
Dilaudid-HP Injection 442
Dilaudid-HP Lyophilized Powder 250 mg . . . 442

SOPHIXIN (Mexico, Venezuela)
CIPROFLOXACIN HYDROCHLORIDE
Ciloxan Ophthalmic Ointment . . . . ⊙204, 559
Ciloxan Ophthalmic Solution . . . . . ⊙206
Cipro Tablets 2977

SOPORIL (Germany)
PROMETHAZINE HYDROCHLORIDE
Phenergan Tablets and Suppositories 3440

SOPROXEN (Singapore, Thailand)
NAPROXEN SODIUM
Anaprox DS Tablets 2761
Anaprox Tablets 2761

SORBIMON (Austria, Czech Republic, Hungary)
ISOSORBIDE MONONITRATE
Imdur Tablets 3018

SOREDINE (Greece)
RANITIDINE HYDROCHLORIDE
Zantac 25 EFFERdose Tablets 1624
Zantac 150 EFFERdose Tablets 1624
Zantac 150 Tablets 1624
Zantac 300 Tablets 1624
Zantac Injection 1619
Zantac Injection Premixed 1619
Zantac Syrup 1624

SOREN (Hong Kong)
NAPROXEN SODIUM
Anaprox DS Tablets 2761
Anaprox Tablets 2761

SORIATANE (Canada, France)
ACITRETIN
Soriatane Capsules 1013

SORMON (Irish Republic)
ISOSORBIDE MONONITRATE
Imdur Tablets 3018

SORTAL (Venezuela)
LOSARTAN POTASSIUM
Cozaar Tablets 1935

SORTIS (Austria, Czech Republic, Hungary, Switzerland)
ATORVASTATIN CALCIUM
Lipitor Tablets 2483

SOSTRIL (Germany, Venezuela)
RANITIDINE HYDROCHLORIDE
Zantac 25 EFFERdose Tablets 1624
Zantac 150 EFFERdose Tablets 1624
Zantac 150 Tablets 1624
Zantac 300 Tablets 1624
Zantac Injection 1619
Zantac Injection Premixed 1619
Zantac Syrup 1624

SOTAZIDEN N (Germany)
NADOLOL
Nadolol Tablets 2159

SOTOVASTIN (Greece)
SIMVASTATIN
Zocor Tablets 2105

SP 54 (Hong Kong, Hungary)
PENTOSAN POLYSULFATE SODIUM
Elmiron Capsules 2415

SPAN-K (Australia, Hong Kong, New Zealand)
POTASSIUM CHLORIDE
K-Dur Extended-Relase Tablets 3033
K-Lor Oral Solution 474
K-Tab Tablets 475

SPARKAL (Denmark, Finland, Sweden)
AMILORIDE HYDROCHLORIDE/HYDROCHLOROTHIAZIDE
Moduretic Tablets 2028

SPATANIL (Greece)
CETIRIZINE HYDROCHLORIDE
Zyrtec Syrup 2594
Zyrtec Tablets 2594

SPECINOR (Greece)
RANITIDINE HYDROCHLORIDE
Zantac 25 EFFERdose Tablets 1624
Zantac 150 EFFERdose Tablets 1624
Zantac 150 Tablets 1624
Zantac 300 Tablets 1624
Zantac Injection 1619
Zantac Injection Premixed 1619
Zantac Syrup 1624

SPECTROBAK (Spain)
GENTAMICIN SULFATE
Garamycin Injectable 3014

SPECTROFLEX (Mexico)
CIPROFLOXACIN
Cipro Oral Suspension 2977

SPECTROXYL (Switzerland)
AMOXICILLIN
Amoxil Pediatric Drops for Oral Suspension 1343
Amoxil Tablets 1343

SPECTRUM (Italy)
CEFTAZIDIME
Fortaz for Injection 1453

SPERSACET (Hong Kong, Switzerland)
SULFACETAMIDE SODIUM
Klaron Lotion 10% 2909

SPERSAMIDE (South Africa)
SULFACETAMIDE SODIUM
Klaron Lotion 10% 2909

SPIROLAIR (Belgium)
PIRBUTEROL ACETATE
Maxair Autohaler 1852

SPIRON (Chile)
RISPERIDONE
Risperdal Oral Solution 1676
Risperdal Tablets 1676

SPOFALYT-KALIUM (Czech Republic)
POTASSIUM CHLORIDE
K-Dur Extended-Relase Tablets 3033
K-Lor Oral Solution 474
K-Tab Tablets 475

SPONIF (Czech Republic)
NIFEDIPINE
Adalat CC Tablets 2964

SPOPHYLLIN (Czech Republic)
THEOPHYLLINE
Uniphyl Tablets 2710

SPREDIOL (Italy)
ESTRADIOL
Climara Transdermal System 771
Estring Vaginal Ring 2635

SRM-RHOTARD (Singapore, South Africa)
MORPHINE SULFATE
Kadian Capsules 577
MS Contin Tablets 2701

STACER (Portugal)
RANITIDINE HYDROCHLORIDE
Zantac 25 EFFERdose Tablets 1624
Zantac 150 EFFERdose Tablets 1624
Zantac 150 Tablets 1624
Zantac 300 Tablets 1624
Zantac Injection 1619
Zantac Injection Premixed 1619
Zantac Syrup 1624

STACIN (Thailand)
ERYTHROMYCIN
Ery-Tab Tablets 449
Erythromycin Base Filmtab Tablets 455
Erythromycin Delayed-Release Capsules, USP 457
PCE Dispertab Tablets 515

STACORT-A (Hong Kong)
TRIAMCINOLONE ACETONIDE
Azmacort Inhalation Aerosol 1726
Nasacort AQ Nasal Spray 2922

STADELANT (Greece)
ENALAPRIL MALEATE
Vasotec I.V. Injection 2103

STARCEF (Italy)
CEFTAZIDIME
Fortaz for Injection 1453

STAREZIN (Greece)
SIMVASTATIN
Zocor Tablets 2105

STARVAL (India)
VALSARTAN
Diovan Tablets 2193

STASIVA (Greece)
SIMVASTATIN
Zocor Tablets 2105

STATEX (Canada, Singapore)
MORPHINE SULFATE
Kadian Capsules 577
MS Contin Tablets 2701

STATICIN (Canada)
ERYTHROMYCIN
Ery-Tab Tablets 449
Erythromycin Base Filmtab Tablets 455
Erythromycin Delayed-Release Capsules, USP 457
PCE Dispertab Tablets 515

STATICINE (Switzerland)
ERYTHROMYCIN
Ery-Tab Tablets 449
Erythromycin Base Filmtab Tablets 455
Erythromycin Delayed-Release Capsules, USP 457
PCE Dispertab Tablets 515

STATINAL (Greece)
SIMVASTATIN
Zocor Tablets 2105

STATIVER (Greece)
SIMVASTATIN
Zocor Tablets 2105

STAURODORM (Austria)
FLURAZEPAM HYDROCHLORIDE
Dalmane Capsules 3342

STAZEPINE (Hungary)
CARBAMAZEPINE
Carbatrol Capsules 3171
Tegretol Chewable Tablets 2295
Tegretol Suspension 2295
Tegretol Tablets 2295
Tegretol-XR Tablets 2295

STEDON (Greece)
DIAZEPAM
Diastat Rectal Delivery System 3343
Valium Tablets 2819

STEINACLOX (Greece)
NORFLOXACIN
Noroxin Tablets 2032

STENOCOR (Italy)
DIPYRIDAMOLE
Persantine Tablets 868

STERICEF (India, Russia)
CEFTRIAXONE SODIUM
Rocephin Injectable Vials, ADD-Vantage, Galaxy, Bulk . . . 2800

STERIGIN (Austria)
ESTRADIOL
Climara Transdermal System . . . 771
Estring Vaginal Ring . . . 2635

STERODOME (Greece)
ETIDRONATE DISODIUM
Didronel Tablets . . . 2697

STERONASE AQ (Israel)
TRIAMCINOLONE ACETONIDE
Azmacort Inhalation Aerosol . . . 1726
Nasacort AQ Nasal Spray . . . 2922

STEROPOTASSIUM (Belgium)
POTASSIUM CHLORIDE
K-Dur Extended-Release Tablets . . . 3033
K-Lor Oral Solution . . . 474
K-Tab Tablets . . . 475

STEROSTATINE (Belgium)
NYSTATIN
Nystop Topical Powder USP . . . 2478
Paddock Nystatin USP for Oral Suspension . . . 2478

STESOLID (Austria, Czech Republic, Denmark, Finland, Germany, Greece, Hong Kong, Hungary, Irish Republic, Israel, Norway, Portugal, Singapore, Spain, Sweden, Switzerland, Thailand, The Netherlands, United Kingdom)
DIAZEPAM
Diastat Rectal Delivery System . . . 3343
Valium Tablets . . . 2819

STEVENCILLIN (Greece)
AMOXICILLIN
Amoxil Pediatric Drops for Oral Suspension . . . 1343
Amoxil Tablets . . . 1343

STIBENYL (Greece)
RAMIPRIL
Altace Capsules . . . 1702

STIEFCORTIL (Argentina, Brazil)
HYDROCORTISONE
Hydrocortone Tablets . . . 1989

STIEFOTREX (Greece)
ISOTRETINOIN
Accutane Capsules . . . 2731

STIEMAZOL (Germany, South Africa)
CLOTRIMAZOLE
Lotrimin Cream . . . 3039
Lotrimin Lotion 1% . . . 3039
Lotrimin Topical Solution 1% . . . 3039

STIEMYCIN (Argentina, Brazil, Hong Kong, Irish Republic, Malaysia, Mexico, New Zealand, Singapore, South Africa, Thailand, The Netherlands, United Kingdom)
ERYTHROMYCIN
Ery-Tab Tablets . . . 449
Erythromycin Base Filmtab Tablets . . . 455
Erythromycin Delayed-Release Capsules, USP . . . 457
PCE Dispertab Tablets . . . 515

STIEMYCINE (Austria, Germany, Switzerland)
ERYTHROMYCIN
Ery-Tab Tablets . . . 449
Erythromycin Base Filmtab Tablets . . . 455
Erythromycin Delayed-Release Capsules, USP . . . 457
PCE Dispertab Tablets . . . 515

STIEVA-A (Australia, Canada, Chile, Hong Kong, Malaysia, Mexico, Singapore, Thailand)
TRETINOIN
Vesanoid Capsules . . . 2820

STIEVAMYCIN (Argentina, Canada, Mexico)
TRETINOIN
Vesanoid Capsules . . . 2820

STIGMICARPIN (Greece)
NIMODIPINE
Nimotop Capsules . . . 749

STILL (Brazil, Mexico)
DICLOFENAC SODIUM
Voltaren Tablets . . . 2307
Voltaren-XR Tablets . . . 2310

STILLINE (United Kingdom)
SELEGILINE HYDROCHLORIDE
Eldepryl Capsules . . . 3208

STILOZ (India)
CILOSTAZOL
Pletal Tablets . . . 2455

STILUX (Brazil)
NAPHAZOLINE HYDROCHLORIDE
Albalon Ophthalmic Solution . . . ⊙218

STIMOLCARDIO (Italy)
DIPYRIDAMOLE
Persantine Tablets . . . 868

STIMULOTON (Hungary, Russia)
SERTRALINE HYDROCHLORIDE
Zoloft Tablets . . . 2586

STIMYCINE (France)
ERYTHROMYCIN
Ery-Tab Tablets . . . 449
Erythromycin Base Filmtab Tablets . . . 455
Erythromycin Delayed-Release Capsules, USP . . . 457
PCE Dispertab Tablets . . . 515

STIOXYL (Sweden)
BENZOYL PEROXIDE
Brevoxyl-4 Creamy Wash . . . 3210
Brevoxyl-4 Gel . . . 3210
Brevoxyl-8 Creamy Wash . . . 3210
Brevoxyl-8 Gel . . . 3210
Triaz Cleanser . . . 1892
Triaz Gel . . . 1892

STIVATE (Thailand)
CLOBETASOL PROPIONATE
Temovate Cream . . . 2668
Temovate E Emollient . . . 2671
Temovate Gel . . . 2669
Temovate Ointment . . . 2668
Temovate Scalp Application . . . 2670

STOCRIN (Argentina, Australia, Austria, Belgium, Brazil, Chile, Czech Republic, Denmark, Finland, Greece, Hong Kong, Israel, Malaysia, Mexico, New Zealand, Norway, Portugal, Russia, Singapore, South Africa, Sweden, Switzerland, Thailand, The Netherlands, Venezuela)
EFAVIRENZ
Sustiva Capsules . . . 930

STOP ESPINILLA NORMADERM (Spain)
BENZOYL PEROXIDE
Brevoxyl-4 Creamy Wash . . . 3210
Brevoxyl-4 Gel . . . 3210
Brevoxyl-8 Creamy Wash . . . 3210
Brevoxyl-8 Gel . . . 3210
Triaz Cleanser . . . 1892
Triaz Gel . . . 1892

STOVAREN (Italy)
CEFOXITIN SODIUM
Mefoxin Premixed Intravenous Solution . . . 2016
Mefoxin for Injection . . . 2012

STRIMOX (Venezuela)
AMOXICILLIN
Amoxil Pediatric Drops for Oral Suspension . . . 1343
Amoxil Tablets . . . 1343

STROMECTOL (Australia, France, Japan, The Netherlands)
IVERMECTIN
Stromectol Tablets . . . 2083

STRONAZON (United Kingdom)
TAMSULOSIN HYDROCHLORIDE
Flomax Capsules . . . 850

STROX (India)
CIPROFLOXACIN HYDROCHLORIDE
Ciloxan Ophthalmic Ointment . . . ⊙204, 559
Ciloxan Ophthalmic Solution . . . ⊙206
Cipro Tablets . . . 2977

STUD (United Kingdom)
LIDOCAINE
Lidoderm Patch . . . 1118

STUD 100 (Australia, Israel)
LIDOCAINE
Lidoderm Patch . . . 1118

SUADIAN (Italy)
NAFTIFINE HYDROCHLORIDE
Naftin Cream . . . 2126
Naftin Gel . . . 2126

SUBELAN (Chile)
VENLAFAXINE HYDROCHLORIDE
Effexor Tablets . . . 3411
Effexor XR Capsules . . . 3417

SUBLIMAZE (Argentina, Australia, Canada, Irish Republic, New Zealand, South Africa, United Kingdom)
FENTANYL CITRATE
Actiq . . . 979

SUBSTITOL (Austria)
ESTRADIOL
Climara Transdermal System . . . 771
Estring Vaginal Ring . . . 2635
MORPHINE SULFATE
Kadian Capsules . . . 577
MS Contin Tablets . . . 2701

SUBSYDE (Thailand)
DICLOFENAC SODIUM
Voltaren Tablets . . . 2307
Voltaren-XR Tablets . . . 2310

SUBUTEX (Australia, Austria, Belgium, Czech Republic, Denmark, Finland, France, Germany, Greece, Hong Kong, Israel, Italy, Malaysia, Norway, Portugal, Singapore, South Africa, Spain, Sweden, Switzerland, United Kingdom)
BUPRENORPHINE HYDROCHLORIDE
Buprenex Injectable . . . 2716

SUCARI (Hong Kong)
SUCRALFATE
Carafate Suspension . . . 701
Carafate Tablets . . . 701

SUCCOSA (Sweden)
SUCRALFATE
Carafate Suspension . . . 701
Carafate Tablets . . . 701

SUCRABEST (Germany)
SUCRALFATE
Carafate Suspension . . . 701
Carafate Tablets . . . 701

SUCRAFEN (Thailand)
SUCRALFATE
Carafate Suspension . . . 701
Carafate Tablets . . . 701

SUCRAFILM (Brazil)
SUCRALFATE
Carafate Suspension . . . 701
Carafate Tablets . . . 701

SUCRAGER (Italy)
SUCRALFATE
Carafate Suspension . . . 701
Carafate Tablets . . . 701

SUCRAL (Italy, Thailand)
SUCRALFATE
Carafate Suspension . . . 701
Carafate Tablets . . . 701

SUCRALAN (Austria, Czech Republic)
SUCRALFATE
Carafate Suspension . . . 701
Carafate Tablets . . . 701

SUCRALBENE (Austria)
SUCRALFATE
Carafate Suspension . . . 701
Carafate Tablets . . . 701

SUCRALFIN (Italy)
SUCRALFATE
Carafate Suspension . . . 701
Carafate Tablets . . . 701

SUCRALMAX (Argentina)
SUCRALFATE
Carafate Suspension . . . 701
Carafate Tablets . . . 701

SUCRALOSE (PREPARATION) (United Arab Emirates)
SUCRALFATE
Carafate Suspension . . . 701
Carafate Tablets . . . 701

SUCRALSTAD (Austria)
SUCRALFATE
Carafate Suspension . . . 701
Carafate Tablets . . . 701

SUCRALUM (Portugal)
SUCRALFATE
Carafate Suspension . . . 701
Carafate Tablets . . . 701

SUCRAMAL (Italy)
SUCRALFATE
Carafate Suspension . . . 701
Carafate Tablets . . . 701

SUCRAMED (Austria)
SUCRALFATE
Carafate Suspension . . . 701
Carafate Tablets . . . 701

SUCRAPHIL (Germany)
SUCRALFATE
Carafate Suspension . . . 701
Carafate Tablets . . . 701

SUCRASE (India)
SUCRALFATE
Carafate Suspension . . . 701
Carafate Tablets . . . 701

SUCRATE (Greece, Italy, Thailand)
SUCRALFATE
Carafate Suspension . . . 701
Carafate Tablets . . . 701

SUCRATYROL (Austria)
SUCRALFATE
Carafate Suspension . . . 701
Carafate Tablets . . . 701

SUCRORIL (Italy)
SUCRALFATE
Carafate Suspension . . . 701
Carafate Tablets . . . 701

SUDAC (Italy)
SULINDAC
Clinoril Tablets . . . 1924

SUFORTAN (Italy, Mexico)
PENICILLAMINE
Cuprimine Capsules . . . 1947

SUFORTANON (Spain)
PENICILLAMINE
Cuprimine Capsules . . . 1947

SUGAR (Italy)
SUCRALFATE
Carafate Suspension . . . 701
Carafate Tablets . . . 701

SUGAST (Italy)
SUCRALFATE
Carafate Suspension . . . 701
Carafate Tablets . . . 701

SUIFLOX (Mexico)
CIPROFLOXACIN HYDROCHLORIDE
Ciloxan Ophthalmic Ointment . . . ⊙204, 559
Ciloxan Ophthalmic Solution . . . ⊙206
Cipro Tablets . . . 2977

SUL 10 (Mexico)
SULFACETAMIDE SODIUM
Klaron Lotion 10% . . . 2909

SULAR (Belgium, Mexico, Spain, The Netherlands)
NISOLDIPINE
Sular Tablets . . . 3122

SULARTRENE (Italy)
SULINDAC
Clinoril Tablets . . . 1924

SULCRAN (Chile)
SUCRALFATE
Carafate Suspension . . . 701
Carafate Tablets . . . 701

SULCRATE (Canada)
SUCRALFATE
Carafate Suspension . . . 701
Carafate Tablets . . . 701

SULEN (Italy)
SULINDAC
Clinoril Tablets . . . 1924

SULEXON (Spain)
DICLOFENAC SODIUM
Voltaren Tablets . . . 2307
Voltaren-XR Tablets . . . 2310

SULFA 10 (Belgium)
SULFACETAMIDE SODIUM
Klaron Lotion 10% . . . 2909

SULFABLEPH N LIQUIFILM (Germany)
SULFACETAMIDE SODIUM
Klaron Lotion 10% . . . 2909

SULFACET (Spain, Venezuela)
SULFACETAMIDE SODIUM
Klaron Lotion 10% . . . 2909

SULFACETA (Spain)
SULFACETAMIDE SODIUM
Klaron Lotion 10% . . . 2909

SULFACETAM (Spain)
SULFACETAMIDE SODIUM
Klaron Lotion 10% . . . 2909

SULFACID (Israel)
SULFACETAMIDE SODIUM
Klaron Lotion 10% . . . 2909

SULFACOLLYRE (Belgium)
SULFACETAMIDE SODIUM
Klaron Lotion 10% . . . 2909

SULFACORT (Venezuela)
SULFACETAMIDE SODIUM
Klaron Lotion 10% . . . 2909

SULFACYL (Russia)
SULFACETAMIDE SODIUM
Klaron Lotion 10% . . . 2909

SULFAMYLON (Canada, United Kingdom)
MAFENIDE ACETATE
Sulfamylon Cream . . . 2162
Sulfamylon for 5% Topical Solution . . . 2162

SULFEX (Canada, Hong Kong)
SULFACETAMIDE SODIUM
Klaron Lotion 10% . . . 2909

SULFINAV (Argentina)
EFAVIRENZ
Sustiva Capsules . . . 930

SULFONA (Portugal, Spain)
DAPSONE
Dapsone Tablets USP . . . 1673

SULFO-SELENIUM (Belgium)
HYDROCORTISONE
Hydrocortone Tablets . . . 1989

SULFOXYL (Canada)
BENZOYL PEROXIDE
Brevoxyl-4 Creamy Wash . . . 3210
Brevoxyl-4 Gel . . . 3210
Brevoxyl-8 Creamy Wash . . . 3210
Brevoxyl-8 Gel . . . 3210
Triaz Cleanser . . . 1892
Triaz Gel . . . 1892

SULIFUR (Mexico)
SULINDAC
Clinoril Tablets . . . 1924

SULINDAL (Spain)
SULINDAC
Clinoril Tablets . . . 1924

SULINOL (Italy)
SULINDAC
Clinoril Tablets . . . 1924

SULIX (Chile)
TAMSULOSIN HYDROCHLORIDE
Flomax Capsules . . . 850

SULMYCIN (Austria, Germany)
GENTAMICIN SULFATE
Garamycin Injectable . . . 3014

SULOCTEN (Argentina)
ENALAPRIL MALEATE
Vasotec I.V. Injection . . . 2103

SULOTIL (Chile)
NIFEDIPINE
Adalat CC Tablets . . . 2964

SULPHAMIDE (Israel)
SULFACETAMIDE SODIUM
Klaron Lotion 10% . . . 2909

SULREUMA (Italy)
SULINDAC
Clinoril Tablets . . . 1924

SULVI (Mexico)
NAPHAZOLINE HYDROCHLORIDE
Albalon Ophthalmic Solution . . . ⊙218

SUMACLINA (Portugal)
SIMVASTATIN
Zocor Tablets . . . 2105

SUMADOL (Italy)
SUMATRIPTAN SUCCINATE
Imitrex Injection . . . 1463
Imitrex Tablets . . . 1471

SUMAX (Brazil)
SUMATRIPTAN SUCCINATE
Imitrex Injection . . . 1463
Imitrex Tablets . . . 1471

SUMIAL (Spain)
PROPRANOLOL HYDROCHLORIDE
Inderal LA Long-Acting Capsules . . . 3429

SUMIGRENE (Italy)
SUMATRIPTAN SUCCINATE
Imitrex Injection . . . 1463
Imitrex Tablets . . . 1471

SUMINAT (India)
SUMATRIPTAN SUCCINATE
Imitrex Injection . . . 1463
Imitrex Tablets . . . 1471

SUMITREX (Mexico)
SUMATRIPTAN
Imitrex Nasal Spray . . . 1467

SUNITON (Malaysia)
ORPHENADRINE CITRATE
Norflex Injection . . . 1856

SUNPROX (Malaysia, Singapore)
NAPROXEN SODIUM
Anaprox DS Tablets . . . 2761
Anaprox Tablets . . . 2761

SUPARTZ (United Kingdom)
SODIUM HYALURONATE
Hyalgan Solution . . . 2901

SUPERAMIN (Greece)
LEVOCARNITINE
Carnitor Injection . . . 3188
Carnitor Tablets and Oral Solution . . . 3190

SUPERO (Italy)
CEFUROXIME SODIUM
Zinacef Injection . . . 1631

SUPEUDOL (Canada)
OXYCODONE HYDROCHLORIDE
OxyContin Tablets . . . 2703
OxyFast Oral Concentrate Solution . . . 2708
OxyIR Capsules . . . 2708

SUPIROCIN (India)
MUPIROCIN
Bactroban Ointment . . . 1395

SUPIROCIN-B (India)
MUPIROCIN
Bactroban Ointment . . . 1395

SUPLASYN (Canada, France, Germany, United Kingdom)
SODIUM HYALURONATE
Hyalgan Solution . . . 2901

SUPOTRON (Greece)
ENALAPRIL MALEATE
Vasotec I.V. Injection . . . 2103

SUPPLIN (Hungary)
METRONIDAZOLE
MetroGel-Vaginal Gel . . . 1855

SUPRACEF (Finland)
CEFIXIME
Suprax . . . 1843

SUPRACOF (Mexico)
BENZONATATE
Tessalon Perles . . . 1199

SUPRACORDIN (Czech Republic)
NIFEDIPINE
Adalat CC Tablets . . . 2964

SUPRAGENTA (Spain)
GENTAMICIN SULFATE
Garamycin Injectable . . . 3014

SUPRAHYAL (Chile, Mexico)
SODIUM HYALURONATE
Hyalgan Solution . . . 2901

SUPRALIP (Thailand, United Kingdom)
FENOFIBRATE
Tricor Tablets . . . 527

SUPRAMOX (Switzerland)
AMOXICILLIN
Amoxil Pediatric Drops for Oral Suspension . . . 1343
Amoxil Tablets . . . 1343

SUPRAN (Israel)
CEFIXIME
Suprax . . . 1843

SUPRAX (Canada, Czech Republic, Germany, Hungary, Irish Republic, Italy, Russia, United Kingdom)
CEFIXIME
Suprax . . . 1843

SUPRIMOX (India)
AMOXICILLIN
Amoxil Pediatric Drops for Oral Suspension . . . 1343
Amoxil Tablets . . . 1343

SURAZEM (The Netherlands)
DILTIAZEM HYDROCHLORIDE
Cardizem LA Extended Release Tablets . . . 1728
Tiazac Capsules . . . 1201

SURFAZ (India)
CLOTRIMAZOLE
Lotrimin Cream . . . 3039
Lotrimin Lotion 1% . . . 3039
Lotrimin Topical Solution 1% . . . 3039

SURIL (Italy)
SUCRALFATE
Carafate Suspension . . . 701
Carafate Tablets . . . 701

SUSTAC (Argentina)
RANITIDINE HYDROCHLORIDE
Zantac 25 EFFERdose Tablets . . . 1624
Zantac 150 EFFERdose Tablets . . . 1624
Zantac 150 Tablets . . . 1624
Zantac 300 Tablets . . . 1624
Zantac Injection . . . 1619
Zantac Injection Premixed . . . 1619
Zantac Syrup . . . 1624

SUSTIVA (Canada, France, Germany, Irish Republic, Italy, Spain, United Kingdom)
EFAVIRENZ
Sustiva Capsules . . . 930

SUTAC (Thailand)
CETIRIZINE HYDROCHLORIDE
Zyrtec Syrup . . . 2594
Zyrtec Tablets . . . 2594

SUTIF (Spain)
TERAZOSIN HYDROCHLORIDE
Hytrin Capsules . . . 471

SUTRICO (Argentina)
FINASTERIDE
Propecia Tablets . . . 2060
Proscar Tablets . . . 2067

SUVALAN (Australia)
SUMATRIPTAN SUCCINATE
Imitrex Injection . . . 1463
Imitrex Tablets . . . 1471

SVELTANET (Greece)
RANITIDINE HYDROCHLORIDE
Zantac 25 EFFERdose Tablets . . . 1624
Zantac 150 EFFERdose Tablets . . . 1624
Zantac 150 Tablets . . . 1624
Zantac 300 Tablets . . . 1624
Zantac Injection . . . 1619
Zantac Injection Premixed . . . 1619
Zantac Syrup . . . 1624

SVIROXIT (Greece)
ETIDRONATE DISODIUM
Didronel Tablets . . . 2697

SWISS-KAL SR (South Africa)
POTASSIUM CHLORIDE
K-Dur Extended-Relase Tablets . . . 3033
K-Lor Oral Solution . . . 474
K-Tab Tablets . . . 475

SYLADOR (Brazil)
TRAMADOL HYDROCHLORIDE
Ultram ER Tablets . . . 2392

SYMBYAX (Argentina, Mexico)
OLANZAPINE
Zyprexa Tablets . . . 1830

SYMMETREL (Australia, Austria, Canada, Germany, Greece, Hong Kong, Irish Republic, Israel, New Zealand, Norway, Singapore, South Africa, Sweden, Switzerland, The Netherlands, United Kingdom, Venezuela)
AMANTADINE HYDROCHLORIDE
Symmetrel Tablets . . . 1135

SYMOXYL (India)
AMOXICILLIN
Amoxil Pediatric Drops for Oral Suspension . . . 1343
Amoxil Tablets . . . 1343

SYNAGIS (Argentina, Australia, Belgium, Brazil, Canada, Chile, Czech Republic, Denmark, Finland, France, Germany, Greece, Hong Kong, Hungary, Irish Republic, Italy, Malaysia, Mexico, New Zealand, Norway, Singapore, South Africa, Spain, Sweden, Switzerland, The Netherlands, United Kingdom, Venezuela)
PALIVIZUMAB
Synagis Intramuscular Powder . . . 1897

SYNAPROSYN (Venezuela)
NAPROXEN
EC-Naprosyn Delayed-Release Tablets . . . 2761
Naprosyn Suspension . . . 2761
Naprosyn Tablets . . . 2761

SYNCLAR (India)
CLARITHROMYCIN
Biaxin Filmtab Tablets . . . 402
Biaxin Granules . . . 402

SYNERPRIL (Austria)
ENALAPRIL MALEATE
Vasotec I.V. Injection . . . 2103

SYNFLEX (Australia, Canada, Hong Kong, Irish Republic, Italy, New Zealand, Singapore, South Africa, Thailand, United Kingdom)
NAPROXEN SODIUM
Anaprox DS Tablets . . . 2761
Anaprox Tablets . . . 2761

SYNITIDINE (Hong Kong)
RANITIDINE HYDROCHLORIDE
Zantac 25 EFFERdose Tablets . . . 1624
Zantac 150 EFFERdose Tablets . . . 1624
Zantac 150 Tablets . . . 1624
Zantac 300 Tablets . . . 1624
Zantac Injection . . . 1619
Zantac Injection Premixed . . . 1619
Zantac Syrup . . . 1624

SYNOGIL (Germany)
NATAMYCIN
Natacyn Antifungal Ophthalmic Suspension . . . ⊙208

SYNOGIN (Thailand)
NAPROXEN
EC-Naprosyn Delayed-Release Tablets . . . 2761
Naprosyn Suspension . . . 2761
Naprosyn Tablets . . . 2761

SYNTARIS (Austria, Belgium, Czech Republic, Germany, Irish Republic, Italy, South Africa, Switzerland, The Netherlands, United Kingdom)
FLUNISOLIDE
Aerobid Inhaler System . . . 1171
Aerobid-M Inhaler System . . . 1171

SYNTHOMANET (Greece)
RANITIDINE HYDROCHLORIDE
Zantac 25 EFFERdose Tablets . . . 1624
Zantac 150 EFFERdose Tablets . . . 1624
Zantac 150 Tablets . . . 1624
Zantac 300 Tablets . . . 1624
Zantac Injection . . . 1619
Zantac Injection Premixed . . . 1619
Zantac Syrup . . . 1624

SYNTHROID (Brazil, Canada)
LEVOTHYROXINE SODIUM
Levothroid Tablets . . . 1186
Levoxyl Tablets . . . 1712
Synthroid Tablets . . . 520

SYNTONOL (Thailand)
PROPRANOLOL HYDROCHLORIDE
Inderal LA Long-Acting Capsules . . . 3429

SYNURETIC (United Kingdom)
AMILORIDE HYDROCHLORIDE/HYDROCHLOROTHIAZIDE
Moduretic Tablets . . . 2028

SYPROL (United Kingdom)
PROPRANOLOL HYDROCHLORIDE
Inderal LA Long-Acting Capsules . . . 3429

SYSCOR (Austria, Belgium, Brazil, Czech Republic, Finland, Greece, Italy, Mexico, New Zealand, South Africa, Spain, Sweden, Switzerland, The Netherlands, United Kingdom)
NISOLDIPINE
Sular Tablets 3122

SYSTEN (Austria, Belgium, Brazil, Czech Republic, France, Hungary, Italy, Mexico, Switzerland, The Netherlands)
ESTRADIOL
Climara Transdermal System 771
Estring Vaginal Ring 2635

SYSTEN CONTI (Brazil, Czech Republic)
ESTRADIOL
Climara Transdermal System 771
Estring Vaginal Ring 2635

SYSTEPIN (Irish Republic)
NIFEDIPINE
Adalat CC Tablets 2964

SYSTRAL HYDROCORT (Germany)
HYDROCORTISONE
Hydrocortone Tablets 1989

T.O.VIR (Thailand)
ZIDOVUDINE
Retrovir Capsules 1560
Retrovir IV Infusion 1564
Retrovir Syrup 1560
Retrovir Tablets 1560

T/H-BASAN (Switzerland)
HYDROCHLOROTHIAZIDE/TRIAMTERENE
Dyazide Capsules 1423

T3 (Greece)
LIOTHYRONINE SODIUM
Cytomel Tablets 1710

T4 (Argentina, Greece)
LEVOTHYROXINE SODIUM
Levothroid Tablets 1186
Levoxyl Tablets 1712
Synthroid Tablets 520

TA OSOTH (Thailand)
TRIAMCINOLONE ACETONIDE
Azmacort Inhalation Aerosol 1726
Nasacort AQ Nasal Spray 2922

TABPHYN (United Kingdom)
TAMSULOSIN HYDROCHLORIDE
Flomax Capsules 850

TABULAN (Venezuela)
CAPTOPRIL
Captopril Tablets 2149

TACEX (Mexico)
CEFTRIAXONE SODIUM
Rocephin Injectable Vials, ADD-Vantage, Galaxy, Bulk 2800

TACHYFENON (Germany)
PROPAFENONE HYDROCHLORIDE
Rythmol SR Capsules 2727

TACICUL (Argentina)
LOSARTAN POTASSIUM
Cozaar Tablets 1935

TACINOL (Thailand)
TRIAMCINOLONE ACETONIDE
Azmacort Inhalation Aerosol 1726
Nasacort AQ Nasal Spray 2922

TACRAF (Argentina)
TACROLIMUS
Prograf Capsules and Injection 632

TACRON (Singapore, Spain)
TICLOPIDINE HYDROCHLORIDE
Ticlid Tablets 2810

TACRO-TIC (Argentina)
TACROLIMUS
Prograf Capsules and Injection 632

TACROZ (India)
TACROLIMUS
Prograf Capsules and Injection 632

TAFENIL (Mexico)
FLUTAMIDE
Eulexin Capsules 3009

TAFLOC (South Africa)
OFLOXACIN
Floxin Otic Solution 1049

TAFLOX (Portugal)
NORFLOXACIN
Noroxin Tablets 2032

TAGAL (Mexico)
CEFTAZIDIME
Fortaz for Injection 1453

TAGREN (Czech Republic)
TICLOPIDINE HYDROCHLORIDE
Ticlid Tablets 2810

TAHOR (France)
ATORVASTATIN CALCIUM
Lipitor Tablets 2483

TAIRAL (Spain)
FAMOTIDINE
Pepcid Injection 2040
Pepcid Injection Premixed 2040
Pepcid Tablets 2038
Pepcid for Oral Suspension 2038

TAKADOL (France)
TRAMADOL HYDROCHLORIDE
Ultram ER Tablets 2392

TAKEPRON (Hong Kong, Japan)
LANSOPRAZOLE
Prevacid Delayed-Release Capsules 3271

TAKS (Malaysia, Thailand)
DICLOFENAC SODIUM
Voltaren Tablets 2307
Voltaren-XR Tablets 2310

TALAM (Australia)
CITALOPRAM HYDROBROMIDE
Celexa Tablets 1176

TALEMA (Venezuela)
DIAZEPAM
Diastat Rectal Delivery System 3343
Valium Tablets 2819

TALGESIL (Malaysia)
FENTANYL
Duragesic Transdermal System 2373

TALICIX (Spain)
CLARITHROMYCIN
Biaxin Filmtab Tablets 402
Biaxin Granules 402

TALIRAX (Greece)
FLUOROMETHOLONE
FML Ophthalmic Ointment . . . . ⊙228

TALIZER (Mexico)
THALIDOMIDE
Thalomid Capsules 965

TALLITON (Hungary, Russia)
CARVEDILOL
Coreg Tablets 1414

TALNUR (Argentina)
FENTANYL
Duragesic Transdermal System 2373

TALOFILINA (Brazil)
THEOPHYLLINE
Uniphyl Tablets 2710

TALOHEXAL (Australia)
CITALOPRAM HYDROBROMIDE
Celexa Tablets 1176

TALOKEN (Mexico)
CEFTAZIDIME
Fortaz for Injection 1453

TALOMIL (South Africa)
CITALOPRAM HYDROBROMIDE
Celexa Tablets 1176

TALZIC (Venezuela)
CETIRIZINE HYDROCHLORIDE
Zyrtec Syrup 2594
Zyrtec Tablets 2594

TAM (Spain)
CIPROFLOXACIN HYDROCHLORIDE
Ciloxan Ophthalmic Ointment . . . . ⊙204, 559
Ciloxan Ophthalmic Solution . . . . ⊙206
Cipro Tablets 2977

TAMBAC (India)
CEFPODOXIME PROXETIL
Vantin Tablets and Oral Suspension 2645

TAMBOCOR (Argentina, Australia, Belgium, Canada, Chile, Czech Republic, Denmark, Finland, Germany, Hong Kong, Irish Republic, Israel, Malaysia, Mexico, New Zealand, Norway, Singapore, South Africa, Sweden, Switzerland, Thailand, The Netherlands, United Kingdom)
FLECAINIDE ACETATE
Tambocor Tablets 1856

TAMERAN (Spain)
FAMOTIDINE
Pepcid Injection 2040
Pepcid Injection Premixed 2040
Pepcid Tablets 2038
Pepcid for Oral Suspension 2038

TAMIN (Spain)
FAMOTIDINE
Pepcid Injection 2040
Pepcid Injection Premixed 2040
Pepcid Tablets 2038
Pepcid for Oral Suspension 2038

TAMIRAM (Brazil)
LEVOFLOXACIN
Levaquin Injection 2384
Levaquin Tablets 2384

TAMOLAN (Thailand)
TRAMADOL HYDROCHLORIDE
Ultram ER Tablets 2392

TAMSUNA (Argentina)
TAMSULOSIN HYDROCHLORIDE
Flomax Capsules 850

TANAVAT (Argentina)
SIMVASTATIN
Zocor Tablets 2105

TANDAX (Mexico)
NAPROXEN SODIUM
Anaprox DS Tablets 2761
Anaprox Tablets 2761

TANDIAL (Mexico)
DIAZEPAM
Diastat Rectal Delivery System 3343
Valium Tablets 2819

TANDIX (Portugal)
INDAPAMIDE
Indapamide Tablets 2156

TANFEDIN (Venezuela)
CARBAMAZEPINE
Carbatrol Capsules 3171
Tegretol Chewable Tablets 2295
Tegretol Suspension 2295
Tegretol Tablets 2295
Tegretol-XR Tablets 2295

TANIDINA (Spain)
RANITIDINE HYDROCHLORIDE
Zantac 25 EFFERdose Tablets 1624
Zantac 150 EFFERdose Tablets 1624
Zantac 150 Tablets 1624
Zantac 300 Tablets 1624
Zantac Injection 1619
Zantac Injection Premixed 1619
Zantac Syrup 1624

TANIZONA (Mexico)
NAPROXEN
EC-Naprosyn Delayed-Release Tablets 2761
Naprosyn Suspension 2761
Naprosyn Tablets 2761

TANYL (Israel, South Africa)
FENTANYL CITRATE
Actiq 979

TAPRODEX (Mexico)
DEXAMETHASONE
Decadron Tablets 1951

TARATEN (Thailand)
CLOTRIMAZOLE
Lotrimin Cream 3039
Lotrimin Lotion 1% 3039
Lotrimin Topical Solution 1% 3039

TARDOTOL (Denmark)
CARBAMAZEPINE
Carbatrol Capsules 3171
Tegretol Chewable Tablets 2295
Tegretol Suspension 2295
Tegretol Tablets 2295
Tegretol-XR Tablets 2295

TAREG (Brazil, Chile, France, Italy, Portugal)
VALSARTAN
Diovan Tablets 2193

TAREG-D (Chile)
HYDROCHLOROTHIAZIDE/VALSARTAN
Diovan HCT Tablets 2196

TAREMIS (Argentina)
METRONIDAZOLE
MetroGel-Vaginal Gel 1855

TARICIN (Russia)
OFLOXACIN
Floxin Otic Solution 1049

TARIFLOX (India)
OFLOXACIN
Floxin Otic Solution 1049

TARIFLOX PLUS (India)
OFLOXACIN
Floxin Otic Solution 1049

TARIVID (Czech Republic, Denmark, Finland, Hungary, India, Israel, Malaysia, Russia, Singapore, South Africa, Sweden, Switzerland, Thailand)
OFLOXACIN
Floxin Otic Solution 1049

TARJEN (Thailand)
DICLOFENAC SODIUM
Voltaren Tablets 2307
Voltaren-XR Tablets 2310

TARJENA (Thailand)
DICLOFENAC SODIUM
Voltaren Tablets 2307
Voltaren-XR Tablets 2310

TARKA (Argentina, Austria, Brazil, Canada, Czech Republic, Denmark, Finland, France, Germany, Greece, Hungary, Italy, Mexico, Russia, South Africa, Spain, Sweden, Switzerland, The Netherlands, United Kingdom, Venezuela)
VERAPAMIL HYDROCHLORIDE
Covera-HS Tablets 3139
Verelan PM Extended-Release Capsules, Controlled-Onset 3106

TAROFLOX (Czech Republic)
OFLOXACIN
Floxin Otic Solution 1049

TARON (Venezuela)
ALBENDAZOLE
Albenza Tablets 1338

TASEDAN (Mexico)
ESTAZOLAM
ProSom Tablets 517

TASMAR (Argentina, Austria, Brazil, Chile, Denmark, France, Greece, Hong Kong, Irish Republic, Mexico, New Zealand, Norway, Singapore, South Africa, Sweden, Switzerland, Thailand, United Kingdom)
TOLCAPONE
Tasmar Tablets 3358

TATIG (Italy)
SERTRALINE HYDROCHLORIDE
Zoloft Tablets 2586

TAUCOR (Spain)
LOVASTATIN
Mevacor Tablets 2021

TAVANIC (Argentina, Austria, Belgium, Brazil, Chile, Czech Republic, Finland, France, Germany, Greece, Hungary, India, Irish Republic, Israel, Italy, Mexico, Portugal, Russia, South Africa, Spain, Sweden, Switzerland, The Netherlands, United Kingdom, Venezuela)
LEVOFLOXACIN
Levaquin Injection 2384
Levaquin Tablets 2384

TAVAN-SP 54 (South Africa)
PENTOSAN POLYSULFATE SODIUM
Elmiron Capsules 2415

TAVER (Malaysia, Thailand)
CARBAMAZEPINE
Carbatrol Capsules 3171
Tegretol Chewable Tablets 2295
Tegretol Suspension 2295
Tegretol Tablets 2295
Tegretol-XR Tablets 2295

(⊙ Described in PDR For Ophthalmic Medicines™)

TAVOR (Mexico, Venezuela)
OXYBUTYNIN CHLORIDE
Ditropan XL Extended-Release Tablets . . . 2413

TAXENAN (Mexico)
NAPROXEN
EC-Naprosyn Delayed-Release Tablets 2761
Naprosyn Suspension 2761
Naprosyn Tablets 2761

TAXIFUR (Mexico)
CEFTAZIDIME
Fortaz for Injection 1453

TAXOTERE (Argentina, Australia, Austria, Belgium, Brazil, Canada, Chile, Czech Republic, Denmark, Finland, France, Germany, Greece, Hong Kong, Hungary, Irish Republic, Israel, Italy, Japan, Malaysia, Mexico, New Zealand, Norway, Portugal, Russia, Singapore, South Africa, Spain, Sweden, Switzerland, Thailand, The Netherlands, United Kingdom, Venezuela)
DOCETAXEL
Taxotere Injection Concentrate 2932

TAXYL (Mexico)
DEXAMETHASONE
Decadron Tablets 1951

TAZEPIN (Brazil)
RANITIDINE HYDROCHLORIDE
Zantac 25 EFFERdose Tablets 1624
Zantac 150 EFFERdose Tablets 1624
Zantac 150 Tablets 1624
Zantac 300 Tablets 1624
Zantac Injection 1619
Zantac Injection Premixed 1619
Zantac Syrup 1624

TAZIDEM (Brazil)
CEFTAZIDIME
Fortaz for Injection 1453

TAZIDIME (Canada)
CEFTAZIDIME
Fortaz for Injection 1453

TAZOBAC (Germany, Italy, Portugal, Switzerland)
PIPERACILLIN SODIUM/TAZOBACTAM SODIUM
Zosyn 3492

TAZOCILLINE (France)
PIPERACILLIN SODIUM/TAZOBACTAM SODIUM
Zosyn 3492

TAZOCIN (Belgium, Denmark, Finland, Greece, Hong Kong, Irish Republic, Israel, Italy, Mexico, New Zealand, Singapore, South Africa, Sweden, Thailand, The Netherlands)
PIPERACILLIN SODIUM/TAZOBACTAM SODIUM
Zosyn 3492

TAZONAM (Austria, Chile)
PIPERACILLIN SODIUM/TAZOBACTAM SODIUM
Zosyn 3492

TAZUSIN (Spain)
TERAZOSIN HYDROCHLORIDE
Hytrin Capsules 471

TEALEP (Argentina)
FINASTERIDE
Propecia Tablets 2060
Proscar Tablets 2067

TEBEGRAN (Mexico)
SUMATRIPTAN SUCCINATE
Imitrex Injection 1463
Imitrex Tablets 1471

TECFLU (Mexico)
FLUOROURACIL
Efudex Topical Cream 3363
Efudex Topical Solutions 3363

TECHNIPHYLLINE (Monaco)
THEOPHYLLINE
Uniphyl Tablets 2710

TECNOFLUT (Brazil)
FLUTAMIDE
Eulexin Capsules 3009

TECNOLIP (Portugal)
LOVASTATIN
Mevacor Tablets 2021

TECNOMAX (Argentina)
SILDENAFIL CITRATE
Viagra Tablets 2573

TECNOTECAN (Brazil)
IRINOTECAN HYDROCHLORIDE
Camptosar Injection 2604

TECPRAZIN (Mexico)
PRAZIQUANTEL
Biltricide Tablets 2976

TEDICUMAR (Spain)
WARFARIN SODIUM
Coumadin Tablets 898
Coumadin for Injection 898

TEDRAL (The Netherlands)
THEOPHYLLINE
Uniphyl Tablets 2710

TEDRALAN (Monaco)
THEOPHYLLINE
Uniphyl Tablets 2710

TEFLUT (Brazil)
FLUTAMIDE
Eulexin Capsules 3009

TEGRETAL (Chile, Germany)
CARBAMAZEPINE
Carbatrol Capsules 3171
Tegretol Chewable Tablets 2295
Tegretol Suspension 2295
Tegretol Tablets 2295
Tegretol-XR Tablets 2295

TEGRETARD (Brazil)
CARBAMAZEPINE
Carbatrol Capsules 3171
Tegretol Chewable Tablets 2295
Tegretol Suspension 2295
Tegretol Tablets 2295
Tegretol-XR Tablets 2295

TEGRETOL (Argentina, Australia, Austria, Belgium, Brazil, Canada, Czech Republic, Denmark, Finland, France, Greece, Hong Kong, Hungary, Irish Republic, Israel, Italy, Malaysia, Mexico, New Zealand, Norway, Portugal, Russia, Singapore, South Africa, Spain, Sweden, Switzerland, Thailand, The Netherlands, United Kingdom, Venezuela)
CARBAMAZEPINE
Carbatrol Capsules 3171
Tegretol Chewable Tablets 2295
Tegretol Suspension 2295
Tegretol Tablets 2295
Tegretol-XR Tablets 2295

TEGREX (Brazil)
CARBAMAZEPINE
Carbatrol Capsules 3171
Tegretol Chewable Tablets 2295
Tegretol Suspension 2295
Tegretol Tablets 2295
Tegretol-XR Tablets 2295

TEGREZIN (Brazil)
CARBAMAZEPINE
Carbatrol Capsules 3171
Tegretol Chewable Tablets 2295
Tegretol Suspension 2295
Tegretol Tablets 2295
Tegretol-XR Tablets 2295

TEGRITAL (India)
CARBAMAZEPINE
Carbatrol Capsules 3171
Tegretol Chewable Tablets 2295
Tegretol Suspension 2295
Tegretol Tablets 2295
Tegretol-XR Tablets 2295

TELARIX (Greece)
CETIRIZINE HYDROCHLORIDE
Zyrtec Syrup 2594
Zyrtec Tablets 2594

TELFAST (Australia, Austria, Belgium, Czech Republic, Denmark, Finland, France, Hong Kong, Hungary, Irish Republic, Israel, Italy, Malaysia, New Zealand, Norway, Portugal, Russia, Singapore, South Africa, Spain, Switzerland, Thailand, The Netherlands, United Kingdom)
FEXOFENADINE HYDROCHLORIDE
Allegra Capsules 2844

TELFAST DECONGESTANT (New Zealand)
FEXOFENADINE HYDROCHLORIDE/PSEUDOEPHEDRINE HYDROCHLORIDE
Allegra-D 12 Hour Extended-Release Tablets 2846

TELFAST-D (Malaysia, Singapore)
FEXOFENADINE HYDROCHLORIDE/PSEUDOEPHEDRINE HYDROCHLORIDE
Allegra-D 12 Hour Extended-Release Tablets 2846

TELMA (India)
TELMISARTAN
Micardis Tablets 854

TELNASE (Australia, New Zealand)
TRIAMCINOLONE ACETONIDE
Azmacort Inhalation Aerosol 1726
Nasacort AQ Nasal Spray 2922

TELSOMET (Venezuela)
DIAZEPAM
Diastat Rectal Delivery System 3343
Valium Tablets 2819

TELUGREN (Chile)
CLOTRIMAZOLE
Lotrimin Cream 3039
Lotrimin Lotion 1% 3039
Lotrimin Topical Solution 1% 3039

TEMACO (Thailand)
THEOPHYLLINE
Uniphyl Tablets 2710

TEMGESIC (Argentina, Australia, Austria, Belgium, Czech Republic, Denmark, Finland, France, Germany, Irish Republic, Italy, Malaysia, Mexico, New Zealand, Norway, Singapore, South Africa, Sweden, Switzerland, Thailand, The Netherlands, United Kingdom)
BUPRENORPHINE HYDROCHLORIDE
Buprenex Injectable 2716

TEMGESIC-NX (New Zealand)
BUPRENORPHINE HYDROCHLORIDE
Buprenex Injectable 2716

TEMISARTAN (Argentina)
LOSARTAN POTASSIUM
Cozaar Tablets 1935

TEMPERAX (Chile)
CITALOPRAM HYDROBROMIDE
Celexa Tablets 1176

TEMPOROL (Irish Republic, South Africa)
CARBAMAZEPINE
Carbatrol Capsules 3171
Tegretol Chewable Tablets 2295
Tegretol Suspension 2295
Tegretol Tablets 2295
Tegretol-XR Tablets 2295

TEMSERIN (Germany, Greece)
TIMOLOL MALEATE
Blocadren Tablets 1916
Timoptic Sterile Ophthalmic Solution 2088
Timoptic in Ocudose 2091
Timoptic-XE Sterile Ophthalmic Gel Forming Solution 2092

TENACID (Italy)
CILASTATIN SODIUM/IMIPENEM
Primaxin I.M. 2045
Primaxin I.V. 2048

TENCAS (Argentina)
ENALAPRIL MALEATE
Vasotec I.V. Injection 2103

TENESCAN (Mexico)
CLOTRIMAZOLE
Lotrimin Cream 3039
Lotrimin Lotion 1% 3039
Lotrimin Topical Solution 1% 3039

TENIBEX (Mexico)
ALBENDAZOLE
Albenza Tablets 1338

TENIKEN (Mexico)
PRAZIQUANTEL
Biltricide Tablets 2976

TENKAFRUSE (United Kingdom)
FUROSEMIDE
Furosemide Tablets 2154

TENOCARD (Argentina)
NIMODIPINE
Nimotop Capsules 749

TENOPRES (Argentina)
LOSARTAN POTASSIUM
Cozaar Tablets 1935

TENOPRES D (Argentina)
LOSARTAN POTASSIUM
Cozaar Tablets 1935

TENOPT (Australia)
TIMOLOL MALEATE
Blocadren Tablets 1916
Timoptic Sterile Ophthalmic Solution 2088
Timoptic in Ocudose 2091
Timoptic-XE Sterile Ophthalmic Gel Forming Solution 2092

TENOVATE (India)
CLOBETASOL PROPIONATE
Temovate Cream 2668
Temovate E Emollient 2671
Temovate Gel 2669
Temovate Ointment 2668
Temovate Scalp Application 2670

TENOVATE G (India)
CLOBETASOL PROPIONATE
Temovate Cream 2668
Temovate E Emollient 2671
Temovate Gel 2669
Temovate Ointment 2668
Temovate Scalp Application 2670

TENOVATE M (India)
CLOBETASOL PROPIONATE
Temovate Cream 2668
Temovate E Emollient 2671
Temovate Gel 2669
Temovate Ointment 2668
Temovate Scalp Application 2670

TENPRIL (Italy)
CAPTOPRIL
Captopril Tablets 2149

TENSADIUR (Italy)
BENAZEPRIL HYDROCHLORIDE/HYDROCHLOROTHIAZIDE
Lotensin HCT Tablets 2246

TENSANIL (Italy)
BENAZEPRIL HYDROCHLORIDE
Lotensin Tablets 2243

TENSAZOL (Portugal)
ENALAPRIL MALEATE
Vasotec I.V. Injection 2103

TENSERPIL (Venezuela)
LOSARTAN POTASSIUM
Cozaar Tablets 1935

TENSIKEY (Spain)
LISINOPRIL
Prinivil Tablets 2052

TENSIKEY COMPLEX (Spain)
LISINOPRIL
Prinivil Tablets 2052

TENSIL (Mexico)
CAPTOPRIL
Captopril Tablets 2149

TENSIOMIN (Czech Republic, Germany, Hong Kong, Hungary, Thailand)
CAPTOPRIL
Captopril Tablets 2149

TENSIOMIN-COR (Germany)
CAPTOPRIL
Captopril Tablets 2149

TENSIPINE (United Kingdom)
NIFEDIPINE
Adalat CC Tablets 2964

TENSIUM (United Kingdom)
DIAZEPAM
Diastat Rectal Delivery System 3343
Valium Tablets 2819

TENSOBON (Germany, Switzerland)
CAPTOPRIL
Captopril Tablets 2149

TENSOBON COMP (Germany)
CAPTOPRIL
Captopril Tablets 2149

TENSOMAX (Venezuela)
NIFEDIPINE
Adalat CC Tablets 2964

TENSOPIN (Venezuela)
NIFEDIPINE
Adalat CC Tablets 2964

TENSOPREL (Singapore, Spain)
CAPTOPRIL
Captopril Tablets 2149

TENSOPRIL (Argentina, Irish Republic, Israel, Portugal, United Kingdom)
LISINOPRIL
Prinivil Tablets 2052

TENSOPRIL D (Argentina)
LISINOPRIL
Prinivil Tablets 2052

TENSOSTAD (Germany)
CAPTOPRIL
Captopril Tablets 2149

TENSO-TIMELETS (Germany)
CLONIDINE HYDROCHLORIDE
Catapres Tablets 843

TENSURIL (Brazil)
DIAZOXIDE
Hyperstat I.V. 3017

TENUALAX (Argentina)
LACTULOSE
Kristalose for Oral Solution 1034

TEOBID (Italy, Venezuela)
THEOPHYLLINE
Uniphyl Tablets 2710

TEODELIN (Spain)
THEOPHYLLINE
Uniphyl Tablets 2710

TEODOSIS (Argentina)
THEOPHYLLINE
Uniphyl Tablets 2710

TEOFILAB (Brazil)
THEOPHYLLINE
Uniphyl Tablets 2710

TEOGEL (Spain)
THEOPHYLLINE
Uniphyl Tablets 2710

TEOLIXIR (Spain)
THEOPHYLLINE
Uniphyl Tablets 2710

TEOLONG (Brazil, Mexico)
THEOPHYLLINE
Uniphyl Tablets 2710

TEONIBSA (Portugal)
THEOPHYLLINE
Uniphyl Tablets 2710

TEONOVA (Italy)
THEOPHYLLINE
Uniphyl Tablets 2710

TEOPHYL (Brazil)
THEOPHYLLINE
Uniphyl Tablets 2710

TEOPLUS (Italy)
THEOPHYLLINE
Uniphyl Tablets 2710

TEOSONA (Argentina)
THEOPHYLLINE
Uniphyl Tablets 2710

TEOSONA SOL (Argentina)
THEOPHYLLINE
Uniphyl Tablets 2710

TEOSTON (Brazil)
THEOPHYLLINE
Uniphyl Tablets 2710

TEOTARD (Czech Republic, Russia)
THEOPHYLLINE
Uniphyl Tablets 2710

TEOVAL/R (Italy)
THEOPHYLLINE
Uniphyl Tablets 2710

TEOVENT (Portugal)
THEOPHYLLINE
Uniphyl Tablets 2710

TERA (Germany)
TERAZOSIN HYDROCHLORIDE
Hytrin Capsules 471

TERAFLUSS (Italy)
TERAZOSIN HYDROCHLORIDE
Hytrin Capsules 471

TERANAR (Germany)
TERAZOSIN HYDROCHLORIDE
Hytrin Capsules 471

TERAPROST (Italy)
TERAZOSIN HYDROCHLORIDE
Hytrin Capsules 471

TERAUMON (Spain)
TERAZOSIN HYDROCHLORIDE
Hytrin Capsules 471

TERAZID (Germany)
TERAZOSIN HYDROCHLORIDE
Hytrin Capsules 471

TERAZOFLO (Germany)
TERAZOSIN HYDROCHLORIDE
Hytrin Capsules 471

TERBAC (Mexico)
CEFTRIAXONE SODIUM
Rocephin Injectable Vials, ADD-Vantage, Galaxy, Bulk 2800

TERBAFIN (New Zealand)
TERBINAFINE HYDROCHLORIDE
Lamisil Tablets 2232

TERBIDERM (The Netherlands)
TERBINAFINE HYDROCHLORIDE
Lamisil Tablets 2232

TERBIFIN (India)
TERBINAFINE HYDROCHLORIDE
Lamisil Tablets 2232

TERBIGRAM (Greece)
TERBINAFINE HYDROCHLORIDE
Lamisil Tablets 2232

TERBISIL (Czech Republic, Hungary)
TERBINAFINE HYDROCHLORIDE
Lamisil Tablets 2232

TEREKOL (Argentina)
TERBINAFINE HYDROCHLORIDE
Lamisil Tablets 2232

TERFEX (Chile)
TERBINAFINE HYDROCHLORIDE
Lamisil Tablets 2232

TERFIN (Argentina)
TERBINAFINE HYDROCHLORIDE
Lamisil Tablets 2232

TERIAM (France)
TRIAMTERENE
Dyrenium Capsules 3400

TERIL (Australia, Hong Kong, Israel, New Zealand, United Kingdom)
CARBAMAZEPINE
Carbatrol Capsules 3171
Tegretol Chewable Tablets 2295
Tegretol Suspension 2295
Tegretol Tablets 2295
Tegretol-XR Tablets 2295

TERODUL (Mexico)
RANITIDINE HYDROCHLORIDE
Zantac 25 EFFERdose Tablets 1624
Zantac 150 EFFERdose Tablets 1624
Zantac 150 Tablets 1624
Zantac 300 Tablets 1624
Zantac Injection 1619
Zantac Injection Premixed 1619
Zantac Syrup 1624

TEROL (India)
TOLTERODINE TARTRATE
Detrol Tablets 2628

TEROLINAL (Greece)
LISINOPRIL
Prinivil Tablets 2052

TEROMOL (Spain)
THEOPHYLLINE
Uniphyl Tablets 2710

TEROST (Brazil)
ALENDRONATE SODIUM
Fosamax Tablets 1969

TERPOSEN (Spain)
RANITIDINE HYDROCHLORIDE
Zantac 25 EFFERdose Tablets 1624
Zantac 150 EFFERdose Tablets 1624
Zantac 150 Tablets 1624
Zantac 300 Tablets 1624
Zantac Injection 1619
Zantac Injection Premixed 1619
Zantac Syrup 1624

TERRAMYCIN N (Germany)
GENTAMICIN SULFATE
Garamycin Injectable 3014

TERSIF (Argentina)
LISINOPRIL
Prinivil Tablets 2052

TERTENSIF (Czech Republic, Spain)
INDAPAMIDE
Indapamide Tablets 2156

TERTROXIN (Australia, Czech Republic, Irish Republic, New Zealand, South Africa, Thailand, United Kingdom, Venezuela)
LIOTHYRONINE SODIUM
Cytomel Tablets 1710

TERVESON (Greece)
LOVASTATIN
Mevacor Tablets 2021

TERZINE (Thailand)
CETIRIZINE HYDROCHLORIDE
Zyrtec Syrup 2594
Zyrtec Tablets 2594

TESALON (Mexico)
BENZONATATE
Tessalon Perles 1199

TESOPEN (Mexico)
BENZONATATE
Tessalon Perles 1199

TESOREN (Venezuela)
ENALAPRIL MALEATE
Vasotec I.V. Injection 2103

TESS (India)
TRIAMCINOLONE ACETONIDE
Azmacort Inhalation Aerosol 1726
Nasacort AQ Nasal Spray 2922

TESSALON (Canada)
BENZONATATE
Tessalon Perles 1199

TESTAC (Germany)
FLUTAMIDE
Eulexin Capsules 3009

TESTOTARD (Germany)
FLUTAMIDE
Eulexin Capsules 3009

TETACID (Austria)
FAMOTIDINE
Pepcid Injection 2040
Pepcid Injection Premixed 2040
Pepcid Tablets 2038
Pepcid for Oral Suspension 2038

TETROID (Brazil)
LEVOTHYROXINE SODIUM
Levothroid Tablets 1186
Levoxyl Tablets 1712
Synthroid Tablets 520

TEXA (South Africa)
CETIRIZINE HYDROCHLORIDE
Zyrtec Syrup 2594
Zyrtec Tablets 2594

TEXACORT (Canada)
HYDROCORTISONE
Hydrocortone Tablets 1989

TEXOT (Argentina)
DOCETAXEL
Taxotere Injection Concentrate 2932

TEXOVEN (Mexico)
BENZONATATE
Tessalon Perles 1199

TEYLOR (Spain)
SIMVASTATIN
Zocor Tablets 2105

THAIS (France)
ESTRADIOL
Climara Transdermal System 771
Estring Vaginal Ring 2635

THALIX (India)
THALIDOMIDE
Thalomid Capsules 965

THELBAN (Malaysia)
ALBENDAZOLE
Albenza Tablets 1338

THEO (Germany)
THEOPHYLLINE
Uniphyl Tablets 2710

THEO MAX (Spain)
THEOPHYLLINE
Uniphyl Tablets 2710

THEO PA (India)
THEOPHYLLINE
Uniphyl Tablets 2710

THEO2 (The Netherlands)
THEOPHYLLINE
Uniphyl Tablets 2710

THEO-24 (Italy)
THEOPHYLLINE
Uniphyl Tablets 2710

THEOBID (India)
THEOPHYLLINE
Uniphyl Tablets 2710

THEO-BROS (Greece)
THEOPHYLLINE
Uniphyl Tablets 2710

THEOCHRON (Canada)
THEOPHYLLINE
Uniphyl Tablets 2710

THEODAY (India)
THEOPHYLLINE
Uniphyl Tablets 2710

THEODUR (Japan)
THEOPHYLLINE
Uniphyl Tablets 2710

THEO-DUR (Argentina, Australia, Belgium, Canada, Czech Republic, Denmark, Finland, Greece, Hong Kong, Irish Republic, Italy, New Zealand, Norway, Singapore, South Africa, Spain, Sweden, Thailand, United Kingdom)
THEOPHYLLINE
Uniphyl Tablets 2710

THEOFOL (Finland)
THEOPHYLLINE
Uniphyl Tablets 2710

THEOFOL COMP (Finland)
THEOPHYLLINE
Uniphyl Tablets 2710

THEOHEXAL (Austria)
THEOPHYLLINE
Uniphyl Tablets 2710

THEOLAIR (Belgium, Canada, France, Germany, Italy, Spain, Switzerland, The Netherlands)
THEOPHYLLINE
Uniphyl Tablets 2710

THEOLAN (Irish Republic)
THEOPHYLLINE
Uniphyl Tablets 2710

THEOLIN (Malaysia, Singapore, The Netherlands)
THEOPHYLLINE
Uniphyl Tablets 2710

THEOLONG (Japan)
THEOPHYLLINE
Uniphyl Tablets 2710

THEON (Switzerland)
THEOPHYLLINE
Uniphyl Tablets 2710

THEOPED (India)
THEOPHYLLINE
Uniphyl Tablets 2710

THEOPEXINE (France)
THEOPHYLLINE
Uniphyl Tablets 2710

THEOPHAR (United Arab Emirates)
THEOPHYLLINE
Uniphyl Tablets 2710

THEOPHTARD (Hungary)
THEOPHYLLINE
Uniphyl Tablets 2710

THEOPHYLLARD (Belgium, Czech Republic, Germany)
THEOPHYLLINE
Uniphyl Tablets 2710

THEOPHYLLINE SEDATIVE BRUNEAU (Belgium)
THEOPHYLLINE
Uniphyl Tablets 2710

THEOPLUS (Czech Republic, South Africa, Spain)
THEOPHYLLINE
Uniphyl Tablets 2710

THEOSPIREX (Hungary)
THEOPHYLLINE
Uniphyl Tablets 2710

THEO-SR (Canada)
THEOPHYLLINE
Uniphyl Tablets 2710

THEOTARD (Israel)
THEOPHYLLINE
Uniphyl Tablets 2710

THEOTRIM (Hong Kong, Israel, Thailand)
THEOPHYLLINE
Uniphyl Tablets 2710

THEOVENT (Hong Kong)
THEOPHYLLINE
Uniphyl Tablets 2710

THERACORT (Brazil)
TRIAMCINOLONE ACETONIDE
Azmacort Inhalation Aerosol 1726
Nasacort AQ Nasal Spray 2922

THERADERM (United Kingdom)
BENZOYL PEROXIDE
Brevoxyl-4 Creamy Wash 3210
Brevoxyl-4 Gel 3210
Brevoxyl-8 Creamy Wash 3210
Brevoxyl-8 Gel 3210
Triaz Cleanser 1892
Triaz Gel 1892

THERADOL (The Netherlands)
TRAMADOL HYDROCHLORIDE
Ultram ER Tablets 2392

THERAPAS (United Kingdom)
AMINOSALICYLIC ACID
Paser Granules 1674

THERAPSOR (Brazil)
CLOBETASOL PROPIONATE
Temovate Cream 2668
Temovate E Emollient 2671
Temovate Gel 2669
Temovate Ointment 2668
Temovate Scalp Application 2670

THERASONA (Brazil)
HYDROCORTISONE
Hydrocortone Tablets 1989

THEVIER (Germany)
LEVOTHYROXINE SODIUM
Levothroid Tablets 1186
Levoxyl Tablets 1712
Synthroid Tablets 520

THIAZID-COMP (Germany)
HYDROCHLOROTHIAZIDE/TRIAMTERENE
Dyazide Capsules 1423

THILO-MICINE (Greece)
TOBRAMYCIN
TOBI Solution for Inhalation 2298

THILOMICINE DEX (Greece)
TOBRAMYCIN
TOBI Solution for Inhalation 2298

THILOTIM (Greece)
TIMOLOL MALEATE
Blocadren Tablets 1916
Timoptic Sterile Ophthalmic Solution 2088
Timoptic in Ocudose 2091
Timoptic-XE Sterile Ophthalmic Gel Forming Solution 2092

THILOXEDINE (Greece)
DEXAMETHASONE
Decadron Tablets 1951

THIODAZINE (Russia)
THIORIDAZINE HYDROCHLORIDE
Thioridazine Hydrochloride Tablets 2163

THIOMED (Thailand)
THIORIDAZINE HYDROCHLORIDE
Thioridazine Hydrochloride Tablets 2163

THIORIL (India)
THIORIDAZINE HYDROCHLORIDE
Thioridazine Hydrochloride Tablets 2163

THIOSIA (Thailand)
THIORIDAZINE HYDROCHLORIDE
Thioridazine Hydrochloride Tablets 2163

THIOZINE (Irish Republic)
THIORIDAZINE HYDROCHLORIDE
Thioridazine Hydrochloride Tablets 2163

THRIONIPEN (Greece)
NIMODIPINE
Nimotop Capsules 749

THRIUSEDON (Greece)
LISINOPRIL
Prinivil Tablets 2052

THROMBOCID (Germany, Spain)
PENTOSAN POLYSULFATE SODIUM
Elmiron Capsules 2415

THROMBODINE (Austria)
TICLOPIDINE HYDROCHLORIDE
Ticlid Tablets 2810

THROMBOHEXAL (Austria)
DIPYRIDAMOLE
Persantine Tablets 868

THROMBOREDUCTIN (Austria)
ANAGRELIDE HYDROCHLORIDE
Agrylin Capsules 3169

THYRADIN-S (Japan)
LEVOTHYROXINE SODIUM
Levothroid Tablets 1186
Levoxyl Tablets 1712
Synthroid Tablets 520

THYRAX (Belgium, Czech Republic, Portugal, Spain, The Netherlands, Venezuela)
LEVOTHYROXINE SODIUM
Levothroid Tablets 1186
Levoxyl Tablets 1712
Synthroid Tablets 520

THYREX (Austria)
LEVOTHYROXINE SODIUM
Levothroid Tablets 1186
Levoxyl Tablets 1712
Synthroid Tablets 520

THYRO-4 (Greece)
LEVOTHYROXINE SODIUM
Levothroid Tablets 1186
Levoxyl Tablets 1712
Synthroid Tablets 520

THYROGEN (Austria, Brazil, Canada, Denmark, Germany, Greece, Israel, Italy, Norway, Spain, Sweden, United Kingdom)
THYROTROPIN ALFA
Thyrogen for Injection 1286

THYROHORMONE (Greece)
LEVOTHYROXINE SODIUM
Levothroid Tablets 1186
Levoxyl Tablets 1712
Synthroid Tablets 520

THYROSIT (Thailand)
LEVOTHYROXINE SODIUM
Levothroid Tablets 1186
Levoxyl Tablets 1712
Synthroid Tablets 520

TIADEN (Greece)
AMILORIDE HYDROCHLORIDE/HYDROCHLOROTHIAZIDE
Moduretic Tablets 2028

TIADIL (Portugal, The Netherlands)
DILTIAZEM HYDROCHLORIDE
Cardizem LA Extended Release Tablets 1728
Tiazac Capsules 1201

TIADYL (Argentina)
CANDESARTAN CILEXETIL
Atacand Tablets 649

TIADYL PLUS (Argentina)
CANDESARTAN CILEXETIL
Atacand Tablets 649

TIAKEM (Czech Republic, Italy)
DILTIAZEM HYDROCHLORIDE
Cardizem LA Extended Release Tablets 1728
Tiazac Capsules 1201

TIAL (Germany)
TRAMADOL HYDROCHLORIDE
Ultram ER Tablets 2392

TIALIN (Venezuela)
SERTRALINE HYDROCHLORIDE
Zoloft Tablets 2586

TIANAK (Mexico)
RANITIDINE HYDROCHLORIDE
Zantac 25 EFFERdose Tablets 1624
Zantac 150 EFFERdose Tablets 1624
Zantac 150 Tablets 1624
Zantac 300 Tablets 1624
Zantac Injection 1619
Zantac Injection Premixed 1619
Zantac Syrup 1624

TIARIX (Argentina)
PAROXETINE HYDROCHLORIDE
Paxil Oral Suspension 1530
Paxil Tablets 1530

TIAZAC (Canada)
DILTIAZEM HYDROCHLORIDE
Cardizem LA Extended Release Tablets 1728
Tiazac Capsules 1201

TIAZEN (Italy)
DILTIAZEM HYDROCHLORIDE
Cardizem LA Extended Release Tablets 1728
Tiazac Capsules 1201

TIBLEX (Spain)
SUCRALFATE
Carafate Suspension 701
Carafate Tablets 701

TICAVENT (Italy)
FLUTICASONE PROPIONATE
Cutivate Cream 2662
Cutivate Ointment 2665
Flonase Nasal Spray 1440

TICDINE (Thailand)
TICLOPIDINE HYDROCHLORIDE
Ticlid Tablets 2810

TICLID (Argentina, Australia, Belgium, Brazil, Canada, Chile, Czech Republic, France, Greece, Hong Kong, Hungary, Malaysia, Mexico, New Zealand, Norway, Singapore, South Africa, Sweden, Switzerland, Thailand, United Kingdom, Venezuela)
TICLOPIDINE HYDROCHLORIDE
Ticlid Tablets 2810

TICLIDIL (Israel)
TICLOPIDINE HYDROCHLORIDE
Ticlid Tablets 2810

TICLO (Thailand)
TICLOPIDINE HYDROCHLORIDE
Ticlid Tablets 2810

TICLOBAL (Brazil)
TICLOPIDINE HYDROCHLORIDE
Ticlid Tablets 2810

TICLOBEST (India)
TICLOPIDINE HYDROCHLORIDE
Ticlid Tablets 2810

TICLODIX (Portugal)
TICLOPIDINE HYDROCHLORIDE
Ticlid Tablets 2810

TICLODONE (Austria, Greece, Italy, Spain)
TICLOPIDINE HYDROCHLORIDE
Ticlid Tablets 2810

TICLOGI (Italy)
TICLOPIDINE HYDROCHLORIDE
Ticlid Tablets 2810

TICLOMED (France)
TICLOPIDINE HYDROCHLORIDE
Ticlid Tablets 2810

TICLOP (India)
TICLOPIDINE HYDROCHLORIDE
Ticlid Tablets 2810

TICLOPAT (Portugal)
TICLOPIDINE HYDROCHLORIDE
Ticlid Tablets 2810

TICLOPID (India)
TICLOPIDINE HYDROCHLORIDE
Ticlid Tablets 2810

TICLOPIN (Venezuela)
TICLOPIDINE HYDROCHLORIDE
Ticlid Tablets 2810

TICLOPROGE (Italy)
TICLOPIDINE HYDROCHLORIDE
Ticlid Tablets 2810

TICLOSAN (Italy)
TICLOPIDINE HYDROCHLORIDE
Ticlid Tablets 2810

TICOPAR (United Arab Emirates)
TICLOPIDINE HYDROCHLORIDE
Ticlid Tablets 2810

TIDACT (Malaysia, Singapore)
CLINDAMYCIN HYDROCHLORIDE
Cleocin Vaginal Ovules 2616

TIENAM (Chile, France, Italy, Norway, Singapore, South Africa, Spain, Sweden, Switzerland, Thailand, The Netherlands)
CILASTATIN SODIUM/IMIPENEM
Primaxin I.M. 2045
Primaxin I.V. 2048

TIFINIDAT (The Netherlands)
METHYLPHENIDATE HYDROCHLORIDE
Ritalin Hydrochloride Tablets 2269
Ritalin-SR Tablets 2269

TIFOX (Italy)
CEFOXITIN SODIUM
Mefoxin Premixed Intravenous Solution 2016
Mefoxin for Injection 2012

TIKALAC (Sweden)
LACTULOSE
Kristalose for Oral Solution 1034

TIKLEEN (India, Russia)
TICLOPIDINE HYDROCHLORIDE
Ticlid Tablets 2810

TIKLID (Austria, Italy, Spain)
TICLOPIDINE HYDROCHLORIDE
Ticlid Tablets 2810

TIKLYD (Germany, Portugal)
TICLOPIDINE HYDROCHLORIDE
Ticlid Tablets 2810

TIKOL (Thailand)
TICLOPIDINE HYDROCHLORIDE
Ticlid Tablets 2810

TILALGIN (The Netherlands)
TRAMADOL HYDROCHLORIDE
Ultram ER Tablets 2392

TILAZEM (Argentina, Chile, Mexico, South Africa, Venezuela)
DILTIAZEM HYDROCHLORIDE
Cardizem LA Extended Release Tablets 1728
Tiazac Capsules 1201

TILDIEM (Belgium, Chile, France, Greece, Hong Kong, Irish Republic, Italy, Singapore, Switzerland, Thailand, The Netherlands, United Kingdom)
DILTIAZEM HYDROCHLORIDE
Cardizem LA Extended Release Tablets 1728
Tiazac Capsules 1201

TILENE (Italy)
FENOFIBRATE
Tricor Tablets 527

TILEXIM (Italy)
CEFUROXIME AXETIL
Ceftin Tablets 1407
Ceftin for Oral Suspension 1407

TILFERAN (Greece)
ETIDRONATE DISODIUM
Didronel Tablets 2697

TILIOS (Argentina)
ALENDRONATE SODIUM
Fosamax Tablets 1969

TILKER (Denmark, Norway, Spain)
DILTIAZEM HYDROCHLORIDE
Cardizem LA Extended Release Tablets 1728
Tiazac Capsules 1201

TILMAT (New Zealand)
TIMOLOL MALEATE
Blocadren Tablets 1916
Timoptic Sterile Ophthalmic Solution 2088
Timoptic in Ocudose 2091
Timoptic-XE Sterile Ophthalmic Gel Forming Solution 2092

TILODENE (Australia)
TICLOPIDINE HYDROCHLORIDE
Ticlid Tablets 2810

TILOETCA COMBI (United Kingdom)
ETIDRONATE DISODIUM
Didronel Tablets 2697

TILOFYL (United Kingdom)
FENTANYL
Duragesic Transdermal System 2373

TILOPIN (Thailand)
TICLOPIDINE HYDROCHLORIDE
Ticlid Tablets ... **2810**

TILOPTIC (Israel)
TIMOLOL MALEATE
Blocadren Tablets ... **1916**
Timoptic Sterile Ophthalmic Solution ... **2088**
Timoptic in Ocudose ... **2091**
Timoptic-XE Sterile Ophthalmic Gel Forming Solution ... **2092**

TILORYTH (United Kingdom)
ERYTHROMYCIN
Ery-Tab Tablets ... **449**
Erythromycin Base Filmtab Tablets ... **455**
Erythromycin Delayed-Release Capsules, USP ... **457**
PCE Dispertab Tablets ... **515**

TILTAB (Brazil)
ROSIGLITAZONE MALEATE
Avandia Tablets ... **1384**

TILTIS (Argentina)
BENZOYL PEROXIDE
Brevoxyl-4 Creamy Wash ... **3210**
Brevoxyl-4 Gel ... **3210**
Brevoxyl-8 Creamy Wash ... **3210**
Brevoxyl-8 Gel ... **3210**
Triaz Cleanser ... **1892**
Triaz Gel ... **1892**

TIMAB (Argentina)
DIAZEPAM
Diastat Rectal Delivery System ... **3343**
Valium Tablets ... **2819**

TIMABAK (Austria, Brazil, Chile, France, Greece, Hong Kong, Singapore, Spain)
TIMOLOL MALEATE
Blocadren Tablets ... **1916**
Timoptic Sterile Ophthalmic Solution ... **2088**
Timoptic in Ocudose ... **2091**
Timoptic-XE Sterile Ophthalmic Gel Forming Solution ... **2092**

TIMACAR (Denmark)
TIMOLOL MALEATE
Blocadren Tablets ... **1916**
Timoptic Sterile Ophthalmic Solution ... **2088**
Timoptic in Ocudose ... **2091**
Timoptic-XE Sterile Ophthalmic Gel Forming Solution ... **2092**

TIMACOR (France)
TIMOLOL MALEATE
Blocadren Tablets ... **1916**
Timoptic Sterile Ophthalmic Solution ... **2088**
Timoptic in Ocudose ... **2091**
Timoptic-XE Sterile Ophthalmic Gel Forming Solution ... **2092**

TIM-AK (Canada)
TIMOLOL MALEATE
Blocadren Tablets ... **1916**
Timoptic Sterile Ophthalmic Solution ... **2088**
Timoptic in Ocudose ... **2091**
Timoptic-XE Sterile Ophthalmic Gel Forming Solution ... **2092**

TIMAROL (Chile)
TRAMADOL HYDROCHLORIDE
Ultram ER Tablets ... **2392**

TIMASEN (Brazil)
TRAMADOL HYDROCHLORIDE
Ultram ER Tablets ... **2392**

TIMAX (Austria)
TIMOLOL MALEATE
Blocadren Tablets ... **1916**
Timoptic Sterile Ophthalmic Solution ... **2088**
Timoptic in Ocudose ... **2091**
Timoptic-XE Sterile Ophthalmic Gel Forming Solution ... **2092**

TIMED (Argentina)
TIMOLOL MALEATE
Blocadren Tablets ... **1916**
Timoptic Sterile Ophthalmic Solution ... **2088**
Timoptic in Ocudose ... **2091**
Timoptic-XE Sterile Ophthalmic Gel Forming Solution ... **2092**

TIMED D (Argentina)
TIMOLOL MALEATE
Blocadren Tablets ... **1916**
Timoptic Sterile Ophthalmic Solution ... **2088**
Timoptic in Ocudose ... **2091**
Timoptic-XE Sterile Ophthalmic Gel Forming Solution ... **2092**

TIMISOL (Switzerland)
TIMOLOL MALEATE
Blocadren Tablets ... **1916**
Timoptic Sterile Ophthalmic Solution ... **2088**
Timoptic in Ocudose ... **2091**
Timoptic-XE Sterile Ophthalmic Gel Forming Solution ... **2092**

TIMO-COMOD (Czech Republic, France, Germany, Malaysia, The Netherlands)
TIMOLOL MALEATE
Blocadren Tablets ... **1916**
Timoptic Sterile Ophthalmic Solution ... **2088**
Timoptic in Ocudose ... **2091**
Timoptic-XE Sterile Ophthalmic Gel Forming Solution ... **2092**

TIMOCORT (United Kingdom)
HYDROCORTISONE
Hydrocortone Tablets ... **1989**

TIMODINE (United Kingdom)
NYSTATIN
Nystop Topical Powder USP ... **2478**
Paddock Nystatin USP for Oral Suspension ... **2478**

TIMODOSE (Greece)
TIMOLOL MALEATE
Blocadren Tablets ... **1916**
Timoptic Sterile Ophthalmic Solution ... **2088**
Timoptic in Ocudose ... **2091**
Timoptic-XE Sterile Ophthalmic Gel Forming Solution ... **2092**

TIMODROP (Thailand)
TIMOLOL MALEATE
Blocadren Tablets ... **1916**
Timoptic Sterile Ophthalmic Solution ... **2088**
Timoptic in Ocudose ... **2091**
Timoptic-XE Sterile Ophthalmic Gel Forming Solution ... **2092**

TIMOEDO (Germany)
TIMOLOL MALEATE
Blocadren Tablets ... **1916**
Timoptic Sterile Ophthalmic Solution ... **2088**
Timoptic in Ocudose ... **2091**
Timoptic-XE Sterile Ophthalmic Gel Forming Solution ... **2092**

TIMOFTAL (Austria)
TIMOLOL MALEATE
Blocadren Tablets ... **1916**
Timoptic Sterile Ophthalmic Solution ... **2088**
Timoptic in Ocudose ... **2091**
Timoptic-XE Sterile Ophthalmic Gel Forming Solution ... **2092**

TIMOFTOL (Spain)
TIMOLOL MALEATE
Blocadren Tablets ... **1916**
Timoptic Sterile Ophthalmic Solution ... **2088**
Timoptic in Ocudose ... **2091**
Timoptic-XE Sterile Ophthalmic Gel Forming Solution ... **2092**

TIMOGAL (Czech Republic)
TIMOLOL MALEATE
Blocadren Tablets ... **1916**
Timoptic Sterile Ophthalmic Solution ... **2088**
Timoptic in Ocudose ... **2091**
Timoptic-XE Sterile Ophthalmic Gel Forming Solution ... **2092**

TIMOGEL (Spain)
TIMOLOL MALEATE
Blocadren Tablets ... **1916**
Timoptic Sterile Ophthalmic Solution ... **2088**
Timoptic in Ocudose ... **2091**
Timoptic-XE Sterile Ophthalmic Gel Forming Solution ... **2092**

TIMOGLAU (Portugal)
TIMOLOL MALEATE
Blocadren Tablets ... **1916**
Timoptic Sterile Ophthalmic Solution ... **2088**
Timoptic in Ocudose ... **2091**
Timoptic-XE Sterile Ophthalmic Gel Forming Solution ... **2092**

TIMOHEXAL (Austria, Czech Republic, Germany, Russia)
TIMOLOL MALEATE
Blocadren Tablets ... **1916**
Timoptic Sterile Ophthalmic Solution ... **2088**
Timoptic in Ocudose ... **2091**
Timoptic-XE Sterile Ophthalmic Gel Forming Solution ... **2092**

TIMOLABAK (Italy)
TIMOLOL MALEATE
Blocadren Tablets ... **1916**
Timoptic Sterile Ophthalmic Solution ... **2088**
Timoptic in Ocudose ... **2091**
Timoptic-XE Sterile Ophthalmic Gel Forming Solution ... **2092**

TIMOLEN (Portugal)
TIMOLOL MALEATE
Blocadren Tablets ... **1916**
Timoptic Sterile Ophthalmic Solution ... **2088**
Timoptic in Ocudose ... **2091**
Timoptic-XE Sterile Ophthalmic Gel Forming Solution ... **2092**

TIMOLER (Argentina)
TIMOLOL MALEATE
Blocadren Tablets ... **1916**
Timoptic Sterile Ophthalmic Solution ... **2088**
Timoptic in Ocudose ... **2091**
Timoptic-XE Sterile Ophthalmic Gel Forming Solution ... **2092**

TIMOLIDE (Canada)
HYDROCHLOROTHIAZIDE/TIMOLOL MALEATE
Timolide Tablets ... **2086**

TIMOLO (India)
TIMOLOL MALEATE
Blocadren Tablets ... **1916**
Timoptic Sterile Ophthalmic Solution ... **2088**
Timoptic in Ocudose ... **2091**
Timoptic-XE Sterile Ophthalmic Gel Forming Solution ... **2092**

TIMOLUX (Italy)
TIMOLOL MALEATE
Blocadren Tablets ... **1916**
Timoptic Sterile Ophthalmic Solution ... **2088**
Timoptic in Ocudose ... **2091**
Timoptic-XE Sterile Ophthalmic Gel Forming Solution ... **2092**

TIMOMANN (Germany)
TIMOLOL MALEATE
Blocadren Tablets ... **1916**
Timoptic Sterile Ophthalmic Solution ... **2088**
Timoptic in Ocudose ... **2091**
Timoptic-XE Sterile Ophthalmic Gel Forming Solution ... **2092**

TIMONIL (Czech Republic, Germany, Hong Kong, Hungary, Israel, Switzerland, United Kingdom)
CARBAMAZEPINE
Carbatrol Capsules ... **3171**
Tegretol Chewable Tablets ... **2295**
Tegretol Suspension ... **2295**
Tegretol Tablets ... **2295**
Tegretol-XR Tablets ... **2295**

TIMO-OPTAL (Thailand)
TIMOLOL MALEATE
Blocadren Tablets ... **1916**
Timoptic Sterile Ophthalmic Solution ... **2088**
Timoptic in Ocudose ... **2091**
Timoptic-XE Sterile Ophthalmic Gel Forming Solution ... **2092**

TIMOP (Chile)
TIMOLOL MALEATE
Blocadren Tablets ... **1916**
Timoptic Sterile Ophthalmic Solution ... **2088**
Timoptic in Ocudose ... **2091**
Timoptic-XE Sterile Ophthalmic Gel Forming Solution ... **2092**

TIM-OPHTAL (Austria, Germany)
TIMOLOL MALEATE
Blocadren Tablets ... **1916**
Timoptic Sterile Ophthalmic Solution ... **2088**
Timoptic in Ocudose ... **2091**
Timoptic-XE Sterile Ophthalmic Gel Forming Solution ... **2092**

TIMOPOS COMOD (Germany)
TIMOLOL MALEATE
Blocadren Tablets ... **1916**
Timoptic Sterile Ophthalmic Solution ... **2088**
Timoptic in Ocudose ... **2091**
Timoptic-XE Sterile Ophthalmic Gel Forming Solution ... **2092**

TIMOPTIC (Argentina, Austria, Canada, Switzerland)
TIMOLOL MALEATE
Blocadren Tablets ... **1916**
Timoptic Sterile Ophthalmic Solution ... **2088**
Timoptic in Ocudose ... **2091**
Timoptic-XE Sterile Ophthalmic Gel Forming Solution ... **2092**

TIMOPTOL (Australia, Belgium, Brazil, Czech Republic, France, Hong Kong, Irish Republic, Italy, Japan, Malaysia, Mexico, New Zealand, Portugal, Singapore, South Africa, Thailand, The Netherlands, United Kingdom, Venezuela)
TIMOLOL MALEATE
Blocadren Tablets ... **1916**
Timoptic Sterile Ophthalmic Solution ... **2088**
Timoptic in Ocudose ... **2091**
Timoptic-XE Sterile Ophthalmic Gel Forming Solution ... **2092**

TIMOPTOL-XE (Australia, Chile)
TIMOLOL MALEATE
Blocadren Tablets ... **1916**
Timoptic Sterile Ophthalmic Solution ... **2088**
Timoptic in Ocudose ... **2091**
Timoptic-XE Sterile Ophthalmic Gel Forming Solution ... **2092**

TIMOSAN (Denmark, Finland, Norway, Sweden)
TIMOLOL MALEATE
Blocadren Tablets ... **1916**
Timoptic Sterile Ophthalmic Solution ... **2088**
Timoptic in Ocudose ... **2091**
Timoptic-XE Sterile Ophthalmic Gel Forming Solution ... **2092**

TIMOSIL (Thailand)
TIMOLOL MALEATE
Blocadren Tablets ... **1916**
Timoptic Sterile Ophthalmic Solution ... **2088**
Timoptic in Ocudose ... **2091**
Timoptic-XE Sterile Ophthalmic Gel Forming Solution ... **2092**

TIMOSINE (Germany)
TIMOLOL MALEATE
Blocadren Tablets ... **1916**
Timoptic Sterile Ophthalmic Solution ... **2088**
Timoptic in Ocudose ... **2091**
Timoptic-XE Sterile Ophthalmic Gel Forming Solution ... **2092**

TIMOSOFT (Italy)
TIMOLOL MALEATE
Blocadren Tablets ... **1916**
Timoptic Sterile Ophthalmic Solution ... **2088**
Timoptic in Ocudose ... **2091**
Timoptic-XE Sterile Ophthalmic Gel Forming Solution ... **2092**

TIMO-STULLN (Germany)
TIMOLOL MALEATE
Blocadren Tablets ... **1916**
Timoptic Sterile Ophthalmic Solution ... **2088**
Timoptic in Ocudose ... **2091**
Timoptic-XE Sterile Ophthalmic Gel Forming Solution ... **2092**

TIMOZZARD (Mexico)
TIMOLOL MALEATE
Blocadren Tablets ... **1916**
Timoptic Sterile Ophthalmic Solution ... **2088**
Timoptic in Ocudose ... **2091**
Timoptic-XE Sterile Ophthalmic Gel Forming Solution ... **2092**

TIMPILO (Argentina, Australia, Czech Republic, Malaysia)
TIMOLOL MALEATE
Blocadren Tablets ... **1916**
Timoptic Sterile Ophthalmic Solution ... **2088**
Timoptic in Ocudose ... **2091**
Timoptic-XE Sterile Ophthalmic Gel Forming Solution ... **2092**

TIMPRON (United Kingdom)
NAPROXEN
EC-Naprosyn Delayed-Release Tablets ... **2761**
Naprosyn Suspension ... **2761**
Naprosyn Tablets ... **2761**

TIMSOPT (Austria)
DORZOLAMIDE HYDROCHLORIDE/TIMOLOL MALEATE
Cosopt Sterile Ophthalmic Solution ... ⊙**268, 1931**

TINACEF (Argentina)
CEFTAZIDIME
Fortaz for Injection ... **1453**

TINADERM EXTRA (Australia)
CLOTRIMAZOLE
Lotrimin Cream ... **3039**
Lotrimin Lotion 1% ... **3039**
Lotrimin Topical Solution 1% ... **3039**

TINAGEL (Belgium, The Netherlands)
BENZOYL PEROXIDE
Brevoxyl-4 Creamy Wash ... **3210**

Brevoxyl-4 Gel 3210
Brevoxyl-8 Creamy Wash 3210
Brevoxyl-8 Gel 3210
Triaz Cleanser 1892
Triaz Gel 1892

TINASIN (Venezuela)
SIMVASTATIN
Zocor Tablets 2105

T-INMUN (Chile)
TACROLIMUS
Prograf Capsules and Injection 632

TIOF (Chile, Mexico)
TIMOLOL MALEATE
Blocadren Tablets 1916
Timoptic Sterile Ophthalmic Solution 2088
Timoptic in Ocudose 2091
Timoptic-XE Sterile Ophthalmic Gel Forming Solution 2092

TIONER (Spain)
TRAMADOL HYDROCHLORIDE
Ultram ER Tablets 2392

TIOSALIS (Argentina)
ONDANSETRON
Zofran ODT Orally Disintegrating Tablets . . 1639

TIPAC (Chile)
RANITIDINE HYDROCHLORIDE
Zantac 25 EFFERdose Tablets 1624
Zantac 150 EFFERdose Tablets 1624
Zantac 150 Tablets 1624
Zantac 300 Tablets 1624
Zantac Injection 1619
Zantac Injection Premixed 1619
Zantac Syrup 1624

TIPAROL (Sweden)
TRAMADOL HYDROCHLORIDE
Ultram ER Tablets 2392

TIPERAL (Irish Republic)
PROPRANOLOL HYDROCHLORIDE
Inderal LA Long-Acting Capsules 3429

TIPIDIN (Hong Kong, Malaysia, Singapore)
TICLOPIDINE HYDROCHLORIDE
Ticlid Tablets 2810

TIPIDINE (Thailand)
TICLOPIDINE HYDROCHLORIDE
Ticlid Tablets 2810

TIPODEX (Spain)
FAMOTIDINE
Pepcid Injection 2040
Pepcid Injection Premixed 2040
Pepcid Tablets 2038
Pepcid for Oral Suspension 2038

TIRACRIN (Italy)
LEVOTHYROXINE SODIUM
Levothroid Tablets 1186
Levoxyl Tablets 1712
Synthroid Tablets 520

TIRIZIN (Austria)
CETIRIZINE HYDROCHLORIDE
Zyrtec Syrup 2594
Zyrtec Tablets 2594

TIROCAL (Mexico)
CALCITRIOL
Calcijex Injection 411
Rocaltrol Capsules 2798
Rocaltrol Oral Solution 2798

TIROIDIN (Brazil)
LEVOTHYROXINE SODIUM
Levothroid Tablets 1186
Levoxyl Tablets 1712
Synthroid Tablets 520

TIROIDINE (Mexico)
LEVOTHYROXINE SODIUM
Levothroid Tablets 1186
Levoxyl Tablets 1712
Synthroid Tablets 520

TIROSINT (Italy)
LEVOTHYROXINE SODIUM
Levothroid Tablets 1186
Levoxyl Tablets 1712
Synthroid Tablets 520

TISOGEN (Argentina)
TOPOTECAN HYDROCHLORIDE
Hycamtin for Injection 1458

TISOREK (Argentina)
CELECOXIB
Celebrex Capsules 3134

TITANOX (Greece, Thailand)
PROMETHAZINE HYDROCHLORIDE
Phenergan Tablets and Suppositories 3440

TITRANE (Spain)
ISOSORBIDE MONONITRATE
Imdur Tablets 3018

TI-TRE (Italy)
LIOTHYRONINE SODIUM
Cytomel Tablets 1710

TI-U-LAC HC (Canada)
HYDROCORTISONE
Hydrocortone Tablets 1989

TIVIRLON (Greece)
LISINOPRIL
Prinivil Tablets 2052

TIXYLIX (Malaysia)
PROMETHAZINE HYDROCHLORIDE
Phenergan Tablets and Suppositories 3440

TIXYLIX NIGHTIME (Australia)
PROMETHAZINE HYDROCHLORIDE
Phenergan Tablets and Suppositories 3440

T-LONG (Germany)
TRAMADOL HYDROCHLORIDE
Ultram ER Tablets 2392

TOBACIN (India)
TOBRAMYCIN
TOBI Solution for Inhalation 2298

TOBAZON (India)
TOBRAMYCIN
TOBI Solution for Inhalation 2298

TOBI (Argentina, Australia, Austria, Belgium, Canada, Denmark, Finland, France, Germany, Greece, Irish Republic, Israel, Italy, New Zealand, Norway, Spain, Sweden, Switzerland, United Kingdom)
TOBRAMYCIN
TOBI Solution for Inhalation 2298

TOBIN (Switzerland)
CETIRIZINE HYDROCHLORIDE
Zyrtec Syrup 2594
Zyrtec Tablets 2594

TOBRABACT (Italy, Spain)
TOBRAMYCIN
TOBI Solution for Inhalation 2298

TOBRABIOTIC (Argentina)
TOBRAMYCIN
TOBI Solution for Inhalation 2298

TOBRABIOTIC D (Argentina)
TOBRAMYCIN
TOBI Solution for Inhalation 2298

TOBRACIN (Brazil)
TOBRAMYCIN
TOBI Solution for Inhalation 2298

TOBRACIN D (Brazil)
TOBRAMYCIN
TOBI Solution for Inhalation 2298

TOBRACORT (Argentina, Brazil)
TOBRAMYCIN
TOBI Solution for Inhalation 2298

TOBRADEX (Argentina, Austria, Belgium, Brazil, Canada, Chile, Czech Republic, France, Greece, Hong Kong, Hungary, Italy, Malaysia, Mexico, New Zealand, Russia, Singapore, South Africa, Spain, Switzerland, Thailand, The Netherlands, United Kingdom, Venezuela)
TOBRAMYCIN
TOBI Solution for Inhalation 2298

TOBRADICLO (Argentina)
TOBRAMYCIN
TOBI Solution for Inhalation 2298

TOBRAFEN (Switzerland)
DICLOFENAC SODIUM
Voltaren Tablets 2307
Voltaren-XR Tablets 2310

TOBRAGAN (Argentina, Brazil, Chile)
TOBRAMYCIN
TOBI Solution for Inhalation 2298

TOBRAGAN D (Argentina, Chile)
TOBRAMYCIN
TOBI Solution for Inhalation 2298

TOBRAL (Italy)
TOBRAMYCIN
TOBI Solution for Inhalation 2298

TOBRALEX (Irish Republic, United Kingdom)
TOBRAMYCIN
TOBI Solution for Inhalation 2298

TOBRA-M (Brazil)
TOBRAMYCIN
TOBI Solution for Inhalation 2298

TOBRAMAXIN (Germany)
TOBRAMYCIN
TOBI Solution for Inhalation 2298

TOBRANOM (Brazil)
TOBRAMYCIN
TOBI Solution for Inhalation 2298

TOBRASOL (Venezuela)
TOBRAMYCIN
TOBI Solution for Inhalation 2298

TOBRASTILL (Italy)
TOBRAMYCIN
TOBI Solution for Inhalation 2298

TOBRATLAS (Argentina)
DICLOFENAC SODIUM
Voltaren Tablets 2307
Voltaren-XR Tablets 2310

TOBREX (Argentina, Australia, Austria, Belgium, Brazil, Canada, Chile, Czech Republic, Denmark, Finland, France, Greece, Hong Kong, Hungary, Israel, Malaysia, Mexico, New Zealand, Norway, Portugal, Russia, Singapore, South Africa, Spain, Sweden, Switzerland, Thailand, The Netherlands, Venezuela)
TOBRAMYCIN
TOBI Solution for Inhalation 2298

TOBRIDAVI (Portugal)
TOBRAMYCIN
TOBI Solution for Inhalation 2298

TOBRIN (Chile)
TOBRAMYCIN
TOBI Solution for Inhalation 2298

TOBRIN-D (Chile)
DEXAMETHASONE/TOBRAMYCIN
TobraDex Ophthalmic Ointment . . . 562, ⊙212
TobraDex Ophthalmic Suspension . 563, ⊙211

TOCODERM (Mexico)
TRETINOIN
Vesanoid Capsules 2820

TODEX (Venezuela)
TOBRAMYCIN
TOBI Solution for Inhalation 2298

TODEXONA (Chile)
DEXAMETHASONE/TOBRAMYCIN
TobraDex Ophthalmic Ointment . . . 562, ⊙212
TobraDex Ophthalmic Suspension . 563, ⊙211

TOFLAMIXINA (Argentina, Brazil)
TOBRAMYCIN
TOBI Solution for Inhalation 2298

TOFLAMIXINA PLUS (Argentina)
TOBRAMYCIN
TOBI Solution for Inhalation 2298

TOLBIN (Argentina)
METRONIDAZOLE
MetroGel-Vaginal Gel 1855

TOLERABIOTICO (Spain)
ERYTHROMYCIN STEARATE
Erythrocin Stearate Filmtab Tablets 453

TOLOXIN (Thailand)
DIGOXIN
Lanoxicaps Capsules 1490
Lanoxin Injection 1494
Lanoxin Injection Pediatric 1497
Lanoxin Tablets 1500

TOLREST (Brazil)
SERTRALINE HYDROCHLORIDE
Zoloft Tablets 2586

TOLTEM (Argentina)
TOLTERODINE TARTRATE
Detrol Tablets 2628

TOLYDOL (India)
TRAMADOL HYDROCHLORIDE
Ultram ER Tablets 2392

TOMAG (Argentina)
RANITIDINE HYDROCHLORIDE
Zantac 25 EFFERdose Tablets 1624
Zantac 150 EFFERdose Tablets 1624
Zantac 150 Tablets 1624
Zantac 300 Tablets 1624
Zantac Injection 1619
Zantac Injection Premixed 1619
Zantac Syrup 1624

TOMPRIL (Brazil)
CAPTOPRIL
Captopril Tablets 2149

TOMYCINE (Canada)
TOBRAMYCIN
TOBI Solution for Inhalation 2298

TONDEX (Mexico)
GENTAMICIN SULFATE
Garamycin Injectable 3014

TONOBEXOL (Argentina)
BETAXOLOL HYDROCHLORIDE
Betoptic S Ophthalmic Suspension . ⊙203, 558

TONOFTAL-N (Germany)
NYSTATIN
Nystop Topical Powder USP 2478
Paddock Nystatin USP for Oral Suspension 2478

TONOTEN (Venezuela)
LISINOPRIL
Prinivil Tablets 2052

TONOTENSIL (Chile)
LISINOPRIL
Prinivil Tablets 2052

TONOTENSIL D (Chile)
HYDROCHLOROTHIAZIDE/LISINOPRIL
Prinzide Tablets 2056

TONOVIT (Greece)
LEVOCARNITINE
Carnitor Injection 3188
Carnitor Tablets and Oral Solution 3190

TOPACE (Australia)
CAPTOPRIL
Captopril Tablets 2149

TOPALGIC (France)
TRAMADOL HYDROCHLORIDE
Ultram ER Tablets 2392

TOPAMAC (Argentina, Greece, India)
TOPIRAMATE
Topamax Sprinkle Capsules 2404
Topamax Tablets 2404

TOPAMATE (India)
TOPIRAMATE
Topamax Sprinkle Capsules 2404
Topamax Tablets 2404

TOPAMAX (Australia, Austria, Belgium, Brazil, Canada, Chile, Czech Republic, Germany, Hong Kong, Hungary, Irish Republic, Israel, Italy, Malaysia, Mexico, New Zealand, Portugal, Russia, Singapore, South Africa, Spain, Switzerland, Thailand, The Netherlands, United Kingdom, Venezuela)
TOPIRAMATE
Topamax Sprinkle Capsules 2404
Topamax Tablets 2404

TOPCORT (India)
MOMETASONE FUROATE
Elocon Cream 0.1% 3005
Elocon Lotion 0.1% 3006
Elocon Ointment 0.1% 3007
Nasonex Nasal Spray 3043

TOPERIT (Argentina)
ERYTHROMYCIN
Ery-Tab Tablets 449
Erythromycin Base Filmtab Tablets 455
Erythromycin Delayed-Release Capsules, USP 457
PCE Dispertab Tablets 515

TOPESTIN (Argentina)
TOPOTECAN HYDROCHLORIDE
Hycamtin for Injection 1458

TOPEX (Australia)
BENZOYL PEROXIDE
Brevoxyl-4 Creamy Wash 3210
Brevoxyl-4 Gel 3210

Brevoxyl-8 Creamy Wash 3210
Brevoxyl-8 Gel 3210
Triaz Cleanser 1892
Triaz Gel 1892

TOPFANS (Italy)
DICLOFENAC SODIUM
Voltaren Tablets 2307
Voltaren-XR Tablets 2310

TOPICTAL (Argentina)
TOPIRAMATE
Topamax Sprinkle Capsules 2404
Topamax Tablets 2404

TOPIFORT (India)
CLOBETASOL PROPIONATE
Temovate Cream 2668
Temovate E Emollient 2671
Temovate Gel 2669
Temovate Ointment 2668
Temovate Scalp Application 2670

TOPILONE (Thailand)
TRIAMCINOLONE ACETONIDE
Azmacort Inhalation Aerosol 1726
Nasacort AQ Nasal Spray 2922

TOPIMAX (Denmark, Finland, Norway, Sweden)
TOPIRAMATE
Topamax Sprinkle Capsules 2404
Topamax Tablets 2404

TOPISTIN (Greece)
CIPROFLOXACIN
Cipro Oral Suspension 2977

TOPIZOL (Australia)
CLOTRIMAZOLE
Lotrimin Cream 3039
Lotrimin Lotion 1% 3039
Lotrimin Topical Solution 1% 3039

TOPLA (South Africa)
LIDOCAINE
Lidoderm Patch 1118

TOPOKEBIR (Argentina)
TOPOTECAN HYDROCHLORIDE
Hycamtin for Injection 1458

TOPOTAG (Argentina)
TOPOTECAN HYDROCHLORIDE
Hycamtin for Injection 1458

TOPOTEL (India)
TOPOTECAN HYDROCHLORIDE
Hycamtin for Injection 1458

TOPREL (Chile)
TOPIRAMATE
Topamax Sprinkle Capsules 2404
Topamax Tablets 2404

TOPRILEM (Mexico)
CAPTOPRIL
Captopril Tablets 2149

TOPROL (Australia)
METOPROLOL SUCCINATE
Toprol-XL Tablets 668

TOPROMEL (Irish Republic)
METOPROLOL TARTRATE
Lopressor Tablets 2238

TORACIN (Hong Kong)
TOBRAMYCIN
TOBI Solution for Inhalation 2298

TORIO (Thailand)
SIMVASTATIN
Zocor Tablets 2105

TORIOL (Spain)
RANITIDINE HYDROCHLORIDE
Zantac 25 EFFERdose Tablets 1624
Zantac 150 EFFERdose Tablets 1624
Zantac 150 Tablets 1624
Zantac 300 Tablets 1624
Zantac Injection 1619
Zantac Injection Premixed 1619
Zantac Syrup 1624

TORIVAS (Argentina)
ATORVASTATIN CALCIUM
Lipitor Tablets 2483

TORLOS (Brazil)
LOSARTAN POTASSIUM
Cozaar Tablets 1935

TORLOS H (Brazil)
LOSARTAN POTASSIUM
Cozaar Tablets 1935

TORVAST (Italy)
ATORVASTATIN CALCIUM
Lipitor Tablets 2483

TORVIC (Mexico)
CLARITHROMYCIN
Biaxin Filmtab Tablets 402
Biaxin Granules 402

TORYXIL (Germany)
DICLOFENAC SODIUM
Voltaren Tablets 2307
Voltaren-XR Tablets 2310

TOTALIP (Italy)
ATORVASTATIN CALCIUM
Lipitor Tablets 2483

TOTATROM (Mexico)
ERYTHROMYCIN
Ery-Tab Tablets 449
Erythromycin Base Filmtab Tablets 455
Erythromycin Delayed-Release Capsules, USP 457
PCE Dispertab Tablets 515

TOTELLE (Sweden)
ESTRADIOL
Climara Transdermal System 771
Estring Vaginal Ring 2635

TOTELLE CONTINUO (Argentina, Chile, Mexico)
ESTRADIOL
Climara Transdermal System 771
Estring Vaginal Ring 2635

TOTELMIN (Brazil)
ALBENDAZOLE
Albenza Tablets 1338

TRABAR (Czech Republic, Israel)
TRAMADOL HYDROCHLORIDE
Ultram ER Tablets 2392

TRABILIN (Brazil)
TRAMADOL HYDROCHLORIDE
Ultram ER Tablets 2392

TRACINE (Thailand)
TRAMADOL HYDROCHLORIDE
Ultram ER Tablets 2392

TRACIX (Spain)
CILASTATIN SODIUM/IMIPENEM
Primaxin I.M. 2045
Primaxin I.V. 2048

TRADEA (Mexico)
METHYLPHENIDATE HYDROCHLORIDE
Ritalin Hydrochloride Tablets 2269
Ritalin-SR Tablets 2269

TRADELIA (Germany)
ESTRADIOL
Climara Transdermal System 771
Estring Vaginal Ring 2635

TRADOL (Germany, Irish Republic, Mexico, Singapore)
TRAMADOL HYDROCHLORIDE
Ultram ER Tablets 2392

TRADOLAN (Austria, Denmark, Finland, Norway, Sweden)
TRAMADOL HYDROCHLORIDE
Ultram ER Tablets 2392

TRADOLGESIC (Thailand)
TRAMADOL HYDROCHLORIDE
Ultram ER Tablets 2392

TRADONAL (Belgium, Hong Kong, Italy, Spain, Thailand, The Netherlands)
TRAMADOL HYDROCHLORIDE
Ultram ER Tablets 2392

TRADOX (Chile)
LAMOTRIGINE
Lamictal Chewable Dispersible Tablets 1481
Lamictal Tablets 1481

TRAFLOXAL (Belgium, The Netherlands)
OFLOXACIN
Floxin Otic Solution 1049

TRALGIOL (Spain)
TRAMADOL HYDROCHLORIDE
Ultram ER Tablets 2392

TRALGIT (Czech Republic)
TRAMADOL HYDROCHLORIDE
Ultram ER Tablets 2392

TRALIC (Mexico)
TRAMADOL HYDROCHLORIDE
Ultram ER Tablets 2392

TRAMA (Germany)
TRAMADOL HYDROCHLORIDE
Ultram ER Tablets 2392

TRAMABENE (Austria, Czech Republic)
TRAMADOL HYDROCHLORIDE
Ultram ER Tablets 2392

TRAMABETA (Germany)
TRAMADOL HYDROCHLORIDE
Ultram ER Tablets 2392

TRAMACET (Argentina, Canada, Mexico, South Africa, United Kingdom)
TRAMADOL HYDROCHLORIDE
Ultram ER Tablets 2392

TRAMACIP (India)
TRAMADOL HYDROCHLORIDE
Ultram ER Tablets 2392

TRAMACIP PLUS (India)
TRAMADOL HYDROCHLORIDE
Ultram ER Tablets 2392

TRAMADA (Malaysia)
TRAMADOL HYDROCHLORIDE
Ultram ER Tablets 2392

TRAMADEX (Israel)
TRAMADOL HYDROCHLORIDE
Ultram ER Tablets 2392

TRAMADIN (Finland)
TRAMADOL HYDROCHLORIDE
Ultram ER Tablets 2392

TRAMADOC (Germany)
TRAMADOL HYDROCHLORIDE
Ultram ER Tablets 2392

TRAMADOL-DOLGIT (Germany)
TRAMADOL HYDROCHLORIDE
Ultram ER Tablets 2392

TRAMADOLOR (Austria, Germany, Hungary, Switzerland)
TRAMADOL HYDROCHLORIDE
Ultram ER Tablets 2392

TRAMADON (Brazil)
TRAMADOL HYDROCHLORIDE
Ultram ER Tablets 2392

TRAMA-DORSCH (Germany)
TRAMADOL HYDROCHLORIDE
Ultram ER Tablets 2392

TRAMADURA (Germany)
TRAMADOL HYDROCHLORIDE
Ultram ER Tablets 2392

TRAMAGETIC (Finland, Germany, Norway, The Netherlands)
TRAMADOL HYDROCHLORIDE
Ultram ER Tablets 2392

TRAMAGIT (Czech Republic, Germany)
TRAMADOL HYDROCHLORIDE
Ultram ER Tablets 2392

TRAMAHEXAL (Australia, South Africa)
TRAMADOL HYDROCHLORIDE
Ultram ER Tablets 2392

TRAMAKE (Irish Republic, United Kingdom)
TRAMADOL HYDROCHLORIDE
Ultram ER Tablets 2392

TRAMA-KLOSIDOL (Argentina)
TRAMADOL HYDROCHLORIDE
Ultram ER Tablets 2392

TRAMAL (Argentina, Australia, Austria, Brazil, Chile, Finland, Germany, Hong Kong, Israel, Malaysia, New Zealand, Portugal, Russia, Singapore, South Africa, Switzerland, Thailand, The Netherlands, Venezuela)
TRAMADOL HYDROCHLORIDE
Ultram ER Tablets 2392

TRAMALAN (Argentina, Thailand)
TRAMADOL HYDROCHLORIDE
Ultram ER Tablets 2392

TRAMALGIC (Hungary)
TRAMADOL HYDROCHLORIDE
Ultram ER Tablets 2392

TRAMAMED (Austria, Thailand)
TRAMADOL HYDROCHLORIDE
Ultram ER Tablets 2392

TRAMAMERCK (Germany)
TRAMADOL HYDROCHLORIDE
Ultram ER Tablets 2392

TRAMAPINE (Irish Republic)
TRAMADOL HYDROCHLORIDE
Ultram ER Tablets 2392

TRAMASTAD (Austria)
TRAMADOL HYDROCHLORIDE
Ultram ER Tablets 2392

TRAMATYROL (Austria)
TRAMADOL HYDROCHLORIDE
Ultram ER Tablets 2392

TRAMAX (Thailand)
TRAMADOL HYDROCHLORIDE
Ultram ER Tablets 2392

TRAMAZAC (India)
TRAMADOL HYDROCHLORIDE
Ultram ER Tablets 2392

TRAMBO (Finland)
TRAMADOL HYDROCHLORIDE
Ultram ER Tablets 2392

TRAMEDPHANO (Germany)
TRAMADOL HYDROCHLORIDE
Ultram ER Tablets 2392

TRAMELENE (The Netherlands)
TRAMADOL HYDROCHLORIDE
Ultram ER Tablets 2392

TRAMEX (Irish Republic)
TRAMADOL HYDROCHLORIDE
Ultram ER Tablets 2392

TRAMIUM (Belgium)
TRAMADOL HYDROCHLORIDE
Ultram ER Tablets 2392

TRAMO (Hong Kong)
TRAMADOL HYDROCHLORIDE
Ultram ER Tablets 2392

TRAMODA (Thailand)
TRAMADOL HYDROCHLORIDE
Ultram ER Tablets 2392

TRAMSILIONE (Thailand)
TRIAMCINOLONE ACETONIDE
Azmacort Inhalation Aerosol 1726
Nasacort AQ Nasal Spray 2922

TRAMUNDAL (Austria)
TRAMADOL HYDROCHLORIDE
Ultram ER Tablets 2392

TRAMUNDIN (Austria, Czech Republic, Germany, Switzerland)
TRAMADOL HYDROCHLORIDE
Ultram ER Tablets 2392

TRANCOCARD (Italy)
DIPYRIDAMOLE
Persantine Tablets 868

TRANGINA (United Kingdom)
ISOSORBIDE MONONITRATE
Imdur Tablets 3018

TRANQUASE (Germany)
DIAZEPAM
Diastat Rectal Delivery System 3343
Valium Tablets 2819

TRANQUILYN (United Kingdom)
METHYLPHENIDATE HYDROCHLORIDE
Ritalin Hydrochloride Tablets 2269
Ritalin-SR Tablets 2269

TRANQUIRIT (Italy)
DIAZEPAM
Diastat Rectal Delivery System 3343
Valium Tablets 2819

TRANQUO (Germany)
DIAZEPAM
Diastat Rectal Delivery System 3343
Valium Tablets 2819

TRANSDERMA H (Argentina)
HYDROCORTISONE
Hydrocortone Tablets 1989

TRANSDIOL (Argentina)
ESTRADIOL
Climara Transdermal System 771
Estring Vaginal Ring 2635

TRANSIPEN (Greece)
INDAPAMIDE
Indapamide Tablets 2156

TRANSPULMINA RINO (Italy)
NAPHAZOLINE HYDROCHLORIDE
Albalon Ophthalmic Solution . . . . ⊙218

TRANSVITAL (Chile)
ESTRADIOL
Climara Transdermal System 771
Estring Vaginal Ring 2635

TRANTIL (Mexico)
CARBAMAZEPINE
Carbatrol Capsules 3171
Tegretol Chewable Tablets 2295
Tegretol Suspension 2295
Tegretol Tablets 2295
Tegretol-XR Tablets 2295

TRASEDAL (France)
TRAMADOL HYDROCHLORIDE
Ultram ER Tablets 2392

TRASTOCIR (Argentina)
CILOSTAZOL
Pletal Tablets 2455

TRASYLOL (Australia, Austria, Belgium, Brazil, Canada, Chile, Czech Republic, Denmark, Finland, France, Germany, Greece, Hong Kong, Hungary, Irish Republic, Italy, Malaysia, Mexico, New Zealand, Russia, Singapore, South Africa, Spain, Sweden, Switzerland, Thailand, The Netherlands, United Kingdom, Venezuela)
APROTININ
Trasylol Injection 754

TRATACNE (Argentina)
TRETINOIN
Vesanoid Capsules 2820

TRAUMOX (South Africa)
NAPROXEN
EC-Naprosyn Delayed-Release Tablets 2761
Naprosyn Suspension 2761
Naprosyn Tablets 2761

TRAVEX (Portugal)
TRAMADOL HYDROCHLORIDE
Ultram ER Tablets 2392

TRAVIATA (Chile)
PAROXETINE HYDROCHLORIDE
Paxil Oral Suspension 1530
Paxil Tablets 1530

TRAVILAN (Greece)
CEFTRIAXONE SODIUM
Rocephin Injectable Vials, ADD-Vantage, Galaxy, Bulk 2800

TRAZIL (Venezuela)
TOBRAMYCIN
TOBI Solution for Inhalation 2298

TRAZOTEVA (Argentina)
DOCETAXEL
Taxotere Injection Concentrate 2932

TRD-CONTIN (India)
TRAMADOL HYDROCHLORIDE
Ultram ER Tablets 2392

TRECIFAN (Greece)
ISOTRETINOIN
Accutane Capsules 2731

TREMAX (Mexico)
GENTAMICIN SULFATE
Garamycin Injectable 3014

TREMEXAL (Greece)
FLUTAMIDE
Eulexin Capsules 3009

TREMOREX (Denmark)
SELEGILINE HYDROCHLORIDE
Eldepryl Capsules 3208

TREPINA (Mexico)
CARBAMAZEPINE
Carbatrol Capsules 3171
Tegretol Chewable Tablets 2295
Tegretol Suspension 2295
Tegretol Tablets 2295
Tegretol-XR Tablets 2295

TREPOL (Mexico)
DIPYRIDAMOLE
Persantine Tablets 868

TRESLEEN (Austria)
SERTRALINE HYDROCHLORIDE
Zoloft Tablets 2586

TRETIN (Greece)
ISOTRETINOIN
Accutane Capsules 2731

TRETINAX (Venezuela)
TRETINOIN
Vesanoid Capsules 2820

TRETINODERM (Argentina)
TRETINOIN
Vesanoid Capsules 2820

TRETINOINE KEFRANE (France)
TRETINOIN
Vesanoid Capsules 2820

TRETINON (Malaysia, Mexico)
TRETINOIN
Vesanoid Capsules 2820

TREVILOR (Germany)
VENLAFAXINE HYDROCHLORIDE
Effexor Tablets 3411
Effexor XR Capsules 3417

TREWILOR (Austria)
VENLAFAXINE HYDROCHLORIDE
Effexor Tablets 3411
Effexor XR Capsules 3417

TREXOFIN (Singapore)
CEFTRIAXONE SODIUM
Rocephin Injectable Vials, ADD-Vantage, Galaxy, Bulk 2800

TREXOL (Mexico)
TRAMADOL HYDROCHLORIDE
Ultram ER Tablets 2392

TRIACORT (Italy, Russia)
TRIAMCINOLONE ACETONIDE
Azmacort Inhalation Aerosol 1726
Nasacort AQ Nasal Spray 2922

TRIADERM (Canada)
TRIAMCINOLONE ACETONIDE
Azmacort Inhalation Aerosol 1726
Nasacort AQ Nasal Spray 2922

TRIAKEN (Mexico)
CEFTRIAXONE SODIUM
Rocephin Injectable Vials, ADD-Vantage, Galaxy, Bulk 2800

TRIAKLIM (Hungary)
ESTRADIOL
Climara Transdermal System 771
Estring Vaginal Ring 2635

TRIAL GEL (Argentina)
ESTRADIOL
Climara Transdermal System 771
Estring Vaginal Ring 2635

TRIAL GEST (Argentina)
ESTRADIOL
Climara Transdermal System 771
Estring Vaginal Ring 2635

TRIAL SAT (Argentina)
ESTRADIOL
Climara Transdermal System 771
Estring Vaginal Ring 2635

TRIALIX (Austria, Irish Republic)
RAMIPRIL
Altace Capsules 1702

TRIALONA (Spain)
FLUTICASONE PROPIONATE
Cutivate Cream 2662
Cutivate Ointment 2665
Flonase Nasal Spray 1440

TRIAM (Hong Kong, Singapore)
TRIAMCINOLONE ACETONIDE
Azmacort Inhalation Aerosol 1726
Nasacort AQ Nasal Spray 2922

TRIAMA (Thailand)
TRIAMCINOLONE ACETONIDE
Azmacort Inhalation Aerosol 1726
Nasacort AQ Nasal Spray 2922

TRIAMAXCO (United Kingdom)
HYDROCHLOROTHIAZIDE/TRIAMTERENE
Dyazide Capsules 1423

TRIAMCINOLON COMPOSITUM (Czech Republic)
TRIAMCINOLONE ACETONIDE
Azmacort Inhalation Aerosol 1726
Nasacort AQ Nasal Spray 2922

TRIAMCINOLON E (Czech Republic)
TRIAMCINOLONE ACETONIDE
Azmacort Inhalation Aerosol 1726
Nasacort AQ Nasal Spray 2922

TRIAMCINOLON S (Czech Republic)
TRIAMCINOLONE ACETONIDE
Azmacort Inhalation Aerosol 1726
Nasacort AQ Nasal Spray 2922

TRIAMCO (United Kingdom)
HYDROCHLOROTHIAZIDE/TRIAMTERENE
Dyazide Capsules 1423

TRIAM-CO (Hong Kong, Russia)
HYDROCHLOROTHIAZIDE/TRIAMTERENE
Dyazide Capsules 1423

TRIAMCORT (Switzerland)
TRIAMCINOLONE ACETONIDE
Azmacort Inhalation Aerosol 1726
Nasacort AQ Nasal Spray 2922

TRIAMCREME (Germany)
TRIAMCINOLONE ACETONIDE
Azmacort Inhalation Aerosol 1726
Nasacort AQ Nasal Spray 2922

TRIAMGALEN (Germany)
TRIAMCINOLONE ACETONIDE
Azmacort Inhalation Aerosol 1726
Nasacort AQ Nasal Spray 2922

TRIAMHEXAL (Germany)
TRIAMCINOLONE ACETONIDE
Azmacort Inhalation Aerosol 1726
Nasacort AQ Nasal Spray 2922

TRIAMIZIDE (New Zealand)
HYDROCHLOROTHIAZIDE/TRIAMTERENE
Dyazide Capsules 1423

TRIAMPUR COMPOSITUM (Germany, Russia)
HYDROCHLOROTHIAZIDE/TRIAMTERENE
Dyazide Capsules 1423

TRIAMSALBE (Germany)
TRIAMCINOLONE ACETONIDE
Azmacort Inhalation Aerosol 1726
Nasacort AQ Nasal Spray 2922

TRIAMTEREN COMP (Austria, Germany)
HYDROCHLOROTHIAZIDE/TRIAMTERENE
Dyazide Capsules 1423

TRIAMTEREN/HCT (Austria)
TRIAMTERENE
Dyrenium Capsules 3400

TRIAMTEREN-H (Germany)
HYDROCHLOROTHIAZIDE/TRIAMTERENE
Dyazide Capsules 1423

TRIAMTERIL COMPLEX (Italy)
HYDROCHLOROTHIAZIDE/TRIAMTERENE
Dyazide Capsules 1423

TRIAMTHIAZID (Germany)
HYDROCHLOROTHIAZIDE/TRIAMTERENE
Dyazide Capsules 1423

TRIAM-TIAZIDA R (Portugal)
HYDROCHLOROTHIAZIDE/TRIAMTERENE
Dyazide Capsules 1423

TRIAMVIRGI (Italy)
TRIAMCINOLONE ACETONIDE
Azmacort Inhalation Aerosol 1726
Nasacort AQ Nasal Spray 2922

TRIAN (Greece)
LEVOCARNITINE
Carnitor Injection 3188
Carnitor Tablets and Oral Solution 3190

TRIANCIL (Brazil)
TRIAMCINOLONE ACETONIDE
Azmacort Inhalation Aerosol 1726
Nasacort AQ Nasal Spray 2922

TRI-ANEMUL (Germany)
TRIAMCINOLONE ACETONIDE
Azmacort Inhalation Aerosol 1726
Nasacort AQ Nasal Spray 2922

TRIARESE (Germany)
HYDROCHLOROTHIAZIDE/TRIAMTERENE
Dyazide Capsules 1423

TRIASTAD HCT (Austria)
HYDROCHLOROTHIAZIDE/TRIAMTERENE
Dyazide Capsules 1423

TRIATEC (Brazil, Chile, Denmark, France, Greece, Italy, Norway, Portugal, Sweden, Switzerland)
RAMIPRIL
Altace Capsules 1702

TRIATEC COMP (Denmark)
RAMIPRIL
Altace Capsules 1702

TRIATEC COMPOSTO (Portugal)
RAMIPRIL
Altace Capsules 1702

TRIATEC D (Brazil)
RAMIPRIL
Altace Capsules 1702

TRIATEC HCT (Italy)
RAMIPRIL
Altace Capsules 1702

TRIAX (Israel)
CEFTRIAXONE SODIUM
Rocephin Injectable Vials, ADD-Vantage, Galaxy, Bulk 2800

TRIAXON (Brazil)
CEFTRIAXONE SODIUM
Rocephin Injectable Vials, ADD-Vantage, Galaxy, Bulk 2800

TRIAXONE (United Arab Emirates)
CEFTRIAXONE SODIUM
Rocephin Injectable Vials, ADD-Vantage, Galaxy, Bulk 2800

TRIAXTON (Brazil)
CEFTRIAXONE SODIUM
Rocephin Injectable Vials, ADD-Vantage, Galaxy, Bulk 2800

TRIAZID (Germany)
HYDROCHLOROTHIAZIDE/TRIAMTERENE
Dyazide Capsules 1423

TRICEF (Austria, Chile, Portugal, Sweden)
CEFIXIME
Suprax 1843

TRICEFIN (Singapore)
CEFTRIAXONE SODIUM
Rocephin Injectable Vials, ADD-Vantage, Galaxy, Bulk 2800

TRICEN (Spain)
TRANDOLAPRIL/VERAPAMIL HYDROCHLORIDE
Tarka Tablets 524

TRICEPHIN (Thailand)
CEFTRIAXONE SODIUM
Rocephin Injectable Vials, ADD-Vantage, Galaxy, Bulk 2800

TRICHAZOLE (South Africa)
METRONIDAZOLE
MetroGel-Vaginal Gel 1855

TRICHEX (Austria)
METRONIDAZOLE
MetroGel-Vaginal Gel 1855

TRICHO CORDES (Germany)
METRONIDAZOLE
MetroGel-Vaginal Gel 1855

TRICHOPOL (Russia)
METRONIDAZOLE
MetroGel-Vaginal Gel 1855

TRICHOZOLE (Australia, New Zealand)
METRONIDAZOLE
MetroGel-Vaginal Gel 1855

TRICLODERM (Hong Kong)
CLOTRIMAZOLE
Lotrimin Cream 3039
Lotrimin Lotion 1% 3039
Lotrimin Topical Solution 1% 3039

TRICOCET (Brazil)
NYSTATIN
Nystop Topical Powder USP 2478

Paddock Nystatin USP for Oral Suspension ... 2478

TRICODAZOLE (Greece)
METRONIDAZOLE
MetroGel-Vaginal Gel ... 1855

TRICOFARMA (Argentina)
FINASTERIDE
Propecia Tablets ... 2060
Proscar Tablets ... 2067

TRICOFIN (Argentina)
METRONIDAZOLE
MetroGel-Vaginal Gel ... 1855

TRICOMED (Thailand)
METRONIDAZOLE
MetroGel-Vaginal Gel ... 1855

TRICOR (Chile)
ADENOSINE
Adenoscan ... 619
Adenocard Injection ... 617

TRICORTONE (Australia)
TRIAMCINOLONE ACETONIDE
Azmacort Inhalation Aerosol ... 1726
Nasacort AQ Nasal Spray ... 2922

TRICOSTEN (Brazil)
CLOTRIMAZOLE
Lotrimin Cream ... 3039
Lotrimin Lotion 1% ... 3039
Lotrimin Topical Solution 1% ... 3039

TRICOWAS B (Spain)
METRONIDAZOLE
MetroGel-Vaginal Gel ... 1855

TRIFAMOX (Argentina)
AMOXICILLIN
Amoxil Pediatric Drops for Oral Suspension ... 1343
Amoxil Tablets ... 1343

TRIGEN (Mexico)
CIPROFLOXACIN HYDROCHLORIDE
Ciloxan Ophthalmic Ointment ... ⊙204, 559
Ciloxan Ophthalmic Solution ... ⊙206
Cipro Tablets ... 2977

TRIGGER (Italy)
RANITIDINE HYDROCHLORIDE
Zantac 25 EFFERdose Tablets ... 1624
Zantac 150 EFFERdose Tablets ... 1624
Zantac 150 Tablets ... 1624
Zantac 300 Tablets ... 1624
Zantac Injection ... 1619
Zantac Injection Premixed ... 1619
Zantac Syrup ... 1624

TRIGON DEPOT (Spain)
TRIAMCINOLONE ACETONIDE
Azmacort Inhalation Aerosol ... 1726
Nasacort AQ Nasal Spray ... 2922

TRIIODOTHYRONINE INJECTION (United Kingdom)
LIOTHYRONINE SODIUM
Cytomel Tablets ... 1710

TRIKACIDE (Canada)
METRONIDAZOLE
MetroGel-Vaginal Gel ... 1855

TRIKOZOL (Finland)
METRONIDAZOLE
MetroGel-Vaginal Gel ... 1855

TRILOSIL (Thailand)
TRIAMCINOLONE ACETONIDE
Azmacort Inhalation Aerosol ... 1726
Nasacort AQ Nasal Spray ... 2922

TRIM (Malaysia, Thailand)
TRIAMCINOLONE ACETONIDE
Azmacort Inhalation Aerosol ... 1726
Nasacort AQ Nasal Spray ... 2922

TRIMASONE (Thailand)
TRIAMCINOLONE ACETONIDE
Azmacort Inhalation Aerosol ... 1726
Nasacort AQ Nasal Spray ... 2922

TRIMAZE (South Africa)
CLOTRIMAZOLE
Lotrimin Cream ... 3039
Lotrimin Lotion 1% ... 3039
Lotrimin Topical Solution 1% ... 3039

TRIMAZOL (Argentina, Malaysia)
CLOTRIMAZOLE
Lotrimin Cream ... 3039
Lotrimin Lotion 1% ... 3039
Lotrimin Topical Solution 1% ... 3039

TRIMEBA (Mexico)
CLARITHROMYCIN
Biaxin Filmtab Tablets ... 402
Biaxin Granules ... 402

TRIMOLEX (South Africa)
AMILORIDE HYDROCHLORIDE/HYDROCHLOROTHIAZIDE
Moduretic Tablets ... 2028

TRIMONIL (Denmark, Finland, Norway, Sweden)
CARBAMAZEPINE
Carbatrol Capsules ... 3171
Tegretol Chewable Tablets ... 2295
Tegretol Suspension ... 2295
Tegretol Tablets ... 2295
Tegretol-XR Tablets ... 2295

TRIMOX (Brazil)
AMOXICILLIN
Amoxil Pediatric Drops for Oral Suspension ... 1343
Amoxil Tablets ... 1343

TRIMSTAT (Argentina)
METRONIDAZOLE
MetroGel-Vaginal Gel ... 1855

TRIMYSTEN (France)
CLOTRIMAZOLE
Lotrimin Cream ... 3039
Lotrimin Lotion 1% ... 3039
Lotrimin Topical Solution 1% ... 3039

TRINALIN (Greece)
LEVOCARNITINE
Carnitor Injection ... 3188
Carnitor Tablets and Oral Solution ... 3190

TRINALION (Portugal)
NIMODIPINE
Nimotop Capsules ... 749

TRINOLONE (Singapore)
TRIAMCINOLONE ACETONIDE
Azmacort Inhalation Aerosol ... 1726
Nasacort AQ Nasal Spray ... 2922

TRINOTECAN (Argentina)
IRINOTECAN HYDROCHLORIDE
Camptosar Injection ... 2604

TRIOMUNE (India)
LAMIVUDINE
Epivir Oral Solution ... 1427
Epivir Tablets ... 1427
Epivir-HBV Oral Solution ... 1432
Epivir-HBV Tablets ... 1432

TRIORAL/HCT (Austria)
TRIAMTERENE
Dyrenium Capsules ... 3400

TRIOSULES (Argentina)
FLUOROURACIL
Efudex Topical Cream ... 3363
Efudex Topical Solutions ... 3363

TRIOX (Mexico)
CEFTRIAXONE SODIUM
Rocephin Injectable Vials, ADD-Vantage, Galaxy, Bulk ... 2800

TRIOX NF (Chile)
NAPROXEN SODIUM
Anaprox DS Tablets ... 2761
Anaprox Tablets ... 2761

TRI-PLEN (South Africa)
RAMIPRIL
Altace Capsules ... 1702

TRISORCIN (Germany)
PENICILLAMINE
Cuprimine Capsules ... 1947

TRITACE (Argentina, Australia, Austria, Belgium, Hong Kong, Hungary, Irish Republic, Israel, Malaysia, Mexico, New Zealand, Singapore, South Africa, Thailand, The Netherlands, United Kingdom)
RAMIPRIL
Altace Capsules ... 1702

TRITACE COMP (Israel)
RAMIPRIL
Altace Capsules ... 1702

TRITACE-HCT (Argentina)
RAMIPRIL
Altace Capsules ... 1702

TRITAZIDE (Belgium, Czech Republic, Mexico, The Netherlands)
RAMIPRIL
Altace Capsules ... 1702

TRI-THIAZID (Germany)
HYDROCHLOROTHIAZIDE/TRIAMTERENE
Dyazide Capsules ... 1423

TRI-THIAZID RESERPIN (Germany)
HYDROCHLOROTHIAZIDE/TRIAMTERENE
Dyazide Capsules ... 1423

TRIVORIN (Mexico)
RIBAVIRIN
Virazole for Inhalation Solution ... 3370

TRIVUDIN (Argentina)
LAMIVUDINE
Epivir Oral Solution ... 1427
Epivir Tablets ... 1427
Epivir-HBV Oral Solution ... 1432
Epivir-HBV Tablets ... 1432

TRIXNE (Argentina)
ERYTHROMYCIN
Ery-Tab Tablets ... 449
Erythromycin Base Filmtab Tablets ... 455
Erythromycin Delayed-Release Capsules, USP ... 457
PCE Dispertab Tablets ... 515

TRIXONE (Thailand)
CEFTRIAXONE SODIUM
Rocephin Injectable Vials, ADD-Vantage, Galaxy, Bulk ... 2800

TRIXOTENE (Argentina)
DOCETAXEL
Taxotere Injection Concentrate ... 2932

TRIYOTEX (Mexico)
LIOTHYRONINE SODIUM
Cytomel Tablets ... 1710

TRIZ (Thailand)
CETIRIZINE HYDROCHLORIDE
Zyrtec Syrup ... 2594
Zyrtec Tablets ... 2594

TRIZELE (Hong Kong)
METRONIDAZOLE
MetroGel-Vaginal Gel ... 1855

TRIZID (Hong Kong, New Zealand)
HYDROCHLOROTHIAZIDE/TRIAMTERENE
Dyazide Capsules ... 1423

TRIZOLIN (Malaysia, Singapore, Thailand)
NORFLOXACIN
Noroxin Tablets ... 2032

TROFENTYL (India)
FENTANYL CITRATE
Actiq ... 979

TROKEN (Argentina)
CLOPIDOGREL BISULFATE
Plavix Tablets ... 917, 2926

TROLIP (Hong Kong)
FENOFIBRATE
Tricor Tablets ... 527

TROLOVOL (Czech Republic, France, Germany)
PENICILLAMINE
Cuprimine Capsules ... 1947

TROMAGESIC (India)
DICLOFENAC SODIUM
Voltaren Tablets ... 2307
Voltaren-XR Tablets ... 2310

TROMAX (India)
DICLOFENAC SODIUM
Voltaren Tablets ... 2307
Voltaren-XR Tablets ... 2310

TROMBENAL (Argentina)
TICLOPIDINE HYDROCHLORIDE
Ticlid Tablets ... 2810

TROMBENOX (Italy)
ENOXAPARIN SODIUM
Lovenox Injection ... 2915

TROMBONOT (Argentina)
CILOSTAZOL
Pletal Tablets ... 2455

TROMBOPAT (Portugal)
TICLOPIDINE HYDROCHLORIDE
Ticlid Tablets ... 2810

TROMBOXANIL (Brazil)
DIPYRIDAMOLE
Persantine Tablets ... 868

TROMIGAL (Mexico)
ERYTHROMYCIN
Ery-Tab Tablets ... 449
Erythromycin Base Filmtab Tablets ... 455
Erythromycin Delayed-Release Capsules, USP ... 457
PCE Dispertab Tablets ... 515

TROMPERSANTIN (Mexico)
DIPYRIDAMOLE
Persantine Tablets ... 868

TROMPHYLLIN (Germany)
THEOPHYLLINE
Uniphyl Tablets ... 2710

TROPHARMA (Mexico)
ERYTHROMYCIN STEARATE
Erythrocin Stearate Filmtab Tablets ... 453

TROPICUR (Argentina)
MEFLOQUINE HYDROCHLORIDE
Lariam Tablets ... 2786

TROPIOVENT (United Kingdom)
IPRATROPIUM BROMIDE
Atrovent Inhalation Solution ... 835
Atrovent Nasal Spray 0.03% ... 837
Atrovent Nasal Spray 0.06% ... 839

TROPISOL (Mexico)
CAPTOPRIL
Captopril Tablets ... 2149

TROPIUM (United Kingdom)
CHLORDIAZEPOXIDE HYDROCHLORIDE
Librium Capsules ... 3347

TROPIX-HC (Mexico)
CAPTOPRIL
Captopril Tablets ... 2149

TROPOCER (Venezuela)
NIMODIPINE
Nimotop Capsules ... 749

TRORIX (Chile)
ONDANSETRON
Zofran ODT Orally Disintegrating Tablets ... 1639

TROSIC (Thailand)
TRAMADOL HYDROCHLORIDE
Ultram ER Tablets ... 2392

TROZOLET (Chile)
ANASTROZOLE
Arimidex Tablets ... 673

TROZOLITE (Argentina)
ANASTROZOLE
Arimidex Tablets ... 673

TRUMSAL (Spain)
DILTIAZEM HYDROCHLORIDE
Cardizem LA Extended Release Tablets ... 1728
Tiazac Capsules ... 1201

TRUOXIN (Irish Republic)
CIPROFLOXACIN
Cipro Oral Suspension ... 2977

TRUSOPT (Argentina, Australia, Austria, Belgium, Brazil, Canada, Chile, Czech Republic, Denmark, Finland, France, Germany, Greece, Hong Kong, Hungary, Irish Republic, Israel, Italy, Malaysia, Mexico, New Zealand, Norway, Portugal, Russia, Singapore, South Africa, Spain, Sweden, Switzerland, Thailand, The Netherlands, United Kingdom, Venezuela)
DORZOLAMIDE HYDROCHLORIDE
Trusopt Sterile Ophthalmic Solution ... 2095

T-STAT (Canada, Mexico, Singapore)
ERYTHROMYCIN
Ery-Tab Tablets ... 449
Erythromycin Base Filmtab Tablets ... 455
Erythromycin Delayed-Release Capsules, USP ... 457
PCE Dispertab Tablets ... 515

TUBERBUT (Argentina)
TOBRAMYCIN
TOBI Solution for Inhalation ... 2298

TULIP (Mexico, Russia)
SIMVASTATIN
Zocor Tablets ... 2105

TULOTRACT (Germany)
LACTULOSE
Kristalose for Oral Solution . . . 1034

TUNDRA (Argentina)
NAPROXEN
EC-Naprosyn Delayed-Release Tablets . . . 2761
Naprosyn Suspension . . . 2761
Naprosyn Tablets . . . 2761

TUPAST (Greece)
RANITIDINE HYDROCHLORIDE
Zantac 25 EFFERdose Tablets . . . 1624
Zantac 150 EFFERdose Tablets . . . 1624
Zantac 150 Tablets . . . 1624
Zantac 300 Tablets . . . 1624
Zantac Injection . . . 1619
Zantac Injection Premixed . . . 1619
Zantac Syrup . . . 1624

TURFA (Germany)
HYDROCHLOROTHIAZIDE/TRIAMTERENE
Dyazide Capsules . . . 1423

TURIMONIT (Germany)
ISOSORBIDE MONONITRATE
Imdur Tablets . . . 3018

TURIMYCIN (Germany)
CLINDAMYCIN HYDROCHLORIDE
Cleocin Vaginal Ovules . . . 2616

TURIXIN (Germany)
MUPIROCIN CALCIUM
Bactroban Cream . . . 1394
Bactroban Nasal . . . 1394

TUSEHLI (Mexico)
BENZONATATE
Tessalon Perles . . . 1199

TUSICAL (Mexico)
BENZONATATE
Tessalon Perles . . . 1199

TUSITATO (Mexico)
BENZONATATE
Tessalon Perles . . . 1199

TUZZIL (Mexico)
BENZONATATE
Tessalon Perles . . . 1199

TWICE (Italy)
MORPHINE SULFATE
Kadian Capsules . . . 577
MS Contin Tablets . . . 2701

TWINA (Thailand)
CLOTRIMAZOLE
Lotrimin Cream . . . 3039
Lotrimin Lotion 1% . . . 3039
Lotrimin Topical Solution 1% . . . 3039

TYKLID (India)
TICLOPIDINE HYDROCHLORIDE
Ticlid Tablets . . . 2810

TYMASIL (United Kingdom)
NATAMYCIN
Natacyn Antifungal Ophthalmic Suspension . . . ⊙208

T-ZA (Thailand)
ZIDOVUDINE
Retrovir Capsules . . . 1560
Retrovir IV Infusion . . . 1564
Retrovir Syrup . . . 1560
Retrovir Tablets . . . 1560

UBICOR (Switzerland)
DILTIAZEM HYDROCHLORIDE
Cardizem LA Extended Release Tablets . . . 1728
Tiazac Capsules . . . 1201

UBIZOL (Portugal)
FLUTICASONE PROPIONATE
Cutivate Cream . . . 2662
Cutivate Ointment . . . 2665
Flonase Nasal Spray . . . 1440

UDIMA ERY (Germany)
ERYTHROMYCIN
Ery-Tab Tablets . . . 449
Erythromycin Base Filmtab Tablets . . . 455
Erythromycin Delayed-Release Capsules, USP . . . 457
PCE Dispertab Tablets . . . 515

UDRAMIL (Germany)
TRANDOLAPRIL/VERAPAMIL HYDROCHLORIDE
Tarka Tablets . . . 524

UDRIK (Germany)
TRANDOLAPRIL
Mavik Tablets . . . 486

UGOTREX (Greece)
CEFTRIAXONE SODIUM
Rocephin Injectable Vials, ADD-Vantage, Galaxy, Bulk . . . 2800

ULCAID (South Africa)
RANITIDINE HYDROCHLORIDE
Zantac 25 EFFERdose Tablets . . . 1624
Zantac 150 EFFERdose Tablets . . . 1624
Zantac 150 Tablets . . . 1624
Zantac 300 Tablets . . . 1624
Zantac Injection . . . 1619
Zantac Injection Premixed . . . 1619
Zantac Syrup . . . 1624

ULCAR (France)
SUCRALFATE
Carafate Suspension . . . 701
Carafate Tablets . . . 701

ULCECUR (Portugal)
RANITIDINE HYDROCHLORIDE
Zantac 25 EFFERdose Tablets . . . 1624
Zantac 150 EFFERdose Tablets . . . 1624
Zantac 150 Tablets . . . 1624
Zantac 300 Tablets . . . 1624
Zantac Injection . . . 1619
Zantac Injection Premixed . . . 1619
Zantac Syrup . . . 1624

ULCEDIN (Mexico)
RANITIDINE HYDROCHLORIDE
Zantac 25 EFFERdose Tablets . . . 1624
Zantac 150 EFFERdose Tablets . . . 1624
Zantac 150 Tablets . . . 1624
Zantac 300 Tablets . . . 1624
Zantac Injection . . . 1619
Zantac Injection Premixed . . . 1619
Zantac Syrup . . . 1624

ULCEFATE (South Africa, Thailand)
SUCRALFATE
Carafate Suspension . . . 701
Carafate Tablets . . . 701

ULCEKON (India)
SUCRALFATE
Carafate Suspension . . . 701
Carafate Tablets . . . 701

ULCELAC (Argentina)
FAMOTIDINE
Pepcid Injection . . . 2040
Pepcid Injection Premixed . . . 2040
Pepcid Tablets . . . 2038
Pepcid for Oral Suspension . . . 2038

ULCENOL (Venezuela)
FAMOTIDINE
Pepcid Injection . . . 2040
Pepcid Injection Premixed . . . 2040
Pepcid Tablets . . . 2038
Pepcid for Oral Suspension . . . 2038

ULCERAL (Austria)
SUCRALFATE
Carafate Suspension . . . 701
Carafate Tablets . . . 701

ULCERAN (Czech Republic, Hong Kong, Hungary, Malaysia, Russia, Singapore, Thailand)
FAMOTIDINE
Pepcid Injection . . . 2040
Pepcid Injection Premixed . . . 2040
Pepcid Tablets . . . 2038
Pepcid for Oral Suspension . . . 2038

ULCERIT (Brazil)
RANITIDINE HYDROCHLORIDE
Zantac 25 EFFERdose Tablets . . . 1624
Zantac 150 EFFERdose Tablets . . . 1624
Zantac 150 Tablets . . . 1624
Zantac 300 Tablets . . . 1624
Zantac Injection . . . 1619
Zantac Injection Premixed . . . 1619
Zantac Syrup . . . 1624

ULCERLMIN (Japan)
SUCRALFATE
Carafate Suspension . . . 701
Carafate Tablets . . . 701

ULCERMIN (Portugal, Spain)
SUCRALFATE
Carafate Suspension . . . 701
Carafate Tablets . . . 701

ULCEROL (Portugal)
RANITIDINE HYDROCHLORIDE
Zantac 25 EFFERdose Tablets . . . 1624
Zantac 150 EFFERdose Tablets . . . 1624
Zantac 150 Tablets . . . 1624
Zantac 300 Tablets . . . 1624
Zantac Injection . . . 1619
Zantac Injection Premixed . . . 1619
Zantac Syrup . . . 1624

ULCERTEC (Malaysia, Portugal, Singapore)
SUCRALFATE
Carafate Suspension . . . 701
Carafate Tablets . . . 701

ULCETAB (South Africa)
SUCRALFATE
Carafate Suspension . . . 701
Carafate Tablets . . . 701

ULCETIC (South Africa)
SUCRALFATE
Carafate Suspension . . . 701
Carafate Tablets . . . 701

ULCETRAX (Spain)
FAMOTIDINE
Pepcid Injection . . . 2040
Pepcid Injection Premixed . . . 2040
Pepcid Tablets . . . 2038
Pepcid for Oral Suspension . . . 2038

ULCEVIT (Mexico)
RANITIDINE HYDROCHLORIDE
Zantac 25 EFFERdose Tablets . . . 1624
Zantac 150 EFFERdose Tablets . . . 1624
Zantac 150 Tablets . . . 1624
Zantac 300 Tablets . . . 1624
Zantac Injection . . . 1619
Zantac Injection Premixed . . . 1619
Zantac Syrup . . . 1624

ULCEX (Italy)
RANITIDINE HYDROCHLORIDE
Zantac 25 EFFERdose Tablets . . . 1624
Zantac 150 EFFERdose Tablets . . . 1624
Zantac 150 Tablets . . . 1624
Zantac 300 Tablets . . . 1624
Zantac Injection . . . 1619
Zantac Injection Premixed . . . 1619
Zantac Syrup . . . 1624

ULCIDINE (Canada, Switzerland)
FAMOTIDINE
Pepcid Injection . . . 2040
Pepcid Injection Premixed . . . 2040
Pepcid Tablets . . . 2038
Pepcid for Oral Suspension . . . 2038

ULCIMAX (India)
FAMOTIDINE
Pepcid Injection . . . 2040
Pepcid Injection Premixed . . . 2040
Pepcid Tablets . . . 2038
Pepcid for Oral Suspension . . . 2038

ULCIRAM (Venezuela)
SUCRALFATE
Carafate Suspension . . . 701
Carafate Tablets . . . 701

ULCIREX (France)
RANITIDINE HYDROCHLORIDE
Zantac 25 EFFERdose Tablets . . . 1624
Zantac 150 EFFERdose Tablets . . . 1624
Zantac 150 Tablets . . . 1624
Zantac 300 Tablets . . . 1624
Zantac Injection . . . 1619
Zantac Injection Premixed . . . 1619
Zantac Syrup . . . 1624

ULCOFAM (Thailand)
FAMOTIDINE
Pepcid Injection . . . 2040
Pepcid Injection Premixed . . . 2040
Pepcid Tablets . . . 2038
Pepcid for Oral Suspension . . . 2038

ULCOGANT (Austria, Belgium, Czech Republic, Germany, Hungary, Switzerland, The Netherlands)
SUCRALFATE
Carafate Suspension . . . 701
Carafate Tablets . . . 701

ULCOLIND METRO (Germany)
METRONIDAZOLE
MetroGel-Vaginal Gel . . . 1855

ULCOLIND RANI (Germany)
RANITIDINE HYDROCHLORIDE
Zantac 25 EFFERdose Tablets . . . 1624
Zantac 150 EFFERdose Tablets . . . 1624
Zantac 150 Tablets . . . 1624
Zantac 300 Tablets . . . 1624
Zantac Injection . . . 1619
Zantac Injection Premixed . . . 1619
Zantac Syrup . . . 1624

ULCONA (Spain)
SUCRALFATE
Carafate Suspension . . . 701
Carafate Tablets . . . 701

ULCOREN (Brazil)
RANITIDINE HYDROCHLORIDE
Zantac 25 EFFERdose Tablets . . . 1624
Zantac 150 EFFERdose Tablets . . . 1624
Zantac 150 Tablets . . . 1624
Zantac 300 Tablets . . . 1624
Zantac Injection . . . 1619
Zantac Injection Premixed . . . 1619
Zantac Syrup . . . 1624

ULCOSIN (Hungary)
RANITIDINE HYDROCHLORIDE
Zantac 25 EFFERdose Tablets . . . 1624
Zantac 150 EFFERdose Tablets . . . 1624
Zantac 150 Tablets . . . 1624
Zantac 300 Tablets . . . 1624
Zantac Injection . . . 1619
Zantac Injection Premixed . . . 1619
Zantac Syrup . . . 1624

ULCOTENK (Argentina)
RANITIDINE HYDROCHLORIDE
Zantac 25 EFFERdose Tablets . . . 1624
Zantac 150 EFFERdose Tablets . . . 1624
Zantac 150 Tablets . . . 1624
Zantac 300 Tablets . . . 1624
Zantac Injection . . . 1619
Zantac Injection Premixed . . . 1619
Zantac Syrup . . . 1624

ULCRAFATE (Thailand)
SUCRALFATE
Carafate Suspension . . . 701
Carafate Tablets . . . 701

ULCRAST (Italy)
SUCRALFATE
Carafate Suspension . . . 701
Carafate Tablets . . . 701

ULCUFATO (Spain)
SUCRALFATE
Carafate Suspension . . . 701
Carafate Tablets . . . 701

ULCUSAN (Austria)
FAMOTIDINE
Pepcid Injection . . . 2040
Pepcid Injection Premixed . . . 2040
Pepcid Tablets . . . 2038
Pepcid for Oral Suspension . . . 2038

ULCYTE (Australia)
SUCRALFATE
Carafate Suspension . . . 701
Carafate Tablets . . . 701

ULDAPRIL (Mexico)
LANSOPRAZOLE
Prevacid Delayed-Release Capsules . . . 3271

ULFAMET (Thailand)
FAMOTIDINE
Pepcid Injection . . . 2040
Pepcid Injection Premixed . . . 2040
Pepcid Tablets . . . 2038
Pepcid for Oral Suspension . . . 2038

ULFAMID (Czech Republic, Russia)
FAMOTIDINE
Pepcid Injection . . . 2040
Pepcid Injection Premixed . . . 2040
Pepcid Tablets . . . 2038
Pepcid for Oral Suspension . . . 2038

ULGARINE (Spain)
FAMOTIDINE
Pepcid Injection . . . 2040
Pepcid Injection Premixed . . . 2040
Pepcid Tablets . . . 2038
Pepcid for Oral Suspension . . . 2038

ULKOBRIN (Italy)
RANITIDINE HYDROCHLORIDE
Zantac 25 EFFERdose Tablets . . . 1624
Zantac 150 EFFERdose Tablets . . . 1624
Zantac 150 Tablets . . . 1624
Zantac 300 Tablets . . . 1624
Zantac Injection . . . 1619
Zantac Injection Premixed . . . 1619
Zantac Syrup . . . 1624

ULKODIN (Mexico)
RANITIDINE HYDROCHLORIDE
Zantac 25 EFFERdose Tablets . . . 1624
Zantac 150 EFFERdose Tablets . . . 1624
Zantac 150 Tablets . . . 1624
Zantac 300 Tablets . . . 1624
Zantac Injection . . . 1619
Zantac Injection Premixed . . . 1619
Zantac Syrup . . . 1624

ULPAX (Mexico)
LANSOPRAZOLE
Prevacid Delayed-Release Capsules . . . 3271

ULRAN (Czech Republic, Russia)
RANITIDINE HYDROCHLORIDE
Zantac 25 EFFERdose Tablets 1624
Zantac 150 EFFERdose Tablets. 1624
Zantac 150 Tablets 1624
Zantac 300 Tablets 1624
Zantac Injection 1619
Zantac Injection Premixed 1619
Zantac Syrup 1624

ULSAL (Austria)
RANITIDINE HYDROCHLORIDE
Zantac 25 EFFERdose Tablets 1624
Zantac 150 EFFERdose Tablets. 1624
Zantac 150 Tablets 1624
Zantac 300 Tablets 1624
Zantac Injection 1619
Zantac Injection Premixed 1619
Zantac Syrup 1624

ULSANIC (Hong Kong, Israel, South Africa, Thailand)
SUCRALFATE
Carafate Suspension 701
Carafate Tablets 701

ULSAVEN (Mexico)
RANITIDINE HYDROCHLORIDE
Zantac 25 EFFERdose Tablets 1624
Zantac 150 EFFERdose Tablets. 1624
Zantac 150 Tablets 1624
Zantac 300 Tablets 1624
Zantac Injection 1619
Zantac Injection Premixed 1619
Zantac Syrup 1624

ULTAK (South Africa)
RANITIDINE HYDROCHLORIDE
Zantac 25 EFFERdose Tablets 1624
Zantac 150 EFFERdose Tablets. 1624
Zantac 150 Tablets 1624
Zantac 300 Tablets 1624
Zantac Injection 1619
Zantac Injection Premixed 1619
Zantac Syrup 1624

ULTICADEX (Greece)
ENALAPRIL MALEATE
Vasotec I.V. Injection 2103

ULTIDIN (Mexico)
FAMOTIDINE
Pepcid Injection 2040
Pepcid Injection Premixed 2040
Pepcid Tablets 2038
Pepcid for Oral Suspension 2038

ULTRA (Belgium)
SULFACETAMIDE SODIUM
Klaron Lotion 10%. 2909

ULTRA CLEARASIL (United Kingdom)
BENZOYL PEROXIDE
Brevoxyl-4 Creamy Wash 3210
Brevoxyl-4 Gel 3210
Brevoxyl-8 Creamy Wash 3210
Brevoxyl-8 Gel 3210
Triaz Cleanser 1892
Triaz Gel 1892

ULTRA HEARTBURN RELIEF (United Kingdom)
FAMOTIDINE
Pepcid Injection 2040
Pepcid Injection Premixed 2040
Pepcid Tablets 2038
Pepcid for Oral Suspension 2038

ULTRABETA (Portugal)
SALMETEROL XINAFOATE
Serevent Diskus 1568

ULTRABIOTIC (Chile)
MUPIROCIN
Bactroban Ointment 1395

ULTRACELE (India)
CELECOXIB
Celebrex Capsules. 3134

ULTRACET (Thailand)
TRAMADOL HYDROCHLORIDE
Ultram ER Tablets 2392

ULTRA-CLEAR-A-MED (Austria)
BENZOYL PEROXIDE
Brevoxyl-4 Creamy Wash. 3210
Brevoxyl-4 Gel 3210
Brevoxyl-8 Creamy Wash. 3210
Brevoxyl-8 Gel 3210
Triaz Cleanser 1892
Triaz Gel 1892

ULTRADERMIS (Argentina)
GENTAMICIN SULFATE
Garamycin Injectable 3014

ULTRAFINA (India)
FINASTERIDE
Propecia Tablets 2060
Proscar Tablets. 2067

ULTRAMICINA (Spain)
CIPROFLOXACIN HYDROCHLORIDE
Ciloxan Ophthalmic Ointment . . . . ⊙204, 559
Ciloxan Ophthalmic Solution . . . . ⊙206
Cipro Tablets 2977

ULTRAMICINA PLUS (Spain)
CIPROFLOXACIN
Cipro Oral Suspension 2977

ULTRAMOP (Canada)
METHOXSALEN
Oxsoralen Lotion 1% 3352
Oxsoralen-Ultra Capsules. 3353

ULTRAMOX (Brazil)
AMOXICILLIN
Amoxil Pediatric Drops for Oral Suspension. 1343
Amoxil Tablets 1343

ULTRANEURAL (Argentina)
GABAPENTIN
Neurontin Capsules 2487

ULTRASE (Brazil, Canada)
PANCRELIPASE
Ultrase Capsules. 708
Ultrase MT Capsules 709

ULTRAVIRAL (Argentina)
LAMIVUDINE
Epivir Oral Solution 1427
Epivir Tablets 1427
Epivir-HBV Oral Solution 1432
Epivir-HBV Tablets 1432

ULTRAVIRAL DUO (Argentina)
LAMIVUDINE
Epivir Oral Solution 1427
Epivir Tablets 1427
Epivir-HBV Oral Solution 1432
Epivir-HBV Tablets 1432

ULTRAZAC (India)
TRAMADOL HYDROCHLORIDE
Ultram ER Tablets 2392

ULTROXIM (Italy)
CEFUROXIME SODIUM
Zinacef Injection 1631

UMAN-SERUM (Italy)
PLASMA PROTEIN FRACTION
Plasmanate 3255

UMAREN (Hungary)
RANITIDINE HYDROCHLORIDE
Zantac 25 EFFERdose Tablets 1624
Zantac 150 EFFERdose Tablets. 1624
Zantac 150 Tablets 1624
Zantac 300 Tablets 1624
Zantac Injection 1619
Zantac Injection Premixed 1619
Zantac Syrup 1624

UMBRIUM (Austria)
DIAZEPAM
Diastat Rectal Delivery System. 3343
Valium Tablets 2819

UMINE (New Zealand, Singapore)
PHENTERMINE HYDROCHLORIDE
Adipex-P Capsules. 1215
Adipex-P Tablets 1215

UNDERACID (Spain)
RANITIDINE HYDROCHLORIDE
Zantac 25 EFFERdose Tablets 1624
Zantac 150 EFFERdose Tablets. 1624
Zantac 150 Tablets 1624
Zantac 300 Tablets 1624
Zantac Injection 1619
Zantac Injection Premixed 1619
Zantac Syrup 1624

UNDERAN (Chile)
MUPIROCIN
Bactroban Ointment. 1395

UNDEX (Switzerland)
CLOTRIMAZOLE
Lotrimin Cream. 3039
Lotrimin Lotion 1%. 3039
Lotrimin Topical Solution 1% 3039

UNI CARBAMAZ (Brazil)
CARBAMAZEPINE
Carbatrol Capsules 3171
Tegretol Chewable Tablets 2295
Tegretol Suspension. 2295
Tegretol Tablets 2295
Tegretol-XR Tablets 2295

UNI DIAZEPAX (Brazil)
DIAZEPAM
Diastat Rectal Delivery System 3343
Valium Tablets 2819

UNI MASDIL (Spain)
DILTIAZEM HYDROCHLORIDE
Cardizem LA Extended Release Tablets. . . 1728
Tiazac Capsules 1201

UNI MIST (Spain)
MORPHINE SULFATE
Kadian Capsules 577
MS Contin Tablets 2701

UNI PROPRALOL (Brazil)
PROPRANOLOL HYDROCHLORIDE
Inderal LA Long-Acting Capsules 3429

UNICLAR (Argentina, Chile, Italy, Mexico, Venezuela)
MOMETASONE FUROATE
Elocon Cream 0.1%. 3005
Elocon Lotion 0.1% 3006
Elocon Ointment 0.1% 3007
Nasonex Nasal Spray 3043

UNICLOPHEN (Czech Republic)
DICLOFENAC SODIUM
Voltaren Tablets 2307
Voltaren-XR Tablets 2310

UNICONTIN (India, Portugal)
THEOPHYLLINE
Uniphyl Tablets 2710

UNICORT (Canada)
HYDROCORTISONE
Hydrocortone Tablets 1989

UNIDERM (Denmark, Finland, Hong Kong, Singapore, Sweden)
HYDROCORTISONE
Hydrocortone Tablets 1989

UNIDET (Canada)
TOLTERODINE TARTRATE
Detrol Tablets. 2628

UNIDIPIN (Austria)
NIFEDIPINE
Adalat CC Tablets 2964

UNIDIPINE (Switzerland)
NIFEDIPINE
Adalat CC Tablets 2964

UNIDROL (India)
METHYLPREDNISOLONE ACETATE
Depo-Medrol Injectable Suspension 2617

UNI-DUR (Czech Republic, Italy, Mexico, South Africa)
THEOPHYLLINE
Uniphyl Tablets 2710

UNIF (Thailand)
TRIAMCINOLONE ACETONIDE
Azmacort Inhalation Aerosol. 1726
Nasacort AQ Nasal Spray 2922

UNIFLOX (Argentina, France)
LEVOFLOXACIN
Levaquin Injection 2384
Levaquin Tablets 2384

UNIFYL (Austria, Switzerland)
THEOPHYLLINE
Uniphyl Tablets 2710

UNIGET (Germany)
TIMOLOL MALEATE
Blocadren Tablets 1916
Timoptic Sterile Ophthalmic Solution 2088
Timoptic in Ocudose 2091
Timoptic-XE Sterile Ophthalmic Gel Forming Solution 2092

UNIGO (Hong Kong)
METRONIDAZOLE
MetroGel-Vaginal Gel 1855

UNIKET (Spain)
ISOSORBIDE MONONITRATE
Imdur Tablets 3018

UNILAIR (Czech Republic, Germany)
THEOPHYLLINE
Uniphyl Tablets 2710

UNILONG (Spain)
THEOPHYLLINE
Uniphyl Tablets 2710

UNIMEZOL (India, Thailand)
METRONIDAZOLE
MetroGel-Vaginal Gel 1855

UNIMOX (South Africa)
AMOXICILLIN
Amoxil Pediatric Drops for Oral Suspension. 1343
Amoxil Tablets 1343

UNIPHYL (Canada, Hong Kong, South Africa)
THEOPHYLLINE
Uniphyl Tablets 2710

UNIPHYLLIN (Germany, Greece)
THEOPHYLLINE
Uniphyl Tablets 2710

UNIPHYLLIN CONTINUS (Irish Republic, United Kingdom)
THEOPHYLLINE
Uniphyl Tablets 2710

UNIPINE XL (United Kingdom)
NIFEDIPINE
Adalat CC Tablets 2964

UNIPRIL (Italy)
RAMIPRIL
Altace Capsules 1702

UNIPRILDIUR (Italy)
RAMIPRIL
Altace Capsules 1702

UNIRELAXED (Mexico)
NAPROXEN
EC-Naprosyn Delayed-Release Tablets. . . . 2761
Naprosyn Suspension. 2761
Naprosyn Tablets 2761

UNIREN (Hong Kong)
DICLOFENAC SODIUM
Voltaren Tablets 2307
Voltaren-XR Tablets 2310

UNISAL (Switzerland)
DIFLUNISAL
Dolobid Tablets. 1955

UNISEDIL (Portugal)
DIAZEPAM
Diastat Rectal Delivery System. 3343
Valium Tablets 2819

UNITIMOFTOL (Spain)
TIMOLOL MALEATE
Blocadren Tablets 1916
Timoptic Sterile Ophthalmic Solution . . . 2088
Timoptic in Ocudose 2091
Timoptic-XE Sterile Ophthalmic Gel Forming Solution 2092

UNIVAL (Chile, Mexico)
LANSOPRAZOLE
Prevacid Delayed-Release Capsules 3271

UNIVATE (Malaysia, Singapore)
CLOBETASOL PROPIONATE
Temovate Cream. 2668
Temovate E Emollient. 2671
Temovate Gel. 2669
Temovate Ointment 2668
Temovate Scalp Application 2670

UNIVER (Spain, United Kingdom)
VERAPAMIL HYDROCHLORIDE
Covera-HS Tablets 3139
Verelan PM Extended-Release Capsules, Controlled-Onset 3106

UNIWARFIN (India)
WARFARIN SODIUM
Coumadin Tablets 898
Coumadin for Injection 898

UNIXAN (Denmark)
THEOPHYLLINE
Uniphyl Tablets 2710

UNIXIME (Italy)
CEFIXIME
Suprax 1843

UNO (Czech Republic)
DICLOFENAC SODIUM
Voltaren Tablets 2307
Voltaren-XR Tablets 2310

UNOCARDIL (Denmark)
DILTIAZEM HYDROCHLORIDE
Cardizem LA Extended Release Tablets. . . 1728

Tiazac Capsules **1201**

UNOPROST (Italy)
TERAZOSIN HYDROCHLORIDE
Hytrin Capsules. **471**

UPHASTATIN (Malaysia)
NYSTATIN
Nystop Topical Powder USP. **2478**
Paddock Nystatin USP for Oral Suspension. **2478**

U-PROXYN (Thailand)
NAPROXEN
EC-Naprosyn Delayed-Release Tablets. . . . **2761**
Naprosyn Suspension. **2761**
Naprosyn Tablets **2761**

URASIN (Thailand)
FUROSEMIDE
Furosemide Tablets **2154**

URASIX (Brazil)
FUROSEMIDE
Furosemide Tablets **2154**

URBAL (Spain)
SUCRALFATE
Carafate Suspension **701**
Carafate Tablets **701**

UREKOLIN (Chile)
NORFLOXACIN
Noroxin Tablets. **2032**

UREMIDE (Australia, South Africa)
FUROSEMIDE
Furosemide Tablets **2154**

UREN (Chile)
HYDROCHLOROTHIAZIDE/TRIAMTERENE
Dyazide Capsules **1423**

URETIC (South Africa)
FUROSEMIDE
Furosemide Tablets **2154**

UREX (Australia, Hong Kong)
FUROSEMIDE
Furosemide Tablets **2154**

URGENDOL (India)
TRAMADOL HYDROCHLORIDE
Ultram ER Tablets **2392**

URGINOL (Argentina)
TOLTERODINE TARTRATE
Detrol Tablets. **2628**

URIBETA (Mexico)
INTERFERON BETA-1B
Betaseron for SC Injection **767**

URIFRON (Mexico)
INTERFERON ALFA-2B
Intron A for Injection. **3024**

URIGON (Greece)
DICLOFENAC SODIUM
Voltaren Tablets **2307**
Voltaren-XR Tablets **2310**

URIMAX (Greece, India)
OFLOXACIN
Floxin Otic Solution **1049**

URIMAX F (India)
TAMSULOSIN HYDROCHLORIDE
Flomax Capsules. **850**

URINOX (Malaysia, Thailand)
NORFLOXACIN
Noroxin Tablets. **2032**

URITOL (Canada)
FUROSEMIDE
Furosemide Tablets **2154**

URITRAT (Brazil)
NORFLOXACIN
Noroxin Tablets. **2032**

URIZIDE (South Africa)
HYDROCHLOROTHIAZIDE/TRIAMTERENE
Dyazide Capsules **1423**

UROBACID (Austria, Greece, Malaysia, Singapore)
NORFLOXACIN
Noroxin Tablets. **2032**

UROCAUDAL (Spain)
TRIAMTERENE
Dyrenium Capsules **3400**

UROCAUDAL TIAZIDA (Spain)
HYDROCHLOROTHIAZIDE/TRIAMTERENE
Dyazide Capsules **1423**

URO-CEPHORAL (Germany)
CEFIXIME
Suprax **1843**

UROCIT-K (Australia, Hong Kong, Malaysia, Singapore)
POTASSIUM CITRATE
Urocit-K Tablets. **2144**

UROCTAL (Hong Kong, Spain)
NORFLOXACIN
Noroxin Tablets. **2032**

URODIE (Italy)
TERAZOSIN HYDROCHLORIDE
Hytrin Capsules. **471**

URODIXIN (Greece)
CIPROFLOXACIN
Cipro Oral Suspension **2977**

UROFIN (Argentina)
FINASTERIDE
Propecia Tablets **2060**
Proscar Tablets. **2067**

UROFLO (Austria)
TERAZOSIN HYDROCHLORIDE
Hytrin Capsules. **471**

UROFLOX (Brazil, Portugal)
NORFLOXACIN
Noroxin Tablets. **2032**

UROFOS (Argentina)
NORFLOXACIN
Noroxin Tablets. **2032**

UROKIT (Argentina)
POTASSIUM CITRATE
Urocit-K Tablets. **2144**

URO-LINFOL (Argentina)
NORFLOXACIN
Noroxin Tablets. **2032**

UROLOSIN (Spain)
TAMSULOSIN HYDROCHLORIDE
Flomax Capsules. **850**

UROMETRON (South Africa)
METRONIDAZOLE
MetroGel-Vaginal Gel **1855**

UROMYKOL (Germany)
CLOTRIMAZOLE
Lotrimin Cream. **3039**
Lotrimin Lotion 1%. **3039**
Lotrimin Topical Solution 1% **3039**

URONEFREX (Belgium, France, Spain)
ACETOHYDROXAMIC ACID
Lithostat Tablets **2140**

URONOVAG (Argentina)
NORFLOXACIN
Noroxin Tablets. **2032**

UROPLEX (Brazil)
NORFLOXACIN
Noroxin Tablets. **2032**

UROSEPTAL (Argentina, Brazil)
NORFLOXACIN
Noroxin Tablets. **2032**

UROSPES-N (Greece)
NORFLOXACIN
Noroxin Tablets. **2032**

URO-TARIVID (Germany, Israel)
OFLOXACIN
Floxin Otic Solution **1049**

UROTEM (Argentina)
NORFLOXACIN
Noroxin Tablets. **2032**

UROTRICEF (Chile)
CEFIXIME
Suprax **1843**

UROTROL (Spain)
TOLTERODINE TARTRATE
Detrol Tablets. **2628**

UROXACIN (Argentina)
NORFLOXACIN
Noroxin Tablets. **2032**

UROXAZOL-N (Brazil)
NORFLOXACIN
Noroxin Tablets. **2032**

UROXIN (Hong Kong, Singapore, Thailand, United Arab Emirates)
CIPROFLOXACIN HYDROCHLORIDE
Ciloxan Ophthalmic Ointment . . . . ⊙**204, 559**
Ciloxan Ophthalmic Solution . . . . ⊙**206**
Cipro Tablets **2977**

URPROSAN (Spain)
FINASTERIDE
Propecia Tablets **2060**
Proscar Tablets. **2067**

UTAC (Thailand)
RANITIDINE HYDROCHLORIDE
Zantac 25 EFFERdose Tablets **1624**
Zantac 150 EFFERdose Tablets. **1624**
Zantac 150 Tablets **1624**
Zantac 300 Tablets **1624**
Zantac Injection **1619**
Zantac Injection Premixed **1619**
Zantac Syrup **1624**

UTAHZONE (Hong Kong)
CIPROFLOXACIN HYDROCHLORIDE
Ciloxan Ophthalmic Ointment . . . . ⊙**204, 559**
Ciloxan Ophthalmic Solution . . . . ⊙**206**
Cipro Tablets **2977**

UTICINA (Italy)
NORFLOXACIN
Noroxin Tablets. **2032**

UTIN (South Africa)
NORFLOXACIN
Noroxin Tablets. **2032**

UTINOR (Italy, United Kingdom)
NORFLOXACIN
Noroxin Tablets. **2032**

UTORAL (Brazil)
FLUOROURACIL
Efudex Topical Cream. **3363**
Efudex Topical Solutions **3363**

UTROGESTAN (Argentina, Austria, Belgium, Brazil, Czech Republic, France, Greece, Hong Kong, Hungary, Irish Republic, Israel, Malaysia, Mexico, Portugal, Russia, Singapore, South Africa, Spain, Switzerland, Thailand)
PROGESTERONE
Prometrium Capsules (100 mg, 200 mg) . **3203**

UV IX (Mexico)
CIPROFLOXACIN
Cipro Oral Suspension **2977**

V DAY ZEPAM (Thailand)
DIAZEPAM
Diastat Rectal Delivery System **3343**
Valium Tablets **2819**

VACINOLONE (Thailand)
TRIAMCINOLONE ACETONIDE
Azmacort Inhalation Aerosol. **1726**
Nasacort AQ Nasal Spray **2922**

VADINAR (Mexico)
DIPYRIDAMOLE
Persantine Tablets **868**

VADITON (Spain)
FLUVASTATIN SODIUM
Lescol Capsules **2233**

VAGIFEM (Australia, Austria, Belgium, Canada, Chile, Czech Republic, Denmark, Finland, Germany, Greece, Hungary, Irish Republic, Israel, Italy, New Zealand, Norway, Portugal, Singapore, South Africa, Spain, Sweden, Switzerland, Thailand, The Netherlands, United Kingdom)
ESTRADIOL
Climara Transdermal System **771**
Estring Vaginal Ring. **2635**

VAGIL (Thailand)
METRONIDAZOLE
MetroGel-Vaginal Gel **1855**

VAGILEN (Italy)
METRONIDAZOLE
MetroGel-Vaginal Gel **1855**

VAGIMAX (Brazil)
METRONIDAZOLE
MetroGel-Vaginal Gel **1855**

VAGIMID (Germany)
METRONIDAZOLE
MetroGel-Vaginal Gel **1855**

VAGINYL (United Kingdom)
METRONIDAZOLE
MetroGel-Vaginal Gel **1855**

VAGISIL (United Kingdom)
LIDOCAINE
Lidoderm Patch **1118**

VAGOSTAL (Spain)
FAMOTIDINE
Pepcid Injection **2040**
Pepcid Injection Premixed **2040**
Pepcid Tablets **2038**
Pepcid for Oral Suspension **2038**

VAGRAN (Venezuela)
VANCOMYCIN HYDROCHLORIDE
Vancocin HCl Capsules, USP **3380**

VAGYL (Thailand)
METRONIDAZOLE
MetroGel-Vaginal Gel **1855**

VALAPLEX (Chile)
VALSARTAN
Diovan Tablets **2193**

VALAPLEX-D (Chile)
VALSARTAN
Diovan Tablets **2193**

VALAXONA (Denmark, Germany)
DIAZEPAM
Diastat Rectal Delivery System **3343**
Valium Tablets **2819**

VALCAPS (Mexico)
VALPROIC ACID
Depakene Capsules **417**
Depakene Oral Solution. **417**

VALCLAIR (United Kingdom)
DIAZEPAM
Diastat Rectal Delivery System **3343**
Valium Tablets **2819**

VALCOTE (Argentina)
VALPROIC ACID
Depakene Capsules **417**
Depakene Oral Solution. **417**

VALDERMA ACTIVE (United Kingdom)
BENZOYL PEROXIDE
Brevoxyl-4 Creamy Wash. **3210**
Brevoxyl-4 Gel **3210**
Brevoxyl-8 Creamy Wash. **3210**
Brevoxyl-8 Gel **3210**
Triaz Cleanser **1892**
Triaz Gel **1892**

VALENAC (United Kingdom)
DICLOFENAC SODIUM
Voltaren Tablets **2307**
Voltaren-XR Tablets **2310**

VALENIUM (Thailand)
DIAZEPAM
Diastat Rectal Delivery System **3343**
Valium Tablets **2819**

VALIQUID (Germany)
DIAZEPAM
Diastat Rectal Delivery System **3343**
Valium Tablets **2819**

VALITRAN (Italy)
DIAZEPAM
Diastat Rectal Delivery System **3343**
Valium Tablets **2819**

VALIUM (Argentina, Australia, Austria, Belgium, Brazil, Canada, Denmark, France, Germany, India, Irish Republic, Israel, Italy, Mexico, Norway, Portugal, Singapore, South Africa, Spain, Sweden, Switzerland, Thailand, The Netherlands, United Kingdom, Venezuela)
DIAZEPAM
Diastat Rectal Delivery System **3343**
Valium Tablets **2819**

VALIX (Brazil)
DIAZEPAM
Diastat Rectal Delivery System **3343**
Valium Tablets **2819**

VALKEN (Mexico)
VALPROIC ACID
Depakene Capsules **417**
Depakene Oral Solution. **417**

VALMETOL-3 (Mexico)
CALCITRIOL
Calcijex Injection **411**
Rocaltrol Capsules. **2798**

Rocaltrol Oral Solution **2798**

VALOCORDIN-DIAZEPAM (Germany)
DIAZEPAM
Diastat Rectal Delivery System **3343**
Valium Tablets **2819**

VALOXIN (Brazil)
DIGOXIN
Lanoxicaps Capsules **1490**
Lanoxin Injection **1494**
Lanoxin Injection Pediatric **1497**
Lanoxin Tablets **1500**

VALPAM (Australia)
DIAZEPAM
Diastat Rectal Delivery System **3343**
Valium Tablets **2819**

VALPAX (Chile)
CLONAZEPAM
Klonopin Tablets **2778**

VALPEX (Argentina)
DONEPEZIL HYDROCHLORIDE
Aricept Tablets **1094**

VALPRESSION (Italy)
VALSARTAN
Diovan Tablets **2193**

VALPROLIM (Portugal)
VALPROIC ACID
Depakene Capsules **417**
Depakene Oral Solution **417**

VALPRON (Venezuela)
VALPROIC ACID
Depakene Capsules **417**
Depakene Oral Solution **417**

VALROX (United Kingdom)
NAPROXEN
EC-Naprosyn Delayed-Release Tablets **2761**
Naprosyn Suspension **2761**
Naprosyn Tablets **2761**

VALS (Spain)
VALSARTAN
Diovan Tablets **2193**

VALSARTAN/HCTZ (Austria)
VALSARTAN
Diovan Tablets **2193**

VAMAZOLE (Thailand)
CLOTRIMAZOLE
Lotrimin Cream **3039**
Lotrimin Lotion 1% **3039**
Lotrimin Topical Solution 1% **3039**

VAMISTOL (Greece)
VANCOMYCIN HYDROCHLORIDE
Vancocin HCl Capsules, USP **3380**

VANAURUS (Mexico)
VANCOMYCIN HYDROCHLORIDE
Vancocin HCl Capsules, USP **3380**

VANCAM (Mexico)
VANCOMYCIN HYDROCHLORIDE
Vancocin HCl Capsules, USP **3380**

VANCLOMIN (Brazil)
VANCOMYCIN HYDROCHLORIDE
Vancocin HCl Capsules, USP **3380**

VANCO (Germany, Italy)
VANCOMYCIN HYDROCHLORIDE
Vancocin HCl Capsules, USP **3380**

VANCOABBOTT (Brazil)
VANCOMYCIN HYDROCHLORIDE
Vancocin HCl Capsules, USP **3380**

VANCOBEHR (Venezuela)
VANCOMYCIN HYDROCHLORIDE
Vancocin HCl Capsules, USP **3380**

VANCOCID (Brazil)
VANCOMYCIN HYDROCHLORIDE
Vancocin HCl Capsules, USP **3380**

VANCOCIN (Argentina, Australia, Belgium, Canada, Czech Republic, Denmark, Finland, Hong Kong, Hungary, India, Irish Republic, Israel, Malaysia, Mexico, New Zealand, Norway, South Africa, Sweden, Switzerland, Thailand, The Netherlands, United Kingdom)
VANCOMYCIN HYDROCHLORIDE
Vancocin HCl Capsules, USP **3380**

VANCOCINA (Chile, Italy, Portugal)
VANCOMYCIN HYDROCHLORIDE
Vancocin HCl Capsules, USP **3380**

VANCOCINE (France)
VANCOMYCIN HYDROCHLORIDE
Vancocin HCl Capsules, USP **3380**

VANCOLED (Australia, Czech Republic, Israel, Sweden, Switzerland)
VANCOMYCIN HYDROCHLORIDE
Vancocin HCl Capsules, USP **3380**

VANCOLON (United Arab Emirates)
VANCOMYCIN HYDROCHLORIDE
Vancocin HCl Capsules, USP **3380**

VANCOPLUS (Brazil)
VANCOMYCIN HYDROCHLORIDE
Vancocin HCl Capsules, USP **3380**

VANCO-SAAR (Germany)
VANCOMYCIN HYDROCHLORIDE
Vancocin HCl Capsules, USP **3380**

VANCOSCAND (Sweden)
VANCOMYCIN HYDROCHLORIDE
Vancocin HCl Capsules, USP **3380**

VANCOSON (Brazil)
VANCOMYCIN HYDROCHLORIDE
Vancocin HCl Capsules, USP **3380**

VANCOTENK (Argentina)
VANCOMYCIN HYDROCHLORIDE
Vancocin HCl Capsules, USP **3380**

VANCO-TEVA (Hong Kong, Israel)
VANCOMYCIN HYDROCHLORIDE
Vancocin HCl Capsules, USP **3380**

VANCOTEX (Italy)
VANCOMYCIN HYDROCHLORIDE
Vancocin HCl Capsules, USP **3380**

VANCOX (Mexico)
VANCOMYCIN HYDROCHLORIDE
Vancocin HCl Capsules, USP **3380**

VANDRAL (Spain)
VENLAFAXINE HYDROCHLORIDE
Effexor Tablets **3411**
Effexor XR Capsules **3417**

VANESTEN (Singapore, Thailand)
CLOTRIMAZOLE
Lotrimin Cream **3039**
Lotrimin Lotion 1% **3039**
Lotrimin Topical Solution 1% **3039**

VANESTRIN-V (Mexico)
METRONIDAZOLE
MetroGel-Vaginal Gel **1855**

VANMICINA (Mexico)
VANCOMYCIN HYDROCHLORIDE
Vancocin HCl Capsules, USP **3380**

VANTICON (Argentina)
ZAFIRLUKAST
Accolate Tablets **671**

VANTIN (Mexico)
NAPROXEN
EC-Naprosyn Delayed-Release Tablets **2761**
Naprosyn Suspension **2761**
Naprosyn Tablets **2761**

VANZOR (Mexico)
DIAZEPAM
Diastat Rectal Delivery System **3343**
Valium Tablets **2819**

VAPRESAN (Argentina)
ENALAPRIL MALEATE
Vasotec I.V. Injection **2103**

VARAXIL (Mexico)
CAPTOPRIL
Captopril Tablets **2149**

VARFINE (Portugal)
WARFARIN SODIUM
Coumadin Tablets **898**
Coumadin for Injection **898**

VARTALAN (Chile)
VALSARTAN
Diovan Tablets **2193**

VARTALAN D (Chile)
HYDROCHLOROTHIAZIDE/VALSARTAN
Diovan HCT Tablets **2196**

VARTELON (Hong Kong)
DICLOFENAC SODIUM
Voltaren Tablets **2307**
Voltaren-XR Tablets **2310**

VASAD (United Kingdom)
NIFEDIPINE
Adalat CC Tablets **2964**

VASCAL (Germany)
ISRADIPINE
DynaCirc CR Tablets **2721**

VASCARD (South Africa)
NIFEDIPINE
Adalat CC Tablets **2964**

VASCOR (Malaysia, Singapore, Thailand)
SIMVASTATIN
Zocor Tablets **2105**

VASCORD (Brazil)
VERAPAMIL HYDROCHLORIDE
Covera-HS Tablets **3139**
Verelan PM Extended-Release Capsules, Controlled-Onset **3106**

VASCORIM (Portugal)
SIMVASTATIN
Zocor Tablets **2105**

VASDALAT (Singapore)
NIFEDIPINE
Adalat CC Tablets **2964**

VASDILAT (Italy)
ISOSORBIDE MONONITRATE
Imdur Tablets **3018**

VASETIC (United Kingdom)
AMILORIDE HYDROCHLORIDE/HYDROCHLOROTHIAZIDE
Moduretic Tablets **2028**

VASILIP (Czech Republic, Russia)
SIMVASTATIN
Zocor Tablets **2105**

VASLAN (Spain)
ISRADIPINE
DynaCirc CR Tablets **2721**

VASLIP (Brazil)
SIMVASTATIN
Zocor Tablets **2105**

VASOCARDIN (Czech Republic)
METOPROLOL TARTRATE
Lopressor Tablets **2238**

VASOCARDOL (Australia)
DILTIAZEM HYDROCHLORIDE
Cardizem LA Extended Release Tablets . . . **1728**
Tiazac Capsules **1201**

VASOCON (Canada)
NAPHAZOLINE HYDROCHLORIDE
Albalon Ophthalmic Solution . . . . ⊙**218**

VASOCONSTRICTOR PENSA (Spain)
NAPHAZOLINE HYDROCHLORIDE
Albalon Ophthalmic Solution . . . . ⊙**218**

VASOCOR (Switzerland)
ENALAPRIL MALEATE
Vasotec I.V. Injection **2103**

VASODIPINA (Brazil)
NIMODIPINE
Nimotop Capsules **749**

VASOFED (Irish Republic, South Africa)
NIFEDIPINE
Adalat CC Tablets **2964**

VASOFLEX (Chile)
NIMODIPINE
Nimotop Capsules **749**

VASOGARD (Brazil)
CILOSTAZOL
Pletal Tablets **2455**

VASOJET (Brazil)
LISINOPRIL
Prinivil Tablets **2052**

VASOLAN (Japan)
VERAPAMIL HYDROCHLORIDE
Covera-HS Tablets **3139**
Verelan PM Extended-Release Capsules, Controlled-Onset **3106**

VASOLAT (Chile)
ENALAPRIL MALEATE
Vasotec I.V. Injection **2103**

VASOMED (Chile)
SIMVASTATIN
Zocor Tablets **2105**

VASOMIL (South Africa)
VERAPAMIL HYDROCHLORIDE
Covera-HS Tablets **3139**
Verelan PM Extended-Release Capsules, Controlled-Onset **3106**

VASOPRIL (Brazil)
ENALAPRIL MALEATE
Vasotec I.V. Injection **2103**

VASOPRIL PLUS (Brazil)
ENALAPRIL MALEATE
Vasotec I.V. Injection **2103**

VASOPTEN (Thailand)
VERAPAMIL HYDROCHLORIDE
Covera-HS Tablets **3139**
Verelan PM Extended-Release Capsules, Controlled-Onset **3106**

VASOTENAL (Argentina, Chile, Venezuela)
SIMVASTATIN
Zocor Tablets **2105**

VASOTOP (India)
NIMODIPINE
Nimotop Capsules **749**

VASTATIL (Brazil)
SIMVASTATIN
Zocor Tablets **2105**

VASTATIN (Greece)
SIMVASTATIN
Zocor Tablets **2105**

VASTIN (Australia, New Zealand)
FLUVASTATIN SODIUM
Lescol Capsules **2233**

VASTRIPINE (Greece)
NIMODIPINE
Nimotop Capsules **749**

VASTUS (Argentina, Chile)
ALBENDAZOLE
Albenza Tablets **1338**

VASYROL (United Kingdom)
DIPYRIDAMOLE
Persantine Tablets **868**

VATRAN (Italy)
DIAZEPAM
Diastat Rectal Delivery System **3343**
Valium Tablets **2819**

VATRIX-S (Mexico)
METRONIDAZOLE
MetroGel-Vaginal Gel **1855**

VECLAM (Italy)
CLARITHROMYCIN
Biaxin Filmtab Tablets **402**
Biaxin Granules **402**

VEENAC (Thailand)
DICLOFENAC SODIUM
Voltaren Tablets **2307**
Voltaren-XR Tablets **2310**

VEFRON (Greece)
ONDANSETRON
Zofran ODT Orally Disintegrating Tablets . . **1639**

VEKFAZOLIN (Greece)
CEFUROXIME SODIUM
Zinacef Injection **1631**

VELAMOX (Brazil)
AMOXICILLIN
Amoxil Pediatric Drops for Oral Suspension **1343**
Amoxil Tablets **1343**

VELARIL (Venezuela)
CLONIDINE
Catapres-TTS **844**

VELDROL (Mexico)
TRAMADOL HYDROCHLORIDE
Ultram ER Tablets **2392**

VELKALOV (Greece)
LOVASTATIN
Mevacor Tablets **2021**

VELMONIT (Spain)
CIPROFLOXACIN HYDROCHLORIDE
Ciloxan Ophthalmic Ointment . . . . ⊙**204, 559**

(⊙ Described in PDR For Ophthalmic Medicines™)

Ciloxan Ophthalmic Solution ⊙206
Cipro Tablets 2977

VELPRO (Mexico)
BENZONATATE
Tessalon Perles 1199

VELSAY (Mexico)
NAPROXEN
EC-Naprosyn Delayed-Release Tablets 2761
Naprosyn Suspension 2761
Naprosyn Tablets 2761

VELSAY-S COMPUESTO (Mexico)
NAPROXEN
EC-Naprosyn Delayed-Release Tablets 2761
Naprosyn Suspension 2761
Naprosyn Tablets 2761

VELTEX (South Africa)
DICLOFENAC SODIUM
Voltaren Tablets 2307
Voltaren-XR Tablets 2310

VELTION (Greece)
MUPIROCIN
Bactroban Ointment 1395

VEMIZOL (Malaysia)
ALBENDAZOLE
Albenza Tablets 1338

VENDAZOL (Venezuela)
ALBENDAZOLE
Albenza Tablets 1338

VENDREX (Brazil)
DICLOFENAC SODIUM
Voltaren Tablets 2307
Voltaren-XR Tablets 2310

VENLA (Israel)
VENLAFAXINE HYDROCHLORIDE
Effexor Tablets 3411
Effexor XR Capsules 3417

VENLIFT (Brazil)
VENLAFAXINE HYDROCHLORIDE
Effexor Tablets 3411
Effexor XR Capsules 3417

VENLOR (India)
VENLAFAXINE HYDROCHLORIDE
Effexor Tablets 3411
Effexor XR Capsules 3417

VENOGYL (Israel)
METRONIDAZOLE
MetroGel-Vaginal Gel 1855

VENOPRIL (Brazil)
CAPTOPRIL
Captopril Tablets 2149

VENT RETARD (Spain)
THEOPHYLLINE
Uniphyl Tablets 2710

VENTER (Czech Republic, Hungary, Russia)
SUCRALFATE
Carafate Suspension 701
Carafate Tablets 701

VENTOFLU (Italy)
FLUNISOLIDE
Aerobid Inhaler System 1171
Aerobid-M Inhaler System 1171

VERABETA (Germany)
VERAPAMIL HYDROCHLORIDE
Covera-HS Tablets 3139
Verelan PM Extended-Release Capsules, Controlled-Onset 3106

VERACAPS (Australia)
VERAPAMIL HYDROCHLORIDE
Covera-HS Tablets 3139
Verelan PM Extended-Release Capsules, Controlled-Onset 3106

VERACIM (Switzerland)
VERAPAMIL HYDROCHLORIDE
Covera-HS Tablets 3139
Verelan PM Extended-Release Capsules, Controlled-Onset 3106

VERACOL (Greece)
CEFTRIAXONE SODIUM
Rocephin Injectable Vials, ADD-Vantage, Galaxy, Bulk 2800

VERACOR (Israel, Venezuela)
VERAPAMIL HYDROCHLORIDE
Covera-HS Tablets 3139
Verelan PM Extended-Release Capsules, Controlled-Onset 3106

VERACORON (Brazil)
VERAPAMIL HYDROCHLORIDE
Covera-HS Tablets 3139
Verelan PM Extended-Release Capsules, Controlled-Onset 3106

VERADAY (Austria)
VERAPAMIL HYDROCHLORIDE
Covera-HS Tablets 3139
Verelan PM Extended-Release Capsules, Controlled-Onset 3106

VERADIL (Australia)
VERAPAMIL HYDROCHLORIDE
Covera-HS Tablets 3139
Verelan PM Extended-Release Capsules, Controlled-Onset 3106

VERADOL (Argentina)
NAPROXEN
EC-Naprosyn Delayed-Release Tablets 2761
Naprosyn Suspension 2761
Naprosyn Tablets 2761

VERADURAT (Germany)
VERAPAMIL HYDROCHLORIDE
Covera-HS Tablets 3139
Verelan PM Extended-Release Capsules, Controlled-Onset 3106

VERAGAMMA (Germany)
VERAPAMIL HYDROCHLORIDE
Covera-HS Tablets 3139
Verelan PM Extended-Release Capsules, Controlled-Onset 3106

VERAHEXAL (Australia, Czech Republic, Germany, South Africa)
VERAPAMIL HYDROCHLORIDE
Covera-HS Tablets 3139
Verelan PM Extended-Release Capsules, Controlled-Onset 3106

VERAKARD (Norway)
VERAPAMIL HYDROCHLORIDE
Covera-HS Tablets 3139
Verelan PM Extended-Release Capsules, Controlled-Onset 3106

VERAL (Argentina, Czech Republic, Hungary)
VERAPAMIL HYDROCHLORIDE
Covera-HS Tablets 3139
Verelan PM Extended-Release Capsules, Controlled-Onset 3106

VERALAN (Mexico)
VERAPAMIL HYDROCHLORIDE
Covera-HS Tablets 3139
Verelan PM Extended-Release Capsules, Controlled-Onset 3106

VERA-LICH (Germany)
VERAPAMIL HYDROCHLORIDE
Covera-HS Tablets 3139
Verelan PM Extended-Release Capsules, Controlled-Onset 3106

VERALOC (Denmark, Sweden)
VERAPAMIL HYDROCHLORIDE
Covera-HS Tablets 3139
Verelan PM Extended-Release Capsules, Controlled-Onset 3106

VERAMEX (Germany)
VERAPAMIL HYDROCHLORIDE
Covera-HS Tablets 3139
Verelan PM Extended-Release Capsules, Controlled-Onset 3106

VERAMIL (Brazil, Irish Republic)
VERAPAMIL HYDROCHLORIDE
Covera-HS Tablets 3139
Verelan PM Extended-Release Capsules, Controlled-Onset 3106

VERANORM (Germany)
VERAPAMIL HYDROCHLORIDE
Covera-HS Tablets 3139
Verelan PM Extended-Release Capsules, Controlled-Onset 3106

VERANZOL (Mexico)
ALBENDAZOLE
Albenza Tablets 1338

VERAP (Irish Republic)
VERAPAMIL HYDROCHLORIDE
Covera-HS Tablets 3139
Verelan PM Extended-Release Capsules, Controlled-Onset 3106

VERAPABENE (Austria)
VERAPAMIL HYDROCHLORIDE
Covera-HS Tablets 3139
Verelan PM Extended-Release Capsules, Controlled-Onset 3106

VERAPAL (Argentina)
VERAPAMIL HYDROCHLORIDE
Covera-HS Tablets 3139
Verelan PM Extended-Release Capsules, Controlled-Onset 3106

VERAPAM (Switzerland)
VERAPAMIL HYDROCHLORIDE
Covera-HS Tablets 3139
Verelan PM Extended-Release Capsules, Controlled-Onset 3106

VERAPIN (Thailand)
VERAPAMIL HYDROCHLORIDE
Covera-HS Tablets 3139
Verelan PM Extended-Release Capsules, Controlled-Onset 3106

VERAPLEX (Argentina, Malaysia, Russia)
MEDROXYPROGESTERONE ACETATE
Depo-Medrol Single-Dose Vial 2619

VERAPRESS (Israel, United Kingdom)
VERAPAMIL HYDROCHLORIDE
Covera-HS Tablets 3139
Verelan PM Extended-Release Capsules, Controlled-Onset 3106

VERAPTIN (Italy, Switzerland)
VERAPAMIL HYDROCHLORIDE
Covera-HS Tablets 3139
Verelan PM Extended-Release Capsules, Controlled-Onset 3106

VERASAL (Germany)
VERAPAMIL HYDROCHLORIDE
Covera-HS Tablets 3139
Verelan PM Extended-Release Capsules, Controlled-Onset 3106

VERASIFAR (Switzerland)
VERAPAMIL HYDROCHLORIDE
Covera-HS Tablets 3139
Verelan PM Extended-Release Capsules, Controlled-Onset 3106

VERASPIR (Portugal)
SALMETEROL XINAFOATE
Serevent Diskus 1568

VERASTAD (Austria)
VERAPAMIL HYDROCHLORIDE
Covera-HS Tablets 3139
Verelan PM Extended-Release Capsules, Controlled-Onset 3106

VERATEN (Argentina)
CARVEDILOL
Coreg Tablets 1414

VERATENSIN (Spain)
VERAPAMIL HYDROCHLORIDE
Covera-HS Tablets 3139
Verelan PM Extended-Release Capsules, Controlled-Onset 3106

VERATYROL (Austria)
VERAPAMIL HYDROCHLORIDE
Covera-HS Tablets 3139
Verelan PM Extended-Release Capsules, Controlled-Onset 3106

VERAVAL (Brazil)
VERAPAMIL HYDROCHLORIDE
Covera-HS Tablets 3139
Verelan PM Extended-Release Capsules, Controlled-Onset 3106

VERCOL (Greece)
LISINOPRIL
Prinivil Tablets 2052

VERDAZOL (Brazil)
ALBENDAZOLE
Albenza Tablets 1338

VERELAIT (Italy)
LACTULOSE
Kristalose for Oral Solution 1034

VERELAN (Canada, Irish Republic)
VERAPAMIL HYDROCHLORIDE
Covera-HS Tablets 3139
Verelan PM Extended-Release Capsules, Controlled-Onset 3106

VEREXAMIL (Austria)
VERAPAMIL HYDROCHLORIDE
Covera-HS Tablets 3139
Verelan PM Extended-Release Capsules, Controlled-Onset 3106

VERIDERM MEDROL (France)
METHYLPREDNISOLONE ACETATE
Depo-Medrol Injectable Suspension 2617

VERISOP (Irish Republic)
VERAPAMIL HYDROCHLORIDE
Covera-HS Tablets 3139
Verelan PM Extended-Release Capsules, Controlled-Onset 3106

VERLOST (Greece)
RANITIDINE HYDROCHLORIDE
Zantac 25 EFFERdose Tablets 1624
Zantac 150 EFFERdose Tablets 1624
Zantac 150 Tablets 1624
Zantac 300 Tablets 1624
Zantac Injection 1619
Zantac Injection Premixed 1619
Zantac Syrup 1624

VERMECTIL (Brazil)
IVERMECTIN
Stromectol Tablets 2083

VERMICLASE (Brazil)
ALBENDAZOLE
Albenza Tablets 1338

VERMILAN (Mexico)
ALBENDAZOLE
Albenza Tablets 1338

VERMIN (Finland)
VERAPAMIL HYDROCHLORIDE
Covera-HS Tablets 3139
Verelan PM Extended-Release Capsules, Controlled-Onset 3106

VERMIN PLUS (Mexico)
ALBENDAZOLE
Albenza Tablets 1338

VERMINE (Thailand)
VERAPAMIL HYDROCHLORIDE
Covera-HS Tablets 3139
Verelan PM Extended-Release Capsules, Controlled-Onset 3106

VERMISEN (Mexico)
ALBENDAZOLE
Albenza Tablets 1338

VERMITAL (Brazil)
ALBENDAZOLE
Albenza Tablets 1338

VERMIXIDE (Thailand)
ALBENDAZOLE
Albenza Tablets 1338

VERMOIL (Chile)
ALBENDAZOLE
Albenza Tablets 1338

VERNTHOL (South Africa)
THEOPHYLLINE
Uniphyl Tablets 2710

VEROGALID (Hungary, Russia)
VERAPAMIL HYDROCHLORIDE
Covera-HS Tablets 3139
Verelan PM Extended-Release Capsules, Controlled-Onset 3106

VEROPTINSTADA (Germany)
VERAPAMIL HYDROCHLORIDE
Covera-HS Tablets 3139
Verelan PM Extended-Release Capsules, Controlled-Onset 3106

VEROXIL (Greece, Italy)
LISINOPRIL
Prinivil Tablets 2052

VERPACOR (Finland)
VERAPAMIL HYDROCHLORIDE
Covera-HS Tablets 3139
Verelan PM Extended-Release Capsules, Controlled-Onset 3106

VERPAMIL (Finland, Malaysia, New Zealand, Singapore, South Africa)
VERAPAMIL HYDROCHLORIDE
Covera-HS Tablets 3139
Verelan PM Extended-Release Capsules, Controlled-Onset 3106

VERRUMAL (Portugal)
FLUOROURACIL
Efudex Topical Cream 3363
Efudex Topical Solutions 3363

VERTAB (United Kingdom)
VERAPAMIL HYDROCHLORIDE
Covera-HS Tablets 3139

(⊙ Described in PDR For Ophthalmic Medicines™)

Verelan PM Extended-Release Capsules, Controlled-Onset 3106

VERYTRACIN (Mexico)
ERYTHROMYCIN
Ery-Tab Tablets 449
Erythromycin Base Filmtab Tablets 455
Erythromycin Delayed-Release Capsules, USP 457
PCE Dispertab Tablets 515

VESALION FLEX (Argentina)
DICLOFENAC SODIUM
Voltaren Tablets 2307
Voltaren-XR Tablets 2310

VESANOID (Argentina, Australia, Austria, Belgium, Brazil, Canada, Chile, Czech Republic, Finland, France, Germany, Greece, Hong Kong, Hungary, Irish Republic, Israel, Italy, Mexico, New Zealand, Norway, Portugal, Singapore, South Africa, Spain, Sweden, Switzerland, Thailand, The Netherlands, United Kingdom, Venezuela)
TRETINOIN
Vesanoid Capsules 2820

VESDIL (Switzerland)
RAMIPRIL
Altace Capsules 1702

VESIX (Finland, The Netherlands)
FUROSEMIDE
Furosemide Tablets 2154

VESTACLAV (Malaysia)
AMOXICILLIN
Amoxil Pediatric Drops for Oral Suspension 1343
Amoxil Tablets 1343

VETAMOL (Greece)
NORFLOXACIN
Noroxin Tablets 2032

VETANSIL (Brazil)
DIAZEPAM
Diastat Rectal Delivery System 3343
Valium Tablets 2819

VETIPROST (Argentina)
FINASTERIDE
Propecia Tablets 2060
Proscar Tablets 2067

VEXURAT (Greece)
FAMOTIDINE
Pepcid Injection 2040
Pepcid Injection Premixed 2040
Pepcid Tablets 2038
Pepcid for Oral Suspension 2038

VIAFUROX (Argentina)
FUROSEMIDE
Furosemide Tablets 2154

VIAGRA (Argentina, Australia, Austria, Belgium, Brazil, Canada, Chile, Czech Republic, Denmark, Finland, France, Germany, Greece, Hong Kong, Hungary, Irish Republic, Israel, Italy, Japan, Malaysia, Mexico, New Zealand, Norway, Portugal, Russia, Singapore, South Africa, Spain, Sweden, Switzerland, Thailand, United Kingdom, Venezuela)
SILDENAFIL CITRATE
Viagra Tablets 2573

VIARTRIL NF (Argentina)
DICLOFENAC SODIUM
Voltaren Tablets 2307
Voltaren-XR Tablets 2310

VIATOPIN (Hungary)
TOPOTECAN HYDROCHLORIDE
Hycamtin for Injection 1458

VIAVOX (Venezuela)
DICLOFENAC SODIUM
Voltaren Tablets 2307
Voltaren-XR Tablets 2310

VIAZEM (Denmark, Sweden, United Kingdom)
DILTIAZEM HYDROCHLORIDE
Cardizem LA Extended Release Tablets 1728
Tiazac Capsules 1201

VIBUZOL (Argentina)
RIBAVIRIN
Virazole for Inhalation Solution 3370

VICARD (Austria, Switzerland)
TERAZOSIN HYDROCHLORIDE
Hytrin Capsules 471

VICK-ZYRT (Hong Kong)
CETIRIZINE HYDROCHLORIDE
Zyrtec Syrup 2594
Zyrtec Tablets 2594

VI-CLARO (Chile)
NAPHAZOLINE HYDROCHLORIDE
Albalon Ophthalmic Solution ⊙218

VICNAS (Spain)
NORFLOXACIN
Noroxin Tablets 2032

VICORTIN (Mexico)
HYDROCORTISONE
Hydrocortone Tablets 1989

VIDA FAMODINE (Hong Kong)
FAMOTIDINE
Pepcid Injection 2040
Pepcid Injection Premixed 2040
Pepcid Tablets 2038
Pepcid for Oral Suspension 2038

VIDALAT (Hong Kong)
NIFEDIPINE
Adalat CC Tablets 2964

VIDAPRIL (Portugal)
CAPTOPRIL
Captopril Tablets 2149

VIDOX (Argentina)
MUPIROCIN
Bactroban Ointment 1395

VIEPAX (Israel)
VENLAFAXINE HYDROCHLORIDE
Effexor Tablets 3411
Effexor XR Capsules 3417

VIFLOXINA (Mexico)
CIPROFLOXACIN
Cipro Oral Suspension 2977

VIGICER (Argentina)
MODAFINIL
Provigil Tablets 988

VIGIL (Czech Republic, Germany)
MODAFINIL
Provigil Tablets 988

VIKING (Greece)
LOVASTATIN
Mevacor Tablets 2021

VIKROL (Mexico)
CLARITHROMYCIN
Biaxin Filmtab Tablets 402
Biaxin Granules 402

VILACRIL (Greece)
DICLOFENAC SODIUM
Voltaren Tablets 2307
Voltaren-XR Tablets 2310

VILADIL (Thailand)
TICLOPIDINE HYDROCHLORIDE
Ticlid Tablets 2810

VILONA (Mexico)
RIBAVIRIN
Virazole for Inhalation Solution 3370

VILONIT (Greece)
DICLOFENAC SODIUM
Voltaren Tablets 2307
Voltaren-XR Tablets 2310

VIMAX (Argentina)
SILDENAFIL CITRATE
Viagra Tablets 2573

VINCOSEDAN (Spain)
DIAZEPAM
Diastat Rectal Delivery System 3343
Valium Tablets 2819

VINDACIN (Mexico)
SULINDAC
Clinoril Tablets 1924

VINGIONAL (Argentina)
RANITIDINE HYDROCHLORIDE
Zantac 25 EFFERdose Tablets 1624
Zantac 150 EFFERdose Tablets 1624
Zantac 150 Tablets 1624
Zantac 300 Tablets 1624
Zantac Injection 1619
Zantac Injection Premixed 1619
Zantac Syrup 1624

VINSEN (Thailand)
NAPROXEN
EC-Naprosyn Delayed-Release Tablets 2761
Naprosyn Suspension 2761
Naprosyn Tablets 2761

VIOKASE (Belgium, Canada)
PANCRELIPASE
Ultrase Capsules 708
Ultrase MT Capsules 709

VIOTISONE (Hong Kong, Thailand)
OFLOXACIN
Floxin Otic Solution 1049

VIPLUS (Mexico)
NAPROXEN SODIUM
Anaprox DS Tablets 2761
Anaprox Tablets 2761

VIPRES (Spain)
ENALAPRIL MALEATE
Vasotec I.V. Injection 2103

VIRAFERON (France, Mexico, Spain)
INTERFERON ALFA-2B
Intron A for Injection 3024

VIRAMID (Brazil, Italy)
RIBAVIRIN
Virazole for Inhalation Solution 3370

VIRAZID (Spain)
RIBAVIRIN
Virazole for Inhalation Solution 3370

VIRAZIDE (Australia, Italy, Mexico)
RIBAVIRIN
Virazole for Inhalation Solution 3370

VIRAZOLE (Belgium, Brazil, Canada, Germany, Hong Kong, Hungary, Irish Republic, Italy, Singapore, Spain, Sweden, Switzerland, The Netherlands, United Kingdom)
RIBAVIRIN
Virazole for Inhalation Solution 3370

VIR-COMPLEX (Brazil)
LAMIVUDINE
Epivir Oral Solution 1427
Epivir Tablets 1427
Epivir-HBV Oral Solution 1432
Epivir-HBV Tablets 1432

VIRDOX (Spain)
CETIRIZINE HYDROCHLORIDE
Zyrtec Syrup 2594
Zyrtec Tablets 2594

VIREGYT (Germany, Hungary)
AMANTADINE HYDROCHLORIDE
Symmetrel Tablets 1135

VIREGYT-K (Czech Republic)
AMANTADINE HYDROCHLORIDE
Symmetrel Tablets 1135

VIRFEN (Greece)
ENALAPRIL MALEATE
Vasotec I.V. Injection 2103

VIRFLUTAM (Italy)
FLUTAMIDE
Eulexin Capsules 3009

VIRILON (Argentina)
SILDENAFIL CITRATE
Viagra Tablets 2573

VIRIPOTENS (Argentina)
SILDENAFIL CITRATE
Viagra Tablets 2573

VIRLIX (Austria, Czech Republic, Denmark, France, Italy, Mexico, Norway, Portugal, Spain, Venezuela)
CETIRIZINE HYDROCHLORIDE
Zyrtec Syrup 2594
Zyrtec Tablets 2594

VIROBRON NF (Argentina)
DICLOFENAC SODIUM
Voltaren Tablets 2307
Voltaren-XR Tablets 2310

VIROFRAL (Denmark, Sweden)
AMANTADINE HYDROCHLORIDE
Symmetrel Tablets 1135

VIRORREVER (Argentina)
EFAVIRENZ
Sustiva Capsules 930

VIROSOL (Argentina)
AMANTADINE HYDROCHLORIDE
Symmetrel Tablets 1135

VIROZID (Brazil)
ZIDOVUDINE
Retrovir Capsules 1560
Retrovir IV Infusion 1564
Retrovir Syrup 1560
Retrovir Tablets 1560

VIRUCID (Austria)
AMANTADINE HYDROCHLORIDE
Symmetrel Tablets 1135

VIRUSTAT (Brazil)
ZIDOVUDINE
Retrovir Capsules 1560
Retrovir IV Infusion 1564
Retrovir Syrup 1560
Retrovir Tablets 1560

VISCARD (Greece)
NIFEDIPINE
Adalat CC Tablets 2964

VISCOR (Italy)
DIPYRIDAMOLE
Persantine Tablets 868

VISCOSEAL (Germany, Malaysia, Switzerland, United Kingdom)
SODIUM HYALURONATE
Hyalgan Solution 2901

VISIAL (India)
SODIUM HYALURONATE
Hyalgan Solution 2901

VISINE ALLERGY (New Zealand)
NAPHAZOLINE HYDROCHLORIDE
Albalon Ophthalmic Solution ⊙218

VISINE ALLERGY WITH ANTIHISTAMINE (Australia)
NAPHAZOLINE HYDROCHLORIDE
Albalon Ophthalmic Solution ⊙218

VISIOL (Germany, Malaysia)
SODIUM HYALURONATE
Hyalgan Solution 2901

VISLUBE (Germany, Malaysia, Switzerland)
SODIUM HYALURONATE
Hyalgan Solution 2901

VISMED (Australia, France, Germany, Hong Kong, Italy, Switzerland)
SODIUM HYALURONATE
Hyalgan Solution 2901

VISTALBALON (Germany)
NAPHAZOLINE HYDROCHLORIDE
Albalon Ophthalmic Solution ⊙218

VISTHESIA (Germany)
SODIUM HYALURONATE
Hyalgan Solution 2901

VISUMETAZONE (Italy)
DEXAMETHASONE
Decadron Tablets 1951

VITACID (Portugal)
TRETINOIN
Vesanoid Capsules 2820

VITAMIN A ACID (Hong Kong)
TRETINOIN
Vesanoid Capsules 2820

VITANOL (Spain)
TRETINOIN
Vesanoid Capsules 2820

VITANOL-A (Argentina, Brazil)
TRETINOIN
Vesanoid Capsules 2820

VITASEPTINE (France)
SULFACETAMIDE SODIUM
Klaron Lotion 10% 2909

VITINOIN (Canada)
TRETINOIN
Vesanoid Capsules 2820

VITOBEL (Greece)
ENALAPRIL MALEATE
Vasotec I.V. Injection 2103

VITRAX (France)
SODIUM HYALURONATE
Hyalgan Solution 2901

VITULPAS (Chile)
HYDROCORTISONE
Hydrocortone Tablets 1989

VIVAL (Norway)
DIAZEPAM
Diastat Rectal Delivery System 3343
Valium Tablets 2819

VIVAPRYL (United Kingdom)
SELEGILINE HYDROCHLORIDE
Eldepryl Capsules 3208

VIVATEC (Denmark, Finland, Norway, Sweden)
LISINOPRIL
Prinivil Tablets 2052

VIVATEC COMP (Finland, Norway)
HYDROCHLOROTHIAZIDE/LISINOPRIL
Prinzide Tablets 2056

VIVAZID (Denmark)
HYDROCHLOROTHIAZIDE/LISINOPRIL
Prinzide Tablets 2056

VIVELLE (Belgium, Canada)
ESTRADIOL
Climara Transdermal System 771
Estring Vaginal Ring 2635

VIVELLE DOT (Denmark)
ESTRADIOL
Climara Transdermal System 771
Estring Vaginal Ring 2635

VIVELLEDOT (France)
ESTRADIOL
Climara Transdermal System 771
Estring Vaginal Ring 2635

VIVERDAL (Brazil)
RISPERIDONE
Risperdal Oral Solution 1676
Risperdal Tablets 1676

VIVIDRIN AKUT AZELASTIN (Germany)
AZELASTINE HYDROCHLORIDE
Astelin Nasal Spray 1904

VIVOL (Canada)
DIAZEPAM
Diastat Rectal Delivery System 3343
Valium Tablets 2819

VIXCEF (Argentina)
CEFIXIME
Suprax 1843

VIXIDERM E (Argentina)
BENZOYL PEROXIDE
Brevoxyl-4 Creamy Wash 3210
Brevoxyl-4 Gel 3210
Brevoxyl-8 Creamy Wash 3210
Brevoxyl-8 Gel 3210
Triaz Cleanser 1892
Triaz Gel 1892

VIXIDONE (Argentina)
DEXAMETHASONE
Decadron Tablets 1951

VIXIDONE T (Argentina)
DEXAMETHASONE
Decadron Tablets 1951

VIZERUL (Argentina, Venezuela)
RANITIDINE HYDROCHLORIDE
Zantac 25 EFFERdose Tablets 1624
Zantac 150 EFFERdose Tablets. 1624
Zantac 150 Tablets 1624
Zantac 300 Tablets 1624
Zantac Injection 1619
Zantac Injection Premixed 1619
Zantac Syrup 1624

VOFENAL (Canada)
DICLOFENAC SODIUM
Voltaren Tablets 2307
Voltaren-XR Tablets 2310

VOKER (Malaysia)
FAMOTIDINE
Pepcid Injection 2040
Pepcid Injection Premixed 2040
Pepcid Tablets 2038
Pepcid for Oral Suspension 2038

VOLCIDOL-S (Thailand)
TRAMADOL HYDROCHLORIDE
Ultram ER Tablets 2392

VOLDAL (France)
DICLOFENAC SODIUM
Voltaren Tablets 2307
Voltaren-XR Tablets 2310

VOLFENAC (Thailand)
DICLOFENAC SODIUM
Voltaren Tablets 2307
Voltaren-XR Tablets 2310

VOLNAC (Thailand)
DICLOFENAC SODIUM
Voltaren Tablets 2307
Voltaren-XR Tablets 2310

VOLOGEN (Irish Republic)
DICLOFENAC SODIUM
Voltaren Tablets 2307
Voltaren-XR Tablets 2310

VOLON A (Austria, Germany)
TRIAMCINOLONE ACETONIDE
Azmacort Inhalation Aerosol. 1726
Nasacort AQ Nasal Spray 2922

VOLONIMAT (Germany)
TRIAMCINOLONE ACETONIDE
Azmacort Inhalation Aerosol. 1726
Nasacort AQ Nasal Spray 2922

VOLONIMAT N (Germany)
TRIAMCINOLONE ACETONIDE
Azmacort Inhalation Aerosol. 1726
Nasacort AQ Nasal Spray 2922

VOLRAMAN (United Kingdom)
DICLOFENAC SODIUM
Voltaren Tablets 2307
Voltaren-XR Tablets 2310

VOLSAID (United Kingdom)
DICLOFENAC SODIUM
Voltaren Tablets 2307
Voltaren-XR Tablets 2310

VOLTA (Thailand)
DICLOFENAC SODIUM
Voltaren Tablets 2307
Voltaren-XR Tablets 2310

VOLTAFLEX (Brazil)
DICLOFENAC SODIUM
Voltaren Tablets 2307
Voltaren-XR Tablets 2310

VOLTAMICIN (Austria, Brazil, Czech Republic, Hungary, Singapore)
DICLOFENAC SODIUM
Voltaren Tablets 2307
Voltaren-XR Tablets 2310

VOLTAREN (Brazil, Greece, Norway, Sweden)
DICLOFENAC SODIUM
Voltaren Tablets 2307
Voltaren-XR Tablets 2310

VOLTAREN COLIRIO (Argentina, Brazil)
DICLOFENAC SODIUM
Voltaren Tablets 2307
Voltaren-XR Tablets 2310

VOLTAREN FLEX (Argentina)
DICLOFENAC SODIUM
Voltaren Tablets 2307
Voltaren-XR Tablets 2310

VOLTAREN FORTE (Argentina, Mexico)
DICLOFENAC SODIUM
Voltaren Tablets 2307
Voltaren-XR Tablets 2310

VOLTAREN OPHTA (Hungary, Switzerland)
DICLOFENAC SODIUM
Voltaren Tablets 2307
Voltaren-XR Tablets 2310

VOLTAREN OPHTHA (Australia, Canada, Germany, Hong Kong, Israel, New Zealand, Norway, Singapore, South Africa, Sweden)
DICLOFENAC SODIUM
Voltaren Tablets 2307
Voltaren-XR Tablets 2310

VOLTAREN PLUS (Germany)
DICLOFENAC SODIUM
Voltaren Tablets 2307
Voltaren-XR Tablets 2310

VOLTARENE (France)
DICLOFENAC SODIUM
Voltaren Tablets 2307
Voltaren-XR Tablets 2310

VOLTAROL OPHTHA (Irish Republic, United Kingdom)
DICLOFENAC SODIUM
Voltaren Tablets 2307
Voltaren-XR Tablets 2310

VOLTEN (Venezuela)
DICLOFENAC SODIUM
Voltaren Tablets 2307
Voltaren-XR Tablets 2310

VOLTRIC (Spain)
CETIRIZINE HYDROCHLORIDE
Zyrtec Syrup 2594
Zyrtec Tablets 2594

VOLUTINE (Italy)
FENOFIBRATE
Tricor Tablets 527

VOLUTOL (Mexico)
CARBAMAZEPINE
Carbatrol Capsules 3171
Tegretol Chewable Tablets 2295
Tegretol Suspension. 2295
Tegretol Tablets 2295
Tegretol-XR Tablets 2295

VOLVERAC (Thailand)
DICLOFENAC SODIUM
Voltaren Tablets 2307
Voltaren-XR Tablets 2310

VOMITRON (Thailand)
ONDANSETRON HYDROCHLORIDE
Zofran Injection. 1634
Zofran Injection Premixed 1634
Zofran Oral Solution. 1639
Zofran Tablets 1639

VONAU (Brazil)
ONDANSETRON HYDROCHLORIDE
Zofran Injection. 1634
Zofran Injection Premixed 1634
Zofran Oral Solution. 1639
Zofran Tablets 1639

V-OPTIC (Israel)
TIMOLOL MALEATE
Blocadren Tablets 1916
Timoptic Sterile Ophthalmic Solution 2088
Timoptic in Ocudose 2091
Timoptic-XE Sterile Ophthalmic Gel Forming Solution 2092

VOREN (Malaysia, Thailand)
DICLOFENAC SODIUM
Voltaren Tablets 2307
Voltaren-XR Tablets 2310

VOREN PLUS (Malaysia)
DICLOFENAC SODIUM
Voltaren Tablets 2307
Voltaren-XR Tablets 2310

VORST (Argentina)
SILDENAFIL CITRATE
Viagra Tablets 2573

VOSTAR (Denmark)
DICLOFENAC SODIUM
Voltaren Tablets 2307
Voltaren-XR Tablets 2310

VOTAMED (Thailand)
DICLOFENAC SODIUM
Voltaren Tablets 2307
Voltaren-XR Tablets 2310

VOTAXIL (Venezuela)
DICLOFENAC SODIUM
Voltaren Tablets 2307
Voltaren-XR Tablets 2310

VOXIN (Greece)
VANCOMYCIN HYDROCHLORIDE
Vancocin HCl Capsules, USP 3380

VUCLODIR (Argentina)
LAMIVUDINE
Epivir Oral Solution 1427
Epivir Tablets 1427
Epivir-HBV Oral Solution 1432
Epivir-HBV Tablets 1432

VUDIRAX (Brazil)
LAMIVUDINE
Epivir Oral Solution 1427
Epivir Tablets 1427
Epivir-HBV Oral Solution 1432
Epivir-HBV Tablets 1432

VURDON (Greece)
DICLOFENAC SODIUM
Voltaren Tablets 2307
Voltaren-XR Tablets 2310

WARAN (Sweden)
WARFARIN SODIUM
Coumadin Tablets 898
Coumadin for Injection 898

WARF (India)
WARFARIN SODIUM
Coumadin Tablets 898
Coumadin for Injection 898

WARFILONE (Canada)
WARFARIN SODIUM
Coumadin Tablets 898
Coumadin for Injection 898

WARI-DICLOWAL (Malaysia)
DICLOFENAC SODIUM
Voltaren Tablets 2307
Voltaren-XR Tablets 2310

WARIDIPIN (Hong Kong)
NIFEDIPINE
Adalat CC Tablets 2964

WARIMAZOL (Hong Kong)
CLOTRIMAZOLE
Lotrimin Cream. 3039
Lotrimin Lotion 1%. 3039
Lotrimin Topical Solution 1% 3039

WASPEZE HYDROCORTISONE (United Kingdom)
HYDROCORTISONE
Hydrocortone Tablets 1989

WAUCOSIN (Greece)
TIMOLOL MALEATE
Blocadren Tablets 1916
Timoptic Sterile Ophthalmic Solution 2088
Timoptic in Ocudose 2091
Timoptic-XE Sterile Ophthalmic Gel Forming Solution 2092

WAYCITAL (Mexico)
PRAZIQUANTEL
Biltricide Tablets 2976

WAYTRAX (Mexico)
CEFTAZIDIME
Fortaz for Injection 1453

WELLBUTRIN (Argentina, Brazil, Canada, Chile, Czech Republic, Hungary, Mexico)
BUPROPION HYDROCHLORIDE
Wellbutrin SR Sustained-Release Tablets . . 1607
Wellbutrin Tablets 1603
Zyban Sustained-Release Tablets 1644

WELLVONE (Australia, Austria, Belgium, Denmark, France, Germany, Greece, Italy, South Africa, Spain, Sweden, Switzerland, The Netherlands, United Kingdom)
ATOVAQUONE
Mepron Suspension 1521

WENFLOX (Argentina)
NORFLOXACIN
Noroxin Tablets. 2032

WEPOX (India)
EPOETIN ALFA
Epogen for Injection. 591
Procrit for Injection 2364

WINOL (Argentina)
IRINOTECAN HYDROCHLORIDE
Camptosar Injection. 2604

WITROMIN (Mexico)
ERYTHROMYCIN
Ery-Tab Tablets 449
Erythromycin Base Filmtab Tablets. 455
Erythromycin Delayed-Release Capsules, USP 457
PCE Dispertab Tablets 515

WONTIZEM (Hong Kong)
DILTIAZEM HYDROCHLORIDE
Cardizem LA Extended Release Tablets. . . 1728
Tiazac Capsules 1201

WORMICIDE (Thailand)
PRAZIQUANTEL
Biltricide Tablets 2976

WYMESONE (India)
DEXAMETHASONE
Decadron Tablets 1951

XACIN (Thailand)
NORFLOXACIN
Noroxin Tablets. 2032

(⊙ Described in PDR For Ophthalmic Medicines™)

XADAREN (Czech Republic)
FLUTAMIDE
Eulexin Capsules . . . 3009

XAGRID (France, Switzerland, United Kingdom)
ANAGRELIDE HYDROCHLORIDE
Agrylin Capsules . . . 3169

XALACOM (Argentina, Australia, Austria, Belgium, Brazil, Canada, Czech Republic, France, Germany, Greece, Hong Kong, Hungary, Irish Republic, Israel, Italy, Malaysia, Mexico, New Zealand, Portugal, Singapore, South Africa, Spain, Switzerland, Thailand, The Netherlands, United Kingdom)
LATANOPROST
Xalatan Ophthalmic Solution . . . ⊙291

XALATAN (Argentina, Australia, Austria, Belgium, Brazil, Canada, Chile, Czech Republic, Denmark, Finland, France, Germany, Greece, Hong Kong, Hungary, Irish Republic, Israel, Italy, Malaysia, Mexico, New Zealand, Norway, Portugal, Russia, Singapore, South Africa, Spain, Sweden, Switzerland, Thailand, The Netherlands, United Kingdom, Venezuela)
LATANOPROST
Xalatan Ophthalmic Solution . . . ⊙291

XALCOM (Denmark, Finland, Norway, Sweden)
LATANOPROST
Xalatan Ophthalmic Solution . . . ⊙291

XALOTINA (Argentina)
AMOXICILLIN
Amoxil Pediatric Drops for Oral Suspension . . . 1343
Amoxil Tablets . . . 1343

XANAES (Argentina)
AZELASTINE HYDROCHLORIDE
Astelin Nasal Spray . . . 1904

XANIDINE (Thailand)
RANITIDINE HYDROCHLORIDE
Zantac 25 EFFERdose Tablets . . . 1624
Zantac 150 EFFERdose Tablets . . . 1624
Zantac 150 Tablets . . . 1624
Zantac 300 Tablets . . . 1624
Zantac Injection . . . 1619
Zantac Injection Premixed . . . 1619
Zantac Syrup . . . 1624

XANOMEL (Hungary, Irish Republic)
RANITIDINE HYDROCHLORIDE
Zantac 25 EFFERdose Tablets . . . 1624
Zantac 150 EFFERdose Tablets . . . 1624
Zantac 150 Tablets . . . 1624
Zantac 300 Tablets . . . 1624
Zantac Injection . . . 1619
Zantac Injection Premixed . . . 1619
Zantac Syrup . . . 1624

XANTHIUM (France, Thailand)
THEOPHYLLINE
Uniphyl Tablets . . . 2710

XANTIVENT (Switzerland)
THEOPHYLLINE
Uniphyl Tablets . . . 2710

XAO T (Argentina)
TOBRAMYCIN
TOBI Solution for Inhalation . . . 2298

XAO-DEX (Argentina)
TOBRAMYCIN
TOBI Solution for Inhalation . . . 2298

XARATOR (Italy)
ATORVASTATIN CALCIUM
Lipitor Tablets . . . 2483

XASMUN (Spain)
NORFLOXACIN
Noroxin Tablets . . . 2032

XEDENOL (Argentina)
DICLOFENAC SODIUM
Voltaren Tablets . . . 2307
Voltaren-XR Tablets . . . 2310

XEDENOL FLEX (Argentina)
DICLOFENAC SODIUM
Voltaren Tablets . . . 2307
Voltaren-XR Tablets . . . 2310

XELODA (Argentina, Australia, Austria, Belgium, Brazil, Canada, Chile, Czech Republic, Denmark, Finland, France, Germany, Greece, Hong Kong, Hungary, Irish Republic, Israel, Italy, Mexico, New Zealand, Norway, Portugal, Singapore, South Africa, Spain, Sweden, Switzerland, Thailand, United Kingdom, Venezuela)
CAPECITABINE
Xeloda Tablets . . . 2822

XENAR (Italy)
NAPROXEN
EC-Naprosyn Delayed-Release Tablets . . . 2761
Naprosyn Suspension . . . 2761
Naprosyn Tablets . . . 2761

XENICAL (Argentina, Australia, Austria, Belgium, Brazil, Canada, Chile, Czech Republic, Denmark, Finland, France, Germany, Greece, Hong Kong, Hungary, Irish Republic, Israel, Italy, Mexico, New Zealand, Norway, Portugal, Singapore, South Africa, Spain, Sweden, Switzerland, Thailand, The Netherlands, United Kingdom, Venezuela)
ORLISTAT
Xenical Capsules . . . 2831

XENOBID (India)
NAPROXEN
EC-Naprosyn Delayed-Release Tablets . . . 2761
Naprosyn Suspension . . . 2761
Naprosyn Tablets . . . 2761

XENOPAN (Austria)
NAPROXEN
EC-Naprosyn Delayed-Release Tablets . . . 2761
Naprosyn Suspension . . . 2761
Naprosyn Tablets . . . 2761

XENOVATE (South Africa)
CLOBETASOL PROPIONATE
Temovate Cream . . . 2668
Temovate E Emollient . . . 2671
Temovate Gel . . . 2669
Temovate Ointment . . . 2668
Temovate Scalp Application . . . 2670

XEPAGAN (Singapore)
PROMETHAZINE HYDROCHLORIDE
Phenergan Tablets and Suppositories . . . 3440

XERASPOR (South Africa)
CLOTRIMAZOLE
Lotrimin Cream . . . 3039
Lotrimin Lotion 1% . . . 3039
Lotrimin Topical Solution 1% . . . 3039

XERGIC (Australia)
FEXOFENADINE HYDROCHLORIDE
Allegra Capsules . . . 2844

XETIN (Spain)
PAROXETINE HYDROCHLORIDE
Paxil Oral Suspension . . . 1530
Paxil Tablets . . . 1530

XICANE (Argentina)
NAPROXEN
EC-Naprosyn Delayed-Release Tablets . . . 2761
Naprosyn Suspension . . . 2761
Naprosyn Tablets . . . 2761

XILANIC (Argentina)
PAROXETINE HYDROCHLORIDE
Paxil Oral Suspension . . . 1530
Paxil Tablets . . . 1530

XILOCLER (Argentina)
LIDOCAINE
Lidoderm Patch . . . 1118

XILONIBSA (Portugal)
LIDOCAINE
Lidoderm Patch . . . 1118

XILOPAR (Austria, Germany, Italy, Portugal)
SELEGILINE HYDROCHLORIDE
Eldepryl Capsules . . . 3208

XIM (India)
CEFIXIME
Suprax . . . 1843

XIMAKEN (Mexico)
CEFUROXIME SODIUM
Zinacef Injection . . . 1631

XINA (Argentina)
DICLOFENAC SODIUM
Voltaren Tablets . . . 2307
Voltaren-XR Tablets . . . 2310

XINDER (Chile)
CLOBETASOL PROPIONATE
Temovate Cream . . . 2668
Temovate E Emollient . . . 2671
Temovate Gel . . . 2669
Temovate Ointment . . . 2668
Temovate Scalp Application . . . 2670

XINSIDONA (Spain)
PAMIDRONATE DISODIUM
Aredia for Injection . . . 2179

XIPROCAN (Mexico)
AMOXICILLIN
Amoxil Pediatric Drops for Oral Suspension . . . 1343
Amoxil Tablets . . . 1343

XISMOX (United Kingdom)
ISOSORBIDE MONONITRATE
Imdur Tablets . . . 3018

XOLOF (Chile)
TOBRAMYCIN
TOBI Solution for Inhalation . . . 2298

XOLOF D (Chile)
DEXAMETHASONE/TOBRAMYCIN
TobraDex Ophthalmic Ointment . . . 562, ⊙212
TobraDex Ophthalmic Suspension . . . 563, ⊙211

XONATIL (Mexico)
CEFTRIAXONE SODIUM
Rocephin Injectable Vials, ADD-Vantage, Galaxy, Bulk . . . 2800

XORIM (Hungary, Venezuela)
CEFUROXIME SODIUM
Zinacef Injection . . . 1631

XSERT (India)
SERTRALINE HYDROCHLORIDE
Zoloft Tablets . . . 2586

X'TAC (Malaysia)
RANITIDINE HYDROCHLORIDE
Zantac 25 EFFERdose Tablets . . . 1624
Zantac 150 EFFERdose Tablets . . . 1624
Zantac 150 Tablets . . . 1624
Zantac 300 Tablets . . . 1624
Zantac Injection . . . 1619
Zantac Injection Premixed . . . 1619
Zantac Syrup . . . 1624

XTENDROL (Mexico)
OXANDROLONE
Oxandrin Tablets . . . 2962

X'TOR (India)
ATORVASTATIN CALCIUM
Lipitor Tablets . . . 2483

XYDEP (Australia)
SERTRALINE HYDROCHLORIDE
Zoloft Tablets . . . 2586

XYLESTESIN (Czech Republic)
LIDOCAINE
Lidoderm Patch . . . 1118

XYLOCAINA (Chile, Venezuela)
LIDOCAINE
Lidoderm Patch . . . 1118

XYLOCAINE (Czech Republic, Greece, India, Israel, Malaysia, South Africa, United Kingdom)
LIDOCAINE
Lidoderm Patch . . . 1118

XYLODASE (United Kingdom)
LIDOCAINE
Lidoderm Patch . . . 1118

XYLOPROCT (Hong Kong)
LIDOCAINE
Lidoderm Patch . . . 1118

XYMEL (Irish Republic)
TRAMADOL HYDROCHLORIDE
Ultram ER Tablets . . . 2392

YANURAX (Argentina)
NORFLOXACIN
Noroxin Tablets . . . 2032

YARA (Greece)
RANITIDINE HYDROCHLORIDE
Zantac 25 EFFERdose Tablets . . . 1624
Zantac 150 EFFERdose Tablets . . . 1624
Zantac 150 Tablets . . . 1624
Zantac 300 Tablets . . . 1624
Zantac Injection . . . 1619
Zantac Injection Premixed . . . 1619
Zantac Syrup . . . 1624

YATROX (Spain)
ONDANSETRON HYDROCHLORIDE
Zofran Injection . . . 1634
Zofran Injection Premixed . . . 1634
Zofran Oral Solution . . . 1639
Zofran Tablets . . . 1639

YECTAMICINA (Mexico, Venezuela)
GENTAMICIN SULFATE
Garamycin Injectable . . . 3014

YEDOC (Switzerland)
GENTAMICIN SULFATE
Garamycin Injectable . . . 3014

YEPOTIN (Mexico)
EPOETIN ALFA
Epogen for Injection . . . 591
Procrit for Injection . . . 2364

YESAN (Greece)
TIMOLOL MALEATE
Blocadren Tablets . . . 1916
Timoptic Sterile Ophthalmic Solution . . . 2088
Timoptic in Ocudose . . . 2091
Timoptic-XE Sterile Ophthalmic Gel Forming Solution . . . 2092

YOKEL (Greece)
CEFUROXIME SODIUM
Zinacef Injection . . . 1631

YRELAN (Brazil)
ENALAPRIL MALEATE
Vasotec I.V. Injection . . . 2103

YUREMID (Mexico)
FUROSEMIDE
Furosemide Tablets . . . 2154

ZAARPRESS (Brazil)
LOSARTAN POTASSIUM
Cozaar Tablets . . . 1935

ZAART-H (India)
LOSARTAN POTASSIUM
Cozaar Tablets . . . 1935

ZADINE (Brazil)
RANITIDINE HYDROCHLORIDE
Zantac 25 EFFERdose Tablets . . . 1624
Zantac 150 EFFERdose Tablets . . . 1624
Zantac 150 Tablets . . . 1624
Zantac 300 Tablets . . . 1624
Zantac Injection . . . 1619
Zantac Injection Premixed . . . 1619
Zantac Syrup . . . 1624

ZADIPINA (Italy)
NISOLDIPINE
Sular Tablets . . . 3122

ZADOLINA (Mexico)
CEFTAZIDIME
Fortaz for Injection . . . 1453

ZADSTAT (Israel, United Kingdom)
METRONIDAZOLE
MetroGel-Vaginal Gel . . . 1855

ZAEDOC (United Kingdom)
RANITIDINE HYDROCHLORIDE
Zantac 25 EFFERdose Tablets . . . 1624
Zantac 150 EFFERdose Tablets . . . 1624
Zantac 150 Tablets . . . 1624
Zantac 300 Tablets . . . 1624
Zantac Injection . . . 1619
Zantac Injection Premixed . . . 1619
Zantac Syrup . . . 1624

ZAFIMIDA (Mexico)
FUROSEMIDE
Furosemide Tablets . . . 2154

ZAFIRASMAL (Argentina)
ZAFIRLUKAST
Accolate Tablets . . . 671

ZAFIRST (Italy)
ZAFIRLUKAST
Accolate Tablets . . . 671

ZAGORINE (Greece)
CEFUROXIME AXETIL
Ceftin Tablets . . . 1407
Ceftin for Oral Suspension . . . 1407

ZAGYL (South Africa)
METRONIDAZOLE
MetroGel-Vaginal Gel . . . 1855

ZALDIAR (Mexico, Spain, Switzerland, The Netherlands)
TRAMADOL HYDROCHLORIDE
Ultram ER Tablets 2392

ZAMACORT (Mexico)
TRIAMCINOLONE ACETONIDE
Azmacort Inhalation Aerosol. 1726
Nasacort AQ Nasal Spray 2922

ZAMADOL (United Kingdom)
TRAMADOL HYDROCHLORIDE
Ultram ER Tablets 2392

ZAMOCILLINE (France)
AMOXICILLIN
Amoxil Pediatric Drops for Oral Suspension. 1343
Amoxil Tablets 1343

ZAMUDOL (France)
TRAMADOL HYDROCHLORIDE
Ultram ER Tablets 2392

ZANDINE (Irish Republic)
RANITIDINE HYDROCHLORIDE
Zantac 25 EFFERdose Tablets 1624
Zantac 150 EFFERdose Tablets. 1624
Zantac 150 Tablets 1624
Zantac 300 Tablets 1624
Zantac Injection 1619
Zantac Injection Premixed 1619
Zantac Syrup 1624

ZANIDEX (Israel)
RANITIDINE HYDROCHLORIDE
Zantac 25 EFFERdose Tablets 1624
Zantac 150 EFFERdose Tablets. 1624
Zantac 150 Tablets 1624
Zantac 300 Tablets 1624
Zantac Injection 1619
Zantac Injection Premixed 1619
Zantac Syrup 1624

ZANIDIN (New Zealand)
RANITIDINE HYDROCHLORIDE
Zantac 25 EFFERdose Tablets 1624
Zantac 150 EFFERdose Tablets. 1624
Zantac 150 Tablets 1624
Zantac 300 Tablets 1624
Zantac Injection 1619
Zantac Injection Premixed 1619
Zantac Syrup 1624

ZANOCIN (Czech Republic, Hungary, India, Malaysia, Russia, South Africa)
OFLOXACIN
Floxin Otic Solution 1049

ZANTAB (Israel)
RANITIDINE HYDROCHLORIDE
Zantac 25 EFFERdose Tablets 1624
Zantac 150 EFFERdose Tablets. 1624
Zantac 150 Tablets 1624
Zantac 300 Tablets 1624
Zantac Injection 1619
Zantac Injection Premixed 1619
Zantac Syrup 1624

ZANTAC (Australia, Austria, Belgium, Chile, Czech Republic, Denmark, Finland, Greece, Hong Kong, Hungary, Irish Republic, Israel, Italy, Malaysia, New Zealand, Norway, Portugal, Russia, Singapore, South Africa, Spain, Sweden, Thailand, The Netherlands, United Kingdom, Venezuela)
RANITIDINE HYDROCHLORIDE
Zantac 150 EFFERdose Tablets. 1624
Zantac 150 Tablets 1624
Zantac 25 EFFERdose Tablets 1624
Zantac 300 Tablets 1624
Zantac Injection 1619
Zantac Injection Premixed 1619
Zantac Syrup 1624

ZANTARAC (Austria)
RANITIDINE HYDROCHLORIDE
Zantac 25 EFFERdose Tablets 1624
Zantac 150 EFFERdose Tablets. 1624
Zantac 150 Tablets 1624
Zantac 300 Tablets 1624
Zantac Injection 1619
Zantac Injection Premixed 1619
Zantac Syrup 1624

ZANTIC (Switzerland)
RANITIDINE HYDROCHLORIDE
Zantac 25 EFFERdose Tablets 1624
Zantac 150 EFFERdose Tablets. 1624
Zantac 150 Tablets 1624
Zantac 300 Tablets 1624
Zantac Injection 1619
Zantac Injection Premixed 1619
Zantac Syrup 1624

ZAPONEX (United Kingdom)
CLOZAPINE
Clozaril Tablets 2184

ZAPTO (South Africa)
CAPTOPRIL
Captopril Tablets 2149

ZAPTO CO (South Africa)
CAPTOPRIL
Captopril Tablets 2149

ZARATOR (Argentina, Chile, Denmark, Greece, Portugal, Spain)
ATORVASTATIN CALCIUM
Lipitor Tablets 2483

ZAREX (Israel)
FAMOTIDINE
Pepcid Injection 2040
Pepcid Injection Premixed 2040
Pepcid Tablets 2038
Pepcid for Oral Suspension 2038

ZARGUS (Brazil)
RISPERIDONE
Risperdal Oral Solution 1676
Risperdal Tablets. 1676

ZART (India)
LOSARTAN POTASSIUM
Cozaar Tablets 1935

ZAXEM (Austria)
BUTENAFINE HYDROCHLORIDE
Mentax Cream 2158

ZAYASEL (Spain)
TERAZOSIN HYDROCHLORIDE
Hytrin Capsules. 471

Z-BEC (Greece)
LISINOPRIL
Prinivil Tablets 2052

ZEBEN (Thailand)
ALBENDAZOLE
Albenza Tablets. 1338

ZECLAR (Czech Republic, Finland, France)
CLARITHROMYCIN
Biaxin Filmtab Tablets 402
Biaxin Granules 402

ZECLAREN (Greece)
CLARITHROMYCIN
Biaxin Filmtab Tablets 402
Biaxin Granules 402

ZEDDAN (Italy)
TRANDOLAPRIL
Mavik Tablets 486

ZEFAXONE (Thailand)
CEFTRIAXONE SODIUM
Rocephin Injectable Vials, ADD-Vantage, Galaxy, Bulk 2800

ZEFFIX (Argentina, Australia, Austria, Belgium, Brazil, Czech Republic, Denmark, Finland, France, Germany, Greece, Hong Kong, Hungary, Irish Republic, Israel, Italy, Malaysia, New Zealand, Portugal, Russia, Singapore, Spain, Sweden, Switzerland, Thailand, United Kingdom)
LAMIVUDINE
Epivir Oral Solution 1427
Epivir Tablets 1427
Epivir-HBV Oral Solution 1432
Epivir-HBV Tablets 1432

ZEFTAM (Thailand)
CEFTAZIDIME
Fortaz for Injection 1453

ZEID (Mexico)
SIMVASTATIN
Zocor Tablets. 2105

ZEISIN (Germany)
PIRBUTEROL ACETATE
Maxair Autohaler 1852

ZELAPAR (United Kingdom)
SELEGILINE HYDROCHLORIDE
Eldepryl Capsules 3208

ZELFIN (Mexico)
ALBENDAZOLE
Albenza Tablets. 1338

ZEM (Greece)
DILTIAZEM HYDROCHLORIDE
Cardizem LA Extended Release Tablets. . . 1728
Tiazac Capsules 1201

ZEMON (United Kingdom)
ISOSORBIDE MONONITRATE
Imdur Tablets 3018

ZEMOX (Germany)
SIMVASTATIN
Zocor Tablets 2105

ZEMPLAR (Austria, Greece, Portugal, Spain, United Kingdom)
PARICALCITOL
Zemplar Injection. 543

ZEMTARD (United Kingdom)
DILTIAZEM HYDROCHLORIDE
Cardizem LA Extended Release Tablets. . . 1728
Tiazac Capsules 1201

ZEMURON (Argentina, Canada)
ROCURONIUM BROMIDE
Zemuron Injection 2346

ZENAXIN (Mexico)
ALBENDAZOLE
Albenza Tablets. 1338

ZENDHIN (Hong Kong, Malaysia, Singapore)
RANITIDINE HYDROCHLORIDE
Zantac 25 EFFERdose Tablets 1624
Zantac 150 EFFERdose Tablets. 1624
Zantac 150 Tablets 1624
Zantac 300 Tablets 1624
Zantac Injection 1619
Zantac Injection Premixed 1619
Zantac Syrup 1624

ZENGAC (Italy)
VANCOMYCIN HYDROCHLORIDE
Vancocin HCl Capsules, USP 3380

ZENODIAN (Italy)
SUCRALFATE
Carafate Suspension 701
Carafate Tablets 701

ZENOXONE (United Kingdom)
HYDROCORTISONE
Hydrocortone Tablets 1989

ZENSIL (Thailand)
CETIRIZINE HYDROCHLORIDE
Zyrtec Syrup 2594
Zyrtec Tablets 2594

ZENTEL (Australia, Brazil, Chile, Czech Republic, France, India, Italy, Malaysia, Mexico, Portugal, Singapore, South Africa, Switzerland, Thailand, Venezuela)
ALBENDAZOLE
Albenza Tablets. 1338

ZENTIUS (Argentina, Chile)
CITALOPRAM HYDROBROMIDE
Celexa Tablets 1176

ZENUSIN (Portugal, Thailand)
NIFEDIPINE
Adalat CC Tablets 2964

ZENZERA (Thailand)
ALBENDAZOLE
Albenza Tablets. 1338

ZEPAN (Mexico)
DIAZEPAM
Diastat Rectal Delivery System 3343
Valium Tablets 2819

ZEPHOLIN (Greece, Irish Republic)
CETIRIZINE HYDROCHLORIDE
Zyrtec Syrup 2594
Zyrtec Tablets 2594

ZEPIKEN (Mexico)
CARBAMAZEPINE
Carbatrol Capsules 3171
Tegretol Chewable Tablets 2295
Tegretol Suspension. 2295
Tegretol Tablets 2295
Tegretol-XR Tablets 2295

ZEPOSE (India)
DIAZEPAM
Diastat Rectal Delivery System 3343
Valium Tablets 2819

ZEPRAT (Mexico)
DIAZEPAM
Diastat Rectal Delivery System 3343
Valium Tablets 2819

ZEPTOL (Russia, Thailand)
CARBAMAZEPINE
Carbatrol Capsules 3171
Tegretol Chewable Tablets 2295
Tegretol Suspension. 2295
Tegretol Tablets 2295
Tegretol-XR Tablets 2295

ZERA (Portugal)
SIMVASTATIN
Zocor Tablets. 2105

ZERELLA (Austria, Italy)
ESTRADIOL
Climara Transdermal System 771
Estring Vaginal Ring 2635

ZERLUBRON (Greece)
FENOFIBRATE
Tricor Tablets 527

ZERMED (Thailand)
CETIRIZINE HYDROCHLORIDE
Zyrtec Syrup 2594
Zyrtec Tablets 2594

ZEROPENEM (Argentina)
MEROPENEM
Merrem I.V. 686

ZERTINE (Hong Kong, Thailand)
CETIRIZINE HYDROCHLORIDE
Zyrtec Syrup 2594
Zyrtec Tablets 2594

ZESGER (Irish Republic)
LISINOPRIL
Prinivil Tablets 2052

ZESTAN (Irish Republic)
LISINOPRIL
Prinivil Tablets 2052

ZESTOMAX (South Africa)
LISINOPRIL
Prinivil Tablets 2052

ZESTORETIC (Argentina, Austria, Belgium, Brazil, Canada, Chile, Denmark, France, Hong Kong, Irish Republic, Italy, Mexico, New Zealand, Norway, Portugal, South Africa, Spain, Sweden, Switzerland, The Netherlands, United Kingdom)
LISINOPRIL
Prinivil Tablets 2052

ZESTRIL (Argentina, Australia, Belgium, Brazil, Canada, Chile, Denmark, Finland, France, Greece, Hong Kong, Irish Republic, Italy, Malaysia, Mexico, New Zealand, Norway, Portugal, Singapore, South Africa, Spain, Sweden, Switzerland, Thailand, The Netherlands, United Kingdom)
LISINOPRIL
Prinivil Tablets 2052

ZETAGAL (Greece)
CEFUROXIME SODIUM
Zinacef Injection 1631

ZETALERG (Brazil)
CETIRIZINE HYDROCHLORIDE
Zyrtec Syrup 2594
Zyrtec Tablets 2594

ZETAVUDIN (Argentina)
ZIDOVUDINE
Retrovir Capsules 1560
Retrovir IV Infusion. 1564
Retrovir Syrup 1560
Retrovir Tablets. 1560

ZETIR (Brazil, Germany)
CETIRIZINE HYDROCHLORIDE
Zyrtec Syrup 2594
Zyrtec Tablets 2594

ZETOMAX (South Africa)
LISINOPRIL
Prinivil Tablets 2052

ZETOP (South Africa)
CETIRIZINE HYDROCHLORIDE
Zyrtec Syrup 2594
Zyrtec Tablets 2594

ZETRON (Thailand)
ONDANSETRON HYDROCHLORIDE
Zofran Injection. 1634

Zofran Injection Premixed . . . 1634
Zofran Oral Solution . . . 1639
Zofran Tablets . . . 1639

ZETROTAX (Argentina)
ZIDOVUDINE
Retrovir Capsules . . . 1560
Retrovir IV Infusion . . . 1564
Retrovir Syrup . . . 1560
Retrovir Tablets . . . 1560

ZIAGEN (Australia, Austria, Belgium, Canada, Chile, Czech Republic, Denmark, Finland, France, Germany, Greece, Hong Kong, Irish Republic, Israel, Italy, New Zealand, Norway, Portugal, Russia, Singapore, South Africa, Spain, Sweden, Switzerland, United Kingdom)
ABACAVIR SULFATE
Ziagen Oral Solution . . . 1626
Ziagen Tablets . . . 1626

ZIAGENAVIR (Argentina, Brazil, Mexico, Thailand)
ABACAVIR SULFATE
Ziagen Oral Solution . . . 1626
Ziagen Tablets . . . 1626

ZIAXEL (Greece, New Zealand)
TRANDOLAPRIL/VERAPAMIL HYDROCHLORIDE
Tarka Tablets . . . 524

ZICET (Hong Kong)
CETIRIZINE HYDROCHLORIDE
Zyrtec Syrup . . . 2594
Zyrtec Tablets . . . 2594

ZIDAC (France)
RANITIDINE HYDROCHLORIDE
Zantac 25 EFFERdose Tablets . . . 1624
Zantac 150 EFFERdose Tablets . . . 1624
Zantac 150 Tablets . . . 1624
Zantac 300 Tablets . . . 1624
Zantac Injection . . . 1619
Zantac Injection Premixed . . . 1619
Zantac Syrup . . . 1624

ZIDA-CO (United Kingdom)
AMILORIDE HYDROCHLORIDE/HYDROCHLOROTHIAZIDE
Moduretic Tablets . . . 2028

ZIDEPRIL (Greece)
CAPTOPRIL
Captopril Tablets . . . 2149

ZIDIC-C (Mexico)
ZIDOVUDINE
Retrovir Capsules . . . 1560
Retrovir IV Infusion . . . 1564
Retrovir Syrup . . . 1560
Retrovir Tablets . . . 1560

ZIDICEF (Mexico)
CEFTAZIDIME
Fortaz for Injection . . . 1453

ZIDIMA (Argentina)
CEFTAZIDIME
Fortaz for Injection . . . 1453

ZIDIS (Thailand)
ZIDOVUDINE
Retrovir Capsules . . . 1560
Retrovir IV Infusion . . . 1564
Retrovir Syrup . . . 1560
Retrovir Tablets . . . 1560

ZIDIX (Brazil)
ZIDOVUDINE
Retrovir Capsules . . . 1560
Retrovir IV Infusion . . . 1564
Retrovir Syrup . . . 1560
Retrovir Tablets . . . 1560

ZIDOLAM (Brazil)
LAMIVUDINE
Epivir Oral Solution . . . 1427
Epivir Tablets . . . 1427
Epivir-HBV Oral Solution . . . 1432
Epivir-HBV Tablets . . . 1432

ZIDOREX (India)
ZIDOVUDINE
Retrovir Capsules . . . 1560
Retrovir IV Infusion . . . 1564
Retrovir Syrup . . . 1560
Retrovir Tablets . . . 1560

ZIDOVAL (Denmark, Finland, Israel, Italy, Norway, Spain, Sweden, United Kingdom)
METRONIDAZOLE
MetroGel-Vaginal Gel . . . 1855

ZIDOVIR (Brazil, India, Mexico)
ZIDOVUDINE
Retrovir Capsules . . . 1560
Retrovir IV Infusion . . . 1564
Retrovir Syrup . . . 1560
Retrovir Tablets . . . 1560

ZIDOVUSAN (Brazil)
ZIDOVUDINE
Retrovir Capsules . . . 1560
Retrovir IV Infusion . . . 1564
Retrovir Syrup . . . 1560
Retrovir Tablets . . . 1560

ZIENAM (Austria)
CILASTATIN SODIUM/IMIPENEM
Primaxin I.M. . . . 2045
Primaxin I.V. . . . 2048

ZIFARTEL (Mexico)
PRAZIQUANTEL
Biltricide Tablets . . . 2976

ZILACTIN-L (Canada)
LIDOCAINE
Lidoderm Patch . . . 1118

ZILAK (Brazil)
RANITIDINE HYDROCHLORIDE
Zantac 25 EFFERdose Tablets . . . 1624
Zantac 150 EFFERdose Tablets . . . 1624
Zantac 150 Tablets . . . 1624
Zantac 300 Tablets . . . 1624
Zantac Injection . . . 1619
Zantac Injection Premixed . . . 1619
Zantac Syrup . . . 1624

ZILAST (India)
CILOSTAZOL
Pletal Tablets . . . 2455

ZILDEM (South Africa)
DILTIAZEM HYDROCHLORIDE
Cardizem LA Extended Release Tablets . . . 1728
Tiazac Capsules . . . 1201

ZILDEN (Greece, Italy)
DILTIAZEM HYDROCHLORIDE
Cardizem LA Extended Release Tablets . . . 1728
Tiazac Capsules . . . 1201

ZILION (India)
ZIDOVUDINE
Retrovir Capsules . . . 1560
Retrovir IV Infusion . . . 1564
Retrovir Syrup . . . 1560
Retrovir Tablets . . . 1560

ZILISTEN (Greece)
CEFUROXIME SODIUM
Zinacef Injection . . . 1631

ZIMMEX (Thailand)
SIMVASTATIN
Zocor Tablets . . . 2105

ZIMSTAT (Australia)
SIMVASTATIN
Zocor Tablets . . . 2105

ZINACEF (Belgium, Brazil, Canada, Czech Republic, Denmark, Finland, Germany, Greece, Hong Kong, Hungary, Irish Republic, Israel, Malaysia, New Zealand, Norway, Russia, Singapore, South Africa, Sweden, Switzerland, Thailand, The Netherlands, United Kingdom, Venezuela)
CEFUROXIME SODIUM
Zinacef Injection . . . 1631

ZINADIUR (Italy)
BENAZEPRIL HYDROCHLORIDE/HYDROCHLOROTHIAZIDE
Lotensin HCT Tablets . . . 2246

ZINADOL (Greece)
CEFUROXIME AXETIL
Ceftin Tablets . . . 1407
Ceftin for Oral Suspension . . . 1407

ZINADRIL (Italy)
BENAZEPRIL HYDROCHLORIDE
Lotensin Tablets . . . 2243

ZINAT (Switzerland)
CEFUROXIME AXETIL
Ceftin Tablets . . . 1407
Ceftin for Oral Suspension . . . 1407

ZINCO SULPHA (India)
SULFACETAMIDE SODIUM
Klaron Lotion 10% . . . 2909

ZINECARD (Canada)
DEXRAZOXANE
Zinecard for Injection . . . 2650

ZINERYT (Belgium, Czech Republic, Hungary, Irish Republic, Portugal, South Africa, Spain)
ERYTHROMYCIN
Ery-Tab Tablets . . . 449
Erythromycin Base Filmtab Tablets . . . 455
Erythromycin Delayed-Release Capsules, USP . . . 457
PCE Dispertab Tablets . . . 515

ZINETAC (India)
RANITIDINE HYDROCHLORIDE
Zantac 25 EFFERdose Tablets . . . 1624
Zantac 150 EFFERdose Tablets . . . 1624
Zantac 150 Tablets . . . 1624
Zantac 300 Tablets . . . 1624
Zantac Injection . . . 1619
Zantac Injection Premixed . . . 1619
Zantac Syrup . . . 1624

ZINNAT (Australia, Austria, Belgium, Brazil, Chile, Czech Republic, Denmark, Finland, Germany, Hong Kong, Hungary, Irish Republic, Israel, Italy, Malaysia, New Zealand, Russia, Singapore, South Africa, Spain, Sweden, Thailand, The Netherlands, United Kingdom, Venezuela)
CEFUROXIME AXETIL
Ceftin Tablets . . . 1407
Ceftin for Oral Suspension . . . 1407

ZINOCEP (Italy)
CEFUROXIME SODIUM
Zinacef Injection . . . 1631

ZINOPRIL (Brazil)
LISINOPRIL
Prinivil Tablets . . . 2052

ZIPOS (Portugal)
CEFUROXIME AXETIL
Ceftin Tablets . . . 1407
Ceftin for Oral Suspension . . . 1407

ZIPRA (Mexico)
CIPROFLOXACIN HYDROCHLORIDE
Ciloxan Ophthalmic Ointment . . . ⊙204, 559
Ciloxan Ophthalmic Solution . . . ⊙206
Cipro Tablets . . . 2977

ZIPRAX (India)
CEFIXIME
Suprax . . . 1843

ZIPTEK (Greece)
CETIRIZINE HYDROCHLORIDE
Zyrtec Syrup . . . 2594
Zyrtec Tablets . . . 2594

ZIREMEX (Greece)
NIMODIPINE
Nimotop Capsules . . . 749

ZIRPINE (Irish Republic)
CETIRIZINE HYDROCHLORIDE
Zyrtec Syrup . . . 2594
Zyrtec Tablets . . . 2594

ZIRTEC (Italy)
CETIRIZINE HYDROCHLORIDE
Zyrtec Syrup . . . 2594
Zyrtec Tablets . . . 2594

ZIRTEK (Austria, Greece, Irish Republic, United Kingdom)
CETIRIZINE HYDROCHLORIDE
Zyrtec Syrup . . . 2594
Zyrtec Tablets . . . 2594

ZIZ (United Kingdom)
PROMETHAZINE HYDROCHLORIDE
Phenergan Tablets and Suppositories . . . 3440

ZNUPRIL (Greece)
CETIRIZINE HYDROCHLORIDE
Zyrtec Syrup . . . 2594
Zyrtec Tablets . . . 2594

ZOBACIDE (South Africa)
METRONIDAZOLE
MetroGel-Vaginal Gel . . . 1855

ZOBEN (Malaysia)
ALBENDAZOLE
Albenza Tablets . . . 1338

ZOCOLIP (Denmark)
SIMVASTATIN
Zocor Tablets . . . 2105

ZOCOR (Argentina, Australia, Belgium, Brazil, Canada, Chile, Czech Republic, Denmark, Finland, France, Germany, Greece, Hong Kong, Hungary, Irish Republic, Italy, Malaysia, Mexico, New Zealand, Norway, Portugal, Russia, Singapore, South Africa, Spain, Switzerland, Thailand, The Netherlands, United Kingdom, Venezuela)
SIMVASTATIN
Zocor Tablets . . . 2105

ZOCORD (Austria, Sweden)
SIMVASTATIN
Zocor Tablets . . . 2105

ZODAC (Czech Republic)
CETIRIZINE HYDROCHLORIDE
Zyrtec Syrup . . . 2594
Zyrtec Tablets . . . 2594

ZODERM (India)
OXICONAZOLE NITRATE
Oxistat Cream . . . 2667
Oxistat Lotion . . . 2667

ZODOL (Chile)
TRAMADOL HYDROCHLORIDE
Ultram ER Tablets . . . 2392

ZOFLUT (India)
FLUTICASONE PROPIONATE
Cutivate Cream . . . 2662
Cutivate Ointment . . . 2665
Flonase Nasal Spray . . . 1440

ZOFRAN (Argentina, Australia, Belgium, Brazil, Czech Republic, Germany, Hong Kong, Hungary, Irish Republic, Israel, Italy, Malaysia, Mexico, New Zealand, Norway, Portugal, Russia, Singapore, South Africa, Spain, Sweden, Switzerland, The Netherlands, United Kingdom, Venezuela)
ONDANSETRON HYDROCHLORIDE
Zofran Injection . . . 1634
Zofran Injection Premixed . . . 1634
Zofran Oral Solution . . . 1639
Zofran Tablets . . . 1639

ZOFRON (Greece)
ONDANSETRON HYDROCHLORIDE
Zofran Injection . . . 1634
Zofran Injection Premixed . . . 1634
Zofran Oral Solution . . . 1639
Zofran Tablets . . . 1639

ZOLAPIN (Brazil)
CLOZAPINE
Clozaril Tablets . . . 2184

ZOLBEN (Brazil)
ALBENDAZOLE
Albenza Tablets . . . 1338

ZOLDAN (Brazil)
ALBENDAZOLE
Albenza Tablets . . . 1338

ZOLEROL (South Africa)
METRONIDAZOLE
MetroGel-Vaginal Gel . . . 1855

ZOLIDEN (Greece)
RANITIDINE HYDROCHLORIDE
Zantac 25 EFFERdose Tablets . . . 1624
Zantac 150 EFFERdose Tablets . . . 1624
Zantac 150 Tablets . . . 1624
Zantac 300 Tablets . . . 1624
Zantac Injection . . . 1619
Zantac Injection Premixed . . . 1619
Zantac Syrup . . . 1624

ZOLINA (Venezuela)
CIPROFLOXACIN
Cipro Oral Suspension . . . 2977

ZOLOFT (Argentina, Australia, Austria, Brazil, Canada, Czech Republic, Denmark, Finland, France, Greece, Hong Kong, Hungary, Italy, Malaysia, New Zealand, Portugal, Russia, Singapore, South Africa, Sweden, Switzerland, Thailand, The Netherlands, Venezuela)
SERTRALINE HYDROCHLORIDE
Zoloft Tablets . . . 2586

ZOLT (Finland)
LANSOPRAZOLE
Prevacid Delayed-Release Capsules . . . 3271

ZOLTEROL (Malaysia, Singapore)
DICLOFENAC SODIUM
Voltaren Tablets **2307**
Voltaren-XR Tablets **2310**

ZOLVERA (United Kingdom)
VERAPAMIL HYDROCHLORIDE
Covera-HS Tablets **3139**
Verelan PM Extended-Release Capsules, Controlled-Onset **3106**

ZOMORPH (United Kingdom)
MORPHINE SULFATE
Kadian Capsules **577**
MS Contin Tablets **2701**

ZONAKER (Mexico)
SODIUM HYALURONATE
Hyalgan Solution **2901**

ZONATIAN (Argentina)
ISOTRETINOIN
Accutane Capsules **2731**

ZOPAM (Thailand)
DIAZEPAM
Diastat Rectal Delivery System **3343**
Valium Tablets **2819**

ZOPIROL (Argentina)
TIMOLOL MALEATE
Blocadren Tablets **1916**
Timoptic Sterile Ophthalmic Solution **2088**
Timoptic in Ocudose **2091**
Timoptic-XE Sterile Ophthalmic Gel Forming Solution **2092**

ZORAIL (Spain)
ENALAPRIL MALEATE
Vasotec I.V. Injection **2103**

ZORAN (Russia, Singapore, Venezuela)
RANITIDINE HYDROCHLORIDE
Zantac 25 EFFERdose Tablets **1624**
Zantac 150 EFFERdose Tablets. **1624**
Zantac 150 Tablets **1624**
Zantac 300 Tablets **1624**
Zantac Injection **1619**
Zantac Injection Premixed **1619**
Zantac Syrup **1624**

ZORCED (Mexico)
SIMVASTATIN
Zocor Tablets. **2105**

ZOREF (Italy, Portugal)
CEFUROXIME AXETIL
Ceftin Tablets. **1407**
Ceftin for Oral Suspension. **1407**

ZOROXIN (Austria, Belgium, Denmark)
NORFLOXACIN
Noroxin Tablets. **2032**

ZOTON (Australia, Irish Republic, Israel, Italy, New Zealand, United Kingdom)
LANSOPRAZOLE
Prevacid Delayed-Release Capsules **3271**

ZUMALGIC (France)
TRAMADOL HYDROCHLORIDE
Ultram ER Tablets **2392**

ZUMENON (Australia, Austria, Belgium, Finland, Portugal, Switzerland, The Netherlands, United Kingdom)
ESTRADIOL
Climara Transdermal System **771**
Estring Vaginal Ring **2635**

ZURFIX (Greece)
RANITIDINE HYDROCHLORIDE
Zantac 25 EFFERdose Tablets **1624**
Zantac 150 EFFERdose Tablets. **1624**
Zantac 150 Tablets **1624**
Zantac 300 Tablets **1624**
Zantac Injection **1619**
Zantac Injection Premixed **1619**
Zantac Syrup **1624**

ZUROCID (Greece)
SIMVASTATIN
Zocor Tablets. **2105**

ZUVAIR (India)
ZAFIRLUKAST
Accolate Tablets **671**

ZYBAN (Australia, Austria, Belgium, Brazil, Canada, Czech Republic, Denmark, Finland, France, Germany, Greece, Hong Kong, Hungary, India, Irish Republic, Israel, Italy, New Zealand, Norway, Portugal, Singapore, South Africa, Sweden, Switzerland, The Netherlands, United Kingdom, Venezuela)
BUPROPION HYDROCHLORIDE
Wellbutrin SR Sustained-Release Tablets . . **1607**
Wellbutrin Tablets **1603**
Zyban Sustained-Release Tablets. **1644**

ZYCEL (India)
CELECOXIB
Celebrex Capsules. **3134**

ZYDOL (Australia, Irish Republic, United Kingdom)
TRAMADOL HYDROCHLORIDE
Ultram ER Tablets **2392**

ZYDOWIN (India)
ZIDOVUDINE
Retrovir Capsules **1560**
Retrovir IV Infusion. **1564**
Retrovir Syrup **1560**
Retrovir Tablets. **1560**

ZYGIUM (Mexico)
CALCITRIOL
Calcijex Injection **411**
Rocaltrol Capsules. **2798**
Rocaltrol Oral Solution **2798**

ZYLIUM (Brazil)
RANITIDINE HYDROCHLORIDE
Zantac 25 EFFERdose Tablets **1624**
Zantac 150 EFFERdose Tablets. **1624**
Zantac 150 Tablets **1624**
Zantac 300 Tablets **1624**
Zantac Injection **1619**
Zantac Injection Premixed **1619**
Zantac Syrup **1624**

ZYLLERGY (Israel)
CETIRIZINE HYDROCHLORIDE
Zyrtec Syrup **2594**
Zyrtec Tablets **2594**

ZYMED (Thailand)
CETIRIZINE HYDROCHLORIDE
Zyrtec Syrup **2594**
Zyrtec Tablets **2594**

ZYNACE (Malaysia)
ENALAPRIL MALEATE
Vasotec I.V. Injection **2103**

ZYNAL (Singapore)
NAPROXEN SODIUM
Anaprox DS Tablets **2761**
Anaprox Tablets **2761**

ZYNOR (Irish Republic)
CETIRIZINE HYDROCHLORIDE
Zyrtec Syrup **2594**
Zyrtec Tablets **2594**

ZYNTABAC (Spain, The Netherlands)
BUPROPION HYDROCHLORIDE
Wellbutrin SR Sustained-Release Tablets . . **1607**
Wellbutrin Tablets **1603**
Zyban Sustained-Release Tablets. **1644**

ZYOMET (United Kingdom)
METRONIDAZOLE
MetroGel-Vaginal Gel **1855**

ZYPREXA (Argentina, Australia, Austria, Belgium, Brazil, Canada, Chile, Czech Republic, Denmark, Finland, France, Germany, Greece, Hong Kong, Hungary, Irish Republic, Israel, Italy, Malaysia, Mexico, New Zealand, Norway, Portugal, Russia, Singapore, South Africa, Spain, Sweden, Switzerland, Thailand, The Netherlands, United Kingdom, Venezuela)
OLANZAPINE
Zyprexa Tablets **1830**

ZYRAC (Thailand)
CETIRIZINE HYDROCHLORIDE
Zyrtec Syrup **2594**
Zyrtec Tablets **2594**

ZYRAZINE (Thailand)
CETIRIZINE HYDROCHLORIDE
Zyrtec Syrup **2594**
Zyrtec Tablets **2594**

ZYRCON (Thailand)
CETIRIZINE HYDROCHLORIDE
Zyrtec Syrup **2594**
Zyrtec Tablets **2594**

ZYREX (Thailand)
CETIRIZINE HYDROCHLORIDE
Zyrtec Syrup **2594**
Zyrtec Tablets **2594**

ZYRLEX (Sweden)
CETIRIZINE HYDROCHLORIDE
Zyrtec Syrup **2594**
Zyrtec Tablets **2594**

ZYRTEC (Argentina, Australia, Austria, Belgium, Brazil, Canada, Chile, Czech Republic, Denmark, Finland, France, Germany, Hong Kong, Hungary, India, Israel, Japan, Malaysia, Mexico, New Zealand, Norway, Portugal, Russia, Singapore, South Africa, Spain, Switzerland, Thailand, The Netherlands, Venezuela)
CETIRIZINE HYDROCHLORIDE
Zyrtec Syrup **2594**
Zyrtec Tablets **2594**

ZYRZINE (Thailand)
CETIRIZINE HYDROCHLORIDE
Zyrtec Syrup **2594**
Zyrtec Tablets **2594**

ZYTAZ (India)
CEFTAZIDIME
Fortaz for Injection **1453**

ZYTINE (Thailand)
CETIRIZINE HYDROCHLORIDE
Zyrtec Syrup **2594**
Zyrtec Tablets **2594**

ZYTRAM (New Zealand, Spain)
TRAMADOL HYDROCHLORIDE
Ultram ER Tablets **2392**

SECTION 7

GENERIC AVAILABILITY GUIDE

This section allows you to quickly determine which forms and strengths of a brand-name drug are also available generically. The entries are organized alphabetically by brand name and dosage form, with strengths in ascending order. Generic availability is indicated by a mark in the "Yes" column. Included are all prescription products described in *PDR®* and *PDR for Ophthalmic Medicines™*. Generic availability information is drawn from the *Red Book® Drug Database* maintained by *PDR*'s parent organization, Thomson Healthcare.

STRENGTH	GENERIC YES	GENERIC NO
Abelcet Injection		
5 mg/ml	■	
Abilify Tablets		
5 mg		■
10 mg		■
15 mg		■
20 mg		■
30 mg		■
5 mg		■
10 mg		■
15 mg		■
30 mg		■
Accolate Tablets		
10 mg		■
20 mg		■
AccuNeb Inhalation Solution		
0.021%		■
0.042%	■	
Accutane Capsules		
10 mg	■	
20 mg	■	
40 mg	■	
Accuzyme Debriding Ointment		
1.1 million u/gm-100 mg/	■	
Accuzyme SE Spray Emulsion		
830000 u/gm-10%		■
Aceon Tablets		
2 mg		■
4 mg		■
8 mg		■
Acetadote Injection		
200 mg/ml		■
Aclovate Cream		
0.05%	■	
Actimmune		
2 million iu/0.5 ml		■
Actiq		
0.2 mg		■
0.4 mg		■
0.6 mg		■
0.8 mg		■
1.2 mg		■
1.6 mg		■
Activase I.V.		
20 mg		■
50 mg		■
100 mg		■
Actonel Tablets		
5 mg		■
30 mg		■
35 mg		■
Actos Tablets		
15 mg		■
30 mg		■
45 mg		■
Acular Ophthalmic Solution		
0.5%		■
Acular LS Ophthalmic Solution		
0.4%		■
ADACEL Vaccine		
2 lf u/0.5 ml-2.5 mcg/0		■
Adalat CC Tablets		
30 mg	■	
60 mg	■	
90 mg	■	
Adderall Tablets		
5 mg	■	
7.5 mg	■	
10 mg	■	
12.5 mg	■	
15 mg	■	
20 mg	■	
30 mg	■	
Adderall XR Capsules		
5 mg		■
10 mg		■
15 mg		■
20 mg		■
25 mg		■
30 mg		■
Adenocard Injection		
3 mg/ml	■	
Adenoscan		
3 mg/ml	■	
Adipex-P Capsules		
37.5 mg	■	
Adipex-P Tablets		
37.5 mg	■	
Advair Diskus 100/50		
0.1 mg/actuation-0.05 mg		■
Advair Diskus 250/50		
0.25 mg/actuation-0.05 m		■
Advair Diskus 500/50		
0.5 mg/actuation-0.05 mg		■
Advair HFA Inhalation Aerosol		
45 mcg/actuation-30.45 m		■
115 mcg/actuation-30.45		■
230 mcg/actuation-30.45		■
Advate Injection		
1 iu		■
Advicor Tablets		
20 mg-1000 mg		■
20 mg-500 mg		■
20 mg-750 mg		■
Aerobid Inhaler System		
0.25 mg/actuation		■
Aerobid-M Inhaler System		
0.25 mg/actuation		■
Agenerase Capsules		
50 mg		■
150 mg		■
Agenerase Oral Solution		
15 mg/ml		■
Aggrastat Injection		
0.05 mg/ml		■
0.25 mg/ml		■
Aggrastat Injection Premixed		
0.05 mg/ml		■
Aggrenox Capsules		
25 mg-200 mg		■
Agrylin Capsules		
0.5 mg	■	
1 mg	■	
Alamast Ophthalmic Solution		
0.1%		■
0.1%		■
Albalon Ophthalmic Solution		
0.1%	■	
Albenza Tablets		
200 mg		■
Albutein 5%, Albumin (Human)		
5%	■	
Albutein 25% , Albumin (Human)		
25%	■	

STRENGTH	GENERIC YES	GENERIC NO
Aldara Cream, 5%		
5%		■
Aldoril Tablets		
15 mg-250 mg	■	
25 mg-250 mg	■	
Aldurazyme for Intravenous Infusion		
0.58 mg/ml		■
Alferon N Injection		
5 million iu/ml		■
Alimta for Injection		
500 mg		■
Alinia for Oral Suspension		
100 mg/5 ml		■
Alinia Tablets		
500 mg		■
Allegra Capsules		
60 mg	■	
Allegra Tablets		
30 mg	■	
60 mg	■	
180 mg	■	
Allegra-D 24 Hour Extended-Release Tablets		
180 mg-240 mg		■
Allegra-D Extended Release Tablets		
60 mg-120 mg	■	
Aloprim for Injection		
500 mg	■	
Aloxi Injection		
0.05 mg/ml		■
Alphagan P Ophthalmic Solution		
0.15%		■
Alphanate, Antihemophilic Factor (Human)		
1 iu	■	
AlphaNine SD, Coagulation Factor IX (Human)		
1 iu	■	
Alrex Ophthalmic Suspension		
0.2%		■
Altace Capsules		
1.25 mg		■
2.5 mg		■
5 mg		■
10 mg		■
Altoprev Extended-Release Tablets		
10 mg		■
20 mg		■
40 mg		■
60 mg		■
Alupent Inhalation Aerosol		
0.4%	■	
0.6%	■	
0.65 mg/actuation	■	
Ambien Tablets		
5 mg		■
10 mg		■
Ambien CR Tablets		
6.25 mg		■
12.5 mg		■
AmBisome for Injection		
50 mg		■
Amerge Tablets		
1 mg		■
2.5 mg		■
Aminohippurate Sodium PAH Injection		
20%		■
Amitiza Capsules		
24 mcg		■
Amoxil Capsules		
250 mg	■	
500 mg	■	
Amoxil Chewable Tablets		
125 mg	■	
200 mg	■	
250 mg	■	
400 mg	■	
Amoxil Pediatric Drops for Oral Suspension		
50 mg/ml	■	
125 mg/5 ml	■	
200 mg/5 ml	■	
250 mg/5 ml	■	
400 mg/5 ml	■	
Amoxil Powder for Oral Suspension		
125 mg/5 ml	■	
200 mg/5 ml	■	
250 mg/5 ml	■	
400 mg/5 ml	■	
Amoxil Tablets/Capsules		
250 mg	■	
500 mg	■	
875 mg	■	
Analpram HC Cream, 1% and 2.5%		
1%-1%	■	
2.5%-1%	■	
Analpram HC Lotion, 2.5%		
2.5%-1%	■	
Anaprox Tablets		
275 mg	■	
Anaprox DS Tablets		
550 mg	■	
AndroGel		
1%	■	
Antivenin (Black Widow Spider Antivenin)		
6000 u		■
Anzemet Injection		
20 mg/ml	■	
Anzemet Tablets		
50 mg		■
100 mg		■
Apexicon E Cream		
0.05%	■	
Appearex Tablets		
2.5 mg	■	
Aptivus Capsules		
250 mg		■
Aralast		
1 mg	■	
Aranesp for Injection		
0.025 mg/ml		■
0.04 mg/ml		■
0.06 mg/0.3 ml		■
0.06 mg/ml		■
0.1 mg/ml		■
0.15 mg/0.75 ml		■
0.2 mg/ml		■
0.3 mg/ml		■
Aredia for Injection		
30 mg	■	
60 mg		■
90 mg	■	
Argatroban Injection		
100 mg/ml		■
Aricept ODT Tablets		
5 mg		■
10 mg		■
Arimidex Tablets		
1 mg		■
Aromasin Tablets		
25 mg		■
Arranon Injection		
5 mg/ml		■
Arthrotec Tablets		
50 mg-0.2 mg		■
75 mg-0.2 mg		■
Asacol Delayed-Release Tablets		
400 mg		■
Astelin Nasal Spray		
137 mcg/actuation		■
Atacand Tablets		
4 mg		■
8 mg		■
16 mg		■
32 mg		■
Atacand HCT		
16 mg-12.5 mg		■
32 mg-12.5 mg		■
Atripla Tablets		
600 mg-200 mg-300 mg		■
Atrovent Inhalation Solution		
0.02%	■	
Atrovent HFA Inhalation Aerosol		
0.017 mg/actuation		■
Atrovent Nasal Spray 0.03%		
0.03%	■	
Atrovent Nasal Spray 0.06%		
0.06%	■	
Attenuvax		
1000 tcid50		■
Augmentin Chewable Tablets		
125 mg-31.25 mg		■
200 mg-28.5 mg	■	
250 mg-62.5 mg		■
400 mg-57 mg	■	
Augmentin Powder for Oral Suspension		
125 mg/5 ml-31.25 mg/5 m		■
200 mg/5 ml-28.5 mg/5 ml	■	
250 mg/5 ml-62.5 mg/5 ml		■
400 mg/5 ml-57 mg/5 ml	■	
Augmentin Tablets		
250 mg-125 mg		■
500 mg-125 mg	■	
875 mg-125 mg	■	
Augmentin XR Extended-Release Tablets		
1000 mg-62.5 mg		■
Augmentin ES-600 Powder for Oral Suspension		
600 mg/5 ml-42.9 mg/5 ml	■	
Avalide Tablets		
12.5 mg-150 mg		■
12.5 mg-300 mg		■
Avandamet Tablets		
500 mg-1 mg		■
500 mg-2 mg		■
500 mg-4 mg		■
1000 mg-2 mg		■
1000 mg-4 mg		■
Avandaryl Tablets		
1 mg-4 mg		■
2 mg-4 mg		■
4 mg-4 mg		■
Avandia Tablets		
2 mg		■
4 mg		■
8 mg		■
Avapro Tablets		
75 mg		■
150 mg		■
300 mg		■
Avar Cleanser		
10%-5%	■	
Avar Gel		
10%-5%	■	
Avar Green Gel		
10%-5%	■	
Avastin IV		
25 mg/ml		■
Avelox Tablets		
400 mg		■
Avinza Capsules		
30 mg		■
60 mg		■
90 mg		■
120 mg		■
Avodart Soft Gelatin Capsules		
0.5 mg		■
Axert Tablets		
6.25 mg		■
12.5 mg		■
Axid Oral Solution		
150 mg	■	
300 mg	■	
Azilect Tablets		
0.5 mg		■
1 mg		■
Azopt Ophthalmic Suspension		
1%		■
1%		■
Bactroban Cream		
2%		■
Bactroban Nasal		
2%		■
Bactroban Ointment		
2%	■	
Baraclude Tablets		
0.5 mg		■
Beconase AQ Nasal Spray		
0.042 mg/actuation		■
BeneFIX Vials		
1 iu		■
Benicar Tablets		
5 mg		■
20 mg		■
40 mg		■
Benicar HCT Tablets		
12.5 mg-20 mg		■
12.5 mg-40 mg		■
25 mg-40 mg		■
Benzaclin Topical Gel		
5%-1%	■	
Betadine 5% Ophthalmic Solution		
5%	■	
Betagan Ophthalmic Solution, USP		
0.25%	■	
0.5%	■	
Betaseron for SC Injection		
0.3 mg		■
Betimol Ophthalmic Solution		
0.25%		■
0.5%		■
Betoptic S Ophthalmic Suspension		
0.25%		■
Biaxin Filmtab Tablets		
250 mg		■
500 mg		■
Biaxin XL Filmtab Tablets		
500 mg		■
Biaxin Granules		
125 mg/5 ml		■
187.5 mg/5 ml		■
250 mg/5 ml		■
BiDil Tablets		
37.5 mg-20 mg		■
Biltricide Tablets		
600 mg		■
Bleph-10 Ophthalmic Solution 10%		
10%	■	
Blephamide Ophthalmic Ointment		
0.2%-10%		■

STRENGTH	GENERIC YES	GENERIC NO
Blephamide Ophthalmic Suspension		
0.2%-10%		■
Blephamide Sterile Ophthalmic Ointment		
0.2%-10%		■
Blephamide Ophthalmic Suspension		
0.2%-10%		■
Blocadren Tablets		
5 mg	■	
10 mg	■	
20 mg	■	
Boniva Tablets		
2.5 mg		■
150 mg		■
Boostrix		
2.5 lf u/0.5 ml-18.5 mcg		■
BOTOX Purified Neurotoxin Complex		
100 u		■
Brevoxyl-4 Creamy Wash		
4%		■
Brevoxyl-4 Gel		
4%		■
Brevoxyl-8 Creamy Wash		
8%		■
Brevoxyl-8 Gel		
8%		■
Brimonidine Tartrate Ophthalmic Solution 0.2%		
0.2%	■	
Bumex Tablets		
0.25 mg/ml	■	
0.5 mg	■	
1 mg	■	
2 mg	■	
Buprenex Injectable		
0.3 mg/ml	■	
Byetta Injection		
250 mcg/ml		■
Caduet Tablets		
2.5 mg-10 mg		■
2.5 mg-20 mg		■
2.5 mg-40 mg		■
5 mg-10 mg		■
5 mg-20 mg		■
5 mg-40 mg		■
5 mg-80 mg		■
10 mg-10 mg		■
10 mg-20 mg		■
10 mg-40 mg		■
10 mg-80 mg		■
Calcijex Injection		
1 mcg/ml	■	
2 mcg/ml	■	
Calcium Disodium Versenate Injection		
200 mg/ml		■
Campath Ampules		
10 mg/ml		■
Camptosar Injection		
20 mg/ml		■
Canasa Rectal Suppositories		
500 mg	■	
Cancidas for Injection		
50 mg		■
70 mg		■
Captopril Tablets		
12.5 mg	■	
25 mg	■	
50 mg	■	
100 mg	■	
Carac Cream, 0.5%		
0.5%		■
Carafate Suspension		
1 gm/10 ml	■	
Carafate Tablets		
1 gm	■	
Carbatrol Capsules		
100 mg		■
200 mg		■
300 mg		■
Cardene I.V.		
2.5 mg/ml		■
Cardizem Injection		
25 mg/vial		■
Cardizem LA Extended Release Tablets		
120 mg		■
180 mg		■
240 mg		■
300 mg		■
360 mg		■
420 mg		■
Carnitor Injection		
100 mg/ml		■
200 mg/ml	■	
Carnitor Tablets and Oral Solution		
100 mg/ml		■
330 mg	■	
Carteolol Hydrochloride Ophthalmic Solution USP, 1%		
1%	■	
Catapres Tablets		
0.1 mg	■	
0.2 mg	■	
0.3 mg	■	
Catapres-TTS		
0.1 mg/24 hr		■
0.2 mg/24 hr		■
0.3 mg/24 hr		■
Cathflo Activase		
2 mg		■
Caverject Impulse Injection		
10 mcg	■	
20 mcg	■	
Ceftin for Oral Suspension		
125 mg/5 ml		■
250 mg/5 ml		■
Ceftin Tablets		
125 mg	■	
250 mg	■	
500 mg	■	
Celebrex Capsules		
100 mg		■
200 mg		■
400 mg		■
Celexa Oral Solution		
10 mg/5 ml	■	
Celexa Tablets		
10 mg	■	
20 mg	■	
40 mg	■	
CellCept Capsules		
250 mg		■
CellCept Intravenous		
500 mg		■
CellCept Oral Suspension		
200 mg/ml		■
CellCept Tablets		
500 mg		■
Cerezyme for Injection		
200 u		■
400 u		■
Cervidil Vaginal Insert		
0.3 mg/hr		■
Cesamet Capsules		
1 mg		■
Cetacaine Topical Anesthetic		
14%-2%-2%		■
Chantix Tablets		
0.5 mg		■
1 mg		■
Chemet Capsules		
100 mg		■
Cialis Tablets		
5 mg		■
10 mg		■
20 mg		■
Ciloxan Ophthalmic Ointment		
0.3%	■	
0.3%		■
Ciloxan Ophthalmic Solution		
0.3%	■	
Cipro Oral Suspension		
250 mg/5 ml		■
500 mg/5 ml		■
Cipro Tablets		
100 mg		■
250 mg	■	
500 mg	■	
750 mg	■	
Cipro XR Tablets		
500 mg		■
1000 mg		■
Citracal Prenatal + DHA Tablets and Capsules		
120 mg-125 mg-2 mg-250 m		■
Citracal Prenatal Rx Tablets		
120 mg-125 mg-2 mg-50 mg	■	
Clarinex Syrup		
0.5 mg/ml		■
Clarinex Tablets		
5 mg		■
Clarinex-D 24-Hour Extended-Release Tablets		
5 mg-240 mg		■
Claripel Cream		
4%	■	
Cleocin Vaginal Ovules		
75 mg	■	
150 mg	■	
300 mg	■	
Climara Transdermal System		
0.025 mg/24 hr	■	
0.0375 mg/24 hr	■	
0.05 mg/24 hr	■	
0.06 mg/24 hr		■
0.075 mg/24 hr	■	
0.1 mg/24 hr	■	
Clindagel		
1%	■	
Clinoril Tablets		
1 mg/ml		■
150 mg	■	
200 mg	■	
Clobevate Gel		
0.05%	■	
Clobex Spray		
0.05%		■
Clolar for Intravenous Infusion		
1 mg/ml		■
Clorpres Tablets		
15 mg-0.1 mg	■	
15 mg-0.2 mg	■	
15 mg-0.3 mg	■	
Clozaril Tablets		
25 mg	■	
100 mg	■	
Colazal Capsules		
750 mg		■
Colyte with Flavor Packs for Oral Solution		
240 gm-2.98 gm-6.72 gm-5	■	
Combivent Inhalation Aerosol		
0.09 mg/actuation-0.018		■
Combivir Tablets		
150 mg-300 mg		■
Comtan Tablets		
200 mg		■
Comvax		
7.5 mcg/0.5 ml-5 mcg/0.5		■
Concerta Extended-Release Tablets		
18 mg		■
27 mg		■
36 mg		■
54 mg		■
Copaxone for Injection		
20 mg/ml		■
Copegus Tablets		
200 mg	■	
Coreg Tablets		
3.125 mg		■
6.25 mg		■
12.5 mg		■
25 mg		■
Cosopt Sterile Ophthalmic Solution		
2%-0.5%		■
Coumadin for Injection		
5 mg		■
Coumadin Tablets		
1 mg	■	
2 mg	■	
2.5 mg	■	
3 mg	■	
4 mg	■	
5 mg	■	
6 mg	■	
7.5 mg	■	
10 mg	■	
Covera-HS Tablets		
180 mg		■
240 mg		■
Cozaar Tablets		
25 mg		■
50 mg		■
100 mg		■
Creon 5 Capsules		
16600 u-5000 u-18750 u	■	
Creon 10 Capsules		
33200 u-10000 u-37500 u	■	
Creon 20 Capsules		
66400 u-20000 u-75000 u	■	
Crixivan Capsules		
100 mg		■
200 mg		■
333 mg		■
400 mg		■
Cubicin for Injection		
500 mg		■
Cuprimine Capsules		
125 mg		■
250 mg		■
Curosurf Intratracheal Suspension		
80 mg/ml		■
Cutivate Cream		
0.05%	■	
Cutivate Ointment		
0.005%	■	
Cytomel Tablets		
0.005 mg		■
0.025 mg		■
0.05 mg		■
Dacogen Injection		
50 mg		■
Dalmane Capsules		
15 mg	■	
30 mg	■	
Dantrium Capsules		
25 mg	■	
50 mg	■	
100 mg	■	
Dapsone Tablets USP		
25 mg		■
100 mg		■
DAPTACEL Vaccine		
15 lf u/0.5 ml-23 mcg/0		■
Daranide Tablets		
50 mg		■

STRENGTH	GENERIC YES	GENERIC NO
Daraprim Tablets		
25 mg		■
Daytrana Transdermal Patch		
10 mg/9 hr		■
15 mg/9 hr		■
20 mg/9 hr		■
30 mg/9 hr		■
Decadron Tablets		
0.5 mg	■	
0.75 mg	■	
4 mg	■	
Demadex Injection		
10 mg/ml		■
Demadex Tablets		
5 mg	■	
10 mg	■	
10 mg/ml		■
20 mg	■	
100 mg	■	
Demser Capsules		
250 mg		■
Denavir Cream		
1%		■
Depacon Injection		
100 mg/ml	■	
Depakene Capsules		
250 mg	■	
Depakene Oral Solution		
250 mg/5 ml	■	
Depakote Sprinkle Capsules		
125 mg		■
Depakote Tablets		
125 mg		■
250 mg		■
500 mg		■
Depakote ER Tablets		
250 mg		■
500 mg		■
DepoCyt Injection		
10 mg/ml		■
DepoDur Extended-Release Injection		
10 mg/ml		■
Depo-Medrol Injectable Suspension		
20 mg/ml	■	
40 mg/ml	■	
80 mg/ml	■	
Depo-Medrol Single-Dose Vial		
400 mg/ml		■
Desoxyn Tablets, USP		
15 mg		■
Detrol Tablets		
1 mg		■
2 mg		■
Detrol LA Capsules		
2 mg		■
4 mg		■
Dexedrine Spansule Capsules		
5 mg	■	
10 mg	■	
15 mg	■	
Dexedrine Tablets		
5 mg	■	
DextroStat Tablets		
5 mg	■	
10 mg	■	
Diastat Rectal Delivery System		
15 mg	■	
Dibenzyline Capsules		
10 mg		■
Didronel Tablets		
200 mg	■	
400 mg	■	
Differin Cream		
0.1%		■
Differin Gel		
0.1%		■
Digibind for Injection		
38 mg		■
Dilaudid Ampules		
1 mg/ml	■	
2 mg/ml	■	
4 mg/ml	■	
Dilaudid Multiple Dose Vials		
2 mg/ml	■	
Dilaudid Oral Liquid		
1 mg/ml	■	
Dilaudid Rectal Suppositories		
3 mg	■	
Dilaudid Tablets		
2 mg	■	
4 mg	■	
Dilaudid Tablets - 8 mg		
8 mg	■	
Dilaudid-HP Injection		
10 mg/ml	■	
Dilaudid-HP Lyophilized Powder 250 mg		
250 mg		■
Diovan Tablets		
40 mg		■
80 mg		■
160 mg		■
320 mg		■
Diovan HCT Tablets		
12.5 mg-160 mg		■
12.5 mg-80 mg		■
25 mg-160 mg		■
Diprolene Gel 0.05%		
0.05%	■	
Diprolene Lotion 0.05%		
0.05%		■
Diprolene Ointment 0.05%		
0.05%	■	
Diprolene AF Cream 0.05%		
0.05%	■	
Diprosone Cream, USP 0.05%		
0.05%	■	
Ditropan XL Extended-Release Tablets		
5 mg	■	
10 mg	■	
15 mg	■	
Diuril Oral Suspension		
250 mg/5 ml		■
Diuril Sodium Intravenous		
0.5 gm		■
Dolobid Tablets		
250 mg	■	
500 mg	■	
Donnatal Extentabs		
0.0582 mg-0.3111 mg-48.6	■	
Doxil Injection		
2 mg/ml		■
Drysol Solution		
20%	■	
Duac Topical Gel		
5%-1%	■	
DuoNeb Inhalation Solution		
3 mg/3 ml-0.5 mg/3 ml		■
Duragesic Transdermal System		
12.5 mcg/hr		■
25 mcg/hr	■	
50 mcg/hr	■	
75 mcg/hr	■	
100 mcg/hr	■	
Dyazide Capsules		
25 mg-37.5 mg	■	
25 mg-50 mg	■	
DynaCirc CR Tablets		
5 mg		■
10 mg		■
Dyrenium Capsules		
50 mg	■	
100 mg	■	
EC-Naprosyn Delayed-Release Tablets		
500 mg	■	
Edecrin Tablets		
25 mg		■
50 mg		■
Edecrin Sodium Intravenous		
50 mg		■
Edex Injection		
10 mcg	■	
20 mcg	■	
40 mcg	■	
E.E.S. 200 Liquid		
200 mg/5 ml	■	
E.E.S. 400 Liquid		
400 mg/5 ml	■	
E.E.S. 400 Filmtab Tablets		
400 mg	■	
E.E.S. Granules		
200 mg/5 ml	■	
Effexor Tablets		
25 mg	■	
37.5 mg	■	
50 mg	■	
75 mg	■	
100 mg	■	
Effexor XR Capsules		
37.5 mg		■
75 mg		■
150 mg		■
Efudex Topical Cream		
5%		■
Efudex Topical Solutions		
2%	■	
5%	■	
Eldepryl Capsules		
5 mg	■	
Elidel Cream 1%		
1%		■
Eligard 7.5 mg		
7.5 mg		■
22.5 mg		■
30 mg		■
45 mg		■
Elitek		
1.5 mg		■
Elmiron Capsules		
100 mg		■
Elocon Cream 0.1%		
0.1%	■	
Elocon Lotion 0.1%		
0.1%		■
Elocon Ointment 0.1%		
0.1%	■	
Eloxatin for Injection		
50 mg		■
100 mg		■
Elspar for Injection		
10000 iu		■
Emcyt Capsules		
140 mg		■
Emend Capsules		
80 mg		■
125 mg		■
Emsam Transdermal System		
6 mg/24 hr		■
9 mg/24 hr		■
12 mg/24 hr		■
Emtriva Capsules		
200 mg		■
Enbrel for Injection		
25 mg		■
Engerix-B Vaccine		
20 mcg/ml		■
Enjuvia Tablets		
0.3 mg		■
0.45 mg		■
0.625 mg		■
1.25 mg		■
Entocort EC Capsules		
3 mg		■
EpiPen Auto-Injector		
1 mg/ml		■
EpiPen Jr. Auto-Injector		
0.5 mg/ml		■
Epivir Oral Solution		
10 mg/ml		■
Epivir Tablets		
300 mg		■
Epivir-HBV Oral Solution		
5 mg/ml		■
Epivir-HBV Tablets		
100 mg		■
Epogen for Injection		
2000 u/ml	■	
3000 u/ml	■	
4000 u/ml	■	
10000 u/ml	■	
20000 u/ml	■	
40000 u/ml	■	
Equetro Extended-Release Capsules		
100 mg		■
200 mg		■
300 mg		■
Eraxis for Injection		
50 mg		■
Erbitux		
2 mg/ml		■
EryPed 200 & EryPed 400 Oral Suspension		
200 mg/5 ml	■	
400 mg/5 ml		■
EryPed Drops		
100 mg/2.5 ml		■
EryPed Chewable Tablets		
200 mg		■
Ery-Tab Tablets		
250 mg	■	
333 mg	■	
500 mg	■	
Erythrocin Stearate Filmtab Tablets		
250 mg	■	
500 mg	■	
Erythromycin Base Filmtab Tablets		
250 mg	■	
500 mg	■	
Erythromycin Delayed-Release Capsules, USP		
250 mg	■	
Estrasorb Topical Emulsion		
2.5 mg/gm		■
Estratest Tablets		
1.25 mg-2.5 mg	■	
Estratest H.S. Tablets		
0.625 mg-1.25 mg	■	
Estring Vaginal Ring		
0.0075 mg/24 hr		■
Ethyol for Injection		
500 mg	■	
Euflexxa		
10 mg/ml		■
Eulexin Capsules		
125 mg	■	

Strength	Generic Yes	Generic No
Evista Tablets		
60 mg		■
Evoclin Foam, 1%		
1%		■
Evoxac Capsules		
30 mg		■
Exelon Capsules		
1.5 mg		■
3 mg		■
4.5 mg		■
6 mg		■
Fabrazyme for Intravenous Infusion		
35 mg		■
Famvir Tablets		
125 mg		■
250 mg		■
500 mg		■
Fansidar Tablets		
25 mg-500 mg		■
Faslodex Injection		
50 mg/ml		■
Feiba VH		
1 iu	■	
Femara Tablets		
2.5 mg		■
Ferrlecit Injection		
62.5 mg/5 ml		■
Finacea Gel		
15%		■
Flexbumin I.V.		
25%	■	
Flomax Capsules		
0.4 mg		■
Flonase Nasal Spray		
0.05 mg/actuation	■	
Flovent Diskus 100 mcg		
0.088 mg/actuation		■
Flovent Diskus 250 mcg		
0.22 mg/actuation		■
Flovent HFA 44 mcg Inhalation Aerosol		
0.044 mg/actuation		■
Flovent HFA 110 mcg Inhalation Aerosol		
0.11 mg/actuation		■
Flovent HFA 220 mcg Inhalation Aerosol		
0.22 mg/actuation		■
Floxin Otic Solution		
0.3%		■
Fluarix		
45 mcg/0.5 ml	■	
Flumadine Syrup		
50 mg/5 ml		■
Flumadine Tablets		
100 mg	■	
Fluorescite Injection		
10%	■	
25%	■	
Fluor-I-Strip A.T. Ophthalmic Strips 1 mg		
1 mg	■	
FML Ophthalmic Ointment		
0.1%		■
FML Ophthalmic Suspension		
0.1%	■	
FML Forte Ophthalmic Suspension		
0.25%		■
FML-S Ophthalmic Suspension		
0.1%-10%		■
Folgard RX Tablets		
0.5 mg-2.2 mg-25 mg	■	
Foradil Aerolizer		
0.012 mg		■
Fortamet Extended-Release Tablets		
500 mg	■	
1000 mg	■	
Fortaz Injection		
1 gm	■	
2 gm	■	
2 gm/50 ml-1.6 gm/50 ml		■
6 gm	■	
500 mg	■	
Fortaz for Injection		
1 gm/50 ml-2.2 gm/50 ml		■
2 gm/50 ml-1.6 gm/50 ml		■
Forteo for Injection		
250 mcg/ml		■
Fortical Nasal Spray		
200 iu/actuation		■
Fosamax Oral Solution		
70 mg/75 ml		■
Fosamax Tablets		
5 mg		■
10 mg		■
35 mg		■
40 mg		■
70 mg		■
Fosamax Plus D Tablets		
70 mg-2800 iu		■
Fosrenol Chewable Tablets		
250 mg		■
500 mg		■
Furosemide Tablets		
20 mg	■	
40 mg	■	
80 mg	■	
Fuzeon Injection		
90 mg		■
Gabitril Tablets		
2 mg		■
4 mg		■
12 mg		■
16 mg		■
20 mg		■
Gammagard Liquid		
100 mg/ml	■	
Gammagard S/D		
0.5 gm	■	
2.5 gm	■	
5 gm	■	
10 gm	■	
Gantrisin Pediatric Suspension		
500 mg/5 ml		■
Garamycin Injectable		
40 mg/ml	■	
Gemzar for Injection		
1 gm		■
200 mg		■
Gengraf Capsules		
25 mg	■	
100 mg	■	
Genotropin Lyophilized Powder		
1.5 mg		■
5.8 mg		■
13.8 mg		■
Geodon Capsules		
20 mg		■
40 mg		■
60 mg		■
80 mg		■
Geodon for Injection		
20 mg		■
Gleevec Tablets		
100 mg		■
400 mg		■
GlucaGen		
1 mg	■	
Glucagon for Injection Vials and Emergency Kit		
1 mg	■	
Gordochom Solution		
3%-25%	■	
Gris-PEG Tablets		
125 mg	■	
250 mg	■	
Guanidine Hydrochloride Tablets		
125 mg		■
Havrix Vaccine		
1440 el u/ml		■
Hectorol Capsules		
2.5 mcg		■
Hectorol Injection		
2 mcg/ml		■
Hepsera Tablets		
10 mg		■
Herceptin I.V.		
440 mg		■
HibTITER		
10 mcg	■	
100 mcg		■
Humalog-Pen		
100 u/ml		■
Humalog Mix 50/50-Pen		
50 u/ml-50 u/ml		■
Humalog Mix 75/25-Pen		
75 u/ml-25 u/ml		■
Humate-P		
1 iu-1 iu		■
Humatrope Vials and Cartridges		
5 mg	■	
6 mg		■
12 mg		■
24 mg		■
Humira Injection		
40 mg/0.8 ml		■
Hyalgan Solution		
10 mg/ml	■	
Hycamtin for Injection		
4 mg		■
Hycodan Syrup		
1.5 mg/5 ml-5 mg/5 ml	■	
Hycodan Tablets		
1.5 mg-5 mg	■	
Hycotuss Expectorant Syrup		
100 mg/5 ml-5 mg/5 ml	■	
Hydrocortone Tablets		
10 mg	■	
20 mg	■	
HyperRAB		
150 iu/ml	■	
Hyperstat I.V.		
15 mg/ml		■
HyperTET		
250 u		■
Hytrin Capsules		
1 mg	■	
2 mg	■	
5 mg	■	
10 mg	■	
Hyzaar 50-12.5 Tablets		
12.5 mg-50 mg		■
25 mg-100 mg		■
Imdur Tablets		
30 mg	■	
60 mg	■	
120 mg	■	
Imitrex Injection		
6 mg/0.5 ml		■
Imitrex Nasal Spray		
5 mg		■
20 mg		■
Imitrex Tablets		
25 mg		■
50 mg		■
100 mg		■
Indapamide Tablets		
1.25 mg	■	
2.5 mg	■	
Inderal LA Long-Acting Capsules		
60 mg	■	
80 mg	■	
120 mg	■	
160 mg	■	
Indocin Capsules		
25 mg	■	
50 mg	■	
Indocin I.V.		
1 mg		■
Indocin Oral Suspension		
25 mg/5 ml	■	
Indocin Suppositories		
50 mg	■	
Infanrix Vaccine		
25 lf u/0.5 ml-58 mcg/0		■
Infasurf Intratracheal Suspension		
35 mg/ml		■
Infed Injection		
50 mg/ml	■	
Infergen		
30 mcg/ml		■
Inspra Tablets		
25 mg		■
50 mg		■
Integrilin Injection		
0.75 mg/ml		■
2 mg/ml		■
Intron A for Injection		
3 million iu		■
3 million iu/0.2 ml		■
3 million iu/0.5 ml		■
5 million iu		■
5 million iu/0.2 ml		■
5 million iu/0.5 ml		■
6 million iu/ml		■
10 million iu		■
10 million iu/0.2 ml		■
10 million iu/ml		■
18 million iu		■
25 million iu		■
50 million iu		■
Invanz for Injection		
1 gm		■
Iressa Tablets		
250 mg		■
Kaletra Oral Solution		
80 mg/ml-20 mg/ml		■
Kaletra Tablets		
133.3 mg-33.3 mg		■
K-Dur Extended-Relase Tablets		
10 meq	■	
20 meq	■	
Kepivance		
6.25 mg		■
Keppra Oral Solution		
100 mg/ml		■
Keppra Tablets		
250 mg		■
500 mg		■
750 mg		■
Ketek Tablets		
400 mg		■
Kineret Injection		
100 mg/0.67 ml		■
Klaron Lotion 10%		
10%	■	

STRENGTH	GENERIC YES	GENERIC NO
Klonopin Tablets		
0.5 mg	■	
1 mg	■	
2 mg	■	
Klonopin Wafers		
0.125 mg		■
0.25 mg		■
0.5 mg		■
1 mg		■
2 mg		■
K-Lor Oral Solution		
15 meq	■	
20 meq	■	
Koate-DVI		
1 iu	■	
Kogenate FS		
1 iu	■	
Kogenate FS with Bio-Set		
1 iu	■	
K-Phos Original (Sodium Free) Tablets		
500 mg		■
K-Phos Neutral Tablets		
155 mg-852 mg-130 mg	■	
Kristalose for Oral Solution		
10 gm/packet		■
20 gm/packet		■
K-Tab Tablets		
10 meq	■	
Kytril Injection		
1 mg/ml		■
Kytril Oral Solution		
2 mg/10 ml		■
Lacrisert Sterile Ophthalmic Insert		
5 mg		■
Lamictal Chewable Dispersible Tablets		
5 mg		■
25 mg		■
Lamictal Tablets		
25 mg		■
100 mg		■
150 mg		■
200 mg		■
Lamisil Tablets		
250 mg		■
Lanoxicaps Capsules		
0.05 mg		■
0.1 mg		■
0.2 mg		■
Lanoxin Injection		
0.25 mg/ml	■	
Lanoxin Injection Pediatric		
0.1 mg/ml	■	
Lanoxin Tablets		
0.125 mg	■	
0.25 mg	■	
0.5 mg	■	
Lantus Injection		
100 u/ml		■
Lariam Tablets		
250 mg	■	
Lescol Capsules		
20 mg		■
40 mg		■
Lescol XL Tablets		
80 mg		■
Leukeran Tablets		
2 mg		■
Leukine		
250 mcg		■
500 mcg/ml		■
Leustatin Injection		
1 mg/ml	■	
Levaquin Oral Solution		
25 mg/ml		■
Levaquin Injection		
5 mg/ml		■
25 mg/ml		■
Levaquin Tablets		
250 mg		■
500 mg		■
750 mg		■
Levaquin in 5% Dextrose Injection		
5 mg/ml		■
Levemir Injection		
100 u/ml		■
Levitra Tablets		
2.5 mg		■
5 mg		■
10 mg		■
20 mg		■
Levothroid Tablets		
0.025 mg	■	
0.05 mg	■	
0.075 mg	■	
0.088 mg	■	
0.1 mg	■	
0.112 mg	■	
0.125 mg	■	
0.137 mg	■	
0.15 mg	■	
0.175 mg	■	
0.2 mg	■	
0.3 mg	■	
Levoxyl Tablets		
0.025 mg	■	
0.05 mg	■	
0.075 mg	■	
0.088 mg	■	
0.1 mg	■	
0.112 mg	■	
0.125 mg	■	
0.137 mg	■	
0.15 mg	■	
0.175 mg	■	
0.2 mg	■	
0.3 mg	■	
Levulan Kerastick for Topical Solution, 20%		
20%		■
Lexapro Oral Solution		
5 mg/5 ml		■
Lexapro Tablets		
5 mg		■
10 mg		■
20 mg		■
Lexiva Tablets		
700 mg		■
Librium Capsules		
5 mg	■	
10 mg	■	
25 mg	■	
Lidoderm Patch		
5%		■
Limbrel Capsules		
250 mg		■
500 mg		■
Lipitor Tablets		
10 mg		■
20 mg		■
40 mg		■
80 mg		■
Lithobid Tablets		
300 mg	■	
Lithostat Tablets		
250 mg		■
Locoid Lipocream Cream		
0.1%		■
Lofibra Tablets		
67 mg	■	
134 mg	■	
200 mg	■	
Lopressor Injection		
1 mg/ml	■	
Lopressor Tablets		
50 mg	■	
100 mg	■	
Lopressor HCT 50/25 Tablets		
25 mg-50 mg		■
Lopressor HCT 100/25 Tablets		
25 mg-100 mg		■
Lopressor HCT 100/50 Tablets		
50 mg-100 mg		■
Loprox Shampoo		
1%		■
Lotemax Ophthalmic Suspension 0.5%		
0.5%		■
Lotensin Tablets		
5 mg	■	
10 mg	■	
20 mg	■	
40 mg	■	
Lotensin HCT Tablets		
5 mg-6.25 mg	■	
10 mg-12.5 mg	■	
20 mg-12.5 mg	■	
20 mg-25 mg	■	
Lotrel Capsules		
2.5 mg-10 mg		■
5 mg-10 mg		■
5 mg-20 mg		■
10 mg-20 mg		■
Lotrimin Cream		
1%	■	
Lotrimin Lotion 1%		
1%	■	
Lotrimin Topical Solution 1%		
1%	■	
Lotrisone Cream		
0.05%-1%	■	
Lotronex Tablets		
1 mg		■
Lovenox Injection		
30 mg/0.3 ml		■
40 mg/0.4 ml		■
60 mg/0.6 ml		■
80 mg/0.8 ml		■
100 mg/ml		■
120 mg/0.8 ml		■
150 mg/ml		■
Lucentis Injection		
0.5 mg/0.05 ml		■
Lumigan Ophthalmic Solution		
0.03%		■
Lunesta Tablets		
1 mg		■
2 mg		■
3 mg		■
Lupron Depot 3.75 mg		
3.75 mg		■
Lupron Depot 7.5 mg		
7.5 mg		■
Lupron Depot--3 Month 11.25 mg		
11.25 mg		■
Lupron Depot-PED 7.5 mg, 11.25 mg and 15 mg		
7.5 mg		■
11.25 mg		■
15 mg		■
Lustra Cream		
4%	■	
Lustra-AF Cream		
4%	■	
Lustra-Ultra Cream		
4%	■	
Luxiq Foam		
0.12%		■
Lyrica Capsules		
25 mg		■
50 mg		■
75 mg		■
100 mg		■
150 mg		■
200 mg		■
225 mg		■
300 mg		■
Macugen Injection		
0.3 mg/0.09 ml		■
Malarone Pediatric Tablets		
62.5 mg-25 mg		■
Malarone Tablets		
250 mg-100 mg		■
Marinol Capsules		
2.5 mg		■
5 mg		■
10 mg		■
Matulane Capsules		
50 mg		■
Mavik Tablets		
1 mg		■
2 mg		■
4 mg		■
Maxair Autohaler		
0.2 mg/actuation		■
Maxalt Tablets		
5 mg		■
10 mg		■
Maxalt-MLT Orally Disintegrating Tablets		
5 mg		■
10 mg		■
Mefoxin for Injection		
1 gm	■	
2 gm	■	
10 gm	■	
Mefoxin Premixed Intravenous Solution		
1 gm/50 ml		■
2 gm/50 ml		■
Megace ES Oral Suspension		
625 mg/5 ml		■
Menactra Vaccine		
16 mcg/0.5 ml		■
Mentax Cream		
1%		■
Mephyton Tablets		
5 mg		■
Mepron Suspension		
750 mg/5 ml		■
Meridia Capsules		
5 mg		■
10 mg		■
15 mg		■
Merrem I.V.		
1 gm		■
500 mg		■
Meruvax II		
1000 tcid50		■
Metadate CD Capsules		
10 mg	■	
20 mg	■	
30 mg	■	
Metrogel		
0.75%		■
1%		■
MetroGel-Vaginal Gel		
0.75%	■	
Mevacor Tablets		
10 mg	■	
20 mg	■	
40 mg	■	
Miacalcin Injection		
200 iu/ml	■	
Miacalcin Nasal Spray		
200 iu/actuation		■
Micardis Tablets		
20 mg		■
40 mg		■

STRENGTH	GENERIC YES	GENERIC NO
80 mg		■
Micardis HCT Tablets		
12.5 mg-40 mg		■
12.5 mg-80 mg		■
Midamor Tablets		
5 mg	■	
Migranal Nasal Spray		
0.5 mg/actuation		■
Mintezol Suspension		
500 mg/5 ml		■
Mintezol Chewable Tablets		
500 mg		■
Mirapex Tablets		
0.125 mg		■
0.25 mg		■
0.5 mg		■
1 mg		■
1.5 mg		■
Mirena Intrauterine System		
52 mg		■
Mivacron Injection		
2 mg/ml	■	
Moban Tablets		
5 mg		■
10 mg		■
25 mg		■
50 mg		■
100 mg		■
Mobic Tablets		
7.5 mg		■
15 mg		■
Moduretic Tablets		
5 mg-50 mg	■	
MS Contin Tablets		
15 mg	■	
30 mg	■	
60 mg	■	
100 mg	■	
200 mg	■	
Mumpsvax		
20000 tcid50		■
Mustargen for Injection		
10 mg		■
Mycamine for Injection		
50 mg		■
Myfortic Tablets		
180 mg		■
360 mg		■
Mylotarg for Injection		
5 mg		■
Myobloc Injection		
2500 u/0.5 ml		■
5000 u/ml		■
Myozyme for Intravenous Infusion		
50 mg		■
Nadolol Tablets		
20 mg	■	
40 mg	■	
80 mg	■	
Naftin Cream		
1%		■
Naftin Gel		
1%		■
Naprosyn Suspension		
25 mg/ml	■	
Naprosyn Tablets		
250 mg	■	
375 mg	■	
500 mg	■	
Nasacort AQ Nasal Spray		
55 mcg/actuation		■
Nasonex Nasal Spray		
0.05 mg/actuation		■
Natacyn Antifungal Ophthalmic Suspension		
5%		■

STRENGTH	GENERIC YES	GENERIC NO
Natrecor for Injection		
1.5 mg		■
Naturethroid Tablets		
32.4 mg	■	
64.8 mg	■	
129.6 mg	■	
194.4 mg		■
Nembutal Sodium Solution, USP		
50 mg/ml	■	
NeoProfen Injection		
10 mg/ml		■
Neoral Oral Solution		
100 mg/ml	■	
Neoral Soft Gelatin Capsules		
25 mg	■	
100 mg	■	
Neulasta Injection		
6 mg/0.6 ml		■
Neumega for Injection		
5 mg		■
Neupogen for Injection		
300 mcg/0.5 ml		■
300 mcg/ml		■
480 mcg/0.8 ml		■
480 mcg/1.6 ml		■
Neurontin Capsules		
100 mg	■	
300 mg	■	
400 mg	■	
Neurontin Oral Solution		
250 mg/5 ml		■
Neurontin Tablets		
600 mg	■	
800 mg	■	
Nexavar Tablets		
200 mg		■
Nexium Delayed-Release Capsules		
20 mg		■
40 mg		■
Nexium I.V.		
20 mg		■
40 mg		■
Niaspan Extended-Release Tablets		
500 mg	■	
750 mg	■	
1000 mg	■	
Nicomide Tablets		
0.5 mg-750 mg-25 mg	■	
Nimotop Capsules		
30 mg		■
Niravam Orally Disintegrating Tablets		
0.25 mg		■
0.5 mg		■
1 mg		■
2 mg		■
Nitro-Dur Transdermal Infusion System		
0.1 mg/hr	■	
0.2 mg/hr	■	
0.3 mg/hr	■	
0.4 mg/hr	■	
0.6 mg/hr	■	
0.8 mg/hr	■	
Nitrolingual Pumpspray		
0.4 mg/actuation		■
Norditropin Cartridges		
5 mg/1.5 ml		■
15 mg/1.5 ml		■
Norflex Injection		
30 mg/ml	■	
Noroxin Tablets		
400 mg		■
Norvasc Tablets		
2.5 mg		■
5 mg		■

STRENGTH	GENERIC YES	GENERIC NO
10 mg		■
Norvir Soft Gelatin Capsules		
100 mg		■
Norvir Oral Solution		
80 mg/ml		■
NovoLog Injection		
100 u/ml		■
NovoLog Mix 70/30		
70 u/ml-30 u/ml		■
NovoSeven		
1 mcg		■
Numorphan Injection		
1 mg/ml		■
1.5 mg/ml		■
Nutropin for Injection		
5 mg	■	
10 mg		■
Nutropin AQ Injection		
5 mg/ml		■
Nutropin AQ Pen Cartridge		
5 mg/ml		■
NuvaRing		
0.015 mg/24 hr-0.12 mg/2		■
Nystop Topical Powder USP		
100000 u/gm	■	
Ocufen Ophthalmic Solution		
0.03%	■	
Ocuvite Lutein Vitamin and Mineral Supplement		
60 mg-2 mg-5 mg-30 iu-15		■
Olux Foam		
0.05%		■
Omacor Capsules		
1 gm		■
Omnicef Capsules		
300 mg	■	
Omnicef for Oral Suspension		
125 mg/5 ml	■	
250 mg/5 ml		■
Ontak Vials		
150 mcg/ml		■
Opana Tablets		
5 mg		■
10 mg		■
Opana ER Tablets		
5 mg		■
10 mg		■
20 mg		■
40 mg		■
Ophthetic Ophthalmic Solution		
0.5%	■	
OptiPranolol Metipranolol Ophthalmic Solution		
0.3%	■	
Oracea Capsules		
40 mg		■
Orencia Powder for Intravenous Infusion		
250 mg		■
Ortho-Cyclen Tablets		
35 mcg-0.25 mg	■	
Ortho Evra Transdermal System		
0.02 mg/24 hr-0.15 mg/24		■
Ortho Micronor Tablets		
0.35 mg	■	
Orthoclone OKT3 Sterile Solution		
1 mg/ml		■
OsmoPrep Tablets		
0.398 gm-1.102 gm	■	
Oxandrin Tablets		
2.5 mg		■

STRENGTH	GENERIC YES	GENERIC NO
10 mg		■
Oxistat Cream		
1%		■
Oxistat Lotion		
1%		■
Oxsoralen Lotion 1%		
1%		■
Oxsoralen-Ultra Capsules		
10 mg	■	
OxyContin Tablets		
10 mg	■	
15 mg		■
20 mg	■	
30 mg		■
40 mg	■	
60 mg		■
80 mg	■	
160 mg		■
OxyFast Oral Concentrate Solution		
20 mg/ml	■	
OxyIR Capsules		
5 mg	■	
Oxytrol Transdermal System		
3.9 mg/24 hr		■
Panafil Ointment		
0.5%-10%-10%	■	
10%-10%		■
Panafil SE Spray Emulsion		
0.5%-10%	■	
Parcopa Orally Disintegrating Tablets		
10 mg-100 mg		■
25 mg-100 mg		■
25 mg-250 mg		■
Parnate Tablets		
10 mg		■
Paser Granules		
4 gm/packet		■
Patanol Ophthalmic Solution		
0.1%		■
0.1%		■
Paxil CR Controlled-Release Tablets		
12.5 mg		■
25 mg		■
37.5 mg		■
Paxil Oral Suspension		
10 mg/5 ml		■
Paxil Tablets		
10 mg	■	
20 mg	■	
30 mg	■	
40 mg	■	
PCE Dispertab Tablets		
333 mg		■
500 mg		■
Liquid PedvaxHIB		
7.5 mcg/0.5 ml		■
Pegasys		
180 mcg/0.5 ml		■
180 mcg/ml		■
Penlac Nail Lacquer, Topical Solution		
8%		■
Pentasa Capsules		
250 mg	■	
Pepcid Injection		
0.4 mg/ml	■	
10 mg/ml	■	
Pepcid Injection Premixed		
0.4 mg/ml	■	
Pepcid for Oral Suspension		
0.4 mg/ml	■	
40 mg/5 ml		■
Pepcid Tablets		
20 mg	■	
40 mg	■	

STRENGTH	GENERIC YES	GENERIC NO
Percocet Tablets		
325 mg-10 mg	■	
325 mg-2.5 mg		■
325 mg-5 mg	■	
325 mg-7.5 mg	■	
500 mg-7.5 mg	■	
650 mg-10 mg	■	
Percodan Tablets		
325 mg-4.5 mg-0.38 mg	■	
Permax Tablets		
0.05 mg	■	
0.25 mg	■	
Persantine Tablets		
25 mg	■	
50 mg	■	
75 mg	■	
Pexeva Tablets		
30 mg		■
Phenergan Tablets and Suppositories		
12.5 mg	■	
25 mg	■	
50 mg	■	
Phenytek Capsules		
200 mg		■
300 mg		■
PhosLo GelCaps		
667 mg		■
Photofrin for Injection		
75 mg		■
Plasbumin-5		
5%	■	
Plasbumin-20		
20%	■	
Plasbumin-25		
25%	■	
Plasmanate		
5%	■	
Plavix Tablets		
75 mg		■
Pletal Tablets		
50 mg	■	
Plexion Cleanser		
10%-5%	■	
Plexion Cleansing Cloths		
10%-5%		■
Plexion SCT		
10%-5%	■	
Plexion Topical Suspension		
10%-5%	■	
Pneumovax 23		
575 mcg/0.5 ml	■	
Podocon-25 Liquid		
75%-25%	■	
Poly-Pred Ophthalmic Suspension		
0.35%-10000 u/ml-0.5%		■
Polytrim Ophthalmic Solution		
10000 u/ml-1 mg/ml	■	
Potaba Envules		
2 gm/packet	■	
Potaba Tablets		
0.5 gm	■	
Pramosone Cream		
1%-1%	■	
2.5%-1%	■	
Pramosone Lotion		
1%-1%	■	
2.5%-1%	■	
Pramosone Ointment		
1%-1%		■
2.5%-1%		■
Precose Tablets		
25 mg		■
50 mg		■
100 mg		■
Pred Forte Ophthalmic Suspension		
1%	■	
Pred-G Ophthalmic Ointment		
0.12%	■	
Pred-G Ophthalmic Suspension		
0.3%-1%		■
Pred Mild Ophthalmic Suspension		
0.12%		■
Premarin Intravenous		
25 mg		■
Premarin Tablets		
0.3 mg		■
0.45 mg		■
0.625 mg		■
0.9 mg		■
1.25 mg		■
2.5 mg		■
Premarin Vaginal Cream		
0.625 mg/gm		■
Premphase Tablets		
0.625 mg-5 mg		■
Prempro Tablets		
0.625 mg-2.5 mg		■
0.625 mg-5 mg		■
Prenate Elite Tablets		
120 mg-0.03 mg-200 mg-6	■	
Prevacid Delayed-Release Capsules		
15 mg		■
30 mg		■
Prevacid for Delayed-Release Oral Suspension		
15 mg/packet		■
30 mg/packet		■
Prevacid I.V. for Injection		
30 mg		■
Prevacid NapraPAC 375		
15 mg-375 mg		■
Prevacid NapraPAC 500		
15 mg-500 mg		■
Prevacid SoluTab Delayed-Release Orally Disintegrating Tablets		
15 mg		■
30 mg		■
Prevnar for Injection		
16 mcg/0.5 ml		■
PREVPAC		
500 mg-500 mg-30 mg		■
Prezista Tablets		
300 mg		■
Primaxin I.M.		
500 mg-500 mg		■
750 mg-750 mg		■
Primaxin I.V.		
250 mg-250 mg		■
500 mg-500 mg		■
Prinivil Tablets		
2.5 mg	■	
5 mg	■	
10 mg	■	
20 mg	■	
40 mg	■	
Prinzide Tablets		
12.5 mg-10 mg	■	
12.5 mg-20 mg	■	
25 mg-20 mg	■	
ProAmatine Tablets		
2.5 mg	■	
5 mg	■	
10 mg	■	
Prochieve		
4%	■	
8%	■	
Procrit for Injection		
2000 u/ml	■	
3000 u/ml	■	
4000 u/ml	■	
10000 u/ml	■	
20000 u/ml	■	
40000 u/ml	■	
ProctoFoam-HC		
1%-1%	■	
Profilnine SD, Factor IX Complex (Human)		
1 iu	■	
Prograf Capsules and Injection		
0.5 mg		■
1 mg		■
5 mg		■
5 mg/ml		■
Prolastin		
1 mg	■	
Proleukin for Injection		
22 million iu		■
Prometrium Capsules		
100 mg		■
200 mg		■
Propecia Tablets		
1 mg		■
Propine Ophthalmic Solution		
0.1%	■	
Proquin XR Tablets		
500 mg		■
Proscar Tablets		
5 mg		■
Prosed/DS Tablets		
0.06 mg-9 mg-0.06 mg-81.	■	
9 mg-0.12 mg-81.6 mg-10.		■
ProSom Tablets		
1 mg	■	
2 mg	■	
Protonix I.V.		
40 mg		■
Protonix Tablets		
20 mg		■
40 mg		■
Protopic Ointment		
0.03%		■
0.1%		■
Proventil Inhalation Aerosol		
0.09 mg/actuation	■	
Proventil HFA Inhalation Aerosol		
0.09 mg/actuation	■	
Provigil Tablets		
100 mg		■
200 mg		■
Provocholine Powder for Inhalation		
100 mg	■	
Prozac Pulvules and Liquid		
10 mg	■	
20 mg	■	
20 mg/5 ml	■	
40 mg	■	
Psoriatec Cream		
1%	■	
Pulmicort Respules		
0.25 mg/2 ml		■
0.5 mg/2 ml		■
Pulmozyme Inhalation Solution		
2.5 mg/2.5 ml		■
Quadramet Injection		
50 mci/ml		■
Quixin Ophthalmic Solution		
0.5%		■
Qvar Inhalation Aerosol		
0.04 mg/actuation		■
0.08 mg/actuation		■
Ranexa Tablets		
500 mg		■
Raniclor Tablets, Chewable		
250 mg		■
375 mg		■
Rapamune Oral Solution and Tablets		
1 mg		■
1 mg/ml		■
2 mg		■
Raptiva for Injection		
125 mg	■	
Razadyne ER Extended-Release Capsules		
8 mg		■
16 mg		■
24 mg		■
Razadyne Tablets		
4 mg		■
8 mg		■
12 mg		■
Rebetol Capsules		
200 mg	■	
Rebetron Combination Therapy		
3 million iu/0.2 ml-200		■
3 million iu/0.5 ml-200		■
Rebif Prefilled Syringe for Injection		
22 mcg/0.5 ml		■
44 mcg/0.5 ml		■
Recombinate		
1 iu	■	
Recombivax HB		
10 mcg/ml		■
40 mcg/ml		■
ReFacto Vials		
1 iu	■	
Refludan for Injection		
50 mg		■
Relenza Rotadisk		
5 mg/actuation		■
Relpax Tablets		
20 mg		■
40 mg		■
Remicade for IV Injection		
100 mg		■
Renagel Tablets		
400 mg		■
800 mg		■
ReoPro Vials		
2 mg/ml		■
Requip Tablets		
0.25 mg		■
0.5 mg		■
1 mg		■
2 mg		■
3 mg		■
4 mg		■
5 mg		■
Rescriptor Tablets		
100 mg		■
200 mg		■
Restasis Ophthalmic Emulsion		
0.05%		■
Restoril Capsules		
7.5 mg	■	
15 mg	■	
30 mg	■	
Retisert Implant		
0.59 mg		■
Retrovir Capsules		
100 mg		■

STRENGTH	GENERIC YES	GENERIC NO
Retrovir IV Infusion		
10 mg/ml		■
Retrovir Syrup		
50 mg/5 ml		■
Retrovir Tablets		
300 mg	■	
Revatio Tablets		
20 mg		■
Revlimid Capsules		
5 mg		■
10 mg		■
15 mg		■
25 mg		■
Reyataz Capsules		
100 mg		■
150 mg		■
200 mg		■
R-Gene 10 for Intravenous Use		
10%		■
Rhinocort Aqua Nasal Spray		
0.032 mg/actuation		■
Rilutek Tablets		
50 mg		■
Risperdal Consta Long-Acting Injection		
25 mg		■
37.5 mg		■
50 mg		■
Risperdal M-Tab Orally Disintegrating Tablets		
0.5 mg		■
1 mg		■
2 mg		■
Risperdal Oral Solution		
1 mg/ml		■
Risperdal Tablets		
0.25 mg		■
0.5 mg		■
1 mg		■
2 mg		■
3 mg		■
4 mg		■
Ritalin Hydrochloride Tablets		
5 mg	■	
10 mg	■	
20 mg	■	
Ritalin LA Capsules		
20 mg	■	
30 mg	■	
40 mg		■
Ritalin-SR Tablets		
20 mg	■	
Rituxan I.V.		
10 mg/ml		■
Rocaltrol Capsules		
0.25 mcg	■	
0.5 mcg	■	
Rocaltrol Oral Solution		
1 mcg/ml	■	
Rocephin Injectable Vials, ADD-Vantage, Galaxy, Bulk		
1 gm	■	
1 gm/50 ml		■
2 gm	■	
2 gm/50 ml		■
10 gm		■
250 mg	■	
500 mg	■	
Romazicon Injection		
0.1 mg/ml	■	
Rozerem Tablets		
8 mg		■
Rythmol SR Capsules		
150 mg	■	
225 mg	■	
300 mg	■	
Sanctura Tablets		
20 mg		■
Sandimmune I.V. Ampuls for Infusion		
50 mg/ml	■	
Sandimmune Oral Solution		
100 mg/ml		■
Sandimmune Soft Gelatin Capsules		
25 mg		■
50 mg		■
100 mg		■
Sandostatin Injection		
50 mcg/ml		■
100 mcg/ml		■
200 mcg/ml		■
500 mcg/ml		■
1000 mcg/ml		■
Sandostatin LAR Depot		
10 mg		■
20 mg		■
30 mg		■
Sensipar Tablets		
30 mg		■
60 mg		■
90 mg		■
Seroquel Tablets		
25 mg		■
100 mg		■
200 mg		■
300 mg		■
Simulect for Injection		
10 mg		■
20 mg		■
Singulair Tablets		
10 mg		■
Singulair Chewable Tablets		
4 mg		■
5 mg		■
Singulair Oral Granules		
4 mg/packet		■
Skelaxin Tablets		
400 mg	■	
800 mg		■
Solodyn Extended Release Tablets		
45 mg		■
90 mg		■
135 mg		■
Somavert Injection		
10 mg	■	
15 mg	■	
20 mg	■	
Sonata Capsules		
5 mg		■
Soriatane Capsules		
30 mg	■	
Spiriva HandiHaler		
18 mcg		■
Stalevo Tablets		
12.5 mg-200 mg-50 mg		■
Strattera Capsules		
10 mg		■
18 mg		■
25 mg		■
40 mg		■
60 mg		■
Striant Mucoadhesive		
30 mg		■
Stromectol Tablets		
3 mg		■
Suboxone Tablets		
2 mg-0.5 mg		■
8 mg-2 mg		■
Subutex Tablets		
2 mg	■	
8 mg	■	
Sular Tablets		
10 mg		■
20 mg		■
30 mg		■
40 mg		■
Sulfamylon Cream		
85 mg/gm		■
Sulfamylon for 5% Topical Solution		
50 gm/packet		■
Suprax		
100 mg/5 ml		■
Sustiva Capsules		
50 mg		■
100 mg		■
200 mg		■
Sutent Capsules		
12.5 mg		■
25 mg		■
50 mg		■
Symbyax Capsules		
25 mg-12 mg		■
25 mg-6 mg		■
50 mg-12 mg		■
50 mg-6 mg		■
Symlin Injection		
0.6 mg/ml		■
Symmetrel Tablets		
100 mg	■	
Synagis Intramuscular Powder		
50 mg		■
100 mg		■
Synera Topical Patch		
70 mg-70 mg		■
Synthroid Tablets		
0.025 mg	■	
0.05 mg	■	
0.075 mg	■	
0.088 mg	■	
0.1 mg	■	
0.112 mg	■	
0.125 mg	■	
0.137 mg	■	
0.15 mg	■	
0.175 mg	■	
0.2 mg	■	
0.3 mg	■	
Syprine Capsules		
250 mg		■
Tabloid Tablets		
40 mg		■
Tambocor Tablets		
50 mg	■	
100 mg	■	
150 mg	■	
Tamiflu Capsules		
75 mg		■
Tamiflu Oral Suspension		
12 mg/ml		■
Tarceva Tablets		
25 mg		■
100 mg		■
150 mg		■
Targretin Capsules		
75 mg		■
Tarka Tablets		
1 mg-240 mg		■
2 mg-180 mg		■
2 mg-240 mg		■
4 mg-240 mg		■
Taxotere Injection Concentrate		
20 mg/0.5 ml		■
Tegretol Chewable Tablets		
100 mg	■	
Tegretol-XR Tablets		
100 mg		■
200 mg		■
400 mg		■
Temodar Capsules		
5 mg		■
20 mg		■
100 mg		■
250 mg		■
Temovate Cream		
0.05%	■	
Temovate Gel		
0.05%	■	
Temovate Ointment		
0.05%	■	
Temovate Scalp Application		
0.05%	■	
Temovate E Emollient		
0.05%	■	
Tequin Injection		
2 mg/ml		■
10 mg/ml		■
Tessalon Capsules		
100 mg	■	
Tessalon Perles		
100 mg	■	
200 mg	■	
Testim 1% Gel		
1%	■	
Teveten Tablets		
400 mg		■
600 mg		■
Tev-Tropin for Injection		
5 mg	■	
Thalomid Capsules		
50 mg		■
100 mg		■
200 mg		■
Thioridazine Hydrochloride Tablets		
10 mg	■	
25 mg	■	
50 mg	■	
100 mg	■	
Thiothixene Capsules		
1 mg	■	
2 mg	■	
5 mg	■	
10 mg	■	
Thrombate III		
1 iu	■	
Thymoglobulin for Intravenous Infusion		
25 mg		■
Thyrogen for Injection		
1.1 mg		■
Tiazac Capsules		
120 mg	■	
180 mg	■	
240 mg	■	
300 mg	■	
360 mg	■	
420 mg		■
Ticlid Tablets		
250 mg	■	
Timentin ADD-Vantage		
100 mg-3 gm		■
100 mg/100 ml-3 gm/100 m		■
Timentin IV Infusion		
100 mg-3 gm		■
Timentin Pharmacy Bulk Package		
1 gm-30 gm		■
Timolide Tablets		
25 mg-10 mg		■
Timoptic Sterile Ophthalmic Solution		
0.25%	■	
0.5%	■	
0.25%	■	
0.5%	■	
Timoptic in Ocudose		
0.25%	■	
0.5%	■	
Timoptic-XE Sterile Ophthalmic Gel Forming Solution		
0.25%	■	
0.5%	■	

STRENGTH	GENERIC YES	GENERIC NO
0.25%	■	
0.5%	■	
Tindamax Tablets		
250 mg		■
500 mg		■
TNKase I.V.		
50 mg		■
TOBI Solution for Inhalation		
60 mg/ml		■
TobraDex Ophthalmic Ointment		
0.1%-0.3%		■
TobraDex Ophthalmic Suspension		
0.1%-0.3%		■
Topamax Sprinkle Capsules		
15 mg		■
25 mg		■
Topamax Tablets		
25 mg		■
100 mg		■
200 mg		■
Toprol-XL Tablets		
25 mg	■	
50 mg		■
100 mg		■
200 mg		■
Tracleer Tablets		
62.5 mg		■
125 mg		■
Transderm Scop Transdermal Therapeutic System		
0.33 mg/24 hr		■
Tranxene T-TAB Tablets		
3.75 mg	■	
7.5 mg	■	
15 mg	■	
Tranxene-SD Tablets		
22.5 mg		■
Trasylol Injection		
10000 kiu/ml		■
Travatan Ophthalmic Solution		
0.004%		■
Trecator Tablets		
250 mg		■
Trelstar Depot		
3.75 mg		■
Triaz Cleanser		
3%		■
6%	■	
10%	■	
Triaz Gel		
3%		■
6%	■	
10%	■	
Triaz Pads		
3%		■
6%		■
9%		■
Tricor Tablets		
54 mg		■
160 mg	■	
Triglide Tablets		
50 mg		■
160 mg	■	
Trileptal Tablets		
150 mg		■
300 mg		■
600 mg		■
Trileptal Oral Suspension		
300 mg/5 ml		■
Tri-Luma Cream		
0.01%-4%-0.05%		■
TriLyte with Flavor Packs for Oral Solution		
420 gm-1.48 gm-5.72 gm-1		■
Trisenox Injection		
1 mg/ml		■
Trizivir Tablets		
300 mg-150 mg-300 mg		■
Trusopt Sterile Ophthalmic Solution		
2%		■
2%		■
Truvada Tablets		
200 mg-300 mg		■
Tussionex Pennkinetic Extended-Release Suspension		
8 mg/5 ml-10 mg/5 ml		■
Twinject 0.3		
1 mg/ml	■	
Twinject 0.15		
1 mg/ml	■	
Twinrix Vaccine		
720 el u/ml-20 mcg/ml		■
Tygacil for Injection		
50 mg		■
Tylenol with Codeine Tablets		
300 mg-15 mg	■	
300 mg-30 mg	■	
300 mg-60 mg	■	
300 mg-7.5 mg	■	
Ultane Liquid for Inhalation		
100%		■
Ultrase Capsules		
20000 u-4500 u-25000 u	■	
Ultrase MT Capsules		
39000 u-12000 u-39000 u	■	
58500 u-18000 u-58500 u	■	
65000 u-20000 u-65000 u	■	
Uniphyl Tablets		
400 mg	■	
600 mg	■	
Uniretic Tablets		
12.5 mg-15 mg		■
12.5 mg-7.5 mg		■
25 mg-15 mg		■
Univasc Tablets		
7.5 mg	■	
15 mg	■	
Urocit-K Tablets		
5 meq		■
10 meq		■
Uroqid-Acid No. 2 Tablets		
500 mg-500 mg		■
Uroxatral Tablets		
10 mg		■
Vagifem Tablets		
25 mcg	■	
Valcyte Tablets		
450 mg		■
Valium Tablets		
2 mg	■	
5 mg	■	
10 mg	■	
Valtrex Caplets		
1 gm		■
500 mg		■
Vancocin HCl Capsules, USP		
125 mg		■
250 mg		■
Vandazole Vaginal Gel		
0.75%	■	
Vanos Cream		
0.1%		■
Vantas		
50 mg		■
Vantin Tablets and Oral Suspension		
50 mg/5 ml		■
100 mg	■	
100 mg/5 ml		■
200 mg	■	
Vaprisol		
20 mg/4 ml		■
Vaqta		
50 u/ml		■
Varivax		
1350 pfu		■
Velcade for Injection		
3.5 mg		■
Ventavis Inhalation Solution		
10 mcg/ml		■
Ventolin HFA Inhalation Aerosol		
0.09 mg/actuation	■	
Verelan PM Extended-Release Capsules, Controlled-Onset		
100 mg		■
200 mg		■
300 mg		■
Vesanoid Capsules		
10 mg		■
VFEND I.V.		
200 mg		■
VFEND Oral Suspension		
40 mg/ml		■
VFEND Tablets		
50 mg		■
200 mg		■
Viadur Implant		
65 mg		■
Viagra Tablets		
25 mg		■
50 mg		■
100 mg		■
Vicodin Tablets		
500 mg-5 mg	■	
Vicodin ES Tablets		
750 mg-7.5 mg	■	
Vicodin HP Tablets		
660 mg-10 mg	■	
Vicoprofen Tablets		
7.5 mg-200 mg	■	
Vigamox Ophthalmic Solution		
0.5%		■
Viokase Powder		
70000 u/0.7 gm-16800 u/0		■
Viokase Tablets		
30000 u-8000 u-30000 u	■	
60000 u-16000 u-60000 u	■	
Viracept Oral Powder		
50 mg/gm		■
Viracept Tablets		
250 mg		■
Viramune Oral Suspension		
50 mg/5 ml		■
Viramune Tablets		
200 mg		■
Virazole for Inhalation Solution		
6 gm		■
Viread Tablets		
300 mg		■
Viroptic Ophthalmic Solution		
1%	■	
Visudyne for Injection		
15 mg		■
Vivaglobin		
160 mg/ml		■
Vivitrol		
380 mg		■
Voltaren Ophthalmic Solution		
0.1%	■	
Voltaren Tablets		
25 mg	■	
50 mg	■	
75 mg	■	
Voltaren-XR Tablets		
100 mg	■	
VoSpire ER Tablets		
4 mg	■	
8 mg	■	
WelChol Tablets		
625 mg		■
Wellbutrin Tablets		
75 mg	■	
100 mg	■	
Wellbutrin SR Sustained-Release Tablets		
100 mg	■	
150 mg	■	
200 mg	■	
Wellbutrin XL Extended-Release Tablets		
150 mg		■
300 mg		■
Westhroid Tablets		
60 mg	■	
64.8 mg	■	
129.6 mg	■	
180 mg	■	
240 mg	■	
WinRho SDF		
600 iu		■
1500 iu		■
5000 iu		■
Xalatan Sterile Ophthalmic Solution		
0.005%		■
Xalatan Ophthalmic Solution		
0.005%		■
Xeloda Tablets		
150 mg		■
500 mg		■
Xenaderm Ointment		
788 mg/gm-87 mg/gm-90 u/		■
Xenical Capsules		
120 mg		■
Xerac AC Solution		
6.25%		■
Xifaxan Tablets		
200 mg		■
Xigris Powder for Intravenous Infusion		
5 mg		■
20 mg		■
Xolair		
150 mg		■
Xopenex Inhalation Solution		
1.25 mg/3 ml		■
Xopenex Inhalation Solution Concentrate		
1.25 mg/0.5 ml		■
Xyrem Oral Solution		
500 mg/ml		■
Yasmin 28 Tablets		
3 mg-0.03 mg		■
Yaz Tablets		
3 mg-0.02 mg		■
Zantac 25 EFFERdose Tablets		
150 mg		■
150 mg/packet		■
Zantac 150 EFFERdose Tablets		
150 mg		■
Zantac Injection		
25 mg/ml	■	
Zantac Injection Premixed		
1 mg/ml		■
Zantac Syrup		
15 mg/ml	■	

STRENGTH	GENERIC YES	GENERIC NO
Zantac 150 Tablets		
150 mg	■	
Zantac 300 Tablets		
300 mg	■	
Zegerid Powder for Oral Solution		
20 mg/packet-1680 mg/pac		■
Zelapar Tablets		
1.25 mg		■
Zelnorm Tablets		
2 mg		■
6 mg		■
Zemaira		
1 mg	■	
Zemplar Injection		
0.002 mg/ml		■
0.005 mg/ml		■
Zemuron Injection		
10 mg/ml		■
Ziagen Oral Solution		
20 mg/ml		■
Ziagen Tablets		
300 mg		■
Zinacef Injection		
1.5 gm	■	
1.5 gm/50 ml	■	
7.5 gm	■	
750 mg	■	
750 mg/50 ml	■	
Zinecard for Injection		
250 mg		■
500 mg		■
Zmax for Oral Suspension		
2 gm/60 ml		■
Zocor Tablets		
5 mg	■	
10 mg	■	
20 mg	■	
40 mg	■	
80 mg	■	
Zofran Injection		
2 mg/ml		■
32 mg/50 ml		■
Zofran Injection Premixed		
32 mg/50 ml		■
Zofran Oral Solution		
4 mg/5 ml		■
Zofran Tablets		
4 mg		■
8 mg		■
24 mg		■
Zofran ODT Orally Disintegrating Tablets		
4 mg		■
8 mg		■
Zoloft Oral Concentrate		
20 mg/ml	■	
Zoloft Tablets		
25 mg	■	
50 mg	■	
100 mg	■	
Zometa for Intravenous Infusion		
4 mg		■
4 mg/5 ml		■
Zostavax Injection		
19400 pfu		■
Zosyn		
2 gm-0.25 gm		■
3 gm-0.375 gm		■
4 gm-0.5 gm		■
4 gm/100 ml-0.5 gm/100 m		■
36 gm-4.5 gm		■
40 mg/ml-5 mg/ml		■
60 mg/ml-7.5 mg/ml		■
Zovirax Capsules		
200 mg	■	
Zovirax Cream		
5%		■
Zovirax Ointment		
5%		■
Zovirax Suspension		
200 mg/5 ml	■	
Zovirax Tablets		
400 mg	■	
800 mg	■	
Zyban Sustained-Release Tablets		
150 mg	■	
Zydone Tablets		
400 mg-10 mg		■
400 mg-5 mg		■
400 mg-7.5 mg		■
Zyflo Tablets		
600 mg		■
Zymar Ophthalmic Solution		
0.3%		■
0.3%		■
Zyprexa Tablets		
2.5 mg		■
5 mg		■
7.5 mg		■
10 mg		■
15 mg		■
20 mg		■
Zyprexa IntraMuscular		
10 mg		■
Zyprexa ZYDIS Orally Disintegrating Tablets		
5 mg		■
10 mg		■
15 mg		■
20 mg		■
Zyrtec Syrup		
1 mg/ml		■
Zyrtec Tablets		
5 mg		■
10 mg		■
Zyrtec-D 12 Hour Extended Release Tablets		
5 mg-120 mg		■
Zyvox for Oral Suspension		
100 mg/5 ml		■
Zyvox Injection		
2 mg/ml		■
Zyvox Tablets		
600 mg		■

SECTION 8

IMPRINT IDENTIFICATION GUIDE

Too often, patients on multiple medications have no idea what they're taking; and a "brown-bag inventory" may not help if it confronts you with a collection of unfamiliar tablets and capsules. This section of the *PDR Guide to Drug Interactions, Side Effects, and Indications*™ provides you with a handy solution.

The convenient table below allows you to identify thousands of solid oral medications by imprint alone. Imprints beginning with a number are listed first, in ascending order. All numbers with leading zeros, as in "053", are listed before numbers without leading zeros. Imprints beginning with a letter follow in alphabetical order. Virtually all commonly prescribed drugs are represented.

Each entry includes the full imprint code, the product's brand or generic name, and, to confirm identification, its strength, color, form, and shape. The name of the product's manufacturer completes each listing. The information is extracted, with permission, from the Identidex System produced by Micromedex, Inc.

IMPRINT	BRAND/GENERIC NAME	STRENGTH	COLOR	FORM	SHAPE	MANUFACTURER
0 8 ; A	Mirtazapine	15 mg	Yellow	Tablet	Capsule-Shape	Aurobindo Pharma
0 9 ; A	Mirtazapine	30 mg	Reddish-Brown	Tablet	Capsule-Shape	Aurobindo Pharma
0.1; RPR ;	Ddavp	0.1 mg	White	Tablet	Oval	Sanofi-Aventis U.S.
0038; G	Etodolac	200 mg	Light Gray	Capsule		Par Pharmaceutical
0039; G	Etodolac	300 mg	Gray	Capsule		Par Pharmaceutical
0040; G	Etodolac	400 mg	Orange	Tablet	Oval	Par Pharmaceutical
0093; HY-PAM 25 MG	HY-Pam	25 mg	Black or Lavender	Capsule		Teva Pharmaceuticals
0093; HY-PAM 50 MG	HY-Pam 50	50 mg	Dark Green and White Opaque	Capsule		Teva Pharmaceuticals
03; 0088 ;	Allegra	30 mg	Peach	Tablet		Sanofi-Aventis U.S.
06; 0088 ;	Allegra	60 mg	Peach	Tablet	Oblong	Sanofi-Aventis U.S.
018; 0088 ;	Allegra	180 mg	Peach	Tablet		Sanofi-Aventis U.S.
019; DMSP	Cimetidine	200 mg	White	Tablet	Oval	Bristol-Myers Squibb
026; G	Piroxicam	10 mg	Opaque Olive and Dark Green	Capsule		Par Pharmaceutical
027; G	Piroxicam	20 mg	Opaque Dark Green	Capsule		Par Pharmaceutical
028; ALPHA SYMBOL	Guaifenesin	1200 mg	White	Tablet		Alphagen Laboratories
050; DMSP	Cimetidine	300 mg	White	Tablet	Oval	Bristol-Myers Squibb
057; DMSP	Cimetidine	400 mg	White	Tablet	Oval	Bristol-Myers Squibb
058; DMSP	Cimetidine	800 mg	White	Tablet	Oval	Bristol-Myers Squibb
081 IMPAX/10	Omeprazole Delayed-Release	10 mg	Lavender, Light Brown	Capsule, Delayed Release		Teva Pharmaceuticals
082 IMPAX 20 ;	Omeprazole Delayed-Release	20 mg	Lavender	Capsule, Delayed Release		Teva Pharmaceuticals
082; OHM	Sudal-12	30 mg/5 ml; 6 mg/5 ml	Red	Suspension		Atley Pharmaceuticals
083 ; KALI	Tramadol Hydrochloride and Acetaminophen	37.5 mg; 325 mg	Orange	Tablet	Capsule-Shape	Par Pharmaceutical
0145; P200	Pacerone	400 mg	Light Yellow	Tablet	Oval, Scored	Upsher-Smith Laboratories
0665; 4120 ;	Valproic Acid	250 mg	Orange	Capsule, Liquid Filled	Oval	Novartis Generics
0665; 4160	Lithium Carbonate	300 mg	White	Capsule		Novartis Generics
1	Fentora	100 mcg		Tablet		Cephalon
1	Lo-Ten	0.1 mg; 25 mg; 15 mg		Tablet		Teva Pharmaceuticals
1	Nitrogard	1 mg	Off-White	Sustained-Release Tablet	Circle, Standard Convex	Forest Pharmaceuticals
1 ; 4 ; A	Metformin Hydrochloride	1000 mg	White	Tablet	Oval	Aurobindo Pharma
1/90; JC; E2/N; OM	Prefest Estradiol/norgestimate	1 mg; 0.09 mg	White	Tablet		Monarch Pharmaceuticals
1; 4036 ;	Estazolam	1 mg	White	Tablet	Square, Flat-Faced, Beveled-Edge, Scored	Ivax Pharmaceuticals
1; JC; E2; OM	Prefest Estradiol	1 mg	Pink	Tablet		Monarch Pharmaceuticals
2	Detrol LA	2 mg	Blue-Green	Capsule, Extended Release		Pharmacia & Upjohn
2	Fentora	200 mcg		Tablet		Cephalon
2	Nitrogard	2 mg	Off-White	Sustained-Release Tablet	Circle, Standard Convex	Forest Pharmaceuticals

IMPRINT	BRAND/GENERIC NAME	STRENGTH	COLOR	FORM	SHAPE	MANUFACTURER
2; 93; 50	Acetaminophen and Codeine No. 2	300 mg; 15 mg	White	Tablet	Circle, Flat, Beveled Edge	Teva Pharmaceuticals
2; 4037 ;	Estazolam	2 mg	Salmon	Tablet	Square, Flat-Faced, Beveled-Edge, Scored	Ivax Pharmaceuticals
2; VALIUM; R; ROCHE	Valium	2 mg	White	Tablet	Circle, Scored	Roche Products
2 1/2; U; 121	Loniten	2.5 mg	White	Tablet	Circle, Scored	Pharmacia & Upjohn
3	Nitrogard	3 mg	Off-White	Sustained-Release Tablet	Circle, Standard Convex	Forest Pharmaceuticals
3	Nitroglycerin	0.3 mg	White	Tablet		Endo Laboratories
3; 93; 150	Acetaminophen and Codeine No. 3	300 mg; 30 mg	White	Tablet	Circle, Flat Beveled Edge	Teva Pharmaceuticals
3M; 107 ;	Alu-Tab	500 mg	Green	Tablet		3M Pharmaceuticals
3M; 221	Norflex	100 mg	White	Tablet	Circle	3M Pharmaceuticals
3M; 221	Orphenadrine Citrate ER	100 mg	White	Extended-Release Tablet	Circle	Mylan Pharmaceuticals
3M; 342	Theolair	125 mg	White	Tablet	Circle, Scored	3M Pharmaceuticals
3M; ALU-CAP ;	Alu-Cap	400 mg	Red and Green	Capsule		3M Pharmaceuticals
3M; SR; 200	Theolair-SR	200 mg	White	Sustained-Release Tablet	Circle, Scored	3M Pharmaceuticals
3M; SR; 250 ;	Theolair-SR	250 mg	White	Sustained-Release Tablet	Circle, Scored	3M Pharmaceuticals
3M; SR; 300 ;	Theolair-SR	300 mg	White	Sustained-Release Tablet	Oval, Scored	3M Pharmaceuticals
3M; SR; 500 ;	Theolair-SR	500 mg	White	Sustained-Release Tablet	Capsule-Shape, Scored	3M Pharmaceuticals
3M; THEOLAIR; 250	Theolair	250 mg	White	Tablet	Capsule-Shape, Scored	3M Pharmaceuticals
3M; TITRALAC ;	Titralac	420 mg	White	Tablet, Chewable	Circle	3M Pharmaceuticals
3M; TR; 100	Tambocor	100 mg	White	Tablet	Circle, Scored	3M Pharmaceuticals
3M; TR; 150	Tambocor	150 mg	White	Tablet	Oval, Scored	3M Pharmaceuticals
3M; UREX	Urex	1 G	White	Tablet	Capsule-Shape, Scored	3M Pharmaceuticals
4	Detrol LA	4 mg	Blue	Capsule, Extended Release		Pharmacia & Upjohn
4	Fentora	400 mcg		Tablet		Cephalon
4	Nitroglycerin	0.4 mg	White	Tablet		Endo Laboratories
4; 93; 350	Acetaminophen and Codeine No. 4	300 mg; 60 mg	White	Tablet	Circle, Flat Beveled Edge	Teva Pharmaceuticals
5	Rhinspec	300 mg; 100 mg; 5 mg	Pink	Tablet		Teva Pharmaceuticals
5	Zyprexa Zydis	5 mg	Yellow	Tablet, Disintegrating	Circle	Eli Lilly
5 ; ARICEPT	Aricept	5 mg	White	Tablet	Circle	Eisai
5 ; ARICEPT	Aricept	5 mg	White	Tablet	Circle	Pfizer
5 ; ARICEPT	Aricept Odt	5 mg	White	Tablet, Disintegrating		Eisai
5 ; ARICEPT	Aricept Odt	5 mg	White	Tablet, Disintegrating		Pfizer
5 MG ; WATSON 369	Loxapine Succinate	5 mg	White	Capsule		Watson Laboratories
5 MG 3512 5 MG SB	Dexedrine Spansule	5 mg	Brown, Clear	Capsule, Extended Release		Glaxosmithkline
5 MG SONATA	Sonata	5 mg	Green, Light Green	Capsule		King Pharmaceuticals
5 MG SONATA	Sonata	5 mg	Green, Light Green	Capsule		Wyeth Pharmaceuticals
5 XL	Ditropan XL	5 mg	Pale Yellow	Tablet, Extended Release	Circle	Ortho-Mcneil Pharmaceutical
5; ARICEPT	Aricept Odt	5 mg	White	Disintegrating Tablet		Eisai
5; ARICEPT	Aricept Odt	5 mg	White	Disintegrating Tablet		Pfizer
5; VALIUM; R; ROCHE	Valium	5 mg	Yellow	Tablet	Circle, Scored	Roche Products
6	Bevitone	20 mg; 3 mcg; 150 mg; 5 mg; 20 mg	Pink	Tablet		Teva Pharmaceuticals
6	Fentora	600 mcg		Tablet		Cephalon
6	Nitroglycerin	0.6 mg	White	Tablet		Endo Laboratories
7.5; DF	Enablex	7.5 mg	White	Tablet, Extended Release	Circle	Novartis Pharmaceuticals
8	Fentora	800 mcg		Tablet		Cephalon
8 HOUR	Tylenol 8 Hour Extended Release Caplet	650 mg	Red	Tablet, Extended Release	Capsule-Shape	Mcneil Consumer Products
8 HOUR	Tylenol 8 Hour Extended Release Geltabs	650 mg	Red, White	Tablet, Extended Release		Mcneil Consumer Products
9 3 ; 1174	Penicillin-VK	500 mg	Mottled White to Off-White	Tablet	Oval	Teva Pharmaceuticals
9 3 ; 7380	Venlafaxine Hydrochloride	37.5 mg	Mottled Peach	Tablet	Circle	Teva Pharmaceuticals
9 3 ; 7381	Venlafaxine Hydrochloride	50 mg	Mottled Peach	Tablet	Circle	Teva Pharmaceuticals
9 3 ; 7382	Venlafaxine Hydrochloride	75 mg	Mottled Peach	Tablet	Circle	Teva Pharmaceuticals
9 3 ; 7383	Venlafaxine Hydrochloride	100 mg	Mottled Peach	Tablet	Circle	Teva Pharmaceuticals
9; 3; 27	Torsemide	5 mg	White to Off-White	Tablet	Oval, Scored	Teva Pharmaceuticals
9; 3; 28	Torsemide	10 mg	White to Off-White	Tablet	Oval, Scored	Teva Pharmaceuticals
9; 3; 29	Torsemide	20 mg	White to Off-White	Tablet	Oval, Scored	Teva Pharmaceuticals
9; 3; 30	Torsemide	100 mg	White to Off-White	Tablet	Oval	Teva Pharmaceuticals
9; 3; 7127	Torsemide	5 mg	White to Off-White	Tablet	Oval, Scored	Teva Pharmaceuticals
9; 3; 7128	Torsemide	10 mg	White to Off-White	Tablet	Oval, Scored	Teva Pharmaceuticals
9; 3; 7129	Torsemide	20 mg	White to Off-White	Tablet	Oval, Scored	Teva Pharmaceuticals
9; 3; 7130	Torsemide	100 mg	White to Off-White	Tablet	Oval, Scored	Teva Pharmaceuticals
9; 3; 7159	Pergolide Mesylate	0.25 mg	Mottled Green	Tablet	Capsule-Shape, Scored	Teva Pharmaceuticals
9; 3; 7160	Pergolide Mesylate	0.05 mg	Ivory	Tablet	Capsule-Shape, Scored	Teva Pharmaceuticals
9; 3; 7161	Pergolide Mesylate	1 mg	Mottled Pink	Tablet	Capsule-Shape, Scored	Teva Pharmaceuticals
10	Zyprexa Zydis	10 mg	Yellow	Tablet, Disintegrating	Circle	Eli Lilly
10/100; SP; 341	Parcopa	10 mg; 100 mg	Blue	Disintegrating Tablet	Circle, Flat-Faced, Scored	Schwarz Pharma
10 ;	Ceenu	10 mg	Two-Tone White	Capsule		Bristol-Myers Oncology
10 ; 0013	Pravastatin Sodium	10 mg	Pink to Peach	Tablet	Ovoid-Rectangular	Watson Laboratories
10 ; A	Mirtazapine	45 mg	White	Tablet	Capsule-Shape	Aurobindo Pharma

IMPRINT	BRAND/GENERIC NAME	STRENGTH	COLOR	FORM	SHAPE	MANUFACTURER
10 ; ARICEPT	Aricept	10 mg	Yellow	Tablet	Circle	Eisai
10 ; ARICEPT	Aricept	10 mg	Yellow	Tablet	Circle	Pfizer
10 ; ARICEPT	Aricept Odt	10 mg	Yellow	Tablet, Disintegrating		Eisai
10 ; ARICEPT	Aricept Odt	10 mg	Yellow	Tablet, Disintegrating		Pfizer
10 MG ; WATSON 370	Loxapine Succinate	10 mg	White and Yellow	Capsule		Watson Laboratories
10 MG SONATA	Sonata	10 mg	Green, Light Green	Capsule		King Pharmaceuticals
10 MG SONATA	Sonata	10 mg	Green, Light Green	Capsule		Wyeth Pharmaceuticals
10 XL	Ditropan XL	10 mg	Pink	Tablet, Extended Release		Ortho-Mcneil Pharmaceutical
10; ARICEPT	Aricept Odt	10 mg	Yellow	Disintegrating Tablet		Eisai
10; ARICEPT	Aricept Odt	10 mg	Yellow	Disintegrating Tablet		Pfizer
10; GILEAD; LIVER SYMBOL	Hepsera	10 mg	White	Tablet		Gilead Sciences
10; VALIUM; R; ROCHE	Valium	10 mg	Blue	Tablet		Roche Products
10MG 3513 10MG SB	Dexedrine Spansule	10 mg	Brown, Clear	Capsule, Extended Release		Glaxosmithkline
11	Akineton	2 mg	White	Tablet	Circle	Par Pharmaceutical
11 ; A	Mirtazapine	7.5 mg	White	Tablet	Capsule-Shape	Aurobindo Pharma
15	Zyprexa Zydis	15 mg	Yellow	Tablet, Disintegrating	Circle	Eli Lilly
15 ; M	Meloxicam	15 mg	Pastel Yellow	Tablet	Oblong	Roxane Laboratories
15 ; M	Mobic	15 mg	Pastel Yellow	Tablet	Oblong	Boehringer Ingelheim Pharmaceuticals
15 XL	Ditropan XL	15 mg	Gray	Tablet, Extended Release	Circle	Ortho-Mcneil Pharmaceutical
15; DF	Enablex	15 mg	Light Peach	Tablet, Extended Release	Circle	Novartis Pharmaceuticals
15MG 3514 15MG SB	Dexedrine Spansule	15 mg	Brown, Clear	Capsule, Extended Release		Glaxosmithkline
17	Moexipril Hydrochloride	7.5 mg	Pink	Tablet	Oval, Scored	Teva Pharmaceuticals
20	Neospect	100 mg; 25 mg; 15 mg; 100 mg	Green	Tablet		Teva Pharmaceuticals
20	Zyprexa Zydis	20 mg	Yellow	Tablet, Disintegrating	Circle	Eli Lilly
20 ; 0014	Pravastatin Sodium	20 mg	Yellow	Tablet	Ovoid-Rectangular	Watson Laboratories
20 MG	Nexium	20 mg	Amethyst with Two Yellow Bars	Timed-Release Capsule		Astra Zeneca
20 MG; LILLY; 3235	Cymbalta	20 mg	Opaque Green	Delayed-Release Capsule		Eli Lilly
22	Rhinex	150 mg; 1.25 mg; 2.5 mg	Pink and White	Tablet		Teva Pharmaceuticals
25 MG ; WATSON 371	Loxapine Succinate	25 mg	White and Green	Capsule		Watson Laboratories
25/100; SP; 342	Parcopa	25 mg; 100 mg	Yellow	Disintegrating Tablet	Circle, Flat-Faced, Scored	Schwarz Pharma
25/250; SP; 343	Parcopa	25 mg; 250 mg	Blue	Disintegrating Tablet	Circle, Flat-Faced, Scored	Schwarz Pharma
25; LL; A; 13	Asendin	25 mg	Off-White	Tablet	Seven-Sided	Lederle Laboratories
25; T4	Levothroid	25 mcg	Orange	Tablet	Capsule-Shape	Forest Pharmaceuticals
30 MG; LILLY; 3240	Cymbalta	30 mg	Opaque White and Opaque Blue	Delayed-Release Capsule		Eli Lilly
30/2 ; 4833G ;	Duetact	30 mg; 2 mg	Off-White to White	Tablet	Circle	Takeda Pharmaceuticals
30/4 ; 4833G ;	Duetact	30 mg; 4 mg	Off-White to White	Tablet	Circle	Takeda Pharmaceuticals
31; BONE IMAGE	Fosamax	70 mg	White	Tablet	Oval	Merck
38AV	Ketek	300 mg	Light Orange	Tablet	Oval	Sanofi-Aventis U.S.
40 ;	Ceenu	40 mg	White and Green	Capsule		Bristol-Myers Oncology
40 ; 0016	Pravastatin Sodium	40 mg	Green	Tablet	Ovoid-Rectangular	Watson Laboratories
40 MG	Nexium	40 mg	Amethyst with Three Yellow Bars	Timed-Release Capsule		Astra Zeneca
42	Neosorb Plus	300 mg; 150 mg	Green and White	Tablet		Teva Pharmaceuticals
44	Vicks 44 Cold, Flu & Cough	250 mg; 2 mg; 30 mg; 10 mg	Blue	Capsule		Procter & Gamble
44	Vicks 44 Liquicaps Cold, Flu & Cough	250 mg; 2 mg; 30 mg; 10 mg	Blue	Capsule		Procter & Gamble
44	Vicks 44 Liquidaps Cough, Cold & Flu Relief	250 mg; 2 mg; 30 mg; 10 mg	Transparent Blue	Gel/jelly		Procter & Gamble
44	Vicks 44 Liquicaps Non-Drowsy Cold & Cough	30 mg; 60 mg	Transparent Red	Capsule		Procter & Gamble
44	Vicks 44 Liquicaps Non-Drowsy Cough & Cold Relief	30 mg; 60 mg	Transparent Red	Gel/jelly		Procter & Gamble
50 MG ; WATSON 372	Loxapine Succinate	50 mg	White and Blue	Capsule		Watson Laboratories
50; LL; A; 15	Asendin	50 mg	Orange	Tablet	Seven-Sided	Lederle Laboratories
50; T4	Levothroid	50 mcg	White	Tablet	Capsule-Shape	Forest Pharmaceuticals
54 005	Anagrelide Hydrochloride	0.5 mg	White	Capsule		Roxane Laboratories
54 015	Torsemide	5 mg	White to Off-White	Tablet	Circle	Roxane Laboratories
54 016	Torsemide	10 mg	White to Off-White	Tablet	Circle	Roxane Laboratories
54 017	Torsemide	20 mg	White to Off-White	Tablet	Circle	Roxane Laboratories
54 104	Fluconazole	100 mg	Pink	Tablet	Circle	Roxane Laboratories
54 107	Lithium Carbonate	300 mg	Beige	Tablet, Extended Release	Circle	Roxane Laboratories
54 111	Mefloquine Hydrochloride	250 mg	Off-White to Yellow	Tablet	Circle	Roxane Laboratories
54 163	Meperidine Hydrochloride	100 mg	White	Tablet		Roxane Laboratories
54 200	Fluconazole	150 mg	Pink	Tablet	Circle	Roxane Laboratories
54 213	Lithium Carbonate	150 mg	White Opaque	Capsule		Roxane Laboratories
54 271	Clarithromycin	250 mg	White	Tablet	Circle	Roxane Laboratories
54 312	Clarithromycin	500 mg	White	Tablet	Capsule-Shape	Roxane Laboratories
54 334	Fluconazole	200 mg	Pink	Tablet	Circle	Roxane Laboratories
54 409 ;	Oramorph SR	30 mg	White	Sustained-Release Tablet	Circle	Roxane Laboratories
54 420	Mercaptopurine	50 mg	Pale Yellow	Tablet	Biconvex	Roxane Laboratories

IMPRINT	BRAND/GENERIC NAME	STRENGTH	COLOR	FORM	SHAPE	MANUFACTURER
54 452	Lithium Carbonate	300 mg	White	Tablet		Roxane Laboratories
54 463	Lithium Carbonate	300 mg	Flesh	Capsule		Roxane Laboratories
54 521	Cilostazol	50 mg	White	Tablet	Triangle	Roxane Laboratories
54 552	Clotrimazole Troche	10 mg	White	Lozenge/troche		Roxane Laboratories
54 609 ;	Hydromorphone Hydrochloride	4 mg	White	Tablet	Circle	Roxane Laboratories
54 647	Pilocarpine Hydrochloride	5 mg	White	Tablet		Roxane Laboratories
54 702	Lithium Carbonate	600 mg	Flesh, White Opaque	Capsule		Roxane Laboratories
54 743 ;	Hydromorphone Hydrochloride	2 mg	White	Tablet	Circle	Roxane Laboratories
54 757	Cilostazol	100 mg	White	Tablet	Circle	Roxane Laboratories
54 777	Zidovudine	300 mg	White	Tablet	Circle	Roxane Laboratories
54 782 ;	Oramorph SR	15 mg	White	Sustained-Release Tablet	Circle	Roxane Laboratories
54 840	Furosemide	20 mg	White	Tablet		Roxane Laboratories
54 862 ;	Oramorph SR	100 mg	White	Tablet, Extended Release	Circle	Roxane Laboratories
54 879	Meperidine Hydrochloride	50 mg	White	Tablet		Roxane Laboratories
54 923	Acyclovir	200 mg		Capsule		Roxane Laboratories
54 996	Fluconazole	50 mg	Pink	Tablet	Circle	Roxane Laboratories
54 998	Anagrelide Hydrochloride	1 mg	Gray	Capsule		Roxane Laboratories
54; 007	Mirtazapine	45 mg	White	Tablet	Circle	Roxane Laboratories
54; 009	Propranolol Hydrochloride	20 mg	White	Tablet	Circle	Roxane Laboratories
54; 010	Diflunisal	250 mg	Orange	Coated Tablet	Capsule-Shape, Biconvex	Roxane Laboratories
54; 012	Amitriptyline Hydrochloride	25 mg	White	Tablet		Roxane Laboratories
54; 013	Leucovorin Calcium	25 mg	Yellow	Tablet	Circle, Scored	Roxane Laboratories
54; 019	Chlorpheniramine Maleate	4 mg	Yellow	Tablet		Roxane Laboratories
54; 024	Flecainide Acetate	50 mg	White	Tablet	Circle	Roxane Laboratories
54; 039	Naproxen	500 mg	Beige	Tablet	Capsule-Shape	Roxane Laboratories
54; 042	Nefazodone Hydrochloride	100 mg	White	Tablet	Oval	Roxane Laboratories
54; 042	Nefazodone Hydrochloride	100 mg	White	Tablet	Oval, Scored	Roxane Laboratories
54; 043	Azathioprine	50 mg	Yellow	Tablet	Circle, Scored	Roxane Laboratories
54; 050	Haloperidol	1 mg		Tablet		Roxane Laboratories
54; 053	Quinidine Sulfate	300 mg	White	Tablet		Roxane Laboratories
54; 062	Propranolol Hydrochloride	60 mg	White	Tablet	Circle	Roxane Laboratories
54; 063	Acetaminophen	325 mg	White	Tablet		Roxane Laboratories
54; 070	Flecainide Acetate	100 mg	White	Tablet	Circle	Roxane Laboratories
54; 072	Hydroxyurea	500 mg	Dark Green and Light Pink	Capsule		Roxane Laboratories
54; 080	Prednisone	25 mg		Tablet		Roxane Laboratories
54; 090	Roxanol SR	30 mg	White	Sustained-Release Tablet		Roxane Laboratories
54; 092	Prednisone	1 mg	White	Tablet		Roxane Laboratories
54; 093	Diflunisal	500 mg	Orange	Coated Tablet	Capsule-Shape, Biconvex	Roxane Laboratories
54; 099	Amitriptyline Hydrochloride	50 mg	White	Tablet		Roxane Laboratories
54; 103	Bisacodyl	5 mg	Orange	Tablet		Roxane Laboratories
54; 133	Calcium Carbonate	1250 mg	Off-White	Tablet, Chewable	Circle	Roxane Laboratories
54; 142	Methadone Hydrochloride	10 mg	White	Tablet		Roxane Laboratories
54; 143	Amitriptyline Hydrochloride	100 mg	White	Tablet		Roxane Laboratories
54; 150	Flecainide Acetate	150 mg	White	Tablet	Capsule-Shape	Roxane Laboratories
54; 162	Dolophine Hydrochloride	5 mg	White	Tablet	Circle	Roxane Laboratories
54; 169	Haloperidol	0.5 mg		Tablet		Roxane Laboratories
54; 172	Isoxsuprine Hydrochloride	10 mg	White	Tablet		Roxane Laboratories
54; 179	Chloral Hydrate	500 mg	Red	Capsule		Roxane Laboratories
54; 180	Naproxen Sodium Film-Coated	275 mg	Light Blue	Tablet	Oval	Roxane Laboratories
54; 183	Prednisolone	5 mg	White	Tablet		Roxane Laboratories
54; 193	Viramune	200 mg	White	Tablet	Oval, Biconvex, Bisected Scored	Boehringer Ingelheim Pharmaceuticals
54; 193	Viramune	200 mg	White	Tablet	Oval, Biconvex, Bisected Scored	Roxane Laboratories
54; 199	Roxicodone	30 mg	Blue	Tablet		Roxane Laboratories
54; 201	Mirtazapine	15 mg	Yellow	Tablet	Circle	Roxane Laboratories
54; 210	Methadone Hydrochloride	5 mg	White	Tablet		Roxane Laboratories
54; 212	Neomycin Sulfate	500 mg	Off-White	Tablet		Roxane Laboratories
54; 223	Diphenhydramine Hydrochloride	50 mg	Pink	Capsule		Roxane Laboratories
54; 249	Propranolol Hydrochloride	80 mg	White	Tablet	Circle	Roxane Laboratories
54; 252	Acetaminophen	500 mg		Tablet		Roxane Laboratories
54; 253	Sulfamethoxazole and Trimethoprim	400 mg; 80 mg	White	Tablet	Capsule-Shape, Scored	Roxane Laboratories
54; 259	Ferrous Sulfate	300 mg	Red	Tablet		Roxane Laboratories
54; 262	Morphine Sulfate	30 mg	White	Tablet		Roxane Laboratories
54; 263	Phenobarbital	100 mg	White	Tablet		Roxane Laboratories
54; 280	Dht	0.125 mg	White	Tablet		Roxane Laboratories
54; 293	Leucovorin Calcium	5 mg	Off-White	Tablet	Circle, Scored	Roxane Laboratories
54; 299	Dexamethasone	0.5 mg	Yellow	Tablet		Roxane Laboratories
54; 302	Calcium Carbonate	1250 mg	White	Tablet	Capsule-Shape	Roxane Laboratories
54; 303	Propantheline Bromide	15 mg	White	Tablet		Roxane Laboratories
54; 310	Nefazodone Hydrochloride	200 mg	Speckled Yellow	Tablet	Oval	Roxane Laboratories
54; 310	Nefazodone Hydrochloride	200 mg	Yellow	Tablet	Oval	Roxane Laboratories
54; 323	Methotrexate	2.5 mg	Yellow	Tablet	Circle, Scored	Roxane Laboratories
54; 329	Indomethacin	50 mg	Light Green	Capsule		Roxane Laboratories
54; 333	Propranolol Hydrochloride	40 mg	White	Tablet	Circle	Roxane Laboratories
54; 339	Prednisone	2.5 mg	White	Tablet		Roxane Laboratories
54; 343	Prednisone	50 mg	White	Tablet		Roxane Laboratories
54; 346	Lithium Carbonate	450 mg	Off-White to Yellow	Extended-Release Tablet		Roxane Laboratories
54; 352	Megestrol Acetate	40 mg	White	Tablet	Circle, Scored	Roxane Laboratories
54; 353	Mirtazapine	30 mg	Biege	Tablet	Circle	Roxane Laboratories
54; 360	Amitriptyline Hydrochloride	75 mg	White	Tablet		Roxane Laboratories
54; 363	Mirtazapine	30 mg	Beige	Tablet	Circle	Roxane Laboratories
54; 369	Loperamide Hydrochloride	2 mg	Light Green	Capsule		Roxane Laboratories
54; 372	Calcium Gluconate	500 mg	White	Tablet		Roxane Laboratories
54; 379	Docusate Sodium	50 mg	Red	Capsule		Roxane Laboratories

IMPRINT	BRAND/GENERIC NAME	STRENGTH	COLOR	FORM	SHAPE	MANUFACTURER
54; 382	Haloperidol	10 mg		Tablet		Roxane Laboratories
54; 383	Methyldopa	500 mg		Tablet		Roxane Laboratories
54; 392	Oxycodone and Acetaminophen	500 mg; 5 mg		Capsule		Roxane Laboratories
54; 392	Roxilox	5 mg; 500 mg		Capsule		Roxane Laboratories
54; 403	Hydromorphone Hydrochloride	8 mg	White	Tablet	Circle, Scored	Roxane Laboratories
54; 409; 30	Morphine Sulfate SR	30 mg	White	Sustained-Release Tablet	Circle, Scored	Roxane Laboratories
54; 410	Levorphanol Tartrate	2 mg	White	Tablet	Circle, Scored	Roxane Laboratories
54; 412	Codeine Sulfate	60 mg	White	Tablet		Roxane Laboratories
54; 422	Indomethacin	25 mg	Light Green	Capsule		Roxane Laboratories
54; 460	Cimetidine	800 mg		Tablet		Roxane Laboratories
54; 472	Piroxicam	10 mg		Capsule		Roxane Laboratories
54; 479	Piroxicam	20 mg	Dark Blue	Capsule		Roxane Laboratories
54; 482	Tamoxifen	20 mg	White	Tablet	Circle	Roxane Laboratories
54; 489	Dexamethasone	1 mg	Yellow	Tablet		Roxane Laboratories
54; 492	Amitriptyline Hydrochloride	150 mg	White	Tablet		Roxane Laboratories
54; 499	Hydrochlorothiazide	50 mg	Peach	Tablet		Roxane Laboratories
54; 503	Phenobarbital	15 mg	White	Tablet		Roxane Laboratories
54; 512	Alprazolam	0.25 mg	White	Tablet	Oval, Scored	Roxane Laboratories
54; 519	Triazolam	0.125 mg	White	Tablet	Oval	Roxane Laboratories
54; 523	Mexiletine Hydrochloride	150 mg		Capsule		Roxane Laboratories
54; 529	Torecan	10 mg	Yellow	Tablet		Roxane Laboratories
54; 532	Pseudoephedrine Hydrochloride	60 mg	White	Tablet		Roxane Laboratories
54; 533	Furosemide	80 mg	White	Tablet	Circle	Roxane Laboratories
54; 539	Ascorbic Acid	250 mg	White	Tablet		Roxane Laboratories
54; 543	Roxicet	5 mg; 325 mg	White	Tablet		Roxane Laboratories
54; 549	Dolophine Hydrochloride	10 mg	White	Tablet	Circle	Roxane Laboratories
54; 570	Haloperidol	2 mg		Tablet		Roxane Laboratories
54; 572	Phenobarbital	30 mg	White	Tablet		Roxane Laboratories
54; 579	Isoxsuprine Hydrochloride	20 mg	White	Tablet		Roxane Laboratories
54; 583	Furosemide	40 mg	White	Tablet		Roxane Laboratories
54; 592	Diclofenac Sodium	50 mg	White	Timed-Release Tablet	Circle	Roxane Laboratories
54; 599	Alprazolam	0.5 mg	White	Tablet	Oval, Scored	Roxane Laboratories
54; 603	Naproxen Sodium Film-Coated	550 mg	Dark Blue	Tablet	Capsule-Shape	Roxane Laboratories
54; 612	Prednisone	5 mg	White	Tablet		Roxane Laboratories
54; 613	Codeine Sulfate	15 mg		Tablet		Roxane Laboratories
54; 620	Triazolam	0.25 mg	Light Blue	Tablet	Oval, Scored	Roxane Laboratories
54; 622	Methyldopa	250 mg		Tablet		Roxane Laboratories
54; 623	Acetaminophen and Codeine Phosphate	300 mg; 30 mg	White	Tablet		Roxane Laboratories
54; 632	Mexiletine Hydrochloride	200 mg		Capsule		Roxane Laboratories
54; 639	Cyclophosphamide	25 mg	Light Blue	Tablet	Circle	Roxane Laboratories
54; 643	Naproxen	250 mg	Beige	Tablet	Circle	Roxane Laboratories
54; 650	Leucovorin Calcium	15 mg	Yellow	Tablet	Circle, Scored	Roxane Laboratories
54; 659	Pseudoephedrine Hydrochloride and Triprolidine Hydrochloride	60 mg; 2.5 mg	White	Tablet		Roxane Laboratories
54; 659	Triprolidine with Pseudoephedrine Hydrochloride	2.5 mg; 60 mg		Tablet		Roxane Laboratories
54; 662	Dexamethasone	2 mg	White	Tablet		Roxane Laboratories
54; 663	Docusate Sodium	100 mg	Red	Capsule		Roxane Laboratories
54; 680	Ascorbic Acid	500 mg	White	Tablet		Roxane Laboratories
54; 690	Haloperidol	20 mg		Tablet		Roxane Laboratories
54; 699	Niacin	50 mg	White	Tablet		Roxane Laboratories
54; 703	Imipramine Hydrochloride	50 mg	Coral	Tablet		Roxane Laboratories
54; 710	Roxicodone	15 mg	Green	Tablet		Roxane Laboratories
54; 713	Nefazodone Hydrochloride	50 mg	Speckled Peach	Tablet	Oval	Roxane Laboratories
54; 713	Nefazodone Hydrochloride	50 mg	Peach	Tablet	Oval	Roxane Laboratories
54; 720	Docusate Sodium with Casanthranol	100 mg; 30 mg	Dark Red	Capsule		Roxane Laboratories
54; 730	Roxicet	5 mg; 500 mg	White	Tablet	Capsule-Shape	Roxane Laboratories
54; 732	Diphenoxylate Hydrochloride and Atropine Sulfate	2.5 mg; 0.025 mg	White	Tablet		Roxane Laboratories
54; 733	Morphine Sulfate	15 mg	White	Tablet		Roxane Laboratories
54; 749	Nefazodone Hydrochloride	150 mg	Speckled Peach	Tablet	Oval, Scored	Roxane Laboratories
54; 749	Nefazodone Hydrochloride	150 mg	Peach	Tablet	Oval	Roxane Laboratories
54; 760	Prednisone	20 mg	White	Tablet		Roxane Laboratories
54; 763	Megestrol Acetate	20 mg	White	Tablet	Circle, Scored	Roxane Laboratories
54; 769	Dexamethasone	6 mg	Aqua	Tablet		Roxane Laboratories
54; 772	Dht	0.4 mg		Tablet		Roxane Laboratories
54; 773	Haloperidol	5 mg	White	Tablet	Six-Sided, Scored	Roxane Laboratories
54; 779	Phenobarbital	60 mg	White	Tablet		Roxane Laboratories
54; 780	Tamoxifen	10 mg	White	Tablet	Circle	Roxane Laboratories
54; 783	Codeine Sulfate	30 mg	White	Tablet		Roxane Laboratories
54; 799	Cimetidine	400 mg		Tablet		Roxane Laboratories
54; 810	Propranolol Hydrochloride	90 mg	White	Tablet	Circle	Roxane Laboratories
54; 812	Hydrochlorothiazide	25 mg	Peach	Tablet		Roxane Laboratories
54; 819	Acetaminophen	650 mg	White	Tablet		Roxane Laboratories
54; 822	Sulfamethoxazole and Trimethoprim Double Strength	800 mg; 160 mg	White	Tablet	Capsule-Shape, Scored	Roxane Laboratories
54; 823	Pseudoephedrine Hydrochloride	30 mg	White	Tablet		Roxane Laboratories
54; 833	Nefazodone Hydrochloride	250 mg	White	Tablet	Oval	Roxane Laboratories
54; 839	Diclofenac Sodium	75 mg	White	Timed-Release Tablet	Circle	Roxane Laboratories
54; 843	Methadone Hydrochloride	40 mg	White	Tablet	Square with Rounded Corners; Cross-Scored	Roxane Laboratories
54; 853	Methyldopa	125 mg		Tablet		Roxane Laboratories
54; 859	Aminophylline	100 mg	White	Tablet		Roxane Laboratories
54; 860	Alprazolam	1 mg	White	Tablet	Oval, Scored	Roxane Laboratories
54; 880	Imipramine Hydrochloride	25 mg	Coral	Tablet		Roxane Laboratories
54; 883	Methadone Hydrochloride	40 mg	Peach	Tablet		Roxane Laboratories

IMPRINT	BRAND/GENERIC NAME	STRENGTH	COLOR	FORM	SHAPE	MANUFACTURER
54; 892	Dexamethasone	4 mg	Green	Tablet		Roxane Laboratories
54; 899	Prednisone	10 mg	White	Tablet		Roxane Laboratories
54; 902	Roxiprin	4.5 mg; 0.38 mg; 325 mg	White	Tablet	Circle	Roxane Laboratories
54; 903	Dht	0.2 mg	Pink	Tablet		Roxane Laboratories
54; 912	Cimetidine	300 mg		Tablet		Roxane Laboratories
54; 930	Aminophylline	200 mg	White	Tablet		Roxane Laboratories
54; 932	Acetaminophen and Codeine No. 4	300 mg; 60 mg	White	Tablet		Roxane Laboratories
54; 939	Imipramine Hydrochloride	10 mg	Coral	Tablet		Roxane Laboratories
54; 942	Leucovorin Calcium	10 mg	Off-White	Tablet	Circle, Scored	Roxane Laboratories
54; 943	Dexamethasone	1.5 mg	Pink	Tablet		Roxane Laboratories
54; 959	Mexiletine Hydrochloride	250 mg		Tablet		Roxane Laboratories
54; 960	Dexamethasone	0.75 mg	Pale Blue	Tablet		Roxane Laboratories
54; 969	Diazepam	2 mg	Peach	Tablet	Circle, Scored	Roxane Laboratories
54; 970	Propranolol Hydrochloride	10 mg	White	Tablet	Circle	Roxane Laboratories
54; 972	Propoxyphene Hydrochloride	65 mg	Pink	Capsule		Roxane Laboratories
54; 973	Diazepam	5 mg	Peach	Tablet	Circle, Scored	Roxane Laboratories
54; 979	Quinidine Sulfate	200 mg	White	Tablet		Roxane Laboratories
54; 980	Cyclophosphamide	50 mg	Light Blue	Tablet	Circle	Roxane Laboratories
54; 982	Diazepam	10 mg	Peach	Tablet	Circle, Scored	Roxane Laboratories
54; 983	Amitriptyline Hydrochloride	10 mg	White	Tablet		Roxane Laboratories
54; 992	Naproxen	375 mg	Pink	Tablet	Capsule-Shape	Roxane Laboratories
54; 997	Mirtazapine	45 mg	White	Tablet	Circle	Roxane Laboratories
56; 105	Symmetrel	100 mg	Red	Capsule, Liquid Filled		Endo Laboratories
57	Zorprin	800 mg	White	Extended-Release Tablet	Oblong	Par Pharmaceutical
60	Terazosin Hydrochloride	1 mg	Grey	Capsule		Teva Pharmaceuticals
60 MG; LILLY; 3237	Cymbalta	60 mg	Opaque Green and Opaque Blue	Delayed-Release Capsule		Eli Lilly
60-60 ; IMDUR	Imdur	60 mg	White	Tablet, Extended Release	Capsule-Shape	Schering
61	Terazosin Hydrochloride	2 mg	Yellow	Capsule		Teva Pharmaceuticals
62	Terazosin Hydrochloride	5 mg	Red	Capsule		Teva Pharmaceuticals
62.5	Tracleer	62.5 mg	Orange-White	Coated Tablet	Circle, Biconvex	Genentech
63	Terazosin Hydrochloride	10 mg	Blue	Capsule		Teva Pharmaceuticals
68; 7	Norpramin	10 mg	Blue	Tablet		Sanofi-Aventis U.S.
70	Adipex 8	8 mg	Blue and White	Tablet		Teva Pharmaceuticals
74; XX	Potassium Chloride	750 mg	Light Brown	Tablet	Oval	Abbott Laboratories
75	Slo-Bid Gyrocaps	75 mg	White and Clear	Extended-Release Capsule		Aventis Pharmaceuticals
75; 1171	Plavix	75 mg	Pink	Coated Tablet	Circle, Biconvex	Bristol-Myers Squibb
75; 1171	Plavix	75 mg	Pink	Coated Tablet	Circle, Biconvex	Sanofi-Synthelabo
75; T4	Levothroid	75 mcg	Violet	Tablet	Capsule-Shape	Forest Pharmaceuticals
77 ; E	Frova	2.5 mg	White	Tablet	Circle	Endo Laboratories
77; BONE IMAGE	Fosamax	35 mg	White	Tablet	Oval	Merck
78/212; 10 ;	Metaprel	10 mg	White	Tablet	Circle, Compressed	Novartis Pharmaceuticals
78/213; 20	Metaprel	20 mg	White	Tablet	Circle, Compressed	Novartis Pharmaceuticals
78; 28 ;	Belladenal	0.25 mg; 50 mg	White	Tablet	Cross-Scored	Novartis Pharmaceuticals
78; 31	Bellergal-S	40 mg; 0.6 mg; 0.2 mg	Dark Green, Orange, Yellow	Tablet	Circle, Compressed	Novartis
78; 52; SANDOZ S ;	Mesantoin	100 mg	Pink	Tablet		Novartis Pharmaceuticals
80 ; 0019	Pravastatin Sodium	80 mg	Yellow	Tablet	Oval	Watson Laboratories
80 INNOPRANXL LOGO	Innopran XL	80 mg	Gray, White	Capsule, Extended Release		Reliant Pharmaceuticals
81	Bayer Low Dose Aspirin Regimen	81 mg	Yellow	Delayed Release Tablet	Circle	Bayer Consumer Care
85; 05; M	Flecainide Acetate	50 mg	Round	Tablet	Circle, White	Mylan Pharmaceuticals
85; 10; M	Flecainide Acetate	100 mg	White	Tablet	Circle	Mylan Pharmaceuticals
85; 15; M	Flecainide Acetate	150 mg	White	Tablet	Capsule-Shape	Mylan Pharmaceuticals
85; WMH; 231	Disophrol Chronotab	6 mg; 120 mg	Red	Extended-Release Tablet		Schering-Plough
86; 62; C ;	Skelaxin	400 mg	Pale Rose	Tablet	Circle, Scored	King Pharmaceuticals
86; 67; S ;	Skelaxin	800 mg	Pink	Tablet	Oval, Scored	King Pharmaceuticals
87	Terramycin with Polymyxin B Sulfate	100 mg; 100000 U	Yellow	Tablet		Pfizer
88; T4	Levothroid	88 mcg	Mint Green	Tablet	Capsule-Shape	Forest Pharmaceuticals
93 ; 0863	Ciprofloxacin	250 mg	White to Off White	Tablet	Circle	Teva Pharmaceuticals
93 ; 0864	Ciprofloxacin	500 mg	White to Off White	Tablet	Capsule-Shape	Teva Pharmaceuticals
93 ; 0865	Ciprofloxacin	750 mg	White to Off White	Tablet	Capsule-Shape	Teva Pharmaceuticals
93 ; 24 ;	Oxycodone Hydrochloride Extended Release	10 mg	White	Tablet, Extended Release	Oval	Teva Pharmaceuticals
93 ; 31 ;	Oxycodone Hydrochloride Extended Release	20 mg	Pink	Tablet, Extended Release	Oval	Teva Pharmaceuticals
93 ; 32 ;	Oxycodone Hydrochloride Extended Release	40 mg	Yellow	Tablet, Extended Release	Oval	Teva Pharmaceuticals
93 ; 33 ;	Oxycodone Hydrochloride Extended Release	80 mg	Green	Tablet, Extended Release	Oval	Teva Pharmaceuticals
93 ; 132	Lamotrigine	25 mg	White to Off-White	Tablet, Chewable	Oval	Teva Pharmaceuticals
93 ; 688	Lamotrigine	5 mg	White to Off-White	Tablet, Chewable	Circle	Teva Pharmaceuticals
93 ; 1172	Penicillin-VK	250 mg	White to Off-White	Tablet	Oval	Teva Pharmaceuticals
93 ; 5124	Benazepril Hydrochloride	5 mg	Light Yellow	Tablet	Triangle	Teva Pharmaceuticals
93 ; 5125	Benazepril Hydrochloride	10 mg	Mustard Yellow	Tablet	Triangle	Teva Pharmaceuticals
93 ; 5126	Benazepril Hydrochloride	20 mg	Pink	Tablet	Triangle	Teva Pharmaceuticals
93 ; 5127	Benazepril Hydrochloride	40 mg	Pink to Light Red	Tablet	Triangle	Teva Pharmaceuticals
93 ; 7114	Paroxetine	10 mg	Yellow	Tablet	Circle	Teva Pharmaceuticals
93 ; 7115	Paroxetine	20 mg	Pink	Tablet	Circle	Teva Pharmaceuticals
93 ; 7116	Paroxetine	30 mg	Blue	Tablet	Circle	Teva Pharmaceuticals
93 ; 7121	Paroxetine	40 mg	Green	Tablet	Circle	Teva Pharmaceuticals
93 ; 7146	Azithromycin	250 mg	Mottled Pink	Tablet	Oval	Teva Pharmaceuticals
93 ; 7147	Azithromycin	600 mg	White to Off-White	Tablet	Capsule-Shape	Teva Pharmaceuticals
93 ; 7157	Clarithromycin	250 mg	Yellow	Tablet	Oval	Teva Pharmaceuticals

IMPRINT	BRAND/GENERIC NAME	STRENGTH	COLOR	FORM	SHAPE	MANUFACTURER
93 ; 7158	Clarithromycin	500 mg	Light Yellow	Tablet	Oval	Teva Pharmaceuticals
93 ; 7169	Azithromycin	500 mg	Mottled Pink	Tablet	Oval	Teva Pharmaceuticals
93 ; 7175	Sertraline Hydrochloride	25 mg	Light Green	Tablet	Oval	Teva Pharmaceuticals
93 ; 7176	Sertraline Hydrochloride	50 mg	Light Blue	Tablet	Oval	Teva Pharmaceuticals
93 ; 7177	Sertraline Hydrochloride	100 mg	Light Yellow	Tablet	Oval	Teva Pharmaceuticals
93 ; 7215	Metolazone	2.5 mg	Mottled Pink	Tablet	Capsule-Shape	Teva Pharmaceuticals
93 ; 7217	Metolazone	10 mg	Yellow	Tablet	Circle	Teva Pharmaceuticals
93 ; 7230	Cilostazol	50 mg	White to Off White	Tablet	Rectangle	Teva Pharmaceuticals
93 ; 7231	Cilostazol	100 mg	White to Off White	Tablet	Circle	Teva Pharmaceuticals
93 ; 7232	Ribavirin	200 mg	Light Pink to Pink	Tablet	Circle	Teva Pharmaceuticals
93 ; 7234	Meloxicam	7.5 mg	Mottled Yellow	Tablet	Capsule-Shape	Teva Pharmaceuticals
93 ; 7251	Fexofenadine Hydrochloride	30 mg	Peach	Tablet	Capsule-Shape	Teva Pharmaceuticals
93 ; 7252	Fexofenadine Hydrochloride	60 mg	Peach	Tablet	Circle	Teva Pharmaceuticals
93 ; 7253	Fexofenadine Hydrochloride	180 mg	Peach	Tablet	Circle	Teva Pharmaceuticals
93 ; 7254 ;	Glimepiride	1 mg	Mottled Pink	Tablet	Circle	Teva Pharmaceuticals
93 ; 7255 ;	Glimepiride	2 mg	Mottled Green	Tablet	Circle	Teva Pharmaceuticals
93 ; 7256 ;	Glimepiride	4 mg	Mottled Light Blue	Tablet	Circle	Teva Pharmaceuticals
93 ; 7299	Meloxicam	15 mg	Mottled Yellow	Tablet	Rectangle	Teva Pharmaceuticals
93 11; 2	Aspirin and Codeine No. 2	325 mg; 15 mg	White	Tablet	Circle, Convex	Teva Pharmaceuticals
93 38	Gabapentin	100 mg	Grey	Capsule		Teva Pharmaceuticals
93 39	Gabapentin	300 mg	Orange	Capsule		Teva Pharmaceuticals
93 40	Gabapentin	400 mg	Caramel	Capsule		Teva Pharmaceuticals
93 778	Carbamazepine	100 mg	Pink, Red	Tablet, Chewable	Circle	Teva Pharmaceuticals
93 2238 ;	Cephalexin	250 mg	White	Tablet	Capsule-Shape	Teva Pharmaceuticals
93 2240 ;	Cephalexin	500 mg	White	Tablet	Capsule-Shape	Teva Pharmaceuticals
93 3145 ;	Cephalexin	250 mg	Gray, Swedish Orange	Capsule		Teva Pharmaceuticals
93 5160	Tizanidine Hydrochloride	4 mg	White to Off-White	Tablet	Circle	Teva Pharmaceuticals
93 5163	Tizanidine Hydrochloride	2 mg	White to Off-White	Tablet	Circle	Teva Pharmaceuticals
93 7162	Zonisamide	100 mg	Flesh Colored Opaque, Pink Opaque	Capsule		Teva Pharmaceuticals
93 7508	Zonisamide	25 mg	White Opaque	Capsule		Teva Pharmaceuticals
93 7509	Zonisamide	50 mg	Iron Gray Opaque	Capsule		Teva Pharmaceuticals
93 9380	Ursodiol	300 mg	Red Opaque, White Opaque	Capsule		Teva Pharmaceuticals
93; 027	Dipyridamole	25 mg		Tablet		Teva Pharmaceuticals
93; 068	Meprobamate	200 mg		Tablet		Teva Pharmaceuticals
93; 069	Meprobamate	400 mg		Tablet		Teva Pharmaceuticals
93; 088	Sulfamethoxazole and Trimethoprim	400 mg; 80 mg	White	Tablet	Circle, Convex, Scored	Teva Pharmaceuticals
93; 089	Sulfamethoxazole and Trimethoprim Double Strength	800 mg; 160 mg	White	Tablet	Oval, Convex, Scored	Teva Pharmaceuticals
93; 0924	Oxaprozin	600 mg	White to Off-White	Tablet	Capsule-Shape	Teva Pharmaceuticals
93; 5	Naproxen Delayed-Release	375 mg	White	Enteric-Coated Tablet	Capsule-Shape	Teva Pharmaceuticals
93; 6	Naproxen Delayed-Release	500 mg	White	Enteric-Coated Tablet	Capsule-Shape	Teva Pharmaceuticals
93; 7	Chlorpropamide	250 mg	Blue	Tablet	Circle, Convex, Scored	Teva Pharmaceuticals
93; 8	Indapamide	2.5 mg	White	Coated Tablet	Circle	Teva Pharmaceuticals
93; 10	Chlorpropamide	100 mg	Blue	Tablet	Circle, Convex, Scored	Teva Pharmaceuticals
93; 12; 3	Aspirin and Codeine No. 3	325 mg; 30 mg	White	Tablet	Circle, Convex	Teva Pharmaceuticals
93; 13; 4	Aspirin and Codeine No. 4	325 mg; 60 mg	White	Tablet	Circle, Convex	Teva Pharmaceuticals
93; 15	Nabumetone	500 mg	White	Tablet	Oval	Teva Pharmaceuticals
93; 16	Nabumetone	750 mg	Beige	Tablet	Oval	Teva Pharmaceuticals
93; 21	Diltiazem ER	60 mg	Pink and White	Extended-Release Capsule		Teva Pharmaceuticals
93; 22	Diltiazem ER	90 mg	Pink and Yellow	Extended-Release Capsule		Teva Pharmaceuticals
93; 23	Diltiazem ER	120 mg	Pink and Orange	Extended-Release Capsule		Teva Pharmaceuticals
93; 26	Enalapril Maleate	2.5 mg	Yellow	Tablet	Oval, Scored	Teva Pharmaceuticals
93; 27	Enalapril Maleate	5 mg	White	Tablet	Oval, Scored	Teva Pharmaceuticals
93; 28	Enalapril Maleate	10 mg		Tablet		Teva Pharmaceuticals
93; 29	Enalapril Maleate	20 mg	Orange	Tablet	Oblong	Teva Pharmaceuticals
93; 41	Clomiphene Citrate	50 mg	White	Tablet	Circle, Flat, Beveled Edge, Scored	Teva Pharmaceuticals
93; 42	Fluoxetine Hydrochloride	10 mg	Light Blue	Capsule		Teva Pharmaceuticals
93; 43	Fluoxetine Hydrochloride	20 mg	Blue and White	Capsule		Teva Pharmaceuticals
93; 53	Buspirone Hydrochloride	5 mg		Tablet		Teva Pharmaceuticals
93; 54	Buspirone Hydrochloride	10 mg		Tablet		Teva Pharmaceuticals
93; 58	Tramadol Hydrochloride	50 mg	White	Tablet	Oval	Teva Pharmaceuticals
93; 61	Sotalol Hydrochloride	80 mg	Light Blue	Tablet	Oblong	Teva Pharmaceuticals
93; 62	Sotalol Hydrochloride	160 mg	Light Blue	Tablet	Oval, Scored	Teva Pharmaceuticals
93; 63	Sotalol Hydrochloride	240 mg	Light Blue	Tablet	Oval, Scored	Teva Pharmaceuticals
93; 76	Isosorbide Mononitrate	20 mg	Yellow	Tablet	Circle, Scored	Teva Pharmaceuticals
93; 91	Captopril	12.5 mg	White	Tablet	Oval, Scored	Teva Pharmaceuticals
93; 92	Captopril	25 mg	White	Tablet	Round, Quadrisected Scored	Teva Pharmaceuticals
93; 97	Captopril	50 mg	White	Tablet	Circle, Scored	Teva Pharmaceuticals
93; 98	Captopril	100 mg	White	Tablet	Circle, Scored	Teva Pharmaceuticals
93; 100	Labetalol Hydrochloride	100 mg		Tablet		Teva Pharmaceuticals
93; 102	Labetalol Hydrochloride	200 mg		Tablet		Teva Pharmaceuticals
93; 106	Labetalol Hydrochloride	300 mg		Tablet		Teva Pharmaceuticals
93; 111	Cimetidine	200 mg	White	Coated Tablet	Circle	Teva Pharmaceuticals
93; 112	Cimetidine	300 mg	White	Coated Tablet	Circle	Teva Pharmaceuticals
93; 113	Cimetidine	400 mg	White	Coated Tablet	Oblong, Scored	Teva Pharmaceuticals
93; 115	Haloperidol	0.5 mg	White	Tablet	Circle	Teva Pharmaceuticals
93; 116	Haloperidol	1 mg	Yellow	Tablet	Circle	Teva Pharmaceuticals
93; 117	Haloperidol	2 mg	Pink	Tablet	Circle	Teva Pharmaceuticals
93; 118	Haloperidol	5 mg	Green	Tablet	Circle	Teva Pharmaceuticals
93; 122	Cimetidine	800 mg	White	Coated Tablet	Oblong, Scored	Teva Pharmaceuticals
93; 129	Estazolam	1 mg	White	Tablet	Oval	Teva Pharmaceuticals
93; 130	Estazolam	2 mg	Coral	Tablet	Oval, Scored	Teva Pharmaceuticals

IMPRINT	BRAND/GENERIC NAME	STRENGTH	COLOR	FORM	SHAPE	MANUFACTURER
93; 132	Acetaminophen and Codeine No. 2	300 mg; 15 mg	Carmel Opaque and White	Capsule		Teva Pharmaceuticals
93; 138	Diphenhydramine Hydrochloride	25 mg	Pink Transparent and Clear	Capsule		Teva Pharmaceuticals
93; 139	Diphenhydramine Hydrochloride	50 mg	Pink Transparent	Capsule		Teva Pharmaceuticals
93; 147	Naproxen	250 mg	Mottled Light Brick Red	Tablet	Circle, Biconvex	Teva Pharmaceuticals
93; 148	Naproxen	375 mg	Mottled Peach	Tablet	Oval	Teva Pharmaceuticals
93; 149	Naproxen	500 mg	Mottled Light Brick Red	Tablet	Oval	Teva Pharmaceuticals
93; 152	Acetaminophen and Codeine No. 3	300 mg; 30 mg	Coral and Scarlet, Opaque	Capsule		Teva Pharmaceuticals
93; 153	Phendimetrazine Tartrate	35 mg	Pink	Tablet	Oblong	Teva Pharmaceuticals
93; 154	Ticlopidine Hydrochloride	250 mg	White	Coated Tablet	Oval	Teva Pharmaceuticals
93; 157	Diethylpropion Hydrochloride	25 mg	White	Tablet	Circle, Flat Beveled Edge	Teva Pharmaceuticals
93; 172	Acetaminophen and Codeine No. 4	300 mg; 60 mg	Brown and Iron Gray, Opaque	Capsule		Teva Pharmaceuticals
93; 176	Captopril and Hydrochlorothiazide	25 mg; 15 mg	White	Tablet	Round, Quadrisected Scored	Teva Pharmaceuticals
93; 177	Captopril and Hydrochlorothiazide	25 mg; 25 mg	Tan	Tablet	Round, Quadrisected Scored	Teva Pharmaceuticals
93; 181	Captopril and Hydrochlorothiazide	50 mg; 15 mg	White	Tablet	Oval, Scored	Teva Pharmaceuticals
93; 182	Captopril and Hydrochlorothiazide	50 mg; 25 mg	Tan	Tablet	Oval, Scored	Teva Pharmaceuticals
93; 205; LEMMON	Donphen	0.02 mg; 0.1 mg; 15 mg; 6 mcg	Pink	Tablet	Circle, Convex, Scored	Teva Pharmaceuticals
93; 214	Tolmetin Sodium	600 mg	Orange	Tablet	Oblong	Teva Pharmaceuticals
93; 290	Bupropion Hydrochloride	100 mg		Coated Tablet		Teva Pharmaceuticals
93; 292	Carbidopa and Levodopa	10 mg; 100 mg	Mottled Blue	Tablet	Circle, Scored	Teva Pharmaceuticals
93; 293	Carbidopa and Levodopa	25 mg; 100 mg	Mottled Yellow	Tablet	Circle, Scored	Teva Pharmaceuticals
93; 294	Carbidopa and Levodopa	25 mg; 250 mg	Mottled Blue	Tablet	Circle, Scored	Teva Pharmaceuticals
93; 307	Clemastine Fumarate	1.34 mg	White	Tablet	Circle, Convex, Scored	Teva Pharmaceuticals
93; 308	Clemastine Fumarate	2.68 mg	White	Tablet	Circle, Convex, Scored	Teva Pharmaceuticals
93; 311	Loperamide Hydrochloride	2 mg	Light Brown and Dark Brown	Capsule		Teva Pharmaceuticals
93; 318	Diltiazem Hydrochloride	30 mg	Faint Orange	Coated Tablet	Circle, Biconvex	Teva Pharmaceuticals
93; 319	Diltiazem Hydrochloride	60 mg	Orange	Coated Tablet	Circle, Biconvex, Scored	Teva Pharmaceuticals
93; 320	Diltiazem Hydrochloride	90 mg	Faint Orange	Coated Tablet	Oblong, Scored	Teva Pharmaceuticals
93; 321	Diltiazem Hydrochloride	120 mg	Orange	Coated Tablet	Oblong, Scored	Teva Pharmaceuticals
93; 431	Chlorthalidone	50 mg	Blue	Tablet	Circle, Flat, Beveled Edge	Teva Pharmaceuticals
93; 433	Chlorthalidone	100 mg	White	Tablet	Circle, Flat Beveled Edge, Scored	Teva Pharmaceuticals
93; 490	Acetaminophen and Propoxyphene Napsylate	650 mg; 100 mg	White	Coated Tablet	Oblong, Convex	Teva Pharmaceuticals
93; 494	Clonidine Hydrochloride	0.1 mg	Green	Tablet	Circle	Teva Pharmaceuticals
93; 495	Clonidine Hydrochloride	0.2 mg	Yellow	Tablet		Teva Pharmaceuticals
93; 496	Clonidine Hydrochloride	0.3 mg	Peach	Tablet	Circle	Teva Pharmaceuticals
93; 525	Amitriptyline Hydrochloride	10 mg	Pink	Coated Tablet	Circle, Biconvex	Teva Pharmaceuticals
93; 527	Amitriptyline Hydrochloride	25 mg	Green	Coated Tablet	Circle, Biconvex	Teva Pharmaceuticals
93; 529	Amitriptyline Hydrochloride	50 mg	Brown	Coated Tablet	Circle, Biconvex	Teva Pharmaceuticals
93; 531	Amitriptyline Hydrochloride	75 mg	Purple	Coated Tablet	Circle, Biconvex	Teva Pharmaceuticals
93; 533	Amitriptyline Hydrochloride	100 mg	Orange	Coated Tablet	Circle, Biconvex	Teva Pharmaceuticals
93; 535	Amitriptyline Hydrochloride	150 mg	Peach	Coated Tablet	Circle, Biconvex	Teva Pharmaceuticals
93; 536	Naproxen Sodium	275 mg	White to Off-White	Coated Tablet	Oval	Teva Pharmaceuticals
93; 539	Mepro Compound	150 mg; 250 mg; 75 mg		Tablet	Three-Layered	Teva Pharmaceuticals
93; 542	Chlorzoxazone	500 mg	White	Tablet	Oblong, Scored, Convex	Teva Pharmaceuticals
93; 545	Chlorzoxazone and Acetaminophen	300 mg; 250 mg	Light Green	Tablet	Circle, Flat, Beveled Edge, Scored	Teva Pharmaceuticals
93; 576	Lovastatin	20 mg	Blue	Tablet	Circle	Teva Pharmaceuticals
93; 613	Amoxicillin	250 mg	Carmel and Ivory, Opaque	Capsule		Teva Pharmaceuticals
93; 615	Amoxicillin	500 mg	Ivory Opaque	Capsule		Teva Pharmaceuticals
93; 617	Chlordinum Sealets	5 mg; 2.5 mg	White Opaque	Capsule		Teva Pharmaceuticals
93; 620	Propranolol Hydrochloride	20 mg	Blue	Tablet	Circle, Scored	Teva Pharmaceuticals
93; 637	Trazodone Hydrochloride	50 mg	White to Off-White	Tablet	Circle	Teva Pharmaceuticals
93; 638	Trazodone Hydrochloride	100 mg	White to Off-White	Tablet	Circle	Teva Pharmaceuticals
93; 640	Propranolol Hydrochloride	40 mg	Green	Tablet	Circle, Scored	Teva Pharmaceuticals
93; 653	Doxycycline Hyclate	100 mg	Aqua Blue Opaque	Capsule		Teva Pharmaceuticals
93; 657	Calcitriol	0.25 mcg	Red-Brown, Yellow-Brown	Capsule, Liquid Filled	Oval	Teva Pharmaceuticals
93; 658	Calcitriol	0.5 mcg	Brown and Pink	Capsule, Liquid Filled	Oval	Teva Pharmaceuticals
93; 665	Albuterol Sulfate	2 mg	White	Tablet	Circle, Scored	Teva Pharmaceuticals
93; 666	Albuterol	4 mg	White	Tablet	Circle, Scored	Teva Pharmaceuticals
93; 670	Gemcor	600 mg	White to Off-White	Coated Tablet	Oval, Scored	Upsher-Smith Laboratories
93; 670	Gemfibrozil	600 mg	White	Coated Tablet	Oval, Scored	Teva Pharmaceuticals
93; 686	Propoxyphene Compound	389 mg; 32.4 mg; 65 mg	Gray and Red	Capsule		Teva Pharmaceuticals
93; 711	Flurbiprofen	100 mg	Deep Sky Blue	Coated Tablet	Circle, Convex	Teva Pharmaceuticals
93; 727	Papaverine Hydrochloride	150 mg	Brown and Clear	Timed-Release Capsule		Teva Pharmaceuticals
93; 728	Sulindac	150 mg	Yellow	Tablet	Circle, Convex	Teva Pharmaceuticals
93; 729	Sulindac	200 mg	Yellow	Tablet	Circle, Convex, Scored	Teva Pharmaceuticals
93; 733	Metoprolol Tartrate	50 mg	Mottled-Red	Coated Tablet	Circle, Biconvex, Scored	Teva Pharmaceuticals
93; 741; 93; 741	Propoxyphene Hydrochloride	65 mg	Opaque Pink	Capsule		Teva Pharmaceuticals
93; 742	Doxy-Lemmon	50 mg	White and Aqua Blue, Opaque	Capsule		Teva Pharmaceuticals
93; 742	Doxycycline Hyclate	50 mg	White and Aqua Blue, Opaque	Capsule		Teva Pharmaceuticals
93; 743	Doxy-Lemmon	50 mg	Aqua Blue Opaque	Capsule		Teva Pharmaceuticals

IMPRINT	BRAND/GENERIC NAME	STRENGTH	COLOR	FORM	SHAPE	MANUFACTURER
93; 752	Atenolol	50 mg	White	Tablet	Circle, Flat, Scored	Teva Pharmaceuticals
93; 753	Atenolol	100 mg	White	Tablet	Circle, Flat	Teva Pharmaceuticals
93; 754	Diflunisal	250 mg	Blue/lavender	Tablet	Capsule-Shape	Teva Pharmaceuticals
93; 755	Diflunisal	500 mg	Blue	Coated Tablet	Oblong	Teva Pharmaceuticals
93; 756	Piroxicam	10 mg	Dark Green and Olive	Capsule		Teva Pharmaceuticals
93; 757	Piroxicam	20 mg	Dark Green	Capsule		Teva Pharmaceuticals
93; 777	Hydrochlorothiazide	25 mg	Peach	Tablet	Circle, Flat, Beveled Edge, Scored	Teva Pharmaceuticals
93; 779	Hydrochlorothiazide	50 mg	Peach	Tablet	Circle, Flat, Beveled Edge, Scored	Teva Pharmaceuticals
93; 782	Tamoxifen	20 mg	White to Off-White	Tablet	Circle	Teva Pharmaceuticals
93; 782	Tamoxifen Citrate	20 mg	White	Tablet	Circle	Teva Pharmaceuticals
93; 784	Tamoxifen	10 mg	White	Tablet	Circle	Teva Pharmaceuticals
93; 784	Tamoxifen Citrate	10 mg	White	Tablet	Circle	Teva Pharmaceuticals
93; 788	Selegiline Hydrochloride	5 mg	White to Off-White	Tablet	Circle, Flat, Beveled Edge	Teva Pharmaceuticals
93; 793	Nicardipine	20 mg	Opaque White and Aqua Blue	Capsule, Liquid Filled		Teva Pharmaceuticals
93; 794	Nicardipine	30 mg	Opaque White and Light Blue	Capsule, Liquid Filled		Teva Pharmaceuticals
93; 798	Indomethacin	25 mg	Light Green Opaque	Capsule		Teva Pharmaceuticals
93; 799	Indomethacin	50 mg	Light Green Opaque	Capsule		Teva Pharmaceuticals
93; 802	Antispasmodic	16.2 mg; 0.1037 mg; 0.0194 mg; 0.0065 mg	Transparent Green and Clear	Capsule		Teva Pharmaceuticals
93; 804	Phentermine Hydrochloride Black and Scarlet	30 mg	Black and Scarlet, Opaque	Capsule		Teva Pharmaceuticals
93; 808	Phentermine Hydrochloride	8 mg	Green	Tablet	Circle	Teva Pharmaceuticals
93; 809	Phentermine Hydrochloride	8 mg	Peach	Tablet	Circle	Teva Pharmaceuticals
93; 810	Nortriptyline Hydrochloride	10 mg	White and Orange	Capsule		Teva Pharmaceuticals
93; 811	Nortriptyline Hydrochloride	25 mg	White and Orange	Capsule		Teva Pharmaceuticals
93; 812	Nortriptyline	50 mg	White	Capsule		Teva Pharmaceuticals
93; 812	Nortriptyline Hydrochloride	50 mg	White	Capsule		Teva Pharmaceuticals
93; 813	Nortriptyline Hydrochloride	75 mg	Orange	Capsule		Teva Pharmaceuticals
93; 816	Belladonna Alkaloids with Phenobarbital	16.2 mg; 0.1037 mg; 0.0194 mg; 0.0065 mg	White	Tablet	Circle, Convex, Scored	Teva Pharmaceuticals
93; 821	Reserpine	0.25 mg	White	Tablet	Circle, Flat, Beveled Edge, Scored	Teva Pharmaceuticals
93; 823	Uridon	0.03 mg; 0.03 mg; 50 mg; 5.5 mg; 20 mg; 5 mg	Blue	Coated Tablet		Teva Pharmaceuticals
93; 824	Pseudoephedrine Hydrochloride	60 mg	White	Tablet	Circle, Convex	Teva Pharmaceuticals
93; 827	Reserpine	0.1 mg	White	Tablet	Circle, Flat, Beveled Edge, Scored	Teva Pharmaceuticals
93; 828	Urinary Anteseptic No. 3	0.06 mg; 0.03 mg; 120 mg; 6 mg; 30 mg; 7.5 mg	Blue	Coated Tablet	Circle	Teva Pharmaceuticals
93; 828	Uritin´	0.06 mg; 0.03 mg; 120 mg; 30 mg; 6 mg; 7.5 mg		Tablet		Teva Pharmaceuticals
93; 832	Clonazepam	0.5 mg	Yellow	Tablet	Circle, Single-Scored	Teva Pharmaceuticals
93; 833	Clonazepam	1 mg	Mottled Green	Tablet	Circle, Single-Scored	Teva Pharmaceuticals
93; 834	Clonazepam	2 mg	White to Off-White	Tablet	Circle, Single-Scored	Teva Pharmaceuticals
93; 838	Dicyclomine Hydrochloride with Phenobarbital	10 mg; 15 mg	Blue and Clear	Capsule		Teva Pharmaceuticals
93; 841	Dicyclomine Hydrochloride	10 mg	Blue Transparent	Capsule		Teva Pharmaceuticals
93; 845	Atrosept	0.03 mg; 0.03 mg; 40.8 mg; 18.1 mg; 4.5 mg; 5.4 mg	Dark Blue	Coated Tablet	Circle	Teva Pharmaceuticals
93; 845	Urinary Antiseptic No. 2	0.03 mg; 0.03 mg; 40.8 mg; 5.4 mg; 18.1 mg; 4.5 mg	Purple	Coated Tablet	Circle	Teva Pharmaceuticals
93; 845	Uroblue	0.03 mg; 0.03 mg; 40.8 mg; 5.4 mg; 18.1 mg; 4.5 mg	Purple	Tablet		Teva Pharmaceuticals
93; 846	Belladonna Extract and Phenobarbital	0.167 Gr; 0.25 Gr	Green	Tablet	Circle	Teva Pharmaceuticals
93; 848	Triphed	2.5 mg; 60 mg	White	Tablet	Circle, Convex, Scored	Teva Pharmaceuticals
93; 851	Metronidazole	250 mg	White	Tablet	Circle, Convex	Teva Pharmaceuticals
93; 853	Phentermine Hydrochloride	30 mg	Blue and Clear with Blue and White Pellets	Capsule		Teva Pharmaceuticals
93; 858	VI-Forte	12500 IU; 50 IU; 150 mg; 80 mg; 70 mg; 25 mg; 10 mg; 10 mg; 5 mg; 4 mg; 2 mg	Black and Orange	Capsule		Teva Pharmaceuticals
93; 859	Phentermine Hydrochloride	30 mg	Brown and Clear with Orange and White Pellets	Capsule		Teva Pharmaceuticals
93; 860	Phentermine Hydrochloride Yellow	30 mg	Yellow Opaque	Capsule		Teva Pharmaceuticals
93; 861	Phentermine Hydrochloride	8 mg	Yellow	Capsule		Teva Pharmaceuticals
93; 862	Phentermine Hydrochloride	8 mg	Black	Capsule		Teva Pharmaceuticals
93; 866	Phendimetrazine Tartrate	35 mg	Black	Capsule		Teva Pharmaceuticals
93; 867	Phendimetrazine Tartrate	35 mg	Brown and Clear	Capsule		Teva Pharmaceuticals
93; 868	Phendimetrazine Tartrate	30 mg	Red and Yellow	Capsule		Teva Pharmaceuticals
93; 869	Phendimetrazine Tartrate	35 mg	Green and Clear	Capsule		Teva Pharmaceuticals
93; 872	Butabarbital Sodium	15 mg	Purple	Tablet	Circle, Convex, Scored	Teva Pharmaceuticals
93; 873	Butabarbital Sodium	30 mg	Green	Tablet	Circle, Convex, Scored	Teva Pharmaceuticals
93; 882	Phentermine Hydrochloride	15 mg	Gray and Yellow	Capsule		Teva Pharmaceuticals
93; 886	Drummergal	20 mg; 0.3 mg; 0.1 mg	Tan	Coated Tablet	Circle	Teva Pharmaceuticals

IMPRINT	BRAND/GENERIC NAME	STRENGTH	COLOR	FORM	SHAPE	MANUFACTURER
93; 886	Ergobel	0.3 mg; 0.1 mg; 20 mg		Tablet		Teva Pharmaceuticals
93; 888	Phentermine Hydrochloride Black	30 mg	Black Opaque	Capsule		Teva Pharmaceuticals
93; 890	Acetaminophen and Propoxyphene Napsylate	650 mg; 100 mg	Pink	Coated Tablet	Oblong, Convex	Teva Pharmaceuticals
93; 891	Dicyclomine Hydrochloride	20 mg	Blue	Tablet	Circle, Flat Beveled Edge	Teva Pharmaceuticals
93; 892	Etodolac	400 mg	Pink	Tablet	Capsule-Shape	Teva Pharmaceuticals
93; 896	Famotidine	20 mg	Beige	Tablet	Circle	Teva Pharmaceuticals
93; 897	Famotidine	40 mg	Tan	Tablet	Circle	Teva Pharmaceuticals
93; 899	Phentermine Hydrochloride	30 mg	Red and Yellow	Capsule		Teva Pharmaceuticals
93; 900	Ketoconazole	200 mg	White	Tablet	Circle	Teva Pharmaceuticals
93; 911; 10	Isoxsuprine Hydrochloride	10 mg	White	Tablet	Circle, Convex	Teva Pharmaceuticals
93; 913; 20	Isoxsuprine Hydrochloride	20 mg	White	Tablet	Circle, Convex, Scored	Teva Pharmaceuticals
93; 926	Lovastatin	10 mg		Tablet		Teva Pharmaceuticals
93; 928	Lovastatin	40 mg		Tablet		Teva Pharmaceuticals
93; 943	Nystatin	100,000 units	Light Yellow	Tablet	Diamond	Teva Pharmaceuticals
93; 948	Diclofenac Potassium	50 mg	Orange	Tablet	Circle	Teva Pharmaceuticals
93; 956	Clomipramine Hydrochloride	25 mg	White and Orange	Capsule		Teva Pharmaceuticals
93; 957	Chlordiazepoxide Hydrochloride	5 mg	Light Green and Yellow, Opaque	Capsule		Teva Pharmaceuticals
93; 958	Clomipramine Hydrochloride	50 mg	White and Light Blue	Capsule		Teva Pharmaceuticals
93; 959	Chlordiazepoxide Hydrochloride	10 mg	Black and Light Green, Opaque	Capsule		Teva Pharmaceuticals
93; 960	Clomipramine Hydrochloride	75 mg	White and Tan	Capsule		Teva Pharmaceuticals
93; 961	Chlordiazepoxide Hydrochloride	25 mg	Light Green and White, Opaque	Capsule		Teva Pharmaceuticals
93; 968	Famotidine	10 mg	Pink	Coated Tablet	Circle, Biconvex	Teva Pharmaceuticals
93; 983	Nystatin	500,000 units	Brown	Coated Tablet	Circle, Convex	Teva Pharmaceuticals
93; 1003; 5	Buspirone Hydrochloride	15 mg		Tablet		Teva Pharmaceuticals
93; 1024	Nefazodone Hydrochloride	100 mg	White	Tablet	Capsule-Shape, Scored	Teva Pharmaceuticals
93; 1025	Nefazodone Hydrochloride	200 mg	Yellow	Tablet	Capsule-Shape, Scored	Teva Pharmaceuticals
93; 1026	Nefazodone Hydrochloride	250 mg	White	Tablet	Capsule-Shape, Scored	Teva Pharmaceuticals
93; 1035	Hydrochlorothiazide and Lisinopril	12.5 mg; 10 mg	Peach	Tablet	Circle	Teva Pharmaceuticals
93; 1036	Hydrochlorothiazide and Lisinopril	12.5 mg; 20 mg	White	Tablet	Circle	Teva Pharmaceuticals
93; 1037	Hydrochlorothiazide and Lisinopril	25 mg; 20 mg	Peach	Tablet	Circle	Teva Pharmaceuticals
93; 1041	Diclofenac Sodium	100 mg	Pink	Extended-Release Tablet	Circle	Teva Pharmaceuticals
93; 1044	Enalapril and Hydrochlorothiazide	5 mg; 12.5 mg	White	Tablet	Capsule-Shape	Teva Pharmaceuticals
93; 1052	Enalapril and Hydrochlorothiazide	10 mg; 25 mg	Rust	Tablet	Capsule-Shape	Teva Pharmaceuticals
93; 1060	Sotalol Hydrochloride	120 mg	Light Blue	Tablet	Oval, Scored	Teva Pharmaceuticals
93; 1087	Cefaclor	500 mg	Blue	Tablet	Oval	Teva Pharmaceuticals
93; 1111	Lisinopril	2.5 mg	White	Tablet	Circle	Teva Pharmaceuticals
93; 1112	Lisinopril	5 mg	Red	Tablet	Circle, Scored	Teva Pharmaceuticals
93; 1113	Lisinopril	10 mg	Red	Tablet	Circle	Teva Pharmaceuticals
93; 1114	Lisinopril	20 mg	Red	Tablet	Capsule-Shape	Teva Pharmaceuticals
93; 1115	Lisinopril	40 mg	Yellow	Tablet	Capsule-Shape	Teva Pharmaceuticals
93; 1118	Etodolac	600 mg	Light Blue	Extended-Release Tablet	Oval	Teva Pharmaceuticals
93; 1122	Etodolac ER	400 mg	Orange	Extended-Release Tablet	Oval	Teva Pharmaceuticals
93; 1177	Neomycin Sulfate	500 mg	Off-White	Tablet	Circle	Novartis Generics
93; 1177	Neomycin Sulfate	500 mg	Off-White	Tablet	Circle	Teva Pharmaceuticals
93; 1215	Cefaclor	375 mg	Blue	Tablet	Oval	Teva Pharmaceuticals
93; 1893	Etodolac	500 mg	Blue	Tablet	Oval	Teva Pharmaceuticals
93; 2264	Amoxicillin	875 mg	Off White	Tablet	Capsule-Shape, Scored	Teva Pharmaceuticals
93; 2268	Amoxicillin	250 mg	Off White	Tablet, Chewable	Capsule-Shape	Teva Pharmaceuticals
93; 2274	Amoxicillin and Clavulanate Potassium	500 mg; 125 mg	White	Tablet	Oblong	Teva Pharmaceuticals
93; 2275 ;	Amoxicillin and Clavulanate Potassium	875 mg; 125 mg	White	Tablet	Oblong	Teva Pharmaceuticals
93; 3107 ;	Amoxicillin	250 mg	Caramel and Buff	Capsule		Teva Pharmaceuticals
93; 3109	Amoxicillin	500 mg	Buff	Capsule		Teva Pharmaceuticals
93; 3111 ;	Ampicillin	250 mg	Scarlet and Grey	Capsule		Teva Pharmaceuticals
93; 3113 ;	Ampicillin	500 mg	Scarlet and Gray	Capsule		Teva Pharmaceuticals
93; 3115 ;	Oxacillin Sodium	250 mg	Blue Opaque	Capsule		Teva Pharmaceuticals
93; 3117 ;	Oxacillin Sodium	500 mg	Blue Opaque	Capsule		Novartis Generics
93; 3117 ;	Oxacillin Sodium	500 mg	Blue Opaque	Capsule		Teva Pharmaceuticals
93; 3119 ;	Cloxacillin	250 mg	Dark Green and Scarlet	Capsule		Teva Pharmaceuticals
93; 3121 ;	Cloxacillin	500 mg	Dark Green and Scarlet	Capsule		Teva Pharmaceuticals
93; 3123 ;	Dicloxacillin Sodium	250 mg	Green and Light Green	Capsule		Novartis Generics
93; 3123 ;	Dicloxacillin Sodium	250 mg	Green and Light Green	Capsule		Teva Pharmaceuticals
93; 3125 ;	Dicloxacillin Sodium	500 mg	Green and Light Green	Capsule		Novartis Generics
93; 3125 ;	Dicloxacillin Sodium	500 mg	Green and Light Green	Capsule		Teva Pharmaceuticals
93; 3127 ;	Disopyramide Phosphate	100 mg	Blue and Scarlet	Capsule		Teva Pharmaceuticals
93; 3129 ;	Disopyramide Phosphate	150 mg	Buff and Scarlet	Capsule		Teva Pharmaceuticals
93; 3153 ;	Cephradine	250 mg	Light Green and Pink	Capsule		Novartis
93; 3153 ;	Cephradine	250 mg	Light Green and Pink	Capsule		Teva Pharmaceuticals
93; 3155 ;	Cephradine	500 mg	Light Green	Capsule		Teva Pharmaceuticals
93; 3165 ;	Minocycline Hydrochloride	50 mg	Pink	Capsule		Teva Pharmaceuticals
93; 3167 ;	Minocycline Hydrochloride	100 mg	Pink and Maroon	Capsule		Teva Pharmaceuticals
93; 3171	Clindamycin Hydrochloride	150 mg	Red and Blue	Capsule		Teva Pharmaceuticals
93; 3193 ;	Ketoprofen	50 mg	Blue and Light Blue	Capsule		Teva Pharmaceuticals
93; 3195 ;	Ketoprofen	75 mg	Blue and White	Capsule		Teva Pharmaceuticals
93; 5150	Moexipril Hydrochloride	15 mg	Pink	Tablet	Oval, Scored	Teva Pharmaceuticals
93; 5157	Lisinopril	30 mg	White	Tablet	Circle	Teva Pharmaceuticals
93; 5194	Penicillin V Potassium	250 mg	White	Tablet	Oval	Teva Pharmaceuticals

IMPRINT	BRAND/GENERIC NAME	STRENGTH	COLOR	FORM	SHAPE	MANUFACTURER
93; 7113	Nefazodone Hydrochloride	150 mg	Peach	Tablet	Capsule-Shape, Scored	Teva Pharmaceuticals
93; 7120	Flutamide	125 mg	Beige	Capsule		Teva Pharmaceuticals
93; 7172	Etodolac	500 mg	Gray	Extended-Release Tablet	Oval	Teva Pharmaceuticals
93; 7178	Nefazodone Hydrochloride	50 mg	Light Pink	Tablet	Capsule-Shape, Scored	Teva Pharmaceuticals
93; 7180	Ofloxacin	200 mg	Light Yellow	Tablet	Oval	Teva Pharmaceuticals
93; 7181	Ofloxacin	300 mg	White to Off-White	Tablet	Oval	Teva Pharmaceuticals
93; 7182	Ofloxacin	400 mg	Pale Gold	Tablet	Oval	Teva Pharmaceuticals
93; 7188	Fluoxetine Hydrochloride	10 mg	Blue	Tablet	Oval, Scored	Teva Pharmaceuticals
93; 7198	Fluoxetine Hyrochloride	40 mg	Blue and Orange	Capsule		Teva Pharmaceuticals
93; 7206	Mirtazapine	15 mg	Yellow	Tablet	Circle	Teva Pharmaceuticals
93; 7207	Mirtazapine	30 mg	Reddish Brown	Tablet	Circle	Teva Pharmaceuticals
93; 7208	Mirtazapine	45 mg	White to Off-White	Tablet	Circle	Teva Pharmaceuticals
93; 7223	Fosinopril Sodium	20 mg	White to Off-White	Tablet	Rectangle	Teva Pharmaceuticals
93; 7224	Fosinopril Sodium	40 mg	White to Off-White	Tablet	Circle	Teva Pharmaceuticals
93; 7267	Metformin Hydrochloride	500 mg	White to Off-White	Extended-Release Tablet	Oval	Teva Pharmaceuticals
93; 9133	Amiodarone Hydrochloride	200 mg	Pink	Tablet	Circle, Scored	Teva Pharmaceuticals
93; 9158	Multivitamins with Fluoride	2500 IU; 60 mg; 400 IU; 15 IU; 1.05 mg; 1.2 mg; 13.5 mg; 1.05 mg; 0.3 mg; 4.5 mcg; 0.5 mg	Pink, Purple, Orange	Tablet, Chewable	Square	Teva Pharmaceuticals
93; 9159	Multivitamins with Fluoride and Iron	2500 IU; 60 mg; 400 IU; 15 IU; 1.05 mg; 1.2 mg; 13.5 mg; 1.05 mg; 0.3 mg; 4.5 mcg; 12 mg; 10 mg; 1 mg; 1 mg	Purple	Tablet, Chewable	Square	Teva Pharmaceuticals
93; 9166	Multivitamins with Fluoride	2500 IU; 60 mg; 400 IU; 15 IU; 1.05 mg; 1.2 mg; 13.5 mg; 1.05 mg; 0.3 mg; 4.5 mcg; 1 mg	Pink, Purple, Orange	Tablet, Chewable	Square	Teva Pharmaceuticals
93; 9197	Multivitamins with Fluoride and Iron	2500 IU; 60 mg; 400 IU; 15 IU; 1.05 mg; 1.2 mg; 13.5 mg; 1.05 mg; 0.3 mg; 4.5 mcg; 12 mg; 10 mg; 1 mg; 0.5 mg	Pink	Tablet, Chewable	Square	Teva Pharmaceuticals
93; 9411	Methazolamide	25 mg	White	Tablet	Square	Teva Pharmaceuticals
93; 9643	Prochlorperazine Maleate	5 mg	Yellow	Tablet	Circle	Teva Pharmaceuticals
93; 9652	Prochlorperazine Maleate	10 mg	Yellow	Tablet	Circle	Teva Pharmaceuticals
93; DOXY	Doxycycline Hyclate	100 mg	Orange	Coated Tablet	Circle	Teva Pharmaceuticals
93; DOXY	Doxy-Lemmon	100 mg	Orange	Coated Tablet	Circle	Teva Pharmaceuticals
93; SOFARIN; 2 ;	Sofarin	2 mg	Lavender	Tablet	Circle, Scored	Teva Pharmaceuticals
93; SOFARIN; 2 1/2 ;	Sofarin	2.5 mg	Orange	Tablet	Circle, Scored	Teva Pharmaceuticals
93; SOFARIN; 5	Sofarin	5 mg	Pink	Tablet	Circle, Scored	Teva Pharmaceuticals
93;307	Clemastine Fumarate	1.34 mg	White	Tablet	Circle, Convex, Scored	Teva Pharmaceuticals
93-93; 852	Metronidazole	500 mg	White	Tablet	Oblong, Scored, Debossed	Teva Pharmaceuticals
99	Adipex 8	8 mg	Blue and White	Capsule		Teva Pharmaceuticals
99	Vibra-Tabs	100 mg	Peach	Coated Tablet	Circle	Pfizer Laboratories
100	Dicumarol	100 mg		Tablet		Abbott Laboratories
100 ;	Ceenu	100 mg	Two-Tone Green	Capsule		Bristol-Myers Oncology
100 DS	Norvir	100 mg	White	Capsule, Liquid Filled		Abbott Laboratories
100; LARODOPA; ROCHE	Larodopa	100 mg	Pink	Tablet	Oval, Scored	Roche Pharmaceuticals
100; LL; A; 17	Asendin	100 mg	Blue	Tablet	Seven-Sided	Lederle Laboratories
100; T4	Levothroid	100 mcg	Yellow	Tablet	Capsule-Shape	Forest Pharmaceuticals
101	Azulfidine	500 mg	Yellow	Tablet	Circle	Pharmacia & Upjohn
103	Oxoids	20 mg; 0.3 mg; 8 mg	Blue	Tablet		Teva Pharmaceuticals
107	Nu'leven	100 mg; 10 mg; 150 mg	Aqua	Tablet	Circle, Concave	Teva Pharmaceuticals
108	Lemidyne with Codeine	30 mg; 230 mg; 150 mg; 30 mg	White	Tablet		Teva Pharmaceuticals
110	Amnesteem	10 mg	Reddish Brown	Capsule		Mylan Bertek Pharmaceuticals
110	Rhinex DM	2 mg; 10 mg; 5 mg	White	Tablet		Teva Pharmaceuticals
112	Januvia	50 mg	Light Beige	Tablet	Circle	Merck & Company
112; T4	Levothroid	112 mcg	Rose	Tablet	Capsule-Shape	Forest Pharmaceuticals
120	Amnesteem	20 mg	Reddish Brown and Cream	Capsule		Mylan Bertek Pharmaceuticals
120 INNOPRANXL LOGO	Innopran XL	120 mg	Gray, Off-White	Capsule, Extended Release		Reliant Pharmaceuticals
123	Atripla	600 mg; 200 mg; 300 mg	Pink	Tablet	Capsule-Shape	Bristol-Myers Squibb & Gilead Sciences
125	Slo-Bid Gyrocaps	125 mg	White	Extended-Release Capsule		Aventis Pharmaceuticals
125	Tracleer	125 mg	Orange-White	Coated Tablet	Oval, Biconvex	Genentech
125; T4	Levothroid	125 mcg	Brown	Tablet	Capsule-Shape	Forest Pharmaceuticals
131; 07	Prednicen-M Tablet 5 mg	5 mg	Red	Coated Tablet	Capsule-Shape	Schwarz Pharma
140	Amnesteem	40 mg	Orange and Brown	Capsule		Mylan Bertek Pharmaceuticals
141 ;	Trilafon Repetab	8 mg	Gray	Timed-Release Tablet		Schering
150 ; AXID ; RELIANT	Axid	150 mg	Opaque Dark Yellow, Opaque Pale Yellow	Capsule		Reliant Pharmaceuticals
150; LL; A; 18	Asendin	150 mg	Peach	Tablet	Seven-Sided	Lederle Laboratories

IMPRINT	BRAND/GENERIC NAME	STRENGTH	COLOR	FORM	SHAPE	MANUFACTURER
150; T4	Levothroid	150 mcg	Blue	Tablet	Capsule-Shape	Forest Pharmaceuticals
155	Lemidyne with Codeine	15 mg; 230 mg; 150 mg; 30 mg	White	Tablet		Teva Pharmaceuticals
157 157 ; GG	Benazepril Hydrochloride and Hydrochlorothiazide	5 mg; 6.25 mg	White	Tablet	Oval	Par Pharmaceutical
158 158 ; GG	Benazepril Hydrochloride and Hydrochlorothiazide	10 mg; 12.5 mg	White	Tablet	Oval	Par Pharmaceutical
159 159 ; GG	Benazepril Hydrochloride and Hydrochlorothiazide	20 mg; 12.5 mg	White	Tablet	Oval	Par Pharmaceutical
160 160 ; GG	Benazepril Hydrochloride and Hydrochlorothiazide	20 mg; 25 mg	White	Tablet	Oval	Par Pharmaceutical
166	Mandelamine	500 mg	Brown	Coated Tablet	Capsule-Shape	Warner Chilcott
167	Mandelamine	1000 mg	Purple	Coated Tablet		Warner Chilcott
170	Sulindac	150 mg	Yellow	Tablet	Six-Sided	Endo Laboratories
172 ;	Meticorten	5 mg	White	Tablet		Schering
175	Synthroid	175 mcg	Lilac	Tablet		Abbott Laboratories
175; T4	Levothroid	175 mcg	Lilac	Tablet	Capsule-Shape	Forest Pharmaceuticals
200 ; 3RP	Ribavirin	200 mg	Light Blue	Tablet	Capsule-Shape	Par Pharmaceutical
200; T4	Levothroid	200 mcg	Pink	Tablet	Capsule-Shape	Forest Pharmaceuticals
204	Amobarbital D-Lay	60 mg	Orange and White	Tablet		Teva Pharmaceuticals
207	Corgard	40 mg		Tablet		Monarch Pharmaceuticals
207; LEMMON; 207	Mepriam	400 mg	Yellow	Tablet	Oblong, Scored	Teva Pharmaceuticals
208	Corgard	120 mg		Tablet		Monarch Pharmaceuticals
221	Januvia	25 mg	Pink	Tablet	Circle	Merck & Company
227; 555	Erythromycin Estolate	250 mg	Orange	Capsule		Teva Pharmaceuticals
231	Ferrocol	150 mg	Blue	Capsule		Teva Pharmaceuticals
232	Corgard	20 mg		Tablet		Monarch Pharmaceuticals
235	Thyrocrine	2.5 Gr	Tan	Tablet		Teva Pharmaceuticals
235	Thyroid	2.5 Gr	Tan	Tablet		Teva Pharmaceuticals
241	Corgard	80 mg		Tablet		Monarch Pharmaceuticals
246 ;	Corgard	160 mg	Blue	Tablet	Oblong, Scored	Monarch Pharmaceuticals
250	Slo-Niacin	250 mg	Pink	Extended-Release Tablet	Capsule-Shape, Scored	Upsher-Smith Laboratories
250 ; K	Tranylcypromine Sulfate	10 mg	Red	Tablet	Circle	Par Pharmaceutical
250; LARODOPA; ROCHE	Larodopa	250 mg	Pink	Tablet	Circle, Scored	Roche Pharmaceuticals
251; DMSP	Carbidopa and Levodopa	25 mg; 250 mg	Light Dapple-Blue	Tablet	Oval, Scored	Bristol-Myers Squibb
261	Codone	5 mg	White	Tablet		Teva Pharmaceuticals
271; DMSP	Carbidopa and Levodopa	10 mg; 100 mg	Dark Dapple-Blue	Tablet	Oval, Scored	Bristol-Myers Squibb
272; DMSP	Carbidopa and Levodopa	25 mg; 100 mg	Yellow	Tablet	Oval, Scored	Bristol-Myers Squibb
277	Januvia	100 mg	Beige	Tablet	Circle	Merck & Company
283; 200 MCG	Baycol	0.2 mg	Light Yellow	Tablet		Bayer Pharmaceutical
284; 300 MCG	Baycol	0.3 mg	Yellow-Brown	Tablet		Bayer Pharmaceutical
285; 400 MCG	Baycol	0.4 mg	Ocher	Tablet		Bayer Pharmaceutical
286; 800 MCG	Baycol	0.8 mg	Brown-Orange	Tablet		Bayer Pharmaceutical
296	Phyldrox	100 mg; 25 mg; 15 mg	White	Tablet		Teva Pharmaceuticals
300 ; AXID ; RELIANT	Axid	300 mg	Opaque Brown, Opaque Pale Yellow	Capsule		Reliant Pharmaceuticals
300 ; TMC114	Prezista	300 mg	Orange	Tablet	Oval	Tibotec Therapeutics
300; M30; MOVA	Cimetidine	300 mg	White	Coated Tablet	Round, Bisected Scored	Par Pharmaceutical
300; T4	Levothroid	300 mcg	Green	Tablet	Capsule-Shape	Forest Pharmaceuticals
304	Pyradyne	210 mg; 30 mg; 150 mg; 15 mg	Red	Tablet		Teva Pharmaceuticals
306	Pyradyne Compound	15 mg; 120 mg; 100 mg; 8 mg; 10 mg; 0.12 mg; 8 mg;	Yellow	Tablet		Teva Pharmaceuticals
308AV	Allegra-D 24 Hour	180 mg; 240 mg	White	Tablet, Extended Release	Circle	Sanofi-Aventis U.S.
311	Vytorin 10/10	10 mg; 10 mg	White to Off-White	Tablet	Capsule-Shape	Merck
312	Vytorin 10/20	10 mg; 20 mg	White to Off-White	Tablet	Capsule-Shape	Merck
313	Vytorin 10/40	10 mg; 40 mg	White to Off-White	Tablet	Capsule-Shape	Merck
315	Vytorin 10/80	10 mg; 80 mg	White to Off-White	Tablet	Capsule-Shape	Merck
322	Lemivite	16 mg; 71 mg; 1.6 mg; 1 mcg; 3.33 mg; 0.33 mg; 55 mg; 0.166 mg; 1 mg; 1 mg; 0.4 mg; 0.4 IU; 1666 IU; 1.7 mg; 8 mg; 1 mg; 66 IU; 0.33 mg	Red	Tablet		Teva Pharmaceuticals
322 ; M	Ciprofloxacin	250 mg	Orange	Tablet	Circle	Mylan Pharmaceuticals
323 ; MYLAN	Ciprofloxacin	500 mg	Orange	Tablet	Capsule-Shape	Mylan Pharmaceuticals
324 ; MYLAN	Ciprofloxacin	750 mg	Orange	Tablet	Capsule-Shape	Mylan Pharmaceuticals
333	Campral	333 mg	White	Enteric-Coated Tablet	Circle	Forest Pharmaceuticals
336	Diagnex Blue Test Sodium Benzoate and Caffeine	250 mg;		Tablet		Bristol-Myers Squibb
348	Glucoron with B12	250 mg; 1 mg; 0.5 mg; 1 mg; 2 mg; 3 mcg	Pink	Tablet		Teva Pharmaceuticals
351; RPR	Slo-Phyllin	100 mg	White	Tablet	Circle	Aventis Pharmaceuticals
355	Aluprin	300 mg;	Green and White	Tablet		Teva Pharmaceuticals
386; ORGANON	Cotazym	8000 U; 30000 U; 30000 U; 25 mg	Red	Capsule		Organon
393	Diabinese	100 mg	Blue	Tablet	D-Shape, Scored	Pfizer Laboratories
394	Diabinese	250 mg	Blue	Tablet	D-Shape, Scored	Pfizer Laboratories
400 ; 3RP	Ribapak	400 mg	Medium Blue	Tablet	Capsule-Shape	Par Pharmaceutical
400 ; 3RP	Ribatab	400 mg	Medium Blue	Tablet	Capsule-Shape	Par Pharmaceutical

IMPRINT	BRAND/GENERIC NAME	STRENGTH	COLOR	FORM	SHAPE	MANUFACTURER
400; M40; MOVA	Cimetidine	400 mg	White	Coated Tablet	Capsule-Shaped, Bisected Scored	Par Pharmaceutical
414	Zetia	10 mg	Off-White	Tablet	Capsule-Shape	Schering
461; 80 MG	Emend	80 mg	White	Capsule		Merck & Company
462; 125 MG	Emend	125 mg	Pink, White	Capsule		Merck & Company
464 40MG ;	Emend	40 mg	Opaque Mustard Yellow, Opaque White	Capsule	Capsule-Shape	Merck & Company
499; SCHERING ;	Oreton Methyl	25 mg	Peach	Tablet		Schering
500	Anacin Maximum Strength	500 mg; 32 mg	White	Coated Tablet	Circle	Whitehall Laboratories
500	Glumetza	500 mg	White	Tablet, Extended Release	Oval	Biovail Laboratories
500	Niacor B3	500 mg	White	Tablet	Oblong, Scored	Upsher-Smith Laboratories
500	Slo-Niacin	500 mg	Pink	Extended-Release Tablet	Capsule-Shape, Scored	Upsher-Smith Laboratories
500 MG; A5; LEDERLE	Achromycin V	500 mg	Yellow and Blue	Capsule		Lederle Laboratories
500; BAYER	Bayer Maximum	500 mg		Tablet		Bayer Consumer Care
500; LARODOPA; ROCHE	Larodopa	500 mg	Pink	Tablet	Oblong, Scored	Roche Pharmaceuticals
500; MG	Mono-Gesic	500 mg	Pink	Coated Tablet	Circle	Schwarz Pharma
502	Azene	6.5 mg	Orange	Tablet	Oblong	Endo Laboratories
511; 0.5	Lorazepam	0.5 mg	White	Tablet	Five-Sided, Small	Esi Lederle
511; 1	Lorazepam	1 mg	White	Tablet	Five-Sided, Scored	Esi Lederle
511; 1 MG	Lorazepam	1 mg	White	Tablet	Five-Sided	Wyeth Pharmaceuticals
511; 2	Lorazepam	2 mg	White	Tablet	Five-Sided, Scored	Esi Lederle
511; 2 MG	Lorazepam	2 mg	White	Tablet	Five-Sided	Wyeth Pharmaceuticals
511; 3620; 400	Etodolac	400 mg	Light Orange	Extended-Release Tablet	Oval	Esi Lederle
511; 3621; 500	Etodolac	500 mg	Light Green	Extended-Release Tablet	Oval	Esi Lederle
511; 3622; 600	Etodolac	600 mg	White	Extended-Release Tablet	Oval	Esi Lederle
511; 7065	Bisoprolol and Hydrochlorothiazide	2.5 mg; 6.25 mg	Off-White to Yellow	Tablet	Circle	Esi Lederle
511; M; X	Methotrexate Sodium	2.5 mg	Yellow	Tablet	Circle	Esi Lederle
511; P77	Pentoxifylline	400 mg	White	Sustained-Release Tablet	Oval	Esi Lederle
521; SINEMET CR	Sinemet Cr 50-200	50 mg; 200 mg	Peach	Sustained-Release Tablet	Oval, Scored, Biconvex, Compressed	Bristol-Myers Squibb
543; 80 ;	Zocor	80 mg	Brick Red	Coated Tablet	Capsule-Shape	Merck & Company
547	Wigrettes	2 mg	White	Tablet		Organon
555; 030	Colchicine	0.65 mg	White	Tablet		Barr Laboratories
555; 19	Hydrochlorothiazide Hydrochloride	25 mg	Peach	Tablet	Circle, Scored	Barr Laboratories
555; 20	Hydrochlorothiazide Hydrochloride	50 mg	Peach	Tablet	Circle, Scored	Barr Laboratories
555; 126	Dicyclomine Hydrochloride	20 mg	Blue	Tablet	Circle	Barr Laboratories
555; 429	Trimethoprim	100 mg	White	Tablet	Circle, Scored	Barr Laboratories
555; 430	Trimethoprim	200 mg		Tablet		Barr Laboratories
591; A	Meprobamate	400 mg	White	Tablet	Circle, Scored	Watson Laboratories
591; B	Meprobamate	200 mg	White	Tablet	Scored, Circle	Watson Laboratories
600 ; 3RP	Ribapak	600 mg	Dark Blue	Tablet	Capsule-Shape	Par Pharmaceutical
600 ; 3RP	Ribatab	600 mg	Dark Blue	Tablet	Capsule-Shape	Par Pharmaceutical
600 ; ADAMS	Mucinex-DM	30 mg; 600 mg	White, Yellow	Tablet, Extended Release	Oval	Adams Laboratories
600; 4141 ;	Fenoprofen Calcium	600 mg	Peach	Coated Tablet	Oval, Bisected Scored	Ivax Pharmaceuticals
601; SINEMET CR	Sinemet Cr 25-100	25 mg; 100 mg	Pink	Sustained-Release Tablet	Oval, Biconvex, Compressed	Bristol-Myers Squibb
603	Sumycin	500 mg	Pink	Tablet	Capsule-Shape	Par Pharmaceutical
603	Sumycin 500	500 mg	Pink	Tablet	Capsule-Shape	Par Pharmaceutical
627	Belap Se	10.8 mg	Green	Tablet		Teva Pharmaceuticals
644	Prednisolone	5 mg	Orange	Tablet		Teva Pharmaceuticals
645	Prednisone	5 mg	White	Tablet		Teva Pharmaceuticals
647 SINEMET	Sinemet 10-100	10 mg; 100 mg	Dark Dapple-Blue	Tablet	Oval, Scored	Bristol-Myers Squibb
650; SINEMET	Sinemet 25-100	25 mg; 100 mg	Yellow	Tablet	Scored, Oval	Bristol-Myers Squibb
654; SINEMET	Sinemet 25-250	25 mg; 250 mg	Light Dapple-Blue	Tablet	Oval, Scored	Bristol-Myers Squibb
663	Sumycin	250 mg	Pink	Tablet	Capsule-Shape	Par Pharmaceutical
663	Sumycin 250	250 mg	Light Pink	Tablet	Capsule-Shape	Par Pharmaceutical
707; SP; 7.5	Univasc	7.5 mg	Pink	Coated Tablet	Circle, Biconvex, Scored	Schwarz Pharma
710 ; LOGO	Fosamax Plus D	70 mg; 2800 IU	White to Off White	Tablet	Capsule-Shape	Merck & Company
715; SP; 15	Univasc	15 mg	Salmon	Coated Tablet	Circle, Biconvex, Scored	Schwarz Pharma
720 / 1/2 ; WC	Estrace	0.5 mg	White to Off-White	Tablet	Oval	Warner Chilcott
721 / 1 ; WC	Estrace	1 mg	Light Purple	Tablet	Oval	Warner Chilcott
722 / 2 ; WC	Estrace	2 mg	Green	Tablet	Oval	Warner Chilcott
730 ;	Tamoxifen	10 mg	White	Tablet	Circle, Biconvex	Astra Zeneca
731 ;	Tamoxifen	20 mg	White	Tablet	Circle, Biconvex	Astra Zeneca
733; 54	Morphine Sulfate	15 mg	White	Tablet		Roxane Laboratories
745	Hyzaar 100-12.5	12.5 mg; 100 mg	White	Tablet	Oval	Merck
750	Slo-Niacin	750 mg	Pink	Extended-Release Tablet	Capsule-Shape, Scored	Upsher-Smith Laboratories
752; 2	Hydromorphone Hydrochloride	2 mg	White	Tablet	Circle	Endo Laboratories
753; TRIANGLE	Mirtazapine	15 mg	Yellow	Tablet	Circle, Scored	Andrx Pharmaceuticals
754; TRIANGLE	Mirtazapine	30 mg	Beige	Tablet	Circle, Scored	Andrx Pharmaceuticals
755; TRIANGLE	Mirtazapine	45 mg	White	Tablet	Circle, Scored	Andrx Pharmaceuticals
757; 4	Hydromorphone Hydrochloride	4 mg	Light Yellow	Tablet	Circle	Endo Laboratories
800; M80; MOVA	Cimetidine	800 mg	White	Coated Tablet	Capsule-Shaped, Bisected Scored	Par Pharmaceutical
810	Thyroid Green	5 Gr	Green	Tablet		Teva Pharmaceuticals
812	Thyroid	3 Gr	Blue	Tablet		Teva Pharmaceuticals
830 ;	Proglycem	100 mg	Orange	Capsule		Schering
832 86	Androxy	10 mg	Green	Tablet	Circle	Upsher-Smith Laboratories
844	Thyroid	2 Gr	Red	Tablet		Teva Pharmaceuticals
854	Thyroid Tan	5 Gr	Tan	Tablet		Teva Pharmaceuticals
861; SCHERING	Chlor-Trimeton Non-Drowsy Decongestant 4 Hour	60 mg	Light Tan	Tablet	Circle, Scored	Schering-Plough Healthcare Products

IMPRINT	BRAND/GENERIC NAME	STRENGTH	COLOR	FORM	SHAPE	MANUFACTURER
866	Disophrol	2 mg; 120 mg	Blue and White Mottled	Tablet	Circle	Schering-Plough
879; 525	Doxycycline Hyclate	50 mg	Blue and White	Capsule		Novartis Generics
879; 526	Doxycycline Hyclate	100 mg	Blue	Capsule		Novartis Generics
901	Chlor-Trimeton Allergy Decongestant 4 Hour	4 mg; 60 mg	Light Blue	Tablet		Schering-Plough Healthcare Products
955	Famotidine	20 mg	White	Tablet	Circle	Andrx Pharmaceuticals
968 ;	Tindal	20 mg	Salmon	Tablet		Schering
989	Femcare	100 mg	White	Tablet	Torpedo-Shaped	Schering-Plough Healthcare Products
1000	Glumetza	1000 mg	White	Tablet, Extended Release	Oval	Biovail Laboratories
1077 ; 93	Cefprozil	250 mg	Light Orange	Tablet	Circle	Teva Pharmaceuticals
1078 ; 93	Cefprozil	500 mg	White	Tablet	Capsule-Shape	Teva Pharmaceuticals
1492	Monopril HCT	10 mg; 12.5 mg	Peach	Tablet	Circle	Bristol-Myers Squibb
1493	Monopril HCT	20 mg; 12.5 mg	Peach	Tablet	Circle, Scored	Bristol-Myers Squibb
2080	Axert	6.25 mg	White with Red Ink	Tablet	Circle, Compressed, Biconvex	Pharmacia & Upjohn
2729; 20	Fosinopril Sodium	20 mg	White to Off-White	Tablet	Oval	Sandoz
2732; 40	Fosinopril Sodium	40 mg	White to Off-White	Tablet	Six-Sided	Sandoz
2737; 10	Fosinopril Sodium	10 mg	White to Off-White	Tablet	Diamond	Sandoz
2771; HEART SHAPE	Avapro	75 mg	White	Tablet	Oval, Biconvex	Bristol-Myers Squibb
2771; HEART SHAPE	Avapro	75 mg	White	Tablet	Oval, Biconvex	Sanofi Pharmaceuticals
2772; HEART SHAPE	Avapro	150 mg	White	Tablet	Oval, Biconvex	Bristol-Myers Squibb
2772; HEART SHAPE	Avapro	150 mg	White	Tablet	Oval, Biconvex	Sanofi Pharmaceuticals
2773; HEART SHAPE	Avapro	300 mg	White	Tablet	Oval, Biconvex	Bristol-Myers Squibb
2773; HEART SHAPE	Avapro	300 mg	White	Tablet	Oval, Biconvex	Sanofi Pharmaceuticals
2775; HEART	Avalide	150 mg; 12.5 mg	Peach	Tablet	Oval, Biconvex	Bristol-Myers Squibb
3000	Quinidine Gluconate	324 mg		Sustained-Release Tablet		Roxane Laboratories
3125 VANCOCIN HCL 125 MG	Vancocin	125 mg	Blue, Brown	Capsule		Eli Lilly
3126 VANCOCIN HCL 125 MG	Vancocin	250 mg	Blue, Lavender	Capsule		Eli Lilly
3230 WPI	Meloxicam	7.5 mg	Yellow	Tablet	Circle	Watson Laboratories
3231 WPI	Meloxicam	15 mg	Yellow	Tablet	Circle	Watson Laboratories
3344; SB; 10 MG	Compazine Spansule	10 mg	Black and Natural	Sustained-Release Capsule		Glaxosmithkline
3346; SB; 15 MG	Compazine Spansule	15 mg	Black and Natural	Sustained-Release Capsule		Glaxosmithkline
3984; 3 ;	Aspirin and Codeine Phosphate	325 mg; 30 mg	White	Tablet	Circle	Ivax Pharmaceuticals
3985; 4 ;	Aspirin and Codeine Phosphate	325 mg; 60 mg	White	Tablet	Circle	Ivax Pharmaceuticals
4266; 200	Acyclovir	200 mg	White	Capsule		Watson Laboratories
4364; 100	Labetalol	100 mg	Yellow	Tablet	Circle, Bisected	Ivax Pharmaceuticals
4365; 200	Labetalol	200 mg	White	Tablet	Circle, Bisected	Ivax Pharmaceuticals
4366; 300	Labetalol	300 mg	Green	Tablet	Circle	Ivax Pharmaceuticals
4440 ; 100 ;	Gabapentin	100 mg	White	Tablet	Circle	Ivax Pharmaceuticals
4441 ; 300 ;	Gabapentin	300 mg	White	Tablet	Circle	Ivax Pharmaceuticals
4442 ; 400 ;	Gabapentin	400 mg	White	Tablet	Oval	Ivax Pharmaceuticals
4443 ; 600 ;	Gabapentin	600 mg	White	Tablet	Oval	Ivax Pharmaceuticals
4444 ; 800 ;	Gabapentin	800 mg	White	Tablet	Oval	Ivax Pharmaceuticals
4833M ; 15/500	Actoplus Met	15 mg; 500 mg	White to Off-White	Tablet	Oblong	Takeda Pharmaceuticals
4833M ; 15/850	Actoplus Met	15 mg; 850 mg	White to Off-White	Tablet	Oblong	Takeda Pharmaceuticals
5161	Hydrocodone Bitartrate and Ibuprofen	7.5 mg; 200 mg	White	Tablet	Circle	Teva Pharmaceuticals
5270 93	Bisoprolol Fumarate	5 mg	Pink	Tablet	Circle	Teva Pharmaceuticals
5271 93	Bisoprolol Fumarate	10 mg	White	Tablet	Circle	Teva Pharmaceuticals
5510 ; 93 ;	Mercaptopurine	50 mg	Pale Yellow to Buff	Tablet	Circle	Teva Pharmaceuticals
5538 ; DAN	Quinidine Gluconate	324 mg	Off White	Tablet, Extended Release	Circle	Watson Laboratories
5623; 150 MG ;	Nizatidine	150 mg	Yellow and White	Capsule		Ivax Pharmaceuticals
5636; DAN	Meclofenamate Sodium	50 mg	Pink	Capsule		Watson Laboratories
5656; 10; HOURGLASS	Tamoxifen	10 mg	White	Tablet	Circle	Ivax Pharmaceuticals
5657; 20; HOURGLASS	Tamoxifen	20 mg	White	Tablet	Circle	Ivax Pharmaceuticals
5777; DAN; 50	Atenolol	50 mg	White	Tablet	Circle, Scored	Watson Laboratories
5778; DAN; 100	Atenolol	100 mg	White	Tablet	Circle	Watson Laboratories
6057	Glyburide and Metformin Hydrochloride	1.25 mg; 250 mg	Pale Yellow	Coated Tablet	Capsule-Shape	Par Pharmaceutical
6058	Glyburide and Metformin Hydrochloride	2.5 mg; 500 mg	Pale Orange	Coated Tablet	Capsule-Shape	Par Pharmaceutical
6059	Glyburide and Metformin Hydrochloride	5 mg; 500 mg	Yellow	Coated Tablet	Capsule-Shape	Par Pharmaceutical
6855	Cold Medicine Plus	325 mg; 2 mg; 30 mg	Blue	Capsule, Liquid Filled	Oblong	Ivax Pharmaceuticals
6857	Cold & Cough Medicine Plus	325 mg; 2 mg; 10 mg; 30 mg	Purple	Capsule, Liquid Filled	Oblong	Ivax Pharmaceuticals
7066; 511	Bisoprolol and Hydrochlorothiazide	5 mg; 6.25 mg		Tablet		Esi Lederle
7067; 511	Bisoprolol and Hydrochlorothiazide	10 mg; 6.25 mg	White	Tablet	Circle, Scored	Esi Lederle
7117; 300 ;	Cimetidine	300 mg	White	Coated Tablet	Circle	Ivax Pharmaceuticals
7171; 400 ;	Cimetidine	400 mg	White	Tablet	Capsule-Shape, Scored	Ivax Pharmaceuticals
7489	Ampicillin	250 mg	Brown and White	Capsule		Bristol-Myers Squibb
7499	Ampicillin	500 mg	Brown and White	Capsule		Bristol-Myers Squibb
7663	Aromasin	25 mg	Off-White to Slightly Gray	Tablet	Circle	Pharmacia & Upjohn
7711; 800 ;	Cimetidine	800 mg	White to Off White	Tablet	Oval, Scored	Ivax Pharmaceuticals
7720; 250 ;	Cefzil	250 mg	Light Orange	Coated Tablet		Bristol-Myers Squibb

IMPRINT	BRAND/GENERIC NAME	STRENGTH	COLOR	FORM	SHAPE	MANUFACTURER
7721; 500 ;	Cefzil	500 mg	White	Coated Tablet		Bristol-Myers Squibb
7767 100	Celebrex	100 mg	White with Blue Band	Capsule		Searle
7767 200	Celebrex	200 mg	White with Gold Band	Capsule		Searle
7767 400	Celebrex	400 mg	White with Green Band	Capsule		Searle
59911; 60	Propranolol Hydrochloride, Long-Acting	60 mg	White	Capsule		Esi Lederle
59911; 80	Propranolol Hydrochloride, Long-Acting	80 mg	White and Light Blue	Capsule		Esi Lederle
59911; 120	Propranolol Hydrochloride, Long-Acting	120 mg	White and Dark Blue	Capsule		Esi Lederle
59911; 160	Propranolol Hydrochloride, Long-Acting	160 mg	White/dark-Blue	Capsule		Esi Lederle
59911; 3606; 200	Etodolac	200 mg	White with Red Ink	Capsule		Esi Lederle
59911; 3607; 300	Etodolac	300 mg	White with Red Ink	Capsule		Esi Lederle
59911; 3608	Etodolac	400 mg	White	Tablet	Oblong	Esi Lederle
59911; 5806	Griseofulvin Ultra	330 mg	White	Tablet	Oblong, Scored	Esi Lederle
59911; 5808	Griseofulvin	500 mg	White	Tablet	Circle	Esi Lederle
59911; 5815	Metoclopramide	10 mg	White	Tablet	Oval, Scored	Esi Lederle
59911; 5869	Minocycline Hydrochloride	50 mg	Yellow and Clear Yellow	Capsule		Esi Lederle
59911; 5870	Minocycline Hydrochloride	100 mg	Green and Yellow	Capsule		Esi Lederle
59911; 5871	Promethazine Hydrochloride	12.5 mg	White	Tablet		Esi Lederle
59911; 5872	Promethazine Hydrochloride	25 mg	White	Tablet		Esi Lederle
59911; 5873	Promethazine Hydrochloride	50 mg	White	Tablet		Esi Lederle
59911; 5876	Oxazepam	10 mg	Pink and White	Capsule		Esi Lederle
59911; 5877	Oxazepam	15 mg	Orange and White	Capsule		Esi Lederle
59911; 5878	Oxazepam	30 mg	Blue and White	Capsule		Esi Lederle
59911; 5885	Potassium Chloride	8 meq	White	Extended-Release Capsule		Esi Lederle
59911; 5899	Potassium Chloride	10 meq	White	Extended-Release Capsule		Esi Lederle
59911; PLUS	Prenatal Plus	65 mg; 4000 IU; 400 IU; 11 mg; 120 mg; 1 mg; 1.5 mg; 3 mg; 20 mg; 10 mg; 12 mcg; 200 mg; 2 mg; 25 mg		Tablet		Esi Lederle
60274; 120MG	Verapamil Hydrochloride	120 mg	Yellow Opaque	Capsule		Watson Laboratories
60274; 180MG	Verapamil Hydrochloride	180 mg	Light Gray Yellow Opaque	Capsule		Watson Laboratories
60274; 240MG	Verapamil Hydrochloride	240 mg	Dark Blue and Yellow Opaque	Capsule		Watson Laboratories
60274; 360MG	Verapamil Hydrochloride	360 mg	Lavender and Yellow Opaque	Capsule		Watson Laboratories
A	Axert	12.5 mg	White with Blue Ink	Tablet	Circle, Compressed, Biconvex	Ortho-Mcneil Pharmaceutical
A	Cefol	750 mg; 100 mg; 20 mg; 15 mg; 10 mg; 5 mg; 0.5 mg; 6 mcg; 30 IU	Green	Coated Tablet	Oval	Abbott Laboratories
A	Children's Aspirin	75 mg	Bright Pink	Tablet, Chewable		Abbott Laboratories
A	Ephedrine and Nembutal 25	25 mg; 25 mg	Black	Capsule		Abbott Laboratories
A	Fero-Gradumet	525 mg	Red	Tablet		Abbott Laboratories
A	Gerilets	27 mg; 5000 IU; 400 IU; 45 IU; 0.4 mg; 2.25 mg; 2.6 mg; 30 mg; 0.45 mg; 15 mg; 90 mg; 3 mg; 9 mcg	Green	Tablet		Abbott Laboratories
A	Iberet-500	525 mg; 500 mg; 25 mcg; 6 mg; 6 mg; 30 mg; 5 mg; 10 mg	Red	Coated Tablet	Oblong	Abbott Laboratories
A	Lidone	5 mg	Cream and Blue	Capsule		Abbott Laboratories
A	Lidone	10 mg	Cream and Red	Capsule		Abbott Laboratories
A	Lidone	25 mg	Cream and Brown	Capsule		Abbott Laboratories
A	Surbex T	15 mg; 10 mg; 100 mg; 5 mg; 10 mcg; 20 mg; 500 mg	Orange	Tablet	Oblong	Abbott Laboratories
A	Tral with Phenobarbital Gradumet	50 mg; 30 mg	Blue	Tablet		Abbott Laboratories
A ;	Clarinex Reditabs	5 mg	Light Red	Tablet, Disintegrating	Circle	Schering-Plough
A ; 0 6	Citalopram Hydrobromide	20 mg	Light Pink	Tablet	Capsule-Shape	Aurobindo Pharma
A ; 0 7	Citalopram Hydrobromide	40 mg	White	Tablet	Capsule-Shape	Aurobindo Pharma
A ; 05	Citalopram Hydrobromide	10 mg	Peach	Tablet	Circle	Aurobindo Pharma
A ; 12	Metformin Hydrochloride	500 mg	White	Tablet	Circle	Aurobindo Pharma
A ; 13	Metformin Hydrochloride	850 mg	White	Tablet	Circle	Aurobindo Pharma
A ; 14	Metformin Hydrochloride	1000 mg	White	Tablet	Oval	Aurobindo Pharma
A ; BPI 63	Ativan	0.5 mg	White	Tablet	Five-Sided	Biovail Pharmaceuticals
A ; BPI 64	Ativan	1 mg	White	Tablet	Five-Sided	Biovail Pharmaceuticals
A 2 ; BPI 65	Ativan	2 mg	White	Tablet	Five-Sided	Biovail Pharmaceuticals
A 24 ;	Children's Dimetapp Nd Non-Drowsy Allergy	10 mg	White	Tablet, Disintegrating	Circle	Wyeth Consumer Healthcare
A 640 ; 10	Abilify Discmelt	10 mg	Pink	Tablet, Disintegrating	Circle	Bristol-Myers Squibb
A 640 ; 10	Abilify Discmelt	10 mg	Pink	Tablet, Disintegrating	Circle	Otsuka America Pharmaceutical
A 641 ; 15	Abilify Discmelt	15 mg	Yellow	Tablet, Disintegrating	Circle	Bristol-Myers Squibb

IMPRINT	BRAND/GENERIC NAME	STRENGTH	COLOR	FORM	SHAPE	MANUFACTURER
A 641 ; 15	Abilify Discmelt	15 mg	Yellow	Tablet, Disintegrating	Circle	Otsuka America Pharmaceutical
A 642 ; 20	Abilify Discmelt	20 mg	White	Tablet, Disintegrating	Circle	Bristol-Myers Squibb
A 642 ; 20	Abilify Discmelt	20 mg	White	Tablet, Disintegrating	Circle	Otsuka America Pharmaceutical
A 643 ; 30	Abilify Discmelt	30 mg	Pink	Tablet, Disintegrating	Circle	Bristol-Myers Squibb
A 643 ; 30	Abilify Discmelt	30 mg	Pink	Tablet, Disintegrating	Circle	Otsuka America Pharmaceutical
A IH	Dutoprol	25 mg; 12.5 mg	Yellow	Tablet, Extended Release	Circle	Astra Zeneca
A IK	Dutoprol	50 mg; 12.5 mg	Light Orange	Tablet, Extended Release	Circle	Astra Zeneca
A IL	Dutoprol	100 mg; 12.5 mg	Yellow	Tablet, Extended Release	Circle	Astra Zeneca
A; 002	Aquatab DM	1200 mg; 60 mg	Light Blue	Coated Tablet	Circle, Scored	Adams Laboratories
A; 003 ;	Phenazopyridine Hydrochloride	100 mg	Maroon	Tablet	Circle	Geneva Generics
A; 004 ;	Phenazopyridine Hydrochloride	200 mg	Maroon	Tablet	Circle	Geneva Generics
A; 018	Chlordiazepoxide Hydrochloride with Clidinium Bromide	5 mg; 2.5 mg	Green	Capsule		Watson Laboratories
A; 2	Dilaudid	2 mg	Orange	Tablet	Circle	Abbott Laboratories
A; 4	Dilaudid	4 mg	Yellow	Tablet	Circle	Abbott Laboratories
A; 21	Acetaminophen	325 mg	White	Tablet		Lederle Laboratories
A; 40	Dimenhydrinate	50 mg	White	Tablet	Circle, Scored	Novartis Generics
A; 50; G	Atenolol	50 mg	White	Tablet	Circle, Flat; Bevelled Edge; Scored	Par Pharmaceutical
A; 100; G	Atenolol	100 mg	White	Tablet	Circle, Flat; Bevelled Edge	Par Pharmaceutical
A; 273	Tramadol Hydrochloride	50 mg	White to Off-White	Tablet	Circle	Ivax Pharmaceuticals
A; 500	Salsalate	500 mg	Light Turquoise	Coated Tablet	Circle	Novartis Generics
A; 554	Carbamazepine	200 mg	White	Tablet	Circle, Flat, Scored	Teva Pharmaceuticals
A; 585	Atamet	25 mg; 100 mg	Mottled Yellow	Tablet	Circle, Scored	Elan Pharma
A; 585	Carbidopa and Levodopa	25 mg; 100 mg	Mottled Yellow	Tablet	Circle, Scored	Teva Pharmaceuticals
A; 587	Atamet	25 mg; 250 mg	Mottled Blue	Tablet	Circle, Scored	Elan Pharma
A; 587	Carbidopa and Levodopa	25 mg; 250 mg	Mottled Blue	Tablet	Circle, Scored	Teva Pharmaceuticals
A; 615	Permax	0.05 mg	Ivory	Tablet	Rectangle, Modified	Elan Pharma
A; 625	Permax	0.25 mg	Green	Tablet	Rectangle, Modified	Elan Pharma
A; 630	Permax	1 mg	Pink	Tablet	Rectangle, Modified	Elan Pharma
A; 750	Salsalate	750 mg	Light Turquoise	Coated Tablet	Capsule-Shape	Novartis Generics
A; 750	Salsalate	750 mg	Blue or Yellow	Tablet		Novartis Generics
A; A; 8	Dilaudid	8 mg	White	Tablet	Triangle	Abbott Laboratories
A; AA	Chlorthalidone	25 mg		Tablet		Abbott Laboratories
A; AB	Chlorthalidone	50 mg		Tablet		Abbott Laboratories
A; AD ;	Peganone	250 mg	White	Tablet	Circle, Scored	Abbott Laboratories
A; AE ;	Peganone	500 mg	White	Tablet	Circle, Scored	Abbott Laboratories
A; AF	Colchicine	0.6 mg		Tablet		Abbott Laboratories
A; AF; 500	Anacin Maximum Strength, Aspirin Free	500 mg	White	Coated Tablet		Whitehall Laboratories
A; AM	Tridione	300 mg		Capsule		Abbott Laboratories
A; AN	Dicumarol	25 mg		Tablet		Abbott Laboratories
A; ANTABUSE; 250	Antabuse	250 mg	White to Off-White	Tablet	Eight-Sided, Scored, Compressed	Wyeth Pharmaceuticals
A; ANTABUSE; 500	Antabuse	500 mg	White to Off-White	Tablet	Eight-Sided, Scored, Compressed	Wyeth Pharmaceuticals
A; AO	Dicumarol	50 mg		Tablet		Abbott Laboratories
A; B	Toprol XL	25 mg		Extended-Release Tablet		Astra Zeneca
A; CE	Nembutal Sodium	30 mg	Yellow	Capsule		Abbott Laboratories
A; CP	A-Poxide	5 mg	Yellow and Green	Capsule		Abbott Laboratories
A; CS	A-Poxide	10 mg	Green and Evergreen	Capsule		Abbott Laboratories
A; CT	A-Poxide	25 mg		Capsule		Abbott Laboratories
A; EC	Ery-Tab	250 mg	White	Enteric-Coated Tablet	Oval	Abbott Laboratories
A; EE	E.E.S.-400 Filmtab	400 mg	Pink	Coated Tablet	Oblong	Abbott Laboratories
A; EH	Ery-Tab	333 mg	White	Enteric-Coated Tablet		Abbott Laboratories
A; FI	Tricor	48 mg	Yellow	Tablet		Abbott Laboratories
A; FO	Tricor	145 mg	White	Tablet		Abbott Laboratories
A; FT ;	Mavik	1 mg	Salmon	Tablet	Circle, Scored	Abbott Laboratories
A; FX ;	Mavik	2 mg	Yellow	Tablet	Circle, Compressed	Abbott Laboratories
A; FZ ;	Mavik	4 mg	Rose	Tablet	Circle, Compressed	Abbott Laboratories
A; IA	Cartrol	2.5 mg	Gray	Tablet	Oval	Abbott Laboratories
A; II	Phenurone	500 mg	White	Tablet		Abbott Laboratories
A; KJ	Biaxin XL	500 mg	Yellow	Extended-Release Tablet	Capsule-Shape	Abbott Laboratories
A; KL	Biaxin	500 mg	Yellow	Coated Tablet	Oval	Abbott Laboratories
A; KT	Biaxin	250 mg	Yellow	Coated Tablet	Oval	Abbott Laboratories
A; LE	Tridione Dulcet	150 mg		Tablet, Chewable		Abbott Laboratories
A; LF ;	Panwarfin	10 mg	White	Tablet		Abbott Laboratories
A; LJ ;	Harmonyl	0.1 mg	Light Yellow	Tablet		Abbott Laboratories
A; LK ;	Harmonyl	0.25 mg	Salmon	Tablet		Abbott Laboratories
A; LM ;	Panwarfin	2 mg	Purple	Tablet		Abbott Laboratories
A; LN ;	Panwarfin	2.5 mg	Orange	Tablet		Abbott Laboratories
A; LO ;	Panwarfin	5 mg	Salmon	Tablet		Abbott Laboratories
A; LR ;	Panwarfin	7.5 mg	Yellow	Tablet		Abbott Laboratories
A; MC	Desoxyn Gradumet	5 mg	White	Tablet		Abbott Laboratories
A; ME	Desoxyn Gradumet	10 mg	Light Orange	Tablet		Abbott Laboratories
A; MF	Desoxyn Gradumet	15 mg	Yellow	Tablet		Abbott Laboratories
A; MO	Toprol XL	50 mg	White	Sustained-Release Tablet	Circle, Biconvex, Scored	Astra Zeneca
A; MS	Toprol XL	100 mg	White	Sustained-Release Tablet	Circle, Biconvex, Scored	Astra Zeneca
A; MY	Toprol XL	200 mg	White	Sustained-Release Tablet	Oval, Biconvex, Scored	Astra Zeneca
A; NC	Nicobid	125 mg	Black and Clear	Capsule		Aventis Behring
A; ND	Nicobid	250 mg	Green and Clear	Capsule		Aventis Behring
A; NE	Nicolar	500 mg	Yellow	Tablet		Aventis Behring

IMPRINT	BRAND/GENERIC NAME	STRENGTH	COLOR	FORM	SHAPE	MANUFACTURER
A; NJ	Cefol	750 mg; 100 mg; 20 mg; 15 mg; 10 mg; 5 mg; 50 mcg; 6 mcg; 30 IU	Green	Coated Tablet	Oval	Abbott Laboratories
A; NR	Depakote	250 mg	Peach	Enteric-Coated Tablet		Abbott Laboratories
A; NS ;	Depakote	500 mg	Lavender	Enteric-Coated Tablet		Abbott Laboratories
A; NT ;	Depakote	125 mg	Salmon Pink	Enteric-Coated Tablet		Abbott Laboratories
A; P; ALOR; 5	Alor 5/500	5 mg; 500 mg	Pink	Tablet	Round with Rectangular Side, Bisected Scored	Atley Pharmaceuticals
A; TC	Armour Thyroid 1/4 grain	15 mg	Light Tan	Tablet	Circle, Convex	Forest Pharmaceuticals
A; TC	Desoxyn	2.5 mg	White	Tablet		Abbott Laboratories
A; TD	Armour Thyroid 1/2 grain	30 mg	Light Tan	Tablet	Circle, Convex	Forest Pharmaceuticals
A; TE	Armour Thyroid 1 grain	60 mg	Light Tan	Tablet	Circle, Convex	Forest Pharmaceuticals
A; TE	Desoxyn	5 mg	White	Tablet		Abbott Laboratories
A; TF	Armour Thyroid 2 grains	120 mg	Light Tan	Tablet	Circle, Convex	Forest Pharmaceuticals
A; TG	Armour Thyroid 3 grains	180 mg	Light Tan	Tablet	Round, Bisected Scored	Forest Pharmaceuticals
A; TH	Armour Thyroid 4 grains	240 mg	Light Tan	Tablet	Circle, Convex	Forest Pharmaceuticals
A; TI	Armour Thyroid 5 grains	300 mg	Light Tan	Tablet	Round, Bisected Scored	Forest Pharmaceuticals
A; TJ	Armour Thyroid 1-1/2 grains	90 mg	Light Tan	Tablet	Circle, Convex	Forest Pharmaceuticals
A; TL	Tranxene T-Tab	3.75 mg	Blue	Tablet	T-Shaped, Scored	Abbott Laboratories
A; TM	Tranxene T-Tab	7.5 mg	Peach	Tablet	T-Shaped, Scored	Abbott Laboratories
A; TN	Tranxene T-Tab	15 mg	Lavender	Tablet	T-Shaped, Scored	Abbott Laboratories
A; TX	Tranxene-Sd Half Strength	11.25 mg	Blue	Tablet	Circle	Abbott Laboratories
A; YC	Thyrolar-1/4	3.1 mcg; 12.5 mcg	Violet and White	Tablet		Forest Pharmaceuticals
A; YD	Thyrolar-1/2	6.25 mcg; 25 mcg	Peach and White	Tablet		Forest Pharmaceuticals
A; YE	Thyrolar-1	12.5 mcg; 50 mcg	Pink and White	Tablet		Forest Pharmaceuticals
A; YF	Thyrolar-2	25 mcg; 100 mcg	Green and White	Tablet		Forest Pharmaceuticals
A; YH	Thyrolar-3	37.5 mcg; 150 mcg	Yellow and White	Tablet		Forest Pharmaceuticals
A; Z	Azathioprine	50 mg	Yellow	Tablet	Circle	Sandoz
A; Z	Azathioprine	50 mg	Yellow	Tablet	Circle, Scored	Mylan Pharmaceuticals
A~	Ambien Cr	12.5 mg	Blue	Tablet, Extended Release	Circle	Sanofi-Aventis U.S.
A~	Ambien Cr	6.25 mg	Pink	Tablet, Extended Release	Circle	Sanofi-Aventis U.S.
A-006 2	Abilify	2 mg	Green	Tablet	Rectangle	Bristol-Myers Squibb
A-007 5	Abilify	5 mg	Blue	Tablet	Rectangle	Bristol-Myers Squibb
A-008 10	Abilify	10 mg	Pink	Tablet	Rectangle	Bristol-Myers Squibb
A-009 15	Abilify	15 mg	Yellow	Tablet	Circle	Bristol-Myers Squibb
A-010 20	Abilify	20 mg	White	Tablet	Circle	Bristol-Myers Squibb
A-011 30	Abilify	30 mg	Pink	Tablet	Circle	Bristol-Myers Squibb
A2C	Lanoxicaps	0.05 mg	Red	Capsule, Liquid Filled	Oblong, Small	Glaxosmithkline
A32	Cefuroxime Axetil	125 mg	White to Off-White	Tablet	Capsule-Shape	Aurobindo Pharma
A33	Cefuroxime Axetil	250 mg	White to Off-White	Tablet	Capsule-Shape	Aurobindo Pharma
A34	Cefuroxime Axetil	500 mg	White to Off-White	Tablet	Capsule-Shape	Aurobindo Pharma
A75; 511	Acyclovir	400 mg	White	Tablet	Circle	Esi Lederle
A77; 511	Acyclovir	800 mg		Tablet		Esi Lederle
ABBOTT LOGO; 25 MG; OR	Gengraf	25 mg	White with Blue Ink	Capsule		Abbott Laboratories
ABBOTT LOGO; 100 MG; OT	Gengraf	100 mg	White, 2 Blue Stripes, Blue Ink	Capsule		Abbott Laboratories
ABBOTT LOGO; AR	Tricor, Micronized	134 mg	White	Capsule		Abbott Laboratories
ABBOTT LOGO; FR	Tricor, Micronized	67 mg	Yellow	Capsule		Abbott Laboratories
ABBOTT LOGO; HC	Depakote ER	500 mg	Gray	Extended-Release Tablet		Abbott Laboratories
ABBOTT LOGO; HF	Depakote ER	250 mg	White	Extended-Release Tablet	Oval	Abbott Laboratories
ABBOTT LOGO; HH	Hytrin	1 mg	Grey	Capsule		Abbott Laboratories
ABBOTT LOGO; HK	Hytrin	5 mg	Red	Capsule		Abbott Laboratories
ABBOTT LOGO; HN	Hytrin	10 mg	Blue	Capsule		Abbott Laboratories
ABBOTT LOGO; HY	Hytrin	2 mg	Yellow	Capsule		Abbott Laboratories
ABBOTT LOGO; SR	Tricor, Micronized	200 mg	Orange	Capsule		Abbott Laboratories
ABG ; 10	Oxycodone Hydrochloride	10 mg	White	Controlled-Release Tablet	Circle	Ivax Pharmaceuticals
ABG ; 10	Oxycodone Hydrochloride Controlled-Release	10 mg	White	Controlled Release Tablet	Circle	Ivax Pharmaceuticals
ABG ; 20	Oxycodone Hydrochloride	20 mg	Pink	Controlled-Release Tablet	Circle	Ivax Pharmaceuticals
ABG ; 20	Oxycodone Hydrochloride Controlled-Release	20 mg	Pink	Controlled Release Tablet	Circle	Ivax Pharmaceuticals
ABG ; 40	Oxycodone Hydrochloride	40 mg	Yellow	Controlled-Release Tablet	Circle	Ivax Pharmaceuticals
ABG ; 40	Oxycodone Hydrochloride Controlled-Release	40 mg	Yellow	Controlled Release Tablet	Circle	Ivax Pharmaceuticals
ABG ; 80	Oxycodone Hydrochloride	80 mg	Green	Controlled-Release Tablet	Circle	Ivax Pharmaceuticals
ABG ; 80	Oxycodone Hydrochloride Controlled-Release	80 mg	Green	Controlled Release Tablet	Circle	Ivax Pharmaceuticals
ABG 15	Morphine Sulfate	15 mg	Blue	Tablet, Extended Release	Circle	Watson Laboratories
ABG 30	Morphine Sulfate	30 mg	Lavender	Tablet, Extended Release	Circle	Watson Laboratories
ABG 60	Morphine Sulfate	60 mg	Orange	Tablet, Extended Release	Circle	Watson Laboratories
ABG 100	Morphine Sulfate	100 mg	Gray	Tablet, Extended Release	Circle	Watson Laboratories
ABG 200	Morphine Sulfate	200 mg	Green	Tablet, Extended Release	Circle	Watson Laboratories
AC; 200; G	Acebutolol Hydrochloride	200 mg	Lavender and Orange	Capsule		Par Pharmaceutical

IMPRINT	BRAND/GENERIC NAME	STRENGTH	COLOR	FORM	SHAPE	MANUFACTURER
AC; 200; G	Acebutolol Hydrochloride	200 mg	Orange and Purple	Capsule		Alpharma
AC; 400; G	Acebutolol Hydrochloride	400 mg	Lavender and Orange	Capsule		Par Pharmaceutical
AC; 1000; 62.5	Augmentin Xr	1000 mg; 62.5 mg	White	Extended-Release Tablet	Oval	Glaxosmithkline
ACCUTANE; 10; ROCHE	Accutane	10 mg	Light Pink	Capsule	Oval	Roche Laboratories
ACCUTANE; 20; ROCHE	Accutane	20 mg	Maroon	Capsule	Oval	Roche Laboratories
ACCUTANE; 40; ROCHE	Accutane	40 mg	Yellow	Capsule	Oval	Roche Laboratories
ACF; 004	Atacand	4 mg	White	Tablet	Circle, Biconvex	Astra Zeneca
ACG; 008	Atacand	8 mg	Pink	Tablet	Biconvex, Circle	Astra Zeneca
ACH; 016	Atacand	16 mg	Pink	Tablet	Circle, Biconvex	Astra Zeneca
ACIPHEX; 20 ;	Aciphex	20 mg	Light Yellow	Delayed-Release Tablet		Eisai
ACJ; 322	Atacand HCT	32 mg; 12.5 mg	Yellow	Tablet	Oval, Biconvex	Astra Zeneca
ACL; 032	Atacand	32 mg	Pink	Tablet	Circle, Biconvex	Astra Zeneca
ACS; 162	Atacand HCT	16 mg; 12.5 mg	Peach	Tablet	Oval, Biconvex	Astra Zeneca
ACTIFED C-S	Actifed Cold and Sinus Maximum Strength	500 mg; 30 mg; 2 mg		Tablet		Pfizer Consumer Health Care
ACTIFED DAY	Actifed Sinus Daytime/nighttime Daytime Tablet	30 mg; 325 mg	White	Tablet	Circle	Pfizer Consumer Health Care
ACTIFED NIGHT	Actifed Sinus Daytime/nighttime Nighttime Tablet	30 mg; 500 mg; 25 mg	Blue	Tablet	Circle	Pfizer Consumer Health Care
ACTIFED; 12-HOUR	Actifed 12 Hour	120 mg; 5 mg	Yellow and Clear	Controlled-Release Capsule		Pfizer Consumer Health Care
ACTIFED; M2A	Actifed Tablet	2.5 mg; 60 mg	White	Tablet	Biconvex, Scored	Pfizer Consumer Health Care
ACTIFED; WELLCOME	Actifed Capsule	60 mg; 2.5 mg	Yellow and Orange	Capsule		Pfizer Consumer Health Care
ACTIGALL; 300 MG ;	Actigall	300 mg	Pink and White	Capsule		Watson Laboratories
ACTOS; 15	Actos	15 mg	White to Off White	Tablet	Circle, Convex	Eli Lilly
ACTOS; 15	Actos	15 mg	White to Off White	Tablet	Circle, Convex	Takeda Pharmaceuticals
ACTOS; 30	Actos	30 mg	White to Off White	Tablet	Circle, Flat	Eli Lilly
ACTOS; 30	Actos	30 mg	White to Off White	Tablet	Circle, Flat	Takeda Pharmaceuticals
ACTOS; 45	Actos	45 mg	White to Off White	Tablet	Circle, Flat	Eli Lilly
ACTOS; 45	Actos	45 mg	White to Off White	Tablet	Circle, Flat	Takeda Pharmaceuticals
ACY; 200	Acyclovir	200 mg		Tablet		Mylan Pharmaceuticals
ACY; 400	Acyclovir	400 mg	White	Tablet	Oval	Mylan Pharmaceuticals
ACY; 800	Acyclovir	800 mg		Tablet		Mylan Pharmaceuticals
AD; 5	Adderall 5 mg Tablet	1.25 mg; 1.25 mg; 1.25 mg; 1.25 mg	Blue	Tablet	Double-Scored	Shire Pharmaceuticals
AD; 7.5	Adderall 7.5 mg Tablet	1.875 mg; 1.875 mg; 1.875 mg; 1.875 mg	Blue	Tablet	Circle, Double-Scored	Shire Pharmaceuticals
AD; 10	Adderall 10 mg Tablet	2.5 mg; 2.5 mg; 2.5 mg; 2.5 mg	Blue	Tablet	Double-Scored	Shire Pharmaceuticals
AD; 12.5	Adderall 12.5 mg Tablet	3.125 mg; 3.125 mg; 3.125 mg; 3.125 mg	Orange	Tablet	Circle, Double-Scored	Shire Pharmaceuticals
AD; 15	Adderall 15 mg Tablet	3.75 mg; 3.75 mg; 3.75 mg; 3.75 mg	Orange	Tablet	Oval, Double-Scored	Shire Pharmaceuticals
AD; 20	Adderall 20 mg Tablet	5 mg; 5 mg; 5 mg; 5 mg	Orange	Tablet	Double-Scored	Shire Pharmaceuticals
AD; 30	Adderall 30 mg Tablet	7.5 mg; 7.5 mg; 7.5 mg; 7.5 mg	Orange	Tablet	Double-Scored	Shire Pharmaceuticals
AD; RPR	Maalox Anti-Diarrheal	2 mg	Light Green	Tablet	Oblong	Novartis Consumer
ADALAT CC; 30	Adalat CC	30 mg	Pink	Tablet, Extended Release	Circle	Bayer Pharmaceutical
ADALAT CC; 30	Adalat CC	30 mg	Pink	Tablet, Extended Release	Circle	Schering
ADALAT CC; 60	Adalat CC	60 mg	Salmon	Tablet, Extended Release	Circle	Bayer Pharmaceutical
ADALAT CC; 60	Adalat CC	60 mg	Salmon	Tablet, Extended Release	Circle	Schering
ADALAT CC; 90	Adalat CC	90 mg	Dark Red	Tablet, Extended Release	Circle	Bayer Pharmaceutical
ADALAT CC; 90	Adalat CC	90 mg	Dark Red	Tablet, Extended Release	Circle	Schering
ADALAT; 10	Adalat	20 mg	Orange and Light Brown	Capsule, Liquid Filled		Bayer Pharmaceutical
ADALAT; 20	Adalat	10 mg	Orange	Capsule, Liquid Filled		Bayer Pharmaceutical
ADAMS ; 006	Allerx-D	2.5 mg; 120 mg	Yellow	Tablet, Extended Release		Adams Laboratories
ADAMS; 063	Aquatab C	60 mg; 1200 mg; 120 mg	Light Yellow	Extended-Release Tablet	Oval, Scored	Adams Laboratories
ADAMS; 068	Aquatab D	1200 mg; 75 mg	Light Green	Extended-Release Tablet	Oval, Scored	Adams Laboratories
ADDERALL XR 10 MG ;	Adderall Xr - 10 mg Capsule	2.5 mg; 2.5 mg; 2.5 mg; 2.5 mg	Blue	Capsule, Extended Release		Shire Pharmaceuticals
ADDERALL XR 15 MG	Adderall Xr - 15 mg Capsule	3.75 mg; 3.75 mg; 3.75 mg; 3.75 mg	White/blue	Capsule, Extended Release		Shire Pharmaceuticals
ADDERALL XR 20 MG ;	Adderall Xr - 20 mg Capsule	5 mg; 5 mg; 5 mg; 5 mg	Orange	Capsule, Extended Release		Shire Pharmaceuticals
ADDERALL XR 25 MG	Adderall Xr - 25 mg Capsule	6.25 mg; 6.25 mg; 6.25 mg; 6.25 mg	Orange/white	Capsule, Extended Release		Shire Pharmaceuticals
ADDERALL XR 30 MG ;	Adderall Xr - 30 mg Capsule	7.5 mg; 7.5 mg; 7.5 mg; 7.5 mg	Natural/orange	Capsule, Extended Release		Shire Pharmaceuticals
ADDERALL XR; 5 MG	Adderall Xr - 5 mg Capsule	1.25 mg; 1.25 mg; 1.25 mg; 1.25 mg	Clear/blue	Capsule, Extended Release		Shire Pharmaceuticals

IMPRINT	BRAND/GENERIC NAME	STRENGTH	COLOR	FORM	SHAPE	MANUFACTURER
ADEFLOR; CHEWABLE; 0.5	Adeflor	5 mg; 2 mcg; 18 mg; 2 mg; 0.5 mg; 4000 IU; 400 IU; 2 mg; 75 mg; 1 mg	Light Brown	Tablet, Chewable	Circle	Pharmacia & Upjohn
ADEFLOR; CHEWABLE; 1.0	Adeflor	5 mg; 2 mcg; 18 mg; 2 mg; 1 mg; 4000 IU; 400 IU; 2 mg; 75 mg; 1 mg	Brown	Tablet, Chewable	Circle	Pharmacia & Upjohn
ADEFLOR; M	Adeflor M	250 mg; 10 mg; 2 mcg; 20 mg; 1 mg; 100 mg; 2.5 mg; 400 IU; 6000 IU; 1.5 mg; 10 mg; 30 mg; 0.1 mg;	Pink	Tablet	Oval	Pharmacia & Upjohn
ADVIL	Advil	200 mg	Light Brown	Tablet		Wyeth Consumer Healthcare
ADVIL	Advil	200 mg	Light Brown	Coated Tablet	Circle	Wyeth Consumer Healthcare
ADVIL	Advil Liqui-Gels	200 mg	Green	Capsule, Liquid Filled	Oblong	Wyeth Consumer Healthcare
ADVIL C&S	Advil Cold & Sinus Tablet	200 mg; 30 mg	Buff	Coated Tablet	Circle	Wyeth Consumer Healthcare
ADVIL COLD & SINUS	Advil Cold & Sinus Caplet	200 mg; 30 mg	Brown	Tablet	Oblong, Coated	Wyeth Consumer Healthcare
ADVIL FLU	Advil Flu & Body Ache	200 mg; 30 mg	White	Tablet	Oval, Film-Coated	Wyeth Consumer Healthcare
ADVIL; 50	Children's Advil Fruit Flavored Chewables	50 mg	Red	Tablet, Chewable	Circle	Wyeth Consumer Healthcare
ADVIL; 50	Children's Advil Grape Flavored Chewables	50 mg	Purple	Tablet, Chewable	Circle	Wyeth Consumer Healthcare
ADVIL; 100	Junior Strength Advil	100 mg	Orange-Brown	Coated Tablet	Circle	Wyeth Consumer Healthcare
ADVIL; 100	Junior Strength Advil Fruit Flavor	100 mg	Red	Tablet, Chewable	Circle	Wyeth Consumer Healthcare
ADVIL; 100	Junior Strength Advil Grape Flavor	100 mg	Purple	Tablet, Chewable	Circle	Wyeth Consumer Healthcare
ADX; 1; A	Arimidex	1 mg	White	Coated Tablet	Biconvex	Astra Zeneca
AEY; 420	Deronil	0.75 mg	Amber-Yellow	Tablet		Schering
AF ANACIN	Anacin Aspirin Free Maximum Strength	500 mg	White	Tablet	Oblong	Whitehall Laboratories
AF; ANACIN	Anacin Maximum Strength, Aspirin Free	500 mg	White	Tablet	Capsule-Shape	Whitehall Laboratories
AFRINOL; 258 ;	Afrinol	120 mg	Blue	Tablet		Schering-Plough Healthcare Products
AHR	Cough Calmers	52.5 mg; 7.5 mg	Red	Lozenge/troche	Square	Wyeth Consumer Healthcare
AHR	Dimacol	10 mg; 100 mg; 30 mg	Orange	Tablet	Oval	Wyeth Consumer Healthcare
AHR	Robalate	500 mg	White	Tablet, Chewable		Wyeth Pharmaceuticals
AHR ;	Z-Bec	45 IU; 600 mg; 15 mg; 10.2 mg; 100 mg; 10 mg; 6 mcg; 25 mg; 22.5 mg	Green	Coated Tablet	Capsule-Shape	Wyeth Consumer Healthcare
AHR; 1535	Mitrolan	500 mg	Pale Yellow	Tablet, Chewable	Circle	Wyeth Pharmaceuticals
AHR; 1650	Dimacol	100 mg; 30 mg; 15 mg	Orange and Green	Capsule		Wyeth Consumer Healthcare
AHR; 2245	Dimetapp Decongestant Non-Drowsy Liqui-Gels	30 mg	Dark Blue	Capsule, Liquid Filled	Oval	Wyeth Consumer Healthcare
AHR; 2250	Dimetapp Allergy Liqui-Gels	4 mg	Green	Capsule, Liquid Filled	Oval	Wyeth Consumer Healthcare
AHR; 5449	Exna	50 mg	Yellow	Tablet	Circle, Scored	Wyeth Pharmaceuticals
AHR; 5650	Imavate	50 mg	Pink	Tablet	Circle	Wyeth Consumer Healthcare
AHR; 6447	Pondimin	20 mg	Orange	Tablet	Scored, Compressed	Whitehall-Robins Healthcare
AHR; 8501	Robitussin Cold Severe Congestion Liquigels	200 mg; 30 mg	Aqua	Capsule, Liquid Filled	Oval	Wyeth Consumer Healthcare
AHR; 8600	Robitussin Cold & Cough Liquigels	10 mg; 200 mg; 30 mg	Red	Capsule, Liquid Filled	Oval	Wyeth Consumer Healthcare
AHR; 8601	Robitussin Severe Congestion Non-Drowsy Formula	200 mg; 30 mg	Aqua	Capsule, Liquid Filled	Oval	Wyeth Consumer Healthcare
AHR; 8831	Silain	50 mg		Tablet		Wyeth Pharmaceuticals
AHR; AHR	Robitussin Cough Calmers Cherry Flavor	5 mg	Red	Lozenge/troche	Square	Wyeth Consumer Healthcare
AHR; ROBICAP; 8417	Robitet-250 Robicaps	250 mg	Pink and Brown	Capsule		Wyeth Pharmaceuticals
AHR; ROBICAP; 8427	Robitet-500 Robicaps	500 mg	Cream and Brown	Capsule		Wyeth Pharmaceuticals
AKH; 892 ;	Tremin	2 mg	White	Tablet		Schering
AKJ; 596 ;	Tremin	5 mg	Gray	Tablet		Schering
AL	Clorazepate Dipotassium	3.75 mg	Blue	Tablet	Circle, Scored, Compressed	Novartis Generics
AL 0.5; G	Alprazolam	0.5 mg	Dark Yellow	Tablet	Oval, Scored	Par Pharmaceutical
AL; 1.0; G ;	Alprazolam	1 mg	White	Tablet	Oval, Scored	Par Pharmaceutical
ALBAMYCIN	Albamycin	250 mg	White and Maroon	Capsule		Pharmacia & Upjohn
ALEVE	Aleve	220 mg	Light Blue	Tablet	Oblong	Bayer Consumer Care
ALEVE CS	Aleve Cold & Sinus Non-Drowsy	220 mg; 120 mg		Tablet, Extended Release, 12 Hr	Capsule-Shape	Bayer Consumer Care
ALEVE SH	Aleve Sinus & Headache Non-Drowsy	220 mg; 120 mg		Tablet, Extended Release, 12 Hr	Capsule-Shape	Bayer Consumer Care
ALKA SELTZER	Alka-Seltzer Original	325 mg; 1916 mg; 1000 mg	White	Tablet, Effervescent	Circle	Bayer Consumer Care
ALKA SELTZER; AF	Alka-Seltzer Advanced Formula	325 mg; 280 mg; 900 mg; 300 mg; 465 mg	White	Effervescent Tablet		Bayer Consumer Care
ALKA SELTZER; PM	Alka-Seltzer Pm	325 mg; 38 mg	White	Tablet, Effervescent	Circle	Bayer Consumer Care
ALKA-MINTS	Alka-Mints	850 mg	White	Tablet, Chewable	Circle	Bayer Consumer Care

IMPRINT	BRAND/GENERIC NAME	STRENGTH	COLOR	FORM	SHAPE	MANUFACTURER
ALKA-SELTZER HR	Alka-Seltzer Heartburn Relief	1000 mg; 1940 mg	White	Tablet, Effervescent	Circle	Bayer Consumer Care
ALKA-SELTZER MR	Alka-Seltzer Morning Relief	500 mg; 65 mg	White	Tablet, Effervescent	Circle	Bayer Consumer Care
ALLEGRA; 60 MG	Allegra	60 mg	White and Pink	Capsule		Aventis Pharmaceuticals
ALLEGRA-D	Allegra-D 12 Hour	60 mg; 120 mg	White and Tan	Tablet, Extended Release	Oblong	Sanofi-Aventis U.S.
ALPHA; 028	Guaifenesin	1200 mg	White	Tablet	Oblong, Scored	Eli Lilly
ALTACE; 1.25; HOECHST	Altace	1.25 mg	Yellow	Capsule		Monarch Pharmaceuticals
ALTACE; 2.5 MG; HOECHST	Altace	2.5 mg	Orange	Capsule		Monarch Pharmaceuticals
ALTACE; 5 MG; HOECHST	Altace	5 mg	Red	Capsule		Monarch Pharmaceuticals
ALTACE; 10 MG; HOECHST	Altace	10 mg	Blue	Capsule		Monarch Pharmaceuticals
AM	Tridione	300 mg	White	Capsule		Abbott Laboratories
AM; 200; G	Amiodarone Hydrochloride	200 mg	White	Tablet	Circle, Scored	Par Pharmaceutical
AMARYL	Amaryl	1 mg	Pink	Tablet	Oblong	Sanofi-Aventis U.S.
AMARYL	Amaryl	2 mg	Green	Tablet	Oblong	Sanofi-Aventis U.S.
AMARYL	Amaryl	4 mg	Blue	Tablet	Oblong	Sanofi-Aventis U.S.
AMB 5 ; 5401	Ambien	5 mg	Pink	Tablet	Capsule-Shape	Sanofi-Aventis U.S.
AMB 10 ; 5421	Ambien	10 mg	White	Tablet	Capsule-Shape	Sanofi-Aventis U.S.
AMGEN; 30	Sensipar	30 mg	Light Green	Tablet	Oval	Amgen
AMGEN; 60	Sensipar	60 mg	Light Green	Tablet	Oval	Amgen
AMGEN; 90	Sensipar	90 mg	Light Green	Tablet	Oval	Amgen
AMIDE; 014	Dexchlorpheniramine Maleate	4 mg	Yellow	Tablet	Oval	Watson Laboratories
AMIDE; 015	Dexchlorpheniramine Maleate	6 mg	White	Tablet	Oval	Watson Laboratories
AMITONE	Amitone	350 mg	White	Tablet, Chewable	Circle	Glaxosmithkline Consumer
AMOXIL; 125	Amoxil	125 mg	Pink	Tablet, Chewable	Oval	Glaxosmithkline
AMOXIL; 200	Amoxil	200 mg	Pale Pink	Tablet, Chewable	Circle	Glaxosmithkline
AMOXIL; 250	Amoxil	250 mg	Pink	Tablet, Chewable	Oval	Glaxosmithkline
AMOXIL; 250	Amoxil	250 mg	Royal Blue and Pink	Capsule		Glaxosmithkline
AMOXIL; 400	Amoxil	400 mg	Pale Pink	Tablet, Chewable	Circle	Glaxosmithkline
AMOXIL; 500	Amoxil	500 mg	Royal Blue and Pink	Capsule		Glaxosmithkline
AMOXIL; 500	Amoxil	500 mg	Pink	Coated Tablet	Capsule-Shape	Glaxosmithkline
AMOXIL; 875	Amoxil	875 mg	Pink	Coated Tablet	Capsule-Shape, Scored	Glaxosmithkline
AMP; 500	Ampicillin	500 mg	Blue and White	Capsule		Teva Pharmaceuticals
AMT; 832	Amantadine Hydrochloride	100 mg	Peach	Tablet	Circle	Upsher-Smith Laboratories
AMX; 500	Amoxicillin	500 mg	Orange and White	Capsule		Par Pharmaceutical
ANACIN	Anacin	400 mg; 32 mg	White	Tablet	Capsule-Shape	Whitehall Laboratories
ANAPROX DS; ROCHE ;	Anaprox DS	550 mg	Dark Blue	Coated Tablet	Oblong	Roche Laboratories
ANDRX 605	Allergy and Congestion Relief	10 mg; 240 mg	White	Tablet, Extended Release	Oval	Andrx Pharmaceuticals
ANDRX 710	Potassium Chloride Extended-Release	10 meq	Off-White	Tablet, Extended Release	Capsule-Shape	Andrx Pharmaceuticals
ANDRX 720	Potassium Chloride Extended-Release	20 meq	Off-White	Tablet, Extended Release	Capsule-Shape	Andrx Pharmaceuticals
ANDRX LOGO ; 935	Fosinopril Sodium	10 mg	White	Tablet	Capsule-Shape	Andrx Pharmaceuticals
ANDRX LOGO ; 936	Fosinopril Sodium	20 mg	White	Tablet	Oval	Andrx Pharmaceuticals
ANDRX LOGO ; 937	Fosinopril Sodium	40 mg	White	Tablet	Circle	Andrx Pharmaceuticals
ANDRX LOGO 10	Altoprev	10 mg	Dark Orange	Tablet, Extended Release	Circle	Andrx Pharmaceuticals
ANDRX LOGO 20	Altoprev	20 mg	Orange	Tablet, Extended Release	Circle	Andrx Pharmaceuticals
ANDRX LOGO 40	Altoprev	40 mg	Peach	Tablet, Extended Release	Circle	Andrx Pharmaceuticals
ANDRX LOGO 60	Altoprev	60 mg	Light Peach	Tablet, Extended Release	Circle	Andrx Pharmaceuticals
ANDRX LOGO 574	Fortamet	500 mg	White	Tablet, Extended Release		Andrx Pharmaceuticals
ANDRX LOGO 575	Fortamet	1000 mg	White	Tablet, Extended Release		Andrx Pharmaceuticals
ANDRX LOGO; 524	Hydrocodone Bitartrate and Ibuprofen	7.5 mg; 200 mg	White	Tablet		Andrx Pharmaceuticals
ANDRX; 333 ;	Entex LA	400 mg; 30 mg	Yellow and Blue	Capsule		Andrx Pharmaceuticals
ANDRX; 510; 100 MG	Ketoprofen	100 mg	White	Extended-Release Capsule		Andrx Pharmaceuticals
ANDRX; 515; 150 MG	Ketoprofen	150 mg	Light Turquoise Blue and White	Extended-Release Capsule		Andrx Pharmaceuticals
ANDRX; 520; 200 MG	Ketoprofen	200 mg	Light Turquoise Blue	Extended-Release Capsule		Andrx Pharmaceuticals
ANDRX; 548	Diltia Xt	120 mg	White	Extended-Release Capsule		Andrx Pharmaceuticals
ANDRX; 549	Diltia Xt	180 mg	Gray and White	Extended-Release Capsule		Andrx Pharmaceuticals
ANDRX; 550	Diltia Xt	240 mg	Gray	Extended-Release Capsule		Andrx Pharmaceuticals
ANDRX; 597	Cartia Xt	120 mg	Orange and White	Extended-Release Capsule		Andrx Pharmaceuticals
ANDRX; 598	Cartia Xt	180 mg	Orange and Yellow	Extended-Release Capsule		Andrx Pharmaceuticals
ANDRX; 599	Cartia Xt	240 mg	Orange and Brown	Extended-Release Capsule		Andrx Pharmaceuticals
ANDRX; 600	Cartia Xt	300 mg	Orange	Extended-Release Capsule		Andrx Pharmaceuticals
ANDRX; 674; 500	Metformin Hydrochloride	500 mg	White	Tablet	Circle	Andrx Pharmaceuticals
ANDRX; 675; 850	Metformin Hydrochloride	850 mg	White	Tablet	Circle	Andrx Pharmaceuticals
ANDRX; 676; 1000	Metformin Hydrochloride	1000 mg	White	Tablet	Circle	Andrx Pharmaceuticals

IMPRINT	BRAND/GENERIC NAME	STRENGTH	COLOR	FORM	SHAPE	MANUFACTURER
ANDRX; 696; 120 MG	Taztia Xt	120 mg	Pink	Capsule		Andrx Pharmaceuticals
ANDRX; 697; 180 MG	Taztia Xt	180 mg	Blue and Cream	Capsule		Andrx Pharmaceuticals
ANDRX; 698; 240 MG	Taztia Xt	240 mg	Pink and Blue	Capsule		Andrx Pharmaceuticals
ANDRX; 699; 300 MG	Taztia Xt	300 mg	Pink and Cream	Capsule		Andrx Pharmaceuticals
ANDRX; 700; 360 MG	Taztia Xt	360 mg	Light Blue	Capsule		Andrx Pharmaceuticals
ANDRX; 827	Generic Entex LA	30 mg; 400 mg	Opaque Orange	Extended-Release Capsule		Andrx Pharmaceuticals
ANK; SP ;	Miradon	50 mg	Pink	Tablet	Oval, Scored	Schering
ANSAID; 50 MG	Ansaid	50 mg	White	Coated Tablet	Oval	Pharmacia & Upjohn
ANSAID; 100 MG	Ansaid	100 mg	Blue	Coated Tablet	Oval	Pharmacia & Upjohn
ANSPOR; 250; SKF	Anspor	250 mg	Red and White	Capsule		Glaxosmithkline
ANSPOR; 500; SKF	Anspor	500 mg	Red	Capsule		Glaxosmithkline
ANZEMET; 50	Anzemet	50 mg	Light Pink	Tablet	Circle	Sanofi-Aventis U.S.
ANZEMET; 100	Anzemet	100 mg	Pink	Tablet	Oval	Sanofi-Aventis U.S.
AP ; 110	Cephadyn	650 mg; 50 mg	Blue	Tablet	Capsule-Shape	Atley Pharmaceuticals
AP; 026	Estradiol	1 mg	Lavender	Tablet	Circle	Bristol-Myers Squibb
AP; 027	Estradiol	2 mg	Green	Tablet	Circle	Bristol-Myers Squibb
AP; 5160	Captopril and Hydrochlorothiazide	25 mg; 15 mg	White and Orange Mottled	Tablet	Rounded Square, Quadrisected Scored	Bristol-Myers Squibb
AP; 5161	Captopril and Hydrochlorothiazide	25 mg; 25 mg	Peach	Tablet	Rounded Square, Quadrisected Scored	Bristol-Myers Squibb
AP; 5162	Captopril and Hydrochlorothiazide	50 mg; 15 mg	White and Orange Mottled	Tablet	Oval, Scored	Bristol-Myers Squibb
AP; 5163	Captopril and Hydrochlorothiazide	50 mg; 25 mg	Peach	Tablet	Oval, Scored	Bristol-Myers Squibb
AP; 7045 ;	Captopril	12.5 mg	White	Tablet	Circle, Scored	Sandoz
AP; 7046	Captopril	25 mg	White	Tablet	Circle, Scored	Sandoz
AP; 7047	Captopril	50 mg	White	Tablet	Circle, Scored	Sandoz
AP; 7048	Captopril	100 mg	White	Tablet	Circle, Scored	Sandoz
APSE	Pseudoephedrine Hydrochloride and Guaifenesin	120 mg; 600 mg	Yellow	Tablet	Oval	Duramed Pharmaceuticals
ARE	Mol-Iron Panhemic	500 mg; 7.5 mcg; 75 mg; 2 mg; 2 mg; 10 mg	Orange and Black	Capsule		Schering-Plough Healthcare Products
ARROW ;	Anacin	400 mg; 32 mg	White	Coated Tablet	Circle	Whitehall Laboratories
ARROW; LIFT CAP UP	Feverall Sprinkle Caps	80 mg	White and Clear	Capsule		Upsher-Smith Laboratories
ARROW; LIFT CAP UP	Feverall Sprinkle Caps Powder, Junior Strength	160 mg	Red and Clear	Capsule		Upsher-Smith Laboratories
AS	Comtrex Allergy/sinus Formula	500 mg; 30 mg; 2 mg	Green	Tablet		Bristol-Myers Squibb
AS	Isoclor	4 mg; 60 mg	White	Tablet	Circle	Novartis Consumer
AS 200 ;	Amiodarone Hydrochloride	200 mg	Yellow	Tablet	Circle	Aurobindo Pharma
AS 400	Amiodarone Hydrochloride	400 mg	Yellow	Tablet	Oval	Aurobindo Pharma
AS+C&C	Alka-Seltzer Plus Cold & Cough Medicine Liqui-Gels	10 mg; 2 mg; 30 mg; 325 mg	Purple	Capsule, Liquid Filled		Bayer Consumer Care
AS+COLD	Alka-Seltzer Plus Cold Medicine Liqui-Gels	2 mg; 30 mg; 325 mg	Clear Blue	Capsule, Liquid Filled		Bayer Consumer Care
AS+NT	Alka-Seltzer Plus Night-Time Cold Medicine Liqui-Gels	10 mg; 6.25 mg; 30 mg; 325 mg	Clear Green	Capsule, Liquid Filled	Oblong	Bayer Consumer Care
ASACOL; NE	Asacol	400 mg	Red-Brown	Timed-Release Tablet	Capsule-Shape	Procter & Gamble Pharmaceuticals
ASB	Bufferin Arthritis Strength	500 mg;	White	Tablet		Bristol-Myers Squibb
	Bufferin Tri-Buffered Arthritis Strength	500 mg; 222.3 mg; 88.9 mg; 55.6 mg		Tablet		Bristol-Myers Squibb
ASBRON; G; 78/202 ;	Asbron G	100 mg; 300 mg	Green with White Inlay	Tablet		Novartis Pharmaceuticals
ASPIRIN	Aspirin	325 mg	White	Tablet	Circle	Baxter Healthcare
ATARAX; 10	Atarax	10 mg	Orange	Tablet	Triangle	Pfizer
ATARAX; 25	Atarax	25 mg	Green	Tablet	Triangle	Pfizer Laboratories
ATARAX; 50	Atarax	50 mg	Yellow	Tablet	Triangle	Pfizer Laboratories
ATARAX; 100	Atarax	100 mg	Red	Tablet	Triangle	Pfizer Laboratories
ATHENA LOGO	Carbatrol	200 mg	Light Gray and Blue-Green	Extended-Release Capsule		Shire Pharmaceuticals
ATHENA LOGO	Carbatrol	300 mg	Black and Blue-Green	Extended-Release Capsule		Shire Pharmaceuticals
ATRAL; 250	Cephalexin	250 mg	Opaque Scarlet and Grey	Capsule		Duramed Pharmaceuticals
ATRAL; 250	Tetracycline Hydrochloride	250 mg	Opaque Yellow and Orange	Capsule		Duramed Pharmaceuticals
ATRAL; 500	Tetracycline Hydrochloride	500 mg	Opaque Black and Yellow	Capsule		Duramed Pharmaceuticals
ATROMID-S; 500	Atromid-S	500 mg	Orange	Capsule, Liquid Filled	Oblong	Wyeth Pharmaceuticals
AUGMENTIN ; 250/ 125	Augmentin	125 mg; 250 mg	White	Tablet	Oval	Glaxosmithkline
AUGMENTIN ; 500/ 125	Augmentin	125 mg; 500 mg	White	Tablet	Oval	Glaxosmithkline
AUGMENTIN XR	Augmentin Xr	1000 mg; 62.5 mg	White	Extended-Release Tablet	Oval, Bl-Layered	Glaxosmithkline
AUGMENTIN; 200	Augmentin	28.5 mg; 200 mg	Mottled Pink	Tablet, Chewable	Circle	Glaxosmithkline
AUGMENTIN; 250/ 125	Augmentin	125 mg; 250 mg	White	Coated Tablet	Oval	Glaxosmithkline
AUGMENTIN; 400	Augmentin	57 mg; 400 mg	Mottled Pink	Tablet, Chewable	Circle, Biconvex	Glaxosmithkline
AUGMENTIN; 875 ;	Augmentin	125 mg; 875 mg	White	Tablet	Capsule-Shape	Glaxosmithkline

IMPRINT	BRAND/GENERIC NAME	STRENGTH	COLOR	FORM	SHAPE	MANUFACTURER
AXID; 150; RELIANT ;	Axid	150 mg	Opaque Dark Yellow and Opaque Pale Yellow	Capsule		Eli Lilly
AXID; 300; RELIANT ;	Axid	300 mg	Opaque Brown and Opaque Pale Yellow	Capsule		Eli Lilly
AXID; AR	Axid AR	75 mg	Yellow	Tablet		Wyeth Consumer Healthcare
AYERST; 878	Premarin with Methyltestosterone	0.625 mg; 5 mg	White	Tablet	Circle	Wyeth Pharmaceuticals
AYERST; 879	Premarin with Methyltestosterone	1.25 mg; 10 mg	Yellow	Tablet	Circle	Wyeth Pharmaceuticals
AYERST; 880	Pmb-200	0.45 mg; 200 mg	Green	Tablet	Oblong	Wyeth Pharmaceuticals
AYERST; 881	Pmb-400	0.45 mg; 400 mg	Pink	Tablet	Oblong	Wyeth Pharmaceuticals
AYGESTIN; 5	Aygestin	5 mg	White	Tablet	Oval, Scored	Barr Laboratories
AYGESTIN; 5	Aygestin	5 mg	White	Tablet	Oval, Scored	Duramed Pharmaceuticals
B	Bufferin	325 mg	White	Tablet	Circle	Bristol-Myers Squibb
B	Bufferin	325 mg	White, Opaque	Tablet	Capsule-Shape	Bristol-Myers Squibb
B	Bufferin Tri-Buffered	325 mg; 158 mg; 63 mg; 34 mg	White	Coated Tablet	Circle, Scored	Bristol-Myers Squibb
B ; 60	Nifediac CC	60 mg	Mustard Yellow	Tablet, Extended Release	Circle	Teva Pharmaceuticals
B ; 90	Nifediac CC	90 mg	Yellow	Tablet, Extended Release	Circle	Teva Pharmaceuticals
B ; 120	Cardizem LA	120 mg	White	Tablet, Extended Release	Capsule-Shape	Biovail Pharmaceuticals
B ; 120	Cardizem LA	120 mg	White	Tablet, Extended Release	Capsule-Shape	Kos Pharmaceuticals
B ; 154	Loestrin 21 1/20	1 mg; 20 mcg	White	Tablet	Circle	Duramed Pharmaceuticals
B ; 154	Loestrin Fe 1/20 - White Tablet	1 mg; 20 mcg	White	Tablet	Circle	Duramed Pharmaceuticals
B ; 155	Loestrin 21 1.5/30	1.5 mg; 30 mcg	Green	Tablet	Circle	Duramed Pharmaceuticals
B ; 155	Loestrin Fe 1.5/30 - Green Tablet	1.5 mg; 30 mcg	Green	Tablet	Circle	Duramed Pharmaceuticals
B ; 156	Loestrin Fe 1/20 - Brown Tablet	75 mg	Brown	Tablet	Circle	Duramed Pharmaceuticals
B ; 156	Loestrin Fe 1.5/30 - Brown Tablet	75 mg	Brown	Tablet	Circle	Duramed Pharmaceuticals
B ; 180	Cardizem LA	180 mg	White	Tablet, Extended Release	Capsule-Shape	Biovail Pharmaceuticals
B ; 180	Cardizem LA	180 mg	White	Tablet, Extended Release	Capsule-Shape	Kos Pharmaceuticals
B ; 240	Cardizem LA	240 mg	White	Tablet, Extended Release	Capsule-Shape	Biovail Pharmaceuticals
B ; 240	Cardizem LA	240 mg	White	Tablet, Extended Release	Capsule-Shape	Kos Pharmaceuticals
B ; 247	Junel Fe 1/20 - Brown Tablet	75 mg	Brown	Tablet	Circle	Barr Laboratories
B ; 247	Junel Fe 1.5/30 - Brown Tablet	75 mg	Brown	Tablet	Circle	Barr Laboratories
B ; 300	Cardizem LA	300 mg	White	Tablet, Extended Release	Capsule-Shape	Biovail Pharmaceuticals
B ; 300	Cardizem LA	300 mg	White	Tablet, Extended Release	Capsule-Shape	Kos Pharmaceuticals
B ; 332	Velivet - Orange Tablet	0.125 mg; 0.025 mg	Orange	Tablet	Circle	Barr Laboratories
B ; 333	Velivet - Beige Tablet	0.1 mg; 0.025 mg	Beige	Tablet	Circle	Barr Laboratories
B ; 335	Velivet - Pink Tablet	0.15 mg; 0.025 mg	Pink	Tablet	Circle	Barr Laboratories
B ; 360	Cardizem LA	360 mg	White	Tablet, Extended Release	Capsule-Shape	Kos Pharmaceuticals
B ; 420	Cardizem LA	420 mg	White	Tablet, Extended Release	Capsule-Shape	Biovail Pharmaceuticals
B ; 420	Cardizem LA	420 mg	White	Tablet, Extended Release	Capsule-Shape	Kos Pharmaceuticals
B ; 555	Seasonique - Light Blue-Green Tablet	0.15 mg; 0.03 mg	Light Blue-Green	Tablet	Circle	Duramed Pharmaceuticals
B ; 556	Seasonique - Yellow Tablet	0.01 mg	Yellow	Tablet	Circle	Duramed Pharmaceuticals
B ; 977	Junel Fe 1/20 - Light Yellow Tablet	1 mg; 20 mcg	Light Yellow	Tablet	Circle	Barr Laboratories
B ; 978	Junel Fe 1.5/30 - Pink Tablet	1.5 mg; 30 mcg	Pink	Tablet	Circle	Barr Laboratories
B ; 992	Jolessa - Pink Tablet	0.15 mg; 0.03 mg	Pink	Tablet	Circle	Barr Laboratories
B 491 ; 0.5	Alprazolam	0.5 mg	White	Tablet, Extended Release	Circle	Barr Laboratories
B 492 ; 1	Alprazolam	1 mg	Yellow	Tablet, Extended Release	Circle	Barr Laboratories
B 493 ; 2	Alprazolam	2 mg	Blue	Tablet, Extended Release	Circle	Barr Laboratories
B 494 ; 3	Alprazolam	3 mg	Green	Tablet, Extended Release	Circle	Barr Laboratories
B; 066; 100	Isoniazid	100 mg	White	Tablet	Circle, Scored, Flat-Faced	Barr Laboratories
B; 071; 300	Isoniazid	300 mg	White	Tablet	Circle, Scored, Flat-Faced	Barr Laboratories
B; 11 ;	Zagam	200 mg	White	Coated Tablet	Circle, Biconvex	Mylan Bertek Pharmaceuticals
B; 21	Levlen 21	0.15 mg; 30 mcg	Orange	21-Day Tablet Pack	Circle	Berlex Laboratories
B; 21	Levlen 28 Orange Tablet	0.15 mg; 30 mcg	Orange	28-Day Tablet Pack	Circle	Berlex Laboratories
B; 25	Benadryl Allergy Tablet	25 mg	Bright Pink	Tablet	Capsule-Shape, Small	Pfizer Consumer Health Care
B; 30	Nifedical XL	30 mg	Reddish Brown	Extended-Release Tablet	Circle	Teva Pharmaceuticals
B; 50; 902	Naltrexone Hydrochloride	50 mg	Beige	Tablet	Circle, Scored	Barr Laboratories
B; 60	Nifedical XL	60 mg	Reddish Brown	Extended-Release Tablet	Circle	Teva Pharmaceuticals
B; 60	Nifedipine	60 mg	Yellow	Extended-Release Tablet	Circle	Teva Pharmaceuticals
B; 95	Tri-Levlen 21 Brown Tablet	0.05 mg; 0.03 mg	Brown	21-Day Tablet Pack	Circle	Berlex Laboratories
B; 95	Tri-Levlen 28 Brown Tablet	0.05 mg; 0.03 mg	Brown	28-Day Tablet Pack	Circle	Berlex Laboratories
B; 96	Tri-Levlen 21 White Tablet	0.075 mg; 0.04 mg	White	21-Day Tablet Pack	Circle	Berlex Laboratories
B; 96	Tri-Levlen 28 White Tablet	0.075 mg; 0.04 mg	White	28-Day Tablet Pack	Circle	Berlex Laboratories
B; 97	Tri-Levlen 21 Light Yellow Tablet	0.125 mg; 0.03 mg	Light Yellow	21-Day Tablet Pack	Circle	Berlex Laboratories

IMPRINT	BRAND/GENERIC NAME	STRENGTH	COLOR	FORM	SHAPE	MANUFACTURER
B; 97	Tri-Levlen 28 Light Yellow Tablet	0.125 mg; 0.03 mg	Light Yellow	28-Day Tablet Pack	Circle	Berlex Laboratories
B; 133	Pyridostigmine Bromide	60 mg	White	Tablet	Round, Quadrisected Scored	Barr Laboratories
B; 145	Digitek	0.125 mg	Yellow	Tablet	Circle, Scored in Imprinted Side	Mylan Bertek Pharmaceuticals
B; 146	Digitek	0.25 mg	White	Tablet	Circle, Scored on Imprinted Side	Mylan Bertek Pharmaceuticals
B; 171	Mefloquine Hydrochloride	250 mg	White	Tablet	Oval	Barr Laboratories
B; 201; 10	Fluoxetine Hydrochloride	10 mg	Beige	Tablet	Scored, Oval	Barr Laboratories
B; 211; 5	Norethindrone Acetate	5 mg	White	Tablet	Oval	Barr Laboratories
B; 241	Mirtazapine	15 mg	White	Disintegrating Tablet	Circle	Barr Laboratories
B; 241	Mirtazapine	15 mg	White to Off White	Disintegrating Tablet	Circle	Barr Laboratories
B; 242	Mirtazapine	30 mg	White	Disintegrating Tablet	Circle	Barr Laboratories
B; 242	Mirtazapine	30 mg	White to Off White	Disintegrating Tablet	Circle	Barr Laboratories
B; 252	Dipyridamole	25 mg	White	Coated Tablet	Circle, Biconvex	Barr Laboratories
B; 275; REVIA	Revia	50 mg	Beige	Tablet	Circle, Scored	Barr Laboratories
B; 285	Dipyridamole	50 mg	White	Coated Tablet	Circle, Biconvex	Barr Laboratories
B; 298	Hydroxyzine Hydrochloride	25 mg	Orange	Tablet	Circle	Barr Laboratories
B; 301	Hydroxyzine Hydrochloride	10 mg	Yellow	Tablet	Circle	Barr Laboratories
B; 302; 2 ;	Acetaminophen and Codeine	300 mg; 15 mg	White	Tablet	Circle, Scored	Barr Laboratories
B; 303; 3 ;	Acetaminophen and Codeine	300 mg; 30 mg	White	Tablet	Circle, Scored	Barr Laboratories
B; 304; 4 ;	Acetaminophen and Codeine	300 mg; 60 mg	White	Tablet	Circle, Scored	Barr Laboratories
B; 344	Errin	0.35 mg	Yellow	Tablet	Circle	Barr Laboratories
B; 345	Lithium Carbonate	300 mg	Off-White	Extended-Release Tablet	Circle	Barr Laboratories
B; 357	Methyldopa	125 mg	White	Coated Tablet	Circle	Barr Laboratories
B; 381 ;	Meperidine Hydrochloride	50 mg	White	Tablet	Circle	Barr Laboratories
B; 385; 500	Metformin Hydrochloride	500 mg	White	Tablet	Oval	Barr Laboratories
B; 386; 850	Metformin Hydrochloride	850 mg	White	Tablet	Oval	Barr Laboratories
B; 387; 10; 00	Metformin Hydrochloride	1000 mg	White	Tablet	Oval	Barr Laboratories
B; 484	Leucovorin Calcium	5 mg	White	Tablet	Circle	Barr Laboratories
B; 485	Leucovorin Calcium	25 mg	Green	Tablet	Circle	Barr Laboratories
B; 555; 424	Metoclopramide	10 mg	White	Tablet	Circle, Scored, Convex	Barr Laboratories
B; 555; 606	Megestrol Acetate	20 mg	White	Tablet	Round, Flat-Faced, Beveled-Edge, Scored	Barr Laboratories
B; 555; 779	Medroxyprogesterone Acetate	10 mg	White	Tablet	Circle, Biconvex, Scored	Barr Laboratories
B; 555; 872	Medroxyprogesterone Acetate	2.5 mg	White	Tablet	Circle, Biconvex, Scored	Barr Laboratories
B; 555; 873	Medroxyprogesterone Acetate	5 mg	White	Tablet	Circle, Biconvex, Scored	Barr Laboratories
B; 572	Methotrexate	2.5 mg	Yellow	Tablet	Oval, Scored	Barr Laboratories
B; 715	Camila	0.35 mg	Light Pink	Tablet	Circle	Barr Laboratories
B; 775; 7; 1/2	Dextroamphetamine Saccharate, Amphetamine Aspartate, Dextroamphetamine Sulfate, Amphetamine Sulfate 7.5 mg Tablet	1.875 mg; 1.875 mg; 1.875 mg; 1.875 mg	Blue	Tablet	Oval	Barr Laboratories
B; 776; 12; 1/2	Dextroamphetamine Saccharate, Amphetamine Aspartate, Dextroamphetamine Sulfate, Amphetamine Sulfate 12.5 mg Tablet	3.125 mg; 3.125 mg; 3.125 mg; 3.125 mg	Peach	Tablet	Oval	Barr Laboratories
B; 777; 1; 5	Dextroamphetamine Saccharate, Amphetamine Aspartate, Dextroamphetamine Sulfate, Amphetamine Sulfate 15 mg Tablet	3.75 mg; 3.75 mg; 3.75 mg; 3.75 mg	Peach	Tablet	Circle	Barr Laboratories
B; 814; 250	Ciprofloxacin	250 mg	Yellow	Tablet	Circle	Barr Laboratories
B; 815; 500	Ciprofloxacin	500 mg	Yellow	Tablet	Capsule-Shape	Barr Laboratories
B; 816; 750	Ciprofloxacin	750 mg	Yellow	Tablet	Capsule-Shape	Barr Laboratories
B; 859	Flecainide Acetate	50 mg	White to Off White	Tablet	Circle	Barr Laboratories
B; 860; 100	Flecainide Acetate	100 mg	White to Off White	Tablet	Oval, Scored	Barr Laboratories
B; 861; 150	Flecainide Acetate	150 mg	White to Off White	Tablet	Oval, Scored	Barr Laboratories
B; 886; 1	Estradiol	1 mg		Tablet		Barr Laboratories
B; 887; 2	Estradiol	2 mg	Green	Tablet	Oval	Barr Laboratories
B; 899; 1/2	Estradiol	0.5 mg		Tablet		Barr Laboratories
B; 917; 200	Amiodarone Hydrochloride	200 mg	White	Tablet	Circle, Scored	Barr Laboratories
B; 923; 400	Ethambutol Hydrochloride	400 mg	White	Tablet	Oval, Scored	Barr Laboratories
B; 927; 5	Trexall	5 mg	Green	Tablet	Oval	Barr Laboratories
B; 928; 7 1/2	Trexall	7.5 mg	Blue	Tablet	Oval, Scored	Barr Laboratories
B; 929; 10	Trexall	10 mg	Pink	Tablet	Oval, Scored	Barr Laboratories
B; 941	Nortrel .5/35	35 mcg; 0.5 mg	Light Yellow	Tablet	Circle	Barr Laboratories
B; 942	Nortrel 7/7/7 Blue Tablet	0.75 mg; 0.035 mg	Blue	28-Day Tablet Pack	Circle	Barr Laboratories
B; 943	Nortrel 7/7/7 Peach Tablet	1 mg; 0.035 mg	Peach	28-Day Tablet Pack	Circle	Barr Laboratories
B; 945; 15	Trexall	15 mg	Purple	Tablet	Oval	Barr Laboratories
B; 949	Nortrel 1/35	35 mcg; 1 mg	Yellow	Tablet	Circle	Barr Laboratories
B; 951	Nortrel 7/7/7 Light Yellow Tablet	0.5 mg; 0.035 mg	Light Yellow	28-Day Tablet Pack	Circle	Barr Laboratories
B; 952; 5	Dextroamphetamine Sulfate	5 mg	Peach	Tablet	Circle	Barr Laboratories
B; 953; 10	Dextroamphetamine Sulfate	10 mg	Pink	Tablet	Circle, Scored	Barr Laboratories
B; 965	Lessina 28 Pink Tablet	0.1 mg; 0.02 mg	Pink	Tablet	Circle	Barr Laboratories
B; 967	Fluvoxamine Maleate	25 mg	Off-White	Tablet	Oval	Barr Laboratories
B; 968; 50	Fluvoxamine Maleate	50 mg	Yellow	Tablet	Oval, Scored	Barr Laboratories
B; 969; 100	Fluvoxamine Maleate	100 mg	Brown	Tablet	Oval, Scored	Barr Laboratories
B; 971; 5	Dextroamphetamine Saccharate, Amphetamine Aspartate, Dextroamphetamine Sulfate, Amphetamine Sulfate 5 mg Tablet	1.25 mg; 1.25 mg; 1.25 mg; 1.25 mg	Blue	Tablet	Oval	Barr Laboratories
B; 972; 1; 0	Dextroamphetamine Saccharate, Amphetamine Aspartate, Dextroamphetamine Sulfate, Amphetamine Sulfate 10 mg Tablet	2.5 mg; 2.5 mg; 2.5 mg; 2.5 mg	Blue	Tablet	Oval, Scored, with Partial Bisects	Barr Laboratories

IMPRINT	BRAND/GENERIC NAME	STRENGTH	COLOR	FORM	SHAPE	MANUFACTURER
B; 973; 2; 0	Dextroamphetamine Saccharate, Amphetamine Aspartate, Dextroamphetamine Sulfate, Amphetamine Sulfate 20 mg Tablet	5 mg; 5 mg; 5 mg; 5 mg	Peach	Tablet	Oval	Barr Laboratories
B; 974; 3; 0	Dextroamphetamine Saccharate, Amphetamine Aspartate, Dextroamphetamine Sulfate, Amphetamine Sulfate 30 mg Tablet	7.5 mg; 7.5 mg; 7.5 mg; 7.5 mg	Peach	Tablet	Oval	Barr Laboratories
B; 987	Sprintec	35 mcg; 0.25 mg	Blue	Tablet	Circle	Barr Laboratories
B; 992	Portia 28 Pink Tablet	0.15 mg; 30 mcg	Pink	28-Day Tablet Pack	Circle	Barr Laboratories
B; 997; 1/10	Fludrocortisone Acetate	0.1 mg	Yellow	Tablet	Oval	Barr Laboratories
B; WL; 28	Benadryl Severe Allergy and Sinus Headache	500 mg; 25 mg; 30 mg		Tablet		Warner Lambert Consumer Health Products
B237	Mindal	60 mg; 500 mg	White	Extended-Release Tablet	Capsule-Shape	Duramed Pharmaceuticals
B2C	Lanoxicaps	0.1 mg	Yellow	Capsule, Liquid Filled	Oval, Small	Glaxosmithkline
B3; LL	Zebeta	10 mg	White	Coated Tablet	Heart-Shape, Biconvex	Lederle Laboratories
BACTRIM; ROCHE	Bactrim	80 mg; 400 mg	Light Green	Tablet	Capsule-Shape, Scored	Roche Laboratories
BACTRIM-DS; ROCHE	Bactrim DS	160 mg; 800 mg	White	Tablet	Capsule-Shape	Roche Laboratories
BARR 827 25 MG	Zonisamide	25 mg	White Opaque	Capsule		Barr Laboratories
BARR 828 50 MG	Zonisamide	50 mg	Grey Opaque	Capsule		Barr Laboratories
BARR 829 100 MG	Zonisamide	100 mg	Orange Opaque	Capsule		Barr Laboratories
BARR/454 ;	Claravis	30 mg	Orange Opaque	Capsule, Liquid Filled		Barr Laboratories
BARR/934 ;	Claravis	10 mg	Light Gray, Light Gray Opaque	Capsule, Liquid Filled		Barr Laboratories
BARR/935 ;	Claravis	20 mg	Brown Opaque, Brown Orange Opaque	Capsule, Liquid Filled		Barr Laboratories
BARR/936 ;	Claravis	40 mg	Light Orange	Capsule, Liquid Filled		Barr Laboratories
BARR; 010	Tetracycline Hydrochloride	500 mg	Black and Yellow	Capsule		Barr Laboratories
BARR; 011	Tetracycline Hydrochloride	250 mg	Orange and Yellow	Capsule		Barr Laboratories
BARR; 033	Chlordiazepoxide Hydrochloride	10 mg	Black and Green	Capsule		Barr Laboratories
BARR; 059 ;	Diphenhydramine Hydrochloride	50 mg	Pink	Capsule		Barr Laboratories
BARR; 128	Dicyclomine Hydrochloride	10 mg	Blue	Capsule		Barr Laboratories
BARR; 158	Chlordiazepoxide Hydrochloride	5 mg	Green and Yellow	Capsule		Barr Laboratories
BARR; 159	Chlordiazepoxide Hydrochloride	25 mg	Green and White	Capsule		Barr Laboratories
BARR; 281	Aminophylline	200 mg	White	Tablet	Circle	Barr Laboratories
BARR; 282	Aminophylline	100 mg	White	Tablet	Circle	Barr Laboratories
BARR; 286 ;	Dipyridamole	75 mg	White	Coated Tablet	Circle, Biconvex	Barr Laboratories
BARR; 299	Hydroxyzine Hydrochloride	50 mg	Orange	Tablet	Circle	Barr Laboratories
BARR; 300	Hydroxyzine Hydrochloride	100 mg	Orange	Tablet	Circle	Barr Laboratories
BARR; 302; 50	Hydroxyzine Pamoate	50 mg	Opaque Yellow and Opaque Maroon with Yellow Powder	Capsule, Liquid Filled		Barr Laboratories
BARR; 323; 25	Hydroxyzine Pamoate	25 mg	Opaque Yellow and Opaque Pink with Yellow Powder	Capsule, Liquid Filled		Barr Laboratories
BARR; 324; 100	Hydroxyzine Pamoate	100 mg	Opaque Yellow and Opaque Pink Filled with Yellow Powder	Capsule, Liquid Filled		Barr Laboratories
BARR; 325	Hydrocodone Bitartrate and Acetaminophen	5 mg; 500 mg	White	Tablet	Capsule-Shape, Scored	Barr Laboratories
BARR; 382 ;	Meperidine Hydrochloride	100 mg	White	Tablet	Circle, Biconvex	Barr Laboratories
BARR; 407	Doxepin Hydrochloride	100 mg	White and Green	Capsule		Barr Laboratories
BARR; 442	Acetohexamide	250 mg	White	Tablet	Oval, Biconvex, Scored	Barr Laboratories
BARR; 443	Acetohexamide	500 mg	White	Tablet	Capsule-Shape, Biconvex, Scored	Barr Laboratories
BARR; 446	Tamoxifen Citrate	10 mg	White	Tablet	Circle, Biconvex	Barr Laboratories
BARR; 555; 163	Diazepam	2 mg	White	Tablet	Round, Flat-Faced, Beveled-Edge, Scored	Barr Laboratories
BARR; 555; 164	Diazepam	10 mg	Blue	Tablet	Round, Flat-Faced, Beveled-Edge, Scored	Barr Laboratories
BARR; 555; 192	Hydrochlorothiazide Hydrochloride	100 mg	Peach	Tablet	Circle, Scored	Barr Laboratories
BARR; 555; 271	Sulfinpyrazone	100 mg	White	Tablet	Round, Flat-Faced, Beveled-Edge, Scored	Barr Laboratories
BARR; 555; 293	Oxycodone with Aspirin	4.5 mg; 0.38 mg; 325 mg	Yellow	Tablet	Circle, Scored	Barr Laboratories
BARR; 555; 363	Diazepam	5 mg	Yellow	Tablet	Round, Flat-Faced, Beveled-Edge, Scored	Barr Laboratories
BARR; 555; 444	Hydrochlorothiazide and Triamterene	50 mg; 75 mg	Yellow	Tablet	Oval	Barr Laboratories
BARR; 555; 444	Triamterene and Hydrochlorothiazide	75 mg; 50 mg	Yellow	Tablet	Oval, Biconvex, Scored	Barr Laboratories
BARR; 555; 483 ;	Amiloride Hydrochloride and Hydrochlorothiazide	5 mg; 50 mg	Light Yellow	Tablet	Circle, Biconvex, Scored	Barr Laboratories
BARR; 555; 489	Trazodone Hydrochloride	50 mg	White	Tablet	Circle, Biconvex, Scored	Barr Laboratories
BARR; 555; 490	Trazodone Hydrochloride	100 mg	White	Tablet	Circle, Biconvex, Scored	Barr Laboratories
BARR; 555; 585	Chlorzoxazone	500 mg	Light Green	Tablet	Circle, Scored	Barr Laboratories
BARR; 555; 607 ;	Megestrol Acetate	40 mg	White	Tablet	Round, Flat-Faced, Beveled-Edge, Scored	Barr Laboratories
BARR; 555; 643	Hydrochlorothiazide and Triamterene	25 mg; 37.5 mg	Green	Tablet	Oval	Barr Laboratories
BARR; 555; 643	Triamterene and Hydrochlorothiazide	37.5 mg; 25 mg	Green	Tablet	Oval, Scored	Barr Laboratories
BARR; 555; 727	Estropipate	0.75 mg	Yellow	Tablet	Circle, Scored	Barr Laboratories
BARR; 555; 728	Estropipate	1.5 mg	Peach	Tablet	Circle	Barr Laboratories
BARR; 555; 729	Estropipate	3 mg	Blue	Tablet	Circle, Scored	Barr Laboratories

IMPRINT	BRAND/GENERIC NAME	STRENGTH	COLOR	FORM	SHAPE	MANUFACTURER
BARR; 633	Danazol	50 mg	Yellow and White	Capsule		Barr Laboratories
BARR; 634	Danazol	100 mg	Yellow	Capsule		Barr Laboratories
BARR; 635	Danazol	200 mg	Opaque Orange and Transparent Orange	Capsule, Liquid Filled		Barr Laboratories
BARR; 658	Oxycodone and Acetaminophen	5 mg; 500 mg	Red and White	Capsule		Barr Laboratories
BARR; 732; 50 50 50	Trazodone Hydrochloride	150 mg	White	Tablet	Oblong	Barr Laboratories
BARR; 733; 100 100 100	Trazodone Hydrochloride	300 mg	White	Tablet	Oval	Barr Laboratories
BARR; 831; 1 ;	Warfarin Sodium	1 mg	Pink	Tablet	Oval, Flat-Faced, Beveled-Edge, Scored	Barr Laboratories
BARR; 832; 2 1/2 ;	Warfarin Sodium	2.5 mg	Green	Tablet	Oval, Flat-Faced, Beveled-Edge, Scored	Barr Laboratories
BARR; 833; 5	Warfarin Sodium	5 mg	Peach	Tablet	Oval, Flat-Faced, Beveled-Edge, Scored	Barr Laboratories
BARR; 834; 7 1/2 ;	Warfarin Sodium	7.5 mg	Yellow	Tablet	Oval, Flat-Faced, Beveled-Edge, Scored	Barr Laboratories
BARR; 835; 10 ;	Warfarin Sodium	10 mg	White	Tablet	Oval, Flat-Faced, Beveled-Edge, Scored	Barr Laboratories
BARR; 869; 2 ;	Warfarin Sodium	2 mg	Lavender	Tablet	Oval, Flat-Faced, Beveled-Edge, Scored	Barr Laboratories
BARR; 870	Flutamide	125 mg	Brown and White	Capsule		Barr Laboratories
BARR; 874; 4 ;	Warfarin Sodium	4 mg	Blue	Tablet	Oval, Flat-Faced, Beveled-Edge, Scored	Barr Laboratories
BARR; 882	Hydroxyurea	500 mg	Pink and Purple	Capsule		Barr Laboratories
BARR; 904	Tamoxifen Citrate	20 mg	White	Tablet	Circle, Biconvex	Barr Laboratories
BARR; 925; 3	Warfarin Sodium	3 mg	Tan	Tablet	Oval	Barr Laboratories
BARR; 926; 6	Warfarin Sodium	6 mg	Teal	Tablet	Oval	Barr Laboratories
BARR; 954	Dextroamphetamine Sulfate	5 mg	Beige	Extended-Release Capsule		Barr Laboratories
BARR; 955	Dextroamphetamine Sulfate	10 mg	Brown and Clear	Extended-Release Capsule		Barr Laboratories
BARR; 956	Dextroamphetamine Sulfate	15 mg	Brown and Clear	Extended-Release Capsule		Barr Laboratories
BAYER	Bayer 8-Hour Extended Release	650 mg	White	Sustained-Release Tablet	Oblong, Scored	Bayer Consumer Care
BAYER	Bayer Children's Low Dose Aspirin Regimen - Orange	81 mg	Orange	Tablet, Chewable	Circle	Bayer Consumer Care
BAYER	Bayer Children's Low Dose Aspirin Regiment - Cherry	81 mg	Pink	Tablet, Chewable	Circle	Bayer Consumer Care
BAYER	Bayer Genuine Aspirin	325 mg	White	Coated Tablet	Circle	Bayer Consumer Care
BAYER	Bayer Genuine Aspirin	325 mg	White	Tablet		Bayer Consumer Care
BAYER BUFFERED	Bayer Buffered	325 mg;	White	Coated Tablet	Circle	Bayer Consumer Care
BAYER C500 QD	Cipro Xr	500 mg	White to Light Yellow	Tablet, Extended Release	Oblong	Bayer Pharmaceutical
BAYER C500 QD	Cipro Xr	500 mg	White to Light Yellow	Tablet, Extended Release	Oblong	Schering
BAYER CROSS ; 200	Nexavar	200 mg	Red	Tablet	Circle	Bayer Pharmaceutical Division
BAYER PLUS	Aspirin Plus	160 mg; 63 mg; 34; 325 mg		Tablet		Bayer Consumer Care
BAYER PLUS; 500	Bayer Plus	500 mg;	White	Tablet		Bayer Consumer Care
BAYER SELECT	Bayer Select Pain Relief Formula	200 mg	White	Tablet		Bayer Consumer Care
BAYER SELECT HEADACHE	Bayer Select	500 mg; 65 mg	White	Tablet	Capsule-Shape	Bayer Consumer Care
BAYER SELECT MENSTRUAL	Bayer Select Menstrual Maximum Strength Multi-Symptom	500 mg; 25 mg	Pink	Tablet	Capsule-Shape	Bayer Consumer Care
BAYER SELECT NIGHT TIME	Bayer Select Night Time Pain Relief	500 mg; 25 mg	Light Blue	Tablet		Bayer Consumer Care
BAYER SELECT SINUS	Bayer Select Sinus Pain Relief Formula	500 mg; 30 mg	Green	Tablet		Bayer Consumer Care
BAYER SELECT; ALLERGY SINUS	Bayer Select Allergy Sinus	500 mg; 30 mg; 2 mg		Tablet	Oval	Bayer Consumer Care
BAYER SELECT; BACKACHE	Bayer Select Backache	580 mg	Yellow	Tablet		Bayer Consumer Care
BAYER SELECT; CHEST COLD	Bayer Select Chest Cold	500 mg; 15 mg	Light Purple	Tablet		Bayer Consumer Care
BAYER SELECT; FLU RELIEF	Bayer Select Flu Relief	500 mg; 2 mg; 30 mg; 15 mg	Red	Tablet		Bayer Consumer Care
BAYER SELECT; HEAD COLD	Bayer Select Head Cold	500 mg; 30 mg	Light Green	Tablet		Bayer Consumer Care
BAYER SELECT; HEAD/CHEST COLD	Bayer Select Head & Chest Cold	325 mg; 10 mg; 100 mg; 30 mg	Light Orange	Tablet		Bayer Consumer Care
BAYER SELECT; NIGHT TIME COLD	Bayer Select Night Time Cold	500 mg; 15 mg; 1.25 mg; 30 mg	Light Blue	Tablet	Oblong	Bayer Consumer Care
BAYER; 5	Levitra	5 mg	Orange	Tablet	Circle	Bayer Pharmaceutical
BAYER; 5	Levitra	5 mg	Orange	Tablet	Circle	Schering
BAYER; 10	Levitra	10 mg	Orange	Tablet	Circle	Bayer Pharmaceutical
BAYER; 10	Levitra	10 mg	Orange	Tablet	Circle	Schering
BAYER; 20	Levitra	20 mg	Orange	Tablet	Circle	Bayer Pharmaceutical
BAYER; 20	Levitra	20 mg	Orange	Tablet	Circle	Schering
BAYER; 325	Bayer Regular Strength Enteric Coated	325 mg	Yellow	Tablet, Extended Release	Capsule-Shape	Bayer Consumer Care
BAYER; 500	Bayer Enteric 500	500 mg	Yellow	Delayed-Release Tablet		Bayer Consumer Care
BAYER; C1000; QD	Cipro Xr	1000 mg	White to Light Yellow	Extended-Release Tablet	Oblong	Bayer Pharmaceutical
BAYER; LG ;	Biltricide	600 mg	White to Orange Tinged	Coated Tablet	Oblong, Triscored	Bayer Pharmaceutical
BAYER; M400	Avelox	400 mg	Red	Tablet	Oblong	Bayer
BAYER; M400	Avelox	400 mg	Red	Tablet	Oblong	Schering-Plough
BAYER; PM	Extra Strength Bayer Pm	500 mg; 25 mg	Light Blue	Tablet	Capsule-Shape	Bayer Consumer Care
BB	Bufferin Tri-Buffered	325 mg		Tablet		Bristol-Myers Squibb
BCI	Hectorol	0.5 mcg	Citrus Orange	Capsule, Liquid Filled	Oval	Genzyme
BCI	Hectorol	2.5 mcg	Sunshine Yellow	Capsule, Liquid Filled	Oval	Genzyme
BEECHAM; 185	Beepen - VK	250 mg	White	Tablet	Oval	Glaxosmithkline
BEECHAM; 186	Beepen - VK	500 mg	White	Tablet	Oval	Glaxosmithkline
BENADRYL; 12.5	Benadryl Allergy Chewable Tablet	12.5 mg	Purple	Tablet, Chewable	Circle, Scored	Pfizer Consumer Health Care

IMPRINT	BRAND/GENERIC NAME	STRENGTH	COLOR	FORM	SHAPE	MANUFACTURER
BENADRYL; ALLERGY SINUS HEADACHE	Benadryl Allergy Sinus Headache	500 mg; 12.5 mg; 30 mg	Light Green	Tablet	Oblong	Pfizer Consumer Health Care
BENADRYL; D	Benadryl Allergy Sinus	25 mg; 60 mg	Blue	Tablet	Capsule-Shape	Pfizer Consumer Health Care
BENTYL; 10 ;	Bentyl	10 mg	Blue	Capsule		Aventis Pharmaceuticals
BENTYL; 20 ;	Bentyl	20 mg	Blue	Tablet	Circle	Aventis Pharmaceuticals
BERLEX	Elixophyllin SR	250 mg	Clear	Extended-Release Capsule		Forest Pharmaceuticals
BERLEX; 100	Elixophyllin	100 mg	White	Capsule		Forest Pharmaceuticals
BERLEX; 120 MG	Betapace Af	120 mg	White	Tablet	Capsule-Shape, Scored	Berlex Laboratories
BERLEX; 129	Elixophyllin SR	125 mg	White	Extended-Release Capsule		Forest Pharmaceuticals
BERLEX; 131	Aminodur Dura-Tabs	300 mg	White to Off-White	Tablet		Berlex Laboratories
BERLEX; 160 MG	Betapace Af	160 mg	White	Tablet	Capsule-Shape, Scored	Berlex Laboratories
BERLEX; 162	Bilivist	500 mg	Yellow-Tan	Capsule, Liquid Filled		Berlex Laboratories
BERLEX; 200	Elixophyllin	200 mg	White	Capsule		Forest Pharmaceuticals
BEROCCA; PLUS; ROCHE	Berocca Plus	5000 IU; 30 IU; 100 mg; 0.15 mg; 25 mg; 0.8 mg; 27 mg; 0.1 mg; 50 mg; 5 mg; 3 mg; 22.5 mg; 500 mg; 20; 20 mg; 25 mg; 50 mg	Yellow-Gold	Tablet	Oblong	Roche Pharmaceuticals
BEROCCA; ROCHE	Berocca	100 mg; 18 mg; 0.5 mg; 500 mg; 15 mg; 15 mg; 4 mg; 5 mcg	Light Green	Tablet	Capsule-Shape	Roche Pharmaceuticals
BERTEK; 560	Phenytoin	100 mg		Capsule		Mylan Bertek Pharmaceuticals
BERTEK; 670	Phenytek	200 mg	Dark Blue Cap, Blue Body	Extended-Release Capsule		Mylan Bertek Pharmaceuticals
BERTEK; 750	Phenytek	300 mg	Blue Cap and Body	Extended-Release Capsule		Mylan Bertek Pharmaceuticals
BETAPACE; 80 MG	Betapace	80 mg	Light Blue	Tablet	Capsule-Shape, Scored	Berlex Laboratories
BETAPACE; 120 MG	Betapace	120 mg	Light Blue	Tablet	Capsule-Shape, Scored	Berlex Laboratories
BETAPACE; 160 MG	Betapace	160 mg	Light Blue	Tablet	Capsule-Shape, Scored	Berlex Laboratories
BETAPACE; 240 MG	Betapace	240 mg	Light Blue	Tablet	Capsule-Shape, Scored	Berlex Laboratories
BI ; 83	Mirapex	0.125 mg	White	Tablet	Circle	Boehringer Ingelheim Pharmaceuticals
BI BI ; 84 84	Mirapex	0.25 mg	White	Tablet	Oval	Boehringer Ingelheim Pharmaceuticals
BI BI ; 85 85	Mirapex	0.5 mg	White	Tablet	Oval	Boehringer Ingelheim Pharmaceuticals
BI BI ; 90 90	Mirapex	1 mg	White	Tablet	Circle	Boehringer Ingelheim Pharmaceuticals
BI BI ; 91 91	Mirapex	1.5 mg	White	Tablet	Circle	Boehringer Ingelheim Pharmaceuticals
BI; 6	Catapres	0.1 mg	Tan	Tablet	Oval, Scored	Boehringer Ingelheim Pharmaceuticals
BI; 7	Catapres	0.2 mg	Orange	Tablet	Oval, Scored	Boehringer Ingelheim Pharmaceuticals
BI; 8	Combipres	0.1 mg; 15 mg	Pink	Tablet	Oval, Scored	Boehringer Ingelheim Pharmaceuticals
BI; 9	Combipres	0.2 mg; 15 mg	Blue	Tablet	Oval, Scored	Boehringer Ingelheim Pharmaceuticals
BI; 10	Combipres	0.3 mg; 15 mg	White	Tablet	Oval, Scored	Boehringer Ingelheim Pharmaceuticals
BI; 11	Catapres	0.3 mg	Orange	Tablet	Oval, Scored	Boehringer Ingelheim Pharmaceuticals
BI; 12	Dulcolax	5 mg	Tan	Enteric-Coated Tablet	Circle	Boehringer Ingelheim Pharmaceuticals
BI; 12	Dulcolax Bowel Prep Kit Tablet	5 mg	Tan	Enteric-Coated Tablet	Circle	Novartis Consumer
BI; 17	Persantine	25 mg	Orange	Coated Tablet	Circle	Boehringer Ingelheim Pharmaceuticals
BI; 18	Persantine	50 mg	Orange	Tablet	Circle	Boehringer Ingelheim Pharmaceuticals
BI; 19	Persantine	75 mg	Orange	Coated Tablet	Circle	Boehringer Ingelheim Pharmaceuticals
BI; 20	Serentil	10 mg	Red	Coated Tablet		Boehringer Ingelheim Pharmaceuticals
BI; 28	Torecan	10 mg	Yellow	Tablet	Circle	Boehringer Ingelheim Pharmaceuticals
BI; 48	Respbid	250 mg	White	Extended-Release Tablet		Boehringer Ingelheim Pharmaceuticals
BI; 49	Respbid	500 mg	White	Extended-Release Tablet		Boehringer Ingelheim Pharmaceuticals
BI; 49	Respid	500 mg	White	Tablet	Capsule-Shape	3M Pharmaceuticals
BI; 62	Preludin	75 mg	Pink	Tablet		Boehringer Ingelheim Pharmaceuticals
BI; 64	Prelu-2	105 mg	Light and Dark Green	Extended-Release Capsule		Boehringer Ingelheim Pharmaceuticals
BI; 66	Mexitil	150 mg	Red and Tan	Capsule		Boehringer Ingelheim Pharmaceuticals
BI; 67	Mexitil	200 mg	Red	Capsule		Boehringer Ingelheim Pharmaceuticals
BI; 68	Mexitil	250 mg	Red and Aqua Green	Capsule		Boehringer Ingelheim Pharmaceuticals
BI; 79	Preludin	50 mg	White	Tablet	Circle	Boehringer Ingelheim Pharmaceuticals

IMPRINT	BRAND/GENERIC NAME	STRENGTH	COLOR	FORM	SHAPE	MANUFACTURER
BI; 100	Serentil	100 mg	Red	Coated Tablet		Boehringer Ingelheim Pharmaceuticals
BIOCAL	Biocal Calcium Supplement	625 mg	White	Tablet, Chewable		Bayer Consumer Care
BIOCAL	Biocal Calcium Supplement	1250 mg	White	Tablet		Bayer Consumer Care
BIOCRAFT; 16	Penicillin VK	250 mg	White	Tablet	Oval	Teva Pharmaceuticals
BIOCRAFT; 32	Sulfamethoxazole and Trimethoprim Single Strength	400 mg; 80 mg	White	Tablet	Circle, Scored	Teva Pharmaceuticals
BIOCRAFT; 33	Smz-Tmp DS	800 mg; 160 mg	White	Tablet	Oval, Scored	Teva Pharmaceuticals
BIOCRAFT; 34	Trimethoprim	100 mg	White	Tablet	Circle	Teva Pharmaceuticals
BIOCRAFT; 49	Penicillin-VK	500 mg	White	Tablet	Oval, Scored	Teva Pharmaceuticals
BIOCRAFT; 94	Cyclacillin	250 mg	White	Tablet	Capsule-Shape	Teva Pharmaceuticals
BIOCRAFT; 95	Cyclacillin	500 mg	White	Tablet	Capsule-Shape	Teva Pharmaceuticals
BIOCRAFT; 105 105	Sucralfate	1 G	White	Tablet	Capsule-Shape, Scored	Teva Pharmaceuticals
BIOCRAFT; 148	Clindamycin Hydrochloride	75 mg	Red	Capsule		Teva Pharmaceuticals
BIOCRAFT; 163	Cinoxacin	250 mg	Blue and Yellow	Capsule		Teva Pharmaceuticals
BIOCRAFT; 164	Cinoxacin	500 mg	Blue and Yellow	Capsule		Teva Pharmaceuticals
BIOCRAFT; 177	Potassium Chloride	600 mg	Opaque Blue and White	Extended-Release Capsule		Teva Pharmaceuticals
BIOCRAFT; 178	Potassium Chloride	750 mg	Opaque Blue	Extended-Release Capsule		Teva Pharmaceuticals
BIOCRAFT; 185	Ketoprofen	25 mg	White	Capsule		Teva Pharmaceuticals
BIOCRAFT; 223	Cefaclor	250 mg	Opaque White and Gray	Capsule		Teva Pharmaceuticals
BIOCRAFT; 224	Cefaclor	500 mg	Opaque Red and White	Capsule		Teva Pharmaceuticals
BJ; 675 ;	Oreton Propionate	10 mg	Pink	Tablet		Schering
BL 01	Ocuvite Preservision	Less Than 15%; Less Than 0.1%; Less Than 20%; Less Than 35%; Less Than 1%; Less Than 10%; Less Than 1%; Less Than 25%; Less Than 10%; Less Than 5%; Less Than 1%; Less Than 10%; Greater Than 89%	Orange	Tablet	Oval	Bausch & Lomb
BL; 07	Penicillin G Potassium	200,000 units	White	Tablet	Circle	Teva Pharmaceuticals
BL; 09	Penicillin G Potassium	250,000 units	White	Tablet	Circle	Teva Pharmaceuticals
BL; 10	Penicillin G Potassium	400,000 units	White	Tablet	Circle	Teva Pharmaceuticals
BL; 15	Penicillin-VK	250 mg	White	Tablet	Circle, Scored	Teva Pharmaceuticals
BL; 17	Penicillin-VK	500 mg	White	Tablet	Circle, Scored	Novartis Generics
BL; 17	Penicillin-VK	500 mg	White	Tablet	Circle, Scored	Teva Pharmaceuticals
BL; 19	Imipramine Hydrochloride	10 mg	Yellow	Tablet	Circle	Teva Pharmaceuticals
BL; 20	Imipramine Hydrochloride	25 mg	Salmon	Tablet	Circle	Teva Pharmaceuticals
BL; 21	Imipramine Hydrochloride	50 mg	Green	Tablet	Circle	Teva Pharmaceuticals
BL; 22	Amitriptyline Hydrochloride	10 mg	Pink	Tablet	Circle	Teva Pharmaceuticals
BL; 23	Amitriptyline Hydrochloride	25 mg	Light Green	Tablet	Circle	Teva Pharmaceuticals
BL; 24	Amitriptyline Hydrochloride	50 mg	Brown	Tablet	Circle	Teva Pharmaceuticals
BL; 25	Amitriptyline Hydrochloride	75 mg	Lavender	Tablet	Circle	Teva Pharmaceuticals
BL; 26	Amitriptyline Hydrochloride	100 mg	Orange	Tablet	Circle	Teva Pharmaceuticals
BL; 32	Smz-Tmp	400 mg; 80 mg	White	Tablet	Circle	Teva Pharmaceuticals
BL; 35	Trimethoprim	200 mg	White	Tablet	Circle	Teva Pharmaceuticals
BL; 42	Thioridazine Hydrochloride	10 mg	Green	Tablet	Oval	Teva Pharmaceuticals
BL; 46	Thioridazine Hydrochloride	100 mg	Light-Green	Tablet	Oval	Teva Pharmaceuticals
BL; 52	Amiloride Hydrochloride and Hydrochlorothiazide	5 mg; 50 mg	Yellow	Tablet	Circle, Scored	Teva Pharmaceuticals
BL; 52	Amiloride Hydrochloride and Hydrochlorothiazide	5 mg; 50 mg	Yellow	Tablet	Circle, Scored	Warner Chilcott
BL; 82 ;	Saluron	50 mg	White	Tablet	Circle, Scored	Bristol-Myers Squibb
BL; 92	Metoclopramide	5 mg	White	Tablet	Circle	Teva Pharmaceuticals
BL; 93	Metoclopramide	10 mg	White	Tablet	Circle, Scored	Duramed Pharmaceuticals
BL; 93	Metoclopramide	10 mg	White	Tablet	Circle, Scored	Teva Pharmaceuticals
BL; 130	Albuterol Sulfate	2 mg	White	Tablet	Circle	Teva Pharmaceuticals
BL; 131	Albuterol	4 mg	White	Tablet	Round, Bisected Scored	Teva Pharmaceuticals
BL; 132	Metaproterenol	10 mg	White	Tablet	Circle, Scored	Teva Pharmaceuticals
BL; 133	Metaproterenol	20 mg	White	Tablet	Circle	Teva Pharmaceuticals
BL; 141	Baclofen	10 mg	White	Tablet	Circle, Scored	Teva Pharmaceuticals
BL; 142	Baclofen	20 mg	White	Tablet	Circle, Scored	Teva Pharmaceuticals
BL; 207 ;	Corgard	40 mg	Blue	Tablet	Circle, Scored	Bristol Laboratories
BL; 208 ;	Corgard	120 mg	Blue	Tablet	Oblong, Scored	Bristol-Myers Squibb
BL; 221	Amoxicillin	125 mg	White to Off-White	Tablet, Chewable	Capsule-Shape	Teva Pharmaceuticals
BL; 222	Amoxicillin	250 mg	White	Tablet, Chewable	Capsule-Shape	Teva Pharmaceuticals
BL; 232 ;	Corgard	20 mg	Blue	Tablet	Circle, Scored	Bristol-Myers Squibb
BL; 241 ;	Corgard	80 mg	Blue	Tablet	Circle, Scored	Bristol-Myers Squibb
BL; C1	Ultracef	1 GM	White or Yellow	Tablet	Capsule-Shape	Bristol-Myers Squibb
BL; E1 ;	Bristamycin	250 mg	Orange	Tablet	Circle	Bristol-Myers Squibb
BL; L1	Lysodren	500 mg	White	Tablet	Circle, Scored	Bristol-Myers Squibb
BL; N2	Naldagesic	325 mg; 15 mg	Blue	Tablet	Capsule-Shape	Bristol-Myers Squibb
BL; V1 ;	Betapen-VK	250 mg	White	Coated Tablet		Bristol-Myers Squibb
BMP; 108	Cotrol-D	60 mg; 4 mg	Green	Tablet		Glaxosmithkline
BMP; 109	Dasikon	2 mg; 32 mg; 195 mg; 130 mg; 0.065 mg	Natural and Blue	Capsule		Glaxosmithkline
BMP; 119	Hybephen	15 mg; 0.1277 mg; 0.0233 mg; 0.0094 mg	Green	Tablet		Glaxosmithkline

IMPRINT	BRAND/GENERIC NAME	STRENGTH	COLOR	FORM	SHAPE	MANUFACTURER
BMP; 121	Livitamin	100 mg; 3 mg; 3 mg; 10 mg; 100 mg; 3 mg; 5 mcg; 0.66 mg; 2 mg; 150 mg	Pink	Capsule		Glaxosmithkline
BMP; 122	Livitamin-If	3 mg; 10 mg; 100 mg; 3 mg; 5 mcg; 0.66 mg; 2 mg; 150 mg; 0.33 NI U; 100 mg; 3 mg	Green	Capsule		Glaxosmithkline
BMP; 123	Livitamin	100 mg; 2 mg; 0.33 mg; 50 mg; 3 mg; 3 mg; 3 mg; 10 mg; 5 mcg	Orange	Tablet, Chewable		Glaxosmithkline
BMP; 124	Livitamin Prenatal	6000 U.S.P. units; 400 U.S.P. units; 100 mg; 20 mg; 10 mg; 5 mg; 3 Mgg; 3 mg; 0.5 mg; 5 mcg; 350 mg; 50 mg	Yellow	Tablet		Glaxosmithkline
BMP; 135	Semets	3 mg	Red	Troche		Glaxosmithkline
BMP; 139	Thalfed	8 mg; 0.12 G; 25 mg	White	Tablet		Glaxosmithkline
BMP; 140	Totacillin	250 mg	Brown and Orange	Capsule		Glaxosmithkline
BMP; 141	Totacillin	500 mg	Brown and Orange	Capsule		Glaxosmithkline
BMP; 143	Bactocill	250 mg	Brown and Yellow	Capsule		Glaxosmithkline
BMP; 144	Bactocill	500 mg	Brown and Yellow	Capsule		Glaxosmithkline
BMP; 145	Daricon	10 mg	White	Tablet	Circle, Grooved	Glaxosmithkline
BMP; 146	Daricon PB	5 mg; 15 mg	Pink	Tablet		Glaxosmithkline
BMP; 150	Obedrin-LA	10 mg		Tablet		Glaxosmithkline
BMP; 165	Dycill	250 mg	Light Blue and Creme	Capsule		Glaxosmithkline
BMP; 166	Dycill	500 mg	Light Blue and Creme	Capsule		Glaxosmithkline
BMP; 167	Actol Expectorant Tablet	30 mg; 200 mg	Red	Coated Tablet		Glaxosmithkline
BMP; 169	Cloxapen	250 mg	Lime and Beige	Capsule		Glaxosmithkline
BMP; 170	Cloxapen	500 mg	Lime and Beige	Capsule		Glaxosmithkline
BMP; 189	Augmentin	125 mg; 31.25 mg	Mottled Yellow	Tablet, Chewable	Circle	Glaxosmithkline
BMP; 190	Augmentin	250 mg; 62.5 mg	Mottled Yellow	Tablet, Chewable	Circle	Glaxosmithkline
BMP; 192	Maxolon	10 mg	Blue	Tablet	Circle, Scored	Glaxosmithkline
BMP; 194	Enarax White	5 mg; 25 mg	White	Tablet		Glaxosmithkline
BMP; 195	Enarax Black and White	10 mg; 25 mg	Black and White	Tablet		Glaxosmithkline
BMP; 211	Larotid	250 mg	Caramel and Buff	Capsule		Glaxosmithkline
BMS ; 524	Sprycel	70 mg	White to Off-White	Tablet	Circle	Bristol-Myers Squibb
BMS ; 527	Sprycel	20 mg	White to Off-White	Tablet	Circle	Bristol-Myers Squibb
BMS ; 528	Sprycel	50 mg	White to Off-White	Tablet	Oval	Bristol-Myers Squibb
BMS ; 1611	Baraclude	0.5 mg	White to Off White	Tablet	Triangle	Bristol-Myers Squibb
BMS ; 1612	Baraclude	1 mg	Pink	Tablet	Triangle	Bristol-Myers Squibb
BMS 1964; 15	Zerit	15 mg	Light Yellow and Dark Red	Capsule		Bristol-Myers Squibb
BMS 1965; 20	Zerit	20 mg	Light Brown	Capsule		Bristol-Myers Squibb
BMS 1966; 30	Zerit	30 mg	Light Orange and Dark Orange	Capsule		Bristol-Myers Squibb
BMS 1967; 40	Zerit	40 mg	Dark Orange	Capsule		Bristol-Myers Squibb
BMS; 37.5 MG; 1555	Zerit Xr	37.5 mg	Red and Yellow	Extended-Release Capsule		Bristol-Myers Squibb
BMS; 50 MG; 1656	Zerit Xr	50 mg	Orange	Extended-Release Capsule		Bristol-Myers Squibb
BMS; 50; 31	Serzone	50 mg	Light Pink	Tablet	Six-Sided	Bristol-Myers Squibb
BMS; 75 MG; 1557	Zerit Xr	75 mg	Red	Extended-Release Capsule		Bristol-Myers Squibb
BMS; 80	Pravachol	80 mg	Yellow	Tablet	Oval	Bristol-Myers Squibb
BMS; 80 ;	Pravigard Pac	325 mg; 80 mg	Yellow Oval Tablet and White Tablet	Tablet		Bristol-Myers Squibb
BMS; 80 ;	Pravigard Pac	81 mg; 80 mg	Yellow Oval Tablet and White Tablet	Tablet		Bristol-Myers Squibb
BMS; 100 MG; 1558	Zerit Xr	100 mg	Yellow	Extended-Release Capsule		Bristol-Myers Squibb
BMS; 100 MG; 3623	Reyataz	100 mg	Blue and White	Capsule		Bristol-Myers Squibb
BMS; 100; 32	Serzone	100 mg	White	Tablet	Hexagonal, Bisected, Scored Scored	Bristol-Myers Squibb
BMS; 125 MG; 6671	Videx Ec	125 mg	White with Tan Ink	Capsule, Delayed Release		Bristol-Myers Squibb
BMS; 150; 39	Serzone	150 mg	Peach	Tablet	Six-Sided, Bisect Scored	Bristol-Myers Squibb
BMS; 200 MG; 3631	Reyataz	200 mg	Blue	Capsule		Bristol-Myers Squibb
BMS; 200 MG; 6672	Videx Ec	200 mg	White with Green Ink	Capsule, Delayed Release		Bristol-Myers Squibb
BMS; 200; 33	Serzone	200 mg	Light Yellow	Tablet	Six-Sided	Bristol-Myers Squibb
BMS; 250 MG; 6673	Videx Ec	250 mg	White with Blue Ink	Capsule, Delayed Release		Bristol-Myers Squibb
BMS; 250; 41	Serzone	250 mg	White	Tablet	Six-Sided	Bristol-Myers Squibb
BMS; 400 MG; 6674	Videx Ec	400 mg	White with Red Ink	Capsule, Delayed Release		Bristol-Myers Squibb
BMS; 6060; 500	Glucophage	500 mg	White	Coated Tablet		Bristol-Myers Squibb
BMS; 6063; 500	Glucophage Xr	500 mg	White	Extended-Release Tablet	Capsule-Shape, Biconvex	Bristol-Myers Squibb
BMS; 6070; 850	Glucophage	850 mg	White	Coated Tablet		Bristol-Myers Squibb
BMS; 6071; 1000	Glucophage	1000 mg	White	Tablet	Oblong, Scored	Bristol-Myers Squibb
BMS; 6072	Glucovance	1.25 mg; 250 mg	Pale Yellow	Coated Tablet	Capsule-Shape, Bevel-Edged, Biconvex	Bristol-Myers Squibb
BMS; 6073	Glucovance	2.5 mg; 500 mg	Pale Orange	Coated Tablet	Capsule-Shape, Bevel-Edged, Biconvex	Bristol-Myers Squibb
BMS; 6074	Glucovance	5 mg; 500 mg	Yellow	Coated Tablet	Capsule-Shape, Bevel-Edged, Biconvex	Bristol-Myers Squibb
BMS; 6077	Metaglip	2.5 mg; 500 mg	White	Tablet	Oval	Bristol-Myers Squibb

IMPRINT	BRAND/GENERIC NAME	STRENGTH	COLOR	FORM	SHAPE	MANUFACTURER
BMS; 6078	Metaglip	5 mg; 500 mg	Pink	Tablet	Oval	Bristol-Myers Squibb
BMS; 6081	Metaglip	2.5 mg; 250 mg	Pink	Tablet	Oval	Bristol-Myers Squibb
BMS; MONOPRIL; 10 ;	Monopril	10 mg	White to Off-White	Tablet	Diamond, Biconvex Flat-End, Compressed, Partially Scored	Bristol-Myers Squibb
BMS; MONOPRIL; 20 ;	Monopril	20 mg	White to Off-White	Tablet	Oval, Compressed	Bristol-Myers Squibb
BMS; MONOPRIL; 40 ;	Monopril	40 mg	White to Off-White	Tablet	Six-Sided, Biconvex Hexagonal Shaped, Compressed	Bristol-Myers Squibb
BMS; TEQUIN; 200	Tequin	200 mg	White	Coated Tablet	Oval, Biconvex	Bristol-Myers Squibb
BMS; TEQUIN; 400	Tequin	400 mg	White	Coated Tablet	Oval, Biconvex	Bristol-Myers Squibb
BNVA ; 150	Boniva	150 mg	White	Tablet	Oblong	Glaxosmithkline
BNVA ; 150	Boniva	150 mg	White	Tablet	Oblong	Roche Laboratories
BOCK; 460	Zephrex	400 mg; 60 mg	White	Coated Tablet	Oval; Bisected Scored	Sanofi Pharmaceuticals
BOCK; HS 33	Hemaspan	110 mg; 20 mg; 200 mg	Tan	Tablet	Oblong	Sanofi Pharmaceuticals
BOCK; P; N	Prenate Ultra Prenatal Vitamins	90 mg; 1 mg; 2700 I.U.; 30 I.U.; 400 IU	White	Tablet	Oval, Scored	Sanofi Pharmaceuticals
BOEHRINGER INGELHEIM LOGO; 01A	Aggrenox	200 mg; 25 mg	Red and Ivory with Yellow Pellets	Capsule		Boehringer Ingelheim Pharmaceuticals
BOEHRINGER MANNHEIM LOGO; 102; 5	Demadex	5 mg	White	Tablet	Oval, Scored	Roche Laboratories
BOEHRINGER MANNHEIM LOGO; 103; 10	Demadex	10 mg	White	Tablet	Oval, Scored	Boehringer Mannheim
BOEHRINGER MANNHEIM LOGO; 103; 10	Demadex	10 mg	White	Tablet	Oval, Scored	Roche Laboratories
BOEHRINGER MANNHEIM LOGO; 104; 20	Demadex	20 mg	White	Tablet	Oval, Scored	Boehringer Mannheim
BOEHRINGER MANNHEIM LOGO; 104; 20	Demadex	20 mg	White	Tablet	Oval, Scored	Roche Laboratories
BOEHRINGER MANNHEIM LOGO; 105; 100	Demadex	100 mg	White	Tablet	Capsule-Shape, Scored	Boehringer Mannheim
BOEHRINGER MANNHEIM LOGO; 105; 100	Demadex	100 mg	White	Tablet	Capsule-Shape, Scored	Roche Laboratories
BREON; 100	Bronkodyl	100 mg	Brown and White	Capsule		Sanofi Winthrop Pharmaceuticals
BREON; 200	Bronkodyl	200 mg	Green and White	Capsule		Sanofi Winthrop Pharmaceuticals
BREON; SR300	Bronkodyl SR	300 mg	Blue and White	Sustained-Release Capsule		Sanofi Winthrop Pharmaceuticals
BRICANYL; 2 1/2 ;	Bricanyl	2.5 mg	White	Tablet	Circle	Aventis Pharmaceuticals
BRICANYL; 5 ;	Bricanyl	5 mg	White	Tablet	Square, Scored	Aventis Pharmaceuticals
BRISTOL	Bristacycline	250 mg	Green and Yellow	Capsule		Bristol-Myers Squibb
BRISTOL	Tetrex	100 mg	Yellow and Orange	Capsule		Bristol-Myers Squibb
BRISTOL	Tetrex-F	250 mg; 250000 U		Capsule		Bristol-Myers Squibb
BRISTOL; 500	Bristacycline	500 mg	Green and Yellow	Capsule		Bristol-Myers Squibb
BRISTOL; 518 ;	Quibron Plus	150 mg; 100 mg; 25 mg; 20 mg		Capsule		Bristol-Myers Squibb
BRISTOL; 732	Enkaid	25 mg	Green and Yellow	Capsule		Bristol-Myers Squibb
BRISTOL; 734	Enkaid	35 mg	Green and Orange	Capsule		Bristol-Myers Squibb
BRISTOL; 735	Enkaid	50 mg	Green and Brown	Capsule		Bristol-Myers Squibb
BRISTOL; 3091	Vepesid	50 mg	Pink	Capsule, Liquid Filled		Bristol-Myers Squibb
BRISTOL; 7271	Cefadroxil	500 mg	Blue and Black	Capsule		Sandoz
BRISTOL; 7278	Trimox	250	Maroon and Pink	Capsule		Bristol-Myers Squibb
BRISTOL; 7279	Trimox	500 mg	Maroon and Pink	Capsule		Bristol-Myers Squibb
BRISTOL-MYERS; COMTREX	Comtrex Multi-Symptom Cold Reliever	500 mg; 30 mg; 2 mg; 15 mg	Orange and Yellow	Capsule, Liquid Filled		Bristol-Myers Squibb
BRISTOL-MYERS; DATRIL; 500MG	Datril Extra Strength	500 mg	Green and White	Capsule		Bristol-Myers Squibb
BRONKAID	Bronkaid Dual Action Formula	25 mg; 400 mg	White	Tablet		Bayer Consumer Care
BVF; 0117	Pentoxifylline	400 mg		Extended-Release Tablet	Oblong, Compressed	Teva Pharmaceuticals
BVF; 120	Diltiazem Hydrochloride	120 mg	Clear Light Green	Extended-Release Capsule		Teva Pharmaceuticals
BVF; 180	Diltiazem Hydrochloride	180 mg	Dark Green and Light Green	Extended-Release Capsule		Teva Pharmaceuticals
BVF; 240	Diltiazem Hydrochloride	240 mg	Clear Dark Green	Extended-Release Capsule		Teva Pharmaceuticals
BVF; 300	Diltiazem Hydrochloride	300 mg	Ivory and Dark Green	Extended-Release Capsule		Teva Pharmaceuticals
C	Comtrex Maximum Strength	500 mg; 2 mg; 30 mg; 15 mg	Yellow	Tablet		Bristol-Myers Squibb
C	Comtrex Maximum Strength Day/night - Capsule & Liquid	500 mg; 15 mg; 30 mg	Orange	Tablet		Bristol-Myers Squibb
C	Comtrex Maximum Strength Day/night - Tablet & Capsule	500 mg; 15 mg; 30 mg	Blue	Tablet	Circle	Bristol-Myers Squibb
C	Comtrex Maximum Strength Day/night - Tablet & Capsule	500 mg; 2 mg; 30 mg; 15 mg	Orange	Tablet	Capsule-Shape	Bristol-Myers Squibb
C	Comtrex Maximum Strength Non-Drowsy	500 mg; 15 mg; 30 mg	Orange	Tablet	Capsule-Shape	Bristol-Myers Squibb
C	Comtrex Multi-Symptom Cold Reliever	30 mg; 2 mg; 10 mg; 325 mg	Yellow	Tablet		Bristol-Myers Squibb

IMPRINT	BRAND/GENERIC NAME	STRENGTH	COLOR	FORM	SHAPE	MANUFACTURER
C	Congespirin Children	1.25 mg; 81 mg	Orange	Tablet, Chewable		Bristol-Myers Squibb
C	Myfortic	180 mg;	Lime Green	Enteric-Coated Tablet	Circle	Novartis
C	Prempro White Tablet	2.5 mg	White	Tablet	Oval, Scored	Wyeth-Ayerst Laboratories
C 402	Gabitril	2 mg	Orange-Peach	Tablet	Circle	Cephalon
C 404	Gabitril	4 mg	Yellow	Tablet	Circle	Cephalon
C 412	Gabitril	12 mg	Green	Tablet	Oval	Cephalon
C 416	Gabitril	16 mg	Blue	Tablet	Oval	Cephalon
C C	Robitussin Cold Cold & Congestion	200 mg; 30 mg; 10 mg	Red	Tablet	Film-Coated	Wyeth Consumer Healthcare
C F	Robitussin Cold Multi-Symptom Cold & Flu	325 mg; 200 mg; 30 mg; 10 mg	Yellow	Tablet	Film-Coated	Wyeth Consumer Healthcare
C S	Robitussin Cold Sinus & Congestion	325 mg; 200 mg; 30 mg	Light Blue	Tablet		Wyeth Consumer Healthcare
C; 5	Cialis	5 mg	Yellow	Tablet	Teardrop-Shape	Eli Lilly
C; 10	Cialis	10 mg	Yellow	Tablet	Teardrop-Shape	Eli Lilly
C; 20	Cialis	20 mg	Yellow	Tablet	Teardrop-Shape	Eli Lilly
C; 83; LL	Centrum Singles	500 mg	White	Coated Tablet	Oval, Convex	Wyeth Consumer Healthcare
C; 119	Famotidine	20 mg	Pale Yellow	Tablet	Circle	Par Pharmaceutical
C; 120	Famotidine	40 mg	Yellow	Tablet	Circle	Par Pharmaceutical
C; 3227	Nifedipine	10 mg	Tan	Capsule		Warner Chilcott
C; 3453	Nifedipine	20 mg	White	Capsule	Oval	Warner Chilcott
C; C+C	Coricidin Hbp Cough & Cold	4 mg; 30 mg	Red	Tablet	Circle	Schering-Plough Healthcare Products
C; CLOCK DESIGN	Quinaglute Dura-Tabs	324 mg	White	Extended-Release Tablet	Circle	Berlex Laboratories
C; DAY	Contac Day & Night Cold & Flu	650 mg; 30 mg; 60 mg	Yellow	Tablet		Glaxosmithkline
C2C	Lanoxicaps	0.2 mg	Green	Capsule, Liquid Filled	Oblong	Glaxosmithkline
C5	Clarinex	5 mg	Light Blue	Tablet	Circle	Schering-Plough
CALAN; 40	Calan	40 mg	Pink	Coated Tablet	Circle	Searle
CALAN; 80	Calan	80 mg	Peach	Coated Tablet	Oval, Scored	Searle
CALAN; 120	Calan	120 mg	Brown	Coated Tablet	Oval, Scored	Searle
CALAN; SR; 120	Calan SR	120 mg	Light Violet	Sustained-Release Tablet	Oval	Searle
CALAN; SR; 180	Calan SR	180 mg	Light Pink	Sustained-Release Tablet	Oval, Scored	Searle
CALAN; SR; 240	Calan SR	240 mg	Light Green	Tablet, Extended Release	Capsule-Shape	Searle
CALTRATE	Caltrate 600 Plus D	200 IU; 600 mg	Light Pink	Tablet	Oval	Wyeth Consumer Healthcare
CALTRATE; M; 600	Caltrate Plus Calcium	600 mg; 200 IU; 40 mg; 7.5 mg; 1 mg; 1.8 mg;	Dusty Rose	Coated Tablet	Oval, Scored	Wyeth Consumer Healthcare
CAMA 500; DORSEY	Cama Arthritis Pain Reliever	150 mg; 500 mg; 150 mg	White with Salmon Inlay	Tablet	Oblong	Novartis Consumer
CAMA 500; DORSEY	Cama Arthritis Pain Reliever	150 mg; 500 mg; 150 mg	White with Salmon Inlay	Tablet	Oblong	Sandoz Consumer Pharmaceuticals
CAPOTEN; 12.5 MG ;	Capoten	12.5 mg	White	Tablet	Oval, Biconvex, Partially Bisected Scored	Bristol-Myers Squibb
CAPOTEN; 25 MG ;	Capoten	25 mg	White	Tablet	Oval, Biconvex with a Quadrisect Bar Scored	Bristol-Myers Squibb
CAPOTEN; 50 MG ;	Capoten	50 mg	White	Tablet	Oval, Biconvex, Scored	Bristol-Myers Squibb
CAPOTEN; 100 MG ;	Capoten	100 mg	White	Tablet	Oval, Biconvex, Scored	Bristol-Myers Squibb
CAPOZIDE 25/15	Capozide 25/15	25 mg; 15 mg	White with Orange Mottling	Tablet	Square	Par Pharmaceutical
CAPOZIDE 25/25	Capozide 25/25	25 mg; 25 mg	Peach	Tablet	Square	Par Pharmaceutical
CAPOZIDE 50/15	Capozide 50/15	50 mg; 15 mg	White with Orange Mottling	Tablet	Oval	Par Pharmaceutical
CAPOZIDE 50/25	Capozide 50/25	50 mg; 25 mg	Peach	Tablet	Oval	Par Pharmaceutical
CARACO LOGO; 872	Nifedipine	10 mg	Yellow	Capsule, Liquid Filled		Geneva Generics
CARACO LOGO; 873	Nifedipine	20 mg	Orange and Brown	Capsule, Liquid Filled		Geneva Generics
CARAFATE; 1712 ;	Carafate	1 G	Light Pink	Tablet	Capsule-Shape, Scored, Embossed	Aventis Pharmaceuticals
CARBEX	Carbex	5 mg	White	Tablet	Oval	Endo Laboratories
CARDENE SR; 30 MG; SYNTEX; 2440	Cardene SR	30 mg	Pink	Sustained-Release Capsule		Roche Laboratories
CARDENE SR; 45 MG; SYNTEX; 2441	Cardene SR	45 mg	Powder Blue	Sustained-Release Capsule		Roche Laboratories
CARDENE SR; 60 MG; SYNTEX; 2442	Cardene SR	60 mg	Light Blue and White	Sustained-Release Capsule		Roche Laboratories
CARDENE; 20 MG; ROCHE	Cardene	20 mg	White with Blue Band	Capsule		Roche Laboratories
CARDENE; 30 MG; ROCHE	Cardene	30 mg	Light Blue with Blue Band	Capsule		Roche Laboratories
CARDILATE; X7A	Cardilate	10 mg	White	Tablet	Square	Glaxosmithkline
CARDIZEM CD; 120 MG	Cardizem Cd	120 mg	Light Turquoise	Extended-Release Capsule		Biovail Pharmaceuticals
CARDIZEM CD; 180 MG	Cardizem Cd	180 mg	Light Turquoise and Blue	Extended-Release Capsule		Biovail Pharmaceuticals
CARDIZEM CD; 240 MG	Cardizem Cd	240 mg	Blue	Extended-Release Capsule		Biovail Pharmaceuticals
CARDIZEM CD; 300 MG	Cardizem Cd	300 mg	Light Gray and Blue	Extended-Release Capsule		Biovail Pharmaceuticals
CARDIZEM CD; 360 MG	Cardizem Cd	360 mg	Light Blue and White	Extended-Release Capsule		Biovail Pharmaceuticals
CARDIZEM SR; 120 MG	Cardizem SR	120 mg	Caramel and Brown	Sustained-Release Capsule		Biovail Pharmaceuticals
CARDIZEM; 90 MG	Cardizem	90 mg	Green	Tablet	Oblong, Scored	Biovail Pharmaceuticals
CARDIZEM; 120 MG	Cardizem	120 mg	Yellow	Tablet	Oblong, Scored	Biovail Pharmaceuticals

IMPRINT	BRAND/GENERIC NAME	STRENGTH	COLOR	FORM	SHAPE	MANUFACTURER
CARDIZEM; SR; 60 MG	Cardizem SR	60 mg	Ivory and Brown	Sustained-Release Capsule		Biovail Pharmaceuticals
CARDIZEM; SR; 90 MG	Cardizem SR	90 mg	Gold and Brown	Sustained-Release Capsule		Biovail Pharmaceuticals
CARDURA; 1 MG	Cardura	1 mg	White	Tablet	Oblong, Scored	Pfizer Laboratories
CARDURA; 2 MG	Cardura	2 mg	Light Orange	Tablet	Oblong, Scored	Pfizer Laboratories
CARDURA; 4 MG	Cardura	4 mg	Orange	Tablet	Oblong, Scored	Pfizer Laboratories
CARDURA; 8 MG	Cardura	8 mg	Green	Tablet	Oblong, Scored	Pfizer Laboratories
CATAFLAM; 25	Cataflam	25 mg	Light Pink	Tablet	Circle, Biconvex	Novartis Pharmaceuticals
CB; 300	Cimetidine	300 mg	Light Yellow	Coated Tablet	Circle	Lederle Laboratories
CB; 400	Cimetidine	400 mg	Light Yellow	Coated Tablet	Oval	Lederle Laboratories
CB; 800	Cimetidine	800 mg	Light Yellow	Coated Tablet	Oval	Lederle Laboratories
CBP ; 01	Allerx - AM Dose	120 mg; 2.5 mg	Yellow	Tablet, Extended Release	Oblong	Adams Laboratories
CBP ; 02	Allerx - Pm Dose	8 mg; 2.5 mg	Blue	Tablet, Extended Release	Oblong	Adams Laboratories
CC	Cycrin	2.5 mg	White	Tablet	Oval, Scored	Esi Pharma
CC; 108	Hydrochlorothiazide	50 mg	Peach	Tablet	Circle	Novartis Generics
CC; 116	Hydrochlorothiazide	25 mg	Peach	Tablet	Circle	Novartis Generics
CC; CYCRIN	Cycrin	5 mg	Light Purple	Tablet	Oval, Scored	Esi Lederle
CC; CYCRIN	Cycrin	10 mg	Peach	Tablet	Oval, Scored	Esi Pharma
CD 129	Ranitidine Hydrochloride	150 mg	Opaque Light Brown	Capsule		Par Pharmaceutical
CD 130	Ranitidine Hydrochloride	300 mg	Opaque Light Brown	Capsule		Par Pharmaceutical
CDX50	Casodex	50 mg	White	Coated Tablet		Astra Zeneca
CEDAX; 400 MG	Cedax	400 mg	White	Capsule		Biovail Pharmaceuticals
CEG	Correctol Extra Gentle Stool Softener	100 mg	Red	Capsule, Liquid Filled	Oval	Schering-Plough Healthcare Products
CELLCEPT; 250; ROCHE	Cellcept	250 mg	Blue and Brown	Capsule, Liquid Filled		Roche
CELLCEPT; 500; ROCHE	Cellcept	500 mg	Lavender	Coated Tablet	Capsule-Shape	Roche Laboratories
CENTRAL; 40	Codimal-L.A.	8 mg; 120 mg	Clear and Red with Blue Beads	Extended-Release Capsule		Schwarz Pharma
CENTRAL; 130 MG	Theoclear LA	130 mg	Clear	Timed-Release Capsule		Schwarz Pharma
CENTRAL; 260 MG	Theoclear LA	260 mg	Clear	Timed-Release Capsule		Schwarz Pharma
CENTRUM ; LL	Centrum Silver with Lycopene	3500 IU; 60 mg; 400 IU; 45 IU; 10 mcg; 1.5 mg; 1.7 mg; 20 mg; 3 mg; 400 mcg; 25 mcg; 30 mcg; 10 mg; 200 mg; 48 mg; 150 mcg; 100 mg; 15 mg; 20 mcg; 2 mg; 2 mg; 150 mcg; 75 mcg; 72 mg; 80 mg; 150 mcg; 5 mcg; 2 mg; 10 mcg; 250 mcg; 300 mcg	Peach	Tablet	Oval	Novartis Consumer Health
CENTRUM; C;1	Centrum Advanced Formula	18 mg; 5000 IU; 30 IU; 400 mcg; 20 mg; 400 IU; 30 mcg; 10 mg; 162 mg; 125 mg; 150 mcg; 100 mg; 2 mg; 15 mg; 2.5 mg; 40 mg; 25 mcg; 25 mcg; 25 mcg; 5 mcg; 10 mcg; 60 mg; 1.5 mg; 1.7 mg; 2 mg; 6 mcg; 25 mcg	Peach	Coated Tablet	Oblong, Scored	Wyeth Consumer Healthcare
CF 250 ; G	Ciprofloxacin	250 mg	White to Off-White	Tablet	Circle	Par Pharmaceutical
CF 500 ; G	Ciprofloxacin	500 mg	White to Off-White	Tablet	Capsule-Shape	Par Pharmaceutical
CF 750 ; G	Ciprofloxacin	750 mg	White to Off-White	Tablet	Capsule-Shape	Par Pharmaceutical
CF; A	Nembutal Sodium	50 mg	Orange and White	Capsule		Abbott Laboratories
CG ; HGH	Diovan HCT	12.5 mg; 80 mg	Light Orange	Tablet	Oval	Novartis Pharmaceuticals
CG ; HHH	Diovan HCT	12.5 mg; 160 mg	Dark Red	Tablet	Oval	Novartis
CG ; HHH	Diovan HCT	12.5 mg; 160 mg	Dark Red	Tablet	Oval	Novartis Pharmaceuticals
CG; FXF	Foradil Aerolizer	12 mcg	Clear	Capsule		Novartis
CH; A	Nembutal Sodium	100 mg	Yellow	Capsule		Abbott Laboratories
CHARACTER IMPRINT	Sesame Street Complete Vitamins and Minerals	10 mg; 2250 IU; 500 IU; 200 IU; 10 mg; 5 mg; 10 IU; 200 mcg; 15 mcg; 75 mcg; 8 mg; 1 mg; 80 mg; 20 mg; 0.75 mg; 0.85 mg; 0.7 mg; 3 mcg; 40 mg		Tablet	Character-Shape	Johnson & Johnson
CHARACTER IMPRINT	Sesame Street Extra C Vitamins	2250 IU; 500 IU; 200 IU; 0.75 mg; 0.85 mg; 10 mg; 5 mg; 0.7 mg; 3 mcg; 80 mg; 10 IU; 200 mcg		Tablet	Character-Shape	Johnson & Johnson

IMPRINT	BRAND/GENERIC NAME	STRENGTH	COLOR	FORM	SHAPE	MANUFACTURER
CHEMET; 100	Chemet	100 mg	Opague White with Medicated Beads	Capsule		Sanofi Winthrop Pharmaceuticals
CHEW; EZ	Eryped	200 mg	White	Tablet, Chewable	Circle, Scored	Abbott Laboratories
CHILDREN; A; 3	Anacin-3 Children's	80 mg	Pink	Tablet, Chewable	Circle, Scored	Wyeth Consumer Healthcare
CIBA	Pyribenzamine Lontabs	50 mg	Light Green	Tablet		Novartis
CIBA NR	Slow Fe	160 mg	Yellowish-White	Extended-Release Tablet	Circle	Novartis Consumer Health
CIBA; 3	Ritalin	10 mg	Pale Green	Tablet	Circle, Scored	Novartis Pharmaceuticals
CIBA; 7	Ritalin	5 mg	Yellow	Tablet	Circle	Novartis Pharmaceuticals
CIBA; 13	Serpasil-Esidrix No. 1	25 mg; 0.1 mg	Light Orange	Tablet	Circle	Novartis
CIBA; 16	Ritalin SR	20 mg	White	Sustained-Release Tablet	Circle, Coated	Novartis Pharmaceuticals
CIBA; 22	Esidrix	25 mg	Pink	Tablet	Circle, Scored	Novartis
CIBA; 24	Cytadren	250 mg	White	Tablet	Circle, Cross-Scored	Novartis
CIBA; 26	Ludiomil	50 mg	Dark Orange	Tablet	Circle, Scored	Novartis
CIBA; 31 (ORANGE) ;	Forhistal	1 mg	Orange or Green	Tablet		Novartis
CIBA; 32	Metandren	25 mg	Yellow	Tablet	Circle, Scored	Novartis
CIBA; 33 ;	Pyribenzamine	50 mg	Light Blue	Tablet		Novartis
CIBA; 34	Ritalin	20 mg	Pale Yellow	Tablet	Circle, Scored	Novartis Pharmaceuticals
CIBA; 35	Serpasil	0.1 mg	White	Tablet	Circle	Novartis
CIBA; 36	Serpasil	0.25 mg	White	Tablet	Circle, Scored	Novartis
CIBA; 40	Serpasil-Apresoline No. 1	25 mg; 0.1 mg	Yellow	Tablet	Circle	Novartis
CIBA; 45	Forhistal Lontabs	2.5 mg	Orange	Tablet	Oblong	Novartis
CIBA; 47	Esimil	10 mg; 25 mg	White	Tablet	Circle, Scored	Novartis
CIBA; 49	Ismelin	10 mg	Yellow	Tablet	Circle, Scored	Novartis
CIBA; 64	Metandren Linguets	10 mg	Yellow	Tablet	Capsule-Shape	Novartis
CIBA; 65	Lithobid	300 mg	Peach	Sustained-Release Tablet		Novartis
CIBA; 71	Ser-AP-Es	25 mg; 15 mg; 0.1 mg	Pink	Tablet	Circle	Novartis
CIBA; 92	Gammacorten	0.75 mg		Tablet		Novartis
CIBA; 95	Pyribenzamine	25 mg	Green	Tablet		Novartis
CIBA; 96	Ultandren	5 mg	Lavender	Tablet		Novartis
CIBA; 103	Ismelin	25 mg	White	Tablet	Circle, Scored	Novartis
CIBA; 104	Serpasil-Apresoline No. 2	50 mg; 0.2 mg	Yellow	Tablet	Circle	Novartis
CIBA; 105	Dialog	300 mg; 15 mg	White	Tablet	Circle, Scored	Novartis
CIBA; 110	Ludiomil	25 mg	Dark Orange	Tablet	Oval, Scored	Novartis
CIBA; 110	Ludiomil	25 mg	Orange	Tablet	Oval, Scored	Novartis
CIBA; 130	Metopirone	250 mg	White	Tablet	Circle, Scored	Novartis
CIBA; 134	Pyribenzamine with Ephedrine	12 mg; 25 mg	White	Tablet		Novartis
CIBA; 135	Ludiomil	75 mg	White	Coated Tablet	Oval	Novartis
CIBA; 135	Ludiomil	75 mg	White	Tablet	Oval, Scored	Novartis
CIBA; 152	Regitine	50 mg	White	Tablet		Novartis
CIBA; 154	Rimactane	300 mg	Scarlet and Caramel	Capsule		Geneva Generics
CIBA; 192	Esidrex	100 mg	Blue	Tablet	Circle, Scored	Novartis
CIBA; 192	Esidrix	100 mg	Blue	Tablet	Circle, Scored	Novartis
CIPRO 250	Cipro	250 mg	White to Slightly Yellow	Tablet	Circle	Bayer Pharmaceutical
CIPRO 250	Cipro	250 mg	White to Slightly Yellow	Tablet	Circle	Schering
CIPRO 500	Cipro	500 mg	White to Slightly Yellow	Tablet	Capsule-Shape	Bayer Pharmaceutical
CIPRO 500	Cipro	500 mg	White to Slightly Yellow	Tablet	Capsule-Shape	Schering
CIPRO 750	Cipro	750 mg	White to Slightly Yellow	Tablet	Capsule-Shape	Bayer Pharmaceutical
CIPRO 750	Cipro	750 mg	White to Slightly Yellow	Tablet	Capsule-Shape	Schering
CIR; 3 MG	Entocort Ec	3 mg	Light Grey and Pink	Capsule		Astra Zeneca
CK	Angeliq	0.5 mg; 1 mg	Pink	Tablet	Circle	Berlex
CL; 101	Methocarbamol	750 mg		Tablet		Roxane Laboratories
CL; 127	Regal-AM	260 mg	White	Tablet	Circle	Geneva Generics
CL; 190	Methocarbamol	500 mg		Tablet		Roxane Laboratories
CL; 400	Ercaf	100 mg; 1 mg	Beige	Coated Tablet	Circle, Scored	Novartis Generics
CL; 418	Phenylbutazone	100 mg	Red	Coated Tablet		Novartis Generics
CL; 503	Papaverine Hydrochloride	150 mg	Brown and Clear	Extended-Release Capsule		Roxane Laboratories
CL; 751	Methyldopa	250 mg		Tablet		Novartis Generics
CL; 752	Methyldopa	500 mg		Tablet		Novartis Generics
CL; 753	Methyldopa and Hydrochlorothiazide	250 mg; 15 mg		Tablet		Novartis Generics
CL; 754	Methyldopa and Hydrochlorothiazide	250 mg; 25 mg		Tablet		Novartis Generics
CLARITIN 10; 458	Claritin	10 mg	White to Off-White	Tablet	Circle, Compressed	Schering
CLARITIN-D	Claritin-D 12 Hour	5 mg; 120 mg	White	Extended-Release Tablet		Schering
CLARITIN-D; 24 HOUR	Claritin-D 24 Hour	10 mg; 240 mg	White to Off-White	Extended-Release Tablet		Schering
CLEOCIN; 75 MG	Cleocin	75 mg	Green	Capsule		Pharmacia & Upjohn
CLEOCIN; 150 MG	Cleocin	150 mg	Blue and Green	Capsule		Pharmacia & Upjohn
CLEOCIN; 300 MG	Cleocin	300 mg	Blue	Capsule		Pharmacia & Upjohn
CLISTIN; MCNEIL	Clistin	4 mg	Pink	Tablet	Circle, Scored	Mcneil Pharmaceutical
CLOMID; 50 ;	Clomid	50 mg	White to Pale Yellow	Tablet	Circle	Sanofi-Aventis U.S.
CLOZARIL; 25	Clozaril	25 mg	Pale Yellow	Tablet	Circle, Compressed, Embossed	Novartis Pharmaceuticals
CLOZARIL; 100	Clozaril	100 mg	Pale Yellow	Tablet	Circle, Compressed	Novartis Pharmaceuticals
CM	Children's Mylanta	400 mg	Pink	Tablet, Chewable	Circle, Scored	Johnson & Johnson Merck
CN; 0.5; G	Clonazepam	0.5 mg	Light Yellow	Tablet	Circle, Scored	Par Pharmaceutical
CN; 1; G	Clonazepam	1 mg	Dark Yellow	Tablet	Circle, Scored	Par Pharmaceutical
CN; 2; G	Clonazepam	2 mg	White	Tablet	Circle, Scored	Par Pharmaceutical
C-NIGHT	Contac Day & Night Cold & Flu	650 mg; 60 mg; 50 mg; 30 mg	Blue	Tablet		Glaxosmithkline Consumer

IMPRINT	BRAND/GENERIC NAME	STRENGTH	COLOR	FORM	SHAPE	MANUFACTURER
COADVIL	CO-Advil	200 mg; 30 mg	Tan	Tablet		Whitehall
COMBID; SKF	Combid	5 mg; 10 mg	Yellow and Clear	Capsule		Glaxosmithkline
COMHIST LA; 01490466	Comhist LA	4 mg; 50 mg; 20 mg	Yellow and Clear	Capsule		Procter & Gamble Pharmaceuticals
COMTAN	Comtan	200 mg	Brown-Orange	Coated Tablet	Oval	Novartis
COMTREX	Comtrex Maximum Strength	500 mg; 2 mg; 30 mg; 15 mg	Yellow	Tablet		Bristol-Myers Squibb
COMTREX; A S	Comtrex Allergy and Sinus	500 mg; 30 mg; 2 mg	Green	Tablet		Bristol-Myers Squibb
CONTAC; S	Contac Sinus	500 mg; 30 mg	Pink	Tablet	Capsule-Shape	Glaxosmithkline Consumer
COPLEY 158 ;	Multivitamins with Fluoride	2500 IU; 400 IU; 15 IU; 0.3 mg; 1.05 mg; 1.2 mg; 13.5 mg; 0.5 mg; 60 mg; 1.05 mg; 4.5 mcg	Multi-Colored	Tablet, Chewable	Square	Novartis Generics
COPLEY; 0519	Vitamins with Fluoride	2500 IU; 400 IU; 15 IU; 0.3 mg; 13.5 mg; 1 mg; 60 mg; 1.05 mg; 1.2 mg; 1.05 mg; 4.5 mcg	Multi-Colored	Tablet, Chewable	Square	Novartis Generics
COPLEY; 107	Mebendazole	100 mg	Light Peach	Tablet, Chewable	Circle	Teva Pharmaceuticals
COPLEY; 111	Prenatal 1+1	65 mg; 4000 IU; 400 IU; 11 mg; 1 mg; 1.5 mg; 3 mg; 20 mg; 200 mg; 2 mg; 25 mg; 120 mg; 10 mg; 12 mcg	Yellow	Coated Tablet	Capsule-Shape	Novartis Generics
COPLEY; 131	Sodium Fluoride	2.2 mg	Pink	Tablet, Chewable	Circle	Novartis Generics
COPLEY; 225	Potassium Chloride	600 mg	Peach	Extended-Release Tablet	Circle	Teva Pharmaceuticals
COPLEY; 225	Potassium Chloride	8 meq	Orange	Extended-Release Tablet	Circle	Teva Pharmaceuticals
COR 140	Glyburide and Metformin Hydrochloride	1.25 mg; 250 mg	Pale Yellow	Tablet	Circle	Sandoz
COR 141	Glyburide and Metformin Hydrochloride	2.5 mg; 500 mg	Orange	Tablet	Circle	Sandoz
COR 142	Glyburide and Metformin Hydrochloride	5 mg; 500 mg	Yellow	Tablet	Circle	Sandoz
COR 152	Doxycycline Hyclate	20 mg	White	Tablet	Circle	Sandoz
COR 153	Clindamycin Hydrochloride	150 mg	Light Blue Opaque	Capsule		Sandoz
COR 154	Clindamycin Hydrochloride	300 mg	Light Blue Opaque	Capsule		Sandoz
COR 164	Glimepiride	1 mg	Pink	Tablet	Circle	Sandoz
COR 165	Glimepiride	2 mg	Green	Tablet	Circle	Sandoz
COR 166	Glimepiride	4 mg	Blue	Tablet	Circle	Sandoz
COR 175	Meloxicam	7.5 mg	Pastel Yellow	Tablet	Circle	Sandoz
COR 176	Meloxicam	15 mg	Pastel Yellow	Tablet	Circle	Sandoz
COR; 103	Carisoprodol	350 mg	White	Tablet	Circle	Geneva Generics
COR; 103 ;	Carisoprodol	350 mg	White	Tablet	Circle	Sandoz
COR; 111	Rimantadine Hydrochloride	100 mg	Orange	Tablet	Circle	Geneva Generics
COR; 123	Glyburide	1.25 mg	White	Tablet	Circle, Scored	Sandoz
COR; 124	Glyburide	2.5 mg	Yellow	Tablet	Circle, Scored	Sandoz
COR; 125	Glyburide	5 mg	Green	Tablet	Circle, Scored	Sandoz
COR; 128	Pyridostigmine Bromide	60 mg	White	Tablet	Round, Quadrisected Scored	Geneva Generics
CORRECTOL	Correctol	5 mg	Bright Pink	Tablet	Oblong	Schering-Plough Healthcare Products
CORRECTOL IN A HALF MOON	Correctol	5 mg	Bright Pink	Tablet	Circle	Schering-Plough Healthcare Products
CORTEF; 5	Cortef	5 mg	White	Tablet	Circle, Scored	Pharmacia & Upjohn
CORTEF; 10	Cortef	10 mg	White	Tablet	Circle, Scored	Pharmacia & Upjohn
CORTEF; 20	Cortef	20 mg	White	Tablet	Circle, Scored	Pharmacia & Upjohn
CORZIDE; 40/5; 283 ;	Corzide 40/5	5 mg; 40 mg	White to Bluish White with Dark Blue Specks	Tablet	Circle, Biconvex	Monarch Pharmaceuticals
CORZIDE; 80/5; 284 ;	Corzide 80/5	5 mg; 80 mg	White to Bluish White with Dark Blue Specks	Tablet	Circle, Biconvex	Monarch Pharmaceuticals
COTRIM DS; 93 93	Cotrim DS	800 mg; 160 mg	White	Tablet	Oval, Convex, Scored	Teva Pharmaceuticals
COTRIM; 93 93	Cotrim	400 mg; 80 mg	White	Tablet	Circle, Convex, Scored	Teva Pharmaceuticals
COTYLENOL	Cotylenol Cold Medication	2 mg; 30 mg; 15 mg; 325 mg	Yellow	Tablet	Oblong	Mcneil Consumer Products
COUMADIN 2 ;	Coumadin	2 mg	Lavender	Tablet	Circle	Bristol-Myers Squibb
COUMADIN 2 1/2 ;	Coumadin	2.5 mg	Green	Tablet	Circle	Bristol-Myers Squibb
COUMADIN 3 ;	Coumadin	3 mg	Tan	Tablet	Circle	Bristol-Myers Squibb
COUMADIN 4 ;	Coumadin	4 mg	Blue	Tablet	Circle	Bristol-Myers Squibb
COUMADIN 5 ;	Coumadin	5 mg	Peach	Tablet	Circle	Bristol-Myers Squibb
COUMADIN 6 ;	Coumadin	6 mg	Teal	Tablet	Circle	Bristol-Myers Squibb
COUMADIN 7 1/2 ;	Coumadin	7.5 mg	Yellow	Tablet	Circle	Bristol-Myers Squibb
COUMADIN 10 ;	Coumadin	10 mg	White	Tablet	Circle	Bristol-Myers Squibb
COVERA-HS; 2011	Covera-Hs	180 mg	Lavender	Tablet, Extended Release	Circle	Searle
COVERA-HS; 2021	Covera-Hs	240 mg	Pale Yellow	Tablet, Extended Release	Circle	Searle
CP; 253; NOTRIPTYLINE; 75 MG	Nortriptyline Hydrochloride	75 mg	Green	Capsule		Geneva Generics
CRESTOR ; 40	Crestor	40 mg	Pink	Tablet	Oval	Astra Zeneca
CRESTOR 5	Crestor	5 mg	Yellow	Tablet	Circle	Astra Zeneca
CRESTOR 10	Crestor	10 mg	Pink	Tablet	Circle	Astra Zeneca

IMPRINT	BRAND/GENERIC NAME	STRENGTH	COLOR	FORM	SHAPE	MANUFACTURER
CRESTOR 20	Crestor	20 mg	Pink	Tablet	Circle	Astra Zeneca
CRIXIVAN; 100 MG	Crixivan	100 mg	White Semi-Translucent	Capsule		Merck
CRIXIVAN; 200 MG	Crixivan	200 mg	White Semi-Translucent	Capsule		Merck & Company
CRIXIVAN; 333 MG	Crixivan	333 mg	White with a Red Band	Capsule		Merck & Company
CRIXIVAN; 400 MG	Crixivan	400 mg	White Semi-Translucent	Capsule		Merck
CT	Myfortic	360 mg	Pale Orange-Red	Enteric-Coated Tablet	Oval	Novartis
CTA	Children's Tylenol Allergy-D	80 mg; 6.25 mg; 7.5 mg	Pink	Tablet, Chewable	Circle	Mcneil Consumer Products
CTS	Children's Tylenol Sinus	80 mg; 7.5 mg	Pink	Tablet, Chewable	Circle	Mcneil Consumer Products
CVT 500	Ranexa	500 mg	Light Orange	Tablet, Extended Release	Oblong	Cv Therapeutics
CXL 4	Cardura XL	4 mg	White	Tablet, Extended Release		Pfizer
CXL 8	Cardura XL	8 mg	White	Tablet, Extended Release		Pfizer
CY	Cyklokapron	500 mg	White	Tablet	Circle, Flat, with Beveled Edges	Pharmacia & Upjohn
CYCRIN; C	Premphase Medroxyprogesterone	5 mg	Light Purple	Tablet	Oval, Scored	Wyeth Pharmaceuticals
CYSTA; 50; MYLAN	Cystagon	50 mg	White, Opaque	Capsule		Mylan Pharmaceuticals
CYSTAGON; 150; MYLAN	Cystagon	150 mg	White, Opaque	Capsule		Mylan Pharmaceuticals
D	Bronkaid	24 mg; 400 mg; 100 mg	White	Coated Tablet	Circle, Scored	Bayer Consumer Care
D	Doan's Ibuprofen Backache Pills	200 mg	White	Tablet		Novartis Consumer
D	Dristan Cold Multi-Symptom	325 mg; 2 mg; 5 mg		Tablet		Wyeth Consumer Healthcare
D ; 24	Clarinex-D 24 Hour	5 mg; 240 mg	Light Blue	Tablet, Extended Release	Oval	Schering
D; 2.5 MG	Focalin	2.5 mg	Blue	Tablet	D-Shape	Novartis
D; 5 MG	Focalin	5 mg	Yellow	Tablet	D-Shape	Novartis
D; 10 MG	Focalin	10 mg	White	Tablet	D-Shape	Novartis
D; 31	Demerol Apap	50 mg; 300 mg	Red	Tablet	Circle	Sanofi Winthrop Pharmaceuticals
D; 92	Drisdol	50000 IU	Green	Capsule, Liquid Filled		Sanofi-Aventis U.S.
D0	Yasmin Light Yellow Tablet	3 mg; 0.03 mg	Light Yellow	Coated Tablet	Circle	Berlex Laboratories
D12	Clarinex-D 12 Hour	2.5 mg; 120 mg	Blue, White	Tablet, Extended Release	Oval	Schering
D35 W	Demerol Hydrochloride	50 mg	White	Tablet	Circle	Sanofi Winthrop Pharmaceuticals
D35 W	Demerol Hydrochloride	50 mg	White	Tablet	Circle	Sanofi-Aventis U.S.
D37 W	Demerol Hydrochloride	100 mg	White	Tablet	Circle	Sanofi-Aventis U.S.
D75	Doryx	75 mg	White, Yellow (Pellets)	Tablet, Delayed Release	Oval	Warner Chilcott
D100	Doryx	100 mg	White, Yellow (Pellets)	Tablet, Delayed Release	Oval	Warner Chilcott
DAN ; 5052	Prednisone	5 mg	White	Tablet	Circle	Watson Laboratories
DAN ; 5442	Prednisone	10 mg	White	Tablet	Circle	Watson Laboratories
DAN ; 5443	Prednisone	20 mg	Peach	Tablet	Circle	Watson Laboratories
DAN 5440 DAN 5440	Doxycycline Hyclate	100 mg	Blue	Capsule		Watson Laboratories
DAN 5658	Cyclobenzaprine Hydrochloride	10 mg	White	Tablet	Circle	Watson Laboratories
DAN 5726	Hydroxyzine Pamoate	25 mg	Dark Green, Light Green	Capsule		Watson Laboratories
DAN DAN 5325	Probenecid and Colchicine	0.5 mg; 500 mg	White	Tablet	Capsule-Shape	Watson Laboratories
DAN DAN; 5600 ;	Trazodone Hydrochloride	50 mg	White	Coated Tablet	Circle, Scored	Watson Laboratories
DAN; 2; 5621	Diazepam	2 mg	White	Tablet	Circle, Scored	Watson Laboratories
DAN; 5; 5619	Diazepam	5 mg	Yellow	Tablet	Circle, Scored	Watson Laboratories
DAN; 5; 5882	Methylphenidate Hydrochloride	5 mg	Light Purple	Tablet	Circle	Watson Laboratories
DAN; 5; 5882	Methylphenidate Hydrochloride	5 mg	Purple	Tablet	Circle	Watson Laboratories
DAN; 10; 5554	Propranolol Hydrochloride	10 mg	Orange	Tablet	Circle, Scored	Watson Laboratories
DAN; 10; 5620	Diazepam	10 mg	Light Blue	Tablet	Circle, Scored	Watson Laboratories
DAN; 10; 5883	Methylphenidate Hydrochloride	10 mg	Green	Tablet	Circle	Watson Laboratories
DAN; 10; 5883	Methylphenidate Hydrochloride	10 mg	Light Green	Tablet	Circle, Scored	Watson Laboratories
DAN; 20; 5884	Methylphenidate Hydrochloride	20 mg	Peach	Tablet	Circle	Watson Laboratories
DAN; 20; 5884	Methylphenidate Hydrochloride	20 mg	Peach	Tablet	Circle, Scored	Watson Laboratories
DAN; 50; 5777	Atenolol	50 mg	White	Tablet	Circle	Watson Laboratories
DAN; 5059 DAN	Prednisolone	5 mg	Peach	Tablet	Circle, Scored	Watson Laboratories
DAN; 5216; DAN	Folic Acid	1 mg	Yellow	Tablet	Circle, Scored	Watson Laboratories
DAN; 5307; DAN	Promethazine Hydrochloride	25 mg	White	Tablet	Circle, Scored	Watson Laboratories
DAN; 5319	Promethazine Hydrochloride	50 mg	White	Tablet	Circle	Watson Laboratories
DAN; 5321; DAN	Primidone	250 mg	White	Tablet	Circle, Scored	Watson Laboratories
DAN; 5335; DAN	Trihexyphenidyl Hydrochloride	2 mg	White	Tablet	Circle, Scored	Watson Laboratories
DAN; 5337; DAN	Trihexyphenidyl Hydrochloride	5 mg	White	Tablet	Circle, Scored	Watson Laboratories
DAN; 5347; DAN	Probenecid	500 mg	Yellow	Coated Tablet	Capsule-Shape, Scored	Watson Laboratories
DAN; 5430; DAN	Acetazolamide	250 mg	White	Tablet	Circle, Scored	Watson Laboratories
DAN; 5438 DAN	Quinidine Sulfate	200 mg	White	Tablet	Scored, Circle	Watson Laboratories
DAN; 5440	Doxycycline Hyclate	100 mg	Light Blue	Capsule		Watson Laboratories
DAN; 5454; DAN	Quinidine Sulfate	300 mg	White	Tablet	Circle, Scored	Watson Laboratories
DAN; 5513	Carisoprodol	350 mg	White	Tablet	Circle	Watson Laboratories
DAN; 5522 ;	Hydroxyzine Hydrochloride	10 mg	Orange	Coated Tablet	Circle	Watson Laboratories
DAN; 5523	Hydroxyzine Hydrochloride	25 mg	Green	Coated Tablet	Circle	Watson Laboratories
DAN; 5535 ;	Doxycycline Hyclate	50 mg	LT. Blue and White	Capsule		Watson Laboratories
DAN; 5540	Metronidazole	250 mg	White to Off-White	Tablet	Circle	Watson Laboratories
DAN; 5543; DAN	Allopurinol	100 mg	White	Tablet	Circle, Scored	Watson Laboratories
DAN; 5544; DAN	Allopurinol	300 mg	Orange	Tablet	Circle, Scored	Watson Laboratories
DAN; 5552; DAN	Metronidazole	500 mg	White to Off-White	Tablet	Circle, Scored	Watson Laboratories
DAN; 5553	Doxycycline Hyclate	100 mg	Orange	Coated Tablet	Circle	Watson Laboratories

IMPRINT	BRAND/GENERIC NAME	STRENGTH	COLOR	FORM	SHAPE	MANUFACTURER
DAN; 5555; 20	Propranolol Hydrochloride	20 mg	Light Blue	Tablet	Circle, Scored	Watson Laboratories
DAN; 5556; 40	Propranolol Hydrochloride	40 mg	Light Green	Tablet	Circle, Scored	Watson Laboratories
DAN; 5557; 80	Propranolol Hydrochloride	80 mg	Yellow	Tablet	Circle, Scored	Watson Laboratories
DAN; 5560	Disopyramide Phosphate	100 mg	Opaque Orange	Capsule		Watson Laboratories
DAN; 5561	Disopyramide Phosphate	150 mg	Opaque Brown	Capsule		Watson Laboratories
DAN; 5599; DAN	Trazodone Hcl	100 mg	White	Coated Tablet	Circle, Scored	Watson Laboratories
DAN; 5629	Doxepin Hydrochloride	10 mg	Buff	Capsule		Watson Laboratories
DAN; 5630	Doxepin Hydrochloride	25 mg	White and Ivory	Capsule		Watson Laboratories
DAN; 5631	Doxepin Hydrochloride	50 mg	Ivory	Capsule		Watson Laboratories
DAN; 5632	Doxepin Hydrochloride	75 mg	Light Green	Capsule		Watson Laboratories
DAN; 5633	Doxepin Hydrochloride	100 mg	Green and White	Capsule		Watson Laboratories
DAN; 5642; 2.5	Minoxidil	2.5 mg	White	Tablet	Circle, Scored	Watson Laboratories
DAN; 5643; 10	Minoxidil	10 mg	White	Tablet	Circle, Scored	Watson Laboratories
DAN; 5660; DAN	Sulindac	200 mg	Yellow	Tablet	Circle, Scored	Watson Laboratories
DAN; 5661	Sulindac	150 mg	Yellow	Tablet	Circle	Watson Laboratories
DAN; 5730; 10	Baclofen	10 mg	White	Tablet	Circle, Scored	Watson Laboratories
DAN; 5731; 20	Baclofen	20 mg	White	Tablet	Circle, Scored	Watson Laboratories
DAN; 5778; 100	Atenolol	100 mg	White	Tablet	Circle	Watson Laboratories
DAN; 5782	Atenolol and Chlorthalidone	50 mg; 25 mg	White	Tablet	Circle, Scored	Watson Laboratories
DAN; 5783	Atenolol and Chlorthalidone	100 mg; 25 mg	White	Tablet	Circle	Watson Laboratories
DAN; DAN; 5382	Methocarbamol	750 mg	White	Tablet	Oval, Scored	Watson Laboratories
DAN; DAN; 5543	Allopurinol	100 mg	White	Tablet	Circle, Scored	Watson Laboratories
DAN; DAN; 5544	Allopurinol	300 mg	Orange	Tablet	Circle, Scored	Watson Laboratories
DANTRIUM 25 MG; 0149 0030	Dantrium	25 mg	Opaque, Orange and Tan	Capsule		Procter & Gamble Pharmaceuticals
DANTRIUM 50 MG; 0149 0031	Dantrium	50 mg	Opaque, Orange and Tan	Capsule		Procter & Gamble Pharmaceuticals
DANTRIUM 100 MG; 0149 0033	Dantrium	100 mg	Opaque, Orange and Tan	Capsule		Procter & Gamble Pharmaceuticals
DARAPRIM; A3A	Daraprim	25 mg	White	Tablet		Glaxosmithkline
DARVON COMP	Darvon Compound	32 mg; 389 mg; 32.4 mg	Pink	Capsule		Eli Lilly
DAYPRO; 1381	Daypro	600 mg	White	Coated Tablet	Capsule-Shape, Scored	Searle
DAYQUIL; SINUS PAIN	Dayquil Sinus Pressure and Pain Relief with Ibuprofen	30 mg; 200 mg	White	Tablet		Procter & Gamble
DDAVP; 0.2; RPR ;	Ddavp	0.2 mg	White	Tablet	Circle	Sanofi-Aventis U.S.
DELTASONE; 2.5	Deltasone	2.5 mg	Pink	Tablet	Circle, Scored	Pharmacia & Upjohn
DELTASONE; 5	Deltasone	5 mg	White	Tablet	Circle, Scored	Pharmacia & Upjohn
DELTASONE; 10	Deltasone	10 mg	White	Tablet	Circle, Scored	Pharmacia & Upjohn
DELTASONE; 20	Deltasone	20 mg	Peach	Tablet	Circle, Scored	Pharmacia & Upjohn
DELTASONE; 50 ;	Deltasone	50 mg	White	Tablet	Circle, Scored	Pharmacia & Upjohn
DEPAKENE	Depakene	250 mg	Orange	Capsule, Liquid Filled		Abbott Laboratories
DEPAKOTE SPRINKLE 125 MG; THIS END UP	Depakote Sprinkle	125 mg	White Opaque/blue	Capsule		Abbott Laboratories
DERMIK; 044	Durrax	10 mg	Lavender	Tablet	Circle	Dermik Laboratories
DERMIK; 045	Durrax	25 mg	Lavender	Tablet	Circle	Dermik Laboratories
DIA; B	Diabeta	2.5 mg	Peach	Tablet	Oblong	Sanofi-Aventis U.S.
DIA; B	Diabeta	1.25 mg	Peach	Tablet	Oblong	Sanofi-Aventis U.S.
DIA; B	Diabeta	2.5 mg	Peach	Tablet	Oblong	Aventis Pharmaceuticals
DIA; B	Diabeta	5 mg	Light Green	Tablet	Oblong	Aventis Pharmaceuticals
DIA; B	Diabeta	5 mg	Light Green	Tablet	Oblong	Sanofi-Aventis U.S.
DIFLUCAN; 50; ROERIG	Diflucan	50 mg	Pink	Tablet	Four-Sided	Pfizer Roerig
DIFLUCAN; 100; ROERIG	Diflucan	100 mg	Pink	Tablet	Four-Sided	Pfizer Roerig
DIFLUCAN; 150; ROERIG	Diflucan	150 mg	Pink	Tablet	Oval	Pfizer Roerig
DIFLUCAN; 200; ROERIG	Diflucan	200 mg	Pink	Tablet	Four-Sided	Pfizer Roerig
DI-GEL	Di-Gel	25 mg; 280 mg; 128 mg	Yellow and White	Tablet		Schering-Plough
DILANTIN; 100 MG	Dilantin Kapseals	100 mg	White with Orange Band	Extended-Release Capsule		Parke-Davis
DIPENTUM; 250 MG	Dipentum	250 mg	Beige	Capsule		Pharmacia & Upjohn
DISALCID; 3M	Disalcid	500 mg	Aqua	Coated Tablet	Round, Bisected Scored	3M Pharmaceuticals
DISALCID; 3M	Disalcid	500 mg	Aqua and White	Capsule		3M Pharmaceuticals
DISALCID; 750; 3M	Disalcid	750 mg	Aqua	Coated Tablet	Capsule-Shaped, Bisected Scored	3M Pharmaceuticals
DIUCARDIN; 50	Diucardin	50 mg	White	Tablet	Oval, Scored	Wyeth Pharmaceuticals
DOAN'S	Doan's, Extra Strength	467.2 mg	White	Tablet	Capsule-Shape	Novartis Consumer
DOAN'S PM	Extra Strength Doan's Pm	580 mg; 25 mg	Light Blue	Tablet	Capsule-Shape	Novartis Consumer
DORMALIN; 722	Dormalin	15 mg	Light Orange	Tablet	Capsule-Shape	Schering
DORSEY	Kanulase	9 mg; 500 mg; 200 mg; 100 mg; 150 mg	Pink	Tablet		Novartis Consumer
DORSEY	Kanulase	9 mg; 500 mg; 200 mg; 100 mg; 150 mg	Pink	Tablet		Sandoz Consumer Pharmaceuticals
DORSEY	Rautensin	2 mg	Orange	Tablet	Circle, Scored	Novartis Pharmaceuticals
DORSEY	Wilpo	8 mg	Green	Tablet		Novartis Pharmaceuticals
DOW; 11	Novahistine Fortis	10 mg; 2 mg	Green and White	Capsule		Glaxosmithkline Consumer
DOW; 71	Novahistine Sinus	325 mg; 30 mg; 2 mg	White	Tablet	Circle	Glaxosmithkline Consumer
DOW; 603	Phenoxene	50 mg	Beige	Tablet	Circle	Aventis Pharmaceuticals
DOXIDAN	Doxidan	30 mg; 100 mg	Dark Red	Capsule		Pharmacia & Upjohn
DP 41	Cenestin	0.3 mg	Green	Tablet	Circle	Duramed Pharmaceuticals
DP 42	Cenestin	0.625 mg	Red	Tablet	Circle	Duramed Pharmaceuticals
DP 43	Cenestin	0.9 mg	White	Tablet	Circle	Duramed Pharmaceuticals

IMPRINT	BRAND/GENERIC NAME	STRENGTH	COLOR	FORM	SHAPE	MANUFACTURER
DP 44	Cenestin	1.25 mg	Blue	Tablet	Circle	Duramed Pharmaceuticals
DP 46	Cenestin	0.45 mg	Orange	Tablet	Circle	Duramed Pharmaceuticals
DP; 10	Propranolol Hydrochloride	10 mg	Orange	Tablet	Circle, Scored	Duramed Pharmaceuticals
DP; 11	Trifluoperazine Hydrochloride	1 mg	Lavender	Coated Tablet		Duramed Pharmaceuticals
DP; 12	Trifluoperazine Hydrochloride	2 mg	Lavender	Coated Tablet		Duramed Pharmaceuticals
DP; 13	Trifluoperazine Hydrochloride	5 mg	Lavender	Coated Tablet		Duramed Pharmaceuticals
DP; 14	Trifluoperazine Hydrochloride	10 mg	Lavender	Coated Tablet		Duramed Pharmaceuticals
DP; 20	Propranolol Hydrochloride	20 mg	Blue	Tablet	Circle, Scored	Duramed Pharmaceuticals
DP; 25	Dipyridamole	25 mg	White	Tablet	Circle	Duramed Pharmaceuticals
DP; 25	Levoxyl	25 mcg	Orange	Tablet	Oval, Notched	Monarch Pharmaceuticals
DP; 30	Conjugated Estrogens	0.3 mg		Tablet		Duramed Pharmaceuticals
DP; 31	Conjugated Estrogens	0.625 mg		Tablet		Duramed Pharmaceuticals
DP; 32	Conjugated Estrogens	1.25 mg		Tablet		Duramed Pharmaceuticals
DP; 33	Conjugated Estrogen	2.5 mg		Tablet		Duramed Pharmaceuticals
DP; 41	Cenestin	0.3 mg	Green	Tablet	Circle	Barr Laboratories
DP; 41	Cenestin	0.3 mg	Green	Tablet	Circle	Duramed Pharmaceuticals
DP; 43	Cenestin	0.9 mg	White	Tablet	Circle	Barr Laboratories
DP; 43	Cenestin	0.9 mg	White	Tablet	Circle	Duramed Pharmaceuticals
DP; 44	Cenestin	1.25 mg	Blue	Tablet	Circle	Barr Laboratories
DP; 44	Cenestin	1.25 mg	Blue	Tablet	Circle	Duramed Pharmaceuticals
DP; 50 ;	Levoxyl	50 mcg	White	Tablet	Oval, Notched	Monarch Pharmaceuticals
DP; 50	Dipyridamole	50 mg	White	Tablet	Circle	Duramed Pharmaceuticals
DP; 60	Propranolol Hydrochloride	60 mg	Pink	Tablet	Circle, Scored	Duramed Pharmaceuticals
DP; 75	Dipyridamole	75 mg	White	Tablet	Circle	Duramed Pharmaceuticals
DP; 75	Levoxyl	75 mcg	Purple	Tablet	Oval, Notched	Monarch Pharmaceuticals
DP; 80	Propranolol Hydrochloride	80 mg	Yellow	Tablet	Scored, Circle	Duramed Pharmaceuticals
DP; 88	Levoxyl	88 mcg	Olive	Tablet	Oval, Notched	Monarch Pharmaceuticals
DP; 90	Propranolol Hydrochloride	90 mg	Lavender	Tablet	Circle, Scored	Duramed Pharmaceuticals
DP; 100	Levoxyl	100 mcg	Yellow	Tablet	Oval, Notched	Monarch Pharmaceuticals
DP; 112	Levoxyl	112 mcg	Rose	Tablet	Oval, Notched	Monarch Pharmaceuticals
DP; 125	Levoxyl	125 mcg	Brown	Tablet	Oval, Notched	Monarch Pharmaceuticals
DP; 137	Levoxyl	137 mcg	Dark Blue	Tablet	Oval, Notched	Monarch Pharmaceuticals
DP; 150	Levoxyl	150 mcg	Blue	Tablet	Oval, Notched	Monarch Pharmaceuticals
DP; 175	Levoxyl	175 mcg	Turquoise	Tablet	Oval, Notched	Monarch Pharmaceuticals
DP; 200	Levoxyl	200 mcg	Pink	Tablet	Oval, Notched	Monarch Pharmaceuticals
DP; 215	Chlorzoxazone and Acetaminophen	250 mg; 300 mg		Tablet		Duramed Pharmaceuticals
DP; 223	Aminophylline	100 mg	White	Tablet	Circle, Scored	Duramed Pharmaceuticals
DP; 224	Aminophylline	200 mg	White	Tablet	Circle, Scored	Duramed Pharmaceuticals
DP; 225	Haloperidol	0.5 mg	White	Tablet	Circle, Scored	Duramed Pharmaceuticals
DP; 226	Haloperidol	1 mg	Yellow	Tablet	Circle, Scored	Duramed Pharmaceuticals
DP; 227	Haloperidol	2 mg	Lavender	Tablet	Circle, Scored	Duramed Pharmaceuticals
DP; 228	Haloperidol	5 mg	Green	Tablet	Circle, Scored	Duramed Pharmaceuticals
DP; 246	Cyproheptadine Hydrochloride	4 mg	White	Tablet	Circle	Duramed Pharmaceuticals
DP; 249	Iodoquinol	650 mg		Tablet		Duramed Pharmaceuticals
DP; 251	Chlorpropamide	250 mg	Blue	Tablet	Circle, Scored	Duramed Pharmaceuticals
DP; 252	Chlorpropamide	100 mg	Blue	Tablet	Circle, Scored	Duramed Pharmaceuticals
DP; 265	Hydroxyzine Pamoate	25 mg	Green	Capsule		Duramed Pharmaceuticals
DP; 266	Hydroxyzine Pamoate	50 mg	White and Green	Capsule		Duramed Pharmaceuticals
DP; 267	Hydroxyzine Pamoate	100 mg	Gray and Green	Capsule		Duramed Pharmaceuticals
DP; 274	Isoniazid	100 mg	White	Tablet	Circle, Scored	Duramed Pharmaceuticals
DP; 275	Indomethacin	25 mg		Capsule		Duramed Pharmaceuticals
DP; 276	Indomethacin	50 mg		Capsule		Duramed Pharmaceuticals
DP; 277	Isoniazid	300 mg	White	Tablet	Circle, Scored	Duramed Pharmaceuticals
DP; 296	Salsalate	500 mg	Blue or Yellow	Tablet	Circle	Duramed Pharmaceuticals
DP; 297	Salsalate	750 mg	Blue or Yellow	Tablet	Capsule-Shape, Scored	Duramed Pharmaceuticals
DP; 300	Levoxyl	300 mcg	Green	Tablet	Oval	Monarch Pharmaceuticals
DP; 301	Methylprednisolone	4 mg	White	Tablet	Oval, Scored	Barr Laboratories
DP; 305	Papaverine Hydrochloride	150 mg		Timed-Release Capsule		Duramed Pharmaceuticals
DP; 311	Prednisone	5 mg	White	Tablet	Circle, Scored	Duramed Pharmaceuticals
DP; 312	Prednisone	10 mg	White	Tablet	Circle, Scored	Duramed Pharmaceuticals
DP; 313	Prednisone	20 mg	Orange	Tablet	Circle, Scored	Duramed Pharmaceuticals
DP; 314	Prochlorperazine Maleate	5 mg	Yellow	Tablet	Circle	Duramed Pharmaceuticals
DP; 315	Prochlorperazine Maleate	10 mg	Yellow	Tablet	Circle	Duramed Pharmaceuticals
DP; 316	Prochlorperazine Maleate	25 mg		Tablet		Duramed Pharmaceuticals
DP; 325	Tolazamide	100 mg	White	Tablet	Circle, Scored	Duramed Pharmaceuticals
DP; 326	Tolazamide	250 mg	White	Tablet	Circle, Scored	Duramed Pharmaceuticals
DP; 327	Tolazamide	500 mg	White	Tablet	Circle, Scored	Duramed Pharmaceuticals
DP; 332	Propranolol Hydrochloride and Hydrochlorothiazide	40 mg; 25 mg	Pale Yellow	Tablet	Scored, Circle	Duramed Pharmaceuticals
DP; 333	Propranolol Hydrochloride and Hydrochlorothiazide	80 mg; 25 mg		Tablet		Duramed Pharmaceuticals
DP; 371	Methyldopa	250 mg	White	Tablet	Circle	Duramed Pharmaceuticals
DP; 372	Methyldopa	500 mg	White	Tablet	Circle	Duramed Pharmaceuticals
DP; 401	Guaifenesin and Pseudoephedrine Hydrochloride	600 mg; 120 mg	Yellow	Extended-Release Tablet	Capsule-Shape, Scored	Duramed Pharmaceuticals
DP; 417	Guaifenesin	600 mg	Green	Extended-Release Tablet	Capsule-Shape, Scored	Duramed Pharmaceuticals
DP; 417	S-Pack P.M. Treatment Phase	600 mg	Green	Controlled-Release Tablet	Capsule-Shape, Scored	Duramed Pharmaceuticals
DP; 420	Guaifenesin DM	600 mg; 30 mg	White	Tablet	Capsule-Shape, Scored	Duramed Pharmaceuticals
DP; 420	S-Pack-DM P.M. Treatment Phase	600 mg; 30 mg	White	Controlled-Release Tablet	Capsule-Shape, Scored	Duramed Pharmaceuticals
DP; 480	Verapamil Hydrochloride SR	120 mg	Light Pink	Sustained-Release Tablet	Capsule-Shape	Duramed Pharmaceuticals
DP; 482	Verapamil Hydrochloride SR	240 mg	Light Tan	Sustained-Release Tablet	Capsule-Shape	Duramed Pharmaceuticals
DP; 501	Estradiol	0.5 mg	Lavender	Tablet	Round, Bisected Scored	Duramed Pharmaceuticals
DP; 502	Estradiol	1 mg	Rose	Tablet	Round, Bisected Scored	Duramed Pharmaceuticals
DP; 504	Estradiol	2 mg	Blue	Tablet	Round, Bisected Scored	Duramed Pharmaceuticals

IMPRINT	BRAND/GENERIC NAME	STRENGTH	COLOR	FORM	SHAPE	MANUFACTURER
DP; 509	Methotrexate Sodium	2.5 mg	Yellow	Tablet	Oval, Scored	Duramed Pharmaceuticals
DP; 510	Enpresse 28 Pink Tablets	0.03 mg; 0.05 mg	Pink	Tablet	Circle	Barr Laboratories
DP; 511	Enpresse 28 White Tablets	0.04 mg; 0.075 mg	White	28-Day Tablet Pack	Circle	Barr Laboratories
DP; 512	Enpresse 28 Orange Tablets	0.03 mg; 0.125 mg	Orange	28-Day Tablet Pack	Circle	Barr Laboratories
DP; 521	Prochlorperazine Maleate	5 mg	Orange	Tablet	Circle	Barr Laboratories
DP; 521	Prochlorperazine Maleate	5 mg	Orange	Tablet	Circle	Duramed Pharmaceuticals
DP; 522	Prochlorperazine Maleate	10 mg	Yellow	Tablet	Circle	Barr Laboratories
DP; 541	Medroxyprogesterone Acetate	5 mg	Yellow	Tablet	Circle, Scored	Duramed Pharmaceuticals
DP; 543	Cryselle 28 White Tablet	0.3 mg; 0.03 mg	White	Tablet	Circle	Barr Laboratories
DP; 548	Hydroxyurea	500 mg	Buff and Dark Green	Capsule		Duramed Pharmaceuticals
DP; 575	Apri 28 Pink Tablets	0.15 mg; 0.03 mg	Pink	Tablet		Barr Laboratories
DP; 610	Acetaminophen and Oxycodone	325 mg; 5 mg	White to Off-White	Tablet	Round, Bisected Scored	Duramed Pharmaceuticals
DP; 651	Phentermine Hydrochloride	30 mg	Blue and Clear	Capsule		Duramed Pharmaceuticals
DP; 660	Temazepam	15 mg	Green and White	Capsule		Duramed Pharmaceuticals
DP; 661	Temazepam	30 mg	White	Capsule		Duramed Pharmaceuticals
DP; 825	Triotann	25 mg; 8 mg; 25 mg	Beige	Tablet	Capsule-Shape, Scored	Duramed Pharmaceuticals
DP; 832	Choline Magnesium Trisalicylate	500 mg	Pale Pink	Tablet	Capsule-Shape	Duramed Pharmaceuticals
DP; 833	Choline Magnesium Trisalicylate	750 mg	White	Tablet	Capsule-Shape	Duramed Pharmaceuticals
DP; 840 ;	Amoxicillin	250 mg	Ivory or Buff Opaque and Brown	Capsule		Duramed Pharmaceuticals
DP; 841 ;	Amoxicillin	500 mg	Ivory or Buff Opaque	Capsule		Duramed Pharmaceuticals
DP; 842	Cephalexin	250 mg	Opaque Scarlet and Gray	Capsule		Duramed Pharmaceuticals
DP; 843 ;	Cephalexin	500 mg	Opaque Scarlet	Capsule		Duramed Pharmaceuticals
DP; 844	Tetracycline Hydrochloride	250 mg	Yellow and Orange Opaque	Capsule		Duramed Pharmaceuticals
DP; 845	Tetracycline Hydrochloride	500 mg	Black and Yellow Opaque	Capsule		Duramed Pharmaceuticals
DP; 857	Guaifenesin	1200 mg		Extended-Release Tablet		Duramed Pharmaceuticals
DP; 896	Durasal II	600 mg; 60 mg	Blue	Extended-Release Tablet	Capsule-Shape	Duramed Pharmaceuticals
DP; 896	S-Pack A.M. Treatment Phase	600 mg; 60 mg	Blue	Controlled-Release Tablet	Capsule-Shape, Scored	Duramed Pharmaceuticals
DP; 896	S-Pack-DM A.M. Treatment Phase	600 mg; 60 mg	Blue	Controlled-Release Tablet	Capsule-Shape, Scored	Duramed Pharmaceuticals
DP; 907	Duragal-S	0.2 mg; 0.6 mg; 40 mg	Green	Tablet	Round, Quadrisected Scored	Duramed Pharmaceuticals
DP; 932	Hyoscyamine Sulfate	0.125 mg	White	Tablet	Circle	Duramed Pharmaceuticals
DP; 933	Hyoscyamine Sulfate	0.375 mg	Orange	Extended-Release Tablet	Capsule-Shape	Duramed Pharmaceuticals
DP; 933	Hyoscyamine Sulfate	0.375 mg	White	Extended-Release Tablet	Capsule-Shape, Scored	Duramed Pharmaceuticals
DP; 935	Hyocyamine Sulfate SL	0.125 mg	Blue	Tablet	Circle	Duramed Pharmaceuticals
DP; 970	Digoxin	0.125 mg	Yellow	Tablet	Circle, Scored	Duramed Pharmaceuticals
DP; 971	Digoxin	0.25 mg	White	Tablet	Circle, Scored	Duramed Pharmaceuticals
DP; 972	Digoxin	0.5 mg	Green	Tablet	Circle, Scored	Duramed Pharmaceuticals
DPI; 2	Acetaminophen and Codeine Phosphate	300 mg; 15 mg	White	Tablet	Circle	Duramed Pharmaceuticals
DPI; 3	Acetaminophen and Codeine Phosphate	300 mg; 30 mg	White	Tablet	Circle	Duramed Pharmaceuticals
DPI; 4	Acetaminophen and Codeine Phosphate	300 mg; 60 mg	White	Tablet	Circle	Duramed Pharmaceuticals
DPI; 125	Estropipate	1.5 mg	White	Tablet	Diamond, Scored	Duramed Pharmaceuticals
DPI; 288	Triamterene and Hydrochlorothiazide	37.5 mg; 25 mg	White	Capsule		Barr Laboratories
DPI; 364	Duradrin	325 mg; 65 mg; 100 mg	White and Scarlet	Capsule		Barr Laboratories
DPI; 488	Hydrochlorothiazide and Triamterene	25 mg; 37.5 mg	White	Capsule		Barr Laboratories
DPI; 488	Triamterene and Hydrochlorothiazide	37.5 mg; 25 mg	White and Clear	Capsule		Duramed Pharmaceuticals
DPI; 625	Estropipate	0.75 mg	Light Orange	Tablet	Diamond, Scored	Duramed Pharmaceuticals
DPI; 644	Acetaminophen and Oxycodone	5 mg; 500 mg	Red and White	Capsule		Duramed Pharmaceuticals
DPI; 658	Acetaminophen and Oxycodone	5 mg; 500 mg	Red and White	Capsule		Duramed Pharmaceuticals
DPI; 855	Pseudoephderine and Guaifenesin	120 mg; 250 mg	White and Clear	Timed-Release Capsule		Duramed Pharmaceuticals
DPI; 856	Pseudoephedrine and Guaifenesin	60 mg; 300 mg	Blue and Clear	Timed-Release Capsule		Duramed Pharmaceuticals
DQSP	Vicks Dayquil Sinus Pressure & Pain Relief	500 mg; 30 mg	Red	Tablet		Procter & Gamble
DRISTAN ALLERGY	Dristan Allergy	60 mg; 4 mg	Green	Tablet		Whitehall Laboratories
DRISTAN COLD	Dristan Cold Multi-Symptom	500 mg; 30 mg; 2 mg	White and Red	Capsule, Liquid Filled	Oblong	Whitehall Laboratories
DRISTAN COLD ND	Dristan Cold NO-Drowsiness	500 mg; 30 mg	Yellow	Tablet	Oblong	Whitehall Laboratories
DRISTAN SINUS	Dristan Sinus	200 mg; 30 mg	White	Tablet	Oval	Whitehall Laboratories
DRISTAN; COLD; ND	Dristan Cold NO Drowsiness Formula	500 mg; 30 mg	Brick Red and Yellow	Capsule, Liquid Filled		Wyeth Consumer Healthcare
DRISTAN; ULTRA	Dristan Ultra Colds Formula	500 mg; 30 mg; 15 mg; 2 mg	Orange and White	Capsule		Whitehall-Robins Healthcare
DRIXORAL	Drixoral Cold & Allergy	120 mg; 6 mg	Polished Dark Green	Extended-Release Tablet	Circle	Schering-Plough Healthcare Products
DRIXORAL ;	Drixoral	6 mg; 120 mg	Green	Coated Tablet		Schering-Plough Healthcare Products
DRIXORAL A/S	Drixoral Allergy Sinus	3 mg; 60 mg; 500 mg	Bright Yellow	Sustained-Release Tablet	Oblong	Schering-Plough Healthcare Products
DRIXORAL C+F	Drixoral Cold & Flu	60 mg; 3 mg; 500 mg	Green	Sustained-Release Tablet	Oval	Schering-Plough Healthcare Products
DRIXORAL COUGH	Drixoral Cough	30 mg	Purple	Capsule	Oval	Schering-Plough Healthcare Products

IMPRINT	BRAND/GENERIC NAME	STRENGTH	COLOR	FORM	SHAPE	MANUFACTURER
DRIXORAL; C&C	Drixoral Cough & Congestion	30 mg; 60 mg	Red	Capsule	Oval	Schering-Plough Healthcare Products
DRIXORAL; C&ST	Drixoral Cough & Sore Throat	325 mg; 15 mg	Blue	Capsule	Oval	Schering-Plough Healthcare Products
DRIXORAL; NDF	Drixoral Non-Drowsy	120 mg	Polished Blue	Sustained-Release Tablet	Circle	Schering-Plough Healthcare Products
DRIXORAL; PLUS	Drixoral Plus	500 mg; 3 mg; 60 mg	Green	Sustained-Release Tablet		Schering-Plough Healthcare Products
DRL; 50; 1	Nefazodone Hydrochloride	50 mg	White	Tablet	Oval	Par Pharmaceutical
DRL; 100; 2	Nefazodone Hydrochloride	100 mg	White	Tablet	Oval	Par Pharmaceutical
DRL; 150; 3	Nefazodone Hydrochloride	150 mg	White	Tablet	Oval	Par Pharmaceutical
DRL; 200; 4	Nefazodone Hydrochloride	200 mg	White	Tablet	Oval	Par Pharmaceutical
DRL; 250; 5	Nefazodone Hydrochloride	250 mg	White	Tablet	Oval	Par Pharmaceutical
DROXIA; 6335	Droxia	200 mg	Blue-Green	Capsule		Bristol-Myers Squibb
DROXIA; 6336	Droxia	300 mg	Purple	Capsule		Bristol-Myers Squibb
DROXIA; 6337	Droxia	400 mg	Red-Orange	Capsule		Bristol-Myers Squibb
DS	Yaz - Pink Tablet	3 mg; 0.02 mg	Light Pink	Tablet	Circle	Berlex Laboratories
DT	Detrol	2 mg	White	Tablet	Circle	Pharmacia & Upjohn
DT; I	Pec-Dec	60 mg	Light Brown	Tablet	Circle	Glaxosmithkline
DUPONT; 1 1 ;	Revia	50 mg	Pale Yellow	Coated Tablet	Capsule-Shape, Scored	Bristol-Myers Squibb
DUPONT; TREXAN	Trexan	50 mg	White	Tablet	Circle, Scored	Bristol-Myers Squibb
DUPONT; VALPIN	Valpin 50	50 mg	Beige	Tablet		Bristol-Myers Squibb
DURA; 009	Fenesin	600 mg	Light Blue	Tablet		Biovail Pharmaceuticals
DURA; 015	Guai-Vent/pse	600 mg; 120 mg	White	Sustained-Release Tablet		Biovail Pharmaceuticals
DURA; CHEW	D.A. Chewable	2 mg; 1.25 mg; 10 mg	Orange	Tablet, Chewable		Biovail Pharmaceuticals
DURA; DA	Dura-Vent/da	8 mg; 2.5 mg; 20 mg	Light Brown	Tablet		Biovail Pharmaceuticals
DURA; DA II	D.A. II	4 mg; 10 mg; 1.25 mg	White	Extended-Release Tablet	Capsule-Shape	Biovail Pharmaceuticals
DURA; FDM; 014	Fenesin DM	600 mg; 30 mg	Dark Blue	Tablet		Biovail Pharmaceuticals
DURACT	Duract	25 mg	Opaque Light Yellow Body and Opaque Red Cap with 2 Blue Bands	Capsule		Wyeth-Ayerst Laboratories
DURATION	Duration 12-Hour	120 mg	Blue	Tablet	Circle	Schering-Plough Healthcare Products
DX 41	Diclofenac Sodium	100 mg	Pink	Tablet, Extended Release	Circle	Watson Laboratories
DX; 2; G	Doxazosin Mesylate	2 mg	White	Tablet	Capsule-Shape, Scored	Par Pharmaceutical
DX; 4; G	Doxazosin Mesylate	4 mg	White	Tablet	Capsule-Shape, Scored	Par Pharmaceutical
DX; 8; G	Doxazosin Mesylate	8 mg	White	Tablet	Capsule-Shape, Scored	Par Pharmaceutical
DX1; G	Doxazosin Mesylate	1 mg	White	Tablet	Circle	Par Pharmaceutical
DYAZIDE; SB	Dyazide	25 mg; 37.5 mg	Red and White	Capsule		Glaxosmithkline
DYFLEX; 400	Dyflex	400 mg	White	Tablet	Circle, Concave, Scored	Teva Pharmaceuticals
DYNACIRC CR; 5	Dynacirc Cr	5 mg	Light Pink	Timed-Release Tablet	Circle, Biconvex	Sandoz
DYNACIRC CR; 10	Dynacirc Cr	10 mg	Beige	Timed-Release Tablet	Circle, Biconvex	Sandoz
DYNACIRC; 2.5; S	Dynacirc	2.5 mg	White	Capsule		Novartis Pharmaceuticals
DYNACIRC; 5; S	Dynacirc	5 mg	Light Pink	Capsule		Novartis Pharmaceuticals
DYNACIRCCR 5	Dynacirc Cr	5 mg	Light Pink	Tablet	Circle	Reliant Pharmaceuticals
DYNACIRCCR 10	Dynacirc Cr	10 mg	Beige	Tablet	Circle	Reliant Pharmaceuticals
DYRENIUM; SKF; 50	Dyrenium	50 mg	Opaque Red	Capsule		Glaxosmithkline
DYRENIUM; SKF; 100	Dyrenium	100 mg	Opaque Red	Capsule		Glaxosmithkline
E	Excedrin Extra Strength	250 mg; 250 mg; 65 mg	White	Tablet		Bristol-Myers Squibb
E	Excedrin Migraine	250 mg; 250 mg; 65 mg	White	Caplet		Bristol-Myers Squibb
E ; 1	Enjuvia	0.3 mg	White	Tablet	Oval	Duramed Pharmaceuticals
E ; 2	Enjuvia	0.45 mg	Mauve	Tablet	Oval	Duramed Pharmaceuticals
E ; 3	Enjuvia	0.625 mg	Pink	Tablet	Oval	Duramed Pharmaceuticals
E ; 4	Enjuvia	1.25 mg	Yellow	Tablet	Oval	Duramed Pharmaceuticals
E 123	Cilostazol	50 mg	White	Tablet	Circle	Sandoz
E 193	Zonisamide	25 mg	Light Gray Opaque, Reddish Orange Opaque	Capsule		Sandoz
E 195	Alprazolam	0.5 mg	White	Tablet, Extended Release	Circle	Sandoz
E 196	Alprazolam	1 mg	Yellow	Tablet, Extended Release	Capsule-Shape	Sandoz
E 197	Alprazolam	2 mg	Blue	Tablet, Extended Release	Capsule-Shape	Sandoz
E 198	Alprazolam	3 mg	Green	Tablet, Extended Release	Circle	Sandoz
E 199	Zonisamide	50 mg	Light Gray Opaque	Capsule		Sandoz
E 200	Zonisamide	100 mg	Reddish Orange Opaque	Capsule		Sandoz
E 223	Cilostazol	100 mg	White	Tablet	Circle	Sandoz
E; 5	Zydone 5/400	5 mg; 400 mg	Yellow	Tablet	Eight-Sided, Elongated, Convex	Endo Laboratories
E; 7.5	Zydone 7.5/400	7.5 mg; 400 mg	Blue	Tablet	Eight-Sided, Elongated, Convex	Endo Laboratories
E; 10	Zydone 10/400	10 mg; 400 mg	Red	Tablet	Eight-Sided, Elongated, Convex	Endo Laboratories
E; 32 ;	Reserpine	0.1 mg	White	Tablet	Circle, Scored, Compressed	Novartis Generics
E; 121	Captopril	12.5 mg	White	Tablet	Circle, Scored	Par Pharmaceutical
E; 122	Captopril	25 mg	White	Tablet	Round, Quadrisected Scored	Par Pharmaceutical
E; 123	Captopril	50 mg	White	Tablet	Circle, Scored	Par Pharmaceutical
E; 124	Captopril	100 mg	White	Tablet	Circle, Scored	Par Pharmaceutical
E; 134 ;	Reserpine	0.25 mg	White	Tablet	Circle, Scored, Compressed	Novartis Generics

IMPRINT	BRAND/GENERIC NAME	STRENGTH	COLOR	FORM	SHAPE	MANUFACTURER
E; 220 ;	Urinary Antiseptic No. 2	0.03 mg; 4.5 mg; 40.8 mg; 18.1 mg; 5.4 mg; 0.03 mg	Dark Blue	Coated Tablet	Circle	Geneva Generics
E; 613 ;	Hydroxyzine Pamoate	25 mg	Light Green and Dark Green	Capsule		Novartis Generics
E; 615 ;	Hydroxyzine Pamoate	50 mg	Dark Green and White	Capsule		Novartis Generics
E; 652; 15	Morphine Sulfate ER	15 mg	Blue	Extended-Release Tablet	Circle	Endo Laboratories
E; 653; 30	Morphine Sulfate ER	30 mg	Green	Extended-Release Tablet	Circle	Endo Laboratories
E; 655; 60	Morphine Sulfate ER	60 mg	Orange	Extended-Release Tablet	Capsule-Shape	Endo Laboratories
E; 658; 100	Morphine Sulfate ER	100 mg	Blue	Extended-Release Tablet	Capsule-Shape	Endo Laboratories
E; 659; 200	Morphine Sulfate ER	200 mg	Green	Extended-Release Tablet	Oval	Endo Laboratories
E; 660	Oxycodone and Acetaminophen	5 mg; 500 mg	Red-Orange	Capsule		Endo Laboratories
E; 675	Aspirin, Butalbital, Caffeine and Codeine	325 mg; 50 mg; 40 mg; 30 mg	Yellow and Blue	Capsule		Endo Laboratories
E; 700; 7.5/325	Endocet	325 mg; 7.5 mg	Peach	Tablet	Capsule-Shape	Endo Laboratories
E; 712; 10/325	Endocet	325 mg; 10 mg	Yellow	Tablet	Oval	Endo Laboratories
E; 796; 7.5	Endocet	500 mg; 7.5 mg	Peach	Tablet	Capsule-Shape	Endo Laboratories
E; 797; 10	Endocet	650 mg; 10 mg	Yellow	Tablet	Oval, Large	Endo Laboratories
E; 5000 ;	Phentermine Hydrochloride Blue/ clear	30 mg	Blue and Clear	Capsule		Novartis Generics
E; 5380 ;	Contrin	0.5 mg; 110 mg; 240 mg; 15 mcg; 75 mg	Maroon and Red	Capsule		Novartis Generics
E1 07 ;	Gabapentin	600 mg	Yellow	Tablet	Oval	Sandoz
E1 13 ;	Gabapentin	800 mg	Yellow	Tablet	Oval	Sandoz
E50	Etoposide	50 mg	Dark Pink with Black Ink	Capsule	Oblong	Mylan Pharmaceuticals
E612 5	Opana	5 mg	Blue	Tablet	Circle	Endo Pharmaceuticals
E613 10	Opana	10 mg	Red	Tablet	Circle	Endo Pharmaceuticals
E617 20	Opana ER	20 mg	Light Green	Tablet, Extended Release	Eight-Sided	Endo Pharmaceuticals
E674 10	Opana ER	10 mg	Light Orange	Tablet, Extended Release	Eight-Sided	Endo Pharmaceuticals
E693 40	Opana ER	40 mg	Yellow	Tablet, Extended Release	Eight-Sided	Endo Pharmaceuticals
E702 ; 10	Oxycodone Hydrochloride	10 mg	White	Tablet, Extended Release	Circle	Endo Generics
E703 ; 20	Oxycodone Hydrochloride	20 mg	Pink	Tablet, Extended Release	Circle	Endo Generics
E705 ; 40	Oxycodone Hydrochloride	40 mg	Yellow	Tablet, Extended Release	Circle	Endo Generics
E710 ; 80	Oxycodone Hydrochloride	80 mg	Green	Tablet, Extended Release	Circle	Endo Generics
E814	Doxycycline Hyclate	75 mg	Dark Green Opaque, Green Transparent	Capsule, Delayed Release		Sandoz
E815	Doxycycline Hyclate	100 mg	Green Transparent, Light Green Opaque	Capsule, Delayed Release		Sandoz
E907 5	Opana ER	5 mg	Pink	Tablet, Extended Release	Eight-Sided	Endo Pharmaceuticals
EA	Erythromycin	500 mg	Pink	Coated Tablet	Capsule-Shape	Abbott Laboratories
EATON; 036	Furadantin	50 mg	Yellow	Tablet		Procter & Gamble Pharmaceuticals
EB; ABBOTT LOGO	Erythromycin	250 mg	Pink	Coated Tablet	Capsule-Shape	Abbott Laboratories
EC-NAPROSYN; 375	Ec-Naprosyn	375 mg	White	Delayed-Release Tablet	Capsule-Shape	Roche Laboratories
EC-NAPROSYN; 500	Ec-Naprosyn	500 mg	White	Delayed-Release Tablet	Capsule-Shape	Roche Laboratories
ECOTRIN MAX	Ecotrin	500 mg	Orange	Enteric-Coated Tablet	Circle	Glaxosmithkline Consumer
ECOTRIN REG	Ecotrin	325 mg	Orange	Tablet		Glaxosmithkline Consumer
ECOTRIN; LOW	Ecotrin Adult Low Strength	81 mg	Orange	Enteric-Coated Tablet		Glaxosmithkline Consumer
ECOTRIN; REG	Ecotrin	325 mg	Orange	Tablet	Circle	Glaxosmithkline Consumer
ED; A	Ery-Tab	500 mg	Pink	Enteric-Coated Tablet		Abbott Laboratories
E-DUAL	Excedrin Dual Aspirin Free	500 mg	Pink	Tablet		Bristol-Myers Squibb
EF	E.E.S.	200 mg	White	Tablet, Chewable	Circle, Scored	Abbott Laboratories
EK; ABBOTT LOGO	Pce Dispertab	500 mg	White	Tablet	Oval	Abbott Laboratories
ELAVIL; 40	Elavil	10 mg	Blue	Coated Tablet	Circle	Astra Zeneca
ELAVIL; 41	Elavil	50 mg	Beige	Coated Tablet	Circle	Astra Zeneca
ELAVIL; 42	Elavil	75 mg	Orange	Coated Tablet	Circle	Astra Zeneca
ELAVIL; 43	Elavil	100 mg	Mauve	Coated Tablet	Circle	Astra Zeneca
ELAVIL; 45	Elavil	25 mg	Yellow	Coated Tablet	Circle	Astra Zeneca
ELAVIL; 47	Elavil	150 mg	Blue	Coated Tablet	Capsule-Shape	Astra Zeneca
ELN; 30	Afeditab Cr	30 mg	Brick Red	Extended-Release Tablet	Circle	Watson Laboratories
ELN; 30	Nifedipine	30 mg	Red-Brown	Extended-Release Tablet	Circle	Teva Pharmaceuticals
ELN; 30	Nifedipine	30 mg	Red-Brown	Extended-Release Tablet	Circle	Watson Laboratories
ELN; 60	Afeditab Cr	60 mg	Brick Red	Extended-Release Tablet	Circle	Watson Laboratories
ELN; 60	Nifedipine ER	60 mg	Red-Brown	Extended-Release Tablet	Circle	Watson Laboratories
EM	Dyflex 200	200 mg	White	Tablet	Circle, Concave, Scored	Teva Pharmaceuticals
EM; SP	Estinyl	0.05 mg	Pink	Coated Tablet		Schering
EMCYT; PHARMACIA; 132	Emcyt	140 mg	White	Capsule		Pharmacia & Upjohn
EMPIRIN; 3	Empirin with Codeine No. 3	30 mg; 325 mg	White	Tablet		Glaxosmithkline
EMPIRIN; 4	Empirin with Codeine No. 4	60 mg; 325 mg	White	Tablet		Glaxosmithkline
E-MYCIN; 250 MG	E-Mycin	250 mg	Orange	Timed-Release Tablet	Circle	Pharmacia & Upjohn
E-MYCIN; 333 MG	E-Mycin	333 mg	White	Timed-Release Tablet	Circle	Pharmacia & Upjohn
EN; 2.5; G	Enalapril Maleate	2.5 mg	White	Tablet	Circle	Par Pharmaceutical
EN; 5; G; G	Enalapril Maleate	5 mg	White	Tablet	Oval	Par Pharmaceutical
EN; 10; G	Enalapril Maleate	10 mg	Rusty Red	Tablet	Oval	Par Pharmaceutical
EN; 20; G	Enalapril Maleate	20 mg	Peach	Tablet	Oval	Par Pharmaceutical
ENDEP; 50; ROCHE	Endep	50 mg	Orange	Coated Tablet	Circle, Scored	Roche Laboratories
ENDEP; 75; ROCHE	Endep	75 mg	Yellow	Coated Tablet	Circle, Scored	Roche Laboratories

IMPRINT	BRAND/GENERIC NAME	STRENGTH	COLOR	FORM	SHAPE	MANUFACTURER
ENDO	Selegiline	5 mg	White	Tablet	Oblong	Endo Laboratories
ENDO 610	Endodan	4.8355 mg; 325 mg	Yellow	Tablet	Circle	Endo Pharmaceuticals
ENDO; 048	Hycomine Compound	250 mg; 2 mg; 10 mg; 5 mg; 30 mg	Pink	Tablet	Circle, Scored	Endo Laboratories
ENDO; 051	Remsed	50 mg	Light Blue	Tablet		Dupont Merck
ENDO; 501	Azene	3.25 mg	Tan	Capsule		Endo Laboratories
ENDO; 502	Clorazepate	6.5 mg	Orange	Capsule		Endo Laboratories
ENDO; 503	Azene	13 mg	Blue	Capsule		Endo Laboratories
ENDO; 570	Percobarb	4.5 mg; 0.38 mg; 100 mg; 224 mg; 160 mg; 32 mg	Blue and Yellow	Capsule		Endo Laboratories
ENDO; 602	Oxycodone and Acetaminophen	5 mg; 325 mg	White	Tablet		Endo Laboratories
ENDO; 603	Carbidopa and Levodopa	10 mg; 100 mg	Dark Dapple-Blue	Tablet	Oval, Scored	Endo Laboratories
ENDO; 605	Carbidopa and Levodopa	25 mg; 100 mg	Yellow	Tablet	Oval, Scored	Endo Laboratories
ENDO; 607	Carbidopa and Levodopa	25 mg; 250 mg	Light Dapple-Blue	Tablet	Oval, Scored	Endo Laboratories
ENDO; 610	Endodan	4.5 mg; 0.38 mg; 325 mg	Yellow	Tablet		Endo Laboratories
ENDO; 630	Cimetidine	200 mg	White	Coated Tablet	Oval	Endo Laboratories
ENDO; 631	Cimetidine	300 mg	White	Coated Tablet	Oval	Endo Laboratories
ENDO; 633	Cimetidine	800 mg	White	Coated Tablet	Oval	Endo Laboratories
ENDO; 714	Glipizide	10 mg	White	Tablet	Circle, Scored	Endo Laboratories
ENDO; 731	Captopril and Hydrochlorothiazide	50 mg; 25 mg	Peach	Tablet	Round, Bisected on One Side Scored	Endo Laboratories
ENDO; 733	Captopril and Hydrochlorothiazide	25 mg; 15 mg	White	Tablet	Round, Quadrisected on One Side Scored	Endo Laboratories
ENDO; 739	Captopril and Hydrochlorothiazide	50 mg; 15 mg	White	Tablet	Round, Bisected on One Side Scored	Endo Laboratories
ENDO; 741	Captopril and Hydrochlorothiazide	25 mg; 25 mg	Peach	Tablet	Round, Quadrisected on One Side Scored	Endo Laboratories
ENDO; 744	Etodolac	400 mg	Pale Yellow	Tablet	Oval	Bristol-Myers Squibb
ENDURON	Enduron	2.5 mg	Orange	Tablet	Square, Scored	Abbott Laboratories
ENDURON	Enduron	5 mg	Salmon	Tablet	Square, Scored	Abbott Laboratories
ENTEX PSE; 032 032	Entex Pse	600 mg; 120 mg	Yellow	Sustained-Release Tablet	Oval, Elongated, Scored	Andrx Pharmaceuticals
ENTEX; ER; 334	Entex ER	300 mg; 10 mg		Extended-Release Tablet		Andrx Pharmaceuticals
ENTOLASE; AHR	Entolase	25,000 USP units; 20,000 USP units; 4000 USP units		Capsule		Wyeth Pharmaceuticals
ENTOLASE-HP; AHR	Entolase-Hp	40,000 USP units; 8000 USP units; 50,000 USP units		Capsule		Wyeth Pharmaceuticals
EPI; 132	Percolone	5 mg	White	Tablet	Round, Biconvex, Bisected, Debossed Scored	Endo Laboratories
EPITOL; 93; 93	Epitol	200 mg	White	Tablet	Circle, Scored, Flat	Teva Pharmaceuticals
EPITOL; 93; 758	Epitol	100 mg	Pink with Red Speckles	Tablet, Chewable	Circle, Flat, Beveled Edge, Scored	Teva Pharmaceuticals
ER; ABBOTT LOGO	Erythromycin Delayed-Release	250 mg	Clear and Maroon with Pink and Yellow Particles	Capsule		Abbott Laboratories
ER; SP	Estinyl	0.02 mg	Beige	Coated Tablet		Schering
ES	Erythrocin Stearate Filmtab	250 mg	Pink	Coated Tablet	Circle	Abbott Laboratories
ES ;	Excedrin Sinus	500 mg; 30 mg	Orange	Tablet	Capsule-Shape	Bristol-Myers Squibb
ESB	Bufferin Extra Strength	500 mg; 222.3 mg; 88.9 mg; 55.6 mg	White	Coated Tablet	Oval	Bristol-Myers Squibb
ESKALITH; SB	Eskalith	300 mg	Gray, Yellow	Capsule		Glaxosmithkline
ESR; 1174; MARION	Gaviscon	160 mg; 105 mg	White	Tablet, Chewable	Circle	Glaxosmithkline Consumer
ESTRADIOL 0.025 MG/DAY (ONCE WEEKLY)	Estradiol	0.025 mg/24 Hr	Peach	Patch, Extended Release	Circle	Mylan Pharmaceuticals
ESTRADIOL 0.0375 MG/DAY (ONCE WEEKLY)	Estradiol	0.0375 mg/24 Hr	Peach	Patch, Extended Release	Circle	Mylan Pharmaceuticals
ESTRADIOL 0.05 MG/DAY (ONCE WEEKLY)	Estradiol	0.05 mg/24 Hr	Peach	Patch, Extended Release	Circle	Mylan Pharmaceuticals
ESTRADIOL 0.06 MG/DAY (ONCE WEEKLY)	Estradiol	0.06 mg/24 Hr	Peach	Patch, Extended Release	Circle	Mylan Pharmaceuticals
ESTRADIOL 0.075 MG/DAY (ONCE WEEKLY)	Estradiol	0.075 mg/24 Hr	Peach	Patch, Extended Release	Circle	Mylan Pharmaceuticals
ESTRADIOL 0.1 MG/ DAY (ONCE WEEKLY)	Estradiol	0.1 mg/24 Hr	Peach	Patch, Extended Release	Circle	Mylan Pharmaceuticals
ET	Erythrocin Stearate Filmtab	500 mg	Pink	Coated Tablet	Oblong	Abbott Laboratories
ETH	Excedrin Tension Headache	500 mg; 65 mg	Red	Tablet	Circle	Novartis Consumer Health
ETO 300	Etodolac	300 mg	Pink	Capsule		Taro Pharmaceuticals
ETP 200	Etodolac	200 mg	Dark Pink	Capsule		Taro Pharmaceuticals
EVOXAC; 30 MG	Evoxac	30 mg	White	Capsule		Daiichi Sankyo
EXCEDRIN	Excedrin Tri-Buffered Arthritis Strength	500 mg	White	Tablet		Bristol-Myers Squibb
EXCEDRIN IB	Excedrin Ib Caplet	200 mg	White	Tablet		Bristol-Myers Squibb
EXCEDRIN IB	Excedrin Ib Tablet	200 mg	White	Tablet	Circle	Bristol-Myers Squibb
EXCEDRIN PM	Excedrin Pm Aspirin Free Caplet	500 mg; 38 mg	Light Blue	Tablet		Bristol-Myers Squibb
EXCEDRIN PM	Excedrin Pm Aspirin Free Tablet	500 mg; 38 mg	Light Blue	Tablet	Circle	Bristol-Myers Products
EXCEDRIN; AF	Aspirin Free Excedrin Extra Strength Geltab	500 mg; 65 mg	Red	Geltab	Capsule-Shape	Bristol-Myers Squibb

IMPRINT	BRAND/GENERIC NAME	STRENGTH	COLOR	FORM	SHAPE	MANUFACTURER
EXELON 1.5 MG	Exelon	1.5 mg	Yellow	Capsule		Novartis
EXELON 3 MG	Exelon	3 mg	Orange	Capsule		Novartis
EXELON 4.5 MG	Exelon	4.5 mg	Red	Capsule		Novartis
EXELON 6 MG	Exelon	6 mg	Orange, Red	Capsule		Novartis
EX-LAX	Ex-Lax	100 mg	Green	Tablet	Oblong	Sandoz Consumer
F; 66; LL	Fibercon	500 mg	Clear	Coated Tablet		Lederle Laboratories
F2F	Actifed Plus Extra Strength	500 mg; 60 mg; 2.5 mg	White	Tablet		Pfizer Consumer Health Care
FAMVIR; 125	Famvir	125 mg	White	Coated Tablet	Circle	Novartis
FAMVIR; 250	Famvir	250 mg	White	Coated Tablet	Circle	Novartis
FAMVIR; 500	Famvir	500 mg	White	Coated Tablet	Oval	Novartis
FANSIDAR; ROCHE	Fansidar	25 mg; 500 mg	White	Tablet	Circle, Scored	Roche Laboratories
FASTIN; BEECHAM	Fastin	30 mg	Blue and Clear with Blue and White Beads	Capsule		Glaxosmithkline
FC; 50; G	Flecainide Acetate	50 mg	White	Tablet	Circle	Par Pharmaceutical
FC; 100; G	Flecainide Acetate	100 mg	White	Tablet	Circle, Scored	Par Pharmaceutical
FC; 150; G	Flecainide Acetate	150 mg	White	Tablet	Oval, Scored	Par Pharmaceutical
FE	Feratab	300 mg	Red	Tablet	Circle	Upsher-Smith Laboratories
FE	Ferrous Gluconate	300 mg	Green	Coated Tablet	Circle	Upsher-Smith Laboratories
FEEN-A-MINT	Feen-A-Mint	5 mg	White	Enteric-Coated Tablet	Circle	Schering-Plough Healthcare Products
FELDENE; PFIZER 322	Feldene	10 mg	Maroon and Blue	Capsule		Pfizer Laboratories
FELDENE; PFIZER 323	Feldene	20 mg	Maroon	Capsule		Pfizer Laboratories
FEOSOL	Feosol	159 mg		Extended-Release Capsule		Glaxosmithkline Consumer
FIORICET WATSON ;	Fioricet	50 mg; 40 mg; 325 mg	Light Blue	Tablet	Circle	Watson Laboratories
FIORICET; CODEINE; FOUR-HEAD PROFILE	Fioricet with Codeine	30 mg; 50 mg; 40 mg; 325 mg	Dark Blue and Gray	Capsule		Watson Laboratories
FIORINAL CODEINE; WATSON 956	Fiorinal with Codeine	30 mg; 50 mg; 40 mg; 325 mg	Blue, Yellow	Capsule		Watson Laboratories
FIORINAL; 78; 103	Fiorinal	325 mg; 50 mg; 40 mg	Kelly Green and Lime Green	Capsule		Watson Laboratories
FL ; 5 ;	Lexapro	5 mg	White to Off White	Tablet	Circle	Forest Pharmaceuticals
FL ; 5 ;	Namenda	5 mg	Tan	Tablet	Capsule-Shape	Forest Pharmaceuticals
FL ; 10 ;	Lexapro	10 mg	White to Off White	Tablet	Circle	Forest Pharmaceuticals
FL ; 10 ;	Namenda	10 mg	Gray	Tablet	Capsule-Shape	Forest Pharmaceuticals
FL ; 20 ;	Lexapro	20 mg	White to Off White	Tablet	Circle	Forest Pharmaceuticals
FL; 10; G	Fluoxetine Hydrochloride	10 mg	White	Tablet	Oval	Par Pharmaceutical
FL; 20; G	Fluoxetine Hydrochloride	20 mg	White	Tablet	Oval	Par Pharmaceutical
FL; 1033	Spastrin	40 mg; 0.6 mg; 0.2 mg	Blue	Tablet	Circle, Scored	Novartis Generics
FLAGYL; 375	Flagyl 375	375 mg	Grey and Green	Capsule	Oblong	Searle
FLAGYL; 500	Flagyl	500 mg	Blue	Coated Tablet	Oblong	Searle
FLOMAX 0.4 MG ; BI 58	Flomax	0.4 mg	Olive Green Opaque Cap and Orange Opaque Body	Capsule		Boehringer Ingelheim Pharmaceuticals
FLOXIN; 200 MG	Floxin	200 mg	Pale Yellow	Coated Tablet		Ortho-Mcneil Pharmaceutical
FLOXIN; 300 MG	Floxin	300 mg	White	Coated Tablet		Ortho-Mcneil Pharmaceutical
FLOXIN; 400 MG	Floxin	400 mg	Pale Gold	Coated Tablet		Ortho-Mcneil Pharmaceutical
FLUMADINE 100; FOREST	Flumadine	100 mg	Orange	Coated Tablet	Oval	Forest Pharmaceuticals
FLUOXETINE; R; 149	Fluoxetine Hydrochloride	40 mg	White	Capsule		Par Pharmaceutical
FOREST; 0372; ESGIC PLUS	Esgic-Plus	500 mg; 50 mg; 40 mg	Red	Capsule		Forest Pharmaceuticals
FOREST; 372 ;	Feostat	100 mg	Brown	Tablet, Chewable	Circle	Forest Pharmaceuticals
FOREST; 610A	Bancap Hc	500 mg; 5 mg	Yellow and Orange	Capsule		Forest Pharmaceuticals
FOREST; 610A	Hydrocodone Bitartrate and Acetaminophen	5 mg; 500 mg	Orange and Yellow	Capsule		Forest Pharmaceuticals
FOREST; 642	Elixophyllin Df 100	100 mg	White	Gel/jelly		Forest Pharmaceuticals
FOREST; 643	Elixophyllin Df 200	200 mg	White	Capsule, Liquid Filled		Forest Pharmaceuticals
FOREST; 678	Esgic-Plus	50 mg; 500 mg; 40 mg	White	Tablet	Capsule-Shape, Scored	Forest Pharmaceuticals
FP ; 5400	Combunox	5 mg; 400 mg	Off White, White	Tablet	Capsule-Shape	Forest Pharmaceuticals
FP; 10 MG	Celexa	10 mg	Beige	Coated Tablet	Oval	Forest Pharmaceuticals
FP; 20 MG	Celexa	20 mg	Pink	Coated Tablet	Oval, Scored	Forest Pharmaceuticals
FP; 40 MG	Celexa	40 mg	White	Coated Tablet	Oval, Scored	Forest Pharmaceuticals
FULVICIN; P/G; 352	Fulvicin P/g	330 mg	White	Tablet	Oval, Compressed, Scored	Schering
FULVICIN; P/G; 654	Fulvicin P/g	165 mg	White	Tablet	Oval, Compressed, Scored	Schering
FV ; CG	Femara	2.5 mg	Dark Yellow	Tablet	Circle	Novartis
G	Geritol Extend	1250 IU; 130 mg; 150 mcg; 35 mg; 100 mg; 3333 IU; 15 mg; 15 IU; 200 IU; 70 mcg; 15 mg; 10 mg; 0.2 mg; 2 mcg; 1.4 mg; 2 mg; 80 mcg; 60 mg; 1.2 mg	Maroon	Tablet	Oblong	Glaxosmithkline Consumer
G ; 2442 ;	Budeprion SR	100 mg	Yellow	Tablet, Extended Release	Circle	Teva Pharmaceuticals
G ; 2444	Buproban	150 mg	Light Yellow	Tablet, Extended Release	Circle	Teva Pharmaceuticals
G ; FL 50	Fluconazole	50 mg	Pink	Tablet	Rectangle	Par Pharmaceutical

IMPRINT	BRAND/GENERIC NAME	STRENGTH	COLOR	FORM	SHAPE	MANUFACTURER
G ; FL 100	Fluconazole	100 mg	Pink	Tablet	Rectangle	Par Pharmaceutical
G ; FL 150	Fluconazole	150 mg	Pink	Tablet	Oval	Par Pharmaceutical
G ; FL 200 ;	Fluconazole	200 mg	Pink	Tablet	Rectangle	Par Pharmaceutical
G ; P1 ;	Paroxetine Hydrochloride	10 mg	White	Tablet	Circle	Andrx Pharmaceuticals
G ; P4 ;	Paroxetine Hydrochloride	40 mg	White	Tablet	Circle	Andrx Pharmaceuticals
G 11 ; MYLAN ;	Glimepiride	1 mg	White	Tablet	Oval	Mylan Pharmaceuticals
G 12 ; MYLAN ;	Glimepiride	2 mg	Yellow	Tablet	Oval	Mylan Pharmaceuticals
G 13 ; MYLAN ;	Glimepiride	4 mg	Peach	Tablet	Oval	Mylan Pharmaceuticals
G; 00; 30	Ranitidine Hydrochloride	150 mg	White	Tablet	Circle	Mylan Pharmaceuticals
G; 00; 53	Oxaprozin	600 mg	White	Tablet	Oval	Par Pharmaceutical
G; 0031	Ranitidine Hydrochloride	300 mg	White	Tablet	Capsule-Shape	Mylan Pharmaceuticals
G; 0034	Acyclovir	200 mg	Blue, Opaque	Capsule		Par Pharmaceutical
G; 0036	Acyclovir	400 mg	White	Tablet	Five-Sided	Par Pharmaceutical
G; 0037	Acyclovir	800 mg	Blue	Tablet	Oval	Par Pharmaceutical
G; 0041	Nicardipine Hydrochloride	20 mg	White and Blue	Capsule		Par Pharmaceutical
G; 0042	Nicardipine Hydrochloride	30 mg	Light Blue	Capsule		Par Pharmaceutical
G; 2	Genac	2.5 mg; 60 mg	White	Tablet	Circle	Ivax Pharmaceuticals
G; 25	Atenolol	25 mg	White	Tablet	Circle, Flat; Bevelled Edge; Scored	Par Pharmaceutical
G; 50; BAYER LOGO	Glucobay	50 mg	White to Brown Tinged	Tablet	Circle, Convex	Bayer Pharmaceutical
G; 100; BAYER LOGO	Glucobay	100 mg	White to Brown Tinged	Tablet	Circle, Convex, Scored	Bayer Pharmaceutical
G; 2444	Budeprion SR	150 mg	Light Yellow	Extended-Release Tablet	Circle	Teva Pharmaceuticals
G; 3327; 4	Methylprednisolone Acetate	4 mg	White	Tablet	Oval	Pharmacia & Upjohn
G; ET; 500	Etodolac	500 mg	Light Blue	Tablet	Oval	Par Pharmaceutical
G; FL; 10	Fluoxetine Hydrochloride	10 mg	Purple and Green	Capsule		Par Pharmaceutical
G; FL; 20	Fluoxetine Hydrochloride	20 mg	Purple and Green	Capsule		Par Pharmaceutical
G; GU; 1	Guanfacine Hydrochloride	1 mg	White	Tablet	Oval	Par Pharmaceutical
G; GU; 2	Guanfacine Hydrochloride	2 mg	White	Tablet	Oval	Par Pharmaceutical
G; S; 80	Sotalol Hydrochloride	80 mg	White	Tablet	Capsule-Shape	Par Pharmaceutical
G; S; 120	Sotalol Hydrochloride	120 mg	White	Tablet	Capsule-Shape	Par Pharmaceutical
G; S; 160	Sotalol Hydrochloride	160 mg	White	Tablet	Capsule-Shape	Par Pharmaceutical
G; S; 240	Sotalol Hydrochloride	240 mg	White	Tablet	Capsule-Shape	Par Pharmaceutical
G; SE; 5	Selegiline Hydrochloride	5 mg	White	Tablet	Circle	Par Pharmaceutical
G; T250	Ticlopidine Hydrochloride	250 mg	White to Off-White	Tablet	Oval	Par Pharmaceutical
GAL 8	Razadyne ER	8 mg	White Opaque	Capsule, Extended Release		Ortho-Mcneil Neurologics
GAL 16	Razadyne ER	16 mg	Pink Opaque	Capsule, Extended Release		Ortho-Mcneil Neurologics
GAL 24	Razadyne ER	24 mg	Caramel Opaque	Capsule, Extended Release		Ortho-Mcneil Neurologics
GANTANOL; ROCHE	Gantanol	0.5 G	Pale Green	Tablet	Circle, Scored	Roche Laboratories
GANTANOL-DS; ROCHE	Gantanol-DS	1 G	Light Orange	Tablet	Capsule-Shape, Scored	Roche Laboratories
GAS-X	Gas-X	80 mg	White	Tablet, Chewable		Novartis Consumer
GAS-X	Gas-X Extra Strength	125 mg		Tablet, Chewable		Novartis Consumer
GDC; 127	Antacid Extra Strength	750 mg	Multi	Tablet, Chewable		Ivax Pharmaceuticals
GEIGY ; 51 51	Lopressor	50 mg	Pink	Tablet	Capsule-Shape	Novartis
GEIGY ; 71 71	Lopressor	100 mg	Light Blue	Tablet	Capsule-Shape	Novartis
GEIGY GM	Lamprene	50 mg	Brown	Capsule	Oblong	Novartis
GEIGY; 14	Butazolidin	100 mg	Red	Coated Tablet	Circle	Novartis
GEIGY; 35 35	Lopressor HCT	25 mg; 50 mg	White and Blue	Tablet		Novartis
GEIGY; 44; BUTAZOLIDIN; 100 MG	Butazolidin	100 mg	Orange and White	Capsule		Novartis
GEIGY; 48	Pbz-SR	100 mg	Lavender	Extended-Release Tablet	Circle	Novartis
GEIGY; 111	Pbz	25 mg	White	Tablet	Circle, Scored	Novartis
GEIGY; 117	Pbz	50 mg	White	Tablet	Circle, Scored	Novartis
GEIGY; GM	Lamprene	100 mg	Brown	Capsule	Oblong	Novartis
GERITOL	Geritol Complete	45 mcg; 162 mg; 2 mg; 150 mcg; 100 mg; 15 mcg; 10 mg; 25 mcg; 125 mg; 400 IU; 60 mg; 1.7 mg; 2 mg; 6 mcg; 1.5 mg; 6000 IU; 15 mcg; 15 mg; 30 IU; 37.5 mg; 20 mg; 2.5 mg; 18 mg; 400 mcg; 15 mcg	Red	Coated Tablet	Oblong	Glaxosmithkline Consumer
GG ; 226	Lovastatin	20 mg	Blue	Tablet	Oval	Sandoz
GG ; 770	Lovastatin	10 mg	White	Tablet	Circle	Sandoz
GG ; 773	Lovastatin	40 mg	Green	Tablet	Oval	Sandoz
GG ; 993	Leflunomide	10 mg	White	Tablet	Circle	Sandoz
GG ; 994	Leflunomide	20 mg	White	Tablet	Circle	Sandoz
GG 181	Methazolamide	50 mg	White	Tablet	Circle	Sandoz
GG 202	Paroxetine Hydrochloride	20 mg	White	Tablet	Circle	Sandoz
GG 203	Paroxetine Hydrochloride	30 mg	White	Tablet	Circle	Sandoz
GG 288 ;	Cyclobenzaprine Hydrochloride	10 mg	Butterscotch	Tablet	Circle	Sandoz
GG 330 ; 137	Levothyroxine Sodium	0.137 mg	Turquoise	Tablet	Capsule-Shape	Sandoz
GG 331 ; 25	Levothyroxine Sodium	0.025 mg	Orange	Tablet	Capsule-Shape	Sandoz
GG 332 ; 50	Levothyroxine Sodium	0.05 mg	White	Tablet		Sandoz
GG 332 ; 50 ;	Levothyroxine Sodium	50 mcg	White	Tablet	Capsule-Shape	Sandoz
GG 333 ; 75	Levothyroxine Sodium	0.075 mg	Dark Blue	Tablet	Capsule-Shape	Sandoz
GG 334 ; 88	Levothyroxine Sodium	0.088 mg	Olive Green	Tablet	Capsule-Shape	Sandoz
GG 335 ; 100	Levothyroxine Sodium	0.1 mg	Yellow	Tablet	Capsule-Shape	Sandoz
GG 336 ; 112	Levothyroxine Sodium	0.112 mg	Rose	Tablet	Capsule-Shape	Sandoz

IMPRINT	BRAND/GENERIC NAME	STRENGTH	COLOR	FORM	SHAPE	MANUFACTURER
GG 337 ; 125	Levothyroxine Sodium	0.125 mg	Brown	Tablet	Capsule-Shape	Sandoz
GG 338 ; 150	Levothyroxine Sodium	0.15 mg	Blue	Tablet	Capsule-Shape	Sandoz
GG 339 ; 175	Levothyroxine Sodium	0.175 mg	Lilac	Tablet	Capsule-Shape	Sandoz
GG 340 ; 200	Levothyroxine Sodium	0.2 mg	Pink	Tablet	Capsule-Shape	Sandoz
GG 341 ; 300	Levothyroxine Sodium	0.3 mg	Green	Tablet	Capsule-Shape	Sandoz
GG 537 ;	Bromocriptine Mesylate	5 mg	White, Yellow	Capsule		Sandoz
GG 781	Paroxetine Hydrochloride	10 mg	White	Tablet	Circle	Sandoz
GG 793	Paroxetine Hydrochloride	40 mg	White	Tablet	Oval	Sandoz
GG 901	Bupropion Hydrochloride SR	150 mg	Brown	Tablet, Extended Release	Circle	Sandoz
GG D6	Azithromycin	250 mg	White	Tablet	Oval	Sandoz
GG D8	Azithromycin	500 mg	White	Tablet	Oval	Sandoz
GG; 3	Phenobarbital	15 mg	White	Tablet	Circle	Geneva Generics
GG; 4 ;	Lonox	0.025 mg; 2.5 mg	White	Tablet	Circle	Sandoz
GG; 9 ;	Dexamethasone	0.75 mg	Blue	Tablet	Five-Sided	Novartis Generics
GG; 11 ;	Chlorthalidone	25 mg	Yellow	Tablet	Circle	Novartis Generics
GG; 12	Medroxyprogesterone	10 mg	White	Tablet	Circle, Scored	Novartis Generics
GG; 13 ;	Chlorthalidone	50 mg	Green	Tablet	Circle, Scored	Novartis Generics
GG; 14 ;	Prednisolone	5 mg	Peach	Tablet	Circle, Scored	Novartis Generics
GG; 15	Nylidrin Hydrochloride	12 mg	White	Tablet	Circle	Geneva Generics
GG; 17	Chlorthalidone and Reserpine	50 mg; 0.25 mg		Tablet		Novartis Generics
GG; 18	Perphenazine	2 mg	White	Coated Tablet	Circle, Debossed	Geneva Generics
GG; 21 ;	Furosemide	20 mg	White	Tablet	Circle, Scored	Sandoz
GG; 22 ;	Pseudoephedrine Hydrochloride	60 mg	White	Tablet	Circle, Scored	Geneva Generics
GG; 23	T.E.P.	130 mg; 24.3 mg; 8.1 mg	White	Tablet	Circle	Novartis Generics
GG; 24 ;	T.E.H.	25 mg; 10 mg; 130 mg	White	Tablet	Circle, Scored; Compressed	Novartis Generics
GG; 26	Isdn	10 mg	White	Tablet	Circle, Scored, Debossed	Sandoz
GG; 27 ;	Hydrochlorothiazide	50 mg	Peach	Tablet	Circle, Scored	Novartis Generics
GG; 28 ;	Hydrochlorothiazide	25 mg	Peach	Tablet	Circle, Scored	Novartis Generics
GG; 29 ;	Triamcinolone	4 mg	White	Tablet	Capsule-Shape	Novartis Generics
GG; 30	Thioridazine Hydrochloride	10 mg	Orange	Coated Tablet	Circle	Geneva Generics
GG; 31; 15	Thioridazine Hydrochloride	15 mg	Orange	Coated Tablet	Circle	Geneva Generics
GG; 32; 25	Thioridazine Hydrochloride	25 mg	Orange	Coated Tablet	Circle	Geneva Generics
GG; 33; 50	Thioridazine Hydrochloride	50 mg	Orange	Coated Tablet	Circle	Geneva Generics
GG; 34; 100	Thioridazine Hydrochloride	100 mg	Orange	Coated Tablet	Circle	Geneva Generics
GG; 35	Thioridazine Hydrochloride	150 mg	Orange	Coated Tablet	Circle	Geneva Generics
GG; 36	Thioridazine Hydrochloride	200 mg	Orange	Coated Tablet	Circle	Geneva Generics
GG; 37	Hydroxyzine Hydrochloride	10 mg	Lavender	Coated Tablet		Novartis Generics
GG; 38	Hydroxyzine Hydrochloride	25 mg	Lavender	Coated Tablet	Circle	Novartis Generics
GG; 39	Hydroxyzine Hydrochloride	50 mg	Purple	Coated Tablet		Novartis Generics
GG; 40 ;	Amitriptyline Hydrochloride	10 mg	Pink with White Core	Coated Tablet	Circle	Sandoz
GG; 41	Imipramine Hydrochloride	10 mg	Yellow	Coated Tablet	Circle, Debossed	Sandoz
GG; 42	Imipramine Hydrochloride	50 mg	Green	Coated Tablet	Circle, Debossed	Sandoz
GG; 45 ;	Dipyridamole	50 mg	White	Coated Tablet	Circle	Novartis Generics
GG; 47	Imipramine Hydrochloride	25 mg	Beige	Coated Tablet	Circle, Debossed	Sandoz
GG; 48 ;	Pseudoephedrine Hydrochloride	30 mg	Red	Coated Tablet	Circle	Geneva Generics
GG; 49	Dipyridamole	25 mg	White	Coated Tablet	Circle	Novartis Generics
GG; 51; 1	Trifluoperazine Hydrochloride	1 mg	Lavender	Coated Tablet	Circle	Geneva Generics
GG; 53; 2	Trifluoperazine Hydrochloride	2 mg	Lavender	Coated Tablet	Circle	Geneva Generics
GG; 55; 5	Trifluoperazine Hydrochloride	5 mg	Lavender	Coated Tablet	Circle	Geneva Generics
GG; 56	Disopyramide Phosphate	100 mg	Opaque Orange	Capsule		Novartis Generics
GG; 57	Disopyramide Phosphate	150 mg		Capsule		Novartis Generics
GG; 58; 10	Trifluoperazine Hydrochloride	10 mg	Lavender	Coated Tablet	Circle	Geneva Generics
GG; 61	Chlorpropamide	100 mg	White	Tablet	Circle, Scored	Novartis Generics
GG; 62	Sodium Fluoride	2.2 mg	Pink	Tablet	Circle	Novartis Generics
GG; 63	Desipramine Hydrochloride	10 mg	White	Coated Tablet	Circle, Debossed	Sandoz
GG; 64	Desipramine Hydrochloride	25 mg	White	Coated Tablet	Circle, Debossed	Sandoz
GG; 65	Desipramine Hydrochloride	50 mg	White	Coated Tablet	Circle, Debossed	Sandoz
GG; 66	Diazepam	2 mg	White	Tablet	Circle, Scored	Novartis Generics
GG; 67	Diazepam	5 mg	Orange	Tablet	Circle, Scored	Novartis Generics
GG; 68	Diazepam	10 mg	Green	Tablet	Circle, Scored	Novartis Generics
GG; 70	Propranolol Hydrochloride	90 mg		Tablet		Novartis Generics
GG; 71	Propranolol Hydrochloride	10 mg	Peach Colored	Tablet	Circle, Scored	Novartis Generics
GG; 72	Propranolol Hydrochloride	20 mg	Blue	Tablet	Circle, Scored	Novartis Generics
GG; 73	Propranolol Hydrochloride	40 mg	Green	Tablet	Circle, Scored	Novartis Generics
GG; 74	Propranolol Hydrochloride	60 mg	Salmon Colored	Tablet	Circle, Scored	Novartis Generics
GG; 75	Propranolol Hydrochloride	80 mg	Yellow	Tablet	Circle, Scored	Novartis Generics
GG; 78	Methazolamide	25 mg	White	Tablet	Circle, Scored, Debossed	Sandoz
GG; 79	Prednisone	5 mg	White	Tablet	Circle, Scored	Novartis Generics
GG; 80	Furosemide	80 mg	White	Tablet	Circle, Scored, Beveled-Edge	Sandoz
GG; 81	Clonidine Hydrochloride	0.1 mg	Light Green	Tablet	Circle, Scored	Novartis Generics
GG; 82	Clonidine Hydrochloride	0.2 mg	Yellow	Tablet	Circle, Scored	Novartis Generics
GG; 83	Clonidine Hydrochloride	0.3 mg	Blue	Tablet	Circle, Scored	Novartis Generics
GG; 84	Timolol Maleate	5 mg	White	Tablet	Circle	Novartis Generics
GG; 85	Spironolactone	25 mg	White	Tablet	Circle, Scored, Debossed	Geneva Generics
GG; 86	Clonidine Hydrochloride and Chlorthalidone	15 mg; 0.1 mg		Tablet		Novartis Generics
GG; 87	Clonidine Hydrochloride and Chlorthalidone	15 mg; 0.2 mg		Tablet		Novartis Generics
GG; 88	Clonidine Hydrochloride and Chlorthalidone	15 mg; 0.3 mg		Tablet		Novartis Generics
GG; 91	Lorazepam	0.5 mg	White	Tablet	Circle	Sandoz
GG; 92	Lorazepam	1 mg	White	Tablet	Circle, Scored	Sandoz
GG; 93	Lorazepam	2 mg	White	Tablet	Circle, Scored	Sandoz
GG; 95	Spironolactone and Hydrochlorothiazide	25 mg; 25 mg	White	Coated Tablet	Circle, Scored	Geneva Generics
GG; 96	Clorazepate Dipotassium	3.75 mg	Blue	Tablet	Circle, Scored, Compressed	Novartis Generics

IMPRINT	BRAND/GENERIC NAME	STRENGTH	COLOR	FORM	SHAPE	MANUFACTURER
GG; 97	Fluphenazine Hydrochloride	1 mg	Rust	Coated Tablet	Circle	Sandoz
GG; 98	Clorazepate Dipotassium	7.5 mg	Peach	Tablet	Circle, Scored, Compressed	Novartis Generics
GG; 99	Clorazepate Dipotassium	15 mg	White	Tablet	Circle, Scored, Compressed	Novartis Generics
GG; 101 ;	Methocarbamol	750 mg	White	Tablet	Oblong	Novartis Generics
GG; 103 ;	Metronidazole	250 mg	White	Coated Tablet	Circle, Scored	Novartis Generics
GG; 104	Methyldopa	125 mg	White	Coated Tablet	Circle	Novartis Generics
GG; 105	Haloperidol	0.5 mg	White	Tablet	Circle, Partially Scored	Sandoz
GG; 107	Perphenazine	4 mg	White	Coated Tablet	Circle, Debossed	Geneva Generics
GG; 108	Perphenazine	8 mg	White	Coated Tablet	Circle, Debossed	Geneva Generics
GG; 109	Perphenazine	16 mg	White	Coated Tablet	Circle, Debossed	Geneva Generics
GG; 111	Methyldopa	250 mg	White	Coated Tablet	Circle	Novartis Generics
GG; 113	Metoclopramide Hydrochloride	10 mg	White	Tablet	Circle, Scored	Novartis Generics
GG; 119 ;	Butal Compound	50 mg; 325 mg; 40 mg	White	Tablet	Circle	Novartis Generics
GG; 122	Sulfasalazine	500 mg	Butterscotch	Tablet	Circle	Novartis Generics
GG; 123	Haloperidol	1 mg	Yellow	Tablet	Circle, Partially Scored	Sandoz
GG; 124	Haloperidol	2 mg	Pink	Tablet	Circle, Scored	Sandoz
GG; 125	Haloperidol	5 mg	Green	Tablet	Circle, Partially Scored	Sandoz
GG; 126	Haloperidol	10 mg	Light Green	Tablet	Circle, Scored	Sandoz
GG; 127	Quiphile	260 mg	White	Tablet	Circle	Novartis Generics
GG; 128	Oxazepam	10 mg		Tablet		Geneva Generics
GG; 129	Oxazepam	30 mg		Tablet		Geneva Generics
GG; 131	Oxazepam	15 mg		Tablet		Geneva Generics
GG; 132	Verapamil Hydrochloride	80 mg	White	Coated Tablet	Circle, Scored	Geneva Generics
GG; 133	Verapamil Hydrochloride	120 mg	White	Coated Tablet	Circle, Scored	Geneva Generics
GG; 134	Haloperidol	20 mg	Coral	Tablet	Circle, Scored	Sandoz
GG; 135	Clorazepate Dipotassium	11.25 mg		Sustained-Release Tablet		Novartis Generics
GG; 136	Clorazepate Dipotassium	22.5 mg		Sustained-Release Tablet		Novartis Generics
GG; 138 ;	Sulfamethoxazole	500 mg	Green	Tablet	Circle, Scored	Novartis Generics
GG; 139	Buspirone Hydrochloride	5 mg		Tablet		Novartis Generics
GG; 140	Buspirone Hydrochloride	10 mg		Tablet		Novartis Generics
GG; 141	Meclizine Hydrochloride Otc	12.5 mg	Blue	Tablet	Oval, Scored	Sandoz
GG; 141	Meclizine Hydrochloride RX	12.5 mg	Blue	Tablet	Oval, Scored	Sandoz
GG; 144	Chlorpropamide	250 mg	White	Tablet	Circle, Scored	Novartis Generics
GG; 145 ;	Dimenhydrinate	50 mg	Yellow	Tablet	Circle, Scored	Novartis Generics
GG; 146	Hydrochlorothiazide and Reserpine	50 mg; 0.125 mg		Tablet		Novartis Generics
GG; 150 ;	Meprobamate	400 mg	White	Tablet	Circle, Scored	Novartis Generics
GG; 153	Propranolol Hydrochloride and Hydrochlorothiazide	25 mg; 40 mg	White	Tablet	Circle, Scored	Novartis Generics
GG; 154	Propranolol Hydrochloride and Hydrochlorothiazide	80 mg; 25 mg	White	Tablet	Circle, Scored	Novartis Generics
GG; 155 ;	Prednisone	20 mg	Peach-Colored	Tablet	Circle, Scored	Novartis Generics
GG; 156	Prednisone	10 mg	White	Tablet	Circle	Novartis Generics
GG; 157	Prednisone	50 mg	White	Tablet	Circle, Scored	Novartis Generics
GG; 158 ;	Sulfisoxazole	500 mg	White	Tablet	Circle	Novartis Generics
GG; 159	Clemastine Fumarate	1.34 mg	White	Tablet	Capsule-Shape, Scored, Debossed	Sandoz
GG; 160	Clemastine Fumarate	2.68 mg	White	Tablet	Circle, Scored, Debossed	Sandoz
GG; 162	Triazolam	0.125 mg	White	Tablet		Geneva Generics
GG; 163	Triazolam	0.25 mg	Blue	Tablet		Geneva Generics
GG; 164	Triazolam	0.5 mg		Tablet		Geneva Generics
GG; 165	Triamterene and Hydrochlorothiazide	25 mg; 37.5 mg	Green	Tablet	Circle, Scored	Geneva Generics
GG; 166	Desipramine Hydrochloride	75 mg	White	Coated Tablet	Circle, Debossed	Sandoz
GG; 167	Desipramine Hydrochloride	100 mg	White	Coated Tablet	Circle, Debossed	Sandoz
GG; 168	Desipramine Hydrochloride	150 mg	White	Coated Tablet	Circle, Debossed	Sandoz
GG; 169	Verapamil Hydrochloride	40 mg	White	Coated Tablet	Circle	Geneva Generics
GG; 172	Triamterene and Hydrochlorothiazide	50 mg; 75 mg	Yellow	Tablet	Circle, Scored	Geneva Generics
GG; 173	Methotrexate	2.5 mg		Tablet		Novartis Generics
GG; 174	Sulfamethoxazole and Trimethoprim	400 mg; 80 mg	White	Tablet	Circle, Scored	Geneva Generics
GG; 175	Sulfamethoxazole and Trimethoprim	800 mg; 160 mg	White	Tablet	Oval	Geneva Generics
GG; 177	Captopril	25 mg		Tablet		Novartis Generics
GG; 178	Captopril	50 mg		Tablet		Novartis Generics
GG; 179	Captopril	100 mg		Tablet		Novartis Generics
GG; 182	Timolol Maleate	10 mg	White	Tablet	Circle, Scored	Novartis Generics
GG; 183	Timolol Maleate	20 mg	Blue	Tablet	Circle, Scored	Novartis Generics
GG; 184	Oxybutynin Chloride	5 mg	Light Blue	Tablet	Round, Convex, Bisected Scored	Novartis Generics
GG; 186	Metaproterenol Sulfate	10 mg		Tablet		Novartis Generics
GG; 187	Metaproterenol Sulfate	20 mg		Tablet		Novartis Generics
GG; 188	Guanabenz Acetate	4 mg		Tablet		Novartis Generics
GG; 189	Guanabenz Acetate	8 mg		Tablet		Novartis Generics
GG; 190 ;	Methocarbamol	500 mg	White	Tablet	Circle, Scored	Novartis Generics
GG; 193	Naloxone and Pentazocine	0.5 mg; 50 mg		Tablet		Novartis Generics
GG; 194	Indapamide	2.5 mg		Tablet		Novartis Generics
GG; 195 ;	Metronidazole	500 mg	White	Coated Tablet	Oblong	Novartis Generics
GG; 201	Furosemide	40 mg	White	Tablet	Circle, Scored	Sandoz
GG; 204	Tolmetin Sodium	200 mg		Tablet		Novartis Generics
GG; 206	Captopril and Hydrochlorothiazide	25 mg; 15 mg		Tablet		Novartis Generics
GG; 207	Captopril and Hydrochlorothiazide	25 mg; 25 mg		Tablet		Novartis Generics
GG; 208	Captopril and Hydrochlorothiazide	50 mg; 15 mg		Tablet		Novartis Generics

IMPRINT	BRAND/GENERIC NAME	STRENGTH	COLOR	FORM	SHAPE	MANUFACTURER
GG; 209	Captopril and Hydrochlorothiazide	50 mg; 25 mg		Tablet		Novartis Generics
GG; 211	Bromocriptine Mesylate	2.5 mg	White	Tablet	Scored, Circle	Sandoz
GG; 213	Perphenazine and Amitriptyline Hydrochloride	10 mg; 2 mg	Blue	Coated Tablet	Circle, Debossed	Geneva Generics
GG; 214	Perphenazine and Amitriptyline Hydrochloride	25 mg; 2 mg	Orange	Coated Tablet	Circle, Debossed	Geneva Generics
GG; 215	Perphenazine and Amitriptyline Hydrochloride	10 mg; 4 mg	Salmon	Coated Tablet	Circle, Debossed	Geneva Generics
GG; 216	Perphenazine and Amitriptyline Hydrochloride	4 mg; 25 mg	Yellow	Coated Tablet	Circle	Geneva Generics
GG; 217	Perphenazine and Amitriptyline Hydrochloride	50 mg; 4 mg	Orange	Coated Tablet	Circle	Geneva Generics
GG; 219	Methyldopa and Hydrochlorothiazide	15 mg; 250 mg	Light Green	Coated Tablet	Circle	Novartis Generics
GG; 221	Theophylline	100 mg		Tablet		Novartis Generics
GG; 222	Theophylline	200 mg		Tablet		Novartis Generics
GG; 223	Theophylline	300 mg		Tablet		Novartis Generics
GG; 225	Promethazine Hydrochloride	25 mg	White	Tablet	Circle, Scored, Debossed	Geneva Generics
GG; 227	Isdn	20 mg	Green	Tablet	Circle, Scored, Debossed	Sandoz
GG; 227	Isoxsuprine Hydrochloride	10 mg	Green	Tablet	Circle, Scored	Sandoz
GG; 234	Methylprednisolone	4 mg	White	Tablet	Oval, Scored	Novartis Generics
GG; 235	Promethazine Hydrochloride	50 mg	Pink	Tablet	Circle	Geneva Generics
GG; 236	Sulindac	150 mg	Yellow	Tablet	Circle, Scored, Debossed	Geneva Generics
GG; 237	Sulindac	200 mg	Yellow	Tablet	Circle, Scored, Debossed	Geneva Generics
GG; 238	Glyburide	1.25 mg	White	Tablet	Circle, Scored	Novartis Generics
GG; 239	Glyburide	2.5 mg	Dark Pink	Tablet	Circle	Geneva Generics
GG; 240	Glyburide	5 mg	Blue	Tablet	Circle, Scored	Novartis Generics
GG; 242	Methyclothiazide	5 mg	Salmon-Colored	Tablet	Circle, Scored	Novartis Generics
GG; 243	Methyldopa and Hydrochlorothiazide	30 mg; 500 mg	Light Green	Coated Tablet	Circle	Novartis Generics
GG; 244	Methyclothiazide	2.5 mg	Orange	Tablet	Circle, Scored	Novartis Generics
GG; 246	Bumetanide	0.5 mg		Tablet		Novartis Generics
GG; 247	Bumetanide	1 mg		Tablet		Novartis Generics
GG; 248	Bumetanide	2 mg		Tablet		Novartis Generics
GG; 249	Alprazolam	2 mg	White	Tablet	Rectangle, Tri-Scored	Sandoz
GG; 250	Quinidine Gluconate	324 mg	White	Sustained-Release Tablet	Circle	Novartis Generics
GG; 251	Carbidopa and Levodopa	10 mg; 100 mg	Blue	Tablet	Circle, Scored	Novartis Generics
GG; 252	Carbidopa and Levodopa	25 mg; 100 mg	Yellow	Tablet	Circle, Scored	Novartis Generics
GG; 253	Carbidopa and Levodopa	25 mg; 250 mg	Light Blue	Tablet	Circle, Scored	Novartis Generics
GG; 254	Fenoprofen Calcium	600 mg	White	Coated Tablet	Oval, Scored, Embossed	Novartis Generics
GG; 255	Disobrom	6 mg; 120 mg	White	Timed-Release Tablet	Circle	Novartis Generics
GG; 256	Alprazolam	0.25 mg	White	Tablet	Oval, Scored	Sandoz
GG; 257	Alprazolam	0.5 mg	Peach	Tablet	Oval, Scored	Sandoz
GG; 258	Alprazolam	1 mg	Blue	Tablet	Oval, Scored	Sandoz
GG; 259	Isdn	5 mg	Pink	Tablet	Circle, Scored, Debossed	Sandoz
GG; 260	Hydroxychloroquine Sulfate	200 mg	White	Coated Tablet	Circle, Scored	Sandoz
GG; 261	Meclizine Hydrochloride Otc	25 mg	Yellow	Tablet	Oval, Scored	Sandoz
GG; 261	Meclizine Hydrochloride RX	25 mg	Yellow	Tablet	Oval, Scored	Sandoz
GG; 263	Atenolol	50 mg	White	Tablet	Circle, Scored	Sandoz
GG; 264	Atenolol	100 mg	White	Tablet	Circle	Sandoz
GG; 265	Methyldopa and Hydrochlorothiazide	25 mg; 250 mg	White	Coated Tablet	Circle	Novartis Generics
GG; 268	Oxaprozin	600 mg		Tablet		Geneva Generics
GG; 270	Tolazamide	100 mg	White	Tablet	Circle, Scored	Novartis Generics
GG; 271	Tolazamide	250 mg	White	Tablet	Circle, Scored	Novartis Generics
GG; 272	Tolazamide	500 mg	White	Tablet	Circle, Scored	Novartis Generics
GG; 273	Quinidine Sulfate	300 mg		Sustained-Release Tablet		Novartis Generics
GG; 277	Sucralfate	1 GM		Tablet		Novartis Generics
GG; 280	Minocycline	50 mg		Tablet		Novartis Generics
GG; 281	Minocycline	100 mg		Tablet		Novartis Generics
GG; 284	Isoxsuprine Hydrochloride	20 mg	White	Tablet	Circle, Scored	Sandoz
GG; 285 ;	Quinidine Sulfate	200 mg	White	Tablet	Circle, Scored	Novartis Generics
GG; 286	Quinidine Sulfate	300 mg	White	Tablet	Circle, Scored	Novartis Generics
GG; 289	Methyldopa and Hydrochlorothiazide	50 mg; 500 mg	White	Coated Tablet	Circle	Novartis Generics
GG; 296	Loratadine	10 mg	White	Tablet	Circle	Sandoz
GG; 297	Doxycycline Hyclate	100 mg		Tablet		Novartis Generics
GG; 364	Benazepril and Hydrochlorothiazide	5 mg; 6.25 mg	White	Tablet	Oval	Sandoz
GG; 365	Benazepril and Hydrochlorothiazide	10 mg; 12.5 mg	Light Pink	Tablet	Oval	Sandoz
GG; 366	Benazepril and Hydrochlorothiazide	20 mg; 12.5 mg	Grayish Violet	Tablet	Oval	Sandoz
GG; 367	Benazepril and Hydrochlorothiazide	20 mg; 25 mg	Red	Tablet	Oval	Sandoz
GG; 406	Probucol	250 mg		Tablet		Novartis Generics
GG; 407 ;	Chlorpromazine Hydrochloride	50 mg	Off-White	Coated Tablet	Circle	Novartis Generics
GG; 407; 50	Chlorpromazine Hydrochloride	50 mg	Butterscotch	Coated Tablet	Circle	Sandoz
GG; 409	Leucovorin Calcium	5 mg		Tablet		Novartis Generics
GG; 410	Leucovorin Calcium	25 mg		Tablet		Novartis Generics
GG; 412	Carisoprodol Compound	325 mg; 200 mg		Tablet		Novartis Generics
GG; 414	Metoprolol Tartrate	50 mg	White	Coated Tablet	Circle, Scored	Geneva Generics
GG; 414	Probenecid	500 mg	Yellow	Coated Tablet	Capsule-Shape	Novartis Generics
GG; 415	Metoprolol Tartrate	100 mg	White	Coated Tablet	Circle, Scored	Geneva Generics
GG; 417	Naproxen Sodium	275 mg	Yellow	Tablet	Oval, Debossed	Geneva Generics
GG; 418	Naproxen Sodium	550 mg	White	Coated Tablet	Oval, Debossed	Geneva Generics

IMPRINT	BRAND/GENERIC NAME	STRENGTH	COLOR	FORM	SHAPE	MANUFACTURER
GG; 419	Trazodone Hydrochloride	50 mg	White	Coated Tablet	Circle, Scored	Geneva Generics
GG; 420	Trazodone Hydrochloride	100 mg	White	Coated Tablet	Circle, Scored	Geneva Generics
GG; 421	Chlorzoxazone	250 mg	Orange	Tablet	Circle, Scored	Novartis Generics
GG; 422	Chlorzoxazone	500 mg	Orange	Tablet	Circle, Scored	Novartis Generics
GG; 425	Erythromycin Ethylsuccinate	400 mg		Coated Tablet		Novartis Generics
GG; 431 ;	Amitriptyline Hydrochloride	50 mg	Brown with White Core	Coated Tablet	Circle	Sandoz
GG; 436	Nystatin	500,000 units	Brown	Coated Tablet	Circle	Novartis Generics
GG; 437 ;	Chlorpromazine Hydrochloride	100 mg	Off-White	Coated Tablet	Circle	Novartis Generics
GG; 437; 100	Chlorpromazine Hydrochloride	100 mg	Butterscotch	Coated Tablet	Circle	Sandoz
GG; 438	Pindolol	5 mg	White	Tablet	Circle, Scored, Debossed	Geneva Generics
GG; 439	Pindolol	10 mg	White	Tablet	Circle, Scored, Debossed	Geneva Generics
GG; 442	Ranitidine Hydrochloride	150 mg		Tablet		Geneva Generics
GG; 443	Ranitidine Hydrochloride	300 mg		Tablet		Geneva Generics
GG; 447	Pentoxifylline	400 mg		Sustained-Release Tablet		Novartis Generics
GG; 449	Verapamil Hydrochloride	240 mg		Sustained-Release Tablet		Geneva Generics
GG; 450 ;	Amitriptyline Hydrochloride	150 mg	Light Green	Coated Tablet	Circle	Sandoz
GG; 451 ;	Amitriptyline Hydrochloride	75 mg	Purple with White Core	Coated Tablet	Circle	Sandoz
GG; 452	Orphenadrine Citrate, Aspirin and Caffeine	385 mg; 30 mg; 25 mg		Tablet		Novartis Generics
GG; 453	Orphenadrine Citrate, Aspirin and Caffeine	770 mg; 60 mg; 50 mg		Tablet		Novartis Generics
GG; 454	Diflunisal	250 mg		Tablet		Novartis Generics
GG; 455 ;	Chlorpromazine Hydrochloride	10 mg	Off-White	Coated Tablet	Circle	Novartis Generics
GG; 455; 10	Chlorpromazine Hydrochloride	10 mg	Butterscotch	Coated Tablet	Circle	Sandoz
GG; 456	Diflunisal	500 mg		Tablet		Novartis Generics
GG; 457 ;	Chlorpromazine Hydrochloride	200 mg	Off-White	Coated Tablet	Circle	Novartis Generics
GG; 457; 200	Chlorpromazine Hydrochloride	200 mg	Butterscotch	Coated Tablet	Circle	Sandoz
GG; 461 ;	Amitriptyline Hydrochloride	100 mg	Orange with White Core	Coated Tablet	Circle	Sandoz
GG; 462	Tocainide	400 mg		Tablet		Novartis Generics
GG; 463	Tocainide	600 mg		Tablet		Novartis Generics
GG; 464 ;	Dipyridamole	75 mg	White	Coated Tablet	Circle	Novartis Generics
GG; 465	Nadolol	20 mg		Tablet		Novartis Generics
GG; 466	Nadolol	40 mg		Tablet		Novartis Generics
GG; 467	Nadolol	80 mg		Tablet		Novartis Generics
GG; 468	Nadolol	120 mg		Tablet		Novartis Generics
GG; 469	Nadolol	160 mg		Tablet		Novartis Generics
GG; 471	Methyldopa	500 mg	White	Coated Tablet	Circle	Novartis Generics
GG; 472	Procainamide Hydrochloride	250 mg	White	Sustained-Release Tablet	Oblong	Novartis Generics
GG; 473	Procainamide Hydrochloride	500 mg	White	Sustained-Release Tablet	Oblong, Scored	Novartis Generics
GG; 476 ;	Chlorpromazine Hydrochloride	25 mg	Off-White	Coated Tablet	Circle	Novartis Generics
GG; 476; 25	Chlorpromazine Hydrochloride	25 mg	Butterscotch	Coated Tablet	Circle	Sandoz
GG; 487	Probenecid and Colchicine	0.5 mg; 500 mg	White	Tablet	Oblong	Novartis Generics
GG; 488	Fluphenazine Hydrochloride	2.5 mg	Beige	Coated Tablet	Circle	Sandoz
GG; 489	Fluphenazine Hydrochloride	5 mg	Light Rust	Coated Tablet	Circle	Sandoz
GG; 490	Fluphenazine Hydrochloride	10 mg	Rust	Coated Tablet	Circle, Debossed	Sandoz
GG; 492	Divalproex Sodium	125 mg		Tablet		Novartis Generics
GG; 493	Divalproex Sodium	250 mg		Tablet		Novartis Generics
GG; 494	Divalproex Sodium	500 mg		Tablet		Novartis Generics
GG; 501 ;	Nitroglycerin	6.5 mg	Blue and Dark Yellow	Sustained-Release Capsule		Novartis Generics
GG; 503	Papaverine Hydrochloride	150 mg	Brown and Clear	Sustained-Release Capsule		Geneva Generics
GG; 504	Tolmetin Sodium	400 mg		Capsule		Novartis Generics
GG; 505	Oxazepam	10 mg	White with Pink and Black Bands	Capsule		Geneva Generics
GG; 506	Oxazepam	15 mg	White with Red and Black Bands	Capsule		Geneva Generics
GG; 507	Oxazepam	30 mg	Opaque White with Maroon and Black Bands	Capsule		Geneva Generics
GG; 508 ;	Pseudoephedrine Hydrochloride	120 mg	Brown and Orange	Sustained-Release Capsule		Geneva Generics
GG; 509 ;	Cyclandelate	400 mg	Blue and Red	Capsule		Novartis Generics
GG; 510	Sulfinpyrazone	200 mg		Capsule		Novartis Generics
GG; 511 ;	Nitroglycerin	2.5 mg	Lavender and Clear	Sustained-Release Capsule		Novartis Generics
GG; 512 ;	Nitroglycerin SR	9 mg	Clear Yellow and Green	Sustained-Release Capsule		Novartis Generics
GG; 513	Gemfibrozil	300 mg		Capsule		Novartis Generics
GG; 514 ;	Phenylbutazone	100 mg	Light Blue	Capsule		Novartis Generics
GG; 515	Quinidine Sulfate	325 mg		Tablet		Novartis Generics
GG; 516 ;	Phendimetrazine	105 mg	Blue and Clear with Blue Beads	Sustained-Release Capsule		Novartis Generics
GG; 517	Indomethacin	25 mg	Light Green	Capsule		Novartis Generics
GG; 518	Indomethacin	50 mg	Light Green	Capsule		Novartis Generics
GG; 519	Indomethacin	75 mg		Extended-Release Capsule		Novartis Generics
GG; 520 ;	Butal Compound	50 mg; 325 mg; 40 mg		Capsule		Novartis Generics
GG; 522	Flurazepam	15 mg	Powder Blue and White	Capsule		Novartis Generics
GG; 523	Flurazepam	30 mg	Powder Blue	Capsule		Novartis Generics

IMPRINT	BRAND/GENERIC NAME	STRENGTH	COLOR	FORM	SHAPE	MANUFACTURER
GG; 524	Meclofenamate Sodium	50 mg	Maroon and Pink	Capsule		Novartis Generics
GG; 525	Meclofenamate Sodium	100 mg	Maroon and White	Capsule		Novartis Generics
GG; 526	Clorazepate Dipotassium	3.75 mg	Opaque White with Bands	Capsule		Novartis Generics
GG; 527	Clorazepate	7.5 mg	Opaque White with Bands	Capsule		Novartis Generics
GG; 528	Clorazepate	15 mg	Opaque White with Bands	Capsule		Novartis Generics
GG; 529 ;	Cyclandelate	200 mg	Powder Blue	Capsule		Novartis Generics
GG; 531	Temazepam	15 mg	Dark Green and White	Capsule		Geneva Generics
GG; 532	Temazepam	30 mg	White	Capsule		Geneva Generics
GG; 533 ;	Diphenhydramine Hydrochloride	25 mg	Pink and Clear with White Powder	Capsule		Novartis Generics
GG; 534	Clofibrate	500 mg		Capsule		Novartis Generics
GG; 538	Nitrofurantoin Macrocrystals	25 mg	Opaque White	Capsule		Geneva Generics
GG; 540	Fluoxetine Hydrochloride	40 mg	White with a Single Orange Band	Capsule		Sandoz
GG; 541 ;	Diphenhydramine Hydrochloride	50 mg	Pink	Capsule		Novartis Generics
GG; 542	Prazepam	5 mg		Capsule		Novartis Generics
GG; 543	Prazepam	10 mg		Capsule		Novartis Generics
GG; 544	Prazepam	20 mg		Capsule		Novartis Generics
GG; 545	Cephalexin	250 mg	Opaque Orange and Gray	Capsule		Novartis Generics
GG; 546	Cephalexin	500 mg	Opaque Orange and Gray	Capsule		Novartis Generics
GG; 549	Ursodiol	300 mg		Capsule		Geneva Generics
GG; 550	Fluoxetine Hydrochloride	20 mg	White with a Single Black Band	Capsule		Sandoz
GG; 554 ;	Niacin	125 mg	Black and Clear	Sustained-Release Capsule		Novartis Generics
GG; 555	Cephalexin	500 mg	Swedish Orange	Capsule		Novartis Generics
GG; 556	Cephalexin	250 mg	Swedish Orange and Gray	Capsule		Novartis Generics
GG; 557	Nifedipine	10 mg		Capsule		Geneva Generics
GG; 558	Fenoprofen Calcium	200 mg	White with Gold and Black Bands	Capsule		Novartis Generics
GG; 559	Fenoprofen Calcium	300 mg	White with Gold Bands	Capsule		Novartis Generics
GG; 560	Ferrous Sulfate	250 mg		Sustained-Release Capsule		Novartis Generics
GG; 560 ;	Ferrous Sulfate	250 mg	Red and Clear with Brown and White Beads	Sustained-Release Capsule		Novartis Generics
GG; 561	Danazol	50 mg		Capsule		Novartis Generics
GG; 564 ;	Niacin	250 mg	Green and Clear	Sustained-Release Capsule		Novartis Generics
GG; 571	Clinoxide	5 mg; 2.5 mg	Opaque White	Capsule		Novartis Generics
GG; 572	Doxepin Hydrochloride	25 mg	Opaque White with Pink and Gold Bands	Capsule		Novartis Generics
GG; 573	Doxepin Hydrochloride	50 mg	Opaque White with Pink and Green Bands	Capsule		Novartis Generics
GG; 574	Doxepin Hydrochloride	75 mg	Opaque White with Black and Gold Bands	Capsule		Novartis Generics
GG; 575	Fluoxetine Hydrochloride	10 mg	White with Green Band	Capsule		Sandoz
GG; 576	Doxepin Hydrochloride	10 mg	White with Red and Gold Band	Capsule		Novartis Generics
GG; 577	Doxepin Hydrochloride	100 mg	White with Blue and Green Bands	Capsule		Novartis Generics
GG; 578	Doxepin Hydrochloride	150 mg		Capsule		Novartis Generics
GG; 580	Triamterene and Hydrochlorothiazide	25 mg; 50 mg	Red	Capsule		Geneva Generics
GG; 582	Hydroxyzine Pamoate	25 mg	Two-Toned Green	Capsule		Novartis Generics
GG; 583	Hydroxyzine Pamoate	50 mg	Opaque White and Green	Capsule		Novartis Generics
GG; 584	Hydroxyzine Pamoate	100 mg		Capsule		Novartis Generics
GG; 585	Loxapine Succinate	5 mg		Capsule		Novartis Generics
GG; 586	Loxapine Succinate	10 mg		Capsule		Novartis Generics
GG; 587	Loxapine Succinate	25 mg		Capsule		Novartis Generics
GG; 588	Loxapine Succinate	50 mg		Capsule		Novartis Generics
GG; 589	Thiothixene	1 mg	White, Orange and Gold	Capsule		Geneva Generics
GG; 591 ;	Propoxyphene Hydrochloride	65 mg	Opaque Pale Pink	Capsule		Novartis Generics
GG; 592	Prazosin Hydrochloride	1 mg	White with Black Ink Bands	Capsule		Novartis Generics
GG; 593	Prazosin Hydrochloride	2 mg	White with Pink and Black Ink Bands	Capsule		Novartis Generics
GG; 594	Prazosin Hydrochloride	5 mg	White with Blue and Black Ink Bands	Capsule		Novartis Generics
GG; 596	Thiothixene	2 mg	White, Blue and Gold	Capsule		Geneva Generics
GG; 597	Thiothixene	5 mg	Opaque White, Orange and Black	Capsule		Geneva Generics
GG; 598	Thiothixene	10 mg	Black and Blue	Capsule		Geneva Generics
GG; 599	Thiothixene	20 mg		Capsule		Geneva Generics
GG; 601	Isotretinoin	10 mg		Capsule		Novartis Generics
GG; 602	Isotretinoin	20 mg		Capsule		Novartis Generics

IMPRINT	BRAND/GENERIC NAME	STRENGTH	COLOR	FORM	SHAPE	MANUFACTURER
GG; 603	Isotretinoin	40 mg		Capsule		Novartis Generics
GG; 604	Cyclosporine	25 mg		Capsule		Novartis Generics
GG; 605	Cyclosporine	100 mg		Capsule		Novartis Generics
GG; 614	Ranitidine Hydrochloride	150 mg	Opaque Caramel	Capsule		Geneva Generics
GG; 615	Ranitidine Hydrochloride	300 mg	Opaque Caramel	Capsule		Geneva Generics
GG; 616	Ranitidine Hydrochloride	150 mg		Capsule		Geneva Generics
GG; 617	Ranitidine Hydrochloride	300 mg		Capsule		Geneva Generics
GG; 621	Terazosin Hydrochloride	1 mg		Capsule		Geneva Generics
GG; 622	Terazosin Hydrochloride	2 mg		Capsule		Geneva Generics
GG; 623	Terazosin Hydrochloride	5 mg		Capsule		Geneva Generics
GG; 624	Terazosin Hydrochloride	10 mg		Capsule		Geneva Generics
GG; 625	Flutamide	125 mg		Capsule		Novartis Generics
GG; 633 ;	Rifampin	300 mg	Scarlet, Caramel	Capsule		Geneva Generics
GG; 634	Amantadine Hydrochloride	100 mg	Red and White	Capsule, Liquid Filled		Sandoz
GG; 702	Isosorbide Mononitrate	20 mg		Tablet		Novartis Generics
GG; 704	Tolmetin Sodium	600 mg		Tablet		Novartis Generics
GG; 705	Ranitidine Hydrochloride	150 mg	Pink	Coated Tablet	Circle	Geneva Generics
GG; 706	Ranitidine Hydrochloride	300 mg	Orange	Coated Tablet	Circle	Geneva Generics
GG; 714	Erythromycin Stearate	250 mg		Tablet		Novartis Generics
GG; 715	Erythromycin Stearate	500 mg		Tablet		Novartis Generics
GG; 721	Terazosin Hydrochloride	1 mg		Tablet		Geneva Generics
GG; 722	Terazosin Hydrochloride	2 mg		Tablet		Geneva Generics
GG; 723	Terazosin Hydrochloride	5 mg		Tablet		Geneva Generics
GG; 724	Naproxen	250 mg	Yellow	Tablet	Circle	Geneva Generics
GG; 725	Naproxen	375 mg	Orange	Tablet	Capsule-Shape	Geneva Generics
GG; 726	Naproxen	500 mg	Yellow	Tablet	Capsule-Shape	Geneva Generics
GG; 730	Pseudoephedrine and Terfenadine	60 mg; 120 mg		Sustained-Release Tablet		Novartis Generics
GG; 731	Trazodone Hydrochloride	150 mg		Tablet		Geneva Generics
GG; 733	Salsalate	500 mg	Light Green	Coated Tablet	Circle	Novartis Generics
GG; 734	Salsalate	750 mg		Coated Tablet	Capsule-Shape, Scored	Novartis Generics
GG; 737	Diclofenac Sodium	25 mg	Yellow	Timed-Release Tablet	Circle	Sandoz
GG; 738	Diclofenac Sodium	50 mg	Light Brown	Timed-Release Tablet	Circle	Sandoz
GG; 739	Diclofenac Sodium	75 mg	Pink	Delayed-Release Tablet	Circle	Sandoz
GG; 741	Ciprofloxacin	250 mg	White	Tablet	Circle	Sandoz
GG; 742	Ciprofloxacin	500 mg	White	Tablet	Capsule-Shape	Sandoz
GG; 743	Ciprofloxacin	750 mg	White	Tablet	Capsule-Shape	Sandoz
GG; 744	Verapamil Hydrochloride	120 mg		Sustained-Release Tablet		Geneva Generics
GG; 745	Verapamil Hydrochloride	180 mg		Sustained-Release Tablet		Geneva Generics
GG; 746	Benazepril	5 mg	Yellow	Tablet	Circle	Sandoz
GG; 747	Benazepril	10 mg	Dark Yellow	Tablet	Circle	Sandoz
GG; 748	Benazepril	20 mg	Pink	Tablet	Circle	Sandoz
GG; 749	Benazepril	40 mg	Dark Rose	Tablet	Circle	Sandoz
GG; 755	Doxazosin	1 mg		Tablet		Novartis Generics
GG; 756	Doxazosin	2 mg		Tablet		Novartis Generics
GG; 757	Doxazosin	4 mg		Tablet		Novartis Generics
GG; 758	Doxazosin	8 mg		Tablet		Novartis Generics
GG; 771	Glipizide	5 mg	White	Tablet	Circle, Scored, Debossed	Sandoz
GG; 772	Glipizide	10 mg	White	Tablet	Circle, Scored, Debossed	Sandoz
GG; 774	Etodolac	400 mg		Tablet		Novartis Generics
GG; 801	Ketoprofen	75 mg		Capsule		Novartis Generics
GG; 802	Ketoprofen	50 mg		Capsule		Novartis Generics
GG; 805	Piroxicam	10 mg		Capsule		Novartis Generics
GG; 806	Piroxicam	20 mg		Capsule		Novartis Generics
GG; 808	Tetracycline Hydrochloride	250 mg	Yellow and Orange	Capsule		Novartis Generics
GG; 809	Tetracycline Hydrochloride	500 mg	Yellow and Black	Capsule		Novartis Generics
GG; 810	Oxytetracycline	250 mg		Capsule		Novartis Generics
GG; 811	Erythromycin Estolate	250 mg	Orange and Buff	Capsule		Novartis Generics
GG; 812	Minocycline	50 mg		Capsule		Novartis Generics
GG; 813	Minocycline	100 mg		Capsule		Novartis Generics
GG; 814	Doxycycline	50 mg	Blue and White	Capsule		Novartis Generics
GG; 815	Doxycycline	100 mg	Blue	Capsule		Novartis Generics
GG; 816	Nizatidine	150 mg		Capsule		Novartis Generics
GG; 817	Nizatidine	300 mg		Capsule		Novartis Generics
GG; 818	Propranolol	60 mg		Sustained-Release Capsule		Novartis Generics
GG; 819	Propranolol	80 mg		Sustained-Release Capsule		Novartis Generics
GG; 820	Propranolol	120 mg		Sustained-Release Capsule		Novartis Generics
GG; 821	Propranolol	160 mg		Sustained-Release Capsule		Novartis Generics
GG; 822	Clomipramine Hydrochloride	25 mg	White and Orange with Yellow Band	Capsule		Sandoz
GG; 823	Clomipramine Hydrochloride	50 mg	Opaque White	Capsule		Sandoz
GG; 824	Clomipramine Hydrochloride	75 mg	Dark Yellow with Yellow Band	Capsule		Sandoz
GG; 828	Rifampin	150 mg		Capsule		Geneva Generics
GG; 832	Etodolac	200 mg		Capsule		Novartis Generics
GG; 833	Etodolac	300 mg		Capsule		Novartis Generics
GG; 835	Erythromycin	250 mg		Capsule		Novartis Generics
GG; 842	Nicardipine Hydrochloride	20 mg		Capsule		Novartis Generics
GG; 843	Nicardipine Hydrochloride	30 mg		Capsule		Novartis Generics
GG; 850	Ampicillin	250 mg	White	Capsule		Sandoz
GG; 851	Ampicillin	500 mg	White	Capsule		Sandoz
GG; 855	Dicloxacillin	500 mg	Blue	Capsule		Sandoz
GG; 904	Diclofenac Sodium	100 mg	Light Pink	Extended-Release Tablet	Circle	Sandoz

IMPRINT	BRAND/GENERIC NAME	STRENGTH	COLOR	FORM	SHAPE	MANUFACTURER
GG; 929	Bupropion Hydrochloride	75 mg	Lavender	Coated Tablet	Circle	Sandoz
GG; 930	Bupropion Hydrochloride	100 mg	Lavender	Coated Tablet	Circle	Sandoz
GG; 931	Orphenadrine Citrate	100 mg	White	Extended-Release Tablet	Circle	Geneva Generics
GG; 932	Pemoline	18.75 mg	White	Tablet	Circle, Scored	Geneva Generics
GG; 933	Pemoline	37.5 mg	White	Tablet	Circle, Scored	Geneva Generics
GG; 934	Pemoline	75 mg	White	Tablet	Circle, Scored	Geneva Generics
GG; 935	Naproxen Delayed-Release	375 mg	White	Delayed-Release Tablet	Capsule-Shape	Geneva Generics
GG; 936	Naproxen Delayed-Release	500 mg	White	Delayed-Release Tablet	Capsule-Shape	Geneva Generics
GG; 952; 5	Prochlorperazine Maleate	5 mg	Light Yellow	Tablet	Circle	Geneva Generics
GG; 953; 10	Prochlorperazine Maleate	10 mg	Pale Yellow	Tablet	Circle	Geneva Generics
GG; 957	Methylprednisolone	4 mg	White	Tablet	Oval, Quadrisect Scored on Blank Side	Geneva Generics
GG; 958 ;	Metoclopramide	5 mg	White	Tablet	Circle	Novartis Generics
GG; 963; 250	Cefuroxime Axetil	250 mg	White to Off-White	Tablet	Oval	Sandoz
GG; 964; 500	Cefuroxime Axetil	500 mg	White to Off-White	Tablet	Oval	Sandoz
GG; 977	Diclofenac Potassium	50 mg	White	Coated Tablet	Circle	Sandoz
GG; C1	Terazosin Hydrochloride	10 mg		Tablet		Geneva Generics
GG; D5	Selegiline Hydrochloride	5 mg		Tablet		Novartis Generics
GG; L7	Atenolol	25 mg	White	Tablet	Circle	Sandoz
GG; M1	Metoclopramide Hydrochloride	1 mg		Tablet		Novartis Generics
GG; N2	Amoxicillin and Clavulanate Potassium	200 mg; 28.5 mg	Pink	Tablet, Chewable	Circle	Sandoz
GG; N4	Amoxicillin and Clavulanate Potassium	400 mg; 57 mg	Pink	Tablet, Chewable	Circle	Sandoz
GG; N6	Amoxicillin and Clavulanate Potassium	500 mg; 125 mg	White to Slight Yellow	Tablet	Oblong	Sandoz
GG; N7	Amoxicillin and Clavulanate Potassium	875 mg; 125 mg	White to Slight Yellow	Tablet	Oblong	Sandoz
GG949; PVK250	Penicillin V Potassium	250 mg	Off White	Tablet	Circle	Geneva Generics
GG949; PVK250	Penicillin VK	250 mg	White	Tablet	Circle, Scored	Geneva Generics
GG950; PVK500	Penicillin VK Potassium	500 mg	Off White	Tablet	Oblong	Geneva Generics
GIL 0.5	Azilect	0.5 mg	White to Off-White	Tablet	Circle	Eisai
GIL 0.5	Azilect	0.5 mg	White to Off-White	Tablet	Circle	Teva Pharmaceuticals
GIL 1	Azilect	1 mg	White to Off-White	Tablet	Circle	Eisai
GIL 1	Azilect	1 mg	White to Off-White	Tablet	Circle	Teva Pharmaceuticals
GILEAD ; 701	Truvada	200 mg; 300 mg	Blue	Tablet	Capsule-Shape	Gilead Sciences
GILEAD; 200 MG	Emtriva	200 mg	Blue and White	Capsule		Gilead Sciences
GILEAD; 4331; 300	Viread	300 mg	Light Blue	Coated Tablet	Teardrop-Shape	Gilead Sciences
GLAXO	Vicon Plus	4000 IU; 50 IU; 150 mg; 80 mg; 70 mg; 25 mg; 10 mg; 10 mg; 5 mg; 4 mg; 2 mg	Red and Beige	Capsule		Glaxosmithkline
GLAXO	Vicon-C	100 mg; 80 mg; 70 mg; 20 mg; 20 mg; 10 mg; 5 mg; 300 mg	Orange and Yellow	Capsule		Glaxosmithkline
GLAXO	VI-Zac	5000 IU; 80 mg; 50 IU; 500 mg	Orange	Capsule		Glaxosmithkline
GLAXO; 268	Theobid Duracap	260 mg	Blue and Clear	Sustained-Release Capsule		Glaxosmithkline
GLAXO; 316	Vicon Forte	8000 IU; 50 IU; 150 mg; 80 mg; 70 mg; 25 mg; 10 mg; 10 mg; 5 mg; 4 mg; 2 mg; 1 mg; 10 mg	Orange and Black	Capsule		Glaxosmithkline
GLAXO; 371	Trandate HCT	100 mg; 25 mg	Pale Peach	Coated Tablet	Oval	Glaxosmithkline
GLAXO; 372	Trandate HCT	200 mg; 25 mg	White	Coated Tablet	Oval	Glaxosmithkline
GLAXO; 373	Trandate HCT	300 mg; 25 mg	Medium Peach	Coated Tablet	Oval	Glaxosmithkline
GLAXO; AMESEC	Amesec	130 mg; 25 mg	Orange and Blue	Capsule		Glaxosmithkline
GLAXO; TRINSICON	Trinsicon	0.5 mg; 75 mg; 110 mg; 240 mg; 15 mcg	Dark Pink and Dark Red	Capsule		Glaxosmithkline
GLAXO; VENTOLIN; 2	Ventolin	2 mg	White	Tablet	Circle, Compressed	Glaxosmithkline
GLAXO; ZANTAC; 150	Zantac 150 Maximum Strength	150 mg	Peach	Coated Tablet	Five-Sided	Glaxosmithkline
GLAXO; ZANTAC; 300	Zantac 300	300 mg	Yellow	Coated Tablet	Capsule-Shape	Glaxosmithkline
GLUCOTROL XL; 2.5	Glucotrol XL	2.5 mg	Blue	Extended-Release Tablet		Pfizer Laboratories
GLUCOTROL XL; 5	Glucotrol XL	5 mg	White	Extended-Release Tablet	Circle, Biconvex	Pfizer Laboratories
GLUCOTROL XL; 10	Glucotrol XL	10 mg	White	Extended-Release Tablet	Circle, Biconvex	Pfizer Laboratories
GLYBUR 364; 364	Glyburide	5 mg	Blue	Tablet	Oblong	Teva Pharmaceuticals
GLYBUR 433; 433	Glyburide	2.5 mg	Pink	Tablet	Oblong, Scored	Teva Pharmaceuticals
GLYNASE 1.5; PT; PT	Glynase Prestab	1.5 mg	White	Tablet	Egg-Shape, Contour, Scored	Pharmacia & Upjohn
GLYNASE 3; PT; PT	Glynase Prestab	3 mg	Blue	Tablet	Egg-Shape, Contour, Scored	Pharmacia & Upjohn
GLYNASE 6; PT; PT	Glynase Prestab	6 mg	Yellow	Tablet	Egg-Shape, Contour, Scored	Pharmacia & Upjohn
GLYSET; 25	Glyset	25 mg	White	Coated Tablet	Circle	Pharmacia & Upjohn
GLYSET; 50	Glyset	50 mg	White	Tablet	Circle	Pharmacia & Upjohn
GLYSET; 100	Glyset	100 mg	White	Tablet	Circle	Pharmacia & Upjohn
GP 5; G	Glipizide	5 mg	White	Tablet	Oval, Convex	Par Pharmaceutical
GP 10; G	Glipizide	10 mg	White	Tablet	Oval, Convex	Par Pharmaceutical
GP; 111	Lisinopril	2.5 mg	White	Coated Tablet	Circle	Sandoz
GP; 112	Lisinopril	5 mg	Pink	Coated Tablet	Circle	Sandoz
GP; 113	Lisinopril	10 mg	White	Coated Tablet	Circle	Sandoz
GP; 114	Lisinopril	20 mg	Peach	Coated Tablet	Circle	Sandoz
GP; 115	Lisinopril	40 mg	Rose	Coated Tablet	Circle	Sandoz
GP; 118	Mefloquine Hydrochloride	250 mg	White	Tablet	Circle, Scored	Sandoz

IMPRINT	BRAND/GENERIC NAME	STRENGTH	COLOR	FORM	SHAPE	MANUFACTURER
GP; 124	Metformin Hydrochloride	500 mg	White	Tablet	Circle	Sandoz
GP; 127	Metformin Hydrochloride	850 mg	White	Coated Tablet	Circle	Sandoz
GP; 128	Metformin Hydrochloride	1000 mg	White	Tablet	Oval	Sandoz
GP; 142	Fluvoxamine Maleate	50 mg	White	Tablet	Circle	Sandoz
GP; 150	Lisinopril	30 mg	Peach	Coated Tablet	Circle	Sandoz
GRISACTIN ULTRA; 125	Grisactin Ultra	125 mg	White	Tablet		Wyeth Pharmaceuticals
GRISACTIN ULTRA; 250	Grisactin Ultra	250 mg	White	Tablet		Wyeth Pharmaceuticals
GRISACTIN ULTRA; 330	Grisactin Ultra	330 mg	White	Tablet		Wyeth Pharmaceuticals
GRISACTIN; 125	Grisactin	125 mg	Orange	Capsule, Liquid Filled		Wyeth Pharmaceuticals
GRISACTIN; 250	Grisactin	250 mg	Yellow	Capsule, Liquid Filled		Wyeth Pharmaceuticals
GRISACTIN; 500	Grisactin	500 mg	Pink	Tablet	Circle	Wyeth Pharmaceuticals
GS; 25C	Zantac 25 Efferdose	25 mg	White to Pale Yellow	Effervescent Tablet	Circle, Flat-Faced, Bevel-Edged	Glaxosmithkline
GS; FC2	Epzicom	600 mg; 300 mg	Orange	Tablet	Capsule-Shape, Modified	Glaxosmithkline
GSK ; 2/1000	Avandamet	2 mg; 1000 mg	Yellow	Tablet	Oval	Glaxosmithkline
GSK ; 4/1 ;	Avandaryl	4 mg; 1 mg	Yellow	Tablet	Triangle	Glaxosmithkline
GSK ; 4/2 ;	Avandaryl	4 mg; 2 mg	Orange	Tablet	Triangle	Glaxosmithkline
GSK ; 4/4 ;	Avandaryl	4 mg; 4 mg	Pink	Tablet	Triangle	Glaxosmithkline
GSK ; 4/500	Avandamet	4 mg; 500 mg	Orange	Tablet	Oval	Glaxosmithkline
GSK ; 4/1000	Avandamet	4 mg; 1000 mg	Pink	Tablet	Oval	Glaxosmithkline
GUAIMAX-D; SP; 2055	Guaimax-D	600 mg; 120 mg	White	Extended-Release Tablet	Capsule-Shape, Scored	Schwarz Pharma
GX CC1	Agenerase	50 mg	Off White to Cream	Capsule, Liquid Filled		Glaxosmithkline
GX CE2	Avodart	0.5 mg	Dull Yellow	Capsule, Liquid Filled		Glaxosmithkline
GX CF7 24	Zofran	24 mg	Pink	Tablet	Oval	Glaxosmithkline
GX CL2	Lamictal	5 mg	White to Off White	Tablet, Chewable	Capsule-Shape	Glaxosmithkline
GX CL5	Lamictal	25 mg	White	Tablet, Chewable	Oval	Glaxosmithkline
GX CW3 ; 300	Retrovir	300 mg	White	Tablet	Circle	Glaxosmithkline
GX EF3 ; M	Myleran	2 mg	White	Tablet	Circle	Glaxosmithkline
GX; 623	Ziagen	300 mg	Yellow	Coated Tablet	Capsule-Shape, Biconvex	Glaxosmithkline
GX; CE3	Amerge	1 mg	White	Coated Tablet	D-Shape	Glaxosmithkline
GX; CE5	Amerge	2.5 mg	Green	Coated Tablet	D-Shape	Glaxosmithkline
GX; CG5	Epivir-Hbv	100 mg	Butterscotch	Coated Tablet	Capsule-Shape, Biconvex	Glaxosmithkline
GX; CG7	Malarone Pediatric	62.5 mg; 25 mg	Pink	Coated Tablet	Circle, Biconvex	Glaxosmithkline
GX; CJ7; 150 ;	Epivir	150 mg	White	Coated Tablet	Diamond, Modified	Glaxosmithkline
GX; CK3	Raxar	200 mg	White to Pale Yellow	Coated Tablet	Circle, Biconvex, Bevel-Edged	Glaxosmithkline
GX; CM3	Malarone	250 mg; 100 mg	Pink	Coated Tablet	Circle, Biconvex	Glaxosmithkline
GX; CT1	Lotronex	1 mg	Blue	Coated Tablet	Oval	Glaxosmithkline
GX; EG2	Ceftin	500 mg	White	Tablet	Capsule-Shape	Glaxosmithkline
GX; EG3; L	Leukeran	2 mg	Brown	Tablet	Circle, Biconvex	Glaxosmithkline
GX; EH3; A	Alkeran	2 mg	White	Coated Tablet	Circle, Biconvex	Glaxosmithkline
GX; EJ7	Epivir	300 mg	Gray	Coated Tablet	Diamond, Modified	Glaxosmithkline
GX; ES7	Ceftin	250 mg	White	Tablet	Capsule-Shape	Glaxosmithkline
GX; EX1	Lotronex	0.5 mg	White	Coated Tablet	Oval	Glaxosmithkline
GX; LL1	Trizivir	300 mg; 150 mg; 300 mg	Blue-Green	Coated Tablet	Capsule-Shape	Glaxosmithkline
GX; LL7	Lexiva	700 mg	Pink	Tablet	Capsule-Shape	Glaxosmithkline
GXFC3	Combivir	150 mg; 300 mg	White	Coated Tablet	Capsule-Shape	Glaxosmithkline
H; 1	Captopril	12.5 mg	White	Tablet	Circle, Scored	Duramed Pharmaceuticals
H; 1; LL	Hydromox	50 mg	White	Tablet	Circle, Flat, Scored, Beveled	Lederle Laboratories
H; 12	Captopril	100 mg	White	Tablet	Circle, Scored	Duramed Pharmaceuticals
H; 111	Captopril	50 mg	White	Tablet	Circle, Scored	Duramed Pharmaceuticals
H; 114	Glipizide	5 mg	White	Tablet	Round, Bisected Scored	Duramed Pharmaceuticals
H; 115	Glipizide	10 mg	White	Tablet	Round, Bisected Scored	Duramed Pharmaceuticals
H; 302; 2	Acetaminophen and Codeine	300 mg; 15 mg	White	Tablet	Circle	Duramed Pharmaceuticals
H; 303	Acetaminophen and Codeine Phosphate	300 mg; 30 mg	White	Tablet	Circle	Duramed Pharmaceuticals
H; 304; 4	Acetaminophen and Codeine Phosphate	300 mg; 60 mg	White	Tablet	Circle	Duramed Pharmaceuticals
H4	Micardis HCT	12.5 mg; 40 mg	White and Red	Tablet	Oblong	Boehringer Ingelheim Pharmaceuticals
H8	Micardis HCT	12.5 mg; 80 mg	White and Red	Tablet	Oblong	Boehringer Ingelheim Pharmaceuticals
H9	Micardis HCT	25 mg; 80 mg	White and Yellow	Tablet	Oblong	Boehringer Ingelheim Pharmaceuticals
HALCION; 0.25 ;	Halcion	0.25 mg	Powder-Blue	Tablet	Oval, Scored	Pharmacia & Upjohn
HALCION; 0.5	Halcion	0.5 mg	White	Tablet	Oval, Scored	Pharmacia & Upjohn
HALDOL; 1; MCNEIL	Haldol	1 mg	Yellow	Tablet	U-Shape, with "h" Cut Out in Center, Scored	Ortho-Mcneil Pharmaceutical
HALDOL; 2; MCNEIL	Haldol	2 mg	Pink	Tablet	U-Shape, with "h" Cut Out in Center, Scored	Ortho-Mcneil Pharmaceutical
HALDOL; 5; MCNEIL	Haldol	5 mg	Green	Tablet	U-Shape, with "h" Cut Out in Center, Scored	Ortho-Mcneil Pharmaceutical
HALDOL; 10; MCNEIL	Haldol	10 mg	Aqua	Tablet	U-Shape, with "h" Cut Out in Center, Scored	Ortho-Mcneil Pharmaceutical
HALDOL; 20; MCNEIL	Haldol	20 mg	Salmon	Tablet	U-Shape, with "h" Cut Out in Center, Scored	Ortho-Mcneil Pharmaceutical
HALFAN	Halfan	250 mg	White	Tablet	Capsule-Shape	Glaxosmithkline
HALOTESTIN; 2 ;	Halotestin	2 mg	Peach	Tablet	Circle, Scored	Pharmacia & Upjohn
HALOTESTIN; 5 ;	Halotestin	5 mg	Light Green	Tablet	Circle, Scored	Pharmacia & Upjohn
HALOTESTIN; 10 ;	Halotestin	10 mg	Green	Tablet	Circle, Scored	Pharmacia & Upjohn
HB; 93; 614	Belap	16.2 mg; 10.8 mg	Green	Tablet	Circle, Convex	Teva Pharmaceuticals
HD 567	Butalbital, Acetaminophen and Caffeine	50 mg; 325 mg; 40 mg	White	Tablet	Circle	Watson Laboratories
HD 813	Atuss HD	5 mg; 30 mg; 2 mg	Maroon	Capsule		Atley Pharmaceuticals

IMPRINT	BRAND/GENERIC NAME	STRENGTH	COLOR	FORM	SHAPE	MANUFACTURER
HD; 532	Roxilox	5 mg; 500 mg	Scarlet Red and Buff White	Capsule		Roxane Laboratories
HD; 544	Diazepam	5 mg	Yellow	Tablet	Circle, Scored	Warner Chilcott
HD; 546	Diazepam	2 mg	White	Tablet	Circle, Scored	Warner Chilcott
HD; 549	Diazepam	10 mg	Blue	Tablet	Circle, Scored	Warner Chilcott
HD; 725	Doxycycline Hyclate	100 mg	Beige	Coated Tablet	Circle	Novartis Generics
HEART ; 2776	Avalide	300 mg; 12.5 mg	Peach	Tablet	Oval	Bristol-Myers Squibb
HIVID; 0.375; ROCHE	Hivid	0.375 mg	Beige	Coated Tablet	Oval	Roche Pharmaceuticals
HIVID; 0.750; ROCHE	Hivid	0.75 mg	Gray	Coated Tablet	Oval	Roche Pharmaceuticals
HOECHST; 73	Festalan	30,000 units; 6000 units; 20,000 units; 1 mg	Orange	Tablet	Circle	Aventis Pharmaceuticals
HOECHST; LASIX	Lasix	20 mg	White	Tablet	Oval	Aventis Pharmaceuticals
HOECHST; LASIX	Lasix	20 mg	White	Tablet	Oval	Sanofi-Aventis U.S.
HOURGLASS ; 75	Ranitidine Hydrochloride	75 mg	Peach	Tablet	Circle	Ivax Pharmaceuticals
HOURGLASS 4330 ; 850	Metformin Hydrochloride	850 mg	White	Tablet	Oval	Ivax Pharmaceuticals
HOURGLASS 4331 ; 500	Metformin Hydrochloride	500 mg	White	Tablet	Oval	Ivax Pharmaceuticals
HOURGLASS 4331 ; 500	Metformin Hydrochloride	500 mg	White	Tablet	Oval	Teva Pharmaceuticals
HOURGLASS 4335 ; 500	Metformin Hydrochloride ER	500 mg	White to Off White	Tablet, Extended Release	Oval	Ivax Pharmaceuticals
HOURGLASS 4346 40 MG	Fluoxetine Hydrochloride	40 mg	Light Blue Opaque	Capsule		Ivax Pharmaceuticals
HOURGLASS 4356 20 MG ;	Fluoxetine Hydrochloride	20 mg	Aqua Blue	Capsule		Ivax Pharmaceuticals
HOURGLASS 4357 ; 150	Ranitidine Hydrochloride	150 mg	Beige	Tablet	Circle	Ivax Pharmaceuticals
HOURGLASS 4363 10 MG ;	Fluoxetine Hydrochloride	10 mg	Aqua Blue, Opaque White	Capsule		Ivax Pharmaceuticals
HOURGLASS 4432 ; 1000	Metformin Hydrochloride	1000 mg	White	Tablet	Oval	Ivax Pharmaceuticals
HOURGLASS 4740 ; 10	Citalopram Hydrobromide	10 mg	Light Beige	Tablet	Capsule-Shape	Ivax Pharmaceuticals
HOURGLASS 4741 ; 20	Citalopram Hydrobromide	20 mg	Light Pink	Tablet	Capsule-Shape	Ivax Pharmaceuticals
HOURGLASS 4742 ; 40	Citalopram Hydrobromide	40 mg	White	Tablet	Capsule-Shape	Ivax Pharmaceuticals
HOURGLASS; 56; 65; 5; 5; 5	Buspirone Hydrochloride	15 mg	White	Tablet	Capsule-Shape	Ivax Pharmaceuticals
HOURGLASS; 120	Verapamil Hydrochloride	120 mg	Ivory	Extended-Release Tablet	Circle	Ivax Pharmaceuticals
HOURGLASS; 200 ;	Cimetidine	200 mg	White	Tablet	Circle	Ivax Pharmaceuticals
HOURGLASS; 3667	Perphenazine	2 mg	White	Coated Tablet	Circle	Ivax Pharmaceuticals
HOURGLASS; 3668	Perphenazine	4 mg	White	Coated Tablet	Oval	Ivax Pharmaceuticals
HOURGLASS; 3669	Perphenazine	8 mg	White	Coated Tablet	Circle	Ivax Pharmaceuticals
HOURGLASS; 3670	Perphenazine	16 mg	White	Coated Tablet	Oval	Ivax Pharmaceuticals
HOURGLASS; 3685; 1	Doxazosin Mesylate	1 mg	White	Tablet	Circle	Ivax Pharmaceuticals
HOURGLASS; 3686; 2	Doxazosin Mesylate	2 mg	White	Tablet	Circle	Ivax Pharmaceuticals
HOURGLASS; 3687; 4	Doxazosin Mesylate	4 mg	Orange	Tablet	Circle	Ivax Pharmaceuticals
HOURGLASS; 3688; 8	Doxazosin Mesylate	8 mg	Green	Tablet	Circle	Ivax Pharmaceuticals
HOURGLASS; 3757	Lisinopril	2.5 mg	White	Tablet	Circle	Ivax Pharmaceuticals
HOURGLASS; 3758	Lisinopril	5 mg	White	Tablet	Square	Ivax Pharmaceuticals
HOURGLASS; 3759	Lisinopril	10 mg	White	Tablet	Oval	Ivax Pharmaceuticals
HOURGLASS; 3760	Lisinopril	20 mg	White	Tablet	Five-Sided	Ivax Pharmaceuticals
HOURGLASS; 3761	Lisinopril	40 mg	White	Tablet	Circle	Ivax Pharmaceuticals
HOURGLASS; 3762	Lisinopril	30 mg	White	Tablet	Oval	Ivax Pharmaceuticals
HOURGLASS; 3966	Diphenoxylate Hydrochloride and Atropine Sulfate	2.5 mg; 0.025 mg	White	Tablet	Circle	Ivax Pharmaceuticals
HOURGLASS; 4058	Cefadroxil	500 mg	Clear and White	Capsule		Ivax Pharmaceuticals
HOURGLASS; 4059 ;	Cefadroxil	1000 mg	White	Tablet		Ivax Pharmaceuticals
HOURGLASS; 4194; 500	Cefaclor Extended-Release	500 mg	Blue	Extended-Release Tablet	Oval	Ivax Pharmaceuticals
HOURGLASS; 4195; 2.5	Enalapril Maleate	2.5 mg	Yellow	Tablet	Circle, Scored	Ivax Pharmaceuticals
HOURGLASS; 4196; 5	Enalapril Maleate	5 mg	White	Tablet	Circle, Scored	Ivax Pharmaceuticals
HOURGLASS; 4197; 10	Enalapril Maleate	10 mg	Salmon	Tablet	Circle	Ivax Pharmaceuticals
HOURGLASS; 4198; 20	Enalapril Maleate	20 mg	Peach	Tablet	Circle	Ivax Pharmaceuticals
HOURGLASS; 4267; 400 ;	Acyclovir	400 mg	White	Tablet	Circle, Flat-Faced, Beveled-Edge	Ivax Pharmaceuticals
HOURGLASS; 4268; 800 ;	Acyclovir	800 mg	White	Tablet	Oval	Ivax Pharmaceuticals
HOURGLASS; 4303	Clozapine	12.5 mg	Pale Yellow	Tablet	Oval	Ivax Pharmaceuticals
HOURGLASS; 4332; 100	Nefazodone Hydrochloride	100 mg	Peach	Tablet	Oval	Ivax Pharmaceuticals
HOURGLASS; 4333; 150	Nefazodone Hydrochloride	150 mg	Peach	Tablet	Circle	Ivax Pharmaceuticals
HOURGLASS; 4334; 200	Nefazodone Hydrochloride	200 mg	Peach	Tablet	Oval	Ivax Pharmaceuticals
HOURGLASS; 4335; 250	Nefazodone Hydrochloride	250 mg	Peach	Tablet	Circle	Ivax Pharmaceuticals

IMPRINT	BRAND/GENERIC NAME	STRENGTH	COLOR	FORM	SHAPE	MANUFACTURER
HOURGLASS; 4343; 50	Nefazodone Hydrochloride	50 mg	Peach	Tablet	Oval	Ivax Pharmaceuticals
HOURGLASS; 4359; 25 ;	Clozapine	25 mg	Pale Yellow	Tablet	Circle	Ivax Pharmaceuticals
HOURGLASS; 4360; 100 ;	Clozapine	100 mg	Pale Yellow	Tablet	Circle	Ivax Pharmaceuticals
HOURGLASS; 4389	Fluvoxamine Maleate	25 mg	White	Tablet	Circle	Ivax Pharmaceuticals
HOURGLASS; 4391	Fluvoxamine Maleate	50 mg	Yellow	Tablet	Circle, Scored	Ivax Pharmaceuticals
HOURGLASS; 4392	Fluvoxamine Maleate	100 mg	Beige	Tablet	Circle	Ivax Pharmaceuticals
HOURGLASS; 4430; 100	Misoprostol	100 mcg		Tablet		Ivax Pharmaceuticals
HOURGLASS; 4431; 200	Misoprostol	200 mcg	White	Tablet	Circle, Scored	Ivax Pharmaceuticals
HOURGLASS; 4510	Fluoxetine Hydrochloride	10 mg	Light Green	Tablet	Oval	Ivax Pharmaceuticals
HOURGLASS; 4960	Flutamide	125 mg	Light Brown Opaque	Capsule		Ivax Pharmaceuticals
HOURGLASS; 4980	Propoxyphene Napsylate and Acetaminophen	100 mg; 650 mg	Pink	Coated Tablet	Capsule-Shape	Ivax Pharmaceuticals
HOURGLASS; 5032; 20/25	Lisinopril and Hydrochlorothiazide	20 mg; 25 mg	Peach	Tablet	Circle	Ivax Pharmaceuticals
HOURGLASS; 5033; 10/12.5	Lisinopril and Hydrochlorothiazide	10 mg; 12.5 mg	Blue	Tablet	Circle	Ivax Pharmaceuticals
HOURGLASS; 5034; 20/12.5	Lisinopril and Hydrochlorothiazide	20 mg; 12.5 mg	Yellow	Tablet	Circle	Ivax Pharmaceuticals
HOURGLASS; 5663; 5	Buspirone Hydrochloride	5 mg	White	Tablet	Oval	Ivax Pharmaceuticals
HOURGLASS; 5664; 10	Buspirone Hydrochloride	10 mg	White	Tablet	Oval	Ivax Pharmaceuticals
HOURGLASS; 5675; 15	Mirtazapine	15 mg	Yellow	Tablet	Circle, Scored	Ivax Pharmaceuticals
HOURGLASS; 5676; 30	Mirtazapine	30 mg	Tan	Tablet	Circle, Scored	Ivax Pharmaceuticals
HOURGLASS; 5695; 45	Mirtazapine	45 mg	White	Tablet	Circle	Ivax Pharmaceuticals
HOURGLASS; 7300 ;	Verapamil Hydrochloride	240 mg	Ivory	Extended-Release Tablet	Oblong	Ivax Pharmaceuticals
HOURGLASS; 9200	Glipizide	10 mg	White	Tablet	Circle, Scored	Ivax Pharmaceuticals
HOURGLASS; 9201	Glipizide	5 mg	White	Tablet	Circle	Ivax Pharmaceuticals
HOURLASS; 7301 ;	Verapamil Hydrochloride	180 mg	Orange	Extended-Release Tablet	Oblong, Scored	Ivax Pharmaceuticals
HTI; 77 ;	Thalitone	15 mg	White	Tablet	Kidney-Shape, Compressed	Monarch Pharmaceuticals
HX 814 ;	Atuss Hx	5 mg; 300 mg	Maroon, White	Capsule		Atley Pharmaceuticals
HYCODAN	Hycodan	5 mg; 1.5 mg	White	Tablet	Circle, Scored	Dupont Pharma
HYCODAN	Hycodan	5 mg; 1.5 mg	White	Tablet	Circle, Scored	Endo Laboratories
HYDERGINE; 0.5; S ;	Hydergine	0.167 mg; 0.167 mg; 0.167 mg	White	Tablet	Circle	Novartis
HYDREA; 830	Hydrea	500 mg	Pink and Green	Capsule		Bristol-Myers Squibb
HZ	Halls Zinc Defense Cold Season Dietary Supplement	5 mg		Lozenge/troche		Pfizer Consumer Health Care
I; 25	Imitrex	25 mg	White	Coated Tablet	Triangle	Glaxosmithkline
IBU; 400	Ibuprofen	400 mg	White	Tablet		Warner Chilcott
IBU; 600	Ibuprofen	600 mg	White	Coated Tablet		Warner Chilcott
IBU; 800	Ibuprofen	800 mg	White	Tablet		Warner Chilcott
IC	Cartrol	5 mg	White	Tablet	Oval	Abbott Laboratories
IE; 1.25; G	Indapamide	1.25 mg	Orange	Tablet	Circle	Par Pharmaceutical
IE; 2.5; G	Indapamide	2.5 mg	White	Tablet	Circle	Par Pharmaceutical
IKA	Serophene	50 mg	White	Tablet		Serono
IL; 3581	Theochron	300 mg	White	Extended-Release Tablet	Capsule-Shape, Scored	Forest Pharmaceuticals
IL; 3583	Theochron	200 mg	White	Extended-Release Tablet	Oval, Convex, Scored	Forest Pharmaceuticals
IL; 3584	Theochron	100 mg	White	Extended-Release Tablet	Circle, Convex, Scored	Forest Pharmaceuticals
IL; 3609	Propranolol Hydrochloride	60 mg	Brown and Clear	Extended-Release Capsule		Novartis Generics
IL; 3610	Propranolol Hydrochloride	80 mg	Opaque Blue and Clear	Extended-Release Capsule		Novartis Generics
IL; 3611	Propranolol Hydrochloride	120 mg	Opaque Blue and Clear	Extended-Release Capsule		Novartis Generics
IL; 3612	Propranolol Hydrochloride	160 mg	Opaque Blue and Clear	Extended-Release Capsule		Novartis Generics
IL; 3613	Isochron	40 mg	Peach	Capsule, Extended Release	Circle	Forest Pharmaceuticals
IL; 3625	Theocap	300 mg	Clear with Off-White Beads	Capsule		Forest Pharmaceuticals
IL; 3634	Theocap	200 mg	Clear and White with Off-White Beads	Capsule		Forest Pharmaceuticals
IL; 3638	Theocap	125 mg	Clear with Off-White Beads	Capsule		Forest Pharmaceuticals
IMDUR	Imdur	30 mg	White	Tablet, Extended Release	Capsule-Shape	Schering
IMDUR ; 120	Imdur	120 mg	White	Tablet, Extended Release	Capsule-Shape	Schering
IMITREX 50 LOGO	Imitrex	50 mg	White	Tablet	Triangle	Glaxosmithkline
IMITREX 100 LOGO	Imitrex	100 mg	Pink	Tablet	Triangle	Glaxosmithkline
IMO ; 2 125	Imodium Advanced	2 mg; 125 mg	White	Tablet	Oblong	Mcneil Consumer Products
IMODIUM AD; 2 MG	Imodium A-D Antidiarrheal	2 mg	Pale Green	Tablet		Mcneil Consumer Products
IMODIUM; 2/125	Imodium Advanced	2 mg; 125 mg	Light Green	Tablet, Chewable	Circle, Scored	Mcneil Consumer Products
INDERAL; 40 ;	Inderal	40 mg	Green	Tablet	Six-Sided, Scored	Wyeth Pharmaceuticals
INDERAL; 60; I	Inderal	60 mg	Pink	Tablet	Six-Sided, Scored	Wyeth Pharmaceuticals
INDERAL; 80; I	Inderal	80 mg	Yellow	Tablet	Six-Sided, Scored	Wyeth Pharmaceuticals
INDERAL; 90; I	Inderal	90 mg	Lavender	Tablet	Six-Sided, Scored	Wyeth Pharmaceuticals
INDERAL; LA; 60	Inderal LA	60 mg	White and Light Blue	Capsule		Wyeth Pharmaceuticals
INDERAL; LA; 80	Inderal LA	80 mg	Light Blue	Capsule		Wyeth Pharmaceuticals

IMPRINT	BRAND/GENERIC NAME	STRENGTH	COLOR	FORM	SHAPE	MANUFACTURER
INDERAL; LA; 120	Inderal LA	120 mg	Light Blue and Dark Blue	Capsule		Wyeth Pharmaceuticals
INDERAL; LA; 160	Inderal LA	160 mg	Dark Blue	Capsule		Wyeth Pharmaceuticals
INDERIDE LA; 80/50	Inderide LA	80 mg; 50 mg	Beige with 4 Gold Bands	Extended-Release Capsule		Wyeth Pharmaceuticals
INDERIDE LA; 120/50	Inderide LA	120 mg; 50 mg	Beige and Brown with 4 Gold Bands	Extended-Release Capsule		Wyeth Pharmaceuticals
INDERIDE LA; 160/50	Inderide LA	160 mg; 50 mg	Brown with 4 Gold Bands	Extended-Release Capsule		Wyeth Pharmaceuticals
INDERIDE; 40/25; I	Inderide	25 mg; 40 mg	Off-White	Tablet	Six-Sided, Scored	Wyeth Pharmaceuticals
INDERIDE; 80/25; I	Inderide	80 mg; 25 mg	Off-White	Tablet	Six-Sided, Scored	Wyeth Pharmaceuticals
INOR	Plan B	0.75 mg	White	Tablet	Circle	Duramed Pharmaceuticals
INV; 258	Iodur	30 mg	White	Tablet	Circle, Scored	Duramed Pharmaceuticals
INV; 290	Naproxen DR	500 mg	White	21-Day Tablet Pack	Capsule-Shape	Geneva Generics
INV; 309	Warfarin Sodium	1 mg	Pink	Tablet	Square	Geneva Generics
INV; 310; 5	Warfarin Sodium	2 mg	Light Purple	Tablet	Square	Geneva Generics
INV; 311; 2.5	Warfarin Sodium	2.5 mg	Green	Tablet	Square	Geneva Generics
INV; 312; 4	Warfarin Sodium	4 mg	Blue	Tablet	Square	Geneva Generics
INV; 313; 5	Warfarin Sodium	5 mg	Peach	Tablet	Square	Geneva Generics
INV; 314; 7.5	Warfarin Sodium	7.5 mg	Yellow	Tablet	Square	Geneva Generics
INV; 315; 10	Warfarin Sodium	10 mg	White	Tablet	Square	Geneva Generics
INV; 375	Ticlopidine Hcl	250 mg	Light Orange	Coated Tablet	Circle	Geneva Generics
INV; 423; 3	Warfarin Sodium	3 mg	Tan	Tablet	Square, Scored	Geneva Generics
INV; 424; 6	Warfarin Sodium	6 mg	Teal	Tablet	Square	Geneva Generics
IP 131 ; 400	Ibuprofen	400 mg	White	Tablet	Circle	Watson Laboratories
IP 132 ; 600	Ibuprofen	600 mg	White	Tablet	Oval	Watson Laboratories
IP 137 ; 800	Ibuprofen	800 mg	White	Tablet	Capsule-Shape	Watson Laboratories
IP 146	Reprexain	5 mg; 200 mg	White	Tablet	Oval	Watson Laboratories
ISMO; 20	Ismo	20 mg	Orange	Coated Tablet	Circle, Scored	Wyeth Pharmaceuticals
IT ; L3	Boniva	2.5 mg	White	Tablet	Oblong	Glaxosmithkline
IT ; L3	Boniva	2.5 mg	White	Tablet	Oblong	Roche Laboratories
J 125 ; NVR	Exjade	125 mg	Off-White	Tablet for Suspension	Circle	Novartis
J 250 ; NVR	Exjade	250 mg	Off-White	Tablet for Suspension	Circle	Novartis
J 500 ; NVR	Exjade	500 mg	Off-White	Tablet for Suspension	Circle	Novartis
J; 19	Potassium Permanganate	300 mg		Tablet		Eli Lilly
J; 37	Phenobarbital	60 mg	White	Tablet	Circle	Eli Lilly
J05	Caffeine, Citrated	65 mg		Tablet		Eli Lilly
J75 ;	Isuprel	10 mg	White	Tablet		Sanofi Winthrop Pharmaceuticals
J77 ;	Isuprel	15 mg	White	Tablet		Sanofi Winthrop Pharmaceuticals
JANSSEN ; G4 ;	Razadyne	4 mg	Off-White	Tablet		Ortho-Mcneil Neurologics
JANSSEN ; G8 ;	Razadyne	8 mg	Pink	Tablet		Ortho-Mcneil Neurologics
JANSSEN ; G12 ;	Razadyne	12 mg	Orange-Brown	Tablet		Ortho-Mcneil Neurologics
JANSSEN R 1	Risperdal	1 mg	White	Tablet		Janssen Pharmaceutica Products
JANSSEN R 2	Risperdal	2 mg	Orange	Tablet		Janssen Pharmaceutica Products
JANSSEN R 3	Risperdal	3 mg	Yellow	Tablet		Janssen Pharmaceutica Products
JANSSEN R 4	Risperdal	4 mg	Green	Tablet		Janssen Pharmaceutica Products
JANSSEN RIS 0.25	Risperdal	0.25 mg	Dark Yellow	Tablet		Janssen Pharmaceutica Products
JANSSEN RIS 0.5	Risperdal	0.5 mg	Red-Brown	Tablet		Janssen Pharmaceutica Products
JANSSEN; AST; 10	Hismanal	10 mg	White	Tablet		Janssen Pharmaceutica Products
JANSSEN; CIS; 10	Prepulsid	10 mg		Tablet		Janssen Pharmaceutica Products
JANSSEN; IMODIUM	Imodium	2 mg	Light Green and Dark Green	Capsule		Mcneil Consumer Products
JANSSEN; L; 50	Ergamisol	50 mg	White	Coated Tablet		Janssen Pharmaceutica Products
JANSSEN; NIZORAL	Nizoral	200 mg	White	Tablet		Janssen Pharmaceutica Products
JANSSEN; P; 10	Propulsid	10 mg	White	Tablet	Circle, Small, Scored	Janssen Pharmaceutica Products
JANSSEN; P; 20	Propulsid	20 mg	Blue	Tablet	Oval	Janssen Pharmaceutica Products
JANSSEN; R; 2	Risperdal	2 mg	Orange	Tablet		Janssen Pharmaceutica Products
JANSSEN; R; 3	Risperdal	3 mg	Yellow	Tablet		Janssen Pharmaceutica Products
JANSSEN; R; 4	Risperdal	4 mg	Green	Tablet		Janssen Pharmaceutica Products
JANSSEN; SPORANOX; 100	Sporanox	100 mg	Blue and Pink	Capsule		Janssen Pharmaceutica Products
JANSSEN; VERMOX	Vermox	100 mg	Orange	Tablet, Chewable		Mcneil Consumer Products
JSP; 507	Aspirin, Butalbital, Caffeine and Codeine	325 mg; 50 mg; 40 mg; 30 mg	Yellow and Blue	Capsule		Duramed Pharmaceuticals
JSP; 513	Unithroid	25 mcg	Peach	Tablet	Round, Partially Bisected Scored	Watson Laboratories
JSP; 514	Unithroid	50 mcg	White	Tablet	Round, Partially Bisected Scored	Watson Laboratories
JSP; 515	Unithroid	75 mcg	Purple	Tablet	Round, Partially Bisected Scored	Watson Laboratories
JSP; 516	Unithroid	100 mcg	Yellow	Tablet	Round, Partially Bisected Scored	Watson Laboratories
JSP; 519	Unithroid	125 mcg	Tan	Tablet	Round, Partially Bisected Scored	Watson Laboratories
JSP; 520	Unithroid	150 mcg	Blue	Tablet	Round, Partially Bisected Scored	Watson Laboratories
JSP; 522	Unithroid	200 mcg	Pink	Tablet	Round, Partially Bisected Scored	Watson Laboratories
JSP; 523	Unithroid	300 mcg	Green	Tablet	Round, Partially Bisected Scored	Watson Laboratories

IMPRINT	BRAND/GENERIC NAME	STRENGTH	COLOR	FORM	SHAPE	MANUFACTURER
JSP; 561	Unithroid	88 mcg	Olive	Tablet	Round, Partially Bisected Scored	Watson Laboratories
JSP; 562	Unithroid	112 mcg	Rose	Tablet	Round, Partially Bisected Scored	Watson Laboratories
JSP; 563	Unithroid	175 mcg	Lilac	Tablet	Round, Partially Bisected Scored	Watson Laboratories
JSP; 873	Thyrox	25 mcg	Peach	Tablet		Watson Laboratories
JSP; 874	Thyrox	50 mcg	White	Tablet		Watson Laboratories
JSP; 875	Thyrox	75 mcg	Purple	Tablet		Watson Laboratories
JSP; 876	Thyrox	88 mcg	Olive	Tablet		Watson Laboratories
JSP; 877	Thyrox	100 mcg	Yellow	Tablet		Watson Laboratories
JSP; 878	Thyrox	112 mcg	Rose	Tablet		Watson Laboratories
JSP; 879	Thyrox	125 mcg	Tan	Tablet		Watson Laboratories
JSP; 880	Thyrox	150 mcg	Blue	Tablet		Watson Laboratories
JSP; 881	Thyrox	175 mcg	Lilac	Tablet		Watson Laboratories
JSP; 882	Thyrox	200 mcg	Pink	Tablet		Watson Laboratories
JSP; 883	Thyrox	300 mcg	Green	Tablet		Watson Laboratories
K	Clarinex Reditabs	2.5 mg	Light Red	Tablet, Disintegrating		Schering-Plough
K ; 220	Leflunomide	10 mg	White	Tablet	Circle	Par Pharmaceutical
K ; 221	Leflunomide	20 mg	White	Tablet	Triangle	Par Pharmaceutical
K 39 ;	Acetaminophen	325 mg	White	Tablet	Circle	Ivax Pharmaceuticals
K 400 ;	Glycopyrrolate	1 mg	White	Tablet	Circle	Par Pharmaceutical
K 401 ;	Glycopyrrolate	2 mg	White	Tablet	Circle	Par Pharmaceutical
K; ARROW ;	Aspirin	325 mg	Orange	Enteric-Coated Tablet	Circle, Scored	Watson Laboratories
K; U	Levsin Forte	0.25 mg	White	Tablet		Schwarz Pharma
K1	Kytril	1 mg	White	Tablet	Triangle	Roche Laboratories
K5	Clonazepam Odt	0.125 mg	White	Tablet, Disintegrating	Circle	Par Pharmaceutical
K6	Clonazepam Odt	0.25 mg	White	Tablet, Disintegrating	Circle	Par Pharmaceutical
K7	Clonazepam Odt	0.5 mg	White	Tablet, Disintegrating	Circle	Par Pharmaceutical
K8	Clonazepam Odt	1 mg	White	Tablet, Disintegrating	Circle	Par Pharmaceutical
K9	Clonazepam Odt	2 mg	White	Tablet, Disintegrating	Circle	Par Pharmaceutical
KA	Kaletra	200 mg; 50 mg	Yellow	Tablet	Oval	Abbott Laboratories
KADIAN 20MG	Kadian	20 mg	Yellow Opaque	Capsule, Extended Release		Alpharma
KADIAN 30MG	Kadian	30 mg	Blue-Violet Opaque	Capsule, Extended Release		Alpharma
KADIAN 50MG	Kadian	50 mg	Blue Opaque	Capsule, Extended Release		Alpharma
KADIAN 60MG	Kadian	60 mg	Pink Opaque	Capsule, Extended Release		Alpharma
KADIAN 100MG	Kadian	100 mg	Green Opaque	Capsule, Extended Release		Alpharma
KC; M10	Klor-Con M10	10 meq	White	Extended-Release Tablet	Oblong	Upsher-Smith Laboratories
KC; M20	Klor-Con M20	20 meq	White	Extended-Release Tablet	Oblong, Scored	Upsher-Smith Laboratories
KC; M20	Klor-Con M20	1500 mg	White	Tablet	Oblong	Upsher-Smith Laboratories
KEFLEX 250 MG	Keflex	250 mg	Opaque Dark Green, Opaque White	Capsule		Advancis Pharmaceutical
KEFLEX 333 MG	Keflex	333 mg	Opaque Light Green	Capsule		Advancis Pharmaceutical
KEFLEX 500 MG	Keflex	500 mg	Opaque Dark Green, Opaque Light Green	Capsule		Advancis Pharmaceutical
KEFLEX 750 MG	Keflex	750 mg	Opaque Dark Green	Capsule		Advancis Pharmaceutical
KEFTAB; 500	Keftab	500 mg	Dark Green	Tablet	Circle	Biovail Pharmaceuticals
KEMADRIN; S3A	Kemadrin	5 mg	White	Tablet		Glaxosmithkline
KERLONE; 10	Kerlone	10 mg	White	Tablet	Circle	Sanofi-Aventis U.S.
KERLONE; 10	Kerlone	10 mg	White	Tablet	Circle	Searle
KERLONE; 20; B	Kerlone	20 mg	White	Tablet	Circle	Sanofi-Aventis U.S.
KERLONE; 20; B	Kerlone	20 mg	White	Tablet	Circle	Searle
KLOR-CON 10	Klor-Con 10	750 mg	Yellow	Coated Tablet	Circle	Upsher-Smith Laboratories
KLOR-CON; 8	Klor-Con 8	600 mg	Blue	Coated Tablet	Circle, Bevel-Edged	Upsher-Smith Laboratories
KLOTRIX; BL; 10MEQ; 770	Klotrix	750 mg	Orange	Timed-Release Tablet	Circle	Bristol-Myers Squibb
KOS ; 502	Advicor	500 mg; 20 mg	Light Yellow	Tablet, Extended Release	Capsule-Shape	Kos Pharmaceuticals
KOS ; 752	Advicor	750 mg; 20 mg	Light Orange	Tablet, Extended Release	Capsule-Shape	Kos Pharmaceuticals
KOS ; 1002	Advicor	1000 mg; 20 mg	Light Purple/dark Pink	Tablet, Extended Release	Capsule-Shape	Kos Pharmaceuticals
KOS ; 1004	Advicor	1000 mg; 40 mg	Reddish Brown	Tablet, Extended Release	Capsule-Shape	Kos Pharmaceuticals
KOS; 500	Niaspan	500 mg	Off-White	Extended-Release Tablet	Capsule-Shape	Kos Pharmaceuticals
KOS; 750	Niaspan	750 mg	Off-White	Extended-Release Tablet	Capsule-Shape	Kos Pharmaceuticals
KOS; 1000	Niaspan	1000 mg	Off-White	Extended-Release Tablet	Capsule-Shape	Kos Pharmaceuticals
KPH; 102	Azulfidine En-Tabs	500 mg	Gold	Enteric-Coated Tablet	Oval	Pharmacia & Upjohn
KPI; 1	Acetaminophen and Hydrocodone Bitartrate	500 mg; 5 mg		Tablet		King Pharmaceuticals
KPI; 2	Acetaminophen and Hydrocodone Bitartrate	750 mg; 7.5 mg	Light Blue	Tablet	Circle	King Pharmaceuticals
KREMERS URBAN; 320	Nitrocine Timecaps	2.5 mg	Violet and Clear	Sustained-Release Capsule		Schwarz Pharma
KREMERS URBAN; 330	Nitrocine Timecaps	6.5 mg	Blue and Orange	Sustained-Release Capsule		Schwarz Pharma
KREMERS URBAN; 340	Nitrocine Timecaps	9 mg	Clear	Sustained-Release Capsule		Schwarz Pharma
KU; 114	Omeprazole	10 mg	White	Delayed-Release Capsule		Schwarz Pharma
KU; 118	Omeprazole	20 mg	White and Gold	Delayed-Release Capsule		Schwarz Pharma
L 438	Pain Reliever Sinus Maximum Strength	500 mg; 30 mg	Light Green	Tablet		Teva Pharmaceuticals
L; 4; M	Levothyroxine Sodium	25 mcg	Orange	Tablet	Capsule-Shape, Scored	Mylan Pharmaceuticals
L; 5; M	Levothyroxine Sodium	50 mcg	White	Tablet	Capsule-Shape, Scored	Mylan Pharmaceuticals
L; 6; M	Levothyroxine Sodium	75 mcg	Purple	Tablet	Capsule-Shape, Scored	Mylan Pharmaceuticals

IMPRINT	BRAND/GENERIC NAME	STRENGTH	COLOR	FORM	SHAPE	MANUFACTURER
L; 7; M	Levothyroxine Sodium	88 mcg	Light Green	Tablet	Capsule-Shape, Scored	Mylan Pharmaceuticals
L; 8; M	Levothyroxine Sodium	100 mcg	Yellow	Tablet	Capsule-Shape, Scored	Mylan Pharmaceuticals
L; 9; LL	Ledercillin VK	500 mg	White	Tablet	Round, Convex, Bisected Scored	Lederle Laboratories
L; 9; M	Levothyroxine Sodium	112 mcg	Rose	Tablet	Capsule-Shape, Scored	Mylan Pharmaceuticals
L; 10; LL	Ledercillin VK	250 mg	White	Tablet	Round, Convex, Bisected Scored	Lederle Laboratories
L; 10; M	Levothyroxine Sodium	125 mcg	Gray	Tablet	Capsule-Shape, Scored	Mylan Pharmaceuticals
L; 11; M	Levothyroxine Sodium	150 mcg	Blue	Tablet	Capsule-Shape, Scored	Mylan Pharmaceuticals
L; 12; M	Levothyroxine Sodium	175 mcg	Light Purple	Tablet	Capsule-Shape, Scored	Mylan Pharmaceuticals
L; 13; M	Levothyroxine Sodium	200 mcg	Pink	Tablet	Capsule-Shape, Scored	Mylan Pharmaceuticals
L; 14; M	Levothyroxine Sodium	300 mcg	Green	Tablet	Capsule-Shape, Scored	Mylan Pharmaceuticals
LA; CTM; D	Chlor-Trimeton Allergy Decongestant 12 Hour	8 mg; 120 mg	Polished Medium Green	Tablet	Circle	Schering-Plough Healthcare Products
LA; CTM; D ;	Chlor-Trimeton Long-Acting Decongestant Repetabs	120 mg; 8 mg	Green	Timed-Release Tablet		Schering-Plough Healthcare Products
LAMICTAL; 25	Lamictal	25 mg	White	Tablet	Shield-Shape	Glaxosmithkline
LAMICTAL; 100	Lamictal	100 mg	Peach	Tablet	Shield-Shape	Glaxosmithkline
LAMICTAL; 150	Lamictal	150 mg	Cream	Tablet	Shield-Shape	Glaxosmithkline
LAMICTAL; 200	Lamictal	200 mg	Blue	Tablet	Shield-Shape	Glaxosmithkline
LAMISIL; 250	Lamisil	250 mg	White to Yellow-Tinged	Tablet	Circle, BI-Convex, Bevelled	Novartis
LAN; 0586	Dicyclomine Hydrochloride	10 mg	Blue	Capsule		Duramed Pharmaceuticals
LANOXIN; T9A	Lanoxin	0.5 mg	Green	Tablet	Circle, Scored	Glaxosmithkline
LANOXIN; X3A	Lanoxin	0.25 mg	White	Tablet	Circle, Scored	Glaxosmithkline
LANOXIN; Y3B	Lanoxin	0.125 mg	Yellow	Tablet	Circle, Scored	Glaxosmithkline
LARIAM; 250; ROCHE	Lariam	250 mg	White	Tablet	Circle, Scored	Roche Pharmaceuticals
LAROBEC; ROCHE	Larobec	100 mg; 18 mg; 0.5 mg; 500 mg; 15 mg; 15 mg; 5 mcg	Orange	Coated Tablet	Oblong	Roche Pharmaceuticals
LARODOPA; ROCHE; 100	Larodopa	100 mg	Pink and Scarlet	Capsule		Roche Pharmaceuticals
LARODOPA; ROCHE; 250	Larodopa	250 mg	Pink and Beige	Capsule		Roche Pharmaceuticals
LARODOPA; ROCHE; 500	Larodopa	500 mg	Pink	Capsule		Roche Pharmaceuticals
LAROTID; 500; BMP; 212	Larotid	500 mg	Buff	Capsule		Glaxosmithkline
LASIX; 40; HOECHST	Lasix	40 mg	White	Tablet	Circle	Aventis Pharmaceuticals
LASIX; 40; HOECHST	Lasix	40 mg	White	Tablet	Circle	Sanofi-Aventis U.S.
LASIX; 80; HOECHST	Lasix	80 mg	White	Tablet	Circle	Aventis Pharmaceuticals
LASIX; 80; HOECHST	Lasix	80 mg	White	Tablet	Circle	Sanofi-Aventis U.S.
LCE; 50	Stalevo 50	12.5 mg; 50 mg; 200 mg	Brown or Grey	Tablet	Circle	Novartis
LCE; 100	Stalevo 100	25 mg; 100 mg; 200 mg	Brown or Grey	Tablet	Oval	Novartis
LCE; 150	Stalevo 150	37.5 mg; 150 mg; 200 mg	Brown or Grey	Tablet	Oblong	Novartis
LCH	Protegra	200 IU; 250 mg; 3 mg; 7.5 mg; 1 mg; 15 mcg; 1.5 mg	Orange	Capsule, Liquid Filled	Oval, Scored	Lederle Laboratories
LE	Tridione	150 mg	White	Tablet, Chewable		Abbott Laboratories
LEDERLE; A; 20	Acetaminophen	500 mg	Blue	Capsule		Lederle Laboratories
LEDERLE; A3; 250 MG	Achromycin V	250 mg	Yellow and Blue	Capsule		Lederle Laboratories
LEDERLE; A31	Ampicillin Trihydrate	250 mg	Green and White	Capsule		Lederle Laboratories
LEDERLE; A32	Ampicillin Trihydrate	500 mg	Green and White	Capsule		Lederle Laboratories
LEDERLE; A33	Amoxicillin	250 mg	Grey and Green	Capsule		Lederle Laboratories
LEDERLE; A34	Amoxicillin	500 mg	Gray and Green	Capsule		Lederle Laboratories
LEDERLE; C; 61	Cephradine	250 mg	Green and Light Pink	Capsule		Lederle Laboratories
LEDERLE; C; 62	Cephradine	500 mg	Light Green	Capsule		Lederle Laboratories
LEDERLE; C; 64	Cephalexin	250 mg	Grey and Red	Capsule		Esi Lederle
LEDERLE; C; 65	Cephalexin	500 mg	Red	Capsule		Esi Lederle
LEDERLE; C54; CEFACLOR; 250MG	Cefaclor	250 mg	Opaque Pink and Blue	Capsule		Lederle Laboratories
LEDERLE; C55	Clorazepate Dipotassium	3.75 mg	White and Lavender	Capsule		Lederle Laboratories
LEDERLE; C56	Clorazepate Dipotassium	7.5 mg	Lavender and Maroon	Capsule		Lederle Laboratories
LEDERLE; C57	Clorazepate Dipotassium	15 mg	Lavender	Capsule		Lederle Laboratories
LEDERLE; C58; CEFACLOR; 500MG	Cefaclor	500 mg	Opaque Lavender and Blue	Capsule		Lederle Laboratories
LEDERLE; D16	Dicloxacillin Sodium	250 mg	Green	Capsule		Lederle Laboratories
LEDERLE; D17	Dicloxacillin Sodium	500 mg	Light Green	Capsule		Lederle Laboratories
LEDERLE; D25	Doxycycline Hyclate	100 mg	Blue	Capsule		Lederle Laboratories
LEDERLE; D36	Dolene	65 mg	Pink	Capsule		Lederle Laboratories
LEDERLE; D47	Doxepin Hydrochloride	25 mg	Ivory and Yellow	Capsule		Lederle Laboratories
LEDERLE; D48	Doxepin Hydrochloride	50 mg	Lavendar and Dark Red	Capsule		Lederle Laboratories
LEDERLE; D49	Doxepin Hydrochloride	75 mg	Purple and Dark Pink	Capsule		Lederle Laboratories
LEDERLE; D50	Doxepin Hydrochloride	10 mg	Buff or Blue	Capsule		Lederle Laboratories
LEDERLE; D54	Doxepin Hydrochloride	100 mg	Green and White	Capsule		Lederle Laboratories
LEDERLE; D55	Doxepin Hydrochloride	150 mg	Gray and Orange	Capsule		Lederle Laboratories
LEDERLE; D62	Disopyramide	100 mg	Dark Red and Blue	Capsule		Lederle Laboratories
LEDERLE; I19 ;	Indomethacin	25 mg	Pink and White	Capsule		Lederle Laboratories
LEDERLE; I20 ;	Indomethacin	50 mg	Opaque Pink and Opaque White	Capsule		Lederle Laboratories
LEDERLE; K1	Ketoprofen	25 mg	Dark Green	Capsule		Lederle Laboratories

IMPRINT	BRAND/GENERIC NAME	STRENGTH	COLOR	FORM	SHAPE	MANUFACTURER
LEDERLE; K2	Ketoprofen	50 mg	Light Green	Capsule		Lederle Laboratories
LEDERLE; K3	Ketoprofen	75 mg	White	Capsule		Lederle Laboratories
LEDERLE; O; P69	Prazosin Hydrochloride	1 mg	Flesh	Capsule		Lederle Laboratories
LEDERLE; O; P70	Prazosin Hydrochloride	2 mg	Pink	Capsule		Lederle Laboratories
LEDERLE; O; P71	Prazosin Hydrochloride	5 mg	Blue	Capsule		Lederle Laboratories
LEDERLE;C2; CENTRUM JR	Centrum JR. Plus Iron	18 mg; 5000 IU; 400 IU; 30 IU; 60 mg; 400 mcg; 1.5 mg; 1.7 mg; 20 mg; 2 mg; 6 mcg; 40 mg; 2 mg; 15 mg; 1 mg; 45 mcg; 150 mg; 20 mcg; 20 mcg; 10 mg; 10 mcg; 50 mg; 108 mg	Various	Tablet, Chewable	Oval	Wyeth Consumer Healthcare
LEMMON	Dralserp	25 mg; 0.1 mg	Orange	Tablet		Teva Pharmaceuticals
LEMMON	Promethazine Hydrochloride	25 mg	Blue	Tablet	Circle, Convex, Scored	Teva Pharmaceuticals
LEMMON; 30	Neothylline	200 mg	White	Tablet	Circle, Convex, Scored	Teva Pharmaceuticals
LEMMON; 37	Neothylline	400 mg	White	Tablet	Oblong, Scored	Teva Pharmaceuticals
LEMMON; 52	Uristat	0.03 mg; 5 mg; 0.03 mg; 5.5 mg; 20 mg; 50 mg	Blue	Tablet		Teva Pharmaceuticals
LEMMON; 71; 71	Statobex	35 mg	Green and White	Tablet	Oblong, Convex; Scored	Teva Pharmaceuticals
LEMMON; 77	Statobex-G	35 mg	Green	Tablet	Oblong, Scored	Teva Pharmaceuticals
LEMMON; 86; 86	S.B.P.	30 mg; 15 mg; 50 mg	White	Tablet	Circle, Flat, Beveled Edge, Scored	Teva Pharmaceuticals
LEMMON; 93-10; GLUCAMIDE; 100	Glucamide	100 mg	Blue	Tablet	Circle, Convex, Scored	Teva Pharmaceuticals
LEMMON; 105	Dralzine	25 mg	Yellow	Tablet	Oblong	Teva Pharmaceuticals
LEMMON; 123	Sed-Tens S.E.	10 mg	Red and White Speckled	Tablet	Oblong	Teva Pharmaceuticals
LEMMON; 128 128	Neothylline GG	200 mg; 200 mg	White	Tablet	Circle, Flat, Beveled Edge, Scored	Teva Pharmaceuticals
LEMMON; 133	Dexampex	15 mg	Green Transparent and Clear	Capsule		Teva Pharmaceuticals
LEMMON; 137	Dipav	150 mg	Brown and Clear	Capsule		Teva Pharmaceuticals
LEMMON; 169	B.P.P.	1.2 mg; 120 mg; 15 mg; 120 mg; 15 mg	Yellow	Tablet	Circle, Convex	Teva Pharmaceuticals
LEMMON; 178 178	Methampex	10 mg	Pink	Tablet	Oblong, Scored	Teva Pharmaceuticals
LEMMON; 179	Dexampex	15 mg	Blue	Tablet	Oblong	Teva Pharmaceuticals
LEMMON; 180	Dexampex	10 mg	Pink	Tablet	Oblong	Teva Pharmaceuticals
LEMMON; 211	Lexor	50 mg	Peach	Tablet		Teva Pharmaceuticals
LEMMON; 238	Diacin	200 mg	Red and Clear with Red and White Pellets Inside	Capsule		Teva Pharmaceuticals
LEMMON; 277	Statobex	35 mg	Green and White, Opaque	Capsule		Teva Pharmaceuticals
LEMMON; 341	Ruhexatal with Reserpine	30 mg; 10 mg; 0.1 mg; 20 mg		Tablet		Teva Pharmaceuticals
LESCOL XL; 80	Lescol XL	80 mg	Yellow	Extended-Release Tablet	Circle	Novartis
LEVAQUIN; 250	Levaquin	250 mg	Terra Cotta Pink	Coated Tablet		Ortho-Mcneil Pharmaceutical
LEVAQUIN; 500	Levaquin	500 mg	Peach	Coated Tablet		Ortho-Mcneil Pharmaceutical
LEVAQUIN; 750	Levaquin	750 mg	White	Coated Tablet	Rectangle, Modified	Ortho-Mcneil Pharmaceutical
LEXXEL 2; 5-2.5	Lexxel	5 mg; 2.5 mg	White	Extended-Release Tablet	Circle, Biconvex, Film-Coated	Astra Zeneca
LEXXEL; 1; 5-5	Lexxel	5 mg; 5 mg	White	Extended-Release Tablet	Circle, Biconvex	Astra Zeneca
LIBRITABS; 5; ROCHE	Libritabs	5 mg	Green	Coated Tablet	Circle, Scored	Roche Products
LIBRITABS; 10; ROCHE	Libritabs	10 mg	Green	Coated Tablet	Circle, Scored	Roche Products
LIBRITABS; 25; ROCHE	Libritabs	25 mg	Green	Coated Tablet	Circle, Scored	Roche Products
LILLY 3227 ; 10 MG	Strattera	10 mg	White	Capsule		Eli Lilly
LILLY 3228 ; 25 MG	Strattera	25 mg	Blue, White	Capsule		Eli Lilly
LILLY 3229 ; 40 MG	Strattera	40 mg	Blue	Capsule		Eli Lilly
LILLY 3238 ; 18 MG	Strattera	18 mg	Gold, White	Capsule		Eli Lilly
LILLY 3239 ; 60 MG	Strattera	60 mg	Blue, Gold	Capsule		Eli Lilly
LILLY F04 ; LILLY F04	Seromycin	250 mg	Opaque Gray, Opaque Red	Capsule		Eli Lilly
LILLY F40	Seconal	100 mg	Orange or Red	Capsule		Eli Lilly
LILLY F77	Becotin with Vitamin C	10 mg; 10 mg; 4.1 mg; 50 mg; 25 mg; 1 mcg; 150 mg	Green and Blue	Capsule		Eli Lilly
LILLY T03	Novacebrin with Fluoride	1 mg; 1.2 mg; 10 mcg; 60 mg; 1.5 mg; 2 mg; 1 mg; 3 mcg; 12 mg; 2.5 mg	Orange	Tablet, Chewable		Eli Lilly
LILLY; 3004; 90 MG	Prozac Weekly	90 mg	Green and Clear with White Enteric-Coated Pellets	Timed-Release Capsule		Eli Lilly
LILLY; 3061	Ceclor	250 mg	White and Purple	Capsule		Eli Lilly
LILLY; 3062	Ceclor	500 mg	Gray and Purple	Capsule		Eli Lilly
LILLY; 3075	Histadyl and A.S.A. Compound	4 mg; 325 mg	White and Red	Capsule		Eli Lilly
LILLY; 3110; DARVON COMP	Darvon Compound	32 mg; 389 mg; 32.4 mg	Pink and Gray	Capsule		Eli Lilly

IMPRINT	BRAND/GENERIC NAME	STRENGTH	COLOR	FORM	SHAPE	MANUFACTURER
LILLY; 3111; DARVON COMP 65	Darvon Compound 65	389 mg; 32.4 mg; 65 mg	Red and Grey	Capsule		Eli Lilly
LILLY; 3132; PINDAC; 12.5	Pindac	12.5 mg	Blue and Clear with Orange Beads	Capsule		Eli Lilly
LILLY; 3133; PINDAC; 25	Pindac	25 mg	Blue and Clear with White Beads	Capsule		Eli Lilly
LILLY; 3170	Lorabid Pulvules	200 mg	Blue and Gray	Capsule		Monarch Pharmaceuticals
LILLY; 3210; 10 MG	Sarafem	10 mg	Lavender	Capsule		Eli Lilly
LILLY; 3220; 20 MG	Sarafem	20 mg	Lavender and Pink	Capsule		Eli Lilly
LILLY; 3231; 6/25	Symbyax	6 mg; 25 mg	Mustard and Light Yellow	Capsule		Eli Lilly
LILLY; 3232; 12/25	Symbyax	12 mg; 25 mg	Red and Light Yellow	Capsule		Eli Lilly
LILLY; 3233; 6/50	Symbyax	6 mg; 50 mg	Mustard and Light Grey	Capsule		Eli Lilly
LILLY; 3234; 12/50	Symbyax	12 mg; 50 mg	Red and Light Grey	Capsule		Eli Lilly
LILLY; 4112	Zyprexa	2.5 mg	White	Tablet	Circle	Eli Lilly
LILLY; 4115	Zyprexa	5 mg	White	Tablet	Circle	Eli Lilly
LILLY; 4116	Zyprexa	7.5 mg	White	Tablet	Circle	Eli Lilly
LILLY; 4117	Zyprexa	10 mg	White	Tablet	Circle	Eli Lilly
LILLY; 4165	Evista	60 mg	White with Blue Ink	Coated Tablet	Circle	Eli Lilly
LILLY; 4415	Zyprexa	15 mg	Blue	Tablet	Egg-Shape	Eli Lilly
LILLY; 4420	Zyprexa	20 mg	Pink	Tablet	Egg-Shape	Eli Lilly
LILLY; A01	Ammonium Chloride	500 mg		Sustained-Release Tablet		Eli Lilly
LILLY; A02	Ferrous Sulfate	325 mg	Red	Sustained-Release Tablet		Eli Lilly
LILLY; A04	Pancreatin, Triple Strength	1 G		Sustained-Release Tablet		Eli Lilly
LILLY; A05	Potassium Chloride	300 mg		Tablet		Eli Lilly
LILLY; A06	Potassium Iodide	300 mg		Enteric-Coated Tablet		Eli Lilly
LILLY; A09	Sodium Chloride	1 GM		Enteric-Coated Tablet		Eli Lilly
LILLY; A10	Sodium Salicylate	325 mg		Coated Tablet		Eli Lilly
LILLY; A11	Sodium Salicylate	650 mg		Enteric-Coated Tablet		Eli Lilly
LILLY; A12	Ammonium Chloride	15 Gr		Sustained-Release Tablet		Eli Lilly
LILLY; A14	Thyroid	30 mg		Enteric-Coated Tablet		Eli Lilly
LILLY; A15	Thyroid	60 mg		Enteric-Coated Tablet		Eli Lilly
LILLY; A16	Thyroid	120 mg		Enteric-Coated Tablet		Eli Lilly
LILLY; A17	Thyroid	200 mg		Enteric-Coated Tablet		Eli Lilly
LILLY; A25	A.S.A.	325 mg		Enteric-Coated Tablet		Eli Lilly
LILLY; A27	Amesec	130 mg; 25 mg; 25 mg		Sustained-Release Tablet		Eli Lilly
LILLY; A30	Aminosalicylic Acid	500 mg		Sustained-Release Tablet		Eli Lilly
LILLY; A31	Potassium Chloride	1 GM		Enteric-Coated Tablet		Eli Lilly
LILLY; A32	A.S.A.	650 mg		Enteric-Coated Tablet		Eli Lilly
LILLY; A36	Ferrous Sulfate	325 mg	Green	Sustained-Release Tablet		Eli Lilly
LILLY; A39	Quinidine Sulfate	200 mg		Enteric-Coated Tablet		Eli Lilly
LILLY; B51	Alphalin	7.5 mg		Capsule		Eli Lilly
LILLY; B52	Alphalin	15 mg		Capsule		Eli Lilly
LILLY; B60	Deltalin	1.25 mg		Capsule, Liquid Filled		Eli Lilly
LILLY; C06	Cascara	325 mg	Chocolate	Coated Tablet		Eli Lilly
LILLY; C07	Cascara Compound	16 mg; 16 mg; 10 mg; 8 mg; 4 mg	Pink	Coated Tablet		Eli Lilly
LILLY; C11	Rhinitis, Full Strength	32.5 mg; 32.5 mg; 5.8 mg	Chocolate	Coated Tablet		Eli Lilly
LILLY; C13	Ferrous Sulfate	325 mg	Chocolate	Coated Tablet		Eli Lilly
LILLY; C27	V-Cillin K	125 mg	White	Tablet		Eli Lilly
LILLY; C29	V-Cillin K	250 mg	White	Tablet		Eli Lilly
LILLY; C31	Anhydron K	2 mg; 500 mg		Coated Tablet		Eli Lilly
LILLY; C32	Anhydron Kr	2 mg; 500 mg; 0.25 mg		Coated Tablet		Eli Lilly
LILLY; C36	Quinine Sulfate	325 mg	Chocolate	Coated Tablet		Eli Lilly
LILLY; C46	V-Cillin K	500 mg	White	Tablet		Eli Lilly
LILLY; C47	Hepicebrin	1.5 mg; 10 mcg; 20 mg; 75 mg; 2 mg; 3 mg		Coated Tablet		Eli Lilly
LILLY; C71	Multi-Cebrin	5 mg; 25 mg; 6 mg; 3 mg; 25 mcg; 3 mg; 3 mg; 1.2 mg; 3 mcg; 75 mg	Dark Red	Tablet		Eli Lilly
LILLY; DARVOCET-N 100	Darvocet-N 100	100 mg; 650 mg	Dark Orange	Coated Tablet	Capsule-Shape	Eli Lilly
LILLY; DARVON-N; 100 ;	Darvon-N	100 mg	Buff	Tablet	Oblong	Eli Lilly
LILLY; DARVON-N; ASA	Darvon-N with A.S.A.	100 mg; 325 mg	Orange	Tablet	Circle	Eli Lilly
LILLY; F09	Seromycin with Isoniazid	250 mg; 150 mg		Capsule		Eli Lilly
LILLY; F11 ;	A.S.A.	325 mg	Clear or Pink	Capsule		Eli Lilly
LILLY; F13	A.S.A. Compound	227 mg; 32.5 mg; 160 mg	White Opaque	Capsule		Eli Lilly
LILLY; F14	Ephedrine and Amytal	25 mg; 50 mg	Yellow	Capsule		Eli Lilly
LILLY; F20	Ephedrine and Seconal Sodium	25 mg; 50 mg	Scarlet	Capsule		Eli Lilly
LILLY; F23	Amytal Sodium No. 4	65 mg	Blue	Capsule		Eli Lilly
LILLY; F24	Ephedrine Sulfate	25 mg	Pink	Capsule		Eli Lilly
LILLY; F25	Ephedrine Sulfate	50 mg	Pink	Capsule		Eli Lilly

IMPRINT	BRAND/GENERIC NAME	STRENGTH	COLOR	FORM	SHAPE	MANUFACTURER
LILLY; F26	Quinine Sulfate	130 mg	White Opaque	Capsule		Eli Lilly
LILLY; F27	Quinine Sulfate	200 mg	White Opaque	Capsule		Eli Lilly
LILLY; F29	Quinine Sulfate	325 mg	White Opaque	Capsule		Eli Lilly
LILLY; F30	A.S.A. Compound	227 mg; 160 mg; 32.5 mg	Pink	Capsule		Eli Lilly
LILLY; F33	Amytal Sodium No. 2	200 mg	Blue	Capsule		Eli Lilly
LILLY; F36	Copavin	15 mg; 15 mg	Clear	Capsule		Eli Lilly
LILLY; F39	Quinidine Sulfate	200 mg		Capsule		Eli Lilly
LILLY; F41	Bilron	300 mg	Green	Capsule		Eli Lilly
LILLY; F42	Seconal Sodium	50 mg	Red	Capsule		Eli Lilly
LILLY; F43	Betalin Compound	3.333 mg; 10 mg; 1 mg; 2 mg; 0.4 mg; 1 mcg	Pink	Capsule		Eli Lilly
LILLY; F45	Epragen	22 mg; 130 mg; 227 mg; 50 mg	Yellow and Brown	Capsule		Eli Lilly
LILLY; F47	Amesec	130 mg; 25 mg; 25 mg	Blue and Orange	Capsule		Eli Lilly
LILLY; F50	A.S.A. and Codeine, No. 2	230 mg; 30 mg; 15 mg; 150 mg	White and Light Gray	Capsule		Eli Lilly
LILLY; F51	A.S.A. and Codeine, No. 3	30 mg; 150 mg; 230 mg; 30 mg	White and Dark Gray	Capsule		Eli Lilly
LILLY; F52	Dibasic Calcium Phosphate with Vitamin D	500 mg; 0.825 mg	Clear	Capsule		Eli Lilly
LILLY; F53	Trisogel	4 1/2 grains	Pink	Capsule		Eli Lilly
LILLY; F56	Calcium Gluconate with Vitamin D	325 mg; 0.825 mcg	Opaque White	Capsule		Eli Lilly
LILLY; F57	Dicalcium Phosphate and Calcium Gluconate with Vitamin D	8.25 mcg; 290 mg; 200 mg	White Opaque	Capsule		Eli Lilly
LILLY; F61	Bilron	150 mg	Green	Capsule		Eli Lilly
LILLY; F62	Becotin	10 mg; 10 mg; 4.1 mg; 50 mg; 25 mg; 1 mcg	Dark Blue	Capsule		Eli Lilly
LILLY; F63	Dicalcium Phosphate with Vitamin D and Iron	500 mg; 33 IU; 10 mg	Pink	Capsule		Eli Lilly
LILLY; F64	Tuinal	25 mg; 25 mg	Blue and Orange	Capsule		Eli Lilly
LILLY; F67	A.S.A. and Codeine, No. 4	230 mg; 30 mg; 60 mg; 150 mg	Dark Gray	Capsule		Eli Lilly
LILLY; F76	Prenalac	0.25 mg; 0.5 mg; 1.25 mcg; 16.6 mg; 2.5 mg; 0.3 mg; 1.7 mcg; 2.5 mg; 0.8 mg; 1 mg;	Pink and Light Blue	Capsule		Eli Lilly
LILLY; F97	CO-Elorine	8 mg	Yellow and Turquoise	Capsule		Eli Lilly
LILLY; G01	Alphalin	3 mg		Capsule		Eli Lilly
LILLY; H03; DARVON	Darvon	65 mg	Pink	Capsule	Capsule-Shape	Eli Lilly
LILLY; H04; DARVON; C; ASA	Darvon with Asa	65 mg; 325 mg	Red and Light Pink	Capsule		Eli Lilly
LILLY; H10	En-Cebrin F	1.2 mg; 3 mg; 2 mg; 10 mg; 2 mg; 1 mg; 5 mcg; 5 mg; 50 mg; 10 mcg; 250 mg; 30 mg; 0.15 mg; 1 mg; 5 mg; 1 mg; 1.5 mg	Pink and Blue	Capsule		Eli Lilly
LILLY; H12	En-Cebrin	1.2 mg; 10 mg; 5 mg; 10 mcg; 250 mg; 30 mg; 0.15 mg; 1 mg; 5 mg; 1 mg; 1.5 mg; 3 mg; 2 mg; 1.7 mg; 5 mcg; 50 mg	Pink and Blue	Capsule		Eli Lilly
LILLY; H13	Novrad	50 mg	Ivory and Light Brown	Capsule		Eli Lilly
LILLY; H14	Novrad	100 mg	Ivory and Light Brown	Capsule		Eli Lilly
LILLY; H15	Novrad with A.S.A.	50 mg; 300 mg	Ivory and Dark Brown	Capsule		Eli Lilly
LILLY; H17	Aventyl	10 mg	White and Yellow	Capsule		Eli Lilly
LILLY; H19	Aventyl	25 mg	White and Yellow	Capsule		Eli Lilly
LILLY; H72	Theracebrin	150 mg; 20 mg; 150 mg; 12.5 mg; 7.5 mg; 37.5 mcg; 15 mg; 10 mg; 2.5 mg; 10 mcg	Black	Capsule		Eli Lilly
LILLY; H91	Doloxene Compound	375 mg; 30 mg; 100 mg	Red and Gray	Capsule		Eli Lilly
LILLY; HO2	Darvon	32 mg	Light Pink	Capsule		Eli Lilly
LILLY; J01	Ammonium Chloride	325 mg		Tablet	Compressed	Eli Lilly
LILLY; J02	Atropine Sulfate	0.4 mg		Tablet		Eli Lilly
LILLY; J03	Belladonna Extract	15 mg		Tablet	Compressed	Eli Lilly
LILLY; J05	Caffeine, Citrated	65 mg		Tablet	Compressed	Eli Lilly
LILLY; J09	Codeine Sulfate	15 mg		Tablet		Eli Lilly
LILLY; J11	Codeine Sulfate	60 mg		Tablet		Eli Lilly
LILLY; J13	Colchicine	0.6 mg		Tablet	Compressed	Eli Lilly
LILLY; J20	Quinidine Sulfate	200 mg		Tablet	Compressed	Eli Lilly
LILLY; J23	Soda Mint	5 Gr		Tablet	Compressed	Eli Lilly

IMPRINT	BRAND/GENERIC NAME	STRENGTH	COLOR	FORM	SHAPE	MANUFACTURER
LILLY; J24	Sodium Bicarbonate	325 mg		Tablet		Eli Lilly
LILLY; J25	Thyroid	60 mg		Tablet	Compressed	Eli Lilly
LILLY; J26	Thyroid	120 mg		Tablet	Compressed	Eli Lilly
LILLY; J29	Thyroid	30 mg		Tablet	Compressed	Eli Lilly
LILLY; J30	Thyroid	15 mg		Tablet	Compressed	Eli Lilly
LILLY; J31	Phenobarbital	15 mg		Tablet		Eli Lilly
LILLY; J32	Phenobarbital	30 mg		Tablet		Eli Lilly
LILLY; J33	Phenobarbital	100 mg	White	Tablet	Circle, Scored	Eli Lilly
LILLY; J36	Ergotrate Maleate	0.2 mg		Tablet		Eli Lilly
LILLY; J41	Niacin	20 mg		Tablet	Compressed	Eli Lilly
LILLY; J43	Niacin	50 mg		Tablet	Compressed, Scored	Eli Lilly
LILLY; J45	Hexa-Betalin	25 mg; 0.5%		Tablet	Compressed	Eli Lilly
LILLY; J46	Niacinamide	50 mg		Tablet	Compressed	Eli Lilly
LILLY; J47	Riboflavin	5 mg		Tablet	Compressed	Eli Lilly
LILLY; J49	Diethylstilbestrol	0.1 mg		Tablet		Eli Lilly
LILLY; J53	Pantholin	10 mg		Tablet	Compressed	Eli Lilly
LILLY; J55	Phenobarbital and Belladonna, No. 1	30 mg; 8 mg		Tablet	Compressed, Scored	Eli Lilly
LILLY; J56	Hexa-Betalin	10 mg		Tablet	Compressed	Eli Lilly
LILLY; J57	Crystodigin	0.2 mg	White	Tablet		Eli Lilly
LILLY; J59	Phenobarbital and Belladonna, No. 2	15 mg; 4 mg		Tablet	Compressed	Eli Lilly
LILLY; J60	Crystodigin	0.1 mg	Pink	Tablet		Eli Lilly
LILLY; J61	Papaverine Hydrochloride	30 mg		Tablet	Compressed	Eli Lilly
LILLY; J62	Papaverine Hydrochloride	60 mg		Tablet		Eli Lilly
LILLY; J63	Riboflavin	10 mg		Tablet		Eli Lilly
LILLY; J64	Dolophine Hydrochloride	5 mg		Tablet		Eli Lilly
LILLY; J66	Folic Acid	5 mg		Tablet	Compressed	Eli Lilly
LILLY; J69	Propylthiouracil	50 mg		Tablet	Compressed, Scored	Eli Lilly
LILLY; J70	Phenobarbital and Belladonna, No. 3	15 mg; 8 mg		Tablet	Compressed	Eli Lilly
LILLY; J72	Dolophine Hydrochloride	10 mg		Tablet		Eli Lilly
LILLY; J73	Methyltestosterone	10 mg		Tablet	Compressed, Scored	Eli Lilly
LILLY; J74	Methyltestosterone	25 mg		Tablet		Eli Lilly
LILLY; J75	Crystodigin	0.05 mg	Orange	Tablet		Eli Lilly
LILLY; J76	Crystodigin	0.15 mg	Yellow	Tablet		Eli Lilly
LILLY; J99	Sandril	0.1 mg	Orange	Tablet	Compressed	Eli Lilly
LILLY; L01	Sandril	0.25 mg	Green	Tablet	Compressed, Scored	Eli Lilly
LILLY; L02	Tylandril	0.25 mg; 5 mg; 0.1 mg		Tablet	Compressed	Eli Lilly
LILLY; S04	Metycaine Hydrochloride and Zinc Oxide Compound	12.5 mg; 125 mg; 250 mg		Suppository		Eli Lilly
LILLY; S05	Seconal Sodium Suppositories	120 mg		Suppository		Eli Lilly
LILLY; S06	Amytal Sodium	200 mg		Suppository		Eli Lilly
LILLY; S11	Seconal Sodium Suppositories	200 mg		Suppository		Eli Lilly
LILLY; S14	Seconal Sodium Suppositories	60 mg		Suppository		Eli Lilly
LILLY; S17	Seconal Sodium Suppositories	30 mg		Suppository		Eli Lilly
LILLY; T02	Novacebrin	4000 IU; 400 IU; 60 mg; 1.5 mg; 2 mg; 0.8 mg; 3 mcg; 12 mg; 2.5 mg	Yellow	Tablet, Chewable	Compressed	Eli Lilly
LILLY; T05	A.S.A.	325 mg		Tablet	Compressed	Eli Lilly
LILLY; T06	A.S.A.	325 mg	Pink	Tablet	Compressed	Eli Lilly
LILLY; T07	A.S.A. Compound	227 mg; 160 mg; 32.5 mg	White	Tablet	Compressed	Eli Lilly
LILLY; T13	Calcium Lactate	325 mg		Tablet	Compressed	Eli Lilly
LILLY; T14	Calcium Lactate	650 mg		Tablet	Compressed	Eli Lilly
LILLY; T19	Methenamine	325 mg		Tablet	Compressed	Eli Lilly
LILLY; T20	Methenamine	500 mg		Tablet	Compressed	Eli Lilly
LILLY; T21	Methenamine and Sodium Biphosphate	325 mg; 325 mg		Tablet	Compressed	Eli Lilly
LILLY; T23	Sodium Chloride	2.25 GM		Tablet	Compressed	Eli Lilly
LILLY; T24	Sodium Chloride	1 GM		Tablet	Compressed	Eli Lilly
LILLY; T26	Pancreatin	325 mg		Tablet	Compressed	Eli Lilly
LILLY; T29	Sodium Bicarbonate	650 mg		Tablet	Compressed	Eli Lilly
LILLY; T32	Amytal	100 mg	Pink	Tablet		Eli Lilly
LILLY; T35	Calcium Carbonate, Aromatic	650 mg		Tablet	Compressed	Eli Lilly
LILLY; T36	Calcium Gluconate	1 GM		Tablet	Compressed	Eli Lilly
LILLY; T37	Amytal	50 mg	Orange	Tablet		Eli Lilly
LILLY; T39	Calcium Gluconate	500 mg		Tablet	Compressed	Eli Lilly
LILLY; T40	Amytal	15 mg	Green	Tablet	Capsule-Shape	Eli Lilly
LILLY; T42	A.S.A. and Codeine, N0. 2	230 mg; 30 mg; 15 mg; 150 mg		Tablet	Compressed	Eli Lilly
LILLY; T44	Calcium Gluconate with Vitamin D	1 GM; 1.65 mcg		Tablet	Compressed	Eli Lilly
LILLY; T46	Sulfapyridine	0.5 GM		Tablet	Compressed	Eli Lilly
LILLY; T49	A.S.A. and Codeine, No. 3	230 mg; 30 mg; 30 mg; 150 mg		Tablet	Compressed	Eli Lilly
LILLY; T50	A.S.A. Compound	227 mg; 160 mg; 32.5 mg	Pink	Tablet	Compressed	Eli Lilly
LILLY; T52	Betalin S	10 mg		Tablet	Compressed	Eli Lilly
LILLY; T55	Papaverine Hydrochloride	100 mg		Tablet	Compressed	Eli Lilly
LILLY; T56	Amytal	30 mg	Yellow	Tablet		Eli Lilly
LILLY; T59	Betalin S	25 mg		Tablet	Compressed	Eli Lilly
LILLY; T61	Dicalcium Phosphate	500 mg		Tablet	Compressed	Eli Lilly
LILLY; T62	Betalin S	50 mg		Tablet	Compressed	Eli Lilly
LILLY; T63	Betalin S	100 mg		Tablet	Compressed	Eli Lilly

IMPRINT	BRAND/GENERIC NAME	STRENGTH	COLOR	FORM	SHAPE	MANUFACTURER
LILLY; T71	Sulfonamides Triplex	0.167 GM; 0.167 GM; 0.167 GM		Tablet	Compressed	Eli Lilly
LILLY; T72	Hexa-Betalin	50 mg		Tablet	Compressed	Eli Lilly
LILLY; T73	Papaverine Hydrochloride	200 mg		Tablet	Compressed	Eli Lilly
LILLY; T75	Neotrizine	167 mg; 167 mg; 167 mg		Tablet	Compressed, Scored	Eli Lilly
LILLY; T77	Neopenzine 150	167 mg; 167 mg; 167 mg; 150,000 units		Tablet	Compressed	Eli Lilly
LILLY; T92	Neopenzine 300	167 mg; 167 mg; 167 mg; 300,000 units		Tablet		Eli Lilly
LILLY; T95	V-Cillin Sulfa	167 mg; 167 mg; 167 mg; 125 mg		Tablet		Eli Lilly
LILLY; T96	Neomycin Sulfate	500 mg		Tablet		Eli Lilly
LILLY; U; 29	Sandril	0.25 mg		Tablet		Eli Lilly
LILLY; U02	Sandril	1 mg		Tablet		Eli Lilly
LILLY; U03	Dymelor	250 mg	White	Tablet	Capsule-Shape, Scored	Eli Lilly
LILLY; U04	V-Cillin K Sulfa	0.167 GM; 0.167 GM; 0.167 GM; 125 mg		Tablet		Eli Lilly
LILLY; U07	Dymelor	500 mg	Yellow	Tablet	Capsule-Shape, Scored	Eli Lilly
LILLY; U09	Anhydron	2 mg	Pink	Tablet		Eli Lilly
LILLY; U30	Tylandril	0.25 mg; 5 mg; 0.1 mg	Green	Tablet		Eli Lilly
LILLY; U56	Folic Acid	1 mg		Tablet		Eli Lilly
LILLY; Y18	Penicillin G Potassium Solvets	100,000 units		Tablet		Eli Lilly
LILLY; Y23	Castor Oil	0.62 ml		Capsule		Eli Lilly
LILLY; Y40	Apomorphine Hydrochloride	6 mg		Tablet		Eli Lilly
LILLY; Y41	Atropine Sulfate Hypodermic Tablet	0.3 mg		Tablet		Eli Lilly
LILLY; Y42	Atropine Sulfate Hypodermic Tablet	0.4 mg		Tablet		Eli Lilly
LILLY; Y43	Atropine Sulfate Hypodermic Tablet	0.6 mg		Tablet		Eli Lilly
LILLY; Y52	Morphine and Atropine Hypodermic	15 mg; 0.4 mg		Tablet		Eli Lilly
LILLY; Y53	Scopolamine Hydrobromide Hypodermic	0.6 mg		Tablet		Eli Lilly
LILLY; Y54	Scopolamine Hydrobromide Hypodermic	0.4 mg		Tablet		Eli Lilly
LILLY; Y56	Codeine Phosphate Hypodermic Tablet	15 mg		Tablet		Eli Lilly
LILLY; Y57	Codeine Phosphate	30 mg		Tablet		Eli Lilly
LINCOCIN; 250 MG ;	Lincocin Pediatric	250 mg	Light Blue	Capsule		Pharmacia & Upjohn
LINCOCIN; 500 MG ;	Lincocin	500 mg	Light Blue and Dark Blue	Capsule		Pharmacia & Upjohn
LIORESAL; 10/10	Lioresal	10 mg	White	Tablet	Oval, Scored	Novartis
LIORESAL; 20/20	Lioresal	20 mg	White	Tablet	Capsule-Shape, Scored	Novartis
LL A4	Aristocort	4 mg	White	Tablet	Oblong	Astellas Pharma
LL A4	Aristocort	4 mg	White	Tablet	Oblong	Lederle Laboratories
LL; 10; C; 12	Leucovorin Calcium	10 mg	Light Yellow	Tablet	Square with Rounded Corners, Convex, Bisected Scored	Lederle Laboratories
LL; A 24	Amitriptyline Hydrochloride	10 mg	Pink	Coated Tablet	Circle	Lederle Laboratories
LL; A 25	Amitriptyline Hydrochloride	25 mg	Green	Coated Tablet	Circle	Lederle Laboratories
LL; A 26	Amitriptyline Hydrochloride	50 mg	Brown	Coated Tablet	Circle	Lederle Laboratories
LL; A; 7	Atenolol	25 mg	White	Tablet	Circle	Lederle Laboratories
LL; A; 27	Amitriptyline Hydrochloride	75 mg	Light Purple	Coated Tablet	Circle	Lederle Laboratories
LL; A; 28	Amitriptyline Hydrochloride	100 mg	Red-Orange	Coated Tablet	Circle	Lederle Laboratories
LL; A; 45	Albuterol Sulfate	2 mg	White	Tablet	Round, Flat, Bisected Scored	Lederle Laboratories
LL; A; 46	Albuterol Sulfate	4 mg	White	Tablet	Round, Flat, Bisected Scored	Lederle Laboratories
LL; A; 49	Atenolol	50 mg	White	Tablet	Circle, Scored	Lederle Laboratories
LL; A; 51	Alprazolam	0.25 mg	White	Tablet	Oval, Convex, Scored	Lederle Laboratories
LL; A; 52	Alprazolam	0.5 mg	Yellow	Tablet	Oval, Convex, Scored	Lederle Laboratories
LL; A; 53	Alprazolam	1 mg	Green	Tablet	Oval, Convex, Scored	Lederle Laboratories
LL; A; 54	Alprazolam	2 mg	Green	Tablet	Oblong, Convex	Lederle Laboratories
LL; A; 71	Atenolol	100 mg	White	Tablet	Circle	Esi Lederle
LL; A1 ;	Aristocort	1 mg	Yellow	Tablet	Oblong, Flat; Scored	Lederle Laboratories
LL; A2 ;	Triamcinolone	2 mg	Pink	Tablet	Oblong, Flat, Scored	Lederle Laboratories
LL; A8 ;	Aristocort	8 mg	Yellow	Tablet	Oblong, Flat, Scored	Lederle Laboratories
LL; A11; ARTANE; 2	Artane	2 mg	White	Tablet	Circle, Flat, Scored	Lederle Laboratories
LL; A12; ARTANE; 5	Artane	5 mg	White	Tablet	Circle, Flat, Scored	Lederle Laboratories
LL; B; 10	Benztropine Mesylate	1 mg	White	Tablet	Oval, Scored	Lederle Laboratories
LL; B; 11	Benztropine Mesylate	2 mg	White	Tablet	Circle, Scored	Lederle Laboratories
LL; B1	Zebeta	5 mg	Pink	Coated Tablet	Heart-Shape	Lederle Laboratories
LL; C; 15	Chlorthalidone	50 mg	Dark Blue	Tablet	Circle, Scored	Lederle Laboratories
LL; C; 40	Caltrate 600 Plus Vitamin D	125 IU; 600 mg	Light Brown	Coated Tablet	Oblong, Scored	Wyeth Consumer Healthcare
LL; C; 42	Clonidine Hydrochloride	0.1 mg	Blue	Tablet	Circle, Convex	Lederle Laboratories
LL; C; 43	Clonidine Hydrochloride	0.2 mg	Light Yellow	Tablet	Circle, Convex	Lederle Laboratories
LL; C; 44	Clonidine Hydrochloride	0.3 mg	Light Green	Tablet	Circle, Convex	Lederle Laboratories
LL; C; 45	Caltrate 600 Plus Iron and Vitamin D	600 mg; 18 mg; 125 IU	Red	Tablet	Oblong, Scored	Wyeth Consumer Healthcare
LL; C; 67	Chlordiazepoxide and Amitriptyline Hydrochloride	5 mg; 12.5 mg	Green	Coated Tablet	Circle	Lederle Laboratories
LL; C; 68	Chlordiazepoxide and Amitriptyline Hydrochloride	10 mg; 25 mg	White	Coated Tablet	Circle	Lederle Laboratories
LL; C; 69	Clorazepate Dipotassium	3.75 mg	Blue	Tablet	Circle, Scored	Lederle Laboratories
LL; C; 70	Clorazepate Dipotassium	7.5 mg	Peach	Tablet	Circle, Scored	Lederle Laboratories
LL; C; 71	Clorazepate Dipotassium	15 mg	White	Tablet	Circle, Scored	Lederle Laboratories

IMPRINT	BRAND/GENERIC NAME	STRENGTH	COLOR	FORM	SHAPE	MANUFACTURER
LL; C; 81	Cephalexin	250 mg	White	Coated Tablet	Oblong	Lederle Laboratories
LL; C; 82	Cephalexin	500 mg	White	Coated Tablet	Oblong	Lederle Laboratories
LL; C;7	Chlorthalidone	25 mg	Dark Orange	Tablet	Circle, Scored	Lederle Laboratories
LL; C37	Chlorpropamide	100 mg	White	Tablet	Circle, Scored	Lederle Laboratories
LL; C38	Chlorpropamide	250 mg	White	Tablet	Circle, Scored	Lederle Laboratories
LL; C60; CENTRUM JR	Centrum JR. with Extra Calcium	18 mg; 5000 IU; 400 IU; 30 IU; 400 mcg; 45 mcg; 1.5 mg; 10 mg; 1.7 mg; 20 mg; 40 mg; 150 mcg; 2 mg; 50 mg; 160 mg; 15 mg; 1 mg; 20 mcg; 20 mcg; 60 mg; 2 mg; 6 mcg; 10 mcg	Red	Tablet	Oblong, Scored	Wyeth Consumer Healthcare
LL; D; 31	Diphenoxylate Hydrochloride and Atropine Sulfate	2.5 mg; 0.025 mg	White	Tablet	Circle	Lederle Laboratories
LL; D; 41	Doxycycline Hyclate	100 mg	Green	Coated Tablet	Circle	Lederle Laboratories
LL; D; 44	Dipyridamole	25 mg	Purple or White	Coated Tablet	Circle	Lederle Laboratories
LL; D; 45	Dipyridamole	50 mg	Purple or White	Coated Tablet	Circle	Lederle Laboratories
LL; D; 46	Dipyridamole	75 mg	Purple or White	Coated Tablet	Circle	Lederle Laboratories
LL; D; 51	Diazepam	2 mg	White	Tablet	Circle, Scored	Lederle Laboratories
LL; D; 72	Diltiazem	60 mg	Blue	Coated Tablet	Round, Convex, Bisected Scored	Lederle Laboratories
LL; D; 75	Diltiazem	90 mg	Blue	Coated Tablet	Oblong, Convex, Bisected Scored	Lederle Laboratories
LL; D; 77	Diltiazem	120 mg	Blue	Coated Tablet	Oblong, Convex, Bisected Scored	Lederle Laboratories
LL; D11	Declomycin	150 mg	Red	Coated Tablet	Circle, Convex	Lederle Laboratories
LL; D12	Declomycin	300 mg	Red	Coated Tablet	Circle, Convex	Lederle Laboratories
LL; D32	Docusate Sodium	100 mg	Red and Orange-Red	Capsule		Lederle Laboratories
LL; D34	Docusate Sodium with Casanthranol	100 mg; 30 mg	Maroon	Capsule		Lederle Laboratories
LL; D52	Diazepam	5 mg	Light Brown	Tablet	Circle, Scored	Lederle Laboratories
LL; D53	Diazepam	10 mg	Light Green	Tablet	Circle, Scored	Lederle Laboratories
LL; D71	Diltiazem	30 mg	Blue	Coated Tablet	Circle, Convex	Lederle Laboratories
LL; E2	Erythromycin Stearate	250 mg	Yellow	Coated Tablet	Circle	Lederle Laboratories
LL; E5 ;	Erythromycin Stearate	500 mg	Yellow	Coated Tablet	Oval	Lederle Laboratories
LL; E10	Erythromycin Ethylsuccinate	400 mg	Beige	Tablet	Oval	Lederle Laboratories
LL; EXTRA C; C39; CENTRUM JR	Centrum JR. Plus Extra C, Advanced Formula	18 mg; 5000 IU; 400 IU; 30 IU; 400 mcg; 45 mcg; 1.5 mg; 10 mg; 1.7 mg; 20 mg; 40 mg; 150 mcg; 2 mg; 50 mg; 108 mg; 15 mg; 1 mg; 20 mcg; 20 mcg; 300 mg; 2 mg; 6 mcg; 10 mcg		Tablet, Chewable	Oblong, Scored	Wyeth Consumer Healthcare
LL; F; 12	Furosemide	40 mg	White to Off-White	Tablet	Circle, Scored	Lederle Laboratories
LL; F; 13	Furosemide	80 mg	White to Off-White	Tablet	Circle, Scored	Lederle Laboratories
LL; F; 22	Fenoprofen Calcium	600 mg	White	Coated Tablet	Capsule-Shape, Scored	Lederle Laboratories
LL; F11	Furosemide	20 mg	White to Off-White	Tablet	Circle	Lederle Laboratories
LL; F21	Ferrous Gluconate	300 mg	Green	Coated Tablet	Circle	Lederle Laboratories
LL; G2	Gevral T	27 mg; 5000 IU; 400 IU; 45 IU; 90 mg; 0.4 mg; 2.25 mg; 2.6 mg; 30 mg; 3 mg; 9 mcg; 162 mg; 225 mcg; 100 mg; 1.5 mg; 22.5 mg	Maroon	Coated Tablet	Oblong	Lederle Laboratories
LL; G17	Gemfibrozil	600 mg	White to Off-White	Coated Tablet	Oval, Scored	Lederle Laboratories
LL; H; 2	Hydromox R	50 mg; 0.125 mg	Yellow	Tablet	Circle, Scored	Lederle Laboratories
LL; H; 14	Hydrochlorothiazide	25 mg	Peach	Tablet	Circle, Scored	Lederle Laboratories
LL; H11	Hydralazine Hydrochloride	25 mg	Red	Coated Tablet	Circle, Convex	Lederle Laboratories
LL; H12	Hydralazine Hydrochloride	50 mg	Red	Coated Tablet	Circle, Convex	Lederle Laboratories
LL; HEART; B; 12	Ziac	2.5 mg; 6.25 mg	Yellow	Coated Tablet	Circle, Convex	Wyeth Pharmaceuticals
LL; HEART; B; 13	Ziac	5 mg; 6.25 mg	Pink	Coated Tablet	Circle, Convex	Wyeth Pharmaceuticals
LL; HEART; B; 14	Ziac	10 mg; 6.25 mg	White	Coated Tablet	Circle, Convex	Wyeth Pharmaceuticals
LL; I; 27	Aches-N-Pain 200	200 mg	Orange	Coated Tablet	Circle, Convex	Lederle Laboratories
LL; I11	Imipramine Hydrochloride	10 mg	Yellow	Tablet	Circle	Lederle Laboratories
LL; I12	Imipramine Hydrochloride	25 mg	Rust	Tablet	Circle	Lederle Laboratories
LL; I13	Imipramine Hydrochloride	50 mg	Green	Tablet	Circle	Lederle Laboratories
LL; J1	Methazolamide	25 mg	White	Tablet	Square, Convex	Lederle Laboratories
LL; J2	Methazolamide	50 mg	White	Tablet	Circle, Convex	Lederle Laboratories
LL; M; 1	Methotrexate	2.5 mg	Yellow	Tablet	Round, Convex, Bisected Scored	Lederle Laboratories
LL; M; 7	Myambutol	400 mg	White	Coated Tablet	Circle, Convex, Scored	Lederle Laboratories
LL; M; 19	Methocarbamol	500 mg	White	Tablet	Circle, Scored	Lederle Laboratories
LL; M; 20	Methocarbamol	750 mg	White	Tablet	Capsule-Shape, Scored	Lederle Laboratories
LL; M; 36	Methyldopa and Hydrochlorothiazide	250 mg; 15 mg	Yellow	Coated Tablet	Circle	Lederle Laboratories
LL; M; 37	Methyldopa and Hydrochlorothiazide	250 mg; 25 mg	Pink	Coated Tablet	Circle	Lederle Laboratories
LL; M1	Rheumatrex	2.5 mg	Yellow	Tablet	Circle, Convex, Scored	Lederle Laboratories
LL; M3	Minocin	50 mg	Orange	Coated Tablet	Circle, Convex	Lederle Laboratories
LL; M5	Minocin	100 mg	Orange	Coated Tablet	Circle, Convex, Scored	Lederle Laboratories
LL; M6	Myambutol	100 mg	White	Coated Tablet	Circle, Convex	Lederle Laboratories
LL; M8; MAXZIDE	Maxzide	50 mg; 75 mg	Yellow	Tablet	Bowtie	Lederle Laboratories
LL; M22	Methyldopa	250 mg	Peach	Coated Tablet	Circle	Lederle Laboratories

IMPRINT	BRAND/GENERIC NAME	STRENGTH	COLOR	FORM	SHAPE	MANUFACTURER
LL; M23	Methyldopa	500 mg	Peach	Coated Tablet	Circle	Lederle Laboratories
LL; M28	Metoclopramide Hydrochloride	10 mg	White		Circle, Scored	Lederle Laboratories
LL; N; 11	Naproxen	250 mg	Light Green	Tablet	Circle	Lederle Laboratories
LL; N; 17	Naproxen	375 mg	White	Tablet	Capsule-Shape	Lederle Laboratories
LL; N; 77	Naproxen	500 mg	Light Green	Tablet	Capsule-Shape	Lederle Laboratories
LL; N6	Nilstat	100,000 units	Yellow	Tablet	Oval, Convex	Lederle Laboratories
LL; P; 33	Propylthiouracil	50 mg	White	Tablet	Circle, Scored	Lederle Laboratories
LL; P; 36	Pyrazinamide	500 mg	White	Tablet	Circle, Scored, Convex	Lederle Laboratories
LL; P; 44	Propranolol Hydrochloride	10 mg	Gray	Tablet	Circle, Scored	Lederle Laboratories
LL; P; 45	Propranolol Hydrochloride	20 mg	Purple	Tablet	Circle, Scored	Lederle Laboratories
LL; P; 46	Propranolol Hydrochloride	40 mg	Light Brown	Tablet	Circle	Lederle Laboratories
LL; P; 47	Propranolol Hydrochloride	80 mg	Light Blue	Tablet	Circle, Scored	Lederle Laboratories
LL; P; 48	Procainamide Hydrochloride SR	250 mg	Light Blue	Coated Tablet	Oval, Scored	Lederle Laboratories
LL; P; 65	Propranolol Hydrochloride	60 mg	White	Tablet	Circle	Lederle Laboratories
LL; P; 76	Perphenazine and Amitriptyline Hydrochloride	4 mg; 50 mg	Orange	Coated Tablet	Circle	Lederle Laboratories
LL; P9	Pronemia	75 mg; 115 mg; 150 mg; 1 mg; 15 mcg	Red	Capsule		Lederle Laboratories
LL; P72	Perphenazine and Amitriptyline Hydrochloride	2 mg; 10 mg	Blue	Coated Tablet	Circle	Lederle Laboratories
LL; P73	Perphenazine with Amitriptyline Hydrochloride	2 mg; 25 mg	Orange	Coated Tablet	Circle	Lederle Laboratories
LL; P74	Perphenazine and Amitriptyline Hydrochloride	4 mg; 10 mg	Light Peach	Coated Tablet	Circle	Lederle Laboratories
LL; P75	Perphenazine and Amitriptyline Hydrochloride	4 mg; 25 mg	Yellow	Coated Tablet	Circle	Lederle Laboratories
LL; Q; 11	Quinidine Sulfate	200 mg	White	Tablet	Circle, Convex, Scored	Lederle Laboratories
LL; S; 1	Advanced Formula Stresstabs 600	45 mcg; 400 mcg; 100 mg; 30 IU; 20 mg; 15 mg; 5 mg; 500 mg; 15 mg; 12 mcg	Orange	Tablet	Oblong	Lederle Laboratories
LL; S; 1	Stresstabs	45 mcg; 400 mcg; 20 mg; 30 IU; 100 mg; 12 mcg; 10 mg; 500 mg; 5 mg; 10 mg	Orange	Tablet	Oblong, Scored	Lederle Laboratories
LL; S; 3	Stresstabs 600 Plus Zinc	30 IU; 600 mg; 400 mcg; 20 mg; 10 mg; 100 mg; 5 mg; 12 mcg; 45 mcg; 25 mg; 3 mg; 23.9 mg	Peach	Tablet	Oblong, Scored	Lederle Laboratories
LL; S; 3	Stresstabs Plus Zinc	30 IU; 500 mg; 400 mcg; 10 mg; 10 mg; 100 mg; 5 mg; 12 mcg; 45 mcg; 20 mg; 3 mg; 23.9 mg	Peach	Tablet	Oblong, Scored	Lederle Laboratories
LL; S; 14	Sulfasalazine	500 mg	Brown	Tablet	Circle, Scored	Lederle Laboratories
LL; S; 16	Sulindac	150 mg	Yellow	Tablet	Circle, Scored	Lederle Laboratories
LL; S; 17	Sulindac	200 mg	Yellow	Tablet	Circle, Scored	Lederle Laboratories
LL; S11	Selegiline Hydrochloride	5 mg	White	Tablet	Circle	Esi Lederle
LL; T; 29	Trazodone Hydrochloride	50 mg	White	Tablet	Circle, Scored	Lederle Laboratories
LL; T; 30	Trazodone Hydrochloride	100 mg	White	Tablet	Circle, Scored	Lederle Laboratories
LL; T; 34	Theophylline C.R.	100 mg	White	Timed-Release Tablet	Circle, Convex	Lederle Laboratories
LL; T1	Tri-Hemic 600	30 IU; 75 mg; 1 mg; 115 mg; 50 mg; 600 mg; 25 mcg	Red	Coated Tablet	Oblong	Lederle Laboratories
LL; T13	Sulfamethoxazole and Trimethoprim	400 mg; 80 mg	White	Tablet	Circle, Scored	Lederle Laboratories
LL; T16	Sulfamethoxazole and Trimethoprim	800 mg; 160 mg	White	Tablet	Oblong	Lederle Laboratories
LL; T31; 50; 100	Trazodone Hydrochloride	150 mg	White	Tablet	Four-Sided, Scored	Lederle Laboratories
LL; V; 5	Verapamil Hydrochloride	120 mg	White	Coated Tablet	Circle, Scored	Lederle Laboratories
LL;A 14	Amiloride and Hydrochlorothiazide	5 mg; 50 mg	Yellow	Tablet	Circle	Lederle Laboratories
LL;CA85	Calcium Centrum Singles	500 mg	White	Tablet	Oblong	Lederle Laboratories
LODINE XL; 400	Lodine XL	400 mg	Orange-Red	Extended-Release Tablet	Capsule-Shape, Biconvex	Wyeth Pharmaceuticals
LODINE XL; 500	Lodine XL	500 mg	Grey-Green	Extended-Release Tablet	Capsule-Shape, Biconvex	Wyeth Pharmaceuticals
LODINE XL; 600	Lodine XL	600 mg	Light Grey	Extended-Release Tablet	Capsule-Shape, Biconvex	Wyeth Pharmaceuticals
LODINE; 200	Lodine	200 mg	Light Grey with a Wide Red Band	Capsule		Wyeth Pharmaceuticals
LODINE; 300	Lodine	300 mg	Light Gray with a Wide Red Band, Light Gray with 2 Narrow Red Bands	Capsule		Wyeth Pharmaceuticals
LODINE; 400	Lodine	400 mg	Yellow-Orange	Coated Tablet	Oval	Wyeth Pharmaceuticals
LODINE; 500	Lodine	500 mg	Blue	Coated Tablet	Oval	Wyeth Pharmaceuticals
LOGO ; 50H	Micardis	20 mg	White or Off-White	Tablet	Circle	Boehringer Ingelheim Pharmaceuticals
LOGO ; 51H	Micardis	40 mg	White or Off-White	Tablet	Oblong	Boehringer Ingelheim Pharmaceuticals
LOGO ; 52H	Micardis	80 mg	White or Off-White	Tablet	Oblong	Boehringer Ingelheim Pharmaceuticals
LOGO ; 746	Tri-Previfem - White Tablet	0.035 mg; 0.18 mg	White	Tablet	Circle	Teva Pharmaceuticals

IMPRINT	BRAND/GENERIC NAME	STRENGTH	COLOR	FORM	SHAPE	MANUFACTURER
LOGO ; 747	Tri-Previfem - Light Blue Tablet	0.215 mg; 0.035 mg	Light Blue	Tablet	Circle	Teva Pharmaceuticals
LOGO ; 748	Previfem - Blue Tablet	0.25 mg; 0.035 mg	Blue	Tablet	Circle	Teva Pharmaceuticals
LOGO ; 748	Tri-Previfem - Blue Tablet	0.25 mg; 0.035 mg	Blue	Tablet	Circle	Teva Pharmaceuticals
LOGO ; 5825	Finasteride	5 mg	Light Blue	Tablet	Circle	Teva Pharmaceuticals
LOGO ; M	Meloxicam	7.5 mg	Pastel Yellow	Tablet	Circle	Roxane Laboratories
LOGO ; M	Mobic	7.5 mg	Pastel Yellow	Tablet	Circle	Boehringer Ingelheim Pharmaceuticals
LOGO 20 ; 5728 ;	Famotidine	20 mg	Beige	Tablet	Circle	Ivax Pharmaceuticals
LOGO 225	Rythmol SR	225 mg	White	Capsule		Reliant Pharmaceuticals
LOGO 325 ; A 325	Rythmol SR	325 mg	White	Capsule		Reliant Pharmaceuticals
LOGO 425 ; A 425	Rythmol SR	425 mg	White	Capsule		Reliant Pharmaceuticals
LOGO 571 ; 500	Metformin Hydrochloride	500 mg	White to Off White	Tablet, Extended Release	Capsule-Shape	Andrx Pharmaceuticals
LOGO 577 ; 750	Metformin Hydrochloride	750 mg	Light Yellow	Tablet, Extended Release	Capsule-Shape	Andrx Pharmaceuticals
LOGO 701 ; 150	Demeclocycline Hydrochloride	150 mg	Pink	Tablet	Circle	Barr Laboratories
LOGO 702 ; 300	Demeclocycline Hydrochloride	300 mg	Pink	Tablet	Circle	Barr Laboratories
LOGO 5710 ; 1.25/ 250	Glyburide (Micronized) and Metformin Hydrochloride	1.25 mg; 250 mg	Light Yellow	Tablet	Oval	Ivax Pharmaceuticals
LOGO 5711 ; 2.5/500	Glyburide (Micronized) and Metformin Hydrochloride	2.5 mg; 500 mg	Light Yellow	Tablet	Oval	Ivax Pharmaceuticals
LOGO 5712 ; 5/500	Glyburide (Micronized) and Metformin Hydrochloride	5 mg; 500 mg	Yellow	Tablet	Oval	Ivax Pharmaceuticals
LOGO DYNACIRC ; RELIANT 2.5	Dynacirc	2.5 mg	White	Capsule		Reliant Pharmaceuticals
LOGO DYNACIRC ; RELIANT 5	Dynacirc	5 mg	Light Pink	Capsule		Reliant Pharmaceuticals
LOGO JC	Rythmol	150 mg		Tablet	Circle	Reliant Pharmaceuticals
LOGO JI	Rythmol	225 mg		Tablet	Circle	Reliant Pharmaceuticals
LOGO JN	Rythmol	300 mg		Tablet	Circle	Reliant Pharmaceuticals
LOGO ZA	Zemplar	1 mcg	Gray	Capsule, Liquid Filled	Oval	Abbott Laboratories
LOGO ZF	Zemplar	2 mcg	Orange-Brown	Capsule, Liquid Filled	Oval	Abbott Laboratories
LOGO ZK	Zemplar	4 mcg	Gold	Capsule, Liquid Filled	Oval	Abbott Laboratories
LONITEN; 10 ;	Loniten	10 mg	White	Tablet	Circle, Scored	Pharmacia & Upjohn
LORTREL 2265	Lotrel	5 mg; 20 mg	Pink, White	Capsule		Novartis
LOTENSIN HCT; 57 ;	Lotensin HCT	5 mg; 6.25 mg	White	Tablet	Oblong, Scored	Novartis Pharmaceuticals
LOTENSIN HCT; 72 ;	Lotensin HCT	10 mg; 12.5 mg	Light Pink	Tablet	Oblong, Scored	Novartis Pharmaceuticals
LOTENSIN HCT; 74 ;	Lotensin HCT	20 mg; 12.5 mg	Grayish-Violet	Tablet	Oblong, Scored	Novartis Pharmaceuticals
LOTENSIN HCT; 75 ;	Lotensin HCT	20 mg; 25 mg	Red	Tablet	Scored, Oblong	Novartis Pharmaceuticals
LOTENSIN; 5 ;	Lotensin	5 mg	Light Yellow	Tablet	Circle	Novartis Pharmaceuticals
LOTENSIN; 10 ;	Lotensin	10 mg	Dark Yellow	Tablet	Circle	Novartis Pharmaceuticals
LOTENSIN; 20 ;	Lotensin	20 mg	Tan	Tablet	Circle	Novartis Pharmaceuticals
LOTENSIN; 40 ;	Lotensin	40 mg	Dark Rose	Tablet	Circle	Novartis Pharmaceuticals
LOTREL 0364	Lotrel	10 mg; 20 mg	Purple, White	Capsule		Novartis
LOTREL 0379	Lotrel	10 mg; 40 mg	Dark Blue, White	Capsule		Novartis
LOTREL 0384	Lotrel	5 mg; 40 mg	Light Blue, White	Capsule		Novartis
LOTREL 2255	Lotrel	2.5 mg; 10 mg	Gold, White	Capsule		Novartis
LOTREL 2260	Lotrel	5 mg; 10 mg	Light Brown, White	Capsule		Novartis
LTG; 2	Lamictal	2 mg	White to Off White	Tablet, Chewable	Circle	Glaxosmithkline
LUPIN; 302	Cefuroxime Axetil	250 mg	White to Off-White	Tablet	Capsule-Shape	Watson Laboratories
LV; 10; G	Lovastatin	10 mg	Peach	Tablet	Circle	Par Pharmaceutical
LV; 20; G	Lovastatin	20 mg	Light Blue	Tablet	Circle	Par Pharmaceutical
LV; 40; G	Lovastatin	40 mg	Green	Tablet	Circle	Par Pharmaceutical
M	Momentum	500 mg; 15 mg	White	Tablet	Oval	Whitehall Laboratories
M	Mylanta Soothing Antacid Cherry Creme	600 mg	Pink	Lozenge/troche		Johnson & Johnson Merck Consumer Pharmaceuticals
M	Mylanta Soothing Antacid Cool Mint Creme	600 mg		Lozenge/troche		Johnson & Johnson Merck Consumer Pharmaceuticals
M ; 633	Nifedipine	90 mg	Brown	Tablet, Extended Release	Circle	Andrx Pharmaceuticals
M ; 751 ;	Cyclobenzaprine Hydrochloride	10 mg	Butterscotch Yellow	Tablet	Circle	Mylan Pharmaceuticals
M ; 771 ;	Cyclobenzaprine Hydrochloride	5 mg	Blue	Tablet	Circle	Mylan Pharmaceuticals
M ; A21	Alprazolam	0.5 mg	White	Tablet, Extended Release	Circle	Mylan Pharmaceuticals
M ; A22	Alprazolam	1 mg	Light Orange	Tablet, Extended Release	Circle	Mylan Pharmaceuticals
M ; A23	Alprazolam	2 mg	Light Lavender	Tablet, Extended Release	Circle	Mylan Pharmaceuticals
M ; A24	Alprazolam	3 mg	Light Pink	Tablet, Extended Release	Circle	Mylan Pharmaceuticals
M ; C 21	Citalopram Hydrobromide	10 mg	Yellow	Tablet	Circle	Mylan Pharmaceuticals
M ; C 22	Citalopram Hydrobromide	20 mg	Yellow	Tablet	Circle	Mylan Pharmaceuticals
M ; C 24	Citalopram Hydrobromide	40 mg	Yellow	Tablet	Circle	Mylan Pharmaceuticals
M 18	Metoprolol Tartrate	25 mg	White	Tablet	Circle	Mylan Pharmaceuticals
M 32	Metoprolol Tartrate	50 mg	Pink	Tablet	Circle	Mylan Pharmaceuticals
M 44	Cyproheptadine Hydrochloride	4 mg	White	Tablet	Circle, Scored, Flat Beveled Edge	Mylan Pharmaceuticals
M 47	Metoprolol Tartrate	100 mg	Light Blue	Tablet	Circle	Mylan Pharmaceuticals
M 54; 10	Thioridazine Hydrochloride	10 mg		Tablet		Roxane Laboratories
M 66	Meloxicam	7.5 mg	Yellow	Tablet	Circle	Mylan Pharmaceuticals
M 89	Meloxicam	15 mg	Yellow	Tablet	Circle	Mylan Pharmaceuticals
M 350	Metformin Hydrochloride	750 mg	Tan	Tablet, Extended Release	Oval	Mylan Pharmaceuticals
M 352	Metformin Hydrochloride	500 mg	Tan	Tablet, Extended Release	Oval	Mylan Pharmaceuticals
M 724	Tizanidine Hydrochloride	4 mg	White to Off-White	Tablet		Mylan Pharmaceuticals
M C41	Cilostazol	50 mg	White to Off-White	Tablet	Circle	Mylan Pharmaceuticals

IMPRINT	BRAND/GENERIC NAME	STRENGTH	COLOR	FORM	SHAPE	MANUFACTURER
M C42	Cilostazol	100 mg	White to Off-White	Tablet	Circle	Mylan Pharmaceuticals
M; 018 ;	Nucofed	20 mg; 60 mg	Green and Clear	Capsule		Monarch Pharmaceuticals
M; 019 ;	Quibron-T/SR	300 mg	White	Sustained-Release Tablet	Accudose (Triple-Scored)	Monarch Pharmaceuticals
M; 020	Quibron-T	300 mg	Ivory	Tablet	Accudose (Triple-Scored)	Monarch Pharmaceuticals
M; 022 ;	Quibron	150 mg; 90 mg	Clear Yellow	Capsule, Liquid Filled		Monarch Pharmaceuticals
M; 4	Fluphenazine Hydrochloride	1 mg	White	Coated Tablet	Triangle	Mylan Pharmaceuticals
M; 9	Fluphenazine Hydrochloride	2.5 mg	Yellow	Coated Tablet	Triangle	Mylan Pharmaceuticals
M; 11	Penicillin V Potassium	250 mg	White	Tablet	Oval	Mylan Pharmaceuticals
M; 12	Penicillin V Potassium	500 mg	White	Tablet	Circle, Scored	Mylan Pharmaceuticals
M; 12	Penicillin VK	500 mg		Tablet		Teva Pharmaceuticals
M; 13	Tolbutamide	500 mg	White	Tablet	Circle, Scored	Mylan Pharmaceuticals
M; 14	Methotrexate Sodium	2.5 mg	Orange	Tablet	Circle, Scored	Mylan Pharmaceuticals
M; 15	Atropine Sulfate and Diphenoxylate Hydrochloride	0.025 mg; 2.5 mg	White	Tablet	Circle	Mylan Pharmaceuticals
M; 15	Klor-Con M15	1125 mg	White	Tablet	Oblong	Upsher-Smith Laboratories
M; 23	Diltiazem Hydrochloride	30 mg	White	Coated Tablet	Circle	Mylan Pharmaceuticals
M; 25	L-Thyroxine	0.025 mg	Blue	Tablet	Circle, Scored	Warner Chilcott
M; 27	Clonidine Hydrochloride and Chlorthalidone	0.2 mg; 15 mg	Yellow	Tablet	Circle, Scored, Biconvex	Mylan Pharmaceuticals
M; 27	Clorpres	15 mg; 0.2 mg	Yellow	Tablet	Circle, Scored	Mylan Bertek Pharmaceuticals
M; 28	Nadolol	20 mg	Yellow	Tablet	Circle, Scored	Mylan Pharmaceuticals
M; 29	Methyclothiazide	5 mg	Blue	Tablet	Circle, Scored	Mylan Pharmaceuticals
M; 31	Allopurinol	100 mg	White	Tablet	Circle, Scored	Mylan Pharmaceuticals
M; 33	Chlorothiazide and Reserpine	0.125 mg; 250 mg	Light Orange	Tablet	Circle, Scored, Flat Beveled Edge	Mylan Pharmaceuticals
M; 35	Chlorthalidone	25 mg	Yellow	Tablet	Circle	Mylan Pharmaceuticals
M; 36	Amitriptyline Hydrochloride	50 mg	Brown	Coated Tablet	Circle	Mylan Pharmaceuticals
M; 37	Amitriptyline Hydrochloride	75 mg	Blue	Coated Tablet	Circle	Mylan Pharmaceuticals
M; 38	Amitriptyline Hydrochloride	100 mg	Orange	Coated Tablet	Circle	Mylan Pharmaceuticals
M; 39	Amitriptyline Hydrochloride	150 mg	Flesh	Coated Tablet	Capsule-Shape	Mylan Pharmaceuticals
M; 40	Clorazepate Dipotassium	7.5 mg	Peach	Tablet	Circle, Scored, Flat Beveled Edge	Mylan Pharmaceuticals
M; 40; MATERNA	Materna Prenatal Vitamin and Mineral	100 mg; 30 mcg; 25 mcg; 1 mg; 60 mg; 5 mg; 20 mg; 5000 IU; 10 mg; 25 mg; 30 IU; 400 IU; 3.4 mg; 10 mg; 12 mcg; 3 mg; 25 mcg; 25 mg; 150 mcg; 2 mg; 250 mg	Off-White	Coated Tablet	Oval, Scored	Lederle Laboratories
M; 40; MATERNA	Materna Prenatal Vitamin and Mineral	100 mg; 30 mcg; 25 mcg; 1 mg; 60 mg; 5 mg; 20 mg; 5000 IU; 10 mg; 25 mg; 30 IU; 400 IU; 3.4 mg; 10 mg; 12 mcg; 3 mg; 25 mcg; 25 mg; 150 mcg; 2 mg; 250 mg	Off-White	Coated Tablet	Oval, Scored	Wyeth Pharmaceuticals
M; 40; MATERNA	Materna Prenatal Vitamin and Mineral	100 mg; 30 mcg; 25 mcg; 1 mg; 60 mg; 5 mg; 20 mg; 5000 IU; 10 mg; 25 mg; 30 IU; 400 IU; 3.4 mg; 10 mg; 12 mcg; 3 mg; 25 mcg; 25 mg; 150 mcg; 2 mg; 250 mg	Off-White	Coated Tablet	Oval, Scored	Wyeth-Ayerst Laboratories
M; 41	Spironolactone and Hydrochlorothiazide	25 mg; 25 mg	Ivory	Tablet	Circle, Scored, Compressed	Mylan Pharmaceuticals
M; 43	Chlorothiazide and Reserpine	0.125 mg; 500 mg	Light Orange	Tablet	Circle, Scored, Flat Beveled Edge	Mylan Pharmaceuticals
M; 45	Diltiazem Hydrochloride	60 mg	White	Coated Tablet	Circle, Scored	Mylan Pharmaceuticals
M; 46	Spironolactone	25 mg	Orange	Tablet		Mylan Pharmaceuticals
M; 50	L-Thyroxine	0.05 mg	Blue	Tablet	Circle, Scored	Warner Chilcott
M; 50	Chlorothiazide	250 mg	White	Tablet	Circle, Scored	Mylan Pharmaceuticals
M; 51	Amitriptyline Hydrochloride	25 mg	Light Green	Coated Tablet	Circle	Mylan Pharmaceuticals
M; 52	Pindolol	5 mg	White	Tablet	Circle, Scored, Biconvex	Mylan Pharmaceuticals
M; 53	Cimetidine	200 mg	Green	Coated Tablet	Five-Sided, House Shaped, Biconvex, Beveled Edge	Mylan Pharmaceuticals
M; 55	Timolol Maleate	5 mg	Green	Tablet	Circle, Flat Beveled Edge	Mylan Pharmaceuticals
M; 58; 25	Thioridazine Hydrochloride	25 mg		Tablet		Roxane Laboratories
M; 58; 25	Thioridazine Hydrochloride	25 mg	Orange	Coated Tablet	Circle	Mylan Pharmaceuticals
M; 59; 50	Thioridazine Hydrochloride	50 mg		Tablet		Roxane Laboratories
M; 59; 50	Thioridazine Hydrochloride	50 mg	Orange	Coated Tablet	Circle	Mylan Pharmaceuticals
M; 60	Maprotiline Hydrochloride	25 mg	White	Coated Tablet	Circle, Scored, Biconvex, Beveled Edge	Mylan Pharmaceuticals
M; 61; 100	Thioridazine Hydrochloride	100 mg		Tablet		Roxane Laboratories
M; 61; 100	Thioridazine Hydrochloride	100 mg	Orange	Coated Tablet	Circle	Mylan Pharmaceuticals
M; 63	Atenolol and Chlorthalidone	50 mg; 25 mg	White	Tablet	Circle, Scored, Biconvex	Mylan Pharmaceuticals
M; 64	Atenolol and Chlorthalidone	100 mg; 25 mg	White	Tablet	Circle, Biconvex	Mylan Pharmaceuticals
M; 65	Acetaminophen and Propoxyphene Hydrochloride	65 mg; 650 mg	Orange	Capsule		Mylan Pharmaceuticals
M; 69	Indapamide	1.25 mg		Tablet		Mylan Pharmaceuticals
M; 70	Clorazepate Dipotassium	15 mg	White	Tablet	Circle, Scored, Flat Beveled Edge	Mylan Pharmaceuticals
M; 71	Allopurinol	300 mg	White	Tablet	Circle, Scored	Mylan Pharmaceuticals
M; 72	Clonidine Hydrochloride and Chlorthalidone	0.3 mg; 15 mg	Yellow	Tablet	Circle, Scored, Biconvex	Mylan Pharmaceuticals

IMPRINT	BRAND/GENERIC NAME	STRENGTH	COLOR	FORM	SHAPE	MANUFACTURER
M; 72	Clorpres	15 mg; 0.3 mg	Yellow	Tablet	Circle, Scored	Mylan Bertek Pharmaceuticals
M; 72	Menest	0.3 mg	Yellow	Coated Tablet	Oblong	Monarch Pharmaceuticals
M; 73	Menest	0.625 mg	Orange	Coated Tablet	Oblong	Monarch Pharmaceuticals
M; 74	Fluphenazine Hydrochloride	5 mg	Green	Coated Tablet	Triangle	Mylan Pharmaceuticals
M; 74	Menest	1.25 mg	Green	Coated Tablet	Oblong	Monarch Pharmaceuticals
M; 75	Chlorthalidone	50 mg	Green	Tablet	Circle, Scored	Mylan Pharmaceuticals
M; 75	L-Thyroxine	0.075 mg	Blue	Tablet	Circle, Scored	Warner Chilcott
M; 75	Menest	2.5 mg	Pink	Coated Tablet	Oblong	Monarch Pharmaceuticals
M; 76	Flurbiprofen	50 mg	Beige	Coated Tablet	Circle	Mylan Pharmaceuticals
M; 77	Amitriptyline Hydrochloride	10 mg	White	Coated Tablet	Circle, Biconvex	Mylan Pharmaceuticals
M; 80	Indapamide	2.5 mg	White	Coated Tablet	Circle, Biconvex, Beveled Edge	Mylan Pharmaceuticals
M; 81	Captopril and Hydrochlorothiazide	25 mg; 15 mg	White	Tablet	Circle, Scored	Mylan Pharmaceuticals
M; 83	Captopril and Hydrochlorothiazide	25 mg; 25 mg	Peach	Tablet	Circle, Scored	Mylan Pharmaceuticals
M; 84	Captopril and Hydrochlorothiazide	50 mg; 15 mg	White	Tablet	Capsule-Shape, Scored	Mylan Pharmaceuticals
M; 86	Captopril and Hydrochlorothiazide	50 mg; 25 mg	Peach	Tablet	Capsule-Shape, Scored	Mylan Pharmaceuticals
M; 87	Maprotiline Hydrochloride	50 mg	Blue	Coated Tablet	Circle, Scored, Biconvex, Beveled Edge	Mylan Pharmaceuticals
M; 92	Maprotiline Hydrochloride	75 mg	White	Coated Tablet	Circle, Scored, Biconvex, Beveled Edge	Mylan Pharmaceuticals
M; 93	Flurbiprofen	100 mg	Beige	Coated Tablet	Circle	Mylan Pharmaceuticals
M; 95	Penicillin V Potassium	250 mg	White	Tablet	Circle, Scored	Mylan Pharmaceuticals
M; 97	Fluphenazine Hydrochloride	10 mg	Orange	Coated Tablet	Triangle	Mylan Pharmaceuticals
M; 98	Penicillin V Potassium	500 mg	White	Tablet	Oval	Mylan Pharmaceuticals
M; 100	L-Thyroxine	0.1 mg	Blue	Tablet	Circle, Scored	Warner Chilcott
M; 100	Motrin	100 mg	White	Tablet	Capsule-Shape, Scored	Mcneil Consumer Products
M; 100; LEVO; T	L-Thyroxine	0.1 mg	Yellow	Tablet	Circle, Scored	Novartis Generics
M; 113	Glyburide, Micronized	1.5 mg	White	Tablet	Oval, Scored	Mylan Pharmaceuticals
M; 125	Glyburide, Micronized	3 mg	Light Yellow	Tablet	Oval, Scored	Mylan Pharmaceuticals
M; 125	L-Thyroxine	0.125 mg	Blue	Tablet	Circle, Scored	Warner Chilcott
M; 127	Pindolol	10 mg	White	Tablet	Circle, Scored, Biconvex	Mylan Pharmaceuticals
M; 132	Nadolol	80 mg	Yellow	Tablet	Circle, Scored	Mylan Pharmaceuticals
M; 134	Ketorolac Tromethamine	10 mg	White	Tablet	Circle	Mylan Pharmaceuticals
M; 135	Diltiazem Hydrochloride	90 mg	White	Coated Tablet	Capsule-Shape, Scored	Mylan Pharmaceuticals
M; 142	Glyburide	6 mg	Green	Tablet	Oval, Scored	Mylan Pharmaceuticals
M; 144	Tamoxifen Citrate	10 mg	White	Tablet	Circle	Mylan Pharmaceuticals
M; 146	Spironolactone	25 mg	White	Coated Tablet	Circle, Biconvex, Bevel-Edged	Mylan Pharmaceuticals
M; 150	L-Thyroxine	0.15 mg	Blue	Tablet	Circle, Scored	Warner Chilcott
M; 150; LEVO; T	L-Thyroxine	0.15 mg	Blue	Tablet	Circle, Scored	Novartis Generics
M; 171	Nadolol	40 mg	Yellow	Tablet	Circle, Scored	Mylan Pharmaceuticals
M; 172	Metolazone	2.5 mg	Peach	Tablet	Circle	Mylan Pharmaceuticals
M; 200	L-Thyroxine	0.2 mg	Blue	Tablet	Circle, Scored	Warner Chilcott
M; 200; LEVO; T	L-Thyroxine	0.2 mg	Pink	Tablet	Circle, Scored	Novartis Generics
M; 221	Timolol Maleate	10 mg	Green	Tablet	Circle, Scored, Flat Beveled Edge	Mylan Pharmaceuticals
M; 231	Atenolol	50 mg	White	Tablet	Circle, Scored	Mylan Pharmaceuticals
M; 234	Metformin Hydrochloride	500 mg	White	Coated Tablet	Circle, Biconvex, Bevel Edged	Mylan Pharmaceuticals
M; 240	Metformin Hydrochloride	850 mg	White	Coated Tablet	Circle, Biconvex, Bevel Edged	Mylan Pharmaceuticals
M; 243	Spironolactone	50 mg	White	Coated Tablet	Circle, Biconvex, Bevel-Edged, Scored	Mylan Pharmaceuticals
M; 244	Metformin Hydrochloride	1000 mg	White	Coated Tablet	Oval, Biconvex, Bevel Edged	Mylan Pharmaceuticals
M; 253	Acyclovir	400 mg	White	Tablet	Circle	Mylan Pharmaceuticals
M; 255	Albuterol	2 mg	White	Tablet	Circle, Scored	Mylan Pharmaceuticals
M; 261	Ketoconazole	200 mg	White	Tablet	Circle	Mylan Pharmaceuticals
M; 273	Penicillin V Potassium	250 mg	White	Coated Tablet	Circle, Biconvex, Scored	Mylan Pharmaceuticals
M; 274	Tamoxifen Citrate	20 mg	White to Off-White	Tablet	Circle	Mylan Pharmaceuticals
M; 275	Penicillin V Potassium	500 mg	White	Coated Tablet	Oblong, Biconvex, Scored on Both Sides	Mylan Pharmaceuticals
M; 300	L-Thyroxine	0.3 mg	Blue	Tablet	Circle, Scored	Warner Chilcott
M; 300; LEVO; T	L-Thyroxine	0.3 mg	Green	Tablet	Circle, Scored	Novartis Generics
M; 302	Acyclovir	800 mg	White	Tablet	Oval	Mylan Pharmaceuticals
M; 305	Sotalol Hydrochloride	80 mg	Orange	Tablet	Circle, Scored	Mylan Pharmaceuticals
M; 310	Sotalol Hydrochloride	120 mg	Orange	Tablet	Circle, Scored	Mylan Pharmaceuticals
M; 312	Verapamil Hydrochloride	180 mg	Blue	Extended-Release Tablet	Oval, Scored	Mylan Pharmaceuticals
M; 313	Tolmetin Sodium	600 mg	Beige	Coated Tablet	Oval	Mylan Pharmaceuticals
M; 314	Sotalol Hydrochloride	160 mg	Orange	Tablet	Circle, Scored	Mylan Pharmaceuticals
M; 316	Sotalol Hydrochloride	240 mg	Orange	Tablet	Circle, Scored	Mylan Pharmaceuticals
M; 317	Cimetidine	300 mg	Green	Coated Tablet	Five-Sided	Mylan Pharmaceuticals
M; 321	Lorazepam	0.5 mg	White	Tablet	Circle	Mylan Pharmaceuticals
M; 355	Diclofenac Sodium	100 mg	Yellow	Extended-Release Tablet	Circle, Biconvex, Bevel-Edged	Mylan Pharmaceuticals
M; 365	Procet	5 mg; 325 mg	White	Tablet	Capsule-Shape, Scored	Andrx Pharmaceuticals
M; 366	Procet	7.5 mg; 325 mg	White	Tablet	Oval, Scored	Andrx Pharmaceuticals
M; 372	Cimetidine	400 mg	Green	Coated Tablet	Five-Sided, House Shaped	Mylan Pharmaceuticals
M; 373	Hydroxychloroquine Sulfate	200 mg	White	Tablet	Circle	Mylan Pharmaceuticals
M; 400	Erythromycin Ethylsuccinate	400 mg	Beige	Coated Tablet	Capsule-Shape, Biconvex, Beveled Edge	Mylan Pharmaceuticals
M; 407	Fluvoxamine Maleate	25 mg	Orange	Tablet	Oval	Mylan Pharmaceuticals
M; 407	Fluvoxamine Maleate	25 mg	Off-White to Yellow	Tablet	Oval	Mylan Pharmaceuticals
M; 411	Verapamil Hydrochloride	240 mg	Blue	Extended-Release Tablet	Capsule-Shape, Modified	Mylan Pharmaceuticals
M; 412	Fluvoxamine Maleate	50 mg	Orange	Tablet	Oval, Scored	Mylan Pharmaceuticals
M; 412	Fluvoxamine Maleate	50 mg	Off-White to Yellow	Tablet	Oval, Scored	Mylan Pharmaceuticals
M; 414	Fluvoxamine Maleate	100 mg	Off-White to Yellow	Tablet	Oval, Scored	Mylan Pharmaceuticals
M; 414	Fluvoxamine Maleate	100 mg	Orange	Tablet	Oval, Scored	Mylan Pharmaceuticals
M; 433	Bupropion Hydrochloride	75 mg	Peach	Tablet	Circle	Mylan Pharmaceuticals
M; 435	Bupropion Hydrochloride	100 mg	Light Blue	Tablet	Circle	Mylan Pharmaceuticals
M; 437	Spironolactone	100 mg	White	Coated Tablet	Circle, Biconvex, Bevel-Edged, Scored	Mylan Pharmaceuticals
M; 441	Benazepril Hydrochloride	5 mg	White	Tablet	Circle	Mylan Pharmaceuticals
M; 443	Benazepril Hydrochloride	10 mg	White	Tablet	Circle	Mylan Pharmaceuticals
M; 444	Benazepril Hydrochloride	20 mg	White	Tablet	Circle	Mylan Pharmaceuticals
M; 447	Benazepril Hydrochloride	40 mg	White	Tablet	Oval	Mylan Pharmaceuticals

IMPRINT	BRAND/GENERIC NAME	STRENGTH	COLOR	FORM	SHAPE	MANUFACTURER
M; 471	Fenoprofen Calcium	600 mg	Orange	Coated Tablet	Capsule-Shape, Scored	Mylan Pharmaceuticals
M; 475	Nifedipine ER	30 mg	Rose-Pink	Extended-Release Tablet	Circle	Mylan Pharmaceuticals
M; 482	Nifedipine ER	60 mg	Rose-Pink	Extended-Release Tablet	Circle	Mylan Pharmaceuticals
M; 495	Nifedipine ER	90 mg	Rose-Pink	Extended-Release Tablet	Circle	Mylan Pharmaceuticals
M; 501	Bisoprolol and Hydrochlorothiazide	2.5 mg; 6.25 mg	Orange	Tablet	Circle	Mylan Pharmaceuticals
M; 503	Bisoprolol and Hydrochlorothiazide	5 mg; 6.25 mg	Blue	Tablet	Circle	Mylan Pharmaceuticals
M; 505	Bisoprolol and Hydrochlorothiazide	10 mg; 6.25 mg	White	Tablet	Circle	Mylan Pharmaceuticals
M; 515	Mirtazapine	15 mg	Beige	Tablet	Circle	Mylan Pharmaceuticals
M; 525	Diltiazem Hydrochloride	120 mg	White with Clear Film Coat	Coated Tablet	Capsule-Shape, Scored	Mylan Pharmaceuticals
M; 530	Mirtazapine	30 mg	Beige	Tablet	Circle	Mylan Pharmaceuticals
M; 537	Naproxen Sodium	275 mg	Light Blue	Coated Tablet	Circle	Mylan Pharmaceuticals
M; 541	Cimetidine	800 mg	Green	Coated Tablet	Oval, Scored	Mylan Pharmaceuticals
M; 545	Mirtazapine	45 mg	Beige	Tablet	Circle	Mylan Pharmaceuticals
M; 572	Albuterol	4 mg	White	Tablet	Circle, Scored, Flat Beveled Edge	Mylan Pharmaceuticals
M; 577	Amiloride Hydrochloride and Hydrochlorothiazide	5 mg; 50 mg	Orange	Tablet	Circle, Scored	Mylan Pharmaceuticals
M; 712	Enalapril and Hydrochlorothiazide	5 mg; 12.5 mg	White	Tablet	Circle, Biconvex	Mylan Pharmaceuticals
M; 715	Timolol Maleate	20 mg	Green	Tablet	Capsule-Shape, Scored, Biconvex, Beveled Edge	Mylan Pharmaceuticals
M; 723	Enalapril and Hydrochlorothiazide	10 mg; 25 mg	White	Tablet	Circle, Biconvex	Mylan Pharmaceuticals
M; 725	Benazepril Hydrochloride and Hydrochlorothiazide	5 mg; 6.25 mg	Beige	Tablet	Oval, Scored	Mylan Pharmaceuticals
M; 735	Benazepril Hydrochloride and Hydrochlorothiazide	10 mg; 12.5 mg	Beige	Tablet	Circle, Scored	Mylan Pharmaceuticals
M; 745	Benazepril Hydrochloride and Hydrochlorothiazide	20 mg; 12.5 mg	Beige	Tablet	Capsule-Shape, Scored	Mylan Pharmaceuticals
M; 757	Atenolol	100 mg	White	Tablet	Circle	Mylan Pharmaceuticals
M; 775	Benazepril Hydrochloride and Hydrochlorothiazide	20 mg; 25 mg	Beige	Tablet	Oval, Scored	Mylan Pharmaceuticals
M; A2	Atenolol	25 mg	White	Tablet	Circle	Mylan Pharmaceuticals
M; B1	Buspirone Hydrochloride	5 mg	White	Tablet	Oval, Biconvex, Scored	Mylan Pharmaceuticals
M; B2	Buspirone Hydrochloride	10 mg	White	Tablet	Oval, Biconvex, Scored	Mylan Pharmaceuticals
M; B3; 5 5 5	Buspirone Hydrochloride	15 mg	White	Tablet	Capsule-Shape, Flat, Beveled Edge, Tri-Sected	Mylan Pharmaceuticals
M; B4; 10 10 10	Buspirone Hydrochloride	30 mg	White	Tablet	Capsule-Shape, Bevel-Edged,trisected	Mylan Pharmaceuticals
M; C; 11	Clozapine	100 mg	Green	Tablet	Circle, Scored	Mylan Pharmaceuticals
M; C; 13	Clonazepam	0.5 mg	Yellow	Tablet	Circle, Scored	Mylan Pharmaceuticals
M; C; 14	Clonazepam	1 mg	Green	Tablet	Circle, Scored	Mylan Pharmaceuticals
M; C; 15	Clonazepam	2 mg	White	Tablet	Circle, Scored	Mylan Pharmaceuticals
M; C; 7	Clozapine	25 mg	Peach	Tablet	Circle, Scored	Mylan Pharmaceuticals
M; C1	Captopril	12.5 mg	White	Tablet	Oval, Partially Scored	Mylan Pharmaceuticals
M; C2	Captopril	25 mg	White	Tablet	Circle, Scored	Mylan Pharmaceuticals
M; C3	Captopril	50 mg	White	Tablet	Circle, Scored	Mylan Pharmaceuticals
M; C4	Captopril	100 mg	White	Tablet	Circle, Scored	Mylan Pharmaceuticals
M; D5	Diclofenac Potassium	50 mg	White	Coated Tablet	Circle, Biconvex	Mylan Pharmaceuticals
M; D6	Dicyclomine Hydrochloride	20 mg	Blue	Tablet	Circle, Flat-Faced, Beveled Edge	Mylan Pharmaceuticals
M; D9	Doxazosin Mesylate	1 mg	White	Tablet	Circle, Scored	Mylan Pharmaceuticals
M; D10	Doxazosin Mesylate	2 mg	Pink	Tablet	Circle, Scored	Mylan Pharmaceuticals
M; D11	Doxazosin Mesylate	4 mg	Blue	Tablet	Circle, Scored	Mylan Pharmaceuticals
M; D12	Doxazosin Mesylate	8 mg	Purple	Tablet	Circle, Scored	Mylan Pharmaceuticals
M; E3	Estradiol	0.5 mg	White	Tablet	Circle	Mylan Pharmaceuticals
M; E4	Estradiol	1 mg	Pink	Tablet	Circle	Mylan Pharmaceuticals
M; E5	Estradiol	2 mg	Blue	Tablet	Circle	Mylan Pharmaceuticals
M; E7	Estropipate	0.75 mg	Yellow	Tablet	Circle	Mylan Pharmaceuticals
M; E8	Estropipate	1.5 mg	Peach	Tablet	Circle	Mylan Pharmaceuticals
M; E9	Estropipate	3 mg	Blue	Tablet	Circle	Mylan Pharmaceuticals
M; E15	Enalapril Maleate	2.5 mg	White	Tablet	Circle, Scored	Mylan Pharmaceuticals
M; E16	Enalapril Maleate	5 mg	White	Tablet	Circle, Scored	Mylan Pharmaceuticals
M; E17	Enalapril Maleate	10 mg	Light Blue	Tablet	Circle	Mylan Pharmaceuticals
M; E18	Enalapril Maleate	20 mg	Blue	Tablet	Circle	Mylan Pharmaceuticals
M; F1	Famotidine	20 mg	Yellow	Coated Tablet	Circle, Biconvex, Bevel-Edgied	Mylan Pharmaceuticals
M; F2	Famotidine	40 mg	Green	Coated Tablet	Circle, Biconvex, Bevel-Edged	Mylan Pharmaceuticals
M; G4	Guanfacine	1 mg	White	Tablet	Circle	Mylan Pharmaceuticals
M; G5	Guanfacine	2 mg	Blue	Tablet	Circle	Mylan Pharmaceuticals
M; IB ;	Midol Ib	200 mg	White	Coated Tablet		Bayer Consumer Care
M; L19	Lovastatin	10 mg	White to Off-White	Tablet	Circle, Flat-Faced, Bevel-Edged	Mylan Pharmaceuticals
M; L20	Lovastatin	20 mg	Yellow	Tablet	Circle, Flat-Faced, Bevel-Edged	Mylan Pharmaceuticals
M; L21	Lovastatin	40 mg	Pink	Tablet	Circle, Flat-Faced, Bevel-Edged	Mylan Pharmaceuticals
M; L22	Lisinopril	2.5 mg	Light Blue	Tablet	Circle	Mylan Pharmaceuticals
M; L23	Lisinopril	5 mg	Peach	Tablet	Circle	Mylan Pharmaceuticals
M; L24	Lisinopril	10 mg	White	Tablet	Circle	Mylan Pharmaceuticals
M; L25	Lisinopril	20 mg	Light Yellow	Tablet	Circle	Mylan Pharmaceuticals
M; L26	Lisinopril	40 mg	Light Green	Tablet	Circle	Mylan Pharmaceuticals
M; L27	Lisinopril	30 mg	Light Blue	Tablet	Circle	Mylan Pharmaceuticals
M; LH1	Hydrochlorothiazide and Lisinopril	12.5 mg; 10 mg		Tablet		Mylan Pharmaceuticals
M; LH2	Hydrochlorothiazide and Lisinopril	12.5 mg; 20 mg		Tablet		Mylan Pharmaceuticals
M; LH3	Hydrochlorothiazide and Lisinopril	25 mg; 20 mg		Tablet		Mylan Pharmaceuticals
M; N; 52	Nefazodone Hydrochloride	100 mg	White	Tablet	Circle	Mylan Pharmaceuticals
M; N; 53	Nefazodone Hydrochloride	150 mg	White	Tablet	Circle	Mylan Pharmaceuticals
M; N; 54	Nefazodone Hydrochloride	200 mg	White	Tablet	Circle	Mylan Pharmaceuticals
M; N; 55	Nefazodone Hydrochloride	250 mg	White	Tablet	Circle	Mylan Pharmaceuticals
M; P1	Prochlorperazine Maleate	5 mg	Maroon	Tablet	Circle	Mylan Pharmaceuticals
M; P2	Prochlorperazine Maleate	10 mg	Maroon	Tablet	Circle	Mylan Pharmaceuticals
M; T3	Trifluoperazine Hydrochloride	1 mg	White	Coated Tablet	Circle	Mylan Pharmaceuticals
M; T4	Trifluoperazine Hydrochloride	2 mg	White	Coated Tablet	Circle	Mylan Pharmaceuticals

IMPRINT	BRAND/GENERIC NAME	STRENGTH	COLOR	FORM	SHAPE	MANUFACTURER
M; T5	Trifluoperazine Hydrochloride	5 mg	Lavender	Coated Tablet	Circle	Mylan Pharmaceuticals
M; T6	Trifluoperazine Hydrochloride	10 mg	Lavender	Coated Tablet	Circle	Mylan Pharmaceuticals
M; T7	Tramadol Hydrochloride	50 mg	White	Tablet	Circle	Mylan Pharmaceuticals
M03; 1.5; MOVA	Glyburide Micronized	1.5 mg	White	Tablet	Oval, Bisected Scored	Watson Laboratories
M04; 3.0; MOVA	Glyburide Micronized	3 mg	Blue	Tablet	Oval, Bisected Scored	Watson Laboratories
M07; 6.0; MOVA	Glyburide Micronized	6 mg	Light Yellow	Tablet	Oval, Bisected Scored	Watson Laboratories
M2 ;	Furosemide	20 mg	Light Pink	Tablet	Circle	Mylan Pharmaceuticals
M4	Mesnex	400 mg	White	Coated Tablet	Oblong, Scored Biconvex	Bristol-Myers Squibb
M30 ;	Clorazepate Dipotassium	3.75 mg	Blue	Tablet	Circle	Mylan Pharmaceuticals
M45; LEDERLE; 50 MG	Minocin	50 mg	Yellow and Green	Capsule		Wyeth Pharmaceuticals
M46; LEDERLE; 100 MG	Minocin	100 mg	Light Green and Green	Capsule		Wyeth Pharmaceuticals
MAALOX PLUS; RPR	Maalox Plus	200 mg; 200 mg; 25 mg		Tablet, Chewable		Novartis Consumer
MAALOX; RPR	Maalox	200 mg; 200 mg	White	Tablet, Chewable	Circle	Novartis Consumer
MACROBID; NORWICH EATON	Macrobid	100 mg	Opaque, Black and Yellow	Capsule		Procter & Gamble Pharmaceuticals
MACRODANTIN; 25 MG; 0149; 0007	Macrodantin	25 mg	Opaque, White	Capsule		Procter & Gamble Pharmaceuticals
MACRODANTIN; 50 MG; 0149-0008	Macrodantin	50 mg	Opaque, Yellow and White	Capsule		Procter & Gamble Pharmaceuticals
MACRODANTIN; 100 MG; 0149; 0009	Macrodantin	100 mg	Opaque, Yellow	Capsule		Procter & Gamble Pharmaceuticals
MAOLATE	Maolate	400 mg	Tan	Tablet	Circle, Scored	Upjohn
MAREZINE; T4A	Marezine	50 mg	White	Tablet		Glaxosmithkline
MARION; 1525	Duotrate	30 mg	Black and Clear with White Pellets	Capsule		Aventis Pharmaceuticals
MARION; 1530	Duotrate	45 mg	Black and Light Blue with White Pellets	Capsule		Aventis Pharmaceuticals
MARION; 1555	Pavabid	150 mg		Extended-Release Capsule		Aventis Pharmaceuticals
MARION; 1555	Pavabid Plateau	150 mg		Timed-Release Capsule		Aventis Pharmaceuticals
MARION; 1555; PAVABID	Pavabid	150 mg	Black and White	Capsule		Aventis Pharmaceuticals
MARION; 1656	Os-Cal-Gesic	400 mg; 100 mg; 50 U	Blue-Green	Tablet	Oblong	Aventis Pharmaceuticals
MARION; 1771	Cardizem	30 mg	Green	Tablet	Circle	Biovail Pharmaceuticals
MARION; 1772	Cardizem	60 mg	Yellow	Tablet	Circle, Scored	Biovail Pharmaceuticals
MARION; GAVISCON; 1175	Gaviscon	80 mg; 20 mg	White	Tablet, Chewable	Circle	Glaxosmithkline Consumer
MARION; OS-CAL; 1650	Os-Cal 250	625 mg; 250 mg; 125 U;	Light Green	Tablet	Circle	Aventis Pharmaceuticals
MARION; OS-CAL; 1650	Os-Cal 250 + D	625 mg; 125 units		Tablet		Aventis Pharmaceuticals
MARION; PAVABID HP	Pavabid Hp Capsulets	300 mg	Light Orange	Tablet		Aventis Pharmaceuticals
MARION; PAVABID; HP	Pavabid Hp	300 mg	Light Orange	Capsule		Aventis Pharmaceuticals
MARION; PRETTS; 1177	Pretts Diet Aid	200 mg; 100 mg; 70 mg	Yellow	Tablet	Circle	Aventis Pharmaceuticals
MAXALT; MRK; 267	Maxalt	10 mg	Pink	Tablet	Capsule-Shape	Merck
MAXAQUIN; 400	Maxaquin	400 mg	White	Coated Tablet	Oval, Scored	Searle
MAXIDONE; 634	Maxidone	750 mg; 10 mg	Yellow	Tablet	Capsule-Shape, Scored	Watson Laboratories
MAXZIDE; B; M8	Maxzide	75 mg; 50 mg	Yellow	Tablet	Bowtie	Mylan Bertek Pharmaceuticals
MAXZIDE; B; M9	Maxzide	37.5 mg; 25 mg	Green	Tablet	Bowtie	Mylan Bertek Pharmaceuticals
MC	Desoxyn	5 mg	White	Sustained-Release Tablet		Abbott Laboratories
MCNEIL; 058 ;	Butibel-Zyme	15 mg; 15 mg	Pink	Tablet		Mcneil Pharmaceutical
MCNEIL; 1/2; HALDOL	Haldol	0.5 mg	White	Tablet	U-Shape, with "h" Cut Out in Center, Scored	Ortho-Mcneil Pharmaceutical
MCNEIL; 151	Clistin-Ra	8 mg	Orange	Coated Tablet		Mcneil Pharmaceutical
MCNEIL; 153	Clistin-Ra	12 mg	Yellow	Coated Tablet		Mcneil Pharmaceutical
MCNEIL; 659 ;	Ultram	50 mg	White	Coated Tablet	Capsule-Shape, Scored	Ortho-Mcneil Pharmaceutical
MCNEIL; BUTIBEL ;	Butibel	15 mg; 15 mg	Red	Tablet		Mcneil Pharmaceutical
MCNEIL; BUTICAPS ;	Buticaps	15 mg	Lavender and White	Capsule		Mcneil Pharmaceutical
MCNEIL; BUTICAPS ;	Buticaps	30 mg	Aqua-Green and White	Capsule		Mcneil Pharmaceutical
MCNEIL; BUTICAPS ;	Buticaps	50 mg	Orange and White	Capsule		Mcneil Pharmaceutical
MCNEIL; BUTICAPS ;	Buticaps	100 mg	Pink and White	Capsule		Mcneil Pharmaceutical
MCNEIL; BUTISOL SODIUM ;	Butisol Sodium	30 mg	Green	Tablet	Circle, Scored	Mcneil Pharmaceutical
MCNEIL; BUTISOL SODIUM ;	Butisol Sodium	50 mg	Orange	Tablet	Circle, Scored	Mcneil Pharmaceutical
MCNEIL; BUTISOL SODIUM ;	Butisol Sodium	100 mg	Pink	Tablet		Mcneil Pharmaceutical
MCNEIL; PANCREASE	Pancrease	4500 U; 20000 U; 25000 U	White	Capsule		Ortho-Mcneil Pharmaceutical
MCNEIL; PANCREASE; MT 4	Pancrease Mt 4	4000 USP units; 12,000 USP units; 12,000 USP units	Yellow and Clear	Capsule		Mcneil Pharmaceutical
MCNEIL; PANCREASE; MT 10	Pancrease Mt 10	10,000 USP units; 30,000 USP units; 30,000 USP units	Pink and Clear	Capsule		Mcneil Pharmaceutical

IMPRINT	BRAND/GENERIC NAME	STRENGTH	COLOR	FORM	SHAPE	MANUFACTURER
MCNEIL; PANCREASE; MT 16	Pancrease Mt 16	16,000 USP units; 48,000 USP units; 48,000 USP units	Salmon and Clear	Capsule		Mcneil Pharmaceutical
MCNEIL; PANCREASE; MT 25	Pancrease Mt 25	25000 U; 75000 U; 75000 U	White	Capsule		Mcneil Pharmaceutical
MCNEIL; PANCREASE; MT 32	Pancrease Mt 32	32000 U; 90000 U; 70000 U	White	Capsule		Mcneil Pharmaceutical
MCNEIL; TYLENOL CODEINE 2 ;	Tylenol with Codeine No. 2	15 mg; 300 mg	White	Tablet		Mcneil Pharmaceutical
MCNEIL; TYLENOL; CODEINE 1 ;	Tylenol with Codeine No. 1	7.5 mg; 300 mg	White	Tablet	Circle	Mcneil Pharmaceutical
MD; 518	Diethylpropion Hydrochloride	25 mg	Medium Blue		Circle	Novartis Generics
MD; 531	Methylphenidate Ir	5 mg	Yellow	Tablet	Circle, Scored	Sandoz
MD; 562	Methylphenidate ER	20 mg	White	Tablet	Circle	Sandoz
ME	Desoxyn	10 mg	Orange	Sustained-Release Tablet		Abbott Laboratories
MEDACID	Medacid Antacid	223 mg; 127 mg; 59 mg	Blue	Tablet		Bristol-Myers Squibb
MEDIPREN	Medipren	200 mg	White	Tablet		Mcneil Consumer Products
MEDROL; 2	Medrol	2 mg	Pink	Tablet	Oval, Scored	Pharmacia & Upjohn
MEDROL; 4 ;	Medrol	4 mg	White	Tablet	Oval, Scored	Pharmacia & Upjohn
MEDROL; 8 ;	Medrol	8 mg	Peach	Tablet	Oval, Scored	Pharmacia & Upjohn
MEDROL; 16 ;	Medrol	16 mg	White	Tablet	Oval, Scored	Pharmacia & Upjohn
MEDROL; 24 ;	Medrol	24 mg	Yellow	Tablet	Oval, Scored	Pharmacia & Upjohn
MEDROL; 32 ;	Medrol	32 mg	Peach	Tablet	Oval, Scored	Pharmacia & Upjohn
MERIDIA; 5	Meridia	5 mg	Blue and Yellow	Capsule		Abbott Laboratories
MERIDIA; 10	Meridia	10 mg	Blue and White	Capsule		Abbott Laboratories
MERIDIA; 15	Meridia	15 mg	Yellow and White	Capsule		Abbott Laboratories
MERRELL; 37	Cantil	25 mg	Yellow	Tablet		Sanofi-Aventis U.S.
MERRELL; 62	Metahydrin	2 mg	Pink	Tablet	Circle, Debossed	Aventis Pharmaceuticals
MERRELL; 63	Metahydrin	4 mg	Aqua Blue	Tablet	Circle, Debossed	Aventis Pharmaceuticals
MERRELL; 64	Metatensin	2 mg; 0.1 mg	Yellow	Tablet		Aventis Pharmaceuticals
MERRELL; 65	Metatensin	4 mg; 0.1 mg	Lavender	Tablet		Aventis Pharmaceuticals
METRYL; 93	Metryl	250 mg	White	Tablet	Circle, Convex	Teva Pharmaceuticals
METRYL; 500; 93; 93	Metryl	500 mg	White	Tablet	Oblong, Scored	Teva Pharmaceuticals
MF	Desoxyn	15 mg	Yellow	Sustained-Release Tablet		Abbott Laboratories
MF; 1; G	Metformin Hydrochloride	500 mg	White	Tablet	Circle	Par Pharmaceutical
MF; 2; G	Metformin Hydrochloride	850 mg	White	Tablet	Circle	Par Pharmaceutical
MF; 3; G	Metformin Hydrochloride	1000 mg	White	Tablet	Oblong	Par Pharmaceutical
MH; 1; M	Midodrine Hydrochloride	2.5 mg	White to Off White	Tablet	Circle, Scored	Mylan Pharmaceuticals
MH; 2; M	Midodrine Hydrochloride	5 mg	White to Off White	Tablet	Circle, Scored	Mylan Pharmaceuticals
MH; 3; M	Midodrine Hydrochloride	10 mg	White to Off White	Tablet	Circle, Scored	Mylan Pharmaceuticals
MIA; 110	Butalbital, Acetaminophen and Caffeine	325 mg; 50 mg; 40 mg	White	Tablet	Capsule-Shape, Scored	Novartis Generics
MICRONASE; 1.25	Micronase	1.25 mg	White	Tablet	Circle, Scored	Pharmacia & Upjohn
MICRONASE; 2.5	Micronase	2.5 mg	Dark Pink	Tablet	Circle, Scored	Pharmacia & Upjohn
MICRONASE; 5	Micronase	5 mg	Blue	Tablet	Circle, Scored	Pharmacia & Upjohn
MICROZIDE; 12.5	Microzide	12.5 mg	Opaque Teal	Capsule, Liquid Filled		Watson Laboratories
MIDOL	Midol Multi-Symptom Formula Regular Strength	325 mg; 12.5 mg	White	Tablet		Bayer Consumer Care
MIDOL	Midol Maximum Strength Multi-Symptom	500 mg; 60 mg; 15 mg	Light Blue and Dark Blue	Capsule, Liquid Filled		Bayer Consumer Care
MIDOL MAXIMUM	Midol Multi-Symptom Formula Maximum Strength	500 mg; 15 mg; 60 mg	White	Tablet		Bayer Consumer Care
MIDOL PM	Midol Pm Night Time Formula	500 mg; 25 mg	Blue	Tablet	Capsule-Shape	Bayer Consumer Care
MIDOL PMS	Midol Pre-Menstrual Syndrome Maximum Strength	500 mg; 25 mg; 15 mg		Tablet	Capsule-Shape	Bayer Consumer Care
MIDOL; MENSTRUAL	Midol Maximum Strength Menstrual Formula	500 mg; 60 mg; 15 mg	White	Tablet	Oblong	Bayer Consumer Care
MIDRIN	Midrin	65 mg; 100 mg; 325 mg	Red with Pink Band	Capsule		Women First Healthcare
MILES; 093	Mycelex-G	100 mg	White	Tablet		Bayer Consumer Care
MILES; 121	Decholin	250 mg	White	Tablet		Bayer Pharmaceutical
MILES; 721	Niclocide	500 mg		Tablet		Bayer Pharmaceutical
MILES; 951	Lithane	300 mg	Green	Tablet	Circle, Scocred(Scored)	Bayer Pharmaceutical
MINOCYCLINE 50 DAN 5694 ;	Minocycline Hydrochloride	50 mg	Opaque Yellow	Capsule		Watson Laboratories
MINOCYCLINE 75 WPI ;	Minocycline Hydrochloride	75 mg	Opaque White, Opaque Yellow	Capsule		Watson Laboratories
MINOCYCLINE 100 DAN 5695 ;	Minocycline Hydrochloride	100 mg	Opaque Dark Gray, Opaque Yelllow	Capsule		Watson Laboratories
MJ; 021	Estrace	0.5 mg		Tablet		Warner Chilcott
MJ; 503; 50	Cytoxan	50 mg	White with Blue Speckles	Tablet		Bristol-Myers Squibb
MJ; 504; 25	Cytoxan	25 mg	White with Blue Speckles	Tablet		Bristol-Myers Squibb
MJ; 543	Vasodilan	10 mg	White	Tablet		Bristol-Myers Squibb
MJ; 583	Ovcon-35-21	0.4 mg; 35 mcg	Peach	21-Day Tablet Pack	Circle	Warner Chilcott
MJ; 584	Ovcon-50 Yellow Tablet	1 mg; 50 mcg	Yellow	28-Day Tablet Pack	Circle	Warner Chilcott
MJ; 755	Estrace	1 mg	Lavender	Tablet		Warner Chilcott
MJ; 784; DURICEF; 500MG ;	Duricef	500 mg	Maroon and White	Capsule		Bristol-Myers Squibb
MJ; 785	Duricef	1 G	White	Tablet		Bristol-Myers Squibb
MJ; 822; 5	Buspar Dividose	15 mg	White	Tablet		Bristol-Myers Squibb
ML; 824; 10	Buspar Dividose	30 mg	Pink	Tablet	Trisected	Bristol-Myers Squibb
MOBAN; 5	Moban	5 mg	Orange	Tablet	Circle, Biconvex	Endo Laboratories

IMPRINT	BRAND/GENERIC NAME	STRENGTH	COLOR	FORM	SHAPE	MANUFACTURER
MOBAN; 10	Moban	10 mg	Lavender	Tablet	Circle, Biconvex	Endo Laboratories
MOBAN; 25	Moban	25 mg	Green	Tablet	Circle, Biconvex, Scored	Endo Laboratories
MOBAN; 50	Moban	50 mg	Blue	Tablet	Circle, Biconvex, Scored	Endo Laboratories
MOBAN; 100	Moban	100 mg	Tan	Tablet	Circle, Biconvex, Scored	Endo Laboratories
MONODOX; 50; M260	Monodox	50 mg	Yellow and White	Capsule		Watson Laboratories
MOTRIN COLD & FLU	Motrin Cold & Flu Non-Drowsy Formula	200 mg; 30 mg	Yellow	Tablet	Film-Coated	Mcneil Consumer Products
MOTRIN; 50	Motrin	50 mg	Orange	Tablet, Chewable	Circle, Scored	Mcneil Consumer Products
MOTRIN; 100	Motrin	100 mg	Orange	Tablet, Chewable	Circle, Scored	Mcneil Consumer Products
MOTRIN; 300 MG	Motrin	300 mg	White	Coated Tablet	Circle	Pharmacia & Upjohn
MOTRIN; 400 MG	Motrin	400 mg	Orange	Coated Tablet	Circle	Pharmacia & Upjohn
MOTRIN; 600 MG	Motrin	600 mg	Peach	Coated Tablet	Oval	Pharmacia & Upjohn
MOTRIN; 800 MG	Motrin	800 mg	Apricot	Coated Tablet	Oblong	Pharmacia & Upjohn
MOTRIN; IB; SINUS	Motrin Ib Sinus	200 mg; 30 mg	White	Tablet	Circle	Mcneil Consumer Products
MPC; 100	Tussend	5 mg; 60 mg; 4 mg	Yellow	Tablet	Capsule-Shape, Scored	Monarch Pharmaceuticals
MR; 15; G	Mirtazapine	15 mg	Yellow	Tablet	Circle	Par Pharmaceutical
MR; 30; G	Mirtazapine	30 mg	Buff	Tablet	Circle	Par Pharmaceutical
MR; 45; G	Mirtazapine	45 mg	White	Tablet	Circle	Par Pharmaceutical
MRK 117 ; SINGULAIR	Singulair	10 mg	Beige	Tablet	Square	Merck & Company
MRK 275 ; SINGULAIR	Singulair	5 mg	Pink	Tablet, Chewable	Circle	Merck & Company
MRK 711 ; SINGULAIR	Singulair	4 mg	Pink	Tablet, Chewable	Oval	Merck & Company
MRK 717 ; HYZAAR	Hyzaar 50-12.5	12.5 mg; 50 mg	Yellow	Tablet	Teardrop-Shape	Merck
MRK 747 ; HYZAAR	Hyzaar 100-25	25 mg; 100 mg	Light Yellow	Tablet	Teardrop-Shape	Merck
MRK; 212; FOSAMAX	Fosamax	40 mg	White	Tablet	Triangle	Merck & Company
MRK; 266	Maxalt	5 mg	Pink	Tablet	Capsule-Shape, Compressed	Merck
MRK; 925	Fosamax	5 mg	White	Tablet	Circle	Merck & Company
MRK; 936	Fosamax	10 mg	White	Tablet	Oval	Merck & Company
MRK; 951	Cozaar	25 mg	Light Green	Coated Tablet	Teardrop-Shape	Merck
MRK; 952; COZAAR	Cozaar	50 mg	Green	Coated Tablet	Teardrop-Shape	Merck
MRK; 960	Cozaar	100 mg	Dark Green	Coated Tablet	Teardrop-Shape	Merck
MSAP	Arthritis Pain Formula	500 mg; 27 mg; 100 mg	Light Brown or White	Tablet		Wyeth Consumer Healthcare
MSD 65 ; EDECRIN	Edecrin	25 mg	White	Tablet	Capsule-Shape	Merck & Company
MSD; 14; VASOTEC	Vasotec	2.5 mg	Yellow	Tablet	Barrel, Biconvex, Scored, Compressed	Merck & Company
MSD; 15	Prinivil	2.5 mg	White	Tablet	Circle, Small	Merck Sharp & Dohme
MSD; 19; PRINIVIL	Prinivil	5 mg	White	Tablet	Shield-Shape, Compressed, Scored	Merck & Company
MSD; 20	Decadron	0.25 mg	Orange	Tablet	Five-Sided, Compressed, Scored	Merck & Company
MSD; 21	Cogentin	0.5 mg	White	Tablet	Circle, Scored	Merck & Company
MSD; 25	Indocin	25 mg	Opaque Blue and White	Capsule		Merck & Company
MSD; 41	Decadron	0.5 mg	Yellow	Tablet	Five-Sided, Compressed, Score	Merck & Company
MSD; 42	Hydrodiuril	25 mg	Peach	Tablet	Circle, Scored, Compressed	Merck & Company
MSD; 43	Mephyton	5 mg	Yellow	Tablet	Circle, Scored, Compressed	Merck & Company
MSD; 50	Indocin	50 mg	Opaque Blue and White	Capsule		Merck & Company
MSD; 53	Hydropres-25	25 mg; 0.125 mg	Green	Tablet	Circle, Scored	Merck & Company
MSD; 59; BLOCADREN	Blocadren	5 mg	Light Blue	Tablet	Circle, Compressed	Merck & Company
MSD; 60	Cogentin	2 mg	White	Tablet	Circle, Scored, Compressed	Merck & Company
MSD; 62	Periactin	4 mg	White	Tablet	Circle, Compressed, Scored	Merck & Company
MSD; 63	Decadron	0.75 mg	Bluish-Green	Tablet	Five-Sided, Compressed, Scored	Merck & Company
MSD; 67	Timolide	10 mg; 25 mg	Light Blue	Tablet		Merck & Company
MSD; 72; PROSCAR	Proscar	5 mg	Blue	Coated Tablet	Character-Shape, Modified Apple	Merck & Company
MSD; 92	Midamor	5 mg	Yellow	Tablet	Diamond-Shaped, Compressed	Merck & Company
MSD; 95	Decadron	1.5 mg	Pink	Tablet	Five-Sided, Compressed, Scored	Merck & Company
MSD; 97	Decadron	4 mg	White	Tablet	Five-Sided, Compressed, Scored	Merck & Company
MSD; 105	Hydrodiuril	50 mg	Peach	Tablet	Circle, Scored, Compressed	Merck & Company
MSD; 106; PRINIVIL	Prinivil	10 mg	Light Yellow	Tablet	Shield-Shape, Compressed	Merck & Company
MSD; 127	Hydropres-50	50 mg; 0.125 mg	Green	Tablet	Circle, Scored	Merck & Company
MSD; 135	Aldomet	125 mg	Yellow	Coated Tablet	Circle	Merck & Company
MSD; 136; BLOCADREN	Blocadren	10 mg	Light Blue	Tablet	Circle, Scored, Compressed	Merck & Company
MSD; 139	Stromectol	6 mg	White	Tablet	Scored, Beveled-Edge	Merck & Company
MSD; 140; PRINZIDE	Prinzide	12.5 mg; 20 mg	Yellow	Tablet	Circle, Fluted-Edge	Merck & Company
MSD; 142; PRINZIDE	Prinzide	25 mg; 20 mg	Peach	Tablet	Circle, Fluted-Edge	Merck & Company
MSD; 145; PRINZIDE	Prinzide	12.5 mg; 10 mg	Blue	Tablet	Six-Sided	Merck & Company
MSD; 147	Decadron	6 mg	Green	Tablet	Five-Sided, Compressed, Scored	Merck & Company
MSD; 173	Vaseretic	5 mg; 12.5 mg	Green	Tablet	Capsule-Shape, Squared, Compressed	Merck & Company
MSD; 207; PRINIVIL	Prinivil	20 mg	Peach	Tablet	Shield-Shape, Compressed	Merck & Company
MSD; 214	Diuril	250 mg	White	Tablet	Circle, Scored, Compressed	Merck & Company
MSD; 219	Cortone Acetate	25 mg	White	Tablet	Circle, Scored, Compressed	Merck & Company
MSD; 230	Diupres-250	250 mg; 0.125 mg	Pink	Tablet	Circle, Scored	Merck & Company
MSD; 237; PRINIVIL	Prinivil	40 mg	Rose-Red	Tablet	Shield-Shape, Compressed	Merck & Company
MSD; 401	Aldomet	250 mg	Yellow	Coated Tablet	Circle	Merck & Company
MSD; 403	Urecholine	5 mg	White	Tablet	Circle, Scored, Compressed	Merck & Company
MSD; 405	Diupres-500	500 mg; 0.125 mg	Pink	Tablet	Circle, Scored	Merck & Company
MSD; 410	Hydrodiuril	100 mg	Peach	Tablet	Circle, Scored, Compressed	Merck & Company
MSD; 412	Urecholine	10 mg	Pink	Tablet	Circle, Compressed, Scored	Merck & Company
MSD; 423	Aldoril-15	250 mg; 15 mg	Salmon	Coated Tablet	Circle	Merck & Company
MSD; 432	Diuril	500 mg	White	Tablet	Circle, Scored, Compressed	Merck & Company
MSD; 437; BLOCADREN	Blocadren	20 mg	Light Blue	Tablet	Capsule-Shape, Scored, Compressed	Merck & Company
MSD; 456	Aldoril-25	250 mg; 25 mg	White	Coated Tablet	Circle	Merck & Company

IMPRINT	BRAND/GENERIC NAME	STRENGTH	COLOR	FORM	SHAPE	MANUFACTURER
MSD; 457	Urecholine	25 mg	Yellow	Tablet	Circle, Compressed, Scored	Merck & Company
MSD; 460	Urecholine	50 mg	Yellow	Tablet	Circle, Compressed, Scored	Merck & Company
MSD; 501	Benemid	500 mg	Yellow	Coated Tablet	Capsule-Shape, Scored	Merck & Company
MSD; 516	Aldomet	500 mg	Yellow	Coated Tablet	Circle	Merck & Company
MSD; 517	Triavil 4-50	4 mg; 50 mg	Orange	Coated Tablet	Diamond	Merck & Company
MSD; 602	Cuprimine	250 mg	Ivory	Capsule		Merck & Company
MSD; 612	Aldoclor 150	250 mg; 150 mg	Beige	Coated Tablet	Oval	Merck & Company
MSD; 614	Colbenemid	0.5 GM; 0.5 mg	White to Off-White	Tablet	Capsule-Shape, Scored	Merck & Company
MSD; 619	Hydrocortone	10 mg	White	Tablet	Oval, Compressed, Scored	Merck & Company
MSD; 634	Aldoclor 250	250 mg; 250 mg	Green	Coated Tablet	Oval	Merck & Company
MSD; 635	Cogentin	1 mg	White	Tablet	Oval, Scored, Compressed	Merck & Company
MSD; 661	Syprine	250 mg	Light Brown, Opaque	Capsule		Merck & Company
MSD; 672	Cuprimine	125 mg	Opaque Ivory and Grey	Capsule		Merck & Company
MSD; 675	Dolobid	250 mg	Peach	Coated Tablet	Capsule-Shape	Merck & Company
MSD; 690; DEMSER	Demser	250 mg	Opaque Two-Tone Blue	Capsule		Merck & Company
MSD; 693	Indocin SR	75 mg	Blue and Clear with White Pellets	Extended-Release Capsule		Merck & Company
MSD; 694	Aldoril D30	500 mg; 30 mg	Salmon	Coated Tablet	Oval	Merck & Company
MSD; 697	Dolobid	500 mg	Orange	Coated Tablet	Capsule-Shape	Merck & Company
MSD; 705; NOROXIN	Noroxin	400 mg	Dark Pink	Coated Tablet	Oval	Merck Sharp & Dohme
MSD; 712; VASOTEC	Vasotec	5 mg	White	Tablet	Barrel, Scored, Compressed	Merck & Company
MSD; 713; VASOTEC	Vasotec	10 mg	Salmon	Tablet	Barrel, Compressed	Merck & Company
MSD; 714; VASOTEC	Vasotec	20 mg	Peach	Tablet	Barrel, Compressed	Merck & Company
MSD; 720; VASERETIC	Vaseretic	10 mg; 25 mg	Rust	Tablet	Capsule-Shape, Squared, Compressed	Merck & Company
MSD; 726; ZOCOR	Zocor	5 mg	Buff	Coated Tablet	Shield-Shape	Merck & Company
MSD; 730; MEVACOR	Mevacor	10 mg	Peach	Tablet	Eight-Sided	Merck & Company
MSD; 731; MEVACOR	Mevacor	20 mg	Light Blue	Tablet	Eight-Sided	Merck & Company
MSD; 732; MEVACOR	Mevacor	40 mg	Green	Tablet	Eight-Sided	Merck & Company
MSD; 735; ZOCOR	Zocor	10 mg	Peach	Coated Tablet	Shield-Shape	Merck & Company
MSD; 740; ZOCOR	Zocor	20 mg	Tan	Coated Tablet	Shield-Shape	Merck & Company
MSD; 749; ZOCOR	Zocor	40 mg	Brick Red	Coated Tablet	Shield-Shape	Merck & Company
MSD; 907	Mintezol	500 mg	White	Tablet, Chewable	Circle, Scored	Merck & Company
MSD; 914	Triavil 2-10	2 mg; 10 mg	Blue	Coated Tablet	Triangle	Merck & Company
MSD; 917	Moduretic	5 mg; 50 mg	Peach	Tablet	Diamond	Merck & Company
MSD; 921	Triavil 2-25	2 mg; 25 mg	Orange	Coated Tablet	Triangle	Merck & Company
MSD; 934	Triavil 4-10	4 mg; 10 mg	Salmon	Coated Tablet	Triangle	Merck & Company
MSD; 935	Aldoril D50	500 mg; 50 mg	White	Coated Tablet	Oval	Merck & Company
MSD; 941	Clinoril	150 mg	Yellow	Tablet	Six-Sided, Compressed	Merck & Company
MSD; 942	Clinoril	200 mg	Yellow	Tablet	Six-Sided, Scored, Compressed	Merck & Company
MSD; 946	Triavil 4-25	4 mg; 25 mg	Yellow	Coated Tablet	Triangle	Merck & Company
MSD; 963	Pepcid	20 mg	Beige	Coated Tablet	U-Shape	Merck & Company
MSD; 964	Pepcid	40 mg	Light Brownish-Orange	Coated Tablet	U-Shape	Merck & Company
MYCOBUTIN; PHARMACIA	Mycobutin	150 mg	Red-Brown	Capsule		Pharmacia & Upjohn
MYL; GAS; 80	Mylanta Gas	80 mg	White or Pink	Tablet, Chewable	Circle, Scored	Johnson & Johnson Merck Consumer Pharmaceuticals
MYL; GAS; 125	Mylanta Gas Maximum Strength	125 mg	White or Pink	Tablet, Chewable	Circle, Scored	Johnson & Johnson Merck Consumer Pharmaceuticals
MYLAN 1560 ;	Extended Phenytoin Sodium	100 mg	Lavender , White	Capsule, Extended Release		Mylan Pharmaceuticals
MYLAN 1650	Nitrofurantoin Macrocrystals	50 mg	Light Brown Opaque	Capsule		Mylan Pharmaceuticals
MYLAN 1700	Nitrofurantoin Macrocrystals	100 mg	Gray Opaque	Capsule		Mylan Pharmaceuticals
MYLAN 7005	Loxapine	5 mg	Olive	Capsule		Mylan Pharmaceuticals
MYLAN 7010	Loxapine	10 mg	Olive, Yellow	Capsule		Mylan Pharmaceuticals
MYLAN 7025	Loxapine	25 mg	Light Green, Olive	Capsule		Mylan Pharmaceuticals
MYLAN 7050	Loxapine	50 mg	Light Blue, Olive	Capsule		Mylan Pharmaceuticals
MYLAN 7065	Propoxyphene Hydrochloride	65 mg	Rose	Capsule		Mylan Pharmaceuticals
MYLAN; 9; 4	Carbidopa and Levodopa	50 mg; 200 mg	Purple	Extended-Release Tablet	Oval, Scored, Biconvex	Mylan Pharmaceuticals
MYLAN; 11; 77	Oxaprozin	600 mg	White	Coated Tablet	Oval, Biconvex, Bevel-Edged, Scored	Mylan Pharmaceuticals
MYLAN; 43	Reserpine and Chlorothiazide	500 mg; 0.125 mg	Peach	Tablet	Circle, Scored	Mylan Pharmaceuticals
MYLAN; 73	Perphenazine and Amitriptyline Hydrochloride	50 mg; 4 mg	Purple	Coated Tablet	Circle, Biconvex, Beveled Edge	Mylan Pharmaceuticals
MYLAN; 88	Carbidopa and Levodopa	25 mg; 100 mg	Purple	Extended-Release Tablet	Oval	Mylan Pharmaceuticals
MYLAN; 101	Tetracycline Hydrochloride	250 mg	Orange and Yellow	Capsule		Mylan Pharmaceuticals
MYLAN; 102	Tetracycline Hydrochloride	500 mg	Black and Yellow	Capsule		Mylan Pharmaceuticals
MYLAN; 106; 250	Erythromycin Stearate	250 mg	Yellow	Coated Tablet	Circle, Biconvex	Mylan Pharmaceuticals
MYLAN; 107; 500	Erythromycin Stearate	500 mg	Yellow	Coated Tablet	Oval, Biconvex	Mylan Pharmaceuticals
MYLAN; 115	Ampicillin Trihydrate	250 mg	Scarlet and Light Gray	Capsule		Mylan Pharmaceuticals
MYLAN; 116	Ampicillin Trihydrate	500 mg	Scarlet and Light Gray	Capsule		Mylan Pharmaceuticals
MYLAN; 131	Propoxyphene Compound	389 mg; 32.4 mg; 65 mg	Red and Grey	Capsule		Mylan Pharmaceuticals
MYLAN; 143	Indomethacin	25 mg	Light Green	Capsule		Mylan Pharmaceuticals
MYLAN; 145	Doxycycline Hyclate	50 mg	Aqua Blue and White	Capsule		Mylan Pharmaceuticals
MYLAN; 147	Indomethacin	50 mg	Light Green	Capsule		Mylan Pharmaceuticals
MYLAN; 148	Doxycycline Hyclate	100 mg	Aqua Blue	Capsule		Mylan Pharmaceuticals
MYLAN; 152	Clonidine Hydrochloride	0.1 mg	White	Tablet	Circle, Scored	Mylan Pharmaceuticals
MYLAN; 155	Acetaminophen and Propoxyphene Napsylate	650 mg; 100 mg	Pink	Coated Tablet	Capsule-Shape	Mylan Pharmaceuticals
MYLAN; 156; 500	Probenecid	500 mg	Yellow	Coated Tablet	Capsule-Shape	Mylan Pharmaceuticals
MYLAN; 162	Chlorothiazide	500 mg	White	Tablet	Circle, Scored, Flat Beveled Edge	Mylan Pharmaceuticals

IMPRINT	BRAND/GENERIC NAME	STRENGTH	COLOR	FORM	SHAPE	MANUFACTURER
MYLAN; 167; 100	Doxycycline Hyclate	100 mg	Beige	Coated Tablet	Circle, Biconvex, Beveled Edge	Mylan Pharmaceuticals
MYLAN; 182; 10	Propranolol Hydrochloride	10 mg	Orange	Tablet	Circle, Scored, Flat Beveled Edge	Mylan Pharmaceuticals
MYLAN; 183; 20	Propranolol Hydrochloride	20 mg	Blue	Tablet	Circle, Scored, Flat Beveled Edge	Mylan Pharmaceuticals
MYLAN; 184; 40	Propranolol Hydrochloride	40 mg	Green	Tablet	Circle, Scored, Flat, Beveled Edge	Mylan Pharmaceuticals
MYLAN; 185; 80	Propranolol Hydrochloride	80 mg	Yellow	Tablet	Circle, Scored, Flat Beveled Edge	Mylan Pharmaceuticals
MYLAN; 186	Clonidine Hydrochloride	0.2 mg	White	Tablet	Circle, Scored	Mylan Pharmaceuticals
MYLAN; 197; 100	Chlorpropamide	100 mg	Green	Tablet	Circle, Scored	Mylan Pharmaceuticals
MYLAN; 199	Clonidine Hydrochloride	0.3 mg	White	Tablet	Circle, Scored	Mylan Pharmaceuticals
MYLAN; 204	Amoxicillin Trihydrate	250 mg	Caramel and Buff	Capsule		Mylan Pharmaceuticals
MYLAN; 205	Amoxicillin Trihydrate	500 mg	Buff	Capsule		Mylan Pharmaceuticals
MYLAN; 210; 250	Chlorpropamide	250 mg	Green	Tablet	Circle, Scored	Mylan Pharmaceuticals
MYLAN; 211	Chlordiazepoxide and Amitriptyline Hydrochloride	12.5 mg; 5 mg	Green	Coated Tablet	Circle, Biconvex	Mylan Pharmaceuticals
MYLAN; 214	Haloperidol	2 mg	Orange	Tablet	Circle, Scored	Mylan Pharmaceuticals
MYLAN; 216; 40	Furosemide	40 mg	White	Tablet	Circle, Scored, Flat Beveled Edge	Mylan Pharmaceuticals
MYLAN; 217; 250	Tolazamide	250 mg	White	Tablet	Circle, Scored, Biconvex	Mylan Pharmaceuticals
MYLAN; 232; 80	Furosemide	80 mg	White	Tablet	Circle, Scored, Flat Beveled Edge	Mylan Pharmaceuticals
MYLAN; 237	Etodolac	400 mg	White	Tablet	Oval	Mylan Pharmaceuticals
MYLAN; 242	Etodolac	500 mg	Pink	Coated Tablet	Oval, Biconvex	Mylan Pharmaceuticals
MYLAN; 244	Verapamil Hydrochloride	120 mg	Blue	Extended-Release Tablet	Oval	Mylan Pharmaceuticals
MYLAN; 245	Bumetanide	0.5 mg	Light Green	Tablet	Oval, Scored	Mylan Pharmaceuticals
MYLAN; 251	Trazodone Hydrochloride	50 mg	Clear	Coated Tablet	Circle, Scored, Biconvex, Beveled Edge	Mylan Pharmaceuticals
MYLAN; 252	Trazodone Hydrochloride	100 mg	Clear	Coated Tablet	Circle, Scored, Biconvex, Beveled Edge	Mylan Pharmaceuticals
MYLAN; 257	Haloperidol	1 mg	Orange	Tablet	Circle, Scored	Mylan Pharmaceuticals
MYLAN; 271	Diazepam	2 mg	White	Tablet	Circle, Scored, Flat Beveled Edge	Mylan Pharmaceuticals
MYLAN; 277	Chlordiazepoxide and Amitriptyline Hydrochloride	25 mg; 10 mg	White	Coated Tablet	Circle, Biconvex	Mylan Pharmaceuticals
MYLAN; 327	Haloperidol	5 mg	Orange	Tablet	Circle, Scored	Mylan Pharmaceuticals
MYLAN; 330	Perphenazine and Amitriptyline Hydrochloride	2 mg; 10 mg	White	Coated Tablet	Circle, Biconvex, Beveled Edge	Mylan Pharmaceuticals
MYLAN; 345	Diazepam	5 mg	Orange	Tablet	Circle, Scored, Flat Beveled Edge	Mylan Pharmaceuticals
MYLAN; 347	Propranolol Hydrochloride and Hydrochlorothiazide	80 mg; 25 mg	White	Tablet	Circle, Scored, Biconvex	Mylan Pharmaceuticals
MYLAN; 351	Haloperidol	0.5 mg	Orange	Tablet	Circle, Scored	Mylan Pharmaceuticals
MYLAN; 357	Pentoxifylline	400 mg	Lavender	Sustained-Release Tablet	Capsule-Shape	Mylan Pharmaceuticals
MYLAN; 370	Bumetanide	1 mg	Yellow	Tablet	Oval, Scored	Mylan Pharmaceuticals
MYLAN; 377	Naproxen	250 mg	White	Tablet	Circle	Mylan Pharmaceuticals
MYLAN; 417	Bumetanide	2 mg	Peach	Tablet	Oval, Scored	Mylan Pharmaceuticals
MYLAN; 421	Methyldopa	500 mg	Beige	Coated Tablet	Capsule-Shape, Biconvex, Beveled Edge	Mylan Pharmaceuticals
MYLAN; 427	Sulindac	150 mg	Yellow-Orange	Tablet	Circle, Biconvex	Mylan Pharmaceuticals
MYLAN; 442	Perphenazine and Amitriptyline Hydrochloride	2 mg; 25 mg	Purple	Coated Tablet	Circle, Biconvex, Beveled Edge	Mylan Pharmaceuticals
MYLAN; 451	Naproxen	500 mg	White	Tablet	Capsule-Shape	Mylan Pharmaceuticals
MYLAN; 457	Lorazepam	1 mg	White	Tablet	Circle, Scored	Mylan Pharmaceuticals
MYLAN; 477	Diazepam	10 mg	Green	Tablet	Circle, Scored	Mylan Pharmaceuticals
MYLAN; 507	Methyldopa and Hydrochlorothiazide	250 mg; 15 mg	Green	Coated Tablet	Circle, Biconvex, Beveled Edge	Mylan Pharmaceuticals
MYLAN; 512	Verapamil Hydrochloride	80 mg	White	Tablet	Circle	Mylan Pharmaceuticals
MYLAN; 517	Gemfibrozil	600 mg	White	Coated Tablet	Oval, Partially Scored	Mylan Pharmaceuticals
MYLAN; 521	Acetaminophen and Propoxyphene Napsylate	650 mg; 100 mg	White	Coated Tablet	Capsule-Shape, Biconvex, Beveled Edge	Mylan Pharmaceuticals
MYLAN; 531	Sulindac	200 mg	Yellow-Orange	Tablet	Circle, Scored, Biconvex	Mylan Pharmaceuticals
MYLAN; 551	Tolazamide	500 mg	White	Tablet	Circle, Scored, Biconvex	Mylan Pharmaceuticals
MYLAN; 555	Naproxen	375 mg	White	Tablet	Capsule-Shape	Mylan Pharmaceuticals
MYLAN; 574	Perphenazine and Amitriptyline Hydrochloride	25 mg; 4 mg	Orange	Coated Tablet	Circle, Biconvex, Beveled Edge	Mylan Pharmaceuticals
MYLAN; 611	Methyldopa	250 mg	Beige	Coated Tablet	Circle, Biconvex, Beveled Edge	Mylan Pharmaceuticals
MYLAN; 711	Methyldopa and Hydrochlorothiazide	250 mg; 25 mg	Green	Coated Tablet	Capsule-Shape, Biconvex	Mylan Pharmaceuticals
MYLAN; 727	Perphenazine and Amitriptyline Hydrochloride	4 mg; 10 mg	Blue	Coated Tablet	Circle, Biconvex, Beveled Edge	Mylan Pharmaceuticals
MYLAN; 731	Propranolol Hydrochloride and Hydrochlorothiazide	40 mg; 25 mg	White	Tablet	Circle, Scored, Biconvex	Mylan Pharmaceuticals
MYLAN; 733	Naproxen Sodium	550 mg	Light Blue	Coated Tablet	Oval, Modified	Mylan Pharmaceuticals
MYLAN; 772	Verapamil Hydrochloride	120 mg	White	Coated Tablet	Circle, Scored	Mylan Pharmaceuticals
MYLAN; 777	Lorazepam	2 mg	White	Tablet	Circle, Scored	Mylan Pharmaceuticals
MYLAN; 810	Hydrochlorothiazide	12.5 mg	White	Capsule		Mylan Pharmaceuticals
MYLAN; 1001	Thiothixene	1 mg	Tan and Blue	Capsule		Mylan Pharmaceuticals
MYLAN; 1010	Piroxicam	10 mg	Green and Olive	Capsule		Mylan Pharmaceuticals
MYLAN; 1020	Nicardipine Hydrochloride	20 mg	Opaque Blue-Green and Yellow	Capsule		Mylan Pharmaceuticals
MYLAN; 1049	Doxepin Hydrochloride	10 mg	Buff	Capsule		Mylan Pharmaceuticals
MYLAN; 1101	Prazosin Hydrochloride	1 mg	Green and Brown	Capsule		Mylan Pharmaceuticals
MYLAN; 1155	Acetaminophen and Propoxyphene Napsylate	100 mg; 650 mg	White	Tablet	Capsule-Shape	Mylan Pharmaceuticals
MYLAN; 1155	Acetaminophen and Propoxyphene Napsylate	650 mg; 100 mg	White	Tablet	Capsule-Shape, Biconvex, Beveled Edge	Mylan Pharmaceuticals
MYLAN; 1200	Acebutolol Hydrochloride	200 mg	Medium Orange Opaque	Capsule		Mylan Pharmaceuticals
MYLAN; 1204	Amoxicillin	250 mg	Yellow	Capsule		Mylan Pharmaceuticals
MYLAN; 1205	Amoxicillin	500 mg	Yellow	Capsule		Mylan Pharmaceuticals
MYLAN; 1400	Acebutolol Hydrochloride	400 mg	Medium Orange Opaque	Capsule		Mylan Pharmaceuticals
MYLAN; 1401	Ibuprofen	400 mg	White	Coated Tablet	Circle	Mylan Pharmaceuticals
MYLAN; 1401 ;	Ibuprofen	400 mg	White	Coated Tablet	Circle, Biconvex, Beveled Edge	Mylan Pharmaceuticals
MYLAN; 1410	Nortriptyline Hydrochloride	10 mg	Opaque Swedish Orange	Capsule		Mylan Pharmaceuticals

IMPRINT	BRAND/GENERIC NAME	STRENGTH	COLOR	FORM	SHAPE	MANUFACTURER
MYLAN; 1430	Nicardipine Hydrochloride	30 mg	Opaque Blue-Green and Yellow	Capsule		Mylan Pharmaceuticals
MYLAN; 1570	Terazosin Hydrochloride	10 mg	Lavender	Capsule		Mylan Pharmaceuticals
MYLAN; 1601	Ibuprofen	600 mg	White	Coated Tablet	Oval	Mylan Pharmaceuticals
MYLAN; 1601 ;	Ibuprofen	600 mg	White	Coated Tablet	Capsule-Shape, Biconvex, Beveled Edge	Mylan Pharmaceuticals
MYLAN; 1610	Dicyclomine Hydrochloride	10 mg	Light Turquoise Blue	Capsule		Mylan Pharmaceuticals
MYLAN; 1801	Ibuprofen	800 mg	White	Coated Tablet	Capsule-Shape	Mylan Pharmaceuticals
MYLAN; 1801 ;	Ibuprofen	800 mg	White	Coated Tablet	Oval, Biconvex, Beveled Edge	Mylan Pharmaceuticals
MYLAN; 2002	Thiothixene	2 mg	Tan and Yellow	Capsule		Mylan Pharmaceuticals
MYLAN; 2020	Piroxicam	20 mg	Green	Capsule		Mylan Pharmaceuticals
MYLAN; 2100	Loperamide Hydrochloride	2 mg	Brown	Capsule		Mylan Pharmaceuticals
MYLAN; 2115	Ampicillin	250 mg	White Opaque	Capsule		Mylan Pharmaceuticals
MYLAN; 2116	Ampicillin	500 mg	White	Capsule		Mylan Pharmaceuticals
MYLAN; 2150	Meclofenamate Sodium	50 mg	Coral	Capsule		Mylan Pharmaceuticals
MYLAN; 2200	Acyclovir	200 mg	Purple	Capsule		Mylan Pharmaceuticals
MYLAN; 2252	Selegiline Hydrochloride	5 mg	Light Blue Opaque and Aqua Blue	Capsule		Mylan Pharmaceuticals
MYLAN; 2260	Terazosin Hydrochloride	1 mg	Rich Yellow and Light Lavender	Capsule		Mylan Pharmaceuticals
MYLAN; 2264	Terazosin Hydrochloride	2 mg	Black and Light Lavender	Capsule		Mylan Pharmaceuticals
MYLAN; 2268	Terazosin Hydrochloride	5 mg	Gray and Lavender	Capsule		Mylan Pharmaceuticals
MYLAN; 2302	Prazosin Hydrochloride	2 mg	Brown	Capsule		Mylan Pharmaceuticals
MYLAN; 2325	Nortriptyline Hydrochloride	25 mg	Opaque Orange and Opaque Swedish Orange	Capsule		Mylan Pharmaceuticals
MYLAN; 2537	Triamterene and Hydrochlorothiazide	25 mg; 37.5 mg	Olive and Yellow	Capsule		Mylan Pharmaceuticals
MYLAN; 3000	Meclofenamate Sodium	100 mg	Coral and White	Capsule		Mylan Pharmaceuticals
MYLAN; 3005	Thiothixene	5 mg	Tan and White	Capsule		Mylan Pharmaceuticals
MYLAN; 3025	Clomipramine Hydrochloride	25 mg	Orange and Flesh	Capsule		Mylan Pharmaceuticals
MYLAN; 3050	Clomipramine Hydrochloride	50 mg	Yellow and Flesh	Capsule		Mylan Pharmaceuticals
MYLAN; 3075	Clomipramine Hydrochloride	75 mg	Orange and Flesh	Capsule		Mylan Pharmaceuticals
MYLAN; 3125	Doxepin Hydrochloride	25 mg	Ivory and White	Capsule		Mylan Pharmaceuticals
MYLAN; 3205	Prazosin Hydrochloride	5 mg	Blue and Brown	Capsule		Mylan Pharmaceuticals
MYLAN; 3250	Nortriptyline Hydrochloride	50 mg	Opaque Yellow and Opaque Swedish Orange	Capsule		Mylan Pharmaceuticals
MYLAN; 3422	Nitrofurantoin Monohydrate/macrocrystals	25 mg; 75 mg	Light Gray and Light Brown	Capsule		Mylan Pharmaceuticals
MYLAN; 4010	Temazepam	15 mg	Peach	Capsule		Mylan Pharmaceuticals
MYLAN; 4070	Ketoprofen	50 mg	Light Green	Capsule		Mylan Pharmaceuticals
MYLAN; 4175	Nortriptyline Hydrochloride	75 mg	Brown and Orange	Capsule		Mylan Pharmaceuticals
MYLAN; 4210	Fluoxetine Hydrochloride	10 mg	White and Flesh	Capsule		Mylan Pharmaceuticals
MYLAN; 4220	Fluoxetine Hydrochloride	20 mg	Turquoise and Flesh	Capsule		Mylan Pharmaceuticals
MYLAN; 4250	Doxepin Hydrochloride	50 mg	Ivory	Capsule		Mylan Pharmaceuticals
MYLAN; 4415	Flurazepam Hydrochloride	15 mg	White and Blue	Capsule		Mylan Pharmaceuticals
MYLAN; 4430	Flurazepam Hydrochloride	30 mg	Blue	Capsule		Mylan Pharmaceuticals
MYLAN; 4700	Gemfibrozil	300 mg	Swedish Orange and White	Capsule		Mylan Pharmaceuticals
MYLAN; 5010	Thiothixene	10 mg	Tan and Peach	Capsule		Mylan Pharmaceuticals
MYLAN; 5050	Temazepam	30 mg	Yellow	Capsule		Mylan Pharmaceuticals
MYLAN; 5200	Tolmetin Sodium	400 mg	Light Blue	Capsule		Mylan Pharmaceuticals
MYLAN; 5211	Omeprazole	10 mg	Dark Green	Delayed-Release Capsule		Mylan Pharmaceuticals
MYLAN; 5220	Diltiazem Hydrochloride	120 mg	Light Pink and Flesh	Extended-Release Capsule		Mylan Pharmaceuticals
MYLAN; 5280	Diltiazem Hydrochloride	180 mg	Lavender and Flesh	Extended-Release Capsule		Mylan Pharmaceuticals
MYLAN; 5340	Diltiazem Hydrochloride	240 mg	Light Blue and Flesh	Extended-Release Capsule		Mylan Pharmaceuticals
MYLAN; 5375	Doxepin Hydrochloride	75 mg	Brite Light Green	Capsule		Mylan Pharmaceuticals
MYLAN; 5750	Ketoprofen	75 mg		Capsule		Mylan Pharmaceuticals
MYLAN; 6025	Cephalexin	250 mg	Dark Blue and Opaque White	Capsule		Mylan Pharmaceuticals
MYLAN; 6050	Cephalexin	500 mg	Dark Blue and Light Blue	Capsule		Mylan Pharmaceuticals
MYLAN; 6060	Diltiazem Hydrochloride	60 mg	Coral and White	Extended-Release Capsule		Mylan Pharmaceuticals
MYLAN; 6090	Diltiazem Hydrochloride	90 mg	Coral and Ivory	Extended-Release Capsule		Mylan Pharmaceuticals
MYLAN; 6120	Diltiazem Hydrochloride	120 mg	Coral	Extended-Release Capsule		Mylan Pharmaceuticals
MYLAN; 6150	Omeprazole	20 mg	Dark Green and Blue Green	Delayed-Release Capsule		Mylan Pharmaceuticals
MYLAN; 6320	Verapamil Hydrochloride	120 mg	Blue-Green and White	Extended-Release Capsule		Mylan Pharmaceuticals
MYLAN; 6380	Verapamil Hydrochloride	180 mg	Blue-Green and Light Green	Extended-Release Capsule		Mylan Pharmaceuticals
MYLAN; 6410	Doxepin Hydrochloride	100 mg	Bright Light Green and White	Capsule		Mylan Pharmaceuticals
MYLAN; 6440	Verapamil Hydrochloride	240 mg	Blue-Green	Extended-Release Capsule		Mylan Pharmaceuticals
MYLAN; 7200	Etodolac	200 mg	Brown Opaque	Capsule		Mylan Pharmaceuticals
MYLAN; 7233	Etodolac	300 mg	Light Brown Opaque	Capsule		Mylan Pharmaceuticals
MYLAN; 7250	Cefaclor	250 mg	Pink and White	Capsule		Mylan Pharmaceuticals
MYLAN; 7500	Cefaclor	500 mg	Pink and Grey	Capsule		Mylan Pharmaceuticals
MYLAN; A	Alprazolam	0.25 mg	White	Tablet	Circle, Scored	Mylan Pharmaceuticals

IMPRINT	BRAND/GENERIC NAME	STRENGTH	COLOR	FORM	SHAPE	MANUFACTURER
MYLAN; A1	Alprazolam	1 mg	Blue	Tablet	Circle	Mylan Pharmaceuticals
MYLAN; A3	Alprazolam	0.5 mg	Peach	Tablet	Circle	Mylan Pharmaceuticals
MYLAN; A4	Alprazolam	2 mg	White	Tablet	Circle	Mylan Pharmaceuticals
MYLAN; G1	Glipizide	5 mg	White	Tablet	Circle, Scored, Biconvex	Mylan Pharmaceuticals
MYLAN; G2	Glipizide	10 mg	White	Tablet	Circle, Scored, Biconvex	Mylan Pharmaceuticals
MYLAN; TH; 2	Triamterene and Hydrochlorothiazide	50 mg; 75 mg	Yellow	Tablet	Circle, Scored	Mylan Pharmaceuticals
MYLANTA DS	Mylanta Double Strength	700 mg; 300 mg	Red or Green	Tablet, Chewable		Johnson & Johnson Merck
MYLANTA; GELCAP	Mylanta Gelcaps	550 mg; 125 mg	Light Blue and White	Capsule, Liquid Filled		Johnson & Johnson Merck Consumer Pharmaceuticals
MYLICON; 125	Mylicon 125	125 mg	Pink	Tablet, Chewable		Johnson & Johnson Merck
N; 1.5; 034	Glyburide	1.5 mg		Tablet		Teva Pharmaceuticals
N; 3	Nitrostat	0.3 mg	White	Tablet	Circle, Flat-Faced	Parke-Davis
N; 3; 035	Glyburide	3 mg	Pale Blue	Tablet	Oval, Scored	Teva Pharmaceuticals
N; 4	Nitrostat	0.4 mg	White	Tablet	Circle, Flat-Faced	Parke-Davis
N; 6	Nitrostat	0.6 mg	White	Tablet	Circle, Flat-Faced	Parke-Davis
N; 126; 0.25	Alprazolam	0.25 mg	White	Tablet	Circle, Scored	Warner Chilcott
N; 127; 0.5	Alprazolam	0.5 mg	Orange	Tablet	Circle, Scored	Warner Chilcott
N; 131; 1.0	Alprazolam	1 mg	Blue	Tablet	Circle, Scored	Warner Chilcott
N; 132; 12.5	Captopril	12.5 mg	White	Tablet	Oval, Scored	Teva Pharmaceuticals
N; 134; 50	Captopril	50 mg	White	Tablet	Oval, Scored	Teva Pharmaceuticals
N; 135; 100	Captopril	100 mg	White	Tablet	Oval, Scored	Teva Pharmaceuticals
N; 171; 10	Nifedipine	10 mg	Brown	Capsule		Teva Pharmaceuticals
N; 181; 200	Cimetidine	200 mg	Green	Coated Tablet	Oval	Teva Pharmaceuticals
N; 192; 300	Cimetidine	300 mg	Green	Coated Tablet	Oval	Teva Pharmaceuticals
N; 204; 400	Cimetidine	400 mg	Green	Coated Tablet	Oval, Scored	Teva Pharmaceuticals
N; 235; 800	Cimetidine	800 mg	Green	Coated Tablet	Oval, Scored	Teva Pharmaceuticals
N; 240; 67	Fenofibrate	67 mg	Pink	Capsule		Teva Pharmaceuticals
N; 342; 1.25	Glyburide	1.25 mg	White	Tablet	Circle, Scored	Teva Pharmaceuticals
N; 343; 2.5	Glyburide	2.5 mg	Peach	Tablet	Circle, Scored	Teva Pharmaceuticals
N; 344; 5	Glyburide	5 mg	Light Green	Tablet	Circle, Scored	Teva Pharmaceuticals
N; 397; 300	Etodolac	300 mg	Red	Capsule		Teva Pharmaceuticals
N; 411; 134	Fenofibrate	134 mg	Light Blue	Capsule		Teva Pharmaceuticals
N; 412; 200	Fenofibrate	200 mg	Orange	Capsule		Teva Pharmaceuticals
N; 544; 150	Ranitidine Hydrochloride	150 mg	White	Tablet	Circle	Teva Pharmaceuticals
N; 547; 300	Ranitidine Hydrochloride	300 mg	White	Tablet	Capsule-Shape	Teva Pharmaceuticals
N; 590; 1	Doxazosin Mesylate	1 mg	White to Off-White	Tablet	Circle, Scored	Teva Pharmaceuticals
N; 593; 2	Doxazosin Mesylate	2 mg	White to Off-White	Tablet	Capsule-Shape	Teva Pharmaceuticals
N; 596; 4	Doxazosin Mesylate	4 mg	White to Off-White	Tablet	Diamond, Scored	Teva Pharmaceuticals
N; 598; 8	Doxazosin Mesylate	8 mg	White to Off-White	Tablet	Circle	Teva Pharmaceuticals
N; 739; 150	Mexiletine Hydrochloride	150 mg	Light Orange and Tan	Capsule		Teva Pharmaceuticals
N; 740; 200	Mexiletine Hydrochloride	200 mg	Light Orange	Capsule		Teva Pharmaceuticals
N; 741; 250	Mexiletine Hydrochloride	250 mg	Light Orange and Dark Green	Capsule		Teva Pharmaceuticals
N; 815; 400	Tolmetin Sodium	400 mg	Red	Capsule		Teva Pharmaceuticals
N; 894; 150	Nizatidine	150 mg	Tan and White	Capsule		Teva Pharmaceuticals
N; 899; 300	Nizatidine	300 mg	Tan	Capsule		Teva Pharmaceuticals
N; 940; 200	Acyclovir	200 mg		Capsule		Teva Pharmaceuticals
N; 943; 400	Acyclovir	400 mg		Tablet		Teva Pharmaceuticals
N; 947; 800	Acyclovir	800 mg		Tablet		Teva Pharmaceuticals
N5; LL	Nilstat	500,000 units	Pink	Coated Tablet	Circle, Convex	Lederle Laboratories
NAPROSYN; 250; ROCHE ;	Naprosyn	250 mg	Yellow	Tablet	Circle, Biconvex	Roche Laboratories
NAPROSYN; 375 ;	Naprosyn	375 mg	Peach	Tablet	Capsule-Shape	Roche Laboratories
NAPROSYN; 500 ;	Naprosyn	500 mg	Yellow	Tablet	Capsule-Shape	Roche Laboratories
NATAFORT	Natafort	1000 IU; 400 IU; 11 IU; 120 mg; 1 mg; 2 mg; 3 mg; 20 mg; 10 mg; 12 mcg; 60 mg	White	Coated Tablet		Warner Chilcott
N-BACK	Nuprin Backache	500 mg	White	Tablet	Capsule-Shape	Bristol-Myers Squibb
ND; A ;	Janimine	10 mg	Orange	Coated Tablet		Abbott Laboratories
ND; SCF	Contac Severe Cold & Flu Non-Drowsy Formula	325 mg; 30 mg; 15 mg	White	Tablet		Glaxosmithkline Consumer
NE 2	Actonel with Calcium (Calcium Carbonate Tablets)	1250 mg	Light Blue	Tablet	Oval	Procter & Gamble
NE; 406	Didronel	400 mg	White	Tablet	Capsule-Shape, Scored	Procter & Gamble Pharmaceuticals
NE; A ;	Janimine	25 mg	Yellow	Coated Tablet		Abbott Laboratories
NEORAL; 25 MG	Neoral	25 mg	Blue-Gray	Capsule, Liquid Filled	Oval	Novartis
NEORAL; 100 MG	Neoral	100 mg	Blue-Gray	Capsule, Liquid Filled	Oblong	Novartis
NEO-SYNEPHRINOL	Neo-Synephrinol	120 mg	Clear with White Pellets	Capsule		Sanofi Winthrop
NICOTINE; 7 MG/ DAY	Nicotine Transdermal System	7 mg/24 Hours	Tan, Opaque	Patch	Square, Round Edges	Watson Laboratories
NICOTINE 14 MG/ DAY	Nicotine Transdermal System	14 mg/24 Hr	Opaque Tan	Patch, Extended Release	Square	Watson Laboratories
NICOTINE; 21 MG/ DAY	Nicotine Transdermal System	21 mg/24 Hours	Tan, Opaque	Patch	Square, Round Edges	Watson Laboratories
NIMOTOP	Nimotop	30 mg	Ivory	Capsule, Liquid Filled		Bayer Pharmaceutical
NL 750	Isoxsuprine Hydrochloride	10 mg	White	Tablet	Circle	Alphagen Laboratories
NL 751	Isoxsuprine Hydrochloride	20 mg	White	Tablet	Circle	Alphagen Laboratories
NL; A ;	Janimine	50 mg	Peach	Coated Tablet		Abbott Laboratories
NM	K-Tab	10 meq	Yellow	Extended-Release Tablet		Abbott Laboratories
NMI	Fe50	50 mg	Off White	Tablet		Ucb Pharma
NO DOZ	NO Doz	100 mg	White	Tablet	Circle	Bristol-Myers Squibb
NO DOZ	NO Doz Maximum Strength	200 mg	White	Tablet	Capsule-Shape	Bristol-Myers Squibb
NO DOZ; CHEW	NO Doz	100 mg	White	Tablet, Chewable		Bristol-Myers Squibb
NOLUDAR	Noludar	300 mg	Amethyst and White	Capsule		Roche Laboratories

IMPRINT	BRAND/GENERIC NAME	STRENGTH	COLOR	FORM	SHAPE	MANUFACTURER
NORCO; 539	Norco 10/325	10 mg; 325 mg	Yellow	Tablet	Capsule-Shape, Scored	Watson Laboratories
NORCO; 729	Norco 7.5/325	7.5 mg; 325 mg	Light Orange	Tablet	Capsule-Shape, Scored	Watson Laboratories
NORGESIC; 3M	Norgesic	25 mg; 385 mg; 30 mg	Light Green, White and Yellow	Tablet	Circle, Three-Layered	3M Pharmaceuticals
NORGESIC; FORTE; 3M	Norgesic Forte	770 mg; 60 mg; 50 mg	Light Green, White and Yellow	Tablet	Capsule-Shape, Three-Layered	3M Pharmaceuticals
NORMOZIDE; 227	Normozide	200 mg; 25 mg	White	Coated Tablet	Capsule-Shape, Scored	Schering
NORMOZIDE; 235	Normozide	100 mg; 25 mg	Light Brown	Coated Tablet	Capsule-Shape, Scored	Schering
NORMOZIDE; 391 ;	Normozide	300 mg; 25 mg	Blue	Coated Tablet	Capsule-Shape, Scored	Schering
NORPRAMIN; 25 ;	Norpramin	25 mg	Yellow	Tablet		Sanofi-Aventis U.S.
NORPRAMIN; 50 ;	Norpramin	50 mg	Green	Tablet		Sanofi-Aventis U.S.
NORPRAMIN; 75 ;	Norpramin	75 mg	Orange	Tablet		Sanofi-Aventis U.S.
NORPRAMIN; 100 ;	Norpramin	100 mg	Peach	Tablet		Sanofi-Aventis U.S.
NORPRAMIN; 150 ;	Norpramin	150 mg	White	Tablet		Sanofi-Aventis U.S.
NORTRIPTYLINE; DAN; 10 MG	Nortriptyline Hydrochloride	10 mg	Opaque Deep Green and Opaque White	Capsule		Watson Laboratories
NORTRIPTYLINE; DAN; 25 MG	Nortriptyline Hydrochloride	25 mg	Opaque Deep Green and Opaque White	Capsule		Watson Laboratories
NORTRIPTYLINE; DAN; 50 MG	Nortriptyline Hydrochloride	50 mg	Opaque White	Capsule		Watson Laboratories
NORTRIPTYLINE; DAN; 75 MG	Nortriptyline Hydrochloride	75 mg	Opaque Deep Green	Capsule		Watson Laboratories
NORVASC; 2.5 ;	Norvasc	2.5 mg	White	Tablet	Diamond-Shaped, Flat-Faced, Beveled Edge	Pfizer
NORVASC; 5 ;	Norvasc	5 mg	White	Tablet	Eight-Sided, Elongated, Flat-Aced, Beveled Edge	Pfizer
NORVASC; 10 ;	Norvasc	10 mg	White	Tablet	Circle, Flat-Faced, Beveled Edge	Pfizer
NOVAFED A ;	Novafed A	120 mg; 8 mg	Red and Orange	Extended-Release Capsule	Capsule-Shape, Red Opaque with Orange Transparent Body	Aventis Pharmaceuticals
NOVAFED; 104	Novafed	120 mg	Orange and Brown	Controlled-Release Capsule	Capsule-Shape	Aventis Pharmaceuticals
NOVO NORDISK LOGO	Prandin	1 mg	Yellow	Tablet	Biconvex	Novo Nordisk
NOVO NORDISK LOGO (BULL)	Prandin	0.5 mg	White	Tablet	Biconvex	Novo Nordisk
NOVO NORDISK LOGO (BULL)	Prandin	2 mg	Peach	Tablet	Biconvex	Novo Nordisk
NOVO; 288; APIS BULL LOGO	Activella	1 mg; 0.5 mg	White	Coated Tablet	Circle, BI-Convex	Pharmacia & Upjohn
NPR LE 375	Prevacid Naprapac 375 - Naprosyn	375 mg	Pink	Tablet	Oval	Tap Pharmaceuticals
NPR LE 500	Prevacid Naprapac 500 - Naprosyn	500 mg	Yellow	Tablet	Capsule-Shape	Tap Pharmaceuticals
NPR; LE; 375	Naprosyn	375 mg	Pink	Tablet	Oval	Roche Laboratories
NT 26 ;	Neurontin	800 mg	White	Coated Tablet	Oval	Parke-Davis
NT; 16 ;	Neurontin	600 mg	White	Coated Tablet	Circle	Parke-Davis
NUPRIN	Nuprin	200 mg	Yellow	Tablet	Capsule-Shape	Bristol-Myers Squibb
NUPRIN; 200	Nuprin	200 mg	Yellow	Tablet	Circle	Bristol-Myers Squibb
NVR R20	Ritalin LA	20 mg	White	Capsule, Extended Release		Novartis Pharmaceuticals
NVR ; CTI	Diovan HCT	25 mg; 320 mg	Yellow	Tablet	Oval	Novartis Pharmaceuticals
NVR ; DO	Diovan	40 mg	Yellow	Tablet	Oval	Novartis
NVR ; DV	Diovan	80 mg	Pale Red	Tablet	Teardrop-Shape	Novartis
NVR ; DX	Diovan	160 mg	Grey-Orange	Tablet	Teardrop-Shape	Novartis
NVR ; DXL	Diovan	320 mg	Dark Grey-Violet	Tablet	Teardrop-Shape	Novartis
NVR ; HIL	Diovan HCT	12.5 mg; 320 mg	Pink	Tablet	Oval	Novartis Pharmaceuticals
NVR ; HXH	Diovan HCT	25 mg; 160 mg	Brown Orange	Tablet	Oval	Novartis Pharmaceuticals
NVR D10	Focalin Xr	10 mg	Light Caramel	Capsule, Extended Release		Novartis Pharmaceuticals
NVR D15	Focalin Xr	15 mg	Green	Capsule, Extended Release		Novartis Pharmaceuticals
NVR D20	Focalin Xr	20 mg	White	Capsule, Extended Release		Novartis Pharmaceuticals
NVR R10	Ritalin LA	10 mg	Light Brown, White	Capsule, Extended Release		Novartis Pharmaceuticals
NVR R30	Ritalin LA	30 mg	Yellow	Capsule, Extended Release		Novartis Pharmaceuticals
NVR R40	Ritalin LA	40 mg	Light Brown	Capsule, Extended Release		Novartis Pharmaceuticals
NVR SI	Gleevec	100 mg	Orange with Red Ink	Capsule		Novartis
NVR; DL	Zelnorm	2 mg	White to Yellow Marbled	Tablet	Circle, Flat	Novartis
NVR; EH	Zelnorm	6 mg	White to Yellow Marbled	Tablet	Circle, Flat	Novartis
NVR; EH	Zelnorm	6 mg	White to Yellow Marbled	Tablet	Circle, Flat	Novartis Pharmaceuticals
NVR; SA	Gleevec	100 mg	Dark Yellow to Brownish Orange	Tablet	Circle, Scored	Novartis
NVR; SL	Gleevec	400 mg	Dark Yellow to Brownish Orange	Tablet	Oval	Novartis
NYQUIL	Vicks Nyquil Multi-Symptom Cold/flu Relief	250 mg; 10 mg; 30 mg; 6.25 mg	Transparent Green	Capsule, Liquid Filled		Procter & Gamble
NZ; 150; G	Nizatidine	150 mg	Light Yellow and Dark Yellow	Capsule		Par Pharmaceutical
NZ; 300; G	Nizatidine	300 mg	Light Brown	Capsule		Par Pharmaceutical
OC; 10	Oxycontin	10 mg	White	Controlled-Release Tablet	Circle, Convex	Purdue
OC; 20	Oxycontin	20 mg	Pink	Controlled-Release Tablet	Circle, Convex	Purdue

IMPRINT	BRAND/GENERIC NAME	STRENGTH	COLOR	FORM	SHAPE	MANUFACTURER
OC; 40	Oxycontin	40 mg	Yellow	Controlled-Release Tablet	Circle, Convex	Purdue
OC; 80	Oxycontin	80 mg	Green	Controlled-Release Tablet	Circle, Convex	Purdue
OC; 160	Oxycontin	160 mg	Blue	Controlled-Release Tablet	Capsule-Shape, Convex	Purdue
O-IR; PF5MG	Oxyir	5 mg	Beige and Orange	Capsule		Purdue Pharmaceutical Products
O-M; 180	Ortho Tri-Cyclen Lo White Tablet	0.18 mg; 0.025 mg	White	28-Day Tablet Pack	Circle	Ortho-Mcneil Pharmaceutical
O-M; 215	Ortho Tri-Cyclen Lo Light Blue Tablet	0.215 mg; 0.025 mg	Light Blue	28-Day Tablet Pack	Circle	Ortho-Mcneil Pharmaceutical
O-M; 250	Ortho Tri-Cyclen Lo Dark Blue Tablet	0.25 mg; 0.025 mg	Dark Blue	28-Day Tablet Pack	Circle	Ortho-Mcneil Pharmaceutical
O-M; 650	Ultracet	325 mg; 37.5 mg	Light Yellow	Coated Tablet	Capsule-Shape	Ortho-Mcneil Pharmaceutical
OMACOR	Omacor	900 mg	Light Yellow Oil	Capsule, Liquid Filled		Reliant Pharmaceuticals
OME 10 ; OME 10	Omeprazole	10 mg	Opaque Light-Brown	Capsule, Delayed Release		Sandoz
OME 20	Omeprazole	20 mg	Opaque White	Capsule, Delayed Release		Sandoz
OMNICEF	Omnicef	300 mg	Lavender and Turquoise	Capsule		Abbott Laboratories
ONE A DAY	One-A-Day Plus Extra C Adult Formula	5000 IU; 1.5 mg; 1.7 mg; 20 mg; 400 IU; 15 IU; 0.4 mg; 500 mg; 2 mg; 6 mcg		Tablet		Bayer Consumer Care
ONE-A-DAY	One-A-Day Multivitamin Supplement	5,000 units; 400 units; 1.5 mg; 1.7 mg; 20 mg; 15 units; 0.4 mg; 2 mg; 6 mcg; 60 mg	Red	Coated Tablet	Circle	Bayer Consumer Care
ORETIC	Oretic	25 mg	White	Tablet	Circle	Abbott Laboratories
ORETIC	Oretic	50 mg	White	Tablet	Circle, Scored	Abbott Laboratories
ORG; 07	Jenest 28 White Tablet	35 mcg; 0.5 mg	White	28-Day Tablet Pack	Circle	Organon Teknika
ORG; 14	Jenest 28 Peach Tablet	35 mcg; 1 mg	Peach	28-Day Tablet Pack	Circle	Organon Teknika
ORGANON ; TZ5	Remeron	30 mg	Red-Brown	Tablet	Oval	Organon
ORGANON; 388	Cotazyme-S	5,000 USP units; 20,000 USP units; 20,000 USP units		Capsule		Organon
ORGANON; 393	Zymase	12,000 USP units; 24,000 USP units; 24,000 USP units	White and Green	Capsule		Organon
ORGANON; 542	Wigraine	1 mg; 100 mg	White	Tablet	Circle	Organon
ORGANON; 790	Hexadrol	1.5 mg	Peach	Tablet		Organon
ORGANON; 791	Hexadrol	0.75 mg	White	Tablet		Organon
ORGANON; 792	Hexadrol	0.5 mg	Yellow	Tablet		Organon
ORGANON; 798	Hexadrol	4 mg	Green	Tablet		Organon
ORGANON; K2S	Mircette Yellow Tablet	0.01 mg	Yellow	Tablet	Circle	Organon
ORGANON; T4R ;	Mircette White Tablet	0.15 mg; 0.02 mg	White	28-Day Tablet Pack	Circle	Organon
ORGANON; TR5	Desogen White Tablet	0.15 mg; 0.03 mg	White	28-Day Tablet Pack	Circle	Organon
ORGANON; TZ3 ;	Remeron	15 mg	Yellow	Coated Tablet	Oval, Scored	Organon
ORGANON; TZ5 ;	Remeron	30 mg	Red-Brown	Coated Tablet	Oval, Scored	Organon
ORGANON; TZ7	Remeron	45 mg	White	Coated Tablet	Oval	Organon
ORINASE; 250	Orinase	250 mg	White	Tablet	Circle, Scored	Upjohn
ORINASE; 500	Orinase	500 mg	White	Tablet	Circle, Scored	Pharmacia & Upjohn
ORTHO; 0.35	Micronor	0.35 mg	Light Green	28-Day Tablet Pack	Circle	Ortho-Mcneil Pharmaceutical
ORTHO; 0214	Grifulvin V	500 mg	White	Tablet		Ortho-Mcneil Pharmaceutical
ORTHO; 75	Ortho-Novum 7/7/7-21 Light Peach Tablet	35 mcg; 0.75 mg	Light Peach	21-Day Tablet Pack	Circle	Ortho-Mcneil Pharmaceutical
ORTHO; 75	Ortho-Novum 7/7/7-28 Light Peach Tablet	35 mcg; 0.75 mg	Light Peach	28-Day Tablet Pack	Circle	Ortho-Mcneil Pharmaceutical
ORTHO; 135	Ortho-Novum 1/35-21	1 mg; 35 mcg	Peach	21-Day Tablet Pack	Circle	Ortho-Mcneil Pharmaceutical
ORTHO; 135	Ortho-Novum 1/35-28 Peach Tablet	1 mg; 35 mcg	Peach	28-Day Tablet Pack	Circle	Ortho-Mcneil Pharmaceutical
ORTHO; 135	Ortho-Novum 10/11-21 Peach Tablet	1 mg; 35 mcg	Peach	21-Day Tablet Pack	Circle	Ortho-Mcneil Pharmaceutical
ORTHO; 135	Ortho-Novum 10/11-28 Peach Tablet	1 mg; 35 mcg	Peach	28-Day Tablet Pack	Circle	Ortho-Mcneil Pharmaceutical
ORTHO; 135	Ortho-Novum 7/7/7-21 Peach Tablet	1 mg; 35 mcg	Peach	21-Day Tablet Pack	Circle	Ortho-Mcneil Pharmaceutical
ORTHO; 135	Ortho-Novum 7/7/7-28 Peach Tablet	1 mg; 35 mcg	Peach	28-Day Tablet Pack	Circle	Ortho-Mcneil Pharmaceutical
ORTHO; 150	Ortho-Novum 1/50-21	1 mg; 50 mcg	Yellow	21-Day Tablet Pack	Circle	Ortho-Mcneil Pharmaceutical
ORTHO; 150	Ortho-Novum 1/50-28 Yellow Tablet	1 mg; 50 mcg	Yellow	28-Day Tablet Pack	Circle	Ortho-Mcneil Pharmaceutical
ORTHO; 180	Ortho Tri-Cyclen 21 White Tablet	0.18 mg; 0.035 mg	White	21-Day Tablet Pack	Circle	Ortho-Mcneil Pharmaceutical
ORTHO; 180	Ortho Tri-Cyclen 28 White Tablet	0.18 mg; 0.035 mg	White	28-Day Tablet Pack	Circle	Ortho-Mcneil Pharmaceutical
ORTHO; 211	Grifulvin V	250 mg	White	Tablet		Ortho-Mcneil Pharmaceutical
ORTHO; 215	Ortho Tri-Cyclen 21 Light Blue Tablet	0.215 mg; 0.035 mg	Light Blue	21-Day Tablet Pack	Circle	Ortho-Mcneil Pharmaceutical
ORTHO; 215	Ortho Tri-Cyclen 28 Light Blue Tablet	0.215 mg; 0.035 mg	Light Blue	28-Day Tablet Pack	Circle	Ortho-Mcneil Pharmaceutical
ORTHO; 250	Ortho-Cyclen 21	0.25 mg; 0.035 mg	Blue	21-Day Tablet Pack	Circle	Ortho-Mcneil Pharmaceutical

IMPRINT	BRAND/GENERIC NAME	STRENGTH	COLOR	FORM	SHAPE	MANUFACTURER
ORTHO; 250	Ortho-Cyclen 28 Blue Tablet	0.25 mg; 0.035 mg	Blue	28-Day Tablet Pack	Circle	Ortho-Mcneil Pharmaceutical
ORTHO; 250	Ortho Tri-Cyclen 21 Blue Tablet	0.25 mg; 0.035 mg	Blue	21-Day Tablet Pack	Circle	Ortho-Mcneil Pharmaceutical
ORTHO; 250	Ortho Tri-Cyclen 28 Blue Tablet	0.25 mg; 0.035 mg	Blue	28-Day Tablet Pack	Circle	Ortho-Mcneil Pharmaceutical
ORTHO; 535	Ortho-Novum 10/11-21 White Tablet	0.5 mg; 35 mcg	White	21-Day Tablet Pack	Circle	Ortho-Mcneil Pharmaceutical
ORTHO; 535	Ortho-Novum 10/11-28 White Tablet	0.5 mg; 35 mcg	White	28-Day Tablet Pack	Circle	Ortho-Mcneil Pharmaceutical
ORTHO; 535	Modicon 21	0.5 mg; 35 mcg	White	21-Day Tablet Pack	Circle	Ortho-Mcneil Pharmaceutical
ORTHO; 535	Modicon 28 White Tablet	0.5 mg; 35 mcg	White	28-Day Tablet Pack	Circle	Ortho-Mcneil Pharmaceutical
ORTHO; 535	Ortho-Novum 7/7/7-21 White Tablet	0.5 mg; 35 mcg	White	21-Day Tablet Pack	Circle	Ortho-Mcneil Pharmaceutical
ORTHO; 535	Ortho-Novum 7/7/7-28 White Tablet	0.5 mg; 35 mcg	White	28-Day Tablet Pack	Circle	Ortho-Mcneil Pharmaceutical
ORTHO; 1570	Protostat	250 mg	White	Tablet	Capsule-Shape	Ortho-Mcneil Pharmaceutical
ORTHO; 1571	Protostat	500 mg	White	Tablet	Capsule-Shape	Ortho-Mcneil Pharmaceutical
ORTHO; 1800	Ortho-Est	1.5 mg	Lavender	Tablet	Diamond, Scored	Women First Healthcare
ORTHO; 1801	Ortho-Est	0.75 mg	White	Tablet	Diamond, Scored	Women First Healthcare
ORTHO; D; 150	Ortho-Cept 21	0.15 mg; 0.03 mg	Orange	21-Day Tablet Pack	Circle	Ortho-Mcneil Pharmaceutical
ORTHO; D; 150	Ortho-Cept 28 Orange Tablet	0.15 mg; 0.03 mg	Orange	28-Day Tablet Pack	Circle	Ortho-Mcneil Pharmaceutical
ORUDIS; KT	Orudis Kt	12.5 mg	Lime Green	Tablet		Wyeth Consumer Healthcare
ORUVAIL; 100	Oruvail	100 mg	Pink and Dark Green with Two Radial Bands	Capsule		Wyeth Pharmaceuticals
ORUVAIL; 150	Oruvail	150 mg	Pink and Light Green with Two Radial Bands	Capsule		Wyeth Pharmaceuticals
ORUVAIL; 200	Oruvail	200 mg	Pink and White with Two Radial Bands	Capsule		Wyeth Pharmaceuticals
OS CAL	Os-Cal 500	500 mg		Tablet, Chewable		Aventis Pharmaceuticals
OV; 12	Desoxyn	5 mg	White	Tablet		Ovation Pharmaceuticals
OV; 31; T	Tranxene T-Tab	3.75 mg	Blue	Tablet	T-Shaped, Scored	Ovation Pharmaceuticals
OV; 32; T	Tranxene T-Tab	7.5 mg	Peach	Tablet	T-Shaped, Scored	Ovation Pharmaceuticals
OV; 33; T	Tranxene T-Tab	15 mg	Lavender	Tablet	T-Shaped, Scored	Ovation Pharmaceuticals
OV; 44	Tranxene-Sd Half Strength	11.25 mg	Blue	Tablet		Ovation Pharmaceuticals
OV; 45	Tranxene-Sd	22.5 mg	Tan	Extended-Release Tablet		Ovation Pharmaceuticals
OXYROL; 3.9 MG/DAY	Oxytrol	3.9 mg/24 Hours		Patch	Rectangle	Watson Laboratories
P	Children's Pepto - Bubble Gum	400 mg	Pink	Tablet, Chewable		Procter & Gamble
P	Children's Pepto - Watermelon	400 mg	Pink	Tablet, Chewable		Procter & Gamble
P	Panadol Junior	160 mg	White	Tablet	Oval	Bayer Consumer Care
P	Panadol, Children's Aspirin Free	80 mg	Pink	Tablet, Chewable		Bayer Consumer Care
P	Primatene P	130 mg; 24 mg; 8 mg	Yellow	Tablet		Whitehall
P	Senokot S	8.6 mg; 50 mg	Yellow-Orange	Tablet	Circle	Purdue Pharmaceutical Products
P	Senokot S	8.6 mg; 50 mg	Yellow-Orange	Tablet	Circle	
P 771	Diphenoxylate Hydrochloride and Atropine Sulfate	2.5 mg; 0.025 mg	White	Tablet	Circle	Par Pharmaceutical
P&G; 402	Didronel	200 mg	White	Tablet	Rectangle	Procter & Gamble Pharmaceuticals
P; 02	Mercaptopurine	50 mg	Light Yellow	Tablet	Diamond	Par Pharmaceutical
P; 054	Peri-Colace	50 mg; 8.6 mg	Dark Red	Tablet	Circle	Purdue Pharmaceutical Products
P; 53; LEDERLE	Ext Phenytoin Sodium	100 mg	Clear	Capsule		Lederle Laboratories
P; 500	Panadol Maximum Strength	500 mg	White	Tablet		Bayer Consumer Care
P; 542	Naproxen Sodium	220 mg	Light Blue	Tablet	Circle	Par Pharmaceutical
P; 543	Naproxen Sodium	220 mg	Blue	Tablet	Oblong	Par Pharmaceutical
P; 771	Atropine and Diphenoxylate Hydrochloride	0.025 mg; 2.5 mg	White	Tablet	Circle	Par Pharmaceutical
P; 4600	Benzonatate	100 mg	Yellow	Capsule, Liquid Filled	Oval	Warner Chilcott
P; PRAVACOL 20; ;	Pravigard Pac	81 mg; 20 mg	Yellow Tablet and White Tablet	Tablet		Bristol-Myers Squibb
P; PRAVACOL 20; ;	Pravigard Pac	325 mg; 20 mg	Yellow Tablet and White Tablet	Tablet		Bristol-Myers Squibb
P; PRAVACOL 40; ;	Pravigard Pac	81 mg; 40 mg	Green Tablet and White Tablet	Tablet		Bristol-Myers Squibb
P; PRAVACOL 40; ;	Pravigard Pac	325 mg; 40 mg	Green Tablet and White Tablet	Tablet		Bristol-Myers Squibb
P; UNDERSCORED	Prilosec Otc	20 mg	Salmon/pink	Tablet	Oval	Procter & Gamble
P; US; 144	Amiodarone Hydrochloride	100 mg	White	Tablet	Circle	Upsher-Smith Laboratories
P2 ; G	Paroxetine Hydrochloride	20 mg	White	Tablet	Circle	Andrx Pharmaceuticals
P2 ; G ;	Paroxetine Hydrochloride	20 mg	White	Tablet	Circle	Andrx Pharmaceuticals
P3 ; G	Paroxetine Hydrochloride	30 mg	White	Tablet	Circle	Andrx Pharmaceuticals
P3 ; G ;	Paroxetine Hydrochloride	30 mg	White	Tablet	Circle	Andrx Pharmaceuticals
P4; LL	Pathilon	25 mg	Pink	Coated Tablet	Circle, Convex	Lederle Laboratories
P5; G	Pindolol	5 mg	White	Tablet	Circle	Par Pharmaceutical
P10; G	Pindolol	10 mg	White	Tablet	Circle	Par Pharmaceutical
P20	Protonix	20 mg	Yellow with Brown Ink	Delayed-Release Tablet	Oval, Biconvex	Wyeth Pharmaceuticals
P46 ;	Amytal Sodium	250 mg/ampule		Solution for Injection		Eli Lilly
PANADOL PLUS	Panadol Plus	500 mg; 65 mg	White	Tablet		Bayer Consumer Care
PANADOL; 500 ;	Panadol Maximum Strength	500 mg	White	Coated Tablet	Circle	Bayer Consumer Care
PANMYCIN; 250 MG	Panmycin	250 mg	Yellow and Gray	Capsule		Upjohn
PAR ; 091	Doxycycline	50 mg	Yellow	Tablet	Circle	Par Pharmaceutical
PAR ; 092	Doxycycline	75 mg	Light Orange	Tablet	Circle	Par Pharmaceutical
PAR ; 093	Doxycycline	100 mg	Yellow	Tablet	Circle	Par Pharmaceutical

IMPRINT	BRAND/GENERIC NAME	STRENGTH	COLOR	FORM	SHAPE	MANUFACTURER
PAR ; 511	Minocycline Hydrochloride	50 mg	White	Tablet	Capsule-Shape	Par Pharmaceutical
PAR ; 512	Minocycline Hydrochloride	75 mg	White	Tablet	Capsule-Shape	Par Pharmaceutical
PAR ; 513	Minocycline Hydrochloride	100 mg	White	Tablet	Capsule-Shape	Par Pharmaceutical
PAR ; 850	Meloxicam	7.5 mg	Off-White to Yellow	Tablet	Circle	Par Pharmaceutical
PAR ; 851	Meloxicam	15 mg	Off-White to Yellow	Tablet	Oval	Par Pharmaceutical
PAR ; 958	Chlordiazepoxide Hydrochloride	5 mg	Opaque Green , Opaque Yellow	Capsule		Par Pharmaceutical
PAR ; 959	Chlordiazepoxide Hydrochloride	10 mg	Opaque Black, Opaque Green	Capsule		Par Pharmaceutical
PAR ; 960	Chlordiazepoxide Hydrochloride	25 mg	Opaque Green , Opaque White	Capsule		Par Pharmaceutical
PAR 256; MINOXIDIL; 2 1/2	Minoxidil	2.5 mg	White	Tablet	Round; Bisected Scored	Par Pharmaceutical
PAR 257; MINOXIDIL 10	Minoxidil	10 mg	White	Tablet	Round; Bisected Scored	Par Pharmaceutical
PAR 845	Glimepiride	1 mg	Pink	Tablet	Rectangle	Par Pharmaceutical
PAR 846	Glimepiride	2 mg	Green	Tablet	Rectangle	Par Pharmaceutical
PAR 847	Glimepiride	4 mg	Blue	Tablet	Rectangle	Par Pharmaceutical
PAR; 009	Isosorbide Dinitrate	30 mg	Blue	Tablet	Circle	Par Pharmaceutical
PAR; 015	Meclizine Hydrochloride	50 mg	Yellow and Blue	Tablet	Oval, Scored; Multiple Layered	Par Pharmaceutical
PAR; 016	Chlorzoxazone	250 mg	Orange	Tablet	Circle, Scored	Par Pharmaceutical
PAR; 020	Isosorbide Dinitrate	5 mg	White	Tablet	Circle, Scored	Par Pharmaceutical
PAR; 021	Isosorbide Dinitrate	10 mg	White	Tablet	Circle, Scored	Par Pharmaceutical
PAR; 022	Isosorbide Dinitrate	20 mg	Green	Tablet	Circle, Scored	Par Pharmaceutical
PAR; 027	Hydralazine Hydrochloride	25 mg	Peach	Tablet	Circle, Convex	Par Pharmaceutical
PAR; 028	Hydralazine Hydrochloride	50 mg	Peach or Blue	Tablet	Round or Oval	Par Pharmaceutical
PAR; 029	Hydralazine Hydrochloride	10 mg	Pink	Tablet	Circle	Par Pharmaceutical
PAR; 034	Meclizine Hydrochloride	12.5 mg	Blue and White	Tablet	Oval	Par Pharmaceutical
PAR; 035	Meclizine Hydrochloride	25 mg	Yellow and White	Tablet	Teardrop-Shape	Par Pharmaceutical
PAR; 043	Cyproheptadine Hydrochloride	4 mg	White	Tablet	Circle, Scored; Compressed	Par Pharmaceutical
PAR; 054	Imipramine Hydrochloride	10 mg	Yellow	Tablet	Triangle	Par Pharmaceutical
PAR; 055	Imipramine Hydrochloride	25 mg	Brown	Tablet	Circle	Par Pharmaceutical
PAR; 056	Imipramine Hydrochloride	50 mg	Green	Coated Tablet		Par Pharmaceutical
PAR; 056	Imipramine Hydrochloride	50 mg	Green	Tablet	Circle	Par Pharmaceutical
PAR; 061	Fluphenazine Hydrochloride	1 mg	White	Coated Tablet	Circle	Par Pharmaceutical
PAR; 062	Fluphenazine Hydrochloride	2.5 mg	Blue	Coated Tablet	Circle	Par Pharmaceutical
PAR; 064	Fluphenazine Hydrochloride	10 mg	Orange	Coated Tablet	Circle	Par Pharmaceutical
PAR; 067	Indomethacin	25 mg	Light Green or White and Blue	Capsule		Par Pharmaceutical
PAR; 068	Indomethacin	50 mg	Light Green or White and Blue	Capsule		Par Pharmaceutical
PAR; 076	Fluphenazine Hydrochloride	5 mg	Dark Pink	Coated Tablet	Circle	Par Pharmaceutical
PAR; 083	Dexamethasone	0.25 mg	Pale Orange	Tablet	Five-Sided, Scored	Par Pharmaceutical
PAR; 084	Dexamethasone	0.5 mg	Pale Yellow	Tablet	Five-Sided, Scored	Par Pharmaceutical
PAR; 085	Dexamethasone	0.75 mg	Pale Blue	Tablet	Five-Sided, Scored	Par Pharmaceutical
PAR; 086	Dexamethasone	1.5 mg	Pale Pink	Tablet	Five-Sided, Scored	Par Pharmaceutical
PAR; 087	Dexamethasone	4 mg	White	Tablet	Five-Sided, Scored	Par Pharmaceutical
PAR; 095	Metronidazole	250 mg	White	Coated Tablet	Circle	Par Pharmaceutical
PAR; 104	Allopurinol	100 mg	White	Tablet	Circle, Flat Bevel	Par Pharmaceutical
PAR; 105	Allopurinol	300 mg	Orange	Tablet	Circle	Par Pharmaceutical
PAR; 110	Clonidine Hydrochloride	0.1 mg	Green	Tablet	Round; Bisected Scored	Par Pharmaceutical
PAR; 111	Clonidine Hydrochloride	0.2 mg	Yellow	Tablet	Round; Bisected Scored	Par Pharmaceutical
PAR; 112	Clonidine Hydrochloride	0.3 mg	Blue	Tablet	Round; Bisected Scored	Par Pharmaceutical
PAR; 113	Clonidine Hydrochloride and Chlorthalidone	15 mg; 0.1 mg	White	Tablet	Round; Flat-Faced; Beveled Edge; Bisected Scored	Par Pharmaceutical
PAR; 114	Metronidazole	500 mg	White	Tablet	Capsule-Shape	Par Pharmaceutical
PAR; 115	Clonidine Hydrochloride and Chlorthalidone	15 mg; 0.2 mg	Blue	Tablet	Circle, Flat-Faced; Beveled Edge	Par Pharmaceutical
PAR; 116	Clonidine Hydrochloride and Chlorthalidone	15 mg; 0.3 mg	White	Tablet	Round; Concave; Bisected Scored	Par Pharmaceutical
PAR; 117	Amiloride Hydrochloride	5 mg	Yellow	Tablet	Circle, Compressed	Par Pharmaceutical
PAR; 118	Propantheline Bromide	15 mg	Light Peach	Tablet	Circle	Par Pharmaceutical
PAR; 119	Nystatin	500,000 units	Brown	Coated Tablet	Circle	Par Pharmaceutical
PAR; 121	Hydralazine Hydrochloride	100 mg	Peach	Tablet	Circle	Par Pharmaceutical
PAR; 129	Dexamethasone	6 mg	Pale Green	Tablet	Five-Sided, Scored	Par Pharmaceutical
PAR; 133	Amitriptyline Hydrochloride	10 mg	Pink	Tablet	Circle	Par Pharmaceutical
PAR; 134	Amitriptyline Hydrochloride	25 mg	Green	Tablet	Circle	Par Pharmaceutical
PAR; 135	Amitriptyline Hydrochloride	50 mg	Brown	Tablet	Circle	Par Pharmaceutical
PAR; 136	Amitriptyline Hydrochloride	75 mg	Purple	Tablet	Circle	Par Pharmaceutical
PAR; 137	Amitriptyline Hydrochloride	100 mg	Orange	Tablet	Circle	Par Pharmaceutical
PAR; 138	Amitriptyline Hydrochloride	150 mg	Peach	Tablet	Circle	Par Pharmaceutical
PAR; 139	Sulfamethoxazole and Trimethoprim	400 mg; 80 mg	White	Tablet		Par Pharmaceutical
PAR; 140	Sulfamethoxazole and Trimethoprim	800 mg; 160 mg	White	Tablet		Par Pharmaceutical
PAR; 143	Hydralazine Hydrochloride and Hydrochlorothiazide	25 mg; 25 mg	White	Capsule		Par Pharmaceutical
PAR; 144	Hydralazine Hydrocloride and Hydrochlorothiazide	50 mg; 50 mg	White and Black	Capsule		Par Pharmaceutical
PAR; 145	Hydralazine Hydrochloride and Hydrochlorothiazide	100 mg; 50 mg	Powder Blue and Light Blue	Capsule		Par Pharmaceutical
PAR; 162; 400	Ibuprofen	400 mg	White	Coated Tablet	Circle	Par Pharmaceutical
PAR; 163; 600	Ibuprofen	600 mg	White	Coated Tablet	Oval	Par Pharmaceutical
PAR; 164	Benztropine Mesylate	0.5 mg	White	Tablet	Circle, Scored	Par Pharmaceutical
PAR; 165	Benztropine Mesylate	1 mg	White	Tablet	Oval, Scored	Par Pharmaceutical
PAR; 166	Benztropine Mesylate	2 mg	White	Tablet	Circle, Scored	Par Pharmaceutical
PAR; 181	Perphenazine and Amitriptyline Hydrochloride	2 mg; 10 mg	Blue	Coated Tablet	Circle	Par Pharmaceutical

IMPRINT	BRAND/GENERIC NAME	STRENGTH	COLOR	FORM	SHAPE	MANUFACTURER
PAR; 182	Perphenazine and Amitriptyline Hydrochloride	2 mg; 25 mg	Orange	Coated Tablet	Circle	Par Pharmaceutical
PAR; 183	Perphenazine and Amitriptyline Hydrochloride	4 mg; 10 mg	Salmon	Coated Tablet	Circle	Par Pharmaceutical
PAR; 184	Perphenazine and Amitriptyline Hydrochloride	4 mg; 25 mg	Yellow	Coated Tablet	Circle	Par Pharmaceutical
PAR; 185	Perphenazine and Amitriptyline Hydrochloride	4 mg; 50 mg	Orange	Coated Tablet	Circle	Par Pharmaceutical
PAR; 186	Methyldopa and Hydrochlorothiazide	250 mg; 15 mg	Green	Coated Tablet	Circle	Par Pharmaceutical
PAR; 187	Methyldopa and Hydrochlorothiazide	250 mg; 25 mg	White	Coated Tablet	Capsule-Shape	Par Pharmaceutical
PAR; 188	Methyldopa and Hydrochlorothiazide	30 mg; 500 mg	Yellow	Coated Tablet	Oval	Par Pharmaceutical
PAR; 189	Methyldopa and Hydrochlorothiazide	50 mg; 500 mg	Pink	Coated Tablet	Oval	Par Pharmaceutical
PAR; 193	Flurazepam Hydrochloride	15 mg	White and Powder Blue	Capsule		Par Pharmaceutical
PAR; 194	Flurazepam Hydrochloride	30 mg	Powder Blue	Capsule		Par Pharmaceutical
PAR; 200; 682	Ofloxacin	200 mg	White	Tablet	Capsule-Shape	Par Pharmaceutical
PAR; 202	Methyldopa and Chlorothiazide	250 mg; 150 mg	Beige	Coated Tablet	Circle	Par Pharmaceutical
PAR; 203	Methyldopa and Chlorothiazide	250 mg; 250 mg	Green	Coated Tablet	Circle	Par Pharmaceutical
PAR; 213	Orphengesic	25 mg; 30 mg; 385 mg	White and Green	Tablet	Circle, Flat; Double Layered	Par Pharmaceutical
PAR; 214	Orphengesic Forte	50 mg; 60 mg; 770 mg	White and Green	Tablet	Capsule-Shaped; Bisected; Double Layered Scored	Par Pharmaceutical
PAR; 216; 800	Ibuprofen	800 mg	White	Coated Tablet	Capsule-Shape	Par Pharmaceutical
PAR; 217	Doxepin Hydrochloride	10 mg	Opaque Buff	Capsule		Par Pharmaceutical
PAR; 218	Doxepin Hydrochloride	25 mg	Opaque Ivory and White	Capsule		Par Pharmaceutical
PAR; 219	Doxepin Hydrochloride	50 mg	Opaque Ivory	Capsule		Par Pharmaceutical
PAR; 220	Doxepin Hydrochloride	75 mg	Bright Light Green	Capsule		Par Pharmaceutical
PAR; 221	Doxepin Hydrochloride	100 mg	White and Bright Light Green	Capsule		Par Pharmaceutical
PAR; 222	Doxepin Hydrochloride	150 mg	Opaque White and Blue	Capsule		Par Pharmaceutical
PAR; 223	Haloperidol	0.5 mg	White	Tablet	Circle, Scored; Flat; Compressed	Par Pharmaceutical
PAR; 224	Haloperidol	1 mg	Yellow	Tablet	Circle, Scored; Flat; Compressed	Par Pharmaceutical
PAR; 225	Haloperidol	2 mg	Pink	Tablet	Circle, Scored; Flat; Compressed	Par Pharmaceutical
PAR; 226	Haloperidol	5 mg	Green	Tablet	Circle, Scored; Flat; Compressed	Par Pharmaceutical
PAR; 227	Haloperidol	10 mg	Aqua	Tablet	Circle, Scored; Flat; Compressed	Par Pharmaceutical
PAR; 240	Temazepam	15 mg	Opaque White and Dark Green	Capsule		Par Pharmaceutical
PAR; 241	Temazepam	30 mg	Opaque White	Capsule		Par Pharmaceutical
PAR; 246	Carisoprodol and Aspirin	325 mg; 200 mg	White and Light Lavender	Tablet	Circle, Double-Layered	Par Pharmaceutical
PAR; 249	Methocarbamol and Aspirin	325 mg; 400 mg	White and Pink	Tablet	Circle, Double Layered; Compressed	Par Pharmaceutical
PAR; 258	Metaproterenol Sulfate	10 mg	White	Tablet	Circle, Scored; Compressed	Par Pharmaceutical
PAR; 259	Metaproterenol Sulfate	20 mg	White	Tablet	Circle, Scored; Compressed	Par Pharmaceutical
PAR; 289	Megestrol Acetate	20 mg	White	Tablet	Round, Bisected Scored	Par Pharmaceutical
PAR; 290	Megestrol Acetate	40 mg	White	Tablet	Round, Bisected Scored	Par Pharmaceutical
PAR; 300; 683	Ofloxacin	300 mg	White	Tablet	Capsule-Shape	Par Pharmaceutical
PAR; 400; 684	Ofloxacin	400 mg	White	Tablet	Capsule-Shape	Par Pharmaceutical
PAR; 412	Metoprolol Tartrate	50 mg	Light Pink	Coated Tablet	Circle	Par Pharmaceutical
PAR; 413	Metoprolol Tartrate	100 mg	Light Blue	Coated Tablet	Circle	Par Pharmaceutical
PAR; 444	Captopril	12.5 mg	White	Tablet	Oval	Par Pharmaceutical
PAR; 445	Captopril	25 mg	White	Tablet	Circle	Par Pharmaceutical
PAR; 446	Captopril	50 mg	White	Tablet	Circle	Par Pharmaceutical
PAR; 447	Captopril	100 mg	White	Tablet	Circle	Par Pharmaceutical
PAR; 448 ;	Alprazolam	0.25 mg	Light Yellow	Tablet	Oval, Scored	Par Pharmaceutical
PAR; 449	Alprazolam	0.5 mg	Dark Yellow	Tablet	Oval	Par Pharmaceutical
PAR; 467	Ibuprofen	400 mg	White	Coated Tablet	Capsule-Shape	Par Pharmaceutical
PAR; 468	Ibuprofen	600 mg	White	Coated Tablet	Capsule-Shape	Par Pharmaceutical
PAR; 473	Orphengesic Forte	100 mg; 60 mg; 770 mg	Blue and White	Tablet	Capsule-Shape, BI-Layered, Scored	Par Pharmaceutical
PAR; 544	Ranitidine Hydrochloride	150 mg		Tablet		Par Pharmaceutical
PAR; 545	Ranitidine Hydrochloride	300 mg		Tablet		Par Pharmaceutical
PAR; 556	Lisinopril	2.5 mg	White	Tablet	Oval	Par Pharmaceutical
PAR; 557	Lisinopril	5 mg	White	Tablet	Capsule-Shape	Par Pharmaceutical
PAR; 558	Lisinopril	10 mg	White	Tablet	Circle	Par Pharmaceutical
PAR; 559	Lisinopril	20 mg	White	Tablet	Circle	Par Pharmaceutical
PAR; 560	Lisinopril	40 mg	White	Tablet	Circle	Par Pharmaceutical
PAR; 635	Lisinopril	30 mg	White	Tablet	Circle	Par Pharmaceutical
PAR; 651; 5	Torsemide	5 mg	White	Tablet	Circle, Scored	Par Pharmaceutical
PAR; 652; 10	Torsemide	10 mg	White	Tablet	Circle, Scored	Par Pharmaceutical
PAR; 653; 20	Torsemide	20 mg	White	Tablet	Circle, Scored	Par Pharmaceutical
PAR; 654; 100	Torsemide	100 mg	White	Tablet	Circle, Scored	Par Pharmaceutical
PAR; 701	Clomiphene Citrate	50 mg	White	Tablet	Circle, Scored	Par Pharmaceutical
PAR; 707; 5	Buspirone Hydrochloride	5 mg	Peach	Tablet	Oval	Par Pharmaceutical
PAR; 708; 10	Buspirone Hydrochloride	10 mg	Peach	Tablet	Oval	Par Pharmaceutical
PAR; 721; 555	Buspirone Hydrochloride	15 mg	Peach	Tablet	Rectangle, Scored	Par Pharmaceutical
PAR; 724	Hydroxyurea	500 mg		Capsule		Par Pharmaceutical
PAR; 725; 7.5	Buspirone Hydrochloride	7.5 mg	Peach	Tablet	Oval	Par Pharmaceutical
PAR; 726	Doxycycline Hyclate	50 mg	Buff and White	Capsule		Par Pharmaceutical
PAR; 727	Doxycycline Hyclate	100 mg	Brown and Cream	Capsule		Par Pharmaceutical
PAR; 876	Paroxetine Hydrochloride	10 mg	White	Tablet		Par
PAR; 877	Paroxetine Hydrochloride	20 mg	White	Tablet		Par
PAR; 878	Paroxetine Hydrochloride	30 mg	White	Tablet		Par
PAR; 879	Paroxetine Hydrochloride	40 mg	White	Tablet		Par

IMPRINT	BRAND/GENERIC NAME	STRENGTH	COLOR	FORM	SHAPE	MANUFACTURER
PAR; 962	Chlordiazepoxide and Amitriptyline Hydrochloride	10 mg; 25 mg	White	Coated Tablet		Par Pharmaceutical
PARAFLEX; MCNEIL	Paraflex	250 mg	Orange or Peach	Tablet		Ortho-Mcneil Pharmaceutical
PARAFON FORTE DSC; MCNEIL	Parafon Forte Dsc	500 mg	Light Green	Tablet		Mcneil Pharmaceutical
PARLODEL; 2 1/2 ;	Parlodel	2.5 mg	White	Tablet	Square, Scored	Novartis
PARLODEL; 5 MG; TRIANGLE(S)	Parlodel	5 mg	Caramel and White	Capsule, Liquid Filled		Novartis
PARNATE; SKF	Parnate	10 mg	Rose-Red	Tablet	Circle	Glaxosmithkline
PAXIL CR; 12.5	Paxil Cr	12.5 mg	Yellow	Controlled-Release Tablet	Circle	Glaxosmithkline
PAXIL CR; 25	Paxil Cr	25 mg	Pink	Controlled-Release Tablet	Circle	Glaxosmithkline
PAXIL CR; 37.5	Paxil Cr	37.5 mg	Blue	Controlled-Release Tablet	Circle	Glaxosmithkline
PAXIL; 10	Paxil	10 mg	Yellow	Film-Coated Tablet	Oval	Glaxosmithkline
PAXIL; 20	Paxil	20 mg	Pink	Film-Coated Tablet	Oval	Glaxosmithkline
PAXIL; 30	Paxil	30 mg	Blue	Film-Coated Tablet	Oval	Glaxosmithkline
PAXIL; 40	Paxil	40 mg	Green	Film-Coated Tablet	Oval	Glaxosmithkline
PBA ;	Proglycem	50 mg	Orange and Clear	Capsule		Schering
PCE; ABBOTT LOGO	Pce Dispertab	333 mg	White with Pink Speckles	Tablet	Oval	Abbott Laboratories
PD 144	Femhrt	1 mg; 5 mcg	White	Tablet	D-Shape	Warner Chilcott
PD 145	Femhrt	0.5 mg; 2.5 mcg	White	Tablet	Oval	Warner Chilcott
PD 155 ; 10	Lipitor	10 mg	White	Coated Tablet	Circle	Parke-Davis
PD 156 ; 20	Lipitor	20 mg	White	Coated Tablet	Circle	Parke-Davis
PD 157 ; 40	Lipitor	40 mg	White	Coated Tablet	Circle	Parke-Davis
PD 158 ; 80	Lipitor	80 mg	White	Coated Tablet	Circle	Parke-Davis
PD 622	Ovcon 35 Fe - Brown Tablet	75 mg	Brown	Tablet	Circle	Warner Chilcott
PD; 220	Accuretic	20 mg; 12.5 mg	Pink	Coated Tablet	Triangle, Scored	Parke-Davis
PD; 222	Accuretic	10 mg; 12.5 mg	Pink	Coated Tablet	Biconvex, Elliptical, Scored	Parke-Davis
PD; 223	Accuretic	20 mg; 25 mg	Pink	Coated Tablet	Circle, Biconvex	Parke-Davis
PD; 352; 200	Rezulin	200 mg	Yellow	Coated Tablet	Oval	Parke-Davis
PD; 353; 400	Rezulin	400 mg	Tan	Coated Tablet	Oval	Parke-Davis
PD; 357; 300	Rezulin	300 mg	White	Coated Tablet	Oval	Parke-Davis
PD; 527; 5	Accupril	5 mg	Brown	Coated Tablet	Circle, Scored	Parke-Davis
PD; 530; 10	Accupril	10 mg	Brown	Coated Tablet	Triangle	Parke-Davis
PD; 532; 20	Accupril	20 mg	Brown	Coated Tablet	Circle	Parke-Davis
PD; 535; 40	Accupril	40 mg	Brown	Coated Tablet	Circle	Parke-Davis
PD; NEURONTIN 100 MG	Neurontin	100 mg	White	Capsule		Parke-Davis
PD; NEURONTIN 300 MG	Neurontin	300 mg	Yellow	Capsule		Parke-Davis
PD; NEURONTIN 400 MG	Neurontin	400 mg	Orange	Capsule		Parke-Davis
P-D ; CENTRAX; 553	Centrax	10 mg	Aqua	Capsule		Parke-Davis
P-D 390	Natabec	30 mg; 4000 IU; 400 IU; 50 mg; 3 mg; 2 mg; 3 mg; 5 mcg; 10 mg; 600 mg	Pink and Blue	Capsule		Parke-Davis Consumer Health Products
P-D 915 ;	Loestrin 24 Fe - White Tablet	1 mg; 20 mcg	White	Tablet	Circle	Warner Chilcott
P-D; 007	Dilantin Infatabs	50 mg	Yellow	Tablet, Chewable	Triangle, Scored	Parke-Davis
P-D; 043	Gelusil-II Chewable Tablet	400 mg; 400 mg; 30 mg	White and Orange	Tablet, Chewable		Pfizer Consumer Health Care
P-D; 045	Gelusil-M Chewable Tablet	300 mg; 200 mg; 25 mg	White	Tablet, Chewable		Pfizer Consumer Health Care
P-D; 141; 2	Diazepam	2 mg	White	Tablet	Oval	Parke-Davis
P-D; 142; 5	Diazepam	5 mg		Tablet	Triangle	Parke-Davis
P-D; 143; 10	Diazepam	10 mg	White	Tablet	Circle	Parke-Davis
P-D; 160	Pyridium Plus	150 mg; 0.3 mg; 15 mg		Tablet		Warner Chilcott
P-D; 200	Brondecon	200 mg; 100 mg		Tablet		Parke-Davis
P-D; 201	Brondecon	200 mg; 100 mg	Pink	Tablet		Parke-Davis
P-D; 202	Procan SR	250 mg	Green	Sustained-Release Tablet	Circle	Parke-Davis
P-D; 207	Procan SR	1000 mg	Red	Sustained-Release Tablet	Circle, Scored	Parke-Davis
P-D; 214	Choledyl SA	400 mg	Pink	Extended-Release Tablet		Parke-Davis
P-D; 221	Choledyl SA	600 mg	Tan	Extended-Release Tablet		Parke-Davis
P-D; 237	Zarontin	250 mg	Orange	Capsule		Parke-Davis
P-D; 248	D-S-S Plus	30 mg; 100 mg		Capsule		Parke-Davis Consumer Health Products
P-D; 260	Euthroid-1/2	30 mcg; 7.5 mcg		Tablet		Parke-Davis
P-D; 261	Euthroid-1	60 mcg; 15 mcg		Tablet		Parke-Davis
P-D; 262	Euthroid-2	120 mcg; 30 mcg		Tablet		Parke-Davis
P-D; 263	Euthroid-3	180 mcg; 45 mcg		Tablet		Parke-Davis
P-D; 270	Nardil	15 mg	Orange	Coated Tablet	Circle, Biconvex	Parke-Davis
P-D; 271	Amitril	100 mg	Brown and Mustard	Coated Tablet		Parke-Davis
P-D; 272	Amitril	10 mg	Tan	Coated Tablet		Parke-Davis
P-D; 273	Amitril	25 mg	Coral	Coated Tablet		Parke-Davis
P-D; 274	Amitril	50 mg	Blue-Purple	Coated Tablet		Parke-Davis
P-D; 275	Amitril	75 mg	Green	Coated Tablet		Parke-Davis
P-D; 276	Centrax	10 mg	Blue	Tablet		Parke-Davis
P-D; 278	Amitril	150 mg	Orange	Coated Tablet		Parke-Davis
P-D; 365 ;	Dilantin Kapseals	30 mg	White with Pink Band	Extended-Release Capsule		Parke-Davis
P-D; 373	Benadryl Capsule	50 mg	Pink	Capsule		Pfizer Consumer Health Care

IMPRINT	BRAND/GENERIC NAME	STRENGTH	COLOR	FORM	SHAPE	MANUFACTURER
P-D; 382	Geriplex	30 mg; 1.5 mg; 20 mg; 15 mg; 5 IU; 4 mg; 4 mg; 2 mg; 200 mg; 2.5 Gr; 50 mg; 5 mg; 5 mg; 2 mcg		Capsule		Parke-Davis Consumer Health Products
P-D; 393	Milontin	500 mg		Capsule		Parke-Davis
P-D; 407	Cyclopar	250 mg	Scarlet and Flesh	Capsule		Parke-Davis
P-D; 471	Benadryl Capsule	25 mg	Pink and White	Capsule		Pfizer Consumer Health Care
P-D; 525	Celontin	300 mg	Yellow with Orange Band	Capsule		Parke-Davis
P-D; 529	Humatin	250 mg		Capsule		Monarch Pharmaceuticals
P-D; 531	Dilantin with Phenobarbital	100 mg; 32 mg	White and Purple with Black Band	Capsule		Parke-Davis
P-D; 537	Celontin	150 mg	Yellow with Brown Band	Capsule		Parke-Davis
P-D; 541	Natabec-FA	30 mg; 4000 IU; 0.1 mg; 10 mg; 600 mg; 50 mg; 3 mg; 2 mg; 3 mg; 5 mcg; 400 IU		Capsule		Parke-Davis Consumer Health Products
P-D; 557	Verapamil Hydrochloride	80 mg		Tablet		Warner Chilcott
P-D; 573	Verapamil Hydrochloride	120 mg		Tablet		Warner Chilcott
P-D; 697	Cyclopar	500 mg	Orange and Flesh	Capsule		Warner Chilcott
P-D; 737; LOPID	Lopid	600 mg	White	Coated Tablet	Circle, Scored	Parke-Davis
P-D; 849	Quinidine Sulfate	200 mg		Tablet		Parke-Davis
P-D; CENTRAX; 552	Centrax	5 mg	Celery	Capsule		Parke-Davis
P-D; CENTRAX; 554	Centrax	20 mg	Yellow	Capsule		Parke-Davis
PE	Sudafed Pe	10 mg	Red	Tablet	Circle	Pfizer
PEDIACARE; 3	Pediacare Cough-Cold	0.5 mg; 2.5 mg; 7.5 mg	Pink	Tablet, Chewable		Pharmacia & Upjohn
PEDIACARE; CC	Pediacare for Ages 6-12 Cough-Cold	1 mg; 5 mg; 15 mg	Pink	Tablet, Chewable		Pharmacia & Upjohn
PEPCID AC	Pepcid Ac	10 mg	Peach	Tablet	Square	Johnson & Johnson Merck
PEPTO-BISMOL	Pepto Bismol	262 mg	Pink	Tablet, Chewable	Oval	Procter & Gamble
PEPTO-BISMOL	Pepto-Bismol	262 mg	Pink	Tablet, Chewable	Circle	Procter & Gamble Pharmaceuticals
PERCOCET; 10	Percocet 10/650	650 mg; 10 mg	Yellow	Tablet	Oval	Endo Laboratories
PERCOCET; 2.5	Percocet 2.5/325	325 mg; 2.5 mg	Pink	Tablet	Oval	Endo Laboratories
PERCOCET; 5	Percocet 5/325	325 mg; 5 mg	Blue	Tablet	Circle, Scored	Endo Laboratories
PERCOCET; 7.5	Percocet 7.5/500	500 mg; 7.5 mg	Peach	Tablet	Capsule-Shape	Endo Laboratories
PERCOCET; 7.5/325	Percocet 7.5/325	325 mg; 7.5 mg	Peach	Tablet	Oval	Endo Laboratories
PERCODAN	Percodan	325 mg; 4.5 mg; 0.38 mg	Yellow	Tablet		Endo Laboratories
PF; 100 ;	Ms Contin	100 mg	Gray	Tablet, Extended Release	Circle	Purdue Pharmaceutical Products
PF; C275	Cardioquin	275 mg	White	Tablet		Purdue Pharmaceutical Products
PF; M15	Ms Contin	15 mg	Blue	Tablet, Extended Release	Circle	Purdue Pharmaceutical Products
PF; M30	Ms Contin	30 mg	Lavender	Tablet, Extended Release	Circle	Purdue Pharmaceutical Products
PF; M60	Ms Contin	60 mg	Orange	Tablet, Extended Release	Circle	Purdue Pharmaceutical Products
PF; M200	Ms Contin	200 mg	Green	Tablet, Extended Release	Capsule-Shape	Purdue Pharmaceutical Products
PF; MI; 15	Msir	15 mg	White	Tablet	Circle, Scored	Purdue Pharmaceutical Products
PF; MI; 30	Msir	30 mg	White	Tablet	Capsule-Shape, Scored	Purdue Pharmaceutical Products
PF; MSIR; 15; THIS END UP	Msir	15 mg	White and Blue	Capsule		Purdue Pharmaceutical Products
PF; MSIR; 30; THIS END UP	Msir	30 mg	Gray and Lavender	Capsule		Purdue Pharmaceutical Products
PF; T; 500	Trilisate 500 mg	293 mg; 362 mg	Salmon	Coated Tablet		Purdue Pharmaceutical Products
PF; T; 750	Trilisate 750 mg	440 mg; 544 mg	White	Coated Tablet		Purdue Pharmaceutical Products
PF; T; 1000	Trilisate 1000 mg	587 mg; 725 mg	Red	Coated Tablet		Purdue Pharmaceutical Products
PF; U; 200	Uniphyl	200 mg	White	Controlled-Release Tablet	Circle	Purdue Pharmaceutical Products
PF; U; 400	Uniphyl	400 mg	White	Timed-Release Tablet		Purdue Pharmaceutical Products
PF; U; 600	Uniphyl	600 mg		Extended-Release Tablet		Purdue Pharmaceutical Products
PF; U200	T-Phyl	200 mg	White	Extended-Release Tablet		Purdue Pharmaceutical Products
PFIZER ; CDT 051 ;	Caduet	5 mg; 10 mg	White	Tablet		Pfizer
PFIZER ; CDT 052 ;	Caduet	5 mg; 20 mg	White	Tablet		Pfizer
PFIZER ; CDT 054 ;	Caduet	5 mg; 40 mg	White	Tablet		Pfizer
PFIZER ; CDT 058 ;	Caduet	5 mg; 80 mg	White	Tablet		Pfizer
PFIZER ; CDT 101 ;	Caduet	10 mg; 10 mg	Blue	Tablet		Pfizer
PFIZER ; CDT 102 ;	Caduet	10 mg; 20 mg	Blue	Tablet		Pfizer
PFIZER ; CDT 104 ;	Caduet	10 mg; 40 mg	Blue	Tablet		Pfizer
PFIZER ; CDT 108 ;	Caduet	10 mg; 80 mg	Blue	Tablet		Pfizer
PFIZER ; CDT 251 ;	Caduet	2.5 mg; 10 mg	White	Tablet		Pfizer
PFIZER ; CDT 252 ;	Caduet	2.5 mg; 20 mg	White	Tablet		Pfizer
PFIZER ; CDT 254 ;	Caduet	2.5 mg; 40 mg	White	Tablet		Pfizer

IMPRINT	BRAND/GENERIC NAME	STRENGTH	COLOR	FORM	SHAPE	MANUFACTURER
PFIZER ; CHX 0.5	Chantix	0.5 mg	Off-White to White	Tablet	Capsule-Shape	Pfizer
PFIZER ; CHX 1.0	Chantix	1 mg	Light Blue	Tablet	Capsule-Shape	Pfizer
PFIZER ; ZTM500	Zithromax	500 mg	Pink	Tablet	Capsule-Shape	Pfizer
PFIZER 306	Zithromax	250 mg	Pink	Tablet	Capsule-Shape	Pfizer
PFIZER 432; MINIZIDE	Minizide 2	2 mg; 0.5 mg	Blue-Green, Pink	Capsule		Pfizer
PFIZER PGN 25	Lyrica	25 mg	White	Capsule		Pfizer
PFIZER PGN 50	Lyrica	50 mg	White	Capsule		Pfizer
PFIZER PGN 75	Lyrica	75 mg	Orange, White	Capsule		Pfizer
PFIZER PGN 100	Lyrica	100 mg	Orange	Capsule		Pfizer
PFIZER PGN 150	Lyrica	150 mg	White	Capsule		Pfizer
PFIZER PGN 200	Lyrica	200 mg	Light Orange	Capsule		Pfizer
PFIZER PGN 225	Lyrica	225 mg	Light Orange, White	Capsule		Pfizer
PFIZER PGN 300	Lyrica	300 mg	Orange, White	Capsule		Pfizer
PFIZER STN 12.5 MG	Sutent	12.5 mg	Orange	Capsule		Pfizer
PFIZER STN 25 MG	Sutent	25 mg	Caramel, Orange	Capsule		Pfizer
PFIZER STN 50 MG	Sutent	50 mg	Caramel	Capsule		Pfizer
PFIZER; 095; VIBRA ;	Vibramycin	100 mg	Blue	Capsule		Pfizer
PFIZER; 015	Tetracyn	250 mg	Black and White	Capsule		Pfizer
PFIZER; 016	Tetracyn	500 mg	Blue and White	Capsule		Pfizer
PFIZER; 072; TERRAMYCIN	Terramycin	125 mg		Capsule		Pfizer
PFIZER; 073	Terramycin	250 mg	Clear Yellow	Capsule		Pfizer
PFIZER; 073; TERRAMYCIN	Terramycin	250 mg	Yellow	Capsule		Pfizer
PFIZER; 084	Terramycin	250 mg	Yellow	Coated Tablet		Pfizer
PFIZER; 088	Terrastatin	250 mg; 250000 U	Pink and Yellow	Capsule		Pfizer
PFIZER; 094	Vibramycin Hyclate	50 mg	Blue and White	Capsule		Pfizer
PFIZER; 094; VIBRA	Vibramycin	50 mg	Blue and White	Capsule		Pfizer Laboratories
PFIZER; 095	Vibramycin Hyclate	100 mg	Blue	Capsule		Pfizer
PFIZER; 099; VIBRA-TABS ;	Vibra-Tabs	100 mg		Coated Tablet	Circle	Pfizer
PFIZER; 105	Pfizerpen VK	250 mg	White	Tablet		Pfizer
PFIZER; 106	Pfizerpen VK	500 mg	White	Tablet		Pfizer
PFIZER; 180	Vistrax 5	5 mg; 25 mg	White	Tablet		Pfizer
PFIZER; 181	Vistrax 10	10 mg; 25 mg	Black and White	Tablet		Pfizer
PFIZER; 220; SUSTAIRE ;	Sustaire	100 mg	White	Delayed-Release Tablet		Pfizer
PFIZER; 221; SUSTAIRE ;	Sustaire	300 mg	White	Delayed-Release Tablet		Pfizer
PFIZER; 308	Zithromax	600 mg	White	Coated Tablet	Oval, Modified	Pfizer Laboratories
PFIZER; 335	Sterane	5 mg	White	Tablet	Oval	Pfizer Laboratories
PFIZER; 375	Renese	1 mg	White	Tablet	Circle, Scored	Pfizer
PFIZER; 376	Renese	2 mg	Yellow	Tablet	Circle, Scored	Pfizer
PFIZER; 377	Renese	4 mg	White	Tablet	Circle, Scored	Pfizer
PFIZER; 378	Trovan	100 mg	Blue	Coated Tablet	Circle	Pfizer
PFIZER; 378	Trovan/zithromax Compliance Pak Trovafloxacin	100 mg	Blue	Coated Tablet	Circle	Pfizer Laboratories
PFIZER; 379	Trovan	200 mg	Blue	Coated Tablet	Oval	Pfizer
PFIZER; 396	Geodon	20 mg	Blue and White	Capsule		Pfizer Laboratories
PFIZER; 397	Geodon	40 mg	Blue	Capsule		Pfizer Laboratories
PFIZER; 398	Geodon	60 mg	White	Capsule		Pfizer Laboratories
PFIZER; 399	Geodon	80 mg	Blue and White	Capsule		Pfizer Laboratories
PFIZER; 411	Glucotrol	5 mg	White	Tablet	Diamond Shaped, Scored	Pfizer Us Pharmaceuticals Group
PFIZER; 412	Glucotrol	10 mg	White	Tablet	Diamond Shaped, Scored	Pfizer Us Pharmaceuticals Group
PFIZER; 430; MINIZIDE	Minizide 1	1 mg; 0.5 mg	Blue-Green	Capsule		Pfizer
PFIZER; 431; MINIPRESS	Minipress	1 mg	White	Capsule		Pfizer
PFIZER; 437; MINIPRESS	Minipress	2 mg	Pink and White	Capsule		Pfizer
PFIZER; 438; MINIPRESS	Minipress	5 mg	Blue and White	Capsule		Pfizer
PFIZER; 441	Moderil	0.25 mg	Yellow	Tablet	Oval, Scored	Pfizer
PFIZER; 442	Moderil	0.5 mg	Salmon; Orange	Tablet	Oval, Scored	Pfizer
PFIZER; 446	Renese-R	2 mg; 0.25 mg	White	Tablet		Pfizer
PFIZER; 541; VISTARIL ;	Vistaril	25 mg	Dark Green and Light Green	Capsule		Pfizer
PFIZER; 542; VISTARIL ;	Vistaril	50 mg	Dark Green and White	Capsule		Pfizer
PFIZER; 543; VISTARIL ;	Vistaril	50 mg	Dark Green and Pink	Capsule		Pfizer
PFIZER; 550	Zyrtec	5 mg	White	Coated Tablet	Rectangle, Rounded-Off	Pfizer Laboratories
PFIZER; 551 ;	Zyrtec	10 mg	White	Coated Tablet	Rectangle, Rounded-Off	Pfizer Laboratories
PFIZER; NSR; 25 ;	Inspra	25 mg	Yellow	Tablet	Diamond	Pfizer
PFIZER; NSR; 25 ;	Inspra	25 mg	Yellow	Tablet	Diamond	Searle
PFIZER; NSR; 50 ;	Inspra	50 mg	Pink	Tablet	Diamond	Pfizer
PFIZER; NSR; 50 ;	Inspra	50 mg	Pink	Tablet	Diamond	Searle
PFIZER; TKN; 125	Tikosyn	125 mcg	Light Orange and White	Capsule		Pfizer Laboratories
PFIZER; TKN; 250	Tikosyn	250 mcg	Peach	Capsule		Pfizer Laboratories
PFIZER; TKN; 500	Tikosyn	500 mcg	Peach and White	Capsule		Pfizer Laboratories
PFIZER;VOR50	Vfend	50 mg	White	Coated Tablet	Circle	Pfizer Laboratories
PFIZER;VOR200	Vfend	200 mg	White	Coated Tablet	Capsule-Shape	Pfizer Laboratories

IMPRINT	BRAND/GENERIC NAME	STRENGTH	COLOR	FORM	SHAPE	MANUFACTURER
PG; 11	Helidac Therapy: Part I	262.4 mg	Pink	Tablet, Chewable	Circle	Procter & Gamble Pharmaceuticals
PG; 12	Helidac Therapy: Part Iii	500 mg	Pale Orange and White	Capsule		Procter & Gamble Pharmaceuticals
PHA; 1730	Inspra	100 mg	Red	Tablet	Diamond	Searle
PHILLIPS	Phillips' Gelcaps	90 mg; 83 mg	White	Capsule, Liquid Filled		Bayer Consumer Care
PK	Kaletra	133.3 mg; 33.3 mg	Orange	Capsule		Abbott Laboratories
PL 500	Amoxicillin/clavulanate Potassium	500 mg; 125 mg	White	Tablet	Oval	Par Pharmaceutical
PL 875	Amoxicillin/clavulanate Potassium	875 mg; 125 mg	White	Tablet	Capsule-Shape	Par Pharmaceutical
PL AT8	Amoxicillin	875 mg	Pink	Tablet	Capsule-Shape	Par Pharmaceutical
PL C40	Amoxicillin/clavulanate Potassium	400 mg; 57 mg	Mottled Pink	Tablet, Chewable	Circle	Par Pharmaceutical
PL CT4	Amoxicillin	400 mg	Pale Pink	Tablet, Chewable	Circle	Par Pharmaceutical
PL; AT8	Amoxicillin	875 mg	Pink	Tablet	Capsule-Shape	Ivax Pharmaceuticals
PLACIDYL; 500	Placidyl	500 mg	Red	Capsule, Liquid Filled		Abbott Laboratories
PLACIDYL; 750	Placidyl	750 mg	Green	Capsule, Liquid Filled		Abbott Laboratories
PLAQUENIL	Hydroxychloroquine Sulfate	200 mg	White with Black Ink	Tablet	Oval	Sanofi-Aventis U.S.
PLAQUENIL; P62	Plaquenil	200 mg	White	Tablet	Capsule-Shape	Sanofi-Aventis U.S.
PLEGINE; 35	Plegine	35 mg		Tablet		Wyeth Pharmaceuticals
PLENDIL; 450	Plendil	2.5 mg	Sage Green	Extended-Release Tablet	Circle, Convex	Astra Zeneca
PLENDIL; 451	Plendil	5 mg	Red-Brown	Extended-Release Tablet	Circle, Convex	Astra Zeneca
PLENDIL; 452	Plendil	10 mg	Red-Brown	Extended-Release Tablet	Circle, Convex	Astra Zeneca
PLETAL; 50	Pletal	50 mg	White	Tablet	Triangle	Otsuka America Pharmaceutical
PLETAL; 100	Pletal	100 mg	White	Tablet	Circle	Otsuka America Pharmaceutical
PN; SANOFI	Prenatal Vitamin Ultra	90 mg; 0.15 mg; 250 mg; 2 mg; 25 mg; 1 mg; 4000 IU; 400 IU; 30 IU; 20 mg; 50 mg; 120 mg; 3 mg; 3.4 mg; 20 mg; 12 mcg	Beige	Coated Tablet	Egg-Shape	Sanofi Pharmaceuticals
PP; 1304	Pseudo-Chlor SR	8 mg; 120 mg	Blue and Clear	Sustained-Release Capsule		Novartis Generics
PPP; 784; DURICEF; 500 MG	Duricef	500 mg	Maroon and Whtie	Capsule		Bristol-Myers Squibb
PPP; 785	Duricef	1 GM	White to Off White	Tablet	Oval	Bristol-Myers Squibb
PRAVACHOL; 10; P ;	Pravachol	10 mg	Pale Pink or Peach	Tablet	Rectangle, Biconvex, Rounded	Bristol-Myers Squibb
PRAVACHOL; 20; P ;	Pravachol	20 mg	Yellow	Tablet	Rectangle, Rounded, Biconvex	Bristol-Myers Squibb
PRAVACHOL; 40; P ;	Pravachol	40 mg	Green	Tablet	Rectangle, Rounded, Biconvex	Bristol-Myers Squibb
PRECOSE; 25	Precose	25 mg	White	Tablet	Circle	Bayer Pharmaceutical
PRECOSE; 50	Precose	50 mg	White to Yellow	Tablet		Bayer Pharmaceutical
PRECOSE; 100	Precose	100 mg	White to Yellow	Tablet		Bayer Pharmaceutical
PREMARIN 0.3	Premarin	0.3 mg	Green	Tablet	Oval	Wyeth Pharmaceuticals
PREMARIN 0.45	Premarin	0.45 mg	Blue	Tablet	Oval	Wyeth Pharmaceuticals
PREMARIN 0.625	Premarin	0.625 mg	Maroon	Tablet	Oval	Wyeth Pharmaceuticals
PREMARIN 0.9	Premarin	0.9 mg	White	Tablet	Oval	Wyeth Pharmaceuticals
PREMARIN 1.25	Premarin	1.25 mg	Yellow	Tablet	Oval	Wyeth Pharmaceuticals
PREMPRO	Premphase Conjugated Estrogens and Medroxyprogesterone	0.625 mg; 5 mg	Light-Blue	Coated Tablet	Oval	Wyeth Pharmaceuticals
PREMPRO	Prempro Single Tablet	0.625 mg; 2.5 mg	Peach	Coated Tablet	Oval	Wyeth Pharmaceuticals
PRILOSEC; 10; 606	Prilosec	10 mg	Apricot and Amethyst	Enteric-Coated Tablet		Astra Zeneca
PRILOSEC; 20; 742	Prilosec	20 mg	Amethyst	Timed-Release Capsule		Astra Zeneca
PROCANBID; 1000	Procanbid	1000 mg	Gray	Extended-Release Tablet	Circle	Monarch Pharmaceuticals
PROCARDIA 20; PFIZER 261	Procardia	20 mg	Orange and Light Brown	Capsule, Liquid Filled		Pfizer Laboratories
PROCARDIA XL; 30	Procardia XL	30 mg	Rose Pink	Extended-Release Tablet	Circle, Biconvex	Pfizer Laboratories
PROCARDIA XL; 60	Procardia XL	60 mg	Rose Pink	Extended-Release Tablet	Circle, Biconvex	Pfizer Laboratories
PROCARDIA XL; 90	Procardia XL	90 mg	Rose Pink	Extended-Release Tablet	Circle, Biconvex	Pfizer Laboratories
PROCARDIA; PFIZER 260	Procardia	10 mg	Orange	Capsule, Liquid Filled		Pfizer Laboratories
PROLOPRIM; 09A	Proloprim	100 mg	White	Tablet	Circle, Scored	Monarch Pharmaceuticals
PROPACET	Propacet 100	650 mg; 100 mg	White	Coated Tablet	Oblong, Convex	Teva Pharmaceuticals
PROPACET; 100; LEMMON	Propacet	650 mg; 100 mg	White	Coated Tablet	Oblong	Teva Pharmaceuticals
PROPECIA; P	Propecia	1 mg	Tan	Coated Tablet	Eight-Sided, Convex	Merck & Company
PROTONIX	Protonix	40 mg	Yellow with Brown Ink	Enteric-Coated Tablet	Oval, Biconvex	Wyeth Pharmaceuticals
PROTOPAM; 500	Protopam	500 mg	White	Tablet	Circle	Wyeth Pharmaceuticals
PROVENTIL; 2; 252	Proventil	2 mg	White	Tablet	Circle	Schering
PROVENTIL; 4; 573	Proventil	4 mg	White	Tablet	Circle, Scored, Compressed	Schering
PROVERA; 2.5	Provera	2.5 mg	Orange	Tablet	Circle, Scored	Pharmacia & Upjohn
PROVERA; 5	Provera	5 mg	White	Tablet	Six-Sided, Scored	Pharmacia & Upjohn
PROVERA; 10	Provera	10 mg	White	Tablet	Circle	Pharmacia & Upjohn
PROVIGIL; 100 MG	Provigil	100 mg	White	Tablet	Capsule-Shape	Cephalon
PROVIGIL; 200 MG	Provigil	200 mg	White	Tablet	Capsule-Shape, Scored	Cephalon
PROZAC; 10	Prozac	10 mg	Green	Tablet	Elliptical-Shaped, Scored	Eli Lilly
PU; 700	Dostinex	0.5 mg	White	Tablet	Capsule-Shape, Scored	Pharmacia & Upjohn
PURDUE	Dhc Plus	16 mg; 256.4 mg; 30 mg	Light Aqua and Bluish-Green	Capsule		Purdue Pharmaceutical Products
PURDUE; 200 MG	Spectracef	200 mg	White with Blue Ink	Tablet	Circle	Purdue
PVK; 250; GG; 949	Penicillin-VK	250 mg	White	Tablet	Circle	Geneva Generics
PVK; 500; GG; 950	Penicillin VK	500 mg	White	Tablet	Oblong	Geneva Generics
P-XL; 12 MG	Palladone	12 mg	Cinnamon	Extended-Release Capsule		Purdue Pharma
P-XL; 16 MG	Palladone	16 mg	Pink	Extended-Release Capsule		Purdue Pharma

IMPRINT	BRAND/GENERIC NAME	STRENGTH	COLOR	FORM	SHAPE	MANUFACTURER
P-XL; 24 MG	Palladone	24 mg	Blue	Extended-Release Capsule		Purdue Pharma
P-XL; 32 MG	Palladone	32 mg	White	Extended-Release Capsule		Purdue Pharma
QD 111	Qdall AR	12 mg	Blue, White	Capsule, Extended Release	Capsule-Shape	Atley Pharmaceuticals
QD 112	Qdall	100 mg; 12 mg	Blue, Yellow	Capsule, Extended Release	Capsule-Shape	Atley Pharmaceuticals
QD; 112	Pseudoephedrine Hydrochloride and Chlorpheniramine Maleate	12 mg; 100 mg	Blue and Yellow with Off-White Beads	Extended-Release Capsule		Atley Pharmaceuticals
QUARZAN; 2.5; ROCHE	Quarzan	2.5 mg	Green and Red Opaque	Capsule		Roche Products
QUARZAN; 5; ROCHE	Quarzan	5 mg	Green and Grey Opaque	Capsule		Roche Products
QUINIDEX; AHR	Quinidex Extentabs	300 mg	White	Extended-Release Tablet		Wyeth Consumer Healthcare
R 179	Tizanidine Hydrochloride	2 mg	White to Off White	Tablet	Oval	Par Pharmaceutical
R 180	Tizanidine Hydrochloride	4 mg	White to Off White	Tablet		Par Pharmaceutical
R 5726	Rondec	4 mg; 60 mg	Orange	Tablet		Biovail Pharmaceuticals
R 6240	Rondec-TR	8 mg; 120 mg	Blue	Timed-Release Tablet		Biovail Pharmaceuticals
R; 8	Lozol	2.5 mg	White	Coated Tablet	Eight-Sided	Aventis Pharmaceuticals
R; 224; 2.5	Minoxidil	2.5 mg	White	Tablet	Circle, Scored	Watson Laboratories
R; 225; 10	Minoxidal	10 mg	White	Tablet	Circle, Scored	Watson Laboratories
R; 229; 0.5	Haloperidol	0.5 mg	White	Tablet	Circle	Watson Laboratories
R; 230; 1	Haloperidol	1 mg	Yellow	Tablet	Circle	Watson Laboratories
R; 231; 2	Haloperidol	2 mg	Purple	Tablet	Circle	Watson Laboratories
R; 232; 5	Haloperidol	5 mg	Green	Tablet	Circle	Watson Laboratories
R; 233; 10	Haloperidol	10 mg	Green-Blue	Tablet	Circle	Watson Laboratories
R; 234; 20	Haloperidol	20 mg	Salmon	Tablet	Circle	Watson Laboratories
R; 316	Phentermine Hydrochloride	37.5 mg	White	Tablet	Capsule-Shape	Alpharma
R; 4374	Propoxyphene with Aspirin and Caffeine	389 mg; 32.4 mg; 65 mg		Capsule		Teva Pharmaceuticals
R; 4956	Triamterene and Hydrochlorothiazide	75 mg; 50 mg	Yellow	Tablet		Watson Laboratories
R0.5 ;	Risperdal M-Tab	0.5 mg	Light Coral	Tablet, Disintegrating	Circle	Janssen Pharmaceutica Products
R1 ;	Risperdal M-Tab	1 mg	Light Coral	Tablet, Disintegrating	Square	Janssen Pharmaceutica Products
R2 ;	Risperdal M-Tab	2 mg	Coral	Tablet, Disintegrating	Square	Janssen Pharmaceutica Products
R3 ;	Risperdal M-Tab	3 mg	Coral	Tablet, Disintegrating	Circle	Janssen Pharmaceutica Products
R4 ;	Risperdal M-Tab	4 mg	Coral	Tablet, Disintegrating	Circle	Janssen Pharmaceutica Products
RAPAMUNE 1 MG	Rapamune	1 mg	White	Tablet	Triangle	Wyeth Pharmaceuticals
RAPAMUNE 2 MG	Rapamune	2 mg	Yellow to Beige	Tablet	Triangle	Wyeth Pharmaceuticals
RD; 12	Nephro-Vite RX Vitamin B Complex and C Supplement	1 mg; 300 mcg; 20 mg; 10 mg; 10 mg; 1.5 mg; 60 mcg; 1.7 mg; 60 mg	Yellow	Tablet	Circle	Watson Laboratories
RD; 13	Nephro-Fer	350 mg	Brown	Capsule		Watson Laboratories
REBETOL; 200 MG; SCHERING LOGO	Rebetol	200 mg	White	Capsule		Schering
REDUX	Redux	15 mg	Opaque White	Capsule		Wyeth-Ayerst Laboratories
REGLAN ; SP 10	Reglan	10 mg	White	Tablet	Capsule-Shape	Schwarz Pharma
REGLAN 5 ; SP	Reglan	5 mg	Green	Tablet	Oval	Schwarz Pharma
REGLAN; 5; SP ;	Reglan	5 mg	Green	Tablet	Circle	Schwarz Pharma
REGLAN; SP; 10 ;	Reglan	10 mg	Pink	Tablet	Capsule-Shape	Schwarz Pharma
RELAFEN 500	Relafen	500 mg	White	Tablet	Oval	Glaxosmithkline
RELAFEN 750	Relafen	750 mg	Beige	Tablet	Oval	Glaxosmithkline
RENAGEL; 400	Renagel	400 mg	White	Coated Tablet	Oval	Genzyme
RENAGEL; 800	Renagel	800 mg	White	Coated Tablet	Oval	Genzyme
REP; 20; PFIZER	Relpax	20 mg	Orange	Tablet	Circle	Pfizer Laboratories
REP; 40; PFIZER	Relpax	40 mg	Orange	Tablet	Circle	Pfizer Laboratories
RG; F50	Fluconazole	50 mg	White or Almost White	Tablet	Rounded Rectangle	Barr Laboratories
RG; F100	Fluconazole	100 mg	White or Almost White	Tablet	Rounded Rectangle	Barr Laboratories
RG; F150	Fluconazole	150 mg	White or Almost White	Tablet	Oblong, Convex	Barr Laboratories
RG; F200	Fluconazole	200 mg	White or Almost White	Tablet	Rounded Rectangle	Barr Laboratories
RHEABAN	Rheaban Maximum Strength	750 mg	White	Tablet		Pfizer Consumer Health Care
RIB; 200; ROCHE	Copegus	200 mg	Light Pink	Tablet	Oval	Roche Laboratories
RIBA 200	Ribasphere	200 mg	White	Capsule		Par Pharmaceutical
RIBAVIRIN 200 ; GG 608	Ribavirin	200 mg	White	Capsule		Sandoz
RIFADIN; 150 ;	Rifadin	150 mg	Maroon and Scarlet	Capsule		Sanofi-Aventis U.S.
RIFADIN; 300 ;	Rifadin	300 mg	Maroon and Scarlet	Capsule		Sanofi-Aventis U.S.
RIFAMATE	Rifamate	300 mg; 150 mg	Red	Capsule		Sanofi-Aventis U.S.
RIFATER	Rifater	50 mg; 300 mg; 120 mg	Light Beige	Tablet	Circle	Sanofi-Aventis U.S.
RIKER; 125; PLUS	Theolair-Plus	125 mg; 100 mg		Tablet	Circle	3M Pharmaceuticals
RIKER; 161	Disipal	50 mg	Green	Tablet	Circle	3M Pharmaceuticals
RIKER; 193	Estomul-M	500 mg; 45 mg	Pink	Tablet	Capsule-Shape	3M Pharmaceuticals
RIKER; 250; PLUS	Theolair-Plus	250 mg; 200 mg		Tablet		3M Pharmaceuticals
RIKER; 265	Rauwiloid	2 mg	Brown	Tablet	Circle	3M Pharmaceuticals
RIKER; TEPANIL	Tepanil	25 mg	White	Tablet		3M Pharmaceuticals

IMPRINT	BRAND/GENERIC NAME	STRENGTH	COLOR	FORM	SHAPE	MANUFACTURER
RIKER; TEPANIL; TEN-TAB	Tepanil Ten-Tab	75 mg	White	Timed-Release Tablet		3M Pharmaceuticals
RIOPAN	Riopan	480 mg		Tablet, Chewable		Wyeth Consumer Healthcare
RIOPAN ;	Riopan	480 mg		Tablet		Wyeth Consumer Healthcare
RIOPAN PLUS	Riopan Plus	480 mg; 20 mg		Tablet, Chewable		Wyeth Consumer Healthcare
RL	Marinol	2.5 mg	White	Capsule, Liquid Filled	Circle	Roxane Laboratories
RL	Marinol	5 mg	Dark Brown	Capsule, Liquid Filled	Circle	Roxane Laboratories
RL	Marinol	10 mg	Orange	Capsule, Liquid Filled	Circle	Roxane Laboratories
RLI 54 698	Zonisamide	50 mg	Gray, White Opaque	Capsule		Roxane Laboratories
RLI 54 889	Zonisamide	100 mg	Gray Opaque, Red	Capsule		Roxane Laboratories
RLI 54 944	Zonisamide	25 mg	White, White Opaque	Capsule		Roxane Laboratories
RO; L3	Boniva	2.5 mg	White	Tablet	Oblong	Roche Laboratories
ROBAXIN; 500; SP	Robaxin	500 mg	Light Orange	Coated Tablet	Circle	Schwarz Pharma
ROBAXIN; 750; SP	Robaxin-750	750 mg	Orange	Coated Tablet	Capsule-Shape	Schwarz Pharma
ROBITAB; 8217	Robicillin VK	250 mg	White	Tablet	Circle, Scored	Wyeth Consumer Healthcare
ROBITAB; 8227	Robicillin VK	500 mg	White	Tablet	Circle, Scored	Wyeth Consumer Healthcare
ROBITAB; 8317	Robimycin	250 mg	Green	Enteric-Coated Tablet		Wyeth Consumer Healthcare
ROCALTROL; 0.25; ROCHE ;	Rocaltrol	0.25 mcg	Light Orange	Capsule, Liquid Filled	Oval	Roche Laboratories
ROCALTROL; 0.5; ROCHE ;	Rocaltrol	0.5 mcg	Dark Orange	Capsule, Liquid Filled	Oblong	Roche Laboratories
ROCHE 0245	Invirase	200 mg	Green Opaque, Light Brown	Capsule		Roche Laboratories
ROCHE SQV 500	Invirase	500 mg	Light Orange to Greyish or Brownish Orange	Tablet	Oval	Roche Laboratories
ROCHE; 0246	Fortovase	200 mg	Opaque Beige	Capsule, Liquid Filled		Roche Laboratories
ROCHE; 05; KLONOPIN	Klonopin	0.5 mg	Orange	Tablet	Circle, K-Shaped Perforation	Roche Pharmaceuticals
ROCHE; 1; KLONOPIN	Klonopin	1 mg	Blue	Tablet	Circle, K-Shaped Perforation	Roche Pharmaceuticals
ROCHE; 16	Noludar	50 mg	White	Tablet		Roche Laboratories
ROCHE; 17	Noludar	200 mg	White	Tablet		Roche Laboratories
ROCHE; 19	Noludar	50 mg	Purple and White	Capsule		Roche Laboratories
ROCHE; 136	Valcaps	2 mg	Blue and White	Capsule		Roche Pharmaceuticals
ROCHE; 137	Valcaps	5 mg	Blue and Yellow	Capsule		Roche Pharmaceuticals
ROCHE; 139	Valcaps	10 mg	Black and Blue	Capsule		Roche Pharmaceuticals
ROCHE; 274	Anaprox	275 mg	Blue	Tablet	Oval, Biconvex	Roche Laboratories
ROCHE; AZO; GANTANOL	Azo Gantanol	0.5 GM; 100 mg	Red	Coated Tablet		Roche Pharmaceuticals
ROCHE; AZO; GANTRISIN	Azo Gantrisin	500 mg; 50 mg	Red	Coated Tablet		Roche Pharmaceuticals
ROCHE; BUMEX 0.5	Bumex	0.5 mg	Light Green	Tablet	Oval	Roche Pharmaceuticals
ROCHE; BUMEX 1	Bumex	1 mg	Yellow	Tablet	Oval	Roche Pharmaceuticals
ROCHE; BUMEX 2	Bumex	2 mg	Peach	Tablet	Oval	Roche Pharmaceuticals
ROCHE; CYTOVENE; 250	Cytovene	250 mg	Opaque Green	Capsule		Roche Laboratories
ROCHE; GANTRISIN	Gantrisin	0.5 GM	White	Tablet	Circle, Scored	Roche Pharmaceuticals
ROCHE; POSICOR; 50	Posicor	50 mg	Pale Yellow	Tablet	Biconvex, Hexagon	Roche Laboratories
ROCHE; POSICOR; 100	Posicor	100 mg	Light Orange	Tablet	Biconvex, Hexagon	Roche Laboratories
ROCHE; PROSTIGMIN	Prostigmin	15 mg	White	Tablet		Roche Laboratories
ROCHE; XENICAL; 120	Xenical	120 mg	Dark Blue	Capsule		Roche Laboratories
ROERIG; 201	Bonine	25 mg		Tablet, Chewable		Pfizer Consumer Health Care
ROERIG; 627	Vitamin E	200 IU	Clear Yellow	Capsule, Liquid Filled		Pfizer Roerig
ROERIG; 628	Vitamin E	400 IU	Light Yellow	Capsule, Liquid Filled		Pfizer Roerig
ROERIG; 991	Vitamin E	600 IU	Light Yellow	Capsule, Liquid Filled		Pfizer Roerig
RORER; 82	Lozol	2.5 mg	White	Tablet	Circle	Aventis Pharmaceuticals
RP; 51	Dextrostat	5 mg	Yellow	Tablet	Circle, Scored	Shire Pharmaceuticals
RP; 52	Dextrostat	10 mg	Yellow	Tablet	Circle, Double-Scored	Shire Pharmaceuticals
RPC; 052	Colace	50 mg	Clear Dark Red with Clear Pink Fill	Capsule, Liquid Filled	Oval	Purdue
RPC; 053	Colace	100 mg	Pink-Red and Light Beige	Capsule, Liquid Filled	Oval	Purdue
RPR; 0514	Combipatch	0.05 mg/day; 0.14 mg/day		Patch	Square	Novartis
RPR; 0525	Combipatch	0.05 mg/day; 0.25 mg/day		Patch	Square	Novartis
RPR; 202	Rilutek	50 mg	White	Tablet	Capsule-Shape	Sanofi-Aventis U.S.
RPR; 352	Slo-Phyllin	200 mg	White	Tablet	Circle	Aventis Pharmaceuticals
RPR; 5100	Penetrex	200 mg	Light Blue	Coated Tablet	Circle	Aventis Pharmaceuticals
RPR; 5140	Penetrex	400 mg	Dark Blue	Coated Tablet	Circle	Aventis Pharmaceuticals
RS; 117	Ergoloid Mesylate	0.5 mg	White	Tablet	Oval	3M Pharmaceuticals
RS; 119	Ergoloid Mesylate	1 mg	White	Tablet	Oval	3M Pharmaceuticals
RS; 142 ;	Diethylpropion Hydrochloride	75 mg	White	Tablet	Oval	3M Pharmaceuticals
RSN ; 5 MG	Actonel	5 mg	Yellow	Tablet	Oval	Procter & Gamble
RSN ; 30 MG	Actonel	30 mg	White	Tablet	Oval	Procter & Gamble
RSN ; 35 MG	Actonel	35 mg	Orange	Tablet	Oval	Procter & Gamble
RSN ; 35 MG	Actonel with Calcium (Risedronate Sodium Tablets)	35 mg	Orange	Tablet	Oval	Procter & Gamble
RUSS; 702	Femcet	50 mg; 325 mg; 40 mg	Lavender	Capsule		Ucb Pharma
RVT20	Revatio	20 mg	White	Tablet	Circle	Pfizer
S	Senokot	8.6 mg	Brown	Tablet		Purdue Pharmaceutical Products
S	Sleep-Eze 3	25 mg	Yellow	Tablet		Whitehall Laboratories

IMPRINT	BRAND/GENERIC NAME	STRENGTH	COLOR	FORM	SHAPE	MANUFACTURER
S	Sominex Maximum Strength Formula	50 mg	Light Blue	Tablet	Oblong	Glaxosmithkline Consumer
S	Sominex Original Formula	25 mg	Light Blue	Tablet	Circle	Glaxosmithkline Consumer
S 063	Agrylin	0.5 mg	White	Capsule		Shire Pharmaceuticals
S 064	Agrylin	1 mg	Gray	Capsule		Shire Pharmaceuticals
S CAFERGOT; P-B 78/35 SUPPOSITORY	Cafergot P-B	2 mg; 100 mg; 0.25 mg; 60 mg		Suppository		Novartis Pharmaceuticals
S/T; DS; 911	Sulfamethoxazole and Trimethoprim	800 mg; 160 mg	White	Tablet	Oval, Convex, Scored	Teva Pharmaceuticals
S; 5	Selegiline Hydrochloride	5 mg	White	Tablet	Shield-Shape	Mylan Pharmaceuticals
S; 20; LESCOL	Lescol	20 mg	Brown and Light Brown	Capsule		Novartis Pharmaceuticals
S; 40; LESCOL	Lescol	40 mg	Brown and Gold	Capsule		Novartis Pharmaceuticals
S; 62	Seasonale	0.15 mg; 0.03 mg	Pink	Tablet	Circle	Barr Laboratories
S; 78/22 ;	Bellergal	20 mg; 0.3 mg; 0.1 mg	Pink	Coated Tablet	Circle	Novartis Pharmaceuticals
S; 78; 240	Sandimmune	25 mg	Pink	Capsule	Oval	Novartis Pharmaceuticals
S; 78; 241	Sandimmune	100 mg	Dusty Rose	Capsule	Oblong	Novartis Pharmaceuticals
S; 78; 242	Sandimmune	50 mg	Yellow	Capsule	Oblong	Novartis Pharmaceuticals
S; 78-2	Mellaril	10 mg	Bright Chartreuse	Coated Tablet		Novartis
S; 78-8	Mellaril	15 mg	Pink	Coated Tablet		Novartis
S; 374	Chlor-Trimeton Allergy	8 mg	Yellow	Sustained-Release Tablet		Schering-Plough Healthcare Products
S; 770	Sorbitrate	5 mg	Green	Tablet	Oval, Scored	Astra Zeneca
S; 780	Sorbitrate	10 mg	Yellow	Tablet	Oval, Scored	Astra Zeneca
S; 810	Sorbitrate	5 mg	Green	Tablet, Chewable	Circle, Scored	Astra Zeneca
S; 820	Sorbitrate	20 mg	Blue	Tablet	Oval, Scored	Astra Zeneca
S; AHG ;	Naqua	2 mg	Pink	Tablet	Character-Shape, Scored	Schering
S; AHH ;	Naqua	4 mg	Aqua	Tablet	Character-Shape, Scored	Schering
S; ANB ;	Etrafon-A	4 mg; 10 mg	Orange	Coated Tablet		Schering
S; ANE ;	Etrafon-Forte	25 mg; 4 mg	Red	Coated Tablet		Schering-Plough
S; HYDERGINE 1 ;	Hydergine	1 mg	White	Tablet	Circle	Novartis
S; HYDERGINE; LC; 1 MG	Hydergine Lc	1 mg	Off White	Capsule		Novartis
S; MELLARIL; 25	Mellaril	25 mg	Light Tan	Coated Tablet		Novartis
S; MELLARIL; 50	Mellaril	50 mg	White	Coated Tablet		Novartis
S; MELLARIL; 100	Mellaril	100 mg	Light Green	Coated Tablet		Novartis
S; MELLARIL; 150	Mellaril	150 mg	Yellow	Coated Tablet		Novartis
S; MELLARIL; 200	Mellaril	200 mg	Pink	Coated Tablet		Novartis
S190	Lunesta	1 mg	Light Blue	Tablet	Circle	Sepracor
S191	Lunesta	2 mg	White	Tablet	Circle	Sepracor
S193	Lunesta	3 mg	Dark Blue	Tablet	Circle	Sepracor
S405 250	Fosrenol	250 mg	White to Off-White	Tablet, Chewable	Circle	Shire Us
S405 500	Fosrenol	500 mg	White to Off- White	Tablet, Chewable	Circle	Shire Us
S405 750	Fosrenol	750 mg	White to Off- White	Tablet, Chewable	Circle	Shire Us
S405 1000	Fosrenol	1000 mg	White to Off-White	Tablet, Chewable	Circle	Shire Us
SANDOZ; 78/71 ;	Sanorex	1 mg	White	Tablet	Elliptical; Scored	Novartis Pharmaceuticals
SANDOZ; 78; 36 ;	Cafergot P-B	0.125 mg; 100 mg; 1 mg; 30 mg	Green	Coated Tablet		Novartis Pharmaceuticals
SANDOZ; 78; 38	Cedilanid	0.5 mg	Salmon	Coated Tablet		Novartis Pharmaceuticals
SANDOZ; 78; 45 ;	Glysennid	12 mg	Rose	Coated Tablet		Novartis Consumer
SANDOZ; 78; 45 ;	Glysennid	12 mg	Rose	Coated Tablet		Sandoz Consumer Pharmaceuticals
SANDOZ; 78; 48	Gynergen	1 mg	Ivory Gray	Coated Tablet		Novartis
SANDOZ; 78; 54	Methergine	0.2 mg	Purple	Tablet		Novartis Pharmaceuticals
SANDOZ; 78; 58	Sansert	2 mg	Yellow	Coated Tablet	Circle	Novartis Pharmaceuticals
SANDOZ; 78; 64	Torecan	10 mg	Yellow	Tablet		Novartis Consumer
SANDOZ; 78; 64	Torecan	10 mg	Yellow	Tablet		Sandoz Consumer Pharmaceuticals
SANDOZ; 78; 66	Sanorex	2 mg	White	Tablet	Circle, Scored	Novartis Pharmaceuticals
SANDOZ; S	Belladenal Spacetabs	0.25 mg; 50 mg	Multi-Colored	Tablet		Novartis Pharmaceuticals
SANDOZ-S ;	Bellergal Spacetabs	0.2 mg; 0.6 mg; 40 mg	Multi-Colored	Tablet		Novartis
SANDOZ-S; 78; 33	Caffergot	2 mg; 100 mg;		Suppository		Novartis Pharmaceuticals
SANKYO; C; 12	Benicar	5 mg	Yellow	Tablet	Circle	Daiichi Sankyo
SANKYO; C; 14	Benicar	20 mg	White	Tablet	Circle	Daiichi Sankyo
SANKYO; C01	Welchol	625 mg	White	Tablet		Daiichi Sankyo
SANKYO; C22	Benicar HCT	20 mg; 12.5 mg	Reddish-Yellow	Tablet	Circle	Daiichi Sankyo
SANKYO; C23	Benicar HCT	40 mg; 12.5 mg	Reddish-Yellow	Tablet	Oval	Daiichi Sankyo
SANKYO; C25	Benicar HCT	40 mg; 25 mg	Pink	Tablet	Oval	Daiichi Sankyo
SB 4890	Requip	0.25 mg	White	Tablet	Five-Sided	Glaxosmithkline
SB 4891	Requip	0.5 mg	Yellow	Tablet	Five-Sided	Glaxosmithkline
SB 4892	Requip	1 mg	Green	Tablet	Five-Sided	Glaxosmithkline
SB 4893	Requip	2 mg	Pale Yellowish-Pink	Tablet	Five-Sided	Glaxosmithkline
SB 4894	Requip	5 mg	Blue	Tablet	Five-Sided	Glaxosmithkline
SB 4895	Requip	3 mg	Pale to Moderate Reddish-Purple	Tablet	Five-Sided	Glaxosmithkline
SB 4896	Requip	4 mg	Pale Brown	Tablet	Five-Sided	Glaxosmithkline
SB; 2	Avandia	2 mg	Pink	Coated Tablet	Five-Sided	Glaxosmithkline
SB; 4	Avandia	4 mg	Orange	Coated Tablet	Five-Sided	Glaxosmithkline
SB; 8	Avandia	8 mg	Red-Brown	Coated Tablet	Five-Sided	Glaxosmithkline
SB; 39	Coreg	3.125 mg	White	Coated Tablet	Oval	Glaxosmithkline
SB; 4140	Coreg	6.25 mg	White	Coated Tablet	Oval	Glaxosmithkline
SB; 4141	Coreg	12.5 mg	White	Coated Tablet	Oval	Glaxosmithkline
SB; 4142	Coreg	25 mg	White	Coated Tablet	Oval	Glaxosmithkline
SB; 5500	Albenza	200 mg	White to Off-White	Coated Tablet	Circle, Biconvex, Bevel-Edged	Glaxosmithkline
SCF	Contac Severe Cold and Flu	500 mg; 15 mg; 30 mg; 2 mg	Blue	Tablet		Glaxosmithkline Consumer

IMPRINT	BRAND/GENERIC NAME	STRENGTH	COLOR	FORM	SHAPE	MANUFACTURER
SCHERING 402 ;	Theovent Long-Acting	125 mg	Dark Green and Yellow	Timed-Release Capsule		Schering
SCHERING LOGO	Children's Coricidin Medilets	1 mg; 80 mg	Pink with Green Speckles	Tablet		Schering-Plough Healthcare Products
SCHERING; 011	Celestone	0.6 mg	Pink	Tablet	Circle, Compressed, Scored	Schering
SCHERING; 080	Chlor-Trimeton Allergy	4 mg		Tablet		Schering-Plough Healthcare Products
SCHERING; 095 ;	Polaramine Repetabs	4 mg	Light Red	Timed-Release Tablet	Oval	Schering
SCHERING; 148 ;	Polaramine Repetabs	6 mg	Bright Red	Timed-Release Tablet	Oval	Schering
SCHERING; 228	Fulvicin P/g	125 mg	White	Tablet	Scored, Compressed	Schering
SCHERING; 251	Paxipam	20 mg	Orange	Tablet	Compressed, Scored	Schering
SCHERING; 311 ;	Oreton Methyl	10 mg	White	Tablet	Circle	Schering
SCHERING; 394 ;	Naquival	4 mg; 0.1 mg	Peach	Tablet		Schering-Plough Healthcare Products
SCHERING; 432 ;	Coriforte	190 mg; 130 mg; 30 mg; 500 G; 4 mg	Red and Yellow	Capsule		Schering
SCHERING; 507	Fulvicin P/g	250 mg	White	Tablet	Scored, Compressed	Schering
SCHERING; 522	Coricidin Hbp Cold & Flu	2 mg; 325 mg	Dark Pink	Tablet	Oblong	Schering-Plough Healthcare Products
SCHERING; 525	Eulexin	125 mg	Opaque, Two-Toned Brown	Capsule		Schering
SCHERING; 538	Paxipam	40 mg	White	Tablet	Compressed, Scored	Schering
SCHERING; 734	Gyne-Lotrimin	100 mg	White	Insert	Tombstone	Schering-Plough Healthcare Products
SCHERING; 753 ;	Theovent Long-Acting	250 mg	Dark Green and Clear	Timed-Release Capsule		Schering
SCHERING; 820	Polaramine	2 mg	Red	Tablet	Oval, Compressed	Schering
SCHERING; 901	Chlor-Trimeton Decongestant	4 mg; 60 mg	Blue	Tablet		Schering-Plough
SCHERING; 970 ;	Oreton Methyl	10 mg	Pink to Lavender	Tablet	Oval	Schering
SCHERING; AGT ;	Polaramine Repetabs	2 mg	Red	Tablet	Oval, Compressed	Schering
SCHERING; AUF ;	Fulvicin-U/f	250 mg	White	Tablet	Compressed, Scored	Schering
SCHERING; AUG ;	Fulvicin-U/f	500 mg	White	Tablet	Compressed, Scored	Schering
SCHERING; JE ;	Oreton Methyl	25 mg	Peach	Tablet	Circle	Schering
SCHERING; KEM ;	Meticorten	1 mg	White	Tablet	Compressed	Schering
SCHWARZ 620; 20	Monoket	20 mg	White	Tablet	Circle, Scored	Schwarz Pharma
SCHWARZ; 053 ;	Fedahist Gyrocaps	10 mg; 65 mg	White and Yellow	Timed-Release Capsule		Schwarz Pharma
SCHWARZ; 055 ;	Fedahist Timecaps	8 mg; 120 mg	Clear	Timed-Release Capsule		Schwarz Pharma
SCHWARZ; 0920	Dilatrate-SR	40 mg	Pink and Clear with White Beads	Sustained-Release Capsule		Schwarz Pharma
SCHWARZ; 525	Ku-Zyme Hp	30000 U; 8000 U; 30000 U	White	Capsule		Schwarz Pharma
SCHWARZ; 531	Levsin	0.125 mg	White	Tablet	Circle, Scored	Schwarz Pharma
SCHWARZ; 532	Levsin SL	0.125 mg	White or Pale Blue-Green	Tablet	Eight-Sided, Scored	Schwarz Pharma
SCHWARZ; 532	Levsin/SL	0.125 mg	White	Tablet	Eight-Sided, Scored	Schwarz Pharma
SCHWARZ; 534 ;	Levsin-PB	0.125 mg; 15 mg	Pink	Tablet	Circle, Scored	Schwarz Pharma
SCHWARZ; 537	Levsinex	0.375 mg	Brown and White	Extended-Release Capsule		Schwarz Pharma
SCHWARZ; 610; 10	Monoket	10 mg	White	Tablet	Circle, Scored	Schwarz Pharma
SCHWARZ; 2489; VERELAN; 180 MG	Verelan	180 mg	Yellow and Gray	Sustained-Release Capsule		Schwarz Pharma
SCHWARZ; 2490; VERELAN; 120 MG	Verelan	120 mg	Yellow	Sustained-Release Capsule		Schwarz Pharma
SCHWARZ; 2491; VERELAN; 240 MG	Verelan	240 mg	Blue and Yellow	Sustained-Release Capsule		Schwarz Pharma
SCHWARZ; 2495; VERELAN; 360 MG	Verelan	360 mg	Lavender and Yellow	Sustained-Release Capsule		Schwarz Pharma
SCHWARZ; 4085; 100 MG	Verelan Pm	100 mg	White and Amethyst	Extended-Release Capsule		Schwarz Pharma
SCHWARZ; 4086; 200 MG	Verelan Pm	200 mg	Amethyst	Extended-Release Capsule		Schwarz Pharma
SCHWARZ; 4087; 300 MG	Verelan Pm	300 mg	Lavender and Amethyst	Extended-Release Capsule		Schwarz Pharma
SCHWARZ; 4122	Ku-Zyme	1200 U; 15000 U; 15000 U	Yellow and White	Capsule		Schwarz Pharma
SCHWARZ; 4175	Kutrase	2400 U; 30000 U; 30000 U	Green and White	Capsule		Schwarz Pharma
SCS; 3; 30	Low-Ogestrel White Tablet	0.3 mg; 0.03 mg	White	28-Day Tablet Pack	Circle	Watson Laboratories
SEARLE; 1/2	Haloperidol	0.5 mg	White	Tablet	Circle	Searle
SEARLE; 6	Tri-Norinyl 21-Day	0.5 mg; 35 mcg	Blue	21-Day Tablet Pack	Circle	Watson Laboratories
SEARLE; 7	Tri-Norinyl 21 Day Yellow-Green Tablet	1 mg; 35 mcg	Yellow-Green	21-Day Tablet Pack	Circle	Watson Laboratories
SEARLE; 51; 5	Enovid	5 mg; 75 mcg	Tan	Tablet	Circle	Searle
SEARLE; 61	Lomotil Tablet	2.5 mg; 0.025 mg	White	Tablet	Circle	Searle
SEARLE; 71	Demulen 1/50-21	1 mg; 50 mcg	White	21-Day Tablet Pack	Circle	Searle
SEARLE; 101; 10	Enovid	10 mg; 75 mcg	Brown	Tablet	Circle	Searle
SEARLE; 531	Chlorthalidone	25 mg	Yellow	Tablet	Circle, Scored	Searle
SEARLE; 541	Chlorthalidone	50 mg	Green	Tablet	Circle, Scored	Searle
SEARLE; 571	Furosemide	20 mg	White	Tablet	Circle, Scored	Searle
SEARLE; 581	Furosemide	40 mg	White	Tablet	Circle, Scored	Searle
SEARLE; 631	Pro-Banthine with Phenobarbital	15 mg; 15 mg	Ivory	Tablet		Searle
SEARLE; 651	Pro-Banthine P.A.	30 mg	Peach	Tablet	Capsule-Shape	Searle
SEARLE; 661	Probital	7.5 mg; 15 mg	Pink	Tablet		Searle
SEARLE; 841; 1	Haloperidol	1 mg	White	Tablet	Circle, Scored	Searle
SEARLE; 871; 10	Haloperidol	10 mg	White	Tablet	Circle, Scored	Searle

IMPRINT	BRAND/GENERIC NAME	STRENGTH	COLOR	FORM	SHAPE	MANUFACTURER
SEARLE; 881; 20	Haloperidol	20 mg	White	Tablet	Circle, Scored	Searle
SEARLE; 1001; ALDACTONE; 25	Aldactone	25 mg	Light Yellow	Coated Tablet	Circle	Searle
SEARLE; 1011; ALDACTAZIDE; 25	Aldactazide	25 mg; 25 mg	Tan	Tablet	Circle	Searle
SEARLE; 1021; ALDACTAZIDE; 50	Aldactazide	50 mg; 50 mg	Tan	Coated Tablet	Circle, Scored	Searle
SEARLE; 1031; ALDACTONE; 100	Aldactone	100 mg	Peach	Coated Tablet	Circle, Scored	Searle
SEARLE; 1041; ALDACTONE; 50	Aldactone	50 mg	Light Orange	Coated Tablet	Oval, Scored	Searle
SEARLE; 1231	Aminophyllin	100 mg	White	Tablet	Circle, Scored	Searle
SEARLE; 1251	Aminophyllin	200 mg	White	Tablet	Oval, Scored	Searle
SEARLE; 1291	Amodrine	100 mg; 25 mg; 8 mg	Salmon	Tablet	Oval	Searle
SEARLE; 1301	Kiophyllin	150 mg; 15 mg; 125 mg	White	Tablet	Circle	Searle
SEARLE; 1401	Anavar	2.5 mg	White	Tablet	Oval, Scored	Searle
SEARLE; 1411; AAAA; 50	Arthrotec	50 mg; 200 mcg	White	Tablet	Circle	Searle
SEARLE; 1421; AAAA; 75	Arthrotec	75 mg; 200 mcg	White	Tablet	Circle	Searle
SEARLE; 1451	Cytotec	100 mcg	White	Tablet	Circle	Searle
SEARLE; 1461; STOMACH (2 STOMACHS LAYERED)	Cytotec	200 mcg	White	Tablet	Scored, Six-Sided	Searle
SEARLE; 1501 ;	Pro-Banthine	50 mg	Peach	Tablet	Circle, Scored	Searle
SEARLE; 151	Demulen 1/35 - 28 White Tablet	1 mg; 35 mcg	White	Tablet	Circle	Searle
SEARLE; 151	Demulen 1/35-21	1 mg; 0.035 mg	White	21-Day Tablet Pack	Circle	Searle
SEARLE; 1611	Floraquin	60 mg; 20 mg; 100 mg		Tablet		Searle
SEARLE; 1831; FLAGYL; 250	Flagyl	250 mg	Blue	Coated Tablet	Circle	Searle
SEARLE; 1961; FLAGYL ER	Flagyl ER	750 mg	Blue	Extended-Release Tablet	Oval	Searle
SEARLE; 2101	Ketochol	250 mg	Red	Tablet		Searle
SEARLE; 2732, NORPACE CR; 100 MG	Norpace Cr	100 mg	Green, White	Capsule, Extended Release		Searle
SEARLE; 2742, NORPACE CR; 150 MG	Norpace Cr	150 mg	Green and Brown	Controlled-Release Capsule		Searle
SEARLE; 2752, NORPACE; 100 MG	Norpace	100 mg	Orange, White	Capsule		Searle
SEARLE; 2762, NORPACE; 150 MG	Norpace	150 mg	Brown and Orange	Capsule		Searle
SEARLE; E; 131	Enovid-E	2.5 mg; 0.1 mg	Pink	Tablet	Circle	Searle
SEROQUEL ; 300	Seroquel	300 mg	White	Tablet	Capsule-Shape	Astra Zeneca
SEROQUEL ; 400	Seroquel	400 mg	Yellow	Tablet	Capsule-Shape	Astra Zeneca
SEROQUEL 25	Seroquel	25 mg	Peach	Tablet	Circle	Astra Zeneca
SEROQUEL 50	Seroquel	50 mg	White	Tablet	Circle	Astra Zeneca
SEROQUEL 100	Seroquel	100 mg	Yellow	Tablet	Circle	Astra Zeneca
SEROQUEL 200	Seroquel	200 mg	White	Tablet	Circle	Astra Zeneca
SINAREST	Sinarest Sinus	325 mg; 30 mg; 2 mg	Yellow	Tablet	Circle	Novartis Consumer
SINE-AID; IB	Sine-Aid Ib, Ibuprofen Strength	200 mg; 30 mg	Light Yellow with Red Ink	Tablet		Mcneil Consumer Products
SINE-OFF	Sine-Off Allergy/sinus Maximum Strength	2 mg; 30 mg; 500 mg	Yellow	Tablet		Glaxosmithkline Consumer
SINE-OFF	Sine-Off Maximum Strength	30 mg; 500 mg		Tablet		Glaxosmithkline Consumer
SINEQUAN; ROERIG; 534	Sinequan	10 mg	Pink and Red	Capsule		Pfizer Roerig
SINEQUAN; ROERIG; 535	Sinequan	25 mg	Pink and Blue	Capsule		Pfizer Roerig
SINEQUAN; ROERIG; 536	Sinequan	50 mg	Pink and White	Capsule		Pfizer Roerig
SINEQUAN; ROERIG; 537	Sinequan	150 mg	Blue	Capsule		Pfizer Roerig
SINEQUAN; ROERIG; 538	Sinequan	100 mg	Blue and White	Capsule		Pfizer Roerig
SINEQUAN; ROERIG; 539	Sinequan	75 mg	White	Capsule		Pfizer Roerig
SINGLES; 1	Beta Carotene Centrum Singles	25000 IU	Brown	Gel/jelly	Oblong	Lederle Laboratories
SINGLES; 2	Vitamin E Centrum Singles	400 IU	Pale Clear Yellow	Capsule, Liquid Filled	Oblong	Lederle Laboratories
SINUS; EXCEDRIN	Excedrin Extra Strength Sinus	30 mg; 500 mg	Orange	Tablet	Circle	Bristol-Myers Squibb
SINUTAB	Sinutab Non-Drying Liquid-Capsule	30 mg; 200 mg	Blue	Capsule	Oval	Pfizer Consumer Health Care
SKF S73	Teldrin	12 mg	Green & Clear with Pink & White Pellets	Timed-Release Capsule		Glaxosmithkline Consumer
SKF; 25	Vontrol	25 mg	Orange	Tablet	Circle	Glaxosmithkline
SKF; 101	SK-Ampicillin	250 mg	Yellow and White	Capsule		Glaxosmithkline
SKF; 102	SK-Ampicillin	500 mg	Yellow and White	Capsule		Glaxosmithkline
SKF; 107	SK-Ampicillin	125 mg	White, Scored	Tablet, Chewable		Glaxosmithkline
SKF; 111	SK-Penicillin G	400,000 units	White	Tablet		Glaxosmithkline

IMPRINT	BRAND/GENERIC NAME	STRENGTH	COLOR	FORM	SHAPE	MANUFACTURER
SKF; 112	SK-Penicillin G	800000 U	White	Tablet	Capsule-Shape	Glaxosmithkline
SKF; 116	SK-Penicillin VK	250 mg	White	Tablet		Glaxosmithkline
SKF; 117	SK-Penicillin VK	500 mg		Tablet		Glaxosmithkline
SKF; 120	SK-Amitriptyline	10 mg	White	Tablet		Glaxosmithkline
SKF; 121	SK-Amitriptyline	25 mg	Green	Tablet		Glaxosmithkline
SKF; 122	SK-Digoxin	0.25 mg	White	Tablet		Glaxosmithkline
SKF; 123	SK-Amitriptyline	50 mg	Yellow	Tablet		Glaxosmithkline
SKF; 124	SK-Amitriptyline	75 mg	Green	Tablet		Glaxosmithkline
SKF; 126	SK-Tetracycline	250 mg	Pink and White	Capsule		Glaxosmithkline
SKF; 127	SK-Tetracycline	500 mg	Pink and White	Capsule		Glaxosmithkline
SKF; 129	SK-Niacin	50 mg	White	Tablet		Glaxosmithkline
SKF; 130	SK-Niacin	100 mg	White	Tablet		Glaxosmithkline
SKF; 131	SK-Amitriptyline	100 mg	Yellow	Tablet		Glaxosmithkline
SKF; 132	SK-Amitriptyline	150 mg	White	Tablet		Glaxosmithkline
SKF; 133	SK-Bamate	200 mg		Tablet		Glaxosmithkline
SKF; 134	SK-Bamate	400 mg	White	Tablet		Glaxosmithkline
SKF; 136	SK-Phenobarbital	15 mg	White	Tablet		Glaxosmithkline
SKF; 137	SK-Phenobarbital	30 mg	White	Tablet		Glaxosmithkline
SKF; 163	SK-Soxazole	500 mg	White	Tablet		Glaxosmithkline
SKF; 169	SK-Reserpine	0.25 mg	White	Tablet		Glaxosmithkline
SKF; 171	SK-Quinidine Sulfate	200 mg	White	Tablet		Glaxosmithkline
SKF; 173	SK-Apap	650 mg	White	Tablet	Capsule-Shape	Glaxosmithkline
SKF; 174	SK-Apap	325 mg	White	Tablet		Glaxosmithkline
SKF; 176	SK-Chloral Hydrate	500 mg	Green	Tablet		Glaxosmithkline
SKF; 303	SK-Diphenhydramine	25 mg	Green	Capsule		Glaxosmithkline
SKF; 304	SK-Diphenhydramine	50 mg	White and Green	Capsule		Glaxosmithkline
SKF; 310	SK-Propantheline	15 mg	White	Tablet	Circle	Glaxosmithkline
SKF; 316	SK-Petn	10 mg	White	Tablet		Glaxosmithkline
SKF; 317	SK-Petn	20 mg	White	Tablet		Glaxosmithkline
SKF; 319	SK-Oxycodone with Aspirin	325 mg; 4.5 mg; 0.38 mg	White	Tablet	Oval	Glaxosmithkline
SKF; 320	SK-Oxycodone with Acetaminophen	325 mg; 5 mg	White	Tablet	Circle	Glaxosmithkline
SKF; 321	SK-Pramine	10 mg	Blue	Tablet		Glaxosmithkline
SKF; 322	SK-Pramine	25 mg	Blue	Tablet		Glaxosmithkline
SKF; 323	SK-Pramine	50 mg	Blue	Tablet		Glaxosmithkline
SKF; 324	SK-Apap	325 mg; 15 mg	White	Tablet		Glaxosmithkline Consumer
SKF; 326	SK-Apap	325 mg; 30 mg	White	Tablet		Glaxosmithkline
SKF; 327	SK-Apap	325 mg; 60 mg	White	Tablet		Glaxosmithkline
SKF; 339	SK-Prednisone	5 mg	White	Tablet		Glaxosmithkline
SKF; 340	SK-Furosemide	20 mg		Tablet		Glaxosmithkline
SKF; 341	SK-Furosemide	40 mg		Tablet		Glaxosmithkline
SKF; 363	SK-Hydrochlorothiazide	25 mg		Tablet		Glaxosmithkline
SKF; 364	SK-Hydrochlorothiazide	50 mg		Tablet		Glaxosmithkline
SKF; 367	SK-Erythromycin	250 mg	Yellow	Tablet		Glaxosmithkline
SKF; 369	SK-Erythromycin	500 mg	Yellow	Coated Tablet	Capsule-Shape	Glaxosmithkline
SKF; 371	SK-Thioridazine Hydrochloride	10 mg		Tablet		Glaxosmithkline
SKF; 372	SK-Thioridazine	25 mg		Tablet		Glaxosmithkline
SKF; 373	SK-Thioridazine	50 mg		Tablet		Glaxosmithkline
SKF; 374	SK-Dexamethasone	0.5 mg	Light Yellow	Tablet		Glaxosmithkline
SKF; 375	SK-Thioridazine Hydrochloride	100 mg		Tablet		Glaxosmithkline
SKF; 376	SK-Dexamethasone	0.75 mg	Light Blue	Tablet		Glaxosmithkline
SKF; 377	SK-Dexamethasone	1.5 mg	Pink	Tablet		Glaxosmithkline
SKF; 379	SK-Dipyridamole	25 mg		Tablet		Glaxosmithkline
SKF; 380; 50MG	SK-Dipyridamole	50 mg		Tablet		Glaxosmithkline
SKF; 381; 75MG	SK-Dipyridamole	75 mg		Tablet		Glaxosmithkline
SKF; 403	SK-Triamcinolone	2 mg	Pink	Tablet		Glaxosmithkline
SKF; 404	SK-Triamcinolone	4 mg	White	Tablet		Glaxosmithkline
SKF; 406	SK-Triamcinolone	8 mg	Yellow	Tablet		Glaxosmithkline
SKF; 409	SK-Tolbutamide	500 mg	Peach-Orange	Tablet	Circle	Glaxosmithkline
SKF; 419	SK-Chlorothiazide	250 mg	White	Tablet	Circle	Glaxosmithkline
SKF; 420	SK-Chlorothiazide	500 mg	White	Tablet	Circle	Glaxosmithkline
SKF; 423	SK-Diphenoxylate	0.025 mg; 2.5 mg	White	Tablet		Glaxosmithkline
SKF; 426	SK Metronidazole	250 mg	Off-White	Tablet		Glaxosmithkline
SKF; 441	SK-Lygen	5 mg	Pink	Capsule		Glaxosmithkline
SKF; 442	SK-Lygen	10 mg	Pink and Orange	Capsule		Glaxosmithkline
SKF; 443	SK-Lygen	25 mg	Orange	Capsule		Glaxosmithkline
SKF; 463	SK-65	65 mg	Gray and White	Capsule		Glaxosmithkline
SKF; 468	SK-65 Compound	32.4 mg; 65 mg; 389 mg	Orange and Gray	Capsule		Glaxosmithkline
SKF; 470	SK-Methocarbamol	500 mg	White	Tablet	Oval	Glaxosmithkline
SKF; 471	SK-Methocarbamol	750 mg	White	Tablet	Oval	Glaxosmithkline
SKF; 474	SK-65	650 mg; 65 mg	Orange	Tablet	Capsule-Shape	Glaxosmithkline
SKF; 494	SK-Apap	300 mg; 15 mg	White	Tablet	Circle	Glaxosmithkline
SKF; 499	SK-Probenecid	500 mg	White	Coated Tablet		Glaxosmithkline
SKF; 499	SK-Probenecid	500 mg	White	Tablet	Capsule-Shape, Scored	Glaxosmithkline
SKF; A70	Anspor	250 mg	Orange and White	Capsule		Glaxosmithkline Consumer
SKF; A71	Anspor	500 mg	Orange	Capsule		Glaxosmithkline
SKF; A90	Benzedrine	15 mg	Purple and Clear	Capsule		Glaxosmithkline
SKF; A91	Benzedrine	5 mg		Tablet		Glaxosmithkline
SKF; A92	Benzedrine	10 mg	Peach	Tablet		Glaxosmithkline
SKF; C26	Combid	10 mg; 5 mg	Yellow & Clear	Capsule		Glaxosmithkline Consumer
SKF; C66	Compazine	5 mg	Yellow-Green	Coated Tablet	Circle	Glaxosmithkline
SKF; C67	Compazine	10 mg	Yellow-Green	Coated Tablet	Circle	Glaxosmithkline
SKF; D14	Cytomel	5 mcg	White	Tablet	Circle	Glaxosmithkline
SKF; D16	Cytomel	25 mcg	White	Tablet	Circle, Scored	Glaxosmithkline
SKF; D17	Cytomel	50 mcg	White	Tablet	Circle, Scored	Glaxosmithkline
SKF; D62	Darbid	5 mg	Pink	Tablet	Circle	Glaxosmithkline
SKF; E33	Dibenzyline	10 mg	Red, Coral	Capsule		Glaxosmithkline Consumer

IMPRINT	BRAND/GENERIC NAME	STRENGTH	COLOR	FORM	SHAPE	MANUFACTURER
SKF; H06	Dyrenium	50 mg		Capsule		Glaxosmithkline Consumer
SKF; H07	Dyrenium	100 mg	Red	Capsule		Glaxosmithkline Consumer
SKF; H24	Ecotrin	325 mg	Orange	Enteric-Coated Tablet		Glaxosmithkline Consumer
SKF; H26	Ecotrin	10 Gr	Orange	Enteric-Coated Tablet		Glaxosmithkline
SKF; H74	Eskabarb	65 mg		Capsule		Glaxosmithkline Consumer
SKF; H76	Eskabarb	97 mg	Blue & Clear	Capsule		Glaxosmithkline Consumer
SKF; J10	Eskalith Cr	450 mg	Yellow	Controlled-Release Tablet	Circle	Glaxosmithkline
SKF; J20	Eskaphen B	0.25 Gr; 5 mg	Peach	Tablet		Glaxosmithkline
SKF; J66	Eskatrol	15 mg; 7.5 mg	White and Clear	Capsule		Glaxosmithkline
SKF; K32	Feosol	200 mg	Green	Tablet	Triangle	Glaxosmithkline Consumer
SKF; K33	Feosol Plus	2 mg; 1.7 mcg; 200 mg; 0.4 mg; 50 mg; 2 mg; 2 mg; 1 mg; 325 mg; 10 mg	Green and Red	Capsule		Glaxosmithkline
SKF; K60	Fortespan	6 mg; 6 mg; 6 mg; 15 mcg; 60 mg; 150 mg; 10,000 USP units; 400 USP units	Red and Clear	Capsule		Glaxosmithkline
SKF; P36	Prydon	0.4 mg; 0.305 mg; 0.06 mg; 0.035 mg; 1 Gr	Blue and Clear	Capsule		Glaxosmithkline
SKF; S03	Stelazine	1 mg	Blue	Coated Tablet	Circle	Glaxosmithkline
SKF; S04	Stelazine	2 mg	Blue	Coated Tablet	Circle	Glaxosmithkline
SKF; S06	Stelazine	5 mg	Blue	Coated Tablet	Circle	Glaxosmithkline
SKF; S07	Stelazine	10 mg	Blue	Coated Tablet	Circle	Glaxosmithkline
SKF; S72	Teldrin	8 mg	Green & Clear with Pink & White Pellets	Timed-Release Capsule		Glaxosmithkline Consumer
SKF; T63	Thorazine	30 mg	Orange and Natural	Sustained-Release Capsule		Glaxosmithkline
SKF; T64	Thorazine	75 mg	Orange and Natural	Sustained-Release Capsule		Glaxosmithkline
SKF; T66	Thorazine	150 mg	Orange and Natural	Sustained-Release Capsule		Glaxosmithkline
SKF; T67	Thorazine	200 mg	Opaque Orange Cap and Natural Body	Sustained-Release Capsule		Glaxosmithkline
SKF; T69	Thorazine	300 mg	Opaque Orange Cap and Natural Body	Sustained-Release Capsule		Glaxosmithkline
SKF; T73	Thorazine	10 mg	Orange	Coated Tablet	Circle	Glaxosmithkline
SKF; T74	Thorazine	25 mg	Orange	Coated Tablet	Circle	Glaxosmithkline
SKF; T76	Thorazine	50 mg	Orange	Coated Tablet	Circle	Glaxosmithkline
SKF; T77	Thorazine	100 mg	Orange	Coated Tablet	Circle	Glaxosmithkline
SKF; T79	Thorazine	200 mg	Orange	Coated Tablet	Circle	Glaxosmithkline
SKF; V23	Trophite	10 mg; 25 mcg	Pink	Tablet		Glaxosmithkline
SKF; V24	Troph-Iron	10 mg; 25 mcg	Pink	Tablet		Glaxosmithkline
SL	Simply Sleep	25 mg	Blue	Tablet		Mcneil Consumer Products
SL	Tylenol Simply Sleep	25 mg	Light Blue	Tablet	Capsule-Shape	Mcneil Consumer Products
SL; 433	Trazodone	50 mg	White	Tablet	Circle, Scored	Warner Chilcott
SL; 434	Trazodone	100 mg	White	Tablet	Circle, Scored	Warner Chilcott
SL; 459	Theophylline	300 mg	White	Sustained-Release Tablet	Capsule-Shaped, Bisected Scored	Novartis Generics
SLO-BID; 50 MG; RPR	Slo-Bid Gyrocaps	50 mg	White and Clear with White Pellets	Capsule	Oblong	Aventis Pharmaceuticals
SLO-BID; 75 MG; RPR	Slo-Bid Gyrocaps	75 mg	White and Clear with White Pellets	Extended-Release Capsule	Oblong	Aventis Pharmaceuticals
SLO-BID; 100 MG; RPR	Slo-Bid Gyrocaps	100 mg	White and Clear with White Pellets	Capsule	Oblong	Aventis Pharmaceuticals
SLO-BID; 125 MG; RPR	Slo-Bid Gyrocaps	125 mg	White and Clear with White Pellets	Extended-Release Capsule	Oblong	Aventis Pharmaceuticals
SLO-BID; 200 MG; RPR	Slo-Bid Gyrocaps	200 mg	White and Clear with White Pellets	Capsule	Oblong	Aventis Pharmaceuticals
SLO-BID; 300 MG; RPR	Slo-Bid Gyrocaps	300 mg	White and Clear with White Pellets	Extended-Release Capsule	Oblong	Aventis Pharmaceuticals
SLOW-MAG	Slow-Mag	64 mg	White with Blue Ink	Enteric-Coated Tablet	Circle, Biconvex	Purdue
SMS	Sudafed Cold & Cough Liquid-Capsule	250 mg; 10 mg; 100 mg; 30 mg	Orange	Capsule	Oval	Pfizer Consumer Health Care
SOLATENE; ROCHE	Solatene	30 mg	Blue and Green	Capsule		Roche Pharmaceuticals
SOLVAY ; 5044	Teveten	400 mg	Pink	Tablet	Oval	Kos Pharmaceuticals
SOLVAY ; 5046	Teveten	600 mg	White	Tablet	Capsule-Shape	Kos Pharmaceuticals
SOLVAY ; 5147	Teveten HCT	600 mg; 12.5 mg	Butterscotch	Tablet	Capsule-Shape	Kos Pharmaceuticals
SOLVAY ; 5150	Teveten HCT	600 mg; 25 mg	Brick Red	Tablet	Capsule-Shape	Kos Pharmaceuticals
SP 321 ; 0.25	Niravam	0.25 mg	Yellow	Tablet, Disintegrating	Circle	Schwarz Pharma
SP 322 ; 0.5	Niravam	0.5 mg	Yellow	Tablet, Disintegrating	Circle	Schwarz Pharma
SP 323 ; 1	Niravam	1 mg	White	Tablet, Disintegrating	Circle	Schwarz Pharma
SP 324 ; 2	Niravam	2 mg	White	Tablet, Disintegrating	Circle	Schwarz Pharma
SP; 111	Nulev	0.125 mg	White	Tablet	Circle	Schwarz Pharma
SP; 351	Kemstro	10 mg	White	Disintegrating Tablet	Circle	Schwarz Pharma
SP; 352	Kemstro	20 mg	White	Disintegrating Tablet	Circle	Schwarz Pharma
SP; 431 ;	Proventil Repetabs	4 mg	White	Timed-Release Tablet	Circle	Schering
SP; 538	Levbid	0.375 mg	Light Orange	Extended-Release Tablet	Capsule-Shape, Scored	Schwarz Pharma
SP; 712	Uniretic	12.5 mg; 7.5 mg	Yellow	Coated Tablet	Oval, Scored	Schwarz Pharma
SP; 720	Uniretic	12.5 mg; 15 mg	White	Coated Tablet	Oval, Scored	Schwarz Pharma
SP; 725	Uniretic	25 mg; 15 mg	Yellow	Coated Tablet	Oval, Scored	Schwarz Pharma
SP; 2104; 500; 5	CO-Gesic	5 mg; 500 mg	White	Tablet	Oval, Compressed, Scored	Schwarz Pharma
SP; 2164; 750 MG	Mono-Gesic	750 mg	Pink	Coated Tablet	Oval, Scored	Schwarz Pharma
SP; ADH ;	Trilafon	2 mg	Gray	Coated Tablet		Schering
SP; ADJ ;	Trilafon	8 mg	Gray	Coated Tablet		Schering

IMPRINT	BRAND/GENERIC NAME	STRENGTH	COLOR	FORM	SHAPE	MANUFACTURER
SP; ADK ;	Trilafon	4 mg	Gray	Coated Tablet		Schering
SP; ADM ;	Trilafon	16 mg	Gray	Coated Tablet		Schering
SP; ANA ;	Etrafon 2-10	10 mg; 2 mg	Deep Yellow	Coated Tablet		Schering
SP; ANC ;	Etrafon	25 mg; 2 mg	Pink	Coated Tablet		Schering
SP; WDR ;	Permitil	2.5 mg	Light Orange	Tablet	Oval, Compressed, Scored	Schering
SP; WEG ;	Permitil	10 mg	Light Red	Tablet	Oval, Compressed, Scored	Schering
SP; WFF ;	Permitil	5 mg	Purple-Pink	Tablet	Oval, Compressed, Scored	Schering
SP22 ;	Levatol	20 mg	Yellow	Tablet	Capsule-Shape, Scored	Schwarz Pharma
SP371; 20	Fluxid	20 mg	White	Disintegrating Tablet	Circle, Biconvex	Schwarz Pharma
SP372; 40	Fluxid	40 mg	White	Disintegrating Tablet	Circle, Biconvex	Schwarz Pharma
SPD417 100 MG	Equetro	100 mg	Bluish Green, Yellow	Capsule, Extended Release		Shire
SPD417 200 MG	Equetro	200 mg	Blue, Yellow	Capsule, Extended Release		Shire
SPD417 300 MG	Equetro	300 mg	Blue, Yellow	Capsule, Extended Release		Shire
SPI	Amitiza	24 mcg	Orange	Capsule, Liquid Filled	Oval	Takeda Pharmaceuticals
SQUARE	Maxalt-Mlt	10 mg	White	Tablet	Circle	Merck
SQUIBB 842	Theragran	5000 IU; 3 mg; 9 mcg; 90 mg; 400 IU; 30 IU; 30 mg; 0.4 mg; 10 mg; 30 mcg		Tablet		Bristol-Myers Squibb
SQUIBB; 28	Imipramine Hydrochloride	25 mg		Tablet		Bristol-Myers Squibb
SQUIBB; 39	Imipramine Hydrochloride	10 mg		Tablet		Bristol-Myers Squibb
SQUIBB; 40	Imipramine Hydrochloride	50 mg		Tablet		Bristol-Myers Squibb
SQUIBB; 45	Desipramine Hydrochloride	25 mg		Tablet		Bristol-Myers Squibb
SQUIBB; 63	Ergoloid Mesylates	1 mg		Tablet		Bristol-Myers Squibb
SQUIBB; 105	Sulindac	150 mg		Tablet		Bristol-Myers Squibb
SQUIBB; 107	Sulindac	200 mg		Tablet		Bristol-Myers Squibb
SQUIBB; 109	Vitamin A	25000 IU		Capsule		Bristol-Myers Squibb
SQUIBB; 110	Vitamin A	50000 IU		Capsule		Bristol-Myers Squibb
SQUIBB; 111	Vitamin A	10000 IU		Capsule		Bristol-Myers Squibb
SQUIBB; 112	Vitamin C	250 mg		Tablet		Bristol-Myers Squibb
SQUIBB; 133	Clorazepate	3.75 mg		Tablet		Bristol-Myers Squibb
SQUIBB; 138	Smz-Tmp 400/80	400 mg; 80 mg	White	Tablet	Circle, Scored	Bristol-Myers Squibb
SQUIBB; 139	Chlorpropamide	100 mg	Blue	Tablet	Circle	Bristol-Myers Squibb
SQUIBB; 152	Chlorpropamide	250 mg	Blue	Tablet	Circle	Bristol-Myers Squibb
SQUIBB; 157	Clorazepate Dipotassium	7.5 mg	Peach	Tablet	Circle, Scored	Bristol-Myers Squibb
SQUIBB; 159	Oxazepam	30 mg		Capsule		Bristol-Myers Squibb
SQUIBB; 160	Ethril	250 mg	Pink	Tablet		Bristol-Myers Squibb
SQUIBB; 161	Ethril	500 mg	Pink	Tablet		Bristol-Myers Squibb
SQUIBB; 162	Chlorthalidone	25 mg	Yellow	Tablet	Circle	Bristol-Myers Squibb
SQUIBB; 163	Clorazepate	15 mg	Pink	Tablet	Circle, Scored	Bristol-Myers Squibb
SQUIBB; 171	Smz-Tmp 800/160	800 mg; 160 mg	White	Tablet	Oval, Scored	Bristol-Myers Squibb
SQUIBB; 180	Chlorthalidone	50 mg		Tablet		Bristol-Myers Squibb
SQUIBB; 187	Chlorthalidone	100 mg	White	Tablet	Circle	Bristol-Myers Squibb
SQUIBB; 192	Ascorbic Acid	50 mg		Tablet		Bristol-Myers Squibb
SQUIBB; 193	Perphenazine with Amitriptyline 2/10	2 mg; 10 mg	Blue	Coated Tablet	Circle	Bristol-Myers Squibb
SQUIBB; 195	Tolazamide	100 mg	White	Tablet	Circle	Bristol-Myers Squibb
SQUIBB; 196	Ascorbic Acid	250 mg		Tablet		Bristol-Myers Squibb
SQUIBB; 202	Dicloxacillin Sodium	250 mg	Blue and White or Green and Light Green	Capsule		Bristol-Myers Squibb
SQUIBB; 203	Dicloxacillin Sodium	500 mg	Blue and White or Green and Light Green	Capsule		Bristol-Myers Squibb
SQUIBB; 204	B Complex Vitamin	9 mg; 0.7 mg; 0.7 mg; 0.9 mg; 2 mcg		Tablet		Bristol-Myers Squibb
SQUIBB; 211	Cloxacillin Sodium	250 mg		Capsule		Bristol-Myers Squibb
SQUIBB; 212	Cloxacillin Sodium	500 mg		Capsule		Bristol-Myers Squibb
SQUIBB; 230	Trimox	250 mg	Green	Capsule		Bristol-Myers Squibb
SQUIBB; 243	Corgard	100 mg		Tablet		Bristol-Myers Squibb
SQUIBB; 259	Perphenazine and Amitriptyline 2/25	2 mg; 25 mg	Orange	Coated Tablet	Circle	Bristol-Myers Squibb
SQUIBB; 267	Perphenazine and Amitriptyline 4/10	4 mg; 10 mg	Salmon	Coated Tablet	Circle	Bristol-Myers Squibb
SQUIBB; 271	Perphenazine and Amitriptyline 4/25	4 mg; 25 mg	Yellow	Coated Tablet	Circle	Bristol-Myers Squibb
SQUIBB; 274	Trazodone	50 mg	White	Tablet	Circle	Bristol-Myers Squibb
SQUIBB; 275	Triamterene and Hydrochlorothiazide	25 mg; 50 mg		Capsule		Bristol-Myers Squibb
SQUIBB; 277	Tolazamide	250 mg		Tablet		Bristol-Myers Squibb
SQUIBB; 279	Isosorbide Dinitrate	40 mg		Tablet		Bristol-Myers Squibb
SQUIBB; 280	Indomethacin	25 mg	Green	Capsule		Bristol-Myers Squibb
SQUIBB; 286	Quinidine Gluconate	324 mg	White	Sustained-Release Tablet	Circle	Bristol-Myers Squibb
SQUIBB; 289	Clonidine	0.1 mg		Tablet		Bristol-Myers Squibb
SQUIBB; 295	Indomethacin	50 mg	Green	Capsule		Bristol-Myers Squibb
SQUIBB; 297	Engran	6000 U; 400 U; 3 mg; 3 mg; 2 mg; 2 mcg; 20 mg; 5 mg; 75 mg; 100 mg; 0.15 mg; 45 mg; 1 mg; 1 mg; 1.5 mg	Blue	Tablet		Bristol-Myers Squibb
SQUIBB; 298	Lorazepam	0.5 mg	White	Tablet	Circle	Bristol-Myers Squibb

IMPRINT	BRAND/GENERIC NAME	STRENGTH	COLOR	FORM	SHAPE	MANUFACTURER
SQUIBB; 300	Prazosin Hydrochloride	1 mg		Capsule		Bristol-Myers Squibb
SQUIBB; 325	Trifluoperazine	10 mg	Lavender	Coated Tablet	Circle	Bristol-Myers Squibb
SQUIBB; 327	Triamterene and Hydrochlorothiazide	25 mg; 50 mg		Tablet		Bristol-Myers Squibb
SQUIBB; 341	Theragran-Z	12 mg; 10000 IU; 400 IU; 15 mg; 100 mg; 20 mg; 150 mcg; 2 mg; 22.5 mg; 1 mg; 0.6 mg; 0.68 mg; 200 mg; 10 mg; 10 mg; 5 mg; 5 mcg	Brown	Tablet	Capsule-Shape	Bristol-Myers Squibb
SQUIBB; 348	Indomethacin SR	75 mg	Green and Clear	Capsule		Bristol-Myers Squibb
SQUIBB; 355	Valadol	325 mg	White	Tablet		Bristol-Myers Squibb
SQUIBB; 357	Valadol	120 mg	Yellow	Tablet, Chewable		Bristol-Myers Squibb
SQUIBB; 359	Furosemide	20 mg	White	Tablet	Oval	Bristol-Myers Squibb
SQUIBB; 360	Furosemide	40 mg	White	Tablet	Circle	Bristol-Myers Squibb
SQUIBB; 365	Trifluoperazine	1 mg	Lavender	Coated Tablet	Circle	Bristol-Myers Squibb
SQUIBB; 368	Trifluoperazine	2 mg	Lavender	Coated Tablet	Circle	Bristol-Myers Squibb
SQUIBB; 371	Digitoxin	0.1 mg		Tablet		Bristol-Myers Squibb
SQUIBB; 386	Carisoprodol	350 mg	White	Tablet	Circle	Bristol-Myers Squibb
SQUIBB; 399	Trifluoperazine	5 mg	Lavender	Coated Tablet	Circle	Bristol-Myers Squibb
SQUIBB; 400	Prazosin Hydrochloride	2 mg		Capsule		Bristol-Myers Squibb
SQUIBB; 408	Lorazepam	1 mg	White	Tablet	Circle	Bristol-Myers Squibb
SQUIBB; 433	Methyldopa	500 mg	White	Coated Tablet	Circle	Bristol-Myers Squibb
SQUIBB; 447	Methyldopa	250 mg	White	Coated Tablet	Circle	Bristol-Myers Squibb
SQUIBB; 457	Mycostatin	100000 U	Ivory	Tablet		Bristol-Myers Squibb
SQUIBB; 476 ;	Engram-Hp	9 mg; 4000 IU; 200 IU; 10 mg; 0.4 mg; 325 mg; 75 mcg; 50 mg; 0.85 mg; 1.25 mg; 4 mcg; 30 mg		Tablet		Bristol-Myers Squibb
SQUIBB; 487	Lorazepam	2 mg	White	Tablet	Circle	Bristol-Myers Squibb
SQUIBB; 488	Metronidazole	250 mg	White	Tablet	Circle	Bristol-Myers Squibb
SQUIBB; 500	Prazosin Hydrochloride	5 mg		Capsule		Bristol-Myers Squibb
SQUIBB; 504	Kenacort	2 mg	White	Tablet		Bristol-Myers Squibb
SQUIBB; 511	Kenacort	1 mg	White	Tablet		Bristol-Myers Squibb
SQUIBB; 512	Kenacort	4 mg	White	Tablet		Bristol-Myers Squibb
SQUIBB; 518	Kenacort	8 mg	Yellow	Tablet		Bristol-Myers Squibb
SQUIBB; 520	B Complex with Vitamin C	10 mg; 10 mg; 2 mg; 4 mcg; 300 mg; 100 mg		Tablet		Bristol-Myers Squibb
SQUIBB; 534	Clonidine	0.3 mg		Tablet		Bristol-Myers Squibb
SQUIBB; 538	Rautrax-N Modified	50 mg; 2 mg; 400 mg		Tablet		Bristol-Myers Squibb
SQUIBB; 539	Rautrax-N	50 mg; 4 mg; 400 mg		Tablet		Bristol-Myers Squibb
SQUIBB; 549	Iron with Vitamin C	50 mg; 25 mg		Tablet		Bristol-Myers Squibb
SQUIBB; 560	Disopyramide	100 mg		Capsule		Bristol-Myers Squibb
SQUIBB; 567	Disopyramide	150 mg		Capsule		Bristol-Myers Squibb
SQUIBB; 572	Metronidazole	500 mg	White	Tablet	Oblong	Bristol-Myers Squibb
SQUIBB; 573	Ora-Testryl	5 mg		Tablet		Bristol-Myers Squibb
SQUIBB; 574	Oxazepam	10 mg		Capsule		Bristol-Myers Squibb
SQUIBB; 598	Neomycin Sulfate	350 mg		Tablet		Bristol-Myers Squibb
SQUIBB; 599	Oxazepam	15 mg		Capsule		Bristol-Myers Squibb
SQUIBB; 602	Naturetin with K	2.5 mg; 500 mg		Tablet		Bristol-Myers Squibb
SQUIBB; 615	Propoxyphene Hydrochloride	65 mg	Green and Orange	Capsule		Bristol-Myers Squibb
SQUIBB; 619	Propoxyphene Hydrochloride and A.P.C.	65 mg; 227 mg; 162 mg; 32.4 mg	Green and Gray	Capsule		Bristol-Myers Squibb
SQUIBB; 622	Meclofenamate	50 mg	Maroon and Pink	Capsule		Bristol-Myers Squibb
SQUIBB; 623	Noctec	250 mg	Red	Capsule		Bristol-Myers Squibb
SQUIBB; 626	Noctec	500 mg	Red	Capsule		Bristol-Myers Squibb
SQUIBB; 629	Meclofenamate	100 mg	Maroon and White	Capsule		Bristol-Myers Squibb
SQUIBB; 630	Methyldopa and Hydrochlorothiazide	250 mg; 15 mg	Red	Coated Tablet	Circle	Bristol-Myers Squibb
SQUIBB; 637	Nydrazid	100 mg		Tablet		Bristol-Myers Squibb
SQUIBB; 645	Methyldopa and Hydrochlorothiazide	250 mg; 25 mg	Pink	Coated Tablet	Circle	Bristol-Myers Squibb
SQUIBB; 649	Trigot	0.5 mg	White	Tablet		Bristol-Myers Squibb
SQUIBB; 652	Methyldopa and Hydrochlorothiazide	500 mg; 30 mg	Red	Coated Tablet	Oval	Bristol-Myers Squibb
SQUIBB; 654	Trigot	1 mg	White	Tablet		Bristol-Myers Squibb
SQUIBB; 671	Methyldopa and Hydrochlorothiazide	500 mg; 50 mg	Pink	Coated Tablet	Oval	Bristol-Myers Squibb
SQUIBB; 685	Rautrax	50 mg; 400 mg; 400 mg		Tablet		Bristol-Myers Squibb
SQUIBB; 690	Teslac	50 mg	White	Tablet	Biconvex	Bristol-Myers Squibb
SQUIBB; 692	Tolbutamide	500 mg	White	Tablet		Bristol-Myers Squibb
SQUIBB; 693 ;	Hydrochlorothiazide	25 mg	White	Tablet		Bristol-Myers Squibb
SQUIBB; 694 ;	Hydrochlorothiazide	50 mg	White	Tablet		Bristol-Myers Squibb
SQUIBB; 718	Chlordiazepoxide Hydrochloride	5 mg	Carmel and Yellow	Capsule		Bristol-Myers Squibb
SQUIBB; 723	Phenytoin Sodium	100 mg	White	Extended-Release Capsule		Bristol-Myers Squibb
SQUIBB; 727	Chlordiazepoxide Hydrochloride	10 mg	Carmel and Black	Capsule		Bristol-Myers Squibb
SQUIBB; 736	Chlordiazepoxide Hydrochloride	25 mg	Carmel and White	Capsule		Bristol-Myers Squibb
SQUIBB; 738	Temazepam	15 mg	Pink	Capsule		Bristol-Myers Squibb

IMPRINT	BRAND/GENERIC NAME	STRENGTH	COLOR	FORM	SHAPE	MANUFACTURER
SQUIBB; 749 ;	Cephalexin	250 mg	Swedish Orange and Gray	Capsule		Bristol-Myers Squibb
SQUIBB; 780	Rau-Sed	0.25 mg		Tablet		Bristol-Myers Squibb
SQUIBB; 788	Vitamin B-12	25 mcg		Capsule		Bristol-Myers Squibb
SQUIBB; 802	Clorazepate Dipotassium	3.75 mg	White	Capsule		Bristol-Myers Squibb
SQUIBB; 829	Chlorothiazide	500 mg	White	Tablet	Compressed	Bristol-Myers Squibb
SQUIBB; 831	Vitamin E	200 mg		Tablet		Bristol-Myers Squibb
SQUIBB; 838	Clorazepate	7.5 mg		Capsule		Bristol-Myers Squibb
SQUIBB; 845	Allopurinol	100 mg	White	Tablet	Circle	Bristol-Myers Squibb
SQUIBB; 849	Multiple Vitamins and Minerals	5000 IU; 30 IU; 500 mg; 20 mg; 20 mg; 100 mg; 25 mg; 0.15 mg; 25 mg; 0.8 mg; 50 mcg; 27 mg; 0.1 mg; 50 mg; 5 mg; 3 mg; 22.5 mg		Tablet		Bristol-Myers Squibb
SQUIBB; 851	Triamterene and Hydrochlorothiazide	75 mg; 50 mg	Yellow	Tablet	Circle, Scored	Bristol-Myers Squibb
SQUIBB; 876	Trigesic	125 mg; 230 mg; 30 mg		Tablet		Bristol-Myers Squibb
SQUIBB; 883	Doxycycline Hyclate	50 mg	White and Brown	Capsule, Liquid Filled		Bristol-Myers Squibb
SQUIBB; 884	Doxycycline Hyclate	100 mg	Brown	Capsule, Liquid Filled		Bristol-Myers Squibb
SQUIBB; 889	Vitamin E	74 mg		Capsule		Bristol-Myers Squibb
SQUIBB; 897	Doxycycline Hyclate	100 mg	Orange	Coated Tablet		Bristol-Myers Squibb
SQUIBB; 915	Vitamin B-1	50 mg		Tablet		Bristol-Myers Squibb
SQUIBB; 916	Vitamin B-1	100 mg		Tablet		Bristol-Myers Squibb
SQUIBB; 921	Vesprin	10 mg	Pink	Tablet		Bristol-Myers Squibb
SQUIBB; 922	Vesprin	25 mg	White and Orange	Tablet		Bristol-Myers Squibb
SQUIBB; 923	Vesprin	50 mg	Green	Tablet		Bristol-Myers Squibb
SQUIBB; 963	Trazodone	100 mg		Tablet		Bristol-Myers Squibb
SQUIBB; 1535	Loxapine Succinate	50 mg		Capsule		Bristol-Myers Squibb
SQUIBB; E.T.	E.T. the Extraterrestrial Children's Chewable Vitamins	5000 IU; 400 IU; 30 IU; 0.4 mg; 1.5 mg; 1.7 mg; 20 mg; 60 mg; 2 mg; 6 mcg	Purple, Orange and Pink	Tablet, Chewable		Bristol-Myers Squibb
SQUIBB; E.T.	E.T. the Extraterrestrial Children's Chewable Vitamins with Iron	5000 IU; 400 IU; 30 IU; 0.4 mg; 1.5 mg; 1.7 mg; 20 mg; 18 mg; 60 mg; 2 mg; 6 mcg	Purple, Orange and Pink	Tablet, Chewable		Bristol-Myers Squibb
SQUIBB; W048	Dicloxacillin	250 mg	Blue	Capsule		Sandoz
SQUIBB; W048	Dicloxacillin Sodium	250 mg		Capsule		Bristol-Myers Squibb
SQUIBB; W058	Dicloxacillin Sodium	500 mg		Capsule		Bristol-Myers Squibb
SQUIBB; W134	Lithium Carbonate	300 mg		Capsule		Bristol-Myers Squibb
SQUIBB; W470	Desipramine Hydrochloride	75 mg		Tablet		Bristol-Myers Squibb
STARLIX; 60	Starlix	60 mg	Pink	Tablet	Circle, Bevel Edged	Novartis
STARLIX; 120	Starlix	120 mg	Yellow	Tablet	Oval	Novartis
STASON; 1020	Selegiline Hydrochloride	5 mg	White	Tablet	Circle	Duramed Pharmaceuticals
STUART	Orexin Softab	10 mg; 5 mg; 25 mcg	Pink	Tablet	Circle, Biconvex	Johnson & Johnson Merck Consumer Pharmaceuticals
STUART; 380	Kasof	240 mg	Brown	Capsule		Johnson & Johnson Merck Consumer Pharmaceuticals
STUART; 450	Mylicon	40 mg	White	Tablet	Circle, Biconvex	Johnson & Johnson Merck Consumer Pharmaceuticals
STUART; 650	Ferancee	3.1 Gr; 150 mg	Brown and Gold	Tablet, Chewable		Johnson & Johnson Merck Consumer Pharmaceuticals
STUART; 851	Mylanta II	400 mg; 400 mg; 40 mg	Green and White	Tablet, Chewable		Johnson & Johnson Merck Consumer Pharmaceuticals
STUART; 858	Mylicon 80	80 mg	Pink	Tablet, Chewable	Circle, Beveled	Johnson & Johnson Merck Consumer Pharmaceuticals
SU	Sudafed	30 mg	Red	Coated Tablet		Pfizer Consumer Health Care
SU; 24	Sudafed 24 Hour	240 mg		Extended-Release Tablet	Oval	Pfizer Consumer Health Care
SUDAFED 12 HOUR; H9B	Sudafed 12 Hour	120 mg	Red and Clear	Extended-Release Capsule		Pfizer Consumer Health Care
SUDAFED C&S	Sudafed Cold and Sinus Liquid Caps	325 mg; 30 mg	Blue	Capsule, Liquid Filled	Oval	Pfizer Consumer Health Care
SUDAFED PLUS ;	Sudafed Plus Tablet	60 mg; 4 mg		Tablet		Pfizer Consumer Health Care
SUDAFED; 60	Sudafed	60 mg	Red	Tablet		Pfizer Consumer Health Care
SUDAFED; SCF	Sudafed Severe Cold Formula	500 mg; 15 mg; 30 mg	White	Coated Tablet	Circle	Pfizer Consumer Health Care
SUDAFED; SCF	Sudafed Severe Cold Formula	500 mg; 15 mg; 30 mg	White	Tablet	Circle	Pfizer Consumer Health Care
SUDAFED; SINUS	Sudafed Non-Drying Sinus Liquid Caps	200 mg; 30 mg	Clear Turquoise	Capsule		Pfizer Consumer Health Care
SUDAFED; SINUS	Sudafed Sinus Headache	500 mg; 30 mg	Peach	Tablet		Pfizer Consumer Health Care
SUDAL; 60; A; P	Sudal 60/500	60 mg; 500 mg	White	Tablet	Capsule-Shape, Scored	Atley Pharmaceuticals
SUDAL; SR; A; P	Sudal SR	50 mg; 1200 mg	White	Extended-Release Tablet	Capsule-Shape	Atley Pharmaceuticals
SUNKIST 60, SUNKIST LOGO, ORANGE SLICE	Sunkist Vitamin C	60 mg	White	Tablet, Chewable	Circle	Novartis Consumer
SUNKIST 250, SUNKIST LOGO, ORANGE SLICE	Sunkist Vitamin C	250 mg	White, Flat	Tablet, Chewable	Circle	Novartis Consumer
SUNKIST 500, SUNKIST LOGO, ORANGE SLICE	Sunkist Vitamin C	500 mg	White	Tablet, Chewable	Circle	Novartis Consumer

IMPRINT	BRAND/GENERIC NAME	STRENGTH	COLOR	FORM	SHAPE	MANUFACTURER
SUNKIST V	Sunkist Multivitamins, Children's Regular	2500 IU; 15 IU; 0.3 mg; 13.5 mg; 400 IU; 60 mg; 1.05 mg; 4.5 mcg; 1.05 mg; 1.2 mg; 5 mcg	Orange, Yellow and Pinkish-Rose	Tablet, Chewable	Circle, Flat	Novartis Consumer
SUNKIST V+M	Sunkist Multivitamins Children's	10 mg; 5000 IU; 400 IU; 30 IU; 60 mg; 0.4 mg; 40 mcg; 10 mg; 20 mg; 2 mg; 6 mcg; 1.5 mg; 1.7 mg; 10 mcg; 20 mg; 150 mcg; 10 mg; 1 mg; 100 mg; 78 mg; 2 mg	Yellow, Orange and Pinkish-Rose	Tablet, Chewable	Circle	Novartis Consumer
SUNKIST XC	Sunkist Multivitamins Plus Extra C	2500 IU; 400 IU; 15 IU; 250 mg; 0.3 mg; 13.5 mg; 1.05 mg; 4.5 mcg; 1.05 mg; 1.2 mg; 5 mcg	Yellow, Orange and Pinkish-Rose	Tablet	Circle, Flat	Novartis Consumer
SUNKIST; 500	Sunkist Vitamin C	500 mg	White to Off-White	Tablet		Novartis Consumer
SUNKIST; V+FE	Sunkist Multivitamins with Iron Children's	15 mg; 2500 IU; 15 IU; 0.3 mg; 13.5 mg; 400 IU; 60 mg; 1.05 mg; 4.5 mcg; 1.05 mg; 1.2 mg; 5 mcg	Orange, Yellow and Pinkish-Rose	Tablet, Chewable	Circle	Novartis Consumer
SUPRAX; LL; 200	Suprax	200 mg	White	Coated Tablet	Rectangle, Scored, Convex	Lederle Laboratories
SUPRAX; LL; 400	Suprax	400 mg	White	Coated Tablet	Rectangle, Scored, Convex	Lederle Laboratories
SURFAK	Surfak Liqui-Gels	240 mg	Dark Purple	Capsule, Liquid Filled	Oblong	Pharmacia & Upjohn
SUSTIVA; 50 MG	Sustiva	50 mg	Gold and White	Capsule		Bristol-Myers Squibb
SUSTIVA; 100 MG	Sustiva	100 mg	White	Capsule		Bristol-Myers Squibb
SUSTIVA; 200 MG	Sustiva	200 mg	Gold	Capsule		Bristol-Myers Squibb
SUSTIVA; SUSTIVA	Sustiva	600 mg	Yellow	Coated Tablet	Capsule-Shape	Bristol-Myers Squibb
SW; 200	Skelid	200 mg	White to Off-White	Tablet	Circle	Sanofi Winthrop Pharmaceuticals
SW; 200	Skelid	200 mg	White to Off-White	Tablet	Circle	Sanofi-Aventis U.S.
SYMMETREL	Symmetrel	100 mg	Light Orange	Tablet	Triangle, Convex	Endo Laboratories
SYNTEX	Norminest Fe-28 Blue Tablet	0.5 mg; 0.035 mg	Blue	28-Day Tablet Pack		Roche Laboratories
SYNTEX; 2902	Anadrol	50 mg	White	Tablet		Roche Laboratories
SYNTEX; TORADOL; T	Toradol Oral	10 mg		Coated Tablet	Circle	Roche Laboratories
SYNTHROID; 25 ;	Synthroid	25 mcg	Orange	Tablet		Abbott Laboratories
SYNTHROID; 50 ;	Synthroid	50 mcg	White	Tablet		Abbott Laboratories
SYNTHROID; 75 ;	Synthroid	75 mcg	Violet	Tablet		Abbott Laboratories
SYNTHROID; 88 ;	Synthroid	88 mcg	Olive	Tablet	Circle, Scored	Abbott Laboratories
SYNTHROID; 100 ;	Synthroid	100 mcg	Yellow	Tablet		Abbott Laboratories
SYNTHROID; 112 ;	Synthroid	112 mcg	Rose	Tablet		Abbott Laboratories
SYNTHROID; 125 ;	Synthroid	125 mcg	Brown	Tablet		Abbott Laboratories
SYNTHROID; 137	Synthroid	137 mcg	Turquoise	Tablet		Abbott Laboratories
SYNTHROID; 150 ;	Synthroid	150 mcg	Blue	Tablet		Abbott Laboratories
SYNTHROID; 175	Synthroid	175 mcg	Lilac	Tablet		Abbott Laboratories
SYNTHROID; 200 ;	Synthroid	200 mcg	Pink	Tablet		Abbott Laboratories
SYNTHROID; 300 ;	Synthroid	300 mcg	Green	Tablet		Abbott Laboratories
SZ 183	Cafergot	1 mg; 100 mg	Beige	Tablet	Circle	Novartis Pharmaceuticals
SZ 183	Cafergot	1 mg; 100 mg	Beige	Tablet	Circle	Sandoz
SZ 301 ;	Cyclobenzaprine Hydrochloride	5 mg	Orange	Tablet	Circle	Sandoz
T	Potassium Bicarbonate	25 meq	Orange	Effervescent Tablet	Circle	Watson Laboratories
T	Teldrin	4 mg	Green	Tablet	Circle	Glaxosmithkline Consumer
T	Tessalon Perles	100 mg	Yellow	Capsule		Forest Pharmaceuticals
T 25	Tarceva	25 mg	White	Tablet	Circle	Genentech
T 100	Tarceva	100 mg	White	Tablet	Circle	Genentech
T 150	Tarceva	150 mg	White	Tablet	Circle	Genentech
T D ; C G	Trileptal	150 mg	Pale Grey-Green	Tablet	Oval	Novartis
T; 2	Enalapril Maleate	2.5 mg	Yellow	Tablet	Circle, Scored	Taro Pharmaceuticals
T; 5	Enalapril Maleate	5 mg	Yellow	Tablet	Circle, Scored	Taro Pharmaceuticals
T; 20	Enalapril Maleate	20 mg	Orange	Tablet	Circle	Taro Pharmaceuticals
T; 31	Warfarin Sodium	1 mg	Pink	Tablet	Capsule-Shape, Scored	Taro Pharmaceuticals
T; 32	Warfarin Sodium	2 mg	Lavender	Tablet	Capsule-Shape, Scored	Taro Pharmaceuticals
T; 33	Warfarin Sodium	2.5 mg	Green	Tablet	Capsule-Shape, Scored	Taro Pharmaceuticals
T; 34	Warfarin Sodium	4 mg	Blue	Tablet	Capsule-Shape, Scored	Taro Pharmaceuticals
T; 35	Warfarin Sodium	5 mg	Peach	Tablet	Capsule-Shape, Scored	Taro Pharmaceuticals
T; 36	Warfarin Sodium	7.5 mg	Yellow	Tablet	Capsule-Shape, Scored	Taro Pharmaceuticals
T; 37	Warfarin Sodium	10 mg	White	Tablet	Capsule-Shape, Scored	Taro Pharmaceuticals
T; 38	Warfarin Sodium	3 mg	Tan	Tablet	Capsule-Shape, Scored	Taro Pharmaceuticals
T; 39	Warfarin Sodium	6 mg	Greenish-Yellow	Tablet	Capsule-Shape, Scored	Taro Pharmaceuticals
T; 45	Clorazepate Dipotassium	3.75 mg	Pale Violet	Tablet	Circle, Flat, Scored	Taro Pharmaceuticals
T; 46	Clorazepate Dipotassium	7.5 mg	Orange	Tablet	Circle, Flat, Scored	Taro Pharmaceuticals
T; 47	Clorazepate Dipotassium	15 mg	Pale Pink	Tablet	Circle, Flat, Scored	Taro Pharmaceuticals
T; 52	Acetazolamide	125 mg	White	Tablet	Circle, Scored	Taro Pharmaceuticals
T; 53	Acetazolamide	250 mg	White	Tablet	Round, Quadrisected Scored	Taro Pharmaceuticals
T; 57	Ketoconazole	200 mg	White to Off-White	Tablet	Flat, Scored	Taro Pharmaceuticals
T; 93	Isoniazid	100 mg		Tablet		Eli Lilly
T; 100 MG	Tegretol-Xr	100 mg	Yellow	Extended-Release Tablet	Circle	Novartis
T; 107	Tenormin	25 mg	White	Tablet	Circle, Flat	Astra Zeneca
T; 109	Carbamazepine	200 mg	White	Tablet	Circle, Single Scored	Teva Pharmaceuticals
T; 200 MG	Tegretol-Xr	200 mg	Pink	Extended-Release Tablet	Circle	Novartis

IMPRINT	BRAND/GENERIC NAME	STRENGTH	COLOR	FORM	SHAPE	MANUFACTURER
T; 400 MG	Tegretol-Xr	400 mg	Brown	Extended-Release Tablet	Circle	Novartis
T0R; ORGANON	Cyclessa Light Yellow Tablet	0.1 mg; 0.025 mg	Light Yellow	Coated Tablet	Circle	Organon
T1R; ORGANON	Cyclessa Red Tablet	0.15 mg; 0.025 mg	Red	Coated Tablet	Circle	Organon
T3	Enalapril and Hydrochlorothiazide	10 mg; 25 mg	Peach	Tablet	Capsule-Shape	Taro Pharmaceuticals
T4	Enalapril and Hydrochlorothiazide	5 mg; 12.5 mg	Ivory	Tablet	Capsule-Shape	Taro Pharmaceuticals
T6R; ORGANON	Cyclessa Orange Tablet	0.125 mg; 0.025 mg	Orange	Coated Tablet	Circle	Organon
T36	Calcium Gluconate	1 GM		Tablet		Eli Lilly
T88	Etodolac	400 mg	Peach	Tablet	Oval	Taro Pharmaceuticals
T400	Etodolac	400 mg	Pink	Tablet, Extended Release	Circle	Taro Pharmaceuticals
T500	Etodolac	500 mg	Green	Tablet, Extended Release	Oblong	Taro Pharmaceuticals
T600	Etodolac	600 mg	Grey	Tablet, Extended Release	Oval	Taro Pharmaceuticals
TAGAMET HB; 200	Tagamet Hb 200	200 mg	White	Tablet	Diamond	Glaxosmithkline Consumer
TAGAMET; 200; SKF	Tagamet	200 mg	Light-Green	Coated Tablet	Circle	Glaxosmithkline
TAGAMET; 300; SB	Tagamet	300 mg	Light-Green	Coated Tablet	Circle	Glaxosmithkline
TAGAMET; 800; SB	Tagamet	800 mg	Light-Green	Coated Tablet	Oval	Glaxosmithkline
TAGAMET; HB; SB	Tagamet Hb	100 mg	White	Coated Tablet	Circle	Glaxosmithkline
TAK RAM-8	Rozerem	8 mg	Pale Orange-Yellow	Tablet	Circle	Takeda Pharmaceuticals
TAP LOGO; PREVACID 15	Prevacid Naprapac 375 - Prevacid	15 mg	Green, Pink	Capsule, Delayed Release		Tap Pharmaceuticals
TAP LOGO; PREVACID 15	Prevacid Naprapac 500 - Prevacid	15 mg	Green, Pink	Capsule, Delayed Release		Tap Pharmaceuticals
TAP; 200 MG	Spectracef	200 mg	White with Blue Ink	Coated Tablet	Circle	Tap Pharmaceuticals
TAP; PREVACID; 15	Prevacid	15 mg	Pink and Green	Delayed-Release Capsule		Tap Pharmaceuticals
TAP; PREVACID; 30	Prevacid	30 mg	Pink and Black	Delayed-Release Capsule		Tap Pharmaceuticals
TARACTAN; ROCHE 10	Taractan	10 mg	Light Coral	Coated Tablet		Roche Pharmaceuticals
TARACTAN; ROCHE 25	Taractan	25 mg	Coral	Coated Tablet		Roche Pharmaceuticals
TARACTAN; ROCHE 50	Taractan	50 mg	Pinkish Orange	Coated Tablet		Roche Pharmaceuticals
TARACTAN; ROCHE 100	Taractan	100 mg	Reddish Brown	Coated Tablet		Roche Pharmaceuticals
TARKA; 182; KNOLL TRIANGLE	Tarka 2/180 mg	2 mg; 180 mg	Pink	Sustained-Release Tablet	Oval	Abbott Laboratories
TARKA; 241; KNOLL TRIANGLE ;	Tarka 1/240 mg	1 mg; 240 mg	White	Sustained-Release Tablet	Oval	Abbott Laboratories
TARKA; 242; KNOLL TRIANGLE ;	Tarka 2/240 mg	2 mg; 240 mg	Gold	Sustained-Release Tablet	Oval	Abbott Laboratories
TARKA; 244; KNOLL TRIANGLE ;	Tarka 4/240 mg	4 mg; 240 mg	Red-Brown	Sustained-Release Tablet	Oval	Abbott Laboratories
TARO ; 89	Etodolac	500 mg	Blue	Tablet	Oval	Taro Pharmaceuticals
TARO 56	Amiodarone Hydrochloride	200 mg	Light Orange	Tablet	Circle	Taro Pharmaceuticals
TARO 59	Amiodarone Hydrochloride	400 mg	Light Yellow	Tablet	Circle	Taro Pharmaceuticals
TARO NTP 10	Nortriptyline Hydrochloride	10 mg	Opaque Light Green	Capsule		Taro Pharmaceuticals
TARO NTP 25	Nortriptyline Hydrochloride	25 mg	Opaque Ivory	Capsule		Taro Pharmaceuticals
TARO NTP 50	Nortriptyline Hydrochloride	50 mg	Opaque Dark Green, Opaque White	Capsule		Taro Pharmaceuticals
TARO NTP 75	Nortriptyline Hydrochloride	75 mg	Opaque Dark Green	Capsule		Taro Pharmaceuticals
TARO; 11	Carbamazepine	200 mg	White	Tablet	Circle, Flat Beveled-Edge, Scored	Taro Pharmaceuticals
TARO; 11	Carbamazepine	200 mg	White	Tablet	Circle, Scored	Taro Pharmaceuticals
TARO; 16	Carbamazepine	100 mg	White, Pink	Tablet, Chewable	Circle, Scored	Taro Pharmaceuticals
TARO; 25	Clomipramine Hydrochloride	25 mg	Dark Blue and Light Blue	Capsule		Taro Pharmaceuticals
TARO; 50	Clomipramine Hydrochloride	50 mg	Yellow	Capsule		Taro Pharmaceuticals
TARO; 75	Clomipramine Hydrochloride	75 mg	White	Capsule		Taro Pharmaceuticals
TAVIST	Tavist Sinus	500 mg; 30 mg	Red and White	Capsule, Liquid Filled		Novartis Consumer
TAVIST; 78/72 ;	Tavist	2.68 mg	White	Tablet	Circle, Scored	Novartis Pharmaceuticals
TAVIST; ALLERGY	Tavist Allergy	1.34 mg	White	Tablet	Oblong, Scored	Novartis Consumer
TC; TYLENOL COLD	Children's Tylenol Cold	80 mg; 0.5 mg; 7.5 mg	Purple	Tablet, Chewable	Circle	Mcneil Consumer Products
TE TE ; CG CG	Trileptal	300 mg	Yellow	Tablet	Oval	Novartis
TEGISON; 10; ROCHE	Tegison	10 mg	Brown and Green	Capsule	Oval	Roche Pharmaceuticals
TEGISON; 25; ROCHE	Tegison	25 mg	Brown and Caramel	Capsule	Oval	Roche Pharmaceuticals
TEGRETOL; 27; 27 ;	Tegretol	200 mg	Pink	Tablet	Capsule-Shape, Single-Scored	Novartis
TEGRETOL; 52 52 ;	Tegretol	100 mg	Pink with Red Speckles	Tablet, Chewable	Circle, Scored	Novartis
TELDRIN; 12 MG	Teldrin	12 mg	Clear, Green	Timed-Release Capsule		Glaxosmithkline Consumer
TEMAZEPAM; 7.5 MG; 271; CP	Temazepam	7.5 mg	White and Pink	Capsule		Geneva Generics
TEMOZOLOMIDE 5 MG SP	Temodar	5 mg	Off-White with Green Ink	Capsule		Schering
TEMOZOLOMIDE; 20 MG; SP	Temodar	20 mg	Off-White with Brown Ink	Capsule		Schering
TEMOZOLOMIDE; 100 MG; SP	Temodar	100 mg	Off-White with Blue Ink	Capsule		Schering
TEMOZOLOMIDE; 250 MG; SP	Temodar	250 mg	Off-White with Black Ink	Capsule		Schering
TEN K	Ten-K	750 mg	White	Timed-Release Tablet	Capsule-Shape, Scored	Novartis
TENORETIC; 115	Tenoretic 50	25 mg; 50 mg	White	Tablet	Round, Biconvex, Bisected Scored	Astra Zeneca
TENORETIC; 117 ;	Tenoretic 100	25 mg; 100 mg	White	Tablet	Circle, Biconvex	Astra Zeneca

IMPRINT	BRAND/GENERIC NAME	STRENGTH	COLOR	FORM	SHAPE	MANUFACTURER
TENORMIN; 101	Tenormin	100 mg	White	Tablet	Circle, Flat	Astra Zeneca
TENORMIN; 105	Tenormin	50 mg	White	Tablet	Round, Flat, Bisected Scored	Astra Zeneca
TENUATE; 25	Tenuate	25 mg	White	Tablet	Circle	Sanofi-Aventis U.S.
TENUATE; 75	Tenuate Dospan	75 mg	White	Tablet, Extended Release	Capsule-Shape	Sanofi-Aventis U.S.
TF TF ; CG CG	Trileptal	600 mg	Light Pink	Tablet	Oval	Novartis
TF TF ; CG CG	Trileptal	600 mg	Light Pink	Tablet	Oval	Novartis Pharmaceuticals
TH; A	Cylert	18.75 mg	White	Tablet	Monogrammed, Grooved	Abbott Laboratories
THEO-24; 100 MG; UCB; 2832 ;	Theo-24	100 mg	Yellow-Orange and Clear	Extended-Release Capsule		Ucb Pharma
THEO-24; 200 MG; UCB; 2842 ;	Theo-24	200 mg	Red-Orange and Clear	Extended-Release Capsule		Ucb Pharma
THEO-24; 300 MG; UCB; 2852 ;	Theo-24	300 mg	Red and Clear	Extended-Release Capsule		Ucb Pharma
THEO-24; 400 MG; UCB; 2902 ;	Theo-24	400 mg	Pink and Clear	Extended-Release Capsule		Ucb Pharma
THEOBID; 130 ;	Theobid Duracap JR.	130 mg	Clear with White Beads	Capsule		Ucb Pharma
THEOBID; 260 ;	Theobid Duracap	260 mg	Clear with White Beads	Capsule		Ucb Pharma
THEO-BID; 260	Theo-Bid Duracap	260 mg	Clear	Extended-Release Capsule		Ucb Pharma
THEOPHYL	Theophyl-SR	250 mg	Green and Clear	Timed-Release Capsule		Mcneil Pharmaceutical
THEOPHYL; 100	Theophyl Chewable	100 mg	White	Tablet, Chewable	Circle	Mcneil Pharmaceutical
THEOPHYL; 125	Theophyl-SR	125 mg	Yellow and Clear	Timed-Release Capsule		Mcneil Pharmaceutical
THEOPHYL; 225	Theophyl-225	225 mg	White	Tablet	Triangle, Scored	Mcneil Pharmaceutical
THERAFLU	Theraflu Maximum Strength Flu, Cold & Cough Non-Drowsy Formula	500 mg; 15 mg; 30 mg	Yellow	Tablet		Novartis Consumer
THERAFLU	Theraflu Maximum Strength Nighttime Flu, Cold & Cough	500 mg; 30 mg; 15 mg; 2 mg	Green	Tablet		Novartis Consumer
THERAFLU	Thera-Flu Maximum Strength Nighttime Formula	500 mg; 30 mg; 15 mg; 2 mg	Green	Tablet	Oblong	Sandoz Consumer
TI; 01	Spiriva	18 mcg	Light Green	Capsule		Pfizer
TI; A	Cylert	37.5 mg	Orange	Tablet	Monogrammed, Grooved	Abbott Laboratories
TIAZAC; 120	Tiazac	120 mg	Lavender	Extended-Release Capsule		Forest Pharmaceuticals
TIAZAC; 180	Tiazac	180 mg	White and Blue-Green	Extended-Release Capsule		Forest Pharmaceuticals
TIAZAC; 240	Tiazac	240 mg	Blue-Green and Lavender	Extended-Release Capsule		Forest Pharmaceuticals
TIAZAC; 300	Tiazac	300 mg	White and Lavender	Extended-Release Capsule		Forest Pharmaceuticals
TIAZAC; 360	Tiazac	360 mg	Blue-Green	Extended-Release Capsule		Forest Pharmaceuticals
TIAZAC; 420	Tiazac	420 mg	White	Extended-Release Capsule		Forest Pharmaceuticals
TIGAN; M079	Tigan	300 mg	Purple	Capsule		Monarch Pharmaceuticals
TITRALAC PLUS	Titralac Plus	420 mg; 21 mg		Tablet, Chewable		3M Pharmaceuticals
TITRALAC; EXTRA	Titralac Extra Strength	750 mg	White	Tablet, Chewable	Circle	3M Pharmaceuticals
TJ; A	Cylert	75 mg	Tan	Tablet	Monogrammed, Grooved	Abbott Laboratories
TK; A	Cylert	37.5 mg	Orange	Tablet, Chewable	Monogrammed, Grooved	Abbott Laboratories
TL; 113	Prochlorperazine Maleate	5 mg	Yellow-Green	Tablet	Circle, Scored	Par Pharmaceutical
TL; 115	Prochlorperazine Maleate	10 mg	Light Green	Tablet	Circle, Scored	Par Pharmaceutical
TL; Q	Tramadol Hydrochloride	50 mg	White	Tablet		Par Pharmaceutical
TO	Detrol	1 mg	White	Tablet	Circle	Pharmacia & Upjohn
TO; 60	Fareston	60 mg	White to Off-White	Tablet	Circle, Convex	Schering
TOLECTIN DS; MCNEIL	Tolectin DS	400 mg	Orange	Capsule		Ortho-Mcneil Pharmaceutical
TOLECTIN; 200; MCNEIL	Tolectin	200 mg	White	Tablet		Ortho-Mcneil Pharmaceutical
TOLECTIN; 600; MCNEIL	Tolectin 600	600 mg	Orange	Tablet	Oval	Ortho-Mcneil Pharmaceutical
TOLINASE; 100 ;	Tolinase	100 mg	White	Tablet	Circle, Scored	Pharmacia & Upjohn
TOLINASE; 250 ;	Tolinase	250 mg	White	Tablet	Circle, Scored	Pharmacia & Upjohn
TOLINASE; 500 ;	Tolinase	500 mg	White	Tablet	Circle, Scored	Pharmacia & Upjohn
TOLMETIN; 200	Tolmetin Sodium	200 mg	White	Tablet	Circle, Scored	Duramed Pharmaceuticals
TOLMETIN; 400	Tolmetin Sodium	400 mg	Orange	Capsule		Duramed Pharmaceuticals
TOLMETIN; 600	Tolmetin Sodium	600 mg	Orange	Tablet	Egg-Shape, Scored	Duramed Pharmaceuticals
TONOCARD; 707	Tonocard	400 mg	Yellow	Coated Tablet	Oval, Scored	Astra Zeneca
TONOCARD; 709	Tonocard	600 mg	Yellow	Coated Tablet	Oblong, Scored	Astra Zeneca
TOP ; 25	Topamax	25 mg	White	Tablet	Circle	Ortho-Mcneil Pharmaceutical
TOP; 15 MG	Topamax Sprinkle Capsule	15 mg	White and Clear with White Spheres	Capsule		Ortho-Mcneil Pharmaceutical
TOP; 25 MG	Topamax Sprinkle Capsule	25 mg	White and Clear with White Spheres	Capsule		Ortho-Mcneil Pharmaceutical
TOPAMAX ; 50	Topamax	50 mg	White	Tablet	Circle	Ortho-Mcneil Pharmaceutical
TOPAMAX ; 100	Topamax	100 mg	Yellow	Tablet	Circle	Ortho-Mcneil Pharmaceutical
TOPAMAX ; 200	Topamax	200 mg	Salmon	Tablet	Circle	Ortho-Mcneil Pharmaceutical
TORADOL; ROCHE	Toradol	10 mg	White	Tablet	Circle	Roche Laboratories
TPV 250	Aptivus	250 mg	Pink	Capsule, Liquid Filled	Oblong	Boehringer Ingelheim Pharmaceuticals
TR; 125; G	Triazolam	0.125 mg	White	Tablet	Oval	Par Pharmaceutical
TR; 250; G	Triazolam	0.25 mg	Pale Yellow	Tablet	Oval, Scored	Par Pharmaceutical
TRANDATE; 100	Trandate	100 mg	Orange	Coated Tablet	Circle, Scored	Glaxosmithkline
TRANDATE; 200	Trandate	200 mg	White	Coated Tablet	Circle, Scored	Glaxosmithkline
TRANDATE; 300	Trandate	300 mg	Peach	Coated Tablet	Circle, Scored	Glaxosmithkline
TRANSDERM-NITRO; 0.1 MG/HR	Transderm-Nitro	0.1 mg/hr	Tan	Patch	Circle	Novartis Generics

IMPRINT	BRAND/GENERIC NAME	STRENGTH	COLOR	FORM	SHAPE	MANUFACTURER
TRANSDERM-NITRO; 0.2 MG/HR	Transderm-Nitro	0.2 mg/hr	Tan	Patch	Oblong	Novartis Generics
TRANSDERM-NITRO; 0.4 MG/HR	Transderm-Nitro	0.4 mg/hr	Tan	Patch	Oblong	Novartis Generics
TRANSDERM-NITRO; 0.6 MG/HR	Transderm-Nitro	0.6 mg/hr	Tan	Patch	Oblong	Novartis Generics
TRANSDERM-NITRO; 0.8 MG/HR	Transderm-Nitro	0.8 mg/hr	Tan	Patch	Circle	Novartis Generics
TRAVIST; SINUS	Tavist Sinus	500 mg; 30 mg	White	Tablet		Novartis Consumer
TRENTAL	Trental	400 mg	Pink	Tablet, Extended Release	Oblong	Aventis Pharmaceuticals
TRENTAL	Trental	400 mg	Pink	Tablet, Extended Release	Oblong	Sanofi-Aventis U.S.
TRIANGEL; 567	Hydrocodone Bitartrate and Acetaminophen	10 mg; 660 mg	White	Tablet	Capsule-Shape, Scored	Andrx Pharmaceuticals
TRIANGLE	Maxalt-Mlt	5 mg	White	Tablet	Circle	Merck
TRIANGLE; 516	Benazepril Hydrochloride	5 mg	Light Orange	Tablet	Circle	Andrx Pharmaceuticals
TRIANGLE; 517	Benazepril Hydrochloride	10 mg	Orange	Tablet	Circle	Andrx Pharmaceuticals
TRIANGLE; 518	Benazepril Hydrochloride	20 mg	Peach	Tablet	Circle	Andrx Pharmaceuticals
TRIANGLE; 519	Benazepril Hydrochloride	40 mg	Orange-Red	Tablet	Circle	Andrx Pharmaceuticals
TRIANGLE; 521; 3	Acetaminophen and Codeine Phosphate	300 mg; 15 mg	White	Tablet	Circle, Scored	Andrx Pharmaceuticals
TRIANGLE; 522; 3	Acetaminophen and Codeine Phosphate	300 mg; 30 mg	White	Tablet	Circle, Scored	Andrx Pharmaceuticals
TRIANGLE; 523; 4	Acetaminophen and Codeine Phosphate	300 mg; 60 mg	White	Tablet	Circle, Scored	Andrx Pharmaceuticals
TRIANGLE; 756	Benazepril Hydrochloride and Hydrochlorothiazide	5 mg; 6.25 mg	White	Tablet		Andrx Pharmaceuticals
TRIANGLE; 757	Benazepril Hydrochloride and Hydrochlorothiazide	10 mg; 12.5 mg	Purple	Tablet		Andrx Pharmaceuticals
TRIANGLE; 758	Benazepril Hydrochloride and Hydrochlorothiazide	20 mg; 12.5 mg	Pink	Tablet		Andrx Pharmaceuticals
TRIANGLE; 759	Benazepril Hydrochloride and Hydrochlorothiazide	20 mg; 25 mg	Red	Tablet		Andrx Pharmaceuticals
TRIANGLE; 791	Lovastatin	10 mg	White to Off-White	Tablet	Circle	Andrx Pharmaceuticals
TRIANGLE; 792	Lovastatin	20 mg	White to Off-White	Tablet	Circle	Andrx Pharmaceuticals
TRIANGLE; 793	Lovastatin	40 mg	White to Off-White	Tablet	Circle	Andrx Pharmaceuticals
TRIANGLE; 871	Glipizide Extended-Release	2.5 mg	Blue	Extended-Release Tablet	Circle	Andrx Pharmaceuticals
TRIANGLE; 872	Glipizide Extended-Release	5 mg	White	Extended-Release Tablet	Circle	Andrx Pharmaceuticals
TRIANGLE; 873	Glipizide Extended-Release	10 mg	White	Extended-Release Tablet	Circle	Andrx Pharmaceuticals
TRIMPEX; 100; ROCHE	Trimpex	100 mg	White	Tablet	Circle, Scored	Roche Pharmaceuticals
TRIMPEX; 100; ROCHE	Trimpex	100 mg	White	Tablet	Oval, Scored	Roche Laboratories
TRINSICON-M; GLAXO	Trinsicon M	75 mg; 110 mg; 240 mg; 15 mcg	Dark Pink and Dark Red	Capsule		Glaxosmithkline
TRITEC; STOMACH-SHAPED LOGO	Tritec	400 mg	Blue	Coated Tablet	Eight-Sided, Elongated	Glaxosmithkline
TUMS	Tums Anti-Gas/antacid	500 mg; 20 mg	Assorted	Tablet	Circle	Glaxosmithkline Consumer
TUMS	Tums Assorted Flavors	500 mg	Pink, Orange, Yellow or Green	Tablet, Chewable	Circle	Glaxosmithkline Consumer
TY 500	Tylenol Extra Strength Rapid Release Gels	500 mg	Grey (Band), Light Blue, Red	Capsule		Mcneil Consumer Products
TY C365 ;	Tylenol Cold Relief Nighttime	500 mg; 25 mg	Light Blue	Tablet	Capsule-Shape	Mcneil Consumer Products
TY; 80	Children's Tylenol Soft-Chews Bubblegum Flavor	80 mg	Pink	Tablet, Chewable	Oval	Mcneil Consumer Products
TY; 80	Children's Tylenol Soft-Chews Fruit Flavor	80 mg	Pink	Tablet, Chewable	Oval	Mcneil Consumer Products
TY; 80	Children's Tylenol Soft-Chews Grape Flavor	80 mg	Purple	Tablet, Chewable	Oval	Mcneil Consumer Products
TY; A	Tranxene-Sd	22.5 mg	Peach	Extended-Release Tablet	Circle	Abbott Laboratories
TYLENOL	Children's Tylenol Bubblegum Flavor	80 mg	Pink	Tablet, Chewable	Circle, Scored	Mcneil Consumer Products
TYLENOL	Children's Tylenol Fruit-Flavored	80 mg	Pink	Tablet, Chewable		Mcneil Consumer Products
TYLENOL	Children's Tylenol Grape Flavored	80 mg	Purple	Tablet, Chewable		Mcneil Consumer Products
TYLENOL	Children's Tylenol Meltaways - Bubble Gum Burst	80 mg		Disintegrating Tablet	Circle	Mcneil Consumer Products
TYLENOL	Children's Tylenol Meltaways - Grape Punch	80 mg		Disintegrating Tablet	Circle	Mcneil Consumer Products
TYLENOL	Children's Tylenol Meltaways - Wacky Watermelon	80 mg		Disintegrating Tablet	Circle	Mcneil Consumer Products
TYLENOL	JR. Tylenol Meltaways - Bubble Gum Burst	160 mg		Tablet, Disintegrating	Circle	Mcneil Consumer Products
TYLENOL	JR. Tylenol Meltaways - Grape Punch	160 mg		Tablet, Disintegrating	Circle	Mcneil Consumer Products
TYLENOL	Tylenol Extra Strength	500 mg	White	Tablet	Circle	Mcneil Consumer Products
TYLENOL	Tylenol Regular Strength	325 mg	White	Tablet	Circle	Mcneil Consumer Products
TYLENOL 500	Tylenol Extra Strength Cool Caplets	500 mg	White	Tablet	Capsule-Shape	Mcneil Consumer Products
TYLENOL C/C TC/C	Children's Tylenol Plus Cold & Cough	80 mg; 0.5 mg; 7.5 mg; 2.5 mg	Pink	Tablet, Chewable		Mcneil Consumer Products
TYLENOL CODEINE 3 ; MCNEIL ;	Tylenol with Codeine No. 3	300 mg; 30 mg	White	Tablet	Circle	Mcneil Pharmaceutical
TYLENOL COLD	Tylenol Cold Multi-Symptom Non-Drowsy Caplets	325 mg; 15 mg; 30 mg	White	Tablet	Oblong	Mcneil Consumer Products
TYLENOL COLD	Tylenol Cold Multi-Symptom Non-Drowsy Gelcaps	325 mg; 15 mg; 30 mg	Yellow and Orange	Capsule, Liquid Filled		Mcneil Consumer Products
TYLENOL COOL CAPLET	Tylenol Extra Strength Cool Caplets	500 mg	White	Caplet	Capsule-Shape	Mcneil Consumer Products

IMPRINT	BRAND/GENERIC NAME	STRENGTH	COLOR	FORM	SHAPE	MANUFACTURER
TYLENOL EZTAB	Tylenol Extra Strength Ez Tabs	500 mg	Red	Tablet	Circle	Mcneil Consumer Products
TYLENOL FLU	Extra Strength Tylenol Flu Convenience Pack Daytime Relief	500 mg; 30 mg; 15 mg	Red and White	Capsule, Liquid Filled	Capsule-Shape	Mcneil Consumer Products
TYLENOL FLU	Extra Strength Tylenol Flu Daytime Relief	500 mg; 30 mg; 15 mg	Red and White	Capsule, Liquid Filled	Capsule-Shape	Mcneil Consumer Products
TYLENOL FLU	Tylenol Flu Maximum Strength	500 mg; 15 mg; 30 mg	Burgundy and White	Capsule, Liquid Filled		Mcneil Consumer Products
TYLENOL FLU; NT	Tylenol Flu Nighttime Maximum Strength	500 mg; 30 mg; 25 mg	White and Dark Blue	Capsule, Liquid Filled		Mcneil Consumer Products
TYLENOL PM ;	Tylenol Pm Extra Strength Caplets	500 mg; 25 mg	Light Blue	Tablet	Capsule-Shape	Mcneil Consumer Products
TYLENOL PM	Tylenol Pm Extra Strength - Gelcaps	500 mg; 25 mg	Blue and White	Capsule, Liquid Filled		Mcneil Consumer Products
TYLENOL PM	Tylenol Pm Extra Strength Geltabs	500 mg; 25 mg	Blue and White	Geltab	Circle	Mcneil Consumer Products
TYLENOL SINUS	Tylenol Sinus Maximum Strength Non-Drowsy Geltabs	30 mg; 500 mg	Green and White	Geltab	Circle	Mcneil Consumer Products
TYLENOL; 160	Junior Strength Tylenol	160 mg	White	Tablet		Mcneil Consumer Products
TYLENOL; 160	Junior Strength Tylenol Fruit Flavor	160 mg	Pink	Tablet, Chewable	Circle	Mcneil Consumer Products
TYLENOL; 160	Junior Strength Tylenol Grape Flavor	160 mg	Purple	Tablet, Chewable	Circle	Mcneil Consumer Products
TYLENOL; 325	Tylenol Regular Strength	325 mg	White	Tablet		Mcneil Consumer Products
TYLENOL; 500	Tylenol Extra Strength Caplets	500 mg	White	Tablet		Mcneil Consumer Products
TYLENOL; 500	Tylenol Extra Strength Gelcaps	500 mg	Yellow and Red	Capsule, Liquid Filled		Mcneil Consumer Products
TYLENOL; 500	Tylenol Extra Strength Geltabs	500 mg	Yellow and Red	Geltab		Mcneil Consumer Products
TYLENOL; A/S	Tylenol Allergy Sinus Maximum Strength Gelcaps	2 mg; 30 mg; 500 mg	Green and Yellow	Capsule, Liquid Filled		Mcneil Consumer Products
TYLENOL; A/S	Tylenol Allergy Sinus Maximum Strength Geltabs	2 mg; 30 mg; 500 mg	Green and Yellow	Geltab	Circle	Mcneil Consumer Products
TYLENOL; A/S; NIGHT TIME	Tylenol Allergy Sinus Nighttime Maximum Strength	500 mg; 30 mg; 25 mg	Light Blue	Capsule, Liquid Filled		Mcneil Consumer Products
TYLENOL; ALLERGY SINUS	Tylenol Allergy Sinus Maximum Strength Caplets	2 mg; 30 mg; 500 mg	Dark Yellow	Tablet	Oblong	Mcneil Consumer Products
TYLENOL; CODEINE; 2	Tylenol with Codeine No. 2	300 mg; 15 mg	White	Tablet	Circle	Mcneil Pharmaceutical
TYLENOL; CODEINE; 4 ;	Tylenol with Codeine No. 4	300 mg; 60 mg	White	Tablet	Circle	Mcneil Pharmaceutical
TYLENOL; COLD	Tylenol Cold Multi-Symptom	325 mg; 2 mg; 30 mg; 15 mg	Light Yellow	Tablet		Mcneil Consumer Products
TYLENOL; COLD	Tylenol Cold Multi-Symptom	325 mg; 2 mg; 30 mg; 15 mg	Yellow	Tablet	Circle	Mcneil Consumer Products
TYLENOL; COLD; DM; 80	Children's Tylenol Cold DM	0.5 mg; 80 mg; 3.75 mg; 7.5 mg		Tablet, Chewable	Flat-Faced, Beveled	Mcneil Consumer Products
TYLENOL; COLD; SC	Tylenol Cold Severe Congestion Non-Drowsy	30 mg; 200 mg; 15 mg; 325 mg	Yellow	Tablet	Capsule-Shape	Mcneil Consumer Products
TYLENOL; ER	Tylenol Arthritis Extended Relief	650 mg	White	Extended-Release Capsule	Oblong	Mcneil Consumer Products
TYLENOL; HEADACHE PLUS	Tylenol Extra Strength Headache Plus Tablet	500 mg; 250 mg	White	Tablet		Mcneil Consumer Products
TYLENOL; SEVERE ALLERGY	Tylenol Severe Allergy Fast Relief	500 mg; 12.5 mg	Bright Yellow	Tablet	Oblong	Mcneil Consumer Products
TYLENOL; SINUS	Tylenol Sinus Maximum Strength Non-Drowsy	500 mg; 30 mg	Light Green	Tablet	Circle	Mcneil Consumer Products
TYLENOL; SINUS	Tylenol Sinus Maximum Strength Non-Drowsy Caplets	500 mg; 30 mg	Light Green	Tablet		Mcneil Consumer Products
TYLENOL; SINUS	Tylenol Sinus Maximum Strength Non-Drowsy Gelcaps	30 mg; 500 mg	Green and White	Capsule, Liquid Filled		Mcneil Consumer Products
TYLOX; MCNEIL	Tylox	5 mg; 500 mg	Red	Capsule		Ortho-Mcneil Pharmaceutical
TYME	Tylenol Women's Menstrual Relief	500 mg; 25 mg	White	Tablet		Mcneil Consumer Products
TZ; 1	Remeron Soltab	15 mg	White	Tablet	Circle	Organon
TZ; 2	Remeron Soltab	30 mg	White	Tablet	Circle	Organon
TZ; 4	Remeron Soltab	45 mg	White	Tablet	Circle	Organon
U	Colestid	1 GM	Yellow	Coated Tablet	Circle	Pharmacia & Upjohn
U	Unicap	5000 IU; 400 IU; 15 IU; 60 mg; 0.4 mg; 1.5 mg; 1.7 mg; 20 mg; 2 mg; 6 mcg	Yellow	Capsule		Upjohn
U	Unicap M	5000 IU; 400 IU; 15 IU; 60 mg; 0.4 mg; 1.5 mg; 1.7 mg; 20 mg; 2 mg; 6 mcg; 10 mg; 150 mcg; 18 mg; 2 mg; 15 mg; 1 mg; 5 mg	Tan	Coated Tablet		Upjohn
U	Unicap M Plus Iron	6 mg; 5 mg; 35 mg; 1.5 mg; 10 mcg; 2.5 mg; 2.5 mg; 50 mg; 20 mg; 0.5 mg; 5 mg; 2 mcg; 10 IU; 50 mg; 0.15 mg; 1 mg; 1 mg	Tan	Coated Tablet		Upjohn

IMPRINT	BRAND/GENERIC NAME	STRENGTH	COLOR	FORM	SHAPE	MANUFACTURER
U	Unicap Plus Iron	18 mg; 5000 IU; 400 IU; 15 IU; 0.4 mg; 1.5 mg; 1.7 mg; 20 mg; 10 mg; 60 mg; 2 mg; 6 mcg	Red	Coated Tablet		Upjohn
U	Uristat	95 mg	Red-Brown	Tablet	Circle	Ortho Advanced
U	Unicap Senior	10 mg; 5000 IU; 15 IU; 0.4 mg; 1.2 mg; 1.7 mg; 14 mg; 10 mg; 150 mcg; 2 mg; 15 mg; 1 mg; 5 mg; 60 mg; 2 mg; 6 mcg	Blue	Coated Tablet		Upjohn
U; 26 ;	Sandril	0.25 mg	Green	Tablet		Eli Lilly
U; 60	Keflex	1 GM	Green	Tablet		Eli Lilly
U; 94 ;	Xanax	2 mg	White	Tablet	Oblong, Multi-Scored	Pharmacia & Upjohn
U; 3617	Vantin	100 mg	Light Orange	Coated Tablet	Circle	Pharmacia & Upjohn
U; 3618	Vantin	200 mg	Coral Red	Coated Tablet	Circle	Pharmacia & Upjohn
UC; ABBOTT LOGO	Prosom	1 mg	White	Tablet		Abbott Laboratories
UCB 579 10 MG	Metadate Cd	10 mg	Green, White	Capsule, Extended Release		Ucb Pharma
UCB 580 20 MG	Metadate Cd	20 mg	Blue, White	Capsule, Extended Release		Ucb Pharma
UCB 581 30 MG	Metadate Cd	30 mg	Reddish-Brown, White	Capsule, Extended Release		Ucb Pharma
UCB 582 40 MG	Metadate Cd	40 mg	White, Yellow Ivory	Capsule, Extended Release		Ucb Pharma
UCB 583 50 MG	Metadate Cd	50 mg	Purple, White	Capsule, Extended Release		Ucb Pharma
UCB 584 60 MG	Metadate Cd	60 mg	White	Capsule, Extended Release		Ucb Pharma
UCB UCB ;	VI-Zac	5000 IU; 18 mg; 50 IU; 500 mg	Orange with Blue Band	Capsule		Ucb Pharma
UCB; 250	Keppra	250 mg	Blue	Coated Tablet	Oblong, Scored	Ucb Pharma
UCB; 364 ;	Trinsicon	0.5 mg; 240 mg; 110 mg; 15 mcg; 75 mg	Dark Pink and Dark Red	Capsule		Ucb Pharma
UCB; 500	Keppra	500 mg	Yellow	Coated Tablet	Oblong, Scored	Ucb Pharma
UCB; 500 ;	Lortab Asa	500 mg; 5 mg	Dark Pink	Tablet	Capsule-Shape	Ucb Pharma
UCB; 612 ;	Duratuss	600 mg; 120 mg	White	Extended-Release Tablet	Oval, Scored	Ucb Pharma
UCB; 620 ;	Duratuss G	1200 mg	White	Extended-Release Tablet	Capsule-Shape, Scored	Ucb Pharma
UCB; 640	Duratuss Gp	1200 mg; 120 mg	White	Extended-Release Tablet	Oval, Coated, Scored	Ucb Pharma
UCB; 750	Keppra	750 mg	Orange	Coated Tablet	Oblong, Scored	Ucb Pharma
UCB; 901 ;	Lortab 2.5/500	500 mg; 2.5 mg	White with Pink Specks	Tablet	Capsule-Shaped, Bisected Scored	Ucb Pharma
UCB; 902 ;	Lortab 5/500	500 mg; 5 mg	White with Blue Specks	Tablet	Capsule-Shaped, Bisected Scored	Ucb Pharma
UCB; 903 ;	Lortab 7.5/500	500 mg; 7.5 mg	White with Green Specks	Tablet	Capsule-Shaped; Bisected Scored	Ucb Pharma
UCB; 910 ;	Lortab 10/500	500 mg; 10 mg	Pink	Tablet	Capsule-Shape	Ucb Pharma
UCB; UCB ;	Vicon-C	300 mg; 7 mg; 18 mg; 10 mg; 18 mg; 20 mg; 4 mg; 99 mg	Orange and Yellow with Blue Band	Capsule		Ucb Pharma
UCB; UCB ;	Vicon Plus	150 mg; 10 mg; 4 mg; 2 mg; 10 mg; 50 IU; 80 mg; 4000 IU; 5 mg; 25 mg; 70 mg	Red and Light Yellow with Blue Band	Capsule		Ucb Pharma
UCBB; 316 ;	Vicon Forte	150 mg; 10 mg; 70 mg; 25 mg; 5 mg; 8000 IU; 50 IU; 80 mg; 10 mcg; 10 mg; 2 mg; 4 mg; 1 mg	Orange and Black	Capsule		Ucb Pharma
UD; ABBOTT LOGO	Prosom	2 mg	Pink	Tablet		Abbott Laboratories
UNISOM	Unisom	25 mg	Blue	Tablet	Oval, Bisected Scored	Pfizer Consumer Health Care
UNISOM	Unisom Sleepgels	50 mg	Clear Blue	Capsule	Oval	Pfizer Consumer Health Care
UPJOHN	Uticillin K	250 mg		Tablet		Upjohn
UPJOHN 949	Uracil Mustard	1 mg	Yellow and Dark Blue	Capsule		Upjohn
UPJOHN; 15	Cortisone Acetate	5 mg	White	Tablet	Circle, Scored	Pharmacia & Upjohn
UPJOHN; 23	Cortisone Acetate	10 mg	White	Tablet	Circle, Scored	Pharmacia & Upjohn
UPJOHN; 34	Cortisone Acetate	25 mg	White	Tablet	Circle, Scored	Pharmacia & Upjohn
UPJOHN; 243	Alkets	780 mg; 130 mg; 65 mg	Pink	Tablet, Chewable		Pharmacia & Upjohn
UPR	Unisom with Pain Relief	650 mg; 50 mg	Pale Blue	Coated Tablet	Capsule-Shape	Pfizer Consumer Health Care
US ; 191	Folgard RX	1; 2.2 mg; 25 mg;	Yellow	Tablet	Oval	Upsher-Smith Laboratories
US; 016	Folgard RX 2.2	2.2 mg; 25 mg; 0.5 mg	Yellow	Tablet	Oval	Upsher-Smith Laboratories
US; 017	Folgard	0.8 mg; 10 mg; 0.115 mg	Green	Tablet	Circle	Upsher-Smith Laboratories
US; 027	Pentoxil	400 mg	Light Pink	Extended-Release Tablet	Capsule-Shape	Upsher-Smith Laboratories
US; 12; 80	Sorine	80 mg	White	Tablet	Capsule-Shape	Upsher-Smith Laboratories
US; 13; 120	Sorine	120 mg	White	Tablet	Capsule-Shape	Upsher-Smith Laboratories
US; 14; 160	Sorine	160 mg	White	Tablet	Capsule-Shape	Upsher-Smith Laboratories
US; 15; 240	Sorine	240 mg	White	Tablet	Capsule-Shape	Upsher-Smith Laboratories
US; 67; 500	Niacor	500 mg	White	Tablet	Oval, Scored	Upsher-Smith Laboratories

IMPRINT	BRAND/GENERIC NAME	STRENGTH	COLOR	FORM	SHAPE	MANUFACTURER
US; 200; A ;	Amiodarone Hydrochloride	200 mg	White	Tablet	Circle, Scored	Sandoz
US; 500	Salsitab	500 mg	Blue	Tablet	Circle	Upsher-Smith Laboratories
US; 750	Salsitab	750 mg	Blue	Tablet	Capsule-Shape	Upsher-Smith Laboratories
USL; 8	Potassium Chloride	600 mg	Blue	Sustained-Release Tablet	Circle	Upsher-Smith Laboratories
USL; 8	Potassium Chloride	600 mg	Blue	Sustained-Release Tablet	Circle	Geneva Generics
USL; 10	Potassium Chloride	10 meq	White	Extended-Release Tablet	Circle	Geneva Generics
USL; 10	Potassium Chloride	750 mg	White	Sustained-Release Tablet	Circle	Geneva Generics
USL; 10	Potassium Chloride	750 mg	White	Sustained-Release Tablet	Circle	Upsher-Smith Laboratories
USL; 80	Zinc Sulfate	220 mg	Pink	Capsule		Upsher-Smith Laboratories
USV; 82	Lozol	2.5 mg	White	Tablet	Circle	Aventis Pharmaceuticals
V	Vivarin	200 mg	Yellow	Tablet		Glaxosmithkline Consumer
VALPROIC; 250; 0364	Valproic Acid	250 mg	Off-White	Capsule		Watson Laboratories
VALRELEASE 15; ROCHE	Valrelease	15 mg	Yellow and Blue	Sustained-Release Capsule		Roche Pharmaceuticals
VALTREX; 1 GRAM	Valtrex	1 G	Blue	Tablet	Film-Coated	Glaxosmithkline
VALTREX; 500 MG	Valtrex	500 mg	Blue	Tablet	Film-Coated	Glaxosmithkline
VANQUISH	Vanquish	227 mg; 194 mg; 33 mg		Tablet		Bayer Consumer Care
VENTOLIN; 4; GLAXO	Ventolin	4 mg	White	Tablet	Circle, Compressed	Glaxosmithkline
VENTOLIN; 200; GLAXO	Ventolin Rotacaps	200 mcg	Light Blue and Clear	Capsule, Liquid Filled		Glaxosmithkline
VESANOID 10; ROCHE	Vesanoid	10 mg	Orange-Yellow and Red-Brown	Capsule		Roche Laboratories
VGC; 450	Valcyte	450 mg	Pink	Tablet	Oval, Convex	Roche Laboratories
VGR; 25; PFIZER	Viagra	25 mg	Blue	Coated Tablet	Diamond, Rounded	Pfizer Laboratories
VGR; 50; PFIZER	Viagra	50 mg	Blue	Coated Tablet	Diamond, Rounded	Pfizer Laboratories
VGR; 100; PFIZER	Viagra	100 mg	Blue	Coated Tablet	Diamond, Rounded	Pfizer Laboratories
VICODIN	Vicodin	5 mg; 500 mg	White	Tablet		Abbott Laboratories
VICODIN HP	Vicodin Hp	10 mg; 660 mg	White	Tablet	Oval	Abbott Laboratories
VICODIN; ES	Vicodin Es	7.5 mg; 750 mg	White	Tablet	Oval, Scored	Abbott Laboratories
VISKEN; 5; 78/111	Visken	5 mg	White	Tablet	Circle, Scored	Novartis Pharmaceuticals
VISKEN; 10; 78/73	Visken	10 mg	White	Tablet	Circle, Scored	Novartis Pharmaceuticals
VP; A ;	Vicoprofen	7.5 mg; 200 mg	White	Coated Tablet	Circle, Convex	Abbott Laboratories
W ; 4117	Trecator	250 mg	Orange	Tablet		Wyeth Pharmaceuticals
W ; A77	Aralen	500 mg	White	Film-Coated, Discoid Tablet	Circle	Sanofi-Aventis U.S.
W 25 ; 701 ;	Effexor	25 mg	Peach	Tablet	Shield-Shape	Wyeth Pharmaceuticals
W 37.5 ; 781 ;	Effexor	37.5 mg	Peach	Tablet	Shield-Shape	Wyeth Pharmaceuticals
W 50 ; 703 ;	Effexor	50 mg	Peach	Tablet	Shield-Shape	Wyeth Pharmaceuticals
W 75 ; 704 ;	Effexor	75 mg	Peach	Tablet	Shield-Shape	Wyeth Pharmaceuticals
W 100 ; 705 ;	Effexor	100 mg	Peach	Tablet	Shield-Shape	Wyeth Pharmaceuticals
W 764	Nefazodone	100 mg	White to Off White	Tablet	Capsule-Shape	Watson Laboratories
W 765	Nefazodone	150 mg	Orange	Tablet	Capsule-Shape	Watson Laboratories
W 766	Nefazodone	200 mg	Yellow	Tablet	Capsule-Shape	Watson Laboratories
W 767	Nefazodone	250 mg	White to Off White	Tablet	Capsule-Shape	Watson Laboratories
W C ; 581	Ovcon 35 Fe - White Tablet	0.4 mg; 0.035 mg	White	Tablet, Chewable	Circle	Warner Chilcott
W EFFEXOR XR 37.5	Effexor Xr	37.5 mg	Grey, Peach	Capsule, Extended Release		Wyeth Pharmaceuticals
W EFFEXOR XR 75	Effexor Xr	75 mg	Peach	Capsule, Extended Release		Wyeth Pharmaceuticals
W; 0.45/1.5	Prempro Single Tablet	0.45 mg; 1.5 mg	Gold	Tablet	Oval	Wyeth Pharmaceuticals
W; 0.625/5	Prempro Single Tablet	0.625 mg; 5 mg	Light Blue	Coated Tablet	Oval	Wyeth Pharmaceuticals
W; 2.5	Isordil	2.5 mg	Yellow	Tablet	Circle	Wyeth Pharmaceuticals
W; 5	Isordil	5 mg	Pink	Tablet	Circle	Wyeth Pharmaceuticals
W; 641	Triphasil-21 Brown Tablet	0.03 mg; 0.05 mg	Brown	21-Day Tablet Pack	Circle	Wyeth Pharmaceuticals
W; 641	Triphasil-28 Brown Tablet	0.03 mg; 0.05 mg	Brown	28-Day Tablet Pack	Circle	Wyeth Pharmaceuticals
W; 642	Triphasil-21 White Tablet	0.04 mg; 75 mcg	White	21-Day Tablet Pack	Circle	Wyeth Pharmaceuticals
W; 642	Triphasil-28 White Tablet	0.04 mg; 75 mcg	White	28-Day Tablet Pack	Circle	Wyeth Pharmaceuticals
W; 643	Triphasil-21 Light Yellow Tablet	0.03 mg; 0.125 mg	Light Yellow	21-Day Tablet Pack	Circle	Wyeth Pharmaceuticals
W; 643	Triphasil-28 Light Yellow Tablet	0.03 mg; 0.125 mg	Light Yellow	28-Day Tablet Pack	Circle	Wyeth Pharmaceuticals
W; 718	Buspirone Hydrochloride	15 mg	White	Tablet	Oval, Scored	Watson Laboratories
W; 912	Alesse 21	20 mcg; 0.1 mg	Pink	21-Day Tablet Pack	Circle	Wyeth Pharmaceuticals
W; 912	Alesse 28 Pink Tablet	20 mcg; 0.1 mg	Pink	28-Day Tablet Pack	Circle	Wyeth Pharmaceuticals
W; 7300	Tacaryl	4 mg	Pink	Tablet, Chewable		Westwood-Squibb Pharmaceuticals
W; 7400	Tacaryl	8 mg	Peach	Tablet		Westwood-Squibb Pharmaceuticals
W; A79	Aralen Phosphate and Primaquine Phosphate	500 mg; 79 mg	Orange	Coated Tablet	Circle	Sanofi Winthrop Pharmaceuticals
W; C; 270	Nardil	15 mg	Orange	Tablet		Pfizer
W; DILACOR XR; 120 MG ;	Dilacor Xr	120 mg	Pink and Flesh	Extended-Release Capsule		Watson Laboratories
W; DILACOR XR; 180 MG ;	Dilacor Xr	180 mg	Lavender and Flesh	Extended-Release Capsule		Watson Laboratories
W; DILACOR XR; 240 MG ;	Dilacor Xr	240 mg	Light Blue and Flesh	Extended-Release Capsule		Watson Laboratories
W; M; 31 ;	Mebaral	32 mg	White	Tablet		Ovation Pharmaceuticals
W; M; 31 ;	Mebaral	32 mg	White	Tablet		Sanofi Winthrop
W; M; 32 ;	Mebaral	50 mg	White	Tablet		Ovation Pharmaceuticals
W; M; 32 ;	Mebaral	50 mg	White	Tablet		Sanofi Winthrop
W; M; 33 ;	Mebaral	100 mg	White	Tablet		Ovation Pharmaceuticals

IMPRINT	BRAND/GENERIC NAME	STRENGTH	COLOR	FORM	SHAPE	MANUFACTURER
W; M; 33 ;	Mebaral	100 mg	White	Tablet		Sanofi Winthrop
W; M; 87	Mytelase Chloride	10 mg	White	Tablet		Sanofi-Aventis U.S.
W; MERRELL; 547	Quinamm	260 mg	White	Tablet	Circle	Aventis Pharmaceuticals
W; T51	Talwin Nx	50 mg; 0.5 mg	Yellow	Tablet	Oblong	Sanofi-Aventis U.S.
W53	Winstrol	2 mg	Pink	Tablet	Circle, Scored	Sanofi Pharmaceuticals
W907	Ranitidine Hydrochloride	300 mg	White	Tablet	Capsule-Shape	Ivax Pharmaceuticals
WATSON 343 ;	Verapamil Hydrochloride	80 mg	White	Tablet	Circle	Watson Laboratories
WATSON ; 243	Leena - Light Blue Tablet	0.5 mg; 0.035 mg	Light Blue	Tablet	Circle	Watson Laboratories
WATSON ; 244	Leena - Light Yellow-Green Tablet	1 mg; 0.035 mg	Light Yellow-Green	Tablet	Circle	Watson Laboratories
WATSON ; 949	Lutera - White Tablet	0.1 mg; 0.02 mg	White	Tablet	Circle	Watson Laboratories
WATSON ; 966	Quasense - White Tablet	0.15 mg; 0.03 mg	White	Tablet	Circle	Watson Pharma
WATSON ; 967	Sronyx - White Tablet	0.1 mg; 0.02 mg	White	Tablet	Circle	Watson Laboratories
WATSON ; 3220	Butalbital, Acetaminophen, Caffeine, and Codeine Phosphate	50 mg; 325 mg; 40 mg; 30 mg	Opaque Dark Blue, Opaque White	Capsule		Watson Laboratories
WATSON ; 3250	Nitrofurantoin Monohydrate/ macrocrystals	25 mg; 75 mg	Opaque Black, Yellow	Capsule		Watson Laboratories
WATSON ; 3253	Nitrofurantoin Macrocrystals	50 mg	White, Yellow	Capsule		Watson Laboratories
WATSON ; 3254	Nitrofurantoin Macrocrystals	100 mg	Yellow	Capsule		Watson Laboratories
WATSON 300	Furosemide	20 mg	White	Tablet	Circle	Watson Laboratories
WATSON 301	Furosemide	40 mg	White	Tablet	Circle	Watson Laboratories
WATSON 302	Furosemide	80 mg	White	Tablet	Circle	Watson Laboratories
WATSON 344 ;	Verapamil Hydrochloride	80 mg	Light Peach	Tablet	Circle	Watson Laboratories
WATSON 345 ;	Verapamil Hydrochloride	120 mg	White	Tablet	Circle	Watson Laboratories
WATSON 346 ;	Verapamil Hydrochloride	120 mg	Peach	Tablet	Circle	Watson Laboratories
WATSON 363	Clorazepate Dipotassium	3.75 mg	Light Blue	Tablet	Circle	Watson Laboratories
WATSON 364	Clorazepate Dipotassium	7.5 mg	Light Beige	Tablet	Circle	Watson Laboratories
WATSON 365	Clorazepate Dipotassium	15 mg	Pink	Tablet	Circle	Watson Laboratories
WATSON 403	Verapamil Hydrochloride	40 mg	White	Tablet	Circle	Watson Laboratories
WATSON 404	Verapamil Hydrochloride	40 mg	Light Peach	Tablet	Circle	Watson Laboratories
WATSON 685; 5-50 ;	Amiloride Hydrochloride and Hydrochlorothiazide	5 mg; 50 mg	Peach	Tablet	Circle	Watson Laboratories
WATSON 706; 2-10 ;	Perphenazine and Amitriptyline Hydrochloride	10 mg; 2.04 mg	Blue	Coated Tablet	Circle	Watson Laboratories
WATSON 707; 2-25	Perphenazine and Amitriptyline Hydrochloride	25 mg; 2 mg	Orange	Coated Tablet	Circle	Watson Laboratories
WATSON 708; 4-10 ;	Perphenazine and Amitriptyline Hydrochloride	10 mg; 4 mg	Salmon	Coated Tablet	Circle	Watson Laboratories
WATSON 709; 4-25 ;	Perphenazine and Amitriptyline Hydrochloride	25 mg; 4 mg	Yellow	Coated Tablet	Circle	Watson Laboratories
WATSON 714; 65-650 ;	Acetaminophen and Propoxyphene Hydrochloride	65 mg; 650 mg	Orange	Coated Tablet	Oblong	Watson Laboratories
WATSON 749	Oxycodone and Acetaminophen	325 mg; 5 mg	White	Tablet	Circle	Watson Laboratories
WATSON 779 ;	Oxybutynin Chloride	5 mg	Pale Blue	Tablet	Circle	Watson Laboratories
WATSON 824	Oxycodone and Acetaminophen	500 mg; 7.5 mg	White	Tablet	Capsule-Shape	Watson Laboratories
WATSON 825	Oxycodone and Acetaminophen	650 mg; 10 mg	White	Tablet	Capsule-Shape	Watson Laboratories
WATSON 932	Oxycodone and Acetaminophen	325 mg; 10 mg	White	Tablet	Circle	Watson Laboratories
WATSON 933	Oxycodone and Acetaminophen	325 mg; 7.5 mg	White	Tablet	Circle	Watson Laboratories
WATSON 3256 ;	Cyclobenzaprine Hydrochloride	5 mg	White	Tablet	Circle	Watson Laboratories
WATSON 3330 ;	Cyclobenzaprine Hydrochloride	7.5 mg	White	Tablet	Circle	Watson Laboratories
WATSON; 15/30	Levora 0.15/30-28 White Tablet	0.15 mg; 30 mcg	White	28-Day Tablet Pack	Circle	Watson Laboratories
WATSON; 15-30	Levora 0.15/30-21	0.15 mg; 30 mcg	White	21-Day Tablet Pack	Circle	Watson Laboratories
WATSON; 75/40	Trivora-21 White Tablet	40 mcg; 75 mcg	White	21-Day Tablet Pack	Circle	Watson Laboratories
WATSON; 75/40	Trivora-28 White Tablet	40 mcg; 75 mcg	White	28-Day Tablet Pack	Circle	Watson Laboratories
WATSON; 125/30	Trivora-21 Pink Tablet	30 mcg; 125 mcg	Pink	21-Day Tablet Pack	Circle	Watson Laboratories
WATSON; 125/30	Trivora-28 Pink Tablet	30 mcg; 125 mcg	Pink	28-Day Tablet Pack	Circle	Watson Laboratories
WATSON; 235 ;	Nor-Qd	0.35 mg	Yellow	Tablet	Circle	Watson Laboratories
WATSON; 240; 0.5 ;	Lorazepam	0.5 mg	White	Tablet	Circle	Watson Laboratories
WATSON; 241; 1 ;	Lorazepam	1 mg	White	Tablet	Circle	Watson Laboratories
WATSON; 242; 2 ;	Lorazepam	2 mg	White	Tablet	Circle, Scored	Watson Laboratories
WATSON; 254	Brevicon 28-Day Blue Tablet	0.5 mg; 0.035 mg	Blue	28-Day Tablet Pack	Circle	Watson Laboratories
WATSON; 254 ;	Tri-Norinyl 28 Day Blue Tablet	0.5 mg; 35 mcg	Blue	28-Day Tablet Pack	Circle	Watson Laboratories
WATSON; 259	Norinyl 1/35 Yellow-Green Tablet	1 mg; 35 mcg	Yellow-Green	28-Day Tablet Pack	Circle	Watson Laboratories
WATSON; 259 ;	Tri-Norinyl 28 Day Yellow-Green Tablet	1 mg; 35 mcg	Yellow-Green	28-Day Tablet Pack	Circle	Watson Laboratories
WATSON; 265	Norinyl 1/50 White Tablet	1 mg; 50 mcg	White	28-Day Tablet Pack	Circle	Watson Laboratories
WATSON; 303	Indomethacin	25 mg	Green	Capsule		Watson Laboratories
WATSON; 304	Indomethacin	50 mg	Green	Capsule		Watson Laboratories
WATSON; 305 ;	Propranolol Hydrochloride	10 mg	Orange	Tablet	Circle	Watson Laboratories
WATSON; 306 ;	Propranolol Hydrochloride	20 mg	Blue	Tablet	Circle	Watson Laboratories
WATSON; 307 ;	Propranolol Hydrochloride	40 mg	Green	Tablet	Circle	Watson Laboratories
WATSON; 308 ;	Propranolol Hydrochloride	80 mg	Yellow	Tablet	Circle	Watson Laboratories
WATSON; 309; 50	Doxycycline	50 mg	Green and Yellow	Capsule		Watson Laboratories
WATSON; 310; 100	Doxycycline	100 mg	Green	Capsule		Watson Laboratories
WATSON; 312	Metoclopramide Hydrochloride	10 mg	White	Tablet	Round; Bisected Scored	Watson Laboratories
WATSON; 332	Lorazepam	0.5 mg	White	Tablet	Circle, Scored	Watson Laboratories
WATSON; 333	Lorazepam	1 mg	White	Tablet	Circle, Scored	Watson Laboratories
WATSON; 334 ;	Lorazepam	2 mg	White	Tablet	Circle, Scored	Watson Laboratories
WATSON; 335	Acyclovir	400 mg	White to Off-White	Tablet	Oval	Watson Laboratories
WATSON; 336	Acyclovir	800 mg	White to Off-White	Tablet	Oval	Watson Laboratories
WATSON; 338	Diclofenac Sodium	50 mg	White to Off-White	Delayed-Release Tablet	Circle, Biconvex, Enteric-Coated	Watson Laboratories
WATSON; 347; 12.5 ;	Hydrochlorothiazide	12.5 mg	Teal and White	Capsule		Watson Laboratories
WATSON; 348 ;	Triamterene and Hydrochlorothiazide	75 mg; 50 mg	Yellow	Tablet	Circle, Scored	Watson Laboratories
WATSON; 349 ;	Hydrocodone Bitartrate and Acetaminophen	500 mg; 5 mg	White	Tablet	Capsule-Shape	Watson Laboratories
WATSON; 352 ;	Propranolol Hydrochloride	60 mg	Pink	Tablet	Circle	Watson Laboratories
WATSON; 353	Propranolol Hydrochloride	90 mg	Lavender	Tablet	Circle	Watson Laboratories

IMPRINT	BRAND/GENERIC NAME	STRENGTH	COLOR	FORM	SHAPE	MANUFACTURER
WATSON; 357	Methyldopa and Hydrochlorothiazide	250 mg; 15 mg	Off-White	Coated Tablet	Circle	Watson Laboratories
WATSON; 358	Methyldopa and Hydrochlorothiazide	250 mg; 25 mg	White	Coated Tablet	Circle	Watson Laboratories
WATSON; 359	Methyldopa and Hydrochlorothiazide	500 mg; 30 mg	Off-White	Coated Tablet	Circle	Watson Laboratories
WATSON; 360	Methyldopa and Hydrochlorothiazide	500 mg; 50 mg	White	Coated Tablet	Circle	Watson Laboratories
WATSON; 366	Fenoprofen Calcium	600 mg	Peach	Coated Tablet	Oblong, Scored	Watson Laboratories
WATSON; 367	Fenoprofen Calcium	200 mg	White and Yellow	Capsule		Watson Laboratories
WATSON; 368	Fenoprofen Calcium	300 mg	Yellow	Capsule		Watson Laboratories
WATSON; 373	Maprotiline Hydrochloride	25 mg	Peach	Coated Tablet	Oval	Watson Laboratories
WATSON; 374	Maprotiline Hydrochloride	50 mg	Peach	Coated Tablet	Circle	Watson Laboratories
WATSON; 375	Maprotiline Hydrochloride	75 mg	White	Coated Tablet	Oval	Watson Laboratories
WATSON; 379 ;	Amoxapine	25 mg	White	Tablet	Circle, Scored	Watson Laboratories
WATSON; 380 ;	Amoxapine	50 mg	Orange	Tablet	Circle, Scored	Watson Laboratories
WATSON; 381 ;	Amoxapine	100 mg	Blue	Tablet	Circle, Scored	Watson Laboratories
WATSON; 382 ;	Amoxapine	150 mg	Orange	Tablet	Circle, Scored	Watson Laboratories
WATSON; 383	Zovia 1/35e-21	1 mg; 35 mcg	Light Pink	21-Day Tablet Pack	Circle	Watson Laboratories
WATSON; 383	Zovia 1/35e-28 Light Pink Tablet	1 mg; 35 mcg	Light Pink	28-Day Tablet Pack	Circle	Watson Laboratories
WATSON; 384	Zovia 1/50e-21	1 mg; 50 mcg	Pink	21-Day Tablet Pack	Circle	Watson Laboratories
WATSON; 384	Zovia 1/50e-28 Pink Tablet	1 mg; 50 mcg	Pink	28-Day Tablet Pack	Circle	Watson Laboratories
WATSON; 385 ;	Hydrocodone Bitartrate and Acetaminophen	500 mg; 7.5 mg	White	Tablet	Capsule-Shape	Watson Laboratories
WATSON; 387 ;	Hydrocodone Bitartrate and Acetaminophen	750 mg; 7.5 mg	White	Tablet	Oblong	Watson Laboratories
WATSON; 388 ;	Hydrocodone Bitartrate and Acetaminophen	2.5 mg; 500 mg	White	Tablet	Oblong	Watson Laboratories
WATSON; 395; 50; 0.5 ;	Pentazocine and Naloxone Hydrochloride	0.5 mg; 50 mg	Green	Tablet	Capsule-Shape	Watson Laboratories
WATSON; 396; 25; 650	Pentazocine and Acetaminophen	25 mg; 650 mg	Light Aqua	Tablet	Capsule-Shape	Watson Laboratories
WATSON; 401	Albuterol Sulfate	2 mg	White	Tablet	Circle	Watson Laboratories
WATSON; 402	Albuterol Sulfate	4 mg	White	Tablet	Circle	Watson Laboratories
WATSON; 405	Lisinopril	2.5 mg	White	Tablet	Circle	Watson Laboratories
WATSON; 406	Lisinopril	5 mg	White	Tablet	Capsule-Shape	Watson Laboratories
WATSON; 407	Lisinopril	10 mg	Light Blue	Tablet	Circle	Watson Laboratories
WATSON; 408	Lisinopril	20 mg	Yellow	Tablet	Circle	Watson Laboratories
WATSON; 409	Lisinopril	40 mg	Yellow	Tablet	Circle	Watson Laboratories
WATSON; 414	Estropipate	0.75 mg	Yellow	Tablet	Circle, Scored	Watson Laboratories
WATSON; 415	Estropipate	1.5 mg	Peach	Tablet	Circle, Scored	Watson Laboratories
WATSON; 416	Estropipate	3 mg	Blue	Tablet	Circle, Scored	Watson Laboratories
WATSON; 424	Triamterene and Hydrochlorothiazide	37.5 mg; 25 mg	Light Green	Tablet	Circle, Scored	Watson Laboratories
WATSON; 425	Butalbital, Aspirin, Caffeine and Codeine Phosphate	50 mg; 325 mg; 40 mg; 30 mg	Blue and Yellow	Capsule		Watson Laboratories
WATSON; 430	Carbidopa and Levodopa	10 mg; 100 mg	Blue	Tablet	Circle, Scored	Watson Laboratories
WATSON; 431	Carbidopa and Levodopa	25 mg; 100 mg	Tan	Tablet	Circle, Scored	Watson Laboratories
WATSON; 432	Carbidopa and Levodopa	25 mg; 250 mg	Blue	Tablet	Circle, Scored	Watson Laboratories
WATSON; 437	Acebutolol Hydrochloride	200 mg	Red and Gray	Capsule		Watson Laboratories
WATSON; 438	Acebutolol Hydrochloride	400 mg	Maroon and Green	Capsule		Watson Laboratories
WATSON; 444	Guanfacine Hydrochloride	1 mg	Pink	Tablet	Circle	Watson Laboratories
WATSON; 451	Guanabenz Acetate	4 mg	Orange	Tablet	Circle	Watson Laboratories
WATSON; 452	Guanabenz Acetate	8 mg	Gray	Tablet	Circle	Watson Laboratories
WATSON; 453	Guanfacine Hydrochloride	2 mg	Peach	Tablet	Circle	Watson Laboratories
WATSON; 454	Gemfibrozil	600 mg	White	Coated Tablet	Oval, Scored	Watson Laboratories
WATSON; 460	Glipizide	5 mg	White	Tablet	Circle, Scored	Watson Laboratories
WATSON; 461	Glipizide	10 mg	White	Tablet	Circle, Scored	Watson Laboratories
WATSON; 462	Metoprolol Tartrate	50 mg	Pink	Tablet	Circle, Scored	Watson Laboratories
WATSON; 463	Metoprolol Tartrate	100 mg	Blue	Tablet	Circle, Scored	Watson Laboratories
WATSON; 466	Tramadol Hydrochloride	50 mg	White	Tablet	Circle	Watson Laboratories
WATSON; 485	Acetaminophen, Butalbital and Caffeine	325 mg; 50 mg; 40 mg	White	Tablet		Watson Laboratories
WATSON; 487	Estradiol	1 mg	Gray	Tablet	Scored, Circle	Watson Laboratories
WATSON; 488	Estradiol	2 mg	Light Green	Tablet	Circle, Scored	Watson Laboratories
WATSON; 491; 150MG	Mexiletine Hydrochloride	150 mg	Brown and Light Brown	Capsule		Watson Laboratories
WATSON; 492; 200MG ;	Mexiletine Hydrochloride	200 mg	Brown	Capsule		Watson Laboratories
WATSON; 493; 250MG ;	Mexiletine Hydrochloride	250 mg	Brown and Light Green	Capsule		Watson Laboratories
WATSON; 498	Doxycycline Hyclate	100 mg	Blue	Capsule		Watson Laboratories
WATSON; 499	Doxycycline Hyclate	100 mg	Beige	Coated Tablet	Circle	Watson Laboratories
WATSON; 500; 50MG ;	Doxycycline Hyclate	50 mg	Blue and White	Capsule		Watson Laboratories
WATSON; 502 ;	Hydrocodone Bitartrate and Acetaminophen	650 mg; 7.5 mg	Pink	Tablet	Capsule-Shape	Watson Laboratories
WATSON; 503 ;	Hydrocodone Bitartrate and Acetaminophen	650 mg; 10 mg	Light Green	Tablet	Capsule-Shape	Watson Laboratories
WATSON; 504	Indapamide	2.5 mg	White	Coated Tablet	Circle	Watson Laboratories
WATSON; 507	Necon 0.5/35-21	0.5 mg; 35 mcg	Light Yellow	21-Day Tablet Pack	Circle	Watson Laboratories
WATSON; 507	Necon 0.5/35-28 Light Yellow Tablet	0.5 mg; 35 mcg	Light Yellow	28-Day Tablet Pack	Circle	Watson Laboratories
WATSON; 507	Necon 10/11-21 Light Yellow Tablet	0.5 mg; 35 mcg	Light Yellow	21-Day Tablet Pack	Circle	Watson Laboratories
WATSON; 507	Necon 10/11-28 Light Yellow Tablet	0.5 mg; 35 mcg	Light Yellow	28-Day Tablet Pack	Circle	Watson Laboratories
WATSON; 508	Necon 1/35-21	1 mg; 35 mcg	Yellow	21-Day Tablet Pack	Circle	Watson Laboratories
WATSON; 508	Necon 1/35-28 Yellow Tablet	1 mg; 35 mcg	Yellow	28-Day Tablet Pack	Circle	Watson Laboratories

IMPRINT	BRAND/GENERIC NAME	STRENGTH	COLOR	FORM	SHAPE	MANUFACTURER
WATSON; 508	Necon 10/11-28 Yellow Tablet	1 mg; 35 mcg	Yellow	28-Day Tablet Pack	Circle	Watson Laboratories
WATSON; 508	Necon 10/11-21 Yellow Tablet	1 mg; 35 mcg	Yellow	21-Day Tablet Pack	Circle	Watson Laboratories
WATSON; 510	Necon 1/50-21	1 mg; 50 mcg	Blue	21-Day Tablet Pack	Circle	Watson Laboratories
WATSON; 510	Necon 1/50-28 Blue Tablet	1 mg; 50 mcg	Blue	28-Day Tablet Pack	Circle	Watson Laboratories
WATSON; 517	Hydrocodone Bitartrate and Acetaminophen	10 mg; 660 mg	White	Tablet	Oval	Watson Laboratories
WATSON; 524	Trinessa White Tablet	0.18 mg; 0.035 mg	White	28-Day Tablet Pack	Circle	Watson Laboratories
WATSON; 525	Trinessa Light Blue Tablet	0.215 mg; 0.035 mg	Light Blue	28-Day Tablet Pack	Circle	Watson Laboratories
WATSON; 526	Mononessa	0.25 mg; 0.035 mg	Blue	Tablet	Circle	Watson Laboratories
WATSON; 526	Trinessa Blue Tablet	0.25 mg; 0.035 mg	Blue	28-Day Tablet Pack	Circle	Watson Laboratories
WATSON; 527	Indapamide	1.25 mg	Orange	Coated Tablet	Circle	Watson Laboratories
WATSON; 528	Estradiol	0.5 mg	White	Tablet	Circle, Scored	Watson Laboratories
WATSON; 540	Hydrocodone Bitartrate and Acetaminophen	10 mg; 500 mg	Blue	Tablet	Capsule-Shape	Watson Laboratories
WATSON; 544 ;	Desipramine Hydrochloride	75 mg	Orange	Coated Tablet	Circle	Watson Laboratories
WATSON; 545 ;	Desipramine Hydrochloride	100 mg	Peach	Coated Tablet	Circle	Watson Laboratories
WATSON; 575	Trihexyphenidyl Hydrochloride	2 mg	White	Tablet	Circle, Scored	Watson Laboratories
WATSON; 576	Trihexyphenidyl Hydrochloride	5 mg	White	Tablet	Circle, Scored	Watson Laboratories
WATSON; 582	Propafenone Hydrochloride	150 mg	White	Coated Tablet	Circle, Scored	Watson Laboratories
WATSON; 583	Propafenone Hydrochloride	225 mg	White	Coated Tablet	Circle, Scored	Watson Laboratories
WATSON; 585	Diclofenac Potassium	50 mg	Brown	Coated Tablet	Circle	Watson Laboratories
WATSON; 594; 25 MG	Clomipramine Hydrochloride	25 mg	Blue	Capsule		Watson Laboratories
WATSON; 595; 50 MG	Clomipramine Hydrochloride	50 mg	Yellow	Capsule		Watson Laboratories
WATSON; 596; 75 MG	Clomipramine Hydrochloride	75 mg	Green	Capsule		Watson Laboratories
WATSON; 605 ;	Labetalol Hydrochloride	100 mg	Beige	Coated Tablet	Circle, Scored	Watson Laboratories
WATSON; 606 ;	Labetalol Hydrochloride	200 mg	White	Coated Tablet	Circle, Scored	Watson Laboratories
WATSON; 607 ;	Labetalol Hydrochloride	300 mg	Blue	Coated Tablet	Circle, Scored	Watson Laboratories
WATSON; 613	Butalbital, Acetaminophen and Caffeine	50 mg; 500 mg; 40 mg	Light Blue	Tablet	Capsule-Shape, Scored	Watson Laboratories
WATSON; 617	Morphine Sulfate	100 mg	Gray	Extended-Release Tablet	Circle	Watson Laboratories
WATSON; 629	Nora-Be	0.35 mg	White	Tablet	Circle	Watson Laboratories
WATSON; 630	Microgestin Fe 1/20 White Tablet	20 mcg; 1 mg	White	28-Day Tablet Pack	Circle	Watson Laboratories
WATSON; 631	Microgestin Fe 1.5/30 Green Tablet	1.5 mg; 30 mcg	Green	28-Day Tablet Pack	Circle	Watson Laboratories
WATSON; 632	Microgestin Fe 1/20 Brown Tablet	75 mg	Brown	28-Day Tablet Pack	Circle	Watson Laboratories
WATSON; 632	Microgestin Fe 1.5/30 Brown Tablet	75 mg	Brown	28-Day Tablet Pack	Circle	Watson Laboratories
WATSON; 632	Microgestin Fe Brown Tablet	75 mg	Brown	Tablet	Circle	Watson Laboratories
WATSON; 637	Pentoxifylline	400 mg	Red	Extended-Release Tablet	Oblong	Andrx Pharmaceuticals
WATSON; 639	Doxazosin Mesylate	1 mg	White	Tablet	Circle, Biconvex, Scored	Watson Laboratories
WATSON; 640	Doxazosin Mesylate	2 mg	Light Orange	Tablet	Circle, Biconvex, Scored	Watson Laboratories
WATSON; 641	Doxazosin Mesylate	4 mg	Light Orange	Tablet	Circle, Biconvex, Scored	Watson Laboratories
WATSON; 642	Doxazosin Mesylate	8 mg	Green	Tablet	Circle, Biconvex, Scored	Watson Laboratories
WATSON; 654	Sotalol Hydrochloride	80 mg	Light Blue	Tablet	Oval, Scored	Watson Laboratories
WATSON; 655	Sotalol Hydrochloride	160 mg	Light Blue	Tablet	Oval, Scored	Watson Laboratories
WATSON; 656	Sotalol Hydrochloride	240 mg	Light Blue	Tablet	Oval, Scored	Watson Laboratories
WATSON; 657	Buspirone Hydrochloride	5 mg	White	Tablet	Oval, Biconvex, Scored	Watson Laboratories
WATSON; 658	Buspirone Hydrochloride	10 mg	White	Tablet	Oval, Biconvex, Scored	Watson Laboratories
WATSON; 662; 120	Diltiazem Hydrochloride	120 mg	Pink and White	Extended-Release Capsule		Watson Laboratories
WATSON; 663; 180	Diltiazem Hydrochloride	180 mg	Pink and White	Extended-Release Capsule		Watson Laboratories
WATSON; 664; 240	Diltiazem Hydrochloride	240 mg	Red and White	Extended-Release Capsule		Watson Laboratories
WATSON; 665	Sotalol Hydrochloride	120 mg	Light Blue	Tablet	Oval, Scored	Watson Laboratories
WATSON; 667; 400 ;	Etodolac	400 mg	Yellow	Coated Tablet	Capsule-Shape	Watson Laboratories
WATSON; 668	Enalapril Maleate	2.5 mg	White to Off-White	Tablet	Circle, Biconvex, Scored	Watson Laboratories
WATSON; 669	Enalapril Maleate	5 mg	White to Off-White	Tablet	Circle, Biconvex	Watson Laboratories
WATSON; 670	Enalapril Maleate	10 mg	Pink with White Speckles	Tablet	Circle, Biconvex	Watson Laboratories
WATSON; 671	Enalapril Maleate	20 mg	Peach with White Speckles	Tablet	Circle, Biconvex	Watson Laboratories
WATSON; 682; 0.25 ;	Alprazolam	0.25 mg	White	Tablet	Oval, BI-Convex	Watson Laboratories
WATSON; 683; 0.5 ;	Alprazolam	0.5 mg	Peach	Tablet	Oval, BI-Convex	Watson Laboratories
WATSON; 684; 1 ;	Alprazolam	1 mg	Blue	Tablet	Oval, BI-Convex	Watson Laboratories
WATSON; 686; 10 ;	Baclofen	10 mg	White	Tablet	Oval	Watson Laboratories
WATSON; 687; 20 ;	Baclofen	20 mg	White	Tablet	Circle	Watson Laboratories
WATSON; 688; 12.5 ;	Captopril	12.5 mg	White	Tablet	Capsule-Shape, Scored	Watson Laboratories
WATSON; 689; 25 ;	Captopril	25 mg	White	Tablet	Circle, Quadrisect-Scored	Watson Laboratories
WATSON; 690; 50 ;	Captopril	50 mg	White	Tablet	Egg-Shape	Watson Laboratories
WATSON; 691; 100 ;	Captopril	100 mg	White	Tablet	Egg-Shape	Watson Laboratories
WATSON; 693; 500 ;	Chlorzoxazone	500 mg	Green	Tablet	Capsule-Shape, Partial-Scored	Watson Laboratories
WATSON; 695; 10 ;	Doxepin Hydrochloride	10 mg	Scarlet and Pink	Capsule		Watson Laboratories
WATSON; 696; 25 ;	Doxepin Hydrochloride	25 mg	Blue and Pink	Capsule		Watson Laboratories
WATSON; 697; 50 ;	Doxepin Hydrochloride	50 mg	Pink and Flesh	Capsule		Watson Laboratories
WATSON; 698; 200 ;	Hydroxychloroquine Sulfate	200 mg	White	Coated Tablet	Oval	Watson Laboratories
WATSON; 700; 25 ;	Hydroxyzine Hydrochloride	25 mg	Green	Coated Tablet	Circle	Watson Laboratories
WATSON; 704; 50 ;	Hydroxyzine Hydrochloride	50 mg	Yellow	Coated Tablet	Circle	Watson Laboratories
WATSON; 710; 5 ;	Pindolol	5 mg	White	Tablet	Circle, Scored	Watson Laboratories
WATSON; 711; 10 ;	Pindolol	10 mg	White	Tablet	Circle, Scored	Watson Laboratories

IMPRINT	BRAND/GENERIC NAME	STRENGTH	COLOR	FORM	SHAPE	MANUFACTURER
WATSON; 712; 10 MG ;	Piroxicam	10 mg	Light Blue and White	Capsule		Watson Laboratories
WATSON; 713; 20 MG ;	Piroxicam	20 mg	Light Blue	Capsule		Watson Laboratories
WATSON; 715; 260 ;	Quinine Sulfate	260 mg	White	Tablet	Circle	Watson Laboratories
WATSON; 716; 325 ;	Quinine Sulfate	325 mg	White	Capsule		Watson Laboratories
WATSON; 726; 50	Meperidine Hydrochloride	50 mg	White	Tablet	Circle, Biconvex	Watson Laboratories
WATSON; 727; 100	Meperidine Hydrochloride	100 mg	White	Tablet	Circle, Biconvex	Watson Laboratories
WATSON; 728; 500	Etodolac	500 mg	Blue	Coated Tablet	Capsule-Shape	Watson Laboratories
WATSON; 735; 200	Etodolac	200 mg	Gray and Brown	Capsule		Watson Laboratories
WATSON; 736; 300	Etodolac	300 mg	Gray and Swedish Orange	Capsule		Watson Laboratories
WATSON; 737; 5; 500 MG	Oxycodone and Acetaminophen	5 mg; 500 mg	White and Red	Capsule		Watson Laboratories
WATSON; 744; 1	Estazolam	1 mg	White	Tablet	Diamond, Scored	Watson Laboratories
WATSON; 745; 2	Estazolam	2 mg	Pink	Tablet	Diamond, Scored	Watson Laboratories
WATSON; 746	Clonazepam	0.5 mg	Yellow	Tablet	Circle, Scored	Watson Laboratories
WATSON; 747	Clonazepam	1 mg	Aqua	Tablet	Circle, Scored	Watson Laboratories
WATSON; 748	Clonazepam	2 mg	White	Tablet	Circle, Scored	Watson Laboratories
WATSON; 760 ;	Ranitidine	150 mg	Beige	Coated Tablet	Circle	Watson Laboratories
WATSON; 761 ;	Ranitidine	300 mg	Beige	Coated Tablet	Capsule-Shape	Watson Laboratories
WATSON; 771; 18.75	Pemoline	75 mg	White	Tablet	Circle, Scored	Watson Laboratories
WATSON; 772; 37.5	Pemoline	37.5 mg	Peach	Tablet	Circle, Scored	Watson Laboratories
WATSON; 773; 18.75	Pemoline	75 mg	Yellow	Tablet	Circle, Scored	Watson Laboratories
WATSON; 774	Oxycodone Hydrochloride	5 mg	White	Tablet	Circle, Scored	Watson Laboratories
WATSON; 775 ;	Diltiazem Hydrochloride	30 mg	Blue	Tablet	Circle, Scored	Watson Laboratories
WATSON; 776 ;	Diltiazem Hydrochloride	60 mg	White	Tablet	Circle	Watson Laboratories
WATSON; 777 ;	Diltiazem Hydrochloride	90 mg	Blue	Tablet	Oblong, Scored	Watson Laboratories
WATSON; 778 ;	Diltiazem Hydrochloride	120 mg	White	Tablet	Oblong, Scored	Watson Laboratories
WATSON; 780 ;	Sucralfate	1 G	Light Blue	Tablet	Oblong	Watson Laboratories
WATSON; 781 ;	Clomiphene	50 mg	White	Tablet	Circle	Watson Laboratories
WATSON; 782 ;	Diethylpropion Hydrochloride	75 mg	White	Extended-Release Tablet	Capsule-Shape	Watson Laboratories
WATSON; 783 ;	Diethylpropion Hydrochloride	25 mg	White	Tablet	Circle	Watson Laboratories
WATSON; 784 ;	Carisoprodol	350 mg	White	Tablet	Circle	Watson Laboratories
WATSON; 785; 5MG ;	Chlordiazepoxide Hydrochloride	5 mg	Green and Yellow	Capsule		Watson Laboratories
WATSON; 786; 10MG ;	Chlordiazepoxide Hydrochloride	10 mg	Green and Black	Capsule		Watson Laboratories
WATSON; 787; 25MG ;	Chlordiazepoxide Hydrochloride	25 mg	Green and White	Capsule		Watson Laboratories
WATSON; 790 ;	Methylprednisolone	4 mg	White	Tablet	Oval, Quadrisect Scored	Watson Laboratories
WATSON; 791 ;	Naproxen	500 mg	White	Tablet	Capsule-Shape	Watson Laboratories
WATSON; 792 ;	Naproxen Sodium	275 mg	White	Coated Tablet	Oval	Watson Laboratories
WATSON; 793 ;	Naproxen Sodium	550 mg	Green	Coated Tablet	Oval	Watson Laboratories
WATSON; 794; 10MG ;	Dicyclomine	10 mg	Dark Blue	Capsule		Watson Laboratories
WATSON; 795 ;	Dicyclomine Hydrochloride	20 mg	Blue	Tablet	Circle	Watson Laboratories
WATSON; 796 ;	Sulfasalazine	500 mg	Mustard	Tablet	Round, Bisected Scored	Watson Laboratories
WATSON; 800; 25 ;	Hydroxyzine Pamoate	25 mg	Dark Green and Light Green	Capsule		Watson Laboratories
WATSON; 801; 50MG ;	Hydroxyzine Pamoate	50 mg	Green and White	Capsule		Watson Laboratories
WATSON; 802 ;	Meclizine Hydrochloride	12.5 mg	Blue and White	Tablet	Oval	Watson Laboratories
WATSON; 803 ;	Meclizine Hydrochloride	25 mg	Yellow and White	Tablet	Oval	Watson Laboratories
WATSON; 804 ;	Meprobamate	200 mg	White	Tablet	Circle	Watson Laboratories
WATSON; 805 ;	Meprobamate	400 mg	White	Tablet	Circle, Convex	Watson Laboratories
WATSON; 806 ;	Methocarbamol	500 mg	White	Tablet	Circle	Watson Laboratories
WATSON; 807 ;	Methocarbamol	750 mg	White	Tablet	Capsule-Shape	Watson Laboratories
WATSON; 808 ;	Desipramine Hydrochloride	25 mg	Yellow	Coated Tablet	Circle	Watson Laboratories
WATSON; 809 ;	Desipramine Hydrochloride	50 mg	Green	Coated Tablet	Circle	Watson Laboratories
WATSON; 820	Oxycodone and Aspirin	4.5 mg; 0.38 mg; 325 mg	Yellow	Tablet	Circle, Scored	Watson Laboratories
WATSON; 821 ;	Naproxen	250 mg	White	Tablet	Circle	Watson Laboratories
WATSON; 822 ;	Naproxen	375 mg	Gray	Tablet	Capsule-Shape	Watson Laboratories
WATSON; 826; 20 MG	Fluoxetine Hydrochloride	10 mg	Light Green	Capsule		Watson Laboratories
WATSON; 827; 20 MG	Fluoxetine Hydrochloride	20 mg	Light Green and White	Capsule		Watson Laboratories
WATSON; 838	Ketorolac Tromethamine	10 mg	White	Coated Tablet	Circle, Convex	Watson Laboratories
WATSON; 841	Bisoprolol and Hydrochlorothiazide	2.5 mg; 6.25 mg	Yellow	Tablet	Circle, Biconvex	Watson Laboratories
WATSON; 842	Bisoprolol and Hydrochlorothiazide	5 mg; 6.25 mg	Pink	Tablet	Circle, Biconvex	Watson Laboratories
WATSON; 843	Bisoprolol and Hydrochlorothiazide	10 mg; 6.25 mg	White	Coated Tablet	Circle, Biconvex	Watson Laboratories
WATSON; 847	Ogestrel White Tablet	0.5 mg; 0.5 mg	White	28-Day Tablet Pack	Circle	Watson Laboratories
WATSON; 848 ;	Ogestrel White Tablet	0.5 mg; 0.05 mg	White	28-Day Tablet Pack	Circle	Watson Laboratories
WATSON; 850 ;	Acetaminophen and Codeine Phosphate	300 mg; 15 mg	White	Tablet	Circle, Flat-Faced, Beveled Edge	Watson Laboratories
WATSON; 851 ;	Acetaminophen and Codeine Phosphate	300 mg; 30 mg	White	Tablet	Circle, Scored	Watson Laboratories
WATSON; 852 ;	Acetaminophen and Codeine Phosphate	300 mg; 60 mg	White	Tablet	Circle, Scored	Watson Laboratories
WATSON; 853	Acetaminophen and Hydrocodone Bitartrate	325 mg; 10 mg	Yellow	Tablet	Capsule-Shape	Watson Laboratories
WATSON; 860	Lisinopril and Hydrochlorothiazide	10 mg; 12.5 mg	Pink	Tablet	Circle	Watson Laboratories
WATSON; 861	Lisinopril and Hydrochlorothiazide	20 mg; 12.5 mg	Light Blue	Tablet	Circle	Watson Laboratories
WATSON; 862	Lisinopril and Hydrochlorothiazide	20 mg; 25 mg	Pink	Tablet	Circle	Watson Laboratories
WATSON; 885	Lisinopril	30 mg	Yellow	Tablet	Circle	Watson Laboratories

IMPRINT	BRAND/GENERIC NAME	STRENGTH	COLOR	FORM	SHAPE	MANUFACTURER
WATSON; 892	Jolivette	0.35 mg	Green	Tablet		Watson Laboratories
WATSON; 913	Norco 5/325	5 mg; 325 mg	White with Orange Specks	Tablet	Capsule-Shape, Scored	Watson Laboratories
WATSON; 3159	Ursodiol	300 mg	White	Capsule		Watson Laboratories
WATSON; 3191	Pyridostigmine Bromide	60 mg	White	Tablet	Round, Quadrisected Scored	Watson Laboratories
WATSON; 3202	Hydrocodone Bitartrate and Acetaminophen	5 mg; 325 mg	White with Orange Specks	Tablet	Capsule-Shape	Watson Laboratories
WATSON; 3203	Hydrocodone Bitartrate and Acetaminophen	7.5 mg; 325 mg	Light Orange	Tablet	Capsule; Bisected Scored	Watson Laboratories
WATSON; 3219	Aspirin, Caffeine and Butalbital	325 mg; 50 mg; 40 mg	Yellow and Green	Capsule		Watson Laboratories
WATSON; LOXITANE; 5 MG ;	Loxitane	5 mg	Opaque Green	Capsule		Watson Laboratories
WATSON; LOXITANE; 10 MG ;	Loxitane	10 mg	Dark Green and Yellow	Capsule		Watson Laboratories
WATSON; LOXITANE; 25 MG ;	Loxitane	25 mg	Dark Green and Light Green	Capsule		Watson Laboratories
WATSON; LOXITANE; 50 MG ;	Loxitane	50 mg	Dark Green and Blue	Capsule		Watson Laboratories
WBA	Mol-Iron with Vitamin C	195 mg; 75 mg	Burgundy	Tablet		Schering-Plough Healthcare Products
WBB	Mol-Iron	195 mg	Brown	Tablet		Schering-Plough Healthcare Products
WC	Tedral Expectorant	130 mg; 24 mg; 8 mg	White	Tablet		Parke-Davis
WC ; 580	Ovcon-35 28 Day - Light Peach Tablet	0.4 mg; 0.035 mg	Light Peach	Tablet	Circle	Warner Chilcott
WC 389	Femtrace	0.45 mg	Cream	Tablet	Circle	Warner Chilcott
WC 390	Femtrace	0.9 mg	White	Tablet	Circle	Warner Chilcott
WC 391	Femtrace	1.8 mg	Yellow	Tablet	Circle	Warner Chilcott
WC; 010	Chlorpromazine Hydrochloride	10 mg		Tablet		Warner Chilcott
WC; 025	Chlorpromazine Hydrochloride	25 mg		Tablet		Warner Chilcott
WC; 030	Methyldopa and Hydrochlorothiazide	250 mg; 15 mg		Tablet		Warner Chilcott
WC; 031	Methyldopa and Hydrochlorothiazide	250 mg; 25 mg		Tablet		Warner Chilcott
WC; 032	Methyldopa and Hydrochlorothiazide	500 mg; 30 mg	Dark Red	Tablet	Circle	Warner Chilcott
WC; 033	Methyldopa and Hydrochlorothiazide	500 mg; 50 mg	Grey	Tablet	Circle	Warner Chilcott
WC; 050	Chlorpromazine Hydrochloride	50 mg		Tablet		Warner Chilcott
WC; 070 ;	Propranolol Hydrochloride	10 mg		Tablet		Warner Chilcott
WC; 071 ;	Propranolol Hydrochloride	20 mg		Tablet		Warner Chilcott
WC; 072 ;	Propranolol Hydrochloride	40 mg		Tablet		Warner Chilcott
WC; 073 ;	Propranolol Hydrochloride	60 mg		Tablet		Warner Chilcott
WC; 074 ;	Propranolol Hydrochloride	80 mg		Tablet		Warner Chilcott
WC; 084	Gemfibrozil	600 mg	White	Coated Tablet	Circle, Scored	Warner Chilcott
WC; 100	Chlorpromazine Hydrochloride	100 mg		Tablet		Warner Chilcott
WC; 117	Diphenoxylate Hydrochloride and Atropine	2.5 mg; 0.025 mg	White	Tablet	Circle	Warner Chilcott
WC; 121	Chlorthalidone	50 mg		Tablet		Warner Chilcott
WC; 123	Chlorthalidone	25 mg		Tablet		Warner Chilcott
WC; 141	Diazepam	2 mg		Tablet		Warner Chilcott
WC; 142	Diazepam	5 mg		Tablet		Warner Chilcott
WC; 201	Chlorpromazine Hydrochloride	200 mg		Tablet		Warner Chilcott
WC; 227	Natachew	1000 IU; 400 IU; 11 IU; 120 mg; 1 mg; 2 mg; 3 mg; 20 mg; 10 mg; 12 mcg; 29 mg	Tan Speckled	Tablet, Chewable	Circle, Scored	Warner Chilcott
WC; 230	Tedral	130 mg; 24 mg; 8 mg	White	Tablet		Parke-Davis
WC; 238	Tedral-25	130 mg; 24 mg; 25 mg	Salmon and Pink	Tablet		Parke-Davis
WC; 242	Carbamazepine	100 mg	Pink Speckled	Tablet, Chewable	Circle, Scored	Warner Chilcott
WC; 243	Carbamazepine	200 mg		Tablet		Warner Chilcott
WC; 271	Amitriptyline	100 mg		Tablet		Warner Chilcott
WC; 272	Amitriptyline	10 mg		Tablet		Warner Chilcott
WC; 273	Amitriptyline	25 mg		Tablet		Warner Chilcott
WC; 274	Amitriptyline	50 mg		Tablet		Warner Chilcott
WC; 275	Amitriptyline	75 mg		Tablet		Warner Chilcott
WC; 278	Amitriptyline	150 mg		Tablet		Warner Chilcott
WC; 402	Amcill	250 mg		Capsule		Warner Chilcott
WC; 404	Amcill	500 mg		Capsule		Warner Chilcott
WC; 420 ;	Quinine Sulfate	5 Gr		Capsule		Warner Chilcott
WC; 440	Furosemide	20 mg	White	Tablet	Oval	Warner Chilcott
WC; 441 ;	Furosemide	40 mg	White	Tablet	Circle	Warner Chilcott
WC; 442 ;	Furosemide	80 mg	White	Tablet	Circle	Warner Chilcott
WC; 443	Clonidine Hydrochloride	0.1 mg		Tablet		Warner Chilcott
WC; 444	Clonidine Hydrochloride	0.2 mg		Tablet		Warner Chilcott
WC; 445	Clonidine Hydrochloride	0.3 mg		Tablet		Warner Chilcott
WC; 451	Clorazepate Dipotassium	3.75 mg		Tablet		Warner Chilcott
WC; 452	Clorazepate Dipotassium	7.5 mg		Tablet		Warner Chilcott
WC; 453	Clorazepate Dipotassium	15 mg		Tablet		Warner Chilcott
WC; 551	Oxazepam	15 mg	Yellow	Tablet	Circle, Biconvex	Warner Chilcott

IMPRINT	BRAND/GENERIC NAME	STRENGTH	COLOR	FORM	SHAPE	MANUFACTURER
WC; 557	Verapamil Hydrochloride	80 mg	White	Tablet		Warner Chilcott
WC; 573	Verapamil Hydrochloride	120 mg	White	Tablet		Warner Chilcott
WC; 606	Aspirin	5 Gr	White	Tablet		Warner Chilcott
WC; 615	Minocycline Hcl	50 mg	Olive and Brown	Capsule		Warner Chilcott
WC; 616	Minocycline Hcl	100 mg	White and Olive	Capsule		Warner Chilcott
WC; 634 ;	Acetaminophen and Codeine No. 2	300 mg; 15 mg		Tablet		Warner Chilcott
WC; 635 ;	Acetaminophen and Codeine No. 3	300 mg; 30 mg	White	Tablet	Circle	Warner Chilcott
WC; 637 ;	Acetaminophen and Codeine No. 4	300 mg; 60 mg	White	Tablet	Flat	Warner Chilcott
WC; 640	Acetaminophen	325 mg	White	Tablet	Circle	Warner Chilcott
WC; 648	Penapar VK	250 mg		Tablet		Warner Chilcott
WC; 672	Erythromycin Stearate	250 mg		Tablet		Warner Chilcott
WC; 673	Penapar VK	500 mg		Tablet		Warner Chilcott
WC; 702	Hydrochlorothiazide	25 mg		Tablet		Warner Chilcott
WC; 710	Hydrochlorothiazide	50 mg		Tablet		Warner Chilcott
WC; 712	Spironolactone with Hydrochlorothiazide	25 mg; 25 mg		Tablet		Warner Chilcott
WC; 713	Spironolactone	25 mg		Tablet		Warner Chilcott
WC; 725	Aspirin with Codeine Phosphate No. 2	15 mg; 325 mg		Tablet		Warner Chilcott
WC; 726	Aspirin with Codeine Phosphate No. 3	30 mg; 325 mg		Tablet		Warner Chilcott
WC; 727	Aspirin with Codeine Phosphate No. 4	60 mg; 325 mg		Tablet		Warner Chilcott
WC; 730	Amoxicillin	250 mg		Capsule		Warner Chilcott
WC; 731	Amoxicillin	500 mg	Red and Pink	Capsule		Warner Chilcott
WC; 784	Potassium Chloride	10 meq		Extended-Release Tablet		Warner Chilcott
WC; 800	Chlordiazepoxide Hydrochloride	5 mg		Capsule		Warner Chilcott
WC; 801	Chlordiazepoxide Hydrochloride	10 mg		Capsule		Warner Chilcott
WC; 802	Chlordiazepoxide Hydrochloride	25 mg		Capsule		Warner Chilcott
WC; 808	Cephradine	250 mg		Capsule		Warner Chilcott
WC; 809	Cephradine	500 mg		Capsule		Warner Chilcott
WC; 813 ;	Doxycycline Hyclate	100 mg		Tablet		Warner Chilcott
WC; 829 ;	Doxycycline Hyclate	50 mg		Capsule		Warner Chilcott
WC; 830 ;	Doxycycline Hyclate	100 mg		Capsule		Warner Chilcott
WC; 832	Amiloride Hydrochloride and Hydrochlorothiazide	5 mg; 50 mg	Yellow	Tablet	Circle	Warner Chilcott
WC; 833	Triamterene and Hydrochlorothiazide	50 mg; 75 mg	Yellow	Tablet	Round, Bisected Scored	Warner Chilcott
WC; 849	Quinidine Sulfate	200 mg		Tablet		Warner Chilcott
WC; 850	Duraquin	330 mg	White	Sustained-Release Tablet		Warner Chilcott
WC; 850	Quinidine Gluconate	330 mg		Tablet		Warner Chilcott
WC; 865 ;	Methyldopa	250 mg	Blue	Tablet	Circle	Warner Chilcott
WC; 866 ;	Methyldopa	500 mg	Blue	Tablet	Circle	Warner Chilcott
WC; 878	Metoclopramide Hydrochloride	10 mg		Tablet		Warner Chilcott
WC; 919	Erythromycin Stearate	500 mg		Tablet		Warner Chilcott
WC; 929	Nelova 0.5/35e-21	0.5 mg; 35 mcg	Light Yellow	21-Day Tablet Pack	Circle	Warner Chilcott
WC; 929	Nelova 0.5/35e-28 Light Yellow Tablet	0.5 mg; 35 mcg	Light Yellow	28-Day Tablet Pack	Circle	Warner Chilcott
WC; 929	Nelova 10/11-21 Light Yellow Tablet	0.5 mg; 35 mcg	Light Yellow	21-Day Tablet Pack	Circle	Warner Chilcott
WC; 929	Nelova 10/11-28 Light Yellow Tablet	0.5 mg; 35 mcg	Light Yellow	28-Day Tablet Pack	Circle	Warner Chilcott
WC; 930	Nelova 1/35e-21	1 mg; 35 mcg	Dark Yellow	21-Day Tablet Pack	Circle	Warner Chilcott
WC; 930	Nelova 1/35e-28 Dark Yellow Tablet	1 mg; 35 mcg	Dark Yellow	28-Day Tablet Pack	Circle	Warner Chilcott
WC; 930	Nelova 10/11-21 Dark Yellow Tablet	1 mg; 35 mcg	Dark Yellow	21-Day Tablet Pack	Circle	Warner Chilcott
WC; 930	Nelova 10/11-28 Dark Yellow Tablet	1 mg; 35 mcg	Dark Yellow	28-Day Tablet Pack	Circle	Warner Chilcott
WC; 940	R-Tannate	25 mg; 8 mg; 25 mg	Buff	Tablet	Capsule-Shape	Warner Chilcott
WC; 942	Nelova 1/50m-21	1 mg; 50 mcg	Light Blue	21-Day Tablet Pack	Circle	Warner Chilcott
WC; 942	Nelova 1/50m-28 Light Blue Tablet	1 mg; 50 mcg	Light Blue	28-Day Tablet Pack	Circle	Warner Chilcott
WC; 945	Dicloxacillin Sodium	250 mg		Capsule		Warner Chilcott
WC; 946	Dicloxacillin Sodium	500 mg		Capsule		Warner Chilcott
WC; 951	Potassium Chloride	8 meq		Extended-Release Capsule		Warner Chilcott
WC; 977	Temazepam	15 mg		Capsule		Warner Chilcott
WC; 978	Temazepam	30 mg		Capsule		Warner Chilcott
WC; 979	Acetaminophen and Propoxyphene Hydrochloride	65 mg; 650 mg		Tablet		Warner Chilcott
WC; 980	Acetaminophen and Propoxyphene Napsylate	100 mg; 650 mg		Tablet		Warner Chilcott
WC; 981	Haloperidol	0.5 mg		Tablet		Warner Chilcott
WC; 982	Haloperidol	1 mg		Tablet		Warner Chilcott
WC; 983	Haloperidol	2 mg		Tablet		Warner Chilcott
WC; 984	Haloperidol	5 mg		Tablet		Warner Chilcott
WC; 985	Clonidine Hydrochloride and Chlorthalidone	0.1 mg; 15 mg		Tablet		Warner Chilcott
WC; 986	Clonidine Hydrochloride and Chlorthalidone	0.2 mg; 15 mg		Tablet		Warner Chilcott
WC; 987	Clonidine Hydrochloride and Chlorthalidone	0.3 mg; 15 mg		Tablet		Warner Chilcott
WC; 988	Flurazepam Hydrochloride	15 mg	Peach and Orange	Capsule		Warner Chilcott

IMPRINT	BRAND/GENERIC NAME	STRENGTH	COLOR	FORM	SHAPE	MANUFACTURER
WC; 989	Flurazepam Hydrochloride	30 mg	Peach and Strawberry	Capsule		Warner Chilcott
WDF	Mol-Iron Chronosule	390 mg	Pink and Red, Clear	Capsule		Schering-Plough Healthcare Products
WELLBUTRIN SR; 100	Wellbutrin SR	100 mg	Blue	Sustained-Release Tablet	Circle, Biconvex	Glaxosmithkline
WELLBUTRIN SR; 150	Wellbutrin SR	150 mg	Purple	Sustained-Release Tablet	Circle, Biconvex	Glaxosmithkline
WELLBUTRIN XL; 150	Wellbutrin XL	150 mg	White to Yellow	Tablet	Circle	Glaxosmithkline
WELLBUTRIN XL; 300	Wellbutrin XL	300 mg	White to Yellow	Tablet	Circle	Glaxosmithkline
WELLBUTRIN; 75	Wellbutrin	75 mg	Yellow-Gold	Coated Tablet	Circle, Biconvex	Glaxosmithkline
WELLBUTRIN; 100	Wellbutrin	100 mg	Red	Coated Tablet	Circle, Biconvex	Glaxosmithkline
WELLBUTRIN; SR; 200	Wellbutrin SR	200 mg	Light Pink	Sustained-Release Tablet	Circle, Biconvex	Glaxosmithkline
WELLBUTRIN; XL; 150	Wellbutrin XL	150 mg	Creamy White to Pale Yellow	Extended-Release Tablet	Circle	Glaxosmithkline
WELLBUTRIN; XL; 300	Wellbutrin XL	300 mg	Creamy White to Pale Yellow	Extended-Release Tablet	Circle	Glaxosmithkline
WELLCOME Y9C ; 100	Retrovir	100 mg	Dark Blue Band, White, Opaque	Capsule		Glaxosmithkline
WELLCOME; U3B	Tabloid	40 mg	Green-Yellow	Tablet	Circle, Scored	Glaxosmithkline
WELLCOME; ZOVIRAX; 200	Zovirax	200 mg	Blue	Capsule		Glaxosmithkline
WER	Mol-Iron Panhemic Chronosule	390 mg; 25 mcg; 150 mg; 6 mg; 6 mg; 5 mg; 30 mg	Clear, Red and Yellow	Capsule		Schering-Plough Healthcare Products
WEST-WARD; 475	Prednisone	5 mg	White	Tablet		Novartis Generics
WEST-WARD; 477	Prednisone	20 mg	Peach	Tablet	Circle, Scored	Novartis Generics
WEST-WARD; 3189	Lithium Carbonate	300 mg	Grey/yellow	Capsule		Ivax Pharmaceuticals
WESTWARD; FLURAZEPAM; 15	Flurazepam Hydrochloride	15 mg	Blue and White	Capsule		Novartis Generics
WESTWARD; FLURAZEPAM; 30	Flurazepam Hydrochloride	30 mg	Blue	Capsule	Oblong	Novartis Generics
WFHC; 91	Equagesic	200 mg; 325 mg	Pink and Yellow	Tablet	Circle, Layered, Scored	Women First Healthcare
WFHC; 4191	Synalgos-Dc	16 mg; 356.4 mg; 30 mg	Blue and Gray	Capsule		Women First Healthcare
WH-SCS; 5752	Piroxicam	10 mg	Opaque Orange and Opaque Light Blue	Capsule		Lederle Laboratories
WH-SCS; 5762	Piroxicam	20 mg	Opaque Orange	Capsule		Lederle Laboratories
WINTHROP; T; 37	Talacen	25 mg; 650 mg	Pale Blue	Tablet		Sanofi-Aventis U.S.
WKJ ;	Permitil Chronotab	1 mg	Yellow	Tablet		Schering
WMM	Mol-Iron with Vitamin C Chronosule	390 mg; 150 mg	Clear, Red and Orange	Capsule		Schering-Plough Healthcare Products
WPI ; 3176	Citalopram Hydrobromide	10 mg	White	Tablet	Circle	Watson Laboratories
WPI 339	Diclofenac Sodium	75 mg	White	Tablet, Delayed Release	Circle	Watson Laboratories
WPI 839	Bupropion Hydrochloride	150 mg	White	Sustained-Release Tablet	Circle	Watson Laboratories
WPI 844	Glipizide	5 mg	Orange	Tablet, Extended Release	Circle	Watson Laboratories
WPI 844	Glipizide Extended-Release	5 mg	Orange	Tablet, Extended Release	Circle	Watson Laboratories
WPI 845	Glipizide	10 mg	White to Off-White	Tablet, Extended Release	Circle	Watson Laboratories
WPI 845	Glipizide Extended-Release	10 mg	White to Off-White	Tablet, Extended Release	Circle	Watson Laboratories
WPI 858	Bupropion Hydrochloride	100 mg	White	Sustained-Release Tablet	Circle	Watson Laboratories
WPI 867	Bupropion Hydrochloride	150 mg	White	Tablet, Extended Release	Circle	Watson Laboratories
WPI 900	Glipizide	2.5 mg	Light Orange	Tablet, Extended Release	Circle	Watson Laboratories
WPI 3177	Citalopram Hydrobromide	20 mg	White	Tablet	Circle	Watson Laboratories
WPI 3178	Citalopram Hydrobromide	40 mg	White	Tablet	Circle	Watson Laboratories
WPI; 1118	Mirtazapine	30 mg	Yellow	Tablet	Oval, Scored	Watson Laboratories
WPI; 1119	Mirtazapine	45 mg	White	Tablet	Oval	Watson Laboratories
WPI; 1117 ;	Mirtazapine	15 mg	White	Tablet	Oval, Scored	Watson Laboratories
WPI; 2455 ;	Metformin Hydrochloride	1000 mg	Light Peach	Coated Tablet	Capsule-Shaped; Bisected Scored	Watson Laboratories
WPI; 2713	Metformin Hydrochloride	500 mg	Light Peach	Coated Tablet	Capsule-Shape	Watson Laboratories
WPI; 2775	Metformin Hydrochloride	850 mg	Light Peach	Coated Tablet	Capsule-Shape	Watson Laboratories
WPI; 3111	Methylphenidate Hydrochloride	20 mg	White	Extended-Release Tablet	Oval	Watson Laboratories
WPI; 3137	Nizatidine	150 mg	Buff	Capsule		Watson Laboratories
WPI; 3138	Nizatidine	300 mg	Light Brown	Capsule		Watson Laboratories
WPPH; 153	Methyldopa and Hydrochlorothiazide	250 mg; 25 mg	White	Coated Tablet	Circle	Endo Laboratories
WPPH; 156	Cyclobenzaprine Hydrochloride	10 mg	Butterscotch Yellow	Coated Tablet	D-Shape	Endo Laboratories
WPPH; 162	Amiloride Hydrochloride and Hydrochlorothiazide	5 mg; 50 mg	Peach	Tablet	Diamond, Scored	Endo Laboratories
WPPH; 179	Methyldopa and Hydrochlorothiazide	250 mg; 15 mg	Salmon	Coated Tablet	Circle	Endo Laboratories
WPPH; 195	Diflunisal	250 mg	Peach	Coated Tablet	Capsule-Shape	Endo Laboratories
WPPH; 196	Diflunisal	500 mg	Orange	Coated Tablet	Capsule-Shape	Endo Laboratories
WYETH; 1	Equanil	400 mg	White	Tablet		Wyeth Pharmaceuticals
WYETH; 2	Equanil	200 mg	White	Tablet		Wyeth Pharmaceuticals
WYETH; 10	Isordil	10 mg	White	Tablet	Circle	Wyeth Pharmaceuticals
WYETH; 13	Amphojel	600 mg	White	Tablet		Wyeth Pharmaceuticals
WYETH; 19	Phenergan	12.5 mg	Orange	Tablet		Wyeth Pharmaceuticals
WYETH; 22	Aludrox	233 mg; 83 mg		Tablet, Chewable		Wyeth Pharmaceuticals

IMPRINT	BRAND/GENERIC NAME	STRENGTH	COLOR	FORM	SHAPE	MANUFACTURER
WYETH; 27	Phenergan	25 mg	White	Tablet		Wyeth Pharmaceuticals
WYETH; 28	Sparine	50 mg	Orange	Coated Tablet	Circle	Wyeth Pharmaceuticals
WYETH; 29	Sparine	25 mg	Yellow	Coated Tablet	Circle	Wyeth Pharmaceuticals
WYETH; 33	Equanil Wyseals	400 mg	Yellow	Coated Tablet	Circle	Wyeth Pharmaceuticals
WYETH; 33	Wyseals	400 mg	Yellow	Coated Tablet		Wyeth Pharmaceuticals
WYETH; 53	Omnipen	250 mg	Violet and Pink	Capsule		Wyeth Pharmaceuticals
WYETH; 56	Ovral	0.5 mg; 50 mcg	White	21-Day Tablet Pack	Circle	Wyeth Pharmaceuticals
WYETH; 57	Unipen	250 mg	Green and Yellow	Capsule		Wyeth Pharmaceuticals
WYETH; 59	Pen-Vee K	250 mg	White	Tablet		Wyeth Pharmaceuticals
WYETH; 62	Ovrette	75 mcg	Yellow	28-Day Tablet Pack	Circle	Wyeth Pharmaceuticals
WYETH; 71	Mazanor	1 mg	White	Tablet	Circle, Scored	Wyeth Pharmaceuticals
WYETH; 73, W; 4	Wytensin	4 mg	Orange	Tablet	Five-Sided	Wyeth Pharmaceuticals
WYETH; 74; W; 8	Wytensin	8 mg	Grey	Tablet	Five-Sided	Wyeth Pharmaceuticals
WYETH; 75	Nordette-21	0.15 mg; 30 mcg	Light Orange	21-Day Tablet Pack	Circle	Wyeth Pharmaceuticals
WYETH; 75	Nordette-28 Light Orange Tablet	0.15 mg; 30 mcg	Light Orange	28-Day Tablet Pack	Circle	Wyeth Pharmaceuticals
WYETH; 78	Lo/ovral	0.3 mg; 30 mcg	White	21-Day Tablet Pack	Circle	Wyeth Pharmaceuticals
WYETH; 78	Lo/ovral-28 White Tablet	0.3 mg; 30 mcg	White	28-Day Tablet Pack	Circle	Wyeth Pharmaceuticals
WYETH; 119	Amphojel	300 mg	White	Tablet	Circle	Wyeth Pharmaceuticals
WYETH; 138	A-M-T	162 mg; 250 mg		Tablet		Wyeth Pharmaceuticals
WYETH; 200	Sparine	100 mg	Pink	Coated Tablet	Circle	Wyeth Pharmaceuticals
WYETH; 227	Phenergan	50 mg	Pink	Tablet		Wyeth Pharmaceuticals
WYETH; 261	Mepergan Fortis	50 mg; 25 mg	Maroon	Capsule		Wyeth Pharmaceuticals
WYETH; 308	Meperidine Hydrochloride	50 mg	Tablet	Tablet	Circle, Scored	Wyeth Pharmaceuticals
WYETH; 309	Omnipen	500 mg	Violet and Pink	Capsule		Wyeth Pharmaceuticals
WYETH; 313	Aspirin	300 mg		Tablet		Wyeth Pharmaceuticals
WYETH; 322	Chloral Hydrate	500 mg	Red	Capsule		Wyeth Pharmaceuticals
WYETH; 360	Pathocil	250 mg	Purple and White	Capsule		Wyeth Pharmaceuticals
WYETH; 389	Tetracycline Hydrochloride	250 mg	Blue and Yellow	Capsule		Wyeth Pharmaceuticals
WYETH; 390	Pen-Vee K	500 mg	White	Tablet		Wyeth Pharmaceuticals
WYETH; 434	Phenergan-D	60 mg; 6.25 mg	Orange and White	Tablet		Wyeth Pharmaceuticals
WYETH; 464	Unipen	500 mg	White	Coated Tablet		Wyeth Pharmaceuticals
WYETH; 471	Tetracycline Hydrochloride	500 mg	Blue and Yellow	Capsule		Wyeth Pharmaceuticals
WYETH; 472	Basaljel	608 mg		Capsule		Wyeth Pharmaceuticals
WYETH; 473	Basaljel	608 mg		Tablet		Wyeth Pharmaceuticals
WYETH; 559	Wymox	250 mg	Gray and Green	Capsule		Wyeth Pharmaceuticals
WYETH; 560	Wymox	500 mg	Gray and Green	Capsule		Wyeth Pharmaceuticals
WYETH; 576	Wyamycin S	250 mg	Yellow	Coated Tablet		Wyeth Pharmaceuticals
WYETH; 578	Wyamycin S	500 mg	Pink	Coated Tablet		Wyeth Pharmaceuticals
WYETH; 593	Pathocil	500 mg	Purple and White	Capsule		Wyeth Pharmaceuticals
WYETH; 614	Cyclapen W	250 mg	Yellow	Tablet	Capsule-Shape, Scored	Wyeth Pharmaceuticals
WYETH; 615	Cyclapen W	500 mg	Yellow	Tablet		Wyeth Pharmaceuticals
WYETH; 794	Stuart Prenatal Multivitamin/ multimineral Supplement	4000 I.U.; 400 I.U.; 11 mg; 0.8 mg; 18 mg; 200 mg; 60 mg; 25 mg; 100 mg; 1.84 mg; 1.7 mg; 2.6 mg; 4 mcg	Pink	Tablet		Wyeth Pharmaceuticals
WYETH; 4120	Cyclospasmol	100 mg	Orange	Coated Tablet		Wyeth Pharmaceuticals
WYETH; 4124	Cyclospasmol	200 mg	Blue	Capsule		Wyeth Pharmaceuticals
WYETH; 4140	Isordil Tembids	40 mg	Clear Blue and Transparent	Capsule		Wyeth Pharmaceuticals
WYETH; 4148	Cyclospasmol	400 mg	Red and Blue	Capsule		Wyeth Pharmaceuticals
WYETH; 4152	Isordil Titradose	5 mg	Pink	Tablet		Wyeth Pharmaceuticals
WYETH; 4153	Isordil Titradose	10 mg	White	Tablet		Wyeth Pharmaceuticals
WYETH; 4154	Isordil Titradose	20 mg	Green	Tablet		Wyeth Pharmaceuticals
WYETH; 4159	Isordil Titradose	30 mg	Blue	Tablet		Wyeth Pharmaceuticals
WYETH; 4169	Synalgos	6.25 mg; 356.4 mg; 30 mg	Maroon and Gray	Capsule		Wyeth Pharmaceuticals
WYETH; 4175	Synalgos-Dc-A	16 mg; 356.4 mg; 30 mg	Green and Gray	Capsule		Wyeth Pharmaceuticals
WYETH; 4177; SECTRAL; 200	Sectral	200 mg	Purple and Orange	Capsule		Wyeth Pharmaceuticals
WYETH; 4179; SECTRAL; 400	Sectral	400 mg	Brown and Orange	Capsule		Wyeth Pharmaceuticals
WYETH; 4181; ORUDIS 50	Orudis	50 mg	Dark Green and Light Green	Capsule		Wyeth Pharmaceuticals
WYETH; 4186; ORUDIS 25	Orudis	25 mg	Dark Green and Red	Capsule		Wyeth Pharmaceuticals
WYETH; 4187; ORUDIS 75	Orudis	75 mg	Dark Green and White	Capsule		Wyeth Pharmaceuticals
WYETH; 4188; C	Cordarone	200 mg	Pink	Tablet	Circle, Convex-Faced	Wyeth Pharmaceuticals
WYETH; 4191	Synalgos-Dc	16 mg; 356.4 mg; 30 mg	Blue and Gray	Capsule		Women First Healthcare
WYETH; 4191	Synalgos-Dc	16 mg; 356.4 mg; 30 mg	Blue and Gray	Capsule		Wyeth Pharmaceuticals
WYETH; 4191	Synalgos-Dc	16 mg; 356.4 mg; 30 mg	Blue and Gray	Capsule		Wyeth-Ayerst Laboratories
WYETH; 4192	Isordil Titradose	40 mg	Green	Tablet		Wyeth Pharmaceuticals
X	Senokot Xtra	17 mg	Tan	Tablet	Circle	Purdue Pharmaceutical Products
X; 0.5	Alprazolam	0.5 mg	White	Extended-Release Tablet	Five-Sided	Pharmacia & Upjohn
X; 0.5	Xanax Xr	0.5 mg	White	Tablet, Extended Release	Five-Sided	Pharmacia & Upjohn
X; 1	Xanax Xr	1 mg	Yellow	Extended-Release Tablet	Square	Pharmacia & Upjohn
X; 2	Xanax Xr	2 mg	Blue	Extended-Release Tablet	Circle	Pharmacia & Upjohn
X; 3	Xanax Xr	3 mg	Green	Extended-Release Tablet	Triangle	Pharmacia & Upjohn
X; 10	Uroxatral	10 mg	White and Yellow	Tablet, Extended Release	Circle	Sanofi-Aventis U.S.

IMPRINT	BRAND/GENERIC NAME	STRENGTH	COLOR	FORM	SHAPE	MANUFACTURER
XANAX; 0.25	Xanax	0.25 mg	White	Tablet	Oval, Scored	Pharmacia & Upjohn
XANAX; 0.5	Xanax	0.5 mg	Peach	Tablet	Oval	Pharmacia & Upjohn
XANAX; 1.0	Xanax	1 mg	Blue	Tablet	Oval, Scored	Pharmacia & Upjohn
XELODA; 150	Xeloda	150 mg	Light Peach	Coated Tablet	Oblong	Roche Laboratories
XELODA; 500	Xeloda	500 mg	Peach	Coated Tablet	Oblong	Roche Laboratories
Z	Zomig-Zmt	2.5 mg	White	Disintegrating Tablet	Circle	Astra Zeneca
Z 4	Zofran Odt	4 mg	White	Tablet, Disintegrating	Circle	Glaxosmithkline
Z 8	Zofran Odt	8 mg	White	Tablet, Disintegrating	Circle	Glaxosmithkline
Z; 5	Zomig-Zmt	5 mg	White	Disintegrating Tablet	Circle, Flat Faced, Bevelled	Astra Zeneca
Z; 75	Zantac 75	75 mg	Pink	Tablet	Five-Sided	Pfizer Consumer Health Care
Z; 2057	Phenytoin Sodium	100 mg	Clear	Capsule		Ivax Pharmaceuticals
Z; 2083	Hydrochlorothiazide	25 mg	Peach	Tablet	Circle	Ivax Pharmaceuticals
Z; 2089	Hydrochlorothiazide	50 mg	Peach	Tablet	Circle	Ivax Pharmaceuticals
Z; 2186	Propoxyphene Hydrochloride	65 mg	Pale Pink	Capsule		Ivax Pharmaceuticals
Z; 2190	Probenecid	500 mg	Yellow	Coated Tablet	Capsule-Shape	Novartis Generics
Z; 2193	Probenecid with Colchicine	0.5 mg; 500 mg	White	Tablet	Capsule-Shape	Novartis Generics
Z; 2218	Sulfisoxazole	500 mg	White	Tablet	Circle, Scored	Ivax Pharmaceuticals
Z; 2345	Procainamide Hydrochloride	250 mg	Yellow	Capsule		Ivax Pharmaceuticals
Z; 2347	Procainamide Hydrochloride	500 mg	Yellow and Orange	Capsule		Ivax Pharmaceuticals
Z; 2485	Hydrochlorothiazide	100 mg	Light Orange	Tablet	Circle	Ivax Pharmaceuticals
Z; 2662; 10	Famotidine	10 mg		Tablet		Ivax Pharmaceuticals
Z; 2907	Furosemide	40 mg	White	Tablet	Circle	Ivax Pharmaceuticals
Z; 2908	Furosemide	20 mg	White	Tablet	Oval	Ivax Pharmaceuticals
Z; 2909	Hydroxyzine Pamoate	50 mg	Green and White	Capsule		Ivax Pharmaceuticals
Z; 2911	Hydroxyzine Pamoate	25 mg	Dark Green and Light Green	Capsule		Ivax Pharmaceuticals
Z; 2929 ;	Cyproheptadine Hydrochloride	4 mg	White	Tablet	Round-Flat, Bisected Scored	Ivax Pharmaceuticals
Z; 2931	Methyldopa	250 mg	White	Coated Tablet	Circle	Ivax Pharmaceuticals
Z; 2932	Methyldopa	500 mg	White	Coated Tablet	Circle	Ivax Pharmaceuticals
Z; 2959	Ergoloid Mesylates SL	1 mg	White	Tablet	Oval	Ivax Pharmaceuticals
Z; 2971	Metronidazole	250 mg	White	Tablet	Circle, Convex	Ivax Pharmaceuticals
Z; 2971 ;	Helidac Therapy: Part II	250 mg	White	Tablet	Circle	Procter & Gamble Pharmaceuticals
Z; 2984	Doxycycline Hyclate	50 mg	Blue and White	Capsule		Ivax Pharmaceuticals
Z; 3001	Quinine Sulfate	260 mg	White	Tablet	Circle	Ivax Pharmaceuticals
Z; 3007	Metronidazole	500 mg	White	Tablet	Oblong, Convex	Ivax Pharmaceuticals
Z; 3626	Doxycycline Hyclate	100 mg	Orange	Coated Tablet	Circle	Ivax Pharmaceuticals
Z; 3690; 5	Prochlorperazine Maleate	5 mg	Gold	Tablet	Circle	Ivax Pharmaceuticals
Z; 3691; 10	Prochlorperazine Maleate	10 mg	Gold	Tablet	Circle	Ivax Pharmaceuticals
Z; 3925; 2	Diazepam	2 mg	White	Tablet	Circle	Ivax Pharmaceuticals
Z; 3926; 5	Diazepam	5 mg	Yellow	Tablet	Circle	Ivax Pharmaceuticals
Z; 3927; 10	Diazepam	10 mg	Light Blue	Tablet	Circle	Ivax Pharmaceuticals
Z; 4029	Indomethacin	25 mg	Green	Capsule		Ivax Pharmaceuticals
Z; 4030	Indomethacin	50 mg	Green	Capsule		Ivax Pharmaceuticals
Z; 4067	Prazosin Hydrochloride	1 mg	Ivory	Capsule		Ivax Pharmaceuticals
Z; 4068	Prazosin Hydrochloride	2 mg	Pink	Capsule		Ivax Pharmaceuticals
Z; 4069	Prazosin Hydrochloride	5 mg	Blue	Capsule		Ivax Pharmaceuticals
Z; 4073	Cephalexin	250 mg	Grey and Red	Capsule		Ivax Pharmaceuticals
Z; 4074	Cephalexin	500 mg	Red	Capsule		Ivax Pharmaceuticals
Z; 4096; 10 ;	Baclofen	10 mg	White	Tablet	Circle, Flat, Scored	Ivax Pharmaceuticals
Z; 4097; 20 ;	Baclofen	20 mg	White	Tablet	Circle, Flat, Scored	Ivax Pharmaceuticals
Z; 4172	Quinine Sulfate	325 mg	White	Capsule		Ivax Pharmaceuticals
Z; 4217; 5	Pindolol	5 mg	White	Tablet	Circle	Ivax Pharmaceuticals
Z; 4218; 10	Pindolol	10 mg	White	Tablet	Circle	Ivax Pharmaceuticals
Z; 4226	Guanabenz Acetate	4 mg	Peach	Tablet	Circle, Compressed	Ivax Pharmaceuticals
Z; 4227	Guanabenz Acetate	8 mg	Grey	Tablet	Round, Compressed, Bisected Scored	Ivax Pharmaceuticals
Z; 4232; 0.5	Bumetanide	0.5 mg	Green	Tablet	Flat, Round, Bevel-Edged, Bisected Scored	Ivax Pharmaceuticals
Z; 4233; 1	Bumetanide	1 mg	Yellow	Tablet	Flat, Round, Bevel-Edged, Bisected Scored	Ivax Pharmaceuticals
Z; 4234; 2	Bumetanide	2 mg	Peach	Tablet	Flat, Round, Bevel-Edged, Bisected Scored	Ivax Pharmaceuticals
Z; 4235; 20	Nadolol	20 mg	White	Tablet	Circle	Ivax Pharmaceuticals
Z; 4236; 40	Nadolol	40 mg	White	Tablet	Circle	Ivax Pharmaceuticals
Z; 4237; 80	Nadolol	80 mg	White	Tablet	Circle	Ivax Pharmaceuticals
Z; 4238; 120	Nadolol	120 mg	White	Tablet	Oblong	Ivax Pharmaceuticals
Z; 4239; 160	Nadolol	160 mg	White	Tablet	Oblong	Ivax Pharmaceuticals
Z; 4259	Indapamide	2.5 mg	White	Coated Tablet	Circle	Ivax Pharmaceuticals
Z; 4262; 1.25	Indapamide	1.25 mg	Orange	Tablet	Circle	Ivax Pharmaceuticals
Z; 4288; 20 MG	Nicardipine Hydrochloride	20 mg	Opaque White	Capsule		Ivax Pharmaceuticals
Z; 4289; 30 MG	Nicardipine Hydrochloride	30 mg	Light Blue Opaque	Capsule		Ivax Pharmaceuticals
Z; 4338; 5 MG	Terazosin Hydrochloride	5 mg	Red and White	Capsule		Ivax Pharmaceuticals
Z; 4348; 600	Oxaprozin	600 mg	White	Tablet	Oval	Ivax Pharmaceuticals
Z; 4804	Oxazepam	10 mg	Blue and White	Capsule		Ivax Pharmaceuticals
Z; 4805	Oxazepam	15 mg	Clear	Capsule		Ivax Pharmaceuticals
Z; 4806	Oxazepam	30 mg	Orange and White	Capsule		Ivax Pharmaceuticals
Z; 5624; 300 MG	Nizatidine	300 mg	Light Brown and White	Capsule		Ivax Pharmaceuticals
Z; LA; BOCK	Zephrex LA	600 mg; 120 mg	Orange	Tablet, Extended Release	Oval	Sanofi Pharmaceuticals
Z; LA; BOCK	Zephrex LA	600 mg; 120 mg	Orange	Tablet, Extended Release	Oval	Sanofi-Aventis U.S.
Z; LA; BOCK	Zephrex LA	600 mg; 120 mg	Orange	Tablet, Extended Release	Oval	Sanofi-Synthelabo
ZANTAC 150 ; GLAXO ;	Zantac 150	150 mg	Peach	Tablet	Five-Sided	Glaxosmithkline
ZANTAC; 150; 427	Zantac 150 Efferdose	150 mg	White to Pale Yellow	Effervescent Tablet	Circle, Flat-Faced, Bevel-Edged	Glaxosmithkline
ZANTAC; 150; GLAXO	Zantac 150 Geldose	150 mg	Beige	Gel/jelly		Glaxosmithkline

IMPRINT	BRAND/GENERIC NAME	STRENGTH	COLOR	FORM	SHAPE	MANUFACTURER
ZANTAC; 300; GLAXO	Zantac 300 Geldose	300 mg	Beige	Gel/jelly		Glaxosmithkline
ZBN	Arava	10 mg	White	Tablet	Circle	Sanofi-Aventis U.S.
ZBO	Arava	20 mg	Yellow	Tablet	Triangle	Sanofi-Aventis U.S.
ZBP	Arava	100 mg	White	Coated Tablet	Circle	Aventis Pharmaceuticals
ZE; 74	Erythromycin Ethylsuccinate	400 mg	Mottled Pink	Tablet	Oval	Abbott Laboratories
ZENECA; ACCOLATE; 10	Accolate	10 mg	White	Coated Tablet	Circle, Biconvex, Mini	Astra Zeneca
ZENECA; ACCOLATE; 20	Accolate	20 mg	White	Coated Tablet	Circle, Biconvex	Astra Zeneca
ZENITH; 50 MG; 2130	Nitrofurantoin Macrocrystals	50 mg	Pink and White	Capsule		Ivax Pharmaceuticals
ZENITH; 100 MG; 2131	Nitrofurantoin Macrocrystals	100 mg	Pink	Capsule		Ivax Pharmaceuticals
ZENITH; 200 MG; 4171	Quinine Sulfate	200 mg	White	Capsule		Ivax Pharmaceuticals
ZENITH; 4266; 200	Acyclovir	200 mg	Opaque White	Capsule		Ivax Pharmaceuticals
ZESTORETIC; 141	Zestoretic	12.5 mg; 10 mg	Peach	Tablet	Circle, Biconvex	Astra Zeneca
ZESTORETIC; 142	Zestoretic	12.5 mg; 20 mg	White	Tablet	Circle, Biconvex	Astra Zeneca
ZESTORETIC; 145	Zestoretic	25 mg; 20 mg	Peach	Tablet	Circle, Biconvex	Astra Zeneca
ZESTRIL; 2 1/2; 135	Zestril	2.5 mg	White	Tablet	Circle, Biconvex	Astra Zeneca
ZESTRIL; 10; 131	Zestril	10 mg	Pink	Tablet	Circle, Biconvex	Astra Zeneca
ZESTRIL; 20; 132	Zestril	20 mg	Red	Tablet	Circle, Biconvex	Astra Zeneca
ZESTRIL; 30; 133	Zestril	30 mg	Red	Tablet	Circle, Biconvex	Astra Zeneca
ZESTRIL; 40; 134	Zestril	40 mg	Yellow	Tablet	Circle, Biconvex	Astra Zeneca
ZESTRIL; 130	Zestril	5 mg	Pink	Tablet	Capsule-Shape, Biconvex, Scored	Astra Zeneca
ZG ZENITH 30MG 4289	Nicardipine Hydrochloride	30 mg	Light Blue Opaque	Capsule		Barr Laboratories
ZOFRAN 4	Zofran	4 mg	White	Tablet	Oval	Glaxosmithkline
ZOFRAN 8	Zofran	8 mg	Yellow	Tablet	Oval	Glaxosmithkline
ZOLOFT; 25 MG	Zoloft	25 mg	Light Green	Coated Tablet	Capsule-Shape, Scored	Pfizer
ZOLOFT; 50 MG	Zoloft	50 mg	Light Blue	Coated Tablet	Capsule-Shape, Scored	Pfizer
ZOLOFT; 100 MG	Zoloft	100 mg	Light Yellow	Coated Tablet	Capsule-Shape, Scored	Pfizer
ZOMIG; 2.5	Zomig	2.5 mg	Yellow	Coated Tablet	Circle, Biconvex, Scored	Astra Zeneca
ZOMIG; 5	Zomig	5 mg	Pink	Coated Tablet	Biconvex	Astra Zeneca
ZONEGRAN; 25	Zonegran	25 mg	White and White	Capsule		Elan Pharma
ZONEGRAN; 50	Zonegran	50 mg	White and Gray	Capsule		Elan Pharma
ZONEGRAN; 100	Zonegran	100 mg	White and Red	Capsule		Elan Pharma
ZONEGRAN; 100; ELAN LOGO	Zonegran	100 mg	White and Red	Capsule		Elan Pharma
ZOVIRAX; 800	Zovirax	800 mg	Light Blue	Tablet	Oval	Glaxosmithkline
ZOVIRAX; TRIANGLE	Zovirax	400 mg	White	Tablet	Shield-Shape	Glaxosmithkline
ZYBAN; 150	Zyban	150 mg	Purple	Sustained-Release Tablet	Circle, Biconvex	Glaxosmithkline
ZYRTEC; C5	Zyrtec Chewable	5 mg	Purple	Tablet	Circle	Pfizer Laboratories
ZYRTEC; C10	Zyrtec Chewable	10 mg	Purple	Tablet	Circle	Pfizer Laboratories
ZYRTEC-D	Zyrtec-D 12 Hour	5 mg; 120 mg	White	Extended-Release Tablet	Biconvex, Bilayer, Circle	Pfizer Laboratories
ZYRTEC-D	Zyrtec-D 12 Hour	5 mg; 120 mg	White	Extended-Release Tablet	Biconvex, Bilayer, Circle	Ucb Pharma
ZYVOX; 400 MG	Zyvox	400 mg	White	Coated Tablet	Oblong, Compressed	Pharmacia & Upjohn
ZYVOX; 600 MG	Zyvox	600 mg	White	Coated Tablet	Capsule-Shape, Compressed	Pharmacia & Upjohn

POISON CONTROL CENTERS

The American Association of Poison Control Centers (AAPCC) uses a single, nationwide emergency number to automatically link callers with their regional poison center. This toll-free number, **800-222-1222**, also works for **teletype lines (TTY)** for the hearing-impaired and **telecommunication devices (TTD)** for individuals who are deaf. However, a few local poison centers and the ASPCA/Animal Poison Control Center are not part of this nationwide system and continue to use separate numbers.

Most of the centers listed below are certified by the AAPCC. **Certified centers are marked by an asterisk after the name**. Each has to meet certain criteria. It must, for example, serve a large geographic area; it must be open 24 hours a day and provide direct-dial or toll-free access; it must be supervised by a medical director; and it must have registered pharmacists or nurses available to answer questions from the public.

Within each state, centers are listed alphabetically by city. Some state poison centers also list their original emergency numbers (including TTY/TDD) that only work within that state. For these listings, callers may use either the state number or the nationwide 800 number.

ALABAMA

BIRMINGHAM

Regional Poison Control Center, The Children's Hospital of Alabama (*)

1600 7th Ave. South
Birmingham, AL 35233-1711
Business: 205-939-9201
Emergency: 800-222-1222
www.chsys.org

TUSCALOOSA

Alabama Poison Center (*)

2503 Phoenix Dr.
Tuscaloosa, AL 35405
Business: 205-345-0600
Emergency: 800-222-1222
800-462-0800 (AL)
www.alapoisoncenter.org

ALASKA

JUNEAU

Alaska Poison Control System

Section of Community Health and EMS
410 Willoughby Ave., Room 103
Box 110616
Juneau, AK 99811-0616
Business: 907-465-3027
Emergency: 800-222-1222
www.chems.alaska.gov

(PORTLAND, OR)

**Oregon Poison Center (*)
Oregon Health Sciences University**

3181 SW Sam Jackson Park Rd.
CB550
Portland, OR 97239
Business: 503-494-8311
Emergency: 800-222-1222
www.oregonpoison.com

ARIZONA

PHOENIX

**Banner Poison Control Center (*)
Banner Good Samaritan Medical Center**

901 E. Willetta St.
Room 2701
Phoenix, AZ 85006
Business: 602-495-4884
Emergency: 800-222-1222
www.bannerpoisoncontrol.com

TUCSON

**Arizona Poison and Drug Information Center (*)
Arizona Health Sciences Center**

1501 N. Campbell Ave.
Room 1156
Tucson, AZ 85724
Business: 520-626-7899
Emergency: 800-222-1222

ARKANSAS

LITTLE ROCK

**Arkansas Poison and Drug Information Center
College of Pharmacy - UAMS**

4301 West Markham St.
Mail Slot 522-2
Little Rock, AR 72205-7122
Business: 501-686-5540
Emergency: 800-222-1222
800-376-4766 (AR)
TDD/TTY: 800-641-3805

ASPCA/ANIMAL POISON CONTROL CENTER

1717 South Philo Rd.
Suite 36
Urbana, IL 61802
Business: 217-337-5030
Emergency: 888-426-4435
800-548-2423
www.napcc.aspca.org

CALIFORNIA

FRESNO/MADERA

**California Poison Control System-Fresno/Madera Div.(*)
Children's Hospital of Central California**

9300 Valley Children's Place
MB 15
Madera, CA 93638-8762
Business: 559-622-2300
Emergency: 800-222-1222
800-876-4766 (CA)
TDD/TTY: 800-972-3323
www.calpoison.org

SACRAMENTO

**California Poison Control System-Sacramento Div.(*)
UC Davis Medical Center**

Room HSF 1024
2315 Stockton Blvd.
Sacramento, CA 95817
Business: 916-227-1400
Emergency: 800-222-1222
800-876-4766 (CA)
TDD/TTY: 800-972-3323
www.calpoison.org

SAN DIEGO

**California Poison Control System-San Diego Div. (*)
UC San Diego Medical Center**

200 West Arbor Dr.
San Diego, CA 92103-8925
Business: 858-715-6300
Emergency: 800-222-1222
800-876-4766 (CA)
TDD/TTY: 800-972-3323
www.calpoison.org

SAN FRANCISCO

**California Poison Control System-San Francisco Div.(*)
San Francisco General Hospital
University of California
San Francisco**

Box 1369
San Francisco, CA 94143-1369
Business: 415-502-6000
Emergency: 800-222-1222
800-876-4766 (CA)
TDD/TTY: 800-972-3323
www.calpoison.org

COLORADO

DENVER

Rocky Mountain Poison and Drug Center (*)

777 Bannock St.
Mail Code 0180
Denver, CO 80204-4507
Business: 303-739-1100
Emergency: 800-222-1222
TDD/TTY: 303-739-1127 (CO)
www.RMPDC.org

CONNECTICUT

FARMINGTON

**Connecticut Regional Poison Control Center (*)
University of Connecticut Health Center**

263 Farmington Ave.
Farmington, CT 06030-5365
Business: 860-679-4540
Emergency: 800-222-1222
TDD/TTY: 866-218-5372
http://poisoncontrol.uchc.edu

DELAWARE

(PHILADELPHIA, PA)

**The Poison Control Center (*)
Children's Hospital of Philadelphia**

34th St. & Civic Center Blvd.
Philadelphia, PA 19104-4303
Business: 215-590-2003
Emergency: 800-222-1222
800-722-7112 (DE)
TDD/TTY: 215-590-8789
www.poisoncontrol.chop.edu

DISTRICT OF COLUMBIA

WASHINGTON, DC

National Capital Poison Center (*)

3201 New Mexico Ave., NW
Suite 310
Washington, DC 20016
Business: 202-362-3867
Emergency: 800-222-1222
www.poison.org

FLORIDA

JACKSONVILLE

Florida Poison Information Center-Jacksonville (*)
SHANDS Hospital

655 West 8th St.
Jacksonville, FL 32209
Business: 904-244-4465
Emergency: 800-222-1222
http://fpicjax.org

MIAMI

Florida Poison Information Center-Miami (*)
University of Miami–Department of Pediatrics

P.O. Box 016960 (R-131)
Miami, FL 33101
Business: 305-585-5250
Emergency: 800-222-1222
www.miami.edu/poison-center

TAMPA

Florida Poison Information Center-Tampa (*)
Tampa General Hospital

P.O. Box 1289
Tampa, FL 33601-1289
Business: 813-844-7044
Emergency: 800-222-1222
www.poisoncentertampa.org

GEORGIA

ATLANTA

Georgia Poison Center (*)
Hughes Spalding Children's Hospital, Grady Health System

80 Jesse Hill Jr. Dr., SE
P.O. Box 26066
Atlanta, GA 30303-3050
Business: 404-616-9237
Emergency: 800-222-1222
404-616-9000 (Atlanta)
TDD: 404-616-9287
www.georgiapoisoncenter.org

HAWAII

(DENVER, CO)

Rocky Mountain Poison and Drug Center (*)

777 Bannock St.
Mail Code 0180
Denver, CO 80204-4507
Business: 303-739-1100
Emergency: 800-222-1222
www.RMPDC.org

IDAHO

(DENVER, CO)

Rocky Mountain Poison and Drug Center (*)

777 Bannock St.
Mail Code 0180
Denver, CO 80204-4507
Business: 303-739-1100
Emergency: 800-222-1222
www.RMPDC.org

ILLINOIS

CHICAGO

Illinois Poison Center (*)

222 South Riverside Plaza
Suite 1900
Chicago, IL 60606
Business: 312-906-6136
Emergency: 800-222-1222
TDD/TTY: 312-906-6185
www.illinoispoisoncenter.org

INDIANA

INDIANAPOLIS

Indiana Poison Control Center (*)
Clarian Health Partners
Methodist Hospital

I-65 at 21st St.
Indianapolis, IN 46206-1367
Business: 317-962-2335
Emergency: 800-222-1222
800-382-9097
317-962-2323 (Indianapolis)
TTY: 317-962-2336
www.clarian.org/poisoncontrol

IOWA

SIOUX CITY

Iowa Statewide Poison Control Center
Iowa Health System and the University of Iowa Hospitals and Clinics

401 Douglas St., Suite 402
Sioux City, IA 51101
Business: 712-279-3710
Emergency: 800-222-1222
712-277-2222 (IA)
www.iowapoison.org

KANSAS

KANSAS CITY

Mid-America Poison Control Center
University of Kansas Medical Center

3901 Rainbow Blvd.
Room B-400
Kansas City, KS 66160-7231
Business: 913-588-6638
Emergency: 800-222-1222
800-332-6633 (KS)
TDD: 913-588-6639
www.kumc.edu/poison

KENTUCKY

LOUISVILLE

Kentucky Regional Poison Center (*)

PO Box 35070
Louisville, KY 40232-5070
Business: 502-629-7264
Emergency: 800-222-1222
502-589-8222 (Louisville)
www.krpc.com

LOUISIANA

MONROE

Louisiana Drug and Poison Information Center (*)
University of Louisiana at Monroe

700 University Ave.
Monroe, LA 71209-6430
Business: 318-342-3648
Emergency: 800-222-1222
www.lapcc.org

MAINE

PORTLAND

Northern New England Poison Center

Maine Medical Center
22 Bramhall St.
Portland, ME 04102
Business: 207-662-7220
Emergency: 800-222-1222
207-871-2879 (ME)
TDD/TTY: 877-299-4447 (ME)
207-871-2879 (ME)
www.nnepc.org

MARYLAND

BALTIMORE

Maryland Poison Center (*)
University of Maryland at Baltimore
School of Pharmacy

20 North Pine St., PH 772
Baltimore, MD 21201
Business: 410-706-7604
Emergency: 800-222-1222
TDD: 410-706-1858
www.mdpoison.com

(WASHINGTON, DC)

National Capital Poison Center (*)

3201 New Mexico Ave., NW
Suite 310
Washington DC 20016
Business: 202-362-3867
Emergency: 800-222-1222
TDD/TTY: 202-362-8563 (MD)
www.poison.org

MASSACHUSETTS

BOSTON

Regional Center for Poison Control and Prevention (*)
(Serving Massachusetts and Rhode Island)

300 Longwood Ave.
Boston, MA 02115
Business: 617-355-6609
Emergency: 800-222-1222
TDD/TTY: 888-244-5313
www.maripoisoncenter.com

MICHIGAN

DETROIT

Regional Poison Control Center (*)
Children's Hospital of Michigan

4160 John R. Harper Professional Office Bldg.
Suite 616
Detroit, MI 48201
Business: 313-745-5335
Emergency: 800-222-1222
TDD/TTY: 800-356-3232
www.mitoxic.org/pcc

GRAND RAPIDS

DeVos Children's Hospital Regional Poison Center (*)

100 Michigan St., NE
Grand Rapids, MI 49503
Business: 616-391-3690
Emergency: 800-222-1222
http://poisoncenter.devoschildrens.org

MINNESOTA

MINNEAPOLIS

Minnesota Poison Control System (*) Hennepin County Medical Center

701 Park Ave.
Mail Code RL
Minneapolis, MN 55415
Business: 612-873-3144
Emergency: 800-222-1222
www.mnpoison.org

MISSISSIPPI

JACKSON

Mississippi Regional Poison Control Center, University of Mississippi Medical Center

2500 North State St.
Jackson, MS 39216
Business: 601-984-1680
Emergency: 800-222-1222

MISSOURI

ST. LOUIS

Missouri Regional Poison Center (*) Cardinal Glennon Children's Hospital

7980 Clayton Rd.
Suite 200
St. Louis, MO 63117
Business: 314-772-5200
Emergency: 800-222-1222
TDD/TTY: 314-612-5705
www.cardinalglennon.com

MONTANA

(DENVER, CO)

Rocky Mountain Poison and Drug Center (*)

777 Bannock St.
Mail Code 0180
Denver, CO 80204-4507
Business: 303-739-1100
Emergency: 800-222-1222
TDD/TTY: 303-739-1127
www.RMPDC.org

NEBRASKA

OMAHA

The Poison Center (*) Children's Hospital

8401 W. Dodge St., Suite 115
Omaha, NE 68114
Business: 402-955-5555
Emergency: 800-222-1222
www.nebraskapoison.com

NEVADA

(DENVER, CO)

Rocky Mountain Poison and Drug Center (*)

777 Bannock St.
Mail Code 0180
Denver, CO 80204-4507
Business: 303-739-1100
Emergency: 800-222-1222
www.RMPDC.org

(PORTLAND, OR)

Oregon Poison Center (*) Oregon Health Sciences University

3181 SW Sam Jackson Park Rd.
Portland, OR 97201
Business: 503-494-8600
Emergency: 800-222-1222
www.oregonpoison.com

NEW HAMPSHIRE

(PORTLAND, ME)

Northern New England Poison Center

Maine Medical Center
22 Bramhall St.
Portland, ME 04102
Business: 207-662-7220
Emergency: 800-222-1222
www.nnepc.org

NEW JERSEY

NEWARK

New Jersey Poison Information and Education System (*) UMDNJ

65 Bergen St.
Newark, NJ 07101
Business: 973-972-9280
Emergency: 800-222-1222
TDD/TTY: 973-926-8008
www.njpies.org

NEW MEXICO

ALBUQUERQUE

New Mexico Poison and Drug Information Center (*)

MSC09-5080
1 University of New Mexico
Albuquerque, NM 87131-0001
Business: 505-272-4261
Emergency: 800-222-1222
http://HSC.UNM.edu/pharmacy/poison

NEW YORK

BUFFALO

Western New York Regional Poison Control Center (*) Children's Hospital of Buffalo

219 Bryant St.
Buffalo, NY 14222
Business: 716-878-7654
Emergency: 800-222-1222
www.fingerlakespoison.org

MINEOLA

Long Island Regional Poison and Drug Information Center (*) Winthrop University Hospital

259 First St.
Mineola, NY 11501
Business: 516-663-2650
Emergency: 800-222-1222
TDD: 516-747-3323 (Nassau)
516-924-8811 (Suffolk)
www.lirpdic.org

NEW YORK CITY

New York City Poison Control Center (*) NYC Dept. of Health

455 First Ave., Room 123
New York, NY 10016
Business: 212-447-8152
Emergency: 800-222-1222
(English) 212-340-4494
212-POISONS
(212-764-7667)

Emergency: 212-VENENOS
(Spanish) (212-836-3667)
TDD: 212-689-9014

ROCHESTER

Finger Lakes Regional Poison and Drug Information Center (*) University of Rochester Medical Center

601 Elmwood Ave.
Box 321
Rochester, NY 14642
Business: 585-273-4155
Emergency: 800-222-1222
TTY: 585-273-3854

SYRACUSE

Central New York Poison Center (*) SUNY Upstate Medical University

750 East Adams St.
Syracuse, NY 13210
Business: 315-464-7078
Emergency: 800-222-1222
www.cnypoison.org

NORTH CAROLINA

CHARLOTTE

Carolinas Poison Center (*) Carolinas Medical Center

PO Box 32861
Charlotte, NC 28232
Business: 704-512-3795
Emergency: 800-222-1222
TDD: 800-735-8262
TTY: 800-735-2962
www.ncpoisoncenter.org

NORTH DAKOTA

(MINNEAPOLIS, MN)

Minnesota Poison Control System (*) Hennepin County Medical Center

701 Park Ave.
Mail Code 820
Minneapolis, MN 55415
Business: 612-873-3144
Emergency: 800-222-1222
www.ndpoison.org

OHIO

CINCINNATI

Cincinnati Drug and Poison Information Center (*) Regional Poison Control System

3333 Burnet Ave.
Vernon Place, 3rd Floor
Cincinnati, OH 45229
Business: 513-636-5111
Emergency: 800-222-1222
TDD/TTY: 800-253-7955
www.cincinnatichildrens.org/dpic

CLEVELAND

Greater Cleveland Poison Control Center

11100 Euclid Ave.
MP 6007
Cleveland, OH 44106-6007
Business: 216-844-1573
Emergency: 800-222-1222
216-231-4455 (OH)

COLUMBUS

**Central Ohio
Poison Center (*)**

700 Children's Dr.
Room L032
Columbus, OH 43205-2696
Business: 614-722-2635
Emergency: 800-222-1222
TTY: 614-228-2272
www.bepoisonsmart.com

OKLAHOMA

OKLAHOMA CITY

**Oklahoma Poison
Control Center (*)
Children's Hospital at OU
Medical Center**

940 Northeast 13th St.
Room 3510
Oklahoma City, OK 73104
Business: 405-271-5062
Emergency: 800-222-1222
www.oklahomapoison.org

OREGON

PORTLAND

**Oregon Poison Center (*)
Oregon Health Sciences
University**

3181 S.W. Sam Jackson Park Rd.,
CB550
Portland, OR 97239
Business: 503-494-8968
Emergency: 800-222-1222
www.oregonpoison.com

PENNSYLVANIA

PHILADELPHIA

**The Poison Control Center (*)
Children's Hospital of
Philadelphia**

34th Street & Civic Center Blvd.
Philadelphia, PA 19104-4399
Business: 215-590-2003
Emergency: 800-222-1222
                     215-386-2100 (PA)
TDD/TTY: 215-590-8789
www.poisoncontrol.chop.edu

PITTSBURGH

**Pittsburgh Poison Center (*)
Children's Hospital of Pittsburgh**

3705 Fifth Ave.
Pittsburgh, PA 15213
Business: 412-390-3300
Emergency: 800-222-1222
                     412-681-6669
www.chp.edu/clinical/03a_
       poison.php

PUERTO RICO

SANTURCE

**San Jorge Children's Hospital
Poison Center**

268 San Jorge St.
Santurce, PR 00912
Business: 787-726-5660
Emergency: 800-222-1222
TTY: 787-641-1934
www.poisoncenter.net

RHODE ISLAND

(BOSTON, MA)

**Regional Center for Poison
Control and Prevention (*)**
(Serving Massachusetts and
Rhode Island)

300 Longwood Ave.
Boston, MA 02115
Business: 617-355-6609
Emergency: 800-222-1222
TDD/TTY: 888-244-5313
www.maripoisoncenter.com

SOUTH CAROLINA

COLUMBIA

**Palmetto Poison Center (*)
College of Pharmacy
University of South Carolina**

Columbia, SC 29208
Business: 803-777-7909
Drug Info: 800-777-7805
Emergency: 800-222-1222
                     803-922-1117 (SC)
www.pharm.sc.edu/PPS/pps.htm

SOUTH DAKOTA

(MINNEAPOLIS, MN)

**Hennepin Regional Poison
Center (*)
Hennepin County Medical
Center**

701 Park Ave.
Minneapolis, MN 55415
Business: 612-873-3144
Emergency: 800-222-1222
www.mnpoison.org

SIOUX FALLS

**Provides education only—Does
not manage exposure cases.**

**Sioux Valley Poison Control
Center (*)**

1305 W. 18th St.
Box 5039
Sioux Falls, SD 57117-5039
Business: 605-328-6670
www.sdpoison.org

TENNESSEE

NASHVILLE

**Tennessee
Poison Center (*)**

1161 21st Ave. South
501 Oxford House
Nashville, TN 37232-4632
Business: 615-936-0760
Emergency: 800-222-1222
www.poisonlifeline.org

TEXAS

AMARILLO

**Texas Panhandle
Poison Center (*)
Northwest Texas Hospital**

1501 S. Coulter Dr.
Amarillo, TX 79106
Business: 806-354-1630
Emergency: 800-222-1222
www.poisoncontrol.org

DALLAS

**North Texas Poison Center (*)
Texas Poison Center Network
Parkland Health and Hospital
System**

5201 Harry Hines Blvd.
Dallas, TX 75235
Business: 214-589-0911
Emergency: 800-222-1222
www.poisoncontrol.org

EL PASO

**West Texas Regional
Poison Center (*)
Thomason Hospital**

4815 Alameda Ave.
El Paso, TX 79905
Business   915-534-3800
Emergency: 800-222-1222
www.poisoncontrol.org

GALVESTON

**Southeast Texas
Poison Center (*)
The University of Texas
Medical Branch**

3.112 Trauma Bldg.
301 University Ave.
Galveston, TX 77555-1175
Business: 409-766-4403
Emergency: 800-222-1222
www.poisoncontrol.org

SAN ANTONIO

**South Texas
Poison Center (*)
The University of Texas Health
Science Center–San Antonio**

7703 Floyd Curl Dr., MC 7849
San Antonio, TX 78229-3900
Business: 210-567-5762
Emergency: 800-222-1222
www.poisoncontrol.org

TEMPLE

**Central Texas Poison Center (*)
Scott & White Memorial Hospital**

2401 South 31st St.
Temple, TX 76508
Business: 254-724-7401
Emergency: 800-222-1222
www.poisoncontrol.org

UTAH

SALT LAKE CITY

Utah Poison Control Center (*)

585 Komas Dr., Suite 200
Salt Lake City, UT 84108
Business: 801-587-0600
Emergency: 800-222-1222
                     801-587-0600 (UT)
http://uuhsc.utah.edu/poison

VERMONT

(PORTLAND, ME)

**Northern New England
Poison Center
Maine Medical Center**
22 Bramhall St.
Portland, ME 04102
Business: 207-662-7220
Emergency: 800-222-1222
www.nnepc.org

VIRGINIA

CHARLOTTESVILLE

Blue Ridge Poison Center (*)
University of Virginia Health System

PO Box 800774
Charlottesville, VA 22908-0774
Business: 434-924-0347
Emergency: 800-222-1222
www.healthsystem.virginia.edu.
 brpc

RICHMOND

Virginia Poison Center (*)
Virginia Commonwealth University

P.O. Box 980522
Richmond, VA 23298-0522
Business: 804-828-4780
Emergency: 800-222-1222
 804-828-9123
www.vcu.edu/mcved/vpc

WASHINGTON

SEATTLE

Washington Poison Center (*)

155 NE 100th St.
Suite 400
Seattle, WA 98125-8011
Business: 206-517-2350
Emergency: 800-222-1222
 206-526-2121 (WA)
TDD: 800-572-0638 (WA)
www.wapc.org

WEST VIRGINIA

CHARLESTON

West Virginia Poison Center (*)

3110 MacCorkle Ave. SE
Charleston, WV 25304
Business: 304-347-1212
Emergency: 800-222-1222
www.wvpoisoncenter.org

WISCONSIN

MILWAUKEE

Children's Hospital of Wisconsin Statewide Poison Center

9000 W. Wisconsin Ave.
P.O. Box 1997, Mail Station 677A
Milwaukee, WI 53226
Business: 414-266-2952
Emergency: 800-222-1222
TDD/TTY: 414-266-2542
www.chw.org

WYOMING

(OMAHA, NE)

The Poison Center (*)
Children's Hospital

8401 W. Dodge St., Suite 115
Omaha, NE 68114
Business: 402-955-5555
Emergency: 800-222-1222
www.nebraskapoison.com

DATE DUE
